Use this card to order your PDR Supplements For 1983

Supplements are published in the Spring and Fall, listing changes and new releases in the preceeding months. They are useful in keeping PDR current between annual editions. While every effort will be made to fill all requests for supplements, orders received late in the year may not receive the Spring supplement if supplies have been exhausted.

☐ Send me 1 copy of each supplement. I understand that I may not receive the Spring supplement if I order late in the year.

OFFER EXPIRES DECEMBER 31, 1983.

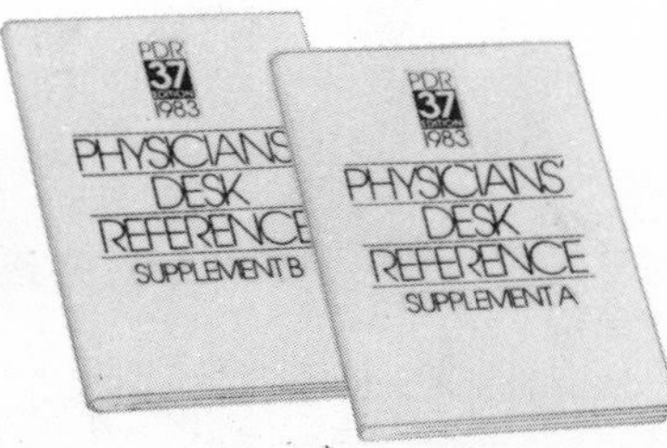

Name __________

Institution __________

Street Address __________

City __________ State __________ Zip __________

Occupation __________

Signature __________

MAIL THIS ORDER FORM, IN AN ENVELOPE, TO: PDR Supplements, Box 58, Oradell, New Jersey 07649

Use this card to order 1983 PDR Supplements

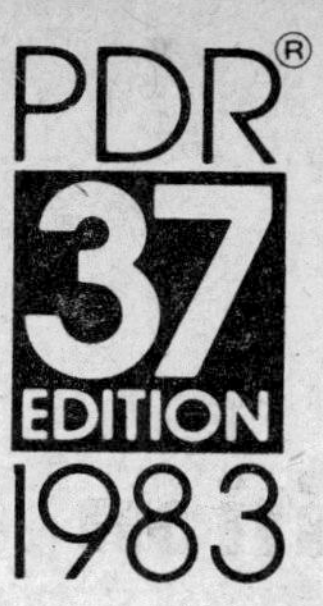

PHYSICIANS' DESK REFERENCE®

Publisher • JACK E. ANGEL

Director of Production
JEROME M. LEVINE

Managing Editor
BARBARA B. HUFF

Medical Consultant
IRVING M. LEVITAS, M.D.

Manager of Production Services
ELIZABETH H. CARUSO

Index Editor
ADELE L. DOWD

Editorial Assistant
F. EDYTHE PATERNITI

Design Director
JOHN NEWCOMB

Art Director
THOMAS DARNSTEADT

Associate Publisher
EDWARD R. BARNHART

Circulation Director
THOMAS S. KRAEMER

Fulfillment Manager
JAMES SCIURBA

Account Managers
ALLAN B. KOLSTEIN
JOHN R. MARMERO
DEBRA E. REYNOLDS

Research Director
ALAN J. FLETCHER

Director of Printing
RALPH G. PELUSO

Copyright © 1983 and published by Medical Economics Company Inc. at Oradell, N.J. 07649. All rights reserved. None of the content of this publication may be reproduced, stored in a retrieval system, or transmitted in any form or by any means (electronic, mechanical, photocopying, recording, or otherwise) without the prior written permission of the publisher.

Officers of Medical Economics Company Inc.: Chairman, Charles P. Daly; President, Carroll V. Dowden; Executive Vice Presidents: Thomas J. McGill, Bartlett R. Rhoades; Senior Vice President: Jack E. Angel; Senior Vice President/Secretary: Stephen J. Sorkenn; Vice Presidents: William J. Reynolds, Lewis A. Scaliti, Kathleen A. Starke, Joseph M. Valenzano Jr.; Treasurer: Charles O. Bennewitz.

ISBN 0-87489-859-5

Foreword to the Thirty-seventh Edition

PHYSICIANS' DESK REFERENCE® is published annually by Medical Economics Company Inc. with the cooperation of the manufacturers whose products appear in the **Product Identification** (Gray Section), in the **Product Information** (White Section) and **Diagnostic Product Information** (Green Section). Intended primarily for physicians, PDR's purpose is to make available essential information on major pharmaceutical and diagnostic products. In addition to this volume, two other editions of PHYSICIANS' DESK REFERENCE will be published in 1983: PDR® For NONPRESCRIPTION DRUGS and PDR® For OPHTHALMOLOGY.

When this edition of PHYSICIANS' DESK REFERENCE® went to press, it included the latest available information on approximately 2,000 products. During the year ahead, however, important new or revised information about these products will be furnished us and will be published periodically in a PDR® Supplement. Retain the Supplement with PDR and before prescribing or administering any product described in PHYSICIANS' DESK REFERENCE, consult the latest PDR Supplement to determine if new or revised information about the product has been published.

This edition includes information concerning the management of overdosage of prescription drugs prepared by the Institute for Clinical Toxicology Department of Medicine, Baylor College of Medicine. It can be found printed inside the back cover. A listing of Poison Control Centers begins on page 444.

The function of the Publisher is the compilation, organization, and distribution of this information. Each product description has been prepared by the manufacturer, and edited and approved by the manufacturer's medical department, medical director, and/or medical consultant. Manufacturers have suggested headings under which their products should be listed in the **Product Category Index** (Blue Section) and in the **Generic and Chemical Name Index** (Yellow Section).

Under the federal Food, Drug & Cosmetic [FD&C] Act, a drug approved for marketing may be labeled, promoted, and advertised by the manufacturer only for those uses for which the drug's safety and effectiveness have been established and which FDA has approved. The Code of Federal Regulations 201.100 (d)(i) pertaining to labeling for prescription products requires that for PDR content, "indications and usage, dosages, routes, methods, and frequency and duration of administration, description, clinical pharmacology and supply and any relevant warnings, hazards, contraindications, adverse reactions, potential for drug abuse and dependence, overdosage and precautions" must be the *"same in language and emphasis"* as the approved labeling for the product. FDA regards the words *"same in language and emphasis"* as requiring VERBATIM use of the approved labeling providing such information. Furthermore, the information in the approved labeling that is emphasized by the use of type set in a box or in capitals, bold face, or italics must be given the same emphasis in PDR.

The FDA has also announced that the FD&C Act "does not, however, limit the manner in which a physician may use an approved drug. Once a product has been approved for marketing, a physician may prescribe it for uses or in treatment regimens or patient populations that are not included in approved labeling." Thus, the FDA states also that "accepted medical practice" often includes drug use that is not reflected in approved drug labeling.

For products which do not have official package circulars, the Publisher has emphasized to manufacturers the necessity of describing such products comprehensively so that physicians would have access to all information essential for intelligent and informed prescribing. In organizing and presenting the material in PHYSICIANS' DESK REFERENCE, the Publisher is providing all the information made available to PDR by manufacturers. Additional information on any product may be obtained from the manufacturer. In making this material available to the medical profession, the Publisher does not advocate the use of any product described herein.

JACK E. ANGEL
Publisher

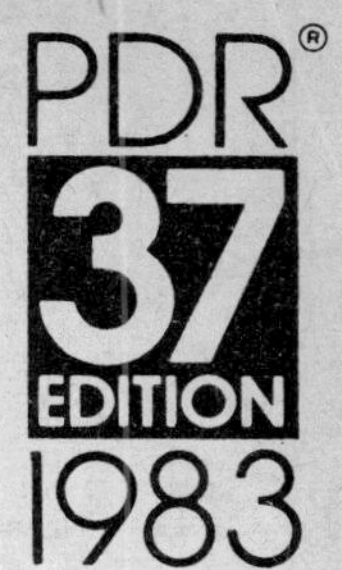

Contents

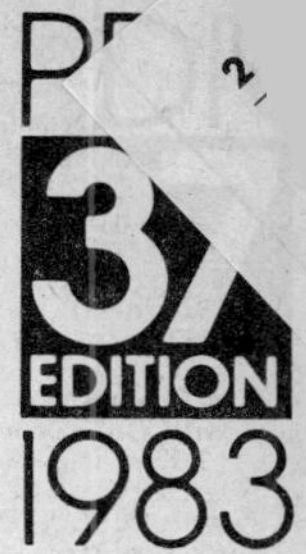

SECTION 1

Manufacturers' Index

The manufacturers appearing in this index (white pages) have provided information concerning their pharmaceutical products in either the Product Information or Diagnostic Product Information Section. It is through their patronage that PHYSICIANS' DESK REFERENCE® is made available to you.

Included in this index are the names and addresses of manufacturers, individuals or departments to whom you may address inquiries, a partial list of products as well as emergency telephone numbers wherever available. The symbol ◆ indicates the product is shown in the Product Identification Section. The symbol ▣ indicates the product is described in PDR® FOR NONPRESCRIPTION DRUGS.

PAGE

ABBOTT LABORATORIES 403, 502
North Chicago, IL 60064

ABBOTT PHARMACEUTICALS, INC.
North Chicago, IL 60064
Address Medical Information Inquiries to:
Pharmaceutical Products Division (312) 937-7069
Hospital Products Division (312) 937-3806
Consumer Products Division (312) 937-3806
Distribution Centers
ATLANTA
Stone Mountain, GA 30302
P.O. Box 5049 (404) 491-7190
CHICAGO
Abbott Park
North Chicago, IL 60064
P.O. Box 68 (312) 937-5153
DALLAS
Dallas, TX 75265
P.O. Box 225295 (214) 398-1350
DENVER
Denver, CO 80217
P.O. Box 5466 (303) 399-7576
HONOLULU
Honolulu, HI 96819
2815 Kilihau Street (808) 833-1691
LOS ANGELES
Los Angeles, CA 90060
60162 Terminal Annex (213) 921-0321
MINNEAPOLIS
Minneapolis, MN 55440
P.O. Box 271 (612) 599-5666
PHILADELPHIA
King of Prussia, PA 19406
920 Eighth Ave., East (215) 265-9100
SEATTLE
Seattle, WA 98124
P.O. Box 24064 (206) 433-0164
Products Available
Abbokinase
◆ Abbo-Pac
Abbott Unit Dose Packages
Dayalets Filmtab
E.E.S. Granules
Enduron Tablets
Enduronyl Tablets
Ery-Tab Tablets
Erythrocin Stearate Filmtab
Erythromycin Base Filmtab
Fero-Grad-500 Filmtab
Iberet-500 Filmtab
K-Lor
K-Tab Filmtab
Nembutal Sodium Capsules
Oretic Tablets
Panwarfin Tablets
Placidyl Capsules
Surbex-T Filmtab
Tranxene Capsules
Acetic Acid Irrigation
Aerohalor
A-hydroCort
Alcohol, Absolute, Ampoules
5% Alcohol & 5% Dextrose Injection
A-methaPred
Aminophyllin 250 mg., 10 ml., Ampul & Vial
Aminophyllin 500 mg., 20 ml., Ampul & Vial
Aminosyn 3.5% M
Aminosyn 5%
Aminosyn 7%
Aminosyn 7% Kit
Aminosyn 7% with Electrolytes
Aminosyn 7% with Electrolytes TPN Kit
Aminosyn 8.5%
Aminosyn 8.5% TPN Kit
Aminosyn 8.5% with Electrolytes
Aminosyn 10%
Aminosyn 10% TPN Kit
Ammonium Chloride
◆ A-Poxide
Atropine 0.1 mg./ml., 5 ml., Abboject, Syringe
Atropine 0.1 mg./ml., 10 ml., Abboject, Syringe
Bupivacaine Hydrochloride Injection, USP, 0.5%
Butesin Picrate Ointment
Butyn Dental Ointment
Calcidrine Syrup
Calcium Chloride 10%, Abboject
Calcium Gluceptate Injection Ampoule & Abboject
Cecon Solution
◆ Cefol Filmtab
Cenolate Ampoules
◆ Chlorthalidone Tablets
Chromium 10 ml. (4 mg./ml.)
Clear Eyes Eye Drops
Colchicine Tablets
Copper 10 ml. (4 mg./ml.)
Covicone Cream
◆ Cylert Chewable Tablets
◆ Cylert Tablets
L-Cysteine Hydrochloride
Dayalets Filmtab
Dayalets plus Iron Filmtab
◆ Depakene Capsules & Syrup
Desoxyn
◆ Desoxyn Gradumet Tablets
6% Dextran w/v & 5% Dextrose Injection
6% Dextran w/v & 0.9% Sodium Chloride Injection
2.5% Dextrose & ½ Str Lact Ringer's Injection
5% Dextrose & Lact Ringer's Injection
5% Dextrose & Ringer's Injection
2.5% Dextrose & 0.45% Sodium Chloride Injection
5% Dextrose & 0.225% Sodium Chloride Injection
5% Dextrose & 0.3% Sodium Chloride Injection
5% Dextrose & 0.45% Sodium Chloride Injection
5% Dextrose & 0.9% Sodium Chloride Injection
10% Dextrose & 0.9% Sodium Chloride Injection
2.5% Dextrose Injection
5% Dextrose Injection
5% Dextrose Injection (Partial fill)
10% Dextrose Injection
20% Dextrose Injection

50% Dextrose Injection
5% Dextrose & 0.075% Pot Chl Injection (10 mEq)
5% Dextrose & 0.15% Pot Chl Injection (20 mEq)
5% Dextrose & 0.224% Pot Chl Injection (30 mEq)
5% Dextrose & 0.3% Pot Chl Injection (40 mEq)
5% Dextrose & 0.225% Sodium Chloride with 0.075% Potassium Chloride Injection (10 mEq)
5% Dextrose & 0.225% Sodium Chloride with 0.15% Potassium Chloride Injection (20 mEq)
5% Dextrose & 0.225% Sodium Chloride with 0.224% Potassium Chloride Injection (30 mEq)
5% Dextrose & 0.225% Sodium Chloride with 0.3% Potassium Chloride Injection (40 mEq)
5% Dextrose & 0.45% Sodium Chloride with 0.075% Potassium Chloride Injection (10 mEq)
5% Dextrose & 0.45% Sodium Chloride with 0.15% Potassium Chloride Injection (20 mEq)
5% Dextrose & 0.45% Sodium Chloride with 0.224% Potassium Chloride Injection (30 mEq)
5% Dextrose & 0.45% Sodium Chloride with 0.3% Potassium Chloride Injection (40 mEq)
10% Dextrose Injection
20% Dextrose Injection
30% Dextrose Injection
40% Dextrose Injection
50% Dextrose Injection
60% Dextrose Injection
70% Dextrose Injection
Diasone Sodium Enterab Tablets
Dical-D Capsules & Wafers
Dical-D with Iron Capsules
Dical-D with Vitamin C Capsules
◆ Dicumarol Tablets
◆ E.E.S. Chewable Tablets
E.E.S. Drops
E.E.S. Granules
E.E.S. 200 Liquid
◆ E.E.S. 400 Filmtab
E.E.S. 400 Liquid
Ear Drops by Murine
  See Murine Ear Wax Removal System/Murine Ear Drops
Empty Evacuated Container
Endrate Solution, Ampoules
◆ Enduron Tablets
◆ Enduronyl Forte Tablets
◆ Enduronyl Tablets
Ephedrine Sulfate, Injection
Epinephrine 1:10,000, 10 ml., Abboject
◆ EryDerm
EryPed Granules
◆ Ery-Tab Tablets
Erythrocin Lactobionate-I.V.
◆ Erythrocin Piggyback
◆ Erythrocin Stearate Filmtab
◆ Erythromycin Base Filmtab
◆ Eutonyl Filmtab
◆ Eutron Filmtab Tablets
◆ Fero-Folic-500 Filmtab
◆ Fero-Grad-500 Filmtab
Fero-Gradumet Filmtab
10% Fructose Injection
Gemonil Tablets
Gerilets Filmtab
Gerix Elixir
Glycine Solution, 1.5%, Irrigation/Aqualite
Halazone Tablets
Halothane
Harmonyl Tablets
Hydron Wound Dressing
Hydroxyzine HCl Injection, Abbojects, Ampuls, Vials, Syringes
Iberet Filmtab
◆ Iberet-500 Filmtab
Iberet-500 Liquid
◆ Iberet-Folic-500 Filmtab
Iberet Liquid
Iberol Filmtab
Iberol-F Filmtab
Inpersol & 1.5% Dextrose
Inpersol & 4.25% Dextrose
10% Invert Sugar Injection
Ionosol B & 5% Dextrose Injection
Ionosol B & 10% Invert Sugar Injection
Ionosol D & 10% Invert Sugar Injection
Ionosol D-CM & 5% Dextrose Injection
Ionosol G & 10% Dextrose Injection
Ionosol G & 10% Invert Sugar Injection
Ionosol MB & 5% Dextrose Injection
Ionosol T & 5% Dextrose Injection
Isoproterenol HCl 1:5,000 1 mg. Pintop
Isoproterenol HCl 1:5,000 2 mg. Pintop
Isoproterenol HCl 1:5,000 5 ml., Universal Add Syringe
Isoproterenol HCl 1:5,000 10 ml., Universal Add Syringe
Isoproterenol HCl 1:50,000, 10 ml., Abboject
◆ Janimine Filmtab
◆ K-Lor Powder
◆ K-Tab Filmtab
10% LMD w/v in 5% Dextrose Injection
10% LMD w/v with 0.9% Sodium Chloride Injection
LTA Kit, Preattached
LTA II Kit
LTA Pediatric Kit
Lactated Ringer's Injection
Lidocaine 0.2% in 5% Dextrose in water
Lidocaine 0.4% in 5% Dextrose in water
Lidocaine 1%, 5 ml., Abboject
Lidocaine 1%, 5 ml., Sterile Pack Abboject
Lidocaine 2%, 5 ml., Abboject
Lidocaine 2%, 5 ml., Sterile Pack Abboject
Lidocaine 20%, 5 ml., 1 gram-Pintop, U.A.S.
Lidocaine 20%, 10 ml., 2 gram-Pintop, U.A.S.
Lidocaine HCl, 5%, with 7.5% Dextrose
Lidocaine Hydrochloride Injection, U.S.P.
Liposyn 10%, 50, 100, 500, 200 ml.
Lubritine
Magnesium Sulfate 12.5%, 8 ml., Pintop
Magnesium Sulfate 50% w/v Ampoules & Abboject
Mammol Ointment
Manganese 10 ml. (1 mg./ml.)
5% Mannitol Injection
10% Mannitol Injection
15% Mannitol Injection
20% Mannitol Injection
25% Mannitol Injection
Murine Ear Wax Removal System/Murine Ear Drops
Murine Eye Drops
Murine Plus Eye Drops
◆ Nembutal Sodium Capsules
Nembutal Sodium Solution
Nembutal Sodium Suppositories
Neut Abbo-Vial & Pintop
Niacin Tablets
Nitropress
Norisodrine Aerotrol
Norisodrine Sulfate Aerohalor
Norisodrine w/Calcium Iodide Syrup
Normosol-M 900 CAL
Normosol-M & 5% Dextrose Injection
Normosol-M & Surbex-T & 5% Dextrose Injection
Normosol-R & 5% Dextrose Injection
Normosol-R/K +& 5% Dextrose Injection
◆ Ogen Tablets
Ogen Vaginal Cream
◆ Optilets-500 Filmtab
◆ Optilets-M-500 Filmtab
◆ Oretic Tablets
Oreticyl Tablets
Oreticyl Forte Tablets
Panheprin
Panheprin Vials
◆ Panwarfin Tablets
◆ Paradione Capsules & Oral Solution
◆ Peganone Tablets
Penthrane
Pentothal Kit
Pentothal Rectal Suspension in Syringe
Pentothal Sodium Thiopental for Injection
Pentothal, (Sterile Powder)
Pentothal Syringe
Phenobarbital Sodium Ampoules
Phenurone Tablets
Physiosol Irrigation/Aqualite
◆ Placidyl Capsules
Potassium Acetate 40 mEq Vial, Pintop & Fliptop
Potassium Chloride Injection Ampoules & Vials, Pintop & Universal Additive Syringe
Potassium Chloride 20 mEq. in D-5 W in Abbo-Vac
Potassium Phosphate 15 mM Vial, Pintop & Fliptop
Potassium Phosphate 45 mM Vial
Procaine Hydrochloride Injection 1% & 2% Vial
Quelicin (Succinylcholine Chloride Injection) Ampul & Vial, Pintop
Quelidrine Syrup
Ringer's Injection
Selsun Blue Lotion
Selsun Lotion
Selsun Suspension
Sodium Acetate 40 mEq Vial
5% Sodium Bicarbonate Injection
0.45% Sodium Chloride
5% Sodium Chloride
20% Sodium Chloride
0.9% Sodium Chloride Injection
Sorbital-Mannitol Irrigating Solution/Aqualite
Sterile Urea
Sulfadiazine Dulcet Tablets
Surbex Filmtab
Surbex w/C Filmtab
◆ Surbex-750 with Iron Filmtab
◆ Surbex-750 with Zinc Filmtab
◆ Surbex-T Filmtab
Surbex-T & 5% Dextrose Injection
TPN Electrolytes
Tham E
Tham Solution
Tral Filmtab
Tral Gradumet
◆ Tranxene Capsules & Tablets
◆ Tranxene-SD Half Strength Tablets
◆ Tranxene-SD Tablets
◆ Tridione Capsules
◆ Tridione Dulcet Tablets
Tridione Solution
Tronolane Anesthetic Hemorrhoidal Cream & Suppositories
Tronothane Hydrochloride Cream & Jelly
Tubocurarine Chloride Injection, USP
Ureaphil
Urological Solution G
Vercyte Tablets
Vita-Kaps Filmtab
Vita-Kaps M Filmtab
Vitamin C Filmtab
Water for Injection, Ampoules, Vial
Water for Injection Bacteriostatic 30 ml. Fliptop
Water for Injection, Sterile, Sterile Water
Water, for Irrigation, Sterile/Aqualite
Zinc 10 ml. (1 mg./1 ml.)

Gamma Counting Systems
Automatic and Manual
Auto-Logic 50
Auto-Logic 100
System Options
Logic 201
Logic 211
Logic 221
Hepatitis
Ausab Hepatitis B Surface Antigen ^{125}I (Human) Radioimmunoassay Diagnostic Kit
Ausab Hepatitis B Surface Antigen ^{125}I (Human) Radioimmunoassay Confirmatory Test
Auscell Antibody to Hepatitis B Surface Antigen (Guinea Pig) Reversed Passive Hemagglutination (RPHA) Diagnostic Kit
Auscell Antibody to Hepatitis B Surface Antigen (Human) Reversed Passive Hemagglutination (RPHA) Confirmatory Test Kit
Ausria II-125 Antibody to Hepatitis B Surface Antigen ^{125}I (Human) Radioimmunoassay Diagnostic Kit
Ausria II-125 Antibody to Hepatitis B Surface Antigen (Human) Radioimmunoassay Confirmatory Test
Aus-tect Test System, Rheophoresis Procedure
Thyroid
HTSH•RIA Diagnostic Kit
Prolactin RIA Diagnostic Kit
Quantisorb-125 T4N Diagnostic Kit
T3RIA (PEG) Diagnostic Kit
T4RIA (PEG) Diagnostic Kit
Thypinone (Protirelin) Synthetic TRH
Thyroscreen T4 Neonate
Triobead T3 Diagnostic Kit
Radiopharmaceuticals
Sensor [Radionuclide-Labeled (^{125}I) Fibrinogen (Human)Glofil]
Diagnostics, General
Digoxin I 125 Imusay Diagnostic Kit
Reptilase-R (Bothrops atrox) (Lyophilized) Coagulation Test
Ruba-tect Rubella Diagnostic Test Systems (Kaolin or Heparin-Manganese Chloride)
Rubacell Rubella Screening Test
Strep-tect FA Group A Beta Hemolytic Streptococcus Fluorescent Antibody Detection System
UTI-tect Bacteriuria Diagnostic Test System

ABBOTT LABORATORIES **3002**
DIAGNOSTICS DIVISION
Abbott Park
North Chicago, IL 60064
Outside Illinois call toll free (800) 323-9100
In Illinois, call collect (312) 937-6161
Address inquiries to:
Marketing Services Dept. 49B
Products Available
Thypinone

ADRIA LABORATORIES INC. **404, 564, 3003**
Administrative Offices:
5000 Post Road
Dublin, OH 43017
Mailing Address:
P. O. Box 16529
Columbus, OH 43216
Address inquiries to:
Medical Department (614) 764-8100
Products Available
(Includes products formerly marketed by Warren-Teed Laboratories)
Adriamycin
Adrucil
Axotal

Epsilan-M Capsules
Evac-Q-Kit
Evac-Q-Kwik
Fluidil
Ilopan Injection (Ampuls & Vials)
Ilopan Stat-Pak (Disposable Syringes)
Ilopan-Choline Tablets
Ilozyme Tablets
Kaochlor 10% Liquid
Kaochlor-Eff Tablets
Kaochlor S-F 10% Liquid
◆ Kaon Cl-10
Kaon Elixir, Grape Flavor
Kaon Elixir, Lemon-Lime Flavor
◆ Kaon Tablets
◆ Kaon-Cl
Kaon-Cl 20%
Magan Tablets
Modane Bulk
Modane Liquid
Modane Mild Tablets
Modane Plus
Modane Soft
Modane Tablets
Myoflex Creme
Neosar for Injection
Pektamalt
Ratio Tablets
Taloin Ointment
Thi-Cin Capsules
Tympagesic Otic Solution
Tymtran Injection
W-T Lotion
Xylo-Pfan

ALBION LABORATORIES, INC. 577
101 N. Main Street
Clearfield, Utah 84015
Address inquiries to:
(800) 453-2406
For Medical Emergencies Contact:
(800) 453-2407
Products Available
▣ Chelated Calcium Tablets
▣ Chelated Iron Tablets
▣ Chelated Magnesium Tablets
▣ Chelated Manganese Capsules
▣ Chelated Manganese Tablets
▣ Chelated Multi-Min Tablets
▣ Chelated Tri-Mins Tablets
▣ Chelated Zinc Capsules
▣ Chelated Zinc Tablets
▣ Complexed Potassium Tablets
▣ Iron Plex Tablets
▣ Multi-Vita-Min Capsules

ALCON LABORATORIES, INC. 577
Alcon Laboratories, Inc.
And its affiliates Inc.
Corporate Headquarters
P.O. Box 1959
6201 South Freeway
Fort Worth, TX 76134
Address inquiries to:
Sales Services (817) 293-0450
Products Available
Adsorbocarpine
Adsorbonac
Adsorbotear
Alcaine
Cetamide Ointment
Cetapred Ointment
Cyclogyl
Cyclomydril
Duratears
Econochlor Solution & Ointment
Econopred
Econopred Plus
Epinal
Eye Stream
Fluorescite
Glaucon
Gonioscopic Prism Solution
Isopto Atropine
Isopto Carbachol
Isopto Carpine
Isopto Cetamide
Isopto Cetapred
Isopto Homatropine
Isopto Hyoscine
Maxidex Suspension & Ointment
Maxitrol Suspension & Ointment
Mydfrin 2.5%
Mydriacyl
Naphcon
Naphcon Forte
Naphcon-A
Natacyn
Schirmer Tear Test Strips
Statrol Solution & Ointment
Tears Naturale
Tobrex Solution & Ointment
Zincfrin

Alcon Lens Care
Adapettes
BoilnSoak
Flex-Care
Opti-clean
Preflex
Soaclens

ALCON (PUERTO RICO) INC. 578
P.O. Box 3000
Humacao, Puerto Rico 00661
Address inquiries to:
Medical Department
P.O. Box 1629
Fort Worth, TX 76101
(817) 293-0450
Products Available
Avitene

ALLERGAN PHARMACEUTICALS, INC. 578
2525 Dupont Drive
Irvine, CA 92713
Address inquiries to:
(714) 752-4500
(See also Herbert Laboratories)
Products Available
Albalon Liquifilm ophthalmic solution
Albalon-A Liquifilm ophthalmic solution
Allergan Cleaning & Disinfecting Solution
Allergan Hydrocare Preserved Saline Solution
Atropine Sulfate ½% S.O.P. ophthalmic ointment
Atropine Sulfate 1.0% S.O.P. ophthalmic ointment
Atropine Sulfate Ophthalmic Solution 1%, 2%
Bleph-10 Liquifilm ophthalmic solution
Blephamide Liquifilm ophthalmic suspension
Blephamide S.O.P. sterile ophthalmic ointment
Blink-N-Clean hard contact lens solution
Chloroptic ophthalmic solution
Chloroptic S.O.P. ophthalmic ointment
Chloroptic-P S.O.P. ophthalmic ointment
Clean-N-Soak hard contact lens solution
Clean-N-Soakit hard contact lens storage case
Clean-N-Stow hard contact lens storage case
Epifrin ophthalmic solution
FML Liquifilm ophthalmic suspension
Genoptic S.O.P. sterile ophthalmic ointment
Genoptic sterile ophthalmic solution
HMS Liquifilm ophthalmic suspension
Herplex Liquifilm ophthalmic solution
LC-65 daily contact lens cleaner
Lacril artificial tears
Lacri-Lube S.O.P. ophthalmic ointment
Lensrins preserved saline solution
Lens-Wet lubricating & rewetting solution
Liquifilm Forte enhanced artificial tears
Liquifilm Tears artificial tears
Liquifilm Wetting Solution hard contact lens solution
Ophthetic ophthalmic solution
P.V. Carpine Liquifilm ophthalmic solution
Poly-Pred Liquifilm ophthalmic suspension
Pred Forte ophthalmic suspension
Pred Mild ophthalmic suspension
Prefrin Liquifilm eye drops
Prefrin-A ophthalmic solution
Prefrin-Z Liquifilm ophthalmic solution
Pre-Sert hard contact lens cushioning solution
Propine ophthalmic solution
Soakare hard contact lens soaking solution
Soflens Enzymatic Contact Lens Cleaner
Tears Plus artificial tears
Total all-in-one hard contact lens solution
Wet-N-Soak wetting and soaking solution for hard contact lenses & Polycon Gas permeable lenses

ALMAY HYPOALLERGENIC COSMETICS & TOILETRIES 578
Almay Inc.
850 Third Avenue
New York, NY 10022
Address inquiries to:
Professional Service Dept.
Apex, NC 27502 (919) 362-7422
Products Available
▣ Cheq Anti-Perspirant Deodorant Spray (Non-Aerosol)
▣ Cheq Extra-Dry Anti-Perspirant Deodorant Spray (Aerosol)
▣ Cheq Roll-On Anti-Perspirant Deodorant
▣ Cheq Soft Powder Extra-Dry Anti-Perspirant Deodorant Spray (Aerosol)
▣ Chip Resistant Top Coat
▣ Clean and Gentle Daily Shampoo
▣ Clean and Gentle Oil-Free Conditioner
▣ Colorplus by Almay Cheekcolor
▣ Colorplus by Almay Eyecolor
▣ Colorplus by Almay Lengthening Lashcolor
▣ Colorplus by Almay Lipcolor (creams & frosts)
▣ Colorplus by Almay Lipgloss
▣ Colorplus by Almay Nailcolor (creams & frosts)
▣ Colorplus by Almay Thickening Lashcolor
▣ Cuticle Treatment Oil
▣ Deep Cleansing Cold Cream
▣ Deep Mist Cleansing Cream for Dry Skin
▣ Deep Mist Cleansing Lotion for Normal/Combination Skin
▣ Deep Mist Extra Light Night Cream for Normal/Combination Skin
▣ Deep Mist Eye Cream
▣ Deep Mist Moisture Cream for Dry Skin
▣ Deep Mist Moisture Lotion for Dry Skin
▣ Deep Mist Purifying Freshener for Dry Skin
▣ Deep Mist Purifying Toner for Normal/Combination Skin
▣ Deep Mist Ultrarich Night Cream for Dry Skin
▣ Deep Pore Cleansing Mask for Normal to Oily Skin
▣ Enamel Quick Dry
▣ Enriched Formula Ultralight Moisture Lotion for Normal/Combination Skin
▣ Extra Cover Cream Makeup
▣ Extra Light Formula Facial Cleanser for Oily Skin
▣ Extra Long Lashes Lengthening Mascara
▣ Extra Mositurizing Under Eye Cover Creme (Ivory & Natural)
▣ Fine Line Brush-On Eyeliner
▣ Fresh Color Blush-On Blush
▣ Fresh Finish Balanced Makeup for Normal/Combination Skin
▣ Fresh Glow Moisturizing Makeup for Dry Skin
▣ Fresh Look Oil-Free Makeup for Oily Skin
▣ Gentle Action Nail Enamel Remover
▣ Gentle Cleansing Facial Soap for Dry Skin
▣ Gentle Cleansing Facial Soap for Normal/Combination Skin
▣ Gentle Cleansing Facial Soap for Oily Skin
▣ Gentle Gel Mask for Normal to Dry Skin
▣ High Gloss Nail Guard
▣ Lasting Glow Brush-On Blush
▣ Longer Lasting Lashes Waterproof Mascara
▣ LongWearing Eye Color (Single, Duo & Trio)
▣ Lush 'N Healthy Conditioning Mascara
▣ Mineral Oil Jelly
▣ Moisture Rich Lipstick (creams & frosts)
▣ Moisturizing Eye Makeup Remover Pads
▣ Natural Blush Cream Cheek Color
▣ Natural Look Cover-Up Stick (light, medium & dark)
▣ Non-Oily Eye Makeup Remover
▣ Oil Control Facial Cleanser for Oily Skin
▣ Oil Control Purifying Pore Lotion for Oily Skin
▣ Oil-Free Moisture Lotion for Oily Skin
▣ Perfect Control Lip Liner Pencils
▣ Professional Formula Eyebrow & Liner Pencils
▣ Protective Base Coat
▣ Protective Formula Nail Enamel (creams & frosts)
▣ Protein Conditioning Hair Spray - Aerosol - Regular and Extra Hold
▣ Protein Conditioning Hair Spray - Non-Aerosol
▣ Pure and Gentle Everday Conditioning Shampoo
▣ Pure Castile Shampoo
▣ Ridge Filling Pre-Coat
▣ Sheer Finish Translucent Pressed Powder
▣ Shine-Free Blotting Powder for Oily Skin
▣ Soft Blending Eye Color Pencils
▣ Super Rich Lash Thickening Mascara
▣ Translucent Finish Face Powder
▣ Wet and Dry Blushing Rouge
▣ Wrinkle Smoothing Moisture Stick

ALTO PHARMACEUTICALS, INC. 404, 578
15509 Casey Rd. Ext.
Tampa, FL 33624
Address inquiries to:
Professional Services
P.O. Box 271369
Tampa, FL 33688 (813) 961-1010
Products Available
Akne Drying Lotion
Akne Kaps
Akne pH Lotion
Alto-Pred Soluble Injection
Anabolin IM Injection
Anabolin LA-100 Injection
Cefinal II Tablets
D'Alpha-E Capsules
Dexamethasone Injection
Dimethyl Sulfoxide Cream, Gel, Liquid, Spray
◆ Efed II Capsules
Efed Tablets
Herp-Ez Drops
Herp-Ez Tablets
Lotio-P Lotion
Microcort Lotion
◆ Zinc-220 Capsules (Zinc Sulfate Capsules)

ALZA CORPORATION 579
950 Page Mill Road
Palo Alto, California 94304
Address inquiries to:
Marie E. Barry, Product Manager
(415) 494-5575
For Medical Emergencies Contact:
Virgil A. Place, Medical Director
(415) 494-5310

(◆ Shown in Product Identification Section) (▣ Described in PDR For Nonprescription Drugs)

Products Available
Ocusert Ocular Therapeutic Systems
Pilo-20
Pilo-40
Progestasert

AMERICAN CRITICAL CARE 581
Div. of American Hospital Supply Corp.
McGaw Park, IL 60085
Address inquiries to:
Medical Director or in Emergency
Call: (312) 473-3000
Products Available
Bretylol Injection
Hespan Injection
Intropin Injection
Inulin Solution, Purified
Isoclor Timesule Capsules
Tridil

AMERICAN DERMAL CORPORATION 586
12 Worlds Fair Drive
Somerset New Jersey 08873
Address Inquiries to:
Professional Services Department (800) 526-0199
In New Jersey call: (201) 356-5544
Products Available
Drithocreme
Viranol

AMERICAN PHARMACEUTICAL COMPANY 587
245 Fourth St.
Passaic, N.J. 07055
Address Inquiries to:
Harvey A. Collins (201) 779-5300
Products Available
Ampicillin Trihydrate Capsules
Aphco Hemorrhoidal Ointment, Suppositories
Bacitracin Ointment
Bisacodyl Tablets, Suppositories
Codanol A&D Ointment
Corticream
Daily Dose 1 Vitamins
B-Complex Liver & Iron Tablets
Belaxa B-Complex & C Capsules
Fe-ritol Tablets
Gerifort Plus
Multiple Vitamins with Iron Tablets
Multiple Vitamins with Minerals Tablets
Nutri Drops
Spectrum
Super Stress-600 Tablets
Super Stress-600 with Iron Tablets
Super Z Stress-600 Tablets
Thera-Amcaps
Thera-Amcaps M
Vitamin E Capsules
Diphenhydramine Capsules, Elixir, Expectorant
Fendon Tablets, Elixir
Ferrous Gluconate Tablets
Ferrous Sulfate Tablets, Capsules
Gelumina Plus Liquid
Gelumina Tablets
Gelumina with Simethicone, Liquid
Iso-Lo Eye Wash, Drops
Isoxsuprine HCl Tablets
Ka-Pek Suspension
Methocarbamol Tablets
Neo-Mist Nasal Spray
Neomycin Tablets
Penicillin V Potassium Tablets
Pertinex Cream, Spray
Phendex Elixir, Tablets
Prednisolone Tablets
Prednisone Tablets
Prenacaps
Promethazine Tablets, Expectorant
Rhusticon Lotion
Romex Decongestant Cough, Cold
SPD Analgesic Cream, Lotion
Spectro-Biotic Ointment
Tetracycline Capsules
Triprolidine w/Pseudoephedrine Tablets, Syrup

AMES DIVISION 3004
Miles Laboratories, Inc.
1127 Myrtle Street
P.O. Box 70
Elkhart, IN 46515
Order/Pricing Information:
(219) 264-8645
Customer Services
(219) 264-8901
Products Available
Ames Instruments
Ames Fluoro-Colorimeter
Ames Seralyzer Reflectance Photometer
Clini-Tek Reflectance Photometer
Dextrometer Reflectance Colorimeter
Glucometer Reflectance Photometer
Urin-Tek System for Urine Specimen Collection and Transportation
Ames Tests
Ames Seralyzer Solid Phase Reagent Strips for: Glucose, Uric Acid, Cholesterol, BUN, LDH, CK Total Bilirubin & Creatinine
Ames TDA Therapeutic Drug Assays
Dextrostix Reagent Strips
Diastix Reagent Strips
Glucola Carbonated Preparation for Postprandial & Glucose Tolerance Test
Hema-Chek Fecal Occult Blood Test
Keto-Diastix Reagent Strips
Microcult-GC
Microstix-3 Reagent Strips
Microstix-Candida
Microstix-Nitrite
N-Multistix Reagent Strips
N-Multistix SG
N-Uristix Reagent Strips
Tek-Chek Controls for Routine Urinalysis
Visidex Reagent Strips

ANBEX, INC. 587
15 West 75th Street
New York, New York 10023
Products Available
Iosat Tablets

ARCO PHARMACEUTICALS, INC. 588
105 Orville Drive
Bohemia, NY 11716
Address inquiries to:
Professional Service Dept. (516) 567-9500
Products Available
Arco-Cee Tablets
Arco-Lase Tablets
Arco-Lase Plus Tablets
Arcoret Tablets
Arcoret w/Iron Tablets
Arcotinic Liquid
Arcotinic Tablets
C-B Time Capsules
C-B Time 500 Tablets
C-B Time Liquid
◆◻ Codexin Capsules
Co-Gel Tablets
Mega-B
Megadose
Spantuss Liquid
Spantuss Tablets

AR-EX PRODUCTS CO. 588
1036 West Van Buren St.
Chicago, IL 60607
Address inquiries to:
Robert W. Francke (312) 226-5241
Products Available
Ar-Ex Hypo-Allergenic Cosmetics
Bath Oil - unscented
Body Lotion - unscented
Brush-On Complexion Coloring - unscented
Brush-On Eyeshadow - unscented
Chap Cream - scented & unscented
Cleansing Cream - scented & unscented
Cold Cream - scented & unscented
Compact Powder - unscented
Cream for Dry Skin - scented & unscented
Cream for Oily Skin - unscented
Deodorant (Cream, Spray, Roll-On) unscented
Disappear (Blemish Stick) - unscented
Eye Cream - unscented
Eye Makeup Remover Pads - unscented
Eye Pencil - unscented
Eye Shadow Stick - unscented
Face Powder - unscented
Foundation Lotion - unscented
Lip Gloss & Sun Screen Stick - unscented
Moisture Cream - unscented
Moisture Lotion - scented & unscented
Night Cream - scented & unscented
Roll-On Mascara - unscented
Shampoo - unscented
Special Formula Lipstick - unscented
Superfatted Soap - unscented
Safe Suds - unscented

ARMOUR PHARMACEUTICAL COMPANY 404, 589
Executive Office
303 South Broadway
Tarrytown, NY 10591 (914) 631-8888
Eastern Distribution Center
P.O. Box 383
South Plainfield, NJ 07080 (201) 668-0110
Midwest Distribution Center
P.O. Box 511
Kankakee, IL 60901 (815) 932-6771
Western Distribution Center
P.O. Box 63249
Los Angeles, CA 90063 (213) 263-9359
Products Available
Acthar
◆ Armour Thyroid (Tablets)
Biopar Forté
◆ Biozyme-C
◆ Calcimar Solution
DDAVP
Dialume
Flexinet
HP Acthar Gel
◆ Levothroid
◆ Levothroid Injectables
◆ Nicobid
Nicolar
Pentritol-60 mg.
Posterior Pituitary Capsules
Thyrar
◆ Thyrolar
Thytropar
Tussar DM
Tussar SF
Tussar-2
Protein Reagents
Bovine Albumin
Crystallized Bovine Plasma Albumin
Bovine Albumin Powder
Protein Standard Solution
Plasma Derivative Products
Albuminar-5, Normal Serum Albumin (Human) U.S.P. 5%
Albuminar-25, Normal Serum Albumin (Human) U.S.P. 25%
Factorate, Antihemophilic Factor (Human) Dried
Factorate, Generation II
Gammar, Immune Serum Globulin (Human) U.S.P.
Gamulin Rh
Mini-Gamulin Rh

B. F. ASCHER & COMPANY, INC. 598
15501 W 109th St.
Lenexa, KS 66219
Address inquiries to:
Product Information Dept. (913) 888-1880
Products Available
Adipost Capsules
Anaspaz PB Tablets
Anaspaz Tablets
◆◻ Ayr Saline Nasal Drops
◆◻ Ayr Saline Nasal Mist
Converspaz Improved Capsules
Converzyme Improved Capsules
◆◻ Dalca Tablets
Drize Capsules
Drotic Ear Drops
Ethaquin Tablets
Hycodaphen Tablets
Mobidin Tablets
◆◻ Mobigesic Tablets
◆◻ Mobisyl Creme
◆◻ Soft 'N Soothe Creme
Tolfrinic Tablets
◆◻ Unilax Tablets

ASTRA PHARMACEUTICAL PRODUCTS INC. 599
7 Neponset St.
Worcester, MA 01606
Address inquiries to:
Professional Information Department
(617) 852-6351
Products Available
Citanest Solutions
Duranest Solutions
Sensorcaine Solutions
Xylocaine Intramuscular Injection for Ventricular Arrhythmias
Xylocaine Intravenous Injection for Cardiac Arrhythmias
Xylocaine 2% Jelly
Xylocaine 2.5% Ointment
Xylocaine 5% Ointment
Xylocaine 10% Oral Spray
Xylocaine Solutions
Xylocaine 1.5% Solution with Dextrose 7.5%
Xylocaine 4% Sterile Solution
Xylocaine 5% Solution with Glucose 7.5%
Xylocaine 4% Topical Solution
Xylocaine 2% Viscous Solution
Yutopar Intravenous Injection
Yutopar Tablets

AYERST LABORATORIES 404, 616, 3006
Division of American Home Products Corp.
685 Third Ave.
New York, NY 10017
For Medical Information
Business hours only (9:00 a.m. to 5:00 p.m. EST), call (212) 878-5900
For Medical Emergency Information After Hours or On Weekends, call
(212) 986-1000
(212) 878-5900
(212) 878-5000
Regional Sales Offices
Burlingame, CA 94010
Suite 100
840 Hinckley Road (415) 692-4258
Chamblee, GA (Atlanta) 30341
3600 American Drive (404) 451-9578
Rockville, MD 20852
6252 Montrose Rd. (301) 984-9140
Chicago, IL 60648
7545 N. Natchez Ave. (312) 647-8948
Lakewood, OH 44107
Suite 795
14701 Detroit Ave. (216) 226-4128
Los Angeles, CA 90061
12833 S. Spring St. (213) 321-5550/1/2
Mesquite, TX (Dallas) 75149
3601 Executive Blvd. (214) 285-8741

Rockville, MD 20852
6252 Montrose Rd. (301) 984-9140
South Plainfield, NJ 07080
4000 Hadley Rd. (201) 754-6220 (NJ)
(212) 964-3903 (NY)

Distribution Centers

Chamblee—3600 American Drive
Chamblee, GA 30341 (404) 457-2518
Chicago—7545 N. Natchez Ave.
Chicago, IL 60648
(312) 763-0888 (Chicago)
(312) 647-8840 or 8841 (Niles)
Cleveland—15620 Industrial Parkway
Cleveland, OH 44135 (216) 267-9090
Lenexa—10700 Pflumm Road
Lenexa, KS 66210 (913) 888-4310
Los Angeles—12833 S. Spring St.
Los Angeles, CA 90061
(213) 321-5550-1-2
Mesquite—3601 Executive Blvd.
Mesquite, TX 75149 (214) 285-8741
Seattle—405 Baker Blvd., Andover Park
Seattle, WA 98188 (206) 244-1921
South Plainfield—4000 Hadley Road
South Plainfield, NJ 07080
(201) 754-6220 (NJ)
(212) 964-3903 (NY)

Products Available

A.P.L.
Almocarpine
◆ Antabuse
◆ Atromid-S
Auralgan Otic Solution
Avlosulfon
◆ Aygestin
◆ Beminal-500
Beminal Forte w/Vitamin C
Beminal Fortified w/Iron & Liver
◆ Beminal Stress Plus
Clusivol Capsules
Clusivol Syrup
Clusivol 130 Tablets
Cytoferin Hematinic Tablets
Dermoplast
◆ Diucardin
Enzactin Cream
Ayerst Epitrate
Estradurin
Estrogenic Substance (estrone) In Aqueous Suspension
Factrel
Fluor-I-Strip Applicators
Fluor-I-Strip-A.T. Applicators
Fluothane
◆ Grisactin
◆ Grisactin Ultra
◆ Inderal
◆ Inderide
Kerodex Cream (water-miscible)
Kerodex Cream (water-repellent)
Larylgan Throat Spray
◆ Mediatric Capsules
Mediatric Liquid
◆ Mediatric Tablets
Mysoline Suspension
◆ Mysoline Tablets
Ophthalgan
◆ PMB 200 & PMB 400
Peptavlon
Phospholine Iodide
◆ Plegine
Premarin Intravenous
◆ Premarin Tablets
◆ Premarin Vaginal Cream
◆ Premarin w/Methyltestosterone
Protopam Chloride for Injection
Protopam Chloride Tablets
◆ Riopan Antacid Chew Tablets
Riopan Antacid Suspension
◆ Riopan Antacid Swallow Tablets
◆ Riopan Plus Chew Tablets
Riopan Plus Suspension
Sonacide
Thiosulfil Duo-Pak Package
◆ Thiosulfil Forte Tablets
◆ Thiosulfil Tablets
◆ Thiosulfil-A Forte Tablets
◆ Thiosulfil-A Tablets
Turgasept Aerosol

BAKER/CUMMINS 659
Dermatological Div. of Key Pharmaceuticals, Inc.
50 N.W. 176th Street
Miami, FL 33169 (305) 652-2276

Products Available

Acno Lotion
Acticort Lotion 100
◘ Complex 15
◘ P&S Liquid
◘ P&S Plus Gel
◘ P&S Shampoo
Panscol Lotion & Ointment
Ultra Derm Moisturizer
◘ Ultra Mide 25
◘ Xseb Shampoo
◘ Xseb-T Shampoo

BARNES-HIND/HYDROCURVE, INC. 659
895 Kifer Road
Sunnyvale, CA 94086

Address inquiries to:

Mr. James Tasker
Sales Services Dept. (408) 736-5462
(800) 538-1562

Products Available

Barnes-Hind Germicidal Solution
Barseb HC Scalp Lotion
Barseb Thera=Spray
HEB Cream Base
Komed Acne Lotion
Komed HC Lotion
Komex
Pro-Cort Cream
Pro-Cort M Cream
Tinver Lotion
The following Barium Products now sold by Armour Pharmaceuticals
Barotrast
Clysodrast
Esophotrast
Oratrast

A. J. BART, INC. 405, 660
P.O. Box 628
Munoz Rivera 938
Penuelas, Puerto Rico 00724
(809) 836-1157

Address inquiries to:

Mr. Alberto Bartolomei, Jr.
(809) 836-1157

Products Available

Alba-3 Ointment
Alba-Ce Liquid, Drops, Capsules
Albacort Cream
Albacort Injectable
Alba-Dex Injectable, Liquid & Tablets
Albadryl Injectable
Albaform-HC Cream
◆ Albafort Injectable
Alba-Gyn Vaginal Cream
◆ Alba-Lybe
Alba-Temp Suppositories, Liquid, Tablets & Drops
Albatussin (Sugar Free)
Albazine Injectable
Alvimin
Asmex KI Liquid
Asmex Liquid
Benzotic Ear Drops
Dramatrol Injectable
Myoforte Tablets
Myophen Injectable
Pasmin Injectable, Liquid, Capsules
Sedaril
◆ Tia-Doce Injectable Monovial

BAY PHARMACEUTICALS, INC. 661
1111 Francisco Blvd.
San Rafael, CA 94901

Address inquiries to:

Professional Services Dept. (415) 459-7600

For Medical Emergencies Contact:

(415) 459-7600

Products Available

ACTH
BayBee-1
BayBee-12
BayBee Complex
BayCaine-1
BayCaine-2
BayCaine-E-1
BayCaine-E-2
BayDex
BayDryl
BayEstros
BayGent
BayHCG
BayMep
BayMeth
BayProgest
BayRox
BaySaline
BayTac-3
BayTac-40
BayTac-D
BayTestone-50
BayTestone-100
BayWater

BEACH PHARMACEUTICALS 405, 662
Division of Beach Products, Inc.

Executive Office

5220 S. Manhattan Ave.
Tampa, FL 33611 (813) 839-6565

Manufacturing and Distribution

Main St. at Perimeter Rd.
Conestee, SC 29605
Toll Free 1-(800) 845-8210

Address inquiries to:

Raymond LaForge, Ph.D. (803) 277-7282
Richard Stephen Jenkins (813) 839-6565

Products Available

◆ Beelith Tablets
Citrolith Tablets
Fer-Bid Improved
◆ K-Phos M.F. (Modified Formula) Tablets
◆ K-Phos Neutral
◆ K-Phos No. 2 Tablets
◆ K-Phos Original Formula 'Sodium Free' Tablets
K-Phos w/S.A.P.
◆ Thiacide Tablets
◆ Uroqid-Acid
◆ Uroqid-Acid No. 2

BEECHAM PRODUCTS 663
Division of Beecham Inc.
P.O. Box 1467
Pittsburgh, PA 15230

Address inquiries to:

Ms. Dona L. Fundis,
Professional Services Dept.
(412) 928-1055

Products Available

Massengill Disposable Douche
Massengill Disposable Medicated Douche
Massengill Liquid Concentrate
Massengill Powder

BEECHAM LABORATORIES 406, 664
Division of Beecham, Inc.
Bristol, TN 37620

Address inquiries to:

Medical Director
Beecham Laboratories
501 Fifth Street
Bristol, TN 37620 (615) 764-5141

Distributing Divisions

Arlington, TX 76011
2118 E. Randol Mill Rd. (817) 261-6626
Bristol, TN 37620
501 Fifth Street (615) 764-5141
Elmhurst, IL 60126
449 West Wrightwood Avenue
Mourekson Industrial Center
(312) 530-2424
Orlando, FL 32859
P.O. Box 13770 (305) 859-9300
Piscataway, NJ 08854
101 Possumtown Road (201) 469-5441
or (201) 469-5449
Sacramento, CA 95826
5900 Warehouse Way (916) 381-4030

Products Available

Actol Expectorant Liquid
Actol Expectorant Tablets
Adrenosem Injectable, Syrup & Tablets
◆ Amoxil Capsules For Oral Suspension & Chewable Tablets
Amoxil Pediatric Drops for Oral Suspension
Anexsia w/Codeine Tablets
Anexsia-D Tablets
◆ Bactocill Capsules
Bactocill for Injection
C M w/Paregoric
Celbenin for Injection
◆ Cloxapen Capsules
Conar Expectorant Syrup
Conar Suspension
Conar-A Suspension
Conar-A Tablets
Corrective Mixture
Corrective Mixture w/Paregoric
Cotrol-D Tablets
Daricon
Daricon PB
Dasikon Capsules
Dasin Capsules
◆ Dycill Capsules
Enarax Tablets
◆ Fastin Capsules
Guaifenesin Syrup
Hybephen Tablets
Hycal Liquid
Livitamin Capsules
Livitamin Capsules w/Intrinsic Factor
Livitamin Chewable Tablets
Livitamin Liquid
Livitamin Prenatal Tablets
Menest Tablets
Morphine & Atropine Injectable
Nucofed Capsules
Nucofed Expectorant
Nucofed Syrup
Pyopen Injectable
Semets Troches
Thalfed Tablets
Theralax Suppositories
Ticar for Injection
◆ Tigan Capsules
Tigan Injectable
Tigan Suppositories
Totacillin Capsules
Totacillin For Oral Suspension
Totacillin-N Injectable

BERLEX LABORATORIES INC. 406, 672
Cedar Knolls, NJ 07927

Address inquiries to:

Professional Services
110 East Hanover Avenue
Cedar Knolls, NJ 07927 (201) 540-8700

For Medical Information
Medical Department
110 East Hanover Avenue
Cedar Knolls, NJ 07927
(201) 540-8700
Products Available
Aminodur Dura-Tabs
Anodynos DHC Tablets
Deconamine Elixir
◆ Deconamine SR Capsules
Deconamine Syrup
◆ Deconamine Tablets
◆ Elixicon Suspension
◆ Elixophyllin Capsules
Elixophyllin Elixir
◆ Elixophyllin SR Capsules
Elixophyllin-KI Elixir
Enuretrol Tablets
Kay Ciel Elixir
◆ Kay Ciel Powder
L-Glutavite Capsules
◆ Pyocidin-Otic Solution
◆ Quinaglute Dura-Tabs
Stomaseptine Douche Powder
◆ Sus-Phrine Injection
Therapav Capsules
Vi-Twel Injection

BEUTLICH, INC. 678
7006 N. Western Ave.
Chicago, IL 60645 (312) 262-7900
Products Available
Ceo-Two Rectal Suppositories
Hurricaine Liquid 1/4cc Unit Dose
Hurricaine Oral, Topical Anesthetic Gel
Hurricaine Oral, Topical Anesthetic Liquid
Hurricaine Topical Anesthetic Spray
Hurricaine Spray Extension Tubes
Mevanin-C Capsules
Mevatinic-C Tablets
Peridin-C Tablets
Pregent Tablets

BIOCRAFT LABORATORIES, INC. 678
92 Route 46
Elmwood Park, N.J. 07407
Address Inquiries to:
(201) 796-3434
Products Available
Amitriptyline HCl Tablets
Amoxicillin Capsules
Amoxicillin Suspension
Ampicillin Capsules
Ampicillin Suspension
Ampicillin-Probenecid Suspension
Chloroquine Phosphate Tablets
Cloxacillin Capsules
Cloxacillin Solution
Dicloxacillin Capsules
Imipramine HCl Tablets
Neomycin Sulfate Tablets
Oxacillin Capsules
Oxacillin Solution
Penicillin G Potassium Solution
Penicillin G Potassium Tablets
Penicillin V Potassium Solution
Penicillin V Potassium Tablets
Sulfamethoxazole and Trimethoprim Tablets
Trimethoprim Tablets

BIO-DYNAMICS 3008
A Boehringer Mannheim Company
9115 Hague Road
Indianapolis, IN 46250 (317) 845-2000
Products Available
Chemstrip bG Blood Glucose Test
Chemstrip Urine Testing System

BOCK PHARMACAL COMPANY 679
5435 Highland Park Drive
St. Louis, MO 63110
Address inquiries to:
Professional Services Dept. (314) 535-4060
Products Available
Amobell Capsules
Broncholate Syrup
Broncholate Tablets
Demasone Injectable
Demasone-LA Injectable
G-200 Capsules
Hemaspan Capsules
Hemaspan-FA Capsules
Limit Tablets
Onset-5 Tablets
Onset-10 Tablets
Pavadyl Capsules
Poly-Histine Capsules
Poly-Histine Elixir
Poly-Histine Expectorant Plain
Poly-Histine Expectorant with Codeine
Poly-Histine-D Capsules
Poly-Histine-D Elixir
Poly-Histine-DX Capsules
Poly-Histine-DX Syrup
Prenate 90 Tablets
Theon Elixir
Theon-300 Capsules
Zephrex Tablets

BOEHRINGER INGELHEIM LTD. 406, 679
90 East Ridge
P.O. Box 368
Ridgefield, CT 06877
Address inquiries to:
Medical Services Dept. (203) 438-0311
Products Available
Alupent Inhalent Solution 5%
Alupent Metered Dose Inhaler
Alupent Syrup
◆ Alupent Tablets
◆ Catapres Tablets
◆ Combipres Tablets
◆ Dulcolax Suppositories
◆ Dulcolax Tablets
◆ Persantine Tablets
◆ Prelu-2 Capsules
◆ Preludin Endurets
◆ Preludin Tablets
◆ Respbid
Serentil Ampuls
Serentil Concentrate
◆ Serentil Tablets
Torecan Ampuls
Torecan Suppositories
◆ Torecan Tablets

BOOTS PHARMACEUTICALS, INC. 406, 690
6540 Line Avenue
Shreveport, LA 71106
Address inquiries to:
Medical Director (318) 869-3551
Products Available
F-E-P Creme
◆ Lopurin Tablets
P-200 Tablets
◆ Rufen Tablets
Ru-Tuss Expectorant
Ru-Tuss Plain
◆ Ru-Tuss Tablets
Ru-Tuss with Hydrocodone
Ru-Vert Liquid
Su-Tinic Liquid
Su-Ton
Su-Zol
Twin-K Liquid
Twin-K-Cl Liquid
◆ Zorprin Tablets

BOWMAN PHARMACEUTICALS 698
Division of Bowman, Inc.
5801 Mayfair Road, N.W.
North Canton OH 44720
Address inquiries to:
C. Richard Chaddock (216) 497-1632
Branch Offices
6405 49th St. N
Pinellas Park, FL. 33565
(phone) (813) 527-7221
111 Liberty St.
Columbus, Ohio 43215
(614) 224-4157
Products Available
APC Tablets
Acetaminophen Tablets
Al-ay Tablets
Analgesic Liquid
Asperbuf (Varicolor)
Aspirin Tablets, 10 gr.
Bowtussin Syrup
Buffets (Haberle)
Charcoal (Activated) USP in Liquid Base
Charcoal Suspension
Dimentabs
Guistrey Fortis Tablets
Histagesic (Haberle)
Histrey Syrup & Tablets
Hiwolfia Tablets
Hospital Lotion
Ipecac Syrup
Ivy-Chex (Non-Aerosol)
Multagen-12 + E Bocaps
Niacal (Haberle)
Niacin Tablets
Phenobarbital ⅛ gr Tablets
Sinexin Capsules
Sinoze Tablets
Stulex Tablets
Theophed Tablets
Therevac Disposable Enema
Thyroid Tablets
Tymatro Lozenges

BOYLE & COMPANY 698
13260 Moore St.
Cerritos, CA 90701
Address inquiries to:
Susan M. Boyle (213) 926-8250
Products Available
Citra Capsules
Citra Forte Capsules
Citra Forte Syrup
Digolase Capsules
Glytinic Liquid
Glytinic Tablets
Triva Combination
Triva Douche Powder
Triva Jel

BREON LABORATORIES INC. 406, 699
90 Park Ave.
New York, NY 10016
Address inquiries to:
Medical Department (212) 907-2705
Main Office
90 Park Avenue
New York, NY 10016 (212) 907-2000
Branch Offices
Atlanta, GA 30336
5090 MacDougall Drive, S.W.
(404) 696-4480
Dallas, TX 75235
6627 Maple Ave. (214) 357-4015
Des Plaines, IL 60018
200 E. Oakton St. (312) 296-8141
Menlo Park, CA 94025
160 Scott Drive (415) 324-4721
Products Available
Breokinase
◆ Breonesin
Bronkephrine Injection
◆ Bronkodyl
◆ Bronkodyl S-R
Bronkolixir
Bronkometer Aerosol
Bronkosol
Bronkosol Unit Dose
◆ Bronkotabs Tablets
Carbocaine Hydrochloride Injection
◆ Demerol APAP Tablets
Dextrose Injection, 10%
◆ Fergon Capsules
Fergon Elixir
Fergon Plus Caplets
◆ Fergon Tablets
Isuprel Hydrochloride Compound Elixir
◆ Isuprel Hydrochloride Glossets
Isuprel Hydrochloride 1:200 & 1:100
Isuprel Hydrochloride Injection 1:5000
Isuprel Hydrochloride Mistometer
Kayexalate
Levophed Bitartrate Injection
Marcaine Hydrochloride Injection
Marcaine Hydrochloride with Epinephrine 1:200,000
Measurin Tablets
◆ Mebaral Tablets
Novocain Hydrochloride for Spinal Anesthesia
Novocain Hydrochloride Injection
Pediacof Cough Syrup
Pontocaine Hydrochloride Eye Ointment
Pontocaine Hydrochloride for Spinal Anesthesia
Pontocaine Hydrochloride Topical Solution
◆ Trancopal Caplets

BRISTOL LABORATORIES 407, 725
(Div. of Bristol-Myers Co.)
Thompson Rd., P.O. Box 657
Syracuse, NY 13201 (315) 432-2000
Address medical inquiries to:
Dept. of Medical Services (315) 432-2838
or (315) 432-2000
Orders may be placed by calling the following toll free numbers:
Within New York State 1-(800) 962-7200
Continental U.S. 1-(800) 448-7700
Alaska - Hawaii 1-(800) 448-1100
Mail orders and all inquiries should be sent to:
Bristol Laboratories
Order Entry Department
P.O. Box 657
Syracuse, NY 13201
Products Available
Amikin
Azotrex Capsules
◆ Betapen-VK Tablets and Oral Solution
BiCNU
Blenoxane
Bristagen
◆ Bristamycin Tablets
Bristoject Products
Atropine Sulfate
Calcium Chloride
Dextrose
Diphenhydromine HCl
Epinephrine
Lidocaine HCl
Magnesium Sulfate
Metaraminol Bitartrate
Sodium Bicarbonate
Bufferin with Codeine No. 3
◆ CeeNU
Cefadyl for Intramuscular or Intravenous Injection
◆ Dynapen Capsules and Powder for Oral Suspension
◆ Kantrex Capsules
Kantrex Injection and Pediatric Injection
Ketaject
◆ Lysodren
Mexate
Mutamycin

Nafcil
◆ Naldecon Syrup, Tablets, Pediatric Drops and Pediatric Syrup
▣ Naldecon-CX Suspension
▣ Naldecon-DX Pediatric Syrup
▣ Naldecon-EX Pediatric Drops
◆ Naldegesic Tablets
Pallace
Platinol
◆ Polycillin Capsules, for Oral Suspension, and Pediatric Drops
Polycillin-N for Intramuscular or Injection
Polycillin-PRB (ampicillin-probenecid) for Oral Suspension
◆ Polymox Capsules, for Oral Suspension, and Pediatric Drops
◆ Prostaphlin Capsules, Oral Solution
Prostaphlin for Injection
◆ Saluron
◆ Salutensin/Salutensin-Demi
Stadol
Staphcillin Injection—Buffered
◆ Tegopen Capsules and For Oral Solution
◆ Tetrex Capsules & *bid* CAPS
◆ Ultracef Capsules, Tablets & Oral Suspension
Versapen Oral Suspension and Pediatric Drops
◆ Versapen-K Capsules

BRISTOL-MYERS PRODUCTS 766
(Div. of Bristol-Myers Co.)
345 Park Avenue
New York, NY 10154
Address inquiries to:
Dr. George Blewitt (201) 926-6758
Products Available
Ammens medicated powder
Arthritis Strength Bufferin analgesic
B.Q. cold tablets
Ban Basic antiperspirant
Ban Big Ball antiperspirant
Ban cream antiperspirant
Ban roll-on antiperspirant
Ban Super Solid antiperspirant
Body on Tap
Bufferin analgesic tablets
Comtrex capsules
Comtrex liquid
Comtrex tablets
Congespirin cold tablets
Congespirin cough syrup
Congespirin liquid cold medicine
Datril acetaminophen tablets
Excedrin analgesic capsules
Excedrin analgesic tablets
Excedrin P.M. analgesic tablets
Extra-Strength Bufferin Capsules & Tablets
Extra-Strength Datril
4-Way cold tablets
4-Way long acting mentholated nasal spray
4-Way long acting nasal spray
4-Way mentholated nasal spray
4-Way nasal spray
Minit-Rub analgesic balm
Multi-Scrub everyday scrubbing lotion with particles
Multi-Scrub medicated cleansing scrub
Mum cream deodorant
No Doz keep alert tablets
Pazo hemorrhoid ointment/suppositories
Score hair cream
Tickle antiperspirant
Ultra Ban roll-on
Ultra Ban II antiperspirant
Vitalis Dry Texture hair groom
Vitalis hair groom liquid
Vitalis hair groom tube
Vitalis Regular Hold hair spray
Vitalis Super Hold hair spray

THE BROWN PHARMACEUTICAL COMPANY, INC. 407, 769
2500 West Sixth St.
P.O. Box 57925
Los Angeles, CA 90057
(213) 389-1394-1395
Address inquiries to:
Professional Service Department
Products Available
◆ Android-5 Buccal
◆ Android-10 Tablets
◆ Android-25 Tablets
◆ Android-F Tablets
Brohembione
Calphosan B-12 I.M.
Calphosan I.M.
Lipo-Nicin/100 mg.
Lipo-Nicin/250 mg. Tablets
Lipo-Nicin/300 mg. Caps Timed
Vivikon I.M.

BURROUGHS WELLCOME CO. 407, 770
3030 Cornwallis Road
Research Triangle Park, NC 27709
(919) 541-9090
Address inquiries to:
Mr. C. A. Parish, Jr. (919) 541-9090
Branch Office
Burlingame, CA 94010
1760 Rollins Rd. (415) 697-5630
Products Available
◆ A.P.C. with Codeine, Tabloid brand
◆ Actidil Tablets & Syrup
◆ Actifed Tablets & Syrup
Actifed-C Expectorant
Aerosporin Powder
◆ Alkeran Tablets
Ammonia Aromatic, Vaporole
Amyl Nitrite, Vaporole
Anectine Flo-Pack
Anectine Injection
◆ Antepar Syrup & Tablets
Atropine Sulfate Injection, Wellcome
Borofax Ointment
◆ Cardilate Chewable Tablets
◆ Cardilate Oral/Sublingual Tablets
Cortisporin Cream
Cortisporin Ointment
Cortisporin Ophthalmic Ointment
Cortisporin Ophthalmic Suspension
Cortisporin Otic Solution
Cortisporin Otic Suspension
◆ Daraprim Tablets
Digoxin (See Lanoxin)
◆ Empirin Aspirin Tablets
◆ Empirin w/Codeine Phosphate Nos. 2, 3 & 4
◆ Empracet with Codeine Phosphate Nos. 3 & 4
◆ Emprazil Tablets
◆ Emprazil-C Tablets
Erythrityl Tetranitrate (See Cardilate)
◆ Fedrazil Tablets
Imuran Injection
◆ Imuran Tablets
◆ Kemadrin Tablets
Lanoline, Wellcome
Lanoxicaps
◆ Lanoxin—Tablets, Injection & Elixir Pediatric
◆ Leukeran Tablets
Lidosporin Otic Solution
Lubafax Surgical Lubricant, Sterile
Mantadil Cream
◆ Marezine Tablets & Injection
◆ Myleran Tablets
Neosporin Aerosol
Neosporin G.U. Irrigant
Neosporin Ointment
Neosporin Ointment Ophthalmic
Neosporin Ophthalmic Solution
Neosporin Topical Powder
Neosporin-G Cream
Polymyxin B Sulfate
Polysporin Ointment
Polysporin Ophthalmic Ointment
◆ Proloprim Tablets
◆ Purinethol Tablets
Scopolamine Hydrobromide Injection, Wellcome
◆ Septra DS Tablets
Septra I.V. Infusion
Septra Suspension
◆ Septra Tablets
▣ Sudafed Cough Syrup
◆ Sudafed Plus Syrup & Tablets
◆ Sudafed Pseudoephedrine Hydrochloride Syrup & Tablets
◆ Sudafed S.A. Capsules
◆ Tabloid Brand Thioguanine
Vasoxyl Injection
Viroptic Ophthalmic Solution
Zincofax Soothing Skin Cream
Zovirax Ointment 5%
Zovirax Sterile Powder
◆ Zyloprim Tablets

BURTON, PARSONS & COMPANY 827
A Division of Alcon Laboratories, Inc.
6201 South Freeway
Fort Worth, TX 76134
Address inquiries to:
Professional Services Dept.
(817) 293-0450
(See also Alcon/bp)
Products Available
Konsyl
L. A. Formula

C & M PHARMACAL, INC. 827
1519 E. Eight Mile Rd.
Hazel Park, MI 48030-2696
Address Inquires to:
C & M Pharmacal, Inc. (313) 548-7846
For Medical Emergencies Contact:
C & M Pharmacal, Inc. (313) 548-7846
Or any Poison Control Center (All products have full ingredient disclosure)
Products Available
Acnesarb
Acnotex
Aquaderm
Colladerm
Cortin 1% Cream
Drytergent
Drytex
Duplex
Duplex T
Finac
HI-COR 1.0
HI-COR 2.5
Hydropel
Neomark
Schamberg's Lotion
Seale's Lotion Modified
Sebisol
Soltex
Sulfoil
Therac
Theracort
Verr-Canth
Verrex
Verrusol

CAMPBELL LABORATORIES, INC. 828
300 East 51st Street
New York, NY 10022 (212) 688-7684
Address inquiries to:
Richard C. Zahn, President
Post Office Box 812, FDR Station
New York, NY 10150
Products Available
Herpecin-L Cold Sore Lip Balm

THE CARLTON CORPORATION 828
83 N. Summit Street
Tenafly, NJ 07670
Address inquiries to:
Professional Service Dept. (201) 569-0050
Products Available
Calphosan
Calphosan B-12

CARNRICK LABORATORIES, INC. 408, 829
65 Horse Hill Road
Cedar Knolls, NJ 07927 (201) 267-2670
Address inquiries to:
Medical Director (201) 267-2670
Products Available
◆ Amen
◆ Bontril PDM
◆ Bontril Slow Release
◆ Capital with Codeine Suspension
◆ Capital with Codeine Tablets
◆ Midrin
◆ Nolahist
◆ Nolamine
◆ Phrenilin
◆ Phrenilin Forte
◆ Propagest & Propagest Syrup
◆ Sinulin

CENTER LABORATORIES 835
Division of EM Industries, Inc.
35 Channel Drive
Port Washington, NY 11050
Address Inquiries to:
Customer Services
Call Toll Free (800) 645-6335
In N.Y. (516) 767-1800
For Medical Emergencies Contact:
Technical Services (516) 767-1800
Products Available
Center-Al—Allergenic Extracts Alum Precipitated
EpiPen—Epinephrine Auto-Injector

CENTRAL PHARMACEUTICALS, INC. 409, 835
112-128 East Third St.
Seymour, IN 47274
Address inquiries to:
Norman B. Kolbe (812) 522-3915
Products Available
Analbalm, Liquid
Biotres Ointment
Cenadex Capsules
Cenocort A-40 Sterile Suspension
Cenocort Forte Sterile Suspension
Codiclear DH Syrup
Codimal DH Syrup
Codimal DM Syrup
Codimal Expectorant
Codimal PH Syrup
Codimal Tablets & Capsules
◆ Codimal-L.A. Cenules
Co-Xan Syrup
Dexacen LA-8 Sterile Suspension
Dexacen-4 Injectable
Dia-Eze
◆ Di-Gesic
Di-Pred Sterile Suspension
Dramocen Injectable
Estronol Aqueous Sterile Suspension
GG-Cen Syrup/Capsules
Hexalol Tablets
Lifolbex Injectable
Neocylate Tablets
Neolax Tablets
Niferex Elixir
Niferex Forte Elixir
Niferex Tablets
Niferex w/Vitamin C Tablets
◆ Niferex-150 Capsules

(◆ Shown in Product Identification Section)

(▣ Described in PDR For Nonprescription Drugs)

◆ Niferex-150 Forte Capsules
◆ Niferex-PN Tablets
Pavacen Cenules
Phencen-50 Injectable
Prednicen-M Tablets
Prednisolone Acetate Sterile Suspension
Rep-Pred 40 Sterile Suspension
Rep-Pred 80 Sterile Suspension
Rubesol-1000 Injectable
Synophylate Elixir
Synophylate Tablets
Synophylate-GG Syrup
Synophylate-GG Tablets
◆ Theoclear L.A.-130 Cenules
◆ Theoclear L.A.-260 Cenules
Theoclear-80 Syrup
Theoclear-100 & Theoclear-200 Tablets

CETYLITE INDUSTRIES, INC. 838
P.O. Box CN6
9051 River Road
Pennsauken, NJ 08110
Address inquiries to:
Mr. Stanley L. Wachman, President
(609) 665-6111
(800) 257-7740
Products Available
Cetacaine Topical Anesthetic
Cetylcide Germicidal Concentrate
Protexin Oral Breath Spray
Protexin Oral Rinse Concentrate
Skin Screen Protective Skin Lotion

CIBA PHARMACEUTICAL COMPANY 409, 839
Division of CIBA-GEIGY Corporation
Address inquiries to:
556 Morris Avenue
Summit, NJ 07901
New Jersey (201) 277-5000
New York (212) 267-6615
Division Offices
Warehouse Offices and Shipping Branches
Eastern
14 Henderson Drive
West Caldwell, NJ 07006 (201) 575-6510
New York (212) 267-6640
Central
7530 No. Natchez Ave.
Niles, IL 60648 Niles (312) 647-9332
Chicago (312) 763-8700
Western
12850 Moore St.
P.O. Box 6300
Cerritos, CA 90701
Cerritos (213) 404-2651
Products Available
◆ Antrenyl Tablets
◆ Anturane Capsules
◆ Anturane Tablets
◆ Apresazide Capsules
Apresoline Ampuls
◆ Apresoline Tablets
◆ Apresoline-Esidrix Tablets
Cibalith Syrup
Coramine Ampuls
Coramine Oral Solution
◆ Cytadren Tablets
Desferal Vials
◆ Esidrix Tablets
◆ Esimil Tablets
INH Tablets
◆ Ismelin Tablets
◆ Lithobid Tablets, Cibalith-S
Locorten Cream
◆ Ludiomil Tablets
◆ Metandren Linquets & Tablets
◆ Metopirone Tablets
Nupercainal Cream
Nupercainal Ointment
Nupercainal Suppositories
Nupercaine Ampuls 1:200
Nupercaine Ampuls 1:1500
Nupercaine (Heavy) Ampuls
Ocular Therapeutic System
Ocusert
Percorten Pellets
Percorten pivalate Multiple-dose Vials
Priscoline Multiple-dose Vials
Privine Nasal Solution
Privine Nasal Spray
◆ Regitine Hydrochloride Tablets
Regitine mesylate Vials
◆ Rimactane Capsules
Rimactane/INH Dual Pack
◆ Ritalin Tablets
◆ Ritalin SR Tablets
◆ Ser-Ap-Es Tablets
Serpasil Parenteral Solution
◆ Serpasil Tablets
◆ Serpasil-Apresoline Tablets
◆ Serpasil-Esidrix Tablets
◆ Slow-K Tablets
◆ Transderm-Nitro Transdermal Therapeutic System
◆ Transderm-Scōp Transdermal Therapeutic System
Vioform Cream
Vioform Ointment
Vioform-Hydrocortisone Cream
Vioform-Hydrocortisone Lotion
Vioform-Hydrocortisone Mild Cream
Vioform-Hydrocortisone Mild Ointment
Vioform-Hydrocortisone Ointment

CIRCLE PHARMACEUTICALS, INC. 877
10377 Hague Road
Indianapolis, IN 46256
Address inquiries to:
Ross A. Deardorff, R.Ph. (317) 849-4210
Products Available
Amcap
Circavite T
Paxarel
Restora
Septa Ointment
Suspen
Tetracap
Tusquelin

CONNAUGHT LABORATORIES, INC. 877
Swiftwater, PA 18370
Address inquiries to:
Biologicals Product Mgr. (717) 839-7187
For Medical Emergencies Contact:
Medical Director (717) 839-7187
Direct orders & returns to:
Elkins-Sinn, Inc./A.H. Robins Co.
Customer Services (800) 257-8349
or (609) 424-3700
Distributed in the Continental U.S.A. by:
Elkins-Sinn, Inc.
A subsidiary of A.H. Robins Co.
2 Esterbrook Lane
Cherry Hill, NJ 08034
Products Available
Diphtheria Antitoxin (Purified, Concentrated Globulin-Equine)
Diphtheria & Tetanus Toxoids & Pertussis Vaccine Adsorbed (For Pediatric Use)
Fluzone (Influenza Virus Vaccine)
Menomune (Meningococcal Polysaccharide Vaccine, Groups A,C,Y,W-135 Combined, Groups A & C Combined, Group A or Group C)
Tetanus Toxoid
Tetanus Toxoid Adsorbed
Tetanus & Diphtheria Toxoids Adsorbed (For Adult Use)
YF-VAX (Yellow Fever Vaccine)(Live, 17D Virus, Avian Leukosis-Free, Stabilized)

CONNAUGHT LABORATORIES, LTD. 877
1755 Steeles Avenue West
Willowdale, Ontario M2R3T4 Canada
Address inquiries to:
Manager, International Customer Services (416) 667-2967
For Medical Emergencies Contact:
Medical Director (416) 667-2622
Direct orders & returns to:
Elkins-Sinn, Inc./A.H. Robins Co.
Customer Services (800) 257-8349
or (609) 424-3700
Distributed in the Continental U.S.A. by:
Elkins-Sinn, Inc.
A subsidiary of A.H. Robins Co.
2 Esterbrook Lane
Cherry Hill, NJ 08034
Products Available
Poliomyelitis Vaccine (Purified) (For the Prevention of Poliomyelitis)
Tuberculin Purified Protein Derivative (Concentrated Solution in 50% Glycerine for Multiple Puncture Test [Heaf])
Tubersol (Tuberculin Purified Protein Derivative [Mantoux])

COOK-WAITE LABORATORIES, INC. 877
90 Park Avenue
New York, NY 10016 (212) 907-2712
Products Available
Carbocaine Hydrochloride 3% Injection
Carbocaine Hydrochloride 2% with Neo-Cobefrin 1:20,000 Injection

COOPERCARE, INC. 878
Dermatology Products
3145 Porter Drive
Palo Alto, CA 94304
Products Available
A-Fil Cream Neutral & Dark
Aveeno Bath Oilated
Aveeno Bath Regular
Aveenobar Medicated
Aveenobar Oilated
Aveenobar Regular
Benisone Gel/Cream/Lotion/Ointment
D-Seb Skin Cleanser
Maxifil Cream
Meted Shampoo
Nu-Flow Shampoo
Packer's Pine Tar Shampoo
Packer's Pine Tar Soap
Pentrax Tar Shampoo
Sebaveen Shampoo
sunDare Clear
sunDare Creamy
sunStick
Texacort Scalp Lotion

COOPERVISION PHARMACEUTICALS INC 880
San German, Puerto Rico 00753
Address inquiries to:
Professional Services
San German, Puerto Rico or call
(except California) (800) 227-8313
(California only) (800) 982-6194
For Medical or Contact Lens Solution Information
Write: Medical Department
455 East Middlefield Road
Mountain View, CA 94043
Call: *(Business Hours Only)*
Joseph Krezanoski, Ph.D. (800) 227-8082
For Medical Emergency Information After Hours or on Weekends, call
Jerome F. Grattan (201) 821-8846
Products Available
Argyrol Stabilized Solution 10%
Atropisol Ophthalmic Solution 1%
Catarase 1:5,000 & 1:10,000
Cystex Tablets
Dacriose Ophthalmic Irrigating Solution
Dropperettes:
Argyrol S.S. 20%
Atropisol 0.5%, 1%, 2%
Epinephrine 1:1000
Fluorescein Sodium 2%
Homatropine HBr 2%, 5%
Phenylephrine HCl 10%
Pilocar 1%, 2%, 4%
Sulf-10 (Sodium Sulfacetamide 10%)
Tetracaine HCl 0.5%
E-Pilo Ophthalmic Solutions 1, 2, 3, 4, 6
Eserine Sulfate Ophthalmic Ointment ¼%
Funduscein-10 or -25 (Fluorescein sodium I.V.)
Glucose Ophthalmic Ointment 40%
Glyrol Solution
Goniosol Solution
Homatropine Hydrobromide Ophthalmic Solution 2%, 5%
Hypotears Moisturizing Eye Drops
Inflamase Forte 1% Ophthalmic Solution
Inflamase ⅛% Ophthalmic Solution
Lens Care Products:
Clerz
Contactisol
d-Film
duo-Flow
hy-Flow
Lensine-5
Lensine Extra Strength Cleaner
Mirasol
Pliagel
Unisol
Lipoflavonoid Vitamin Supplement (Capsule)
Lipotriad Vitamin Supplement (Capsule, Liquid)
Lydia Pinkham (Capsule, Liquid)
Miochol Intraocular
Phenylzin Ophthalmic Solution
Pilocar Ophthalmic Solutions 0.5%, 1%, 2%, 3%, 4%, 6%
Pilocar Ophthalmic Solutions Twin Pack 0.5%, 1%, 2%, 3%, 4%, 6%
Pilomiotin 1%, 2%, 4%
Schirmer Tear Test
Sulf-10 Ophthalmic Solution
Tear-Efrin Ophthalmic Solution
Tearisol Ophthalmic Solution
Vasocidin Ophthalmic Ointment
Vasocidin Ophthalmic Solution
VasoClear Ophthalmic Decongestant Eye Drops
VasoClear A Decongestant Astrigent Lubricating Eye Drops
Vasocon Regular Ophthalmic Solution
Vasocon-A Ophthalmic Solution
Vasosulf Ophthalmic Solution

CUTTER BIOLOGICAL 880
Div. Cutter Laboratories, Inc
2200 Powell Street
Emeryville, CA 94608
Address inquiries to:
Professional Services Manager
(415) 420-4167
Branch Offices
Baltimore, MD 21224
1900 Portal Street
(301) 633-8100
Chattanooga, TN 37421
5910 Quintus Loop (615) 624-4661
Chicago Office
725 Golf Lane
Bensenville, IL 60106 (312) 595-3620

Dallas, TX 75240
P.O. Box 400358 (214) 661-5850
Los Angeles Office
15320 East Salt Lake Avenue
City of Industry, CA 91744
(213) 968-8561
New Orleans Office
2631 Delaware St.
Kenner, LA 70062 (504) 469-8479
New York Office
40 E. Cotters Lane
East Brunswick, NJ 08816
(201) 238-0140
Ogden, UT 84404
475 W. Cutter Way (801) 626-4515
Seattle Office
1147 Andover Park West
Tukwila, WA 98188 (206) 575-0490

Products Available

Antihemophilic Factor (Human) (Factor VIII, AHF, AHG) Koāte
Factor IX Complex (Human) (Factors II, VII, IX, and X) Konȳne
Gamastan (Immune Serum Globulin-Human)
Gamimune (Immune Globulin Intraveneous, 5% in 10% Maltose)
Hepatitis B Immune Globulin (Human) HyperHep
Hyperab (Rabies Immune Globulin-Human)
HyperHep (Hepatitis B Immune Globulin-Human)
Hyper-Tet (Tetanus Immune Globulin-Human)
HypRho-D (Rh_0-D Immune Globulin-Human)
Immune Globulin Intravenous, 5% (In 10% Maltose) Gamimune
Immune Serum Globulin (Human) Gamastan
Koāte (Factor VIII, Antihemophilic Factor-Human)
Konȳne (Factor IX Complex-Human) (Factors II, VII, IX and X)
Pertussis Immune Globulin (Human) Hypertussis
Plague Vaccine (Human)
Rh_0-D Immune Globulin (Human) HypRho-D
Rabies Immune Globulin (Human) Hyperab
Tetanus Immune Globulin (Human) Hyper-Tet

DALIN PHARMACEUTICALS, INC. 882
74-80 Marine Street
Farmingdale, NY 11735

Address inquiries to:

Professional Services Dept. (516) 454-9282
Subsidiaries:
DG Packaging

Branch Offices

Dagoberto Rivera, Inc.
Salud 23 Int.
Station 6, Box 233
Ponce, Puerto Rico 00731
(809) 842-6263

Products Available

Audax Ear Drops
Ban Itch
Celluzyme Chewable Tablets
Cremesone
Dalex Capsules & Lozenges
Dalex Pediatric Syrup
Dalex Syrup
Dalex Syrup Forte
Dalicote Lotion
Dalicreme
Daliderm Liquid
Dalidyne
Dalidyne Jel
Dalidyne Spray (Mouth and Throat)
Dalifort Tablets
Daligesic Liniment
Dalimycin Capsules
Dalisept Ointment
Dalivim Forte Liquid & Tablets
Pentacort Cream
Phenagesic Capsules
Phenarex Syrup
Phenatuss Expectorant
Polysept Ointment
Sorbutuss
Spandecon Capsules
Spasmid Elixir & Capsules

DANBURY PHARMACAL, INC. 883
131 West Street
P.O. Box 296
Danbury, CT 06810

Address Inquiries to:

Nessim Maleh
Ira Sacks
Milton Blitz (203) 744-7200

Products Available

Bethanechol Chloride Tablets
Butalbital with Acetaminophen Tablets
Carisoprodol Compound Tablets
Carisoprodol Tablets
Chloroquine Phosphate Tablets
Chlorothiazide Tablets
Chlorpheniramine Maleate T.D. Capsules
Chlorpheniramine Maleate T.D. Tablets
Chlorthalidone Tablets
Chlorzoxazone Tablets
Chlorzoxazone with APAP Tablets
Colchicine Tablets
Col-Probenecid Tablets
Cyproheptadine HCl Tablets
Dicyclomine HCl Capsules
Dicyclomine HCl Tablets
Diphenhydramine HCl Capsules
Dipyridamole Tablets
Disulfiram Tablets
Doxycycline Hyclate Capsules
Ergoloid Mesylates Oral Tablets
Ergoloid Mesylates Sublingual Tablets
Erythromycin Estolate Capsules
Folic Acid Tablets
Glutethimide Tablets
Glycopyrrolate Tablets
Hydralazine HCl Tablets
Hydrochlorothiazide, Hydralazine HCl, Reserpine Tablets
Hydrochlorothiazide/Reserpine Tablets
Hydrochlorothiazide Tablets
Hydrocortisone Tablets
Hydroxyzine Pamoate Capsules
Isoniazid Tablets
Isosorbide Dinitrate Oral Tablets
Isosorbide Dinitrate Sublingual Tablets
Isoxsuprine HCl Tablets
Meprobamate Tablets
Methocarbamol Tablets
Metronidazole Tablets
Nylidrin HCl Tablets
Papaverine HCl T.D. Tablets
Phenobarbital Tablets
Phenylbutazone Tablets
Prednisolone Tablets
Prednisone Tablets
Primidone Tablets
Probenecid Tablets
Procainamide HCl Capsules
Propantheline Bromide Tablets
Pseudoephedrine HCl Tablets
Quindan Tablets
Quinidine Gluconate Sustained Action Tablets
Quinidine Sulfate Tablets
Spironolactone/Hydrochlorothiazide Tablets
Sulfasalazine Tablets
Sulfinpyrazone Tablets
Tetracycline HCl Capsules
Theofedral Tablets
Tolbutamide Tablets
Triamcinolone Tablets
Trihexyphenidyl HCl Tablets
Tripelennamine HCl Tablets
Tripodrine Tablets

DELMONT LABORATORIES, INC. 884
P.O. Box AA
Swarthmore, PA 19081

Address inquiries to:

(215) 543-3365

Products Available

Staphage Lysate (SPL)

DERMIK LABORATORIES, INC. 884
1777 Walton Road, Dublin Hall
Blue Bell, PA 19422

Address inquiries to:

Albert M. Packman, D.Sc. (215) 641-1962

Distribution Centers

Langhorne, PA 19047
P.O. Box 247 (215) 752-1211
Oak Forest, IL 60452
P.O. Box 280 (800) 323-4474
San Leandro, CA 94577
1550 Factor Avenue (415) 357-9741
Tucker, GA 30084
4660 Hammermill Road (800) 241-9120

Products Available

Anthra-Derm Ointment 1%, ½%, ¼%, 1/10%
5 Benzagel (5% benzoyl peroxide) & 10 Benzagel (10% benzoyl peroxide), Acne Gels, Microgel Formula
Comfortine Ointment
Drest
Fomac Foam
Hytone Cream ½%, 1%, 2½%
Hytone Lotion 1%, 2½%
Hytone Ointment ½%, 1%
Jeri-Bath
Jeri-Lotion
Klaron Acne Lotion
Loroxide Acne Lotion
Loroxide-HC Acne Lotion
Post Acne Lotion
Rezamid Acne Lotion
Shepard's Cream Lotion
Shepard's Dry Skin Cream
Shepard's Moisturizing Soap
Shepard's Skin Cream
Sulfacet-R Acne Lotion
Vanoxide Acne Lotion
Vanoxide-HC Acne Lotion
Vlemasque
Vytone Cream ½%, 1%
Zetar Emulsion
Zetar Shampoo

DISTA PRODUCTS COMPANY 410, 887
Division of Eli Lilly and Company
General Offices
307 East McCarty Street
Indianapolis, IN 46285

For Medical Information, Write:

Medical Department
307 East McCarty Street
Indianapolis, IN 46285 (317) 261-4000

Sales Offices

Aurora, CO 80014
3131 South Vaughn Way (303) 695-7733
Bloomington, MN 55420
Suite 1142, One Appletree Square
(612) 854-0214
*Chicago, IL 60631
Suite 270, O'Hare Plaza
5735 East River Road (312) 693-8360
Cincinnati, OH 45241
4055 Executive Park Drive
(513) 563-7010
Cleveland, OH 44130
16600 West Sprague Road (216) 243-3600
Dallas, TX 75234
4404 Beltwood Parkway, South
(214) 661-5669
Dedham, MA 02026
990 Washington Street (617) 329-6858
Indianapolis, IN 46268
Suite 235, Northwest Plaza (317) 261-5770
or (317) 261-5794
Memphis, TN 38117
755 Crossover Lane (901) 767-0360
Metairie, LA 70002
4900 Veterans Memorial Boulevard
Security Homestead Bldg (504) 455-0339
Nashville, TN 37217
1101 Kermit Drive (615) 361-5971
*Norcross, GA 30091
5944 Peachtree Corners East
Post Office Box 628 (404) 449-4928
*Pasadena, CA 91101
301 East Colorado Blvd. (213) 792-3197
Pittsburgh, PA 15220
1910 Cochran Road (412) 561-5044
Raleigh, NC 27604
3109 Poplarwood Court (919) 872-5210
Silver Spring, MD 20903
1734 Elton Road (301) 439-1109
Southfield, MI 48075
3000 Town Center (313) 358-2278
*Stamford, CT 06905
1600 Summer St. (203) 357-8872
Tampa, FL 33609
5401 West Kennedy Boulevard
(813) 870-3086
Wynnewood, PA 19096
Seven Wynnewood Road (215) 477-8739
*Regional Office also

Products Available

Becotin Pulvules
Becotin with Vitamin C Pulvules
Becotin-T Tablets
◆ Cinobac
Co-Pyronil Pulvules, Pediatric Pulvules, and Suspension
Cordran Ointment & Lotion
Cordran SP Cream
Cordran Tape
Cordran-N Cream and Ointment
Ilosone Chewable Tablets
Ilosone, for Oral Suspension
Ilosone Liquids, Oral Suspensions
◆ Ilosone Pulvules & Tablets
Ilosone Ready-Mixed Drops
Ilotycin Gluceptate, I.V., Vials
Ilotycin Ointment
Ilotycin Sterile Ophthalmic Ointment
Ilotycin Tablets
Keflex, for Oral Suspension
Keflex, for Pediatric Drops
◆ Keflex, Pulvules & Tablets
Mi-Cebrin Tablets
Mi-Cebrin T Tablets
◆ Nalfon Pulvules & Tablets
◆ Nalfon 200 Pulvules
Nebcin Vials & Hyporets
◆ Valmid Pulvules

DOAK PHARMACAL CO., INC. 904
700 Shames Drive
Westbury, NY 11590

Address inquiries to:

Director of Physician Services
(516) 333-7222

Branch Offices

Obergfel Brothers
2660 East 37th Street
Vernon, CA 90058 (213) 583-8981

Products Available

Buro-Sol Antiseptic Powder
Diasporal Cream
▣ Doak Oil & Doak Oil Forte
▣ Doak Tar Lotion
▣ Doak Tar Shampoo
▣ Formula 405 Skin Care Products
Enriched Cream
Eye Cream

(◆ Shown in Product Identification Section) (▣ Described in PDR For Nonprescription Drugs)

Light Textured Moisturizer
Moisturizing Lotion
Moisturizing Soap
Skin Cleanser & Patented Buffing Mitt
Solar Cream
Therapeutic Bath Oil
▣ Lavatar Tar Bath
Lotio Alsulfa
Normaderm Cream
Normaderm Lotion
Petro-Phylic Soap Cake
Tar Distillate "Doak"
▣ Tarpaste
▣ Tersaseptic Hygienic Skin Cleanser
▣ Tersa-Tar
Unguentum Bossi

DORSEY LABORATORIES 410, 904
Division of Sandoz, Inc.
P.O. Box 83288
Lincoln, NB 68501
Address inquiries to:
Medical Department (402) 464-6311
Products Available
Acid Mantle Creme & Lotion
Cama Inlay-Tabs
Chexit Tablets
Dorcol Pediatric Cough Syrup
Kanulase Tablets
Pabirin Buffered Tablets
Triaminic Expectorant
Triaminic Syrup
Triaminic-DM Cough Formula
Triaminic-12 Tablets
▣ Triaminicin Tablets
Triaminicol Syrup
▣ Tussagesic Tablets & Suspension
▣ Ursinus Inlay-Tabs

DORSEY PHARMACEUTICALS 410, 906
Division of Sandoz, Inc.
East Hanover, NJ 07936
Address inquiries to:
Medical Department
Products Available
◆ Asbron G Elixir & Inlay-Tabs
◆ Bellergal Tablets
◆ Bellergal-S Tablets
Gris-PEG Tablets
◆ Hydergine Tablets, Sublingual Tablets, & Liquid
◆ Klorvess Effervescent Granules/Tablets
Klorvess 10% Liquid
Metaprel Inhalant Solution 5%
◆ Metaprel MDI, Syrup, Tablets
Neo-Calglucon Syrup
◆ Tavist Tablets
◆ Tavist-1 Tablets
Trest Tablets
Triaminic Expectorant w/Codeine
Triaminic Juvelets
Triaminic Oral Infant Drops
◆ Triaminic Tablets

DRUG INDUSTRIES CO., INC. 915
3237 Hilton Road
Ferndale, MI 48220
Address inquiries to:
John Hadd (313) 547-3784
Products Available
Al-Vite
BC-Vite
Bilax
C-Caps 500
Calfer-Vite
Day-Vite
Di-Sosul
Di-Sosul Forte
E-Plus
Hemo-Vite
Hemo-Vite Liquid
Sinovan Timed
Trilax
Vanodonnal Timed
Vicef

DURA PHARMACEUTICALS, INC 916
P.O. Box 28331
San Diego, CA 92128
Address inquiries to:
Same as above (714) 789-6840
For Medical Emergencies Contact:
Craig Wheeler (714) 789-6840
Tom Evangelisti
Products Available
Dura Tap-PD
Dura-Vent
Dura-Vent/A
Dura-Vent/DA

EDWARDS PHARMACAL, INC. 918
100 East Hale
Osceola, AR 72370
Address inquiries to:
Mr. John Newcomb (501) 563-1144
For Medical Emergencies Contact:
Mr. John Newcomb (501) 563-5757
Branch Offices None
Products Available
Blanex Capsules
▣ C-Span Capsules
Double-A
▣ ECEE Plus Capsules
Nico-Vert Capsules
Rymed Capsules
Rymed-JR Capsules
Rymed Liquid
Rymed-TR Capsules
Slyn-LL
Urogesic Tablets
Uromide Tablets

ELDER PHARMACEUTICALS, INC. 410, 918
705 E. Mulberry Street
Bryan, OH 43506
Address inquiries to:
P.O. Box 31 (800) 537-4294
Bryan, OH
In Ohio (800) 472-4588
Products Available
Benoquin Cream
Elaqua XX Cream
Eldecort Cream
Elder Psoralite
Eldopaque Cream
Eldopaque Forte Cream
Eldoquin Cream
Eldoquin Lotion
Eldoquin Forte Cream
Eloxyl-5 Gel
Eloxyl-10 Gel
Fototar Cream
HQC Kit
HyCort Cream
◆ Oxsoralen Capsule
Oxsoralen Lotion 1%
Pabanol Lotion
RVP Ointment
RVPaba Lip Stick
RVPaque Cream
Solaquin Cream
Solaquin Forte Cream
◆ Trisoralen Tablet
Vitadye Lotion

ELKINS-SINN, INC. 926
A subsidiary of A.H. Robins Company
2 Esterbrook Lane
Post Office Box 5483
Cherry Hill, NJ 08034
(609) 424-3700
Address price and packaging inquiries to:
Marketing Department
Address scientific information inquiries to:
Professional Services
Products Available
Aminocaproic Acid Injection
Aminophylline Injection
Atropine Sulfate Injection
Calcium Chloride Injection
Calcium Gluconate Injection
Chlorpromazine HCl Injection
Codeine Phosphate Injection
Cyanocobalamin (Vit. B_{12}) Injection
Dexamethasone Sodium Phosphate Injection
Dexpanthenol Injection
Dextrose Injection
Digoxin Injection
Diphenhydramine HCl Injection
Dopamine HCl Injection
Epinephrine Injection
Furosemide Injection
Gentamicin Sulfate Injection
Heparin Sodium Injection
Hep-Lock (Heparin Sodium for IV Flush)
Hydrocortisone Sodium Succinate for Injection
Hydromorphone HCl Injection
Hydroxyzine HCl Intramuscular Injection
Isoproterenol HCl Injection
Lidocaine HCl Injection
Lidocaine Hydrochloride Injection for Cardiac Arrhythmias
Lidocaine HCl & Epinephrine Injection
Magnesium Sulfate Injection
Meperidine HCl Injection
Metaraminol Bitartrate Injection
Methylene Blue Injection
Methylprednisolone Sodium Succinate for Injection
Mineral Oil, Sterile
Morphine Sulfate Injection
Neostigmine Methylsulfate Injection
Paraldehyde (Sterile)
Pentobarbital Sodium Injection
Phenobarbital Sodium Injection
Phenytoin Sodium Injection
Potassium Chloride Injection
Procaine HCl Injection
Prochlorperazine Edisylate Injection
Promethazine HCl Injection
Scopolamine Hydrobromide Injection
Sodium Chloride Injection
Sodium Nitroprusside Injection
Sotradecol (Sodium Tetradecyl Sulfate Injection)
Sterile Empty Vials
Thiamine HCl Injection
Water For Injection

ENDO LABORATORIES, INC. 410, 927
Sub. of the DuPont Company
One Rodney Square
Wilmington, Delaware 19898
Address inquiries to:
Director, Professional Services
(302) 773-3652
Emergency No. (302) 773-3652
Branch Offices
Chicago, IL 60641
4956 W. Belmont Ave. (312) 282-0440
Claremont, CA 91711
1480 N. Claremont Blvd.
(714) 621-7986, 7987

ENDO INC. 410, 927
Manati, Puerto Rico 00701
Subsidiary of Endo Laboratories, Inc.
Subsidiary of the DuPont Company
Address inquiries to:
Endo Laboratories, Inc.
Sub. of the DuPont Company
One Rodney Square
Wilmington, Delaware 19898
Director, Professional Services
(302) 773-3652
Products Available

ENDO PHARMACEUTICALS, INC. 410, 927
Manati, Puerto Rico 00701
Subsidiary of Endo Laboratories, Inc.
Subsidiary of the DuPont Company
Address Inquiries to:
Endo Laboratories, Inc.
Subsidiary of the DuPont Company
One Rodney Square
Wilmington, Delaware 19898
Director, Professional Services
(302) 773-3652
Products Available
◆ Coumadin Injection & Tablets
Endecon Tablets
Endotussin-NN Pediatric Syrup
Endotussin-NN Syrup
Hycodan Syrup, Tablets
◆ Hycomine Compound Tablets
Hycomine Pediatric Syrup
Hycomine Syrup
Hycotuss Expectorant Syrup
◆ Moban Tablets & Concentrate
◆ Narcan Injection
Narcan Neonatal Injection
◆ Nubain Injection
Numorphan Hydrochloride Injection, Suppositories
◆ Percocet-5 Tablets
◆ Percodan Tablets
◆ Percodan-Demi Tablets
Percogesic with Codeine Tablets
Remsed Tablets
◆ Symmetrel Capsules & Syrup
◆ Tessalon Perles
Valpin 50 Tablets
Valpin 50-PB Tablets

EVERETT LABORATORIES, INC. 945
76 Franklin Street
East Orange, NJ 07017
Address inquiries to:
Professional Service Dept. (201) 674-8455
Products Available
Anafed Capsules & Syrup
Florvite Chewable Tablets
Florvite Drops
Florvite + Iron Chewable Tablets
Florvite + Iron Drops
Folic Acid Tablets
Libidinal Capsules
Nicotym Capsules
Pavatym Capsules
Repan Tablets
Vitafol Tablets

FERNDALE LABORATORIES, INC. 945
780 W. Eight Mile Road
Ferndale, MI 48220
Address inquiries to:
Professional Service Dept. (313) 548-0900
Products Available
Adphen Tablets
Aquaphyllin Sugarbeads Capsules
Aquaphyllin Syrup
Bellkatal Tablets
Benase Tablets
Betuline Liniment
Dapa Tablets
Dapa & Codeine Tablets
Dapacin Capsules
Delaxin Tablets
Detachol Adhesive Remover
Doss 300 Capsule

Fastamine Tablets
Ferndex Tablets
Fernisolone-P-Tablets
Flavitab Tablets
Kronofed-A Jr. Kronocaps
Kronofed-A Kronocaps
Kronohist Kronocaps
Liqui-Doss
Livonamine Tablets
Lixaminol AT Elixir
Lixaminol Elixir
Maigret Tablets
Mastisol Liquid Adhesive
Niapent Tablets
Obestin-30 Capsules
Oxychinol Tablets
Phenobella Tablets
Pramosone Cream, Lotion & Ointment
Prax Cream & Lotion
Procute Cream & Lotion
Rauserpin Tablets
Rhinocaps Capsules
Salatin Capsules
Strifon Forte Tablets
Tin-Ben Dispenser
Tin-Co-Ben Dispenser
Vio-Pramosone Cream
Vio-Pramosone Lotion

FISONS CORPORATION 946
Pharmaceutical Division
Two Preston Court
Bedford, MA 01730
Address inquiries to:
Professional Services Dept. (617) 275-1000
Distribution Centers
ATLANTA
James M. Hogan Co., Inc.
5356 Ponce de Leon Ave.
Stone Mountain, GA 30083
(404) 938-7901
BEDFORD
Fisons Corporation
2 Preston Court
Bedford, MA 01730 (617) 275-1000
LOS ANGELES
Obergfel Brothers
2660 East 37th Street
Vernon, CA 90058 (213) 583-8981
Products Available
Bacid Capsules
Ergomar
Intal
Intal Nebulizer Solution
Kondremul
Kondremul with Cascara
Kondremul with Phenolphthalein
Neo-Cultol
Persistin
Proferdex
Somophyllin Oral Liquid
Somophyllin Rectal Solution
Somophyllin-CRT Capsules
Somophyllin-DF Liquid
Somophyllin-T Capsules
Tusscapine
Vapo-Iso Solution
Vaponefrin Solution
Vitron-C
Vitron-C-Plus

C. B. FLEET CO., INC. 950
4615 Murray Pl.
Lynchburg, VA 24506
Address inquiries to:
Fred T. Wickis, Jr. (804) 528-4000
Products Available
Fleet Babylax
Fleet Bisacodyl Enema
Fleet Enema
Fleet Enema Pediatric
Fleet Flavored Castor Oil Emulsion
Fleet Mineral Oil Enema
Fleet Phospho-Soda
Fleet Prep Kits
Summer's Eve Medicated Douche
Summer's Eve Medicated Vaginal Suppositories

FLEMING & COMPANY 952
1600 Fenpark Dr.
Fenton, MO 63026
Address inquiries to:
John J. Roth, M.D. (314) 343-8200
Products Available
Aerolate Liquid
Aerolate III T.D. Capsules
Aerolate Jr. T.D. Capsules
Aerolate Sr. T.D. Capsules
Alumadrine Tablets
Congess Jr. T.D. Capsules
Congess Sr. T.D. Capsules
Ectasule Minus III T.D. Capsules
Ectasule Minus Jr. T.D. Capsules
Ectasule Minus Sr. T.D. Capsules
Ectasule III T.D. Capsules
Ectasule Jr. T.D. Capsules
Ectasule Sr. T.D. Capsules
Extendryl Chewable Tablets
Extendryl Sr. & Jr. T.D. Capsules
Extendryl Syrup
Impregon Concentrate
Magonate Tablets
■ Marblen Suspension Peach/Apricot
■ Marblen Suspension Unflavored
■ Marblen Tablets
Nephrocaps
■ Nephrox Suspension
■ Nicotinex Elixir
■ Ocean Nasal Mist
Ocean-Plus Mist
Pima Syrup
■ Purge Liquid
Rum-K Syrup
S-P-T "Liquid" Capsules

FLINT LABORATORIES 411, 953
Division of Travenol Laboratories, Inc.
Deerfield, IL 60015 (312) 940-5211
Address inquiries to:
Professional Services Dept.
Products Available
◆ Choloxin
◆ Silver Sulfadiazine Cream
◆ Synthroid Injection
◆ Synthroid Tablets
◆ Travase Ointment

FLUORITAB CORPORATION 957
P.O. Box 381
Flint, MI 48501
Address inquiries to Main Office:
M. L. Cleveland, Manager (1-313) 239-9770
Howard D. Vogt, Research & Promotion (1-813) 439-1652
Post Office Box 263
Lake Hamilton, FL 33851
Products Available
Fluoritab Liquid
Fluoritab Tablets

FOREST LABORATORIES, INC. 957
919 Third Avenue
New York, NY 10022
Address inquiries to:
Professional Service Dept. (212) 421-7850
Products Available
Brocon C.R. Tablets

GEIGY PHARMACEUTICALS 411, 958
Division of CIBA-GEIGY Corporation
Ardsley, NY 10502
Address inquiries to:
Medical Services Dept. (201) 277-5000
Products Available
Brethine Ampuls
◆ Brethine Tablets
◆ Butazolidin Capsules & Tablets
◆ Constant-T Tablets
◆ Lioresal Tablets
◆ Lopressor Tablets
Otrivin Nasal Spray
Otrivin Nasal Solution
Otrivin Pediatric Solution
PBZ Elixir
PBZ Hydrochloride Cream
PBZ Lontabs
◆ PBZ Tablets
PBZ Tablets w/Ephedrine
◆ PBZ-SR Tablets
◆ Tandearil
◆ Tegretol Chewable Tablets
◆ Tegretol Tablets
Tofranil Ampuls
◆ Tofranil Tablets
◆ Tofranil-PM

GENEVA GENERICS 977
2599 W. Midway Blvd.
Broomfield, CO 80020
Address inquiries to:
Professional Services Department
(303) 466-2341
Products Available
APAP w/Codeine Tablets
Aminophylline Tablets
Amitriptyline HCl Tablets
Antibiotic Ear Drops
Aspirin w/Codeine Tablets
Azo-Sulfisoxazole Tablets
Bisacodyl Suppositories
Caltro Tablets
Carisoprodol Compound Tablets
Carisoprodol Tablets
Chloral Hydrate Capsules
Chlordiazepoxide Capsules
Chlorothiazide Tablets
Chlorothiazide w/Reserpine Tablets
Chlorpheniramine Maleate T.D. Capsules
Chlorpromazine Tablets & Concentrate Syrup
Chlorzoxasone w/APAP Tablets
Conjugated Estrogens Tablets
Cyclandelate Capsules
Cyproheptadine HCl Tablets
DSS Capsules & Syrup
DSS w/Casanthranol Capsules
Deproist Expectorant w/Codeine
Diphenhydramine Capsules
Dipyridamole Tablets
Disobrom Tablets
Disulfiram Tablets
Ergoloid Mesylates Tablets
Furosemide Tablets
Glutethimide Tablets
Hydralazine HCl Tablets
Hydrochorothiazide Tablets
Hydrochlorothiazide w/Reserpine Tablets
Hydroxyzine Tablets
Imipramine Tablets
Isosorbide Dinitrate Tablets
Isosorbide Dinitrate T.D. Capsules & Tablets
Isoxsuprine Tablets
Lonox Tablets
Meclizine HCl Tablets
Meprobamate Tablets
Methocarbamol Tablets
Methocarbomal with Aspirin Tablets
Metronidazole Tablets
Mygel Suspension
Nitrofurantoin Capsules & Tablets
Nitroglycerin T.D. Capsules
Nylidrin Tablets
P.E.T.N. S.R. Tablets
Papaverine T.D. Capsules
Phenylbutazone Capsules
Phenylbutazone Tablets
Polyvite with Fluoride Drops
Potassium Chloride Elixir
Potassium Gluconate Elixir (K-G Elixir)
Prednisolone Tablets
Prednisone Tablets
Primidone Tablets
Probenecid Tablets
Probenecid w/Colchicine Tablets
Procainamide Capsules
Prochlorperazine Tablets
Pro-Iso Capsules
Promethazine DM (Ped) Expectorant
Promethazine Expectorant Plain
Promethazine w/Codeine Expectorant
Promethazine VC Expectorant
Promethazine VC w/Codeine Expectorant
Propantheline Bromide Tablets
Propox 65 w/APAP Tablets
Propoxyphene Compound 65 Capsules
Propoxyphene HCl Capsules
Pseudoephedrine S.R. Capsules
Pseudoephedrine Tablets
Quinidine Gluconate S.R. Tablets
Quinidine Sulfate Tablets
Quinine Capsules
Quinine Sulfate Tablets
Quiphile Tablets
Resaid T.D. Capsules
Rescaps-D T.D. Capsules
Spironolactone Tablets
Spironolactone w/Hydrochlorothiazide Tablets
Sulfamethoxazole Tablets
Sulfasalazine Tablets
Sulfisoxazole Tablets
T.E.H. Tablets
T.E.P. Tablets
Tamine Elixir, Expectorant & Expectorant DC
Tamine S.R. Tablets
Theophylline Elixir
Tolbutamide Tablets
Triamcinolone Tablets
Trichlormethiazide Tablets
Trifed Tablets & Syrup
Trifed-C Syrup
Trifluoperazine Tablets
Triplevite w/Fluoride Drops
Uroblue Tablets

GERBER PRODUCTS COMPANY 978
Fremont, MI 49412 (616) 928-2000
Address inquiries to:
Professional Communications Department
Products Available
Gerber Cereals
Barley Cereal
Cereals with Fruit
High Protein Cereal
Mixed Cereal
Oatmeal Cereal
Rice Cereal
Gerber High Meat Dinners (Strained & Junior)
Gerber Junior Cookies
Gerber Junior Foods
Gerber Junior Meats
Gerber Strained Egg Yolks
Gerber Strained Foods
Gerber Strained Juices
Gerber Strained Meats
Gerber Teething Biscuits
Gerber Toddler Meals
MBF (Meat Base Formula) Liquid

GERIATRIC PHARM. CORP. 979
397 Jericho Turnpike
Floral Park, NY 11001 (516) 354-1121
Products Available
B-C-Bid Capsules (sustained release)

(◆ Shown in Product Identification Section)
(■ Described in PDR For Nonprescription Drugs)

Bilezyme Tablets
Bilezyme-Plus Tablets
Cevi-Bid Capsules (sustained release)
Cevi-Fer Capsules (sustained release)
Gaysal-S Tablets
Geritinic Tablets
Geritonic Liquid
Ger-O-Foam Aerosol
Gustalac Tablets
Gustase Tablets
Gustase-Plus Tablets
Iso-Bid Capsules (sustained release)
Stimulax Capsules
Testand-B Injectable

GILBERT LABORATORIES 411, 979
31 Fairmount Avenue
Chester NJ 07930
Address inquiries to:
Professional Service Dept. (201) 879-7374
Products Available
◆ Esgic Tablets & Capsules

GLAXO INC. 412, 981
1900 West Commercial Blvd.
Fort Lauderdale, FL 33309
(305) 776-5300
Address inquiries to:
Professional Service Department
Products Available
Amesec Capsules
Atrocholin Tablets
BCG Vaccine
◆ Beclovent Inhaler
◆ Beclovent Inhaler Refill
◆ Beconase Nasal Inhaler
Bronchobid Duracap Capsules
◆ Corticaine Cream
◆ Corticaine Suppositories
Doctate Tablets
Doctate-P Tablets
Duragesic Tablets
◆ Ethatab Tablets
Ferrobid Duracap Capsules
◆ Histabid Duracap Capsules
Renalgin Tablets
Sinacon Tablets
◆ Theobid Duracap Capsules
◆ Theobid Jr. Duracap Capsules
◆ Tri-Cone Capsules
◆ Tri-Cone Plus Capsules
Trinsicon/Trinsicon M Capsules
◆ Ventolin Inhaler
◆ Ventolin Inhaler Refill
◆ Ventolin Tablets
◆ Vicon Forte Capsules
◆ Vicon with Iron
◆ Vicon-C Capsules
◆ Vicon-Plus Capsules
◆ Vi-Zac Capsules
Vi-Zinc Capsules

GLENBROOK LABORATORIES 990
Division of Sterling Drug Inc.
90 Park Avenue
New York, NY 10016
Address inquiries to:
Medical Director (212) 972-4141
Products Available
Bayer Aspirin
Bayer Children's Chewable Aspirin
Bayer Children's Cold Tablets
Bayer Cough Syrup for Children
Bayer Timed-Release Aspirin
Breacol
Cope
Diaparene Line
Dr. Caldwell's Laxative
Fizrin
Fletcher's Castoria
Midol
Phillips' Milk of Magnesia Liquid
Phillips' Milk of Magnesia Tablets
Vanquish

GLENWOOD, INC. 412, 992
83 North Summit Street
Tenafly, NJ 07670
Address inquiries to:
Professional Service Dept. (201) 569-0050
Products Available
Amid-Sal Tablets
◆ Myotonachol
◆ Potaba
Potaba Plus 6
Pyridoxine HCl
◆ Yodoxin
Zinc-Glenwood

GRAY PHARMACEUTICAL CO. 993
Affiliate, The Purdue Frederick Company
100 Connecticut Avenue
Norwalk, CT 06854
Address inquiries to:
Medical Department (203) 853-0123
Products Available
X-Prep Bowel Evacuant Kit
X-Prep Bowel Evacuant Kit #2
X-Prep Liquid

GUARDIAN CHEMICAL 993
A Division of United-Guardian, Inc.
230 Marcus Boulevard
P.O. Box 2500
Smithtown, NY 11787
(516) 273-0900
(800) 645-5566 Address inquiries to:
Director of Medical Research
Products Available
Clorpactin WCS-90
Clorpactin XCB
Lubrajel
Lubrajel HC
Lubraseptic Jelly
pHos-pHaid Tablets
Renacidin
Warexin

W. E. HAUCK, INC. 994
P.O. Box 1065
Roswell, GA 30075
Address inquiries to:
Warren E. Hauck (404) 475-4758
Products Available
Besta Capsules
Cantri Vaginal Cream
Chlorafed H.S. Timecelles
Chlorafed Liquid
Chlorafed Timecelles
Diaqua Tablets
Entuss Expectorant
Entuss Tablets
G-1 Capsules
G-2 Capsules
G-3 Capsules
Geravite Elixir
Histor-D Syrup
Histor-D Timecelles
Isotrate Timecelles
MSG-600
Otic-HC Ear Drops
Otic-Plain Ear Drops
Palbar Tablets
Palmiron Forte Tablets
Palmiron-C Tablets
Sinufed Timecelles
Wehless-105 Timecelles

HAWAII DIET PLAN, INC. 994
737 Bishop Street
Suite 2990
Honolulu, Hawaii 96813
Address inquiries to:
737 Bishop Street, Suite 2990
Honolulu, Hawaii 800-521-1072
For Medical Emergencies Contact:
Mr. Peter Nardozzi 800-367-5056
Products Available
▣ The Hawaii Diet

HEALTH CARE PRODUCTS DIVISION 994
of Consolidated Chemical, Inc.
3224 S. Kingshighway Blvd.
St. Louis, MO 63139
Address inquiries to:
John C. Brereton (314) 772-4610
Products Available
CC-500
Consept
Consol Concentrate
Formula Magic
GCP Shampoo
New Consol 20
Perineal/Ostomy Spray Cleaner
Satin
Skin Magic
Staphoclean
Staphosan
Swirlsoft

HERBERT LABORATORIES 995
Dermatology Division of Allergan Pharmaceuticals, Inc.
2525 Dupont Drive
Irvine, CA 92713 (714) 752-4500
Products Available
Aeroseb-Dex Topical Aerosol Spray
Aeroseb-HC Topical Aerosol Spray
▣ Aquacare Dry Skin Cream & Lotion, 2% Urea Cream & Lotion
▣ Aquacare/HP Dry Skin Cream & Lotion, 10% Urea Cream & Lotion
▣ Bluboro Powder Astringent Soaking Solution
Clear By Design, Acne Skin Medication
▣ Danex Protein Enriched Dandruff Shampoo
▣ Eclipse After Sun Lotion
▣ Eclipse Sunscreen Gel, Original, SPF 10
▣ Eclipse Sunscreen Lip & Face Protectant, SPF6; SPF15
▣ Eclipse Sunscreen Lotion, Original, SPF10
▣ Eclipse Sunscreen Lotion, Total, Alcohol Base or Moisturizing Base, SPF15
▣ Eclipse Suntan Lotion, Partial, SPF5
Exsel Lotion
Fluonid Ointment, Cream & Topical Solution
Fluoroplex Topical Solution & Cream
Maxiflor Cream
Maxiflor Ointment
▣ Vanseb Cream Dandruff Shampoo
▣ Vanseb Lotion Dandruff Shampoo
▣ Vanseb-T Cream Tar Shampoo
▣ Vanseb-T Lotion Tar Shampoo

DOW B. HICKAM, INC. 999
P.O. Box 35413
Houston, TX 77035
Address inquiries to:
Professional Service Dept. (713) 723-0690
Products Available
Granulex
Proderm Topical Dressing

HIGH CHEMICAL COMPANY 1000
Div. Day & Frick, Inc.
1760 N. Howard St.
Philadelphia, PA 19122
Address inquiries to:
Professional Service Dept. (215) 634-2224
Products Available
Amo-Derm
Klorlyptus
Mus-L-Tone
Sarapin

HILL DERMACEUTICALS, INC. 1000
P.O. Box 19283
Orlando, Florida 32814
Address inquiries to:
Mr. Jerry S. Roth, President
(305) 896-8280
Products Available
Burdeo
Derma-Smoothe/FS
Derma-Smoothe Oil
Derma-Sone Cream
Florida Foam Improved
Hill Cortac Lotion
Hill-Shade Lotion
R.S. Lotion No. 2

HOECHST-ROUSSEL PHARMACEUTICALS INC. 412, 1000
Route 202-206 North
Somerville, NJ 08876
Address inquiries to:
Medical Dept. (201) 231-2000
Products Available
◆ A/T/S
Claforan
Doxan
◆ Doxidan
Doxinate
Doxinate Solution
Duadacin
◆ Festal
◆ Festalan
◆ Lasix Oral Solution
◆ Lasix Tablets and Injection
Streptase
◆ Surfak
◆ Topicort
◆ Topicort LP

HOFFMANN-LA ROCHE INC.
(See Roche Laboratories & Roche Products Inc.)

HOLLAND-RANTOS COMPANY, INC. 1009
Post Office Box 385
865 Centennial Avenue
Piscataway, NJ 08854
See YOUNGS DRUG PRODUCTS CORPORATION

HOYT LABORATORIES 413, 1009
Division of Colgate-Palmolive Co.
575 University Avenue
Norwood MA 02062
Address inquiries to:
Professional Services Dept. (617) 769-6850
Products Available
Luride Drops
◆ Luride Lozi-Tabs Tablets
◆ Full-strength 1.0 mg F
◆ Luride-SF (no artificial flavor or color) 1.0 mg F
◆ Half-strength 0.5 mg F
◆ Quarter-strength 0.25 mg F
Orabase HCA Oral Paste
Orabase Plain Oral Protective Paste
Orabase with Benzocaine Analgesic Oral Protective Paste
PerOxyl Mouthrinse
Phos-Flur Oral Rinse/Supplement
Point-Two Dental Rinse
Thera-Flur Topical Gel-Drops
Thera-Flur-N Topical Gel-Drops

HYLAND THERAPEUTICS DIVISION 1012
Travenol Laboratories, Inc.
444 W. Glenoaks Blvd.
Glendale, CA 91202
Address inquiries to:
Product Management
(toll free) (800) 423-2862
For Medical Emergencies Contact:
Medical Director
Parenteral Div. (312) 480-5303
Medical Director,
Hyland Therapeutics Div. (213) 956-3200
Branch Offices
Los Angeles, CA
4501 Colorado (800) 423-2862
(213) 240-5600
Coagulation Products Distributed By:
Hyland Therapeutics Division
Travenol Laboratories, Inc.
Glendale, CA 91202
(800) 423-2862
Plasma Extenders & Gamma Globulin Products
Distributed By:
Parenteral Products Div.
Travenol Laboratories, Inc.
Deerfield, IL 60015 (800) 323-6474
Products Available
Autoplex, Anti-Inhibitor Coagulant Complex, Dried
Buminate 5%, Normal Serum Albumin (Human), U.S.P., 5% Solution
Buminate 25%, Normal Serum Albumin (Human), U.S.P., 25% Solution
Hemofil, Antihemophilic Factor (Human), Method Four, Dried
Hu-Tet, Tetanus Immune Globulin (Human), U.S.P.
Immune Serum Globulin (Human), U.S.P. Gamma Globulin
Proplex, Factor IX Complex (Human) (Factors II, VII, IX & X), Dried
Protenate 5%, Plasma Protein Fraction (Human), U.S.P., 5% Solution

HYNSON, WESTCOTT & DUNNING 1013
Division of Becton Dickinson and Co.
Charles & Chase Sts.
Baltimore, MD 21201 (301) 837-0890
Products Available
BAL in Oil Ampules
Cardio-Green Vials & Single Use Units
Indigo Carmine Ampules
◘ Lactinex Tablets & Granules
Phenolsulfonphthalein Solution Ampules
Thantis Lozenges

HYREX PHARMACEUTICALS 1013
3494 Democrat Road
Memphis, TN 38118
Address inquiries to:
Professional Service Dept. (901) 794-9050
Products Available
Atropine Sulfate Injection
C & T
Chorex
Cortisone Acetate Injection
Depogen
Depotest
Depotestogen
Dermarex Cream
Efedron Nasal Jelly
Everone
Glukor Injection
Hybolin Decanoate
Hydrate Injection
Hylate Tablets
Hyrex-105
Hytinic Capsules & Elixir
Hytinic Injection
Hytuss Tablets
Hytuss-2X Capsules
Hyzine-50 Injection
Kavrin Capsules
Kestrin Injection
Key-Plex Capsules
Key-Pred
Key-Pred SP
Lipoderm Capsules
ND-Gesic Tablets
ND-Hist Capsules
ND-Stat Injection
Nicozol Capsules & Elixir
Panzyme Tablets
Prorex Injection
Pylora Tablets
Solurex Injection
Trac Tablets
Trac Tablets 2X
Two-Dyne Capsules
Valergen
Valertest #2

ICN PHARMACEUTICALS, INC. 1014
222 N. Vincent Avenue
Covina, CA 91722
Address inquiries to:
Professional Service Dept. (213) 967-5121
Products Available
Testred Capsules

I.C.P. PHARMACEUTICALS 1015
A Division of Wisconsin Medical Enterprises, Inc.
P.O. Box 294
Cudahy, Wisconsin 53110
Address inquiries to:
C. Jrolf (414) 931-6299
Products Available
Decubitex Ointment
Decubitex Powder
Historal Capsules
Historal Liquid
Historal Pediatric Oral Drops

IVES LABORATORIES INC. 413, 1015
685 Third Ave.
New York, NY 10017
Address medical inquiries to:
Clarence Denton, M.D.
(Day) (212) 878-5166
Night Emergency (914) 769-9060
General Information (212) 878-5125
Branch Warehouses
Andover, MA 01810
7 Lowell Junction Rd. Connector
(617) 475-7227
Atlanta, GA 30324
221 Armour Dr., N.E. (404) 875-8380
Baltimore, MD 21224
101 Kane St. (301) 633-4005
Buena Park, CA 90620
6530 Altura Blvd. (714) 523-5110
Dallas, TX 75247
8717 Directors Row (214) 631-7865
Denver, CO 80216
4345 Oneida St. (303) 377-0233
Honolulu, HI 96814
1013 Kawaiahao St. (808) 538-1988
N. Kansas City, MO 64116
1340 Taney St. (816) 842-3680
Memphis, TN 38127
4171 Steele Road (901) 353-5040
St. Paul, MN 55121
935 Apollo Road
Eagandale Center Indus. Pk.
(612) 454-1613
Kent, WA 98031
19255 80th Ave. South (206) 872-8166
Skokie, IL 60076
3435 Madison St. (312) 267-1700
Strongsville, OH 44136
17647 Foltz Industrial Parkway
(216) 238-3820
Products Available
Cerose Compound Capsules
Cerose-DM
Cerubidine
Cetro-Cirose
◆ Cyclospasmol Capsules & Tablets
◆ Isordil Chewable
◆ Isordil Oral Titradose Tablets
◆ Isordil Sublingual Tablets
◆ Isordil Tembids Capsules
◆ Isordil Tembids Tablets
◆ Isordil w/Phenobarbital
◆ Surmontil Capsules
◆ Synalgos Capsules
◆ Synalgos-DC Capsules
Trecator-SC Tablets

JACOBUS PHARMACEUTICAL CO., INC. 1021
37 Cleveland Lane
Princeton, NJ 08540
Address inquiries to:
Professional Services (609) 921-7447
For Medical Emergencies Contact:
Medical Department (609) 799-8221
Products Available
Dapsone

JAMOL LABORATORIES INC. 1022
13 Ackerman Avenue
Emerson, NJ 07630 (201) 262-6363
Products Available
Bahim Foot-Aide
Bahim Oil
Otide
Ponaris Nasal Mucosal Emollient
Prep-Aide
Roma-Nol Antiseptic

JANSSEN PHARMACEUTICA INC. 413, 1022
501 George Street
New Brunswick, NJ 08903
Products Available
Droperidol, See Inapsine
Fentanyl, See Sublimaze
◆ Imodium Capsules
Inapsine Injection
Innovar Injection
◆ Monistat I.V.
◆ Nizoral Tablets
◆ Sublimaze Injection
◆ Vermox Chewable Tablets

JOHNSON & JOHNSON PRODUCTS INC. 1030
Patient Care Division
501 George Street
New Brunswick, NJ 08903
(201) 524-0400
Products Available
Debrisan Wound Cleaning Beads
Debrisan Wound Cleaning Paste
Surgicel Absorbable Hemostat

KEIGHLEY PROCTOLOGICAL INSTRUMENTS, INC. 1033
359 Forest Ave.
Dayton, Oh. 45405
Address Inquiries to:
Ms. Lowana G. Looper, General Manager
(513) 222-9347
Products Available
K-HC Rectal Suppositories

KENWOOD LABORATORIES, INC. 1033
490-A Main Street
New Rochelle, NY 10801 (914) 632-1002
Products Available
Apatate Liquid
Bonacal Plus Tablets
Cebral Capsules
Ferrous-G Elixir
Glutofac Tablets
I.L.X. B_{12} Elixir
I.L.X. B_{12} Tablets
I.L.X. Elixir
Kenpectin
Kenpectin-P
Kenwood Therapeutic Liquid
Ominal Tablets
Papavatral L.A. Capsules
Papavatral L.A. with Phenobarbital Capsules
Papavatral Tablets
Papavatral 20 Tablets
Posterisan Ointment
Posterisan Suppositories
Therapeutic Liquid
Tossecol

KEY PHARMACEUTICALS, INC. 413, 1033
18425 N.W. 2nd Ave.
Miami, FL 33169
Address inquiries to:
Professional Service Dept. (305) 652-2276
Products Available
Casafru
Genapax
Geriliquid
Guanidine HCl Tablets
Ipsatol Expectorant Syrup
Ipsatol-DM Expectorant/Antitussive
Ircon Tablets
Ircon-FA Tablets
Nico-Span Capsules
◆ Nitro-Dur Transdermal Infusion System
◆ Nitroglyn Tablets
Pavakey Capsules
Pavakey-300 Capsules
Quinora Tablets
◆ Theo-Dur Sprinkle
◆ Theo-Dur Tablets
Tyzine Nasal Solution
Tyzine Pediatric Nasal Drops

KNOLL PHARMACEUTICAL COMPANY 414, 1038
30 North Jefferson Road
Whippany, NJ 07981 (201) 887-8300
Address inquiries to:
Professional Services Department
Products Available
Akineton Injection
◆ Akineton Tablets
Codeine Phosphate Injection
Codeine Sulfate Tablets
Dicodid Tablets
Dilaudid Cough Syrup
Dilaudid Injection
Dilaudid Multiple Dose Vials (Sterile Solution)
Dilaudid Powder
Dilaudid Rectal Suppositories
◆ Dilaudid Tablets
◆ Isoptin for Intravenous Injection
◆ Isoptin Oral Tablets
Meperidine Hydrochloride Injection
Metrazol Injection
Metrazol Liquidum
Metrazol Tablets
Morphine Sulfate Injection
Nico-Metrazol Elixir & Tablets
Promethazine Hydrochloride Injection
Quadrinal Suspension
◆ Quadrinal Tablets
◆ Santyl Ointment
Theokin Elixir
Theokin Tablets
Verequad Suspension
Verequad Tablets

◆ Vicodin Tablets
Vita-Metrazol Elixir

KREMERS-URBAN COMPANY 414, 1049
P.O. Box 2038
Milwaukee, WI 53201
Address inquiries to:
Professional Service Dept. (414) 354-4300
Products Available
Calciferol Drops (Oral Solution)
Calciferol in Oil, Injection
◆ Calciferol Tablets
Kudrox Suspension (Double Strength)
Kutapressin Injection
◆ Kutrase Capsules
◆ Ku-Zyme Capsules
◆ Ku-Zyme HP Capsules
◆ Levsin Drops
◆ Levsin Elixir
◆ Levsin Injection
◆ Levsin Tablets
Levsin-PB Drops
Levsin/Phenobarbital Elixir
Levsin/Phenobarbital Tablets
◆ Levsinex Timecaps
Levsinex/Phenobarbital Timecaps
Milkinol
◆ Nitrol Ointment
Pre-Pen
Salimeph Forte

LACTAID INC. 414, 1054
600 Fire Road P.O. Box 111
Pleasantville, NJ 08232-0111
Address inquiries to:
Alan E. Kligerman (609) 645-7500
Products Available
◆ LactAid brand lactase enzyme

LAMBDA PHARMACAL CORPORATION 1054
Sub. of A. J. Bart, Inc.
Plainview, NY 11803 (516) 931-3300
Address inquiries to:
In the United States
Mr. Tony Zimardo (516) 931-3300
In Puerto Rico
Dr. L.O. Bartolomei (809) 844-3506
Products Available
Dextrotussin Syrup
Feraplex Injectable
Feraplex Liquid
Migralam Capsules
Neuro B-12 Forte Injectable
Neuro B-12 Injectable
Vita-Numonyl Injectable

THE LANNETT COMPANY, INC. 1055
9000 State Road
Philadelphia, PA 19136
Address inquiries to:
Medical Service Dept. (215) 333-9000
Products Available
Acetazolamide Tablets
▣ Acnederm Lotion & Soap
Adalan Lanatabs
Alphamul Suspension
Amtren Tablets
Arithmin Tablets
Baroflave Powder
Bellafedrol AH Tablets
Bethanechol Chloride
Bisacodyl Suppositories & Tablets
Brompheniramine Maleate Tablets
Castaderm
Chlorpromazine Tablets
Chlorulan Tablets
Codalan
Diphenoxylate & Atropine Tablets
Disanthrol Capsules
Disolan Capsules
Disonate Capsules & Liquid
Efricon Expectorant
Glutethimide Tablets
Hydrochlorulan Tablets
Kaylixir
Lanacillin "400"
Lanahex Liquid
Lanamin Capsules
Lanatuss Expectorant
Lanorinal Capsules & Tablets
Lanvisone Cream
Lofene Tablets
Lycolan Elixir
▣ Magnatril Suspension & Tablets
Nitrofurantoin Tablets
Obalan Tablets
Orcophen Capsules
P-I-N Forte Tablets
Paverolan Lanacaps
Potasalan Elixir
Primidone Tablets
Probenecid Tablets
Promethazine Expectorant
Promethazine Tablets
Pyrralan Expectorant DM
Rufolex Capsules
S-A-C Tablets
Salatar Cream
Sedragesic Tablets
Trichlorex Tablets
Trichlormethiazide Tablets
Veltane Tablets & Expectorant

LASALLE LABORATORIES, INC. 1055
Subsidiary of Mallard, Inc.
3021 Wabash Avenue
Detroit, MI 48216
Address inquiries to:
Mallard, Inc. (313) 964-3910
Products Available
Allercort
Aquex Tablets
Dytuss
Fetrin
Orabex-TF Tablets
Pacaps
Protid Tablets
Spasmatol Elixir & Tablets
Sul-Azo Tablets

LASER, INC. 1055
2000 N. Main Street,
P.O. Box 905, Crown Point, IN 46307
Address inquiries to:
Donald A. Laser (219) 663-1165
Products Available
Dallergy Capsules
Dallergy Syrup
Dallergy Tablets
Donatussin DC Syrup
Donatussin Drops
Donatussin Syrup
Fumatinic Capsules
Fumerin Tablets
KIE Syrup
Lactocal-F Tablets
Myobid Capsules
Respaire-SR Capsules
Theospan-SR Capsules
Theostat 80 Syrup
Theostat Tablets
Trimstat Tablets

LEDERLE LABORATORIES 414, 1056, 3009
Division of American Cyanamid Co.
One Cyanamid Plaza
Wayne, NJ 07470
LEDERLE PARENTERALS, INC.
Carolina, Puerto Rico 00630
LEDERLE PIPERACILLIN, INC.
Carolina, Puerto Rico 00630
Address inquiries on medical matter to:
Professional Services Dept.
Lederle Laboratories
Pearl River, NY 10965 (914) 735-5000
Distribution Centers
ATLANTA
Bulk Address
Chamblee (Atlanta), GA 30341
5180 Peachtree Industrial Blvd.
Mail Address
Atlanta, GA 30302
P.O. Box 4272 (404) 455-0320
(GA Only) (800) 282-0399
(All Other) (800) 241-3043
CHICAGO
Bulk Address
Rosemont, IL 60018
10401 W. Touhy Ave.
Mail Address
Chicago, IL 60666
P.O. Box 66189 (312) 827-8871
(IL Only) (800) 942-1493
(All Other) (800) 323-9744
DALLAS
Bulk Address
Dallas, TX 75247
7611 Carpenter Freeway
Mail Address
Dallas, TX 75265
P.O. Box 225731 (214) 631-2130
(TX Only) (800) 442-7510
(All Other) (800) 527-9770
LOS ANGELES
Bulk Address
Los Angeles, CA 90040
2300 S. Eastern Ave.
Mail Address
Los Angeles, CA 90051
T.A. Box 2202 (213) 726-1016
(CA Only) (800) 372-6325
(All Other) (800) 423-4120
PHILADELPHIA
Fort Washington, PA 19034
185 Commerce Drive
(PA Only) (800) 562-6924
(NY-NJ-MD-DE) (800) 523-6610
(CT-VA-WV-DC) (800) 523-6230
(Phila. Only) (215) 248-3900
(All Other) (215) 646-7000
Products Available
◆ Acetaminophen Capsules, Tablets, Elixir
Achromycin Intramuscular
Achromycin Intravenous
Achromycin Ophthalmic Ointment 1%
Achromycin Ophthalmic Suspension 1%
Achromycin 3% Ointment
◆ Achromycin V Capsules
Achromycin V Oral Suspension
Achrostatin V Capsules
◆ Amicar Intravenous, Syrup & Tablets
◆ Amitriptyline HCl
◆ Ampicillin Trihydrate
◆ Aristocort A Topical Cream
◆ Aristocort A Topical Ointment
Aristocort Forte Parenteral
Aristocort Intralesional
Aristocort Syrup
◆ Aristocort Tablets
◆ Aristocort Topical Cream
◆ Aristocort Topical Ointment
Aristospan Suspension (Intraarticular)
Aristospan Suspension (Intralesional)
Artane Elixir
◆ Artane Sequels
◆ Artane Tablets
Ascorbic Acid Tablets
◆ Asendin
Aureomycin Ointment 3%
Aureomycin Ointment (Ophthalmic) 1%
Brompheniramine Maleate, Phenylephrine & Phenylpropanolamine Sequels
Caramiphen Edisylate & Phenylpropanolamine Sequels
▣ Centrum
▣ Centrum, Jr. (Childrens' Chewable)
Chlordiazepoxide HCl
Chlorothiazide
◆ Chlorpheniramine Maleate
Chlorpheniramine Maleate & Phenylpropanolamine Sequels
◆ Chlorpromazine HCl
◆ Chlorthalidone Tablets
Chlorzoxazone
Cholera Vaccine (India Strains)
Cloxacillin
◆ Cyclocort Cream
◆ Cyclocort Ointment
◆ Declomycin Capsules, Tablets
Diamox Parenteral
◆ Diamox Sequels, Tablets
Dicyclomine HCl
Dihydroergotoxine Methanesulfonate Sublingual Tablets
Diluting Fluid
Diphenhydramine HCl
Diphenoxylate HCl
Diphtheria & Tetanus Toxoids, Combined
Diphtheria & Tetanus Toxoids & Pertussis Vaccine, Adsorbed
◆ Dipyridamole Tablets
◆ Docusate Sodium, USP (DSS)
◆ Docusate Sodium, USP w/Casanthranol
Dolene AP-65 Tablets
Dolene Capsules
Dolene Compound-65 Capsules
Ergoloid Mesylates
Erythromycin Ethylsuccinate Oral Suspension
◆ Erythromycin Stearate Tablets
◆ Ferro-Sequels
Ferrous Gluconate Iron Supplement
Ferrous Sulfate
◆ Filibon F.A. Prenatal Vitamin Tablets
◆ Filibon Forte
◆ Filibon OT
◆ Filibon Prenatal Vitamin Tablets
Folbesyn Tablets
Folbesyn Vitamins, Parenteral
Folvite Parenteral & Tablets
Folvron Capsules
◆ Furosemide Tablets
▣ Gevrabon Liquid
Gevral Protein Powder
▣ Gevral T Tablets
▣ Gevral Tablets
Gevrite Tablets
Guaifenesin
Guaifenesin w/D-Methorphan Hydrobromide
Hetrazan Tablets
Hydralazine HCl
◆ Hydrochlorothiazide
◆ Hydromox R Tablets
◆ Hydromox Tablets
◆ Imipramine HCl Tablets
▣ Incremin w/Iron Syrup
Isosorbide Dinitrate
Isosorbide Dinitrate, Sublingual
Ledercillin VK Oral Solution & Tablets
▣ Lederplex Capsules, Liquid & Tablets
Leucovorin Calcium
Levoprome
Levothyroxine Sodium
Liver Injection
◆ Loxitane C Oral Concentrate
◆ Loxitane Capsules
◆ Loxitane IM
◆ Materna 1•60 Tablets
◆ Meclizine HCl
Methenamine Mandelate
Methocarbamol
◆ Methotrexate Tablets & Parenteral
◆ Minocin Capsules
Minocin Intravenous
Minocin Oral Suspension
Myambutol Tablets

(◆ Shown in Product Identification Section) (▣ Described in PDR For Nonprescription Drugs)

▣ Neoloid Emulsified Castor Oil
Neomycin Sulfate
◆ Neptazane Tablets
Niacin
Nilstat Oral Suspension
Nilstat Oral Tablets
Nilstat Topical Cream, Ointment
Nilstat Vaginal Tablets
◆ Nitroglycerin
Nylidrin HCl
Orimune Poliovirus Vaccine, Live, Oral, Trivalent
◆ Papaverine HCl
◆ Pathibamate Tablets
Pathilon Sequels
◆ Pathilon Tablets
Pathilon w/Phenobarbital Tablets
Penicillin G Potassium
Penicillin V Potassium
Perihemin Capsules
▣ Peritinic Tablets
Phenobarbital
◆ Pipracil
Pnu-Imune Pneumococcal Vaccine Polyvalent
Potassium Chloride Liquid
Potassium Gluconate
Prednisone
◆ Probenecid
◆ Procainamide HCl
Promethazine HCl Expectorant, Plain
Promethazine HCl Expectorant V.C. Plain
Promethazine HCl Expectorant V.C. w/Codeine
Promethazine HCl Expectorant w/Codeine
Pronemia Capsules
Propantheline Bromide
Propoxyphene HCl
Propylthiouracil Tablets
Pseudoephedrine HCl Tablets & Syrup
◆ Pyrazinamide Tablets
Pyridoxine HCl
◆ Quinidine Sulfate
Quinine Sulfate
▣ Rhulicaine
▣ Rhulicort
▣ Rhulicream
▣ Rhuligel
▣ Rhulispray
◆ Spironolactone Tablets
◆ Spironolactone with Hydrochlorothiazide Tablets
▣ Stresscaps Capsules
▣ Stresstabs 600 Tablets, Advanced Formula
▣ Stresstabs 600 with Iron, Advanced Formula
▣ Stresstabs 600 with Zinc, Advanced Formula
Sulfadiazine-Sulfamerazine-Sulfamethazine
Sulfasalazine
Sulfisoxazole
Tetanus Toxoid, Adsorbed
Tetanus Toxoid Purogenated
Tetanus & Diphtheria Toxoids, Combined Purogenated
Thiamine HCl (Vitamin B-1) Tablets
Thiotepa Parenteral
Thyroid
Tolbutamide Tablets
◆ TriHemic 600 Tablets
Tri-Immunol
Tuberculin, Old, Tine Test
Tuberculin Purified Protein Derivative Tine Test (PPD)
Vi-Magna Capsules
Vitamin A, Natural
Vitamin C Chewable
Vitamin E, Natural USP
Vitamin E USP
▣ Zincon Dandruff Shampoo, Improved Richer Formula

LEEMING DIVISION 1099
Pfizer Inc.
100 Jefferson Rd.
Parsippany, NJ 07054
Address inquiries to:
Research and Development Dept.
(201) 887-2100
Products Available
▣ Ben Gay External Analgesic Products
▣ Desitin Ointment
Rheaban Tablets & Liquid
Unisom Nighttime Sleep-Aid
Visine A.C. Eye Drops
Visine Eye Drops

LEGERE PHARMACEUTICALS, INC. 1099
7326 E. Evans Road
Scottsdale, Az. 85260 (602) 991-4033
Address Inquiries to:
Customer Service & Product Information
Toll Free 1(800) 528-3144
Products Available
ACE + Z Tablets
Acetaco Tablets
Adenosine
Allerphen 12 Tablets
Aquamed Tablets
B Complex 100
Brosema
Cafamine T.D. 2X Capsules
Cee-500
Cee-1000 T.D. Tablets
chorionic 10,000 IU
Cinalone 40
Cinonide 40
Depo-Cobolin
Depo-Predate 80
Dexasone 4
Dexasone L.A.
Dexol T.D. Tablets
Dextraron-50
Di-Atro Tablets
Dieutrim Capsules
E-Cypionate
E.D.T.A.
Hydrochlor 50 Tablets
Ironex #2
Kabolin
Lipo-B-C
Livolex
Mag-5
Megaplex Tablets
Menaval-10
Menaval 20
Myotrol
Neucalm 50
P T 105 Capsules
Phenazine Tablets & Capsules
Predate-100
Predate-L.A.S.A.
Predate S
Prevenzyme Tablets
Probahist Capsules
Probocon
Rodex
Rodex Forte Tablets
Rodex T.D. Capsules
Spasgesic Tablets
T-Cypionate
T.E.-Cypionate
Teramine Capsules & Tablets
Testaval 90/4
Vagimide Cream

LEMMON COMPANY 416, 1099
Ethical Division
Post Office Box 30
Sellersville, PA 18960
Address inquiries to:
Professional Services Department
Toll Free (800) 523-6542
In Pennsylvania (215) 723-5544
Products Available
Acetaminophen Capsules
Acetaminophen Tablets
Acetaminophen with Codeine Tablets
◆ Adipex-P Tablets
Allerstat Capsules
B.P.P.-Lemmon
Belap Tablets
Chlordiazepoxide Hydrochloride Capsules
Chlorpromazine Hydrochloride
Dexampex Capsules
Dexampex Tablets
Diacin
Dipav
Diphenhydramine Hydrochloride Capsules
Donphen Tablets
Dralserp Tablets
Dralzine Tablets
Glucoron with B_{12} Tablets
Hydrap-ES Tablets
KEFF
Lexor
Lidocaine Hydrochloride
Lidocaine Hydrochloride with Epinephrine
Mepriam Tablets
Mequin
Methampex Tablets
◆ Metryl
Myco Triacet Cream
Myco Triacet Ointment
Nandrolone Decanoate
Neothylline Elixir
Neothylline Injection
Neothylline Tablets
Neothylline-GG Elixir
Neothylline-GG Tablets
Neutralox Suspension
Nu'Leven Tablets
Nystatin Cream
Nystatin Oral Tablets
Nystatin Vaginal Tablets
Obestat 75
Otocort Sterile Ear Drops
Oxymetazoline Hydrochloride Nasal Spray
Parest
Phentermine HCl Capsules
◆ Potage
Pyracort-D Nasal Spray
Pyridoxine Hydrochloride
Quāālude
Quin III (Iodochlorhydroxyquin 3%)
Racet Cream
Racet LCD Cream
Racet-1% Cream
Rhinex D•Lay Tablets
Rhinex DM Syrup
Rhinspec Tablets
Rhus Tox Antigen Injection
Ruhexatal w/Reserpine Tablets
S.B.P. Plus Tablets
Sed-Tens SE Tablets
Statobex Capsules
Statobex Tablets
Statobex-G Tablets
Sulfisoxazole Tablets
Tetracycline Hydrochloride Capsules
Triacet Cream
Triamcinolone Diacetate
Trimethoprim & Sulfmethazoxazole
Trimethoprim & Sulfmethazoxazole, D.S.
Uristat Tablets
◆ Vagilia Cream
Vagilia Suppositories
Vagitrol Vaginal Cream
Vagitrol Vaginal Suppositories

ELI LILLY AND COMPANY 416, 1103, 3011
For Medical Information, Write
Medical Department (317) 261-2000
307 E. McCarty St.
Indianapolis, IN 46285
Lilly Regional & District Offices
*Aurora, CO 80014
3131 South Vaughn Way (303) 695-7730
Birmingham, AL 35223
3300 Cahaba Road (205) 879-2441
Bloomington, MN 55420
One Appletree Square
(612) 854-3505
Charlotte, NC 28209
1515 Mockingbird Lane (704) 525-8905
*Chicago, IL 60631
5735 East River Road (312) 693-8740
Cincinnati, OH 45241
4055 Executive Park Dr. (513) 563-0720
Cleveland, OH 44130
16600 W. Sprague Rd. (216) 243-3600
*Dallas, TX 75234
4404 Beltwood Parkway, South
(214) 661-5620
*Dedham, MA 02026
990 Washington St. (617) 329-2816
(617) 329-4320
Enfield, CT 06082
150 Freshwater Boulevard
(203) 741-2055
Grand Rapids, MI 49506
3040 Charlevoix Dr., S.E.
(616) 949-0876
Hasbrouck Heights, NJ 07604
377 Route 17 South (201) 288-3321
(201) 288-3324
Honolulu, HI 96825
912 Puuomao Place (808) 395-2488
Houston, TX 77042
9800 Richmond Ave. (713) 975-6766
Indianapolis, IN 46268
3901 West 86th Street (317) 261-2512
Jacksonville, FL 32216
7825 Baymeadows Way (904) 731-7124
Kansas City, MO 64112
9200 Ward Parkway (816) 361-6116
(816) 361-6117
Louisville, KY 40223
10170 Linn Station (502) 425-2372
Melville, NY 11747
1 Huntington Quadrangle (516) 752-9797
Memphis, TN 38117
755 Crossover Lane (901) 767-0360
Metarie, LA 70002
4900 Veterans Memorial Blvd.
(504) 885-9645
Miami, FL 33143
8603 S. Dixie Highway (305) 661-2787
Nashville, TN 37217
1101 Kermit Drive (615) 361-0639
*Norcross, GA 30091
5944 Peachtree Corners East
(404) 441-5400
Oklahoma City, OK 73112
5400 N.W. Grand Blvd. (405) 947-2482
Omaha, NE 68103
5600 South 42d St. (402) 734-4635
*Pasadena, CA 91101
301 E. Colorado Blvd. (213) 792-5121
Pittsburgh, PA 15220
1910 Cochran Rd. (412) 922-9770
Portland, OR 97205
720 S.W. Washington St. (503) 223-8298
Raleigh, NC 27604
3109 Poplarwood Ct. (919) 872-4863
Redmond, WA 98052
11811 Willows Road (206) 881-5796
Richmond, VA 23229
2800 Parham Rd. (804) 747-7160
St. Louis, MO 63131
1633 Des Peres Road (314) 821-0190
Sacramento, CA 95814
555 Capitol Mall (916) 444-2173
San Antonio, TX 78216
800 N.W. Loop 410 (512) 341-2211
San Diego, CA 92103
2550 Fifth Ave. (714) 234-6664

San Francisco, CA 94111
100 California St. (415) 362-0559
Silver Spring, MD 20903
1734 Elton Road (301) 439-7991
(301) 439-7992
*Southfield, MI 48075
3000 Town Center
(313) 358-2206
(313) 358-2207
(313) 358-2208
*Stamford, CT 06905
1600 Summer St. (203) 357-1422
Tampa, FL 33609
5401 W. Kennedy Blvd. (813) 870-2036
Williamsville, NY 14221
5820 Main St. (716) 634-0178
Worthington, OH 43085
300 E. Wilson Bridge Rd.
(614) 846-5090
Wynnewood, PA 19096
Seven Wynnewood Rd. (215) 296-2575
(215) 477-8739

*Regional office also

Products Available

A.S.A. Compound Pulvules & Tablets
◆ A.S.A. & Codeine Compound Pulvules & Tablets
A.S.A. Enseals, Pulvules, Suppositories & Tablets
Acidulin Pulvules
Aerolone Solution
Alphalin Gelseals & Pulvules
Amertan Jelly
Aminosalicylic Acid Enseals
Ammoniated Mercury Ointments
Ammonium Chloride Enseals
Amyl Nitrite, Aspirols
◆ Amytal Elixir & Tablets
◆ Amytal Sodium Pulvules
Amytal Sodium Vials
Analgesic Balm Ointment
Anhydron Tablets
Apomorphine Hydrochloride Soluble Tablets
Arnica Tincture
Aromatic Ammonia Aspirols & Spirit
Aromatic Elixir
Atropine Sulfate Vials, Sterile Ophthalmic Ointment, Tablets & Soluble Tablets
◆ Aventyl HCl Liquid & Pulvules
Bacitracin Ointment & Sterile Ophthalmic Ointment
Belladonna Extract Tablets
Belladonna Powdered Extract & Tincture
Benzoin Tincture
Betalin Complex Ampoules, Vials & Elixir
Betalin Complex F.C. Ampoules & Vials
Betalin Compound Pulvules
Betalin S Ampoules, Vials, Elixir & Tablets
Betalin 12 Crystalline Vials
Bilron Pulvules
Bismuth Subcarbonate Tablets
Blank (Placebo) Soluble Tablets
Boric Acid Ointment & Sterile Ophthalmic Ointments
Brevital Sodium Vials
Buchu, Juniper & Potassium Acetate Elixir
Caffeine & Sodium Benzoate, Ampoules
Calcium Carbonate Tablets, Aromatic
Calcium Gluceptate, Ampoules
Calcium Gluconate Tablets
Calcium Gluconate w/Vitamin D Pulvules & Tablets
Calcium Hydroxide Powder
Calcium Lactate Tablets
Camphor Spirit
Capastat Sulfate Vials
Capsules, Empty Gelatin
Carbarsone Capsules
Cascara, Aromatic, Fluid Extract
Cascara Compound Tablets
Cascara Sagrada Fluid Extract
Cascara Tablets
Castor Oil Elastic Filled Capsules
Ceclor Pulvules & Suspension
Cevalin Ampoules & Tablets
Citrated Caffeine Tablets
Cocaine Hydrochloride Solvets
Coco-Quinine Suspension
Codeine Phosphate Vials & Soluble Tablets
Codeine Sulfate Tablets & Soluble Tablets
Colchicine Ampoules & Tablets
Cold Cream, for Compounding Prescriptions, Ointment
Cologel Liquid
Compound Benzoin Tincture
Copavin, Pulvules
Crystodigin Ampoules
◆ Crystodigin Tablets
Cyanide Antidote Package
◆ Darvocet-N 50 Tablets
◆ Darvocet-N 100 Tablets
◆ Darvon Pulvules
◆ Darvon Compound Pulvules
◆ Darvon Compound-65 Pulvules
◆ Darvon with A.S.A. Pulvules
◆ Darvon-N Suspension & Tablets
◆ Darvon-N with A.S.A. Tablets
Deltalin Gelseals
Dextrose (Buffered) Ampoules
Dibasic Calcium Phosphate Tablets
Dibasic Calcium Phosphate w/Vitamin D Pulvules
Dibasic Calcium Phosphate w/Vitamin D & Iron Pulvules
Dicumarol Pulvules
Diethylstilbestrol Enseals, Suppositories & Tablets
Digiglusin Tablets
Digitalis Pulvules
Dobutrex Vials
Dolophine Hydrochloride Ampoules, Vials & Tablets
Drolban Vials
◆ Dymelor Tablets
Emetine Hydrochloride Ampoules
En-Cebrin Pulvules
En-Cebrin F Pulvules
Ephedrine & Amytal Pulvules
Ephedriine & Seconal Sodium Pulvules
Ephedrine Sulfate Ampoules, Pulvules, Solution & Syrups
Eprolin Gelseals
Ergotrate Maleate Ampoules & Tablets
Extralin B Pulvules
Extralin F Pulvules
Extralin Pulvules
Ferrous Gluconate Pulvules
Ferrous Sulfate Enseals & Tablets
Folic Acid Tablets
Glucagon for Injection Vials
Green Soap Tincture
Haldrone Tablets
Heparin Sodium Vials
Hepicebrin Tablets
Hexa-Betalin Vials & Tablets
Histalog, Ampoules
Histamine Phosphate (For Gastric Test)
Histamine Phosphate (Histamine Test for Pheochromocytoma)
Homicebrin
Hydriodic Acid Syrup
Ichthammol Ointments
Lente Iletin I, 40 & 100 units
Regular Iletin I, 40 & 100 units
Regular Iletin II (Concentrated), 500 units
Semilente Iletin I, 40 & 100 units
Ultralente Iletin I, 40 & 100 units
NPH Iletin I, 40 & 100 units
Protamine, Zinc & Iletin I, 40 & 100 units
Beef Regular Iletin II, 100 units
Beef Lente Iletin II, 100 units
Beef NPH Iletin II, 100 units
Beef Protamine Zinc & Iletin II, 100 units
Pork Regular Iletin II, 100 units
Pork Lente Iletin II, 100 units
Pork NPH Iletin II, 100 units
Pork Protamine, Zinc & Iletin II, 100 units
Iodine, Strong, Tincture
Ipecac Syrup
Isoniazid Tablets
Isopropyl Alcohol, Lilly, 91%
Keflin, Neutral, Vials
Kefzol Vials
Lactated Pepsin Elixir
Lexavite Vials
Lextron F.G. Pulvules
Lextron Ferrous Pulvules
Lextron Pulvules
Liver Vials
Magnesium Sulfate Ampoules
Mandol Vials
Menadione Tablets
Mercuric Oxide, Yellow, Sterile Ophthalmic Ointments
Merthiolate, Aeropump, Cream, Glycerite, Ophthalmic Ointment, Powder, Solution & Tincture
◆ Methadone Hydrochloride Diskets
Methenamine Tablets
Methenamine & Sodium Biphosphate Tablets
Methyltestosterone Tablets
Metubine Iodide Vials
Metycaine Hydrochloride Vials & Powder
Milk of Bismuth
Morphine & Atropine Vials
Morphine Sulfate Vials & Soluble Tablets
Moxam Vials
Multicebrin Tablets
Mumps Skin-Test Antigen
Myrrh Tincture
Neomycin Sulfate Ointment & Tablets
Neotrizine Suspension & Tablets
Niacin Ampoules & Tablets
Niacinamide Vials & Tablets
Nitroglycerin Sublingual Tablets
Novrad, Pulvules
Oncovin Vials
Opium (Deodorized) Tincture
Ouabain, Ampoules
Ox Bile Extract Enseals
Pagitane Hydrochloride Tablets
Pancebrin Vials
Pancreatin Enseals, Powder & Tablets
Pantholin Tablets
Papaverine Hydrochloride, Ampoules, Powder, Tablets & Vials
Paregoric Tincture
Penicillin G Potassium Vials (Buffered)
Penicillin G Procaine Suspension, Sterile, Vials
Phenobarbital Elixir & Tablets
Phenobarbital Sodium Vials
Potassium Chloride Ampoules & Enseals
Potassium Iodide Enseals
Potassium Permanganate Tablets
Powder Papers
Progesterone Vials
Propylthiouracil Tablets
Protamine Sulfate Ampoules & Vials
Prunicodeine
Pyridoxine Hydrochloride Tablets
Quinidine Gluconate Vials
Quinidine Sulfate Pulvules & Tablets
Quinine Sulfate Pulvules & Tablets
Reserpine Tablets
Reticulex Pulvules
Reticulogen Vials
Reticulogen Fortified Vials
Rhinitis, Full Strength, Tablets
Riboflavin Tablets
Rose, Soluble, for Making Artificial Rose Water
Saccharin Sodium Tablets
Sandril, Vials
Scarlet Red Ointment
Scopolamine Hydrobromide Soluble Tablets
Seconal Elixir
◆ Seconal Sodium Vials, Pulvules & Suppositories
Seromycin Pulvules
Silver Nitrate Wax Ampoules
Soda Mint Tablets
Sodium Bicarbonate Tablets
Sodium Chloride Vials, Enseals & Tablets
Sodium Iodide Ampoules
Sodium Salicylate Enseals
Streptomycin Sulfate Vials
Sulfadiazine Tablets
Sulfapyridine Tablets
Sulfur Ointment
Surfacaine Cream, Jelly & Ointment
Surfadil Cream & Lotion
Tapazole Tablets
Terpin Hydrate & Codeine Elixir
Terpin Hydrate Elixir
Tes-Tape
Testosterone Propionate Vials
Theracebrin Pulvules
Thiamine Hydrochloride, Elixir & Tablets
Thyroid Enseals & Tablets
Trikates, Liquid
Tubocurarine Chloride Vials
◆ Tuinal Pulvules
Tycopan Pulvules
Tylosterone, Tablets
V-Cillin K for Oral Solution & Tablets
Valerian Tincture
Vancocin HCl, for Oral Solution
Vancocin HCl, Vials
Velban Vials
Vitamin A, Gelseals & Pulvules
Vitamin B Complex, Elixir & Pulvules
Vitamin C, Tablets
Vitamin D, Gelseals
Vitamin E, Gelseals
Water for Injection Ampoules
Whitfield's Ointment (Double Strength)
Wild Cherry Syrup
Zentinic Pulvules
Zentron Chewable Tables & Liquid
Zinc Oxide Ointments
Zinc Oxide Paste Ointment
Zinc Sulfate Compound Powder
M² - Lacto

MACSIL, INC. 1172
1326 Frankford Avenue
Philadelphia, PA 19125 (215) 739-7300

Products Available

◘ Balmex Baby Powder
◘ Balmex Emollient Lotion
◘ Balmex Ointment

MALLARD INCORPORATED 1172
3021 Wabash Ave.
Detroit, MI 48216

Address inquiries to:

Sales Department (313) 964-3910

Products Available

Allersone
Anaphen
Bexomal-C
Bexophene
Buffex
Chlorohist L.A.
Coldrine
Coltab
Condrin-LA
Copan
Coracin
Coryza Brengle
Dermal Rub
Dermolin
Diaral

(◆ Shown in Product Identification Section)

(◘ Described in PDR For Nonprescription Drugs)

Dimotal
Di-Phos D
Ditan
Dynosal
Eazol
Enzobile Improved Formula
Evac-U-Lax
Fenylhist
Fenylhist-25
Fynex
Gelazine
Halercol
Hematinic
Histex
Hydromal
Hysone
Iromal
Ivy-Rid
Laxinate 100
Lipotrol
Lixolin
Magnagel
Malatal
Malatal Elixir
Mallamint
Mallergan
Mallisol
Mallopress
Malotuss
Metho-500
Minro-Plex
Neomixin
Neotal
Nitrofurazone
Obephen
Obetrim
Panex
Pavased
Phenate
Phenzine
Predoxine-5
Prenabex
Presalin
Respirol
Saleto
Saleto-D
Salphenyl
Sedabamate
Serfolia
Tetrasine
Thyro-teric
Trocaine
Trocal
Tyrobenz
Urazide
Uremide
Uro-Ves
Vera-67
Vitamin A & D
Vitamin-C
Vitamin-E
Vitasol
Zoxaphen

A. G. MARIN PHARMACEUTICALS 1172
Post Office Box 174
Miami, FL 33144
Address inquiries to:
Ricardo Mayo (305) 264-1241
Products Available
Codegesic Tablets
Colidrops Pediatric Drops
Dranochol Tablets
Intestinex Capsules
MarEPA Capsules
Orlenta Capsules
Otocidin Otic Drops
Otomycet-HC Otic Solution
Siderol Syrup
Solu-Phyllin Liquid
Support Liquid
Support-500 Capsules
Tolerase Tablets
Uretron D/S Tablets
Vigorex Capsules
Vigorex Injection

MARION LABORATORIES, INC. 417, 1173
Pharmaceutical Division
Marion Industrial Park
10236 Bunker Ridge Rd.
Kansas City, MO 64137
Address inquiries to:
Medical Director
P.O. Box 9627
Kansas City, MO 64134 (816) 761-2500
Products Available
Ambenyl Expectorant
Ambenyl-D
◆ Carafate Tablets
◆ Cardizem Tablets
Debrox Drops
Ditropan Syrup
◆ Ditropan Tablets
◆ Duotrate Plateau Caps
◆ Duotrate 45 Plateau Caps
◆ Gaviscon Liquid
◆ Gaviscon Tablets
◆ Gaviscon-2 Tablets
Gly-Oxide Liquid
◆ Nico-400
Nitro-Bid IV
◆ Nitro-Bid Ointment
◆ Nitro-Bid 2.5 Plateau Caps
◆ Nitro-Bid 6.5 Plateau Caps
◆ Nitro-Bid 9 Plateau Caps
◆ Os-Cal 500 Tablets
◆ Os-Cal Forte Tablets
◆ Os-Cal Plus Tablets
◆ Os-Cal Tablets
◆ Os-Cal-Gesic Tablets
◆ Pavabid Capsules
◆ Pavabid HP Capsulets
Silvadene Cream
Throat Discs Throat Lozenges
◆ Thyroid Strong Tablets
◆ Thyroid Tablets
Triten Tablets

MARLYN PHARMACEUTICAL CO., INC. 1183
350 Pauma Place
Escondido, CA 92025 (714) 489-6115
Products Available
Albumin 500 Tablets
C Speridin Tablets, Sustained Release
Daily Nutritional Paks
..... Care-4
..... Pro-Formance
Hep-Forte Capsules
Marbec Tablets
Marlyn Formula 50 Capsules
Marlyn Prolonged Release Vitamins
Balanced B 125
Clock E
Iron-L
Niacin
Super One Daily
Super Citro Cee
Ultimate One
Vitamin B 12, 1000 mcg.
Vitamin C, 1000 mg.

MASON PHARMACEUTICALS, INC. 1184
P.O. Box 8330
Newport Beach, CA 92660 (714) 851-9388
Products Available
Damason-P

MASTAR PHARMACEUTICAL CO., INC. 1185
P.O. Box 1122
Bethlehem, PA 18016
Address inquiries to:
Joseph C. Mastriani, President (215) 258-8770
Products Available
Adatuss DC Expectorant Cough Syrup
Maxigesic Capsules

MAYRAND, INC. 1186
P.O. Box 8869
4 Dundas Circle
Greensboro, NC 27419 (919) 292-5347
Products Available
Anamine Syrup
Anamine T.D. Caps
Anatuss Syrup
Anatuss Syrup w/Codeine
Anatuss Tablets
Anatuss Tablets w/Codeine
Asproject
Becomject-100
Benoject-10
Benoject-50
Buff-A Comp Caps
Buff-A Comp Tablets
Buff-A Comp No. 3 Tablets (with Codeine)
Buff-A Tablets
Corgonject-5
Cyanoject
Decaject
Decaject-L.A.
Dramoject
Eldercaps
Eldertonic Elixir
Estroject-2
Estroject-LA
Flexoject
Glytuss Tabs
Histaject
Hydrotensin-50 Tablets
Hydro-Z-50 Tablets
Lidoject-1
Lidoject-2
Lifoject
Menoject-LA
Nu-Iron Elixir
Nu-Iron 150 Caps
Nu-Iron-Plus Elixir
Nu-Iron-V Tablets
Penalate Elixir
Phenoject-50
Predaject-50
Progestaject-50
Sedapap-10 Tablets
Selestoject
Soluject
Sorbide T.D. Caps
Spasmoject
Stera-Form Cream
Steramine Otic
Sterapred Tablets
Sterapred Uni-Pak
Testoject-50
Testoject-E.P.
Testoject-L.A.
Trimcaps
Trimtabs
Tristoject
Vistaject

McGREGOR PHARMACEUTICALS 1187
32580 Grand River Avenue
Farmington, MI 48024
Address inquiries to:
Mr. Edward McGregor (313) 474-8727
Products Available
Rhinafed Capsules
Rhinafed-EX Capsules
Rhindecon Capsules
Rhindecon-G Capsules
Rhinolar Capsules
Rhinolar-EX Capsules
Rhinolar-EX 12 Capsules

McNEIL CONSUMER PRODUCTS CO. 418, 1187
McNEILAB, INC.
Fort Washington, PA 19034
Address inquiries to:
Professional Relations Department
Fort Washington, PA 19034
Manufacturing Divisions
Fort Washington, PA 19034
Southwest Manufacturing Plant
4001 N. I-35
Round Rock, TX 78664
Distribution Centers
Order Services
Fort Washington, PA 19034
Camp Hill Road
Local Area (215) 233-7000
Pennsylvania (800) 822-3978
Out of State (800) 523-3484
Arlington, TX 76010
3129 Pinewood Drive (817) 640-1167
Glendale, CA 91201
512 Paula Avenue (213) 245-1491
Montgomeryville, PA 18936
1390 Welsh Road (215) 641-1420
Products Available
◆ Children's CoTylenol Liquid Cold Formula
◆ Children's Tylenol acetaminophen Chewable Tablets, Elixir & Drops
◆ CoTylenol Cold Formula Tablets & Capsules
CoTylenol Liquid Cold Formula
◆ Extra-Strength Tylenol acetaminophen Capsules, Tablets & Liquid
◆ Infants' Tylenol Drops
◆ Maximum-Strength Tylenol Sinus Medication Tablets & Capsules
◆ Regular Strength Tylenol acetaminophen Tablets & Capsules
Sine-Aid Sinus Headache Tablets

McNEIL PHARMACEUTICAL 418, 1191
McNEILAB, INC.
Spring House, PA 19477
Address inquiries to:
Professional Services Department
Spring House, PA 19477
(215) 628-5000
Manufacturing Affiliate
Dorado, Puerto Rico 00646
P.O. Box P
Fort Washington, PA 19034
Distribution Divisions
Arlington, TX 76010
3129 Pinewood Drive
P.O. Box 699 (817) 640-0871
Broadview, IL 60153
2122 Roberts Drive (312) 344-3187
Doraville, GA 30360
2801 Bankers Industrial Drive
(404) 447-8600
Glendale, CA 91201
512 Paula Avenue (213) 245-0217
Montgomeryville PA 18936
2 Progress Drive (215) 699-3551
Products Available
Butibel-Zyme Tablets
Carbinoxamine Maleate, see Clistin
Chlorzoxazone, see Paraflex
Clistin Tablets
Clistin-D Tablets
◆ Haldol Injection, Tablets & Concentrate
Haloperidol, see Haldol
◆ Pancrease
Paraflex Tablets
◆ Parafon Forte Tablets
◆ Theophyl Chewable Tablets
◆ Theophyl-SR
Theophyl-225 Elixir
◆ Theophyl-225 Tablets
◆ Tolectin Tablets & DS Capsules

Tolmetin Sodium, see Tolectin Tablets
◆ Tylenol w/Codeine Capsules, Tablets & Elixir
◆ Tylox Capsules
◆ Zomax Tablets
Zomepirac Sodium, see Zomax Tablets

MEAD JOHNSON NUTRITIONAL DIVISION 1205
Mead Johnson & Company
2404 W. Pennsylvania St.
Evansville, IN 47721 (812) 426-6000
Address inquiries to:
Scientific Information Section
Medical Department
Products Available
◘ Casec
◘ Ce-Vi-Sol
◘ Criticare HN
◘ Enfamil
◘ Enfamil Nursette
◘ Enfamil Ready-To-Use
◘ Enfamil w/Iron
◘ Enfamil w/Iron Ready-To-Use
◘ Fer-In-Sol
◘ Isocal
Isocal HCN
◘ Lofenalac
◘ Lonalac
◘ Lytren
◘ MCT Oil
◘ Moducal
◘ Nutramigen
Poly-Vi-Flor 1.0 mg Vitamins w/Fluoride Chewable Tablets
Poly-Vi-Flor 1.0 Vitamins w/Iron & Fluoride Chewable Tablets
Poly-Vi-Flor 0.25 mg Vitamins w/Fluoride Drops
Poly-Vi-Flor 0.25 mg Vitamins w/Iron & Fluoride Drops
Poly-Vi-Flor 0.5 mg Vitamins w/Fluoride Chewable Tablets & Drops
Poly-Vi-Flor 0.5 mg Vitamins w/Iron & Fluoride Chewable Tablets & Drops
◘ Poly-Vi-Sol Vitamins Chewable Tablets & Drops
◘ Poly-Vi-Sol Vitamins w/Iron Chewable Tablets & Drops
◘ Portagen
◘ Pregestimil
◘ ProSobee
◘ Sustacal
◘ Sustacal HC
◘ Sustagen
◘ Tempra
◘ Traumacal
◘ Trind
◘ Trind-DM
Tri-Vi-Flor 1.0 mg Vitamins w/Fluoride Chewable Tablets
Tri-Vi-Flor 0.5 mg Vitamins w/Fluoride Drops
Tri-Vi-Flor 0.25 mg Vitamins w/Fluoride Drops
Tri-Vi-Flor 0.25 mg Vitamins w/Iron & Fluoride Drops
◘ Tri-Vi-Sol Vitamins, Chewable Tablets & Drops
◘ Tri-Vi-Sol Vitamins w/Iron, Drops

MEAD JOHNSON PHARMACEUTICAL DIVISION 418, 1214
Mead Johnson & Company
2404 W. Pennsylvania St.
Evansville, IN 47721 (812) 426-6000
Address inquiries to:
Scientific Information Section
Medical Department
Products Available
◆ Colace
◆ Cytoxan
◆ Deapril-ST
◆ Desyrel
◆ Duricef
◆ Estrace
◆ K-Lyte & K-Lyte DS
◆ K-Lyte/Cl & K-Lyte/Cl 50
◆ Klotrix
◆ Megace Tablets
Mucomyst
Mucomyst with Isoproterenol
◆ Natalins
◆ Natalins Rx
◆ Ovcon-35
◆ Ovcon-50
◆ Peri-Colace
Questran
◆ Quibron & Quibron-300
◆ Quibron Plus
◆ Quibron-T & Quibron-T/SR
◆ Vasodilan

MEDICAL PRODUCTS PANAMERICANA, INC. 1241
Post Office Box 771
Coral Gables, Florida 33134
Address inquiries to:
Professional Services Dept. (305) 545-6524
Branch and Distribution Division
San Juan, Puerto Rico (809) 783-6736
Products Available
Aminobrain Capsules
Aminobrain Injection
Aminobrain Plus Capsules
Aminobrain Tablets
Atoximetrin-B Capsules
Broncopectol Syrup
Digesplen Elixir
Digesplen Tablets
Ferlivit Capsules
Ferlivit Injection
Ferlivit Syrup
Flebomedic
Folisplen B-12 Capsules
Folisplen B-12 Injection
Medispray
Neurodep Injection Lyophilized
Novaflor Capsules
Rubroben-1000 Injection Lyophilized
Rutiplen-C
Tempotest 225
Trilycal-12
VG Capsules
Varidin Capsules

MEDICONE COMPANY 419, 1241
225 Varick St.
New York, NY 10014
Address inquiries to:
Professional Service Dept. (212) 924-5166
Products Available
◘ Derma Medicone Ointment
Derma Medicone-HC
◘ DioMedicone Tablets
◘ Medicone Dressing Cream
◘ Mediconet
◆ Rectal Medicone Suppositories
◘ Rectal Medicone Unguent
◆ Rectal Medicone-HC Suppositories

MENLEY & JAMES LABORATORIES
a SmithKline company
P.O. Box 8082
Philadelphia, PA 19101
Address inquiries to:
Medical Department (215) 751-5000
For Products Available, see Smith Kline & French Laboratories

MERCK SHARP & DOHME 419, 1242
Division of Merck & Co., Inc.
West Point, PA 19486 (215) 661-5000
For Medical or Drug Information
Write: Professional Information
Business hours only (8:30 a.m. to 4:45 p.m. EST), call (215) 661-7300
For Medical Emergency Information after hours or on weekends, call (215) 661-5000
Address other inquiries to:
Professional Service Department
West Point, PA 19486
Branch Offices
Arlington, TX 76011
Great Southwest Industrial District
925-111th Street (817) 261-7527
Atlanta, GA 30354
3415 Empire Blvd., S.W. (404) 765-1700
Baltimore Area:
see Columbia, MD
Boston Area:
see Needham Heights, MA
Chicago Area:
see Oak Brook, IL
Columbia, MD 21045
9199 Red Branch Rd. (301) 730-8240
Columbus, OH 43228
4242 Janitrol Road (614) 276-5308
Commerce, CA 90040
6409 E. Gayhart Street (213) 723-9661
Dallas/Ft. Worth Area:
see Arlington, TX
Denver, CO 80216
4900 Jackson Street (303) 355-1601
Kansas City area:
see Overland Park, KS
Kenner, LA 70062
1431 E. Airline Highway (504) 464-0111
King of Prussia, PA 19406
1045 First Avenue (215) 278-2550
Los Angeles Area:
see Commerce, CA
Memphis, TN 38106
1980 Latham Street (901) 948-8501
Minneapolis, MN 55441
12955 State Highway 55 (612) 559-4445
Needham Heights, MA 02194
40 A Street (617) 444-5510
New Orleans Area:
see Kenner, LA
New York Area:
see Teterboro, NJ
Oak Brook, IL 60521
2010 Swift Drive (312) 920-2160
Overland Park, KS 66215
9001 Quivira Rd. (913) 888-1110
Philadelphia Area:
see King of Prussia, PA
Portland, OR 97211
717 N.E. Lombard St. (503) 285-2582
S. San Francisco, CA 94080
340 Shaw Road (415) 583-4330
Teterboro, NJ 07608
111 Central Avenue (201) 288-2275
Products Available
◆ Aldoclor Tablets
Aldomet Ester HCl Injection
Aldomet Oral Suspension
◆ Aldomet Tablets
◆ Aldoril Tablets
alphaRedisol Injection
Aminohippurate Sodium Injection
Antivenin (Black Widow Spider)
AquaMEPHYTON Injection
Aramine Injection
Attenuvax
◆ Benemid Tablets
Biavax_{II}
◆ Blocadren Tablets
◆ Clinoril Tablets
Cogentin Injection
◆ Cogentin Tablets
◆ ColBENEMID Tablets
Cortone Saline Suspension
Cortone Tablets
Cosmegen Injection
◆ Cuprimine Capsules
Cyclaine Topical Solution
Daranide Tablets
Decaderm
Decadron Elixir
Decadron Phosphate Injection
Decadron Phosphate Respihaler
Decadron Phosphate Sterile Ophthalmic Ointment
Decadron Phosphate Sterile Ophthalmic Solution
Decadron Phosphate Topical Cream
Decadron Phosphate Turbinaire
Decadron Phosphate w/Xylocaine Injection
◆ Decadron Tablets
Decadron-LA Suspension
Decaspray Topical Aerosol
◆ Demser Capsules
◆ Diupres Tablets
Diuril Oral Suspension
◆ Diuril Tablets
◆ Dolobid Tablets
◆ Edecrin Tablets
Elavil Injection
◆ Elavil Tablets
Elspar
◆ Flexeril Tablets
Floropryl Sterile Ophthalmic Ointment
Fluax
Hep-B-Gammagee
Heptavax-B
Humorsol Sterile Ophthalmic Solution
Hydeltrasol Injection
Hydeltrasol Sterile Ophthalmic Solution
Hydeltra-T.B.A. Suspension
Hydrocortone Phosphate Injection
Hydrocortone Saline Suspension
Hydrocortone Sterile Ophthalmic Ointment
Hydrocortone Sterile Ophthalmic Suspension
Hydrocortone Tablets
Hydrocortone Topical Ointment
◆ HydroDIURIL Tablets
◆ Hydropres Tablets
◆ Indocin Capsules
◆ Indocin SR Capsules
Inversine Tablets
Lacrisert Sterile Ophthalmic Insert
M-M-R_{II}
M-R-VAX_{II}
Mefoxin
Meningovax-AC
Mephyton Tablets
Meruvax_{II}
◆ Midamor Tablets
◆ Mintezol Chewable Tablets
Mintezol Suspension
◆ Moduretic Tablets
Mumpsvax
Mustargen
Myochrysine Injection
Neodecadron Sterile Ophthalmic Ointment
Neodecadron Sterile Ophthalmic Solution
Neodecadron Topical Cream
Neo-Hydeltrasol Sterile Ophthalmic Solution
◆ Periactin Syrup
◆ Periactin Tablets
Pneumovax
Propadrine Capsules
Propadrine Elixir
Redisol Injection
Redisol Tablets
Respihaler (see Decadron Phosphate Respihaler)
◆ Sinemet Tablets
Sodium Diuril Intravenous
Sodium Edecrin Intravenous
◆ Timolide Tablets
Timoptic Sterile Ophthalmic Solution

(◆ Shown in Product Identification Section) (◘ Described in PDR For Nonprescription Drugs)

◆ Triavil Tablets
Turbinaire (see Decadron Phosphate Turbinaire)
Urecholine Injection
◆ Urecholine Tablets
◆ Vivactil Tablets

MERICON INDUSTRIES, INC. 1344
Post Office Box 5759
Peoria, IL 61601
Address inquiries to:
Thomas P. Morrissey (309) 676-0744
Products Available
▣ Orazinc Capsules
▣ Zinc Tablets

MERIEUX INSTITUTE, INC. 1344, 3013
1200 N.W. 78th Avenue
Suite 109
Miami, FL 33126
Address inquiries to:
1200 N.W. 78th Avenue
Suite 109
Miami, FL (305) 593-9577
For Medical Emergencies Contact:
Merieux Institute, Inc. (800) 327-2842
Alaska, FL, & HI, call Collect
(305) 593-9577
Products Available
Mono-Vacc
Rabies Immune Globulin (Human), Imogam Rabies
Rabies Vaccine Human Diploid Cell, Imovax Rabies
Tuberculin, Mono-Vacc Test

MERRELL DOW PHARMACEUTICALS INC. 420, 1344
Subsidiary of The Dow Chemical Company
Cincinnati, OH 45215
Address inquiries to:
Manager Professional Services
(513) 948-9111
Products Available
AVC Suppositories
AVC Vaginal Cream
AVC/Dienestrol Cream
AVC/Dienestrol Suppositories
Accurbron
Bacimycin Ointment
◆ Bendectin Tablets
◆ Bentyl 10 mg Capsules
Bentyl 10 mg w/Phenobarbital Capsules
Bentyl Injection
Bentyl Syrup
Bentyl w/Phenobarbital Syrup
◆ Bentyl 20 mg Tablets
Bentyl 20 mg Tablets w/Phenobarbital
Bricanyl Injection
Bricanyl Tablets
◆ Cantil Tablets
Cantil w/Phenobarbital Tablets
▣ Cēpacol Anesthetic Lozenges (Troches)
▣ Cēpacol Mouthwash/Gargle
▣ Cēpacol Throat Lozenges
▣ Cēpastat Sore Throat Spray
▣ Cēpastat Sore Throat Lozenges
▣ Cēpastat Sore Throat Lozenges, Cherry Flavor
◆ Cephulac Syrup
◆ Chronulac Syrup
Clomid Tablets
Consotuss Antitussive Syrup
Cotussis Syrup
Cyanocobalamin Injection
DV Cream/DV Suppositories
Decapryn Syrup & Tablets
Delcid
Diothane Ointment
Dow-Isoniazid
Ganatrex Elixir
Hedulin Tablets
◆ Hiprex Tablets
Imferon
Kolantyl Gel
Kolantyl Tablets
Kolantyl Wafers
◆ Lorelco
Mercodol Cough Syrup w/Decapryn
◆ Metahydrin
◆ Metatensin
Neocholan
Neo-Polycin Topical Antibiotic
◆ Norpramin
◆ Novafed A Capsules
Novafed A Liquid
◆ Novafed Capsules
Novafed Liquid
▣ Novahistine Cold Tablets
▣ Novahistine Cough Formula
▣ Novahistine Cough & Cold Formula
▣ Novahistine DH
▣ Novahistine DMX
▣ Novahistine Elixir
◆ Novahistine Expectorant
▣ Novahistine Sinus Tablets
Orenzyme
Orenzyme Bitabs
Phenoxene
Pyridoxine Hydrochloride Tablets
Quide Tablets
◆ Quinamm Tablets
▣ Resolve Cold Sore & Fever Blister Relief
◆ Rifadin
◆ Rifamate
Sedadrops
Simron Capsules
Simron Plus Capsules
◆ Singlet
Sterile Hydroxystilbamidine Isethionate
◆ Susadrin Transmucosal Tablets
2/G
2/G-DM
◆ TACE 12 mg Capsules
◆ TACE 25 mg Capsules
◆ TACE 72 mg Capsules
◆ Tenuate Dospan Tablets
◆ Tenuate Tablets
Terpin Hydrate & Codeine Elixir
◆ Triclos Tablets & Liquid
◆ Tussend Expectorant
◆ Tussend Liquid & Tablets
Vanobid Vaginal Ointment
Vanobid Vaginal Tablets

MEYER LABORATORIES, INC. 411, 1379
1900 West Commercial Blvd.
Fort Lauderdale, FL 33309
(305) 776-5300
See product listing under Glaxo Inc.

MILES LABORATORIES, INC. 1379
P.O. Box 340
Elkhart, IN 46515
Address inquiries to:
Medical Dept. (219) 262-7886
Consumer Health Care Division only
Products Available
▣ Alka-Seltzer Effervescent Antacid
▣ Alka-Seltzer Effervescent Pain Reliever and Antacid
▣ Alka-Seltzer Plus Cold Medicine
▣ Alka-2 Chewable Antacid Tablets
▣ Bactine Antiseptic-Anesthetic First Aid Spray
▣ Bactine Hydrocortisone Skin Care Cream
▣ Bugs Bunny Multivitamin Supplement
▣ Bugs Bunny Plus Iron Multivitamin Supplement
▣ Bugs Bunny With Extra C
▣ Flintstones Multivitamin Supplement
▣ Flintstones Plus Iron Multivitamin Supplement
▣ Flintstones With Extra C
▣ Miles Nervine Nighttime Sleep-Aid
▣ One-A-Day Core C 500 Vitamins
▣ One-A-Day Plus Extra C
▣ One-A-Day Stressguard Vitamins
▣ One-A-Day Vitamins
▣ One-A-Day Vitamins Plus Iron
▣ One-A-Day Vitamins Plus Minerals

MILES PHARMACEUTICALS 421, 1379
Division of Miles Laboratories, Inc.
400 Morgan Lane
West Haven, CT 06516
Address Inquiries to:
Director, Medical Services (203) 934-9221
Products Available
Acne-Dome Creme & Lotion
Acne-Dome Medicated Cleanser
Allpyral Allergenic Extracts
Azlin
Candex Lotion
Cort-Dome ⅛%, ¼%, ½%, and 1% Creme
Cort-Dome ⅛%, ¼%, ½%, and 1% Lotion
Cort-Dome Suppositories
DTIC-Dome
◆ Decholin Tablets
◆ Domeboro Powder Packets, Effervescent Tablets
Dome-Paste Bandage (Unna's Boot)
Domol Bath & Shower Oil
Exzit Medicated Cleanser
Exzit Medicated Creme and Lotion
Lidaform-HC Creme
◆ Lithane Tablets
Mezlin
Mithracin
Mycelex 1% Cream
Mycelex 1% Solution
◆ Mycelex-G Vaginal Tablets
Mycelex-G 1% Vaginal Cream
◆ Niclocide Chewable Tablets
Nystaform Ointment
Otic Domeboro Solution
Otic Neo-Cort-Dome Suspension
Otic Tridesilon Solution
◆ Stilphostrol Tablets and Ampuls
Tridesilon Creme 0.05%
Tridesilon Ointment 0.05%

MILEX PRODUCTS, INC. 1398
5915 Northwest Highway
Chicago, IL 60631 (312) 631-6484
Shipping Offices
Milex Western
Post Office Box 46030
Los Angeles, CA 90046 (213) 651-4301
Milex Central
1873 Grove Street
Glenview, IL 60025 (312) 729-5253
Milex Michigan
Post Office Box 20264
Ferndale, MI 48220 (313) 399-9223
Milex Puerto Rico
GPO Box 554
San Juan, Puerto Rico 00936
(809) 791-3309
Milex Hawaii
Box 6337
Honolulu, HI 96818 (808) 422-9581
Milex Southeastern
Post Office Drawer 4647
Clearwater, FL 33518 (813) 461-1949
Milex Southern
Post Office Drawer "M"
Weatherford, TX 76086 (817) 594-6865
Milex Carolinas
Post Office Box 23060
Charlotte, NC 28212 (704) 545-4567
Milex Delaware Valley
350 White Horse Pike
Atco, NJ 08004 (609) 767-4818
Milex Delta
Post Office Drawer 5684
Shreveport, LA 71105 (318) 797-1554
Products Available
Amino-Cerv
Basal Thermometers
Breast Self-Examination Kit
Cannula Curette with Swivel Handle
Dilateria
Endometrial Suction Curettes
Fertility Cannula
Fertilo-Pak
Laminaria Japonica
Oligospermia Cups
Pessaries
Pro-Ception
Seminal Pouches
Shur-Seal Gel
Spatula
Sufamal
Tis-U-Trap
Trimo-San
Wide-Seal Diaphragm

MISSION PHARMACAL COMPANY 1399
1325 E. Durango
San Antonio, TX 78210
Address inquiries to:
Professional Service Dept. (512) 533-7118
Post Office Box 1676
San Antonio, TX 78296
Products Available
Calcet
Compete
Dilax-100
Dilax-250
Equilet
Ferralet
Fosfree
Homapin-5
Homapin-10
Iromin-G
Mission Prenatal
Mission Prenatal F.A.
Mission Prenatal H.P.
Mission Pre-Surgical
Prulet
Prulet Liquitab
Supac
Therabid
Thera-Gesic

MURO PHARMACEUTICAL, INC. 1401
890 East Street
Tewksbury, MA 01876
Address inquiries to:
Professional Service Dept.
1-(800) 225-0974
(617) 851-5981
Products Available
Bromfed Capsules (Timed Release)
Bromfed-PD Capsules (Timed Release)
Bromfed Tablets
Duolube Ophthalmic Ointment
Gonio-Gel
Guaifed Capsules (Timed Release)
Liquid Pred Syrup
Muro 128 Ophthalmic Ointment
Muro 128 Ophthalmic Solution
Murocel - Ophthalmic Solution
Murocoll-2 Ophthalmic Solution
Muro's Opcon Ophthalmic Solution
Muro's Opcon-A Ophthalmic Solution
Muro Tears Ophthalmic Solution
▣ Salinex Nasal Mist and Drops
Sulphrin Ophthalmic Suspension

NEUTROGENA CORPORATION 1402
5755 West 96th Street
P.O. Box 45036
Los Angeles, CA 90045 (800) 421-6857
In CA (213) 776-5223

(◆ Shown in Product Identification Section) (▣ Described in PDR For Nonprescription Drugs)

Products Available
Neutrogena Acne Cleansing Formula Soap
Neutrogena Acne-Drying Gel
Neutrogena Baby Soap
Neutrogena Body Lotion
Neutrogena Dry Skin Formula Soap
Neutrogena Melanex
Neutrogena Norwegian Formula Hand Cream
Neutrogena Original Formula Soap
Neutrogena Rainbath Shower and Bath Gel
Neutrogena Sesame Seed Body Oil
Neutrogena Shampoo
Neutrogena Solid Soap Shampoo
Neutrogena T/Derm Therapeutic Tar Body Oil
Neutrogena T/Gel Therapeutic Shampoo
Neutrogena Vehicle/N
Neutrogena Vehicle/N Mild

NORCLIFF THAYER INC. 421, 1404
One Scarsdale Road
Tuckahoe, NY 10707 (914) 631-0033
Products Available
◆ A-200 Pyrinate Liquid, Gel
⊡ Esotérica Medicated Fade Cream
⊡ Liquiprin Acetaminophen
⊡ Nature's Remedy Laxative
⊡ NoSalt Salt Alternative
⊡ Oxy Wash Antibacterial Skin Wash
⊡ Oxy-5 Lotion
⊡ Oxy-10 Lotion
⊡ Oxy-Scrub Abradant Cleanser
⊡ Tums Antacid Tablets

NORDISK-USA 1404
7315 Wisconsin Avenue
Suite 851W
Bethesda, MD 20814
Address inquiries to:
Medical Director (301) 656-5411
(301) 656-7232
Products Available
Insulatard NPH
Mixtard
Velosulin

NORGINE LABORATORIES, INC. 1406
420 Lexington Avenue
New York, NY 10170 (212) 697-1513
Products Available
Bilamide Tablets
Enzypan Tablets
Fybranta Tablets
Hepp-Iron Drops
Movicol Granules
Muripsin Tablets

NORTHEAST UNIT-DOSE & REPACKING CO., INC. 1406
Post Office Box 2896
Laurel, MD 20708
Address inquiries to:
Leonard Bramson (301) 792-0956
Products Available
Circubid Capsules

NORWICH EATON PHARMACEUTICALS, INC. 421, 1407, 3013
Professional Products Group
(formerly Eaton Laboratories)
Consumer Products Group
(formerly Norwich Products)
13-27 Eaton Avenue
Norwich, NY 13815
Address medical inquiries to:
Medical Department
Norwich Eaton Pharmaceuticals
Norwich, NY 13815 (607) 335-2565
Sales Offices
CHICAGO
Elk Grove Village, IL 60007
1350 Greenleaf Avenue (312) 593-0100
DALLAS
Dallas, TX 75265
P.O. Box 225490, Terminal Annex
(214) 337-4794
GREENVILLE
Greenville, SC 29602
P.O. Box 2468 (803) 277-7110
LOS ANGELES
Los Angeles, CA 90051
P.O. Box 2171, Terminal Annex
(213) 726-0505
NORWICH
Norwich, NY 13815
13-27 Eaton Avenue (607) 335-2121
Products Available
Alphaderm Cream
Chloraseptic Preparations
Children's Chloraseptic Lozenges
Chloraseptic Liquid-Menthol or Cherry
Chloraseptic Liquid-Nitrogen Propelled Spray
Chloraseptic Lozenges
Chloraseptic Cough Control Lozenges
Chloraseptic Gel
Comhist LA Capsules
Comhist Liquid
Comhist Tablets
Dantrium Capsules
Dantrium Intravenous
Dopar Capsules
Duvoid Tablets
Entex Capsules
Entex LA Tablets
Entex Liquid
Furacin Preparations
Furacin Soluble Dressing
Furacin Topical Cream
Furadantin Oral Suspension
Furadantin Tablets
Furoxone Liquid
Furoxone Tablets
Ivadantin
LāBID 250 mg Tablets
◆ Macrodantin Capsules
Pepto-Bismol Liquid & Tablets
Sarenin
Vivonex
Standard Vivonex Diet
High Nitrogen Vivonex Diet
Flavor Packets
Devices
Vivonex Acutrol Enteral Feeding System
Vivonex Decompression Tube
Vivonex Delivery System
Vivonex Jejunostomy Kit
Vivonex Moss Tube
Vivonex Tungsten Tip Feeding Tube
Vivonex Tungsten Tip Tube Stylet

OLC LABORATORIES, INC. 1421
99 N.W. Miami Gardens Dr.
Miami, FL 33169
Toll Free WATS Line 1-(800) 327-7914
Address inquiries to:
OLC Laboratories, Inc
Herman H. Orlove
6770 N. Lincoln Ave.
Lincolnwood, IL 60646
Toll Free WATS Line
1-(800) 327-7914
Branch Offices
Orlove's Lincoln Crawford
6770 N. Lincoln Ave.
Lincolnwood, IL 60646
Toll Free WATS Line
1-(800) 327-7914
Products Available
⊡ Tryptacin Tablets
L. Tryptophan Tablets

OBETROL PHARMACEUTICALS 1421
(Division of Rexar Pharmacal Corp.)
396 Rockaway Avenue
Valley Stream, NY 11581
Address inquiries to:
Ellen Zivitz (516) 561-7662
Products Available
Dextroamphetamine Sulfate, 5mg. & 10mg.
Methamphetamine Hydrochloride, 5mg. & 10mg.
Obetrol-10
Obetrol-20
Oby-Trim 30 Capsules
X-Trozine Capsules & Tablets
X-Trozine LA-105 Capsules

O'NEAL, JONES & FELDMAN PHARMACEUTICALS 421, 1421
2510 Metro Blvd.
Maryland Heights, MO 63043
(314) 569-3610
Products Available
A.C.T.H. "40" Injectable
A.C.T.H. "80" Injectable
Acetycol Tablets
Adeno Injectable
Almora Tablets
Amonidrin Tablets
Anaids Tablets
Andro L.A. "200" Injectable
Andro "100" Injectable
Androgyn L.A. Injectable
Anergan "25" & "50" Injectable
Antilirium Injectable
Arbon Injectable
Arbon Tablets
Asminyl Injectable
Asminyl Tablets
B-12 Plus Injectable
◆ Banalg Hospital Strength Arthritic Pain Reliever
◆ Banalg Liniment
Bancap Capsules
Bancap c̄ Codeine Capsules
Bancaps HC Capsules
Banesin Tablets
Banflex Injectable
Beesix Injectable
Belfer Tablets
Betaprone Liquid
Biamine Injectable
Breonex Injectable
Calcium Gluconate Injectable
Calscorbate Tablets & Injectable
Canz Tablets
Caquin Cream
Cebocap
Cetane Injection
Cetane Injection (w/o preservative)
Cetane Timed Capsules
Choron "10" Injectable Pak
Codroxomin Injectable
Conex DA Tablet
Conex Liquid
Conex Lozenges
Conex Plus Tablets
Conex Tablets
Conex c̄ Codeine Liquid
Cyomin Injectable
Dalalone Injectable
Dalalone D.P. Injectable
Dalanone I.L. Injectable
Dalalone L.A. Injectable
Dalcaine Injection
Dehist Capsules
Dehist Injectable
depAndro "100" & "200" Injectable
depAndrogyn Injectable
depGynogen Injectable
depMedalone "40" Injectable
depMedalone "80" Injectable
depPredalone "40" & "80" Injectable
Derfule Capsules
Diabismul Suspension
Diabismul Tablets
Disotate Injectable
Dommanate Injectable
Duradyne DHC Tablets
Duradyne Forte Tablets
Duradyne Tablets
Dureze Drops
Eferol Injectable
Eferol Ointment
Eferol Succinate Capsules
Enzymet Tablet
Feostat Drops
Feostat Injectable
Feostat Suspension
Feostat Tablets
Feostim Tablets
G.B.S. Tablets
Gest Tablets
Gesterol in Oil "100" Injectable
Gesterol L.A. "250" Injectable
Glycate Tablets
Gynogen Injectable
Gynogen L.A. "10" & "20" Injectable
Gynogen R.P. Injectable
Heparin Sodium Injectable
Heparin Sodium w/o preservative Injectable
Hista-Derfule Capsules
Iodo-Niacin Injectable
◆ Iodo-Niacin Tablets
KBP/O Capsules
Lidocaine 1% & 2% Injectable
Livroben Injectable
Magnesium Chloride Injectable
Magnesium Sulfate Injectable
Metra Tablets
N.B.P. Ointment
Nandrobolic Injectable
Nandrobolic L.A. Injectable
Neoquess Injectable
Neoquess Tablets
Neo-Rhiban Tablets
Neurogyn Injectable
Niac Capsules
Nobese Tablets
Obermine Capsules
Osteolate Injectable
Oxymycin Injectable
Panol Injectable
Panvitex Prenatal Tablets
Paral Injectable
Paral Liquid
◆ Pedameth Capsules
Pedameth Liquid
Petameth Capsules
Philject Injectable
Predalone R.P. Injectable
Predalone T.B.A. Injectable
Proklar Tablets
Psychozine Injectable
Queltuss Tablets
Quiess Injectable
Rauverid Tablets
Rogenic Injectable
Rogenic Tablets
Solu-Eze Solvent
soluPredalone Injectable
Soniphen Tablets
Sulfaloid "500" Tablets
Sulfaloid Suspension
Tanurol Ointment
Tetracycline HCl Capsules
Tralmag Suspension
Triamolone "40" Injectable
Triamonide "40" Injectable
Uri-Pak Unit
Urithol Tablets
Verazinc Capsules
Wolfina "50" & "100" Tablets

(◆ Shown in Product Identification Section) **(⊡ Described in PDR For Nonprescription Drugs)**

ORGANON PHARMACEUTICALS 421, 1424
375 Mount Pleasant Ave.
West Orange, NJ 07052 (201) 325-4500
Products Available
Accelerase
Accelerase-PB
Bilogen
Cortrophin Gel
Cortrophin-Zinc
Cortrosyn
◆ Cotazym
Cotazym-B
◆ Cotazym-S
◆ Cotazym-65B
Deca-Durabolin
Doca Acetate
Dodex Injectable
Durabolin
Heparin Sodium (from Beef Lung Sources)
◆ Hexadrol Tablets
Hexadrol Cream
Hexadrol Phosphate Injection
◆ Hexadrol Therapeutic Pack
Liquaemin Sodium
◆ Liquamar
▣ Magnacal
◆ Maxibolin
Medache
▣ Microlipid
Orgatrax
Pavulon
Pernaemon
Pregnyl
▣ Propac
Regonol
▣ Renu
Succinylcholine
▣ Sumacal
▣ Vitaneed
◆ Wigraine
Wigrettes

ORTHO DIAGNOSTIC SYSTEMS INC. 1432
Route 202
Raritan, NJ 08869
Address inquiries to:
Professional Service Div. (201) 524-1732
(201) 524-2374
Products Available
Activated Thrombofax Reagent-Optimized
Affirmagen Reagent Red Blood Cells
Anti-Human Serum, Anti-C3d Serum (Mouse Hybridoma) Bio Clone
EluAid System for Antibody Elution
Fetaldex Quantitative Test for Fetal Red Blood Cells in the Maternal Blood Circulation
Fetalscreen Qualitative Screening Test for D(Rho) Postive Fetal Red Blood Cells in the Maternal Circulation
Fibrindex Thrombin (Human)
Gravindex Slide Test for Pregnancy
Gravindex Tube Test for Pregnancy
MICRhoGAM Rh$_o$ (D) Immune Globulin (Human), Micro-Dose
Monospot Slide Test for Infectious Mononucleosis
Ortho A$_2$ Cells Reagent Red Blood Cells
Ortho Abnormal Plasma Coagulation Control
Ortho Antibody Enhancement Solution
Ortho Anti-Human Serum (Rabbit)
Ortho Anti-IgG Serum (Rabbit)
Ortho Antithrombin III Assay
Ortho Blood Grouping Sera
Ortho Blood Group Substances
Ortho Bovine Albumin and Ortho Polymerized Bovine Albumin
Ortho Brain Thromboplastin
Ortho Coombs Control
Ortho Papanicolaou Smear Stains
Ortho Plasma Coagulation Control
Ortho Pregnancy Test Control Urines
Ortho Reagent Confidence Sera
Ortho Rh-hr Control
Resolve Panel A & B Reagent Red Blood Cells
RhoGAM Rh$_o$ (D) Immune Globulin (Human)
Selectogen Reagent Red Blood Cells
Sickledex Tube Test for Hemoglobin S
Surgiscreen Reagent Red Blood Cells
Thrombofax Reagent

ORTHO PHARMACEUTICAL CORPORATION 422, 1434
Raritan, NJ 08869
Address inquiries to:
Director of Medical Services,
Medical Research Dept. (201) 524-0400
Products Available
Aci-Jel Therapeutic Vaginal Jelly
▣ Conceptrol Birth Control Cream
▣ Conceptrol Contraceptive Gel Disposable
▣ Conceptrol Shields
▣ Conceptrol Supreme
▣ Delfen Contraceptive Foam
▣ Gynol II Contraceptive Jelly
Lippes Loop Intrauterine Double-S
▣ Massé Breast Cream
◆ Micronor Tablets
◆ Modicon 21 Tablets
Modicon 28 Tablets
Monistat 7 Vaginal Cream
Monistat 7 Vaginal Suppositories
Ortho Diaphragm Kit-All Flex
Ortho Diaphragm Kit-Coil Spring
Ortho Diaphragm Kit-Flat Spring
Ortho Dienestrol Cream
▣ Ortho Disposable Applicator
▣ Ortho Personal Lubricant
▣ Ortho-Creme Contraceptive Cream
▣ Ortho-Gynol Contraceptive Jelly
◆ Ortho-Novum 1/35□21
Ortho-Novum 1/35□28
◆ Ortho-Novum 1/50□21
Ortho-Novum 1/50□28
◆ Ortho-Novum 1/80□21
Ortho-Novum 1/80□28
◆ Ortho-Novum 10/11□.. 21 Tablets
Ortho-Novum 10/11□.. 28 Tablets
◆ Ortho-Novum Tablets 2 mg□21
Sultrin Triple Sulfa Cream
Sultrin Triple Sulfa Vaginal Tablets

ORTHO PHARMACEUTICAL CORPORATION, 1450
Dermatological Division
Route 202
Raritan, NJ 08869
(201) 524-0400
Products Available
Cloderm (clocortolone pivalate) Cream
Grifulvin V (griseofulvin microsize)
Meclan (meclocycline sulfosalicylate) Cream
Monistat-Derm (miconazole nitrate) Cream & Lotion
Persa-Gel (benzoyl peroxide)
Persa-Gel W (benzoyl peroxide)
▣ Purpose Dry Skin Cream
▣ Purpose Shampoo
▣ Purpose Soap
Retin-A (tretinoin)

PARKE-DAVIS 422, 1453, 3015
Division of Warner-Lambert Company
201 Tabor Road
Morris Plains, NJ 07950 (201) 540-2000
Regional Sales Offices
Atlanta, GA 30328
1140 Hammond Drive (404) 396-4080
Baltimore (Hunt Valley), MD 21031
11350 McCormick Road (301) 666-7810
Chicago (Schaumburg), IL. 60195
1111 Plaza Drive (312) 884-6990
Dallas, TX 75234
12200 Ford Drive (214) 484-5566
Detroit (Troy), MI 48084
Suite 412
500 Stephenson Highway(313) 589-3292
Los Angeles (Tustin), CA 92680
17822 East 17th Street (714) 731-3441
Memphis, TN 38138
1355 Lynnfield Road (901) 767-1921
New York (East Hartford, CT) 06108
111 Founders Plaza (203) 528-9601
Pittsburgh, PA 15220
Manor Oak Two
1910 Cochran Road (412) 343-9855
Seattle (Bellevue), WA 98004
301-116th Ave, Southeast
(206) 451-1119

PARKE-DAVIS 422, 1453, 3015
Division Warner-Lambert Inc
Santurce, PR 00911
Direct Medical Inquiries to:
Parke-Davis
Div Warner-Lambert Inc
201 Tabor Road
Morris Plains, NJ 07950
Attn: Medical Affairs Department
Products Available
ACTH Steri-Vials
Abdec Baby Vitamin Drops
Abdec Kapseals
Abdec with Fluoride Baby Vitamin Drops
Abdol with Minerals Capsules
Acetaminophen (Tapar)
Acetaminophen with Codeine Phosphate Tablets, No. 2
Acetaminophen with Codeine Phosphate Tablets, No. 3
Acetaminophen with Codeine Phosphate Tablets, No. 4
Adrenalin Chloride Solution 1:100 & 1:1,000
Agoral, Liquid, Plain
Agoral, Marshmallow Flavor
Agoral, Raspberry Flavor
Alcohol, Rubbing (Lavacol)
Alophen Pills
Ambodryl Hydrochloride Kapseals
◆ Amcill Capsules
Amcill for Oral Suspension
Amcill Pediatric Drops
◆ Amitriptyline Hydrochloride Tablets (Amitril)
Amoxicillin for Oral Suspension
◆ Amoxicillin (Utimox) Capsules
Antibiotics
◆ Amcill Products
◆ Amoxicillin Products
◆ Chloromycetin Products
◆ Erythromycin Stearate Tablets (Erypar)
Humatin
Oxytetracycline Hydrochloride Capsules (Oxlopar)
Penicillin Products
Penicillin V Potassium Products (Penapar VK)
◆ Tetracycline Hydrochloride Capsules, (Cyclopar) (Cyclopar 500)
Anusol Ointment
◆ Anusol Suppositories
◆ Anusol-HC Cream
◆ Anusol-HC Suppositories
Aplisol (tuberculin PPD, diluted)
Aplitest (tuberculin PPD, multiple-puncture device)
Aspirin Compound Tablets
Aspirin Compound with Codeine Phosphate Tablets, No. 2 & No. 3
Aspirin Tablets
Aspirin with Codeine Phosphate Tablets, No. 2, No. 3 & No. 4
◆ Benadryl Capsules
Benadryl Cream
Benadryl Elixir
◆ Benadryl Kapseals
Benadryl Steri-Vials, Ampoules, and Steri-Dose Syringe
Benylin Cough Syrup
▣ Benylin DM Cough Syrup
Betapar
Brondecon Elixir
◆ Brondecon Tablets
Caladryl Cream, Lotion
Caladryl-HC Cream, Lotion
Calcium Gluconate Injection
Calcium Lactate Tablets
Cascara Sagrada Extract Filmseals
Celontin (Half Strength) Kapseals
◆ Celontin Kapseals
◆ Centrax Capsules, Tablets
Cherry Syrup
Chloramphenicol (Chloromycetin)
Chlordiazepoxide Hydrochloride Capsules
Chloromycetin Cream, 1%
Chloromycetin Hydrocortisone Ophthalmic
◆ Chloromycetin Kapseals
Chloromycetin Ophthalmic
Chloromycetin Ophthalmic Ointment, 1%
Chloromycetin Ophthalmic Solution (Ophthochlor)
Chloromycetin Otic
Chloromycetin Palmitate, Oral Suspension
Chloromycetin Sodium Succinate
Chloromycetin-Polymyxin-Hydrocortisone Acetate Ophthalmic Ointment (Ophthocort)
Chloromyxin
Chlorpromazine Hydrochloride Tablets (Promapar)
Choledyl Elixir
Choledyl Pediatric Syrup
◆ Choledyl SA Tablets
◆ Choledyl Tablets
Coly-Mycin M Parenteral
Coly-Mycin S For Oral Suspension
Coly-Mycin S Otic w/Neomycin & Hydrocortisone
Combex Kapseals
Combex with Vitamin C Kapseals
Corticotropin Injection (ACTH)
Cyanocobalamin Injection (Sytobex)
Cyclopar Capsules (tetracycline hydrochloride)
Digifortis Kapseals
◆ Dilantin Infatabs
◆ Dilantin Kapseals
Dilantin, Parenteral
◆ Dilantin with Phenobarbital Kapseals
Dilantin-30 Pediatric/Dilantin-125 Suspension
Diphenhydramine Hydrochloride (Benadryl)
Dispos-A-Med Flow Path Kit
Dispos-A-Med, isoetharine hydrochloride; isoproterenol hydrochloride
Dispos-A-Med Vials, Empty
Dispos-A-Vial: Sterile Water, Normal Saline, Half Normal Saline
Docusate Sodium Capsules (D-S-S Capsules)
Docusate Sodium with Casanthranol Capsules (D-D-S Plus Capsules)
Dolonil (Pyridium Plus)
Dopamine Hydrochloride Ampoules (Dopastat)
◆ Duraquin
◆ Easprin
Elase
Elase Ointment
V-Applicator (for Elase Ointment)
Elase-Chloromycetin Ointment
◆ Eldec Kapseals
Epinephrine (Adrenalin)
◆ Ergostat
◆ ERYC
◆ Erythromycin Stearate Tablets (Erypar)

(◆ Shown in Product Identification Section) (▣ Described in PDR For Nonprescription Drugs)

◆ Estrovis
Ethosuximide (see Zarontin)
◆ Euthroid
Ferrous Sulfate Filmseals
Fluogen (influenza virus vaccine)
Furosemide Injection, USP
◆ Gelusil Liquid & Tablets
Gelusil-M Liquid & Tablets
◆ Gelusil-II Liquid & Tablets
Geriplex Kapseals
◆ Geriplex-FS Kapseals
Geriplex-FS Liquid
Heparin Sodium Injection
Histoplasmin, Diluted
Humatin Capsules
Hydrochlorothiazide Tablets, USP (Thiuretic)
Hydrogen Peroxide Solution
Infatabs (Dilantin)
Influenza Virus Vaccine (Fluogen)
Ketalar
Ketamine Hydrochloride Injection (Ketalar)
Lavacol
◆ Loestrin [21] 1/20
◆ Loestrin [Fe] 1/20
◆ Loestrin [21] 1.5/30
◆ Loestrin [Fe] 1.5/30
◆ Lopid Capsules
Mandelamine Granules
Mandelamine Suspension
Mandelamine Suspension Forte
◆ Mandelamine Tablets
◆ Meclomen
Meprednisone (Betapar)
Meprobamate Tablets
Methsuximide (Celontin)
Milk of Bismuth
◆ Milontin Kapseals
Myadec
◆ Nardil
◆ Natabec Kapseals
◆ Natabec Rx Kapseals
Natabec with Fluoride Kapseals
Natabec-FA Kapseals
◆ Natafort Filmseal
Nema Worm Capsules
Nitroglycerin Tablets (Nitrostat)
◆ Nitrostat Tablets
Nitrostat IV Ampoules
Nitrostat IV Infusion Kit
◆ Nitrostat SR Capsules
Norethindrone Acetate and Ethinyl Estradiol Tablets (Loestrin, Norlestrin)
◆ Norlestrin [21] 1/50
◆ Norlestrin [21] 2.5/50
Norlestrin [28] 1/50
◆ Norlestrin [Fe] 1/50
◆ Norlestrin [Fe] 2.5/50
◆ Norlutate
◆ Norlutin
◆ Ophthochlor Ophthalmic Solution, 0.5%
Ophthocort Ophthalmic Ointment
Oxymetholone (Adroyd)
Oxytocin Injection (Pitocin)
Paladac
Paladac with Minerals Tablets
Panteric Filmseals, Granules
◆ Papase
Paromomycin (Humatin)
◆ Parsidol
Penicillin G Potassium for Injection
Penicillin G Procaine
Penicillin V Potassium for Oral Solution
◆ Penicillin V Potassium Tablets (Penapar VK)
◆ Peritrate Sustained Action
◆ Peritrate Tablets
Peroxide, Hydrogen
Phenobarbital Tablets
Phensuximide (Milontin)
Phenytoin Sodium (Dilantin)
Pitocin Injection, Ampoules, Steri-Dose Syringes
Pitressin, Synthetic, Ampoules
Pitressin Tannate in Oil Ampoules
Pituitrin-S Ampoules
Poison Ivy Extract
◆ Ponstel
◆ Povan Filmseals
Prazepam Capsules
◆ Procainamide Hydrochloride Capsules
◆ Procan SR Tablets
◆ Proloid Tablets
Propoxyphene Compound 65
Propoxyphene Hydrochloride Capsules
◆ Pyridium
◆ Pyridium Plus
Pyrvinium Pamoate (Povan)
Quinidine Sulfate Tablets
Quinine Sulfate Capsules
◆ Renoquid Tablets
Rubbing Alcohol (Lavacol)
Saf-Tip Enema
Siblin Granules
◆ Sinubid
◆ Sulfacytine Tablets (Renoquid)
Surital Ampoules, Steri-Vials
Syntobex (Cyanocobalamin Injection)
◆ Tabron Filmseal
◆ Tedral
Tedral Elixir
Tedral Expectorant
◆ Tedral SA
Tedral Suspension
◆ Tedral-25
Terpin Hydrate & Codeine Elixir
◆ Tetracycline HCl Capsules (Cyclopar)
◆ Tetracycline HCl Capsules, (Cyclopar 500)
Theelin Aqueous Suspension
◆ Thera-Combex H-P Kapseals
Thiamylal Sodium (Surital)
Thiuretic (Hydrochlorothiazide Tablets)
Thrombostat
Tolbutamide Tablets
Tuberculin, Aplisol and Aplitest
Tucks Cream
Tucks Ointment
Tucks Premoistened Pads
Tucks Take-Alongs
Unibase
◆ Uticort Cream, Gel, Lotion & Ointment
V-Applicators for Elase Ointment
Vakutage
Vasopressin Injection (Pitressin)
Vira-A for Infusion
◆ Vira-A Ophthalmic Ointment, 3%
Water for Injection, Steri-Vials
◆ Zarontin Capsules
Zarontin Syrup
Ziradryl Lotion

PEDINOL PHARMACAL INC. 1548
110 Bell Street
W. Babylon, NY 11704
Address inquiries to:
Director of Professional Services
(516) 293-9500
Products Avaiable
Alginate Styptic Gauze
Breezee Mist Foot Powder
Castellani Paint
Fungoid Creme & Solution
Fungoid Tincture
Hydrisalic Gel
Hydrisea Lotion
Hydrisinol Creme & Lotion
Osti-Derm Lotion
PNS Unna Boot
Pedi-Bath Salts
Pedi-Boro Soak Paks
Pedi-Cort V Creme
Pedi-Dri Foot Powder
Pedi-Vit A Creme
Salactic Film
Steri Unna Boot
Ureacin Lotion & Creme

PENNWALT PHARMACEUTICAL DIVISION 425, 1548
Pennwalt Corporation
755 Jefferson Road
Rochester, NY 14623

Prescription Division
755 Jefferson Road
Rochester, NY 14623
Address inquiries to:
Director of Professional Relations
P.O. Box 1766
Rochester, NY 14603 (716) 475-9000
PHARMACRAFT
755 Jefferson Road
Rochester, NY 14623
Address inquiries to:
Professional Services Department
P.O. Box 1212
Rochester, NY 14603
Products Available
◆ Adapin Capsules
◆ Biphetamine Capsules
Cholan HMB
Cholan-DH
Emul-O-Balm
Infalyte
◆ Ionamin Capsules
Kolyum Liquid and Powder
Nesacaine
Nesacaine-CE
Tussionex Capsules
Tussionex Suspension
Tussionex Tablets
◆ Zaroxolyn Tablets

PERSŌN & COVEY, INC. 1554
616 Allen Avenue
Glendale, CA 91201
Address inquiries to:
Lorne V. Persōn, President (213) 240-1030
Products Available
•□ A.C.N. Tablets
•□ DHS Conditioning Rinse
•□ DHS Shampoo
•□ DHS Tar Shampoo
•□ DHS Zinc Dandruff Shampoo
DOB Bath & Shower Oil (Formerly Tolakol)
Drysol
•□ Enisyl Tablets
•□ Solbar Plus 15 Sun Protectant Cream
•□ Solbar Sun Protective Cream
•□ Xerac
Xerac AC
Xerac BP5
Xerac BP10
Z-Pro-C Tablets

PFIPHARMECS DIVISION 425, 1555
Pfizer Inc.
235 E. 42nd St.
New York, NY 10017
Address inquiries to:
Professional Services Dept. (212) 573-2323
Address Export inquiries to:
Pfizer International Inc. (212) 573-2323
Distribution Centers
Doraville, GA 30340
4360 Northeast Expressway
(404) 448-6666
Hoffman Estates, IL 60196
2400 W. Central Road (312) 381-9500
Clifton, NJ 07012
230 Brighton Rd. (201) 546-7700
Grand Prairie, TX 75050
502 Fountain Parkway (817) 261-9131
Irvine, CA 92705
16700 Red Hill Ave. (714) 540-9180
Products Available
◆ Antiminth Oral Suspension
Bacitracin Sterile
Bacitracin Topical Ointment
Bonine Tablets
Cortril Topical Ointment
Coryban-D Capsules
Coryban-D Cough Syrup
Isoject Vistaril Intramuscular Solution
Li-Ban Lice Control Spray
Neobiotic Tablets
◆ Permapen Isoject
Pfizer-E Film Coated Tablets
Pfizerpen for Injection
◆ Pfizerpen G Tablets
Pfizerpen VK Powder For Oral Solution
◆ Pfizerpen VK Tablets
◆ Pfizerpen-A Capsules
Pfizerpen-A Powder For Oral Suspension
◆ Pfizerpen-AS Aqueous Suspension
◆ Pfizerpen-AS Aqueous Suspension, Isoject
Polymixin B Sulfate Sterile
◆ RID Pediculicide
Sterane Tablets
Streptomycin Sulfate Injection
TerraCortril Ophthalmic Suspension
◆ Terra-Cortril Topical Ointment
◆ Terramycin Capsules
Terramycin Film-coated Tablets
◆ Terramycin Intramuscular Solution
Terramycin Topical Ointment
Terramycin Syrup
◆ Terramycin with Polymyxin B Sulfate Ophthalmic Ointment
◆ Terrastatin Capsules
◆ Tetracyn & Tetracyn 500 Capsules
Tetrastatin Capsules
Vansil Capsules
Vistaril Intramuscular Solution
Wart-Off Wart Remover

PFIZER LABORATORIES DIVISION 425, 1572
Pfizer Inc.
235 E. 42nd St.
New York, NY 10017
Address inquiries to:
Professional Services Dept. (212) 573-2422
Medical Emergency Calls
(Day or Night) (212) 573-2422
Address Export inquiries to:
Pfizer International Inc. (212) 573-2323
Distribution Centers
Doraville, GA 30340
4360 Northeast Expressway
(404) 448-6666
Hoffman Estates, IL 60196
2400 W. Central Road (312) 381-9500
Clifton, NJ 07012
230 Brighton Rd. (201) 546-7700
Grand Prairie, TX 75050
502 Fountain Parkway (214) 647-0222
Irvine, CA 92714
16700 Red Hill Ave. (714) 540-9180
Products Available
Bonine Chewable Tablets
Cortril Acetate Aqueous Suspension
◆ Diabinese Tablets
◆ Feldene Capsules
◆ Minipress Capsules
◆ Minizide Capsules
◆ Moderil Tablets
◆ Procardia Capsules
◆ Renese Tablets
◆ Renese-R Tablets
Vibramycin Calcium Syrup
◆ Vibramycin Hyclate Capsules
Vibramycin Hyclate Intravenous
Vibramycin Monohydrate for Oral Suspension
◆ Vibra-Tabs Film Coated Tablets
◆ Vistaril Capsules

(◆ Shown in Product Identification Section) **(•□ Described in PDR For Nonprescription Drugs)**

Vistaril Oral Suspension
◆ Vistrax Tablets

PHARMACIA LABORATORIES **426, 1587**
Division of Pharmacia Inc.
800 Centennial Ave.
Piscataway, NJ 08854
Address inquiries to:
Medical Director (201) 457-8162
Products Available
◆ Azulfidine Tablets, EN-tabs, Oral Suspension
Crescormon
Healon
Hyskon Hysteroscopy Fluid
Kabikinase
Macrodex
Rheomacrodex
Secretin-Kabi

PHARMACRAFT DIVISION **1590**
Pennwalt Corporation
755 Jefferson Road
Rochester, NY 14623
Address inquiries to:
Professional Service Department
P.O. Box 1212
Rochester, NY 14603 (716) 475-9000
Products Available
▣ Allerest Tablets, Childrens Chewable Tablets & Headache Strength Tablets
▣ Allerest Timed Release Allergy Capsules
▣ CaldeCORT Hydrocortisone Multi-Purpose Anti-Itch Cream, Spray, Ointment & Towelettes
▣ Caldesene Medicated Ointment
▣ Caldesene Medicated Baby Powder
▣ Cruex Antifungal Cream
▣ Cruex Antifungal Powder
▣ Desenex Antifungal Ointment, Powder, Soap & Solution
▣ Desenex Antifungal Spray Powder
▣ Sinarest Tablets

WM. P. POYTHRESS & CO., INC. **426, 1590**
16 N. 22nd St.
Post Office Box 26946
Richmond, VA 23261 (804) 644-8591
Address inquiries to:
Special Services Department
Products Available
Antrocol Elixir
◆ Antrocol Tablets & Capsules
Bensulfoid
▣ Bensulfoid Lotion
◆ Lodrane Tablets-130 & 260
Mudrane GG Elixir
◆ Mudrane GG Tablets
◆ Mudrane GG-2 Tablets
◆ Mudrane Tablets
◆ Mudrane-2 Tablets
Panalgesic
◆ Solfoton Tablets, Capsules & S/C (Sugar-Coated) Tablets
◆ Trocinate Tablets
◆ Uro-Phosphate Tablets

PROCTER & GAMBLE **426, 1593**
P.O. Box 171
Cincinnati, OH 45201
Address inquiries to:
Arnold P. Austin (800) 543-0299
In Ohio (800) 582-2684
Products Available
◆ Didronel
▣ Head & Shoulders
◆ Topicycline

THE PURDUE FREDERICK COMPANY **426, 1595**
100 Connecticut Avenue
Norwalk, CT 06854 (203) 853-0123
Address inquiries to:
Medical Department
Products Available
Arthropan Liquid
Betadine Aerosol Spray
Betadine Antiseptic Gauze Pad
Betadine Douche
Betadine Douche Kit
Betadine Hēlafoam Solution
Betadine Mouthwash/Gargle
Betadine Ointment
Betadine Perineal Wash Concentrate
Betadine Shampoo
Betadine Skin Cleanser
Betadine Skin Cleanser Foam
Betadine Solution
Betadine Solution Swab Aid
Betadine Solution Swabsticks
Betadine Surgical Scrub
Betadine Surgi-Prep Sponge-Brush
Betadine Viscous Formula Antiseptic Gauze Pad
Betadine Whirlpool Concentrate
◆ Cardioquin Tablets
◆ Cerumenex Drops
◆ Fibermed Supplements
Parelixir Liquid
◆ Phyllocontin Tablets
◆ Prioderm Lotion
Senokap DSS Capsules
Senokot Suppositories
Senokot Syrup
◆ Senokot Tablets/Granules
Senokot Tablets Unit Strip Pack
◆ Senokot-S Tablets
◆ Trilisate Tablets/Liquid

BLAIR LABORATORIES, INC.
Calamatum Lotion
Calamatum Ointment
Calamatum Spray
Fungacetin Ointment
Gertlax B Granules
Gertlax S Tablets
Isodine Antiseptic Solution
Isodine Concentrate Gargle/Mouthwash
Kerid Ear Drops
Riasol Lotion
Saratoga Ointment

SHIELD LABORATORIES, INC.
Central Venous Catheter Dressing Change Set
Urinary Catheter Care Set

REED & CARNRICK **427, 1601**
1 New England Avenue
Piscataway, NJ 08854
Address inquiries to:
Professional Service Dept. (201) 272-6600
Products Available
Alphosyl Lotion, Cream
Alphosyl-HC Lotion & Cream
◆ Cortifoam
◆ Dilatrate-SR
◆ Epifoam
Kwell Cream
Kwell Lotion
Kwell Shampoo
Peptenzyme Elixir
◆ Phazyme
◆ Phazyme-95
◆ Phazyme-PB Tablets
◆ Proctofoam-HC
◆ proctoFoam/non-steroid
Proxigel
R&C Spray
Trichotine Liquid, Vaginal Douche
Trichotine Powder, Vaginal Douche
Trichotine-D Disposable Vaginal Douche

REID-PROVIDENT LABORATORIES, INC. **427, 1605**
Scientific Affairs and Manufacturing
25 Fifth Street, N.W.
Atlanta, GA 30308
Executive Offices
640 Tenth Street, N.W.
Atlanta, GA 30318 (404) 898-1000
Address inquiries to:
Medical Director
Products Available
Anduracaine Injection
◆ Calinate-FA
Chloramate Unicelles
Crystimin-1000
Curretab Tablets
Dentavite Chewable Tablets
Dentavite Drops
Estraguard Vaginal Cream
◆ Estratab Tablets
◆ Estratest H.S.
◆ Estratest Tablets
Eugel Liquid
Femguard Vaginal Cream
Fumatrin Forte
Histalet DM Syrup
◆ Histalet Forte Tablets
Histalet Syrup
Histalet X Syrup
◆ Histalet X Tablets
◆ Melfiat Tablets
◆ Melfiat 105 Unicelles
Mity-Mycin Ointment
Mity-Quin Cream
Otoreid-HC Ear Drops
P-V-Tussin Syrup
◆ P-V-Tussin Tablets
Pavacap Unicelles
Proaqua Tablets
Proval #3 Capsules
Provigan Injection
RP-Mycin Tablets
Reidamine Injection
Repen-VK Suspensions
Repen-VK Tablets
Retet-250 Capsules
Retet-500 Capsules
Spalix Tablets
Sumox Capsules
Sumox Oral Suspensions
Supen Capsules
Supen Oral Suspensions
Tranmep Tablets
Tusstrol Syrup
Unifast Unicelles
◆ Unipres Tablets
Vaso-80 Unicelles
◆ Zenate Tablets

REID-PROVIDENT LABORATORIES, INC. **427, 1608**
DIRECT DIVISION (Formerly TUTAG)
640 Tenth Street, N.W.
Atlanta GA 30318
Address inquiries to:
Professional Service Dept. (404) 898-1000
Products Available
Acetospan Injection
Alermine Tablets
Ampicillin Capsules, Suspension
Analone Injection
Andriol Injection
Aquatag Tablets
Arthrolate Injection
Asminorel Improved Tablets
◆ Bacarate Tablets
Baltron Injection
Bendylate Capsules, Elixir
Bendylate Injection
C-BE Zinc Tablets
Cino-40 Injection
Codap Tablets
Cotropic-Gel 40 Injection
Cotropic-Gel 80 Injection
Cyvaso Capsules
Depletite-25 Tablets
Dezone Injectable
Dimate Injection
Droxomin Injection
Dua-Pred Injection
Duoval P.A. Injection
E-Ionate P.A. Injection
Enoxa Tablets
Escot Capsules
Estraval 2X Injection
Estraval 4X Injection
Estraval-P.A. Injection
Fenbutal Tablets
Ganphen Injection
Hyproval P.A. Injection
I.D. 50 Injection
Irolong II
L.A. Dezone Injection
Murcil Capsules
Nandrolin Injection
Neotep Granucaps
Neozyl
Nospaz Injection
1000 BC Injection
P.S.P. IV (four) Injection
Penicillin G Tablets
Piracaps Capsules
Pre-Dep 40 Injection
Pre-Dep 80 Injection
Prednisolone Acetate Injection
Pre-Enthus FA Capsules
Quadnite Tablets
Quinite Tablets
Rauserpa Tablets
SPRX-1
SPRX-3 Capsules
◆ SPRX-105 Capsules
Sanicide Liquid
Sorquad Tablets
Suladyne Tablets
T.D. Alermine Granucaps
T.D. Therals Granucaps
T-E Ionate P.A. Injection
T-Ionate P.A. Injection
Tagafed Tablets
Tagatap Tablets & Elixir
Testostroval P.A. Injection
Tora Tablets
Tora-I & -II Capsules
Tora-30 Capsules
Trates Granucaps
Tuzon Tablets
Unproco Capsules
Vagimine Cream
Vasal Granucaps
Vernate II Granucaps
Viotag Cream
X-Otag Injection
◆ X-Otag S.R. Tablets
Zide Tablets

RESEARCH INDUSTRIES CORPORATION **1609**
Pharmaceutical Division
1847 West 2300 South
Salt Lake City, UT 84119
(800) 453-8432
(801) 972-5500
Products Available
Rimso-50
Rimso-100

RHO MU CORPORATION **1610**
Subsidiary of RICHARDSON-VICKS INC.
10 Westport Road
Wilton, CT 06897

Address inquiries to:
Vicks Research Center (203) 929-2500
For Medical Emergencies Contact:
Medical Director
Vicks Research Center (203) 929-2500
Products Available
Percogesic Analgesic Tablets

RIKER LABORATORIES, INC. **428, 1610**
Subsidiary of 3M Company
19901 Nordhoff Street
Northridge, CA 91324
For medical information, address inquiries to:
Associate Director, Medical Services
(213) 709-3137
Customer Service and other inquiries:
(800) 423-5197
For medical emergency information only after hours
(213) 341-1300
Products Available
Alu-Cap Capsules
Alu-Tab Tablets
Calcium Disodium Versenate Injection
Cal-Sup
◆ Circanol Tablets
Deaner Tablets
Deaner-250 Tablets
◆ Disalcid Capsules
◆ Disalcid Tablets
Disipal Tablets
Duo-Medihaler Aerosol
Estomul-M Liquid & Tablets
Heparin Sodium Injection, Aqueous (Lipo-Hepin)
Lipo-Hepin (Heparin Sodium Injection USP)
Medihaler Ergotamine Aerosol
Medihaler-Epi Aerosol
Medihaler-Iso Aerosol
Norflex Injectable
◆ Norflex Tablets
◆ Norgesic Tablets
◆ Norgesic Forte Tablets
Rauwiloid Tablets
Sodium Versenate Injection
◆ Tepanil Tablets
◆ Tepanil Ten-tab Tablets
Theolair Liquid
◆ Theolair Tablets
◆ Theolair-Plus
◆ Theolair-SR Tablets
Ulo Syrup
◆ Urex Tablets

THE ROBERTSON/TAYLOR CO. **1619**
A division of Intra-Medic Formulations, Inc.
135 E. Oakland Park Boulevard
Fort Lauderdale, Florida 33334
Address inquiries to:
Mitchell K. Friedlander (305) 566-2287
Products Available
Medi-Tec 90 Therapeutic Conditioner with Strengthening Agents
Medi-Tec 90 Therapeutic Scalp Stimulant with Strengthening Agents
Medi-Tec 90 Therapeutic Shampoo & Scalp Conditioner with Strengthening Agents

A. H. ROBINS COMPANY **428, 1620**
Pharmaceutical Division
1407 Cummings Drive
Richmond, VA 23220
Address inquiries to:
The Medical Dept. (804) 257-2000
Medical Emergency calls (day or night) (804) 257-2000
If no answer, call answering service (804) 257-7788
Products Available
▣ Allbee C-800 Plus Iron Tables
▣ Allbee C-800 Tablets
◆ Allbee w/C Capsules
◆ Allbee-T Tablets
Arthralgen Tablets
Cough Calmers
◆ Dimacol Capsules
Dimacol Liquid
▣ Dimetane Decongestant Elixir
▣ Dimetane Decongestant Tablets
Dimetane Elixir
Dimetane Expectorant
Dimetane Expectorant-DC
◆ Dimetane Extentabs
◆ Dimetane Tablets
Dimetane-Ten Injectable
Dimetapp Elixir
◆ Dimetapp Extentabs
Donnagel
Donnagel-PG
◆ Donnatal Capsules
Donnatal Elixir
◆ Donnatal Extentabs
Donnatal No. 2 Tablets
◆ Donnatal Tablets
◆ Donnazyme Tablets
Dopram Injectable
◆ Entozyme Tablets
◆ Exna Tablets
Exna-R Tablets
Imavate Tablets
◆ Micro-K Extencaps
◆ Mitrolan Chewable Tablets
◆ Pabalate Tablets
◆ Pabalate-SF Tablets
◆ Phenaphen Capsules
◆ Phenaphen w/Codeine Capsules
◆ Phenaphen-650 with Codeine Tablets
◆ Pondimin Tablets
◆ Quinidex Extentabs
Reglan Injectable
◆ Reglan Tablets
Robaxin Injectable
◆ Robaxin Tablets
◆ Robaxin-750 Tablets
◆ Robaxisal Tablets
Robicillin VK for Oral Solution
◆ Robicillin VK Robitabs
◆ Robimycin Robitabs
◆ Robinul Forte Tablets
Robinul Injectable
◆ Robinul Tablets
◆ Robitet '250' Hydrochloride Robicaps
◆ Robitet '500' Hydrochloride Robicaps
▣ Robitussin
Robitussin A-C
▣ Robitussin-CF
Robitussin-DAC
▣ Robitussin-DM
▣ Robitussin-PE
Silain Tablets
Silain-Gel Liquid
Skelaxin Tablets
Tybatran Capsules
◆ Z-Bec Tablets

ROCHE LABORATORIES **429, 1643, 3017**
Division of Hoffmann-La Roche Inc.
Nutley, NJ 07110 (201) 235-5000
For Medical Information
Write: Professional Services Department
Business hours only (8:30 a.m. to 5:00 p.m. EST), call (201) 235-2355
For Medical Emergency Information only after hours or on weekends, call (201) 235-2355
Branch Warehouses
Belvidere, NJ 07823
Water Street (201) 475-5337
Des Plaines, IL 60018
105 E. Oakton St. (312) 299-0021
(Chicago) (312) 775-0733
San Leandro, CA 94577
1599 Factor Ave. (415) 352-1660
◆ Accutane
Alurate Elixir
◆ Ancobon Capsules
Arfonad Ampuls
◆ Azo Gantanol Tablets
◆ Azo Gantrisin Tablets
◆ Bactrim DS Tablets
Bactrim I.V. Infusion
Bactrim Pediatric Suspension
Bactrim Suspension
◆ Bactrim Tablets
◆ Berocca Plus Tablets
◆ Berocca Tablets
Berocca-C & Berocca-C 500
Berocca-WS Injectable
◆ Clonopin Tablets
Efudex Cream
Efudex Solution
◆ Emcyt Capsules
◆ Endep Tablets
FUDR Injectable
◆ Fansidar Tablets
Fluorouracil Ampuls
◆ Gantanol DS Tablets
Gantanol Suspension
◆ Gantanol Tablets
Gantrisin Injectable
Gantrisin Ophthalmic Ointment/Solution
Gantrisin Pediatric Suspension
Gantrisin Syrup
◆ Gantrisin Tablets
Konakion Injectable
◆ Larobec Tablets
◆ Larodopa Capsules
◆ Larodopa Tablets
◆ Larotid Capsules
Larotid for Oral Suspension
Larotid Pediatric Drops
Levo-Dromoran Injectable
◆ Levo-Dromoran Tablets
Lipo Gantrisin
Lorfan Injectable
◆ Marplan Tablets
◆ Matulane Capsules
◆ Menrium Tablets
Mestinon Injectable
Mestinon Syrup
◆ Mestinon Tablets
◆ Mestinon Timespan
Nipride Injectable
Nisentil Injectable
◆ Noludar Tablets
◆ Noludar 300 Capsules
Pantopon Injectable
Prostigmin Injectable
◆ Prostigmin Tablets
◆ Quarzan Capsules
◆ Rocaltrol Capsules
Roniacol Elixir
◆ Roniacol Tablets
◆ Roniacol Timespan
◆ Solatene Capsules
Synkayvite Injectable
◆ Synkayvite Tablets
Taractan Concentrate
Taractan Injectable
◆ Taractan Tablets
◆ Tel-E-Dose (unit dose) Products:
Bactrim Tablets
Bactrim DS Tablets
Endep Tablets
Gantanol DS Tablets
Gantanol Tablets
Gantrisin Tablets
Larotid Capsules
Larotid Oral Suspension
Trimpex Tablets
Tensilon Injectable
◆ Trimpex Tablets
◆ Valium Injectable
◆ Valium Tel-E-Ject
◆ Valrelease Capsules
◆ Vi-Penta F Chewables
Vi-Penta F Infant Drops
Vi-Penta F Multivitamin Drops
Vi-Penta Infant Drops
Vi-Penta Multivitamin Drops
Vitamin K—see Synkayvite
Vitamin K_1—see Konakion

ROCHE PRODUCTS INC. **429, 1696**
Manati, Puerto Rico 00701
Address inquiries to:
Roche Laboratories (see above)
Products Available
◆ Dalmane Capsules
◆ Librax Capsules
◆ Libritabs Tablets
◆ Librium Capsules
Librium Injectable
◆ Limbitrol Tablets
◆ Tel-E-Dose (unit dose) Products:
Dalmane Capsules
Librax Capsules
Librium Capsules
Limbitrol Tablets
Valium Tablets
◆ Valium Tablets

ROERIG **431, 1703**
A division of Pfizer Pharmaceuticals
235 E. 42nd St.
New York, NY 10017
Address inquiries to:
Medical Department (212) 573-2187
Branch Offices
Doraville, GA 30340
4360 N.E. Expressway
(Southern Region) (404) 448-6666
Hoffman Estates, IL 60196
2400 W. Central Road (312) 381-9500
(Midwestern & Great Lakes Regions)
Clifton, NJ 07012
230 Brighton Road
(Metro Region) (201) 546-7700
Dallas, TX 75222
P.O. Box 22249
(Southwestern Region) (214) 647-0222
Irvine, CA 92705
16700 Red Hill Ave.
(Western Region) (714) 540-9180
Products Available
◆ Antivert, Antivert/25 Tablets & Antivert/25 Chewable Tablets
◆ Atarax Tablets & Syrup
Cartrax Tablets
Emete-con Intramuscular/Intravenous
◆ Geocillin Tablets
Geopen Intramuscular/Intravenous
◆ Heptuna Plus Capsules
◆ Marax Tablets & DF Syrup
◆ Navane Capsules and Concentrate
Navane Intramuscular
◆ Sinequan Capsules
Sinequan Oral Concentrate
◆ Spectrobid Tablets & Oral Suspension
◆ Sustaire Tablets
◆ Tao Capsules & Oral Suspension
◆ Urobiotic-250 Capsules

WILLIAM H. RORER, INC. **431, 1720**
500 Virginia Drive
Fort Washington, PA 19034
For Medical Emergencies Contact:
John F. A. Vance, M.D.
Medical Director (215) 628-6761
For Quality Matters Contact:
William E. Kinas, Vice President,
Quality Assurance (215) 628-6420
For Product Information Contact:
Ronald A. Amey
Services Manager (215) 628-6492

Branch Offices
Langhorne, PA 19047
2201 Cabot Blvd. West (215) 752-8555
Oak Forest, IL 60452
P.O. Box 280
4325 Frontage Rd. (312)687-7440
San Leandro, CA 94577
P.O. Box 1569
1550 Factor Avenue (415) 357-9741
Tucker, GA 30084
4660 Hammermill Road (404) 934-3091
Products Available
◆ Ananase Tablets
◆ Ascriptin Tablets
◆ Ascriptin A/D Tablets
◆ Ascriptin w/Codeine Tablets
Camalox Suspension
◆ Camalox Tablets
◆ Chardonna-2 Tablets
Emetrol Solution
Fedahist Expectorant
◆ Fedahist Gyrocaps
Fedahist Syrup
◆ Fedahist Tablets
◆ Fermalox Tablets
◆ Gemnisyn
◆ Maalox No. 1 Tablets
◆ Maalox No. 2 Tablets
Maalox Plus Suspension
◆ Maalox Plus Tablets
Maalox Suspension
Maalox TC
Parepectolin Suspension
◆ Perdiem Granules
◆ Slo-bid Gyrocaps
◆ Slo-Phyllin Gyrocaps
◆ Slo-Phyllin Tablets
Slo-Phyllin 80 Syrup
◆ Slo-Phyllin GG Capsules
Slo-Phyllin GG Syrup

ROSS LABORATORIES 432, 1731
Div. Abbott Laboratories
Columbus, OH 43216
Address inquiries to:
Henry S. Sauls, M.D., Vice President,
Medical Affairs (614) 227-3333
Products Available
Advance
Component Nipple System
Ensure
Ensure Plus
Flexiflo Enteral Delivery System
Flexiflo Enteral Nutrition Container
Flexiflo Enteral Nutrition Pump
Flexiflo Enteral Pump Set
Flexiflo Gravity Gavage Set
Forta Pudding
Glucose Water 5% & 10%
Isomil
Isomil SF
Isomil SF 20
Osmolite
Pediaflor
Pedialyte
Pediamycin
Pediazole
Polycose
◆ Pramet FA
◆ Pramilet FA
RCF
Redi-Nurser System
Rondec Drops
Rondec Syrup
◆ Rondec Tablet
Rondec-DM Drops
Rondec-DM Syrup
◆ Rondec-TR Tablet
Ross Hospital Formula System
Similac
Similac PM 60/40
Similac 13
Similac 20
Similac 24
Similac 24 LBW
Similac 27
Similac Special Care 20
Similac Special Care 24
Similac With Iron
Similac With Iron 13
Similac With Iron 20
Similac With Iron 24
Similac With Whey
Similac With Whey 20
Sterilized Water
Vari-Flavors Flavor Pacs
Vi-Daylin ADC Drops
◆ Vi-Daylin Chewable
Vi-Daylin Drops
Vi-Daylin Liquid
Vi-Daylin Plus Iron ADC Drops
◆ Vi-Daylin Plus Iron Chewable
Vi-Daylin Plus Iron Drops
Vi-Daylin Plus Iron Liquid
Vi-Daylin/F ADC Drops
Vi-Daylin/F ADC + Iron Drops
◆ Vi-Daylin/F Chewable
Vi-Daylin/F Drops
◆ Vi-Daylin/F + Iron Chewable
Vi-Daylin/F + Iron Drops
Vital/High Nitrogen
Volu-Feed

ROTEX PHARMACEUTICALS, INC. 1749
P.O. Box 19283
Orlando, FL 32814
Address inquiries to:
Mr. Jerry S. Roth, President
(305) 896-8280
Products Available
Arthrogesic
Nasalspan Capsules
Nasalspan Expectorant
Podiliquid
Rogesic Capsules
Rogesic #3 Tablets
Ropres
Rothav-150
Rovite
Rovite Tonic

ROWELL LABORATORIES, INC. 1750
210 Main Street, W.
Baudette, MN 56623
Toll Free (800) 346-5040
In Minn. Call (800) 542-5012
Address inquiries to:
Professional Service Dept.
Products Available
Balneol
C-Ron
C-Ron FA
C-Ron Forte
C-Ron Freckles
Cin-Quin
Colrex Capsules
Colrex Compound Capsules
Colrex Compound Elixir
Colrex Decongestant
Colrex Expectorant
Colrex Syrup
Colrex Troches
Cortenema
Dermacort Cream
Dermacort Lotion-0.5%, 1%
Dexone 0.5, 0.75, 1.5, 4
Hydrocil Fortified
Hydrocil Instant
Hydrocil Plain
Lithonate
Lithotabs
Multivitamins Rowell
Norlac
Norlac RX
Orasone 1, 5, 10, 20, 50
Perifoam
Prednisone Tablets
Proctocort
Proctodon
Quine Capsules
Quinidine Sulfate Capsules & Tablets
Ro-Bile
S.A.S.-500
Vio-Bec
Vio-Bec Forte
Vio-Geric

ROXANE LABORATORIES, INC. 1755
330 Oak St., Columbus, OH 43216
Address inquiries to:
Professional Services Department
P.O. 16532
Columbus, OH 43216
(Toll Free) (800) 848-0120
(In Ohio call) (614) 228-5403
Products Available
Acetaminophen Elixir
Acetaminophen Suppositories
Acetaminophen Tablets
Acetaminophen with Codeine Phosphate Elixir
Acetaminophen with Codeine Phosphate Tablets
Aluminum Hydroxide, Concentrate
Aluminum Hydroxide Gel
Aluminum & Magnesium Hydroxides with Simethicone I
Aluminum & Magnesium Hydroxides with Simethicone II
Aminophylline Tablets
Amitriptyline Hydrochloride Tablets
Aromatic Cascara Fluidextract
Ascorbic Acid Tablets
Aspirin Suppositories
Basic Aluminum Carbonate Gel
Bisacodyl Patient Pack
Bisacodyl Suppositories
Bisacodyl Tablets
Calcium Gluconate Tablets
Castor Oil
Castor Oil Flavored
Chloral Hydrate Capsules
Chloral Hydrate Syrup
Chlordiazepoxide Hydrochloride Capsules
Chlorpheniramine Maleate Tablets
Chlorpromazine Hydrochloride Tablets
Cocaine Hydrochloride Topical Solution
Codeine Sulfate Tablets
Dexamethasone Tablets
Dihydrotachysterol Tablets
Diluent (Flavored) for Oral Use
Diphenhydramine Hydrochloride Capsules
Diphenhydramine Hydrochloride Elixir
Diphenoxylate Hydrochloride & Atropine Sulfate Tablets & Oral Solution
Docusate Sodium Capsules
Docusate Sodium Syrup
Docusate Sodium with Casanthranol Capsules
Dovamide Capsules
Ferrous Sulfate Liquid
Ferrous Sulfate Tablets
Gentz Wipes
Glycerin Oral Solution
Guaiahist Tablets
Guaiahist T.T. Tablets
Guaifenesin Syrup
Hydrochlorothiazide Tablets
Imipramine Hydrochloride Tablets
Ipecac Syrup
Isoetharine Hydrochloride
Isoxsuprine Hydrochloride Tablets
Kaolin-Pectin Suspension
Kaolin-Pectin Suspension Concentrated
Lithium Carbonate Capsules & Tablets
Lithium Citrate Syrup
Magnesia & Alumina Oral Suspension
Methadone Hydrochloride Oral Solution
Milk of Magnesia
Milk of Magnesia-Concentrated
Milk of Magnesia-Cascara Suspension Concentrated
Milk of Magnesia-Mineral Oil Emulsion & Emulsion (Flavored)
Mineral Oil
Mineral Oil-Light Sterile
Morphine Sulfate Oral Solution
Morphine Sulfate Tablets
Neomycin Sulfate Tablets
Niacin Tablets
Oxycodone Hydrochloride Oral Solution
Oxycodone Hydrochloride Tablets
Oxycodone Hydrochloride & Acetaminophen Tablets
Oxycodone Hydrochloride, Oxycodone Terephthalate & Aspirin Tablets
Papaverine Hydrochloride Capsules
Paregoric
Phenobarbital Elixir
Phenobarbital Tablets
Potassium Chloride for Oral Solution (Flavored)
Potassium Chloride Oral Solution
Potassium Chloride Powder Unflavored
Potassium Gluconate Elixir
Potassium Iodide Liquid
Potassium Iodide Oral Solution
Potassium Phosphates Oral Solution
Prednisolone Tablets
Prednisone Tablets
Propantheline Bromide Tablets
Propoxyphene Hydrochloride Capsules
Pseudoephedrine Hydrochloride & Triprolidine Hydrochloride Syrup
Pseudoephedrine Hydrochloride & Triprolidine Hydrochloride Tablets
Pseudoephedrine Hydrochloride Tablets, Syrup
Quinidine Sulfate Tablets
Quinine Sulfate Capsules
Saliva Substitute
Sodium Chloride Inhalation
Sodium Phosphates Oral Solution
Sulfisoxazole Tablets
Terpin Hydrate & Codeine Elixir
Theophylline Elixir

RYSTAN COMPANY, INC. 1761
470 Mamaroneck Avenue
White Plains, NY 10605
Address inquiries to:
Professional Service Dept. (914) 761-0044
Products Available
Chloresium Dental Ointment
▣ Chloresium Ointment
▣ Chloresium Solution
Chloresium Tablets
▣ Derifil Tablets & Powder
Panafil Ointment
Panafil-White Ointment
Prophyllin Ointment
Prophyllin Powder

SDA PHARMACEUTICALS, INC. 1761
919 Third Avenue
New York, NY 10022
Address inquiries to:
Dr. Edward L. Steinberg (212) 688-4420
Products Available
Anorexin Capsules
Anorexin One-Span Capsules

SANDOZ PHARMACEUTICALS 432, 1761
(Division of Sandoz, Inc.)
Route 10, East Hanover, NJ 07936
Address inquiries to:
William F. Westlin, M.D. (201) 386-7500
New York City (212) 349-1212

(◆ Shown in Product Identification Section)

(▣ Described in PDR For Nonprescription Drugs)

Products Available
◆ Belladenal Tablets
◆ Belladenal-S Tablets
Bellafoline Injection & Tablets
Cafergot Suppositories
◆ Cafergot Tablets
Cafergot P-B Suppositories
◆ Cafergot P-B Tablets
Cedilanid-D Injection
D.H.E. 45 Injection
Diapid Nasal Spray
◆ Fiogesic Tablets
◆ Fiorinal Capsules
◆ Fiorinal Tablets
◆ Fiorinal w/Codeine Capsules
Gynergen Tablets
◆ Hydergine Tablets & Sublingual Tablets
Mellaril Concentrate
Mellaril-S Suspension
◆ Mellaril Tablets
◆ Mesantoin Tablets
Methergine Injection
◆ Methergine Tablets
◆ Pamelor Capsules
Pamelor Solution
◆ Parlodel Capsules
◆ Parlodel Tablets
◆ Plexonal Tablets
◆ Restoril Capsules
◆ Sanorex Tablets
◆ Sansert Tablets
Syntocinon Injection
Syntocinon Nasal Spray
Visken

SARON PHARMACAL CORP. 1777
1640 Central Ave.
St. Petersburg, FL 33712
Address inquiries to:
Gary M. Posey
1640 Central Ave.
St. Petersburg, FL 33712
(813) 898-8525
Products Available
AL-R TD Capsules
AL-R TD, Pediatric
Aural Acute II
Butabell HMB Tablets
Butabell HMB Elixir
Cardabid TD
Cerebid TD
Cerebid-200 TD
Emfaseem Capsules
Emfaseem Elixir
HCV Creme
Hycoff Caps
Hycoff-A NN
Hycoff-X NN
Mega-Vita Tablets
Mega-Vita Hematinic
Mega-Vita Tonic
Otall
Pulm 100 mg. TD
Pulm 200 mg. TD
Pulm 300 mg. TD
Sarocycline
Saroflex
Sarolax
Symptrol Liquid
Symptrol TD

SAVAGE LABORATORIES 432, 1778
a division of Byk-Gulden, Inc.
1000 Main Street
Post Office Box 1000
Missouri City, TX 77459 (713) 499-4547
Products Available
Alpha-Ruvite
Aridose-R
◆ Brexin Capsules & Liquid
◆ Brexin L.A. Capsules
◆ Chromagen Capsules
Chromagen Injection
Cortigel-40
Cortigel-80
Dilor Elixir
◆ Dilor Injectable
◆ Dilor Tablets
◆ Dilor-400 Tablets
◆ Dilor-G Tablets & Liquid
Ditate
Ditate-DS
Estate
Estrone
Ethiodol
Homo-Tet
Hydroxyzine Hydrochloride
Immuglobin
Libigen 10,000 & Diluent
Mepred-40
Mepred-80
Mytrex Cream & Ointment
Negatan
Physpan & Physpan-130
Ruvite 1000
◆ Sätric
Savacort-50
Savacort-100
Savacort-D
Testate
Testosterone
Thiodyne
Tracilon
Trymex
Trysul
ZiPan-25 & ZiPan-50

THE R. SCHATTNER COMPANY 1782
Pharmaceutical Division
4000 Massachusetts Ave., N.W.
Washington, DC 20016
Address inquiries to:
Dr. Robert I. Schattner, President
(202) 244-6606
Products Available
Chloraderm
Derma La Douche
Gynaseptic
Hot Lips
Oraderm
Permacide
Ristex
Sporicidin

HENRY SCHEIN, INC. 1782
5 Harbor Park Drive
Port Washington, NY 11050
Address inquiries to:
Peter Schwartz (516) 621-4300
Products Available
Acetazolamide Tablets
Allopurinol Tablets
Aminophylline Oral Liquid, Suppositories & Tabs
Amitriptyline HCl Tablets
Amoxicillin Trihydrate Capsules & Powder for Oral Suspension
Ampicillin Trihydrate Capsules & Powder for Oral Suspension
Antispasmodic Elixir & Tablets
Apap Extra Strength Capsules & Tablets
Apap Tablets
Apap 300 mg. with Codeine Tabs
Apap with Codeine Elixir
Aspirin 325 mg. with Codeine Tabs
Azo-Sulfisoxazole Tablets
Bromanyl Expectorant
Bromphen Compound Elixir - Sugar Free
Bromphen Compound Tablets
Bromphen DC Expectorant
Bromphen Expectorant
Cafetrate-PB Suppositories
Cardec DM Drops & Syrup
Chloral Hydrate Capsules
Chlordiazepoxide HCl Capsules
Chloroserpine 250 & 500 Tablets
Chlorthiazide Tablets
Chlorpromazine HCl Tablets
Chlorthalidone Tablets
Chlorzone Forte Tablets
Clipoxide Capsules
Cloxacillin Sodium Capsules
Conjugated Estrogens Tablets - Coated
Cyclandelate Capsules
Cyproheptadine HCl Syrup & Tablets
D.S.S. Syrup - Docusate Sodium
Decongestant Elixir
Decongestant Expectorant
Decongestant-AT (Antitussive) Liquid
Detussin Expectorant
Detussin Liquid
Dexamethasone Tablets
Dexchlor Repeat Action Tablets
Dicloxacillin Sodium Capsules
Diethylpropion HCl Tablets & Timed Tablets
Dihydrocodeine Compound Tablets
Dioctocal Capsules - Docusate Calcium USP
Diphenhydramine Cough Syrup & Elixir
Diphenhydramine HCl Caps
Diphenoxylate & Atropine Liquid (DPXL) & Tabs
Dipyridamole Tablets
Disulfiram Tablets
Docusate Sodium Capsules (D.S.S.)
Docusate Sodium with Casanthranol (D.S.S.)
Doxycycline Tablets
Doxycycline Hyclate Capsules
Duo-Hist Timed Release Tablets
Effervescent Potassium Tablets
Erythromycin Estolate Capsules
Erythromycin Ethylsuccinate Granules, Suspension & Tablets
Fluocinolone Acetonide Cream
Furosemide Tablets
Gentamicin Cream 0.1% & Ointment 0.1%
Glutethimide Tablets
Guiatuss Syrup
Guiatuss A-C Syrup
Guiatuss D-M Syrup
H-H-R Tablets
Hydralazine HCl Tablets
Hydralazine-Thiazide Capsules & Tablets
Hydrochlorothiazide Tablets
Hydrocodone Syrup
Hydro-Ergoloid Oral & Sublingual Tablets
Hydroserpine Tablets #1 & #2
Hydroxyzine HCl Syrup & Tablets
Hydroxyzine Pamoate
Imipramine HCl Tablets
Iophen-C Liquid
Isosorbide Dinitrate Tablets - Oral & Sublingual
Isosorbide Dinitrate Timed Capsules & Tablets
Isoxsuprine HCl Tablets
Kaolin, Pectin, Belladonna Mixture
Kaolin-Pectin Mixture
Kaolin-Pectin PG Mixture
Lidocaine HCl 2% Viscous Solution
Lindane Lotion & Shampoo
Liothyronine Sodium Tablets
Meclizine HCl MLT Tablets
Mepro Compound Tablets
Meprobamate Tablets
Methenamine Mandelate Forte Suspension & Tablets
Methocarbamol Tablets
Methocarbamol with Aspirin Tablets
Methyclothiazide Tablets
Methylprednisolone Tablets
Metronidazole Oral Tablets
Nitrofurantoin Capsules & Tablets
Nitroglycerin Ointment 2%
Nitrolin Timed Capsules
Nylidrin HCl Tablets
Nystatin Cream, Oral & Vaginal Tablets
Nyst-olone Cream & Ointment
Oxacillin Sodium Capsules & Tablets
Oxymeta-12 Nasal Spray
Oxytetracycline HCl Capsules
Papaverine HCl Timed Capsules
Penicillin VK Powder for Oral Solution & Tablets
Pentaerythritol Tetranitrate Tabs, Timed Capsules & Tablets
Phenobarbital Elixir & Tablets
Phentermine HCl Capsules
Phenylbutazone Capsules & Tablets
Phenytoin Sodium Capsules-Prompt Action
Polyvitamin-Fluoride Drops & Tablets
Potassium Chloride Concentrate & Liquid
Potassium Gluconate Elixir
Prednisolone Tablets
Prednisone Tablets
Primidone Tablets
Probenecid Tablets
Probenecid with Colchicine Tablets
Procainamide HCl Capsules
Prochlor-Iso Timed Release Capsules
Propantheline Bromide Tablets
Propoxyphene & Apap Tablets 65/650
Propoxyphene Compound 65
Propoxyphene HCl Capsules
Pseudoephedrine Syrup
Pseudoephedrine HCl Tablets
Pyrinal Liquid
Quadra-Hist Pediatric Syrup, Syrup & Timed Release Tablets
Quinidine Gluconate Tablets
Quinidine Sulfate Capsules
Quinine Sulfate Capsules & Tablets
Reserpine Tablets
Selenium Sulfide Lotion 2½%
Soprodol Compound Tablets
Soprodol Tablets (Carisoprodol)
Spironazide Tablets
Spironolactone Tablets
Sulfasalazine Tablets
Sulfatrim & Sulfatrim D/S Tablets
Sulfinpyrazone Tablets
Sulfisoxazole Tablets
T-E-P Tablets
Tetracycline HCl Capsules & Syrup
Theophylline Elixir & KI Elixir
Theozine Syruo & Tablets - Dye-Free
L-Thyroxine Tablets
Tolbutamide Tablets
Triafed Syrup & Tablets
Triafed-C Expectorant
Triamcinolone Tablets
Triamcinolone Acetonide Cream
Trichlormethiazide Tablets
Trifluoperazine Tablets
Trimethobenzamide HCl Suppositories
Triple Sulfa Vaginal Cream
Tuss-Ade Timed Capsules
Vaginal Sulfa Suppositories
Warfarin Sodium Tablets

SCHERING CORPORATION 433, 1786
Galloping Hill Road
Kenilworth, NJ 07033 (201) 558-4000
Address inquiries to:
Professional Services Department
Galloping Hill Road
Kenilworth, NJ 07033 (201) 558-4000
Branch Offices
Southeast Branch
5884 Peachtree Rd., N.E.
Chamblee, GA 30341 (404) 457-6315

Midwest Branch
7500 N. Natchez Ave.
Niles, IL 60648 (312) 647-9363
Southwest Branch
1921 Gateway Dr.
Irving, TX 75062 (214) 258-3545
West Coast Branch
14775 Wicks Blvd.
San Leandro, CA 94577 (415) 357-3125

Products Available

◘A and D Hand Cream*
◘A and D Ointment*
◘Afrin Menthol Nasal Spray, 0.05%
◘Afrin Nasal Spray 0.05%
◘Afrin Nose Drops 0.05%
◘Afrin Pediatric Nose Drops 0.025%
◆ Afrinol Repetabs Tablets Long-Acting Nasal Decongestant
Akrinol Cream
Celestrone Cream
Celestone Phosphate Injection
Celestone 0.6 mg. Six-Day Pack
Celestone Soluspan Suspension
Celestone Syrup
◆ Celestone Tablets
◘Chlor-Trimeton Allergy Syrup
◆ Chlor-Trimeton Allergy Tablets
◆ Chlor-Trimeton Decongestant Tablets
◘Chlor-Trimeton Expectorant
Chlor-Trimeton Injection
◆ Chlor-Trimeton Long-Acting Allergy Repetabs Tablets
◆ Chlor-Trimeton Long-Acting Decongestant Repetabs Tablets
◆ Chlor-Trimeton Repetabs Tablets & Injection
◆ Cod Liver Oil Concentrate Capsules*
◆ Cod Liver Oil Concentrate Tablets*
◆ Cod Liver Oil Concentrate Tablets w/Vitamin C*
◘Coricidin Cough Syrup
◆ Corcidin "D" Decongestant Tablets
◘Corcidin Decongestant Nasal Mist
◆ Coricidin Demilets Tablets For Children
◆ Coricidin Extra Strength Sinus Headache Tablets
◆ Coricidin Medilets Tablets For Children
◆ Coricidin Tablets
Coriforte Capsules
Corilin Infant Liquid
◆ Demazin Repetabs Tablets
◘Demazin Syrup
◘Dermolate Anal-Itch Ointment
◘Dermolate Anti-Itch Cream
◘Dermolate Anti-Itch Spray
◘Dermolate Scalp-Itch Lotion
Diprosone Cream 0.05%
Diprosone Lotion 0.05% w/w
Diprosone Ointment 0.05%
Diprosone Topical Aerosol 0.1% w/w
◘Dismiss Douche
◆ Disophrol Chronotab Tablets*
◆ Disophrol Tablets*
◆ Drixoral Sustained-Action Repetabs Tablets
◘Emko Because Contraceptor Vaginal Contraceptive Foam
◘Emko Pre-Fil Vaginal Contraceptive Foam
◘Emko Vaginal Contraceptive Foam
◆ Estinyl Tablets
◆ Etrafon A Tablets (4-10)
◆ Etrafon 2-10 Tablets (2-10)
◆ Etrafon Tablets (2-25)
◆ Etrafon Forte Tablets (4-25)
◆ Fulvicin P/G Tablets
◆ Fulvicin P/G 165 & 330 Tablets
◆ Fulvicin-U/F Tablets
Garamycin Cream 0.1%
Garamycin Injectable
Garamycin Injectable Disposable Syringes
Garamycin Intrathecal Injection
Garamycin I.V. Piggyback Injection
Garamycin Ointment 0.1%
Garamycin Ophthalmic Ointment
Garamycin Ophthalmic Solution
Garamycin Pediatric Injectable
Gitaligin Tablets
Gyne-Lotrimin Vaginal Cream 1%
◆ Gyne-Lotrimin Vaginal Tablets
Hyperstat I.V. Injection
Lotrimin Cream 1%
Lotrimin Solution 1%
Meticortelone Acetate Aqueous Suspension
◆ Meticorten Tablets
Meti-Derm Cream 0.5%
Metimyd Ophthalmic Ointment
Metimyd Ophthalmic Suspension
Metreton Ophthalmic/Otic Solution-Sterile
◆ Mol-Iron Chronosule Capsules*
◘Mol-Iron Liquid
◆ Mol-Iron Tablets*
◆ Mol-Iron Tablets w/Vitamin C
◆ Mol-Iron w/Vitamin C Tablets
◆ Naqua Tablets
◆ Naquival Tablets
◆ Optimine Tablets
Optimyd Ophthalmic Solution
◆ Oreton Methyl Buccal Tablets
◆ Oreton Methyl Tablets
Oreton Pellets for Subcutaneous Implantation
Otobione Otic Suspension*
Otobiotic Sterile Otic Solution*
◆ Paxipam Tablets
◆ Permitil Chronotab Tablets*
Permitil Oral Concentrate*
◆ Permitil Tablets*
Polaramine Expectorant
◆ Polaramine Repetabs Tablets
Polaramine Syrup
◆ Polaramine Tablets
◆ Proglycem Capsules
Proglycem Suspension
◆ Proventil Inhaler
Proventil Syrup
◆ Proventil Tablets
◆ Rela Tablets
Sebizon Lotion
Sodium Sulamyd Ophthalmic Ointment 10%
Sodium Sulamyd Ophthalmic Solution 10%
Sodium Sulamyd Ophthalmic Solution 30%
Solganal Suspension
◘Sunril Premenstrual Capsules
◆ Theovent Long-Acting Capsules
◘Tinactin Cream 1%
◘Tinactin Powder 1%
◘Tinactin Powder 1% Aerosol
◘Tinactin Solution 1%
Tindal Tablets
Tremin Tablets
Trilafon Concentrate
Trilafon Injection
◆ Trilafon Repetabs Tablets
◆ Trilafon Tablets
◆ Trinalin Repetabs Tablets
Valisone Cream 0.1%
Valisone Lotion 0.1%
Valisone Ointment 0.1%
Valisone Reduced Strength Cream 0.01%
◆ Vancenase Nasal Inhaler
◆ Vanceril Inhaler
*Schering/White Product Line

SCHMID PRODUCTS COMPANY **1840**
Division of Schmid Laboratories, Inc.
Route 46 West
Little Falls, NJ 07424

Address inquiries to:
Professional Service Dept. (201) 256-5500

Products Available
Ramses Bendex Flexible Cushioned Diaphragm
Ramses Contraceptive Vaginal Jelly
Ramses Flexible Cushioned Diaphragm
Saf-T-Coil 33-S, 32-S and 25-S Nullip Intra-Uterine Contraceptive Devices
Vagisec Medicated Liquid Douche Concentrate
Vagisec Plus Suppositories

SCLAVO INC. **1843, 3018**
5 Mansard Court
Wayne, NJ 07470

Address inquiries to:
Francis J. O'Grady (800) 526-5260

Products Available
Antirabies Serum (equine), Purified
Cholera Vaccine
Diphtheria Antitoxin (equine), Refined
Diphtheria & Tetanus Toxoids, Adsorbed (For Pediatric Use)
Diphtheria Toxoid, Adsorbed
SclavoTest-PPD, Tuberculin PPD Multiple Puncture Device
Tetanus Antitoxin (equine), Refined
Tetanus Toxoid, Adsorbed
Tetanus & Diphtheria Toxoids, Adsorbed (For Adult Use)

SCOT-TUSSIN PHARMACAL CO., INC. **1843**
50 Clemence Street
Post Office Box 8217
Cranston, RI 02920

Address inquiries to:
Professional Service Dept. (401) 942-8555

Products Available
Chlorpheniramine Maleate Syrup, USP
Ferro-Bob Tablets
S-T Cort Lotion
S-T Decongest Sugar-Free & Dye-Free
S-T Expectorant Sugar-Free & Dye-Free
S-T Expectorant w/Codeine S-F & Dye-Free
S-T Febrol Tablets & Elixir
S-T Forte Sugar-Free
S-T Forte Syrup
Scot–Tussin DM Syrup
Scot-Tussin Sugar-Free
Scot-Tussin Syrup
Tussirex Sugar-Free Liquid
Tussirex w/Codeine Syrup
Vita-Bob Capsules
Vita-Natal Capsules
Vita-Plus B 12, 10 ml. Vials, 1000 mcgm./ml.
Vita-Plus D (diet) Capsules
Vita-Plus E Capsules Natural 400 I.U.
Vita-Plus G (geriatric) Capsules
Vita-Plus H (hematinic) Capsules
Vita-Plus H (hematinic) Sugar-Free, Liquid

SEARLE PHARMACEUTICALS INC. **434, 1843**
Box 5110
Chicago, IL 60680

Address medical inquiries to:
Medical Communications Department
G.D. Searle & Co., Box 5110, Chicago, IL 60680
(within IL) (312) 982-7000
(outside IL) (800) 323-4397

Products Available
Aminophyllin Injection
◆ Calan for IV Injection
◆ Calan Tablets
◆ Cu-7
◆ Diulo
Dramamine Injection
Dramamine Liquid
◆ Dramamine Tablets
◆ Flagyl I.V.
◆ Flagyl I.V. RTU
◆ Nitrodisc
◆ Tatum-T

SEARLE CONSUMER PRODUCTS **1859**
Division of Searle Pharmaceuticals Inc.
Box 5110
Chicago, IL 60680

Address medical inquiries to:
Medical Communications Department
G.D. Searle & Co., Box 5110, Chicago, IL 60680
(312) 982-7000

Products Available
◘Comfolax
◘Comfolax-*plus*
◘Equal
◘Icy Hot Balm
◘Icy Hot Rub
Metamucil
Metamucil, Instant Mix
Metamucil, Orange Flavor
Metamucil, Orange Flavor Instant Mix
◘Prompt

SEARLE & CO. **434, 1859**
San Juan, Puerto Rico 00936

Address medical inquiries to:
G.D. Searle & Co.
Medical Communications Department,
Box 5110
Chicago, IL 60680

Products Available
◆ Aldactazide
◆ Aldactone
◆ Aminophyllin Tablets
◆ Amodrine
◆ Anavar
◆ Banthine Tablets
◆ Demulen
◆ Demulen 1/35-21
◆ Demulen 1/35-28
Demulen-28
◆ Enovid 5 mg
◆ Enovid 10 mg
◆ Enovid-E 21
◆ Flagyl Tablets
Lomotil Liquid
◆ Lomotil Tablets
◆ Norpace Capsules
◆ Norpace CR Capsules
◆ Ovulen-21
◆ Ovulen-28
◆ Pro-Banthine Tablets
Pro-Banthine for Injection
◆ Pro-Banthine w/Phenobarbital Tablets

THE SEATRACE COMPANY **1881**
P.O. Box 363
Gadsden, Alabama 35902

Address Inquiries to:
R. L. Richardson, Jr. (205) 442-5023

For Medical Emergencies Contact:
R. L. Richardson, Jr. (205) 442-5023

Products Available
Acucron Tablets
Akshun Tablets
Andrest 90-4 Injection
Articulose-50 Injection
Articulose L.A. Injection
B-12-1000 Injection
B-13 Injection
B-Complex 100 Injection
Bena-D 10 Injection
Bena-D 50 Injection
Bionate 50-2 Injection
Cyclonil Injection
Dekasol 5cc Injection
Dekasol 10cc Injection
Dekasol L.A. Injection
Dinol Tablets
Durasal Tablets
Durasil Tablets
Dyline GG Liquid
Dyline GG Tablets
E-Vista Injection

Geritone-S Injection
Isofil T.D. Tablets
Lobac Capsules
Methylpred-40 Injection
Myosal Injection
N D Clear T.D. Capsules
O-Flex Injection
Panasol Tablets
Prednisolone TBA Injection
Prometh-50 Injection
Seatra-Gesic Tablets
Solu-Sone R.P. Injection
Tesionate 100 mg/cc Injection
Tesionate 200 mg/cc Injection
Testosterone Aqueous
Trancaps T.D. Capsules
Trianide 40 mg/cc Injection
Venstat Injection
Ventabs
Versacaps
Z-Tec Injection

SERES LABORATORIES, INC. 1882
3331 Industrial Drive
Box 470
Santa Rosa, CA 95402
Address inquiries to:
Kathryn M. MacLeod, Ph.D. (707) 526-4526
Products Available
Cantharone
Cantharone Plus

SERONO LABORATORIES, INC. 1882
280 Pond Street
Randolph, MA 02368
Address inquiries to:
Director, Sales and Marketing
(outside MA) (800) 225-5185
(within MA) (617) 963-8154
For Medical Emergencies Contact:
Director, Research and Development
(outside MA) (800) 225-5185
(within MA) (617) 963-8154
Products Available
Asellacrin (somatropin)
Pergonal (menotropins)
Profasi HP
Serophene (clomiphene citrate USP)

SMITH KLINE & FRENCH LABORATORIES 435, 1888
Division of SmithKline Beckman Corporation
1500 Spring Garden St.
P.O. Box 7929
Philadelphia, PA 19101
Address inquiries to:
Medical Dept. (215) 751-4000

SK&F CO. 435, 1888
Carolina, Puerto Rico 00630
Subsidiary of SmithKline Beckman Corporation
Address inquiries to:
Smith Kline & French Laboratories (see above)

SK&F LAB CO. 435, 1888
Carolina, Puerto Rico 00630
Subsidiary of SmithKline Beckman Corporation
Address inquiries to:
Smith Kline & French Laboratories (see above)

MENLEY & JAMES LABORATORIES 435, 1888
a SmithKline company
P.O. Box 8082
Philadelphia, PA 19101
Address inquiries to
Medical Department (215) 751-5000
Products Available
▣ Acnomel Cream*
Ancef Injection
◆ Anspor Capsules
Anspor for Oral Suspension
▣ Benzedrex Inhaler*
◆ Combid Spansule Capsules
Compazine Injection
◆ Compazine Spansule Capsules
◆ Compazine Suppositories
Compazine Syrup
◆ Compazine Tablets
◆ Cytomel Tablets
◆ Darbid Tablets
Dexedrine Elixir
◆ Dexedrine Spansule Capsules
◆ Dexedrine Tablets
◆ Dibenzyline Capsules
◆ Dyazide Capsules
◆ Dyrenium Capsules
Ecotrin Duentric Coated Aspirin*
Ecotrin, Maximum Strength Tablets
◆ Eskalith Capsules
◆ Eskalith Tablets
◆ Eskalith CR Controlled Release Tablets
Feosol Elixir*
Feosol Plus Capsules*
Feosol Spansule Capsules*
Feosol Tablets*
Fortespan Capsules*
◆ Hispril Spansule Capsules
▣ Ornacol Capsules*
▣ Ornacol Liquid*
◆ Ornade Spansule Capsules
Ornade 2 Liquid
▣ Ornex Capsules*
Paredrine 1% w/Boric Acid, Ophthalmic Solution
◆ Parnate Tablets
▣ Pragmatar w/Sulfur & Salicylic Acid Ointment*
SK-Amitriptyline Tablets
SK-Ampicillin Capsules
SK-Ampicillin For Oral Suspension
SK-Ampicillin-N For Injection
SK-APAP Elixir
SK-APAP Tablets
SK-APAP with Codeine Tablets
SK-Bamate Tablets
SK-Chloral Hydrate Capsules
SK-Chlorothiazide Tablets
SK-Dexamethasone Tablets
SK-Diphenhydramine Capsules
SK-Diphenhydramine Elixir
SK-Diphenoxylate Tablets
SK-Erythromycin Tablets
SK-Furosemide Tablets
SK-Hydrochlorothiazide Tablets
SK-Lygen Capsules
SK-Methocarbamol Tablets
SK-Penicillin G For Oral Solution
SK-Penicillin G Tablets
SK-Penicillin VK For Oral Solution
SK-Penicillin VK Tablets
SK-Phenobarbital Tablets
SK-Potassium Chloride Oral Solution
SK-Pramine Tablets
SK-Prednisone Tablets
SK-Probenecid Tablets
SK-Propantheline Bromide Tablets
SK-Quinidine Sulfate Tablets
SK-Reserpine Tablets
SK-65 APAP Tablets
SK-65 Capsules
SK-65 Compound Capsules
SK-Soxazole Tablets
SK-Terpin Hydrate & Codeine Elixir
SK-Tetracycline Capsules
SK-Tetracycline Syrup
SK-Tolbutamide Tablets
Spansule, sustained release capsules:
◆ 'Combid' Spansule Capsules
◆ 'Compazine' Spansule Capsules
◆ 'Dexedrine' Spansule Capsules
◆ 'Feosol' Spansule Capsules
◆ 'Hispril' Spansule Capsules
◆ 'Ornade' Spansule Capsules
◆ 'Temaril' Spansule Capsules
◆ 'Thorazine' Spansule Capsules
◆ 'Tuss-Ornade' Spansule Capsules
Stelazine Concentrate
Stelazine Injection
◆ Stelazine Tablets
Tagamet Injection
Tagamet Liquid
◆ Tagamet Tablets
▣ Teldrin Multi-Symptom Allergy Reliever Capsules*
▣ Teldrin Timed-Release Capsules*
◆ Temaril Spansule Capsules
Temaril Syrup
◆ Temaril Tablets
Thorazine Concentrate
Thorazine Injection
◆ Thorazine Spansule Capsules
◆ Thorazine Suppositories
Thorazine Syrup
◆ Thorazine Tablets
▣ Troph-Iron Liquid & Tablets*
▣ Trophite Liquid & Tablets*
Tuss-Ornade Liquid
◆ Tuss-Ornade Spansule Capsules
◆ Urispas Tablets
◆ Vontrol Tablets
*A product of Menley & James Laboratories, a SmithKline company

SPRINGBOK PHARMACEUTICALS, INC. 1921
12502 South Garden Street
Houston, Texas 77071
Address inquiries to:
Ralph Berson (713) 988-7373
For Medical Emergencies Contact:
Ralph Berson (713) 988-7373
Products Available
E.N.T. Syrup
E.N.T. Tablets
Stopayne Capsules
Stopayne Syrup

E. R. SQUIBB & SONS INC. 436, 1921, 3018
General Offices
Post Office Box 4000
Princeton, NJ 08540 (609) 921-4000
Address inquiries to:
Squibb Professional Services Dept.
Lawrenceville-Princeton Road
Princeton, NJ 08540 (609) 921-4006
Distribution Centers
ATLANTA, GEORGIA
Post Office Box 16503
Atlanta, GA 30321
State of Ga. Customers Call (800) 282-9103
Customers in States of Ala., Fla., Miss., N.C., S.C., and Tenn. Call (800) 241-1744
All others call (800) 241-5364
CHICAGO, ILLINOIS
Post Office Box 788
Arlington Heights, IL 60006
State of IL Customers Call (800) 942-0674
All others call (800) 323-0665
KANSAS CITY, KANSAS
Mail or telephone orders and customer service inquiries should be directed to Chicago, IL (see above)
State of IL Customers Call (800) 942-0674
All others call (800) 323-0665
LOS ANGELES, CALIFORNIA
Post Office Box 428
La Mirada, CA 90638
State of CA Customers Call (800) 422-4254
State of HI Customers Call (714) 521-7050
All others call (800) 854-3050
SEATTLE, WASHINGTON
Mail or telephone orders and customer service inquiries should be directed to Los Angeles, CA (see above)
State of AK and MT Customers Call (714) 521-7050
State of CA Customers Call (800) 422-4254
All others call (800) 854-3050
NEW YORK AREA
E. R. Squibb & Sons, Inc.
Post Office Box 2013
New Brunswick, NJ 08903
New York City Area Customers Call (212) 227-1371
States of ME and NC Customers Call (201) 469-5400
State of NJ Customers Call (800) 352-4865
All others call (800) 631-5244
HOUSTON, TEXAS
Mail or telephone orders and customer service inquiries should be directed to Atlanta, GA (see above)
State of MS Customers call (800) 241-1744
All others call (800) 241-5364
SQUIBB LABORATORIES
E. R. Squibb & Sons, Inc.
Georges Road
New Brunswick, NJ 08903
Products Available
Actrapid Pork Insulin Injection
Amitid Tablets
Aspirin Tablets USP
B Complex Vitamin Tablets
Brewer's Yeast Tablets
Broxodent Automatic-Action Toothbrush
Calcium, Phosphate and Vitamin D Tablets
◆ Capoten (Captopril Tablets)
Cardiografin
Castor Oil USP
Chlordiazepoxide Hydrochloride Capsules USP
Chlorothiazide Tablets USP
Cholografin Meglumine
Cholografin Meglumine for Infusion
Cholovue
Cholovue for Infusion
ClearAid Cream, Lotion, Ointment
Cod Liver Oil Capsules
Cod Liver Oil Plain & Mint Flavored
◆ Corgard
Crysticillin 300 A.S. & 600 A.S.
Cystografin
Deladumone
Deladumone OB
Delalutin
Delatestryl
Delestrogen
Diatrizoate Meglumine Injection USP 76%
Engran-HP Tablets
◆ Ethril '250' and Ethril '500' Tablets
Florinef Acetate Tablets
Follutein
Fungizone Cream, Lotion and Ointment
Fungizone for Tissue Culture
Fungizone Intravenous
Gastrografin
Halciderm Cream
Halog Cream, Ointment & Solution
◆ Hydrea Capsules
Hydrochlorothiazide Tablets USP
Insulin, Isophane Insulin (NPH)
Insulin, Isophane Purified Beef Insulin Suspension (NPH)
Insulin, Lente
Insulin, Protamine Zinc Insulin
Insulin, Purified Beef Insulin Zinc Suspension (Lente)

Insulin, Purified Pork Insulin Injection (Regular)
Insulin (Regular)
Insulin, Semilente
Insulin, Ultralente
Iron and Vitamin C Tablets
Kenacort Diacetate Syrup
Kenacort Tablets
Kenalog Cream, Lotion, Ointment, Spray
Kenalog in Orabase
Kenalog-H Cream
Kenalog-10 Injection
Kenalog-40 Injection
Kinevac
Lentard Purified Pork & Beef Insulin Zinc Suspension
Medotopes (Radiopharmaceuticals)
- A-C-D Solution Modified
- Albumotope I 131 (Diagnostic Injection)
- Chromitope Sodium (Diagnostic Injection)
- Cobatope-57 Reference Standard Solution
- Cobatope-60 Reference Standard Solution
- Hipputope I 131 (Diagnostic Injection)
- Intrinsic Factor Concentrate Capsules
- Iodotope Diagnostic Capsules (I 131)
- Iodotope Therapeutic Capsules (I 131)
- Iodotope Therapeutic Oral Solution (I 131)
- MDP-Squibb
- Minitec
- Phosphotec
- Robengatope Diagnostic Injection
- Rubratope-57 Diagnostic Capsules
- Rubratope-57 Diagnostic Kit
- Rubratope-60 Diagnostic Capsules
- Rubratope-60 Diagnostic Kit
- Sethotope
- Techneplex Diagnostic Kit
- Tesuloid Diagnostic Kit

Milk of Magnesia Liquid & Tablets
Mineral Oil
Monotard Purified Pork Insulin Zinc Suspension
Mycolog Cream, Ointment
Mycostatin Cream, Ointment
Mycostatin Oral Suspension
◆ Mycostatin Oral Tablets
Mycostatin Powder (for laboratory use)
Mycostatin Topical Powder
◆ Mycostatin Vaginal Tablets
◆ Mysteclin-F Capsules
Mysteclin-F Syrup
◆ Naturetin Tablets
Neomycin Sulfate Tablets USP
Niacin Tablets
Nitrazine Paper
◆ Noctec Capsules
Noctec Syrup
Nydrazid Injection, Tablets
O-V Statin
Ophthaine Solution
Oragrafin Calcium Granules
◆ Oragrafin Sodium Capsules
Ora-Testryl Tablets
Penicillin G Potassium for Injection USP
Penicillin G Sodium for Injection USP
Pentids for Syrup
Pentids '400' for Syrup
◆ Pentids '400' & '800' Tablets
◆ Pentids Tablets
◆ Principen Capsules '250' & '500'
Principen for Oral Suspension '125' & '250'
Principen with Probenecid Capsules
Prolixin Decanoate
Prolixin Enanthate
Prolixin Elixir
Prolixin Injection
◆ Prolixin Tablets
◆ Pronestyl Capsules and Tablets
Pronestyl Injection
◆ Pronestyl-SR Tablets
Propoxyphene Hydrochloride Capsules USP
Propoxyphene Hydrochloride and APC Capsules, USP
Protaphane NPH (Isophane Purified Pork Insulin Suspension)
Protein Powder & Tablets
◆ Raudixin Tablets
Rau-Sed Tablets
◆ Rauzide Tablets
Renografin-60
Renografin-76
Reno-M-DIP
Reno-M-30
Reno-M-60
Renovist
Renovist II
Renovue-65
Renovue-DIP
Rubramin PC
Saccharin Tablets
Semitard Prompt Purified Pork Insulin Zinc Suspension
Serenium Tablets
Sinografin
Spec-T Sore Throat Anesthetic Lozenges
Spec-T Sore Throat/Cough Suppressant Lozenges
Spec-T Sore Throat/Decongestant Lozenges
Spectrocin Ointment
Stomahesive
Stomahesive Paste
Stomahesive Protective Powder
Stomahesive Sterile Wafer
Stomahesive Wafer with Sur-Fit Flange
Sucostrin Injection, High Potency
◆ Sumycin '250' & '500' Capsules
◆ Sumycin '250' and '500' Tablets
Sumycin Syrup
Suppositories, Glycerin
Sur-Fit Disposable Convex Inserts
Sur-Fit Flange Cap
Sur-Fit Irrigation Sleeve
Sur-Fit O.R. Loop Ostomy Sets
Sur-Fit O.R. Set 1 (Urostomy)
Sur-Fit O.R. Set 2 (Colo-ileo)
Sur-Fit Pouch Covers
Sur-Fit Pouches
Sur-Fit Preoperation Set
Sweeta Liquid & Tablets
Terfonyl Tablets, Oral Suspension
Teslac Tablets
◆ Theragran Hematinic Tablets
Theragran Liquid
◆ Theragran Tablets
◆ Theragran-M Tablets
◆ Theragran-Z Tablets
Tolbutamide Tablets USP
Trigesic Tablets
Trigot Tablets
◆ Trimox '250' & '500' Capsules
Trimox '125' & '250' For Oral Suspension
Tubocurarine Chloride Injection USP
Ultratard Extended Purified Beef Insulin Zinc Suspension
Urihesive Strips
Urihesive System
Valadol Liquid
Valadol Tablets, Liquid
Veetids '125' & '250' for Oral Solution
◆ Veetids '250' & '500' Tablets
◆ Velosef '250' & '500' Capsules
Velosef for Infusion
Velosef for Injection
Velosef '125' & '250' for Oral Suspension
◆ Velosef Tablets
Vesprin Injection, Tablets, High-Potency Suspension
Vigran Chewables
Vigran plus Iron Tablets
Vigran Tablets
Vitamin A Capsules
Vitamin B_1 Tablets USP
Vitamin B_{12} Capsules
Vitamin C Tablets
Vitamin E Capsules & Tablets
Wheat Germ Oil Capsules
Yeast Tablets & Flavored Powder
Zinc Oxide Ointment USP

STANDARD PROCESS LABORATORIES, INC. **1975**
2023 West Wisconsin Avenue
Milwaukee, WI 53201 (414) 933-2100

Branch Offices

Campbell, CA 95008
501-C Vandell Way (408) 866-0707
Chilton, WI 53014
253 East Main (414) 849-9014
Columbus, OH 43227
5195 Ivyhurst Drive (614) 866-5520
Dallas, TX 75211
9103 Highway 67, South (214) 298-1417
Denver, CO 80222
2179 South Ash (303) 758-6321
Harrisburg, PA 17112
5145 Jonestown Road (717) 545-9264
Honolulu, HI 96818
1106 Ukana Street (808) 423-1616
Kansas City, MO 64111
3711 Southwest Trafficway (816) 561-5550
(Los Angeles)
City of Commerce, CA 90040
2401 S. Atlantic Blvd. (213) 263-6133
Oklahoma City, OK 73112
3419 Roff Ave., North (405) 943-1056
Orlando, FL 32859
7653 Currency Drive (305) 851-6610
Portland, OR 97220
10704 N.E. Wygant St. (503) 252-2405
St. Joseph, MI 49085
413 State Street (616) 983-3014
Seattle, WA 98101
930 Terminal Sales Building (206) 622-6381
Watertown, MA 02172
76 Coolidge Hill Rd. (617) 923-2330

Products Available

Allorganic Trace Minerals-B12
Antronex
Betaine Hydrochloride
Biost Powder
Cal-Amo
Calcium Lactate (Fortified)
Cardio-Plus
Cardiotrophin (Heart)
Catalyn
Cataplex A-F & Betaris
Cataplex E-2
Cataplex F
Chlorophyll Complex Ointment (Fat Soluble)
Chlorophyll Complex Perles (Fat Soluble)
Choline
Comfrey, Pepsin—Formula E-3
Ferroplus
Inositol
Multizyme
Niacinamide B6
Ovex
Pneumotrophin (Lung)
Prost-X
Ribo-Nucleic Acid (RNA)
Thymex
Vasculin
Vitamin B-6 w/Niacinamide
Zypan Tablets

STAR PHARMACEUTICALS, INC. **1975**
16499 North East 19th Avenue
North Miami Beach, FL 33160

Address inquiries to:

Scott L. Davidson, President
(305) 949-1612

Branch Offices

Panamerican Pharmaceutical Distributors, Inc.
Reparada Industrial Park
Estacion #6
Ponce, PR 00731 (809) 842-6263

Products Available

Microsul Tablets
Microsul-A
Nitrex Tablets
Prosed
◘ Star-Otic
Uro-KP-Neutral
Urolene Blue
Vesicholine Tablets
Virilon

STERI-MED INC. **1975**
P.O. Box 459
Lindenhurst, NY 11757

Address inquiries to:

Director, Professional Services Dept.
(516) 842-4209

Products Available

A.P.C. Tablets w/Codeine
Acetazolamide Tablets
Aminophylline Tablets
Amitriptyline HCl Tablets
Amoxicillin Capsules
Ampicillin Capsules
Ampicillin Powder for Suspension
Antispasmodic Elixir
Atropine Sulfate
Azo Sulfisoxazole Tablets
Belladonna with Phenobarbital Tablets
Bromenate Elixir
Bromenate Expectorant
Chlordiazepoxide Capsules
Chlorothiazide Tablets
Chlorpheniramine Maleate Tablets
Chlorpheniramine Syrup
Chlorpromazine HCl Tablets
Chlorzoxazone with APAP Tablets
Chorionic G Vial/with Diluent Vial
Colchicine Tablets
Conjugated Estrogen Tablets
Cortisone Acetate Tablets
Cyproheptadine HCl Tablets
Dexamethasone Tablets & Elixir
Dicyclomine HCl Capsules
Digitoxin Tablets
Digoxin Tablets
Dimenhydrinate Tablets
Diphenhydramine Elixir
Diphenhydramine HCl Capsules
Diphenoxylate HCl & Atropine Sulfate Tablets
Doxycycline Hyclate Capsules
Ergonovine Maleate Tablets
Erythromycin Stearate Tablets
Estrone
Folic Acid Tablets
Hydralazine HCl Tablets
Hydrochlorothiazide Tablets
Hydrocortisone Cream
Hydrocortisone Tablets
Hydroxyzine Compound Tablets
Imipramine HCl Tablets
Isoniazid Tablets
Isosorbide Dinitrate Tablets
Isoxsuprine HCl Tablets
Levodopa Capsules
Lidocaine HCl Injectable Solution
Meclizine HCl Tablets
Meprobamate Tablets
Methenamine Mandelate Tablets, E.C.
Methocarbamol Tablets
Methyltestosterone Tablets
Neomycin Sulfate Tablets
Nitrofurantoin Tablets

Nitroglycerin Capsules, T.D.
Nylidrin HCl Tablets
Oxytetracycline HCl Capsules
PETN Tablets
Papaverine HCl Capsules, T.D.
Penicillin G Buffered Tablets
Penicillin G Powder for Suspension
Penicillin V Oval Tablets
Penicillin V Powder for Suspension
Phenytoin Sodium Capsules
Pilocarpine HCl Ophthalmic Solution
Potassium Chloride Liquid
Potassium Gluconate Elixir (sugar-free)
Potassium Iodide Solution
Prednisolone Tablets
Prednisone Tablets
Probenecid Tablets
Procainamide HCl Capsules
Promethazine Expectorant
Promethazine Expectorant VC
Promethazine Expectorant with Codeine
Promethazine HCl Tablets
Propantheline Bromide
Propoxyphene HCl Capsules
Propoxyphene HCl Compound Capsules
Propylthiouracil
Pseudoephedrine Tablets
Quinidine Sulfate Tablets
Quinine Sulfate Capsules
Reserpine Tablets
Selenium Sulfide
Sodium Flouride Tablets
Sodium Sulfacetamide Ophthalmic Solution
Spironolactone Tablets
Spironolactone w/Hydrochlorothiazide Tablets
Sulfisoxazole Tablets
Testosterone
Tetracaine HCl
Tetracycline HCl Capsules
Theofedral Tablets
Theophylline Elixir
Thyroid Tablets, CT
l-Thyroxin Tablets
Tolbutamide Tablets
Triamcinolone Tablets
Trichlormethiazide Tablets
Triple Antibiotic Ointment
Triplennamine HCl Tablets
Vaginal Sulfa Cream (w/applicator)
Vitamin B-1
Vitamin B-12
Zinc Sulfate Tablets

STIEFEL LABORATORIES, INC. 1975
2801 Ponce de Leon Blvd.
Coral Gables, FL 33134
Address inquiries to:
Werner K. Stiefel (305) 443-3807
Branch Offices
CALIFORNIA
P.O. Box 375
Gardena, CA 90247 (213) 321-4006
GEORGIA
Post Office Box 47789
Doraville, GA 30340 (404) 455-1896
NEW YORK
Route 145
Oak Hill, NY 12460 (518) 239-6901
PUERTO RICO
P.O. Box 387
Mayaguez, Puerto Rico 00708
(809) 832-1376
Products Available
Acne-Aid Cream
Acne-Aid Detergent Soap
Acne-Aid Lotion
Benoxyl-5 Lotion
Benoxyl-10 Lotion
Brasivol Base
Brasivol Fine
Brasivol Medium
Brasivol Rough
Duofilm
Ichthyol Ointment
LactiCare Lotion
Lasan Unguent
Oilatum Soap
PanOxyl 5, PanOxyl 10 Gels
PanOxyl AQ 2½, 5 & 10 Acne Gel
PanOxyl Bar
Polytar Bath
Polytar Shampoo
Polytar Soap
Salicylic Acid Soap
Salicylic Acid & Sulfur Soap
Saligel
Sarna Lotion
SAStid (AL)
SAStid (Plain)
SAStid Soap
Scabene Lotion
Sulfoxyl Lotion Regular
Sulfoxyl Lotion Strong
Sulfur Soap
Surfol
Zeasorb Powder

STUART PHARMACEUTICALS 437, 1976
Div. of ICI Americas Inc.
Wilmington, DE 19897
Address inquiries to:
Yvonne Graham, Manager
Professional Services (302) 575-2231
For Medical Emergencies Contact:
After Hours or Weekends (302) 575-3000
Products Available
◆ ALternaGEL Liquid
◆ Bucladin-S Softab
Cari-Tab Softab
◆ Dialose Capsules
◆ Dialose Plus Capsules
Effersyllium Instant Mix
◆ Ferancee Tablets
◆ Ferancee-HP Tablets
◆ Hibiclens
◆ Hibistat
◆ Hibitane Tincture
◆ Kasof Capsules
◆ Kinesed Tablets
◆ Mulvidren-F Softab
◆ Mylanta Liquid
◆ Mylanta Tablets
◆ Mylanta-II Liquid
◆ Mylanta-II Tablets
◆ Mylicon (Tablets & Drops)
◆ Mylicon-80 Tablets
◆ Nolvadex Tablets
Orexin Softab
◆ Probec-T Tablets
◆ Sorbitrate Chewable Tablets
◆ Sorbitrate Oral Tablets
◆ Sorbitrate Sublingual Tablets
◆ Sorbitrate Sustained Action Tablets
◆ Stuart Formula (tablets), The
◆ Stuart Prenatal Tablets
◆ Stuart Prenatal w/Folic Acid Tablets
◆ Stuartinic Tablets
◆ Stuartnatal 1+1 Tablets
◆ Tenormin Tablets

SWEEN CORPORATION 1984
Sween Building
P.O. Box 980
Lake Crystal, MN 56055
(507) 726-6200
Products Available
Fordustin'
Gentle Rain
Medicated Soft Touch
Micro-Guard
Peri-Care
Peri-Wash
Puri-Clens
Surgi-Kleen
Sween Cream
Whirl-Sol
Xtracare II

SYNTEX (F.P.) INC. 439, 1986
Humacao, Puerto Rico 00661
Address inquiries to:
Syntex Laboratories, Inc. (see below)
Products Available
◆ Brevicon 21-Day Tablets
◆ Brevicon 28-Day Tablets
◆ Norinyl 1+35 21-Day Tablets
◆ Norinyl 1+35 28-Day Tablets
◆ Norinyl 1+50 21-Day Tablets
◆ Norinyl 1+50 28-Day Tablets
◆ Norinyl 1+80 21-Day Tablets
◆ Norinyl 1+80 28-Day Tablets
◆ Norinyl 2 mg. Tablets
◆ Nor-Q.D. Tablets

SYNTEX LABORATORIES, INC. 439, 1986
3401 Hillview Ave.
Palo Alto, CA 94304
Address Medical inquiries on marketed products to:
Medical Services Dept. (415) 855-5545
Other inquiries to:
(415) 855-5050
Products Available
◆ Anadrol-50 Tablets
Carmol HC Cream
▣ Carmol 10 Lotion
▣ Carmol 20 Cream
Evex Tablets
Lidex Cream
Lidex Ointment
Lidex-E Cream
Nasalide Nasal Solution
Neo-Synalar Cream
Synacort Creams
Synalar Creams, Ointment and Topical Solution
Synalar-HP Cream
Synemol Cream
▣ Topic Gel
Topsyn Gel

SYNTEX PUERTO RICO, INC. 439, 1986
Humacao, Puerto Rico 00661
Address Medical inquires to: Syntex Laboratories, Inc. (see above)
Products Available
◆ Anaprox Tablets
Kato Powder
◆ Naprosyn Tablets

THOMPSON MEDICAL COMPANY, INC. 2007
919 Third Avenue
New York, NY 10022
Address inquiries to:
Dr. Edward L. Steinberg (212) 688-4420
Products Available
Appedrine, Maximum Strength
Aspercreme
Control Capsules
Dexatrim Capsules
Dexatrim Capsules, Extra Strength
Dexatrim Capsules, Extra Strength, Caffeine-Free
Dexatrim Capsules, Extra Strength, Plus Vitamins
Prolamine Capsules, Maximum Strength

TRAVENOL LABORATORIES, INC. 2008
Parenteral Products
One Baxter Parkway
Deerfield, IL 60015
Address inquiries to:
Marketing Communications (312) 940-5387
Products Available
Travasol, 5.5% and 8.5% (Amino Acid) Injection with Electrolytes
Travasol, 5.5% and 8.5% (Amino Acid) Injection without Electrolytes
Travasol, 10% (Amino Acid) Injection without Electrolytes

TRIMEN LABORATORIES, INC. 2011
80 - 26th Street
Pittsburgh, PA 15222
Address inquiries to:
Professional Service Dept. (412) 261-0339
Products Available
Allerid-D.C. Capsules
Allerid-O.D.-8 Capsules
Allerid-O.D.-12 Capsules
Amaphen Capsules
Amaphen with Codeine #3
Bellermine-O.D. Capsules
Deltamycin Capsules
Deltapen-VK Solution
Deltapen-VK Tablets
Deltavac Cream
Dilart Capsules
Dyrexan-OD Capsules
Fe-O.D. Tablets
Flexaphen Capsules
Hydrex Tablets
Korigesic Tablets
Laxatyl Tablets
Natacomp-FA Tablets
Neurate-400 Tablets
Sorate-5 Chewable Tablets
Sorate-2.5 Sublingual Tablets
Sorate-5 Sublingual Tablets
Sorate-10 Chewable Tablets
Sorate-40 Capsules
Titracid Tablets
Trimedine Expectorant
Viopan-T Tablets

TYSON and ASSOCIATES, INC. 2012
19725 Sherman Way, Suite 270
Canoga Park, CA 91306
Address Inquiries to:
Professional Services Dept. (213) 998-2161
Products Available
Amino B Plex Tablets
Amino Dox Tablets
Aminoform Capsules & Powder
Amino GTF Tablets
Amino K Tablets
Amino Lac Tablets
Amino Min D Tablets
Aminoplex Capsules & Powder
Aminotate Capsules & Powder
Amino Vi Min Tablets
Amino Zn Tablets
Bromelain Forte
Colloidal Trace Minerals
Enteric Coated Enzymes
Optivite Tablets
Selenicel
Tyson Amino-Silica
Tyson L-Alanine Powder
Tyson L-Arginine Capsules & Powder
Tyson L-Aspartic Acid Powder
Tyson L-Citrulline Powder
Tyson L-Cysteine HCl Capsules & Powder
Tyson L-Cystine Capsules & Powder
Tyson L-Glycine Powder
Tyson L-Glutamic Acid Powder
Tyson L-Glutamine Powder
Tyson L-Histidine Powder
Tyson L-Isoleucine Powder

Tyson L-Leucine Powder
Tyson L-Lysine Powder
Tyson L-Methionine Powder
Tyson L-Phenylalanine Capsules & Powder
Tyson L-Proline Powder
Tyson L-Serine Powder
Tyson L-Threonine Powder
Tyson L-Tryptophan Capsules & Powder
Tyson L-Tyrosine Capsules & Powder
Tyson L-Valine Powder
Vitamin E Succinate 400IU

U. S. CHEMICAL MARKETING GROUP, INC. 2012
203 Rio Circle
Decatur, GA 30030
Mailing Address:
P.O. Box 1165
Decatur, GA 30030
Office of the President:
1826 Clairmont Road
Decatur, GA 30033 (404) 325-5910
Address inquiries to:
Marketing Director (404) 371-1957
Products Available
Cervex Vaginal Cream
Hemocyte Injection
Hemocyte Plus Tabules
Hemocyte Tablets
Hemocyte-F Tablets
Isovex Capsules
Magsal Tablets
Medigesic Plus Capsules
Mediplex Tabules
Medizinc Tablets
Norel Plus Capsules

U. S. ETHICALS INC.
37-02 48th Avenue
Long Island City, NY 11101
Address inquiries to:
Medical Director (212) 786-8607
Products Available
Azlytal Tablets
Azmadrine Elixir & Tablets
Azmadrine S.A. Capsules
Bellastal Capsules
Bellastal Elixir & Tablets
Capa Tablets
Eclabron Capsules & Elixir
Eclabron-T/SR Capsules
Eclamide Capsules
Eclasufed Capsules
Eclasufed SR Capsules
Etnapa Elixir
Etnergan Syrup
Ferbetrin Tablets & Syrup
Gastrical Tablets
Geristone Capsules
Hepaferron Syrup
Histabs Tablets
Klavikordal Tablets
Natalac Capsules
Natalac Forte Capsules
Neocomplex Injection
Neodex Tablets & Syrup
Nicostrol Capsules
Niong Tablets
Nitromed
Nitronet Tablets
Nitrong Ointment (See Wharton Laboratories)
Nitrong Tablets (See Wharton Laboratories)
Supervim Drops, Tablets & Syrup
Ulcinal Tablets
Vitacoms Capsules

U. S. PRODUCT, INC. 2012
16636 N.W. 54th Avenue
Miami Lakes, Florida 33014
Address inquiries to:
(305) 620-9540
For Medical Emergencies Contact:
Bob Brooks, Vice President
(305) 620-9540
Products Available
Amebaquin Tablets
Charcoal-Antidose Suspension
Charcoal-Anti-Dote Powder

USV LABORATORIES, DIVISION USV PHARMACEUTICAL CORP. 439, 2013
1 Scarsdale Road
Tuckahoe, NY 10707
Address inquiries to:
Medical Department (914) 631-8500
Nights, Weekends and Holidays, call
(914) 779-6300

USV LABORATORIES Inc. 439, 2013
Manati, Puerto Rico 00701
Address inquiries to:
USV Pharmaceutical Corp. (see above)

USV (P.R.) DEVELOPMENT CORP. 439, 2013
Manati, Puerto Rico 00701
Address inquiries to:
USV Pharmaceutical Corp. (see above)
Products Available
◆ Aquasol A Capsules
Aquasol A Drops
Aquasol A Parenteral
◆ Aquasol E Capsules
◆ Aquasol E Drops
◆ Arlidin Tablets
◆ Azolid Capsules & Tablets
Bi-K
C-B Vone Capsules
◆ Cerespan Capsules
◆ Chrometrace
◆ Coppertrace
◆ Demi-Regroton Tablets
◆ Doriden Tablets
◆ Histaspan-D Capsules
◆ Histaspan-Plus Capsules
◆ Hygroton Tablets
Lufa Capsules
◆ M.V.I. (Multi-Vitamin Infusion)
◆ M.V.I. Concentrate
◆ M.V.I.-12 (Multi-Vitamin Infusion)
◆ Mangatrace
Methischol Capsules
◆ Nitrospan Capsules
◆ Oxalid Tablets
Panthoderm Lotion and Cream
◆ Pertofrane Capsules
◆ Regroton Tablets
◆ Trace Elements
...Chrometrace
...Coppertrace
...Mangatrace
...Zinctrace
Vi-Aqua Forte Capsules
Vi-Aquamin Forte Capsules
◆ Zinctrace

ULMER PHARMACAL COMPANY 2027
(Division of Physicians & Hospitals Supply Co.)
2440 Fernbrook Lane
Minneapolis, MN 55441
Address inquiries to:
Professional Service Dept. (612) 559-3333
Products Available
Aerosan
Andoin Ointment
Aspirin Tablets
Auto-Kler
Bacitracin Ointment
Bi-Amine
Bu-Lax Capsules
Bu-Lax Plus Capsules
Cal-Zo Ointment
Cardio-Gel
Chloral Methylol Ointment
Cobalin Injection
Col-Vi-Nol Ointment
Dextro-Tuss GG
Dibucaine Ointment
Gentle Shampoo
Hematovals
Hiscatabs
Iodocort Cream
Kler-ro Liquid
Kler-ro Powder
L.F.B. 12-100 Injection
▣ Lobana Bath Oil
▣ Lobana Body Lotion
▣ Lobana Body Powder
▣ Lobana Body Shampoo
▣ Lobana Conditioning Shampoo
▣ Lobana Derm-ade Cream
▣ Lobana Liquid Hand Soap
▣ Lobana Peri-Gard
▣ Lobana Perineal Cleanse
Milk of Magnesia
Mineral Oil
Pentazyme Tablets
Pheneen Solution
Reagent Alcohol
Surgel Liquid
Ta-Poff
Ta-Poff Aerosol
Theolixir
Tokols Capsules
Ulcort Cream
Ulcort Lotion
Ultar Cream
Ultracaine Injection
Ulvical SG
Vasospan Capsules
Versa-Quat
Vitamin A & D Ointment
Vitamin B 12 Crystalline Injection
▣ Vleminckx' Solution
Zinc Oxide Ointment

THE UPJOHN COMPANY 439, 2027
7000 Portage Road
Kalamazoo, MI 49001
(616) 323-4000

THE UPJOHN MANUFACTURING COMPANY
Barceloneta, Puerto Rico 00617
(809) 846-4900
THE UPJOHN MANUFACTURING COMPANY M
Barceloneta, Puerto Rico 00617
(809) 846-4900
Emergency Medical Information
(616) 323-6615
Address inquiries to:
Medical Information Unit
The Upjohn Company
Kalamazoo, MI 49001
Pharmaceutical Sales Areas and Distribution Centers
Atlanta (Chamblee), GA 30341 (404) 451-4822
Boston (Needham Heights), MA 02194 (617) 449-0320
Buffalo (Cheektowaga), NY 14225 (716) 681-7160
Chicago (Oak Brook), IL 60521 (312) 654-3300
Cincinnati, OH 45214 (513) 242-4574
Dallas, TX 75265 (214) 824-3028
Denver, CO 80217 (303) 399-3113
Honolulu, HI 96809 (808) 538-1181
Kalamazoo, MI 49001 (616) 323-7222
Kansas City, MO 64141 (816) 361-2286
Los Angeles, CA 90051 (213) 463-8101
Memphis, TN 38122 (901) 761-4170
Miami, FL 33152 (305) 758-3317
Minneapolis, MN 55440 (612) 588-2786
New York Long Island, NY 11514
(516) 747-1970
Philadelphia (Wayne) PA 19087 (215) 265-2100
Pittsburgh, (Bridgeville) PA 15017
(412) 257-0200
Portland, OR 97208 (503) 232-2133
St. Louis, MO 63177 (314) 872-8626
San Francisco (Palo Alto) CA 94304 (415) 493-8080
Washington, DC 20013 (202) 882-6163
Products Available
◆ Adeflor Chewable Tablets
Adeflor Drops
Adeflor M Tablets
Albamycin Capsules
Alkets Tablets
Alphadrol Tablets
Atgam Sterile Solution
▣ Baciguent Antibiotic Ointment
Baciguent Ophthalmic Ointment
Bacitracin, USP, Sterile Powder
Berubigen Sterile Solution
Calcium Chloride Injection, USP, Sterile Solution
Calcium Gluconate Injection, USP, Sterile Solution
Calcium Gluconate Tablets, USP
Calcium Lactate Tablets, USP
◆ Calderol Capsules
Casyllium Granules
Cebefortis Tablets
Cebenase Tablets
Cheracol Cough Syrup
▣ Cheracol D Cough Syrup
Cheracol D Cough Syrup (Bilingual) (English & Spanish labeling)
▣ Cheracol Plus Cough Syrup
▣ Citrocarbonate, Antacid
◆ Cleocin HCl Capsules*
Cleocin Pediatric Flavored Granules*
◆ Cleocin Phosphate Sterile Solution*
◆ Cleocin T Topical Solution*
Clocream Skin Cream
◆ Colestid Granules
▣ Cortaid Cream
▣ Cortaid Lotion
▣ Cortaid Ointment
▣ Cortaid Spray
Cortef Acetate Ointment
Cortef Acetate Sterile Suspensiion
▣ Cortef Feminine Itch Cream
Cortef Oral Suspension
▣ Cortef Rectal Itch Ointment
Cortef Sterile Suspension IM
Cortef Tablets
Cortisone Acetate Tablets, USP
Cytosar-U Sterile Powder
Delta-Cortef Tablets
◆ Deltasone Tablets
Depo-Estradiol Sterile Solution
◆ Depo-Medrol Sterile Aqueous Suspension
Depo-Provera Sterile Aqueous Suspension
Depo-Testadiol Sterile Solution
Depo-Testosterone Sterile Solution
◆ Didrex Tablets
Diostate D Tablets
◆ E-Mycin E Liquid
◆ E-Mycin Tablets
Epinephricaine Rectal Ointment
Ergophene Skin Ointment
◆ Erythromycin Tablets (E-Mycin)
Feminone Tablets
Florone Cream
Florone Ointment

Gelfilm Sterile Film
Gelfilm Sterile Ophthalmic Film
Gelfoam Dental Packs
Gelfoam Packs
Gelfoam Prostatectomy Cones
Gelfoam Sterile Compressed Sponge
Gelfoam Sterile Powder
Gelfoam Sterile Sponge
Gerizyme Liquid
Halcion Tablets
Halodrin Tablets
◆ Halotestin Tablets
Heparin Sodium Injection, USP, Sterile Solution
Hydrocortisone Acetate, U.S.P.; Micronized, Nonsterile Powder (For Prescription Compounding)
Hydrocortisone, U.S.P. Micronized, Nonsterile Powder (For Prescription Compounding)
▣ Kaopectate Anti-Diarrhea Medicine
Kaopectate Anti-Diarrhea Medicine (Bilingual) (English & Spanish labeling)
▣ Kaopectate Concentrate Anti-Diarrhea Medicine
Lincocin Capsules
Lincocin Pediatric Capsules
Lincocin Sterile Solution
Lipomul Oral Liquid
◆ Loniten Tablets
◆ Maolate Tablets
Medrol Acetate Topical
Medrol Enpak Kit
Medrol Enpak (Refill)
Medrol ADT Pak Unit of Use
◆ Medrol Dosepak Unit of Use
◆ Medrol Tablets
Mercresin Tincture
◆ Motrin Tablets**
Mycifradin Oral Solution
Mycifradin Sterile Powder
Mycifradin Tablets
▣ Myciguent Antibiotic Cream & Ointment
▣ Mycitracin Antibiotic Ointment
Mycitracin Ophthalmic Ointment
Myringacaine Ear Drops
Neo-Cortef Cream
Neo-Cortef Ointment
Neo-Cortef Ophthalmic Ointment
Neo-Cortef Ophthalmic Suspension
Neo-Delta-Cortef Ointment
Neo-Delta-Cortef Ophthalmic Suspension
Neo-Medrol Acetate Topical
Neo-Medrol Ophthalmic Ointment
Neo-Oxylone Ointment
Orinase Diagnostic Sterile Powder
◆ Orinase Tablets
Orthoxicol Cough Syrup
Oxylone Cream
P-A-C Compound Tablets
P-A-C w/Codeine Tablets
Pamine Tablets
Panmycin Capsules
Panmycin Tablets
Pentacresol Instrument Disinfecting Solution
Pentacresol Oral Solution
Phenolax Wafers
Prostin VR Pediatric Sterile Solution
Protamine Sulfate for Injection, USP, Sterile Powder
Protamine Sulfate for Injection, USP, Sterile Solution
◆ Provera Tablets
◆▣ Pyrroxate Capsules
Reserpoid Tablets
Sigtab Tablets
Sodium Chloride Injection, (Bacteriotstic) USP, Sterile Solution
Solu-B Sterile Powder
Solu-B w/Ascorbic Acid Sterile Powder
Solu-Cortef Sterile Powder
◆ Solu-Medrol Mix-O-Vials & Vials
◆ Solu-Medrol Sterile Powder
Super D Perles
◆ Tolinase Tablets
Trobicin Sterile Powder
▣ Unicap Capsules & Tablets
▣ Unicap Chewable Tablets
▣ Unicap M Tablets
▣ Unicap Plus Iron Tablets
▣ Unicap Senior Tablets
▣ Unicap T Tablets
Upjohn Vitamin C Tablets, 250 mg
Upjohn Vitamin E Capsules, 200 I.U.
Uracil Mustard Capsules
Uticillin VK Tablets
Water for Injection (Bacteriostatic), USP, Sterile Solution
◆ Xanax Tablets
Zanosar Sterile Powder
Zymacap Capsules
Zymalixir Fluid
*Product of the Upjohn Manufacturing Company
**Product of the Upjohn Manufacturing Company M
[Products without reference marks are products of the Upjohn Company]

UPSHER-SMITH LABORATORIES, INC. 2077
14905 23rd Ave. North
Minneapolis, MN 55441
(612) 473-4412
Address inquiries to:
Professional Service Department
Products Available
Acetaminophen Uniserts Suppositories
Aspirin Uniserts Suppositories
Bisacodyl Tablets
Bisacodyl Uniserts Suppositories
Daily-M Tablets
Dexamethasone Tablets
Docusate Sodium Capsules
Docusate Sodium with Casanthranol Capsules
Ferrous Gluconate Tablets
Ferrous Sulfate Tablets
Hemorrhoidal Uniserts Suppositories
Hemorrhoidal-HC Uniserts Suppositories
Hexavitamin Tablets
Histatapp Elixir
Histatapp T.D. Tablets
Hydrochlorothiazide Tablets
Kerasol Therapeutic Bath Oil
Klor-Con Powder
Klor-Con/25 Powder
Klor-Con 20% Solution
Klor-10% Solution
Methocarbamol Tablets
Papaverine Hydrochloride T.R. Capsules
Prednisone Tablets
SSKI
Sorbitol Solution
Spironolactone Tablets
Spironolactone w/Hydrochlorothiazide Tablets
Stress-600 Tablets
Stress-600 with Zinc
Suhist Tablets
Theobron SR Capsules
Therapeutic B Complex with C Capsules
Therapeutic Multivitamin Tablets
Therapeutic Multivitamin & Mineral Tablets
Trofan Tablets (L-Tryptophan)
Zinc Sulfate Capsules

THE VALE CHEMICAL CO., INC. 2078
1201 Liberty St.
Allentown, PA 18102
Address inquiries to:
Elliot R. Davis (215) 433-7579
Products Available
Acedoval Tablets
Acedyne Tablets
Alkaline Aromatic Tablets
Aluminum Hydroxide Gel, Tablets
Aminophyllin Tablets
Ammonium Chloride Tablets
Antrin Tablets
Antussal Syrup
Aquabase (Beeler's) Hydrophyllic Ointment Base
Ascorbic Acid Tablets
Asmacol Tablets
Aspirin Tablets, 5 gr. & 10 gr.
Aspir-10 Tablets
Barbeloid Tablets
Belexal Tablets
Benzo-Menth Lozenges
Biothesin Tablets
Bipectol Wafers
Bismapec Tablets
Butalix
Calcium Gluconate Tablets
Calfos-D Tablets
Coraval Improved Tablets
Dermaval Cream
Double-Sal Tablets
Duphrene Syrup & Tablets
Ephedrine & Sodium Phenobarbital Tablets
Extract of Ox Bile Tablets
Ferate-C Tablets
Glucovite Tablets
Glycofed
▣ Glycotuss Syrup & Tablets
Glycotuss-dM Syrup & Tablets
Guiosan Syrup
Hydra-Mag Tablets
Ironco-B Tablets
Magmalin Tablets & Suspension
Mandex Tablets
Methenamine & Acid Sodium Phosphate Tablets
Methiokap Capsules
Neocet Tablets
Neofed
Neogesic Tablets
Neo-Tab Tablets
Nevrotose Capsutabs
Niacin Tablets
Nisaval Tablets
Nyral Lozenges
Obeval Tablets
Oxynitral w/Veratrum Viride Tablets
Pedric Elixir & Tablets
Pedric Senior Tablets
Phenobarbital Tablets
Potassium Iodide Tablets
Rauval Tablets
Rhinogesic Tablets
Rhinogesic-GG Tablets
Riboflavin Tablets
Serpate Tablets
Sodium Salicylate Tablets
Soothogel Cream
Synthetar Cream
Taurophyllin Tablets
Taystron Tablets
Terphan Elixir
Theolix Elixir
Thiamine Hydrochloride Tablets
Thyroid Tablets
Tono-B, Wafers
Trioval Tablets
Triple Sulfoid Tablets
Valacet Tablets
Valax Tablets
Valcaine Ointment
Valcreme Lotion
Valdeine Tablets
Valdrene Expectorant Syrup
Valdrene Tablets
Val-Tep Tablets

VEREX LABORATORIES, INC. 2078
5241 South Quebec Street
Englewood, CO 80111
(303) 741-3277
For Medical Emergencies Contact:
James M. Dunn, M.D. (303) 741-3277
Products Available
Help
Verin

VICKS TOILETRY PRODUCTS DIVISION 2079
Richardson-Vicks Inc.
10 Westport Road
Wilton, CT 06897
Address inquiries to:
Vicks Research Center (203) 929-2500
For Medical Emergencies Contact
Medical Director
Vicks Research Center (203) 929-2500
Products Available
▣ Clearasil 5% Benzoyl Peroxide Lotion Acne Treatment
▣ Clearasil Pore Deep Cleanser (Salicylic Acid 0.5%)
▣ Clearasil Super Strength Acne Treatment Cream (10% Benzoyl Peroxide)
▣ Denquel Sensitive Teeth Toothpaste
▣ Topex 10% Benzoyl Peroxide Lotion Buffered Acne Medication

VICKS HEALTH CARE DIVISION 2079
Richardson-Vicks Inc.
10 Westport Road
Wilton, CT 06897
Address inquiries to:
Vicks Research Center (203) 929-2500
For Medical Emergencies Contact
Medical Director
Vicks Research Center (203) 929-2500
Products Available
Daycare Daytime Colds Medicine-liquid
Daycare Multi-Symptom Colds Medicine-capsules
Formula 44 Cough Control Discs
Formula 44 Cough Mixture
Formula 44D Decongestant Cough Mixture
Headway Capsules
Headway Tablets
Nyquil Nighttime Colds Medicine
Oracin Cherry Flavor Cooling Throat Lozenges
Oracin Cooling Throat Lozenges
Sinex Decongestant Nasal Spray
Sinex Long-Acting Decongestant Nasal Spray
Tempo Antacid with Antigas Action
Vaposteam
Vatronol Nose Drops
Vicks Cough Silencers Cough Drops
Vicks Cough Syrup
Vicks Formula 44 Cough Control Discs
Vicks Formula 44 Cough Mixture
Vicks Formula 44D Decongestant Cough Mixture
Vicks Inhaler
Vicks Nyquil Nighttime Colds Medicine
Vicks Sinex Decongestant Nasal Spray
Vicks Sinex Long-Acting Decongestant Nasal Spray
Vicks Throat Lozenges
Vicks Vaporub
Vicks Vaposteam
Vicks Vatronol Nose Drops

VIOBIN CORPORATION 2082
a Subsidiary of A. H. Robins Co
226 W. Livingston St.
Monticello, IL 61856
Address inquiries to:
W. E. Melby (217) 762-2561
Products Available
Viobin Wheat Germ Oil, Liquid & Capsules
Viokase

VITALINE FORMULAS 2082
P.O. Box 6757
Incline Village, NV 89450
Address inquiries to:
Jed D. Meese,
Technical Director (702) 831-5656
Products Available
Alka Aid
B6 Tablets
B Complex "50" & "100" Tablets
B Complex "50" & "100" Time Release Tablets
Calcium Carbonate (chewable)
Calcium, Oyster Shell
Chromium Tablets
Compound Hematinic
Digestive Enzymes (chewable)
Digestive Supplement
Enviro-Stress with Zinc & Selenium
Fructose Wafers
Lipo Plus (lipotropics) Tablets
Magna Zinc Tablets
Magnesium Tablets
Manganese Tablets
Multimineral Plus Tablets
NoRX Tablets
Pancreatin Tablets 2400 mg. N.F. (High Lipase)
Potassium Gluconate
Selenium Tablets
StimuLean Tablets
Total Formula
Vitamin C
Vitamin C Time Release Tablets 1000 mg.
Vitamin E (d-alpha tocopherol acetate) 400 I.U.
Vitamin E (d-alpha tocopherol succinate) 400 I.U.
Zinc Tablets 220 mg.

WALKER, CORP & CO., INC. 2083
Easthampton Pl. & N. Collingwood Ave.
Syracuse, NY 13206
Address inquiries to:
P.O. Drawer 1320
Syracuse, NY 13201 (315) 463-4511
Products Available
Evac-U-Gen

WALKER PHARMACAL COMPANY 2083
4200 Laclede Avenue
St. Louis, MO 63108
Address inquiries to:
Customer Service (314) 533-9600
Products Available
Succus Cineraria Maritima

WALLACE LABORATORIES 441, 2083
P.O. Box 1
Cranbury, NJ 08512
Address inquiries to:
Professional Services (609) 655-6000
Night and Weekend Emergencies
(609) 799-1167
Send all orders to:
Wallace Laboratories
Div. of Carter-Wallace, Inc.
Post Office Drawer 5
Cranbury, NJ 08512
Products Available
◆ Aquatensen Tablets
Avazyme/Avazyme-100 Tablets
Barbidonna Elixir & Tablets
Barbidonna No. 2 Tablets
Butibel Elixir & Tablets
Buticaps
◆ Butisol Sodium Elixir & Tablets
Covanamine Liquid
Covangesic Tablets
Dainite Tablets
Dainite-KI Tablets
Depen Titratabs
Deprol Tablets
Diutensen Tablets
◆ Diutensen-R Tablets
Lufyllin Elixir
◆ Lufyllin Injection
◆ Lufyllin & Lufyllin-400 Tablets
Lufyllin-EPG Elixir & Tablets
◆ Lufyllin-GG Elixir & Tablets
Maltsupex Liquid, Powder & Tablets
Meprospan Capsules
◆ Micrainin
◆ Milpath Tablets
Milprem Tablets
◆ Miltown Tablets
◆ Miltown 600 Tablets
Miltrate Tablets
◆ Organidin Elixir, Solution & Tablets
◆ Rondomycin Capsules
Ryna Liquid
Ryna-C Liquid
Ryna-CX Liquid
Rynatan Pediatric Suspension
◆ Rynatan Tablets
Rynatuss Pediatric Suspension
◆ Rynatuss Tablets
◆ Soma Tablets
◆ Soma Compound Tablets
◆ Soma Compound w/Codeine Tablets
Syllact Powder
Syllamalt Powder
Theo-Organidin Elixir
Tussi-Organidin DM Elixir
Tussi-Organidin Elixir
Unitensen Aqueous Injection
◆ Unitensen Tablets
◆ VōSol HC Otic Solution
◆ VōSol Otic Solution

WARREN-TEED LABORATORIES 404, 2105
Warren-Teed products are now marketed by Adria Laboratories Inc.
Please see Adria Laboratories Inc. in this index for Warren-Teed product listing.

WEBCON PHARMACEUTICALS 2105
Division of Alcon (Puerto Rico) Inc.
Post Office Box 3000
Humacao, Puerto Rico 00661
Address inquiries to:
Medical Department
Post Office Box 1629
Fort Worth, TX 76101 (817) 293-0450
Products Available
Alconefrin 12 Drops
Alconefrin 25 Drops
Alconefrin 50 Drops
Alconefrin 25 Spray
Anestacon Sterile Solution
Aquachloral
Azo-Standard Tablets
B & O No. 15A & No. 16A Supprettes
Cystospaz Tablets
Cystospaz-M Capsules
Neopap Supprettes
*Oxiphen Tablets
Urised Tablets
Urisedamine Tablets
WANS Children Supprettes
WANS No. 1 & No. 2 Supprettes
*TM The Dow Chemical Co.

THE WESLEY PHARMACAL COMPANY, INC. 2108
9984 Gantry Road
Philadelphia, PA 19115
Address inquiries to:
Professional Service Dept. (215) 698-2900
Products Available
Alkaline Gargle
Allee
Aqwadril
Aqweside
Aqwesine
Auralcort
Auralgesic Drops
Avasol
Bee 12 Injection
Bilagog
Bilox Tablets
Bioplex
Calfoject Injection
Cee w/Bee
Ceeject
Ceespan T.D. Capsules
Cetacet Capsules
Cinolone
Cobaldrox-12
Codasol
Codinets Tablets
Deco-Disc Lozenges
Decodult Tablets
Decofed
Decogest Tablets
Decolate Tablets
Decominic
Deco-Mist Spray
Decospan
Decostat, Improved
Decotussin Tablets
Dexadrol
Diotabs
Duolate-Q
EDTA Injection
Eisenzucker Tablets
Eramycin
Estralate
Flatulence Tabs
Flexon
Foli-B
Gasticans
Gastomins
Gonadoplex
Hydocaine
Hytrophen
Infer
K-Glucon
Kaogoric
Kaybiotic Cream
Kaycort H.C. Cream
Kaytar Cream
Kryzen Tablets
Lactoease
Liferavite
Megabee
Merculyn
Metabol
Niaspan
Nicosine
Optozine
P.D.P. Capsules
P.D.P. Liquid
P.D.P. Powder
P.D.P. Wafers
Panitone Liquid
Panitone Tablets
Panivon
Pecadine Tablets
Peritrol
Phenterspan
Prednasol
Prednaspan Forte
Prednoid
Protobol
Pulsaphen Tablets
Quadramin
Reposans-10
Ribozime
Robinetts
Romazine Cough Syrup
Romazine Injection
Salisicol Tablets
Sedastat
Sterozone Cream
Sweet-Ups
Tenalate Ointment
Testostal
Testralate-200
Theolate
Thyrodine
Thyrodoxine
Triacillin
Trimette Tablets
Trimette TD Capsules
Triptos
Uracid
Uratin Tablets
Urisal
Verescorite Tablets
Wescaldrin
Wescoid Tablets
Wescolates Tablets
Wescophen-S Tablets
Wesdex-T
Weslin
Wesmatic Forte Tablets
Wesmatic Tablets
Wesplex
Wesplex, Liver w/B_{12}
Wesprin Buffered Tablets
Westrol
Westron Tablets
Z-Glucon

WESTWOOD PHARMACEUTICALS INC. 2109
468 Dewitt St.
Buffalo, NY 14213
Address inquiries to:
Consumer Affairs Department
(716) 887-3773
Products Available
Alpha Keri Bath Oil
Alpha Keri Soap
Alpha Keri Spray
Balnetar
Capitrol Cream Shampoo
Desquam-X 5 Gel
Desquam-X 10 Gel
Desquam-X Wash
Desquam-X 10 Wash
Estar Gel
Eurax Cream & Lotion
Fostex Medicated Cleansing Bar
Fostex Medicated Cleansing Cream
Fostex 5% Benzoyl Peroxide Gel
Fostex 10% Benzoyl Peroxide Cleansing Bar
Fostex 10% Benzoyl Peroxide Wash
Fostril
Halotex Cream & Solution
Keralyt Gel
Keri Creme
Keri Facial Soap
Keri Lotion
Lowila Cake
Pernox Lotion
Pernox Medicated Lathering Scrub
Pernox Shampoo
PreSun 4 Creamy Sunscreen
PreSun 8 Lotion, Creamy & Gel
PreSun 15 Creamy Sunscreen
PreSun 15 Sunscreen Lotion
Sebucare
Sebulex & Sebulex Cream Shampoo
Sebulex Conditioning Shampoo with Protein
Sebutone & Sebutone Cream Shampoo
Staticin (erythromycin) 1.5% Topical Solution
Tacaryl Chewable Tablets
Tacaryl Syrup & Tablets
Transact
Westcort Cream

WHARTON LABORATORIES, INC. **2118**
37-02 48th Ave.
Long Island City, NY 11101
Address inquiries to:
Medical Director (212) 786-8607
Products Available
Nitrong Ointment
Nitrong Ointment, Unit Dose
Nitrong Tablets
Nitrong SR Tablets

WILLEN DRUG COMPANY **2118**
18 North High St.
Baltimore, MD 21202 (301) 752-1865
Products Available
Bicitra—Sugar-Free
Neutra-Phos Powder & Capsules
Neutra-Phos-K Powder & Capsules
Polycitra Syrup
Polycitra-K Syrup
Polycitra-LC—Sugar-Free

T. E. WILLIAMS PHARMACEUTICALS, INC. **2120**
P.O. Box 1860
Edmond, Oklahoma 73034
Address Inquiries to:
(405) 348-5010
For Medical Emergencies Contact:
(405) 348-5010
Products Available
A P Cream
Artha-G
Mus-Lax Capsules
Pre-H-Cal
T-Circ Capsules
T-Diet Capsules
T-Dry Capsules
T-Dry Jr. Capsules
T-Gesic Capsules
T-Koff Syrup
T-Moist Tablets
T-Ritis
Theo-Tuss
Theo-Tuss-S
Vag-All

WINTHROP LABORATORIES **441, 2122, 3047**
90 Park Avenue
New York, NY 10016 (212) 907-2000

Professional Services Department
(212) 907-2525
Products Available
A.P.C. w/Demerol
Amipaque
Anti-Rust Tablets
Aralen Hydrochloride Injection
◆ Aralen Phosphate Tablets
Aralen Phosphate w/Primaquine Phosphate
Atabrine Hydrochloride Tablets
◆ Bilopaque Sodium
Codeine Phosphate Carpuject
◆ Danocrine
Demerol Carpuject
Demerol Hydrochloride Injection
Demerol Hydrochloride Syrup
◆ Demerol Hydrochloride Tablets
Demerol Uni-Amp
Drisdol 50,000 Unit Capsules
Drisdol in Propylene Glycol
Hydromorphone Carpuject
Hydroxyzine Carpuject
Hydroxyzine Hydrochloride Injection
Hypaque Meglumine 30%
Hypaque Meglumine 60%
Hypaque Sodium Oral Powder & Liquid
Hypaque Sodium 20%
Hypaque Sodium 25%
Hypaque Sodium 50% Injection
Hypaque-Cysto
Hypaque-M, 75% Injection
Hypaque-M, 90% Injection
Hypaque-76 Injection
Hytakerol Capsules & Liquid
Lotusate Caplets
Luminal Ovoids
Luminal Sodium Injection
Morphine Sulfate Carpuject
Mytelase Chloride Caplets
◆ NegGram Caplets
NegGram Suspension
Neo-Synephrine Hydrochloride 1% Injection
Neo-Synephrine Hydrochloride (Ophthalmic)
phisoDerm
pHisoHex
pHisoScrub
◆ Plaquenil Sulfate Tablets
Primaquine Phosphate Tablets
Sulfamylon Acetate Cream
◆ Talacen
Talwin Carpuject
Talwin Compound
◆ Talwin 50 Tablets
Talwin Injection
◆ Talwin Nx
Talwin Uni-Amp
◆ Telepaque Tablets
Vitamins
Vitamin D, USP
Drisdol 50,000 Unit Capsules
Drisdol in Propylene Glycol
◆ Winstrol Tablets
Zephiran Chloride Aqueous Solution
Zephiran Chloride Concentrate Solution
Zephiran Chloride Spray
Zephiran Chloride Tinted Tincture
Zephiran Towelettes

CONSUMER PRODUCTS DIVISION
Astring-o-sol
▣ Bronkaid Mist
▣ Bronkaid Mist Suspension
▣ Bronkaid Tablets
▣ Campho-Phenique Lip Balm
▣ Campho-Phenique Liquid & Gel
Caroid Laxative
Caroid Tooth Powder
Creamalin Tablets
▣ Haley's M-O, Regular & Flavored
Mucilose Flakes & Granules
▣ NTZ Drops & Spray
Neocurtasal
Neo-Synephrine Hydrochloride Jelly
▣ Neo-Synephrine Nasal Spray (Mentholated)
▣ Neo-Synephrine Nasal Sprays
▣ Neo-Synephrine Nose Drops
▣ Neo-Synephrine 12 Hour Nasal Spray
▣ Neo-Synephrine 12 Hour Nose Drops (Adult & Children Strengths)
▣ Neo-Synephrine 12 Hour Vapor Nasal Spray
▣ Neo-Synephrine II Long Acting Nasal Spray
▣ Neo-Synephrine II Long Acting Nose Drops (Adult & Pediatric Strengths)
▣ Neo-Synephrine II Long Acting Vapor Nasal Spray
▣ Neo-Synephrinol Day Relief Capsules
pHisoAc
pHisoDan
▣ pHisoDerm Regular & Fresh Scent
phisoPuff
▣ WinGel Liquid & Tablets

WYETH LABORATORIES **442, 2143**
Division of American Home Products Corporation
P.O. Box 8299
Philadelphia, PA 19101
Address inquiries to:
Professional Service (215) 688-4400
For Medical Emergency Information
Day or night call (215) 688-4400
Wyeth Distribution Centers:
Andover, MA 01810
P.O. Box 1776 (617) 475-9075
Atlanta, GA 30302
P.O. Box 4365 (404) 873-1681
Baltimore, MD 21224
101 Kane St. (301) 633-4000
Boston Distribution Center, see under Andover, MA
Buena Park, CA 90620
P.O. Box 5000 (714) 523-5500
(Los Angeles) (213) 627-5374
Chicago Distribution Center, see under Evanston, IL
Cleveland, OH 44101
P.O. Box 91549 (216) 238-9450
Dallas, TX 75235
P.O. Box 35213 (214) 631-4360
Denver, CO 80201
P.O. Box 2107 (303) 388-3635
Evanston, IL 60204
P.O. Box 1659 (Skokie) (312) 675-1400
(Chicago) (312) 463-2400
Honolulu, HI 96814
1013 Kawaiahao St. (808) 538-1988
Kansas City Distribution Center, see under North Kansas City, MO
Kent, WA 98031
P.O. Box 5609 (206) 872-8790
Los Angeles Distribution Center, see under Buena Park, CA
Memphis, TN 38101
P.O. Box 1698 (901) 353-4680
North Kansas City, MO 64116
P.O. Box 7588 (816) 842-0680
Philadelphia Distribution Center
Paoli, PA 19301,
P.O. Box 61 (215) 644-8000
Philadelphia (215) 878-9500
St. Paul, MN 55164
P.O. Box 43034 (612) 454-6270
Seattle Distribution Center, see under Kent, WA
Products Available
Alcohol Sponges
Aludrox Suspension
Aludrox Tablets
Aminophylline Rectal Suppositories
Amphojel Suspension
Amphojel Suspension w/o Flavor
Amphojel Tablets
Antisnakebite Serum (see Antivenin)
Antivenin (Crotalidae) Polyvalent
Antivenin (Micrurus Fulvius)
Aspirin Rectal Suppositories
Aspirin Tablets, Redipak
Ativan Injection
◆ Ativan Tablets
Atropine Sulfate Injection
Basaljel Capsules
Basaljel Suspension
Basaljel Suspension, Extra Strength
Basaljel Swallow Tablets
Benzathine Penicillin G (see Bicillin)
Bewon Elixir
Bicillin C-R Injection
Bicillin C-R 900/300 Injection
Bicillin Long-Acting Injection
Bicillin Tablets
Biologicals
Bisacodyl Suppositories
Chloral Hydrate Capsules, Redipak
Chlorpromazine HCl Injection
Cholera Vaccine
Codeine Phosphate Injection
Codeine Sulfate Tablets, Redipak
Collyrium Eye Lotion
Collyrium w/Ephedrine Eye Drops
Cyanocobalamin Injection
Cyclapen-W Oral Suspension
◆ Cyclapen-W Tablets
Dexamethasone Sodium Phosphate Injection
Digitoxin (see Purodigin)
Digoxin Injection
Dimenhydrinate Injection
Diphenhydramine HCl Injection
Diphtheria and Tetanus Toxoids Adsorbed (Adult Use) (see Tetanus and Diphtheria Toxoids Adsorbed)
Diphtheria & Tetanus Toxoids Adsorbed, Pediatric
Diphtheria & Tetanus Toxoids & Pertussis Vaccine Adsorbed (see Triple Antigen)
Dryvax, Dried Smallpox Vaccine
Epinephrine Injection (1:1000)
◆ Equagesic Tablets
◆ Equagesic-M Tablets
◆ Equanil Capsules
◆ Equanil Tablets
◆ Equanil Wyseals
Equanitrate 10 & 20 Tablets
Ergonovine Maleate Injection
Erythromycin Ethylsuccinate Oral Suspension (See Wyamycin E Liquid)
Erythromycin Stearate Tablets (see Wyamycin S Tablets)
Furosemide Injection USP
Heparin Lock Flush Solution
Heparin Sodium Injection
Hydromorphone HCl Injection
Hydroxyzine HCl Injection
Immune Serum Globulin (Human)
Influenza Virus Vaccine Subvirion Type
Largon Injection
Lidocaine HCl Injection
◆ Lo/Ovral Tablets
◆ Lo/Ovral-28 Tablets
◆ Mazanor
◆ Mepergan Fortis Capsules
Mepergan Injection
Meperidine HCl Injection
Meperidine HCl Tablets, Redipak
Morphine Sulfate Injection
◆ Nordette Tablets
◆ Nordette-28 Tablets
Nursoy, Soy Protein Formula for Infants, Concentrated Liquid & Ready-to-Feed
◆ Omnipen Capsules
Omnipen Oral Suspension
Omnipen Pediatric Drops
Omnipen-N Injection
Opium & Belladonna Rectal Suppositories
◆ Ovral Tablets
◆ Ovral-28 Tablets
Ovrette Tablets
Oxaine M Suspension
Oxytocin Injection, Synthetic
◆ Pathocil Capsules
Pathocil Oral Suspension
Pediatric Phenergan Expectorant w/Dextromethorphan
Penicillin Preparations:
Bicillin Products
Penicillin G Potassium Tablets
Pen•Vee K Products
Wycillin Products
Pentobarbital Sodium Capsules, Redipak
Pentobarbital Sodium Injection
Pen•Vee K for Oral Solution
◆ Pen•Vee K Tablets
Petrogalar, Phenolphthalein
Petrogalar, Plain
◆ Phenergan Compound Tablets
Phenergan Expectorant, Plain
Phenergan Expectorant, w/Codeine
Phenergan Expectorant, w/Dextromethorphan, Pediatric
Phenergan Injection
Phenergan Syrup Fortis
◆ Phenergan Tablets, Syrup & Rectal Suppositories

Phenergan VC Expectorant, Plain
Phenergan VC Expectorant, w/Codeine
◆ Phenergan-D Tablets
Phenobarbital Sodium Injection
Phenobarbital Tablets, Redipak
Phosphaljel
Plebex Injection
Polymagma Plain Tablets
Potassium Penicillin G Tablets, Buffered
Prochlorperazine Edisylate Injection
Proketazine Tablets
Purodigin Tablets
Redipak Unit Dose Medications (Strip Pack and/or Individually Wrapped) Products:
- Aspirin Tablets
- Ativan Tablets
- Chloral Hydrate Capsules
- Codeine Sulfate Tablets
- Equagesic Tablets
- Equanil Tablets
- Meperidine HCl Tablets
- Omnipen Capsules
- Penicillin G Potassium Tablets, Buffered
- Pentobarbital Sodium Capsules
- Pen•Vee K Tablets
- Phenergan Tablets
- Phenobarbital Tablets
- Secobarbital Sodium Capsules
- Serax Capsules
- Unipen Capsules
- Wygesic Tablets
- Zactirin Compound-100 Tablets

Redipak (Liquid Unit Dose) Products:
- Omnipen Oral Suspension
- Pen•Vee K Solution

Redipak (Unit of Use Suppository Pack) Products:
- Aminophylline Rectal Suppositories
- Aspirin Rectal Suppositories
- Phenergan Rectal Suppositories
- Wyanoids HC Rectal Suppositories w/Hydrocortisone

Redipak (Respiratory Therapy Unit) Products:
- Sodium Chloride 0.9% and 0.45%
- Sterile Distilled Water

RediTemp-C, Disposable Cold Pack
SMA Infant Formula, Liquid Concentrated
SMA Infant Formula, Powder
SMA Infant Formula, Ready-to-Feed
Saline Solution (see Sodium Chloride Injection)
Secobarbital Sodium Capsules, Redipak
Secobarbital Sodium Injection
◆ Serax Capsules
◆ Serax Tablets
Simeco Suspension
Smallpox Vaccine, Dried (see Dryvax)
Snakebite Serum (see Antivenin)
Sodium Chloride Injection, Bacteriostatic
Sopronol Ointment, Powder & Solution
Sparine Concentrate
Sparine Syrup
◆ Sparine Tablets
Tetanus & Diphtheria Toxoids Adsorbed (Adults)
Tetanus & Diphtheria Toxoids Adsorbed (Pediatric) (see Diphtheria & Tetanus Toxoids Adsorbed)
Tetanus Immune Globulin (Human)
Tetanus Toxoid Adsorbed, Aluminum Phosphate
Tetanus Toxoid Fluid, Purified
◆ Tetracycline HCl Capsules
Thiamine HCl Injection
Triple Antigen
Tubex Closed Injection System Products:
- Ativan
- Bicillin C-R
- Bicillin C-R 900/300
- Bicillin L-A
- Chlorpromazine HCl
- Codeine Phosphate
- ◆ Cyanocobalamin (Vitamin B_{12})
- Dexamethasone Sodium Phosphate
- Digoxin
- Dimenhydrinate
- Diphenhydramine HCl
- Diphtheria & Tetanus Toxoids Adsorbed, Pediatric
- Epinephrine
- Ergonovine Maleate
- Furosemide
- Heparin Lock Flush Solution
- Heparin Sodium
- Hydromorphone HCl
- Hydroxyzine HCl
- Immune Serum Globulin (Human)
- Influenza Virus Vaccine, Purified, Subvirion
- Largon
- Lidocaine HCl
- Mepergan
- Meperidine HCl
- Morphine Sulfate
- Oxytocin, Synthetic
- Pentobarbital Sodium
- Phenergan
- Phenobarbital Sodium
- Prochlorperazine Edisylate
- Secobarbital Sodium
- Sodium Chloride, Bacteriostatic
- Sparine
- Tetanus & Diphtheria Toxoids Adsorbed (Adult)
- Tetanus Immune Globulin (Human)
- Tetanus Toxoid, Aluminum Phosphate Adsorbed
- Tetanus Toxoid Fluid, Purified
- Thiamine HCl
- Triple Antigen
- Vitamin B_{12} (Cyanocobalamin)
- Wyamine Sulfate
- Wycillin

◆ Tubex Hypodermic Syringe
Tubex Sterile Cartridge-Needle Unit Empty
Typhoid Vaccine
◆ Unipen Capsules
Unipen Injection
Unipen Oral Solution
◆ Unipen Tablets
Vitamin B Complex (see Plebex)
Vitamin B_{12} Injection (see Cyanocobalamin)
Wyamine Sulfate Injection
Wyamycin E Liquid
◆ Wyamycin S Tablets
Wyanoid Ointment
◆ Wyanoids HC Rectal Suppositories w/Hydrocortisone
◆ Wyanoids Hemorrhoidal Suppositories
Wycillin Injection
Wycillin Injection & Probenecid Tablets
Wydase, Lyophilized
Wydase, Stabilized Solution
◆ Wygesic Tablets
◆ Wymox Capsules
Wymox Oral Suspension
Wyseals (see Equanil)
◆ Wytensin Tablets
Wyvac Rabies Vaccine
Zactane Tablets
◆ Zactirin Compound-100 Tablets
◆ Zactirin Tablets

YOUNGS DRUG PRODUCTS CORP. **2205**
Post Office Box 385
865 Centennial Avenue
Piscataway, NJ 08854

Address inquiries to:
Mr. Phillip L. Frank or
Mr. Murray H. Glantz (201) 885-5777
*Sole Distributor for products manufactured by
Holland-Rantos Company, Inc.
865 Centennial Avenue
Piscataway, NJ 08854

Products Available
H-R Sterile Lubricating Jelly
Koro-Flex Arcing Spring Diaphragm
Koro-Flex Arcing Spring Diaphragm Compact Set
Koro-Flex Fitting Rings, Set of
Koromex Coil Spring Diaphragm
Koromex Coil Spring Diaphragm Compact Set
◘ Koromex Contraceptive Foam
Koromex Diaphragm Introducer
Koromex Fitting Rings, Set of
Koromex Jelly/Cream Applicator
◘ Koromex‖ Contraceptive Cream
◘ Koromex‖ Contraceptive Jelly
◘ Koromex‖-A Contraceptive Jelly
Korostatin (Nystatin) Vaginal Tablets
Koro-Sulf (Sulfisoxazole) Vaginal Cream
◘ Nylmerate‖ Solution Concentrate
Rantex Personal Cloth Wipes
◘ Transi-Lube
◘ Triple X

PDR 37 EDITION 1983

SECTION 2

Product Name Index

Part 1—In this section products are listed in alphabetical sequence by brand name or (if described) generic name. Only described products have page numbers to assist you in locating additional information. For additional information on other products, you may wish to contact the manufacturer directly.
The symbol ◆ indicates the product is shown in the Product Identification Section. The symbol ▣ indicates the product is described in PDR® FOR NONPRESCRIPTION DRUGS.

Part 2—A list of products that have been discontinued by manufacturers during the past year.

Part 1

A

▣ **A and D Hand Cream** (Schering)
▣ **A and D Ointment** (Schering)
ACE + Z Tablets (Legere) p 1099
▣ **A.C.N. Tablets** (Person & Covey)
ACTH (Bay)
A.C.T.H. "40" Injectable (O'Neal, Jones & Feldman) p 1421
A.C.T.H. "80" Injectable (O'Neal, Jones & Feldman) p 1421
A-Fil Cream Neutral & Dark (CooperCare)
AL-R TD Capsules (Saron) p 1777
AL-R TD, Pediatric (Saron)
A P Cream (Williams)
APAP w/Codeine Tablets (Geneva) p 977
APC Tablets (Bowman)
◆ **A.P.C. with Codeine, Tabloid brand** (Burroughs Wellcome) p 407, 775
A.P.C. w/Demerol (Winthrop)
A.P.L. (Ayerst) p 617
A.S.A. Compound Pulvules & Tablets (Lilly)
◆ **A.S.A. & Codeine Compound Pulvules & Tablets** (Lilly) p 417
A.S.A. Enseals, Pulvules, Suppositories & Tablets (Lilly)
◆ **A/T/S** (Hoechst-Roussel) p 412, 1000
◆ **A-200 Pyrinate Liquid, Gel** (Norcliff Thayer) p 421, 1404
AVC Cream (Merrell Dow) p 1344
AVC Suppositories (Merrell Dow) p 1344
AVC Vaginal Cream (Merrell Dow)
AVC/Dienestrol Cream (Merrell Dow)
AVC/Dienestrol Suppositories (Merrell Dow)
Abbokinase (Abbott) p 503
◆ **Abbo-Pac** (Abbott) p 403, 502
Abdec Baby Vitamin Drops (Parke-Davis)
Abdec Kapseals (Parke-Davis)
Abdec with Fluoride Baby Vitamin Drops (Parke-Davis)
Abdol with Minerals Capsules (Parke-Davis)
Accelerase (Organon)
Accelerase-PB (Organon)
Accurbron (Merrell Dow) p 1345
◆ **Accutane** (Roche) p 429, 1643
Acedoval Tablets (Vale)
Acedyne Tablets (Vale)
Acetaco Tablets (Legere) p 1099
◆ **Acetaminophen Capsules, Tablets, Elixir** (Lederle) p 415
Acetaminophen Elixir, Tablets, Suppositories (Roxane) p 1755
Acetaminophen Uniserts Suppositories (Upsher-Smith) p 2077
Acetaminophen with Codeine Phosphate Tablets (Roxane) p 1755
Acetazolamide Tablets (Schein) p 1782
Acetospan Injection (Reid-Provident, Direct Div.)
Acetycol Tablets (O'Neal, Jones & Feldman)
Achromycin Intramuscular (Lederle) p 1058
Achromycin Intravenous (Lederle) p 1058
Achromycin Ophthalmic Ointment (Lederle) p 1060
Achromycin Ophthalmic Suspension 1% (Lederle) p 1060
Achromycin 3% Ointment (Lederle) p 1060
◆ **Achromycin V Capsules** (Lederle) p 414, 1058
Achromycin V Oral Suspension (Lederle) p 1058
Achrostatin V Capsules (Lederle)
Acid Mantle Creme & Lotion (Dorsey Laboratories) p 904
Acidulin (Lilly) p 1108
Aci-Jel Therapeutic Vaginal Jelly (Ortho Pharmaceutical) p 1434
Acne-Aid Cream (Stiefel)
Acne-Aid Detergent Soap (Stiefel)
Acne-Aid Lotion (Stiefel)
▣ **Acnederm Lotion & Soap** (Lannett)
Acne-Dome Creme & Lotion (Miles Pharmaceuticals) p 1379
Acne-Dome Medicated Cleanser (Miles Pharmaceuticals) p 1379
Acnesarb (C & M)
Acno Lotion (Baker/Cummins)
▣ **Acnomel Cream** (Smith Kline & French)
Acnotex (C & M)
Acthar (Armour) p 589
Acticort Lotion 100 (Baker/Cummins)
◆ **Actidil Tablets & Syrup** (Burroughs Wellcome) p 407
◆ **Actifed Tablets & Syrup** (Burroughs Wellcome) p 407
Actifed-C Expectorant (Burroughs Wellcome) p 770
Activated Thrombofax Reagent-Optimized (Ortho Diagnostic)
Actol Expectorant Liquid (Beecham Laboratories)
Actol Expectorant Tablets (Beecham Laboratories)
Actrapid (Squibb) p 1934
Acucron Tablets (Seatrace) p 1881
Adalan Lanatabs (Lannett)
Adapettes (Alcon Lens Care)
◆ **Adapin** (Pennwalt) p 425, 1548
Adatuss DC Expectorant Cough Syrup (Mastar) p 1185
◆ **Adeflor Chewable Tablets** (Upjohn) p 439, 2029
Adeflor Drops (Upjohn) p 2029
Adeflor M Tablets (Upjohn)
Adeno Injectable (O'Neal, Jones & Feldman) p 1421
Adenosine (Legere) p 1099
◆ **Adipex-P Tablets** (Lemmon) p 416, 1099
Adipost Capsules (Ascher)
Adphen Tablets (Ferndale)
Adrenalin Chloride Solution, Injectable (Parke-Davis) p 1457
Adrenosem Injectable, Syrup & Tablets (Beecham Laboratories)
Adriamycin (Adria) p 564
Adrucil Injectable (Adria) p 565
Adsorbocarpine (Alcon Labs.)
Adsorbonac (Alcon Labs.)
Adsorbotear (Alcon Labs.)
Advance (Ross) p 1731
Aerohalor (Abbott)
Aerolate Liquid (Fleming) p 952
Aerolate Sr. & Jr. & III Capsules (Fleming) p 952
Aerolone Solution (Lilly) p 1108
Aerosan (Ulmer)
Aeroseb-Dex Topical Aerosol Spray (Herbert) p 995
Aeroseb-HC Topical Aerosol Spray (Herbert) p 996
Aerosporin Powder (Burroughs Wellcome) p 771
Affirmagen Reagent Red Blood Cells (Ortho Diagnostic)
▣ **Afrin Menthol Nasal Spray, 0.05%** (Schering)
▣ **Afrin Nasal Spray 0.05%** (Schering)
▣ **Afrin Nose Drops 0.05%** (Schering)
▣ **Afrin Pediatric Nose Drops 0.025%** (Schering)
◆ **Afrinol Repetabs Tablets Long-Acting Nasal Decongestant** (Schering) p 433
Agoral, Plain (Parke-Davis) p 1457
Agoral, Raspberry & Marshmallow Flavors (Parke-Davis) p 1457
A-hydroCort (Abbott) p 505
◆ **Akineton** (Knoll) p 414, 1038
Akne Drying Lotion (Alto)
Akne Kaps (Alto)
Akne pH Lotion (Alto)
Akrinol Cream (Schering)
Akshun Tablets (Seatrace)
Al-ay Tablets (Bowman)
Alba-3 Ointment (Bart)
Alba-Ce Liquid, Drops, Capsules (Bart)
Albacort Cream (Bart)
Albacort Injectable (Bart)
Alba-Dex Injectable, Liquid & Tablets (Bart)
Albadryl Injectable (Bart)
Albaform-HC Cream (Bart)
◆ **Albafort Injectable** (Bart) p 405, 660
Alba-Gyn Vaginal Cream (Bart)
Albalon Liquifilm ophthalmic solution (Allergan)
Albalon-A Liquifilm ophthalmic solution (Allergan)

(◆ Shown in Product Identification Section) (▣ Described in PDR For Nonprescription Drugs) (Products without page numbers are not described)

B

(◆ Shown in Product Identification Section) (▣ Described in PDR For Nonprescription Drugs) (Products without page numbers are not described)

C

D

(◆ Shown in Product Identification Section) (▣ Described in PDR For Nonprescription Drugs) (Products without page numbers are not described)

F

H

(◆ Shown in Product Identification Section) (▣ Described in PDR For Nonprescription Drugs) (Products without page numbers are not described)

Malatal (Mallard)
Malatal Elixir (Mallard)
Mallamint (Mallard)
Mallergan (Mallard)
Mallisol (Mallard)
Mallopress (Mallard)
Malotuss (Mallard)
Maltsupex (Wallace) p 2094
Mammol Ointment (Abbott)
◆ Mandelamine (Parke-Davis) p 423, 1513
Mandex Tablets (Vale)
Mandol (Lilly) p 1147
◆ Mangatrace (USV Pharmaceutical) p 439, 2021
Mantadil Cream (Burroughs Wellcome) p 804
◆ Maolate Tablets (Upjohn) p 440, 2058
◆ Marax Tablets & DF Syrup (Roerig) p 431, 1711
Marbec Tablets (Marlyn)
▣ Marblen Suspension Peach/Apricot (Fleming)
▣ Marblen Suspension Unflavored (Fleming)
▣ Marblen Tablets (Fleming)
Marcaine Hydrochloride (Breon) p 716
Marcaine Hydrochloride with Epinephrine 1:200,000 (Breon) p 716
MarEPA Capsules (Marin) p 1172
◆ Marezine (Burroughs Wellcome) p 408, 805
Marlyn Formula 50 (Marlyn) p 1184
Marlyn Prolonged Release Vitamins (Marlyn)
◆ Marplan Tablets (Roche) p 430, 1669
▣ Massé Breast Cream (Ortho Pharmaceutical)
Massengill Disposable Douche (Beecham Products) p 663
Massengill Disposable Medicated Douche (Beecham Products) p 664
Massengill Liquid Concentrate (Beecham Products) p 663
Massengill Powder (Beecham Products) p 663
Mastisol Liquid Adhesive (Ferndale)
◆ Materna 1•60 (Lederle) p 415, 1080
◆ Matulane Capsules (Roche) p 430, 1670
Maxifil Cream (CooperCare)
◆ Maxibolin (Organon) p 422
Maxidex Suspension & Ointment (Alcon Labs.)
Maxiflor Cream (Herbert) p 998
Maxiflor Ointment (Herbert) p 999
Maxigesic Capsules (Mastar) p 1185
Maxitrol Suspension & Ointment (Alcon Labs.)
◆ Mazanor (Wyeth) p 442, 2170
Measurin Tablets (Breon)
◆ Mebaral (Breon) p 407, 717
Meclan (Ortho Pharmaceutical (Dermatological Div.)) p 1451
◆ Meclizine HCl (Lederle) p 416
Meclizine HCl MLT Tablets (Schein) p 1782
Meclizine HCl Tablets (Geneva) p 977
◆ Meclomen (Parke-Davis) p 423, 1513
Medache (Organon)
◆ Mediatric Capsules, Tablets & Liquid (Ayerst) p 405, 633
Medicated Soft Touch (Sween) p 1985
▣ Medicone Dressing Cream (Medicone)
▣ Mediconet (Medicone)
Medigesic Plus Capsules (U.S. Chemical) p 2012
Medihaler Ergotamine Aerosol (Riker) p 1614
Medihaler-Epi (Riker) p 1614
Medihaler-Iso (Riker) p 1614
Mediplex Tabules (U.S. Chemical) p 2012
Medispray (Medical Products)
Medi-Tec 90 Therapeutic Conditioner with Strengthening Agents (Robertson/Taylor) p 1619
Medi-Tec 90 Therapeutic Scalp Stimulant with Strengthening Agents (Robertson/Taylor) p 1619
Medi-Tec 90 Therapeutic Shampoo & Scalp Conditioner with Strengthening Agents (Robertson/Taylor) p 1620
Medizinc Scored Tablets (U.S. Chemical) p 2012
Medotopes (Squibb) p 3028
Medrol Acetate Topical (Upjohn) p 2058
Medrol Enpak Kit (Upjohn)
◆ Medrol Dosepak Unit of Use (Upjohn) p 440
◆ Medrol Tablets (Upjohn) p 440, 2058
Mefoxin (Merck Sharp & Dohme) p 1314
Mega-B (Arco) p 588
Megabee (Wesley)
◆ Megace Tablets (Mead Johnson Pharmaceutical) p 419, 1224
Megadose (Arco) p 588
Megaplex Tablets (Legere)
Mega-Vita Tablets (Saron) p 1778
Mega-Vita Hematinic (Saron)
Mega-Vita Tonic (Saron)
◆ Melfiat Tablets (Reid-Provident) p 427, 1606
◆ Melfiat 105 Unicelles (Reid-Provident) p 427, 1606
◆ Mellaril (Sandoz) p 432, 1766
Mellaril-S (Sandoz) p 1766
Menadione Tablets (Lilly)
Menaval-10 (Legere)
Menaval 20 (Legere) p 1099
Menest Tablets (Beecham Laboratories)
Meningovax-AC (Merck Sharp & Dohme)
Menoject-LA (Mayrand)
Menomune (Meningococcal Polysaccharide Vaccine, Groups A,C,Y,W-135 Combined, Groups A & C Combined, Group A or Group C) (Connaught Laboratories, Inc.) p 877
◆ Menrium Tablets (Roche) p 430, 1671
◆ Mepergan Fortis Capsules (Wyeth) p 442
Mepergan Injection (Wyeth) p 2171
Meperidine HCl in Tubex (Wyeth) p 2192
Meperidine HCl Injection (Elkins-Sinn) p 926
Mephyton Tablets (Merck Sharp & Dohme)
Mepred-40 (Savage)
Mepred-80 (Savage)
Mepriam Tablets (Lemmon)
Mepro Compound Tablets (Schein) p 1782
Meprobamate Tablets (Danbury) p 883
Meprobamate Tablets (Geneva) p 977
Meprobamate Tablets (Schein) p 1782
Meprobamate Tablets (Steri-Med) p 1975
Meprospan (Wallace) p 2094
Mequin (Lemmon)
Mercodol Cough Syrup w/Decapryn (Merrell Dow)
Mercresin Tincture (Upjohn)
Merculyn (Wesley)
Merthiolate, Aeropump, Cream, Glycerite, Ophthalmic Ointment, Powder, Solution & Tincture (Lilly)
Meruvax$_{II}$ (Merck Sharp & Dohme) p 1317
◆ Mesantoin (Sandoz) p 432, 1767
Mestinon Injectable (Roche) p 1675
Mestinon Syrup (Roche) p 1676
◆ Mestinon Tablets (Roche) p 430, 1676
◆ Mestinon Timespan Tablets (Roche) p 430, 1676
Metabol (Wesley)
◆ Metahydrin (Merrell Dow) p 421, 1356
Metamucil, Instant Mix (Searle Consumer Products) p 1859
Metamucil, Orange Flavor (Searle Consumer Products) p 1859
Metamucil, Orange Flavor Instant Mix (Searle Consumer Products) p 1859
Metamucil Powder (Searle Consumer Products) p 1859
◆ Metandren Linquets & Tablets (CIBA) p 409, 856
Metaprel Inhalant Solution 5% (Dorsey Pharmaceuticals) p 911
Metaprel Metered Dose Inhaler (Dorsey Pharmaceuticals) p 910
◆ Metaprel Syrup/Tablets (Dorsey Pharmaceuticals) p 410, 910
Metaraminol Bitartrate Injection (Bristol) p 735
Metaraminol Bitartrate Injection (Elkins-Sinn) p 926
◆ Metatensin (Merrell Dow) p 421, 1357
Meted Shampoo (CooperCare)
◆ Methadone Hydrochloride Diskets (Lilly) p 417, 1150
Methadone Hydrochloride Oral Solution (Roxane) p 1757
Methamphetamine Hydrochloride, 5mg. & 10mg. (Obetrol) p 1421
Methenamine Mandelate Forte Suspension & Tablets (Schein) p 1782
◆ Methergine (Sandoz) p 432, 1768
Methiokap Capsules (Vale)
Methischol Capsules (USV Pharmaceutical)
Methocarbamol Tablets (American Pharmaceutical) p 587
Methocarbamol Tablets (Danbury) p 883
Methocarbamol Tablets (Geneva) p 977
Methocarbamol Tablets (Schein) p 1782
Methocarbamol with Aspirin Tablets (Schein) p 1782
Metho-500 (Mallard)
◆ Methotrexate Tablets & Parenteral (Lederle) p 415, 1080
Methyclothiazide Tablets (Schein) p 1782
Methylene Blue Injection (Elkins-Sinn) p 926
Methylpred-40 Injection (Seatrace)
Methylprednisolone Tablets (Schein) p 1782
Methylprednisolone Sodium Succinate for Injection (Elkins-Sinn) p 926
Meticortelone Acetate Aqueous Suspension (Schering)
◆ Meticorten Tablets (Schering) p 433
Meti-Derm Cream 0.5% (Schering)
Metimyd Ophthalmic Ointment - Sterile (Schering) p 1813
Metimyd Ophthalmic Suspension (Schering) p 1813
◆ Metopirone (CIBA) p 409, 857
Metra Tablets (O'Neal, Jones & Feldman)
Metrazol Injection (Knoll)
Metrazol Liquidum (Knoll)
Metrazol Tablets (Knoll)
Metreton Ophthalmic/Otic Solution-Sterile (Schering) p 1814
Metronidazole Oral Tablets (Schein) p 1782
Metronidazole Tablets (Danbury) p 883
Metronidazole Tablets (Geneva) p 977
◆ Metryl (Lemmon) p 416, 1100
Metubine Iodide (Lilly) p 1152
Metycaine Hydrochloride Vials & Powder (Lilly)
Mevanin-C Capsules (Beutlich) p 678
Mevatinic-C Tablets (Beutlich)
Mexate (Bristol) p 745
Mezlin (Miles Pharmaceuticals) p 1388
Mi-Cebrin (Dista) p 898
Mi-Cebrin T (Dista) p 898
◆ Micrainin (Wallace) p 441
MICRhoGAM (Ortho Diagnostic) p 1432
Microcort Lotion (Alto)
Microcult-GC (Ames) p 3005
Micro-Guard (Sween) p 1985
◆ Micro-K Extencaps (Robins) p 428, 1628
▣ Microlipid (Organon)
◆ Micronor Tablets (Ortho Pharmaceutical) p 422, 1440
Microstix-Candida (Ames) p 3005
Microstix-Nitrite (Ames) p 3006
Microstix-3 (Ames) p 3005
Microsul Tablets (Star) p 1975
Microsul-A (Star) p 1975
◆ Midamor Tablets (Merck Sharp & Dohme) p 420, 1318
Midol (Glenbrook) p 991
◆ Midrin Capsules (Carnrick) p 408, 832
Migralam Capsules (Lambda) p 1054
▣ Miles Nervine Nighttime Sleep-Aid (Miles Laboratories)
Milk of Magnesia, Milk of Magnesia-Concentrated (Roxane) p 1755
Milk of Magnesia-Cascara Suspension Concentrated (Roxane) p 1755
Milk of Magnesia-Mineral Oil Emulsion & Emulsion (Flavored) (Roxane) p 1755
Milkinol (Kremers-Urban) p 1052
◆ Milontin Kapseals (Parke-Davis) p 423, 1515
◆ Milpath (Wallace) p 441, 2095
Milprem Tablets (Wallace)
◆ Miltown (Wallace) p 441, 2097
◆ Miltown 600 (Wallace) p 441, 2097
Miltrate Tablets (Wallace)
▣ Mineral Oil Jelly (Almay)
Mineral Oil-Light Sterile, Mineral Oil (Roxane) p 1755
Mini-Gamulin Rh (Armour) p 598
◆ Minipress (Pfizer) p 425, 1576
Minit-Rub analgesic balm (Bristol-Myers)
◆ Minizide Capsules (Pfizer) p 426, 1577
◆ Minocin (Lederle) p 415, 1083
Minro-Plex (Mallard)
◆ Mintezol Chewable Tablets & Suspension (Merck Sharp & Dohme) p 420, 1320
Miochol Intraocular (CooperVision)
MiraSol (CooperVision)
Mission Prenatal (Mission) p 1400
Mission Prenatal F.A. (Mission) p 1400
Mission Prenatal H.P. (Mission) p 1400
Mission Pre-Surgical (Mission) p 1400
Mithracin (Miles Pharmaceuticals) p 1391
◆ Mitrolan (Robins) p 428, 1629
Mity-Mycin Ointment (Reid-Provident)
Mity-Quin Cream (Reid-Provident)
Mixtard (Nordisk-USA) p 1405
◆ Moban Tablets & Concentrate (Endo Pharmaceuticals) p 410, 934
Mobidin Tablets (Ascher)
▣ Mobigesic Tablets (Ascher)
▣ Mobisyl Creme (Ascher)
Modane Bulk (Adria) p 573
Modane Plus (Adria) p 575
Modane Soft (Adria) p 573
Modane, Tablets & Liquid (Adria) p 574
◆ Moderil (Pfizer) p 426, 1579
◆ Modicon 21 Tablets (Ortho Pharmaceutical) p 422, 1440
Modicon 28 Tablets (Ortho Pharmaceutical) p 1440
▣ Moducal (Mead Johnson Nutritional)
◆ Moduretic Tablets (Merck Sharp & Dohme) p 420, 1321
▣ Moisture Rich Lipstick (creams & frosts) (Almay)
▣ Moisturizing Eye Makeup Remover Pads (Almay)
◆ Mol-Iron Chronosule Capsules (Schering) p 433
▣ Mol-Iron Liquid (Schering)
◆ Mol-Iron Tablets (Schering) p 433
◆ Mol-Iron Tablets w/Vitamin C (Schering) p 433
◆ Mol-Iron w/Vitamin C Tablets (Schering) p 433
Monistat-Derm (miconazole nitrate) Cream & Lotion (Ortho Pharmaceutical (Dermatological Div.)) p 1452
◆ Monistat I.V. (Janssen) p 413, 1026
Monistat 7 Vaginal Cream (Ortho Pharmaceutical) p 1436
Monistat 7 Vaginal Suppositories (Ortho Pharmaceutical) p 1436
Monospot Slide Test for Infectious Mononucleosis (Ortho Diagnostic)
Mono-Vacc (Merieux) p 1344
Monotard (Squibb) p 1934
Morphine Sulfate Carpuject (Winthrop)
Morphine Sulfate Injection (Elkins-Sinn) p 926
Morphine Sulfate Oral Solution (Roxane) p 1758
Morphine Sulfate Tablets (Roxane) p 1758
Morphine Sulfate in Tubex (Wyeth) p 2192
◆ Motrin Tablets•• (Upjohn) p 440, 2060
Movicol (Norgine) p 1406
Moxam Vials (Lilly) p 1153
Mucilose Flakes & Granules ((Consumer Products Division) (Winthrop))
Mucomyst (Mead Johnson Pharmaceutical) p 1225
Mucomyst with Isoproterenol (Mead Johnson Pharmaceutical) p 1226
Mudrane GG Elixir (Poythress) p 1592
◆ Mudrane GG Tablets (Poythress) p 426, 1592
◆ Mudrane GG-2 Tablets (Poythress) p 426, 1592

N

(◆ Shown in Product Identification Section) (◘ Described in PDR For Nonprescription Drugs) (Products without page numbers are not described)

O

Q

R

(◆ Shown in Product Identification Section) (▣ Described in PDR For Nonprescription Drugs) (Products without page numbers are not described)

S

U

V

W

X

Y

Z

Discontinued Products

A list, supplied to us by manufacturers, of products discontinued this past year.

Part 2

A-M-T (Wyeth)
Acticort Lotion 25 (Baker/Cummins)
Adroyal (Parke-Davis)
Aerosporin Otic Solution (Burroughs Wellcome)
Aminobrain-PT (Medical Prods. Panamerica)
Aridose (Savage)
Athrombin-K (Purdue Frederick)
Atoximetin-B Inj. (Medical Products Panamerica)
Azo-Mandelamine (Parke-Davis)
Belladonna Alkaloids w/Phenobarbital 16.2 mg. (Danbury)
Benadryl w/Epinephrine Sulfate Kapseals (Parke-Davis)
Betadine Vaginal Gel (Purdue Frederick)
Bisacodyl Tabs., USP, 5 mg. (Lederle)
Buren (Improved) (Asher)
Camphorated Tincture of Opium (Paregoric) (Parke-Davis)
Capsolin (Parke-Davis)
Carbrital (Parke-Davis)
Cascara Aromatic Fluidextract (Parke-Davis)
Cas-Evac (Parke-Davis)
Cerebid-300 mg. TD (Saron)
Cerebro-Nicin (Brown)
Chloral Hydrate Caps., USP, 500 mg. (Lederle)
Cobalamed-100 U.S. Chemical)
Cobalamen-1000 (U.S. Chemical)
Co-Gel (Ulmer)
Coricidin Children's Cough Syrup (Schering)
Danbade T.D. (Danbury)
Declostatin for Oral Use (Lederle)
Decongestcaps (Ulmer)
Dianabol (CIBA)
Duo-Dezone (Tutag Direct)
Dyclone 0.5%, 1% (Merrell Dow)
Erythromycin Ethylsuccinate Oral Susp. (Parke-Davis)
Febrigesic (Seatrace)
Feminins (Mead Johnson Nutritional)
Flexical (Mead Johnson Nutritional)
G-B Prep Emulsion (Gray)
Gentamicin Sulfate Injection (Wyeth)
Gentamicin Sulfate Injection, Pediatric (Wyeth)
Geritag (Tutag Direct)
Glucotropin-Forte (U.S. Chemical)
Hetrazan (Lederle)
Imodium (Ortho Pharmaceutical)
Ketochol (Searle Laboratories)
Lidosporin Otic (Burroughs Wellcome)
Meclizine HCl (Lederle)
Menic (Geriatric)
Meni-D (Seatrace)
Meperidine HCl (Parke-Davis)
Meprobamate 200 mg., 400 mg. (Lederle)
Meprobamate (Tutag Direct)
Migral (Burroughs Wellcome)
Miradon (Schering)
Mol-Iron w/Vit. C. Chronosule Caps. (Schering)
Mulvitab (Reid-Provident)
Neopavrin Forte (Savage)
Nioric (Ascher)
Nu-Natal w/Fluoride (Marlyn)
Omega-P.A. (U.S. Chemical)
Otomedic (Medical Products Panamerica)
PBZ Expectorant w/Epinephrine (Geigy)
Pan Ultra Sun Lotion, Stick (Baker/Cummins)
Peritrate w/Phenobarbital (Parke-Davis)
Peritrate w/Phenobarbital Sustained Action (Parke-Davis)
Pheneen Sanitizer (Ulmer)
Pheneen Solution N.R.I. (Ulmer)
Phenoxene (Merrell Dow)
Phenylpropanolamine HCl T.D. Caps (Geneva Generics)
Phenytoin Sodium Caps, USP, 100 mg. (Lederle)
Polysorbin (Reid-Provident)
Polysorbin-F (Reid-Provident)
Povan Suspension (Parke-Davis)
Prantal (Schering)
Prednisone 1 mg. Tablets (Geneva Generics)
Pre-Sate (Parke-Davis)
Probilagol (Purdue Frederick)
Proct-Kit (Parke-Davis)
Proprion Gel (Wyeth)
Proternol (Key)
Prov-U-Sep (Reid-Provident)
Prov-U-Sep Forte (Reid-Provident)
Reserpine Tabs, USP, 0.25 mg. (Lederle)
Repro Compound-65 (Reid-Provident)
Rhulihist (Lederle)
Robalate (Robins)
Robamox (Robins)
Robitet Syrup (Robins)
Rondec w/Hydrocodone (Ross)
Ruc-Dane (Boots)
Ru-Hy-T (Boots)
Ru-K-N (Boots)
Ru-Lor-N (Boots)

Senokot w/Psyllium (Purdue Frederick)
Setamine (Tutag Direct)
Sodestrin (Tutag Direct)
Sodestrin-H (Tutag Direct)
Spalix (Reid-Provident)
Spanestrin P (Savage)
Supertah (Purdue Frederick)
Surg-C (Saron)
Symptom 1, 2, 3 and Multi-Symptom (Parke-Davis)

Taka-Combex Kapseals (Parke-Davis)
Tenax (Reid-Provident)
Theo-Nar 200 (Key)
Therapads (Parke-Davis)
Therapads Plus (Parke-Davis)
Thiamine HCl Inj. (Parke-Davis)
Thyroid Tabs., USP, 200 mg. (Lederle)
Trisorbin (Reid-Provident)
Trisorbin F (Reid-Provident)
Trisureid (Reid-Provident)
Tucks Cream HC (Parke-Davis)

Uropeutic (Circle)

Valisone Topical Aerosol 0.15% w/w (Schering)
Verstat (Saron)
Verstran (Centrax Tablets) (Parke-Davis)
Vitamin B w B_{12}, Injection (Wyeth)
Voranil (USV)

Wellcortin (Burroughs Wellcome)

X-Prep Powder (Gray)

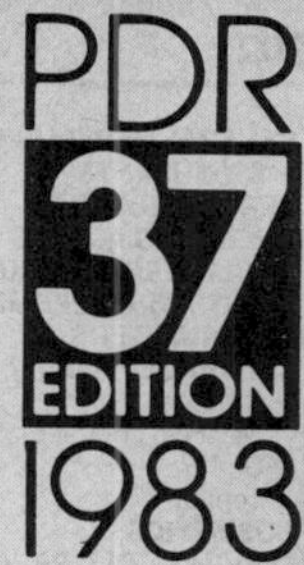

SECTION 3

Product Category Index

Products described in the Product Information (White) or Diagnostic Product Information (Green) Sections are listed according to their classifications. The headings and sub-headings have been determined by the Publisher with the cooperation of the individual manufacturers. In cases where there were differences of opinion or where the manufacturer had no opinion, the Publisher made the final decision. A QUICK-REFERENCE INDEX of headings and sub-headings can be found below.

Product Category Quick-Reference

Product Category Index

A

Urinary Antibacterial

Urinary Antibacterial with Analgesics

ANTIBIOTICS

Amebicides

Antifungal

Antituberculosis

Antiviral

Broad & Medium Spectrum

URICOSURIC AGENTS

Pediatric with Fluoride

Prenatal

Therapeutic

Other

X

X-RAY CONTRAST MEDIA

PDR 37 EDITION 1983

SECTION 4

Generic and Chemical Name Index

In this section the products described in the Product Information (White) and Diagnostic Product Information (Green) Sections are listed under generic and chemical name headings according to the principal ingredient(s). The headings under which products are listed have been determined by the Publisher with the cooperation of the individual manufacturers.

A

B

BCG Vaccine
BCG Vaccine (Glaxo) p 981

Bacampicillin Hydrochloride
Spectrobid Tablets & Oral Suspension (Roerig) p 431, 1716

Bacitracin
Bacitracin Ointment (American Pharmaceutical) p 587
Bacitracin Topical Ointment (Pfipharmecs) p 1556

Bacitracin Zinc
Cortisporin Ointment (Burroughs Wellcome) p 780
Cortisporin Ophthalmic Ointment (Burroughs Wellcome) p 780
Neo-Polycin (Merrell Dow) p 1358
Neosporin Aerosol (Burroughs Wellcome) p 808
Neosporin Ointment (Burroughs Wellcome) p 809
Neosporin Ointment Ophthalmic (Burroughs Wellcome) p 810
Neosporin Powder (Burroughs Wellcome) p 810
Polysporin Ointment (Burroughs Wellcome) p 811
Polysporin Ophthalmic Ointment (Burroughs Wellcome) p 811

Baclofen
Lioresal Tablets (Geigy) p 411, 963

BAL
BAL in Oil Ampules (Hynson, Westcott & Dunning) p 1013

Balsam Peru
Anusol Ointment (Parke-Davis) p 1461
Anusol Suppositories (Parke-Davis) p 422, 1461
Decubitex Ointment (I.C.P.) p 1015
Granulex (Hickam) p 999
Rectal Medicone-HC Suppositories (Medicone) p 419, 1242
Wyanoids HC Rectal Suppositories (Wyeth) p 443, 2197

Barbiturate Preparations
Alurate Elixir (Roche) p 1644
Buff-A Comp Tablets (Mayrand) p 1186
Buff-A Comp No. 3 Tablets (with Codeine) (Mayrand) p 1186
Donnatal Capsules (Robins) p 428, 1623
Donnatal Elixir (Robins) p 1623
Donnatal Extentabs (Robins) p 428, 1623
Donnatal Tablets (Robins) p 428, 1623
G-1 Capsules (Hauck) p 994
G-2 Capsules (Hauck) p 994
G-3 Capsules (Hauck) p 994
Kinesed Tablets (Stuart) p 438, 1978
Levsin/Phenobarbital Tablets, Elixir & Drops (Kremers-Urban) p 1051
Levsinex/Phenobarbital Timecaps (Kremers-Urban) p 1051
Lotusate Caplets (Winthrop) p 2128
Mebaral (Breon) p 407, 717
Nembutal Sodium Capsules (Abbott) p 403, 534
Nembutal Sodium Solution (Abbott) p 536
Nembutal Sodium Suppositories (Abbott) p 539
Plexonal (Sandoz) p 432, 1771
Repan Tablets (Everett) p 945

Barley Malt Extract
Maltsupex (Wallace) p 2094

Basic Fuchsin
Castellani Paint (Pedinol) p 1548

Beclomethasone Dipropionate
Beclovent Inhaler (Glaxo) p 412, 981
Beconase Nasal Inhaler (Glaxo) p 412, 983
Vancenase Nasal Inhaler (Schering) p 434, 1837
Vanceril Inhaler (Schering) p 434, 1838

Belladonna Ergotamine
Bellergal Tablets (Dorsey Pharmaceuticals) p 410, 908
Bellergal-S Tablets (Dorsey Pharmaceuticals) p 410, 908

Belladonna Extract
Chardonna-2 (Rorer) p 431, 1722

Belladonna Preparations
Belladenal & Belladenal-S (Sandoz) p 432, 1761
Bellermine-O.D. Capsules (Trimen) p 2011
Chardonna-2 (Rorer) p 431, 1722
Comhist LA Capsules (Norwich Eaton) p 1408
Donnagel (Robins) p 1622
Donnagel-PG (Robins) p 1622
Donnatal Capsules (Robins) p 428, 1623
Donnatal Elixir (Robins) p 1623
Donnatal Extentabs (Robins) p 428, 1623
Donnatal Tablets (Robins) p 428, 1623
Donnazyme Tablets (Robins) p 428, 1624
Kaolin, Pectin, Belladonna Mixture (Schein) p 1782
Kinesed Tablets (Stuart) p 438, 1978
Trac Tabs (Hyrex) p 1014
Trac Tabs 2X (Hyrex) p 1014
Wyanoids HC Rectal Suppositories (Wyeth) p 443, 2197

Benactyzine Hydrochloride
Deprol (Wallace) p 2089

Bendroflumethiazide
Naturetin Tablets (Squibb) p 437, 1944
Rauzide Tablets (Squibb) p 437, 1959

Benzalkonium Chloride
Amino-Cerv (Milex) p 1398
Cetylcide Solution (Cetylite) p 839
Florida Foam Improved (Hill Dermaceuticals) p 1000
Ivy-Chex (Non-Aerosol) (Bowman) p 698
Zephiran Chloride 1:750 (Winthrop) p 2141
Zephiran Chloride Spray (Winthrop) p 2141
Zephiran Chloride Tinted Tincture (Winthrop) p 2141

Benzethonium Chloride
Dalidyne (Dalin) p 882

Benzocaine
Auralgan Otic Solution (Ayerst) p 619
Cetacaine Topical Anesthetic (Cetylite) p 838
Children's Chloraseptic Lozenges (Norwich Eaton) p 1407
Dalidyne (Dalin) p 882
Derma Medicone-HC Ointment (Medicone) p 1241
Dermoplast Aerosol Spray (Ayerst) p 622
Dieutrim Capsules (Legere) p 1099
Formula 44 Cough Control Discs (Vicks Health Care) p 2079
Ger-O-Foam (Geriatric) p 979
Hurricaine Liquid 1/4cc Unit Dose (Beutlich) p 678
Hurricaine Oral, Topical Anesthetic Gel, Liquid, Spray (Beutlich) p 678
Orabase with Benzocaine Analgesic Oral Protective Paste (Hoyt) p 1010
Pazo Hemorrhoid Ointment/Suppositories (Bristol-Myers) p 769
Rectal Medicone-HC Suppositories (Medicone) p 419, 1242
Tympagesic Otic Solution (Adria) p 576
Vicks Cough Silencers Cough Drops (Vicks Health Care) p 2081
Vicks Formula 44 Cough Control Discs (Vicks Health Care) p 2079
Vicks Throat Lozenges (Vicks Health Care) p 2081
Wyanoids Hemorrhoidal Suppositories (Wyeth) p 443, 2197

Benzoic Acid
Trac Tabs (Hyrex) p 1014
Trac Tabs 2X (Hyrex) p 1014
Uretron D/S Tablets (Marin) p 1172

Benzonatate
Tessalon (Endo Pharmaceuticals) p 411, 943

Benzoyl Peroxide
5 Benzagel (5% benzoyl peroxide) & 10 Benzagel (10% benzoyl peroxide), Acne Gels, Microgel Formula (Dermik) p 884
Desquam-X 5 Gel (Westwood) p 2109
Desquam-X 10 Gel (Westwood) p 2109
Desquam-X Wash (Westwood) p 2110
Desquam-X 10 Wash (Westwood) p 2111
Fostex 5% Benzoyl Peroxide Gel (Westwood) p 2112
Fostex 10% Benzoyl Peroxide Cleansing Bar (Westwood) p 2112
Fostex 10% Benzoyl Peroxide Wash (Westwood) p 2112
Loroxide-HC Acne Lotion (Dermik) p 886
Persa-Gel 5% & 10% (Ortho Pharmaceutical (Dermatological Div.)) p 1452
Persa-Gel W 5% & 10% (Ortho Pharmaceutical (Dermatological Div.)) p 1452
Vanoxide-HC Acne Lotion (Dermik) p 886
Xerac BP5 & Xerac BP10 (Person & Covey) p 1555

Benzphetamine Hydrochloride
Didrex Tablets (Upjohn) p 440, 2047

Benzquinamide Hydrochloride
Emete-con (Roerig) p 1705

Benzthiazide
Aquatag (Reid-Provident, Direct Div.) p 1608
Aquex (LaSalle) p 1055
Exna Tablets (Robins) p 428, 1627
Hydrex Tablets (Trimen) p 2012

Benztropine Mesylate
Cogentin (Merck Sharp & Dohme) p 419, 1262

Benzylpenicilloyl-Polylysine
Pre-Pen (Kremers-Urban) p 1053

Beta-carotene
Solatene Capsules (Roche) p 430, 1685

Betaine Hydrochloride
Zypan Tablets (Standard Process) p 1975

Betamethasone
Celestone Syrup & Tablets (Schering) p 433, 1787

Betamethasone Acetate
Celestone Soluspan Suspension (Schering) p 1790

Betamethasone Benzoate
Benisone Gel/Cream/Lotion/Ointment (CooperCare) p 879
Uticort Cream, Gel, Lotion & Ointment (Parke-Davis) p 425, 1543

Betamethasone Dipropionate
Diprosone Cream 0.05% (Schering) p 1792
Diprosone Lotion 0.05% w/w (Schering) p 1792
Diprosone Ointment 0.05% (Schering) p 1792
Diprosone Topical Aerosol 0.1% w/w (Schering) p 1792

Betamethasone Sodium Phosphate
Celestone Phosphate Injection (Schering) p 1788
Celestone Soluspan Suspension (Schering) p 1790

Betamethasone Valerate
Valisone Cream 0.1% (Schering) p 1836
Valisone Lotion 0.1% (Schering) p 1836
Valisone Ointment 0.1% (Schering) p 1836
Valisone Reduced Strength Cream 0.01% (Schering) p 1836

Bethanechol Chloride
Bethanechol Chloride Tablets (Danbury) p 883
Duvoid (Norwich Eaton) p 1411
Myotonachol (Glenwood) p 412, 992
Urecholine (Merck Sharp & Dohme) p 420, 1342
Vesicholine (Star) p 1975

Bioflavonoids
Mevanin-C Capsules (Beutlich) p 678
Peridin-C (Beutlich) p 678

Biotin
Berocca Plus Tablets (Roche) p 429, 1654
Mega-B (Arco) p 588
Megadose (Arco) p 588

Biperiden
Akineton (Knoll) p 414, 1038

Bisacodyl
Bisacodyl Patient Pack, Suppositories, Tablets (Roxane) p 1755
Bisacodyl Suppositories (Geneva) p 977
Bisacodyl Tablets, Suppositories (American Pharmaceutical) p 587
Dulcolax Suppositories (Boehringer Ingelheim) p 406, 683
Dulcolax Tablets (Boehringer Ingelheim) p 406, 683
Evac-Q-Kwik (Adria) p 567
Fleet Bisacodyl Enema (Fleet) p 950
Fleet Prep Kits (Fleet) p 951

Bishydroxycoumarin (see under Dicumarol)

Bismuth Aluminate
Escot Capsules (Reid-Provident, Direct Div.) p 1608

Bismuth Oxyiodide
Wyanoids HC Rectal Suppositories (Wyeth) p 443, 2197
Wyanoids Hemorrhoidal Suppositories (Wyeth) p 443, 2197

C

Os-Cal Tablets (Marion) p 418, 1180
Os-Cal-Gesic Tablets (Marion) p 418, 1180

Calcium Pantothenate
Al-Vite (Drug Industries) p 915
B-C-Bid Capsules (Geriatric) p 979
Besta Capsules (Hauck) p 994
Eldercaps (Mayrand) p 1186
Hemo-Vite (Drug Industries) p 916
Megadose (Arco) p 588
Rovite (Rotex) p 1749
Therabid (Mission) p 1401

Calcium & Calcium-Phosphorus Preparations
Calphosan (Carlton) p 828
Calphosan B-12 (Carlton) p 828
Dical-D Capsules & Wafers (Abbott) p 514

Calcium Polycarbophil
Mitrolan (Robins) p 428, 1629

Camphor
Panalgesic (Poythress) p 1593
Sinex Decongestant Nasal Spray (Vicks Health Care) p 2080
Vaposteam (Vicks Health Care) p 2081
Vatronol Nose Drops (Vicks Health Care) p 2081
Vicks Inhaler (Vicks Health Care) p 2081
Vicks Sinex Decongestant Nasal Spray (Vicks Health Care) p 2080
Vicks Throat Lozenges (Vicks Health Care) p 2081
Vicks Vaporub (Vicks Health Care) p 2082
Vicks Vaposteam (Vicks Health Care) p 2081
Vicks Vatronol Nose Drops (Vicks Health Care) p 2081

Candicidin
Vanobid Vaginal Ointment (Merrell Dow) p 1378
Vanobid Vaginal Tablets (Merrell Dow) p 1378

Cantharidin
Cantharone (Seres) p 1882
Cantharone Plus (Seres) p 1882
Verr-Canth (C & M) p 827
Verrusol (C & M) p 828

Capreomycin Sulfate
Capastat Sulfate (Lilly) p 1114

Captopril
Capoten (Captopril Tablets) (Squibb) p 436, 1922

Caramiphen Edisylate
Rescaps-D T.D. Capsules (Geneva) p 977
Tuss-Ade Timed Capsules (Schein) p 1782
Tuss-Ornade Liquid (Smith Kline & French) p 1918
Tuss-Ornade Spansule Capsules (Smith Kline & French) p 436, 1919

Carbamazepine
Tegretol Chewable Tablets (Geigy) p 411, 971
Tegretol Tablets (Geigy) p 411, 971

Carbamide Peroxide
Ear Drops by Murine
See Murine Ear Wax Removal System/Murine Ear Drops (Abbott) p 514
Murine Ear Wax Removal System/Murine Ear Drops (Abbott) p 533
Proxigel (Reed & Carnrick) p 1605

Carbamide Preparations
Carmol HC Cream (Syntex) p 1997
Debrox Drops (Marion) p 1176
Gly-Oxide Liquid (Marion) p 1177

Carbarsone (Arsenic Derivative)
Carbarsone Capsules (Lilly) p 1115

Carbenicillin Disodium (see under Disodium Carbenicillin)

Carbenicillin Indanyl Sodium
Geocillin Tablets (Roerig) p 431, 1706

Carbetapentane Tannate
Rynatuss Tablets & Pediatric Suspension (Wallace) p 441, 2100

Carbidopa
Sinemet Tablets (Merck Sharp & Dohme) p 420, 1333

Carbinoxamine Maleate
Brexin Capsules & Liquid (Savage) p 432, 1778
Cardec DM Drops & Syrup (Schein) p 1782
Rondec Drops (Ross) p 1742
Rondec Syrup (Ross) p 1742
Rondec Tablet (Ross) p 432, 1742
Rondec-DM Drops (Ross) p 1741
Rondec-TR Tablet (Ross) p 432, 1742

Carbohydrates
Emetrol (Rorer) p 1723

Carbon Dioxide
Evac-Q-Kit (Adria) p 566

Carboxymethylcellulose Sodium
Dieutrim Capsules (Legere) p 1099

Carisoprodol
Carisoprodol Compound Tablets (Danbury) p 883
Carisoprodol Compound Tablets (Geneva) p 977
Carisoprodol Tablets (Danbury) p 883
Carisoprodol Tablets (Geneva) p 977
Soma (Wallace) p 441, 2101
Soma Compound (Wallace) p 441, 2101
Soma Compound w/Codeine (Wallace) p 441, 2102
Soprodol Compound Tablets (Schein) p 1782
Soprodol Tablets (Carisoprodol) (Schein) p 1782

Carmustine (BCNU)
BiCNU (Bristol) p 729

Casanthranol
DSS w/Casanthranol Capsules (Geneva) p 977
Dialose Plus Capsules (Stuart) p 438, 1977
Docusate Sodium with Casanthranol Capsules (Roxane) p 1755
Docusate Sodium with Casanthranol (D.S.S.) (Schein) p 1782
Peri-Colace (Mead Johnson Pharmaceutical) p 419, 1235

Cascara Sagrada
Aromatic Cascara Fluidextract (Roxane) p 1755
Milk of Magnesia-Cascara Suspension Concentrated (Roxane) p 1755
Peri-Colace (Mead Johnson Pharmaceutical) p 419, 1235

Castor Oil
Castor Oil, Castor Oil Favored (Roxane) p 1755
Decubitex Ointment (I.C.P.) p 1015
Fleet Flavored Castor Oil Emulsion (Fleet) p 951
Fleet Prep Kits (Fleet) p 951
Granulex (Hickam) p 999
Hydrisinol Creme & Lotion (Pedinol) p 1548
Neoloid (Lederle) p 1087

Cefaclor
Ceclor (Lilly) p 1116

Cefadroxil Monohydrate
Duricef (Mead Johnson Pharmaceutical) p 419, 1218
Ultracef Capsules, Tablets & Oral Suspension (Bristol) p 407, 764

Cefamandole Nafate
Mandol (Lilly) p 1147

Cefazolin Sodium
Ancef (Smith Kline & French) p 1888
Kefzol (Lilly) p 1145

Cefotaxime Sodium
Claforan (Hoechst-Roussel) p 1000

Cefoxitin Sodium
Mefoxin (Merck Sharp & Dohme) p 1314

Cellulase
Celluzyme Chewable Tablets (Dalin) p 882
Kanulase (Dorsey Laboratories) p 905
Tolerase Tablets (Marin) p 1172

Cellulolytic Enzyme
Arco-Lase (Arco) p 588
Arco-Lase Plus (Arco) p 588
Celluzyme Chewable Tablets (Dalin) p 882
Festal (Hoechst-Roussel) p 412, 1003
Festalan (Hoechst-Roussel) p 412, 1003
Gustase (Geriatric) p 979
Kutrase Capsules (Kremers-Urban) p 414, 1050
Ku-Zyme Capsules (Kremers-Urban) p 414, 1051

Cephalexin
Keflex Oral Preparations (Dista) p 410, 897

Cephalothin Sodium
Keflin, Neutral, Vials (Lilly) p 1143

Cephapirin Sodium
Cefadyl (Bristol) p 737

Cephradine
Anspor (Smith Kline & French) p 435, 1891
Velosef Capsules (Squibb) p 437, 1967
Velosef for Infusion (Sodium-Free) (Squibb) p 1968
Velosef for Injection (Squibb) p 1970
Velosef for Oral Suspension (Squibb) p 1967
Velosef Tablets (Squibb) p 437, 1967

Ceruletide diethylamine
Tymtran Injection (Adria) p 3003

Cervical Caps (Rubber)
Koro-Flex Arcing Spring Diaphragm (Youngs) p 2205
Koromex Coil Spring Diaphragm (Youngs) p 2205

Cetyl Dimethyl Ethyl Ammonium Bromide
Cetylcide Solution (Cetylite) p 839

Cetylpyridinium Chloride
Fungoid Creme & Solution (Pedinol) p 1548
Fungoid Tincture (Pedinol) p 1548
Sinex Decongestant Nasal Spray (Vicks Health Care) p 2080
Vicks Sinex Decongestant Nasal Spray (Vicks Health Care) p 2080
Vicks Throat Lozenges (Vicks Health Care) p 2081

Charcoal, Activated
Charcoal (Activated) USP in Liquid Base (Bowman) p 698
Charcoal-Antidose Suspension (U. S. Products) p 2013
Charcoal-Anti-Dote Powder (U. S. Products) p 2013

Chlophedianol Hydrochloride
Ulo Syrup (Riker) p 1619

Chloral Hydrate
Chloral Hydrate Capsules (Geneva) p 977
Chloral Hydrate Capsules, Syrup (Roxane) p 1755
Chloral Hydrate Capsules (Schein) p 1782
Noctec Capsules & Syrup (Squibb) p 437, 1945
SK-Chloral Hydrate Capsules (Smith Kline & French) p 1909

Chlorambucil
Leukeran (Burroughs Wellcome) p 408, 803

Chloramphenicol
Chloromycetin Cream, 1% (Parke-Davis) p 1465
Chloromycetin Kapseals (Parke-Davis) p 423, 1465
Chloromycetin Ophthalmic Ointment, 1% (Parke-Davis) p 1467
Chloromycetin Otic (Parke-Davis) p 1467
Chloromyxin (Parke-Davis) p 1471
Ophthochlor, 0.5% (Parke-Davis) p 424, 1530
Ophthocort (Parke-Davis) p 1530

Chloramphenicol Palmitate
Chloromycetin Palmitate (Parke-Davis) p 1468

Chloramphenicol Sodium Succinate
Chloromycetin Sodium Succinate (Parke-Davis) p 1469

Chlorcyclizine Hydrochloride
Mantadil Cream (Burroughs Wellcome) p 804

Chlordiazepoxide
Libritabs Tablets (Roche) p 430, 1698
Limbitrol Tablets (Roche) p 430, 1700
Menrium Tablets (Roche) p 430, 1671

Chlordiazepoxide Hydrochloride
A-Poxide (Abbott) p 403, 509
Chlordiazepoxide Capsules (Geneva) p 977
Chlordiazepoxide Hydrochloride Capsules (Roxane) p 1755
Chlordiazepoxide HCl Capsules (Schein) p 1782
Clipoxide Capsules (Schein) p 1782
Librax Capsules (Roche) p 429, 1697
Librium Capsules (Roche) p 430, 1698
Librium Injectable (Roche) p 1699
SK-Lygen Capsules (Smith Kline & French) p 1909

E

N

P

Q

R

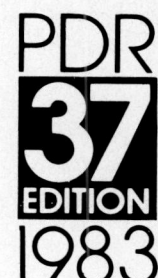

Product Identification Section

Designed to help you identify products, this section contains actual size, full-color reproductions selected for inclusion by participating manufacturers. Because tablets and capsules, for the most part, are shown here, you should not infer that these are the only dosage forms. Where other dosage forms are available, the product name is preceded by the † symbol. Refer to the product's description in the PRODUCT INFORMATION (White Section) or check directly with manufacturer.

While every effort has been made to reproduce products faithfully, this section should be considered only as a quick reference identification aid.

If overdosage is suspected, the user may wish to consult Guide to Management of Drug Overdose printed inside the back cover.

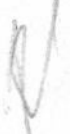

INDEX BY MANUFACTURER

This section is made possible through the courtesy of the manufacturers whose products appear on the following pages. Page numbers of individual products included can be found in the Product Name, Generic and Product Category Indices.

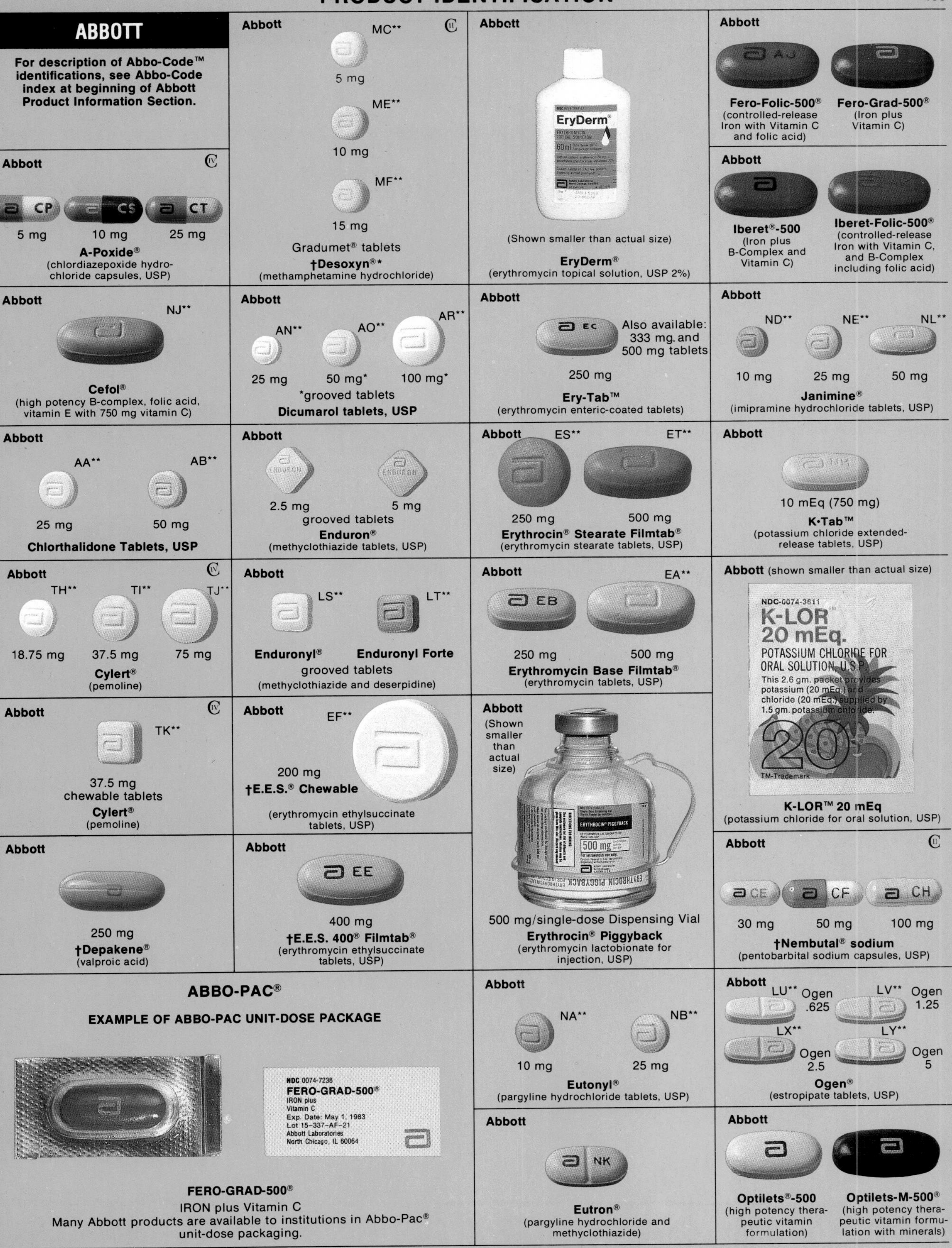

†Other dosage forms available. See Product Information section or check directly with manufacturer.
*Logo only may appear on tablet. **Abbott identification letters. ®Filmtab—Film-sealed tablets, Abbott.

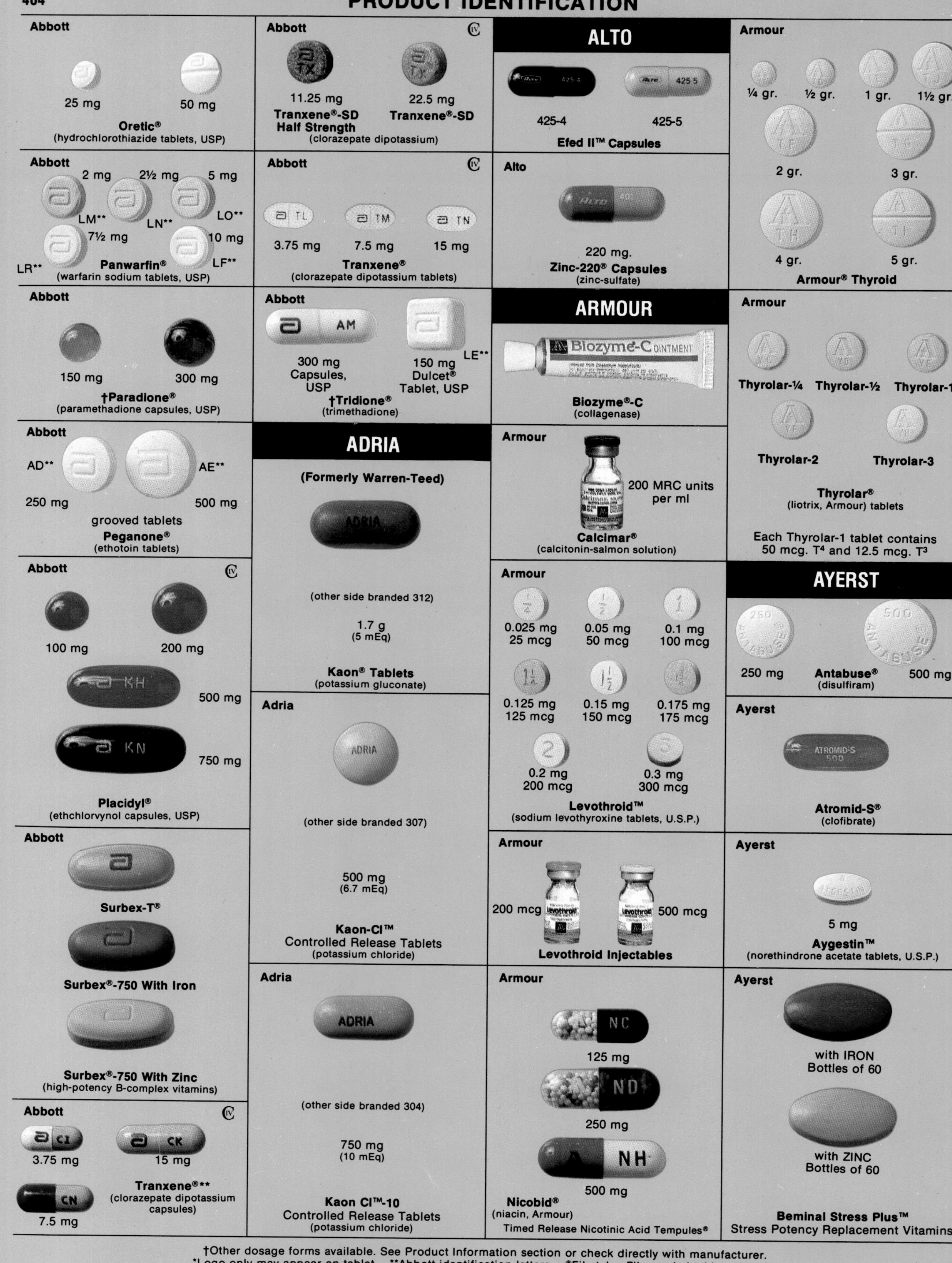
Abbott
25 mg
50 mg
Oretic®
(hydrochlorothiazide tablets, USP)
Abbott
2 mg
2½ mg
5 mg
LM**
LN**
LO**
7½ mg
10 mg
LR**
LF**
Panwarfin®
(warfarin sodium tablets, USP)
Abbott
150 mg
300 mg
†Paradione®
(paramethadione capsules, USP)
Abbott
AD**
AE**
250 mg
500 mg
grooved tablets
Peganone®
(ethotoin tablets)
Abbott
100 mg
200 mg
KH
500 mg
KN
750 mg
Placidyl®
(ethchlorvynol capsules, USP)
Abbott
Surbex-T®
Surbex®-750 With Iron
Surbex®-750 With Zinc
(high-potency B-complex vitamins)
Abbott
CI
3.75 mg
CK
15 mg
CN
7.5 mg
Tranxene®**
(clorazepate dipotassium capsules)
Abbott
TX
11.25 mg
Tranxene®-SD Half Strength
22.5 mg
Tranxene®-SD
(clorazepate dipotassium)
Abbott
TL
TM
TN
3.75 mg
7.5 mg
15 mg
Tranxene®
(clorazepate dipotassium tablets)
Abbott
AM
300 mg Capsules, USP
LE**
150 mg Dulcet® Tablet, USP
†Tridione®
(trimethadione)
ADRIA
(Formerly Warren-Teed)
ADRIA
(other side branded 312)
1.7 g
(5 mEq)
Kaon® Tablets
(potassium gluconate)
Adria
ADRIA
(other side branded 307)
500 mg
(6.7 mEq)
Kaon-Cl™
Controlled Release Tablets
(potassium chloride)
Adria
ADRIA
(other side branded 304)
750 mg
(10 mEq)
Kaon Cl™-10
Controlled Release Tablets
(potassium chloride)
ALTO
425-4
425-5
Efed II™ Capsules
Alto
ALTO
401
220 mg.
Zinc-220® Capsules
(zinc-sulfate)
ARMOUR
Biozyme-C OINTMENT
Biozyme®-C
(collagenase)
Armour
200 MRC units per ml
Calcimar®
(calcitonin-salmon solution)
Armour
0.025 mg 25 mcg
0.05 mg 50 mcg
0.1 mg 100 mcg
0.125 mg 125 mcg
0.15 mg 150 mcg
0.175 mg 175 mcg
0.2 mg 200 mcg
0.3 mg 300 mcg
Levothroid™
(sodium levothyroxine tablets, U.S.P.)
Armour
200 mcg
Levothroid
500 mcg
Levothroid Injectables
Armour
NC
125 mg
ND
250 mg
NH
500 mg
Nicobid®
(niacin, Armour)
Timed Release Nicotinic Acid Tempules®
Armour
¼ gr.
½ gr.
1 gr.
1½ gr.
2 gr.
3 gr.
4 gr.
5 gr.
Armour® Thyroid
Armour
Thyrolar-¼
Thyrolar-½
Thyrolar-1
Thyrolar-2
Thyrolar-3
Thyrolar®
(liotrix, Armour) tablets
Each Thyrolar-1 tablet contains 50 mcg. T4 and 12.5 mcg. T3
AYERST
250 ANTABUSE
500 ANTABUSE
250 mg
Antabuse®
(disulfiram)
500 mg
Ayerst
ATROMID-S 500
Atromid-S®
(clofibrate)
Ayerst
AYGESTIN
5 mg
Aygestin™
(norethindrone acetate tablets, U.S.P.)
Ayerst
with IRON
Bottles of 60
with ZINC
Bottles of 60
Beminal Stress Plus™
Stress Potency Replacement Vitamins

†Other dosage forms available. See Product Information section or check directly with manufacturer.
*Logo only may appear on tablet. **Abbott identification letters. ®Filmtab—Film-sealed tablets, Abbott.

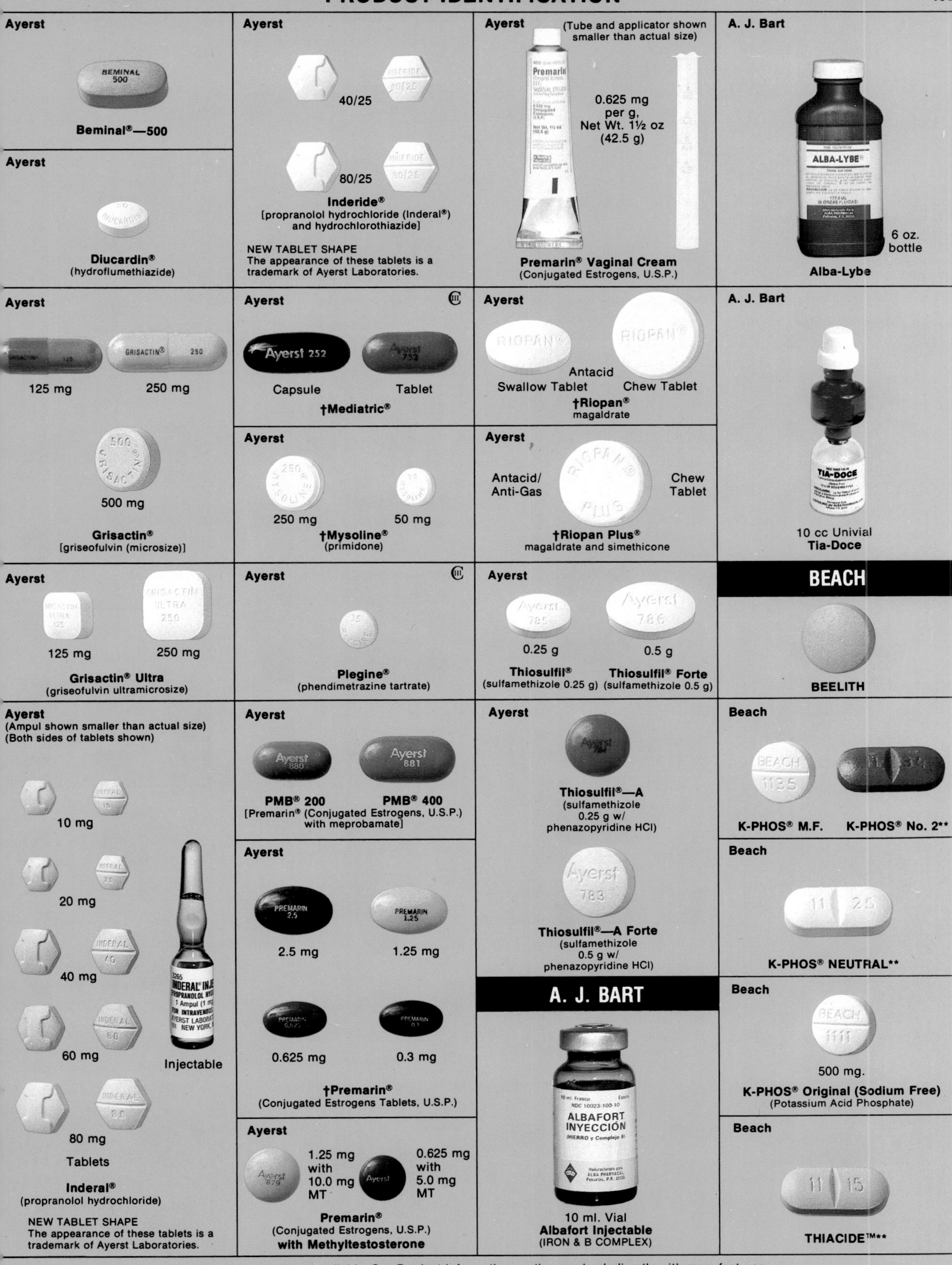

†Other dosage forms available. See Product Information section or check directly with manufacturer.
**The name BEACH appears on the reverse side of these tablets.

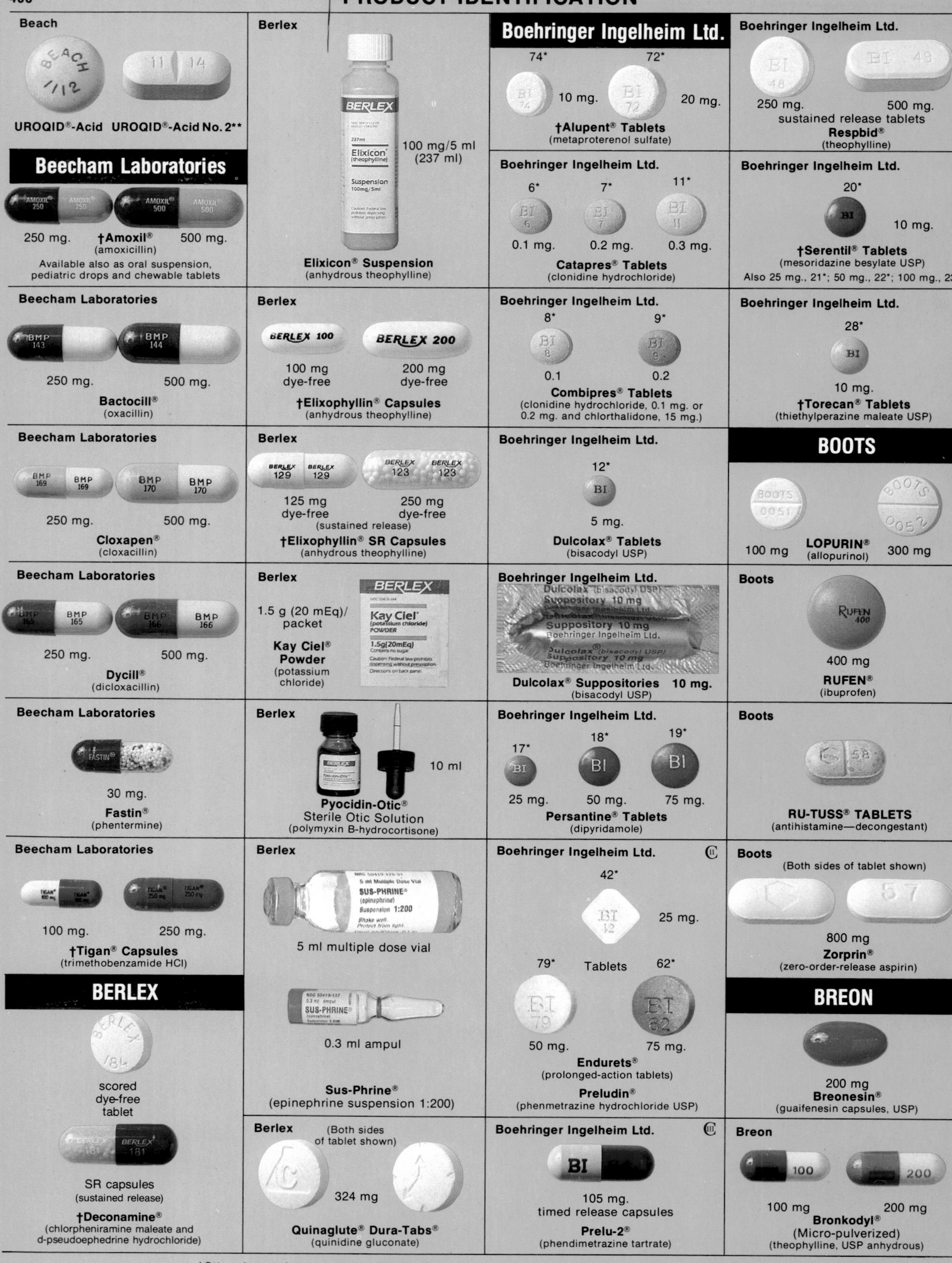

Beach

UROQID®-Acid UROQID®-Acid No. 2**

Beecham Laboratories

250 mg. †Amoxil® 500 mg.
(amoxicillin)
Available also as oral suspension, pediatric drops and chewable tablets

Beecham Laboratories

250 mg. 500 mg.
Bactocill®
(oxacillin)

Beecham Laboratories

250 mg. 500 mg.
Cloxapen®
(cloxacillin)

Beecham Laboratories

250 mg. 500 mg.
Dycill®
(dicloxacillin)

Beecham Laboratories

30 mg.
Fastin®
(phentermine)

Beecham Laboratories

100 mg. 250 mg.
†Tigan® Capsules
(trimethobenzamide HCl)

BERLEX

scored
dye-free
tablet

SR capsules
(sustained release)
†Deconamine®
(chlorpheniramine maleate and d-pseudoephedrine hydrochloride)

Berlex

100 mg/5 ml
(237 ml)
Elixicon® Suspension
(anhydrous theophylline)

Berlex

100 mg dye-free 200 mg dye-free
†Elixophyllin® Capsules
(anhydrous theophylline)

Berlex

125 mg dye-free 250 mg dye-free
(sustained release)
†Elixophyllin® SR Capsules
(anhydrous theophylline)

Berlex

1.5 g (20 mEq)/packet
Kay Ciel® Powder
(potassium chloride)

Berlex

10 ml
Pyocidin-Otic®
Sterile Otic Solution
(polymyxin B-hydrocortisone)

Berlex

5 ml multiple dose vial

0.3 ml ampul

Sus-Phrine®
(epinephrine suspension 1:200)

Berlex (Both sides of tablet shown)

324 mg
Quinaglute® Dura-Tabs®
(quinidine gluconate)

Boehringer Ingelheim Ltd.

74* 10 mg. 72* 20 mg.
†Alupent® Tablets
(metaproterenol sulfate)

Boehringer Ingelheim Ltd.

6* 0.1 mg. 7* 0.2 mg. 11* 0.3 mg.
Catapres® Tablets
(clonidine hydrochloride)

Boehringer Ingelheim Ltd.

8* 0.1 9* 0.2
Combipres® Tablets
(clonidine hydrochloride, 0.1 mg. or 0.2 mg. and chlorthalidone, 15 mg.)

Boehringer Ingelheim Ltd.

12*
5 mg.
Dulcolax® Tablets
(bisacodyl USP)

Boehringer Ingelheim Ltd.

Dulcolax® Suppositories 10 mg.
(bisacodyl USP)

Boehringer Ingelheim Ltd.

17* 25 mg. 18* 50 mg. 19* 75 mg.
Persantine® Tablets
(dipyridamole)

Boehringer Ingelheim Ltd. (C-II)

42* 25 mg.
Endurets®
(prolonged-action tablets)

Tablets
79* 50 mg. 62* 75 mg.
Preludin®
(phenmetrazine hydrochloride USP)

Boehringer Ingelheim Ltd. (C-III)

105 mg.
timed release capsules
Prelu-2®
(phendimetrazine tartrate)

Boehringer Ingelheim Ltd.

250 mg. 500 mg.
sustained release tablets
Respbid®
(theophylline)

Boehringer Ingelheim Ltd.

20* 10 mg.
†Serentil® Tablets
(mesoridazine besylate USP)
Also 25 mg., 21*; 50 mg., 22*; 100 mg., 23

Boehringer Ingelheim Ltd.

28*
10 mg.
†Torecan® Tablets
(thiethylperazine maleate USP)

BOOTS

100 mg LOPURIN® (allopurinol) 300 mg

Boots

400 mg
RUFEN®
(ibuprofen)

Boots

RU-TUSS® TABLETS
(antihistamine—decongestant)

Boots (Both sides of tablet shown)

800 mg
Zorprin®
(zero-order-release aspirin)

BREON

200 mg
Breonesin®
(guaifenesin capsules, USP)

Breon

100 mg 200 mg
Bronkodyl®
(Micro-pulverized)
(theophylline, USP anhydrous)

†Other dosage forms available. See Product Information section or check directly with manufacturer.
*Manufacturers' identification number.
**The name BEACH appears on the reverse side of these tablets.

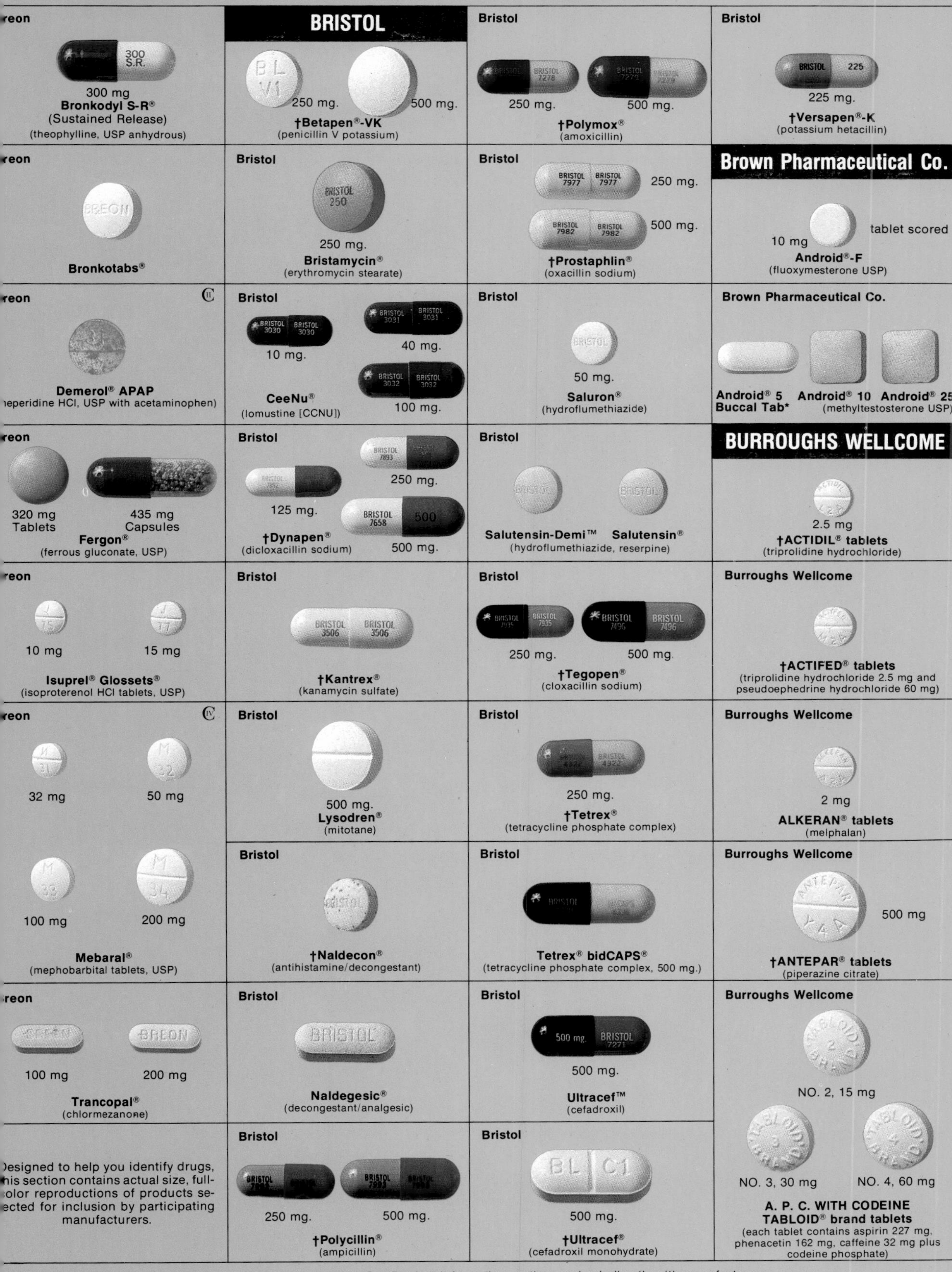

†Other dosage forms available. See Product Information section or check directly with manufacturer.

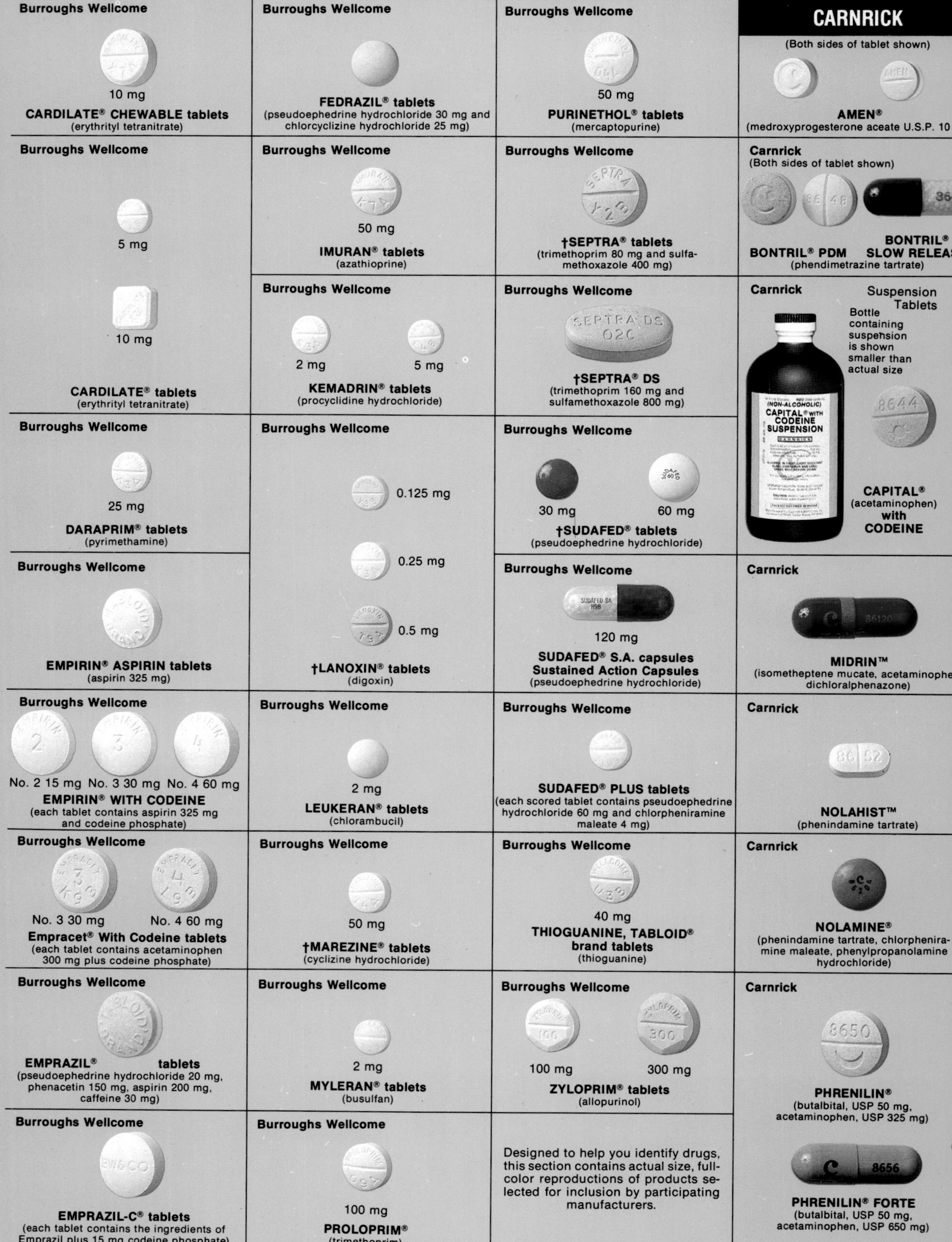

†Other dosage forms available. See Product Information section or check directly with manufacturer.

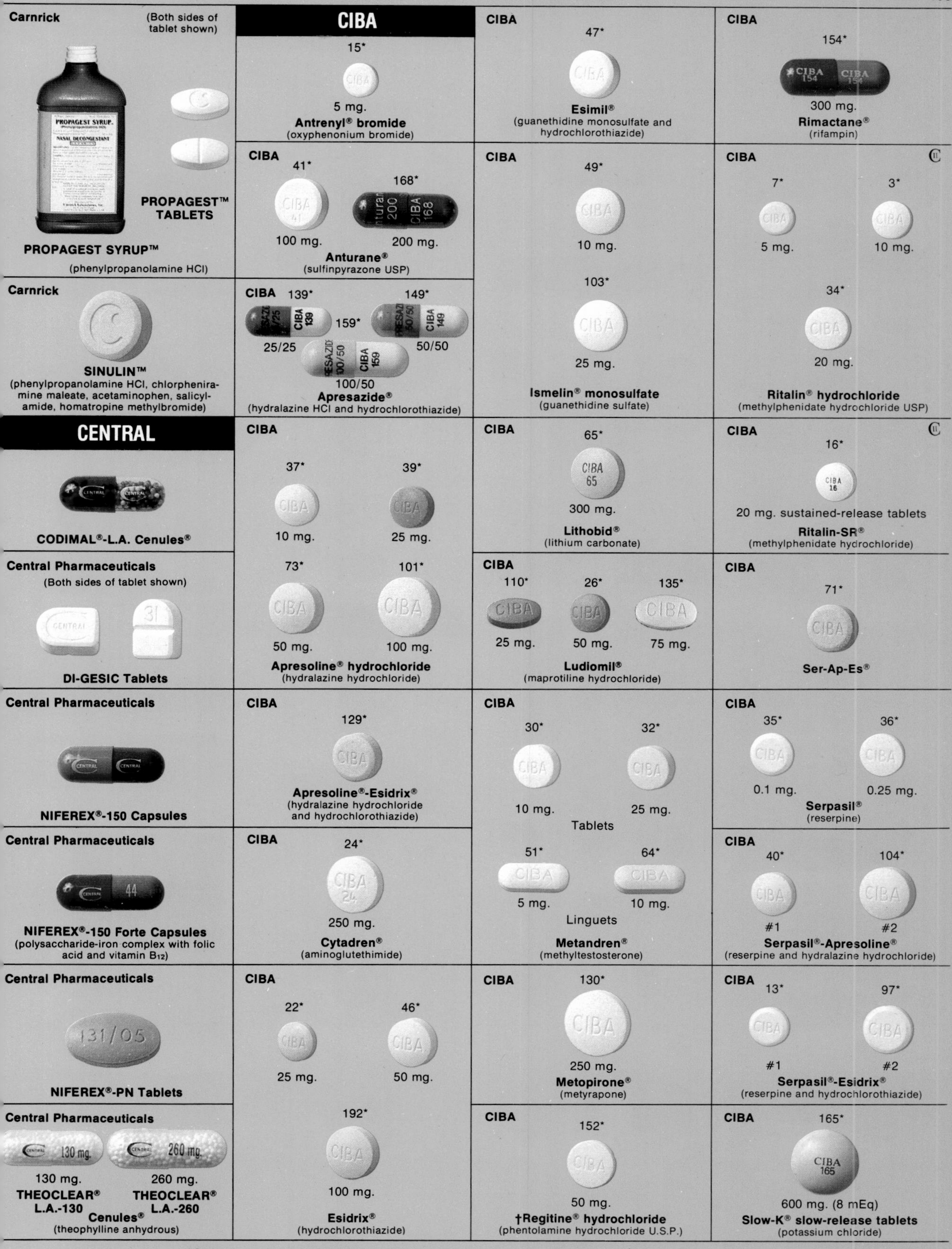

Carnrick (Both sides of tablet shown)

PROPAGEST™ TABLETS

PROPAGEST SYRUP™ (phenylpropanolamine HCl)

Carnrick

SINULIN™ (phenylpropanolamine HCl, chlorpheniramine maleate, acetaminophen, salicylamide, homatropine methylbromide)

CENTRAL

CODIMAL®-L.A. Cenules®

Central Pharmaceuticals (Both sides of tablet shown)

DI-GESIC Tablets

Central Pharmaceuticals

NIFEREX®-150 Capsules

Central Pharmaceuticals

NIFEREX®-150 Forte Capsules (polysaccharide-iron complex with folic acid and vitamin B_{12})

Central Pharmaceuticals

NIFEREX®-PN Tablets

Central Pharmaceuticals

130 mg. THEOCLEAR® L.A.-130 — 260 mg. THEOCLEAR® L.A.-260 Cenules® (theophylline anhydrous)

CIBA

15* 5 mg. **Antrenyl® bromide** (oxyphenonium bromide)

CIBA 41* 100 mg. 168* 200 mg. **Anturane®** (sulfinpyrazone USP)

CIBA 139* 25/25 159* 100/50 149* 50/50 **Apresazide®** (hydralazine HCl and hydrochlorothiazide)

CIBA 37* 10 mg. 39* 25 mg. 73* 50 mg. 101* 100 mg. **Apresoline® hydrochloride** (hydralazine hydrochloride)

CIBA 129* **Apresoline®-Esidrix®** (hydralazine hydrochloride and hydrochlorothiazide)

CIBA 24* 250 mg. **Cytadren®** (aminoglutethimide)

CIBA 22* 25 mg. 46* 50 mg. 192* 100 mg. **Esidrix®** (hydrochlorothiazide)

CIBA 47* **Esimil®** (guanethidine monosulfate and hydrochlorothiazide)

CIBA 49* 10 mg. 103* 25 mg. **Ismelin® monosulfate** (guanethidine sulfate)

CIBA 65* 300 mg. **Lithobid®** (lithium carbonate)

CIBA 110* 25 mg. 26* 50 mg. 135* 75 mg. **Ludiomil®** (maprotiline hydrochloride)

CIBA Tablets: 30* 10 mg. 32* 25 mg. Linguets: 51* 5 mg. 64* 10 mg. **Metandren®** (methyltestosterone)

CIBA 130* 250 mg. **Metopirone®** (metyrapone)

CIBA 152* 50 mg. **†Regitine® hydrochloride** (phentolamine hydrochloride U.S.P.)

CIBA 154* 300 mg. **Rimactane®** (rifampin)

CIBA Ⓒ 7* 5 mg. 3* 10 mg. 34* 20 mg. **Ritalin® hydrochloride** (methylphenidate hydrochloride USP)

CIBA Ⓒ 16* 20 mg. sustained-release tablets **Ritalin-SR®** (methylphenidate hydrochloride)

CIBA 71* **Ser-Ap-Es®**

CIBA 35* 0.1 mg. 36* 0.25 mg. **Serpasil®** (reserpine)

CIBA 40* #1 104* #2 **Serpasil®-Apresoline®** (reserpine and hydralazine hydrochloride)

CIBA 13* #1 97* #2 **Serpasil®-Esidrix®** (reserpine and hydrochlorothiazide)

CIBA 165* 600 mg. (8 mEq) **Slow-K® slow-release tablets** (potassium chloride)

†Other dosage forms available. See Product Information section or check directly with manufacturer.
*Manufacturers' identification number.

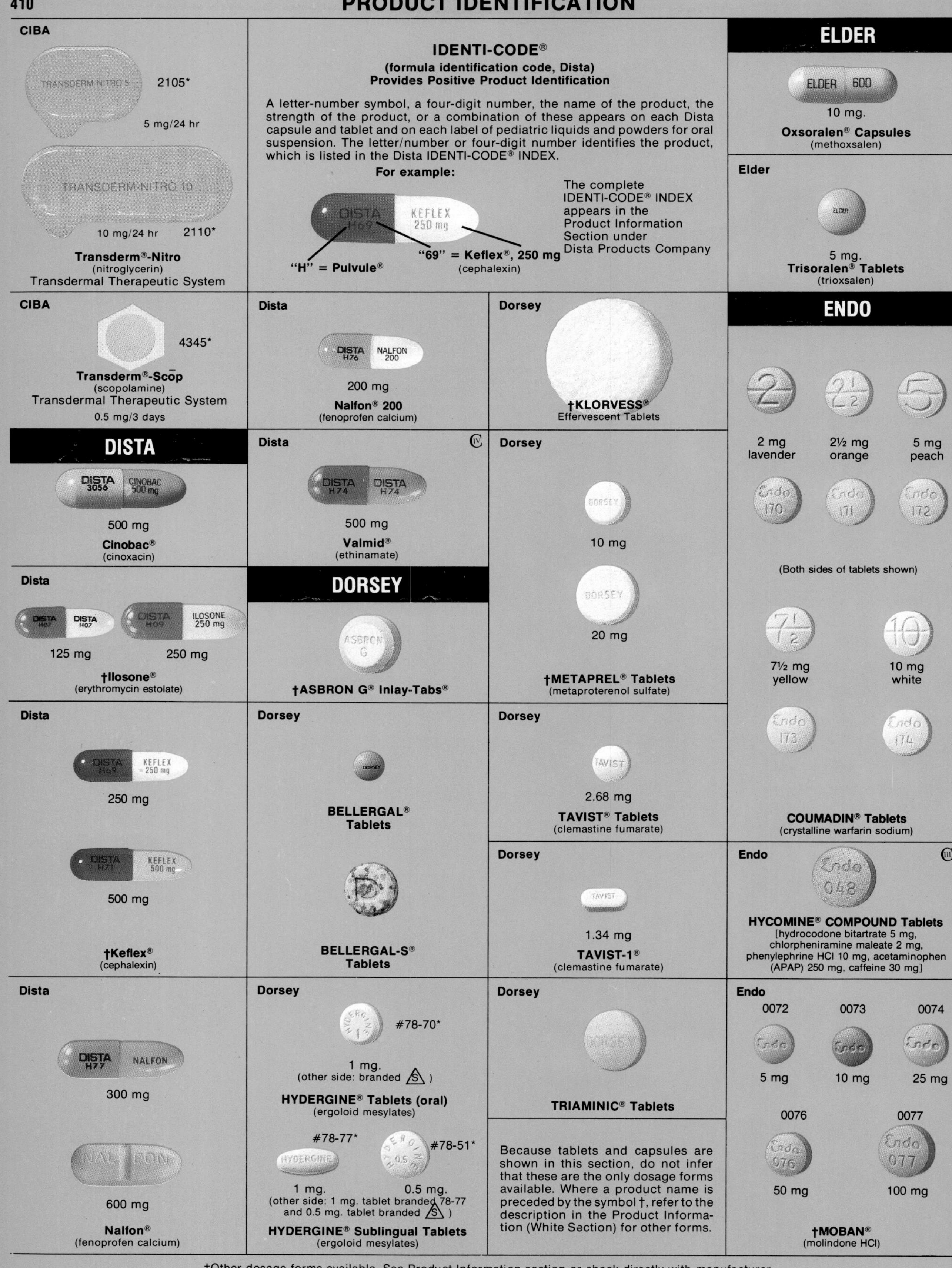
CIBA
TRANSDERM-NITRO 5
2105*
5 mg/24 hr
TRANSDERM-NITRO 10
10 mg/24 hr
2110*
Transderm®-Nitro
(nitroglycerin)
Transdermal Therapeutic System
IDENTI-CODE®
(formula identification code, Dista)
Provides Positive Product Identification
A letter-number symbol, a four-digit number, the name of the product, the strength of the product, or a combination of these appears on each Dista capsule and tablet and on each label of pediatric liquids and powders for oral suspension. The letter/number or four-digit number identifies the product, which is listed in the Dista IDENTI-CODE® INDEX.
For example:
DISTA H69
KEFLEX 250 mg
"H" = Pulvule®
"69" = Keflex®, 250 mg
(cephalexin)
The complete IDENTI-CODE® INDEX appears in the Product Information Section under Dista Products Company
ELDER
ELDER 600
10 mg.
Oxsoralen® Capsules
(methoxsalen)
Elder
ELDER
5 mg.
Trisoralen® Tablets
(trioxsalen)
CIBA
4345*
Transderm®-Scōp
(scopolamine)
Transdermal Therapeutic System
0.5 mg/3 days
Dista
DISTA H76
NALFON 200
200 mg
Nalfon® 200
(fenoprofen calcium)
Dorsey
†KLORVESS®
Effervescent Tablets
ENDO
2 mg
lavender
2½ mg
orange
5 mg
peach
Endo 170
Endo 171
Endo 172
(Both sides of tablets shown)
7½ mg
yellow
10 mg
white
Endo 173
Endo 174
COUMADIN® Tablets
(crystalline warfarin sodium)
DISTA
DISTA 3056
CINOBAC 500 mg
500 mg
Cinobac®
(cinoxacin)
Dista
DISTA H74
500 mg
Valmid®
(ethinamate)
Dorsey
DORSEY
10 mg
DORSEY
20 mg
†METAPREL® Tablets
(metaproterenol sulfate)
Dista
DISTA H07
125 mg
DISTA H09
ILOSONE 250 mg
250 mg
†Ilosone®
(erythromycin estolate)
DORSEY
ASBRON G
†ASBRON G® Inlay-Tabs®
Dista
DISTA H69
KEFLEX 250 mg
250 mg
DISTA H71
KEFLEX 500 mg
500 mg
†Keflex®
(cephalexin)
Dorsey
DORSEY
BELLERGAL® Tablets
BELLERGAL-S® Tablets
Dorsey
TAVIST
2.68 mg
TAVIST® Tablets
(clemastine fumarate)
Dorsey
TAVIST
1.34 mg
TAVIST-1®
(clemastine fumarate)
Endo
Endo 048
HYCOMINE® COMPOUND Tablets
[hydrocodone bitartrate 5 mg, chlorpheniramine maleate 2 mg, phenylephrine HCl 10 mg, acetaminophen (APAP) 250 mg, caffeine 30 mg]
Dista
DISTA H77
NALFON
300 mg
NAL FON
600 mg
Nalfon®
(fenoprofen calcium)
Dorsey
#78-70*
1 mg.
(other side: branded S)
HYDERGINE® Tablets (oral)
(ergoloid mesylates)
#78-77*
#78-51*
HYDERGINE
1 mg.
0.5 mg.
(other side: 1 mg. tablet branded 78-77 and 0.5 mg. tablet branded S)
HYDERGINE® Sublingual Tablets
(ergoloid mesylates)
Dorsey
DORSEY
TRIAMINIC® Tablets
Because tablets and capsules are shown in this section, do not infer that these are the only dosage forms available. Where a product name is preceded by the symbol †, refer to the description in the Product Information (White Section) for other forms.
Endo
0072
0073
0074
5 mg
10 mg
25 mg
0076
0077
Endo 076
Endo 077
50 mg
100 mg
†MOBAN®
(molindone HCl)

†Other dosage forms available. See Product Information section or check directly with manufacturer.
*Manufacturers' identification number.

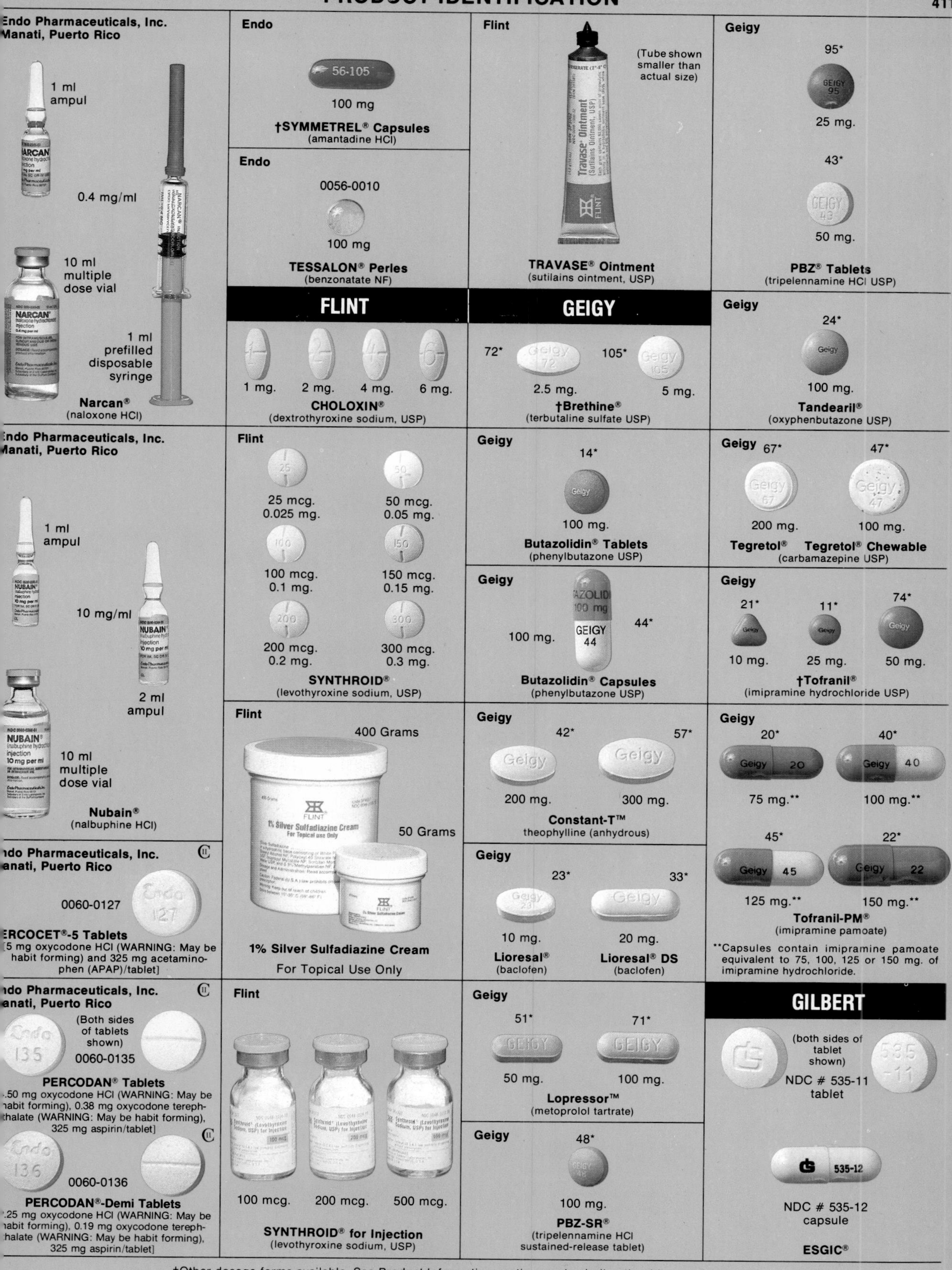
Endo Pharmaceuticals, Inc.
Manati, Puerto Rico
1 ml ampul
0.4 mg/ml
10 ml multiple dose vial
1 ml prefilled disposable syringe
Narcan®
(naloxone HCl)
Endo
56-105
100 mg
†SYMMETREL® Capsules
(amantadine HCl)
Endo
0056-0010
100 mg
TESSALON® Perles
(benzonatate NF)
Flint
(Tube shown smaller than actual size)
Travase® Ointment
TRAVASE® Ointment
(sutilains ointment, USP)
Geigy
95*
25 mg.
43*
50 mg.
PBZ® Tablets
(tripelennamine HCl USP)
FLINT
1 mg.
2 mg.
4 mg.
6 mg.
CHOLOXIN®
(dextrothyroxine sodium, USP)
GEIGY
72*
105*
2.5 mg.
5 mg.
†Brethine®
(terbutaline sulfate USP)
Geigy
24*
100 mg.
Tandearil®
(oxyphenbutazone USP)
Endo Pharmaceuticals, Inc.
Manati, Puerto Rico
1 ml ampul
10 mg/ml
2 ml ampul
10 ml multiple dose vial
Nubain®
(nalbuphine HCl)
Flint
25 mcg. 0.025 mg.
50 mcg. 0.05 mg.
100 mcg. 0.1 mg.
150 mcg. 0.15 mg.
200 mcg. 0.2 mg.
300 mcg. 0.3 mg.
SYNTHROID®
(levothyroxine sodium, USP)
Geigy
14*
100 mg.
Butazolidin® Tablets
(phenylbutazone USP)
Geigy 67*
47*
200 mg.
100 mg.
Tegretol®
Tegretol® Chewable
(carbamazepine USP)
Geigy
100 mg.
GEIGY 44
44*
Butazolidin® Capsules
(phenylbutazone USP)
Geigy
21*
11*
74*
10 mg.
25 mg.
50 mg.
†Tofranil®
(imipramine hydrochloride USP)
Flint
400 Grams
1% Silver Sulfadiazine Cream
For Topical use Only
50 Grams
1% Silver Sulfadiazine Cream
For Topical Use Only
Geigy
42*
57*
200 mg.
300 mg.
Constant-T™
theophylline (anhydrous)
Geigy
20*
40*
75 mg.**
100 mg.**
45*
22*
125 mg.**
150 mg.**
Tofranil-PM®
(imipramine pamoate)
**Capsules contain imipramine pamoate equivalent to 75, 100, 125 or 150 mg. of imipramine hydrochloride.
Endo Pharmaceuticals, Inc.
Manati, Puerto Rico
0060-0127
PERCOCET®-5 Tablets
[5 mg oxycodone HCl (WARNING: May be habit forming) and 325 mg acetaminophen (APAP)/tablet]
Geigy
23*
33*
10 mg.
20 mg.
Lioresal®
(baclofen)
Lioresal® DS
(baclofen)
Endo Pharmaceuticals, Inc.
Manati, Puerto Rico
(Both sides of tablets shown)
0060-0135
PERCODAN® Tablets
[4.50 mg oxycodone HCl (WARNING: May be habit forming), 0.38 mg oxycodone terephthalate (WARNING: May be habit forming), 325 mg aspirin/tablet]
0060-0136
PERCODAN®-Demi Tablets
[2.25 mg oxycodone HCl (WARNING: May be habit forming), 0.19 mg oxycodone terephthalate (WARNING: May be habit forming), 325 mg aspirin/tablet]
Flint
100 mcg.
200 mcg.
500 mcg.
SYNTHROID® for Injection
(levothyroxine sodium, USP)
Geigy
51*
71*
50 mg.
100 mg.
Lopressor™
(metoprolol tartrate)
Geigy
48*
100 mg.
PBZ-SR®
(tripelennamine HCl sustained-release tablet)
GILBERT
(both sides of tablet shown)
NDC # 535-11 tablet
535-12
NDC # 535-12 capsule
ESGIC®

†Other dosage forms available. See Product Information section or check directly with manufacturer.
*Manufacturers' identification number.

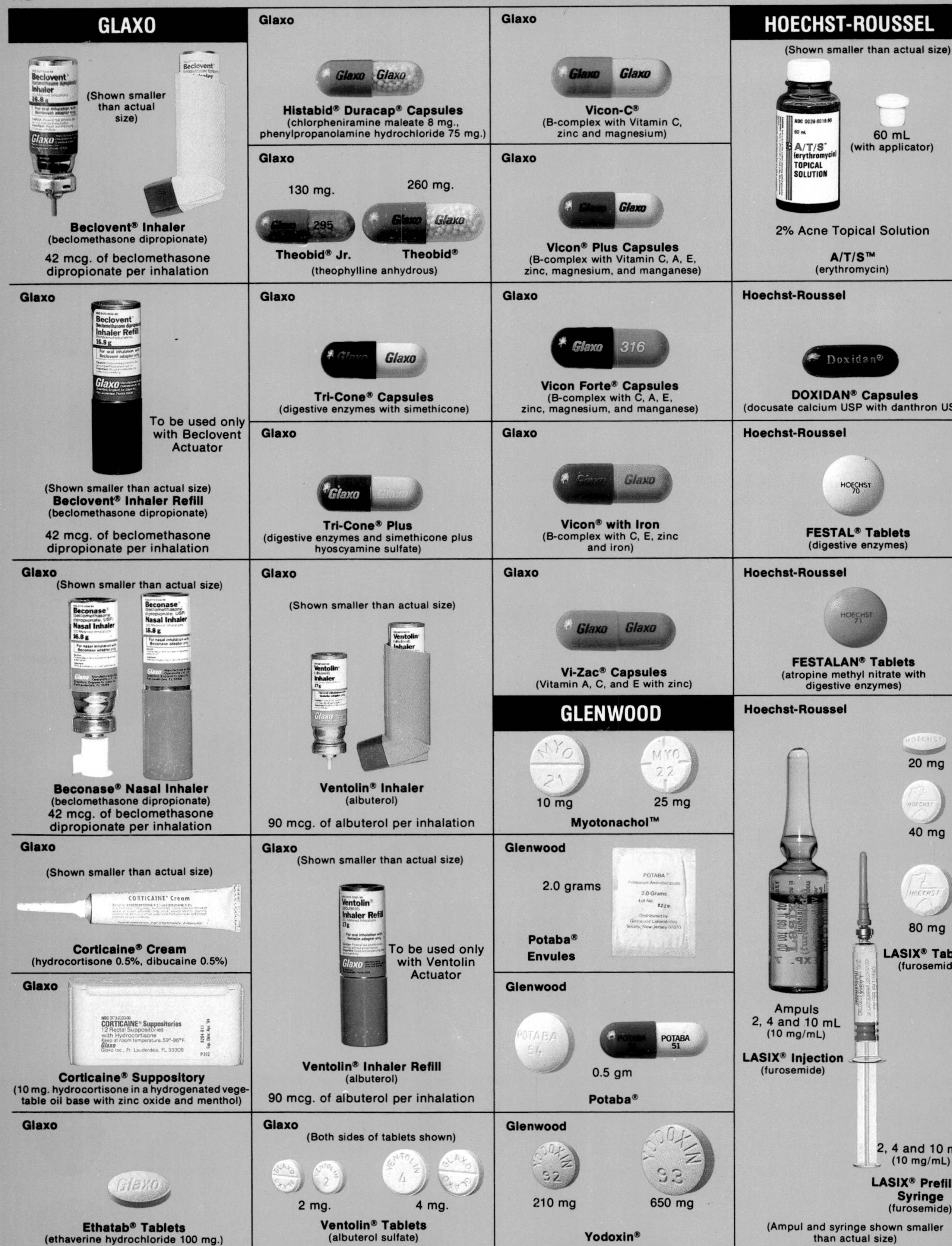

GLAXO

Glaxo

(Shown smaller than actual size)

Beclovent® Inhaler
(beclomethasone dipropionate)

42 mcg. of beclomethasone dipropionate per inhalation

Glaxo

Histabid® Duracap® Capsules
(chlorpheniramine maleate 8 mg., phenylpropanolamine hydrochloride 75 mg.)

Glaxo

Vicon-C®
(B-complex with Vitamin C, zinc and magnesium)

Glaxo

130 mg. 260 mg.

Theobid® Jr. **Theobid®**
(theophylline anhydrous)

Glaxo

Vicon® Plus Capsules
(B-complex with Vitamin C, A, E, zinc, magnesium, and manganese)

Glaxo

To be used only with Beclovent Actuator

(Shown smaller than actual size)

Beclovent® Inhaler Refill
(beclomethasone dipropionate)

42 mcg. of beclomethasone dipropionate per inhalation

Glaxo

Tri-Cone® Capsules
(digestive enzymes with simethicone)

Glaxo

Vicon Forte® Capsules
(B-complex with C, A, E, zinc, magnesium, and manganese)

Glaxo

Tri-Cone® Plus
(digestive enzymes and simethicone plus hyoscyamine sulfate)

Glaxo

Vicon® with Iron
(B-complex with C, E, zinc and iron)

Glaxo

(Shown smaller than actual size)

Beconase® Nasal Inhaler
(beclomethasone dipropionate)
42 mcg. of beclomethasone dipropionate per inhalation

Glaxo

(Shown smaller than actual size)

Ventolin® Inhaler
(albuterol)

90 mcg. of albuterol per inhalation

Glaxo

Vi-Zac® Capsules
(Vitamin A, C, and E with zinc)

Glaxo

(Shown smaller than actual size)

Corticaine® Cream
(hydrocortisone 0.5%, dibucaine 0.5%)

Glaxo

Corticaine® Suppository
(10 mg. hydrocortisone in a hydrogenated vegetable oil base with zinc oxide and menthol)

Glaxo

(Shown smaller than actual size)

To be used only with Ventolin Actuator

Ventolin® Inhaler Refill
(albuterol)

90 mcg. of albuterol per inhalation

Glaxo

Ethatab® Tablets
(ethaverine hydrochloride 100 mg.)

Glaxo

(Both sides of tablets shown)

2 mg. 4 mg.

Ventolin® Tablets
(albuterol sulfate)

GLENWOOD

10 mg 25 mg

Myotonachol™

Glenwood

2.0 grams

Potaba® Envules

Glenwood

0.5 gm

Potaba®

Glenwood

210 mg 650 mg

Yodoxin®

HOECHST-ROUSSEL

(Shown smaller than actual size)

60 mL (with applicator)

2% Acne Topical Solution

A/T/S™
(erythromycin)

Hoechst-Roussel

DOXIDAN® Capsules
(docusate calcium USP with danthron US

Hoechst-Roussel

FESTAL® Tablets
(digestive enzymes)

Hoechst-Roussel

FESTALAN® Tablets
(atropine methyl nitrate with digestive enzymes)

Hoechst-Roussel

20 mg

40 mg

80 mg

LASIX® Tab
(furosemid

Ampuls
2, 4 and 10 mL
(10 mg/mL)

LASIX® Injection
(furosemide)

2, 4 and 10 m
(10 mg/mL)

LASIX® Prefill Syringe
(furosemide)

(Ampul and syringe shown smaller than actual size)

Hoechst-Roussel

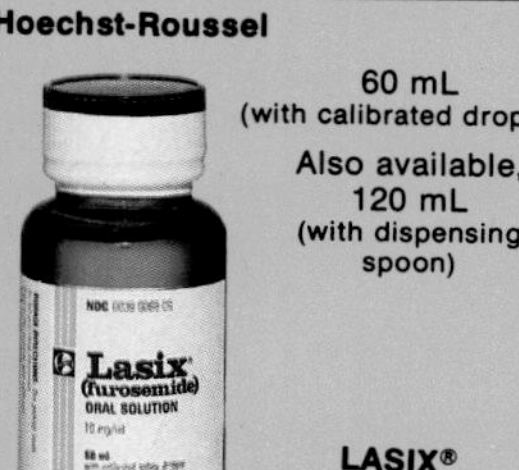

60 mL (with calibrated dropper)

Also available, 120 mL (with dispensing spoon)

LASIX® Oral Solution (furosemide)

(Lasix Oral Solution shown smaller than actual size)

Hoechst-Roussel

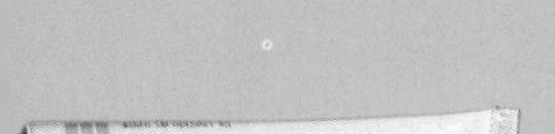

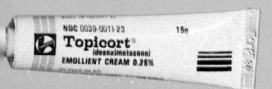

240 mg 50 mg

SURFAK® Capsules (docusate calcium USP)

Hoechst-Roussel (Tubes shown smaller than actual size)

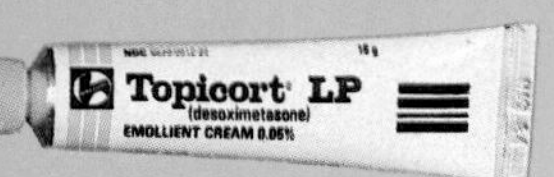

15 and 60 g tubes

TOPICORT® Emollient Cream 0.25% (desoximetasone)

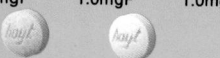

15 and 60 g tubes

TOPICORT® LP Emollient Cream 0.05% (desoximetasone)

HOYT LABORATORIES

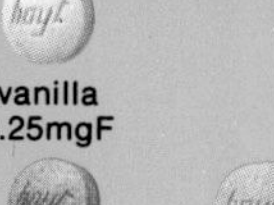

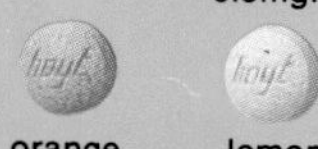

vanilla 0.25mgF — grape 0.5mgF

cherry 1.0mgF — orange 1.0mgF — lemon 1.0mgF

lime 1.0mgF — SF* 1.0mgF (Special Formula)

†LURIDE® (sodium fluoride)

Because tablets and capsules are shown in this section, do not infer that these are the only dosage forms available. Where a product name is preceded by the symbol †, refer to the description in the Product Information (White Section) for other forms.

IVES LABORATORIES

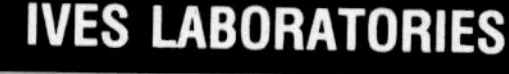

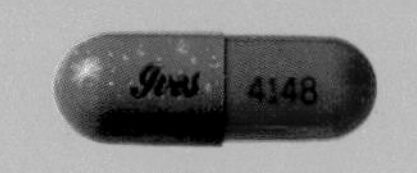

400 mg.

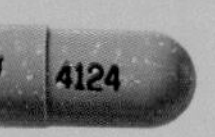

200 mg. 100 mg.

CYCLOSPASMOL® (cyclandelate)

Ives Laboratories

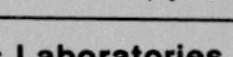

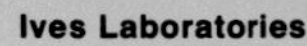

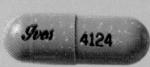

10 mg. 5 mg. 2.5 mg.

Sublingual 4164‡

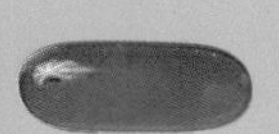

Both sides of tablet shown

Chewable 10 mg.

Oral Titradose® Dosage Forms:

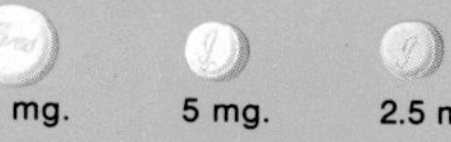

4152‡ 5 mg. Titradose® — 4153‡ 10 mg. Titradose®

4154‡ 20 mg. Titradose® — 4159‡ 30 mg. Titradose®

Both sides of Titradose tablets shown above

ISORDIL® (isosorbide dinitrate)

Ives Laboratories

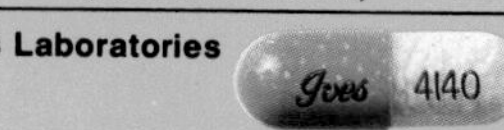

Tembids® Capsules

4125‡

Tembids® Tablets

Sustained Action 40 mg.

4123‡

w/Phenobarbital

(Both sides of Tembids Tablets and w/Phenobarbital are shown)

ISORDIL® (isosorbide dinitrate)

Ives Laboratories

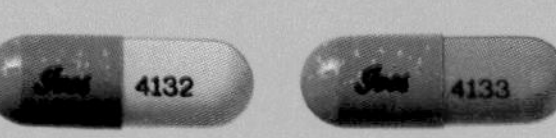

25 mg. 50 mg.

Also available: 100 mg. capsule

SURMONTIL® (trimipramine maleate)

Ives Laboratories

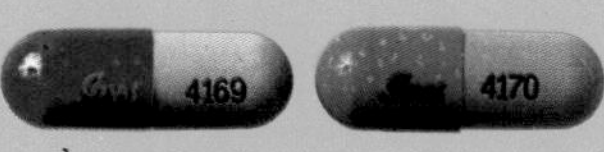

SYNALGOS® — **SYNALGOS®-DC**

JANSSEN

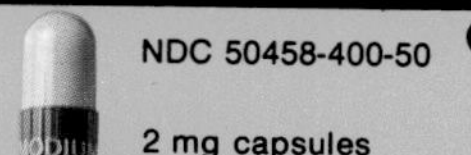

NDC 50458-400-50 Ⓒ V

2 mg capsules

†IMODIUM® (loperamide HCl)

Janssen

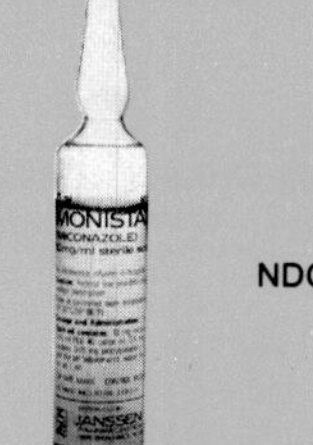

NDC 50458-200-20

20 ml ampoules

MONISTAT i.v.™ (miconazole)

Janssen

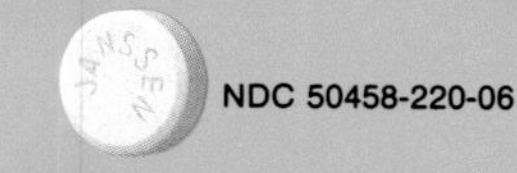

NDC 50458-220-06

200 mg tablets

NIZORAL® (ketoconazole)

Janssen Ⓒ II

NDC 50458-030-20

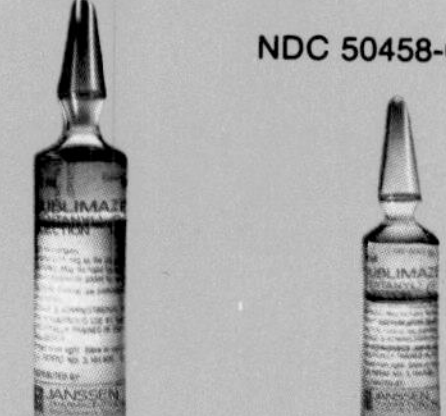

NDC 50458-030-10

20 ml ampoules — 10 ml ampoules

†SUBLIMAZE® Injection (fentanyl)

Janssen

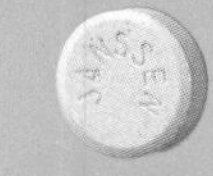

NDC 50458-110-01

100 mg tablet

VERMOX® (mebendazole)

JOHNSON & JOHNSON

McNeil Pharmaceutical

Enteric Coated Microspheres

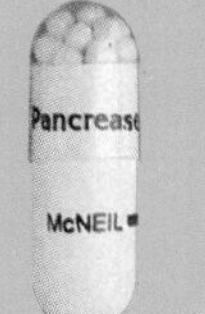

0095*

PANCREASE® Capsules (brand of pancrelipase)

Bottles of 100 and 250

Johnson & Johnson McNeil Pharmaceutical

Also available: Elixir-225

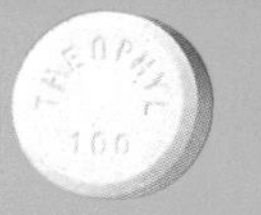

100 mg.

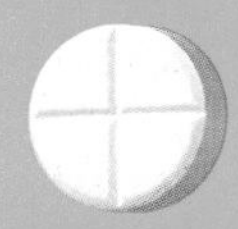

225 mg.

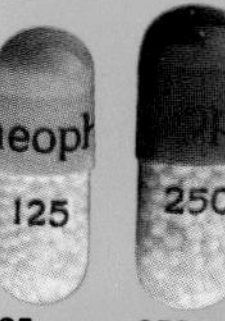

Theophyl® Chewable Tablet (anhydrous theophylline U.S.P.)

Theophyl®-225 Tablet (anhydrous theophylline U.S.P. 225 mg.)

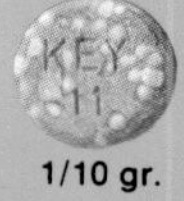

125 mg. 250 mg.

Theophyl®-SR (anhydrous theophylline U.S.P.)

Key Pharmaceuticals

Sustained Action Tablets

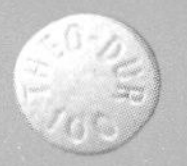

1/10 gr.

1/25 gr.

Nitroglyn® (nitroglycerin)

Key Pharmaceuticals

100 mg. 200 mg.

Sustained Action Tablets

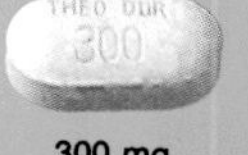

300 mg.

Theo-Dur® (theophylline, anhydrous)

Key Pharmaceuticals

Sustained Action Capsules

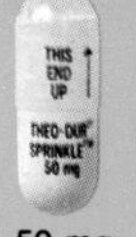

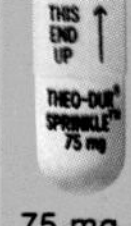

50 mg. 75 mg.

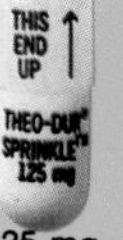

125 mg. 200 mg.

Theo-Dur® Sprinkle (anhydrous theophylline)

†Other dosage forms available. See Product Information section or check directly with manufacturer.

*Manufacturers' identification number.

‡All ISORDIL® tablets, except the sublinguals, bear engraved identification numbers as listed above the tablets.

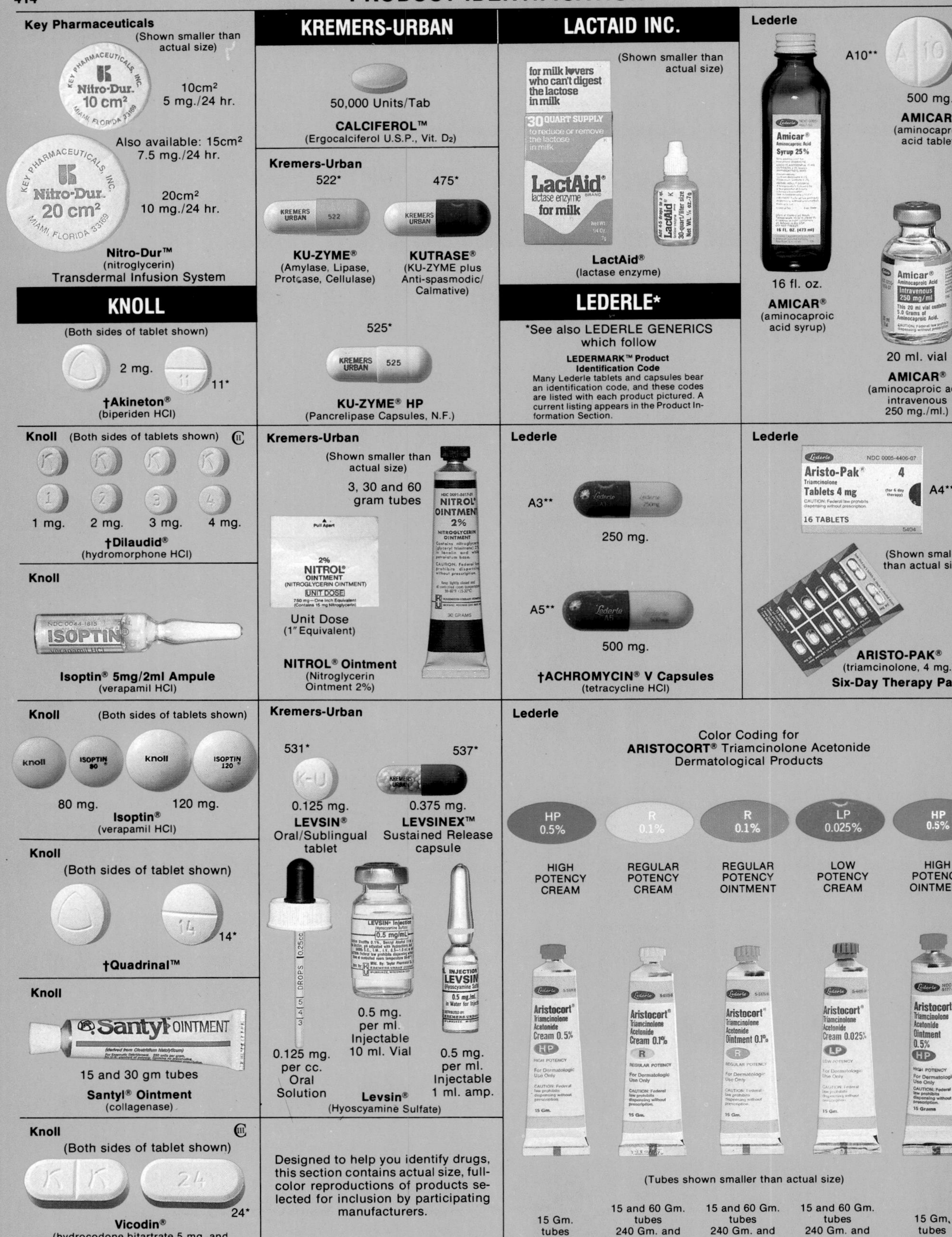
Key Pharmaceuticals
(Shown smaller than actual size)
10cm²
5 mg./24 hr.
Also available: 15cm²
7.5 mg./24 hr.
20cm²
10 mg./24 hr.
Nitro-Dur™
(nitroglycerin)
Transdermal Infusion System
KNOLL
(Both sides of tablet shown)
2 mg.
11*
†Akineton®
(biperiden HCl)
Knoll (Both sides of tablets shown)
1 mg.
2 mg.
3 mg.
4 mg.
†Dilaudid®
(hydromorphone HCl)
Knoll
ISOPTIN
Isoptin® 5mg/2ml Ampule
(verapamil HCl)
Knoll (Both sides of tablets shown)
80 mg.
120 mg.
Isoptin®
(verapamil HCl)
Knoll
(Both sides of tablet shown)
14*
†Quadrinal™
Knoll
Santyl OINTMENT
15 and 30 gm tubes
Santyl® Ointment
(collagenase)
Knoll
(Both sides of tablet shown)
24*
Vicodin®
(hydrocodone bitartrate 5 mg. and acetaminophen 500 mg.)
KREMERS-URBAN
50,000 Units/Tab
CALCIFEROL™
(Ergocalciferol U.S.P., Vit. D2)
Kremers-Urban
522*
475*
KU-ZYME®
(Amylase, Lipase, Protease, Cellulase)
KUTRASE®
(KU-ZYME plus Anti-spasmodic/ Calmative)
525*
KU-ZYME® HP
(Pancrelipase Capsules, N.F.)
Kremers-Urban
(Shown smaller than actual size)
3, 30 and 60 gram tubes
NITROL® OINTMENT 2%
Unit Dose
(1" Equivalent)
NITROL® Ointment
(Nitroglycerin Ointment 2%)
Kremers-Urban
531*
537*
0.125 mg.
LEVSIN®
Oral/Sublingual tablet
0.375 mg.
LEVSINEX™
Sustained Release capsule
0.125 mg. per cc. Oral Solution
0.5 mg. per ml. Injectable 10 ml. Vial
0.5 mg. per ml. Injectable 1 ml. amp.
Levsin®
(Hyoscyamine Sulfate)
Designed to help you identify drugs, this section contains actual size, full-color reproductions of products selected for inclusion by participating manufacturers.
LACTAID INC.
(Shown smaller than actual size)
for milk lovers who can't digest the lactose in milk
30 QUART SUPPLY
LactAid® lactase enzyme for milk
LactAid®
(lactase enzyme)
LEDERLE*
*See also LEDERLE GENERICS which follow
LEDERMARK™ Product Identification Code
Many Lederle tablets and capsules bear an identification code, and these codes are listed with each product pictured. A current listing appears in the Product Information Section.
Lederle
A3**
250 mg.
A5**
500 mg.
†ACHROMYCIN® V Capsules
(tetracycline HCl)
Lederle
Color Coding for
ARISTOCORT® Triamcinolone Acetonide Dermatological Products
HP 0.5%
R 0.1%
R 0.1%
LP 0.025%
HP 0.5%
HIGH POTENCY CREAM
REGULAR POTENCY CREAM
REGULAR POTENCY OINTMENT
LOW POTENCY CREAM
HIGH POTENCY OINTMENT
(Tubes shown smaller than actual size)
15 Gm. tubes 240 Gm. jar
15 and 60 Gm. tubes 240 Gm. and 5¼ lb. jars
15 and 60 Gm. tubes 240 Gm. and 5 lb. jars
15 and 60 Gm. tubes 240 Gm. and 5¼ lb. jars
15 Gm. tubes 240 Gm. jar
Lederle
A10**
500 mg.
AMICAR®
(aminocaproic acid tablet)
Amicar® Aminocaproic Acid Syrup 25%
16 fl. oz.
AMICAR®
(aminocaproic acid syrup)
20 ml. vial
AMICAR®
(aminocaproic acid intravenous 250 mg./ml.)
Lederle
Aristo-Pak® 4
Tablets 4 mg
16 TABLETS
A4**
(Shown smaller than actual size)
ARISTO-PAK®
(triamcinolone, 4 mg.)
Six-Day Therapy Pack

†Other dosage forms available. See Product Information section or check directly with manufacturer.
*Manufacturers' identification number.
**Ledermark Product Identification Codes

Lederle

A1** 1 mg — A2** 2 mg.

A4** 4 mg. — A8** 8 mg. — A16** 16 mg.

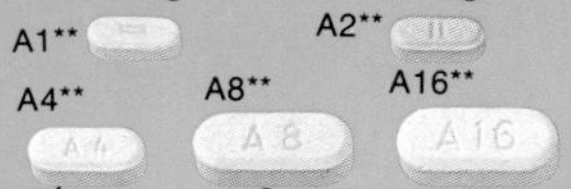

†ARISTOCORT® Tablets
(triamcinolone)

Lederle

(Tubes shown smaller than actual size)

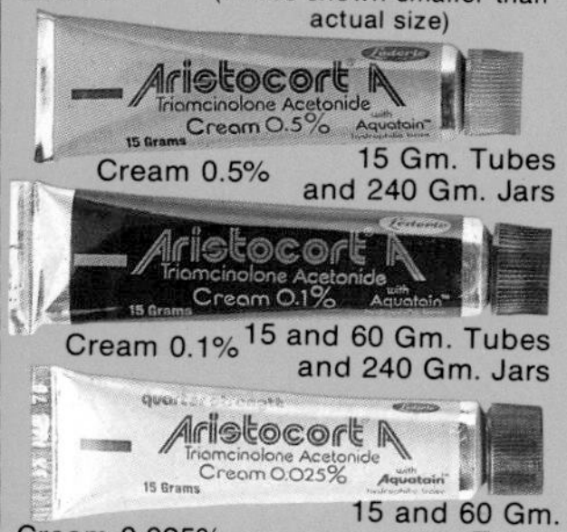

Cream 0.5% — 15 Gm. Tubes and 240 Gm. Jars

Cream 0.1% — 15 and 60 Gm. Tubes and 240 Gm. Jars

Cream 0.025% — 15 and 60 Gm. Tubes

ARISTOCORT A®
(triamcinolone acetonide with AQUATAIN®)

Lederle

(Tubes shown smaller than actual size)

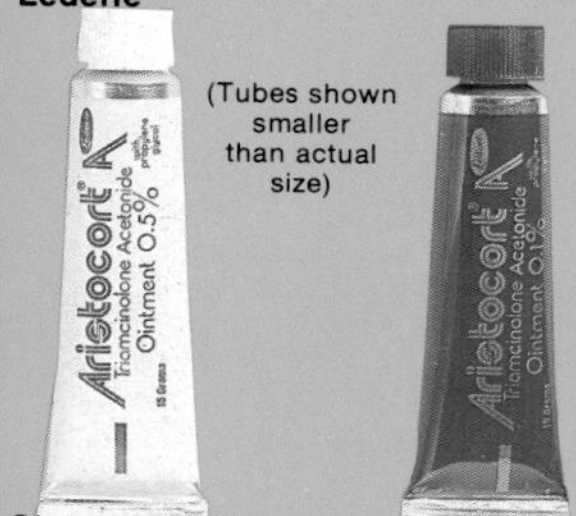

Ointment 0.5% 15 Gm. tubes — Ointment 0.1% 15 and 60 Gm. tubes

ARISTOCORT A®
(triamcinolone acetonide with propylene glycol)

Lederle

A11** 2 mg. — A12** 5 mg. — A9** 5 mg.

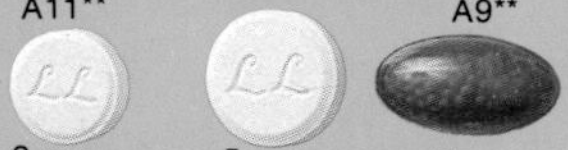

ARTANE® Tablets — **†ARTANE® Sequels®**
(trihexyphenidyl hydrochloride)

Lederle

A15** 50 mg. — A17** 100 mg. — A18** 150 mg.

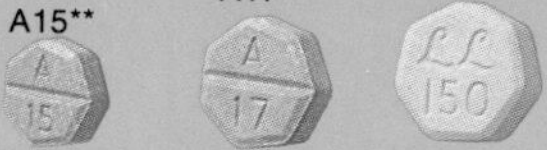

ASENDIN®
(amoxapine)

Lederle

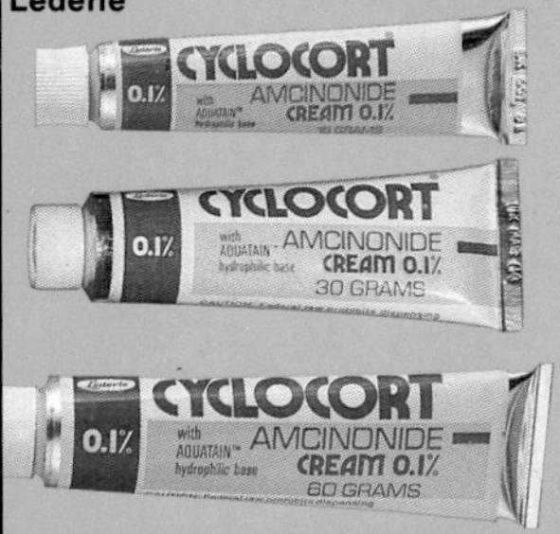

15 Gm., 30 Gm. and 60 Gm. tubes
CYCLOCORT® Cream 0.1%
Amcinonide with AQUATAIN™

Lederle

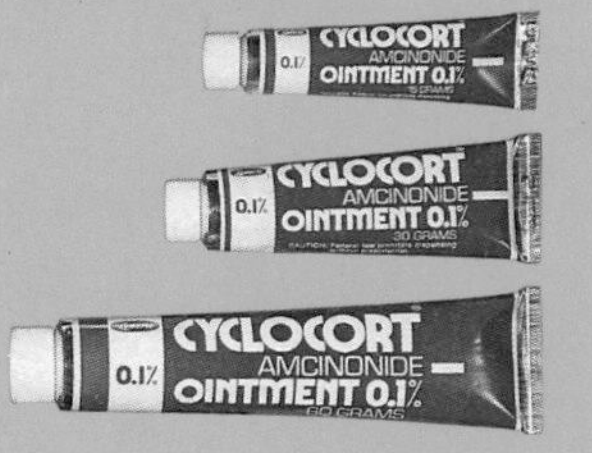

15 Gm., 30 Gm. and 60 Gm. tubes
CYCLOCORT® Amcinonide Ointment 0.1%

Lederle

D9** 150 mg.

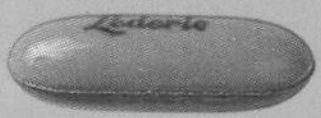

†DECLOMYCIN® Capsules
(demeclocycline HCl)

D12** 300 mg. — D11** 150 mg.

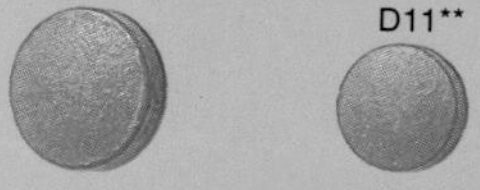

†DECLOMYCIN® Tablets
(demeclocycline HCl)

Lederle

D1** 125 mg. — D2** 250 mg.

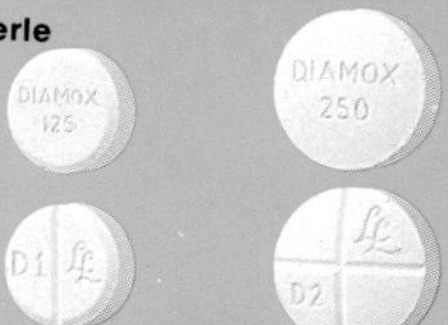

†DIAMOX® Tablets

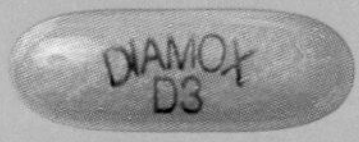

D3** 500 mg.

†DIAMOX® Sequels®
(acetazolamide)

Lederle

F2**

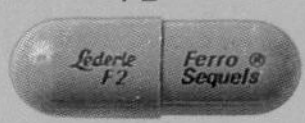

FERRO-SEQUELS®
Sustained Release Iron Capsules
Supplied in bottles of 30, 100, and 1000

Lederle

F4** **FILIBON®**

F5** **FILIBON® F.A.**

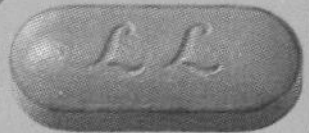

F6** **FILIBON® Forte** Prenatal Tablets

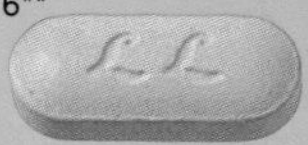

Supplied in bottles of 100

F7** **FILIBON® OT Tablets**

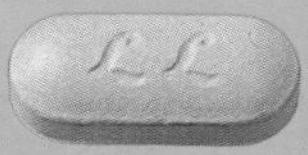

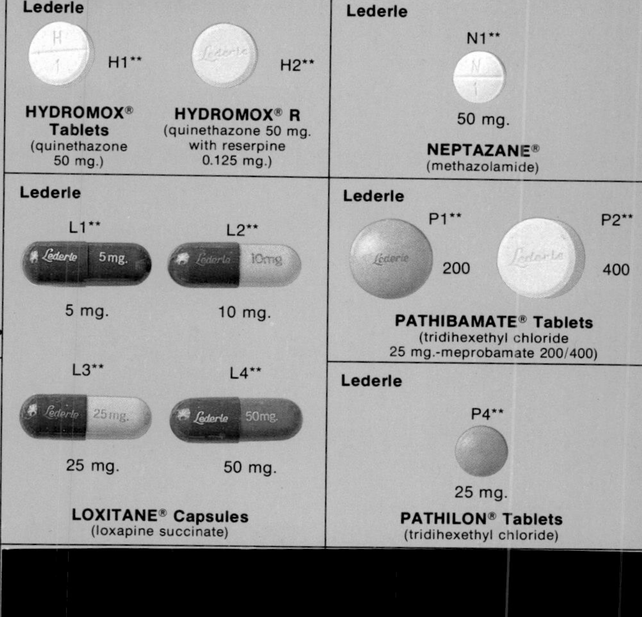

Lederle

H1** **HYDROMOX® Tablets** (quinethazone 50 mg.)

H2** **HYDROMOX® R** (quinethazone 50 mg. with reserpine 0.125 mg.)

Lederle

N1** 50 mg.

NEPTAZANE®
(methazolamide)

Lederle

L1** 5 mg. — L2** 10 mg.

L3** 25 mg. — L4** 50 mg.

LOXITANE® Capsules
(loxapine succinate)

Lederle

P1** 200 — P2** 400

PATHIBAMATE® Tablets
(tridihexethyl chloride 25 mg.-meprobamate 200/400)

Lederle

P4** 25 mg.

PATHILON® Tablets
(tridihexethyl chloride)

†Other dosage forms available. See Product Info[rmation]
**Ledermark Produ[cts]

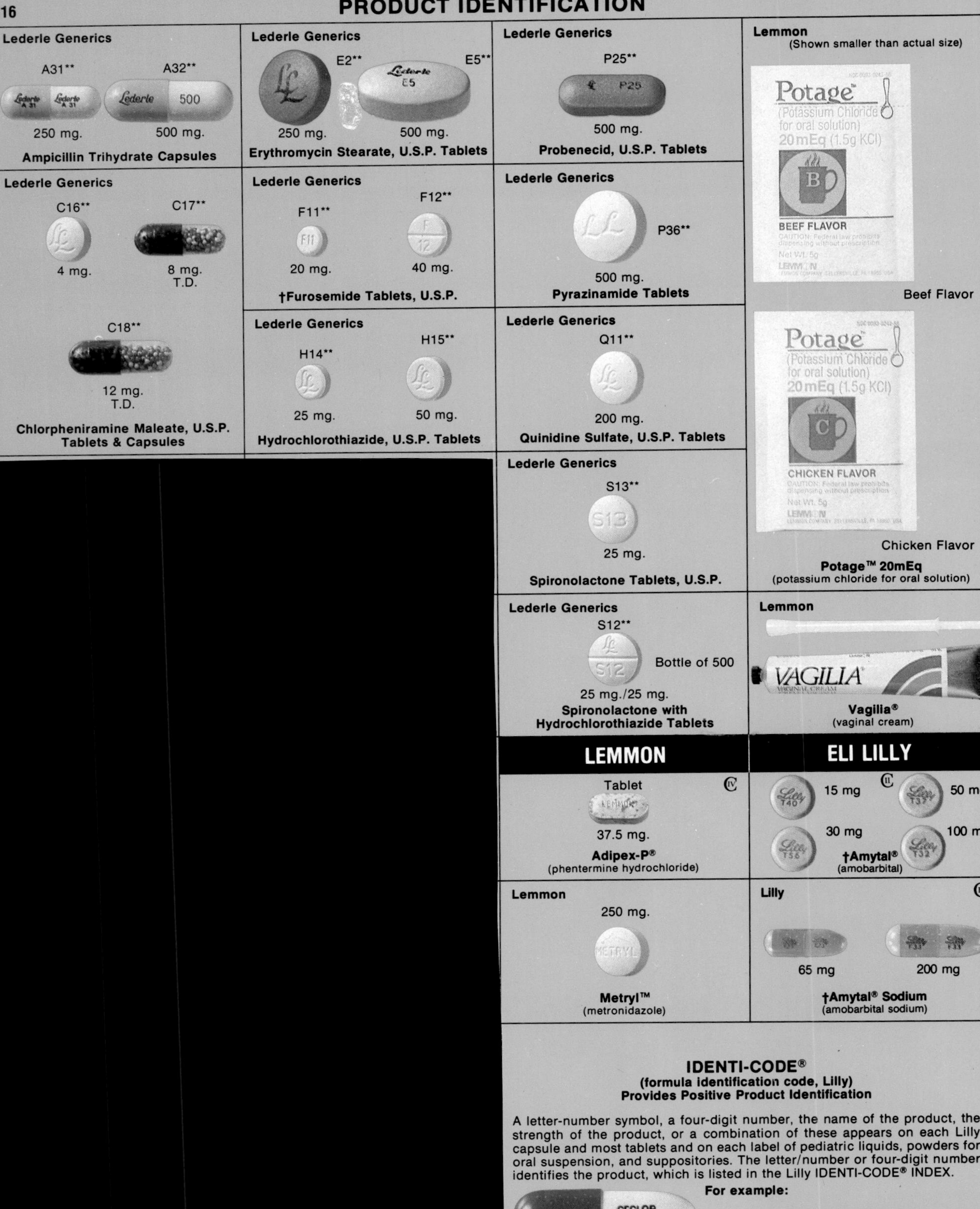
Lederle Generics
A31**
A32**
250 mg.
500 mg.
Ampicillin Trihydrate Capsules
Lederle Generics
E2**
E5**
250 mg.
500 mg.
Erythromycin Stearate, U.S.P. Tablets
Lederle Generics
P25**
500 mg.
Probenecid, U.S.P. Tablets
Lemmon
(Shown smaller than actual size)
Potage
(Potassium Chloride for oral solution)
20 mEq (1.5g KCl)
BEEF FLAVOR
Beef Flavor
Lederle Generics
C16**
C17**
4 mg.
8 mg. T.D.
C18**
12 mg. T.D.
Chlorpheniramine Maleate, U.S.P. Tablets & Capsules
Lederle Generics
F11**
F12**
20 mg.
40 mg.
†Furosemide Tablets, U.S.P.
Lederle Generics
P36**
500 mg.
Pyrazinamide Tablets
Lederle Generics
H14**
H15**
25 mg.
50 mg.
Hydrochlorothiazide, U.S.P. Tablets
Lederle Generics
Q11**
200 mg.
Quinidine Sulfate, U.S.P. Tablets
Potage
(Potassium Chloride for oral solution)
20 mEq (1.5g KCl)
CHICKEN FLAVOR
Chicken Flavor
Potage™ 20mEq
(potassium chloride for oral solution)
Lederle Generics
S13**
25 mg.
Spironolactone Tablets, U.S.P.
Lederle Generics
S12**
Bottle of 500
25 mg./25 mg.
Spironolactone with Hydrochlorothiazide Tablets
Lemmon
VAGILIA
Vagilia®
(vaginal cream)
LEMMON
Tablet
37.5 mg.
Adipex-P®
(phentermine hydrochloride)
ELI LILLY
15 mg
50 mg
30 mg
100 mg
†Amytal®
(amobarbital)
Lemmon
250 mg.
Metryl™
(metronidazole)
Lilly
65 mg
200 mg
†Amytal® Sodium
(amobarbital sodium)
IDENTI-CODE®
(formula identification code, Lilly)
Provides Positive Product Identification
A letter-number symbol, a four-digit number, the name of the product, the strength of the product, or a combination of these appears on each Lilly capsule and most tablets and on each label of pediatric liquids, powders for oral suspension, and suppositories. The letter/number or four-digit number identifies the product, which is listed in the Lilly IDENTI-CODE® INDEX.
For example:
CECLOR 250 mg
Ceclor® (cefaclor)
3061 = Number of product
250 mg = Strength of product
The complete IDENTI-CODE® INDEX appears in the Product Information Section under Eli Lilly and Company

ation section or check directly with manufacturer.
Identification Codes

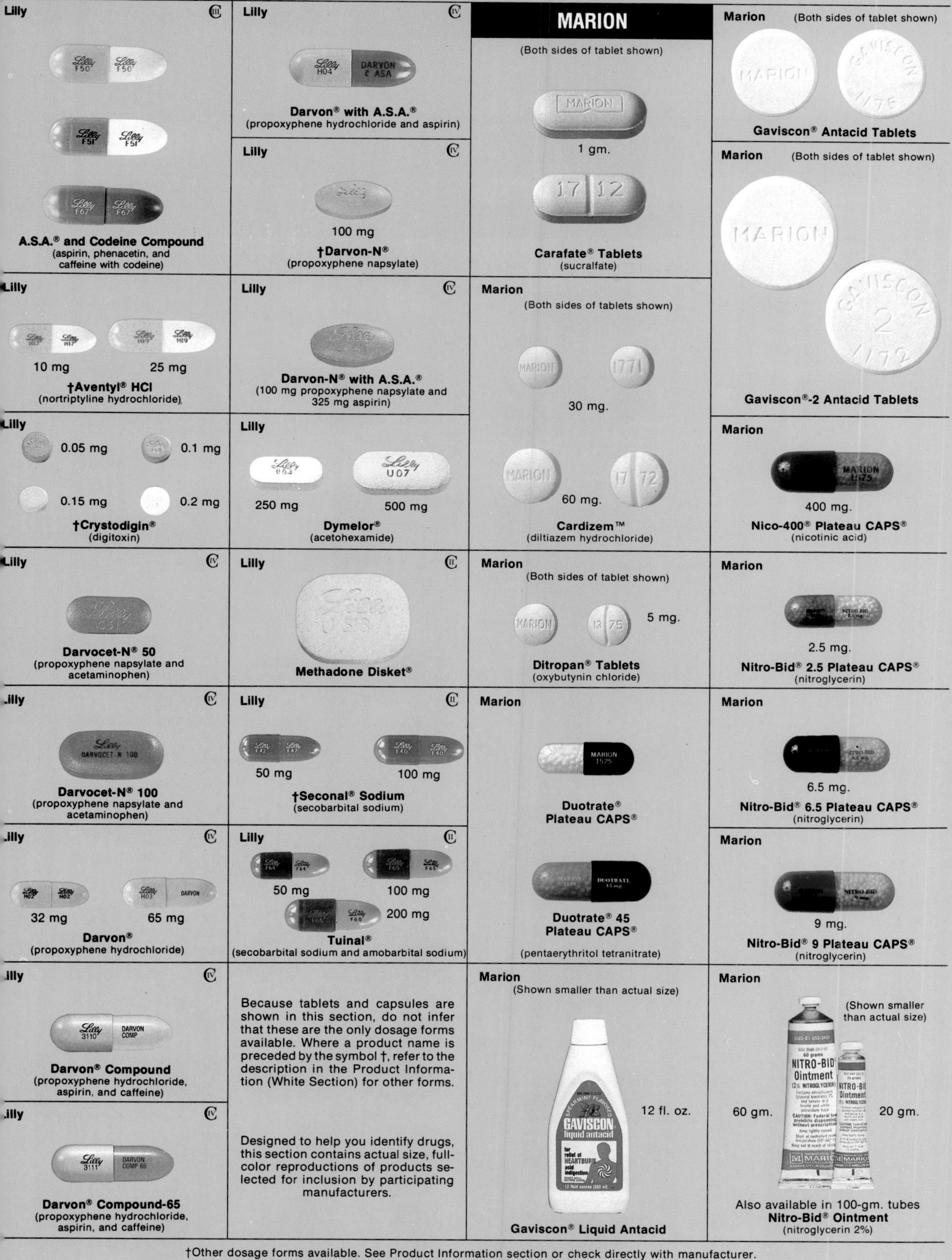

Lilly
A.S.A.® and Codeine Compound
(aspirin, phenacetin, and caffeine with codeine)

Lilly
10 mg 25 mg
†Aventyl® HCl
(nortriptyline hydrochloride)

Lilly
0.05 mg 0.1 mg
0.15 mg 0.2 mg
†Crystodigin®
(digitoxin)

Lilly
Darvocet-N® 50
(propoxyphene napsylate and acetaminophen)

Lilly
Darvocet-N® 100
(propoxyphene napsylate and acetaminophen)

Lilly
32 mg 65 mg
Darvon®
(propoxyphene hydrochloride)

Lilly
Darvon® Compound
(propoxyphene hydrochloride, aspirin, and caffeine)

Lilly
Darvon® Compound-65
(propoxyphene hydrochloride, aspirin, and caffeine)

Lilly
Darvon® with A.S.A.®
(propoxyphene hydrochloride and aspirin)

Lilly
100 mg
†Darvon-N®
(propoxyphene napsylate)

Lilly
Darvon-N® with A.S.A.®
(100 mg propoxyphene napsylate and 325 mg aspirin)

Lilly
250 mg 500 mg
Dymelor®
(acetohexamide)

Lilly
Methadone Disket®

Lilly
50 mg 100 mg
†Seconal® Sodium
(secobarbital sodium)

Lilly
50 mg 100 mg 200 mg
Tuinal®
(secobarbital sodium and amobarbital sodium)

Because tablets and capsules are shown in this section, do not infer that these are the only dosage forms available. Where a product name is preceded by the symbol †, refer to the description in the Product Information (White Section) for other forms.

Designed to help you identify drugs, this section contains actual size, full-color reproductions of products selected for inclusion by participating manufacturers.

MARION

(Both sides of tablet shown)
1 gm.
Carafate® Tablets
(sucralfate)

Marion
(Both sides of tablets shown)
30 mg.
60 mg.
Cardizem™
(diltiazem hydrochloride)

Marion
(Both sides of tablet shown)
5 mg.
Ditropan® Tablets
(oxybutynin chloride)

Marion
Duotrate®
Plateau CAPS®

Duotrate® 45
Plateau CAPS®
(pentaerythritol tetranitrate)

Marion
(Shown smaller than actual size)
12 fl. oz.
Gaviscon® Liquid Antacid

Marion (Both sides of tablet shown)
Gaviscon® Antacid Tablets

Marion (Both sides of tablet shown)
Gaviscon®-2 Antacid Tablets

Marion
400 mg.
Nico-400® Plateau CAPS®
(nicotinic acid)

Marion
2.5 mg.
Nitro-Bid® 2.5 Plateau CAPS®
(nitroglycerin)

Marion
6.5 mg.
Nitro-Bid® 6.5 Plateau CAPS®
(nitroglycerin)

Marion
9 mg.
Nitro-Bid® 9 Plateau CAPS®
(nitroglycerin)

Marion
(Shown smaller than actual size)
60 gm. 20 gm.
Also available in 100-gm. tubes
Nitro-Bid® Ointment
(nitroglycerin 2%)

†Other dosage forms available. See Product Information section or check directly with manufacturer.

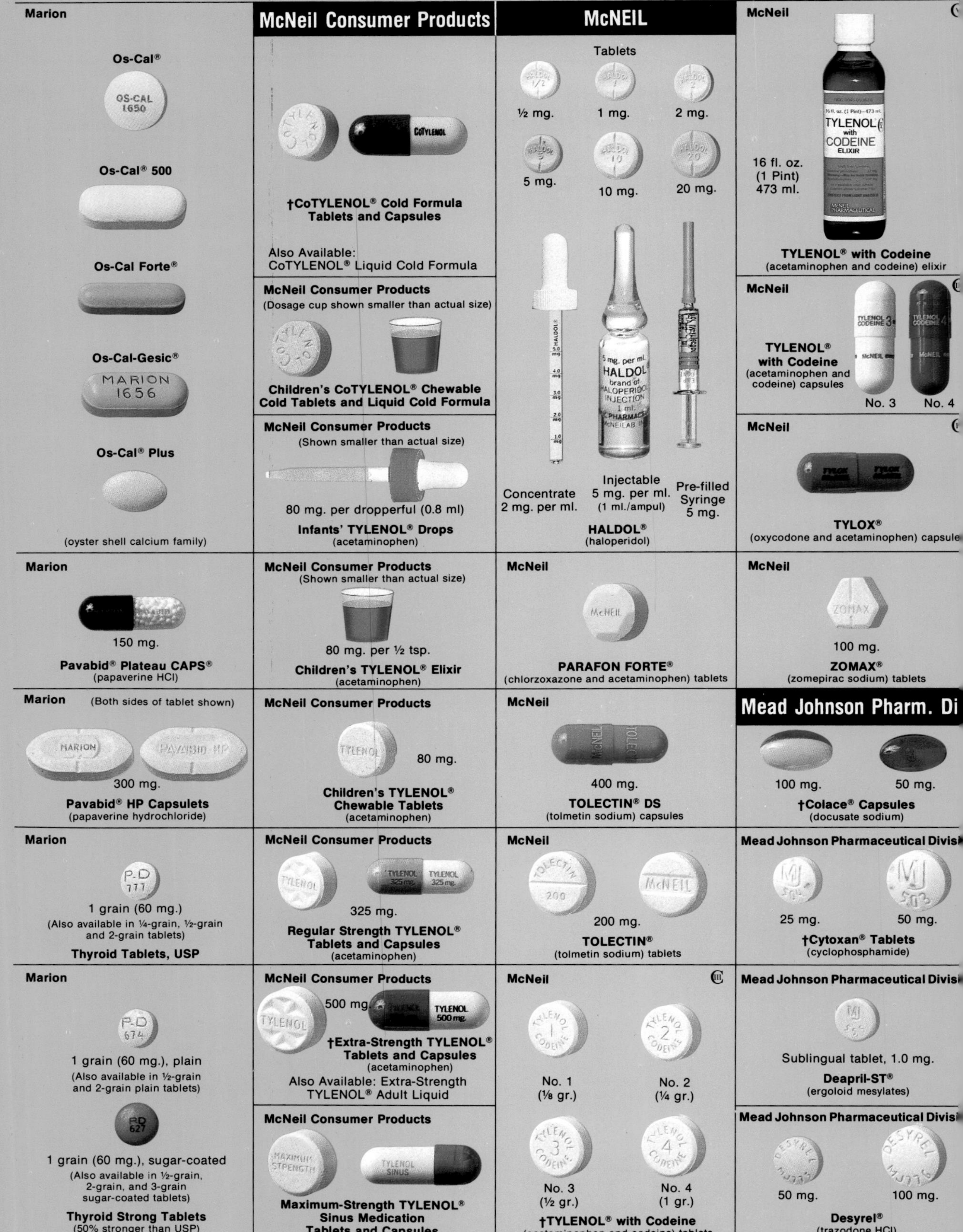

Marion

Os-Cal®

Os-Cal® 500

Os-Cal Forte®

Os-Cal-Gesic®

Os-Cal® Plus

(oyster shell calcium family)

McNeil Consumer Products

†CoTYLENOL® Cold Formula Tablets and Capsules

Also Available:
CoTYLENOL® Liquid Cold Formula

McNEIL

Tablets

½ mg. 1 mg. 2 mg.

5 mg. 10 mg. 20 mg.

Concentrate 2 mg. per ml.

Injectable 5 mg. per ml. (1 ml./ampul)

Pre-filled Syringe 5 mg.

HALDOL®
(haloperidol)

McNeil

16 fl. oz.
(1 Pint)
473 ml.

TYLENOL® with Codeine
(acetaminophen and codeine) elixir

McNeil Consumer Products

(Dosage cup shown smaller than actual size)

Children's CoTYLENOL® Chewable Cold Tablets and Liquid Cold Formula

McNeil

TYLENOL® with Codeine
(acetaminophen and codeine) capsules

No. 3 No. 4

McNeil Consumer Products

(Shown smaller than actual size)

80 mg. per dropperful (0.8 ml)

Infants' TYLENOL® Drops
(acetaminophen)

McNeil

TYLOX®
(oxycodone and acetaminophen) capsule

Marion

150 mg.

Pavabid® Plateau CAPS®
(papaverine HCl)

McNeil Consumer Products

(Shown smaller than actual size)

80 mg. per ½ tsp.

Children's TYLENOL® Elixir
(acetaminophen)

McNeil

PARAFON FORTE®
(chlorzoxazone and acetaminophen) tablets

McNeil

100 mg.

ZOMAX®
(zomepirac sodium) tablets

Marion

(Both sides of tablet shown)

300 mg.

Pavabid® HP Capsulets
(papaverine hydrochloride)

McNeil Consumer Products

80 mg.

Children's TYLENOL® Chewable Tablets
(acetaminophen)

McNeil

400 mg.

TOLECTIN® DS
(tolmetin sodium) capsules

Mead Johnson Pharm. Di

100 mg. 50 mg.

†Colace® Capsules
(docusate sodium)

Marion

1 grain (60 mg.)
(Also available in ¼-grain, ½-grain and 2-grain tablets)

Thyroid Tablets, USP

McNeil Consumer Products

325 mg.

Regular Strength TYLENOL® Tablets and Capsules
(acetaminophen)

McNeil

200 mg.

TOLECTIN®
(tolmetin sodium) tablets

Mead Johnson Pharmaceutical Divis

25 mg. 50 mg.

†Cytoxan® Tablets
(cyclophosphamide)

Marion

1 grain (60 mg.), plain
(Also available in ½-grain and 2-grain plain tablets)

1 grain (60 mg.), sugar-coated
(Also available in ½-grain, 2-grain, and 3-grain sugar-coated tablets)

Thyroid Strong Tablets
(50% stronger than USP)

McNeil Consumer Products

500 mg.

†Extra-Strength TYLENOL® Tablets and Capsules
(acetaminophen)

Also Available: Extra-Strength TYLENOL® Adult Liquid

McNeil Consumer Products

Maximum-Strength TYLENOL® Sinus Medication Tablets and Capsules

McNeil

No. 1 (⅛ gr.) No. 2 (¼ gr.)

No. 3 (½ gr.) No. 4 (1 gr.)

†TYLENOL® with Codeine
(acetaminophen and codeine) tablets

Mead Johnson Pharmaceutical Divis

Sublingual tablet, 1.0 mg.

Deapril-ST®
(ergoloid mesylates)

Mead Johnson Pharmaceutical Divis

50 mg. 100 mg.

Desyrel®
(trazodone HCl)

†Other dosage forms available. See Product Information section or check directly with manufacturer.

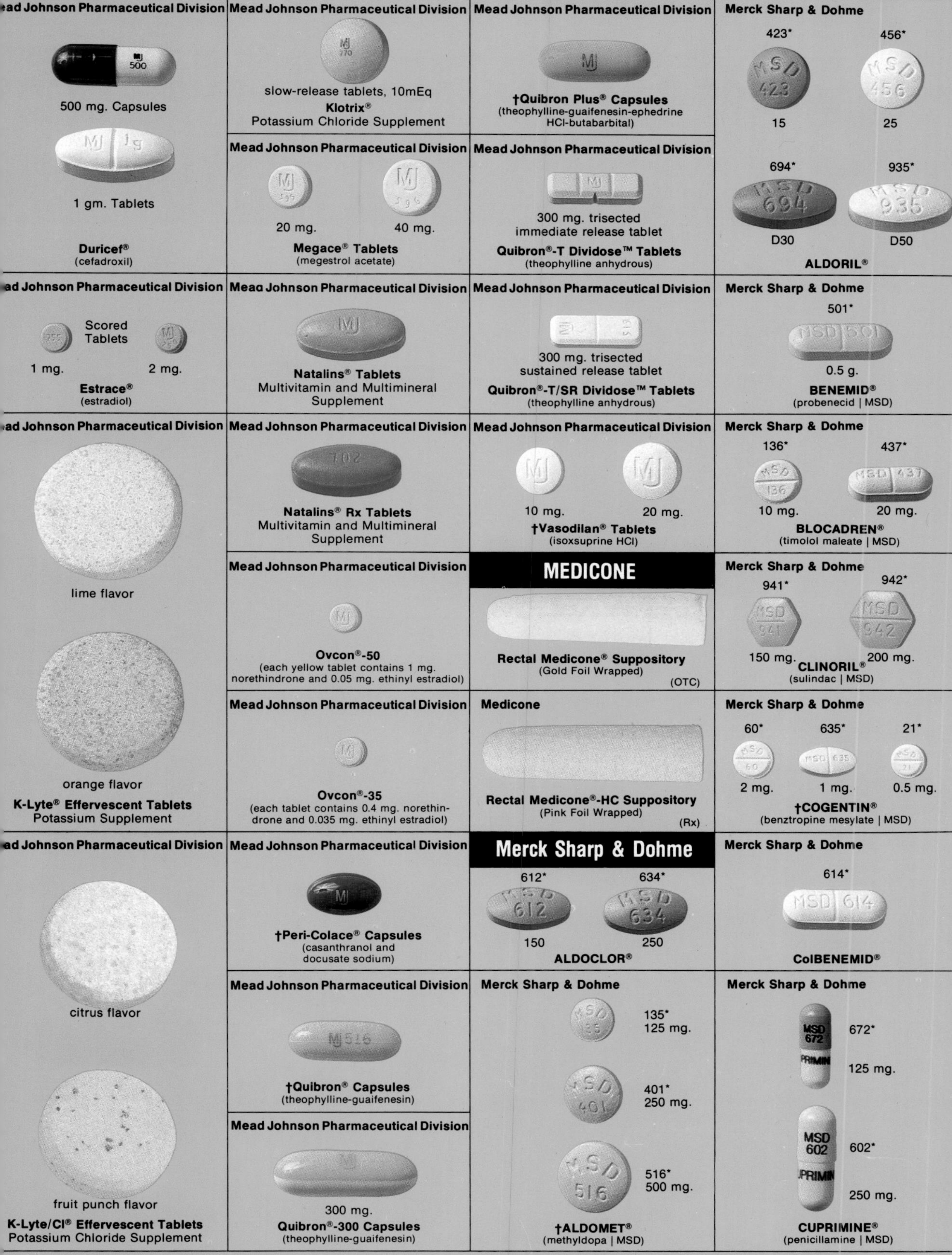

†Other dosage forms available. See Product Information section or check directly with manufacturer.
*Manufacturers' identification number.

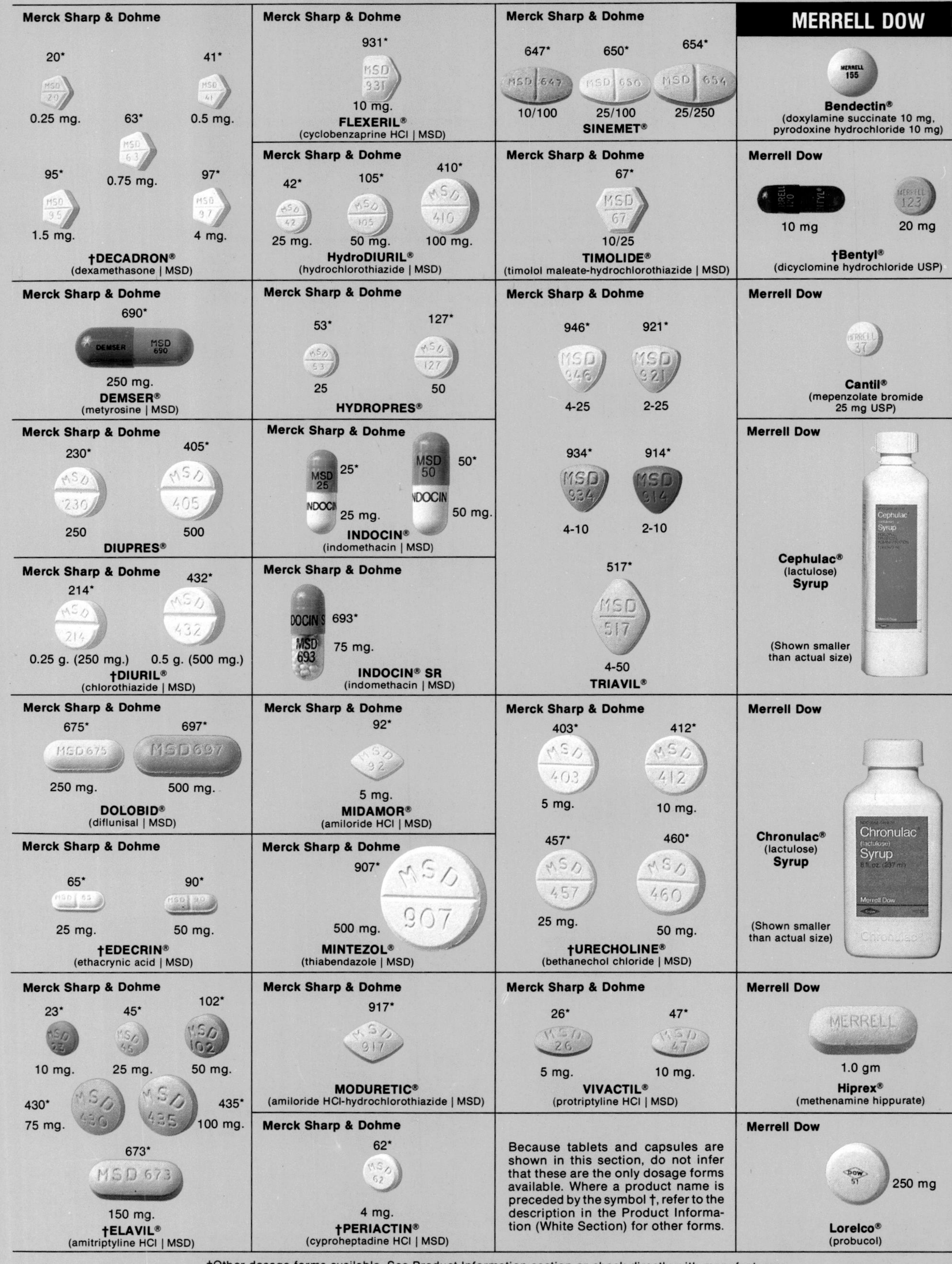

Merck Sharp & Dohme
20* 0.25 mg. · 41* 0.5 mg. · 63* 0.75 mg. · 95* 1.5 mg. · 97* 4 mg.
†DECADRON®
(dexamethasone | MSD)

Merck Sharp & Dohme
931* 10 mg.
FLEXERIL®
(cyclobenzaprine HCl | MSD)

Merck Sharp & Dohme
647* 10/100 · 650* 25/100 · 654* 25/250
SINEMET®

MERRELL DOW
Bendectin®
(doxylamine succinate 10 mg, pyrodoxine hydrochloride 10 mg)

Merck Sharp & Dohme
42* 25 mg. · 105* 50 mg. · 410* 100 mg.
HydroDIURIL®
(hydrochlorothiazide | MSD)

Merck Sharp & Dohme
67* 10/25
TIMOLIDE®
(timolol maleate-hydrochlorothiazide | MSD)

Merrell Dow
10 mg · 20 mg
†Bentyl®
(dicyclomine hydrochloride USP)

Merck Sharp & Dohme
690* 250 mg.
DEMSER®
(metyrosine | MSD)

Merck Sharp & Dohme
53* 25 · 127* 50
HYDROPRES®

Merck Sharp & Dohme
946* 4-25 · 921* 2-25 · 934* 4-10 · 914* 2-10 · 517* 4-50
TRIAVIL®

Merrell Dow
Cantil®
(mepenzolate bromide 25 mg USP)

Merck Sharp & Dohme
230* 250 · 405* 500
DIUPRES®

Merck Sharp & Dohme
25* 25 mg. · 50* 50 mg.
INDOCIN®
(indomethacin | MSD)

Merrell Dow
Cephulac®
(lactulose)
Syrup
(Shown smaller than actual size)

Merck Sharp & Dohme
214* 0.25 g. (250 mg.) · 432* 0.5 g. (500 mg.)
†DIURIL®
(chlorothiazide | MSD)

Merck Sharp & Dohme
693* 75 mg.
INDOCIN® SR
(indomethacin | MSD)

Merck Sharp & Dohme
675* 250 mg. · 697* 500 mg.
DOLOBID®
(diflunisal | MSD)

Merck Sharp & Dohme
92* 5 mg.
MIDAMOR®
(amiloride HCl | MSD)

Merck Sharp & Dohme
403* 5 mg. · 412* 10 mg. · 457* 25 mg. · 460* 50 mg.
†URECHOLINE®
(bethanechol chloride | MSD)

Merrell Dow
Chronulac®
(lactulose)
Syrup
(Shown smaller than actual size)

Merck Sharp & Dohme
65* 25 mg. · 90* 50 mg.
†EDECRIN®
(ethacrynic acid | MSD)

Merck Sharp & Dohme
907* 500 mg.
MINTEZOL®
(thiabendazole | MSD)

Merck Sharp & Dohme
23* 10 mg. · 45* 25 mg. · 102* 50 mg. · 430* 75 mg. · 435* 100 mg. · 673* 150 mg.
†ELAVIL®
(amitriptyline HCl | MSD)

Merck Sharp & Dohme
917*
MODURETIC®
(amiloride HCl-hydrochlorothiazide | MSD)

Merck Sharp & Dohme
26* 5 mg. · 47* 10 mg.
VIVACTIL®
(protriptyline HCl | MSD)

Merrell Dow
1.0 gm
Hiprex®
(methenamine hippurate)

Merck Sharp & Dohme
62* 4 mg.
†PERIACTIN®
(cyproheptadine HCl | MSD)

Because tablets and capsules are shown in this section, do not infer that these are the only dosage forms available. Where a product name is preceded by the symbol †, refer to the description in the Product Information (White Section) for other forms.

Merrell Dow
250 mg
Lorelco®
(probucol)

†Other dosage forms available. See Product Information section or check directly with manufacturer.
*Manufacturers' identification number.

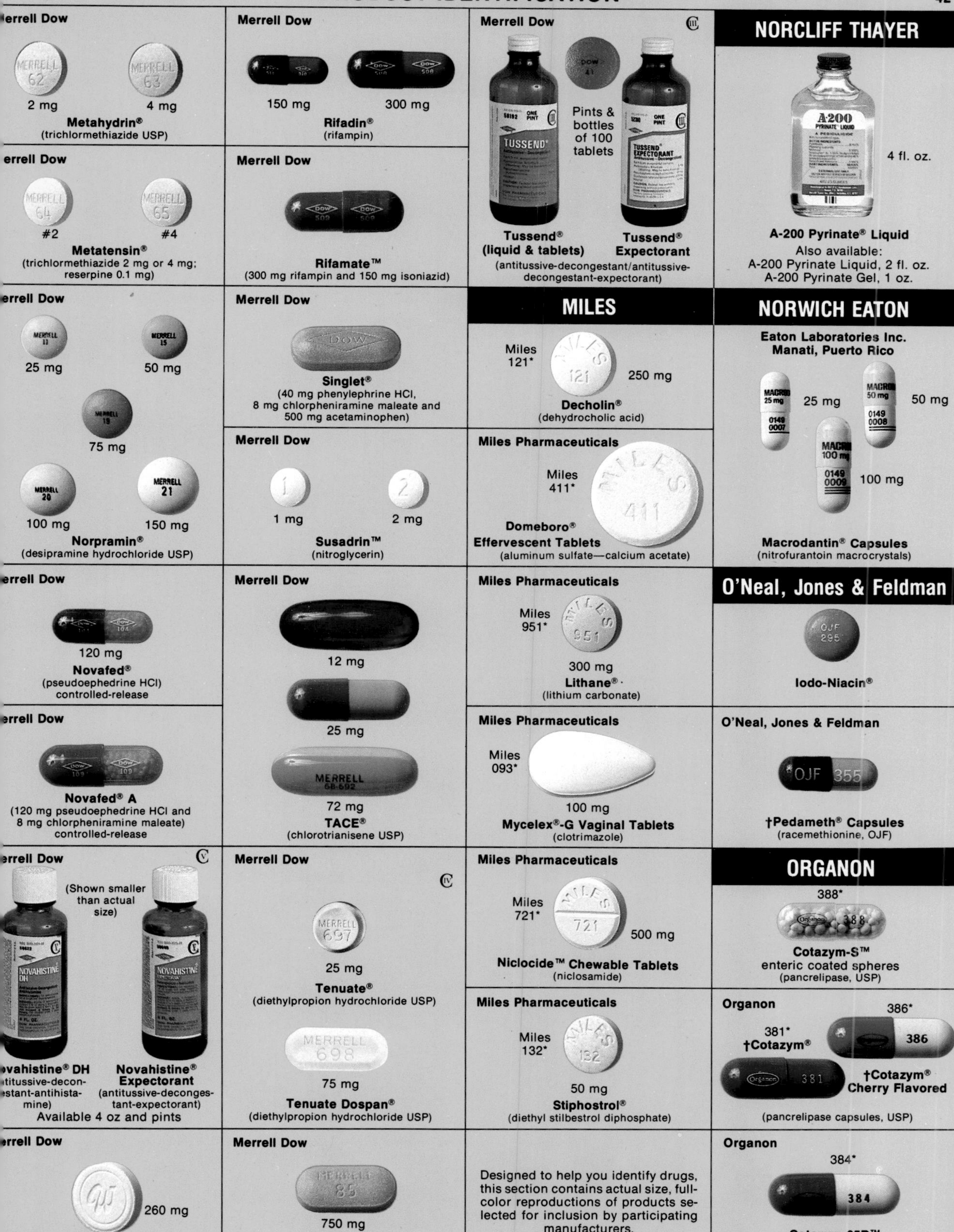
erreIl Dow
2 mg
4 mg
Metahydrin®
(trichlormethiazide USP)
erreIl Dow
#2
#4
Metatensin®
(trichlormethiazide 2 mg or 4 mg; reserpine 0.1 mg)
erreIl Dow
25 mg
50 mg
75 mg
100 mg
150 mg
Norpramin®
(desipramine hydrochloride USP)
erreIl Dow
120 mg
Novafed®
(pseudoephedrine HCl) controlled-release
erreIl Dow
Novafed® A
(120 mg pseudoephedrine HCl and 8 mg chlorpheniramine maleate) controlled-release
erreIl Dow
(Shown smaller than actual size)
ovahistine® DH
titussive-decon-
estant-antihista-
mine)
Novahistine® Expectorant
(antitussive-deconges-tant-expectorant)
Available 4 oz and pints
erreIl Dow
260 mg
Quinamm™
(quinine sulfate tablets)
Merrell Dow
150 mg
300 mg
Rifadin®
(rifampin)
Merrell Dow
Rifamate™
(300 mg rifampin and 150 mg isoniazid)
Merrell Dow
Singlet®
(40 mg phenylephrine HCl, 8 mg chlorpheniramine maleate and 500 mg acetaminophen)
Merrell Dow
1 mg
2 mg
Susadrin™
(nitroglycerin)
Merrell Dow
12 mg
25 mg
72 mg
TACE®
(chlorotrianisene USP)
Merrell Dow
25 mg
Tenuate®
(diethylpropion hydrochloride USP)
75 mg
Tenuate Dospan®
(diethylpropion hydrochloride USP)
Merrell Dow
750 mg
†Triclos®
(triclofos sodium)
Merrell Dow
Pints & bottles of 100 tablets
Tussend®
(liquid & tablets)
Tussend®
Expectorant
(antitussive-decongestant/antitussive-decongestant-expectorant)
MILES
Miles 121*
250 mg
Decholin®
(dehydrocholic acid)
Miles Pharmaceuticals
Miles 411*
Domeboro®
Effervescent Tablets
(aluminum sulfate—calcium acetate)
Miles Pharmaceuticals
Miles 951*
300 mg
Lithane®
(lithium carbonate)
Miles Pharmaceuticals
Miles 093*
100 mg
Mycelex®-G Vaginal Tablets
(clotrimazole)
Miles Pharmaceuticals
Miles 721*
500 mg
Niclocide™ Chewable Tablets
(niclosamide)
Miles Pharmaceuticals
Miles 132*
50 mg
Stiphostrol®
(diethyl stilbestrol diphosphate)
Designed to help you identify drugs, this section contains actual size, full-color reproductions of products selected for inclusion by participating manufacturers.
NORCLIFF THAYER
4 fl. oz.
A-200 Pyrinate® Liquid
Also available:
A-200 Pyrinate Liquid, 2 fl. oz.
A-200 Pyrinate Gel, 1 oz.
NORWICH EATON
Eaton Laboratories Inc.
Manati, Puerto Rico
25 mg
50 mg
100 mg
Macrodantin® Capsules
(nitrofurantoin macrocrystals)
O'Neal, Jones & Feldman
Iodo-Niacin®
O'Neal, Jones & Feldman
†Pedameth® Capsules
(racemethionine, OJF)
ORGANON
388*
Cotazym-S™
enteric coated spheres
(pancrelipase, USP)
Organon
386*
381*
†Cotazym®
†Cotazym®
Cherry Flavored
(pancrelipase capsules, USP)
Organon
384*
Cotazym-65B™
(pancrelipase USP with mixed conjugated bile salts)

†Other dosage forms available. See Product Information section or check directly with manufacturer.
*Manufacturers' identification number.

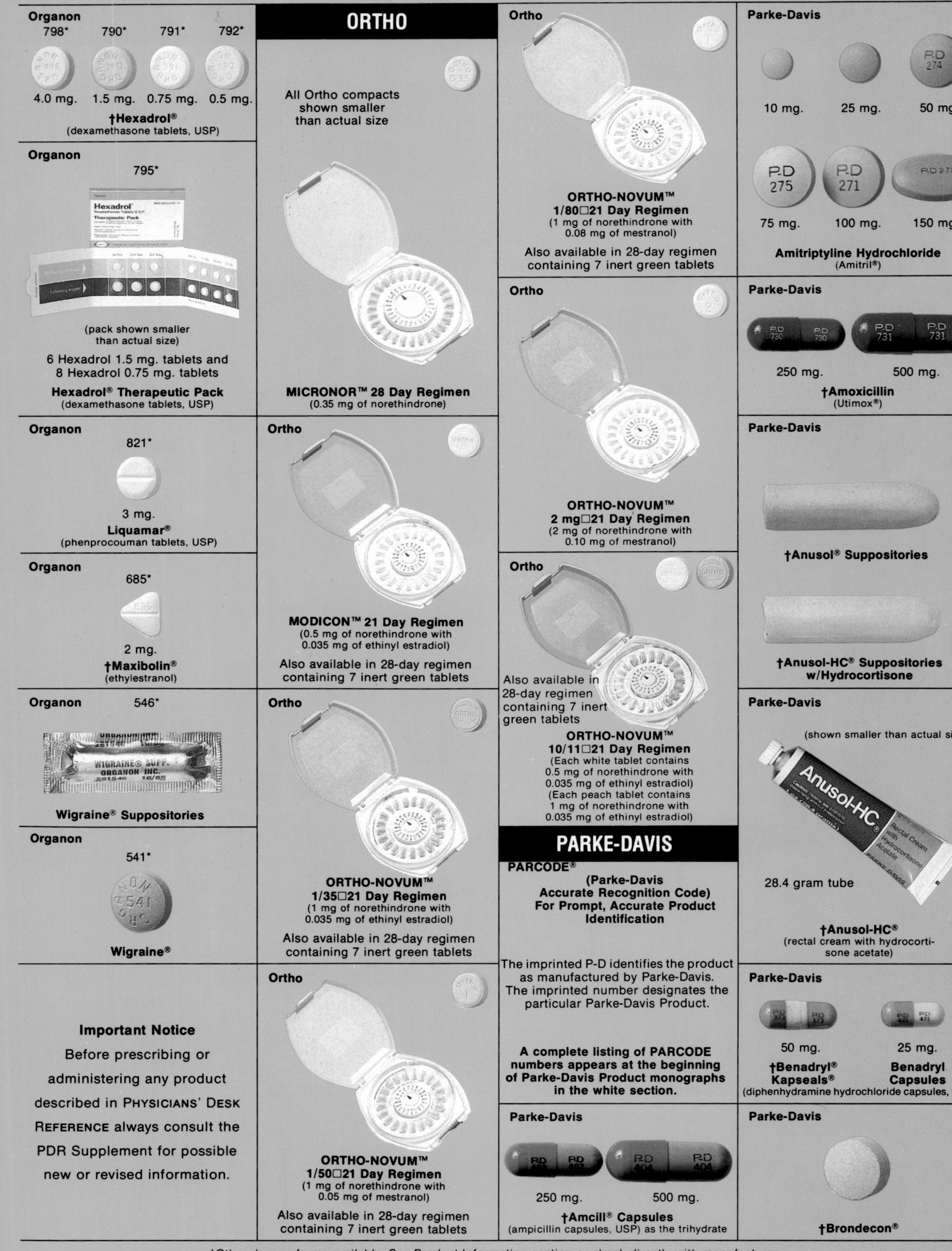

Organon
798* 790* 791* 792*
4.0 mg. 1.5 mg. 0.75 mg. 0.5 mg.
†Hexadrol®
(dexamethasone tablets, USP)

Organon
795*
(pack shown smaller than actual size)
6 Hexadrol 1.5 mg. tablets and 8 Hexadrol 0.75 mg. tablets
Hexadrol® Therapeutic Pack
(dexamethasone tablets, USP)

Organon
821*
3 mg.
Liquamar®
(phenprocouman tablets, USP)

Organon
685*
2 mg.
†Maxibolin®
(ethylestranol)

Organon 546*
Wigraine® Suppositories

Organon
541*
Wigraine®

Important Notice
Before prescribing or administering any product described in PHYSICIANS' DESK REFERENCE always consult the PDR Supplement for possible new or revised information.

ORTHO

All Ortho compacts shown smaller than actual size

MICRONOR™ 28 Day Regimen
(0.35 mg of norethindrone)

Ortho
MODICON™ 21 Day Regimen
(0.5 mg of norethindrone with 0.035 mg of ethinyl estradiol)
Also available in 28-day regimen containing 7 inert green tablets

Ortho
ORTHO-NOVUM™ 1/35□21 Day Regimen
(1 mg of norethindrone with 0.035 mg of ethinyl estradiol)
Also available in 28-day regimen containing 7 inert green tablets

Ortho
ORTHO-NOVUM™ 1/50□21 Day Regimen
(1 mg of norethindrone with 0.05 mg of mestranol)
Also available in 28-day regimen containing 7 inert green tablets

Ortho
ORTHO-NOVUM™ 1/80□21 Day Regimen
(1 mg of norethindrone with 0.08 mg of mestranol)
Also available in 28-day regimen containing 7 inert green tablets

Ortho
ORTHO-NOVUM™ 2 mg□21 Day Regimen
(2 mg of norethindrone with 0.10 mg of mestranol)

Ortho
Also available in 28-day regimen containing 7 inert green tablets
ORTHO-NOVUM™ 10/11□21 Day Regimen
(Each white tablet contains 0.5 mg of norethindrone with 0.035 mg of ethinyl estradiol)
(Each peach tablet contains 1 mg of norethindrone with 0.035 mg of ethinyl estradiol)

PARKE-DAVIS

PARCODE®
(Parke-Davis Accurate Recognition Code) For Prompt, Accurate Product Identification

The imprinted P-D identifies the product as manufactured by Parke-Davis. The imprinted number designates the particular Parke-Davis Product.

A complete listing of PARCODE numbers appears at the beginning of Parke-Davis Product monographs in the white section.

Parke-Davis
250 mg. 500 mg.
†Amcill® Capsules
(ampicillin capsules, USP) as the trihydrate

Parke-Davis
10 mg. 25 mg. 50 mg.
75 mg. 100 mg. 150 mg.
Amitriptyline Hydrochloride
(Amitril®)

Parke-Davis
250 mg. 500 mg.
†Amoxicillin
(Utimox®)

Parke-Davis
†Anusol® Suppositories
†Anusol-HC® Suppositories w/Hydrocortisone

Parke-Davis
(shown smaller than actual siz
28.4 gram tube
†Anusol-HC®
(rectal cream with hydrocortisone acetate)

Parke-Davis
50 mg. 25 mg.
†Benadryl® Kapseals® **Benadryl Capsules**
(diphenhydramine hydrochloride capsules, U

Parke-Davis
†Brondecon®

†Other dosage forms available. See Product Information section or check directly with manufacturer.
*Manufacturers' identification number.

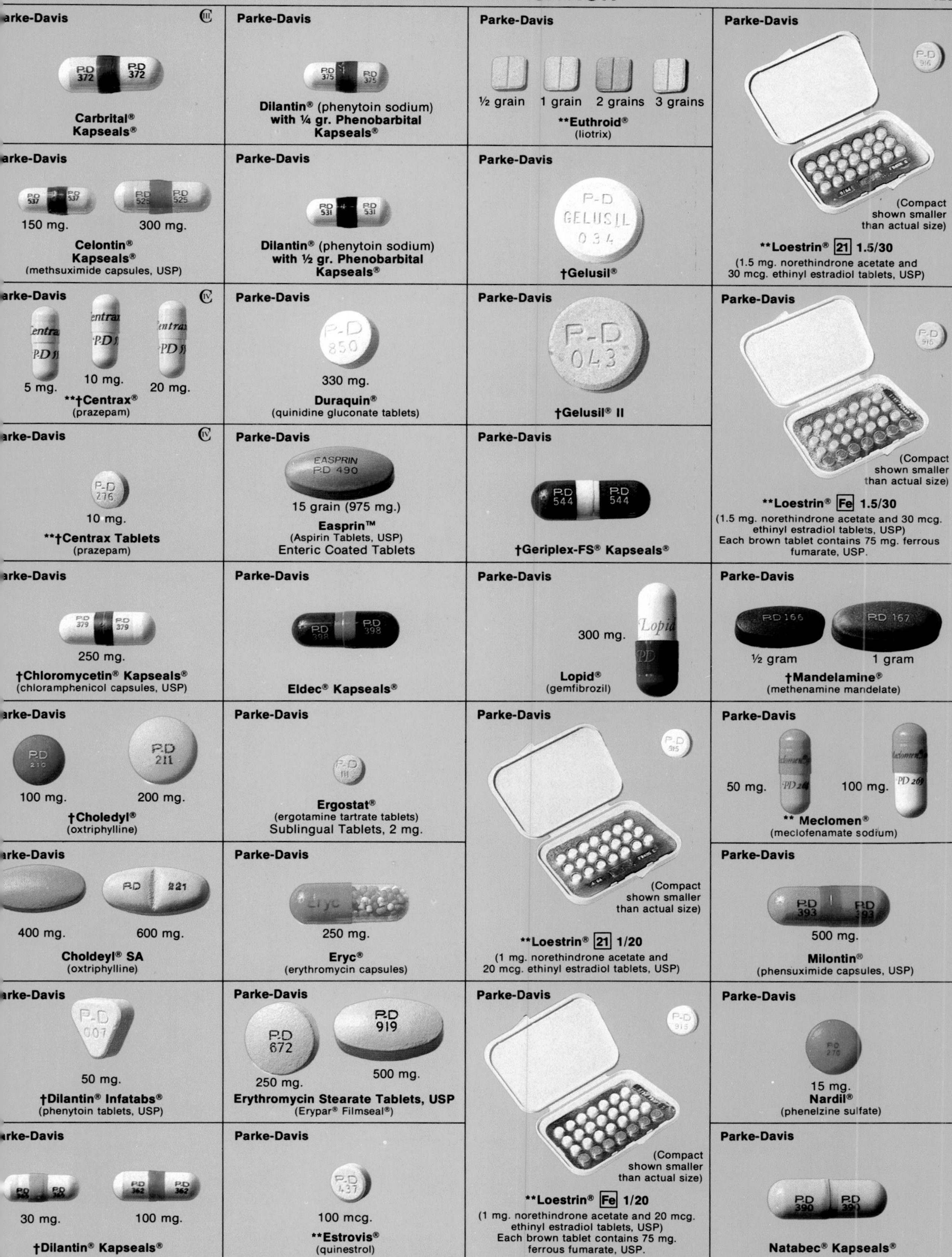

Parke-Davis

Carbrital®
Kapseals®

Parke-Davis

Dilantin® (phenytoin sodium)
with ¼ gr. Phenobarbital
Kapseals®

Parke-Davis

½ grain 1 grain 2 grains 3 grains

**Euthroid®
(liotrix)

Parke-Davis

(Compact shown smaller than actual size)

**Loestrin® 21 1.5/30
(1.5 mg. norethindrone acetate and 30 mcg. ethinyl estradiol tablets, USP)

Parke-Davis

150 mg. 300 mg.

Celontin®
Kapseals®
(methsuximide capsules, USP)

Parke-Davis

Dilantin® (phenytoin sodium)
with ½ gr. Phenobarbital
Kapseals®

Parke-Davis

†Gelusil®

Parke-Davis

5 mg. 10 mg. 20 mg.

**†Centrax®
(prazepam)

Parke-Davis

330 mg.

Duraquin®
(quinidine gluconate tablets)

Parke-Davis

†Gelusil® II

Parke-Davis

(Compact shown smaller than actual size)

**Loestrin® Fe 1.5/30
(1.5 mg. norethindrone acetate and 30 mcg. ethinyl estradiol tablets, USP)
Each brown tablet contains 75 mg. ferrous fumarate, USP.

Parke-Davis

10 mg.

**†Centrax Tablets
(prazepam)

Parke-Davis

15 grain (975 mg.)

Easprin™
(Aspirin Tablets, USP)
Enteric Coated Tablets

Parke-Davis

†Geriplex-FS® Kapseals®

Parke-Davis

250 mg.

†Chloromycetin® Kapseals®
(chloramphenicol capsules, USP)

Parke-Davis

Eldec® Kapseals®

Parke-Davis

300 mg.

Lopid®
(gemfibrozil)

Parke-Davis

½ gram 1 gram

†Mandelamine®
(methenamine mandelate)

Parke-Davis

100 mg. 200 mg.

†Choledyl®
(oxtriphylline)

Parke-Davis

Ergostat®
(ergotamine tartrate tablets)
Sublingual Tablets, 2 mg.

Parke-Davis

(Compact shown smaller than actual size)

**Loestrin® 21 1/20
(1 mg. norethindrone acetate and 20 mcg. ethinyl estradiol tablets, USP)

Parke-Davis

50 mg. 100 mg.

** Meclomen®
(meclofenamate sodium)

Parke-Davis

400 mg. 600 mg.

Choldeyl® SA
(oxtriphylline)

Parke-Davis

250 mg.

Eryc®
(erythromycin capsules)

Parke-Davis

500 mg.

Milontin®
(phensuximide capsules, USP)

Parke-Davis

50 mg.

†Dilantin® Infatabs®
(phenytoin tablets, USP)

Parke-Davis

250 mg. 500 mg.

Erythromycin Stearate Tablets, USP
(Erypar® Filmseal®)

Parke-Davis

(Compact shown smaller than actual size)

**Loestrin® Fe 1/20
(1 mg. norethindrone acetate and 20 mcg. ethinyl estradiol tablets, USP)
Each brown tablet contains 75 mg. ferrous fumarate, USP.

Parke-Davis

15 mg.
Nardil®
(phenelzine sulfate)

Parke-Davis

30 mg. 100 mg.

†Dilantin® Kapseals®

Parke-Davis

100 mcg.

**Estrovis®
(quinestrol)

Parke-Davis

Natabec® Kapseals®

†Other dosage forms available. See Product Information section or check directly with manufacturer.
**Product of PARKE-DAVIS, Div. Warner-Lambert Inc, Santurce, PR 00911.

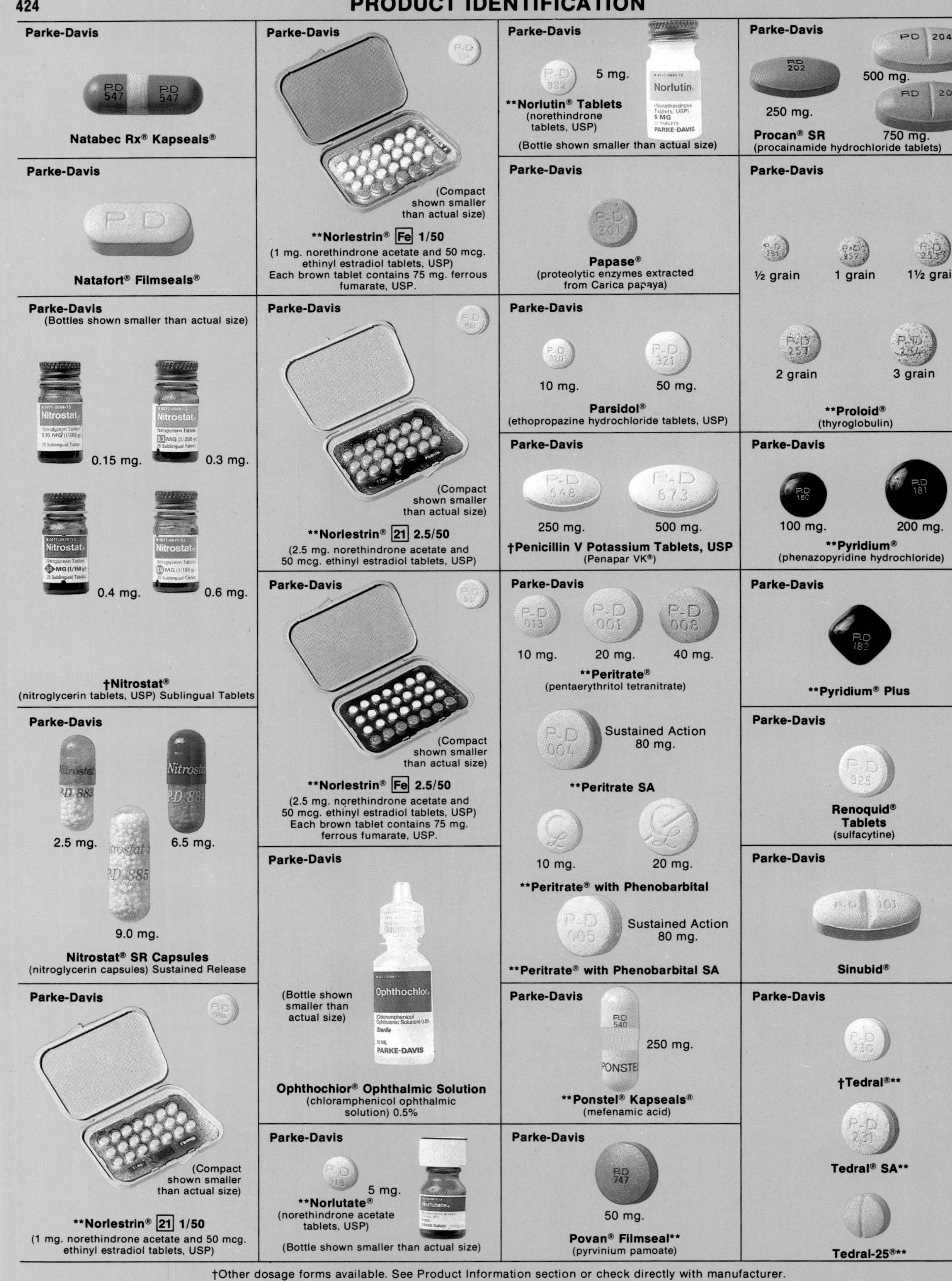

Parke-Davis

Natabec Rx® Kapseals®

Parke-Davis

Natafort® Filmseals®

Parke-Davis
(Bottles shown smaller than actual size)

0.15 mg. 0.3 mg. 0.4 mg. 0.6 mg.

†Nitrostat®
(nitroglycerin tablets, USP) Sublingual Tablets

Parke-Davis

2.5 mg. 6.5 mg. 9.0 mg.

Nitrostat® SR Capsules
(nitroglycerin capsules) Sustained Release

Parke-Davis

(Compact shown smaller than actual size)

****Norlestrin® 21 1/50**
(1 mg. norethindrone acetate and 50 mcg. ethinyl estradiol tablets, USP)

Parke-Davis

(Compact shown smaller than actual size)

****Norlestrin® Fe 1/50**
(1 mg. norethindrone acetate and 50 mcg. ethinyl estradiol tablets, USP)
Each brown tablet contains 75 mg. ferrous fumarate, USP.

Parke-Davis

(Compact shown smaller than actual size)

****Norlestrin® 21 2.5/50**
(2.5 mg. norethindrone acetate and 50 mcg. ethinyl estradiol tablets, USP)

Parke-Davis

(Compact shown smaller than actual size)

****Norlestrin® Fe 2.5/50**
(2.5 mg. norethindrone acetate and 50 mcg. ethinyl estradiol tablets, USP)
Each brown tablet contains 75 mg. ferrous fumarate, USP.

Parke-Davis

(Bottle shown smaller than actual size)

Ophthochlor® Ophthalmic Solution
(chloramphenicol ophthalmic solution) 0.5%

Parke-Davis

5 mg.

****Norlutate®**
(norethindrone acetate tablets, USP)

(Bottle shown smaller than actual size)

Parke-Davis

5 mg.

****Norlutin® Tablets**
(norethindrone tablets, USP)

(Bottle shown smaller than actual size)

Parke-Davis

Papase®
(proteolytic enzymes extracted from Carica papaya)

Parke-Davis

10 mg. 50 mg.

Parsidol®
(ethopropazine hydrochloride tablets, USP)

Parke-Davis

250 mg. 500 mg.

†Penicillin V Potassium Tablets, USP
(Penapar VK®)

Parke-Davis

10 mg. 20 mg. 40 mg.

****Peritrate®**
(pentaerythritol tetranitrate)

Sustained Action 80 mg.

****Peritrate SA**

10 mg. 20 mg.

****Peritrate® with Phenobarbital**

Sustained Action 80 mg.

****Peritrate® with Phenobarbital SA**

Parke-Davis

250 mg.

****Ponstel® Kapseals®**
(mefenamic acid)

Parke-Davis

50 mg.

Povan® Filmseal**
(pyrvinium pamoate)

Parke-Davis

250 mg. 500 mg. 750 mg.

Procan® SR
(procainamide hydrochloride tablets)

Parke-Davis

½ grain 1 grain 1½ grain 2 grain 3 grain

****Proloid®**
(thyroglobulin)

Parke-Davis

100 mg. 200 mg.

****Pyridium®**
(phenazopyridine hydrochloride)

Parke-Davis

****Pyridium® Plus**

Parke-Davis

Renoquid® Tablets
(sulfacytine)

Parke-Davis

Sinubid®

Parke-Davis

†Tedral®**

Tedral® SA**

Tedral-25®**

†Other dosage forms available. See Product Information section or check directly with manufacturer.
*Manufacturers' identification number.
**Product of PARKE-DAVIS, Div. Warner-Lambert Inc, Santurce, PR 00911.

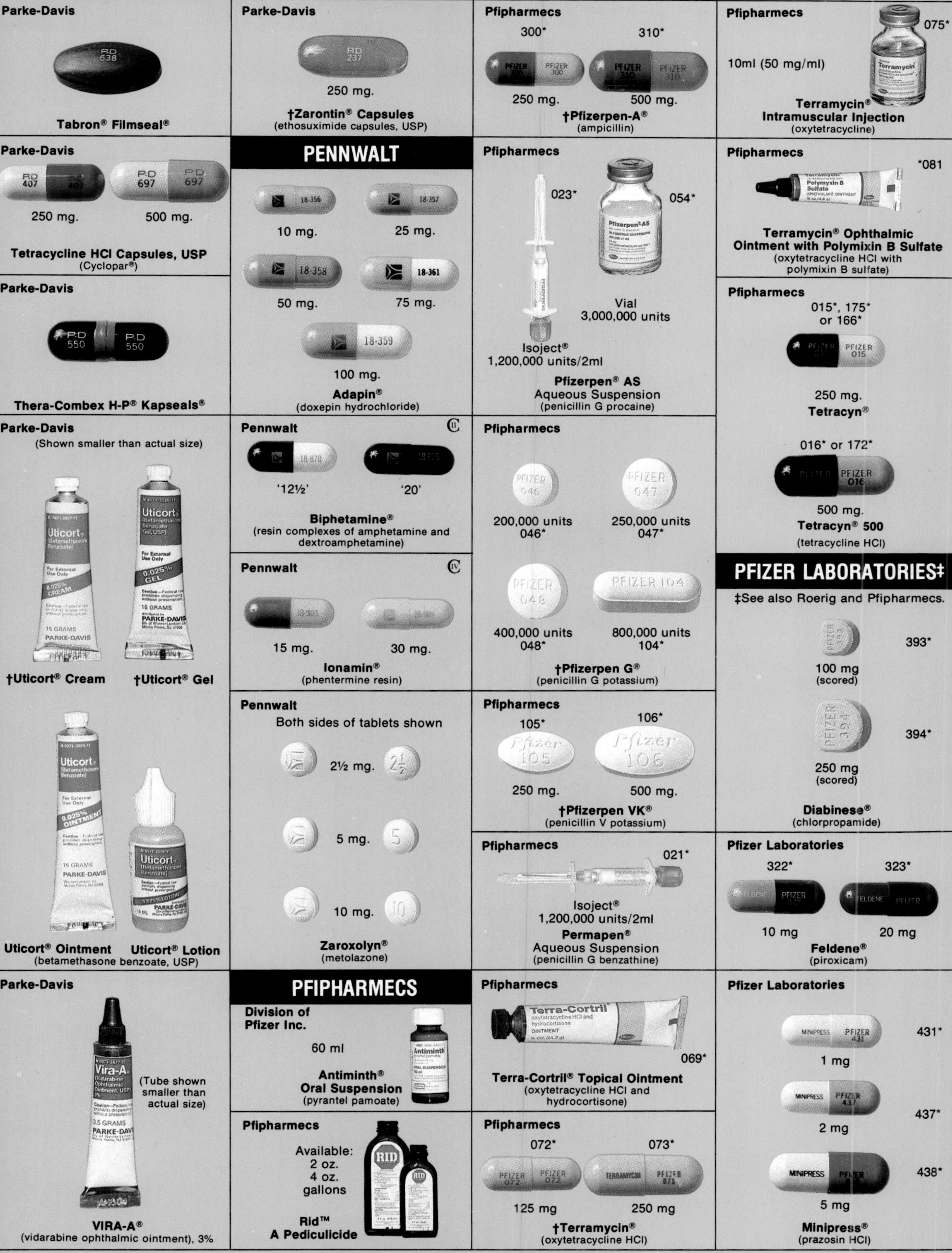
Parke-Davis
Tabron® Filmseal®
Parke-Davis
250 mg.
†Zarontin® Capsules
(ethosuximide capsules, USP)
Pfipharmecs
300* 310*
250 mg. 500 mg.
†Pfizerpen-A®
(ampicillin)
Pfipharmecs
075*
10ml (50 mg/ml)
Terramycin®
Intramuscular Injection
(oxytetracycline)
Parke-Davis
250 mg. 500 mg.
Tetracycline HCl Capsules, USP
(Cyclopar®)
PENNWALT
10 mg. 25 mg.
50 mg. 75 mg.
100 mg.
Adapin®
(doxepin hydrochloride)
Pfipharmecs
023* 054*
Vial
3,000,000 units
Isoject®
1,200,000 units/2ml
Pfizerpen® AS
Aqueous Suspension
(penicillin G procaine)
Pfipharmecs
*081
Terramycin® Ophthalmic
Ointment with Polymyxin B Sulfate
(oxytetracycline HCl with
polymyxin B sulfate)
Parke-Davis
Thera-Combex H-P® Kapseals®
Pfipharmecs
015*, 175*
or 166*
250 mg.
Tetracyn®
016* or 172*
500 mg.
Tetracyn® 500
(tetracycline HCl)
Parke-Davis
(Shown smaller than actual size)
†Uticort® Cream †Uticort® Gel
Uticort® Ointment Uticort® Lotion
(betamethasone benzoate, USP)
Pennwalt
'12½' '20'
Biphetamine®
(resin complexes of amphetamine and
dextroamphetamine)
Pfipharmecs
200,000 units 250,000 units
046* 047*
400,000 units 800,000 units
048* 104*
†Pfizerpen G®
(penicillin G potassium)
PFIZER LABORATORIES‡
‡See also Roerig and Pfipharmecs.
393*
100 mg
(scored)
394*
250 mg
(scored)
Diabinese®
(chlorpropamide)
Pennwalt
15 mg. 30 mg.
Ionamin®
(phentermine resin)
Pennwalt
Both sides of tablets shown
2½ mg.
5 mg.
10 mg.
Zaroxolyn®
(metolazone)
Pfipharmecs
105* 106*
250 mg. 500 mg.
†Pfizerpen VK®
(penicillin V potassium)
Pfipharmecs
021*
Isoject®
1,200,000 units/2ml
Permapen®
Aqueous Suspension
(penicillin G benzathine)
Pfizer Laboratories
322* 323*
10 mg 20 mg
Feldene®
(piroxicam)
Parke-Davis
(Tube shown
smaller than
actual size)
VIRA-A®
(vidarabine ophthalmic ointment), 3%
PFIPHARMECS
Division of
Pfizer Inc.
60 ml
Antiminth®
Oral Suspension
(pyrantel pamoate)
Pfipharmecs
Available:
2 oz.
4 oz.
gallons
Rid™
A Pediculicide
Pfipharmecs
069*
Terra-Cortril® Topical Ointment
(oxytetracycline HCl and
hydrocortisone)
Pfipharmecs
072* 073*
125 mg 250 mg
†Terramycin®
(oxytetracycline HCl)
Pfizer Laboratories
431*
1 mg
437*
2 mg
438*
5 mg
Minipress®
(prazosin HCl)

†Other dosage forms available. See Product Information section or check directly with manufacturer.
*Manufacturers' identification number.

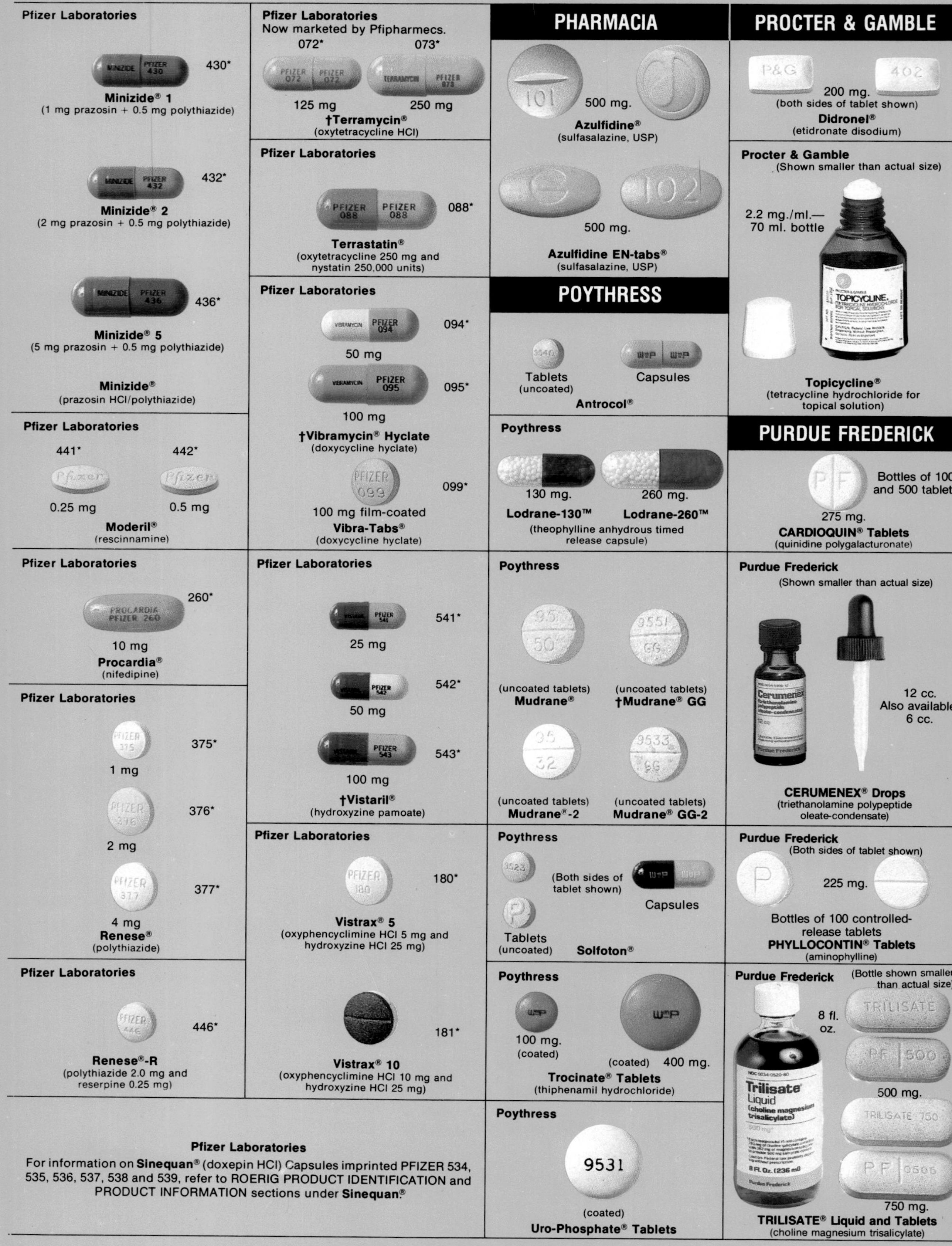
Pfizer Laboratories
430*
Minizide® 1
(1 mg prazosin + 0.5 mg polythiazide)
432*
Minizide® 2
(2 mg prazosin + 0.5 mg polythiazide)
436*
Minizide® 5
(5 mg prazosin + 0.5 mg polythiazide)
Minizide®
(prazosin HCl/polythiazide)
Pfizer Laboratories
441* 442*
0.25 mg 0.5 mg
Moderil®
(rescinnamine)
Pfizer Laboratories
260*
10 mg
Procardia®
(nifedipine)
Pfizer Laboratories
375*
1 mg
376*
2 mg
377*
4 mg
Renese®
(polythiazide)
Pfizer Laboratories
446*
Renese®-R
(polythiazide 2.0 mg and reserpine 0.25 mg)
Pfizer Laboratories
Now marketed by Pfipharmecs.
072* 073*
125 mg 250 mg
†Terramycin®
(oxytetracycline HCl)
Pfizer Laboratories
088*
Terrastatin®
(oxytetracycline 250 mg and nystatin 250,000 units)
Pfizer Laboratories
094*
50 mg
095*
100 mg
†Vibramycin® Hyclate
(doxycycline hyclate)
099*
100 mg film-coated
Vibra-Tabs®
(doxycycline hyclate)
Pfizer Laboratories
541*
25 mg
542*
50 mg
543*
100 mg
†Vistaril®
(hydroxyzine pamoate)
Pfizer Laboratories
180*
Vistrax® 5
(oxyphencyclimine HCl 5 mg and hydroxyzine HCl 25 mg)
181*
Vistrax® 10
(oxyphencyclimine HCl 10 mg and hydroxyzine HCl 25 mg)
Pfizer Laboratories
For information on Sinequan® (doxepin HCl) Capsules imprinted PFIZER 534, 535, 536, 537, 538 and 539, refer to ROERIG PRODUCT IDENTIFICATION and PRODUCT INFORMATION sections under Sinequan®.
PHARMACIA
500 mg.
Azulfidine®
(sulfasalazine, USP)
500 mg.
Azulfidine EN-tabs®
(sulfasalazine, USP)
POYTHRESS
Tablets (uncoated)
Capsules
Antrocol®
Poythress
130 mg. 260 mg.
Lodrane-130™ Lodrane-260™
(theophylline anhydrous timed release capsule)
Poythress
(uncoated tablets) Mudrane®
(uncoated tablets) †Mudrane® GG
(uncoated tablets) Mudrane®-2
(uncoated tablets) Mudrane® GG-2
Poythress
(Both sides of tablet shown)
Capsules
Tablets (uncoated)
Solfoton®
Poythress
100 mg. (coated)
(coated) 400 mg.
Trocinate® Tablets
(thiphenamil hydrochloride)
Poythress
9531
(coated)
Uro-Phosphate® Tablets
PROCTER & GAMBLE
200 mg.
(both sides of tablet shown)
Didronel®
(etidronate disodium)
Procter & Gamble
(Shown smaller than actual size)
2.2 mg./ml.— 70 ml. bottle
TOPICYCLINE
Topicycline®
(tetracycline hydrochloride for topical solution)
PURDUE FREDERICK
Bottles of 100 and 500 tablets
275 mg.
CARDIOQUIN® Tablets
(quinidine polygalacturonate)
Purdue Frederick
(Shown smaller than actual size)
Cerumenex
12 cc.
Also available 6 cc.
CERUMENEX® Drops
(triethanolamine polypeptide oleate-condensate)
Purdue Frederick
(Both sides of tablet shown)
225 mg.
Bottles of 100 controlled-release tablets
PHYLLOCONTIN® Tablets
(aminophylline)
Purdue Frederick
(Bottle shown smaller than actual size)
8 fl. oz.
Trilisate Liquid (choline magnesium trisalicylate)
500 mg.
750 mg.
TRILISATE® Liquid and Tablets
(choline magnesium trisalicylate)

†Other dosage forms available. See Product Information section or check directly with manufacturer.
*Manufacturers' identification number.

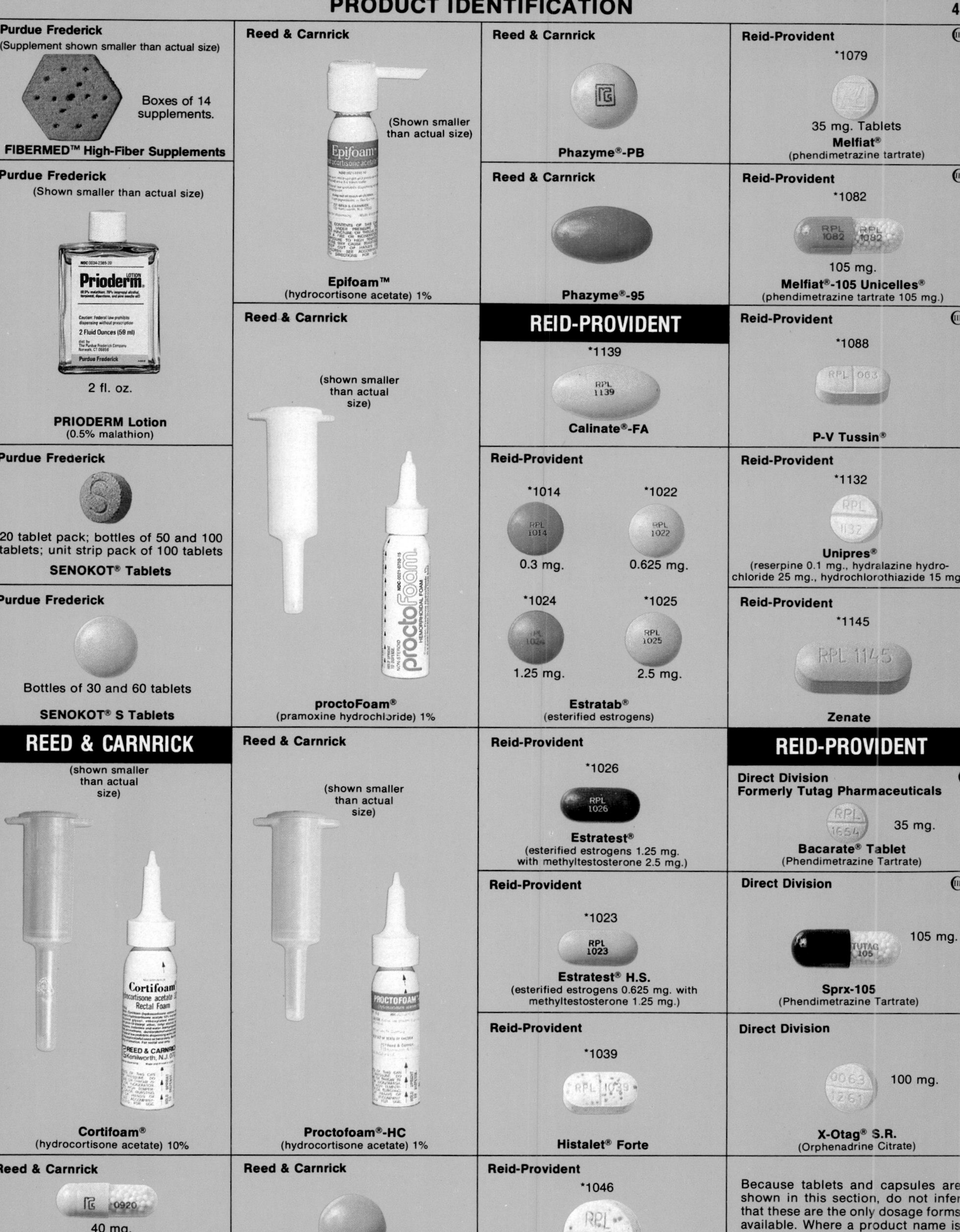

Purdue Frederick
(Supplement shown smaller than actual size)
Boxes of 14 supplements.
FIBERMED™ High-Fiber Supplements
Purdue Frederick
(Shown smaller than actual size)
Prioderm. Lotion
2 Fluid Ounces (59 ml)
Purdue Frederick
2 fl. oz.
PRIODERM Lotion
(0.5% malathion)
Purdue Frederick
20 tablet pack; bottles of 50 and 100 tablets; unit strip pack of 100 tablets
SENOKOT® Tablets
Purdue Frederick
Bottles of 30 and 60 tablets
SENOKOT® S Tablets
REED & CARNRICK
(shown smaller than actual size)
Cortifoam
Rectal Foam
REED & CARNRICK
Kenilworth, N.J.
Cortifoam®
(hydrocortisone acetate) 10%
Reed & Carnrick
0920
40 mg.
Sustained Release Capsules
Dilatrate®-SR
(isosorbide dinitrate)
Reed & Carnrick
(Shown smaller than actual size)
Epifoam
Epifoam™
(hydrocortisone acetate) 1%
Reed & Carnrick
(shown smaller than actual size)
proctoFoam
HEMORRHOIDAL FOAM
proctoFoam®
(pramoxine hydrochloride) 1%
Reed & Carnrick
(shown smaller than actual size)
PROCTOFOAM
Proctofoam®-HC
(hydrocortisone acetate) 1%
Reed & Carnrick
Phazyme®
Reed & Carnrick
Phazyme®-PB
Reed & Carnrick
Phazyme®-95
REID-PROVIDENT
*1139
RPL 1139
Calinate®-FA
Reid-Provident
*1014
RPL 1014
0.3 mg.
*1022
RPL 1022
0.625 mg.
*1024
RPL 1024
1.25 mg.
*1025
RPL 1025
2.5 mg.
Estratab®
(esterified estrogens)
Reid-Provident
*1026
RPL 1026
Estratest®
(esterified estrogens 1.25 mg. with methyltestosterone 2.5 mg.)
Reid-Provident
*1023
RPL 1023
Estratest® H.S.
(esterified estrogens 0.625 mg. with methyltestosterone 1.25 mg.)
Reid-Provident
*1039
RPL 1039
Histalet® Forte
Reid-Provident
*1046
RPL 1046
Histalet® X
Reid-Provident
*1079
35 mg. Tablets
Melfiat®
(phendimetrazine tartrate)
Reid-Provident
*1082
RPL 1082
105 mg.
Melfiat®-105 Unicelles®
(phendimetrazine tartrate 105 mg.)
Reid-Provident
*1088
RPL 063
P-V Tussin®
Reid-Provident
*1132
RPL 1132
Unipres®
(reserpine 0.1 mg., hydralazine hydrochloride 25 mg., hydrochlorothiazide 15 mg.)
Reid-Provident
*1145
RPL 1145
Zenate
REID-PROVIDENT
Direct Division
Formerly Tutag Pharmaceuticals
RPL 1654
35 mg.
Bacarate® Tablet
(Phendimetrazine Tartrate)
Direct Division
TUTAG 105
105 mg.
Sprx-105
(Phendimetrazine Tartrate)
Direct Division
0063 1261
100 mg.
X-Otag® S.R.
(Orphenadrine Citrate)
Because tablets and capsules are shown in this section, do not infer that these are the only dosage forms available. Where a product name is preceded by the symbol †, refer to the description in the Product Information (White Section) for other forms.

*Manufacturers' identification number.

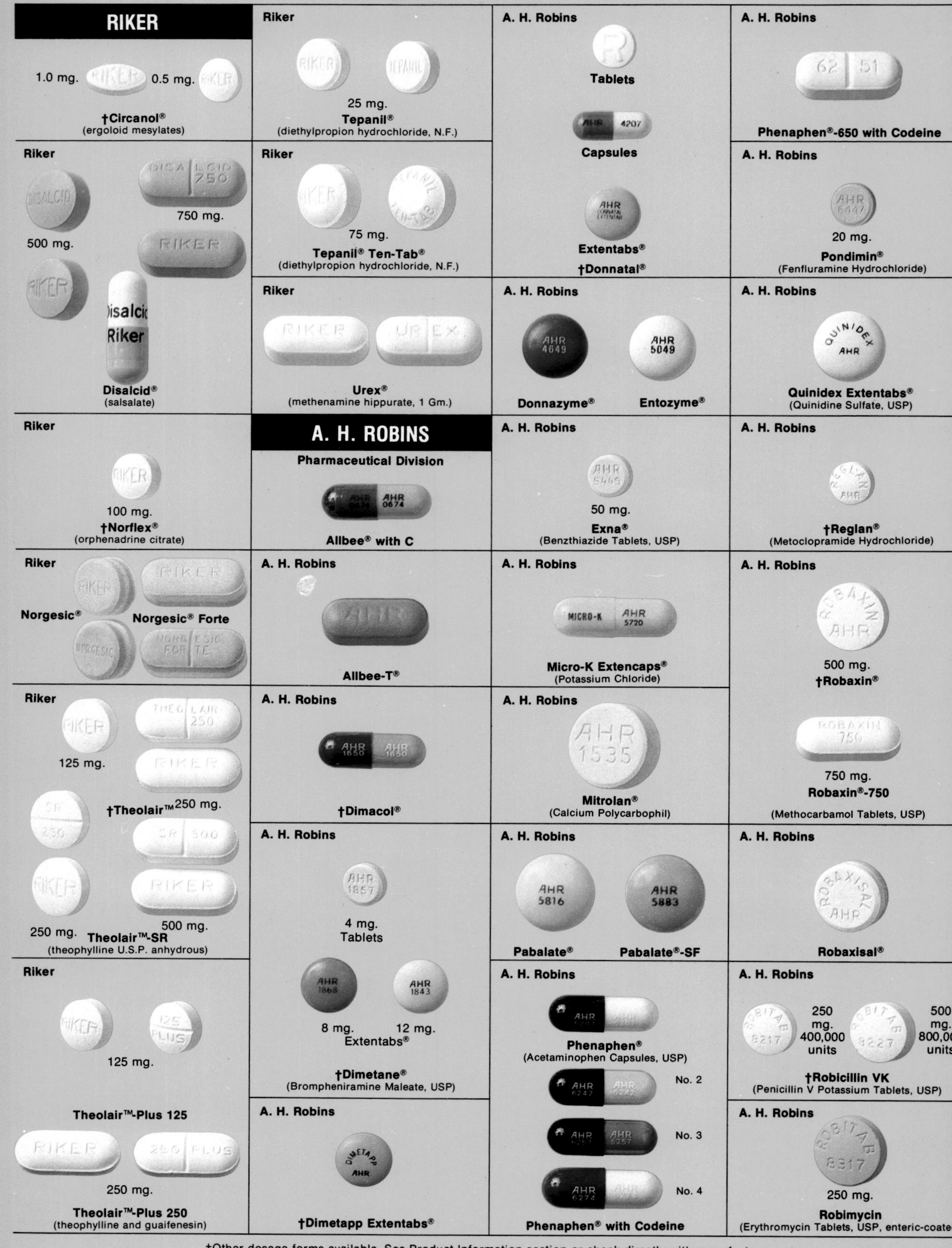

†Other dosage forms available. See Product Information section or check directly with manufacturer.

A. H. Robins

†Robinul® Robinul® Forte
(Glycopyrrolate Tablets, USP)

A. H. Robins

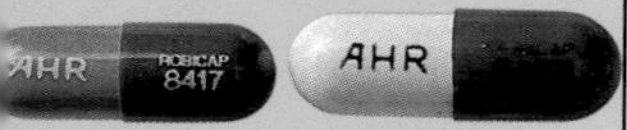

250 mg. 500 mg.
Robitet® '250' Hydrochloride
Robitet® '500' Hydrochloride
Tetracycline Hydrochloride Capsules, USP)

A. H. Robins

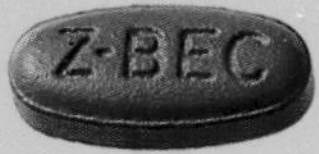

Z-BEC®

ROCHE

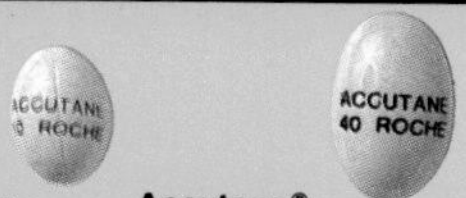

10 mg **Accutane®** 40 mg
(isotretinoin/Roche)

Roche

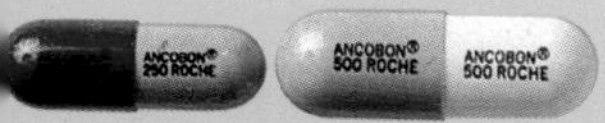

250 mg 500 mg
Ancobon®
(flucytosine/Roche)

Roche

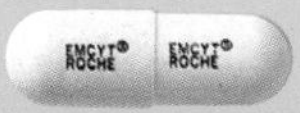

Azo Gantanol®

Roche

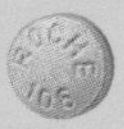

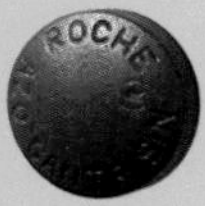

Azo Gantrisin®

Roche

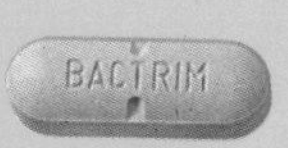

†Bactrim™
(trimethoprim and sulfamethoxazole)

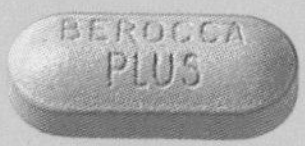

Roche

†Bactrim™ DS
(trimethoprim and sulfamethoxazole)

Roche

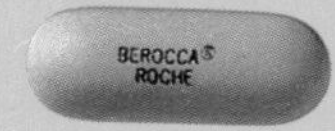

Berocca® Tablets

Roche

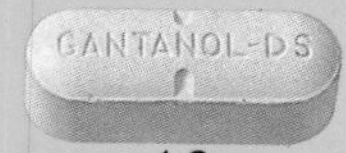

Berocca® Plus

Roche C-IV

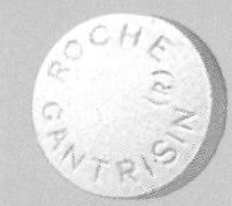

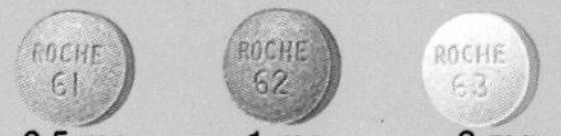

ROCHE 61 ROCHE 62 ROCHE 63
0.5 mg 1 mg 2 mg
Clonopin®
(clonazepam/Roche)

Roche C-IV

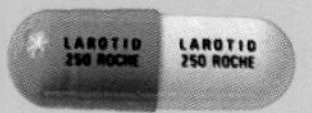

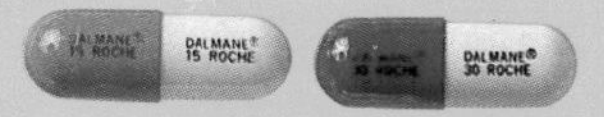

15 mg 30 mg
***Dalmane®**
(flurazepam HCl/Roche)

Roche

140 mg
Emcyt®
(estramustine phosphate sodium/Roche)

Roche

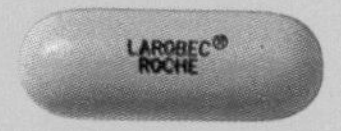

ROCHE 106 — 10 mg
ROCHE 107 — 25 mg 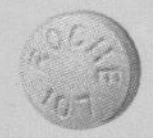
ROCHE 109 — 50 mg 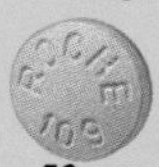
ROCHE 114 — 75 mg 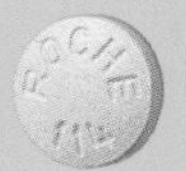
ROCHE 116 — 100 mg 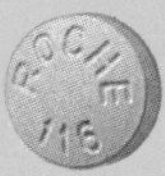
150 mg
Endep®
(amitriptyline HCl/Roche)

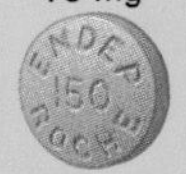

Roche

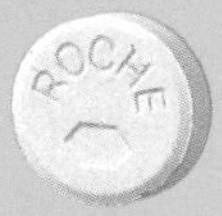

Fansidar®
(sulfadoxine and pyrimethamine)

Roche

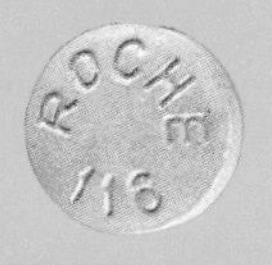

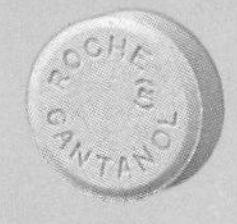

500 mg
†Gantanol®
(sulfamethoxazole/Roche)

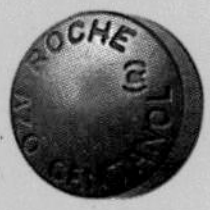

Roche

1 Gm
†Gantanol® DS
(sulfamethoxazole/Roche)

Roche

500 mg
†Gantrisin®
(sulfisoxazole/Roche)

Roche

250 mg

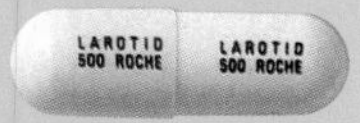

500 mg
†Larotid®
(amoxicillin/Roche)

Roche

Larobec®

Roche

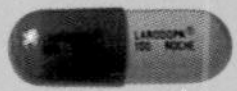

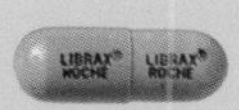

0.1 Gm Capsule
0.25 Gm Capsule 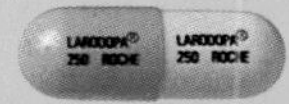
0.5 Gm Capsule 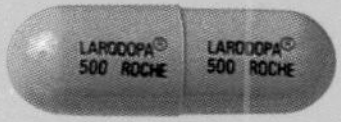
0.1 Gm Tablet 0.25 Gm Tablet
0.5 Gm Tablet 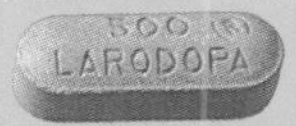
Larodopa®
(levodopa/Roche)

Roche C-II

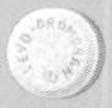

2 mg
†Levo-Dromoran®
(levorphanol tartrate/Roche)

Roche

***Librax®**

ROCHE®
Tel-E-Mark™ System

Example:

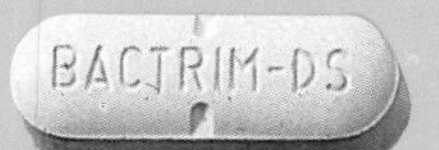

†Bactrim™ DS
(trimethoprim and sulfamethoxazole/Roche)

Quick and simple product identification is provided by the Roche Tel-E-Mark, whereby product and company names and, where applicable, dosage strength are imprinted directly on the tablet or capsule. Eventually, most solid oral dosage forms of Roche products will bear the Tel-E-Mark.

ROCHE®
Tel-E-Code™ System

Example:

Endep® 100 mg
(amitriptyline HCl/Roche)

Based on the National Drug Code, the Roche Tel-E-Code marking includes the Roche name and numbers indicating product and strength. It, too, provides speedy product identification when needed. Solid oral dosage forms of Roche products not phased into the Tel-E-Mark System are marked with this Tel-E-Code.

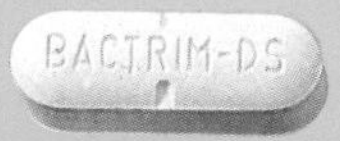

†Other dosage forms available. See Product Information section or check directly with manufacturer.
*Dalmane, Librax, Libritabs, Librium, Limbitrol and Valium tablets are products of Roche Products Inc., Manati, PR 00701.

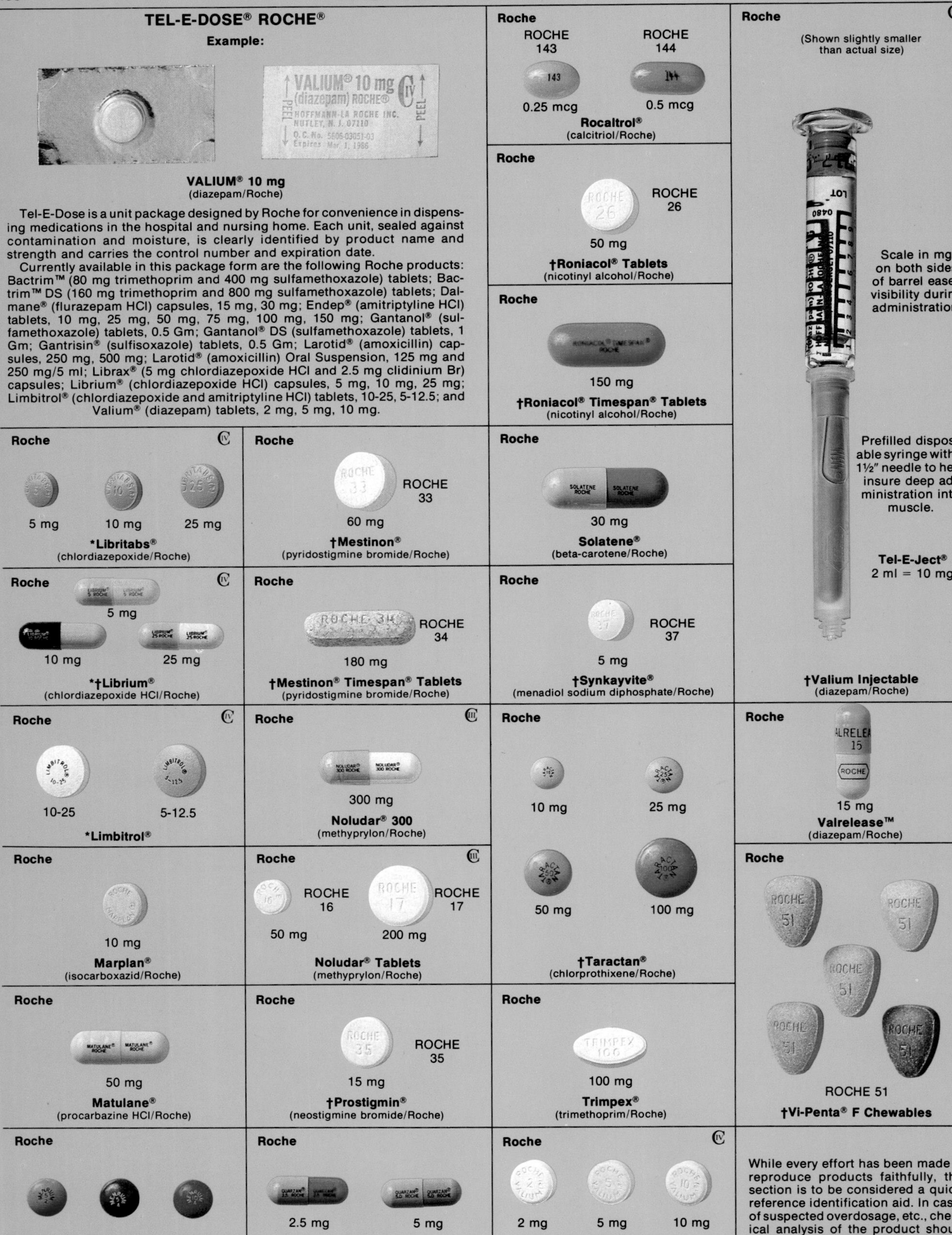

TEL-E-DOSE® ROCHE®

Example:

VALIUM® 10 mg
(diazepam/Roche)

Tel-E-Dose is a unit package designed by Roche for convenience in dispensing medications in the hospital and nursing home. Each unit, sealed against contamination and moisture, is clearly identified by product name and strength and carries the control number and expiration date.

Currently available in this package form are the following Roche products: Bactrim™ (80 mg trimethoprim and 400 mg sulfamethoxazole) tablets; Bactrim™ DS (160 mg trimethoprim and 800 mg sulfamethoxazole) tablets; Dalmane® (flurazepam HCl) capsules, 15 mg, 30 mg; Endep® (amitriptyline HCl) tablets, 10 mg, 25 mg, 50 mg, 75 mg, 100 mg, 150 mg; Gantanol® (sulfamethoxazole) tablets, 0.5 Gm; Gantanol® DS (sulfamethoxazole) tablets, 1 Gm; Gantrisin® (sulfisoxazole) tablets, 0.5 Gm; Larotid® (amoxicillin) capsules, 250 mg, 500 mg; Larotid® (amoxicillin) Oral Suspension, 125 mg and 250 mg/5 ml; Librax® (5 mg chlordiazepoxide HCl and 2.5 mg clidinium Br) capsules; Librium® (chlordiazepoxide HCl) capsules, 5 mg, 10 mg, 25 mg; Limbitrol® (chlordiazepoxide and amitriptyline HCl) tablets, 10-25, 5-12.5; and Valium® (diazepam) tablets, 2 mg, 5 mg, 10 mg.

Roche — ROCHE 143, 0.25 mcg; ROCHE 144, 0.5 mcg
Rocaltrol®
(calcitriol/Roche)

Roche — ROCHE 26, 50 mg
†Roniacol® Tablets
(nicotinyl alcohol/Roche)

Roche — 150 mg
†Roniacol® Timespan® Tablets
(nicotinyl alcohol/Roche)

Roche — (Shown slightly smaller than actual size)
Scale in mg on both sides of barrel eases visibility during administration.
Prefilled disposable syringe with a 1½" needle to help insure deep administration into muscle.
Tel-E-Ject®
2 ml = 10 mg
†Valium Injectable
(diazepam/Roche)

Roche (CIV) — 5 mg, 10 mg, 25 mg
***Libritabs®**
(chlordiazepoxide/Roche)

Roche — ROCHE 33, 60 mg
†Mestinon®
(pyridostigmine bromide/Roche)

Roche — 30 mg
Solatene®
(beta-carotene/Roche)

Roche (CIV) — 5 mg, 10 mg, 25 mg
***†Librium®**
(chlordiazepoxide HCl/Roche)

Roche — ROCHE 34, 180 mg
†Mestinon® Timespan® Tablets
(pyridostigmine bromide/Roche)

Roche — ROCHE 37, 5 mg
†Synkayvite®
(menadiol sodium diphosphate/Roche)

Roche (CIV) — 10-25, 5-12.5
***Limbitrol®**

Roche (CIII) — 300 mg
Noludar® 300
(methyprylon/Roche)

Roche — 10 mg, 25 mg, 50 mg, 100 mg
†Taractan®
(chlorprothixene/Roche)

Roche — 15 mg
Valrelease™
(diazepam/Roche)

Roche — 10 mg
Marplan®
(isocarboxazid/Roche)

Roche (CIII) — ROCHE 16, 50 mg; ROCHE 17, 200 mg
Noludar® Tablets
(methyprylon/Roche)

Roche — ROCHE 51
†Vi-Penta® F Chewables

Roche — 50 mg
Matulane®
(procarbazine HCl/Roche)

Roche — ROCHE 35, 15 mg
†Prostigmin®
(neostigmine bromide/Roche)

Roche — 100 mg
Trimpex®
(trimethoprim/Roche)

Roche — **Menrium® 5-2**, **Menrium® 5-4**, **Menrium® 10-4**

Roche — 2.5 mg, 5 mg
Quarzan®
(clidinium bromide/Roche)

Roche (CIV) — 2 mg, 5 mg, 10 mg
***†Valium®**
(diazepam/Roche)

While every effort has been made to reproduce products faithfully, this section is to be considered a quick reference identification aid. In case of suspected overdosage, etc., chemical analysis of the product should be done.

†Other dosage forms available. See Product Information section or check directly with manufacturer.
*Dalmane, Librax, Libritabs, Librium, Limbitrol and Valium tablets are products of Roche Products Inc., Manati, PR 00701.

ROERIG

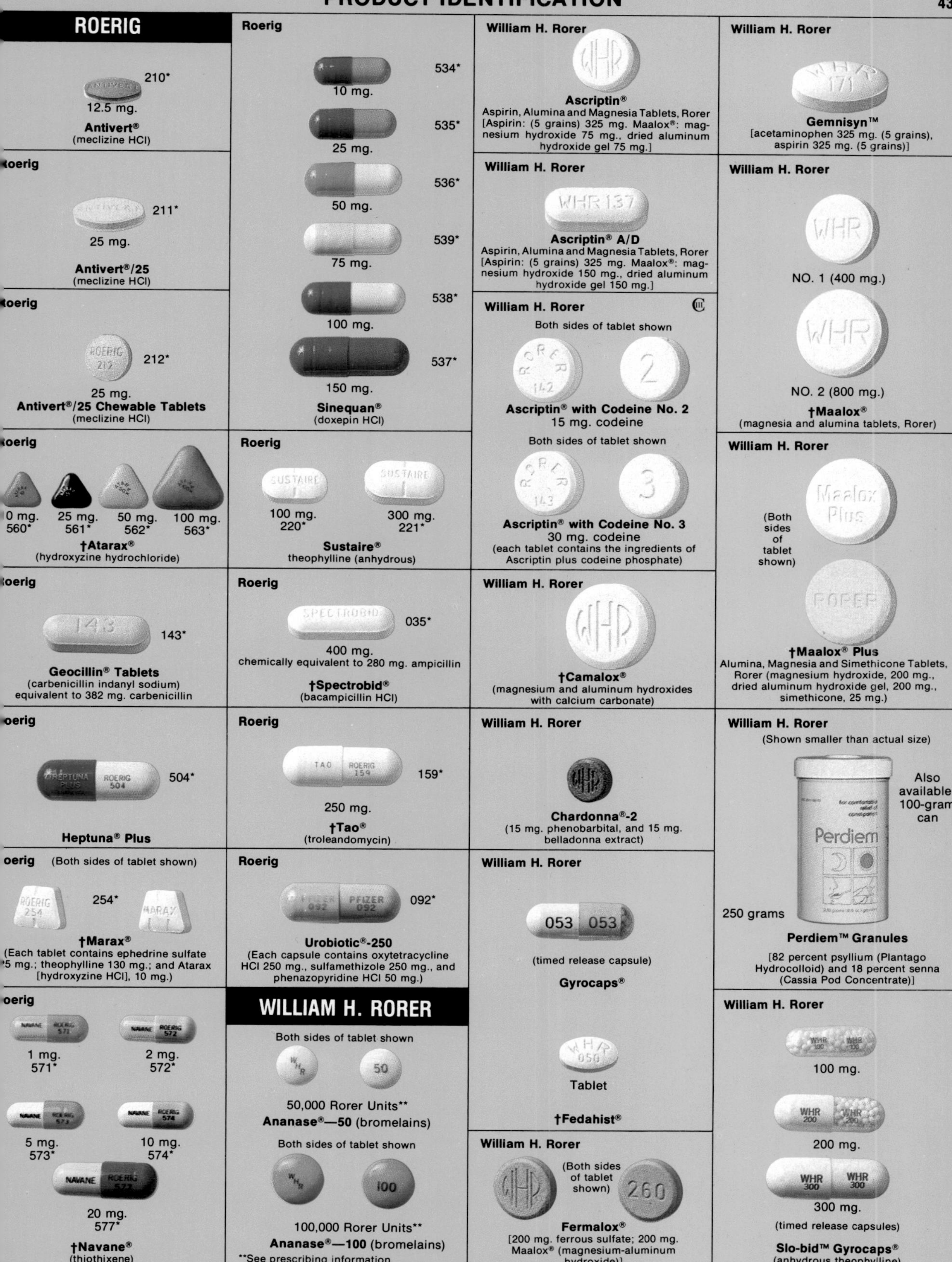

210*
12.5 mg.
Antivert®
(meclizine HCl)

Roerig
211*
25 mg.
Antivert®/25
(meclizine HCl)

Roerig
212*
25 mg.
Antivert®/25 Chewable Tablets
(meclizine HCl)

Roerig
10 mg. 560*
25 mg. 561*
50 mg. 562*
100 mg. 563*
†Atarax®
(hydroxyzine hydrochloride)

Roerig
143*
Geocillin® Tablets
(carbenicillin indanyl sodium)
equivalent to 382 mg. carbenicillin

Roerig
504*
Heptuna® Plus

Roerig (Both sides of tablet shown)
254*
†Marax®
(Each tablet contains ephedrine sulfate 25 mg.; theophylline 130 mg.; and Atarax [hydroxyzine HCl], 10 mg.)

Roerig
1 mg. 571*
2 mg. 572*
5 mg. 573*
10 mg. 574*
20 mg. 577*
†Navane®
(thiothixene)

Roerig
534* 10 mg.
535* 25 mg.
536* 50 mg.
539* 75 mg.
538* 100 mg.
537* 150 mg.
Sinequan®
(doxepin HCl)

Roerig
100 mg. 220*
300 mg. 221*
Sustaire®
theophylline (anhydrous)

Roerig
035*
400 mg.
chemically equivalent to 280 mg. ampicillin
†Spectrobid®
(bacampicillin HCl)

Roerig
159*
250 mg.
†Tao®
(troleandomycin)

Roerig
092*
Urobiotic®-250
(Each capsule contains oxytetracycline HCl 250 mg., sulfamethizole 250 mg., and phenazopyridine HCl 50 mg.)

WILLIAM H. RORER

Both sides of tablet shown
50,000 Rorer Units**
Ananase®—50 (bromelains)

Both sides of tablet shown
100,000 Rorer Units**
Ananase®—100 (bromelains)
**See prescribing information.

William H. Rorer
Ascriptin®
Aspirin, Alumina and Magnesia Tablets, Rorer [Aspirin: (5 grains) 325 mg. Maalox®: magnesium hydroxide 75 mg., dried aluminum hydroxide gel 75 mg.]

William H. Rorer
Ascriptin® A/D
Aspirin, Alumina and Magnesia Tablets, Rorer [Aspirin: (5 grains) 325 mg. Maalox®: magnesium hydroxide 150 mg., dried aluminum hydroxide gel 150 mg.]

William H. Rorer
Both sides of tablet shown
Ascriptin® with Codeine No. 2
15 mg. codeine
Both sides of tablet shown
Ascriptin® with Codeine No. 3
30 mg. codeine
(each tablet contains the ingredients of Ascriptin plus codeine phosphate)

William H. Rorer
†Camalox®
(magnesium and aluminum hydroxides with calcium carbonate)

William H. Rorer
Chardonna®-2
(15 mg. phenobarbital, and 15 mg. belladonna extract)

William H. Rorer
(timed release capsule)
Gyrocaps®
Tablet
†Fedahist®

William H. Rorer
(Both sides of tablet shown)
Fermalox®
[200 mg. ferrous sulfate; 200 mg. Maalox® (magnesium-aluminum hydroxide)]

William H. Rorer
Gemnisyn™
[acetaminophen 325 mg. (5 grains), aspirin 325 mg. (5 grains)]

William H. Rorer
NO. 1 (400 mg.)
NO. 2 (800 mg.)
†Maalox®
(magnesia and alumina tablets, Rorer)

William H. Rorer
(Both sides of tablet shown)
†Maalox® Plus
Alumina, Magnesia and Simethicone Tablets, Rorer (magnesium hydroxide, 200 mg., dried aluminum hydroxide gel, 200 mg., simethicone, 25 mg.)

William H. Rorer
(Shown smaller than actual size)
Also available: 100-gram can
250 grams
Perdiem™ Granules
[82 percent psyllium (Plantago Hydrocolloid) and 18 percent senna (Cassia Pod Concentrate)]

William H. Rorer
100 mg.
200 mg.
300 mg.
(timed release capsules)
Slo-bid™ Gyrocaps®
(anhydrous theophylline)

†Other dosage forms available. See Product Information section or check directly with manufacturer.
*Manufacturers' identification number.

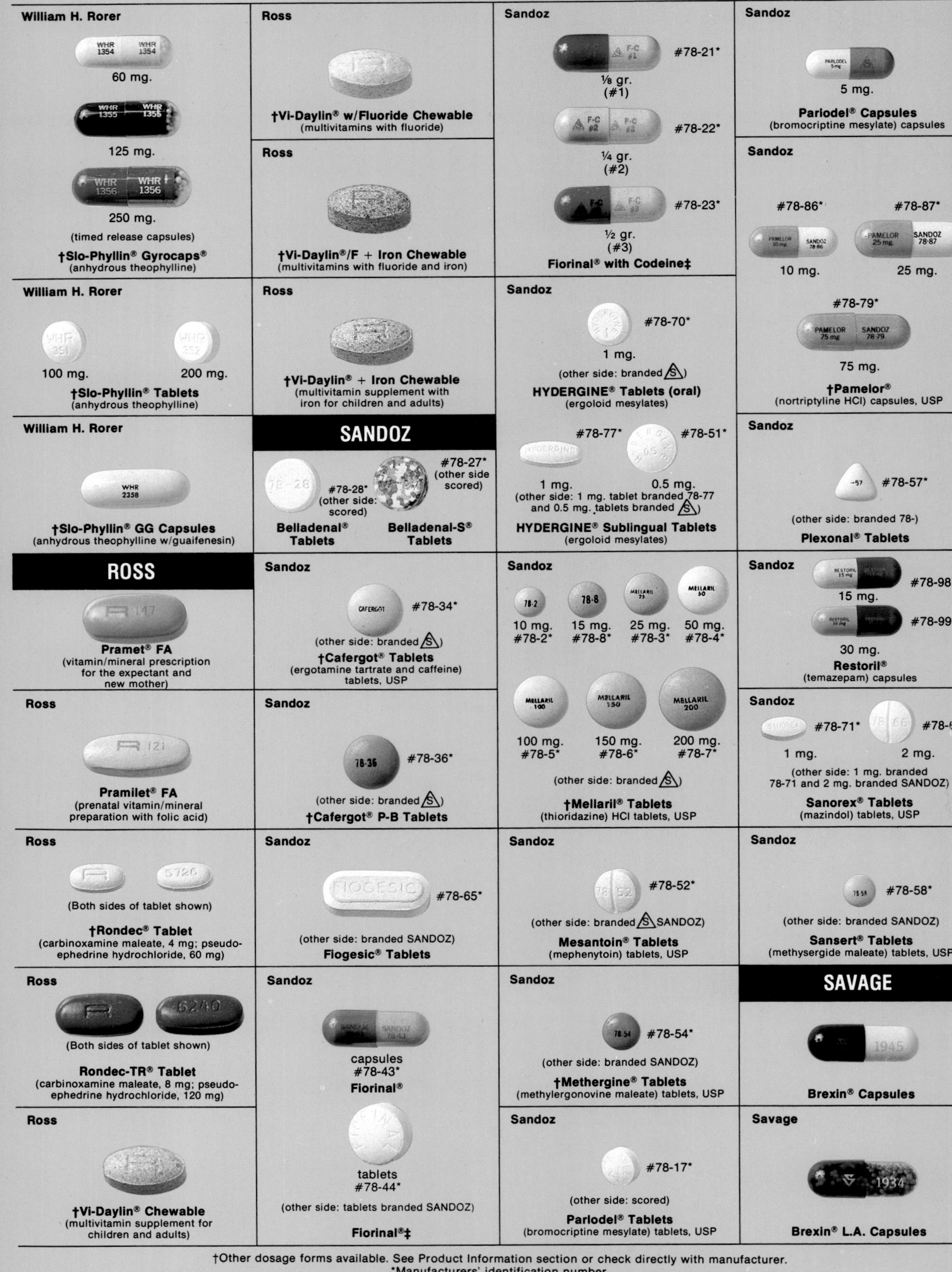

†Other dosage forms available. See Product Information section or check directly with manufacturer.
*Manufacturers' identification number.
‡For changes in branding of Fiorinal and Fiorinal with Codeine effective 1/1/83, see Product Information section.

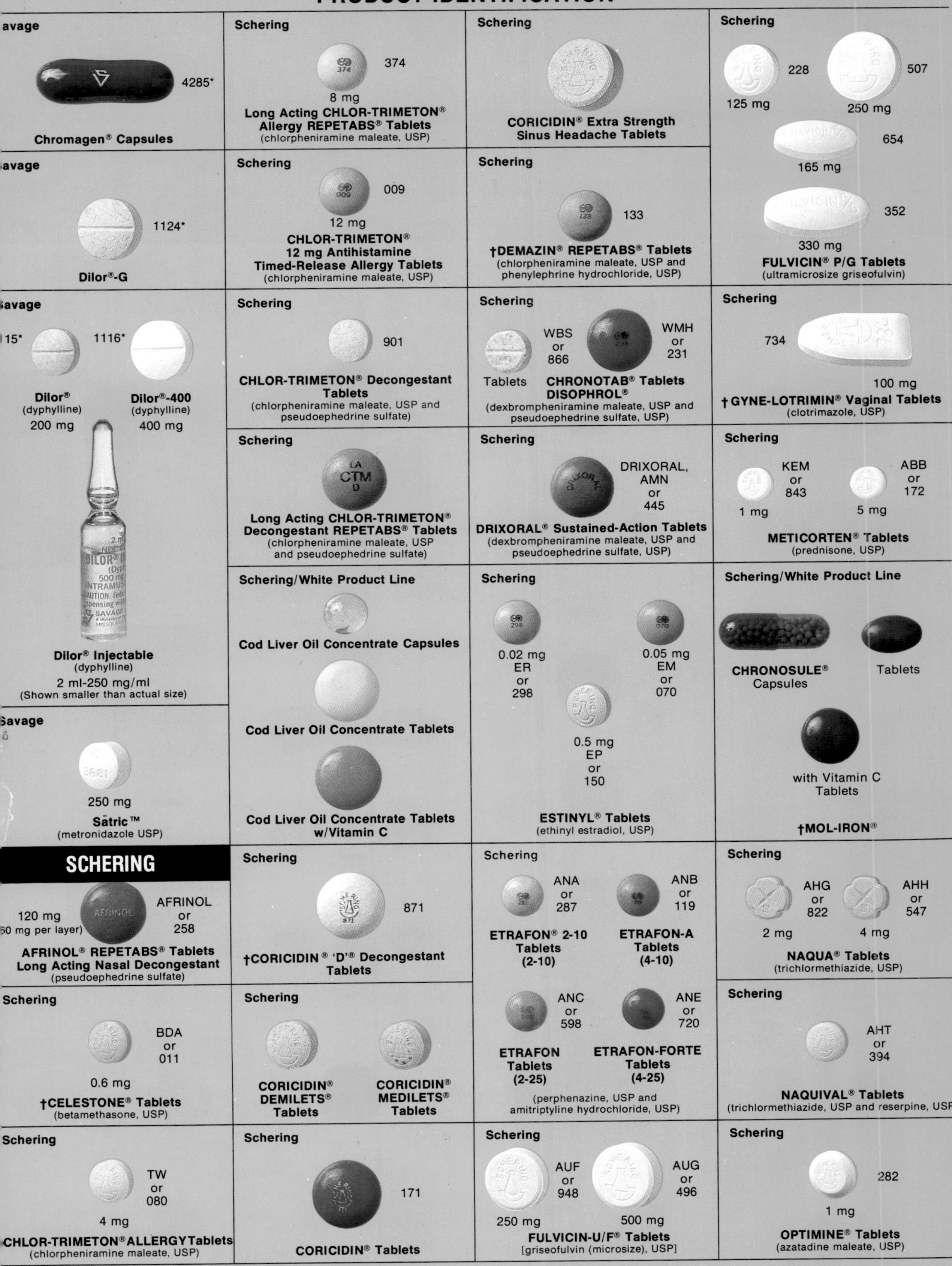

†Other dosage forms available. See Product Information section or check directly with manufacturer.

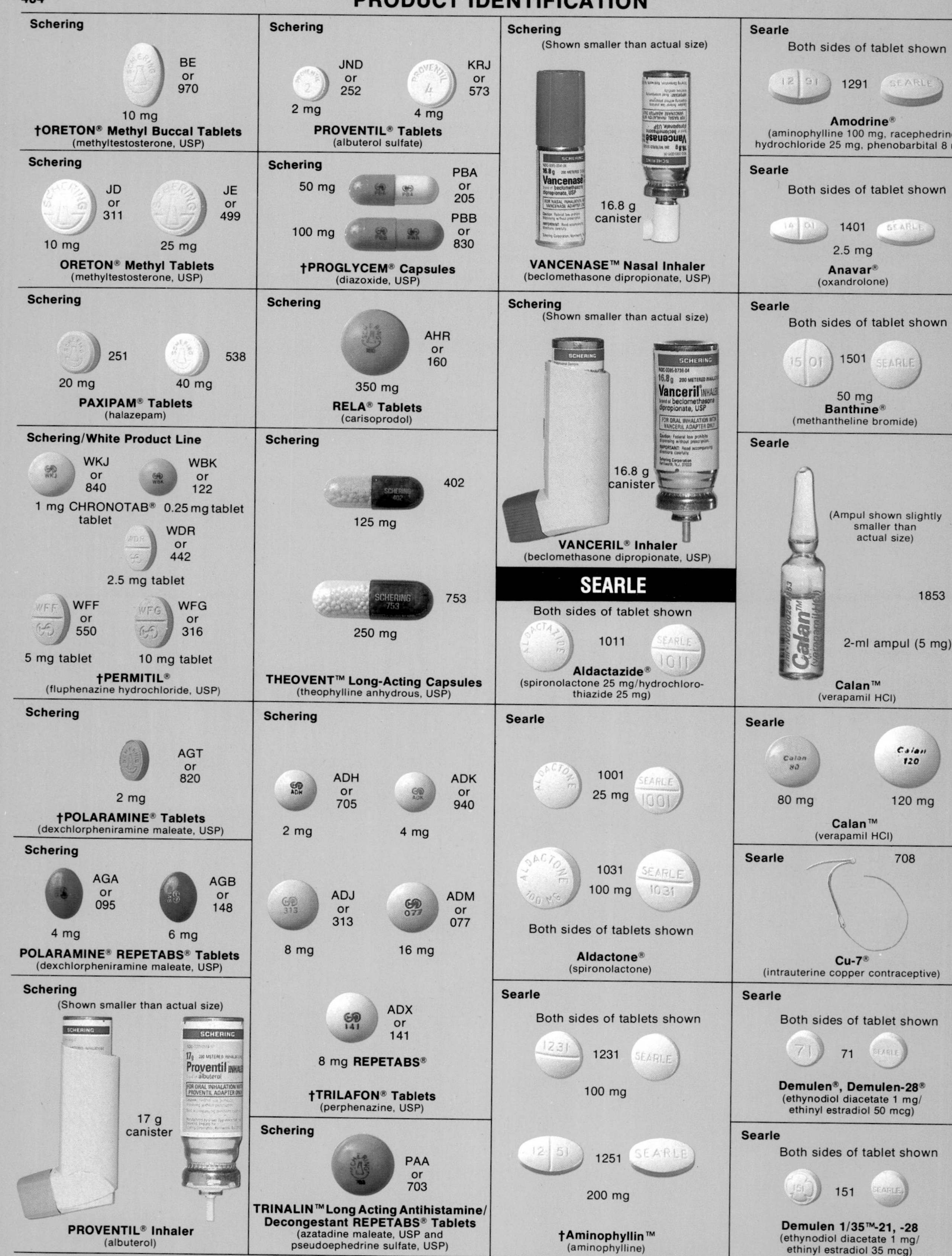

†Other dosage forms available. See Product Information section or check directly with manufacturer.

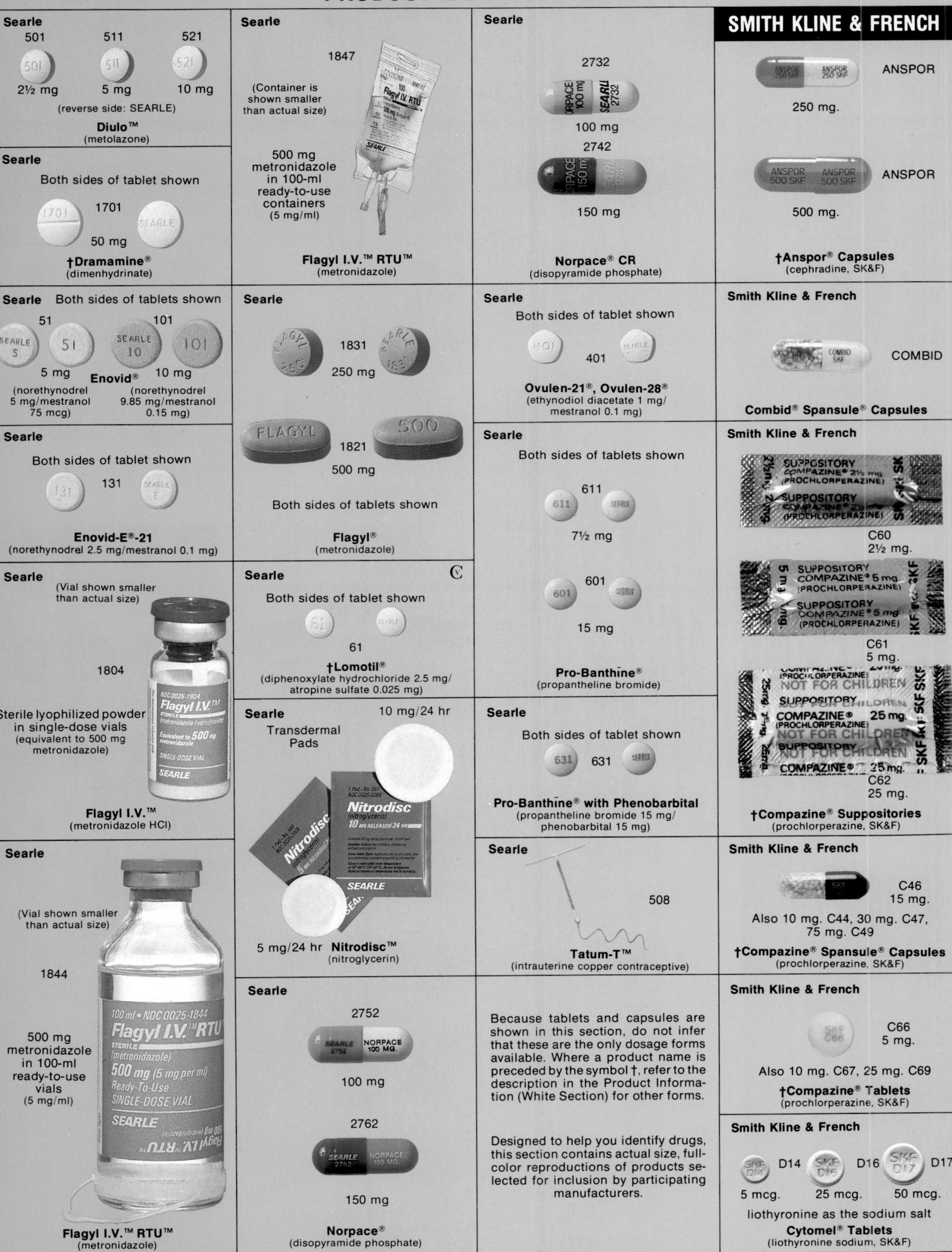

Because tablets and capsules are shown in this section, do not infer that these are the only dosage forms available. Where a product name is preceded by the symbol †, refer to the description in the Product Information (White Section) for other forms.

Designed to help you identify drugs, this section contains actual size, full-color reproductions of products selected for inclusion by participating manufacturers.

†Other dosage forms available. See Product Information section or check directly with manufacturer.

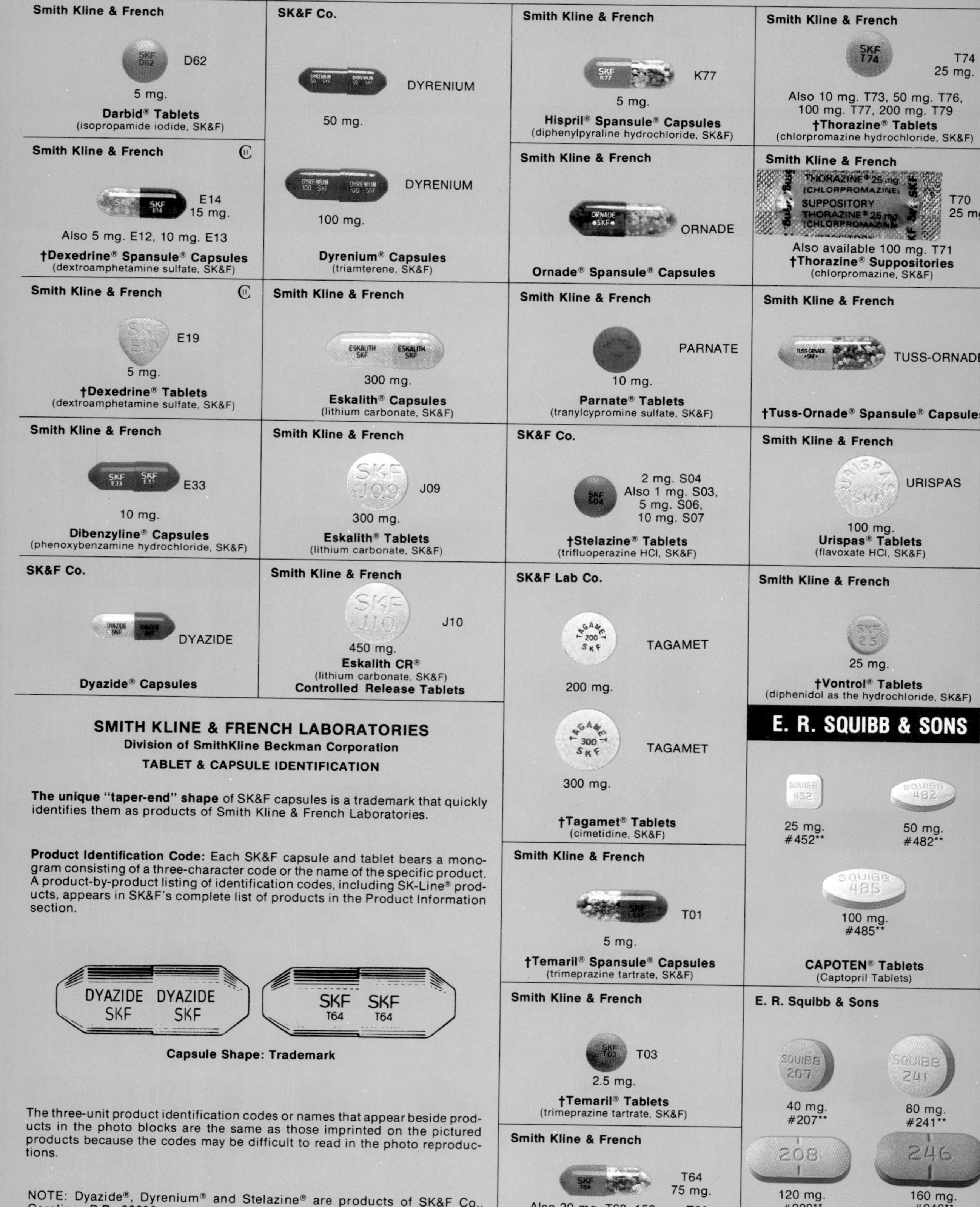

Smith Kline & French

D62
5 mg.
Darbid® Tablets
(isopropamide iodide, SK&F)

Smith Kline & French Ⓒ

E14
15 mg.
Also 5 mg. E12, 10 mg. E13
†Dexedrine® Spansule® Capsules
(dextroamphetamine sulfate, SK&F)

Smith Kline & French Ⓒ

E19
5 mg.
†Dexedrine® Tablets
(dextroamphetamine sulfate, SK&F)

Smith Kline & French

E33
10 mg.
Dibenzyline® Capsules
(phenoxybenzamine hydrochloride, SK&F)

SK&F Co.

DYAZIDE
Dyazide® Capsules

SK&F Co.

DYRENIUM
50 mg.

DYRENIUM
100 mg.
Dyrenium® Capsules
(triamterene, SK&F)

Smith Kline & French

300 mg.
Eskalith® Capsules
(lithium carbonate, SK&F)

Smith Kline & French

J09
300 mg.
Eskalith® Tablets
(lithium carbonate, SK&F)

Smith Kline & French

J10
450 mg.
Eskalith CR®
(lithium carbonate, SK&F)
Controlled Release Tablets

SMITH KLINE & FRENCH LABORATORIES

Division of SmithKline Beckman Corporation

TABLET & CAPSULE IDENTIFICATION

The unique "taper-end" shape of SK&F capsules is a trademark that quickly identifies them as products of Smith Kline & French Laboratories.

Product Identification Code: Each SK&F capsule and tablet bears a monogram consisting of a three-character code or the name of the specific product. A product-by-product listing of identification codes, including SK-Line® products, appears in SK&F's complete list of products in the Product Information section.

DYAZIDE DYAZIDE SKF SKF — SKF SKF T64 T64

Capsule Shape: Trademark

The three-unit product identification codes or names that appear beside products in the photo blocks are the same as those imprinted on the pictured products because the codes may be difficult to read in the photo reproductions.

NOTE: Dyazide®, Dyrenium® and Stelazine® are products of SK&F Co., Carolina, P.R. 00630, a subsidiary of SmithKline Beckman Corporation. Tagamet® is a product of SK&F Lab Co., Carolina, P.R. 00630, a subsidiary of SmithKline Beckman Corporation.

Smith Kline & French

K77
5 mg.
Hispril® Spansule® Capsules
(diphenylpyraline hydrochloride, SK&F)

Smith Kline & French

ORNADE
Ornade® Spansule® Capsules

Smith Kline & French

PARNATE
10 mg.
Parnate® Tablets
(tranylcypromine sulfate, SK&F)

SK&F Co.

2 mg. S04
Also 1 mg. S03,
5 mg. S06,
10 mg. S07
†Stelazine® Tablets
(trifluoperazine HCl, SK&F)

SK&F Lab Co.

TAGAMET
200 mg.

TAGAMET
300 mg.
†Tagamet® Tablets
(cimetidine, SK&F)

Smith Kline & French

T01
5 mg.
†Temaril® Spansule® Capsules
(trimeprazine tartrate, SK&F)

Smith Kline & French

T03
2.5 mg.
†Temaril® Tablets
(trimeprazine tartrate, SK&F)

Smith Kline & French

T64
75 mg.
Also 30 mg. T63, 150 mg. T66,
200 mg. T67, 300 mg. T69
†Thorazine® Spansule® Capsules
(chlorpromazine hydrochloride, SK&F)

Smith Kline & French

T74
25 mg.
Also 10 mg. T73, 50 mg. T76,
100 mg. T77, 200 mg. T79
†Thorazine® Tablets
(chlorpromazine hydrochloride, SK&F)

Smith Kline & French

T70
25 m
Also available 100 mg. T71
†Thorazine® Suppositories
(chlorpromazine, SK&F)

Smith Kline & French

TUSS-ORNADE
†Tuss-Ornade® Spansule® Capsules

Smith Kline & French

URISPAS
100 mg.
Urispas® Tablets
(flavoxate HCl, SK&F)

Smith Kline & French

25 mg.
†Vontrol® Tablets
(diphenidol as the hydrochloride, SK&F)

E. R. SQUIBB & SONS

25 mg. #452**
50 mg. #482**
100 mg. #485**
CAPOTEN® Tablets
(Captopril Tablets)

E. R. Squibb & Sons

40 mg. #207**
80 mg. #241**
120 mg. #208**
160 mg. #246**
CORGARD® Tablets
(Nadolol Tablets)

†Other dosage forms available. See Product Information section or check directly with manufacturer.
**Squibb product identification number.

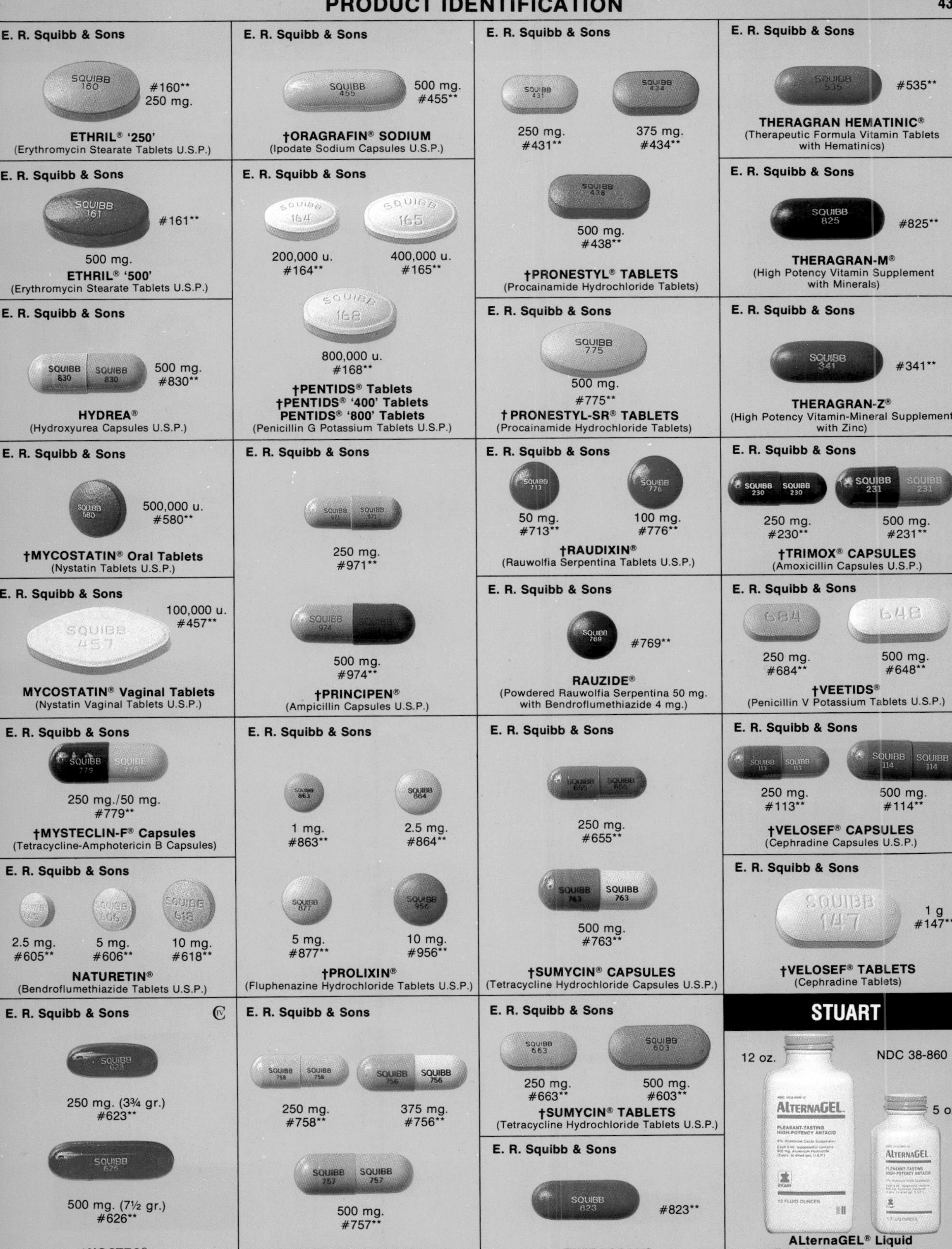

†Other dosage forms available. See Product Information section or check directly with manufacturer.
**Squibb product identification number.

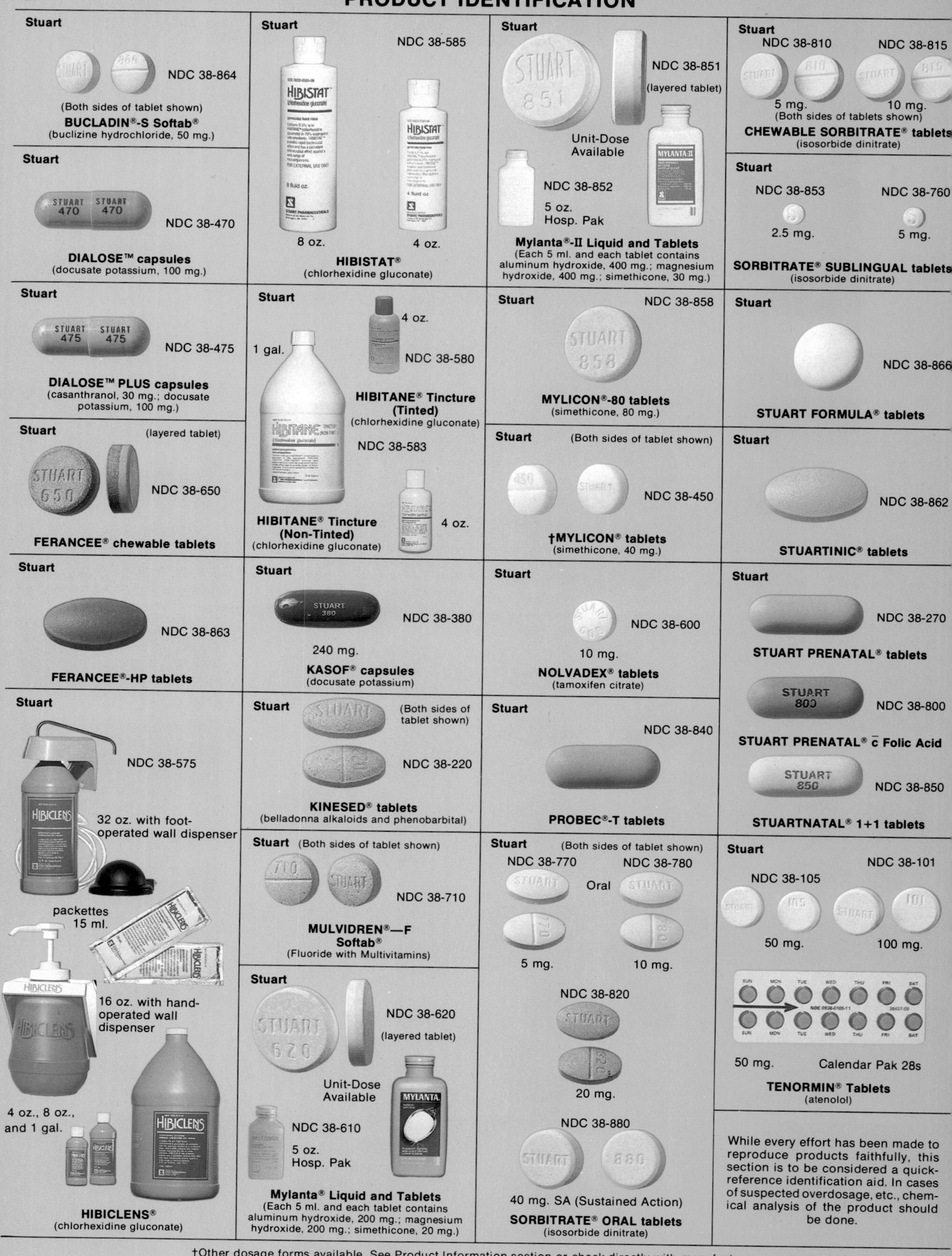

†Other dosage forms available. See Product Information section or check directly with manufacturer.

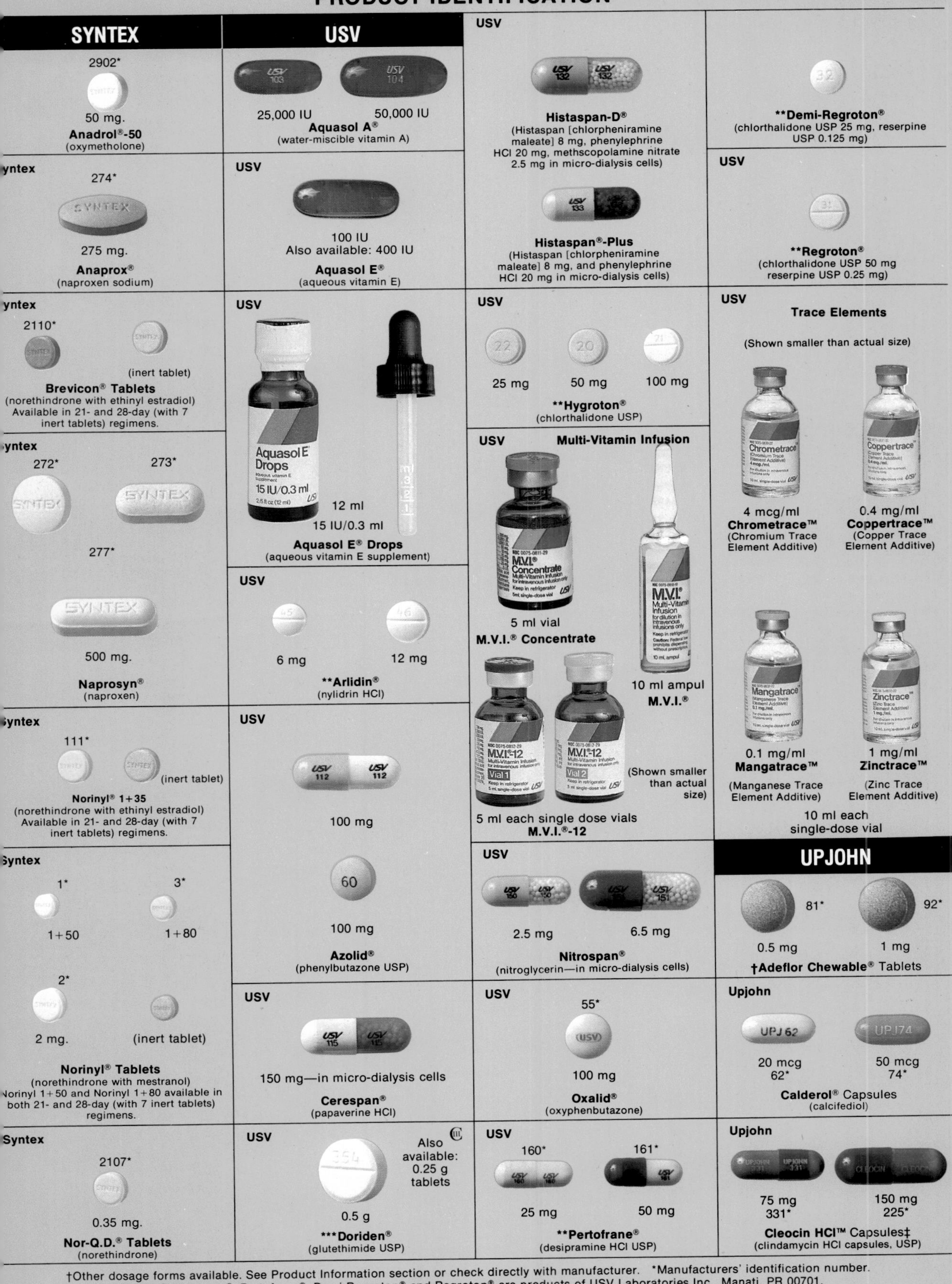

†Other dosage forms available. See Product Information section or check directly with manufacturer. *Manufacturers' identification number.
**Arlidin®, Hygroton®, Pertofrane®, Demi-Regroton® and Regroton® are products of USV Laboratories Inc., Manati, PR 00701.
***Doriden® is a product of USV (PR) Development Corp., Manati, PR 00701. ‡Product of The Upjohn Manufacturing Company, Barceloneta, P.R. 00617.

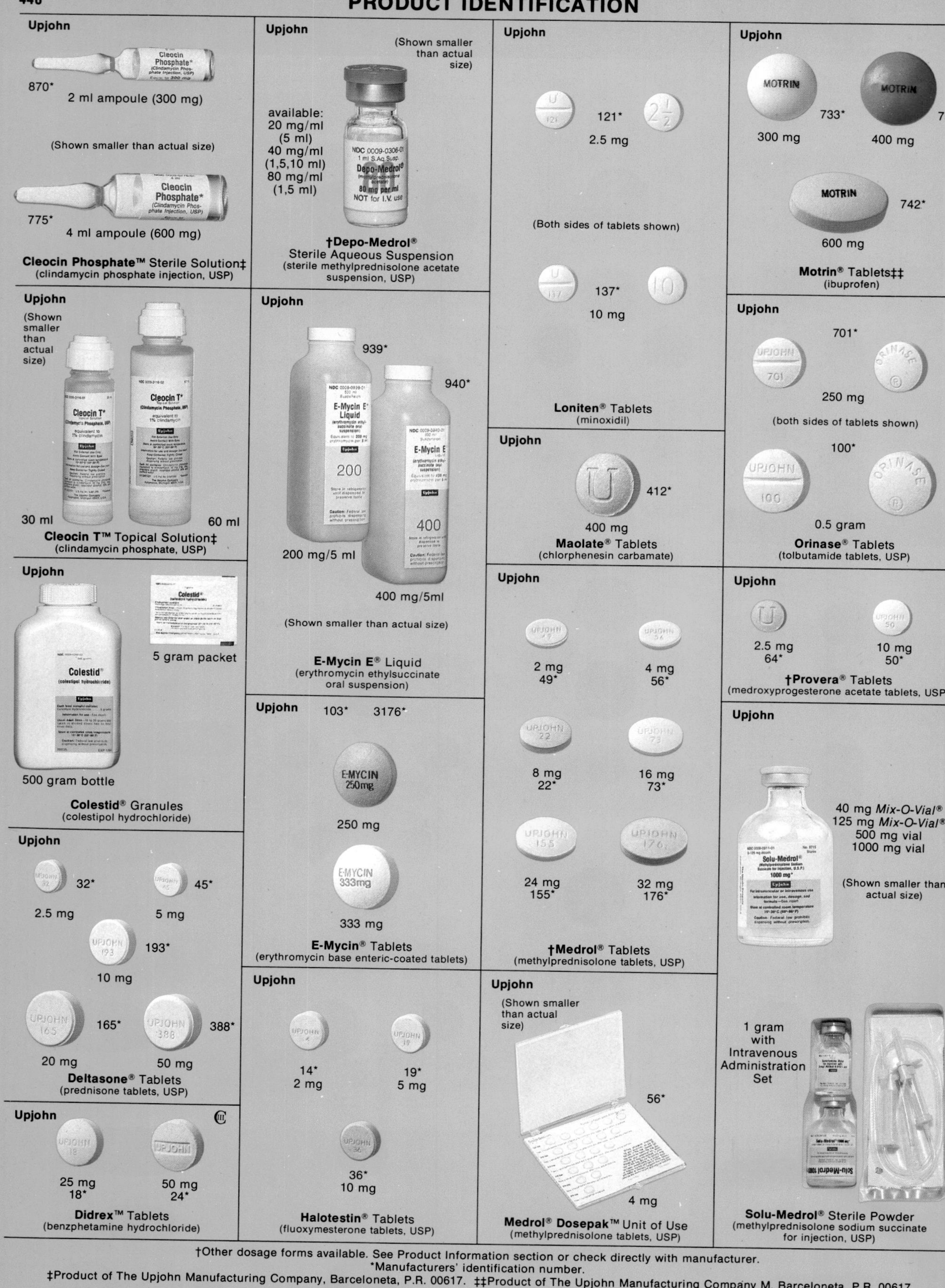
Upjohn
Cleocin Phosphate* (Clindamycin Phosphate Injection, USP)
870*
2 ml ampoule (300 mg)
(Shown smaller than actual size)
775*
4 ml ampoule (600 mg)
Cleocin Phosphate™ Sterile Solution‡
(clindamycin phosphate injection, USP)
Upjohn
(Shown smaller than actual size)
available:
20 mg/ml
(5 ml)
40 mg/ml
(1,5,10 ml)
80 mg/ml
(1,5 ml)
NDC 0009-0306-01
1 ml S.Aq.Susp.
Depo-Medrol®
80 mg per ml
NOT for I.V. use
†Depo-Medrol®
Sterile Aqueous Suspension
(sterile methylprednisolone acetate suspension, USP)
Upjohn
121*
2.5 mg
(Both sides of tablets shown)
137*
10 mg
Loniten® Tablets
(minoxidil)
Upjohn
MOTRIN
300 mg
733*
400 mg
742*
600 mg
Motrin® Tablets‡‡
(ibuprofen)
Upjohn
(Shown smaller than actual size)
Cleocin T*
Cleocin T*
30 ml
60 ml
Cleocin T™ Topical Solution‡
(clindamycin phosphate, USP)
Upjohn
939*
940*
E-Mycin E Liquid
200
400
200 mg/5 ml
400 mg/5ml
(Shown smaller than actual size)
E-Mycin E® Liquid
(erythromycin ethylsuccinate oral suspension)
Upjohn
412*
400 mg
Maolate® Tablets
(chlorphenesin carbamate)
Upjohn
701*
250 mg
(both sides of tablets shown)
100*
0.5 gram
Orinase® Tablets
(tolbutamide tablets, USP)
Upjohn
Colestid®
5 gram packet
Colestid®
(colestipol hydrochloride)
500 gram bottle
Colestid® Granules
(colestipol hydrochloride)
Upjohn
103*
3176*
E-MYCIN 250mg
250 mg
E-MYCIN 333mg
333 mg
E-Mycin® Tablets
(erythromycin base enteric-coated tablets)
Upjohn
2 mg
49*
4 mg
56*
8 mg
22*
16 mg
73*
24 mg
155*
32 mg
176*
†Medrol® Tablets
(methylprednisolone tablets, USP)
Upjohn
2.5 mg
64*
10 mg
50*
†Provera® Tablets
(medroxyprogesterone acetate tablets, USP
Upjohn
40 mg Mix-O-Vial®
125 mg Mix-O-Vial®
500 mg vial
1000 mg vial
(Shown smaller than actual size)
Upjohn
32*
2.5 mg
45*
5 mg
193*
10 mg
165*
20 mg
388*
50 mg
Deltasone® Tablets
(prednisone tablets, USP)
Upjohn
14*
2 mg
19*
5 mg
36*
10 mg
Halotestin® Tablets
(fluoxymesterone tablets, USP)
Upjohn
(Shown smaller than actual size)
56*
4 mg
Medrol® Dosepak™ Unit of Use
(methylprednisolone tablets, USP)
Upjohn
1 gram with Intravenous Administration Set
Solu-Medrol® Sterile Powder
(methylprednisolone sodium succinate for injection, USP)
Upjohn
25 mg
18*
50 mg
24*
Didrex™ Tablets
(benzphetamine hydrochloride)
†Other dosage forms available. See Product Information section or check directly with manufacturer.
*Manufacturers' identification number.
‡Product of The Upjohn Manufacturing Company, Barceloneta, P.R. 00617. ‡‡Product of The Upjohn Manufacturing Company M, Barceloneta, P.R. 00617.

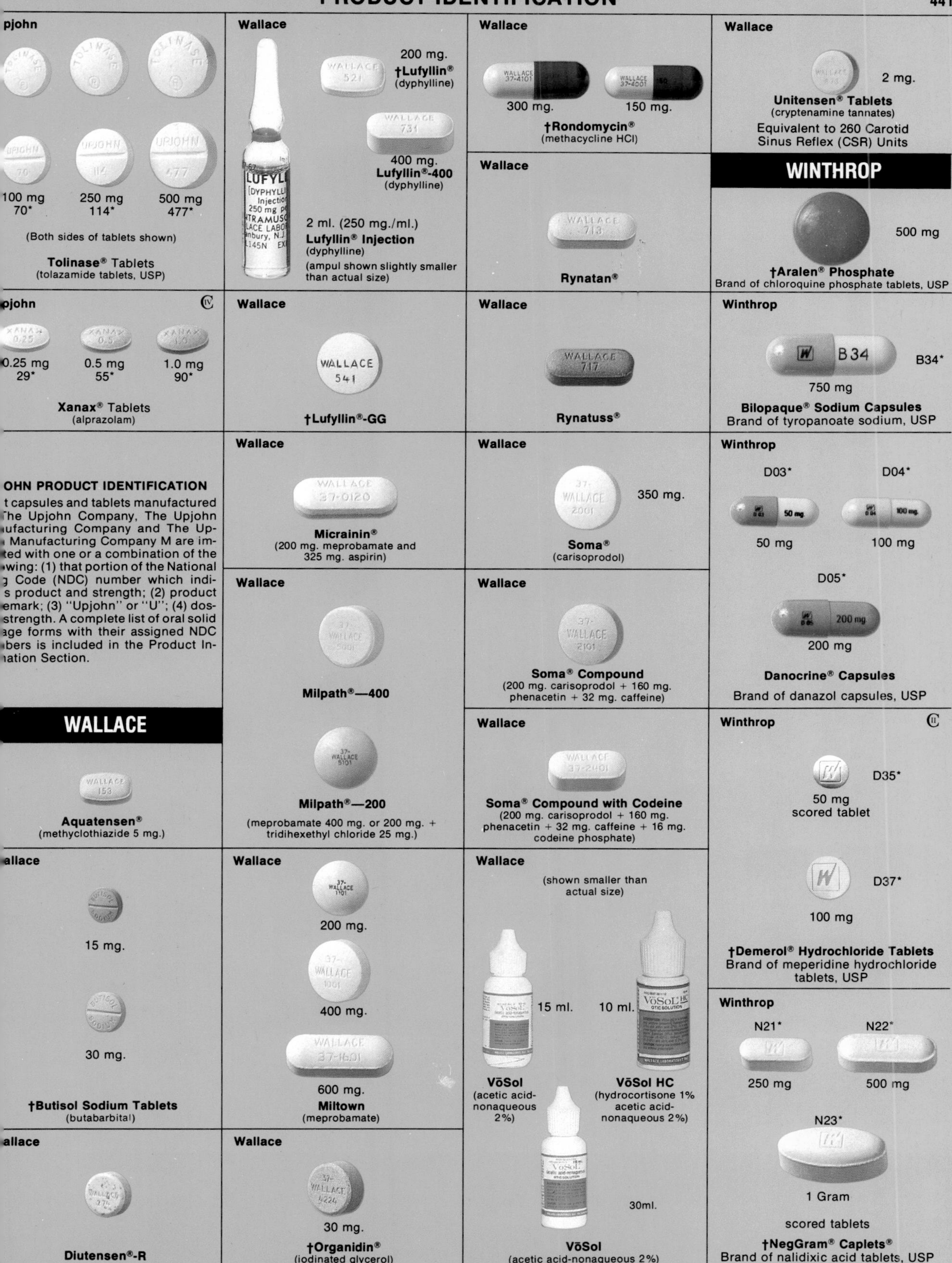

pjohn

100 mg 70* · 250 mg 114* · 500 mg 477*

(Both sides of tablets shown)

Tolinase® Tablets
(tolazamide tablets, USP)

pjohn Ⓒ IV

0.25 mg 29* · 0.5 mg 55* · 1.0 mg 90*

Xanax® Tablets
(alprazolam)

OHN PRODUCT IDENTIFICATION

t capsules and tablets manufactured The Upjohn Company, The Upjohn ufacturing Company and The Up- Manufacturing Company M are im- ted with one or a combination of the wing: (1) that portion of the National g Code (NDC) number which indi- s product and strength; (2) product emark; (3) "Upjohn" or "U"; (4) dos- strength. A complete list of oral solid age forms with their assigned NDC bers is included in the Product In- nation Section.

WALLACE

Aquatensen®
(methyclothiazide 5 mg.)

allace

15 mg. · 30 mg.

†Butisol Sodium Tablets
(butabarbital)

allace

Diutensen®-R

Wallace

200 mg. **†Lufyllin®** (dyphylline)

400 mg. **Lufyllin®-400** (dyphylline)

2 ml. (250 mg./ml.) **Lufyllin® Injection** (dyphylline)
(ampul shown slightly smaller than actual size)

Wallace

†Lufyllin®-GG

Wallace

Micrainin®
(200 mg. meprobamate and 325 mg. aspirin)

Wallace

Milpath®—400

Milpath®—200
(meprobamate 400 mg. or 200 mg. + tridihexethyl chloride 25 mg.)

Wallace

200 mg. · 400 mg. · 600 mg.

Miltown
(meprobamate)

Wallace

30 mg.

†Organidin®
(iodinated glycerol)

Wallace

300 mg. · 150 mg.

†Rondomycin®
(methacycline HCl)

Wallace

Rynatan®

Wallace

Rynatuss®

Wallace

350 mg.

Soma®
(carisoprodol)

Wallace

Soma® Compound
(200 mg. carisoprodol + 160 mg. phenacetin + 32 mg. caffeine)

Wallace

Soma® Compound with Codeine
(200 mg. carisoprodol + 160 mg. phenacetin + 32 mg. caffeine + 16 mg. codeine phosphate)

Wallace

(shown smaller than actual size)

15 ml. **VōSol** (acetic acid-nonaqueous 2%)

10 ml. **VōSol HC** (hydrocortisone 1% acetic acid-nonaqueous 2%)

30ml. **VōSol** (acetic acid-nonaqueous 2%)

Wallace

2 mg.

Unitensen® Tablets
(cryptenamine tannates)
Equivalent to 260 Carotid Sinus Reflex (CSR) Units

WINTHROP

500 mg

†Aralen® Phosphate
Brand of chloroquine phosphate tablets, USP

Winthrop

B34* · 750 mg

Bilopaque® Sodium Capsules
Brand of tyropanoate sodium, USP

Winthrop

D03* 50 mg · D04* 100 mg · D05* 200 mg

Danocrine® Capsules
Brand of danazol capsules, USP

Winthrop Ⓒ II

D35* 50 mg scored tablet

D37* 100 mg

†Demerol® Hydrochloride Tablets
Brand of meperidine hydrochloride tablets, USP

Winthrop

N21* 250 mg · N22* 500 mg

N23* 1 Gram

scored tablets

†NegGram® Caplets®
Brand of nalidixic acid tablets, USP

†Other dosage forms available. See Product Information section or check directly with manufacturer.
*Manufacturers' identification number.

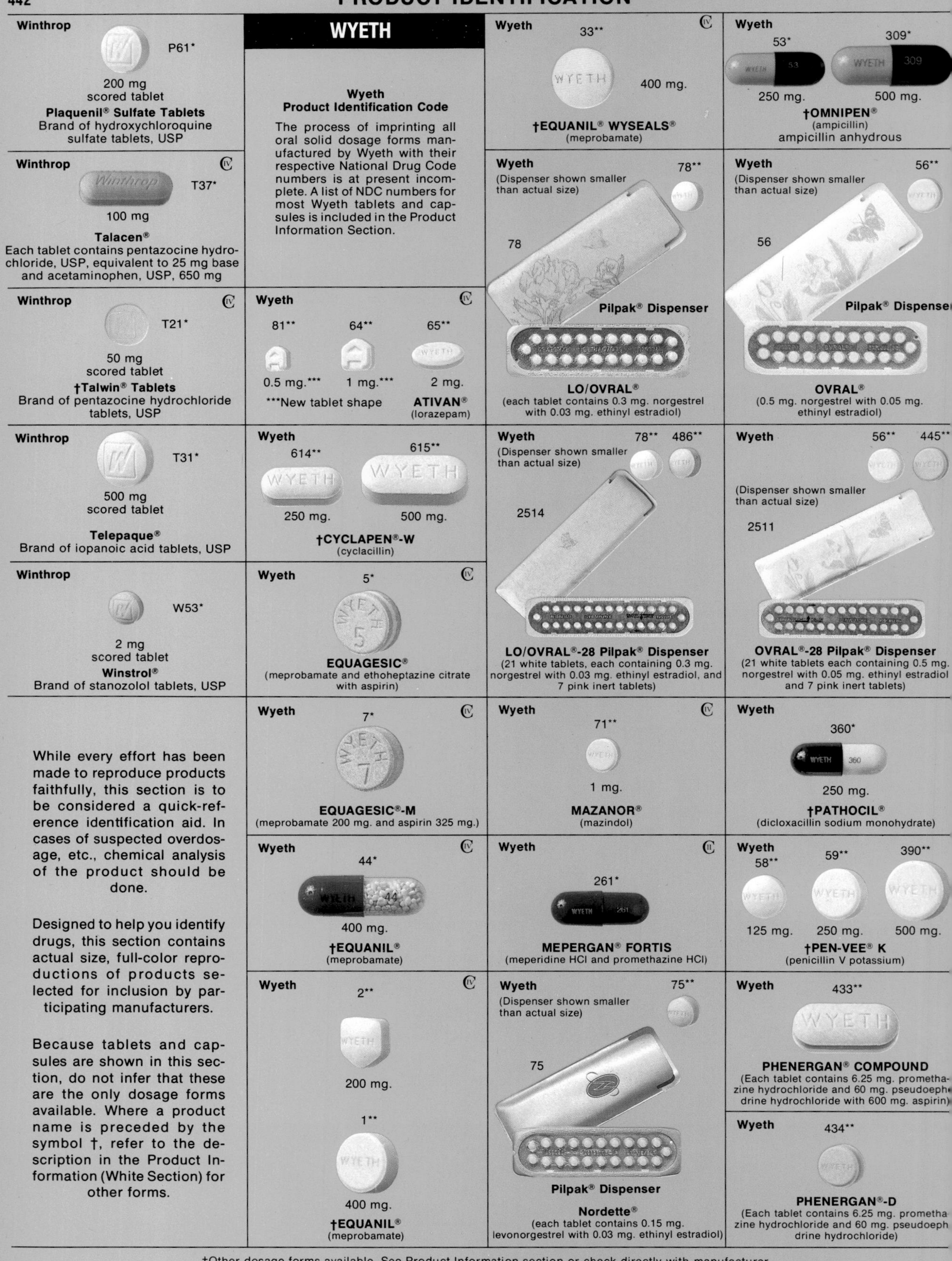

While every effort has been made to reproduce products faithfully, this section is to be considered a quick-reference identification aid. In cases of suspected overdosage, etc., chemical analysis of the product should be done.

Designed to help you identify drugs, this section contains actual size, full-color reproductions of products selected for inclusion by participating manufacturers.

Because tablets and capsules are shown in this section, do not infer that these are the only dosage forms available. Where a product name is preceded by the symbol †, refer to the description in the Product Information (White Section) for other forms.

†Other dosage forms available. See Product Information section or check directly with manufacturer.
*Manufacturers' identification number.
**Product identification number on reverse side of tablet.

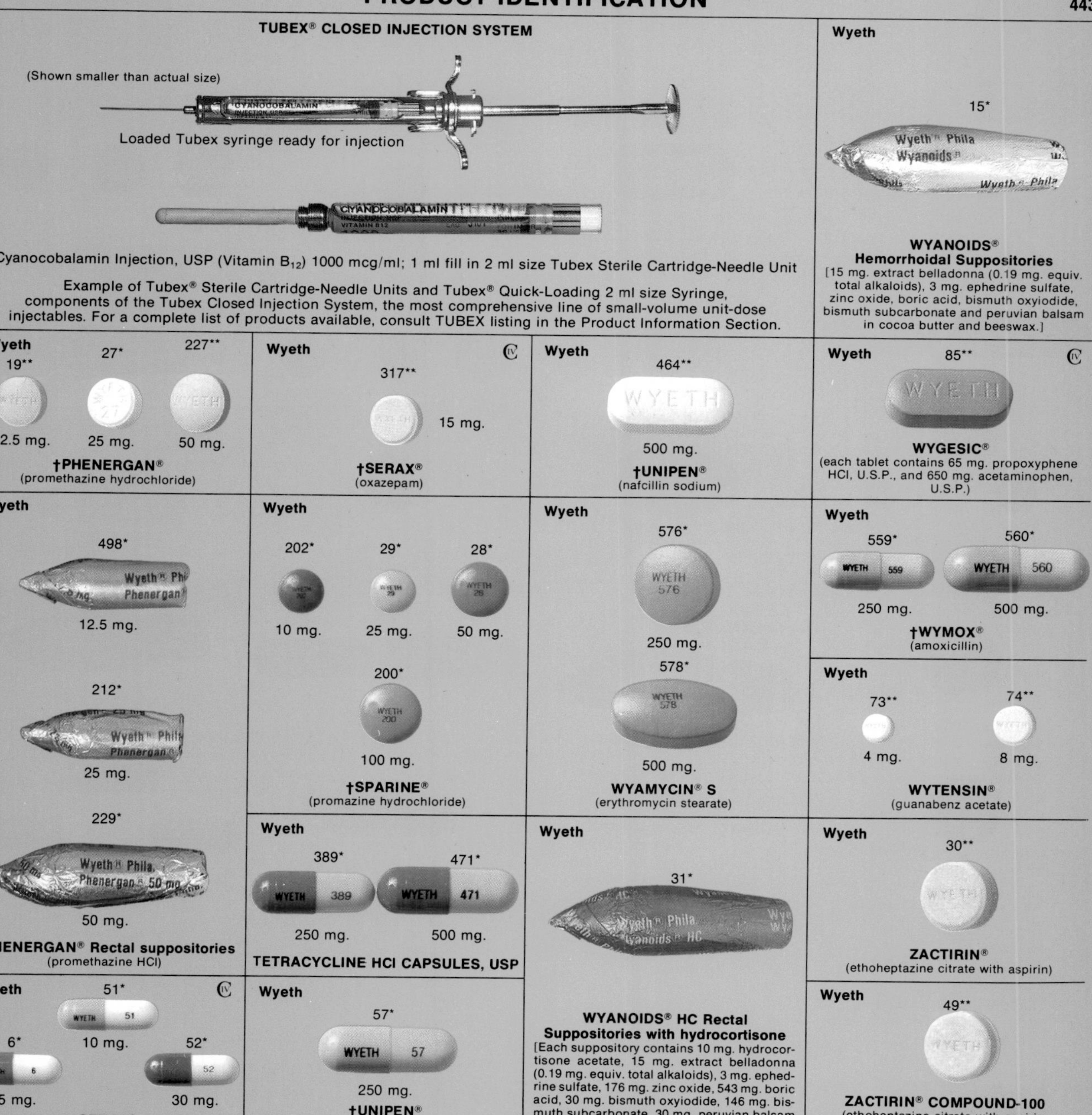
TUBEX® CLOSED INJECTION SYSTEM
(Shown smaller than actual size)
Loaded Tubex syringe ready for injection
Cyanocobalamin Injection, USP (Vitamin B12) 1000 mcg/ml; 1 ml fill in 2 ml size Tubex Sterile Cartridge-Needle Unit
Example of Tubex® Sterile Cartridge-Needle Units and Tubex® Quick-Loading 2 ml size Syringe, components of the Tubex Closed Injection System, the most comprehensive line of small-volume unit-dose injectables. For a complete list of products available, consult TUBEX listing in the Product Information Section.
Wyeth
15*
Wyeth Phila
Wyanoids
WYANOIDS®
Hemorrhoidal Suppositories
[15 mg. extract belladonna (0.19 mg. equiv. total alkaloids), 3 mg. ephedrine sulfate, zinc oxide, boric acid, bismuth oxyiodide, bismuth subcarbonate and peruvian balsam in cocoa butter and beeswax.]
Wyeth
19** 27* 227**
2.5 mg. 25 mg. 50 mg.
†PHENERGAN®
(promethazine hydrochloride)
Wyeth
317**
15 mg.
†SERAX®
(oxazepam)
Wyeth
464**
WYETH
500 mg.
†UNIPEN®
(nafcillin sodium)
Wyeth
85**
WYETH
WYGESIC®
(each tablet contains 65 mg. propoxyphene HCl, U.S.P., and 650 mg. acetaminophen, U.S.P.)
Wyeth
498*
12.5 mg.
212*
25 mg.
229*
Wyeth Phila.
Phenergan 50 mg
50 mg.
PHENERGAN® Rectal suppositories
(promethazine HCl)
Wyeth
202* 29* 28*
10 mg. 25 mg. 50 mg.
200*
100 mg.
†SPARINE®
(promazine hydrochloride)
Wyeth
576*
WYETH 576
250 mg.
578*
500 mg.
WYAMYCIN® S
(erythromycin stearate)
Wyeth
559* 560*
WYETH 559
WYETH 560
250 mg. 500 mg.
†WYMOX®
(amoxicillin)
Wyeth
73** 74**
4 mg. 8 mg.
WYTENSIN®
(guanabenz acetate)
Wyeth
389* 471*
WYETH 389
WYETH 471
250 mg. 500 mg.
TETRACYCLINE HCl CAPSULES, USP
Wyeth
31*
Wyeth Phila
Wyanoids HC
WYANOIDS® HC Rectal Suppositories with hydrocortisone
[Each suppository contains 10 mg. hydrocortisone acetate, 15 mg. extract belladonna (0.19 mg. equiv. total alkaloids), 3 mg. ephedrine sulfate, 176 mg. zinc oxide, 543 mg. boric acid, 30 mg. bismuth oxyiodide, 146 mg. bismuth subcarbonate, 30 mg. peruvian balsam in cocoa butter and beeswax.]
Wyeth
30**
WYETH
ZACTIRIN®
(ethoheptazine citrate with aspirin)
Wyeth
51*
WYETH 51
10 mg.
6* 52*
5 mg. 30 mg.
†SERAX®
Wyeth
57*
WYETH 57
250 mg.
†UNIPEN®
(nafcillin sodium)
Wyeth
49**
WYETH
ZACTIRIN® COMPOUND-100
(ethoheptazine citrate with aspirin, phenacetin and caffeine)

†Other dosage forms available. See Product Information section or check directly with manufacturer.
*Manufacturers' identification number.
**Product identification number on reverse side of tablet.

Directory of Poison Control Centers

The Directory of Poison Control Centers has been compiled from information furnished by the National Clearinghouse for Poison Control Centers, Bureau of Drugs, 5600 Fishers Lane, Room 1347, Rockville, Md. 20857.
It includes those facilities which provide for the medical profession, on a 24-hour basis, information concerning the prevention and treatment of accidents involving ingestion of poisonous and potentially poisonous substances. Unless otherwise noted, inquiries should be addressed to: Poison Control Center

ALABAMA

STATE COORDINATOR
Department of Public Health (205) 832-3194
Montgomery 36117 832-3935
Birmingham
Children's Hospital 933-4050
of Birmingham 800/292-6678
1601 6th Ave., S. 35233 (Statewide)
Tuscaloosa
The Alabama Poison Control Center
Druid City Hospital (205) 345-0600
809 University Blvd., E. (800) 462-0800 (Statewide)

ALASKA

STATE COORDINATOR
Department of Health & (907) 465-3100
Social Services
Juneau 99811
Anchorage
Anchorage Poison Center
Providence Hospital 274-6535
3200 Providence Dr. 99504
Fairbanks
Fairbanks Poison Center (907) 456-7182
Fairbanks Memorial Hospital
1650 Cowles 99701

ARIZONA

STATE COORDINATOR
Arizona Poison Control System
College of Pharmacy (602) 626-6016
University of Arizona 800/362-0101
Tucson 85724 (Statewide)
Flagstaff
Flagstaff Hospital and 779-0555
Medical Center of Northern Arizona
1215 N. Beaver St. 86001
Phoenix
St. Luke's Hospital and 253-3334
Medical Center
525 N. 18th St. 85006
Tucson
Arizona Poison and Drug Information Center
Arizona Hlth. Sciences Ctr. 626-6016
University of Arizona 85724 (800) 362-0101 (Statewide)
Yuma
Yuma Regional Med. Center 344-2000
Avenue A and 24th St. 85364

ARKANSAS

STATE COORDINATOR
Division of Environmental (501) 661-6161
Health Protection 661-2301
Little Rock 72201
El Dorado
Warner Brown Hospital 863-2266
Emergency Room
460 West Oak St. 71730
Fort Smith
St. Edward's Mercy Medical Center 452-5100
Emergency Room Ext. 2401
7301 Rogers Avenue 72903
Emergency Room
Sparks Regional Med. Center 441-5011
1311 S. Eye St. 72901
Harrison
Boone County Hospital 741-6141
Emergency Room
620 N. Willow St. 72601 Ext. 275, 277
Helena
Helena Hospital 338-6411
Emergency Room
Hospital Drive 72342 Ext. 340
Little Rock
Univ. of Arkansas Medical Center 661-6161
Emergency Room
4301 W. Markham St. 72201
Osceola
Osceola Memorial Hospital 563-7180
Emergency Room Ext. 7180/2
611 Lee Ave. West 72370
Pine Bluff
Jefferson Regional Medical Center 541-7111
Emergency Department Ext. 5350
1515 W. 42nd Ave. 71601

CALIFORNIA

STATE COORDINATOR
Emergency Medical Services Authority
1600 Ninth St., Room 460 (916) 322-4336
Sacramento 95814
Fresno
Central Valley Regional 445-1222
Poison Control Ctr.
Fresno Community Hospital and
Medical Center
Fresno & R Sts.
Los Angeles
Los Angeles County
Medical Association 484-5151
Regional Poison Information Center
1925 Wilshire Blvd. 90057
Oakland
Children's Hosp. Medical Center 428-3248
of Northern California
51st & Grove St. 94609
Orange
University of California 634-5988
Irvine Medical Center
101 City Drive, Route 32 92688
Sacramento
Sacramento Medical Center 453-3692
Univ. of California, Davis 800/852-7221
2315 Stockton Blvd. 95817 (N. Cal.)
San Diego
San Diego Regional Poison Center 294-6000
University Calif. at San Diego Medical Center
225 W. Dickinson St. 92103
San Francisco
San Francisco Bay Area
Regional Poison Center
Room IE 86
San Francisco General Hosp. 666-2845
1001 Potrerro Ave. 94102 800/792-0720 (N. Cal.)
San Jose
Central-Coast Counties (800) 662-9886
Regional Poison Control Center (Statewide)
Santa Clara Valley Medical Center 279-5112
751 S. Bascom Ave., 95128

COLORADO

STATE COORDINATOR
Department of Health; (303) 320-8476
Emergency Medical Services Div
4210 E. 11th Ave.
Denver 80220
Denver
Rocky Mountain Poison Center 629-1123
Denver General Hospital 800/332-3073
W. 8th Ave. & Cherokee St. 80204

CONNECTICUT

STATE COORDINATOR
University of Connecticut (203) 674-3456
Health Center
Farmington 06032
Bridgeport
Bridgeport Hospital 384-3566
267 Grant St. 06602
St. Vincent's Medical Center 576-5178
2800 Main St. 06606
Danbury
Danbury Hospital 797-7300
95 Locust Ave. 06810
Farmington
Connecticut Poison Control Center 674-3456
University of Connecticut
Health Center 06032
Middletown
Middlesex Memorial Hospital 344-6684
28 Crescent St. 06457
New Haven
The Hospital of St. Raphael 789-3464
1450 Chapel St. 06511
Dept. of Pediatrics
Yale-New Haven Hospital 436-1960
20 York St. 06504
Norwalk
Department of Emergency Medicine
Norwalk Hospital 852-2160
Maple St. 06856

Waterbury
St. Mary's Hospital 574-6011
Emergency Room
56 Franklin St. 06702

DELAWARE

STATE COORDINATOR
Wilmington Medical Center (302) 655-3389
Delaware Division
Wilmington 19801
Wilmington
Wilmington Medical Center 655-3389
Delaware Division
501 W. 14th St. 19899

DISTRICT OF COLUMBIA

STATE COORDINATOR
Department of Human (202) 673-6741
Services (202) 673-6736
Washington, D.C. 20009
Washington, D.C.
National Capital Poison Center
Georgetown University Hospital 625-3333
3800 Reservoir Rd. 20007

FLORIDA

STATE COORDINATOR
Department of Health and (904) 487-1566
Rehabilitative Office of
Emergency Medical Services
Tallahassee 32301
Bradenton
Manatee Memorial Hospital 748-2121
206 2nd St. E. 33505
Daytona Beach
Halifax Hospital 258-1513
Emergency Department
P.O. Box 1990 32014
Ft. Lauderdale
Broward General Medical Center 463-3131
Poison Control
1600 S. Andrews Ave. 33316 Ext. 1955/6
Fort Myers
Lee Memorial Hospital 334-5287
2776 Cleveland Ave.
P.O. Drawer 2218 33902
Ft. Walton Beach
General Hospital of 862-1111
1000 Mar-Walt Drive Ext. 106
Ft. Walton Beach 32548
Gainesville
Shands Teaching Hosp. 392-3389
and Clinics
University of Florida 32610
Inverness
Citrus Memorial Hosp. 726-2800
502 Highland Blvd. 32650
Jacksonville
St. Vincent's Medical Center 387-7500
P.O. Box 2982 32203 387-7499
Lakeland
Lakeland Regional Medical Center 687-1137
Lakeland General Hospital
Lakeland Hills Blvd.
Drawer 448 33802
Leesburg
Leesburg Regional Medical Center 787-9900
600 E. Dixie 32748
Melbourne
James E. Holmes Regional 727-7000
Medical Center Ext. 675
Emergency Department
1350 S. Hickory St. 32901
Naples
Naples Community Hospital 262-3131
350 7th St. N. 33940
Ocala
Munroe Regional Medical Center 351-7607
131 S.W. 15th St. Ext. 187
P.O. Box 6000 32670
Orlando
Orlando Reg. Med. Ctr. 841-5222
Orange Memorial Division
1414 S. Kuhl Ave. 32806
Pensacola
Gulf Region Poison Center 434-4611
Baptist Hospital (800) 342-3222
P.O. Box 17500 32522 (Statewide)
Punta Gorda
Medical Center Hospital 637-2529
809 E. Marion Ave. 33950
Rockledge
Wuesthoff Memorial Hospital 636-4357
110 Longwood Ave. 32955
St. Petersburg
Bay Front Medical Center, Inc. 282-3171
701 6th St., S. 33701 (Statewide)
Sarasota
Memorial Hospital 953-1332
1901 Arlington Ave. 33579
Tallahassee
Tallahassee Memorial Regional 681-5411
Medical Center
1300 Miccouskee Road 32304
Tampa
Tampa Bay Regional Poison Control Center
Tampa General Hospital 251-6995
Davis Island 33606 (800) 282-3171
(Statewide)
Titusville
Jess Parrish Mem. Hospital 268-6260
P.O. Drawer W
951 N. Washington Ave. 32780
West Palm Beach
Good Samaritan Hospital 655-5511
Flagler Dr. at Ext. 4250
Palm Beach Lakes Blvd. 33402
Winter Haven
Poison Control Center
Winter Haven Hospital, Inc. 299-9701
200 Avenue F., N.E. 33880

GEORGIA

STATE COORDINATOR
Department of Human (404) 894-5170
Resources
Emergency Health Section
Atlanta 30308
Albany
Phoebe Putney Memorial Hosp. 888-4150
417 Third Avenue 31705
Athens
Athens General Hospital 543-5215
1199 Prince Ave. 30613
Atlanta
Georgia Poison Control Center 588-4400
P.O. Box 26066
80 Butler St., S.E. 30335 (800) 282-5846
(Statewide)
(Deaf) 404 525-3323
Augusta 724-5050
University Hospital
1350 Walton Way 30902
Columbus
The Medical Center 571-1080
710 Center Street 31902
Macon
Medical Center of Central Georgia 744-1427
Regional Poison Control Center
777 Hemlock St. 31201
Rome
Floyd Hospital 295-5500
Turner McCall Blvd. 31061
Savannah
Savannah Reg. EMS Poison Ctr. 355-5228
Depart. of Emergency Med.
Memorial Medical Center
P.O. Box 23089 31403
Thomasville
John D. Archbold 226-4121
Memorial Hospital Ext. 169
900 Gordon Ave. 31792
Valdosta
S. Georgia Medical Center 333-1110
P.O. Box 1727 31603
Waycross
Memorial Hospital 283-3030
410 Darling Ave. 31501

HAWAII

STATE COORDINATOR
Department of Health (808) 531-7776
Honolulu 96801
Honolulu
Kapiolani-Childrens Medical Center 941-4411
1319 Punahou St. 96826 (808) 362-3585

IDAHO

STATE COORDINATOR
Department of Health (208) 334-4245
and Welfare
Boise 83720
Boise
Idaho Emergency Medical 334-2241
Poison Center (800) 632-8000
1055 N. Curtis Rd. 83706 (Statewide)
Idaho Falls
Consolidated Hospitals 522-3600
Emergency Department
900 Memorial Dr. 83401
Pocatello
Idaho Drug Information Service 234-0777
and Poison Control Center Ext. 2019
Pocatello Regional (800) 632- 9490
Medical Center (Statewide)
777 Hospital Way 83202

ILLINOIS

STATE COORDINATOR
Division of Emergency Medical (217) 785-2080
Services and Highway Safety
Springfield 62761
Chicago
Rush-Presbyterian-St. Lukes 942-5969
Medical Center 800 942-5969
1753 W. Congress Parkway 60612
Peoria
Peoria Poison Center
St. Francis Hospital & 672-2334
Medical Center 800 322-5330
530 N.E. Glen Oak Avenue 61637
Springfield
Central & Southern Illinois
Resource Center
St. John's Hospital 753-3330
800 East Carpenter 62769 (800) 753-3330
(Statewide)

INDIANA

STATE COORDINATOR
Indiana State Board of Health (317) 633-0332
Hazardous Products Section
and Division of Drug Control
P.O. Box 1964
Indianapolis 46206
Anderson
Community Hospital 646-5143
1515 N. Madison Ave. 46012
St. John's Hickey 646-8222
Memorial Hospital
2015 Jackson St. 46014
Angola
Cameron Memorial Hospital 665-2141
416 East Maumee St. 46703 Ext. 146

Crown Point
St. Anthony Medical Ctr. — 738-2100
Main at Franciscan Rd. 46307 — Ext. 1311

Evansville
Deaconess Hospital — 426-3333
600 Mary St. 47710

Welborn Memorial — 426-8336
Baptist Hospital
401 S.E. 6th St. 47713

Fort Wayne
Lutheran Hospital — 458-2211
Emergency Dept.
3024 Fairfield Ave. 46807

Parkview Memorial Hospital — 484-9711
220 Randalia Dr. 46805

St. Joseph's Hospital — 426-8280
700 Broadway 46802

Gary
Methodist Hospital of Gary, Inc. — 886-4710
600 Grant St. 46402

Hammond
St. Margaret's Hospital — 931-4477
Poison Control Centers
25 Douglas St. 46320

Indianapolis
Indiána Poison Center — 630-7351
1001 West 10th St. 46202 — 800 382-9097

Kokomo
Howard Community Hospital — 453-8444
3500 S. LaFountain St. 46901

Lafayette
Lafayette Home Hospital — 447-6811
2400 South Street 47902

Poison Control Center
St. Elizabeth Hospital — 423-6699
1501 Hartfort St. 47904

Lebanon
Witham Memorial Hospital — 482-2700
1124 N. Lebanon St. 46052 — Ext. 241

Madison
King's Daughter's Hospital — 265-5211
112 Presbyterian Ave. 47250 — Ext. 131

Marion
Marion General Hospital — 662-4693
Wabash & Euclid Ave. 46952

Muncie
Ball Memorial Hospital — 747-4321
2401 University Ave. 47303

Richmond
Reid Memorial Hospital — 983-3148
1401 Chester Blvd. 47374

Shelbyville
Wm. S. Major Hospital — 392-3211
150 W. Washington St. 46176 — Ext. 252

South Bend
St. Joseph's Medical Center — 237-7264
811 E. Madison St. 46622

Terre Haute
Union Hospital, Inc. — 238-7000
1606 N. 7th St. 47804 — Ext. 7523

Valparaiso
Porter Memorial Hosp. — 464-8611
814 LaPorte Ave. 46383 — Ext. 301

Vincennes
The Good Samaritan — 885-3348
Hospital
520 S. 7th St. 47591

IOWA

STATE COORDINATOR
Department of Health — (515) 281-4964
Des Moines 50319

Des Moines
Variety Club Poison and — 283-6254
Drug Information Center — 800 362-2327
Iowa Methodist Medical Center — (Statewide)
1200 Pleasant St. 50308

Dubuque
Mercy Health Center — 589-9099
Mercy Drive 52001

Fort Dodge
Trinity Regional Hospital — 573-3101
Poison Information Center
Kenyon Rd. 50501

Iowa City
Univ. of Iowa Hospitals — 356-2922
and Clinics — 800 272-6477
Poison Control Center 52242 — (Statewide)

Waterloo
Allen Memorial Hospital — 235-3893
Emergency Department
1825 Logan Avenue 50703

KANSAS

STATE COORDINATOR
Department of Health & — (913) 862-9360
Environment — Ext. 541
Topeka 66620

Atchison
Atchison Hospital — 367-2131
1301 N. 2nd St. 66002

Dodge City
Dodge City Reg. Hosp. — 225-9050
Ross & Ave. "A" 67801 — Ext. 381

Emporia
Newman Memorial Hospital — 343-6800
12th & Chestnut Sts. 66801 — Ext. 545

Fort Riley
Irwin Army Hospital — 239-7776
Emergency Room 66442

Fort Scott
Mercy Hospital — 223-2200
821 Burke St. 66701 — Ext. 136

Great Bend
Central Kansas Medical — 792-2511
Center — Ext. 115
3515 Broadway 67530

Hays
Hadley Regional Medical Center — 628-8251
201 E. 7th St. 67601 — Ext. 145

Kansas City
Mid-America Poison Center
University of Kansas — 588-6633
Medical Center — (800) 332-6633
39th & Rainbow Blvd. 66103 — (Statewide)

Lawrence
Lawrence Memorial Hospital — 843-3680
325 Maine St. 66044 — Ext. 162

Salina
St. John's Hospital — 827-3187
139 N. Penn St. 67401

Topeka
Stormont-Vail Regional Med. Ctr. — 354-6100
10th & Washburn Sts. 66606
Northeast Kansas Poison Center
St. Francis Hospital — 295-8094
and Medical Center
1700 W. 7th St. 66606

Wichita
Wesley Medical Center — 688-2277
550 N. Hillside Ave. 67214

KENTUCKY

STATE COORDINATOR
Department For Human — (502) 564-3970
Resources
Frankfort 40601

Fort Thomas
St. Lukes Hospital — 572-3215
85 N. Grand Ave. 41075 — 800 352-9900
(Statewide)

Lexington
Central Baptist Hospital — 278-3411
1740 S. Limestone St. 40503 — Ext. 363

Drug Information Center — 233-5320
University of Kentucky
Medical Center 40536

Louisville
Kentucky Regional Poison Center — 589-8222
of Kosair-Children's Hospital — 800 722-5725
NKC, Inc. — (Statewide)
P.O. Box 35070 40232

Murray
Murray-Calloway County — 753-7588
Hospital
803 Popular 42071

Owensboro
Owensboro-Daviess County — 926-3030
Hospital — Ext. 180
811 Hospital Court 42301

Paducah
Western Baptist Hospital — 444-5180
2501 Kentucky Ave. 42001

Prestonburg
Poison Control Center — 886-8511
Highlands Regional Medical — Ext. 132
Center 41653

LOUISIANA

STATE COORDINATOR
L.S.U. Poison Control and Drug — 425-1524
Abuse Information Center
Louisiana State University Medical Center
P.O. Box 33932 71130

Alexandria
Rapides General Hospital — 445-4665
Poison Control Center
P.O. Box 7146 71301

Lafayette
Our Lady of Lourdes Hosp. — 234-7381
611 St. Landry St. 70501

Lake Charles
Lake Charles Memorial Hosp. — 478-6800
P.O. Drawer M 70601

Monroe
Northeast Louisiana University — 342-3008
School of Pharmacy
700 University Ave. 71209

St. Francis Hospital — 325-6454
P.O. Box 1901 71301

New Orleans
Charity Hospital — 568-5222
1532 Tulane Ave. 70140

Shreveport
Louisiana State University Poison Control
and Drug Abuse Information Center
LSU Medical Center — 425-152
P.O. Box 33932 71130

MAINE

STATE COORDINATOR
Maine Poison Control Center — (207) 871-295
Portland 04102

Portland
Maine Medical Center — 871-238
Emergency Division — 800 442-630
22 Bramhall St. 04102 — (Statewide)

MARYLAND

STATE COORDINATOR
Maryland Poison Information Center
University of Maryland — (301) 528-77
School of Pharmacy — (800) 492-24
636 W. Lombard St. — (Statewid
Baltimore 21201

Baltimore
Maryland Poison Information Center — 528-77
University of Maryland — 800 492-24
(Statewid

School of Pharmacy
636 W. Lombard St. 21201

Cumberland
Tri-State Poison Center
Sacred Heart Hospital — 722-6677
900 Seton Drive 21502

MASSACHUSETTS

STATE COORDINATOR
Department of Public Health — (617) 727-2700
Boston 02111

Boston
Massachusetts Poison Control System — 232-2120, 800 682-9211 (Statewide)
300 Longwood Ave. 02115

MICHIGAN

STATE COORDINATOR
Department of Public Health — (517) 373-1406
Emergency Medical Services
Lansing 48909

Adrian
Emma L. Bixby Hospital — 263-2412
Poison Control Center
818 Riverside Ave. 49221

Ann Arbor
University Hospital — 764-7667
Poison Control Center
1405 E. Ann St. 48104

Battle Creek
Community Hospital — 963-5521
Pharmacy Dept.
183 West St. 49016

Bay City
Bay Medical Center — 894-3131
1900 Columbus Ave. 48706

Coldwater
Community Health Center of Branch County — 278-7361
274 E. Chicago St. 49036

Detroit
Children's Hospital of Michigan — 494-5711
Southeast Regional Poison Center — (800) 572-1655 (Statewide)
3901 Beaubien 48201

Flint
Poison Information Center
Hurley Medical Center — 257-9111
6th Ave & Begole 48502 — (800) 572-5396

Grand Rapids
Western Michigan Regional Poison Center — 774-7854, (800) 632-2727 (Statewide)
1840 Wealthy, S.E. 49506

Jackson
W.A. Foote Memorial Hosp. — 788-4816
Poison Control Center
205 N. East St. 49201

Kalamazoo
Midwest Poison Center — 383-7104
Borgess Medical Center — (800) 632-4177 (Statewide)
1521 Gull Rd. 49001

Great Lakes Poison Center — 383-6409
Bronson Methodist Hospital — 800 442-4112 (Statewide)
252 E. Lovell St. 49006

Lansing
St. Lawrence Hospital — 372-5112
1210 W. Saginaw St. 48914

Marquette
Upper Peninsula Regional Poison Center
Marquette General Hospital — 228-9440
420 W. Magnetic Dr. 49855 — (800) 562-9781
Regional Poison Center
420 W. Magnetic Dr. 49855

Midland
Midland Hospital — 631-8100
Poison Control Center
4005 Orchard 48640

Pontiac
St. Joseph Mercy Hospital — 858-7373
900 S. Woodward Ave. 48053

Port Huron
Port Huron Hospital — 987-5555
Poison Control Center
1001 Kearney St. 48060

Saginaw
Saginaw Region Poison Center
Saginaw General Hospital — 755-1111
1447 N. Harrison 48602

Westland
Wayne County General Hospital — 722-3748, 274-3000
2345 Merriman Rd. 48185

MINNESOTA

STATE COORDINATOR
EMS Section
Minnesota Department of Health — (612) 623-5284
717 S.E. Delaware St.
Minneapolis 55404

Duluth
St. Luke's Hospital — 727-5466
Poison Control Center
915 E. First St. 55805

St. Mary's Hospital — 726-4500
407 E. 3rd St. 55805

Fridley
Unity Medical Center — 786-2200 Ext. 6844
550 Osborne Rd. 55432

Mankato
Immanual - St. Joseph's Hospital — 625-4031 Ext. 2760
Poison Control Center
325 Garden Blvd. 56001

Minneapolis
Hennepin Poison Ctr. — 347-3141
Hennepin County Medical Center
701 Park Ave. 55415

Morris
Stevens County Memorial Hospital 56267 — 589-1313 Ext. 231

Rochester
Southeastern Minnesota Poison Control Ctr. — 285-5123
St. Mary's Hospital
1216 Second St., S.W. 55901

St. Cloud
St. Cloud Hospital — 255-5617
1406 6th Avenue, N. 56301

St. Paul
St. John's Hospital — 228-3132
403 Maria Ave. 55106

United and Children's Hospitals — 298-8402
333 N. Smith 55102

Minnesota Poison Information Center
St. Paul-Ramsey Medical Center — 221-2113
640 Jackson St. 55101

Willmar
Rice Memorial Hospital — 235-4543 Ext. 560
301 Becker Ave., S.W.

Worthington
Worthington Regional Hosp. — 372-2941 Ext. 109
1016 6th Ave. 56187

MISSISSIPPI

STATE COORDINATOR
State Board of Health — (601) 354-7660
Jackson 39205

Biloxi
Gulf Coast Community Hospital — 388-1919
4642 West Beach Blvd. 39531

USAF Hospital Keesler — 377-6555
Keesler Air Force Base
39534

Brandon
Rankin General Hospital — 825-2811
Emergency Department
350 Crossgates Blvd. 39042 — Ext. 405

Columbia
Marion County General Hospital — 736-6303 Ext. 1020
Sumrall Rd. 39429

Greenwood
Greenwood-LeFlore Hosp. — 459-2790
River Road 38930

Hattiesburg
Forrest County General Hosp — 264-4235
400 S. 28th Ave. 39401

Jackson
St. Dominic-Jackson Mem. Hosp — 982-0121 Ext. 2345
969 Lakeland Dr.
39216

University Medical Center — 354-7660
2500 N. State St. 39216

Laurel
Jones County Community Hospital — 649-4000 Ext. 603
Jefferson St. at 13th Ave.
39440

Meridian
Meridian Regional Hosp. — 483-6211 Ext. 440
Highway 39, North 39301

Pascagoula
Singing River Hospital — 938-5162
Emergency Room
2609 Denny Ave. East 39567

University
University of Mississippi — 234-1522
School of Pharmacy
Poison Information Center 38677

MISSOURI

STATE COORDINATOR
Bureau of EMS
Missouri Division of Health — (314) 751-2713
Jefferson City 65102

Cape Girardeau
St. Francis Medical Ctr. — 651-6235
St. Francis Drive 63701

Columbia
University of Missouri Medical Center — 882-8091
807 Stadium Blvd. 65212

Hannibal
St. Elizabeth Hospital, Pharmacy Dept. — 221-0414 Ext. 264
109 Virginia St. 63401

Jefferson City
Charles E. Still Osteopathic Hospital — 635-7141 Ext. 215
1125 Madison 65101

Joplin
St. John's Medical Center — 781-2727 Ext. 2305
2727 McClelland Blvd. 64801

Kansas City
Children's Mercy Hospital — 234-3000
24th & Gillham Rd. 64108

Kirksville
Kirksville Osteopathic Health Center — 626-2266
Box 949
1 Osteopathy Ave.
63501

Poplar Bluff
Lucy Lee Hospital — 785-7721 Ext. 264
2620 N. Westwood Blvd. 63901

Rolla
Phelps County Regional Medical Center. — 364-1322 Ext. 287
1000 W. 10th St. 65401

St. Joseph
Methodist Medical Center — 271-7580, 232-8481
Seventh to Ninth on Faron Sts. 64501

St. Louis
Cardinal Glennon Memorial Hospital for Children — 772-5200
1465 S. Grand Ave. 63104

St. Louis Children's Hosp. — 454-6099
500 S. Kingshighway 63110

Springfield
Ozark Poison Center — 831-9746
Lester E. Cox Medical Center
1423 N. Jefferson St. 65802

West Plains
West Plains Memorial Hosp. — 256-9111 Ext. 258
1103 Alaska Ave. 65775

MONTANA

STATE COORDINATOR
Department of Health and Environmental Sciences — (406) 449-3895
Helena 59620

HELENA
Montana Poison Control System — 442-2480, (800)-525-5042
Cogswell Bldg.
Helena 59620

NEBRASKA

STATE COORDINATOR
Department of Health — (402) 471-2122
Lincoln 68502

Omaha
Mid-Plains Regional Poison Center — 390-5400
Children's Memorial Hospital — 800-642-9999 (Statewide)
8301 Dodge 68114
Nebraska (N.E. Residents) — 800-228-9515 Surrounding States

NEVADA

STATE COORDINATOR
Department of Human Resources — (702) 885-4750
Carson City 89710

Las Vegas
Southern Nevada Memorial Hosp. — 385-1277
1800 W. Charleston Blvd. 89102

Sunrise Hospital Med. Ctr. — 732-4989
3186 South Maryland Parkway 89109

Reno
St. Mary's Hospital — 789-3013
235 W. 6th 89520

Washoe Medical Center — 785-4129
77 Pringle Way 89502

NEW HAMPSHIRE

STATE COORDINATOR
New Hampshire Poison Center — (603) 646-5000
NH-2 Dartmouth Hitchcock Medical Center — (800) 562-8236 (Statewide)
Maynard St. 03756

Hanover
New Hampshire Poison Center — (603) 646-5000
Mary Hitchcock Hospital — (800) 562-8236 (Statewide)
2 Maynard St. 03756

NEW JERSEY

STATE COORDINATOR
Department of Health — (609) 292-5666
Accident Prevention & Poison Control Program
Trenton 08625

Atlantic City
Atlantic City Medical Center — 344-4081 Ext. 2359
1925 Pacific Ave. 08401

Belleville
Clara Maass Medical Center. — 450-2000 Ext. 781
1A Franklin Ave. 07109

Berlin
West Jersey Hospital — 768-6666
South Division 08009

Boonton
Riverside Hospital — 334-5000 Ext. 186
Powerville Rd. 07055

Bridgeton
Bridgeton Hospital — 451-6600 Ext. 251
Irving Ave. 08302

Denville
St. Clare's Hospital — 625-6050 Ext. 6063
Pocono Rd. 07834

East Orange
East Orange General Hospital — 672-8400 Ext. 223
300 Central Ave. 07019

Elizabeth
St. Elizabeth's Hospital — 527-5059
225 Williamson St. 07207

Englewood
Englewood Hospital — 894-3262
350 Engle St. 07631

Flemington
Hunterdon Medical Center — 782-2121 Ext. 369
Route #31 08822

Livingston
St. Barnabas Medical Center — 992-5161
Old Short Hills Rd. 07039

Long Branch
Monmouth Medical Center — 222-2210
Emergency Dept.
Dunbar & 2nd Ave. 07740

Montclair
Mountainside Hospital — 429-6202
Bay & Highland Ave. 07042

Mount Holly
Burlington County Memorial — 267-7877
175 Madison Ave. 08060

Neptune
Jersey Shore Medical Center-Fitkin Hospital — 775-5500, (800) 822-9761 (NJ)
1945 Corlies Ave. 07753

Newark
Newark Beth Israel Medical Center — 926-7240, 926-7241, 926-7242, 926-7243
201 Lyons Ave. 07112

New Brunswick
Middlesex General Hospital — 937-8583
180 Somerset St. 08903

St. Peter's Medical Center — 745-8527
245 Easton Ave. 08903

Newton
Newton Memorial Hospital — 383-2121 Ext. 270, 271
175 High St. 07860

Orange
Hospital Center at Orange — 266-2120
Emergency Dept.
188 S. Essex Ave. 07051

Passaic
St. Mary's Hospital — 473-1000 Ext. 441
211 Pennington Ave. 07055

Perth Amboy
Perth Amboy General Hosp. — 442-3700 Ext. 2501
530 New Brunswick Ave. 08861

Phillipsburg
Warren Hospital — 859-1500 Ext. 222
185 Roseberry St. 08865

Point Pleasant
Point Pleasant Hospital — 892-1100 Ext. 383
Osborn Ave. & River Front 08742

Princeton
Medical Center at Princeton — 734-4554
253 Witherspoon St. 08540

Saddle Brook
Saddle Brook General Hosp. — 368-6025
300 Market St. 07662

Somers Point
Shore Memorial Hospital — 653-3515
Brighton & Sunny Aves. 08244

Somerville
Somerset Medical Center — 725-4000 Ext. 436
Rehill Ave. 08876

Summit
Overlook Hospital — 522-2232
193 Morris Ave. 07901

Teaneck
Holy Name Hospital — 833-3242
718 Teaneck Rd. 07666

Trenton
Helene Fuld Medical Center — 396-1077
750 Brunswick Ave. 08638

Union
Memorial General Hospital — 687-1900 Ext. 3710
1000 Galloping Hill Rd. 07083

Wayne
Greater Paterson General Hospital — 942-6900 Ext. 224
224 Hamburg Tnpk. 07470

NEW MEXICO

STATE COORDINATOR
N.M. Poison, Drug Inf. & Med. Crisis Center — (505) 843-2551, 800-432-6866
University of New Mexico
Albuquerque 87131

NEW YORK

STATE COORDINATOR
Department of Health — (518) 474-3785
Albany 12237

Binghampton
Southern Tier Poison Center
Binghampton General Hospital — 723-892
Mitchell Avenue 13903

Our Lady of Lourdes Memorial Hospital — 798-523
169 Riverside Drive 13905

Buffalo
Western N.Y. Poison Control Center — 878-765
Children's Hospital
219 Bryant St. 14222

Dunkirk
Brooks Memorial Hospital — 366-111 Ext. 41
10 West 6th St. 14048
Ext. 415

East Meadow
Long Island Regional Poison Center — 542-232
Nassau County Medical Ctr. — 542-232
2201 Hempstead Tpk. 11554

Elmira
Arnot Ogden Memorial Hosp. — 737-419
Roe Ave. & Grove 14901

St. Joseph's Hospital Health Center — 734-266
555 E. Market St. 14901

Endicott
Ideal Hospital — 754-717
600 High St. 13760

Glens Falls
Glens Falls Hospital — 761-526 Ext. 45
100 Parks St. 12801

Jamestown
W.C.A. Hospital — 484-864
207 Foote Ave. 14701

Johnson City
Wilson Memorial Hospital — 773-661
33 Harrison St. 13790

Kingston
Kingston Hospital — 331-331
396 Broadway 12401

Listings Continued Following Product Information Section

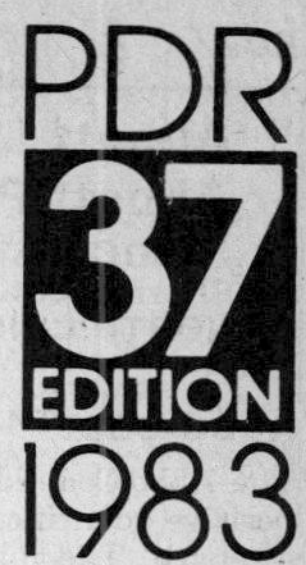

SECTION 6

Product Information Section

This section is made possible through the courtesy of the manufacturers whose products appear on the following pages. The information concerning each product has been prepared, edited and approved by the medical department, medical director, and/or medical counsel of each manufacturer.

Products described in PHYSICIANS' DESK REFERENCE® which have official package circulars must be in full compliance with Food & Drug Administration regulations pertaining to labeling for prescription drugs. These regulations require that for PDR copy, "indications and usage, dosages, routes, methods, and frequency and duration of administration, description, clinical pharmacology and supply and any relevant warnings, hazards, contraindications, adverse reactions, potential for drug abuse and dependence, overdosage and precautions" must be in the *"same language and emphasis"* as the approved labeling for the product. FDA regards the words *"same in language and emphasis"* as requiring VERBATIM use of the approved labeling providing such information. Furthermore, the information in the approved labeling that is emphasized by the use of type set in a box or in capitals, bold face, or italics must be given the same emphasis in PDR. For products which do not have official package circulars, the Publisher has emphasized to manufacturers the necessity of describing such products comprehensively so that physicians would have access to all information essential for intelligent and informed prescribing. In organizing and presenting the material in PHYSICIANS' DESK REFERENCE, the Publisher is providing all the information made available to PDR by manufacturers.

This edition of PHYSICIANS' DESK REFERENCE contains the latest product information available at press-time. During the year, however, new and revised information about the products described herein may be furnished us. This information will be published in the PDR Supplement. Therefore, before prescribing or administering any product described in the following pages, you should first consult the PDR Supplement.

In presenting the following material to the medical profession, the Publisher is not necessarily advocating the use of any product listed.

Abbott Laboratories—Abbott Pharmaceuticals, Inc.

Pharmaceutical Products Division
NORTH CHICAGO, IL 60064

ABBO–CODE™ INDEX

The Abbo-Code identification system provides positive identification of a drug and dosage strength. The following Abbott products are imprinted or debossed with an Abbo-Code designation:

PRODUCT	*ABBO-CODE*
A-poxide® Capsules Ⓒ (chlordiazepoxide hydrochloride capsules, USP)	
5 mg	CP
10 mg	CS
25 mg	CT
Cefol® Filmtab® Tablets B-complex vitamins with folic acid, vitamin E, and vitamin C	NJ
Chlorthalidone Tablets, USP	
25 mg	AA
50 mg	AB
Colchicine Tablets, USP	
0.6 mg	AF
Cylert® Tablets Ⓒ (pemoline)	
18.75 mg	TH
37.5 mg	TI
75 mg	TJ
37.5 mg Chewable	TK
Depakene® Capsules (valproic acid capsules)	
250 mg	HH
Desoxyn® Ⓒ (methamphetamine hydrochloride)	
2.5 mg Tablet	TC
5 mg Tablet	TE
5 mg Gradumet®	MC
10 mg Gradumet	ME
15 mg Gradumet	MF
Diasone® Sodium Enterab® Tablets (sulfoxone sodium tablets, USP)	
165 mg	AS
Dicumarol Tablets, USP	
25 mg	AN
50 mg	AO
100 mg	AR
Ery-Tab® Tablets (erythromycin enteric-coated tablets)	
250 mg	EC
333 mg	EH
500 mg	ED
E.E.S.® Chewable Tablets (erythromycin ethylsuccinate tablets, USP)	
200 mg erythromycin activity	EF
E.E.S. 400® Filmtab® Tablets (erythromycin ethylsuccinate tablets, USP)	
400 mg erythromycin activity	EE
Enduron® Tablets (methyclothiazide tablets, USP)	
2.5 mg	ENDURON
5 mg	ENDURON
Enduronyl® Tablets	
5 mg methyclothiazide and 0.25 mg deserpidine	LS
Enduronyl® Forte Tablets	
5 mg methyclothiazide and 0.5 mg deserpidine	LT
Erythrocin® Stearate Filmtab® Tablets (erythromycin stearate tablets, USP)	
250 mg erythromycin activity	ES
500 mg erythromycin activity	ET
Erythromycin Base Filmtab® Tablets (erythromycin tablets, USP)	
250 mg	EB
500 mg	EA
Eutonyl® Filmtab® Tablets (pargyline hydrochloride tablets, USP)	
10 mg	NA
25 mg	NB
Eutron® Filmtab® Tablets	
25 mg pargyline hydrochloride and 5 mg methyclothiazide	NK
Fero-Folic-500® Filmtab® Tablets controlled-release iron, folic acid, and vitamin C	AJ
Gemonil® Tablets Ⓒ (metharbital tablets, USP)	
100 mg	TF
Harmonyl® Tablets (deserpidine tablets)	
0.1 mg	LJ
0.25 mg	LK
Iberet-Folic-500® Filmtab® Tablets controlled-release iron, B-complex vitamins with folic acid, and vitamin C	AK
Janimine® Filmtab® Tablets (imipramine hydrochloride tablets, USP)	
10 mg	ND
25 mg	NE
50 mg	NL
K·Tab™ Filmtab® Tablets (potassium chloride extended-release tablets, USP)	
10 mEq (750 mg)	NM
Nembutal® Sodium Capsules Ⓒ (pentobarbital sodium capsules, USP)	
30 mg	CE
50 mg	CF
100 mg	CH
Ogen® Tablets (estropipate tablets, USP)	
0.625 tablet (0.75 mg estropipate)	LU
1.25 tablet (1.5 mg estropipate)	LV
2.5 tablet (3 mg estropipate)	LX
5 tablet (6 mg estropipate)	LY
Oretic® Tablets (hydrochlorothiazide tablets, USP)	
25 mg	ORETIC
50 mg	ORETIC
Oreticyl® 25 Tablets	
25 mg hydrochlorothiazide and 0.125 mg deserpidine	AH
Oreticyl® 50 Tablets	
50 mg hydrochlorothiazide and 0.125 mg deserpidine	AI
Oreticyl® Forte Tablets	
25 mg hydrochlorothiazide and 0.25 mg deserpidine	LL
Panwarfin® Tablets (warfarin sodium tablets, USP)	
2 mg	LM
2.5 mg	LN
5 mg	LO
7.5 mg	LR
10 mg	LF
Peganone® Tablets (ethotoin tablets)	
250 mg	AD
500 mg	AE
Phenurone® Tablets (phenacemide tablets, USP)	
500 mg	II
Placidyl® Capsules Ⓒ (ethchlorvynol capsules, USP)	
500 mg	KH
750 mg	KN
Tral® Filmtab® Tablets (hexocyclium methylsulfate tablets)	
25 mg	NF
Tral® Gradumet® Tablets (hexocyclium methylsulfate controlled-release tablets)	
50 mg	AL
Tranxene® Ⓒ (clorazepate dipotassium)	
3.75 mg Capsule	CI
7.5 mg Capsule	CN
15 mg Capsule	CK
3.75 mg Tablet	TL
7.5 mg Tablet	TM
15 mg Tablet	TN
Tranxene®-SD Ⓒ Single Dose Tablets (clorazepate dipotassium)	
22.5 mg	TY
11.25 mg Half Strength	TX
Tridione® Dulcet® Tablets (trimethadione tablets, USP)	
150 mg	LE
Tridione® Capsules (trimethadione capsules, USP)	
300 mg	AM
Vercyte® Tablets (pipobroman tablets, USP)	
25 mg	AT

Code letters were added to many products during 1981; these products may still be available without Abbo-Code markings.

[*Examples shown in Product Identification Section*]

ABBO-PAC®
Unit Dose Packages

Abbott's Abbo-Pac unit dose system offers a wide range of drugs.

Each individual dose is clearly identified by generic name, Abbott name, strength, NDC identification number, expiration date and lot number. Abbo-Pac unit dose containers are designed to accommodate virtually all hospital pharmacy storage racks and to provide maximum accessibility and ease of handling.

The following is a list of products which are now available:

PRODUCT	*DOSAGE STRENGTH*
Dayalets® Filmtab® Multivitamin Supplement	
Depakene® Capsules (valproic acid)	250 mg
Enduron® Tablets (methyclothiazide tablets, USP)	5 mg
Enduronyl® Tablets (methyclothiazide 5 mg and deserpidine 0.25 mg)	
E.E.S. 400® Filmtab (erythromycin ethylsuccinate tablets, USP)	400 mg
E.E.S.® Granules (erythromycin ethylsuccinate for oral suspension, USP)	200 mg/5 ml
EryPed™ Granules (erythromycin ethylsuccinate for oral suspension, USP)	400 mg/5 ml
Ery-Tab® (erythromycin enteric-coated tablets)	250 mg
Ery-Tab	333 mg
Ery-Tab	500 mg
Erythrocin® Stearate Filmtab (erythromycin stearate tablets, USP)	250 mg
Erythromycin Base Film® (erythromycin tablets, USP)	250 mg
Fero-Grad-500® Filmtab Controlled-Release Iron plus Vitamin C	
Iberet®-500 Filmtab Controlled-Release Iron plus B-Complex and Vitamin C	
K-Lor™ 20 mEq (potassium chloride for oral solution, USP)	20 mEq Potassium 20 mEq Chloride/Packet
K-Lor™ 15 mEq	15 mEq Potassium 15 mEq Chloride/Packet
K·Tab™ Filmtab® (potassium chloride extended-release tablets, USP)	10 mEq (750 mg)
Nembutal® Sodium Capsules Ⓒ (pentobarbital sodium capsules, USP)	100 mg
Nembutal Sodium Capsules Ⓒ Disp. Pack (20/25's)	100 mg
Oretic® Tablets (hydrochlorothiazide tablets, USP)	25 mg
Oretic® Tablets	50 mg
Panwarfin® Tablets (warfarin sodium tablets, USP)	2 mg

Panwarfin® Tablets....2.5 mg
Panwarfin® Tablets....5 mg
Panwarfin® Tablets....7.5 mg
Panwarfin® Tablets....10 mg
Placidyl® Capsules Ⓒ
(ethchlorvynol capsules, USP)....500 mg
Placidyl® Capsules Ⓒ....750 mg
Surbex-T® Filmtab
(high-potency vitamin B-complex with vitamin C)
Tranxene® Capsules Ⓒ
(clorazepate dipotassium)....3.75 mg
Tranxene® Capsules Ⓒ....7.5 mg
Tranxene® Capsules Ⓒ....15 mg
[*Examples shown in Product Identification Section*]

ABBOKINASE® ℞
Urokinase For Injection

ABBOKINASE (urokinase for injection) when used in the management of pulmonary embolism should be used in hospitals where the recommended diagnostic and monitoring techniques are available. Thrombolytic therapy should be considered in all situations where the benefits to be achieved outweigh the risk of potentially serious hemorrhage. When internal bleeding does occur, it may be more difficult to manage than that which occurs with conventional anticoagulant therapy.
Urokinase treatment should be instituted as soon as possible after onset of pulmonary embolism, preferably no later than seven days after onset. Any delay in instituting lytic therapy to evaluate the effect of heparin decreases the potential for optimal efficacy.[1]

Description: Urokinase is an enzyme (protein) produced by the kidney, and found in the urine. There are two forms of urokinase differing in molecular weight but having similar clinical effects. ABBOKINASE (urokinase for injection) is a thrombolytic agent obtained from human kidney cells by tissue culture techniques and is primarily the low molecular weight form. It is supplied as a sterile lyophilized white powder containing mannitol (25 mg/vial) and sodium chloride (45 mg/vial).
Following reconstitution with 5.2 ml of Sterile Water for Injection, USP, it is a clear, practically colorless solution; each ml contains 50,000 IU of urokinase activity, 0.5% mannitol, and 0.9% sodium chloride.
The pH of ABBOKINASE is adjusted with sodium hydroxide and/or hydrochloric acid prior to lyophilization. (For intravenous infusion only.)

Clinical Pharmacology: Urokinase acts on the endogenous fibrinolytic system. It converts plasminogen to the enzyme plasmin. Plasmin degrades fibrin clots as well as fibrinogen and other plasma proteins.
Intravenous infusion of urokinase in doses recommended for lysis of pulmonary embolism is followed by increased fibrinolytic activity. This effect disappears within a few hours after discontinuation, but a decrease in plasma levels of fibrinogen and plasminogen and an increase in the amount of circulating fibrin (ogen) degradation products may persist for 12-24 hours.[2,3] There is a lack of correlation between embolus resolution and changes in coagulation and fibrinolytic assay results.
Information is incomplete about the pharmacokinetic properties in man. Urokinase administered by intravenous infusion is cleared rapidly by the liver. The serum half-life in man is 20 minutes or less. Patients with impaired liver function (e.g., cirrhosis) would be expected to show a prolongation in half-life. Small fractions of an administered dose are excreted in bile and urine.

Indications and Usage:
Pulmonary Embolism: ABBOKINASE (urokinase for injection) is indicated in adults:
- For the lysis of acute massive pulmonary emboli, defined as obstruction of blood flow to a lobe or multiple segments.
- For the lysis of pulmonary emboli accompanied by unstable hemodynamics, i.e., failure to maintain blood pressure without supportive measures.

The diagnosis should be confirmed by objective means, such as pulmonary angiography via an upper extremity vein, or non-invasive procedures such as lung scanning.
Angiographic and hemodynamic measurements demonstrate a more rapid improvement with lytic therapy than with heparin therapy.[4,5,6,7,8]
I.V. Catheter Clearance: ABBOKINASE is indicated for the restoration of patency to intravenous catheters, including central venous catheters, obstructed by clotted blood or fibrin.[9,10] (See separate section at end of prescribing information concerning I.V. catheter clearance for information regarding warnings, precautions, adverse reactions, and dosage and administration.)

Contraindications: Because thrombolytic therapy increases the risk of bleeding, urokinase is contraindicated in the following situations: (See WARNINGS.)
- Active internal bleeding
- Recent (within two months) cerebrovascular accident, intracranial or intraspinal surgery
- Intracranial neoplasm

Warnings:
Bleeding: The aim of urokinase is the production of sufficient amounts of plasmin for lysis of intravascular deposits of fibrin; however, fibrin deposits which provide hemostasis, for example, at sites of needle puncture, will also lyse, and bleeding from such sites may occur.
Intramuscular injections and nonessential handling of the patient must be avoided during treatment with urokinase. Venipunctures should be performed carefully and as infrequently as possible.
Should an arterial puncture be necessary, upper extremity vessels are preferable. Pressure should be applied for at least 30 minutes, a pressure dressing applied, and the puncture site checked frequently for evidence of bleeding.
In the following conditions, the risks of therapy may be increased and should be weighed against the anticipated benefits:
- Recent (within 10 days) major surgery, obstetrical delivery, organ biopsy, previous puncture of non-compressible vessels
- Recent (within 10 days) serious gastrointestinal bleeding
- Recent trauma including cardiopulmonary resuscitation
- Severe uncontrolled arterial hypertension
- High likelihood of a left heart thrombus, e.g., mitral stenosis with atrial fibrillation
- Subacute bacterial endocarditis
- Hemostatic defects including those secondary to severe hepatic or renal disease
- Pregnancy
- Cerebrovascular disease
- Diabetic hemorrhagic retinopathy
- Any other condition in which bleeding might constitute a significant hazard or be particularly difficult to manage because of its location

Should serious spontaneous bleeding (not controllable by local pressure) occur, the infusion of urokinase should be terminated immediately, and treatment instituted as described under ADVERSE REACTIONS.
Use of Anticoagulants: Concurrent use of anticoagulants with urokinase is not recommended. Before starting urokinase in patients being treated with heparin, the effects of heparin should be allowed to diminish with time.

Precautions:
Laboratory Tests: Before commencing thrombolytic therapy, obtain a hematocrit, platelet count, and a thrombin time (TT), activated partial thromboplastin time (APTT), or prothrombin time (PT). If heparin has been given, it should be discontinued. TT or APTT should be less than twice the normal control value before thrombolytic therapy is started.
During the infusion, coagulation tests and/or measures of fibrinolytic activity may be performed if desired. Results do not, however, reliably predict either efficacy or a risk of bleeding. The clinical response should be observed frequently, and vital signs, i.e., pulse, temperature, respiratory rate and blood pressure, should be checked at least every four hours. The blood pressure should not be taken in the lower extremities to avoid dislodgment of possible deep vein thrombi.
Following the infusion, *before (re)instituting heparin*, the TT or APTT should be less than twice the upper limits of normal.
Drug Interactions: The interaction of urokinase with other drugs has not been studied. Drugs that alter platelet function should not be used. Common examples are: aspirin, indomethacin and phenylbutazone.
Concomitant use of urokinase and oral anticoagulants or heparin may increase the risk of hemorrhage. Urokinase should not be given concurrently with these drugs. (See "WARNINGS" section.)
Carcinogenicity: Adequate data is not available on the long-term potential for carcinogenicity in animals or humans.
Pregnancy: Pregnancy category B. Reproduction studies have been performed in mice and rats at doses up to 1,000 times the human dose and have revealed no evidence of impaired fertility or harm to the fetus due to urokinase. There are, however, no adequate and well-controlled studies in pregnant women. Because animal reproduction studies are not always predictive of human response, this drug should be used during pregnancy only if clearly needed.
Nursing Mothers: It is not known whether this drug is excreted in human milk. Because many drugs are excreted in human milk, caution should be exercised when urokinase is administered to a nursing woman.
Pediatric Use: Safety and effectiveness in children have not been established.

Adverse Reactions:
Bleeding: The type of bleeding associated with thrombolytic therapy can be placed into two broad categories:
- Superficial or surface bleeding, observed mainly at invaded or disturbed sites (e.g., venous cutdowns, arterial punctures, sites of recent surgical intervention, etc.).
- Internal bleeding, involving, e.g., the gastrointestinal tract, genitourinary tract, vagina, or intramuscular, retroperitoneal, or intracerebral sites.

Several fatalities due to cerebral or retroperitoneal hemorrhage have occurred during thrombolytic therapy.
Should serious bleeding occur, urokinase infusion should be discontinued and, if necessary, blood loss and reversal of the bleeding tendency can be effectively managed with whole blood (fresh blood preferable), packed red blood cells and cryoprecipitate or fresh frozen plasma. Dextran should not be used. Although the use of aminocaproic acid (ACA, AMICAR®) in humans as an antidote for urokinase has not been documented, it may be considered in an emergency situation.
Allergic Reactions: *In vitro* tests with urokinase, as well as intradermal tests in humans, gave no evidence of induced antibody formation. Relatively mild allergic type reactions, e.g., bronchospasm and skin rash, have been reported rarely. When such reactions occur, they usually respond to conventional therapy.

Continued on next page

If desired, additional literature on any Abbott Product will be provided upon request to Abbott Laboratories.

Abbott—Cont.

Fever: Febrile episodes have occurred in approximately 2-3% of treated patients. A cause and effect relationship has not been established. Symptomatic treatment with acetaminophen is usually sufficient to alleviate discomfort. Aspirin is not recommended.

Dosage and Administration:

Preparation: Reconstitute ABBOKINASE (urokinase for injection) by aseptically adding 5.2 ml of Sterile Water for Injection, USP, to the vial (It is important that ABBOKINASE be reconstituted *only* with Sterile Water for Injection, USP, *without* preservatives. Bacteriostatic Water for Injection should not be used.) Each vial should be visually inspected for discoloration (practically colorless solution) and for the presence of particulate material. Because ABBOKINASE contains no preservatives, it should not be reconstituted until immediately before using. Any unused portion of the reconstituted material should be discarded. Reconstituted ABBOKINASE is diluted with 0.9% Sodium Chloride Injection, USP or 5% Dextrose Injection, USP, prior to intravenous infusion. (See Table I, **Dose Preparation.**)

Dosing: ABBOKINASE IS INTENDED FOR INTRAVENOUS INFUSION ONLY.

Administer ABBOKINASE (urokinase for injection) by means of a constant infusion pump that is capable of delivering a total volume of 195 ml. Table I may be used as an aid in the preparation of ABBOKINASE (urokinase for injection) for administration.

A priming dose of 2,000 IU/lb (4,400 IU/kg) of ABBOKINASE is given as the ABBOKINASE-0.9% Sodium Chloride Injection or 5% Dextrose Injection admixture at a rate of 90 ml/hour over a period of 10 minutes. This is followed by a continuous infusion of 2,000 IU/lb/hr (4,400 IU/kg/hr) of ABBOKINASE at a rate of 15 ml/hour for 12 hours. Since some ABBOKINASE admixture will remain in the tubing at the end of an infusion pump delivery cycle, the following flush procedure should be performed to insure that the total dose of ABBOKINASE is administered. A solution of 0.9% Sodium Chloride Injection or 5% Dextrose Injection approximately equal in amount to the volume of the tubing in the infusion set should be administered via the pump to flush the ABBOKINASE admixture from the entire length of the infusion set. The pump should be set to administer the flush solution at the continuous infusion rate of 15 ml/hour.

[See table below].

Anticoagulation After Terminating Urokinase Treatment: At the end of urokinase therapy, treatment with heparin by continuous intravenous infusion is recommended to prevent recurrent thrombosis. Heparin treatment, without a loading dose, should not begin until the thrombin time has decreased to *less than twice* the normal control value (approximately 3 to 4 hours after completion of the infusion). See manufacturer's prescribing information for proper use of heparin. This should then be followed by oral anticoagulants in the conventional manner.

I.V. Catheter Clearance:

Warnings: Excessive pressure should be avoided when ABBOKINASE is injected into the catheter. Such force could cause rupture of the catheter or expulsion of the clot into the circulation.

Precautions: Catheters may be occluded by substances other than blood products, such as drug precipitate. ABBOKINASE is not effective in such a case, and there is the possibility that the precipitate may be forced into the vascular system.

Adverse Reactions: Although there have been no adverse reactions reported as a result of using ABBOKINASE for the removal of clot obstruction from I.V. catheters, the possibility of reactions should nevertheless be considered.

Dosage and Administration:

Preparation: Reconstitute ABBOKINASE (urokinase for injection) by aseptically adding 5.2 ml of Sterile Water for Injection, USP, to the vial. (It is important that ABBOKINASE be reconsituted *only* with Sterile Water for Injection, USP, *without* preservatives. Bacteriostatic Water for Injection should not be used.) Add 1 ml of the reconstituted drug to 9.0 ml Sterile Water for Injection to make a final dilution equivalent to 5,000 IU/ml. One ml of this preparation is to be utilized for each catheter clearing procedure. BECAUSE ABBOKINASE CONTAINS NO PRESERVATIVES, IT SHOULD NOT BE RECONSTITUTED UNTIL IMMEDIATELY BEFORE USING.

Administration: NOTE: When the following procedure is used to clear a central venous catheter, the patient should be instructed to exhale and hold his breath any time the catheter is not connected to I.V. tubing or a syringe. This is to prevent air from entering the open catheter.

Aseptically disconnect the I.V. tubing connection at the catheter hub and attach a 10 ml syringe. Determine occlusion of the catheter by *gently* attempting to aspirate blood from the catheter with the 10 ml syringe. If aspiration is not possible, remove the 10 ml syringe and attach a 1 ml tuberculin syringe filled with prepared ABBOKINASE to the catheter. Slowly and gently inject an amount of ABBOKINASE equal to the volume of the catheter. Aseptically remove the tuberculin syringe and connect a 5 ml syringe to the catheter. Wait at least 5 minutes before attempting to aspirate the drug and residual clot with the 5 ml syringe. Repeat aspiration attempts every 5 minutes. If the catheter is not open within 30 minutes, the catheter may be capped allowing ABBOKINASE to remain in the catheter for 30 to 60 minutes before again attempting to aspirate. A second injection of ABBOKINASE may be necessary in resistant cases.

When patency is restored, aspirate 4 to 5 ml of blood to assure removal of all drug and clot residual. Remove the blood-filled syringe and replace it with a 10 ml syringe filled with 0.9% Sodium Chloride for Injection, USP. The catheter should then be gently irrigated with this solution to assure patency of the catheter. After the catheter has been irrigated, remove the 10 ml syringe and aseptically reconnect sterile I.V. tubing to the catheter hub.

How Supplied: ABBOKINASE (urokinase for injection) is supplied as a sterile lyophilized preparation (**NDC** 0074-6109-05). Each vial contains 250,000 IU urokinase activity, 25 mg mannitol, and 45 mg sodium chloride. Store ABBOKINASE powder at 2°C to 8°C.

TABLE 1
Dose Preparation

Weight (pounds)	Total Dose* Urokinase (I.U.)	Number Vials ABBOKINASE (urokinase for injection)	Volume of ABBOKINASE After Reconstitution (ml)**	+	Volume of Diluent (ml)	=	Final Volume (ml)
81-90	2,250,000	9	45		150		195
91-100	2,500,000	10	50		145		195
101-110	2,750,000	11	55		140		195
111-120	3,000,000	12	60		135		195
121-130	3,250,000	13	65		130		195
131-140	3,500,000	14	70		125		195
141-150	3,750,000	15	75		120		195
151-160	4,000,000	16	80		115		195
161-170	4,250,000	17	85		110		195
171-180	4,500,000	18	90		105		195
181-190	4,750,000	19	95		100		195
191-200	5,000,000	20	100		95		195
201-210	5,250,000	21	105		90		195
211-220	5,500,000	22	110		85		195
221-230	5,750,000	23	115		80		195
231-240	6,000,000	24	120		75		195
241-250	6,250,000	25	125		70		195

	Priming Dose	Dose for 12-Hour Period
Infusion Rate:	15 ml/10 min***	15 ml/hr for 12 hrs

*Priming dose + dose administered during 12-hour period
**After addition of 5.2 ml of Sterile Water for Injection, USP, per vial (See Preparation.)
***Pump rate = 90 ml/hr

References:

1. Sherry, S., *et al:* Thrombolytic Therapy in Thrombosis: A National Institutes of Health Consensus Development Conference. Ann. Intern. Med. *93:*141-144 (1980).
2. Bang, N. U.: Physiology and Biochemistry of Fibrinolysis in *Thrombosis and Bleeding Disorders* (Bang, N. U., Beller, F. K., Deutsch, E., Mammen, E. F., eds.). Academic Press (1971). pp. 292-327.
3. McNicol, G. P.: The Fibrinolytic Enzyme System. Postgrad. Med. J. (August Suppl. 5). *49:*10-12 (1973).
4. Sasahara, A. A., Hyers, T. M., Cole, C. M., *et al.:* The Urokinase Pulmonary Embolism Trial Circulation, (Suppl. II) *47:*1-108 (1973).
5. Urokinase pulmonary embolism trial study group: Urokinase-Streptokinase Embolism Trial. JAMA *229:*1606-1613 (1974).
6. Sasahara, A. A., Bell, W. R., Simon, T. L., Stengle, J. M. and Sherry, S.: The Phase II Urokinase-Streptokinase Pulmonary Embolism Trial. Thrombos. Diathes, Haemorrh. (Stuttg.) *33:*464-476 (1975).
7. Bell, W. R.: Thrombolytic Therapy: A Comparison Between Urokinase and Streptokinase. Sem. Thromb, Hemost, *2:*1-13 (1975).
8. Fratantoni, J. C., Ness, P., Simon, T. L.: Thrombolytic Therapy: Current Status. N. Eng. J. Med., *293:*1073-1078 (1975).
9. Hurtubise, Michel R., M.D., Bottino, Joseph C., M.D., Lawson, Millie, R.N., McCredie, Kenneth B., M.D., Restoring patency of Occluded Central Venous Catheters, Arch. Surg. *115:*212-213 (1980).
10. Glynn, M.F.X., *et al:* Therapy for Thrombotic Occlusion of Long-term Intravenous Alimentation Catheters, Journal of Parenteral and Enteral Nutrition, *4*(4):387-390 (July/Aug. 1980).

Abbott Laboratories
North Chicago, IL 60064
Ref. 01-2230-R4

A-HYDROCORT™ ℞

(hydrocortisone sodium succinate for injection, USP)

For Intravenous or Intramuscular Use

Description: Hydrocortisone sodium succinate, USP, an adrenocortical-like steroid, is the sodium succinate ester of hydrocortisone.

It occurs as a white, or nearly white, odorless hygroscopic amorphous solid. Hydrocortisone sodium succinate is very soluble in water and in alcohol; it is insoluble in chloroform and is very slightly soluble in acetone.

Hydrocortisone sodium succinate is soluble in water and is especially well suited for intravenous use in situations in which high blood levels of hydrocortisone are required rapidly.

A-HYDROCORT (hydrocortisone sodium succinate for injection, USP) is available as:

100 mg Univial®—Each 2 ml (when mixed) contains hydrocortisone sodium succinate equivalent to 100 mg hydrocortisone; also 0.8 mg monobasic sodium phosphate anhydrous; 8.73 mg dibasic sodium phosphate anhydrous; and 18 mg of benzyl alcohol.

250 mg Univial—Each 2 ml (when mixed) contains hydrocortisone sodium succinate equivalent to 250 mg hydrocortisone; also 2 mg monobasic sodium phosphate anhydrous; 21.8 mg dibasic sodium phosphate anhydrous; and 18 mg of benzyl alcohol.

500 mg Univial—Each 4 ml (when mixed) contains hydrocortisone sodium succinate equivalent to 500 mg hydrocortisone; also 4 mg monobasic sodium phosphate anhydrous; 44 mg dibasic sodium phosphate anhydrous; and 36 mg benzyl alcohol.

1000 mg Univial—Each 8 ml (when mixed) contains hydrocortisone sodium succinate equivalent to 1000 mg hydrocortisone; also 8 mg monobasic sodium phosphate anhydrous; 88 mg dibasic sodium phosphate anhydrous; and 72 mg benzyl alcohol.

100 mg Vial with Diluent—Each 2 ml (when mixed) contains hydrocortisone sodium succinate equivalent to 100 mg hydrocortisone; also 0.8 mg monobasic sodium phosphate anhydrous; 8.73 mg dibasic sodium phosphate anhydrous; and 18 mg of benzyl alcohol.

The pH of each formula was adjusted with sodium hydroxide and/or hydrochloric acid.

Important: The solid contents of A-HYDROCORT should not be used with any diluent other than that provided.

Use within 3 days after mixing. Store below 86°F. Protect from light. Avoid freezing. Refrigeration not required.

When reconstituted as directed, the pH of the solutions ranges from 7–8 and the tonicities are: for the 100 mg per ml solution, 0.36 osmolar; for the 250 mg per 2 ml, 500 mg per 4 ml, and 1000 mg per 8 ml solutions, 0.57 osmolar. [Isotonic saline (0.9% Sodium Chloride Injection, USP) = 0.28 osmolar.]

Clinical Pharmacology: Hydrocortisone sodium succinate has potent anti-inflammatory effects. Because it is an adrenocortical-like steroid, hydrocortisone sodium succinate may cause profound and varied metabolic effects in addition to modifying the body's immune response to diverse stimuli.

When given parenterally and in equimolar quantitites, hydrocortisone sodium succinate and hydrocortisone are equivalent in biologic activity.

Following intravenous injection of hydrocortisone sodium succinate, demonstrable effects are evident within one hour and persist for a variable period. Excretion of the administered dose is nearly complete within 12 hours. Thus, if constantly high blood levels are required, injections should be made every four to six hours.

This preparation is also rapidly absorbed when administered intramuscularly and is excreted in a pattern similar to that observed after intravenous injection.

Indications: Sterile A-HYDROCORT (hydrocortisone sodium succinate) is indicated in situations requiring a rapid and intense hormonal effect.

Intravenous administration of A-HYDROCORT is most appropriate for the following indications:

1. **Endocrine disorders:**
   a. Acute adrenocortical insufficiency (hydrocortisone or cortisone is the drug of choice; mineralocorticoid supplementation may be necessary, particularly when synthetic analogs are used).
   b. Preoperatively and in the event of serious trauma or illness, in patients with known adrenal insufficiency or when adrenocortical reserve is doubtful.
   c. Shock unresponsive to conventional therapy if adrenocortical insufficiency exists or is suspected.
2. **Collagen diseases**—During an exacerbation or as maintenance therapy in selected cases of:
   a. Acute rheumatic carditis.
3. **Allergic states**—Control of severe or incapacitating allergic conditions intractable to adequate trials of conventional treatment in:
   a. Bronchial asthma.
   b. Serum sickness.
   c. Drug hypersensitivity reactions.
   d. Urticarial transfusion reactions.
   e. Acute noninfectious laryngeal edema (epinephrine is the drug of first choice).
4. **Hematologic disorders:**
   a. Idiopathic thrombocytopenic purpura in adults (I.M. administration is contraindicated).

Intramuscular administration of A-HYDROCORT is appropriate for the following indications:

1. **Endocrine disorders:**
   a. Primary or secondary adrenocortical insufficiency (hydrocortisone or cortisone is the drug of choice; synthetic analogs may be used in conjunction with mineralocorticoids where applicable; in infancy, mineralocorticoid supplementation is of particular importance).
   b. Acute adrenocortical insufficiency (hydrocortisone or cortisone is the drug of choice; mineralocorticoid supplementation may be necessary, particularly when synthetic analogs are used).
   c. Preoperatively and in the event of serious trauma or illness, in patients with known adrenal insufficiency or when adrenocortical reserve is doubtful.
   d. Shock unresponsive to conventional therapy if adrenocortical insufficiency exists or is suspected.
   e. Congenital adrenal hyperplasia.
   f. Nonsuppurative thyroiditis.
   g. Hypercalcemia associated with cancer.
2. **Rheumatic disorders**—As adjunctive therapy for short-term administration (to tide the patient over an acute episode or exacerbation) in:
   a. Post-traumatic osteoarthritis.
   b. Synovitis of osteoarthritis.
   c. Rheumatoid arthritis, including juvenile rheumatoid arthritis (selected cases may require low-dose maintenance therapy).
   d. Acute and subacute bursitis.
   e. Epicondylitis.
   f. Acute nonspecific tenosynovitis.
   g. Acute gouty arthritis.
   h. Psoriatic arthritis.
   i. Ankylosing spondylitis.
3. **Collagen diseases**—During an exacerbation or as maintenance therapy in selected cases of:
   a. Systemic lupus erythematosus.
   b. Acute rheumatic carditis.
4. **Dermatologic diseases:**
   a. Severe erythema multiforme (Stevens-Johnson syndrome).
   b. Exfoliative dermatitis.
   c. Bullous dermatitis herpetiformis.
   d. Severe seborrheic dermatitis.
   e. Severe psoriasis.
   f. Pemphigus.
   g. Mycosis fungoides.
   h. Systemic dermatomyositis (polymyositis).
5. **Allergic states**—Control of severe or incapacitating allergic conditions intractable to adequate trials of conventional treatment in:
   a. Bronchial asthma.
   b. Contact dermatitis.
   c. Atopic dermatitis.
   d. Serum sickness.
   e. Seasonal or perennial allergic rhinitis.
   f. Drug hypersensitivity reactions.
   g. Urticarial transfusion reactions.
   h. Acute noninfectious laryngeal edema (epinephrine is the drug of first choice).
6. **Ophthalmic diseases**—Severe acute and chronic allergic and inflammatory processes involving the eye, such as:
   a. Herpes zoster ophthalmicus.
   b. Iritis, iridocyclitis.
   c. Chorioretinitis.
   d. Diffuse posterior uveitis and choroiditis.
   e. Optic neuritis.
   f. Sympathetic ophthalmia.
   g. Anterior segment inflammation.
   h. Allergic conjunctivitis.
   i. Allergic corneal marginal ulcers.
7. **Gastrointestinal diseases**—To tide the patient over a critical period of disease in:
   a. Ulcerative colitis—(Systemic therapy).
   b. Regional enteritis—(Systemic therapy).
8. **Respiratory diseases:**
   a. Symptomatic sarcoidosis.
   b. Berylliosis.
   c. Fulminating or disseminated pulmonary tuberculosis when concurrently accompanied by appropriate antituberculous chemotherapy.
   d. Aspiration pneumonitis.
   e. Loeffler's syndrome not manageable by other means.
9. **Hematologic disorders:**
   a. Acquired (autoimmune) hemolytic anemia.
   b. Secondary thrombocytopenia in adults.
   c. Erythroblastopenia (RBC anemia).
   d. Congenital (erythroid) hypoplastic anemia.
10. **Neoplastic diseases**—For palliative management of:
   a. Leukemias and lymphomas in adults.
   b. Acute leukemia of childhood.
11. **Edematous state**—To induce diuresis or remission of proteinuria in the nephrotic syndrome, without uremia, of the idiopathic type or that due to lupus erythematosus.
12. **Nervous system**—Acute exacerbations of multiple sclerosis.
13. **Miscellaneous:**
   a. Tuberculous meningitis with subarachnoid block or impending block

Continued on next page

If desired, additional literature on any Abbott Product will be provided upon request to Abbott Laboratories.

Abbott—Cont.

when used concurrently with appropriate antituberculous chemotherapy.

b. Trichinosis with neurologic or myocardial involvement.

Contraindications: Systemic fungal infections.

Warnings: In patients on corticosteroid therapy subjected to any unusual stress, increased dosage of rapidly acting corticosteroids before, during, and after the stressful situation is indicated.

Corticosteroids may mask some signs of infection, and new infections may appear during their use. There may be decreased resistance and inability to localize infection when corticosteroids are used.

Prolonged use of corticosteroids may produce posterior subcapsular cataracts, glaucoma with possible damage to the optic nerves, and may enhance the establishment of secondary ocular infections due to fungi or viruses.

Average and large doses of cortisone or hydrocortisone can cause elevation of blood pressure, salt and water retention, and increased excretion of potassium. These effects are less likely to occur with the synthetic derivatives except when used in large doses. Dietary salt restriction and potassium supplementation may be necessary. All corticosteroids increase calcium excretion.

While on corticosteroid therapy patients should not be vaccinated against smallpox. Other immunization procedures should not be undertaken in patients who are on corticosteroids, especially on high dose, because of possible hazards of neurological complications and a lack of antibody response.

The use of A-HYDROCORT (hydrocortisone sodium succinate) in active tuberculosis should be restricted to those cases of fulminating or disseminated tuberculosis in which the corticosteroid is used for the management of the disease in conjunction with appropriate antituberculous regimen.

If corticosteroids are indicated in patients with latent tuberculosis or tuberculin reactivity, close observation is necessary as reactivation of the disease may occur. During prolonged corticosteroid therapy, these patients should receive chemoprophylaxis.

Because rare instances of anaphylactoid reactions have occurred in patients receiving parenteral corticosteroid therapy, appropriate precautionary measures should be taken prior to administration, especially when the patient has a history of allergy to any drug.

Usage in Pregnancy: Since adequate human reproduction studies have not been done with corticosteroids, the use of these drugs in pregnancy, nursing mothers, or women of childbearing potential requires that the possible benefits of the drug be weighed against the potential hazards to the mother and embryo or fetus. Infants born of mothers who have received substantial doses of corticosteroids during pregnancy should be carefully observed for signs of hypoadrenalism.

Precautions: Drug-induced secondary adrenocortical insufficiency may be minimized by gradual reduction of dosage. This type of relative insufficiency may persist for months after discontinuation of therapy; therefore, in any situation of stress occurring during that period, hormone therapy should be reinstituted. Since mineralocorticoid secretion may be impaired, salt and/or a mineralocorticoid should be administered concurrently.

There is an enhanced effect of corticosteroids on patients with hypothyroidism and in those with cirrhosis.

Corticosteroids should be used cautiously in patients with ocular herpes simplex because of possible corneal perforation.

The lowest possible dose of corticosteroid should be used to control the condition under treatment, and when reduction in dosage is possible, the reduction should be gradual.

Psychic derangements may appear when corticosteroids are used, ranging from euphoria, insomnia, mood swings, personality changes and severe depression, to frank psychotic manifestations. Also, existing emotional instability or psychotic tendencies may be aggravated by corticosteroids.

Aspirin should be used cautiously in conjunction with corticosteroids in hypoprothrombinemia.

Steroids should be used with caution in nonspecific ulcerative colitis, if there is a probability of impending perforation, abscess or other pyogenic infection; diverticulitis; fresh intestinal anastomoses; active or latent peptic ulcer; renal insufficiency; hypertension; osteoporosis; and myasthenia gravis.

Growth and development of infants and children on prolonged corticosteroid therapy should be carefully observed.

Although controlled clinical trials have shown corticosteroids to be effective in speeding the resolution of acute exacerbations of multiple sclerosis they do not show that they affect the ultimate outcome or natural history of the disease. The studies do show that relatively high doses of corticosteroids are necessary to demonstrate a significant effect. (See "Dosage and Administration" section).

Since complications of treatment with glucocorticoids are dependent on the size of the dose and the duration of treatment a risk/benefit decision must be made in each individual case as to dose and duration of treatment and as to whether daily or intermittent therapy should be used.

Adverse Reactions:

Fluid and Electrolyte Disturbances

Sodium retention
Fluid retention
Congestive heart failure in susceptible patients
Potassium loss
Hypokalemic alkalosis
Hypertension

Musculoskeletal

Muscle weakness
Steroid myopathy
Loss of muscle mass
Osteoporosis
Vertebral compression fractures
Aseptic necrosis of femoral and humeral heads
Pathologic fracture of long bones

Gastrointestinal

Peptic ulcer with possible perforation and hemorrhage
Pancreatitis
Abdominal distention
Ulcerative esophagitis

Dermatologic

Impaired wound healing
Thin fragile skin
Petechiae and ecchymoses
Facial erythema
Increased sweating
May suppress reactions to skin tests

Neurological

Increased intracranial pressure with papilledema (pseudo-tumor cerebri) usually after treatment
Convulsions
Vertigo
Headache

Endocrine

Development of Cushingoid state
Suppression of growth in children
Secondary adrenocortical and pituitary unresponsiveness, particularly in times of stress, as in trauma, surgery or illness
Menstrual irregularities
Decreased carbohydrate tolerance
Manifestations of latent diabetes mellitus
Increased requirements for insulin or oral hypoglycemic agents in diabetics

Ophthalmic

Posterior subcapsular cataracts
Increased intraocular pressure
Glaucoma
Exophthalmos

Metabolic

Negative nitrogen balance due to protein catabolism

The following additional adverse reactions are related to parenteral corticosteroid therapy:

Hyperpigmentation or hypopigmentation
Subcutaneous and cutaneous atrophy
Sterile abscess

Dosage and Administration: This preparation may be administered by intravenous injection, by intravenous infusion, or by intramuscular injection, the preferred method for initial emergency use being intravenous injection. Following the initial emergency period, consideration should be given to employing a longer acting injectable preparation or an oral preparation.

Therapy is initiated by administering hydrocortisone sodium succinate intravenously over a period of 30 seconds (e.g., 100 mg) to 10 minutes (e.g., 500 mg or more). In general, high dose corticosteroid therapy should be continued only until the patient's condition has stabilized—usually not beyond 48 to 72 hours. Although adverse effects associated with high dose, short-term corticoid therapy are uncommon, peptic ulceration may occur. Prophylactic antacid therapy may be indicated.

When high dose hydrocortisone therapy must be continued beyond 48 to 72 hours, hypernatremia may occur. Under such circumstances it may be desirable to replace hydrocortisone sodium succinate with a corticoid which causes little or no sodium retention.

The initial dose of hydrocortisone sodium succinate is 100 mg to 500 mg depending upon the severity of the condition. This dose may be repeated at intervals of 2, 4 or 6 hours as indicated by the patient's response and clinical condition. While the dose may be reduced for infants and children, it is governed more by the severity of the condition and response of the patient than by age or body weight but should not be less than 25 mg daily. Patients subjected to severe stress following corticosteroid therapy should be observed closely for signs and symptoms of adrenocortical insufficiency.

Corticoid therapy is an adjunct to, and not a replacement for, conventional therapy.

Multiple Sclerosis:

In the treatment of acute exacerbations of multiple sclerosis, daily doses of 200 mg of prednisolone for a week followed by 80 mg every other day for one month have been shown to be effective (20 mg of hydrocortisone is equivalent to 5 mg of prednisolone).

Preparation of Solutions:

Univial:

1. Remove protective cap, give the plunger-stopper a quarter turn and press to force diluent into lower compartment.
2. Gently agitate to effect solution. Use solution within 72 hours.
3. Sterilize top of plunger-stopper with a suitable germicide.
4. Insert needle squarely through center of plunger-stopper until tip is just visible. Invert vial and withdraw dose.

100 mg/2 ml Combination Package:

Prepare solution by aseptically adding 2 ml of Bacteriostatic Water for Injection to the vial.

Further dilution is not necessary for intravenous or intramuscular injection.

For Intravenous Infusion:

Prepare solution as described above. The 100 mg solution may then be added to 100 to 1000 ml (but not less than 100 ml) of 5% Dextrose Injection (or 0.9% Sodium Chloride Injection or 5% Dextrose and 0.9% Sodium Chloride Injection if patient is not on sodium restriction). The 250 mg solution may be added to 250 to 1000 ml (but not less than 250 ml), the 500 mg solution may be added to 500 to 1000 ml (but not less than 500 ml) and the 1000 mg solution to not less than 1000 ml of the same diluents.

How Supplied: Sterile A-HYDROCORT (hydrocortisone sodium succinate for injection, USP) is available in the following packages:

100 mg/2 ml Univial **NDC** 0074-5671-02;
250 mg/2 ml Univial **NDC** 0074-5672-02;
500 mg/4 ml Univial **NDC** 0074-5673-04;
1000 mg/8 ml Univial **NDC** 0074-5674-08;
100 mg/2 ml Combination Package **NDC** 0074-5676-02.

Abbott Laboratories
North Chicago, IL 60064
Ref. 01-2248-R6

A–METHAPRED® ℞

(methylprednisolone sodium succinate for injection, USP)
For Intravenous or Intramuscular Use

Description: Methylprednisolone sodium succinate, USP, an adrenocortical-like steroid, is the sodium succinate ester of methylprednisolone.

It occurs as a white, or nearly white, odorless hygroscopic, amorphous solid.

Methylprednisolone sodium succinate is extremely soluble in water and is especially well suited for intravenous use in situations in which high blood levels of methylprednisolone are required rapidly.

A-METHAPRED (methylprednisolone sodium succinate for injection, USP) is available as:

40 mg Univial®—Each 1 ml (when mixed) contains methylprednisolone sodium succinate equivalent to 40 mg methylprednisolone; also 1.6 mg monobasic sodium phosphate anhydrous; 17.46 mg dibasic sodium phosphate anhydrous; 25 mg lactose anhydrous; and 9 mg of benzyl alcohol.

125 mg Univial—Each 2 ml (when mixed) contains methylprednisolone sodium succinate equivalent to 125 mg methylprednisolone; also 1.6 mg monobasic sodium phosphate anhydrous; 17.4 mg dibasic sodium phosphate anhydrous; and 18 mg of benzyl alcohol.

500 mg Vial with Diluent—Each 8 ml (when mixed) contains methylprednisolone sodium succinate equivalent to 500 mg methylprednisolone; also 6.4 mg monobasic sodium phosphate anhydrous; 69.6 mg dibasic sodium phosphate anhydrous; and 72 mg of benzyl alcohol.

1000 mg Vial with Diluent—16 ml (when mixed) contains methylprednisolone sodium succinate equivalent to 1000 mg methylprednisolone; also 12.8 mg monobasic sodium biphosphate anhydrous; 139.2 mg dibasic sodium phosphate anhydrous; and 144 mg of benzyl alcohol.

The pH of each formula was adjusted with sodium hydroxide and/or hydrochloric acid.

Important: The solid contents of A-METHAPRED should not be used with any diluent other than that provided. **Use within 48 hours after mixing.**

When reconstituted as directed, the pH of the solutions ranges from 7–8 and the tonicities are, for the 40 mg per ml solution, 0.50 osmolar; for the 125 mg per 2 ml, 500 mg per 8 ml and 1000 mg per 16 ml solutions, 0.40 osmolar. [Isotonic saline (0.9% Sodium Chloride Injection) = 0.28 osmolar].

Clinical Pharmacology: Methylprednisolone sodium succinate is a potent anti-inflammatory steroid. It has a greater anti-inflammatory potency than prednisolone and even less tendency than prednisolone to induce sodium and water retention. Like the adrenocortical steroids, methylprednisolone sodium succinate may cause profound and varied metabolic effects in addition to modifying the body's immune response to diverse stimuli.

When given parenterally and in equimolar quantities, methylprednisolone sodium succinate and methylprednisolone are equivalent in biologic activity.

The relative potency of methylprednisolone sodium succinate and hydrocortisone sodium succinate, as indicated by depression of eosinophil count, following intravenous administration, is at least four to one. This is in good agreement with the relative oral potency of methylprednisolone and hydrocortisone.

Indications: When oral therapy is not feasible, and the strength, dosage form and route of administration of the drug reasonably lend the preparation to the treatment of the condition, A-METHAPRED (methylprednisolone sodium succinate) is indicated for intravenous or intramuscular use in the following conditions:

1. **Endocrine disorders:**
   a. Primary or secondary adrenocortical insufficiency (hydrocortisone or cortisone is the drug of choice, synthetic analogs may be used in conjunction with mineralocorticoids where applicable; in infancy, mineralocorticoid supplementation is of particular importance).
   b. Acute adrenocortical insufficiency (hydrocortisone or cortisone is the drug of choice; mineralocorticoid supplementation may be necessary, particularly when synthetic analogs are used).
   c. Preoperatively and in the event of serious trauma or illness, in patients with known adrenal insufficiency or when adrenocortical reserve is doubtful.
   d. Shock unresponsive to conventional therapy if adrenocortical insufficiency exists or is suspected.
   e. Congenital adrenal hyperplasia.
   f. Hypercalcemia associated with cancer.
   g. Nonsuppurative thyroiditis.
2. **Rheumatic disorders**—As adjunctive therapy for short-term administration (to tide the patient over an acute episode or exacerbation) in:
   a. Post- traumatic osteoarthritis.
   b. Synovitis of osteoarthritis.
   c. Rheumatoid arthritis, including juvenile rheumatoid arthritis (selected cases may require low-dose maintenance therapy).
   d. Acute and subacute bursitis.
   e. Epicondylitis.
   f. Acute nonspecific tenosynovitis.
   g. Acute gouty arthritis.
   h. Psoriatic arthritis.
   i. Ankylosing spondylitis.
3. **Collagen diseases** — During an exacerbation or as maintenance therapy in selected cases of:
   a. Systemic lupus erythematosus.
   b. Acute rheumatic carditis.
   c. Systemic dermatomyositis (polymyositis).
4. **Dermatologic diseases:**
   a. Severe erythema multiforme (Stevens-Johnson syndrome).
   b. Exfoliative dermatitis.
   c. Bullous dermatitis herpetiformis.
   d. Severe seborrheic dermatitis.
   e. Severe psoriasis.
   f. Pemphigus.
   g. Mycosis fungoides.
5. **Allergic states** — Control of severe or incapacitating allergic conditions intractable to adequate trials of conventional treatment in:
   a. Bronchial asthma.
   b. Contact dermatitis.
   c. Atopic dermatitis.
   d. Serum sickness.
   e. Seasonal or perennial allergic rhinitis.
   f. Drug hypersensitivity reactions.
   g. Urticarial transfusion reactions.
   h. Acute noninfectious laryngeal edema (epinephrine is the drug of first choice).
6. **Ophthalmic diseases** — Severe acute and chronic allergic and inflammatory processes involving the eye, such as:
   a. Herpes zoster ophthalmicus.
   b. Iritis, iridocyclitis.
   c. Chorioretinitis.
   d. Diffuse posterior uveitis and choroiditis.
   e. Optic neuritis.
   f. Sympathetic ophthalmia.
   g. Anterior segment inflammation.
   h. Allergic conjunctivitis.
   i. Allergic corneal marginal ulcers.
   j. Keratitis.
7. **Gastrointestinal diseases** — To tide the patient over a critical period of disease in:
   a. Ulcerative colitis — (Systemic therapy).
   b. Regional enteritis — (Systemic therapy).
8. **Respiratory diseases:**
   a. Symptomatic sarcoidosis.
   b. Berylliosis.
   c. Fulminating or disseminated pulmonary tuberculosis when concurrently accompanied by appropriate antituberculous chemotherapy.
   d. Aspiration pneumonitis.
   e. Loeffler's syndrome not manageable by other means.
9. **Hematologic disorders:**
   a. Acquired (autoimmune) hemolytic anemia.
   b. Idiopathic thrombocytopenic purpura in adults (IV only; IM administration is contraindicated).
   c. Secondary thrombocytopenia in adults.
   d. Erythroblastopenia (RBC anemia).
   e. Congenital (erythroid) hypoplastic anemia.
10. **Neoplastic diseases** — For palliative management of:
    a. Leukemias and lymphomas in adults.
    b. Acute leukemia of childhood.
11. **Edematous state** — To induce diuresis or remission of proteinuria in the nephrotic syndrome, without uremia, of the idiopathic type or that due to lupus erythematosus.
12. **Nervous System:**
    a. Acute exacerbations of multiple sclerosis.
13. **Miscellaneous:**
    a. Tuberculous meningitis with subarachnoid block or impending block when used concurrently with appropriate antituberculous chemotherapy.
    b. Trichinosis with neurologic or myocardial involvement.

Contraindications: Systemic fungal infections.

Warnings: In patients on corticosteroid therapy subjected to any unusual stress, increased dosage of rapidly acting corticosteroids before, during, and after the stressful situation is indicated.

Corticosteroids may mask some signs of infection, and new infections may appear during their use. There may be decreased resistance and inability to localize infection when corticosteroids are used.

Prolonged use of corticosteroids may produce posterior subcapsular cataracts, glaucoma with possible damage to the optic nerves, and may enhance the establishment of secondary ocular infections due to fungi or viruses.

Average and large doses of cortisone or hydrocortisone can cause elevation of blood pressure, salt and water retention, and increased excretion of potassium. These effects are less likely to occur with the synthetic derivatives except when used in large doses. Dietary salt restriction and potassium supplementation may be

Continued on next page

If desired, additional literature on any Abbott Product will be provided upon request to Abbott Laboratories.

Abbott—Cont.

necessary. All corticosteroids increase calcium excretion.

While on corticosteroid therapy patients should not be vaccinated against smallpox. Other immunization procedures should not be undertaken in patients who are on corticosteroids, especially on high dose, because of possible hazards of neurological complications and a lack of antibody response.

The use of A-METHAPRED (methylprednisolone sodium succinate) in active tuberculosis should be restricted to those cases of fulminating or disseminated tuberculosis in which the corticosteroid is used for the management of the disease in conjunction with appropriate antituberculous regimen.

If corticosteroids are indicated in patients with latent tuberculosis or tuberculin reactivity, close observation is necessary as reactivation of the disease may occur. During prolonged corticosteroid therapy, these patients should receive chemoprophylaxis.

Because rare instances of anaphylactoid reactions have occurred in patients receiving parenteral corticosteroid therapy, appropriate precautionary measures should be taken prior to administration, especially when the patient has a history of allergy to any drug.

There are reports of cardiac arrhythmias and/or circulatory collapse and/or cardiac arrest following the rapid administration of large IV doses of methylprednisolone sodium succinate (greater than 0.5 gram administered over a period of less than 10 minutes).

Usage in Pregnancy: Since adequate human reproduction studies have not been done with corticosteroids, the use of these drugs in pregnancy, nursing mothers, or women of childbearing potential requires that the possible benefits of the drug be weighed against the potential hazards to the mother and embryo or fetus. Infants born of mothers who have received substantial doses of corticosteroids during pregnancy should be carefully observed for signs of hypoadrenalism.

Precautions: Drug-induced secondary adrenocortical insufficiency may be minimized by gradual reduction of dosage. This type of relative insufficiency may persist for months after discontinuation of therapy; therefore, in any situation of stress occurring during that period, hormone therapy should be reinstituted. Since mineralocorticoid secretion may be impaired, salt and/or a mineralocorticoid should be administered concurrently.

There is an enhanced effect of corticosteroids on patients with hypothyroidism and in those with cirrhosis.

Corticosteroids should be used cautiously in patients with ocular herpes simplex because of possible corneal perforation.

The lowest possible dose of corticosteroid should be used to control the condition under treatment, and when reduction in dosage is possible, the reduction should be gradual.

Psychic derangements may appear when corticosteroids are used, ranging from euphoria, insomnia, mood swings, personality changes and severe depression, to frank psychotic manifestations. Also, existing emotional instability or psychotic tendencies may be aggravated by corticosteroids.

Aspirin should be used cautiously in conjunction with corticosteroids in hypoprothrombinemia.

Steroids should be used with caution in nonspecific ulcerative colitis, if there is a probability of impending perforation, abscess or other pyogenic infection; diverticulitis; fresh intestinal anastomoses; active or latent peptic ulcer; renal insufficiency; hypertension; osteoporosis, and myasthenia gravis.

Growth and development of infants and children on prolonged corticosteroid therapy should be carefully observed.

Although controlled clinical trials have shown corticosteroids to be effective in speeding the resolution of acute exacerbations of multiple sclerosis, they do not show that corticosteroids affect the ultimate outcome or natural history of the disease. The studies do show that relatively high doses of corticosteroids are necessary to demonstrate a significant effect. (See "Dosage and Administration" section).

Since complications of treatment with glucocorticoids are dependent on the size of the dose and the duration of treatment, a risk/benefit decision must be made in each individual case as to dose and duration of treatment and as to whether daily or intermittent therapy should be used.

Adverse Reactions:

Fluid and Electrolyte Disturbances

- Sodium retention
- Fluid retention
- Congestive heart failure in susceptible patients
- Potassium loss
- Hypokalemic alkalosis
- Hypertension

Musculoskeletal

- Muscle weakness
- Steroid myopathy
- Loss of muscle mass
- Severe arthralgia
- Osteoporosis
- Vertebral compression fractures
- Aseptic necrosis of femoral and humeral heads
- Pathologic fracture of long bones

Gastrointestinal

- Peptic ulcer with possible perforation and hemorrhage
- Pancreatitis
- Abdominal distention
- Ulcerative esophagitis

Dermatologic

- Impaired wound healing
- Thin fragile skin
- Petechiae and ecchymoses
- Facial erythema
- Increased sweating
- May suppress reactions to skin tests

Neurological

- Increased intracranial pressure with papilledema (pseudo-tumor cerebri) usually after treatment
- Convulsions
- Vertigo
- Headache

Endocrine

- Development of Cushingoid state
- Suppression of growth in children
- Secondary adrenocortical and pituitary unresponsiveness particularly in times of stress, as in trauma, surgery or illness
- Menstrual irregularities
- Decreased carbohydrate tolerance
- Manifestations of latent diabetes mellitus
- Increased requirements for insulin or oral hypoglycemic agents in diabetics

Ophthalmic

- Posterior subcapsular cataracts
- Increased intraocular pressure
- Glaucoma
- Exophthalmos

Metabolic

- Negative nitrogen balance due to protein catabolism

The following additional adverse reactions are related to parenteral corticosteroid therapy:

- Hyperpigmentation or hypopigmentation
- Subcutaneous and cutaneous atrophy
- Sterile abscess
- Anaphylactic reaction with or without circulatory collapse, cardiac arrest, bronchospasm
- Urticaria
- Nausea and vomiting
- Cardiac arrhythmias, hypotension or hypertension

Dosage and Administration: When high dose therapy is desired, the recommended dose of methylprednisolone as the sodium succinate is 30 mg/kg administered intravenously over a 10 to 20-minute period. This dose may be repeated every 4 to 6 hours.

In general, high dose corticosteroid therapy should be continued only until the patient's condition has stabilized, usually not beyond 48 to 72 hours.

Although adverse effects associated with high dose short-term corticoid therapy are uncommon, peptic ulceration may occur. Prophylactic antacid therapy may be indicated.

In other indications initial dosage will vary from 10 to 40 mg of methylprednisolone depending on the clinical problem being treated. The larger doses may be required for short-term management of severe, acute conditions. The initial dose usually should be given intravenously over a period of one to several minutes. Subsequent doses may be given intravenously or intramuscularly at intervals dictated by the patient's response and clinical condition. Corticoid therapy is an adjunct to, and not replacement for conventional therapy.

Dosage may be reduced for infants and children but should be governed more by the severity of the condition and response of the patient than by age or size. It should not be less than 0.5 mg/kg every 24 hours.

Dosage must be decreased or discontinued gradually when the drug has been administered for more than a few days. If a period of spontaneous remission occurs in a chronic condition, treatment should be discontinued. Routine laboratory studies, such as urinalysis, two-hour postprandial blood sugar, determination of blood pressure and body weight, and a chest X-ray should be made at regular intervals during prolonged therapy. Upper GI X-rays are desirable in patients with an ulcer history or significant dyspepsia.

Methylprednisolone may be administered intravenously by direct push, or by intermittent or continuous infusion; or by intramuscular injection. The preferred method for initial emergency use is either direct I.V. push or intermittent infusion. To administer by intravenous (or intramuscular) injection, prepare solution as directed. The desired dose may be administered intravenously over a period of one to several minutes (for doses of 40 mg or less).

Multiple Sclerosis: In treatment of acute exacerbations of multiple sclerosis, daily doses of 200 mg of prednisolone for a week followed by 80 mg every other day for 1 month have been shown to be effective (4 mg of methylprednisolone is equivalent to 5 mg of prednisolone).

Preparation of Solutions:

Univial:

1. Remove protective cap, give the plunger-stopper a quarter turn and press to force diluent into the lower compartment.
2. Gently agitate to effect solution. Use solution within 48 hours.
3. Sterilize top of plunger-stopper with a suitable germicide.
4. Insert needle squarely through center of plunger-stopper until tip is just visible. Invert vial and withdraw dose.

500 mg (vial) with Bacteriostatic Water for Injection:

Prepare solution by aseptically adding 8 ml of Bacteriostatic Water for Injection to the vial.

1000 mg (vial) with Bacteriostatic Water for Injection:

Prepare solution by aseptically adding 16 ml of Bacteriostatic Water for Injection to the vial.

For Intravenous Infusion:

To prepare solutions for intravenous infusion, first prepare the solution for injection as directed. This solution may then be added to indicated amounts of 5% Dextrose Injection, 0.9% Sodium Chloride Injection, USP or 5% Dex-

trose and 0.9% Sodium Chloride Injection, USP.
Storage: After mixing, store solution below 86°F; avoid freezing. Refrigeration not required. Use within 48 hours.
How Supplied: Sterile A-METHAPRED (methylprednisolone sodium succinate for injection, USP) is available in the following packages:
40 mg/ml Univial **NDC** 0074-5684-01;
125 mg/2 ml Univial **NDC** 0074-5685-02;
500 mg/8 ml Combination Package **NDC** 0074-5687-08;
1000 mg/16 ml Combination Package **NDC** 0074-5689-16.
Store unreconstituted products below 86°F. Protect from light and avoid freezing.
Abbott Laboratories
North Chicago, IL 60064

A-POXIDE® ℞ Ⓒ
(chlordiazepoxide hydrochloride capsules, USP)

How Supplied: A-POXIDE capsules are supplied in three dosage strengths:
5 mg capsules (yellow and green) in bottles of 500 (**NDC** 0074-2648-53).
10 mg capsules (green and evergreen) in bottles of 500 (**NDC** 0074-2649-53).
25 mg capsules (light and dark green) in bottles of 100 (**NDC** 0074-2650-13).
[*Shown in Product Identification Section*]
Abbott Pharmaceuticals, Inc.
North Chicago, IL 60064

BUTESIN® PICRATE Ointment
(butambem picrate)

Description: Butesin Picrate is an anesthetic ointment containing Butesin Picrate (Butamben Picrate), 1%.
Indication: For temporary relief of pain due to minor burns.
Warning: Certain persons, due to idiosyncrasy, are sensitive to this ointment and may develop a rash following its application. In such cases its use should be discontinued, and the ointment remaining on the skin removed with soap and water.
Precautions: Should not be applied repeatedly or to large areas except under a physician's instructions. As Butesin Picrate stains cannot be removed from animal fibers, contact with silk or wool fabrics and hair should be avoided.
Dosage and Administration: Spread thinly on painful or denuded lesions of the skin, if these are small. Apply a loose bandage to protect the clothing.
How Supplied: 1 oz tube (**NDC** 0074-4392-01).
Abbott Laboratories
North Chicago, IL 60064
Ref. 09-5413-2/R4

CALCIDRINE® SYRUP ℞ Ⓒ

Description: Calcidrine is an oral antitussive, expectorant syrup. Each 5 ml (teaspoonful) contains Codeine, USP, 8.4 mg, (Warning—May be habit forming); Calcium Iodide, anhydrous 152 mg, in a palatable syrup. Alcohol 6%.
The chemical formula for calcium iodide is CaI_2. Codeine is methylmorphine, a natural alkaloid of opium. The chemical formula for codeine is $C_{18}H_{21}NO_3 \cdot H_2O$.
Clinical Pharmacology: The major effects of codeine in man are on the central nervous system. The antitussive effect is produced by depression of the cough reflex. Codeine is rapidly absorbed from the gastrointestinal tract and is metabolized in the liver.
Iodides are readily absorbed from the gastrointestinal tract and are distributed to extracellular fluid as well as gastric and salivary secretions. Iodides are accumulated by the thyroid gland. Excretion occurs mainly through the kidneys.
Indications and Usage: In adults and children as an expectorant, and for symptomatic relief of coughs.
Contraindications: Calcidrine should not be used in patients with a history of iodism, or with known hypersensitivity to iodides or codeine. Long-term use of iodide-containing preparations is contraindicated during pregnancy.
Warnings: Physiological dependence may develop with the use of codeine.
Usage During Pregnancy: Calcidrine Syrup can cause fetal harm when administered to a pregnant woman. Maternal ingestion of large amounts of iodides during pregnancy has been associated with development of fetal goiter and resultant acute respiratory distress of the neonate. If this drug is used during pregnancy, or if the patient becomes pregnant while taking this drug, the patient should be apprised of the potential hazard to the fetus.
Severe and occasionally fatal skin eruptions have been reported rarely in patients receiving prolonged administration of iodides.
Precautions: *Laboratory Tests:* Patients who must receive prolonged iodide therapy should be evaluated periodically for possible depression of thyroid function.
Drug Interactions: The concurrent administration of calcium iodide and lithium carbonate may enhance the hypothyroid and goitrogenic effects of either drug.
Laboratory Test Interactions: Elevated values may be obtained on thyroid function tests or protein-bound iodine tests when iodide-containing compounds have been ingested. False positive results may be obtained if iodides have been ingested prior to guaiac or benzidine testing.
Carcinogenesis: No data is available on long-term carcinogenicity in animals or humans.
Pregnancy: Pregnancy Category D. See "WARNINGS" section.
Nursing Mothers: Iodine is excreted in breast milk. Caution should be exercised when Calcidrine is administered to a nursing woman.
Adverse Reactions: In decreasing order of severity: severe and sometimes fatal skin eruptions (ioderma) occur rarely after the prolonged use of iodides. Iodism can occur. Symptoms of iodism include metallic taste, acneform skin lesions, mucous membrane irritation, salivary gland swelling, and gastric distress. These side effects subside quickly upon discontinuance of the iodide-containing drug.
Codeine may produce vomiting, nausea, and constipation.
Overdosage: Symptoms of acute codeine poisoning include respiratory and central nervous system depression, pinpoint pupils and coma. Blood pressure and body temperature may fall.
Acute iodide poisoning is associated with gastrointestinal irritation. Angioedema with laryngeal swelling may develop. Shock may also occur.
Treatment for overdose of Calcidrine is:
a. Establish a patent airway and ventilate if needed. b. Gastric evacuation. c. Treatment for shock. d. General supportive measures including replacement of fluids and electrolytes may be indicated. e. The use of naloxone to antagonize the narcotic depression of the central nervous system should be considered.
Dosage and Administration: Adults and children over ten years of age, usual dose, 1 to 2 teaspoonfuls every 4 hours. Children 6 to 10 years of age, ½ to 1 teaspoonful every 4 hours. Children 2 to 6 years of age, ½ teaspoonful every 4 hours.
How Supplied: Orange-colored syrup with a pleasant apricot-menthol flavor in 4 fl oz (**NDC** 0074-5763-04), pint (**NDC** 0074-5763-16), and gallon (**NDC** 0074-5763-11) bottles.
Calcidrine must be dispensed in USP tight, light-resistant glass containers.
Abbott Laboratories
North Chicago, IL 60064
Ref. 02-6039-2/R5

CEFOL® Filmtab® Tablets ℞
(B-Complex, folic acid, vitamin E with 750 mg vitamin C)

Description: Each oral Cefol Filmtab vitamin tablet provides:

Ascorbic Acid (C) (as sodium ascorbate)	750 mg
Niacinamide	100 mg
Calcium Pantothenate	20 mg
Thiamine Mononitrate (B_1)	15 mg
Riboflavin (B_2)	10 mg
Pyridoxine Hydrochloride (B_6)	5 mg
Folic Acid	500 mcg
Cyanocobalamin (B_{12})	6 mcg
Vitamin E (as dl-alpha tocopheryl acetate)	30 IU

Clinical Pharmacology: The vitamin components of Cefol are absorbed by the active transport process. All but Vitamin E are rapidly eliminated and not stored in the body. Vitamin E is stored in body tissues.
Indications and Usage: Cefol is indicated in non-pregnant* adults for the treatment of Vitamin C deficiency states with an associated deficient intake or increased need for Vitamin B-Complex, Folic Acid, and Vitamin E.
*Pregnancy may require greater Folic Acid intake.
Contraindications: Rare hypersensitivity to Folic Acid.
Warnings: Folic Acid alone is improper treatment of pernicious anemia and other megaloblastic anemias where Vitamin B_{12} is deficient.
Precautions: Folic Acid above 0.1 mg daily may obscure pernicious anemia (hematologic remission may occur while neurological manifestations remain progressive).
Adverse Reactions: Allergic sensitization has been reported following oral and parenteral administration of Folic Acid.
Dosage: Usual adult dose is one tablet daily.
How Supplied: Cefol is supplied as green Filmtab tablets in bottles of 100 (NDC 0074-6089-13).
Filmtab—Film-sealed tablets, Abbott.
[*Shown in Product Identification Section*]
Abbott Pharmaceuticals, Inc.
North Chicago, IL 60064
Ref. 03-0936-8/R10

CHLORTHALIDONE Tablets, USP ℞

How Supplied: Abbott Chlorthalidone Tablets, USP are available as scored tablets in two dosage strengths:
25 mg, peach-colored:
Bottles of 100 (**NDC** 0074-4325-13).
50 mg, lavender-colored:
Bottles of 100 (**NDC** 0074-4338-13).
Bottles of 500 (**NDC** 0074-4338-53).
[*Shown in Product Identification Section*]

CLEAR EYES® OTC
Eye Drops

Description: Clear Eyes® is a sterile isotonic buffered solution containing naphazoline hydrochloride 0.012%, boric acid, sodium borate, and water. Edetate Disodium 0.1% and benzalkonium chloride 0.01% are added as preservatives.
Indications: Clear Eyes is a decongestant ophthalmic solution specially designed to soothe as it removes redness from irritated eyes. Clear Eyes contains laboratory tested,

Continued on next page

If desired, additional literature on any Abbott Product will be provided upon request to Abbott Laboratories.

Abbott—Cont.

and scientifically blended ingredients including an effective vasoconstrictor which narrows swollen blood vessels and rapidly whitens reddened eyes in a formulation which produces a refreshing, soothing effect. Clear Eyes is a sterile, isotonic solution compatible with the natural fluids of the eye.

Warning: Clear Eyes should only be used for minor eye irritations. If relief is not obtained within 48 hours, or if irritation persists or increases discontinue use and consult your physician.

Clear Eyes should not be used by individuals with glaucoma and serious eye diseases. In some instances redness or inflammation may be due to serious eye conditions such as acute iritis, acute glaucoma, or corneal trauma. When redness, pain, or blurring persist, a physician should be consulted at once.

Dosage and Administration: One or two drops in eye(s) two or three times daily or as directed by physician. Do not touch bottle tip to any surface, since this may contaminate the solution. Remove contact lenses before using. Keep container tightly closed. Keep this and all other medicines out of reach of children.

How Supplied: In 0.5 fl. oz. and 1.5 fl. oz. plastic dropper bottle.

CYLERT® Tablets ℞ Ⓒ
(pemoline)

Description: CYLERT (pemoline) is a central nervous system stimulant. Pemoline is structurally dissimilar to the amphetamines and methylphenidate.

It is an oxazolidine compound and is chemically identified as 2-amino-5-phenyl-2-oxazolin-4-one.

Pemoline is a white, tasteless, odorless powder, relatively insoluble (less than 1 mg/ml) in water, chloroform, ether, acetone, and benzene; its solubility in 95% ethyl alcohol is 2.2 mg/ml. CYLERT (pemoline) is supplied as tablets for oral administration.

Clinical Pharmacology: CYLERT (pemoline) has a pharmacological activity similar to that of other known central nervous system stimulants; however, it has minimal sympathomimetic effects. Although studies indicate that pemoline may act in animals through dopaminergic mechanisms, the exact mechanism and site of action of the drug in man is not known. There is neither specific evidence which clearly establishes the mechanism whereby CYLERT produces its mental and behavioral effects in children, nor conclusive evidence regarding how these effects relate to the condition of the central nervous system.

The serum half-life of pemoline is approximately 12 hours. Peak serum levels of the drug occur within 2 to 4 hours after ingestion of a single dose. Multiple dose studies in adults at several dose levels indicate that steady state is reached in approximately 2 to 3 days.

Metabolites of pemoline include pemoline conjugate, pemoline dione, mandelic acid, and unidentified polar compounds. CYLERT is excreted primarily by the kidneys; approximately 75% of an oral dose is recovered in the urine within 24 hours. Approximately 43% of pemoline is excreted unchanged.

CYLERT (pemoline) has a gradual onset of action. Using the recommended schedule of dosage titration, significant clinical benefit may not be evident until the third or fourth week of drug administration.

Indications: CYLERT is indicated as an integral part of a total treatment program which typically includes other remedial measures (psychological, educational, social) for a stabilizing effect in children with a behavioral syndrome characterized by the following group of developmentally inappropriate symptoms: moderate to severe distractibility, short attention span, hyperactivity, emotional lability, and impulsivity. The diagnosis of this syndrome should not be made with finality when these symptoms are only of comparatively recent origin. Nonlocalizing (soft) neurological signs, learning disability, and abnormal EEG may or may not be present, and a diagnosis of central nervous system dysfunction may or may not be warranted.

Attention Deficit Disorder and Hyperkinetic Syndrome are among the terms being used to describe the above signs and symptoms. In the past, a variety of terms has been associated with these signs and symptoms, including: Minimal Brain Dysfunction, Hyperkinetic Reaction of Childhood, Hyperkinetic Syndrome, Hyperactive Child Syndrome, Minimal Brain Damage, Minimal Cerebral Dysfunction, and Minor Cerebral Dysfunction.

Contraindications: CYLERT (pemoline) is contraindicated in patients with known hypersensitivity or idiosyncrasy to the drug. (See ADVERSE REACTIONS.)

Warnings: CYLERT is not recommended for children less than 6 years of age since its safety and efficacy in this age group have not been established.

Clinical experience suggests that in psychotic children, administration of CYLERT may exacerbate symptoms of behavior disturbance and thought disorder.

Data are inadequate to determine whether chronic administration of CYLERT may be associated with growth inhibition; therefore, growth should be monitored during treatment.

Precautions: Drug treatment is not indicated in all cases of the behavioral syndrome characterized by moderate to severe distractibility, short attention span, hyperactivity, emotional lability and impulsivity. It should be considered only in light of the complete history and evaluation of the child. The decision to prescribe CYLERT should depend on the physician's assessment of the chronicity and severity of the child's symptoms and their appropriateness for his/her age. Prescription should not depend solely on the presence of one or more of the behavioral characteristics.

When these symptoms are associated with acute stress reactions, treatment with CYLERT is usually not indicated.

Long-term effects of CYLERT in children have not been well established.

Liver function tests should be performed prior to and periodically during therapy with CYLERT. The drug should be discontinued if abnormalities are revealed and confirmed by follow-up tests. (See ADVERSE REACTIONS regarding reports of abnormal liver function tests and jaundice.)

CYLERT should be administered with caution to patients with significantly impaired hepatic or renal function.

The interaction of CYLERT with other drugs has not been studied in humans. Patients who are receiving CYLERT concurrently with other drugs, especially drugs with CNS activity, should be monitored carefully.

CYLERT failed to demonstrate a potential for self-administration in primates. However, the pharmacologic similarity of pemoline to other psychostimulants with known dependence liability suggests that psychological and/or physical dependence might also occur with CYLERT. There have been isolated reports of transient psychotic symptoms occurring in adults following the long-term misuse of excessive oral doses of pemoline. CYLERT should be given with caution to emotionally unstable patients who may increase the dosage on their own initiative.

Usage during Pregnancy and Lactation: The safety of CYLERT (pemoline) for use during pregnancy and lactation has not been established. Studies in rats have shown an increased incidence of stillbirths and cannibalization when pemoline was administered at a dose of 37.5 mg/kg/day. Postnatal survival of offspring was reduced at doses of 18.75 and 37.5 mg/kg/day.

Adverse Reactions: Insomnia is the most frequently reported side effect of CYLERT; it usually occurs early in therapy, prior to an optimum therapeutic response. In the majority of cases it is transient in nature or responds to a reduction in dosage.

Anorexia with weight loss may occur during the first weeks of therapy. In the majority of cases it is transient in nature; weight gain usually resumes within three to six months.

Stomach ache, skin rashes, increased irritability, mild depression, nausea, dizziness, headache, drowsiness, and hallucinations have been reported.

Elevations of SGOT, SGPT, and serum LDH have occurred in patients taking CYLERT, usually after several months of therapy. These effects appear to be reversible upon withdrawal of the drug, and are thought to be manifestations of a delayed hypersensitivity reaction. There have also been a few reports of jaundice occurring in patients taking CYLERT; a causal relationship between the drug and this clinical finding has not been established.

The following CNS effects have been reported with the use of CYLERT: dyskinetic movements of the tongue, lips, face and extremities, nystagmus and nystagmoid eye movements, and convulsive seizures. A definite causal relationship between CYLERT and these reactions has not been established.

Mild adverse reactions appearing early during the course of treatment with CYLERT often remit with continuing therapy. If adverse reactions are of a significant or protracted nature, dosage should be reduced or the drug discontinued.

Overdosage: Signs and symptoms of acute CYLERT overdosage may include agitation, restlessness, hallucinations, dyskinetic movements and tachycardia. The treatment for an acute overdosage of pemoline is essentially the same as that for an overdosage of any CNS stimulant. Management is primarily symptomatic and may include induction of emesis or gastric lavage, sedation, and other appropriate supportive measures.

Results of studies in dogs indicate that extracorporeal hemodialysis may be useful in the management of CYLERT overdosage; forced diuresis and peritoneal dialysis appear to be of little value.

Dosage and Administration: CYLERT (pemoline) is administered as a single oral dose each morning. The recommended starting dose is 37.5 mg/day. This daily dose should be gradually increased by 18.75 mg at one week intervals until the desired clinical response is obtained. The effective daily dose for most patients will range from 56.25 to 75 mg. The maximum recommended daily dose of pemoline is 112.5 mg.

Clinical improvement with CYLERT is gradual. Using the recommended schedule of dosage titration, significant benefit may not be evident until the third or fourth week of drug administration.

Where possible, drug administration should be interrupted occasionally to determine if there is a recurrence of behavioral symptoms sufficient to require continued therapy.

How Supplied: CYLERT (pemoline) is supplied as monogrammed, grooved tablets in three dosage strengths:

18.75 mg tablets (white) in bottles of 100 (**NDC** 0074-6025-13)

37.5 mg tablets (orange-colored) in bottles of 100 (**NDC** 0074-6057-13)

75 mg tablets (tan-colored) in bottles of 100 (**NDC** 0074-6073-13)

CYLERT Chewable is supplied as monogrammed, grooved tablets in one dosage strength:

37.5 mg tablets (orange-colored) in bottles of 100 (**NDC** 0074-6088-13)

[*Shown in Product Identification Section*]
Abbott Pharmaceuticals, Inc.
North Chicago, IL 60064
Ref. 03-4196/R3

DAYALETS® Filmtab®
Multivitamin Supplement for adults and children 4 or more years of age
DAYALETS® PLUS IRON Filmtab®
Multivitamin Supplement with Iron for adults and children 4 or more years of age

Description: Dayalets provide 100% of the recommended daily allowances of essential vitamins. Dayalets Plus Iron provides 100% of the recommended daily allowances of essential vitamins plus the mineral iron.
Daily dosage (one Dayalets tablet) provides:

VITAMINS			% U.S. RDA
Vitamin A	(1.5 mg)	5000 IU	100%
Vitamin D	(10 mcg)	400 IU	100%
Vitamin E		30 IU	100%
Vitamin C		60 mg	100%
Folic Acid		0.4 mg	100%
Thiamine (Vitamin B_1)		1.5 mg	100%
Riboflavin (Vitamin B_2)		1.7 mg	100%
Niacin		20 mg	100%
Vitamin B_6		2 mg	100%
Vitamin B_{12}		6 mcg	100%

Ingredients: Ascorbic acid, cellulose, dl-alpha tocopheryl acetate, niacinamide, pyridoxine hydrochloride, riboflavin, thiamine hydrochloride, vitamin A acetate, vitamin A palmitate, folic acid, ergocalciferol, and cyanocobalamin in a film-coated tablet with vanillin flavoring and artificial coloring added.
Each Dayalets Plus Iron Filmtab® represents all the vitamins in the Dayalets formula in the same concentrations, plus the mineral iron 18 mg (100% U.S. R.D.A.), as ferrous sulfate. Dayalets Plus Iron contain the same ingredients as Dayalets plus the ingredient povidone.
These products contain no sugar and essentially no calories.
Indications: Dietary supplement and supplement with iron for adults and children 4 or more years of age.
Administration and Dosage: One Filmtab tablet daily.
How Supplied: In bottles of 100 tablets.
® Filmtab—Film-sealed tablets, Abbott.
Abbott Laboratories
North Chicago, IL 60064
Ref. 02-6004-6/R3, 02-5323-6/R5

DEPAKENE® Capsules and Syrup ℞
(Valproic Acid)

Warning: HEPATIC FAILURE RESULTING IN FATALITIES HAS OCCURRED IN PATIENTS RECEIVING DEPAKENE. THESE INCIDENTS USUALLY HAVE OCCURRED DURING THE FIRST SIX MONTHS OF TREATMENT WITH DEPAKENE. SERIOUS OR FATAL HEPATOTOXICITY MAY BE PRECEDED BY NONSPECIFIC SYMPTOMS SUCH AS LOSS OF SEIZURE CONTROL, MALAISE, WEAKNESS, LETHARGY, ANOREXIA AND VOMITING. LIVER FUNCTION TESTS SHOULD BE PERFORMED PRIOR TO THERAPY AND AT FREQUENT INTERVALS THEREAFTER, ESPECIALLY DURING THE FIRST SIX MONTHS.

Description: DEPAKENE (valproic acid) is a carboxylic acid designated as 2-propylpentanoic acid. It is also known as dipropylacetic acid.
Valproic acid (pKa 4.8) has a molecular weight of 144 and occurs as a colorless liquid with a characteristic odor. It is slightly soluble in water (1.3 mg/ml) and very soluble in organic solvents.
DEPAKENE is supplied as soft elastic capsules and syrup for oral administration. Each capsule contains 250 mg valproic acid. The syrup contains the equivalent of 250 mg valproic acid per 5 ml as the sodium salt.
Clinical Pharmacology: DEPAKENE is an antiepileptic agent which is chemically unrelated to other drugs used to treat seizure disorders. It has no nitrogen or aromatic moiety characteristic of other antiepileptic drugs. The mechanism by which DEPAKENE exerts its antiepileptic effects has not been established. It has been suggested that its activity is related to increased brain levels of gamma-aminobutyric acid (GABA). The effect on the neuronal membrane is unknown.
DEPAKENE is rapidly absorbed after oral administration. Peak serum levels of valproic acid occur approximately one to four hours after a single oral dose of DEPAKENE. The serum half-life ($t_{0.5,\beta}$) of the parent compound is typically in the range of six to sixteen hours. Half-lives in the lower part of the above range are usually found in patients taking other antiepileptic drugs. A slight delay in absorption occurs when the drug is administered with meals but this does not affect the total absorption.
Valproic acid is rapidly distributed and at therapeutic drug concentrations, drug is highly bound (90%) to human plasma proteins. Increases in dose may result in decreases in the extent of protein binding and variable changes in valproate clearance and elimination.
Elimination of DEPAKENE and its metabolites occurs principally in the urine, with minor amounts in the feces and expired air. Very little unmetabolized parent drug is excreted in the urine. The drug is primarily metabolized in the liver and is excreted as the glucuronide conjugate. Other metabolites in the urine are products of beta omega-1, and omega oxidation (C-3, C-4, and C-5 positions). The major oxidative metabolite in the urine is 2-propyl-3-ketopentanoic acid; minor metabolites are 2-propyl-glutaric acid, 2-propyl-5-hydroxypentanoic acid, 2-propyl-3-hydroxypentanoic acid and 2-propyl-4-hydroxypentanoic acid.
Indications: DEPAKENE (valproic acid) is indicated for use as sole and adjunctive therapy in the treatment of simple (petit mal) and complex absence seizures. DEPAKENE may also be used adjunctively in patients with multiple seizure types which include absence seizures.
In accordance with the International Classification of Seizures, simple absence is defined as very brief clouding of the sensorium or loss of consciousness (lasting usually 2–15 seconds), accompanied by certain generalized epileptic discharges without other detectable clinical signs. Complex absence is the term used when other signs are also present.
SEE "WARNINGS" SECTION FOR STATEMENT REGARDING FATAL HEPATIC DYSFUNCTION.
Contraindications: DEPAKENE (valproic acid) should not be administered to patients with hepatic disease or significant dysfunction.
DEPAKENE is contraindicated in patients with known hypersensitivity to the drug.
Warnings: Hepatic failure resulting in fatalities has occurred in patients receiving DEPAKENE. These incidents usually have occurred during the first six months of treatment with DEPAKENE. Serious or fatal hepatotoxicity may be preceded by non-specific symptoms such as loss of seizure control, malaise, weakness, lethargy, anorexia and vomiting. Liver function tests should be performed prior to therapy and at frequent intervals thereafter, especially during the first six months. However, physicians should not rely totally on serum biochemistry since these tests may not be abnormal in all instances, but should also consider the results of careful interim medical history and physical examination. Caution should be observed when administering DEPAKENE to patients with a prior history of hepatic disease. Patients with various unusual congenital disorders, those with severe seizure disorders accompanied by mental retardation, and those with organic brain disease may be at particular risk.
The drug should be discontinued immediately in the presence of significant hepatic dysfunction, suspected or apparent. In some cases, hepatic dysfunction has progressed in spite of discontinuation of drug. The frequency of adverse effects (particularly elevated liver enzymes) may be dose-related. The benefit of improved seizure control which may accompany the higher doses should therefore be weighed against the possibility of a greater incidence of adverse effects.
Usage in Pregnancy: THE EFFECTS OF DEPAKENE IN HUMAN PREGNANCY ARE UNKNOWN. ANIMAL STUDIES HAVE DEMONSTRATED TERATOGENICITY.
Studies in rats and human females demonstrated placental transfer of the drug. Doses greater than 65 mg/kg/day given to pregnant rats and mice produced skeletal abnormalities in the offspring, primarily involving ribs and vertebrae; doses greater than 150 mg/kg/day given to pregnant rabbits produced fetal resorptions and (primarily) soft-tissue abnormalities in the offspring. In rats a dose-related delay in the onset of parturition was noted. Postnatal growth and survival of the progeny were adversely affected, particularly when drug administration spanned the entire gestation and early lactation period.
THERE ARE MULTIPLE REPORTS IN THE CLINICAL LITERATURE WHICH INDICATE THAT THE USE OF ANTIEPILEPTIC DRUGS DURING PREGNANCY RESULTS IN AN INCREASED INCIDENCE OF BIRTH DEFECTS IN THE OFFSPRING. ALTHOUGH DATA ARE MORE EXTENSIVE WITH RESPECT TO TRIMETHADIONE, PARAMETHADIONE, PHENYTOIN, AND PHENOBARBITAL, REPORTS INDICATE A POSSIBLE SIMILAR ASSOCIATION WITH THE USE OF OTHER ANTIEPILEPTIC DRUGS. THEREFORE, ANTIEPILEPTIC DRUGS SHOULD BE ADMINISTERED TO WOMEN OF CHILDBEARING POTENTIAL ONLY IF THEY ARE CLEARLY SHOWN TO BE ESSENTIAL IN THE MANAGEMENT OF THEIR SEIZURES.
Antiepileptic drugs should not be discontinued in patients in whom the drug is administered to prevent major seizures because of the strong possibility of precipitating status epilepticus with attendant hypoxia and threat to life. In individual cases where the severity and frequency of the seizure disorder are such that the removal of medication does not pose a serious threat to the patient, discontinuation of the drug may be considered prior to and during pregnancy, although it cannot be said with any confidence that even minor seizures do not pose some hazard to the developing embryo or fetus.
The prescribing physician will wish to weigh these considerations in treating or counseling epileptic women of childbearing potential.
Precautions:
Hepatic dysfunction: See "Contraindications" and "Warnings" sections.
General: Because of reports of thrombocytopenia and inhibition of the secondary phase of platelet aggregation, platelet counts and bleeding time determination are recommended before initiating therapy and at periodic intervals. It is recommended that patients receiving DEPAKENE be monitored for platelet count prior to planned surgery. Clinical evidence of hemorrhage, bruising or a disorder of hemostasis/

Continued on next page

If desired, additional literature on any Abbott Product will be provided upon request to Abbott Laboratories.

Abbott—Cont.

coagulation is an indication for reduction of DEPAKENE dosage or withdrawal of therapy pending investigation.

Hyperammonemia with or without lethargy or coma has been reported and may be present in the absence of abnormal liver function tests. If elevation occurs, DEPAKENE should be discontinued.

Since DEPAKENE (valproic acid) may interact with concurrently administered antiepileptic drugs, periodic serum level determinations of concomitant antiepileptic drugs are recommended during the early course of therapy. (See "Drug Interactions" section.)

DEPAKENE is partially eliminated in the urine as a keto-metabolite which may lead to a false interpretation of the urine ketone test.

Information For Patients: Since DEPAKENE may produce CNS depression, especially when combined with another CNS depressant (e.g., alcohol), patients should be advised not to engage in hazardous occupations, such as driving an automobile or operating dangerous machinery, until it is known that they do not become drowsy from the drug.

Drug Interactions: DEPAKENE may potentiate the CNS depressant activity of alcohol.

THERE IS EVIDENCE THAT DEPAKENE CAN CAUSE AN INCREASE IN SERUM PHENOBARBITAL LEVELS BY IMPAIRMENT OF NONRENAL CLEARANCE. THIS PHENOMENON CAN RESULT IN SEVERE CNS DEPRESSION. THE COMBINATION OF DEPAKENE AND PHENOBARBITAL HAS ALSO BEEN REPORTED TO PRODUCE CNS DEPRESSION WITHOUT SIGNIFICANT ELEVATIONS OF BARBITURATE OR VALPROATE SERUM LEVELS. ALL PATIENTS RECEIVING CONCOMITANT BARBITURATE THERAPY SHOULD BE CLOSELY MONITORED FOR NEUROLOGICAL TOXICITY. SERUM BARBITURATE LEVELS SHOULD BE OBTAINED, IF POSSIBLE, AND THE BARBITURATE DOSAGE DECREASED, IF APPROPRIATE.

Primidone is metabolized into a barbiturate and, therefore, may also be involved in a similar or identical interaction.

THERE HAVE BEEN REPORTS OF BREAKTHROUGH SEIZURES OCCURRING WITH THE COMBINATION OF DEPAKENE AND PHENYTOIN. MOST REPORTS HAVE NOTED A DECREASE IN TOTAL PLASMA PHENYTOIN CONCENTRATION. HOWEVER, INCREASES IN TOTAL PHENYTOIN SERUM CONCENTRATION HAVE BEEN REPORTED. AN INITIAL FALL IN TOTAL PHENYTOIN LEVELS WITH SUBSEQUENT INCREASE IN PHENYTOIN LEVELS HAS ALSO BEEN REPORTED. IN ADDITION, A DECREASE IN TOTAL SERUM PHENYTOIN WITH AN INCREASE IN THE FREE VS. PROTEIN BOUND PHENYTOIN LEVELS HAS BEEN REPORTED. THE DOSAGE OF PHENYTOIN SHOULD BE ADJUSTED AS REQUIRED BY THE CLINICAL SITUATION.

THE CONCOMITANT USE OF VALPROIC ACID AND CLONAZEPAM MAY PRODUCE ABSENCE STATUS.

Caution is recommended when DEPAKENE (valproic acid) is administered with drugs affecting coagulation, e.g., aspirin and warfarin. (See "Adverse Reactions" section.)

There have been reports of altered thyroid function tests associated with DEPAKENE. The clinical significance of these is unknown.

Carcinogenesis: DEPAKENE was administered to Sprague Dawley rats and ICR (HA/ICR) mice at doses of 0, 80 and 170 mg/kg/day for two years. Although a variety of neoplasms were observed in both species, the chief findings were a statistically significant increase in the incidence of subcutaneous fibrosarcomas in high dose male rats receiving DEPAKENE and a statistically significant dose-related trend for benign pulmonary adenomas in male mice receiving DEPAKENE. The actual incidence of fibrosarcomas in male rats was low with only two low dose and five high dose animals being affected. The presence of these tumors is not considered to be drug-related or of biological significance for the following reasons: (1) the overall low incidence, (2) the published variable incidence of spontaneously occurring fibrosarcomas and pulmonary adenomas in rats and mice respectively, (3) the long latency period of the neoplasms and (4) the fact that statistical significance of tumor incidence was present in males only. The significance of these findings for man is unknown at present.

Mutagenesis: Studies on DEPAKENE have been performed using bacterial and mammalian systems. These studies have provided no evidence of a mutagenic potential for DEPAKENE.

Fertility: Chronic toxicity studies in juvenile and adult rats and dogs demonstrated reduced spermatogenesis and testicular atrophy at doses greater than 200 mg/kg/day in rats and greater than 90 mg/kg/day in dogs. Segment I fertility studies in rats have shown doses up to 350 mg/kg/day for 60 days to have no effect on fertility. THE EFFECT OF DEPAKENE (VALPROIC ACID) ON THE DEVELOPMENT OF THE TESTES AND ON SPERM PRODUCTION AND FERTILITY IN HUMANS IS UNKNOWN.

Pregnancy: See "WARNINGS" section.

Nursing Mothers: DEPAKENE is excreted in breast milk. Concentrations in breast milk have been reported to be 1-10% of serum concentrations. It is not known what effect this would have on a nursing infant. Caution should be exercised when DEPAKENE is administered to a nursing woman.

Adverse Reactions: Since DEPAKENE (valproic acid) has usually been used with other antiepileptic drugs, it is not possible, in most cases, to determine whether the following adverse reactions can be ascribed to DEPAKENE alone, or the combination of drugs.

Gastrointestinal: The most commonly reported side effects at the initiation of therapy are nausea, vomiting and indigestion. These effects are usually transient and rarely require discontinuation of therapy. Diarrhea, abdominal cramps and constipation have been reported. Both anorexia with some weight loss and increased appetite with weight gain have also been reported.

CNS Effects: Sedative effects have been noted in patients receiving valproic acid alone but are found most often in patients receiving combination therapy. Sedation usually disappears upon reduction of other antiepileptic medication. Ataxia, headache, nystagmus, diplopia, asterixis, "spots before eyes", tremor, dysarthria, dizziness, and incoordination have rarely been noted. Rare cases of coma have been noted in patients receiving valproic acid alone or in conjunction with phenobarbital.

Dermatologic: Transient increases in hair loss have been observed. Skin rash and petechiae have rarely been noted.

Psychiatric: Emotional upset, depression, psychosis, aggression, hyperactivity and behavioral deterioration have been reported.

Musculoskeletal: Weakness has been reported.

Hematopoietic: Thrombocytopenia has been reported. Valproic acid inhibits the secondary phase of platelet aggregation. (See "Drug Interactions" section.) This may be reflected in altered bleeding time. Bruising, hematoma formation and frank hemorrhage have been reported. Relative lymphocytosis and hypofibrinogenemia have been noted. Leukopenia and eosinophilia have also been reported. Anemia and bone marrow suppression have been reported.

Hepatic: Minor elevations of transaminases (e.g., SGOT and SGPT) and LDH are frequent and appear to be dose related. Occasionally, laboratory test results include, as well, increases in serum bilirubin and abnormal changes in other liver function tests. These results may reflect potentially serious hepatoxicity. (See "Warnings" section.)

Endocrine: There have been reports of irregular menses and secondary amenorrhea occurring in patients receiving DEPAKENE.

Abnormal thyroid function tests have been reported. (see "Precautions" section.)

Pancreatic: There have been reports of acute pancreatitis occurring in patients receiving DEPAKENE.

Metabolic: Hyperammonemia. (See "Precautions" section.)

Hyperglycinemia has been reported and has been associated with a fatal outcome in a patient with preexistent nonketotic hyperglycinemia.

Overdosage: Overdosage with valproic acid may result in deep coma.

Since DEPAKENE is absorbed very rapidly, the value of gastric evacuation will vary with the time since ingestion. General supportive measures should be applied with particular attention being given to the maintenance of adequate urinary output.

Naloxone has been reported to reverse the CNS depressant effects of DEPAKENE overdosage. Because naloxone could theoretically also reverse the antiepileptic effects of DEPAKENE it should be used with caution.

Dosage and Administration: DEPAKENE (valproic acid) is administered orally. The recommended initial dose is 15 mg/kg/day, increasing at one week intervals by 5 to 10 mg/kg/day, until seizures are controlled or side effects preclude further increases. The maximum recommended dosage is 60 mg/kg/day. If the total daily dose exceeds 250 mg, it should be given in a divided regimen.

The following table is a guide for the initial daily dose of DEPAKENE (valproic acid) (15 mg/kg/day):

(See table left)

Recommended Initial Dosages for DEPAKENE

Weight (kg)	Weight (lb)	Total Daily Dose (mg)	Number of Capsules or Teaspoonfuls of Syrup: Dose 1	Dose 2	Dose 3
10—24.9	22— 54.9	250	0	0	1
25—39.9	55— 87.9	500	1	0	1
40—59.9	88—131.9	750	1	1	1
60—74.9	132—164.9	1,000	1	1	2
75—89.9	165—197.9	1,250	2	1	2

The frequency of adverse effects (particularly elevated liver enzymes) may be dose-related. The benefit of improved seizure control which may accompany the higher doses should therefore be weighed against the possibility of a greater incidence of adverse reactions.

A good correlation has not been established between daily dose, serum level and therapeutic effect, however, therapeutic serum levels for most patients will range from 50 to 100 mcg/ml. Occasional patients may be controlled with serum levels lower or higher than this range.

As the DEPAKENE dosage is titrated upward, blood levels of phenobarbital and/or phenytoin may be affected. (See "Precautions" section.)

Patients who experience G.I. irritation may benefit from administration of the drug with food or by slowly building up the dose from an initial low level.

THE CAPSULES SHOULD BE SWALLOWED WITHOUT CHEWING TO AVOID LOCAL IRRITATION OF THE MOUTH AND THROAT.

How Supplied: DEPAKENE (valproic acid) is available as orange-colored soft gelatin capsules of 250 mg valproic acid in bottles of 100 capsules (**NDC** 0074-5681-13), in ABBO-PAC® unit dose packages of 100 capsules (**NDC** 0074-5681-11), and as a red syrup containing the equivalent of 250 mg valproic acid per 5 ml as the sodium salt in bottles of 16 ounces (**NDC** 0074-5682-16).

[*Shown in Product Identification Section*]

Abbott Laboratories
North Chicago, IL 60064
Ref. 01-2213-R9

DESOXYN® ℞ ©
(methamphetamine hydrochloride)
Tablets—Gradumet® Tablets

METHAMPHETAMINE HAS A HIGH POTENTIAL FOR ABUSE. IT SHOULD THUS BE TRIED ONLY IN WEIGHT REDUCTION PROGRAMS FOR PATIENTS IN WHOM ALTERNATIVE THERAPY HAS BEEN INEFFECTIVE. ADMINISTRATION OF METHAMPHETAMINE FOR PROLONGED PERIODS OF TIME IN OBESITY MAY LEAD TO DRUG DEPENDENCE AND MUST BE AVOIDED. PARTICULAR ATTENTION SHOULD BE PAID TO THE POSSIBILITY OF SUBJECTS OBTAINING METHAMPHETAMINE FOR NON-THERAPEUTIC USE OR DISTRIBUTION TO OTHERS, AND THE DRUG SHOULD BE PRESCRIBED OR DISPENSED SPARINGLY.

Description: DESOXYN (methamphetamine hydrochloride), previously known as *d*-desoxyephedrine, is a member of the amphetamine group of sympathomimetic amines.

DESOXYN is available as Gradumet tablets and as conventional tablets. The Gradumet is an inert, porous, plastic matrix, which is impregnated with DESOXYN. The drug is leached slowly from the Gradumet as it passes through the gastrointestinal tract. The expended matrix is not absorbed and is excreted in the stool.

Actions: DESOXYN is a sympathomimetic amine with CNS stimulant activity. Peripheral actions include elevation of systolic and diastolic blood pressures and weak bronchodilator and respiratory stimulant action. Drugs of this class used in obesity are commonly known as "anorectics" or "anorexigenics." It has not been established, however, that the action of such drugs in treating obesity is primarily one of appetite suppression. Other central nervous system actions, or metabolic effects, may be involved, for example.

Adult obese subjects instructed in dietary management and treated with "anorectic" drugs, lose more weight on the average than those treated with placebo and diet, as determined in relatively short-term clinical trials.

The magnitude of increased weight loss of drug-treated patients over placebo-treated patients is only a fraction of a pound a week. The rate of weight loss is greatest in the first weeks of therapy for both drug and placebo subjects and tends to decrease in succeeding weeks. The origins of the increased weight loss due to the various possible drug effects are not established. The amount of weight loss associated with the use of an "anorectic" drug varies from trial to trial, and the increased weight loss appears to be related in part to variables other than the drug prescribed, such as the physician-investigator, the population treated, and the diet prescribed. Studies do not permit conclusions as to the relative importance of the drug and non-drug factors on weight loss.

The natural history of obesity is measured in years, whereas the studies cited are restricted to a few weeks duration; thus, the total impact of drug-induced weight loss over that of diet alone must be considered clinically limited.

There is neither specific evidence which clearly establishes the mechanism whereby DESOXYN produces its mental and behavioral effects in children, nor conclusive evidence regarding how these effects relate to the condition of the central nervous system.

Indications: *Exogenous Obesity*—as a short-term (i.e., a few weeks) adjunct in a regimen of weight reduction based on caloric restriction, for patients in whom obesity is refractory to alternative therapy, e.g., repeated diets, group programs, and other drugs. The limited usefulness of DESOXYN (see ACTIONS) should be weighed against possible risks inherent in use of the drug, such as those described below.

DESOXYN is indicated as an integral part of a total treatment program which typically includes other remedial measures (psychological, educational, social) for a stabilizing effect in children over 6 years of age with a behavioral syndrome characterized by the following group of developmentally inappropriate symptoms: moderate to severe distractibility, short attention span, hyperactivity, emotional lability, and impulsivity. The diagnosis of this syndrome should not be made with finality when these symptoms are only of comparatively recent origin. Nonlocalizing (soft) neurological signs, learning disability, and abnormal EEG may or may not be present, and a diagnosis of central nervous system dysfunction may or may not be warranted.

Attention Deficit Disorder and Hyperkinetic Syndrome are among the terms being used to describe the above signs and symptoms. In the past, a variety of terms has been associated with these signs and symptoms, including: Minimal Brain Dysfunction, Hyperkinetic Reaction of Childhood, Hyperkinetic Syndrome, Hyperactive Child Syndrome, Minimal Brain Damage, Minimal Cerebral Dysfunction, and Minor Cerebral Dysfunction.

Contraindications: DESOXYN (methamphetamine hydrochloride) is contraindicated during or within 14 days following the administration of monoamine oxidase inhibitors; hypertensive crises may result. It is also contraindicated in patients with glaucoma, advanced arteriosclerosis, symptomatic cardiovascular disease, moderate to severe hypertension, hyperthyroidism or known hypersensitivity or idiosyncrasy to sympathomimetic amines. Methamphetamine should not be given to patients who are in an agitated state or who have a history of drug abuse.

Warnings: Tolerance to the anorectic effect usually develops within a few weeks. When this occurs, the recommended dose should not be exceeded in an attempt to increase the effect; rather, the drug should be discontinued. Methamphetamine may impair the ability of the patient to engage in potentially hazardous activities such as operating machinery or driving a motor vehicle; the patient should therefore be cautioned accordingly.

Drug Dependence—DESOXYN has been extensively abused. Tolerance, extreme psychological dependence, and severe social disability have occurred. There are reports of patients who have increased the dosage to many times that recommended. Abrupt cessation following prolonged high dosage administration results in extreme fatigue and mental depression; changes are also noted on the sleep EEG. Manifestations of chronic intoxication with DESOXYN include severe dermatoses, marked insomnia, irritability, hyperactivity, and personality changes. The most severe manifestation of chronic intoxication is psychosis, often clinically indistinguishable from schizophrenia.

Usage in Pregnancy—Safe use in pregnancy has not been established. Reproduction studies in mammals at high multiples of the human dose have suggested both an embryotoxic and a teratogenic potential. Use of methamphetamine by women who are or who may become pregnant, and especially those in the first trimester of pregnancy, requires that the potential benefit be weighed against the possible hazard to mother and infant.

Usage in Children—Methamphetamine is not recommended for use as an anorectic agent in children under 12 years of age.

Clinical experience suggests that in psychotic children, administration of DESOXYN may exacerbate symptoms of behavior disturbance and thought disorder.

Data are inadequate to determine whether chronic administration of DESOXYN may be associated with growth inhibition: therefore, growth should be monitored during treatment.

Precautions: DESOXYN (methamphetamine hydrochloride) should be used with caution in patients with even mild hypertension.

Methamphetamine should not be used to combat fatigue or to replace rest in normal persons.

Insulin requirements in diabetes mellitus may be altered in association with the use of methamphetamine and the concomitant dietary regimen.

Methamphetamine may decrease the hypotensive effect of guanethidine.

Prescribing and dispensing of methamphetamine should be limited to the smallest amount that is feasible at one time in order to minimize the possibility of overdosage.

Drug treatment is not indicated in all cases of the behavioral syndrome characterized by moderate to severe distractibility, short attention span, hyperactivity, emotional lability and impulsivity. It should be considered only in light of the complete history and evaluation of the child. The decision to prescribe DESOXYN should depend on the physician's assessment of the chronicity and severity of the child's symptoms and their appropriateness for his/her age. Prescription should not depend solely on the presence of one or more of the behavioral characteristics.

When these symptoms are associated with acute stress reactions, treatment with DESOXYN is usually not indicated.

Long-term effects of DESOXYN in children have not been well established.

The 15 mg dosage strength of DESOXYN Gradumet contains FD&C Yellow No. 5 (tartrazine) which may cause allergic-type reactions (including bronchial asthma) in certain susceptible individuals. Although the overall incidence of FD&C Yellow No. 5 (tartrazine) sensitivity in the general population is low, it is frequently seen in patients who also have aspirin hypersensitivity.

Adverse Reactions: Cardiovascular—Palpitation, tachycardia, elevation of blood pressure.

Central Nervous System—Overstimulation, restlessness, dizziness, insomnia, euphoria, dysphoria, tremor, headache; rarely, psychotic episodes at recommended doses.

Gastrointestinal—Dryness of mouth, unpleasant taste, diarrhea, constipation, and other gastrointestinal disturbances.

Continued on next page

If desired, additional literature on any Abbott Product will be provided upon request to Abbott Laboratories.

Abbott—Cont.

Allergic—Urticaria.
Endocrine—Impotence, changes in libido.

Dosage and Administration: DESOXYN (methamphetamine hydrochloride) is given orally.

Methamphetamine should be administered at the lowest effective dosage, and dosage should be individually adjusted. Late evening medication should be avoided because of the resulting insomnia.

For obesity: one Gradumet tablet, 10 or 15 mg, once a day in the morning. When the conventional tablet form is prescribed, 2.5 or 5 mg should be taken one-half hour before each meal. Treatment should not exceed a few weeks in duration. Methamphetamine is not recommended for use as an anorectic agent in children under 12 years of age.

For treatment of children with a behavioral syndrome characterized by moderate to severe distractibility, short attention span, hyperactivity, emotional lability and impulsivity: an initial dose of 2.5 to 5 mg DESOXYN (methamphetamine hydrochloride) once or twice a day is recommended. Daily dosage may be raised in increments of 5 mg at weekly intervals until an optimum clinical response is achieved. The usual effective dose is 20 to 25 mg daily. The total daily dose may be given as conventional tablets in two divided doses daily or once daily using the Gradumet tablet. The Gradumet form should not be utilized for initiation of dosage nor until the conventional titrated daily dosage is equal to or greater than the dosage provided in a Gradumet tablet.

Where possible, drug administration should be interrupted occasionally to determine if there is a recurrence of behavioral symptoms sufficient to require continued therapy.

Overdosage: Manifestations of acute overdosage with methamphetamine include restlessness, tremor, hyperreflexia, rapid respiration, confusion, assaultiveness, hallucinations, and panic states. Fatigue and depression usually follow the central stimulation. Cardiovascular effects include arrhythmias, hypertension or hypotension, and circulatory collapse. Gastrointestinal symptoms include nausea, vomiting, diarrhea, and abdominal cramps. Fatal poisoning usually terminates in convulsions and coma.

Management of acute methamphetamine intoxication is largely symptomatic and includes lavage and sedation with a barbiturate. Experience with hemodialysis or peritoneal dialysis is inadequate to permit recommendations in this regard.

Acidification of urine increases methamphetamine excretion. Intravenous phentolamine (Regitine®) has been suggested for possible acute, severe hypertension, if this complicates methamphetamine overdosage.

How Supplied: DESOXYN (methamphetamine hydrochloride) is supplied as follows:
Gradumet Tablets, 5 mg, white, in bottles of 100 (**NDC** 0074-6941-04); 10 mg, orange, in bottles of 100 (**NDC** 0074-6948-08) and 500 (**NDC** 0074-6948-09); and 15 mg, yellow, in bottles of 100 (**NDC** 0074-6959-07) and 500 (**NDC** 0074-6959-08).
Tablets, 5 mg, white, in bottles of 100 (**NDC** 0074-3377-04) and 1000 (**NDC** 0074-3377-02).

[*Shown in Product Identification Section*]

Abbott Laboratories/
Abbott Pharmaceuticals, Inc.
North Chicago, IL 60064
Ref. 01-2203-R1

DICAL-D® CAPSULES—WAFERS
(Dibasic Calcium Phosphate with Vitamin D)

Description:
Capsules
Daily dosage (three capsules) provides:
Vitamin D .... 399 IU .... 99% USRDA* (10 mcg)
Calcium .... 0.35 Gm ... 35% USRDA
Phosphorous ...... 0.27 Gm ... 27% USRDA
Each gelatin capsule contains:
Dibasic Calcium Phosphate, hydrous (as anhydrous form) .... 500 mg
Vitamin D_2 .... 3.33 mcg (133 IU)
Corn starch added.
Calcium to phosphorous ratio 1.3 to 1.
Wafers
Daily dosage (two wafers) provides:
Vitamin D ...... 400 IU .... 100% USRDA (10 mcg)
Calcium .... 0.464 Gm ..... 46% USRDA
Phosphorous ... 0.36 Gm ...... 36% USRDA
Each wafer contains:
Vitamin D_2 .... 5 mcg (200 IU)
Dibasic Calcium Phosphate, hydrous ... 1 Gm
Added dextrose, sucrose, talc, stearic acid, mineral oil, salt, and natural and artificial flavorings.
Calcium to phosphorous ratio 1.29 to 1.
*% U.S. Recommended Daily Allowance for adults and children 4 or more years of age.

Indications: For those individuals who must restrict their intake of dairy products.

Dosage and Administration: Usual dose for adults and children 4 years and older:
Wafers—Chew 1 wafer twice daily with meals, or as directed by the physician.
Capsules—1 capsule 3 times daily with meals, or as directed by the physician or dentist according to the need of the patient.

How Supplied:
Dical-D Capsules in bottles of 100 (NDC 0074-3594-04) and 500 (NDC 0074-3594-02).
Dical-D Wafers in box of 51 (NDC 0074-3589-01).

Abbott Laboratories/
Abbott Pharmaceuticals, Inc.
North Chicago, IL 60064
Ref. 03-0507-4/R10 & 09-5424-4/R6

DICUMAROL Tablets, USP ℞

How Supplied: Dicumarol tablets are supplied as:
25 mg tablets:
bottles of 100 (**NDC** 0074-3794-01);
bottles of 1000 (**NDC** 0074-3794-06).
50 mg tablets:
bottles of 100 (**NDC** 0074-3773-01);
bottles of 1000 (**NDC** 0074-3773-02).
100 mg tablets:
bottles of 100 (**NDC** 0074-3775-06).

[*Shown in Product Identification Section*]

Abbott Pharmaceuticals, Inc.
North Chicago, IL 60064

EAR DROPS BY MURINE OTC
See Murine Ear Wax Removal System/Murine Ear Drops

ENDURON® ℞
(methyclothiazide tablets, USP)

Description: ENDURON (methyclothiazide) is a member of the benzothiadiazine (thiazide) family of drugs. It is an analogue of hydrochlorothiazide.

Clinically, ENDURON is an oral diuretic-antihypertensive agent.

Actions: The diuretic and saluretic effects of ENDURON result from a drug-induced inhibition of the renal tubular reabsorption of electrolytes. The excretion of sodium and chloride is greatly enhanced. Potassium excretion is also enhanced to a variable degree, as it is with the other thiazides. Although urinary excretion of bicarbonate is increased slightly, there is usually no significant change in urinary pH. Methyclothiazide has a per mg natriuretic activity approximately 100 times that of the prototype thiazide, chlorothiazide. At maximal therapeutic dosages, all thiazides are approximately equal in their diuretic/natriuretic effects.

There is significant natriuresis and diuresis within two hours after administration of a single dose of methyclothiazide. These effects reach a peak in about six hours and persist for 24 hours following oral administration of a single dose.

Like other benzothiadiazines, ENDURON also has antihypertensive properties, and may be used for this purpose either alone or to enhance the antihypertensive action of other drugs. The mechanism by which the benzothiadiazines, including methyclothiazide, produce a reduction of elevated blood pressure is not known. However, sodium depletion appears to be involved.

ENDURON is rapidly absorbed and slowly eliminated by the kidneys as both intact drug and as a metabolite showing no diuretic activity in a rat model.

Indications: ENDURON is indicated in the management of hypertension either as the sole therapeutic agent or to enhance the effect of other antihypertensive drugs in the more severe forms of hypertension.

ENDURON (methyclothiazide) is indicated as adjunctive therapy in edema associated with congestive heart failure, hepatic cirrhosis, and corticosteroid and estrogen therapy.

ENDURON has also been found useful in edema due to various forms of renal dysfunction such as the nephrotic syndrome, acute glomerulonephritis, and chronic renal failure.

Usage in Pregnancy: The routine use of diuretics in an otherwise healthy pregnant woman is inappropriate and exposes mother and fetus to unnecessary hazard. Diuretics do not prevent development of toxemia of pregnancy, and there is no satisfactory evidence that they are useful in the treatment of developed toxemia.

Edema during pregnancy may arise from pathological causes or from the physiological and mechanical consequences of pregnancy. Thiazides are indicated in pregnancy when edema is due to pathological causes, just as they are in the absence of pregnancy (however, see Warnings, below). Dependent edema in pregnancy, resulting from restriction of venous return by the expanded uterus, is properly treated through elevation of the lower extremities and use of support hose; use of diuretics to lower intravascular volume in this case is illogical and unnecessary. There is hypervolemia during normal pregnancy which is harmful to neither the fetus nor the mother (in the absence of cardiovascular disease), but which is associated with edema, including generalized edema, in the majority of pregnant women. If this edema produces discomfort, increased recumbency will often provide relief. In rare instances, this edema may cause extreme discomfort which is not relieved by rest. In these cases, a short course of diuretics may provide relief and may be appropriate.

Contraindications: Renal decompensation. Hypersensitivity to this or other sulfonamide-derived drugs.

Warnings: Methyclothiazide shares with other thiazides the propensity to deplete potassium reserves to an unpredictable degree.

Thiazides should be used with caution in patients with renal disease or significant impairment of renal function, since azotemia may be precipitated and cumulative drug effects may occur.

Thiazides should be used with caution in patients with impaired hepatic function or progressive liver disease, since minor alterations of fluid and electrolyte balance may precipitate hepatic coma.

Thiazides may be additive or potentiative of the action of other antihypertensive drugs. Potentiation occurs with ganglionic or peripheral adrenergic blocking drugs.

Sensitivity reactions may occur in patients with a history of allergy or bronchial asthma.

The possibility of exacerbation or activation of systemic lupus erythematosus has been reported.

Usage in Pregnancy: Thiazides cross the placental barrier and appear in cord blood. The use of thiazides in pregnant women requires that the anticipated benefit be weighed against possible hazards to the fetus. These hazards include fetal or neonatal jaundice, thrombocytopenia, and possible other adverse reactions that have occurred in the adult.

Nursing Mothers: Thiazides appear in breast milk. If use of the drug is deemed essential, the patient should stop nursing.

Precautions: Periodic determinations of serum electrolytes should be performed at appropriate intervals for the purpose of detecting possible electrolyte imbalances such as hyponatremia, hypochloremic alkalosis, and hypokalemia. Serum and urine electrolyte determinations are particularly important when a patient is vomiting excessively or receiving parenteral fluids. All patients should be observed for other clinical signs of electrolyte imbalances such as dryness of mouth, thirst, weakness, lethargy, drowsiness, restlessness, muscle pains or cramps, muscular fatigue, hypotension, oliguria, tachycardia, and gastrointestinal disturbances such as nausea and vomiting.

Hypokalemia may develop with thiazides as with any other potent diuretic, especially when brisk diuresis occurs, severe cirrhosis is present, or when corticosteroids or ACTH are given concomitantly. Interference with the adequate oral intake of electrolytes will also contribute to the possible development of hypokalemia. Potassium depletion, even of a mild degree, resulting from thiazide use, may sensitize a patient to the effects of cardiac glycosides such as digitalis.

Any chloride deficit is generally mild and usually does not require specific treatment except under extraordinary circumstances (as in liver disease or renal disease). Dilutional hyponatremia may occur in edematous patients in hot weather; appropriate therapy is water restriction rather than administration of salt, except in rare instances when the hyponatremia is life threatening.

In actual salt depletion, appropriate replacement is the therapy of choice.

Hyperuricemia may occur or frank gout may be precipitated in certain patients receiving thiazide therapy.

Insulin requirements in diabetic patients may be increased, decreased, or unchanged. Latent diabetes mellitus may become manifest during thiazide administration.

Thiazide drugs may increase the responsiveness to tubocurarine.

The antihypertensive effects of the drug may be enhanced in the postsympathectomy patient.

Thiazides may decrease arterial responsiveness to norepinephrine. This diminution is not sufficient to preclude effectiveness of the pressor agent for therapeutic use.

If progressive renal impairment becomes evident as indicated by a rising nonprotein nitrogen or blood urea nitrogen, a careful reappraisal of therapy is necessary with consideration given to withholding or discontinuing diuretic therapy.

Thiazides may decrease serum PBI levels without signs of thyroid disturbance.

Thiazides have been reported, on rare occasions, to have elevated serum calcium to hypercalcemic levels. The serum calcium levels have returned to normal when the medication has been stopped. This phenomenon may be related to the ability of the thiazide diuretics to lower the amount of calcium excreted in the urine.

Adverse Reactions: Gastrointestinal system reactions: Anorexia, gastric irritation, nausea, vomiting, cramping, diarrhea, constipation, jaundice (intrahepatic cholestatic jaundice), pancreatitis.

Central nervous system reactions: Dizziness, vertigo, paresthesias, headache, xanthopsia.

Hematologic reactions: Leukopenia, agranulocytosis, thrombocytopenia, aplastic anemia.

Dermatologic—hypersensitivity reactions: Purpura, photosensitivity, rash, urticaria, necrotizing angiitis (vasculitis) (cutaneous vasculitis).

Cardiovascular reaction: Orthostatic hypotension may occur and may be aggravated by alcohol, barbiturates, or narcotics.

Other: Hyperglycemia, glycosuria, hypercalcemia, hyperuricemia, muscle spasm, weakness, restlessness.

There have been isolated reports that certain nonedematous individuals developed severe fluid and electrolyte derangements after only brief exposure to normal doses of thiazide and non-thiazide diuretics. The condition is usually manifested as severe dilutional hyponatremia, hypokalemia, and hypochloremia. It has been reported to be due to inappropriately increased ADH secretion and appears to be idiosyncratic. Potassium replacement is apparently the most important therapy in the treatment of this syndrome along with removal of the offending drug.

Whenever adverse reactions are severe, treatment should be discontinued.

Dosage and Administration: ENDURON (methyclothiazide) is administered orally. Therapy should be individualized according to patient response. This therapy should be titrated to gain maximal therapeutic response as well as the minimal dose possible to maintain that therapeutic response.

For edematous conditions: The usual adult dose ranges from 2.5 to 10 mg once daily. Maximum effective single dose is 10 mg; larger single doses do not accomplish greater diuresis, and are not recommended.

For the treatment of hypertension: The usual adult dose ranges from 2.5 to 5 mg once daily. If control of blood pressure is not satisfactory after 8 to 12 weeks of therapy with 5 mg once daily, another antihypertensive drug should be added. Increase of the dosage of ENDURON will usually not result in further lowering of blood pressure.

Methyclothiazide may be either employed alone for mild to moderate hypertension or concurrently with other antihypertensive drugs in the management of more severe forms of hypertension. Combined therapy may provide adequate control of hypertension with lower dosage of the component drugs and fewer or less severe side effects. An enhanced response frequently follows its concurrent administration with Harmonyl® (deserpidine) so that dosage of both drugs may be reduced.

When other antihypertensive agents are to be added to the regimen, this should be accomplished gradually. Ganglionic blocking agents should be given at only half the usual dose since their effect is potentiated by pretreatment with ENDURON.

Overdosage: Symptoms of overdosage include electrolyte imbalance and signs of potassium deficiency such as confusion, dizziness, muscular weakness, and gastrointestinal disturbances. General supportive measures including replacement of fluids and electrolytes may be indicated in treatment of overdosage.

How Supplied: ENDURON (methyclothiazide tablets, USP) is provided in two dosage sizes as monogrammed, grooved, square-shaped tablets:

2.5 mg, orange-colored:
bottles of 100 (**NDC** 0074-6827-01),
bottles of 1000 (**NDC** 0074-6827-02).

5 mg, salmon-colored:
bottles of 100 (**NDC** 0074-6812-01),
bottles of 1000 (**NDC** 0074-6812-02),
bottles of 5000 (**NDC** 0074-6812-03),
Abbo-Pac® unit dose packages of 100 (**NDC** 0074-6812-10).

[*Shown in Product Identification Section*]
Abbott Pharmaceuticals, Inc.
North Chicago, IL 60064
Ref. 03-4235-R8

ENDURONYL® Tablets ℞
(methyclothiazide and deserpidine)

Oral thiazide-rauwolfia therapy for hypertension.

> **Warning:**
> This fixed combination drug is not indicated for initial therapy of hypertension. Hypertension requires therapy titrated to the individual patient. If the fixed combination represents the dosage so determined, its use may be more convenient in patient management. The treatment of hypertension is not static, but must be reevaluated as conditions in each patient warrant.

Description: ENDURONYL is an orally-administered combination of Enduron® (methyclothiazide) and Harmonyl® (deserpidine). Methyclothiazide is an oral diuretic-antihypertensive of the benzothiadiazine (thiazide) class. Deserpidine is a purified rauwolfia alkaloid, chemically identified as 11-desmethoxyreserpine, which produces antihypertensive effects.

Actions: The combined antihypertensive actions of methyclothiazide and deserpidine result in a total clinical antihypertensive effect which is greater than can ordinarily be achieved by either drug given individually.

The diuretic and saluretic effects of methyclothiazide result from a drug-induced inhibition of the renal tubular reabsorption of electrolytes. The excretion of sodium and chloride is greatly enhanced. Potassium excretion is also enhanced to a variable degree, as it is with the other thiazides. Although urinary excretion of bicarbonate is increased slightly, there is usually no significant change in urinary pH. Methyclothiazide has a per mg natriuretic activity approximately 100 times that of the prototype thiazide, chlorothiazide. At maximal therapeutic dosages, all thiazides are approximately equal in their diuretic/natriuretic effects.

There is significant natriuresis and diuresis within two hours after administration of a single dose of methyclothiazide. These effects reach a peak in about six hours and persist for 24 hours following oral administration of a single dose.

Like other benzothiadiazines, methyclothiazide also has antihypertensive properties, and may be used for this purpose either alone or to enhance the antihypertensive action of other drugs. The mechanism by which the benzothiadiazines, including methyclothiazide, produce a reduction of elevated blood pressure is not known. However, sodium depletion appears to be involved.

Methyclothiazide is rapidly absorbed and slowly eliminated by the kidney as both intact drug and as a metabolite showing no diuretic activity in a rat model.

The pharmacologic actions of Harmonyl (deserpidine) are essentially the same as those of other active rauwolfia alkaloids. Deserpidine probably produces its antihypertensive effects through depletion of tissue stores of catecholamines (epinephrine and norepinephrine) from peripheral sites. The antihypertensive effect is often accompanied by bradycardia. There is no significant alteration in cardiac output or re-

Continued on next page

If desired, additional literature on any Abbott Product will be provided upon request to Abbott Laboratories.

Abbott—Cont.

nal blood flow. The carotid sinus reflex is inhibited, but postural hypotension is rarely seen with the use of conventional doses of Harmonyl alone.
Deserpidine, like other rauwolfia alkaloids, is characterized by slow onset of action and sustained effect which may persist following withdrawal of the drug.
Indications: ENDURONYL (methyclothiazide and deserpidine) is indicated in the treatment of mild to moderately severe hypertension (see boxed warning). In many cases ENDURONYL alone produces an adequate reduction of blood pressure. In resistant or unusually severe cases ENDURONYL also may be supplemented by more potent antihypertensive agents. When administered with ENDURONYL, more potent agents can be given at reduced dosage to minimize undesirable side effects.
Contraindications: Methyclothiazide is contraindicated in patients with renal decompensation and in those who are hypersensitive to this or other sulfonamide-derived drugs.
Deserpidine is contraindicated in patients with known hypersensitivity, mental depression especially with suicidal tendencies, active peptic ulcer, and ulcerative colitis. It is also contraindicated in patients receiving electroconvulsive therapy.
Warnings:
Methyclothiazide
Methyclothiazide shares with other thiazides the propensity to deplete potassium reserves to an unpredictable degree.
Thiazides should be used with caution in patients with renal disease or significant impairment of renal function, since azotemia may be precipitated and cumulative drug effects may occur.
Thiazides should be used with caution in patients with impaired hepatic function or progressive liver disease, since minor alterations of fluid and electrolyte balance may precipitate hepatic coma.
Thiazides may be additive or potentiative of the action of other antihypertensive drugs. Potentiation occurs with ganglionic or peripheral adrenergic blocking drugs.
Sensitivity reactions may occur in patients with a history of allergy or bronchial asthma. The possibility of exacerbation or activation of systemic lupus erythematosus has been reported.
Deserpidine
Extreme caution should be exercised in treating patients with a history of mental depression. Discontinue the drug at the first sign of despondency, early morning insomnia, loss of appetite, impotence, or self-deprecation. Drug-induced depression may persist for several months after drug withdrawal and may be severe enough to result in suicide.
Usage in Pregnancy and Lactation:
Methyclothiazide
Thiazides cross the placental barrier and appear in cord blood. The use of thiazides in pregnant women requires that the anticipated benefit be weighed against possible hazards to the fetus. These hazards include fetal or neonatal jaundice, thrombocytopenia, and possible other adverse reactions that have occurred in the adult.
Thiazides appear in breast milk. If use of the drug is deemed essential, the patient should stop nursing.
Deserpidine
The safety of deserpidine for use during pregnancy or lactation has not been established; therefore, it should be used in pregnant women or in women of childbearing potential only when in the judgment of the physician its use is deemed essential to the welfare of the patient. Increased respiratory secretions, nasal congestion, cyanosis, and anorexia may occur in infants born to rauwolfia alkaloid-treated mothers, since these preparations are known to cross the placental barrier to enter the fetal circulation and appear in cord blood. They also are secreted by nursing mothers into breast milk.
Reproductive and teratology studies in rats reduced the mating index and neonatal survival indices; the no-effect dosage has not been established.
Precautions: Periodic determinations of serum electrolytes should be performed at appropriate intervals for the purpose of detecting possible electrolyte imbalances such as hyponatremia, hypochloremic alkalosis, and hypokalemia. Serum and urine electrolyte determinations are particularly important when a patient is vomiting excessively or receiving parenteral fluids. All patients should be observed for other clinical signs of electrolyte imbalances such as dryness of mouth, thirst, weakness, lethargy, drowsiness, restlessness, muscle pains or cramps, muscular fatigue, hypotension, oliguria, tachycardia, and gastrointestinal disturbances such as nausea and vomiting.
Hypokalemia may develop with thiazides as with any other potent diuretic, especially when brisk diuresis occurs, severe cirrhosis is present, or when corticosteroids or ACTH are given concomitantly. Interference with the adequate oral intake of electrolytes will also contribute to the possible development of hypokalemia. Potassium depletion, even of a mild degree, resulting from thiazide use, may sensitize a patient to the effects of cardiac glycosides such as digitalis.
Any chloride deficit is generally mild and usually does not require specific treatment except under extraordinary circumstances (as in liver disease or renal disease). Dilutional hyponatremia may occur in edematous patients in hot weather; appropriate therapy is water restriction rather than administration of salt, except in rare instances when the hyponatremia is life threatening.
In actual salt depletion, appropriate replacement is the therapy of choice.
Hyperuricemia may occur or frank gout may be precipitated in certain patients receiving thiazide therapy.
Insulin requirements in diabetic patients may be increased, decreased, or unchanged. Latent diabetes mellitus may become manifest during thiazide administration.
Thiazide drugs may increase the responsiveness to tubocurarine.
The antihypertensive effects of the drug may be enhanced in the postsympathectomy patient.
Thiazides may decrease arterial responsiveness to norepinephrine. This diminution is not sufficient to preclude effectiveness of the pressor agent for therapeutic use.
If progressive renal impairment becomes evident as indicated by a rising nonprotein nitrogen or blood urea nitrogen, a careful reappraisal of therapy is necessary with consideration given to withholding or discontinuing diuretic therapy.
Thiazides may decrease serum PBI levels without signs of thyroid disturbance.
Thiazides have been reported, on rare occasions, to have elevated serum calcium to hypercalcemic levels. The serum calcium levels have returned to normal when the medication has been stopped. This phenomenon may be related to the ability of the thiazide diuretics to lower the amount of calcium excreted in the urine.
Because rauwolfia preparations increase gastrointestinal motility and secretion, this drug should be used cautiously in patients with a history of peptic ulcer, ulcerative colitis, or gallstones, where biliary colic may be precipitated.
Caution should be exercised when treating hypertensive patients with renal insufficiency since they adjust poorly to lowered blood pressure levels.
Use deserpidine cautiously with digitalis and quinidine since cardiac arrhythmias have occurred with rauwolfia preparations.
Preoperative withdrawal of deserpidine does not assure that circulatory instability will not occur. It is important that the anesthesiologist be aware of the patient's drug intake and consider this in the overall management, since hypotension has occurred in patients receiving rauwolfia preparations. Anticholinergic and/ or adrenergic drugs (metaraminol, norepinephrine) have been employed to treat adverse vagocirculatory effects.
Adverse Reactions:
Methyclothiazide
Gastrointestinal System Reactions: Anorexia, gastric irritation, nausea, vomiting, cramping, diarrhea, constipation, jaundice (intrahepatic cholestatic jaundice), pancreatitis.
Central Nervous System Reactions: Dizziness, vertigo, paresthesias, headache, xanthopsia.
Hematologic Reactions: Leukopenia, agranulocytosis, thrombocytopenia, aplastic anemia.
Dermatologic — Hypersensitivity Reactions: Purpura, photosensitivity, rash, urticaria, necrotizing angiitis (vasculitis) (cutaneous vasculitis).
Cardiovascular Reaction: Orthostatic hypotension may occur and may be aggravated by alcohol, barbiturates, or narcotics.
Other: Hyperglycemia, glycosuria, hypercalcemia, hyperuricemia, muscle spasm, weakness, restlessness.
There have been isolated reports that certain nonedematous individuals developed severe fluid and electrolyte derangements after only brief exposure to normal doses of thiazide and non-thiazide diuretics. The condition is usually manifested as severe dilutional hyponatremia, hypokalemia, and hypochloremia. It has been reported to be due to inappropriately increased ADH secretion and appears to be idiosyncratic. Potassium replacement is apparently the most important therapy in the treatment of this syndrome along with removal of the offending drug.
Whenever adverse reactions are severe, treatment should be discontinued.
Deserpidine
The following adverse reactions have been reported with rauwolfia preparations. These reactions are usually reversible and disappear when the drug is discontinued.
Gastrointestinal: Including hypersecretion, anorexia, diarrhea, nausea, and vomiting.
Cardiovascular: Including angina-like symptoms, arrhythmias (particularly when used concurrently with digitalis or quinidine), and bradycardia.
Central Nervous System: Including drowsiness, depression, nervousness, paradoxical anxiety, nightmares, extrapyramidal tract symptoms, CNS sensitization manifested by dull sensorium, and deafness.
Dermatologic—Hypersensitivity: Including pruritus, rash, and asthma in asthmatic patients.
Ophthalmologic: Including glaucoma, uveitis, optic atrophy, and conjunctival injection.
Hematologic: Thrombocytopenic purpura.
Miscellaneous: Nasal congestion, weight gain, impotence or decreased libido, dysuria, dyspnea, muscular aches, dryness of mouth, dizziness, and headache.
Dosage and Administration: Dosage should be determined by individual titration of ingredients (see boxed warning). Dosage of both components should be carefully adjusted to the needs of the individual patient. Since at least ten days to two weeks may elapse before the full effects of the drugs become manifest, the dosage of the drugs should not be adjusted more frequently.
Two tablet strengths, ENDURONYL (methyclothiazide 5 mg, deserpidine 0.25 mg) and ENDURONYL FORTE (methyclothiazide 5 mg, deser-

pidine 0.5 mg), each grooved, are provided to permit considerable latitude in meeting the dosage requirements of individual patients.*
The following table will help in determining which dose of ENDURONYL or ENDURONYL FORTE best represents the equivalent of the titrated dose.

Daily Dosage of ENDURONYL	methyclothiazide	deserpidine
½ tablet	2.5 mg	0.125 mg
1 tablet	5.0 mg	0.250 mg
1½ tablet	7.5 mg	0.375 mg
2 tablets	10.0 mg	0.500 mg

Daily Dosage of ENDURONYL FORTE	methyclothiazide	deserpidine
½ tablet	2.5 mg	0.250 mg
1 tablet	5.0 mg	0.500 mg
1½ tablet	7.5 mg	0.750 mg
2 tablets	10.0 mg	1.000 mg

The appropriate dose of ENDURONYL is administered orally, once daily. The usual adult dosage is one lower-strength ENDURONYL tablet daily. There is no contraindication to combining the administration of ENDURONYL with other antihypertensive agents. When other antihypertensive agents are to be added to the regimen, this should be accomplished gradually. Ganglionic blocking agents should be given at only half the usual dose since their effect is potentiated by pretreatment with ENDURONYL.

Overdosage: Symptoms of thiazide overdosage include electrolyte imbalance and signs of potassium deficiency such as confusion, dizziness, muscular weakness, and gastrointestinal disturbances. General supportive measures including replacement of fluids and electrolytes may be indicated in treatment of overdosage.
An overdosage of deserpidine is characterized by flushing of the skin, conjunctival injection, and pupillary constriction. Sedation ranging from drowsiness to coma may occur. Hypotension, hypothermia, central respiratory depression and bradycardia may develop in cases of severe overdosage. Treatment consists of the careful evacuation of stomach contents followed by the usual procedures for the symptomatic management of CNS depressant overdosage. If severe hypotension occurs it should be treated with a direct acting vasopressor such as norepinephrine bitartrate injection.

How Supplied: ENDURONYL (methyclothiazide and deserpidine) is supplied as monogrammed, grooved, square-shaped tablets in the following dosage sizes and quantities:
ENDURONYL (5 mg of methyclothiazide and 0.25 mg of deserpidine) yellow tablets in bottles of 100 (**NDC** 0074-6838-01) and 1000 (**NDC** 0074-6838-02). Also available in ABBO-PAC® unit dose packages, 100 tablets (**NDC** 0074-6838-06), in strips of 10 tablets.
ENDURONYL FORTE (5 mg of methyclothiazide and 0.5 mg of deserpidine) gray-colored tablets in bottles of 100 (**NDC** 0074-6854-01) and 1000 (**NDC** 0074-6854-02).

*Each component is separately available as ENDURON (methyclothiazide) and HARMONYL (deserpidine).

[*Shown in Product Identification Section*]
Abbott Pharmaceuticals, Inc.
North Chicago, IL 60064
Ref. 03-4199-R4

ERYDERM® ℞
erythromycin topical solution, 2%

Description: Erythromycin is an antibiotic produced from a strain of *Streptomyces erythraeus*. It is basic and readily forms salts with acids. Each ml of ERYDERM (erythromycin topical solution) contains 20 mg of erythromycin base (2%) in a vehicle consisting of polyethylene glycol, acetone, and alcohol 77%.

Actions: Although the mechanism by which ERYDERM acts in reducing inflammatory lesions of acne vulgaris is unknown, it is presumably due to its antibiotic action.

Indications: ERYDERM is indicated for the topical control of acne vulgaris.

Contraindications: ERYDERM is contraindicated in persons who have shown hypersensitivity to any of its ingredients.

Warnings: The safe use of ERYDERM during pregnancy or lactation has not been established.

Precautions: ERYDERM is for external use only and should be kept away from the eyes and mucous membranes including those of the nose and mouth. Do not allow solution to contact clothing and furniture. Concomitant topical acne therapy should be used with caution because a cumulative irritant effect may occur, especially with the use of peeling, desquamating, or abrasive agents.
The use of antimicrobial agents may be associated with the overgrowth of antibiotic resistant organisms. If this occurs, administration of this drug should be discontinued and appropriate measures taken.

Adverse Reactions: Adverse conditions experienced included dryness, pruritus, erythema, desquamation, and burning sensation.

Dosage and Administration: ERYDERM should be applied to the affected area twice a day after the skin is thoroughly washed with warm water and soap. Use enough solution to cover the affected area lightly.

How Supplied: ERYDERM (erythromycin topical solution) 2%, is supplied in 60 ml bottles (**NDC** 0074-2698-02). Store at temperatures below 86°F (30°C).

[*Shown in product identification section*]
Abbott Laboratories
North Chicago, IL 60064
Ref. 01-2150/R2

ERYPED™ ℞
(erythromycin ethylsuccinate for oral suspension, USP)

Description: Erythromycin is produced by a strain of *Streptomyces erythraeus* and belongs to the macrolide group of antibiotics. It is basic and readily forms salts with acids. The base, the stearate salt, and the esters are poorly soluble in water. Erythromycin ethylsuccinate is an ester of erythromycin suitable for oral administration.
EryPed (erythromycin ethylsuccinate for oral suspension) is for reconstitution with water to form a suspension containing erythromycin ethylsuccinate equivalent to 400 mg of erythromycin per 5 ml (teaspoonful) with an appealing banana flavor. After mixing, EryPed must be stored below 77°F (25°C) and used within 35 days; refrigeration is not required. This product is intended primarily for pediatric use but can also be used in adults.

Actions:
Microbiology: Biochemical tests demonstrate that erythromycin inhibits protein synthesis of the pathogen without directly affecting nucleic acid synthesis. Antagonism has been demonstrated between clindamycin and erythromycin.
NOTE: Many strains of *Hemophilus influenzae* are resistant to erythromycin alone, but are susceptible to erythromycin and sulfonamides together. Staphylococci resistant to erythromycin may emerge during a course of erythromycin therapy. Culture and susceptibility testing should be performed.
Disc Susceptibility Tests: Quantitative methods that require measurement of zone diameters give the most precise estimates of antibiotic susceptibility. One recommended procedure (21 CFR section 460.1) uses erythromycin class discs for testing susceptibility; interpretations correlate zone diameters of this disc test with MIC values for erythromycin. With this procedure, a report from the laboratory of "susceptible" indicates that the infecting organism is likely to respond to therapy. A report of "resistant" indicates, that the infective organism is not likely to respond to therapy. A report of "intermediate susceptibility" suggests that the organism would be susceptible if higher doses were used.

Clinical Pharmacology: Erythromycin binds to the 50 S ribosomal subunits of susceptible bacteria and suppresses protein synthesis.
Orally administered erythromycin ethylsuccinate suspension is readily and reliably absorbed under both fasting and nonfasting conditions.
Erythromycin diffuses readily into most body fluids. Only low concentrations are normally achieved in the spinal fluid, but passage of the drug across the blood-brain barrier increases in meningitis. In the presence of normal hepatic function, erythromycin is concentrated in the liver and excreted in the bile; the effect of hepatic dysfunction on excretion of erythromycin by the liver into the bile is not known. Less than 5 percent of the orally administered dose of erythromycin is excreted in active form in the urine.
Erythromycin crosses the placental barrier and is excreted in breast milk.

Indications: *Streptococcus pyogenes* (Group A beta hemolytic streptococcus): Upper and lower respiratory tract, skin, and soft tissue infections of mild to moderate severity.
Injectable benzathine penicillin G is considered by the American Heart Association to be the drug of choice in the treatment and prevention of streptococcal pharyngitis and in long-term prophylaxis of rheumatic fever.
When oral medication is preferred for treatment of the above conditions, penicillin G, V, or erythromycin are alternate drugs of choice.
When oral medication is given, the importance of strict adherence by the patient to the prescribed dosage regimen must be stressed. A therapeutic dose should be administered for at least 10 days.
Alpha-hemolytic streptococci (viridans group): Although no controlled clinical efficacy trials have been conducted, oral erythromycin has been suggested by the American Heart Association and American Dental Association for use in a regimen for prophylaxis against bacterial endocarditis in patients hypersensitive to penicillin who have congenital heart disease, or rheumatic or other acquired valvular heart disease when they undergo dental procedures and surgical procedures of the upper respiratory tract.[1] Erythromycin is not suitable prior to genitourinary or gastrointestinal tract surgery. NOTE: When selecting antibiotics for the prevention of bacterial endocarditis the physician or dentist should read the full joint statement of the American Heart Association and the American Dental Association.[1]
Staphylococcus aureus: Acute infections of skin and soft tissue of mild to moderate severity. Resistant organisms may emerge during treatment.
Streptococcus pneumoniae (Diplococcus pneumoniae): Upper respiratory tract infections (e.g., otitis media, pharyngitis) and lower respiratory tract infections (e.g., pneumonia) of mild to moderate degree.
Mycoplasma pneumoniae (Eaton agent, PPLO): For respiratory infections due to this organism.
Hemophilus influenzae: For upper respiratory tract infections of mild to moderate sever-

Continued on next page

If desired, additional literature on any Abbott Product will be provided upon request to Abbott Laboratories.

Abbott—Cont.

ity when used concomitantly with adequate doses of sulfonamides. (See sulfonamide labeling for appropriate prescribing information). The concomitant use of the sulfonamides is necessary since not all strains of *Hemophilus influenzae* are susceptible to erythromycin at the concentrations of the antibiotic achieved with usual therapeutic doses.
Treponema pallidum: Erythromycin is an alternate choice of treatment for primary syphilis in patients allergic to the penicillins. In treatment of primary syphilis, spinal fluid examinations should be done before treatment and as part of follow-up after therapy.
Corynebacterium diphtheriae: As an adjunct to antitoxin, to prevent establishment of carriers, and to eradicate the organism in carriers.
Corynebacterium minutissimum: For the treatment of erythrasma.
Entamoeba histolytica: In the treatment of intestinal amebiasis only. Extraenteric amebiasis requires treatment with other agents.
Listeria monocytogenes: Infections due to this organism.
Bordetella pertussis: Erythromycin is effective in eliminating the organism from the nasopharynx of infected individuals, rendering them non-infectious. Some clinical studies suggest that erythromycin may be helpful in the prophylaxis of pertussis in exposed susceptible individuals.
Legionnaires' Disease: Although no controlled clinical efficacy studies have been conducted, *in vitro* and limited preliminary clinical data suggest that erythromycin may be effective in treating Legionnaires' Disease.
Contraindications: Erythromycin is contraindicated in patients with known hypersensitivity to this antibiotic.
Precautions: Erythromycin is principally excreted by the liver. Caution should be exercised in administering the antibiotic to patients with impaired hepatic function. There have been reports of hepatic dysfunction, with or without jaundice occurring in patients receiving oral erythromycin products.
Areas of localized infection may require surgical drainage in addition to antibiotic therapy.
Recent data from studies of erythromycin reveal that its use in patients who are receiving high doses of theophylline may be associated with an increase of serum theophylline levels and potential theophylline toxicity. In case of theophylline toxicity and/or elevated serum theophylline levels, the dose of theophylline should be reduced while the patient is receiving concomitant erythromycin therapy.
Usage during pregnancy and lactation: The safety of erythromycin for use during pregnancy has not been established.
Erythromycin crosses the placental barrier. Erythromycin also appears in breast milk.
Adverse Reactions: The most frequent side effects of erythromycin preparations are gastrointestinal, such as abdominal cramping and discomfort, and are dose related. Nausea, vomiting, and diarrhea occur infrequently with usual oral doses.
During prolonged or repeated therapy, there is a possibility of overgrowth of nonsusceptible bacteria of fungi. If such infections occur, the drug should be discontinued and appropriate therapy instituted.
Allergic reactions ranging from urticaria and mild skin eruptions to anaphylaxis have occurred.
There have been isolated reports of reversible hearing loss occurring chiefly in patients with renal insufficiency and in patients receiving high doses of erythromycin.
Dosage and Administration: EryPed (erythromycin ethylsuccinate for oral suspension) may be administered without regard to meals.
Children: Age, weight, and severity of the infection are important factors in determining the proper dosage. In mild to moderate infections the usual dosage of erythromycin ethylsuccinate for children is 30 to 50 mg/kg/day in equally divided doses. For more severe infections this dosage may be doubled.
The following dosage schedule is suggested for mild to moderate infections:

Body Weight	Total Daily Dose
Under 10 lbs	30-50 mg/kg/day 15-25 mg/lb/day
10 to 15 lbs	200 mg
16 to 25 lbs	400 mg
26 to 50 lbs	800 mg
51 to 100 lbs	1200 mg
over 100 lbs	1600 mg

Adults: 400 mg erythromycin ethylsuccinate every 6 hours is the usual dose. Dosage may be increased up to 4 g per day according to the severity of the infection.
If twice-a-day dosage is desired in either adults or children, one-half of the total daily dose may be given every 12 hours. Doses may also be given three times daily if desired by administering one-third of the total daily dose every 8 hours.
In the treatment of streptococcal infections, a therapeutic dosage of erythromycin ethylsuccinate should be administered for at least 10 days. In continuous prophylaxis against recurrences of streptococcal infections in persons with a history of rheumatic heart disease, the usual dosage is 400 mg twice a day.
For prophylaxis against bacterial endocarditis[1] in patients with congenital heart disease, or rheumatic or other acquired valvular heart disease when undergoing dental procedures or surgical procedures of the upper respiratory tract, give 1.6 g (20 mg/kg for children) orally 1 ½ to 2 hours before the procedure, and then, 800 mg (10 mg/kg for children) orally every 6 hours for 8 doses.
For treatment of primary syphilis: Adults: 48 to 64 g given in divided doses over a period of 10 to 15 days.
For intestinal amebiasis: Adults: 400 mg four times daily for 10 to 14 days. Children: 30 to 50 mg/kg/day in divided doses for 10 to 14 days.
For use in pertussis: Although optimal dosage and duration have not been established, doses of erythromycin utilized in reported clinical studies were 40 to 50 mg/kg/day, given in divided doses for 5 to 14 days.
For treatment of Legionnaires' Disease: Although optimal doses have not been established, doses utilized in reported clinical data were 1.6 to 4 g daily in divided doses.
How Supplied: EryPed (erythromycin ethylsuccinate for oral suspension, USP), 400 mg per 5 ml, is supplied in 100-ml (**NDC** 0074-6305-13) and 200-ml (**NDC** 0074-6305-53) bottles, and 5-ml unit dose in ABBO-PAC® packages of 100 bottles (**NDC** 0074-6305-05). After reconstitution, EryPed must be stored below 77°F (25°C) and used within 35 days; refrigeration not required.

Reference: 1. American Heart Association. 1977. Prevention of bacterial endocarditis. Circulation 56:139A-143A.

TM — Trademark.
Abbott Laboratories
North Chicago, IL 60064
Ref. 07-5222-R2

ERY-TAB® ℞
(erythromycin enteric-coated tablets)

Description: Erythromycin is produced by a strain of *Streptomyces erythraeus* and belongs to the macrolide group of antibiotics. It is basic and readily forms salts with acids. The base is white to off-white crystals or powder slightly soluble in water, soluble in alcohol, in chloroform, and in ether. ERY-TAB (erythromycin enteric-coated tablets) is specially coated to protect the contents from the inactivating effects of gastric acidity and to permit efficient absorption of the antibiotic in the small intestine.
ERY-TAB is available in three dosage strengths containing either 250 mg, 333 mg, or 500 mg of erythromycin as the free base.
Actions: The mode of action of erythromycin is inhibition of protein synthesis without affecting nucleic acid synthesis. Resistance to erythromycin of some strains of *Hemophilus influenzae* and staphylococci has been demonstrated. Culture and susceptibility testing should be done. If the Kirby-Bauer method of disc susceptibility is used, a 15 mcg erythromycin disc should give a zone diameter of at least 18 mm when tested against an erythromycin susceptible organism.
Bioavailability data are available from Abbott Laboratories, Dept. 498.
ERY-TAB is well absorbed and may be given without regard to meals.
After absorption, erythromycin diffuses readily into most body fluids. In the absence of meningeal inflammation, low concentrations are normally achieved in the spinal fluid but passage of the drug across the blood-brain barrier increases in meningitis. In the presence of normal hepatic function, erythromycin is concentrated in the liver and excreted in the bile; the effect of hepatic dysfunction on excretion of erythromycin by the liver into the bile is not known. After oral administration, less than 5 percent of the activity of the administered dose can be recovered in the urine.
Erythromycin crosses the placental barrier but fetal plasma levels are low.
Indications: *Streptococcus pyogenes* (Group A beta hemolytic streptococcus): For upper and lower respiratory tract, skin, and soft tissue infections of mild to moderate severity.
Injectable benzathine penicillin G is considered by the American Heart Association to be the drug of choice in the treatment and prevention of streptococcal pharyngitis and in long-term prophylaxis of rheumatic fever.
When oral medication is preferred for treatment of the above conditions, penicillin G, V, or erythromycin are alternate drugs of choice.
When oral medication is given, the importance of strict adherence by the patient to the prescribed dosage regimen must be stressed. A therapeutic dose should be administered for at least 10 days.
Alpha-hemolytic streptococci (viridans group): Although no controlled clinical efficacy trials have been conducted, oral erythromycin has been suggested by the American Heart Association and American Dental Association for use in a regimen for prophylaxis against bacterial endocarditis in patients hypersensitive to penicillin who have congenital heart disease, or rheumatic or other acquired valvular heart disease when they undergo dental procedures and surgical procedures of the upper respiratory tract.[1] Erythromycin is not suitable prior to genitourinary or gastrointestinal tract surgery. NOTE: When selecting antibiotics for the prevention of bacterial endocarditis the physician or dentist should read the full joint statement of the American Heart Association and the American Dental Association.[1]
Staphylococcus aureus: For acute infections of skin and soft tissue of mild to moderate severity. Resistant organisms may emerge during treatment.
Streptococcus pneumoniae (Diplococcus pneumoniae): For upper respiratory tract infections (e.g., otitis media, pharyngitis) and lower respiratory tract infections (e.g., pneumonia) of mild to moderate degree.
Mycoplasma pneumoniae (Eaton agent, PPLO): For respiratory infections due to this organism.

Hemophilus influenzae: For upper respiratory tract infections of mild to moderate severity when used concomitantly with adequate doses of sulfonamides. Not all strains of this organism are susceptible at the erythromycin concentrations ordinarily achieved (see appropriate sulfonamide labeling for prescribing information).

Treponema pallidum: Erythromycin is an alternate choice of treatment for primary syphilis in patients allergic to the penicillins. In treatment of primary syphilis, spinal fluid examinations should be done before treatment and as part of follow-up after therapy.

Corynebacterium diphtheriae and C. minutissimum: As an adjunct to antitoxin, to prevent establishment of carriers, and to eradicate the organism in carriers.

In the treatment of erythrasma.

Entamoeba histolytica: In the treatment of intestinal amebiasis only. Extra-enteric amebiasis requires treatment with other agents.

Listeria monocytogenes: Infections due to this organism.

Neisseria gonorrhoeae: Erythrocin® Lactobionate-I.V. (erythromycin lactobionate for injection, USP) in conjunction with erythromycin base orally, as an alternative drug in treatment of acute pelvic inflammatory disease caused by *N. gonorrhoeae* in female patients with a history of sensitivity to penicillin. Before treatment of gonorrhea, patients who are suspected of also having syphilis should have a microscopic examination for *T. pallidum* (by immunofluorescence or darkfield) before receiving erythromycin, and monthly serologic tests for a minimum of 4 months.

Bordetella pertussis: Erythromycin is effective in eliminating the organism from the nasopharynx of infected individuals, rendering them non-infectious. Some clinical studies suggest that erythromycin may be helpful in the prophylaxis of pertussis in exposed susceptible individuals.

Legionnaires' Disease: Although no controlled clinical efficacy studies have been conducted, *in vitro* and limited preliminary clinical data suggest that erythromycin can be effective in treating Legionnaires' Disease.

Contraindications: Erythromycin is contraindicated in patients with known hypersensitivity to this antibiotic.

Warning: *Usage in pregnancy:* Safety for use in pregnancy has not been established.

Precautions: Erythromycin is principally excreted by the liver. Caution should be exercised in administering the antibiotic to patients with impaired hepatic function.

There have been reports of hepatic dysfunction, with or without jaundice, occurring in patients receiving oral erythromycin products.

Recent data from studies of erythromycin reveal that its use in patients who are receiving high doses of theophylline may be associated with an increase of serum theophylline levels and potential theophylline toxicity. In cases of theophylline toxicity and/or elevated serum theophylline levels, the dose of theophylline should be reduced while the patient is receiving concomitant erythromycin therapy.

Surgical procedures should be performed when indicated.

Adverse Reactions: The most frequent side effects of erythromycin preparations are gastrointestinal, such as abdominal cramping and discomfort, and are dose-related. Nausea, vomiting, and diarrhea occur infrequently with usual oral doses.

During prolonged or repeated therapy, there is a possibility of overgrowth of nonsusceptible bacteria or fungi. If such infections occur, the drug should be discontinued and appropriate therapy instituted.

Mild allergic reactions such as urticaria and other skin rashes have occurred. Serious allergic reactions, including anaphylaxis, have been reported.

There have been isolated reports of reversible hearing loss occurring chiefly in patients with renal insufficiency and in patients receiving high doses of erythromycin.

Dosage and Administration: ERY-TAB (erythromycin enteric-coated tablets) is well absorbed and may be given without regard to meals.

Adults: The usual dose is 250 mg four times daily in equally spaced doses. The 333 mg tablet is recommended if dosage is desired every 8 hours. If twice-a-day dosage is desired, the recommended dose is 500 mg every 12 hours. Dosage may be increased up to 4 or more grams per day according to the severity of the infection. Twice-a-day dosing is not recommended when doses larger than 1 gram daily are administered.

Children: Age, weight, and severity of the infection are important factors in determining the proper dosage. 30 to 50 mg/kg/day, in divided doses, is the usual dose. For more severe infections, this dose may be doubled.

In the treatment of streptococcal infections, a therapeutic dosage of erythromycin should be administered for at least 10 days. In continuous prophylaxis of streptococcal infections in persons with a history of rheumatic heart disease, the dose is 250 mg twice a day.

For prophylaxis against bacterial endocarditis[1] in patients with congenital heart disease, or rheumatic or other acquired valvular heart disease when undergoing dental procedures or surgical procedures of the upper respiratory tract, give 1 g (20 mg/kg for children) orally 1½ to 2 hours before the procedure, and then, 500 mg (10 mg/kg in children) orally every 6 hours for 8 doses.

For treatment of primary syphilis: 30 to 40 grams given in divided doses over a period of 10 to 15 days.

For treatment of acute pelvic inflammatory disease caused by *N. gonorrhoeae:* After initial treatment with Erythrocin® Lactobionate-I.V. (erythromycin lactobionate for injection, USP) 500 mg every 6 hours for 3 days, the oral dosage recommendation is 250 mg every 6 hours for 7 days.

For dysenteric amebiasis: 250 mg four times daily for 10 to 14 days, for adults; 30 to 50 mg/kg/day in divided doses for 10 to 14 days, for children.

For use in pertussis: Although optimal dosage and duration have not been established, doses of erythromycin utilized in reported clinical studies were 40 to 50 mg/kg/day, given in divided doses for 5 to 14 days.

For treatment of Legionnaires' Disease: Although optimal doses have not been established, doses utilized in reported clinical data were 1 to 4 grams erythromycin base daily in divided doses.

Treatment of Overdosage: The drug is virtually nontoxic, though some individuals may exhibit gastric intolerance to even therapeutic amounts. Allergic reactions associated with acute overdosage should be handled in the usual manner—that is, by the administration of adrenalin, corticosteroids, and antihistamines as indicated, and the prompt elimination of unabsorbed drug, in addition to all needed supportive measures.

How Supplied: ERY-TAB (erythromycin enteric-coated tablets), 250 mg, is supplied as pink tablets in bottles of 100 (**NDC** 0074-6304-13), bottles of 500 (**NDC** 0074-6304-53), and Abbo-Pac® unit dose packages of 100 (**NDC** 0074-6304-11).

ERY-TAB, 333 mg, is supplied as white tablets in bottles of 100 (**NDC** 0074-6320-13), and Abbo-Pac® unit dose packages of 100 (**NDC** 0074-6320-11).

ERY-TAB, 500 mg, is supplied as pink tablets in bottles of 100 (**NDC** 0074-6321-13) and Abbo-Pac unit dose packages of 100 (**NDC** 0074-6321-11).

Reference: 1. American Heart Association, 1977. Prevention of bacterial endocarditis. Circulation 56: 139A–143A.

U.S. Pat. No. 4,340,582.

[*Shown in Product Identification Section*]

Abbott Laboratories
North Chicago, IL 60064
Ref. 01-2261-R6

E.E.S.® ℞
(erythromycin ethylsuccinate)

Description: Erythromycin is produced by a strain of *Streptomyces erythraeus* and belongs to the macrolide group of antibiotics. It is basic and readily forms salts with acids. The base, the stearate salt, and the esters are poorly soluble in water. Erythromycin ethylsuccinate is an ester of erythromycin suitable for oral administration.

The cherry-flavored, chewable tablets are easily ingested and are particularly acceptable for the administration of antibiotic medication to young children who are unable to swallow regular tablets or in whom persuasion of a pleasant taste insures cooperation. Each chewable tablet, providing the equivalent of 200 mg of erythromycin, is conveniently scored for division into half-dose (100 mg) portions.

The granules and drops are intended for reconstitution with water. When reconstituted, they are palatable cherry-flavored suspensions.

The pleasant tasting, fruit-flavored liquids are supplied ready for oral administration.

Granules, drops and ready-made suspensions are intended primarily for pediatric use but can also be used in adults.

The Filmtab® tablets are intended primarily for adults or older children.

Actions: Microbiology: Biochemical tests demonstrate that erythromycin inhibits protein synthesis of the pathogen without directly affecting nucleic acid synthesis. Antagonism has been demonstrated between clindamycin and erythromycin.

NOTE: Many strains of *Hemophilus influenzae* are resistant to erythromycin alone, but are susceptible to erythromycin and sulfonamides together. Staphylococci resistant to erythromycin may emerge during a course of erythromycin therapy. Culture and susceptibility testing should be performed.

Disc Susceptibility Tests: Quantitative methods that require measurement of zone diameters give the most precise estimates of antibiotic susceptibility. One recommended procedure (21 CFR section 460.1) uses erythromycin class discs for testing susceptibility; interpretations correlate zone diameters of this disc test with MIC values for erythromycin. With this procedure, a report from the laboratory of "susceptible" indicates that the infecting organism is likely to respond to therapy. A report of "resistant" indicates that the infective organism is not likely to respond to therapy. A report of "intermediate susceptibility" suggests that the organism would be susceptible if higher doses were used.

Clinical Pharmacology: Erythromycin binds to the 50 S ribosomal subunits of susceptible bacteria and suppresses protein synthesis.

Orally administered erythromycin ethylsuccinate suspensions and Filmtab tablets are readily and reliably absorbed. Erythromycin ethylsuccinate chewable tablets are readily and reliably absorbed when chewed. Comparable serum levels of erythromycin are achieved in the fasting and nonfasting states.

Continued on next page

If desired, additional literature on any Abbott Product will be provided upon request to Abbott Laboratories.

Abbott—Cont.

Erythromycin diffuses readily into most body fluids. Only low concentrations are normally achieved in the spinal fluid, but passage of the drug across the blood-brain barrier increases in meningitis. In the presence of normal hepatic function, erythromycin is concentrated in the liver and excreted in the bile; the effect of hepatic dysfunction on excretion of erythromycin by the liver into the bile is not known. Less than 5 percent of the orally administered dose of erythromycin is excreted in active form in the urine.
Erythromycin crosses the placental barrier and is excreted in breast milk.

Indications: *Streptococcus pyogenes* (Group A beta hemolytic streptococcus): Upper and lower respiratory tract, skin, and soft tissue infections of mild to moderate severity.
Injectable benzathine penicillin G is considered by the American Heart Association to be the drug of choice in the treatment and prevention of streptococcal pharyngitis and in long-term prophylaxis of rheumatic fever.
When oral medication is preferred for treatment of the above conditions, penicillin G, V, or erythromycin are alternate drugs of choice.
When oral medication is given, the importance of strict adherence by the patient to the prescribed dosage regimen must be stressed. A therapeutic dose should be administered for at least 10 days.
Alpha-hemolytic streptococci (viridans group): Although no controlled clinical efficacy trials have been conducted, oral erythromycin has been suggested by the American Heart Association and American Dental Association for use in a regimen for prophylaxis against bacterial endocarditis in patients hypersensitive to penicillin who have congenital heart disease, or rheumatic or other acquired valvular heart disease when they undergo dental procedures and surgical procedures of the upper respiratory tract.[1] Erythromycin is not suitable prior to genitourinary or gastrointestinal tract surgery. NOTE: When selecting antibiotics for the prevention of bacterial endocarditis the physician or dentist should read the full joint statement of the American Heart Association and the American Dental Association.[1]
Staphylococcus aureus: Acute infections of skin and soft tissue of mild to moderate severity. Resistant organisms may emerge during treatment.
Streptococcus pneumoniae (Diplococcus pneumoniae): Upper respiratory tract infections (e.g., otitis media, pharyngitis) and lower respiratory tract infections (e.g., pneumonia) of mild to moderate degree.
Mycoplasma pneumoniae (Eaton agent, PPLO): For respiratory infections due to this organism.
Hemophilus influenzae: For upper respiratory tract infections of mild to moderate severity when used concomitantly with adequate doses of sulfonamides. (See sulfonamide labeling for appropriate prescribing information). The concomitant use of the sulfonamides is necessary since not all strains of *Hemophilus influenzae* are susceptible to erythromycin at the concentrations of the antibiotic achieved with usual therapeutic doses.
Treponema pallidum: Erythromycin is an alternate choice of treatment for primary syphilis in patients allergic to the penicillins. In treatment of primary syphilis, spinal fluid examinations should be done before treatment and as part of follow-up after therapy.
Corynebacterium diphtheriae: As an adjunct to antitoxin, to prevent establishment of carriers, and to eradicate the organism in carriers.
Corynebacterium minutissimum: For the treatment of erythrasma.
Entamoeba histolytica: In the treatment of intestinal amebiasis only. Extraenteric amebiasis requires treatment with other agents.
Listeria monocytogenes: Infections due to this organism.
Bordetella pertussis: Erythromycin is effective in eliminating the organism from the nasopharynx of infected individuals, rendering them non-infectious. Some clinical studies suggest that erythromycin may be helpful in the prophylaxis of pertussis in exposed susceptible individuals.
Legionnaires' Disease: Although no controlled clinical efficacy studies have been conducted, *in vitro* and limited preliminary clinical data suggest that erythromycin may be effective in treating Legionnaires' Disease.

Contraindications: Erythromycin is contraindicated in patients with known hypersensitivity to this antibiotic.

Precautions: Erythromycin is principally excreted by the liver. Caution should be exercised in administering the antibiotic to patients with impaired hepatic function. There have been reports of hepatic dysfunction, with or without jaundice occurring in patients receiving oral erythromycin products.
Areas of localized infection may require surgical drainage in addition to antibiotic therapy.
Recent data from studies of erythromycin reveal that its use in patients who are receiving high doses of theophylline may be associated with an increase of serum theophylline levels and potential theophylline toxicity. In case of theophylline toxicity and/or elevated serum theophylline levels, the dose of theophylline should be reduced while the patient is receiving concomitant erythromycin therapy.

Usage during pregnancy and lactation: The safety of erythromycin for use during pregnancy has not been established.
Erythromycin crosses the placental barrier. Erythromycin also appears in breast milk.

Adverse Reactions: The most frequent side effects of erythromycin preparations are gastrointestinal, such as abdominal cramping and discomfort, and are dose related. Nausea, vomiting, and diarrhea occur infrequently with usual oral doses.
During prolonged or repeated therapy, there is a possibility of overgrowth of nonsusceptible bacteria or fungi. If such infections occur, the drug should be discontinued and appropriate therapy instituted.
Allergic reactions ranging from urticaria and mild skin eruptions to anaphylaxis have occurred.
There have been isolated reports of reversible hearing loss occurring chiefly in patients with renal insufficiency and in patients receiving high doses of erythromycin.

Dosage and Administration: Erythromycin ethylsuccinate suspensions, Filmtab tablets and chewable tablets may be administered without regard to meals. For full therapeutic effect, the chewable tablets must be chewed.
Children: Age, weight, and severity of the infection are important factors in determining the proper dosage. In mild to moderate infections the usual dosage of erythromycin ethylsuccinate for children is 30 to 50 mg/kg/day in equally divided doses. For more severe infections this dosage may be doubled.
The following dosage schedule is suggested for mild to moderate infections:

Body Weight	Total Daily Dose
Under 10 lbs	30–50 mg/kg/day 15–25 mg/lb/day
10 to 15 lbs	200 mg
16 to 25 lbs	400 mg
26 to 50 lbs	800 mg
51 to 100 lbs	1200 mg
over 100 lbs	1600 mg

Adults: 400 mg erythromycin ethylsuccinate every 6 hours is the usual dose. Dosage may be increased up to 4 g per day according to the severity of the infection.
If twice-a-day dosage is desired in either adults or children, one-half of the total daily dose may be given every 12 hours. Doses may also be given three times daily if desired by administering one-third of the total daily dose every 8 hours.
In the treatment of streptococcal infections, a therapeutic dosage of erythromycin ethylsuccinate should be administered for at least 10 days. In continuous prophylaxis against recurrences of streptococcal infections in persons with a history of rheumatic heart disease, the usual dosage is 400 mg twice a day.
For prophylaxis against bacterial endocarditis[1] in patients with congenital heart disease, or rheumatic or other acquired valvular heart disease when undergoing dental procedures or surgical procedures of the upper respiratory tract, give 1.6 g (20 mg/kg for children) orally $1\frac{1}{2}$ to 2 hours before the procedure, and then, 800 mg (10 mg/kg for children) orally every 6 hours for 8 doses.
For treatment of primary syphilis: Adults: 48 to 64 g given in divided doses over a period of 10 to 15 days.
For intestinal amebiasis: Adults: 400 mg four times daily for 10 to 14 days. Children: 30 to 50 mg/kg/day in divided doses for 10 to 14 days.
For use in pertussis: Although optimal dosage and duration have not been established, doses of erythromycin utilized in reported clinical studies were 40 to 50 mg/kg/day, given in divided doses for 5 to 14 days.
For treatment of Legionnaires' Disease: Although optimal doses have not been established, doses utilized in reported clinical data were 1.6 to 4 g daily in divided doses.

How Supplied: E.E.S. 200 LIQUID (erythromycin ethylsuccinate oral suspension, USP) is supplied in 1 pint bottles (**NDC** 0074-6306-16) and in packages of six 100-ml bottles (**NDC** 0074-6306-13). Each 5-ml teaspoonful of fruit-flavored suspension contains activity equivalent to 200 mg of erythromycin.
E.E.S. 400® LIQUID (erythromycin ethylsuccinate oral suspension, USP) is supplied in 1 pint bottles (**NDC** 0074-6373-16) and in packages of six 100-ml bottles (**NDC** 0074-6373-13). Each 5-ml teaspoonful of orange, fruit-flavored suspension contains activity equivalent to 400 mg of erythromycin.
Both liquid products require refrigeration to preserve taste until dispensed. Refrigeration by patient is not required if used within 14 days.
E.E.S. GRANULES (erythromycin ethylsuccinate for oral suspension, USP) is supplied in 60-ml (**NDC** 0074-6369-01), 100-ml (**NDC** 0074-6369-02) and 200-ml (**NDC** 0074-6369-10) size bottles. Each 5-ml teaspoonful of reconstituted cherry-flavored suspension contains activity equivalent to 200 mg of erythromycin. E.E.S. GRANULES is also available in 5-ml bottles (when reconstituted) in the ABBO-PAC® unit dose packages of 100 bottles (**NDC** 0074-6369-05).
E.E.S. DROPS (erythromycin ethylsuccinate for oral suspension, USP) is supplied in 50-ml size bottles (**NDC** 0074-6360-50). Each 2.5-ml drop-

perful (½ teaspoonful) of reconstituted cherry-flavored suspension contains activity equivalent to 100 mg of erythromycin.

E.E.S. CHEWABLE (erythromycin ethylsuccinate tablets, USP) cherry-flavored wafers containing the equivalent of 200 mg of erythromycin are available in packages of 50 (**NDC** 0074-6371-50). Each wafer is individually sealed in a blister package.

E.E.S. 400 Filmtab tablets (erythromycin ethylsuccinate tablets, USP) 400 mg, are available in bottles of 100 (**NDC** 0074-5729-13) and ABBO-PAC® unit dose strip packages of 100 (**NDC** 0074-5729-11). Tablets are pink in color.

Reference: 1. American Heart Association. 1977. Prevention of bacterial endocarditis. Circulation 56: 139A-143A.

[*Shown in Product Identification Section*]

Abbott Laboratories
North Chicago, IL 60064
Ref. 07-5219-R8

ERYTHROCIN® LACTOBIONATE-I.V. ℞

(erythromycin lactobionate for injection, USP)
For I.V. use only

Description: Erythromycin is produced by a strain of *Streptomyces erythraeus* and belongs to the macrolide group of antibiotics. It is basic and readily forms salts with acids.

ERYTHROCIN LACTOBIONATE is a soluble salt of erythromycin suitable for intravenous administration.

Actions: Microbiology: Biochemical tests demonstrate that erythromycin inhibits protein synthesis of the pathogen without directly affecting nucleic acid synthesis. Antagonism has been demonstrated between clindamycin and erythromycin.

NOTE: Many strains of *Hemophilus influenzae* are resistant to erythromycin alone, but are susceptible to erythromycin and sulfonamides together. Staphylococci resistant to erythromycin may emerge during a course of erythromycin therapy. Culture and susceptibility testing should be performed.

Disc Susceptibility Tests: Quantitative methods that require measurement of zone diameters give the most precise estimates of antibiotic susceptibility. One recommended procedure (21 CFR section 460.1) uses erythromycin class discs for testing susceptibility; interpretations correlate zone diameters of this disc test with MIC values for erythromycin. With this procedure, a report from the laboratory of "susceptible" indicates that the infecting organism is likely to respond to therapy. A report of "resistant" indicates that the infective organism is not likely to respond to therapy. A report of "intermediate susceptibility" suggests that the organism would be susceptible if higher doses were used.

Clinical Pharmacology: Erythromycin binds to the 50 S ribosomal subunits of susceptible bacteria and suppresses protein synthesis.

Intravenous infusion of 500 mg erythromycin lactobionate at a constant rate over 1 hour in fasting adults produced a mean serum erythromycin level of approximately 7 mcg/ml at 20 minutes, 10 mcg/ml at 1 hour, 2.6 mcg/ml at 2.5 hours, and 1 mcg/ml at 6 hours.

Erythromycin diffuses readily into most body fluids. Only low concentrations are normally achieved in the spinal fluid, but passage of the drug across the blood-brain barrier increases in meningitis. In the presence of normal hepatic function, erythromycin is concentrated in the liver and excreted in the bile; the effect of hepatic dysfunction on excretion of erythromycin by the liver into the bile is not known. From 12 to 15 percent of intravenously administered erythromycin is excreted in active form in the urine.

Erythromycin crosses the placental barrier and is excreted in breast milk.

Indications: ERYTHROCIN LACTOBIONATE is indicated in the treatment of patients where oral administration is not possible or where the severity of the infection requires immediate high serum levels of erythromycin. Intravenous therapy should be replaced by oral administration at the appropriate time.

Streptococcus pyogenes (Group A beta hemolytic streptococcus): Upper and lower respiratory tract, skin, and soft tissue infections of mild to moderate severity.

Injectable benzathine penicillin G is considered by the American Heart Association to be the drug of choice in the treatment and prevention of streptococcal pharyngitis and in long-term prophylaxis of rheumatic fever.

When oral medication is preferred for treatment of the above conditions, penicillin G, V, or erythromycin are alternate drugs of choice.

Staphylococcus aureus: Acute infections of skin and soft tissue of mild to moderate severity. Resistant organisms may emerge during treatment.

Streptococcus pneumoniae (*Diplococcus pneumoniae*): For upper respiratory tract infections (e.g., otitis media, pharyngitis) and lower respiratory tract infections (e.g., pneumonia) of mild to moderate severity.

Mycoplasma pneumoniae (Eaton agent, PPLO): For respiratory infections due to this organism.

Hemophilus influenzae: For upper respiratory tract infections of mild to moderate severity when used concomitantly with adequate doses of sulfonamides. (See sulfonamide labeling for appropriate prescribing information). The concomitant use of the sulfonamides is necessary since not all strains of *Hemophilus influenzae* are susceptible to erythromycin at the concentrations of the antibiotic achieved with usual therapeutic doses.

Corynebacterium diphtheriae: As an adjunct to antitoxin, to prevent the establishment of carriers, and to eradicate the organism in carriers.

Corynebacterium minutissimum: In the treatment of erythrasma.

Listeria monocytogenes: Infections due to this organism.

Neisseria gonorrhoeae: ERYTHROCIN LACTOBIONATE-I.V. in conjunction with erythromycin stearate or base orally, as an alternative drug in treatment of acute pelvic inflammatory disease caused by *N. gonorrhoeae* in female patients with a history of sensitivity to penicillin. Before treatment of gonorrhea, patients who are suspected of also having syphilis should have a microscopic examination for *T. pallidum* (by immunofluorescence or darkfield) before receiving erythromycin, and monthly serologic tests for a minimum of 4 months.

Legionnaires' Disease: Although no controlled clinical efficacy studies have been conducted, *in vitro* and limited preliminary clinical data suggest that erythromycin may be effective in treating Legionnaires' Disease.

Contraindications: Erythromycin is contraindicated in patients with known hypersensitivity to this antibiotic.

Precautions: Since erythromycin is principally excreted by the liver, caution should be exercised when erythromycin is administered to patients with impaired hepatic function.

Prolonged or repeated use of erythromycin may result in an overgrowth of non-susceptible bacteria or fungi. If superinfection occurs, erythromycin should be discontinued and appropriate therapy instituted.

Areas of localized infection may require surgical drainage in addition to antibiotic therapy.

Recent data from studies of erythromycin reveal that its use in patients who are receiving high doses of theophylline may be associated with an increase of serum theophylline levels and potential theophylline toxicity. In case of theophylline toxicity and/or elevated serum theophylline levels, the dose of theophylline should be reduced while the patient is receiving concomitant erythromycin therapy.

Usage during pregnancy and lactation: The safety of erythromycin for use during pregnancy has not been established.

Erythromycin crosses the placental barrier. Erythromycin also appears in breast milk.

Adverse Reactions: Side effects following the use of intravenous erythromycin are rare. Occasional venous irritation has been encountered, but if the infusion is given slowly, in dilute solution, preferably by continuous intravenous infusion or intermittent infusion in no less than 20 to 60 minutes, pain and vessel trauma are minimized.

Allergic reactions, ranging from urticaria and mild skin eruptions to anaphylaxis, have occurred with intravenously administered erythromycin.

Reversible hearing loss associated with the intravenous infusion of 4 g or more per day of erythromycin lactobionate has been reported rarely.

Dosage and Administration: For the treatment of severe infections in adults and children, the recommended intravenous dose of erythromycin lactobionate is 15 to 20 mg/kg/day. Higher doses, up to 4 g/day, may be given for very severe infections. ERYTHROCIN LACTOBIONATE-I.V. must be administered by continuous or intermittent intravenous infusion only. Due to the irritative properties of erythromycin, I.V. push is an unacceptable route of administration.

Continuous infusion of erythromycin lactobionate is preferable due to the slower infusion rate and lower concentration of erythromycin; however, intermittent infusion at intervals not greater than every six hours is also effective. Intravenous erythromycin should be replaced by oral erythromycin as soon as possible.

For slow continuous infusion: The final diluted solution of erythromycin lactobionate is prepared to give a concentration of 1 g per liter (1 mg/ml).

For intermittent infusion: Administer one-fourth the total daily dose of erythromycin lactobionate by intravenous infusion in 20 to 60 minutes at intervals not greater than every six hours. The final diluted solution of erythromycin lactobionate is prepared to give a concentration of 1 to 5 mg/ml. No less than 100 ml of I.V. diluent should be used. Infusion should be sufficiently slow to minimize pain along the vein.

For treatment of acute pelvic inflammatory disease caused by *N. gonorrhoeae,* in female patients hypersensitive to penicillins, administer 500 mg erythromycin lactobionate every six hours for three days, followed by oral administration of 250 mg erythromycin stearate or base every six hours for seven days.

For treatment of Legionnaires' Disease: Although optimal doses have not been established, doses utilized in reported clinical data were 1 to 4 grams daily in divided doses.

Preparation of Solution:

1. PREPARE THE INITIAL SOLUTION OF ERYTHROCIN® LACTOBIONATE-I.V. BY ADDING 10 ML OF STERILE WATER FOR INJECTION, USP, TO THE 500 MG VIAL OR 20 ML OF STERILE WATER FOR INJECTION, USP, TO THE 1 G VIAL. Use only Sterile Water for Injection, USP, as other diluents may cause precipitation during reconstitution. Do not use diluents containing preservatives or inorganic salts. Note: When the product is reconstituted as directed above, the resulting solution contains an effective microbial preservative.

After reconstitution, each ml contains 50 mg of erythromycin activity. The initial solution is

Continued on next page

If desired, additional literature on any Abbott Product will be provided upon request to Abbott Laboratories.

Abbott—Cont.

stable at refrigerator temperature for two weeks, or for 24 hours at room temperature.

2. ADD THE INITIAL DILUTION TO ONE OF THE FOLLOWING DILUENTS BEFORE ADMINISTRATION to give a concentration of 1 g of erythromycin activity per liter (1 mg/ml) for continuous infusion or 1 to 5 mg/ml for intermittent infusion:

0.9% SODIUM CHLORIDE INJECTION, USP
LACTATED RINGER'S INJECTION, USP
NORMOSOL®-R

3. THE FOLLOWING SOLUTIONS MAY ALSO BE USED PROVIDING THEY ARE FIRST BUFFERED WITH NEUT® (4% SODIUM BICARBONATE, ABBOTT) by adding 1 ml of Neut per 100 ml of solution:

5% DEXTROSE INJECTION, USP
5% DEXTROSE AND LACTATED RINGER'S INJECTION
5% DEXTROSE AND 0.9% SODIUM CHLORIDE INJECTION, USP

Neut® (4% sodium bicarbonate, Abbott) must be added to these solutions so that their pH is in the optimum range for erythromycin lactobionate stability. Acidic solutions of erythromycin lactobionate are unstable and lose their potency rapidly. A pH of at least 5.5 is desirable for the final diluted solution of erythromycin lactobionate.

No drug or chemical agent should be added to an erythromycin lactobionate-I.V. fluid admixture unless its effect on the chemical and physical stability of the solution has first been determined.

Stability: The final diluted solution of erythromycin lactobionate should be completely administered within 8 hours, since it is not suitable for storage.*

How Supplied: ERYTHROCIN LACTOBIONATE-I.V. (erythromycin lactobionate for injection, USP) is supplied as a sterile, lyophilized powder in packages of 5 vials (**NDC** 0074-6342-05), each vial containing the equivalent of 1 g of erythromycin with 180 mg benzyl alcohol added as preservative; and in packages of 5 vials (**NDC** 0074-6365-02), each vial containing the equivalent of 500 mg of erythromycin with 90 mg benzyl alcohol added as preservative.

*Contact Abbott Laboratories, Dept. 498 for additional stability data.

Abbott Laboratories
North Chicago, IL 60064
Ref. 01-2163-R13

ERYTHROCIN® PIGGYBACK ℞

(erythromycin lactobionate for injection, USP)
Single Dose Dispensing Vial
For I.V. use only

Description: Erythromycin is produced by a strain of *Streptomyces erythraeus* and belongs to the macrolide group of antibiotics. It is basic and readily forms salts with acids.

Erythromycin lactobionate is a soluble salt of erthromycin. ERYTHROCIN PIGGYBACK is a dosage form suitable for intermittent intravenous administration.

Actions: Microbiology: Biochemical tests demonstrate that erythromycin inhibits protein synthesis of the pathogen without directly affecting nucleic acid synthesis. Antagonism has been demonstrated between clindamycin and erythromycin.

NOTE: Many strains of *Hemophilus influenzae* are resistant to erythromycin alone, but are susceptible to erythromycin and sulfonamides together. Staphylococci resistant to erythromycin may emerge during a course of erythromycin therapy. Culture and susceptibility testing should be performed.

Disc Susceptibility Tests: Quantitative methods that require measurement of zone diameters give the most precise estimates of antibiotic susceptibility. One recommended procedure (21 CFR section 460.1) uses erythromycin class discs for testing susceptibility; interpretations correlate zone diameters of this disc test with MIC values for erythromycin. With this procedure, a report from the laboratory of "susceptible" indicates that the infecting organism is likely to respond to therapy. A report of "resistant" indicates that the infective organism is not likely to respond to therapy. A report of "intermediate susceptibility" suggests that the organism would be susceptible if higher doses were used.

Clinical Pharmacology: Erythromycin binds to the 50 S ribosomal subunits of susceptible bacteria and suppresses protein synthesis.

Intravenous infusion of 500 mg erythromycin lactobionate at a constant rate over 1 hour in fasting adults produced a mean serum erythromycin level of approximately 7 mcg/ml at 20 minutes, 10 mcg/ml at 1 hour, 2.6 mcg/ml at 2.5 hours, and 1 mcg/ml at 6 hours.

Erythromycin diffuses readily into most body fluids. Only low concentrations are normally achieved in the spinal fluid, but passage of the drug across the blood-brain barrier increases in meningitis. In the presence of normal hepatic function, erythromycin is concentrated in the liver and excreted in the bile; the effect of hepatic dysfunction on excretion of erythromycin by the liver into the bile is not known. From 12 to 15 percent of intravenously administered erythromycin is excreted in active form in the urine.

Erythromycin crosses the placental barrier and is excreted in breast milk.

Indications: ERYTHROCIN PIGGYBACK is indicated in the treatment of patients where oral administration is not possible or where the severity of the infection requires immediate high serum levels of erythromycin. Intravenous therapy should be replaced by oral administration at the appropriate time.

Steptococcus pyogenes (Group A beta hemolytic streptococcus): Upper and lower respiratory tract, skin, and soft tissue infections of mild to moderate severity.

Injectable benzathine penicillin G is considered by the American Heart Association to be the drug of choice in the treatment and prevention of streptococcal pharyngitis and in long-term prophylaxis of rheumatic fever.

When oral medication is preferred for treatment of the above conditions, penicillin G, V, or erythromycin are alternate drugs of choice.

Staphylococcus aureus: Acute infections of skin and soft tissue of mild to moderate severity. Resistant organisms may emerge during treatment.

Streptococcus pneumoniae (Diplococcus pneumoniae): For upper respiratory tract infections (e.g., otitis media, pharyngitis) and lower respiratory tract infections (e.g., pneumonia) of mild to moderate severity.

Mycoplasma pneumoniae (Eaton agent, PPLO): For respiratory infections due to this organism.

Hemophilus influenzae: For upper respiratory tract infections of mild to moderate severity when used concomitantly with adequate doses of sulfonamides. (See sulfonamide labeling for appropriate prescribing information). The concomitant use of the sulfonamides is necessary since not all strains of *Hemophilus influenzae* are susceptible to erythromycin at the concentrations of the antibiotic achieved with usual therapeutic doses.

Corynebacterium diphtheriae: As an adjunct to antitoxin, to prevent the establishment of carriers, and to eradicate the organism in carriers.

Corynebacterium minutissimum: In the treatment of erythrasma.

Listeria monocytogenes: Infections due to this organism.

Neisseria gonorrhoeae: ERYTHROCIN PIGGYBACK in conjunction with erythromycin stearate or base orally, as an alternative drug in treatment of acute pelvic inflammatory disease caused by *N. gonorrhoeae* in female patients with a history of sensitivity to penicillin. Before treatment of gonorrhea, patients who are suspected of also having syphilis should have a microscopic examination for *T. pallidum* (by immunofluorescence or darkfield) before receiving erythromycin, and monthly serologic tests for a minimum of 4 months.

Legionnaires' Disease: Although no controlled clinical efficacy studies have been conducted, *in vitro* and limited preliminary clinical data suggest that erythromycin may be effective in treating Legionnaires' Disease.

Contraindications: Erythromycin is contraindicated in patients with known hypersensitivity to this antibiotic.

Precautions: Since erythromycin is principally excreted by the liver, caution should be exercised when erythromycin is administered to patients with impaired hepatic function.

Prolonged or repeated use of erythromycin may result in an overgrowth of nonsusceptible bacteria or fungi. If superinfection occurs, erythromycin should be discontinued and appropriate therapy instituted.

Areas of localized infection may require surgical drainage in addition to antibiotic therapy.

Recent data from studies of erythromycin reveal that its use in patients who are receiving high doses of theophylline may be associated with an increase of serum theophylline levels and potential theophylline toxicity. In case of theophylline toxicity and/or elevated serum theophylline levels, the dose of theophylline should be reduced while the patient is receiving concomitant erythromycin therapy.

Usage during pregnancy and lactation: The safety of erythromycin for use during pregnancy has not been established.

Erythromycin crosses the placental barrier. Erythromycin also appears in breast milk.

Adverse Reactions: Side effects following the use of intravenous erythromycin are rare. Occasional venous irritation has been encountered.

Allergic reactions, ranging from urticaria and mild skin eruptions to anaphylaxis, have occurred with intravenously administered erythromycin.

Reversible hearing loss associated with the intravenous infusion of 4 g or more per day of erythromycin lactobionate has been reported rarely.

Dosage and Administration: For the treatment of severe infections in adults and children, the recommended intravenous dose of erythromycin lactobionate is 15 to 20 mg/kg/day. Higher doses, up to 4 g/day, may be given for very severe infections. ERYTHROCIN PIGGYBACK should be administered by intravenous infusion. Due to the high concentration of erythromycin, I.V. push is not an acceptable route of administration. Intravenous erythromycin should be replaced by oral erythromycin as soon as possible.

After reconstitution each ml of ERYTHROCIN PIGGYBACK solution contains 5 mg of erythromycin activity (500 mg in 100 ml). The drug may be administered directly from the vial. When this preparation is administered by intermittent infusion one-fourth the total daily dose of erythromycin lactobionate should be administered over a 20 to 60 minute period at intervals not greater than every 6 hours. The infusion should be sufficiently slow to minimize pain along the vein.

For treatment of acute pelvic inflammatory disease caused by *N. gonorrhoeae*, in female patients hypersensitive to penicillins, administer 500 mg erythromycin lactobionate every 6 hours for 3 days, followed by oral administration of 250 mg erythromycin stearate or base every 6 hours for 7 days.

For treatment of Legionnaires' Disease: Although optimal doses have not been established, doses utilized in reported clinical data were 1 to 4 grams daily in divided doses.

Preparation of Solution: Prepare the ERYTHROCIN PIGGYBACK solution by adding 100 ml of

0.9% Sodium Chloride Injection, USP, or Lactated Ringer's Injection, USP, or Normosol®-R Solution to the dispensing vial. Immediately after adding diluent, the product should be shaken well to aid dissolution. Lack of immediate agitation will greatly increase time required for complete dissolution. Reconstitution may also be made using 100 ml of the following solutions to which 1 ml of Neut® (4% sodium bicarbonate, Abbott) has first been added:

5% Dextrose Injection, USP
5% Dextrose and Lactated Ringer's Injection
5% Dextrose and 0.9% Sodium Chloride Injection, USP
Normosol®-M and 5% Dextrose Injection
Normosol®-R and 5% Dextrose Injection

Neut® (4% sodium bicarbonate, Abbott) must be added to these solutions so that their pH is in the optimum range for erythromycin lactobionate stability. Acidic solutions of erythromycin lactobionate are unstable and lose their potency rapidly. A pH of at least 5.5 is desirable.

No drug or chemical agent should be added to an erythromycin lactobionate-I.V. fluid admixture unless its effect on the chemical and physical stability of the solution has first been determined.

Stability: The solution should be used within 8 hours if stored at room temperature and 24 hours if stored in the refrigerator. If the solution is to be frozen, it should be frozen (−10°C to −20°C) within 4 hours of preparation. Frozen solution may be stored for 30 days. Frozen solution should be thawed in the refrigerator and used within 8 hours after thawing is completed. THAWED SOLUTION MUST NOT BE REFROZEN.

How Supplied: ERYTHROCIN PIGGYBACK (erythromycin lactobionate for injection, USP) is supplied as a sterile, lyophilized powder in packages of 5 single dose dispensing vials (**NDC** 0074-6368-13). Each vial contains the equivalent of 500 mg of erythromycin with 90 mg of benzyl alcohol.

[*Shown in Product Identification Section*]
Abbott Laboratories
North Chicago, IL 60064
Ref. 01-2161-R4

ERYTHROCIN® STEARATE ℞
(erythromycin stearate tablets, USP)
Filmtab® Tablets

Description: Erythromycin is produced by a strain of *Streptomyces erythraeus* and belongs to the macrolide group of antibiotics. It is basic and readily forms salts with acids. The base, the stearate salt, and the esters are poorly soluble in water, and are suitable for oral administration.

ERYTHROCIN STEARATE Filmtab tablets contain the stearate salt of the antibiotic in a unique film coating.

Actions: Microbiology: Biochemical tests demonstrate that erythromycin inhibits protein synthesis of the pathogen without directly affecting nucleic acid synthesis. Antagonism has been demonstrated between clindamycin and erythromycin.

NOTE: Many strains of *Hemophilus influenzae* are resistant to erythromycin alone, but are susceptible to erythromycin and sulfonamides together. Staphylococci resistant to erythromycin may emerge during a course of erythromycin therapy. Culture and susceptibility testing should be performed.

Disc Susceptibility Tests: Quantitative methods that require measurement of zone diameters give the most precise estimates of antibiotic susceptibility. One recommended procedure (21 CFR section 460.1) uses erythromycin class discs for testing susceptibility; interpretations correlate zone diameters of this disc test with MIC values for erythromycin. With this procedure, a report from the laboratory of "susceptible" indicates that the infecting organism is likely to respond to therapy. A report of "resistant" indicates that the infective organism is not likely to respond to therapy. A report of "intermediate susceptibility" suggests that the organism would be susceptible if higher doses were used.

Clinical Pharmacology: Erythromycin binds to the 50 S ribosomal subunits of susceptible bacteria and suppresses protein synthesis.

Orally administered ERYTHROCIN STEARATE tablets are readily and reliably absorbed. Optimal serum levels of erythromycin are reached when the drug is taken in the fasting state or immediately before meals.

Erythromycin diffuses readily into most body fluids. Only low concentrations are normally achieved in the spinal fluid, but passage of the drug across the blood-brain barrier increases in meningitis. In the presence of normal hepatic function, erythromycin is concentrated in the liver and excreted in the bile; the effect of hepatic dysfunction on excretion of erythromycin by the liver into the bile is not known. Less than 5 percent of the orally administered dose of erythromycin is excreted in active form in the urine.

Erythromycin crosses the placental barrier and is excreted in breast milk.

Indications: *Streptococcus pyogenes* (Group A beta hemolytic streptococcus): Upper and lower respiratory tract, skin, and soft tissue infections of mild to moderate severity.

Injectable benzathine penicillin G is considered by the American Heart Association to be the drug of choice in the treatment and prevention of streptococcal pharyngitis and in long-term prophylaxis of rheumatic fever.

When oral medication is preferred for treatment of the above conditions, penicillin G, V, or erythromycin are alternate drugs of choice.

When oral medication is given, the importance of strict adherence by the patient to the prescribed dosage regimen must be stressed. A therapeutic dose should be administered for at least 10 days.

Alpha-hemolytic streptococci (viridans group): Although no controlled clinical efficacy trials have been conducted, oral erythromycin has been suggested by the American Heart Association and American Dental Association for use in a regimen for prophylaxis against bacterial endocarditis in patients hypersensitive to penicillin who have congenital heart disease, or rheumatic or other acquired valvular heart disease when they undergo dental procedures and surgical procedures of the upper respiratory tract.[1] Erythromycin is not suitable prior to genitourinary or gastrointestinal tract surgery. NOTE: When selecting antibiotics for the prevention of bacterial endocarditis the physician or dentist should read the full joint statement of the American Heart Association and the American Dental Association.[1]

Staphylococcus aureus: Acute infections of skin and soft tissue of mild to moderate severity. Resistant organisms may emerge during treatment.

Streptococcus pneumoniae (Diplococcus pneumoniae): Upper respiratory tract infections (e.g., otitis media, pharyngitis) and lower respiratory tract infections (e.g., pneumonia) of mild to moderate degree.

Mycoplasma pneumoniae (Eaton agent, PPLO): For respiratory infections due to this organism.

Hemophilus influenzae: For upper respiratory tract infections of mild to moderate severity when used concomitantly with adequate doses of sulfonamides. (See sulfonamide labeling for appropriate prescribing information). The concomitant use of the sulfonamides is necessary since not all strains of *Hemophilus influenzae* are susceptible to erythromycin at the concentrations of the antibiotic achieved with usual therapeutic doses.

Treponema pallidum: Erythromycin is an alternate choice of treatment for primary syphilis in patients allergic to the penicillins. In treatment of primary syphilis, spinal fluid examinations should be done before treatment and as part of follow-up after therapy.

Corynebacterium diphtheriae: As an adjunct to antitoxin, to prevent establishment of carriers, and to eradicate the organism in carriers.

Corynebacterium minutissimum: For the treatment of erythrasma.

Entamoeba histolytica: In the treatment of intestinal amebiasis only. Extra-enteric amebiasis requires treatment with other agents.

Listeria monocytogenes: Infections due to this organism.

Neisseria gonorrhoeae: Erythrocin Lactobionate-I.V. (erythromycin lactobionate for injection) in conjunction with erythromycin stearate orally, as an alternative drug in treatment of acute pelvic inflammatory disease caused by *N. gonorrhoeae* in female patients with a history of sensitivity to penicillin. Before treatment of gonorrhea, patients who are suspected of also having syphilis should have a microscopic examination for *T. pallidum* (by immunofluorescence or darkfield) before receiving erythromycin, and monthly serologic tests for a minimum of 4 months.

Bordetella pertussis: Erythromycin is effective in eliminating the organism from the nasopharynx of infected individuals, rendering them non-infectious. Some clinical studies suggest that erythromycin may be helpful in the prophylaxis of pertussis in exposed susceptible individuals.

Legionnaires' Disease: Although no controlled clinical efficacy studies have been conducted, *in vitro* and limited preliminary clinical data suggest that erythromycin may be effective in treating Legionnaires' Disease.

Contraindications: Erythromycin is contraindicated in patients with known hypersensitivity to this antibiotic.

Precautions: Erythromycin is principally excreted by the liver. Caution should be exercised in administering the antibiotic to patients with impaired hepatic function. There have been reports of hepatic dysfunction, with or without jaundice occurring in patients receiving oral erythromycin products.

Areas of localized infection may require surgical drainage in addition to antibiotic therapy.

Recent data from studies of erythromycin reveal that its use in patients who are receiving high doses of theophylline may be associated with an increase of serum theophylline levels and potential theophylline toxicity. In case of theophylline toxicity and/or elevated serum theophylline levels, the dose of theophylline should be reduced while the patient is receiving concomitant erythromycin therapy.

Usage during pregnancy and lactation: The safety of erythromycin for use during pregnancy has not been established.

Erythromycin crosses the placental barrier. Erythromycin also appears in breast milk.

Adverse Reactions: The most frequent side effects of oral erythromycin preparations are gastrointestinal, such as abdominal cramping and discomfort, and are dose-related. Nausea, vomiting, and diarrhea occur infrequently with usual oral doses.

During prolonged or repeated therapy, there is a possibility of overgrowth of nonsusceptible bacteria or fungi. If such infections occur, the drug should be discontinued and appropriate therapy instituted.

Allergic reactions ranging from urticaria and mild skin eruptions to anaphylaxis have occurred.

There have been isolated reports of reversible hearing loss occurring chiefly in patients with

Continued on next page

If desired, additional literature on any Abbott Product will be provided upon request to Abbott Laboratories.

Abbott—Cont.

renal insufficiency and in patients receiving high doses of erythromycin.

Dosage and Administration: Optimal serum levels of erythromycin are reached when ERYTHROCIN STEARATE (erythromycin stearate) is taken in the fasting state or immediately before meals.

Adults: The usual dosage is 250 mg every 6 hours; or 500 mg every 12 hours, taken in the fasting state or immediately before meals. Up to 4 g per day may be administered, depending upon the severity of the infection.

Children: Age, weight, and severity of the infection are important factors in determining the proper dosage. For the treatment of mild to moderate infections, the usual dosage is 30 to 50 mg/kg/day in 3 or 4 divided doses. When dosage is desired on a twice-a-day schedule, one-half of the total daily dose may be taken every 12 hours in the fasting state or immediately before meals. For the treatment of more severe infections the total daily dose may be doubled.

In the treatment of streptococcal infections, a therapeutic dosage of erythromycin should be administered for at least 10 days. In continuous prophylaxis of streptococcal infections in persons with a history of rheumatic heart disease, the dose is 250 mg twice a day.

For prophylaxis against bacterial endocarditis[1] in patients with congenital heart disease, or rheumatic or other acquired valvular heart disease when undergoing dental procedures or surgical procedures of the upper respiratory tract, give 1 g (20 mg/kg for children) orally 1½ to 2 hours before the procedure, and then, 500 mg (10 mg/kg for children) orally every 6 hours for 8 doses.

For treatment of primary syphilis: 30 to 40 g given in divided doses over a period of 10 to 15 days.

For treatment of acute pelvic inflammatory disease caused by *N. gonorrhoeae:* 500 mg Erythrocin Lactobionate-I.V. (erythromycin lactobionate for injection) every 6 hours for 3 days, followed by 250 mg ERYTHROCIN STEARATE every 6 hours for 7 days.

For intestinal amebiasis: Adults: 250 mg four times daily for 10 to 14 days. Children: 30 to 50 mg/kg/day in divided doses for 10 to 14 days.

For use in pertussis: Although optimal dosage and duration have not been established, doses of erythromycin utilized in reported clinical studies were 40 to 50 mg/kg/day, given in divided doses for 5 to 14 days.

For treatment of Legionnaires' Disease: Although optimal doses have not been established, doses utilized in reported clinical data were 1 to 4 g daily in divided doses.

How Supplied: ERYTHROCIN STEARATE Filmtab Tablets (erythromycin stearate tablets, USP) are supplied as:

Erythrocin Stearate Filmtab, 250 mg
Bottles of 20 ....(**NDC** 0074-6346-23)
Bottles of 100 ....(**NDC** 0074-6346-20)
Bottles of 500 ....(**NDC** 0074-6346-53)
ABBO-PAC® unit dose strip packages of
100 tablets ....(**NDC** 0074-6346-38)

Erythrocin Stearate Filmtab, 500 mg
Bottles of 100 ....(**NDC** 0074-6316-13)

Reference: 1. American Heart Association. 1977. Prevention of bacterial endocarditis. Circulation 56: 139A-143A.

[*Shown in Product Identification Section*]

Abbott Laboratories
North Chicago, IL 60064
Ref. 07-5220-R6

ERYTHROMYCIN BASE FILMTAB® ℞
(Erythromycin Tablets, USP)

Description: Erythromycin is produced by a strain of *Streptomyces erythraeus* and belongs to the macrolide group of antibiotics. It is basic and readily forms salts with acids. The base, the stearate salt, and the esters are poorly soluble in water, and are suitable for oral administration.

ERYTHROMYCIN BASE FILMTAB tablets contain erythromycin, USP, in a unique, nonenteric film coating.

Actions: Microbiology: Biochemical tests demonstrate that erythromycin inhibits protein synthesis of the pathogen without directly affecting nucleic acid synthesis. Antagonism has been demonstrated between clindamycin and erythromycin.

NOTE: Many strains of *Hemophilus influenzae* are resistant to erythromycin alone, but are susceptible to erythromycin and sulfonamides together. Staphylococci resistant to erythromycin may emerge during a course of erythromycin therapy. Culture and susceptibility testing should be performed.

Disc Susceptibility Tests: Quantitative methods that require measurement of zone diameters give the most precise estimates of antibiotic susceptibility. One recommended procedure (21 CFR section 460.1) uses erythromycin class discs for testing susceptibility; interpretations correlate zone diameters of this disc test with MIC values for erythromycin. With this procedure, a report from the laboratory of "susceptible" indicates that the infecting organism is likely to respond to therapy. A report of "resistant" indicates that the infective organism is not likely to respond to therapy. A report of "intermediate susceptibility" suggests that the organism would be susceptible if higher doses were used.

Clinical Pharmacology: Erythromycin binds to the 50 S ribosomal subunits of susceptible bacteria and suppresses protein synthesis.

Orally administered erythromycin is readily absorbed by most patients, especially on an empty stomach, but patient variation is observed. Due to its formulation and nonenteric coating, this erythromycin tablet gives reliable blood levels in the average subject; however, the levels may vary with the individual.

Erythromycin diffuses readily into most body fluids. Only low concentrations are normally achieved in the spinal fluid, but passage of the drug across the blood-brain barrier increases in meningitis. In the presence of normal hepatic function, erythromycin is concentrated in the liver and excreted in the bile; the effect of hepatic dysfunction on excretion of erythromycin by the liver into the bile is not known. Less than 5 percent of the orally administered dose of erythromycin is excreted in active form in the urine.

Erythromycin crosses the placental barrier and is excreted in breast milk.

Indications: *Streptococcus pyogenes* (Group A beta hemolytic streptococcus): Upper and lower respiratory tract, skin, and soft tissue infections of mild to moderate severity.

Injectable benzathine penicillin G is considered by the American Heart Association to be the drug of choice in the treatment and prevention of streptococcal pharyngitis and in long-term prophylaxis of rheumatic fever.

When oral medication is preferred for treatment of the above conditions, penicillin G, V, or erythromycin are alternate drugs of choice.

When oral medication is given, the importance of strict adherence by the patient to the prescribed dosage regimen must be stressed. A therapeutic dose should be administered for at least 10 days.

Alpha-hemolytic streptococci (viridans group): Although no controlled clinical efficacy trials have been conducted, oral erythromycin has been suggested by the American Heart Association and American Dental Association for use in a regimen for prophylaxis against bacterial endocarditis in patients hypersensitive to penicillin who have congenital heart disease, or rheumatic or other acquired valvular heart disease when they undergo dental procedures and surgical procedures of the upper respiratory tract.[1] Erythromycin is not suitable prior to genitourinary or gastrointestinal tract surgery. NOTE: When selecting antibiotics for the prevention of bacterial endocarditis the physician or dentist should read the full joint statement of the American Heart Association and the American Dental Association.[1]

Staphylococcus aureus: Acute infections of skin and soft tissue of mild to moderate severity. Resistant organisms may emerge during treatment.

Streptococcus pneumoniae (Diplococcus pneumoniae): Upper respiratory tract infections (e.g., otitis media, pharyngitis) and lower respiratory tract infections (e.g., pneumonia) of mild to moderate degree.

Mycoplasma pneumoniae (Eaton agent, PPLO): For respiratory infections due to this organism.

Hemophilus influenzae: For upper respiratory tract infections of mild to moderate severity when used concomitantly with adequate doses of sulfonamides. (See sulfonamide labeling for appropriate prescribing information). The concomitant use of the sulfonamides is necessary since not all strains of *Hemophilus influenzae* are susceptible to erythromycin at the concentrations of the antibiotic achieved with usual therapeutic doses.

Treponema pallidum: Erythromycin is an alternate choice of treatment for primary syphilis in patients allergic to the penicillins. In treatment of primary syphilis, spinal fluid examinations should be done before treatment and as part of follow-up after therapy.

Corynebacterium diphtheriae: As an adjunct to antitoxin, to prevent establishment of carriers, and to eradicate the organism in carriers.

Corynebacterium minutissimum: For the treatment of erythrasma.

Entamoeba histolytica: In the treatment of intestinal amebiasis only. Extra-enteric amebiasis requires treatment with other agents.

Listeria monocytogenes: Infections due to this organism.

Neisseria gonorrhoeae: Erythrocin® Lactobionate-I.V. (erythromycin lactobionate for injection) in conjunction with erythromycin base orally, as an alternative drug in treatment of acute pelvic inflammatory disease caused by *N. gonorrhoeae* in female patients with a history of sensitivity to penicillin. Before treatment of gonorrhea, patients who are suspected of also having syphilis should have a microscopic examination for *T. pallidum* (by immunofluorescence or darkfield) before receiving erythromycin, and monthly serologic tests for a minimum of 4 months.

Bordetella pertussis: Erythromycin is effective in eliminating the organism from the nasopharynx of infected individuals, rendering them non-infectious. Some clinical studies suggest that erythromycin may be helpful in the prophylaxis of pertussis in exposed susceptible individuals.

Legionnaires' Disease: Although no controlled clinical efficacy studies have been conducted, *in vitro* and limited preliminary clinical data suggest that erythromycin may be effective in treating Legionnaires' Disease.

Contraindications: Erythromycin is contraindicated in patients with known hypersensitivity to this antibiotic.

Precautions: Erythromycin is principally excreted by the liver. Caution should be exercised in administering the antibiotic to patients with impaired hepatic function. There have been reports of hepatic dysfunction, with or without jaundice occurring in patients receiving oral erythromycin products.

Areas of localized infection may require surgical drainage in addition to antibiotic therapy.

Recent data from studies of erythromycin reveal that its use in patients who are receiving high doses of theophylline may be associated with an increase of serum theophylline levels and potential theophylline toxicity. In case of theophylline toxicity and/or elevated serum theophylline levels, the dose of theophylline should be reduced while the patient is receiving concomitant erythromycin therapy.

Usage during pregnancy and lactation: The safety of erythromycin for use during pregnancy has not been established.

Erythromycin crosses the placental barrier. Erythromycin also appears in breast milk.

Adverse Reactions: The most frequent side effects of oral erythromycin preparations are gastrointestinal, such as abdominal cramping and discomfort, and are dose-related. Nausea, vomiting, and diarrhea occur infrequently with usual oral doses.

During prolonged or repeated therapy, there is a possibility of overgrowth of nonsusceptible bacteria or fungi. If such infections occur, the drug should be discontinued and appropriate therapy instituted.

Allergic reactions ranging from urticaria and mild skin eruptions to anaphylaxis have occurred.

There have been isolated reports of reversible hearing loss occurring chiefly in patients with renal insufficiency and in patients receiving high doses of erythromycin.

Dosage and Administration: Optimum blood levels are obtained when doses are given on an empty stomach.

Adults: 250 mg every 6 hours is the usual dose; or 500 mg every 12 hours one hour before meals. Dosage may be increased up to 4 g per day according to the severity of the infection.

Children: Age, weight, and severity of the infection are important factors in determining the proper dosage. 30 to 50 mg/kg/day, in divided doses, is the usual dose. For more severe infections this dose may be doubled. If dosage is desired on a twice-a-day schedule, one-half of the total daily dose may be given every 12 hours, one hour before meals.

For the treatment of streptococcal infections: a therapeutic dosage should be administered for at least 10 days. In continuous prophylaxis of streptococcal infections in persons with rheumatic heart disease history, the dose is 250 mg twice a day.

For prophylaxis against bacterial endocarditis[1] in patients with congenital heart disease, or rheumatic or other acquired valvular heart disease when undergoing dental procedures or surgical procedures of the upper respiratory tract, give 1 g (20 mg/kg for children) orally 1½ to 2 hours before the procedure, and then, 500 mg (10 mg/kg for children) orally every 6 hours for 8 doses.

For treatment of primary syphilis: 30 to 40 g given in divided doses over a period of 10 to 15 days.

For treatment of acute pelvic inflammatory disease caused by *N. gonorrhoeae:* 500 mg Erythrocin Lactobionate-I.V. (erythromycin lactobionate for injection) every 6 hours for 3 days, followed by 250 mg erythromycin base every 6 hours for 7 days.

For intestinal amebiasis: Adults: 250 mg four times daily for 10 to 14 days. Children: 30 to 50 mg/kg/day in divided doses for 10 to 14 days.

For use in pertussis: Although optimal dosage and duration have not been established, doses of erythromycin utilized in reported clinical studies were 40 to 50 mg/kg/day, given in divided doses for 5 to 14 days.

For treatment of Legionnaires' Disease: Although optimal doses have not been established, doses utilized in reported clinical data were 1 to 4 g daily in divided doses.

How Supplied: ERYTHROMYCIN BASE FILMTAB tablets (erythromycin tablets, USP) are supplied as pink capsule-shaped tablets in two dosage strengths:

250 mg tablets:
Bottles of 100 ....(**NDC** 0074-6326-13)
ABBO-PAC® unit dose strip packages of
100 tablets ....(**NDC** 0074-6326-11)

500 mg tablets:
Bottles of 100 ....(**NDC** 0074-6227-13)

Reference: 1. American Heart Association. 1977. Prevention of bacterial endocarditis. Circulation. 56: 139A-143A.

FILMTAB—Film-sealed tablets, Abbott.
[*Shown in Product Identification Section*]
Abbott Laboratories
North Chicago, IL 60064
Ref. 01-2259-R7

EUTONYL® Filmtab® Tablets ℞
(pargyline hydrochloride tablets, USP)

Description: EUTONYL (pargyline hydrochloride) is a non-hydrazine monoamine oxidase (MAO) inhibitor with hypotensive activity and is chemically identified as N-methyl-N-2-propynylbenzylamine hydrochloride. Clinically, EUTONYL is an effective antihypertensive agent which is primarily useful in the treatment of moderate to severe hypertension.

Actions: EUTONYL (pargyline hydrochloride) is a MAO inhibitor which has a potent antihypertensive action. Its exact mode of action is uncertain. The antihypertensive effect of pargyline is greatest when the patient is in the standing position. In about half of the patients treated, reduction of blood pressure in the sitting and supine positions was nearly as great as in the standing position. An interval of four days to three weeks or more may elapse following initiation of therapy before the full therapeutic effects of a given dosage schedule become manifest. A similar interval may be required for effects to subside after withdrawal of the drug, because the termination of drug effect is dependent on the regeneration of inhibited enzymes.

In rats, about ninety percent of a given dose of pargyline is excreted in the urine within the first twenty-four hours following dosing.

Indications: EUTONYL (pargyline hydrochloride) is indicated in the treatment of moderate to severe hypertension. *It is not recommended for use in patients with mild or labile hypertension.* EUTONYL does not interfere with or obviate the use of diuretic therapy in hypertensive patients who may have an associated edema. EUTONYL may be used alone or concurrently with most other antihypertensive agents. It is often effective at reduced dosage when administered with one of the thiazides and/or rauwolfia alkaloids.

Contraindications:

1. EUTONYL (pargyline hydrochloride) is contraindicated in patients with pheochromocytoma, paranoid schizophrenia, hyperthyroidism, and advanced renal failure.
2. EUTONYL should not be administered to those with malignant hypertension or to children under twelve years of age because significant clinical information concerning the use of the drug in these conditions is not available.
3. In general, the following drugs or agents are contraindicated in patients receiving EUTONYL (pargyline hydrochloride):

a. Centrally acting sympathomimetic amines such as amphetamine and related compounds (includes most anorectic agents).

Peripherally acting sympathomimetic drugs such as ephedrine and its derivatives (also found in nasal decongestants, cold remedies, and hay fever preparations).

b. Aged cheese (e.g., Cheddar, Camembert, and Stilton), processed cheese, beer and wine (especially, Chianti wine), and other foods which require the action of bacteria or molds for their preparation or preservation because of the presence of pressor substances such as tyramine. Other foods which should be avoided during pargyline therapy because of their high pressor amine content include chocolate, yeast extract, avocado, pickled herring, pods of broad beans, ripened bananas, papaya products (including certain meat tenderizers), and chicken livers. Cream cheese, ricotta, and cottage cheese can be allowed in the diet during pargyline therapy since their tyramine content is inconsequential. In some patients receiving pargyline, tyramine may precipitate an abrupt rise in blood pressure accompanied by some or all of the following: severe headache, chest pain, profuse sweating, palpitation, tachycardia or bradycardia, visual disturbances, stertorous breathing, coma, and intracranial bleeding (which could be fatal). Phentolamine may be administered parenterally for treatment of such an acute hypertensive reaction.

c. Parenteral reserpine or guanethidine. Parenteral use of these drugs in patients receiving monoamine oxidase inhibitors results in a sudden release of accumulated catecholamines which may cause a hypertensive reaction. Reserpine and guanethidine should not be given parenterally during, and for at least one week following, treatment with pargyline.

d. Imipramine, amitriptyline, desipramine, nortriptyline, protriptyline, doxepin, or their analogues. The use of these drugs with a monoamine oxidase inhibitor has been reported to cause vascular collapse and hyperthermia which may be fatal. A drug-free interval (about two weeks) should separate therapy with EUTONYL (pargyline hydrochloride) and use of these agents.

e. Other monoamine oxidase inhibitors. These may augment the effects of pargyline.

f. Methyldopa or dopamine. These drugs may cause hyperexcitability in patients receiving pargyline.

g. L-dopa. There have been several reports of potentiation of the pressor effects of this drug by various monoamine oxidase inhibitors. At least one month should elapse after the discontinuation of pargyline before L-dopa is given.

Warnings:

A. PATIENTS

1. PATIENTS SHOULD BE WARNED AGAINST THE USE OF ANY OVER-THE-COUNTER PREPARATIONS, PARTICULARLY "COLD PREPARATIONS" AND ANTIHISTAMINES, OR PRESCRIPTION DRUGS WITHOUT THE KNOWLEDGE AND CONSENT OF THE PHYSICIAN.
2. PATIENTS SHOULD BE CAUTIONED ON THE USE OF CHEESE AND OTHER FOODS WITH HIGH TYRAMINE CONTENT (See *Contraindications*) AND ALCOHOLIC BEVERAGES IN ANY FORM.
3. PATIENTS SHOULD BE WARNED ABOUT THE LIKELIHOOD OF THE OCCURRENCE OF ORTHOSTATIC HYPOTENSION.
4. PATIENTS SHOULD BE INSTRUCTED TO REPORT PROMPTLY THE OCCURRENCE OF SEVERE HEADACHE OR OTHER UNUSUAL SYMPTOMS.
5. PATIENTS WITH ANGINA PECTORIS OR CORONARY ARTERY DISEASE SHOULD BE ESPECIALLY WARNED NOT TO INCREASE THEIR PHYSICAL ACTIVITIES IN RESPONSE TO A DIMINUTION IN ANGINAL SYMPTOMS OR AN INCREASE IN WELL-BEING OCCUR-

Continued on next page

If desired, additional literature on any Abbott Product will be provided upon request to Abbott Laboratories.

Abbott—Cont.

RING DURING TREATMENT WITH EUTONYL.

B. PHYSICIANS
1. WHEN INDICATED THE FOLLOWING SHOULD BE CAUTIOUSLY PRESCRIBED IN REDUCED DOSAGES:
   a. ANTIHISTAMINES
   b. HYPNOTICS, SEDATIVES, OR TRANQUILIZERS
   c. NARCOTICS (MEPERIDINE SHOULD NOT BE USED)
2. DISCONTINUE EUTONYL AT LEAST TWO WEEKS PRIOR TO ELECTIVE SURGERY.
3. IN EMERGENCY SURGERY THE DOSE OF NARCOTICS OR OTHER PREMEDICATIONS SHOULD BE REDUCED TO ¼ TO ⅕ THE USUAL AMOUNT. CLINICAL EXPERIENCE HAS SHOWN THAT RESPONSE TO ALL ANESTHETIC AGENTS CAN BE EXAGGERATED IN PATIENTS RECEIVING EUTONYL. THEREFORE THE DOSE OF THE ANESTHETIC SHOULD BE CAREFULLY ADJUSTED.
4. EUTONYL MAY INDUCE HYPOGLYCEMIA. THEREFORE, EUTONYL SHOULD BE GIVEN WITH CAUTION TO DIABETICS RECEIVING HYPOGLYCEMIC AGENTS BECAUSE SEVERE HYPOGLYCEMIA MAY OCCUR. IF IT IS NECESSARY TO ADMINISTER EUTONYL TO PATIENTS RECEIVING INSULIN OR OTHER HYPOGLYCEMIC AGENTS, THE DOSE OF THESE AGENTS SHOULD BE REDUCED ACCORDINGLY AND THE PATIENT CAREFULLY MONITORED.
5. CARE SHOULD BE EXERCISED IN USING EUTONYL IN PATIENTS WITH IMPAIRED RENAL FUNCTION.

Use In Pregnancy and Lactation: Safe use of EUTONYL (pargyline hydrochloride) during pregnancy or lactation has not yet been established. Before prescribing EUTONYL in pregnancy, lactation, or in women of childbearing age, the potential benefit of the drug should be weighed against its possible hazard to mother and child.

Precautions: The therapeutic response to a variety of drugs may be changed or exaggerated in patients receiving a monoamine oxidase inhibitor such as pargyline hydrochloride. Caffeine, alcohol, antihistamines, barbiturates, chloral hydrate and other hypnotics, sedatives, tranquilizers, and narcotics (meperidine should not be used) should be used cautiously and at reduced dosage in patients who are taking pargyline.

There have been no substantiated reports of hepatotoxicity associated with pargyline therapy. However, since liver damage has resulted from use of certain other monoamine oxidase inhibitors, and since transient alterations in liver enzyme levels have occasionally occurred with pargyline, it is advisable that patients receiving EUTONYL have periodic liver function tests.

All patients with impaired circulation to vital organs from any cause including those with angina pectoris, coronary artery disease, and cerebral arteriosclerosis should be closely observed for symptoms of orthostatic hypotension. If hypotension develops in these patients, EUTONYL (pargyline hydrochloride) dosage should be reduced or therapy discontinued since severe and/or prolonged hypotension may precipitate cerebral or coronary vessel thrombosis.

The hypotensive effect of EUTONYL may be augmented by febrile illnesses. It may be advisable to withdraw the drug during such diseases.

Since pargyline is excreted primarily in the urine, patients with impaired renal function may experience cumulative drug effects. Such patients should also be watched for elevations of blood urea nitrogen and other evidence of progressive renal failure. If such alterations should persist and progress, the drug should be discontinued.

An increased response to central depressants may be manifested by acute hypotension and increased sedative effect. EUTONYL also may augment the hypotensive effects of anesthetic agents, and surgery. For this reason, the drug should be discontinued at least two weeks prior to surgery.

In the event of emergency surgery, ¼ to ⅕ of the usual dose of narcotics, sedatives, analgesics and other premedications should be used. If severe hypotension should occur, this can be controlled by small doses of a vasopressor agent such as norepinephrine bitartrate injection.

EUTONYL should not be used in individuals with hyperactive or hyperexcitable personalities, as some of these patients show an undesirable increase in motor activity with restlessness, confusion, agitation, and disorientation. Clinical studies have shown that pargyline may unmask severe psychotic symptoms such as hallucinations or paranoid delusions in some patients with pre-existing serious emotional problems. This can usually be controlled by judicious administration of chlorpromazine intramuscularly, or other phenothiazines, the patient remaining supine for one hour after administration.

Pargyline should be used with caution in patients with Parkinsonism, as it may increase symptoms. In addition, great care is required if pargyline is administered in conjunction with anti-parkinsonian agents.

Documented cases of eye changes or optic atrophy have not been reported with the use of pargyline as they have with the use of certain other monoamine oxidase inhibitors. However, since non-specific visual disturbances and aggravation of glaucoma have occurred occasionally, it is advisable that patients receiving EUTONYL be examined for changes in color perception, visual fields, fundi, and visual acuity.

Clinical reports state that certain individuals receiving pargyline for a prolonged period of time are refractory to the nerve-blocking effects of local anesthetics, e.g., lidocaine.

The 25 mg dosage strength of EUTONYL tablets contains FD&C Yellow No. 5 (tartrazine) which may cause allergic-type reactions (including bronchial asthma) in certain susceptible individuals. Although the overall incidence of FD&C Yellow No. 5 (tartrazine) sensitivity in the general population is low, it is frequently seen in patients who also have aspirin hypersensitivity.

Adverse Reactions: Generally side effects are not severe or serious when the recommended dosages are used and necessary precautions are observed. If side effects are severe or persist the drug should be discontinued. See also *Warnings* and *Precautions*.

The most frequently occurring side effects are those associated with orthostatic hypotension (dizziness, weakness, palpitation, or fainting). These usually respond to a reduction of dosage. Patients should be warned against rising to a standing position too quickly, especially when getting out of bed. Severe and persistent orthostatic hypotension should be avoided by reduction in dosage or discontinuation of therapy.

Mild constipation, fluid retention with or without edema, dry mouth, sweating, increased appetite, arthralgia, nausea and vomiting, blurred vision, headache, insomnia, difficulty in micturition, nightmares, impotence and delayed ejaculation, rash, and purpura have also been encountered. Hyperexcitability, increased neuromuscular activity (muscle twitching), and other extrapyramidal symptoms have been reported. Gain in weight may be due to either edema or increased appetite. Drug fever is extremely rare. In some patients reduction of blood sugar has been noted. Although the significance of this has not been elucidated, the possibility of hypoglycemic effects should be borne in mind. Congestive heart failure has been reported in patients with reduced cardiac reserve.

Dosage and Administration: EUTONYL (pargyline hydrochloride) is orally administered as a single daily dose; there is no known advantage in prescribing the drug more frequently than once daily. Clinical response to the drug is not immediate. Four days to three weeks or more may be required to produce the full effects of a given daily dosage. *For this reason it is generally unwise to increase dosage more frequently than once a week.* Likewise the effects of the drug may persist following reduction of dosage or withdrawal. If therapy must be interrupted because of undesirable side effects, the drug should be withheld until all such effects have disappeared. Therapy is then reinstituted at a lower dosage. Because the drug exerts an orthostatic effect on blood pressure, dosage adjustments should be based upon the blood pressure response *in the standing position.*

The usual adult dosage for initiating therapy in hypertensive patients not receiving other antihypertensive agents is 25 mg once daily. This dosage may be increased once a week by 10 mg increments until the desired response is obtained. The total daily dose of pargyline should not exceed 200 mg if excessive side effects are to be avoided.

Patients over age 65, or those who have undergone sympathectomy may be unusually sensitive to the antihypertensive properties of the drug. In such patients the initial daily dosage should be 10 to 25 mg. When EUTONYL (pargyline hydrochloride) is added to an established antihypertensive regimen, the initial dose should not exceed 25 mg daily (less in sympathectomized or elderly patients).

EUTONYL should not be administered to children under 12 years of age because of limited experience with the drug in this group.

Reduction of blood pressure is often maintained in hypertensive patients with a daily dose of 25 to 50 mg of EUTONYL alone. Larger doses may be tried in resistant cases. In general, dosage should be kept at the minimum level required to maintain a desirable reduction in blood pressure without encountering undue side effects. A few patients may develop a relative tolerance to the antihypertensive effects of the drug. The administration of additional antihypertensive agents may be considered in cases not controlled by EUTONYL alone.

Overdosage: Reported effects of MAOI overdosage include agitation, hallucinations, hyperreflexia, hyperpyrexia, convulsions, and both hypotension and hypertension.

Management must be attempted with great caution because of the potential for interaction with antidotal drugs. Conservative treatment aimed at the maintenance of normal temperature, respiration, blood pressure, and proper fluid and electrolyte balance has generally been successful.

How Supplied: EUTONYL (pargyline hydrochloride tablets, USP) is available in Filmtab tablet strengths of 10 mg and 25 mg. The tablets are available in the following packages: 10 mg tablets in bottles of 100 (**NDC** 0074-6876-02) and 25 mg tablets in bottles of 100 (**NDC** 0074-6878-01).

Abbott Pharmaceuticals, Inc.
North Chicago, IL 60064

[*Shown in Product Identification Section*]

Ref. 03-4213-R6

FERO-FOLIC-500® Filmtab® Tablets ℞
Controlled-Release Iron with Folic Acid and Vitamin C

IBERET-FOLIC-500® Filmtab® Tablets ℞
Controlled-Release Iron with Vitamin C, and B-Complex, including Folic Acid

Description: FERO-FOLIC-500 Filmtab is a hematinic for oral administration containing 525 mg of ferrous sulfate (equivalent to 105 mg of elemental iron) in a unique controlled-release vehicle, the Gradumet®. In addition, this product contains 800 mcg of folic acid and 500 mg of ascorbic acid present as sodium ascorbate.

IBERET-FOLIC-500 is an Abbott hematinic containing iron in the Gradumet® controlled-release vehicle; vitamin C for enhancement of iron absorption; and the B-Complex vitamins including folic acid. The IBERET-FOLIC-500 Filmtab is for oral use.

Each Filmtab tablet provides:

*Ferrous Sulfate	525 mg
(equivalent to 105 mg of elemental iron)	
Ascorbic Acid (present as sodium ascorbate) (C)	500 mg
Niacinamide	30 mg
Calcium Pantothenate	10 mg
Thiamine Mononitrate (B_1)	6 mg
Riboflavin (B_2)	6 mg
Pyridoxine Hydrochloride (B_6)	5 mg
Folic Acid	800 mcg
Cyanocobalamin (B_{12})	25 mcg

*In controlled-release form (Gradumet)

Controlled-release of iron from the Gradumet protects against gastric side effects. The Gradumet is an inert, porous, plastic matrix which is impregnated with ferrous sulfate. Iron is leached from the Gradumet as it passes through the gastrointestinal tract, and the expended matrix is excreted harmlessly in the stool. Controlled-release iron is particularly helpful in patients who have demonstrated intolerance to oral iron preparations.

Clinical Pharmacology: Oral iron is absorbed most efficiently when it is administered between meals. Conventional iron preparations, however, frequently cause gastric irritation when taken on an empty stomach. Studies with iron in the Gradumet have indicated that relatively little of the iron is released in the stomach, gastric intolerance is seldom encountered, and hematologic response ranks with that obtained from plain ferrous sulfate.

Iron is found in the body principally as hemoglobin. Storage in the form of ferritin occurs in the liver, spleen, and bone marrow. Concentrations of plasma iron and the total iron-binding capacity of plasma vary greatly in different physiological conditions and disease states.

Large amounts of ascorbic acid administered orally with ferrous sulfate have been shown to enhance iron absorption. Apparently this is due to the ability of ascorbic acid to prevent the oxidation of ferrous iron to the less effectively absorbed ferric form.

Folic acid and iron are absorbed in the proximal small intestine, particularly the duodenum. Folic acid is absorbed maximally and rapidly at this site, and iron is absorbed in a descending gradient from the duodenum distally.

After absorption folic acid is rapidly converted into its metabolically active forms. Approximately two-thirds is bound to plasma protein. Half of the folic acid stored in the body is found in the liver. Folic acid is also concentrated in spinal fluid.

Except for the folates ingested in liver, yeast, and egg yolk, the percentage of absorption of food folates averages about 10%.

The B-complex vitamins in IBERET-FOLIC-500 are absorbed by the active transport process. B-complex vitamins are rapidly eliminated and therefore are not stored in the body.

Calcium pantothenate is absorbed readily from the gastrointestinal tract and distributed to all body tissues.

Indications and Usage: FERO-FOLIC-500 is indicated for the treatment of iron deficiency and prevention of concomitant folic acid deficiency in nonpregnant adults. FERO-FOLIC-500 is also indicated in pregnancy for the prevention and treatment of iron deficiency and to supply a maintenance dosage of folic acid.

IBERET-FOLIC-500 is indicated in non-pregnant adults for the treatment of iron deficiency and prevention of concomitant folic acid deficiency where there is an associated deficient intake or increased need for the B-complex vitamins. IBERET-FOLIC-500 is also indicated in pregnancy for the prevention and treatment of iron deficiency where there is a concomitant deficient intake or increased need for the B-complex vitamins (including folic acid).

Contraindications: FERO-FOLIC-500 and IBERET-FOLIC-500 are contraindicated in patients with pernicious anemia.

FERO-FOLIC-500 and IBERET-FOLIC-500 are also contraindicated in the rare instance of hypersensitivity to folic acid.

Warnings: Folic acid alone is improper therapy in the treatment of pernicious anemia and other megaloblastic anemias where vitamin B_{12} is deficient.

Precautions: Where anemia exists, its nature should be established and underlying causes determined.

FERO-FOLIC-500 and IBERET-FOLIC-500 contain 800 mcg of folic acid per tablet. Folic acid especially in doses above 0.1 mg daily may obscure pernicious anemia, in that hematologic remission may occur while neurological manifestations remain progresssive. Concomitant parenteral therapy with vitamin B_{12} may be necessary in patients with deficiency of vitamin B_{12}. Pernicious anemia is rare in women of childbearing age, and the likelihood of its occurrence along with pregnancy is reduced by the impairment of fertility associated with vitamin B_{12} deficiency.

Like other oral iron preparations, FERO-FOLIC-500 and IBERET-FOLIC-500 should be stored out of the reach of children to guard against accidental iron poisoning (see Overdosage).

Laboratory Tests: In older patients and those with conditions tending to lead to vitamin B_{12} depletion, serum B_{12} levels should be regularly assessed during treatment with FERO-FOLIC-500 or IBERET-FOLIC-500.

Drug Interactions: Absorption of iron is inhibited by *magnesium trisilicate* and *antacids containing carbonates.*

Ferrous sulfate may interfere with the absorption of *tetracyclines.*

The antiparkinsonism effects of *levodopa* may be reversed by pyridoxine.

Iron absorption is inhibited by the ingestion of eggs or milk.

Carcinogenesis: Adequate data is not available on long-term potential for carcinogenesis in animals or humans.

Pregnancy: Pregnancy Category A. Studies in pregnant women have not shown that FERO-FOLIC-500 or IBERET-FOLIC-500 increase the risk of fetal abnormalities if administered during pregnancy. If either of these drugs is used during pregnancy, the possibility of fetal harm appears remote. Because studies cannot rule out the possibility of harm, however, FERO-FOLIC-500 or IBERET-FOLIC-500 should be used during pregnancy only if clearly needed.

Nursing Mothers: Folic acid, ascorbic acid, and B-complex vitamins are excreted in breast milk.

Adverse Reactions: The likelihood of gastric intolerance to iron in the controlled-release Gradumet vehicle is remote. If such should occur, the tablet may be taken after a meal. Allergic sensitization has been reported following both oral and parenteral administration of folic acid.

Overdosage: Signs of serious toxicity may be delayed because the iron is in a controlled-release dose form. Increased capillary permeability, reduced plasma volume, increased cardiac output, and sudden cardiovascular collapse may occur in acute iron intoxication. In overdosage, efforts should be made to hasten the elimination of the Gradumet tablets ingested. An emetic should be administered as soon as possible, followed by gastric lavage if indicated. Immediately following emesis, a large dose of a saline cathartic should be used to speed passage through the intestinal tract. X-ray examination may then be considered to determine the position and number of Gradumet tablets remaining in the gastrointestinal tract.

Dosage and Administration: FERO-FOLIC-500 is administered orally and may be taken on an empty stomach.

Adults: For treatment of iron deficiency and prevention of folic acid deficiency, the recommended dose is one tablet daily.

Pregnant Adults: For prevention and treatment of iron deficiency and to supply a maintenance dosage of folic acid, the recommended dose is one tablet daily.

IBERET-FOLIC-500 is administered orally and may be taken on an empty stomach.

Adults: For the treatment of iron deficiency and prevention of concomitant folic acid deficiency where there is an associated deficient intake or increased need for the B-complex vitamins, the recommended dose is one tablet daily.

Pregnant Adults: For the prevention and treatment of iron deficiency where there is a concomitant deficient intake or increased need for the B-complex vitamins including folic acid, the recommended dose is one tablet daily.

How Supplied: FERO-FOLIC-500 is supplied as red Filmtab tablets in bottles of 100 (**NDC** 0074-7079-13) and 500 (**NDC** 0074-7079-53).

IBERET-FOLIC-500 is supplied as red Filmtab tablets in bottles of 60 (**NDC** 0074-7125-60).

Abbott Pharmaceuticals, Inc.
North Chicago, IL 60064
Ref. 03-4240-R3

[*Shown in Product Identification Section*]

FERO-GRAD-500® Filmtab® tablets
IRON plus Vitamin C
Well-tolerated once-daily hematinic with controlled-release iron.
FERO-GRADUMET® Filmtab® tablets
Hematinic supplying controlled-release dose of iron

Description: Each Fero-Gradumet and Fero-Grad-500 tablet contains the equivalent of 105 mg of elemental iron (525 mg of ferrous sulfate) in a unique controlled-release vehicle, the Gradumet®. In addition, each Fero-Grad-500 tablet contains 500 mg of vitamin C (as sodium ascorbate) to improve iron absorption.

The Gradumet, an inert, porous, plastic matrix, is impregnated with ferrous sulfate. Iron is leached from the Gradumet as it passes through the gastrointestinal tract, and the expended matrix is excreted harmlessly in the stool. Controlled-release iron is particularly helpful in patients who have demonstrated intolerance to other oral iron preparations.

Indications: Fero-Grad-500: For the treatment of iron deficiency and iron deficiency anemia. Fero-Gradumet: For the prevention and treatment of iron deficiency.

Precautions: Where anemia exists, its nature should be established and underlying cause determined.

Like other oral iron preparations Fero-Gradumet and Fero-Grad-500 should be stored out of

Continued on next page

If desired, additional literature on any Abbott Product will be provided upon request to Abbott Laboratories.

Abbott—Cont.

the reach of children to protect against accidental iron poisoning. (see Overdosage).

Adverse Reactions: The likehood of gastric intolerance to iron in the controlled-release Gradumet vehicle is slight. If it should occur, the tablet may be taken after a meal.

Dosage and Administration: Fero-Gradumet and Fero-Grad-500 are administered orally and may be taken on an empty stomach. The Gradumet controlled-release vehicle reduces the incidence of gastric side effects by delaying the release of almost all the iron until the tablet has passed the stomach.

Fero-Grad-500: Usual adult dose: One tablet daily, or as directed by the physician.

Fero-Gradumet: Usual adult dose: Prevention: One tablet daily; Treatment: One tablet twice daily, or as directed by the physician.

Overdosage: Signs of serious toxicity may be delayed because the iron is in a controlled-release dose form. Increased capillary permeability, reduced plasma volume, increased cardiac output, and sudden cardiovascular collapse may occur in acute iron intoxication. In overdosage, efforts should be made to hasten the elimination of the Gradumet tablets ingested. An emetic should be administered as soon as possible, followed by gastric lavage if indicated. Immediately following emesis, a large dose of a saline cathartic should be used to speed passage through the intestinal tract. X-ray examination may then be considered to determine the position and number of Gradumet tablets remaining in the gastrointestinal tract.

How Supplied: Fero-Gradumet is supplied as red tablets in bottles of 100 (**NDC** 0074-6852-02); Fero-Grad-500 is supplied as red tablets in bottles of 30 (**NDC** 0074-7238-30), 100 (**NDC** 0074-7238-01) and 500 (**NDC** 0074-7238-02). The ingredients of these products are listed in one or more of the Medicare designated compendia.

Abbott Pharmaceuticals, Inc.
North Chicago, IL 60064

[*Shown in Product Identification Section*]

Ref. 03-0819-7/R24, 03-0956-6/R2

GEMONIL® ℞ ©
(metharbital tablets, USP)

Description: GEMONIL (metharbital) is a synthetic, N-methylated derivative of barbital which is identified chemically as 5,5-diethyl-1-methyl-barbituric acid.

Actions: GEMONIL produces anticonvulsant effects which are similar to those produced by phenobarbital and mephobarbital. In experimental animals the drug has been shown to be unusually effective against pentylenetetrazol-induced convulsions. GEMONIL is less effective against convulsions induced by electroshock. Toxicity studies in mice, rats, cats and dogs indicate that the drug is less toxic and has less sedative effect than phenobarbital.

GEMONIL is adequately absorbed from the gastrointestinal tract following oral administration. It is demethylated in the liver to barbital, and is excreted largely in this form by the kidneys.

Indications: GEMONIL is indicated for the control of grand mal, petit mal, myoclonic and mixed types of seizures.

Contraindications: GEMONIL is contraindicated in patients with known hypersensitivity to barbiturates, and in those with a history of manifest or latent porphyria.

Warnings: Metharbital may be habit forming.

USAGE DURING PREGNANCY AND LACTATION: THERE ARE MULTIPLE REPORTS IN THE CLINICAL LITERATURE WHICH INDICATE THAT THE USE OF ANTICONVULSANT DRUGS DURING PREGNANCY RESULTS IN AN INCREASED INCIDENCE OF BIRTH DEFECTS IN THE OFFSPRING. ALTHOUGH DATA ARE MORE EXTENSIVE WITH RESPECT TO TRIMETHADIONE, PARAMETHADIONE, PHENYTOIN, AND PHENOBARBITAL, REPORTS INDICATE A POSSIBLE SIMILAR ASSOCIATION WITH THE USE OF OTHER ANTICONVULSANT DRUGS. THEREFORE, ANTICONVULSANT DRUGS SHOULD BE ADMINISTERED TO WOMEN OF CHILDBEARING POTENTIAL ONLY IF THEY ARE CLEARLY SHOWN TO BE ESSENTIAL IN THE MANAGEMENT OF THEIR SEIZURES.

ANTICONVULSANT DRUGS SHOULD NOT BE DISCONTINUED IN PATIENTS IN WHOM THE DRUG IS ADMINISTERED TO PREVENT MAJOR SEIZURES BECAUSE OF THE STRONG POSSIBILITY OF PRECIPITATING STATUS EPILEPTICUS WITH ATTENDANT HYPOXIA AND RISK TO BOTH MOTHER AND THE UNBORN CHILD. CONSIDERATION SHOULD, HOWEVER, BE GIVEN TO DISCONTINUATION OF ANTICONVULSANTS PRIOR TO AND DURING PREGNANCY WHEN THE NATURE, FREQUENCY AND SEVERITY OF THE SEIZURES DO NOT POSE A SERIOUS THREAT TO THE PATIENT. IT IS NOT, HOWEVER, KNOWN WHETHER EVEN MINOR SEIZURES CONSTITUTE SOME RISK TO THE DEVELOPING EMBRYO OR FETUS.

REPORTS HAVE SUGGESTED THAT THE MATERNAL INGESTION OF ANTICONVULSANT DRUGS, PARTICULARLY BARBITURATES, IS ASSOCIATED WITH A NEONATAL COAGULATION DEFECT THAT MAY CAUSE BLEEDING DURING THE EARLY (USUALLY WITHIN 24 HOURS OF BIRTH) NEONATAL PERIOD. THE POSSIBILITY OF THE OCCURRENCE OF THIS DEFECT WITH THE USE OF GEMONIL SHOULD BE KEPT IN MIND. THE DEFECT IS CHARACTERIZED BY DECREASED LEVELS OF VITAMIN K-DEPENDENT CLOTTING FACTORS, AND PROLONGATION OF EITHER THE PROTHROMBIN TIME OR THE PARTIAL THROMBOPLASTIN TIME, OR BOTH. IT HAS BEEN SUGGESTED THAT VITAMIN K BE GIVEN PROPHYLACTICALLY TO THE MOTHER ONE MONTH PRIOR TO AND DURING DELIVERY, AND TO THE INFANT, INTRAVENOUSLY, IMMEDIATELY AFTER BIRTH.

THE SAFETY OF GEMONIL FOR USE DURING LACTATION HAS NOT BEEN ESTABLISHED.

THE PHYSICIAN SHOULD WEIGH THESE CONSIDERATIONS IN TREATMENT AND COUNSELING OF EPILEPTIC WOMEN OF CHILDBEARING POTENTIAL.

Precautions: There is evidence that some barbiturates stimulate hepatic microsomal enzymes and therefore may increase the rate of metabolism of some drugs including the coumarin anticoagulants. Although metharbital has not been directly associated with such effect, caution is advised in patients receiving such anticoagulants.

Since metharbital is detoxified primarily in the liver, GEMONIL should be used with caution in patients with hepatic impairment.

In patients with convulsive disorders who have been taking regular daily doses, withdrawal of GEMONIL should be gradual since abrupt discontinuation of barbiturates given for the treatment of epilepsy may result in status epilepticus.

Adverse Reactions: GEMONIL (metharbital) has a low toxicity, and side effects are usually infrequent and mild. Gastric distress, dizziness, increased irritability, skin rash and drowsiness (large doses) may occur. If side effects become severe or cannot be controlled by dosage adjustment, the drug should be gradually withdrawn.

Dosage and Administration: GEMONIL is administered orally. As with all antiepileptic therapy, it is particularly important to adjust the dosage for each patient to obtain optimal effect. For adults, the usual starting dose is 100 mg, one to three times daily. The usual initial pediatric dose should be one-half of a 100 mg tablet, one to three times daily, depending on the age and weight of the patient. A dose of 5 to 15 mg/kg per day has been recommended for children. According to the patient's tolerance these dosages may be gradually increased to the level required to control seizures. In some cases very small doses may be effective, whereas in other instances as much as 600 to 800 mg daily are required for adequate control. GEMONIL may be used alone or in conjunction with other antiepileptic drugs such as Tridione® (trimethadione), Paradione® (paramethadione), Phenurone® (phenacemide), Peganone® (ethotoin), phenytoin sodium, or mephenytoin. Frequently, more effective control of seizures can be achieved by a combination of drugs. When added to an established regimen to replace or supplement other anticonvulsant therapy, the dosage of other medication should be gradually reduced while increasing that of GEMONIL so as to avoid or minimize recurrence of seizures.

Overdosage: Symptoms of overdosage include drowsiness, irritability, dizziness, and gastric distress. Loss of consciousness and coma may occur following very high doses. Treatment is the same as that for barbiturate intoxication.

How Supplied: GEMONIL (metharbital tablets, USP) is supplied as grooved, 100 mg tablets in bottles of 100 (**NDC** 0074-6401-01).

This product is listed in USP, a Medicare designated compendium.

Abbott Laboratories
North Chicago, IL 60064
Ref. 01-2109-R3

HARMONYL® Tablets ℞
(deserpidine)

Description: Harmonyl (deserpidine) is a purified rauwolfia alkaloid chemically identified as 11-desmethoxyreserpine.

Actions: The pharmacologic actions of HARMONYL (deserpidine) are essentially the same as those of other active rauwolfia alkaloids. Deserpidine probably produces its antihypertensive effects through depletion of tissue stores of catecholamines (epinephrine and norepinephrine) from peripheral sites. By contrast, its sedative and tranquilizing properties are thought to be related to depletion of 5 - hydroxytryptamine from the brain.

The antihypertensive effect is often accompanied by bradycardia. There is no significant alteration in cardiac output or renal blood flow. The carotid sinus reflex is inhibited, but postural hypotension is rarely seen with the use of conventional doses of HARMONYL alone. Deserpidine, like other rauwolfia alkaloids, is characterized by slow onset of action and sustained effect which may persist following withdrawal of the drug.

Indications: HARMONYL (deserpidine) is indicated for the treatment of mild essential hypertension. It is also useful as adjunctive therapy with other antihypertensive agents in the more severe forms of hypertension.

The drug is also indicated for the relief of symptoms in agitated psychotic states, e.g., schizophrenia—primarily in those individuals unable to tolerate phenothiazine derivatives or those who also require antihypertensive medication.

Contraindications: HARMONYL (deserpidine) is contraindicated in patients with known hypersensitivity, mental depression especially with suicidal tendencies, active peptic ulcer, and ulcerative colitis. It is also contraindicated in patients receiving electroconvulsive therapy.

Warnings: Extreme caution should be exercised in treating patients with a history of mental depression. Discontinue the drug at the first sign of despondency, early morning insomnia, loss of appetite, impotence, or self-deprecation. Drug-induced depression may persist for several months after drug withdrawal and may be severe enough to result in suicide.

Usage in Pregnancy and Lactation

The safety of deserpidine for use during pregnancy or lactation has not been established; therefore, it should be used in pregnant women or in women of childbearing potential only when, in the judgment of the physician, its use is deemed essential to the welfare of the patient. Increased respiratory secretions, nasal congestion, cyanosis, and anorexia may occur in infants born to rauwolfia alkaloid-treated mothers since these preparations are known to cross the placental barrier to enter the fetal circulation and appear in cord blood. They also are secreted by nursing mothers into breast milk.

Reproductive and teratology studies in rats reduced the mating index and neonatal survival indices; the no-effect dosage has not been established.

Precautions: Because rauwolfia preparations increase gastrointestinal motility and secretion, this drug should be used cautiously in patients with a history of peptic ulcer, ulcerative colitis, or gallstones, where biliary colic may be precipitated.

Caution should be exercised when treating hypertensive patients with renal insufficiency since they adjust poorly to lowered blood pressure levels.

Use HARMONYL (deserpidine) cautiously with digitalis and quinidine since cardiac arrhythmias have occurred with rauwolfia preparations.

Preoperative withdrawal of deserpidine does not assure that circulatory instability will not occur. It is important that the anesthesiologist be aware of the patient's drug intake and consider this in the over-all management, since hypotension has occurred in patients receiving rauwolfia preparations. Anticholinergic and/or adrenergic drugs (metaraminol, norepinephrine) have been employed to treat adverse vagocirculatory effects.

The 0.1 mg dosage strength of HARMONYL contains FD&C Yellow No. 5 (tartrazine) which may cause allergic-type reactions (including bronchial asthma) in certain susceptible individuals. Although the overall incidence of FD&C Yellow No. 5 (tartrazine) sensitivity in the general population is low, it is frequently seen in patients who also have aspirin hypersensitivity.

Adverse Reactions: The following adverse reactions have been reported with rauwolfia preparations. These reactions are usually reversible and disappear when the drug is discontinued.

Gastrointestinal: Including hypersecretion, anorexia, diarrhea, nausea, and vomiting.

Cardiovascular: Including angina-like symptoms, arrhythmias (particularly when used concurrently with digitalis or quinidine), and bradycardia.

Central Nervous System: Including drowsiness, depression, nervousness, paradoxical anxiety, nightmares, extrapyramidal tract symptoms, CNS sensitization manifested by dull sensorium, and deafness.

Dermatologic-Hypersensitivity: Including pruritus, rash, and asthma in asthmatic patients.

Ophthalmologic: Including glaucoma, uveitis, optic atrophy, and conjunctival injection.

Hematologic: Thrombocytopenic purpura.

Miscellaneous: Nasal congestion, weight gain, impotence or decreased libido, dysuria, dyspnea, muscular aches, dryness of mouth, dizziness, and headache.

Water retention with edema in patients with hypertensive vascular disease may occur rarely, but the condition generally clears with cessation of therapy or with the administration of a diuretic agent.

Dosage and Administration: HARMONYL (deserpidine) is administered orally. For the management of mild essential hypertension in the average patient not receiving other antihypertensive agents, the usual initial adult dose is 0.75 to 1 mg daily. Because 10 to 14 days are required to produce the full effects of the drug, adjustments in dosage should not be made more frequently. If the therapeutic response is not adequate, it is generally advisable to add another antihypertensive agent to the regimen. For maintenance, dosage should be reduced. A single daily dose of 0.25 mg of deserpidine may suffice for some patients.

Concomitant use of deserpidine with ganglionic blocking agents, guanethidine, veratrum, hydralazine, methyldopa, chlorthalidone, or thiazides necessitates careful titration of dosage with each agent.

For psychiatric disorders: The average initial oral dose is 0.5 mg daily with a range of 0.1 to 1 mg. Adjust dosage upward or downward according to the patient's response.

Overdosage: An overdosage of deserpidine is characterized by flushing of the skin, conjunctival injection, and pupillary constriction. Sedation ranging from drowsiness to coma may occur. Hypotension, hypothermia, central respiratory depression and bradycardia may develop in cases of severe overdosage.

Treatment consists of the careful evacuation of stomach contents followed by the usual procedures for the symptomatic management of CNS depressant overdosage. If severe hypotension occurs, it should be treated with a direct acting vasopressor such as Levophed® (norepinephrine bitartrate injection, USP).

How Supplied: HARMONYL (deserpidine) Tablets, 0.1 mg, are yellow and supplied in bottles of 100 (**NDC** 0074-6901-01).

HARMONYL (deserpidine) Tablets (grooved), 0.25 mg, are salmon-pink and supplied in bottles of 100 (**NDC** 0074-6906-07) and 1000 (**NDC** 0074-6906-03).

Abbott Laboratories
North Chicago, IL 60064
Ref. 01-2216-R1

IBERET®-500 Filmtab® tablets
IRON plus B-complex and Vitamin C
Well-tolerated once-daily hematinic with controlled-release iron.
IBERET® Filmtab® tablets
Hematinic Supplying Controlled-Release Iron, Vitamin C and Vitamin B-Complex

Description: Each Iberet-500 and Iberet Filmtab tablet contains 525 mg of ferrous sulfate (equivalent to 105 mg elemental iron) in the Gradumet® controlled-release vehicle. To enhance iron absorption, 500 mg of vitamin C has been added to each Iberet-500 Filmtab.

The Gradumet is an inert, porous, plastic matrix which is impregnated with ferrous sulfate. Iron is leached from the Gradumet as it passes through the gastrointestinal tract, and the expended matrix is excreted harmlessly in the stool. Controlled-release iron is particularly helpful in patients who have demonstrated intolerance to other oral iron preparations.

Each Iberet-500 Filmtab tablet contains:

Ferrous Sulfate	525 mg
(equivalent to 105 mg of elemental iron)	
Vitamin C (as Sodium Ascorbate)	500 mg
Niacinamide	30 mg
Calcium Pantothenate	10 mg
Vitamin B_1 (Thiamine Mononitrate)	6 mg
Vitamin B_2 (Riboflavin)	6 mg
Vitamin B_6 (Pyridoxine Hydrochloride)	5 mg
Vitamin B_{12} (Cyanocobalamin)	25 mcg

The formulation of Iberet differs from Iberet-500 only in that it contains a lesser amount of vitamin C, 150 mg per Filmtab tablet.

Indications: Iberet-500: For the treatment of iron deficiency or iron deficiency anemia where there is a deficient intake or increased need for B-complex vitamins.* Iberet: For conditions in which iron deficiency and vitamin C deficiency occur concomitantly with deficient intake or increased need for the B-complex vitamins.*

*Contains no folic acid.

Precautions: Where anemia exists, its nature should be established and underlying cause determined.

Like other oral iron preparations, Iberet-500 and Iberet should be stored out of the reach of children to protect against accidental iron poisoning (see Overdosage).

Adverse Reactions: The likelihood of gastric intolerance to iron in the controlled-release Gradumet vehicle is slight. If it should occur, the tablet may be taken after a meal.

Dosage and Administration: Iberet-500 and Iberet are administered orally and may be taken on an empty stomach. Iberet-500: Usual Adult Dose: One tablet daily, or as directed by the physician. Iberet: Usual Adult Dose: One tablet daily, or as directed by the physician.

Overdosage: Signs of serious iron toxicity may be delayed because the iron is in a controlled-release dose form. Increased capillary permeability, reduced plasma volume, increased cardiac output, and sudden cardiovascular collapse may occur in acute iron intoxication. In overdosage, efforts should be made to hasten the elimination of the Gradumet tablets ingested. An emetic should be administered as soon as possible, followed by gastric lavage if indicated. Immediately following emesis, a saline cathartic should be administered to hasten passage through the intestinal tract. X-ray examination may then be considered to determine the position and number of Gradumet tablets remaining in the gastrointestinal tract.

How Supplied: Iberet-500 is supplied as red, oval shaped tablets in bottles of 30 (**NDC** 0074-7235-30), 60 (**NDC** 0074-7235-01) and 500 (**NDC** 0074-7235-03), and in Abbo-Pac® unit dose packages of 100 (**NDC** 0074-7235-11); Iberet is supplied as red, round tablets in bottles of 60 (**NDC** 0074-6863-01) and 500 (**NDC** 0074-6863-02).

[*Shown in Product Identification Section*]

Abbott Pharmaceuticals, Inc.
North Chicago, IL 60064
Ref. 03-0935-9/R2, 03-0938-7/R17

IBERET-FOLIC-500® ℞
(Controlled-Release Iron with Vitamin C, and B-Complex, including Folic Acid) Filmtab® Tablets

See combined listing under FERO-FOLIC-500.

IBERET®-500 LIQUID
Hematinic Supplying Iron, Vitamin C and Vitamin B-Complex*
IBERET®-LIQUID
Hematinic Supplying Iron, Vitamin C and Vitamin B-Complex*

Description: Iberet-500 Liquid and Iberet-Liquid are hematinic preparations of ferrous sulfate, B-complex vitamins* and ascorbic acid.

Each teaspoonful (5 ml) of Iberet-500 Liquid provides:

Elemental Iron (as ferrous sulfate)	26.25 mg
Vitamin C (Ascorbic Acid)	125 mg
Niacinamide	7.5 mg
Dexpanthenol	2.5 mg
Vitamin B_1 (Thiamine Hydrochloride)	1.5 mg
Vitamin B_2 (Riboflavin)	1.5 mg
Vitamin B_6 (Pyridoxine Hydrochloride)	1.25 mg
Vitamin B_{12} (Cyanocobalamin)	6.25 mcg

In a citrus-flavored vehicle.

Iberet-Liquid has a raspberry-mint flavored vehicle, alcohol 1%; it has the same formula as

Continued on next page

If desired, additional literature on any Abbott Product will be provided upon request to Abbott Laboratories.

Abbott—Cont.

Iberet-500 Liquid except for a smaller amount of ascorbic acid: 37.5 mg per teaspoonful.

Indications: Iberet-500 Liquid: For conditions in which iron deficiency occurs concomitantly with deficient intake or increased need for the B-complex vitamins.* Iberet-Liquid: For conditions in which iron deficiency and vitamin C deficiency occur concomitantly with deficient intake or increased need for the B-complex vitamins.*

*Contains no folic acid.

Precautions: Where anemia exists, its nature should be established and underlying cause determined. Iberet-500 Liquid and Iberet-Liquid should be stored out of the reach of children because of the possibility of iron intoxication from accidental overdosage.

Adverse Reactions: If gastrointestinal symptoms appear as a sign of iron intolerance, smaller individual doses may be given at more frequent intervals to provide the desired daily amount. Administering Iberet-500 Liquid or Iberet-Liquid after meals may also reduce such effects.

Like other liquid iron preparations, Iberet-500 Liquid or Iberet-Liquid may stain the teeth on continued use. Stains may be prevented to a large extent by taking the dose through a straw, first mixing it with water or fruit juice, and by following the dose with a drink of plain water or juice. Brushing the teeth with sodium bicarbonate or hydrogen peroxide will usually remove existing stains.

Dosage and Administration: Iberet-500 Liquid and Iberet-Liquid are administered orally, preferably after meals. Each has a fruit-flavored vehicle, and is suitable for pediatric patients who are unable to take tablets or capsules, and for patients who prefer or can better tolerate liquid medication. Iberet-500 Liquid and Iberet-Liquid may be administered by spoon or incorporated into infant formulas, water, or fruit juices. Iberet-500 Liquid: Usual dosage: Adults and children 4 years of age and older—2 teaspoonfuls (10 ml) twice daily, after meals; Children 1–3 years of age—1 teaspoonful (5 ml) twice daily, after meals. Otherwise as directed by the physician. Iberet-Liquid: Usual dosage: Adults and children 4 years of age and older—2 teaspoonfuls (10 ml) three times daily, after meals; Children 1–3 years of age—1 teaspoonful (5 ml) three times daily, after meals. Otherwise as directed by the physician.

How Supplied: Iberet-500 Liquid (**NDC** 0074-8422-02) and Iberet-Liquid (**NDC** 0074-7173-01) are supplied in 8 fl oz bottles.

Abbott Laboratories
North Chicago, IL 60064
Ref. 02-5560-3/R13, 02-5561-4/R11

JANIMINE® Filmtab® Tablets ℞
(imipramine hydrochloride tablets, USP)

How Supplied: JANIMINE is provided in three dosage sizes as monogrammed tablets:

10 mg, round-shaped, orange-colored, in bottles of 100 (**NDC** 0074-1897-13) and bottles of 1000 (**NDC** 0074-1897-19).

25 mg, round-shaped, yellow, in bottles of 100 (**NDC** 0074-1898-13) and bottles of 1000 (**NDC** 0074-1898-19).

50 mg, ovaloid-shaped, peach-colored, in bottles of 100 (**NDC** 0074-1899-13) and bottles of 1000 (**NDC** 0074-1899-19).

[*Shown in Product Identification Section*]

Abbott Laboratories
North Chicago, IL 60064

K-LOR™ Powder ℞
(potassium chloride for oral solution, USP)

Description: Natural fruit-flavored K-LOR (potassium chloride for oral solution, USP) is an oral potassium supplement offered as a powder for reconstitution in individual packets. Each packet of K-LOR 20 mEq contains potassium 20 mEq and chloride 20 mEq provided by potassium chloride 1.5 Gm. Each packet of K-LOR 15 mEq contains potassium 15 mEq and chloride 15 mEq provided by potassium chloride 1.125 Gm.

Clinical Pharmacology: Potassium ion is the principal intracellular cation of most body tissues. Potassium ions participate in a number of essential physiological processes, including the maintenance of intracellular tonicity, the transmission of nerve impulses, the contraction of cardiac, skeletal, and smooth muscle and the maintenance of normal renal function.

Potassium depletion may occur whenever the rate of potassium loss through renal excretion and/or loss from the gastrointestinal tract exceeds the rate of potassium intake. Such depletion usually develops slowly as a consequence of prolonged therapy with oral diuretics, primary or secondary hyperaldosteronism, diabetic ketoacidosis, severe diarrhea, or inadequate replacement of potassium in patients on prolonged parenteral nutrition. Potassium depletion due to these causes is usually accompanied by a concomitant deficiency of chloride and is manifested by hypokalemia and metabolic alkalosis. Potassium depletion may produce weakness, fatigue, disturbances of cardiac rhythm (primarily ectopic beats), prominent U-waves in the electrocardiogram, and in advanced cases flaccid paralysis and/or impaired ability to concentrate urine.

Potassium depletion associated with metabolic alkalosis is managed by correcting the fundamental causes of the deficiency whenever possible and administering supplemental potassium chloride, in the form of high potassium food or potassium chloride solution or tablets. In rare circumstances, (e.g., patients with renal tubular acidosis) potassium depletion may be associated with metabolic acidosis and hyperchloremia. In such patients potassium replacement should be accomplished with potassium salts other than the chloride, such as potassium bicarbonate, potassium citrate, potassium gluconate, or potassium acetate.

Indications and Usage:

1. For therapeutic use in patients with hypokalemia with or without metabolic alkalosis; in digitalis intoxication and in patients with hypokalemic familial periodic paralysis.
2. For prevention of potassium depletion when the dietary intake of potassium is inadequate in the following conditions: patients receiving digitalis and diuretics for congestive heart failure; hepatic cirrhosis with ascites; states of aldosterone excess with normal renal function; potassium-losing nephropathy, and certain diarrheal states.
3. The use of potassium salts in patients receiving diuretics for uncomplicated essential hypertension is often unnecessary when such patients have a normal dietary pattern. Serum potassium should be checked periodically, however, and, if hypokalemia occurs, dietary supplementation with potassium-containing foods may be adequate to control milder cases. In more severe cases supplementation with potassium salts may be indicated.

Contraindications: Potassium supplements are contraindicated in patients with hyperkalemia since a further increase in serum potassium concentration in such patients can produce cardiac arrest. Hyperkalemia may complicate any of the following conditions: chronic renal failure, systemic acidosis such as diabetic acidosis, acute dehydration, extensive tissue breakdown as in severe burns or adrenal insufficiency. Potassium supplements are contraindicated in patients receiving potassium-sparing diuretics (e.g., spironolactone, triamterene), since such use may produce severe hyperkalemia.

Potassium chloride supplements are contraindicated in hypokalemic patients with metabolic acidosis. These patients should be treated with an alkalinizing potassium salt such as potassium bicarbonate, potassium citrate, potassium gluconate, or potassium acetate.

Warnings: *Hyperkalemia:* In patients with impaired mechanisms for excreting potassium, the administration of potassium salts can produce hyperkalemia and cardiac arrest. This occurs most commonly in patients given potassium by the intravenous route but may also occur in patients given potassium orally. Potentially fatal hyperkalemia can develop rapidly and be asymptomatic.

Interaction with Potassium-Sparing Diuretics: Hypokalemia should not be treated by the concomitant administration of potassium salts and a potassium-sparing diuretic (e.g., spironolactone or triamterene), since the simultaneous administration of these agents can produce severe hyperkalemia.

Precautions: The diagnosis of potassium depletion is ordinarily made by demonstrating hypokalemia in a patient with a clinical history suggesting some cause for potassium depletion. In interpreting the serum potassium level, the physician should bear in mind that acute alkalosis *per se* can produce hypokalemia in the absence of a deficit in total body potassium, while acute acidosis *per se* can increase the serum potassium concentration into the normal range even in the presence of a reduced total body potassium. The treatment of potassium depletion, particularly in the presence of cardiac disease, renal disease, or acidosis, requires careful attention to acid-base balance and appropriate monitoring of serum electrolytes, the electrocardiogram, and the clinical status of the patient.

The use of potassium salts in patients with chronic renal disease, or any other condition which impairs potassium excretion, requires particularly careful monitoring of the serum potassium concentration and appropriate dosage adjustment.

Carcinogenesis: No data are available on long-term potential for carcinogenicity in animals or humans.

Pregnancy: K-LOR is not expected to cause fetal harm when administered in dosages which will not result in hyperkalemia.

Nursing Mothers: Although no studies have been done, it is presumed that potassium chloride is excreted in human milk. Caution should be exercised when K-LOR is administered to a nursing woman.

Pediatric Use: Safety and effectiveness in children have not been established.

Adverse Reactions: One of the most severe adverse effects is hyperkalemia (see CONTRAINDICATIONS, WARNINGS and OVERDOSAGE).

The most common adverse reactions to oral potassium salts are nausea, vomiting, abdominal discomfort, and diarrhea. These symptoms are due to irritation of the gastrointestinal tract and are best managed by diluting the preparation further, taking the dose with meals, or reducing the dose.

Skin rash has been reported rarely.

Overdosage: The administration of oral potassium salts to persons with normal excretory mechanisms for potassium rarely causes serious hyperkalemia. However, if excretory mechanisms are impaired or if potassium is administered too rapidly intravenously, potentially fatal hyperkalemia can result (see Contraindications and Warnings). It is important to recognize that hyperkalemia is usually asymptomatic and may be manifested only by an increased serum potassium concentration and characteristic electrocardiographic changes (peaking of T-waves, loss of P-waves, depression of S-T segments, and prolongation of QT intervals). Late manifestations include muscle paralysis and cardiovascular collapse from cardiac arrest.

Treatment measures for hyperkalemia include the following: (1) elimination of foods and medications containing potassium and of potassium-sparing diuretics; (2) intravenous administration of 300 to 500 ml/hr of dextrose injection (10–25%), containing 10 units of insulin/20 g dextrose; (3) correction of acidosis, if present, with intravenous sodium bicarbonate; (4) use of exchange resins, hemodialysis, or peritoneal dialysis. In treating hyperkalemia, it should be recalled that in patients who have been stabilized on digitalis, too rapid a lowering of the serum potassium concentration can produce digitalis toxicity.

Dosage and Administration: The dosage depends on the severity of the condition. The usual adult dose is 20 to 80 mEq of potassium per day (1 K-LOR 20 mEq packet 1 to 4 times daily after meals, or 1 K-LOR 15 mEq packet 2 to 5 times daily after meals).

Each 20 mEq (one K-LOR 20 mEq packet) of potassium should be dissolved in at least 4 oz (approximately ½ glassful) cold water or juice. Each 15 mEq (one K-LOR 15 mEq packet) of potassium should be dissolved in at least 3 oz (approximately ½ glassful) cold water or juice. These preparations, like other potassium supplements, must be properly diluted to avoid the possibility of gastrointestinal irritation.

How Supplied: K-LOR 20 mEq (potassium chloride for oral solution, USP) is supplied in cartons of 30 packets (**NDC** 0074-3611-01), and cartons of 100 packets (**NDC** 0074-3611-02). Each packet contains potassium, 20 mEq, and chloride, 20 mEq, provided by potassium chloride, 1.5 Gm.

K-LOR 15 mEq (potassium chloride for oral solution, USP) is supplied in cartons of 100 packets (**NDC** 0074-3633-11). Each packet contains potassium, 15 mEq, and chloride, 15 mEq, provided by potassium chloride, 1.125 Gm.

Abbott Laboratories
North Chicago, IL 60064
TM—Trademark

[*Shown in Product Identification Section*]
Ref. 01-2079-R8

K•Tab™ ℞

(Potassium Chloride Slow-Release Tablets)

Description: K-TAB (potassium chloride slow-release tablets) is a film-coated (not enteric-coated) tablet containing 750 mg of potassium chloride (equivalent to 10 mEq) in an inert, porous matrix. This oral potassium supplement formulation is intended to provide a controlled release of potassium from the matrix to minimize the likelihood of producing high localized concentrations of potassium within the gastrointestinal tract. The expended matrix is not absorbed and may be excreted intact in the stool.

Clinical Pharmacology: Potassium ion is the principal intracellular cation of most body tissues. Potassium ions participate in a number of essential physiological processes, including the maintenance of intracellular tonicity, the transmission of nerve impulses, the contraction of cardiac, skeletal, and smooth muscle and the maintenance of normal renal function.

Potassium depletion may occur whenever the rate of potassium loss through renal excretion and/or loss from the gastrointestinal tract exceeds the rate of potassium intake. Such depletion usually develops slowly as a consequence of prolonged therapy with oral diuretics, primary or secondary hyperaldosteronism, diabetic ketoacidosis, severe diarrhea, or inadequate replacement of potassium in patients on prolonged parenteral nutrition. Potassium depletion due to these causes is usually accompanied by a concomitant deficiency of chloride and is manifested by hypokalemia and metabolic alkalosis. Potassium depletion may produce weakness, fatigue, disturbances of cardiac rhythm (primarily ectopic beats), prominent U-waves in the electrocardiogram, and in advanced cases flaccid paralysis and/or impaired ability to concentrate urine.

Potassium depletion associated with metabolic alkalosis is managed by correcting the fundamental causes of the deficiency whenever possible and administering supplemental potassium chloride, in the form of high potassium food or potassium chloride solution or tablets. In rare circumstances, (e.g., patients with renal tubular acidosis) potassium depletion may be associated with metabolic acidosis and hyperchloremia. In such patients potassium replacement should be accomplished with potassium salts other than the chloride, such as potassium bicarbonate, potassium citrate, potassium gluconate, or potassium acetate.

Bioavailability: Studies of urinary potassium excretion in subjects with potassium balance controlled by dietary measures were used to determine bioavailability of K-TAB (potassium chloride slow-release tablets). There were no significant differences in the cumulative amount of potassium excreted over 48 hours between K-TAB and 10% potassium chloride liquid demonstrating the bioequivalence of K-TAB to the 10% liquid.

Indications and Usage: BECAUSE OF REPORTS OF INTESTINAL AND GASTRIC ULCERATION AND BLEEDING WITH SLOW-RELEASE POTASSIUM CHLORIDE PREPARATIONS, THESE DRUGS SHOULD BE RESERVED FOR THOSE PATIENTS WHO CANNOT TOLERATE OR REFUSE TO TAKE LIQUID OR EFFERVESCENT POTASSIUM PREPARATIONS OR FOR PATIENTS IN WHOM THERE IS A PROBLEM OF COMPLIANCE WITH THESE PREPARATIONS.

1. For therapeutic use in patients with hypokalemia with or without metabolic alkalosis; in digitalis intoxication and in patients with hypokalemic familial periodic paralysis.
2. For prevention of potassium depletion when the dietary intake of potassium is inadequate in the following conditions: patients receiving digitalis and diuretics for congestive heart failure; hepatic cirrhosis with ascites; states of aldosterone excess with normal renal function; potassium-losing nephropathy, and certain diarrheal states.
3. The use of potassium salts in patients receiving diuretics for uncomplicated essential hypertension is often unnecessary when such patients have a normal dietary pattern. Serum potassium should be checked periodically, however, and, if hypokalemia occurs, dietary supplementation with potassium-containing foods may be adequate to control milder cases. In more severe cases supplementation with potassium salts may be indicated.

Contraindications: Potassium supplements are contraindicated in patients with hyperkalemia since a further increase in serum potassium concentration in such patients can produce cardiac arrest. Hyperkalemia may complicate any of the following conditions: chronic renal failure, systemic acidosis such as diabetic acidosis, acute dehydration, extensive tissue breakdown as in severe burns, or adrenal insufficiency. Potassium supplements are contraindicated in patients receiving potassium-sparing diuretics (e.g., spironolactone, triamterene), since such use may produce severe hyperkalemia.

Slow-release potassium chloride preparations have produced esophageal ulceration in certain cardiac patients with esophageal compression due to an enlarged left atrium. Their use in such patients is contraindicated.

All solid dosage forms of potassium supplements are contraindicated in any patient in whom there is cause for arrest or delay in tablet passage through the gastrointestinal tract. In these instances, potassium supplementation should be with a liquid preparation.

Potassium chloride supplements are contraindicated in hypokalemic patients with metabolic acidosis. These patients should be treated with an alkalinizing potassium salt such as potassium bicarbonate, potassium citrate, potassium gluconate, or potassium acetate.

Warnings: *Hyperkalemia:* In patients with impaired mechanisms for excreting potassium, the administration of potassium salts can produce hyperkalemia and cardiac arrest. This occurs most commonly in patients given potassium by the intravenous route but may also occur in patients given potassium orally. Potentially fatal hyperkalemia can develop rapidly and be asymptomatic.

Interaction with Potassium-Sparing Diuretics: Hypokalemia should not be treated by the concomitant administration of potassium salts and a potassium-sparing diuretic (e.g., spironolactone or triamterene), since the simultaneous administration of these agents can produce severe hyperkalemia.

Gastrointestinal lesions:

Potassium chloride tablets have produced stenotic and/or ulcerative lesions of the small bowel and deaths. These lesions are caused by a high localized concentration of potassium ion in the region of a rapidly dissolving tablet, which injures the bowel wall and thereby produces obstruction, hemorrhage, or perforation. K-TAB (potassium chloride slow-release tablets) is an inert, porous matrix tablet formulated to provide a controlled rate of release of potassium chloride and thus to minimize the possibility of a high local concentration of potassium ion near the bowel wall. While the reported frequency of small-bowel lesions is much less with slow-release tablets (less than one per 100,000 patient-years) than with enteric-coated potassium chloride tablets (40–50 per 100,000 patient-years), cases associated with slow-release tablets have been reported both in foreign countries and in the United States. In addition, perhaps because the slow-release tablet preparations are not enteric-coated and release potassium in the stomach, there have been reports of upper gastrointestinal bleeding associated with these products. The total number of gastrointestinal lesions remains less than one per 100,000 patient-years. Potassium chloride slow-release tablets should be discontinued immediately and the possibility of bowel obstruction or perforation considered if severe vomiting, abdominal pain, distention, or gastrointestinal bleeding occurs.

Precautions: The diagnosis of potassium depletion is ordinarily made by demonstrating hypokalemia in a patient with a clinical history suggesting some cause for potassium depletion. In interpreting the serum potassium level, the physician should bear in mind that acute alkalosis *per se* can produce hypokalemia in the absence of a deficit in total body potassium, while acute acidosis *per se* can increase the serum potassium concentration into the normal range even in the presence of a reduced total body potassium. The treatment of potassium depletion, particularly in the presence of cardiac disease, renal disease, or acidosis, requires careful attention to acid-base balance and appropriate monitoring of serum electrolytes, the electrocardiogram, and the clinical status of the patient.

The use of potassium salts in patients with chronic renal disease, or any other condition which impairs potassium excretion, requires particularly careful monitoring of the serum potassium concentration and appropriate dosage adjustment.

Continued on next page

If desired, additional literature on any Abbott Product will be provided upon request to Abbott Laboratories.

Abbott—Cont.

Carcinogenesis: No data are available on long-term potential for carcinogenicity in animals or humans.
Pregnancy: K-TAB tablets are not expected to cause fetal harm when administered in dosages which will not result in hyperkalemia.
Nursing Mothers: Although no studies have been done, it is presumed that potassium chloride is excreted in human milk. Caution should be exercised when K-TAB is administered to a nursing woman.
Pediatric use: Safety and effectiveness in children have not been established.

Adverse Reactions: One of the most severe adverse effects is hyperkalemia (see Contraindications, Warnings, and Overdosage). There also have been reports of upper and lower gastrointestinal conditions including obstruction, bleeding, ulceration, and perforation (see Contraindications and Warnings); other factors known to be associated with such conditions were present in many of these patients.
The most common adverse reactions to oral potassium salts are nausea, vomiting, abdominal discomfort, and diarrhea. These symptoms are due to irritation of the gastrointestinal tract and are best managed by diluting the preparation further, taking the dose with meals, or reducing the dose.
Skin rash has been reported rarely.

Overdosage: The administration of oral potassium salts to persons with normal excretory mechanisms for potassium rarely causes serious hyperkalemia. However, if excretory mechanisms are impaired or if potassium is administered too rapidly intravenously, potentially fatal hyperkalemia can result (see Contraindications and Warnings). It is important to recognize that hyperkalemia is usually asymptomatic and may be manifested only by an increased serum potassium concentration and characteristic electrocardiographic changes (peaking of T-waves, loss of P-waves, depression of S-T segments, and prolongation of QT intervals). Late manifestations include muscle paralysis and cardiovascular collapse from cardiac arrest.
Treatment measures for hyperkalemia include the following: (1) elimination of foods and medications containing potassium and of potassium-sparing diuretics; (2) intravenous administration of 300 to 500 ml/hr of dextrose solution (10–25%), containing 10 units of insulin/20 g dextrose; (3) correction of acidosis, if present, with intravenous sodium bicarbonate; (4) use of exchange resins, hemodialysis, or peritoneal dialysis. In treating hyperkalemia, it should be recalled that in patients who have been stabilized on digitalis, too rapid a lowering of the serum potassium concentration can produce digitalis toxicity.

Dosage and Administration: The usual dietary intake of potassium by the average adult is 40 to 80 mEq per day. Potassium depletion sufficient to cause hypokalemia usually requires the loss of 200 or more mEq of potassium from the total body store. Dosage must be adjusted to the individual needs of each patient but the usual adult dose is 20–80 mEq of potassium per day. One K-TAB tablet twice daily provides 20 mEq of potassium and 20 mEq of chloride.
NOTE: K-TAB IS TO BE SWALLOWED WHOLE AND NOT CRUSHED OR CHEWED.

How Supplied: K-TAB (potassium chloride slow-release tablets) contains 750 mg of potassium chloride (equivalent to 10 mEq). K-TAB is provided as yellow, ovaloid, slow-release Filmtab® tablets in bottles of 100 (**NDC** 0074-7804-13) and 1000 (**NDC** 0074-7804-19) and in ABBO-PAC® unit dose packages of 100 (**NDC** 0074-7804-11).
[*Shown in Product Identification Section*]

TM—Trademark
Filmtab—Film-sealed tablets, Abbott
Abbott Pharmaceuticals, Inc.
North Chicago, IL 60064
Ref. 03-4236-R6

LIDOCAINE HYDROCHLORIDE INJECTION, U.S.P. ℞

Aqueous solutions for acute management of cardiac arrhythmias or for local anesthesia.

Description: Lidocaine hydrochloride is designated chemically as 2-(diethylamino)-2′, 6′-acetoxylidide monohydrochloride and is freely soluble in water. Lidocaine occurs as colorless crystals. The injectable preparation is an aqueous solution of the freely soluble hydrochloride salt. pH adjusted with sodium hydroxide and hydrochloric acid.

FOR CARDIAC ARRHYTHMIAS

Actions: Lidocaine reportedly exerts a cardiac antiarrhythmic effect by increasing the electrical stimulation threshold of the ventricle during diastole. At usual doses, lidocaine produces no change in myocardial contractility, in systemic arterial pressure or in absolute refractory period.
About 90% of an administered dose of the drug is metabolized in the liver. The remaining 10% is excreted unchanged in the urine.
Indications: Lidocaine administered intravenously is specifically indicated in the acute management of (1) ventricular arrhythmias occurring during cardiac manipulation, such as cardiac surgery; and (2) life-threatening arrhythmias, particularly those which are ventricular in origin, such as occur during acute myocardial infarction.
Contraindications: Lidocaine is contraindicated in patients with a known hypersensitivity to local anesthetics of the amide type.
Intravenous injection is contraindicated in patients with Adams-Stokes syndrome or with severe degrees of sinoatrial, atrioventricular or intraventricular heart block.
Warnings: Constant monitoring with an electrocardiograph is essential for proper intravenous administration of lidocaine. Signs of excessive depression of cardiac conductivity, such as prolongation of PR interval and QRS complex and appearance or aggravation of arrhythmias, should be followed by prompt cessation of intravenous injection or infusion of this agent. It is mandatory to have emergency equipment and drugs immediately available to manage possible adverse reactions involving the cardiovascular, respiratory or central nervous systems. Evidence for proper use in children is limited.
Precautions: Caution should be exercised with repeated use of lidocaine in patients with severe liver or renal disease because accumulation may lead to toxic phenomena, since the drug is metabolized mainly in the liver and partially excreted unchanged by the kidney. The drug also should be used with caution in patients with hypovolemia and shock, and all forms of heart block (see CONTRAINDICATIONS and WARNINGS).
In patients with sinus bradycardia the intravenous administration of lidocaine for the elimination of ventricular ectopic beats without prior acceleration in heart rate (e.g., by isoproterenol or by electric pacing) may provoke more frequent and serious ventricular arrhythmias.
Adverse Reactions: Systemic reactions of the following types have been reported:

1. Central Nervous System: Light-headedness; drowsiness; dizziness; apprehension; euphoria; tinnitus; blurred or double vision; vomiting; sensation of heat, cold or numbness; twitching; tremors; convulsions; unconsciousness and respiratory depression and arrest.
2. Cardiovascular System: Hypotension; cardiovascular collapse and bradycardia which may lead to cardiac arrest.

There have been no reports of cross sensitivity between lidocaine and procainamide or between lidocaine and quinidine.
Management of Adverse Reactions:

1. In case of severe reaction, discontinue use of the drug.
2. Institute the emergency resuscitative procedures and administer the emergency drugs necessary to manage the severe reaction.
3. For severe convulsions, small doses of an ultrashort-acting barbiturate or a short-acting muscle relaxant (if the patient is under anesthesia) may be used.

Dosage and Administration: For direct intravenous injection, the usual adult dose is 50 to 100 mg. administered at an approximate rate of 25 to 50 mg./minute. Sufficient time should be allowed to enable a slow circulation to carry the drug to the site of action. If the initial injection of 50 to 100 mg. does not produce the desired response, a second dose may be repeated after five minutes.
NO MORE THAN 200 TO 300 MG. OF LIDOCAINE SHOULD BE ADMINISTERED DURING A ONE-HOUR PERIOD.
Patients with reduced hepatic function or diminished hepatic blood flow (as in heart failure and after cardiac surgery), or those over 70 years of age, should receive half the usual loading dose and also receive lower maintenance doses of intravenous lidocaine.
In children, experience with the drug is limited.
For continuous intravenous infusion in patients whose arrhythmia tends to recur following a temporary response to a single or once repeated direct injection, and who are incapable of receiving oral antiarrhythmic therapy, lidocaine hydrochloride may be infused continuously in a concentration of 0.1% (1 mg./ml.) at a rate of 1 to 4 ml./minute (20 to 50 micrograms/kg./minute in the average 70 kg. adult). A 0.2% solution (2 mg./ml.) can be given at a rate of 0.5 to 2 ml./minute. I.V. infusion of the drug must be administered under constant ECG monitoring to avoid potential overdosage and toxicity. I.V. infusion should be terminated as soon as the patient's basic cardiac rhythm appears to be stable or at the earliest signs of toxicity. As soon as possible, and when indicated, patients should be changed to an oral antiarrhythmic agent for maintenance therapy.
When administering lidocaine hydrochloride (or any potent medication) by continuous intravenous infusion, it is advisable to use a precision volume control I.V. set.
A 0.1% solution (1 mg./ml.) for I.V. infusion may be prepared by the addition of one gram of lidocaine hydrochloride injected through the rubber stopper of a 1000 ml bottle of 5% Dextrose Injection (preferred diluent). Infusion of such solution at a rate of 1 to 4 ml./minute will provide approximately 1 to 4 mg./minute.
A 0.2% solution can be prepared by adding two grams of lidocaine hydrochloride to 1000 ml of 5% Dextrose Injection. The rate of administration sufficient to provide 1 to 4 mg./minute is 0.5 to 2 ml./minute.

FOR LOCAL ANESTHESIA

Actions: Lidocaine stabilizes the neuronal membrane and prevents the initiation and transmission of nerve impulses, thereby effecting local anesthetic action.
The onset of action is rapid and the blockade may last from one to one and one-half hours.

Lidocaine, because of its non-ester structure, is not detoxified by the circulating plasma esterases. The liver is the chief site of biotransformation of the drug, and both free and conjugated forms of the drug are excreted in the urine.

Lidocaine does not ordinarily produce irritation or tissue damage following parenteral administration.

Anesthesia may be extended and absorption retarded by the addition of a dilute concentration of epinephrine or other appropriate vasoconstrictor drugs.

Indications: Lidocaine hydrochloride injection USP is indicated for production of local anesthesia by nerve block, infiltration injection, caudal or other epidural blocks.

Contraindications: Lidocaine is contraindicated in patients with a known hypersensitivity to local anesthetics of the amide type.

Local anesthetic agents should not be used in patients with severe shock or heart block. Local anesthetic procedures should not be used when there is inflammation in the region of the proposed injection.

Warnings: RESUSCITATIVE EQUIPMENT AND DRUGS SHOULD BE IMMEDIATELY AVAILABLE WHEN ANY LOCAL ANESTHETIC IS USED.

Solutions which contain a vasoconstrictor should be used with extreme caution in patients whose medical history and physical evaluation suggest the existence of hypertension, arteriosclerotic heart disease, cerebral vascular insufficiency, heart block, thyrotoxicosis and diabetes, etc.

Solutions mixed with epinephrine or other vasopressor agents should be used with extreme caution in patients receiving drugs known to produce blood pressure alterations (i.e., MAO inhibitors, tricyclic antidepressants, phenothiazines, etc.) as either severe and sustained hypotension or hypertension may occur.

Usage in Pregnancy: Safe use of lidocaine has not been established with respect to possible adverse effects upon fetal development. Therefore, lidocaine should not be used in women of childbearing potential and particularly during early pregnancy unless, in the judgment of the clinician the potential benefits outweigh the unknown hazards.

This does not exclude use of the drug at term for obstetrical analgesia. Lidocaine has been used effectively for obstetrical analgesia. Adverse effects on the fetus, course of labor or delivery are rare when proper dosage and technique are used. For paracervical block during labor or pudendal block during delivery, the use of local anesthesia without epinephrine is recommended.

In obstetrics, if vasopressor drugs are used either to correct hypotension or added to the local anesthetic solution, it should be noted that some oxytocic drugs may cause severe persistent hypertension and even rupture of a cerebral blood vessel may occur during the postpartum period.

Precautions: The safety and effectiveness of lidocaine depends upon proper dosage, correct technique, adequate precautions and readiness for emergencies.

The lowest dosage that results in effective anesthesia should be used to avoid high plasma levels and serious undesirable systemic side effects.

Injection of repeated doses of lidocaine may cause significant increases in blood levels with each repeated dose due to slow accumulation of the drug or its metabolites or due to slow metabolic degradation. Tolerance varies with the status of the patient. Debilitated, elderly patients, acutely ill patients and children should be given doses commensurate with their age and physical status.

Injections should always be made slowly after aspiration to avoid or reduce the possibility of inadvertent intravascular injection. Intravascular injection may result in serious adverse reactions as well as anesthetic failure.

Lidocaine should be used cautiously in patients with known drug allergies or sensitivities. Patients allergic to a para-aminobenzoic acid ester type of local anesthetic (e.g., procaine, tetracaine, etc.) have not shown cross sensitivity to lidocaine.

Caudal or other epidural block anesthesia should be used with extreme caution in patients with existing neurological disease, spinal deformities, septicemia or severe hypertension and in very young patients.

Solutions admixed with epinephrine or other vasopressor agents should be used with caution in the presence of diseases which may adversely affect the patient's cardiovascular system.

Solutions containing a vasoconstrictor should be used cautiously and in carefully circumscribed quantities in areas of the body supplied by end arteries or having otherwise compromised blood supply (e.g., digits, nose, external ear, penis, etc.).

The decision whether or not to use local anesthesia in the following conditions depends on the physician's appraisal of the advantages as opposed to the risk:

1. Paracervical block when fetal distress is anticipated or when predisposing factors causative of fetal distress are present (i.e., toxemia, prematurity, diabetes, etc.). Fetal bradycardia frequently follows paracervical block and may be associated with fetal acidosis. Fetal heart rate should always be monitored during paracervical anesthesia. When the recommended dose is exceeded the incidence of fetal bradycardia increases.
2. Serious cardiac arrhythmias may occur if preparations containing a vasoconstrictor are employed in patients following the administration of chloroform, trichloroethylene, halothane, etc.

Adverse Reactions: Adverse reactions result from high plasma levels due to rapid absorption, inadvertent intravascular injection, or excessive dosage. Other causes of reactions are hypersensitivity, idiosyncrasy or diminished tolerance.

Reactions due to overdosage (high plasma levels) are systemic and involve the central nervous system and the cardiovascular system.

Reactions involving the central nervous system are characterized by excitation and/or depression. Nervousness, dizziness, blurred vision or tremors may occur followed by drowsiness, convulsions, unconsciousness and possible respiratory arrest. Excitement may be transient or absent, and the first manifestations may be drowsiness merging into unconsciousness and respiratory arrest.

Reactions involving the cardiovascular system include depression of the myocardium, hypotension, bradycardia, and even cardiac arrest.

Allergic reactions are characterized by cutaneous lesions of delayed onset, or urticaria, edema and other manifestations of allergy. The detection of sensitivity by skin testing is of doubtful value.

Treatment of a patient with toxic manifestations consists of maintaining an airway, and supporting ventilation using oxygen and assisted or controlled respiration is required. Supportive treatment of the cardiovascular system consists of using vasopressors, preferably those that stimulate the myocardium (e.g., epinephrine, metaraminol, etc.) and intravenous fluids and, when necessary, external cardiac massage. Convulsions may be controlled by the intravenous administration of small increments of an anticonvulsive agent such as benzodiazepine (e.g., diazepem) or an ultrashort-acting barbiturate (i.e., thiopental, thiamylal) or a short-acting barbiturate (secobarbital, pentobarbital) or, if these are not available, a short-acting muscle relaxant (succinylcholine), together with oxygen. Muscle relaxants and intravenous barbiturates should only be used by those familiar with their use.

Dosage and Administration: The dosage varies and depends upon the area to be anesthetized, vascularity of the tissues, number of neuronal segments to be blocked, individual tolerance and the technique of anesthesia. The lowest dosage needed to provide effective anesthesia should be administered. For specific techniques and procedures refer to standard textbooks.

THE USUAL INITIAL ADULT DOSE OF LIDOCAINE HYDROCHLORIDE WITHOUT EPINEPHRINE SHOULD NOT EXCEED 2 MG PER POUND.

THE USUAL INITIAL ADULT DOSE WITH EPINEPHRINE SHOULD NOT EXCEED 3 MG PER POUND.

Use of 0.5 or 1% concentrations of lidocaine is recommended in children to minimize the possibility of toxic reactions and the total dose should be reduced in proportion to body weight or surface area.

FOR EPIDURAL OR SPINAL ANESTHESIA, USE ONLY SOLUTIONS WITHOUT PRESERVATIVES

How Supplied: Lidocaine Hydrochloride Injection, U.S.P. is available in a variety of dosage strengths, containers and sizes. Consult Abbott Laboratories for a current listing.

Ref. 06-2704-R13

MURINE EAR WAX REMOVAL SYSTEM/MURINE EAR DROPS — OTC

Description: Carbamide peroxide 6.5% in anhydrous glycerin and a 1.0 fl. oz. soft rubber ear syringe. The MURINE EAR WAX REMOVAL SYSTEM is the only self-treatment method on the market for complete ear wax removal. Application of carbamide peroxide drops followed by warm water irrigation is the only effective, medically recommended way to remove hardened ear wax.

Actions: The carbamide peroxide formula in MURINE EAR DROPS is an aid in the removal of hardened cerumen from the ear canal. Anhydrous glycerin penetrates and softens wax while the release of oxygen from carbamide peroxide provides a mechanical action resulting in the loosening of the softened wax accumulation. It is usually necessary to remove the loosened wax by gentle irrigation with warm water using the soft rubber ear syringe provided.

Indications: The MURINE EAR WAX REMOVAL SYSTEM is indicated as an aid in the removal of hardened or tightly packed cerumen from the ear canal or as an aid in the prevention of ceruminosis.

Caution: If redness, tenderness, pain, dizziness or ear drainage is present or develops, the medication should not be used or continued until a physician is seen. Do not use if ear drum is known to be perforated.

Dosage and Administration: For wax removal, place five drops into affected ear twice daily for three or four days. Tip of bottle should not enter ear canal. Remove softened wax after each application by gently flushing ear with warm (body temperature) water using the soft rubber ear syringe provided. Tip of syringe should be at the edge of the ear canal.

The ear canal can be kept free from accumulated hardened cerumen by regular usage of the MURINE EAR WAX REMOVAL SYSTEM.

How Supplied: The MURINE EAR WAX REMOVAL SYSTEM contains 0.5 fl. oz. drops and a 1.0 fl. oz. soft rubber ear syringe.

Continued on next page

If desired, additional literature on any Abbott Product will be provided upon request to Abbott Laboratories.

Abbott—Cont.

Also available in 0.5 fl. oz. drops only, MURINE EAR DROPS

MURINE® OTC
Eye Drops

Description: Murine® Regular Formula is a sterile isotonic buffered solution containing glycerin, potassium chloride, sodium chloride, sodium phosphate (monobasic and dibasic), and water. Edetate disodium 0.05% and benzalkonium chloride 0.01% are added as preservatives.

Indications: Murine is non-staining, clear solution formulated to closely match the natural fluid of the eye for gentle, soothing relief from minor eye irritation. Murine Regular Formula is the only leading eye drop formulated with a pH that closely matches the pH of the eye. Murine, which contains no vasoconstrictor, compliments the eye's natural cleaning, lubricating process. Use whenever desired to cleanse or refresh the eyes and to relieve minor irritation due to smog, sun glare, wind, dust, wearing contact lenses and overuse of the eyes in reading, driving, TV and close work.

Warning: Murine Regular Formula should only be used for minor eye irritations. If irritation persists or increases, discontinue use and consult your physician.

Dosage and Administration: Two or three drops into each eye several times a day or as directed by a physician. Do not touch bottle tip to any surface since this may contaminate solution. Remove contact lenses before using. Keep container tightly closed. Keep this and all medications out of reach of children.

How Supplied: In 0.5 fl. oz. and 1.5 fl. oz. plastic dropper bottle.

MURINE® PLUS OTC
Eye Drops

Description: Murine® Plus is a sterile isotonic buffered solution containing tetrahydrozoline hydrochloride 0.05%, boric acid, sodium borate and water. Edetate disodium 0.1% and benzalkonium chloride 0.01% are added as preservatives.

Indications: Murine Plus is a decongestant ophthalmic solution designed to refresh and soothe as it removes redness from irritated eyes. Murine Plus contains laboratory tested, and scientifically blended ingredients including an effective vasoconstrictor which narrows swollen blood vessels and rapidly whitens reddened eyes in a formulation which produces a refreshing, soothing effect. Murine Plus is a sterile, isotonic solution compatible with the natural fluids of the eye.

Warning: Murine Plus should only be used for minor eye irritations. If relief is not obtained within 48 hours, or if irritation persists or increases, discontinue use and consult your physician.

Murine Plus should not be used by individuals with glaucoma and serious eye diseases. In some instances redness or inflammation may be due to serious eye conditions such as acute iritis, acute glaucoma, or corneal trauma. When redness, pain, or blurring persist, a physician should be consulted at once.

Dosage and Administration: One or two drops in eye(s) two or three times daily or as directed by physician. Do not touch bottle tip to any surface, since this may contaminate the solution. Remove contact lenses before using. Keep container tightly closed. Keep this and all other medicines out of reach of children.

How Supplied: In 0.5 fl. oz. and 1.5 fl. oz. plastic dropper bottle.

NEMBUTAL® SODIUM CAPSULES ℞ Ⓒ
(pentobarbital sodium capsules, USP)

WARNING: MAY BE HABIT FORMING

Description: The barbiturates are nonselective central nervous system depressants which are primarily used as sedative hypnotics. The barbiturates and their sodium salts are subject to control under the Federal Controlled Substances Act (See "Drug Abuse and Dependence" section).

Barbiturates are substituted pyrimidine derivatives in which the basic structure common to these drugs is barbituric acid, a substance which has no central nervous system (CNS) activity. CNS activity is obtained by substituting alkyl, alkenyl, or aryl groups on the pyrimidine ring. Nembutal (pentobarbital sodium) is chemically represented by sodium 5-ethyl-5-(1-methylbutyl) barbiturate.

The sodium salt of pentobarbital occurs as a white, slightly bitter powder which is freely soluble in water and alcohol but practically insoluble in benzene and ether. Nembutal Sodium capsules for oral administration contain either 30 mg, 50 mg, or 100 mg of pentobarbital sodium.

Clinical Pharmacology: Barbiturates are capable of producing all levels of CNS mood alteration from excitation to mild sedation, to hypnosis, and deep coma. Overdosage can produce death. In high enough therapeutic doses, barbiturates induce anesthesia.

Barbiturates depress the sensory cortex, decrease motor activity, alter cerebellar function, and produce drowsiness, sedation, and hypnosis.

Barbiturate-induced sleep differs from physiological sleep. Sleep laboratory studies have demonstrated that barbiturates reduce the amount of time spent in the rapid eye movement (REM) phase of sleep or dreaming stage. Also, Stages III and IV sleep are decreased. Following abrupt cessation of barbiturates used regularly, patients may experience markedly increased dreaming, nightmares, and/or insomnia. Therefore, withdrawal of a single therapeutic dose over 5 or 6 days has been recommended to lessen the REM rebound and disturbed sleep which contribute to drug withdrawal syndrome (for example, decrease the dose from 3 to 2 doses a day for 1 week).

In studies, secobarbital sodium and pentobarbital sodium have been found to lose most of their effectiveness for both inducing and maintaining sleep by the end of 2 weeks of continued drug administration at fixed doses. The short-, intermediate-, and, to a lesser degree, long-acting barbiturates have been widely prescribed for treating insomnia. Although the clinical literature abounds with claims that the short-acting barbiturates are superior for producing sleep while the intermediate-acting compounds are more effective in maintaining sleep, controlled studies have failed to demonstrate these differential effects. Therefore, as sleep medications, the barbiturates are of limited value beyond short-term use.

Barbiturates have little analgesic action at subanesthetic doses. Rather, in subanesthetic doses these drugs may increase the reaction of painful stimuli. All barbiturates exhibit anticonvulsant activity in anesthetic doses. However, of the drugs in this class, only phenobarbital, mephobarbital, and metharbital have been clinically demonstrated to be effective as oral anticonvulsants in subhypnotic doses.

Barbiturates are respiratory depressants. The degree of respiratory depression is dependent upon dose. With hypnotic doses, respiratory depression produced by barbiturates is similar to that which occurs during physiologic sleep with slight decrease in blood pressure and heart rate.

Studies in laboratory animals have shown that barbiturates cause reduction in the tone and contractility of the uterus, ureters, and urinary bladder. However, concentrations of the drugs required to produce this effect in humans are not reached with sedative-hypnotic doses.

Barbiturates do not impair normal hepatic function, but have been shown to induce liver microsomal enzymes, thus increasing and/or altering the metabolism of barbiturates and other drugs. (See "Precautions—*Drug Interactions*" section).

Pharmacokinetics: Barbiturates are absorbed in varying degrees following oral, rectal, or parenteral administration. The salts are more rapidly absorbed than are the acids. The rate of absorption is increased if the sodium salt is ingested as a dilute solution or taken on an empty stomach.

The onset of action for oral or rectal administration varies from 20 to 60 minutes.

Duration of action, which is related to the rate at which the barbiturates are redistributed throughout the body, varies among persons and in the same person from time to time. In Table 1, the barbiturates are classified according to their duration of action. This classification should not be used to predict the exact duration of effect, but the grouping of drugs should be used as a guide in the selection of barbiturates.

No studies have demonstrated that the different routes of administration are equivalent with respect to bioavailability.

[See table 1 shown in Nembutal Elixir prescribing information.]

Barbiturates are weak acids that are absorbed and rapidly distributed to all tissues and fluids with high concentrations in the brain, liver, and kidneys. Lipid solubility of the barbiturates is the dominant factor in their distribution within the body. The more lipid soluble the barbiturate, the more rapidly it penetrates all tissues of the body. Barbiturates are bound to plasma and tissue proteins to a varying degree with the degree of binding increasing directly as a function of lipid solubility. The plasma half-life for pentobarbital in adults is 15 to 50 hours and appears to be dose dependent.

Barbiturates are metabolized primarily by the hepatic microsomal enzyme system, and the metabolic products are excreted in the urine, and less commonly, in the feces. Approximately 25 to 50 percent of a dose of aprobarbital or phenobarbital is eliminated unchanged in the urine, whereas the amount of other barbiturates excreted unchanged in the urine is negligible. The excretion of unmetabolized barbiturate is one feature that distinguishes the long-acting category from those belonging to other categories which are almost entirely metabolized. The inactive metabolites of the barbiturates are excreted as conjugates of glucuronic acid.

Indications and Usage: *Oral:*

a. Sedatives.

b. Hypnotics, for the short-term treatment of insomnia, since they appear to lose their effectiveness for sleep induction and sleep maintenance after 2 weeks (See "Clinical Pharmacology" section).

c. Preanesthetics.

Contraindications: Barbiturates are contraindicated in patients with known barbiturate sensitivity. Barbiturates are also contraindicated in patients with a history of manifest or latent porphyria.

Warnings:

1. *Habit forming:* Barbiturates may be habit forming. Tolerance, psychological and physical dependence may occur with continued use. (See "Drug Abuse and Dependence" and "Pharmacokinetics" sections). Patients who have psychological dependence on barbiturates may increase the dosage or decrease the dosage interval without consulting a physician and may subsequently develop a physical dependence on barbiturates. To minimize the possibility of overdosage or the development of dependence, the prescribing

and dispensing of sedative-hypnotic barbiturates should be limited to the amount required for the interval until the next appointment. Abrupt cessation after prolonged use in the dependent person may result in withdrawal symptoms, including delirium, convulsions, and possibly death. Barbiturates should be withdrawn gradually from any patient known to be taking excessive dosage over long periods of time. (See "Drug Abuse and Dependence" section).

2. *Acute or chronic pain:* Caution should be exercised when barbiturates are administered to patients with acute or chronic pain, because paradoxical excitement could be induced or important symptoms could be masked. However, the use of barbiturates as sedatives in the postoperative surgical period and as adjuncts to cancer chemotherapy is well established.
3. *Use in pregnancy:* Barbiturates can cause fetal damage when administered to a pregnant woman. Retrospective, case-controlled studies have suggested a connection between the maternal consumption of barbiturates and a higher than expected incidence of fetal abnormalities. Following oral or parenteral administration, barbiturates readily cross the placental barrier and are distributed throughout fetal tissues with highest concentrations found in the placenta, fetal liver, and brain.
   Withdrawal symptoms occur in infants born to mothers who receive barbiturates throughout the last trimester of pregnancy. (See "Drug Abuse and Dependence" section). If this drug is used during pregnancy, or if the patient becomes pregnant while taking this drug, the patient should be apprised of the potential hazard to the fetus.
4. *Synergistic effects:* The concomitant use of alcohol or other CNS depressants may produce additive CNS depressant effects.

Precautions:

General: Barbiturates may be habit forming. Tolerance and psychological and physical dependence may occur with continuing use. (See "Drug Abuse and Dependence" section). Barbiturates should be administered with caution, if at all, to patients who are mentally depressed, have suicidal tendencies, or a history of drug abuse.

Elderly or debilitated patients may react to barbiturates with marked excitement, depression, and confusion. In some persons, barbiturates repeatedly produce excitement rather than depression.

In patients with hepatic damage, barbiturates should be administered with caution and initially in reduced doses. Barbiturates should not be administered to patients showing the premonitory signs of hepatic coma.

The 30 mg and 100 mg capsules of Nembutal Sodium contain FD&C Yellow No. 5 (tartrazine) which may cause allergic-type reactions (including bronchial asthma) in certain susceptible individuals. Although the overall incidence of FD&C Yellow No. 5 (tartrazine) sensitivity in the general population is low, it is frequently seen in patients who also have aspirin hypersensitivity.

Information for the patient: Practitioners should give the following information and instructions to patients receiving barbiturates.

1. The use of barbiturates carries with it an associated risk of psychological and/or physical dependence. The patient should be warned against increasing the dose of the drug without consulting a physician.
2. Barbiturates may impair mental and/or physical abilities required for the performance of potentially hazardous tasks (e.g., driving, operating machinery, etc.).
3. Alcohol should not be consumed while taking barbiturates. Concurrent use of the barbiturates with other CNS depressants (e.g., alcohol, narcotics, tranquilizers, and antihistamines) may result in additional CNS depressant effects.

Laboratory tests: Prolonged therapy with barbiturates should be accompanied by periodic laboratory evaluation of organ systems, including hematopoietic, renal, and hepatic systems. (See "Precautions—*General*" and "Adverse Reactions" sections).

Drug interactions: Most reports of clinically significant drug interactions occurring with the barbiturates have involved phenobarbital. However, the application of these data to other barbiturates appears valid and warrants serial blood level determinations of the relevant drugs when there are multiple therapies.

1. *Anticoagulants:* Phenobarbital lowers the plasma levels of dicumarol (name previously used: bishydroxycoumarin) and causes a decrease in anticoagulant activity as measured by the prothrombin time. Barbiturates can induce hepatic microsomal enzymes resulting in increased metabolism and decreased anticoagulant response of oral anticoagulants (e.g., warfarin, acenocoumarol, dicumarol, and phenprocoumon). Patients stabilized on anticoagulant therapy may require dosage adjustments if barbiturates are added to or withdrawn from their dosage regimen.
2. *Corticosteroids:* Barbiturates appear to enhance the metabolism of exogenous corticosteroids probably through the induction of hepatic microsomal enzymes. Patients stabilized on corticosteroid therapy may require dosage adjustments if barbiturates are added to or withdrawn from their dosage regimen.
3. *Griseofulvin:* Phenobarbital appears to interfere with the absorption of orally administered griseofulvin, thus decreasing its blood level. The effect of the resultant decreased blood levels of griseofulvin on therapeutic response has not been established. However, it would be preferable to avoid concomitant administration of these drugs.
4. *Doxycycline:* Phenobarbital has been shown to shorten the half-life of doxycycline for as long as 2 weeks after barbiturate therapy is discontinued.
   This mechanism is probably through the induction of hepatic microsomal enzymes that metabolize the antibiotic. If phenobarbital and doxycycline are administered concurrently, the clinical response to doxycycline should be monitored closely.
5. *Phenytoin, sodium valproate, valproic acid:* The effect of barbiturates on the metabolism of phenytoin appears to be variable. Some investigators report an accelerating effect, while others report no effect. Because the effect of barbiturates on the metabolism of phenytoin is not predictable, phenytoin and barbiturate blood levels should be monitored more frequently if these drugs are given concurrently. Sodium valproate and valproic acid appear to decrease barbiturate metabolism; therefore, barbiturate blood levels should be monitored and appropriate dosage adjustments made as indicated.
6. *Central nervous system depressants:* The concomitant use of other central nervous system depressants including other sedatives or hypnotics, antihistamines, tranquilizers, or alcohol, may produce additive depressant effects.
7. *Monoamine oxidase inhibitors (MAOI):* MAOI prolong the effects of barbiturates probably because metabolism of the barbiturate is inhibited.
8. *Estradiol, estrone, progesterone and other steroidal hormones:* Pretreatment with or concurrent administration of phenobarbital may decrease the effect of estradiol by increasing its metabolism. There have been reports of patients treated with antiepileptic drugs (e.g., phenobarbital) who became pregnant while taking oral contraceptives. An alternate contraceptive method might be suggested to women taking phenobarbital.

Carcinogenesis: Adequate data are not available on long-term potential for carcinogenicity in humans or animals for pentobarbital.

Data from one retrospective study of 235 children in which the types of barbiturates are not identified suggested an association between exposure to barbiturates prenatally and an increased incidence of brain tumor. (Gold, E., et al., "Increased Risk of Brain Tumors in Children Exposed to Barbiturates," Journal of National Cancer Institute, 61:1031–1034, 1978).

Pregnancy: 1. *Teratogenic effects.* Pregnancy Category D—See "Warnings—Use in Pregnancy" section.

2. *Nonteratogenic effects.* Reports of infants suffering from long-term barbiturate exposure in utero included the acute withdrawal syndrome of seizures and hyperirritability from birth to a delayed onset of up to 14 days. (See "Drug Abuse and Dependence" section).

Labor and delivery: Hypnotic doses of these barbiturates do not appear to significantly impair uterine activity during labor. Full anesthetic doses of barbiturates decrease the force and frequency of uterine contractions. Administration of sedative-hypnotic barbiturates to the mother during labor may result in respiratory depression in the newborn. Premature infants are particularly susceptible to the depressant effects of barbiturates. If barbiturates are used during labor and delivery, resuscitation equipment should be available.

Data are currently not available to evaluate the effect of these barbiturates when forceps delivery or other intervention is necessary. Also, data are not available to determine the effect of these barbiturates on the later growth, development, and functional maturation of the child.

Nursing mothers: Caution should be exercised when a barbiturate is administered to a nursing woman since small amounts of barbiturates are excreted in the milk.

Adverse Reactions: The following adverse reactions and their incidence were compiled from surveillance of thousands of hospitalized patients. Because such patients may be less aware of certain of the milder adverse effects of barbiturates, the incidence of these reactions may be somewhat higher in fully ambulatory patients.

More than 1 in 100 patients. The most common adverse reaction estimated to occur at a rate of 1 to 3 patients per 100 is: *Nervous System:* Somnolence.

Less than 1 in 100 patients. Adverse reactions estimated to occur at a rate of less than 1 in 100 patients listed below, grouped by organ system, and by decreasing order of occurrence are:

Nervous system: Agitation, confusion, hyperkinesia, ataxia, CNS depression, nightmares, nervousness, psychiatric disturbance, hallucinations, insomnia, anxiety, dizziness, thinking abnormality.

Respiratory system: Hypoventilation, apnea.

Cardiovascular system: Bradycardia, hypotension, syncope.

Digestive system: Nausea, vomiting, constipation.

Other reported reactions: Headache, injection site reactions, hypersensitivity reactions (angioedema, skin rashes, exfoliative dermatitis), fever, liver damage, megaloblastic anemia following chronic phenobarbital use.

Drug Abuse and Dependence: Pentobarbital sodium capsules are subject to control by the Federal Controlled Substances Act under DEA schedule II.

Continued on next page

If desired, additional literature on any Abbott Product will be provided upon request to Abbott Laboratories.

Abbott—Cont.

Barbiturates may be habit forming. Tolerance, psychological dependence, and physical dependence may occur especially following prolonged use of high doses of barbiturates. Daily administration in excess of 400 mg of pentobarbital or secobarbital for approximately 90 days is likely to produce some degree of physical dependence. A dosage of from 600 to 800 mg taken for at least 35 days is sufficient to produce withdrawal seizures. The average daily dose for the barbiturate addict is usually about 1.5 grams. As tolerance to barbiturates develops, the amount needed to maintain the same level of intoxication increases; tolerance to a fatal dosage, however, does not increase more than two-fold. As this occurs, the margin between an intoxicating dosage and fatal dosage becomes smaller.

Symptoms of acute intoxication with barbiturates include unsteady gait, slurred speech, and sustained nystagmus. Mental signs of chronic intoxication include confusion, poor judgment, irritability, insomnia, and somatic complaints.

Symptoms of barbiturate dependence are similar to those of chronic alcoholism. If an individual appears to be intoxicated with alcohol to a degree that is radically disproportionate to the amount of alcohol in his or her blood the use of barbiturates should be suspected. The lethal dose of a barbiturate is far less if alcohol is also ingested.

The symptoms of barbiturate withdrawal can be severe and may cause death. Minor withdrawal symptoms may appear 8 to 12 hours after the last dose of a barbiturate. These symptoms usually appear in the following order: anxiety, muscle twitching, tremor of hands and fingers, progressive weakness, dizziness, distortion in visual perception, nausea, vomiting, insomnia, and orthostatic hypotension. Major withdrawal symptoms (convulsions and delirium) may occur within 16 hours and last up to 5 days after abrupt cessation of these drugs. Intensity of withdrawal symptoms gradually declines over a period of approximately 15 days. Individuals susceptible to barbiturate abuse and dependence include alcoholics and opiate abusers, as well as other sedative-hypnotic and amphetamine abusers.

Drug dependence to barbiturates arises from repeated administration of a barbiturate or agent with barbiturate-like effect on a continuous basis, generally in amounts exceeding therapeutic dose levels. The characteristics of drug dependence to barbiturates include: (a) a strong desire or need to continue taking the drug; (b) a tendency to increase the dose; (c) a psychic dependence on the effects of the drug related to subjective and individual appreciation of those effects; and (d) a physical dependence on the effects of the drug requiring its presence for maintenance of homeostasis and resulting in a definite, characteristic, and self-limited abstinence syndrome when the drug is withdrawn.

Treatment of barbiturate dependence consists of cautious and gradual withdrawal of the drug. Barbiturate-dependent patients can be withdrawn by using a number of different withdrawal regimens. In all cases withdrawal takes an extended period of time. One method involves substituting a 30 mg dose of phenobarbital for each 100 to 200 mg dose of barbiturate that the patient has been taking. The total daily amount of phenobarbital is then administered in 3 to 4 divided doses, not to exceed 600 mg daily. Should signs of withdrawal occur on the first day of treatment, a loading dose of 100 to 200 mg of phenobarbital may be administered IM in addition to the oral dose. After stabilization on phenobarbital, the total daily dose is decreased by 30 mg a day as long as withdrawal is proceeding smoothly. A modification of this regimen involves initiating treatment at the patient's regular dosage level and decreasing the daily dosage by 10 percent if tolerated by the patient.

Infants physically dependent on barbiturates may be given phenobarbital 3 to 10 mg/kg/day. After withdrawal symptoms (hyperactivity, disturbed sleep, tremors, hyperreflexia) are relieved, the dosage of phenobarbital should be gradually decreased and completely withdrawn over a 2 week period.

Overdosage: The toxic dose of barbiturates varies considerably. In general, an oral dose of 1 g of most barbiturates produces serious poisoning in an adult. Death commonly occurs after 2 to 10 g of ingested barbiturate. Barbiturate intoxication may be confused with alcoholism, bromide intoxication, and with various neurological disorders.

Acute overdosage with barbiturates is manifested by CNS and respiratory depression which may progress to Cheyne-Stokes respiration, areflexia, constriction of the pupils to a slight degree (though in severe poisoning they may show paralytic dilation), oliguria, tachycardia, hypotension, lowered body temperature, and coma. Typical shock syndrome (apnea, circulatory collapse, respiratory arrest, and death) may occur.

In extreme overdose, all electrical activity in the brain may cease, in which case a "flat" EEG normally equated with clinical death cannot be accepted. This effect is fully reversible unless hypoxic damage occurs. Consideration should be given to the possibility of barbiturate intoxication even in situations that appear to involve trauma.

Complications such as pneumonia, pulmonary edema, cardiac arrhythmias, congestive heart failure, and renal failure may occur. Uremia may increase CNS sensitivity to barbiturates. Differential diagnosis should include hypoglycemia, head trauma, cerebrovascular accidents, convulsive states, and diabetic coma. Blood levels from acute overdosage for some barbiturates are listed in Table 2.

[See table 2 shown in Nembutal Elixir prescribing information.]

Treatment of overdosage is mainly supportive and consists of the following:

1. Maintenance of an adequate airway, with assisted respiration and oxygen administration as necessary.
2. Monitoring of vital signs and fluid balance.
3. If the patient is conscious and has not lost the gag reflex, emesis may be induced with ipecac. Care should be taken to prevent pulmonary aspiration of vomitus. After completion of vomiting, 30 g activated charcoal in a glass of water may be administered.
4. If emesis is contraindicated, gastric lavage may be performed with a cuffed endotracheal tube in place with the patient in the face down position. Activated charcoal may be left in the emptied stomach and a saline cathartic administered.
5. Fluid therapy and other standard treatment for shock, if needed.
6. If renal function is normal, forced diuresis may aid in the elimination of the barbiturate. Alkalinization of the urine increases renal excretion of some barbiturates, especially phenobarbital, also aprobarbital, and mephobarbital (which is metabolized to phenobarbital).
7. Although not recommended as a routine procedure, hemodialysis may be used in severe barbiturate intoxications or if the patient is anuric or in shock.
8. Patient should be rolled from side to side every 30 minutes.
9. Antibiotics should be given if pneumonia is suspected.
10. Appropriate nursing care to prevent hypostatic pneumonia, decubiti, aspiration, and other complications of patients with altered states of consciousness.

Dosage and Administration: *Adults:* Daytime sedation can ordinarily be provided by one 30 mg capsule of Nembutal Sodium (pentobarbital sodium) taken 3 or 4 times per day. The usual hypnotic dose consists of 100 mg.

Children: Daytime sedation can be provided by 2 to 6 mg/kg/24 hours (maximum 100 mg), depending on age, weight, and the desired degree of sedation.

The proper hypnotic dose for children must be judged on the basis of individual age and weight.

Dosages of barbiturates must be individualized with full knowledge of their particular characteristics and recommended rate of administration. Factors of consideration are the patient's age, weight, and condition.

Special patient population: Dosage should be reduced in the elderly or debilitated because these patients may be more sensitive to barbiturates. Dosage should be reduced for patients with impaired renal function or hepatic disease.

How Supplied: Nembutal Sodium Capsules (pentobarbital sodium capsules, USP) are supplied as follows:

30 mg yellow capsules in bottles of 100 (**NDC** 0074-3120-01);

50 mg transparent and orange-colored capsules in bottles of 100 (**NDC** 0074-3150-11), 500 (**NDC** 0074-3150-02), and 1000 (**NDC** 0074-3150-03);

100 mg yellow capsules in bottles of 100 (**NDC** 0074-3114-01), 500 (**NDC** 0074-3114-02), and 1000 (**NDC** 0074-3114-03), in reverse-numbered strip packages of 25 (**NDC** 0074-3114-10), and in the Abbo-Pac® unit dose packages of 100 (**NDC** 0074-3114-21).

Abbott Pharmaceuticals, Inc.
North Chicago, IL 60064

[*Shown in Product Identification Section*]

Ref. 03-4246-R3

NEMBUTAL® SODIUM SOLUTION ℞ Ⓒ
(pentobarbital sodium injection, USP)
Ampuls—Vials

WARNING: MAY BE HABIT FORMING. DO NOT USE IF MATERIAL HAS PRECIPITATED.

Description: The barbiturates are nonselective central nervous system depressants which are primarily used as sedative hypnotics and also anticonvulsants in subhypnotic doses. The barbiturates and their sodium salts are subject to control under the Federal Controlled Substances Act (See "Drug Abuse and Dependence" section).

The sodium salts of amobarbital, pentobarbital, phenobarbital, and secobarbital are available as sterile parenteral solutions.

Barbiturates are substituted pyrimidine derivatives in which the basic structure common to these drugs is barbituric acid, a substance which has no central nervous system (CNS) activity. CNS activity is obtained by substituting alkyl, alkenyl, or aryl groups on the pyrimidine ring.

Nembutal Sodium Solution (pentobarbital sodium injection) is a sterile solution for intravenous or intramuscular injection. Each ml contains pentobarbital sodium 50 mg, in a vehicle of propylene glycol, 40%, alcohol, 10% and water for injection, to volume. The pH is adjusted to approximately 9.5 with hydrochloric acid and/or sodium hydroxide.

Nembutal Sodium is a short-acting barbiturate, chemically designated as sodium 5-ethyl-5-(1-methylbutyl) barbiturate.

The sodium salt occurs as a white, slightly bitter powder which is freely soluble in water and alcohol but practically insoluble in benzene and ether.

Clinical Pharmacology: Barbiturates are capable of producing all levels of CNS mood alteration from excitation to mild sedation, to hypnosis, and deep coma. Overdosage can produce death. In high enough therapeutic doses, barbiturates induce anesthesia.

Barbiturates depress the sensory cortex, decrease motor activity, alter cerebellar function, and produce drowsiness, sedation, and hypnosis.

Barbiturate-induced sleep differs from physiological sleep. Sleep laboratory studies have demonstrated that barbiturates reduce the amount of time spent in the rapid eye movement (REM) phase of sleep or dreaming stage. Also, Stages III and IV sleep are decreased. Following abrupt cessation of barbiturates used regularly, patients may experience markedly increased dreaming, nightmares, and/or insomnia. Therefore, withdrawal of a single therapeutic dose over 5 or 6 days has been recommended to lessen the REM rebound and disturbed sleep which contribute to drug withdrawal syndrome (for example, decrease the dose from 3 to 2 doses a day for 1 week).

In studies, secobarbital sodium and pentobarbital sodium have been found to lose most of their effectiveness for both inducing and maintaining sleep by the end of 2 weeks of continued drug administration at fixed doses. The short-, intermediate-, and, to a lesser degree, long-acting barbiturates have been widely prescribed for treating insomnia. Although the clinical literature abounds with claims that the short-acting barbiturates are superior for producing sleep while the intermediate-acting compounds are more effective in maintaining sleep, controlled studies have failed to demonstrate these differential effects. Therefore, as sleep medications, the barbiturates are of limited value beyond short-term use.

Barbiturates have little analgesic action at subanesthetic doses. Rather, in subanesthetic doses these drugs may increase the reaction to painful stimuli. All barbiturates exhibit anticonvulsant activity in anesthetic doses. However, of the drugs in this class, only phenobarbital, mephobarbital, and metharbital have been clinically demonstrated to be effective as oral anticonvulsants in subhypnotic doses.

Barbiturates are respiratory depressants. The degree of respiratory depression is dependent upon dose. With hypnotic doses, respiratory depression produced by barbiturates is similar to that which occurs during physiologic sleep with slight decrease in blood pressure and heart rate.

Studies in laboratory animals have shown that barbiturates cause reduction in the tone and contractility of the uterus, ureters, and urinary bladder. However, concentration of the drugs required to produce this effect in humans are not reached with sedative-hypnotic doses.

Barbiturates do not impair normal hepatic function, but have been shown to induce liver microsomal enzymes, thus increasing and/or altering the metabolism of barbiturates and other drugs. (See "Precautions—*Drug Interactions*" section).

Pharmacokinetics: Barbiturates are absorbed in varying degrees following oral, rectal, or parenteral administration. The salts are more rapidly absorbed than are the acids.

The onset of action for oral or rectal administration varies from 20 to 60 minutes. For IM administration, the onset of action is slightly faster. Following IV administration, the onset of action ranges from almost immediately for pentobarbital sodium to 5 minutes for phenobarbital sodium. Maximal CNS depression may not occur until 15 minutes or more after IV administration for phenobarbital sodium.

Duration of action, which is related to the rate at which the barbiturates are redistributed throughout the body, varies among persons and in the same person from time to time.

No studies have demonstrated that the different routes of administration are equivalent with respect to bioavailability.

Barbiturates are weak acids that are absorbed and rapidly distributed to all tissues and fluids with high concentration in the brain, liver, and kidneys. Lipid solubility of the barbiturates is the dominant factor in their distribution within the body. The more lipid soluble the barbiturate, the more rapidly it penetrates all tissues of the body. Barbiturates are bound to plasma and tissue proteins to a varying degree with the degree of binding increasing directly as a function of lipid solubility. The plasma half-life for pentobarbital in adults is 15 to 50 hours and appears to be dose-dependent.

Barbiturates are metabolized primarily by the hepatic microsomal enzyme system, and the metabolic products are excreted in the urine, and less commonly, in the feces. Approximately 25 to 50 percent of a dose of aprobarbital or phenobarbital is eliminated unchanged in the urine, whereas the amount of other barbiturates excreted unchanged in the urine is negligible. The excretion of unmetabolized barbiturate is one feature that distinguishes the long-acting category from those belonging to other categories which are almost entirely metabolized. The inactive metabolities of the barbiturates are excreted as conjugates of glucuronic acid.

Indications and Usage:

Parenteral:

a. Sedatives.
b. Hypnotics, for the short-term treatment of insomnia, since they appear to lose their effectiveness for sleep induction and sleep maintenance after 2 weeks (See "Clinical Pharmacology" section).
c. Preanesthetics.
d. Anticonvulsant, in anesthetic doses, in the emergency control of certain acute convulsive episodes, e.g., those associated with status epilepticus, cholera, eclampsia, meningitis, tetanus, and toxic reactions to strychnine or local anesthetics.

Contraindications: Barbiturates are contraindicated in patients with known barbiturate sensitivity. Barbiturates are also contraindicated in patients with a history of manifest or latent porphyria.

Warnings: 1. *Habit forming:* Barbiturates may be habit forming. Tolerance, psychological and physical dependence may occur with continued use. (See "Drug Abuse and Dependence" and "Pharmacokinetics" sections). Patients who have psychological dependence on barbiturates may increase the dosage or decrease the dosage interval without consulting a physician and may subsequently develop a physical dependence on barbiturates. To minimize the possibility of overdosage or the development of dependence, the prescribing and dispensing of sedative-hypnotic barbiturates should be limited to the amount required for the interval until the next appointment. Abrupt cessation after prolonged use in the dependent person may result in withdrawal symptoms, including delirium, convulsions, and possibly death. Barbiturates should be withdrawn gradually from any patient known to be taking excessive dosage over long periods of time. (See "Drug Abuse and Dependence" section).

2. *IV administration:* Too rapid administration may cause respiratory depression, apnea, laryngospasm, or vasodilation with fall in blood pressure.
3. *Acute or chronic pain:* Caution should be exercised when barbiturates are administered to patients with acute or chronic pain, because paradoxical excitement could be induced or important symptoms could be masked. However, the use of barbiturates as sedatives in the postoperative surgical period and as adjuncts to cancer chemotherapy is well established.
4. *Use in pregnancy:* Barbiturates can cause fetal damage when administered to a pregnant woman. Retrospective, case-controlled studies have suggested a connection between the maternal consumption of barbiturates and a higher than expected incidence of fetal abnormalities. Following oral or parenteral administration, barbiturates readily cross the placental barrier and are distributed throughout fetal tissues with highest concentrations found in the placenta, fetal liver, and brain. Fetal blood levels approach maternal blood levels following parenteral administration.

   Withdrawal symptoms occur in infants born to mothers who receive barbiturates throughout the last trimester of pregnancy. (See "Drug Abuse and Dependence" section). If this drug is used during pregnancy, or if the patient becomes pregnant while taking this drug, the patient should be apprised of the potential hazard to the fetus.
5. *Synergistic effects:* The concomitant use of alcohol or other CNS depressants may produce additive CNS depressant effects.

Precautions: *General:* Barbiturates may be habit forming. Tolerance and psychological and physical dependence may occur with continuing use. (See "Drug Abuse and Dependence" section). Barbiturates should be administered with caution, if at all, to patients who are mentally depressed, have suicidal tendencies, or a history of drug abuse.

Elderly or debilitated patients may react to barbiturates with marked excitement, depression, and confusion. In some persons, barbiturates repeatedly produce excitement rather than depression.

In patients with hepatic damage, barbiturates should be administered with caution and initially in reduced doses. Barbiturates should not be administered to patients showing the premonitory signs of hepatic coma.

Parenteral solutions of barbiturates are highly alkaline. Therefore, extreme care should be taken to avoid perivascular extravasation or intra-arterial injection. Extravascular injection may cause local tissue damage with subsequent necrosis; consequences of intra-arterial injection may vary from transient pain to gangrene of the limb. Any complaint of pain in the limb warrants stopping the injection.

Information for the patient: Practitioners should give the following information and instructions to patients receiving barbiturates.

1. The use of barbiturates carries with it an associated risk of psychological and/or physical dependence. The patient should be warned against increasing the dose of the drug without consulting a physician.
2. Barbiturates may impair mental and/or physical abilities required for the performance of potentially hazardous tasks (e.g., driving, operating machinery, etc.).
3. Alcohol should not be consumed while taking barbiturates. Concurrent use of the barbiturates with other CNS depressants (e.g., alcohol, narcotics, tranquilizers, and antihistamines) may result in additional CNS depressant effects.

Laboratory tests: Prolonged therapy with barbiturates should be accompanied by periodic laboratory evaluation of organ systems, including hematopoietic, renal, and hepatic systems. (See "Precautions-*General*" and "Adverse Reactions" sections).

Drug interactions: Most reports of clinically significant drug interactions occurring with the barbiturates have involved phenobarbital. However, the application of these data to other barbiturates appears valid and warrants serial blood level determinations of the relevant drugs when there are multiple therapies.

Continued on next page

If desired, additional literature on any Abbott Product will be provided upon request to Abbott Laboratories.

Abbott—Cont.

1. *Anticoagulants:* Phenobarbital lowers the plasma levels of dicumarol (name previously used: bishydroxycoumarin) and causes a decrease in anticoagulant activity as measured by the prothrombin time. Barbiturates can induce hepatic microsomal enzymes resulting in increased metabolism and decreased anticoagulant response of oral anticoagulants (e.g., warfarin, acenocoumarol, dicumarol, and phenprocoumon). Patients stabilized on anticoagulant therapy may require dosage adjustments if barbiturates are added to or withdrawn from their dosage regimen.
2. *Corticosteroids:* Barbiturates appear to enhance the metabolism of exogenous corticosteroids probably through the induction of hepatic microsomol enzymes. Patients stabilized on corticosteroid therapy may require dosage adjustments if barbiturates are added to or withdrawn from their dosage regimen.
3. *Griseofulvin:* Phenobarbital appears to interfere with the absorption of orally administered griseofulvin, thus decreasing its blood level. The effect of the resultant decreased blood levels of griseofulvin on therapeutic response has not been established. However, it would be preferable to avoid concomitant administration of these drugs.
4. *Doxycycline:* Phenobarbital has been shown to shorten the half-life of doxycycline for as long as 2 weeks after barbiturate therapy is discontinued.

This mechanism is probably through the induction of hepatic microsomal enzymes that metabolize the antibiotic. If phenobarbital and doxycycline are administered concurrently, the clincial response to doxycycline should be monitored closely.

5. *Phenytoin, sodium valproate, valproic acid:* The effect of barbiturates on the metabolism of phenytoin appears to be variable. Some investigators report an accelerating effect, while others report no effect. Because the effect of barbiturates on the metabolism of phenytoin is not predictable, phenytoin and barbiturate blood levels should be monitored more frequently if these drugs are given concurrently. Sodium valproate and valproic acid appear to decrease barbiturate metabolism; therefore, barbiturate blood levels should be monitored and appropriate dosage adjustments made as indicated.
6. *Central nervous system depressants:* The concomitant use of other central nervous system depressants, including other sedatives or hypnotics, antihistamines, tranquilizers, or alcohol, may produce additive depressant effects.
7. *Monoamine oxidase inhibitors (MAOI):* MAOI prolong the effects of barbiturates probably because metabolism of the barbiturate is inhibited.
8. *Estradiol, estrone, progesterone and other steroidal hormones:* Pretreatment with or concurrent administration of phenobarbital may decrease the effect of estradiol by increasing its metabolism. There have been reports of patients treated with antiepileptic drugs (e.g., phenobarbital) who became pregnant while taking oral contraceptives. An alternate contraceptive method might be suggested to women taking phenobarbital.

Carcinogenesis: Adequate data are not available on long-term potential for carcinogenicity in humans or animals for pentobarbital.

Data from one retrospective study of 235 children in which the types of barbiturates are not identified suggested an association between exposure to barbiturates prenatally and an increased incidence of brain tumor. (Gold, E., et al., "Increased Risk of Brain Tumors in Children Exposed to Barbiturates," Journal of National Cancer Institute, 61:1031–1034, 1978).

Pregnancy: 1. *Teratogenic effects.* Pregnancy Category D—See "Warnings—Use in Pregnancy" section.

2. *Nonteratogenic effects.* Reports of infants suffering from long-term barbiturate exposure in utero included the acute withdrawal syndrome of seizures and hyperirritability from birth to a delayed onset of up to 14 days. (See "Drug Abuse and Dependence" section).

Labor and delivery: Hypnotic doses of these barbiturates do not appear to significantly impair uterine activity during labor. Full anesthetic doses of barbiturates decrease the force and frequency of uterine contractions. Administration of sedative-hypnotic barbiturates to the mother during labor may result in respiratory depression in the newborn. Premature infants are particularly susceptible to the depressant effects of barbiturates. If barbiturates are used during labor and delivery, resuscitation equipment should be available.

Data are currently not available to evaluate the effect of these barbiturates when forceps delivery or other intervention is necessary. Also, data are not available to determine the effect of these barbiturates on the later growth, development, and functional maturation of the child.

Nursing mothers: Caution should be exercised when a barbiturate is administered to a nursing woman since small amounts of barbiturates are excreted in the milk.

Adverse Reactions: The following adverse reactions and their incidence were compiled from surveillance of thousands of hospitalized patients. Because such patients may be less aware of certain of the milder adverse effects of barbiturates, the incidence of these reactions may be somewhat higher in fully ambulatory patients.

More than 1 in 100 patients. The most common adverse reaction estimated to occur at a rate of 1 to 3 patients per 100 is: *Nervous System:* Somnolence.

Less than 1 in 100 patients. Adverse reactions estimated to occur at a rate of less than 1 in 100 patients listed below, grouped by organ system, and by decreasing order of occurrence are:

Nervous system: Agitation, confusion, hyperkinesia, ataxia, CNS depression, nightmares, nervousness, psychiatric disturbance, hallucinations, insomnia, anxiety, dizziness, thinking abnormality.

Respiratory system: Hypoventilation, apnea.

Cardiovascular system: Bradycardia, hypotension, syncope.

Digestive system: Nausea, vomiting, constipation.

Other reported reactions: Headache, injection site reactions, hypersensitivity reactions (angioedema, skin rashes, exfoliative dermatitis), fever, liver damage, megaloblastic anemia following chronic phenobarbital use.

Drug Abuse and Dependence: Pentobarbital sodium injection is subject to control by the Federal Controlled Substances Act under DEA schedule II.

Barbiturates may be habit forming. Tolerance, psychological dependence, and physical dependence may occur especially following prolonged use of high doses of barbiturates. Daily administration in excess of 400 mg of pentobarbital or secobarbital for approximately 90 days is likely to produce some degree of physical dependence. A dosage of from 600 to 800 mg taken for at least 35 days is sufficient to produce withdrawal seizures. The average daily dose for the barbiturate addict is usually about 1.5 g. As tolerance to barbiturate develops, the amount needed to maintain the same level of intoxication increases; tolerance to a fatal dosage, however, does not increase more than twofold. As this occurs, the margin between an intoxicating dosage and fatal dosage becomes smaller.

Symptoms of acute intoxication with barbiturates include unsteady gait, slurred speech, and sustained nystagmus. Mental signs of chronic intoxication include confusion, poor judgment, irritability, insomnia, and somatic complaints.

Symptoms of barbiturate dependence are similar to those of chronic alcoholism. If an individual appears to be intoxicated with alcohol to a degree that is radically disproportionate to the amount of alcohol in his or her blood the use of barbiturates should be suspected. The lethal dose of a barbiturate is far less if alcohol is also ingested.

The symptoms of barbiturate withdrawal can be severe and may cause death. Minor withdrawal symptoms may appear 8 to 12 hours after the last dose of a barbiturate. These symptoms usually appear in the following order: anxiety, muscle twitching, tremor of hands and fingers, progressive weakness, dizziness, distortion in visual perception, nausea, vomiting, insomnia, and orthostatic hypotension. Major withdrawal symptoms (convulsions and delirium) may occur within 16 hours and last up to 5 days after abrupt cessation of these drugs. Intensity of withdrawal symptoms gradually declines over a period of approximately 15 days. Individuals susceptible to barbiturate abuse and dependence include alcoholics and opiate abusers, as well as other sedative-hypnotic and amphetamine abusers.

Drug dependence to barbiturates arises from repeated administration of a barbiturate or agent with barbiturate-like effect on a continuous basis, generally in amounts exceeding therapeutic dose levels. The characteristics of drug dependence to barbiturates include: (a) a strong desire or need to continue taking the drug; (b) a tendency to increase the dose; (c) a psychic dependence on the effects of the drug related to subjective and individual appreciation of those effects; and (d) a physical dependence on the effects of the drug requiring its presence for maintenance of homeostasis and resulting in a definite, characteristic, and self-limited abstinence syndrome when the drug is withdrawn.

Treatment of barbiturate dependence consists of cautious and gradual withdrawal of the drug. Barbiturate-dependent patients can be withdrawn by using a number of different withdrawal regimens. In all cases withdrawal takes an extended period of time. One method involves substituting a 30 mg dose of phenobarbital for each 100 to 200 mg dose of barbiturate that the patient has been taking. The total daily amount of phenobarbital is then administered in 3 to 4 divided doses, not to exceed 600 mg daily. Should signs of withdrawal occur on the first day of treatment, a loading dose of 100 to 200 mg of phenobarbital may be administered IM in addition to the oral dose. After stabilization on phenobarbital, the total daily dose is decreased by 30 mg a day as long as withdrawal is proceeding smoothly. A modification of this regimen involves initiating treatment at the patient's regular dosage level and decreasing the daily dosage by 10 percent if tolerated by the patient.

Infants physically dependent on barbiturates may be given phenobarbital 3 to 10 mg/kg/day. After withdrawal symptoms (hyperactivity, disturbed sleep, tremors, hyperreflexia) are relieved, the dosage of phenobarbital should be gradually decreased and completely withdrawn over a 2-week period.

Overdosage: The toxic dose of barbiturates varies considerably. In general, an oral dose of 1 g of most barbiturates produces serious poisoning in an adult. Death commonly occurs after 2 to 10 g of ingested barbiturates. Barbiturate intoxication may be confused with alcoholism, bromide intoxication, and with various neurological disorders.

Acute overdosage with barbiturates is manifested by CNS and respiratory depression which may progress to Cheyne-Stokes respiration, areflexia, constriction of the pupils to a slight degree (though in severe poisoning they may show paralytic dilation), oliguria, tachycardia, hypotension, lowered body temperature, and coma. Typical shock syndrome (apnea, circulatory collapse, respiratory arrest, and death) may occur.

In extreme overdose, all electrical activity in the brain may cease, in which case a "flat" EEG normally equated with clinical death cannot be accepted. This effect is fully reversible unless hypoxic damage occurs. Consideration should be given to the possibility of barbiturate intoxication even in situations that appear to involve trauma.

Complications such as pneumonia, pulmonary edema, cardiac arrhythmias, congestive heart failure, and renal failure may occur. Uremia may increase CNS sensitivity to barbiturates. Differential diagnosis should include hypoglycemia, head trauma, cerebrovascular accidents, convulsive states, and diabetic coma. Blood levels from acute overdosage for some barbiturates are listed in Table 2.

[See Table 2 shown in Nembutal Elixir prescribing information.]

Treatment of overdosage is mainly supportive and consists of the following:

1. Maintenance of an adequate airway, with assisted respiration and oxygen administration as necessary.
2. Monitoring of vital signs and fluid balance.
3. Fluid therapy and other standard treatment for shock, if needed.
4. If renal function is normal, forced diuresis may aid in the elimination of the barbiturate. Alkalinization of the urine increases renal excretion of some barbiturates, especially phenobarbital, also aprobarbital, and mephobarbital (which is metabolized to phenobarbital).
5. Although not recommended as a routine procedure, hemodialysis may be used in severe barbiturate intoxications or if the patient is anuric or in shock.
6. Patient should be rolled from side to side every 30 minutes.
7. Antibiotics should be given if pneumonia is suspected.
8. Appropriate nursing care to prevent hypostatic pneumonia, decubiti, aspiration, and other complications of patients with altered states of consciousness.

Dosage and Administration: Dosages of barbiturates must be individualized with full knowledge of their particular characteristics and recommended rate of administration. Factors of consideration are the patient's age, weight, and condition. Parenteral route should be used only when oral administration is impossible or impractical.

Intramuscular Administration: IM injection of the sodium salts of barbiturates should be made deeply into a large muscle, and a volume of 5 ml should not be exceeded at any one site because of possible tissue irritation. After IM injection of a hypnotic dose, the patient's vital signs should be monitored. The usual adult dosage of NEMBUTAL Sodium Solution is 150 to 200 mg as a single IM injection; the recommended pediatric dosage ranges from 2 to 6 mg/kg as a single IM injection not to exceed 100 mg.

Intravenous Administration: IV injection is restricted to conditions in which other routes are not feasible, either because the patient is unconscious (as in cerebral hemorrhage, eclampsia, or status epilepticus, or because the patient resists (as in delirium), or because prompt action is imperative. Slow IV injection is essential and patients should be carefully observed during administration. This requires that blood pressure, respiration, and cardiac function be maintained, vital signs be recorded, and equipment for resuscitation and artificial ventilation be available. The rate of IV injection should not exceed 50 mg/min for pentobarbital sodium.

There is no average intravenous dose of NEMBUTAL Sodium Solution (pentobarbital sodium injection) that can be relied on to produce similar effects in different patients. The possibility of overdose and respiratory depression is remote when the drug is injected slowly in fractional doses.

A commonly used initial dose for the 70 kg adult is 100 mg. Proportional reduction in dosage should be made for pediatric or debilitated patients. At least one minute is necessary to determine the full effect of intravenous pentobarbital. If necessary, additional small increments of the drug may be given up to a total of from 200 to 500 mg for normal adults.

Anticonvulsant use: In convulsive states, dosage of NEMBUTAL Sodium Solution should be kept to a minimum to avoid compounding the depression which may follow convulsions. The injection must be made slowly with due regard to the time required for the drug to penetrate the blood-brain barrier.

Special patient population: Dosage should be reduced in the elderly or debilitated because these patients may be more sensitive to barbiturates. Dosage should be reduced for patients with impaired renal function or hepatic disease.

Inspection: Parenteral drug products should be inspected visually for particulate matter and discoloration prior to administration, whenever solution containers permit. Solutions for injection showing evidence of precipitation should not be used.

How Supplied: NEMBUTAL Sodium Solution (pentobarbital sodium injection, USP) is available in the following sizes:

2-ml ampul, 100 mg (1½ gr), in boxes of 25 (**NDC** 0074-6899-04); 20-ml multiple-dose vial, 1 g, in boxes of 5 (**NDC** 0074-3778-04); and 50-ml multiple-dose vial, 2.5 g, in boxes of 5 (**NDC** 0074-3778-05).

Each ml contains:
Pentobarbital Sodium,
derivative of barbituric acid ....50 mg (¾ gr)
Warning—May be habit forming.
Propylene glycol ....40% v/v
Alcohol 10%
Water for Injection ....qs
(pH adjusted to approximately 9.5 with hydrochloric acid and/or sodium hydroxide.)

Abbott Laboratories
North Chicago, IL 60064
Ref. 07-5165-R1

NEMBUTAL® SODIUM SUPPOSITORIES ℞ Ⓒ

(pentobarbital sodium suppositories)

WARNING: MAY BE HABIT FORMING

Description: The barbiturates are nonselective central nervous system depressants which are primarily used as sedative hypnotics. The barbiturates and their sodium salts are subject to control under the Federal Controlled Substances Act (See "Drug Abuse and Dependence" section).

Barbiturates are substituted pyrimidine derivatives in which the basic structure common to these drugs is barbituric acid, a substance which has no central nervous system (CNS) activity. CNS activity is obtained by substituting alkyl, alkenyl, or aryl groups on the pyrimidine ring. Nembutal (pentobarbital sodium) is chemically represented by sodium 5-ethyl-5-(1-methylbutyl) barbiturate.

The sodium salt of pentobarbital occurs as a white, slightly bitter powder which is freely soluble in water and alcohol but practically insoluble in benzene and ether. Each rectal suppository contains either 30 mg, 60 mg, 120 mg, or 200 mg of pentobarbital sodium.

Clinical Pharmacology: Barbiturates are capable of producing all levels of CNS mood alteration from excitation to mild sedation, to hypnosis, and deep coma. Overdosage can produce death. In high enough therapeutic doses, barbiturates induce anesthesia.

Barbiturates depress the sensory cortex, decrease motor activity, alter cerebellar function, and produce drowsiness, sedation, and hypnosis.

Barbiturate-induced sleep differs from physiological sleep. Sleep laboratory studies have demonstrated that barbiturates reduce the amount of time spent in the rapid eye movement (REM) phase of sleep or dreaming stage. Also, Stages III and IV sleep are decreased. Following abrupt cessation of barbiturates used regularly, patients may experience markedly increased dreaming, nightmares, and/or insomnia. Therefore, withdrawal of a single therapeutic dose over 5 or 6 days has been recommended to lessen the REM rebound and disturbed sleep which contribute to drug withdrawal syndrome (for example, decrease the dose from 3 to 2 doses a day for 1 week).

In studies, secobarbital sodium and pentobarbital sodium have been found to lose most of their effectiveness for both inducing and maintaining sleep by the end of 2 weeks of continued drug administration at fixed doses. The short-, intermediate-, and, to a lesser degree, long-acting barbiturates have been widely prescribed for treating insomnia. Although the clinical literature abounds with claims that the short-acting barbiturates are superior for producing sleep while the intermediate-acting compounds are more effective in maintaining sleep, controlled studies have failed to demonstrate these differential effects. Therefore, as sleep medications, the barbiturates are of limited value beyond short-term use.

Barbiturates have little analgesic action at subanesthetic doses. Rather, in subanesthetic doses these drugs may increase the reaction to painful stimuli. All barbiturates exhibit anticonvulsant activity in anesthetic doses. However, of the drugs in this class, only phenobarbital, mephobarbital, and metharbital have been clinically demonstrated to be effective as oral anticonvulsants in subhypnotic doses.

Barbiturates are respiratory depressants. The degree of respiratory depression is dependent upon dose. With hypnotic doses, respiratory depression produced by barbiturates is similar to that which occurs during physiologic sleep with slight decrease in blood pressure and heart rate.

Studies in laboratory animals have shown that barbiturates cause reduction in the tone and contractility of the uterus, ureters, and urinary bladder. However, concentrations of the drugs required to produce this effect in humans are not reached with sedative-hypnotic doses.

Barbiturates do not impair normal hepatic function, but have been shown to induce liver microsomal enzymes, thus increasing and/or altering the metabolism of barbiturates and other drugs. (See "Precautions—*Drug Interactions*" section).

Pharmacokinetics: Barbiturates are absorbed in varying degrees following oral, rectal, or parenteral administration.

The onset of action for oral or rectal administration varies from 20 to 60 minutes.

Duration of action, which is related to the rate at which the barbiturates are redistributed throughout the body, varies among persons and in the same person from time to time.

No studies have demonstrated that the different routes of administration are equivalent with respect to bioavailability.

Continued on next page

If desired, additional literature on any Abbott Product will be provided upon request to Abbott Laboratories.

Abbott—Cont.

Barbiturates are weak acids that are absorbed and rapidly distributed to all tissues and fluids with high concentrations in the brain, liver, and kidneys. Lipid solubility of the barbiturates is the dominant factor in their distribution within the body. The more lipid soluble the barbiturate, the more rapidly it penetrates all tissues of the body. Barbiturates are bound to plasma and tissue proteins to a varying degree with the degree of binding increasing directly as a function of lipid solubility. The plasma half-life for pentobarbital in adults is 15 to 50 hours and appears to be dose dependent.

Barbiturates are metabolized primarily by the hepatic microsomal enzyme system, and the metabolic products are excreted in the urine, and less commonly, in the feces. Approximately 25 to 50 percent of a dose of aprobarbital or phenobarbital is eliminated unchanged in the urine, whereas the amount of other barbiturates excreted unchanged in the urine is negligible. The excretion of unmetabolized barbiturate is one feature that distinguishes the long-acting category from those belonging to other categories which are almost entirely metabolized. The inactive metabolites of the barbiturates are excreted as conjugates of glucuronic acid.

Indications and Usage: *Rectal:* Barbiturates administered rectally are absorbed from the colon and are used when oral or parenteral administration may be undesirable.

1. Sedative.
2. Hypnotic, for the short-term treatment of insomnia, since they appear to lose their effectiveness for sleep induction and sleep maintenance after 2 weeks (See "Clinical Pharmacology" section).

Contraindications: Barbiturates are contraindicated in patients with known barbiturate sensitivity. Barbiturates are also contraindicated in patients with a history of manifest or latent porphyria.

Warnings: 1. *Habit forming:* Barbiturates may be habit forming. Tolerance, psychological and physical dependence may occur with continued use. (See "Drug Abuse and Dependence" and "Pharmacokinetics" sections). Patients who have psychological dependence on barbiturates may increase the dosage or decrease the dosage interval without consulting a physician and may subsequently develop a physical dependence on barbiturates. To minimize the possibility of overdosage or the development of dependence, the prescribing and dispensing of sedative-hypnotic barbiturates should be limited to the amount required for the interval until the next appointment. Abrupt cessation after prolonged use in the dependent person may result in withdrawal symptoms, including delirium, convulsions, and possibly death. Barbiturates should be withdrawn gradually from any patient known to be taking excessive dosage over long periods of time. (See "Drug Abuse and Dependence" section).

2. *Acute or chronic pain:* Caution should be exercised when barbiturates are administered to patients with acute or chronic pain, because paradoxical excitement could be induced or important symptoms could be masked. However, the use of barbiturates as sedatives in the postoperative surgical period and as adjuncts to cancer chemotherapy is well established.

3. *Use in pregnancy:* Barbiturates can cause fetal damage when administered to a pregnant woman. Retrospective, case-controlled studies have suggested a connection between the maternal consumption of barbiturates and a higher than expected incidence of fetal abnormalities. Following oral or parenteral administration, barbiturates readily cross the placental barrier and are distributed throughout fetal tissues with highest concentrations found in the placenta, fetal liver, and brain. It is presumed that this effect will also be seen following rectal administration.

Withdrawal symptoms occur in infants born to mothers who receive barbiturates throughout the last trimester of pregnancy. (See "Drug Abuse and Dependence" section). If this drug is used during pregnancy, or if the patient becomes pregnant while taking this drug, the patient should be apprised of the potential hazard to the fetus.

4. *Synergistic effects:* The concomitant use of alcohol or other CNS depressants may produce additive CNS depressant effects.

Precautions: *General:* Barbiturates may be habit forming. Tolerance and psychological and physical dependence may occur with continuing use. (See "Drug Abuse and Dependence" section). Barbiturates should be administered with caution, if at all, to patients who are mentally depressed, have suicidal tendencies, or a history of drug abuse.

Elderly or debilitated patients may react to barbiturates with marked excitement, depression, and confusion. In some persons, barbiturates repeatedly produce excitement rather than depression.

In patients with hepatic damage, barbiturates should be administered with caution and initially in reduced doses. Barbiturates should not be administered to patients showing the premonitory signs of hepatic coma.

Information for the patient: Practitioners should give the following information and instructions to patients receiving barbiturates.

1. The use of barbiturates carries with it an associated risk of psychological and/or physical dependence. The patient should be warned against increasing the dose of the drug without consulting a physician.
2. Barbiturates may impair mental and/or physical abilities required for the performance of potentially hazardous tasks (e.g., driving, operating machinery, etc.)
3. Alcohol should not be consumed while taking barbiturates. Concurrent use of the barbiturates with other CNS depressants (e.g., alcohol, narcotics, tranquilizers, and antihistamines) may result in additional CNS depressant effects.

Laboratory tests: Prolonged therapy with barbiturates should be accompanied by periodic laboratory evaluation of organ systems, including hematopoietic, renal, and hepatic systems. (See "Precautions — *General*" and "Adverse Reactions" sections).

Drug interactions: Most reports of clinically significant drug interactions occurring with the barbiturates have involved phenobarbital. However, the application of these data to other barbiturates appears valid and warrants serial blood level determinations of the relevant drugs when there are multiple therapies.

1. *Anticoagulants:* Phenobarbital lowers the plasma levels of dicumarol (name previously used: bishydroxycoumarin) and causes a decrease in anticoagulant activity as measured by the prothrombin time. Barbiturates can induce hepatic microsomal enzymes resulting in increased metabolism and decreased anticoagulant response of oral anticoagulants (e.g., warfarin, acenocoumarol, dicumarol, and phenprocoumon). Patients stabilized on anticoagulant therapy may require dosage adjustments if barbiturates are added to or withdrawn from their dosage regimen.
2. *Corticosteroids:* Barbiturates appear to enhance the metabolism of exogenous corticosteroids probably through the induction of hepatic microsomal enzymes. Patients stabilized on corticosteroid therapy may require dosage adjustments if barbiturates are added to or withdrawn from their dosage regimen.
3. *Griseofulvin:* Phenobarbital appears to interfere with the absorption of orally administered griseofulvin, thus decreasing its blood level. The effect of the resultant decreased blood levels of griseofulvin on therapeutic response has not been established. However, it would be preferable to avoid concomitant administration of these drugs.
4. *Doxycycline:* Phenobarbital has been shown to shorten the half-life of doxycycline for as long as 2 weeks after barbiturate therapy is discontinued.
   This mechanism is probably through the induction of hepatic microsomal enzymes that metabolize the antibiotic. If phenobarbital and doxycycline are administered concurrently, the clinical response to doxycycline should be monitored closely.
5. *Phenytoin, sodium valproate, valproic acid:* The effect of barbiturates on the metabolism of phenytoin appears to be variable. Some investigators report an accelerating effect, while others report no effect. Because the effect of barbiturates on the metabolism of phenytoin is not predictable, phenytoin and barbiturate blood levels should be monitored more frequently if these drugs are given concurrently. Sodium valproate and valproic acid appear to decrease barbiturate metabolism; therefore, barbiturate blood levels should be monitored and appropriate dosage adjustments made as indicated.
6. *Central nervous system depressants:* The concomitant use of other central nervous system depressants, including other sedatives or hypnotics, antihistamines, tranquilizers, or alcohol, may produce additive depressant effects.
7. *Monoamine oxidase inhibitors (MAOI):* MAOI prolong the effects of barbiturates probably because metabolism of the barbiturate is inhibited.
8. *Estradiol, estrone, progesterone and other steroidal hormones:* Pretreatment with or concurrent administration of phenobarbital may decrease the effect of estradiol by increasing its metabolism. There have been reports of patients treated with antiepileptic drugs (e.g., phenobarbital) who became pregnant while taking oral contraceptives. An alternate contraceptive method might be suggested to women taking phenobarbital.

Carcinogenesis: Adequate data are not available on long-term potential for carcinogenicity in humans or animals for pentobarbital.

Data from one retrospective study of 235 children in which the types of barbiturates are not identified suggested an association between exposure to barbiturates prenatally and an increased incidence of brain tumor. (Gold, E., et al, "Increased Risk of Brain Tumors in Children Exposed to Barbiturates," Journal of National Cancer Institute, 61:1031–1034, 1978).

Pregnancy: 1. Teratogenic effects. Pregnancy Category D — See "Warnings — Use in Pregnancy" section.

2. *Nonteratogenic effects.* Reports of infants suffering from long-term barbiturate exposure in utero included the acute withdrawal syndrome of seizures and hyperirritability from birth to a delayed onset of up to 14 days. (See "Drug Abuse and Dependence" section).

Labor and delivery: Hypnotic doses of these barbiturates do not appear to significantly impair uterine activity during labor. Full anesthetic doses of barbiturates decrease the force and frequency of uterine contractions. Administration of sedative-hypnotic barbiturates to the mother during labor may result in respiratory depression in the newborn. Premature infants are particularly susceptible to the depressant effects of barbiturates. If barbiturates are used during labor and delivery, resuscitation equipment should be available.

Data are currently not available to evaluate the effect of these barbiturates when forceps delivery or other intervention is necessary.

Also, data are not available to determine the effect of these barbiturates on the later growth, development, and functional maturation of the child.

Nursing mothers: Caution should be exercised when a barbiturate is administered to a nursing woman since small amounts of barbiturates are excreted in the milk.

Adverse Reactions: The following adverse reactions and their incidence were compiled from surveillance of thousands of hospitalized patients. Because such patients may be less aware of certain of the milder adverse effects of barbiturates, the incidence of these reactions may be somewhat higher in fully ambulatory patients.

More than 1 in 100 patients. The most common adverse reaction estimated to occur at a rate of 1 to 3 patients per 100 is: *Nervous System:* Somnolence.

Less than 1 in 100 patients. Adverse reactions estimated to occur at a rate of less than 1 in 100 patients listed below, grouped by organ system, and by decreasing order of occurrence are:

Nervous system: Agitation, confusion, hyperkinesia, ataxia, CNS depression, nightmares, nervousness, psychiatric disturbance, hallucinations, insomnia, anxiety, dizziness, thinking abnormality.

Respiratory system: Hypoventilation, apnea.

Cardiovascular system: Bradycardia, hypotension, syncope.

Digestive system: Nausea, vomiting, constipation.

Other reported reactions: Headache, injection site reactions, hypersensitivity reactions (angioedema, skin rashes, exfoliative dermatitis), fever, liver damage, megaloblastic anemia following chronic phenobarbital use.

Drug Abuse and Dependence: Pentobarbital sodium suppositories are subject to control by the Federal Controlled Substances Act under DEA schedule III.

Barbiturates may be habit forming. Tolerance, psychological dependence, and physical dependence may occur especially following prolonged use of high doses of barbiturates. Daily administration in excess of 400 mg of pentobarbital or secobarbital for approximately 90 days is likely to produce some degree of physical dependence. A dosage of from 600 to 800 mg taken for at least 35 days is sufficient to produce withdrawal seizures. The average daily dose for the barbiturate addict is usually about 1.5 grams. As tolerance to barbiturates develops, the amount needed to maintain the same level of intoxication increases; tolerance to a fatal dosage, however, does not increase more than two-fold. As this occurs, the margin between an intoxicating dosage and fatal dosage becomes smaller.

Symptoms of acute intoxication with barbiturates include unsteady gait, slurred speech, and sustained nystagmus. Mental signs of chronic intoxication include confusion, poor judgment, irritability, insomnia, and somatic complaints.

Symptoms of barbiturate dependence are similar to those of chronic alcoholism. If an individual appears to be intoxicated with alcohol to a degree that is radically disproportionate to the amount of alcohol in his or her blood the use of barbiturates should be suspected. The lethal dose of a barbiturate is far less if alcohol is also ingested.

The symptoms of barbiturate withdrawal can be severe and may cause death. Minor withdrawal symptoms may appear 8 to 12 hours after the last dose of a barbiturate. These symptoms usually appear in the following order: anxiety, muscle twitching, tremor of hands and fingers, progressive weakness, dizziness, distortion in visual perception, nausea, vomiting, insomnia, and orthostatic hypotension. Major withdrawal symptoms (convulsions and delirium) may occur within 16 hours and last up to 5 days after abrupt cessation of these drugs. Intensity of withdrawal symptoms gradually declines over a period of approximately 15 days. Individuals susceptible to barbiturate abuse and dependence include alcoholics and opiate abusers, as well as other sedative-hypnotic and amphetamine abusers.

Drug dependence to barbiturates arises from repeated administration of a barbiturate or agent with barbiturate-like effect on a continuous basis, generally in amounts exceeding therapeutic dose levels. The characteristics of drug dependence to barbiturates include: (a) a strong desire or need to continue taking the drug; (b) a tendency to increase the dose; (c) a psychic dependence on the effects of the drug related to subjective and individual appreciation of those effects; and (d) a physical dependence on the effects of the drug requiring its presence for maintenance of homeostasis and resulting in a definite, characteristic, and self-limited abstinence syndrome when the drug is withdrawn.

Treatment of barbiturate dependence consists of cautious and gradual withdrawal of the drug. Barbiturate-dependent patients can be withdrawn by using a number of different withdrawal regimens. In all cases withdrawal takes an extended period of time. One method involves substituting a 30 mg dose of phenobarbital for each 100 to 200 mg dose of barbiturate that the patient has been taking. The total daily amount of phenobarbital is then administered in 3 to 4 divided doses, not to exceed 600 mg daily. Should signs of withdrawal occur on the first day of treatment, a loading dose of 100 to 200 mg of phenobarbital may be administered IM in addition to the oral dose. After stabilization on phenobarbital, the total daily dose is decreased by 30 mg a day as long as withdrawal is proceeding smoothly. A modification of this regimen involves initiating treatment at the patient's regular dosage level and decreasing the daily dosage by 10 percent if tolerated by the patient.

Infants physically dependent on barbiturates may be given phenobarbital 3 to 10 mg/kg/day. After withdrawal symptoms (hyperactivity, disturbed sleep, tremors, hyperreflexia) are relieved, the dosage of phenobarbital should be gradually decreased and completely withdrawn over a 2 week period.

Overdosage: The toxic dose of barbiturates varies considerably. In general, an oral dose of 1 g of most barbiturates produces serious poisoning in an adult. Death commonly occurs after 2 to 10 g of ingested barbiturate. Barbiturate intoxication may be confused with alcoholism, bromide intoxication, and with various neurological disorders.

Acute overdosage with barbiturates is manifested by CNS and respiratory depression which may progress to Cheyne-Stokes respiration, areflexia, constriction of the pupils to a slight degree (though in severe poisoning they may show paralytic dilation), oliguria, tachycardia, hypotension, lowered body temperature, and coma. Typical shock syndrome (apnea, circulatory collapse, respiratory arrest, and death) may occur.

In extreme overdose, all electrical activity in the brain may cease, in which case a "flat" EEG normally equated with clinical death cannot be accepted. This effect is fully reversible unless hypoxic damage occurs. Consideration should be given to the possibility of barbiturate intoxication even in situations that appear to involve trauma.

Complications such as pneumonia, pulmonary edema, cardiac arrhythmias, congestive heart failure, and renal failure may occur. Uremia may increase CNS sensitivity to barbiturates. Differential diagnosis should include hypoglycemia, head trauma, cerebrovascular accidents, convulsive states, and diabetic coma. Blood levels from acute overdosage for some barbiturates are listed in Table 2. [See Table 2 shown in Nembutal Elixir prescribing information.]

Treatment of overdosage is mainly supportive and consists of the following:

1. Maintenance of an adequate airway, with assisted respiration and oxygen administration as necessary.
2. Monitoring of vital signs and fluid balance.
3. Fluid therapy and other standard treatment for shock, if needed.
4. If renal function is normal, forced diuresis may aid in the elimination of the barbiturate. Alkalinization of the urine increases renal excretion of some barbiturates, especially phenobarbital, also aprobarbital, and mephobarbital (which is metabolized to phenobarbital).
5. Although not recommended as a routine procedure, hemodialysis may be used in severe barbiturate intoxications or if the patient is anuric or in shock.
6. Patient should be rolled from side to side every 30 minutes.
7. Antibiotics should be given if pneumonia is suspected.
8. Appropriate nursing care to prevent hypostatic pneumonia, decubiti, aspiration, and other complications of patients with altered states of consciousness.

Dosage and Administration: Typical hypnotic doses for adults and children are given below. These are intended only as a guide, and administration should be adjusted to the individual needs of each patient. For sedation, in children 5–14 years and in adults, reduce dose appropriately.

Adults (average to above average weight)—one 120 mg or one 200 mg suppository.

Children —

12–14 years (80–110 lbs)	one 60 mg or one 120 mg suppository
5–12 years (40–80 lbs)	one 60 mg suppository
1–4 years (20–40 lbs)	one 30 mg or one 60 mg suppository
2 months–1 year (10–20 lbs)	one 30 mg suppository

Suppositories should not be divided.

Dosages of barbiturates must be individualized with full knowledge of their particular characteristics and recommended rate of administration. Factors of consideration are the patient's age, weight, and condition.

Special patient population: Dosage should be reduced in the elderly or debilitated because these patients may be more sensitive to barbiturates. Dosage should be reduced for patients with impaired renal function or hepatic disease.

How Supplied: NEMBUTAL Sodium Suppositories (pentobarbital sodium suppositories) are available as suppositories containing pentobarbital sodium in the amount of 30 mg (½ gr) (NDC 0074-3272-01); 60 mg (1 gr) (NDC 0074-3148-01); 120 mg (2 gr) (NDC 0074-3145-01) and 200 mg (3 gr) (NDC 0074-3164-01). Supplied in boxes of 12 suppositories.

Semi-synthetic glycerides provide the base for each suppository.

Store in a refrigerator (36°–46°F).

Abbott Laboratories
North Chicago, IL 60064
Ref. 07-5174-R9

NITROPRESS™ ℞

(sterile sodium nitroprusside, USP)

NITROPRESS is only to be used as an infusion with sterile 5% dextrose injection. Not for direct injection.

Continued on next page

If desired, additional literature on any Abbott Product will be provided upon request to Abbott Laboratories.

Abbott—Cont.

NITROPRESS should be used only when the necessary facilities and equipment for continuous monitoring of blood pressure are available.
If at infusion rates of up to 10 mcg/kg/minute, an adequate reduction of blood pressure is not obtained within ten minutes, administration of NITROPRESS should be stopped.
The instructions included herein should be reviewed thoroughly before administration of NITROPRESS.

Description: This antihypertensive agent is for intravenous infusion only. NITROPRESS (sterile sodium nitroprusside, USP) in injectable form contains the equivalent of 50 mg of sodium nitroprusside dihydrate (sodium nitrosylpentacyanoferrate [III]) in an amber-colored, single dose Univial.®
Chemically, sodium nitroprusside is $Na_2[Fe(CN)_5NO] \cdot 2H_2O$. It is a reddish-brown powder which is soluble in water. In aqueous solution, it is photosensitive and should be protected from light.
Clinical Pharmacology: NITROPRESS is a potent, immediate acting, intravenous hypotensive agent. This action is probably due to the nitroso (NO) group. Its effect is almost immediate and ends when the IV infusion is stopped. Generally, NITROPRESS is rapidly metabolized to cyanide and subsequently converted to thiocyanate through the mediation of a hepatic enzyme, rhodanase. The rate of conversion from cyanide to thiocyanate is dependent on the availability of sulfur, usually thiosulfate. The hypotensive effect is augmented by ganglionic blocking agents, volatile liquid anesthetics (such as halothane and enflurane), and by most other circulatory depressants.
The hypotensive effects of NITROPRESS are caused by peripheral vasodilation as a result of a direct action on the blood vessels, independent of autonomic innervation. No relaxation is seen in the smooth muscle of the uterus or duodenum *in situ* in animals.
Sodium nitroprusside administered intravenously to hypertensive and normotensive patients produced a marked lowering of the arterial blood pressure, slight increase in heart rate, a mild decrease in cardiac output and a moderate diminution in calculated total peripheral vascular resistance.
The decrease in calculated total peripheral vascular resistance suggests arteriolar vasodilatation. The decreases in cardiac and stroke index noted may be due to the peripheral vascular pooling of blood.
In hypertensive patients, moderate depressor doses induce renal vasodilatation roughly equivalent to the decrease in pressure without an appreciable increase in renal blood flow or a decrease in glomerular filtration.
In normotensive subjects, acute reduction of mean arterial pressure to 60 to 75 mmHg by infusion of sodium nitroprusside caused a significant increase in renin activity of renal venous plasma in correlation with the degree of reduction in pressure. Renal response to reduction in pressure was more striking in renovascular hypertensive patients, with significant increase in renin release occurring from the involved kidney at mean arterial pressures ranging from 90 to 137 mmHg. Furthermore, the magnitude of renin release from the involved kidney was significantly greater when compared with that in normotensive subjects, while in the contralateral, uninvolved kidney, no significant release of renin was detected during the reduction of pressure.
Indications and Usage: NITROPRESS (sterile sodium nitroprusside) is indicated for the immediate reduction of blood pressure of patients in hypertensive crises. Concomitant oral antihypertensive medication should be started while the hypertensive emergency is being brought under control with NITROPRESS.
NITROPRESS is also indicated for producing controlled hypotension during anesthesia in order to reduce bleeding in surgical procedures where surgeon and anesthesiologist deem it appropriate.
Contraindications: NITROPRESS should not be used in the treatment of compensatory hypertension, *e.g.*, arteriovenous shunt or coarctation of the aorta.
The use of NITROPRESS to produce controlled hypotension during surgery is contraindicated in patients with known inadequate cerebral circulation. NITROPRESS is not intended for use during emergency surgery in moribund patients (A.S.A. Class 5E).
Warnings:

If excessive amounts of NITROPRESS are used and/or sulfur—usually thiosulfate—supplies are depleted, cyanide toxicity can occur. (See Overdosage.)
If sodium nitroprusside infusion is to be extended, particularly if renal impairment is present, close attention should be given to not exceeding the recommended maximum infusion rate of 10 mcg/kg/min. If in the course of therapy increased tolerance to the drug (as shown by the need for higher infusion rate) develops, it is essential to monitor blood acid-base balance, as metabolic acidosis is the earliest and most reliable evidence of cyanide toxicity. If signs of metabolic acidosis appear, NITROPRESS should be discontinued and an alternate drug administered.
Serum thiocyanate levels do not reflect cyanide toxicity. However, serum thiocyanate levels should be monitored daily if treatment is to be extended, especially in patients with renal dysfunction. Thiocyanate accumulation and toxicity may manifest itself as tinnitus, blurred vision, delirium.

The following warnings apply to use of NITROPRESS for controlled hypotension during anesthesia:

1. Tolerance to blood loss, anemia and hypovolemia may be diminished. If possible, preexisting anemia and hypovolemia should be corrected prior to employing controlled hypotension.
2. Hypotensive anesthetic techniques may alter pulmonary ventilation perfusion ratio. Patients intolerant of additional dead air space at ordinary oxygen partial pressure may benefit from higher oxygen partial pressure.
3. Extreme caution should be exercised in patients who are especially poor surgical risks (A.S.A. Class 4 and 4E).

NITROPRESS IS ONLY TO BE USED AS AN INFUSION WITH 5% DEXTROSE INJECTION. NOT FOR DIRECT INJECTION.
Infusion rates greater than 10 mcg/kg/minute are rarely required. If, at this rate, an adequate reduction in blood pressure is not obtained within 10 minutes, administration of NITROPRESS (sterile sodium nitroprusside) should be stopped.
Precautions:
General: Adequate facilities, equipment and personnel should be available for frequent and vigilant monitoring of blood pressure, since the hypotensive effect of NITROPRESS occurs rapidly.
When the infusion is slowed or stopped, blood pressure usually begins to rise immediately and returns to pretreatment levels within one to ten minutes. It should be used with caution and initially in low doses in elderly patients, since they may be more sensitive to the hypotensive effects of the drug. Young, vigorous males may require somewhat larger than ordinary doses of sodium nitroprusside for hypotensive anesthesia; however, the infusion rate of 10 mcg/kg/minute should not be exceeded. Deepening of anesthesia, if indicated, might permit satisfactory conditions to exist within the recommended dosage range.
Because of the rapid onset of action and potency of NITROPRESS, it should preferably be administered with the use of an infusion pump, micro-drip regulator, or any similar device that would allow precise measurement of the flow rate.
Since cyanide is converted into thiocyanate through the mediation of a hepatic enzyme, rhodanase, NITROPRESS should be used with caution in patients with hepatic insufficiency.
Since thiocyanate inhibits both the uptake and binding of iodine, caution should be exercised in using NITROPRESS in patients with hypothyroidism or severe renal impairment.
Hypertensive patients are more sensitive to the intravenous effect of sodium nitroprusside than are normotensive subjects. Patients who are receiving concomitant antihypertensive medications are more sensitive to the hypotensive effect of sodium nitroprusside and the dosage should be adjusted accordingly.
Once dissolved in solution, NITROPRESS tends to deteriorate in the presence of light. Therefore, it must be protected from light by wrapping the container of the prepared solution with aluminum foil, the foil sheet supplied in product carton, or other opaque materials. If properly protected from light, the reconstituted solution is stable for 24 hours.
NITROPRESS in aqueous solution yields the nitroprusside ion which reacts with even minute quantities of a wide variety of inorganic and organic substances to form usually highly colored reaction products (blue, green or dark red). If this occurs, the infusion should be replaced.
Drug Interactions: The hypotensive effect of sodium nitroprusside is augmented by *ganglionic blocking agents. Volatile liquid anesthetics* (such as halothane and enflurane) also augment the hypotensive effect. Most other *circulatory depressants* will augment the hypotensive effect of sodium nitroprusside.
Carcinogenesis: No data are available on long-term potential for carcinogenicity in animals or humans for sodium nitroprusside.
Usage During Pregnancy: Pregnancy Category C. Animal reproduction studies have not been conducted with NITROPRESS. It is also not known whether NITROPRESS (sterile sodium nitroprusside) can cause fetal harm when administered to a pregnant woman or can affect reproduction capacity. NITROPRESS should be given to a pregnant woman only if clearly needed.
Nursing Mothers: It is not known whether this drug is excreted in human milk. Because many drugs are excreted in human milk, caution should be exercised when NITROPRESS is administered to a nursing woman.
Adverse Reactions: Nausea, retching, diaphoresis, apprehension, headache, restlessness, muscle twitching, retrosternal discomfort, palpitations, dizziness and abdominal pain have been noted with too rapid reduction in blood pressure, but these symptoms rapidly disappeared with slowing of the rate of the infusion or temporary discontinuation of infusion and did not reappear with continued slower rate of administration. Irritation at the infusion site may occur.
One case of hypothyroidism following prolonged therapy with intravenous sodium nitroprusside has been reported. A patient with severe hypertension with uremia received 3900 mg of sodium nitroprusside intravenously over a period of 21 days. This is one of the longest reported intravenous uses of this agent. There was no tachyphylaxis, but the patient developed evidence of hypothyroidism, together with retention of thiocyanate (9.5 mg/100 ml). With peritoneal dialysis the thiocyanate level

diminished and the signs of hypothyroidism subsided.

Overdosage: The first signs of sodium nitroprusside overdosage are those of profound hypotension. As with instances of depletion of thiosulfate supplies, overdosage may lead to cyanide toxicity. Metabolic acidosis and increasing tolerance to the drug are early indications of overdosage. These may be associated with or followed by dyspnea, headache, vomiting, dizziness, ataxia and loss of consciousness. Sodium nitroprusside should then be immediately discontinued. Other signs of cyanide poisoning are coma, imperceptible pulse, absent reflexes, widely dilated pupils, pink color, distant heart sounds, and shallow breathing. Oxygen alone will not provide relief. Nitrites should be administered to induce methemoglobin formation. Methemoglobin, in turn, combines with cyanide bound to cytochrome oxidase to liberate cytochrome oxidase and form a non-toxic complex, cyanmethemoglobin. Cyanide then gradually dissociates from the latter and is converted by administration of thiosulfate to sodium thiocyanate in the presence of rhodanase.

Treatment: In cases of massive overdosage when signs of cyanide toxicity are present use the following regimen:

1. Discontinue administration of NITROPRESS.
2. Administer amyl nitrite inhalations for 15 to 30 seconds each minute until 3% sodium nitrite solution can be prepared for I.V. administration.
3. Sodium nitrite 3% solution should be injected intravenously at a rate not exceeding 2.5 to 5 ml/minute up to a total dose of 10 to 15 ml with careful monitoring of the blood pressure.
4. Following the above steps, inject sodium thiosulfate intravenously, 12.5 Gm in 50 ml of 5% dextrose injection over a ten-minute period.
5. Since signs of overdosage may reappear, the patient must be observed for several hours.
6. If signs of overdosage reappear, sodium nitrite and sodium thiosulfate injections are repeated in one-half of the above doses.
7. During the administration of nitrites and later when thiocyanate formation is taking place, blood pressure may drop but can be corrected with vasopressor agents.

Dosage and Administration:
Reconstitution Directions for Univial:

1. Remove protective cap.
   Turn plunger-stopper a quarter turn and press to force diluent into lower chamber.
2. Shake gently to effect solution.
   Use only a clear solution.
3. Sterilize top of stopper with a suitable germicide.
4. Insert needle through the center of stopper until tip is barely visible. Invert vial and withdraw contents.

Depending on the desired concentration, all of the reconstituted Univial solution should be diluted in 250 to 1000 ml of 5% dextrose injection and promptly wrapped in aluminum foil, the foil sheet supplied in product carton, or other opaque materials to protect from light. *If properly protected from light, the reconstituted solution is stable for 24 hours.* The freshly prepared solution for infusion has a very faint brownish tint. If it is highly colored, it should be discarded (see Precautions). *The infusion fluid used for the administration of NITROPRESS should not be employed as a vehicle for simultaneous administration of any other drug.*

In patients who are not receiving antihypertensive drugs, the average dose of NITROPRESS (sterile sodium nitroprusside) for both adults and children is 3 mcg/kg/minute (range of 0.5 to 10 mcg/kg/minute). Usually, at 3 mcg/kg/minute, blood pressure can be lowered by about 30 to 40% below the pretreatment diastolic levels and maintained. In hypertensive patients receiving concomitant antihypertensive medication, smaller doses are required. In order to avoid excessive levels of thiocyanate and lessen the possibility of a precipitous drop in blood pressure, infusion rates greater than 10 mcg/kg/minute should rarely be used. If, at this rate, an adequate reduction of blood pressure is not obtained within 10 minutes, administration of NITROPRESS should be stopped.

One Univial (50 mg) NITROPRESS in 1000 ml 5% dextrose injection provides a concentration of 50 mcg/ml.

One Univial (50 mg) NITROPRESS in 500 ml 5% dextrose injection provides a concentration of 100 mcg/ml.

One Univial (50 mg) NITROPRESS in 250 ml 5% dextrose injection provides a concentration of 200 mcg/ml.

Dose	mcg/kg/min.
Average	3
Range	0.5 to 10

The intravenous infusion of NITROPRESS should be administered by an infusion pump, microdrip regulator or any similar device that will allow precise measurement of the flow rate. Care should be taken to avoid extravasation. The rate of administration should be adjusted to maintain the desired antihypertensive or hypotensive effect, as determined by frequent blood pressure determinations. It is recommended that the blood pressure should not be allowed to drop at a too rapid rate and the systolic pressure not be lowered below 60 mmHg. In hypertensive emergencies NITROPRESS infusion may be continued until the patient can safely be treated with oral antihypertensive medications.

How Supplied: NITROPRESS (sterile sodium nitroprusside, USP) is supplied in an amber-colored, single dose Univial (**NDC** 0074-3019-02), each vial containing the equivalent of 50 mg sodium nitroprusside dihydrate. Store below 86°F (30°C). Protect from light—store in carton until use. Avoid freezing.

Univial®—Sterile two-compartment vial, Abbott.
TM—Trademark
Abbott Laboratories
North Chicago, IL 60064
Ref. 01-2255-R2

NORISODRINE® AEROTROL® ℞

**(isoproterenol hydrochloride inhalation aerosol, USP)
In a Controlled-Dose Nebulizer**

Description: Isoproterenol HCl 0.25% w/w (=2.8 mg/ml) in inert chlorofluorohydrocarbon propellants; alcohol 33%; ascorbic acid 0.1% as preservative; and artificial and natural flavors.

Each depression of the valve delivers approximately 0.12 mg to the patient.

Actions: Isoproterenol is a short-acting sympathomimetic drug. It produces pharmacologic response in the cardiovascular system and on the smooth muscles of the bronchial tree. The drug will prevent or overcome histamine-induced asthma in both experimental animals and man, and is effective when used prophylactically. It is one of the most potent bronchodilators known and can be used in patients who do not respond to the bronchodilating action of epinephrine. Isoproterenol has a cardio-accelerating effect, but its vasoconstricting action is less pronounced than that of epinephrine. Therapeutic doses may produce a slight increase in systolic blood pressure, but a slight decrease in diastolic. Larger doses may cause peripheral vasodilatation in the renal, mesenteric and femoral beds and some patients respond with a decrease in diastolic, but no change in systolic pressure. Such effects are usually of very short duration.

Indications: For the treatment of bronchospasm associated with acute and chronic bronchial asthma, pulmonary emphysema, bronchitis, and bronchiectasis.

Contraindications: Use of isoproterenol in patients with pre-existing cardiac arrhythmias associated with tachycardia is contraindicated because the cardiac stimulant effects of the drug may aggravate such disorders.

Warnings: Excessive use of an adrenergic aerosol should be discouraged, as it may lose its effectiveness. Occasional patients have been reported to develop severe paradoxical airway resistance with repeated excessive use of isoproterenol inhalation preparations. The cause of this refractory state is unknown. It is advisable that in such instances the use of this preparation be discontinued immediately and alternative therapy instituted, since in the reported cases the patients did not respond to other forms of therapy until the drug was withdrawn.

Deaths have been reported following excessive use of isoproterenol inhalation preparations and the exact cause is unknown. Cardiac arrest was noted in several instances.

Precautions: Isoproterenol and epinephrine may be used interchangeably if the patient becomes unresponsive to one or the other but should not be used concurrently. If desired, these drugs may be alternated, provided an interval of at least four hours has elapsed.

As with all sympathomimetic drugs, isoproterenol should be used with great caution in the presence of cardiovascular disorders, including coronary insufficiency, hypertension, hyperthyroidism and diabetes, or when there is a sensitivity to sympathomimetic amines.

Although there has been no evidence of teratogenic effects with this drug, use of any drug in pregnancy, lactation, or in women of childbearing age requires that the potential benefit of the drug be weighed against its possible hazard to the mother and child.

Adverse Reactions: Only a small percentage of patients experience any side effects following oral inhalation of aerosolized isoproterenol. Overdosage may produce tachycardia with resultant coronary insufficiency, palpitations, vertigo, nausea, tremors, headache, insomnia, central excitation, and blood pressure changes. These reactions are similar to those produced by other sympathomimetic agents.

Dosage and Administration: The usual dose for the relief of dyspnea in the acute episode is 1 to 2 inhalations. Start with one inhalation. If no relief is evident after 2 to 5 minutes, a second inhalation may be taken. For daily maintenance, use 1 to 2 inhalations 4 to 6 times daily, or as directed by the physician. The physician should be careful to instruct the patient in the proper technique of administration so that the number of inhalations per treatment and the frequency of treatment may be titrated to the patient's response.

No more than two inhalations should be taken at any one time, or more than 6 inhalations in any hour during a 24-hour period, unless advised by physician.

Directions for Use: Before each use, remove cap and assemble.

1. Breathe out fully. Place mouthpiece well into the mouth, aimed at the back of the throat.
2. As you begin to breathe in deeply, press the vial firmly down into the adapter. This releases one dose. Continue to breathe in until your lungs are completely filled.
3. Remove from mouth. Hold your breath for several seconds, then breathe out slowly.

Continued on next page

If desired, additional literature on any Abbott Product will be provided upon request to Abbott Laboratories.

Abbott—Cont.

Warning: Do not exceed the dose prescribed by your physician. If difficulty in breathing persists, contact your physician immediately.
How Supplied: NORISODRINE AEROTROL (isoproterenol hydrochloride inhalation aerosol, USP), 0.25% w/w, is supplied in a 15 ml controlled-dose nebulizer (**NDC** 0074-6869-03).
Manufactured for
Abbott Laboratories
North Chicago, IL 60064
Ref. 01-2149-R3

NORISODRINE® SULFATE ℞
(isoproterenol sulfate)
For Oral Use With The Aerohalor®
To Control Bronchospasm

Description: Isoproterenol sulfate is a white, odorless, crystalline powder which darkens on exposure to air. It is chemically identified as 1,2-Benzenediol,4-[1-hydroxy-2-[(1-methylethyl)amino]ethyl]-, sulfate (2:1) (salt), dihydrate.
Each Aerohalor Cartridge 10% contains 10 mg isoproterenol sulfate and 90 mg lactose as a diluent. Each Aerohalor Cartridge 25% contains 25 mg isoproterenol sulfate and 75 mg lactose as a diluent.
Actions: Isoproterenol is classified as a catecholamine which acts predominantly on beta receptor sites of peripheral inhibitory and cardiac excitatory sympathetic nerves. Therefore, its primary pharmacological actions are to increase both the rate and force of cardiac contraction and to relax the smooth muscle of the bronchi, alimentary tract, and skeletal muscle vasculature. Isoproterenol can prevent or relieve bronchospasm due to drugs, as well as that due to disease. The drug lowers peripheral vascular resistance and reduces the diastolic blood pressure. Systolic pressure is unchanged or slightly increased as a consequence of increased cardiac output.
The calorigenic effects of isoproterenol are similar to those of epinephrine; however, it causes less hyperglycemia than epinephrine. Isoproterenol can also cause central excitation.
Isoproterenol is readily absorbed following inhalation. The duration of action of isoproterenol is the same as that of epinephrine and it is probably metabolized and excreted by the same routes.
Indications: NORISODRINE (isoproterenol) is indicated for the treatment of bronchospasm associated with acute and chronic bronchial asthma, pulmonary emphysema, bronchitis, and bronchiectasis.
Contraindications: NORISODRINE should not be used in those rare instances in which a patient has demonstrated hypersensitivity to isoproterenol or other sympathomimetic amines.
The use of isoproterenol is contraindicated in patients with pre-existing cardiac arrythmias, because the cardiac stimulant effect of the drug may aggravate such disorders.
Warnings: Occasional patients have been reported to develop severe, paradoxical airway resistance of unknown etiology with repeated, excessive use of isoproterenol inhalation preparations. Because of the frequent development of such refractoriness, excessive use of any adrenergic aerosol should be discouraged. Should the refractory state develop, it is advisable to discontinue isoproterenol immediately and institute alternative therapy, since in the reported cases the patients did not respond to other forms of therapy until isoproterenol was withdrawn.
Deaths have been reported following excessive use of isoproterenol inhalation preparations. The exact cause is unknown. Cardiac arrhythmia or cardiac arrest has been noted.
Bronchial asthma may mask the presence of cardiac asthma (pulmonary edema). A differential diagnosis should be made before instituting therapy.
This product is a powdered formulation which may irritate the oropharynx and tracheobronchial tree. Therefore, its use should be considered secondary to formulations in solution or suspension.
Usage in Pregnancy: Use of isoproterenol in women of childbearing age or during pregnancy or lactation requires that the potential benefit of the drug be weighed against its possible hazards to mother and child.
Precautions: Isoproterenol should be used cautiously in patients with heart disease, hypertension, hyperthyroidism, diabetes, or unstable vasomotor systems.
The concomitant use of NORISODRINE SULFATE (isoproterenol sulfate) AEROHALOR and a parenteral or inhalation form of epinephrine or other adrenergic agent should be avoided since it may result in excessive response and the occurrence of serious cardiovascular symptoms.
Caution should be exercised when NORISODRINE SULFATE AEROHALOR is administered concomitantly with an oral form of adrenergic agent since the effects of these drugs are additive.
In neutral or alkaline solution, isoproterenol may become red on exposure to air. Accordingly, the saliva or sputum may appear pink or red in color after oral inhalation of the drug. This is not harmful but should be explained to patients to allay possible apprehension or confusion with bleeding.
Adverse Reactions: As with other sympathomimetic drugs, NORISODRINE (isoproterenol) may produce undesirable side effects such as nervousness, dizziness, palpitation, nausea, vomiting, headache, tremor, flushing, sweating, weakness, precordial distress and anginal-type pain, and tachycardia. Cardiac arrhythmias may occur, and death from cardiac arrest has been reported with excessive use of isoproterenol.
Swelling of the parotid glands has been reported with the prolonged use of isoproterenol. In such cases the drug should be withdrawn.
Dosage and Administration: NORISODRINE (isoproterenol) SULFATE is administered by oral inhalation. This method is rapidly effective for controlling acute attacks of bronchospasm and is suitable for adults or older children.
Tests done in a mechanical breathing apparatus indicate that one inhalation of the 10% concentration yields about 0.045 mg of isoproterenol sulfate. One inhalation of the 25% concentration yields about 0.11 mg of isoproterenol sulfate.
For the mild or moderate acute attack, 2 to 4 inhalations of normal depth of the 10% concentration, through the AEROHALOR, are usually sufficient. The patient should be cautioned not to take a forced, deep inhalation. If the first two to four inhalations do not provide relief within five minutes this dose may be repeated. If relief is still not apparent, a third dose may be taken after an interval of 10 minutes. When therapy has been unsuccessful following three doses the medication should be discontinued as ineffective for that particular attack.
If the 10% concentration does not afford relief and does not induce undesired side effects, the 25% concentration may be used in the same manner.
Symptoms and Treatment of Overdosage: Symptoms may include palpitation, tachycardia, restlessness, tremor, sweating, headache, dizziness, weakness, nausea, and vomiting. Blood pressure may at first be elevated slightly. Later, blood pressure may fall and the general picture of "shock" may develop.
Treatment includes general supportive measures. Sedatives (barbiturates) may be given for restlessness.
How Supplied: NORISODRINE SULFATE (isoproterenol sulfate) 10% (**NDC** 0074-3867-12) and 25% (**NDC** 0074-3882-12) are supplied in bottles containing 12 AEROHALOR cartridges.
Abbott Laboratories
North Chicago, IL 60064
Ref. 01-2828-R6

NORISODRINE® WITH CALCIUM IODIDE SYRUP ℞
(isoproterenol sulfate and calcium iodide)

How Supplied: Each teaspoonful of NORISODRINE WITH CALCIUM IODIDE SYRUP contains 3 mg of isoproterenol sulfate, 150 mg of anhydrous calcium iodide and 6% alcohol in a palatable syrup. Norisodrine with Calcium Iodide Syrup is supplied in pint (**NDC** 0074-6953-01) bottles.
Abbott Laboratories
North Chicago, IL 60064

OGEN® ℞
(estropipate tablets and vaginal cream, USP)

WARNING:
1. ESTROGENS HAVE BEEN REPORTED TO INCREASE THE RISK OF ENDOMETRIAL CARCINOMA.
Three independent case control studies have shown an increased risk of endometrial cancer in postmenopausal women exposed to exogenous estrogens for prolonged periods.[1–3] This risk was independent of the other known risk factors for endometrial cancer. These studies are further supported by the finding that incidence rates of endometrial cancer have increased sharply since 1969 in eight different areas of the United States with population-based cancer reporting systems, an increase which may be related to the rapidly expanding use of estrogens during the last decade.[4]
The three case control studies reported that the risk of endometrial cancer in estrogen users was about 4.5 to 13.9 times greater than in nonusers. The risk appears to depend on both duration of treatment[1] and on estrogen dose.[3] In view of these findings, when estrogens are used for the treatment of menopausal symptoms, the lowest dose that will control symptoms should be utilized and medication should be discontinued as soon as possible. When prolonged treatment is medically indicated, the patient should be reassessed on at least a semiannual basis to determine the need for continued therapy. Although the evidence must be considered preliminary, one study suggests that cyclic administration of low doses of estrogen may carry less risk than continuous administration;[3] it therefore appears prudent to utilize such a regimen.
Close clinical surveillance of all women taking estrogens is important. In all cases of undiagnosed persistent or recurring abnormal vaginal bleeding, adequate diagnostic measures should be undertaken to rule out malignancy.
There is no evidence at present that "natural" estrogens are more or less hazardous than "synthetic" estrogens at equiestrogenic doses.
2. OGEN SHOULD NOT BE USED DURING PREGNANCY.
According to some investigators, the use of female sex hormones, both estrogens and progestogens, during early pregnancy may seriously damage the offspring. Studies have reported that females exposed in utero to diethylstilbestrol, a non-steroidal estrogen, have an increased risk of developing in later life a form of vaginal or cervical cancer that is ordinarily extremely rare.[5,6] In one of these studies, this risk was estimated as not greater than 4 per 1000 exposures.[7] Furthermore, there are reports that a high percentage of such exposed women (from 30 to 90 percent) have been found to have vaginal adenosis,[8–12]

epithelial changes of the vagina and cervix. Although these reported changes are histologically benign, the investigators have not determined whether they are precursors of adenocarcinoma.

Several reports suggest an association between intrauterine exposure to female sex hormones and congenital anomalies in the offspring, including heart defects and limb reduction defects.[13–16] One case control study[16] estimated a 4.7 fold increased risk of limb reduction defects in infants exposed in utero to sex hormones (oral contraceptives, hormone withdrawal tests for pregnancy, or attempted treatment for threatened abortion). Some of these exposures were very short and involved only a few days of treatment. The data suggest that the risk of limb reduction defects in exposed fetuses is somewhat less than 1 per 1000.

In the past, female sex hormones have been used during pregnancy in an attempt to treat threatened or habitual abortion. OGEN (estropipate) is not intended for these uses, nor has it been studied for these uses, and therefore should not be used during pregnancy. There is no evidence from well controlled studies that progestogens are effective for these uses.

If OGEN is used during pregnancy, or if the patient becomes pregnant while taking this drug, she should be apprised of the potential risks to the fetus, and the question of continuation of the pregnancy should be addressed.

Description: OGEN (estropipate) is a preparation of pure, crystalline estrone, solubilized as the sulfate and stabilized with piperazine. It is appreciably soluble in water and has almost no odor or taste. The amount of piperazine in OGEN is not sufficient to exert a pharmacological action. Its addition ensures solubility, stability, and uniform potency of the estrone sulfate.

OGEN Tablets are available in four dosage strengths: OGEN .625 (0.75 mg estropipate), OGEN 1.25 (1.5 mg estropipate), OGEN 2.5 (3 mg estropipate) and OGEN 5 (6 mg estropipate). The tablets are standardized to provide uniform estrone activity and are grooved (Divide-Tab®) to provide dosage flexibility.

Each gram of OGEN Vaginal Cream contains 1.5 mg estropipate in a base composed of the following ingredients: glycerin, mineral oil, glyceryl monostearate, polyethylene glycol ether complex of higher fatty alcohols, cetyl alcohol, anhydrous lanolin, sodium biphosphate, cis-N-(3-chloroallyl)hexaminium chloride, propylparaben, methylparaben, piperazine hexahydrate, citric acid and water.

Clinical Pharmacology: Estropipate owes its therapeutic action to estrone, one of the three principal estrogenic steroid hormones of man: estradiol, estrone, and estriol. Estradiol is rapidly hydrolyzed in the body to estrone, which in turn may be hydrated to the less active estriol. These transformations occur readily, mainly in the liver, where there is also free interconversion between estrone and estradiol. These hormones are responsible for the development and maintenance of the female reproductive system and the primary and secondary female sex characteristics. They stimulate endometrial growth, promote the thickening, stratification, and cornification of the vagina, and cause the growth of mammary gland ducts.

Gastrointestinal absorption of orally administered estrogens is usually prompt and complete. Inactivation of estrogens in the body occurs mainly in the liver. During cyclic passage through the liver, estrogens are degraded to less active estrogenic compounds and conjugated with sulfuric and glucuronic acids. Estrone is loosely bound to protein as it circulates in the blood, usually as a conjugate with sulfate.

The topical application of an estrogen hormone such as OGEN Vaginal Cream may alleviate the signs and symptoms of atrophic changes in the vaginal and vulval epithelia.

OGEN Vaginal Cream may be absorbed transmucosally and may produce systemic estrogenic effects.

Indications: OGEN (estropipate) Tablets are indicated for the treatment of estrogen deficiency associated with:

1. Moderate to severe *vasomotor* symptoms of menopause. (There is no evidence that estrogens are effective for nervous symptoms or depression which might occur during menopause, and they should not be used to treat these conditions.)
2. Atrophic vaginitis.
3. Kraurosis vulvae.
4. Female hypogonadism.
5. Female castration.
6. Primary ovarian failure.

OGEN Vaginal Cream is indicated for the treatment of atrophic vaginitis or kraurosis vulvae.

OGEN (estropipate) HAS NOT BEEN TESTED FOR EFFICACY FOR ANY PURPOSE DURING PREGNANCY. SINCE ITS EFFECT UPON THE FETUS IS UNKNOWN, IT CANNOT BE RECOMMENDED FOR ANY CONDITION DURING PREGNANCY (SEE BOXED WARNING).

Contraindications: OGEN should not be used in women with any of the following conditions:

1. Known or suspected cancer of the breast.
2. Known or suspected estrogen dependent neoplasia.
3. Known or suspected pregnancy (See Boxed Warning).
4. Undiagnosed abnormal genital bleeding.
5. Active thrombophlebitis or thromboembolic disorders.
6. A past history of thrombophlebitis, thrombosis, or thromboembolic disorders associated with previous estrogen use.

OGEN (estropipate) is contraindicated in patients hypersensitive to its ingredients.

Warnings:

1. *Induction of malignant neoplasms.* Long-term continuous administration of natural and synthetic estrogens in certain animal species has been reported by some investigators to increase the frequency of carcinomas of the breast, cervix, vagina, and liver. There is now evidence that estrogens increase the risk of carcinoma of the endometrium in humans. (See Boxed Warning).

At the present time there is no satisfactory evidence that estrogens given to postmenopausal women increase the risk of cancer of the breast,[17] although a recent long-term follow-up of a single physician's practice has raised this possibility.[18] Therefore, caution should be exercised when administering estrogens to women with a strong family history of breast cancer or who have breast nodules, fibrocystic disease, or abnormal mammograms. Careful breast examinations should be performed periodically.

2. *Gallbladder disease.* A recent study has reported a 2 to 3 fold increase in the risk of surgically confirmed gallbladder disease in women receiving postmenopausal estrogens,[17] similar to the 2-fold increase previously noted in users of oral contraceptives.[19,22] In the case of oral contraceptives, the increased risk appeared after two years of use.[22]

3. *Effects similar to those caused by estrogen-progestogen oral contraceptives.* There are several serious adverse effects of oral contraceptives, most of which have not, up to now, been documented as consequences of postmenopausal estrogen therapy. This may reflect the comparatively low doses of estrogen used in postmenopausal women. It would be expected that the larger doses of estrogen used to treat postpartum breast engorgement would be more likely to result in these adverse effects, and, in fact, it has been shown that there is an increased risk of thrombosis in women receiving estrogens for postpartum breast engorgement.[20,21]

a. *Thromboembolic disease.* It is now well established that users of oral contraceptives have an increased risk of various thromboembolic and thrombotic vascular diseases, such as thrombophlebitis, pulmonary embolism, stroke, and myocardial infarction.[22–29] Cases of retinal thrombosis, mesenteric thrombosis, and optic neuritis have been reported in oral contraceptive users. There is evidence that the risk of several of these adverse reactions is related to the dose of the drug.[30,31] An increased risk of post-surgery thromboembolic complications has also been reported in users of oral contraceptives.[32,33] If feasible, estrogen should be discontinued at least 4 weeks before surgery of the type associated with an increased risk of thromboembolism; it should also be discontinued during periods of prolonged immobilization.

While an increased rate of thromboembolic and thrombotic disease in postmenopausal users of estrogens has not been found[17,34] this does not rule out the possibility that such an increase may be present or that subgroups of women who have underlying risk factors or who are receiving relatively large doses of estrogens may have increased risk. Therefore, estrogens should not be used in persons with active thrombophlebitis or thromboembolic disorders, and they should not be used in persons with a history of such disorders in association with estrogen use. They should be used with caution in patients with cerebral vascular or coronary artery disease and only for those in whom estrogens are clearly needed.

Large doses of estrogen (5 mg conjugated estrogens per day), comparable to those used to treat cancer of the prostate and breast, have been shown in a large prospective clinical trial in men[35] to increase the risk of nonfatal myocardial infarction, pulmonary embolism and thrombophlebitis. When estrogen doses of this size are used, any of the thromboembolic and thrombotic adverse effects associated with oral contraceptive use should be considered a clear risk.

b. *Hepatic adenoma.* Benign hepatic adenomas appear to be associated with the use of oral contraceptives.[36–38] Although benign, and rare, these may rupture and cause death through intraabdominal hemorrhage. Such lesions have not yet been reported in association with other estrogen or progestogen preparations but should be considered in estrogen users having abdominal pain and tenderness, abdominal mass, or hypovolemic shock. Hepatocellular carcinoma has also been reported in women taking estrogen-containing oral contraceptives.[37] The relationship of this malignancy to these drugs is not known at this time.

c. *Elevated blood pressure.* Increased blood pressure is not uncommon in women using oral contraceptives. There is now a report that this may occur with use of estrogens in the menopause[39] and blood pressure should be monitored with estrogen use, especially if high doses are used.

d. *Glucose tolerance.* A worsening of glucose tolerance has been observed in a significant percentage of patients on estrogen-containing oral contraceptives. For this reason, diabetic patients should be carefully observed while receiving estrogen.

4. *Hypercalcemia.* Administration of estrogens may lead to severe hypercalcemia in patients with breast cancer and bone metastases.

Continued on next page

If desired, additional literature on any Abbott Product will be provided upon request to Abbott Laboratories.

Abbott—Cont.

Precautions:
A. General Precautions.
1. A complete medical and family history should be taken prior to the initiation of any estrogen therapy. The pretreatment and periodic physical examinations should include special reference to blood pressure, breasts, abdomen, and pelvic organs, and should include a Papanicolau smear. As a general rule, estrogen should not be prescribed for longer than one year without another physical examination being performed.
2. Diagnostic measures should be taken to rule out gonorrhea or neoplasia before prescribing OGEN Vaginal Cream. Trichomonal, monilial, or bacterial infection should be treated by appropriate anti-microbial therapy.
3. Fluid retention—Estrogens may cause some degree of fluid retention. Therefore, patients with conditions such as epilepsy, migraine, and cardiac or renal dysfunction, which might be influenced by this factor, require careful observation.
4. Certain patients may develop undesirable manifestations of excessive estrogenic stimulation, such as abnormal or excessive uterine bleeding, mastodynia, etc.
5. Oral contraceptives appear to be associated with an increased incidence of mental depression.[22] Although it is not clear whether this is due to the estrogenic or progestogenic component of the contraceptive, patients with a history of depression should be carefully observed.
6. Preexisting uterine leiomyomata may increase in size during estrogen use.
7. The pathologist should be advised of the patient's use of estrogen therapy when relevant specimens are submitted.
8. Patients with a past history of jaundice during pregnancy have an increased risk of recurrence of jaundice while receiving estrogen containing oral contraceptive therapy. If jaundice develops in any patient receiving estrogen, the medication should be discontinued while the cause is investigated.
9. Estrogens may be poorly metabolized in patients with impaired liver function and they should be administered with caution in such patients.
10. Because estrogens influence the metabolism of calcium and phosphorus, they should be used with caution in patients with metabolic bone diseases that are associated with hypercalcemia or in patients with renal insufficiency.
11. Because of the effects of estrogens on epiphyseal closure, they should be used judiciously in young patients in whom bone growth is not complete.
12. Certain endocrine and liver function tests may be affected by estrogen-containing oral contraceptives. The following similar changes may be expected with larger doses of estrogen:
a. Increased sulfobromophthalein retention.
b. Increased prothrombin and factors VII, VIII, IX, and X; decreased antithrombin 3; increased norepinephrine-induced platelet aggregability.
c. Increased thyroid binding globulin (TBG) leading to increased circulating total thyroid hormone, as measured by PBI, T4 by column, or T4 by radioimmunoassay. Free T3 resin uptake is decreased, reflecting the elevated TBG; free T4 concentration is unaltered.
d. Impaired glucose tolerance.
e. Decreased pregnanediol excretion.
f. Reduced response to metyrapone test.
g. Reduced serum folate concentration.
h. Increased serum triglyceride and phospholipid concentration.
B. Information for the Patient. See text of Patient Package Insert which appears after Physician References.
C. OGEN (estropipate) cannot be recommended for use during pregnancy. See Contraindications and Boxed Warning.
D. Nursing Mothers. Estrogens have been reported to be excreted in human breast milk.

Adverse Reactions: Hypersensitivity reactions, systemic effects such as breast tenderness, and rarely, withdrawal bleeding, have occurred with the use of topical estrogens.
The following additional adverse reactions have been reported with estrogenic therapy, including oral contraceptives (See Warnings regarding reports of possible induction of neoplasia, unknown effects upon the fetus, increased incidence of gallbladder disease, and adverse effects similar to those of oral contraceptives, including thromboembolism):
1. *Genitourinary system.*
Breakthrough bleeding, spotting, change in menstrual flow.
Dysmenorrhea.
Premenstrual-like syndrome.
Amenorrhea during and after treatment.
Increase in size of uterine fibromyomata.
Vaginal candidiasis.
Change in cervical eversion and in degree of cervical secretion.
Cystitis-like syndrome.
2. *Breast.*
Tenderness, enlargement, secretion.
3. *Gastrointestinal.*
Nausea, vomiting.
Abdominal cramps, bloating.
Cholestatic jaundice.
4. *Skin.*
Chloasma or melasma which may persist when drug is discontinued.
Erythema multiforme.
Erythema nodosum.
Hemorrhagic eruption.
Loss of scalp hair.
Hirsutism.
5. *Eyes.*
Steepening of corneal curvature.
Intolerance to contact lenses.
6. *CNS.*
Headache, migraine, dizziness.
Mental depression.
Chorea.
7. *Miscellaneous.*
Increase or decrease in weight.
Reduced carbohydrate tolerance.
Aggravation of porphyria.
Edema.
Changes in libido.

Acute Overdosage: Numerous reports of ingestion of large doses of estrogen-containing oral contraceptives by young children indicate that serious ill effects do not occur. Overdosage of oral estrogen may cause nausea and withdrawal bleeding may occur in females.

Dosage and Administration: OGEN (estropipate) Tablets:
1. *Given cyclically for short-term use:*
For treatment of moderate to severe *vasomotor* symptoms, atrophic vaginitis, or kraurosis vulvae associated with the menopause.
The lowest dose that will control symptoms should be chosen and medication should be discontinued as promptly as possible.
Administration should be cyclic (e.g., 3 weeks on and 1 week off).
Attempts to discontinue or taper medication should be made at 3 to 6 month intervals.
The usual dosage range is one OGEN .625 Tablet to one OGEN 5 Tablet per day.
2. *Given cyclically.*
Female hypogonadism. Female castration. Primary ovarian failure. The lowest dose that will control symptoms should be chosen. A daily dose of one OGEN 1.25 Tablet to three OGEN 2.5 Tablets may be given for the first three weeks of a theoretical cycle, followed by a rest period of eight to ten days. The same schedule is repeated if bleeding does not occur by the end of the rest period. The duration of cyclic estrogen therapy necessary to produce withdrawal bleeding will vary according to the responsiveness of the endometrium. If satisfactory withdrawal bleeding does not occur, an oral progestogen may be given in addition to estrogen during the third week of the cycle.
Treated patients with an intact uterus should be monitored closely for signs of endometrial cancer and appropriate diagnostic measures should be taken to rule out malignancy in the event of persistent or recurring abnormal vaginal bleeding.
OGEN (estropipate) Vaginal Cream:
To be adminstered cyclically for short-term use only:
For treatment of atropic vaginitis or kraurosis vulvae.
The lowest dose that will control symptoms should be chosen and medication should be discontinued as promptly as possible.
Administration should be cyclic (e.g., three weeks on and one week off).
Attempts to discontinue or taper medication should be made at three to six month intervals.
Usual dosage intravaginally, 2 to 4 g of OGEN Vaginal Cream daily, depending upon the severity of the condition.
The following instructions for use are intended for the patient and are printed on the carton label for OGEN Vaginal Cream (estropipate):
1. Remove cap from tube.
2. Make sure plunger of applicator is all the way into the barrel.
3. Screw nozzle end of applicator onto the tube.
4. Squeeze tube to force sufficient cream into applicator so that number on plunger indicating prescribed dose is level with top of barrel.
5. Unscrew applicator from tube and replace cap on tube.
6. To deliver medication, insert end of applicator into vagina and push plunger all the way down.
Between uses, pull plunger out of barrel and wash applicator in warm, soapy water. DO NOT PUT APPLICATOR IN HOT OR BOILING WATER.

How Supplied: OGEN (estropipate tablets, USP) is supplied as OGEN .625 (0.75 mg estropipate), yellow tablets, **NDC** 0074-3943-04; OGEN 1.25 (1.5 mg estropipate), peach-colored tablets, **NDC** 0074-3946-04; OGEN 2.5 (3 mg estropipate), blue tablets, **NDC** 0074-3951-04; and OGEN 5 (6 mg estropipate), light green tablets, **NDC** 0074-3958-13. Tablets of all four dosage levels are standardized to provide uniform estrone activity and are grooved (Divide-Tab®) to provide dosage flexibility. All tablet sizes of OGEN are available in bottles of 100.
OGEN (estropipate vaginal cream, USP), 1.5 mg estropipate per gram, is available in packages containing a 1½ oz (42.5 Gm) tube with one plastic applicator calibrated at 2, 3, and 4 g levels. (**NDC** 0074-2467-42).
[*Shown in Product Identification Section*]

Physician References:

[1]Ziel, H. K. and W. D. Finkel, "Increased Risk of Endometrial Carcinoma Among Users of Conjugated Estrogens," *New England Journal of Medicine*, 293:1167-1170, 1975
[2]Smith, D. C., R. Prentic, D. J. Thompson and W. L. Hermann, "Association of Exogenous Estrogen and Endometrial Carcinoma," *New England Journal of Medicine*, 293:1164-1167, 1975.
[3]Mack, T. M., M. C. Pike, B. E. Henderson, R. I. Pfeffer, V. R. Gerkins, M. Arthur and S. E. Brown, "Estrogens and Endometrial Cancer in a Retirement Community," *New England Journal of Medicine*, 294:1262-1267, 1976.
[4]Weiss, N. S., D. R. Szekely and D. F. Austin, "Increasing Incidence of Endometrial Cancer in the United States," *New England Journal of Medicine*. 294:1259-1262, 1976.
[5]Herbst, A. L., H. Ulfelder and D. C. Poskanzer, "Adenocarcinoma of Vagina," *New England Journal of Medicine*, 284:878-881, 1971.
[6]Greenwald, P., J. Barlow, P. Nasca and W. Burnett, "Vaginal Cancer after Maternal

Treatment with Synthetic Estrogens," *New England Journal of Medicine,* 285:390-392, 1971.

[7]Lanier, A., K. Noller, D. Decker, L. Elveback and L. Kurland, "Cancer and Stilbestrol, A Follow Up of 1719 Persons Exposed to Estrogens In Utero and Born 1943-1959," *Mayo Clinic Proceedings,* 48:793-799, 1973.

[8]Herbst, A., R. Kurman and R. Scully, "Vaginal and Cervical Abnormalities After Exposure to Stilbestrol In Utero," *Obstetrics and Gynecology,* 40:287-298, 1972.

[9]Herbst, A., S. Robboy, G. Macdonald and R. Scully, "The Effects of Local Progesterone on Stilbestrol Associated Vaginal Adenosis," *American Journal of Obstetrics and Gynecology,* 118:607-615, 1974.

[10]Herbst, A., D. Poskanzer, S. Robboy, L. Friedlander and R. Scully, "Prenatal Exposure to Stilbestrol, A Prospective Comparison of Exposed Female Offspring with Unexposed Controls," *New England Journal of Medicine,* 292:334-339, 1975.

[11]Stafl, A., R. Mattingly, D. Foley and W. Fetherston, "Clinical Diagnosis of Vaginal Adenosis," *Obstetrics and Gynecology,* 43:118-128, 1974.

[12]Sherman, A. I., M. Goldrath, A. Berlin, V. Vakhariya, F. Banooni, W. Michaels, P. Goodman and S. Brown, "Cervical Vaginal Adenosis After *In Utero* Exposure to Synthetic Estrogens," *Obstetrics and Gynecology,* 44:531-545, 1974.

[13]Gal, I., B. Kirman and J. Stern, "Hormone Pregnancy Tests and Congenital Malformation," *Nature,* 216:83, 1967.

[14]Levy, E. P., A. Cohen and F. C. Fraser, "Hormone Treatment During Pregnancy and Congenital Heart Defects," *Lancet,* 1:611, 1973.

[15]Nora, J. and A. Nora, "Birth Defects and Oral Contraceptives," *Lancet,* 1:941-942, 1973.

[16]Janerich, D. T., J. M. Piper and D. M. Glebatis, "Oral Contraceptives and Congenital Limb Reducton Defects," *New England Journal of Medicine,* 291:697-700, 1974.

[17]Boston Collaborative Drug Surveillance Program "Surgically Confirmed Gall Bladder Disease, Venous Thromboembolism and Breast Tumors in Relation to Post Menopausal Estrogen Therapy," *New England Journal of Medicine,* 290:15-19, 1974.

[18]Hoover, R., L. A. Gray, Sr., P. Cole and B. MacMahon, "Menopausal Estrogens and Breast Cancer," *New England Journal of Medicine,* 295:401-405, 1976.

[19]Boston Collaborative Drug Surveillance Program, "Oral Contraceptives and Venous Thromboembolic Disease, Surgically Confirmed Gall Bladder Disease and Breast Tumors," *Lancet* 1:1399-1404, 1973.

[20]Daniel, D.G., H. Campbell and A. C. Turnbull, "Puerperal Thromboembolism and Suppression of Lactation," *Lancet* 2:287-289, 1967.

[21]Bailar, J. C., "Thromboembolism and Oestrogen Therapy," *Lancet* 2:560, 1967.

[22]Royal College of General Practitioners, "Oral Contraception and Thromboembolic Disease," *Journal of the Royal College of General Practitioners,* 13:267-279, 1967.

23 Inman, W. H. W. and M. P. Vessey, "Investigation of Deaths from Pulmonary, Coronary, and Cerebral Thrombosis and Embolism in Women of Child Bearing Age," *British Medical Journal,* 2:193-199, 1968.

[24]Vessey, M. P. and R. Doll, "Investigation of Relation Between Use of Oral Contraceptives and Thromboembolic Disease, A Further Report," *British Medical Journal,* 2:651-657, 1969.

[25]Sartwell, P. E., A. T. Masi, F. G. Arthes, G. R. Greene and H. E. Smith, "Thromboembolism and Oral Contraceptives: An Epidemiological Case Control Study," *American Journal of Epidemiology,* 90:365-380, 1969.

[26]Collaborative Group for the Study of Stroke in Young Women, "Oral Contraception and Increased Risk of Cerebral Ischemia or Thrombosis," *New England Journal of Medicine,* 288:871-878, 1973.

[27]Collaborative Group for the Study of Stroke in Young Women, "Oral Contraceptives and Stroke in Young Women: Associated Risk Factors," *Journal of American Medical Association,* 231:718-722, 1975.

[28]Mann, J. I. and W. H. W. Inman, "Oral Contraceptives and Death from Myocardial Infarction," *British Medical Journal,* 2:245-248, 1975.

[29]Mann, J. I., M. P. Vessey, M. Thorogood and R. Doll, "Myocardial Infarction in Young Women with Special Reference to Oral Contraceptives Practice," *British Medical Journal,* 2:241-245, 1975.

[30]Inman, W. H. W., V. P. Vessey, B. Westerholm and A. Engelund, "Thromboembolic Disease and the Steroidal Content of Oral Contraceptives," *British Medical Journal,* 2:203-209, 1970.

[31]Stolley, P. D., J. A. Tonascia, M. S. Tockman, P. E. Sartwell, A. H. Rutledge and M. P. Jacobs, "Thrombosis with Low-Estrogen Oral Contraceptives," *American Journal of Epidemiology,* 102:197-208, 1975.

[32]Vessey, M. P., R. Doll, A. S. Fairbairn and G. Glober, "Post Operative Thromboembolism and the Use of the Oral Contraceptives," *British Medical Journal,* 3:123-126, 1970.

[33]Greene, G. R. and P. E. Sartwell, "Oral Contraceptive Use in Patients with Thromboembolism Following Surgery, Trauma or Infection," *American Journal of Public Health,* 62:680-685, 1972.

[34]Rosenberg, L. M., B. Armstrong and H. Jick, "Myocardial Infarction and Estrogen Therapy in Postmenopausal Women," *New England Journal of Medicine,* 294:1256-1259, 1976.

[35]Coronary Drug Project Research Group, "The Coronary Drug Project: Initial Findings Leading to Modifications of Its Research Protocol," *Journal of the American Medical Association,* 214:1303-1313, 1970.

[36]Baum, J., F. Holtz, J. J. Bookstein and E. W. Klein, "Possible Association Between Benign Hepatomas and Oral Contraceptives," *Lancet,* 2:926-928, 1973.

[37]Mays, E. T., W. M. Christopherson, M. M. Mahr and H. C. Williams, "Hepatic Changes in Young Women Ingesting Contraceptive Steroids, Hepatic Hemorrhage and Primary Hepatic Tumors," *Journal of the American Medical Association,* 235:730-782, 1976.

[38]Edmondson, H. A., B. Henderson and B. Benton, "Liver Cell Adenomas Associated with the Use of Oral Contraceptives," *New England Journal of Medicine,* 294:470-472, 1976.

[39]Pfeffer, R. I. and S. Van Den Noort, "Estrogen Use and Stroke Risk in Postmenopausal Women," *American Journal of Epidemiology,* 103:445-456, 1976.

PATIENT LABELING
OGEN®
(estropipate tablets and vaginal cream, USP)

The discussion that follows is about estrogens that are taken internally for the treatment of symptoms of estrogen deficiency. Some or all of the information below on the systemic use of estrogens may also apply to the estrogen cream.

WHAT YOU SHOULD KNOW ABOUT ESTROGENS

Estrogens are female hormones produced by the ovaries. The ovaries make several different kinds of estrogens. In addition, scientists have been able to make a variety of synthetic estrogens. As far as we know, all these estrogens have similar properties and therefore much the same usefulness, side effects, and risks. This leaflet is intended to help you understand what estrogens are used for, the risks involved in their use, and how to use them as safely as possible.

This leaflet includes the most important information about estrogens, but not all the information. If you want to know more, you can ask your doctor or pharmacist to let you read the package insert prepared for the doctor.

Uses of Estrogen: Estrogens are prescribed by doctors for a number of purposes, including:

1. To provide estrogen during a period of adjustment when a woman's ovaries no longer produce it, in order to prevent certain uncomfortable symptoms of estrogen deficiency. (All women normally stop producing estrogens, generally between the ages of 45 and 55; this is called the menopause.)
2. To prevent symptoms of estrogen deficiency when a woman's ovaries have been removed surgically before the natural menopause.
3. To prevent pregnancy. (Estrogens are given along with a progestogen, another female hormone; these combinations are called oral contraceptives or birth control pills. Patient labeling is available to women taking oral contraceptives and they will not be discussed in this leaflet.)

THERE IS NO PROPER USE OF OGEN (ESTROPIPATE) IN A PREGNANT WOMAN.

Estrogens in the menopause: In the natural course of their lives, all women eventually experience a decrease in estrogen production. This usually occurs between ages 45 and 55 but may occur earlier or later. Sometimes the ovaries may need to be removed before natural menopause by an operation, producing a "surgical menopause."

When the amount of estrogen in the blood begins to decrease, many women may develop typical symptoms: Feelings of warmth in the face, neck, and chest or sudden intense episodes of heat or sweating throughout the body (called "hot flashes" or "hot flushes"). These symptoms are sometimes very uncomfortable. A few women eventually develop changes in the vagina (called "atrophic vaginitis") which cause discomfort, especially during and after intercourse.

Estrogens can be prescribed to treat these symptoms of the menopause. It is estimated that considerably more than half of all women undergoing the menopause have only mild symptoms or no symptoms at all and therefore do not need estrogens. Other women may need estrogens for a few months, while their bodies adjust to lower estrogen levels. Sometimes the need will be for periods longer than six months. In an attempt to avoid overstimulation of the uterus (womb), oral estrogens are usually given cyclically during each month of use, that is three weeks of pills followed by one week without pills.

Sometimes women experience nervous symptoms or depression during menopause. There is no evidence that estrogens are effective for such symptoms and they should not be used to treat them, although other treatment may be needed.

You may have heard that taking estrogens for long periods (years) after the menopause will keep your skin soft and supple and keep you feeling young. There is no evidence that this is so, however, and such long-term treatment carries important risks.

The Dangers of Estrogens:

1. *Cancer of uterus.* If estrogens are used in the postmenopausal period for more than a year, there is an increased risk of *endometrial cancer* (cancer of the uterus). Women taking estrogens have roughly 5 to 10 times as great a chance of getting this cancer as women who take no estrogens. To put this another way, while a postmenopausal woman not taking estrogens has 1 chance in 1,000 each year of getting cancer of the uterus, a woman taking

Continued on next page

If desired, additional literature on any Abbott Product will be provided upon request to Abbott Laboratories.

Abbott—Cont.

estrogens has 5 to 10 chances in 1,000 each year. For this reason *it is important to take estrogens only when you really need them.*
The risk of this cancer is greater the longer estrogens are used and also seems to be greater when larger doses are taken. For this reason *it is important to take the lowest dose of estrogen that will control symptoms and to take it only as long as it is needed.* If estrogens are needed for longer periods of time, your doctor will want to reevaluate your need for estrogens at least every six months.
Women using estrogens should report any irregular vaginal bleeding to their doctors; such bleeding may be of no importance, but it can be an early warning of cancer of the uterus. If you have undiagnosed vaginal bleeding, you should not use estrogens until a diagnosis is made and you are certain there is no cancer of the uterus. If you have had your uterus completely removed (total hysterectomy), there is no danger of developing cancer of the uterus.
2. *Other possible cancers.* Estrogens can cause development of other tumors in animals, such as tumors of the breast, cervix, vagina, or liver, when given for a long time. At present there is no good evidence that women using estrogen in the menopause have an increased risk of such tumors, but there is no way yet to be sure they do not; and one study raises the possibility that use of estrogens in the menopause may increase the risk of breast cancer many years later. This is a further reason to use estrogens only when clearly needed. While you are taking estrogens, it is important that you go to your doctor at least once a year for a physical examination. Also, if members of your family have had breast cancer or if you have breast nodules or abnormal mammograms (breast x-rays), your doctor may wish to carry out more frequent examinations of your breasts.
3. *Gallbladder disease.* Women who use estrogens after menopause are more likely to develop gallbladder disease needing surgery than women who do not use estrogens. Birth control pills have a similar effect.
4. *Abnormal blood clotting.* Oral contraceptives increase the risk of blood clotting in various parts of the body. This can result in a stroke (if the clot is in the brain), a heart attack (clot in a blood vessel of the heart), or a pulmonary embolus (a clot which forms in the legs or pelvis, then breaks off and travels to the lungs). Any of these can be fatal.
At this time use of estrogens in the menopause is not known to cause such blood clotting, but this has not been fully studied and there could still prove to be such a risk. It is recommended that if you have had clotting in the legs or lungs or a heart attack or stroke while you were using estrogens or birth control pills, you should not use estrogens. If you have had a stroke or heart attack or if you have angina pectoris, estrogens should be used with great caution and only if clearly needed (for example, if you have severe symptoms of the menopause.)
Special Warning About Pregnancy: You should not receive OGEN (estropipate) if you are pregnant. Some scientists have reported that, if estrogens are used during pregnancy, there may be a greater than usual chance that the developing baby will be born with a birth defect, although the risk remains small. In addition, other scientists have reported that there is an association between another estrogen-type product (diethylstilbestrol) and appearance of a particular cancer of the vagina or cervix (adenocarcinoma) in young women whose mothers took that drug in pregnancy. Every effort should be made to avoid exposure to OGEN in pregnancy. If exposure occurs, see your doctor.

Other Effects of Estrogens: In addition to the serious known risks of estrogens described above, estrogens have the following side effects and potential risks:
1. *Nausea and vomiting.* The most common side effect of estrogen therapy is nausea. Vomiting is less common.
2. *Effects on breasts.* Estrogens may cause breast tenderness or enlargement and may cause the breasts to secrete a liquid. These effects are not dangerous.
3. *Effects on the uterus.* Estrogens may cause benign fibroid tumors of the uterus to get larger.
Some women will have menstrual bleeding when estrogens are stopped. But if the bleeding occurs on days you are still taking estrogens you should report this to your doctor.
4. *Effects on liver.* Women taking oral contraceptives develop on rare occasions a tumor of the liver which can rupture and bleed into the abdomen. So far, these tumors have not been reported in women using estrogens in the menopause, but you should report any swelling or unusual pain or tenderness in the abdomen to your doctor immediately.
Women with a past history of jaundice (yellowing of the skin and white parts of the eyes) may get jaundice again during estrogen use. If this occurs, stop taking estrogens and see your doctor.
5. *Other effects.* Estrogens may cause excess fluid to be retained in the body. This may make some conditions worse, such as epilepsy, migraine, heart disease, or kidney disease.
Summary: Estrogens have important uses, but they have serious risks as well. You must decide, with your doctor, whether the risks are acceptable to you in view of the benefits of treatment. You should not use OGEN if you have cancer of the breast or uterus, are pregnant, have undiagnosed abnormal vaginal bleeding, clotting in the legs or lungs, or have had a stroke, heart attack or angina, or clotting in the legs or lungs in the past while you were taking estrogens.
You can use estrogens as safely as possible by understanding that your doctor will require regular physical examinations while you are taking them and will try to discontinue the drug as soon as possible and use the smallest dose possible. Be alert for signs of trouble including:
1. Abnormal bleeding from the vagina.
2. Pains in the calves or chest or sudden shortness of breath, or coughing blood (indicating possible clots in the legs, heart, or lungs).
3. Severe headache, dizziness, faintness, or changes in vision (indicating possible developing clots in the brain or eye).
4. Breast lumps (you should ask your doctor how to examine your own breasts).
5. Jaundice (yellowing of the skin).
6. Mental depression.
Based on his or her assessment of your medical needs, your doctor has prescribed this drug for you. Do not give the drug to anyone else.
Abbott Laboratories/
Abbott Pharmaceuticals, Inc.
North Chicago, IL 60064

OPTILETS®-500

High potency multivitamin for use in treatment of multivitamin deficiency.*

OPTILETS-M-500®

High potency multivitamin for use in treatment of multivitamin deficiency.* Mineral supplementation added.**

Description: A therapeutic formula of ten important vitamins, with and without minerals, in a small tablet with the Abbott Filmtab® coating. Each Optilets-500 tablet provides:
Vitamin C (as sodium ascorbate) .... 500 mg
Niacinamide .... 100 mg
Calcium Pantothenate .... 20 mg
Vitamin B_1 (thiamine mononitrate) .... 15 mg
Vitamin B_2 (riboflavin) .... 10 mg
Vitamin B_6 (pyridoxine hydrochloride) ... 5 mg
Vitamin A (as palmitate 1.5 mg, as acetate 1.5 mg—total 3 mg) .... 10,000 IU
Vitamin B_{12} (cyanocobalamin) .... 12 mcg
Vitamin D (ergocalciferol) ...... (10 mcg) 400 IU
Vitamin E (as dl-alpha tocopheryl acetate) .... 30 IU
Each Optilets-M-500 Filmtab contains all the vitamins in the same quantities provided in Optilets-500, plus the following minerals:
Magnesium (as oxide) .... 80 mg**
Iron (as dried ferrous sulfate) .... 20 mg
Copper (as sulfate) .... 2 mg
Zinc (as sulfate) .... 1.5 mg**
Manganese (as sulfate) .... 1 mg
Iodine (as calcium iodate) .... 0.15 mg
* These products contain no folic acid and only dietary supplement levels of vitamins D and E.
** Below USRDA levels.
Dosage and Administration: Usual adult dosage is one Filmtab tablet daily, or as directed by physician.
How Supplied: Optilets-500 tablets are supplied in bottles of 30 (**NDC** 0074-4287-30) and 100 (**NDC** 0074-4287-13). Optilets-M-500 tablets are supplied in bottles of 30 (**NDC** 0074-4286-30) and 100 (**NDC** 0074-4286-13).
[*Shown in Product Identification Section*]
Abbott Laboratories
North Chicago, IL 60064
Ref. 02-5861-4/R9, 02-5551-4/R8

ORETIC® ℞

(hydrochlorothiazide tablets, USP)

Description: ORETIC (hydrochlorothiazide) is a member of the benzothiadiazine (thiazide) family of drugs. It is closely related to chlorothiazide. Clinically, ORETIC is an orally active diuretic-antihypertensive agent.
Actions: The diuretic and saluretic effects of ORETIC result from a drug-induced inhibition of the renal tubular reabsorption of electrolytes. The excretion of sodium and chloride is greatly enhanced. Potassium excretion is also enhanced to a variable degree, as it is with the other thiazides. Although urinary excretion of bicarbonate is increased slightly, there is usually no significant change in urinary pH. Hydrochlorothiazide has a per mg natriuretic activity approximately 10 times that of the prototype thiazide, chlorothiazide. At maximal therapeutic dosages, all thiazides are approximately equal in their diuretic/natriuretic effects.
There is significant natriuresis and diuresis within two hours after administration of a single oral dose of hydrochlorothiazide. These effects reach a peak in about six hours and persist for about 12 hours following oral administration of a single dose.
Like other benzothiadiazines, ORETIC also has antihypertensive properties, and may be used for this purpose either alone or to enhance the antihypertensive action of other drugs. The mechanism by which the benzothiadiazines, including hydrochlorothiazide, produce a reduction of elevated blood pressure is not known. However, sodium depletion appears to be involved.
ORETIC (hydrochlorothiazide) is readily absorbed from the gastrointestinal tract and is excreted unchanged by the kidneys.
Indications: ORETIC is indicated in the management of hypertension either as the sole therapeutic agent or to enhance the effect of other antihypertensive drugs in the more severe forms of hypertension.
ORETIC is indicated as adjunctive therapy in edema associated with congestive heart failure, hepatic cirrhosis, and corticosteroid and estrogen therapy.
ORETIC has also been found useful in edema due to various forms of renal dysfunction such as the nephrotic syndrome, acute glomerulonephritis and chronic renal failure.

Usage in Pregnancy: The routine use of diuretics in an otherwise healthy pregnant woman is inappropriate and exposes mother and fetus to unnecessary hazard. Diuretics do not prevent development of toxemia of pregnancy, and there is no satisfactory evidence that they are useful in the treatment of developed toxemia.

Edema during pregnancy may arise from pathological causes or from the physiological and mechanical consequences of pregnancy. Thiazides are indicated in pregnancy when edema is due to pathological causes, just as they are in the absence of pregnancy (however, see Warnings, below). Dependent edema in pregnancy, resulting from restriction of venous return by the expanded uterus, is properly treated through elevation of the lower extremities and use of support hose; use of diuretics to lower intravascular volume in this case is illogical and unnecessary. There is hypervolemia during normal pregnancy which is harmful to neither the fetus nor the mother (in the absence of cardiovascular disease), but which is associated with edema, including generalized edema, in the majority of pregnant women. If this edema produces discomfort, increased recumbency will often provide relief. In rare instances, this edema may cause extreme discomfort which is not relieved by rest. In these cases, a short course of diuretics may provide relief and may be appropriate.

Contraindications: Renal decompensation. Hypersensitivity to this or other sulfonamide-derived drugs.

Warnings: Hydrochlorothiazide shares with other thiazides the propensity to deplete potassium reserves to an unpredictable degree.

Thiazides should be used with caution in patients with renal disease or significant impairment of renal function, since azotemia may be precipitated and cumulative drug effects may occur.

Thiazides should be used with caution in patients with impaired hepatic function or progressive liver disease, since minor alterations of fluid and electrolyte balance may precipitate hepatic coma.

Thiazides may be additive or potentiative of the action of other antihypertensive drugs. Potentiation occurs with ganglionic or peripheral adrenergic blocking drugs.

Sensitivity reactions may occur in patients with a history of allergy or bronchial asthma. The possibility of exacerbation or activation of systemic lupus erythematosus has been reported.

Usage in Pregnancy: Thiazides cross the placental barrier and appear in cord blood. The use of thiazides in pregnant women requires that the anticipated benefit be weighed against possible hazards to the fetus. These hazards include fetal or neonatal jaundice, thrombocytopenia, and possible other adverse reactions that have occurred in the adult.

Nursing Mothers: Thiazides appear in breast milk. If use of the drug is deemed essential, the patient should stop nursing.

Precautions: Periodic determinations of serum electrolytes should be performed at appropriate intervals for the purpose of detecting possible electrolyte imbalances such as hyponatremia, hypochloremic alkalosis, and hypokalemia. Serum and urine electrolyte determinations are particularly important when a patient is vomiting excessively or receiving parenteral fluids. All patients should be observed for other clinical signs of electrolyte imbalances such as dryness of mouth, thirst, weakness, lethargy, drowsiness, restlessness, muscle pains or cramps, muscular fatigue, hypotension, oliguria, tachycardia, and gastrointestinal disturbances such as nausea and vomiting.

Hypokalemia may develop with thiazides as with any other potent diuretic, especially when brisk diuresis occurs, severe cirrhosis is present, or when corticosteroids or ACTH are given concomitantly. Interference with the adequate oral intake of electrolytes will also contribute to the possible development of hypokalemia. Potassium depletion, even of a mild degree, resulting from thiazide use, may sensitize a patient to the effects of cardiac glycosides such as digitalis.

Any chloride deficit is generally mild and usually does not require specific treatment except under extraordinary circumstances (as in liver disease or renal disease). Dilutional hyponatremia may occur in edematous patients in hot weather; appropriate therapy is water restriction rather than administration of salt, except in rare instances when the hyponatremia is life threatening.

In actual salt depletion, appropriate replacement is the therapy of choice.

Hyperuricemia may occur or frank gout may be precipitated in certain patients receiving thiazide therapy.

Insulin requirements in diabetic patients may be increased, decreased, or unchanged. Latent diabetes mellitus may become manifest during thiazide administration.

Thiazide drugs may increase the responsiveness to tubocurarine.

The antihypertensive effects of the drug may be enhanced in the postsympathectomy patient.

Thiazides may decrease arterial responsiveness to norepinephrine. This diminution is not sufficient to preclude effectiveness of the pressor agent for therapeutic use.

If progressive renal impairment becomes evident as indicated by a rising-nonprotein nitrogen or blood urea nitrogen, a careful reappraisal of therapy is necessary with consideration given to withholding or discontinuing diuretic therapy.

Thiazides may decrease serum PBI levels without signs of thyroid disturbance.

Thiazides have been reported, on rare occasions, to have elevated serum calcium to hypercalcemic levels. The serum calcium levels have returned to normal when the medication has been stopped. This phenomenon may be related to the ability of the thiazide diuretics to lower the amount of calcium excreted in the urine.

Adverse Reactions: Gastrointestinal system reactions: Anorexia, gastric irritation, nausea, vomiting, cramping, diarrhea, constipation, jaundice (intrahepatic cholestatic jaundice), pancreatitis.

Central nervous system reactions: Dizziness, vertigo, paresthesias, headache, xanthopsia.

Hematologic reactions: Leukopenia, agranulocytosis, thrombocytopenia, aplastic anemia.

Dermatologic — hypersensitivity reactions: Purpura, photosensitivity, rash, urticaria, necrotizing angiitis (vasculitis) (cutaneous vasculitis).

Cardiovascular reaction: Orthostatic hypotension may occur and may be aggravated by alcohol, barbiturates, or narcotics.

Other: Hyperglycemia, glycosuria, hypercalcemia, hyperuricemia, muscle spasm, weakness, restlessness.

There have been isolated reports that certain nonedematous individuals developed severe fluid and electrolyte derangements after only brief exposure to normal doses of thiazide and non-thiazide diuretics. The condition is usually manifested as severe dilutional hyponatremia, hypokalemia, and hypochloremia. It has been reported to be due to inappropriately increased ADH secretion and appears to be idiosyncratic. Potassium replacement is apparently the most important therapy in the treatment of this syndrome along with removal of the offending drug.

Whenever adverse reactions are severe, treatment should be discontinued.

Dosage and Administration: ORETIC (hydrochlorothiazide) is administered orally. Therapy should be individualized according to patient response. This therapy should be titrated to gain maximal therapeutic response as well as the minimal dose possible to maintain that therapeutic response.

For the management of edema the adult dosage ranges from 25 to 200 mg daily and may be given in single or divided doses. Usually 75 to 100 mg will produce the desired diuretic effect.

For the management of hypertension the usual initial adult dosage is 25 to 50 mg two times daily. The dosage may be increased if necessary to a maximum of 100 mg twice daily.

When therapy is prolonged or large doses are used, particular attention should be given to the patient's electrolyte status. Supplemental potassium may be required.

In the treatment of hypertension hydrochlorothiazide may be either employed alone or concurrently with other antihypertensive drugs. Combined therapy may provide adequate control of hypertension with lower dosage of the component drugs and fewer or less severe side effects. An enhanced response frequently follows its concurrent administration with Harmonyl® (deserpidine) so that dosage of both drugs may be reduced.

For treatment of moderately severe or severe hypertension, supplemental use of other more potent antihypertensive agents such as Eutonyl® (pargyline hydrochloride) may be indicated.

When other antihypertensive agents are to be added to the regimen, this should be accomplished gradually. Additional potent antihypertensive agents should be given at only half the usual dose since their effect is potentiated by pretreatment with ORETIC.

Overdosage: Symptoms of overdosage include electrolyte imbalance and signs of potassium deficiency such as confusion, dizziness, muscular weakness, and gastrointestinal disturbances. General supportive measures including replacement of fluids and electrolytes may be indicated in treatment of overdosage.

How Supplied: ORETIC (hydrochlorothiazide tablets, USP) is provided in two dosage sizes as white tablets:

25 mg tablets:
bottles of 100 (**NDC** 0074-6978-01),
bottles of 1000 (**NDC** 0074-6978-02),
Abbo-Pac® unit dose packages, 100 tablets (**NDC** 0074-6978-05).

50 mg tablets:
bottles of 100 (**NDC** 0074-6985-01),
bottles of 1000 (**NDC** 0074-6985-02),
Abbo-Pac unit dose packages, 100 tablets (**NDC** 0074-6985-06).

[*Shown in Product Identification Section*]

Abbott Laboratories
North Chicago, IL 60064
Ref. 01-2131-R3

ORETICYL® ℞

(hydrochlorothiazide and deserpidine tablets)

Oral thiazide-rauwolfia therapy for hypertension.

Warning:
This fixed combination drug is not indicated for initial therapy of hypertension. Hypertension requires therapy titrated to the individual patient. If the fixed combination represents the dosage so determined, its use may be more convenient in patient management. The treatment of hypertension is not static, but must be reevaluated as conditions in each patient warrant.

Continued on next page

If desired, additional literature on any Abbott Product will be provided upon request to Abbott Laboratories.

Abbott—Cont.

Description: ORETICYL is an orally administered combination of Oretic® (hydrochlorothiazide) and Harmonyl® (deserpidine). Hydrochlorothiazide is a diuretic-antihypertensive agent of the benzothiadiazine (thiazide) class. Deserpidine is a purified rauwolfia alkaloid, chemically identified as 11-desmethoxyreserpine, which produces antihypertensive effects.

Actions: The combined antihypertensive actions of hydrochlorothiazide and deserpidine result in a total clinical antihypertensive effect which is greater than can ordinarily be achieved by either drug given individually.

The diuretic and saluretic effects of hydrochlorothiazide result from a drug-induced inhibition of the renal tubular reabsorption of electrolytes. The excretion of sodium and chloride is greatly enhanced. Potassium excretion is also enhanced to a variable degree, as it is with the other thiazides. Although urinary excretion of bicarbonate is increased slightly, there is usually no significant change in urinary pH. Hydrochlorothiazide has a per mg natriuretic activity approximately 10 times that of the prototype thiazide, chlorothiazide. At maximal therapeutic dosages, all thiazides are approximately equal in their diuretic/natriuretic effects.

There is significant natriuresis and diuresis within two hours after administration of a single oral dose of hydrochlorothiazide. These effects reach a peak in about six hours and persist for about 12 hours following oral administration of a single dose.

Like other benzothiadiazines, hydrochlorothiazide also has antihypertensive properties, and may be used for this purpose either alone or to enhance the antihypertensive action of other drugs. The mechanism by which the benzothiadiazines, including hydrochlorothiazide, produce a reduction of elevated blood pressure is not known. However, sodium depletion appears to be involved.

Hydrochlorothiazide is readily absorbed from the gastrointestinal tract and is excreted unchanged by the kidneys.

The pharmacologic actions of Harmonyl (deserpidine) are essentially the same as those of other active rauwolfia alkaloids. Deserpidine probably produces its antihypertensive effects through depletion of tissue stores of catecholamines (epinephrine and norepinephrine) from peripheral sites. The antihypertensive effect is often accompanied by bradycardia. There is no significant alteration in cardiac output or renal blood flow. The carotid sinus reflex is inhibited, but postural hypotension is rarely seen with the use of conventional doses of Harmonyl alone.

Deserpidine, like other rauwolfia alkaloids, is characterized by slow onset of action and sustained effect which may persist following withdrawal of the drug.

Indications: ORETICYL (hydrochlorothiazide and deserpidine) is indicated in the treatment of patients with mild to moderately severe hypertension (see boxed warning). It may be used alone for this purpose or added to other antihypertensive agents for the management of more severe hypertension. When administered with ORETICYL, more potent agents can be given at reduced dosage to minimize undesirable side effects.

Contraindications: Hydrochlorothiazide is contraindicated in patients with renal decompensation and in those who are hypersensitive to this or other sulfonamide-derived drugs.

Deserpidine is contraindicated in patients with known hypersensitivity, mental depression especially with suicidal tendencies, active peptic ulcer, and ulcerative colitis. It is also contraindicated in patients receiving electroconvulsive therapy.

Warnings:

Hydrochlorothiazide

Hydrochlorothiazide shares with other thiazides the propensity to deplete potassium reserves to an unpredictable degree.

Thiazides should be used with caution in patients with renal disease or significant impairment of renal function, since azotemia may be precipitated and cumulative drug effects may occur.

Thiazides should be used with caution in patients with impaired hepatic function or progressive liver disease, since minor alterations of fluid and electrolyte balance may precipitate hepatic coma.

Thiazides may be additive or potentiative of the action of other antihypertensive drugs. Potentiation occurs with ganglionic or peripheral adrenergic blocking drugs.

Sensitivity reactions may occur in patients with a history of allergy or bronchial asthma. The possibility of exacerbation or activation of systemic lupus erythematosus has been reported.

Deserpidine

Extreme caution should be exercised in treating patients with a history of mental depression. Discontinue the drug at the first sign, of despondency, early morning insomnia, loss of appetite, impotence, or self-deprecation. Drug-induced depression may persist for several months after drug withdrawal and may be severe enough to result in suicide.

Usage in Pregnancy and Lactation:

Hydrochlorothiazide

Thiazides cross the placental barrier and appear in cord blood. The use of thiazides in pregnant women requires that the anticipated benefit be weighed against possible hazards to the fetus. These hazards include fetal or neonatal jaundice, thrombocytopenia, and possible other adverse reactions that have occurred in the adult.

Thiazides appear in breast milk. If use of the drug is deemed essential, the patient should stop nursing.

Deserpidine

The safety of deserpidine for use during pregnancy or lactation has not been established; therefore, it should be used in pregnant women or in women of childbearing potential only when in the judgment of the physician its use is deemed essential to the welfare of the patient. Increased respiratory secretions, nasal congestion, cyanosis, and anorexia may occur in infants born to rauwolfia alkaloid-treated mothers, since these preparations are known to cross the placental barrier to enter the fetal circulation and appear in cord blood. They also are secreted by nursing mothers into breast milk.

Reproductive and teratology studies in rats reduced the mating index and neonatal survival indices. The no-effect dosage has not been established.

Precautions: Periodic determinations of serum electrolytes should be performed at appropriate intervals for the purpose of detecting possible electrolyte imbalances such as hyponatremia, hypochloremic alkalosis, and hypokalemia. Serum and urine electrolyte determinations are particularly important when a patient is vomiting excessively or receiving parenteral fluids. All patients should be observed for other clinical signs of electrolyte imbalances such as dryness of mouth, thirst, weakness, lethargy, drowsiness, restlessness, muscle pains or cramps, muscular fatigue, hypotension, oliguria, tachycardia, and gastrointestinal disturbances such as nausea and vomiting.

Hypokalemia may develop with thiazides as with any other potent diuretic, especially when brisk diuresis occurs, severe cirrhosis is present, or when corticosteroids or ACTH are given concomitantly. Interference with the adequate oral intake of electrolytes will also contribute to the possible development of hypokalemia. Potassium depletion, even of a mild degree, resulting from thiazide use, may sensitize a patient to the effects of cardiac glycosides such as digitalis.

Any chloride deficit is generally mild and usually does not require specific treatment except under extraordinary circumstances (as in liver disease or renal disease). Dilutional hyponatremia may occur in edematous patients in hot weather; appropriate therapy is water restriction rather than administration of salt, except in rare instances when the hyponatremia is life threatening.

In actual salt depletion, appropriate replacement is the therapy of choice.

Hyperuricemia may occur or frank gout may be precipitated in certain patients receiving thiazide therapy.

Insulin requirements in diabetic patients may be increased, decreased, or unchanged. Latent diabetes mellitus may become manifest during thiazide administration.

Thiazide drugs may increase the responsiveness to tubocurarine.

The antihypertensive effects of the drug may be enhanced in the postsympathectomy patient.

Thiazides may decrease arterial responsiveness to norepinephrine. This diminution is not sufficient to preclude effectiveness of the pressor agent for therapeutic use.

If progressive renal impairment becomes evident as indicated by a rising-nonprotein nitrogen or blood urea nitrogen, a careful reappraisal of therapy is necessary with consideration given to withholding or discontinuing diuretic therapy.

Thiazides may decrease serum PBI levels without signs of thyroid disturbance.

Thiazides have been reported, on rare occasions, to have elevated serum calcium to hypercalcemic levels. The serum calcium levels have returned to normal when the medication has been stopped. This phenomenon may be related to the ability of the thiazide diuretics to lower the amount of calcium excreted in the urine.

Because rauwolfia preparations increase gastrointestinal motility and secretion, this drug should be used cautiously in patients with a history of peptic ulcer, ulcerative colitis, or gallstones, where biliary colic may be precipitated.

Caution should be exercised when treating hypertensive patients with renal insufficiency since they adjust poorly to lowered blood pressure levels.

Use deserpidine cautiously with digitalis and quinidine since cardiac arrhythmias have occurred with rauwolfia preparations.

Preoperative withdrawal of deserpidine does not assure that circulatory instability will not occur. It is important that the anesthesiologist be aware of the patient's drug intake and consider this in the overall management, since hypotension has occurred in patients receiving rauwolfia preparations. Anticholinergic and/or adrenergic drugs (metaraminol, norepinephrine) have been employed to treat adverse vagocirculatory effects.

Adverse Reactions:

Hydrochlorothiazide

Gastrointestinal System Reactions: Anorexia, gastric irritation, nausea, vomiting, cramping, diarrhea, constipation, jaundice (intrahepatic cholestatic jaundice), pancreatitis.

Central Nervous System Reactions: Dizziness, vertigo, paresthesias, headache, xanthopsia.

Hematologic Reactions: Leukopenia, agranulocytosis, thrombocytopenia, aplastic anemia.

Dermatologic — Hypersensitivity Reactions: Purpura, photosensitivity, rash, urticaria, necrotizing angitis (vasculitis) (cutaneous vasculitis).

Cardiovascular Reaction: Orthostatic hypotension may occur and may be aggravated by alcohol, barbiturates, or narcotics.

Other: Hyperglycemia, glycosuria, hypercalcemia, hyperuricemia, muscle spasm, weakness, restlessness.

There have been isolated reports that certain nonedematous individuals developed severe fluid and electrolyte derangements after only brief exposure to normal doses of thiazide and non-thiazide diuretics. The condition is usually manifested as severe dilutional hyponatremia, hypokalemia, and hypochloremia. It has been reported to be due to inappropriately increased ADH secretion and appears to be idiosyncratic. Potassium replacement is apparently the most important therapy in the treatment of this syndrome along with the removal of the offending drug.

Whenever adverse reactions are severe, treatment should be discontinued.

Deserpidine

The following adverse reactions have been reported with rauwolfia preparations. These reactions are usually reversible and disappear when the drug is discontinued.

Gastrointestinal: Including hypersecretion, anorexia, diarrhea, nausea, and vomiting.

Cardiovascular: Including angina-like symptoms, arrhythmias (particularly when used concurrently with digitalis or quinidine), and bradycardia.

Central Nervous System: Including drowsiness, depression, nervousness, paradoxical anxiety, nightmares, extrapyramidal tract symptoms, CNS sensitization manifested by dull sensorium, and deafness.

Dermatologic—Hypersensitivity: Including pruritus, rash, and asthma in asthmatic patients.

Ophthalmologic: Including glaucoma, uveitis, optic atrophy, and conjunctival injection.

Hematologic: Thrombocytopenic purpura.

Miscellaneous: Nasal congestion, weight gain, impotence or decreased libido, dysuria, dyspnea, muscular aches, dryness of mouth, dizziness and headache.

Dosage and Administration: Dosage should be determined by individual titration of ingredients (see boxed warning). Dosage of both components should be carefully adjusted to the needs of the individual patient. Since at least ten days to two weeks may elapse before the full effects of the drugs become manifest, the dosage should not be adjusted more frequently. Three tablet strengths, ORETICYL 25 (hydrochlorothiazide 25 mg, deserpidine 0.125 mg); ORETICYL 50 (hydrochlorothiazide 50 mg, deserpidine 0.125 mg); and ORETICYL FORTE (hydrochlorothiazide 25 mg, deserpidine 0.25 mg), all grooved, are provided to permit considerable latitude in meeting the dosage requirements of individual patients.

The table below will help in determining which dose of ORETICYL 25, ORETICYL 50, or ORETICYL FORTE best represents the equivalent of the titrated dose.

ORETICYL 25	hydro-chlorothiazide	deserpidine
1 tablet bid	25.0 mg bid	0.125 mg bid
1½ tablet bid	37.5 mg bid	0.188 mg bid
2 tablets bid	50.0 mg bid	0.250 mg bid

ORETICYL 50	hydro-chlorothiazide	deserpidine
1 tablet bid	50 mg bid	0.125 mg bid
1½ tablet bid	75 mg bid	0.188 mg bid
2 tablets bid	100 mg bid	0.250 mg bid

ORETICYL FORTE	hydro-chlorothiazide	deserpidine
1 tablet bid	25.0 mg bid	0.250 mg bid
1½ tablet bid	37.5 mg bid	0.375 mg bid
2 tablets bid	50.0 mg bid	0.500 mg bid

The usual adult dosage is one ORETICYL 50 two times daily.

When other antihypertensive agents are to be added to the regimen, this should be accomplished gradually. Ganglionic blocking agents should be given at only half the usual dose since their effect is potentiated by pretreatment with ORETICYL (hydrochlorothiazide and deserpidine).

Overdosage: Symptoms of thiazide overdosage include electrolyte imbalance and signs of potassium deficiency such as confusion, dizziness, muscular weakness, and gastrointestinal disturbances. General supportive measures including replacement of fluids and electrolytes may be indicated in treatment of overdosage.

An overdosage of deserpidine is characterized by flushing of the skin, conjunctival injection, and pupillary constriction. Sedation ranging from drowsiness to coma may occur. Hypotension, hypothermia, central respiratory depression and bradycardia may develop in cases of severe overdosage. Treatment consists of the careful evacuation of stomach contents followed by the usual procedures for the symptomatic management of CNS depressant overdosage. If severe hypotension occurs it should be treated with a direct acting vasopressor such as norepinephrine bitartrate injection.

How Supplied: ORETICYL is supplied as grooved tablets in the following dosage sizes:

Rose-colored ORETICYL 25, contains hydrochlorothiazide 25 mg, deserpidine 0.125 mg, in bottles of 100 (**NDC** 0074-6922-01) and bottles of 1000 (**NDC** 0074-6922-02).

Rose-colored ORETICYL 50, contains hydrochlorothiazide 50 mg, deserpidine 0.125 mg, in bottles of 100 (**NDC** 0074-6931-01) and bottles of 1000 (**NDC** 0074-6931-02).

Gray-colored ORETICYL FORTE, contains hydrochlorothiazide 25 mg, deserpidine 0.25 mg, in bottles of 100 (**NDC** 0074-6927-01) and bottles of 1000 (**NDC** 0074-6927-02).

Abbott Laboratories
North Chicago, IL 60064
Ref. 01-2020-R4

PANWARFIN® ℞
(warfarin sodium tablets, USP)

How Supplied: PANWARFIN (warfarin sodium tablets, USP) for oral administration, grooved and bearing dosage strength numerals are available as follows:

2 mg, lavender-colored: bottles of 100 (**NDC** 0074-6626-03), and ABBO-PAC® unit dose packages of 100 tablets (**NDC** 0074-6626-07).

2½ mg, orange-colored: bottles of 100 (**NDC** 0074-7202-01), and ABBO-PAC unit dose packages of 100 tablets (**NDC** 0074-7202-05).

5 mg, peach-colored: bottles of 100 (**NDC** 0074-7210-01), 500 (**NDC** 0074-7210-09), and ABBO-PAC unit dose packages of 100 tablets (**NDC** 0074-7210-05).

7½ mg, yellow: bottles of 100 (**NDC** 0074-6638-03), and ABBO-PAC unit dose packages of 100 tablets (**NDC** 0074-6638-07).

10 mg, white: bottles of 100 (**NDC** 0074-7218-01), and ABBO-PAC unit dose packages of 100 tablets (**NDC** 0074-7218-05).

[*Shown in Product Identification Section*]

Abbott Pharmaceuticals, Inc.
North Chicago, IL 60064

PARADIONE® ℞
(paramethadione)
Capsules and Oral Solution

BECAUSE OF ITS POTENTIAL TO PRODUCE FETAL MALFORMATIONS AND SERIOUS SIDE EFFECTS, PARADIONE (paramethadione) SHOULD ONLY BE UTILIZED WHEN OTHER LESS TOXIC DRUGS HAVE BEEN FOUND INEFFECTIVE IN CONTROLLING ABSENCE (PETIT MAL) SEIZURES.

Description: PARADIONE (paramethadione) is an antiepileptic agent. An oxazolidinedione compound, it is chemically identified as 5-Ethyl-3,5-dimethyl-2,4-oxazolidinedione. PARADIONE is a synthetic, oily, slightly water-soluble liquid. It is supplied in capsular and liquid forms for oral use only. The capsules are available in two dosage strengths. One strength contains 150 mg the other 300 mg of paramethadione per capsule. Each ml of the liquid contains 300 mg of paramethadione; alcohol 65%.

Clinical Pharmacology: PARADIONE has been shown to prevent pentylenetetrazol-induced and thujone-induced seizures in experimental animals; the drug has a less marked effect on seizures induced by picrotoxin, procaine, cocaine, or strychnine. Unlike the hydantoins and antiepileptic barbiturates, PARADIONE does not modify the maximal seizure pattern in patients undergoing electroconvulsive therapy. PARADIONE has a sedative effect that may increase to the point of ataxia when excessive doses are used. A toxic dose of the drug in animals (approximately 1 Gm/kg) produced sleep, unconsciousness, and respiratory depression.

Paramethadione is rapidly absorbed from the gastrointestinal tract. It is demethylated by liver microsomes to an active N-demethylated metabolite, and is excreted slowly in this form by the kidney; almost no unmetabolized PARADIONE is excreted.

Indications and Usage: PARADIONE (paramethadione) is indicated for the control of absence (petit mal) seizures that are refractory to treatment with other drugs.

Contraindications: PARADIONE is contraindicated in patients with a known hypersensitivity to the drug.

Warnings: PARADIONE may cause serious side effects. Strict medical supervision of the patient is mandatory, especially during the initial year of therapy.

USAGE DURING PREGNANCY: THERE ARE MULTIPLE REPORTS IN THE CLINICAL LITERATURE WHICH INDICATE THAT THE USE OF ANTIEPILEPTIC DRUGS DURING PREGNANCY RESULTS IN AN INCREASED INCIDENCE OF BIRTH DEFECTS IN THE OFFSPRING. DATA ARE MORE EXTENSIVE WITH RESPECT TO TRIMETHADIONE, PARAMETHADIONE, PHENYTOIN AND PHENOBARBITAL THAN WITH OTHER ANTIEPILEPTIC DRUGS.

THEREFORE, ANTIEPILEPTIC DRUGS SUCH AS PARADIONE (PARAMETHADIONE) SHOULD BE ADMINISTERED TO WOMEN OF CHILDBEARING POTENTIAL ONLY IF THEY ARE CLEARLY SHOWN TO BE ESSENTIAL IN THE MANAGEMENT OF THEIR SEIZURES. EFFECTIVE MEANS OF CONTRACEPTION SHOULD ACCOMPANY THE USE OF PARADIONE IN SUCH PATIENTS. IF A PATIENT BECOMES PREGNANT WHILE TAKING PARADIONE, TERMINATION OF THE PREGNANCY SHOULD BE CONSIDERED. A PATIENT WHO REQUIRES THERAPY WITH PARADIONE AND WHO WISHES TO BECOME PREGNANT SHOULD BE ADVISED OF THE RISKS.

REPORTS HAVE SUGGESTED THAT THE MATERNAL INGESTION OF ANTIEPILEPTIC DRUGS, PARTICULARLY BARBITURATES, IS ASSOCIATED WITH A NEONATAL COAGULATION DEFECT THAT MAY CAUSE BLEEDING DURING THE EARLY (USUALLY WITHIN 24 HOURS OF BIRTH) NEONATAL PERIOD. THE POSSIBILITY OF THE OCCURRENCE OF THIS DEFECT WITH THE USE OF PARADIONE SHOULD

Continued on next page

If desired, additional literature on any Abbott Product will be provided upon request to Abbott Laboratories.

Abbott—Cont.

BE KEPT IN MIND. THE DEFECT IS CHARACTERIZED BY DECREASED LEVELS OF VITAMIN K-DEPENDENT CLOTTING FACTORS, AND PROLONGATION OF EITHER THE PROTHROMBIN TIME OR THE PARTIAL THROMBOPLASTIN TIME, OR BOTH. IT HAS BEEN SUGGESTED THAT PROPHYLACTIC VITAMIN K BE GIVEN TO THE MOTHER ONE MONTH PRIOR TO, AND DURING DELIVERY, AND TO THE INFANT, INTRAVENOUSLY, IMMEDIATELY AFTER BIRTH.

Precautions: *General:* Abrupt discontinuation of PARADIONE may precipitate absence (petit mal) status. PARADIONE (paramethadione) should always be withdrawn gradually unless serious adverse effects dictate otherwise. In the latter case, another antiepileptic may be substituted to protect the patient.

PARADIONE (paramethadione) should be withdrawn promptly if skin rash appears, because of the grave possibility of the occurrence of exfoliative dermatitis or severe forms of erythema multiforme. Even a minor acneiform or morbilliform rash should be allowed to clear completely before treatment with PARADIONE is resumed; reinstitute therapy cautiously.

PARADIONE should ordinarily not be used in patients with severe blood dyscrasias.

Hepatitis has been associated rarely with the use of oxazolidinediones. Jaundice or other signs of liver dysfunction are an indication for withdrawal of PARADIONE. PARADIONE should ordinarily not be used in patients with severe hepatic impairment.

Fatal nephrosis has been reported with the use of oxazolidinediones. Persistent or increasing albuminuria, or the development of any other significant renal abnormality, is an indication for withdrawal of the drug. PARADIONE should ordinarily not be used in patients with severe renal dysfunction.

Hemeralopia has occurred with the use of oxazolidinedione compounds; this appears to be an effect of the drugs on the neural layers of the retina, and usually can be reversed by a reduction in dosage. Scotomata are an indication for withdrawal of the drug. Caution should be observed when treating patients who have diseases of the retina or optic nerve.

Manifestations of systemic lupus erythematosus have been associated with the use of the oxazolidinediones, as they have with the use of certain other antiepileptics. Lymphadenopathies simulating malignant lymphoma have also occurred. Lupus-like manifestations or lymph node enlargement are indications for withdrawal of PARADIONE. Signs and symptoms may disappear after discontinuation of therapy, and specific treatment may be unnecessary.

A myasthenia gravis-like syndrome has been associated with the chronic use of the oxazolidinediones. Symptoms suggestive of this condition are indications for withdrawal of PARADIONE.

The 300 mg capsule of PARADIONE contains FD&C Yellow No. 5 (tartrazine) which may cause allergic-type reactions (including bronchial asthma) in certain susceptible individuals. Although the overall incidence of FD&C Yellow No. 5 (tartrazine) sensitivity in the general population is low, it is frequently seen in patients who also have aspirin hypersensitivity.

Information for Patients: Patients should be advised to report immediately such signs and symptoms as sore throat, fever, malaise, easy-bruising, petechiae, or epistaxis, or others that may be indicative of an infection or bleeding tendency.

Laboratory Tests: A complete blood count should be done prior to initiating therapy with PARADIONE, and at monthly intervals thereafter. A marked depression of the blood count is an indication for withdrawal of the drug. If no abnormality appears within 12 months, the interval between blood counts may be extended. A moderate degree of neutropenia with or without a corresponding drop in the leukocyte count is not uncommon. Therapy need not be withdrawn unless the neutrophil count is 2500 or less; more frequent blood examinations should be done when the count is less than 3,000. Other blood dyscrasias, including leukopenia, eosinophilia, thrombocytopenia, pancytopenia, agranulocytosis, hypoplastic anemia, and fatal aplastic anemia, have occurred with the use of oxazolidinediones.

Liver function tests should be done prior to initiating therapy with PARADIONE, and at monthly intervals thereafter.

A urinalysis should be done prior to initiating therapy with PARADIONE and at monthly intervals thereafter.

Drug Interactions: Drugs known to cause toxic effects similar to those of the oxazolidinediones should be avoided or used only with extreme caution during therapy with PARADIONE.

Carcinogenesis: No data are available on long-term potential for carcinogenicity in animals or humans.

Pregnancy: Pregnancy Category D. See "Warnings" section.

Nursing Mothers: It is not known whether this drug is excreted in human milk. Because many drugs are excreted in human milk and because of the potential for serious adverse reactions in nursing infants from PARADIONE, a decision should be made whether to discontinue nursing or to discontinue the drug, taking into account the importance of the drug to the mother.

Adverse Reactions: The following side effects, in decreasing order of severity, have been associated with the use of oxazolidinedione compounds. Although not all of them have been reported with the use of PARADIONE, the possibility of their occurrence should be kept in mind when the drug is prescribed.

Renal: Fatal nephrosis has occurred. Albuminuria.

Hematologic: Fatal aplastic anemia, hypoplastic anemia, pancytopenia, agranulocytosis, leukopenia, neutropenia, thrombocytopenia, eosinophilia, retinal and petechial hemorrhages, vaginal bleeding, epistaxis, and bleeding gums.

Hepatic: Hepatitis has been reported rarely.

Dermatologic: Acneiform or morbilliform skin rash that may progress to severe forms of erythema multiforme or to exfoliative dermatitis. Hair loss.

CNS/Neurologic: A myasthenia gravis-like syndrome has been reported. Precipitation of tonic-clonic (grand mal) seizures, vertigo, personality changes, increased irritability, drowsiness, headache, parasthesias, fatigue, malaise, and insomnia.

Drowsiness usually subsides with continued therapy. If it persists, a reduction in dosage is indicated.

Ophthalmologic: Diplopia, hemeralopia, and photophobia.

Cardiovascular: Changes in blood pressure.

Gastrointestinal: Vomiting, abdominal pain, gastric distress, nausea, anorexia, weight loss, and hiccups.

Other: Lupus erythematosus, and lymphadenopathies simulating malignant lymphoma, have been reported. Pruritus associated with lymphadenopathy and hepatosplenomegaly has occurred in hypersensitive individuals.

Overdosage: Symptoms of acute PARADIONE overdosage include drowsiness, nausea, dizziness, ataxia, visual disturbances. Coma may follow massive overdosage.

Gastric evacuation, either by induced emesis, or by lavage, or both, should be done immediately. General supportive care, including frequent monitoring of the vital signs and close observation of the patient, are required.

It has been reported that alkalinization of the urine may be expected to increase the excretion of the N-demethylated metabolite of PARADIONE.

A blood count and a careful evaluation of hepatic and renal function should be done following recovery.

Dosage and Administration: PARADIONE is administered orally.

Because PARADIONE Oral Solution contains alcohol 65%, it may be desirable to dilute the preparation with water before administering it to small children.

Usual Adult Dosage: 0.9–2.4 Gm daily in 3 or 4 equally divided doses (i.e., 300–600 mg 3 or 4 times daily).

Initially, give 0.9 Gm daily; increase this dose by 300 mg at weekly intervals until therapeutic results are seen or until toxic symptoms appear.

Maintenance dosage should be the least amount of drug required to maintain control.

Children's Dosage: Usually 0.3–0.9 Gm daily in 3 or 4 equally divided doses.

How Supplied: PARADIONE Capsules (paramethadione capsules, USP) are round capsules supplied as 150 mg (orange color) (**NDC** 0074-3976-01), and 300 mg (green color) (**NDC** 0074-3838-01) in bottles of 100.

[*Shown in Product Identification Section*]

PARADIONE Solution (paramethadione oral solution, USP), 300 mg per ml, is supplied in 50-ml bottles (**NDC** 0074-3860-01). A dropper is provided with each bottle, which is marked to permit easy measurement of 0.5 ml and 1 ml doses. The solution is clear and colorless.

Abbott Laboratories
North Chicago, IL 60064
Ref. 01-2200/R5

PEGANONE® ℞
(ethotoin tablets)

Description: PEGANONE (ethotoin) is an oral antiepileptic of the hydantoin series and is chemically identified as 3-ethyl-5-phenyl-2, 4-imidazolidinedione. PEGANONE tablets are available in two dosage strengths of 250 mg and 500 mg respectively.

Clinical Pharmacology: PEGANONE (ethotoin) exerts an antiepileptic effect without causing general central nervous system depression. The mechanism of action is probably very similar to that of phenytoin. The latter drug appears to stabilize rather than to raise the normal seizure threshold, and to prevent the spread of seizure activity rather than to abolish the primary focus of seizure discharges.

In laboratory animals, the drug was found effective against electroshock convulsions, and to a lesser extent, against complex partial (psychomotor) and pentylenetetrazol-induced seizures.

In mice, the duration of antiepileptic activity was prolonged by hepatic injury but not by bilateral nephrectomy; the drug is apparently biotransformed by the liver.

Ethotoin is fairly rapidly absorbed; the extent of oral absorption is not known. The drug exhibits saturable metabolism with respect to the formation of N-deethyl and p-hydroxyl-ethotoin, the major metabolites. Where plasma concentrations are below about 8 mg/l, the elimination half-life of ethotoin is in the range of 3 to 9 hours. Above this concentration, the dose-dependent, nonlinear kinetics of the drug preclude definition of any conventional half-life. Experience suggests that therapeutic plasma concentrations fall in the range of 15 to 50 mg/l; however, this range is not as extensively documented as those quoted for other antiepileptics.

Indications and Usage: PEGANONE (ethotoin) is indicated for the control of tonic-clonic (grand mal) and complex partial (psychomotor) seizures.

Contraindications: PEGANONE (ethotoin) is contraindicated in patients with hepatic abnormalities or hematologic disorders.

Warnings: USAGE DURING PREGNANCY—THERE ARE MULTIPLE REPORTS IN THE CLINICAL LITERATURE WHICH INDICATE THAT THE USE OF ANTIEPILEPTIC DRUGS DURING PREGNANCY RESULTS IN AN INCREASED INCIDENCE OF BIRTH DEFECTS IN THE OFFSPRING. ALTHOUGH DATA ARE MORE EXTENSIVE WITH RESPECT TO TRIMETHADIONE, PARAMETHADIONE, PHENYTOIN, AND PHENOBARBITAL, REPORTS INDICATE A POSSIBLE SIMILAR ASSOCIATION WITH THE USE OF OTHER ANTIEPILEPTIC DRUGS.

THEREFORE, ANTIEPILEPTIC DRUGS SHOULD BE ADMINISTERED TO WOMEN OF CHILDBEARING POTENTIAL ONLY IF THEY ARE CLEARLY SHOWN TO BE ESSENTIAL IN THE MANAGEMENT OF THEIR SEIZURES.

ANTIEPILEPTIC DRUGS SHOULD NOT BE DISCONTINUED IN PATIENTS IN WHOM THE DRUG IS ADMINISTERED TO PREVENT MAJOR SEIZURES BECAUSE OF THE STRONG POSSIBILITY OF PRECIPITATING STATUS EPILEPTICUS WITH ATTENDANT HYPOXIA AND RISK TO BOTH MOTHER AND THE UNBORN CHILD. CONSIDERATION SHOULD, HOWEVER, BE GIVEN TO DISCONTINUATION OF ANTIEPILEPTICS PRIOR TO AND DURING PREGNANCY WHEN THE NATURE, FREQUENCY AND SEVERITY OF THE SEIZURES DO NOT POSE A SERIOUS THREAT TO THE PATIENT. IT IS NOT, HOWEVER, KNOWN WHETHER EVEN MINOR SEIZURES CONSTITUTE SOME RISK TO THE DEVELOPING EMBRYO OR FETUS.

REPORTS HAVE SUGGESTED THAT THE MATERNAL INGESTION OF ANTIEPILEPTIC DRUGS, PARTICULARLY BARBITURATES, IS ASSOCIATED WITH A NEONATAL COAGULATION DEFECT THAT MAY CAUSE BLEEDING DURING THE EARLY (USUALLY WITHIN 24 HOURS OF BIRTH) NEONATAL PERIOD. THE POSSIBILITY OF THE OCCURRENCE OF THIS DEFECT WITH THE USE OF PEGANONE SHOULD BE KEPT IN MIND. THE DEFECT IS CHARACTERIZED BY DECREASED LEVELS OF VITAMIN K-DEPENDENT CLOTTING FACTORS, AND PROLONGATION OF EITHER THE PROTHROMBIN TIME OR THE PARTIAL THROMBOPLASTIN TIME, OR BOTH. IT HAS BEEN SUGGESTED THAT VITAMIN K BE GIVEN PROPHYLACTICALLY TO THE MOTHER ONE MONTH PRIOR TO, AND DURING DELIVERY, AND TO THE INFANT, INTRAVENOUSLY, IMMEDIATELY AFTER BIRTH.

THE PHYSICIAN SHOULD WEIGH THESE CONSIDERATIONS IN TREATMENT AND COUNSELING OF EPILEPTIC WOMEN OF CHILDBEARING POTENTIAL.

Precautions: *General:* Blood dyscrasias have been reported in patients receiving PEGANONE. Although the etiologic role of PEGANONE has not been definitely established, physicians should be alert for general malaise, sore throat and other symptoms indicative of possible blood dyscrasia.

There is some evidence suggesting that hydantoin-like compounds may interfere with folic acid metabolism, precipitating a megaloblastic anemia. If this should occur during gestation, folic acid therapy should be considered.

Information for Patients: Patients should be advised to report immediately such signs and symptoms as sore throat, fever, malaise, easy bruising, petechiae, epistaxis, or others that may be indicative of an infection or bleeding tendency.

Laboratory Tests: Liver function tests should be performed if clinical evidence suggests the possibility of hepatic dysfunction. Signs of liver damage are indication for withdrawal of the drug.

It is recommended that blood counts and urinalyses be performed when therapy is begun and at monthly intervals for several months thereafter. As in patients receiving other hydantoin compounds and other antiepileptic drugs, blood dyscrasias have been reported in patients receiving PEGANONE (ethotoin). Marked depression of the blood count is indication for withdrawal of the drug.

Drug Interactions: PEGANONE used in combination with other drugs known to adversely affect the hematopoietic system should be avoided if possible.

Considerable caution should be exercised if PEGANONE is administered concurrently with *Phenurone (phenacemide)* since paranoid symptoms have been reported during therapy with this combination.

A two-way interaction between the hydantoin antiepileptic, *phenytoin*, and the *coumarin anticoagulants* has been suggested. Presumably, phenytoin acts as a stimulator of coumarin metabolism and has been reported to cause decreased serum levels of the coumarin anticoagulants and increased prothrombin-proconvertin concentrations. Conversely, the coumarin anticoagulants have been reported to increase the serum levels and prolong the serum half-life of phenytoin by inhibiting its metabolism. Although there is no documentation of such, a similar interaction between ethotoin and the coumarin anticoagulants may occur. Caution is therefore advised when administering PEGANONE to patients receiving coumarin anticoagulants.

Carcinogenesis: No data are available on long-term potential for carcinogenicity in animals or humans.

Pregnancy: Pregnancy Category C. See "Warnings" section.

Nursing Mothers: Ethotoin is excreted in breast milk. Because of the potential for serious adverse reactions in nursing infants from ethotoin, a decision should be made whether to discontinue nursing or to discontinue the drug, taking into account the importance of the drug to the mother.

Adverse Reactions: Adverse reactions associated with PEGANONE, in decreasing order of severity, are:

Isolated cases of lymphadenopathy and systemic lupus erythematosus have been reported in patients taking hydantoin compounds, and lymphadenopathy has occurred with PEGANONE. Withdrawal of therapy has resulted in remission of the clinical and pathological findings. Therefore, if a lymphoma-like syndrome develops, the drug should be withdrawn and the patient should be closely observed for regression of signs and symptoms before treatment is resumed.

Ataxia and gum hypertrophy have occurred only rarely—usually only in patients receiving an additional hydantoin derivative. It is of interest to note that ataxia and gum hypertrophy have subsided in patients receiving other hydantoins when PEGANONE was given as a substitute antiepileptic.

Occasionally, vomiting or nausea after ingestion of PEGANONE has been reported, but if the drug is administered after meals, the incidence of gastric distress is reduced. Other side effects have included chest pain, nystagmus, diplopia, fever, dizziness, diarrhea, headache, insomnia, fatigue, numbness and skin rash.

Overdosage: Symptoms of acute overdosage include drowsiness, visual disturbance, nausea and ataxia. Coma is possible at very high dosage.

Treatment should be begun by inducing emesis; gastric lavage may be considered as an alternative. General supportive measures will be necessary. A careful evaluation of blood-forming organs should be made following recovery.

Dosage and Administration: PEGANONE is administered orally in 4 to 6 divided doses daily. The drug should be taken after food, and doses should be spaced as evenly as practicable. Initial dosage should be conservative. For adults, the initial daily dose should be 1 g or less, with subsequent gradual dosage increases over a period of several days. The optimum dosage must be determined on the basis of individual response. The usual adult maintenance dose is 2 to 3 g daily. Less than 2 g daily has been found ineffective in most adults.

Pediatric dosage depends upon the age and weight of the patient. The initial dose should not exceed 750 mg daily. The usual maintenance dose in children ranges from 500 mg to 1 g daily, although occasionally 2 or (rarely) 3 g daily may be necessary.

If a patient is receiving another antiepileptic drug, it should not be discontinued when PEGANONE therapy is begun. The dosage of the other drug should be reduced gradually as that of PEGANONE is increased. PEGANONE may eventually replace the other drug or the optimal dosage of both antiepileptics may be established.

PEGANONE is compatible with all commonly employed antiepileptic medications with the possible exception of Phenurone® (phenacemide). In tonic-clonic (grand mal) seizures, use of the drug with Gemonil® (metharbital) or phenobarbital may be beneficial. PEGANONE may be used in combination with drugs such as Tridione® (trimethadione) or Paradione® (paramethadione), as an adjunct in those patients with absence (petit mal) associated with tonic-clonic (grand mal).

How Supplied: PEGANONE (ethotoin) grooved, white tablets are supplied in two dosage strengths: 250 mg, bottles of 100 (**NDC** 0074-6902-01); 500 mg, bottles of 100 (**NDC** 0074-6905-04).

This product is listed in N.D., a Medicare designated compendium.

Abbott Laboratories
North Chicago, IL 60064

[*Shown in Product Identification Section*]

Ref. 01-2206-R4

PENTHRANE® ℞

(methoxyflurane, USP)

Description: PENTHRANE (methoxyflurane, USP) is 2,2-dichloro-1, 1-difluoroethyl methyl ether with the structural formula:

```
     Cl  F       H
     |   |       |
H —  C — C — O — C — H
     |   |       |
     Cl  F       H
```

Certain of the physical constants are:

Molecular weight	164.97
Boiling point at 760 mm Hg	104.65°C
Partition coefficients at 37°C	
water/gas	4.5
blood/gas (mean range)	10.20 to 14.06*
oil/gas	825
Vapor Pressure 17.7°C	20 mm Hg
Flash points	
in air	62.8°C
in oxygen (closed system)	32.8°C
in nitrous oxide 50% with 50% oxygen	28.2°C
Lower limits of flammability of vapor concentration	
in air	7.0%
in oxygen	5.4%
in N_2O 50%	4.6%

* As reported by different investigators.

If desired, additional literature on any Abbott Product will be provided upon request to Abbott Laboratories.

Continued on next page

Abbott—Cont.

PENTHRANE (methoxyflurane, USP) is stable and does not decompose in contact with soda lime. It has a mildly pungent odor. An antioxidant, butylated hydroxytoluene 0.01% w/w, is added to insure stability on standing. This slowly oxidizes to a yellow pigment that progressively turns to brown, and which may accumulate on the vaporizer wick. The colored matter may be removed by rinsing the wick with diethyl ether. The wick must be dried after cleaning to avoid introducing diethyl ether into the system.

Polyvinyl chloride plastics are extracted by PENTHRANE; therefore, contact should be avoided. PENTHRANE does not extract polyethylene plastics, polypropylene plastics, fluorinated hydrocarbon plastics or nylon. It is very soluble in rubber and soda lime. Disposable conductive plastic circuits should be discarded after a single use to avoid cross contamination and because PENTHRANE may reduce conductivity of such materials below safe limits for subsequent administration of a flammable anesthetic.

The vapor concentration of PENTHRANE is limited by its vapor pressure at room temperature to a maximum of about 3.5% at 23°C. In practice, this concentration is not easily reached due to the cooling effect of vaporization. PENTHRANE is not flammable except at vapor concentrations well above those recommended for its use. Recommended concentrations are nonflammable and nonexplosive in air, oxygen and nitrous oxide mixtures at ordinary room temperature.

Actions: PENTHRANE provides anesthesia and/or analgesia.
After surgical anesthesia with PENTHRANE analgesia and drowsiness may persist after consciousness has returned. This may obviate or reduce the need for narcotics in the immediate postoperative period.
When used alone in safe concentration, PENTHRANE (methoxyflurane, USP) will not produce appreciable skeletal muscle relaxation. A muscle relaxing agent, e.g., succinylcholine chloride (Quelicin®) or tubocurarine should be used as an adjunct.
Bronchiolar constriction or laryngeal spasm is not ordinarily provoked by PENTHRANE.
During PENTHRANE anesthesia, the cardiac rhythm is usually regular. The myocardium is only minimally sensitized by PENTHRANE to epinephrine. Some decrease in blood pressure often accompanies light planes of anesthesia. This may be accompanied by bradycardia. The hypotension noted is accompanied by reduced cardiac contractile force and reduced cardiac output.
When used for obstetrical delivery, light planes of PENTHRANE anesthesia have little effect on uterine contractions. There are no known contraindications to the concomitant use of PENTHRANE and oxytocic agents.
Biotransformation of PENTHRANE in man results in the formation of several metabolites which include inorganic fluoride, methoxydifluoracetic acid, dichloroacetic acid, and probably, oxalic acid. See WARNINGS.

Indications:

1. PENTHRANE is indicated, usually in combination with oxygen and nitrous oxide, to provide anesthesia for surgical procedures in which the total duration of PENTHRANE administration is anticipated to be 4 hours or less, and in which PENTHRANE is not to be used in concentrations that will provide skeletal muscle relaxation; see WARNINGS regarding time and dose relationships.
2. PENTHRANE (methoxyflurane, USP) may be used alone with hand-held inhalers or in combination with oxygen and nitrous oxide for analgesia in obstetrics and in minor surgical procedures.

Contraindications: See WARNINGS.
Warnings: SEQUENTIAL ANESTHESIA WITH PENTHRANE (METHOXYFLURANE, USP) AND HALOTHANE, OR HALOTHANE AND PENTHRANE, IN EITHER ORDER, HAS BEEN FOLLOWED BY JAUNDICE IN A FEW RARE CASES. WHEN A PREVIOUS EXPOSURE TO PENTHRANE OR HALOTHANE HAS BEEN FOLLOWED BY UNEXPLAINED JAUNDICE, CONSIDERATION SHOULD BE GIVEN TO THE USE OF OTHER AGENTS.
THE NEPHROTOXICITY ASSOCIATED WITH PENTHRANE ADMINISTRATION APPEARS TO BE RELATED TO THE TOTAL DOSE (TIME AND CONCENTRATIONS). SEE PARAGRAPH 5. THE MANIFESTATIONS RANGE IN SEVERITY FROM REVERSIBLE ALTERATIONS IN LABORATORY FINDINGS TO POLYURIC OR OLIGURIC RENAL FAILURE, SOMETIMES FATAL.
POLYURIC RENAL FAILURE IS CHARACTERIZED BY THE DEVELOPMENT, EARLY IN THE POSTOPERATIVE PERIOD, OF THE FOLLOWING:
WEIGHT LOSS.
URINE: LOW SPECIFIC GRAVITY, LARGE VOLUME EQUAL TO OR IN EXCESS OF FLUID INTAKE, DECREASED OSMOLALITY.
SERUM/BLOOD: ELEVATION OF SODIUM, CHLORIDE, URIC ACID, BUN, CREATININE.
THIS SYNDROME IS BELIEVED TO BE RELATED TO RELEASE OF THE FLUORIDE ION, A METABOLIC PRODUCT OF PENTHRANE AND TO BE RELATED TO THE TOTAL DOSAGE ADMINISTERED. THEREFORE, THE LOWEST EFFECTIVE DOSAGE SHOULD BE ADMINISTERED, ESPECIALLY IN AGED OR OBESE PATIENTS AND IN SURGICAL PROCEDURES OF LONG DURATION, BEARING IN MIND THAT THE TOTAL DOSE DELIVERED TO THE PATIENT IS A FACTOR OF DURATION OF ADMINISTRATION AND CONCENTRATION OF VAPOR.
OXALATE CRYSTALS AND/OR ACUTE TUBULAR NECROSIS HAVE BEEN NOTED AT AUTOPSY.
The guiding principles in minimizing the possibility of renal injury are:

1. AVOID USING PENTHRANE (METHOXYFLURANE, USP) AS THE SOLE OR PRINCIPAL AGENT TO ACHIEVE MUSCULAR RELAXATION.
2. PATIENTS WITH PRE-EXISTING RENAL DISEASE, IMPAIRMENT OF RENAL FUNCTION, TOXEMIA OF PREGNANCY, AND PATIENTS UNDERGOING VASCULAR SURGERY AT OR NEAR THE RENAL VESSELS SHOULD NOT RECEIVE PENTHRANE UNLESS, IN THE JUDGMENT OF THE PHYSICIAN, THE BENEFITS OUTWEIGH THE INCREASED RISK OF NEPHROTOXIC EFFECT.
3. URINARY OUTPUT SHOULD BE MONITORED IN ALL PATIENTS. IF EXCESSIVE URINE OUTPUT OCCURS, APPROPRIATE LABORATORY STUDIES SHOULD BE DONE TO ASSESS RENAL FUNCTION. IN HIGH RISK PATIENTS (SEE 2, ABOVE) SERIAL TESTS OF RENAL FUNCTION AND MEASUREMENTS OF FLUID AND ELECTROLYTE BALANCE ARE IMPERATIVE. ALL FLUID AND ELECTROLYTE LOSSES SHOULD BE PROMPTLY REPLACED.
4. THE CONCURRENT USE OF TETRACYCLINE AND PENTHRANE HAS BEEN REPORTED TO RESULT IN FATAL RENAL TOXICITY. THE POSSIBILITY EXISTS THAT PENTHRANE MAY ENHANCE THE ADVERSE RENAL EFFECTS OF OTHER DRUGS INCLUDING CERTAIN ANTIBIOTICS OF KNOWN NEPHROTOXIC POTENTIAL SUCH AS GENTAMICIN, KANAMYCIN, COLISTIN, POLYMYXIN B, CEPHALORIDINE AND AMPHOTERICIN B. THIS SHOULD BE CAREFULLY CONSIDERED WHEN PRESCRIBING SUCH DRUGS DURING THE PREOPERATIVE, OPERATIVE AND POSTOPERATIVE PERIODS.
5. BECAUSE OF THE DOSE-RELATED NEPHROTOXICITY POTENTIAL OF PENTHRANE (METHOXYFLURANE, USP), IT IS SUGGESTED THAT THE TOTAL DURATION OF LIGHT ANESTHETIC DEPTH WITH PENTHRANE NOT EXCEED APPROXIMATELY 4 HOURS AT A SINGLE ADMINISTRATION.

Usage in Pregnancy: Safe use of PENTHRANE (methoxyflurane, USP) other than for obstetrics has not been established with respect to adverse effects upon fetal development. Therefore, PENTHRANE should not be used in women of childbearing potential and particularly during early pregnancy unless, in the judgment of the physician, the potential benefits outweigh the possible hazards.
Usage in Obstetrics: Attention should be given to the directions for dosage and administration shown below. Fluoride levels in cord blood are usually less than, but may equal those of the mother at delivery. The effect of inorganic fluoride on the infant is not known. However, clinical experience has demonstrated that cases of high output renal failure in either mother or child must be considered unlikely.
Precautions: Diabetic patients may have an increased likelihood of developing nephropathy if they have impaired renal function or polyuria, are obese, or are not optimally controlled.
Caution should be exercised in using PENTHRANE in patients under treatment with enzyme inducing drugs (e.g., barbiturates) as such agents may enhance the metabolism of PENTHRANE resulting in increased fluoride levels.
Ventilation should be assessed carefully and, if depressed, should be augmented to insure adequate oxygenation and carbon dioxide removal. Parenteral anesthetic adjuncts (ex. barbiturates, narcotics and neuromuscular blocking agents) may also cause depression of respiration requiring assisted or controlled ventilation. A sufficient reduction in respiratory minute volume occurs during deep anesthesia to produce a significant respiratory acidosis if ventilation is not adequately assisted. PENTHRANE (methoxyflurane, USP) causes a slight metabolic acidosis.
PENTHRANE augments the effect of nondepolarizing muscle relaxants so that their usual dosage should be reduced by approximately one-half.
Epinephrine or levarterenol (norepinephrine) should be employed cautiously during PENTHRANE anesthesia.
When PENTHRANE is used under the conditions of dosage and administration shown below, in surgery or obstetrics, inorganic fluoride levels may infrequently reach those at which changes in renal laboratory values have been seen.
Adverse Reactions: Renal dysfunction—see WARNINGS.
Hepatic dysfunction, jaundice, and fatal hepatic necrosis have occurred following PENTHRANE anesthesia. Also as with other anesthetics, transient alterations in liver function tests may follow PENTHRANE administration. Hepatic complications rarely have involved reported cross reactions between PENTHRANE and Halothane.

Some patients exhibit pallor during recovery from PENTHRANE anesthesia.
Other adverse reactions which have been reported include: cardiac arrest, malignant hyperpyrexia, prolonged postoperative somnolence, respiratory depression, laryngospasm, bronchospasm, nausea, vomiting, postoperative headache, hypotension and emergence delirium.

Dosage and Administration: THE LOWEST EFFECTIVE DOSAGE OF PENTHRANE (METHOXYFLURANE, USP) SHOULD BE USED IN ORDER TO MINIMIZE THE POSSIBILITY OF NEPHROPATHY AND TO ALLOW FOR OPTIMAL RECOVERY TIME. IN CASES OF UNUSUALLY HIGH MAINTENANCE REQUIREMENTS, THE USE OF ANESTHETIC ADJUNCTS OR ANOTHER AGENT MAY BE INDICATED. THE ABSENCE OF HYPOTENSION CANNOT BE RELIED UPON AS EVIDENCE THAT DOSAGE HAS NOT BEEN EXCESSIVE DURING MAINTENANCE.

Analgesia: For analgesia, intermittent inhalation of vapor concentrations in the range of 0.3 to 0.8% are recommended. PENTHRANE may be self-administered by hand-held inhalers (e.g., Analgizer, Cyprane) if the patient is kept under close observation.
For intermittent administration from the hand-held inhaler, dosage for each patient is limited to not more than a single 15 ml. charge of liquid PENTHRANE. Such analgesia in labor should not be instituted before relief becomes necessary. Use of the hand-held inhaler does not preclude transfer of the patient to a conventional anesthesia machine for inhalation anesthesia, but concentrations should be kept at the lowest effective dosage. Total time for anesthesia combined with analgesia should be as short as possible, bearing in mind the recommended duration for continuous anesthesia (four hours).

Anesthesia: A light level of anesthesia should be used. The use of deeper levels to achieve muscle relaxation should be avoided.
Apparatus: PENTHRANE should be vaporized by calibrated, temperature compensated, out-of-circle vaporizers (e.g., Pentec II, Pentomatic) or other methods which provide accurate delivered vapor concentration. Anesthetic up-take by rubber tubing, bags, and soda lime which may prolong induction and recovery time can be reduced by the use of nonabsorptive plastic circuit material (not polyvinyl chloride) and fresh moist Baralyme. The fresh gas inlet should be located downstream of the CO_2 absorber in order to avoid excessive anesthetic absorption, and the rebreathing bag and pop-off valve should be located on the expiratory side.
Premedication: The usual preanesthetic medications may be administered prior to PENTHRANE (methoxyflurane, USP) anesthesia: see PRECAUTIONS.
Induction: Use of a parenteral induction agent (such as an ultra-short acting barbiturate) is recommended unless contraindicated in an individual patient.
Carrier gases: For general surgery, PENTHRANE should usually be administered with a carrier gas flow consisting of oxygen and at least 50% nitrous oxide in order to minimize the total PENTHRANE doses unless nitrous oxide is contraindicated.
Muscle relaxation: PENTHRANE should not be administered at levels required to achieve muscle relaxation. Adequate relaxation should be obtained from adjunctive use of a muscle relaxant, e.g., succinylcholine chloride (Quelicin®) or tubocurarine. The usual dosage of nondepolarizing muscle relaxants should be reduced by approximately one-half.
Vapor concentrations: Initially: PENTRANE concentrations may be increased as tolerated to a maximum of approximately 2.0%. This concentration should only be continued for about two to five minutes, or until the patient signs of light anesthesia are evident. The concentration of PENTHRANE should then be reduced by frequent decrements to the lowest possible levels consistent with the maintenance of adequate anesthesia. For example, in a 70 kg. patient, the following sequential reduction in the delivered vapor concentration of PENTHRANE (methoxyflurane, USP) may be appropriate: [See table above].

Elapsed Minutes	0 to 5	5 to 20	20 to 60	60 to 120	120 to 240
Vapor Conc.*	2.0%	0.6%	0.4%	0.2%	0.1%

* Concentrations are approximate and subject to adjustment according to patient signs of anesthesia. Based on 5 liters per minute gas flow and ventilation rate throughout procedure, 50/50 N_2 and oxygen.

Concentration may be increased or decreased according to the requirements of the individual patient. Four hours of 0.25% delivered methoxyflurane should not be exceeded in normal adult patients unless, in the opinion of the clinician, the anticipated benefits outweigh the increased risk of dose related nephrotoxicity. The product of these two factors (four hours of 0.25% delivered methoxyflurane) may be used to estimate other combinations of time and dose: thus two hours of 0.5%, for example, should not ordinarily be exceeded. In sufficiently long cases, PENTHRANE should be discontinued 30 to 40 minutes before the end of surgery. Rapid flushing will not remove PENTHRANE absorbed by rubber circuit components.
Patient signs and levels: The PENTHRANE level of conscious analgesia is suited for pain relief, as in labor and uncomplicated vaginal deliveries. The level of unconscious analgesia is suitable for many minor surgical procedures. The level of light anesthesia is recommended for general surgical use. Deep anesthesia with PENTHRANE (methoxyflurane, USP) is not recommended.
Appropriate patient signs of PENTHRANE anesthesia should be observed closely as a guide to proper depth. A blood pressure decrease of about 20 mm. Hg may be seen during induction. A greater decrease may occur in hypertensive patients. Blood pressure usually recovers as a level of light anesthesia is reached. The absence of hypotension cannot be relied upon as evidence that dosage has not been excessive during maintenance.

How Supplied: PENTHRANE (methoxyflurane, USP), is supplied in 125 and 15 ml bottles, List 6864. Butylated hydroxytoluene, 0.01% w/w, is present as an antioxidant.
Caution: Federal (USA) law prohibits dispensing without prescription.
Protect from light. Protect from freezing and extreme heat.
Marketed by
Abbott Laboratories
North Chicago, IL 60064, USA
Ref. 06-3029-R25-2/81

PENTOTHAL® Ⓒ III
(thiopental sodium for injection, USP)

Description: Pentothal (Thiopental Sodium for Injection, USP) is a thiobarbiturate, the sulfur analogue of sodium pentobarbital.
The drug is prepared as a sterile powder and after reconstitution with an appropriate diluent is administered by the intravenous route. Pentothal is chemically designated sodium 5-ethyl-5-(1-methylbutyl)-2-thiobarbiturate.
The drug is a yellowish, hygroscopic powder, stabilized with anhydrous sodium carbonate as a buffer (60 mg/g of thiopental sodium).

Clinical Pharmacology: Pentothal (Thiopental Sodium for Injection, USP) is an ultra-short-acting depressant of the central nervous system which induces hypnosis and anesthesia, but not analgesia. It produces hypnosis within 30 to 40 seconds of intravenous injection. Recovery after a small dose is rapid, with some somnolence and retrograde amnesia. Repeated intravenous doses lead to prolonged anesthesia because fatty tissues act as a reservoir; they accumulate Pentothal in concentrations 6 to 12 times greater than the plasma concentration, and then release the drug slowly to cause prolonged anesthesia.
The half-life of the elimination phase after a single intravenous dose is three to eight hours.
The distribution and fate of Pentothal (as with other barbiturates) is influenced chiefly by its lipid solubility (partition coefficient), protein binding and extent of ionization. Pentothal has a partition coefficient of 580.
Approximately 80% of the drug in the blood is bound to plasma protein. Pentothal is largely degraded in the liver and to a smaller extent in other tissues, especially the kidney and brain. It has a pK_a of 7.4.
Pentothal readily crosses the placental barrier and small amounts may appear in the milk of nursing mothers following ingestion of large doses. Concentration in spinal fluid is slightly less than in the plasma.
Biotransformation products of thiopental are pharmacologically inactive and mostly excreted in the urine.

Indications and Usage: Pentothal (Thiopental Sodium for Injection USP) is indicated (1) as the sole anesthetic agent for brief (15 minute) procedures, (2) for induction of anesthesia prior to administration of other anesthetic agents, (3) to supplement regional anesthesia, (4) to provide hypnosis during balanced anesthesia with other agents for analgesia or muscle relaxation, (5) for the control of convulsive states during or following inhalation anesthesia, local anesthesia, or other causes, (6) in neurosurgical patients with increased intracranial pressure, if adequate ventilation is provided, and (7) for narcoanalysis and narcosynthesis in psychiatric disorders.

Contraindications:
Absolute Contraindications:
(1) Absence of suitable veins for intravenous administration, (2) hypersensitivity (allergy) to barbiturates, (3) status asthmaticus, and (4) latent or manifest porphyria.
Relative Contraindications:
(1) Severe cardiovascular disease, (2) hypotension or shock, (3) conditions in which the hypnotic effect may be prolonged or potentiated —excessive premedication, Addison's disease, hepatic or renal dysfunction, myxedema, increased blood urea, severe anemia, asthma and myasthenia gravis.

Warnings: KEEP RESUSCITATIVE AND ENDOTRACHEAL INTUBATION EQUIPMENT AND OXYGEN READILY AVAILABLE. MAINTAIN PATENCY OF THE AIRWAY AT ALL TIMES.
This drug should be administered only by persons qualified in the use of intravenous anesthetics.
Avoid extravasation or intra-arterial injection.
WARNING: May be habit forming.

Precautions: Observe aseptic precautions at all times in preparation and handling of Pento-

Continued on next page

If desired, additional literature on any Abbott Product will be provided upon request to Abbott Laboratories.

Abbott—Cont.

thal (Thiopental Sodium for Injection, USP) solutions.
If used in conditions involving relative contraindications, reduce dosage and administer slowly.
Care should be taken in administering the drug to patients with advanced cardiac disease, increased intracranial pressure, asthma, myasthenia gravis and endocrine insufficiency (pituitary, thyroid, adrenal, pancreas).
Pregnancy Category C. Animal reproduction studies have not been conducted with Pentothal. It is also not known whether Pentothal can cause fetal harm when administered to a pregnant woman or can affect reproduction capacity. Pentothal should be given to a pregnant woman only if clearly needed.
Adverse Reactions: Adverse reactions include respiratory depression, myocardial depression, cardiac arrhythmias, prolonged somnolence and recovery, sneezing, coughing, bronchospasm, laryngospasm and shivering. Hypersensitivity reactions to barbiturates, including Pentothal (Thiopental Sodium for Injection, USP), have been reported.
Drug Abuse and Dependence: None known.
Overdosage: Overdosage may occur from too rapid or repeated injections. Too rapid injection may be followed by an alarming fall in blood pressure even to shock levels. Apnea, occasional laryngospasm, coughing and other respiratory difficulties with excessive or too rapid injections may occur. In the event of suspected or apparent overdosage, the drug should be discontinued, a patent airway established (intubate if necessary) or maintained, and oxygen should be administered, with assisted ventilation if necessary. The lethal dose of barbiturates varies and cannot be stated with certainty. Lethal blood levels may be as low as 1 mg/100 ml for short-acting barbiturates; less if other depressant drugs or alcohol are also present.
Dosage and Administration: Pentothal (Thiopental Sodium for Injection, USP) is administered by the intravenous route only. Individual response to the drug is so varied that there can be no fixed dosage. The drug should be titrated against patient requirements as governed by age, sex and body weight. Younger patients require relatively larger doses than middle-aged and elderly persons; the latter metabolize the drug more slowly. Pre-puberty requirements are the same for both sexes, but adult females require less than adult males. Dose is usually proportional to body weight and obese patients require a larger dose than relatively lean persons of the same weight.

Premedication
Premedication usually consists of atropine or scopolamine to suppress vagal reflexes and inhibit secretions. In addition, a barbiturate or an opiate is often given. Sodium pentobarbital injection (Nembutal®) is suggested because it provides a preliminary indication of how the patient will react to barbiturate anesthesia. Ideally, the peak effect of these medications should be reached shortly before the time of induction.

Test Dose
It is advisable to inject a small "test" dose of 25 to 75 mg (1 to 3 ml of a 2.5% solution) of Pentothal (Thiopental Sodium for Injection, USP) to assess tolerance or unusual sensitivity to Pentothal, and pausing to observe patient reaction for at least 60 seconds. If unexpectedly deep anesthesia develops or if respiratory depression occurs, consider these possibilities: (1) the patient may be unusually sensitive to Pentothal, (2) the solution may be more concentrated than had been assumed, or (3) the patient may have received too much premedication.

Use in Anesthesia
Moderately slow induction can usually be accomplished in the "average" adult by injection of 50 to 75 mg (2 to 3 ml of a 2.5% solution) at intervals of 20 to 40 seconds, depending on the reaction of the patient. Once anesthesia is established, additional injections of 25 to 50 mg can be given whenever the patient moves.
Slow injection is recommended to minimize respiratory depression and the possibility of overdosage. The smallest dose consistent with attaining the surgical objective is the desired goal. Momentary apnea following each injection is typical, and progressive decrease in the amplitude of respiration appears with increasing dosage. Pulse remains normal or increases slightly and returns to normal. Blood pressure usually falls slightly but returns toward normal. Muscles usually relax about 30 seconds after unconsciousness is attained, but this may be masked if a skeletal muscle relaxant is used. The tone of jaw muscles is a fairly reliable index. The pupils may dilate but later contract; sensitivity to light is not usually lost until a level of anesthesia deep enough to permit surgery is attained. Nystagmus and divergent strabismus are characteristic during early stages, but at the level of surgical anesthesia, the eyes are central and fixed. Corneal and conjunctival reflexes disappear during surgical anesthesia.
When Pentothal (Thiopental Sodium for Injection, USP) is used for induction in balanced anesthesia with a skeletal muscle relaxant and an inhalation agent, the total dose of Pentothal can be estimated and then injected in two to four fractional doses. With this technique, brief periods of apnea may occur which may require assisted or controlled pulmonary ventilation. As an initial dose, 210 to 280 mg (3 to 4 mg/kg) of Pentothal is usually required for rapid induction in the average adult (70 kg).
When Pentothal (Thiopental Sodium for Injection, USP) is used as the sole anesthetic agent, the desired level of anesthesia can be maintained by injection of small repeated doses as needed or by using a continuous intravenous drip in a 0.2% or 0.4% concentration. (Sterile water should not be used as the diluent in these concentrations, since hemolysis will occur.) With continuous drip, the depth of anesthesia is controlled by adjusting the rate of infusion.

Use in Convulsive States
For the control of convulsive states following anesthesia (inhalation or local) or other causes, 75 to 125 mg (3 to 5 ml of a 2.5% solution) should be given as soon as possible after the convulsion begins. Convulsions following the use of a local anesthetic may require 125 to 250 mg of Pentothal (Thiopental Sodium for Injection), given over a ten minute period. If the convulsion is caused by a local anesthetic, the required dose of Pentothal will depend upon the amount of local anesthetic given and its convulsant properties.

Use in Neurosurgical Patients with Increased Intracranial Pressure
In neurosurgical patients, intermittent bolus injections of 1.5 to 3.5 mg/kg of body weight may be given to reduce intraoperative elevations of intracranial pressure, if adequate ventilation is provided.

Use in Psychiatric Disorders
For narcoanalysis and narcosynthesis in psychiatric disorders, premedication with an anticholinergic agent may precede administration of Pentothal. After a test dose, Pentothal is injected at a slow rate of 100 mg/min (4 ml/min of a 2.5% solution) with the patient counting backwards from 100. Shortly after counting becomes confused but before actual sleep is produced, the injection is discontinued. Allow the patient to return to a semidrowsy state where conversation is coherent. Alternatively, Pentothal (Thiopental Sodium for Injection, USP) may be administered by rapid I.V. drip using a 0.2% concentration in 5% dextrose and water. At this concentration, the rate of administration should not exceed 50 ml/min.

Management of Some Complications:
Respiratory depression (hypoventilation, apnea), which may result from either unusual responsiveness to Pentothal (Thiopental Sodium for Injection, USP) or overdosage, is managed as stated above. Pentothal should be considered to have the same potential for producing respiratory depression as an inhalation agent, and patency of the airway must be protected at all times.
Laryngospasm may occur with light Pentothal narcosis at intubation, or in the absence of intubation if foreign matter or secretions in the respiratory tract create irritation. Laryngeal and bronchial vagal reflexes can be suppressed, and secretions minimized by giving atropine or scopolamine premedication and a barbiturate or opiate. Use of a skeletal muscle relaxant or positive pressure oxygen will usually relieve laryngospasm. Tracheostomy may be indicated in difficult cases.
Myocardial depression, proportional to the amount of drug in direct contact with the heart, can occur and may cause hypotension, particularly in patients with an unhealthy myocardium. Arrhythmias may appear if Pco_2 is elevated, but they are uncommon with adequate ventilation. Management of myocardial depression is the same as for overdosage. Pentothal (Thiopental Sodium for Injection, USP) does not sensitize the heart to epinephrine or other sympathomimetic amines.
Extravascular infiltration should be avoided. Care should be taken to insure that the needle is within the lumen of the vein before injection of Pentothal. Extravascular injection may cause chemical irritation of the tissues varying from slight tenderness to venospasm, extensive necrosis and sloughing. This is due primarily to the high alkaline pH (10 to 11) of clinical concentrations of the drug. If extravasation occurs, the local irritant effects can be reduced by injection of 1% procaine locally to relieve pain and enhance vasodilatation. Local application of heat also may help to increase local circulation and removal of the infiltrate.
Intra-arterial injection can occur inadvertently, especially if an aberrant superficial artery is present at the medial aspect of the antecubital fossa. The area selected for intravenous injection of the drug should be palpated for detection of an underlying pulsating vessel. Accidental intra-arterial injection can cause arteriospasm and severe pain along the course of the artery with blanching of the arm and fingers. Appropriate corrective measures should be instituted promptly to avoid possible development of gangrene. Any patient complaint of pain warrants stopping the injection. Methods suggested for dealing with this complication vary with the severity of symptoms. The following have been suggested:

1. Dilute the injected Pentothal (Thiopental Sodium for Injection, USP) by removing the tourniquet and any restrictive garments.
2. Leave the needle in place, if possible.
3. Inject the artery with a dilute solution of papaverine, 40 to 80 mg, or 10 ml of 1% procaine, to inhibit smooth muscle spasm.
4. If necessary, perform sympathetic block of the brachial plexus and/or stellate ganglion to relieve pain and assist in opening collateral circulation. Papaverine can be injected into the subclavian artery, if desired.
5. Unless otherwise contraindicated, institute immediate heparinization to prevent thrombus formation.
6. Consider local infiltration of an alpha-adrenergic blocking agent such as phentolamine into the vasospastic area.
7. Provide additional symptomatic treatment as required.

Shivering after Pentothal anesthesia, manifested by twitching face muscles and occasional progression to tremors of the arms, head, shoulder and body, is a thermal reaction due to increased sensitivity to cold. Shivering appears if the room environment is cold and if a large ventilatory heat loss has been sustained with balanced inhalation anesthesia employing nitrous oxide. Treatment consists of warming the patient with blankets, maintaining room temperature near 22° C (72° F), and administration of chlorpromazine or methylphenidate.

Preparation of Solutions: Pentothal (Thiopental Sodium for Injection, USP) is supplied as a yellowish, hygroscopic powder in a variety of different containers. Solutions should be prepared aseptically with one of the three following diluents; Sterile Water for Injection, USP, Sodium Chloride Injection, USP or 5% Dextrose Injection, USP. Clinical concentrations used for intermittent intravenous administration vary between 2.0 and 5.0%. A 2.0 or 2.5% solution is most commonly used. A 3.4% concentration in sterile water for injection is isotonic; concentrations less than 2.0% in this diluent are not used because they cause hemolysis. For continuous intravenous drip administration, concentrations of 0.2 or 0.4% are used. Solutions may be prepared by adding Pentothal to 5% Dextrose Injection, USP, Sodium Chloride Injection, USP or Normosol®-R pH 7.4.

Since Pentothal (Thiopental Sodium for Injection, USP) contains no added bacteriostatic agent, extreme care in preparation and handling should be exercised at all times to prevent the introduction of microbial contaminants. Solutions should be freshly prepared and used promptly; when reconstituted for administration to several patients, unused portions should be discarded after 24 hours. Sterilization by heating should not be attempted.

Warning: The 2.5 g and larger sizes contain adequate medication for several patients

Compatibility: Any solution of Pentothal (Thiopental Sodium for Injection, USP) with a visible precipitate should not be administered. The stability of Pentothal solutions depends upon several factors, including the diluent, temperature of storage and the amount of carbon dioxide from room air that gains access to the solution. Any factor or condition which tends to lower pH (increase acidity) of Pentothal solutions will increase the likelihood of precipitation of thiopental acid. Such factors include the use of diluents which are too acid and the absorption of carbon dioxide which can combine with water to form carbonic acid.

Solutions of succinycholine, tubocurarine or other drugs which have an acid pH should not be mixed with Pentothal solutions. The most stable solutions are those reconstituted in water or isotonic saline, kept under refrigeration and tightly stoppered. The presence or absence of a visible precipitate offers a practical guide to the physical compatibility of prepared solutions of Pentothal (Thiopental Sodium for Injection, USP).

Calculations for Various Concentrations:

Concentration Desired		Amounts to Use	
Percent	mg/ml	Pentothal g	Diluent ml
0.2	2	1	500
0.4	4	1	250
		2	500
2.0	20	5	250
		10	500
2.5	25	1	40
		5	200
5	50	1	20
		5	100

Reconstituted solutions of Pentothal should be inspected visually for particulate matter and discoloration, whenever solution and container permit.

How Supplied: Pentothal (Thiopental Sodium for Injection, USP) is available in a variety of sizes and containers in combination packages with diluent as shown at the end of this insert.

Caution: Federal (USA) law prohibits dispensing without prescription.

Ref. No. 06-4000-R1-10/79

PHENURONE® ℞

(phenacemide tablets, USP)

Description: PHENURONE (phenacemide) is a valuable antiepileptic drug for use in selected patients with epilepsy. Since therapy with PHENURONE involves certain risks, *physicians should thoroughly familiarize themselves with the undesirable side effects which may occur and the precautions to be observed.* PHENURONE (phenacemide) is a substituted acetylurea derivative. Chemically PHENURONE is identified as N-(aminocarbonyl)-benzeneacetamide. PHENURONE tablets contain 500 mg phenacemide for oral administration.

Clinical Pharmacology: In experimental animals, PHENURONE in doses well below those causing neurological signs, elevates the threshold for minimal electroshock convulsions and abolishes the tonic phase of maximal electroshock seizures. The drug prevents or modifies seizures induced by pentylenetetrazol or other convulsants. In comparative tests, PHENURONE was found to be equal or more effective than other commonly used antiepileptics against complex partial (psychomotor) seizures which were induced in mice by low frequency stimulation of the cerebral cortex. Studies in mice have shown that PHENURONE exerts a synergistic antiepileptic effect with mephenytoin, phenobarbital, or trimethadione.

Given orally to laboratory animals, PHENURONE has a low acute toxicity. In mice, slight ataxia appears at 400 mg/kg and light sleep occurs at 800 mg/kg. In high doses the drug causes marked ataxia and coma, the fatal dose being in the range of 3 to 5 g/kg for mice, rats, and cats.

PHENURONE is metabolized by the liver, however, further definition of human pharmacokinetics has not been determined.

Indications and Usage: PHENURONE (phenacemide) is indicated for the control of severe epilepsy, particularly mixed forms of complex partial (psychomotor) seizures, refractory to other drugs.

Contraindications: PHENURONE should not be administered unless other available antiepileptics have been found to be ineffective in satisfactorily controlling seizures.

Warnings: PHENURONE (phenacemide) can produce serious side effects as well as direct organ toxicity. As a consequence its use entails the assumption of certain risks which must be weighed against the benefit to the patient. *Ordinarily PHENURONE should not be administered unless other available antiepileptics have been found to be ineffective in controlling seizures.*

Death attributable to liver damage during therapy with PHENURONE has been reported. PHENURONE should be used with caution in patients with a history of previous liver dysfunction. If jaundice or other signs of hepatitis appear, the drug should be discontinued.

Aplastic anemia has occurred in association with PHENURONE therapy and death from this condition has been reported. PHENURONE should ordinarily not be used in patients with severe blood dyscrasias. Marked depression of the blood count is an indication for withdrawal of the drug.

Usage During Pregnancy: PHENURONE can cause fetal harm when administered to a pregnant woman. There are multiple reports in the clinical literature which indicate that the use of antiepileptic drugs during pregnancy results in an increased incidence of birth defects in the offspring. Reports have also suggested that the maternal ingestion of antiepileptic drugs, particularly barbiturates, is associated with a neonatal coagulation defect that may cause bleeding during the early (usually within 24 hours of birth) neonatal period. The possibility of the occurrence of this defect with the use of PHENURONE should be kept in mind. The defect is characterized by decreased levels of vitamin K-dependent clotting factors, and prolongation of either the prothrombin time or the partial thromboplastin time, or both. It has been suggested that vitamin K be given prophylactically to the mother one month prior to and during delivery, and to the infant, intravenously, immediately after birth. If this drug is used during pregnancy, or if the patient becomes pregnant while taking this drug, the patient should be apprised of the potential hazard to the fetus.

Precautions: *General:* Extreme caution must be exercised in treating patients who previously have shown personality disorders. It may be advisable to hospitalize such patients during the first week of treatment. Personality changes, including attempts at suicide and the occurrence of psychoses requiring hospitalization, have been reported during therapy with PHENURONE (phenacemide). Severe or exacerbated personality changes are an indication for withdrawal of the drug.

PHENURONE (phenacemide) should be used with caution in patients with a history of previous liver dysfunction.

PHENURONE should be administered with caution to patients with a history of allergy, particularly in association with the administration of other antiepileptics. The drug should be discontinued at the first sign of a skin rash or other allergic manifestation.

Information for Patients: The patient and his family should be aware of the possibility of personality changes so the family can watch for changes in the behavior of the patient such as decreased interest in surroundings, depression, or aggressiveness.

The patient should be told to report immediately any symptoms indicative of a developing blood dyscrasia such as malaise, sore throat, or fever.

Laboratory Tests: Liver function tests should be performed before and during therapy. Death attributable to liver damage during therapy with PHENURONE has been reported. If jaundice or other signs of hepatitis appear, the drug should be discontinued.

Complete blood counts should be made before instituting PHENURONE, and at monthly intervals thereafter. If no abnormality appears within 12 months, the interval between blood counts may be extended. Blood changes have been reported with leukopenia (leukocyte count of 4,000 or less per cubic millimeter of blood) as the most commonly observed effect. However, aplastic anemia has occurred in association with PHENURONE therapy, and death from this condition has been reported. *The total number of each cellular element per cubic millimeter is a better index of possible blood dyscrasia than the percentage of cells.* Marked depression of the blood count is an indication for withdrawal of the drug.

Similarly, as nephritis has occasionally occurred in patients on PHENURONE, the urine should be examined at regular intervals. Abnormal urinary findings are an indication for discontinuance of therapy.

Drug Interactions: Extreme caution is essential if PHENURONE is administered with any other antiepileptic which is known to cause similar toxic effects.

Considerable caution should be exercised if PHENURONE (phenacemide) is administered concurrently with *Peganone (ethotoin)* since

Continued on next page

If desired, additional literature on any Abbott Product will be provided upon request to Abbott Laboratories.

Abbott—Cont.

paranoid symptoms have been reported during therapy with this combination.
Carcinogenesis: No data are available on long-term potential for carcinogenicity in animals or humans.
Pregnancy: Pregnancy Category D. See "Warnings" section.
Nursing Mothers: It is not known whether this drug is excreted in human milk. Because many drugs are excreted in human milk and because of the potential for serious adverse reactions in nursing infants from PHENURONE, a decision should be made whether to discontinue nursing or to discontinue the drug, taking into account the importance of the drug to the mother.
Pediatric Use: Safety and effectiveness in children below the age of 5 years have not been established.
Adverse Reactions: The following adverse effects associated with PHENURONE are listed by decreasing order of frequency based on data from one large clinical study.[1]
Psychiatric: Psychic changes (17 in 100 patients).
Gastrointestinal: Gastrointestinal disturbances (8 in 100 patients), including anorexia (5 in 100 patients) and weight loss (less than 1 in 100 patients).
Dermatologic: Skin rash (5 in 100 patients).
CNS: Drowsiness (4 in 100 patients), headache (2 in 100 patients), insomnia (1 in 100 patients), dizziness and paresthesias (less than 1 in 100 patients).
Hematopoietic: Blood dyscrasias (primarily leukopenia), including fatal aplastic anemia (2 in 100 patients).
Hepatic: Hepatitis, including fatalities (2 in 100 patients).
Renal: Abnormal urinary findings, including a rise in serum creatinine[2], and nephritis (1 in 100 patients or less).
Other: Fatigue, fever, muscle pain and palpitation (less than 1 in 100 patients).
Overdosage: Symptoms of acute overdosage include excitement or mania, followed by drowsiness, ataxia and coma. In one case of acute overdosage, dizziness was followed by coma which lasted nearly 24 hours. Treatment should be started by inducing emesis; gastric lavage may be considered as an alternative or adjunct. General supportive measures will be necessary. A careful evaluation of liver and kidney function, mental state, and the blood-forming organs should be made following recovery.
Dosage and Administration: PHENURONE is administered orally.
Since PHENURONE may produce serious toxic effects, it is strongly recommended that the dosage be held to the minimum amount necessary to achieve an adequate therapeutic effect.
For adults the usual starting dose is 1.5 g daily, administered in three divided doses of 500 mg each. After the first week, if seizures are not controlled and the drug is well tolerated, an additional 500 mg tablet may be taken upon arising. In the third week, if necessary, the dosage may be further increased by another 500 mg at bedtime. Satisfactory results have been noted in some patients on an initial dose of 250 mg three times per day. The effective total daily dose for adults usually ranges from 2 to 3 g, although some patients have required as much as 5 g daily.
For the pediatric patient from 5 to 10 years of age, approximately one-half the adult dose is recommended. It should be given at the same intervals as for adults.
PHENURONE may be administered alone or in conjunction with other antiepileptics. However, extreme caution must be exercised if other antiepileptics cause toxic effects similar to PHENURONE.
When PHENURONE is to replace other antiepileptic medication, the latter should be withdrawn gradually as the dosage of PHENURONE is increased to maintain seizure control.
How Supplied: PHENURONE (Phenacemide Tablets, USP), grooved, white, 500 mg are supplied in bottles of 100 (**NDC** 0074-3971-05).
References:

1. Tyler, M. W., King, E. Q.: Phenacemide in Treatment of Epilepsy. JAMA 147: 17–21 (1951).
2. Richards, R.K., Bjornsson, T. D., Waterbury, L. D.: Rise in Serum and Urine Creatinine After Phenacemide. Clin. Pharmacol. Ther. 23: 430–437 (1978).

Abbott Laboratories
North Chicago, IL 60064
Ref. 01-2238-R7

PLACIDYL® ℞ Ⓒ
(ethchlorvynol capsules, USP)
Oral hypnotic

Description: PLACIDYL (ethchlorvynol) is a tertiary carbinol. It is chemically designated as ethyl β-chlorovinyl ethynyl carbinol. Ethchlorvynol occurs as a liquid which is immiscible with water and miscible with most organic solvents.
Clinical Pharmacology: The usual hypnotic dose of PLACIDYL induces sleep within 15 minutes to one hour. The duration of the hypnotic effect is about five hours.
PLACIDYL is rapidly absorbed from the gastrointestinal tract with peak plasma concentrations usually occurring within two hours after a single oral fasting dose. The plasma half-life ($t_{1/2}$, β) of the parent compound is approximately ten to twenty hours. Studies with ^{14}C-PLACIDYL have demonstrated that within 24 hours, 33% of a single 500 mg dose is excreted in the urine mostly as metabolites. The major plasma and urinary metabolite is the secondary alcohol of PLACIDYL. The free and conjugated forms of the metabolite in the urine account for about 40% of the dose. Studies with ^{14}C-PLACIDYL in animals indicate that the parent compound and its metabolites undergo extensive enterohepatic recirculation.
Distribution studies indicate that there is extensive tissue localization of ethchlorvynol, particularly in adipose tissue.
Indications: PLACIDYL is indicated as short-term hypnotic therapy for periods up to one week in duration in the management of insomnia. If retreatment becomes necessary, after drug-free intervals of one or more weeks, it should only be undertaken upon further evaluation of the patient.
Contraindications: PLACIDYL is contraindicated in patients with known hypersensitivity to the drug and in patients with porphyria.
Warnings: PLACIDYL SHOULD BE ADMINISTERED WITH CAUTION TO MENTALLY DEPRESSED PATIENTS WITH OR WITHOUT SUICIDAL TENDENCIES. IT SHOULD ALSO BE ADMINISTERED WITH CAUTION TO THOSE WHO HAVE A PSYCHOLOGICAL POTENTIAL FOR DRUG DEPENDENCE. THE LEAST AMOUNT OF DRUG THAT IS FEASIBLE SHOULD BE PRESCRIBED FOR THESE PATIENTS.
Patients should be advised that, for the duration of the effect of PLACIDYL , mental and/or physical abilities required for the performance of potentially hazardous tasks such as the operation of dangerous machinery including motor vehicles, may be impaired.
Usage During Pregnancy and Lactation: PLACIDYL (ethchlorvynol) is not recommended for use during the first and second trimesters of pregnancy. Also clinical experience has indicated that PLACIDYL when taken during the third trimester of pregnancy may produce CNS depression and transient withdrawal symptoms in the newborn.
Studies in rats have shown a higher percentage of stillbirths and a lower survival rate of progeny among animals given 40 mg/kg/day.
The safety of use of PLACIDYL during lactation has not been established.
Drug Interactions: Patients should be cautioned that the concomitant use of PLACIDYL and alcohol, barbiturates, other CNS depressants, or MAO inhibitors may produce exaggerated depressant effects.
Ethchlorvynol may cause a decreased prothrombin time response to coumarin anticoagulants; therefore, the dosage of these drugs may require adjustment when therapy with ethchlorvynol is initiated and after it is discontinued.
Transient delirium has been reported with the concomitant use of PLACIDYL and amitriptyline; therefore, PLACIDYL should be administered with caution to patients receiving tricyclic antidepressants.
Usage in Children: PLACIDYL is not recommended for use in children since its safety and effectiveness in the pediatric age group has not been established.
Psychological and Physical Dependence: PROLONGED USE OF PLACIDYL MAY RESULT IN TOLERANCE AND PSYCHOLOGICAL AND PHYSICAL DEPENDENCE. PROLONGED ADMINISTRATION OF THE DRUG IS NOT RECOMMENDED.
Signs and symptoms of intoxication have been reported with the prolonged use of doses as low as 1 g/day. Signs and symptoms of chronic intoxication may include incoordination, tremors, ataxia, confusion, slurred speech, hyperreflexia, diplopia, and generalized muscle weakness. Toxic amblyopia, scotoma, nystagmus, and peripheral neuropathy have also been reported with prolonged use of ethchlorvynol; these symptoms are usually reversible.
Pulmonary edema of rapid onset has resulted from the I.V. abuse of PLACIDYL (ethchlorvynol).
Severe withdrawal symptoms similar to those seen during barbiturate and alcohol withdrawal have been reported following abrupt discontinuance of prolonged use of PLACIDYL. These symptoms may appear as late as nine days after sudden withdrawal of the drug. Signs and symptoms of PLACIDYL withdrawal may include convulsions, delirium, schizoid reaction, perceptual distortions, memory loss, ataxia, insomnia, slurring of speech, unusual anxiety, irritability, agitation, and tremors. Other signs and symptoms may include anorexia, nausea, vomiting, weakness, dizziness, sweating, muscle twitching, and weight loss.
Management of a patient who manifests withdrawal symptoms from PLACIDYL involves readministration of the drug to approximately the same level of chronic intoxication that existed before the abrupt discontinuance. (Phenobarbital may be substituted for PLACIDYL.) A gradual, stepwise reduction of dosage may then be made over a period of days or weeks. A phenothiazine compound may be used in addition to this regimen for those patients who exhibit psychotic symptoms during the withdrawal period. The patient undergoing withdrawal from PLACIDYL must be hospitalized or closely observed, and given general supportive care as indicated.
Precautions: Elderly or debilitated patients should receive the smallest effective amount of PLACIDYL (ethchlorvynol).
Caution should be exercised when treating patients with impaired hepatic or renal function.
Patients who exhibit unpredictable behavior, or paradoxical restlessness or excitement in response to barbiturates or alcohol may react in this manner to PLACIDYL.
PLACIDYL should not be used for the management of insomnia in the presence of pain unless insomnia persists after pain is controlled with analgesics.

The 750 mg dosage strength of PLACIDYL contains FD&C Yellow No. 5 (tartrazine) which may cause allergic-type reactions (including bronchial asthma) in certain susceptible individuals. Although the overall incidence of FD&C Yellow No. 5 (tartrazine) sensitivity in the general population is low, it is frequently seen in patients who also have aspirin hypersensitivity.

Adverse Reactions: Nausea, vomiting, gastric upset, aftertaste, dizziness, blurred vision, facial numbness, and hypotension have occurred.

Hypersensitivity reactions have included skin rash, urticaria, and occasionally, thrombocytopenia and cholestatic jaundice.

Mild "hangover" has occurred.

The following idiosyncratic responses have been reported occasionally: mild stimulation, marked excitement, hysteria; prolonged hypnosis, profound muscular weakness, syncope without marked hypotension.

Transient giddiness and ataxia have occurred in patients in whom absorption of the drug is especially rapid; these effects can sometimes be controlled by giving PLACIDYL with food.

(See Psychological and Physical Dependence for the signs and symptoms of chronic intoxication.)

Dosage and Administration: The usual adult hypnotic dose of PLACIDYL (ethchlorvynol) is 500 mg taken orally at bedtime. A dose of 750 mg may be required for patients whose sleep response to a 500 mg capsule is inadequate, or for patients being changed from barbiturates or other nonbarbiturate hypnotics. Up to 1000 mg may be given as a single bedtime dose when insomnia is unusually severe. A single supplemental dose of 100 to 200 mg may be given to reinstitute sleep in patients who may awaken after the original bedtime dose of 500 or 750 mg.

For patients whose insomnia is characterized only by untimely awakening during the early morning hours, a single dose of 100 to 200 mg taken upon awakening may be adequate for relief.

The smallest effective dose of PLACIDYL should be given to elderly or debilitated patients.

PLACIDYL should not be prescribed for periods exceeding one week. (See Psychological and Physical Dependence.)

Overdosage: Acute intoxication is characterized by prolonged deep coma, severe respiratory depression, hypothermia, hypotension, and relative bradycardia. Nystagmus and pancytopenia resulting from acute PLACIDYL overdose have been reported.

Although death has occurred following the ingestion of 6 g of PLACIDYL, there have been reports of patients who have survived overdoses of 50 g and more with intensive care.

Management of acute PLACIDYL intoxication is similar to that of acute barbiturate intoxication. Gastric evacuation should be performed immediately. (In the unconscious patient, gastric lavage should be preceded by tracheal intubation with a cuffed tube.) Supportive care (assisted ventilation, frequent and careful monitoring of vital signs, control of blood pressure) is essential. Emphasis should be placed on pulmonary care and monitoring of blood gases. Hemoperfusion utilizing the Amberlite column technique has been reported in the literature to be the most effective method in the management of acute PLACIDYL overdose.[1] In addition, hemodialysis and peritoneal dialysis have each been reported to be of some value in the management of acute PLACIDYL overdose. (Aqueous and oil dialysates have been used. Forced diuresis with maintenance of a high urinary output has also been reported to be of some value.)

(See Psychological and Physical Dependence for the signs and symptoms of chronic intoxication.)

How Supplied: PLACIDYL (ethchlorvynol capsules, USP) is supplied as:

100 mg capsules: Bottles of 100 (**NDC** 0074-6649-04).

200 mg capsules: Bottles of 100 (**NDC** 0074-6661-08).

500 mg capsules: Bottles of 100 (**NDC** 0074-6685-15), Bottles of 500 (**NDC** 0074-6685-02), and ABBO-PAC® unit dose strip packages of 100 (**NDC** 0074-6685-10).

750 mg capsules: Bottles of 100 (**NDC** 0074-6630-01), and ABBO-PAC unit dose strip packages of 100 (**NDC** 0074-6630-10).

Reference

1. Lynn, R.I., et al. Resin Hemoperfusion for Treatment of Ethchlorvynol Overdose, *Annals of Internal Medicine,* 91:549-553, 1979.

[*Shown in Product Identification Section*]

Abbott Laboratories
North Chicago, IL 60064
Ref. 01-2108-R6

QUELIDRINE® SYRUP

(non-narcotic, antihistaminic cough suppressant)

Composition: Each teaspoonful (5 ml) contains:

Dextromethorphan Hydrobromide	10 mg
Chlorpheniramine Maleate	2 mg
Ephedrine Hydrochloride	5 mg
Phenylephrine Hydrochloride	5 mg
Ammonium Chloride	40 mg
Ipecac Fluidextract	0.005 ml
Alcohol	2%

in a palatable, aromatic syrup.

Action and Indications: Quelidrine is designed as an aid in the management of cough associated with acute or subacute simple respiratory infections. Quelidrine provides a wide range of therapeutic action against the cough complex—without the risk of addiction or the production of undue central depression.

Precautions: Quelidrine should be administered with caution to patients with hypertension, serious organic heart disease, angina pectoris, diabetes, thyroid disease, or to persons receiving digitalis. When cough persists or accompanies a high fever, the underlying cause and need for other medication should be reevaluated. Consult your physician if pregnant or nursing, or taking other medication.

Side Effects: Quelidrine is safe for patients of all ages, but professional supervision of dosage for very young patients is essential. Side effects are infrequent. Drowsiness, nausea, vomiting, nervousness, palpitation, blurred vision and insomnia may occur in susceptible patients. Constipation is seldom a problem. If side effects are encountered, dosage should be reduced or medication withdrawn.

Dosage and Administration: *Adults*—1 teaspoonful, one to four times daily. Children 6 years of age or older, ½ teaspoonful, one to four times daily. Children 2 to 6 years old, ¼ teaspoonful one to four times daily. Under 2, as directed by physician. Quelidrine may be diluted with Syrup, NF in order to facilitate pediatric administration. Patients should be warned that this medication should be kept from the reach of children.

How Supplied: Quelidrine Syrup is supplied in bottles of 4 fluid ounces (**NDC** 0074-6883-04), 1 pint (**NDC** 0074-6883-02), and 1 gallon (**NDC** 0074-6883-03) with or without a prescription.

Abbott Laboratories
North Chicago, IL 60064
Ref. 07-5201-4/R18

SELSUN® ℞

(selenium sulfide lotion, USP)

Description: SELSUN (selenium sulfide lotion) is a liquid preparation containing selenium sulfide 2½% w/v in aqueous suspension. The product also contains: bentonite, lauric diethanolamide, ethylene glycol monostearate, titanium dioxide, amphoteric-2, sodium lauryl sulfate, sodium phosphate (monobasic), glyceryl monoricinoleate, citric acid, captan, and perfume.

Indications: For the treatment of dandruff and seborrheic dermatitis of the scalp.

Contraindications: SELSUN (selenium sulfide lotion) should not be used by patients allergic to any of its components.

Warnings: Safety for use on infants has not been established.

Precautions: Cutaneous sensitization of the scalp or adjacent areas has been reported. If sensitivity reactions should occur, the lotion should be discontinued.

Chemical conjunctivitis may result if the preparation enters the eyes.

The product should not be used when acute inflammation or exudation is present as an increase in absorption may occur.

Adverse Reactions: As with other shampoos, oiliness or dryness of the hair and scalp may occur following use and there have been occasional reports of an increase in the amount of normal hair loss. Discoloration of the hair may follow use of the preparation. This can be avoided or minimized by thorough rinsing of the hair after treatment.

Dosage and Administration: For treatment of dandruff or seborrheic dermatitis of the scalp:

1. Massage about 1 or 2 teaspoonfuls of the medicated shampoo into the wet scalp.
2. Allow product to remain on the scalp for 2 to 3 minutes.
3. Rinse the scalp thoroughly.
4. Repeat application and rinse thoroughly.
5. After treatment wash hands.

For the usual case, two applications each weeks for two weeks will afford control. After this, the lotion may be used at less frequent intervals—weekly, every two weeks, or even every 3 or 4 weeks in some cases. The preparation should not be applied more frequently than required to maintain control.

The product may damage jewelry; jewelry should be removed before use.

Accidental Oral Ingestion: Selsun is intended for external use only. There have been no documented reports of serious toxicity in humans resulting from acute ingestion of SELSUN; however, acute toxicity studies in animals suggest that ingestion of large amounts could result in potential human toxicity. For this reason, evacuation of the stomach contents should be considered in cases of acute oral ingestion.

How Supplied: SELSUN (selenium sulfide lotion, USP) is supplied in 4-fluidounce nonbreakable plastic bottles (**NDC** 0074-2660-04).

SELSUN is to be dispensed only on the prescription of a physician.

Abbott Laboratories
North Chicago, IL 60064
Ref. 01-2878-R2

Continued on next page

If desired, additional literature on any Abbott Product will be provided upon request to Abbott Laboratories.

Abbott—Cont.

SELSUN BLUE® OTC
(selenium sulfide)
Lotion

Selsun Blue is a non-prescription anti-dandruff shampoo containing a 1% concentration of selenium sulfide in a freshly scented pH balanced formula to leave hair clean and manageable. Available in formulations for dry, oily or normal hair types.
Recent clinical testing at a major medical school proved that Selsun Blue is significantly more effective at controlling dandruff than any leading brand of dandruff shampoo.
Directions: Shake well before using. Lather, rinse thoroughly and repeat. Use once or twice weekly for effective dandruff control.
Caution: For external use only. Keep this and all shampoos out of children's reach. Avoid getting shampoo in eyes—if this happens, rinse thoroughly with water. When used before or after bleaching, tinting or permanent waving, rinse for at least five minutes in cool running water. If irritation occurs, discontinue use. Protect from heat.
How Supplied: In 4 fl. oz., 7 fl. oz., and 11 fl. oz. bottles.

SURBEX®
Vitamin B-Complex*
SURBEX® with C
Vitamin B-Complex* with Vitamin C

Description: Each Surbex Filmtab tablet provides:

Niacinamide	30 mg
Calcium Pantothenate	10 mg
Vitamin B_1 (thiamine mononitrate)	6 mg
Vitamin B_2 (riboflavin)	6 mg
Vitamin B_6 (pyridoxine hydrochloride)	2.5 mg
Vitamin B_{12} (cyanocobalamin)	5 mcg

Each Surbex with C Filmtab tablet provides the same ingredients as Surbex, plus 250 mg Vitamin C (as sodium ascorbate).
Indications: Surbex is indicated for treatment of Vitamin B-Complex* deficiency.
Surbex with C is indicated for use in treatment of Vitamin B-Complex* with Vitamin C deficiency.
* Contains no folic acid; not for treatment of folate deficiency.
Dosage and Administration: Usual adult dosage is one tablet twice daily or as directed by physician.
How Supplied: Surbex is supplied as bright orange-colored tablets in bottles of 100 (NDC 0074-4876-13).
Surbex with C is supplied as yellow-colored tablets in bottles of 100 (NDC 0074-4877-13) and 500 (NDC 0074-4877-53).
Abbott Pharmaceuticals, Inc.
North Chicago, IL 60064
Ref. 03-0810-3/R6, 03-0811-3/R5

SURBEX-T®
High-Potency Vitamin B-Complex* with 500 mg of Vitamin C

Description: Each Filmtab® tablet provides:

Vitamin C (as sodium ascorbate)	500 mg
Niacinamide	100 mg
Calcium Pantothenate	20 mg
Vitamin B_1 (thiamine mononitrate)	15 mg
Vitamin B_2 (riboflavin)	10 mg
Vitamin B_6 (pyridoxine hydrochloride)	5 mg
Vitamin B_{12} (cyanocobalamin)	10 mcg

Indications: For use in treatment of Vitamin B-Complex* with Vitamin C deficiency.
*Contains no folic acid; not for treatment of folate deficiency.
Dosage and Administration: Usual adult dosage is one Filmtab tablet daily, or as directed by physician.
How Supplied: Orange-colored tablets in bottles of 50 (NDC 0074-4878-50), 100 (NDC 0074-4878-13), and 500 (NDC 0074-4878-53). Also supplied in Abbo-Pac® unit dose packages of 100 tablets in strips of 10 tablets per strip (NDC 0074-4878-11). ®Filmtab—Film-sealed Tablets, Abbott.
[Shown in Product Identification Section]
Abbott Pharmaceuticals, Inc.
North Chicago, IL 60064
Ref. 03-0934-4/R5

SURBEX®-750 with IRON
High-potency B-complex with iron, vitamin E and 750 mg vitamin C

Description: Each Filmtab® tablet provides:

VITAMINS	
Vitamin C (as sodium ascorbate)	750 mg
Niacinamide	100 mg
Vitamin B_6 (pyridoxine hydrochloride)	25 mg
Calcium Pantothenate	20 mg
Vitamin B_1 (thiamine mononitrate)	15 mg
Vitamin B_2 (riboflavin)	15 mg
Vitamin B_{12} (cyanocobalamin)	12 mcg
Folic Acid	400 mcg
Vitamin E (as dl-alpha tocopheryl acetate)	30 IU
MINERAL	
Elemental Iron (as dried ferrous sulfate)	27 mg
equivalent to 135 mg ferrous sulfate	

Indications: For the treatment of vitamin C and B-complex deficiencies and to supplement the daily intake of iron and vitamin E.
Dosage and Administration: Usual adult dosage is one tablet daily or as directed by physician.
How Supplied: Bottles of 50 tablets (NDC 0074-8029-50)
[Shown in Product Identification Section]
Abbott Pharmaceuticals, Inc.
North Chicago, IL 60064
Ref. 03-0920-3/R3

SURBEX®-750 with ZINC
Zinc, vitamin B-complex and vitamins C and E for persons 12 years of age or older

Description: Daily dose (one Filmtab® tablet) provides:

		%U.S. R.D.A.*
VITAMINS		
Vitamin E	30 IU	100%
Vitamin C	750 mg	1250%
Folic Acid	0.4 mg	100%
Thiamine (B_1)	15 mg	1000%
Riboflavin (B_2)	15 mg	882%
Niacin	100 mg	500%
Vitamin B_6	20 mg	1000%
Vitamin B_{12}	12 mcg	200%
Pantothenic Acid	20 mg	200%
MINERAL		
Zinc**	22.5 mg	150%

* % U.S. Recommended Daily Allowance for Adults.
** Equivalent to 100 mg of zinc sulfate.
Ingredients: Sodium ascorbate, niacinamide, zinc sulfate, dl-alpha tocopheryl acetate, povidone, cellulose, pyridoxine hydrochloride, calcium pantothenate, thiamine mononitrate, riboflavin, cyanocobalamin, magnesium stearate, colloidal silicon dioxide, folic acid, in a film-coated tablet with vanillin flavoring and artificial coloring added.
Usual Adult Dose: One tablet daily.
How Supplied: Bottles of 50 tablets (NDC 0074-8152-50).
[Shown in Product Identification Section]
Abbott Pharmaceuticals, Inc.
North Chicago, IL 60064
Ref. 03-0921-3/R4

TRAL® Filmtab® Tablets ℞
(hexocyclium methylsulfate)

Description: TRAL (hexocyclium methylsulfate) is a quaternary ammonium salt. Chemically, it is designated as N-(beta-cyclohexyl-beta-hydroxy-beta-phenylethyl)-N′-methylpiperazine methosulfate. Physically, TRAL is a white powder soluble in water or physiological saline yielding a stable solution.
Actions: Clinically, TRAL is an effective anticholinergic agent which inhibits gastric secretion and gastrointestinal motility.
The drug has an antimuscarinic action similar to that of other quaternary ammonium compounds which produce anticholinergic effects. In experimental animals the drug has been shown to decrease gastric secretion, prevent gastric ulceration, decrease gastrointestinal motility, dilate the pupils, inhibit salivation, increase the heart rate, and counteract the peripheral muscarinic effect of choline esters. With massive overdosage the drug also may produce a peripheral curare-like neuromuscular block and ganglionic blockade. In studies with human subjects, TRAL produced a decrease in gastric acidity, and a decrease in the volume of gastric secretion.
TRAL is absorbed from the gastrointestinal tract but the degree of absorption varies. Following oral administration of a single dose of the drug in conventional tablet form, its effects persist for 3 to 4 hours. The metabolic fate and route of excretion are unknown.
Indications: TRAL is indicated as adjunctive therapy in the treatment of peptic ulcer. IT SHOULD BE NOTED AT THIS POINT IN TIME THAT THERE IS A LACK OF CONCURRENCE AS TO THE VALUE OF ANTICHOLINERGICS IN THE TREATMENT OF GASTRIC ULCER. IT HAS NOT BEEN SHOWN WHETHER ANTICHOLINERGIC DRUGS AID IN THE HEALING OF A PEPTIC ULCER, DECREASE THE RATE OF RECURRENCES OR PREVENT COMPLICATION. To be effective the dosage must be titrated to the individual patient's needs.
Contraindications: TRAL is contraindicated in patients with glaucoma; obstructive uropathy (for example, bladder neck obstruction due to prostatic hypertrophy); obstructive disease of the gastrointestinal tract (as in achalasia, paralytic ileus, pyloroduodenal stenosis, etc.); intestinal atony of the elderly or debilitated patient; unstable cardiovascular status; in acute hemorrhage; severe ulcerative colitis; toxic megacolon complicating ulcerative colitis; myasthenia gravis.
Warnings: In the presence of a high environmental temperature, heat prostration can occur with drug use (fever and heat stroke due to decreased sweating).
TRAL may produce drowsiness or blurred vision. In this event, the patient should be warned not to engage in activities requiring mental alertness such as operating a motor vehicle or other machinery, or perform hazardous work while taking this drug.
Usage in Pregnancy and Lactation: The safety of TRAL for use during pregnancy or lactation has not been established.
When given to pregnant rabbits at daily oral doses of 2.5 and 40 mg/kg/day, which are 1.2 and 20 times the human dose, TRAL increased the rate of abortion and fetal resorption.
As with all anticholinergic drugs, an inhibitory effect on lactation may occur.
Precautions: TRAL should be used with caution in patients with:
- Autonomic neuropathy.
- Hepatic or renal disease.
- Ulcerative colitis—large doses may suppress intestinal motility to the point of producing a paralytic ileus and the use of this drug may precipitate or aggravate the serious complication of toxic megacolon.
- Hyperthyroidism, coronary heart disease, congestive heart failure, cardiac ar-

rhythmias, hypertension and non-obstructing prostatic hypertrophy.
Hiatal hernia associated with reflux esophagitis since anticholinergic drugs may aggravate this condition.

It should be noted that the use of anticholinergic drugs in the treatment of gastric ulcer may produce a delay in gastric emptying time and may complicate such therapy (antral stasis).

Investigate any tachycardia before giving anticholinergic (atropine-like) drugs since they may increase the heart rate.

With overdosage, a curare-like action may occur.

This product contains FD&C Yellow No. 5 (tartrazine) which may cause allergic-type reactions (including bronchial asthma) in certain susceptible individuals. Although the overall incidence of FD&C Yellow No. 5 (tartrazine) sensitivity in the general population is low, it is frequently seen in patients who also have aspirin hypersensitivity.

Adverse Reactions: Adverse reactions may include xerostomia, urinary hesitancy and retention, blurred vision, mydriasis, cycloplegia, increased intra-ocular tension, tachycardia, palpitations, headaches, nervousness, drowsiness, weakness, dizziness, insomnia, nausea, vomiting, impotency, dysphagia, altered taste perception, heartburn, bloated feeling, constipation, paralytic ileus, flushing, decreased sweating, urticaria and other dermal manifestations, severe allergic reaction or drug idiosyncrasies, and some degree of mental confusion and/or excitement especially in elderly persons.

When side effects are severe and cannot be controlled by reduction of dosage, the medication should be withdrawn.

Dosage and Administration: TRAL is administered orally. The usual recommended adult dose of TRAL is one 25 mg Filmtab tablet four times daily, taken before meals and at bedtime.

For optimal therapeutic effect, dosage should be adjusted to the patient's response.

TRAL is not for use in children.

Overdosage: The first sign of overdosage may be indicated by an atropine-like flush, particularly in the blush areas. Other manifestations of overdosage are revealed by the appearance or an increase in intensity of dryness of the mouth or other side effects.

With unusually large doses the quaternary ammonium type of anticholinergic agent may produce a curare-like action and ganglionic blockade manifested by respiratory paralysis and circulatory collapse. This is unlikely to occur with therapeutic doses. Neostigmine methylsulfate at a dose of 0.5 to 2 mg given by slow intravenous injection and repeated as required may be administered as an antidote. Only in exceptional cases should the total dose of neostigmine methylsulfate exceed 5 mg. Artificial respiration and other supportive measures should be applied if needed.

How Supplied: TRAL (hexocyclium methylsulfate) Filmtab tablets, 25 mg, green, (**NDC** 0074-6698-02) are supplied in bottles of 100.

Abbott Laboratories
North Chicago, IL 60064
Ref. 01-2061-R5

TRAL® Gradumet® Tablets ℞
(hexocyclium methylsulfate)

How Supplied: TRAL (hexocyclium methylsulfate) Gradumet, 50 mg, orange-colored tablets, is supplied in bottles of 50 (**NDC** 0074-6920-09).

Abbott Laboratories
North Chicago, IL 60064

TRANXENE® ℞ Ⓒ
(clorazepate dipotassium)
Capsules
Tablets
TRANXENE®-SD & TRANXENE-SD HALF STRENGTH
(clorazepate dipotassium)
Tablets

Description: Chemically, TRANXENE (clorazepate dipotassium) is a benzodiazepine. The empirical formula is $C_{16}H_{11}ClK_2N_2O_4$; the molecular weight is 408.92.

The compound occurs as a fine, light yellow, practically odorless powder. It is insoluble in the common organic solvents, but very soluble in water. Aqueous solutions are unstable, clear, light yellow, and alkaline.

Actions: Pharmacologically, clorazepate dipotassium has the characteristics of the benzodiazepines. It has depressant effects on the central nervous system. The primary metabolite, nordiazepam, quickly appears in the blood stream. The serum half-life is about 2 days. The drug is metabolized in the liver and excreted primarily in the urine. (See ANIMAL AND CLINICAL PHARMACOLOGY section).

Indications: TRANXENE is indicated for the management of anxiety disorders or for the short-term relief of the symptoms of anxiety. Anxiety or tension associated with the stress of everyday life usually does not require treatment with an anxiolytic.

TRANXENE is indicated as adjunctive therapy in the management of partial seizures.

The effectiveness of TRANXENE in long-term management of anxiety, that is, more than 4 months, has not been assessed by systematic clinical studies. Long-term studies in epileptic patients, however, have shown continued therapeutic activity. The physician should reassess periodically the usefulness of the drug for the individual patient.

TRANXENE is indicated for the symptomatic relief of acute alcohol withdrawal.

Contraindications: TRANXENE is contraindicated in patients with a known hypersensitivity to the drug, and in those with acute narrow angle glaucoma.

Warnings: TRANXENE is not recommended for use in depressive neuroses or in psychotic reactions.

Patients on TRANXENE should be cautioned against engaging in hazardous occupations requiring mental alertness, such as operating dangerous machinery including motor vehicles.

Since TRANXENE has a central nervous system depressant effect, patients should be advised against the simultaneous use of other CNS-depressant drugs, and cautioned that the effects of alcohol may be increased.

Because of the lack of sufficient clinical experience, TRANXENE is not recommended for use in patients less than 9 years of age.

Physical and Psychological Dependence: Withdrawal symptoms (similar in character to those noted with barbiturates and alcohol) have occurred following abrupt discontinuance of clorazepate. Symptoms of nervousness, insomnia, irritability, diarrhea, muscle aches and memory impairment have followed abrupt withdrawal after long-term use of high dosage. Withdrawal symptoms have also been reported following abrupt discontinuance of benzodiazepines taken continuously at therapeutic levels for several months. Caution should be observed in patients who are considered to have a psychological potential for drug dependence.

Evidence of drug dependence has been observed in dogs and rabbits which was characterized by convulsive seizures when the drug was abruptly withdrawn or the dose was reduced; the syndrome in dogs could be abolished by administration of clorazepate.

Usage in Pregnancy: **An increased risk of congenital malformations associated with the use of minor tranquilizers (chlordiazepoxide, diazepam, and meprobamate) during the first trimester of pregnancy has been suggested in several studies. TRANXENE, a benzodiazepine derivative, has not been studied adequately to determine whether it, too, may be associated with an increased risk of fetal abnormality. Because use of these drugs is rarely a matter of urgency, their use during this period should almost always be avoided. The possibility that a woman of childbearing potential may be pregnant at the time of institution of therapy should be considered. Patients should be advised that if they become pregnant during therapy or intend to become pregnant they should communicate with their physician about the desirability of discontinuing the drug.**

Usage during Lactation: TRANXENE should not be given to nursing mothers since it has been reported that nordiazepam is excreted in human breast milk.

Precautions: In those patients in which a degree of depression accompanies the anxiety, suicidal tendencies may be present and protective measures may be required. The least amount of drug that is feasible should be available to the patient.

Patients on TRANXENE for prolonged periods should have blood counts and liver function tests periodically. The usual precautions in treating patients with impaired renal or hepatic function should also be observed.

In elderly or debilitated patients, the initial dose should be small, and increments should be made gradually, in accordance with the response of the patient, to preclude ataxia or excessive sedation.

Adverse Reactions: The side effect most frequently reported was drowsiness. Less commonly reported (in descending order of occurrence) were: dizziness, various gastrointestinal complaints, nervousness, blurred vision, dry mouth, headache, and mental confusion. Other side effects included insomnia, transient skin rashes, fatigue, ataxia, genitourinary complaints, irritability, diplopia, depression and slurred speech.

There have been reports of abnormal liver and kidney function tests and of decrease in hematocrit.

Decrease in systolic blood pressure has been observed.

Dosage and Administration: *For the symptomatic relief of anxiety:* TRANXENE capsules and tablets are administered orally in divided doses. The usual daily dose is 30 mg. The dose should be adjusted gradually within the range of 15 to 60 mg daily in accordance with the response of the patient. In elderly or debilitated patients it is advisable to initiate treatment at a daily dose of 7.5 to 15 mg.

TRANXENE capsules and tablets may also be administered in a single dose daily at bedtime; the recommended initial dose is 15 mg. After the initial dose, the response of the patient may require adjustment of subsequent dosage. Lower doses may be indicated in the elderly patient. Drowsiness may occur at the initiation of treatment and with dosage increment.

TRANXENE-SD (22.5 mg tablets) may be administered as a single dose every 24 hours. This tablet is intended as an alternate dosage form for the convenience of patients stabilized on a dose of 7.5 mg capsules or tablets three times a day. TRANXENE-SD should not be used to initiate therapy.

TRANXENE-SD HALF STRENGTH (11.25 mg tablets) may be administered as a single dose every 24 hours.

Continued on next page

If desired, additional literature on any Abbott Product will be provided upon request to Abbott Laboratories.

Abbott—Cont.

For the symptomatic relief of acute alcohol withdrawal:
The following dosage schedule is recommended:

1st 24 hours (Day 1)	30 mg Tranxene, initially; followed by 30 to 60 mg in divided doses
2nd 24 hours (Day 2)	45 to 90 mg in divided doses
3rd 24 hours (Day 3)	22.5 to 45 mg in divided doses
Day 4	15 to 30 mg in divided doses

Thereafter, gradually reduce the daily dose to 7.5 to 15 mg. Discontinue drug therapy as soon as patient's condition is stable.
The maximum recommended total daily dose is 90 mg. Avoid excessive reductions in the total amount of drug administered on successive days.
As an Adjunct to Antiepileptic Drugs:
In order to minimize drowsiness, the recommended initial dosages and dosage increments should not be exceeded.
Adults: The maximum recommended initial dose in patients over 12 years old is 7.5 mg three times a day. Dosage should be increased by no more than 7.5 mg every week and should not exceed 90 mg/day.
Children (9-12 years): The maximum recommended initial dose is 7.5 mg two times a day. Dosage should be increased by no more than 7.5 mg every week and should not exceed 60 mg/day.
Drug Interactions: If TRANXENE is to be combined with other drugs acting on the central nervous system, careful consideration should be given to the pharmacology of the agents to be employed. Animal experience indicates that TRANXENE prolongs the sleeping time after hexobarbital or after ethyl alcohol, increases the inhibitory effects of chlorpromazine, but does not exhibit monoamine oxidase inhibition. Clinical studies have shown increased sedation with concurrent hypnotic medications. The actions of the benzodiazepines may be potentiated by barbiturates, narcotics, phenothiazines, monoamine oxidase inhibitors or other antidepressants.
If TRANXENE is used to treat anxiety associated with somatic disease states, careful attention must be paid to possible drug interaction with concomitant medication.
In bioavailability studies with normal subjects, the concurrent administration of antacids at therapeutic levels did not significantly influence the bioavailability of TRANXENE.
Management of Overdosage: Overdosage is usually manifested by varying degrees of CNS depression ranging from slight sedation to coma. As in the management of overdosage with any drug, it should be borne in mind that multiple agents may have been taken.
There are no specific antidotes for the benzodiazepines. The treatment of overdosage should consist of the general measures employed in the management of overdosage of any CNS depressant. Gastric evacuation either by the induction of emesis, lavage, or both, should be performed immediately. General supportive care, including frequent monitoring of the vital signs and close observation of the patient, is indicated. Hypotension, though rarely reported, may occur with large overdoses. In such cases the use of agents such as Levophed® Bitartrate (norepinephrine bitartrate injection, USP) or Aramine® Injection (metaraminol bitartrate injection, USP) should be considered.
While reports indicate that individuals have survived overdoses of TRANXENE as high as 450 to 675 mg, these doses are not necessarily an accurate indication of the amount of drug absorbed since the time interval between ingestion and the institution of treatment was not always known. Sedation in varying degrees was the most common physiological manifestation of TRANXENE overdosage. Deep coma when it occurred was usually associated with the ingestion of other drugs in addition to TRANXENE.
Animal and Clinical Pharmacology: Studies in rats and monkeys have shown a substantial difference between doses producing tranquilizing, sedative and toxic effects. In rats, conditioned avoidance response was inhibited at an oral dose of 10 mg/kg; sedation was induced at 32 mg/kg; the LD_{50} was 1320 mg/kg. In monkeys aggressive behavior was reduced at an oral dose of 0.25 mg/kg; sedation (ataxia) was induced at 7.5 mg/kg; the LD_{50} could not be determined because of the emetic effect of large doses, but the LD_{50} exceeds 1600 mg/kg. Twenty-four dogs were given TRANXENE orally in a 22-month toxicity study; doses up to 75 mg/kg were given. Drug-related changes occurred in the liver; weight was increased and cholestasis with minimal hepatocellular damage was found, but lobular architecture remained well preserved.
Eighteen rhesus monkeys were given oral doses of TRANXENE from 3 to 36 mg/kg daily for 52 weeks. All treated animals remained similar to control animals. Although total leucocyte count remained within normal limits it tended to fall in the female animals on the highest doses.
Examination of all organs revealed no alterations attributable to TRANXENE. There was no damage to liver function or structure.
Reproduction Studies: Standard fertility, reproduction, and teratology studies were conducted in rats and rabbits. Oral doses in rats up to 150 mg/kg and in rabbits up to 15 mg/kg produced no abnormalities in the fetuses. TRANXENE (clorazepate dipotassium) did not alter the fertility indices or reproductive capacity of adult animals. As expected, the sedative effect of high doses interfered with care of the young by their mothers (see Usage in Pregnancy).
Clinical Pharmacology: Studies in healthy men have shown that TRANXENE has depressant effects on the central nervous system. Prolonged administration of single daily doses as high as 120 mg was without toxic effects. Abrupt cessation of high doses was followed in some patients by nervousness, insomnia, irritability, diarrhea, muscle aches, or memory impairment.
Absorption—Excretion: After oral administration of TRANXENE there is essentially no circulating parent drug. Nordiazepam, its primary metabolite, quickly appears in the blood stream. In 2 volunteers given 15 mg (50 μC) of ^{14}C-Tranxene, about 80% was recovered in the urine and feces within 10 days. Excretion was primarily in the urine with about 1% excreted per day on day 10.

How Supplied: TRANXENE (clorazepate dipotassium) is supplied as:
3.75 mg gray and white capsules:
Bottles of 100 ....(**NDC** 0074-3417-13)
Bottles of 500 ....(**NDC** 0074-3417-53)
ABBO-PAC® unit dose packages:
100 ....(**NDC** 0074-3417-11).
7.5 mg gray and maroon capsules:
Bottles of 100 ....(**NDC** 0074-3418-13)
Bottles of 500 ....(**NDC** 0074-3418-53)
ABBO-PAC unit dose packages:
100 ....(**NDC** 0074-3418-11)
4 cartons of 25
(reverse-numbered) ....(**NDC** 0074-3418-25).
15 mg gray capsules:
Bottles of 100 ....(**NDC** 0074-3419-13)
Bottles of 500 ....(**NDC** 0074-3419-53)
ABBO-PAC unit dose packages:
100 ....(**NDC** 0074-3419-11).
3.75 mg blue-colored, scored tablets:
Bottles of 100 ....(**NDC** 0074-4389-13).
7.5 mg peach-colored, scored tablets:
Bottles of 100 ....(**NDC** 0074-4390-13).
15 mg lavender-colored, scored tablets:
Bottles of 100 ....(**NDC** 0074-4391-13).
TRANXENE-SD 22.5 mg tan-colored, single dose tablets:
Bottles of 100 ....(**NDC** 0074-2997-13).
TRANXENE-SD HALF STRENGTH 11.25 mg blue-colored, single dose tablets:
Bottles of 100 ....(**NDC** 0074-2699-13).
[*Shown in Product Identification Section*]
Abbott Pharmaceuticals, Inc.
North Chicago, IL 60064
Ref. 03-4224-R14

TRIDIONE® ℞
(trimethadione)
Tablets, Capsules, and Oral Solution

BECAUSE OF ITS POTENTIAL TO PRODUCE FETAL MALFORMATIONS AND SERIOUS SIDE EFFECTS, TRIDIONE (trimethadione) SHOULD ONLY BE UTILIZED WHEN OTHER LESS TOXIC DRUGS HAVE BEEN FOUND INEFFECTIVE IN CONTROLLING PETIT MAL SEIZURES.

Description: TRIDIONE (trimethadione) is an antiepileptic agent. An oxazolidinedione compound, it is chemically identified as 3,5,5-trimethyloxazolidine-2,4-dione.
TRIDIONE is a synthetic, water-soluble, white, crystalline powder. It is supplied in capsular, tablet, and liquid forms for oral use only.
Clinical Pharmacology: TRIDIONE has been shown to prevent pentylenetetrazol-induced and thujone-induced seizures in experimental animals; the drug has a less marked effect on seizures induced by picrotoxin, procaine, cocaine, or strychnine. Unlike the hydantoins and antiepileptic barbiturates, TRIDIONE does not modify the maximal seizure pattern in patients undergoing electroconvulsive therapy.
TRIDIONE has a sedative effect that may increase to the point of ataxia when excessive doses are used. A toxic dose of the drug in animals (approximately 2 Gm/kg) produced sleep, unconsciousness, and respiratory depression.
Trimethadione is rapidly absorbed from the gastrointestinal tract. It is demethylated by liver microsomes to the active metabolite, dimethadione.
Approximately 3% of a daily dose of TRIDIONE is recovered in the urine as unchanged drug. The majority of trimethadione is excreted slowly by the kidney in the form of dimethadione.
Indications: TRIDIONE (trimethadione) is indicated for the control of petit mal seizures that are refractory to treatment with other drugs.
Contraindications: TRIDIONE is contraindicated in patients with a known hypersensitivity to the drug.
Warnings: TRIDIONE may cause serious side effects. Strict medical supervision of the patient is mandatory, especially during the initial year of therapy.
TRIDIONE (trimethadione) should be withdrawn promptly if skin rash appears, because of the grave possibility of the occurrence of exfoliative dermatitis or severe forms of erythema multiforme. Even a minor acneiform or morbilliform rash should be allowed to clear completely before treatment with TRIDIONE is resumed; reinstitute therapy cautiously.
A complete blood count should be done prior to initiating therapy with TRIDIONE, and at monthly intervals thereafter. A marked depression of the blood count is an indication for withdrawal of the drug. If no abnormality appears within 12 months, the interval between blood counts may be extended. A moderate

degree of neutropenia with or without a corresponding drop in the leukocyte count is not uncommon. Therapy need not be withdrawn unless the neutrophil count is 2500 or less; more frequent blood examinations should be done when the count is less than 3,000. Other blood dyscrasias, including leukopenia, eosinophilia, thrombocytopenia, pancytopenia, agranulocytosis, hypoplastic anemia, and fatal aplastic anemia, have occurred. Patients should be advised to report immediately such signs and symptoms as sore throat, fever, malaise, easy bruising, petechiae, or epistaxis, or others that may be indicative of an infection or bleeding tendency. TRIDIONE should ordinarily not be used in patients with severe blood dyscrasias.

Liver function tests should be done prior to initiating therapy with TRIDIONE, and at monthly intervals thereafter. Hepatitis has been reported rarely. Jaundice or other signs of liver dysfunction are an indication for withdrawal of the drug. TRIDIONE should ordinarily not be used in patients with severe hepatic impairment.

A urinalysis should be done prior to initiating therapy with TRIDIONE and at monthly intervals thereafter. Fatal nephrosis has been reported. Persistent or increasing albuminuria, or the development of any other significant renal abnormality, is an indication for withdrawal of the drug. TRIDIONE should ordinarily not be used in patients with severe renal dysfunction.

Hemeralopia has occurred; this appears to be an effect of TRIDIONE on the neural layers of the retina, and usually can be reversed by a reduction in dosage. Scotomata are an indication for withdrawal of the drug. Caution should be observed when treating patients who have diseases of the retina or optic nerve.

Manifestations of systemic lupus erythematosus have been associated with the use of TRIDIONE, as they have with the use of certain other anticonvulsants. Lymphadenopathies simulating malignant lymphoma have occurred. Lupus-like manifestations or lymph node enlargement are indications for withdrawal of the drug. Signs and symptoms may disappear after discontinuation of therapy, and specific treatment may be unnecessary.

A myasthenia gravis-like syndrome has been associated with the chronic use of trimethadione. Symptoms suggestive of this condition are indications for withdrawal of the drug.

Drugs known to cause toxic effects similar to those of TRIDIONE should be avoided or used only with extreme caution during therapy with TRIDIONE.

USAGE DURING PREGNANCY AND LACTATION:

THERE ARE MULTIPLE REPORTS IN THE CLINICAL LITERATURE WHICH INDICATE THAT THE USE OF ANTICONVULSANT DRUGS DURING PREGNANCY RESULTS IN AN INCREASED INCIDENCE OF BIRTH DEFECTS IN THE OFFSPRING. DATA ARE MORE EXTENSIVE WITH RESPECT TO TRIMETHADIONE, PARAMETHADIONE, PHENYTOIN AND PHENOBARBITAL THAN WITH OTHER ANTICONVULSANT DRUGS.

THEREFORE, ANTICONVULSANT DRUGS SUCH AS TRIDIONE (TRIMETHADIONE) SHOULD BE ADMINISTERED TO WOMEN OF CHILDBEARING POTENTIAL ONLY IF THEY ARE CLEARLY SHOWN TO BE ESSENTIAL IN THE MANAGEMENT OF THEIR SEIZURES. EFFECTIVE MEANS OF CONTRACEPTION SHOULD ACCOMPANY THE USE OF TRIDIONE IN SUCH PATIENTS. IF A PATIENT BECOMES PREGNANT WHILE TAKING TRIDIONE, TERMINATION OF THE PREGNANCY SHOULD BE CONSIDERED. A PATIENT WHO REQUIRES THERAPY WITH TRIDIONE AND WHO WISHES TO BECOME PREGNANT SHOULD BE ADVISED OF THE RISKS.

REPORTS HAVE SUGGESTED THAT THE MATERNAL INGESTION OF ANTICONVULSANT DRUGS, PARTICULARLY BARBITURATES, IS ASSOCIATED WITH A NEONATAL COAGULATION DEFECT THAT MAY CAUSE BLEEDING DURING THE EARLY (USUALLY WITHIN 24 HOURS OF BIRTH) NEONATAL PERIOD. THE POSSIBILITY OF THE OCCURRENCE OF THIS DEFECT WITH THE USE OF TRIDIONE SHOULD BE KEPT IN MIND. THE DEFECT IS CHARACTERIZED BY DECREASED LEVELS OF VITAMIN K-DEPENDENT CLOTTING FACTORS, AND PROLONGATION OF EITHER THE PROTHROMBIN TIME OR THE PARTIAL THROMBOPLASTIN TIME, OR BOTH. IT HAS BEEN SUGGESTED THAT PROPHYLACTIC VITAMIN K BE GIVEN TO THE MOTHER ONE MONTH PRIOR TO, AND DURING DELIVERY, AND TO THE INFANT, INTRAVENOUSLY, IMMEDIATELY AFTER BIRTH.

THE SAFETY OF TRIDIONE FOR USE DURING LACTATION HAS NOT BEEN ESTABLISHED.

Precautions: Abrupt discontinuation of TRIDIONE may precipitate petit mal status. TRIDIONE should always be withdrawn gradually unless serious adverse effects dictate otherwise. In the latter case, another anticonvulsant may be substituted to protect the patient.

Usage during Pregnancy and Lactation: See WARNINGS.

Adverse Reactions: The following side effects, some of them serious, have been associated with the use of TRIDIONE.

Gastrointestinal: nausea, vomiting, abdominal pain, gastric distress.

CNS/Neurologic: drowsiness, fatigue, malaise, insomnia, vertigo, headache, paresthesias, precipitation of grand mal seizures, increased irritability, personality changes.

Drowsiness usually subsides with continued therapy. If it persists, a reduction in dosage is indicated.

Hematologic: bleeding gums, epistaxis, retinal and petechial hemorrhages, vaginal bleeding; neutropenia, leukopenia, eosinophilia, thrombocytopenia, pancytopenia, agranulocytosis, hypoplastic anemia, and fatal aplastic anemia.

Dermatologic: acneiform or morbilliform skin rash that may progress to exfoliative dermatitis or to severe forms of erythema multiforme.

Other: hiccups, anorexia, weight loss, hair loss, changes in blood pressure, albuminuria, hemeralopia, photophobia, diplopia.

Fatal nephrosis has occurred.

Hepatitis has been reported rarely.

Lupus erythematosus, and lymphadenopathies simulating malignant lymphoma, have been reported.

Pruritus associated with lymphadenopathy and hepatosplenomegaly has occurred in hypersensitive individuals.

A myasthenia gravis-like syndrome has been reported.

Overdosage: Symptoms of acute TRIDIONE overdosage include drowsiness, nausea, dizziness, ataxia, visual disturbances. Coma may follow massive overdosage.

Gastric evacuation, either by induced emesis, or by lavage, or both, should be done immediately. General supportive care, including frequent monitoring of the vital signs and close observation of the patient, are required.

Alkalinization of the urine has been reported to enhance the renal excretion of dimethadione, the active metabolite of TRIDIONE.

A blood count and a careful evaluation of hepatic and renal function should be done following recovery.

Dosage and Administration: TRIDIONE is administered orally.

Usual Adult Dosage: 0.9–2.4 Gm daily in 3 or 4 equally divided doses (i.e. 300–600 mg 3 or 4 times daily).

Initially, give 0.9 Gm daily; increase this dose by 300 mg at weekly intervals until therapeutic results are seen or until toxic symptoms appear.

Maintenance dosage should be the least amount of drug required to maintain control.

Children's Dosage: Usually 0.3–0.9 Gm daily in 3 or 4 equally divided doses.

How Supplied: TRIDIONE Capsules (trimethadione capsules, USP), 300 mg (white) are supplied in bottles of 100 (**NDC** 0074-3709-01).

TRIDIONE Dulcet® Tablets (trimethadione tablets, USP), 150 mg (white) chewable tablets are supplied in bottles of 100 (**NDC** 0074-3753-01).

[*Shown in Product Identification Section*]

TRIDIONE Solution (trimethadione oral solution, USP), 1.2 Gm per fluidounce (40 mg per ml), is supplied in pint bottles (**NDC** 0074-3721-01).

Abbott Laboratories/
Abbott Pharmaceuticals, Inc.
North Chicago, IL 60064
®Dulcet—Sweetened tablets, Abbott.
Ref. 03-4194/R3

TRONOLANE™ OTC
(pramoxine hydrochloride)
Cream, Suppositories

Description: Tronolane contains pramoxine hydrochloride a surface anesthetic agent, chemically unrelated to the benzoate esters of the "caine" type, which is chemically designated as a 4-n-butoxyphenyl gammamorpholinopropyl- ether hydrochloride.

Indications: Tronolane is indicated for use as a topical anesthetic to relieve pain, burning, itching and discomfort that accompanies hemorrhoids. It also has a soothing, lubricant action on mucous membranes.

Tronolane contains an excellent rapidly acting topical anesthetic with surface analgesia that lasts up to 5 hours. It fills a conspicuous gap among anesthetics by combining: prompt and potent relief from surface pain or itching, with almost complete freedom from toxicity and sensitization. Since the drug is chemically unrelated to other anesthetics, cross-sensitization is unlikely. Patients who are already sensitized to the "caine" drugs or other anesthetics can generally use Tronolane with excellent results.

Tronolane provides a desirable combination of properties—low toxicity, low sensitization, and structural individuality, together with prompt and adequate anesthetic effect.

Tronolane provides adjunctive therapy for the symptomatic relief of pain and discomfort in external and internal hemorrhoids.

The special emollient/emulsion base of the cream provides soothing lubrication making bowel movements easier and more comfortable. Tronolane cream is a bland, non-toxic, well balanced formula in a non-drying base which is nongreasy, not messy, and nonstaining to undergarments.

Warnings: If bleeding is present, consult physician. Certain persons can develop allergic reactions to ingredients in this product. During treatment, if condition worsens or persists 7 days, consult physician. For children under 12 years, use only as directed by physician.

Dosage and Administration: CREAM: Apply up to five times daily, especially morning, night and after bowel movements or as directed by physician.

External—Apply liberally to affected area.

Intrarectal—Remove protective cover from clean applicator, lubricate with small amount of Tronolane, gently insert applicator into rectum and squeeze tube. Thoroughly cleanse applicator with soap after use.

Continued on next page

If desired, additional literature on any Abbott Product will be provided upon request to Abbott Laboratories.

Abbott—Cont.

Dosage and Administration: SUPPOSITORIES: Use up to five times daily, especially morning, night, and after bowel movements, or as directed by physician. Detach one suppository from pack. Tear notch at pointed end and remove wrapper before insertion. Insert suppository into the rectum, pointed end first.
How Supplied: Tronolane is available in 1-oz., 2-oz. cream tubes and 10 and 20 count suppository boxes.

TRONOTHANE® HYDROCHLORIDE

(pramoxine hydrochloride)
Cream, Jelly

Description: Tronothane Hydrochloride (pramoxine hydrochloride) is a surface anesthetic agent, chemically unrelated to the benzoate esters of the "caine" type. It is chemically designated as 4-n-butoxyphenyl gammamorpholinopropyl ether hydrochloride.
Indications: Tronothane Hydrochloride is indicated as a surface anesthetic to relieve pain and itching associated with dermatoses, ano-genital pruritis, hemorrhoids, anal fissure and minor burns.
Contraindications: Tronothane Hydrochloride is not suitable for and should not be injected into the tissues. It should not be used in the eye or nose, for bronchoscopy or gastroscopy, or in patients who are hypersensitive to the drug.
Precautions: Tronothane Hydrochloride should not be applied to extensive areas of skin, and is not intended for indefinitely prolonged use. Discontinue use if redness, irritation, swelling or pain occur.
Adverse Reactions: Local skin reactions, e.g. stinging and burning.
Dosage and Administration: Tronothane Hydrochloride 1% Cream and 1% Jelly are applied externally, directly to the area affected every three to four hours as needed. In cases of severe discomfort, the medication may be applied every two hours.
How Supplied: Tronothane Hydrochloride 1% Cream (pramoxine hydrochloride cream, USP), pramoxine hydrochloride 1% in a water miscible base containing cetyl alcohol, cetyl esters wax, glycerin, sodium lauryl sulfate, methylparaben, and propylparaben, is supplied in a 1-oz tube with rectal applicator (**NDC** 0074-6645-01).
Tronothane Hydrochloride 1% Jelly (pramoxine hydrochloride jelly, USP), pramoxine hydrochloride 1% in a water soluble base containing propylene glycol, and hydroxypropyl methylcellulose, is supplied in a 1-oz tube with rectal applicator (**NDC** 0074-6650-01).
These products are listed in USP, a Medicare designated compendium.
Abbott Laboratories
North Chicago, IL 60064

If desired, additional literature on any Abbott Product will be provided upon request to Abbott Laboratories.

Adria Laboratories Inc.

5000 POST ROAD
DUBLIN, OH 43017

(includes products formerly marketed by Warren-Teed Laboratories)

PRODUCT IDENTIFICATION CODES

To provide quick and positive identification of Adria Laboratories Inc. products, we have imprinted the product identification number on one side of all tablets and capsules. The other side of the tablet displays the name "ADRIA".

PRODUCT IDENTIFICATION CODE	NUMERICAL PRODUCT INDEX
200	Ilozyme® (pancrelipase, USP) Tablets
231	Ilopan-Choline® Tablets (dexpanthenol 50 mg./choline bitartrate 25 mg)
304	Kaon CL™-10 (potassium chloride) Controlled Release Tablets, 750 mg. (10 mEq)
305	Kaochlor-Eff® Tablets (potassium and chloride) 20 mEq.
307	Kaon-CL™ (potassium chloride) Controlled Release Tablets, 500 mg (6.7 mEq)
312	Kaon® (potassium gluconate) Tablets, 1.7 g (5 mEq)
412	Magan® (magnesium salicylate) Tablets, 545 mg.
648	Fluidil™ (cyclothiazide, USP) 2 mg.

In order that you may quickly identify a product by its code number, we have compiled below a numerical list of code numbers of prescription products with their corresponding product names:
[See table below].

ADRIAMYCIN™ ℞

(doxorubicin hydrochloride)
for Injection
FOR INTRAVENOUS USE ONLY

WARNINGS

1. Severe local tissue necrosis will occur if there is extravasation during administration.
(See Dosage and Administration.)
Adriamycin must not be given by the intramuscular or subcutaneous route.
2. Serious irreversible myocardial toxicity with delayed congestive failure often unresponsive to any cardiac supportive therapy may be encountered as total dosage approaches 550 mg/m^2. This toxicity may occur at lower cumulative doses in patients with prior mediastinal irradiation or on concurrent cyclophosphamide therapy.
3. Dosage should be reduced in patients with impaired hepatic function.
4. Severe myelosuppression may occur.
5. Adriamycin should be administered only under the supervision of a physician who is experienced in the use of cancer chemotherapeutic agents.

Description: Doxorubicin is a cytotoxic anthracycline antibiotic isolated from cultures of Streptomyces peucetius var. caesius. It is supplied in the hydrochloride form as a freeze-dried powder containing lactose.
Clinical Pharmacology: Though not completely elucidated, the mechanism of action of doxorubicin is related to its ability to bind to DNA and inhibit nucleic acid synthesis. Cell culture studies have demonstrated rapid cell penetration and perinucleolar chromatin binding, rapid inhibition of mitotic activity and nucleic acid synthesis, mutagenesis and chromosomal aberrations. Animal studies have shown activity in a spectrum of experimental tumors, immunosuppression, carcinogenic properties in rodents, induction of a variety of toxic effects, including delayed and progressive cardiac toxicity, myelosuppression in all species and atrophy to testes in rats and dogs.
Pharmacokinetic studies show the intravenous administration of normal or radiolabeled Adriamycin (doxorubicin hydrochloride) for Injection is followed by rapid plasma clearance and significant tissue binding. Urinary excretion, as determined by fluorimetric methods, accounts for approximately 4-5% of the administered dose in five days. Biliary excretion represents the major excretion route, 40-50% of the administered dose being recovered in the bile or the feces in seven days. Impairment of liver function results in slower excretion, and consequently, increased retention and accumulation in plasma and tissues. Adriamycin does not cross the blood brain barrier.
Indications: Adriamycin has been used successfully to produce regression in disseminated neoplastic conditions such as acute lymphoblastic leukemia, acute myeloblastic leukemia, Wilms' tumor, neuroblastoma, soft tissue and bone sarcomas, breast carcinoma, ovarian carcinoma, transitional cell bladder carcinoma, thyroid carcinoma, lymphomas of both Hodgkin and non-Hodgkin types and bronchogenic carcinoma in which the small cell histologic type is the most responsive compared to other cell types. A number of other solid tumors have also shown some responsiveness but in numbers too limited to justify specific recommendation. Studies to date have shown malignant melanoma, kidney carcinoma, large bowel carcinoma, brain tumors and metastases to the central nervous system not to be significantly responsive to Adriamycin therapy.
Contraindications: Adriamycin therapy should not be started in patients who have marked myelosuppression induced by previous treatment with other antitumor agents or by radiotherapy. Conclusive data are not available on pre-existing heart disease as a co-factor of increased risk of Adriamycin induced cardiac toxicity. Preliminary data suggest that in such cases cardiac toxicity may occur at doses lower than the recommended cumulative limit. It is therefore not recommended to start Adriamycin in such cases. Adriamycin treatment is contraindicated in patients who received previous treatment with complete cumulative doses of Adriamycin and/or daunorubicin.
Warnings: Special attention must be given to the cardiac toxicity exhibited by Adriamycin. Although uncommon, acute left ventricular failure has occurred, particularly in patients who have received total dosage of the drug exceeding the currently recommended limit of 550 mg/m^2. This limit appears to be lower (400 mg/m^2) in patients who received radiotherapy to the mediastinal area or concomitant therapy with other potentially cardiotoxic agents such as cyclophosphamide. The total dose of Adriamycin administered to the individual patient should also take into account a previous or concomitant therapy with related compounds such as daunorubicin. Congestive heart failure and/or cardiomyopathy may be encountered several weeks after discontinuation of Adriamycin therapy.
Cardiac failure is often not favorably affected by presently known medical or physical therapy for cardiac support. Early clinical diagnosis of drug induced heart failure appears to be essential for successful treatment with digitalis, diuretics, low salt diet and bed rest. Severe cardiac toxicity may occur precipitously without antecedent EKG changes. A baseline EKG

and EKGs performed prior to each dose or course after 300 mg/m^2 cumulative dose has been given is suggested. Transient EKG changes consisting of T-wave flattening, S-T depression and arrhythmias lasting for up to two weeks after a dose or course of Adriamycin are presently not considered indications for suspension of Adriamycin therapy. Adriamycin cardiomyopathy has been reported to be associated with a persistent reduction in the voltage of the QRS wave, a prolongation of the systolic time interval and a reduction of the ejection fraction as determined by echocardiography or radionuclide angiography. None of these tests have yet been confirmed to consistently identify those individual patients that are approaching their maximally tolerated cumulative dose of Adriamycin. If test results indicate change in cardiac function associated with Adriamycin the benefit of continued therapy must be carefully evaluated against the risk of producing irreversible cardiac damage.
Acute life-threatening arrhythmias have been reported to occur during or within a few hours after Adriamycin administration.
There is a high incidence of bone marrow depression, primarily of leukocytes, requiring careful hematologic monitoring. With the recommended dosage schedule, leukopenia is usually transient, reaching its nadir at 10-14 days after treatment with recovery usually occurring by the 21st day. White blood cell counts as low as 1000/mm^3 are to be expected during treatment with appropriate doses of Adriamycin. Red blood cell and platelet levels should also be monitored since they may also be depressed. Hematologic toxicity may require dose reduction or suspension or delay of Adriamycin therapy. Persistent severe myelosuppression may result in superinfection or hemorrhage.
Adriamycin may potentiate the toxicity of other anticancer therapies. Exacerbation of cyclophosphamide induced hemorrhagic cystitis and enhancement of the hepatotoxicity of 6-mercaptopurine have been reported. Radiation induced toxicity to the myocardium, mucosae, skin and liver have been reported to be increased by the administration of Adriamycin.
Toxicity to recommended doses of Adriamycin is enhanced by hepatic impairment, therefore, prior to the individual dosing, evaluation of hepatic function is recommended using conventional clinical laboratory tests such as SGOT, SGPT, alkaline phosphatase and bilirubin. (See Dosage and Administration.)
On intravenous administration of Adriamycin extravasation may occur with or without an accompanying stinging or burning sensation and even if blood returns well on aspiration of the infusion needle. (See Dosage and Administration.) If any signs or symptoms of extravasation have occurred the injection or infusion should be immediately terminated and restarted in another vein.
Adriamycin and related compounds have also been shown to have mutagenic and carcinogenic properties when tested in experimental models.
Usage in Pregnancy—Safe use of Adriamycin in pregnancy has not been established. Adriamycin is embryotoxic and teratogenic in rats and embryotoxic and abortifacient in rabbits. Therefore, the benefits to the pregnant patient should be carefully weighed against the potential toxicity to fetus and embryo. The possible adverse effects on fertility in males and females in humans or experimental animals have not been adequately evaluated.
Precautions: Initial treatment with Adriamycin requires close observation of the patient and extensive laboratory monitoring. It is recommended, therefore, that patients be hospitalized at least during the first phase of the treatment.
Like other cytotoxic drugs, Adriamycin may induce hyperuricemia secondary to rapid lysis of neoplastic cells. The clinician should monitor the patient's blood uric acid level and be prepared to use such supportive and pharmacologic measures as might be necessary to control this problem.
Adriamycin imparts a red coloration to the urine for 1-2 days after administration and patients should be advised to expect this during active therapy.
Adriamycin is not an anti-microbial agent.
Adverse Reactions: Dose limiting toxicities of therapy are myelosuppression and cardiotoxicity. (See Warnings.) Other reactions reported are:
Cutaneous—Reversible complete alopecia occurs in most cases. Hyperpigmentation of nailbeds and dermal creases, primarily in children, have been reported in a few cases. Recall of skin reaction due to prior radiotherapy has occurred with Adriamycin administration.
Gastrointestinal—Acute nausea and vomiting occurs frequently and may be severe. This may be alleviated by antiemetic therapy. Muscositis (stomatitis and esophagitis) may occur 5-10 days after administration. The effect may be severe leading to ulceration and represent a site of origin for severe infections. The dose regimen consisting of administration of Adriamycin on three successive days results in the greater incidence and severity of mucositis. Anorexia and diarrhea have been occasionally reported.
Vascular—Phlebosclerosis has been reported especially when small veins are used or a single vein is used for repeated administration. Facial flushing may occur if the injection is given too rapidly.
Local—Severe cellulitis, vesication and tissue necrosis will occur if Adriamycin is extravasated during administration. Erythematous streaking along the vein proximal to the site of the injection has been reported. (See Dosage and Administration.)
Hypersensitivity—Fever, chills and urticaria have been reported occasionally. Anaphylaxis may occur. A case of apparent cross sensitivity to lincomycin has been reported.
Other—Conjunctivitis and lacrimation occur rarely.
Dosage and Administration: Care in the administration of Adriamycin will reduce the chance of perivenous infiltration. It may also decrease the chance of local reactions such as urticaria and erythematous streaking. On intravenous administration of Adriamycin, extravasation may occur with or without an accompanying stinging or burning sensation and even if blood returns well on aspiration of the infusion needle. If any signs or symptoms of extravasation have occurred, the injection or infusion should be immediately terminated and restarted in another vein. If it is known or suspected that subcutaneous extravasation has occurred, local infiltration with an injectable corticosteroid and flooding the site with normal saline has been reported to lessen the local reaction. Because of the progressive nature of extravasation reactions, the area of injection should be frequently examined and plastic surgery consultation obtained. If ulceration begins, early wide excision of the involved area should be considered.[1]
The recommended dosage schedule is 60-75 mg/m^2 as a single intravenous injection administered at 21-day intervals. The lower dose should be given to patients with inadequate marrow reserves due to old age, or prior therapy, or neoplastic marrow infiltration. An alternative dose schedule is 30 mg/m^2 on each of three successive days repeated every 4 weeks.
Adriamycin dosage must be reduced if the bilirubin is elevated as follows: Serum Bilirubin 1.2-3.0 mg 100 ml-give ½ normal dose, > 3 mg/100 ml-give ¼ normal dose.
Preparation of Solution: Adriamycin 10 mg vials and 50 mg vials should be reconstituted with 5 ml and 25 ml respectively of Sodium Chloride injection USP (0.9%) or Sterile Water for Injection USP to give a final concentration of 2 mg/ml of doxorubicin hydrochloride. If Sterile Water for Injection USP is used for reconstitution, the resulting solution must be brought towards isotonicity before injection by adding 2 to 3 times the volume of 0.9% Sodium Chloride Injection USP to the aqueous solution. An appropriate volume of air should be withdrawn from the vial during reconstitution to avoid excessive pressure build-up. Bacteriostatic diluents are not recommended.
Skin reactions associated with Adriamycin have been reported. Caution in the handling and preparation of the powder and solution must be exercised and the use of gloves is recommended. If Adriamycin powder or solution contacts the skin or mucosae, immediately wash thoroughly with soap and water.
After adding the diluent, the vial should be shaken and the contents allowed to dissolve. The reconstituted solution is stable for 24 hours at room temperature and 48 hours under refrigeration (4-10°C). It should be protected from exposure to sunlight and any unused solution should be discarded.
It is recommended that Adriamycin be slowly administered into the tubing of a freely running intravenous infusion of Sodium Chloride Injection USP or 5% Dextrose Injection USP. The tubing should be attached to a Butterfly® needle inserted preferably into a large vein. If possible, avoid veins over joints or in extremities with compromised venous or lymphatic drainage. The rate of administration is dependent on the size of the vein and the dosage. However the dose should be administered in not less than 3 to 5 minutes. Local erythematous streaking along the vein as well as facial flushing may be indicative of too rapid an administration. A burning or stinging sensation may be indicative of perivenous infiltration and the infusion should be immediately terminated and restarted in another vein. Perivenous infiltration may occur painlessly.
Adriamycin should not be mixed with heparin or 5-fluorouracil since it has been reported that these drugs are incompatible to the extent that a precipitate may form. Until specific compatibility data are available, it is not recommended that Adriamycin be mixed with other drugs.
Adriamycin has been used in combination with other approved chemotherapeutic agents. Though evidence is available that at least in some types of neoplastic disease combination chemotherapy is superior to single agents, the benefits and risks of such therapy have not yet been fully elucidated.
How Supplied: ADRIAMYCIN^{tm} (doxorubicin hydrochloride) for injection is available in two sizes:
10 mg—Each vial contains 10 mg of doxorubicin HCl and 50 mg of lactose USP as a sterile red-orange lyophilized powder. Packaged and supplied in 10-vial cartons NDC 0013-1006-91.
50 mg—Each vial contains 50 mg of doxorubicin HCl and 250 mg of lactose USP as a sterile red-orange lyophilized powder. Packaged and supplied in a single vial carton NDC 0013-1016-79.
Distributed by: Adria Laboratories Inc., Columbus, Ohio 43215. Manufactured by: Farmitalia Carlo Erba S.p.A., Italy
[1]Rudolph, R. et al: Skin Ulcers Due to Adriamycin. Cancer 38:1087–1094, Sept., 1976

ADRUCIL® ℞
(fluorouracil, USP)
INJECTABLE
FOR INTRAVENOUS USE ONLY

WARNINGS
Adrucil should be administered only by or under the supervision of a qualified physi-

Continued on next page

Adria—Cont.

cian who is experienced in cancer chemotherapy and the use of potent antimetabolites. Because severe toxic reactions may occur, it is recommended that patients be hospitalized during the initial course of therapy. Before administering Adrucil, the contents of this insert should be thoroughly reviewed.

Description: Fluorouracil is a fluorinated pyrimidine belonging to the category of antimetabolites. Fluorouracil resembles the natural uracil molecule except it has been fluorinated in the 5 position.

It is sparingly soluble in water (12.2 mg/ml) at pH 7 and has pK's of 8.0 and 13.0.

Adrucil (Fluorouracil, USP) Injectable is supplied as a sterile aqueous solution for intravenous injection. It has pH of 8.6 to 9.0. The ampules are filled with a 5% excess to permit withdrawal and administration of the labeled volume.

A precipitate may form as a result of exposure to low temperatures. Redissolve by heating to 140°F (60°C) with vigorous shaking, and allow to cool to body temperature prior to use.

Actions: The mechanism of action of fluorouracil is mainly related to competitive inhibition of thymidylate synthetase, the enzyme catalyzing the methylation of deoxyuridylic acid to thymidylic acid. The consequent thymidine deficiency results in inhibition of deoxyribonucleic acid (DNA) synthesis, thus inducing cell death. Also, moderate inhibition of ribonucleic acid (RNA) and incorporation of fluorouracil into RNA have been observed, but these effects do not appear to play a significant role in the determination of the antitumor action of fluorouracil.

The effects of DNA and RNA deprivation are most marked on those cells which grow rapidly and which take up fluorouracil at more rapid pace. Inactive degradation products (e.g., CO_2, urea, α-fluoro-β-alanine) result from the extensive catabolic metabolism of fluorouracil. Following intravenous injection, no intact drug can be detected in the plasma after 3 hours and 60 to 80% of the dose is excreted as respiratory Co_2 in 8 to 12 hours. Within 6 hours approximately 15% of the total drug administered is excreted unchanged in the urine with over 90% of this excretion occurring in the first hour.

Indications: Adrucil is effective in the palliative management of carcinoma of the colon, rectum, breast, stomach and pancreas in patients who are considered incurable by surgery or other means.

Contraindications: Adrucil therapy should not be started in patients with a poor nutritional state, depressed bone marrow function, or potentially serious infections.

Warnings: THE DAILY DOSE OF ADRUCIL IS NOT TO EXCEED 800 MG AND IT IS RECOMMENDED THAT PATIENTS BE HOSPITALIZED DURING THEIR FIRST COURSE OF TREATMENT.

Adrucil (Fluorouracil, USP) should be used with extreme caution in poor risk patients with a history of high-dose pelvic irradiation, previous use of alkylating agents, or who have a widespread involvement of bone marrow by metastatic tumors, or impaired hepatic or renal function. The drug is not intended as an adjuvant to surgery. Although severe toxicity and fatalities are more likely to occur in poor risk patients, these effects have occasionally been encountered in patients in relatively good condition. Severe hematologic toxicity, gastrointestinal hemorrhage, and even death may result from use of Adrucil (Fluorouracil, USP) despite meticulous selection of patients and careful adjustment of dosage.

Usage in Pregnancy: Safe use of Adrucil (Fluorouracil, USP) has not been established with respect to adverse effects on fetal development. Therefore, this drug should not be used during pregnancy, particularly in the first trimester, unless in the judgement of the physician the potential benefits to the patient outweigh the hazards.

Because the risk of mutagenesis has not been evaluated, such possible effects on males and females must be considered.

Combination Therapy: Any form of therapy which adds to the stress of the patient, interfers with nutrition or depresses bone marrow function will increase the toxicity of Adrucil (Fluorouracil, USP).

Precautions: Adrucil (Fluorouracil, USP) is a highly toxic drug with a narrow margin of safety. Special attention must be given to the toxicity exhibited by fluorouracil. Patients should be carefully supervised since it must be recognized that therapeutic response is unlikely to occur without some evidence of toxicity. Patients should be advised of expected toxic effects, especially oral manifestations. White blood counts with differential are recommended before each dose. Knowledge of WBC nadir is necessary for eventual subsequent dosage adjustments.

Administration of Adrucil (Fluorouracil, USP) is to be discontinued promptly when one of the following signs appear:

1. Stomatitis or esophagopharyngitis (at first visible sign)
2. Leukopenia (WBC $<$ 3500 mm^3) or rapidly falling white blood count
3. Vomiting (intractable)
4. Diarrhea (frequent bowel movements or watery stools)
5. Gastrointestinal ulceration and bleeding
6. Thrombocytopenia (platelets $<$ 100,000 mm^3)
7. Hemorrhage (from any site)

Adverse Reactions: Stomatitis and esophagopharyngitis (which may lead to sloughing and ulceration), diarrhea, anorexia, nausea and emesis are common.

Myelosuppression almost uniformly accompanies a course of adequate therapy with fluorouracil. Low WBC counts are usually first observed between the 9th and 14th day after the first course of treatment with nadir occurring during the third week, although at times delayed for as long as 25 days. By the 30th day the count is usually within the normal range. Thrombocytopenia also may occur.

Alopecia and dermatitis are seen in a substantial number of cases and patients should be advised of this consequence of treatment. The alopecia is reported to be reversible. The dermatitis is often a pruritic maculopapular rash generally appearing on the extremities and less frequently on the trunk. It is usually reversible and responsive to symptomatic treatment. Dry skin and fissuring have also been noted.

Photosensitivity, as manifested by erythema or increased pigmentation of the skin, may occasionally occur. Also reported were photophobia, lacrimation, epistaxis, euphoria, acute cerebellar syndrome (which may persist following discontinuation of treatment) and nail changes including loss of nails. Myocardial ischemia has also been reported.

Dosage and Administration:

Note:

The recommended route of administration of Adrucil is only by intravenous injection, using care to avoid extravasation. No dilution of Adrucil is required.

It is recommended that all dosages be based on the patient's actual weight. However, if the patient is obese or if there has been a spurious weight gain due to edema, ascites, or other forms of abnormal fluid retention, then the estimated lean body mass (dry weight) should be used.

Prior to treatment, it is recommended that each patient be carefully evaluated to accurately estimate the optimum initial dosage of Adrucil.

Initial Therapy (See Contraindications, Warnings and Precautions before prescribing):

I. A dose of 12 mg/kg is given intravenously once daily for 4 successive days. The daily dose should not be more than 800 mg. If no toxicity is observed at any time during the course of therapy, 6 mg/kg are given on the 6th, 8th, 10th and 12th days. No therapy is given on the 5th, 7th, 9th or 11th days. Therapy is to be discontinued at the end of the 12th day, even if no toxicity has become apparent.

II. In poor risk patients or those who are not in an adequate nutritional state, a dose level of 6 mg/kg/day for 3 days is recommended. If no toxicity is observed at any time during the treatment, 3 mg/kg may be given on the 5th, 7th and 9th days. No therapy is given on the 4th, 6th or 8th days. The daily dose should not exceed 400 mg.

A sequence of injections on either schedule constitutes a "course of therapy."

Therapy should be discontinued promptly when any of the signs of toxicity listed under PRECAUTIONS appears.

Maintenance Therapy: When toxicity has not been a problem, or after the toxic signs from the initial course of therapy have subsided, therapy should be continued using either of the following schedules:

A. Repeat dosage of the first course, beginning 30 days after the last day of the previous course of treatment.

B. Administer a maintenance dosage of 10 to 15 mg/kg/week. Do not exceed 1 gram per week. Reduced doses should be used for poor risk patients.

The dosage of drug to be used should take into account the patient's reaction to the previous course of therapy and be adjusted accordingly. Some patients have received from 9 to 45 courses of treatment during periods which ranged from 12 to 60 months.

Adrucil (Fluorouracil, USP) should not be mixed with IV additives or chemotherapeutic agents.

How Supplied: Adrucil (Fluorouracil, USP) Injectable is available in 10 ml ampules, as a colorless to faint yellow aqueous solution containing 500 mg of fluorouracil and pH adjusted with sodium hydroxide to 8.6 to 9.0. Packaged and supplied in individual cartons, there are 10 ampules per shelf container NDC 0013-1026-91.

NOTE: Although Adrucil ampule solution may discolor slightly during storage, the potency and safety are not adversely affected. Store at room temperature 59–86°F (15–30°C) and protect from light. If a precipitate occurs due to exposure to low temperatures, re-solubilize by heating to 140°F (60°C) with vigorous shaking; allow to cool to body temperature before using.

Distributed by: Adria Laboratories Inc., Columbus, Ohio 43215

Manufactured by: Taylor Pharmacal Co., Decatur, Illinois 62525

9000100

Revised 3/80

EVAC-Q-KIT®

Description: Each EVAC-Q-KIT® contains:

1. EVAC-Q-MAG®—10 fl. oz. Sugar-Free. Ingredients: magnesium citrate, citric acid and potassium citrate in cherry flavored base. Carbonated.
2. EVAC-Q-TABS® — 2 tablets. Ingredients: Each tablet contains 2 grains (130 mg) of phenophthalein. Contains color additives including FD&C Yellow No. 5 (tartrazine).

3. EVAC-Q-SERT®—2 suppositories. Ingredients: Potassium bitartrate and sodium bicarbonate in polyethylene glycol base.
4. 1 Instruction Sheet (In English and Spanish)

Actions: Bowel Evacuant.

Indications: Preparations of the colon for single and multiple radiology examinations requiring a clean colon.

Contraindications: EVAC-Q-MAG is contraindicated in the presence of severe renal insufficiency.

Warnings: Do not use any of these preparations when abdominal pain, nausea, or vomiting are present. Frequent and continued use may cause dependence upon laxatives. Rectal bleeding or failure to respond may indicate a serious condition. Consult physician. KEEP OUT OF REACH OF CHILDREN.

Precautions: If skin rash appears, do not use this or any other preparation containing phenolphthalein.

Dosage and Administration:
Instructions for Patients—early schedule*
Your physician is preparing you for an X-ray examination that requires thorough clearing of the intestinal tract. He is using this EVAC-Q-KIT® routine to make this procedure more comfortable for you.
BE SURE TO FOLLOW EACH STEP AND COMPLETE ALL INSTRUCTIONS OR ENTIRE X-RAY EXAMINATION MAY HAVE TO BE REPEATED.

DAY BEFORE EXAMINATION

IMPORTANT: A high fluid intake is essential to the success of this regimen. You MUST take a large glass (8 oz.) of fluid at specified times. ([glass]= 8 oz. fluid.) Drink only black coffee, plain tea, strained fruit juice, soft drinks or water at the times indicated. NO MILK OR CREAM.

☐ **Noon.** Light lunch. Clear soup, two hardboiled eggs, plain Jell-O, fluid.
☐ **12:30 P.M.** (or ½ hr. after lunch) Drink entire contents—EVAC-Q-MAG® (#1 in your kit), over Ice.
☐ **1:00 P.M.** + [glass].
☐ **3:00 P.M.** Take two (2) EVAC-Q-TABS® laxative tablets (#2 in your kit) with large glass of water.
☐ **4:00 P.M.** + [glass].
☐ **5:00 P.M.** Liquid dinner. Clear Soup, plain Jell-O + [glass].
☐ **6:00 P.M.** + [glass].
☐ **9:00 P.M.** + [glass].
☐ **10:00 P.M.** Remove cover from EVAC-Q-SERT® suppository (#3 in your kit). Moisten the suppository in tap water. Insert suppository into rectum. Wait at least 10–15 minutes before evacuating, even if urge is strong.
☐ **BEDTIME:** + [glass]

DAY OF TEST. No breakfast.
☐ **6:00 A.M.** (must be at least 2 hours before test).
Use remaining EVAC-Q-SERT® suppository (#4 in your kit). Follow same directions as 10:00 P.M. night before.

BE SURE TO DRINK ALL THE FLUID SPECIFIED.
NOTE: This product information is for professional use only.

How Supplied: Each EVAC-Q-KIT NDC 0013-2199 contains:
1. One 10 fl. oz. EVAC-Q-MAG
2. Two tablets—EVAC-Q-TABS
3. Two suppositories—EVAC-Q-SERT
4. 1 Instruction Sheet

Shipping Unit: 12 EVAC-Q-KIT units per carton.

---

*Late schedule also available. See Instruction Sheet in EVAC-Q-KIT. Instruction sheet printed in both English and Spanish.)

EVAC–Q–KWIK®

Description: Each EVAC-Q-KWIK® contains:
1. EVAC-Q-MAG®—10 fl. oz. Sugar-Free. Ingredients: Magnesium citrate, citric acid and potassium citrate in cherry flavored base. Carbonated.
2. EVAC-Q-TABS® — 2 tablets. Ingredients: Each tablet contains 2 grains (130 mg) of phenophthalein. Contains color additives including FD&C Yellow No. 5 (tartrazine).
3. EVAC-Q-KWIK®Suppository. Suppository contains 10 mg. of bisacodyl.
4. Illustrated Multilingual Instruction Sheet.

Actions: Bowel Evacuant

Indications: Preparation of the colon for single and multiple radiology examinations requiring a clean colon.

Contraindications: EVAC-Q-MAG is contraindicated in the presence of severe renal insufficiency.

Warnings: Do not use any laxative preparations when abdominal pain, nausea, or vomiting are present. Frequent and continued use may cause dependence upon laxatives. Rectal bleeding or failure to respond may indicate a serious condition. Consult physician. KEEP OUT OF REACH OF CHILDREN.

Precautions: If skin rash appears, do not use this or any other preparation containing phenolphthalein.

Dosage and Administration: Your physician is preparing you for an X-ray examination that requires thorough clearing of the intestinal tract. He is using this EVAC-Q-KWIK routine to make the procedure more comfortable for you. BE SURE TO FOLLOW EACH STEP AND COMPLETE ALL INSTRUCTIONS OR ENTIRE X-RAY EXAMINATION MAY HAVE TO BE REPEATED.
IMPORTANT: A high fluid intake is essential to the success of this regimen. You MUST take a large glass (8 oz.) of fluid at specified times. Drink only black coffee, plain tea, strained fruit juice, soft drinks or water at the time indicated. NO MILK OR CREAM.

4:00 P.M.	Drink entire contents—EVAC-Q-MAG® (No. 1 in your kit), over ice.
5:00 P.M.	8 oz. of fluid.
6:00 P.M.	Liquid dinner. Clear soup, plain Jell-O. 8 oz. of fluid.
7:00 P.M.	Take two (2) EVAC-Q-TABS® laxative tablets (No. 2 in your kit) with large glass of water.
8:00 P.M.	8 oz. of fluid.
9:00 P.M.	8 oz. of fluid.
10:00 P.M.	Insert on EVAC-Q-KWIK suppository (No. 3 in your kit) into rectum as far as possible, retain as long as comfort will permit—usually 10–15 minutes—before defecating. Nothing by mouth after 10:00 P.M. until X-ray exam.

BE SURE TO DRINK ALL FLUID SPECIFIED.
See Illustrated Multilingual Instruction Sheet.
NOTE: This product information is for professional use only.

How Supplied: Each EVAC-Q-KWIK® NDC 0013-2189 contains:
1. One 10 fl. oz. EVAC-Q-MAG®
2. Two tablets—EVAC-Q-TABS®
3. One EVAC-Q-KWIK Suppository
4. Instruction Sheet.

Shipping Unit: 12 EVAC-Q-KWIK units per carton.

ILOPAN® INJECTION ℞
(dexpanthenol)

Description: ILOPAN® INJECTION (dexpanthenol) is a derivative of pantothenic acid, a member of the B complex of vitamins. ILOPAN INJECTION is a sterile aqueous solution indicated for use as a gastrointestinal stimulant. The chemical name is D-(+)-2, 4-dihydroxy-N- (3-hydroxpropyl) -3, 3-dimethylbutylramide. The structural formula is

$$HOCH_2-\overset{CH_3}{\underset{CH_3}{C}}-\overset{OH}{\underset{H}{C}}-CONHCH_2CH_2CH_2OH$$

The empirical formula is $C_9H_{19}NO_4$.
Each ml contains dexpanthenol 250 mg in distilled water for injection.

Clinical Pharmacology: Pantothenic acid is a precursor of coenzyme A, which serves as a cofactor for a variety of enzyme-catalyzed reactions involving transfer of acetyl groups. The final step in the synthesis of acetylcholine consists of the choline acetylase transfer of an acetyl group from acetylcoenzyme A to choline. Acetylcholine is the neurohumoral transmitter in the parasympathetic system and as such maintains the normal functions of the intestine. Decrease in acetylcholine content would result in decreased peristalsis and in extreme cases adynamic ileus. The pharmacological mode of action of the drug is unknown. Pharmacokinetic data in humans are unavailable.

Indications and Usage: Prophylactic use immediately after major abdominal surgery to minimize the possibility of paralytic ileus. Intestinal atony causing abdominal distention; postoperative or postpartum retention of flatus, or postoperative delay in resumption of intestinal motility; paralytic ileus.

Contraindications: There are no known contraindications to the use of ILOPAN INJECTION.

Warnings: There have been rare instances of allergic reactions of unknown cause during the concomitant use of ILOPAN INJECTION with drugs such as antibiotics, narcotics and barbiturates.
Administration of ILOPAN INJECTION directly into the vein is not advised (See Dosage and Administration).
ILOPAN INJECTION should not be administered within one hour of succinylcholine.

Precautions:
General—If any signs of a hypersensitivity reaction appear, ILOPAN INJECTION should be discontinued. If ileus is a secondary consequence of mechanical obstruction, primary attention should be directed to the obstruction. The management of adynamic ileus includes the correction of any fluid and electrolyte imbalance (especially hypokalemia), anemia and hypoproteinemia, treatment of infection, avoidance where possible of drugs which are known to decrease gastrointestinal motility and decompression of the gastrointestinal tract when considerably distended by nasogastric suction or use of a long intestinal tube.
Drug Interactions—The effects of succinylcholine appeared to have been prolonged in a woman administered dexpanthenol.
Carcinogenicity, Mutagenicity, and Impairment of Fertility—There have been no studies in animals to evaluate the carcinogenic, mutagenic, or impairment of fertility potential of dexpanthenol.

Continued on next page

Adria—Cont.

Pregnancy—Category C. Animal reproduction studies have not been conducted with ILOPAN INJECTION. It is also not known whether ILOPAN INJECTION can cause fetal harm when administered to a pregnant woman or can affect reproduction capacity. ILOPAN INJECTION should be given to a pregnant woman only if clearly needed.
Nursing Mothers—It is not known whether this drug is excreted in human milk. Because many drugs are excreted in human milk, caution should be exercised when ILOPAN INJECTION is administered to a nursing woman.
Pediatric Use—Safety and effectiveness in children have not been established.
Adverse Reactions: There have been a few reports of allergic reactions and single reports of several other adverse events in association with the administration of dexpanthenol. A causal relationship is uncertain. One patient experienced itching, tingling, difficulty in breathing. Another patient had red patches of skin. Two patients had generalized dermatitis and one patient urticaria.
One patient experienced temporary respiratory difficulty following administration of ILOPAN INJECTION 5 minutes after succinylcholine was discontinued.
One patient experienced a noticeable but slight drop in blood pressure after administration of dexpanthenol while in the recovery room.
One patient experienced intestinal colic one-half hour after the drug was administered.
Two patients vomited following administration and two patients had diarrhea 10 days post-surgery and after ILOPAN INJECTION.
One elderly patient became agitated after administration of the drug.
Dosage and Administration: Prevention of post-operative adynamic ileus: 250 mg (1 ml) or 500 mg (2 ml) intramuscularly. Repeat in 2 hours and then every 6 hours until all danger of adynamic ileus has passed.
Treatment of adynamic ileus: 500 mg (2 ml) intramuscularly. Repeat in 2 hours and then every 6 hours as needed.
Intravenous administration: ILOPAN INJECTION 2 ml (500 mg) may be mixed with bulk I.V. solutions such as glucose or lactate-Ringer's and slowly infused intravenously.
Parenteral drug products should be inspected visually for particulate matter and discoloration prior to administration, whenever solution and container permit.
How Supplied: Each milliliter of ILOPAN INJECTION contains dexpanthenol, 250 mg in Water for Injection. ILOPAN INJECTION is available as follows:
ILOPAN INJECTION
NDC 0013-2356-93 2 ml Ampuls, Box of 12
NDC 0013-2356-95 2 ml Ampuls, Box of 25
NDC 0013-2356-97 2 ml Ampuls, Box of 100
Ampules maufactured by:
TAYLOR PHARMACAL CO.
DECATUR, ILLINOIS 62525
ILOPAN INJECTION
NDC 0013-2356-86 10 ml Vial
ILOPAN INJECTION STAT-PAK® (unit dose)
NDC 0013-2366-95 Disposable Syringe 2 ml, Box of 25
Protect from freezing or excessive heat.

KAOCHLOR® ℞
(Potassium Chloride)
10% Liquid
Contains Sugar

Description: Each 15 ml (tablespoonful) of KAOCHLOR 10% Liquid supplies 20 mEq each of potassium and chloride (as potassium chloride, 1.5 g) with sugar, saccharin, flavoring, and alcohol 5%. Contains FD&C Yellow No. 5 (tartrazine) as a color additive. The chemical name of the drug is potassium chloride.
Clinical Pharmacology: Potassium ion is the principal intracellular cation of most body tissues. Potassium ions participate in a number of essential physiological processes including the maintenance of intracellular tonicity, the transmission of nerve impulses, the contraction of cardiac, skeletal and smooth muscle and the maintenance of normal renal function.
Potassium depletion may occur whenever the rate of potassium loss through renal excretion and/or loss from the gastrointestinal tract exceeds the rate of potassium intake. Such depletion usually develops slowly as a consequence of prolonged therapy with oral diuretics, primary or secondary hyperaldosteronism, diabetic ketoacidosis, or inadequate replacement of potassium in patients on prolonged parenteral nutrition. Such depletion can develop rapidly with severe diarrhea, especially if associated with vomiting. Potassium depletion due to these causes is usually accompanied by a concomitant loss of chloride and is manifested by hypokalemia and metabolic alkalosis. Potassium depletion may produce weakness, fatigue, disturbances of cardiac rhythm (primarily ectopic beats), prominent U-waves in the electrocardiogram, and in advanced cases, flaccid paralysis and/or impaired ability to concentrate urine.
Potassium depletion associated with metabolic alkalosis is managed by correcting the fundamental cause of the deficiency whenever possible and administering supplemental potassium chloride, in the form of high potassium food or potassium chloride solution or tablets. In rare circumstances (e.g., patients with renal tubular acidosis) potassium depletion may be associated with metabolic acidosis and hyperchloremia. In such patients potassium replacement should be accomplished with potassium salts other than the chloride, such as potassium bicarbonate, potassium citrate, potassium acetate, or potassium gluconate.
Indications and Usage:
1. For therapeutic use in patients with hypokalemia with or without metabolic alkalosis, in digitalis intoxication and in patients with hypokalemic familial periodic paralysis.
2. For the prevention of potassium depletion when the dietary intake is inadequate in the following conditions: Patients receiving digitalis and diuretics for congestive heart failure, hepatic cirrhosis with ascites, states of aldosterone excess with normal renal function, potassium-losing nephropathy, and with certain diarrheal states.
3. The use of potassium salts in patients receiving diuretics for uncomplicated essential hypertension is often unnecessary when such patients have a normal dietary pattern. Serum potassium should be checked periodically, however, and if hypokalemia occurs, dietary supplementation with potassium-containing foods may be adequate to control milder cases. In more severe cases supplementation with potassium salts may be indicated.

Contraindications: Potassium supplements are contraindicated in patients with hyperkalemia since a further increase in serum potassium concentration in such patients can produce cardiac arrest. Hyperkalemia may complicate any of the following conditions: Chronic renal failure, systemic acidosis such as diabetic acidosis, acute dehydration, extensive tissue breakdown as in severe burns, adrenal insufficiency, or the administration of a potassium-sparing diuretic (e.g., spironolactone, triamterene).
Warnings: Do not administer full strength. KAOCHLOR 10% Liquid will cause gastrointestinal irritation if administered undiluted. For details regarding adequate dilution, see Dosage and Administration.
Hyperkalemia—In patients with impaired mechanisms for excreting potassium, the administration of potassium salts can produce hyperkalemia and cardiac arrest. This occurs most commonly in patients given potassium by the intravenous route but may also occur in patients given potassium orally. Potentially fatal hyperkalemia can develop rapidly and be asymptomatic. The use of potassium salts in patients with chronic renal disease, or any other condition which impairs potassium excretion, requires particularly careful monitoring of the serum potassium concentration and appropriate dosage adjustment.
Interaction with Potassium Sparing Diuretics—Hypokalemia should not be treated by the concomitant administration of potassium salts and a potassium-sparing diuretic (e.g., spironolactone or triamterene) since the simultaneous administration of these agents can produce severe hyperkalemia.
Metabolic Acidosis—Hypokalemia in patients with metabolic acidosis should be treated with an alkalinizing potassium salt such as potassium bicarbonate, potassium citrate, potassium acetate or potassium gluconate.
Precautions:
General—The diagnosis of potassium depletion is ordinarily made by demonstrating hypokalemia in a patient with a clinical history suggesting some cause for potassium depletion.
This product contains FD&C Yellow No. 5 (tartrazine) which may cause allergic-type reactions (including bronchial asthma) in certain susceptible individuals. Although the overall incidence of FD&C Yellow No. 5 (tartrazine) sensitivity in the general population is low, it is frequently seen in patients who also have aspirin hypersensitivity.
Laboratory Tests—In interpreting the serum potassium level, the physician should bear in mind that acute alkalosis *per se* can produce hypokalemia in the absence of a deficit in total body potassium while acute acidosis *per se* can increase the serum potassium concentration into the normal range even in the presence of a reduced total body potassium. The treatment of potassium depletion, particularly in the presence of cardiac disease, renal disease, or acidosis, requires careful attention to acid-base balance and appropriate monitoring of serum electrolytes, the electrocardiogram, and the clinical status of the patient.
It is important to recognize that hyperkalemia is usually asymptomatic and may be manifested only by an increased serum potassium concentration and characteristic electrocardiographic changes (peaking of T-waves, loss of P-wave, depression of S-T segment, and prolongation of the QT interval). (See Contraindications, Warnings and Overdosage.)
The use of potassium salts in patients with chronic renal disease, or any other condition which impairs potassium excretion, requires particularly careful monitoring of the serum potassium concentration and appropriate dosage adjustment.
When blood is drawn for analysis of plasma potassium levels, it is important to recognize that artifactual elevations do occur after repeated fist clenching to make veins more prominent during application of a tourniquet.
Carcinogenesis, Mutagenesis, Impairment of Fertility—There have been no studies in animals or humans to evaluate the carcinogenesis, mutagenesis or impairment of fertility for potassium.
Pregnancy—Category C. Animal reproduction studies have not been conducted with KAOCHLOR 10% Liquid. It is also not known whether KAOCHLOR 10% Liquid can cause fetal harm when administered to a pregnant woman or can affect reproduction capacity. KAOCHLOR 10% Liquid should be given to a pregnant woman only if clearly needed.
Nursing Mothers—It is not known whether this drug is excreted in human milk. Because many drugs are excreted in human milk, caution should be exercised when KAOCHLOR 10% Liquid is administered to a nursing woman.

Pediatric Use—Safety and effectiveness in children have not been established.

Adverse Reactions: The most severe effect is hyperkalemia (see Contraindications, Warnings and Overdosage).

The most common adverse reactions to oral potassium salts are nausea, vomiting, abdominal discomfort, and diarrhea. These symptoms are due to irritation of the gastrointestinal tract and are best managed by diluting the preparation further, taking the dose with meals, or reducing the dose.

Overdosage: The administration of oral potassium salts to persons with normal excretory mechanisms for potassium rarely causes serious hyperkalemia. However, if excretory mechanisms are impaired or if potassium is administered too rapidly intravenously, potentially fatal hyperkalemia can result (see Contraindications and Warnings). It is important to recognize that hyperkalemia is usually asymptomatic and may be manifested only by an increased serum potassium concentration and characteristic electrocardiographic changes (peaking of T-waves, loss of P-wave, depression of S-T segment, and prolongation of the QT interval). Late manifestations include muscle-paralysis and cardiovascular collapse from cardiac arrest.

Treatment for hyperkalemia includes the following:

1. Elimination of foods and medications containing potassium and potassium-sparing diuretics.
2. Intravenous administration of 300 to 500 ml/hr of 10% dextrose solution containing 10-20 units of crystalline insulin per 1,000 ml.
3. Correction of acidosis, if present, with intravenous sodium bicarbonate.
4. Use of exchange resins, hemodialysis, or peritoneal dialysis.

In treating hyperkalemia, it should be recalled that in patients who have been stabilized on digitalis, too rapid a lowering of the serum potassium concentration can produce digitalis toxicity.

Dosage and Administration: The usual dietary intake of potassium by the average adult is 40 to 80 mEq per day. Potassium depletion sufficient to cause hypokalemia usually requires the loss of 200 or more mEq of potassium from the total body store.

Dosage must be adjusted to the individual needs of each patient but is typically in the range of 20 mEq per day for the prevention of hypokalemia to 40-100 mEq per day or more for the treatment of potassium depletion.

To minimize gastrointestinal irritation, patients must follow directions regarding dilution. Each tablespoonful (15 ml) should be diluted with three (3) fluid ounces or more of water or other liquid.

One (1) tablespoonful (15 ml) twice daily (after morning and evening meals) supplies 40 mEq of potassium. Deviations from this recommendation may be indicated, since no average total daily dose can be defined but must be governed by close observation for clinical effects. However, potassium intoxication may result from any therapeutic dosage. See "Overdosage" and "Precautions".

How Supplied:
KAOCHLOR 10% Liquid supplies 20 mEq each of potassium and chloride per tablespoonful (15 ml).
NDC 0013-3103-51 Pint
NDC 0013-3103-53 Gallon
NDC 0013-3103-56 Bottle of 4 Fl. oz. (36's only)
NDC 0013-3103-58 Bottle of 15 ml, Stat-Pak® (Unit Dose), 100's only.
Storage Conditions—Protect from cold.

KAOCHLOR® S-F ℞
(Potassium Chloride)
10% Liquid
Sugar-Free

Description: Each 15 ml (tablespoonful) of KAOCHLOR S-F 10% Liquid supplies 20 mEq each of potassium and chloride (as potassium chloride, 1.5g) with saccharin, flavoring, and alcohol 5%. The chemical name of the drug is potassium chloride.

Clinical Pharmacology: See KAOCHLOR 10% LIQUID

Indications and Usage: See KAOCHLOR 10% LIQUID

Contraindications: See KAOCHLOR 10% LIQUID

Warnings: See KAOCHLOR 10% LIQUID

Precautions:
General—The diagnosis of potassium depletion is ordinarily made by demonstrating hypokalemia in patients with a clinical history suggesting some cause for potassium depletion.
Laboratory Tests—See KAOCHLOR 10% LIQUID
Carcinogenesis, Mutagenesis, Impairment of Fertility—See KAOCHLOR 10% LIQUID
Pregnancy—See KAOCHLOR 10% LIQUID
Nursing Mothers—See KAOCHLOR 10% LIQUID
Pediatric Use—See KAOCHLOR 10% LIQUID

Adverse Reactions: See KAOCHLOR 10% LIQUID

Overdosage: See KAOCHLOR 10% LIQUID

Dosage and Administration: See KAOCHLOR 10% LIQUID

How Supplied: KAOCHLOR S-F 10% Liquid supplies 20 mEq each of potassium and chloride per tablespoonful (15 ml).
NDC 0013-3093-51 Pint
NDC 0013-3093-53 Gallon
NDC 0013-3093-56 Bottle of 4 Fl. Oz. (36's only).
NDC 0013-3093-58 Bottle of 15 ml Stat-Pak® (Unit Dose) 100's only.
Storage Conditions—Protect from cold.

KAON® ELIXIR ℞
(Potassium Gluconate)
Grape Flavor
Sugar-Free

Description: Each 15 ml (tablespoonful) supplies 20 mEq of potassium (as potassium gluconate, 4.68 g) with saccharin and aromatics and alcohol 5%. The chemical name of the drug is gluconic acid potassium salt. The structural formula is:

```
         H    H    OH   H
         |    |    |    |
HOCH2- C  -  C  -  C  -  C - COOK
         |    |    |    |
         OH   OH   H    OH
```

Clinical Pharmacology: Potassium ion is the principal intracellular cation of most body tissues. Potassium ions participate in a number of essential physiological processes including the maintenance of intracellular tonicity, the transmission of nerve impulses, the contraction of cardiac, skeletal and smooth muscle and the maintenance of normal renal function. Potassium depletion may occur whenever the rate of potassium loss through renal excretion and/or loss from the gastrointestinal tract exceeds the rate of potassium intake. Potassium depletion sufficient to cause hypokalemia usually requires the loss of 200 or more mEq of potassium from the total body store. Such depletion usually develops slowly as a consequence of prolonged therapy with oral diuretics, primary or secondary hyperaldosteronism, diabetic ketoacidosis, or inadequate replacement of potassium in patients on prolonged parenteral nutrition. Such depletion can develop rapidly with severe diarrhea, especially if associated with vomiting. Potassium depletion may produce weakness, fatigue, disturbances of cardiac rhythm (primarily ectopic beats), prominent U-waves in the electrocardiogram, and in advanced cases, flaccid paralysis and/or impaired ability to concentrate urine.

Indications and Usage:

1. For therapeutic use in patients with hypokalemia with or without metabolic alkalosis, in digitalis intoxication and in patients with hypokalemic familial periodic paralysis.
2. For the prevention of potassium depletion when the dietary intake is inadequate in the following conditions: Patients receiving digitalis and diuretics for congestive heart failure; hepatic cirrhosis with ascites, states of aldosterone excess with normal renal function, potassium-losing nephropathy, and with certain diarrheal states.
3. The use of potassium salts in patients receiving diuretics for uncomplicated essential hypertension is often unnecessary when such patients have a normal dietary pattern. Serum potassium should be checked periodically, however, and if hypokalemia occurs, dietary supplementation with potassium-containing foods may be adequate to control milder cases. In more severe cases supplementation with potassium salts may be indicated.
4. Hypokalemia in patients with metabolic acidosis should be treated with an alkalinizing potassium salt such as potassium gluconate.

Contraindications: Potassium supplements are contraindicated in patients with hyperkalemia since a further increase in serum potassium concentration in such patients can produce cardiac arrest. Hyperkalemia may complicate any of the following conditions: Chronic renal failure, systemic acidosis such as diabetic acidosis, acute dehydration, extensive tissue breakdown as in severe burns, adrenal insufficiency, or the administration of a potassium-sparing diuretic (e.g., spironolactone, triamterene).

Warnings: Do not administer full strength. KAON ELIXIR may cause gastrointestinal irritation if administered undiluted. For details regarding adequate dilution, see Dosage and Administration.

Hyperkalemia—In patients with impaired mechanisms for excreting potassium, the administration of potassium salts can produce hyperkalemia and cardiac arrest. This occurs most commonly in patients given potassium by the intravenous route but may also occur in patients given potassium orally. Potentially fatal hyperkalemia can develop rapidly and be asymptomatic. The use of potassium salts in patients with chronic renal disease, or any other condition which impairs potassium excretion, requires particularly careful monitoring of the serum potassium concentration and appropriate dosage adjustment.

Interaction with Potassium Sparing Diuretics—Hypokalemia should not be treated by the concomitant administration of potassium salts and a potassium-sparing diuretic (e.g., spironolactone or triamterene) since the simultaneous administration of these agents can produce severe hyperkalemia.

Precautions:
General—The diagnosis of potassium depletion is ordinarily made by demonstrating hypokalemia in a patient with a clinical history suggesting some cause for potassium depletion. In hypokalemic states, especially in patients on a low-salt diet, hypochloremic alkalosis is a possibility that may require chloride as well as potassium supplementation. In these circumstances, potassium replacement with potassium chloride may be more advantageous than with other potassium salts.
However, KAON ELIXIR can be supplemented with chloride. Ammonium chloride is an excellent source of chloride ion (18.7 mEq per gram)

Continued on next page

Adria—Cont.

but it should not be used in patients with hepatic cirrhosis where ammonium salts are contraindicated.

Laboratory Tests—In interpreting the serum potassium level, the physician should bear in mind that acute alkalosis *per se* can produce hypokalemia in the absence of a deficit in total body potassium while acute acidosis *per se* can increase the serum potassium concentration into the normal range even in the presence of a reduced total body potassium. The treatment of potassium depletion, particularly in the presence of cardiac disease, renal disease, or acidosis, requires careful attention to acid-base balance and appropriate monitoring of serum electrolytes, the electrocardiogram, and the clinical status of the patient.

It is important to recognize that hyperkalemia is usually asymptomatic and may be manifested only by an increased serum potassium concentration and characteristic electrocardiographic changes (peaking of T-waves, loss of P-wave, depression of S-T segment, and prolongation of the QT interval). (See Contraindications, Warnings, and Overdosage.)

The use of potassium salts in patients with chronic renal disease, or any other condition which impairs potassium excretion, requires particularly careful monitoring of the serum potassium concentration and appropriate dosage adjustment.

When blood is drawn for analysis of plasma potassium levels, it is important to recognize that artifactual elevations do occur after repeated fist clenching to make veins more prominent during application of a tourniquet.

Carcinogenesis, Mutagenesis, Impairment of Fertility—There have been no studies in animals or humans to evaluate the carcinogenesis, mutagenesis or impairment of fertility for potassium.

Pregnancy—Category C. Animal reproduction studies have not been conducted with KAON ELIXIR. It is also not known whether KAON ELIXIR can cause fetal harm when administered to a pregnant woman or can affect reproduction capacity. KAON ELIXIR should be given to a pregnant woman only if clearly needed.

Nursing Mothers—It is not known whether this drug is excreted in human milk. Because many drugs are excreted in human milk, caution should be exercised when KAON ELIXIR is administered to a nursing woman.

Pediatric Use—Safety and effectiveness in children have not been established.

Adverse Reactions: The most severe adverse effect is hyperkalemia (see Contraindications, Warnings and Overdosage).

The most common adverse reactions to oral potassium salts are nausea, vomiting, abdominal discomfort, and diarrhea. These symptoms are due to irritation of the gastrointestinal tract and are best managed by diluting the preparation further, taking the dose with meals, or reducing the dose.

Overdosage: The administration of oral potassium salts to persons with normal excretory mechanisms for potassium rarely causes serious hyperkalemia. However, if excretory mechanisms are impaired or if potassium is administered too rapidly intravenously, potentially fatal hyperkalemia can result (see Contraindications and Warnings). It is important to recognize that hyperkalemia is usually asymptomatic and may be manifested only by an increased serum potassium concentration and characteristic electrocardiographic changes (peaking of T-waves, loss of P-wave, depression of S-T segment, and prolongation of the QT interval). Late manifestations include muscle-paralysis and cardiovascular collapse from cardiac arrest.

Treatment for hyperkalemia includes the following:

1. Elimination of foods and medications containing potassium and potassium-sparing diuretics.
2. Intravenous administration of 300 to 500 ml/hr of 10% dextrose solution containing 10–20 units of crystalline insulin per 1,000 ml.
3. Correction of acidosis, if present, with intravenous sodium bicarbonate.
4. Use of exchange resins, hemodialysis, or peritoneal dialysis.

In treating hyperkalemia, it should be recalled that in patients who have been stabilized on digitalis, too rapid a lowering of the serum potassium concentration can produce digitalis toxicity.

Dosage and Administration: The usual dietary intake of potassium by the average adult is 40 to 80 mEq per day. Potassium depletion sufficient to cause hypokalemia usually requires the loss of 200 or more mEq of potassium from the total body store.

Dosage must be adjusted to the individual needs of each patient but is typically in the range of 20 mEq per day for the prevention of hypokalemia to 40–100 mEq per day or more for the treatment of potassium depletion.

To minimize gastrointestinal irritation, patients must follow directions regarding dilution. Each tablespoonful (15 ml) should be diluted with one fluid ounce or more of water or other liquid.

One tablespoonful twice daily (after morning and evening meals) supplies 40 mEq of potassium. Deviations from this recommendation may be indicated, since no average total daily dose can be defined but must be governed by close observation for clinical effects. However, potassium intoxications may result from any therapeutic dosage. See "Overdosage" and "Precautions".

How Supplied: KAON ELIXIR (potassium gluconate), Grape, supplies 20 mEq of potassium (as potassium gluconate, 4.68g) per tablespoonful (15 ml).

NDC 0013-3203-51 Pint
NDC 0013-3203-53 Gallon
NDC 0013-3203-56 Bottle of 4 Fl. Oz. (36's only).
NDC 0013-3203-58 Bottle of 15 ml, Stat-Pak® (Unit Dose) 100's only.

Storage Conditions: Protect from cold.

KAON® TABLETS ℞
(Potassium Gluconate)

Description: Each sugar coated tablet supplies 5 mEq of elemental potassium (as potassium gluconate 1.17 g). KAON Tablets are sugar coated, not enteric coated, which favors dissolution in the stomach and absorption before reaching the small intestine where the lesions with enteric potassium chloride have occurred. The sugar coating merely adds to palatability and ease of swallowing, not to delay absorption as does the enteric coating.

Indications: Oral potassium therapy for the prevention and treatment of hypokalemia which may occur secondary to diuretic or corticosteroid administration. It may be used in the treatment of cardiac arrhythmias due to digitalis intoxication.

Contraindications: Severe renal impairment with oliguria or azotemia, untreated Addison's disease, adynamia episodica hereditaria, acute dehydration, heat cramps and hyperkalemia from any cause.

Warning: There have been several reports, published and unpublished, concerning nonspecific small-bowel lesions consisting of stenosis, with or without ulceration, associated with the administration of enteric-coated thiazides with potassium salts. These lesions may occur with enteric-coated potassium tablets alone or when they are used with nonenteric-coated thiazides or certain other oral diuretics. These small bowel lesions have caused obstruction, hemorrhage and perforation. Surgery was frequently required and deaths have occurred. Available information tends to implicate enteric-coated potassium salts, although lesions of this type also occur spontaneously. Therefore, coated potassium-containing formulations should be administered only when indicated and should be discontinued immediately if abdominal pain, distention, nausea, vomiting, or gastrointestinal bleeding occur. Coated potassium tablets should be used only when adequate dietary supplementation is not practical.

Precautions: In response to a rise in the concentration of body potassium, renal excretion of the ion is increased. With normal kidney function, it is difficult, therefore, to produce potassium intoxication by oral adminstration. However, potassium supplements must be administered with caution, since the amount of the deficiency or daily dosage is not accurately known. Frequent checks of the clinical status of the patient, and periodic ECG and/or serum potassium levels should be made. High serum concentrations of potassium ion may cause death through cardiac depression, arrhythmias or arrest. This drug should be used with caution in the presence of cardiac disease. In hypokalemic states, especially in patients on a salt-free diet, hypochloremic alkalosis is a possibility that may require chloride as well as potassium supplementation. In these circumstances, KAON (potassium gluconate) should be supplemented with chloride. Ammonium chloride is an excellent source of chloride ion (18.7 mEq per Gram), but it should not be used in patients with hepatic cirrhosis where ammonium salts are contraindicated. Other sources for chloride are sodium chloride and Diluted Hydrochloric Acid, NF. It should also be kept in mind that ammonium cycle cation exchange resin, sometimes used to treat hyperkalemia, should not be administered to patients with hepatic cirrhosis.

Adverse Reactions: Nausea, vomiting, diarrhea and abdominal discomfort have been reported. The symptoms and signs of potassium intoxication include paresthesias of the extremities, flaccid paralysis, listlessness, mental confusion, weakness and heaviness of the legs, fall in blood pressure, cardiac arrhythmias and heart block. Hyperkalemia may exhibit the following electrocardiographic abnormalities: disappearance of the P wave, widening and slurring of QRS complex, changes of the S-T segment, tall peaked T waves, etc.

Dosage and Adminstration: The usual adult dosage is 2 tablets four times daily (after meals and at bedtime). This supplies 40 mEq of elemental potassium, the approximate minimum adult daily requirement for potassium. Deviations from this recommendation may be indicated, since no average total daily dose can be defined but must be governed by close observation for clinical effects. However, potassium intoxication may result from any therapeutic dosage. See "Overdosage" and "Precautions."

Overdosage: Potassium intoxication may result from overdosage of potassium or from therapeutic dosage in conditions stated under "Contraindications." Hyperkalemia, when detected, must be treated immediately because lethal levels can be reached in a few hours.

Treatment of Hyperkalemia:

1. Dextrose solution, 10 or 25% containing 10 units of crystalline insulin per 20 g dextrose, given I.V. in a dose of 300 to 500 ml in an hour.
2. Adsorption and exchange of potassium using sodium or ammonium cycle cation exchange resin, orally and as retention enema. See "Precautions."
3. Hemodialysis and peritoneal dialysis.
4. The use of potassium-containing foods or medicaments must be eliminated.

In cases of digitalization too rapid a lowering of plasma potassium concentration can cause digitalis toxicity.

How Supplied:

NDC 0013-3121-17 Bottle of 100 Tablets
NDC 0013-3121-21 Bottle of 500 Tablets
NDC 0013-3121-18 Stat-Pak® (Unit Dose) 100's only

[*Shown in Product Identification Section*]

KAON-CL™ ℞
(Potassium Chloride)
CONTROLLED RELEASE TABLETS

Description: KAON-CL 6.7 mEq is a sugar coated (not enteric-coated) tablet containing 500 mg potassium chloride (equivalent to 6.7 mEq potassium chloride) in a wax matrix. Contains color additives including FD&C Yellow No. 5 (tartrazine). This formulation is intended to provide a controlled release of potassium from the matrix to minimize the likelihood of producing high localized concentrations of potassium within the gastrointestinal tract.

Actions: Potassium ion is the principal intracellular cation of most body tissues. Potassium ions participate in a number of essential physiological processes including the maintenance of intracellular tonicity, the transmission of nerve impulses, the contraction of cardiac, skeletal and smooth muscle and the maintenance of normal renal function.

Potassium depletion may occur whenever the rate of potassium loss through renal excretion and/or loss from the gastrointestinal tract exceeds the rate of potassium intake. Such depletion usually develops slowly as a consequence of prolonged therapy with oral diuretics, primary or secondary hyperaldosteronism, diabetic ketoacidosis, severe diarrhea, or inadequate replacement of potassium in patients on prolonged parenteral nutrition. Potassium depletion due to these causes is usually accompanied by a concomitant deficiency of chloride and is manifested by hypokalemia and metabolic alkalosis. Potassium depletion may produce weakness, fatigue, disturbances of cardiac rhythm (primarily ectopic beats), prominent U-waves in the electrocardiogram, and in advanced cases, flaccid paralysis and/or impaired ability to concentrate urine.

Potassium depletion associated with metabolic alkalosis is managed by correcting the fundamental cause of the deficiency whenever possible and administering supplemental potassium chloride, in the form of high potassium food or potassium chloride solution or tablets. In rare circumstances (e.g., patients with renal tubular acidosis) potassium depletion may be associated with metabolic acidosis and hyperchloremia. In such patients potassium replacement should be accomplished with potassium salts other than the chloride, such as potassium bicarbonate, potassium citrate, potassium acetate, or potassium gluconate.

Indications:

BECAUSE OF REPORTS OF INTESTINAL AND GASTRIC ULCERATION AND BLEEDING WITH SLOW RELEASE POTASSIUM CHLORIDE PREPARATIONS, THESE DRUGS SHOULD BE RESERVED FOR THOSE PATIENTS WHO CANNOT TOLERATE OR REFUSE TO TAKE LIQUIDS OR EFFERVESCENT POTASSIUM PREPARATIONS OR FOR PATIENTS IN WHOM THERE IS A PROBLEM OF COMPLIANCE WITH THESE PREPARATIONS.

1. For therapeutic use in patients with hypokalemia with or without metabolic alkalosis, in digitalis intoxication and in patients with hypokalemic familial periodic paralysis.
2. For the prevention of potassium depletion when the dietary intake is inadequate in the following conditions: Patients receiving digitalis and diuretics for congestive heart failure, hepatic cirrhosis with ascites, states of aldosterone excess with normal renal function, potassium-losing nephropathy, and with certain diarrheal states.
3. The use of potassium salts in patients receiving diuretics for uncomplicated essential hypertension is often unnecessary when such patients have a normal dietary pattern. Serum potassium should be checked periodically, however, and if hypokalemia occurs, dietary supplementation with potassium-containing foods may be adequate to control milder cases. In more severe cases supplementation with potassium salts may be indicated.

Contraindications: Potassium supplements are contraindicated in patients with hyperkalemia since a further increase in serum potassium concentration in such patients can produce cardiac arrest. Hyperkalemia may complicate any of the following conditions: Chronic renal failure, systemic acidosis such as diabetic acidosis, acute dehydration, extensive tissue breakdown as in severe burns, adrenal insufficiency, or the administration of a potassium-sparing diuretic (e.g., spironolactone, triamterene).

Wax-matrix potassium chloride preparations have produced esophageal ulceration in certain cardiac patients with esophageal compression due to enlarged left atrium. Potassium supplementation, when indicated in such patients, should be with a liquid preparation.

All solid dosage forms of potassium chloride supplements are contraindicated in any patient in whom there is cause for arrest or delay in tablet passage through the gastrointestinal tract. In these instances, potassium supplementation should be with a liquid preparation.

Warnings:

Hyperkalemia—In patients with impaired mechanisms for excreting potassium, the administration of potassium salts can produce hyperkalemia and cardiac arrest. This occurs most commonly in patients given potassium by the intravenous route but may also occur in patients given potassium orally. Potentially fatal hyperkalemia can develop rapidly and be asymptomatic. The use of potassium salts in patients with chronic renal disease, or any other condition which impairs potassium excretion, requires particularly careful monitoring of the serum potassium concentration and appropriate dosage adjustment.

Interaction with Potassium Sparing Diuretics—Hypokalemia should not be treated by the concomitant administration of potassium salts and a potassium-sparing diuretic (e.g., spironolactone or triamterene) since the simultaneous administration of these agents can produce severe hyperkalemia.

Gastrointestinal Lesions—Potassium chloride tablets have produced stenotic and/or ulcerative lesions of the small bowel and deaths. These lesions are caused by a high localized concentration of potassium ion in the region of a rapidly dissolving tablet, which injures the bowel wall and thereby produces obstruction hemorrhage or perforation. KAON-CL 6.7 mEq (potassium chloride) is a wax-matrix tablet formulated to provide a controlled rate of release of potassium chloride and thus to minimize the possibility of a high local concentration of potassium ion near the bowel wall. While the reported frequency of small bowel lesions is much less with wax-matrix tablets (less than one per 100,000 patient years) than with enteric-coated potassium chloride tablets (40-50 per 100,000 patient years) cases associated with wax-matrix tablets have been reported both in foreign countries and in the United States. In addition, perhaps because the wax-matrix preparations are not enteric-coated and release potassium in the stomach, there have been reports of upper gastrointestinal bleeding associated with these products. The total number of gastrointestinal lesions remains less than one per 100,000 patient years. KAON-CL 6.7 mEq should be discontinued immediately and the possibility of bowel obstruction or perforation considered if severe vomiting, abdominal pain, distention, or gastrointestinal bleeding occurs.

Metabolic Acidosis—Hypokalemia in patients with metabolic acidosis should be treated with an alkalinizing potassium salt such as potassium bicarbonate, potassium citrate, potassium acetate, or potassium gluconate.

Precautions: The diagnosis of potassium depletion is ordinarily made by demonstrating hypokalemia in a patient with a clinical history suggesting some cause for potassium depletion. In interpreting the serum potassium level, the physician should bear in mind that acute alkalosis *per se* can produce hypokalemia in the absence of a deficit in total body potassium while acute acidosis *per se* can increase the serum potassium concentration into the normal range even in the presence of a reduced total body potassium. The treatment of potassium depletion, particularly in the presence of cardiac arrest, renal disease, or acidosis requires careful attention to acid-base balance and appropriate monitoring of serum electrolytes, the electrocardiogram, and the clinical status of the patient.

This product contains FD&C Yellow No. 5 (tartrazine) which may cause allergic-type reactions (including bronchial asthma) in certain susceptible individuals. Although the overall incidence of FD&C Yellow No. 5 (tartrazine) sensitivity in the general population is low, it is frequently seen in patients who also have aspirin hypersensitivity.

Adverse Reactions: The most common adverse reactions to oral potassium salts are nausea, vomiting, abdominal discomfort and diarrhea. These symptoms are due to irritation of the gastrointestinal tract and are best managed by diluting the preparation further, taking the dose with meals, or reducing the dose. The most severe adverse effects are hyperkalemia (see Contraindications, Warnings and Overdosage) and gastrointestinal obstruction, bleeding or perforation (see Warnings).

Overdosage: The administration of oral potassium salts to persons with normal excretory mechanisms for potassium rarely causes serious hyperkalemia. However, if excretory mechanisms are impaired or if potassium is administered too rapidly intravenously, potentially fatal hyperkalemia can result (see Contraindications and Warnings). It is important to recognize that hyperkalemia is usually asymptomatic and may be manifested only by an increased serum potassium concentration and characteristic electrocardiographic changes (peaking of T-waves, loss of P-wave, depression of S-T segment, and prolongation of the QT interval). Late manifestations include muscle-paralysis and cardiovascular collapse from cardiac arrest.

Treatment measures for hyperkalemia include the following:

1. Elimination of foods and medications containing potassium and of potassium-sparing diuretics.
2. Intravenous administration of 300 to 500 ml/hr of 10% dextrose solution containing 10–20 units of crystalline insulin per 1,000 ml.
3. Correction of acidosis, if present, with intravenous sodium bicarbonate.
4. Use of exchange resins, hemodialysis, or peritoneal dialysis.

In treating hyperkalemia, it should be recalled that in patients who have been stabilized on digitalis, too rapid a lowering of the serum potassium concentration can produce digitalis toxicity.

Dosage and Administration: The usual dietary intake of potassium by the average adult is 40 to 80 mEq per day. Potassium depletion sufficient to cause hypokalemia usually

Continued on next page

Adria—Cont.

requires the loss of 200 or more mEq of potassium from the total body store.
Dosage must be adjusted to the individual needs of each patient but is typically in the range of 20 mEq per day for the prevention of hypokalemia to 40–100 mEq per day or more for the treatment of potassium depletion.
One KAON-CL 6.7 mEq three times daily provides 20 mEq of potassium chloride. Two KAON-CL 6.7 mEq three times daily provides 40 mEq of potassium chloride.
Tablets should be taken with a glass of water or other liquid.
How Supplied:
NDC 0013-3071-17 Bottle of 100 Tablets.
NDC 0013-3071-19 Bottle of 250 Tablets.
NDC 0013-3071-23 Bottle of 1000 Tablets.
NDC 0013-3071-18 Stat-Pak® Unit Dose Box of 100 Tablets
[*Shown in Product Identification Section*]

KAON CL™-10 ℞
(Potassium Chloride)
CONTROLLED RELEASE TABLETS

Description: KAON CL-10 mEq is a sugar coated (not enteric-coated) tablet containing 750 mg potassium chloride (equivalent to 10 mEq potassium chloride) in a wax matrix. This formulation is intended to provide a controlled release of potassium from the matrix to minimize the likelihood of producing high localized concentrations of potassium within the gastrointestinal tract.
Actions: See KAON-CL™ TABLETS
Indications: See KAON-CL TABLETS
Contraindications: See KAON-CL TABLETS
Warnings: See KAON-CL TABLETS
Precautions: The diagnosis of potassium depletion is ordinarily made by demonstrating hypokalemia in a patient with a clinical history suggesting some cause for potassium depletion. In interpreting the serum potassium level, the physician should bear in mind that acute alkalosis *per se* can produce hypokalemia in the absence of a deficit in total body potassium while acute acidosis *per se* can increase the serum potassium concentration into the normal range even in the presence of a reduced total body potassium. The treatment of potassium depletion, particularly in the presence of cardiac disease, renal disease, or acidosis requires careful attention to acid-base balance and appropriate monitoring of serum electrolytes, the electrocardiogram, and the clinical status of the patient.
Adverse Reactions: See KAON-CL TABLETS
Overdosage: See KAON-CL TABLETS
Dosage and Administration: The usual dietary intake of potassium by the average adult is 40 to 80 mEq per day. Potassium depletion sufficient to cause hypokalemia usually requires the loss of 200 or more mEq of potassium from the total body store.
Dosage must be adjusted to the individual needs of each patient but is typically in the range of 20 mEq per day for the prevention of hypokalemia to 40–100 mEq per day or more for the treatment of potassium depletion.
One KAON CL-10 mEq two times daily provides 20 mEq of potassium chloride. Two KAON CL-10 mEq two times daily provides 40 mEq of potassium chloride.
Tablets should be taken with a glass of water or other liquid.
Caution: Federal law prohibits dispensing without prescription.
How Supplied:
NDC 0013-3041-17 Bottles of 100 Tablets
NDC 0013-3041-21 Bottle of 500 Tablets
NDC 0013-3041-18 Stat-Pak® (Unit Dose) Box of 100 Tablets
[*Shown in Product Identification Section*]

KAON-CL 20% ℞
(Potassium Chloride)
Sugar-Free

Description: Each 15 ml (tablespoonful) of KAON-CL 20% supplies 40 mEq each of potassium and chloride (as potassium chloride, 3g) with saccharin, flavoring, and alcohol 5%. The chemical name of the drug is potassium chloride.
Clinical Pharmacology: See KAOCHLOR 10% LIQUID
Indications and Usage: See KAOCHLOR 10% LIQUID
Contraindications: See KAOCHLOR 10% LIQUID
Warnings: See KAOCHLOR 10% LIQUID
Precautions:
General: The diagnosis of potassium depletion is ordinarily made by demonstrating hypokalemia in a patient with a clinical history suggesting some cause for potassium depletion.
Laboratory Tests—See KAOCHLOR 10% LIQUID
Carcinogenesis, Mutagenesis, Impairment of Fertility—See KAOCHLOR 10% LIQUID
Pregnancy—See KAOCHLOR 10% LIQUID
Nursing Mothers:—See KAOCHLOR 10% LIQUID
Pediatric Use:—See KAOCHLOR 10% LIQUID
Adverse Reactions: See KAOCHLOR 10% LIQUID
Overdosage: See KAOCHLOR 10% LIQUID
Dosage and Administration: The usual dietary intake of potassium by the average adult is 40 to 80 mEq per day. Potassium depletion sufficient to cause hypokalemia usually requires the loss of 200 or more mEq of potassium from the total body store.
Dosage must be adjusted to the individual needs of each patient but is typically in the range of 20 mEq per day for the prevention of hypokalemia to 40-100 mEq per day or more for the treatment of potassium depletion.
To minimize gastrointestinal irritation, patients must follow directions regarding dilution. Each tablespoonful (15 ml) should be diluted with six (6) fluid ounces or more of water or other liquid.
One (1) tablespoonful (15 ml) per day (after the morning meal) supplies 40 mEq of potassium. One tablespoonful twice a day, in six (6) or more fluid ounces of water or other fluid, provides 80 mEq potassium chloride. Deviations from these recommendations may be indicated, since no average total daily dose can be defined but must be governed by close observation for clinical effects. However, potassium intoxication may result from any therapeutic dosage. See "Overdosage" and "Precautions".
How Supplied: KAON-CL 20% supplies 40 mEq each of potassium and chloride per tablespoonful (15 ml).
NDC 0013-3113-51 Pint
NDC 0013-3113-53 Gallon
NDC 0013-3113-56 Bottles of 4 Fl. Oz. (36's only).
Storage Conditions: Protect from cold or excessive heat.

MAGAN® ℞
(Magnesium Salicylate)

Description: Each MAGAN uncoated, pink, capsule-shaped tablet for oral administration contains 545 mg of magnesium salicylate equivalent to 500 mg of salicylate. Magnesium salicylate is a non-steroidal, antiinflammatory agent with antipyretic and analgesic properties. Its molecular weight is 298.54. It has the following structural formula:

O ‖ C — O — Mg — O — C ‖ O
OH HO

Magnesium salicylate is a white, odorless, crystalline powder with a sweet taste. It is soluble in water and alcohol.

Clinical Pharmacology: Salicylic acid is the active moiety released into the plasma by MAGAN (magnesium salicylate). Salicylic acid is enzymatically biotransformed through two pathways to salicyluric acid and salicylphenolic glucuronide and eliminated in the urine.
Oral salicylates are absorbed rapidly, partly from the stomach but mostly from the upper intestine. Salicylic acid is rapidly distributed throughout all body tissues and most transcellular fluids, mainly by pH-dependent passive processes. It can be detected in synovial, spinal and peritoneal fluid, in saliva and in milk. It readily crosses the placental barrier. From 50% to 90% of salicylic acid is bound to plasma proteins, especially albumin.
Following the ingestion of a single dose of 524 mg of magnesium salicylate, a peak concentration of 3.6 mg/dl salicylic acid is reached in 1.5 hours with a T ½ of 2 hours. The major biotransformation paths for the elimination of salicylic acid from the plasma become saturated by low doses of salicylic acid. As a result, repeated doses of MAGAN increase the plasma concentration and markedly prolong the plasma half-time. The plasma concentration of salicylic acid is increased by conditions that reduce the glomerular filtration rate or tubular secretion such as renal disease or the presence of inhibitors that compete for the transport system such as probenecid.
Therapeutic plasma concentrations of salicylic acid for an adequate antiinflammatory effect needed for the treatment of rheumatoid arthritis range between 20–30 mg/dl. Effective analgesia is achieved at lower concentrations. Salicylates relieve pain by both a peripheral and a CNS effect. Salicylates inhibit the synthesis of prostaglandins; the importance of this mechanism in analgesia and antiinflammation has not been fully elucidated. Salicylates have a antipyretic effect in febrile patients but little in subjects with normal temperatures. This appears to be due to the inhibition of the synthesis of prostaglandins which are powerful pyrogens that affect the hypothalamus. Higher therapeutic concentrations cause reversible tinnitus and high tone hearing loss. Full therapeutic doses of salicylates increase oxygen consumption and CO_2 production. They cause an extracellular and intracellular respiratory alkalosis which is rapidly compensated. Salicylates irritate the gastric mucosa and frequently lead to blood loss in the stool; this effect is more pronounced with aspirin than magnesium salicylate. Salicylates in large doses (over 6 g/day) reduce the plasma prothrombin level. In contrast to aspirin, magnesium salicylate does not affect platelets. Salicylic acid increases the urinary excretion of urates at higher doses but may decrease excretion at lower doses.

Indications and Usage: MAGAN is indicated for the relief of the signs and symptoms of rheumatoid arthritis, osteoarthritis, bursitis and other musculoskeletal disorders.

Contraindications: MAGAN is contraindicated in patients with advanced chronic renal insufficiency. It may counteract the effect of uricosuric agents and should not be prescribed for patients on such drugs.

Warnings: As with all salicylates, MAGAN should be avoided or administered with caution to patients with liver damage, pre-existing hypoprothrombinemia, vitamin K deficiency and before surgery.

Precautions:
General—Appropriate precautions should be taken in prescribing MAGAN for persons

known to be sensitive to salicylates and in patients with erosive gastritis or peptic ulcer. If a reaction develops, the drug should be discontinued. MAGAN should be used with caution, if at all, concomitantly with anticoagulants. Appropriate precautions should be taken in administering MAGAN to patients with any impairment of renal function including discontinuing other drugs containing magnesium and monitoring serum magnesium levels if dosage levels of MAGAN are high.

Drug Interactions—Even small doses of MAGAN should not be given with uricosuric agents such as probenecid that decrease tubular reabsorption because it counteracts their effect. Large doses of MAGAN cause hypoprothrombinemia. Lower doses enhance the effects of anticoagulants such as coumadin and must be used with caution in patients receiving anticoagulants that affect the prothrombin time. Caution should also be exercised in patients concurrently treated with a sulfonylurea hypoglycemic agent or methotrexate because of the drug's capability of displacing them from the plasma protein binding sites, resulting in enhanced action of these agents. A similar displacement of barbiturates and diphenylhydantoin may occur; diphenylhydantoin intoxication has been precipitated by the consumption of aspirin. Salicylates inhibit the diuretic action of spironolactone.

Carcinogenesis, Mutagenesis, Impairment of Fertility— There have been no studies in animals or humans to evaluate the carcinogenesis, mutagenesis or impairment of fertility for magnesium salicylate. Aspirin causes testicular atrophy and inhibition of spermatogenesis in animals.

Pregnancy—Category C.

1. *Teratogenic effects*—Aspirin has been shown to be teratogenic in animals and to increase the incidence of still births and neonatal deaths in women. There are no adequate or well-controlled studies of MAGAN in pregnant women. MAGAN should be used during pregnancy only if the potential benefit justifies the potential risk to the fetus.
2. *Non-Teratogenic effects*—Chronic, high dose salicylate therapy of pregnant women increases the length of gestation and the frequency of post maturity and prolongs spontaneous labor. It is recommended MAGAN be taken during the last three months of pregnancy only under the close supervision of a physician.

Nursing Mothers—Since salicylates are excreted in human milk, caution should be exercised when MAGAN is administered to a nursing woman.

Pediatric Use—Safety and effectiveness of MAGAN in children have not been established.

Adverse Reactions: Magnesium salicylate in large doses has a hypoprothrombinemic effect and should be given with caution in patients receiving anticoagulant drugs, patients with liver damage, pre-existing hypoprothrombinemia, vitamin K deficiency or before surgery.

Salicylates given in overdose produce stimulation (often manifested as tinnitus) followed by depression of the central nervous system. The dosage should be lowered at the onset of tinnitus.

Salicylates may cause gastric mucosal irritation and bleeding. However, fecal blood loss in patients taking MAGAN is significantly less than in those taking aspirin.

MAGAN should not be given to patients with severe renal damage because of the possibility of hypermagnesemia.

In moderate to high doses, salicylates lower the blood glucose in diabetics. Aspirin-induced hypoglycemia has been described in adults undergoing hemodialysis.

Unlike aspirin, magnesium salicylate is not known to affect the platelet adhesiveness involved in the clotting mechanism; and therefore, does not prolong bleeding time. MAGAN has not been associated with reactions causing asthmatic attacks in susceptible people.

Overdosage: Acute overdosage results in salicylate toxicity. Early signs and symptoms from repeated larger doses as well as a large single dose consist of headache, dizziness, tinnitus (which may be absent in children or the elderly), difficulty in hearing, dimness of vision, mental confusion, lassitude, drowsiness, sweating, thirst, hyperventilation, nausea, vomiting and occasionally diarrhea. More severe salicylate poisoning is manifested by CNS disturbances including EEG abnormalities. Hyperventilation occurs producing initial respiratory alkalosis. This is followed by severe metabolic acidosis with dehydration and loss of potassium. Restlessness, garrulity, incoherent speech, apprehension, vertigo, tremor, diplopia, maniacal delirium, hallucinations, generalized convulsions and coma may occur. Toxic symptoms may occur at serum levels greater than 20 mg/dl in patients over 60 years of age. Hyperventilation may occur at plasma salicylate levels over 35 mg/dl. Death may result from salicylate levels between 45–75 mg/dl. As with other salicylates, 10 to 30 g of the drug may be fatal. Renal or hepatic insufficiency and fever and dehydration in children enhance the acute toxicity of salicylate overdoses. Treatment of acute poisoning is a medical emergency and should be undertaken in a hospital. Serum Na, K, Cl, CO_2 levels, pH, BUN, blood glucose and urine pH and specific gravity should be obtained. Emesis should be induced or gastric lavage performed. Activated charcoal may be administered. Hyperthermia should be controlled with tepid water sponging. Dehydration should be treated and acid-base imbalance corrected. A high concentration of salicylic acid in the brain may be fatal. Correction of acidosis shifts salicylate from the brain to the plasma. A bicarbonate solution should be infused to maintain an alkaline diuresis. Care should be taken to avoid pulmonary edema. The blood pH, plasma pCO_2 and plasma glucose level should be monitored frequently. Ketosis and hypoglycemia may be corrected by glucose infusions and hypokalemia by potassium chloride added to the intravenous infusate. Avoid respiratory depressants. Shock may be combatted by plasma infusions. Hemorrhagic phenomena may necessitate whole blood transfusions or vitamin K_1. In severe intoxication, exchange transfusion, peritoneal dialysis, hemodialysis or hemoperfusion should be performed to remove plasma salicylic acid. Dialysis should be seriously considered if the patient's condition is worsening despite appropriate therapy.

Dosage and Administration: The dosage for MAGAN in the treatment of musculoskeletal disorders such as arthritis should be adjusted according to individual patient's needs. The recommended initial regimen is two tablets three times per day. Dosage may be increased, if necessary, to achieve the desired therapeutic effect. In adjusting the dosage, the physician should monitor the dose limiting parameters such as tinnitus and/or serum salicylate over 30 mg/dl.

How Supplied: Each MAGAN tablet contains 545 mg of magnesium salicylate equivalent to 500 mg salicylate. MAGAN is available for oral administration as uncoated, pink, capsule-shaped tablets coded Adria 412. They are supplied as follows:

NDC 0013-4121-17 in bottles of 100
NDC 0013-4121-21 in bottles of 500
Store at room temperature and protect from light.

MODANE® BULK
(psyllium and dextrose)

Description: MODANE BULK is a powdered mixture of equal parts of psyllium, a bulking agent, and dextrose, as a dispersing agent. Psyllium is a highly efficient dietary fiber derived from the husk of the seed of *Plantago ovata*. Each rounded teaspoonful contains approximately 3.5 g psyllium, 3.5 g dextrose, 2 mg sodium and 37 mg potassium, and provides 14 calories.

Clinical Pharmacology: Psyllium absorbs water and expands. When taken with adequate amounts of water, it increases the water content and bulk volume of the stool. The initial response usually occurs in 12 to 24 hours but, in patients who have used laxatives chronically, up to three days may elapse before the initial response.

Indications and Usage: MODANE BULK is indicated in the treatment of constipation resulting from a diet low in residue. It is used also as adjunctive therapy in patients with diverticular disease, spastic or irritable colon, hemorrhoids, in pregnancy, and in convalescent and senile patients.

Contraindications: Intestinal obstruction, fecal impaction.

Precautions *General*—Impaction or obstruction may occur if the bulk-forming agent is temporarily arrested in its passage through parts of the alimentary canal. In this case, water is absorbed and the bolus may become inspissated. Use of this product in patients with narrowing of the intestinal lumen may be hazardous. Inspissation should not occur in a normal gastrointestinal tract if the product is taken with one or more glasses of water.

Drug Interactions—Psyllium may combine with certain other drugs. Products containing psyllium should not be taken with salicylates, digitalis and other cardiac glycosides, or nitrofurantoin.

Adverse Reactions: Adverse reactions are uncommon, and most often have resulted from inadequate intake of water or from underlying organic disease. Esophageal, gastric, small intestinal and rectal obstruction have resulted from the accumulation of the mucilaginous components of psyllium.

Dosage and Administration: Adults and children over 12 years of age—ONE ROUNDED TEASPOONFUL ONE TO THREE TIMES DAILY STIRRED INTO AN 8 OUNCE GLASS OF WATER, JUICE OR OTHER SUITABLE LIQUID AND PREFERABLY FOLLOWED BY A SECOND GLASSFUL OF LIQUID. Children 6 to 12 years of age —one-half the adult dose in 8 ounces of liquid.

How Supplied: Each rounded teaspoonful of MODANE BULK powder contains approximately 3.5 g psyllium.

NDC 0013-5025-72 14 oz. container.
Store at room temperature.

MODANE® SOFT
(docusate sodium)
Capsules

Description: Each MODANE SOFT capsule contains docusate sodium 120 mg, and color additives including FD&C Yellow No. 5 (tartrazine) in a soft gelatin capsule. Docusate sodium is classified as a stool softener. Chemically, docusate sodium is sulfobutanedioic acid 1,4-bis (2-ethylhexyl) ester sodium salt. The chemical structure is: (See next page)

The empirical formula is $C_{20}H_{37}O_7SNa$ and the molecular weight is 444.56. At 25°C the solubility of docusate sodium in water is 15 g/l.

Clinical Pharmacology: Hydration of the stool has been attributed to the drug's surfactant effect on the intestinal contents which

Continued on next page

Adria—Cont.

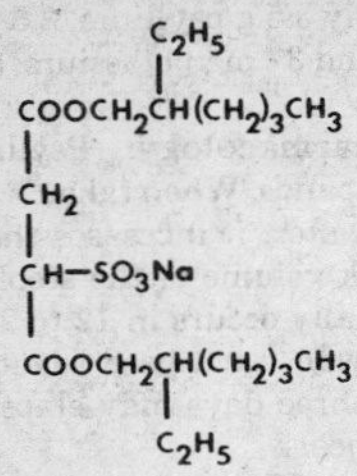

C_2H_5
$COOCH_2CH(CH_2)_3CH_3$
CH_2
$CH—SO_3Na$
$COOCH_2CH(CH_2)_3CH_3$
C_2H_5

docusate sodium

was assumed to facilitate penetration of the fecal mass by water and lipids. Although this emollient effect may exist, there is evidence that mucosal permeability is increased and water absorption is inhibited in the jejunum. Similar concentrations inhibit colonic absorption and/or increase intraluminal water and electrolytes. In these respects, it is similar to bile salts and in this manner, may also be considered as a stimulant laxative.
Docusate sodium is absorbed to some extent in the duodenum and proximal jejunum. It appears in the bile.
Indications and Usage: MODANE SOFT is indicated for the management of functional constipation associated with dry hard stools. It is especially useful when it is desirable to lessen the strain of defecation (e.g. in persons with painful rectal lesions, hernia or cardiovascular disease). The effect on the stools may not be apparent until 1–3 days after the first dose.
Contraindications: Mineral oil administration or when abdominal pain, nausea, vomiting, or other signs and/or symptoms of appendicitis are present.
Precautions: *General*—This product contains FD&C Yellow No. 5 (tartrazine) which may cause allergic-type reactions (including bronchial asthma) in certain susceptible individuals. Although the overall incidence of FD&C Yellow No. 5 (tartrazine) sensitivity in the general population is low, it is frequently seen in patients who also have aspirin hypersensitivity.
Drug Interactions—MODANE SOFT may increase the intestinal absorption of mineral oil and may increase the intestinal absorption and/or hepatic uptake of other drugs administered concurrently.
Carcinogenesis, Mutagenesis, Impairment of Fertility—There have been no long term studies of docusate to evaluate carcinogenic potential. There have been no studies to evaluate mutagenic potential or to determine whether docusate has the potential to impair fertility.
Teratogenic Effects—Pregnancy Category C. Animal reproduction studies have not been conducted with docusate. It is also not known whether MODANE SOFT can cause fetal harm when administered to a pregnant woman or can affect reproductive capacity. MODANE SOFT should be given to a pregnant woman only if clearly needed.
Nursing Mothers—It is not known whether this drug is excreted in human milk. Caution should be exercised when MODANE SOFT is administered to a nursing woman.
Pediatric Use—Because of its dosage size, MODANE SOFT is not recommended for use by children less than 6 years of age.
Adverse Reactions: Adverse reactions are uncommon. Diarrhea, cramping pains and rash have been reported.
Overdosage: Docusates have a low potential for toxicity. Single doses as large as 50 mg/kg have not produced adverse effects in children. Anorexia, vomiting and diarrhea may result from overdosage.
Dosage and Administration: Adults and children over 12 years of age—1 to 3 capsules daily. Children 6–12 years of age—one capsule daily.
How Supplied: Each MODANE SOFT green, soft gelatin capsule contains docusate sodium 120 mg coded 13 503.
NDC 0013-5031-13 Package of 30 Capsules
Store at controlled room temperature (59°–86°F, 15°–30°C).

MODANE®
(danthron)
Tablets and Liquid

Description: MODANE® Tablets (yellow) —Each tablet contains danthron 75 mg and color additives including FD&C Yellow No. 5 (tartrazine).
MODANE® MILD Tablets—Each tablet contains danthron 37.5 mg and color additives including FD&C Yellow No. 5 (tartrazine).
MODANE® Liquid—Each 5 ml (teaspoonful) contains danthron 37.5 mg and alcohol 5%.
Danthron is classified as a stimulant laxative and is chemically 1,8-dihydroxyanthraquinone. Its chemical structure is:

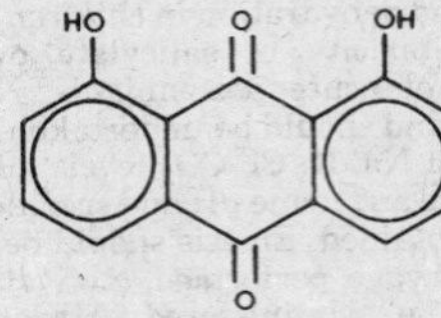

HO O OH
O

danthron

The empirical formula is $C_{14}H_8O_4$ and the molecular weight is 240.21. It is practically insoluble in water.
Clinical Pharmacology: Stimulant cathartics act on the intestinal mucosa and have effects both on the net absorption of electrolytes and water and on motility. This group includes danthron, the docusates, castor oil, and bile acids. Despite similarity of their mechanism of action, there are differences among these drugs which are due, for the most part, to dosage and the major site of action, i.e. small intestine or colon.
Anthraquinone cathartics vary in their effects depending upon their anthraquinone content and the ease of liberation of the active constituents from their inactive precursor glycosides. Danthron, although a free anthraquinone, is similar to the pro-drug glycosides in its pharmacological properties. A soft or semifluid stool is passed 6 to 8 hours after administration of an anthraquinone glycoside cathartic such as danthron.
Danthron is absorbed from the small intestine to a limited extent, circulated through the portal system and into the general circulation and excreted in the bile, urine, saliva, colonic mucosa and milk.
Indications and Usage: MODANE is indicated for the management of constipation. It may be useful in the management of constipation in geriatric, cardiac, surgical and postpartum patients. MODANE may be useful in the management of constipation which may occur with or during the concomitant use of antihypertensive agents, ganglionic blocking agents, antihistamines, tranquilizers, sympathomimetics and anticholinergics. A soft or semifluid stool is passed 6 to 8 hours after administration.
Adequate bulk should be provided in the diet and, if the diet does not provide sufficient bulk, by hydrophilic bulking agents. Poor bowel habits should be corrected.
Contraindications: Should not be used when abdominal pain, nausea, vomiting or other signs and/or symptoms of appendicitis are present.
Precautions: *General*—This product contains FD&C Yellow No. 5 (tartrazine) which may cause allergic-type reactions (including bronchial asthma) in certain susceptible individuals. Although the overall incidence of FD&C Yellow No. 5 (tartrazine) sensitivity in the general population is low, it is frequently seen in patients who also have aspirin hypersensitivity. MODANE may cause harmless pink discoloration of urine (the urine may be pink-red, red-violet or red-brown if alkaline). As with all laxatives, frequent or prolonged use may result in dependence.
Drug Interactions—The absorption of danthron from the gastrointestinal tract and/or its uptake by hepatic cells may be increased by the co-administration of docusate.
Carcinogenesis, Mutagenesis, Impairment of Fertility—There have been no long term studies of MODANE to evaluate carcinogenic potential. There have been no studies to evaluate mutagenic potential or whether MODANE has the potential to impair fertility.
Teratogenic Effects—Pregnancy Category C. Animal reproduction studies have not been conducted with danthron. It is also not known whether danthron can cause fetal harm when administered to a pregnant woman or can affect reproductive capacity. MODANE should be given to a pregnant woman only if clearly needed.
Nursing Mothers—Danthron is excreted in human milk and has been reported to increase bowel activity in infants nursed by women taking it. Caution should be exercised when MODANE is administered to a nursing woman.
Pediatric Use—In general stimulant cathartics should seldom be used in children.
Adverse Reactions: Adverse reactions are uncommon. These are in order of frequency: excessive bowel activity (griping, diarrhea, nausea, vomiting), peri-anal irritation, weakness, dizziness, palpitations and sweating. Temporary brownish mucosal staining has occurred with prolonged use. There has also been reported a suspected allergic reaction with facial swelling, redness and discomfort.
Overdosage: The lowest reported lethal dose in mice and rats is 500 mg/kg. Overdosage may be expected to result in excessive bowel activity. Treatment is symptomatic when the duration of effects is prolonged.
Dosage and Administration: MODANE Tablet (yellow)–Adults—1 tablet with evening meal.
MODANE MILD Tablets (half-strength, pink)–Adults—1 or 2 tablets with the evening meal. For adults who have previously responded with excessive bowel activity to a mild laxative or who are diet-restricted or who are bedfast and for children 6–12 years of age—1 tablet with the evening meal.
MODANE Liquid–Adults—1 to 2 teaspoonfuls with the evening meal. For adults who have previously responded with excessive bowel activity to a mild laxative or who are diet-restricted or who are bedfast and children who are 6–12 years of age—1 teaspoonful with the evening meal.
How Supplied:
Each MODANE Tablet contains danthron 75 mg in a yellow, round, sugar coated tablet, coded 13 501.
NDC 0013-5011-17 Bottle of 100 Tablets
NDC 0013-5011-23 Bottle of 1000 Tablets
NDC 0013-5011-18 STAT-PAK® (unit dose) 100 Tablets
NDC 0013-5011-07 Package of 10 Tablets
NDC 0013-5011-13 Package of 30 Tablets
Store at room temperature.
Each MODANE MILD Tablet contains danthron 37.5 mg in a pink, round, sugar coated tablet, coded 13 502.
NDC 0013-5021-17 Bottle of 100 Tablets
NDC 0013-5021-23 Bottle of 1000 Tablets
Store at room temperature.
Each 5 ml (teaspoonful) of MODANE Liquid contains danthron 37.5 mg in a red liquid.
NDC 0013-5033-51 Pint Bottles
Protect from cold.

MODANE® PLUS

(danthron and docusate sodium)

Tablets

Description: Each MODANE PLUS tablet contains danthron 50 mg and docusate sodium 100 mg and color additives including FD&C Yellow No. 5 (tartrazine). Danthron is classified as a stimulant cathartic and docusate sodium is a stool softener. Chemically docusate sodium is sulfobutanedioic acid 1,4-bis (2-ethylhexyl) ester sodium salt and danthron is 1,8-dihydroxyanthraquinone. The empirical formula of docusate sodium is $C_{20}H_{37}O_7SNa$ and its molecular weight is 444.56. The empirical formula of danthron is $C_{14}H_8O_4$ and its molecular weight is 240.21.

danthron   docusate sodium

Danthron is practically insoluble in water. At 25°C the solubility of docusate sodium in water is 15 g/1.

Clinical Pharmacology: Contact cathartics act on the intestinal mucosa and have effects both on the net absorption of electrolytes and water and on motility. This group includes danthron, the docusates, castor oil, and bile acids. Despite similarity of their mechanism of action, there are differences among these drugs which are due, for the most part, to dosage and the major site of action, i.e. small intestine or colon.

Anthraquinone cathartics vary in their effects depending upon their anthraquinone content and the ease of liberation of the active constituents from their precursor glycosides. Danthron, although a free anthraquinone, is similar to the pro-drug glycosides in its pharmacological properties. A soft or semifluid stool is passed 6 to 8 hours after administration of an anthraquinone glycoside cathartic or danthron.

Hydration of the stool has been attributed to docusate sodium's surfactant effect on the intestinal contents which was assumed to facilitate penetration of the fecal mass by water and lipids. Although this emollient effect may exist, there is evidence that mucosal permeability is increased and water absorption is inhibited in the jejunum. Similar concentrations inhibit colonic absorption and/or increase intraluminal water and electrolytes. In these respects docusate sodium is similar to bile salts and in this manner may also be considered as a stimulant laxative.

Danthron is absorbed from the small intestine to a limited extent, circulated through the portal system and into the general circulation and excreted in the bile, urine, saliva, colonic mucosa and milk.

Docusate sodium is absorbed to some extent in the duodenum and proximal jejunum. It appears in the bile.

Indications and Usage: MODANE PLUS is indicated for the management of constipation where a combination of a stimulant plus a stool softener is needed. It may be useful in geriatric or inactive patients, following surgery, and in patients refractory to other laxatives (see MODANE, MODANE SOFT and MODANE BULK). Adequate bulk should be provided in the diet and, if the diet does not provide sufficient bulk, by hydrophilic bulking agents (MODANE BULK). Poor bowel habits should be corrected.

Contraindications: Mineral oil administration, or when abdominal pain, nausea, vomiting or other signs and/or symptoms of appendicitis are present.

Precautions: *General*—This product contains FD&C Yellow No. 5 (tartrazine) which may cause allergic-type reactions (including bronchial asthma) in certain susceptible individuals. Although the overall incidence of FD&C Yellow No. 5 (tartrazine) sensitivity in the general population is low, it is frequently seen in patients who also have aspirin hypersensitivity. It may cause harmless discoloration of urine (the urine may be pink-red, red-violet or red-brown if alkaline).

As with all laxatives, frequent or prolonged use may result in dependence.

Drug Interactions—Docusate sodium may increase the intestinal absorption and/or hepatic uptake of other drugs administered concurrently.

Carcinogenesis, Mutagenesis, Impairment of Fertility—There have been no long term studies of MODANE PLUS to evaluate carcinogenic potential. There have been no studies to evaluate mutagenic potential or to determine whether MODANE PLUS has the potential to impair fertility.

Teratogenic Effects—Pregnancy Category C. Animal reproduction studies have not been conducted with danthron and docusate sodium. It is also not known whether MODANE PLUS can cause fetal harm when administered to a pregnant woman or can affect reproductive capacity. MODANE PLUS should be given to a pregnant woman only if clearly needed.

Nursing Mothers—Danthron is excreted in human milk and has been reported to increase bowel activity in infants nursed by women taking it. Caution should be exercised when MODANE PLUS is administered to a nursing woman.

Pediatric Use—Because of its dosage size, MODANE PLUS is not recommended for use by children less than 12 years.

Adverse Reactions: Adverse reactions are uncommon. These are in order of frequency: Excessive bowel activity (griping, diarrhea, nausea, vomiting), peri-anal irritation, weakness, dizziness, palpitations and sweating. Temporary brownish mucosal staining has occurred with prolonged use. There have also been reports of rash and a report of facial swelling, redness and discomfort.

Overdosage: Docusates and danthron have low potential for toxicity. The oral LD_{50} values of danthron, docusate sodium and danthron—docusate sodium combination in mice were greater than 7 g/kg, 2.64 g/kg and 3.44 g/kg, respectively. The lowest reported lethal dose of danthron in mice and rats is 500 mg/kg. Single doses of docusate sodium, as large as 50 mg/kg, have not produced adverse effects in children. Overdosage may be expected to result in anorexia, vomiting and diarrhea. Treatment is symptomatic when the duration of effects is prolonged.

Dosage and Administration: Adults and children over 12 years of age—1 tablet daily with evening meal.

How Supplied Each MODANE PLUS tablet contains a combination of danthron 50 mg and docusate sodium 100 mg in a brown, round, sugar coated tablet coded 13 504.

NDC 0013-5041-13 30 Tablet Package

NDC 0013-5041-17 Bottle of 100 Tablets

Store at room temperature

AHFS 56:12

MYOFLEX® CREME

(Triethanolamine Salicylate)

Description: Triethanolamine salicylate 10% in a non-greasy base. Nonirritating, nonburning, odorless, stainless, readily absorbed.

Actions: Topical Analgesic. Penetration assured with maximal salicylate appearing in urine 5 hours after application.

Indications: An effective analgesic rub for sore muscles, joint attachments, stiffness and strains; a helpful topical adjunct in arthritis and rheumatism. Excellent as a hand cream for patients with minor rheumatic stiffness and soreness of the hands. Excellent for sore feet.

Contraindications: Do not use in patients manifesting idiosyncrasy to salicylates.

Warnings: For external use only. Avoid getting into eyes or on mucous membranes. To be used only according to directions. Keep out of the reach of children.

Precautions: Apply to affected parts only. Do not apply to irritated skin or if excessive irritation develops, consult physician. A 2 oz. tube contains the salicylate equivalent of about 56 grains of aspirin.

Adverse Reactions: None reported, but if applied to large skin areas may cause typical salicylate side effects such as tinnitus, nausea, or vomiting.

Dosage and Administration: Adults—Rub into area of soreness two or three times daily. Wrists, elbows, knees and ankles may be wrapped loosely with 2″ or 3″ elastic bandage after liberal application.

How Supplied:

NDC 0013-5404-61 Tubes, 2 oz.

NDC 0013-5404-74 Jars, 1 lb.

NEOSAR™ FOR INJECTION

(cyclophosphamide USP)

Description: NEOSAR is a synthetic antineoplastic drug chemically related to the nitrogen mustards. It is a white crystalline powder which is soluble in water, physiological saline, or alcohol. **Store NEOSAR products at 2–32°C(36–90°F).**

Actions: Although it is classified generally as an alkylating agent, cyclophosphamide itself is not an alkylating agent or irritant. It interferes with the growth of susceptible neoplasms and, to some extent, certain normal tissues. Its mechanism of action is not known. Cyclophosphamide is absorbed from the gastrointestinal tract and parenteral sites. It is metabolized (the details of metabolism are not fully known) and the drug and its metabolites are distributed throughout the body, including the brain. Intravenously administered cyclophosphamide is reported to have a serum half-life of about four hours; however, the drug and /or its metabolites may be detected in plasma up to seventy-two hours. Cyclophosphamide and its metabolites are excreted by the kidneys, but the extent to which they are excreted by other routes is not known. Of three alkylating metabolites found in urine, only one (nornitrogen mustard) has been definitely identified.

Indications: Cyclophosphamide, though effective alone in susceptible malignancies, is more frequently used concurrently or sequentially with other antineoplastic drugs. The following malignancies are often susceptible to cyclophosphamide treatment:

1. Malignant lymphomas (Stages III and IV, Ann Arbor Staging System).
   a. Hodgkin's disease.
   b. Lymphoma (nodular or diffuse).
   c. Mixed-cell type lymphoma.
   d. Histiocytic lymphoma.
   e. Burkitt's lymphoma.
2. Multiple myeloma.
3. Leukemias:
   a. Chronic lymphocytic leukemia.
   b. Chronic granulocytic leukemia (it is ineffective in acute blastic crises).
   c. Acute myelogenous and monocytic leukemia.
   d. Acute lymphoblastic (stem-cell) leukemia in children (cyclophosphamide given during remission is effective in prolonging its duration).

Continued on next page

Adria—Cont.

4. Mycosis fungoides (advanced disease).
5. Neuroblastoma.
6. Adenocarcinoma of the ovary.
7. Retinoblastoma.
8. Carcinoma of the breast.

Warnings: Since cyclophosphamide has been reported to be more toxic in adrenalectomized dogs, adjustment of the doses of both replacement steroids and cyclophosphamide may be necessary for the adrenalectomized patient.
The rate of metabolism and the leukopenic activity of cyclophosphamide reportedly are increased by chronic administration of high doses of phenobarbital. The physician should be alert for possible combined drug actions, desirable or undesirable, involving cyclophosphamide even though cyclophosphamide has been used successfully concurrently with other drugs, including other cytotoxic drugs.
Cyclophosphamide may interfere with normal wound healing.
Usage in Pregnancy: Category C. Cyclophosphamide can be teratogenic or cause fetal resorption in experimental animals. It should not be used in pregnancy, particularly in early pregnancy, unless in the judgment of the physician the potential benefits outweigh the possible risks. Cyclophosphamide is excreted in breast milk and breast-feeding should be terminated prior to institution of cyclophosphamide therapy.
Patients, male or female, capable of conception ordinarily should be advised of the mutagenic potential of cyclophosphamide. Adequate methods of contraception appear desirable for such patients receiving cyclophosphamide.
Precautions: Cyclophosphamide should be given cautiously to patients with any of the following conditions:

1. Leukopenia
2. Thrombocytopenia
3. Tumor cell infiltration of bone marrow
4. Previous X-ray therapy
5. Previous therapy with other cytotoxic agents
6. Impaired hepatic function
7. Impaired renal function

Because cyclophosphamide may exert a suppressive action on immune mechanisms, interruption or modification of dosage should be considered for patients who develop bacterial, fungal or viral infections. This is especially true for patients receiving concomitant steroid therapy and perhaps those with a recent history of steroid therapy, since infections in some of these patients have been fatal. Varicella-zoster infections appear to be particularly dangerous under these circumstances.
Adverse Reactions:
Secondary Neoplasia: Secondary malignancies have developed in some patients treated with cyclophosphamide alone or in association with other antineoplastic drugs and/or modalities. These malignancies most frequently have been urinary bladder, myeloproliferative, and lymphoproliferative malignancies. Secondary malignancies most frequently have developed in the cyclophosphamide-treated patients with primary myeloproliferative and lymphoproliferative malignancies and primary nonmalignant diseases in which immune processes are believed to be involved pathologically. In some cases, the secondary malignancy was detected up to several years after cyclophosphamide treatment was discontinued. The secondary urinary bladder malignancies generally have occurred in patients who previously developed hemorrhagic cystitis (see Genitourinary under Adverse Reactions). Although no cause-effect relationship has been established between cyclophosphamide and the development of malignancy in humans, the possibility of secondary malignancy, based on available data, should be considered in any benefit-to-risk assessment for the use of the drug.
Hematopoietic: Leukopenia is an expected effect and ordinarily is used as a guide to therapy. Thrombocytopenia or anemia may occur in a few patients. These effects are almost always reversible when therapy is interrupted.
Gastrointestinal: Anorexia, nausea, or vomiting are common and related to dose as well as individual susceptibility. There are isolated reports of hemorrhagic colitis, oral mucosal ulceration and jaundice occurring during therapy.
Genitourinary: Sterile hemorrhagic cystitis can result from the administration of cyclophosphamide. THIS CAN BE SEVERE, EVEN FATAL, and is probably due to metabolites in the urine. Nonhemorrhagic cystitis and/or fibrosis of the bladder also have been reported to result from cyclophosphamide administration. Atypical epithelial cells may be found in the urinary sediment. **Ample fluid intake and frequent voiding help to prevent the development of cystitis,** but when it occurs it is ordinarily necessary to interrupt cyclophosphamide therapy. Hematuria usually resolves spontaneously within a few days after cyclophosphamide therapy is discontinued, but may persist for several months. In severe cases replacement of blood loss may be required. The application of electrocautery to telangiectatic areas of the bladder and diversion of urine flow have been successful methods used in treatment of protracted cases. Cryosurgery has also been used. (See also Secondary Neoplasia under Adverse Reactions.) Nephrotoxicity, including hemorrhage and clot formation in the renal pelvis, have been reported.
Gonadal suppression, resulting in amenorrhea or azoospermia, has been reported in a number of patients treated with cyclophosphamide and appears to be related to dosage and duration of therapy. This side effect, possibly irreversible, should be anticipated in patients treated with cyclophosphamide. It is not known to what extent cyclophosphamide may affect prepuberal gonads. Fibrosis of the ovary following cyclophosphamide therapy has been reported also.
Integument: It is ordinarily advisable to inform patients in advance of possible alopecia, a frequent complication of cyclophosphamide therapy. Regrowth of hair can be expected although occasionally the new hair may be of a different color or texture. The skin and fingernails may become darker during therapy. Nonspecific dermatitis has been reported to occur with cyclophosphamide.
Pulmonary: Interstitial pulmonary fibrosis has been reported in patients receiving high doses of cyclophosphamide over a prolonged period.
Dosage and Administration: Chemotherapy with NEOSAR, as with other drugs used in cancer chemotherapy, is potentially hazardous and fatal complications can occur. It is recommended that it be administered only by physicians aware of the associated risks. Therapy may be aimed at either induction or maintenance of remission.
Induction Therapy: The usual initial intravenous loading dose for patients with no hematologic deficiency is 40-50 mg/kg (1500–1800 mg/m^2). This total initial intravenous loading dose usually is given in divided doses over a period of two to five days.
Patients with any previous treatment that may have compromised the functional capacity of the bone marrow, such as X-ray or cytotoxic drugs, and patients with tumor infiltration of the bone marrow may require reduction of the initial loading dose by ⅓ to ½.
A marked leukopenia is usually associated with the above doses, but recovery usually begins after 7–10 days. The white blood cell count should be monitored closely during induction therapy.
Maintenance Therapy: It is frequently necessary to maintain chemotherapy in order to suppress or retard neoplastic growth. A variety of schedules has been used:

1. 10–15 mg/kg (350–550 mg/m^2) i.v. every 7–10 days
2. 3–5 mg/kg (110–185 mg/m^2) i.v. twice weekly

Unless the disease is unusually sensitive to NEOSAR, it is advisable to give the largest maintenance dose that can be reasonably tolerated by the patient. The total leukocyte count is a good objective guide for regulating the maintenance dose. Ordinarily a leukopenia of 3000–4000 cells/mm^3 can be maintained without undue risk of serious infection or other complications.
Preparation and Handling of Solutions: NEOSAR FOR INJECTION should be prepared for parenteral use by adding **Sterile Water for Injection, USP or Bacteriostatic Water for Injection, USP (paraben preserved only)** to the vial and shaking to dissolve. Use 5 ml for the 100 mg vial, 10 ml for the 200 mg vial, or 25 ml for the 500 mg vial. Solutions of NEOSAR FOR INJECTION may be injected intravenously, intramuscularly, intraperitoneally or intrapleurally or they may be infused intravenously in Dextrose Injection, USP (5% dextrose) or Dextrose and Sodium Chloride Injection, USP (5% dextrose and 0.9% sodium chloride). These solutions should be used within 24 hours if stored at room temperature or within 6 days if stored under refrigeration (2–8°C; 36°–46°F). NEOSAR FOR INJECTION does not contain an antimicrobial agent and **care must be taken to insure the sterility of prepared solutions.**
Extemporaneous liquid preparations of NEOSAR for oral administration may be prepared by dissolving NEOSAR FOR INJECTION in Aromatic Elixir, USP. Such preparations should be stored under refrigeration and used within 14 days.
Overdosages: No specific antidote for NEOSAR is known. Management of overdosage would include general supportive measures to sustain the patient through any period of toxicity that might occur.
How Supplied:
NEOSAR FOR INJECTION (cyclophosphamide USP) is available as follows:
NDC 0013-5606-93 100 mg vials, cartons of 12
NDC 0013-5616-93 200 mg vials, cartons of 12
NDC 0013-5626-93 500 mg vials, cartons of 12
Store at 2–32°C (36–90°F).
Manufactured by:
ASTA-WERKE A.G.
BIELEFELD, GERMANY
for:
ADRIA LABORATORIES INC.
COLUMBUS, OHIO 43215

TYMPAGESIC® ℞
Otic Solution

Analgesic-Decongestant Ear Drops

Description: TYMPAGESIC Otic Solution, analgesic-decongestant ear drops, contains phenylephrine hydrochloride USP 0.25%, antipyrine USP 5% and benzocaine USP 5% v/v in propylene glycol USP.
Phenylephrine hydrochloride is a sympathomimetic amine with local vasoconstriction or decongestant action. It is chemically (R)-3-hydroxy-α-[(methylamino)methyl] benzenemethanol hydrochloride and has the following structure:

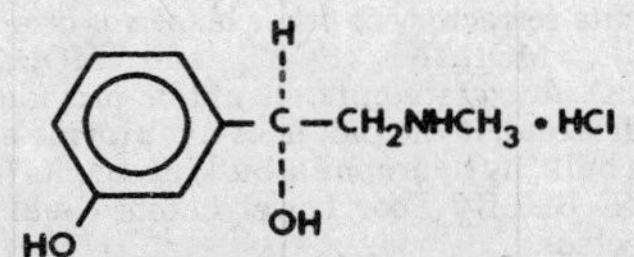

It occurs as white crystals, has bitter taste and

is freely soluble in water and alcohol. Its molecular weight is 203.67.

Antipyrine is an analgesic with local anesthetic action. It is chemically 2:3-dimethyl-1-phenyl-3-pyrazolin-5-one and has the following structure:

Antipyrine occurs as colorless crystals or white powder, has a slightly bitter taste and is soluble in water and alcohol. Its molecular weight is 188.23.

Benzocaine is a local anesthetic. It is chemically ethyl p-aminobenzoate and has the following structure:

It occurs as white crystals or white crystalline powder and is slightly soluble in water and soluble in organic solvents. Its molecular weight is 165.19.

Clinical Pharmacology: Topical application of phenylephrine produces vasoconstriction mainly by a direct effect on α-adrenergic receptors. The effects of phenylephrine are similar to those of epinephrine. However, phenylephrine is considered less CNS and cardiostimulatory than epinephrine. Phenylephrine, after its absorption, is metabolized in the liver and the intestine by the enzyme monoamine oxidase (MAO). The type, route and rate of excretion of metabolites have not been defined.

Like other local anesthetics, benzocaine acts by blocking nerve conduction first in autonomic, then in sensory and finally in motor nerve fibers. Its effect appears to be due to decreased nerve cell membrane permeability to sodium ions or competition with calcium ions for membrane binding sites. A vasoconstrictor, such as phenylephrine, is added to decrease the rate of absorption and prolong the duration of action of the anesthetic. Ester-type anesthetics, which include benzocaine, after absorption are comparatively rapidly degraded by esterases mainly in the liver and excreted in the urine as metabolites and in small amounts as the unchanged drug.

Antipyrine is believed to have analgesic and local anesthetic effects on the nerve endings. After absorption, it is slowly metabolized in the liver by oxidation and conjugation with glucuronic acid and is excreted in the urine mainly in the conjugated form.

Indications and Usage: TYMPAGESIC Otic Solution may be used as a topical anesthetic in the external auditory canal to relieve ear pain. It may be used concomitantly with systemic antibiotics as in the treatment of acute otitis media.

Contraindications: TYMPAGESIC is contraindicated in the presence of a perforated tympanic membrane or ear discharge and in individuals with a history of hypersensitivity to any of its ingredients.

Warnings: As with all drugs containing a sympathomimetic or an anesthetic, systemic reactions may occur after local application. Phenylephrine may cause blanching and a feeling of coolness in the skin. Allergic and idiosyncratic reactions to local anesthetics have been observed infrequently. Such reactions are unlikely because absorption from the skin of the ear drum or the external ear canal is minimal.

Cross-sensitivity reactions between members of the *caine* group of local anesthetics have been reported.

Precautions:

General—Drugs containing a sympathomimetic should be used with caution in the elderly and in patients with hypertension, increased intraocular pressure, diabetes mellitus, ischemic heart disease, hyperthyroidism and prostatic hypertrophy.

High plasma levels of benzocaine and antipyrine may cause CNS stimulation with nausea and vomiting. Such levels, however, are unlikely to be attained following local application in the external ear.

Drug Interactions—MAO inhibitors and β-adrenergic blockers enhance the effects of sympathomimetics. Benzocaine is hydrolyzed in the body to p-aminobenzoic acid which competes with the antibacterial action of sulfonamides. However, these are unlikely to occur because of limited absorption from the external ear canal.

Carcinogenesis, Mutagenesis, Impairment of Fertility—There have been no studies in animals or humans to evaluate the carcinogenesis, mutagenesis or impairment of fertility for Tympagesic.

Pregancy—Category C. Animal reproduction studies have not been conducted with TYMPAGESIC. It is also not known whether TYMPAGESIC can cause fetal harm when administered to a pregnant woman or can effect reproduction capacity. Tympagesic should be given to a pregnant woman only if clearly needed.

Nursing Mothers—It is not known whether this drug is excreted in human milk. Because many drugs are excreted in human milk, caution should be exercised when TYMPAGESIC is administered to a nursing woman.

Pediatric Use—Safety and effectiveness in children below the age of 12 has not been established.

Adverse Reactions: Following its absorption, phenylephrine may produce a pressor response or cause restlessness, anxiety, nervousness, weakness, pallor, headache and dizziness. Absorption of benzocaine and antipyrine in the plasma may cause chills, nausea, vomiting, tinnitus and agranulocytosis. Such reactions are unlikely following application of TYMPAGESIC on the external ear canal.

Benzocaine can cause a hypersensitivity reaction consisting of rash, urticaria and edema. Individuals frequently exposed to ester-type local anesthetics can develop contact dermatitis characterized by erythema and pruritus which may progress to vesiculation and oozing.

Overdosage: It is more likely to be associated with accidental or deliberate ingestion rather than cutaneous absorption. Phenylephrine present in a bottle (13 ml) of TYMPAGESIC, if absorbed, may cause hypertension, headache, vomiting and palpitations. Effects of benzocaine overdosage may include yawning, restlessness, excitement, nausea and vomiting. Antipyrine overdosage may cause giddiness, tremor, sweating and skin eruptions.

Treatment is symptomatic. If ingestion of the contents of a bottle or more of TYMPAGESIC is recent or food is present in the stomach, induction of emesis with ipecac syrup, gastric emptying and lavage and introduction of activated charcoal may be recommended.

Dosage and Administration: Using the dropper, instill TYMPAGESIC Otic Solution in the external ear canal allowing the solution to run into the canal until filled. Insert a cotton pledget into the meatus after moistening with the otic solution. Repeat every 2 to 4 hours, if necessary, until pain is relieved.

Replace dropper in bottle without rinsing.

How Supplied: TYMPAGESIC Otic Solution is supplied in 13 ml amber glass dropper bottles (NDC 0013-7363-39).

Store at 15–30°C (59–86°F).

Albion Laboratories, Inc.
101 N. MAIN STREET
CLEARFIELD, UT 84015

CHELATED CALCIUM TABLETS
(See PDR For Nonprescription Drugs)

CHELATED IRON TABLETS
(See PDR For Nonprescription Drugs)

CHELATED IRON PLEX TABLETS
(See PDR For Nonprescription Drugs)

CHELATED MAGNESIUM TABLETS
(See PDR For Nonprescription Drugs)

CHELATED MANGANESE CAPSULES
(See PDR For Nonprescription Drugs)

CHELATED MANGANESE TABLETS
(See PDR For Nonprescription Drugs)

CHELATED MULTI-MIN TABLETS
(See PDR For Nonprescription Drugs)

CHELATED MULTI-VITA-MIN CAPSULES
(See PDR For Nonprescription Drugs)

CHELATED TRI-MINS TABLETS
(See PDR For Nonprescription Drugs)

CHELATED ZINC CAPSULES
(See PDR For Nonprescription Drugs)

CHELATED ZINC TABLETS
(See PDR For Nonprescription Drugs)

COMPLEXED POTASSIUM TABLETS
(See PDR For Nonprescription Drugs)

Alcon Laboratories, Inc.
and its affiliates
CORPORATE HEADQUARTERS:
PO BOX 1959
6201 SOUTH FREEWAY
FORT WORTH, TX 76134

OPHTHALMIC PRODUCTS
For information on Alcon ophthalmic products, consult the PDR for Ophthalmology. See a complete listing of products in the Manufacturer's Index Section of this book. For information, literature, samples or service items contact Alcon Sales Services.

IDENTIFICATION PROBLEM?

Consult PDR's

Product Identification Section

where you'll find over 900

products pictured actual size

and in full color.

Alcon (Puerto Rico) Inc.
P.O. BOX 3000
HUMACAO, PUERTO RICO 00661

AVITENE® ℞
(Microfibrillar Collagen Hemostat)

Description: Avitene® (Microfibrillar Collagen Hemostat, or MCH), is an absorbable topical hemostatic agent prepared as a dry, sterile, fibrous, water insoluble partial hydrochloric acid salt of purified bovine corium collagen. It is prepared in a loose fibrous form and in a compacted "non-woven" web form. In its manufacture, swelling of the native collagen fibrils is controlled by ethyl alcohol to permit non-covalent attachment of hydrochloric acid to amine groups on the collagen molecule and preservation of the essential morphology of native collagen molecules. Dry heat sterilization causes some cross-linking which is evidenced by reduction of hydrating properties, and a decrease of molecular weight which implies some degradation of collagen molecules. However, the characteristics of collagen which are essential to its effect on the blood coagulation mechanisms are preserved.

Actions: Avitene (MCH), in contact with a bleeding surface, attracts platelets which adhere to the fibrils and undergo the release phenomenon to trigger aggregation of platelets into thrombi in the interstices of the fibrous mass. The effect on platelet adhesion and aggregation is not inhibited by heparin *in vitro*. It has been found effective in heparinized dogs and in eight of nine fully heparinized human subjects. Platelets of patients with clinical thrombasthenia do not adhere to MCH *in vitro*. However, in clinical trials it was effective in 50 of 68 patients receiving aspirin. MCH cannot control bleeding due to systemic coagulation disorders. Appropriate therapy to correct the underlying coagulopathy should be instituted prior to use of the product. MCH is tenaciously adherent to surfaces wet with blood but excess material not involved in the hemostatic clot may be removed by teasing or irrigation, usually without causing rebleeding. In animal and human studies, it has been shown to stimulate a mild, chronic cellular inflammatory response. When implanted in animal tissues, it is absorbed in less than 84 days. In human studies of hemostasis in osteotomy cuts, it has been shown not to interfere with bone regeneration or healing. In animal studies, it has been demonstrated that MCH does not predispose to stenosis at vascular anastomotic sites. These findings have not been confirmed in human use. Studies have been performed using MCH (fibrous form) in experimental wounds contaminated with hemolytic *Staphylococcus aureus*. The presence of MCH does not enhance or initiate staphylococcus wound infections to a greater or lesser extent than control agents employed for the same purpose. The effects of MCH (fibrous form) on experimental wounds contaminated with a gram-negative aerobic rod and an anaerobic non-spore forming bacteria are currently under investigation.

Indications: Avitene (MCH) is used in surgical procedures as an adjunct to hemostasis when control of bleeding by ligature or conventional procedures is ineffective or impractical.

Contraindications: Avitene (MCH) should not be used in the closure of skin incisions as it may interfere with the healing of the skin edges. This is due to simple mechanical interposition of dry collagen and not to any intrinsic interference with wound healing. By filling porosities of cancellous bone, MCH may significantly reduce the bond strength of methylmethacrylate adhesives. MCH should not, therefore, be employed on bone surfaces to which prosthetic materials are to be attached with methylmethacrylate adhesives.

Warnings: Avitene (MCH) is inactivated by autoclaving. Ethylene oxide reacts with bound hydrochloric acid to form ethylene chlorohydrin. This product should not be resterilized. It is not for injection. Moistening MCH or wetting with saline or thrombin impairs its hemostatic efficacy. It should be used dry. Discard any unused portion. As with any foreign substance, use in contaminated wounds may enhance infection.

Precautions: Only that amount of Avitene (MCH) necessary to produce hemostasis should be used. After several minutes, excess material should be removed; this is usually possible without the re-initiation of active bleeding. Failure to remove excess MCH may result in bowel adhesion or mechanical pressure sufficient to compromise the ureter. In otolaryngological surgery, precautions against aspiration should include removal of all excess dry material and thorough irrigation of the pharynx. MCH contains a low, but detectable, level of intercalated bovine serum protein which reacts immunologically as does beef serum albumin. Increases in anti-BSA titer have been observed following treatment with MCH. About two-thirds of individuals exhibit antibody titers because of ingestion of food products of bovine origin. Intradermal skin tests have occasionally shown a weak positive reaction to BSA or MCH but these have not been correlated with IgG titers to BSA. Tests have failed to demonstrate clinically significant elicitation of antibodies of the IgE class against BSA following MCH therapy. Care should be exercised to avoid spillage on nonbleeding surfaces, particularly in abdominal or thoracic viscera. Teratology studies in rats and rabbits have revealed no harm to the animal fetus. There are no well-controlled studies in pregnant women; therefore, MCH should be used in pregnant women only when clearly needed.

Adverse Reactions: The most serious adverse reactions reported which may be related to the use of Avitene (MCH) are potentiation of infection including abscess formation, hematoma, wound dehiscence and mediastinitis. Other reported adverse reactions possibly related are adhesion formation, allergic reaction, foreign body reaction and subgaleal seroma (report of a single case). The use of MCH in dental extraction sockets has been reported to increase the incidence of alveolalgia. Transient laryngospasm due to aspiration of dry material has been reported following use of MCH in tonsillectomy.

Dosage and Administration: Avitene (MCH) must be applied directly to the source of bleeding. Because of its adhesiveness, it may seal over the exit site of deeper hemorrhage and conceal an underlying hematoma as in penetrating liver wounds. Surfaces to be treated should be compressed with dry sponges immediately prior to application of the dry MCH. It is then necessary to apply pressure over the MCH with a dry sponge for a period of time which varies with the force and severity of bleeding. A minute may suffice for capillary bleeding (e.g., skin graft donor sites, dermatologic curettage) but three to five or more minutes may be required for brisk bleeding (e.g., splenic tears) or high pressure leaks in major artery suture holes. For control of oozing from cancellous bone, it should be firmly packed into the spongy bone surface. After five to ten minutes, excess MCH should be teased away (see **Precautions**); this is usually be accomplished with blunt forceps and is facilitated by wetting with sterile 0.9% saline solution and irrigation. If breakthrough bleeding occurs in areas of thin application, additional MCH may be applied. The amount required depends, again, on the severity of bleeding. In capillary bleeding, one gram will usually be sufficient for a 50 cm^2 area. Thicker coverage will be required for more brisk bleeding. MCH will adhere to wet gloves, instruments, or tissue surfaces. To facilitate handling, dry smooth forceps should be used. Gloved fingers should not be used to apply pressure. In neurosurgical and other procedures the non-woven web may conveniently be used by applying small squares to bleeding areas and then covering the sites with moist cottonoid "patties". To prevent wetting of the MCH, and to apply needed pressure, a suction tip should be held against the cottonoid for one to several minutes, depending on the briskness of bleeding. After five to ten minutes excess MCH may be removed by teasing and irrigation.

How Supplied: Fibrous Form; in 1 g and 5 g sterile jars of sterile microfibrillar collagen hemostat all contained in a sealed can. Sterility of the jar exterior cannot be guaranteed if can seal is broken. Content of jar is sterile until opened. Non-woven Web form; as 70 mm × 70 mm × 1 mm (2.75″ × 2.75″ × .04″) and 70 mm × 35 mm × 1 mm (2.75″ × 1.4″ × .04″) sheets, each contained in a sterile blister pack within a foil pouch. Sterility of the blister pack cannot be guaranteed after the pouch is opened. Content of the blister pack is sterile until adhesive backing is removed.

"Avitene" is a registered trademark of Alcon (Puerto Rico) Inc.

Allergan Pharmaceuticals, Inc.
2525 DUPONT DRIVE
IRVINE, CA 92713

OPHTHALMIC PRODUCTS

For information on Allergan prescription and OTC ophthalmic products, consult the Physicians' Desk Reference For Ophthalmology. For literature, service items or sample material, contact Allergan directly. See a complete listing of products in the Manufacturers' Index section of this book.

Almay Hypoallergenic Cosmetics and Toiletries
Almay, Inc.
850 THIRD AVENUE
NEW YORK, NY 10022

Almay Hypoallergenic Cosmetics and Toiletries
Almay, Inc.
PROFESSIONAL SERVICE DEPT.
APEX, NC 27502

ALMAY HYPO-ALLERGENIC COSMETICS, SKIN CARE PRODUCTS AND TOILETRIES
(See PDR For Nonprescription Drugs)

Alto Pharmaceuticals, Inc.
PO BOX 271369
TAMPA, FL 33688

EFED II™

Description: Each Efed II capsule contains: Theionized® ephedrine sulfate 25 mg. and caffeine 150 mg.

Indications: Efed II capsules are safe, effective, and non-habit forming. Efed II fast acting ingredients give immediate relief from fatigue, drowsiness and stuffiness. Use as a stimulant to aid in mental alertness; also as a decongestant and bronchodilator in the management of bronchial asthma.

Warnings: Keep this and all medications out of the reach of small children. Do not exceed recommended dosage. Reduce dosage if nervousness, or restlessness, or sleeplessness occurs. Because of the ephedrine component, this medicine should be used with caution by el-

derly males or those with known prostatic hypertrophy.
Caution: If under medical care do not take without consulting a pharmacist or physician. Individuals with high blood pressure, heart disease, diabetes or thyroid disease, should use only as directed by a physician. Do not take as a substitute for normal sleep. May interfere with sleep if taken within four (4) hours of bedtime.
Adult Dosage: One capsule every four hours, not to exceed four (4) capsules in a 24 hour period. Not recommended for children under 12 years of age.
How Supplied: Packages of 24 capsules and bottles of 100.
[*Shown in Product Identification Section*]

ZINC-220® CAPSULES
(zinc sulfate 220 mg.)

Composition: Each opaque blue and pink capsule contains zinc sulfate 220 mg. delivering 55 mg. of elemental zinc. Zinc-220 Capsules do not contain dextrose or glucose.
Action and Uses: Zinc-220 Capsules are indicated as a dietary supplement. Normal growth and tissue repair are directly dependent upon an adequate supply of zinc in the diet. Zinc functions as an integral part of a number of enzymes important to protein and carbohydrate metabolism. Zinc-220 Capsules are recommended for deficiencies or the prevention of deficiencies of zinc.
Warnings: Zinc-220 if administered in stat dosages of 2 grams (9 capsules) will cause an emetic effect.
Precaution: It is recommended that Zinc-220 Capsules be taken with meals or milk to avoid gastric distress.
Contraindications: None.
Dosage: One capsule daily with milk or meals. One capsule daily provides approximately 5.3 times the recommended adult requirement for zinc.
How Supplied: Bottles of 100 and 1000 capsules and Unit Dose Strips boxes of 100 capsules. (NDC 0731-0401)
[*Shown in Product Identification Section*]

Alza Corporation
950 PAGE MILL ROAD
PALO ALTO, CA 94304

PROGESTASERT® ℞
Intrauterine Progesterone Contraceptive System
Release rated 65 μg/day progesterone for one year

Description: The PROGESTASERT® Intrauterine Progesterone Contraceptive System is a white, T-shaped unit constructed of ethylene/vinyl acetate copolymer (EVA) containing titanium dioxide. The 36-mm tubular stem of the T contains a reservoir of 38 mg of progesterone, USP, together with barium sulfate, USP, for radiopacity; both are dispersed in medical grade silicone fluid. The 32-mm horizontal crossarms are solid EVA. Two monofilament nylon indicator/retrieval threads are fastened to the base of the T stem.

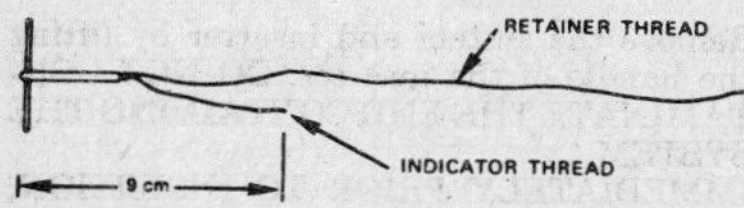

One tip of the shorter indicator thread is 9 cm from the top or leading end of the system and is used to ascertain correct placement at insertion. The long thread extends the length of the inserter where it is anchored by a plug and retains the system in the inserter. This thread is cut to length after insertion.

The PROGESTASERT® system is packaged sterile within its curved, malleable inserter. Progesterone is released from the system at an average rate of 65 μg/day for one year by membrane-controlled diffusion from the reservoir. None of the inert ingredients of the reservoir or membrane—barium sulfate, silicone fluid, titanium dioxide, or EVA—is released from the system.
Action: Available data indicate that the contraceptive effectiveness of the PROGESTASERT® system is enhanced by its continuous release of progesterone at an average rate of 65 μg/day for one year into the uterine cavity. The mechanism by which progesterone enhances the contraceptive effectiveness of the T is local, not systemic. The concentrations of luteinizing hormone, estradiol, and progesterone in systemic venous plasma follow regular cyclic patterns indicative of ovulation during use of the PROGESTASERT® system. Blood chemistry studies related to liver, kidney, and thyroid function also reveal no changes.
During use of the system the endometrium shows progestational influence. Progesterone from the system suppresses proliferation of the endometrial tissue (an anti-estrogenic effect). Following removal of the system, the endometrium rapidly returns to its normal cyclic pattern and can support pregnancy. The local mechanism by which continuously released progesterone enhances the contraceptive effectiveness of the T has not been conclusively demonstrated. The hypotheses that have been offered are: progesteone-induced inhibition of sperm capacitation or survival; and alteration of the uterine milieu so as to prevent nidation.
Indications and Usage: The PROGESTASERT® system is indicated for contraception in parous and nulliparous women.
Contraindications: The PROGESTASERT® system should not be inserted when the following conditions exist:
1. Pregnancy or suspicion of pregnancy.
2. Previous ectopic pregnancy.
3. Presence of, or a history of one or more episodes of, pelvic inflammatory disease.
4. Presence of, or a history of one or more episodes of, venereal disease, including gonorrhea, syphilis, or chlamydial infection of the genital tract.
5. Previous pelvic surgery.
6. Presence of, or a history of one or more episodes of, postpartum endometritis or infected abortion.
7. Abnormalities of the uterus which have resulted in distortion of the uterine cavity.
8. Known or suspected uterine or cervical malignancy including, but not limited to, an unresolved, abnormal "Pap" smear.
9. Genital bleeding of unknown etiology.
10. Acute cervicitis, unless and until infection has been completely controlled and has been shown to be nongonococcal.

Warnings:
1. Pregnancy
a. *Long term effects.* Long term effects on the offspring when pregnancy occurs with the PROGESTASERT® system in place are unknown.
b. *Septic Abortion.* Reports have indicated an increased incidence of septic abortion associated in some instances with septicemia, septic shock and death in patients becoming pregnant with an intrauterine device (IUD) in place. Most of these reports have been associated with the mid-trimester of pregnancy. In some cases, the initial symptoms have been insidious and not easily recognized. If pregnancy should occur with a PROGESTASERT® system *in situ*, it should be removed if the thread is visible or, if removal proves to be or would be difficult, termination of the pregnancy should be considered and offered the patient as an option, bearing in mind that the risks associated with an elective abortion increase with gestational age.
c. *Continuation of pregnancy.* If the patient chooses to continue the pregnancy, she must be warned of the increased risk of spontaneous abortion and of the increased risk of sepsis, including death if the pregnancy continues with the system in place. The patient must be closely observed and she must be advised to report all abnormal symptoms, such as flu-like syndrome, fever, abdominal cramping and pain, bleeding, or vaginal discharge immediately because generalized symptoms of septicemia may be insidious.
2. Ectopic Pregnancy
a. A pregnancy that occurs while a patient is wearing an IUD is much more likely to be ectopic than a pregnancy occurring without an IUD in place. Accordingly, patients in whom pregnancy occurs while wearing the system should be carefully evaluated for the possibility of an ectopic pregnancy.
b. Special attention should be directed toward determining whether ectopic pregnancy has occurred in patients with delayed menses, slight metrorrhagia and/or unilateral pelvic pain, especially when associated with a falling or low hematocrit, and in patients who wish to terminate an unplanned pregnancy.
c. Women who have previously had acute salpingitis (pelvic inflammatory disease) subsequently have an 8-to- 10-fold greater than normal risk of ectopic pregnancy. Data provided to the FDA indicate an estimated incidence of ectopic pregnancy in women previously having had salpingitis of 2.7 per 100 woman years, compared with an estimated risk in normal women of 0.1 to 0.3 per 100 woman years. Since IUD use has little or no effect in preventing ectopic pregnancy, patients considering IUD use should be carefully evaluated for evidence of previous pelvic inflammatory disease. Previous pelvic surgery that has involved the reproductive tract, endometritis, and retrograde menstruation have also been recognized as risk factors for ectopic pregnancy, but the increased degree of risk with respect to each of these factors has not yet been quantified.
d. There are no comparable clinical trial data on the incidence of ectopic pregnancy during use of unmedicated, copper, and progesterone IUDs. Data gathered from separate studies and presented to the FDA, however, indicated that the incidence of ectopic pregnancy was greater in the studies with the PROGESTASERT® system than in studies with other IUDs. These data on uterine and extrauterine pregnancies for the PROGESTASERT® system, unmedicated IUDs, and copper IUDs, given as rates per 100 woman years, are listed below.
[See table above].

	Woman Months	*Intrauterine Pregnancy*	*Extrauterine Pregnancy*
PROGESTASERT® System	126,800	1.7	0.4
Unmedicated IUD	343,365	2.7	0.12
Copper T-200	132,432	3.1	0.05
Cu-7	157,625	2.3	0.04

Factors responsible for the differences in extrauterine pregnancies could include the increased incidence of salpingitis, the selection of patients, the criteria for diagnosing ectopic pregnancies, or other yet unexplained factors.
3. Pelvic infection. An increased risk of pelvic inflammatory disease associated with the use of IUDs has been reported. This risk is greatest for young women who are nulliparous and/or who have a multiplicity of sexual partners.

Continued on next page

Alza—Cont.

Salpingitis can result in tubal damage and occlusion, thereby threatening future fertility, and/or can predispose to ectopic pregnancy as described above. It is recommended that patients be taught to recognize the symptoms of pelvic inflammatory disease and ectopic pregnancy. The decision to use an IUD in a particular case must be made by the physician and patient with the consideration of a possible deleterious effect on future fertility.
Pelvic infection may occur with PROGESTASERT® system *in situ*, and at times result in the development of tubo-ovarian abscesses or general peritonitis. The symptoms of pelvic infection include new development of menstrual disorders (prolonged or heavy bleeding), abnormal vaginal discharge, abdominal or pelvic pain or tenderness, dyspareunia, fever. The symptoms are especially significant if they occur following the first two or three cycles after insertion. Appropriate aerobic and anaerobic bacteriologic studies should be done and antibiotic therapy initiated promptly. The PROGESTASERT® system should be removed and the continuing treatment assessed on the basis of the results of culture and sensitivity tests.
4. Embedment. Partial penetration or lodging of an IUD in the endometrium can result in difficult removals.
5. Perforation. Partial or total perforation of the uterine wall or cervix may occur with the use of IUDs. The possiblity of perforation must be kept in mind during insertion and at the time of any subsequent examination. If perforation occurs, the system should be removed. Adhesions, foreign body reactions, and intestinal obstruction may result if an IUD is left in the peritoneal cavity.
6. Congenital anomalies. Systemically administered sex steroids, including progestational agents, have been associated with an increased risk of congenital anomalies. It is not known whether there is an increased or decreased risk of such anomalies when pregnancy is continued with a PROGESTASERT® system in place.

Precautions:
1. Patient Counseling. Prior to insertion the physician, nurse, or other trained health professional should provide the patient with the Patient Information Leaflet. The patient should be given the opportunity to read the leaflet and discuss fully any questions she may have concerning the PROGESTASERT® system as well as other methods of contraception.
2. Patient Evaluation and Clinical Considerations.

a. A complete medical history should be obtained to determine conditions that might influence the selection of an IUD. Special attention must be given during the history to ascertain if the woman is at a high risk to ectopic pregnancy by virtue of previous pelvic inflammatory disease. Physical examination should include a pelvic examination, a "Pap" smear, gonorrhea culture, and, if indicated, appropriate tests for other forms of venereal disease.

b. The uterus should be carefully sounded prior to insertion to determine the degree of patency of the endocervial canal and the internal os, and the direction and depth of the uterine cavity. In occasional cases, severe cervical stenosis may be encountered. Do not use excessive force to overcome this resistance.

c. The uterus should sound to a depth of 6 to 10 centimeters (cm). Insertion of a PROGESTASERT® system into a uterine cavity measuring less than 6 cm by sounding may increase the incidence of expulsion, bleeding, and pain.

d. The possibility of insertion in the presence of an existing undetermined pregnancy is reduced if insertion is performed during or shortly following a menstrual period. The system should not be inserted postpartum or postabortion until involution of the uterus is completed. The incidence of perforation and expulsion is greater if involution is not completed.

e. IUDs should still be used with caution in those patients who have an anemia or a history of menorrhagia or hypermenorrhea. Patients experiencing menorrhagia and/or metrorrhagia following IUD insertion may be at risk for the development of hypochromic microcytic anemia. Also, IUDs should be used with caution in patients receiving anticoagulants or having a coagulopathy.

f. Syncope, bradycardia or other neurovascular episodes may occur during insertion or removal of IUDs, especially in patients with a previous disposition to these conditions.

g. Patients with valvular or congenital heart disease are more prone to develop subacute bacterial endocarditis than patients who do not have valvular or congenital heart disease. Use of an IUD in these patients may represent a potential source of septic emboli.

h. Use of an IUD in those patients with acute cervicitis should be postponed until proper treatment has cleared up the infection.

i. Since an IUD may be expelled or displaced, patients should be reexamined and evaluated shortly after the first postinsertion menses, but definitely within 3 months after insertion. Thereafter annual examination with appropriate medical and laboratory examination should be carried out. The PROGESTASERT® system should be replaced each year, since the level of contraceptive efficacy of the system after this time has yet to be established.

j. The patient should be told that some bleeding and cramps may occur during the first few weeks after insertion, but if her symptoms continue or are severe she should report them to her physician. She should be instructed on how to check after each menstrual period to make certain that the threads still protrude from the cervix, and she should be cautioned that there is no contraceptive protection if the system is expelled. She should be cautioned not to pull on the threads thus displacing the system. If partial expulsion occurs, removal is indicated and a new system may be inserted. The patient should be told to return in one year for replacement of the system.

Adverse Reactions: These adverse reactions are not listed in any order of frequency or severity.
Reported adverse reactions of IUD use include: endometritis, spontaneous abortion, septic abortion, septicemia, perforation of uterus and cervix, pelvic infection, cervical erosion, vaginitis, leukorrhea, pregnancy, ectopic pregnancy, uterine embedment, difficult removal, complete or partial expulsion, intermenstrual spotting, prolongation of menstrual flow, anemia, amenorrhea or delayed menses, pain and cramping, dysmenorrhea, backaches, dyspareunia, neuro-vascular episodes including bradycardia, and syncope secondary to insertion. Perforation into the abdomen followed by abdominal adhesions, intestinal penetration, intestinal obstruction, and cystic masses in the pelvis has been reported in general IUD use, but these have not been reported with PROGESTASERT® system perforations to date.

Directions For Use: A single PROGESTASERT® system is to be inserted into the uterine cavity (see Precautions section). Present information indicates that the contraceptive effectiveness of the system is retained for one year, and must be replaced one year after insertion.

Insertion Instructions:
NOTE: Physicians are cautioned to become thoroughly familiar with the insertion instructions before attempting placement with the PROGESTASERT® system.

Description of Inserter: The inserter is a malleable, curved tube designed to conform to the anatomical configuration of most cervical-uterine cavities. The horizontal arms of the T are positioned outside of the inserter and are folded by an arm-cocker attachment immediately prior to insertion.

■ DO NOT REMOVE ANY COMPONENT FROM THE INSERTER BEFORE INSERTION OF THE SYSTEM INTO THE UTERUS.

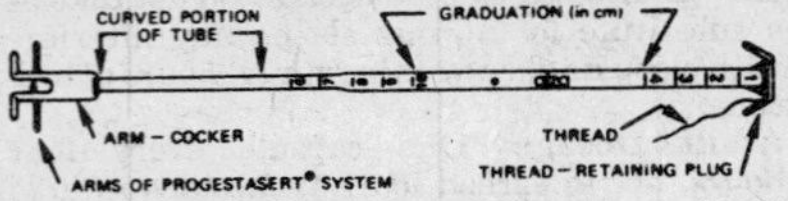

The PROGESTASERT® system inserter is designed to permit determination of the depth of uterine placement of the PROGESTASERT® system. The curvature of the inserter conforms with the usual orientation of the uterus; however, in cases of extreme flexion, the malleable inserter can be shaped gently to the desired curvature.

Preliminary Preparation and Precautions:
1. The completion of a medical history, a cervical Papanicolaou smear, gonorrhea culture, and pelvic examination is recommended prior to insertion of the PROGESTASERT® system.
2. Use of aseptic technique during insertion is essential.
3. Refer to the package insert for CONTRAINDICATIONS, WARNINGS, and PRECAUTIONS.
4. The system should preferably be inserted during or shortly after menstruation to ensure a nonpregnant state. (This approach may not be practical in certain clinical situations.)
5. The endocervix should be cleansed with an antiseptic solution and a tenaculum applied to the cervix with downward traction for correction of the angulation of the cervix and stabilization of the cervix.
6. Prior to insertion, it is desirable to ascertain the depth and position of the uterus and the patency of the cervical canal by uterine sounding. Insertion is not recommended into a uterus which sounds under 6 cm. or more than 10 cm.
7. THE PROGESTASERT® SYSTEM MUST BE USED ONLY WITH ITS SPECIALLY DESIGNED, PLUNGER-FREE INSERTER. This inserter will facilitate fundal placement and is designed to decrease the possibility of uterine perforation. No component should be removed from the inserter before insertion of the system into the uterus.
NOTE: Any intrauterine procedure can result in severe pain, bradycardia and syncope.

System Insertion:
1. Open the PROGESTASERT® system package by COMPLETELY removing the sealed cover starting at the indicated position.

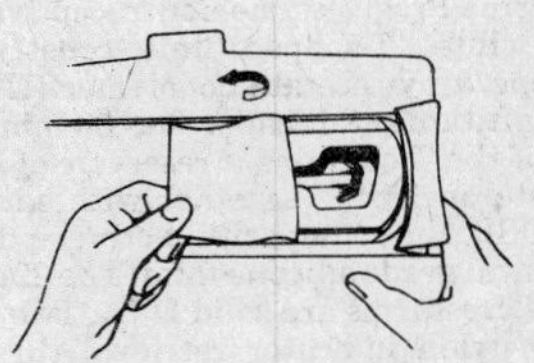

Remove the system and inserter by lifting the handle of the inserter. DO NOT CONTAMINATE THE END CONTAINING THE SYSTEM.
2. IMMEDIATELY PRIOR TO INSERTION, cock the arms of the PROGESTASERT® system by pressing straight down on the inserter onto the tray or other sterile field as shown. This will cause the arms to fold against the side of the inserter.
NOTE: To avoid alteration of system shape, do not leave the system in the folded position for more than a few minutes.

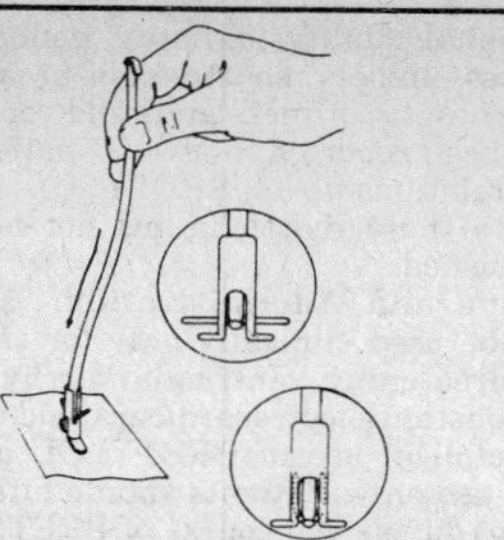

3. After aligning the curvature of the inserter with the direction of uterine flexion, introduce the inserter into the cervical canal. Be certain the thread-retaining plug is still secure in the end of the inserter. The armcocker will slide along the inserter shaft as the inserter moves through the cervical canal.

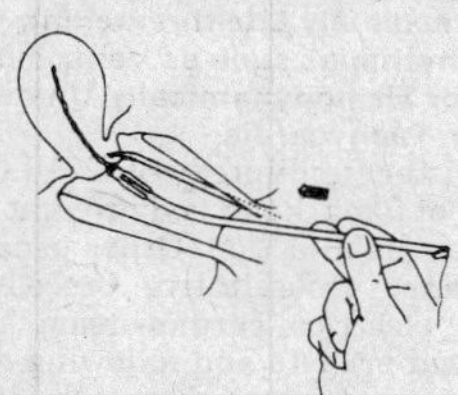

4. Sound steadily but gently with the inserter until the fundus is reached. While the inserter is in this position, note the number seen on the shaft at the base of the armcocker. This number approximates the depth in centimeters of the uterus.

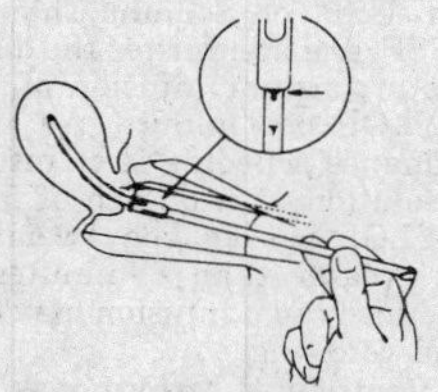

5. With the inserter still at the fundus, release the retaining thread by squeezing the wings of and removing the thread-retaining plug.

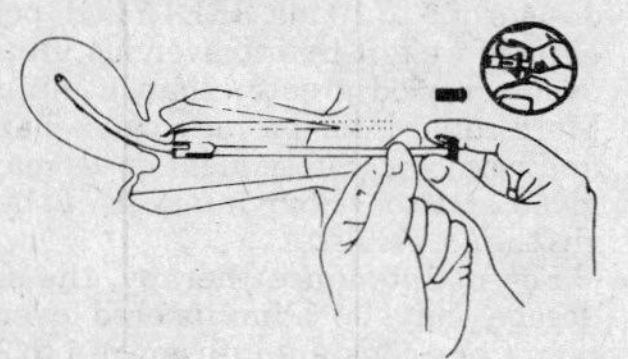

6. Slowly withdraw the inserter. The PROGESTASERT® system is released as the inserter is withdrawn.

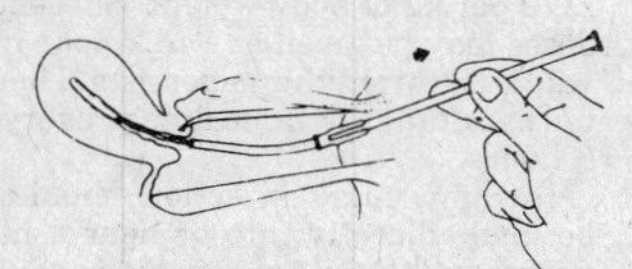

Correct Fundal Placement: To be fully effective, the PROGESTASERT® system must be placed at the fundus.

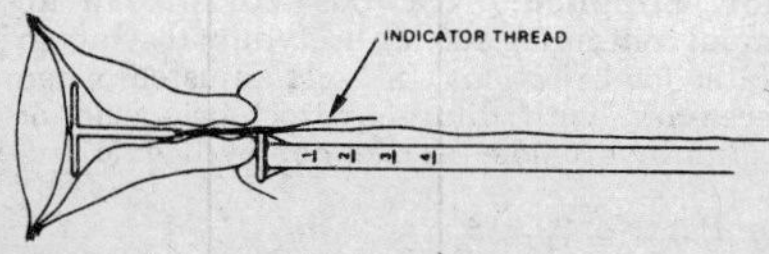

Estimate the length of the short thread protruding from the cervix to determine correct placement. The depth of the uterus, added to the length of the shorter "indicator" thread protruding from the cervix should approximate 9 cm. For example, with a uterine depth of 6 cm, you should see a 3 cm protrusion of the short "indicator" thread.

Trim the long thread to a standard 3 cm length from the cervix. This measurement is used for future reference in determining continued fundal placement.

How Supplied: Available in cartons containing six sterile systems (PROGESTASERT® system with an inserter).

Clinical Studies: Different event rates have been recorded with the use of different contraceptive methods. Inasmuch as these rates are usually derived from separate studies conducted by different investigators in several population groups, they cannot be compared with precision. Furthermore, event rates tend to be lower as clinical experience is expanded, possibly due to retention in the clinical study of those patients who accept the treatment regimen and do not discontinue due to adverse reactions or pregnancy. In clinical trials conducted by ALZA and the World Health Organization with the PROGESTRASERT® system, use-effectiveness was determined as follows for parous and nulliparous women by the life table method. (Rates are expressed as events per 100 women through 12 months of use.) This experience is based on 68,780 woman-months of use with 7,614 women, of whom about 25% were nulliparous; 4,724 women completed 12 months of use.

	Parous	*Nulliparous*
Pregnancy	1.8	2.6
Expulsion	3.1	7.4
Medical Removals	11.2	15.1
Continuation Rate	79.8	71.8

Caution: Federal law prohibits dispensing without prescription.

© ALZA Corporation, 1975, 1977, 1978, 1980

American Critical Care

Division of American Hospital Supply Corporation
McGAW PARK, IL 60085

BRETYLOL® ℞
(bretylium tosylate)
INJECTION

For Intramuscular or Intravenous Use

Description: BRETYLOL (bretylium tosylate) is o-Bromobenzyl ethyl-dimethylammonium p-toluene sulfonate.

BRETYLOL is a white, crystalline powder with an extremely bitter taste. It is freely soluble in water and alcohol. Each ml of sterile, non-pyrogenic solution contains 50 mg bretylium tosylate in Water for Injection, USP. The pH is adjusted when necessary, with dilute hydrochloric acid or sodium hydroxide. BRETYLOL contains no preservative.

Clinical Pharmacology: BRETYLOL (bretylium tosylate) is a bromobenzyl quaternary ammonium compound which selectively accumulates in sympathetic ganglia and their postganglionic adrenergic neurons where it inhibits norepinephrine release by depressing adrenergic nerve terminal excitability.

BRETYLOL also suppresses ventricular fibrillation and ventricular arrhythmias. The mechanisms of the antifibrillatory and antiarrhythmic actions of BRETYLOL are not established. In efforts to define these mechanisms, the following electrophysiologic actions of BRETYLOL have been demonstrated in animal experiments:

1. Increase in ventricular fibrillation threshold.
2. Increase in action potential duration and effective refractory period without changes in heart rate.
3. Little effect on the rate of rise or amplitude of the cardiac action potential (Phase 0) or in resting membrane potential (Phase 4) in normal myocardium. However, when cell injury slows the rate of rise, decreases amplitude, and lowers resting membrane potential, BRETYLOL transiently restores these parameters toward normal.
4. In canine hearts with infarcted areas BRETYLOL decreases the disparity in action potential duration between normal and infarcted regions.
5. Increase in impulse formation and spontaneous firing rate of pacemaker tissue as well as increased ventricular conduction velocity.

The restoration of injured myocardial cell electrophysiology toward normal, as well as the increase of the action potential duration and effective refractory period without changing their ratio to each other, may be important factors in suppressing re-entry of aberrant impulses and decreasing induced dispersion of local excitable states.

BRETYLOL induces a chemical sympathectomy-like state which resembles a surgical sympathectomy. Catecholamine stores are not depleted by BRETYLOL, but catecholamine effects on the myocardium and on peripheral vascular resistance are often seen shortly after administration because BRETYLOL causes an early release of norepinephrine from the adrenergic postganglionic nerve terminals. Subsequently, BRETYLOL blocks the release of norepinephrine in response to neuron stimulation. Peripheral adrenergic blockade regularly causes orthostatic hypotension but has less effect on supine blood pressure. The relationship of adrenergic blockade to the antifibrillatory and antiarrhythmic actions of BRETYLOL is not clear. In a study in patients with frequent ventricular premature beats, peak plasma concentration of BRETYLOL and peak hypotensive effects were seen within one hour of intramuscular administration, presumably reflecting adrenergic neuronal blockade. However, suppression of premature ventricular beats was not maximal until 6–9 hours after dosing, when mean plasma concentration had declined to less than one-half of peak level. This suggests a slower mechanism, other than neuronal blockade, was involved in suppression of the arrhythmia. On the other hand, antifibrillatory effect can be seen within minutes of an intravenous injection, suggesting that the effect on the myocardium may occur quite rapidly.

BRETYLOL has a positive inotropic effect on the myocardium, but it is not yet certain whether this effect is direct or is mediated by catecholamine release.

BRETYLOL is eliminated intact by the kidneys. No metabolites have been identified following administration of BRETYLOL in man and laboratory animals. In man, approximately 70 to 80% of a ^{14}C-labelled intramuscular dose is excreted in the urine during the first 24 hours, with an additional 10% excreted over the next three days.

The terminal half-life in four normal volunteers averaged 7.8 $\pm$ 0.6 hrs (range 6.9–8.1). In one patient with a creatinine clearance of 21.0 ml/min x 1.73 m^2, the half-life was 16 hours. In one patient with a creatinine clearance of 1.0 ml/min x 1.73 m^2 the half-life was 31.5 hours. During hemodialysis, this patient's arterial and venous BRETYLOL concentrations declined rapidly, resulting in a half-life of 13 hours. During dialysis there was a two-fold increase in total BRETYLOL clearance.

Effect on Heart Rate: There is sometimes an initial small increase in heart rate when

Continued on next page

American Critical—Cont.

BRETYLOL is administered, but this is an inconsistent and transient occurrence.

Hemodynamic Effects: Following intravenous administration of 5 mg/kg of BRETYLOL to patients with acute myocardial infarction, there was a mild increase in arterial pressure, followed by a modest decrease, remaining within normal limits throughout. Pulmonary artery pressures, pulmonary capillary wedge pressure, right atrial pressure, cardiac index, stroke volume index, and stroke work index were not significantly changed. These hemodynamic effects were not correlated with antiarrhythmic activity.

Onset of Action: Suppression of ventricular fibrillation is rapid, usually occurring within minutes following intravenous administration. Suppression of ventricular tachycardia and other ventricular arrhythmias develops more slowly, usually 20 minutes to 2 hours after parenteral administration.

Indications: BRETYLOL is indicated in the prophylaxis and therapy of ventricular fibrillation.

BRETYLOL is also indicated in the treatment of life-threatening ventricular arrhythmias, such as ventricular tachycardia, that have failed to respond to adequate doses of a first-line antiarrhythmic agent, such as lidocaine. Use of BRETYLOL should be limited to intensive care units, coronary care units or other facilities where equipment and personnel for constant monitoring of cardiac arrhythmias and blood pressure are available.

Following injection of BRETYLOL there may be a delay of 20 minutes to 2 hours in the onset of antiarrhythmic action, although it appears to act within minutes in ventricular fibrillation. The delay in effect appears to be longer after intramuscular than after intravenous injection.

Contraindications: There are no contraindications to use in treatment of ventricular fibrillation or life-threatening refractory ventricular arrhythmias.

Warnings:

1. **Hypotension**
   Administration of BRETYLOL regularly results in postural hypotension, subjectively recognized by dizziness, light-headedness, vertigo or faintness. Some degree of hypotension is present in about 50% of patients while they are supine. Hypotension may occur at doses lower than those needed to suppress arrhythmias.

   > Patients should be kept in the supine position until tolerance to the hypotensive effect of BRETYLOL develops. Tolerance occurs unpredictably but may be present after several days.

   Hypotension with supine systolic pressure greater than 75 mm Hg need not be treated unless there are associated symptoms. If supine systolic pressure falls below 75 mm Hg, an infusion of dopamine or norepinephrine may be used to raise blood pressure. When catecholamines are administered, a dilute solution should be employed and blood pressure monitored closely because the pressor effects of the catecholamines are enhanced by BRETYLOL. Volume expansion with blood or plasma and correction of dehydration should be carried out where appropriate.
2. **Transient Hypertension and Increased Frequency of Arrhythmias**
   Due to the initial release of norepinephrine from adrenergic postganglionic nerve terminals by BRETYLOL, transient hypertension or increased frequency of premature ventricular contractions and other arrhythmias may occur in some patients.
3. **Caution During Use with Digitalis Glycosides**
   The initial release of norepinephrine caused by BRETYLOL may aggravate digitalis toxicity. When a life-threatening cardiac arrhythmia occurs in a digitalized patient, BRETYLOL should be used only if the etiology of the arrhythmia does not appear to be digitalis toxicity and other antiarrhythmic drugs are not effective. Simultaneous initiation of therapy with digitalis glycosides and BRETYLOL (bretylium tosylate) should be avoided.
4. **Patients with Fixed Cardiac Output**
   In patients with fixed cardiac output (i.e., severe aortic stenosis or severe pulmonary hypertension) BRETYLOL should be avoided since severe hypotension may result from a fall in peripheral resistance without a compensatory increase in cardiac output. If survival is threatened by the arrhythmia, BRETYLOL may be used but vasoconstrictive catecholamines should be given promptly if severe hypotension occurs.

Use in Pregnancy: The safety of BRETYLOL in human pregnancy has not been established. However, as the drug is intended for use only in life-threatening situations, it may be used in pregnant women when its benefits outweigh the potential risk to the fetus.

Use in Children: The safety and efficacy of this drug in children has not been established. BRETYLOL has been administered to a limited number of pediatric patients, but such use has been inadequate to define fully proper dosage and limitations for use.

Precautions:

1. **Dilution for Intravenous Use**
   BRETYLOL should be diluted (one part BRETYLOL with four parts of Dextrose Injection, USP or Sodium Chloride Injection, USP) prior to intravenous use. Rapid intravenous administration may cause severe nausea and vomiting. Therefore, the diluted solution should be infused over a period greater than 8 minutes. In treating existing ventricular fibrillation BRETYLOL should be given as rapidly as possible and may be given without dilution.
2. **Use Various Sites for Intramuscular Injection**
   When injected intramuscularly, not more than 5 ml should be given in a site, and injection sites should be varied since repeated intramuscular injection into the same site may cause atrophy and necrosis of muscle tissue, fibrosis, vascular degeneration and inflammatory changes.
3. **Reduce Dosage in Impaired Renal Function**
   Since BRETYLOL is excreted principally via the kidney, the dosage interval should be increased in patients with impaired renal function. See 'Clinical Pharmacology' section for information on the effect of reduced renal function on half-life.

Adverse Reactions: Hypotension and postural hypotension have been the most frequently reported adverse reactions (see Warnings section). Nausea and vomiting occurred in about three percent of patients, primarily when BRETYLOL was administered rapidly by the intravenous route (see Precautions section). Vertigo, dizziness, light-headedness and syncope, which sometimes accompanied postural hypotension, were reported in about 7 patients in 1000.

Bradycardia, increased frequency of premature ventricular contractions, transitory hypertension, initial increase in arrhythmias (see Warnings section), precipitation of anginal attacks, and sensation of substernal pressure have also been reported in a small number of patients, i.e., approximately 1–2 patients in 1000.

Renal dysfunction, diarrhea, abdominal pain, hiccups, erythematous macular rash, flushing, hyperthermia, confusion, paranoid psychosis, emotional lability, lethargy, generalized tenderness, anxiety, shortness of breath, diaphoresis, nasal stuffiness and mild conjunctivitis, have been reported in about 1 patient in 1000. The relationship of BRETYLOL administration to these reactions has not been clearly established.

Dosage and Administration: BRETYLOL is to be used clinically only for treatment of life-threatening ventricular arrhythmias under constant electrocardiographic monitoring. The clinical use of BRETYLOL is for short-term use only. Patients should either be kept supine during the course of BRETYLOL therapy or be closely observed for postural hypotension. The optimal dose schedule for parenteral administration of BRETYLOL has not been determined. There is comparatively little experience with dosages greater than 40 mg/kg/day, although such doses have been used without apparent adverse effects. The following schedule is suggested.

A. **For immediately Life-threatening Ventricular Arrhythmias such as Ventricular Fibrillation or Hemodynamically Unstable Ventricular Tachycardia:**
   Administer undiluted BRETYLOL at a dosage of 5 mg/kg of body weight by rapid intravenous injection. Other usual cardiopulmonary resuscitative procedures, including electrical cardioversion, should be employed prior to and following the injection in accordance with good medical practice. If ventricular fibrillation persists, the dosage may be increased to 10 mg/kg and repeated as necessary.

   For continuous suppression, dilute contents of one BRETYLOL ampul (10 ml containing 500 mg bretylium tosylate) to a minimum of 50 ml with Dextrose (5%) Injection, USP, or Sodium Chloride Injection, USP, and administer the diluted solution as a constant infusion of 1 to 2 mg BRETYLOL per minute. An alternative maintenance schedule is to infuse the diluted solution at a dosage of 5 to 10 mg BRETYLOL per kg body weight, over a period greater than 8 minutes, every 6 hours. More rapid infusion may cause nausea and vomiting.

B. **Other Ventricular Arrhythmias:**
   1. Intravenous Use: **BRETYLOL must be diluted as described above before intravenous use.**
      Administer the diluted solution at a dosage of 5 to 10 mg BRETYLOL per kg of body weight by intravenous infusion over a period greater than 8 minutes. More rapid infusion may cause nausea and vomiting. Subsequent doses may be given at 1 to 2 hour intervals if the arrhythmia persists.
      For maintenance therapy, the same dosage may be administered every 6 hours, or a constant infusion of 1 to 2 mg BRETYLOL per minute may be given.
   2. For intramuscular Injection: **Do not dilute BRETYLOL prior to intramuscular injection.** Inject 5 to 10 mg BRETYLOL per kg of body weight. Subsequent doses may be given at 1 to 2 hour intervals if the arrhythmia persists. Thereafter maintain the same dosage every 6 to 8 hours.
      Intramuscular injection should not be made directly into or near a major nerve, and the site of injection should be varied on repeated injection.

As soon as possible, and when indicated, patients should be changed to an oral antiarrhythmic agent for maintenance therapy.

How Supplied: NDC 0094-0012-10: 10 ml ampul containing 500 mg bretylium tosylate in Water for Injection, USP. pH adjusted, when necessary, with dilute hydrochloric acid or sodium hydroxide. Sterile, non-pyrogenic.

Re. Pat. No. 29,618

HESPAN® ℞
6% Hetastarch in
0.9% Sodium Chloride Injection

Description:
Composition per 100 ml:
Hetastarch ....6.0 g
Sodium Chloride USP ....0.90 g
Water for Injection USP ....qs
pH adjusted with Sodium Hydroxide
Concentration of Electrolytes (mEq/liter): Sodium 154, Chloride 154
pH: Approx. 5.5
Calculated Osmolarity: Approximately 310 mOsm/liter
Hetastarch is an artificial colloid derived from a waxy starch composed almost entirely of amylopectin. Hydroxyethyl ether groups are introduced into the glucose units of the starch and the resultant material is hydrolyzed to yield a product with a molecular weight suitable for use as a plasma expander. Clinical Hetastarch is characterized by its molecular weight and its degree of substitution. The weight average molecular weight is approximately 450,000 with 90% of the polymer units falling within the range of 10,000 to 1,000,000. The degree of substitution is 0.7 which means Hetastarch has 7 hydroxyethyl groups for every 10 glucose units. The polymerized glucose units in Hetastarch are joined primarily by 1–4 linkages with hydroxyethyl groups being attached primarily at the No. 2 position. The polymer closely resembles glycogen.
Actions: The colloidal properties of 6% Hetastarch approximate those of human albumin. Intravenous infusion of Hetastarch results in expansion of plasma volume slightly in excess of the volume infused which decreases from this maximum over the succeeding 24 to 36 hours. This expansion of plasma volume may improve the hemodynamic status for 24 hours and longer. Hetastarch molecules below 50,000 molecular weight are rapidly eliminated by renal excretion with approximately 40% of a given total dose appearing in the urine in 24 hours. This is a variable process but generally results in an intravascular Hetastarch concentration of less than 1% of the total dose injected by two weeks. The hydroxyethyl group is not cleaved by the body, but remains intact and attached to glucose units when excreted.
The addition of Hetastarch to whole blood increases the erythrocyte sedimentation rate. Therefore, Hetastarch is used to improve the efficiency of granulocyte collection by centrifugal means.
Indications: Hetastarch is indicated when plasma volume expansion is desired as an adjunct in the treatment of shock due to hemorrhage, burns, surgery, sepsis or other trauma. It is not a substitute for blood or plasma.
The adjunctive use of Hetastarch in leukapheresis has also been shown to be safe and efficacious in improving the harvesting and increasing the yield of granulocytes by centrifugal means.
Contraindications: Hetastarch is contraindicated in patients with severe bleeding disorders or with severe congestive cardiac and renal failure with oliguria or anuria.
Warnings: Large volumes may alter the coagulation mechanism. Thus, administration of Hetastarch may result in transient prolongation of prothrombin, partial thromboplastin and clotting times. With administration of large doses, the physician should also be alert to the possibility of transient prolongation of bleeding time.
Hematocrit may be decreased and plasma proteins diluted excessively by administration of large volumes of Hetastarch.
Usage of Leukapheresis: Significant declines in platelet counts and hemoglobin levels have been observed in donors undergoing repeated leukapheresis procedures due to the volume expanding effects of Hetastarch. Hemoglobin levels usually return to normal within 24 hours. Hemodilution by Hetastarch and saline may also result in 24 hour declines of total protein, albumin, calcium and fibrinogen values.
Usage in Pregnancy: Reproduction studies have been done in mice with no evidence of fetal damage. Relevance to humans is not known since Hetastarch has not been given to pregnant women. Therefore, it should not be used in pregnant women, particularly during early pregnancy, unless in the judgment of the physician the potential benefits outweigh the potential hazards.
Usage in Children: No data are available pertaining to use in children.
The safety and compatibility of additives have not been established.
Precautions: The possibility of circulatory overload should be kept in mind. Special care should be exercised in patients who have impaired renal clearance since this is the principal way in which Hetastarch is eliminated. Caution should be used when the risk of pulmonary edema and/or congestive heart failure is increased. Indirect bilirubin levels of 0.83 mg % (normal 0.0–0.7 mg %) have been reported in 2 out of 20 normal subjects who received multiple Hetastarch infusions. Total bilirubin was within normal limits at all times; indirect bilirubin returned to normal by 96 hours following the final infusion. The significance, if any, of these elevations is not known; however, caution should be observed before administering Hetastarch to patients with a history of liver disease.
Regular and frequent clinical evaluation and laboratory determinations are necessary for proper monitoring of Hetastarch use during leukapheresis. Studies should include CBC, total leukocyte and platelet counts, leukocyte differential count, hemoglobin, hematocrit, prothrombin time (PT), and partial thromboplastin time (PTT).
Hetastarch is nonantigenic. However, allergic or sensitivity reactions have been reported (see **Adverse Reactions**). If such reactions occur, they are readily controlled by discontinuation of the drug and, if necessary, administration of an antihistaminic agent.
Adverse Reactions: The following have been reported: vomiting, mild temperature elevation, chills, itching, submaxillary and parotid glandular enlargement, mild influenza-like symptoms, headaches, muscle pains, peripheral edema of the lower extremities, and anaphylactoid reactions consisting of periorbital edema, urticaria, and wheezing.
Dosage and Administration: Dosage in Plasma Volume Expansion: Hetastarch is administered by intravenous infusion only. Total dosage and rate of infusion depend upon the amount of blood lost and the resultant hemoconcentration. In adults, the amount usually administered is 500 to 1000 ml. Total dosage does not usually exceed 1500 ml per day or approximately 20 ml per kg of body weight for the typical 70 kg patient. In acute hemorrhagic shock, an administration rate approaching 20 ml per kg per hour may be used; in burn or septic shock it is usually administered at slower rates.
Dosage in Leukapheresis: In continuous-flow centrifugation (CFC) procedures, 250 to 700 ml Hetastarch is typically infused at a constant fixed ratio, usually 1:8, to venous whole blood. Multiple CFC procedures using Hetastarch of up to 2 per week and a total of 7 to 10 have been reported to be safe and effective. Adequate data are not available to establish the safety of more frequent or a greater number of procedures.
How Supplied: NDC **0094-0037-05-Hespan®** (6% Hetastarch in 0.9% Sodium Chloride Injection) is supplied sterile and nonpyrogenic in 500 ml intravenous infusion bottles.

INTROPIN® ℞
(dopamine HCl)
5 ml VIAL and RAP-ADD® Syringe—
200 mg, 400 mg and 800 mg
5 ml AMPUL—200 mg

Description: INTROPIN (dopamine HCl) is a clear, practically colorless, aqueous, additive solution for intravenous infusion after dilution. Each ml contains either 40 mg, 80 mg or 160 mg dopamine hydrochloride (equivalent to 32.3 mg, 64.6 mg and 129.2 mg dopamine base, respectively) in Water for Injection, USP containing 1% sodium bisulfite as an antioxidant. Hydrochloric acid or sodium hydroxide added to adjust pH when necessary. The solution is sterile and non-pyrogenic. The pH is 2.5-4.5. INTROPIN, a naturally-occurring catecholamine, is an inotropic vasopressor agent. Its chemical name is 3,4 dihydroxyphenethylamine hydrochloride.
INTROPIN is sensitive to alkalis, iron salts and oxidizing agents. **It must be diluted in an appropriate, sterile parenteral solution** (see Dosage and Administration section) **before intravenous administration.**
Actions: INTROPIN exerts an inotropic effect on the myocardium resulting in an increased cardiac output. INTROPIN produces less increase in myocardial oxygen consumption than isoproterenol and its use is usually not associated with a tachyarrhythmia. Clinical studies indicate that INTROPIN usually increases systolic and pulse pressure with either no effect or a slight increase in diastolic pressure. Total peripheral resistance at low and intermediate therapeutic doses is usually unchanged. Blood flow to peripheral vascular beds may decrease while mesenteric flow increases. INTROPIN has also been reported to dilate the renal vasculature presumptively by activation of a "dopaminergic" receptor. This action is accompanied by increases in glomerular filtration rate, renal blood flow, and sodium excretion. An increase in urinary output produced by dopamine is usually not associated with a decrease in osmolality of the urine.
Indications: INTROPIN is indicated for the correction of hemodynamic imbalances present in the shock syndrome due to myocardial infarctions, trauma, endotoxic septicemia, open heart surgery, renal failure, and chronic cardiac decompensation as in congestive failure.
Where appropriate, restoration of blood volume with a suitable plasma expander or whole blood should be instituted or completed prior to administration of INTROPIN.
Patients most likely to respond adequately to INTROPIN are those in whom physiological parameters, such as urine flow, myocardial function, and blood pressure, have not undergone profound deterioration. Multiclinic trials indicate that the shorter the time interval between onset of signs and symptoms and initiation of therapy with volume correction and INTROPIN, the better the prognosis.
Poor Perfusion of Vital Organs—Urine flow appears to be one of the better diagnostic signs by which adequacy of vital organ perfusion can be monitored. Nevertheless, the physician should also observe the patient for signs of reversal of confusion or comatose condition. Loss of pallor, increase in toe temperature, and/or adequacy of nail bed capillary filling may also be used as indices of adequate dosage. Clinical studies have shown that when INTROPIN is administered before urine flow has diminished to levels approximately 0.3 ml/minute, prognosis is more favorable. Nevertheless, in a number of oliguric or anuric patients, administration of INTROPIN has resulted in an increase in urine flow which in some cases reached normal levels. INTROPIN may also increase urine flow in patients whose output is within normal limits and thus may be of value

Continued on next page

American Critical—Cont.

in reducing the degree of pre-existing fluid accumulation. It should be noted that at doses above those optimal for the individual patient, urine flow may decrease, necessitating reduction of dosage. Concurrent administration of INTROPIN and diuretic agents may produce an additive or potentiating effect.

Low Cardiac Output—Increased cardiac output is related to INTROPIN's direct inotropic effect on the myocardium. Increased cardiac output at low or moderate doses appears to be related to a favorable prognosis. Increase in cardiac output has been associated with either static or decreased systemic vascular resistance (SVR). Static or decreased SVR associated with low or moderate increments in cardiac output is believed to be a reflection of differential effects on specific vascular beds with increased resistance in peripheral beds (e.g. femoral) and concomitant decreases in mesenteric and renal vascular beds. Redistribution of blood flow parallels these changes so that an increase in cardiac output is accompanied by an increase in mesenteric and renal blood flow. In many instances the renal fraction of the total cardiac output has been found to increase. Increase in cardiac output produced by INTROPIN is not associated with substantial decreases in systemic vascular resistance as may occur with isoproterenol.

Hypotension—Hypotension due to inadequate cardiac output can be managed by administration of low to moderate doses of INTROPIN, which have little effect on SVR. At high therapeutic doses, INTROPIN's alpha adrenergic activity becomes more prominent and thus may correct hypotension due to diminished SVR. As in the case of other circulatory decompensation states, prognosis is better in patients whose blood pressure and urine flow have not undergone profound deterioration. Therefore, it is suggested that the physician administer INTROPIN as soon as a definite trend toward decreased systolic and diastolic pressure becomes evident.

Contraindications: INTROPIN should not be used in patients with pheochromocytoma.

Warnings: INTROPIN should not be administered in the presence of uncorrected tachyarrhythmias or ventricular fibrillation.

Do **NOT** add INTROPIN to any alkaline diluent solution, since the drug is inactivated in alkaline solution.

Patients who have been treated with monamine oxidase (MAO) inhibitors prior to the administration of INTROPIN will require substantially reduced dosage. Dopamine is metabolized by MAO, and inhibition of this enzyme prolongs and potentiates the effect of INTROPIN. The starting dose in such patients should be reduced to at least one-tenth (1/10) of the usual dose.

Usage in Pregnancy—Animal studies have revealed no evidence of teratogenic effects from INTROPIN. In one study, administration of INTROPIN to pregnant rats resulted in a decreased survival rate of the newborn and a potential for cataract formation in the survivors. The drug may be used in pregnant women when, in the judgment of the physician, the expected benefits outweigh the potential risk to the fetus.

Usage in Children—The safety and efficacy of this drug in children has not been established. INTROPIN has been used in a limited number of pediatric patients, but such use has been inadequate to fully define proper dosage and limitations for use. Further studies are in progress.

Precautions: **Avoid Hypovolemia**—Prior to treatment with INTROPIN, hypovolemia should be fully corrected, if possible, with either whole blood or plasma as indicated.

Decreased Pulse Pressure—If a disproportionate rise in the diastolic pressure (i.e., a marked decrease in the pulse pressure) is observed in patients receiving INTROPIN, the infusion rate should be decreased and the patient observed carefully for further evidence of predominant vasoconstrictor activity, unless such an effect is desired.

Extravasation—INTROPIN should be infused into a large vein whenever possible to prevent the possibility of extravasation into tissue adjacent to the infusion site. Extravasation may cause necrosis and sloughing of surrounding tissue. Large veins of the antecubital fossa are preferred to veins in the dorsum of the hand or ankle. Less suitable infusion sites should be used only if the patient's condition requires immediate attention. The physician should switch to more suitable sites as rapidly as possible. The infusion site should be continuously monitored for free flow.

Occlusive Vascular Disease—Patients with a history of occlusive vascular disease (for example, atherosclerosis, arterial embolism, Raynaud's disease, cold injury, diabetic endarteritis, and Buerger's disease) should be closely monitored for any changes in color or temperature of the skin in the extremities. If a change in skin color or temperature occurs and is thought to be the result of compromised circulation to the extremities, the benefits of continued INTROPIN infusion should be weighed against the risk of possible necrosis. This condition may be reversed by either decreasing or discontinuing the rate of infusion.

IMPORTANT—Antidote for Peripheral Ischemia: To prevent sloughing and necrosis in ischemic areas, the area should be infiltrated as soon as possible with 10 to 15 ml. of saline solution containing from 5 to 10 mg. of Regitine® (brand of phentolamine), an adrenergic blocking agent. A syringe with a fine hypodermic needle should be used, and the solution liberally infiltrated throughout the ischemic area. Sympathetic blockade with phentolamine causes immediate and conspicuous local hyperemic changes if the area is infiltrated within 12 hours. Therefore, phentolamine should be given as soon as possible after the extravasation is noted.

Avoid Cyclopropane or Halogenated Hydrocarbon Anesthetics—Cyclopropane or halogenated hydrocarbon anesthetics increase cardiac autonomic irritability and therefore may sensitize the myocardium to the action of certain intravenously administered catecholamines. This interaction appears to be related both to pressor activity and to beta adrenergic stimulating properties of these catecholamines. Therefore, as with certain other catecholamines, and because of the theoretical arrhythmogenic potential, INTROPIN should be used with EXTREME CAUTION in patients inhaling cyclopropane or halogenated hydrocarbon anesthetics.

Careful Monitoring Required—Close monitoring of the following indices—urine flow, cardiac output and blood pressure—during INTROPIN infusion is necessary as in the case of any adrenergic agent.

Adverse Reactions: The most frequent adverse reactions observed in clinical evaluation of INTROPIN included ectopic beats, nausea, vomiting, tachycardia, anginal pain, palpitation, dyspnea, headache, hypotension, and vasoconstriction. Other adverse reactions which have been reported infrequently were aberrant conduction, bradycardia, piloerection, widened QRS complex, azotemia, and elevated blood pressure.

Dosage and Administration:

WARNING: This is a potent drug: It must be diluted before administration to patient.

Suggested Dilution—Transfer contents of one or more ampuls, vials or additive syringes (5 ml containing 200 mg dopamine HCl) or vials or additive syringes (5 ml containing 400 mg dopamine HCl) by aseptic technique to either a 250 ml or 500 ml bottle of one of the following sterile intravenous solutions:

1) Sodium Chloride Injection, USP
2) Dextrose (5%) Injection, USP
3) Dextrose (5%) and Sodium Chloride (0.9%) Injection, USP
4) Dextrose (5%) in Sodium Chloride (0.45%) Solution
5) Dextrose (5%) in Lactated Ringer's Solution
6) Sodium Lactate (1/6 Molar) Injection, USP
7) Lactated Ringer's Injection, USP

INTROPIN has been found to be stable for a minimum of 24 hours after dilution in the sterile intravenous solutions listed above. However, as with all intravenous admixtures, dilution should be made just prior to administration.

Do **NOT** add INTROPIN to 5% Sodium Bicarbonate or other alkaline intravenous solutions, since the drug is inactivated in alkaline solution.

Rate of Administration—INTROPIN, after dilution, is administered intravenously through a suitable intravenous catheter or needle. An i.v. drip chamber or other suitable metering device is essential for controlling the rate of flow in drops/minute. Each patient must be individually titrated to the desired hemodynamic and/or renal response with INTROPIN. In titrating to the desired increase in systolic blood pressure, the optimum dosage rate for renal response may be exceeded, thus necessitating a reduction in rate after the hemodynamic condition is stablized.

Administration at rates greater than 50 mcg/kg/min has safely been used in advanced circulatory decompensation states. If unnecessary fluid expansion is of concern, adjustment of drug concentration may be preferred over increasing the flow rate of a less concentrated dilution.

Suggested Regimen:

1. When appropriate, increase blood volume with whole blood or plasma until central venous pressure is 10 to 15 cm H_2O or pulmonary wedge pressure is 14–18 mm Hg.
2. Begin administration of diluted solution at doses of 2–5 mcg/kg/minute INTROPIN in patients who are likely to respond to modest increments of heart force and renal perfusion. In more seriously ill patients, begin administration of diluted solution at doses of 5 mcg/kg/minute INTROPIN and increase gradually using 5 to 10 mcg/kg/minute increments up to 20 to 50 mcg/kg/minute as needed. If doses of INTROPIN in excess of 50 mcg/kg/minute are required, it is suggested that urine output be checked frequently. Should urine flow begin to decrease in the absence of hypotension, reduction of INTROPIN dosage should be considered. Multiclinic trials have shown that more than 50% of the patients were satisfactorily maintained on doses of INTROPIN less than 20 mcg/kg/minute. In patients who do not respond to these doses with adequate arterial pressures or urine flow, additional increments of INTROPIN may be employed in an effort to produce an appropriate arterial pressure and central perfusion.
3. Treatment of all patients requires constant evaluation of therapy in terms of the blood volume, augmentation of myocardial contractility, and distribution of peripheral perfusion. Dosage of INTROPIN should be adjusted according to the patient's response, with particular attention to diminution of established urine flow rate, increasing tachycardia or development of new dysrhythmias as indices for decreasing or temporarily suspending the dosage.
4. As with all potent intravenously administered drugs, care should be taken to control the

rate of administration so as to avoid inadvertent administration of a bolus of drug.

Overdosage: In case of accidental overdosage, as evidenced by excessive blood pressure elevation, reduce rate of administration or temporarily discontinue INTROPIN until patient's condition stabilizes. Since INTROPIN's duration of action is quite short, no additional remedial measures are usually necessary. If these measures fail to stabilize the patient's condition, use of the short-acting alpha adrenergic blocking agent, phentolamine, should be considered.

How Supplied:
—200 mg (5 ml containing 40 mg dopamine HCl per ml)
5 ml Ampul
5 ml Single-dose vial (color coded white)
5 ml RAP-ADD® Additive Syringe (color coded white)
—400 mg (5 ml containing 80 mg dopamine HCl per ml)
5 ml Single-dose vial (color coded green)
5 ml RAP-ADD® Additive Syringe (color coded green)
—800 mg (5 ml containing 160 mg dopamine HCl per ml)
5 ml Single-dose vial (color coded yellow)
5 ml RAP-ADD® Additive Syringe (color coded yellow)

Warning: NOT FOR DIRECT INTRAVENOUS INJECTION. MUST BE DILUTED BEFORE USE.

ISOCLOR® Timesule® ℞
Capsules

Description: Each sustained-action Timesule capsule contains 8 mg chlorpheniramine maleate and 120 mg pseudoephedrine HCl in a special form providing a prolonged therapeutic effect.

Indications: For temporary relief of upper respiratory and nasal congestion associated with the common cold, hay fever and allergies, sinusitis, and vasomotor and allergic rhinitis.

Contraindications: Severe hypertension or severe cardiac disease. Sensitivity to antihistamines or sympathomimetic agents.

Precautions: Use with caution in patients with hyperthyroidism. Patients susceptible to the soporific effects of chlorpheniramine should be warned against driving or operating machinery which requires complete mental alertness.

Dosage: *Adults*—1 Timesule capsule every 12 hrs.

Supplied: Bottles of 100 and 500.

TRIDIL® ℞
(nitroglycerin)

NOT FOR DIRECT INTRAVENOUS INJECTION. TRIDIL® MUST BE DILUTED IN DEXTROSE (5%) INJECTION, USP OR SODIUM CHLORIDE (0.9%) INJECTION, USP PRIOR TO ITS INFUSION (SEE DOSAGE AND ADMINISTRATION SECTION). THE ADMINISTRATION SET USED FOR INFUSION WILL AFFECT THE AMOUNT OF TRIDIL DELIVERED TO THE PATIENT. (SEE WARNINGS, AND DOSAGE AND ADMINISTRATION SECTIONS).

Caution SEVERAL PREPARATIONS OF NITROGLYCERIN FOR INJECTION ARE AVAILABLE. THEY DIFFER IN CONCENTRATION AND/OR VOLUME PER VIAL. WHEN SWITCHING FROM ONE PRODUCT TO ANOTHER ATTENTION MUST BE PAID TO THE DILUTION AND DOSAGE AND ADMINISTRATION INSTRUCTIONS.

Description: TRIDIL (nitroglycerin) is a clear, practically colorless additive solution for intravenous infusion after dilution. Each ml of TRIDIL 5 mg contains 0.5 mg Nitroglycerin with 13.6 mg Monobasic Potassium Phosphate, NF (equivalent to 0.1 mEq K+) as a buffer; 10% Alcohol, USP; 4.5 mg Lactose, USP; and Water for Injection, USP. Each ml of TRIDIL 25 mg or 50 mg contains 5 mg Nitroglycerin in 30% Alcohol, USP; 30% Propylene Glycol, USP; and Water for Injection, USP.

The solution is sterile, nonpyrogenic, and nonexplosive. TRIDIL, an organic nitrate, is a vasodilator. The chemical name for nitroglycerin is 1,2,3 propanetriol, trinitrate and its chemical structure is:

$$\begin{array}{l} CH_2 - ONO_2 \\ | \\ CH - ONO_2 \\ | \\ CH_2 - ONO_2 \end{array}$$

$C_3H_5N_3O_9$ MOL. WT. 227.09

Clinical Pharmacology: Relaxation of vascular smooth muscle is the principal pharmacologic action of TRIDIL (nitroglycerin). Although venous effects predominate, nitroglycerin produces, in a dose-related manner, dilation of both arterial and venous beds. Dilation of the post-capillary vessels, including large veins, promotes peripheral pooling of blood and decreases venous return to the heart, reducing left ventricular end-diastolic pressure (pre-load). Arteriolar relaxation reduces systemic vascular resistance and arterial pressure (afterload). Myocardial oxygen consumption or demand (as measured by the pressure-rate product, tension-time index and stroke work index) is decreased by both the arterial and venous effects of nitroglycerin, and a more favorable supply-demand ratio can be achieved. Therapeutic doses of intravenous nitroglycerin reduce systolic, diastolic and mean arterial blood pressure. Effective coronary perfusion pressure is usually maintained, but can be compromised if blood pressure falls excessively or increased heart rate decreases diastolic filling time.

Elevated central venous and pulmonary capillary wedge pressures, pulmonary vascular resistance and systemic vascular resistance are also reduced by nitroglycerin therapy. Heart rate is usually slightly increased, presumably a reflex response to the fall in blood pressure. Cardiac index may be increased, decreased, or unchanged. Patients with elevated left ventricular filling pressure and systemic vascular resistance values in conjunction with a depressed cardiac index are likely to experience an improvement in cardiac index. On the other hand, when filling pressures and cardiac index are normal, cardiac index may be slightly reduced by intravenous nitroglycerin.

Nitroglycerin is widely distributed in the body with an apparent volume of distribution of approximately 200 liters in adult male subjects, and is rapidly metabolized to dinitrates and mononitrates, with a short half-life estimated at 1–4 minutes. This results in a low plasma concentration after intravenous infusion. At plasma concentrations of between 50 and 500 ng/ml, the binding of nitroglycerin to plasma proteins is approximately 60%, while that of 1,2 dinitroglycerin and 1,3 dinitroglycerin is 60% and 30% respectively. The activity and half-life of the dinitroglycerin metabolites are not well characterized. The mononitrate is not active.

Indications and Usage: TRIDIL is indicated for:

1. **Control of blood pressure in perioperative hypertension,** i.e., hypertension associated with surgical procedures, especially cardiovascular procedures, such as the hypertension seen during intratracheal intubation, anesthesia, skin incision, sternotomy, cardiac bypass, and in the immediate postsurgical period.
2. **Congestive Heart Failure Associated with Acute Myocardial Infarction.**
3. **Treatment of Angina Pectoris** in patients who have not responded to recommended doses of organic nitrates and/or a beta blocker.
4. **Production of controlled hypotension during surgical procedures.**

Contraindications: TRIDIL should not be administered to individuals with:

1. A known hypersensitivity to nitroglycerin or a known idiosyncratic reaction to organic nitrates.
2. Hypotension or uncorrected hypovolemia, as the use of TRIDIL in such states could produce severe hypotension or shock.
3. Increased intracranial pressure (e.g., head trauma or cerebral hemorrhage).
4. Constrictive pericarditis and pericardial tamponade.

Warnings:

1. Nitroglycerin readily migrates into many plastics. To avoid absorption of nitroglycerin into plastic parenteral solution containers, the dilution and storage of TRIDIL for intravenous infusion should be made only in *glass* parenteral solution bottles.
2. Some filters absorb nitroglycerin; they should be avoided.
3. Forty to 80% of the total amount of nitroglycerin in the final diluted solution for infusion is absorbed by the polyvinyl chloride (PVC) tubing of the intravenous administration sets currently in general use. The higher rates of absorption occur when flow rates are low, nitroglycerin concentrations are high, and the administration set is long. Although the rate of loss is highest during the early phase of infusion (when flow rates are lowest) the loss is neither constant nor self-limiting; consequently no simple calculation or correction can be performed to convert the theoretical infusion rate (based on the concentration of the infusion solution) to the actual delivery rate.

Because of this problem, American Critical Care has developed TRIDILSET,™ an administration set in which loss of TRIDIL is minimal (less than 1%). TRIDILSET (or a similar administration set) is recommended for infusions of TRIDIL.

DOSING INSTRUCTIONS MUST BE FOLLOWED WITH CARE. IT SHOULD BE NOTED THAT WHEN TRIDILSET IS USED, THE CALCULATED DOSE WILL BE DELIVERED TO THE PATIENT BECAUSE THE LOSS OF TRIDIL DUE TO ABSORPTION IN STANDARD PVC TUBING WILL BE KEPT TO A MINIMUM. NOTE THAT THE DOSAGES COMMONLY USED IN PUBLISHED STUDIES UTILIZED GENERAL-USE PVC ADMINISTRATION SETS AND RECOMMENDED DOSES BASED ON THIS EXPERIENCE ARE TOO HIGH WHEN TRIDILSET IS USED.

Precautions: TRIDIL (nitroglycerin) should be used with caution in patients with severe liver or renal disease.

Excessive hypotension, especially for prolonged periods of time, must be avoided because of possible deleterious effects on the brain, heart, liver, and kidney from poor perfusion and the attendant risk of ischemia, thrombosis, and altered function of these organs. Paradoxical bradycardia and increased angina pectoris may accompany nitroglycerin-induced hypotension. Patients with normal or low pulmonary capillary wedge pressure are especially sensitive to the hypotensive effects of TRIDIL.® If pulmonary capillary wedge pressure is being monitored, it will be noted that a fall in wedge pressure precedes the onset of arterial hypotension, and the pulmonary capillary wedge pressure is thus a useful guide to safe titration of the drug.

Carcinogenesis, mutagenesis, impairment of fertility

No long-term studies in animals were performed to evaluate carcinogenic potential of TRIDIL.

Continued on next page

American Critical—Cont.

Pregnancy
Category C. Animal reproduction studies have not been conducted with TRIDIL. It is also not known whether TRIDIL can cause fetal harm when administered to a pregnant woman or can affect reproduction capacity. TRIDIL should be given to a pregnant woman only if clearly needed.

Nursing Mothers
It is not known whether nitroglycerin is excreted in human milk. Because many drugs are excreted in human milk, caution should be exercised when TRIDIL is administered to a nursing woman.

Pediatric Use
The safety and effectiveness of TRIDIL in children have not been established.

Adverse Reactions: The most frequent adverse reaction in patients treated with TRIDIL is headache, which occurs in approximately 2% of patients. Other adverse reactions occurring in less than 1% of patients are the following: tachycardia, nausea, vomiting, apprehension, restlessness, muscle twitching, retrosternal discomfort, palpitations, dizziness and abdominal pain.
The following additional adverse reactions have been reported with the oral and/or topical use of nitroglycerin: cutaneous flushing, weakness and occasionally drug rash or exfoliative dermatitis.

Overdosage: Accidental overdosage of TRIDIL may result in severe hypotension and reflex tachycardia which can be treated by elevating the legs and decreasing or temporarily terminating the infusion until the patient's condition stabilizes. Since the duration of the hemodynamic effects following TRIDIL administration is quite short, additional corrective measures are usually not required. However, if further therapy is indicated, administration of an intravenous alpha adrenergic agonist (e.g. methoxamine or phenylephrine) should be considered.

Dosage and Administration:
NOT FOR DIRECT INTRAVENOUS INJECTION
TRIDIL IS A CONCENTRATED, POTENT DRUG WHICH MUST BE DILUTED IN DEXTROSE (5%) INJECTION, USP OR SODIUM CHLORIDE (0.9%) INJECTION, USP PRIOR TO ITS INFUSION. TRIDIL SHOULD NOT BE ADMIXED WITH OTHER DRUGS.

1. **Initial Dilution:**
Aseptically transfer the contents of one TRIDIL ampul (containing 5, 25 or 50 mg of nitroglycerin) into a 500 ml *glass* bottle of either Dextrose (5%) Injection, USP or Sodium Chloride Injection (0.9%), USP. This yields a final concentration of 10, 50 or 100 mcg/ml.
2. **Maintenance Dilution:**
It is important to consider the fluid requirements of the patient as well as the expected duration of infusion in selecting the appropriate dilution of TRIDIL.
After the initial dosage titration, the concentration of the admixture solution may be increased, if necessary, to limit fluids given to the patient. The TRIDIL concentration should not exceed 400 mcg/ml. See chart.

Note: If the concentration is adjusted, it is imperative to flush TRIDILSET™ before a new concentration is utilized. The dead-space of the set is approximately 15 ml, and depending on the flow rate it could take from 10 minutes to 3 hours for the new concentration to reach the patient if the set were not flushed.
Invert the glass parenteral bottle several times following admixture to assure uniform dilution of TRIDIL. When stored in *glass* containers, the diluted solution is physically and chemically stable for up to 48 hours at room temperature, and up to seven days under refrigeration.
Dosage is affected by the type of container and administration set used. See WARNINGS.
Although the usual starting adult dose range reported in clinical studies was 25 mcg/min or more, these studies used PVC ADMINISTRATION SETS. THE USE OF NON-ABSORBING TUBING WILL RESULT IN THE NEED FOR REDUCED DOSES.
The dosage for TRIDILSET should initially be 5 mcg/min delivered through an infusion pump capable of exact and constant delivery of the drug. Subsequent titration must be adjusted to the clinical situation, with dose increments becoming more cautious as partial response is seen. Initial titration should be in 5 mcg/min increments with increases every 3–5 minutes until some response is noted. If no response is seen at 20 mcg/min, increments of 10 and later 20 mcg/min can be used. Once a partial blood pressure response is observed, the dose increase should be reduced and the interval between increases should be lengthened.
Some patients with normal or low left ventricular filling pressures or pulmonary capillary wedge pressure (e.g. angina patients without other complications) may be hypersensitive to the effects of TRIDIL and may respond fully to doses as small as 5 mcg/min. These patients require especially careful titration and monitoring.
There is no fixed optimum dose of TRIDIL. Due to variations in the responsiveness of individual patients to the drug, each patient must be titrated to the desired level of hemodynamic function. Therefore, continuous monitoring of physiologic parameters (e.g. blood pressure and heart rate in all patients, other measurement such as pulmonary capillary wedge pressure, as appropriate MUST BE PERFORMED to achieve the correct dose. Adequate systemic blood pressure and coronary perfusion pressure must be maintained.

How Supplied:
NDC 0094-0089-10, 5 mg–10 ml ampul.
NDC 0094-0090-05, 25 mg–5 ml ampul.
NDC 0094-0090-10, 50 mg–10 ml ampul.
Protect from freezing.

TRIDIL DILUTION AND ADMINISTRATION TABLE

	DILUTE 5 MG TRIDIL IN 100 ML OR 25 MG TRIDIL IN 500 ML	5 MG TRIDIL IN 50 ML OR 25 MG TRIDIL IN 250 ML OR 50 MG TRIDIL IN 500 ML	10 MG TRIDIL IN 50 ML OR 50 MG TRIDIL IN 250 ML OR 100 MG TRIDIL IN 500 ML	100 MG TRIDIL IN 250 ML OR 200 MG TRIDIL IN 500 ML
	TO YIELD 50 MCG/ML	100 MCG/ML	200 MCG/ML	400 MCG/ML
ADMIXTURE FLOW RATE MICRO DROPS/MIN = ML/HR	TRIDIL ADMINISTRATION RATE MCG I.V. NITROGLYCERIN/MIN			
3	—	5	10	20
6	5	10	20	40
12	10	20	40	80
24	20	40	80	160
48	40	80	160	320
72	60	120	240	480
96	80	160	320	640

American Dermal Corporation

12 WORLDS FAIR DRIVE
SOMERSET, NJ 08873

DRITHOCREME™ ℞
(anthralin)

Description: Pale yellow cream containing 0.1%, 0.25% or 0.5% anthralin USP in a base containing white petrolatum, ceto-oleyl macrogol, cetostearyl alcohol, ascorbic acid, salicylic acid, chlorocresol and purified water.

Action: Drithocreme provides the inhibitory and anti-mitotic action of anthralin in an aqueous cream formulation which, being available in three strengths, provides a flexibility of treatment to suit most patients.

Indications: For an aid in the topical treatment of quiescent or chronic psoriasis.

Contraindications: Do not use in cases of renal disease. Use only on quiescent or chronic patches and not in acute eruptions.

Precautions: For external use only. Keep out of the reach of children. Avoid contact with the eyes or mucous membranes. Exercise care when applying to the face or intertriginous skin areas. Discontinue use of the product if irritation or redness develops on uninvolved skin adjacent to lesions. Some temporary discoloration of hair or fingernails may arise during the period of treatment but should be minimized by careful application. Always wash hands after use.
To prevent the possibility of staining clothing or bed linen, while gaining experience in using Drithocreme, it may be advisable to use protective dressings.

Adverse Reactions: A small proportion of patients are sensitive to any form of anthralin treatment. If the initial treatment produces excessive soreness or if the lesions spread (particularly when potent topical steroids have recently been used), reduce frequency of application and in extreme cases discontinue use and consult physician.

Dosage and Administration: Where the response to anthralin treatment has not previously been established, always commence treatment for at least one week using 0.1% Drithocreme. Increase to the 0.25% and 0.5% strengths if appropriate.
Treatment should be continued until the skin is entirely clear, i.e. when there is nothing to feel with the fingers and the texture is normal.
For the skin: Drithocreme should be applied sparingly only to the psoriatic lesions, preferably at night, and rubbed gently and carefully into the skin until absorbed. It is most important to avoid applying an excessive quantity which may cause unnecessary soiling and staining of the clothing and/or bed linen. In the morning a bath should be taken to remove any surplus cream, which will have become red/brown in color. The margins of the lesion will gradually become stained purple/brown as treatment progresses, but this will disappear after cessation of treatment.
For the scalp: Shampoo to remove scalar debris and any previous application. Dry the hair, and, after suitably parting, rub the cream well into the lesions. Care should be taken to avoid application of the cream to uninvolved

scalp margins. Remove any unintended residue which may be deposited behind the ears.
How Supplied: 50g tubes.
Drithocreme 0.1% N.D.C. 51201-0029-1
Drithocreme 0.25% N.D.C. 51201-0028-1
Drithocreme 0.5% N.D.C. 51201-0027-1
Caution: Federal law prohibits dispensing without prescription.

VIRANOL™ ℞

Description: Viranol™ is a solution for topical application containing 16.7% Salicylic Acid U.S.P., and 16.7% Lactic Acid U.S.P. in a vehicle of Flexible Collodion U.S.P.
Action: The active ingredients, Salicylic Acid and Lactic Acid are believed to exert a keratolytic action which effects the removal of wart epidermal cells infected by deoxyribonucleic acid viruses.
Indications: Viranol™ is indicated as an aid in the treatment and removal of plantar warts and other common warts.
Contraindications: Viranol™ should not be used by diabetics or individuals with impaired blood circulation.
Warnings: Viranol™ should not be applied to moles, birthmarks, unusual warts with protruding hair, genital warts, or warts on the face.
Precautions: Viranol™ is for external use only. Discontinue use if excessive irritation occurs on normal skin areas. Avoid contact with eyes or on mucous membranes. If contact with eyes or mucous membranes should occur, flush with water to remove Collodion film and continue rinsing for an additional 15 minutes. Viranol™ is highly flammable and should not be used or stored near fire or flame. Avoid inhaling vapors.
Adverse Reactions: Viranol™ may cause local irritation on normal skin. Care should be used to avoid contact with normal surrounding skin areas while applying Viranol™ directly to wart.
Dosage and Administration: Wash affected area and soak wart in hot water for 5 minutes. Dry thoroughly, then gently remove softened area of the wart by rubbing with a pumice stone, emery board or washcloth. Using the special applicator provided, apply 2 to 4 drops to the wart only. Keep Viranol™ away from surrounding skin (preferably by encircling the wart with a ring of petrolatum). Allow to dry before covering with a waterproof bandage. Repeat the above procedure once daily and continue as directed by physician. Discontinue treatment if skin irritation develops or if no improvement occurs after two months' use.
How Supplied: 10 ml bottle with applicator. NDC #51201-5006-1 Keep bottle tightly capped and store in an upright position at controlled room temperature. Keep out of reach of children.
Caution: Federal law prohibits dispensing without prescription.

IDENTIFICATION PROBLEM?

Consult PDR's

Product Identification Section

where you'll find over 900

products pictured actual size

and in full color.

American Pharmaceutical Company

245 FOURTH STREET
PASSAIC, NEW JERSEY 07055

AMPICILLIN TRIHYDRATE ℞
CAPSULES, USP
250 mg., 500 mg.

APHCO™ HEMORRHOIDAL OINTMENT, SUPPOSITORIES

BACITRACIN OINTMENT

BISACODYL
TABLETS AND SUPPOSITORIES

CODANOL® A&D OINTMENT

CORTICREME™ ℞
Hydrocortisone Cream (1/2% & 1%)

DAILY DOSE 1 VITAMINS
B-Complex Liver & Iron Tablets
Belaxa™ B-Complex & C Capsules
Fe-ritol Tablets
Gerifort™ Plus
Multiple Vitamins with Iron Tablets
Multiple Vitamins with Minerals Tablets
Nutri-Drops
Spectrum™
Super Stress-600 Tablets
Super Stress-600 with Iron Tablets
Super Z Stress-600 Tablets
Thera-Amcaps™
Thera-Amcaps™ M
Vitamin E Capsules

DIPHENHYDRAMINE ℞
CAPSULES, ELIXIR, EXPECTORANT

FENDON® TABLETS, ELIXIR
(Acetaminophen)

FERROUS GLUCONATE TABLETS

FERROUS SULFATE TABLETS, CAPSULES

GELUMINA™ PLUS LIQUID

GELUMINA™ TABLETS

GELUMINA™ with SIMETHICONE, LIQUID

ISO-LO™ EYE WASH, DROPS

ISOXSUPRINE HCl TABLETS ℞
10 mg., 20 mg.

KA-PEK™ SUSPENSION

METHOCARBAMOL TABLETS ℞
500 mg., 750 mg.

NEO-MIST™ NASAL SPRAY

NEOMYCIN TABLETS ℞
0.5 mg.

PENICILLIN V POTASSIUM ℞
TABLETS USP
125 mg. 200 MU, 250 mg. 400 MU

PERTINEX™ CREAM, SPRAY
Athlete's Foot Control

PHENDEX® ELIXIR, TABLETS ℞

PREDNISOLONE TABLETS, USP ℞
5 mg.

PREDNISONE TABLETS, USP ℞
5 mg.

PRENACAPS™

PROMETHAZINE ℞
TABLETS, EXPECTORANT

RHUSTICON™ LOTION
Antihistaminic—Antipruritic

ROMEX® DECONGESTANT COUGH, COLD
Preparations: Liquid, Capsules, Troches

SPD® ANALGESIC CREAM, LOTION

SPECTRO-BIOTIC OINTMENT

TETRACYCLINE CAPSULES, USP ℞
250 mg., 500 mg.

TRIPROLIDINE ℞
W/PSEUDOEPHEDRINE
TABLETS, SYRUP

Anbex, Inc.

15 WEST 75TH STREET
NEW YORK, NEW YORK 10023

IOSAT™
(Brand of Potassium Iodide Tablets, U.S.P.)

Description: Each IOSAT tablet contains 130 mg. of potassium iodide.
Indications: Thyroid blocking in a radiation emergency only.
Actions: Because the accidental release of radioactive iodine represents the most serious health threat posed by nuclear power (in terms of the number of people who could be affected by an accident), the FDA has called for the administration of potassium iodide whenever projected thyroid dose levels reach 25 rem. Physicians should be aware that in a serious nuclear accident, this dose level could jeopardize populations hundreds of miles downwind from the reactor site.
Potassium iodide provides almost complete protection from radioactive iodine. If the recommended dose is taken just prior to radiation exposure, the thyroid gland will become saturated (blocked), thus preventing absorption of the radioactive material. Continued use (not expected to exceed 10 to 14 days) will provide protection during the time necessary for the radio-iodine to disappear due to beta decay. Patients should understand that while IOSAT could significantly reduce the number of casualties in a radiation emergency, the drug is not a panacea for all radiation dangers. It should be taken only on the advice of public health officials, and patients should be encouraged to read the product insert which provides additional valuable information.
Warning: Potassium iodide should not be used by people allergic to iodide.
Adverse Reactions: Side effects from IOSAT are unlikely because of the low dose and short period the drug will be taken. However, effects which may appear include skin rashes, swelling of the salivary glands, and iodism. A few people have an allergic reaction with more serious symptoms.
Dosage: Adults and children one year of age: One tablet once a day. Crush for small children. Babies under one year: One half tablet once a day. Crush first. Take for 10 days unless directed otherwise by state or local public health authorities.
How Supplied: IOSAT tablets (potassium iodide, U.S.P.): Bottles of 14 tablets. (NDC 51803-001-01)

Important Notice

Before prescribing or administering

any product described in

PHYSICIANS' DESK REFERENCE

always consult the PDR Supplement for

possible new or revised information.

Arco Pharmaceuticals, Inc.
105 ORVILLE DRIVE
BOHEMIA, NY 11716

ARCO-LASE®
(broad pH spectrum digestant)

Composition: Each soft, mint flavored tablet contains Trizyme*, 38 mg., and Lipase, 25 mg.
*Contains the following standardized enzymes: amylolytic 30 mg.; proteolytic 6 mg.; cellulolytic 2 mg.
Action and Uses: Indicated for most gastrointestinal disorders due to poor digestion. Flatulence, gas and bloating, dyspepsia, distention, fullness, heartburn, or in any condition where normal digestion is impaired by digestive insufficiencies. Arcolase provides the highest standardized enzymatic activity, plus the protective action of the widest pH range. Thus it is effective throughout the entire G.I. tract. Requiring no enteric coating, there is assurance of a positive breakdown of its factors. This is advantageous, because quite often patients with digestive disorders cannot digest their food properly, let alone hard, or enteric coated capsules or tablets.
Side Effects: None.
Administration and Dosage: One tablet with or immediately following meals. Tablet may be swallowed or chewed.
Supplied: Bottles of 50's. NDC 275-4040.

ARCO-LASE® PLUS ℞

Composition: Same as Arco-Lase, plus the addition of Hyoscyamine sulfate 0.10 mg., atropine sulfate 0.02 mg. and phenobarbital 1/8 gr. (Warning: may be habit forming.)
Action and Uses: Gastrointestinal disturbances, such as cramps, bloating, spasms, diarrhea, nausea, vomiting and peptic ulcer. The enzymes correct the digestive insufficiencies. The antispasmodic and phenobarbital contribute to the symptomatic relief of hypermotility and nervous tension, which usually accompanies functional disturbances of the bowel.
Administration and Dosage: One tablet following meals.
Side Effects: May cause rapid pulse, dryness of mouth and blurred vision.
Contraindications: This product is contraindicated in the presence of glaucoma or prostatic hypertrophy.
Supplied: Bottles of 50's. NDC 275-45-45.
Literature Available: Yes.

CODEXIN™ Capsules

(See PDR For Nonprescription Drugs)

MEGA-B®
(super potency vitamin B complex, sugar & starch free)

Composition: Each Mega-B Tablet contains the following Mega Vitamins:

B_1 (Thiamine Mononitrate)	100 mg.
B_2 (Riboflavin)	100 mg.
B_6 (Pyridoxine Hydrochloride)	100 mg.
B_{12} (Cyanocobalamin)	100 mcg.
Choline Bitartrate	100 mg.
Inositol	100 mg.
Niacinamide	100 mg.
Folic Acid	100 mcg.
Pantothenic Acid	100 mg.
d-Biotin	100 mcg.
Para-Aminobenzoic Acid (PABA)	100 mg.

In a base of yeast to provide the identified and unidentified B-Complex Factors.
Advantages: Each Mega-B capsule-shaped tablet provides the highest vitamin B complex available in a single dose.
Mega-B was designed for those patients who require truly Mega vitamin potencies with the convenience of minimum dosage.
Indications: Mega-B is indicated in conditions characterized by depletions or increased demand of the water-soluble B-complex vitamins. It may be useful in the nutritional management of patients during prolonged convalescence associated with major surgery. It is also indicated for stress conditions, as an adjunct to antibiotics and diuretic therapy, pre and post operative cases, liver conditions, gastro-intestinal disorders interferring with intake or absorbtion of water-soluble vitamins, prolonged or wasting diseases, diabetes, burns, fractures, severe infections, and some psychological disorders.
Warning: NOT INTENDED FOR TREATMENT OF PERNICIOUS ANEMIA, OR OTHER PRIMARY OR SECONDARY ANEMIAS.
Dosage: Usual dosage is one Mega-B tablet daily, or varied, depending on clinical needs.
Supplied: Yellow capsule shaped tablets in bottles of 30, 100 and 500.

MEGADOSE™
(multiple mega-vitamin formula with minerals, sugar and starch free)

Composition:

Vitamin A	25,000 USP Units
Vitamin D	1,000 USP Units
Vitamin C w/Rose Hips	250 mg.
Vitamin E	100 IU
Folic Acid	400 mcg.
Vitamin B_1	80 mg.
Vitamin B_2	80 mg.
Niacinamide	80 mg.
Vitamin B_6	80 mg.
Vitamin B_{12}	80 mcg.
Biotin	80 mcg.
Pantothenic Acid	80 mg.
Choline Bitartrate	80 mg.
Inositol	80 mg.
Para-Aminobenzoic Acid	80 mg.
Rutin	30 mg.
Citrus Bioflavonoids	30 mg.
Betaine Hydrochloride	30 mg.
Glutamic Acid	30 mg.
Hesperidin Complex	5 mg.
Iodine (from Kelp)	0.15 mg.
Calcium Gluconate*	50 mg.
Zinc Gluconate*	25 mg.
Potassium Gluconate*	10 mg.
Ferrous Gluconate*	10 mg.
Magnesium Gluconate*	7 mg.
Manganese Gluconate*	6 mg.
Copper Gluconate*	0.5 mg.

*Natural mineral chelates in a base containing natural ingredients.
Dosage: One tablet daily.
Supplied: Capsule shaped tablets in bottles of 30, 100 and 250.

Ar-Ex Products Co.
1036 WEST VAN BUREN STREET
CHICAGO, IL 60607

AR-EX HYPO-ALLERGENIC COSMETICS

Composition: Formulated so you can prescribe cosmetics as you prescribe medications or other therapeutic regimen in dermatological, respiratory, gastrointestinal and other allergies where usual cosmetics are contraindicated.
Action and Uses: To provide safe beauty aids and eliminate a whole field of potential irritants and sensitizers that may aggravate or precipitate allergic conditions, as: skin irritations and erythema, contact dermatitis, photosensitivity, dry, chapped skin, lipstick cheilitis, eyelid dermatitis, chronic coryza, chronic vasomotor rhinitis, chronic conjunctivitis, asthma, urticaria, colitis and other G-I symptoms, also other conditions where cosmetics may be prime or contributing offenders.
Unscented Cosmetics: Perfumes, natural or synthetic, and essential oils are known to be capable of irritating the skin, causing Berloque dermatitis (photosensitivity), and causing or aggravating respiratory symptoms simulating asthma and hay fever. For these persons, all AR-EX Cosmetics are available Unscented, and contain absolutely no perfume, natural or synthetic.
A Complete Line: Following is a list of AR-EX Cosmetics, together with a partial list of potential irritants and allergens which they do NOT contain. When these substances are suspected etiological agents, you can rule them out of your diagnoses when you prescribe AR-EX Cosmetics *by brand name.*
Creams and Lotions: Contain no soap, almond oil, oil of orris, coconut oil, bergamot or other citrus oils, lanolin, cocoa butter, karaya gum, gum arabic, tragacanth, rose water or phenol. Unscented.
Deodorants: Cream, Spray and Roll-On. Contain no aluminum chloride, aluminum chlorhydroxide, aluminum acetate, aluminum sulfate, alum, salicylic acid, formaldehyde, alcohol or hexachlorophene.
Eye Makeup: Contain no lanolin, indelible or aniline dyes, perfume, turpentine, bergamot or other photosensitizers, chromium or nickel compounds, or pharaphenylenediamine.
Hair Preparations: Contain no soap, lanolin, sulfonated oil, palm or coconut oil, gum karaya, gum arabic, tragacanth, resin, lacquer, shellac. Unscented.
Powders: Contain no orris root, oil of orris, bergamot or other citrus oils, corn starch, rice starch, wheat starch, powdered gums or lanolin.
Soap: Low in excess alkali, superfatted. Contains no lanolin, perfumes, essential oils.
Foundation Lotion: Liquid makeup. Contains no gum acacia, karaya or tragacanth, lanolin, corn oil or other vegetable oils, oil of orris, perfumes or essential oils.
AR-EX Special Formula Lipstick: Contains no indelible dyes, eosin, mono-di-tri-or-tetra-bromfluorescein compounds, but achieves shades through use of lake pigments. Contains no perfumes or essential oils, lanolin, almond oil or cocoa butter.
Literature Available: For precise prescription of hypo-allergenic cosmetics in indicated conditions, refer to the AR-EX Professional Formulary. Sent on request.

SAFE SUDS

Composition: Hypo-allergenic, all-purpose detergent for patients whose hands or respiratory membranes are irritated by soaps or detergents. For dishes, laundry, floors, rugs, upholstery, etc. Suds in hard or soft water, with pH approximately 6.8. Contains no enzymes, phosphates, lanolin, fillers or bleaches. Biodegradable. NOT scented.

Important Notice

Before prescribing or administering any product described in PHYSICIANS' DESK REFERENCE always consult the PDR Supplement for possible new or revised information.

Armour Pharmaceutical Company

303 SOUTH BROADWAY
TARRYTOWN, NY 10591

H.P. ACTHAR® GEL* ℞
(repository corticotropin injection)
and
ACTHAR® ℞
(corticotropin for injection)

Description: H.P. ACTHAR® GEL (Repository Corticotropin Injection) is a Highly Purified preparation of CORTICOTROPIN in gelatin which has both rapid onset and prolonged action. Each milliliter contains the labeled activity of Corticotropin U.S.P., 16% Gelatin, 0.5% Phenol, not more than 0.1% Cysteine (added), Sodium Hydroxide and/or Acetic acid to adjust pH, and Water for Injection, q.s.
ACTHAR® (Corticotropin for Injection) is sterile powdered lyophilized ACTH which in the dry form is stable at room temperature. Each vial contains 25 or 40 Units of Corticotropin U.S.P. and approximately 9 and 14 milligrams of hydrolyzed gelatin respectively.
Actions: H.P. ACTHAR® (Repository Corticotropin Injection) and ACTHAR® (Corticotropin for Injection) are the Armour Pharmaceutical Company brands of preparations containing the anterior pituitary hormone. This hormone stimulates the functioning adrenal cortex to produce and secrete the adrenocortical hormones.
Indications: ACTHAR® (Corticotropin for Injection) and H.P. ACTHAR® GEL (Repository Corticotropin Injection) are indicated for diagnostic testing of adrenocortical function.
ACTHAR® (Corticotropin for Injection) and H.P. ACTHAR® GEL (Repository Corticotropin Injection) have limited therapeutic value in those conditions responsive to corticosteroid therapy; in such case, corticosteroid therapy is considered to be the treatment of choice. ACTHAR® (Corticotropin for Injection) and H.P. ACTHAR® GEL (Repository Corticotropin Injection) may be employed in the following disorders:

ENDOCRINE DISORDERS: Nonsuppurative thyroiditis; Hypercalcemia associated with cancer.
NERVOUS SYSTEM DISEASES: Acute exacerbations of multiple sclerosis.
RHEUMATIC DISORDERS: As adjunctive therapy for short-term administration (to tide the patient over an acute episode or exacerbation) in:
Psoriatic arthritis; Rheumatoid arthritis, including juvenile rheumatoid arthritis (selected cases may require low-dose maintenance therapy); Ankylosing spondylitis; Acute and subacute bursitis; Acute nonspecific tenosynovitis; Acute gouty arthritis; Post-traumatic arthritis; Synovitis of osteoarthritis; Epicondylitis.
COLLAGEN DISEASES: During an exacerbation or as maintenance therapy in selected cases of:
Systemic lupus erythematosus; Systemic dermatomyositis (polymyositis); Acute rheumatic carditis.
DERMATOLOGIC DISEASES: Pemphigus; Bullous dermatitis herpetiformis; Severe erythema multiforme (Stevens-Johnson syndrome); Exfoliative dermatitis; Severe psoriasis; Severe seborrheic dermatitis; Mycosis fungoides.
ALLERGIC STATES: Control of severe or incapacitating allergic conditions intractable to adequate trials of conventional treatment—Seasonal or perennial allergic rhinitis; Bronchial asthma; Contact dermatitis; Atopic dermatitis; Serum sickness.
OPHTHALMIC DISEASES: Severe acute and chronic allergic and inflammatory processes involving the eye and its adnexa such as: Allergic conjunctivitis; Keratitis; Herpes zoster ophthalmicus; Iritis and iridocyclitis; Diffuse posterior uveitis and choroiditis; Optic neuritis; Sympathetic ophthalmia; Chorioretinitis; Anterior segment inflammation; Allergic corneal marginal ulcers.
RESPIRATORY DISEASES: Symptomatic sarcoidosis; Loeffler's syndrome not manageable by other means; Berylliosis; Fulminating or disseminated pulmonary tuberculosis when used concurrently with antituberculous chemotherapy; Aspiration pneumonitis.
HEMATOLOGIC DISORDERS: Acquired (autoimmune) hemolytic anemia; Secondary thrombocytopenia in adults; Erythroblastopenia (RBC anemia); Congenital (erythroid) hypoplastic anemia.
NEOPLASTIC DISEASES: For palliative management of:
Leukemias and lymphomas in adults; Acute leukemia of childhood.
EDEMATOUS STATE: To induce a diuresis or a remission of proteinuria in the nephrotic syndrome without uremia of the idiopathic type or that due to lupus erythematosus.
GASTROINTESTINAL DISEASES: To tide the patient over a critical period of the disease in: Ulcerative colitis; Regional enteritis.
MISCELLANEOUS: Tuberculous meningitis with subarachnoid block or impending block when used concurrently with appropriate anti-tuberculous chemotherapy; Trichinosis with neurologic or myocardial involvement.

Contraindications: Corticotropin is contraindicated in patients with scleroderma, osteoporosis, systemic fungal infections, ocular herpes simplex, recent surgery, history of or the presence of a peptic ulcer, congestive heart failure, hypertension, or sensitivity to proteins of porcine origin.
Treatment of conditions listed within the indication section (see above) when they are accompanied by primary adrenocortical insufficiency or adrenocortical hyperfunction.
Intravenous administration of corticotropin is contraindicated for treatment of conditions listed within the indications section.
Warnings: Chronic administration of corticotropin may lead to adverse effects which are not reversible. Corticotropin may only suppress symptoms and signs of chronic disease without altering the natural course of the disease. Neither H.P. ACTHAR® GEL (Repository Corticotropin Injection) nor ACTHAR® (Corticotropin for Injection) should be administered for treatment until adrenal responsiveness has been verified with the route of administration which will be utilized during treatment, intramuscularly or subcutaneously. A rise in urinary and plasma corticosteroid values provides direct evidence of a stimulatory effect. Prolonged administration of corticotropin increases the risk of hypersensitivity reactions. Although the action of corticotropin is similar to that of exogenous adrenocortical steroids the quantity of adrenocorticoid may be variable. In patients who receive prolonged corticotropin therapy the additional use of rapidly acting corticosteroids before, during, and after an unusual stressful situation is indicated.
Prolonged use of corticotropin may produce posterior subcapsular cataracts and glaucoma with possible damage to the optic nerves.
Corticotropin may mask some signs of infection, and new infections including those of the eye due to fungi or viruses may appear during its use. There may be decreased resistance and inability to localize infection when corticotropin is used.
Corticotropin can cause elevation of blood pressure, salt and water retention, and increased excretion of potassium. Dietary salt restriction and potassium supplementation may be necessary. Corticotropin increases calcium excretion.
While on corticotropin therapy, patients should not be vaccinated against smallpox. Other immunization procedures should be undertaken with caution in patients who are receiving corticotropin, especially when high doses are administered because of the possible hazards of neurological complications and lack of antibody response.
Precautions: Patients with latent tuberculosis or tuberculin reactivity who receive corticotropin should be closely observed as reactivation of the disease may occur. During prolonged corticotropin therapy, these patients should receive chemoprophylaxis.
Skin testing should be performed prior to treatment of all patients with suspected sensitivity to porcine proteins. During intravenous or immediately following intramuscular or subcutaneous administration of corticotropin all patients should be observed carefully for sensitivity reactions.
Relative adrenocortical insufficiency induced by prolonged corticotropin therapy may be minimized by gradual reduction of corticotropin dosage. This type of insufficiency may persist for months after discontinuation of therapy; therefore, in any situation of stress during that period, hormone therapy should be reinstituted.
There is an enhanced effect of corticotropin in patients with hypothyroidism and in those with cirrhosis.
The lowest possible dosage of corticotropin should be used to control the condition under treatment, and when reduction in dosage is possible the reduction should be gradual.
Corticotropin should be administered for treatment only when the disease is intractable to more conventional therapy. Corticotropin should be adjunctive and not the sole therapy in the treatment of a disease.
Since maximal corticotropin stimulation of the adrenals may be limited during the first few days of treatment, other drugs should be administered when an immediate therapeutic effect is desirable.
When infection is present appropriate anti-infective therapy should be administered during corticotropin and following discontinuation of corticotropin therapy.
Although controlled clinical trials have shown ACTH to be effective in speeding the resolution of acute exacerbations of multiple sclerosis they do not show that it affects the ultimate outcome or natural history of the disease. The studies do show that relatively high doses of ACTH are necessary to demonstrate a significant effect. (See DOSAGE AND ADMINISTRATION section.)
Treatment of acute gouty arthritis should be limited to a few days. Since rebound attacks may occur when corticotropin is discontinued, conventional concomitant therapy should be administered during corticotropin treatment, and for several days after it is stopped.
Psychic derangements may appear when corticotropin is used, ranging from euphoria, insomnia, mood swings, personality changes, and depression, to frank psychotic manifestations. Also, existing emotional instability or psychotic tendencies may be aggravated by corticotropin.
Aspirin should be used cautiously in conjunction with corticotropin in hypoprothrombinemia. Corticotropin should be used with caution in patients with diabetes, abscess, pyogenic infections, diverticulitis, renal insufficiency, and myasthenia gravis.
Usage in pregnancy: Since fetal abnormalities have been observed in experimental animals, use of this drug in pregnancy, nursing mothers, or women of child bearing potential requires that the potential benefits of the drug be weighed against the potential hazards to the mother and embryo or fetus. Infants born of mothers who have received substantial doses of

Continued on next page

Armour—Cont.

corticotropin during pregnancy should be carefully observed for signs of hypoadrenalism.
Growth and development of infants and children on prolonged corticotropin therapy should be carefully observed.

Adverse Reactions:
Fluid and electrolyte disturbances:
Sodium retention; fluid retention; potassium loss; hypokalemic alkalosis; calcium loss.
Musculoskeletal:
Muscle weakness; steroid myopathy; loss of muscle mass; osteoporosis; vertebral compression fractures; aseptic necrosis of femoral and humeral heads; pathologic fracture of long bones.
Gastrointestinal:
Peptic ulcer with possible perforation and hemorrhage; pancreatitis; abdominal distention; ulcerative esophagitis.
Dermatologic:
Impaired wound healing; thin fragile skin; petechiae and ecchymoses; facial erythema; increased sweating; suppression of skin test reactions; acne; hyperpigmentation.
Cardiovascular:
Hypertension, necrotizing angiitis; congestive heart failure.
Neurological:
Convulsions; increased intracranial pressure with papilledema, (pseudo-tumor cerebri) usually after treatment; headache, vertigo.
Endocrine:
Menstrual irregularities; development of Cushingoid state; suppression of growth in children; secondary adrenocortical pituitary unresponsiveness, particularly in times of stress, as in trauma, surgery or illness; decreased carbohydrate tolerance; manifestations of latent diabetes mellitus; increased requirements for insulin or oral hypoglycemic agents in diabetics; hirsutism.
Ophthalmic:
Posterior subcapsular cataracts; increased intraocular pressure; glaucoma with possible damage to optic nerve; exophthalmos.
Metabolic:
Negative nitrogen balance due to protein catabolism.
Allergic reactions:
Especially in patients with allergic responses to proteins manifesting as dizziness, nausea and vomiting, shock, skin reactions.
Miscellaneous:
Abscess: prolonged use of ACTH may result in antibodies to it and resulting loss of stimulatory effect.

Dosage and Administration: Standard tests for verification of adrenal responsiveness to corticotropin may utilize as much as 80 units as a single injection or one or more injections of a lesser dosage. Verification tests should be performed prior to treatment with corticotropins. The test should utilize the route(s) of administration proposed for treatment. Following verification, dosage should be individualized according to the disease under treatment and the general medical condition of each patient. Frequency and dose of the drug should be determined by considering severity of the disease, plasma and urine corticosteroid levels and the initial response of the patient. Only gradual change in dosage schedules should be attempted, after full drug effects have become apparent.
The chronic administration of more than 40 units daily may be associated with uncontrollable adverse effects.
When reduction in dosage is indicated this should be done gradually by either reducing the amount of each injection, or administering injections at longer intervals, or by a combination of both of the above. During reduction of dosage careful consideration should be given to the disease being treated, the general medical conditions of the patient and the duration over which corticotropin was administered.
Acthar must be reconstituted at the time of use by dissolving in a convenient volume of Sterile Water for Injection or Sodium Chloride Injection in such a manner that the individual dose will be contained in 1–2 ml. of solution. The reconstituted solution should be refrigerated and used in 24 hours.
H.P. ACTHAR® GEL (Repository Corticotropin Injection) and ACTHAR® (Corticotropin for Injection may be administered intramuscularly or subcutaneously.
H.P. ACTHAR® GEL (Repository Corticotropin Injection) is given intramuscularly or subcutaneously every 24-72 hours in doses of 40-80 units.
The usual intramuscular or subcutaneous dose for ACTHAR® (Corticotropin for Injection) is 20 units four times a day.
In the treatment of acute exacerbations of multiple sclerosis daily intramuscular doses of 80–120 units for 2–3 weeks may be administered.
For diagnostic purposes, ACTHAR® (Corticotropin for Injection) may be given intravenously in doses of 10-25 units dissolved in 500 ml. of 5% glucose infused over an 8-hour period.

How Supplied: H.P. ACTHAR® GEL (Repository Corticotropin Injection) is supplied in 5 milliliter multiple dose vials in strengths of 40 and 80 U.S.P. Units per milliliter and 1 milliliter vials containing 40 and 80 U.S.P. Units per milliliter.
ACTHAR® (Corticotropin for Injection) is supplied as a lyophilized powder in vials containing 25 and 40 U.S.P. Units per vial.
H.P. ACTHAR® GEL (Repository Corticotropin Injection) is stable for the period indicated on the label when stored under refrigeration between 2°–8°C (36°–46°F).
ACTHAR® (Corticotropin For Injection) is stable for the period indicated on the label when stored at controlled room temperature between 15°–30°C (59°–86°F).
*U.S. PAT. NO. 2,992,165

BIOZYME®-C Ointment ℞
Collagenase

Description: BIOZYME®-C OINTMENT is a sterile enzymatic debriding ointment which contains 250 collagenase units per gram of white petrolatum USP. The enzyme collagenase is derived from the fermentation by *Clostridium histolyticum*. It possesses the unique ability to digest native and denatured collagen in necrotic tissue.

Action: Since collagen accounts for 75% of the dry weight of skin tissue, the ability of collagenase to digest collagen in the physiological pH range and temperature makes it particularly effective in the removal of detritus.[1] Collagenase thus contributes towards the formation of granulation tissue and subsequent epithelization of dermal ulcers and severely burned areas.[2,3,4,5,6] Collagen in healthy tissue or in newly formed granulation tissue is not attacked.[2,3,4,5,6,7,8]

Indications: BIOZYME®-C OINTMENT is indicated for debriding chronic dermal ulcers[2,3,4,5,6,8,9,10,11,12,13,14,15,16,17,18] and severely burned areas.[3,4,5,7,16,19,20,21]

Contraindications: BIOZYME®-C OINTMENT is contraindicated in patients who have shown local or systemic hypersensitivity to collagenase.

Precautions: The optimal pH range of collagenase is 6 to 8. Higher or lower pH conditions will decrease the enzyme's activity and appropriate precautions should be taken. The enzymatic activity is also adversely affected by detergents, hexachlorophene and heavy metal ions such as mercury and silver which are used in some antiseptics. When it is suspected such materials have been used, the site should be carefully cleansed by repeated washings with normal saline before BIOZYME®-C OINTMENT is applied. Soaks containing metal ions or acidic solutions such as Burow's solution should be avoided because of the metal ion and low pH. Cleansing materials such as hydrogen peroxide, Dakin's solution, and sterile saline are compatible with BIOZYME®-C OINTMENT.
Debilitated patients should be closely monitored for systemic bacterial infections because of the theoretical possibility that debriding enzymes may increase the risk of bacteremia.
A slight transient erythema has been noted occasionally in the surrounding tissue, particularly when BIOZYME®-C OINTMENT was not confined to the lesion. Therefore, the ointment should be applied carefully within the area of the lesion.

Adverse Reactions: No allergic sensitivity or toxic reactions have been noted in the recorded clinical investigations. However, one case of systemic manifestations of hypersensitivity to collagenase in a patient treated for more than one year with a combination of collagenase and cortisone has been reported to us.

Dosage and Administration: BIOZYME®-C OINTMENT should be applied once daily (or more frequently if the dressing becomes soiled, as from incontinence) in the following manner:

(1) Prior to application the lesion should be cleansed of debris and digested material by gently rubbing with a gauze pad saturated with hydrogen peroxide or Dakin's solution followed by sterile normal saline.
(2) Whenever infection is present it is desirable to use an appropriate topical antibacterial agent. Neomycin-Bacitracin-Polymyxin B (Neosporin) powder has been found to be compatible with BIOZYME®-C OINTMENT. The antibiotic should be applied to the lesion prior to the application of BIOZYME®-C OINTMENT. Should the infection not respond, therapy with BIOZYME®-C OINTMENT should be discontinued until remission of the infection.
(3) BIOZYME®-C OINTMENT should be applied directly from the tube. For shallow lesions, BIOZYME®-C OINTMENT may be applied to a sterile gauze pad which is then applied to the wound and properly secured.
(4) Crosshatching thick eschar with a #10 blade allows collagenase more surface contact with necrotic debris. It is also desirable to remove, with forceps and scissors, as much loosened detritus as can be done readily.
(5) All excess ointment should be removed each time dressing is changed.
(6) Use of BIOZYME®-C OINTMENT should be terminated when debridement of necrotic tissue is complete and granulation tissue is well established.

Overdose: Action of the enzyme may be stopped, should this be desired, by the application of Burow's solution USP (pH 3.6-4.4) to the lesion.

How Supplied: BIOZYME®-C OINTMENT contains 250 units of collagenase enzyme per gram of white petrolatum USP. The potency assay of collagenase is based on the digestion of undenatured collagen (from bovine Achilles tendon) at pH 7.2 and 37°C for 24 hours. The number of peptide bonds cleaved are measured by reaction with ninhydrin. Amino groups released by a trypsin digestion control are subtracted. One net collagenase unit will solubilize ninhydrin reactive material equivalent to 4 micromoles of leucine.

References:
1—Mandl, I., Adv. Enzymol. 23:163, 1961.
2—Boxer, A.M., Gottesman, N., Bernstein, H., & Mandl, I., Geriatrics 24:75, 1969.
3—Mazurek, I., Med. Welt 22:150, 1971.
4—Zimmerman, W.E., in "Collagenase," I., Mandl, ed., Gordon & Breach, Science Publishers, New York, 1971, p. 131, p. 185.

5—Vetra, H., & Whittaker, D., Geriatrics 30:53, 1975.
6—Rao, D.B., Sane, P.G., & Georgiev, E.L., J. Am. Geriatrics Soc. 23:22, 1975.
7—Vrabec, R., Moserova, J., Konickova, Z., Behounkova, E., & Blaha, J., J. Hyg. Epidemiol. Microbiol. Immunol. 18:496, 1974.
8—Lippmann, H.I., Arch. Phys. Med. Rehabil. 54:588, 1973.
9—German, F.M., in "Collagenase," I., Mandl, ed., Gordon & Breach, Science Publishers, New York, 1971, p. 165.
10—Haimovici, H. & Strauch, B., in "Collagenase," I. Mandl, ed., Gordon & Breach, Science Publishers, New York, 1971, p. 177.
11—Lee, L.K., & Ambrus, J.L., Geriatrics 30:91, 1975.
12—Locke, R.K., & Heifitz, N.M., J. Am. Pod. Assoc. 65:242, 1975.
13—Varma, A.O., Bugatch, E., & German, F.M., Surg. Gynecol. Obstet. 136:281, 1973.
14—Barrett, D., Jr., & Klibanski, A., Am. J. Nurs. 73:849, 1973.
15—Bardfeld, L.A., J. Pod. Ed. 1:41, 1970.
16—Blum, G., Schweiz. Rundschau Med. Praxis 62:820, 1973. Abstr. in Dermatology Digest, Feb. 1974, p. 36.
17—Zarauba, F., Lettl, A., Brozkova, L., Skrdlantova, H., & Krs. V., J. Hyg. Epidemiol. Microbiol. Immunol. 18:499, 1974.
18—Altman, M.I., Goldstein, L., Horowitz, S., J. Am. Pod. Assoc. 68:11, 1978.
19—Rehn, V.J., Med. Klin. 58:799, 1963.
20—Krauss, H., Koslowski, L., & Zimmermann, W.E., Langenbecks Arch. Klin. Chir. 303:23, 1963.
21—Gruenagel, H.H., Med. Klin. 58:442, 1963.

Manufactured by:
Advance Biofactures Corporation
35 Wilbur Street
Lynbrook, New York 11563
U.S. Gov't. License #383
Distributed by:
Armour Pharmaceutical Company
Kankakee, IL 60901

[*Shown in Product Identification Section*]

CALCIMAR® ℞
(calcitonin-salmon), Armour
SOLUTION

Description: Calcitonin is a polypeptide hormone secreted by the parafollicular cells of the thyroid gland in mammals and by the ultimobranchial gland of birds and fish.

CALCIMAR® (calcitonin-salmon) is a synthetic polypeptide of 32 amino acids in the same linear sequence that is found in calcitonin of salmon origin. This is shown by the following graphic formula:

Cys- Ser- Asn- Leu- Ser-Thr- Cys-Val- Leu-Gly-
1 2 3 4 5 6 7 8 9 10
Lys-Leu- Ser- Gln- Glu- Leu-His- Lys-Leu- Gln-
11 12 13 14 15 16 17 18 19 20
Thr-Tyr- Pro- Arg-Thr- Asn-Thr- Gly- Ser- Gly-
21 22 23 24 25 26 27 28 29 30
Thr-Pro-NH_2
31 32

It is provided in sterile solution for subcutaneous or intramuscular injection. Each milliliter contains 200 I.U. (MRC) of Calcitonin-Salmon, Armour, 5 mg Phenol (as preservative), with Sodium Chloride, Sodium Acetate, Acetic Acid, and Sodium Hydroxide to adjust tonicity and pH.

The activity of CALCIMAR® is stated in International Units (equal to MRC or Medical Research Council units) based on bioassay in comparison with the International Reference Preparation of Calcitonin, Salmon for Bioassay, distributed by the National Institute for Biological Standards and Control, Holly Hill, London.

Clinical Pharmacology: Calcitonin acts primarily on bone, but direct renal effects and actions on the gastrointestinal tract are also recognized. Salmon calcitonin appears to have actions essentially identical to calcitonins of mammalian origin, but its potency per mg is greater and it has a longer duration of action. The actions of calcitonin on bone and its role in normal human bone physiology are still incompletely understood.

Bone—Single injections of calcitonin cause a marked transient inhibition of the ongoing bone resorptive process. With prolonged use, there is a persistent, smaller decrease in the rate of bone resorption. Histologically this is associated with a decreased number of osteoclasts and an apparent decrease in their resorptive activity. Decreased osteocytic resorption may also be involved. There is some evidence that initially bone formation may be augmented by calcitonin through increased osteoblastic activity. However, calcitonin will probably not induce a long-term increase in bone formation.

Animal studies indicate that endogenous calcitonin, primarily through its action on bone, participates with parathyroid hormone in the homeostatic regulation of blood calcium. Thus, high blood calcium levels cause increased secretion of calcitonin which, in turn, inhibits bone resorption. This reduces the transfer of calcium from bone to blood and tends to return blood calcium to the normal level. The importance of this process in humans has not been determined. In normal adults, who have a relatively low rate of bone resorption, the administration of exogenous calcitonin results in only a slight decrease in serum calcium. In normal children and in patients with generalized Paget's disease, bone resorption is more rapid and decreases in serum calcium are more pronounced in response to calcitonin.

Paget's Disease of Bone (osteitis deformans)—Paget's disease is a disorder of uncertain etiology characterized by abnormal and accelerated bone formation and resorption in one or more bones. In most patients only small areas of bone are involved and the disease is not symptomatic. In a small fraction of patients, however, the abnormal bone may lead to bone pain and bone deformity, cranial and spinal nerve entrapment, or spinal cord compression. The increased vascularity of the abnormal bone may lead to high output congestive heart failure.

Active Paget's disease involving a large mass of bone may increase the urinary hydroxyproline excretion (reflecting breakdown of collagen-containing bone matrix) and serum alkaline phosphatase (reflecting increased bone formation).

Salmon calcitonin, presumably by an initial blocking effect on bone resorption, causes a decreased rate of bone turnover with a resultant fall in the serum alkaline phosphatase and urinary hydroxyproline excretion in approximately ⅔ of patients treated. These biochemical changes appear to correspond to changes toward more normal bone, as evidenced by a small number of documented examples of: 1) radiologic regression of Pagetic lesions, 2) improvement of impaired auditory nerve and other neurologic function, 3) decreases (measured) in abnormally elevated cardiac output. These improvements occur extremely rarely, if ever, spontaneously (elevated cardiac output may disappear over a period of years when the disease slowly enters a sclerotic phase; in the cases treated with calcitonin, however, the decreases were seen in less than one year).

Some patients with Paget's disease who have good biochemical and/or symptomatic responses initially, later relapse. Suggested explanations have included the formation of neutralizing antibodies and the development of secondary hyperparathyroidism, but neither suggestion appears to explain adequately the majority of relapses.

Although the parathyroid hormone levels do appear to rise transiently during each hypocalcemic response to calcitonin, most investigators have been unable to demonstrate persistent hypersecretion of parathyroid hormone in patients treated chronically with calcitonin.

Circulating antibodies to calcitonin after 2–18 months' treatment have been reported in about half of the patients with Paget's disease in whom antibody studies were done, but calcitonin treatment remained effective in many of these cases. Occasionally patients with high antibody titers are found. These patients usually will have suffered a biochemical relapse of Paget's disease and are unresponsive to the acute hypocalcemic effects of calcitonin.

Hypercalcemia—In clinical trials, CALCIMAR® has been shown to lower the elevated serum calcium of patients with carcinoma (with or without demonstrated metastases), multiple myeloma or primary hyperparathyroidism (lesser response). Patients with higher values for serum calcium tend to show greater reduction during CALCIMAR® therapy. The decrease in calcium occurs about 2 hours after the first injection ahd lasts for about 6–8 hours. CALCIMAR® given every 12 hours maintained a calcium lowering effect for about 5–8 days, the time period evaluated for most patients during the clinical studies. The average reduction of 8-hour post-injection serum calcium during this period was about 9 percent.

Kidney—Calcitonin increases the excretion of filtered phosphate, calcium, and sodium by decreasing their tubular reabsorption. In some patients the inhibition of bone resorption by calcitonin is of such magnitude that the consequent reduction of filtered calcium load more than compensates for the decrease in tubular reabsorption of calcium. The result in these patients is a decrease rather than an increase in urinary calcium.

Transient increases in sodium and water excretion may occur after the initial injection of calcitonin. In most patients these changes return to pre-treatment levels with continued therapy.

Gastrointestinal tract—Increasing evidence indicates that calcitonin has significant actions on the gastrointestinal tract. Short-term administration results in marked transient decreases in the volume and acidity of gastric juice and in the volume and the trypsin and amylase content of pancreatic juice. Whether these effects continue to be elicited after each injection of calcitonin during chronic therapy has not been investigated.

Metabolism—The metabolism of salmon calcitonin has not yet been studied clinically. Information from animal studies with salmon calcitonin and from clinical studies with calcitonins of porcine and human origin suggest that salmon calcitonin is rapidly metabolized by conversion to smaller inactive fragments, primarily in the kidneys, but also in the blood and peripheral tissues. A small amount of unchanged hormone and its inactive metabolites are excreted in the urine.

It appears that salmon calcitonin cannot cross the placental barrier and its passage to the cerebrospinal fluid or to breast milk has not been determined.

Indications and Usage: CALCIMAR® (Calcitonin-Salmon) is indicated for the treatment of symptomatic Paget's disease of bone and for the treatment of hypercalcemia.

Paget's Disease—At the present time effectiveness has been demonstrated principally in patients with moderate to severe disease characterized by polyostotic involvement with elevated serum alkaline phosphatase and urinary hydroxyproline excretion.

Continued on next page

Armour—Cont.

In these patients, the biochemical abnormalities were substantially improved (more than 30% reduction) in about ⅔ of patients studied, and bone pain was improved in a similar fraction. A small number of documented instances of reversal of neurologic deficits has occurred, including improvement in the basilar compression syndrome, and improvement of spinal cord and spinal nerve lesions. At present there is too little experience to predict the likelihood of improvement of any given neurologic lesion. Hearing loss, the most common neurologic lesion of Paget's disease is improved infrequently (4 of 29 patients studied audiometrically).

Patients with increased cardiac output due to extensive Paget's disease have had measured decreases in cardiac output while receiving calcitonin. The number of treated patients in this category is still too small to predict how likely such a result will be.

The large majority of patients with localized, especially monostotic disease do not develop symptoms and most patients with mild symptoms can be managed with analgesics. There is no evidence that the prophylactic use of calcitonin is beneficial in asymptomatic patients, although treatment may be considered in exceptional circumstances in which there is extensive involvement of the skull or spinal cord with the possibility of irreversible neurologic damage. In these instances treatment would be based on the demonstrated effect of calcitonin on Pagetic bone, rather than on clinical studies in the patient population in question.

Hypercalcemia—CALCIMAR® (Calcitonin-Salmon) is indicated for early treatment of hypercalcemic emergencies, along with other appropriate agents, when a rapid decrease in serum calcium is required, until more specific treatment of the underlying disease can be accomplished. It may also be added to existing therapeutic regimens for hypercalcemia such as intravenous fluids and furosemide, oral phosphate or corticosteroids, or other agents.

Contraindications: Clinical allergy to synthetic salmon calcitonin.

Warnings:

Allergic Reactions

Because calcitonin is protein in nature, the possibility of a systemic allergic reaction cannot be overlooked. The usual provisions should be made for the emergency treatment of such a reaction should it occur. Patients with a positive skin test to CALCIMAR® were excluded from clinical trials.

Skin testing should be considered prior to treatment with calcitonin, particularly for patients with suspected sensitivity to calcitonin. The following procedure is suggested: Prepare a dilution at 10 I.U. (MRC) per ml by withdrawing 1/20 ml (0.05 ml) in a tuberculin syringe and filling it to 1.0 ml with Sodium Chloride Injection, U.S.P. Mix well, discard 0.9 ml and inject intracutaneously 0.1 ml (approximately 1 I.U.) on the inner aspect of the forearm. Observe the injection site 15 minutes after injection. The appearance of more than mild erythema or wheal constitutes a positive response.

The incidence of osteogenic sarcoma is known to be increased in Paget's disease. Pagetic lesions, with or without therapy, may appear by x-ray to progress markedly, possibly with some loss of definition or periosteal margins. Such lesions should be evaluated carefully to differentiate these from osteogenic sarcoma.

Precautions:

1. General

The administration of calcitonin possibly could lead to hypocalcemic tetany under special circumstances although no cases have yet been reported. Provisions for parenteral calcium administration should be available during the first several administrations of calcitonin.

2. Laboratory Tests

Periodic examinations of urine sediment of patients on chronic therapy are recommended. Coarse granular casts and casts containing renal tubular epithelial cells were reported in young adult volunteers at bed rest who were given salmon calcitonin to study the effect on immobilization osteoporosis. There was no other evidence of renal abnormality and the urine sediment became normal after calcitonin was stopped. Urine sediment abnormalities have not been reported by other investigators.

3. Instructions for the patient

Careful instruction in sterile injection technique should be given to the patient, and to other persons who may administer CALCIMAR®.

4. Carcinogenesis

No long-term studies have been performed to evaluate carcinogenic potential of salmon calcitonin.

5. Pregnancy

Salmon calcitonin has been shown to cause decrease in fetal birth weights in rabbits when given in doses 14–56 times the dose recommended for human use. Since calcitonin does not cross the placental barrier, this finding may be due to metabolic effects of calcitonin on the pregnant animal. There are no studies in pregnant women. Salmon calcitonin should be used only when clearly needed in women who are or may become pregnant.

6. Nursing Mothers

It is not known whether this drug is excreted in human milk. As a general rule, nursing should not be undertaken while a patient is on drug since many drugs are excreted in human milk. Calcitonin has been shown to inhibit lactation in animals.

7. Pediatric Use

Disorders of bone in children referred to as juvenile Paget's disease have been reported rarely. The relationship of these disorders to adult Paget's disease has not been established and experience with the use of calcitonin in these disorders is very limited. There are no adequate data to support the use of CALCIMAR® in children.

Adverse Reactions: Nausea with or without vomiting has been noted in about 10% of patients treated with calcitonin. It is most evident when treatment is first initiated and tends to decrease or disappear with continued administration.

Local inflammatory reactions at the site of subcutaneous or intramuscular injection have been reported in about 10% of patients. Flushing of face or hands occurred in about 2 to 5% of patients. Skin rashes have been reported occasionally.

Overdosage: A dose of 1000 I.U. (MRC) subcutaneously may produce nausea and vomiting as the only adverse effects. Doses of 32 units per kg per day for one or two days demonstrate no other adverse effects.

Data on chronic high dose administration are insufficient to judge toxicity.

Dosage and Administration:

Paget's Disease—The recommended starting dose of calcitonin in Paget's disease is 100 I.U. (MRC) (0.5 ml) per day administered subcutaneously (preferred for outpatient self-administration) or intramuscularly. Drug effect should be monitored by periodic measurement of serum alkaline phosphatase and 24-hour urinary hydroxyproline (if available) and evaluation of symptoms. A decrease toward normal of the biochemical abnormalities is usually seen, if it is going to occur, within the first few months. Bone pain may also decrease during that time. Improvement of neurologic lesions, when it occurs, requires a longer period of treatment, often more than one year.

In many patients doses of 50 I.U. (MRC) (0.25 ml) per day or every-other day are sufficient to maintain biochemical and clinical improvement. At the present time, however, there are insufficient data to determine whether this reduced dose will have the same effect as the higher dose on forming more normal bone structure. It appears preferable, therefore, to maintain the higher dose in any patient with serious deformity or neurological involvement.

In any patient with a good response initially who later relapses, either clinically or biochemically, the possibility of antibody formation should be explored. Although specialized tests for antibody titer are not widely available, the patients can be tested for high antibody titer as follows:

> After overnight fasting, a sample of the patient's blood is taken for determination of serum calcium and 100 I.U. (MRC) of CALCIMAR® (Calcitonin-Salmon) are injected IM. The patient is then permitted to eat his usual breakfast. At 3 and 6 hours post-injection additional blood samples are drawn and the patient is released. The serum calcium values are then compared. A decrease of 0.5 mg % or more from fasting level at 3 and 6 hours is usually seen in the responsive patient. Decreases of 0.3 mg % or less constitute an inadequate response to calcitonin in the patient with active Paget's disease. If the hypocalcemic action of calcitonin is lost, further therapy with CALCIMAR® will not be effective.

Patient compliance should also be assessed in the event of relapse.

In patients who relapse, whether because of antibodies or for unexplained reasons, a dosage increase beyond 100 I.U. (MRC) per day does not usually appear to elicit an improved response.

Hypercalcemia—The recommended starting dose of CALCIMAR® (Calcitonin-Salmon) in hypercalcemia is 4 I.U. (MRC)/kg body weight every 12 hours by subcutaneous or intramuscular injection. If the response to this dose is not satisfactory after one or two days, the dose may be increased to 8 I.U. (MRC)/kg every 12 hours. If the response remains unsatisfactory after two more days, the dose may be further increased to a maximum of 8 I.U. (MRC)/kg every 6 hours.

If the volume of CALCIMAR® (Calcitonin-Salmon) to be injected exceeds 2 ml, intramuscular injection is preferable and multiple sites of injection should be used.

How Supplied: CALCIMAR® Solution (Calcitonin-Salmon), Armour is available as a sterile solution in 2 ml vials containing 200 I.U. (MRC) per ml.

STORE IN REFRIGERATOR—Between 2°–8° C (36°–46° F)

[*Shown in Product Identification Section*]

DDAVP® ℞

(desmopressin acetate)

Description: DDAVP (desmopressin acetate) is a synthetic analogue of 8-argininevasopressin. It is chemically defined as follows: Mol. wt. 1183.2. Empirical formula: $C_{48}H_{74}N_{14}O_{17}S_2SCH_2CH_2CO$-Tyr-Phe-Gln-Asn-Cys-Pro-D-Arg-Gly-$NH_2 \cdot C_2H_4O_2 \cdot 3H_2O$ 1-(3-mercaptopropionic acid)-8-D-argininevasopressin monoacetate (salt) trihydrate.

DDAVP (desmopressin acetate) is provided as a sterile, aqueous solution for intranasal use.

Each ml contains:

Desmopressin acetate	0.1 mg
Chlorobutanol	5.0 mg
Sodium Chloride	9.0 mg

Hydrochloric acid to adjust pH to approximately 4

Clinical Pharmacology: DDAVP (desmopressin acetate) contains as active substance 1-(3-mercaptopropionic acid)-8-D-argininevasopressin, which is a synthetic analogue of the natural hormone argininevasopressin. One ml (0.1 mg) of DDAVP (desmopressin acetate) has an antidiuretic activity of about 400 IU as compared with argininevasopressin.

Clinical results obtained thus far indicate that DDAVP (desmopressin acetate) is effective in the management of central diabetes insipidus:
1. The biphasic half-lives for DDAVP (desmopressin acetate) were 7.8 and 75.5 minutes for the fast and slow phases, compared with 2.5 and 14.5 minutes for lysinevasopressin, another form of the hormone used in this condition. As a result, DDAVP (desmopressin acetate) provides a prompt onset of antidiuretic action with a long duration after each administration.
2. The change in structure of arginine vasopressin to DDAVP (desmopressin acetate) has resulted in a decreased vasopressor action and decreased actions on visceral smooth muscle relative to the enhanced antidiuretic activity, so that clinically effective antidiuretic doses are usually below threshold levels for effects on vascular or visceral smooth muscle.

Indications: Antidiuretic replacement therapy in the management of cranial diabetes insipidus and for the temporary polyuria and polydipsia associated with trauma to, or surgery in the pituitary region. DDAVP (desmopressin acetate) is ineffective for the treatment of nephrogenic diabetes insipidus.

Contraindications: Hypersensitivity to DDAVP (desmopressin acetate).

Warnings: 1. For intranasal use only.
2. In very young and elderly patients in particular, fluid intake should be adjusted in order to decrease the potential occurrence of water intoxication and hyponatremia.

Precautions: DDAVP (desmopressin acetate) at high dosage has infrequently produced a slight elevation of blood pressure, which disappeared with a reduction in dosage. The drug should be used with caution in patients with coronary artery insufficiency and/or hypertensive cardiovascular disease.

Use in Pregnancy: Reproduction studies performed in rats and rabbits with doses up to 12.5 times the human intranasal dose have revealed no evidence for a harmful action on the fetus from DDAVP (desmopressin acetate). There are no studies in pregnant women.

Adverse Reactions: Infrequently, high dosages have produced transient headache and nausea. Nasal congestion, rhinitis and flushing have been reported occasionally, as well as mild abdominal cramps and vulval pain. These symptoms disappeared with reduction in dosage.

Overdosage: See adverse reactions above. In case of overdosage, the dosage should be reduced, frequency of administration decreased, or the drug withdrawn according to the severity of the condition.
There is no known specific antidote for DDAVP. If considerable fluid retention is causing concern, a saluretic such as furosemide may induce a diuresis.

Dosage and Administration: This drug is administered into the nose through a soft, flexible plastic nasal tube which has four graduation marks on it that measure 0.2, 0.15, 0.1 and 0.05 ml. DDAVP (desmopressin acetate) dosage must be determined for each individual patient and adjusted according to the diurnal pattern of response. Response should be estimated by two parameters: adequate duration of sleep and adequate, not excessive, water turnover. Patients with nasal congestion and blockage have often responded well to DDAVP (desmopressin acetate). The usual dosage range in adults is 0.1 to 0.4 ml daily, either as a single dose or divided into two or three doses. Most adults require 0.2 ml daily in two divided doses. The morning and evening doses should be separately adjusted for an adequate diurnal rhythm of water turnover. For children aged 3 months to 12 years, the usual dosage range is 0.05 to 0.3 ml daily, either as a single dose or divided into two doses.
About 1/4 to 1/3 of patients can be controlled by a single daily dose.

How Supplied: 2.5 ml per vial, packaged with two applicator tubes per carton. Keep refrigerated at about 4°C.
Issued: January 1978

LEVOTHROID® ℞
(levothyroxine sodium, U.S.P.)

LEVOTHYROXINE TABLETS
for oral use
LEVOTHYROXINE INJECTION
for parenteral use

Description: LEVOTHROID® (Levothyroxine Sodium, U.S.P.) provides crystalline sodium levothyroxine (T_4), a potent thyroid hormone, in eight different strengths to permit easy convenient dosage adjustment.

Clinical Pharmacology: The major thyroid hormones are L-thyroxine (T_4) and L-triiodothyronine (T_3). The amounts of T_4 and T_3 released into the circulation from the normally functioning thyroid gland are regulated by the amount of thyrotropin (TSH) secreted from the anterior pituitary gland. TSH secretion is in turn regulated by the levels of circulating T_4 and T_3 and by secretion of thyrotropin releasing factor (TRH) from the hypothalamus. Recognition of this complex feedback system is important in the diagnosis and treatment of thyroid dysfunction.
The principal effect of exogenous thyroid hormones is to increase the metabolic rate of body tissues.
The thyroid hormones are also concerned with growth and differentiation of tissues. In deficiency states in the young there is retardation of growth and failure of maturation of the skeletal and other body systems, especially in failure of ossification in the epiphyses and in the growth and development of the brain.
The precise mechanism of action by which thyroid hormones affect thermogenesis and cellular growth and differentiation is not known. It is recognized that these physiologic effects are mediated at the cellular level primarily by T_3, a large part of which is derived from T_4 by deiodination in the peripheral tissues. Thyroxine (T_4) is the major component of normal secretions of the thyroid gland and is thus the primary determinant of normal thyroid function. L-thyroxine is readily absorbed from the gastrointestinal tract. In the circulation T_4 is largely bound to plasma proteins and upon release to the tissues it is bound to intracellular proteins. L-thyroxine displays greater binding affinity than L-triiodothyronine, both in the circulation and at the cellular level, which explains its longer duration of action. The half-life of T_4 in normal plasma is 6–7 days while that of T_3 is about 1 day. The plasma half-lives of T_4 and T_3 are decreased in hyperthyroidism and increased in hypothyroidism.

Indications and Usage: LEVOTHROID® (Levothyroxine Sodium, U.S.P.) is indicated as replacement or substitution therapy of diminished or absent thyroid function (e.g., cretinism, myxedema, non-toxic goiter or hypothyroidism generally, including the hypothyroid state in children, in pregnancy and in the elderly) resulting from functional deficiency, primary atrophy, from partial or complete absence of the gland or from the effects of surgery, radiation or anti-thyroid agents. Therapy must be maintained continuously to control the symptoms of hypothyroidism.
It may also be used to suppress the secretion of thyrotropin (TSH) which action may be beneficial in simple nonendemic goiter and in chronic lymphocytic thyroiditis. This may cause a reduction in the goiter size.
Thyroid hormones may also be used with antithyroid drugs to treat thyrotoxicosis. This combination has been used to prevent goitrogenesis and hypothyroidism. This may be particularly useful in the management of thyrotoxicosis during pregnancy.
Symptoms of hypothyroidism including fatigue, weakness, lethargy, cold insensitivity, dry skin, and coarse hair can be expected to subside with replacement therapy. Adequate dose may be determined by clinical symptoms and laboratory evaluation. These tests may include serum thyroxine (T_4), serum triiodothyronine (T_3), free thyroxine index, and thyroid stimulating hormone (TSH) blood level.

Contraindications: LEVOTHROID® administration is contraindicated in thyrotoxicosis and in acute myocardial infarction. LEVOTHROID® is contraindicated in the presence of uncorrected adrenal insufficiency because it increases the tissue demands for adrenocortical hormones and may cause an acute adrenal crisis in such patients. (See Warnings)

Warnings:

> Drugs with thyroid hormone activity, alone or together with other therapeutic agents, have been used for the treatment of obesity. In euthyroid patients, doses within the range of daily hormonal requirements are ineffective for weight reduction. Larger doses may produce serious or even life-threatening manifestations of toxicity, particularly when given in association with sympathomimetic amines such as those used for their anorectic effects.

LEVOTHROID® should be used with caution in patients with cardiovascular disease, including hypertension. The development of chest pain or other aggravation of cardiovascular disease will require a decrease in dosage.
Patients with coronary artery disease should be carefully observed during surgery, since the possibility of precipitating cardiac arrhythmias may be greater in those treated with thyroid hormones.
In patients whose hypothyroidism is secondary to hypopituitarism, adrenal insufficiency will probably also be present. When adrenal insufficiency and hypothyroidism coexist, the adrenal insufficiency should be corrected by corticosteroids before administering thyroid hormones.

Precautions:
General—Patients with hypothyroidism, and especially myxedema, are particularly sensitive to thyroid preparations so that treatment should begin with small doses and increments should be gradual.
Laboratory Tests—The patient's response to thyroid replacement therapy may be followed by laboratory tests such as serum thyroxine (T_4), serum triiodothyronine (T_3), free thyroxine index and thyroid stimulating hormone (TSH) blood levels.
Drug Interactions—In patients with diabetes mellitus, addition of thyroid hormone therapy may cause an increase in the required dosage of insulin or oral hypoglycemic agents. Conversely, decreasing the dose of thyroid hormone may possibly cause hypoglycemic reactions if the dosage of insulin or oral hypoglycemic agents is not adjusted.
Thyroid replacement may potentiate anticoagulant effects with agents such as warfarin or bishydroxycoumarin and reduction of one-third in anticoagulant dosage should be undertaken upon initiation of LEVOTHROID® therapy. Subsequent anticoagulant dosage adjustment should be made on the basis of frequent prothrombin determinations.
Injection of epinephrine in patients with coronary artery disease may precipitate an episode of coronary insufficiency. This may be enhanced in patients receiving thyroid preparations. Careful observation is required if catecholamines are administered to patients in this category.
Pregnancy—Treatment for hypothyroidism should be continued throughout pregnancy and if diagnosed during pregnancy, treatment should be instituted. Serum T_4 levels will be

Continued on next page

Armour—Cont.

lower than normal during pregnancy. The diagnosis should be confirmed by evaluating TSH levels.

Pediatric Use—The diagnosis and institution of therapy for cretinism should be done as soon after birth as feasible to prevent developmental deficiency. Screening tests for serum T_4 and TSH will identify this group of newborn patients.

Adverse Reactions: Patients who are sensitive to lactose may show intolerance to LEVOTHROID® since this substance is used in the manufacture of the product.

Overdosage: Excessive dosage of thyroid medication may result in symptoms of hyperthyroidism. Since, however, the effects do not appear at once, the symptoms may not appear for one to three weeks after the dosage regimen is begun. The most common signs and symptoms of overdosage are weight loss, palpitation, nervousness, diarrhea or abdominal cramps, sweating, tachycardia, cardiac arrhythmias, angina pectoris, tremors, headache, insomnia, intolerance to heat and fever. If symptoms of overdosage appear, discontinue medication for several days and reinstitute treatment at a lower dosage level.

Laboratory tests such as serum T_4, serum T_3 and the free thyroxine index will be elevated during the period of overdosage.

Complications as a result of the induced hypermetabolic state may include cardiac failure and death due to arrhythmia or failure.

Dosage and Administration: The goal of therapy should be the restoration of euthyroidism as judged by clinical response and confirmed by appropriate laboratory values. In adults with no complicating endocrine or cardiovascular disease, the predicted full maintenance dose may be achieved immediately with adjustments made as indicated by clinical evaluation. The usual maintenance dose of LEVOTHROID® is 0.1 mg to 0.2 mg daily.

In patients with known complications or in case of doubt, individual dose titration at 2 to 4 week intervals is recommended. The usual starting dose is 0.05 mg with increases of 0.05 mg at 2 to 4 week intervals until the patient is euthyroid or symptoms ensue which preclude further dose increase.

In adult myxedema or hypothyroid patients with angina, the starting dose should be 0.025 mg with increases at 2 to 4 week intervals of 0.025 to 0.05 mg as determined by clinical response.

In cretinism or severe hypothyroidism in children, the initial dosage should be 0.025 to 0.05 mg with increases of 0.05 to 0.1 mg at 2 week intervals until the child is clinically euthyroid and laboratory values are in the normal range. In growing children, the usual maintenance dose may be as high as 0.3 to 0.4 mg daily. It is essential in children to reach the euthyroid state as rapidly as possible because of the importance of thyroid in growth and maturation.

For treatment of myxedema coma or stupor, LEVOTHROID® (Levothyroxine Sodium, U.S.P.) Injection may be administered intravenously in a dose of 0.2-0.5 mg. The patient response will determine the need for additional parenteral doses. The patient should be placed on oral maintenance therapy as soon as feasible. In the presence of severe heart disease, small incremental doses may be indicated with close patient monitoring.

Tablets should be stored at controlled room temperature—between 15°-30°C (59°-86°F) in capped bottles or unbroken plastic strip packing.

How Supplied: LEVOTHROID® (Levothyroxine Sodium Tablets, U.S.P.) is available in bottles of 100 tablets and larger. The 0.05 mg, 0.1 mg, 0.125 mg, 0.15 mg, 0.175 mg, 0.2 mg, and 0.3 mg potencies are also available in cartons of 100 (10 strips of 10 tablets) packaged in Unit Dose as Armadose®. Each LEVOTHROID® Tablet is distinctively colored and bears identifying markings.

Strength (mg)	Tablets Color	Markings	Approx. Equivalent in Armour Thyroid
0.025	Orange	¼ LK	¼ gr
0.05	White	½ LL	½ gr
0.1	Yellow	1 LM	1 gr
0.125	Purple	1¼ LH	1¼ gr
0.15	Blue	1½ LN	1½ gr
0.175	Turquoise	1¾ LP	1¾ gr
0.2	Pink	2 LR	2 gr
0.3	Green	3 LS	3 gr

LEVOTHROID® (Levothyroxine Sodium, U.S.P.) Injection is supplied in 6 ml vials containing 200 or 500 mcg of drug lyophilized with 15 mg of Mannitol.

Store at room temperature, between 15°-30°C (59°-86°F). Directions for reconstitution: using aseptic technique add 2 ml, 0.9% Sodium Chloride Injection, U.S.P. to the 200 mcg vial and 5 ml, 0.9% Sodium Chloride Injection, U.S.P. to the 500 mcg vial. Note: Do not use Bacteriostatic Sodium Chloride Injection, U.S.P. Shake to dissolve the contents of the vial. Use immediately and discard the unused portion.

[*Shown in Product Identification Section*]

NICOBID® ℞
(niacin, Armour)
Timed Release Nicotinic Acid Supplement Tempules®

Description: Each black-and-clear Tempule (timed-release capsule) contains 125 mg. niacin (nicotinic acid); each green-and-clear Tempule (timed-release capsule) contains 250 mg. niacin (nicotinic acid); and each opaque blue and white Tempule (timed-release capsule) contains 500 mg. niacin (nicotinic acid). Nicobid Tempules® provides the full actions of niacin (nicotinic acid). Portions of the pellets contained in the Tempule are released immediately. The remainder is released over several hours.

Uses: Nicobid (niacin, Armour) is used in all those conditions in which niacin (nicotinic acid) supplementation is indicated. It has the advantage of a slower release of niacin (nicotine acid) than conventional tablet dosage forms. This may permit its use by those who do not tolerate the tablets.

Cautions: Nicobid should not be used by persons with a known sensitivity to niacin (nicotinic acid) and by persons with arterial bleeding, glaucoma, severe diabetes, impaired liver function, peptic ulcer, or by pregnant women.

Side Effects: Temporary flushing and feeling of warmth may be expected. These seldom reach levels so as to necessitate discontinuance. If these symptoms persist, discontinue use and consult a physician. Temporary headache, itching and tingling, gastric disturbances, skin rash and allergies may occur.

Dosage: Usual adult dose—one Tempule, 125 mg., 250 mg. or 500 mg. morning and evening.

KEEP OUT OF THE REACH OF CHILDREN

NICOLAR® ℞
(niacin tablets, Armour)

Description: Nicolar® (niacin tablets, Armour) is a scored yellow colored tablet containing 500 mg. of niacin (nicotinic acid).

Actions: Niacin functions in the body as a component of two hydrogen transporting coenzymes; Coenzyme I (Nicotinamide Adenine Dinucleotide [NAD], sometimes called Diphosphopyridine Nucleotide [DPN]) and Coenzyme II (Nicotinamide Adenine Dinucleotide Phosphate [NADP], sometimes called Triphosphopyridine Nucleotide [TPN]). Niacin in addition to its functions as a vitamin, exerts several distinctive pharmacologic effects which vary according to the dosage level employed.

Niacin, in large doses, causes a reduction in serum lipids. The exact mechanism of this action is unknown.

Indications: Nicolar® is indicated as adjunctive therapy in patients with significant hyperlipidemia (elevated cholesterol and/or triglycerides) who do not respond adequately to diet and weight loss.

Notice: It has not been established whether the drug-induced lowering of serum cholesterol or triglyceride levels has a beneficial effect, no effect, or a detrimental effect on the morbidity or mortality due to atherosclerosis including coronary heart disease. Investigations now in progress may yield an answer to this question.

Contraindications: Niacin is contraindicated in patients with hepatic dysfunction or in patients with active acute peptic ulcer.

Warnings: Use of this drug in pregnancy, lactation or in women of child-bearing age requires that the potential benefits of the drug be weighed against its possible hazards to the mother and child. Although fetal abnormalities have not been reported with this drug, its use as an antilipidemic agent requires high dosages, and animal reproduction or teratology studies have not been done. There are insufficient studies done for usage in children.

Precautions: Patients with gall bladder disease, or those with a past history of jaundice, liver disease or peptic ulcer should be observed closely while taking this medication.

Frequent monitoring of liver function tests and blood glucose should be performed in the initial stage of therapy until it is ascertained that the drug has no adverse effects on these organ systems.

Diabetic or potential diabetic patients should be observed closely in the event of decreased tolerance. Adjustment of diet and/or hypoglycemic therapy may be necessary.

Patients receiving antihypertensive drugs of the adrenal-blocking type may have an additive vasodilating effect and produce postural hypotension.

Elevated uric acid levels have occurred; therefore use with caution in patients predisposed to gout.

This product contains FD&C Yellow No. 5 (tartrazine) which may cause allergic-type reactions (including asthma) in certain susceptible individuals. Although the overall incidence of FD&C Yellow No. 5 (tartrazine) sensitivity in the general population is low, it is frequently seen in patients who also have aspirin hypersensitivity.

Adverse Reactions: Severe generalized flushing
Decreased glucose tolerance
Activation of peptic ulcers
Abnormalities of hepatic functional tests
Jaundice
Gastrointestinal disorders
Dryness of the skin
Keratosis nigricans
Pruritus
Hyperuricemia
Toxic amblyopia
Hypotension
Transient headache

Dosage and Administration: Two to four tablets (1–2 grams) daily with or following meals or as directed by physician.

Since flushing, pruritus and gastrointestinal distress appear frequently, begin therapy with small doses and slowly build up dose in gradual increments observing for adverse effects and efficacy. The usual maximum daily dose is 8 grams.

How Supplied: Nicolar® (niacin tablets, Armour) is available in bottles of 100 scored tablets, each containing 500 mg. of nicotinic acid (identified by the Armacode® NE).

Caution: Federal law prohibits dispensing without prescription.

PENTRITOL®—60 mg. ℞
(pentaerythritol tetranitrate)
timed release tempules® Armour

Description:
Empirical Formula: $C_5H_8N_4O_{12}$
Molecular Weight: 316.15
The pentaerythritol tetranitrate is in a special timed-release base (tempule®) designed to give prolonged systemic effect.
Action: The mechanism of action in the relief of angina pectoris is unknown at this time, although the basic pharmacologic action is to relax smooth muscle.

Indication
Based on a review of this drug by the National Academy of Science—National Research Council and/or other information, FDA has classified the indication as follows:
"Possibly" effective for the relief of angina pectoris (pain of coronary artery disease). It is not intended to abort the acute anginal episode, but is widely regarded as useful in the prophylactic treatment of angina pectoris.
Final classification of the less-than-effective indications requires further investigation.

Contraindications: Idiosyncrasy to this drug.
Warning: Data supporting the use of nitrites during the early days of the acute phase of myocardial infarction (the period during which clinical and laboratory findings are unstable) are insufficient to establish safety.
Precautions: Intraocular pressure is increased; therefore, caution is required in administering to patients with glaucoma. Tolerance to this drug, and cross-tolerance to other nitrites and nitrates may occur.
Adverse Reactions: Cutaneous vasodilation with flushing. Headache is common and may be severe and persistent. Transient episodes of dizziness and weakness, as well as other signs of cerebral ischemia associated with postural hypotension, occasionally may develop. This drug can act as a physiological antagonist to norepinephrine, acetylcholine, histamine, and many other agents. An occasional individual exhibits marked sensitivity to the hypotensive effects of nitrite and severe responses (nausea, vomiting, weakness, restlessness, pallor, perspiration, and collapse) can occur, even with the usual therapeutic dose. Alcohol may enhance this effect. Drug rash and/or exfoliative dermatitis may occasionally occur.
Dosage and Administration: One 60 mg. oral tempule® every 12 hours on an empty stomach. (Not recommended for sublingual use).
Although the onset of effect and the duration of effect of this drug are quite variable, the following are the generally reported ranges for these values:
Onset of effect: estimated to be 30 minutes.
Duration of effect: considered to be up to 12 hours.
How Supplied: Pentritol® 60 mg. tempules® identified by Armacode® PE are available in bottles of 60 and 250. Pentritol® 30 mg. identified by Armacode® PC in bottles of 100 and 250 tempules®.

ARMOUR THYROID (Tablets) ℞

Description: Armour® Thyroid (Thyroid, U.S.P.) Tablets for oral use are prepared by a special process from fresh, dessicated animal thyroid glands. Thus, the active thyroid hormones, L-thyroxine (T_4) and L-triiodothyronine T_3) are available in their natural state and ratio attached to a carrier protein and are available for full therapeutic availability.
Armour® Thyroid is standardized both by the official U.S.P. method for iodine content and biologically assayed to assure full metabolic potency.
Clinical Pharmacology: The amounts of thyroxine (T_4) and triiodothyronine (T_3) released into the circulation from the normally functioning thyroid gland are regulated by the amount of thyrotropin (TSH) secreted from the anterior pituitary gland. TSH secretion is in turn regulated by the levels of circulating T_4 and T_3 and by secretion of thyrotropin releasing factor (TRH) from the hypothalamus. Recognition of this complex feedback system is important in the diagnosis and treatment of thyroid dysfunction.
The principal effect of exogenous thyroid hormones is to increase the metabolic rate of body tissues. This effect develops slowly but is prolonged. It begins within 48 hours and reaches a maximum in 8 to 10 days although full effects of continued administration may not be evident for several weeks.
The thyroid hormones are also concerned with growth and differentiation of tissues. In deficiency states in the young there is retardation of growth and failure of maturation of the skeletal and other body systems, especially in failure of ossification in the epiphyses and in the growth and development of the brain.
The precise mechanism of action by which thyroid hormones affect thermogenesis and cellular growth and differentiation is not known. It is recognized that these physiologic effects are mediated at the cellular level primarily by T_3, a large part of which is derived from T_4 by deiodination in the peripheral tissues. Since T_4 is the major component of thyroid tablets and of normal secretions of the thyroid gland it is the primary determinant of the overall effect of thyroid hormone therapy.
Both T_4 and T_3 are released from Thyroid protein (thyroglubulin) by digestion in the gastrointestinal tract and are readily absorbed. In the circulation they are largely bound to plasma proteins and upon release to the tissues they are bound to intracellular proteins. L-thyroxine displays greater binding affinity than L-triiodothyronine, both in the circulation and at the cellular level, which explains its longer duration of action. The half-life of T_4 in normal plasma is 6-7 days while that of T_3 is about 1 day. The plasma half-lives of T_4 and T_3 are decreased in hyperthyroidism and increased in hypothyroidism.
Indications and Usage: Armour® Thyroid is indicated as replacement or substitution therapy of diminished or absent thyroid function (e.g., cretinism, myxedema, non-toxic goiter or hypothyroidism generally, including the hypothyroid state in children, in pregnancy and in the elderly) resulting from functional deficiency, primary atrophy, from partial or complete absence of the gland or from the effects of surgery, radiation or antithyroid agents. Therapy must be maintained continuously to control the symptoms of hypothyroidism.
It may also be used to suppress the secretion of thyrotropin (TSH) which action may be beneficial in simple nonendemic goiter and in chronic lymphocytic thyroiditis. This may cause a reduction in the goiter size.
Thyroid hormones may also be used with antithyroid drugs to treat thyrotoxicosis. This combination has been used to prevent goitrogenesis and hypothyroidism. This may be particularly useful in the management of thyrotoxicosis during pregnancy.
Symptoms of hypothyroidism including fatique, weakness, lethargy, cold insensitivity, dry skin, and coarse hair can be expected to subside with replacement therapy. Adequate dose may be determined by clinical symptoms and laboratory evaluation. These tests may include serum thyroxine (T_4), serum triiodothyronine (T_3), free thyroxine index, and thyroid stimulating hormone (TSH) blood level.
Contraindications: Armour® Thyroid is contraindicated in the presence of thyrotoxicosis and in acute myocardial infarction uncomplicated by hypothyroidism. However, when hypothyroidism is a complicating or causative factor in myocardial infarction, or heart disease, the judicious use of small doses of Armour® Thyroid should be considered. Where hypothyroidism and hypoadrenalism (Addison's Disease) co-exist, Armour® Thyroid is contraindicated unless treatment of hypoadrenalism with adrenocortical steroids precedes the initiation of Armour® Thyroid therapy. (See Warnings.)

Warnings:

Drugs with thyroid hormone activity, alone or together with other therapeutic agents, have been used for the treatment of obesity. In euthyroid patients, doses within the range of daily hormonal requirements are ineffective for weight reduction. Larger doses may produce serious or even life-threatening manifestations of toxicity, particularly when given in association with sympathomimetic amines such as those used for their anorectic effects.

Armour® Thyroid should be used with caution in patients with cardiovascular disease, including hypertension. The development of chest pain or other aggravation of cardiovascular disease will require a decrease in dosage.
Patients with coronary artery disease should be carefully observed during surgery since the possibility of precipitating cardiac arrhythmias may be greater in thos treated with thyroid hormones.
In patients whose hypothyroidism is secondary to hypopituitarism, adrenal insufficiency will probably also be present. When adrenal insufficiency and hypothyroidism co-exist, the adrenal insufficiency should be corrected by corticosteroids before administering thyroid hormones.
Precautions:
General—Patients with hypothyroidism, and especially myxedema, are particularly sensitive to thyroid preparations so that treatment should begin with small doses and increments should be gradual.
Laboratory Tests—The patient's response to thyroid replacement therapy may be followed by laboratory tests such as serum thyroxine (T_4) serum triiodothyronine (T_3), free thyroxine index and thyroid stimulating hormone (TSH) blood levels.
Drug Interactions—In patients with diabetes mellitus, addition of thyroid hormone therapy may cause an increase in the required dosage of insulin or oral hypoglycemic agents. Conversely, decreasing the dose of thyroid hormone may possibly cause hypoglycemic reactions if the dosage of insulin or oral hypoglycemic agents is not adjusted.
Injection of epinephrine in patients with coronary artery disease may precipitate an episode of coronary insufficiency. This may be enhanced in patients receiving thyroid preparations. Careful observation is required if catecholamines are administered to patients in this category.
Thyroid replacement may potentiate anticoagulant effects with agents such as warfarin or bishydroxycoumarin and reduction of one-third in anticoagulant dosage should be undertaken upon initiation of thyroid therapy. Subsequent anticoagulant dosage adjustment should be made on the basis of frequent prothrombin determinations.
Pregnancy—Treatment for hypothyroidism should be continued throughout pregnancy and if diagnosed during pregnancy, treatment should be instituted. Serum T_4 levels will be lower than normal during pregnancy. The diagnosis should be confirmed by evaluating TSH levels.
Pediatric Use—The diagnosis and institution of therapy for cretinism should be done as soon

Continued on next page

Armour—Cont.

after birth as feasible to prevent developmental deficiency. Screening tests for serum $_4$ and TSH will identify this group of newborn patients.

Adverse Reactions: Gastric intolerance may rarely be seen in those patients highly sensitive to pork products or corn.

Overdosage: Effects of overdosage include palpitation, tachycardia, cardiac arrhythmias, weight loss, angina pectoris, tremors, headache, diarrhea, nervousness, insomnia, sweating, and intolerance to heat and fever. If symptoms of excessive dosage appear, discontinue medication for several days and reinstitute treatment at a lower dosage level.

Laboratory tests such as serum $_4$, serum $_3$ and he free thyroxine index will be elevated during the period of overdosage.

Complications as a result of the induced hypermetabolic state may include cardiac failure and death due to arrhythmia or failure.

Dosage and Administration: As with any type of thyroid administration the dosage of Armour® Thyroid must be individualized to approximate the deficit in the patient's thyroid secretion. The response of the patient is determined by clinical judgment in conjunction with laboratory findings. Generally, thyroid therapy is instituted at relatively low dosage levels and increased in small increments at intervals until the desired response is obtained. Armour® Thyroid is given as a single, daily dose, preferably before breakfast.

Adult Myxedema. In adult myxedema, give 15 mg (¼ gr) of Armour® Thyroid a day. Usually after two weeks the dosage is increased to one 30 mg (½ gr) tablet a day and two weeks later increased to one 60 mg (1 gr) tablet daily. It is suggested that the patient be carefully assessed after one month of treatment with the 60 mg (1 gr) dose and again after an additional month's treatment.

If necessary, daily dosage may then be increased to 120 mg (2 gr) per day for two months and the examination repeated. If the values of the laboratory test used are low or if the clinical response is inadequate, dosage may be increased to 180 mg (3 gr). Further increases, when necessary, may be made in increments of 30 mg (½ gr) or 60 mg (1 gr) a day. The usual maintenance dose is from 60 mg (1 gr) to 180 mg (3 gr) per day, but it may vary, in individual patients.

Adult hypothyroidism without myxedema. The initial dose is usually one 60 mg (1 gr) Armour® Thyroid tablet per day, increasing by 60 mg (1 gr) every 30 days until the desired result is obtained. Clinical examination at monthly intervals and serum T_4, serum T_3, and/or TSH levels will assist in establishing the maintenance dose.

Children's Dosage. In cretinism or severe hypothyroidism in children the dosage regimen is as for adults with myxedema, with, however, each dosage increment made at intervals of two weeks. The final maintenance dose may be greater in the growing child that in the adult. The sleeping pulse and the basal morning temperature are simple, useful guides to treatment.

Tablets should be stored at normal room temperature in capped bottles or unbroken plastic strip packing.

How Supplied: Armour® Thyroid Tablets, U.S.P.: Bottles of 100, 1000 and larger, available in potencies of 30 mg (½ gr), 60 mg (1 gr), and 120 mg (2 gr) tablets; Bottles of 100 and 1000 of 15 mg (¼ gr) and 180 mg (3 gr) tablets; and Bottles of 100 of 90 mg (1½ gr), 240 mg (4 gr), and 300 mg (5 gr) tablets.

The 15 mg (¼ gr), 30 mg (½ gr), 60 mg (1 gr), 90 mg (1½ gr), 120 mg (2 gr), 180 mg (3 gr), 240 mg (4 gr), and 300 mg (5 gr) potencies are available in special dispensing bottles of 100 tablets designated as Handy 100's® (child-resistant closure with tear-off label). The 30 mg (½ gr), 60 mg (1 gr), and 120 mg (2 gr) potencies ae also available in cartons of 100 tablets (10 strips of 10 tablets) packaged in Unit Dose as Armadose.®

[*Shown in Product Identification Section*]

THYROLAR® ℞

(liotrix, Armour)

Description: Thyrolar® tablets provide a combination of the synthetic active thyroid hormones, sodium levothyroxine and sodium liothyronine in a ratio of 4:1 by weight. Thyrolar® is available in five potencies approximately equivalent in therapeutic effect to ¼ gr., ½ gr., 1 gr., 2 gr. and 3 gr. of desiccated thyroid. In Thyrolar® 1 tablets a combination of 50 mcg. of sodium levothyroxine and 12.5 mcg. of sodium liothyronine represent the approximate activity of 1 gr. of desiccated thyroid. The other available potencies are proportional in strength.

Action: Thyrolar® is an effective agent for correcting the hypothyroid state and inducing clinical euthyroidism. The ratio of active hormones present closely simulates the clinical biochemical effects of desiccated thyroid and of the natural endogenous thyroid secretion. Thus, the various thyroid function parameters respond to Thyrolar® as they do to the administration of desiccated thyroid.

The principal effect of thyroid hormones is to increase the metabolic rate of body tissues. Sodium liothyronine is more readily absorbed from the gastrointestinal tract than is sodium levothyroxine. Excretion is rapid so that the action is dissipated more readily than is that of levothyroxine (T_4).

The effects of sodium levothyroxine develop slowly but are more prolonged.

With Thyrolar® the most widely used parameters of thyroid function may be used to aid in the assessment of the response since, when the euthyroid state is achieved, the values may ordinarily be expected to fall within the normal range. This is not true with sodium liothyronine administration alone where subnormal values are present or with sodium levothyroxine alone where abnormally high values are associated with clinical euthyroidism.

Indications: Thyrolar® is indicated in the treatment of hypothyroidism as a source of exogenous thyroid hormone in diminished or absent thyroid function. This may be due to the use of antithyroid agents, radiation therapy, primary atrophy, partial or complete surgical removal of the gland or it may be functional in nature.

Thyrolar® is efficacious in the treatment of hypothyroidism regardless of the etiology. The use of Thyrolar® for suppression therapy in simple (non-toxic) goiter gives prompt results in reducing the size of the gland.

Contraindications: Thyrolar® administration is contraindicated in thyrotoxicosis and in acute myocardial infarction.

Thyrolar® is contraindicated in the presence of uncorrected adrenal insufficiency because it increases the tissue demands for adrenocortical hormones and may cause an acute adrenal crisis in such patients (See Warnings).

Warnings:

> Drugs with thyroid hormone activity, alone or together with other therapeutic agents, have been used for the treatment of obesity. In euthyroid patients, doses within the range of daily hormonal requirements are ineffective for weight reduction. Larger doses may produce serious or even life-threatening manifestations of toxicity, particularly when given in association with sympathomimetic amines such as those used for their anorectic effects.

Thyrolar® should be used with caution in patients with cardiovascular disease, including hypertension. The development of chest pain or other aggravation of cardiovascular disease will require a decrease in dosage.

Injection of epinephrine in patients with coronary artery disease may precipitate an episode of coronary insufficiency. This may be enhanced in patients receiving thyroid preparations. Careful observation is required if catecholamines are administered to patients in this category. Thyrolar® treated patients with concomitant coronary artery disease should be carefully observed during surgery since the possibility of precipitating cardiac arrhythmias may be greater in patients treated with thyroid hormones.

The institution of thyroid replacement therapy may potentiate anticoagulant effects with agents such as warfarin or bishydroxycoumarin and reduction of one-third in anticoagulant dosage should be undertaken upon initiation of Thyrolar® therapy. Subsequent anticoagulant dosage adjustment should be made on the basis of frequent prothrombin determinations.

In patients whose hypothyroidism is secondary to hypopituitarism, adrenal insufficiency will probably also be present. When the adrenal insufficiency and hypothyroidism coexist, the adrenal insufficiency should be corrected by corticosteroids before administering thyroid hormones.

Precautions: Patients with hypothyroidism and especially myxedema are particularly sensitive to thyroid preparations so that treatment should begin with small doses and increments should be gradual. In patients with diabetes mellitus addition of thyroid hormone therapy may cause an increase in the required dosage of insulin or oral hypoglycemic agents. Conversely, decreasing the dose of thyroid hormone may possibly cause hypoglycemic reactions if the dosage of insulin or oral agents is not adjusted.

Adverse Reactions: Excessive dosage of thyroid medication may result in symptoms of hyperthyroidism. Since, however, the effects do not appear at once, the symptoms may not appear for 1 to 3 weeks after the dosage regimen is begun. The most common signs and symptoms of overdosage are weight loss, palpitation, nervousness, diarrhea or abdominal cramps, sweating, tachycardia, cardiac arrhythmias, angina pectoris, tremors, headache, insomnia, intolerance to heat, fever. If symptoms of overdosage appear, discontinue medication for several days and reinstitute treatment at a lower dosage level.

In some individuals who are euthyroid on Thyrolar® headache may appear. Dosage should be decreased. If headache persists or the patient develops signs of hypothyroidism on the lower dosage, another thyroid preparation should be substituted.

Dosage and Administration: As with all thyroid preparations, the dosage of Thyrolar® must be individualized to approximate the deficit in the patient's thyroid secretion. The response of the patient is determined by clinical judgment in conjunction with laboratory findings.

For newly diagnosed or untreated hypothyroidism, therapy may be initiated with one tablet of Thyrolar® ¼ or Thyrolar® ½ daily depending on the patient's status and increased gradually every one or two weeks. In children, increments in dosage should be made every two weeks. For unstabilized hypothyroid patients receiving some form of thyroid therapy direct substitution of Thyrolar® for the current dose of the other product can be made, with gradual increase in dose every one to two weeks.

In patients previously rendered euthyroid with desiccated thyroid, sodium levothyroxine or sodium liothyronine, each Thyrolar®-1 tablet will usually replace 1 grain of desiccated thyroid, 0.1 mg. sodium levothyroxine or 25 mcg.

sodium liothyronine. Dosage adjustments, other than those routinely necessary with any thyroid therapy, are seldom necessary.
Thyrolar® is usually given as a single daily dose preferably before breakfast in the morning.
In the normal euthyroid individual, PBI values range from 4 to 8 micrograms/100 ml. and with Thyrolar® values in this range usually correspond to the clinical euthyroid state. Other useful tests include the T_3-resin uptake tests, T_4 by Column and Free thyroxine. In patients rendered euthyroid with Thyrolar®, these tests usually give values within the normal range.
Tablets should be stored at controlled room temperature—between 15°-30°C (59°-86°F) in a light-resistant container.
How Supplied: Thyrolar® is available in five potencies, coded as follows:
[See table above].
Supplied in bottles of 100, two-layered compressed tablets. Thyrolar®-½, Thyrolar®-1, Thyrolar®-2, and Thyrolar®-3 are also supplied in bottles of 1000.

[*Shown in Product Identification Section*]

Name	Composition (T_4/T_3 per Tablet)	Color	Armacode®	Desiccated Thyroid—Approximate Equivalence
Thyrolar®—¼	12.5 mcg./3.1 mcg.	Violet/White	YC	¼ gr.
Thyrolar®—½	25 mcg./6.25 mcg.	Peach/White	YD	½ gr.
Thyrolar®—1	50 mcg./12.5 mcg.	Pink/White	YE	1 gr.
Thyrolar®—2	100 mcg./25 mcg.	Green/White	YF	2 gr.
Thyrolar®—3	150 mcg./37.5 mcg.	Yellow/White	YH	3 gr.

THYTROPAR® ℞

(thyrotropin for injection)
U.S. PAT. No. 2,871,159

Description:
THYTROPAR® (Thyrotropin for Injection) is a highly purified and lyophilized thyrotropic or thyroid stimulating hormone (TSH) isolated from bovine anterior pituitary. The potency of THYTROPAR® is designated in terms of International Thyrotropin units and is free of significant amounts of adrenocorticotropic, gonadotropic, somatotropic and posterior pituitary hormones. It is soluble throughout a wide pH range and is stable at room temperature when kept in the dry state. It dissolves readily in physiologic saline and will retain its potency when in solution for at least two weeks if refrigerated.
Thytropar® Diluent (Sodium Chloride Injection) contains in each ml 9 mg. of Sodium Chloride, Water for Injection, q.s.
Action:
The action of the thyrotropic hormone may be briefly described as fourfold, the degree of action depending upon the amount of the hormone acting upon the thyroid:
1. Increases iodine uptake by the thyroid.
2. Increases formation of thyroid hormone.
3. Increases secretion or release of thyroid hormone.
4. Causes a hyperplasia of thyroid cells.

When given exogenously as THYTROPAR® the fourth effect is not significant clinically in doses recommended except as it results in the other three desirable effects. The process is rapidly reversible following a given dose or series of doses.
THYTROPAR® offers a safe and useful tool for both diagnosis and treatment of certain types of thyroid disease. The increase in the thyroid gland's uptake of tracer doses of radioactive iodine and of the serum protein-bound iodine following a single injection of THYTROPAR® has enabled its use in diagnostic tests which are sufficiently simple to be practical for routine clinical application. Through its use the ability of the human thyroid gland to respond to stimulation can now be determined, and this property has certain unique diagnostic advantages. Furthermore, THYTROPAR® has been helpful in the treatment of certain disorders of the thyroid gland.
Indications:
A. Diagnostic applications of Thytropar (Thyrotropin for Injection)
   1. To determine subclinical hypothyroidism or low thyroid reserve.
   2. To differentiate between primary and secondary hypothyroidism.
   3. To differentiate between primary hypothyroidism and euthyroidism in patients whose thyroid function has been suppressed by the administration of thyroid replacement therapy.
   4. To aid in detection of remnants and metastases of thyroid carcinoma.

B. Therapeutic application of Thytropar (Thyrotropin for Injection)
   1. As an adjunct in the management of certain types of functioning thyroid carcinoma and resulting metastases.

Contraindications:
1. Hypersensitivity to thyrotropin.
2. Coronary thrombosis.
3. Untreated Addison's disease.

Precautions:
1. Use THYTROPAR® with caution in the presence of angina pectoris or cardiac failure.
2. Use with care in the presence of hypopituitarism since varying degrees of adrenal cortical atrophy are generally present with this condition. Adrenal cortical suppression as may be seen with corticosteroid therapy should not be overlooked.

Adverse Reactions:
Menstrual irregularities, nausea, vomiting, urticaria, transitory hypotension, tachycardia, auricular fibrillation, fever, headache, thyroid swelling, post injection flare, and anaphylactic reactions have been reported. The hypotension appears to be part of an allergic type reaction whereas the thyroid swelling is related to larger doses (10–20 units) which some workers have employed. The swelling is self-limited when the hormone is discontinued.
Dosage and Administration:
Thytropar (Thyrotropin for Injection) is administered intramuscularly or subcutaneously after dissolving the material in sterile physiologic saline solution. Ten International Units of Thytropar per 2 ml. of diluent is a satisfactory ratio of dilution for injection.
1. Use of Thytropar in PBI or I^{131} uptake determinations in the differential diagnosis of subclinical hypothyroidism or low thyroid reserve: 10 International Units.
2. To determine thyroid status in a patient receiving thyroid medication: 10 International Units for 1–3 days.*
3. In the differential diagnosis of primary and secondary hypothyroidism: 10 International Units for 1–3 days.*
4. Diagnosis of thyroid cancer remnant with I^{131} after surgery: 10 International Units for 3–7 days.
5. Therapy of thyroid carcinoma (local tumor or metastases) with I^{131}: 10 International Units for 3–8 days.

Overdosage:
SYMPTOMS—Headache, irritability, nervousness, sweating, tachycardia, increased bowel motility, menstrual irregularities. Angina pectoris or congestive heart failure may be induced or aggravated. Shock may also develop. Excessive doses may result in symptoms resembling thyroid storm. Chronic excessive dosage will produce the signs and symptoms of hyperthyroidism.
TREATMENT—in shock, supportive measures and treatment of unrecognized adrenal insufficiency should be considered. Thyrotropin is discontinued.
How Supplied:
THYTROPAR® is supplied as a sterile lyophilized powder containing 10 International Units of Thyrotropic activity according to the chick thyroid iodine depletion assay method of Piotrowski (Walaszek) Steelman and Koch (Endocrinology 52: 489, 1953) when compared to the International Reference Standard. Each package contains one vial of THYTROPAR® (Thyrotropin for injection) and one vial of Thytropar® Diluent (Sodium Chloride Injection).

*The 3-day schedule may be indicated in those who have received thyroid medication for prolonged periods or in those with long-standing pituitary myxedema.

TUSSAR® DM

Cough Syrup
Non-narcotic, Alcohol Free
Antitussive/Decongestant/Antihistaminic

Each 5 ml (one teaspoonful) contains:
Dextromethorphan
  Hydrobromide, U.S.P. ....15 mg
Chlorpheniramine Maleate, U.S.P. ....2 mg
Phenylephrine Hydrochloride, U.S.P. ....5 mg
Methylparaben, N.F. 0.1%
Indications: For relief of cough due to common cold and minor throat and bronchial irritations. TUSSAR DM provides relief of nasal congestion, running nose and watery eyes as may occur in allergic rhinitis (such as hay fever).
Directions For Use: ADULTS—One or two teaspoonfuls (5 or 10 ml) every six to eight hours, not to exceed eight teaspoonfuls in any 24-hour period.
CHILDREN 6–12 YEARS—One teaspoonful (5 ml) every six to eight hours, not to exceed four teaspoonfuls in any 24-hour period.
CHILDREN UNDER 6 YEARS—Not to be administered unless directed by a physician.
Warnings: Do not take this product for persistent cough which may indicate a serious condition except under the supervision of a physician. Do not take this product if you have high blood pressure, heart disease or thyroid disease unless directed by a physician. Do not exceed recommended dosage.
Cautions: If symptoms persist for more than 7 days or are accompanied by a high fever, rash or persistent headache, consult a physician. If drowsiness occurs, do not drive a car or operate machinery.

TUSSAR®-2 Ⓒ

(exempt narcotic cough syrup)

Each 5 ml (one teaspoonful) contains:
Codeine Phosphate, U.S.P. ....10 mg
(Warning—may be habit-forming)
Carbetapentane Citrate ....7.5 mg
Chlorpheniramine Maleate, U.S.P. ....2.0 mg
Guaifenesin, U.S.P. ....50 mg
Sodium Citrate, U.S.P. ....130 mg
Citric Acid, U.S.P. ....20 mg

Continued on next page

Armour—Cont.

Methylparaben, N.F. 0.1%
Alcohol 5%

Indications: For relief of severe coughs due to respiratory conditions caused by common cold, bronchitis, and influenza.
Dosage: One teaspoonful 3 to 4 times a day as needed for cough, but no more than 8 teaspoonfuls in any 24-hour period.
Cautions: Persistent cough may indicate the presence of a serious condition. Secure medical advice if there is a high fever or if relief does not occur within 3 days. Persons with a high fever or persistent cough should use only on advice of a physician. Not to be administered to infants or children unless directed by a physician. If drowsiness occurs, do not drive a car or operate machinery.

TUSSAR SF (Sugar Free) ©
(exempt narcotic cough syrup)

Formulation identical to Tussar-2, except Tussar SF contains saccharine-sorbitol base for patients who must limit sugar intake. Alcohol content 12 percent instead of 5 percent.

PLASMA DERIVATIVE PRODUCTS

ALBUMINAR®-5 ℞
Normal Serum Albumin
(Human) U.S.P. 5%

ALBUMINAR®-5 Normal Serum Albumin (Human) is supplied as a 5% solution in:
- 50 ml. bottles containing 2.5 grams of albumin
- 250 ml. bottles containing 12.5 grams of albumin
- 500 ml. bottles containing 25.0 grams of albumin
- 1000 ml. bottles containing 50 grams of albumin

For use with intravenous administration set. See directions on set supplied.

ALBUMINAR®-25 ℞
Normal Serum Albumin
(Human) U.S.P. 25%

ALBUMINAR®-25 Normal Serum Albumin (Human), is supplied as a 25% solution in:
- 20 ml. vials containing 5.0 grams of albumin
- 50 ml. vials containing 12.5 grams of albumin
- 100 ml. vials containing 25.0 grams of albumin

For use with intravenous administration set. See directions on set supplied.

FACTORATE® ℞
Antihemophilic Factor
(Human) U.S.P.
Dried

FACTORATE® Antihemophilic Factor (Human)—Dried is supplied in single dose vials (AHF activity is stated on label of each vial) with sterile diluent and needles for reconstitution and withdrawal.

FACTORATE® GENERATION II™ ℞
Antihemophilic Factor (Human) U.S.P. Dried

FACTORATE® GENERATION II™ Antihemophilic Factor (Human) U.S.P. Dried is supplied in single dose vials (AHF) activity is stated on label of each vial) with sterile diluent and needles for reconstitution and withdrawal.

GAMMAR® ℞
Immune Serum Globulin
(Human) U.S.P.

GAMMAR® Immune Serum Globulin (Human) U.S.P. is supplied in 2 ml. and 10 ml. vials.

GAMULIN® Rh ℞
Rh_o (D) Immune Globulin (Human)

A sterile Immune Globulin Solution containing Rh_o (D) antibodies. Supplied with Gamulin Rh, crossmatch solution, laboratory card, and patient ID card.

MINI-GAMULIN™ Rh ℞
Rh_o (D) Immune Globulin (Human)

A sterile Immune Globulin Solution containing Rh_o (D) antibodies. Mini-Gamulin Rh contains one-sixth the quantity of Rh_o (D) antibody contained in a standard dose of Rh_o Immune Globulin (Human).

B.F. Ascher & Company, Inc.
15501 WEST 109TH STREET
LENEXA, KS 66219

ANASPAZ® Tablets ℞
(l-hyoscyamine sulfate)

Description: Each ANASPAZ tablet contains l-hyoscyamine sulfate 0.125 mg. ANASPAZ tablets are compressed, light yellow and scored with the Ascher logo on one side and 225/295 on the other.
Clinical Pharmacology: ANASPAZ is chemically pure l-hyoscyamine sulfate, one of the principal anticholinergic/antispasmodic components of belladonna alkaloids. ANASPAZ inhibits specifically the actions of acetylcholine on structures innervated by postganglionic cholinergic nerves and on smooth muscles that respond to acetylcholine but lack cholinergic innervation. These peripheral cholinergic receptors are present in the autonomic effector cells of smooth muscle, cardiac muscle, the sino-atrial node, the atrioventricular node and exocrine glands. It is completely devoid of any action in the autonomic ganglia. ANASPAZ inhibits gastrointestinal propulsive motility and decreases gastric acid secretion. ANASPAZ also controls excessive pharyngeal, tracheal and bronchial secretions. ANASPAZ is absorbed totally and completely by sublingual administration as well as oral administration. Once absorbed, ANASPAZ disappears rapidly from the blood and is distributed throughout the entire body. The half-life of ANASPAZ is 3.5 hours and the majority of drug is excreted in the urine unchanged within the first 12 hours. Only traces of this drug are found in breast milk.
Indications and Usage: ANASPAZ is effective as adjunctive therapy in the treatment of peptic ulcer and irritable bowel syndrome (irritable colon, spastic colon, mucous colitis), acute entercolitis and other functional gastrointestinal disorders. It can also be used to control gastric secretion, visceral spasm and hypermotility in cystitis, pylorospasm and associated abdominal cramps. May be used in functional intestinal disorders to reduce symptoms such as those seen in mild dysenteries and diverticulitis. ANASPAZ is indicated (along with appropriate analgesics) in symptomatic relief of biliary and renal colic and as a drying agent in the relief of symptoms of acute rhinitis.
Contraindications: Glaucoma, obstructive uropathy (for example, bladder neck obstruction due to prostatic hypertrophy); obstructive disease of the gastrointestinal tract (as in achalasia, pyloroduodenal stenosis); paralytic ileus; intestinal atony of elderly or debilitated patients; unstable cardiovascular status; severe ulcerative colitis; toxic megacolon; myasthenia gravis; myocardial ischemia.
Warnings: In the presence of high environmental temperature, heat prostration can occur with drug use (fever and heat stroke due to decreased sweating). Diarrhea may be an early symptom of incomplete intestinal obstruction, especially in patients with ileostomy or colostomy. In this instance, treatment with this drug would be inappropriate and possibly harmful. Like other anticholinergic agents, ANASPAZ may produce drowsiness or blurred vision. In this event, the patient should be warned not to engage in activities requiring mental alertness such as operating a motor vehicle or other machinery or to perform hazardous work while taking this drug.
Precautions: Use with caution and only when clearly indicated in patients with autonomic neuropathy, hyperthyroidism, coronary heart disease, congestive heart failure and cardiac arrhythmias. Investigate any tachycardia before giving any anticholinergic drugs since they may increase the heart rate. Use with caution in patients with hiatal hernia associated with reflux esophagitis.
Adverse Reactions: Adverse reactions may include dryness of the mouth, urinary hesitancy, urinary retention, blurred vision, mydriasis, cycloplegia, tachycardia, palpitations, increased intraocular pressure, headache, nervousness, drowsiness, weakness, and decreased sweating. Allergic reactions or drug idiosyncrasies such as urticaria and other dermal manifestations may also occur.
Overdosage: The signs and symptoms of overdosage include dry mouth, blurred vision, tachycardia, arrhythmias, dry skin, fever, difficulty in swallowing, excitation, lethargy, stupor, coma, respiratory depression, and paralysis (with large overdoses). General measures such as emesis or gastric lavage and administration of activated charcoal should be undertaken immediately. Supportive therapy is given as needed, including artificial respiration if required. Physostigmine may be given by intravenous injection to reverse severe anticholinergic symptoms.
Dosage and Administration: One or two tablets three or four times a day, according to condition and severity of symptoms. ANASPAZ may be taken orally or sublingually. The dosage of ANASPAZ should be adjusted to the needs of the individual patient to assure symptomatic control with a minimum of adverse effects.
How Supplied: ANASPAZ is available as a compressed, yellow, scored tablet, imprinted with the Ascher logo and 225/295 in bottles of 100 tablets (NDC 0225-0295-15) and 500 tablets (NDC 0225-0295-20).
Also available:
ANASPAZ® PB tablets ℞
l-hyoscyamine sulfate 0.125 mg
Phenobarbital 15.0 mg.
(WARNING: May be habit forming)
Caution: Federal law prohibits dispensing without prescription.
Manufactured for B.F. Ascher & Co., Inc.

AYR® SALINE NASAL DROPS

(See PDR For Nonprescription Drugs)

AYR® SALINE NASAL MIST

(See PDR For Nonprescription Drugs)

DALCA® Tablets

(See PDR For Nonprescription Drugs)

ETHAQUIN® Tablets ℞
(Ethaverine Hydrochloride)

Description: Each compressed ETHAQUIN Tablet contains Ethaverine Hydrochloride 100 mg.
Clinical Pharmacology: ETHAQUIN (Ethaverine Hydrochloride) acts directly on the smooth muscle cells, without involving the autonomic nervous system or its receptors. It produces smooth muscle relaxation, particularly where spasm exists, affecting the larger blood vessels, especially systemic, peripheral

and pulmonary vessels, smooth muscle of the intestines, biliary tree, and ureters.

Indications and Usage: In peripheral vascular insufficiency associated with arterial spasm; also useful as a smooth muscle spasmolytic in spastic conditions of the gastrointestinal and genitourinary tracts.

Contraindications: The use of ETHAQUIN (Ethaverine Hydrochloride) is contraindicated in the presence of complete atrioventricular dissociation.

Precautions: As with all vasodilators, ETHAQUIN (Ethaverine Hydrochloride) should be administered with caution to patients with glaucoma.

The safety of Ethaverine Hydrochloride during pregnancy or lactation has not been established; therefore it should not be used in pregnant women or in women of childbearing age unless, in the judgment of the physician, its use is deemed essential to the welfare of the patient.

Adverse Reactions: Even though the incidence of side effects as reported in the literature is very low, it is possible for a patient to evidence nausea, anorexia, abdominal distress, dryness of the throat, hypotension, malaise, lassitude, drowsiness, flushing, sweating, vertigo, respiratory depression, cardiac depression, cardiac arrhythmia and headache. If these side effects occur, reduce dosage or discontinue medication.

Dosage and Administration: In mild or moderate disease, the usual dose for adults is one tablet three times a day: morning, mid-afternoon, evening. In more difficult cases, dosage may be increased to two tablets three times a day. It is most effective given early in the course of the vascular disorder. Because of the chronic nature of the disease, long-term therapy is required.

How Supplied: ETHAQUIN (Ethaverine Hydrochloride) Tablets in bottles of 100, 500, 1000, 2500 and 5000.

Caution: Federal law prohibits dispensing without prescription.

Keep out of reach of children.

Manufactured for B.F. Ascher & Co., Inc.

MOBIGESIC® Tablets

(See PDR For Nonprescription Drugs)

MOBISYL® Creme

(See PDR For Nonprescription Drugs)

SOFT 'N SOOTHE® Creme

(See PDR For Nonprescription Drugs)

UNILAX® Tablets

(See PDR For Nonprescription Drugs)

Astra Pharmaceutical Products, Inc.

7 NEPONSET ST.
WORCESTER, MA 01606

CITANEST® (prilocaine HCl) SOLUTIONS ℞

Local anesthetic for infiltration and nerve block

Description: Citanest (prilocaine) is a local anesthetic, chemically designated as 2-propylamino-o-propionotoluidide.

Aqueous solutions of Citanest hydrochloride may be autoclaved repeatedly, if necessary.

Please refer to Table 1 for the exact composition of Citanest hydrochloride solutions.

[See table above].

Actions: Citanest stabilizes the neuronal membrane and prevents the initiation and transmission of nerve impulses, thereby effecting local anesthetic action.

TABLE I COMPOSITION OF AVAILABLE CITANEST SOLUTIONS

PRODUCT IDENTIFICATION	FORMULA					
	MULTIPLE DOSE VIALS			AMPULES		
Citanest (prilocaine) Hydrochloride (percent)	Prilocaine Hydrochloride (mg per ml)	Sodium Chloride (mg per ml)	Methylparaben (mg per ml)	Prilocaine Hydrochloride (mg per ml)	Sodium Chloride (mg per ml)
1%	10.0	6.0	1.0	10.0	6.0
2%	20.0	6.0	1.0	20.0	6.0
3%	N.S.	N.S.	N.S.	30.0	6.0

NOTE: All solutions are adjusted to a pH of 6.0–7.0 with sodium hydroxide.
N.S. Not supplied.

Citanest is metabolized in both the liver and the kidney and excreted via the kidney. It is not metabolized by plasma esterases. One of the metabolites of Citanest appears to be o-toluidine. This substance has been found to produce methemoglobin both *in vitro* and *in vivo* (see ADVERSE REACTIONS).

When used for infiltration anesthesia in obstetrical patients, the time of onset of Citanest averages 1–2 minutes with an approximate duration of 60 minutes or longer. For major nerve blocks (e.g. epidural block), the onset of analgesia is approximately two minutes longer for Citanest than for lidocaine, whereas the duration of action is, at least, 30–60 minutes longer for Citanest than for lidocaine.

Indications: Citanest (prilocaine) is indicated for the production of local anesthesia in infiltration procedures, peripheral nerve blocks, and epidural or caudal blocks.

Since Citanest hydrochloride solutions contain no epinephrine, they are particularly useful for patients in whom vasopressor agents may be contraindicated, e.g., patients with hypertension, diabetes, thyrotoxicosis, or other cardiovascular disorders.

Contraindications: Citanest is contraindicated in patients with a known history of hypersensitivity to local anesthetics of the amide type. This agent should not be used in patients with congenital or idiopathic methemoglobinemia.

Local anesthetic agents should not be used in patients with severe shock or heart block. Local anesthetic procedures should not be used when there is inflammation and/or sepsis in the region of the proposed injection.

Warnings:

(1) RESUSCITATIVE EQUIPMENT AND DRUGS SHOULD BE IMMEDIATELY AVAILABLE WHEN ANY LOCAL ANESTHETIC IS USED.

(2) Usage in Pregnancy: The safe use of Citanest (prilocaine) has not been established with respect to adverse effects upon fetal development. Careful consideration should be given to this fact before administering this drug to women of childbearing potential, particularly during early pregnancy. (See ANIMAL STUDIES)

This does not exclude the use of the drug at term for obstetrical analgesia. Adverse effects on the fetus, course of labor, or delivery have rarely been observed when proper dosage and proper technique have been employed.

Precautions: The safety and effectiveness of Citanest depend upon proper dosage, correct technique, adequate precautions, and readiness for emergencies.

The lowest dosage that results in effective anesthesia should be used to avoid high plasma levels and serious adverse effects. Injection of repeated doses of Citanest may cause significant increases in blood levels with each repeated dose due to slow accumulation of the drug or its metabolites. Tolerance varies with the status of the patient. Debilitated, elderly patients, acutely ill patients and children should be given reduced doses commensurate with their age and physical status.

INJECTIONS SHOULD ALWAYS BE MADE SLOWLY AND WITH FREQUENT ASPIRATIONS. Aspiration is advisable since it reduces the possibility of intravascular injection, thereby keeping the incidence of side effects and anesthetic failures at a minimum.

Consult standard textbooks for specific techniques and precautions for various local anesthetic procedures.

Epidural anesthesia and caudal anesthesia should be used with extreme caution in persons with the following conditions: existing neurological disease, spinal deformities, septicemia, severe hypertension, and extreme youth.

The drug should be used with caution in persons with known drug sensitivities.

Local anesthetics react with certain metals and cause the release of their respective ions which, if injected, may cause severe local irritation. Adequate precaution should be taken to avoid this type of interaction.

Adverse Reactions: Adverse reactions may result from high plasma levels due to excessive dosage, rapid absorption or inadvertent intravascular injection, or may result from a hypersensitivity, idiosyncrasy or diminished tolerance on the part of the patient. Such reactions are systemic in nature and involve the central nervous system and/or the cardiovascular system.

CNS reactions are excitatory and/or depressant, and may be characterized by nervousness, dizziness, blurred vision and tremors, followed by drowsiness, convulsions, unconsciousness and possibly respiratory arrest. The excitatory reactions may be very brief or may not occur at all, in which case the first manifestations of toxicity may be drowsiness, merging into unconsciousness and respiratory arrest.

Cardiovascular reactions are depressant, and may be characterized by hypotension, myocardial depression, bradycardia and possibly cardiac arrest.

Treatment of a patient with toxic manifestations consists of assuring and maintaining a patent airway and supporting ventilation using oxygen and assisted or controlled respiration as required. This usually will be sufficient in the management of most reactions. Should circulatory depression occur, vasopressors, such as ephedrine or metaraminol, and intravenous fluids may be used. Should a convulsion persist despite oxygen therapy, small increments of an ultra-short acting barbiturate (thiopental or thiamylal) or a short acting barbiturate (pentobarbital or secobarbital) may be given intravenously.

Allergic reactions are characterized by cutaneous lesions, urticaria, edema or anaphylactoid reactions. The detection of sensitivity by skin testing is of doubtful value.

Swelling and paresthesia of the lips and oral tissues has been reported following injection of 4% solutions of Citanest into the oral cavity.

Continued on next page

Astra—Cont.

Such reactions have not been reported with 1%, 2%, or 3% solutions.

Methemoglobinemia

In vivo o-toluidine apparently is formed from the metabolic degradation of Citanest (prilocaine) with the resultant formation of methemoglobinemia. A dose-response relationship appears to exist between the amount of Citanest administered as a single injection and the incidence and degree of methemoglobin formation.

In studies conducted in man to date, the formation of methemoglobin at a dose of 400 mg Citanest has not been statistically significant. Cases of cyanosis at doses between 400 and 600 mg are extremely rare. At a dose of 600 mg, which is the maximum recommended dose for any anesthetic procedure, methemoglobin formation occurred at levels which were less than 15% of the total hemoglobin content in all patients. At no time was the methemoglobinemia associated with any adverse respiratory, cardiovascular, or CNS symptoms. However, cyanosis has been reported at this dosage level. In addition, blood at the time of surgery has appeared somewhat darker than usual in some cases. Cyanosis is reported to be prevalent when 900 or more mg are administered as a single dose. It should be emphasized that this dose exceeds the recommended single dose.

Methemoglobin levels of less than 20 percent of total hemoglobin content are usually not associated with any clinical symptoms of hypoxia. At levels of 20 to 50 percent, fatigue, weakness, dyspnea, tachycardia, headaches, and dizziness may occur. Only one case exhibiting clinical symptoms of lightheadedness and dizziness, which may have been related to a methemoglobin value in excess of 20%, has been reported. The patient received a single injection of 900 mg. The intravenous use of methylene blue alleviated these symptoms within fifteen minutes.

Methemoglobinemia is rapidly and easily treated by 1–2 mg/kg of a 1% solution of methylene blue administered intravenously over a five-minute period. In most patients in whom the maximum recommended dose of Citanest is not exceeded, the appearance of clinical signs and symptoms of hypoxia is probably related to improper ventilation and should be treated with oxygen. If signs and symptoms of hypoxia persist following adequate alveolar ventilation with oxygen, then methemoglobinemia should be suspected and methylene blue treatment initiated. In patients with anemia or cardiac failure in whom the availability of oxygen has already been decreased, the potential disadvantages of a further hypoxic embarrassment due to the use of large doses of this agent must be carefully considered.

Dosage and Administration:

Infiltration Anesthesia—Citanest may be employed for infiltration anesthesia in any of the cases for which this technique is indicated. Selection of appropriate volumes and concentrations is dependent on the nature and extent of the surgical procedure. For most surgical procedures, 20–30 ml of Citanest hydrochloride 1% or 2% will usually provide adequate operative analgesia. The lowest concentration and smallest volume that will produce the desired results should be given. These suggested doses are for adults. Smaller amounts and weaker concentrations should be used for children depending on their age and weight.

Peripheral Nerve Blocks—For therapeutic nerve blocks (e.g. intercostal or paravertebral blocks), 3–5 ml of Citanest hydrochloride will usually be adequate for the management of pain. Selection of the appropriate concentration depends on the degree and duration of the analgesia required. Both parameters increase proportionally as the volume and concentration of drug is increased.

For blocks such as brachial plexus or sciatic-femoral, 20–30 ml of Citanest hydrochloride 2% or 15–20 ml of Citanest hydrochloride 3% will usually provide adequate operative analgesia for most routine surgical procedures involving the upper or lower extremities.

Central Neural Blocks—Citanest may be employed in epidural anesthesia for any of the surgical procedures for which this anesthetic technique is indicated. Volumes of 20–30 ml of Citanest hydrochloride 2% or 15–20 ml of Citanest hydrochloride 3% will usually provide adequate operative analgesia for both minor and major surgical procedures performed under epidural anesthesia.

Caudal anesthesia is useful for obstetrical analgesia and certain pelvic operative procedures such as hysterectomy, transurethral resection, etc. Citanest hydrochloride 1% in volumes of 20–30 ml will usually provide adequate obstetrical analgesia for most routine vaginal deliveries. For surgical procedures requiring more extensive anesthesia, 20–30 ml of Citanest hydrochloride 2% or 15–20 ml of Citanest hydrochloride 3% are recommended.

IMPORTANT: A test dose of 2–5 ml should be administered at least five minutes prior to injecting the total required volume for central neural blocks (epidural or caudal anesthesia). It is important that a single dose container be employed for epidural anesthesia.

Table II summarizes the recommended volumes and concentrations of Citanest hydrochloride for various types of anesthetic procedures. These recommended doses serve only as a guide to the amount of anesthetic required for most routine procedures. The actual volume and concentrations to be used depend on a number of factors, such as type and extent of surgical procedure, degree of muscular relaxation required, duration of anesthesia required, the physical state of the patient, etc. In all cases the smallest dose that will produce the desired result should be given.

The onset of anesthesia, the duration of anesthesia and the degree of muscular relaxation are proportional to the volume and concentration of local anesthetic used. Thus, an increase in volume and concentration of Citanest will decrease the onset of anesthesia, prolong the duration of anesthesia, provide a greater degree of muscular relaxation and increase the segmental spread of anesthesia. However, increasing the volume and concentration of Citanest may result in a more profound fall in blood pressure when used in epidural anesthesia. Although the incidence of side effects with Citanest is quite low, caution should be exercised particularly when employing large volumes and concentrations of Citanest since the incidence of side effects is directly proportional to the total dose of local anesthetic agent injected.

Maximum Recommended Dosages

Dosages in excess of those listed in Table II have been administered without serious side effects. However, caution should be exercised in the use of larger dosages, and in general, the amount given at any one time should not exceed that recommended in Table II.

[See table below].

Normal Healthy Adults: No more than 600 mg of Citanest hydrochloride should ever be administered as a single injection, i.e. no more than 8 mg/kg or 4 mg/lb should be given as a single injection. For continuous epidural or caudal anesthesia the maximum recommended dosage should not be administered at intervals of less than two hours.

Children: Experience in children under the age of ten is limited. It is difficult to recommend a maximum dose of any drug for children since this varies as a function of age and weight. With respect to Citanest hydrochloride, 400 mg have been used without toxic effects in children of 10–15 years. However, for children of less than 10 years who have a normal lean body mass and normal body development, the use of one of the standard pediatric drug formulas (e.g. Clark's rule or Young's rule) to determine the maximum dose is recommended. For example, in a child of five years weighing 50 lbs, the dose of Citanest hydrochloride should not exceed 150–200 mg when calculated according to Clark's rule or Young's rule. In order to minimize the possibility of toxic reactions in children the use of a 1% concentration of Citanest hydrochloride is recommended.

Patients with Liver Disease and Debilitated Patients: The use of any local anesthetic agent is undesirable in patients with liver disease or severely debilitated patients. However, for emergency or definitive surgical procedures where a local anesthetic is required, care should be taken to use the lowest dose and concentration of Citanest hydrochloride necessary to provide adequate anesthesia. The maximum safe dose of any drug for such patients depends on the degree of liver damage and degree of debilitation. For most anesthetic procedures, it is advisable to use the 1% concentration of Citanest hydrochloride in order to obtain the minimum dose that will provide adequate anesthesia and avoid possible toxic reactions in these patients. In such patients it is not advisable to exceed a maximum dose of 400 mg.

How Supplied:

Multiple dose vials: 30 ml Citanest hydrochloride 1% and 2%.

Ampules: 30 ml Citanest hydrochloride 1% and 2%; 20 ml Citanest hydrochloride 3%.

All solutions contain sodium chloride 6 mg per ml and are adjusted to a pH of 6.0 to 7.0 with

TABLE II RECOMMENDED DOSES OF CITANEST (PRILOCAINE) HYDROCHLORIDE FOR VARIOUS ANESTHETIC PROCEDURES IN NORMAL HEALTHY ADULTS

Anesthetic Procedure	Citanest hydrochloride Conc. (%)	Volume (ml)	Total Dose (mg)
Infiltration	1 or 2	20–30	200–600
Peripheral Nerve Blocks			
(a) Therapeutic Nerve Blocks (e.g. intercostal or paravertebral)	1 or 2	3–5	30–100
(b) For blocks such as Brachial Plexus or Sciatic-femoral	2	20–30	400–600
	3	15–20	450–600
Central Neural Blocks			
(a) Epidural	1	20–30	200–300
	2	20–30	400–600
	3	15–20	450–600
(b) Caudal			
(1) Obstetrical Analgesia	1	20–30	200–300
(2) Surgical Anesthesia	2	20–30	400–600
	3	15–20	450–600

TABLE 1. COMPOSITION OF AVAILABLE SOLUTIONS

Product Identification		Formula						
		Multiple Dose Vials				Single Dose Vials		
Duranest (etidocaine) HCl Concentration	Epinephrine (as the bitartrate) Dilution	Sodium chloride (mg/ml)	Methyl-paraben (mg/ml)	Sodium metabisulfite (mg/ml)	Citric Acid (mg/ml)	Sodium chloride (mg/ml)	Sodium metabisulfite (mg/ml)	Citric Acid (mg/ml)
0.5	None	—	—	—	—	8.07	None	—
0.5	1:200,000	8.07	1.0	0.5	0.2	8.07	0.5	0.2
1.0	None	—	—	—	—	7.1	None	—
1.0	1:200,000	—	—	—	—	7.1	0.5	0.2
1.5	1:200,000	—	—	—	—	6.2	0.5	0.2

NOTE: pH of all solutions adjusted with sodium hydroxide and/or hydrochloric acid. Duranest Solutions with epinephrine are adjusted to pH 3–4.5. Duranest Solutions without epinephrine are adjusted to pH 4.5.

sodium hydroxide. Multiple dose vials contain methylparaben, 1 mg per ml.

Animal Studies: Two studies of the effects of Citanest on reproduction and fetal development have been carried out in animals. In one study, doses of Citanest of 10 and 30 mg/kg (1 to 3 times the maximum human dose) were injected subcutaneously each day for 8 months into male and female rats. During these 8 months the rats were mated three times and the resultant litters were examined. The study revealed no teratogenic effects of Citanest and no adverse effects on the number of litters produced, on the average weight of pups at birth, on the average weight of pups surviving to weaning age, and on the distribution of sex. In the third littering, the average number of pups per litter at birth was lower in the group treated with the high dose of Citanest than in the control group. In all three litterings, the survival of pups in some of the treated groups was less than in their corresponding control groups. Adjustments in the experimental procedure indicated that these differences in survival were at least partially due to experimental artifacts.

In the other study, the effects of Citanest on organogenesis and fetal development was investigated in the rat. Doses ranging from 100 to 300 mg/kg (10 to 30 times the maximum human dose) were injected intramuscularly into pregnant rats from day 7 to day 13 post coitum. On the twenty-first gestational day the fetuses were examined. No external or skeletal malformations were observed and no significant differences were observed in the number of living and dead fetuses among the treated and control groups. The mean fetal weights in the treated groups were, however, less than that of the control group. In addition, hydronephrosis was observed in approximately 1% of the fetuses derived from treated mothers, but in none of the fetuses of the control group. This latter observation was not statistically significant.

DURANEST® (etidocaine hydrochloride) ℞ SOLUTION
STERILE AQUEOUS SOLUTION

Local anesthetic for infiltration and nerve block

Description: Duranest (etidocaine hydrochloride) Solution is a local anesthetic of the amide type, chemically related to lidocaine. Its chemical name is (±)-2-(N-ethylpropylamino)-2′,6′-butyroxylidide monohydrochloride.

The pKa of etidocaine (7.74) is similar to that of lidocaine (7.86). However, etidocaine possesses a greater degree of lipid solubility (partition coefficient of 141 in heptane/7.4 phosphate buffer system) and protein binding capacity (94%) as compared to lidocaine (partition coefficient = 3.6, protein binding = 55%).

Duranest solutions are sterile and except for the 1.5% concentration, are available with or without epinephrine 1:200,000. Duranest solutions without epinephrine may be reautoclaved if necessary.

Please refer to Table 1 for the composition of available solutions.

[See table above].

Actions: Etidocaine stabilizes the neuronal membrane and prevents the initiation and conduction of nerve impulses, thereby effecting local anesthetic action. *In vivo* animal studies have shown that Duranest (etidocaine hydrochloride) Solution has a rapid onset (3–5 minutes) and a prolonged duration of action (5–10 hours). Based on comparative clinical studies of lidocaine and etidocaine, the anesthetic properties of etidocaine in man may be characterized as follows: Initial onset of sensory analgesia and motor blockade is rapid (usually 3–5 minutes) and similar to that produced by lidocaine. Duration of sensory analgesia is 1.5 to 2 times longer than that of lidocaine, by the peridural route. The difference in analgesic duration between etidocaine and lidocaine may be even greater following peripheral nerve blockade than following central neural block. Duration of analgesia in excess of 9 hours is not infrequent when etidocaine is used for peripheral nerve blocks such as brachial plexus blockade. Etidocaine produces a profound degree of motor blockade and abdominal muscle relaxation when used for peridural analgesia.

Following absorption from the site of injection, etidocaine redistributes rapidly and demonstrates a larger volume of distribution than that seen with comparable local anesthetic drugs due to its high tissue solubility.

The rate of metabolism is similar to that of lidocaine. Etidocaine is metabolized in the liver and its metabolites are excreted via the kidneys. Little unchanged drug is recovered in the urine. Animal studies to date indicate that no single metabolite will account for more than 10% of the administered dose.

Clinical trials to date demonstrate that etidocaine does not produce methemoglobinemia or tissue irritation.

Indications: Duranest Solution is indicated for percutaneous infiltration anesthesia, peripheral nerve blocks, and central neural blocks, i.e., caudal or epidural blocks.

Contraindications: Duranest Solution is contraindicated in patients with a known history of hypersensitivity to local anesthetic agents of the amide type.

Warnings:

1. RESUSCITATIVE EQUIPMENT AND DRUGS, INCLUDING OXYGEN, SHOULD BE IMMEDIATELY AVAILABLE WHEN ANY LOCAL ANESTHETIC AGENT IS USED.
2. *Use in Pregnancy:* Reproductive studies have been performed in rats and rabbits without evidence of harm to the animal fetus. However, the safe use of Duranest Solution in humans has not been established with respect to adverse effects upon fetal development. Careful consideration should be given to this fact before administering this drug to women of childbearing potential, particularly during early pregnancy. This does not exclude the use of the drug at term for obstetrical analgesia. Duranest Solution has been used for obstetrical analgesia by the peridural route without evidence of adverse effects on the fetus. The use of Duranest Solution by the paracervical route have *not* been investigated for effects on the fetus.
3. Local anesthetic procedures should be used with caution when there is inflammation and/or sepsis in the region of the proposed injection.
4. Solutions which contain epinephrine or other vasoconstrictor agents should be used with extreme caution in patients receiving drugs known to produce blood pressure alterations (i.e., MAO inhibitors, tricyclic antidepressants, phenothiazines, etc.) as either severe sustained hypertension or hypotension may occur.
5. Vasopressor agents (administered for the treatment of hypotension related to caudal or other epidural blocks) should be used with extreme caution in the presence of oxytocic drugs as they are known to interact and may produce severe persistent hypertension and/or rupture of cerebral blood vessels.
6. The use of Duranest Solution has not been investigated in children under 14 years of age.

Precautions: The safety and effectiveness of Duranest Solutions depend on proper dosage, correct technique, adequate precautions, and readiness for emergencies. Consult standard textbooks for specific techniques and precautions for various regional anesthetic procedures.

The lowest dosage that results in effective anesthesia should be used to avoid high plasma levels and possible adverse effects. Tolerance varies with the status of the patient. For example, debilitated, elderly or acutely ill patients should be given reduced doses commensurate with their physical status. Duranest Solutions should also be used with caution in patients with severe shock or heart block.

INJECTIONS SHOULD ALWAYS BE MADE SLOWLY AND WITH FREQUENT ASPIRATIONS TO AVOID INADVERTENT RAPID INTRAVASCULAR ADMINISTRATION WHICH CAN PRODUCE SYSTEMIC TOXICITY.

Occasionally, duration of motor block may appear to exceed that of sensory block (see ACTIONS). Consideration should be given to the profound motor block and its effect on the need

Continued on next page

Astra—Cont.

for voluntary expulsive muscles when using Duranest for epidural block in obstetrics.
Epidural anesthesia and caudal anesthesia should be used with extreme caution in persons with the following conditions: existing neurological disease, septicemia, severe hypertension, or spinal deformities which may affect the quality of the block.
Solutions which contain a vasoconstrictor agent should be used with caution in the presence of diseases which may adversely affect the patient's cardiovascular system. Serious cardiac arrhythmias may occur if preparations containing a vasoconstrictor drug are employed in patients during or following the administration of chloroform, halothane, cyclopropane, trichlorethylene, or other related agents. Solutions containing epinephrine should be used cautiously in areas with limited blood supply.
Duranest Solutions should be used with caution in persons with known drug sensitivities. Patients allergic to paraaminobenzoic acid derivatives (procaine, tetracaine, benzocaine, etc.) have not shown cross sensitivity to agents of the amide type such as etidocaine. Since etidocaine is metabolized in the liver and excreted via the kidneys, it should be used cautiously in patients with liver and renal disease. Consideration should be given to the long duration of peripheral nerve block (8–10 hours) when using this drug for ambulatory patients.
Adverse Reactions: Reactions to etidocaine are similar in character to those observed with other local anesthetic agents such as lidocaine. Adverse reactions may result from high plasma levels due to excessive dosage, rapid absorption or inadvertent intravascular injection. Such reactions are systemic in nature and involve the central nervous system and/or the cardiovascular system.
A small number of reactions may result from hypersensitivity, idiosyncrasy or diminished tolerance on the part of the patient.
CNS reactions are excitatory and/or depressant, and are usually characterized by nervousness, dizziness, blurred vision and tremors, followed by drowsiness, convulsions, unconsciousness and possibly respiratory arrest. Excitatory CNS effects commonly represent the initial signs of local anesthetic systemic toxicity. However, these reactions may be very brief or absent in some patients in which case the first manifestations of toxicity may be drowsiness, merging into unconsciousness and respiratory arrest.
Hypotension and bradycardia may occur as normal physiological phenomena following sympathetic block with central neural blocks.
Toxic cardiovascular reactions to local anesthetics are usually depressant in nature and are characterized by peripheral vasodilation, hypotension, myocardial depression, bradycardia, and possibly cardiac arrest. However, direct cardiovascular depressant effects have not been seen with etidocaine in the absence of central nervous system toxicity.
Treatment of a patient wth toxic manifestations consists of assuring and maintaining a patent airway and supporting ventilation with oxygen and assisted or controlled respiration as required. This usually will be sufficient in the management of most reactions. Should a convulsion persist despite ventilatory therapy with oxygen, small increments of anticonvulsive agents may be given intravenously such as a benzodiazepine (e.g., diazepam), an ultrashort acting barbiturate (e.g., thiopental or thiamylal) or a short-acting barbiturate (e.g., pentobarbital or secobarbital). Cardiovascular depression may require circulatory assistance with intravenous fluids and/or vasopressor agents as dictated by the clinical situation.
Allergic reactions may occur as a result of sensitivity to the local anesthetic or methylparaben used as a preservative in multiple dose vials and are characterized by cutaneous lesions, urticaria, edema or anaphylactoid type symtomatology. True allergic reactions should be managed by conventional means. The detection of potential sensitivity by skin testing is of limited value.
Dosage and Administration: As with all local anesthetic agents the dose of Duranest Solution to be employed will depend on the area to be anesthetized, the vascularity of the tissues, the number of neuronal segments to be blocked, the type of regional anesthetic technique and the status and tolerance of the individual patient. The maximum dose of Duranest Solution to be employed as a single injection should be determined on the basis of the status of the patient and the type of regional anesthetic technique to be performed. Although single injections of 450 mg have been employed for regional anesthesia without adverse effects, at present it is strongly recommended that the maximal dose of Duranest Solution as a single injection should not exceed 400 mg (approximately 5.5 mg/kg or 2.7 mg/lb) with epinephrine 1:200,000 and 300 mg (approximately 4 mg/kg or 2 mg/lb) without epinephrine. Because etidocaine has been shown to disappear quite rapidly from blood, toxicity is influenced by rapidity of administration, and therefore slow injection in vascular areas is highly recommended. Incremental doses of Duranest Solution may be repeated at 2–3 hour intervals.
The following dosage recommendations are intended as guides for the use of Duranest Solution in the average adult patient. As indicated previously, the dosage should be reduced for elderly or debilitated patients or patients with severe renal disease.
[See table below left].
No information is available on appropriate pediatric doses.

TABLE 2. Recommended Doses of Duranest Solutions For Various Anesthetic Procedures In Normal Healthy Adults

PROCEDURE	Duranest HCl with epinephrine 1:200,000		
	Conc. (%)	Vol. (ml)	Total Dose (mg)
Percutaneous Infiltration	0.5	1–80	5–400
Peripheral Nerve Block	0.5	5–80	25–400
	or		
	1.0	5–40	50–400
Central Neural Block			
Lumbar Peridural			
Intraabdominal or Pelvic Surgery	1.0	10–30	100–300
Lower Limb Surgery	or		
Caesarean Section	1.5	10–20	150–300
	0.5	10–30	50–150
Vaginal Obstetrical and	or		
Gynecologic Procedures	1.0	5–20	50–200
	0.5	10–30	50–150
Caudal	or		
	1.0	10–30	100–300

How Supplied:

Dosage Form and Volume	Duranest Solution Concentration	Epinephine (as the bitartrate) Dilution
Multiple Dose Vials		
50 ml	0.5%	1:200,000
Single Dose Vials		
30 ml	0.5%	None
	0.5%	1:200,000
	1.0%	None
	1.0%	1:200,000
20 ml	1.5%	1:200,000

SENSORCAINE™ ℞
(bupivacaine HCl)
STERILE AQUEOUS SOLUTION
Local anesthetic for infiltration and nerve block

Description: Bupivacaine is a local anesthetic of the amide (aminoacyl) type and is chemically designated as 1-butyl-2′6′-pipecoloxylidide.
The pKa of bupivacaine (7.7) is similar to that of lidocaine (7.86). However, bupivacaine possesses a greater degree of lipid solubility (partition coefficient of 27.5 in heptane/7.4 phosphate buffer system and protein binding capacity 95% as compared to lidocaine partition coefficient =3.6, protein binding 55%).
SENSORCAINE (bupivacaine hydrochloride) solutions are sterile, isotonic solutions for injection. Single dose containers of SENSORCAINE solution without epinephrine may be reautoclaved if necessary.

TABLE 1. COMPOSITION OF AVAILABLE SOLUTIONS

Sensorcaine (bupivacaine HCl) Concentration (percent)	sodium chloride (mg/ml)	pH
0.25	8.0	4.5–6.5
0.50	8.0	4.5–6.5
0.75	8.0	4.5–6.5

NOTE: pH of all solutions adjusted with sodium hydroxide or hydrochloric acid
Clinical Pharmacology: Bupivacaine stabilizes the neuronal membrane and prevents the initiation and conduction of nerve impulses, thereby effecting local anesthetic action.
Onset is rapid and action is prolonged. Anesthesia may persist for several hours. The addition of a dilute concentration of epinephrine (1:200,000 or 5 μg/ml), when necessary and

when the patient's general condition permits such usage of epinephrine, generally delays systemic absorption of bupivacaine hydrochloride and thus permits the use of moderately larger total doses. The duration of action of bupivacaine hydrochloride may be extended by use of epinephrine, but this effect, if any, is minimal. Analgesia often persists after sensation has returned, thereby reducing the need for additional potent analgesics.

In man, peak blood levels of bupivacaine are reached within 30 to 45 minutes following injection for caudal, epidural, or peripheral nerve block and then decline substantially during the next three to six hours.

Detoxification of bupivacaine occurs in the liver where it is conjugated with glucuronic acid.

Bupivacaine hydrochloride, when injected in recommended doses and concentrations, does not ordinarily cause irritation, tissue damage or methemoglobinemia.

Indications and Dosage: Sensorcaine (bupivacaine hydrochloride) solution is indicated for the production of local anesthesia by percutaneous infiltration, peripheral nerve block(s) and central neural block (caudal or epidural), when the accepted procedures for these techniques, as described in standard textbooks, are followed.

Contraindications: Bupivacaine hydrochloride is contraindicated in patients with a known hypersensitivity to local anesthetic agents of the amide type or to other components of the injectable formulation.

Warnings: RESUSCITATIVE EQUIPMENT AND DRUGS SHOULD BE IMMEDIATELY AVAILABLE WHEN ANY LOCAL ANESTHETIC AGENT IS USED.

There are insufficient data concerning safety of Sensorcaine (bupivacaine hydrochloride) solution when used for obstetrical or gynecological paracervical block. Such use is, therefore, not recommended. Fetal bradycardia frequently follows paracervical block with some amide type local anesthetics and may be associated with fetal acidosis. Added risk appears to be present in prematurity, toxemia of pregnancy, and fetal distress.

Case reports of maternal convulsions and cardiovascular collapse following use of some local anesthetics for paracervical block in early pregnancy (as anesthesia for elective abortion) suggest that systemic absorption under these circumstances may be rapid.

There are insufficient data available to support the use of Sensorcaine for the production of spinal anesthesia (subarachnoid block). Such use is, therefore, not recommended.

Local anesthetic procedures should be used with caution when there is inflammation and/or sepsis in the region of the proposed injection.

Vasopressor agents (administered for the treatment of hypotension related to caudal or other epidural blocks) should be used with caution in the presence of oxytocic drugs as a severe persistent hypertension and even rupture of cerebral blood vessels may occur. The solutions which contain a vasoconstrictor should be used with extreme caution for patients whose medical history and physical evaluation suggest the existence of hypertension, arteriosclerotic heart disease, cerebral vascular insufficiency, heart block, thyrotoxicosis or diabetes, etc.

The solutions which contain a vasoconstrictor should also be used with extreme caution in patients receiving drugs known to produce blood pressure alterations (i.e. MAO inhibitors, tricyclic anti-depressants, phenothiazines, etc.) as either severe and sustained hypotension or hypertension may occur.

Precautions: The safety and effectiveness of bupivacaine hydrochloride depend on proper dosage, correct technique, adequate precautions, and readiness for emergencies. Consult standard textbooks for specific techniques and precautions for various regional anesthetic procedures.

The lowest dosage that results in effective anesthesia should be used. Injection of repeated doses of bupivacaine hydrochloride may cause significant increases in blood levels with each repeated dose due to slow accumulation of the drug or its metabolites. Tolerance varies with the status of the patient. Debilitated, elderly or acutely ill patients should be given reduced doses commensurate with their physical status. Bupivacaine hydrochloride should also be used with caution in patients with severe shock or heart block.

INJECTIONS SHOULD ALWAYS BE MADE SLOWLY AND WITH FREQUENT ASPIRATIONS TO AVOID INADVERTENT RAPID INTRAVASCULAR ADMINISTRATION WHICH CAN PRODUCE SYSTEMIC TOXICITY.

Epidural anesthesia and caudal anesthesia should be used with caution in persons with the following conditions: existing neurological disease, spinal deformities, septicemia, severe hypertension, or extreme youth.

Solutions containing a vasoconstrictor should be used cautiously and in carefully circumscribed quantities in areas of the body supplied by end arteries or having otherwise compromised blood supply. (e.g., digits, nose, external ear, penis, etc.). Serious cardiac arrhythmias may occur if preparations containing a vasoconstrictor drug are employed in patients during or following the administration of chloroform, halothane, cyclopropane, trichloroethylene, or other related agents.

Bupivacaine hydrochloride should be used with caution in persons with known drug sensitivities. Patients allergic to para-aminobenzoic acid derivatives (procaine, tetracaine, benzocaine, etc.) have not shown cross-sensitivity to agents of the amide type such as bupivacaine.

Since bupivacaine is metabolized in the liver and excreted via the kidneys, it should be used cautiously in patients with liver and renal disease.

The safety of amide local anesthetics in patients with malignant hyperthermia has not been assessed and, therefore, those agents should be used with caution in such patients.

Drowsiness following bupivacaine hydrochloride injection is *usually*an early indication of a high blood level of the drug and may occur following inadvertent intravascular administration or *rapid absorption* of bupivacaine.

Local anesthetics react with certain metals and cause the release of their respective ions which, if injected, may cause severe local irritation. Adequate precaution should be taken to avoid this type of interaction. (See STERILIZATION, STORAGE AND TECHNICAL PROCEDURES).

Pregnancy Category C. Bupivacaine hydrochloride has been shown to have an embryocidal effect in rats and rabbits when given in doses 13 and 7 times the human dose, respectively. There are no adequate and well-controlled studies in pregnant women of the effect of the drug on the developing fetus. Bupivacaine hydrochloride should be used during pregnancy only if the potential benefit justifies the potential risk to the fetus. This does not exclude the use of the drug at term for obstetrical analgesia. (See LABOR AND DELIVERY).

Bupivacaine hydrochloride solutions have been used for obstetrical analgesia by the peridural route without evidence of adverse effects on the fetus.

LABOR AND DELIVERY

Local anesthetics rapidly cross the placenta, and when used for epidural, paracervical, pudendal or caudal block anesthesia, can cause varying degrees of maternal, fetal and neonatal toxicity. The incidence and degree of toxicity depend upon the procedure performed, the type and amount of drug used, and the technique of drug administration. Adverse reactions in the parturient, fetus and neonate involve alterations of the central nervous system, peripheral vascular tone and cardiac function.

Maternal hypotension has resulted from regional anesthesia. Local anesthetics produce vasodilation by blocking sympathetic nerves. Elevating the patients's legs and positioning her on her left side will help prevent decreases in blood pressure. The fetal heart rate also should be monitored continuously, and electronic fetal monitoring is highly advisable.

Epidural or caudal anesthesia may alter the forces of parturition through changes in uterine contractility or maternal expulsive efforts. Epidural anesthesia has also been reported to prolong the second state of labor by removing the parturient's reflex urge to bear down or by interfering with motor function. The use of obstetrical anesthesia may increase the need for forceps assistance.

The use of some local anesthetic drug products during labor and delivery may be followed by diminished muscles strength and tone for the first day or two of life. The long-term significance of these observations is unknown.

NURSING MOTHERS

It is not known whether bupivacaine is excreted in human milk. Because many drugs are excreted in human milk, caution should be exercised when local anesthetics are administered to a nursing woman.

PEDIATRIC USE

Safety and effectiveness in children below the age of 12 have not been established.

Adverse Reactions: Reactions to bupivacaine hydrochloride are similar in character to those observed with other local anesthetic agents. Adverse reactions may result from high plasma levels as a result of excessive dosage, rapid absorption or inadvertent intravascular injection. Such reactions are systemic in nature and involve the central nervous system and/or cardiovascular system.

A small number of reactions may result from hypersensitivity, idiosyncrasy, or diminished tolerance on the part of the patient.

CNS reactions are excitatory and/or depressant, and may be characterized by nervousness, dizziness, blurred vision and tremors, followed by drowsiness, convulsions, unconsciousness and possibly respiratory arrest. The excitatory reactions may be very brief or may not occur at all, in which case the first manifestations of toxicity may be drowsiness, merging into unconsciousness and respiratory arrest.

Other CNS effects may be nausea, vomiting, chills, miosis, or tinnitus.

Cardiovascular reactions are depressant, and may be characterized by hypotension, myocardial depression, bradycardia and possibly cardiac arrest.

The following reactions may also occur after caudal or epidural anesthesia: Total or high spinal block; fecal incontinence, urinary retention; persistent analgesia, paresthesia and paralysis of the lower extremities; loss of perineal sensation and sexual function; slowing of labor, increased incidence of forceps delivery; headache and backache.

TREATMENT OF A PATIENT WITH TOXIC MANIFESTATIONS consists of assuring and maintaining a patent airway, supporting ventilation with oxygen and assisted or controlled ventilation (respiration) as required. This usually will be sufficient in the management of most reactions. Should a convulsion persist despite ventilatory therapy, small increments of anticonvulsive agents may be given intravenously, such as a benzodiazepine (e.g. diazepam), or ultrashort acting barbiturates (e.g. thiopental or thiamylal) or short acting barbiturates (e.g. pentobarbital or secobarbital). Cardiovascular depression may require circulatory assistance with intravenous fluids and

Continued on next page

Astra—Cont.

vasopressors (e.g. ephedrine) as dictated by the clinical situation.
Allergic reactions may occur as a result of sensitivity to the local anesthetic. Anaphylactoid type symptomatology and reactions, characterized by cutaneous lesions, urticaria, and edema, should be managed by conventional means. The detection of potential sensitivity by skin testing is of limited value.
Dosage and Administration: The dosage varies and depends upon the area to be anesthetized, the vascularity of the tissues, the number of neuronal segments to be blocked, individual tolerance and the technique of anesthesia. The lowest dosage needed to provide effective anesthesia should be administered. For specific techniques and procedures, refer to standard textbooks.
For most indications, the duration of anesthesia with SENSORCAINE (bupivacaine hydrochloride) solution is such that a single dose is sufficient.
In each case, maximum dosage limit must be determined by evaluating the size and physical status of the patient, and considering the usual rate of systemic absorption from a particular injection site. Most experience to date is with single doses up to 175 mg of bupivacaine hydrochloride without epinephrine, more or less drug may be used depending on the status of each case.
The dose may be repeated as often as once every three hours. In studies to date, total daily doses up to 400 mg have been reported. Until further experience is gained, this dose should not be exceeded in 24 hours. The dosages in the following table are recommended as a guide for use in the average adult. For young, elderly or debilitated patients, these dosages should be reduced. Until further experience is gained, SENSORCAINE solution is not recommended for children younger than 12 years.
UNUSED PORTIONS OF THE SOLUTION SHOULD BE DISCARDED SINCE THIS PRODUCT CONTAINS NO PRESERVATIVES.
Table 2. DOSAGE RECOMMENDATIONS
[See table below].
THESE SOLUTIONS OF SENSORCAINE SHOULD NOT BE USED FOR THE PRODUCTION OF SPINAL ANESTHESIA (SUBARACHNOID BLOCK) BECAUSE OF INSUFFICIENT DATA TO SUPPORT SUCH USE.
Sterilization, Storage and Technical procedures: Disinfecting agents containing heavy metals, which cause release of respective ions (mercury, zinc, copper, etc.), should not be used for skin or mucous membrane disinfection as they have been related to incidents of swelling and edema. When chemical disinfection of the container surface is desired, either pure undiluted isopropyl alcohol (91%) or 70% ethyl alcohol U.S.P. is recommended. It is recommended that chemical disinfection be accomplished by wiping the ampule thoroughly with cotton or gauze that has been moistened with the recommended alcohol just prior to use.
How Supplied: SENSORCAINE (bupivacaine hydrochloride) solutions are supplied in 30 ml ampules containing 0.25%, 0.50% or 0.75% bupivacaine hydrochloride.

for
SENSORCAINE
(bupivacaine hydrochloride)

Type of Block	Conc (%)	Each Dose ml.	mg.	Motor Block(1)
Local infiltration	0.25	up to max	up to max	—
Epidural	0.75(2)	10–20	75–150	Complete
	0.50	10–20	50–100	Moderate to complete
	0.25	10–20	25–50	Partial to moderate
Caudal	0.50	15–30	75–150	Moderate to complete
	0.25	15–30	37.5–75	Moderate
Peripheral	0.50	5 to max	25 to max	Moderate to complete
	0.25	5 to max	12.5 to max	Moderate to complete
Sympathetic	0.25	20–50	50–125	—

(1) With continuous (intermittent) techniques, repeat doses increase the degree of motor block. The first repeat dose of 0.50% may produce complete motor block. Intercostal nerve block with 0.25% may also produce complete motor block for intra-abdominal surgery.
(2) For single dose use: not for intermittent techniques.

XYLOCAINE® (lidocaine hydrochloride) ℞ STERILE AQUEOUS SOLUTIONS

Local anesthetic for infiltration and nerve block

Description: Xylocaine® (lidocaine hydrochloride) Solutions are sterile aqueous solutions prepared from lidocaine hydrochloride and water. Lidocaine hydrochloride is a local anesthetic chemically designated as 2-(diethylamino)-N-(2,6-dimethylphenyl)-acetamide monohydrochloride.
Xylocaine Solutions are available with or without epinephrine. Xylocaine Solutions without epinephrine may be reautoclaved if necessary Please refer to Table I for the exact composition of available Xylocaine Solutions.
[See table top next page].
Clinical Pharmacology: Lidocaine stabilizes the neuronal membrane and prevents the initiation and conduction of nerve impulses, thereby effecting local anesthetic action.
Lidocaine is metabolized mainly in the liver and excreted via the kidneys. Approximately 90% of lidocaine administered is excreted in the form of various metabolites, while less than 10% is excreted unchanged.
Indications: Xylocaine Solutions are indicated for production of local or regional anesthesia, by infiltration techniques, including percutaneous injection and intravenous regional anesthesia by peripheral nerve block techniques such as brachial plexus and intercostal blocks and by central neural techniques, including epidural and caudal blocks, when the accepted procedures for these techniques as described in standard textbooks are followed.
Contraindications: Xylocaine (lidocaine hydrochloride) Solutions are containdicated in patients with a known history of hypersensitivity either to local anesthetic agents of the amide type or to other components of the injectable formulations.
Warnings:
(1) RESUSCITATIVE EQUIPMENT AND DRUGS, INCLUDING OXYGEN, SHOULD BE IMMEDIATELY AVAILABLE WHEN ANY LOCAL ANESTHETIC AGENT IS USED.
(2) USE IN PREGNANCY: Reproductive studies have been performed in rats and rabbits without evidence of harm to the animal fetus. However, the safe use of lidocaine in humans has not been established with respect to possible adverse effects upon fetal development. Careful consideration should be given to this fact before administering this drug to women of childbearing potential, particularly during early pregnancy.
This does not exclude the use of the drug at term for obstetrical analgesia. Xylocaine Solution has been used effectively for obstetrical analgesia. Adverse effects on the fetus, course of labor or delivery have rarely been observed when proper dosage and proper technique have been employed.
(3) Local anesthetic procedures should be used with caution when there is inflammation and/or sepsis in the region of the proposed injection.
(4) Vasopressor agents (administered for the treatment of hypotension related to caudal or other epidural blocks) should be used with caution in the presence of oxytocic drugs, as a severe persistent hypertension and even rupture of cerebral blood vessels may occur.
(5) The solutions which contain a vasoconstrictor should be used with extreme caution for patients whose medical history and physical evaluation suggest the existence of hypertension, arteriosclerotic heart disease, cerebral vascular insufficiency, heart block, thyrotoxicosis or diabetes, etc. The solutions which contain a vasoconstrictor should also be used with extreme caution in patients receiving drugs known to produce blood pressure alterations (e.g., MAO inhibitors, tricyclic antidepressants, phenothiazines, etc.) as either sustained hypotension or hypertension may occur.

Precautions: The safety and effectiveness of Xylocaine Solution depends on proper dosage, correct technique, adequate precautions and readiness for emergencies. Standard textbooks should be consulted for specific techniques and precautions for various regional anesthetic procedures.
The lowest dosage that results in effective anesthesia should be used. Injection of repeated doses of Xylocaine Solution may cause significant increases in blood levels with each repeated dose due to slow accumulation of lidocaine or its metabolites. Tolerance varies with the status of the patient. Debilitated, elderly patients, acutely ill patients, and children should be given reduced doses commensurate with their age and physical status. Xylocaine Solution should also be used with caution in patients with severe shock or heart block.
In using Xylocaine Solution for infiltration or regional block anesthesia, injection should always be made slowly and with frequent aspirations. Proper tourniquet technique is essential in the performance of intravenous regional anesthesia. Solutions containing epinephrine or other vasoconstrictors should not be used for this technique.
Epidural anesthesia and caudal anesthesia should be used with extreme caution in persons with the following conditions: existing neurological disease, spinal deformities, septicemia, severe hypertension, and extreme youth.
Fetal bradycardia frequently follows paracervical block and may be associated with fetal acidosis. Fetal heart rate should always be monitored during paracervical anesthesia. Added risk appears to be present in prematurity, postmaturity, toxemia of pregnancy, uteroplacental insufficiency and fetal distress. The physician should weigh the possible advantages against dangers when considering paracervical block in these conditions. When the recommended dose is exceeded, the incidence of fetal bradycardia increases. Short term neonatal neurobehavioral alterations have been observed in association with some local anesthetics administered during labor and delivery. The short term and long term significance of these alterations is not known.
Solutions containing a vasoconstrictor should be used cautiously and in carefully circum-

TABLE I COMPOSITION OF AVAILABLE SOLUTIONS

PRODUCT IDENTIFICATION		FORMULA							
		SINGLE DOSE VIALS			MULTIPLE DOSE VIALS				AMPULES
Xylocaine (lidocaine hydrochloride Solution (Percent)	Epinephrine (dilution)	Sodium Chloride (mg/ml)	Sodium Metabisulfite (mg/ml)	Citric Acid (mg/ml)	Sodium Chloride (mg/ml)	Sodium Metabisulfite (mg/ml)	Citric Acid (mg/ml)	Methyl-Paraben (mg/ml)	Sodium Chloride (mg/ml)
0.5	None	8.0	None	None	8.0	None	None	1.0	N.S.
0.5	1:200,000	N.S.	N.S.	N.S.	8.0	0.5	0.2	1.0	N.S.
1.0	None	7.0	None	None	7.0	None	None	1.0	7.0
1.0	1:200,000	7.0	0.5	0.2	N.S.	N.S.	N.S.	N.S.	N.S.
1.0	1:100,000	N.S.	N.S.	N.S.	7.0	0.5	0.2	1.0	N.S.
1.5	None	6.5	None	None	N.S.	N.S.	N.S.	N.S.	N.S.
1.5	1:200,000	6.5	0.5	0.2	N.S.	N.S.	N.S.	N.S.	N.S.
2.0	None	6.0	None	None	6.0	None	None	1.0	6.0
2.0	1:200,000	6.0	0.5	0.2	N.S.	N.S.	N.S.	N.S.	N.S.
2.0	1:100,000	N.S.	N.S.	N.S.	6.0	0.5	0.2	1.0	N.S.

N.S. Not Supplied
NOTE: the pH of all solutions is adjusted to USP limits with sodium hydroxide and/or hydrochloric acid.

scribed quantities in areas of the body supplied by end arteries or having otherwise compromised blood supply (e.g., digits, nose, external ear, penis, etc.) Serious cardiac arrhythmias may occur if preparations containing a vasoconstrictor are employed in patients during or following the administration of chloroform, halothane, cyclopropane, trichlorethylene, or other related agents.

Xylocaine Solution should be used with caution in persons with known drug sensitivities. Patients allergic to para-aminobenzoic acid derivatives (procaine, tetracaine, benzocaine, etc.) have not shown cross sensitivity to lidocaine.

The safety of amide local anesthetics in patients with malignant hyperthermia has not been assessed, and therefore, these agents should be used with caution in such patients.

Drowsiness following an injection of Xylocaine Solution is usually an early indication of a high blood level of the drug and may occur following inadvertent intravascular administration or rapid absorption of lidocaine.

Local anesthetics react with certain metals and cause the release of their respective ions which, if injected, may cause severe local irritation. Adequate precautions should be taken to avoid this type of interaction (see STERILIZATION, STORAGE AND TECHNICAL PROCEDURES).

Adverse Reactions: Reactions to Xylocaine Solutions are similar in character to those observed with other local anesthetic agents. Adverse reactions may be due to high plasma levels as a result of excessive dosage, rapid absorption or inadvertent intravascular injection. Such reactions are systemic in nature and involve the central nervous system and/or the cardiovascular system.

Rarely reactions may result from hypersensitivity, idiosyncrasy or diminished tolerance on the part of the patient.

CNS reactions are excitatory and/or depressant, and may be characterized by nervousness, dizziness, blurred vision and tremors, followed by drowsiness, convulsions, unconsciousness and, possibly, respiratory arrest. The excitatory reactions may be very brief or may not occur at all, in which case the first manifestations of toxicity may be drowsiness, merging into unconsciousness and respiratory arrest.

Hypotension and bradycardia may occur as normal physiological phenomena following sympathetic block with central neural blocks.

Toxic cardiovascular reactions to local anesthetics are usually depressant in nature and are characterized by peripheral vasodilation, hypotension, myocardial depression, bradycardia and, possibly cardiac arrest.

Treatment of a patient with toxic manifestations consists of assuring and maintaining a patent airway, supporting ventilation with oxygen, and assisted or controlled ventillation (respiration) as required. This usually will be sufficient in the management of most reactions.

Should a convulsion persist despite ventilatory therapy with oxygen, small increments of anticonvulsive agents may be given intravenously. Examples of such agents include a benzodiazepine (e.g. diazepam), ultra-short acting barbiturates (e.g., thiopental or thiamylal) or a short acting barbiturate (e.g. pentobarbital or secobarbital). Cardiovascular depression may require circulatory assistance with intravenous fluids and/or vasopressors (e.g., ephedrine) as dictated by the clinical situation.

Allergic reactions may occur as a result of sensitivity either to local anesthetics or to the methylparaben used as a preservative in multiple dose vials. Anaphylactoid type symptomatology and reactions, characterized by cutaneous lesions, urticaria, and edema, should be managed by conventional means. The detection of potential sensitivity by skin testing of limited value.

Dosage and Administration: Table II (Recommended Dosages) summarizes the recommended volumes and concentrations of Xylocaine (lidocaine hydrochloride) Solutions for various types of anesthetic procedures. The dosages suggested in this table are for normal healthy adults and refer to the use of epinephrine-free solutions. When larger dosages are required, only solutions containing epinephrine should be used except in those cases where vasopressor drugs may be contraindicated.

[See table on next page].

These recommended doses serve only as a guide to the amount of anesthetic required for most routine procedures. The actual volume and concentrations to be used depend on a number of factors, such as type and extent of surgical procedure, degree of muscular relaxation required, duration of anesthesia required, the physical state of the patient, etc. In all cases the lowest concentration and smallest dose that will produce the desired result should be given. Dosages should be reduced for children and for elderly and debilitated patients.

The onset of anesthesia, the duration of anesthesia and the degree of muscular relaxation are proportional to the volume and concentration of local anesthetic solution used. Thus, an increase in concentration and volume of Xylocaine Solution administered will decrease the onset of anesthesia, prolong the duration of anesthesia, provide a greater degree of muscular relaxation and increase the segmental spread of anesthesia. However, increasing the concentration and volume of Xylocaine Solution administered may result in a more profound fall in blood pressure when used in epidural anesthesia. Although the incidence of side effects with Xylocaine Solution is quite low, caution should be exercised particularly when employing large volumes and concentrations of Xylocaine Solutions, since the incidence of side effects is directly related to the total dose of local anesthetic agent injected.

It is important that a single dose container be employed for epidural anesthesia and major peripheral nerve block. For intravenous regional anesthesia, only the single dose containers designated for intravenous regional anesthesia should be used.

Epidural Anesthesia

For epidural anesthesia, only the following dosage forms of Xylocaine Solutions are recommended:

1% without epinephrine ....30 ml ampules
30 ml single dose vials
1% with epinephrine
1:200,000 ....30 ml single dose vials
1.5% without
epinephrine..............20 ml single dose vials
1.5% with epinephrine
1:200,000..................30 ml single dose vials
2% without
epinephrine...............10 ml single dose vials
2% with epinephrine
1:200,000 .... 20 ml single dose vials

Although these solutions are intended specifically for epidural anesthesia, they may also be used for infiltration and peripheral nerve block provided they are employed as single dose units. These solutions contain no bacteriostatic agent.

In epidural anesthesia, the dosage varies with the number of dermatomes to be anesthetized (generally 2-3 ml of the indicated concentration per dermatome).

IMPORTANT: *A test dose of 2-5 ml should be administered at least 5 minutes prior to injecting the total required volume for central neural blocks (e.g., epidural or caudal anesthesia).*

Maximum Recommended Dosages

For normal healthy adults, the individual dose of Xylocaine Solution with epinephrine should be such that the dose of lidocaine hydrochloride is kept below 500 mg and, in any case, should not exceed 7 mg/kg (3.2 mg/lb) of body weight. When used without epinephrine, the amount of Xylocaine Solution administered should be such that the dose of lidocaine hydrochloride is kept below 300 mg and in any case should not exceed 4.5 mg/kg (2.0 mg per lb) of body weight. For continuous epidural or caudal anesthesia, the maximum recommended dos-

Continued on next page

Astra—Cont.

age should not be administered at intervals of less than 90 minutes. For paracervical block for obstetrical analgesia, (including abortion) the maximum recommended dosage (200 mg) should not be administered at intervals of less than 90 minutes. When paracervical block is used for non-obstetrical procedures, more drug may be administered if required to obtain adequate anesthesia. For intravenous regional anesthesia in adults (using Xylocaine 0.5% solution without epinephrine), the dose administered should not exceed 4 mg/kg (1.8 mg/lb) of body weight.

Children:

It is difficult to recommend a maximum dose of any drug for children since this varies as a function of age and weight. For children of less than ten years who have a normal lean body mass and normal body development, the maximum dose may be determined by the application of one of the standard pediatric drug formulas (e.g., Clark's rule). For example, in a child of five years weighing 50 lbs., the dose of lidocaine hydrochloride should not exceed 75–100 mg when calculated according to Clark's rule. In any case, the maximum dose of Xylocaine Solution with epinephrine should not exceed 7 mg/kg (3.2 mg/lb) of body weight. When used without epinephrine, the amount of Xylocaine Solution administered should not exceed 4.5 mg/kg (2.0 mg/lb) of body weight. In order to minimize the possibility of toxic reactions, the use of Xylocaine 0.5% or 1.0% Solution is recommended for most anesthetic procedures involving pediatric patients. The use of even more dilute solutions (i.e., 0.25–0.5%) and total dosages not to exceed 3 mg/kg (1.4 mg/lb) are recommended for induction of intravenous regional anesthesia in children.

Sterilization, Storage and Technical Procedures: Disinfecting agents containing heavy metals, which cause release of respective ions (mercury, zinc, copper, etc.) should not be used for skin or mucous membrane disinfection as they have been related to incidence of swelling and edema. When chemical disinfection of multi-dose vials is desired, either pure undiluted isoprophyl alcohol (91%) or 70% ethyl alcohol U.S.P. is recommended. Many commercially available brands of rubbing alcohol, as well as solutions of ethyl alcohol not of U.S.P. grade, contain denaturants which are injurious to rubber and, therefore, are not to be used. It is recommended that chemical disinfection be accomplished by wiping the vial or ampule thoroughly with cotton or gauze that has been moistened with the recommended alcohol just prior to use.

How Supplied:

[See table on next page].

TABLE II Recommended dosages of Xylocaine (lidocaine hydrochloride) For Various Anesthetic Procedures In Normal Healthy Adults.

PROCEDURE	Xylocaine (lidocaine hydrochloride) Solution (without epinephrine)		
	Conc. (%)	Vol. (ml)	Total Dose (mg)
Infiltration			
Percutaneous	0.5 or 1.0	1–60	5–300
Intravenous regional	0.5	10–60	50–300
Peripheral Nerve Blocks, e.g.			
Brachial	1.5	15–20	225–300
Dental	2.0	1–5	20–100
Intercostal	1.0	3	30
Paravertebral	1.0	3–5	30–50
Pudendal (each side)	1.0	10	100
Paracervical			
Obstetrical analgesia (each side)	1.0	10	100
Sympathetic Nerve Blocks, e.g.			
Cervical (stellate ganglion)	1.0	5	50
Lumbar	1.0	5–10	50–100
Central Neural Blocks			
Epidural*			
Thoracic	1.0	20–30	200–300
Lumbar			
Analgesia	1.0	25–30	250–300
Anesthesia	1.5	15–20	225–300
	2.0	10–15	200–300
Caudal			
Obstetrical analgesia	1.0	20–30	200–300
Surgical anesthesia	1.5	15–20	225–300

*Dose determined by number of dermatomes to be anesthetized (2–3 ml/dermatome).

THE ABOVE SUGGESTED CONCENTRATIONS AND VOLUMES SERVE ONLY AS A GUIDE. OTHER VOLUMES AND CONCENTRATIONS MAY BE USED PROVIDED THE TOTAL MAXIMUM RECOMMENDED DOSE IS NOT EXCEEDED.

XYLOCAINE® (lidocaine hydrochloride) ℞ SOLUTION INTRAMUSCULAR INJECTION FOR VENTRICULAR ARRHYTHMIAS

Description: Xylocaine (lidocaine hydrochloride) Solution, Intramuscular Injection for Ventricular Arrhythmias, is a sterile solution prepared from lidocaine hydrochloride and water. Lidocaine hydrochloride is chemically designated, as 2-(diethylamino)-N-(2,6 dimethylphenyl) acetamide monohydrochloride. Each ml of the sterile solution for intramuscular injection contains 100 mg of lidocaine hydrochloride, and sodium hydroxide or hydrochloric acid to adjust pH to 5.0 to 7.0.

Actions: Lidocaine is reported to increase the electrical stimulation threshold of the ventricle during diastole and, thereby, exert an antiarrhythmic effect. In the dosage recommended, lidocaine produces no change in systolic arterial blood pressure, absolute refractory period, or myocardial contractility.

When an appropriate dose of Xylocaine (lidocaine hydrochloride) Solution is administered by the intramuscular (deltoid) route, effective antiarrhythmic blood levels are usually attained within 5–15 minutes and usually persist for 60–90 minutes. Clinical studies in which cardiac arrhythmias were monitored indicated that the onset and duration of antiarrhythmic activity of intramuscular lidocaine are correlated with the attained blood levels of lidocaine. As with intravenous Xylocaine Solution, the intramuscular use of this agent has been found to exert beneficial antiarrhythmic activity in approximately 80% of treated patients. Approximately 90% of an administered dose of lidocaine is metabolized in the liver. Less than 10% of the drug is excreted unchanged via the kidneys.

Indications: Xylocaine (lidocaine hydrochloride) Solution is indicated in the management of cardiac arrhythmias, particularly those of ventricular origin such as occur with acute myocardial infarction.

Intramuscular administration (single dose) is justified in the following exceptional circumstances:

1. by a physician when ECG equipment is not available to verify the diagnosis but in whose opinion the potential benefits outweigh the possible risks
2. by a physician when facilities for intravenous administration are not readily available
3. by paramedical personnel in a mobile coronary care unit on direction by a physician viewing the transmitted ECG.

Contraindications: Xylocaine (lidocaine hydrochloride) is contraindicated (1) in patients with a known history of hypersensitivity to local anesthetics of the amide type and (2) in patients with Adams-Stokes syndrome or with severe degrees of sinoatrial, atrioventricular or intraventricular block.

Warnings: INJECTIONS SHOULD BE MADE WITH FREQUENT ASPIRATIONS TO AVOID POSSIBLE INADVERTENT INTRAVASCULAR ADMINISTRATION.

Monitoring with an electrocardiograph is recommended when Xylocaine (lidocaine hydrochloride) Solution is administered by the intramuscular route. In emergency situations when a ventricular rhythm disorder is suspected and electrocardiographic equipment is not available, a single dose may be administered when the physician in attendance has determined that the potential benefits outweigh the possible risks. If possible, emergency resuscitative equipment and drugs should be immediately available to manage potential adverse reactions involving the cardiovascular, respiratory or central nervous systems.

The intramuscular use of Xylocaine Solution may result in an increase in creatine phosphokinase levels. Thus, the use of this enzyme determination, without isoenzyme separation, as a diagnostic test for the presence of acute myocardial infarction may be compromised by the use of intramuscular Xylocaine Solution.

The intramuscular administration of Xylocaine Solution is not recommended in pediatrics, since evidence concerning proper use in children is not available.

Precautions: Xylocaine (lidocaine hydrochloride) Solution is metabolized mainly in the liver and excreted by the kidney. Therefore, caution should be employed in the repeated or prolonged use of Xylocaine Solution in patients with severe liver or renal disease due to the possible accumulation of lidocaine or its metabolites which may lead to toxic phenomena. The drug should also be used with caution in patients with hypovolemia and shock, and all forms of heart block.

Adverse Reactions: Serious adverse reactions have been rare following the use of intramuscular Xylocaine (lidocaine hydrochloride) Solution. However, systemic reactions of the following types previously have been reported following Xylocaine Solution administration, usually with excessive doses:

(1) Central Nervous System: lightheadedness; drowsiness; dizziness; apprehension; euphoria; tinnitus; blurred or double vision; vom-

DOSAGE FORM	Xylocaine (lidocaine hydrochloride) Solution (Percent)	Epinephrine (dilution)
Single Dose Vial		
10 ml	2.0%	None
20 ml	1.5%	None
	2.0%	1:200,000
30 ml	1.0%	None
	1.0%	1:200,000
	1.5%	1:200,000
50 ml	0.5%	None

DOSAGE FORM	Xylocaine (lidocaine hydrochloride) Solution (Percent)	Epinephrine (dilution)
Multiple Dose Vial		
20 ml	1.0%	None
	1.0%	1:100,000
	2.0%	None
	2.0%	1:100,000
50 ml	0.5%	None
	0.5%	1:200,000
	1.0%	None
	1.0%	1:100,000
	2.0%	None
	2.0%	1:100,000

DOSAGE FORM	Xylocaine (lidocaine hydrochloride) Solution (Percent)
Ampules	
2 ml	1%
	2%
5 ml	1%
30 ml	1%

iting; sensations of heat, cold or numbness; twitching; tremors; convulsions; unconsciousness; and respiratory depression and arrest.

(2) Cardiovascular System: hypotension; cardiovascular collapse; and bradycardia which may lead to cardiac arrest.

There have been no reports of cross sensitivity between lidocaine and procainamide or between lidocaine and quinidine.

Soreness at the injection site following intramuscular injections has occasionally been reported.

Management of Adverse Reactions:

1. In the case of severe reaction discontinue the use of the drug.
2. Institute the emergency resuscitative procedures, including maintenance of patent airway and assisted respiration, if necessary. Administer the emergency drugs necessary to manage the severe reaction.
3. For severe convulsions, parenteral administration of a rapidly acting anticonvulsant may be used.

Dosage and Administration: The recommended dose of Xylocaine (lidocaine hydrochloride) Solution by the intramuscular route in the average 70 kg or 150 lb man is 300 mg (approximately 4.3 mg/kg or 2.0 mg/lb). The deltoid muscle is recommended as the preferred site of injection, since therapeutic blood levels of lidocaine occur faster and the peak blood level is significantly higher following deltoid administration as compared to injections into the lateral thigh or gluteus. Injections should be made with frequent aspirations to avoid possible inadvertent intravascular injection.

As soon as possible, and when indicated, patients should be changed to an intravenous infusion of Xylocaine Solution or to an oral antiarrhythmic preparation for maintenance therapy. However, if necessary, an additional intramuscular injection may be made after an interval of 60–90 minutes.

How Supplied: Xylocaine (lidocaine hydrochloride) Solution for intramuscular use is supplied in 5 ml ampules, packed 10 to a carton. Each ml of the sterile solution contains 100 mg of lidocaine hydrochloride. Thus, 3 ml of solution will provide the recommended dose.

XYLOCAINE® ℞
(lidocaine hydrochloride) SOLUTION INTRAVENOUS INJECTION FOR CARDIAC ARRHYTHMIAS

Description: Xylocaine (lidocaine hydrochloride) Solution, Intravenous Injection for Ventricular Arrythmias, is a sterile solution prepared from lidocaine hydrochloride and water. Lidocaine hydrochloride is chemically designated as 2-(diethylamino)-N-(2,6 dimethylphenyl) acetamine monohydrochloride. [See table below].

Actions: Lidocaine has been reported to exert an antiarrhythmic effect by increasing the electrical stimulation threshold of the ventricle during disatole. In usual therapeutic doses lidocaine produces no changes in myocardial contractility, in systemic arterial pressure, or in absolute refractory period.

Approximately 90% of an administered dose of lidocaine is metabolized in the liver. The remaining 10% is excreted unchanged via the kidneys.

Indications: Xylocaine (lidocaine hydrochloride) Solution administered intravenously is specifically indicated in the acute management of (1) ventricular arrhythmias occurring during cardiac manipulation such as cardiac surgery, and (2) life-threatening arrhythmias which are ventricular in origin, such as occur during acute myocardial infarction.

Contraindications: Xylocaine (lidocaine hydrochloride) Solution is contraindicated in patients with a known history of hypersensitivity to local anesthetics of the amide type. Xylocaine Solutions should not be used in patients with STOKES-ADAMS syndrome, Wolff-Parkinson-White syndrome, or with severe degrees of sinoatrial, atrioventricular, or intraventricular block.

Warnings: Constant monitoring with an electrocardiograph is essential to the proper intravenous administration of a Xylocaine (lidocaine hydrochloride) Solution. Signs of excessive depression of cardiac conductivity, such as prolongation of PR interval and QRS complex and the appearance or aggravation of arrhythmias, should be followed by prompt cessation of the intravenous infusion of this agent. It is mandatory to have emergency resuscitative equipment and drugs immediately available to manage possible adverse reactions involving cardiovascular, respiratory, or central nervous systems.

Occasional acceleration of ventricular rate may occur when Xylocaine Solution is administered to patients with atrial fibrillation. Evidence for proper usage in children is limited.

Usage in pregnancy: It is not known whether Xylocaine Solution may have adverse effects upon fetal development. The benefits of the drug to the mother should be weighed against possible risk to the fetus.

Precautions: Caution should be employed in the repeated use of Xylocaine (lidocaine hydrochloride) Solution in patients with severe liver or kidney disease because accumulation of lidocaine or its metabolites may occur and lead to toxic phenomena, since lidocaine is metabolized mainly in the liver and excreted by the kidneys. The drug should also be used with caution in patients with hypovolemia and shock, and in all forms of heart block (see CONTRAINDICATIONS and WARNINGS).

In patients with sinus bradycardia or incomplete heart block, the administration of Xylocaine Solution intravenously for the elimination of ventricular ectopic beats without prior acceleration in heart rate (e.g. by isoproterenol or by electric pacing) may promote more frequent and serious ventricular arrhythmias or complete heart block (see CONTRAINDICATIONS).

Adverse Reactions: Systemic reactions of the following types have been reported:

1. Central Nervous System:
   Light-headedness; drowsiness; dizziness; apprehension; euphoria; tinnitus; blurred vision or double vision; vomiting; sensations of heat, cold or numbness; twitching; tremors; convulsions; unconsciousness; respiratory depression and arrest.
2. Cardiovascular System:
   Hypotension; cardiovascular collapse; and bradycardia which may lead to cardiac arrest.
3. Allergic reactions may occur but are infrequent. There have been no reports of cross-sensitivity between lidocaine and procainamide or between lidocaine and quinidine.

TABLE I Composition of available Xylocaine Intravenous Solutions for Cardiac Arrhythmias.

	Dosage Form	Composition* lidocaine HCl (mg per ml)	sodium chloride (mg per ml)
For Direct Injection	5 ml (100 mg) prefilled syringe	20	6
	5 ml (100 mg) ampule	20	6
For Preparation of Infusion Solutions	25 ml (One Gram) single use vial	40	None
	50 ml (Two Grams) single use vial	40	None
	5 ml (One Gram) additive syringe	200	None
	10 ml (Two Grams) additive syringe	200	None

*pH of all solutions adjusted with sodium hydroxide or hydrochloric acid to 5.0–7.0.
All containers are for single use: solutions do not contain preservatives.

Continued on next page

Astra—Cont.

Management of Adverse Reactions:

1. In the case of severe reaction, discontinue the use of Xylocaine (lidocaine hydrochloride) Solution.
2. Institute emergency resuscitative procedures and administer the emergency drugs necessary to manage the severe reaction. For severe convulsions, small increments of diazepam or an ultra-short acting barbiturate (thiopental or thiamylal); or if those are not available, a short-acting barbiturate (pentobarbital or secobarbital); or if the patient is under anesthesia, a short-acting muscle relaxant (succinylcholine) may be given intravenously. Muscle relaxants and intravenous medications should only be used by those familiar with their use. Patency of the airway and adequacy of ventilation must be assured.
3. Should circulatory depression occur, vasopressors, such as ephedrine, or metaraminol may be used.

Dosage and Administration:

Single Direct Intravenous Injection

Only the 5 ml, 100 mg dosage size should be used for direct intravenous injection. The usual dose is 50 to 100 mg administered intravenously under ECG monitoring. This dose may be administered at the rate of approximately 20 to 50 mg/min. Sufficient time should be allowed to enable a slow circulation to carry the drug to the site of action. If the initial injection of 50 to 100 mg does not produce a desired response, a second dose may be repeated after 5 minutes. Activate syringe only when prepared to administer injection. See illustrated instructions for use.

NO MORE THAN 200 TO 300 MG OF XYLOCAINE (LIDOCAINE HYDROCHLORIDE) SOLUTION SHOULD BE ADMINISTERED DURING A ONE HOUR PERIOD.

Evidence for proper usage in children is limited.

Continuous Infusion

Following a single injection, using a 5 ml, 100 mg dosage size, in those patients in whom the arrhythmia tends to recur and who are incapable of receiving oral antiarrhythmic therapy, intravenous infusions of Xylocaine Solution may be administered at the rate of 1 to 4 mg/min. (20 to 50 μg/kg/min. in the average 70 kg man). Intravenous infusions of Xylocaine Solution must be administered under constant ECG monitoring to avoid potential overdosage and toxicity. Intravenous infusion should be terminated as soon as the patient's basic cardiac rhythm appears to be stable or at the earliest signs of toxicity. It should rarely be necessary to continue intravenous infusions beyond 24 hours. As soon as possible, and when indicated, patients should be changed to an oral antiarrhythmic agent for maintenance therapy. The elimination half-life of lidocaine following an intravenous bolus injection is typically 1.5 to 2.0 hours. There are data which indicate that the half-life may be 3 hours or longer following infusions of greater than 24 hours.

Solutions for intravenous infusion may be prepared by the addition of one gram or two grams of Xylocaine Solution to one liter of 5% dextrose in water, the preferred diluent, using aseptic technique. Approximately a 0.1% to 0.2% solution will result from this procedure, that is, each ml will contain approximately 1 to 2 mg of lidocaine hydrochloride. Thus, depending upon whether the final concentration is 0.1% or 0.2%, 1 to 2 ml/min will provide 1 to 4 mg of lidocaine hydrochloride/min.

In those cases in which fluid restriction is medically desirable, a more concentrated solution may be prepared.

Xylocaine Solution has been found to be chemically stable for a minimum of 24 hours after dilution in the sterile intravenous solution recommended above. However, as with all intravenous admixtures, dilution should be made just prior to administration.

NOTE: Xylocaine Solutions containing 40 mg or 200 mg of lidocaine hydrochloride per ml, without sodium chloride or preservatives, are recommended for the preparation of intravenous infusion solutions.

CAUTION: The flow rate of all intravenous infusion solutions must be closely monitored. Xylocaine Solutions should not be added to blood transfusion assemblies.

How Supplied: For direct injection Xylocaine (lidocaine hydrochloride) Solution without preservatives is supplied in 5 ml, 100 mg ampules and in 5 ml, 100 mg prefilled syringes. For preparing intravenous infusion solutions, Xylocaine Solution without sodium chloride or preservatives is supplied in one and two gram additive syringes and in one and two gram single use vials. Each vial is packed with a presterilized transfer unit manufactured by the West Company.

XYLOCAINE® (lidocaine hydrochloride) ℞ 4% STERILE SOLUTION

For transtracheal use, retrobulbar injection, and for topical application

Description: Xylocaine® (lidocaine hydrochloride) 4% Sterile Solution, is a sterile aqueous solution prepared from lidocaine hydrochloride and water. Lidocaine hydrochloride is a local anesthetic chemically designated as 2-(diethylamino)-N-(2,6-dimethylphenyl)-acetamide monohydrochloride.

Xylocaine 4% Sterile Solution in 5 ml ampules may be autoclaved repeatedly, if necessary.

Composition of Xylocaine 4% Sterile Solution

Each ml contains:
2-(diethylamino)-N-(2,6-dimethylphenyl)-acetamide
(lidocaine) hydrochloride .... 40 mg
sodium hydroxide and/or hydrochloric acid to adjust pH to 5.0–7.0.

Actions: Lidocaine stabilizes the neuronal membrane and prevents the initiation and conduction of nerve impulses, thereby effecting local anesthetic action.

Lidocaine is metabolized mainly in the liver and excreted via the kidneys. Approximately 90% of lidocaine administered is excreted in the form of various metabolites; while less than 10% is excreted unchanged.

The onset of action is rapid. For retrobulbar injection, 4 ml of Xylocaine 4% Sterile Solution provides an average duration of action of 1 to 1½ hours. This duration may be extended for ophthalmic surgery by the addition of epinephrine, the usual recommended dilution being 1:50,000 to 1:100,000.

Indications: Xylocaine 4% Sterile Solution is indicated for the production of topical anesthesia of the mucous membranes of the respiratory tract or the genito-urinary tract. It may be injected trans-tracheally to anesthetize the larynx and trachea. It may be administered by retrobulbar injection to provide anesthesia for ophthalmic surgery.

Contraindications: Xylocaine 4% sterile solution is contraindicated in patients with a known history of hypersensitivity either to local anesthetics of the amide type or to other components of the sterile solution.

Warnings:

(1) RESUSCITATIVE EQUIPMENT AND DRUGS, INCLUDING OXYGEN, SHOULD BE IMMEDIATELY AVAILABLE WHEN ANY LOCAL ANESTHETIC IS USED.

(2) *Usage in Pregnancy:* Reproductive studies have been performed in rats and rabbits without evidence of harm to the animal fetus. However, the safe use of lidocaine has not been established with respect to adverse effects upon fetal development. Careful consideration should be given to this fact before administering this drug to women of childbearing potential, particularly during early pregnancy.

(3) Local anesthetic procedures should be used with caution when there is inflammation and/or sepsis in the region of the proposed injection.

(4) If a vasoconstrictor has been added to the solution, it should be used with extreme caution for patients whose medical history and physical evaluation suggest the existence of hypertension, arteriosclerotic heart disease, cerebral vascular insufficiency, heart block, thyrotoxicosis or diabetes, etc. The solutions which contain a vasoconstrictor should also be used with extreme caution in patients receiving drugs known to produce blood pressure alterations (e.g., MAO inhibitors, tricyclic antidepressants, phenothiazines, etc.) as either sustained hypotension or hypertension may occur.

Precautions: The safety and effectiveness of Xylocaine 4% Sterile Solution depend on proper dosage, correct technique, adequate precautions, and readiness for emergencies. Standard textbooks should be consulted for specific techniques and precautions for various anesthetic procedures.

The lowest dosage that results in effective anesthesia should be used. Injection of repeated doses of Xylocaine 4% Sterile Solution may cause significant increases in blood levels with each repeated dose due to slow accumulation of the drug or its metabolites. Tolerance varies with the status of the patient. Debilitated, elderly patients, acutely ill patients, and children should be given reduced doses commensurate with their age and physical status. Xylocaine 4% Sterile Solution should also be used with caution in patients with severe shock or heart block.

As with all injections of local anesthetics, retrobulbar injection should always be made slowly and with frequent aspirations.

Solutions to which a vasoconstrictor has been added should be used with caution in the presence of diseases which may adversely affect the patient's cardiovascular system. Serious cardiac arrhythmias may occur if preparations containing a vasoconstrictor are employed in patients during or following the administration of chloroform, halothane, cyclopropane, trichlorethylene, or other related agents.

Xylocaine 4% Sterile Solution should be used with caution in persons with known drug sensitivities. Patients allergic to para-aminobenzoic acid derivatives (procaine, tetracaine, benzocaine, etc.) have not shown cross sensitivity to lidocaine HCl.

Local anesthetics react with certain metals and cause the release of their respective ions which, if injected, may cause severe local irritation. Adequate precaution should be taken to avoid this type of interaction.

The safety of amide local anesthetics in patients with malignant hyperthermia has not been assessed, and therefore lidocaine should be used with caution in such patients.

Drowsiness following an injection of Xylocaine 4% Sterile Solution is *usually* an early indication of a high blood level of the drug and may occur following inadvertent intravascular administration or *rapid absorption* of lidocaine.

Adverse Reactions: Reactions to Xylocaine 4% Sterile Solution are similar in nature to those observed with other local anesthetic agents. Adverse reactions may result from high plasma levels due to excessive dosage, rapid absorption or inadvertent intravascular injection. Such reactions are systemic in nature and involve the central nervous system and/or the cardiovascular system. A small number of reactions may result from a hypersensitivity, idiosyncrasy or diminished tolerance on the part of the patient. CNS reactions are excitatory and/or depressant, and may be characterized by nervousness, dizziness, blurred vision and tremors, followed by drowsiness, convulsions, unconsciousness and possibly respiratory arrest. The excitatory reactions may be very brief or may not occur at all, in which case the first manifestations of toxicity may be drowsiness, merging into unconsciousness and respiratory arrest.

Toxic cardiovascular reactions to local anesthetics are usually depressant in nature and are characterized by hypotension, myocardial depression, bradycardia and possibly cardiac arrest.

Treatment of a patient with toxic manifestations consists of assuring and maintaining a patent airway, supporting ventilation with oxygen, and assisted or controlled ventillation (respiration) as required. This usually will be sufficient in the management of most reactions. Should a convulsion persist despite ventilatory therapy, small increments of anticonvulsive agents may be given intravenously. Examples of such agents include benzodiazepine (e.g., diazepam), ultrashort acting barbiturates (e.g., thiopental or thiamylal) or a short acting barbiturate (e.g., pentobarbital or secobarbital). Cardiovascular depression may require circulatory assistance with intravenous fluids and/or vasopressors (e.g., ephedrine) as dictated by the clinical situation.

Allergic reactions may occur as a result of sensitivity either to local anesthetics or to other components of the sterile solution. Anaphylactoid type symptomatology and reactions, characterized by cutaneous lesions, urticaria, and edema, should be managed by conventional means. The detection of potential sensitivity by skin testing is of limited value.

Dosage and Administration: The dosage varies and depends upon the area to be anesthetized, vascularity of the tissues, individual tolerance and the technique of anesthesia. The lowest dosage needed to provide effective anesthesia should be administered. Dosages should be reduced for children and for elderly and debilitated patients commensurate with their body weights and physical condition. Although the incidence of adverse effects with Xylocaine 4% Sterile Solution is quite low, caution should be exercised, particularly when employing large volumes of Xylocaine 4% Sterile Solution since the incidence of adverse effects is directly proportional to the total dose of local anesthetic agent administered.

For specific techniques and procedures refer to standard textbooks.

The dosages recommended below are for a normal, healthy 70 kg adult:

RETROBULBAR INJECTION: The suggested dose is 3–5 ml (120–200 mg of lidocaine hydrochloride), i.e. 1.7–3 mg/kg or 0.8–1.3 mg/lb body weight. A portion of this is injected retrobulbarly and the rest may be used to block the facial nerve.

TRANSTRACHEAL INJECTION: For local anesthesia by the transtracheal route 2–3 ml should be injected through a large enough needle so that the injection can be made rapidly. By injecting during inspiration some of the drug will be carried into the bronchi and the resulting cough will distribute the rest of the drug over the vocal cords and the epiglottis. Occasionally it may be necessary to spray the pharynx by oropharyngeal spray to achieve complete analgesia. For the combination of the injection and spray, it should rarely be necessary to utilize more than 5 ml (200 mg of lidocaine hydrochloride) i.e., 3 mg/kg or 1.3 mg/lb body weight.

TOPICAL APPLICATION: For laryngoscopy, bronchoscopy and endotracheal intubation, the pharynx and larynx may be sprayed with 1–5 ml (40–200 mg of lidocaine hydrochloride), i.e. 0.6–3 mg/kg or 0.3–1.3 mg/lb body weight.

Maximum Recommended Dosages:

Normal healthy adults:

The maximum recommended dose of Xylocaine 4% Sterile Solution should be such that the dose of lidocaine hydrochloride is kept below 300 mg and in any case should not exceed 4.3 mg/kg (2 mg/lb) body weight.

Children:

It is difficult to recommend a maximum dose of any drug for children since this varies as a function of age and weight. For children of less than ten years who have a normal lean body mass and normal body development, the maximum dose may be determined by the application of one of the standard pediatric drug formulas (e.g. Clark's rule). For example, in a child of five years weighing 50 lbs., the dose of lidocaine hydrochloride should not exceed 75–100 mg when calculated according to Clark's rule.

How Supplied: Xylocaine (lidocaine hydrochloride) 4% Sterile Solution: 5 ml ampule, package of 10; 5 ml prefilled sterile disposable syringe.

XYLOCAINE® ℞

(lidocaine hydrochloride) 4% TOPICAL SOLUTION

For topical application

Description: Lidocaine is a local anesthetic chemically designated as 2-(diethylamino)-N-(2,6-dimethylphenyl)-acetamide.

The 50 ml screw-cap bottle should not be autoclaved because the closure employed cannot withstand autoclaving temperatures and pressures.

Composition of Xylocaine 4% (lidocaine hydrochloride) Topical Solution

50 ml screw-cap bottle:

Each ml contains:

2-(diethylamino)-N-(2, 6-dimethylphenyl)-acetamide (lidocaine) hydrochloride ....40 mg

methylparaben..1 mg

sodium hydroxide. . .

to adjust pH to..................................6.0–7.0

An aqueous solution. NOT FOR INJECTION.

Actions: Lidocaine stabilizes the neuronal membrane and prevents the initiation and conduction of nerve impulses, thereby effecting local anesthetic action.

Lidocaine is metabolized mainly in the liver and excreted via the kidneys. Approximately 90% of lidocaine administered is excreted in the form of various metabolites, while less than 10% is excreted unchanged.

Indications: Xylocaine 4% (lidocaine hydrochloride) Topical Solution is indicated for the production of topical anesthesia of accessible mucous membranes of the oral and nasal cavities and proximal portions of the digestive tract.

Contraindications: Lidocaine hydrochloride is contraindicated in patients with a known history of hypersensitivity either to local anesthetics of the amide type or to the components of the topical solution.

Local anesthetic agents should not be used in patients with severe shock or heart block. Xylocaine 4% Topical Solution should not be used to anesthetize mucous membranes of the tracheobronchial tree and urinary tract, nor should it be used for ophthalmologic procedures.

Warnings:

1. RESUSCITATIVE EQUIPMENT AND DRUGS SHOULD BE IMMEDIATELY AVAILABLE WHEN ANY LOCAL ANESTHETIC IS USED.
2. *Usage in Pregnancy:* Reproductive studies have been performed in rats and rabbits without evidence of harm to the fetus. However, safe use of lidocaine hydrochloride topical solution has not been established with respect to adverse effects upon fetal development. Careful consideration should be given to this fact before administering this drug to women of childbearing potential, particularly during early pregnancy.

Precautions: The safety and effectiveness of lidocaine hydrochloride topical solution depends on proper dosage, correct technique, adequate precautions, and readiness for emergencies. Standard textbooks should be consulted for specific techniques and precautions for various anesthetic procedures.

The lowest dosage that results in effective anesthesia should be used to avoid high plasma levels and serious adverse effects. Debilitated, elderly patients, acutely ill patients, and children should be given reduced doses commensurate with their age and physical status.

Lidocaine hydrochloride topical solution should be used with caution in patients with severely traumatized mucosa and sepsis in the region of the proposed application.

Lidocaine hydrochloride topical solution should be used with caution in persons with known drug sensitivities. Patients allergic to para-aminobenzoic acid derivatives (procaine, tetracaine, benzocaine, etc.) have not shown cross sensitivity to lidocaine.

Adverse Reactions: Reactions to lidocaine hydrochloride are similar in character to those observed with other local anesthetic agents. Adverse reactions may be due to high plasma levels as a result of excessive dosage, rapid absorption or inadvertent intravascular injection. Such reactions are systemic in nature and involve the central nervous system and/or the cardiovascular system. A small number of reactions may result from hypersensitivity, idiosyncrasy or diminished tolerance on the part of the patient.

CNS reactions are excitatory and/or depressant, and may be characterized by nervousness, dizziness, blurred vision and tremors, followed by drowsiness, convulsions, unconsciousness and possibly respiratory arrest. The excitatory reactions may be very brief or may not occur at all, in which case the first manifestations of toxicity may be drowsiness, merging into unconsciousness and respiratory arrest.

Toxic cardiovascular reactions to local anesthetics are usually depressant in nature and may be characterized by hypotension, myocardial depression, bradycardia and possibly cardiac arrest.

Treatment of a patient with toxic manifestations consists of assuring and maintaining a patent airway, supporting ventilation with oxygen, and assisted or controlled ventilation (respiration) as required. This usually will be sufficient in the management of most reactions. Should a convulsion persist despite ventilatory therapy, small increments of anticonvulsive agents may be given intravenously. Examples of such agents include benzodiazepine (e.g., diazepam), ultrashort acting barbiturates (e.g., thiopental or thiamylal) or a short acting barbiturate (e.g., pentobarbital or secobarbital). Cardiovascular depression may require circulatory assistance with intravenous fluids and/or vasopressors (e.g., ephedrine) as dictated by the clinical situation.

Allergic reactions may occur as a result of sensitivity either to local anesthetics or to other components of the topical solution. Anaphylactoid type symptomatology and reactions, characterized by cutaneous lesions, urticaria, and edema, should be managed by conventional means. The detection of potential sensitivity skin testing is of limited value.

Dosage and Administration: The dosage varies and depends upon the area to be anesthetized, vascularity of the tissues, individual tolerance and the technique of anesthesia. The lowest dosage needed to provide effective anesthesia should be administered. Dosages should be reduced for children and for elderly and debilitated patients. The maximum dose should not exceed 7 mg/kg (3.17 mg/lb) of body

Continued on next page

Astra—Cont.

weight. Although the incidence of adverse effects with Xylocaine 4% (lidocaine hydrochloride) Topical Solution is quite low, caution should be exercised particularly when employing large volumes since the incidence of adverse effects is proportional to the total dose of local anesthetic agent administered.
The dosages recommended below are for normal, healthy adults:
When used as a spray, or when applied by means of cotton applicators or packs, as well as when instilled into a cavity, the suggested dosage of Xylocaine 4% Topical Solution is 1–5 ml (40–200 mg of lidocaine hydrochloride), i.e., 0.6–3.0 mg/kg or 0.3–1.5 mg/lb body weight.
NOTE: The solution may be applied from a sterile swab which should be discarded after use and never reused under any circumstances. When spraying, transfer the solution from the original container to an atomizer.
Maximum recommended dosages
Normal healthy adults:
The maximum recommended dose of Xylocaine 4% (lidocaine hydrochloride) Topical Solution should be such that the dose of lidocaine hydrochloride is kept below 300 mg and in any case should not exceed 4.5 mg/kg (2 mg/lb) body weight.
Children:
It is difficult to recommend a maximum dose of any drug for children since this varies as a function of age and weight. For childen of less than ten years who have a normal lean body mass and normal body development, the maximum dose may be determined by the application of one of the standard pediatric drug formulas (e.g., Clark's rule or Young's rule). For example, in a child of five years weighing 50 lbs., the dose of lidocaine should not exceed 75–100 mg when calculated according to Clark's rule or Young's rule.
How Supplied: Xylocaine 4% (lidocaine hydrochloride) Topical Solution 50 ml screw-cap bottle, cartoned. NOT FOR INJECTION.

XYLOCAINE® (lidocaine) HYDROCHLORIDE 1.5% WITH DEXTROSE 7.5% ℞

Sterile Aqueous Solution Only for Spinal Anesthesia in Obstetrics

Description: Xylocaine Hydrochloride 1.5% solution with Dextrose 7.5% is a hyperbaric solution for use only for spinal anesthesia in obstetrics. Xylocaine is a local anesthetic chemically designated as diethylaminoacet-2,6-xylidide.
Xylocaine Hydrochloride 1.5% with Dextrose 7.5% may be autoclaved at 15 lbs. pressure at 121°C (250°F) for 15 minutes (USP Standard). Since this preparation contains glucose, caramelization may occur under prolonged heating and in some instances prolonged storage. Therefore, this preparation should be resterilized no more than once and should not be permitted to remain in the sterilizer any longer than necessary. The solution should not be used if a precipitate is present.

Composition of Xylocaine Hydrochloride 1.5% with Dextrose 7.5%
Each ml contains:
Diethylaminoacet-2,6-xylidide (lidocaine) hydrochloride ....15 mg
Dextrose (d-glucose) ....75 mg
Sodium Hydroxide....to adjust pH to ...6.0–6.7
Specific gravity, 1.028–1.034

Actions: Xylocaine (lidocaine) stabilizes the neuronal membrane and prevents the initiation and transmission of nerve impulses, thereby effecting local anesthetic action.
Xylocaine is metabolized mainly in the liver and excreted via the kidneys. Approximately 90% of Xylocaine administered is excreted in the form of various metabolites, while less than 10% is excreted unchanged.
The onset of action is rapid, usually within 30 to 60 seconds of administration. The duration of sensory anesthesia obtained is usually adequate for completion of routine, uncomplicated vaginal delivery while motor anesthesia is limited to the levator and perineal muscles.
Indications: Xylocaine (lidocaine) Hydrochloride 1.5% with Dextrose 7.5% is indicated only for low spinal or "saddle block" anesthesia in vaginal delivery when selective sensory anesthesia is desired.
Contraindications: The following conditions preclude the use of spinal anesthesia:
1. Severe hemorrhage, shock, or heart block.
2. Local infection at the site of proposed puncture.
3. Septicemia.
4. Known sensitivity to the anesthetic agent.

The use of this preparation for spinal anesthesia in obstetrics is contraindicated in the presence of pre-existing neurological disease, and disease of the subarachnoid region.
Warnings:
1. RESUSCITATIVE EQUIPMENT AND DRUGS SHOULD BE IMMEDIATELY AVAILABLE WHEN ANY LOCAL ANESTHETIC IS USED.
2. Vasopressor agents should not be used in the presence of oxytocic drugs, as a severe persistent hypertension and even rupture of cerebral blood vessels may occur.

Precautions: The safety and effectiveness of Xylocaine (lidocaine) hydrochloride depends on proper dosage, correct technique, adequate precautions, and readiness for emergencies.
The lowest dosage that results in effective anesthesia should be used to avoid serious adverse effects.
CONSULT STANDARD TEXTBOOKS FOR SPECIFIC TECHNIQUES AND PRECAUTIONS FOR SPINAL ANESTHETIC PROCEDURES.
Xylocaine should be used with caution in persons with known drug sensitivities. Patients allergic to paraaminobenzoic acid derivatives (procaine, tetracaine, benzocaine, etc.) have not shown cross sensitivity to Xylocaine.
Local anesthetics react with certain metals and cause the release of their respective ions which, if injected, may cause severe local irritation. Adequate precaution should be taken to avoid this type of interaction.
Adverse Reactions: Adverse reactions may result from inadvertent intravascular injection, or may result from a hypersensitivity, idiosyncrasy or diminished tolerance on the part of the patient. However, most adverse reactions seen with spinal anesthesia are related to the technique rather than the drug employed. In addition, use of inappropriate doses or techniques (e.g., improper positioning of patient) may result in extensive spinal blockade leading to occurrences such as profound hypotension, respiratory arrest, etc. Adverse effects on the fetus, course of labor, or delivery have rarely been observed when proper dosage and proper techniques have been employed.
Sympathetic block accompanying spinal anesthesia may result in depression of blood pressure and accentuate supine hypotension which is produced by the gravid uterus compressing the inferior vena cava. High levels or total spinal anesthesia may result in respiratory depression and depressed myocardial contractility. Management consists of uterine displacement, fluid replacement with respiratory support and vasoconstrictors when necessary.
CNS reactions are excitatory and/or depressant, and may be characterized by nervousness, dizziness, blurred vision and tremors, followed by drowsiness, convulsions, unconsciousness, and possibly respiratory arrest. The excitatory reactions may be very brief or may not occur at all, in which case the first manifestations of toxicity may be drowsiness, merging into unconsciousness and respiratory arrest.
Cardiovascular reactions are depressant, and may be characterized by hypotension, myocardial depression, bradycardia and possibly cardiac arrest.
Treatment of a patient with toxic manifestations consists of assuring and maintaining a patent airway and supporting ventilation using oxygen and assisted or controlled respiration as required. This usually will be sufficient in the management of most reactions. Should circulatory depression occur, vasopressors, such as ephedrine or metaraminol, and intravenous fluids may be used. Should a convulsion persist despite oxygen therapy, small increments of an ultra-short acting barbiturate (thiopental or thiamylal) or a short acting barbiturate (pentobarbital or secobarbital) may be given intravenously.
UNDER NO CIRCUMSTANCES SHOULD THE PATIENT BE MOVED OR PLACED IN TRENDELENBERG (HEAD DOWN) POSITION IN AN ATTEMPT TO IMPROVE VENOUS RETURN.
Allergic reactions are characterized by cutaneous lesions, urticaria, edema or anaphylactoid reactions. The detection of sensitivity by skin testing is of doubtful value.
Dosage and Administration: Spinal anesthesia with Xylocaine (lidocaine) Hydrochloride 1.5% with Dextrose 7.5% may be induced in the right or left lateral recumbent or the sitting position. Since this is a hyperbaric solution, the anesthetic will tend to move in the direction in which the table is tilted. After the desired level of anesthesia is obtained and the anesthetic has become fixed, usually in 5–10 minutes with Xylocaine, the patient may be positioned according to the requirement of the surgeon or obstetrician.
INJECTIONS SHOULD BE MADE SLOWLY.
Barbotage is not recommended. Consult standard textbooks for specific techniques for spinal anesthetic procedures.
Recommended dosage
The following recommended dosage is for normal healthy adults and serves only as a guide to the amount of anesthetic required for most routine vaginal deliveries. In all cases, the smallest dose that will produce the desired result should be given.
Obstetrical low spinal or "saddle block" anesthesia: The dosage recommended for normal vaginal delivery is approximately 0.6 to 1.0 ml (9–15 mg).
How Supplied: Xylocaine® (lidocaine) Hydrochloride 1.5% solution with Dextrose 7.5% is supplied in 2 ml ampules.

XYLOCAINE® (lidocaine hydrochloride) 5% SOLUTION WITH GLUCOSE 7.5% ℞

Sterile Aqueous Solution for Spinal Anesthesia

Description: Xylocaine (lidocaine hydrochloride) 5% Solution with Glucose 7.5% is a sterile hyperbaric solution for use in spinal anesthesia. Lidocaine hydrochloride is a local anesthetic chemically designated as 2-diethylamino-N-(2,6-dimethylphenyl)-acetamide monohydrochloride.
Xylocaine 5% Solution with Glucose 7.5% may be autoclaved at 15 lbs. pressure at 121°C (250°F) for 15 minutes (USP Standard). Since this preparation contains glucose, caramelization may occur under prolonged heating and in some instances prolonged storage. Therefore, this preparation should be resterilized no more than once or twice and should not be permitted to remain in the sterilizer any longer than necessary. The solution should not be used if a precipitate is present.
Composition of Xylocaine 5% Solution with Glucose 7.5%

Each ml contains:
Lidocaine hydrochloride........................ 50 mg
Dextrose (d-glucose).................................75 mg
Sodium hydroxide or hydrochloric acid to adjust pH to..5.5-7.0
Specific gravity 1.030-1.035

Actions: Lidocaine stabilizes the neuronal membrane and prevents the initiation and transmission of nerve impulses, thereby effecting local anesthetic action.

Lidocaine is metabolized mainly in the liver and excreted via the kidneys. Approximately 90% of the lidocaine administered is excreted in the form of various metabolites while less than 10% is excreted unchanged.

The onset of action is rapid. The duration of perineal anesthesia provided with 1 ml (50 mg) Xylocaine 5% Solution with Glucose 7.5% averages 100 minutes with analgesia continuing for an additional 40 minutes. The duration of surgical anesthesia provided with 1.5 to 2 ml (75-100 mg) of this agent is approximately two hours. The duration of anesthesia may be extended by the addition of epinephrine or other appropriate vasoconstrictor agents.

Indications: Xylocaine (lidocaine hydrochloride) 5% Solution with Glucose 7.5% is indicated for the production of spinal anesthesia.

Contraindications: The following conditions preclude the use of spinal anesthesia:

(1) Severe hemorrhage, shock, or heart block.
(2) Local infection at the site of proposed puncture.
(3) Septicemia.
(4) Known sensitivity to the anesthetic agent.

Warnings:

(1) RESUSCITATIVE EQUIPMENT AND DRUGS SHOULD BE IMMEDIATELY AVAILABLE WHEN ANY LOCAL ANESTHETIC IS USED.
(2) *Usage in Pregnancy:* The safe use of Xylocaine (lidocaine hydrochloride) 5% Solution with Glucose 7.5% has not been established with respect to adverse effects upon fetal development. Careful consideration should be given to this fact before administering this drug to women of childbearing potential, particularly during early pregnancy.
This does not exclude the use of the drug at term for obstetrical analgesia. Xylocaine 5% Solution with Glucose 7.5% has been used effectively for obstetrical analgesia. Adverse effects on the fetus, course of labor, or delivery have rarely been observed when proper dosage and proper techniques have been employed.
(3) Vasopressor agents should not be used in the presence of oxytocic drugs since a severe persistent hypertension and even rupture of cerebral blood vessels may occur.

Precautions: The safety and effectiveness of Xylocaine 5% Solution with Glucose 7.5% depends on proper dosage, correct technique, adequate precautions, and readiness for emergencies.

The lowest dosage that results in effective anesthesia should be used to avoid serious adverse effects.

The following conditions may preclude the use of spinal anesthesia, depending upon the physician's ability to deal with the complications which may occur:

(1) Pre-existing neurological disease such as poliomyelitis, pernicious anemia, paralysis from nerve injuries and syphilis.
(2) Disturbance in blood morphology and/or anticoagulant therapy: In these conditions trauma to a blood vessel during needle puncture may result in uncontrollable hemorrhage into the epidural or subarachnoid space. Also profuse hemorrhage into the soft tissue may occur.
(3) Extremes of age.
(4) Chronic backache and preoperative headache.
(5) Hypotension and hypertension.
(6) Arthritis or spinal deformity.
(7) Technical problems (persistent paresthesias, persistent bloody tap).
(8) Psychotic or uncooperative patients.

CONSULT STANDARD TEXTBOOKS FOR SPECIFIC TECHNIQUES AND PRECAUTIONS FOR SPINAL ANESTHETIC PROCEDURES.

Xylocaine Solutions should be used with caution in persons with known drug sensitivities. Patients allergic to para-aminobenzoic acid derivatives (procaine, tetracaine, benzocaine, etc.) have not shown cross sensitivity to lidocaine.

Local anesthetics react with certain metals and cause the release of their respective ions which, if injected, may cause severe local irritation. Adequate precaution should be taken to avoid this type of interaction.

Adverse Reactions: Adverse reactions may result from inadvertent intravascular injection, or may result from a hypersensitivity, idiosyncrasy or diminished tolerance on the part of the patient. In addition, use of inappropriate doses or techniques (e.g. improper positioning of patient) may result in extensive spinal blockade leading to occurrences such as profound hypotension, respiratory arrest, etc.

CNS reactions are excitatory and/or depressant, and may be characterized by nervousness, dizziness, blurred vision and tremors, followed by drowsiness, convulsions, unconsciousness and possibly respiratory arrest.

The excitatory reactions may be very brief or may not occur at all, in which case the first manifestations of toxicity may be drowsiness, merging into unconsciousness and respiratory arrest.

Cardiovascular reactions are depressant, and may be characterized by hypotension, myocardial depression, bradycardia and possibly cardiac arrest.

Treatment of a patient with toxic manifestations consists of assuring and maintaining a patent airway and supporting ventilation using oxygen and assisted or controlled respiration as required. This usually will be sufficient in the management of most reactions. Should circulatory depression occur, vasopressors, such as ephedrine or metaraminol, and intravenous fluids may be used. Should a convulsion persist despite oxygen therapy, small increments of an ultra-short acting barbiturate (thiopental or thiamylal) or a short acting barbiturate (pentobarbital or secobarbital) may be given intravenously.

Allergic reactions are characterized by cutaneous lesions, urticaria, edema or anaphylactoid reactions. The detection of sensitivity by skin testing is of doubtful value.

Dosage and Administration: Spinal anesthesia with Xylocaine (lidocaine hydrochloride) 5% Solution with Glucose 7.5% may be induced in the right or left lateral recumbent or the sitting position. Since this is a hyperbaric solution, the anesthetic will tend to move in the direction in which the table is tilted. After the desired level of anesthesia is obtained and the anesthetic has become fixed, usually in 5-10 minutes with Xylocaine 5% Solution with Dextrose 7.5%, the patient may be positioned according to the requirement of the surgeon or obstetrician.

INJECTIONS SHOULD BE MADE SLOWLY. Barbotage is not recommended. Consult standard textbooks for specific techniques for spinal anesthetic procedures.

Recommended dosages

The following recommended dosages are for normal healthy adults and serve only as a guide to the amount of anesthetic required for most routine procedures. In all cases, the smallest dose that will produce the desired result should be given.

If the technique is properly performed and the needle is properly placed in the subarachnoid space, it should not be necessary to administer more than one ampule (100 mg).

Obstetrical low spinal or saddle block anesthesia:

The dosage recommended for normal vaginal delivery is approximately 1.0 ml (50 mg). For Cesarean section and those deliveries requiring intrauterine manipulations, 1.5 ml (75 mg) is usually adequate.

Surgical anesthesia:

The dosage recommended for abdominal surgical anesthesia is 1.5-2 ml (75-100 mg).

How Supplied: Xylocaine® (lidocaine hydrochloride) 5% solution with Glucose 7.5% is supplied in 2 ml ampules in packages of 10 and 100.

XYLOCAINE® 2% (lidocaine HCl) JELLY ℞

A Topical Anesthetic for Urological Procedures and Lubrication of Endotracheal Tubes

Description: Lidocaine is a local anesthetic chemically designated as 2-(Diethylamino)-N-(2,6-Dimethylphenyl)-Acetamide. Xylocaine® (lidocaine hydrochloride) 2% Jelly is a sterile, aqueous solution thickened to a suitable viscosity, of the following composition:

Each ml contains:
Lidocaine hydrochloride.................................20mg
Methyl-p-hydroxybenzoate............................0.7mg
Propyl-p-hydroxybenzoate............................0.3mg
Sodium Hydroxide ....to adjust pH
Sodium Carboxymethylcellulose, to adjust to a suitable consistency.

Actions: Lidocaine stabilizes the neuronal membrane and prevents the initiation and conduction of nerve impulses, thereby effecting local anesthetic action.

Xylocaine (lidocaine hydrochloride) 2% Jelly effects local, topical anesthesia. The onset of action is 3–5 minutes. It is ineffective when applied to intact skin.

Lidocaine is metabolized mainly in the liver and excreted via the kidneys. Approximately 90% of lidocaine administered is excreted in the form of various metabolites, while less than 10% is excreted unchanged.

Indications: Xylocaine® (lidocaine hydrochloride) 2% Jelly is indicated for prevention and control of pain in procedures involving the male and female urethra and for topical treatment of painful urethritis.

It is also useful as an anesthetic lubricant for endotracheal intubation.

Contraindications: Xylocaine® (lidocaine hydrochloride) 2% Jelly is contraindicated in patients with a known history of hypersensitivity to local anesthetics of the amide type, or to other components of the jelly formulation.

USE IN PREGNANCY: Reproductive studies have been performed in rats and rabbits without evidence of harm to the animal fetus. However, the safe use of lidocaine in humans has not been established with respect to possible adverse effects upon fetal development. Careful consideration should be given to this fact before administering this drug to women of childbearing potential, particularly during early pregnancy.

Precautions: The safety and effectiveness of lidocaine depends on proper dosage, correct technique, adequate precautions and readiness for emergencies. The lowest dose that results in effective anesthesia should be used to avoid high plasma levels and serious adverse effects. Debilitated, elderly patients, acutely ill patients and children should be given reduced doses commensurate with their age and physical status. Standard textbooks should be consulted for specific technique and precautions. Xylocaine® (lidocaine hydrochloride) 2% Jelly should be used with caution in patients

Continued on next page

Astra—Cont.

with severely traumatized mucosa and/or sepsis in the region of the proposed application. Xylocaine 2% Jelly should be used with caution in persons with known drug sensitivities. Patients with allergic sensitivity to para-aminobenzoic acid derivatives (procaine, tetracaine, benzocaine, etc.) have not shown cross sensitivity to lidocaine.

Adverse Reactions: Systemic adverse reactions are extremely rare with Xylocaine® (lidocaine hydrochloride) 2% Jelly. However, as with any local anesthetic, adverse reactions may result from high plasma levels due to excessive dosage, or rapid absorption, or may result from a hypersensitivity, idiosyncrasy or diminished tolerance.

CNS reactions are excitatory and/or depressant, and may be characterized by nervousness, dizziness, blurred vision and tremors, followed by drowsiness, convulsions, unconsciousness and possibly respiratory arrest. The excitatory reactions may be very brief or may not occur at all, in which case the first manifestations of toxicity may be drowsiness, merging into unconsciousness and respiratory arrest.

Cardiovascular reactions are depressant, and may be characterized by hypotension, myocardial depression, bradycardia and possibly, cardiac arrest.

Treatment of a patient with toxic manifestations consists of assuring and maintaining a patent airway, supporting ventilation with oxygen, and assisted or controlled ventilation (respiration) as required. This usually will be sufficient in the management of most reactions. Should a convulsion persist despite ventilatory therapy, small increments of an anticonvulsive agents may be given intravenously. Examples of such agents include benzodiazepine (e.g. diazepam), ultra-short acting barbiturates (e.g. thiopental or thiamylal) or a short acting barbiturate (e.g. pentobarbital or secobarbital). Cardiovascular depression may require circulatory assistance with intravenous fluids and/or vasopressor (e.g. ephedrine) as dictated by the clinical situation.

Allergic reactions may occur as a result of sensitivity to local anesthetics or other components of the jelly formulation. Anaphylactoid type symptomatology and reactions, characterized by cutaneous lesions, urticaria, and edema, should be managed by conventional means. The detection of potential sensitivity by skin testing is of limited value.

Dosage and Administration:

For surface anesthesia of the male urethra: The outer orifice is washed and cleansed with a disinfectant. The plastic cone is sterilized for 5 minutes in boiling water, cooled, and attached to the tube. The cone may be gas sterilized or cold sterilized, if preferred. The tube key is attached. The jelly is instilled slowly into the urethra by turning the tube key until the patient has a feeling of tension or until almost half the tube (15 ml; 300 mg) is emptied. A penile clamp is then applied for several minutes at the corona and then the remaining contents of the tube are instilled.

Prior to sounding or cystoscopy, a penile clamp should be applied for 5 to 10 minutes to obtain adequate anesthesia. The contents of one tube (30 ml; 600 mg) are usually required to fill and dilate the male urethra.

Prior to catheterization, smaller volumes (5-10 ml; 100-200 mg) are usually adequate.

For surface anesthesia of the female urethra: The outer orifice is washed and cleansed with a disinfectant. The plastic cone is sterilized for 5 minutes in boiling water, cooled, and attached to the tube. The cone may be gas sterilized or cold sterilized, if preferred. The tube key is attached. Three to five ml of the jelly is instilled slowly into the urethra by turning the tube key (approximately 1½ - 2 full turns). If desired, some jelly may be deposited on a cotton swab and introduced into the urethra. In order to obtain adequate anesthesia, several minutes should be allowed prior to performing urological procedures.

For endotracheal intubation: Apply to the catheter, as needed, prior to intubation.

Maximum Dosage: No more than one tube should be given in any 12 hour period.

How Supplied: Collapsible tubes which deliver 30 ml. A detachable applicator cone and a key for expressing contents are included in each package.

XYLOCAINE® (lidocaine) ℞
5% OINTMENT
A Water-Soluble Topical Anesthetic Ointment

Description: Lidocaine is a local anesthetic chemically designated as 2-(Diethylamino-N-(2,6 Dimethylphenyl)-Acetamide.

Composition of Xylocaine 5% (lidocaine) Ointment:

2- (Diethylamino) - N - (2, 6 Dimethylphenyl)-Acetamide 5% in a water miscible ointment vehicle consisting of polyethylene glycols and propylene glycol.

Actions: Lidocaine stabilizes the neuronal membrane and prevents the initiation and conduction of nerve impulses, thereby effecting local anesthetic action. Xylocaine 5% (lidocaine) Ointment effects local, topical anesthesia. The onset of action is 3-5 minutes. It is ineffective when applied to intact skin.

Lidocaine is metabolized mainly in the liver and excreted via the kidneys. Approximately 90% of lidocaine administered is excreted in the form of various metabolites, while less than 10% is excreted unchanged.

Indications: Xylocaine 5% (lidocaine) Ointment is indicated for production of anesthesia of accessible mucous membranes of the oropharynx.

It is also useful as an anesthetic lubricant for endotracheal intubation, and for the temporary relief of pain associated with minor burns and abrasions of the skin.

Contraindications: Xylocaine 5% (lidocaine) Ointment is contraindicated in patients with a known history of hypersensitivity to local anesthetics of the amide type, or to other components of the ointment.

Warnings: *USE IN PREGNANCY:* Reproductive studies have been performed in rats and rabbits without evidence of harm to the animal fetus. However, the safe use of lidocaine in humans has not been established with respect to possible adverse effects upon fetal development. Careful consideration should be given to this fact before administering this drug to women of childbearing potential, particularly during early pregnancy.

Precautions: The safety and effectiveness of lidocaine depends on proper dosage, correct technique, adequate precautions and readiness for emergencies. The lowest dose that results in effective anesthesia should be used to avoid high plasma levels and serious adverse effects. Debilitated, elderly patients, acutely ill patients and children should be given reduced doses commensurate with their age and physical status. Standard textbooks should be consulted for specific techniques and precautions.

Xylocaine 5% (lidocaine) Ointment should be used with caution in patients with severely traumatized mucosa and/or sepsis in the region of the proposed application.

Xylocaine 5% (lidocaine) Ointment should be used with caution in persons with known drug sensitivities. Patients with allergic sensitivity to para-aminobenzoic acid derivatives (procaine, tetracaine, benzocaine, etc.) have not shown cross sensitivity to lidocaine.

Adverse Reactions: Systemic adverse reactions are extremely rare with Xylocaine 5% (lidocaine) Ointment. However, as with any local anesthetic, adverse reactions may result from high plasma levels due to excessive dosage, or rapid absorption, or may result from hypersensitivity, idiosyncrasy, or diminished tolerance.

CNS reactions are excitatory, and/or depressant, and may be characterized by nervousness, dizziness, blurred vision and tremors, followed by drowsiness, convulsions, unconsciousness, and, possibly, respiratory arrest. The excitatory reactions may be very brief or may not occur at all, in which case the first manifestations of toxicity may be drowsiness, merging into unconsciousness and respiratory arrest.

Cardiovascular reactions are depressant, and may be characterized by hypotension, myocardial depression, bradycardia, and, possibly, cardiac arrest.

Treatment of a patient with toxic manifestations consists of assuring and maintaining a patent airway, supporting ventilation with oxygen, and assisted or controlled ventilation (respiration) as required. This usually will be sufficient in the management of most reactions. Should a convulsion persist despite ventilatory therapy, small increments of anticonvulsive agents may be given intravenously. Examples of such agents include benzodiazepine (e.g., diazepam), ultrashort acting barbiturates (e.g., thiopental or thiamylal) or a short acting barbiturate (e.g., pentobarbital or secobarbital). Cardiovascular depression may require circulatory assistance with intravenous fluids and/or vasopressors (e.g., ephedrine) as dictated by the clinical situation.

Allergic reactions may occur as a result of sensitivity to local anesthetics. Anaphylactoid type symptomatology and reactions, characterized by cutaneous lesions, urticaria, and edema, should be managed by conventional means. The detection of potential sensitivity by skin testing is of limited value.

Dosage and Administration: Apply topically for adequate control of symptoms. The use of a sterile gauze pad is suggested for application to broken skin tissue. Apply to the catheter prior to endotracheal intubation.

In dentistry, apply to previously dried oral mucosa. Subsequent removal of excess saliva with cotton rolls or saliva ejector minimizes dilution of the ointment and permits maximum penetration. Avoid cross-contamination between patients by aseptically transferring from its container to a separate plate or small dish the estimated amount of ointment required for each patient. Discard any unused portion. For use in connection with the insertion of new dentures, apply to all denture surfaces contacting mucosa.

IMPORTANT: Patients should consult dentist at intervals not exceeding 36 hours throughout the fitting period.

NOTE: No more than 35 grams should be administered in any one day.

How Supplied: Xylocaine 5% (lidocaine) Ointment is available in 35-gram tubes.

Xylocaine 5% (lidocaine) Ointment Flavored, for application within the oral cavity, is dispensed in 3.5-gram tubes, 10 tubes per carton, and in 35-gram jars.

KEEP CONTAINER TIGHTLY CLOSED AT ALL TIMES WHEN NOT IN USE.

XYLOCAINE® (lidocaine)
2.5% OINTMENT

Composition: Diethylaminoacet-2,6-xylidide 2.5% in a water miscible ointment vehicle consisting of polyethylene glycols and propylene glycol.

Action and Uses: A topical anesthetic ointment for fast, temporary relief of pain and itching due to minor burns, sunburn, minor cuts, abrasions, insect bites and minor skin irritations. The ointment can be easily removed with water. It is ineffective when applied to intact skin.

Administration and Dosage: Apply topically in liberal amounts for adequate control of symptoms. When the anesthetic effect wears off additional ointment may be applied as needed.

Important Warning: *In persistent, severe or extensive skin disorders, advise patient to use only as directed. In case of accidental ingestion advise patient to seek professional assistance or to contact a poison control center immediately. Keep out of the reach of children.*

Caution: *Do not use in the eyes. Not for prolonged use. If the condition for which this preparation is used persists or if a rash or irritation develops, advise patient to discontinue use and consult a physician.*

How Supplied: Available in tube of 35 grams (approximately 1.25 ounces).

XYLOCAINE® (lidocaine) 10% Oral Spray ℞
Flavored Topical Anesthetic For Use In The Oral Cavity

WARNING—CONTENTS UNDER PRESSURE. Read carefully other warnings included in insert.

Name of Drug: Xylocaine 10% (lidocaine) Oral Spray.

Description: Lidocaine is a local anesthetic, chemically designated as diethylaminoacet-2,6-xylidide. It has the following structural formula:

CH_3 / C_2H_5 / $NH-CO-CH_2-N$ / C_2H_5 / CH_3

Composition of Xylocaine 10% Oral Spray: Each actuation of the metered dose (0.1 ml) valve delivers:

Lidocaine	10.0 mg
absolute alcohol	4.92 mg
cetylpyridinium chloride	0.01 mg
saccharin	0.39 mg
flavor	3.27 mg
polyethylene glycol	20.79 mg

And as propellents: trichlorofluoromethane/ dichlorodifluoromethane (65%/35%)

Actions: Xylocaine 10% Oral Spray acts on intact mucous membranes to produce local anesthesia. Anesthesia occurs usually within 1–2 minutes and persists for approximately 10–15 minutes.

Approximately 90% of an administered dose of Xylocaine is metabolized in the liver. The remainder (10%) of the drug is excreted unchanged via the kidneys.

Indications: Xylocaine 10% Oral Spray is indicated for the production of topical anesthesia of the gingival and oral mucous membranes.

Contraindications: Xylocaine is contraindicated in patients with a known history of hypersensitivity to local anesthetics of the amide type.

Warnings: RESUSCITATIVE EQUIPMENT AND DRUGS SHOULD BE IMMEDIATELY AVAILABLE WHEN ANY LOCAL ANESTHETIC IS USED.

Avoid contact with the eyes. Inhalation and swallowing should be avoided. The recommended dosage should not be exceeded because of the possibility of toxicity or side effects. Contents under pressure. Therefore, do not puncture or incincerate container and do not expose to heat or store at temperatures above 120°F. Keep out of the reach of children.

Precautions: The lowest dosage that results in effective anesthesia should be used to avoid high plasma levels and serious undesirable systemic side effects. Tolerance varies with the status of the patient. The debilitated, elderly, and acutely ill patients should be given reduced doses commensurate with their age and physical status.

The safety and effectiveness of Xylocaine depends upon proper dosage, correct technique, adequate precautions, and readiness for emergencies. Xylocaine should be used cautiously in patients with known drug allergies or sensitivities. Patients allergic to para-aminobenzoic acid derivatives (procaine, tetracaine, benzocaine, etc.) have not shown similar sensitivity to Xylocaine.

Adverse Reactions: Adverse reactions result from high plasma levels due to excessive dosage or rapid absorption. Hypersensitivity, idiosyncrasy or diminished tolerance may also be the cause of reactions. Reactions due to overdosage (high plasma levels) are systemic and involve the central nervous system and the cardiovascular system.

Reactions involving the central nervous system are characterized by excitation and/or depression. Nervousness, dizziness, blurred vision or tremors may occur followed by convulsions, drowsiness, unconsciousness and possibly respiratory arrest. Excitement may be transient or absent and the first manifestations may be drowsiness merging into unconsciousness and respiratory arrest.

Reactions involving the cardiovascular system include depression of the myocardium, hypotension, bradycardia, and even cardiac arrest.

The treatment of a patient with toxic manifestations consists of assuring and maintaining a patent airway and supporting ventilation using oxygen and assisted or controlled respiration as required. This will be sufficient in the management of most reactions. Should circulatory depression occur, vasopressors such as ephedrine or metaraminol, and intravenous fluids may be used. Should a convulsion persist despite oxygen therapy small increments of an ultra-short acting barbiturate (thiopental or thiamylal) or a short acting barbiturate (pentobarbital or secobarbital) may be given intravenously.

Allergic reactions are characterized by cutaneous lesions, urticaria, edema, or anaphylactoid reactions. The detection of sensitivity by skin testing is of doubtful value.

Dosage and Administration: Two metered doses are recommended as the upper limit and under no circumstances, should one exceed three metered doses per quadrant of gingiva and oral mucosa over a one-half hour period to produce the desired anesthetic effect. Experience in children is inadequate to recommend a pediatric dose at this time. *Note:* Each actuation of the metered dose valve delivers 10 mg Xylocaine base. It is unnecessary to dry the site prior to application.

How Supplied: An 82.5 gm (60 ml) aerosol container equipped with a metered dose valve.

XYLOCAINE® 2% (lidocaine hydrochloride) VISCOUS SOLUTION ℞
A Topical Anesthetic for the Mucous Membranes of the Mouth and Pharynx

Description: Lidocaine hydrochloride is a local anesthetic chemically designated as 2-(diethylamino) -N- (2,6-dimethylphenyl) -acetamide hydrochloride.

Composition of Xylocaine 2% (lidocaine hydrochloride) Viscous Solution: lidocaine hydrochloride 2% in an aqueous solution adjusted to suitable vicosity and low surface tension with sodium carboxymethylcellulose, and pleasantly flavored.

Actions: Lidocaine hydrochloride stabilizes the neuronal membrane and prevents the initiation and conduction of nerve impulses, thereby effecting local anesthetic action. Lidocaine hydrochloride is metabolized mainly in the liver and excreted via the kidneys. Approximately 90% of lidocaine administered is excreted in the form of various metabolites, while less than 10% is excreted unchanged.

Indications: Xylocaine 2% (lidocaine hydrochloride) Viscous Solution is indicated for the production of topical anesthesia of irritated or inflamed mucous membranes of the mouth and pharynx.

Contraindications: Xylocaine 2% (lidocaine hydrochloride) Viscous Solution is contraindicated in patients with a known history of hypersensitivity to local anesthetics of the amide type or to other components of the solution.

Warnings: *Use in Pregnancy:* Reproductive studies have been performed in rats and rabbits without evidence of harm to the animal fetus. However, the safe use of lidocaine in humans has not been established with respect to possible adverse effects upon fetal development. Careful consideration should be given to this fact before administering this drug to women of childbearing potential, particularly during early pregnancy.

Precautions: The safety and effectiveness of lidocaine depends on proper dosage, correct technique, adequate precautions and readiness for emergencies. The lowest dose that results in effective anesthesia should be used to avoid high plasma levels and serious adverse effects. Debilitated, elderly patients, acutely ill patients and children should be given reduced doses commensurate with their age and physical status. Standard textbooks should be consulted for specific techniques and precautions.

Xylocaine 2% (lidocaine hydrochloride) Viscous Solution should be used with caution in persons with known drug sensitivities. Patients with allergic sensitivity to para-aminobenzoic acid derivatives (procaine, tetracaine, benzocaine, etc.) have not shown cross sensitivity to lidocaine hydrochloride.

The use of oral topical anesthetic agents may interfere with the second stage (pharyngeal stage) of swallowing. Thus, care should be exercised, particularly in children, when food is ingested within 60 minutes following the use of oral topical anesthetics to prevent the possible aspiration of food.

Adverse Reactions: Systemic adverse reactions are extremely rare with Xylocaine 2% (lidocaine hydrochloride) Viscous Solution. However, as with any local anesthetic, adverse reactions may result from high plasma levels due to excessive dosage, or rapid absorption, or may result from a hypersensitivity, idiosyncrasy or diminished tolerance.

CNS reactions are excitatory and/or depressant, and may be characterized by nervousness, dizziness, blurred vision and tremors, followed by drowsiness, convulsions, unconsciousness and possibly respiratory arrest. The excitatory reactions may be very brief or may not occur at all, in which case the first manifestations of toxicity may be drowsiness, merging into unconsciousness and respiratory arrest.

Cardiovascular reactions are depressant, and may be characterized by hypotension, myocardial depression, bradycardia and possibly cardiac arrest.

Treatment of a patient with toxic manifestations consists of assuring and maintaining a patent airway, supporting ventilation with oxygen, and assisted or controlled ventilation (respiration) as required. This usually will be sufficient in the management of most reactions. Should a convulsion persist despite ventilatory therapy, small increments of anticonvulsive agents may be given intravenously. Examples of such agents include benzodiazepine (e.g., diazepam), ultrashort acting barbiturates (e.g., thiopental or thiamylal) or a short acting barbiturate (e.g., pentobarbital or secobarbital). Cardiovascular depression may require circulatory assistance with intravenous fluids and/or vasopressors (e.g., ephedrine) as dictated by the clinical situation.

Allergic reactions may occur as a result of sensitivity to local anesthetics. Anaphyloctoid

Continued on next page

Astra—Cont.

type symptomatology and reactions, characterized by cutaneous lesions, urticaria, and edema, should be managed by conventional means. The detection of potential sensitivity by skin testing is of limited value.

Dosage and Administration: For symptomatic treatment of irritated or inflamed mucous membranes of the mouth and pharynx, the usual adult dose is one 15 ml tablespoonful undiluted. The solution should be swished around in the mouth and can be swallowed without water. It should rarely be necessary to administer this dose at intervals of less than three hours and not more than eight doses should be given in a 24-hour period.

The dosage should be adjusted commensurate with the patient's age and/or physical status (see Precautions).

How Supplied: Xylocaine 2% (lidocaine hydrochloride) Viscous Solution is available in 100 ml and 450 ml polyethylene squeeze bottles, and in unit of use (adult dose) packages of 25 (20 ml) polyethylene bottles.

YUTOPAR® ℞
(ritodrine hydrochloride)

CAUTION: Federal law prohibits dispensing without prescription.

Description: Yutopar, which contains the betamimetic (beta sympathomimetic amine) ritodrine hydrochloride, is available in two dosage forms. Yutopar for parenteral (intravenous) use is a clear, colorless, sterile, aqueous solution; each milliliter contains 10 mg. of ritodrine hydrochloride, 0.44% (w/v) of acetic acid, 0.24% (w/v) of sodium hydroxide, 0.1% (w/v) of sodium metabisulfite, and 0.29% (w/v) of sodium chloride in water for injection USP. Hydrochloric acid or additional sodium hydroxide is used to adjust pH. Each Yutopar tablet contains 10 mg. of ritodine hydrochloride. Ritodrine hydrochloride is a white, odorless crystalline powder, freely soluble in water, with a melting point between 196° and 205° C. The chemical name of ritodrine hydrochloride is erythro-p-hydroxy-α-[1[(p-hydroxyphenethyl)-amino]ethyl]benzyl alcohol hydrochloride and has the chemical structure:

HO–⟨C₆H₄⟩–CH(OH)–CH(CH_3)–NH–CH_2–CH_2–⟨C₆H₄⟩–OH •HCl

Clinical Pharmacology: Yutopar (ritodrine hydrochloride) is a beta-receptor agonist, which has been shown by *in vitro* and *in vivo* pharmacologic studies in animals to exert a preferential effect on the β_2 adrenergic receptors such as those in the uterine smooth muscle. Stimulation of the β_2 receptors inhibits contractility of the uterine smooth muscle.

In humans, intravenous infusions of 0.05 to 0.30 mg./min. or single oral doses of 10 to 20 mg. decreased the intensity and frequency of uterine contractions. These effects were antagonized by beta-blocking compounds. Intravenous administration induced an immediate dose-related elevation of heart rate with maximum mean increases between 19 and 40 beats per minute. Widening of the pulse pressure was also observed; the average increase in systolic blood pressure was also observed; the average increase in systolic blood pressure was 4.0 mm. Hg, and the average decrease in diastolic pressure was 12.3 mm. Hg. With oral intake, the increase in heart rate was mild and delayed.

During intravenous infusion in humans, transient elevations of blood glucose, insulin, and free fatty acids have been observed. Decreased serum potassium has also been found, but effects on other electrolytes have not been reported.

Serum kinetics in humans (non-pregnant females) of an intravenous infusion of 60 minutes duration were determined by measuring serum ritodrine levels by a radioimmunoassay technique. Three half-lives were calculated: the first of 6 to 9 minutes dominated the ascending phase of the serum drug-level curve; the second phase of 1.7 to 2.6 hours dominated the descending curve; and finally, a third phase, with a half-life of more than 10 hours, was discernible. In a study of serum kinetics after oral ingestion (male subjects), the decline of serum drug levels could be described in terms of a two-phase decay with an initial half-life of 1.3 hours and a final half-life of 12 hours. With either route of administration, 90% of the excretion was completed within 24 hours after the dose.

Comparison of ritodrine serum levels after intravenous administration with those after oral dosage indicates the oral bioavailability is about 30%. Intravenous infusion at a rate of 0.15 mg./min. for 1 hour yielded maximum serum levels ranging between 32 and 52 ng./ml. in a group of 6 non-pregnant female volunteers; maximum serum levels following single and repeated (4 × 10 mg./24 hr.) 10 mg. oral doses ranged between 5 and 15 ng./ml. and were obtained within 30 to 60 minutes after ingestion.

Placental transfer was confirmed by measurement of drug concentrations in cord blood showing that ritodrine and its conjugates reach the fetal circulation.

Indications And Usage: Yutopar is indicated for the management of preterm labor in suitable patients.

Administered intravenously, the drug will decrease uterine activity and thus prolong gestation in the majority of such patients. After intravenous Yutopar has arrested the acute episode, oral administration may help to avert relapse. Additional acute episodes may be treated by repeating the intravenous infusion.

The incidence of neonatal mortality and respiratory distress syndrome increases when the normal gestation period is shortened.

Since successful inhibition of labor is more likely with early treatment, therapy with Yutopar should be instituted as soon as the diagnosis of preterm labor is established and contraindications ruled out in pregnancies of 20 or more weeks' gestation. The efficacy and safety of Yutopar in advanced labor, that is, when cervical dilatation is more than 4 cm. or effacement is more than 80%, have not been established.

Contraindications: Yutopar is contraindicated before the 20th week of pregnancy.

Yutopar is also contraindicated in those conditions of the mother or fetus in which continuation of pregnancy is hazardous; specific contraindications include:

1. Antepartum hemorrhage which demands immediate delivery
2. Eclampsia and severe preeclampsia
3. Intrauterine fetal death
4. Chorioamnionitis
5. Maternal cardiac disease
6. Pulmonary hypertension
7. Maternal hyperthyroidism
8. Uncontrolled maternal diabetes mellitus (See PRECAUTIONS.)
9. Pre-existing maternal medical conditions that would be seriously affected by the known pharmacologic properties of a betamimetic drug; such as: hypovolemia, cardiac arrhythmias associated with tachycardia or digitalis intoxication, uncontrolled hypertension, pheochromocytoma, bronchial asthma already treated by betamimetics and/or steroids
10. Known hypersensitivity to any component of the product

Warnings:

Maternal pulmonary edema has been reported in patients treated with Yutopar, sometimes after delivery. It has occurred more often when patients were treated concomitantly with corticosteroids. Maternal death from this condition has been reported with or without corticosteroids given concomitantly with drugs of this class.

Patients so treated must be closely monitored in the hospital. The patient's state of hydration should be carefully monitored; fluid overload must be avoided. (See DOSAGE AND ADMINISTRATION.) Intravenous fluid loading may be aggravated by the use of betamimetics with or without corticosteroids and may turn into manifest circulatory overloading with subsequent pulmonary edema. If pulmonary edema develops during administration, the drug should be discontinueed. Edema should be managed by conventional means.

Intravenous administration of Yutopar should be supervised by persons having knowledge of the pharmacology of the drug and who are qualified to identify and manage complications of drug administration and pregnancy. *Because cardiovascular responses are common and more pronounced during intravenous administration of Yutopar, cardiovascular effects, including maternal pulse rate and blood pressure and fetal heart rate, should be closely monitored. Care should be exercised for maternal signs and symptoms of pulmonary edema. A persistent high tachycardia (over 140 beats per minute) may be one of the signs of impending pulmonary edema with drugs of this class. Occult cardiac disease may be unmasked with the use of Yutopar. If the patient complains of chest pain or tightness of chest, the drug should be temporarily discontinued and an ECG should be done as soon as possible.*

The drug should not be administered to patients with mild to moderate preeclampsia, hypertension, or diabetes unless the attending physician considers that the benefits clearly outweigh the risks.

Precautions: When Yutopar is used for the management of preterm labor in a patient with premature rupture of the membranes, the benefits of delaying delivery should be balanced against the potential risks of development of chorioamnionitis.

Among low birth weight infants, approximately 9% may be growth retarded for gestational age. Therefore, Intra-Uterine Growth Retardation (IUGR) should be considered in the differential diagnosis of preterm labor; this is especially important when the gestational age is in doubt. The decision to continue or reinitiate the administration of Yutopar will depend on an assessment of fetal maturity. In addition to clinical parameters, other studies, such as sonography or amniocentesis, may be helpful in establishing the state of fetal maturity if it is in doubt.

Laboratory Tests

Because intravenous administration of Yutopar has been shown to elevate plasma insulin and glucose and to decrease plasma potassium concentrations, monitoring of glucose and electrolyte levels is recommended during protracted infusions. Decrease of plasma potassium concentrations is usually transient, returning to normal within 24 hours. Special attention should be paid to biochemical variables when treating diabetic patients or those receiving potassium-depleting diuretics.

Serial hemograms may be helpful as an index of state of hydration.

Drug Interactions

Corticosteroids used concomitantly may lead to pulmonary edema. (see WARNINGS)

The effects of other sympathomimetic amines may be potentiated when concurrently administered and these effects may be additive. A sufficient time interval should elapse prior to administration of another sympathomimetic drug. With either oral or intravenous administration, 90% of the excretion of Yutopar is completed within 24 hours after the dose. (See CLINICAL PHARMACOLOGY.)

Beta-adrenergic blocking drugs inhibit the action of Yutopar; coadministration of these drugs should, therefore, be avoided.

With anesthetics used in surgery, the possibility that hypotensive effects may be potentiated should be considered.

Carcinogenesis, Mutagenesis, Impairment of Fertility

In rats given oral doses of 1, 10 and 150 mg./kg./day of ritodrine hydrochloride for 82 weeks, benign and malignant tumors were found in the various dosage groups. Since there were no important differences between untreated controls and treated groups and no dose-related trends, it was concluded that there was no evidence of tumorigenicity. The incidence (2–4%) of tumors of the type found in this study is not unusual in this species.

Reproduction studies in rats and rabbits have revealed no evidence of impaired fertility due to ritodrine hydrochloride.

Pregnancy

Teratogenic Effects

(Pregnancy Category B)

Reproduction studies were performed in rats and rabbits. The doses employed intravenously were 1/9 (1 mg./kg.), 1/3 (3 mg./kg.), and 1 (9 mg./kg.) times the maximum human daily intravenous dose (but given to the animals as a bolus rather than by infusion). The oral doses, 10 and 100 mg./kg. represented 5 and 50 times the maximum human daily oral maintenance dose. The results of these studies have revealed no evidence of impaired fertility or harm to the fetus due to ritodrine hydrochloride.

No adverse fetal effects were encountered when single intravenous doses of 1, 3, and 9 mg./kg./day or oral doses of 10 and 100 mg./kg./day were given to rats and rabbits on Days 6 through 15 and 6 through 18 of gestation, respectively. Intravenous doses of 1 and 8 mg./kg./day or oral doses of 10 and 100 mg./kg./day administered to the mother from Day 15 of pregnancy to Day 21 postpartum did not affect perinatal or postnatal development in rats. A slight increase in fetal weight in the rat was observed. Oral administration to both sexes did not impair fertility or reproductive performance. Lethal doses to pregnant rats did not cause immediate fetal demise. There are no adequate and well-controlled studies of Yutopar effects in pregnant women before 20 weeks' gestation; *therefore, this drug should not be used before the 20th week of pregnancy.* Studies of Yutopar administered to pregnant women from the 20th week of gestation have not shown increased risk of fetal abnormalities. Follow-up of selected variables in a small number of children for up to 2 years has not revealed harmful effects on growth, developmental or functional maturation. Nonetheless, although clinical studies did not demonstrate a risk of permanent adverse fetal effects from Yutopar, the possibility cannot be excluded; therefore, Yutopar should be used only when clearly indicated.

Some studies indicate that infants born before 36 weeks' gestation make up less than 10% of all births but account for as many as 75% of perinatal deaths and one-half of all neurologically handicapped infants. There are data available indicating that infants born at any time prior to full term may manifest a higher incidence of neurologic or other handicaps than occurs in the total population of infants born at or after full term. In delaying or preventing preterm labor, the use of Yutopar should result in an overall increase in neonatal survival. Handicapped infants who might not have otherwise survived may survive.

Adverse Reactions: The unwanted effects of Yutopar are related to its betamimetic activity and usually are controlled by suitable dosage adjustments.

Effects Associated with Intravenous Administration

Usual effects (80–100% of patients)

Intravenous infusion of Yutopar leads almost invariably to dose-related alterations in maternal and fetal heart rates and in maternal blood pressure. During clinical studies in which the maximum infusion rate was limited to 0.35 mg./min. (one patient received 0.40 mg./min.), the maximum maternal and fetal heart rates averaged, respectively, 130 (range 60 to 180) and 164 (range 130 to 200) beats per minute. The maximum maternal systolic blood pressures averaged 128 mm. Hg (range 96 to 162 mm. Hg), an average increase of 12 mm. Hg from pretreatment levels. The minimum maternal diastolic blood pressures averaged 48 mm. Hg (range 0 to 76 mm. Hg), an average decrease of 23 mm. Hg from pretreatment levels. While the more severe effects were usually managed effectively by dosage adjustments, in less than 1% of patients, persistent maternal tachycardia or decreased diastolic blood pressure required withdrawal of the drug. A persistent high tachycardia (over 140 beats per minute) may be one of the signs of impending pulmonary edema. (See WARNINGS.)

Yutopar infusion is associated with transient elevation of blood glucose and insulin, which decreases toward normal values after 48 to 72 hours despite continued infusion. Elevation of free fatty acids and cAMP has been reported. Reduction of potassium levels should be expected; other biochemical effects have not been reported.

Frequent effects (10–50% of patients)

Intravenous Yutopar, in about one-third of the patients, was associated with palpitation. Tremor, nausea, vomiting, headache, or erythema was observed in 10 to 15% of patients.

Occasional effects (5–10% of patients)

Nervousness, jitteriness, restlessness, emotional upset, or anxiety was reported in 5 to 6% of patients and malaise in similar numbers.

Infrequent effects (1–3% of patients)

Cardiac symptoms including chest pain or tightness (rarely associated with abnormalities of ECG) and arrhythmia were reported in 1 to 2% of patients. (See WARNINGS.)

Other infrequently reported maternal effects included: anaphylactic shock, rash, heart murmur, epigastric distress, ileus, bloating, constipation, diarrhea, dyspnea, hyperventilation, hemolytic icterus, glycosuria, lactic acidosis, sweating, chills, drowsiness, and weakness.

Neonatal Effects

Infrequently reported neonatal symptoms include hypoglycemia and ileus. In addition, hypocalcemia and hypotension have been reported in neonates whose mothers were treated with other betamimetic agents.

Effects Associated with Oral Administration

Frequent effects (≤ 50% of patients)

Oral ritodrine in clinical studies was often associated with small increases in maternal heart rate, but little or no effect upon either maternal systolic or diastolic blood pressure or upon fetal heart rate was found.

Oral ritodrine in 10 to 15% of patients was associated with palpitation or tremor. Nausea and jitterness were less frequent (5 to 8%), while rash was observed in some patients (3 to 4%), and arrhythmia was infrequent (about 1%).

Overdosage: The symptoms of overdosage are those of excessive beta-adrenergic stimulation including exaggeration of the known pharmacologic effects, the most prominent being tachycardia (maternal and fetal), palpitation, cardiac arrhythmia, hypotension, dyspnea, nervousness, tremor, nausea, and vomiting. If an excess of ritodrine tablets is ingested, gastric lavage or induction of emesis should be carried out followed by administration of activated charcoal. When symptoms of overdose occur as a result of intravenous administration, ritodrine should be discontinued; an appropriate beta-blocking agent may be used as an antidote. Ritodrine hydrochloride is dialyzable.

Acute intravenous toxicity was studied in rats and rabbits and acute oral toxicity in mice, rats, guinea pigs, and dogs. The LD50 values in the most sensitive of the species used were 64 mg./kg. intravenously in the nonpregnant rabbit and 540 mg./kg. orally in the nonpregnant mouse. The intravenous LD50 value in the pregnant rat was 85 mg./kg. The amount of drug required to produce symptoms of overdose in humans is individually variable. No reports of human mortality due to overdose have been received.

Dosage And Administration: In the management of preterm labor, the initial intravenous treatment should usually be followed by oral administration. The optimum dose of Yutopar is determined by a clinical balance of uterine response and unwanted effects.

Intravenous Therapy

Do not use intravenous Yutopar if the solution is discolored or contains any precipitate or particulate matter. Yutopar solution should be used promptly after preparation, but in no case after 48 hours of preparation.

Method of Administration: To minimize the risks of hypotension, the patient should be maintained in the left lateral position throughout infusion and careful attention given to her state of hydration, but fluid overload must be avoided.

For appropriate control and dose titration, a controlled infusion device is recommended to adjust the rate of flow in drops/minute. An i.v. microdrip chamber (60 drops/ml.) can provide a convenient range of infusion rates within the recommended dose range for Yutopar.

Recommended Dilution: 150 mg. ritodrine hydrochloride (3 ampuls) in 500 ml. fluid yielding a final concentration of 0.3 mg./ml. Ritodrine for intravenous infusion should be diluted with one of the following:

—0.9% w/v sodium chloride solution
—5% w/v dextrose solution
—10% w/v dextran 40 in 0.9% w/v sodium chloride solution
—10% w/v invert sugar solution
—Compound sodium chloride solution (Ringer's solution)
—Hartmann's solution

Intravenous therapy should be started as soon as possible after diagnosis. The usual initial dose is 0.1 mg./minute (0.33 ml./min., 20 drops/min. using a microdrip chamber at the recommended dilution), to be gradually increased according to the results by 0.05 mg./minute (0.17 ml./min., 10 drops/min. using a microdrip chamber at the recommended dilution) every 10 minutes until the desired result is attained. The effective dosage usually lies between 0.15 and 0.35 mg./minute (0.50 to 1.17 ml./min., 30–70 drops/min. using a microdrip chamber at the recommended dilution). Frequent monitoring of maternal uterine contractions, heart rate, and blood pressure, and of fetal heart rate is required, with dosage individually titrated according to response. If other drugs need to be given intravenously, the use of "piggyback" or other site of intravenous administration permits the continued independent control of the rate of infusion of the Yutopar.

The infusion should generally be continued for at least 12 hours after uterine contractions cease. With the recommended dilution, the maximum volume of fluid that might be administered after 12 hours at the highest dose (0.35 mg./min.) will be approximately 840 ml. *The amount of i.v. fluids administered and the rate of administration should be monitored to avoid circulatory fluid overload (over-hydration) or inadequate hydration.* (See PRECAUTIONS, *Laboratory Tests.*)

Oral Maintenance

One tablet (10 mg.) may be given approximately 30 minutes before the termination of intravenous therapy. The usual dosage schedule for the first 24 hours of oral administration

Astra—Cont.

is 1 tablet (10 mg.) every two hours. Thereafter, the usual maintenance is 1 or 2 tablets (10 to 20 mg.) every four to six hours, the dose depending on uterine activity and unwanted effects. The total daily dose of oral ritodrine should not exceed 120 mg. The treatment may be continued as long as the physician considers it desirable to prolong pregnancy.
Recurrence of unwanted preterm labor may be treated with repeated infusion of Yutopar.

How Supplied:

NDC 0186-0599-53: 5 ml. ampuls in boxes of 12. Each ampul contains 50 mg. (10 mg./ml.) of ritodrine hydrochloride.

NDC 0186-0595-60: 10 mg. tablets in bottles of 60. Each round, yellow tablet contains 10 mg. ritodrine hydrochloride and is inscribed YUTOPAR on one side and scored on the other.

Product information as of October, 1982

Both the tablet and intravenous dosage forms should be stored at room temperature, preferably below 86°F. (30°C). Protect from excessive heat.

Parenteral (intravenous) dosage form manufactured by Taylor Pharmacal Company
Decatur, Illinois 62525

Oral dosage form manufactured by Merrell Dow Pharmaceuticals Inc.
Subsidiary of The Dow Chemical Company
Cincinnati, Ohio 45215, U.S.A.

Distributed by:
ASTRA®
Astra Pharmaceuticals Products, Inc.
Worcester, Massachusetts 01606
Yutopar® licensed by Duphar B. V. Amsterdam, Holland

Ayerst Laboratories

Division of American Home Products Corporation
685 THIRD AVE.
NEW YORK, NY 10017

ANTABUSE® ℞
Brand of disulfiram
In Alcoholism

Description: CHEMICAL NAME: bis(diethylthiocarbamoyl) disulfide STRUCTURAL FORMULA:

$$(C_2H_5)_2N-\underset{\underset{S}{\|}}{C}-S-S-\underset{\underset{S}{\|}}{C}-N(C_2H_5)_2$$

ANTABUSE occurs as a white to off-white, odorless, and almost tasteless powder, soluble in water to the extent of about 20 mg in 100 ml, and in alcohol to the extent of about 3.8 g in 100 ml.

Action: ANTABUSE produces a sensitivity to alcohol which results in a highly unpleasant reaction when the patient under treatment ingests even small amounts of alcohol.

ANTABUSE blocks the oxidation of alcohol at the acetaldehyde stage. During alcohol metabolism after ANTABUSE intake, the concentration of acetaldehyde occurring in the blood may be 5 to 10 times higher than that found during metabolism of the same amount of alcohol alone.

Accumulation of acetaldehyde in the blood produces the complex of highly unpleasant symptoms referred to hereinafter as the ANTABUSE-alcohol reaction. This reaction, which is proportional to the dosage of both ANTABUSE (disulfiram) and alcohol, will persist as long as alcohol is being metabolized. ANTABUSE does not appear to influence the rate of alcohol elimination from the body.

ANTABUSE is slowly absorbed from the gastrointestinal tract and is slowly eliminated from the body. One (or even two) weeks after a patient has taken his last dose of ANTABUSE, ingestion of alcohol may produce unpleasant symptoms.

Prolonged administration of ANTABUSE does not produce tolerance; the longer a patient remains on therapy, the more exquisitely sensitive he becomes to alcohol.

Indication: ANTABUSE (disulfiram) is an aid in the management of selected chronic alcoholic patients who want to remain in a state of enforced sobriety so that supportive and psychotherapeutic treatment may be applied to best advantage. (Used alone, without proper motivation and without supportive therapy, ANTABUSE is not a cure for alcoholism, and it is unlikely that it will have more than a brief effect on the drinking pattern of the chronic alcoholic).

Contraindications: Patients who are receiving or have recently received metronidazole, paraldehyde, alcohol, or alcohol-containing preparations, *e.g.* cough syrups, tonics and the like, should not be given ANTABUSE.

ANTABUSE is contraindicated in the presence of severe myocardial disease or coronary occlusion, psychoses, and hypersensitivity to disulfiram or to other thiuram derivatives used in pesticides and rubber vulcanization.

Warnings

> ANTABUSE should never be administered to a patient when he is in a state of alcohol intoxication or without his full knowledge.
> The physician should instruct relatives accordingly.

The patient must be fully informed of the ANTABUSE-alcohol reaction. He must be strongly cautioned against surreptitious drinking while taking the drug and he must be fully aware of possible consequences. He should be warned to avoid alcohol in disguised form, *i.e.* in sauces, vinegars, cough mixtures, and even aftershave lotions and back rubs. He should also be warned that reactions may occur with alcohol up to 14 days after ingesting ANTABUSE.

The ANTABUSE-ALCOHOL REACTION: ANTABUSE plus alcohol, even small amounts, produces flushing, throbbing in head and neck, throbbing headache, respiratory difficulty, nausea, copious vomiting, sweating, thirst, chest pain, palpitation, dyspnea, hyperventilation, tachycardia, hypotension, syncope, marked uneasiness, weakness, vertigo, blurred vision, and confusion. In severe reactions there may be respiratory depression, cardiovascular collapse, arrhythmias, myocardial infarction, acute congestive heart failure, unconsciousness, convulsions, and death.

The intensity of the reaction varies with each individual, but is generally proportional to the amounts of ANTABUSE (disulfiram) and alcohol ingested. Mild reactions may occur in the sensitive individual when the blood alcohol concentration is increased to as little as 5 to 10 mg per 100 ml. Symptoms are fully developed at 50 mg per 100 ml and unconsciousness usually results when the blood alcohol level reaches 125 to 150 mg.

The duration of the reaction varies from 30 to 60 minutes to several hours in the more severe cases, or as long as there is alcohol in the blood.

DRUG INTERACTIONS: Disulfiram appears to decrease the rate at which certain drugs are metabolized and so may increase the blood levels and the possibility of clinical toxicity of drugs given concomitantly.

DISULFIRAM SHOULD BE USED WITH CAUTION IN THOSE PATIENTS RECEIVING PHENYTOIN AND ITS CONGENERS, SINCE THE CONCOMITANT ADMINISTRATION OF THESE TWO DRUGS CAN LEAD TO PHENYTOIN INTOXICATION. PRIOR TO ADMINISTERING DISULFIRAM TO A PATIENT ON PHENYTOIN THERAPY, A BASELINE PHENYTOIN SERUM LEVEL SHOULD BE OBTAINED. SUBSEQUENT TO INITIATION OF DISULFIRAM THERAPY, SERUM LEVELS ON PHENYTOIN SHOULD BE DETERMINED ON DIFFERENT DAYS FOR EVIDENCE OF AN INCREASE OR FOR A CONTINUING RISE IN LEVELS. INCREASED PHENYTOIN LEVELS SHOULD BE TREATED WITH APPROPRIATE DOSAGE ADJUSTMENT.

It may be necessary to adjust the dosage of oral anticoagulants upon beginning or stopping disulfiram, since disulfiram may prolong prothrombin time.

Patients taking isoniazid when disulfiram is given should be observed for the appearance of unsteady gait or marked changes in mental status and the disulfiram discontinued if such signs appear.

In rats, simultaneous ingestion of disulfiram and nitrite in the diet for 78 weeks has been reported to cause tumors, and it has been suggested that disulfiram may react with nitrites in the rat stomach to form a nitrosamine which is tumorigenic. Disulfiram alone in the diet of rats did not lead to such tumors. The relevance of this finding to humans is not known at this time.

CONCOMITANT CONDITIONS: Because of the possibility of an accidental ANTABUSE-alcohol reaction, ANTABUSE (disulfiram) should be used with extreme caution in patients with any of the following conditions: diabetes mellitus, hypothyroidism, epilepsy, cerebral damage, chronic and acute nephritis, hepatic cirrhosis or insufficiency.

USAGE IN PREGNANCY: The safe use of this drug in pregnancy has not been established. Therefore, ANTABUSE should be used during pregnancy only when, in the judgment of the physician, the probable benefits outweigh the possible risks.

Precautions: Patients with a history of rubber contact dermatitis should be evaluated for hypersensitivity to thiuram derivatives before receiving ANTABUSE (See Contraindications).

It is suggested that every patient under treatment carry an Identification Card, stating that he is receiving ANTABUSE and describing the symptoms most likely to occur as a result of the ANTABUSE-alcohol reaction. In addition, this card should indicate the physician or institution to be contacted in emergency. (Cards may be obtained from Ayerst Laboratories upon request.)

Alcoholism may accompany or be followed by dependence on narcotics or sedatives. Barbiturates have been administered concurrently with ANTABUSE without untoward effects, but the possibility of initiating a new abuse should be considered.

Baseline and follow-up transaminase tests (10–14 days) are suggested to detect any hepatic dysfunction that may result with ANTABUSE therapy. In addition, a complete blood count and a sequential multiple analysis-12 (SMA-12) test should be made every six months.

Patients taking ANTABUSE Tablets should not be exposed to ethylene dibromide or its vapors. This precaution is based on preliminary results of animal research currently in progress which suggests a toxic interaction between inhaled ethylene dibromide and ingested disulfiram resulting in a higher incidence of tumors and mortality in rats. Correlation of this finding to humans, however, has not been demonstrated.

Adverse Reactions: (See Contraindications, Warnings, and Precautions.)

OPTIC NEURITIS, PERIPHERAL NEURITIS AND POLYNEURITIS MAY OCCUR FOLLOWING ADMINISTRATION OF ANTABUSE.

Occasional skin eruptions are, as a rule, readily controlled by concomitant administration of an antihistaminic drug.

In a small number of patients, a transient mild drowsiness, fatigability, impotence, headache, acneform eruptions, allergic dermatitis, or a metallic or garlic-like aftertaste may be experienced during the first two weeks of therapy. These complaints usually disappear spontaneously with the continuation of therapy or with reduced dosage.

Psychotic reactions have been noted, attributable in most cases to high dosage, combined toxicity (with metronidazole or isoniazid), or to the unmasking of underlying psychoses in patients stressed by the withdrawal of alcohol.

One case of cholestatic hepatitis has been reported, but its relationship to ANTABUSE has not been unequivocally established.

Dosage and Administration: ANTABUSE (disulfiram) should never be administered until the patient has abstained from alcohol for at least 12 hours.

INITIAL DOSAGE SCHEDULE: In the first phase of treatment, a maximum of 500 mg daily is given in a single dose for one to two weeks. Although usually taken in the morning, ANTABUSE may be taken on retiring by patients who experience a sedative effect. Alternatively, to minimize, or eliminate, the sedative effect, dosage may be adjusted downward.

MAINTENANCE REGIMEN: The average maintenance dose is 250 mg daily (range, 125 to 500 mg); it should not exceed 500 mg daily.

NOTE: Occasional patients, while seemingly on adequate maintenance doses of ANTABUSE, report that they are able to drink alcoholic beverages with impunity and without any symptomatology. All appearances to the contrary, such patients must be presumed to be disposing of their tablets in some manner without actually taking them. Until such patients have been observed reliably taking their daily ANTABUSE tablets (preferably crushed and well mixed with liquid), it cannot be concluded that ANTABUSE is ineffective.

DURATION OF THERAPY: The daily, uninterrupted administration of ANTABUSE (disulfiram) must be continued until the patient is fully recovered socially and a basis for permanent self-control is established. Depending on the individual patient, maintenance therapy may be required for months or even years.

TRIAL WITH ALCOHOL: During early experience with ANTABUSE, it was thought advisable for each patient to have at least one supervised alcohol-drug reaction. More recently, the test reaction has been largely abandoned. Furthermore, such a test reaction should never be administered to a patient over 50 years of age. A clear, detailed, and convincing description of the reaction is felt to be sufficient in most cases.

However, where a test reaction is deemed necessary, the suggested procedure is as follows:

After the first one to two weeks' therapy with 500 mg daily, a drink of 15 ml (½ oz) of 100 proof whiskey or equivalent is taken slowly. This test dose of alcoholic beverage may be repeated once only so that the total dose does not exceed 30 ml (1 oz) of whiskey. Once a reaction develops, no more alcohol should be consumed. Such tests should be carried out only when the patient is hospitalized, or comparable supervision and facilities, including oxygen, are available.

MANAGEMENT OF ANTABUSE-ALCOHOL REACTION: In severe reactions, whether caused by an excessive test dose or by the patient's unsupervised ingestion of alcohol, supportive measures to restore blood pressure and treat shock should be instituted. Other recommendations include: oxygen, carbogen (95 per cent oxygen and 5 per cent carbon dioxide), vitamin C intravenously in massive doses (1 g), and ephedrine sulfate. Antihistamines have also been used intravenously. Potassium levels should be monitored particularly in patients on digitalis since hypokalemia has been reported.

How Supplied: ANTABUSE—Each tablet (scored) contains 250 mg disulfiram, in bottles of 100 (NDC 0046-0809-81)—Each tablet (scored) contains 500 mg disulfiram, in bottles of 50 (NDC 0046-0810-50) and 1,000 (NDC 0046-0810-91).

[*Shown in Product Identification Section*]

A.P.L.® ℞

Brand of chorionic gonadotropin for injection, U.S.P.

For Intramuscular Injection Only

Description: Human chorionic gonadotropin (HCG), a polypeptide hormone produced by the human placenta, is composed of an alpha and a beta subunit. The alpha subunit is essentially identical to the alpha subunits of the human pituitary gonadotropins, luteinizing hormone (LH) and follicle-stimulating hormone (FSH), as well as to the alpha subunit of human thyroid stimulating hormone (TSH). The beta subunits of these hormones differ in amino acid sequence.

A.P.L. (chorionic gonadotropin, U.S.P.) is a gonad-stimulating principle obtained from the urine of pregnant women. It is an amorphous powder prepared by cryodesiccation, and is freely soluble in water.

Actions: The action of HCG is virtually identical to that of pituitary LH, although HCG appears to have a small degree of FSH activity as well. It stimulates production of gonadal steroid hormones by stimulating the interstitial cells (Leydig cells) of the testis to produce androgens and the corpus luteum of the ovary to produce progesterone. Androgen stimulation in the male leads to the development of secondary sex characteristics and may stimulate testicular descent when no anatomical impediment to descent is present. This descent is usually reversible when HCG is discontinued. During the normal menstrual cycle, LH participates with FSH in the development and maturation of the normal ovarian follicle, and the midcycle LH surge triggers ovulation. HCG can substitute for LH in this function.

During a normal pregnancy, HCG secreted by the placenta maintains the corpus luteum after LH secretion decreases, supporting continued secretion of estrogen and progesterone, and preventing menstruation. HCG HAS NO KNOWN EFFECT ON FAT MOBILIZATION, APPETITE OR SENSE OF HUNGER, OR BODY FAT DISTRIBUTION.

Indications: HCG HAS NOT BEEN DEMONSTRATED TO BE EFFECTIVE ADJUNCTIVE THERAPY IN THE TREATMENT OF OBESITY. THERE IS NO SUBSTANTIAL EVIDENCE THAT IT INCREASES WEIGHT LOSS BEYOND THAT RESULTING FROM CALORIC RESTRICTION, THAT IT CAUSES A MORE ATTRACTIVE OR "NORMAL" DISTRIBUTION OF FAT, OR THAT IT DECREASES THE HUNGER AND DISCOMFORT ASSOCIATED WITH CALORIE RESTRICTED DIETS.

1. Cryptorchidism not due to anatomic obstruction. In general, A.P.L. (Chorionic Gonadotropin for Injection, U.S.P.) is thought to induce testicular descent in situations when descent would have occurred at puberty. A.P.L. thus may help to predict whether or not orchiopexy will be needed in the future. Although, in some cases, descent following A.P.L. administration is permanent, in most cases the response is temporary. Therapy is usually instituted between the ages of 4 and 9.
2. Selected cases of male hypogonadism secondary to pituitary failure.
3. Induction of ovulation and pregnancy in the anovulatory, infertile woman in whom the cause of anovulation is secondary and not due to ovarian failure, and who has been appropriately pretreated with human menotropins.

Contraindications: Precocious puberty, prostatic carcinoma or other androgen-dependent neoplasia, prior allergic reaction to chorionic gonadotropin.

Warnings: HCG should be used in conjunction with human menopausal gonadotropins only by physicians experienced with infertility problems who are familiar with the criteria for patient selection, contraindications, warnings, precautions, and adverse reactions described in the package insert for menotropins. The principal serious adverse reactions during this use are: (1) ovarian enlargement, ascites with or without pain, and/or pleural effusion, (2) rupture of ovarian cysts with resultant hemoperitoneum, (3) multiple births, and (4) arterial thromboembolism.

Precautions: Induction of androgen secretion by chorionic gonadotropin may induce precocious puberty in patients treated for cryptorchidism. If signs of precocious puberty occur, therapy should be discontinued.

Since androgens may cause fluid retention, chorionic gonadotropin should be used with caution in patients with epilepsy, migraine, asthma, cardiac or renal disease.

Adverse Reactions:

Headache
Irritability
Restlessness
Depression
Tiredness
Edema
Precocious puberty
Gynecomastia
Pain at site of injection

Dosage and Administration: There is a marked variance of opinion concerning the dosage regimens to be used. Therefore the regimen employed in any particular case will depend upon the indication for use, the age and weight of the patient, and the physician's preference. The following regimens have been advocated by various authorities.

Cryptorchidism: (Therapy is usually instituted between the ages of 4 and 9.)

(1) 4,000 U.S.P. Units three times weekly for three weeks.

(2) 5,000 U.S.P. Units every second day for four injections.

(3) 15 injections of 500 to 1,000 U.S.P. Units over a period of six weeks.

(4) 500 U.S.P. Units three times weekly for four to six weeks. If this course of treatment is not successful, another is begun one month later, giving 1,000 U.S.P. Units per injection.

Selected cases of male hypogonadism secondary to pituitary failure:

(1) 500 to 1,000 U.S.P. Units three times a week for three weeks, followed by the same dose twice a week for three weeks.

(2) 1,000 to 2,000 U.S.P. Units three times weekly.

(3) 4,000 U.S.P. Units three times weekly for six to nine months, following which the dosage may be reduced to 2,000 U.S.P. Units three times weekly for an additional three months.

Induction of ovulation and pregnancy in the anovulatory, infertile woman in whom the cause of anovulation is secondary:

5,000 to 10,000 U.S.P. Units one day following the last dose of menotropins.

How Supplied: A.P.L. (Chorionic Gonadotropin for Injection, U.S.P.)

NDC 0046-0970-10 — Each package provides:
(1) One vial containing 5,000 U.S.P. Units chorionic gonadotropin in dry form, and
(2) One 10 ml ampul sterile diluent.

NDC 0046-0971-10 — Each package provides:
(1) One vial containing 10,000 U.S.P. Units chorionic gonadotropin in dry form, and
(2) One 10 ml ampul sterile diluent.

NDC 0046-0972-10 — Each package provides:
(1) One vial containing 20,000 U.S.P. Units chorionic gonadotropin in dry form, and

Continued on next page

Ayerst—Cont.

(2) One 10 ml ampul sterile diluent.

When reconstituted with 10 ml of accompanying sterile diluent, the resulting solutions also contain 2.0% benzyl alcohol, not more than 0.2% phenol, and the following concentrations of lactose: No. 970, 0.9%; No. 971, 1.8%; No. 972, 3.6%. The pH is adjusted with sodium hydroxide or hydrochloric acid.

MAY BE STORED FOR 90 DAYS IN A REFRIGERATOR AFTER RECONSTITUTION.

ATROMID-S® ℞

Brand of clofibrate

Antilipidemic agent for reduction of elevated serum lipids

Actions: ATROMID-S is an antilipidemic agent. It acts to lower elevated serum lipids by reducing the very low density lipoprotein fraction (S_f20–400) rich in triglycerides. Serum cholesterol, especially the low density lipoprotein fraction (S_f0–20), is also decreased, particularly in those whose cholesterol levels are elevated at the outset.

The mechanism of action has not been established definitively. In man, clofibrate reduces cholesterol formation early in the biosynthetic chain. In addition, clofibrate has been shown to cause increased excretion of neutral sterols.

Animal studies suggest that clofibrate interrupts cholesterol biosynthesis prior to mevalonate formation.

Indications: Drug therapy should not be used for the routine treatment of elevated blood lipids for the prevention of coronary heart disease. Dietary therapy specific for the type of hyperlipidemia is the initial treatment of choice.[1] Excess body weight and alcoholic intake may be important factors in hypertriglyceridemia and should be addressed prior to any drug therapy. Physical exercise can be an important ancillary measure. Contributory diseases such as hypothyroidism or diabetes mellitus should be looked for and adequately treated. The use of drugs should be considered only when reasonable attempts have been made to obtain satisfactory results with non-drug methods. If the decision ultimately is to use drugs, the patient should be instructed that this does not reduce the importance of adhering to diet.

Because ATROMID-S (clofibrate) is associated with certain serious adverse findings reported in two large clinical trials (see WARNINGS), agents other than clofibrate may be more suitable for a particular patient.

ATROMID-S is indicated for Primary Dysbetalipoproteinemia (Type III hyperlipidemia) that does not respond adequately to diet.

ATROMID-S may be considered for the treatment of adult patients with very high serum triglyceride levels (Types IV and V hyperlipidemia) who present a risk of abdominal pain and pancreatitis and who do not respond adequately to a determined dietary effort to control them. Patients with triglyceride levels in excess of 750 mg per deciliter are likely to present such risk.

ATROMID-S has little effect on the elevated cholesterol levels of most subjects with hypercholesterolemia. A minority of subjects show a more pronounced response. However, it must be understood that there is no evidence that use of any lipid-altering agent will be beneficial in preventing death from coronary heart disease (See Warnings). Therefore, the physician should be very selective and confine clofibrate treatment to patients with clearly defined risk due to severe hypercholesterolemia (*e.g.* individuals with familial hypercholesterolemia starting in childhood) who inadequately respond to appropriate diet and more effective cholesterol-lowering drugs.

ATROMID-S is not useful for the hypertriglyceridemia of Type I hyperlipidemia.

The biochemical response to ATROMID-S (clofibrate) is variable, and it is not always possible to predict from the lipoprotein type or other factors which patients will obtain favorable results. It is essential that lipid levels be assessed and that the drug be discontinued in any patient in whom lipids do not show significant improvement.

Contraindications: Clofibrate is contraindicated in pregnant women. While teratogenic studies have not demonstrated any effect attributable to clofibrate, it is known that serum of the rabbit fetus accumulates a higher concentration of clofibrate than that found in maternal serum, and it is possible that the fetus may not have developed the enzyme system required for the excretion of clofibrate.

It is contraindicated in lactating women since it is not known if clofibrate is secreted in the milk.

It is contraindicated in patients with clinically significant hepatic or renal dysfunction.

It is contraindicated in patients with primary biliary cirrhosis since it may raise the already elevated cholesterol in these cases.

Warnings

In a large prospective study involving 5,000 patients in a clofibrate-treated group and 5,000 in a placebo-treated group followed for an average of five years on drug or placebo and one year beyond (the WHO study), there was a statistically significant 36% higher mortality due to noncardiovascular causes in the clofibrate-treated group than in a comparable placebo group. Half of this difference was due to malignancy; other causes of death included post-cholecystectomy complications and pancreatitis.[2] In another prospective study involving 1,000 clofibrate- and 3,000 placebo-treated patients followed for an average of six years on drug or placebo (the Coronary Drug Project study), the noncardiovascular mortality rate, including that of malignancy, was not significantly different in the clofibrate- and placebo-treated groups.[3] This should not be interpreted to mean that clofibrate is not associated with an increased risk of noncardiovascular death because the patients in the Coronary Drug Project were much older than those in the WHO study and they all had had a previous myocardial infarction so that the deaths in the Coronary Drug Project were overwhelmingly due to cardiovascular causes and it would have been very difficult to discern a clofibrate-associated risk of death due to noncardiovascular causes if it existed. Both studies demonstrated that clofibrate users have twice the risk of developing cholelithiasis and cholecystitis requiring surgery as do nonusers.

A potential benefit of clofibrate was, however, reported in the WHO study which involved patients with hypercholesterolemia and no history of myocardial infarction or angina pectoris. In this study, there was noted a statistically significant 25% decrease in subsequent nonfatal myocardial infarctions in the clofibrate-treated group when compared with the placebo group. There was no difference in incidence of fatal myocardial infarction in the two groups. If the study had been continued longer, had included diet, had been restricted to patients who had both hyperlipidemia and increased risk factors *and* who obtained significant clofibrate-induced reduction in serum lipids, it is possible that it may have shown a decrease in fatal myocardial infarctions. In the Coronary Drug Project study, which involved patients with or without hypercholesterolemia and/or hypertriglyceridemia and with a history of previous myocardial infarction, there was no significant difference in incidence of either nonfatal or fatal myocardial infarction between the clofibrate- and placebo-treated groups.[2]

As a result of these and other studies, the following can be stated:

1. Clofibrate, in general, causes a relatively modest reduction of serum cholesterol and a somewhat greater reduction of serum triglycerides. In Type III hyperlipidemia, however, substantial reductions of both cholesterol and triglycerides can occur with use of clofibrate.
2. No study to date has shown a convincing reduction in incidence of *fatal* myocardial infarction.
3. A significantly increased incidence of cholelithiasis has been demonstrated consistently in clofibrate-treated groups, and an increase in morbidity from this complication and mortality from cholecystectomy must be anticipated during clofibrate treatment.
4. Several types of other undesirable events have been associated in a statistically significant way with clofibrate administration in the WHO or the Coronary Drug Project studies. There was an increase in incidence of noncardiovascular deaths reported in the WHO study. There was an increase in cardiac arrhythmias and intermittent claudication and in definite or suspected thromboembolic events and angina reported in the Coronary Drug Project, which was not, however, reported in the WHO study.
5. Administration of clofibrate to mice and rats in long-term studies at eight times the human dose, and to rats at five times the human dose, resulted in a higher incidence of benign and malignant liver tumors than in controls. Lower doses were not included in these studies.

BECAUSE OF THE HEPATIC TUMORIGENICITY OF CLOFIBRATE IN RODENTS AND THE POSSIBLE INCREASED RISK OF MALIGNANCY ASSOCIATED WITH CLOFIBRATE IN THE HUMAN, AS WELL AS THE INCREASED RISK OF CHOLELITHIASIS, AND BECAUSE THERE IS NOT, TO DATE, SUBSTANTIAL EVIDENCE OF A BENEFICIAL EFFECT ON CARDIOVASCULAR MORTALITY FROM CLOFIBRATE, THIS DRUG SHOULD BE UTILIZED ONLY FOR THOSE PATIENTS DESCRIBED IN THE INDICATIONS SECTION, AND SHOULD BE DISCONTINUED IF SIGNIFICANT LIPID RESPONSE IS NOT OBTAINED.

Concomitant Anticoagulants

CAUTION SHOULD BE EXERCISED WHEN ANTICOAGULANTS ARE GIVEN IN CONJUNCTION WITH ATROMID-S (CLOFIBRATE). THE DOSAGE OF THE ANTICOAGULANT SHOULD BE REDUCED USUALLY BY ONE-HALF (DEPENDING ON THE INDIVIDUAL CASE) TO MAINTAIN THE PROTHROMBIN TIME AT THE DESIRED LEVEL TO PREVENT BLEEDING COMPLICATIONS. FREQUENT PROTHROMBIN DETERMINATIONS ARE ADVISABLE UNTIL IT HAS BEEN DEFINITELY DETERMINED THAT THE PROTHROMBIN LEVEL HAS BEEN STABILIZED.

Avoidance of Pregnancy

Strict birth control procedures must be exercised by women of childbearing potential. In patients who plan to become pregnant, clofibrate should be withdrawn several months before conception. Because of the possibility of pregnancy occurring despite birth control precautions in patients taking clofibrate, the possible benefits of the drug to the patient must be weighed against possible hazards to the fetus.

Precautions: Before instituting therapy with clofibrate, attempts should be made to control serum lipids with appropriate dietary regimens, weight loss in obese patients, control of diabetes mellitus, etc.

Because of the long-term administration of a drug of this nature, adequate baseline studies should be performed to determine that the patient has significantly elevated serum lipid levels. Frequent determinations of serum lipids should be obtained during the first few months of ATROMID-S (clofibrate) administration, and periodic determinations thereafter. The drug should be withdrawn after three months if response is inadequate. However, in the case of xanthoma tuberosum, the drug should be employed for longer periods (even up to one year) provided that there is a reduction in the size and/or number of the xanthomata.

Subsequent serum lipid determinations should be done to detect a paradoxical rise in serum cholesterol or triglyceride levels. Clofibrate will not alter the seasonal variations of serum cholesterol peak elevations in midwinter and late summer and decreases in fall and spring. If the drug is discontinued, the patient should be continued on an appropriate hypolipidemic diet, and his serum lipids should be monitored until stabilized, as a rise in these values to or above the original baseline may occur.

During clofibrate therapy, frequent serum transaminase determinations and other liver function tests should be performed since the drug may produce abnormalities in these parameters. These effects are usually reversible when the drug is discontinued. Hepatic biopsies are usually within normal limits. If the hepatic function tests steadily rise or show excessive abnormalities, the drug should be withdrawn. Therefore use with caution in those patients with a past history of jaundice or hepatic disease.

Since cholelithiasis is a possible side effect of clofibrate therapy, appropriate diagnostic procedures should be performed if signs and symptoms related to disease of the biliary system should occur.

Clofibrate may produce "flu like" symptoms (muscular aching, soreness, cramping). The physician should differentiate this from actual viral and/or bacterial disease.

Use with caution in patients with peptic ulcer since reactivation has been reported. Whether this is drug-related is unknown.

Complete blood counts should be done periodically since anemia, and more frequently, leukopenia have been reported in patients who have been taking clofibrate.

Various cardiac arrhythmias have been reported with the use of clofibrate.

Several investigators have observed in their studies that clofibrate may produce a decrease in cholesterol linoleate but an increase in palmitoleate and oleate, the latter being considered atherogenic in experimental animals. The significance of this finding is unknown at this time.

Adverse Reactions: Of the pertinent reactions, the most common is nausea. Less frequently encountered gastrointestinal reactions are vomiting, loose stools, dyspepsia, flatulence, and abdominal distress. Reactions reported less often than gastrointestinal ones are headache, dizziness, and fatigue; muscle cramping, aching, and weakness; skin rash, urticaria, and pruritus; dry brittle hair, and alopecia.

The following reported adverse reactions are listed alphabetically by systems:

Cardiovascular
- Increased or decreased angina
- Cardiac arrhythmias
- Both swelling and phlebitis at site of xanthomas

Dermatologic
- Skin rash
- Alopecia
- Allergic reaction including urticaria
- Dry skin and dry brittle hair
- Puritus

Gastrointestinal
- Nausea
- Diarrhea
- Gastrointestinal upset (bloating, flatulence, abdominal distress)
- Hepatomegaly (not associated with hepatotoxicity)
- Gallstones
- Vomiting
- Stomatitis and gastritis

Genitourinary
- Impotence and decreased libido
- Findings consistent with renal dysfunction as evidenced by dysuria, hematuria, proteinuria, decreased urine output. One patient's renal biopsy suggested "allergic reaction."

Hematologic
- Leukopenia
- Potentiation of anticoagulant effect
- Anemia
- Eosinophilia

Musculoskeletal
- Myalgia (muscle cramping, aching, weakness)
- "Flu like" symptoms
- Arthralgia

Neurologic
- Fatigue, weakness, drowsiness
- Dizziness
- Headache

Miscellaneous
- Weight gain
- Polyphagia

Laboratory Findings
- Abnormal liver function tests as evidenced by increased transaminase (SGOT and SGPT), BSP retention, and increased thymol turbidity
- Proteinuria
- Increased creatine phosphokinase

Reported adverse reactions whose direct relationship with the drug has not been established: peptic ulcer, gastrointestinal hemorrhage, rheumatoid arthritis, tremors, increased perspiration, systemic lupus erythematosus, blurred vision, gynecomastia, thrombocytopenic purpura.

Dosage and Administration:
Initial: The recommended dosage for adults is 2 g daily in divided doses. Some patients may respond to a lower dosage.
Maintenance: Same as for initial dosage.
Note: In children, insufficient studies have been done to show safety and efficacy.

Drug Interactions: Caution should be exercised when anticoagulants are given in conjunction with ATROMID-S (clofibrate). The dosage of the anticoagulant should be reduced usually by one-half (depending on the individual case) to maintain the prothrombin time at the desired level to prevent bleeding complications. Frequent prothrombin determinations are advisable until it has been definitely determined that the prothrombin level has been stabilized.

Management of Overdosage: While there has been no reported case of overdosage, should it occur, symptomatic supportive measures should be taken.

How Supplied: ATROMID-S—Each capsule contains 500 mg clofibrate, in bottles of 100 (NDC 0046-0243-81).

References:

1. Coronary Risk Handbook (1973), American Heart Association.
2. Report from the Committee of Principal Investigators: A cooperative trial in the primary prevention of ischaemic heart disease using clofibrate, Br. Heart J. *40:*1069, 1978.
3. The Coronary Drug Project Research Group: Clofibrate and niacin in coronary heart disease, J.A.M.A. *231:*360, 1975.

[*Shown in Product Identification Section*]

AURALGAN® Otic Solution ℞

Each ml contains:
Antipyrine ....54.0 mg
Benzocaine ....14.0 mg
Glycerin dehydrated q.s. to ....1.0 ml
(contains not more than 0.6% moisture)
(also contains oxyquinoline sulfate)

TOPICAL DECONGESTANT AND ANALGESIC

AURALGAN is an otic solution containing antipyrine, benzocaine, and dehydrated glycerin. The solution congeals at 0° C (32° F), but returns to normal consistency, unchanged, at room temperature.

Clinical Pharmacology: AURALGAN combines the hygroscopic property of dehydrated glycerin with the analgesic action of antipyrine and benzocaine to relieve pressure, reduce inflammation and congestion, and alleviate pain and discomfort in acute otitis media. AURALGAN does not blanch the tympanic membrane or mask the landmarks and, therefore, does not distort the otoscopic picture.

Indications and Usage: *Acute otitis media of various etiologies*
—prompt relief of pain and reduction of inflammation in the congestive and serous stages
—adjuvant therapy during systemic antibiotic administration for resolution of the infection

Because of the close anatomical relationship of the eustachian tube to the nasal cavity, otitis media is a frequent problem, especially in children in whom the tube is shorter, wider, and more horizontal than in adults.

Removal of cerumen
—facilitates the removal of excessive or impacted cerumen.

Contraindications: Hypersensitivity to any of the components or substances related to them.
In the presence of spontaneous perforation or discharge.

Precautions: *Carcinogenesis, Mutagenesis, Impairment of Fertility:* No long-term studies in animals or humans have been conducted.
Pregnancy Category C: Animal reproduction studies have not been conducted with AURALGAN. It is also not known whether AURALGAN can cause fetal harm when administered to a pregnant woman, or can affect reproduction capacity. AURALGAN should be given to a pregnant woman only if clearly needed.
Nursing Mothers: It is not known whether this drug is excreted in human milk. Because many drugs are excreted in human milk, caution should be exercised when AURALGAN is administered to a nursing woman.

Dosage and Administration: *Acute otitis media:* Instill AURALGAN, permitting the solution to run along the wall of the canal until it is filled. Avoid touching the ear with dropper. Then moisten a cotton pledget with AURALGAN and insert into meatus. Repeat every one to two hours until pain and congestion are relieved.

Removal of cerumen
Before: Instill AURALGAN three times daily for two or three days to help detach cerumen from wall of canal and facilitate removal.
After: AURALGAN is useful for drying out the canal or relieving discomfort.

Before and after removal of cerumen, a cotton pledget moistened with AURALGAN should be inserted into the meatus following instillation.

NOTE: Do not rinse dropper after use. Replace in bottle and screw cap tightly.

Continued on next page

Ayerst—Cont.

How Supplied: AURALGAN® Otic Solution, in package containing 15 ml (½ fl oz) bottle with separate dropper-screw cap attachment (NDC 0046-1000-15).

AYGESTIN® ℞
Brand of norethindrone acetate tablets, U.S.P.

> **WARNING:**
> THE USE OF PROGESTATIONAL AGENTS DURING THE FIRST FOUR MONTHS OF PREGNANCY IS NOT RECOMMENDED.
> Progestational agents have been used beginning with the first trimester of pregnancy in an attempt to prevent habitual abortion or treat threatened abortion. There is no adequate evidence that such use is effective and there is evidence of potential harm to the fetus when such drugs are given during the first four months of pregnancy. Furthermore, in the vast majority of women, the cause of abortion is a defective ovum, which progestational agents could not be expected to influence. In addition, the use of progestational agents with their uterine-relaxant properties, in patients with fertilized defective ova may cause a delay in spontaneous abortion. Therefore, the use of such drugs during the first four months of pregnancy is not recommended. Several reports suggest an association between intrauterine exposure to female sex hormones and congenital anomalies, including congenital heart defects and limb reduction defects.[1-5] One study[4] estimated a 4.7-fold increased risk of limb reduction defects in infants exposed in utero to sex hormones (oral contraceptives, hormone withdrawal tests for pregnancy, or attempted treatment for threatened abortion). Some of these exposures were very short and involved only a few days of treatment. The data suggest that the risk of limb reduction defects in exposed fetuses is somewhat less than 1 in 1,000 if the patient is exposed to AYGESTIN® (norethindrone acetate tablets, U.S.P.) during the first four months of pregnancy or if she becomes pregnant while taking this drug, she should be apprised of the potential risks to the fetus.

Description:

AYGESTIN®
(norethindrone acetate tablets, U.S.P.)—
5 mg oral tablets.

AYGESTIN, (17-hydroxy-19-nor-17α-pregn-4-en-20-yn-3-one acetate), a synthetic, orally active progestin, is the acetic acid ester of norethindrone. On a weight basis it is twice as potent as norethindrone. It is a white, or creamy white, crystalline powder.

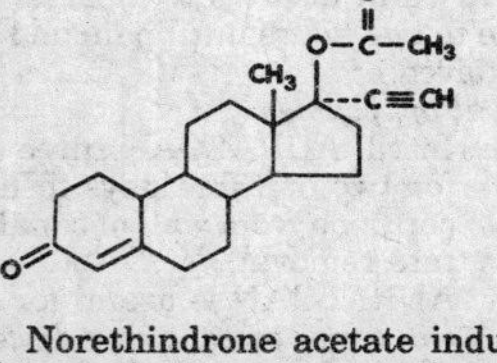

Actions: Norethindrone acetate induces secretory changes in an estrogen-primed endometrium. It acts to inhibit the secretion of pituitary gonadotropins which, in turn, prevent follicular maturation and ovulation.

Indications: AYGESTIN is indicated for the treatment of secondary amenorrhea, endometriosis, and abnormal uterine bleeding due to hormonal imbalance in the absence of organic pathology such as submucous fibroids or uterine cancer.

Contraindications: Thrombophlebitis, thromboembolic disorders, cerebral apoplexy, or a past history of these conditions. Markedly impaired liver function or liver disease.
Known or suspected carcinoma of the breast
Undiagnosed vaginal bleeding
Missed abortion
As a diagnostic test for pregnancy

Warnings:
1. Discontinue medication pending examination if there is a sudden partial or complete loss of vision, or if there is sudden onset of proptosis, diplopia, or migraine. If examination reveals papilledema or retinal vascular lesions, medication should be withdrawn.
2. Detectable amounts of progestogens have been identified in the milk of mothers receiving them. The effect of this on the nursing infant has not been determined.
3. Because of the occasional occurrence of thrombophlebitis and pulmonary embolism in patients taking progestogens, the physician should be alert to the earliest manifestations of the disease.
4. Masculinization of the female fetus has occurred when progestogens have been used in pregnant women.
5. Some beagle dogs treated with medroxy-progesterone acetate developed mammary nodules. Although nodules occasionally appeared in control animals, they were intermittent in nature, whereas nodules in treated animals were larger and more numerous, and persisted. There is no general agreement as to whether the nodules are benign or malignant. Their significance with respect to humans has not been established.

Precautions:
A. General Precautions
1. The pretreatment physical examination should include special reference to breasts and pelvic organs, as well as a Papanicolaou smear.
2. Because this drug may cause some degree of fluid retention, conditions which might be influenced by this factor, such as epilepsy, migraine, asthma, cardiac or renal dysfunctions, require careful observation.
3. In cases of breakthrough bleeding, as in all cases of irregular bleeding per vaginam, nonfunctional causes should be borne in mind. In cases of undiagnosed vaginal bleeding, adequate diagnostic measures are indicated.
4. Patients who have a history of psychic depression should be carefully observed and the drug discontinued if the depression recurs to a serious degree.
5. Any possible influence of prolonged progestogen therapy on pituitary, ovarian, adrenal, hepatic, or uterine functions awaits further study.
6. A decrease in glucose tolerance has been observed in a small percentage of patients on estrogen-progestogen combination drugs. The mechanism of this decrease is obscure. For this reason, diabetic patients should be carefully observed while receiving progestogen therapy.
7. The age of the patient constitutes no absolute limiting factor, although treatment with progestogens may mask the onset of the climacteric.
8. The pathologist should be advised of progestogen therapy when relevant specimens are submitted.

B. Information for the Patient. See text which appears after REFERENCES.

Adverse Reactions: The following adverse reactions have been observed in women taking progestins:
breakthrough bleeding
spotting
change in menstrual flow
amenorrhea
edema
changes in weight (decreases, increases)
changes in cervical erosion and cervical secretions
cholestatic jaundice
rash (allergic) with and without pruritus
melasma or chloasma
mental depression

Progestins may alter the result of pregnanediol determinations. The following laboratory results may be altered by the concomitant use of estrogens with progestins:
hepatic function
coagulation tests—increase in prothrombin, factors VII, VIII, IX, and X
increase in PBI, BEI, and a decrease in T^3 uptake
metyrapone test

A statistically significant association has been demonstrated between use of estrogen-progestogen combination drugs and the following serious adverse reactions: thrombophlebitis, pulmonary embolism, and cerebral thrombosis and embolism. For this reason, patients on progestogen therapy should be carefully observed.
Although available evidence is suggestive of an association, such a relationship has been neither confirmed nor refuted for the following serious adverse reactions:
Neuro-ocular lesions, *e.g.*, retinal thrombosis and optic neuritis.
The following adverse reactions have been observed in patients receiving estrogen-progestogen combination drugs.

1. Rise in blood pressure in susceptible individuals
2. Premenstrual-like syndrome
3. Changes in libido
4. Changes in appetite
5. Cystitis-like syndrome
6. Headache
7. Nervousness
8. Dizziness
9. Fatigue
10. Backache
11. Hirsutism
12. Loss of scalp hair
13. Erythema multiforme
14. Erythema nodosum
15. Hemorrhagic eruption
16. Itching

In view of these observations, patients on progestogen therapy should be carefully observed.

Dosage and Administration: *Therapy with AYGESTIN® must be adapted to the specific indications and therapeutic response of the individual patient.* This dosage schedule assumes the interval between menses to be 28 days.

Secondary amenorrhea, abnormal uterine bleeding due to hormonal imbalance in the absence of organic pathology: 2.5 to 10 mg AYGESTIN may be given daily for from 5 to 10 days during the second half of the theoretical menstrual cycle to produce an optimum secretory transformation of an endometrium that has been adequately primed with either endogenous or exogenous estrogen.

Progestin withdrawal bleeding usually occurs within three to seven days after discontinuing AYGESTIN therapy. Patients with a past history of recurrent episodes of abnormal uterine bleeding may benefit from planned menstrual cycling with AYGESTIN.

Endometriosis:
Initial daily dosage of 5 mg AYGESTIN for two weeks. Dosage should be increased by 2.5 mg per day every two weeks until 15 mg per day of AYGESTIN is reached. Therapy may be held at this level for six to nine months or until annoying breakthrough bleeding demands temporary termination.

How Supplied: Each scored AYGESTIN tablet contains 5 mg norethindrone acetate, U.S.P., in bottles of 50 (NDC 0046-0894-50).

Physician References:

1. Gal I, Kirman B, Stern J: Hormonal pregnancy tests and congenital malformation. Nature *216*:83, 1967.
2. Levy EP, Cohen A, Fraser FC: Hormone treatment during pregnancy and congenital heart defects. Lancet *1*:611, 1973.

3. Nora JJ, Nora AH: Birth defects and oral contraceptives. Lancet *1*:941-942, 1973.
4. Janerich DT, Piper JM, Glebatis DM: Oral contraceptives and congenital limb-reduction defects. N Engl J Med *291*:697-700, 1974.
5. Hernonen OP, Stone D, Monson RR, et al: Cardiovascular birth defects and antenatal exposure to female sex hormones. N Engl J Med *296*:67-70, 1977.

Information for the Patient: Your doctor has prescribed AYGESTIN® (norethindrone acetate tablets, U.S.P.), a progestin, for you. AYGESTIN is similar to the progesterone hormones naturally produced by the body. Progestins are used to treat menstrual disorders and to test if the body is producing certain hormones.

Warning: There is an increased risk of birth defects in children whose mothers take this drug during the first four months of pregnancy.

Progestins have been used as a test for pregnancy but such use is no longer considered safe because of possible damage to a developing baby. Also, more rapid methods for testing for pregnancy are now available.

These drugs have also been used to prevent miscarriage in the first few months of pregnancy. No adequate evidence is available to show that they are effective for this purpose and there is evidence of an increased risk of birth defects, such as heart or limb defects, if these drugs are taken during the first four months of pregnancy. Furthermore, most cases of early miscarriage are due to causes which could not be helped by these drugs.

The exact risk of taking these drugs early in pregnancy and having a baby with a birth defect is not known. However, one study found that babies born to women who had taken sex hormones (such as progesterone-like drugs) during the first three months of pregnancy were 4 to 5 times more likely to have abnormalities of the arms or legs than if their mothers had not taken such drugs. Some of these women had taken these drugs for only a few days. The chance that an infant whose mother had taken this drug will have this type of defect is about 1 in 1,000. If you take AYGESTIN (norethindrone acetate tablets, U.S.P.) and later find you were pregnant when you took it, be sure to discuss this with your doctor as soon as possible.

How Supplied:
AYGESTIN® (norethindrone acetate tablets, U.S.P.)—scored 5 mg tablets, in bottles of 50, for oral administration.

[*Shown in Product Identification Section*]

BEMINAL®-500

Therapeutic vitamin B complex tablets with 500 mg vitamin C

Each tablet contains:

Thiamine mononitrate (Vit. B_1)	25.0 mg
Riboflavin (Vit. B_2)	12.5 mg
Niacinamide (Vit. B_3)	100.0 mg
Calcium pantothenate (Vit. B_5)	20.0 mg
Pyridoxine hydrochloride (Vit. B_6)	10.0 mg
Cyanocobalamin (Vit. B_{12})	5.0 mcg
Ascorbic acid (Vit. C) as sodium ascorbate	500.0 mg

Does not contain saccharin or other sweeteners.

Indications: Whenever the administration of high potency B complex vitamins with vitamin C is needed—in pre- and postoperative care; in acute infection, long term illness, or debilitating disease; in chronic alcoholism, and whenever nutrition is impaired by digestive problems; to supplement restricted diets prescribed in obesity and other conditions; in geriatrics to help provide nutritional support.

Dosage: Adults—1 tablet daily, or as directed by physician.

How Supplied: BEMINAL-500 Tablets, in bottles of 100 (NDC 0046-0832-81).

[*Shown in Product Identification Section*]

BEMINAL® FORTE with VITAMIN C

Therapeutic vitamin B complex capsules with vitamin C

Each capsule contains:

Thiamine mononitrate (Vit. B_1)	25.0 mg
Riboflavin (Vit. B_2)	12.5 mg
Niacinamide (Vit. B_3)	50.0 mg
Calcium pantothenate (Vit. B_5)	10.0 mg
Pyridoxine HCl (Vit. B_6)	3.0 mg
Cyanocobalamin (Vit. B_{12})	2.5 mcg
Ascorbic acid (Vit. C)	250.0 mg

Indications: Whenever the administration of high potency B complex with vitamin C is needed—pre- and postoperatively; during treatment with sulfonamides and antibiotics; etc.

Dosage: Adults—1 capsule daily, or as directed by physician.

How Supplied: BEMINAL Forte with Vitamin C Capsules, in bottles of 100 (NDC 0046-0817-81).

BEMINAL STRESS PLUS™

Stress potency replacement vitamins

BEMINAL STRESS PLUS™ with IRON

Each tablet contains:	% U.S. RDA*
Vitamin B1 as thiamine mononitrate, U.S.P., 25.0 mg	1717%
Vitamin B2 as riboflavin, U.S.P., 12.5 mg	735%
Vitamin B3 as niacinamide, 100.0 mg	504%
Vitamin B5 as calcium pantothenate, U.S.P., 20.0 mg	184%
Vitamin B6 as pyridoxine hydrochloride, U.S.P., 10.0 mg	411%
Vitamin B12 as cyanocobalamin, 25.0 mcg	417%
Vitamin Bc as folic acid, U.S.P., 400.0 mcg	100%
Vitamin C as sodium ascorbate, U.S.P., 787.0 mg	1166%
Vitamin E as *dl-a*-tocopheryl acetate, 45.0 I.U.	150%
Iron as ferrous fumarate, U.S.P., 82.2 mg	150%

*percentage of U.S. recommended daily allowance

BEMINAL STRESS PLUS™ with ZINC

Each tablet contains:	% U.S. RDA*
Vitamin B1 as thiamine mononitrate, U.S.P., 25.0 mg	1717%
Vitamin B2 as riboflavin, U.S.P., 12.5 mg	735%
Vitamin B3 as niacinamide, 100.0 mg	504%
Vitamin B5 as calcium pantothenate, U.S.P., 20.0 mg	184%
Vitamin B6 as pyridoxine hydrochloride, U.S.P., 10.0 mg	411%
Vitamin B12 as cyanocobalamin, 25.0 mcg	417%
Vitamin C as sodium ascorbate, U.S.P., 787.0 mg	1166%
Vitamin E as *dl-a*-tocopheryl acetate, 45.0 I.U.	150%
Zinc as zinc sulfate, 111.1 mg	300%

*percentage of U.S. recommended daily allowance

Indication: Dietary supplement.

Action and Uses: The BEMINAL STRESS PLUS formulas can help replenish the vitamins and minerals depleted by the stress of sickness, infections, and surgery. BEMINAL STRESS PLUS formulas may also be used where the demand on the body's store of vitamins and minerals may be increased by dieting, lack of sleep, the use of alcohol or cigarettes, jogging and other strenuous physical exercise.

Recommended Intake: *Adults*, one tablet daily.

How Supplied: BEMINAL STRESS PLUS with Iron—bottles of 60 tablets. BEMINAL STRESS PLUS with Zinc—bottles of 60 tablets.

[*Shown in Product Identification Section*]

CLUSIVOL® SYRUP

Therapeutic vitamin-mineral syrup for children and adults

Each 5 ml (1 teaspoonful) contains:

Vitamin A (as palmitate)	2,500 U.S.P. Units
Cholecalciferol (Vit. D_3)	400 U.S.P. Units
Ascorbic acid (Vit. C)	15.0 mg
Thiamine HCl (Vit. B_1)	1.0 mg
Riboflavin (Vit. B_2)	1.0 mg
Niacinamide (Vit. B_3)	5.0 mg
d-Panthenol	3.0 mg
Pyridoxine HCl (Vit. B_6)	0.6 mg
Cyanocobalamin (Vit. B_{12})	2.0 mcg
Manganese†	0.5 mg
Zinc†	0.5 mg
Magnesium†	3.0 mg

†Supplied as the gluconates of manganese and magnesium, and zinc lactate.

A comprehensive nutritional formula incorporating essential fat- and water-soluble vitamins together with important minerals. Presented in a candy-flavored syrup base; particularly appealing to children, but also enjoyed by older individuals who prefer a liquid preparation.

Action and Uses: A nutritional safeguard for better health for the entire family.

Dosage: *Children and Adults:* One teaspoonful (5 ml) daily, or as prescribed by the physician.

How Supplied: CLUSIVOL Syrup, in bottles of 8 fl oz (½ pint) (NDC 0046-0920-08), 16 fl oz (1 pint) (NDC 0046-0920-16), and 32 fl oz (1 quart) (NDC 0046-0920-32).

CLUSIVOL® Tablet/Capsule

CLUSIVOL® 130

Therapeutic vitamin-mineral tablets for adults

Each tablet contains:

Vitamin A (as palmitate)	10,000 U.S.P. Units
Ergocalciferol (Vit. D_2)	400 U.S.P. Units
Ascorbic acid (Vit. C) (as sodium ascorbate)	150.0 mg
Thiamine mononitrate (Vit. B_1)	10.0 mg
Riboflavin (Vit. B_2)	5.0 mg
Niacinamide (Vit. B_3)	50.0 mg
d-Panthenol	1.0 mg
Pyridoxine HCl (Vit. B_6)	0.5 mg
Cyanocobalamin (Vit. B_{12})	2.5 mcg
Vitamin E†	0.5 I.U.
Iron†	15.0 mg
Calcium†	120.0 mg
Manganese†	0.5 mg
Zinc†	0.6 mg
Magnesium†	3.0 mg

†Supplied as *dl-a*-tocopheryl acetate, ferrous fumarate, calcium carbonate, manganese gluconate, zinc oxide, and magnesium oxide.

CLUSIVOL® Capsules

Therapeutic vitamin-mineral capsules for adults

Each capsule contains:

Vitamin A (as palmitate)	10,000 U.S.P. Units
Ergocalciferol (Vit. D_2)	400 U.S.P. Units
Ascorbic acid (Vit. C) (as sodium ascorbate)	150.0 mg
Thiamine mononitrate (Vit. B_1)	10.0 mg
Riboflavin (Vit. B_2)	5.0 mg
Niacinamide (Vit. B_3)	50.0 mg
d-Panthenol	1.0 mg
Pyridoxine HCl (Vit. B_6)	0.5 mg

Continued on next page

Ayerst—Cont.

Cyanocobalamin (Vit. B_{12})	2.5 mcg
Vitamin E†	0.5 I.U.
Iron†	15.0 mg
Calcium†	120.0 mg
Manganese†	0.5 mg
Zinc†	0.6 mg
Magnesium†	3.0 mg

†Supplied as *d-α*-tocopheryl acetate concentrate, ferrous sulfate, calcium carbonate, manganous sulfate, zinc sulfate, and magnesium sulfate.

Indications: For use in vitamin deficiencies, especially for patients with generally inadequate or broadly restricted diets.

Dosage and Administration: One tablet (capsule) daily, or as directed by the physician.

How Supplied: CLUSIVOL 130, bottle of 130 tablets (NDC 0046-0270-81). CLUSIVOL Capsules, bottle of 100 (NDC 0046-0293-81).

DERMOPLAST® Aerosol Spray
Topical anesthetic and antipruritic

Contains (exclusive of propellants) 20% benzocaine and 0.5% menthol in a water-dispersible base of TWEEN® 85 and polyethylene glycol 400 monolaurate with methylparaben as a preservative.

A topical anesthetic and antipruritic spray providing soothing, temporary relief of skin pain, itching, and discomfort due to episiotomy, pruritus vulvae, postpartum hemorrhoids, sunburn, abrasions, minor wounds, burns, and insect bites. May be applied without touching sensitive affected areas.

Warnings: FOR EXTERNAL USE ONLY. Avoid spraying in eyes. Contents under pressure. Do not puncture or incinerate. Do not expose to heat or temperatures above 120° F. Do not use near open flame. Use only as directed. Intentional misuse by deliberately concentrating and inhaling the contents can be harmful or fatal.

Do not take orally. Not for prolonged use. If the condition for which this preparation is used persists or if a rash or irritation develops, discontinue use and consult physician.

Directions for Use: Hold can in a convenient position 6-12 inches away from affected area. Point spray nozzle and press button. To apply to face, spray in palm of hand. May be administered three or four times daily, or as directed by physician.

How Supplied: DERMOPLAST Aerosol Spray, in Net Wt 3 oz (85 g)—NDC 0046-1008-03; and in Net Wt 6 oz (170 g)—NDC 0046-1008-06.

DIUCARDIN® ℞
Brand of hydroflumethiazide
A diuretic-antihypertensive agent

Actions: DIUCARDIN is a thiazide diuretic and antihypertensive. DIUCARDIN affects the renal tubular mechanism of electrolyte reabsorption. At maximal therapeutic dosage all thiazides are approximately equal in their diuretic potency.

DIUCARDIN increases excretion of sodium and chloride in approximately equivalent amounts. Natriuresis causes a secondary loss of potassium and bicarbonate.

The mechanism of the antihypertensive effect of DIUCARDIN is unknown. DIUCARDIN does not affect normal blood pressure.

Onset of action of DIUCARDIN occurs in two hours and the peak effect at about four hours. Its action persists for approximately 6 to 12 hours. Thiazides are eliminated rapidly by the kidney.

Indications: DIUCARDIN (hydroflumethiazide) is indicated as adjunctive therapy in edema associated with congestive heart failure, hepatic cirrhosis and corticosteroid and estrogen therapy.

DIUCARDIN has also been found useful in edema due to various forms of renal dysfunction as: nephrotic syndrome; acute glomerulonephritis; and chronic renal failure.

DIUCARDIN is indicated in the management of hypertension either as the sole therapeutic agent or to enhance the effect of other antihypertensive drugs in the more severe forms of hypertension.

Usage in Pregnancy: The routine use of diuretics in an otherwise healthy woman is inappropriate and exposes mother and fetus to unnecessary hazard. Diuretics do not prevent development of toxemia of pregnancy, and there is no satisfactory evidence that they are useful in the treatment of developed toxemia.

Edema during pregnancy may arise from pathological causes or from the physiologic and mechanical consequences of pregnancy. Thiazides are indicated in pregnancy when edema is due to pathologic causes just as they are in the absence of pregnancy (however, see Warnings, below). Dependent edema in pregnancy, resulting from restriction of venous return by the expanded uterus, is properly treated through elevation of the lower extremities and use of support hose. Use of diuretics to lower intravascular volume in this case is illogical and unnecessary. There is hypervolemia during normal pregnancy which is harmful to neither the fetus nor the mother (in absence of cardiovascular disease), but which is associated with edema, including generalized edema, in the majority of pregnant women. If this edema produces discomfort, increased recumbency will often provide relief. In rare instances, this edema may cause extreme discomfort which is not relieved by rest. In these cases, a short course of diuretics may provide relief and may be appropriate.

Contraindications: Anuria.

Hypersensitivity to this or other sulfonamide-derived drugs.

Warnings: Thiazides should be used with caution in severe renal disease. In patients with renal disease, thiazides may precipitate azotemia. Cumulative effects of the drug may develop in patients with impaired renal function.

Thiazides should be used with caution in patients with impaired hepatic function or progressive liver disease, since minor alterations of fluid and electrolyte balance may precipitate hepatic coma.

Thiazides may add to or potentiate the action of other antihypertensive drugs. Potentiation occurs with ganglionic or peripheral adrenergic blocking drugs.

Sensitivity reactions may occur in patients with or without a history of allergy or bronchial asthma.

The possibility of exacerbation or activation of systemic lupus erythematosus has been reported.

Usage in Pregnancy: Thiazides cross the placental barrier and appear in cord blood. The use of thiazides in pregnant women requires that the anticipated benefit be weighed against possible hazards to the fetus. These hazards include fetal or neonatal jaundice, thrombocytopenia, and possibly other adverse reactions which have occurred in the adult.

Nursing Mothers: Thiazides appear in breast milk. If use of the drug is deemed essential, the patient should stop nursing.

Precautions: Periodic determination of serum electrolytes to detect possible electrolyte imbalance should be performed at appropriate intervals.

All patients receiving thiazide therapy should be observed for clinical signs of fluid or electrolyte imbalance: namely, hyponatremia, hypochloremic alkalosis, and hypokalemia. Serum and urine electrolyte determinations are particularly important when the patient is vomiting excessively or receiving parenteral fluids. Medication such as digitalis may also influence serum electrolytes. Warning signs, irrespective of cause are: dryness of mouth, thirst, weakness, lethargy, drowsiness, restlessness, muscle pains or cramps, muscular fatigue, hypotension, oliguria, tachycardia, and gastrointestinal disturbances such as nausea and vomiting.

Hypokalemia may develop, especially with brisk diuresis, when severe cirrhosis is present, or during concomitant use of corticosteroids or ACTH.

Interference with adequate oral electrolyte intake will also contribute to hypokalemia. Hypokalemia can sensitize or exaggerate the response of the heart to the toxic effects of digitalis (*e.g.,* increased ventricular irritability). Hypokalemia may be avoided or treated by use of potassium supplements such as foods with a high potassium content.

Any chloride deficit is generally mild and usually does not require specific treatment except under extraordinary circumstances (as in liver disease or renal disease). Dilutional hyponatremia may occur in edematous patients in hot weather; appropriate therapy is water restriction, rather than administration of salt, except in rare instances when the hyponatremia is life-threatening. In actual salt depletion, appropriate replacement is the therapy of choice.

Hyperuricemia may occur or frank gout may be precipitated in certain patients receiving thiazide therapy.

Insulin requirements in diabetic patients may be increased, decreased, or unchanged. Diabetes mellitus which has been latent may become manifest during thiazide administration.

Thiazide drugs may increase the responsiveness to tubocurarine.

The antihypertensive effects of the drug may be enhanced in the postsympathectomy patient. Thiazides may decrease arterial responsiveness to norepinephrine. This diminution is not sufficient to preclude effectiveness of the pressor agent for therapeutic use.

If progressive renal impairment becomes evident, consider withholding or discontinuing diuretic therapy.

Thiazides may decrease serum PBI levels without signs of thyroid disturbance.

Calcium excretion is decreased by thiazides. Pathological changes in the parathyroid gland with hypercalcemia and hypophosphatemia have been observed in a few patients on prolonged thiazide therapy. The common complications of hyperparathyroidism such as renal lithiasis, bone resorption, and peptic ulceration have not been seen. Thazides should be discontinued before carrying out tests for parathyroid function.

Adverse Reactions: *Gastrointestinal System:* anorexia, gastric irritation, nausea, vomiting, cramping, diarrhea, constipation, jaundice (intrahepatic cholestatic jaundice), pancreatitis, sialadenitis

Central Nervous System: dizziness, vertigo, paresthesias, headache, xanthopsia

Hematologic: leukopenia, agranulocytosis, thrombocytopenia, aplastic anemia

Cardiovascular: orthostatic hypotension (may be aggravated by alcohol, barbiturates, or narcotics)

Hypersensitivity: purpura, photosensitivity, rash, urticaria, necrotizing angiitis (vasculitis, cutaneous vasculitis), fever, respiratory distress including pneumonitis, anaphylactic reactions

Other: hyperglycemia, glycosuria, hyperuricemia, muscle spasm, weakness, restlessness, transient blurred vision

Whenever adverse reactions are moderate or severe, thiazide dosage should be reduced or therapy withdrawn.

Dosage and Administration: Therapy should be individualized according to patient response. Use the smallest dosage necessary to maintain the required response.

The usual daily dosages for antihypertensive and diuretic effect are:

	Diuretic	Antihypertensive
Adult:	25 to 200 mg	50 to 100 mg

Dosage regimens using 25 mg DIUCARDIN (hydroflumethiazide) may be adequate in some cases.
Dosage should not exceed 200 mg per day.
For Diuresis in the Adult:
Initial recommended dose is 50 mg once or twice a day. Daily maintenance dose may be as little as 25 mg or as much as 200 mg, depending on patient's response. With dosages in excess of 100 mg daily, it is generally preferable to administer DIUCARDIN in divided doses.
Many patients with edema respond to intermittent therapy, i.e., administration on alternate days or on three to five days each week. With an intermittent schedule, excessive response and the resulting undesirable electrolyte imbalance are less likely to occur.
For Control of Hypertension in the Adult:
Usual starting dose is 50 mg twice daily. Dosage is increased or decreased according to the blood pressure response of the patient. Usual maintenance dose is 50 mg to 100 mg per day. Dosage should not exceed 200 mg per day.
Careful observations for changes in blood pressure must be made when this compound is used with other antihypertensive drugs, especially during initial therapy. The dosage of other agents must be reduced by at least 50 percent as soon as it is added to the regimen to prevent excessive drop in blood pressure. As the blood pressure falls under the potentiating effect of this agent, a further reduction in dosage, or even discontinuation, of other antihypertensive drugs may be necessary.
Overdosage: The following information is provided to serve as guidelines in treating overdosage.
HYDROFLUMETHIAZIDE
Signs and Symptoms:
Diuresis is to be expected; lethargy of varying degree may appear and may progress to coma within a few hours, with minimal depression of respiration and cardiovascular function, and without significant serum electrolyte changes or dehydration. The mechanism of CNS depression with thiazide overdosage is unknown.
G.I. irritation and hypermotility may occur; temporary elevation of BUN has been reported and serum electrolyte changes could occur, especially in patients with impairment of renal function.
Treatment:
Evacuate gastric contents but take care to prevent aspiration, especially in the stuporous or comatose patient. G.I. effects are usually of short duration, but may require symptomatic treatment.
Monitor serum electrolyte levels and renal function; institute supportive measures as required individually to maintain hydration, electrolyte balance, respiration, and cardiovascular-renal function.
How Supplied: DIUCARDIN—Each scored tablet contains 50 mg hydroflumethiazide, in bottles of 100 (NDC 0046-0702-81) and 1,000 (NDC 0046-0702-91).
[*Shown in Product Identification Section*]

ENZACTIN® Cream
Brand of triacetin

Action: For prevention and treatment of athlete's foot and other superficial fungus infections. The "self-regulating" action of ENZACTIN (triacetin) releases a constant effective level of *free* fatty acid at the site of infection, in a concentration that is nonirritating.
"*Self-regulating*" *action*—At a neutral or higher pH of infected skin and in the presence of the enzyme esterase (found abundantly in skin, serum, and fungi), glycerol and free fatty acid (acetic) are rapidly liberated from triacetin. At this point, the growth of fungi is inhibited by the free acid.
With an accumulation of free acid, the pH drops and esterase activity decreases. Then, as the acid in the skin diffuses or becomes neutralized, the pH rises and esterase is reactivated, to release more free acid for fungistatic control.
Relieves itching and soreness promptly. Helps prevent spread of infection. Nonirritating. Odorless and stainless.
Indications: Athlete's foot and other superficial fungus infections.
Administration: Thoroughly cleanse affected and adjacent areas with dilute alcohol or a mild soap and warm water. Pat dry. Apply cream liberally twice daily, preferably morning and evening.
Note: Rayon fabrics should not come in contact with ENZACTIN (triacetin) Cream. For protection, cover treated areas with clean cotton cloth or bandage. If infection persists, consult a physician.
How Supplied: ENZACTIN *Cream*—250 mg triacetin per gram (in emollient base), in 1 oz (28.35 g) collapsible tubes (NDC 0046-0201-01).

Ayerst

EPITRATE® ℞
Brand of epinephrine bitartrate ophthalmic solution

Description: EPITRATE (epinephrine bitartrate) Ophthalmic Solution is a sterile aqueous solution of levorotatory epinephrine bitartrate, 2% (equivalent to 1.1% base). Inactive ingredients include chlorobutanol (chloral derivative) 0.55%, sodium bisulfite, sodium chloride, polyoxypropylene-polyoxyethylene-diol, and disodium edetate. Epinephrine bitartrate is an adrenergic agent with the chemical name (-)-3,4,-Dihydroxy-α-[(methylamino) methyl] benzyl alcohol (+) tartrate (1:1) salt. It has a low surface tension.
Clinical Pharmacology: EPITRATE lowers intraocular pressure by reducing the rate of aqueous formation. Improvement in outflow facility is also observed in certain cases following prolonged therapy.
Indications and Usage: Useful in management of chronic simple (open-angle) glaucoma, either alone or in combination with miotics. In selected cases, it may also be used with carbonic anhydrase inhibitors.
Contraindications: Prior to peripheral iridectomy, an epinephrine preparation is contraindicated in eyes that are capable of angle closure since its relatively weak mydriatic action may, nevertheless, precipitate angle block. Gonioscopy should be carried out on all patients before initiating therapy.
Warnings: Topical use of epinephrine in any form should be interrupted prior to general anesthesia with certain anesthetics such as cyclopropane or halothane which sensitize the myocardium to sympathomimetics.
Precautions: EPITRATE (epinephrine bitartrate) should be used with caution in the presence of hypertension, diabetes, hyperthyroidism, heart disease, and cerebral arteriosclerosis because of the possibility of systemic action.
Do not use the solution if it is brown or contains a precipitate.
Drug Interactions: See Warnings.
Carcinogenesis, Mutagenesis, Impairment of Fertility: No long-term studies in animals or humans have been conducted.
Pregnancy Category C: Animal reproduction studies have not been conducted with EPITRATE. It is also not known whether EPITRATE can cause fetal harm when administered to a pregnant woman or can affect reproduction capacity. EPITRATE should be given to a pregnant woman only if clearly needed.
Nursing Mothers: It is not known whether this drug is excreted in human milk. Because many drugs are excreted in human milk, caution should be exercised when EPITRATE is administered to a nursing woman.
Pediatric Use: Safety and effectiveness in children have not been established.
Adverse Reactions: As with other epinephrine solutions, transitory stinging on initial instillation may be expected. Headache or browache frequently occur on beginning EPITRATE therapy, but usually diminish as treatment is continued. Conjunctival allergy occurs occasionally. Pigmentary deposits in the lids, conjunctiva or cornea may occur after prolonged use of epinephrine eyedrops. In rare cases, maculopathy with a central scotoma may result from the use of topical epinephrine in aphakic patients; prompt reversal generally follows discontinuance of the drug. Systemic effects have occasionally been reported, such as: palpitation, tachycardia, extrasystoles, hypertension, trembling, sweating, and pallor.
Dosage and Administration: One drop, with frequency of instillation being individualized, from every two or three days to twice daily. More frequent instillation than one drop four times daily does not usually elicit any further improvement in therapeutic response.
How Supplied: EPITRATE—ophthalmic solution of epinephrine bitartrate 2% (equivalent to 1.1% base). Package containing 7.5 ml bottle with separate dropper-screw cap attachment (NDC 0046-1015-07).

ESTRADURIN® ℞
Brand of polyestradiol phosphate
For Intramuscular Injection Only

Description: ESTRADURIN (polyestradiol phosphate) is a water-soluble, high molecular weight polyester of phosphoric acid and 17β-estradiol. It is provided in a SECULE® containing 40 mg polyestradiol phosphate, 0.022 mg phenylmercuric nitrate, and 5.2 mg sodium phosphate. As solubilizing agents for the active ingredient, 25 mg niacinamide and 4 mg propylene glycol are also present. The pH is adjusted with sodium hydroxide.
One 2 ml ampul of sterile diluent is also provided.
Clinical Pharmacology: Estrogens are important in the development and maintenance of the female reproductive system. In responsive tissues estrogens enter the cell and are transported into the nucleus.
In the male patient with androgenic hormone-dependent conditions such as metastatic carcinoma of the prostate gland, estrogens counter the androgenic influence by competing for the receptor sites. As a result of treatment with estrogens, metastatic lesions in the bone may also show improvement.
Biologically active estradiol units are gradually split off from the large parent molecule, thus providing a continuous level of active estrogen over a prolonged period. The liberated estradiol is metabolized by the body in the same manner as the endogenous hormone. There is no depot effect at the site of injection—90 percent of injected dose leaves the bloodstream within 24 hours. Passive storage occurs in the reticuloendothelial system. As circulating levels of estradiol drop, more returns to the bloodstream from the site of storage for an even, continuous therapeutic effect. Increasing the dose acts to prolong the duration of pharmacologic action rather than to increase blood levels.
Metabolism and inactivation occur primarily in the liver. Some estrogens are excreted into the bile; however they are reabsorbed from the intestine and returned to the liver through the portal venous system. Water-soluble estrogen conjugates are strongly acidic and are ionized in body fluids, which favor excretion through

Continued on next page

Ayerst—Cont.

the kidneys since tubular reabsorption is minimal.

Indication: ESTRADURIN (polyestradiol phosphate) is indicated in the treatment of prostatic carcinoma—palliative therapy of advanced disease.

Contraindications: Estrogens should not be used in men with any of the following conditions:

1. Known or suspected cancer of the breast except in appropriately selected patients being treated for metastatic disease.
2. Known or suspected estrogen-dependent neoplasia.
3. Active thrombophlebitis or thromboembolic disorders.

Warnings:

1. *Induction of malignant neoplasms.* Long term continuous administration of natural and synthetic estrogens in certain animal species increases the frequency of carcinomas of the breast, cervix, vagina, and liver.
2. *Gallbladder disease.* A recent study has reported a 2 to 3-fold increase in the risk of surgically confirmed gallbladder disease in women receiving postmenopausal estrogens,[1] similar to the 2-fold increase previously noted in users of oral contraceptives.[2,7a]
3. *Effects similar to those caused by estrogen-progestogen oral contraceptives.* There are several serious adverse effects of oral contraceptives. It has been shown that there is an increased risk of thrombosis in men receiving estrogens for prostatic cancer and women for postpartum breast engorgement.[3–6]

a. *Thromboembolic disease.* It is now well established that users of oral contraceptives have an increased risk of various thromboembolic and thrombotic vascular diseases, such as thrombophlebitis, pulmonary embolism, stroke, and myocardial infarction.[7–14] Cases of retinal thrombosis, mesenteric thrombosis, and optic neuritis have been reported in oral contraceptive users. There is evidence that the risk of several of these adverse reactions is related to the dose of the drug.[15,16] An increased risk of postsurgery thromboembolic complications has also been reported in users of oral contraceptives.[17,18] If feasible, estrogen should be discontinued at least 4 weeks before surgery of the type associated with an increased risk of thromboembolism, or during periods of prolonged immobilization.

Estrogens should not be used in persons with active thrombophlebitis or thromboembolic disorders. They should be used with caution in patients with cerebral vascular or coronary artery disease and only for those in whom estrogens are clearly indicated.

Large doses of estrogen (5 mg conjugated estrogens per day), comparable to those used to treat cancer of the prostate, have been shown in a large prospective clinical trial in men[19] to increase the risk of nonfatal myocardial infarction, pulmonary embolism and thrombophlebitis. When estrogen doses of this size are used, any of the thromboembolic and thrombotic adverse effects associated with oral contraceptive use should be considered a clear risk.

b. *Hepatic adenoma.* Benign hepatic adenomas appear to be associated with the use of oral contraceptives.[20–22] Although benign, and rare, these may rupture and may cause death through intra-abdominal hemorrhage. Such lesions have not yet been reported in association with other estrogen or progestogen preparations but should be considered in estrogen users having abdominal pain and tenderness, abdominal mass, or hypovolemic shock. Hepatocellular carcinoma has also been reported in women taking estrogen-containing oral contraceptives.[21] The relationship of this malignancy to these drugs is not known at this time.

c. *Elevated blood pressure.* Women using oral contraceptives sometimes experience increased blood pressure which, in most cases, returns to normal on discontinuing the drug. There is now a report that this may occur with use of estrogens in the menopause[23] and blood pressure should be monitored with estrogen use, especially if high doses are used.

d. *Glucose tolerance.* A worsening of glucose tolerance has been observed in a significant percentage of patients on estrogen-containing oral contraceptives. For this reason, diabetic patients should be carefully observed while receiving estrogen.

4. *Hypercalcemia.* Administration of estrogens may lead to severe hypercalcemia in patients with breast cancer and bone metastases. If this occurs, the drug should be stopped and appropriate measures taken to reduce the serum calcium level.

Precautions:

1. A complete medical and family history should be taken prior to the initiation of any estrogen therapy. The pretreatment and periodic physical examinations should include special reference to blood pressure, breasts, abdomen, and pelvic organs. As a general rule, estrogen should not be prescribed for longer than one year without another physical examination being performed.
2. Fluid retention—Because estrogens may cause some degree of fluid retention, conditions which might be influenced by this factor such as asthma, epilepsy, migraine, and cardiac or renal dysfunction, require careful observation.
3. Certain patients may develop undesirable manifestations of excessive estrogenic stimulation, such as gynecomastia.
4. Oral contraceptives appear to be associated with an increased incidence of mental depression.[7a] Although it is not clear whether this is due to the estrogenic or progestogenic component of the contraceptive, patients with a history of depression should be carefully observed.
5. The pathologist should be advised of estrogen therapy when relevant specimens are submitted.
6. If jaundice develops in any patient receiving estrogen, the medication should be discontinued while the cause is investigated.
7. Estrogens may be poorly metabolized in patients with impaired liver function and they should be administered with caution in such patients.
8. Because estrogens influence the metabolism of calcium and phosphorus, they should be used with caution in patients with metabolic bone diseases that are associated with hypercalcemia or in patients with renal insufficiency.
9. Because of the effects of estrogens on epiphyseal closure, they should be used judiciously in young patients in whom bone growth is not complete.
10. Certain endocrine and liver function tests may be affected by estrogen-containing oral contraceptives. The following similar changes may be expected with larger doses of estrogen:

a. Increased sulfobromophthalein retention.
b. Increased prothrombin and factors VII, VIII, IX, and X; decreased antithrombin 3; increased norepinephrine-induced platelet aggregability.
c. Increased thyroid binding globulin (TBG) leading to increased circulating total thyroid hormone, as measured by PBI, T4 by column, or T4 by radioimmunoassay. Free T3 resin uptake is decreased, reflecting the elevated TBG; free T4 concentration is unaltered.
d. Impaired glucose tolerance.
e. Reduced response to metyrapone test.
f. Reduced serum folate concentration.
g. Increased serum triglyceride and phospholipid concentration.

Adverse Reactions: (See Warnings regarding induction of neoplasia, increased incidence of gallbladder disease, and adverse effects similar to those of oral contraceptives, including thromboembolism.) The following additional adverse reactions have been reported with estrogenic therapy, including oral contraceptives:

1. *Breasts:* Tenderness, enlargement, secretion.
2. *Gastrointestinal:* Nausea, vomiting; abdominal cramps, bloating; cholestatic jaundice.
3. *Skin:* Chloasma or melasma which may persist when drug is discontinued; erythema multiforme; erythema nodosum; hemorrhagic eruption; loss of scalp hair; hirsutism.
4. *Eyes:* Steepening of corneal curvature; intolerance to contact lenses.
5. *CNS:* Headache, migraine, dizziness; mental depression; chorea.
6. *Miscellaneous:* Increase or decrease in weight; reduced carbohydrate tolerance; aggravation of porphyria; edema; changes in libido.

Acute Overdosage: Numerous reports of ingestion of large doses of estrogen-containing oral contraceptives by young children indicate that acute serious ill effects do not occur. Overdosage of estrogen may cause nausea, and withdrawal bleeding may occur in females.

Dosage and Administration: Inoperable progressing prostatic cancer— 40 mg intramuscularly every two to four weeks or less frequently, depending on clinical response of the patient. If the response is not satisfactory doses up to 80 mg may be used. Experimental evidence indicates that increasing the dose primarily prolongs the duration of action, but the amount of estrogen available at any one time is not significantly increased. The dosage should be adjusted as indicated by careful observation of the patient.

Deep intramuscular injection only is recommended. (Initially, some patients may experience a burning sensation at site of injection. This is transitory, and it may not recur with subsequent injections, or may be obviated by concomitant administration of a local anesthetic.)

If a response to estrogen therapy is going to occur, it will be apparent within three months of the beginning of therapy. If it does occur, the hormone should be continued until the disease is again progressive. The hormone should then be stopped, and the patient may obtain another period of improvement known as "rebound regression." This occurs in 30% of the patients who show objective improvement on estrogens.

DIRECTIONS FOR USE

Reconstitution for use:

1. Introduce sterile diluent into SECULE, preferably with a 20 gauge needle affixed to a 5 ml syringe.
2. Swirl gently until a solution is effected. (DO NOT AGITATE VIOLENTLY.)

Stability: After reconstitution, if storage is desired, the solution should be kept at room temperature and away from direct light. Under these conditions the solution is stable for about 10 days, so long as cloudiness or evidence of a precipitate has not occurred.

How Supplied: NDC 0046-0451-02—Each package provides:

1. One SECULE® containing 40 mg polyestradiol phosphate, 0.022 mg phenylmercuric nitrate, and 5.2 mg sodium phosphate. As solubilizing agents for the active ingredient, 25 mg niacinamide and 4 mg propylene glycol are also present. The pH is adjusted with sodium hydroxide.
2. One 2 ml ampul of sterile diluent.

ESTRADURIN (polyestradiol phosphate) is prepared by cryodesiccation.

Physician References:

1. Boston Collaborative Drug Surveillance Program: N. Engl. J. Med. *290*:15–19, 1974.
2. Boston Collaborative Drug Surveillance Program: Lancet *1*:1399–1404, 1973.

3. Daniel, D. G., *et al.*: Lancet *2*:287–289, 1967.
4. The Veterans Administration Cooperative Urological Research Group: J. Urol. *98*:516–522, 1967.
5. Bailar, J. C.: Lancet *2*:560, 1967.
6. Blackard, C., *et al.*: Cancer *26*:249–256, 1970.
7. Royal College of General Practitioners: J. R. Coll. Gen. Pract. *13*:267–279, 1967.
7a. Royal College of General Practitioners: Oral Contraceptives and Health, New York, Pitman Corp., 1974.
8. Inman, W. H. W., *et al*: Br. Med. J. *2*:193–199, 1968.
9. Vessey, M. P., *et al.*: Br. Med. J. *2*:651–657, 1969.
10. Sartwell, P. E., *et al*: Am. J. Epidemiol. *90*:365–380, 1969.
11. Collaborative Group for the Study of Stroke in Young Women: N. Engl. J. Med. *288*:871–878, 1973.
12. Collaborative Group for the Study of Stroke in Young Women: J.A.M.A. *231*:718–722, 1975.
13. Mann, J. I., *et al.*: Br. Med. J. *2*:245–248, 1975.
14. Mann, J. I., *et al.*: Br. Med. J. *2*:241–245, 1975.
15. Inman, W. H. W., *et al.*: Br. Med. J. *2*:203–209, 1970.
16. Stolley, P. D., *et al.*: Am. J. Epidemiol. *102*:197–208, 1975.
17. Vessey, M. P., *et al.*: Br. Med. J. *3*:123–126, 1970.
18. Greene, G. R., *et al.*: Am. J. Public Health *62*:680–685, 1972.
19. Coronary Drug Project Research Group: J.A.M.A. *214*:1303–1313, 1970.
20. Baum, J., *et al.*: Lancet *2*:926–928, 1973.
21. Mays, E. T., *et al.*: J.A.M.A. *235*:730–732, 1976.
22. Edmondson, H. A., *et al.*: N. Engl. J. Med. *294*:470–472, 1976.
23. Pfeffer, R. I., *et al.*: Am. J. Epidemiol. *103*:445–456, 1976.

SECULE®—Trademark to designate a special vial containing an injectable preparation in dry form.

FACTREL® ℞

(gonadorelin hydrochloride)
Synthetic Luteinizing Hormone Releasing Hormone (LH-RH)
DIAGNOSTIC USE ONLY

Description: An agent for use in evaluating hypothalamicpituitary gonadotropic function. FACTREL (gonadorelin hydrochloride) injectable is available as a sterile lyophylized powder for reconstitution and administration by subcutaneous or intravenous routes.

Chemical Name: 5-oxo-L-prolyl-L-histidyl-L-tryptophyl-L-seryl-L-tyrosyl-glycyl-L-leucyl-L-arginyl-L-prolyl glycinamide hydrochloride [See structural formula above].

FACTREL is $C_{55}H_{75}N_{17}O_{13}HCl$, as the mono- or dihydrochloride, or their mixture. The gonadorelin base has a molecular weight of 1182.33. It is a white powder, soluble in alcohol and water, hygroscopic and moisture-sensitive, and stable at room temperature. The synthetic decapeptide, FACTREL, has a chemical composition and structure identical to the natural hormone, identified from porcine or ovine hypothalami.

Each vial of FACTREL contains 100 or 500 mcg gonadorelin as the hydrochloride, with 100 mg lactose, U.S.P. Each ampul of sterile diluent contains 2% benzyl alcohol and Water for Injection, U.S.P.

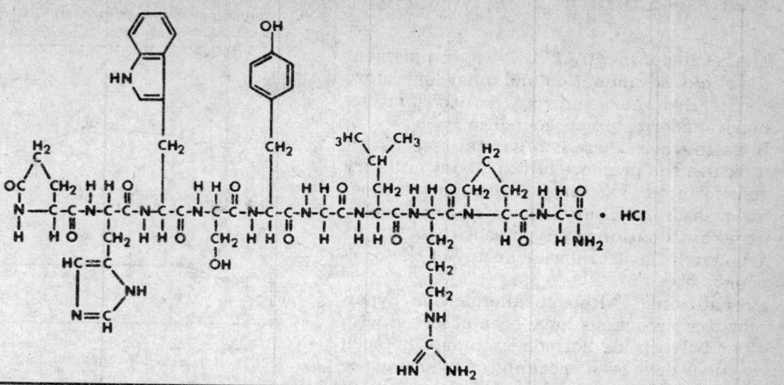

Clinical Pharmacology: FACTREL has been shown to have gonadotropin-releasing effects upon the anterior pituitary. The range for normal baseline LH levels, as determined from the literature, is 5-25 mIU/ml in postpubertal males, and postpubertal and premenopausal females. The standard used is the Second International Reference Preparation—HMC. This range may not correspond in each laboratory performing the assay since the concentration of LH in normal individuals varies with different assay methods. The normal responses to FACTREL analyzed from the results of clinical studies included:

Structural Formula:

(1) LH peak (mIU/ml)
  (highest LH value post-FACTREL administration)
(2) Maximum LH increase (mIU/ml)
  (peak LH value—LH baseline value)
(3) LH percent response
  $\frac{\text{peak LH—baseline LH}}{\text{baseline LH}} \times 100\%$
(4) Time to peak (minutes)
  (time required to reach LH peak value)

Normal adult subjects were shown to have these LH responses following FACTREL administration by subcutaneous or intravenous routes.

I. MALE ADULTS:

A) Subcutaneous Administration
  The results are based on 18 tests in males between the ages of 18–42 years, inclusive:
  (1) LH peak: mean 60.3 ± 26.2 mIU/ml
    100% ≥ 24.0 mIU/ml
    90% ≥ 32.8 mIU/ml
  (2) Maximum LH increase: mean 46.7 ± 20.8 mIU/ml
    100% ≥ 12.3 mIU/ml
    90% ≥ 20.9 mIU/ml
  (3) LH percent response: mean 437 ± 243% range: 68–1853%
    90% ≥ 188%

B) Intravenous Administration
  The results are based on 26 tests in males between the ages of 19–58 years, inclusive:
  (1) LH peak: mean 63.8 ± 40.3 mIU/ml
    100% ≥ 12.6 mIU/ml
    90% ≥ 26.0 mIU/ml
  (2) Maximum LH increase: mean 51.3 ± 35.2 mIU/ml
    100% ≥ 7.4 mIU/ml
    90% ≥ 14.8 mIU/ml
  (3) LH percent response: mean 481 ± 184% range: 67–2139%
    90% ≥ 142%
  (4) Time to peak: mean 27 ± 14 min.

In males older than 50 years, the LH baseline and peak levels tend to be higher; however, the maximum LH increases do not differ in regard to age.

II. FEMALE ADULTS:

A) Subcutaneous Administration
  The results are based on 38 tests in females between the ages of 19–36 years, inclusive:
  (1) LH peak: mean 67.9 ± 27.5 mIU/ml
    100% ≥ 12.5 mIU/ml
    90% ≥ 39.0 mIU/ml
  (2) Maximum LH increase: mean 52.8 ± 26.4 mIU/ml
    100% ≥ 7.5 mIU/ml
    90% ≥ 23.8 mIU/ml
  (3) LH percent response: mean 374 ± 221% range: 108–981%
    90% ≥ 185%
  (4) Time to peak: mean 71.5 ± 49.6 min.

B) Intravenous Administration
  The results are based on 31 tests in females between the ages of 20–35 years inclusive:
  (1) LH peak: mean 57.6 ± 36.7 mIU/ml
    100% ≥ 20.0 mIU/ml
    90% ≥ 24.6mIU/ml
  (2) Maximum LH increase: mean 44.5 ± 31.8 mIU/ml
    100% ≥ 7.5 mIU/ml
    90% ≥ 16.2 mIU/ml
  (3) LH percent response: mean 356 ± 282% range: 60–1300%
    90% ≥ 142%
  (4) Time to peak: mean 36 ± 24 min.

The FACTREL tests on which the normal female responses are based were performed in the early follicular phase of the menstrual cycle (Days 1–7).

In menopausal and postmenopausal females, the baseline LH levels are elevated and the maximum LH increases are exaggerated when compared with the premenopausal levels.

Patients with clinically diagnosed or suspected pituitary and/or hypothalamic dysfunction were often shown to have subnormal or no LH responses following FACTREL administration. For example, in clinical tests of 6 patients with known postpubertal panhypopituitarism, and 11 patients with Prader-Willi Syndrome, 100% showed subnormal responses or no rise in LH. Subnormal responses to the FACTREL test also were observed in 21 (95%) of 22 patients with prepubertal panhypopituitarism. In 19 patients with Sheehan Syndrome, 16 (84%) had a subnormal response. In the FACTREL test in 44 patients with Kallmann Syndrome, 33 (77%) had subnormal LH responses.

Indications and Usage: FACTREL as a single injection is indicated for evaluating the functional capacity and response of the gonadotropes of the anterior pituitary. This single injection test does not measure pituitary gonadotropic reserve for which more prolonged or repeated administration may be required. The LH response is useful in testing patients with suspected gonadotropin deficiency, whether due to the hypothalamus alone or in combination with anterior pituitary failure. FACTREL is also indicated for evaluating residual gonadotropic function of the pituitary following removal of a pituitary tumor by surgery and/or irradiation. In clinical studies to date, however, the single injection test has not been useful in differentiating pituitary disorders from hypothalamic disorders. The FACTREL test can be performed concomitantly with other post-treatment evaluations.

Continued on next page

Ayerst—Cont.

The results of the FACTREL test complement the clinical examination and other laboratory tests used to confirm or substantiate hypogonadotropic hypogonadism.
In cases where there is a normal response, it indicates the presence of functional pituitary gonadotropes. The single injection test does not measure pituitary gonadotropic reserve.
Contraindications: Hypersensitivity to gonadorelin hydrochloride or any of the components.
Precautions: Although allergic and hypersensitivity reactions have been observed with other polypeptide hormones, to date no such reactions have been encountered following the administration of a single 100 mcg dose of FACTREL. Antibody formulation has been rarely reported after chronic administration of large doses of FACTREL.
The FACTREL test should be conducted in the absence of other drugs which directly affect the pituitary secretion of the gonadotropins. These would include a variety of preparations which contain androgens, estrogens, progestins, or glucocorticoids. The gonadotropin levels may be transiently elevated by spironolactone, minimally elevated by levodopa, and suppressed by oral contraceptives and digoxin. The response to FACTREL may be blunted by phenothiazines and dopamine antagonists which cause a rise in prolactin.
Pregnancy Category B. Reproduction studies have been performed in mice, rats, and rabbits at doses up to 50 times the human dose, and have revealed no evidence of harm to the fetus due to FACTREL. There are, however, no adequate and well-controlled studies in pregnant women. Because animal reproduction studies are not always predictive of human response, this drug should be used during pregnancy only if clearly needed.
Appropriate precautions should be taken because the effects of LH-RH on the fetus and developing offspring have not been adequately evaluated. Repetitive, high doses of FACTREL may cause luteolysis and inhibition of spermatogenesis.
Adverse Reactions: Systemic complaints such as headaches, nausea, lightheadedness, abdominal discomfort, and flushing have been reported rarely following administration of 100 mcg of FACTREL. Local swelling, occasionally with pain and pruritus, at the injection site may occur if FACTREL is administered subcutaneously. Local and generalized skin rash have been noted after chronic subcutaneous administration.
Overdosage: FACTREL has been administered parenterally in doses up to 3 mg BID for 28 days without any signs or symptoms of overdosage. In case of overdosage or idiosyncrasy, symptomatic treatment should be administered as required.
Dosage and Administration: Adults: 100 mcg dose, subcutaneously or intravenously. In females for whom the phase of the menstrual cycle can be established, the test should be performed in the early follicular phase (Days 1–7).
Test Methodology: To determine the status of the gonadotropin secretory capacity of the anterior pituitary, a test procedure requiring seven venous blood samples for LH is recommended.

PROCEDURE:

1. Venous blood samples should be drawn at -15 minutes and immediately prior to FACTREL administration. The LH baseline is obtained by averaging the LH values of the two samples.
2. Administer a bolus of 100 mcg of FACTREL subcutaneously or intravenously.
3. Draw venous blood samples at 15, 30, 45, 60, and 120 minutes after administration.

Fig. 1:
Normal Male LH Response After FACTREL 100 mcg, Subcutaneous Administration 10th and 90th percentiles.

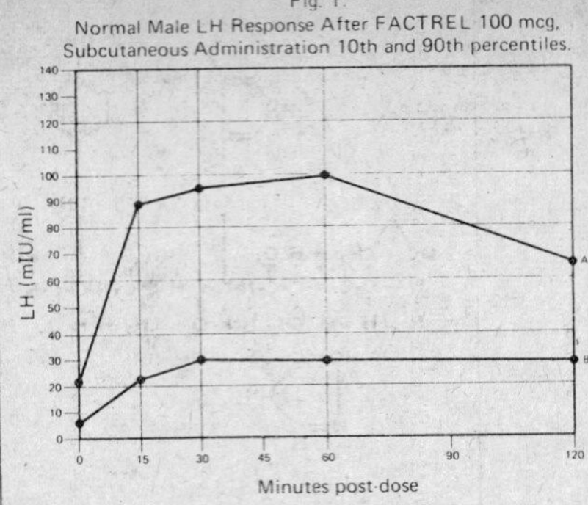

Fig. 2:
Normal Male LH Response After FACTREL 100 mcg, Intravenous Administration 10th and 90th percentiles.

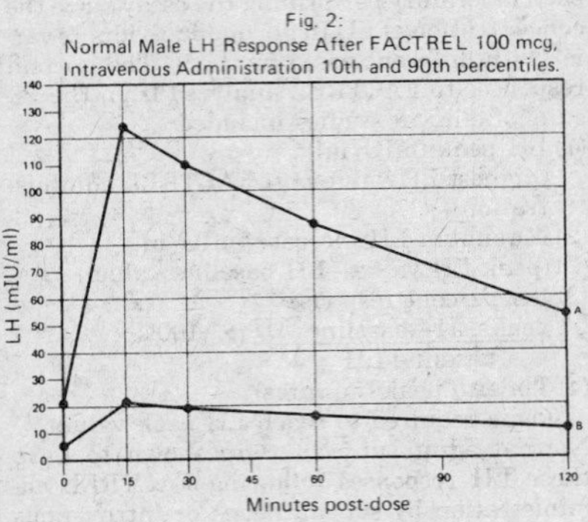

Fig. 3:
Normal Female LH Response After FACTREL 100 mcg, Subcutaneous Administration 10th and 90th percentiles.

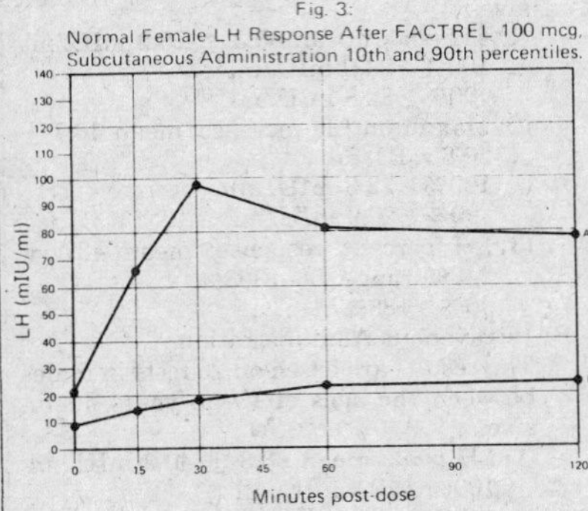

Fig. 4:
Normal Female LH Response After FACTREL 100 mcg, Intravenous Administration 10th and 90th percentiles.

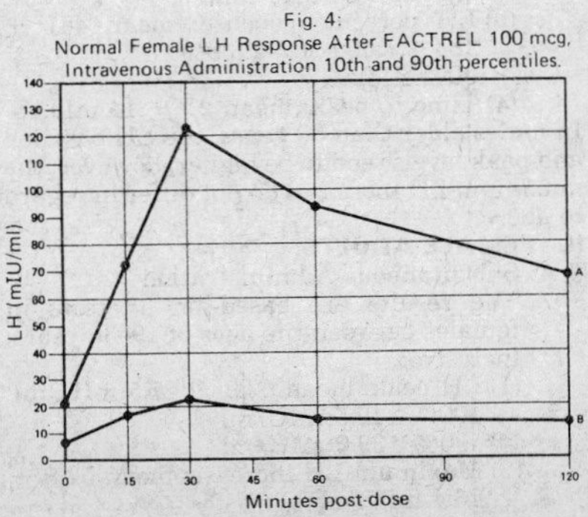

4. Blood samples should be handled as recommended by the laboratory that will determine the LH content. It must be emphasized that the reliability of the test is directly related to the inter-assay and intra-assay reliability of the laboratory performing the assay.

Interpretation of Test Results: Interpretation of the LH response to FACTREL requires an understanding of the hypothalamic-pituitary physiology, knowledge of the clinical status of the individual patient, and familiarity with the normal ranges and the standards used in the laboratory performing the LH assays.
Figures 1 through 4 represent the LH response curves after FACTREL administration in normal subjects. The normal LH response curves were established between the 10th percentile (B line) and 90th percentile (A line) of all LH responses in normal subjects analyzed from the results of clinical studies. LH values are reported in units of mIU/ml and time is displayed in minutes. Individual patient responses should be plotted on the appropriate curve. A subnormal response in patients is defined as three or more LH values which fall below the B line of the normal LH response curve.
In cases where there is a blunted or borderline response, the FACTREL test should be repeated.
The FACTREL test complements the clinical assessment of patients with a variety of endocrine disorders involving the hypothalamic-pituitary axis in cases where there is a normal response, it indicates the presence of functional pituitary gonadotropes. The single injection test does not determine the pathophysiological cause for the subnormal response and does not measure pituitary gonadotropic reserve.
How Supplied: LYOPHILIZED POWDER in single-dose vials containing 100 mcg (NDC 0046-0507-05) and 500 mcg (NDC 0046-0509-05) gonadorelin as the hydrochloride with 100 mg lactose, U.S.P. Each vial is accompanied by one ampul containing 2 ml sterile diluent of 2% benzyl alcohol in Water for Injection, U.S.P.
Directions: Store at room temperature (approximately 25°C).
Reconstitute 100 mcg vial with 1.0 ml of the accompanying sterile diluent.
Reconstitute 500 mcg vial with 2.0 ml of the accompanying sterile diluent.
Prepare solution immediately before use.
After reconstitution, store at room temperature and use within 1 day.
Discard unused reconstituted solution and diluent.
Diagnostic Method of Use Patent 3,947,569

FLUOTHANE® ℞

Brand of halothane, U.S.P.

Description: FLUOTHANE, brand of halothane, U.S.P., is an inhalation anesthetic. It is 2-bromo-2-chloro-1,1,1-trifluoroethane.
The specific gravity is 1.872-1.877 at 20° C, and the boiling point (range) is 49° C-51° C at 760 mm Hg. The vapor pressure is 243 mm Hg at 20° C. The blood/gas coefficient is 2.5 at 37° C, and the olive oil/water coefficient is 220 at 37° C. Vapor concentrations within anesthetic range are nonirritating and have a pleasant odor. FLUOTHANE is nonflammable, and its vapors mixed with oxygen in proportions from 0.5 to 50 per cent (v/v) are not explosive.
FLUOTHANE does not decompose in contact with warm soda lime. When moisture is present, the vapor attacks aluminum, brass, and lead, but not copper. Rubber, some plastics,

and similar materials are soluble in FLUOTHANE; such materials will deteriorate rapidly in contact with FLUOTHANE vapor or liquid. Stability of FLUOTHANE is maintained by the addition of 0.01 per cent thymol (w/w), up to 0.00025% ammonia (w/w), and storage is in amber colored bottles.

FLUOTHANE should not be kept indefinitely in vaporizer bottles not specifically designed for its use. Thymol does not volatilize along with FLUOTHANE, and therefore accumulates in the vaporizer, and may, in time, impart a yellow color to the remaining liquid or to wicks in vaporizers. The development of such discoloration may be used as an indicator that the vaporizer should be drained and cleaned, and the discolored FLUOTHANE (halothane, U.S.P.) discarded. Accumulation of thymol may be removed by washing with diethyl ether. After cleaning a wick or vaporizer, make certain all the diethyl ether has been removed before reusing the equipment to avoid introducing ether into the system.

Actions: FLUOTHANE is an inhalation anesthetic. Induction and recovery are rapid and depth of anesthesia can be rapidly altered. FLUOTHANE progressively depresses respiration. There may be tachypnea with reduced tidal volume and alveolar ventilation. FLUOTHANE is not an irritant to the respiratory tract, and no increase in salivary or bronchial secretions ordinarily occurs. Pharyngeal and laryngeal reflexes are rapidly obtunded. It causes bronchodilation. Hypoxia, acidosis, or apnea may develop during deep anesthesia.

FLUOTHANE reduces the blood pressure, and frequently decreases the pulse rate. The greater the concentration of the drug, the more evident these changes become. Atropine may reverse the bradycardia. FLUOTHANE does not cause the release of catecholamines from adrenergic stores. FLUOTHANE also causes dilation of the vessels of the skin and skeletal muscles.

Cardiac arrhythmias may occur during FLUOTHANE anesthesia. These include nodal rhythm, AV dissociation, ventricular extrasystoles and asystole. FLUOTHANE sensitizes the myocardial conduction system to the action of epinephrine and norepinephrine, and the combination may cause serious cardiac arrhythmias. FLUOTHANE increases cerebral spinal fluid pressure. FLUOTHANE produces moderate muscular relaxation. Muscle relaxants are used as adjuncts in order to maintain lighter levels of anesthesia. FLUOTHANE augments the action of nondepolarizing relaxants and ganglionic blocking agents. FLUOTHANE is a potent uterine relaxant.

Indications: FLUOTHANE (halothane, U.S.P.) is indicated for the induction and maintenance of general anesthesia.

Contraindications: FLUOTHANE is not recommended for obstetrical anesthesia except when uterine relaxation is required.

Warnings: When previous exposure to FLUOTHANE was followed by unexplained jaundice, consideration should be given to the use of other agents.

FLUOTHANE should be used in vaporizers that permit a reasonable approximation of output, and preferably of the calibrated type. The vaporizer should be placed out of circuit in closed circuit rebreathing systems; otherwise overdosage is difficult to avoid. The patient should be closely observed for signs of overdosage, *i.e.*, depression of blood pressure, pulse rate, and ventilation, particularly during assisted or controlled ventilation.

Usage in Pregnancy. Safe use of FLUOTHANE has not been established with respect to possible adverse effects upon fetal development. Therefore, FLUOTHANE should not be used in women where pregnancy is possible and particularly during early pregnancy, unless, in the judgment of the physician, the potential benefits outweigh the unknown hazards to the fetus.

Precautions: The uterine relaxation obtained with FLUOTHANE (halothane, U.S.P.) unless carefully controlled, may fail to respond to ergot derivatives and oxytocic posterior pituitary extract.

FLUOTHANE increases cerebrospinal fluid pressure. Therefore, in patients with markedly raised intracranial pressure, if FLUOTHANE is indicated, administration should be preceded by measures ordinarily used to reduce cerebrospinal fluid pressure. Ventilation should be carefully assessed, and it may be necessary to assist or control ventilation to insure adequate oxygenation and carbon dioxide removal.

Epinephrine or norepinephrine should be employed cautiously, if at all, during FLUOTHANE (halothane, U.S.P.) anesthesia since their simultaneous use may induce ventricular tachycardia or fibrillation.

Nondepolarizing relaxants and ganglionic blocking agents should be administered cautiously, since their actions are augmented by FLUOTHANE.

It has been reported that in genetically susceptible individuals, the use of general anesthetics and the muscle relaxant, succinylcholine, may trigger a syndrome known as malignant hyperthermic crisis. Monitoring temperature during surgery will aid in early recognition of this syndrome. Dantrolene sodium and supportive measures are generally indicated in the management of malignant hyperthermia.

Adverse Reactions: The following adverse reactions have been reported: mild, moderate and severe hepatic dysfunction (including hepatic necrosis), cardiac arrest, hypotension, respiratory arrest, cardiac arrhythmias, hyperpyrexia, shivering, nausea, and emesis.

Dosage and Administration: FLUOTHANE may be administered by the nonrebreathing technic, partial rebreathing, or closed technic. The induction dose varies from patient to patient. The maintenance dose varies from 0.5 per cent to 1.5 per cent.

FLUOTHANE may be administered with either oxygen or a mixture of oxygen and nitrous oxide.

How Supplied: Unit packages of 125 ml (NDC 0046-3125-81) and 250 ml (NDC 0046-3125-82) of halothane, U.S.P., stabilized with 0.01% thymol (w/w) and up to 0.00025% ammonia (w/w).

GRISACTIN® ℞

Brand of griseofulvin (microsize)

Indications: Griseofulvin is indicated for the treatment of ringworm infections of the skin, hair, and nails, namely: *tinea corporis, tinea pedis, tinea cruris, tinea barbae, tinea capitis, tinea unguium* (onychomycosis) when caused by one or more of the following genera of fungi: *Trichophyton rubrum, T. tonsurans, T. mentagrophytes, T. interdigitalis, T. verrucosum, T. megnini, T. gallinae, T. crateriform, T. sulphureum, T. schoenleini, Microsporum audouini, M. canis, M. gypseum, Epidermophyton floccosum.*

NOTE: Prior to therapy, the type of fungi responsible for the infection should be identified.

The use of this drug is not justified in minor or trivial infections which will respond to topical agents alone.

Griseofulvin is *not* effective in the following: Bacterial infections, candidiasis (moniliasis), histoplasmosis, actinomycosis, sporotrichosis, chromoblastomycosis, coccidioidomycosis, North American blastomycosis, cryptococcosis (torulosis), *tinea versicolor,* nocardiosis.

Contraindications: This drug is contraindicated in patients with porphyria, hepatocellular failure, and in individuals with a history of hypersensitivity to griseofulvin.

Warnings: *Prophylactic Usage*—Safety and efficacy of griseofulvin for prophylaxis of fungal infections has not been established.

Animal Toxicology—Chronic feeding of griseofulvin, at levels ranging from 0.5-2.5% of the diet, resulted in the development of liver tumors in several strains of mice, particularly males. Smaller particle sizes result in an enhanced effect. Lower oral dosage levels have not been tested. Subcutaneous administration of relatively small doses of griseofulvin, once a week, during the first three weeks of life has also been reported to induce hepatomata in mice. Although studies in other animal species have not yielded evidence of tumorigenicity, these studies were not of adequate design to form a basis for conclusions in this regard.

In subacute toxicity studies, orally administered griseofulvin produced hepatocellular necrosis in mice, but this has not been seen in other species. Disturbances in porphyrin metabolism have been reported in griseofulvin-treated laboratory animals. Griseofulvin has been reported to have a colchicine-like effect on mitosis and cocarcinogenicity with methylcholanthrene in cutaneous tumor induction in laboratory animals.

Usage in Pregnancy—The safety of this drug during pregnancy has not been established.

Animal Reproduction Studies—It has been reported in the literature that griseofulvin was found to be embryotoxic and teratogenic on oral administration to pregnant rats. Pups with abnormalities have been reported in the litters of a few bitches treated with griseofulvin. Additional animal reproduction studies are in progress.

Suppression of spermatogenesis has been reported to occur in rats, but investigation in man failed to confirm this.

Precautions: Patients on prolonged therapy with any potent medication should be under close observation. Periodic monitoring of organ system function, including renal, hepatic, and hematopoietic, should be done.

Since griseofulvin is derived from species of *Penicillium,* the possibility of cross-sensitivity with penicillin exists; however, known penicillin-sensitive patients have been treated without difficulty.

Since a photosensitivity reaction is occasionally associated with griseofulvin therapy, patients should be warned to avoid exposure to intense natural or artificial sunlight. Should a photosensitivity reaction occur, lupus erythematosus may be aggravated.

Griseofulvin decreases the activity of warfarin-type anticoagulants so that patients receiving these drugs concomitantly may require dosage adjustment of the anticoagulant during and after griseofulvin therapy.

Barbiturates usually depress griseofulvin activity and concomitant administration may require a dosage adjustment of the antifungal agent.

Griseofulvin may augment or potentiate the effects of alcohol.

Adverse Reactions: When adverse reactions occur, they are most commonly of the hypersensitivity type such as skin rashes, urticaria, and rarely, angioneurotic edema, and may necessitate withdrawal of therapy and appropriate countermeasures. Paresthesias of the hands and feet have been reported rarely after extended therapy. Other side effects reported occasionally are oral thrush, nausea, vomiting, epigastric distress, diarrhea, headache, fatigue, dizziness, insomnia, mental confusion, and impairment of performance of routine activities.

Proteinuria and leukopenia have been reported rarely. Administration of the drug should be discontinued if granulocytopenia occurs.

Continued on next page

Ayerst—Cont.

When rare, serious reactions occur with griseofulvin, they are usually associated with high dosages, long periods of therapy, or both.

Dosage and Administration: Accurate diagnosis of the infecting organism is essential. Identification should be made either by direct microscopic examination of a mounting of infected tissue in a solution of potassium hydroxide or by culture on an appropriate medium.

Medication must be continued until the infecting organism is completely eradicated as indicated by appropriate clinical or laboratory examination. Representative treatment periods are—*tinea capitis,* 4 to 6 weeks; *tinea corporis,* 2 to 4 weeks; *tinea pedis,* 4 to 8 weeks; *tinea unguium*—depending on rate of growth—fingernails, at least 4 months: toenails, at least 6 months.

General measures in regard to hygiene should be observed to control sources of infection or reinfection. Concomitant use of appropriate topical agents is usually required, particularly in treatment of *tinea pedis.* In some forms of athlete's foot, yeasts and bacteria may be involved as well as fungi. Griseofulvin will not eradicate the bacterial or monilial infection.

Adults: 0.5 g daily (125 mg q.i.d., 250 mg b.i.d., or 500 mg/day). Patients with less severe or extensive infections may require less, whereas those with widespread lesions may require a starting dose of 0.75 g to 1.0 g a day. This may be reduced gradually to 0.5 g or less after a response has been noted. In all cases, the dosage should be individualized.

Children: A dosage of 10 mg/kg daily is usually adequate (children from 30 to 50 lb, 125 mg to 250 mg daily; children over 50 lb, 250 mg to 500 mg daily, in divided doses). Dosage should be individualized, as with adults.

Clinical relapse will occur if the medication is not continued until the infecting organism is eradicated.

How Supplied: GRISACTIN [griseofulvin (microsize)]—GRISACTIN 125, each capsule contains 125 mg, in bottles of 100 (NDC 0046-0442-81); GRISACTIN 250, each capsule contains 250 mg, in bottles of 100 (NDC 0046-0443-81) and 500 (NDC 0046-0443-85); and GRISACTIN 500, each tablet (scored) contains 500 mg, in bottles of 60 (NDC 0046-0444-60).

[*Shown in Product Identification Section*]

GRISACTIN® Ultra ℞
(griseofulvin ultramicrosize)

Description: Griseofulvin is an oral fungistatic antibiotic for the treatment of superficial mycoses. It is derived from a species of *Penicillium.*

GRISACTIN Ultra (griseofulvin ultramicrosize) tablets contain either 125 mg or 250 mg of griseofulvin ultramicrosize.

Action: Griseofulvin is fungistatic with *in vitro* activity against various species of *Microsporum, Epidermophyton,* and *Trichophyton.* It has no effect on bacteria or on other genera of fungi.

Griseofulvin is deposited in the keratin precursor cells and has a greater affinity for diseased tissue. The drug is tightly bound to the new keratin which becomes highly resistant to fungal invasions.

Controlled bioavailability studies of GRISACTIN Ultra (griseofulvin ultramicrosize) have demonstrated comparable values to blood levels regarded as adequate. The efficiency of gastrointestinal absorption of ultramicrocrystalline griseofulvin is approximately twice that of the conventional microsized griseofulvin. This factor permits the oral intake of half as much griseofulvin per tablet but there is no evidence, at this time, that this confers any significant clinical differences in regard to safety and efficacy.

Indications: Griseofulvin is indicated for the treatment of ringworm infections of the skin, hair, and nails, namely:

Tinea corporis
Tinea pedis
Tinea cruris
Tinea barbae
Tinea capitis

Tinea unguium (onychomycosis) when caused by one or more of the following genera of fungi:

Trichophyton rubrum
Trichophyton tonsurans
Trichophyton mentagrophytes
Trichophyton interdigitalis
Trichophyton verrucosum
Trichophyton megnini
Trichophyton gallinae
Trichophyton crateriform
Trichophyton sulphureum
Trichophyton schoenleini
Microsporum audouini
Microsporum canis
Microsporum gypseum
Epidermophyton floccosum

NOTE: Prior to therapy, the type of fungi responsible for the infection should be identified.

The use of this drug is not justified in minor or trivial infections which will respond to topical agents alone.

Griseofulvin is *not* effective in the following:

Bacterial infections
Candidiasis (Moniliasis)
Histoplasmosis
Actinomycosis
Sporotrichosis
Chromoblastomycosis
Coccidioidomycosis
North American Blastomycosis
Cryptococcosis (Torulosis)
Tinea versicolor
Nocardiosis

Contraindications: This drug is contraindicated in patients with porphyria, hepatocellular failure, and in individuals with a history of hypersensitivity to griseofulvin.

Warnings:

Prophylactic Usage

Safety and efficacy of griseofulvin for prophylaxis of fungal infections has not been established.

Animal Toxicology

Chronic feeding of griseofulvin, at levels ranging from 0.5–2.5% of the diet, resulted in the development of liver tumors in several strains of mice, particularly males. Smaller particle sizes result in an enhanced effect. Lower oral dosage levels have not been tested. Subcutaneous administration of relatively small doses of griseofulvin, once a week, during the first three weeks of life has also been reported to induce hepatomata in mice. Although studies in other animal species have not yielded evidence of tumorigenicity, these studies were not of adequate design to form a basis for conclusions in this regard.

In subacute toxicity studies, orally administered griseofulvin produced hepatocellular necrosis in mice, but this has not been seen in other species. Disturbances in porphyrin metabolism have been reported in griseofulvin-treated laboratory animals. Griseofulvin has been reported to have a colchicine-like effect on mitosis and cocarcinogenicity with methylcholanthrene in cutaneous tumor induction in laboratory animals.

Usage in Pregnancy

The safety of this drug during pregnancy has not been established.

Animal Reproduction Studies

It has been reported in the literature that griseofulvin was found to be embryotoxic and teratogenic on oral administration to pregnant rats. Pups with abnormalities have been reported in the litters of a few bitches treated with griseofulvin. Additional animal reproduction studies are in progress.

Suppression of spermatogenesis has been reported to occur in rats, but investigation in man failed to confirm this.

Precautions: Patients on prolonged therapy with any potent medication should be under close observation. Periodic monitoring of organ system function, including renal, hepatic, and hematopoietic, should be done.

Since griseofulvin is derived from species of *Penicillium,* the possibility of cross-sensitivity with penicillin exists; however, known penicillin-sensitive patients have been treated without difficulty.

Since a photosensitivity reaction is occasionally associated with griseofulvin therapy, patients should be warned to avoid exposure to intense natural or artificial sunlight. Should a photosensitivity reaction occur, lupus erythematosus may be aggravated.

Griseofulvin decreases the activity of warfarin-type anticoagulants so that patients receiving these drugs concomitantly may require dosage adjustment of the anticoagulant during and after griseofulvin therapy.

Barbiturates usually depress griseofulvin activity and concomitant administration may require a dosage adjustment of the antifungal agent.

Griseofulvin may augment or potentiate the effects of alcohol.

Adverse Reactions: When adverse reactions occur, they are most commonly of the hypersensitivity type such as skin rashes, urticaria, and rarely, angioneurotic edema, and may necessitate withdrawal of therapy and appropriate countermeasures. Paresthesias of the hands and feet have been reported rarely after extended therapy. Other side effects reported occasionally are oral thrush, nausea, vomiting, epigastric distress, diarrhea, headache, fatigue, dizziness, insomnia, mental confusion, and impairment of performance of routine activities.

Proteinuria and leukopenia have been reported rarely. Administration of the drug should be discontinued if granulocytopenia occurs.

When rare, serious reactions occur with griseofulvin, they are usually associated with high dosages, long periods of therapy, or both.

Dosage and Administration: Accurate diagnosis of the infecting organism is essential. Identification should be made either by direct microscopic examination of a mounting of infected tissue in a solution of potassium hydroxide or by culture on an appropriate medium.

Medication must be continued until the infecting organism is completely eradicated as indicated by appropriate clinical or laboratory examination. Representative treatment periods are—*tinea capitis,* 4 to 6 weeks; *tinea corporis,* 2 to 4 weeks; *tinea pedis,* 4 to 8 weeks; *tinea unguium*—depending on rate of growth—fingernails, at least 4 months; toenails, at least 6 months.

General measures in regard to hygiene should be observed to control sources of infection or reinfection. Concomitant use of appropriate topical agents is usually required, particularly in treatment of *tinea pedis.* In some forms of athlete's foot, yeasts and bacteria may be involved as well as fungi. Griseofulvin will not eradicate the bacterial or monilial infection.

Adults: Daily administration of 250 mg (as a single dose or in divided doses) will give a satisfactory response in most patients with tinea corporis, tinea cruris, and tinea capitis. For those fungal infections more difficult to eradicate such as tinea pedis and tinea unguium, a divided dose of 500 mg is recommended.

Children: Approximately 2.5 mg per pound of body weight per day is an effective dose for most children. On this basis the following dosage schedule is suggested: Children weighing 30–50 pounds—62.5 mg to 125 mg daily. Children weighing over 50 pounds—125–250 mg daily. Children 2 years of age and younger—

dosage has not been established. Clinical experience with griseofulvin in children with tinea capitis indicates that a single daily dose is effective. Clinical relapse will occur if the medication is not continued until the infecting organism is eradicated.

How Supplied: GRISACTIN® Ultra (griseofulvin ultramicrosize) tablets, 125 mg: white, compressed tablets impressed with the trade name and dosage strength, in bottles of 100 (NDC 0046-0434-81).

GRISACTIN® Ultra tablets, 250 mg: white, compressed tablets impressed with the trade name and dosage strength, in bottles of 100 (NDC 0046-0435-81).

Store at room temperature (approximately 25° C).

[*Shown in Product Identification Section*]

INDERAL® ℞

Brand of propranolol hydrochloride

> BEFORE USING INDERAL (PROPRANOLOL HYDROCHLORIDE), THE PHYSICIAN SHOULD BE THOROUGHLY FAMILIAR WITH THE BASIC CONCEPT OF ADRENERGIC RECEPTORS (ALPHA AND BETA), AND THE PHARMACOLOGY OF THIS DRUG.

Description: *Chemical name:* 1-(Isopropylamino)-3-(1-naphthyloxy)-2-propanol hydrochloride.

Structural formula:

$O\,CH_2CHOHCH_2NHCH(CH_3)_2 \cdot HCl$

INDERAL (propranolol hydrochloride) is a stable, colorless, crystalline solid with a melting point of about 164° C. It is readily soluble in water and ethanol and insoluble in non-polar solvents.

Actions: INDERAL is a beta-adrenergic receptor blocking drug, possessing no other autonomic nervous system activity. It specifically competes with beta-adrenergic receptor stimulating agents for available beta receptor sites. When access to beta receptor sites is blocked by INDERAL, the chronotropic, inotropic, and vasodilator responses to beta-adrenergic stimulation are decreased proportionately.

Propranolol is almost completely absorbed from the gastrointestinal tract, but a portion is immediately bound by the liver. Peak effect occurs in one to one and one-half hours. The biologic half-life is approximately two to three hours. Propranolol is not significantly dialyzable. There is no simple correlation between dose or plasma level and therapeutic effect, and the dose-sensitivity range as observed in clinical practice is wide. The principal reason for this is that sympathetic tone varies widely between individuals. Since there is no reliable test to estimate sympathetic tone or to determine whether total beta blockade has been achieved, proper dosage requires titration.

The mechanisms of the antihypertensive and antimigraine effects of INDERAL (propranolol HCl) have not been established. Among the factors that may be involved in the antihypertensive action are (1) decreased cardiac output, (2) inhibition of renin release by the kidneys, and (3) diminution of tonic sympathetic nerve outflow from vasomotor centers in the brain. The antimigraine effect may be due to inhibition of vasodilation or to the fact that beta-adrenergic receptors have been demonstrated in the pial vessels of the brain and that arteriolar spasms over the cortex can be inhibited with INDERAL.

Propranolol hydrochloride decreases heart rate, cardiac output, and blood pressure. Although total peripheral vascular resistance may increase initially, it readjusts to the pretreatment level, or lower, with chronic usage. Earlier studies indicate that plasma volume remains unchanged or may decrease. However, there are certain more recent studies suggesting that in the absence of sodium restriction, plasma volume may increase.

Beta receptor blockade is useful in conditions in which, because of pathologic or functional changes, sympathetic activity is excessive or inappropriate and detrimental to the patient. But there are also situations in which sympathetic stimulation is vital. For example, in patients with severely damaged hearts, adequate ventricular function is maintained by virtue of sympathetic drive which should be preserved. In the presence of AV block, beta blockade may prevent the necessary facilitating effect of sympathetic activity on conduction. Beta blockade results in bronchial constriction by interfering with adrenergic bronchodilator activity which should be preserved in patients subject to bronchospasm.

The proper objective of beta blockade therapy is to decrease adverse sympathetic stimulation but not to the degree that may impair necessary sympathetic support.

Propranolol exerts its antiarrhythmic effects in concentrations associated with beta-adrenergic blockade and this appears to be its principal antiarrhythmic mechanism of action. The membrane effect also plays a role, particularly, some authorities believe, in digitalis-induced arrhythmias. Beta-adrenergic blockade is of unique importance in the management of arrhythmias due to increased levels of circulating catecholamines or enhanced sensitivity of the heart to catecholamines (arrhythmias associated with pheochromocytoma, thyrotoxicosis, exercise).

In dosages greater than required for beta blockade, INDERAL (propranolol HCl) also exerts a quinidine-like or anesthetic-like membrane action which affects the cardiac action potential and depresses cardiac function.

Propranolol may reduce the oxygen requirement of the heart at any given level of effort by blocking catecholamine-induced increases in heart rate, systolic blood pressure, and the velocity and extent of myocardial contraction. On the other hand, propranolol may increase oxygen requirements by increasing left ventricular fiber length, end diastolic pressure, and systolic ejection period.

If the net physiologic effect of beta-adrenergic blockade in angina is advantageous, it would be expected to manifest itself during exercise by delayed onset of pain due to decreased oxygen requirement.

Indications:

Hypertension

INDERAL is indicated in the management of hypertension. It is usually used in combination with other drugs, particularly a thiazide diuretic. INDERAL is not indicated for treatment of hypertensive emergencies.

Angina Pectoris Due to Coronary Atherosclerosis

The initial treatment of angina pectoris involves weight control, rest, cessation of smoking, use of sublingual nitroglycerin, and avoidance of precipitating circumstances. INDERAL is indicated in selected patients with moderate to severe angina pectoris who have not responded to these conventional measures. Propranolol should not be used in patients with angina which occurs only with considerable effort or with infrequent precipitating factors.

INDERAL exerts both favorable and unfavorable effects, the preponderance of which may be beneficial. (See ACTIONS Section.) INDERAL should not be continued unless there is reduced pain or increased work capacity.

Because of the potential for adverse results, treatment should be carefully monitored. The patient should also be reevaluated periodically since the dosage requirement and the need to continue INDERAL may be altered by clinical exacerbations or remissions. (See DOSAGE AND ADMINISTRATION.)

Additional studies of the effects of INDERAL in angina pectoris patients are in progress to better evaluate and define the proper role of INDERAL in this condition.

Cardiac Arrhythmias

1.) Supraventricular arrhythmias
   a) Paroxysmal atrial tachycardias, particularly those arrhythmias induced by catecholamines or digitalis or associated with the Wolff-Parkinson-White syndrome (See W-P-W under WARNINGS.)
   b) Persistent sinus tachycardia which is noncompensatory and impairs the well-being of the patient.
   c) Tachycardias and arrhythmias due to thyrotoxicosis when causing distress or increased hazard and when immediate effect is necessary as adjunctive, short term (2–4 weeks) therapy.
   May be used with, but not in place of, specific therapy (See Thyrotoxicosis under WARNINGS.)
   d) Persistent atrial extrasystoles which impair the well-being of the patient and not respond to conventional measures.
   e) Atrial flutter and fibrillation when ventricular rate cannot be controlled by digitalis alone, or when digitalis is contraindicated.

2.) Ventricular tachycardias
   Ventricular arrhythmias do not respond to propranolol as predictably as do the supraventricular arrhythmias.
   a) Ventricular tachycardias
   With the exception of those induced by catecholamines or digitalis. INDERAL (propranolol HCl) is not the drug of first choice. In critical situations when cardioversion technics or other drugs are not indicated or are not effective, INDERAL may be considered. If, after consideration of the risks involved, INDERAL is used, it should be given intravenously in low dosage and very slowly. (See DOSAGE AND ADMINISTRATION.) *Care in the administration of INDERAL with constant electrocardiographic monitoring is essential as the failing heart requires some sympathetic drive for maintenance of myocardial tone.*
   b) Persistent premature ventricular extrasystoles which do not respond to conventional measures and impair the well-being of the patient.

3.) Tachyarrhythmias of digitalis intoxication
   If digitalis-induced tachyarrhythmias persist following discontinuance of digitalis and correction of electrolyte abnormalities, they are usually reversible with *oral* INDERAL. Severe bradycardia may occur. (See OVERDOSAGE OR EXAGGERATED RESPONSE.)
   Intravenous propranolol hydrochloride is reserved for life-threatening arrhythmias. Temporary maintenance with oral therapy may be indicated. (See DOSAGE AND ADMINISTRATION.)

4.) Resistant tachyarrhythmias due to excessive catecholamine action during anesthesia
   Tachyarrhythmias due to excessive catecholamine action during anesthesia may sometimes arise because of release of endogenous catecholamines or administration of catecholamines. When usual measures fail in such arrhythmias, INDERAL may be given intravenously to abolish them. All general inhalation anesthetics produce some degree of myocardial depres-

Continued on next page

Ayerst—Cont.

sion. Therefore, when INDERAL is used to treat arrhythmias during anesthesia, it should be used with extreme caution and constant ECG and central venous pressure monitoring. (See WARNINGS.)

Migraine

INDERAL is indicated for the prophylaxis of common migraine headache. The efficacy of INDERAL in the treatment of a migraine attack that has already started has not been established and INDERAL is not indicated for such use.

Vascular headaches of the migraine type are often familial, are recurrent, and vary widely in frequency, duration, and intensity. The attacks are commonly unilateral in onset, and are usually associated with anorexia, and sometimes nausea and vomiting. In females, these headaches often occur premenstrually or early during the menses. Migraine attacks are sometimes preceded by, or associated with, conspicuous sensory, motor, and mood disturbances, but common migraine usually occurs without striking prodromes, and is less often unilateral.

Hypertrophic Subaortic Stenosis

INDERAL (propranolol HCl) is useful in the management of hypertrophic subaortic stenosis, especially for treatment of exertional or other stress-induced angina, palpitations, and syncope. INDERAL also improves exercise performance. The effectiveness of INDERAL in this disease appears to be due to a reduction of the elevated outflow pressure gradient which is exacerbated by beta receptor stimulation. Clinical improvement may be temporary.

Pheochromocytoma

After primary treatment with an alpha-adrenergic blocking agent has been instituted, INDERAL may be useful as *adjunctive* therapy if the control of tachycardia becomes necessary before or during surgery.

It is hazardous to use INDERAL unless alpha-adrenergic blocking drugs are already in use, since this would predispose to serious blood pressure elevation. Blocking only the peripheral dilator (beta) action of epinephrine leaves its constrictor (alpha) action unopposed.

In the event of hemorrhage or shock, there is a disadvantage in having both beta and alpha blockade since the combination prevents the increase in heart rate and peripheral vasoconstriction needed to maintain blood pressure.

With inoperable or metastatic pheochromocytoma, INDERAL may be useful as an adjunct to the management of symptoms due to excessive beta receptor stimulation.

Contraindications: INDERAL is contraindicated in: 1) bronchial asthma; 2) allergic rhinitis during the pollen season; 3) sinus bradycardia and greater than first degree block; 4) cardiogenic shock; 5) right ventricular failure secondary to pulmonary hypertension; 6) congestive heart failure (see WARNINGS) unless the failure is secondary to a tachyarrhythmia treatable with INDERAL; 7) in patients on adrenergic-augmenting psychotropic drugs (including MAO inhibitors), and during the two week withdrawal period from such drugs.

Warnings: CARDIAC FAILURE: Sympathetic stimulation is a vital component supporting circulatory function in congestive heart failure, and inhibition with beta-blockade always carries the potential hazard of further depressing myocardial contractility and precipitating cardiac failure. INDERAL acts selectively without abolishing the inotropic action of digitalis on the heart muscle (*i.e.*, that of supporting the strength of myocardial contractions). In patients already receiving digitalis, the positive inotropic action of digitalis may be reduced by INDERAL's negative inotropic effect. The effects of INDERAL and digitalis are additive in depressing AV conduction.

IN PATIENTS WITHOUT A HISTORY OF CARDIAC FAILURE, continued depression of the myocardium over a period of time can, in some cases, lead to cardiac failure. In rare instances, this has been observed during INDERAL therapy. Therefore, at the first sign or symptom of impending cardiac failure, patients should be fully digitalized and/or given a diuretic, and the response observed closely: a) if cardiac failure continues, despite adequate digitalization and diuretic therapy, INDERAL therapy should be immediately withdrawn; b) if tachyarrhythmia is being controlled, patients should be maintained on combined therapy and the patient closely followed until threat of cardiac failure is over.

IN PATIENTS WITH ANGINA PECTORIS, there have been reports of exacerbation of angina and, in some cases, myocardial infarction, following *abrupt* discontinuation of INDERAL (propranolol HCl) therapy. Therefore, when discontinuance of INDERAL is planned the dosage should be gradually reduced and the patient carefully monitored. In addition, when INDERAL is prescribed for angina pectoris, the patient should be cautioned against interruption or cessation of therapy without the physician's advice. If INDERAL therapy is interrupted and exacerbation of angina occurs, it usually is advisable to reinstitute INDERAL therapy and take other measures appropriate for the management of unstable angina pectoris. Since coronary artery disease may be unrecognized, it may be prudent to follow the above advice in patients considered at risk of having occult atherosclerotic heart disease, who are given propranolol for other indications.

IN PATIENTS WITH THYROTOXICOSIS, possible deleterious effects from long term use have not been adequately appraised. Special consideration should be given to propranolol's potential for aggravating congestive heart failure. Propranolol may mask the clinical signs of developing or continuing hyperthyroidism or complications and give a false impression of improvement. Therefore, abrupt withdrawal of propranolol may be followed by an exacerbation of symptoms of hyperthyroidism, including thyroid storm. This is another reason for withdrawing propranolol slowly. Propranolol does not distort thyroid function tests.

IN PATIENTS WITH WOLFF-PARKINSON-WHITE SYNDROME, several cases have been reported in which, after propranolol, the tachycardia was replaced by a severe bradycardia requiring a demand pacemaker. In one case this resulted after an initial dose of 5 mg propranolol.

IN PATIENTS DURING ANESTHESIA with agents that require catecholamine release for maintenance of adequate cardiac function, beta blockade will impair the desired inotropic effect. Therefore, INDERAL should be titrated carefully when administered for arrhythmias occurring during anesthesia.

IN PATIENTS UNDERGOING MAJOR SURGERY, beta blockade impairs the ability of the heart to respond to reflex stimuli. For this reason, with the exception of pheochromocytoma, INDERAL should be withdrawn 48 hours prior to surgery, at which time all chemical and physiologic effects are gone according to available evidence. However, in case of emergency surgery, since INDERAL is a competitive inhibitor of beta receptor agonists, its effects can be reversed by administration of such agents, *e.g.*, isoproterenol or levarterenol. However, such patients may be subject to protracted severe hypotension. Difficulty in restarting and maintaining the heart beat has also been reported.

IN PATIENTS PRONE TO NONALLERGIC BRONCHOSPASM (*e.g.*, CHRONIC BRONCHITIS, EMPHYSEMA), INDERAL should be administered with caution since it may block bronchodilation produced by endogenous and exogenous catecholamine stimulation of beta receptors.

DIABETICS AND PATIENTS SUBJECT TO HYPOGLYCEMIA: Because of its beta-adrenergic blocking activity, INDERAL may prevent the appearance of premonitory signs and symptoms (pulse rate and pressure changes) of acute hypoglycemia. This is especially important to keep in mind in patients with labile diabetes. Hypoglycemic attacks may be accompanied by a precipitous elevation of blood pressure.

USE IN PREGNANCY: The safe use of INDERAL (propranolol HCl) in human pregnancy has not been established. Use of any drug in pregnancy or women of childbearing potential requires that the possible risk to mother and/ or fetus be weighed against the expected therapeutic benefit. Embryotoxic effects have been seen in animal studies at doses about 10 times the maximum recommended human dose.

Precautions: Patients receiving catecholamine depleting drugs such as reserpine should be closely observed if INDERAL is administered. The added catecholamine blocking action of this drug may then produce an excessive reduction of the resting sympathetic nervous activity. Occasionally, the pharmacologic activity of INDERAL may produce hypotension and/or marked bradycardia resulting in vertigo, syncopal attacks, or orthostatic hypotension.

As with any new drug given over prolonged periods, laboratory parameters should be observed at regular intervals. The drug should be used with caution in patients with impaired renal or hepatic function.

Adverse Reactions: *Cardiovascular:* bradycardia, congestive heart failure; intensification of AV block; hypotension; paresthesia of hands; arterial insufficiency, usually of the Raynaud type; thrombocytopenic purpura

Central Nervous System: lightheadedness; mental depression manifested by insomnia, lassitude, weakness, fatigue; reversible mental depression progressing to catatonia; visual disturbances; hallucinations; an acute reversible syndrome characterized by disorientation for time and place, short term memory loss, emotional lability, slightly clouded sensorium and decreased performance on neuropsychometrics

Gastrointestinal: nausea, vomiting, epigastric distress, abdominal cramping, diarrhea, constipation, mesenteric arterial thrombosis, ischemic colitis

Allergic: pharyngitis and agranulocytosis, erythematous rash, fever combined with aching and sore throat, laryngospasm and respiratory distress

Respiratory: bronchospasm

Hematologic: agranulocytosis, nonthrombocytopenic purpura, thrombocytopenic purpura

Miscellaneous: reversible alopecia. Oculomucocutaneous reactions involving the skin, serous membranes and conjunctivae reported for a beta blocker (practolol) have not been conclusively associated with propranolol.

Clinical Laboratory Test Findings: Elevated blood urea levels in patients with severe heart disease, elevated serum transaminase, alkaline phosphatase, lactate dehydrogenase

Dosage and Administration:

The dosage range for INDERAL is different for each Indication.

ORAL

HYPERTENSION—*Dosage must be individualized.*

The usual initial dosage is 40 mg INDERAL (propranolol HCl) twice daily, whether used alone or added to a diuretic. Dosage may be increased gradually until adequate blood pressure is achieved. The usual dosage is 160 to 480 mg per day. In some instances a dosage of 640 mg may be required. The time needed for full hypertensive response to a given dosage is variable and may range from a few days to several weeks.

While twice-daily dosing is effective and can maintain a reduction in blood pressure throughout the day, some patients, especially when lower doses are used, may experience a modest rise in blood pressure toward the end of the 12 hour dosing interval. This can be evaluated by measuring blood pressure near the end of the dosing interval to determine whether satisfactory control is being maintained throughout the day. If control is not adequate, a larger dose, or 3 times daily therapy may achieve better control.

ANGINA PECTORIS—*Dosage must be individualized.*

Starting with 10–20 mg three or four times daily, before meals and at bedtime, dosage should be gradually increased at three to seven day intervals until optimum response is obtained. Although individual patients may respond at any dosage level, the average optimum dosage appears to be 160 mg per day. In angina pectoris, the value and safety of dosage exceeding 320 mg per day have not been established.

If treatment is to be discontinued, reduce dosage gradually over a period of several weeks. (See WARNINGS.)

ARRHYTHMIAS—10–30 mg three or four times daily, before meals and at bedtime.

MIGRAINE—*Dosage must be individualized.*

The initial oral dose is 80 mg INDERAL daily in divided doses. The usual effective dose range is 160–240 mg per day. The dosage may be increased gradually to achieve optimum migraine prophylaxis.

If a satisfactory response is not obtained within four to six weeks after reaching the maximum dose, INDERAL therapy should be discontinued. It may be advisable to withdraw the drug gradually over a period of two weeks.

HYPERTHROPHIC SUBAORTIC STENOSIS—20–40 mg three or four times daily, before meals and at bedtime.

PHEOCHROMOCYTOMA — *Preoperatively* —60 mg daily in divided doses for three days prior to surgery, concomitantly with an alpha-adrenergic blocking agent.

—*Management of inoperable tumor*—30 mg daily in divided doses.

PEDIATRIC DOSAGE

At this time the data on the use of the drug in this age group are too limited to permit adequate directions for use.

INTRAVENOUS

Intravenous administration is reserved for life-threatening arrhythmias or those occurring under anesthesia. The usual dose is from 1 to 3 mg administered under careful monitoring, *e.g.,* electrocardiographic, central venous pressure. The rate of administration should not exceed 1 mg (1 ml) per minute to diminish the possibility of lowering blood pressure and causing cardiac standstill. Sufficient time should be allowed for the drug to reach the site of action even when a slow circulation is present. If necessary, a second dose may be given after two minutes. Thereafter, additional drug should not be given in less than four hours. Additional INDERAL (propranolol HCl) should not be given when the desired alteration in rate and/or rhythm is achieved.

Transference to oral therapy should be made as soon as possible.

The intravenous administration of INDERAL has not been evaluated adequately in the management of hypertensive emergencies.

Overdosage or Exaggerated Response:

IN THE EVENT OF OVERDOSAGE OR EXAGGERATED RESPONSE, THE FOLLOWING MEASURES SHOULD BE EMPLOYED:

BRADYCARDIA—ADMINISTER ATROPINE (0.25 to 1.0 mg): IF THERE IS NO RESPONSE TO VAGAL BLOCKADE, ADMINISTER ISOPROTERENOL CAUTIOUSLY.

CARDIAC FAILURE—DIGITALIZATION AND DIURETICS

HYPOTENSION—VASOPRESSORS, *e.g.,* LEVARTERENOL OR EPINEPHRINE (THERE IS EVIDENCE THAT EPINEPHRINE IS THE DRUG OF CHOICE.)

BRONCHOSPASM—ADMINISTER ISOPROTERENOL AND AMINOPHYLLINE

How Supplied:

INDERAL

(propranolol hydrochloride)

TABLETS

—Each hexagonal-shaped, orange, scored tablet is embossed with an "I" and imprinted with "INDERAL 10," contains **10 mg** propranolol hydrochloride, in bottles of 100 (NDC 0046-0421-81) and 1,000 (NDC 0046-0421-91). Also in unit dose package of 100 (NDC 0046-0421-99).

—Each hexagonal-shaped, blue, scored tablet is embossed with an "I" and imprinted with "INDERAL 20," contains **20 mg** propranolol hydrochloride, in bottles of 100 (NDC 0046-0422-81) and 1,000 (NDC 0046-0422-91). Also in unit dose package of 100 (NDC 0046-0422-99).

—Each hexagonal-shaped, green, scored tablet is embossed with an "I" and imprinted with "INDERAL 40," contains **40 mg** propranolol hydrochloride, in bottles of 100 (NDC 0046-0424-81) and 1,000 (NDC 0046-0424-91). Also in unit dose package of 100 (NDC 0046-0424-99).

—Each hexagonal-shaped, pink, scored tablet is embossed with an "I" and imprinted with "INDERAL 60," contains **60 mg** propranolol hydrochloride in bottles of 100 (NDC 0046-0426-81) and 1,000 (NDC 0046-0426-91) and in unit dose packages of 100 (NDC 0046-0426-99).

—Each hexagonal-shaped, yellow, scored tablet is embossed with an "I" and imprinted with "INDERAL 80," contains **80 mg** propranolol hydrochloride, in bottles of 100 (NDC 0046-0428-81) and 1,000 (NDC 0046-0428-91). Also in unit dose package of 100 (NDC 0046-0428-99).

The appearance of these tablets is a trademark of Ayerst Laboratories.

Store at room temperature (approximately 25° C).

INJECTABLE

—Each ml contains 1 mg of propranolol hydrochloride in Water for Injection. The pH is adjusted with citric acid. Supplied as: 1 ml ampuls in boxes of 10 (NDC 0046-3265-10).

Store at room temperature (approximately 25° C).

[Shown in Product Identification Section]

INDERIDE® ℞

Brand of propranolol hydrochloride (INDERAL®) and hydrochlorothiazide

No. 484—Each INDERIDE®-40/25 tablet contains:

Propranolol hydrochloride (Inderal®)	40 mg
Hydrochlorothiazide	25 mg

No. 488—Each INDERIDE®-80/25 tablet contains:

Propranolol hydrochloride (INDERAL®)	80 mg
Hydrochlorothiazide	25 mg

Warning

This fixed combination drug is not indicated for initial therapy of hypertension. Hypertension requires therapy titrated to the individual patient. If the fixed combination represents the dosage so determined, its use may be more convenient in patient management. The treatment of hypertension is not static, but must be reevaluated as conditions in each patient warrant.

Description: INDERIDE combines two antihypertensive agents: INDERAL (propranolol hydrochloride), a beta-adrenergic blocking agent, and hydrochlorothiazide, a thiazide diuretic-antihypertensive.

Propranolol hydrochloride is a stable, white to off-white, crystalline powder with a melting point of about 164° C. It is odorless and has a bitter taste. It is readily soluble in water and ethanol, and insoluble in non-polar solvents. Its chemical name is 1-(Isopropylamino)-3-(1-naphthyloxy)-2-propanol hydrochloride.

Hydrochlorothiazide is a white, or practically white, practically odorless, crystalline powder. It is slightly soluble in water, freely soluble in sodium hydroxide solution, sparingly soluble in methanol; insoluble in ether, chloroform, benzene, and dilute mineral acids. Its chemical name is 6-Chloro-3,4-dihydro-2H-1,2,4-benzothiadiazine-7-sulfonamide 1,-1-dioxide.

Clinical Pharmacology:

Propranolol hydrochloride (INDERAL®):

Propranolol hydrochloride is a beta-adrenergic receptor blocking drug, possessing no other autonomic nervous system activity. It specifically competes with beta-adrenergic receptor stimulating agents for available beta-receptor sites. When access to beta-receptor sites is blocked by propranolol, the chronotropic, inotropic, and vasodilator responses to beta-adrenergic stimulation are decreased proportionately.

Propranolol is almost completely absorbed from the gastrointestinal tract, but a portion is immediately bound by the liver. Peak effect occurs in one to one and one-half hours. The biologic half-life is approximately two to three hours. Propranolol is not significantly dialyzable. There is no simple correlation between dose or plasma level and therapeutic effect, and the dose-sensitivity range as observed in clinical practice is wide. The principal reason for this is that sympathetic tone varies widely between individuals. Since there is no reliable test to estimate sympathetic tone or to determine whether total beta blockade has been achieved, proper dosage requires titration.

The mechanism of the antihypertensive effects of propranolol has not been established. Among the factors that may be involved are (1) decreased cardiac output, (2) inhibition of renin release by the kidneys, and (3) diminution of tonic sympathetic nerve outflow from vasomotor centers in the brain.

Propranolol hydrochloride decreases heart rate, cardiac output, and blood pressure. Although total peripheral vascular resistance may increase initially, it readjusts to the pretreatment level or lower with chronic usage. Earlier studies indicate that plasma volume remains unchanged or may decrease. However, there are certain more recent studies suggesting that in the absence of sodium restriction, plasma volume may increase.

Beta-receptor blockade is useful in conditions in which, because of pathologic or functional changes, sympathetic activity is excessive or inappropriate, and detrimental to the patient. But there are also situations in which sympathetic stimulation is vital. For example, in patients with severely damaged hearts, adequate ventricular function is maintained by virtue of sympathetic drive which should be preserved. In the presence of AV block, beta blockade may prevent the necessary facilitating effect of sympathetic activity on conduction. Beta blockade results in bronchial constriction by interfering with adrenergic bronchodilator activity which should be preserved in patients subject to bronchospasm.

Continued on next page

Ayerst—Cont.

The proper objective of beta-blockade therapy is to decrease adverse sympathetic stimulation, but not to the degree that may impair necessary sympathetic support.

Hydrochlorothiazide:
Hydrochlorothiazide is a benzothiadiazine (thiazide) diuretic closely related to chlorothiazide. The mechanism of the antihypertensive effect of the thiazides is unknown. Thiazides do not affect normal blood pressure.

Thiazides affect the renal tubular mechanism of electrolyte reabsorption. At maximal therapeutic dosage, all thiazides are approximately equal in their diuretic potency.

Thiazides increase excretion of sodium and chloride in approximately equivalent amounts. Natriuresis causes a secondary loss of potassium and bicarbonate.

Onset of diuretic action of thiazides occurs in two hours, and the peak effect in about four hours. Its action persists for approximately six to 12 hours. Thiazides are eliminated rapidly by the kidney.

Indication: INDERIDE [propranolol HCl (INDERAL®) and hydrochlorothiazide] is indicated in the management of hypertension. (See boxed warning.)

Contraindications:

Propranolol hydrochloride (INDERAL®):
Propranolol hydrochloride is contraindicated in: 1) bronchial asthma; 2) allergic rhinitis during the pollen season; 3) sinus bradycardia and greater than first degree block; 4) cardiogenic shock; 5) right ventricular failure secondary to pulmonary hypertension; 6) congestive heart failure (see WARNINGS) unless the failure is secondary to a tachyarrhythmia treatable with propranolol; 7) in patients on adrenergic-augmenting psychotropic drugs (including MAO inhibitors), and during the two week withdrawal period from such drugs.

Hydrochlorothiazide:
Hydrochlorothiazide is contraindicated in patients with anuria or hypersensitivity to this or other sulfonamide-derived drugs.

Warnings:

Propranolol hydrochloride (INDERAL®):
CARDIAC FAILURE: Sympathetic stimulation is a vital component supporting circulatory function in congestive heart failure, and inhibition with beta blockade always carries the potential hazard of further depressing myocardial contractility and precipitating cardiac failure. Propranolol acts selectively without abolishing the inotropic action of digitalis on the heart muscle (*i.e.* that of supporting the strength of myocardial contractions). In patients already receiving digitalis, the positive inotropic action of digitalis may be reduced by propranolol's negative inotropic effect. The effects of propranolol and digitalis are additive in depressing AV conduction.

IN PATIENTS WITHOUT A HISTORY OF CARDIAC FAILURE, continued depression of the myocardium over a period of time can, in some cases, lead to cardiac failure. In rare instances, this has been observed during propranolol therapy. Therefore, at the first sign or symptom of impending cardiac failure, patients should be fully digitalized and/or given a diuretic, and the response observed closely: a) if cardiac failure continues, despite adequate digitalization and diuretic therapy, propranolol therapy should be immediately withdrawn; b) if tachyarrhythmia is being controlled, patients should be maintained on combined therapy and the patient closely followed until threat of cardiac failure is over.

IN PATIENTS WITH ANGINA PECTORIS, there have been reports of exacerbation of angina and, in some cases, myocardial infarction, following *abrupt* discontinuation of propranolol therapy. Therefore, when discontinuance of propranolol is planned the dosage should be gradually reduced and the patient carefully monitored. In addition, when propranolol is prescribed for angina pectoris, the patient should be cautioned against interruption or cessation of therapy without the physician's advice. If propranolol therapy is interrupted and exacerbation of angina occurs, it usually is advisable to reinstitute propranolol therapy and take other measures appropriate for the management of unstable angina pectoris. Since coronary artery disease may be unrecognized, it may be prudent to follow the above advice in patients considered at risk of having occult atherosclerotic heart disease, who are given propranolol for other indications.

IN PATIENTS WITH THYROTOXICOSIS, possible deleterious effects from long-term use have not been adequately appraised. Special consideration should be given to propranolol's potential for aggravating congestive heart failure. Propranolol may mask the clinical signs of developing or continuing hyperthyroidism or complications and give a false impression of improvement. Therefore, abrupt withdrawal of propranolol may be followed by an exacerbation of symptoms of hyperthyroidism, including thyroid storm. This is another reason for withdrawing propranolol slowly. Propranolol does not distort thyroid function tests.

IN PATIENTS WITH WOLFF-PARKINSON-WHITE SYNDROME, several cases have been reported in which, after propranolol, the tachycardia was replaced by a severe bradycardia requiring a demand pacemaker. In one case this resulted after an initial dose of 5 mg propranolol.

IN PATIENTS UNDERGOING MAJOR SURGERY, beta blockade impairs the ability of the heart to respond to reflex stimuli. For this reason, with the exception of pheochromocytoma, propranolol should be withdrawn 48 hours prior to surgery, at which time all chemical and physiologic effects are gone according to available evidence. However, in case of emergency surgery, since propranolol is a competitive inhibitor of beta-receptor agonists, its effects can be reversed by administration of such agents, *e.g.* isoproterenol or levarterenol. However, such patients may be subject to protracted severe hypotension. Difficulty in restarting and maintaining the heart beat has also been reported.

IN PATIENTS PRONE TO NONALLERGIC BRONCHOSPASM (*e.g.,* CHRONIC BRONCHITIS, EMPHYSEMA), propranolol should be administered with caution since it may block bronchodilation produced by endogenous and exogenous catecholamine stimulation of beta receptors.

DIABETICS AND PATIENTS SUBJECT TO HYPOGLYCEMIA: Because of its beta-adrenergic blocking activity, propranolol may prevent the appearance of premonitory signs and symptoms (pulse rate and pressure changes) of acute hypoglycemia. This is especially important to keep in mind in patients with labile diabetes. Hypoglycemic attacks may be accompanied by a precipitous elevation of blood pressure.

Hydrochlorothiazide:
Thiazides should be used with caution in severe renal disease. In patients with renal disease, thiazides may precipitate azotemia. In patients with impaired renal function, cumulative effects of the drug may develop.

Thiazides should also be used with caution in patients with impaired hepatic function or progressive liver disease, since minor alterations of fluid and electrolyte balance may precipitate hepatic coma.

Thiazides may add to or potentiate the action of other antihypertensive drugs. Potentiation occurs with ganglionic or peripheral adrenergic blocking drugs.

Sensitivity reactions may occur in patients with a history of allergy or bronchial asthma.

The possibility of exacerbation or activation of systemic lupus erythematosus has been reported.

USE IN PREGNANCY:

Propranolol hydrochloride (INDERAL®):
The safe use of propranolol in human pregnancy has not been established. Use of any drug in pregnancy or women of childbearing potential requires that the possible risk to mother and/or fetus be weighed against the expected therapeutic benefit. Embryotoxic effects have been seen in animal studies at doses about 10 times the maximum recommended human dose.

Hydrochlorothiazide:
Thiazides cross the placental barrier and appear in cord blood. The use of thiazides in pregnant women requires that the anticipated benefit be weighed against possible hazards to the fetus. These hazards include fetal or neonatal jaundice, thrombocytopenia, and possibly other adverse reactions which have occurred in the adult.

Nursing Mothers: Thiazides appear in breast milk. If the use of the drug is deemed essential, the patient should stop nursing.

Precautions:

Propranolol hydrochloride (INDERAL®):
Patients receiving catecholamine-depleting drugs such as reserpine should be closely observed if propranolol is administered. The added catecholamine blocking action of this drug may then produce an excessive reduction of the resting sympathetic nervous activity.

Occasionally, the pharmacologic activity of propranolol may produce hypotension and/or marked bradycardia resulting in vertigo, syncopal attacks, or orthostatic hypotension.

As with any new drug given over prolonged periods, laboratory parameters should be observed at regular intervals. The drug should be used with caution in patients with impaired renal or hepatic function.

Hydrochlorothiazide:
Periodic determination of serum electrolytes to detect possible electrolyte imbalance should be performed at appropriate intervals.

All patients receiving thiazide therapy should be observed for clinical signs of fluid or electrolyte imbalance, namely: hyponatremia, hypochloremic alkalosis, and hypokalemia. Serum and urine electrolyte determinations are particularly important when the patient is vomiting excessively or receiving parenteral fluids. Medication such as digitalis may also influence serum electrolytes. Warning signs, irrespective of cause are: dryness of mouth, thirst, weakness, lethargy, drowsiness, restlessness, muscle pains or cramps, muscular fatigue, hypotension, oliguria, tachycardia, and gastrointestinal disturbances such as nausea and vomiting.

Hypokalemia may develop, especially with brisk diuresis, when severe cirrhosis is present or during concomitant use of corticosteroids or ACTH.

Interference with adequate oral electrolyte intake will also contribute to hypokalemia. Hypokalemia can sensitize or exaggerate the response of the heart to the toxic effects of digitalis (*e.g.,* increased ventricular irritability). Hypokalemia may be avoided or treated by use of potassium supplements such as foods with a high potassium content.

Any chloride deficit is generally mild, and usually does not require specific treatment except under extraordinary circumstances (as in liver or renal disease). Dilutional hyponatremia may occur in edematous patients in hot weather; appropriate therapy is water restriction, rather than administration of salt, except in rare instances when the hyponatremia is life-threatening. In actual salt depletion, appropriate replacement is the therapy of choice.

Hyperuricemia may occur or frank gout may be precipitated in certain patients receiving thiazide therapy.
Insulin requirements in diabetic patients may be increased, decreased, or unchanged. Diabetes mellitus which has been latent may become manifest during thiazide administration.
Thiazide drugs may increase the responsiveness to tubocurarine.
The antihypertensive effects of the drug may be enhanced in the postsympathectomy patient. Thiazides may decrease arterial responsiveness to norepinephrine. This diminution is not sufficient to preclude effectiveness of the pressor agent for therapeutic use.
If progressive renal impairment becomes evident, consider withholding or discontinuing diuretic therapy.
Thiazides may decrease serum PBI levels without signs of thyroid disturbance.
Calcium excretion is decreased by thiazides. Pathologic changes in the parathyroid gland with hypercalcemia and hypophosphatemia have been observed in a few patients on prolonged thiazide therapy. The common complications of hyperparathyroidism such as renal lithiasis, bone resorption, and peptic ulceration, have not been seen. Thiazides should be discontinued before carrying out tests for parathyroid function.

Adverse Reactions:

Propranolol hydrochloride (INDERAL®):

Cardiovascular: bradycardia; congestive heart failure; intensification of AV block; hypotension; paresthesia of hands; arterial insufficiency, usually of the Raynaud type; thrombocytopenic purpura.
Central Nervous System: lightheadedness; mental depression manifested by insomnia, lassitude, weakness, fatigue, reversible mental depression progressing to catatonia; visual disturbances; hallucinations; an acute reversible syndrome characterized by disorientation for time and place, short term memory loss, emotional lability, slightly clouded sensorium, and decreased performance on neuropsychometrics.
Gastrointestinal: nausea, vomiting, epigastric distress, abdominal cramping, diarrhea, constipation, mesenteric arterial thrombosis, ischemic colitis.
Allergic: pharyngitis and agranulocytosis, erythematous rash, fever combined with aching and sore throat, laryngospasm and respiratory distress.
Respiratory: bronchospasm.
Hematologic: agranulocytosis, nonthrombocytopenic purpura, thrombocytopenic purpura.
Miscellaneous: reversible alopecia. Oculomucocutaneous reactions involving the skin, serous membranes and conjunctivae reported for a beta blocker (practolol) have not been conclusively associated with propranolol.
Clinical Laboratory Test Findings: Elevated blood urea levels in patients with severe heart disease, elevated serum transaminase, alkaline phosphatase, lactate dehydrogenase.

Hydrochlorothiazide:

Gastrointestinal: anorexia, gastric irritation, nausea, vomiting, cramping, diarrhea, constipation, jaundice (intrahepatic cholestatic jaundice), pancreatitis, sialadenitis.
Central Nervous System: dizziness, vertigo, paresthesias, headache, xanthopsia.
Hematologic: leukopenia, agranulocytosis, thrombocytopenia, aplastic anemia.
Cardiovascular: orthostatic hypotension (may be aggravated by alcohol, barbiturates, or narcotics).
Hypersensitivity: purpura, photosensitivity, rash, urticaria, necrotizing angiitis (vasculitis, cutaneous vasculitis), fever, respiratory distress including pneumonitis, anaphylactic reactions.
Other: hyperglycemia, glycosuria, hyperuricemia, muscle spasm, weakness, restlessness, transient blurred vision.
Whenever adverse reactions are moderate or severe, thiazide dosage should be reduced or therapy withdrawn.

Dosage and Administration:

The dosage must be determined by individual titration (see boxed warning).
Hydrochlorothiazide is usually given at a dose of 50 to 100 mg per day. The initial dose of propranolol is 40 mg twice daily and it may be increased gradually until optimum blood pressure control is achieved. The usual effective dose is 160 to 480 mg per day.
One to two INDERIDE [propranolol HCl (INDERAL®) and hydrochlorothiazide] tablets twice daily can be used to administer up to 320 mg of propranolol and 100 mg of hydrochlorothiazide. For doses of propranolol greater than 320 mg, the combination products are not appropriate because their use would lead to an excessive dose of the thiazide component.
When necessary, another antihypertensive agent may be added gradually beginning with 50 percent of the usual recommended starting dose to avoid an excessive fall in blood pressure.

Overdosage or Exaggerated Response:

The propranolol hydrochloride (INDERAL) component may cause bradycardia, cardiac failure, hypotension, or bronchospasm.
The hydrochlorothiazide component can be expected to cause diuresis. Lethargy of varying degree may appear and may progress to coma within a few hours, with minimal depression of respiration and cardiovascular function, and in the absence of significant serum electrolyte changes or dehydration. The mechanism of central nervous system depression with thiazide overdosage is unknown. Gastrointestinal irritation and hypermotility can occur; temporary elevation of BUN has been reported, and serum electrolyte changes could occur, especially in patients with impairment of renal function.

TREATMENT

The following measures should be employed:
GENERAL—If ingestion is, or may have been, recent, evacuate gastric contents taking care to prevent pulmonary aspiration.
BRADYCARDIA—Administer atropine (0.25 to 1.0 mg). If there is no response to vagal blockade, administer isoproterenol cautiously.
CARDIAC FAILURE—Digitalization and diuretics.
HYPOTENSION—Vasopressors, *e.g.*, levarterenol or epinephrine.
BRONCHOSPASM—Administer isoproterenol and aminophylline.
STUPOR OR COMA—Administer supportive therapy as clinically warranted.
GASTROINTESTINAL EFFECTS—Though usually of short duration, these may require symptomatic treatment.
ABNORMALITIES IN BUN AND/OR SERUM ELECTROLYTES—Monitor serum electrolyte levels and renal function; institute supportive measures as required individually to maintain hydration, electrolyte balance, respiration, and cardiovascular-renal function.

How Supplied:

—Each hexagonal-shaped, off-white, scored INDERIDE 40/25 tablet is embossed with an "I" and imprinted with "INDERIDE 40/25," contains 40 mg propranolol hydrochloride (INDERAL®) and 25 mg hydrochlorothiazide, in bottles of 100 (NDC 0046-0484-81) and 1,000 (NDC 0046-0484-91). Also in unit dose package of 100 (NDC 0046-0484-99).
—Each hexagonal-shaped, off-white, scored INDERIDE 80/25 tablet is embossed with an "I" and imprinted with "INDERIDE 80/25," contains 80 mg propranolol hydrochloride (INDERAL®) and 25 mg hydrochlorothiazide, in bottles of 100 (NDC 0046-0488-81) and 1,000 (NDC 0046-0488-91). Also in unit dose package of 100 (NDC 0046-0488-99).
The appearance of these tablets is a trademark of Ayerst Laboratories.
Store at room temperature (approximately 25° C).

[Shown in Product Identification Section]

KERODEX®
Skin Barrier Cream

Action and Uses: A specially formulated barrier cream to help protect against potentially irritating chemicals, compounds, and solutions in common use. When applied and used as directed, KERODEX provides a barrier film that helps to block contact with skin irritants. KERODEX No. 71 (water-repellent) is for use in handling or working with *wet* materials; No. 51 is for *dry* or *oily* work. KERODEX is greaseless and stainless.
Application: 1. Wash hands clean and dry *thoroughly*. 2. Squeeze out ½ inch of cream into palm of one hand. Rub hands together with a washing motion until cream is *lightly* and *evenly* distributed, leaving no excess. Make sure cream reaches under nails, around cuticles, between fingers, across wrists and backs of hands (forearms, if necessary). 3. A second application is recommended. **NOTE:** After applying KERODEX 71, "set" by holding hands under cold running water. Pat dry. After applying KERODEX 51, avoid contact with water. If hands become wet during work, reapply.
How Supplied: KERODEX (water-repellent cream for wet work), in 4 oz (113 g) tubes (NDC 0046-0071-04) and 1 lb. jars (NDC 0046-0071-01). KERODEX (water-miscible cream for dry or oily work), in 4 oz (113 g) tubes (NDC 0046-0051-04) and 1 lb. jars (NDC 0046-0051-01).

LARYLGAN® Throat Spray

An aqueous solution containing:

Antipyrine	0.30%
Pyrilamine maleate	0.05%
Sodium caprylate	0.50%

Also contains menthol, gentian violet, methyl salicylate, methylparaben, propylparaben, peppermint oil, spearmint oil, anise oil, cinnamon oil, isobornyl acetate, benzyl alcohol 0.05%, ethyl alcohol 1.00%, glycerin, sodium saccharin, and other aromatics.
Action: The analgesic-like effect of LARYLGAN helps to allay pain of irritated mucosa. The glycerin dehydrated vehicle provides maximum spreading and penetrating properties to help the medication reach the affected areas. It is non-narcotic.
Indications: A soothing and refreshing spray for dry throat and for minor sore throat due to irritants such as smoking or postnasal drip.
Warning: Severe and persistent sore throat or sore throat accompanied by high fever, headache, nausea, and vomiting may be serious. Consult physician promptly. Do not use more than two days or administer to children under 3 years of age unless directed by physician.
Administration: *Instructions for Use:* Adults and children 3 years of age or older. Remove cap. Hold close to mouth. Spray as needed. If throat condition persists, consult a physician.
How Supplied: LARYLGAN Throat Spray, in 0.94 fl oz (28 ml) bottles (NDC 0046-1005-01).

MEDIATRIC® Ⓜ ℞

Each capsule or tablet contains:

Premarin® (Conjugated Estrogens, U.S.P.)	0.25	mg
Methyltestosterone	2.5	mg
Ascorbic acid (Vit. C)*	100.0	mg
Cyanocobalamin	2.5	mcg
Thiamine mononitrate	10.0	mg
Riboflavin	5.0	mg
Niacinamide	50.0	mg
Pyridoxine HCl	3.0	mg

Continued on next page

Ayerst—Cont.

Calc. pantothenate	20.0	mg
Dried ferrous sulfate	30.0	mg
Methamphetamine HCl	1.0	mg

*For Capsules, provided as ascorbic acid, 70 mg, and as sodium ascorbate, 30 mg.

Also available: MEDIATRIC Liquid
Each 15 ml (3 teaspoonfuls) contains:

Premarin® (Conjugated Estrogens, U.S.P.)	0.25	mg
Methyltestosterone	2.5	mg
Thiamine HCl	5.0	mg
Cyanocobalamin	1.5	mcg
Methamphetamine HCl	1.0	mg

Contains 15% alcohol—some loss unavoidable.

1. ESTROGENS HAVE BEEN REPORTED TO INCREASE THE RISK OF ENDOMETRIAL CARCINOMA.

Three independent case control studies have reported an increased risk of endometrial cancer in postmenopausal women exposed to exogenous estrogens for more than one year.[1–3] This risk was independent of the other known risk factors for endometrial cancer. These studies are further supported by the finding that incidence rates of endometrial cancer have increased sharply since 1969 in eight different areas of the United States with population-based cancer reporting systems, an increase which may be related to the rapidly expanding use of estrogens during the last decade.[4]

The three case control studies reported that the risk of endometrial cancer in estrogen users was about 4.5 to 13.9 times greater than in nonusers. The risk appears to depend on both duration of treatment[1] and on estrogen dose.[3] In view of these findings, when estrogens are used for the treatment of menopausal symptoms, the lowest dose that will control symptoms should be utilized and medication should be discontinued as soon as possible. When prolonged treatment is medically indicated, the patient should be reassessed on at least a semiannual basis to determine the need for continued therapy. Although the evidence must be considered preliminary, one study suggests that cyclic administration of low doses of estrogen may carry less risk than continuous administration;[3] it therefore appears prudent to utilize such a regimen.

Close clinical surveillance of all women taking estrogens is important. In all cases of undiagnosed persistent or recurring abnormal vaginal bleeding, adequate diagnostic measures should be undertaken to rule out malignancy.

There is no evidence at present that "natural" estrogens are more or less hazardous than "synthetic" estrogens at equiestrogenic doses.

2. ESTROGENS SHOULD NOT BE USED DURING PREGNANCY.

The use of female sex hormones, both estrogens and progestogens, during early pregnancy may seriously damage the offspring. It has been shown that females exposed in utero to diethylstilbestrol, a non-steroidal estrogen, have an increased risk of developing in later life a form of vaginal or cervical cancer that is ordinarily extremely rare.[5,6] This risk has been estimated as not greater than 4 per 1000 exposures.[7] Furthermore, a high percentage of such exposed women (from 30 to 90 percent) have been found to have vaginal adenosis,[8–12] epithelial changes of the vagina and cervix. Although these changes are histologically benign, it is not known whether they are precursors of malignancy. Although similar data are not available with the use of other estrogens, it cannot be presumed they would not induce similar changes.

Several reports suggest an association between intrauterine exposure to female sex hormones and congenital anomalies, including congenital heart defects and limb reduction defects.[13–16] One case control study[16] estimated a 4.7-fold increased risk of limb reduction defects in infants exposed in utero to sex hormones (oral contraceptives, hormone withdrawal tests for pregnancy, or attempted treatment for threatened abortion). Some of these exposures were very short and involved only a few days of treatment. The data suggest that the risk of limb reduction defects in exposed fetuses is somewhat less than 1 per 1000.

In the past, female sex hormones have been used during pregnancy in an attempt to treat threatened or habitual abortion. There is considerable evidence that estrogens are ineffective for these indications, and there is no evidence from well controlled studies that progestogens are effective for these uses.

If MEDIATRIC is used during pregnancy, or if the patient becomes pregnant while taking this drug, she should be apprised of the potential risks to the fetus, and the advisability of pregnancy continuation.

Description: MEDIATRIC provides estrogen and androgen in small doses, nutritional supplements, together with a mild antidepressant.

Action: MEDIATRIC provides (1) *steroids* to help counteract declining gonadal hormone secretion, and as important regulators of metabolic processes; (2) *nutritional supplements* specially selected to meet the needs of the aged and aging patient, and to act as necessary catalysts for the maintenance of efficient enzyme systems; and (3) *a mild antidepressant* to impart a gentle emotional uplift.

Indication: For use in aging patients of both sexes.

MEDIATRIC HAS NOT BEEN SHOWN TO BE EFFECTIVE FOR ANY PURPOSE DURING PREGNANCY AND ITS USE MAY CAUSE SEVERE HARM TO THE FETUS (SEE BOXED WARNING).

Contraindications: Estrogens should not be used in women (or men) with any of the following conditions:

1. Known or suspected cancer of the breast except in appropriately selected patients being treated for metastatic disease.
2. Known or suspected estrogen-dependent neoplasia.
3. Known or suspected pregnancy (See Boxed Warning).
4. Undiagnosed abnormal genital bleeding.
5. Active thrombophlebitis or thromboembolic disorders.
6. A past history of thrombophlebitis, thrombosis, or thromboembolic disorders associated with previous estrogen use (except when used in treatment of breast or prostatic malignancy).

Methyltestosterone should not be used in persons with any of the following conditions:

1. Known or suspected carcinoma of the prostate and in carcinoma of the male breast.
2. Severe liver damage.
3. Pregnancy or in breast-feeding mothers because of the possibility of masculinization of the female fetus or breast-fed infant.

Warnings:

Associated with Estrogens

1. *Induction of malignant neoplasms.* Long term continuous administration of natural and synthetic estrogens in certain animal species increases the frequency of carcinomas of the breast, cervix, vagina, and liver. There are now reports that estrogens increase the risk of carcinoma of the endometrium in humans. (See Boxed Warning.)

At the present time there is no satisfactory evidence that estrogens given to postmenopausal women increase the risk of cancer of the breast,[17] although a recent long-term followup of a single physician's practice has raised this possibility.[18] Because of the animal data, there is a need for caution in prescribing estrogens for women with a strong family history of breast cancer or who have breast nodules, fibrocystic disease, or abnormal mammograms.

2. *Gallbladder disease.* A recent study has reported a 2 to 3-fold increase in the risk of surgically confirmed gallbladder disease in women receiving postmenopausal estrogens,[17] similar to the 2-fold increase previously noted in users of oral contraceptives.[19,24a]

3. *Effects similar to those caused by estrogen-progestogen oral contraceptives.* There are several serious adverse effects of oral contraceptives, most of which have not, up to now, been documented as consequences of postmenopausal estrogen therapy. This may reflect the comparatively low doses of estrogen used in postmenopausal women. It would be expected that the larger doses of estrogen used to treat prostatic or breast cancer or postpartum breast engorgement are more likely to result in these adverse effects, and, in fact, it has been shown that there is an increased risk of thrombosis in men receiving estrogens for prostatic cancer and women for postpartum breast engorgement.[20–23]

a. *Thromboembolic disease.* It is now well established that users of oral contraceptives have an increased risk of various thromboembolic and thrombotic vascular diseases, such as thrombophlebitis, pulmonary embolism, stroke, and myocardial infarction.[24–31] Cases of retinal thrombosis, mesenteric thrombosis, and optic neuritis have been reported in oral contraceptive users. There is evidence that the risk of several of these adverse reactions is related to the dose of the drug.[32,33] An increased risk of postsurgery thromboembolic complications has also been reported in users of oral contraceptives.[34,35] If feasible, estrogen should be discontinued at least 4 weeks before surgery of the type associated with an increased risk of thromboembolism, or during periods of prolonged immobilization.

While an increased rate of thromboembolic and thrombotic disease in postmenopausal users of estrogens has not been found,[17–24,25–36] this does not rule out the possibility that such an increase may be present or that subgroups of women who have underlying risk factors or who are receiving relatively large doses of estrogens may have increased risk. Therefore estrogens should not be used in persons with active thrombophlebitis or thromboembolic disorders, and they should not be used (except in treatment of malignancy) in persons with a history of such disorders in association with estrogen use. They should be used with caution in patients with cerebral vascular or coronary artery disease and only for those in whom estrogens are clearly needed.

Large doses of estrogen (5 mg conjugated estrogens per day), comparable to those used to treat cancer of the prostate and breast, have been shown in a large prospective clinical trial in men[37] to increase the risk of nonfatal myocardial infarction, pulmonary embolism and thrombophlebitis. When estrogen doses of this size are used, any of the thromboembolic and thrombotic adverse effects associated with oral contraceptive use should be considered a clear risk.

b. *Hepatic adenoma.* Benign hepatic adenomas appear to be associated with the use of oral contraceptives.[38–40] Although benign, and rare, these may rupture and may cause death through intra-abdominal hemorrhage. Such lesions have not yet been reported in association with other estrogen or progestogen preparations but should be considered in estrogen users having abdominal pain and tenderness, abdominal mass, or hypovolemic shock. Hepatocellular carcinoma has also been reported in women taking estrogen-containing oral contraceptives.[39] The relationship of this malignancy to these drugs is not known at this time.

c. *Elevated blood pressure.* Women using oral contraceptives sometimes experience increased blood pressure which, in most cases, returns to normal on discontinuing the drug. There is now a report that this may occur with use of estrogens in the menopause[41] and blood pressure should be monitored with estrogen use, especially if high doses are used.

d. *Glucose tolerance.* A worsening of glucose tolerance has been observed in a significant percentage of patients on estrogen-containing oral contraceptives. For this reason, diabetic patients should be carefully observed while receiving estrogen.

4. *Hypercalcemia.* Administration of estrogens may lead to severe hypercalcemia in patients with breast cancer and bone metastases. If this occurs, the drug should be stopped and appropriate measures taken to reduce the serum calcium level.

Associated with Methyltestosterone

1. Female patients should be watched carefully for symptoms or signs of virilization such as hoarseness or deepening of the voice, oily skin, acne, hirsutism, enlarged clitoris, stimulation of libido, and menstrual irregularities. At the dosage necessary to achieve a tumor response, androgens will cause masculinization of a female, but occasionally a sensitive female may exhibit one or more of these signs on smaller doses. Some of these changes, such as voice changes may be irreversible even after drug is stopped.

2. Cholestatic hepatitis with jaundice and altered liver function tests, such as increased BSP retention and rises in SGOT levels, have been reported with methyltestosterone. These changes appear to be related to dosage of the drug. Therefore, in the presence of any changes in liver function tests, the drug should be discontinued.

Precautions:

Associated with Estrogens

A. General Precautions.

1. A complete medical and family history should be taken prior to the initiation of any estrogen therapy. The pretreatment and periodic physical examinations should include special reference to blood pressure, breasts, abdomen, and pelvic organs, and should include a Papanicolau smear. As a general rule, estrogen should not be prescribed for longer than one year without another physical examination being performed.

2. Fluid retention—Because estrogens may cause some degree of fluid retention, conditions which might be influenced by this factor such as asthma, epilepsy, migraine, and cardiac or renal dysfunction, require careful observation.

3. Certain patients may develop undesirable manifestations of excessive estrogenic stimulation, such as abnormal or excessive uterine bleeding, mastodynia, etc.

4. Oral contraceptives appear to be associated with an increased incidence of mental depression.[24a] Although it is not clear whether this is due to the estrogenic or progestogenic component of the contraceptive, patients with a history of depression should be carefully observed.

5. Preexisting uterine leiomyomata may increase in size during estrogen use.

6. The pathologist should be advised of estrogen therapy when relevant specimens are submitted.

7. Patients with a past history of jaundice during pregnancy have an increased risk of recurrence of jaundice while receiving estrogen-containing oral contraceptive therapy. If jaundice develops in any patient receiving estrogen, the medication should be discontinued while the cause is investigated.

8. Estrogens may be poorly metabolized in patients with impaired liver function and they should be administered with caution in such patients.

9. Because estrogens influence the metabolism of calcium and phosphorus, they should be used with caution in patients with metabolic bone diseases that are associated with hypercalcemia or in patients with renal insufficiency.

10. Because of the effects of estrogens on epiphyseal closure, they should be used judiciously in young patients in whom bone growth is not complete.

11. Certain endocrine and liver function tests may be affected by estrogen-containing oral contraceptives. The following similar changes may be expected with larger doses of estrogen:

a. Increased sulfobromophthalein retention.

b. Increased prothrombin and factors VII, VIII, IX, and X; decreased antithrombin 3; increased norepinephrine-induced platelet aggregability.

c. Increased thyroid binding globulin (TBG) leading to increased circulating total thyroid hormone, as measured by PBI, T4 by column, or T4 by radioimmunoassay. Free T3 resin uptake is decreased, reflecting the elevated TBG; free T4 concentration is unaltered.

d. Impaired glucose tolerance.

e. Decreased pregnanediol excretion.

f. Reduced response to metyrapone test.

g. Reduced serum folate concentration.

h. Increased serum triglyceride and phospholipid concentration.

B. Information for the Patient. See text which appears after the PHYSICIAN REFERENCES.

C. Pregnancy Category X. See CONTRAINDICATIONS and Boxed Warning.

D. Nursing Mothers. As a general principle, the administration of any drug to nursing mothers should be done only when clearly necessary since many drugs are excreted in human milk.

Associated with Methyltestosterone

A. Prolonged dosage of androgen may result in sodium and fluid retention. This may present a problem, especially in patients with compromised cardiac reserve or renal disease.

B. If priapism or other signs of excessive sexual stimulation develop, discontinue therapy.

C. In the male, prolonged administration or excessive dosage may cause inhibition of testicular function, with resultant oligospermia and decrease in ejaculatory volume. Use cautiously in young boys to avoid possible premature epiphyseal closure or precocious sexual development.

D. Hypersensitivity and gynecomastia may occur rarely.

E. PBI may be decreased in patients taking androgens.

F. Hypercalcemia may occur. If this does occur, the drug should be discontinued.

Adverse Reactions:

Associated with Estrogens

(See Warnings regarding induction of neoplasia, adverse effects on the fetus, increased incidence of gallbladder disease, and adverse effects similar to those of oral contraceptives, including thromboembolism.) The following additional adverse reactions have been reported with estrogenic therapy, including oral contraceptives:

1. *Genitourinary system:* Breakthrough bleeding, spotting, change in menstrual flow; dysmenorrhea; premenstrual-like syndrome; amenorrhea during and after treatment; increase in size of uterine fibromyomata; vaginal candidiasis; change in cervical erosion and in degree of cervical secretion; cystitis-like syndrome.

2. *Breasts:* Tenderness, enlargement, secretion.

3. *Gastrointestinal:* Nausea, vomiting; abdominal cramps, bloating; cholestatic jaundice.

4. *Skin:* Chloasma or melasma which may persist when drug is discontinued; erythema multiforme; erythema nodosum; hemorrhagic eruption; loss of scalp hair; hirsutism.

5. *Eyes:* Steepening of corneal curvature; intolerance to contact lenses.

6. *CNS:* Headache, migraine, dizziness; mental depression; chorea.

7. *Miscellaneous:* Increase or decrease in weight; reduced carbohydrate tolerance; aggravation of porphyria; edema; changes in libido.

Associated with Methyltestosterone

Cholestatic jaundice

Hypercalcemia, particularly in patients with metastatic breast carcinoma. This usually indicates progression of bone metastases.

Sodium and water retention

Priapism

Virilization in female patients

Hypersensitivity and gynecomastia

Acute Overdosage: Numerous reports of ingestion of large doses of estrogen-containing oral contraceptives by young children indicate that acute serious ill effects do not occur. Overdosage of estrogen may cause nausea, and withdrawal bleeding may occur in females.

Dosage and Administration: *Male and female*—1 MEDIATRIC Capsule or Tablet daily. (MEDIATRIC Liquid, 3 teaspoonfuls daily.)

In the female: To avoid continuous stimulation of breast and uterus, cyclic therapy is recommended (3 week regimen with 1 week rest period—Withdrawal bleeding may occur during this 1 week rest period).

Treated patients with an intact uterus should be monitored closely for signs of endometrial cancer and appropriate diagnostic measures should be taken to rule out malignancy in the event of persistent or recurring abnormal vaginal bleeding.

In the male: A careful check should be made on the status of the prostate gland when therapy is given for protracted intervals.

How Supplied:

MEDIATRIC Capsules, in bottles of 100 (NDC 0046-0252-81).

MEDIATRIC Tablets, in bottles of 100 (NDC 0046-0752-81).

MEDIATRIC Liquid, in bottles of 16 fluidounces (NDC 0046-0910-16).

Physician References:

1. Ziel, H. K., *et al.:* N. Engl. J. Med. *293*:1167–1170, 1975.
2. Smith, D. C., *et al.:* N. Engl. J. Med. *293*:1164–1167, 1975.
3. Mack, T. M., *et al.:* N. Engl. J. Med. *294*:1262–1267, 1976.
4. Weiss, N. S., *et al.:* N. Engl. J. Med. *294*:1259–1262, 1976.
5. Herbst, A. L., *et al.:* N. Engl. J. Med. *284*:878–881, 1971.
6. Greenwald, P., *et al.:* N. Engl. J. Med. *285*:390–392, 1971.
7. Lanier, A., *et al.:* Mayo Clin. Proc. *48*:793–799, 1973.
8. Herbst, A., *et al.:* Obstet. Gynecol. *40*:287–298, 1972.
9. Herbst, A., *et al.:* Am. J. Obstet. Gynecol. *118*:607–615, 1974.
10. Herbst, A., *et al.:* N. Engl. J. Med. *292*:334–339, 1975.
11. Stafl, A., *et al.:* Obstet. Gynecol. *43*:118–128, 1974.
12. Sherman, A. I., *et al.:* Obstet. Gynecol. *44*:531–545, 1974.
13. Gal, I., *et al.:* Nature *216*:83, 1967.
14. Levy, E. P., *et al.:* Lancet *1*:611, 1973.
15. Nora, J., *et al.:* Lancet *1*:941–942, 1973.
16. Janerich, D. T., *et al.:* N. Engl. J. Med. *291*:697–700, 1974.

Continued on next page

Ayerst—Cont.

17. Boston Collaborative Drug Surveillance Program: N. Engl. J. Med. *290*:15–19, 1974.
18. Hoover, R., *et al.*: N. Engl. J. Med. *295*:401–405, 1976.
19. Boston Collaborative Drug Surveillance Program: Lancet *1*:1399–1404, 1973.
20. Daniel, D. G., *et al.*: Lancet *2*:287–289, 1967.
21. The Veterans Administration Cooperative Urological Research Group: J. Urol. *98*:516–522, 1967.
22. Bailar, J. C.: Lancet *2*:560, 1967.
23. Blackard, C., *et al.*: Cancer *26*:249–256, 1970.
24. Royal College of General Practitioners: J. R. Coll. Gen. Pract. *13*:267–279, 1967.
24a. Royal College of General Practitioners: Oral Contraceptives and Health, New York, Pitman Corp., 1974.
25. Inman, W. H. W., *et al.*: Br. Med. J. *2*:193–199, 1968.
26. Vessey, M. P., *et al.*: Br. Med. J. *2*:651–657, 1969.
27. Sartwell, P. E., *et al.*: Am. J. Epidemiol. *90*:365–380, 1969.
28. Collaborative Group for the Study of Stroke in Young Women: N. Engl. J. Med. *288*:871–878, 1973.
29. Collaborative Group for the Study of Stroke in Young Women: J.A.M.A. *231*:718–722, 1975.
30. Mann, J. I., *et al.*: Br. Med. J. *2*:245–248, 1975.
31. Mann, J. I., *et al.*: Br. Med. J. *2*:241–245, 1975.
32. Inman, W. H. W., *et al.*: Br. Med. J. *2*:203–209, 1970.
33. Stolley, P. D., *et al.*: Am. J. Epidemiol. *102*:197–208, 1975.
34. Vessey, M. P., *et al.*: Br. Med. J. *3*:123–126, 1970.
35. Greene, G. R., *et al.*: Am. J. Public Health *62*:680–685, 1972.
36. Rosenberg, L., *et al.*: N. Engl. J. Med. *294*:1256–1259, 1976.
37. Coronary Drug Project Research Group: J.A.M.A. *214*:1303–1313, 1970.
38. Baum, J., *et al.*: Lancet *2*:926–928, 1973.
39. Mays, E. T., *et al.*: J.A.M.A. *235*:730–732, 1976.
40. Edmondson, H. A., *et al.*: N. Engl. J. Med. *294*:470–472, 1976.
41. Pfeffer, R. I., *et al.*: Am. J. Epidemiol. *103*:445–456, 1976.

INFORMATION FOR THE PATIENT

What You Should Know about Estrogens: Estrogens are female hormones produced by the ovaries. The ovaries make several different kinds of estrogens. In addition, scientists have been able to make a variety of synthetic estrogens. As far as we know, all these estrogens have similar properties and therefore much the same usefulness, side effects, and risks. This leaflet is intended to help you understand what estrogens are used for, the risks involved in their use, and how to use them as safely as possible.

This leaflet includes the most important information about estrogens, but not all the information. If you want to know more, you should ask your doctor for more information or you can ask your doctor or pharmacist to let you read the package insert prepared for the doctor.

Uses of Estrogen: THERE IS NO PROPER USE OF ESTROGENS IN A PREGNANT WOMAN.

Estrogens are prescribed by doctors for a number of purposes, including:

1. To provide estrogen during a period of adjustment when a woman's ovaries stop producing a majority of her estrogens, in order to prevent certain uncomfortable symptoms of estrogen deficiency. (With the menopause, which generally occurs between the ages of 45 and 55, women produce a much smaller amount of estrogens.)
2. To prevent symptoms of estrogen deficiency when a woman's ovaries have been removed surgically before the natural menopause.
3. To prevent pregnancy. (Estrogens are given along with a progestogen, another female hormone; these combinations are called oral contraceptives or birth control pills. Patient labeling is available to women taking oral contraceptives and they will not be discussed in this leaflet.)
4. To treat certain cancers in women and men.
5. To prevent painful swelling of the breasts after pregnancy in women who choose not to nurse their babies.

Estrogens in the Menopause: In the natural course of their lives, all women eventually experience a decrease in estrogen production. This usually occurs between ages 45 and 55 but may occur earlier or later. Sometimes the ovaries may need to be removed before natural menopause by an operation, producing a "surgical menopause."

When the amount of estrogen in the blood begins to decrease, many women may develop typical symptoms: feelings of warmth in the face, neck, and chest or sudden intense episodes of heat and sweating throughout the body (called "hot flashes" or "hot flushes"). These symptoms are sometimes very uncomfortable. Some women may also develop changes in the vagina (called "atrophic vaginitis") which cause discomfort, especially during and after intercourse.

Estrogens can be prescribed to treat these symptoms of the menopause. It is estimated that considerably more than half of all women undergoing the menopause have only mild symptoms or no symptoms at all and therefore do not need estrogens. Other women may need estrogens for a few months, while their bodies adjust to lower estrogen levels. Sometimes the need will be for periods longer than six months. In an attempt to avoid overstimulation of the uterus (womb), estrogens are usually given cyclically during each month of use, such as three weeks of pills followed by one week without pills.

Sometimes women experience nervous symptoms or depression during menopause. There is no evidence that estrogens are effective for such symptoms without associated vasomotor symptoms. In the absence of vasomotor symptoms, estrogens should not be used to treat nervous symptoms, although other treatment may be needed.

You may have heard that taking estrogens for long periods (years) after the menopause will keep your skin soft and supple and keep you feeling young. There is no evidence that this is so, however, and such long-term treatment carries important risks.

Estrogens to Prevent Swelling of the Breasts after Pregnancy: If you do not breast-feed your baby after delivery, your breasts may fill up with milk and become painful and engorged. This usually begins about 3 to 4 days after delivery and may last for a few days to up to a week or more. Sometimes the discomfort is severe, but usually it is not and can be controlled by pain-relieving drugs such as aspirin and by binding the breasts up tightly. Estrogens can be used to try to prevent the breasts from filling up. While this treatment is sometimes successful, in many cases the breasts fill up to some degree in spite of treatment. The dose of estrogens needed to prevent pain and swelling of the breasts is much larger than the dose needed to treat symptoms of the menopause and this may increase your chances of developing blood clots in the legs or lungs (see below). Therefore, it is important that you discuss the benefits and the risks of estrogen use with your doctor if you have decided not to breast-feed your baby.

The Dangers of Estrogens:

1. *Endometrial cancer.* There are reports that if estrogens are used in the postmenopausal period for more than a year, there is an increased risk of *endometrial cancer* (cancer of the lining of the uterus). Women taking estrogens have roughly 5 to 10 times as great a chance of getting this cancer as women who take no estrogens. To put this another way, while a postmenopausal woman not taking estrogens has 1 chance in 1,000 each year of getting endometrial cancer, a woman taking estrogens has 5 to 10 chances in 1,000 each year. For this reason *it is important to take estrogens only when they are really needed.*

The risk of this cancer is greater the longer estrogens are used and when larger doses are taken. Therefore you should not take more estrogen than your doctor prescribes. *It is important to take the lowest dose of estrogen that will control symptoms and to take it only as long as it is needed.* If estrogens are needed for longer periods of time, your doctor will want to reevaluate your need for estrogens at least every six months.

Women using estrogens should report any vaginal bleeding to their doctors; such bleeding may be of no importance, but it can be an early warning of endometrial cancer. If you have undiagnosed vaginal bleeding, you should not use estrogens until a diagnosis is made and you are certain there is no endometrial cancer.

NOTE: If you have had your uterus removed (total hysterectomy), there is no danger of developing endometrial cancer.

2. *Other possible cancers.* Estrogens can cause development of other tumors in animals, such as tumors of the breast, cervix, vagina, or liver, when given for a long time. At present there is no good evidence that women using estrogen in the menopause have an increased risk of such tumors, but there is no way yet to be sure they do not; and one study raises the possibility that use of estrogens in the menopause may increase the risk of breast cancer many years later. This is a further reason to use estrogens only when clearly needed. While you are taking estrogens, it is important that you go to your doctor at least once a year for a physical examination. Also, if members of your family have had breast cancer or if you have breast nodules or abnormal mammograms (breast x-rays), your doctor may wish to carry out more frequent examinations of your breasts.

3. *Gallbladder disease.* Women who use estrogens after menopause are more likely to develop gallbladder disease needing surgery than women who do not use estrogens. Birth control pills have a similar effect.

4. *Abnormal blood clotting.* Oral contraceptives increase the risk of blood clotting in various parts of the body. This can result in a stroke (if the clot is in the brain), a heart attack (clot in a blood vessel of the heart), or a pulmonary embolus (a clot which forms in the legs or pelvis, then breaks off and travels to the lungs). Any of these can be fatal.

At this time use of estrogens in the menopause is not known to cause such blood clotting, but this has not been fully studied and there could still prove to be such a risk. It is recommended that if you have had clotting in the legs or lungs or a heart attack or stroke while you were using estrogens or birth control pills, you should not use estrogens (unless they are being used to treat cancer of the breast or prostate). If you have had a stroke or heart atack or if you have angina pectoris, estrogens should be used with great caution and only if clearly needed (for example, if you have severe symptoms of the menopause).

The larger doses of estrogen used to prevent swelling of the breasts after pregnancy have been reported to cause clotting in the legs and lungs.

Special Warning about Pregnancy: You should not receive estrogen if you are pregnant. If this should occur, there is a greater than usual chance that the developing child will be born with a birth defect, although the possibility remains fairly small. A female child may have an increased risk of developing cancer of the vagina or cervix later in life (in the teens or twenties). Every possible effort should be made to avoid exposure to estrogens during pregnancy. If exposure occurs, see your doctor.

Other Effects of Estrogens: In addition to the serious known risks of estrogens described above, estrogens have the following side effects and potential risks:

1. *Nausea and vomiting.* The most common side effect of estrogen therapy is nausea. Vomiting is less common.
2. *Effects on breasts.* Estrogens may cause breast tenderness or enlargement and may cause the breasts to secrete a liquid. These effects are not dangerous.
3. *Effects on the uterus.* Estrogens may cause benign fibroid tumors of the uterus to get larger.
4. *Effects on liver.* Women taking oral contraceptives develop on rare occasions a tumor of the liver which can rupture and bleed into the abdomen and may cause death. So far, these tumors have not been reported in women using estrogens in the menopause, but you should report any swelling or unusual pain or tenderness in the abdomen to your doctor immediately.

Women with a past history of jaundice (yellowing of the skin and white parts of the eyes) may get jaundice again during estrogen use. If this occurs, stop taking estrogens and see your doctor.

5. *Other effects.* Estrogens may cause excess fluid to be retained in the body. This may make some conditions worse, such as asthma, epilepsy, migraine, heart disease, or kidney disease.

Summary: Estrogens have important uses, but they have serious risks as well. You must decide, with your doctor, whether the risks are acceptable to you in view of the benefits of treatment. Except where your doctor has prescribed estrogens for use in special cases of cancer of the breast or prostate, you should not use estrogens if you have cancer of the breast or uterus, are pregnant, have undiagnosed abnormal vaginal bleeding, clotting in the legs or lungs, or have had a stroke, heart attack or angina, or clotting in the legs or lungs in the past while you were taking estrogens.

You can use estrogens as safely as possible by understanding that your doctor will require regular physical examinations while you are taking them and will try to discontinue the drug as soon as possible and use the smallest dose possible. Be alert for signs of trouble including:

1. Abnormal bleeding from the vagina.
2. Pains in the calves or chest or sudden shortness of breath, or coughing blood.
3. Severe headache, dizziness, faintness, or changes in vision.
4. Breast lumps (you should ask your doctor how to examine your own breasts).
5. Jaundice (yellowing of the skin).
6. Mental depression.

Your doctor has prescribed this drug for you and you alone. Do not give the drug to anyone else.

How Supplied:
MEDIATRIC®—provides estrogen and androgen in small doses, nutritional supplements, and a mild antidepressant. It is supplied as capsules, tablets, and liquid.

[*Shown in Product Identification Section*]

MYSOLINE® ℞

Brand of primidone
Anticonvulsant

Actions: MYSOLINE raises electro- or chemoshock seizure thresholds or alters seizure patterns in experimental animals. The mechanism(s) of primidone's antiepileptic action is not known.

Primidone *per se* has anticonvulsant activity as do its two metabolites, phenobarbital and phenylethylmalonamide (PEMA). In addition to its anticonvulsant activity, PEMA potentiates that of phenobarbital in experimental animals.

Indications: MYSOLINE, either alone or used concomitantly with other anticonvulsants, is indicated in the control of grand mal, psychomotor, and focal epileptic seizures. It may control grand mal seizures refractory to other anticonvulsant therapy.

Contraindications: Primidone is contraindicated in: 1) patients with porphyria and 2) patients who are hypersensitive to phenobarbital (see ACTIONS).

Warnings: The abrupt withdrawal of antiepileptic medication may precipitate status epilepticus.

The therapeutic efficacy of a dosage regimen takes several weeks before it can be assessed.

Usage in pregnancy: The effects of MYSOLINE (primidone) in human pregnancy and nursing infants are unknown.

Recent reports suggest an association between the use of anticonvulsant drugs by women with epilepsy and an elevated incidence of birth defects in children born to these women. Data are more extensive with respect to diphenylhydantoin and phenobarbital, but these are also the most commonly prescribed anticonvulsants; less systematic or anecdotal reports suggest a possible similar association with the use of all known anticonvulsant drugs.

The reports suggesting an elevated incidence of birth defects in children of drug-treated epileptic women cannot be regarded as adequate to prove a definite cause and effect relationship. There are intrinsic methodologic problems in obtaining adequate data on drug teratogenicity in humans; the possibility also exists that other factors, *e.g.*, genetic factors or the epileptic condition itself, may be more important than drug therapy in leading to birth defects. The great majority of mothers on anticonvulsant medication deliver normal infants. It is important to note that anticonvulsant drugs should not be discontinued in patients in whom the drug is administered to prevent major seizures because of the strong possibility of precipitating status epilepticus with attendant hypoxia and threat to life. In individual cases where the severity and frequency of the seizure disorder are such that the removal of medication does not pose a serious threat to the patient, discontinuation of the drug may be considered prior to and during pregnancy, although it cannot be said with any confidence that even minor seizures do not pose some hazard to the developing embryo or fetus.

The prescribing physician will wish to weigh these considerations in treating or counseling epileptic women of childbearing potential.

Neonatal hemorrhage, with a coagulation defect resembling vitamin K deficiency, has been described in newborns whose mothers were taking primidone and other anticonvulsants. Pregnant women under anticonvulsant therapy should receive prophylactic vitamin K_1 therapy for one month prior to, and during, delivery.

Precautions: The total daily dosage should not exceed 2 g. Since MYSOLINE (primidone) therapy generally extends over prolonged periods, a complete blood count and a sequential multiple analysis-12 (SMA-12) test should be made every six months.

In nursing mothers: There is evidence that in mothers treated with primidone, the drug appears in the milk in substantial quantities. Since tests for the presence of primidone in biological fluids are too complex to be carried out in the average clinical laboratory, it is suggested that the presence of undue somnolence and drowsiness in nursing newborns of MYSOLINE-treated mothers be taken as an indication that nursing should be discontinued.

Adverse Reactions: The most frequently occurring early side effects are ataxia and vertigo. These tend to disappear with continued therapy, or with reduction of initial dosage. Occasionally, the following have been reported: nausea, anorexia, vomiting, fatigue, hyperirritability, emotional disturbances, sexual impotency, diplopia, nystagmus, drowsiness, and morbilliform skin eruptions. Occasionally, persistent or severe side effects may necessitate withdrawal of the drug. Megaloblastic anemia may occur as a rare idiosyncrasy to MYSOLINE and to other anticonvulsants. The anemia responds to folic acid without necessity of discontinuing medication.

Dosage and Administration: *Adult Dosage:* Patients 8 years of age and older who have received no previous treatment may be started on MYSOLINE (primidone) according to the following regimen using either 50 mg or scored 250 mg MYSOLINE tablets.

Days 1–3: 100 to 125 mg at bedtime
Days 4–6: 100 to 125 mg b.i.d.
Days 7–9: 100 to 125 mg t.i.d.
Day 10-maintenance: 250 mg t.i.d.

For most adults and children 8 years of age and over, the usual maintenance dosage is three to four 250 mg MYSOLINE tablets daily in divided doses (250 mg t.i.d. or q.i.d.). If required, an increase to five or six 250 mg tablets daily may be made but daily doses should not exceed 500 mg q.i.d.

INITIAL: ADULTS AND CHILDREN OVER 8

KEY: · = 50 mg tablet; ● = 250 mg tablet

DAY	1	2	3	4	5	6
AM				··	··	··
NOON						
PM	··	··	··	··	··	··

DAY	7	8	9	10	11	12
AM	··	··	··	●		
NOON	··	··	··	●	Adjust to	
PM	··	··	··	●	Maintenance	

Dosage should be individualized to provide maximum benefit. In some cases, serum blood level determinations of primidone may be necessary for optimal dosage adjustment. The clinically effective serum level for primidone is between 5–12 μg/ml.

In patients already receiving other anticonvulsants: MYSOLINE should be started at 100 to 125 mg at bedtime and gradually increased to maintenance level as the other drug is gradually decreased. This regimen should be continued until satisfactory dosage level is achieved for the combination, or the other medication is completely withdrawn. When therapy with MYSOLINE (primidone) alone is the objective, the transition from concomitant therapy should not be completed in less than two weeks.

Pediatric Dosage: For children under 8 years of age, the following regimen may be used:

Days 1–3: 50 mg at bedtime
Days 4–6: 50 mg b.i.d.
Days 7–9: 100 mg b.i.d.
Day 10-maintenance: 125 mg t.i.d. to 250 mg t.i.d.

For children under 8 years of age, the usual maintenance dosage is 125 to 250 mg three

Continued on next page

Ayerst—Cont.

times daily, or 10–25 mg/kg/day in divided doses.

How Supplied:
MYSOLINE (primidone) Tablets
Each tablet contains 250 mg of primidone (scored), in bottles of 100 (NDC 0046-0430-81) and 1,000 (NDC 0046-0430-91).
Also in unit dose package of 100 (NDC 0046-0430-99).
Each tablet contains 50 mg of primidone (scored), in bottles of 100 (NDC 0046-0431-81) and 500 (NDC 0046-0431-85).
MYSOLINE Suspension
Each 5 ml (teaspoonful) contains 250 mg of primidone, in bottles of 8 fluidounces (NDC 0046-3850-08).
[*Shown in Product Identification Section*]

PEPTAVLON® ℞
Brand of pentagastrin
A diagnostic agent for evaluation of gastric acid secretory function.

Actions: PEPTAVLON (pentagastrin) contains the C-terminal tetrapeptide responsible for the actions of the natural gastrins and, therefore, acts as a physiologic gastric acid secretagogue. The recommended dose of 6 mcg/kg subcutaneously produces a peak acid output which is reproducible when used in the same individual.

PEPTAVLON stimulates gastric acid secretion approximately ten minutes after subcutaneous injection, with peak responses occurring in most cases twenty to thirty minutes after administration. Duration of activity is usually between sixty and eighty minutes.

Indications: PEPTAVLON (pentagastrin) is used as a diagnostic agent to evaluate gastric acid secretory function. It is useful in testing for:

Anacidity:—as a diagnostic aid in patients with suspected pernicious anemia, atrophic gastritis, or gastric carcinoma.

Hypersecretion:—as a diagnostic aid in patients with suspected duodenal ulcer or postoperative stomal ulcer, and for the diagnosis of Zollinger-Ellison tumor.

PEPTAVLON (pentagastrin) is also useful in determining the adequacy of acid-reducing operations for peptic ulcer.

Contraindications: Hypersensitivity or idiosyncrasy to pentagastrin.

Warnings: *Use in Pregnancy*—The use of pentagastrin in pregnancy has NOT been studied, and the benefit of administration of the drug must be weighed against any possible risk to the mother and/or fetus.

Use in Children—There are insufficient data to recommend the use of, or establish a dosage, in children.

****

In amounts in excess of the recommended dose, pentagastrin may cause inhibition of gastric acid secretion.

Precautions: Use with caution in patients with pancreatic, hepatic, or biliary disease. Like gastrin, pentagastrin could, in some cases, have the physiologic effect of stimulating pancreatic enzyme and bicarbonate secretion, as well as biliary flow.

Adverse Reactions: Pentagastrin causes fewer and less severe cardiovascular and other adverse reactions than histamine or betazole. The majority of reactions to pentagastrin are related to the gastrointestinal tract.
The following reactions associated with the use of pentagastrin have been reported.

Gastrointestinal: abdominal pain, desire to defecate, nausea, vomiting, borborygmi, blood-tinged mucus

Cardiovascular: flushing, tachycardia

Central Nervous System: dizziness, faintness or lightheadedness, drowsiness, sinking feeling, transient blurring of vision, tiredness, headache

Allergic and Hypersensitivity Reactions: May occur in some patients.

Miscellaneous: shortness of breath, heavy sensation in arms and legs, tingling in fingers, chills, sweating, generalized burning sensation, warmth, pain at site of injection, bile in collected specimens

Dosage and Administration: *Adults:* 6 mcg/kg subcutaneously. Effect begins in about ten minutes; peak response usually occurs in twenty to thirty minutes. (For discussion of the test and explicit directions, consult Baron, J.H.: Gastric Function Tests, in Wastell, C.: Chronic Duodenal Ulcer, New York, Appleton-Century-Crofts, 1972, pp. 82–114.)

Note: Data are inadequate to recommend the use of, or establish a dosage, in children.

Overdosage: In case of overdosage or idiosyncrasy, symptomatic treatment should be administered as required.

How Supplied: PEPTAVLON—In 2 ml ampuls. Each ml contains 0.25 mg (250 mcg) pentagastrin. Also contains 0.88% sodium chloride, and Water for Injection U.S.P. The pH is adjusted with ammonium hydroxide. Cartons of 10 (NDC 0046-3290-10).

PHOSPHOLINE IODIDE® ℞
(echothiophate iodide for ophthalmic solution)

Description: PHOSPHOLINE IODIDE occurs as a white, crystalline, water-soluble, hygroscopic solid having a slight mercaptan-like odor. When freeze-dried in the presence of potassium acetate, the mixture appears as a white amorphous deposit on the walls of the bottle.
Each package contains materials for dispensing 5 ml of eyedrops: (1) bottle containing PHOSPHOLINE IODIDE in one of four potencies [1.5 mg (0.03%), 3.0 mg (0.06%), 6.25 mg (0.125%), or 12.5 mg (0.25%)] as indicated on the label, with 40 mg potassium acetate in each case. Sodium hydroxide or acetic acid may have been incorporated to adjust pH during manufacturing. (2) a 5 ml bottle of diluent containing chlorobutanol (chloral derivative), 0.5%; mannitol, 1.2%; boric acid, 0.06%; and exsiccated sodium phosphate, 0.026% (3) sterilized dropper.

Actions: PHOSPHOLINE IODIDE is a long-acting cholinesterase inhibitor for topical use which enhances the effect of endogenously liberated acetylcholine in iris, ciliary muscle, and other parasympathetically innervated structures of the eye. It thereby causes miosis, increase in facility of outflow of aqueous humor, fall in intraocular pressure, and potentiation of accommodation.
PHOSPHOLINE IODIDE (echothiophate iodide) will depress both plasma and erythrocyte cholinesterase levels in most patients after a few weeks of eyedrop therapy.

Indications: GLAUCOMA—Chronic open-angle glaucoma. Subacute or chronic angle-closure glaucoma after iridectomy or where surgery is refused or contraindicated. Certain non-uveitic secondary types of glaucoma, especially glaucoma following cataract surgery.
ACCOMMODATIVE ESOTROPIA—Concomitant esotropias with a significant accommodative component.

Contraindications:
1. Active uveal inflammation.
2. Most cases of angle closure glaucoma, due to the possibility of increasing angle block.
3. Hypersensitivity to the active or inactive ingredients.

Warnings:
1. *Use in Pregnancy:* Safe use of anticholinesterase medications during pregnancy has not been established, nor has the absence of adverse effects on the fetus or on the respiration of the neonate.
2. Succinylcholine should be administered only with great caution, if at all, prior to or during general anesthesia to patients receiving anticholinesterase medication because of possible respiratory or cardiovascular collapse.
3. Caution should be observed in treating glaucoma with PHOSPHOLINE IODIDE (echothiophate iodide) in patients who are at the same time undergoing treatment with systemic anticholinesterase medications for myasthenia gravis, because of possible adverse additive effects.

Precautions:
1. Gonioscopy is recommended prior to initiation of therapy.
2. Where there is a quiescent uveitis or a history of this condition, anticholinesterase therapy should be avoided or used cautiously because of the intense and persistent miosis and ciliary muscle contraction that may occur.
3. While systemic effects are infrequent, proper use of the drug requires digital compression of the nasolacrimal ducts for a minute or two following instillation to minimize drainage into the nasal chamber with its extensive absorption area. The hands should be washed immediately following instillation.
4. Temporary discontinuance of medication is necessary if salivation, urinary incontinence, diarrhea, profuse sweating, muscle weakness, respiratory difficulties, or cardiac irregularities occur.
5. Patients receiving PHOSPHOLINE IODIDE who are exposed to carbamate or organophosphate type insecticides and pesticides (professional gardeners, farmers, workers in plants manufacturing or formulating such products, etc.) should be warned of the additive systemic effects possible from absorption of the pesticide through the respiratory tract or skin. During periods of exposure to such pesticides, the wearing of respiratory masks, and frequent washing and clothing changes may be advisable.
6. Anticholinesterase drugs should be used with extreme caution, if at all, in patients with marked vagotonia, bronchial asthma, spastic gastrointestinal disturbances, peptic ulcer, pronounced bradycardia and hypotension, recent myocardial infarction, epilepsy, parkinsonism, and other disorders that may respond adversely to vagotonic effects.
7. Anticholinesterase drugs should be employed prior to ophthalmic surgery only as a considered risk because of the possible occurrence of hyphema.
8. PHOSPHOLINE IODIDE (echothiophate iodide) should be used with great caution, if at all, where there is a prior history of retinal detachment.

Adverse Reactions:
1. Although the relationship, if any, of retinal detachment to the administration of PHOSPHOLINE IODIDE has not been established, retinal detachment has been reported in a few cases during the use of PHOSPHOLINE IODIDE in adult patients without a previous history of this disorder.
2. Stinging, burning, lacrimation, lid muscle twitching, conjunctival and ciliary redness, browache, induced myopia with visual blurring may occur.
3. Activation of latent iritis or uveitis may occur.
4. Iris cysts may form, and if treatment is continued, may enlarge and obscure vision. This occurrence is more frequent in children. The cysts usually shrink upon discontinuance of the medication, reduction in strength of the drops or frequency of instillation. Rarely, they may rupture or break free into the aqueous. Regular examinations are advis-

able when the drug is being prescribed for the treatment of accommodative esotropia.

5. Prolonged use may cause conjunctival thickening, obstruction of nasolacrimal canals.
6. Lens opacities occurring in patients under treatment for glaucoma with PHOSPHOLINE IODIDE have been reported and similar changes have been produced experimentally in normal monkeys. Routine examinations should accompany clinical use of the drug.
7. Paradoxical increase in intraocular pressure may follow anticholinesterase instillation. This may be alleviated by prescribing a sympathomimetic mydriatic such as phenylephrine.

Dosage and Administration:
GLAUCOMA—
Selection of Therapy: The *medication prescribed* should be that which will control the intraocular pressure around-the-clock with the least risk of side effects or adverse reactions. "Tonometric glaucoma" (ocular hypertension without other evidence of the disease) is frequently not treated with any medication, and PHOSPHOLINE IODIDE (echothiophate iodide) is certainly not recommended for this condition. In early chronic simple glaucoma with field loss or disc changes, pilocarpine is generally used for initial therapy and can be recommended so long as control is thereby maintained over the 24 hours of the day.
When this is not the case, PHOSPHOLINE IODIDE 0.03% may be effective and probably has no greater potential for side effects. If this dosage is inadequate, epinephrine and a carbonic anhydrase inhibitor may be added to the regimen. When still more effective medication is required, the higher strengths of PHOSPHOLINE IODIDE may be prescribed with the recognition that the control of the intraocular pressure should have priority regardless of potential side effects. In secondary glaucoma following cataract surgery, the higher strengths of the drug are frequently needed and are ordinarily very well tolerated.
The *dosage regimen* prescribed should call for the lowest concentration that will control the intraocular pressure around-the-clock. Where tonometry around-the-clock is not feasible, it is suggested that appointments for tension-taking be made at different times of the day so that inadequate control may be more readily detected. Two doses a day are preferred to one in order to maintain as smooth a diurnal tension curve as possible, although a single dose per day or every other day has been used with satisfactory results. Because of the long duration of action of the drug, it is never necessary or desirable to exceed a schedule of twice a day. The daily dose or one of the two daily doses should always be instilled just before retiring to avoid inconvenience due to the miosis.
Early Chronic Simple Glaucoma: PHOSPHOLINE IODIDE (echothiophate iodide) 0.03% instilled twice a day, just before retiring and in the morning, may be prescribed advantageously for cases of early chronic simple glaucoma that are not controlled around-the-clock with pilocarpine. Because of prolonged action, control during the night and early morning hours may then sometimes be obtained. A change in therapy is indicated if, at any time, the tension fails to remain at an acceptable level on this regimen.
Advanced Chronic Simple Glaucoma and Glaucoma Secondary to Cataract Surgery: These cases may respond satisfactorily to PHOSPHOLINE IODIDE 0.03% twice a day as above. When the patient is being transferred to PHOSPHOLINE IODIDE (echothiophate iodide) because of unsatisfactory control with pilocarpine, carbachol, epinephrine, etc., one of the higher strengths, 0.06%, 0.125%, or 0.25% will usually be needed. In this case, a brief trial with the 0.03% eyedrops will be advantageous in that the higher strengths will then be more easily tolerated.
Concomitant Therapy: PHOSPHOLINE IODIDE may be used concomitantly with epinephrine, a carbonic anhydrase inhibitor, or both.
Technic: Good technic in the administration of PHOSPHOLINE IODIDE requires that finger pressure at the inner canthus should be exerted for a minute or two following instillation of the eyedrops, to minimize drainage into the nose and throat. Excess solution around the eye should be removed with tissue and any medication on the hands should be rinsed off.
ACCOMMODATIVE ESOTROPIA—
In Diagnosis: One drop of 0.125% may be instilled once a day in both eyes on retiring, for a period of two or three weeks. If the esotropia is accommodative, a favorable response will usually be noted which may begin within a few hours.
In Treatment: PHOSPHOLINE IODIDE (echothiophate iodide) is prescribed at the lowest concentration and frequency which gives satisfactory results. After the initial period of treatment for diagnostic purposes, the schedule may be reduced to 0.125% every other day or 0.06% every day. These dosages can often be gradually lowered as treatment progresses. The 0.03% strength has proven to be effective in some cases. The maximum usually recommended dosage is 0.125% once a day, although more intensive therapy has been used for short periods.
Technic: See Dosage and Administration, Section on Glaucoma.
Duration of Treatment
In diagnosis, only a short period is required and little time will be lost in instituting other procedures if the esotropia proves to be unresponsive. In therapy, there is no definite limit so long as the drug is well tolerated. However, if the eyedrops, with or without eyeglasses, are gradually withdrawn after about a year or two and deviation recurs, surgery should be considered. As with other miotics, tolerance may occasionally develop after prolonged use. In such cases, a rest period will restore the original activity of the drug.
Overdosage: Antidotes are atropine, 2 mg parenterally; PROTOPAM® CHLORIDE (pralidoxime chloride), 25 mg per kg intravenously; artificial respiration should be given if necessary.

Directions for Preparing Eyedrops

1. Use aseptic technic.
2. Tear off aluminum seals, and remove and discard rubber plugs from both drug and diluent containers.
3. Pour diluent into drug container.
4. Remove dropper assembly from its sterile wrapping. Holding dropper assembly by the screw cap and, WITHOUT COMPRESSING RUBBER BULB, insert into drug container and screw down tightly.
5. Shake for several seconds to ensure mixing.
6. Do not cover nor obliterate instructions to patient regarding storage of eyedrops.

Storage and Stability of Eyedrops
Keep eyedrops in refrigerator to obtain maximum useful life of six months. Room temperature is acceptable if drops will be used up within a month.

How Supplied: Each package contains PHOSPHOLINE IODIDE (echothiophate iodide), diluent, and dropper for dispensing 5 ml eyedrops of the strength indicated on the label. Four potencies are available:
NDC 0046-1062-05 .... 1.5 mg package for 0.03%
NDC 0046-1064-05 .... 3.0 mg package for 0.06%
NDC 0046-1065-05 .... 6.25 mg package for 0.125%
NDC 0046-1066-05 .... 12.5 mg package for 0.25%

PLEGINE® Tablets ℞
Brand of phendimetrazine tartrate
Anorexiant

Actions: PLEGINE is a phenylalkylamine sympathomimetic with pharmacologic activity similar to the prototype drugs of this class used in obesity, the amphetamines. Actions include central nervous system stimulation and elevation of blood pressure. Tachyphylaxis and tolerance have been demonstrated with all drugs of this class in which these phenomena have been looked for.
Drugs of this class used in obesity are commonly known as "anorectics" or "anorexigenics." It has not been established, however, that the action of such drugs in treating obesity is primarily one of appetite suppression. Other central nervous system actions, or metabolic effects, may be involved, for example.
Adult obese subjects instructed in dietary management and treated with "anorectic" drugs, lose more weight on the average than those treated with placebo and diet, as determined in relatively short term clinical trials.
The magnitude of increased weight loss of drug-treated patients over placebo-treated patients is only a fraction of a pound a week. The rate of weight loss is greatest in the first weeks of therapy for both drug and placebo subjects and tends to decrease in succeeding weeks. The possible origins of the increased weight loss due to the various drug effects are not established. The amount of weight loss associated with the use of an "anorectic" drug varies from trial to trial, and the increased weight loss appears to be related in part to variables other than the drug prescribed, such as the physician-investigator, the population treated, and the diet prescribed. Studies do not permit conclusions as to the relative importance of the drug and non-drug factors on weight loss.
The natural history of obesity is measured in years, whereas the studies cited are restricted to a few weeks' duration; thus, the total impact of drug-induced weight loss over that of diet alone must be considered clinically limited.
Indications: PLEGINE (phendimetrazine tartrate) is indicated in the management of exogenous obesity as a short term adjunct (a few weeks) in a regimen of weight reduction based on caloric restriction. The limited usefulness of agents of this class should be measured against possible risk factors inherent in their use (see **Actions**).
Contraindications: Known hypersensitivity or idiosyncratic reactions to sympathomimetics.
Advanced arteriosclerosis, symptomatic cardiovascular disease, moderate and severe hypertension, hyperthyroidism
Highly nervous or agitated patients
Patients with a history of drug abuse
Patients taking other CNS stimulants, including monamine oxidase inhibitors
Warnings: DRUG DEPENDENCE: PLEGINE is related chemically and pharmacologically to the amphetamines. Amphetamines and related stimulant drugs have been extensively abused, and the possibility of abuse of PLEGINE should be kept in mind when evaluating the desirability of including a drug as part of a weight reduction program. Abuse of amphetamines and related drugs may be associated with intense psychological dependence and severe social dysfunction. There are reports of patients who have increased the dosage to many times that recommended. Abrupt cessation following prolonged high dosage administration results in extreme fatigue and mental

Continued on next page

Ayerst—Cont.

depression; changes are also noted on the sleep EEG. Manifestations of chronic intoxication with anorectic drugs include severe dermatoses, marked insomnia, irritability, hyperactivity, and personality changes. The most severe manifestation of chronic intoxications is psychosis, often clinically indistinguishable from schizophrenia.

Tolerance to the anorectic effect of PLEGINE (phendimetrazine tartrate) develops within a few weeks. When this occurs, its use should be discontinued; the maximum recommended dose should not be exceeded.

Use of PLEGINE (phendimetrazine tartrate) within 14 days following the administration of monamine oxidase inhibitors may result in a hypertensive crisis.

Abrupt cessation of administration following prolonged high dosage results in extreme fatigue and depression. Because of the effect on the central nervous system, PLEGINE may impair the ability of the patient to engage in potentially hazardous activities such as operating machinery or driving a motor vehicle; the patient should therefore be cautioned accordingly.

Usage in Pregnancy: Safe use in pregnancy has not been established. Until more information is available, phendimetrazine tartrate should not be taken by women who are or may become pregnant unless, in the opinion of the physician, the potential benefits outweigh the possible hazards.

Usage in Children: PLEGINE is not recommended for use in children under 12 years of age.

Precautions: Caution is to be exercised in prescribing PLEGINE for patients with even mild hypertension.

Insulin requirements in diabetes mellitus may be altered in association with the use of PLEGINE and the concomitant dietary regimen.

PLEGINE may decrease the hypotensive effect of guanethidine.

The least amount feasible should be prescribed or dispensed at one time in order to minimize the possibility of overdosage.

Adverse Reactions: *Central Nervous System:* Overstimulation, restlessness, insomnia, agitation, flushing, tremor, sweating, dizziness, headache, psychotic states, blurring of vision

Cardiovascular: Palpitation, tachycardia, elevated blood pressure

Gastrointestinal: Mouth dryness, nausea, diarrhea, constipation, stomach pain

Genitourinary: Urinary frequency, dysuria, changes in libido

Dosage and Administration: *Usual adult dosage:* 1 tablet (35 mg.) b.i.d. or t.i.d., one hour before meals.

Dosage should be individualized to obtain an adequate response with the lowest effective dosage. In some cases, ½ tablet per dose may be adequate; dosage should not exceed 2 tablets t.i.d.

Overdosage: Acute overdosage of phendimetrazine tartrate may manifest itself by the following signs and symptoms: unusual restlessness, confusion, belligerence, hallucinations, and panic states. Fatigue and depression usually follow the central stimulation. Cardiovascular effects include arrhythmias, hypertension, or hypotension and circulatory collapse. Gastrointestinal symptoms include nausea, vomiting, diarrhea, and abdominal cramps. Poisoning may result in convulsions, coma, and death.

The management of overdosage is largely symptomatic. It includes sedation with a barbiturate. If hypertension is marked, the use of a nitrate or rapid-acting alpha receptor-blocking agent should be considered. Experience with hemodialysis or peritoneal dialysis is inadequate to permit recommendations for its use.

How Supplied: PLEGINE—Each scored tablet contains 35 mg phendimetrazine tartrate, in bottles of 100 (NDC 0046-0755-81) and 1,000 (NDC 0046-0755-91).

[*Shown in Product Identification Section*]

PMB® 200 ℞

Each tablet contains:
Premarin® (Conjugated Estrogens, U.S.P.) ....0.45 mg
Meprobamate ....200.0 mg

PMB® 400

Each tablet contains:
Premarin® (Conjugated Estrogens, U.S.P.) ....0.45 mg
Meprobamate ....400.0 mg

1. ESTROGENS HAVE BEEN REPORTED TO INCREASE THE RISK OF ENDOMETRIAL CARCINOMA.

Three independent case control studies have reported an increased risk of endometrial cancer in postmenopausal women exposed to exogenous estrogens for more than one year.[1–3] This risk was independent of the other known risk factors for endometrial cancer. These studies are further supported by the finding that incidence rates of endometrial cancer have increased sharply since 1969 in eight different areas of the United States with population-based cancer reporting systems, an increase which may be related to the rapidly expanding use of estrogens during the last decade.[4]

The three case control studies reported that the risk of endometrial cancer in estrogen users was about 4.5 to 13.9 times greater than in nonusers. The risk appears to depend on both duration of treatment[1] and on estrogen dose.[3] In view of these findings, when estrogens are used for the treatment of menopausal symptoms, the lowest dose that will control symptoms should be utilized and medication should be discontinued as soon as possible. When prolonged treatment is medically indicated, the patient should be reassessed on at least a semiannual basis to determine the need for continued therapy. Although the evidence must be considered preliminary, one study suggests that cyclic administration of low doses of estrogen may carry less risk than continuous administration;[3] it therefore appears prudent to utilize such a regimen.

Close clinical surveillance of all women taking estrogens is important. In all cases of undiagnosed persistent or recurring abnormal vaginal bleeding, adequate diagnostic measures should be undertaken to rule out malignancy.

There is no evidence at present that "natural" estrogens are more or less hazardous than "synthetic" estrogens at equiestrogenic doses.

2. ESTROGENS SHOULD NOT BE USED DURING PREGNANCY.

The use of female sex hormones, both estrogens and progestogens, during early pregnancy may seriously damage the offspring. It has been shown that females exposed in utero to diethylstilbestrol, a non-steroidal estrogen, have an increased risk of developing in later life a form of vaginal or cervical cancer that is ordinarily extremely rare.[5,6] This risk has been estimated as not greater than 4 per 1000 exposures.[7] Furthermore, a high percentage of such exposed women (from 30 to 90 percent) have been found to have vaginal adenosis,[8–12] epithelial changes of the vagina and cervix. Although these changes are histologically benign, it is not known whether they are precursors of malignancy. Although similar data are not available with the use of other estrogens, it cannot be presumed they would not induce similar changes.

Several reports suggest an association between intrauterine exposure to female sex hormones and congenital anomalies, including congenital heart defects and limb reduction defects.[13–16] One case control study[16] estimated a 4.7-fold increased risk of limb reduction defects in infants exposed in utero to sex hormones (oral contraceptives, hormone withdrawal tests for pregnancy, or attempted treatment for threatened abortion). Some of these exposures were very short and involved only a few days of treatment. The data suggest that the risk of limb reduction defects in exposed fetuses is somewhat less than 1 per 1000.

In the past, female sex hormones have been used during pregnancy in an attempt to treat threatened or habitual abortion. There is considerable evidence that estrogens are ineffective for these indications, and there is no evidence from well controlled studies that progestogens are effective for these uses.

If PMB is used during pregnancy, or if the patient becomes pregnant while taking this drug, she should be apprised of the potential risks to the fetus, and the advisability of pregnancy continuation.

3. THIS FIXED COMBINATION DRUG IS NOT INDICATED FOR INITIAL THERAPY.

In cases where estrogen given alone has not alleviated anxiety and tension existing as part of the menopausal symptom complex, therapy may then consist of separate administration of estrogen and meprobamate in order to determine the appropriate dosage of each drug for the patient. If this fixed combination represents the dosage so determined, its use may be more convenient in patient management. The treatment of such patients is not static, but must be reevaluated as conditions in each patient warrant.

Description: PMB is a combination of PREMARIN® (Conjugated Estrogens, U.S.P.) and meprobamate, a tranquilizing agent, in tablet form for oral administration.

PREMARIN (Conjugated Estrogens, U.S.P.) is a mixture of estrogens, obtained exclusively from natural sources, occurring as the sodium salts of water-soluble estrogen sulfates blended to represent the average composition of material derived from pregnant mares' urine. It contains estrone, equilin, and 17α-dihydroequilin, together with smaller amounts of 17α-estradiol, equilenin, and 17 α-dihydroequilenin as salts of their sulfate esters.

Meprobamate is the dicarbamic acid ester of 2-methyl-2-*n*-propyl-1,3-propanediol.

Clinical Pharmacology: Estrogens are important in the development and maintenance of the female reproductive system and secondary sex characteristics. They promote growth and development of the vagina, uterus, and fallopian tubes, and enlargement of the breasts. Indirectly, they contribute to the shaping of the skeleton, maintenance of tone and elasticity of urogenital structures, changes in the epiphyses of the long bones that allow for the pubertal growth spurt and its termination, growth of axillary and pubic hair, and pigmentation of the nipples and genitals. Decline of estrogenic activity at the end of the menstrual cycle can bring on menstruation, although the cessation of progesterone secretion is the most important factor in the mature ovulatory cycle. However, in the preovulatory or nonovulatory cycle, estrogen is the primary determinant in the onset of menstruation. Estrogens also affect the release of pituitary gonadotropins.

The pharmacologic effects of conjugated estrogens are similar to those of endogenous estrogens. They are soluble in water and are well absorbed from the gastrointestinal tract.

In responsive tissues (female genital organs, breasts, hypothalamus, pituitary) estrogens enter the cell and are transported into the nucleus. As a result of estrogen action, specific RNA and protein synthesis occurs.

Metabolism and inactivation occur primarily in the liver. Some estrogens are excreted into the bile; however they are reabsorbed from the intestine and returned to the liver through the portal venous system. Water soluble estrogen conjugates are strongly acidic and are ionized in body fluids, which favor excretion through the kidneys since tubular reabsorption is minimal.

Meprobamate is used clinically for the reduction of anxiety and tension. The precise mechanism(s) of its action is not known. It is well-absorbed from the gastrointestinal tract and has a physiological half-life of about 10 hours. It is excreted in the urine primarily as hydroxymeprobamate and as a glucuronide.

The combination of PREMARIN (Conjugated Estrogens, U.S.P.) with meprobamate as provided in PMB relieves the underlying estrogen deficiency and affords tranquilizing activity to ameliorate the anxiety and tension not due to estrogen deficiency.

Indication: For the treatment of moderate to severe vasomotor symptoms of the menopause when anxiety and tension are part of the symptom complex and only in those cases in which the use of estrogens alone has not resulted in alleviation of such symptoms.

PMB HAS NOT BEEN SHOWN TO BE EFFECTIVE FOR ANY PURPOSE DURING PREGNANCY AND ITS USE MAY CAUSE SEVERE HARM TO THE FETUS (SEE BOXED WARNING).

Contraindications: Estrogens should not be used in women with any of the following conditions:

1. Known or suspected cancer of the breast.
2. Known or suspected estrogen-dependent neoplasia.
3. Known or suspected pregnancy (See Boxed Warning).
4. Undiagnosed abnormal genital bleeding.
5. Active thrombophlebitis or thromboembolic disorders.
6. A past history of thrombophlebitis, thrombosis, or thromboembolic disorders associated with previous estrogen use.

Meprobamate should not be used in patients with the following conditions:

1. A history of allergic or idiosyncratic reactions to meprobamate or related compounds such as carisoprodol, mebutamate, tybamate, or carbromal.
2. Acute intermittent porphyria.

Warnings:

USAGE IN PREGNANCY AND LACTATION.

An increased risk of congenital malformations associated with the use of minor tranquilizers (meprobamate, chlordiazepoxide, and diazepam) during the first trimester of pregnancy has been suggested in several studies. Because use of these drugs is rarely a matter of urgency, their use during this period should almost always be avoided. The possibility that a woman of childbearing potential may be pregnant at the time of institution of therapy should be considered. Patients should be advised that if they become pregnant during therapy or intend to become pregnant they should communicate with their physicians about the desirability of discontinuing the drug.

Meprobamate passes the placental barrier. It is present both in umbilical cord blood at or near maternal plasma levels and in breast milk of lactating mothers at concentrations two to four times that of maternal plasma. When use of meprobamate is contemplated in breast-feeding patients, the drug's higher concentrations in breast milk as compared to maternal plasma levels should be considered.

Usage in Children—PMB is not intended for use in children.

Associated with Estrogen Administration:

1. *Induction of malignant neoplasms.* Long term continuous administration of natural and synthetic estrogens in certain animal species increases the frequency of carcinomas of the breast, cervix, vagina, and liver. There are now reports that estrogens increase the risk of carcinoma of the endometrium in humans. (See Boxed Warning.)

At the present time there is no satisfactory evidence that estrogens given to postmenopausal women increase the risk of cancer of the breast,[17] although a recent long-term followup of a single physician's practice has raised this possibility.[18] Because of the animal data, there is a need for caution in prescribing estrogens for women with a strong family history of breast cancer or who have breast nodules, fibrocystic disease, or abnormal mammograms.

2. *Gallbladder disease.* A recent study has reported a 2 to 3-fold increase in the risk of surgically confirmed gallbladder disease in women receiving postmenopausal estrogens,[17] similar to the 2-fold increase previously noted in users of oral contraceptives.[19,24a]

3. *Effects similar to those caused by estrogen-progestogen oral contraceptives.* There are several serious adverse effects of oral contraceptives, most of which have not, up to now, been documented as consequences of postmenopausal estrogen therapy. This may reflect the comparatively low doses of estrogen used in postmenopausal women. It would be expected that the larger doses of estrogen used to treat prostatic or breast cancer or postpartum breast engorgement are more likely to result in these adverse effects, and, in fact, it has been shown that there is an increased risk of thrombosis in men receiving estrogens for prostatic cancer and women for postpartum breast engorgement.[20–23]

a. *Thromboembolic disease.* It is now well established that users of oral contraceptives have an increased risk of various thromboembolic and thrombotic vascular diseases, such as thrombophlebitis, pulmonary embolism, stroke, and myocardial infarction.[24–31] Cases of retinal thrombosis, mesenteric thrombosis, and optic neuritis have been reported in oral contraceptive users. There is evidence that the risk of several of these adverse reactions is related to the dose of the drug.[32,33] An increased risk of postsurgery thromboembolic complications has also been reported in users of oral contraceptives.[34,35] If feasible, estrogen should be discontinued at least 4 weeks before surgery of the type associated with an increased risk of thromboembolism, or during periods of prolonged immobilization.

While an increased rate of thromboembolic and thrombotic disease in postmenopausal users of estrogens has not been found,[17–24,25–36] this does not rule out the possibility that such an increase may be present or that subgroups of women who have underlying risk factors or who are receiving relatively large doses of estrogens may have increased risk. Therefore estrogens should not be used in persons with active thrombophlebitis or thromboembolic disorders, and they should not be used (except in treatment of malignancy) in persons with a history of such disorders in association with estrogen use. They should be used with caution in patients with cerebral vascular or coronary artery disease and only for those in whom estrogens are clearly needed.

Large doses of estrogen (5 mg conjugated estrogens per day), comparable to those used to treat cancer of the prostate and breast, have been shown in a large prospective clinical trial in men[37] to increase the risk of nonfatal myocardial infarction, pulmonary embolism and thrombophlebitis. When estrogen doses of this size are used, any of the thromboembolic and thrombotic adverse effects associated with oral contraceptive use should be considered a clear risk.

b. *Hepatic adenoma.* Benign hepatic adenomas appear to be associated with the use of oral contraceptives.[38–40] Although benign, and rare, these may rupture and may cause death through intra-abdominal hemorrhage. Such lesions have not yet been reported in association with other estrogen or progestogen preparations but should be considered in estrogen users having abdominal pain and tenderness, abdominal mass, or hypovolemic shock. Hepatocellular carcinoma has also been reported in women taking estrogen-containing oral contraceptives.[39] The relationship of this malignancy to these drugs is not known at this time.

c. *Elevated blood pressure.* Women using oral contraceptives sometimes experience increased blood pressure which, in most cases, returns to normal on discontinuing the drug. There is now a report that this may occur with use of estrogens in the menopause[41] and blood pressure should be monitored with estrogen use, especially if high doses are used.

d. *Glucose tolerance.* A worsening of glucose tolerance has been observed in a significant percentage of patients on estrogen-containing oral contraceptives. For this reason, diabetic patients should be carefully observed while receiving estrogen.

4. *Hypercalcemia.* Administration of estrogens may lead to severe hypercalcemia in patients with breast cancer and bone metastases. If this occurs, the drug should be stopped and appropriate measures taken to reduce the serum calcium level.

Associated with Meprobamate Administration:

1. *Drug Dependence*—Physical dependence, psychological dependence, and abuse have occurred. When chronic intoxication from prolonged use occurs, it usually involves ingestion of greater than recommended doses and is manifested by ataxia, slurred speech, and vertigo. Therefore, careful supervision of dose and amounts prescribed is advised, as well as avoidance of prolonged administration, especially for alcoholics and other patients with a known propensity for taking excessive quantities of drugs.

Sudden withdrawal of the drug after prolonged and excessive use may precipitate recurrence of preexisting symptoms, such as anxiety, anorexia, or insomnia, or withdrawal reactions, such as vomiting, ataxia, tremors, muscle twitching, confusional states, hallucinosis, and, rarely, convulsive seizures. Such seizures are more likely to occur in persons with central nervous system damage or preexistent or latent convulsive disorders. Onset of withdrawal symptoms occurs usually within 12 to 48 hours after discontinuation of meprobamate; symptoms usually cease within the next 12 to 48 hours.

When excessive dosage has continued for weeks or months, dosage should be reduced gradually over a period of one or two weeks rather than abruptly stopped. Alternatively, a short-acting barbiturate may be substituted, then gradually withdrawn.

2. *Potentially Hazardous Tasks*—Patients should be warned that this drug may impair the mental and/or physical abilities required for the performance of potentially hazardous tasks such as driving a motor vehicle or operating machinery.

3. *Additive Effects*—Since the effects of meprobamate and alcohol or meprobamate and other CNS depressants or psychotropic drugs may be additive, appropriate caution should be exercised with patients who take more than one of these agents simultaneously.

Continued on next page

Ayerst—Cont.

Precautions:

Associated with Estrogen

A. General Precautions.

1. A complete medical and family history should be taken prior to the initiation of any estrogen therapy. The pretreatment and periodic physical examinations should include special reference to blood pressure, breasts, abdomen, and pelvic organs, and should include a Papanicolau smear. As a general rule, estrogen should not be prescribed for longer than one year without another physical examination being performed.
2. Fluid retention—Because estrogens may cause some degree of fluid retention, conditions which might be influenced by this factor such as asthma, epilepsy, migraine, and cardiac or renal dysfunction, require careful observation.
3. Certain patients may develop undesirable manifestations of excessive estrogenic stimulation, such as abnormal or excessive uterine bleeding, mastodynia, etc.
4. Oral contraceptives appear to be associated with an increased incidence of mental depression.[24a] Although it is not clear whether this is due to the estrogenic or progestogenic component of the contraceptive, patients with a history of depression should be carefully observed.
5. Preexisting uterine leiomyomata may increase in size during estrogen use.
6. The pathologist should be advised of estrogen therapy when relevant specimens are submitted.
7. Patients with a past history of jaundice during pregnancy have an increased risk of recurrence of jaundice while receiving estrogen-containing oral contraceptive therapy. If jaundice develops in any patient receiving estrogen, the medication should be discontinued while the cause is investigated.
8. Estrogens may be poorly metabolized in patients with impaired liver function and they should be administered with caution in such patients.
9. Because estrogens influence the metabolism of calcium and phosphorus, they should be used with caution in patients with metabolic bone diseases that are associated with hypercalcemia or in patients with renal insufficiency.
10. Because of the effects of estrogens on epiphyseal closure, they should be used judiciously in young patients in whom bone growth is not complete.
11. Certain endocrine and liver function tests may be affected by estrogen-containing oral contraceptives. The following similar changes may be expected with larger doses of estrogen:

a. Increased sulfobromophthalein retention.
b. Increased prothrombin and factors VII, VIII, IX, and X; decreased antithrombin 3; increased norepinephrine-induced platelet aggregability.
c. Increased thyroid binding globulin (TBG) leading to increased circulating total thyroid hormone, as measured by PBI, T4 by column, or T4 by radioimmunoassay. Free T3 resin uptake is decreased, reflecting the elevated TBG; free T4 concentration is unaltered.
d. Impaired glucose tolerance.
e. Decreased pregnanediol excretion.
f. Reduced response to metyrapone test.
g. Reduced serum folate concentration.
h. Increased serum triglyceride and phospholipid concentration.

B. Information for the Patient. See text which appears after the PHYSICIAN REFERENCES under PREMARIN® (Conjugated Estrogens Tablets, U.S.P.).

C. Pregnancy Category X. See CONTRAINDICATIONS and Boxed Warning.

D. Nursing Mothers. As a general principle, the administration of any drug to nursing mothers should be done only when clearly necessary since many drugs are excreted in human milk.

Associated with Meprobamate

A. The lowest effective dose should be administered, particularly to debilitated patients, in order to preclude oversedation.
B. The possibility of suicide attempts should be considered and the least amount of drug feasible should be dispensed at any one time.
C. Meprobamate is metabolized in the liver and excreted by the kidney; to avoid its excess accumulation, caution should be exercised in administration to patients with compromised liver or kidney function.
D. Meprobamate occasionally may precipitate seizures in epileptic patients.

Adverse Reactions:

Associated with Estrogen Administration

(See Warnings regarding induction of neoplasia, adverse effects on the fetus, increased incidence of gallbladder disease, and adverse effects similar to those of oral contraceptives, including thromboembolism.) The following additional adverse reactions have been reported with estrogenic therapy, including oral contraceptives:

1. *Genitourinary system:* Breakthrough bleeding, spotting, change in menstrual flow; dysmenorrhea; premenstrual-like syndrome; amenorrhea during and after treatment; increase in size of uterine fibromyomata; vaginal candidiasis; change in cervical erosion and in degree of cervical secretion; cystitis-like syndrome.
2. *Breasts:* Tenderness, enlargement, secretion.
3. *Gastrointestinal:* Nausea, vomiting; abdominal cramps, bloating; cholestatic jaundice.
4. *Skin:* Chloasma or melasma which may persist when drug is discontinued; erythema multiforme; erythema nodosum; hemorrhagic eruption; loss of scalp hair; hirsutism.
5. *Eyes:* Steepening of corneal curvature; intolerance to contact lenses.
6. *CNS:* Headache, migraine, dizziness; mental depression; chorea.
7. *Miscellaneous:* Increase or decrease in weight; reduced carbohydrate tolerance; aggravation of porphyria; edema; changes in libido.

The following have been reported with meprobamate therapy:

1. *Central Nervous System*—Drowsiness, ataxia, dizziness, slurred speech, headache, vertigo, weakness, paresthesias, impairment of visual accommodation, euphoria, overstimulation, paradoxical excitement, fast EEG activity.
2. *Gastrointestinal*—Nausea, vomiting, diarrhea.
3. *Cardiovascular*—Palpitations, tachycardia, various forms of arrhythmia, transient ECG changes, syncope; also, hypotensive crises (including one fatal case).
4. *Allergic or Idiosyncratic*—Allergic or idiosyncratic reactions are usually seen within the period of the first to fourth dose in patients having had no previous contact with the drug. Milder reactions are characterized by an itchy, urticarial, or erythematous maculopapular rash which may be generalized or confined to the groin. Other reactions have included leukopenia, acute nonthrombocytopenic purpura, petechiae, ecchymoses, eosinophilia, peripheral edema, adenopathy, fever, fixed drug eruption with cross reaction to carisoprodol, and cross sensitivity between meprobamate/mebutamate and meprobamate/carbromal.

More severe hypersensitivity reactions, rarely reported, include hyperpyrexia, chills, angioneurotic edema, bronchospasm, oliguria, and anuria. Also, anaphylaxis, erythema multiforme, exfoliative dermatitis, stomatitis, proctitis, Stevens-Johnson syndrome, and bullous dermatitis, including one fatal case of the latter, following administration of meprobamate in combination with prednisolone.

In case of allergic or idiosyncratic reactions to meprobamate, discontinue the drug and initiate appropriate symptomatic therapy, which may include epinephrine, antihistamines, and in severe cases corticosteroids. In evaluating possible allergic reactions, also consider allergy to excipients (information on excipients is available to physicians on request).

5. *Hematologic* (See also *Allergic or Idiosyncratic.*)—Agranulocytosis and aplastic anemia have been reported, although no causal relationship has been established. These cases rarely were fatal. Rare cases of thrombocytopenic purpura have been reported.
6. *Other*—Exacerbation of porphyric symptoms.

Overdosage:

Acute overdosage (estrogen alone):

Numerous reports of ingestion of large doses of estrogen-containing oral contraceptives by young children indicate that acute serious ill effects do not occur. Overdosage of estrogen may cause nausea, and withdrawal bleeding may occur in females.

Acute simple overdosage (meprobamate alone): Death has been reported with ingestion of as little as 12 grams meprobamate and survival with as much as 40 grams.

Blood levels:

0.5—2.0 mg% represents the usual blood level range of meprobamate after therapeutic doses. The level may occasionally be as high as 3.0 mg%.

3—10 mg% usually corresponds to findings of mild to moderate symptoms of overdosage, such as stupor or light coma.

10—20 mg% usually corresponds to deeper coma, requiring more intensive treatment. Some fatalities occur.

At levels greater than 20 mg%, more fatalities than survivals can be expected.

Acute combined (alcohol or other CNS depressants or psychotropic drugs) **overdosage:** Since effects can be additive, a history of ingestion of a low dose of meprobamate plus any of these compounds (or of a relatively low blood or tissue level) cannot be used as a prognostic indicator.

In cases where excessive doses have been taken, sleep ensues rapidly and blood pressure, pulse, and respiratory rates are reduced to basal levels. Any drug remaining in the stomach should be removed and symptomatic therapy given. Should respiration or blood pressure become compromised, respiratory assistance, central nervous system stimulants, and pressor agents should be administered cautiously as indicated. Meprobamate is metabolized in the liver and excreted by the kidney. Diuresis, osmotic (mannitol) diuresis, peritoneal dialysis, and hemodialysis have been used successfully. Careful monitoring of urinary output is necessary and caution should be taken to avoid overhydration. Relapse and death, after initial recovery, have been attributed to incomplete gastric emptying and delayed absorption. Meprobamate can be measured in biological fluids by two methods: colorimetric[42] and gas chromatographic.[43]

Dosage and Administration:

Given cyclically for short term use only:

For the treatment of moderate to severe vasomotor symptoms of the menopause when anxiety and tension are part of the symptom complex and only in those cases in which the use of estrogens alone has not resulted in alleviation of such symptoms.

The lowest dose that will control symptoms should be chosen and medication should be discontinued as promptly as possible. The usual dosage of conjugated estrogen is 1.25 milligrams daily. The usual dosage of meprobamate is 1,200 to 1,600 milligrams daily.

Administration should be cyclic (e.g., three weeks on and one week off).
Attempts to discontinue or taper medication should be made at three to six month intervals.

PMB® 200 & PMB® 400: The usual dosage is one tablet of either strength three times daily administered cyclically. Use of meprobamate during the rest period should be considered for those patients who may require continuing medication with tranquilizer. After the first few cycles of therapy, the patient's need for continuing the use of the meprobamate component should be reevaluated.
Daily dosage should be adjusted to individual requirements. The daily dosage should not exceed 6 tablets of PMB 200 per day or 4 tablets of PMB 400 per day.
Treated patients with an intact uterus should be monitored closely for signs of endometrial cancer and appropriate diagnostic measures should be taken to rule out malignancy in the event of persistent or recurring abnormal vaginal bleeding.

How Supplied: PMB® 200, in bottles of 60 (NDC 0046-0880-60).
PMB® 400, in bottles of 60 (NDC 0046-0881-60).

Physician References:

1. Ziel, H. K., *et al.*: N. Engl. J. Med. *293*:1167–1170, 1975.
2. Smith, D. C., *et al.*: N. Engl. J. Med. *293*:1164–1167, 1975.
3. Mack, T. M., *et al.*: N. Engl. J. Med. *294*:1262–1267, 1976.
4. Weiss, N. S., *et al.*: N. Engl. J. Med. *294*:1259–1262, 1976.
5. Herbst, A. L., *et al.*: N. Engl. J. Med. *284*:878–881, 1971.
6. Greenwald, P., *et al.*: N. Engl. J. Med. *285*:390–392, 1971.
7. Lanier, A., *et al.*: Mayo Clin. Proc. *48*:793–799, 1973.
8. Herbst, A., *et al.*: Obstet. Gynecol. *40*:287–298, 1972.
9. Herbst, A., *et al.*: Am. J. Obstet. Gynecol. *118*:607–615, 1974.
10. Herbst, A., *et al.*: N. Engl. J. Med. *292*:334–339, 1975.
11. Stafl, A., *et al.*: Obstet. Gynecol. *43*:118–128, 1974.
12. Sherman, A. I., *et al.*: Obstet. Gynecol. *44*:531–545, 1974.
13. Gal, I., *et al.*: Nature *216*:83, 1967.
14. Levy, E. P., *et al.*: Lancet *1*:611, 1973.
15. Nora, J., *et al.*: Lancet *1*:941–942, 1973.
16. Janerich, D. T., *et al.*: N. Engl. J. Med. *291*:697–700, 1974.
17. Boston Collaborative Drug Surveillance Program N. Engl. J. Med. *290*:15–19, 1974.
18. Hoover, R., *et al.*: N. Engl. J. Med. *295*:401–405, 1976.
19. Boston Collaborative Drug Surveillance Program: Lancet *1*:1399–1404, 1973.
20. Daniel, D. G., *et al.*: Lancet *2*:287–289, 1967.
21. The Veterans Administration Cooperative Urological Research Group: J. Urol. *98*:516–522, 1967.
22. Bailar, J. C.: Lancet *2*:560, 1967.
23. Blackard, C., *et al.*: Cancer *26*:249–256, 1970.
24. Royal College of General Practitioners: J. R. Coll. Gen. Pract. *13*:267–279, 1967.
24a. Royal College of General Practitioners: Oral Contraceptives and Health, New York, Pitman Corp., 1974.
25. Inman, W. H. W., *et al.*: Br. Med. J. *2*:193–199, 1968.
26. Vessey, M. P., *et al.*: Br. Med. J. *2*:651–657, 1969.
27. Sartwell, P. E., *et al.*: Am. J. Epidemiol. *90*:365–380, 1969.
28. Collaborative Group for the Study of Stroke in Young Women: N. Engl. J. Med. *288*:871–878, 1973.
29. Collaborative Group for the Study of Stroke in Young Women: J.A.M.A. *231*:718–722, 1975.
30. Mann, J. I., *et al.*: Br. Med. J. *2*:245–248, 1975.
31. Mann, J. I., *et al.*: Br. Med. J. *2*:241–245, 1975.
32. Inman, W. H. W., *et al.*: Br. Med. J. *2*:203–209, 1970.
33. Stolley, P. D., *et al.*: Am. J. Epidemiol. *102*:197–208, 1975.
34. Vessey, M. P., *et al.*: Br. Med. J. *3*:123–126, 1970.
35. Greene, G. R., *et al.*: Am. J. Public Health *62*:680–685, 1972.
36. Rosenberg, L., *et al.*: N. Engl. J. Med. *294*:1256–1259, 1976.
37. Coronary Drug Project Research Group: J.A.M.A. *214*:1303–1313, 1970.
38. Baum, J., *et al.*: Lancet *2*:926–928, 1973.
39. Mays, E. T., *et al.*: J.A.M.A. *235*:730–732, 1976.
40. Edmondson, H. A., *et al.*: N. Engl. J. Med. *294*:470–472, 1976.
41. Pfeffer, R. I., *et al.*: Am. J. Epidemiol. *103*:445–456, 1976.
42. Hoffman, A. J., *et al.*: J. Am. Pharm. Assoc. *48*:740, 1959.
43. Douglas, J. F., *et al.*: Anal. Chem. *39*:956, 1967.

[*Shown in Product Identification Section*]

PREMARIN® INTRAVENOUS ℞

Brand of Conjugated Estrogens, U.S.P., for Injection
Specially prepared for Intravenous & Intramuscular use

1. ESTROGENS HAVE BEEN REPORTED TO INCREASE THE RISK OF ENDOMETRIAL CARCINOMA.
Three independent case control studies have reported an increased risk of endometrial cancer in postmenopausal women exposed to exogenous estrogens for more than one year.[1–3] This risk was independent of the other known risk factors for endometrial cancer. These studies are further supported by the finding that incidence rates of endometrial cancer have increased sharply since 1969 in eight different areas of the United States with population-based cancer reporting systems, an increase which may be related to the rapidly expanding use of estrogens during the last decade.[4]
The three case control studies reported that the risk of endometrial cancer in estrogen users was about 4.5 to 13.9 times greater than in nonusers. The risk appears to depend on both duration of treatment[1] and on estrogen dose.[3] In view of these findings, when estrogens are used for the treatment of menopausal symptoms, the lowest dose that will control symptoms should be utilized and medication should be discontinued as soon as possible. When prolonged treatment is medically indicated, the patient should be reassessed on at least a semiannual basis to determine the need for continued therapy. Although the evidence must be considered preliminary, one study suggests that cyclic administration of low doses of estrogen may carry less risk than continuous administration;[3] it therefore appears prudent to utilize such a regimen.
Close clinical surveillance of all women taking estrogens is important. In all cases of undiagnosed persistent or recurring abnormal vaginal bleeding, adequate diagnostic measures should be undertaken to rule out malignancy.
There is no evidence at present that "natural" estrogens are more or less hazardous than "synthetic" estrogens at equiestrogenic doses.

2. ESTROGENS SHOULD NOT BE USED DURING PREGNANCY.
The use of female sex hormones, both estrogens and progestogens, during early pregnancy may seriously damage the offspring. It has been shown that females exposed in utero to diethylstilbestrol, a non-steroidal estrogen, have an increased risk of developing in later life a form of vaginal or cervical cancer that is ordinarily extremely rare.[5,6] This risk has been estimated as not greater than 4 per 1000 exposures.[7] Furthermore, a high percentage of such exposed women (from 30 to 90 percent) have been found to have vaginal adenosis,[8–12] epithelial changes of the vagina and cervix. Although these changes are histologically benign, it is not known whether they are precursors of malignancy. Although similar data are not available with the use of other estrogens, it cannot be presumed they would not induce similar changes.
Several reports suggest an association between intrauterine exposure to female sex hormones and congenital anomalies, including congenital heart defects and limb reduction defects.[13–16] One case control study[16] estimated a 4.7-fold increased risk of limb reduction defects in infants exposed in utero to sex hormones (oral contraceptives, hormone withdrawal tests for pregnancy, or attempted treatment for threatened abortion). Some of these exposures were very short and involved only a few days of treatment. The data suggest that the risk of limb reduction defects in exposed fetuses is somewhat less than 1 per 1000.
In the past, female sex hormones have been used during pregnancy in an attempt to treat threatened or habitual abortion. There is considerable evidence that estrogens are ineffective for these indications, and there is no evidence from well controlled studies that progestogens are effective for these uses.
If PREMARIN Intravenous (Conjugated Estrogens, U.S.P., for Injection) is used during pregnancy, or if the patient becomes pregnant while taking this drug, she should be apprised of the potential risks to the fetus, and the advisability of pregnancy continuation.

Description: Each Secule® contains 25 mg of Conjugated Estrogens, U.S.P. in a sterile lyophilized cake which also contains lactose 200 mg, sodium citrate 12.5 mg and simethicone 0.2 mg. The pH is adjusted with sodium hydroxide or hydrochloric acid. A sterile diluent (5 ml) containing 2% benzyl alcohol and Water for Injection, U.S.P. is provided for reconstitution. The reconstituted solution is suitable for intravenous or intramuscular injection.
PREMARIN (Conjugated Estrogens, U.S.P.) is a mixture of estrogens obtained exclusively from natural sources, occurring as the sodium salts of water-soluble estrogen sulfates blended to represent the average composition of material derived from pregnant mares' urine. It contains estrone, equilin, and 17 α-dihydroequilin, together with smaller amounts of 17 α-estradiol, equilenin, and 17 α-dihydroequilenin as salts of their sulfate esters.

Clinical Pharmacology: Estrogens are important in the development and maintenance of the female reproductive system and secondary sex characteristics. They promote growth and development of the vagina, uterus, and fallopian tubes, and enlargement of the breasts. Indirectly, they contribute to the shap-

Continued on next page

Ayerst—Cont.

ing of the skeleton, maintenance of tone and elasticity of urogenital structures, changes in the epiphyses of the long bones that allow for the pubertal growth spurt and its termination, growth of axillary and pubic hair, and pigmentation of the nipples and genitals. Decline of estrogenic activity at the end of the menstrual cycle can bring on menstruation, although the cessation of progesterone secretion is the most important factor in the mature ovulatory cycle. However, in the preovulatory or nonovulatory cycle, estrogen is the primary determinant in the onset of menstruation. Estrogens also affect the release of pituitary gonadotropins.

The pharmacologic effects of conjugated estrogens are similar to those of endogenous estrogens. They are soluble in water and may be administered by intravenous or intramuscular injection.

In responsive tissues (female genital organs, breasts, hypothalamus, pituitary) estrogens enter the cell and are transported into the nucleus. As a result of estrogen action, specific RNA and protein synthesis occurs.

Metabolism and inactivation occur primarily in the liver. Some estrogens are excreted into the bile; however they are reabsorbed from the intestine and returned to the liver through the portal venous system. Water-soluble estrogen conjugates are strongly acidic and are ionized in body fluids, which favor excretion through the kidneys since tubular reabsorption is minimal.

Indication: PREMARIN Intravenous (Conjugated Estrogens, U.S.P., for Injection) is indicated in the treatment of abnormal uterine bleeding due to hormonal imbalance in the absence of organic pathology.

Contraindications: Estrogens should not be used in women with any of the following conditions:

1. Known or suspected cancer of the breast except in appropriately selected patients being treated for metastatic disease.
2. Known or suspected estrogen-dependent neoplasia.
3. Known or suspected pregnancy (See Boxed Warning).
4. Undiagnosed abnormal genital bleeding.
5. Active thrombophlebitis or thromboembolic disorders.
6. A past history of thrombophlebitis, thrombosis, or thromboembolic disorders associated with previous estrogen use (except when used in treatment of breast malignancy).

Warnings:

1. *Induction of malignant neoplasms.* Long term continuous administration of natural and synthetic estrogens in certain animal species increases the frequency of carcinomas of the breast, cervix, vagina, and liver. There are now reports that estrogens increase the risk of carcinoma of the endometrium in humans. (See Boxed Warning.)

At the present time there is no satisfactory evidence that estrogens given to postmenopausal women increase the risk of cancer of the breast,[17] although a recent long-term followup of a single physician's practice has raised this possibility.[18] Because of the animal data, there is a need for caution in prescribing estrogens for women with a strong family history of breast cancer or who have breast nodules, fibrocystic disease, or abnormal mammograms.

2. *Gallbladder disease.* A recent study has reported a 2 to 3-fold increase in the risk of surgically confirmed gallbladder disease in women receiving postmenopausal estrogens,[17] similar to the 2-fold increase previously noted in users of oral contraceptives.[19,24a]

3. *Effects similar to those caused by estrogen-progestogen oral contraceptives.* There are several serious adverse effects of oral contraceptives, most of which have not, up to now, been documented as consequences of postmenopausal estrogen therapy. This may reflect the comparatively low doses of estrogen used in postmenopausal women. It would be expected that the larger doses of estrogen used to treat prostatic or breast cancer or postpartum breast engorgement are more likely to result in these adverse effects, and, in fact, it has been shown that there is an increased risk of thrombosis in men receiving estrogens for prostatic cancer and women for postpartum breast engorgement.[20–23]

a. *Thromboembolic disease.* It is now well established that users of oral contraceptives have an increased risk of various thromboembolic and thrombotic vascular diseases, such as thrombophlebitis, pulmonary embolism, stroke, and myocardial infarction.[24–31] Cases of retinal thrombosis, mesenteric thrombosis, and optic neuritis have been reported in oral contraceptive users. There is evidence that the risk of several of these adverse reactions is related to the dose of the drug.[32,33] An increased risk of postsurgery thromboembolic complications has also been reported in users of oral contraceptives.[34,35] If feasible, estrogen should be discontinued at least 4 weeks before surgery of the type associated with an increased risk of thromboembolism, or during periods of prolonged immobilization.

While an increased rate of thromboembolic and thrombotic disease in postmenopausal users of estrogens has not been found,[17–24,25–36] this does not rule out the possibility that such an increase may be present or that subgroups of women who have underlying risk factors or who are receiving relatively large doses of estrogens may have increased risk. Therefore estrogens should not be used in persons with active thrombophlebitis or thromboembolic disorders, and they should not be used (except in treatment of malignancy) in persons with a history of such disorders in association with estrogen use. They should be used with caution in patients with cerebral vascular or coronary artery disease and only for those in whom estrogens are clearly needed.

Large doses of estrogen (5 mg conjugated estrogens per day), comparable to those used to treat cancer of the prostate and breast, have been shown in a large prospective clinical trial in men[37] to increase the risk of nonfatal myocardial infarction, pulmonary embolism and thrombophlebitis. When estrogen doses of this size are used, any of the thromboembolic and thrombotic adverse effects associated with oral contraceptive use should be considered a clear risk.

b. *Hepatic adenoma.* Benign hepatic adenomas appear to be associated with the use of oral contraceptives.[38–40] Although benign, and rare, these may rupture and may cause death through intra-abdominal hemorrhage. Such lesions have not yet been reported in association with other estrogen or progestogen preparations but should be considered in estrogen users having abdominal pain and tenderness, abdominal mass, or hypovolemic shock. Hepatocellular carcinoma has also been reported in women taking estrogen-containing oral contraceptives.[39] The relationship of this malignancy to these drugs is not known at this time.

c. *Elevated blood pressure.* Women using oral contraceptives sometimes experience increased blood pressure which, in most cases, returns to normal on discontinuing the drug. There is now a report that this may occur with use of estrogens in the menopause[41] and blood pressure should be monitored with estrogen use, especially if high doses are used.

d. *Glucose tolerance.* A worsening of glucose tolerance has been observed in a significant percentage of patients on estrogen-containing oral contraceptives. For this reason, diabetic patients should be carefully observed while receiving estrogen.

4. *Hypercalcemia.* Administration of estrogens may lead to severe hypercalcemia in patients with breast cancer and bone metastases. If this occurs, the drug should be stopped and appropriate measures taken to reduce the serum calcium level.

Precautions:

A. General Precautions.

1. A complete medical and family history should be taken prior to the initiation of any estrogen therapy. The pretreatment and periodic physical examinations should include special reference to blood pressure, breasts, abdomen, and pelvic organs, and should include a Papanicolau smear. As a general rule, estrogen should not be prescribed for longer than one year without another physical examination being performed.
2. Fluid retention—Because estrogens may cause some degree of fluid retention, conditions which might be influenced by this factor such as asthma, epilepsy, migraine, and cardiac or renal dysfunction, require careful observation.
3. Certain patients may develop undesirable manifestations of excessive estrogenic stimulation, such as abnormal or excessive uterine bleeding, mastodynia, etc.
4. Oral contraceptives appear to be associated with an increased incidence of mental depression.[24a] Although it is not clear whether this is due to the estrogenic or progestogenic component of the contraceptive, patients with a history of depression should be carefully observed.
5. Preexisting uterine leiomyomata may increase in size during estrogen use.
6. The pathologist should be advised of estrogen therapy when relevant specimens are submitted.
7. Patients with a past history of jaundice during pregnancy have an increased risk of recurrence of jaundice while receiving estrogen-containing oral contraceptive therapy. If jaundice develops in any patient receiving estrogen, the medication should be discontinued while the cause is investigated.
8. Estrogens may be poorly metabolized in patients with impaired liver function and they should be administered with caution in such patients.
9. Because estrogens influence the metabolism of calcium and phosphorus, they should be used with caution in patients with metabolic bone diseases that are associated with hypercalcemia or in patients with renal insufficiency.
10. Because of the effects of estrogens on epiphyseal closure, they should be used judiciously in young patients in whom bone growth is not complete.
11. Certain endocrine and liver function tests may be affected by estrogen-containing oral contraceptives. The following similar changes may be expected with larger doses of estrogen:

a. Increased sulfobromophthalein retention.
b. Increased prothrombin and factors VII, VIII, IX, and X; decreased antithrombin 3; increased norepinephrine-induced platelet aggregability.
c. Increased thyroid binding globulin (TBG) leading to increased circulating total thyroid hormone, as measured by PBI, T4 by column, or T4 by radioimmunoassay. Free T3 resin uptake is decreased, reflecting the elevated TBG; free T4 concentration is unaltered.
d. Impaired glucose tolerance.
e. Decreased pregnanediol excretion.
f. Reduced response to metyrapone test.
g. Reduced serum folate concentration.
h. Increased serum triglyceride and phospholipid concentration.

B. Information for the Patient. See text which appears after the PHYSICIAN REFERENCES under PREMARIN® (Conjugated Estrogens Tablets, U.S.P.).

C. Pregnancy Category X. See CONTRAINDICATIONS and Boxed Warning.

D. Nursing Mothers. As a general principle, the administration of any drug to nursing mothers should be done only when clearly necessary since many drugs are excreted in human milk.

Adverse Reactions: (See Warnings regarding induction of neoplasia, adverse effects on the fetus, increased incidence of gallbladder disease, and adverse effects similar to those of oral contraceptives, including thromboembolism.) The following additional adverse reactions have been reported with estrogenic therapy, including oral contraceptives:

1. *Genitourinary system:* Breakthrough bleeding, spotting, change in menstrual flow; dysmenorrhea; premenstrual-like syndrome; amenorrhea during and after treatment; increase in size of uterine fibromyomata; vaginal candidiasis; change in cervical erosion and in degree of cervical secretion; cystitis-like syndrome.
2. *Breasts:* Tenderness, enlargement, secretion.
3. *Gastrointestinal:* Nausea, vomiting; abdominal cramps, bloating; cholestatic jaundice.
4. *Skin:* Chloasma or melasma which may persist when drug is discontinued; erythema multiforme; erythema nodosum; hemorrhagic eruption; loss of scalp hair; hirsutism.
5. *Eyes:* Steepening of corneal curvature; intolerance to contact lenses.
6. *CNS:* Headache, migraine, dizziness; mental depression; chorea.
7. *Miscellaneous:* Increase or decrease in weight; reduced carbohydrate tolerance; aggravation of porphyria; edema; changes in libido.

Acute Overdosage: Numerous reports of ingestion of large doses of estrogen-containing oral contraceptives by young children indicate that acute serious ill effects do not occur. Overdosage of estrogen may cause nausea, and withdrawal bleeding may occur in females.

Dosage and Administration:

Abnormal uterine bleeding due to hormonal imbalance: One 25 mg injection, intravenously or intramuscularly. Intravenous use is preferred since more rapid response can be expected from this mode of administration. Repeat in 6 to 12 hours if necessary. The use of PREMARIN Intravenous (Conjugated Estrogens, U.S.P., for Injection) does not preclude the advisability of other appropriate measures.

The usual precautionary measures governing intravenous administration should be adhered to. Injection should be made SLOWLY to obviate the occurrence of flushes.

Infusion of PREMARIN Intravenous (Conjugated Estrogens, U.S.P., for Injection) with other agents is not generally recommended. In emergencies, however, when an infusion has already been started, it may be expedient to make the injection into the tubing just distal to the infusion needle. If so used, compatibility of solutions must be considered.

Compatibility of solutions: PREMARIN Intravenous is compatible with normal saline, dextrose, and invert sugar solutions. IT IS NOT COMPATIBLE WITH PROTEIN HYDROLYSATE, ASCORBIC ACID, OR ANY SOLUTION WITH AN ACID pH.

Treated patients with an intact uterus should be monitored closely for signs of endometrial cancer and appropriate diagnostic measures should be taken to rule out malignancy in the event of persistent or recurring abnormal vaginal bleeding.

Directions for Storage and Reconstitution:

Storage before reconstitution: Store package in refrigerator, 2–8°C (36–46°F).

To reconstitute: First withdraw air from SECULE so as to facilitate introduction of sterile diluent. Then, flow the sterile diluent slowly against side of SECULE and agitate gently. DO NOT SHAKE VIOLENTLY.

Storage after reconstitution: It is common practice to utilize the reconstituted solution within a few hours. If it is necessary to keep the reconstituted solution for more than a few hours, store the reconstituted solution under refrigeration (2–8°C). Under these conditions, the solution is stable for 60 days, and is suitable for use unless darkening or precipitation occurs.

How Supplied: NDC 0046-0552-05-Each package provides: (1)One SECULE® containing 25 mg of Conjugated Estrogens, U.S.P., for Injection (also lactose 200 mg, sodium citrate 12.5 mg, and simethicone 0.2 mg). The pH is adjusted with sodium hydroxide or hydrochloric acid. (2)One 5 ml ampul sterile diluent with benzyl alcohol 2%, and Water for Injection, U.S.P.

PREMARIN Intravenous (Conjugated Estrogens, U.S.P., for Injection) is prepared by cryodesiccation.

Physician References:

1. Ziel, H. K., *et al.*: N. Engl. J. Med. *293*:1167–1170, 1975.
2. Smith, D. C., *et al.*: N. Engl. J. Med. *293*:1164–1167, 1975.
3. Mack, T. M., *et al.*: N. Engl. J. Med. *294*:1262–1267, 1976.
4. Weiss, N. S., *et al.*: N. Engl. J. Med. *294*:1259–1262, 1976.
5. Herbst, A. L., *et al.*: N. Engl. J. Med. *284*:878–881, 1971.
6. Greenwald, P., *et al.*: N. Engl. J. Med. *285*:390–392, 1971.
7. Lanier, A., *et al.*: Mayo Clin. Proc. *48*:793–799, 1973.
8. Herbst, A., *et al.*: Obstet. Gynecol. *40*:287–298, 1972.
9. Herbst, A., *et al.*: Am. J. Obstet. Gynecol. *118*:607–615, 1974.
10. Herbst, A., *et al.*: N. Engl. J. Med. *292*:334–339, 1975.
11. Stafl, A., *et al.*: Obstet. Gynecol. *43*:118–128, 1974.
12. Sherman, A. I., *et al.*: Obstet. Gynecol. *44*:531–545, 1974.
13. Gal, I., *et al.*: Nature *216*:83, 1967.
14. Levy, E. P., *et al.*: Lancet *1*:611, 1973.
15. Nora, J., *et al.*: Lancet *1*:941–942, 1973.
16. Janerich, D. T., *et al.*: N. Engl. J. Med. *291*:697–700, 1974.
17. Boston Collaborative Drug Surveillance Program: N. Engl. J. Med. *290*:15–19, 1974.
18. Hoover, R., *et al.*: N. Engl. J. Med. *295*:401–405, 1976.
19. Boston Collaborative Drug Surveillance Program: Lancet *1*:1399–1404, 1973.
20. Daniel, D. G., *et al.*: Lancet *2*:287–289, 1967.
21. The Veterans Administration Cooperative Urological Research Group: J. Urol. *98*:516–522, 1967.
22. Bailar, J. C.: Lancet *2*:560, 1967.
23. Blackard, C., *et al.*: Cancer *26*:249–256, 1970.
24. Royal College of General Practitioners: J. R. Coll. Gen. Pract. *13*:267–279, 1967.

24a. Royal College of General Practitioners: Oral Contraceptives and Health, New York, Pitman Corp., 1974.

25. Inman, W. H. W., *et al.*: Br. Med. J. *2*:193–199, 1968.
26. Vessey, M. P., *et al.*: Br. Med. J. *2*:651–657, 1969.
27. Sartwell, P. E., *et al.*: Am. J. Epidemiol. *90*:365–380, 1969.
28. Collaborative Group for the Study of Stroke in Young Women: N. Engl. J. Med. *288*:871–878, 1973.
29. Collaborative Group for the Study of Stroke in Young Women: J.A.M.A. *231*:718–722, 1975.
30. Mann, J. I., *et al.*: Br. Med. J. *2*:245–248, 1975.
31. Mann, J. I., *et al.*: Br. Med. J. *2*:241–245, 1975.
32. Inman, W. H. W., *et al.*: Br. Med. J. *2*:203–209, 1970.
33. Stolley, P. D., *et al.*: Am. J. Epidemiol. *102*:197–208, 1975.
34. Vessey, M. P., *et al.*: Br. Med. J. *3*:123–126, 1970.
35. Greene, G. R., *et al.*: Am. J. Public Health *62*:680–685, 1972.
36. Rosenberg, L., *et al.*: N. Engl. J. Med. *294*:1256–1259, 1976.
37. Coronary Drug Project Research Group: J.A.M.A. *214*:1303–1313, 1970.
38. Baum, J., *et al.*: Lancet *2*:926–928, 1973.
39. Mays, E. T., *et al.*: J.A.M.A. *235*:730–732, 1976.
40. Edmondson, H. A., *et al.*: N. Engl. J. Med. *294*:470–472, 1976.
41. Pfeffer, R. I., *et al.*: Am. J. Epidemiol. *103*:445–456, 1976.

PREMARIN® ℞

Brand of Conjugated Estrogens Tablets, U.S.P.

1. ESTROGENS HAVE BEEN REPORTED TO INCREASE THE RISK OF ENDOMETRIAL CARCINOMA.

Three independent case control studies have reported an increased risk of endometrial cancer in postmenopausal women exposed to exogenous estrogens for more than one year.[1–3] This risk was independent of the other known risk factors for endometrial cancer. These studies are further supported by the finding that incidence rates of endometrial cancer have increased sharply since 1969 in eight different areas of the United States with population-based cancer reporting systems, an increase which may be related to the rapidly expanding use of estrogens during the last decade.[4]

The three case control studies reported that the risk of endometrial cancer in estrogen users was about 4.5 to 13.9 times greater than in nonusers. The risk appears to depend on both duration of treatment[1] and on estrogen dose.[3] In view of these findings, when estrogens are used for the treatment of menopausal symptoms, the lowest dose that will control symptoms should be utilized and medication should be discontinued as soon as possible. When prolonged treatment is medically indicated, the patient should be reassessed on at least a semiannual basis to determine the need for continued therapy. Although the evidence must be considered preliminary, one study suggests that cyclic administration of low doses of estrogen may carry less risk than continuous administration;[3] it therefore appears prudent to utilize such a regimen.

Close clinical surveillance of all women taking estrogens is important. In all cases of undiagnosed persistent or recurring abnormal vaginal bleeding, adequate diagnostic measures should be undertaken to rule out malignancy.

There is no evidence at present that "natural" estrogens are more or less hazardous than "synthetic" estrogens at equiestrogenic doses.

2. ESTROGENS SHOULD NOT BE USED DURING PREGNANCY.

The use of female sex hormones, both estrogens and progestogens, during early pregnancy may seriously damage the offspring. It has been shown that females exposed in utero to diethylstilbestrol, a non-steroidal estrogen, have an increased risk of developing in later life a form of vaginal or cervical cancer that is ordinarily extremely rare.[5,6] This risk has

Continued on next page

Ayerst—Cont.

been estimated as not greater than 4 per 1000 exposures.[7] Furthermore, a high percentage of such exposed women (from 30 to 90 percent) have been found to have vaginal adenosis,[8–12] epithelial changes of the vagina and cervix. Although these changes are histologically benign, it is not known whether they are precursors of malignancy. Although similar data are not available with the use of other estrogens, it cannot be presumed they would not induce similar changes.

Several reports suggest an association between intrauterine exposure to female sex hormones and congenital anomalies, including congenital heart defects and limb reduction defects.[13–16] One case control study[16] estimated a 4.7-fold increased risk of limb reduction defects in infants exposed in utero to sex hormones (oral contraceptives, hormone withdrawal tests for pregnancy, or attempted treatment for threatened abortion). Some of these exposures were very short and involved only a few days of treatment. The data suggest that the risk of limb reduction defects in exposed fetuses is somewhat less than 1 per 1000.

In the past, female sex hormones have been used during pregnancy in an attempt to treat threatened or habitual abortion. There is considerable evidence that estrogens are ineffective for these indications, and there is no evidence from well controlled studies that progestogens are effective for these uses.

If PREMARIN is used during pregnancy, or if the patient becomes pregnant while taking this drug, she should be apprised of the potential risks to the fetus, and the advisability of pregnancy continuation.

Description: PREMARIN (Conjugated Estrogens Tablets, U.S.P.) for oral administration contains a mixture of estrogens, obtained exclusively from natural sources, occurring as the sodium salts of water-soluble estrogen sulfates blended to represent the average composition of material derived from pregnant mares' urine. It contains estrone, equilin, and 17 α-dihydroequilin, together with smaller amounts of 17 α-estradiol, equilenin, and 17 α-dihydroequilenin as salts of their sulfate esters.

Clinical Pharmacology: Estrogens are important in the development and maintenance of the female reproductive system and secondary sex characteristics. They promote growth and development of the vagina, uterus, and fallopian tubes, and enlargement of the breasts. Indirectly, they contribute to the shaping of the skeleton, maintenance of tone and elasticity of urogenital structures, changes in the epiphyses of the long bones that allow for the pubertal growth spurt and its termination, growth of axillary and pubic hair, and pigmentation of the nipples and genitals. Decline of estrogenic activity at the end of the menstrual cycle can bring on menstruation, although the cessation of progesterone secretion is the most important factor in the mature ovulatory cycle. However, in the preovulatory or nonovulatory cycle, estrogen is the primary determinant in the onset of menstruation. Estrogens also affect the release of pituitary gonadotropins.

The pharmacologic effects of conjugated estrogens are similar to those of endogenous estrogens. They are soluble in water and are well absorbed from the gastrointestinal tract.

In responsive tissues (female genital organs, breasts, hypothalamus, pituitary) estrogens enter the cell and are transported into the nucleus. As a result of estrogen action, specific RNA and protein synthesis occurs.

Metabolism and inactivation occur primarily in the liver. Some estrogens are excreted into the bile; however they are reabsorbed from the intestine and returned to the liver through the portal venous system. Water soluble estrogen conjugates are strongly acidic and are ionized in body fluids, which favor excretion through the kidneys since tubular reabsorption is minimal.

Indications: Based on a review of PREMARIN Tablets by the National Academy of Sciences—National Research Council and/or other information, FDA has classified the indications for use as follows:

Effective: 1. Moderate to severe *vasomotor* symptoms associated with the menopause. (There is no evidence that estrogens are effective for nervous symptoms or depression without associated vasomotor symptoms, and they should not be used to treat such conditions.)
2. Atrophic vaginitis.
3. Kraurosis vulvae.
4. Female hypogonadism.
5. Female castration.
6. Primary ovarian failure.
7. Breast cancer (for palliation only) in appropriately selected women and men with metastatic disease.
8. Prostatic carcinoma—palliative therapy of advanced disease.
9. Postpartum breast engorgement—Although estrogens have been widely used for the prevention of postpartum breast engorgement, controlled studies have demonstrated that the incidence of significant painful engorgement in patients not receiving such hormonal therapy is low and usually responsive to appropriate analgesic or other supportive therapy. Consequently, the benefit to be derived from estrogen therapy for this indication must be carefully weighed against the potential increased risk of puerperal thromboembolism associated with the use of large doses of estrogens.[20]

PREMARIN (Conjugated Estrogens Tablets, U.S.P.) HAS NOT BEEN SHOWN TO BE EFFECTIVE FOR ANY PURPOSE DURING PREGNANCY AND ITS USE MAY CAUSE SEVERE HARM TO THE FETUS (SEE BOXED WARNING).

"Probably" effective: For estrogen deficiency-induced osteoporosis, and only when used in conjunction with other important therapeutic measures such as diet, calcium, physiotherapy, and good general health-promoting measures. Final classification of this indication requires further investigation.

Contraindications: Estrogens should not be used in women (or men) with any of the following conditions:
1. Known or suspected cancer of the breast except in appropriately selected patients being treated for metastatic disease.
2. Known or suspected estrogen-dependent neoplasia.
3. Known or suspected pregnancy (See Boxed Warning).
4. Undiagnosed abnormal genital bleeding.
5. Active thrombophlebitis or thromboembolic disorders.
6. A past history of thrombophlebitis, thrombosis, or thromboembolic disorders associated with previous estrogen use (except when used in treatment of breast or prostatic malignancy).

Warnings:
1. *Induction of malignant neoplasms.* Long term continuous administration of natural and synthetic estrogens in certain animal species increases the frequency of carcinomas of the breast, cervix, vagina, and liver. There are now reports that estrogens increase the risk of carcinoma of the endometrium in humans. (See Boxed Warning.)

At the present time there is no satisfactory evidence that estrogens given to postmenopausal women increase the risk of cancer of the breast,[17] although a recent long-term followup of a single physician's practice has raised this possibility.[18] Because of the animal data, there is a need for caution in prescribing estrogens for women with a strong family history of breast cancer or who have breast nodules, fibrocystic disease, or abnormal mammograms.

2. *Gallbladder disease.* A recent study has reported a 2 to 3-fold increase in the risk of surgically confirmed gallbladder disease in women receiving postmenopausal estrogens,[17] similar to the 2-fold increase previously noted in users of oral contraceptives.[19,24a]

3. *Effects similar to those caused by estrogen-progestogen oral contraceptives.* There are several serious adverse effects of oral contraceptives, most of which have not, up to now, been documented as consequences of postmenopausal estrogen therapy. This may reflect the comparatively low doses of estrogen used in postmenopausal women. It would be expected that the larger doses of estrogen used to treat prostatic or breast cancer or postpartum breast engorgement are more likely to result in these adverse effects, and, in fact, it has been shown that there is an increased risk of thrombosis in men receiving estrogens for prostatic cancer and women for postpartum breast engorgement.[20–23]

a. *Thromboembolic disease.* It is now well established that users of oral contraceptives have an increased risk of various thromboembolic and thrombotic vascular diseases, such as thrombophlebitis, pulmonary embolism, stroke, and myocardial infarction.[24–31] Cases of retinal thrombosis, mesenteric thrombosis, and optic neuritis have been reported in oral contraceptive users. There is evidence that the risk of several of these adverse reactions is related to the dose of the drug.[32,33] An increased risk of postsurgery thromboembolic complications has also been reported in users of oral contraceptives.[34,35] If feasible, estrogen should be discontinued at least 4 weeks before surgery of the type associated with an increased risk of thromboembolism, or during periods of prolonged immobilization.

While an increased rate of thromboembolic and thrombotic disease in postmenopausal users of estrogens has not been found,[17–24,25–36] this does not rule out the possibility that such an increase may be present or that subgroups of women who have underlying risk factors or who are receiving relatively large doses of estrogens may have increased risk. Therefore estrogens should not be used in persons with active thrombophlebitis or thomboembolic disorders, and they should not be used (except in treatment of malignancy) in persons with a history of such disorders in association with estrogen use. They should be used with caution in patients with cerebral vascular or coronary artery disease and only for those in whom estrogens are clearly needed.

Large doses of estrogen (5 mg conjugated estrogens per day), comparable to those used to treat cancer of the prostate and breast, have been shown in a large prospective clinical trial in men[37] to increase the risk of nonfatal myocardial infarction, pulmonary embolism and thrombophlebitis. When estrogen doses of this size are used, any of the thromboembolic and thrombotic adverse effects associated with oral contraceptive use should be considered a clear risk.

b. *Hepatic adenoma.* Benign hepatic adenomas appear to be associated with the use of oral contraceptives.[38–40] Although benign, and rare, these may rupture and may cause death through intra-abdominal hemorrhage. Such lesions have not yet been reported in association with other estrogen or progestogen preparations but should be considered in estrogen users having abdominal pain and tenderness, abdominal mass, or hypovolemic shock. Hepatocellular carcinoma has also been reported in women taking estrogen-containing oral contraceptives.[39] The relationship of this malignancy to these drugs is not known at this time.

c. *Elevated blood pressure.* Women using oral contraceptives sometimes experience increased blood pressure which, in most cases, returns to normal on discontinuing the drug. There is now a report that this may occur with use of estrogens in the menopause[41] and blood pressure should be monitored with estrogen use, especially if high doses are used.

d. *Glucose tolerance.* A worsening of glucose tolerance has been observed in a significant percentage of patients on estrogen-containing oral contraceptives. For this reason, diabetic patients should be carefully observed while receiving estrogen.

4. *Hypercalcemia.* Administration of estrogens may lead to severe hypercalcemia in patients with breast cancer and bone metastases. If this occurs, the drug should be stopped and appropriate measures taken to reduce the serum calcium level.

Precautions:

A. General Precautions.

1. A complete medical and family history should be taken prior to the initiation of any estrogen therapy. The pretreatment and periodic physical examinations should include special reference to blood pressure, breasts, abdomen, and pelvic organs, and should include a Papanicolau smear. As a general rule, estrogen should not be prescribed for longer than one year without another physical examination being performed.
2. Fluid retention—Because estrogens may cause some degree of fluid retention, conditions which might be influenced by this factor such as asthma, epilepsy, migraine, and cardiac or renal dysfunction, require careful observation.
3. Certain patients may develop undesirable manifestations of excessive estrogenic stimulation, such as abnormal or excessive uterine bleeding, mastodynia, etc.
4. Oral contraceptives appear to be associated with an increased incidence of mental depression.[24a] Although it is not clear whether this is due to the estrogenic or progestogenic component of the contraceptive, patients with a history of depression should be carefully observed.
5. Preexisting uterine leiomyomata may increase in size during estrogen use.
6. The pathologist should be advised of estrogen therapy when relevant specimens are submitted.
7. Patients with a past history of jaundice during pregnancy have an increased risk of recurrence of jaundice while receiving estrogen-containing oral contraceptive therapy. If jaundice develops in any patient receiving estrogen, the medication should be discontinued while the cause is investigated.
8. Estrogens may be poorly metabolized in patients with impaired liver function and they should be administered with caution in such patients.
9. Because estrogens influence the metabolism of calcium and phosphorus, they should be used with caution in patients with metabolic bone diseases that are associated with hypercalcemia or in patients with renal insufficiency.
10. Because of the effects of estrogens on epiphyseal closure, they should be used judiciously in young patients in whom bone growth is not complete.
11. Certain endocrine and liver function tests may be affected by estrogen-containing oral contraceptives. The following similar changes may be expected with larger doses of estrogen:

a. Increased sulfobromophthalein retention.
b. Increased prothrombin and factors VII, VIII, IX, and X; decreased antithrombin 3; increased norepinephrine-induced platelet aggregability.
c. Increased thyroid binding globulin (TBG) leading to increased circulating total thyroid hormone, as measured by PBI, T4 by column, or T4 by radioimmunoassay. Free T3 resin uptake is decreased, reflecting the elevated TBG; free T4 concentration is unaltered.
d. Impaired glucose tolerance.
e. Decreased pregnanediol excretion.
f. Reduced response to metyrapone test.
g. Reduced serum folate concentration.
h. Increased serum triglyceride and phospholipid concentration.

B. Information for the Patient. See text which appears after the PHYSICIAN REFERENCES.

C. Pregnancy Category X. See CONTRAINDICATIONS and Boxed Warning.

D. Nursing Mothers. As a general principle, the administration of any drug to nursing mothers should be done only when clearly necessary since many drugs are excreted in human milk.

Adverse Reactions: (See Warnings regarding induction of neoplasia, adverse effects on the fetus, increased incidence of gallbladder disease, and adverse effects similar to those of oral contraceptives, including thromboembolism.) The following additional adverse reactions have been reported with estrogenic therapy, including oral contraceptives:

1. *Genitourinary system:* Breakthrough bleeding, spotting, change in menstrual flow; dysmenorrhea; premenstrual-like syndrome; amenorrhea during and after treatment; increase in size of uterine fibromyomata; vaginal candidiasis; change in cervical erosion and in degree of cervical secretion; cystitis-like syndrome.
2. *Breasts:* Tenderness, enlargement, secretion.
3. *Gastrointestinal:* Nausea, vomiting; abdominal cramps, bloating; cholestatic jaundice.
4. *Skin:* Chloasma or melasma which may persist when drug is discontinued; erythema multiforme; erythema nodosum; hemorrhagic eruption; loss of scalp hair; hirsutism.
5. *Eyes:* Steepening of corneal curvature; intolerance to contact lenses.
6. *CNS:* Headache, migraine, dizziness; mental depression; chorea.
7. *Miscellaneous:* Increase or decrease in weight; reduced carbohydrate tolerance; aggravation of porphyria; edema; changes in libido.

Acute Overdosage: Numerous reports of ingestion of large doses of estrogen-containing oral contraceptives by young children indicate that acute serious ill effects do not occur. Overdosage of estrogen may cause nausea, and withdrawal bleeding may occur in females.

Dosage and Administration:

1. *Given cyclically for short term use only:*
For treatment of moderate to severe *vasomotor* symptoms, atrophic vaginitis, or kraurosis vulvae associated with the menopause.

The lowest dose that will control symptoms should be chosen and medication should be discontinued as promptly as possible.

Administration should be cyclic (e.g., three weeks on and one week off).

Attempts to discontinue or taper medication should be made at three to six month intervals.

Usual dosage ranges:

Vasomotor symptoms—1.25 mg daily. If the patient has not menstruated within the last two months or more, cyclic administration is started arbitrarily. If the patient is menstruating, cyclic administration is started on day 5 of bleeding.

Atrophic vaginitis and kraurosis vulvae—0.3 mg to 1.25 mg or more daily, depending upon the tissue response of the individual patient. Administer cyclically.

2. *Given cyclically:* Female hypogonadism; female castration; primary ovarian failure; osteoporosis.

Usual dosage ranges:

Female hypogonadism—2.5 to 7.5 mg daily, in divided doses for 20 days, followed by a rest period of 10 days' duration. If bleeding does not occur by the end of this period, the same dosage schedule is repeated. The number of courses of estrogen therapy necessary to produce bleeding may vary depending on the responsiveness of the endometrium.

If bleeding occurs before the end of the 10 day period, begin a 20 day estrogen-progestin cyclic regimen with PREMARIN (Conjugated Estrogens Tablets, U.S.P.), 2.5 to 7.5 mg daily in divided doses, for 20 days. During the last five days of estrogen therapy, give an oral progestin. If bleeding occurs before this regimen is concluded, therapy is discontinued and may be resumed on the fifth day of bleeding.

Female castration and primary ovarian failure—1.25 mg daily, cyclically. Adjust dosage upward or downward according to severity of symptoms and response of the patient. For maintenance, adjust dosage to lowest level that will provide effective control.

Osteoporosis (to retard progression)—1.25 mg daily, cyclically.

3. *Given for a few days:* Prevention of postpartum breast engorgement—3.75 mg every four hours for five doses, or 1.25 mg every four hours for five days.

4. *Given chronically:* Inoperable progressing prostatic cancer—1.25 to 2.5 mg three times daily. The effectiveness of therapy can be judged by phosphatase determinations as well as by symptomatic improvement of the patient.

Inoperable progressing breast cancer in appropriately selected men and postmenopausal women. (See INDICATIONS)—Suggested dosage is 10 mg three times daily for a period of at least three months.

Treated patients with an intact uterus should be monitored closely for signs of endometrial cancer and appropriate diagnostic measures should be taken to rule out malignancy in the event of persistent or recurring abnormal vaginal bleeding.

How Supplied: PREMARIN (Conjugated Estrogens Tablets, U.S.P.)

—Each *purple* tablet contains 2.5 mg, in bottles of 100 (NDC 0046-0865-81) and 1,000 (NDC 0046-0865-91).

—Each *yellow* tablet contains 1.25 mg, in bottles of 100 (NDC 0046-0866-81) and 1,000 (NDC 0046-0866-91). Also in unit dose package of 100 (NDC 0046-0866-99).

—Each *red* tablet contains 0.625 mg, in bottles of 100 (NDC 0046-0867-81) and 1,000 (NDC 0046-0867-91). Also in unit dose package of 100 (NDC 0046-0867-99).

—Each *green* tablet contains 0.3 mg, in bottles of 100 (NDC 0046-0868-81) and 1,000 (NDC 0046-0868-91).

Physician References:

1. Ziel, H. K., *et al.*: N. Engl. J. Med. *293*:1167–1170, 1975.
2. Smith, D. C., *et al.*: N. Engl. J. Med. *293*:1164–1167, 1975.
3. Mack, T. M., *et al.*: N. Engl. J. Med. *294*:1262–1267, 1976.
4. Weiss, N. S., *et al.*: N. Engl. J. Med. *294*:1259–1262, 1976.
5. Herbst, A. L., *et al.*: N. Engl. J. Med. *284*:878–881, 1971.
6. Greenwald, P., *et al.*: N. Engl. J. Med. *285*:390–392, 1971.
7. Lanier, A., *et al.*: Mayo Clin. Proc. *48*: 793–799, 1973.
8. Herbst, A., *et al.*: Obstet. Gynecol. *40*:287–298, 1972.

Continued on next page

Ayerst—Cont.

9. Herbst, A., *et al.*: Am. J. Obstet. Gynecol. *118*:607–615, 1974.
10. Herbst, A., *et al.*: N. Engl. J. Med. *292*: 334–339, 1975.
11. Stafl, A., *et al.*: Obstet. Gynecol. *43*:118–128, 1974.
12. Sherman, A. I., *et al.*: Obstet. Gynecol. *44*:531–545, 1974.
13. Gal, I., *et al.*: Nature *216*:83, 1967.
14. Levy, E. P., *et al.*: Lancet *1*:611, 1973.
15. Nora, J., *et al.*: Lancet *1*:941–942, 1973.
16. Janerich, D. T., *et al.*: N. Engl. J. Med. *291*:697–700, 1974.
17. Boston Collaborative Drug Surveillance Program: N. Engl. J. Med. *290*:15–19, 1974.
18. Hoover, R., *et al.*: N. Engl. J. Med. *295*:401–405, 1976.
19. Boston Collaborative Drug Surveillance Program: Lancet *1*:1399–1404, 1973.
20. Daniel, D. G., *et al.*: Lancet *2*:287–289, 1967.
21. The Veterans Administration Cooperative Urological Research Group: J. Urol. *98*:516–522, 1967.
22. Bailar, J. C.: Lancet *2*:560, 1967.
23. Blackard, C., *et al.*: Cancer *26*:249–256, 1970.
24. Royal College of General Practitioners: J. R. Coll. Gen. Pract. *13*:267–279, 1967.

24a. Royal College of General Practitioners: Oral Contraceptives and Health, New York, Pitman Corp., 1974.

25. Inman, W. H. W., *et al.*: Br. Med. J. *2*:193–199, 1968.
26. Vessey, M. P., *et al.*: Br. Med. J. *2*:651–657, 1969.
27. Sartwell, P. E., *et al.*: Am. J. Epidemiol. *90*:365–380, 1969.
28. Collaborative Group for the Study of Stroke in Young Women: N. Engl. J. Med. *288*:871–878, 1973.
29. Collaborative Group for the Study of Stroke in Young Women: J.A.M.A. *231*:718–722, 1975.
30. Mann, J. I., *et al.*: Br. Med. J. *2*:245–248, 1975.
31. Mann, J. I., *et al.*: Br. Med. J. *2*:241–245, 1975.
32. Inman, W. H. W., *et al.*: Br. Med. J. *2*:203–209, 1970.
33. Stolley, P. D., *et al.*: Am. J. Epidemiol. *102*:197–208, 1975.
34. Vessey, M. P., *et al.*: Br. Med. J. *3*:123–126, 1970.
35. Greene, G. R., *et al.*: Am. J. Public Health *62*:680–685, 1972.
36. Rosenberg, L., *et al.*: N. Engl. J. Med. *294*:1256–1259, 1976.
37. Coronary Drug Project Research Group: J.A.M.A. *214*:1303–1313, 1970.
38. Baum, J., *et al.*: Lancet *2*: 926–928, 1973.
39. Mays, E. T., *et al.*: J.A.M.A. *235*:730–732, 1976.
40. Edmondson, H. A., *et al.*: N. Engl. J. Med. *294*:470–472, 1976.
41. Pfeffer, R. I., *et al.*: Am. J. Epidemiol. *103*:445–456, 1976.

INFORMATION FOR THE PATIENT

What You Should Know about Estrogens: Estrogens are female hormones produced by the ovaries. The ovaries make several different kinds of estrogens. In addition, scientists have been able to make a variety of synthetic estrogens. As far as we know, all these estrogens have similar properties and therefore much the same usefulness, side effects, and risks. This leaflet is intended to help you understand what estrogens are used for, the risks involved in their use, and how to use them as safely as possible.

This leaflet includes the most important information about estrogens, but not all the information. If you want to know more, you should ask your doctor for more information or you can ask your doctor or pharmacist to let you read the package insert prepared for the doctor.

Uses of Estrogen: THERE IS NO PROPER USE OF ESTROGENS IN A PREGNANT WOMAN.

Estrogens are prescribed by doctors for a number of purposes, including:

1. To provide estrogen during a period of adjustment when a woman's ovaries stop producing a majority of her estrogens, in order to prevent certain uncomfortable symptoms of estrogen deficiency. (With the menopause, which generally occurs between the ages of 45 and 55, women produce a much smaller amount of estrogens.)
2. To prevent symptoms of estrogen deficiency when a woman's ovaries have been removed surgically before the natural menopause.
3. To prevent pregnancy. (Estrogens are given along with a progestogen, another female hormone; these combinations are called oral contraceptives or birth control pills. Patient labeling is available to women taking oral contraceptives and they will not be discussed in this leaflet.)
4. To treat certain cancers in women and men.
5. To prevent painful swelling of the breasts after pregnancy in women who choose not to nurse their babies.

Estrogens in the Menopause: In the natural course of their lives, all women eventually experience a decrease in estrogen production. This usually occurs between ages 45 and 55 but may occur earlier or later. Sometimes the ovaries may need to be removed before natural menopause by an operation, producing a "surgical menopause."

When the amount of estrogen in the blood begins to decrease, many women may develop typical symptoms: feelings of warmth in the face, neck, and chest or sudden intense episodes of heat and sweating throughout the body (called "hot flashes" or "hot flushes"). These symptoms are sometimes very uncomfortable. Some women may also develop changes in the vagina (called "atrophic vaginitis") which cause discomfort, especially during and after intercourse.

Estrogens can be prescribed to treat these symptoms of the menopause. It is estimated that considerably more than half of all women undergoing the menopause have only mild symptoms or no symptoms at all and therefore do not need estrogens. Other women may need estrogens for a few months, while their bodies adjust to lower estrogen levels. Sometimes the need will be for periods longer than six months. In an attempt to avoid overstimulation of the uterus (womb), estrogens are usually given cyclically during each month of use, such as three weeks of pills followed by one week without pills.

Sometimes women experience nervous symptoms or depression during menopause. There is no evidence that estrogens are effective for such symptoms without associated vasomotor symptoms. In the absence of vasomotor symptoms, estrogens should not be used to treat nervous symptoms, although other treatment may be needed.

You may have heard that taking estrogens for long periods (years) after the menopause will keep your skin soft and supple and keep you feeling young. There is no evidence that this is so, however, and such long-term treatment carries important risks.

Estrogens to Prevent Swelling of the Breasts after Pregnancy: If you do not breast-feed your baby after delivery, your breasts may fill up with milk and become painful and engorged. This usually begins about 3 to 4 days after delivery and may last for a few days to up to a week or more. Sometimes the discomfort is severe, but usually it is not and can be controlled by pain-relieving drugs such as aspirin and by binding the breasts up tightly. Estrogens can be used to try to prevent the breasts from filling up. While this treatment is sometimes successful, in many cases the breasts fill up to some degree in spite of treatment. The dose of estrogens needed to prevent pain and swelling of the breasts is much larger than the dose needed to treat symptoms of the menopause and this may increase your chances of developing blood clots in the legs or lungs (see below). Therefore, it is important that you discuss the benefits and the risks of estrogen use with your doctor if you have decided not to breast-feed your baby.

The Dangers of Estrogens:

1. *Endometrial cancer.* There are reports that if estrogens are used in the postmenopausal period for more than a year, there is an increased risk of *endometrial cancer* (cancer of the lining of the uterus). Women taking estrogens have roughly 5 to 10 times as great a chance of getting this cancer as women who take no estrogens. To put this another way, while a postmenopausal woman not taking estrogens has 1 chance in 1,000 each year of getting endometrial cancer, a woman taking estrogens has 5 to 10 chances in 1,000 each year. For this reason *it is important to take estrogens only when they are really needed.*

The risk of this cancer is greater the longer estrogens are used and when larger doses are taken. Therefore you should not take more estrogen than your doctor prescribes. *It is important to take the lowest dose of estrogen that will control symptoms and to take it only as long as it is needed.* If estrogens are needed for longer periods of time, your doctor will want to reevaluate your need for estrogens at least every six months.

Women using estrogens should report any vaginal bleeding to their doctors; such bleeding may be of no importance, but it can be an early warning of endometrial cancer. If you have undiagnosed vaginal bleeding, you should not use estrogens until a diagnosis is made and you are certain there is no endometrial cancer.

NOTE: If you have had your uterus removed (total hysterectomy), there is no danger of developing endometrial cancer.

2. *Other possible cancers.* Estrogens can cause development of other tumors in animals, such as tumors of the breast, cervix, vagina, or liver, when given for a long time. At present there is no good evidence that women using estrogen in the menopause have an increased risk of such tumors, but there is no way yet to be sure they do not; and one study raises the possibility that use of estrogens in the menopause may increase the risk of breast cancer many years later. This is a further reason to use estrogens only when clearly needed. While you are taking estrogens, it is important that you go to your doctor at least once a year for a physical examination. Also, if members of your family have had breast cancer or if you have breast nodules or abnormal mammograms (breast x-rays), your doctor may wish to carry out more frequent examinations of your breasts.

3. *Gallbladder disease.* Women who use estrogens after menopause are more likely to develop gallbladder disease needing surgery than women who do not use estrogens. Birth control pills have a similar effect.

4. *Abnormal blood clotting.* Oral contraceptives increase the risk of blood clotting in various parts of the body. This can result in a stroke (if the clot is in the brain), a heart attack (clot in a blood vessel of the heart), or a pulmonary embolus (a clot which forms in the legs or pelvis, then breaks off and travels to the lungs). Any of these can be fatal.

At this time use of estrogens in the menopause is not known to cause such blood clotting, but this has not been fully studied and there could still prove to be such a risk. It is recommended that if you have had clotting in the legs or lungs or a heart attack or stroke while you were using estrogens or birth control pills, you should not use estrogens (unless they are being used to treat cancer of the breast or prostate). If you have had a stroke or heart attack or if you have angina pectoris, estrogens should be used with great caution and only if clearly needed (for example, if you have severe symptoms of the menopause).

The larger doses of estrogen used to prevent swelling of the breasts after pregnancy have been reported to cause clotting in the legs and lungs.

Special Warning about Pregnancy: You should not receive estrogen if you are pregnant. If this should occur, there is a greater than usual chance that the developing child will be born with a birth defect, although the possibility remains fairly small. A female child may have an increased risk of developing cancer of the vagina or cervix later in life (in the teens or twenties). Every possible effort should be made to avoid exposure to estrogens during pregnancy. If exposure occurs, see your doctor.

Other Effects of Estrogens: In addition to the serious known risks of estrogens described above, estrogens have the following side effects and potential risks:

1. *Nausea and vomiting.* The most common side effect of estrogen therapy is nausea. Vomiting is less common.
2. *Effects on breasts.* Estrogens may cause breast tenderness or enlargement and may cause the breasts to secrete a liquid. These effects are not dangerous.
3. *Effects on the uterus.* Estrogens may cause benign fibroid tumors of the uterus to get larger.
4. *Effects on liver.* Women taking oral contraceptives develop on rare occasions a tumor of the liver which can rupture and bleed into the abdomen and may cause death. So far, these tumors have not been reported in women using estrogens in the menopause, but you should report any swelling or unusual pain or tenderness in the abdomen to your doctor immediately.

Women with a past history of jaundice (yellowing of the skin and white parts of the eyes) may get jaundice again during estrogen use. If this occurs, stop taking estrogens and see your doctor.

5. *Other effects.* Estrogens may cause excess fluid to be retained in the body. This may make some conditions worse, such as asthma, epilepsy, migraine, heart disease, or kidney disease.

Summary: Estrogens have important uses, but they have serious risks as well. You must decide, with your doctor, whether the risks are acceptable to you in view of the benefits of treatment. Except where your doctor has prescribed estrogens for use in special cases of cancer of the breast or prostate, you should not use estrogens if you have cancer of the breast or uterus, are pregnant, have undiagnosed abnormal vaginal bleeding, clotting in the legs or lungs, or have had a stroke, heart attack or angina, or clotting in the legs or lungs in the past while you were taking estrogens.

You can use estrogens as safely as possible by understanding that your doctor will require regular physical examinations while you are taking them and will try to discontinue the drug as soon as possible and use the smallest dose possible. Be alert for signs of trouble including:

1. Abnormal bleeding from the vagina.
2. Pains in the calves or chest or sudden shortness of breath, or coughing blood.
3. Severe headache, dizziness, faintness, or changes in vision.
4. Breast lumps (you should ask your doctor how to examine your own breasts).
5. Jaundice (yellowing of the skin).
6. Mental depression.

Your doctor has prescribed this drug for you and you alone. Do not give the drug to anyone else.

How Supplied:

PREMARIN® (Conjugated Estrogens Tablets, U.S.P.)—tablets for oral administration.

PREMARIN® VAGINAL CREAM —PREMARIN® in a nonliquefying base, designed for vaginal use.

PREMARIN® with METHYLTESTOSTERONE —a combination of PREMARIN and methyltestosterone (an androgen) in tablet form for oral administration.

PMB® 200,400—a combination of PREMARIN® and meprobamate (a tranquilizing agent) in tablet form for oral administration.

PREMARIN® INTRAVENOUS —PREMARIN® specially prepared for intravenous and intramuscular use.

ESTROGENIC SUBSTANCE (Estrone) in Aqueous Suspension—a sterile aqueous suspension of estrone, a short-acting estrogen, for intramuscular injection only.

[*Shown in Product Identification Section*]

PREMARIN® ℞
(Conjugated Estrogens, U.S.P.)
VAGINAL CREAM
in a nonliquefying base

1. ESTROGENS HAVE BEEN REPORTED TO INCREASE THE RISK OF ENDOMETRIAL CARCINOMA.

Three independent case control studies have reported an increased risk of endometrial cancer in postmenopausal women exposed to exogenous estrogens for more than one year.[1–3] This risk was independent of the other known risk factors for endometrial cancer. These studies are further supported by the finding that incidence rates of endometrial cancer have increased sharply since 1969 in eight different areas of the United States with population-based cancer reporting systems, an increase which may be related to the rapidly expanding use of estrogens during the last decade.[4]

The three case control studies reported that the risk of endometrial cancer in estrogen users was about 4.5 to 13.9 times greater than in nonusers. The risk appears to depend on both duration of treatment[1] and on estrogen dose.[3] In view of these findings, when estrogens are used for the treatment of menopausal symptoms, the lowest dose that will control symptoms should be utilized and medication should be discontinued as soon as possible. When prolonged treatment is medically indicated, the patient should be reassessed on at least a semiannual basis to determine the need for continued therapy. Although the evidence must be considered preliminary, one study suggests that cyclic administration of low doses of estrogen may carry less risk than continuous administration;[3] it therefore appears prudent to utilize such a regimen.

Close clinical surveillance of all women taking estrogens is important. In all cases of undiagnosed persistent or recurring abnormal vaginal bleeding, adequate diagnostic measures should be undertaken to rule out malignancy.

There is no evidence at present that "natural" estrogens are more or less hazardous than "synthetic" estrogens at equiestrogenic doses.

2. ESTROGENS SHOULD NOT BE USED DURING PREGNANCY.

The use of female sex hormones, both estrogens and progestogens, during early pregnancy may seriously damage the offspring. It has been shown that females exposed in utero to diethylstilbestrol, a non-steroidal estrogen, have an increased risk of developing in later life a form of vaginal or cervical cancer that is ordinarily extremely rare.[5,6] This risk has been estimated as not greater than 4 per 1000 exposures.[7] Furthermore, a high percentage of such exposed women (from 30 to 90 percent) have been found to have vaginal adenosis,[8–12] epithelial changes of the vagina and cervix. Although these changes are histologically benign, it is not known whether they are precursors of malignancy. Although similar data are not available with the use of other estrogens, it cannot be presumed they would not induce similar changes.

Several reports suggest an association between intrauterine exposure to female sex hormones and congenital anomalies, including congenital heart defects and limb reduction defects.[13–16] One case control study[16] estimated a 4.7-fold increased risk of limb reduction defects in infants exposed in utero to sex hormones (oral contraceptives, hormone withdrawal tests for pregnancy, or attempted treatment for threatened abortion). Some of these exposures were very short and involved only a few days of treatment. The data suggest that the risk of limb reduction defects in exposed fetuses is somewhat less than 1 per 1000.

In the past, female sex hormones have been used during pregnancy in an attempt to treat threatened or habitual abortion. There is considerable evidence that estrogens are ineffective for these indications, and there is no evidence from well controlled studies that progestogens are effective for these uses.

If PREMARIN (Conjugated Estrogens, U.S.P.) Vaginal Cream is used during pregnancy, or if the patient becomes pregnant while taking this drug, she should be apprised of the potential risks to the fetus, and the advisability of pregnancy continuation.

Description: Each gram contains 0.625 mg Conjugated Estrogens, U.S.P., in a nonliquefying base containing cetyl esters wax, cetyl alcohol, white wax, glyceryl monostearate, propylene glycol monostearate, methyl stearate, phenylethyl alcohol, sodium lauryl sulfate, glycerin, and mineral oil.

PREMARIN (Conjugated Estrogens, U.S.P.) is a mixture of estrogens, obtained exclusively from natural sources, occurring as the sodium salts of water-soluble estrogen sulfates blended to represent the average composition of material derived from pregnant mares' urine. It contains estrone, equilin, and 17 α-dihydroequilin, together with smaller amounts of 17 α-estradiol, equilenin, and 17 α-dihydroequilenin as salts of their sulfate esters.

Clinical Pharmacology: Estrogens are important in the development and maintenance of the female reproductive system and secondary sex characteristics. They promote growth and development of the vagina, uterus, and fallopian tubes, and enlargement of the breasts. Indirectly, they contribute to the shaping of the skeleton, maintenance of tone and elasticity of urogenital structures, changes in the epiphyses of the long bones that allow for the pubertal growth spurt and its termination, growth of axillary and pubic hair, and pigmentation of the nipples and genitals. Decline of estrogenic activity at the end of the menstrual cycle can bring on menstruation, although the cessation of progesterone secretion is the most important factor in the mature ovulatory cycle. However, in the preovulatory or nonovula-

Continued on next page

Ayerst—Cont.

tory cycle, estrogen is the primary determinant in the onset of menstruation. Estrogens also affect the release of pituitary gonadotropins.

The pharmacologic effects of conjugated estrogens are similar to those of endogenous estrogens. They are soluble in water and may be absorbed from mucosal surfaces after local administration.

In responsive tissues (female genital organs, breasts, hypothalamus, pituitary) estrogens enter the cell and are transported into the nucleus. As a result of estrogen action, specific RNA and protein synthesis occurs.

Metabolism and inactivation occur primarily in the liver. Some estrogens are excreted into the bile; however they are reabsorbed from the intestine and returned to the liver through the portal venous system. Water-soluble estrogen conjugates are strongly acidic and are ionized in body fluids, which favor excretion through the kidneys since tubular reabsorption is minimal.

Indications: PREMARIN (Conjugated Estrogens, U.S.P.) Vaginal Cream is indicated in the treatment of atrophic vaginitis and kraurosis vulvae.

PREMARIN Vaginal Cream HAS NOT BEEN SHOWN TO BE EFFECTIVE FOR ANY PURPOSE DURING PREGNANCY AND ITS USE MAY CAUSE SEVERE HARM TO THE FETUS (SEE BOXED WARNING).

Contraindications: Estrogens should not be used in women with any of the following conditions:

1. Known or suspected cancer of the breast except in appropriately selected patients being treated for metastatic disease.
2. Known or suspected estrogen-dependent neoplasia.
3. Known or suspected pregnancy (See Boxed Warning).
4. Undiagnosed abnormal genital bleeding.
5. Active thrombophlebitis or thromboembolic disorders.
6. A past history of thrombophlebitis, thrombosis, or thromboembolic disorders associated with previous estrogen use (except when used in treatment of breast malignancy).

PREMARIN Vaginal Cream should not be used in patients hypersensitive to its ingredients.

Warnings:

1. *Induction of malignant neoplasms.* Long term continuous administration of natural and synthetic estrogens in certain animal species increases the frequency of carcinomas of the breast, cervix, vagina, and liver. There are now reports that estrogens increase the risk of carcinoma of the endometrium in humans. (See Boxed Warning.)

At the present time there is no satisfactory evidence that estrogens given to postmenopausal women increase the risk of cancer of the breast,[17] although a recent long-term followup of a single physician's practice has raised this possibility.[18] Because of the animal data, there is a need for caution in prescribing estrogens for women with a strong family history of breast cancer or who have breast nodules, fibrocystic disease, or abnormal mammograms.

2. *Gallbladder disease.* A recent study has reported a 2 to 3-fold increase in the risk of surgically confirmed gallbladder disease in women receiving postmenopausal estrogens,[17] similar to the 2-fold increase previously noted in users of oral contraceptives.[19,24a]

3. *Effects similar to those caused by estrogen-progestogen oral contraceptives.* There are several serious adverse effects of oral contraceptives, most of which have not, up to now, been documented as consequences of postmenopausal estrogen therapy. This may reflect the comparatively low doses of estrogen used in postmenopausal women. It would be expected that the larger doses of estrogen used to treat breast cancer or postpartum breast engorgement are more likely to result in these adverse effects, and, in fact, it has been shown that there is an increased risk of thrombosis in men receiving estrogens for prostatic cancer and women for postpartum breast engorgement.[20–23]

a. *Thromboembolic disease.* It is now well established that users of oral contraceptives have an increased risk of various thromboembolic and thrombotic vascular diseases, such as thrombophlebitis, pulmonary embolism, stroke, and myocardial infarction.[24–31] Cases of retinal thrombosis, mesenteric thrombosis, and optic neuritis have been reported in oral contraceptive users. There is evidence that the risk of several of these adverse reactions is related to the dose of the drug.[32,33] An increased risk of postsurgery thromboembolic complications has also been reported in users of oral contraceptives.[34,35] If feasible, estrogen should be discontinued at least 4 weeks before surgery of the type associated with an increased risk of thromboembolism, or during periods of prolonged immobilization.

While an increased rate of thromboembolic and thrombotic disease in postmenopausal users of estrogens has not been found,[17–24,25–36] this does not rule out the possibility that such an increase may be present or that subgroups of women who have underlying risk factors or who are receiving relatively large doses of estrogens may have increased risk. Therefore estrogens should not be used in persons with active thrombophlebitis or thromboembolic disorders, and they should not be used (except in treatment of malignancy) in persons with a history of such disorders in association with estrogen use. They should be used with caution in patients with cerebral vascular or coronary artery disease and only for those in whom estrogens are clearly needed.

Large doses of estrogen (5 mg conjugated estrogens per day), comparable to those used to treat cancer of the prostate and breast, have been shown in a large prospective clinical trial in men[37] to increase the risk of nonfatal myocardial infarction, pulmonary embolism and thrombophlebitis. When estrogen doses of this size are used, any of the thromboembolic and thrombotic adverse effects associated with oral contraceptive use should be considered a clear risk.

b. *Hepatic adenoma.* Benign hepatic adenomas appear to be associated with the use of oral contraceptives.[38–40] Although benign, and rare, these may rupture and may cause death through intra-abdominal hemorrhage. Such lesions have not yet been reported in association with other estrogen or progestogen preparations but should be considered in estrogen users having abdominal pain and tenderness, abdominal mass, or hypovolemic shock. Hepatocellular carcinoma has also been reported in women taking estrogen-containing oral contraceptives.[39] The relationship of this malignancy to these drugs is not known at this time.

c. *Elevated blood pressure.* Women using oral contraceptives sometimes experience increased blood pressure which, in most cases, returns to normal on discontinuing the drug. There is now a report that this may occur with use of estrogens in the menopause[41] and blood pressure should be monitored with estrogen use, especially if high doses are used.

d. *Glucose tolerance.* A worsening of glucose tolerance has been observed in a significant percentage of patients on estrogen-containing oral contraceptives. For this reason, diabetic patients should be carefully observed while receiving estrogen.

4. *Hypercalcemia.* Administration of estrogens may lead to severe hypercalcemia in patients with breast cancer and bone metastases. If this occurs, the drug should be stopped and appropriate measures taken to reduce the serum calcium level.

Precautions:

A. General Precautions.

1. A complete medical and family history should be taken prior to the initiation of any estrogen therapy. The pretreatment and periodic physical examinations should include special reference to blood pressure, breasts, abdomen, and pelvic organs, and should include a Papanicolau smear. As a general rule, estrogen should not be prescribed for longer than one year without another physical examination being performed.
2. Fluid retention—Because estrogens may cause some degree of fluid retention, conditions which might be influenced by this factor such as asthma, epilepsy, migraine, and cardiac or renal dysfunction, require careful observation.
3. Certain patients may develop undesirable manifestations of excessive estrogenic stimulation, such as abnormal or excessive uterine bleeding, mastodynia, etc.
4. Oral contraceptives appear to be associated with an increased incidence of mental depression.[24a] Although it is not clear whether this is due to the estrogenic or progestogenic component of the contraceptive, patients with a history of depression should be carefully observed.
5. Preexisting uterine leiomyomata may increase in size during estrogen use.
6. The pathologist should be advised of estrogen therapy when relevant specimens are submitted.
7. Patients with a past history of jaundice during pregnancy have an increased risk of recurrence of jaundice while receiving estrogen-containing oral contraceptive therapy. If jaundice develops in any patient receiving estrogen, the medication should be discontinued while the cause is investigated.
8. Estrogens may be poorly metabolized in patients with impaired liver function and they should be administered with caution in such patients.
9. Because estrogens influence the metabolism of calcium and phosphorus, they should be used with caution in patients with metabolic bone diseases that are associated with hypercalcemia or in patients with renal insufficiency.
10. Because of the effects of estrogens on epiphyseal closure, they should be used judiciously in young patients in whom bone growth is not complete.
11. Certain endocrine and liver function tests may be affected by estrogen-containing oral contraceptives. The following similar changes may be expected with larger doses of estrogen:
    a. Increased sulfobromophthalein retention.
    b. Increased prothrombin and factors VII, VIII, IX, and X; decreased antithrombin 3; increased norepinephrine-induced platelet aggregability.
    c. Increased thyroid binding globulin (TBG) leading to increased circulating total thyroid hormone, as measured by PBI, T4 by column, or T4 by radioimmunoassay. Free T3 resin uptake is decreased, reflecting the elevated TBG; free T4 concentration in unaltered.
    d. Impaired glucose tolerance.
    e. Decreased pregnanediol excretion.
    f. Reduced response to metyrapone test.
    g. Reduced serum folate concentration.
    h. Increased serum triglyceride and phospholipid concentration.

B. Information for the Patient. See text which appears after the PHYSICIAN REFERENCES under PREMARIN® (Conjugated Estrogens Tablets, U.S.P.).

C. Pregnancy Category X. See CONTRAINDICATIONS and Boxed Warning.

D. Nursing Mothers. As a general principle, the administration of any drug to nursing mothers should be done only when clearly necessary since many drugs are excreted in human milk.

Adverse Reactions: (See Warnings regarding induction of neoplasia, adverse effects on the fetus, increased incidence of gallbladder disease, and adverse effects similar to those of oral contraceptives, including thromboembolism.) The following additional adverse reactions have been reported with estrogenic therapy, including oral contraceptives.

1. *Genitourinary system:* Breakthrough bleeding, spotting, change in menstrual flow; dysmenorrhea; premenstrual-like syndrome; amenorrhea during and after treatment; increase in size of uterine fibromyomata; vaginal candidiasis; change in cervical erosion and in degree of cervical secretion; cystitis-like syndrome.
2. *Breasts:* Tenderness, enlargement, secretion.
3. *Gastrointestinal:* Nausea, vomiting; abdominal cramps, bloating; cholestatic jaundice.
4. *Skin:* Chloasma or melasma which may persist when drug is discontinued; erythema multiforme; erythema nodosum; hemorrhagic eruption; loss of scalp hair; hirsutism.
5. *Eyes:* Steepening of corneal curvature; intolerance to contact lenses.
6. *CNS:* Headache, migraine, dizziness; mental depression; chorea.
7. *Miscellaneous:* Increase or decrease in weight; reduced carbohydrate tolerance; aggravation of porphyria; edema; changes in libido.

Acute Overdosage: Numerous reports of ingestion of large doses of estrogen-containing oral contraceptives by young children indicate that acute serious ill effects do not occur. Overdosage of estrogen may cause nausea, and withdrawal bleeding may occur in females.

Dosage and Administration:
Given cyclically for short-term use only:
For treatment of atrophic vaginitis, or kraurosis vulvae.
The lowest dose that will control symptoms should be chosen and medication should be discontinued as promptly as possible.
Administration should be cyclic (e.g., three weeks on and one week off).
Attempts to discontinue or taper medication should be made at three to six month intervals.
Usual dosage range: 2 to 4 g daily, intravaginally or topically, depending on the severity of the condition.
Treated patients with an intact uterus should be monitored closely for signs of endometrial cancer and appropriate diagnostic measures should be taken to rule out malignancy in the event of persistent or recurring abnormal vaginal bleeding.

How Supplied: PREMARIN (Conjugated Estrogens, U.S.P.) Vaginal Cream—Each gram contains 0.625 mg Conjugated Estrogens, U.S.P. (Also contains cetyl esters wax, cetyl alcohol, white wax, glyceryl monostearate, propylene glycol monostearate, methyl stearate, phenylethyl alcohol, sodium lauryl sulfate, glycerin, and mineral oil.)
Combination package: Each contains Net Wt. 1½ oz (42.5 g) tube with one calibrated plastic applicator (NDC 0046-0872-93).
Also Available—Refill package: Each contains Net Wt. 1½ oz (42.5 g) tube (NDC 0046-0872-01).

Physician References:

1. Ziel, H. K., *et al.*: N. Engl. J. Med. *293*:1167–1170, 1975.
2. Smith, D. C., *et al.*: N. Engl. J. Med. *293*:1164–1167, 1975.
3. Mack, T. M., *et al.*: N. Engl. J. Med *294*:1262–1267, 1976.
4. Weiss, N. S., *et al.*: N. Engl. J. Med. *294*:1259–1262, 1976.
5. Herbst, A. L., *et al.*: N. Engl. J. Med. *284*:878–881, 1971.
6. Greenwald, P., *et al.*: N. Engl. J. Med. *285*:390–392, 1971.
7. Lanier, A., *et al.*: Mayo Clin. Proc. *48*:793–799, 1973.
8. Herbst, A., *et al.*: Obstet. Gynecol. *40*:287–298, 1972.
9. Herbst, A., *et al.*: Am. J. Obstet. Gynecol. *118*:607–615, 1974.
10. Herbst, A., *et al.*: N. Engl. J. Med. *292*:334–339, 1975.
11. Stafl, A., *et al.*: Obstet. Gynecol. *43*:118–128, 1974.
12. Sherman, A. I., *et al.*: Obstet. Gynecol. *44*:531–545, 1974.
13. Gal, I., *et al.*: Nature *216*:83, 1967.
14. Levy, E. P., *et al.*: Lancet *1*:611, 1973.
15. Nora, J., *et al.*:Lancet *1*:941–942, 1973.
16. Janerich, D. T., *et al.*: N. Engl. J. Med. *291*:697–700, 1974.
17. Boston Collaborative Drug Surveillance Program: N. Engl. J. Med. *290*:15–19, 1974.
18. Hoover, R., *et al.*: N. Engl. J. Med. *295*:401–405, 1976.
19. Boston Collaborative Drug Surveillance Program: Lancet *1*:1399–1404, 1973.
20. Daniel, D. G., *et al.*: Lancet *2*:287–289, 1967.
21. The Veterans Administration Cooperative Urological Research Group: J. Urol. *98*:516–522, 1967.
22. Bailar, J. C.: Lancet *2*:560, 1967.
23. Blackard, C., *et al.*: Cancer *26*:249–256, 1970.
24. Royal College of General Practitioners: J. R. Coll. Gen. Pract. *13*:267–279, 1967.
24a. Royal College of General Practitioners: Oral Contraceptives and Health, New York, Pitman Corp., 1974.
25. Inman, W. H. W., *et al.*: Br. Med. J. *2*:193–199, 1968.
26. Vessey, M. P., *et al.*: Br. Med. J. *2*:651–657, 1969.
27. Sartwell, P. E., *et al.*: Am. J. Epidemiol. *90*:365–380, 1969.
28. Collaborative Group for the Study of Stroke in Young Women: N. Engl. J. Med. *288*:871–878, 1973.
29. Collaborative Group for the Study of Stroke in Young Women: J.A.M.A. *231*:718–722, 1975.
30. Mann, J. I., *et al.*: Br. Med. J. *2*:245–248, 1975.
31. Mann, J. I., *et al.*: Br. Med. J. *2*:241–245, 1975.
32. Inman, W. H. W., *et al.*: Br. Med. J. *2*:203–209, 1970.
33. Stolley, P. D., *et al.*: Am. J. Epidemiol. *102*:197–208, 1975.
34. Vessey, M. P., *et al.*: Br. Med. J. *3*:123–126, 1970.
35. Greene, G. R., *et al.*: Am. J. Public Health *62*:680–685, 1972.
36. Rosenberg, L., *et al.*: N. Engl. J. Med. *294*:1256–1259, 1976.
37. Coronary Drug Project Research Group: J.A.M.A. *214*:1303–1313, 1970.
38. Baum, J., *et al.*: Lancet *2*:926–928, 1973.
39. Mays, E. T., *et al.*: J.A.M.A. *235*:730–732, 1976.
40. Edmondson, H. A., *et al.*: N. Engl. J. Med. *294*:470–472, 1976.
41. Pfeffer, R. I., *et al.*: Am. J. Epidemiol. *103*:445–456, 1976.

[*Shown in Product Identification Section*]

PREMARIN® ℞
(Conjugated Estrogens, U.S.P.)
with METHYLTESTOSTERONE

No. 879—Each yellow tablet contains:
Premarin® (Conjugated Estrogens, U.S.P.) ....1.25 mg
Methyltestosterone ....10.0 mg
No. 878—Each red tablet contains:
Premarin® (Conjugated Estrogens, U.S.P.) ....0.625 mg
Methyltestosterone ....5.0 mg

1. ESTROGENS HAVE BEEN REPORTED TO INCREASE THE RISK OF ENDOMETRIAL CARCINOMA.
Three independent case control studies have reported an increased risk of endometrial cancer in postmenopausal women exposed to exogenous estrogens for more than one year.[1–3] This risk was independent of the other known risk factors for endometrial cancer. These studies are further supported by the finding that incidence rates of endometrial cancer have increased sharply since 1969 in eight different areas of the United States with population-based cancer reporting systems, an increase which may be related to the rapidly expanding use of estrogens during the last decade.[4]
The three case control studies reported that the risk of endometrial cancer in estrogen users was about 4.5 to 13.9 times greater than in nonusers. The risk appears to depend on both duration of treatment[1] and on estrogen dose.[3] In view of these findings, when estrogens are used for the treatment of menopausal symptoms, the lowest dose that will control symptoms should be utilized and medication should be discontinued as soon as possible. When prolonged treatment is medically indicated, the patient should be reassessed on at least a semiannual basis to determine the need for continued therapy. Although the evidence must be considered preliminary, one study suggests that cyclic administration of low doses of estrogen may carry less risk than continuous administration;[3] it therefore appears prudent to utilize such a regimen.
Close clinical surveillance of all women taking estrogens is important. In all cases of undiagnosed persistent or recurring abnormal vaginal bleeding, adequate diagnostic measures should be undertaken to rule out malignancy.
There is no evidence at present that "natural" estrogens are more or less hazardous than "synthetic" estrogens at equiestrogenic doses.

2. ESTROGENS SHOULD NOT BE USED DURING PREGNANCY.
The use of female sex hormones, both estrogens and progestogens, during early pregnancy may seriously damage the offspring. It has been shown that females exposed in utero to diethylstilbestrol, a non-steroidal estrogen, have an increased risk of developing in later life a form of vaginal or cervical cancer that is ordinarily extremely rare.[5,6] This risk has been estimated as not greater than 4 per 1000 exposures.[7] Furthermore, a high percentage of such exposed women (from 30 to 90 percent) have been found to have vaginal adenosis,[8–12] epithelial changes of the vagina and cervix. Although these changes are histologically benign, it is not known whether they are precursors of malignancy. Although similar data are not available with the use of other estrogens, it cannot be presumed they would not induce similar changes.
Several reports suggest an association between intrauterine exposure to female sex hormones and congenital anomalies, including congenital heart defects and limb reduction defects.[13–16] One case control study[16] estimated a 4.7-fold increased risk of limb reduction defects in infants exposed in utero to sex hormones (oral contraceptives, hormone withdrawal tests for pregnancy, or attempted treatment for threatened abortion). Some of these expo-

Continued on next page

Ayerst—Cont.

sures were very short and involved only a few days of treatment. The data suggest that the risk of limb reduction defects in exposed fetuses is somewhat less than 1 per 1000.
In the past, female sex hormones have been used during pregnancy in an attempt to treat threatened or habitual abortion. There is considerable evidence that estrogens are ineffective for these indications, and there is no evidence from well controlled studies that progestogens are effective for these uses.
If PREMARIN with METHYLTESTOSTERONE is used during pregnancy, or if the patient becomes pregnant while taking this drug, she should be apprised of the potential risks to the fetus, and the advisability of pregnancy continuation.

Description: PREMARIN (Conjugated Estrogens, U.S.P.) with METHYLTESTOSTERONE is provided in tablets for oral administration.
PREMARIN (Conjugated Estrogens, U.S.P.) is a mixture of estrogens, obtained exclusively from natural sources, occurring as the sodium salts of water-soluble estrogen sulfates blended to represent the average composition of material derived from pregnant mares' urine. It contains estrone, equilin, and 17 α-dihydroequilin, together with smaller amounts of 17 α-estradiol, equilenin, and 17 α-dihydroequilenin as salts of their sulfate esters.
Methyltestosterone is an androgen. It is a white to light yellow crystalline substance that is virtually insoluble in water but soluble in organic solvents. It is stable in air but decomposes in light.
Clinical Pharmacology: Estrogens are important in the development and maintenance of the female reproductive system and secondary sex characteristics. They promote growth and development of the vagina, uterus, and fallopian tubes, and enlargement of the breasts. Indirectly, they contribute to the shaping of the skeleton, maintenance of tone and elasticity of urogenital structures, changes in the epiphyses of the long bones that allow for the pubertal growth spurt and its termination, growth of axillary and pubic hair, and pigmentation of the nipples and genitals. Decline of estrogenic activity at the end of the menstrual cycle can bring on menstruation, although the cessation of progesterone secretion is the most important factor in the mature ovulatory cycle. However, in the preovulatory or nonovulatory cycle, estrogen is the primary determinant in the onset of menstruation. Estrogens also affect the release of pituitary gonadotropins.
The pharmacologic effects of conjugated estrogens are similar to those of endogenous estrogens. They are soluble in water and are well absorbed from the gastrointestinal tract.
In responsive tissues (female genital organs, breasts, hypothalamus, pituitary) estrogens enter the cell and are transported into the nucleus. As a result of estrogen action, specific RNA and protein synthesis occurs.
Metabolism and inactivation occur primarily in the liver. Some estrogens are excreted into the bile; however they are reabsorbed from the intestine and returned to the liver through the portal venous system. Water soluble estrogen conjugates are strongly acidic and are ionized in body fluids, which favor excretion through the kidneys since tubular reabsorption is minimal.
Androgens are male sex hormones which mediate the development of the male genital organs and the secondary sex characteristics. Methyltestosterone is also an anabolic agent and promotes the retention of nitrogen, potassium, and phosphate, and increases in protein, skeletal muscle, and body mass. In the female, androgen generally opposes the action of estrogen on the female genital tissues by competing for estrogen-binding receptors.
Methyltestosterone is readily absorbed from the intestine. It is metabolized primarily in the liver and excreted primarily in the urine.
Indications: PREMARIN (Conjugated Estrogens, U.S.P.) with Methyltestosterone is indicated in the treatment of:
1. Moderate to severe *vasomotor* symptoms associated with the menopause in those patients not improved by estrogens alone. (There is no evidence that estrogens are effective for nervous symptoms or depression without associated vasomotor symptoms, and they should not be used to treat such conditions.)
2. Postpartum breast engorgement—Although estrogens have been widely used for the prevention of postpartum breast engorgement, controlled studies have demonstrated that the incidence of significant painful engorgement in patients not receiving such hormonal therapy is low and usually responsive to appropriate analgesic or other supportive therapy. Consequently, the benefit to be derived from estrogen therapy for this indication must be carefully weighed against the potential increased risk of puerperal thromboembolism associated with the use of large doses of estrogens.[20,22]
PREMARIN with METHYLTESTOSTERONE HAS NOT BEEN SHOWN TO BE EFFECTIVE FOR ANY PURPOSE DURING PREGNANCY AND ITS USE MAY CAUSE SEVERE HARM TO THE FETUS (SEE BOXED WARNING).
Contraindications: Estrogens should not be used in women with any of the following conditions:
1. Known or suspected cancer of the breast except in appropriately selected patients being treated for metastatic disease.
2. Known or suspected estrogen-dependent neoplasia.
3. Known or suspected pregnancy (See Boxed Warning).
4. Undiagnosed abnormal genital bleeding.
5. Active thrombophlebitis or thromboembolic disorders.
6. A past history of thrombophlebitis, thrombosis, or thromboembolic disorders associated with previous estrogen use (except when used in treatment of breast malignancy).
Methyltestosterone should not be used in:
1. The presence of severe liver damage.
2. Pregnancy and in breast-feeding mothers because of the possibility of masculinization of the female fetus or breast-fed infant.
Warnings:
Associated with Estrogens
1. *Induction of malignant neoplasms.* Long term continuous administration of natural and synthetic estrogens in certain animal species increases the frequency of carcinomas of the breast, cervix, vagina, and liver. There are now reports that estrogens increase the risk of carcinoma of the endometrium in humans. (See Boxed Warning.)
At the present time there is no satisfactory evidence that estrogens given to postmenopausal women increase the risk of cancer of the breast,[17] although a recent long-term followup of a single physician's practice has raised this possibility.[18] Because of the animal data, there is a need for caution in prescribing estrogens for women with a strong family history of breast cancer or who have breast nodules, fibrocystic disease, or abnormal mammograms.
2. *Gallbladder disease.* A recent study has reported a 2 to 3-fold increase in the risk of surgically confirmed gallbladder disease in women receiving postmenopausal estrogens,[17] similar to the 2-fold increase previously noted in users of oral contraceptives.[19,24a]
3. *Effects similar to those caused by estrogen-progestogen oral contraceptives.* There are several serious adverse effects of oral contraceptives, most of which have not, up to now, been documented as consequences of postmenopausal estrogen therapy. This may reflect the comparatively low doses of estrogen used in postmenopausal women. It would be expected that the larger doses of estrogen used to treat prostatic or breast cancer or postpartum breast engorgement are more likely to result in these adverse effects, and, in fact, it has been shown that there is an increased risk of thrombosis in men receiving estrogens for prostatic cancer and women for postpartum breast engorgement.[20–23]
a. *Thromboembolic disease.* It is now well established that users of oral contraceptives have an increased risk of various thromboembolic and thrombotic vascular diseases, such as thrombophlebitis, pulmonary embolism, stroke, and myocardial infarction.[24–31] Cases of retinal thrombosis, mesenteric thrombosis, and optic neuritis have been reported in oral contraceptive users. There is evidence that the risk of several of these adverse reactions is related to the dose of the drug.[32,33] An increased risk of postsurgery thromboembolic complications has also been reported in users of oral contraceptives.[34,35] If feasible, estrogen should be discontinued at least 4 weeks before surgery of the type associated with an increased risk of thromboembolism, or during periods of prolonged immobilization.
While an increased rate of thromboembolic and thrombotic disease in postmenopausal users of estrogens has not been found,[17–24,25–36] this does not rule out the possibility that such an increase may be present or that subgroups of women who have underlying risk factors or who are receiving relatively large doses of estrogens may have increased risk. Therefore estrogens should not be used in persons with active thrombophlebitis or thromboembolic disorders, and they should not be used (except in treatment of malignancy) in persons with a history of such disorders in association with estrogen use. They should be used with caution in patients with cerebral vascular or coronary artery disease and only for those in whom estrogens are clearly needed.
Large doses of estrogen (5 mg conjugated estrogens per day), comparable to those used to treat cancer of the prostate and breast, have been shown in a large prospective clinical trial in men[37] to increase the risk of nonfatal myocardial infarction, pulmonary embolism and thrombophlebitis. When estrogen doses of this size are used, any of the thromboembolic and thrombotic adverse effects associated with oral contraceptive use should be considered a clear risk.
b. *Hepatic adenoma.* Benign hepatic adenomas appear to be associated with the use of oral contraceptives.[38–40] Although benign, and rare, these may rupture and may cause death through intra-abdominal hemorrhage. Such lesions have not yet been reported in association with other estrogen or progestogen preparations but should be considered in estrogen users having abdominal pain and tenderness, abdominal mass, or hypovolemic shock. Hepatocellular carcinoma has also been reported in women taking estrogen-containing oral contraceptives.[39] The relationship of this malignancy to these drugs is not known at this time.
c. *Elevated blood pressure.* Women using oral contraceptives sometimes experience increased blood pressure which, in most cases, returns to normal on discontinuing the drug. There is now a report that this may occur with use of estrogens in the menopause[41] and blood pressure should be monitored with estrogen use, especially if high doses are used.
d. *Glucose tolerance.* A worsening of glucose tolerance has been observed in a significant percentage of patients on estrogen-containing oral contraceptives. For this reason, diabetic patients should be carefully observed while receiving estrogen.

4. *Hypercalcemia.* Administration of estrogens may lead to severe hypercalcemia in patients with breast cancer and bone metastases. If this occurs, the drug should be stopped and appropriate measures taken to reduce the serum calcium level.

Associated with Methyltestosterone

1. Female patients should be watched carefully for symptoms or signs of virilization such as hoarseness or deepening of the voice, oily skin, acne, hirsutism, enlarged clitoris, stimulation of libido, and menstrual irregularities. At the dosage necessary to achieve a tumor response, androgens will cause masculinization of a female, but occasionally a sensitive female may exhibit one or more of these signs on smaller doses. Some of these changes, such as voice changes may be irreversible even after drug is stopped.
2. Cholestatic hepatitis with jaundice and altered liver function tests, such as increased BSP retention and rises in SGOT levels, have been reported with methyltestosterone. These changes appear to be related to dosage of the drug. Therefore, in the presence of any changes in liver function tests, the drug should be discontinued.

Precautions:

Associated with Estrogens

A. General Precautions.

1. A complete medical and family history should be taken prior to the initiation of any estrogen therapy. The pretreatment and periodic physical examinations should include special reference to blood pressure, breasts, abdomen, and pelvic organs, and should include a Papanicolau smear. As a general rule, estrogen should not be prescribed for longer than one year without another physical examination being performed.
2. Fluid retention—Because estrogens may cause some degree of fluid retention, conditions which might be influenced by this factor such as asthma, epilepsy, migraine, and cardiac or renal dysfunction, require careful observation.
3. Certain patients may develop undesirable manifestations of excessive estrogenic stimulation, such as abnormal or excessive uterine bleeding, mastodynia, etc.
4. Oral contraceptives appear to be associated with an increased incidence of mental depression.[24a] Although it is not clear whether this is due to the estrogenic or progestogenic component of the contraceptive, patients with a history of depression should be carefully observed.
5. Preexisting uterine leiomyomata may increase in size during estrogen use.
6. The pathologist should be advised of estrogen therapy when relevant specimens are submitted.
7. Patients with a past history of jaundice during pregnancy have an increased risk of recurrence of jaundice while receiving estrogen-containing oral contraceptive therapy. If jaundice develops in any patient receiving estrogen, the medication should be discontinued while the cause is investigated.
8. Estrogens may be poorly metabolized in patients with impaired liver function and they should be administered with caution in such patients.
9. Because estrogens influence the metabolism of calcium and phosphorus, they should be used with caution in patients with metabolic bone diseases that are associated with hypercalcemia or in patients with renal insufficiency.
10. Because of the effects of estrogens on epiphyseal closure, they should be used judiciously in young patients in whom bone growth is not complete.
11. Certain endocrine and liver function tests may be affected by estrogen-containing oral contraceptives. The following similar changes may be expected with larger doses of estrogen:

a. Increased sulfobromophthalein retention.
b. Increased prothrombin and factors VII, VIII, IX, and X; decreased antithrombin 3; increased norepinephrine-induced platelet aggregability.
c. Increased thyroid binding globulin (TBG) leading to increased circulating total thyroid hormone, as measured by PBI, T4 by column, or T4 by radioimmunoassay. Free T3 resin uptake is decreased, reflecting the elevated TBG; free T4 concentration is unaltered.
d. Impaired glucose tolerance.
e. Decreased pregnanediol excretion.
f. Reduced response to metyrapone test.
g. Reduced serum folate concentration.
h. Increased serum triglyceride and phospholipid concentration.

B. Information for the Patient. See text which appears after the PHYSICIAN REFERENCES under PREMARIN® (Conjugated Estrogens Tablets, U.S.P.).

C. Pregnancy Category X. See CONTRAINDICATIONS and Boxed Warning.

D. Nursing Mothers. As a general principle, the administration of any drug to nursing mothers should be done only when clearly necessary since many drugs are excreted in human milk.

Associated with Methyltestosterone

A. Prolonged dosage of androgen may result in sodium and fluid retention. This may present a problem, especially in patients with compromised cardiac reserve or renal disease.
B. Hypersensitivity may occur rarely.
C. PBI may be decreased in patients taking androgens.
D. Hypercalcemia may occur. If this does occur, the drug should be discontinued.

Adverse Reactions:

Associated with Estrogens

(See Warnings regarding induction of neoplasia, adverse effects on the fetus, increased incidence of gallbladder disease and adverse effects similar to those of oral contraceptives, including thromboembolism.) The following additional adverse reactions have been reported with estrogenic therapy, including oral contraceptives:

1. *Genitourinary system:* Breakthrough bleeding, spotting, change in menstrual flow; dysmenorrhea; premenstrual-like syndrome; amenorrhea during and after treatment; increase in size of uterine fibromyomata; vaginal candidiasis; change in cervical erosion and in degree of cervical secretion; cystitis-like syndrome.
2. *Breasts:* Tenderness, enlargement, secretion.
3. *Gastrointestinal:* Nausea, vomiting; abdominal cramps, bloating; cholestatic jaundice.
4. *Skin:* Chloasma or melasma which may persist when drug is discontinued; erythema multiforme; erythema nodosum; hemorrhagic eruption; loss of scalp hair; hirsutism.
5. *Eyes:* Steepening of corneal curvature; intolerance to contact lenses.
6. *CNS:* Headache, migraine, dizziness; mental depression; chorea.
7. *Miscellaneous:* Increase or decrease in weight; reduced carbohydrate tolerance; aggravation of porphyria; edema; changes in libido.

Associated with Methyltestosterone

Cholestatic jaundice
Hypercalcemia, particularly in patients with metastatic breast carcinoma. This usually indicates progression of bone metastases.
Sodium and water retention
Virilization in female patients
Hypersensitivity

Acute Overdosage: Numerous reports of ingestion of large doses of estrogen-containing oral contraceptives by young children indicate that acute serious ill effects do not occur. Overdosage of estrogen may cause nausea, and withdrawal bleeding may occur in females.

Dosage and Administration:

1. *Given cyclically for short-term use only:*
For treatment of moderate to severe *vasomotor* symptoms associated with the menopause in patients not improved by estrogen alone.
The lowest dose that will control symptoms should be chosen and medication should be discontinued as promptly as possible.
Administration should be cyclic (e.g., three weeks on and one week off).
Attempts to discontinue or taper medication should be made at three to six month intervals.

Usual dosage range:

1.25 mg Conjugated Estrogens, U.S.P. and 10.0 mg Methyltestosterone (1 yellow tablet, No. 879, or 2 red tablets, No. 878) daily and cyclically.

2. Given for a few days.
Prevention of postpartum breast engorgement

Usual dosage range:

Using No. 879 (yellow) tablets containing 1.25 mg Conjugated Estrogens, U.S.P. and 10.0 mg Methyltestosterone, either
(a) 3 tablets every four hours for 5 doses, then 2 tablets daily for balance of the week, or
(b) 1 tablet three times each day for the first four days postpartum, then 1 tablet daily for the next 10 days.

Treated patients with an intact uterus should be monitored closely for signs of endometrial cancer and appropriate diagnostic measures should be taken to rule out malignancy in the event of persistent or recurring abnormal vaginal bleeding.

How Supplied: PREMARIN (Conjugated Estrogens, U.S.P.) with Methyltestosterone Tablets
—Each *yellow* tablet contains 1.25 mg PREMARIN and 10.0 mg Methyltestosterone, in bottles of 100 (NDC 0046-0879-81) and 1,000 (NDC 0046-0879-91).
—Each *red* tablet contains 0.625 mg PREMARIN and 5.0 mg Methyltestosterone, in bottles of 100 (NDC 0046-0878-81) and 1,000 (NDC 0046-0878-91).

Physician References:

1. Ziel, H. K., *et al.*: N. Engl. J. Med. *293*:1167–1170, 1975.
2. Smith, D. C., *et al.*: N. Engl. J. Med. *293*:1164–1167, 1975.
3. Mack, T. M., *et al.*: N. Engl. J. Med. *294*:1262–1267, 1976.
4. Weiss, N. S., *et al.*: N. Engl. J. Med. *294*:1259–1262, 1976.
5. Herbst, A. L., *et al.*: N. Engl. J. Med. *284*:878–881, 1971.
6. Greenwald, P., *et al.*: N. Engl. J. Med. *285*:390–392, 1971.
7. Lanier, A., *et al.*: Mayo Clin. Proc. *48*:793–799, 1973.
8. Herbst, A., *et al.*: Obstet. Gynecol. *40*:287–298, 1972.
9. Herbst, A., *et al.*: Am. J. Obstet. Gynecol. *118*:607–615, 1974.
10. Herbst, A., *et al.*: N. Engl. J. Med. *292*:334–339, 1975.
11. Stafl, A., *et al.*: Obstet. Gynecol. *43*:118–128, 1974.
12. Sherman, A. I., *et al.*: Obstet. Gynecol. *44*:531–545, 1974.
13. Gal. I., *et al.*: Nature *216*:83, 1967.
14. Levy, E. P., *et al.*: Lancet *1*:611, 1973.
15. Nora, J., *et al.*: Lancet *1*:941–942, 1973.
16. Janerich, D. T., *et al.*: N. Engl. J. Med. *291*:697–700, 1974.
17. Boston Collaborative Drug Surveillance Program: N. Engl. J. Med. *290*:15–19, 1974.
18. Hoover, R., *et al.*: N. Engl. J. Med. 295: 401–405, 1976.
19. Boston Collaborative Drug Surveillance Program: Lancet *1*:1399–1404, 1973.
20. Daniel, D. G., *et al.*: Lancet *2*:287–289, 1967.

Continued on next page

Ayerst—Cont.

21. The Veterans Administration Cooperative Urological Research Group: J. Urol. *98*:516–522, 1967.
22. Bailar, J. C.: Lancet *2*:560, 1967.
23. Blackard, C., *et al.*: Cancer *26*:249–256, 1970.
24. Royal College of General Practitioners: J. R. Coll. Gen. Pract. *13*:267–279, 1967.
24a. Royal College of General Practitioners: Oral Contraceptives and Health, New York, Pitman Corp., 1974.
25. Inman, W. H. W., *et al.*: Br. Med. J. *2*:193–199, 1968.
26. Vessey, M. P., *et al.*: Br. Med. J. *2*:651–657, 1969.
27. Sartwell, P. E., *et al.*: Am. J. Epidemiol. *90*:365–380, 1969.
28. Collaborative Group for the Study of Stroke in Young Women: N. Engl. J. Med. *288*:871–878, 1973.
29. Collaborative Group for the Study of Stroke in Young Women: J.A.M.A. *231*: 718–722, 1975.
30. Mann, J. I., *et al.*: Br. Med. J. *2*:245–248, 1975.
31. Mann, J. I., *et al.*: Br. Med. J. *2*:241–245, 1975.
32. Inman, W. H. W., *et al.*: Br. Med. J. *2*:203–209, 1970.
33. Stolley, P. D., *et al.*: Am. J. Epidemiol. *102*:197–208, 1975.
34. Vessey, M. P., *et al.*: Br. Med. J. *3*:123–126, 1970.
35. Greene, G. R., *et al.*: Am. J. Public Health *62*:680–685, 1972.
36. Rosenberg, L., *et al.*: N. Engl. J. Med. *294*: 1256–1259, 1976.
37. Coronary Drug Project Research Group: J.A.M.A. *214*:1303–1313, 1970.
38. Baum, J., *et al.*: Lancet *2*:926–928, 1973.
39. Mays, E. T., *et al.*: J.A.M.A. *235*:730–732, 1976.
40. Edmondson, H. A., *et al.*: N. Engl. J. Med. *294*:470–472, 1976.
41. Pfeffer, R. I., *et al.*: Am. J. Epidemiol. *103*:445–456, 1976.

[*Shown in Product Identification Section*]

PROTOPAM® CHLORIDE ℞
Brand of pralidoxime chloride

Description: PROTOPAM CHLORIDE (pralidoxime chloride) is a cholinesterase reactivator. Chemically, it is 2-formyl-1-methylpyridinium chloride oxime (pyridine-2-aldoxime methochloride), and has the generic name pralidoxime chloride. It has also been referred to as 2-PAM Chloride.

PROTOPAM CHLORIDE occurs as a white, nonhygroscopic, crystalline powder which is soluble in water to the extent of 1 g in less than 1 ml.

The specific activity of the drug resides in the 2-formyl-1-methylpyridinium ion and is independent of the particular salt employed.

Actions: The principal action of PROTOPAM (pralidoxime) is to reactivate cholinesterase (mainly outside of the central nervous system) which has been inactivated by phosphorylation due to an organophosphate pesticide or related compound. The destruction of accumulated acetylcholine can then proceed and neuromuscular junctions will again function normally. PROTOPAM also slows the process of "aging" of phosphorylated cholinesterase to a non-reactivatable form, and detoxifies certain organophosphates by direct chemical reaction. The drug has its most critical effect in relieving paralysis of the muscles of respiration. Because PROTOPAM is less effective in relieving depression of the respiratory center, atropine is always required concomitantly to block the effect of accumulated acetylcholine at this site. PROTOPAM relieves muscarinic signs and symptoms, salivation, bronchospasm, etc., but this action is relatively unimportant since atropine is adequate for this purpose.

PROTOPAM antagonizes the effects on the neuromuscular junction of the carbamate anticholinesterases, neostigmine, pyridostigmine and ambenonium, used in the treatment of myasthenia gravis. However, it is not nearly as effective as an antidote to these drugs as it is to the organophosphates.

PROTOPAM (pralidoxime) is distributed throughout the extracellular water; it is not bound to plasma protein. The drug is rapidly excreted in the urine partly unchanged, and partly as a metabolite produced by the liver. Consequently. PROTOPAM is relatively short acting and repeated doses may be needed, especially where there is any evidence of continuing absorption of the poison.

Indications: PROTOPAM is indicated as an antidote: (1) in the treatment of poisoning due to those pesticides and chemicals of the organophosphate class which have anticholinesterase activity, and (2) in the control of overdosage by anticholinesterase drugs used in the treatment of myasthenia gravis.

Warnings: Use of PROTOPAM should always be under supervision of the subject's personal physician or of the medical department of his employer.

PROTOPAM is not effective in the treatment of poisoning due to phosphorus, inorganic phosphates or organophosphates not having anticholinesterase activity.

Until further information is available, no recommendation is made as to the use of PROTOPAM in intoxication by pesticides of the carbamate class.

Precautions: PROTOPAM (pralidoxime) has been very well tolerated in most cases, but it must be remembered that the desperate condition of the organophosphate-poisoned patient will generally mask such minor signs and symptoms as have been noted in normal subjects.

Intravenous administration of PROTOPAM should be carried out slowly and, preferably, by infusion, since certain side effects, such as tachycardia, laryngospasm, and muscle rigidity, have been attributed in a few cases to a too rapid rate of injection. (See Dosage and Administration.)

Because PROTOPAM is excreted in the urine, a decrease in renal function will result in increased blood levels of the drug. Thus, the dosage of PROTOPAM should be reduced in the presence of renal insufficiency.

PROTOPAM should be used with great caution in treating organophosphate overdosage in cases of myasthenia gravis since it may precipitate a myasthenic crisis.

The following precautions should be kept in mind in the treatment of anticholinesterase poisoning, although they do not bear directly on the use of PROTOPAM (pralidoxime): since barbiturates are potentiated by the anticholinesterases, they should be used cautiously in the treatment of convulsions; morphine, theophylline, aminophylline, succinylcholine, reserpine, and phenothiazine-type tranquilizers should be avoided in patients with organophosphate poisoning.

Adverse Reactions: Dizziness, blurred vision, diplopia and impaired accommodation, headache, drowsiness, nausea, tachycardia, hyperventilation, and muscular weakness have been reported after the use of PROTOPAM, but it is very difficult to differentiate the toxic effects produced by atropine or the organophosphate compounds from those of the drug. When atropine and PROTOPAM are used together, the signs of atropinization may occur earlier than might be expected when atropine is used alone. This is especially true if the total dose of atropine has been large and the administration of PROTOPAM has been delayed. Excitement and manic behavior immediately following recovery of consciousness have been reported in several cases. However, similar behavior has occurred in cases of organophosphate poisoning that were not treated with PROTOPAM.

Dosage and Administration:

Organophosphate poisoning

Initial measures should include removal of secretions, maintenance of a patent airway and, if necessary, artificial ventilation.

In the absence of cyanosis, atropine should be given intravenously in doses of 2 to 4 mg; where cyanosis is present, this dose of atropine should be given intramuscularly while simultaneously initiating measures for improving ventilation. Atropine administration should be repeated at 5 to 10 minute intervals until signs of atropine toxicity appear. Some degree of atropinization should be maintained for at least 48 hours.

PROTOPAM (pralidoxime) administration should be started at the same time as atropine.

In adults, inject an initial dose of 1 to 2 g of PROTOPAM, preferably as an infusion in 100 ml of saline, over a 15 to 30 minute period. If this is not practicable or if pulmonary edema is present, the dose should be given slowly by intravenous injection as a 5 percent solution in water over not less than five minutes. After about an hour, a second dose of 1 to 2 g will be indicated if muscle weakness has not been relieved. Additional doses may be given cautiously if muscle weakness persists. If intravenous administration is not feasible, intramuscular or subcutaneous injection should be used.

In children, the dose should be 20 to 40 mg per kg.

Treatment will be most effective if given within a few hours after poisoning has occurred. Usually, little will be accomplished if the drug is first administered more than 48 hours after exposure, but in severe poisoning, it is, nevertheless, indicated since occasionally patients have responded after such an interval.

In severe cases, especially after ingestion of the poison, it may be desirable to monitor the effect of therapy electrocardiographically because of the possibility of heart block due to the anticholinesterase. Where the poison has been ingested, it is particularly important to take into account the likelihood of continuing absorption from the lower bowel since this constitutes new exposure. In such cases, additional doses of PROTOPAM (pralidoxime) may be needed every three to eight hours. In effect, the patient should be "titrated" with PROTOPAM as long as signs of poisoning recur.

In the absence of severe gastrointestinal symptoms, resulting from the anticholinesterase intoxication, PROTOPAM (pralidoxime) may be administered orally in doses of 1 to 3 g (2 to 6 tablets) every five hours. As in all cases of organophosphate poisoning, care should be taken to keep the patient under observation for at least 24 hours.

If convulsions interfere with respiration, sodium thiopental (2.5 percent solution) may be given intravenously with care.

Anticholinesterase overdosage

As an antagonist to such anticholinesterases as neostigmine, pyridostigmine, and ambenonium, which are used in the treatment of myasthenia gravis, PROTOPAM may be given in a dosage of 1 to 2 g intravenously followed by increments of 250 mg every five minutes.

Overdosage: Artificial respiration and other supportive therapy should be administered as needed.

How Supplied: NDC 0046-0375-98—*Emergency Kit:* This contains one 20 ml vial of 1 g of sterile PROTOPAM CHLORIDE (pralidoxime chloride) white to off white porous cake*; one 20 ml ampul of Sterile Water for Injection, U.S.P. without preservative to be used as diluent; sterile, disposable 20 ml syringe; needle; alcohol swab. This is a single dose kit for intravenous administration. Intramuscular or subcutaneous injection may be used when intravenous injection is not feasible.

NDC 0046-0374-06—*Hospital Package:* This contains six 20 ml vials of 1 g each of sterile PROTOPAM CHLORIDE (pralidoxime chloride) white to off white porous cake*, without diluent or syringe. Solution may be prepared by adding 20 ml of Sterile Water for Injection, U.S.P. These are single dose vials for intravenous injection or for intravenous infusion after further dilution with physiologic saline. Intramuscular or subcutaneous injection may be used when intravenous injection is not feasible.

*When necessary, sodium hydroxide is added during processing to adjust the pH.

PROTOPAM CHLORIDE for Injection is prepared by cryodesiccation.

NDC 0046-0376-81—*Tablets:* Each tablet contains 500 mg of pralidoxime chloride, in bottles of 100.

A FULL DISCUSSION OF THE ACTIONS AND USES OF PROTOPAM (PRALIDOXIME) IS GIVEN IN A PROFESSIONAL BROCHURE WHICH IS AVAILABLE FROM AYERST LABORATORIES ON REQUEST.

Animal Pharmacology and Toxicology: The following table lists chemical and trade or generic names of pesticides, chemicals, and drugs against which PROTOPAM (usually administered in conjunction with atropine) has been found to have antidotal activity on the basis of animal experiments. All compounds listed are organophosphates having anticholinesterase activity. A great many additional substances are in industrial use but have been omitted because of lack of specific information. The use of PROTOPAM should, nevertheless, be considered in any life-threatening situation resulting from poisoning by these compounds, since the limited and arbitrary conditions of pharmacologic screening do not always accurately reflect the usefulness of PROTOPAM in the clinical situation.

AAT—see PARATHION

AFLIX®—see FORMOTHION

ALKRON®—see PARATHION

AMERICAN CYANAMID 3422—see PARATHION

AMITON—diethyl -S- (2-diethyl-aminoethyl) phosphorothiolate

ANTHIO®—see FORMOTHION

APHAMITE—see PARATHION

ARMIN—ethyl-4-nitrophenyl-ethylphosphonate

AZINPHOS-METHYL—dimethyl-S- (4-oxo-1, 2, 3, -benzotriazin-3 (4 H) -ylmethyl) phosphorodithioate

AZODRIN—dimethyl phosphate of 3-hydroxy-N-methyl-cis-crotonamide

BAYER 16259—see ETHYL GUTHION

BAYER 19639—see DISULFOTON

BAYER 25141 — diethyl-4-methyl-sulfinyl-phenylphosphorothionate

BAYER 29493—see FENTHION

BAYER L13/59—see TRICHLOROFON

BAYER E605—see PARATHION

BAYTEX®—see FENTHION

CHIPMAN R6199—see AMITON

COMPOUND 3422—see PARATHION

COMPOUND 4049—see MALATHION

COMPOUND 4072—2-chloro-1-(2,4-dichlorophenyl) vinyl diethyl-phosphate

CO-RAL®—see COUMAPHOS

COROTHION—see PARATHION

COUMAPHOS—3-chloro-4-methyl coumarin-7-yl-diethyl-phosphorothionate

DBD —see AZINPHOS-METHYL

DDVP—see DICHLORVOS

DELNAV—see DIOXATHION

DEMETON—Mixture of SYSTOX® and ISOSYSTOX®

DEMETON-S—see ISOSYSTOX®

DFP—see ISOFLUROPHATE

DIAZINON—diethyl- (2- isopropyl -4- methyl - 6- pyrimidyl) phosphorothionate

DICHLORVOS—dimethyl-2, 2-dichloro vinyl phosphate

DIETHYL-p-NITROPHENYL-PHOSPHOROTHIONATE—see PARATHION

DIETHYL -p- NITROPHENYL - THIONOPHOSPHATE—see PARATHION

DIOXATHION—2, 3-p-dioxanedithio-S, S-bis (0, 0-diethyl phosphorodithioate)

DIPTEREX®—see TRICHLOROFON

DISULFOTON—diethyl -S- (2-ethylthioethyl) phosphorodiothiate

DISYSTON®—see DISULFOTON

DITHIOSYSTOX—see DISULFOTON

DNTP—see PARATHION

DPP—see PARATHION

DSDP—see AMITON

DYFLOS—see DFP

DYLOX®—see TRICHLOROFON

E 600—see PARAOXON

E 601—see METHYL PARATHION

E 605—see PARATHION

E 1059—see SYSTOX

ECHOTHIOPHATE IODIDE—diethoxyphosphinylthio-choline iodide

EKATIN®—see MORPHOTHION

ENDOTHION—2- (dimethoxyphosphinylthio-methyl)-5-methoxy-4-pyrone

ENT 15108—see PARATHION

ENTEX®—see FENTHION

EPN—ethyl -4- nitrophenyl - phenylphosphonothionate

ETHION—0,0,0',0'-tetraethyl-S,S'-methylene-bis-phosphoro dithioate

ETHYL GUSATHION—see ETHYL GUTHION

ETHYL GUTHION®—diethyl-S-(4-oxo-1,2,3,-benzotriazinyl-3-methyl) phosphorodithioate

ETILON—see PARATHION

FENTHION—dimethyl-(4-methylthio-3-tolyl) phosphorothionate

FLOROPRYL®—see DFP

FOLIDOL®—see PARATHION

FORMOTHION—dimethyl -S- (N-formyl -N-methylcarbamyl-methyl) phosphorodithioate

G 24480—see DIAZINON

GB—see SARIN

GENITHION—see PARATHION

GUSATHION®—see AZINPHOSMETHYL

GUTHION®—see AZINPHOSMETHYL

HETP—see TEPP

I-ARMIN—isopropyl -4- nitro-phenyl methyl-phosphonate

ISOFLUROPHATE—diisopropyl - phosphorofluoridate

ISOSYSTOX®— diethyl-S-(2-ethylmercapto-ethyl)-phosphorothiolate

LEBACYD®—see FENTHION

MACKOTHION—see PARATHION

MALATHION—dimethyl -S- (1, 2-dicarbeth-oxyethyl) -phosphorodithioate

MALATHON—see MALATHION

M-ARMIN—ethyl-4-nitrophenyl methylphosphonate

MECARBAM—0, 0-dimethyl -S- (N-ethoxycarbonyl-N-methyl carbamoylmethyl) phosphorodithioate

METACIDE—see METHYL PARATHION

METASYSTOX®—see METHYL DEMETON

METASYSTOX I®—dimethyl -2- ethyl-mercaptoethylphos-phorothiolate

METASYSTOX R®—see OXYDEMETON-METHYL

METHYL DEMETON—mixture of dimethyl(2-ethylmercapto-ethyl) phosphorothionate and dimethyl-S-(2-ethylmercapto-ethyl) phosphorothiolate

METHYL PARATHION—dimethyl - (4-nitrophenyl) phosphorothionate

MEVINPHOS—1- carbomethoxy-1- propen-2-yl-dimethylphosphate

MINTACOL®—see PARAOXON

Continued on next page

Ayerst—Cont.

ML 97—see PHOSPHAMIDON

MORPHOTHION—dimethyl -S- 2-keto-2- (N-morpholyl ethyl-phosphorodithioate

NEGUVON®—see TRICHLOROFON

NIRAN®—see PARATHION

NITROSTIGMINE—see PARATHION

0, 0-DIETHYL -O- p-NITRO-PHENYL PHOSPHOROTHIOATE—see PARATHION

0, 0-DIETHYL -O- p-NITRO-PHENYLTHIOPHOSPHATE —see PARATHION

OR 1191—see PHOSPHAMIDON

OS 1836—see VINYLPHOS

OXYDEMETONMETHYL—dimethyl -S- 2-(ethylsulfinyl) ethyl phosphorothiolate

PARAOXON—diethyl (4 - nitro - phenyl) phosphate.

PARATHION—diethyl (4-nitro-phenyl) phosphorothionate

PENPHOS—see PARATHION

PHENCAPTON—diethyl -S- (2, 5-dichlorophenylmercaptomethyl) phosphorodithioate

PHOSDRIN®—see MEVINPHOS

PHOS-KIL—see PARATHION

PHOSPHAMIDON—1-chloro -1- diethylcarbamoyl -1- propen -2- yl-dimethylphosphate

PHOSPHOLINE IODIDE®—see echothiophate iodide

PHOSPHOROTHIOIC ACID, 0,0-DIETHYL-0-p-NITRO-PHENYL ESTER—see PARATHION

PLANTHION—see PARATHION

QUELETOX—see FENTHION

RHODIATOX®—see PARATHION

RUELENE®— 4- tert-butyl -2- chlorophenyl-methyl-N-methyl-phosphoroamidate

SARIN— isopropyl - methylphos - phonofluoridate

SHELL OS 1836—see VINYLPHOS

SHELL 2046—see MEVINPHOS

SNP—see PARATHION

SOMAN—pinacolyl - methyl - phosphonofluoridate

SYSTOX®—diethyl - (2-ethyl-mercaptoethyl) phosphorothionate

TEP—see TEPP

TEPP—tetraethylpyro phosphate

THIOPHOS®—see PARATHION

TIGUVON—see FENTHION

TRICHLOROFON—dimethyl -1- hydroxy-2, 2, 2-trichloro ethylphosphonate

VAPONA®—see DICHLORVOS

VAPOPHOS—see PARATHION

VINYLPHOS—diethyl -2- chloro - vinylphosphate

PROTOPAM appears to be ineffective, or marginally effective, against poisoning by:
CIODRIN® (alpha-methylbenzyl-3-[dimethoxyphosphinyloxy]-cis-crotonate)
DIMEFOX (tetramethylphosphorodiamidic fluoride)
DIMETHOATE (dimethyl-S-[N-methylcarbamoylmethyl]phosphorodithioate)
METHYL DIAZINON (dimethyl-[2-isopropyl-4-methylpyrimidyl]-phosphorothionate)
METHYL PHENCAPTON (dimethyl-S- [2, 5-dichlorophenylmercaptomethyl] phosphorodithioate)
PHORATE (diethyl-S-ethylmercaptomethyl-phosphorodithioate)
SCHRADAN (octamethylpyrophosphoramide)
WEPSYN® (5-amino-1-[bis-(dimethylamino)-phosphinyl]-3-phenyl-1,2,4-triazole)

Clinical Studies: The use of PROTOPAM (pralidoxime) has been reported in the treatment of human cases of poisoning by the following substances:

Azodrin
Diazinon
Dichlorvos (DDVP) with chlordane
Disulfoton
EPN
Isoflurophate
Malathion
Metasystox I® and Fenthion
Methyl demeton
Methyl parathion
Mevinphos
Parathion
Parathion and Mevinphos
Phosphamidon
Sarin
Systox®
TEPP

Of these cases, over 100 were due to parathion, about a dozen each to malathion, diazinon, and mevinphos, and a few to each of the other compounds.

RIOPAN®
magaldrate
Antacid

RIOPAN is a chemical entity (not a physical mixture), providing the advantages of a true buffer-antacid (not simply a neutralizing agent): (1) rapid action; (2) uniform buffering action; (3) high acid-consuming capacity; (4) no alkalinization or acid rebound.

Low Sodium Content: Not more than 0.3 mg of sodium—per teaspoonful (5 ml) suspension—per chew tablet—per swallow tablet.

Acid-neutralizing Capacity—13.5 mEq/5 ml or tablet.

Indications: For the relief of upset stomach associated with heartburn, sour stomach, and/or acid indigestion. For symptomatic relief of hyperacidity associated with the diagnosis of peptic ulcer, gastritis, peptic esophagitis, gastric hyperacidity, and hiatal hernia.

Directions: RIOPAN (magaldrate) Antacid *Suspension*—Recommended dosage, one or two teaspoonfuls, between meals and at bedtime, or as directed by the physician. RIOPAN Antacid *Chew Tablets*—Recommended dosage, one or two tablets, between meals and at bedtime, or as directed by the physician. Chew before swallowing. RIOPAN Antacid *Swallow Tablets*—Recommended dosage, one or two tablets, between meals and at bedtime, or as directed by the physician. Take with enough water to swallow promptly.

Drug Interaction Precaution: Do not use in patients taking a prescription antibiotic drug containing any form of tetracycline.

Warnings: Patients should not take more than 20 teaspoonfuls (or 20 tablets) in a 24-hour period or use this maximum dosage for more than two weeks, except under the advice and supervision of a physician. If you have kidney disease, do not use this product except under the advice and supervision of a physician.

How Supplied: RIOPAN Antacid *Suspension*—Each teaspoonful (5 ml) contains 480 mg magaldrate, in 12 fl oz (355 ml) bottles (NDC 0046-0933-12). Individual Cups, 1 fl oz (30 ml) ea., tray of 10—10 trays per packer (NDC 0046-0933-99). RIOPAN Antacid *Chew Tablets*—Each tablet contains 480 mg magaldrate. Packages of 60 (NDC 0046-0928-60) and 100 (NDC 0046-0928-81) in individual film strips (10 x 6 and 10 x 10, respectively). RIOPAN Antacid *Swallow Tablets*—Each tablet contains 480 mg magaldrate. Packages of 60 (NDC 0046-0927-60) and 100 (NDC 0046-0927-81) in individual film strips (6 x 10 and 10 x 10, respectively).

[*Shown in Product Identification Section*]

RIOPAN PLUS®
magaldrate and SIMETHICONE
Antacid/Anti-Gas

Each teaspoonful (5 ml) of Suspension contains:
Magaldrate .... 480 mg
Simethicone .... 20 mg
Each Chew Tablet contains:
Magaldrate .... 480 mg
Simethicone .... 20 mg

Low Sodium Content: Not more than 0.3 mg per teaspoonful (5 ml) or Chew Tablet.

Acid-neutralizing Capacity—13.5 mEq/5 ml or Chew Tablet.

Indications: For the relief of upset stomach associated with heartburn, sour stomach, and/or acid indigestion, accompanied by the symptoms of gas. For symptomatic relief of hyperacidity associated with the diagnosis of peptic ulcer, gastritis, peptic esophagitis, gastric hyperacidity, and hiatal hernia. For postoperative gas pain or for use in endoscopic examinations.

Directions: RIOPAN PLUS (magaldrate and SIMETHICONE) *Suspension*—Recommended dosage, one or two teaspoonfuls between meals and at bedtime, or as directed by the physician.
RIOPAN PLUS *Chew Tablets*—Recommended dosage, one or two tablets, between meals and at bedtime, or as directed by the physician. Chew before swallowing.

Drug Interaction Precaution: Do not use in patients taking a prescription antibiotic drug containing any form of tetracycline.

Warnings: Patients should not take more than 20 teaspoonfuls (or 20 tablets) in a 24-hour period or use this maximum dosage for more than two weeks, except under the advice and supervision of a physician. If you have kidney disease, do not use this product except under the advice and supervision of a physician.

How Supplied: RIOPAN PLUS *Suspension*—in 12 fl oz (355 ml) plastic bottles (NDC 0046-0937-12). Individual Cups, 1 fl oz (30 ml) ea., tray of 10—10 trays per packer (NDC 0046-0937-99).
RIOPAN PLUS *Chew Tablets*—in bottles of 60 (NDC 0046-0930-60).

[*Shown in Product Identification Section*]

THIOSULFIL® ℞
(sulfamethizole)
DUO-PAK®
Package

This package contains 2 products:

Bottle No. 1—24 Tablets (*yellow*)

THIOSULFIL®-A Forte
(sulfamethizole 0.5 g with phenazopyridine HCl)

Each tablet contains:
Sulfamethizole.. 0.5 g
Phenazopyridine HCl .... 50.0 mg

Bottle No. 2—32 Tablets (*white*)

THIOSULFIL® Forte
(sulfamethizole 0.5 g)
Each tablet contains:
Sulfamethizole.. 0.5 g

Clinical Pharmacology: The combination of sulfamethizole and phenazopyridine in THIOSULFIL-A Forte (sulfamethizole 0.5 g with phenazopyridine HCl) acts to eradicate urinary tract infections due to susceptible organisms, and relieve pain and discomfort associated with infection. Following relief of pain, THIOSULFIL Forte (sulfamethizole 0.5 g), containing only sulfamethizole, provides continuing antibacterial therapy.

PHENAZOPYRIDINE HCl: Phenazopyridine HCl is an analgesic that acts on the mucosa of the urinary tract to provide relief of pain and discomfort caused by inflammation associated with urinary tract infection.

SULFAMETHIZOLE:

Mechanism of sulfonamide bacteriostatic action: The primary mechanism of bacteriostatic action by THIOSULFIL (sulfamethizole) is the same as that of most sulfonamides. By competing with the precursor para-aminobenzoic acid, sulfonamides inhibit bacterial synthesis of folic (pteroylglutamic) acid which is required for bacterial growth. Resistant strains are capable of utilizing folic acid precursors of preformed folic acid.

Sulfonamide antibacterial spectrum: The antibacterial spectrum of all sulfonamides is similar. *In vitro* sensitivity of bacteria to sulfonamides does not always reflect *in vivo* sensitivity. Therefore, efficacy must be carefully evaluated with bacteriologic and clinical responses in the individual patient. (See Warnings)

Factors determining antibacterial efficacy: Efficacy of antimicrobial therapy is dependent upon a number of factors including the *in vivo* sensitivity of the involved organisms, the concentration of the drug required for bacteriostasis, and the achievable concentration of the sulfonamide at the desired site of action.

Because of the very rapid renal clearance of sulfamethizole, the blood levels attained are low, and accumulation of the drug in tissues outside the urinary tract is very limited. Therefore, sulfamethizole is not appropriate for treatment of systemic infections such as nocardiosis or for local lesions outside the urinary tract such as chancroid and trachoma. However, its low degree of acetylation and its rapid renal clearance permit high concentrations of active sulfamethizole to occur in the urinary tract, making it especially applicable for the treatment of infections of this tract. In addition, the possibility of crystalluria is minimized because of the high solubility of the drug in urine.

Approximately 95 percent of a given dose of sulfamethizole is not metabolized; less than 5 percent is acetylated. As a consequence, almost all of a given dose of THIOSULFIL (sulfamethizole) is present in its active form in the body.

Approximately 80 percent of an administered dose is recoverable within eight hours; approximately 98 percent is cleared within 15 to 24 hours. Sulfamethizole is cleared by the kidney at a rate only 10 to 20 percent lower than that for creatinine.

Indications and Usage: THIOSULFIL-A Forte (sulfamethizole 0.5 g with phenazopyridine HCl)—Bottle No. 1.—is indicated for pain, burning, frequency, and urgency due to inflammation associated with urinary tract infection.

THIOSULFIL Forte (sulfamethizole 0.5 g)—Bottle No. 2—is indicated for continuing antibacterial therapy after pain and discomfort have been relieved.

THIOSULFIL is indicated in the treatment of urinary tract infections (primarily pyelonephritis, pyelitis, and cystitis) in the absence of obstructive uropathy or foreign bodies, when these infections are caused by susceptible strains of the following organisms: *Escherichia coli, Klebsiella-Enterobacter, Staphylococcus aureus, Proteus mirabilis,* and *Proteus vulgaris.*

Important note, *In vitro* sulfonamide sensitivity tests are not always reliable. The test must be carefully coordinated with bacteriologic and clinical response. When the patient is already taking sulfonamides, follow-up cultures should have aminobenzoic acid added to the culture media.

Currently, the increasing frequency of resistant organisms is a limitation of the usefulness of antibacterial agents, including the sulfonamides, especially in the treatment of recurrent and complicated urinary tract infections.

Wide variation in blood levels may result with identical doses. Blood levels should be measured in patients receiving sulfonamides for serious infections. Free sulfonamide blood levels of 5–15 mg per 100 ml may be considered therapeutically effective for most infections, with blood levels of 12–15 mg per 100 ml optimal for serious infections; 20 mg per 100 ml should be the maximal total sulfonamide level, as adverse reactions occur more frequently above this level.

Contraindications: Sulfonamides should not be used in patients hypersensitive to sulfa drugs. They should not be used in infants less than two months of age, in pregnancy at term, and during the nursing period because sulfonamides pass the placenta and are excreted in the milk and may cause kernicterus.

Phenazopyridine HCl is contraindicated in renal or hepatic failure, glomerulonephritis, and pyelonephritis of pregnancy with gastrointestinal disturbances.

Warnings: Sulfonamides should not be used to treat group A streptococci infections or their sequelae. The occurrence of sore throat, fever, pallor, purpura, or jaundice during sulfonamide administration may be an early indication of serious blood dyscrasias.

Deaths associated with the administration of sulfonamides have been reported from hypersensitivity reactions, agranulocytosis, aplastic anemia, and other blood dyscrasias.

Frequent blood counts and renal function tests should be carried out during sulfonamide treatment, especially during prolonged administration. Microscopic urinalyses should be done once a week when a patient is treated for longer than two weeks. Urine cultures should be made to confirm eradication of bacteriuria.

Precautions: To allay any possible apprehension, patients should be told that this medication may color the urine orange or red.

The usual precautions used in sulfonamide therapy should be observed, including the maintenance of an adequate fluid intake. Sulfonamides should be used with caution in patients with severe allergy or bronchial asthma, severe impairment of hepatic or renal function, and in patients with glucose-6-phosphate dehydrogenase deficiency since sulfas may cause hemolysis in this latter group.

Carcinogenesis: Rats appear to be especially susceptible to the goitrogenic effects of sulfonamides, and long-term administration has produced thyroid malignancies in the species.

Mutagenesis or Impairment of Fertility: No long-term studies in animals or humans have been conducted.

Pregnancy Category C.: Certain sulfonamides of the short-, intermediate-, and long-acting types, when given to rats and mice in doses 7 to 25 times the human dose, have been associated with a significant increase in the incidence of cleft palate and other bony abnormalities of the offspring. There are no adequate and well-controlled studies in pregnant women. THIOSULFIL® Forte (sulfamethizole 0.5 g) and THIOSULFIL®-A Forte (sulfamethizole 0.5 g with phenazopyridine HCl) should be used during pregnancy only if the potential benefit justifies the potential risk to the fetus.

Nursing Mothers: See Contraindications.

Adverse Reactions:

Blood dyscrasias. Agranulocytosis, aplastic anemia, thrombocytopenia, leukopenia, hemolytic anemia, purpura, hypoprothrombinemia, and methemoglobinemia.

Allergic reactions. Erythema multiforme (Stevens-Johnson Syndrome), generalized skin eruptions, epidermal necrolysis, urticaria, serum sickness, pruritus, exfoliative dermatitis, anaphylactoid reactions, periorbital edema, conjunctival and scleral injection, photosensitization, arthralgia, and allergic myocarditis.

Gastrointestinal reactions. Nausea, emesis, abdominal pains, hepatitis, diarrhea, anorexia, pancreatitis, and stomatitis.

C.N.S. reactions. Headache, peripheral neuritis, mental depression, convulsions, ataxia, hallucinations, tinnitus, vertigo, and insomnia.

Miscellaneous reactions. Drug fever, chills, and toxic nephrosis with oliguria and anuria. Periarteritis nodosum and L.E. phenomenon have occurred.

The sulfonamides bear certain chemical similarities to some goitrogens, diuretics (acetazolamide and the thiazides), and oral hypoglycemic agents. Goiter production, diuresis, and hypoglycemia have occurred rarely in patients receiving sulfonamides. Cross-sensitivity may exist with these agents.

Dosage and Administration: *Adult dosage regimen:*

Start—Bottle No. 1 THIOSULFIL-A Forte (sulfamethizole 0.5 g with phenazopyridine HCl)—Two *yellow* tablets (1 g) four times daily for three days.

Continue—Bottle No. 2 THIOSULFIL Forte (sulfamethizole 0.5 g)—Two *white* tablets (1 g) four times daily for four days. Continue medication as recommended by physician.

If pain persists after a course of THIOSULFIL-A Forte, causes for the discomfort other than infection should be investigated.

How Supplied: THIOSULFIL® (sulfamethizole) DUO-PAK®—NDC 0046-0780-98.

Bottle No. 1—THIOSULFIL®-A Forte: 24 tablets (yellow).

Bottle No. 2—THIOSULFIL® Forte: 32 tablets (white).

[*Shown in Product Identification Section*]

THIOSULFIL® FORTE ℞
Brand of sulfamethizole 0.5 g
and
THIOSULFIL®
Brand of sulfamethizole 0.25 g

Bacteriostatic agent for use in Urinary Tract Infection (due to susceptible organisms)

Description: Chemical name: N′-(5-Methyl-1,3,4-thiadiazol-2-yl) sulfanilamide.
Structural formula:

$H_2N-C_6H_4-SO_2-NH-C_4N_2S-CH_3$ (1,3,4-thiadiazole ring: N—N, C, C, S)

Sulfamethizole is a 5-membered heterocyclic sulfanilamide, occurring as a white or light buff-colored crystalline powder. Solubility in water is dependent upon the pH (1 g/5 ml at pH 7.5; 1 g/4000 ml at pH 6.5). It is soluble in alcohol, and practically insoluble in benzene.

Actions:

Mechanism of sulfonamide bacteriostatic action: The primary mechanism of bacteriostatic action by THIOSULFIL (sulfamethizole) is the same as that of most sulfonamides. By competing with the precursor para-aminobenzoic acid, sulfonamides inhibit bacterial syn-

Continued on next page

Ayerst—Cont.

thesis of folic (pteroylglutamic) acid which is required for bacterial growth. Resistant strains are capable of utilizing folic acid precursors or preformed folic acid.
Antibacterial spectrum: The antibacterial spectrum of all sulfonamides is similar. *In vitro* sensitivity of bacteria to sulfonamides does not always reflect *in vivo* sensitivity. Therefore, efficacy must be carefully evaluated with bacteriologic and clinical responses in the individual patient. (See Warnings)
Factors determining efficacy: Efficacy of antimicrobial therapy is dependent upon a number of factors including the *in vivo* sensitivity of the involved organisms, the concentration of the drug required for bacteriostasis, and the achievable concentration of the sulfonamide at the desired site of action.
Because of the very rapid renal clearance of sulfamethizole, the blood levels attained are low, and accumulation of the drug in tissues outside the urinary tract is very limited. Therefore, sulfamethizole is not appropriate for treatment of systemic infections such as nocardiosis or for local lesions outside the urinary tract such as chancroid and trachoma. However, its low degree of acetylation and its rapid renal clearance permit high concentrations of active sulfamethizole to occur in the urinary tract, making it especially applicable for the treatment of infections of this tract. In addition, the possibility of crystalluria is minimized because of the high solubility of the drug in urine.
Approximately 95 per cent of a given dose of sulfamethizole is not metabolized; less than 5 per cent is acetylated. As a consequence, almost all of a given dose of THIOSULFIL (sulfamethizole) is present in its active form in the body.
Approximately 80 per cent of an administered dose is recoverable within eight hours; approximately 98 per cent is cleared within 15 to 24 hours. Sulfamethizole is cleared by the kidney at a rate only 10 to 20 per cent lower than that for creatinine.
Indications: THIOSULFIL (sulfamethizole) is indicated in the treatment of urinary tract infections (primarily pyelonephritis, pyelitis, and cystitis) in the absence of obstructive uropathy or foreign bodies, when these infections are caused by susceptible strains of the following organisms: *Escherichia coli, Klebsiella-Enterobacter, Staphylococcus aureus, Proteus mirabilis,* and *Proteus vulgaris.*
Important note, *In vitro* sulfonamide sensitivity tests are not always reliable. The test must be carefully coordinated with bacteriologic and clinical reponse. When the patient is already taking sulfonamides, follow-up cultures should have aminobenzoic acid added to the culture media.
Currently, the increasing frequency of resistant organisms is a limitation of the usefulness of antibacterial agents, including the sulfonamides, especially in the treatment of recurrent and complicated urinary tract infections.

Wide variation in blood levels may result with identical doses. Blood levels should be measured in patients receiving sulfonamides for serious infections. Free sulfonamide blood levels of 5–15 mg per 100 ml may be considered therapeutically effective for most infections, with blood levels of 12–15 mg per 100 ml optimal for serious infections; 20 mg per 100 ml should be the maximum total sulfonamide level, as adverse reactions occur more frequently above this level.
Contraindications: Sulfonamides should not be used in patients hypersensitive to sulfa drugs. They should not be used in infants less than two months of age, in pregnancy at term, and during the nursing period because sulfonamides pass the placenta and are excreted in the milk and may cause kernicterus.
Warnings: Sulfonamides should not be used to treat group A streptococci infections or their sequelae. The occurrence of sore throat, fever, pallor, purpura, or jaundice during sulfonamide administration may be an early indication of serious blood dyscrasias.
Deaths associated with the administration of sulfonamides have been reported from hypersensitivity reactions, agranulocytosis, aplastic anemia, and other blood dyscrasias.
Frequent blood counts and renal function tests should be carried out during sulfonamide treatment, especially during prolonged administration. Microscopic urinalyses should be done once a week when a patient is treated for longer than two weeks. Urine cultures should be made to confirm eradication of bacteriuria.

Usage in Pregnancy: The safe use of sulfonamides in pregnancy has not been established. The teratogenicity potential of most sulfonamides has not been thoroughly investigated in either animals or humans. However, a significant increase in the incidence of cleft palate and other bony abnormalities of offspring has been observed when certain sulfonamides of the short-, intermediate-, and long-acting types were given to pregnant rats and mice at high oral doses (7 to 25 times the human dose).
Precautions: The usual precautions used in sulfonamide therapy should be observed, including the maintenance of an adequate fluid intake. Sulfonamides should be used with caution in patients with severe allergy or bronchial asthma, severe impairment of hepatic or renal function, and in patients with glucose-6-phosphate dehydrogenase deficiency since sulfas may cause hemolysis in this latter group.
Adverse Reactions: *Blood dyscrasias.* Agranulocytosis, aplastic anemia, thrombocytopenia, leukopenia, hemolytic anemia, purpura, hypoprothrombinemia, and methemoglobinemia.
Allergic reactions. Erythema multiforme (Stevens-Johnson Syndrome), generalized skin eruptions, epidermal necrolysis, urticaria, serum sickness, pruritus, exfoliative dermatitis, anaphylactoid reactions, periorbital edema, conjunctival and scleral injection, photosensitization, arthralgia, and allergic myocarditis.
Gastrointestinal reactions. Nausea, emesis, abdominal pains, hepatitis, diarrhea, anorexia, pancreatitis, and stomatitis.
C.N.S. reactions. Headache, peripheral neuritis, mental depression, convulsions, ataxia, hallucinations, tinnitus, vertigo, and insomnia.
Miscellaneous reactions. Drug fever, chills, and toxic nephrosis with oliguria and anuria. Periarteritis nodosum and L.E. phenomenon have occurred.
The sulfonamides bear certain chemical similarities to some goitrogens, diuretics (acetazolamide and the thiazides), and oral hypoglycemic agents. Goiter production, diuresis, and hypoglycemia have occurred rarely in patients receiving sulfonamides. Cross-sensitivity may exist with these agents.
Rats appear to be especially susceptible to the goitrogenic effects of sulfonamides, and long term administration has produced thyroid malignancies in the species.
Dosage and Administration: Usual dosage: *Adults:* 0.5 to 1.0 g three or four times daily. *Children and infants* (over 2 months of age): 30 to 45 mg/kg/24 hours, divided into 4 doses.
How Supplied: THIOSULFIL Forte—Each tablet contains sulfamethizole 0.5 g (scored), in bottles of 100 (NDC 0046-0786-81) and 1,000 (NDC 0046-0786-91).
Also in unit dose package of 100 (NDC 0046-0786-99).
THIOSULFIL—Each tablet contains sulfamethizole 0.25 g (scored), in bottles of 100 (NDC 0046-0785-81).
[*Shown in Product Identification Section*]

THIOSULFIL®-A Forte ℞
(sulfamethizole 0.5 g with phenazopyridine HCl)

Each tablet contains:
Sulfamethizole....0.5 g
Phenazopyridine HCl....50.0 mg

and

THIOSULFIL®-A
(sulfamethizole 0.25 g with phenazopyridine HCl)

Each tablet contains:
Sulfamethizole....0.25 g
Phenazopyridine HCl....50.0 mg

Where pain is part of the problem in Urinary Tract Infection (due to susceptible organisms)

Clinical Pharmacology: The combination of sulfamethizole and phenazopyridine HCl acts to eradicate urinary tract infections caused by susceptible organisms and to relieve associated pain and discomfort.
PHENAZOPYRIDINE HCl:
Phenazopyridine HCl is an analgesic that acts on the mucosa of the urinary tract providing relief of pain and discomfort caused by inflammation associated with urinary tract infection.
SULFAMETHIZOLE:
MECHANISM OF SULFONAMIDE BACTERIOSTATIC ACTION: The primary mechanism of bacteriostatic action by THIOSULFIL (sulfamethizole) is the same as that of most sulfonamides. By competing with the precursor para-aminobenzoic acid, sulfonamides inhibit bacterial synthesis of folic (pteroylglutamic) acid which is required for bacterial growth. Resistant strains are capable of utilizing folic acid precursors or preformed folic acid.
SULFONAMIDE ANTIBACTERIAL SPECTRUM: The antibacterial spectrum of all sulfonamides is similar. *In vitro* sensitivity of bacteria to sulfonamides does not always reflect *in vivo* sensitivity. Therefore, efficacy must be carefully evaluated with bacteriologic and clinical responses in the individual patient. (See Warnings)
FACTORS DETERMINING ANTIBACTERIAL EFFICACY: Efficacy of antimicrobial therapy is dependent upon a number of factors including the *in vivo* sensitivity of the involved organisms, the concentration of the drug required for bacteriostasis, and the achievable concentration of the sulfonamide at the desired site of action.
Because of the very rapid renal clearance of sulfamethizole, the blood levels attained are low, and accumulation of the drug in tissues outside the urinary tract is very limited. Therefore, sulfamethizole is not appropriate for treatment of systemic infections such as nocardiosis or for local lesions outside the urinary tract such as chancroid and trachoma. However, its low degree of acetylation and its rapid renal clearance permit high concentrations of active sulfamethizole to occur in the urinary tract, making it especially applicable for the treatment of infections of this tract. In addition, the possibility of crystalluria is minimized because of the high solubility of the drug in urine.
Approximately 95 per cent of a given dose of sulfamethizole is not metabolized; less than 5 per cent is acetylated. As a consequence, almost all of a given dose of THIOSULFIL (sulfamethizole) is present in its active form in the body.
Approximately 80 per cent of an administered dose is recoverable within eight hours; approximately 98 per cent is cleared within 15 to 24 hours. Sulfamethizole is cleared by the kidney at a rate only 10 to 20 per cent lower than that for creatinine.

Indications and Usage: Phenazopyridine HCl is indicated for the treatment of pain, burning, frequency, and urgency caused by the inflammation associated with urinary tract infection.

THIOSULFIL (sulfamethizole) is indicated in the treatment of urinary tract infections (primarily pyelonephritis, pyelitis, and cystitis) in the absence of obstructive uropathy or foreign bodies, when these infections are caused by susceptible strains of the following organisms: *Escherichia coli, Klebsiella-Enterobacter, Staphylococcus aureus, Proteus mirabilis,* and *Proteus vulgaris.*

Important note. *In vitro* sulfonamide sensitivity tests are not always reliable. The test must be carefully coordinated with bacteriologic and clinical reponse. When the patient is already taking sulfonamides, follow-up cultures should have aminobenzoic acid added to the culture media.

Currently, the increasing frequency of resistant organisms is a limitation of the usefulness of antibacterial agents, including the sulfonamides, especially in the treatment of recurrent and complicated urinary tract infections.

Wide variation in blood levels may result with identical doses. Blood levels should be measured in patients receiving sulfonamides for serious infections. Free sulfonamide blood levels of 5–15 mg per 100 ml may be considered therapeutically effective for most infections, with blood levels of 12–15 mg per 100 ml optimal for serious infections; 20 mg per 100 ml should be the maximum total sulfonamide level, as adverse reactions occur more frequently above this level.

Contraindications: Sulfonamides should not be used in patients hypersensitive to sulfa drugs. They should not be used in infants less than two months of age, in pregnancy at term, and during the nursing period because sulfonamides pass the placenta and are excreted in the milk and may cause kernicterus.

Phenazopyridine HCl is contraindicated in renal or hepatic failure, glomerulonephritis, and pyelonephritis of pregnancy with gastrointestinal disturbances.

Warnings: Sulfonamides should not be used to treat group A streptococci infections or their sequelae. The occurrence of sore throat, fever, pallor, purpura, or jaundice during sulfonamide administration may be an early indication of serious blood dyscrasias.

Deaths associated with the administration of sulfonamides have been reported from hypersensitivity reactions, agranulocytosis, aplastic anemia, and other blood dyscrasias.

Frequent blood counts and renal function tests should be carried out during sulfonamide treatment, especially during prolonged administration. Microscopic urinalyses should be done once a week when a patient is treated for longer than two weeks. Urine cultures should be made to confirm eradication of bacteriuria.

Precautions: To allay any possible apprehension, patients should be told that this medication may color the urine orange or red.

The usual precautions used in sulfonamide therapy should be observed, including the maintenance of an adequate fluid intake. Sulfonamides should be used with caution in patients with severe allergy or bronchial asthma, severe impairment of hepatic or renal function, and in patients with glucose-6-phosphate dehydrogenase deficiency since sulfas may cause hemolysis in this latter group.

Carcinogenesis: Rats appear to be especially susceptible to the goitrogenic effects of sulfonamides, and long-term administration has produced thyroid malignancies in the species.

Mutagenesis or Impairment of Fertility: No long-term studies in animals or humans have been conducted.

Pregnancy Category C: Certain sulfonamides of the short-, intermediate-, and long-acting types, when given to rats and mice in doses 7 to 25 times the human dose, have been associated with a significant increase in the incidence of cleft palate and other bony abnormalities of the offspring. There are no adequate and well-controlled studies in pregnant women. THIOSULFIL®-A (sulfamethizole 0.25 g with phenazopyridine HC1 and THIOSULFIL®-A Forte (sulfamethizole 0.5 g with phenazopyridine HCl) should be used during pregnancy only if the potential benefit justifies the potential risk to the fetus.

Nursing Mothers: See Contraindications.

Adverse Reactions:

Blood dyscrasias. Agranulocytosis, aplastic anemia, thrombocytopenia, leukopenia, hemolytic anemia, purpura, hypoprothrombinemia, and methemoglobinemia.

Allergic reactions. Erythema multiforme (Stevens-Johnson Syndrome), generalized skin eruptions, epidermal necrolysis, urticaria, serum sickness, pruritus, exfoliative dermatitis, anaphylactoid reactions, periorbital edema, conjunctival and scleral injection, photosensitization, arthralgia, and allergic myocarditis.

Gastrointestinal reactions. Nausea, emesis, abdominal pains, hepatitis, diarrhea, anorexia, pancreatitis, and stomatitis.

C.N.S. reactions. Headache, peripheral neuritis, mental depression, convulsions, ataxia, hallucinations, tinnitus, vertigo, and insomnia.

Miscellaneous reactions. Drug fever, chills, and toxic nephrosis with oliguria and anuria. Periarteritis nodosum and L.E. phenomenon have occurred.

The sulfonamides bear certain chemical similarities to some goitrogens, diuretics (acetazolamide and the thiazides), and oral hypoglycemic agents. Goiter production, diuresis, and hypoglycemia have occurred rarely in patients receiving sulfonamides. Cross-sensitivity may exist with these agents.

Dosage and Administration: Usual dosage (based on sulfamethizole content): *Adults:* 0.5 to 1.0 g three or four times daily.

THIOSULFIL-A Forte and THIOSULFIL-A are recommended for use in the initial phase of urinary tract infection when there is associated pain. After relief of pain has been obtained, treatment of the infection with sulfamethizole alone should be considered. If pain persists, other causes for the discomfort should be investigated.

How Supplied: THIOSULFIL-A Forte (sulfamethizole 0.5 g, phenazopyridine HCl 50.0 mg) Tablets, in bottles of 100 (NDC 0046-0783-81). THIOSULFIL-A (sulfamethizole 0.25 g, phenazopyridine HCl 50.0 mg) Tablets, in bottles of 100 (NDC 0046-0784-81).

[*Shown in Product Identification Section*]

Baker/Cummins

Dermatological Div. of Key Pharmaceuticals, Inc.
50 N.W. 176TH STREET
MIAMI, FLORIDA 33169

COMPLEX 15

(See PDR For Nonprescription Drugs)

P&S® LIQUID

(See PDR For Nonprescription Drugs)

P&S® PLUS GEL

(See PDR For Nonprescription Drugs)

P&S® SHAMPOO
Antiseborrheic Shampoo

(See PDR For Nonprescription Drugs)

ULTRA MIDE 25

(See PDR For Nonprescription Drugs)

XSEB® SHAMPOO

(See PDR For Nonprescription Drugs)

XSEB®-T SHAMPOO

(See PDR For Nonprescription Drugs)

Barnes-Hind/Hydrocurve, Inc.

895 KIFER ROAD
SUNNYVALE, CA 94086

BARSEB® HC SCALP LOTION ℞
(hydrocortisone)

BARSEB® THERA=SPRAY® ℞
Topical Aerosol

Description: BARSEB® HC contains hydrocortisone 1%, salicylic acid 0.5%, isopropyl alcohol 45%, isopropyl myristate, propylene glycol, ascorbic acid, and citric acid.

BARSEB® THERA=SPRAY—Each 84g bottle contains 360 mg. hydrocortisone, 288 mg. salicylic acid, 14 mg. benzalkonium chloride, propylene glycol, isopropyl myristate, 46 g. alcohol, and butane (propellant). After evaporation of the propellant, the vehicle contains 0.6% hydrocortisone, 0.48% salicylic acid, and 0.024% benzalkonium chloride.

Actions: Primarily effective because of the anti-inflammatory, antipruritic, and vasoconstrictive actions of hydrocortisone, and salicylic acid aids in loosening and removing adherent sebum, crusts, and epithelial debris.

Indications: BARSEB® THERA=SPRAY® and BARSEB® HC are indicated for the relief of the inflammatory manifestations of corticosteroid-responsive dermatoses of the scalp.

Contraindications: Topical steroids are contraindicated in those patients with a history of hypersensitivity to any of the components of the preparations.

Precautions: If irritation develops, discontinue use and institute appropriate therapy.

In the presence of an infection, use of an appropriate antifungal or antibacterial agent should be instituted. If a favorable response does not occur promptly, application of Barseb should be discontinued until the infection has been adequately controlled.

If extensive areas are treated or if the occlusive technique is used, there will be increased systemic absorption of the corticosteroid and suitable precautions should be taken, particularly with children and infants.

Avoid inhalation, ingestion or contact with the eyes or nose. If spray accidentally gets into eyes, flush with copious amounts of water.

Although topical steroids have not been reported to have an adverse effect on human pregnancy, the safety of their use in pregnant women has not absolutely been established. In laboratory animals, increases in incidence of fetal abnormalities have been associated with exposure of gestating females to topical corticosteroids, in some cases at rather low dosage levels. Therefore, drugs of this class should not be used extensively on pregnant patients, in large amounts, or for prolonged periods of time.

These preparations are not for ophthalmic use or use around the eyes. Do not spray BARSEB® THERA-SPRAY toward an open flame. Contents under pressure. Do not puncture or or incinerate. Keep out of reach of children.

Adverse Reactions: The following local adverse reactions have been reported with topical corticosteroids, especially under occlusive

Continued on next page

Barnes-Hind/Hydrocurve—Cont.

dressings: burning, itching, irritation, dryness, folliculitis, hypertrichosis, acneform eruptions, hypopigmentation, perioral dermatitis, allergic contact dermatitis, maceration of the skin, secondary infection, skin atrophy, striae, and miliaria.
Transient discomfort may occur when first applied to an inflamed scalp.
Dosage and Administration: BARSEB® THERA=SPRAY should be applied once daily during the acute phase or as directed by a physician. A maintenance schedule may be adjusted to the patient's response to therapy.
Directions For Use: BARSEB® HC—Part hair, apply once or twice a day with gentle rubbing. Use BARSEB® HC sparingly. BARSEB® THERA=SPRAY-shake well. Hold the bottle upright (being careful not to spray forehead or eyes); insert applicator tube through hair to scalp at front hairline. Then start spraying and moving applicator tube slowly toward the back of the head. Repeat this procedure until all affected areas of the scalp are treated. Because of the spreading and penetrating properties of BARSEB® THERA=SPRAY it is not necessary to rub or massage medication into the scalp. Assembly directions are provided.
How Supplied: BARSEB® THERA=SPRAY is supplied in 84g aerosol bottles with applicator tube.
BARSEB® HC is supplied in 1¾ fl. oz. (52 ml.) plastic squeeze bottles.
Store at room temperature, avoid excessive heat (104°F).

KOMED® Acne Lotion — OTC

Sodium thiosulfate	8%
Salicylic acid	2%
Isopropyl alcohol	25%

The above product also contains menthol, camphor, colloidal alumina, edetate disodium, and purified water.
Indications: Primarily indicated for the treatment of acne associated with oily skin. KOMED Acne Lotion is indicated in more severe conditions or where stronger keratolytic effect is desired. Komed Lotion features a thixotropic gel of colloidal alumina. It is greaseless and dries to an almost invisible film, forming a medicated base over which non-oily cosmetics may be applied.
Precautions: Do not use Komed Lotion on or near the eyes.
Dosage and Administration: Wash affected areas thoroughly. Shake lotion well and apply a thin film twice a day.
How Supplied: 1¾ fl. oz. (52.5 ml.) plastic squeeze bottles.

KOMED® HC Lotion — ℞
(hydrocortisone)

Description: Contains hydrocortisone acetate 0.5%, sodium thiosulfate 8%, salicylic acid 2%, isopropyl alcohol 25%, menthol, camphor, colloidal alumina, edetate disodium, and purified water.
Indications: KOMED HC Acne Lotion is indicated for topical treatment of acne conditions when accompanied by inflammation. KOMED HC features a thixotropic gel of colloidal alumina. The lotion is greaseless and dries to an almost invisible film, forming a medicated base over which non-oily cosmetics may be applied.
Contraindications: Topical steroids are contraindicated in those patients with a history of hypersensitivity to any of the components of the preparation.
Precautions: If irritation develops, the product should be discontinued and appropriate therapy instituted.
In the presence of an infection, the use of an appropriate antifungal or antibacterial agent should be instituted. If a favorable response does not occur promptly, the corticosteroid should be discontinued until the infection has been adequately controlled.
If extensive areas are treated or if the occlusive technique is used, there will be increased systemic absorption of the corticosteroid and suitable precautions should be taken, particularly in children and infants.
Although topical steroids have not been reported to have an adverse effect on human pregnancy, the safety of their use in pregnant women has not been absolutely established. In laboratory animals, increases in incidence of fetal abnormalities have been associated with exposure of gestating females to topical corticosteroids. Therefore, drugs of this class should not be used extensively on pregnant patients, in large amounts, or for prolonged periods of time.
Not for Ophthalmic Use or Use Around the Eyes.
Adverse Reactions: The following local adverse reactions have been reported with topical corticosteroids especially under occlusive dressings: burning, itching, irritation, dryness, folliculitis, hypertrichosis, acneform eruptions, hypopigmentation, perioral dermatitis, allergic contact dermatitis, maceration of the skin, secondary infection, skin atrophy, striae, and miliaria.
Dosage and Administration: Wash affected areas thoroughly. Shake lotion well and apply a thin film twice a day, or as directed.
How Supplied: 1¾ fl. oz. (52.5 ml.) plastic squeeze bottles. Store at room temperature, avoid excessive heat.

KOMEX® — OTC
(Scrub for Oily Skin and Acne)

Description: KOMEX® is a dissolving cleanser useful as an aid in reducing oily skin conditions associated with acne.
Contents: SCRUBULES, Barnes-Hind brand of dissolving particles (sodium tetraborate decahydrate), in a preserved base containing a unique combination of surface active soapless cleaning agents, and skin conditioners.
Directions: Use Komex in place of your usual soap or cleanser.
Skin Cleansing: Wet the face with warm water. Squeeze Komex onto your fingertips, and gently massage into the face. Continue scrubbing and adding water until Scrubules are completely dissolved (about one minute). Rinse thoroughly and dry. Use once or twice daily.
Caution: Avoid contact with eyes. If granules get into the eyes, flush thoroughly with water and avoid rubbing eyes. If skin irritation or excessive dryness develops, or increases, discontinue use. For external use only. Keep out of reach of children. Not to be used on infants. Do not use on inflamed skin.
How Supplied: 2.65 oz. (75 g.) plastic squeeze tube in unit carton.

PRO-CORT™ — OTC
(Hydrocortisone ½% Cream–Unscented)

PRO-CORT M™ — OTC
(Hydrocortisone ½% Cream–Scented)

Description: Pro-Cort and Pro-Cort M medication, with hydrocortisone ½%, is blended with a cooling, soothing emollient skin cream base (scented or unscented).
Indications: Pro-Cort's cooling, soothing and anti-itching properties offer effective, temporary relief of minor skin irritations, itching and rashes due to eczema, dermatitis, insect bites, poison ivy, poison sumac, soaps, detergents, cosmetics, and jewelry and for itchy genital and anal areas.
Directions for Use: For adults and children 2 years of age and older—apply to affected area not more than 3 to 4 times daily. For children under 2 years of age, there is no recommended dosage except under the advice and supervision of a physician.
Warnings: For external use only. Avoid contact with the eyes. Keep out of the reach of children.
How Supplied: Pro-Cort ½% is supplied in ½ oz. (15 g) tube or 1 oz. (30 g) tube in unit carton. Pro-Cort M ½% is supplied in 1 oz. (30 g) tube in unit carton.

TINVER® LOTION — ℞

Description: Sodium thiosulfate 25%, salicylic acid 1%, isopropyl alcohol 10%, propylene glycol, menthol, edetate disodium, colloidal alumina, purified water.
Indications: For topical use in treatment of tinea versicolor infections.
Precautions: Discontinue use if irritation or sensitivity develops. Do not use on or about the eyes.
Dosage and Administration: Thoroughly wash, rinse, and dry affected and susceptible areas before application. Apply thin film of TINVER twice a day. Although diagnostic evidence of the disease may disappear in a few days, it is advisable to continue treatment for a much longer period. Clothing should be boiled to prevent reinfection.
How Supplied: 6 fl. oz. (180 ml.) plastic squeeze bottles. Store at room temperature, avoid excessive heat.

A. J. Bart, Inc.
POST OFFICE BOX 628
MUNOZ RIVERA 938
PENUELAS, PUERTO RICO 00724

ALBAFORT® INJECTABLE — ℞
(Iron and B Complex)

Composition: Each ml of Albafort (Iron and B Complex) Injection contains: Iron as ferrous gulconate 50 mg; Vit. B_{12} 100 mcg; 20% Liver Extract N.F., (Vit. B_{12} eq. 10 mcq/ml); Thiamine HCl 12.5 mg; Riboflavin 0.5 mg; Pyridoxine HCl 2.0 mg, Panthenol 1.0 mg; Niacinamide 12.5 mg, with phenol 0.5% and Benzyl alcohol 1.5% as preservatives, water for injection q.s.
Actions: Albafort (Iron and B Complex) provides a combination of the hematinic effect of iron and the hematopoietic effect of liver.
Indications: Albafort (Iron and B Complex) is indicated in the treatment of hypochromic and macrocytic anemias, pernicious anemia and sprue that responds to B_{12} therapy. Hypochromic anemias are mostly due to prolonged loss of blood of the gastrointestinal tract, urinary tract and uterus. In addition, iron requirements must be increased at certain times of life such as, infancy and childhood, puberty (especially in females), during pregnancy and menopause. Albafort offers a balanced and stable formula for the treatment of hypochromic anemias.
Advantages: Iron in Albafort does not stain the skin. A Z-track technique need not be used nor deep needle injection in the gluteal area. No soft-tissue sarcomas have developed at site of injection as with iron dextran; no iron bound permanently to muscle and no fibromyositis. Due to the presence of 20% liver (ferritin present in liver) an excellent iron binding capacity occurs so there is more stimulation of the bone marrow to produce more erythrocites and greater levels of hemoglobin are obtained.
Warnings: As with other iron compounds toxic symptoms may occur at injection. The immediate reactions most frequently found are vomiting, nausea, lowering of blood pressure and pallor. These reactions are transitory and not frequent with ferrous gluconate. Some patients are sensitive to liver. Keep in a dark place at low temperature. DO NOT USE IF

SEDIMENTATION OR PRECIPITATION SHOWS.
Contraindication: Individuals who have shown hypersensitivity to any of its components.
Dosage: Children—½ to 1 ml once or twice a week. Adults—1 to 2 ml once or twice a week or as the physician thinks necessary. For intramuscular use only.
How Supplied: 10 ml multidose vials (NDC 10023-100-10).
[*Shown in Product Identification Section*]

ALBA-LYBE® OTC

Composition: Each 5 cc contains: Lysine Monohydrochloride 275 mg., Vit. B_{12} Crystalline 10 mcq., Thiamine HCl 5 mg., Riboflavin 4 mg., Pyridoxine HCl 1 mg., Niacinamide 35 mg., Calcium Pantothenate 7 mg., Sorbitol q.s. (imitation sherry wine flavor).
Actions: Alba-Lybe provides lysine as an appetite stimulant and sorbitol q.s. to provide greater absorption of B_{12} and lysine.
Indications: As dietetic supplement of all ages, especially in states of anorexia and convalescence.
Advantages: Alba-Lybe can be administered to patients including the diabetic patient since it contains sorbitol. Sorbitol q.s. base has the advantage over the alcohol base since sorbitol is absorbed much more rapidly than alcohol, as well as the fact that the molecules of lysine and B_{12} adhere to sorbitol. This results in greater appetite and fixing of proteins producing weight increase and better anabolic results.
Dosage: Children—½ to 1 teaspoonful three times a day. Adults—1 tablespoonful three times a day.
How Supplied: 6 oz. bottle (NDC 10023-101-06).
[*Shown in Product Identification Section*]

ALBATUSSIN® OTC
(Antitussive, Expectorant, Sugar Free)

Composition: Each 5 cc contains: Dextromethorphan HBr 10 mg., pyrilamine maleate 8.33 mg., potassium guaiacolsulfonate 75 mg., phenylephrine HBr 5 mg., sodium citrate 215 mg., citric acid 50 mg., alcohol 4% with menthol, thymol and tolu in a sugar free base.
Actions: Albatussin suppresses coughing, helps in nasal decongestion, sneezing and expectoration.
Indications: For coughing relief due to colds or allergy, as well as an expectorant.
Advantages: Albatussin has a nice, pleasing flavor and can be given to diabetic patients and children of all ages as well as adults.
Dosage: Adults and older children—1 or 2 teaspoonfuls; Children six to twelve years—1 teaspoonful; four to six years—½ to 1 teaspoonful; one to four years—½ teaspoonful; under one year—¼ to ½ teaspoonful. These dosages should be given every four hours.
How Supplied: 4 oz bottle (NDC 10023-104-04).

TIA-DOCE® INJECTABLE MONOVIAL ℞
(B_{12}—B_1)

Composition: Each cc in the univial, after reconstitution, contains: Cyanocobalamin (Vit. B_{12}) 1000 mcq., Thiamine HCl (Vit. B_1) 100 mg. in bacteriostatic water for injection, 0.9% Benzyl Alcohol, NaOH and HCl for pH control.
Actions and Indications: Tia-Doce Univial is intended for the prevention and treatment of a variety of disorders associated with Vitamin B_1 deficiency as well as for the managment of certain sensory neuropathies responding to massive doses of Vit. B_{12}. Specifically Vitamin B_1 is indicated in the prevention and treatment of beriberi and in the correction of anorexia of dietary origin.
Advantages: Tia-Doce is a stable combination of Vit. B_{12} and Vit. B_1. Since they are separated in the univial there is no reaction between them, resulting in less oxidation of the vitamins and no reduction of vitamin potency. Tia-Doce can be administered either intramuscularly, intravenously, or subcutaneously.
Warnings: Allergic and anaphilactic reactions may occur after frequent I.V. dosage. Contraindicated in persons who are hypersensitive to any of its components.
Dosage: Tia-Doce is administered 0.5 to 1 cc intramuscularly or intravenously daily or as needed. Can be used 1 cc/500 ml of dextrose for I.V. difusion.
How Supplied: Tia-Doce is supplied in 10 cc univials containing the freeze dried Vit. B_1 in the lower chamber and Vit. B_{12} in bacteriostatic water in the upper chamber (NDC 10023-126-10).
[*Shown in Product Identification Section*]

Bay Pharmaceuticals, Inc.
1111 FRANCISCO BLVD.
SAN RAFAEL, CA 94901

BAYTAC™-3 ℞
(Sterile Triamcinolone Acetonide Suspension)
3 mg./ml.
NOT FOR INTRAVENOUS USE
FOR INTRALESIONAL AND INTRADERMAL USE

Description: BayTac-3 is a white to cream-colored, crystalline powder, having not more than a slight odor.
It is practically insoluble in water, very soluble in dehydrated alcohol, in chloroform, and in methanol.

$C_{24}H_{31}FO_6$ 434.50

Pregna-1,4-diene-3,20-dione, 9-fluoro-11,21-dihydroxy-16,17-[(1-methylethylidene)bis(oxy)]-, (11β,16α)-.
9-Fluro-11β,16α17,21-tetrahydroxypregna-1, 4-diene-3,20-dione cyclic 16,17-acetal with acetone [*76-25-5*].
Each ml. of aqueous suspension contains: Triamcinolone Acetonide 3 mg., Sodium Chloride 2 mg., Carboxymethylcellulose Sodium 7.5 mg., Polysorbate 80-0.4 mg., Benzyl Alcohol 0.9% as preservative in Water for Injection q.s. Sodium Hydroxide and/or Hydrochloric Acid used to adjust pH.
Clinical Pharmacology: Naturally occurring glucocorticoids (hydrocortisone), which also have salt-retaining properties, are used as replacement therapy in adrenocortical deficiency states. Their synthetic analogs are primarily used for their potent anti-inflammatory effects in disorders of many organ systems. Glucocorticoids cause profound and varied metabolic effects. In addition, they modify the body's immune responses to diverse stimuli.
Indications and Usage: Intradermal—Intralesional administration is indicated for the treatment of keloids, discoid lupus erythematosus, necrobiosis lipoidica diabeticorum, alopecia areata, and localized hypertrophic, infiltrated, inflammatory lesions of: lichen planus, psoriatic plaques, granuloma annulare, and lichen simplex chronicus (neurodermatitis).
Contraindications: Systemic fungal infections.
Warnings: In patients on corticosteroid therapy subjected to any unusual stress, increased dosage of rapidly acting corticosteroids before, during, and after the stressful situation is indicated.
Corticosteroids may mask some signs of infection, and new infections may appear during their use. There may be decreased resistance and inability to localize infection when corticosteroids are used.
Prolonged use of corticosteroids may produce posterior subcapsular cataracts, glaucoma with possible damage to the optic nerves and may enhance the establishment of secondary ocular infections due to fungi or viruses.
Usage in pregnancy: Since adequate human reproduction studies have not been done with corticosteroids, the use of these drugs in pregnancy, nursing mothers, or women of childbearing potential requires that the possible benefits of the drug be weighed against the potential hazards to the mother and embryo or fetus. Infants born of mothers who have received substantial doses of corticosteroids during pregnancy should be carefully observed for signs of hypoadrenalism.
Average and large doses of cortisone or hydrocortisone can cause elevation of blood pressure, salt and water retention, and increased excretion of potassium. These effects are less likely to occur with the synthetic derivatives except when used in large doses. Dietary salt restriction and potassium supplementation may be necessary. All corticosteroids increase calcium excretion.
While on Corticosteroid Therapy Patients Should Not Be Vaccinated Against Smallpox. Other Immunization Procedures Should Not be Undertaken in Patients Who Are on Corticosteroids, Especially in High Doses, Because of Possible Hazards of Neurological Complications and Lack of Antibody Response.
The use of Triamcinolone Acetonide in active tuberculosis should be restricted to those cases of fulminating or disseminated tuberculosis in which the corticosteroid is used for the management of the disease in conjunction with appropriate antituberculous regimen.
If corticosteroids are indicated in patients with latent tuberculosis or tuberculin reactivity, close observation is necessary as reactivation of the disease may occur. During prolonged corticosteroid therapy, these patients should receive chemoprophylaxis.
Because rare instances of anaphylactoid reactions have occurred in patients receiving parenteral corticosteroid therapy, appropriate precautionary measures should be taken prior to administration, especially when the patient has a history of allergy to any drug.
Precautions: Drug-induced secondary adrenocortical insufficiency may be minimized by gradual reduction of dosage. This type of relative insufficiency may persist for months after discontinuation of therapy; therefore, in any situation of stress occurring during that period, hormone therapy should be reinstituted. Since mineralocorticoid secretion may be impaired, salt and/or a mineralocorticoid should be administered concurrently.
There is an enhanced effect of corticosteroids in patients with hypethyroidism and in those with cirrhosis.
Corticosteroids should be used cautiously in patients with ocular herpes simplex for fear of corneal perforation.
The lowest possible dose of corticosteroid should be used to control the condition under treatment, and when reduction in dosage is possible, the reduction must be gradual.
Psychic derangements may appear when corticosteroids are used, ranging from euphoria, insomnia, mood swings, personality changes, and severe depression to frank psychotic manifestations. Also, existing emotional instability or psychotic tendencies may be aggravated by corticosteroids.
Aspirin should be used cautiously in conjunction with corticosteroids in hypoprothrombinemia.

Continued on next page

Bay Pharm.—Cont.

Although controlled clinical trials have shown corticosteroids to be effective in speeding the resolution of acute exacerbations of multiple sclerosis they do not show that they affect the ultimate outcome or natural history of the disease. The studies do show that relatively high doses of corticosteroids are necessary to demonstrate a significant effect (See DOSAGE AND ADMINISTRATION Section).

Since complications of treatment with glucocorticoids are dependent on the size of the dose and the duration of treatment a risk/benefit decision must be made in each individual case as to dose and duration of treatment and as to whether daily or intermittent therapy should be used.

Steroids should be used with caution in nonspecific ulcerative colitis, if there is a probability of impending perforation, abscess or other pyogenic infection, also in diverticulitis, fresh intestinal anastomoses, active or latent peptic ulcer, renal insufficiency, hypertension, osteoporosis, and myasthenia gravis.

Growth and development of infants and children on prolonged corticosteroid therapy should be carefully followed.

The following additional precautions apply for parenteral corticosteroids. Intra-articular injection of a corticosteroids may produce systemic as well as local effects. Appropriate examination of any joint fluid present is necessary to exclude a septic process.

A marked increase in pain accompanied by local swelling, further restriction of joint motion, fever, and malaise are suggestive of septic arthritis. If this complication occurs and the diagnosis of sepsis is confirmed, appropriate antimicrobial therapy should be instituted.

Local injection of a steroid into a previously infected joint is to be avoided.

Corticosteroids should not be injected into unstable joints.

The slower rate of absorption by intramuscular administration should be recognized.

Adverse Reactions: Fluid and electrolyte disturbances: Sodium retention; fluid retention; congestive heart failure in susceptible patients; potassium loss; hypokalemic alkalosis; hypertension.

Musculoskeletal: Muscle weakness; steroid myopathy; loss of muscle mass; osteoporosis; vertebral compression fractures; aseptic necrosis of femoral and humeral heads; pathologic fracture of long bones.

Gastrointestinal: Peptic ulcer with possible subsequent perforation and hemorrhage; pancreatitis; abdominal distention; ulcerative esophagitis.

Dermatologic: Impaired wound healing, thin fragile skin; petechiae and ecchymoses, facial erythemia; increased sweating; may suppress reactions to skin tests.

Neurological: Increased intracranial pressure with papilledema (pseudotumor cerebri) usually after treatment; convulsions; vertigo; headache.

Endocrine: Menstrual irregularities; development of Cushingoid state; suppression of growth in children; secondary adrenocortical and pituitary unresponsiveness, particularly in times of stress, as in trauma, surgery, or illness; decreased carbohydrate tolerance; manifestations of latent diabetes mellitus; increased requirements for insulin or oral hypoglycemic agents in diabetes.

Ophthalmic: Posterior subcapsular cataracts; increased intraocular pressure; glaucoma; exophthalmos.

Metabolic: Negative nitrogen balance due to protein catabolism.

The following additional adverse reactions are related to parenteral corticosteroid therapy: Rare instances of blindness associated with intralesional therapy around the face and head; hyperpigmentation and hypopigmentation; subcutaneous and cutaneous atrophy; sterile abscess; postinjection flare, (following intra-articular use); charcot-like arthropathy.

Drug Abuse and Dependence: (See WARNINGS Section).

Overdosage: (See ADVERSE REACTIONS Section).

Dosage and Administration: For intradermal administration, the initial dose of BayTac-3 will vary depending upon the specific disease entity being treated but should be limited to 1.0 mg. per injection site, since larger volumes are more likely to produce cutaneous atrophy. Multiple sites (separated by one centimeter or more) may be so injected, keeping in mind that the greater the *total* volume employed the more corticosteroid becomes available for possible systemic absorption and subsequent corticosteroid effects. Such injections may be repeated, if necessary, at weekly or less frequent intervals. Dosage requirements are variable and must be individualized on the basis of the disease under treatment and the response of the patient. Dosage in children under 12 has not been established.

For treatment of dermal lesions, inject directly into the lesion, i.e. intradermally or sometimes subcutaneously. For accuracy of dosage measurement and ease of administration, it is preferable to employ a tuberculin syringe and a small bore needle (23- to 25-gauge). Ethyl chloride spray may be used to alleviate the discomfort of the injection.

How Supplied: Multiple dose vials of 5 ml. containing Triamcinolone Acetonide 3 mg. per ml.

STORE AT ROOM TEMPERATURE
AVOID FREEZING

Caution: Federal law prohibits dispensing without prescription.

Beach Pharmaceuticals

Division of BEACH PRODUCTS, INC.
5220 SOUTH MANHATTAN AVE.
TAMPA, FL 33611

BEELITH Tablets — OTC

Description: Each tablet contains magnesium oxide 600 mg and pyridoxine hydrochloride (Vitamin B_6) 25 mg equivalent to B_6 20 mg.

Warning: Keep this and all drugs out of the reach of children. In case of accidental overdose, seek professional assistance or contact a Poison Control Center immediately.

Actions and Uses: BEELITH is a dietary supplement for patients deficient in magnesium and/or pyridoxine. Each tablet yields approximately 362 mg. of elemental magnesium & supplies 1000% of the Adult U.S. Recommended Daily Allowance (RDA) for Vitamin B_6 & 90% of the RDA for magnesium.

Dosage: The usual adult dose is one or two tablets daily.

Precaution: Excessive dosage might cause laxation.

Caution: Use only under the supervision of a physician. Use with caution in renal insufficiency.

Drug Interaction Precautions: Do not take this product if you are presently taking a prescription antibiotic drug containing any form of tetracycline.

Storage: Keep tightly closed. Store at controlled room temperature 15°C–30°C (59°F–86°F).

[*Shown in Product Identification Section*]

K-PHOS® M.F. (Modified Formula) — ℞

Urinary Acidifier
Phosphorus Supplement

Description: Each tablet contains potassium acid phosphate 155 mg and sodium acid phosphate, anhydrous 350 mg. Each tablet yields approximately 125.6 mg of phosphorus, 44.5 mg of potassium or 1.14 mEq and 67 mg of sodium or 2.9 mEq. Two K-PHOS® M.F. tablets supply approximately 25% of the U.S. Recommended Daily Allowance (U.S. RDA) of phosphorus for adults and children 4 or more years of age and 19% of the U.S. RDA for pregnant or lactating women.

Actions: K-PHOS M.F. is a highly effective urinary acidifier. Also, the phosphate component reduces urinary calcium and increases urinary orthophosphate.

Indications: For use in patients with elevated urinary pH. Also, helps keep calcium soluble and reduces odor and rash caused by ammoniacal urine. Also, by acidifying the urine it increases the antibacterial activity of methenamine mandelate and methenamine hippurate.

Contraindications: Renal insufficiency, severe hepatic disease, Addison's disease and hyperkalemia.

Side Effects: Some patients may experience mild laxation which will usually subside by reducing the dosage. If laxation persists, the drug should be discontinued. Hyperacidity and nausea may also occur.

Precaution: Use with caution if the patient is on a sodium restricted diet.

Dosage and Administration: K-PHOS® (Modified Formula). Two tablets four times daily with a full glass of water.

Caution: Federal law prohibits dispensing without prescription.

Storage: Keep tightly closed. Store at controlled room temperature, 15°C–30°C (59°F–86°F).

How Supplied: Bottles of 100 and 500 tablets.

Diets Available: Beach's Acid Ash Guide and Beach's Low Calcium Acid Ash Guide Diets with literature available upon request.

[*Shown in Product Identification Section*]

K-PHOS® No. 2 — ℞

Urinary Acidifier
Phosphorus Supplement

Description: Each tablet contains potassium acid phosphate 305 mg and sodium acid phosphate, anhydrous 700 mg. Each tablet yields approximately 250 mg of phosphorus, 88 mg of potassium or 2.25 mEq and 134 mg of sodium or 5.83 mEq. Each tablet supplies approximately 25% of the U.S. Recommended Daily Allowance (U.S. RDA) of phosphorus for adults and children 4 or more years of age and 19% of the U.S. RDA for pregnant or lactating women.

Actions: K-PHOS No. 2 is a highly effective urinary acidifier. Also, the phosphate component reduces urinary calcium and increases urinary orthophosphate.

Indications: For use in patients with elevated urinary pH. Also, helps keep calcium soluble and reduce odor and rash caused by ammoniacal urine. Also, by acidifying the urine it increases the antibacterial activity of methenamine mandelate and methenamine hippurate.

Contraindications: Renal insufficiency, severe hepatic disease, Addison's disease and hyperkalemia.

Side Effects: Some patients may experience mild laxation which will usually subside by reducing the dosage. If laxation persists, the drug should be discontinued. Hyperacidity and nausea may also occur.

Precaution: Use with caution if the patient is on a sodium restricted diet.

Dosage and Administration: One tablet four times daily with a full glass of water. When the urine is difficult to acidify administer one tablet every two hours not to exceed eight tablets in a 24 hour period.

Caution: Federal law prohibits dispensing without prescription.

Storage: Keep tightly closed. Store at controlled room temperature, 15°C–30°C (59°F–86°F).
How Supplied: Bottles of 100 and 500 tablets.
Diets Available: Beach's Acid Ash Guide and Beach's Low Calcium Acid Ash Guide Diets with literature available upon request.
[*Shown in Product Identification Section*]

K-PHOS® NEUTRAL Tablets ℞
Phosphorus Supplement

Description: Each tablet contains dibasic sodium phosphate, anhydrous 852 mg, potassium acid phosphate 155 mg and sodium acid phosphate, monohydrate 130 mg. Each tablet yields approximately 250 mg of phosphorus, 298 mg of sodium or 12.6 mEq and 45 mg of potassium or 1.15 mEq.
Actions and Uses: K-PHOS NEUTRAL lowers urinary calcium levels and increases phosphate and pyrophosphate. As a phosphorous supplement, each tablet supplies 25% of the U.S. Recommended Daily Allowance (U.S. RDA) of phosphorus for adults and children 4 or more years of age and 19% of the U.S. RDA for pregnant or lactating women.
Precaution: Use with caution if on a sodium restricted diet.
Side Effects: Some patients may experience mild laxation which will usually subside by reducing the dosage. If laxation persists, the drug should be discontinued.
Contraindications: Addison's disease and hyperkalemia.
Administration and Dosage: One or two tablets four times a day with a full glass of water.
Caution: Federal law prohibits dispensing without prescription.
Storage: Keep tightly closed. Store at controlled room temperature, 15°C–30°C (59°F–86°F).
How Supplied: Bottles of 100 and 500 tablets.
[*Shown in Product Identification Section*]

K-PHOS® ORIGINAL (Sodium Free) ℞
(Potassium Acid Phosphate)

Description: Each tablet contains potassium acid phosphate 500 mg. Each tablet yields 114 mg of phosphorus and 144 mg of potassium or 3.67 mEq.
Actions: K-PHOS ORIGINAL is a highly effective urinary acidifier. Also, the phosphate component reduces urinary calcium and increases urinary orthophosphate.
Indications: For use in patients with elevated urinary pH. Also, helps keep calcium soluble and reduces odor and rash caused by ammoniacal urine. Also, by acidifying the urine it increases the antibacterial activity of methenamine mandelate and methenamine hippurate.
Contraindications: Renal insufficiency, severe hepatic disease, Addison's disease and hyperkalemia.
Side Effects: Some patients may experience mild laxation which will usually subside by reducing the dosage if laxation persists, the drug should be discontinued. Hyperacidity and nausea may also occur.
Warning: There have been several reports, published and unpublished, concerning nonspecific small-bowel lesions consisting of stenosis, with or without ulceration, associated with the administration of enteric-coated thiazides with potassium salts. These lesions may occur with enteric-coated potassium tablets alone or when they are used with nonenteric coated thiazides or certain other oral diuretics. These small-bowel lesions have caused obstruction, hemorrhage, and perforation. Surgery was frequently required and deaths have occurred. Based on a large survey of physicians and hospitals, both United States and foreign, the incidence of these lesions is low, and a causal relationship in man has not been definitely established. Available information tends to implicate enteric-coated potassium salts, although lesions of this type also occur spontaneously. Therefore, coated potassium-containing formulations should be administered only when indicated and should be discontinued immediately if abdominal pain, distension, nausea, vomiting or gastrointestinal bleeding occur. Coated potassium tablets should be used only when adequate dietary supplementation is not practicable.
When prescribing this product for patients who are receiving concurrent potassium supplementation (e.g., to replace potassium excreted during thiazide therapy), it should be kept in mind that this product also contains potassium. A decrease in supplemental potassium dosage should be considered in order to help avoid hyperkalemia. Administer with caution in digitalized patients.
Dosage and Administration: Two tablets dissolved in 6–8 oz. of water 4 times daily with meals and at bedtime. For best results let the tablets soak in the water for 2–5 minutes, stir vigorously and swallow.
Caution: Federal law prohibits dispensing without prescription.
Storage: Keep tightly closed. Store at controlled room temperature, 15°C–30°C (59°F–86°F).
How Supplied: Bottles of 100 and 500 tablets.
[*Shown in Product Identification Section*]

THIACIDE TABLETS ℞

Description: Each tablet contains methenamine mandelate 500 mg. and potassium acid phosphate 250 mg.
[*Shown in Product Identification Section*]

UROQID–Acid® tablets ℞
UROQID–Acid® No. 2 tablets
Urinary acidifier-Antibacterial

Description: Each UROQID-Acid tablet contains methenamine mandelate 350 mg., sodium acid phosphate, monohydrate 200 mg. Each UROQID-Acid No. 2 tablet contains methenamine mandelate 500 mg., sodium acid phosphate, monohydrate 500 mg.
Actions and Uses: Methenamine mandelate is rapidly absorbed and excreted in the urine. Formaldehyde is released by acid hydrolysis from methenamine with bactericidal levels rapidly reached at pH 5.0. Proportionally less formaldehyde is released as urinary pH approaches 6.0 and insufficient quantities are released above this level for therapeutic response. Since infected urines are frequently above pH 5.0 additional acidification is beneficial. Formaldehyde is 'cidal' against nearly all uropathogens.
Long Term Prophylactic Use: For prevention of reinfection of a sterile urine by converting the urine into an antibacterial medium. Especially useful for long term administration because bacterial resistance will not develop and the components are exceptionally safe.
General Indications: Particularly useful in those infections which are often incurable because of stone or other obstruction, inlying catheter drainage or residual urine in the bladder in neurological disorders. Specifically recommended for the management of chronic urinary tract infections including pyelitis, pyelonephritis, cystitis and infections accompanying neurogenic bladder. Not recommended for acute infections with parenchymal involvement.
Rationale: Methenamine mandelate should not be used unless urinary pH below 6.0 can be maintained. Sodium acid phosphate is a safe, dependable urinary acidifier. The concomitant use of sodium acid phosphate with methenamine mandelate is recommended when the urinary pH is above 6.0. (See U.S. Dispensatory, 1960 Ed., pp 846–847).
Administration and Dosage: UROQID-Acid: initially, 3 tablets 4 times daily. For maintenance, 1 or 2 tablets 4 times daily. UROQID-Acid No. 2: initially, 2 tablets 4 times daily. For maintenance, 2 to 4 tablets daily, in divided doses.
Side Effects: A mild laxative effect may be noted in an occasional patient. Methenamine mandelate may cause gastrointestinal upset and/or dysuria.
Precautions: Urine must be kept acid (on the average below 6.0) or therapy should be discontinued as methenamine mandelate is not effective at higher pH. Frequent urine pH tests are essential. This drug is a urine acidifier and can cause metabolic acidosis. Allergic reactions to methenamine mandelate have been reported.
Use with caution if the patient is on a sodium restricted diet.
Contraindications: Moderate to severe renal insufficiency with acidosis. Severe hepatic disease.
How Supplied: Bottles of 100 and 500.
Literature Available: Literature and Beach's Low Calcium Acid Ash Guide Diet pads are available on request.
[*Shown in Product Identification Section*]

Beecham Products
DIVISION OF BEECHAM INC.
POST OFFICE BOX 1467
PITTSBURGH, PA 15230

MASSENGILL® DISPOSABLE DOUCHE
MASSENGILL® LIQUID CONCENTRATE
MASSENGILL® POWDER

Composition: LIQUID DISPOSABLE DOUCHES: Vinegar and Water Disposable Douche—Water and vinegar.
Country Flowers—Water, SD Alcohol 40, Lactic Acid, Sodium Lactate, Octoxynol-9, Cetylpyridinium Chloride, Sorbic Acid, Disodium EDTA, Fragrance, D&C Red #19.
Mountain Herbs—Water, Octoxynol-9, SD Alcohol 40, Lactic Acid, Sodium Lactate, Cetylpyridinium Chloride, Sorbic Acid, Fragrance, Disodium EDTA, D&C Yellow #10, FD&C Blue #1.
LIQUID CONCENTRATE—Water, Lactic Acid, Sodium Lactate, Octoxynol-9, Methyl Salicylate, menthol, eucalyptus oil, Thymol, D&C Yellow #10, FD&C Yellow #6. Alcohol 25%.
POWDER—Sodium chloride, ammonium alum, PEG-8, phenol, methyl salicylate, eucalyptus oil, menthol, thymol, and color.
Action and Uses: Massengill Disposable Douche, Liquid, and Powder are valuable adjuncts to specific vaginal therapy, following the prescribed use of vaginal medications or contraceptives and in feminine hygiene.
Directions for Use:
LIQUID DISPOSABLE DOUCHE—Twist off tab from bottle containing premixed solution, attach nozzle supplied and use. Unit completely disposable after use.
LIQUID CONCENTRATE—Fill cap three quarters full, to measuring line, and pour contents into douche bag containing one quart of warm water. Mix thoroughly.
POWDER—Dissolve two rounded teaspoonfuls in a quart of warm water and mix thoroughly.
Warning: Vaginal douches should not be used more than twice weekly except on the advice of a physician. If irritation occurs, discontinue use.
How Supplied: LIQUID DISPOSABLE DOUCHE, 6 oz.
LIQUID, 4 oz., 8 oz., plastic bottles. Packettes, 12's.

Continued on next page

Beecham Products—Cont.

POWDER, 4 oz., 8 oz., 16 oz., 22 oz. Packettes, 10's, 12's.
Is This Product O.T.C.: Yes.

MASSENGILL® DISPOSABLE MEDICATED DOUCHE

Active Ingredient: CEPTICIN™ (0.23% povidone-iodine).
Indications: For temporary relief of minor irritation and itching associated with vaginitis due to *Candida albicans, Trichomonas vaginalis* and *Gardnerella vaginalis.*
Actions: Povidone-iodine is widely recognized as an effective broad spectrum microbicide against both gram negative and gram positive bacteria, fungi, yeasts and protozoa. While remaining active in the presence of blood, serum or bodily secretions, it possesses virtually none of the irritating properties of iodine.
Warnings: If symptoms persist after seven days of use, or if redness, swelling or pain develop during treatment, consult a physician. Women with iodine-sensitivity should not use this product. Women may douche during menstruation if they douche gently. Do not douche during pregnancy unless directed by a physician. Douching does not prevent pregnancy. Keep out of the reach of children.
Dosage and Administration: Dosage is provided as a single unit concentrate to be added to 6 oz. of sanitized water supplied in a disposable bottle. A specially designed nozzle is provided. After use the unit is discarded. Use once daily for up to 7 days.
How Supplied: 6 oz. bottle of sanitized water with 0.17 oz. vial of povidone-iodine and nozzle.

Beecham Laboratories

DIV. OF BEECHAM INC.,
501 FIFTH STREET
BRISTOL, TN 37620

PRODUCT IDENTIFICATION CODES

To provide quick and positive identification of Beecham Laboratories' products, we have imprinted a code number or brand name on tablet and capsule products. In order that you may identify a product by its code and number, we have compiled below a numerical list of code numbers with their corresponding product names. The code number as it appears on tablets and capsules bears the letters BMP plus the numerical code. Amoxil® and Fastin® capsules, and Amoxil® Chewable Tablets bear the brand name only.

BMP Code No.	Product
100	ADRENOSEM® SALICYLATE (Carbazochrome Salicylate) Tablets 2.5 mg.
105	ANEXSIA® w/Codeine Tablets
106	ANEXSIA®-D Tablets
107	CONAR®-A Tablets
108	COTROL-D Tablets
109	DASIKON Capsules
112	DASIN® Capsules
119	HYBEPHEN® Tablets
121	LIVITAMIN® Capsules
122	LIVITAMIN® w/INTRINSIC FACTOR Capsules
123	LIVITAMIN® CHEWABLE Tablets
124	LIVITAMIN® PRENATAL Tablets
125	MENEST™ (Esterified Estrogens, U.S.P.) Tablets 0.3 mg.
126	MENEST™ (Esterified Estrogens, U.S.P.) Tablets 0.625 mg.
127	MENEST™ (Esterified Estrogens, U.S.P.) Tablets 1.25 mg.
128	MENEST™ (Esterified Estrogens, U.S.P.) Tablets 2.5 mg.
135	SEMETS®
139	THALFED® Tablets
140	TOTACILLIN® (Ampicillin) Capsules 250 mg.
141	TOTACILLIN® (Ampicillin) Capsules 500 mg.
143	BACTOCILL® (Oxacillin Sodium) Capsules 250 mg.
144	BACTOCILL® (Oxacillin Sodium) Capsules 500 mg.
145	DARICON® (Oxyphencyclimine HCl) Tablets 10 mg.
146	DARICON®-PB (Oxyphencyclimine HCl, 5 mg. and Phenobarbital, 15 mg.) Tablets
156	TIGAN® (Trimethobenzamide HCl) Capsules 100 mg.
157	TIGAN® (Trimethobenzamide HCl) Capsules 250 mg.
165	DYCILL® (Dicloxacillin Sodium) Capsules 250 mg.
166	DYCILL® (Dicloxacillin Sodium) Capsules 500 mg.
167	ACTOL EXPECTORANT® Tablets
169	CLOXAPEN® (Cloxacillin Sodium) Capsules 250 mg.
170	CLOXAPEN® (Cloxacillin Sodium) Capsules 500 mg.
182	NUCOFED® Capsules
194	ENARAX®5 (Oxphencyclimine HCl, 5 mg. and Hydroxyzine HCl, 25 mg.) Tablets
195	ENARAX®10 (Oxphencyclimine HCl, 10 mg, and Hydroxyzine HCl, 25 mg.) Tablets

AMOXIL® ℞
(amoxicillin)
capsules, for oral suspension and chewable tablets

Description: AMOXIL (Amoxicillin) is a semisynthetic antibiotic, an analog of ampicillin, with a broad spectrum of bactericidal activity against many Gram-positive and Gram-negative microorganisms. Chemically it is D-(-)-α-amino-p-hydroxybenzyl penicillin trihydrate.
Actions:
PHARMACOLOGY
Amoxicillin is stable in the presence of gastric acid and may be given without regard to meals. It is rapidly absorbed after oral administration. It diffuses readily into most body tissues and fluids, with the exception of brain and spinal fluid, except when meninges are inflamed. The half-life of amoxicillin is 61.3 minutes. Most of the amoxicillin is excreted unchanged in the urine; its excretion can be delayed by concurrent administration of probenecid. Amoxicillin is not highly protein-bound. In blood serum, Amoxicillin is approximately 20% protein-bound as compared to 60% for penicillin G.
Orally administered doses of 250 mg and 500 mg Amoxicillin capsules result in average peak blood levels one to two hours after administration in the range of 3.5 mcg/ml to 5.0 mcg/ml and 5.5 mcg/ml to 7.5 mcg/ml respectively.
Orally administered doses of Amoxicillin suspension 125 mg/5 ml and 250 mg/5 ml result in average peak blood levels one to two hours after administration in the range of 1.5 mcg/ml to 3.0 mcg/ml and 3.5 mcg/ml to 5.0 mcg/ml respectively. Amoxicillin chewable tablets, 125 mg and 250 mg, produced blood levels similar to those achieved with the corresponding doses of Amoxicillin oral suspensions.
Detectable serum levels are observed up to 8 hours after an orally administered dose of Amoxicillin. Following a 1 Gm dose and utilizing a special skin window technique to determine levels of the antibiotic, it was noted that therapeutic levels were found in the interstitial fluid. Approximately 60 percent of an orally administered dose of Amoxicillin is excreted in the urine within six to eight hours.
MICROBIOLOGY:
AMOXIL (Amoxicillin) is similar to ampicillin in its bactericidal action against susceptible organisms during the stage of active multiplication. It acts through the inhibition of biosynthesis of cell wall mucopeptide. *In vitro* studies have demonstrated the susceptibility of most strains of the following Gram-positive bacteria: alpha- and beta-hemolytic streptococci, *Diplococcus pneumoniae,* nonpenicillinase-producing staphylococci, and *Streptococcus faecalis.* It is active *in vitro* against many strains of *Haemophilus influenzae, Neisseria gonorrhoeae, Escherichia coli* and *Proteus mirabilis.* Because it does not resist destruction by penicillinase, it is not effective against penicillinase-producing bacteria, particularly resistant staphylococci. All strains of Pseudomonas and most strains of Klebsiella and Enterobacter are resistant.
DISC SUSCEPTIBILITY TESTS: Quantitative methods that require measurement of zone diameters give the most precise estimates of antibiotic susceptibility. One such procedure* has been recommended for use with discs for testing susceptibility to ampicillin-class antibiotics. Interpretations correlate diameters of the disc test with MIC values for Amoxicillin. With this procedure, a report from the laboratory of "susceptible" indicates that the infecting organism is likely to respond to therapy. A report of "resistant" indicates that the infecting organism is not likely to respond to therapy. A report of "intermediate susceptibility" suggests that the organism would be susceptible if high dosage is used, or if the infection is confined to tissues and fluids (e.g., urine), in which high antibiotic levels are attained.

*Bauer, A. W., Kirby, W. M. M., Sherris, J. C., and Turck, M.: Antibiotic Testing by a Standardized Single Disc Method, Am. J. Clin. Pathol., 45:493, 1966. Standardized Disc Susceptibility Test, FEDERAL REGISTER 37:20527-29, 1972.

Indications: AMOXIL (Amoxicillin) is indicated in the treatment of infections due to susceptible strains of the following:
Gram-negative organisms—*H. influenzae, E. coli, P. mirabilis* and *N. gonorrhoeae.*
Gram-positive organisms—Streptococci (including *Streptococcus faecalis*), *D. pneumoniae* and nonpenicillinase-producing staphylococci.
Therapy may be instituted prior to obtaining results from bacteriological and susceptibility studies to determine the causative organisms and their susceptibility to Amoxicillin. Indicated surgical procedures should be performed.
Contraindications: A history of allergic reaction to any of the penicillins is a contraindication.
Warnings: SERIOUS AND OCCASIONALLY FATAL HYPERSENSITIVITY (ANAPHYLACTOID) REACTIONS HAVE BEEN

REPORTED IN PATIENTS ON PENICILLIN THERAPY. ALTHOUGH ANAPHYLAXIS IS MORE FREQUENT FOLLOWING PARENTERAL THERAPY, IT HAS OCCURRED IN PATIENTS ON ORAL PENICILLINS. THESE REACTIONS ARE MORE LIKELY TO OCCUR IN INDIVIDUALS WITH A HISTORY OF SENSITIVITY TO MULTIPLE ALLERGENS. THERE HAVE BEEN REPORTS OF INDIVIDUALS WITH A HISTORY OF PENICILLIN HYPERSENSITIVITY WHO HAVE EXPERIENCED SEVERE REACTIONS WHEN TREATED WITH CEPHALOSPORINS. BEFORE THERAPY WITH ANY PENICILLIN, CAREFUL INQUIRY SHOULD BE MADE CONCERNING PREVIOUS HYPERSENSITIVITY REACTIONS TO PENICILLINS, CEPHALOSPORINS, OR OTHER ALLERGENS. IF AN ALLERGIC REACTION OCCURS, APPROPRIATE THERAPY SHOULD BE INSTITUTED AND DISCONTINUANCE OF AMOXICILLIN THERAPY CONSIDERED. **SERIOUS ANAPHYLACTOID REACTIONS REQUIRE IMMEDIATE EMERGENCY TREATMENT WITH EPINEPHRINE. OXYGEN, INTRAVENOUS STEROIDS, AND AIRWAY MANAGEMENT, INCLUDING INTUBATION, SHOULD ALSO BE ADMINISTERED AS INDICATED.**

USAGE IN PREGNANCY

Safety for use in pregnancy has not been established.

Precautions: As with any potent drug, periodic assessment of renal, hepatic and hematopoietic function should be made during prolonged therapy.

The possibility of superinfections with mycotic or bacterial pathogens should be kept in mind during therapy. If superinfections occur (usually involving Enterobacter, Pseudomonas or Candida), the drug should be discontinued and/or appropriate therapy instituted.

Adverse Reactions: As with other penicillins, it may be expected that untoward reactions will be essentially limited to sensitivity phenomena. They are more likely to occur in individuals who have previously demonstrated hypersensitivity to penicillins and in those with a history of allergy, asthma, hay fever or urticaria. The following adverse reactions have been reported as associated with the use of the penicillins:

Gastrointestinal: Nausea, vomiting and diarrhea.

Hypersensitivity Reactions: Erythematous maculopapular rashes and urticaria have been reported.

NOTE: Urticaria, other skin rashes and serum sickness-like reactions may be controlled with antihistamines and, if necessary, systemic corticosteroids. Whenever such reactions occur, Amoxicillin should be discontinued unless, in the opinion of the physician, the condition being treated is life-threatening and amenable only to Amoxicillin therapy.

Liver: A moderate rise in serum glutamic oxaloacetic transaminase (SGOT) has been noted, but the significance of this finding is unknown.

Hemic and Lymphatic Systems: Anemia, thrombocytopenia, thrombocytopenic purpura, eosinophilia, leukopenia and agranulocytosis have been reported during therapy with the penicillins. These reactions are usually reversible on discontinuation of therapy and are believed to be hypersensitivity phenomena.

Dosage and Administration:

Infections of the ear, nose and throat due to streptococci, pneumococci, nonpenicillinase-producing staphylococci and *H. influenzae;*

Infections of the genitourinary tract due to *E. coli, Proteus mirabilis* and *Streptococcus faecalis;*

Infections of the skin and soft-tissues due to streptococci, susceptible staphylococci and *E. coli.*

USUAL DOSAGE:

Adults: 250 mg every 8 hours.

Children: 20 mg/kg/day in divided doses every 8 hours.

Children weighing 20 kg or more should be dosed according to the adult recommendations.

In severe infections or those caused by less susceptible organisms:

500 mg every 8 hours for adults, and 40 mg/kg/day in divided doses every 8 hours for children may be needed.

Infections of the lower respiratory tract due to streptococci, pneumococci, nonpenicillinase-producing staphylococci and *H. influenzae:*

USUAL DOSAGE:

Adults: 500 mg every 8 hours.

Children: 40 mg/kg/day in divided doses every 8 hours.

Children weighing 20 kg or more should be dosed according to the adult recommendations.

Gonorrhea, acute uncomplicated ano-genital and urethral infections due to *N. gonorrhoeae* (males and females):

USUAL DOSAGE:

Adults: 3 grams as a single oral dose.

Prepubertal children: 50 mg/kg amoxicillin combined with 25 mg/kg probenecid as a single dose.

NOTE: SINCE PROBENECID IS CONTRAINDICATED IN CHILDREN UNDER 2 YEARS, THIS REGIMEN SHOULD NOT BE USED IN THESE CASES.

Cases of gonorrhea with a suspected lesion of syphilis should have dark-field examinations before receiving Amoxicillin, and monthly serological tests for a minimum of four months.

Larger doses may be required for stubborn or severe infections.

The children's dosage is intended for individuals whose weight will not cause a dosage to be calculated greater than that recommended for adults.

It should be recognized that in the treatment of chronic urinary tract infections, frequent bacteriological and clinical appraisals are necessary. Smaller doses than those recommended above should not be used. Even higher doses may be needed at times. In stubborn infections, therapy may be required for several weeks. It may be necessary to continue clinical and/or bacteriological follow-up for several months after cessation of therapy. Except for gonorrhea, treatment should be continued for a minimum of 48 to 72 hours beyond the time that the patient becomes asymptomatic or evidence of bacterial eradication has been obtained. It is recommended that there be at least 10 days' treatment for any infection caused by hemolytic streptococci to prevent the occurrence of acute rheumatic fever or glomerulonephritis.

Dosage and Administration of Pediatric Drops:

Usual dosage for all indications except infections of the lower respiratory tract:

Under 6 kg (13 lbs): 0.75 ml every 8 hours.
6—7 kg (13—15 lbs): 1.0 ml every 8 hours.
8 kg (16—18 lbs): 1.5 ml every 8 hours.

Infections of the lower respiratory tract:

Under 6 kg (13 lbs): 1.75 ml every 8 hours.
6—7 kg (13—15 lbs): 2.0 ml every 8 hours.
8 kg (16—18 lbs): 2.5 ml every 8 hours.

Children weighing more than 8 kg (18 lbs) should receive the appropriate dose of the Oral Suspension 125 mg or 250 mg/5 ml.

After reconstitution, the required amount of suspension should be placed directly on the child's tongue for swallowing. Alternate means of administration are to add the required amount of suspension to formula, milk, fruit juice, water, ginger ale or cold drinks. These preparations should then be taken immediately. To be certain the child is receiving full dosage, such preparations should be consumed in entirety.

Directions For Mixing Oral Suspension:

Prepare suspension at time of dispensing as follows: Tap bottle until all powder flows freely. Add approximately ⅓ of the total amount of water for reconstitution (see table below) and shake vigorously to wet powder. Add remainder of the water and again shake vigorously.

125 mg per 5 ml

Bottle Size	Amount of Water Required for Reconstitution
80 ml	62 ml
100 ml	78 ml
150 ml	116 ml

Each teaspoonful (5 ml) will contain 125 mg Amoxicillin.

125 mg unit dose	5 ml

250 mg per 5 ml

Bottle Size	Amount of Water Required for Reconstitution
80 ml	59 ml
100 ml	74 ml
150 ml	111 ml

Each teaspoonful (5 ml) will contain 250 mg Amoxicillin.

250 mg unit dose	5 ml
3 Gm single dose	40 ml

Directions For Mixing Pediatric Drops:

Prepare pediatric drops at time of dispensing as follows: Add the required amount of water (see table below) to the bottle and shake vigorously. Each ml of suspension will then contain Amoxicillin Trihydrate equivalent to 50 mg Amoxicillin.

Bottle Size	Amount of Water Required for Reconstitution
15 ml	12 ml
30 ml	23 ml

NOTE: SHAKE BOTH ORAL SUSPENSION AND PEDIATRIC DROPS WELL BEFORE USING. Keep bottle tightly closed. Any unused portion of the reconstituted suspension must be discarded after 14 days. Refrigeration preferable, but not required.

How Supplied:

AMOXIL (Amoxicillin) **Capsules.** Each capsule contains 250 mg or 500 mg Amoxicillin as the trihydrate.

250 mg/Capsule

NDC 0029-6006-24 ....bottles of 15
NDC 0029-6006-30 ....bottles of 100
NDC 0029-6006-32 ....bottles of 500
NDC 0029-6006-31 ......unit dose carton of 100

500 mg/Capsule

NDC 0029-6007-24 ....bottles of 15
NDC 0029-6007-29 ....bottles of 50
NDC 0029-6007-32 ....bottles of 500
NDC 0029-6007-31 ....unit dose cartons of 100

[*Shown in Product Identification Section*]

Therapy Pack:

NDC 0029-6007-79 ....6 × 500 mg Capsules (3 packs per carton)

AMOXIL (Amoxicillin) **Chewable Tablets.** Each scored tablet contains 125 mg or 250 mg Amoxicillin as the trihydrate.

125 mg/Tablet

NDC 0029-6004-39 ....bottles of 60

250 mg/Tablet

NDC 0029-6005-39 ....bottles of 60

AMOXIL (Amoxicillin) **for Oral Suspension.**

125 mg/5 ml

NDC 0029-6008-21 ....80 ml bottle
NDC 0029-6008-23 ....100 ml bottle
NDC 0029-6008-22 ....150 ml bottle

250 mg/5 ml

NDC 0029-6009-21 ....80 ml bottle
NDC 0029-6009-23 ....100 ml bottle
NDC 0029-6009-22 ....150 ml bottle

Each 5 ml of reconstituted suspension contains 125 mg or 250 mg Amoxicillin as the trihydrate.

NDC 0029-6008-18 .....125 mg unit dose bottle
NDC 0029-6009-18 .....250 mg unit dose bottle

3 Gm for Oral Suspension:

NDC 0029-6037-28 ....single dose bottle

Each single dose bottle contains 3 grams Amoxicillin as the trihydrate.

Continued on next page

Beecham Laboratories—Cont.

AMOXIL (Amoxicillin) **Pediatric Drops for Oral Suspension.**
Each ml of reconstituted suspension contains 50 mg Amoxicillin as the trihydrate.
NDC 0029-6035-20 ....15 ml bottle
NDC 0029-6038-39 ....30 ml bottle
REV. MAY, 1981

FASTIN® Capsules℮
(phentermine hydrochloride)

Description: Each Fastin (phentermine hydrochloride) capsule contains phentermine hydrochloride, 30 mg (equivalent to 24 mg phentermine).
Phentermine Hydrochloride is a white crystalline powder, very soluble in water and alcohol. Chemically, the product is phenyl-tertiary-butyl-amine hydrochloride.
Actions: FASTIN is a sympathomimetic amine with pharmacologic activity similar to the prototype drugs of this class used in obesity, the amphetamines. Actions include central nervous system stimulation and elevation of blood pressure. Tachyphylaxis and tolerance have been demonstrated with all drugs of this class in which these phenomena have been looked for.
Drugs of this class used in obesity are commonly known as "anorectics" or "anorexigenics." It has not been established that the action of such drugs in treating obesity is primarily one of appetite suppression. Other central nervous system actions, or metabolic effects may be involved, for example.
Adult obese subjects instructed in dietary management and treated with "anorectic" drugs, lose more weight on the average than those treated with placebo and diet, as determined in relatively short-term clinical trials.
The magnitude of increased weight loss of drug-treated patients over placebo-treated patients is only a fraction of a pound a week. The rate of weight loss is greatest in the first weeks of therapy for both drug and placebo subjects and tends to decrease in succeeding weeks. The possible origins of the increased weight loss due to the various drug effects are not established. The amount of weight loss associated with the use of an "anorectic" drug varies from trial to trial, and the increased weight loss appears to be related in part to variables other than the drugs prescribed, such as the physician-investigator, the population treated, and the diet prescribed. Studies do not permit conclusions as to the relative importance of the drug and nondrug factors on weight loss.
The natural history of obesity is measured in years, whereas the studies cited are restricted to a few weeks duration; thus, the total impact of drug-induced weight loss over that of diet alone must be considered clinically limited.
Indication: FASTIN is indicated in the management of exogenous obesity as a short term (a few weeks) adjunct in a regimen of weight reduction based on caloric restriction. The limited usefulness of agents of this class (see ACTIONS) should be measured against possible risk factors inherent in their use such as those described below.
Contraindications: Advanced arteriosclerosis, symptomatic cardiovascular disease, moderate to severe hypertension, hyperthyroidism, known hypersensitivity, or idiosyncrasy to the sympathomimetic amines, glaucoma.
Agitated states.
Patients with a history of drug abuse.
During or within 14 days following the administration of monoamine oxidase inhibitors (hypertensive crises may result).
Warnings: Tolerance to the anorectic effect usually develops within a few weeks. When this occurs, the recommended dose should not be exceeded in an attempt to increase the effect; rather, the drug should be discontinued. FASTIN may impair the ability of the patient to engage in potentially hazardous activities such as operating machinery or driving a motor vehicle; the patient should therefore be cautioned accordingly.
Drug Dependence: FASTIN is related chemically and pharmacologically to the amphetamines. Amphetamines and related stimulant drugs have been extensively abused, and the possibility of abuse of FASTIN should be kept in mind when evaluating the desirability of including a drug as part of a weight reduction program. Abuse of amphetamines and related drugs may be associated with intense psychological dependence and severe social dysfunction. There are reports of patients who have increased the dosage to many times that recommended. Abrupt cessation following prolonged high dosage administration results in extreme fatigue and mental depression; changes are also noted on the sleep EEG. Manifestations of chronic intoxication with anorectic drugs include severe dermatoses, marked insomnia, irritability, hyperactivity, and personality changes. The most severe manifestation of chronic intoxications is psychosis, often clinically indistinguishable from schizophrenia.
Usage in Pregnancy: Safe use in pregnancy has not been established. Use of FASTIN by women who are or who may become pregnant, and those in the first trimester of pregnancy, requires that the potential benefit be weighed against the possible hazard to mother and infant.
Usage in Children: FASTIN is not recommended for use in children under 12 years of age.
Usage with Alcohol: Concomitant use of alcohol with FASTIN may result in an adverse drug interaction.
Precautions: Caution is to be exercised in prescribing FASTIN for patients with even mild hypertension.
Insulin requirements in diabetes mellitus may be altered in association with the use of FASTIN and the concomitant dietary regimen.
FASTIN may decrease the hypotensive effect of guanethidine.
The least amount feasible should be prescribed or dispensed at one time in order to minimize the possibility of overdosage.
Adverse Reactions:
Cardiovascular: Palpitation, tachycardia, elevation of blood pressure.
Central Nervous System: Overstimulation, restlessness, dizziness, insomnia, euphoria, dysphoria, tremor, headache, rarely psychotic episodes at recommended doses.
Gastrointestinal: Dryness of the mouth, unpleasant taste, diarrhea, constipation, other gastrointestinal disturbances.
Allergic: Urticaria.
Endocrine: Impotence, changes in libido.
Dosage and Administration:
Exogenous Obesity: One capsule at approximately 2 hours after breakfast for appetite control. Late evening medication should be avoided because of the possibility of resulting insomnia.
Administration of one capsule (30 mg.) daily has been found to be adequate in depression of the appetite for twelve to fourteen hours.
FASTIN is not recommended for use in children under 12 years of age.
Overdosage: Manifestations of acute overdosage with phentermine include restlessness, tremor, hyperreflexia, rapid respiration, confusion, assaultiveness, hallucinations, panic states. Fatigue and depression usually follow the central stimulation. Cardiovascular effects include arrhythmias, hypertension or hypotension, and circulatory collapse. Gastrointestinal symptoms include nausea, vomiting, diarrhea, and abdominal cramps. Fatal poisoning usually terminates in convulsions and coma.
Management of acute phentermine intoxication is largely symptomatic and includes lavage and sedation with a barbiturate. Experience with hemodialysis or peritoneal dialysis is inadequate to permit recommendations in this regard. Acidification of the urine increases phentermine excretion. Intravenous phentolamine (REGITINE) has been suggested for possible acute, severe hypertension, if this complicates phentermine overdosage.
Caution: Federal law prohibits dispensing without prescription.
How Supplied: Blue and white capsules containing 30 mg. phentermine hydrochloride (equivalent to 24 mg. Phentermine).
NDC 0029-2205-30 ....bottles of 100
NDC 0029-2205-39 ....bottles of 450
[*Shown in Product Identification Section*]

NUCOFED® ℮
SYRUP and CAPSULES

Description: Nucofed Syrup and Capsules is an antitussive-decongestant containing in each 5 ml (teaspoonful) and each capsule: Codeine Phosphate, 20 mg (Warning: May Be Habit Forming); Pseudoephedrine Hydrochloride, 60 mg. Nucofed Syrup contains no alcohol and contains 2.25 gm of sucrose per 5 ml (teaspoonful).
Clinical Pharmacology:
Nucofed Syrup and Capsules
The clinical pharmacology of this formulated product is thought to be due to the action of its ingredients, Codeine Phosphate and Pseudoephedrine Hydrochloride.
Codeine Phosphate. Codeine causes suppression of the cough reflex by a direct effect on the cough center in the medulla and appears to exert a drying effect on respiratory tract mucosa and to increase viscosity of bronchial secretions.
Codeine is well absorbed from the gastrointestinal tract. Following oral administration, peak antitussive effects usually can be expected to occur within 1–2 hours and may persist for a period of four hours. Codeine is metabolized in the liver. The drug undergoes O-demethylation, N-demethylation, and partial conjugation with glucuronic acid, and is excreted mainly in the urine as norcodeine and morphine in the free and conjugated forms.
Codeine appears in breast milk of nursing mothers and has been reported to cross the placental barrier.
Pseudoephedrine Hydrochloride. Pseudoephedrine is a physiologically active stereoisomer of ephedrine which acts directly on *alpha*, and, to a lesser degree, *beta*-adrenergic receptors. The *alpha*-adrenergic effects are believed to result from the reduced production of cyclic adenosine-3′,5′ monophosphate (cyclic 3′,5′-AMP) by inhibition of the enzyme adenyl cyclase, where *beta*-adrenergic effects appear to be caused by the stimulation of adenyl cyclase activity.
Pseudoephedrine acts directly on *alpha*-adrenergic receptors in the respiratory tract mucosa producing vasoconstriction resulting in shrinkage of swollen nasal mucous membranes, reduction of tissue hyperemia, edema, and nasal congestion, and an increase in nasal airway patency. Drainage of sinus secretions is increased and obstructed eustachian ostia may be opened. Relaxation of bronchial smooth muscle by stimulation of $beta_2$ adrenergic receptors may also occur. Following oral administration significant broncho-dilation has not been demonstrated consistently.
Nasal decongestion usually occurs within 30 minutes and persists for 4–6 hours after oral administration of 60 mg of Pseudoephedrine Hydrochloride.
Although specific information is not available, Pseudoephedrine is presumed to cross the placenta and to enter cerebrospinal fluid. It is incompletely metabolized in the liver by N-demethylation to an inactive metabolite. Both are excreted in the urine with 55%–75% of a dose being unchanged.

Indications and Usage: NUCOFED is indicated for symptomatic relief when both coughing and congestion are associated with upper respiratory infections and related conditions such as common cold, bronchitis, influenza, and sinusitis.
Contraindications: Hypersensitivity to product's active ingredients.
Warnings: Persons with persistent cough such as occurs with smoking, asthma, emphysema, or where cough is accompanied by excessive secretions should not take this product except under the advice and supervision of a physician.
May cause or aggravate constipation.
Do not give this product to children taking other drugs except under the advice and supervision of a physician.
Persons with a chronic pulmonary disease or shortness of breath, high blood pressure, heart disease, diabetes or thyroid disease should not take this product except under the advice and supervision of a physician.
Do not exceed recommended dosage because at higher doses nervousness, dizziness, or sleeplessness may occur.
If symptoms do not improve within 7 days or are accompanied by high fever, consult a physician before continuing use.
Precautions:
General
Inasmuch as the active ingredients of Nucofed Syrup and Capsules consist of Codeine Phosphate and Pseudoephedrine Hydrochloride, this medication should be used with caution in the presence of the following:
- Cardiovascular disease (of any etiology)
- Diabetes mellitus
- Hypertension (of any severity)
- Abnormal thyroid function
- Prostatic hypertrophy
- Addison's disease
- Chronic ulcerative colitis
- History of drug abuse or dependence
- Chronic respiratory disease or impairment
- Functional impairment of the liver or kidney

Patients taking Nucofed Syrup and Capsules should be cautioned when driving or doing jobs requiring alertness and to get up slowly from a lying or sitting position, or to lie down if nausea occurs.
Possible Drug Interactions
Because of the potential for drug interactions, persons currently taking any of the following medications should take Nucofed Syrup and Capsules on the advice and under the supervision of a physician.
- Beta adrenergic blockers—concurrent use may increase the pressor effect of pseudoephedrine.
- Digitalis glycosides—concurrent use with pseudoephedrine may increase the possibility of cardiac arrhythmias.
- Antihypertensive agents including Veratrum alkaloids—hypotensive effects may be decreased by the concurrent use of pseudoephedrine.
- Monoamine oxidase (MAO) inhibitors—these agents may potentiate the pressor effect of Pseudoephedrine and may result in a hypertensive crisis; pseudoephedrine should not be administered during or within 14 days of MAO inhibitors.
- Sympathomimetics, other — sympathomimetics used concurrently may increase the effects either of these agents or of pseudoephedrine, thereby increasing the potential for side effects.
- Tricyclic antidepressants—the concurrent use of tricyclic antidepressants may antagonize the effects of pseudoephedrine and may increase the effects either of the antidepressants themselves or of the codeine component.
- CNS depressants
- Alcohol
- General anesthetics
- Anticholinergics—concurrent use may result in paralytic ileus.

Drug/Laboratory Test Interactions
- Codeine may cause an elevation in serum amylase levels due to the spasm producing potential of narcotic analgesics on the sphincter of Oddi.

Pregnancy: Category C
Animal reproduction studies of the components of Nucofed Syrup and Capsules (Codeine, Pseudoephedrine) have not been conducted. Thus, it is not known whether these agents can cause fetal harm when administered to pregnant women or whether they affect reproductive capacity. Accordingly, Nucofed Syrup and Capsules should be given to pregnant women only where clearly needed.
Nursing Mothers
Codeine and Pseudoephedrine are excreted in breast milk; therefore, caution should be exercised when this medication is prescribed for a nursing mother.
Pediatric Use
Do not give Nucofed Syrup and Capsules to children under two years of age except on the advice and under the supervision of a physician.
Adverse Reactions: Based on the composition of Nucofed Syrup and Capsules the following side effects may occur: nervousness, restlessness, trouble in sleeping, drowsiness, difficult or painful urination, dizziness or lightheadedness, headache, nausea and vomiting, constipation, trembling, troubled breathing, increase in sweating, unusual paleness, weakness, changes in heart rate.
Drug Abuse and Dependence: NUCOFED is placed in Schedule III of the Controlled Substances Act.
Overdosage: Nucofed Syrup and Capsules contain Codeine Phosphate and Pseudoephedrine Hydrochloride. Overdosage as a result of this product should be treated based upon the symptomatology of the patient as it relates to the individual ingredient. Treatment of acute overdosage would probably be based upon treating the patient for codeine toxicity which may be manifested as:
- Gradual drowsiness, dizziness, heaviness of the head, weariness, diminution of sensibility, loss of pain and other modalities of sensation.
- Nausea and vomiting.
- A transient excitement stage, characterized by extreme restlessness, delirium, and rarely epileptiform convulsions, is sometimes seen in children and rarely in adult women.
- Bilateral miosis, progressing to pinpoint pupils, which do not react to light or accommodation. The pupils may dilate during terminal asphyxia.
- Itching of the skin and nose, sometimes with skin rashes and urticaria.
- Coma, with muscular relaxation and depressed or absent superficial and deep reflexes. A Babinski toe sign may appear.
- Marked slowing of the respiratory rate with inadequate pulmonary ventilation and consequent cyanosis. Breathing becomes stertorous and irregular (Cheyne-Stokes or Biot).
- The pulse is slow and the blood pressure gradually falls to shock levels. Urine formation ceases or is reduced to a very low rate.

The lethal dose of codeine for an adult is about 0.5–1.0 gm. Treatment is as recommended for narcotics.
Dosage and Administration:
Recommended Dosage: Capsule
Adults: 1 capsule every 6 hours, not to exceed 4 capsules in 24 hours.
Recommended Dosage: Syrup
Adults: 1 teaspoonful every 6 hours, not to exceed 4 teaspoonfuls in 24 hours.
Children:
6 to under 12 years: ½ teaspoonful every 6 hours, not to exceed 2 teaspoonfuls in 24 hours.
2 to under 6 years: ¼ teaspoonful every 6 hours, not to exceed 1 teaspoonful in 24 hours.
Do not give this product to children under 2 years, except under the advice and supervision of a physician.
How Supplied:
Nucofed Syrup, Green, Mint Flavored
NDC 0029-3135-34 Pints
Nucofed Capsules, Green Top, Clear Bottom
NDC 0029-3138-39 Bottles of 60
Caution: Federal law prohibits dispensing without prescription.
Revised July, 1981

NUCOFED® EXPECTORANT SYRUP Ⓒ

Description: Nucofed Expectorant is an antitussive-decongestant-expectorant syrup for oral administration containing in each 5 ml (teaspoonful): Codeine Phosphate, 20 mg (Warning: May Be Habit Forming); Pseudoephedrine HCl, 60 mg; Guaifenesin, 200 mg; alcohol, 12.5%.
Clinical Pharmacology:
Nucofed Expectorant
The clinical pharmacology of this formulated product is thought to be due to the action of its ingredients, Codeine Phosphate, Pseudoephedrine Hydrochloride and Guaifenesin.
Codeine Phosphate. Codeine causes suppression of the cough reflex by a direct effect on the cough center in the medulla and appears to exert a drying effect on respiratory tract mucosa and to increase viscosity of bronchial secretions.
Codeine is well absorbed from the gastrointestinal tract. Following oral administration, peak antitussive effects can be expected to occur within one to two hours and may persist for a period of four hours. Codeine is metabolized in the liver. The drug undergoes O-demethylation, N-demethylation, and partial conjugation with glucuronic acid, and is excreted mainly in the urine as norcodeine and morphine in the free and conjugated forms. Codeine appears in breast milk of nursing mothers and has been reported to cross the placental barrier.
Pseudoephedrine Hydrochloride. Pseudoephedrine is a physiologically active stereoisomer of ephedrine which acts directly on *alpha*, and to a lesser degree, *beta*-adrenergic receptors. The *alpha*-adrenergic effects are believed to result from the reduced production of cyclic adenosine-3′,5′ monophosphate (cyclic 3′,5′-AMP) by inhibition of the enzyme adenyl cyclase, whereas *beta*-adrenergic effects appear to be caused by the stimulation of adenyl cyclase activity.
Pseudoephedrine acts directly on *alpha*-adrenergic receptors in the respiratory tract mucosa producing vasoconstriction resulting in shrinkage of swollen nasal mucous membranes, reduction of tissue hyperemia, edema, and nasal congestion, and an increase in nasal airway patency. Drainage of sinus secretions is increased and obstructed eustachian ostia may be opened. Relaxation of bronchial smooth muscle by stimulation of $beta_2$ adrenergic receptors may also occur. Following oral administration significant broncho-dilation has not been demonstrated consistently.
Nasal decongestion usually occurs within 30 minutes and persists for 4–6 hours after oral administration of 60 mg of pseudoephedrine hydrochloride.
Although specific information is not available, pseudoephedrine is presumed to cross the placenta and to enter cerebrospinal fluid. It is incompletely metabolized in the liver by N-demethylation to an inactive metabolite. Both are excreted in the urine with 55%–75% of a dose being unchanged.

Continued on next page

Beecham Laboratories—Cont.

Guaifenesin. Guaifenesin, by increasing respiratory tract fluid, reduces the viscosity of tenacious secretions and acts as an expectorant. Guaifenesin is excreted in the urine mainly as glucuronates and sulfonates.

Indications and Usage: NUCOFED EXPECTORANT is indicated for symptomatic relief when both coughing and congestion are associated with upper respiratory infections and related conditions such as common colds, bronchitis, influenza, and sinusitis.

Contraindications: Hypersensitivity to product's active ingredients.

Warnings: Persons with persistent cough such as occurs with smoking, asthma, emphysema, or where cough is accompanied by excessive secretions should not take this product except under the advice and supervision of a physician.

Do not give this product to children taking other drugs except under the advice and supervision of a physician.

Persons with a chronic pulmonary disease or shortness of breath, high blood pressure, heart disease, diabetes or thyroid disease should not take this product except under the advice and supervision of a physician.

Do not exceed recommended dosage because at higher doses nervousness, dizziness, or sleeplessness may occur.

If symptoms do not improve within 7 days or are accompanied by high fever, consult a physician before continuing use.

Precautions:

General. Inasmuch as the active ingredient of Nucofed Expectorant consist of Codeine Phosphate, Pseudoephedrine Hydrochloride and Guaifenesin, this medication should be used with caution in the presence of the following:

- Cardiovascular disease (of any etiology)
- Diabetes mellitus
- Hypertension (of any severity)
- Abnormal thyroid function
- Prostatic hypertrophy
- Addison's disease
- Chronic ulcerative colitis
- History of drug abuse or dependence
- Chronic respiratory disease or impairment
- Functional impairment of the liver or kidney

Patients taking Nucofed Expectorant should be cautioned when driving or doing jobs requiring alertness and to get up slowly from a lying or sitting position, or to lie down if nausea occurs.

Possible Drug Interactions. Because of the potential for drug interactions, persons currently taking any of the following medications should take Nucofed Expectorant only on the advice and under the supervision of a physician.

- Beta adrenergic blockers—concurrent use may increase the pressor effect of pseudoephedrine.
- Digitalis glycosides—concurrent use with pseudoephedrine may increase the possibility of cardiac arrhythmias.
- Antihypertensive agents including Veratrum alkaloids—hypotensive effects may be decreased by the concurrent use of pseudoephedrine.
- Monoamine oxidase (MAO) inhibitors—these agents may potentiate the pressor effect of pseudoephedrine and may result in a hypertensive crisis; pseudoephedrine should not be administered during or within 14 days of MAO inhibitors.
- Sympathomimetics, other — sympathomimetics used concurrently may increase the effects either of these agents or of pseudoephedrine, thereby increasing the potential for side effects.
- Tricyclic antidepressants—the concurrent use of tricyclic antidepressants may antagonize the effects of pseudoephedrine and may increase the effects either of the antidepressants themselves or of the codeine component.
- CNS depressants
- Alcohol
- General anesthetics
- Anticholinergics—concurrent use may result in paralytic ileus.

Drug/Laboratory Test Interactions

- Codeine may cause an elevation in serum amylase levels due to the spasm producing potential of narcotic analgesics on the sphincter of Oddi.
- Guaifenesin in known to interfere with the colorimetric determination of 5-hydroxy-indole-acetic acid (5-HIAA) and vanilmandelic acid (VMA).

Pregnancy: Category C

Animal reproduction studies of the components of Nucofed Expectorants (codeine, pseudoephedrine and guaifenesin) have not been conducted. Thus, it is not known whether these agents can cause fetal harm when administered to pregnant women or whether they affect reproductive capacity. Accordingly, Nucofed Expectorant should be given to pregnant women only where clearly needed.

Nursing Mothers

Codeine and Pseudoephedrine, two of the ingredients in Nucofed Expectorant, are excreted in breast milk; therefore, caution should be exercised when this medication is prescribed for a nursing mother.

Pediatric Use

Do not give Nucofed Expectorant to Children under two years of age except on the advice and under the supervision of a physician.

Adverse Reactions: Based on the composition of Nucofed Expectorant the following side effects may occur: nervousness, restlessness, trouble in sleeping, drowsiness, difficult or painful urination, dizziness or lightheadedness, headache, nausea or vomiting, constipation, trembling, troubled breathing, increase in sweating, unusual paleness, weakness, changes in heart rate.

Drug Abuse and Dependence: Nucofed Expectorant has been placed in Schedule III of the Controlled Substances Act.

Overdosage: Nucofed Expectorant contains Codeine Phosphate, Pseudoephedrine Hydrochloride and Guaifenesin. Overdosage as a result of this product should be treated based upon the symptomatology of the patient as it relates to the individual ingredient. Treatment of acute overdosage would probably be based upon treating the patient for codeine toxicity which may be manifested as:

- Gradual drowsiness, dizziness, heaviness of the head, weariness, diminution of sensibility, loss of pain and other modalities of sensation.
- Nausea and vomiting.
- A transient excitement stage, characterized by extreme restlessness, delirium, and rarely epileptiform convulsions, is sometimes seen in children and rarely in adult women.
- Bilateral miosis, progressing to pinpoint pupils, which do not react to light or accommodation. The pupils may dilate during terminal asphyxia.
- Itching of the skin and nose, sometimes with skin rashes and urticaria.
- Coma, with muscular relaxation and depressed or absent superficial and deep reflexes. A Babinski toe sign may appear.
- Marked slowing of the respiratory rate with inadequate pulmonary ventilation and consequent cyanosis. Breathing becomes stertorous and irregular (Cheyne-Stokes or Biot).
- The pulse is slow and the blood pressure gradually falls to shock levels. Urine formation ceases or is reduced to a very low rate.

The lethal dose of codeine for an adult is about 0.5–1.0 gram. Treatment is as recommended for narcotics.

Dosage and Administration:

Recommended Dosage:

Adults: 1 teaspoonful every 6 hours, not to exceed 4 teaspoonfuls in 24 hours.

Children:

6 to under 12 years: ½ teaspoonful every 6 hours, not to exceed 2 teaspoonfuls in 24 hours.

2 to under 6 years: ¼ teaspoonful every 6 hours, not to exceed 1 teaspoonful in 24 hours.

Do not give this product to children under 2 years, except under the advice and supervision of a physician.

How Supplied:

Red, Wintergreen Flavored Syrup

NDC 0029-3142-34 Pints

Caution: Federal law prohibits dispensing without prescription.

TICAR® ℞

(sterile ticarcillin disodium for Intramuscular or Intravenous Use

Description: TICAR (Ticarcillin Disodium) is a semisynthetic injectable penicillin derived from the penicillin nucleus, 6-amino-penicillanic acid. Chemically, it is 6-[(Carboxy-3-thienylacetyl) amino]-3,3-dimethyl-7-oxo-4-thia-1-aza-bicyclo [3.2.0] heptane-2-carboxylic acid disodium salt.

It is supplied as a white to pale yellow powder or lyophilized cake for reconstitution. The reconstituted solution is clear, colorless or pale yellow, having a pH of 6.0-8.0. Ticarcillin is very soluble in water, its solubility is greater than 600 mg/ml.

Actions:

PHARMACOLOGY

Ticarcillin is not absorbed orally, therefore, it must be given intravenously or intramuscularly. Following intramuscular administration, peak serum concentrations occur within ½-1hour. Somewhat higher and more prolonged serum levels can be achieved with the concurrent administration of probenecid. The minimum inhibitory concentrations (MIC) for many strains of *Pseudomonas* are relatively high by usual standards; serum levels of 60 mcg/ml or greater are required. However, the low degree of toxicity of Ticarcillin permits the use of doses large enough to achieve inhibitory levels for these strains in serum of tissues. Other susceptible organisms usually require serum levels in the 10–25 mcg/ml range. [See table on next page].

As with other penicillins, Ticarcillin is eliminated by glomerular filtration and tubular secretion. It is not highly bound to serum protein (approximately 45%) and is excreted unchanged in high concentrations in the urine. After the administration of a 1–2 Gm I.M. dose, a urine concentration of 2000–4000 mcg/ml may be obtained in patients with normal renal function. The serum half-life of Ticarcillin in normal individuals is approximately 70 minutes.

An inverse relationship exists between serum half-life and creatinine clearance, but the dosage of TICAR need only be adjusted in cases of severe renal impairment (see DOSAGE AND ADMINISTRATION). The administered Ticarcillin may be removed from patients undergoing dialysis; the actual amount removed depends on the duration and type of dialysis.

Ticarcillin can be detected in tissues and interstitial fluid following parenteral administration. Penetration into the cerebrospinal fluid, bile and pleural fluid has been demonstrated.

MICROBIOLOGY

Ticarcillin is bactericidal and demonstrates substantial *in vitro* activity against both Gram-positive and Gram-negative organisms. Many strains of the following organisms were found to be susceptible to Ticarcillin *in vitro:*

Pseudomonas aeruginosa (and other species)
Escherichia coli
Proteus mirabilis
Proteus morganii
Proteus rettgeri

Proteus vulgaris
Enterbacter species
Haemophilus influenzae
Neisseria species
Salmonella species
Staphylococcus aureus (non-penicillinase producing)
Staphylococcus epidermidis
Beta-hemolytic streptococci (Group A)
Streptococcus faecalis (Enterococcus)
Streptococcus pneumoniae
Anaerobic bacteria, including:
Bacteroides species including *B. fragilis*
Fusobacterium species
Veillonella species
Clostridium species
Eubacterium species
Peptococcus species
Peptostreptococcus species

In vitro synergism between Ticarillin and gentamicin sulfate, tobramycin sulfate or amikacin sulfate against certain strains of *Pseudomonas aeruginosa* has been demonstrated.

Some strains of such microorganisms as *Mima-Herellea (Acinetobacter), Citrobacter* and *Serratia* have shown susceptibility.

Ticarcillin is not stable in the presence of penicillinase.

Some strains of *Pseudomonas* have developed resistance fairly rapidly.

DISC SUSCEPTIBILITY TESTS

Quantitative methods that require measurement of zone diameters give the most precise estimates of antibiotic susceptibility. One such procedure* has been recommended for use with discs for testing susceptibility to carbenicillin class antibiotics. With this procedure, a report from the laboratory of "susceptible" indicates that the infecting organism is likely to respond to therapy. A report of "resistant" indicates that the infecting organism is not likely to respond to therapy. A report of "intermediate susceptibility" suggests that the organism would be susceptible if high dosage is used, or if the infection is confined to tissues and fluids (e.g., urine) in which high antibiotic levels are attained.

At present, only dilution methods can be recommended for testing antibiotic susceptibility of obligate anaerobes.

---

* Bauer, A.W., Kirby, W.M.M., Sherris, J.C., and Turck, M.: Antibiotic Testing by a Standardized Single Disc Method, Am. J. Clin. Pathol., 45:493, 1966. Standardized Disc Susceptibility Test, FEDERAL REGISTER 73:20527–29, 1972.

Indications: TICAR (Ticarcillin Disodium) is indicated for the treatment of the following infections:

Bacterial septicemia (†)
Skin and soft-tissue infections (†)
Acute and chronic respiratory tract infections (†)(‡)

(†) caused by susceptible strains of *Pseudomonas aeruginosa, Proteus* species (both indole-positive and indole-negative) and *Escherichia coli.*

(‡) (Though clinical improvement has been shown, bacteriological cures cannot be expected in patients with chronic respiratory disease or cystic fibrosis.)

Genitourinary tract infections (complicated and uncomplicated) due to susceptible strains of Pseudomonas aeruginosa. Proteus species (both indole-positive and indole-negative), *Escherichia coli, Enterobacter* and *Streptococcus faecalis* (enterococcus).

Ticarcillin is also indicated in the treatment of the following infections due to susceptible anaerobic bacteria:

1. Bacterial septicemia.
2. Lower respiratory tract infections such as empyema, anaerobic pneumonitis and lung abscess.
3. Intra-abdominal infections such as peritonitis and intra-abdominal abscess (typically resulting from anaerobic organisms resident in the normal gastrointestinal tract).
4. Infections of the female pelvis and genital tract, such as endometritis, pelvic inflammatory disease, pelvic abscess and salpingitis.
5. Skin and soft-tissue infections.

TICARCILLIN SERUM LEVELS
mcg/ml

Dosage	Route	¼ hr.	½ hr.	1 hr.	2 hr.	3 hr.	4 hr.	6 hr.
Adults:								
500 mg	IM	—	7.7	8.6	6.0	4.0	—	2.9
1 Gm	IM	—	31.0	18.7	15.7	9.7	—	3.4
2 Gm	IM	—	63.6	39.7	32.3	18.9	—	3.4
3 Gm	IV	190.0	140.0	107.0	52.2	31.3	13.8	4.2
5 Gm	IV	327.0	280.0	175.0	106.0	63.0	28.5	9.6
3 Gm + 1 Gm Probenecid	IV Oral	223.0	166.0	123.0	78.0	54.0	35.4	17.1

Neonates:		**½ hr.**	**1 hr.**	**1½ hr.**	**2 hr.**	**4 hr.**	**8 hr.**
50 mg/kg	IM	64.0	70.7	63.7	60.1	33.2	11.6

Although Ticarcillin is primarily indicated in Gram-negative infections, its *in vitro* activity against Gram-positive organisms should be considered in treating infections caused by both Gram-negative and Gram-positive organisms (see MICROBIOLOGY).

Based on the *in vitro* synergism between Ticarcillin and gentamicin sulfate, tobramycin sulfate or amikacin sulfate against certain strains of *Pseudomonas aeruginosa,* combined therapy has been successful, using full therapeutic dosages. (For additional prescribing information, see the gentamicin sulfate, tobramycin sulfate and amikacin sulfate package inserts.)

NOTE: Culturing and susceptibilty testing should be performed initially and during treatment to monitor the effectiveness of therapy and the susceptibility of the bacteria.

Contraindications: A history of allergic reaction to any of the penicillins is a contraindication.

Warnings: Serious and occasionally fatal hypersensitivity (anaphylactoid) reactions have been reported in patients receiving penicillin. These reactions are more likely to occur in persons with a history of sensitivity to multiple allergens.

There are reports of patients with a history of penicillin hypersensitivity reactions who experience severe hypersensitivity reactions when treated with a cephalosporin. Before therapy with a penicillin, careful inquiry should be made about previous hypersensitivity reactions to penicillins, cephalosporins, and other allergens. If a reaction occurs, the drug should be discontinued unless, in the opinion of the physician, the condition being treated is life-threatening and amenable only to Ticarcillin therapy. **Serious anaphylactoid reactions require immediate emergency treatment with epinephrine. Oxygen, intravenous steroids, airway management, including intubation, should also be administered as indicated.**

Some patients receiving high doses of Ticarcillin may develop hemorrhagic manifestations associated with abnormalities of coagulation tests, such as bleeding time and platelet aggregation. On withdrawal of the drug, the bleeding should cease and coagulation abnormalities revert to normal. Other causes of abnormal bleeding should also be considered. Patients with renal impairment, in whom excretion of Ticarcillin is delayed, should be observed for bleeding manifestations. Such patients should be dosed strictly according to recommendations (see DOSAGE AND ADMINISTRATION). If bleeding manifestations appear, Ticarcillin treatment should be discontinued and appropriate therapy instituted.

Precautions: Although TICAR (Ticarcillin Disodium) exhibits the characteristic low toxicity of the penicillins, as with any other potent agent, it is advisable to check periodically for organ system dysfunction (including renal, hepatic and hematopoietic) during prolonged treatment. If overgrowth of resistant organisms occurs, the appropriate therapy should be initiated.

Since the theoretical sodium content is 5.2 milequivalents (120 mg) per gram of Ticarcillin, and the actual vial content can be as high as 6.5 mEq/Gm, electrolyte and cardiac status should be monitored carefully.

In a few patients receiving intravenous Ticarcillin, hypokalemia has been reported. Serum potassium should be measured periodically, and, if necessary, corrective therapy should be implemented.

As with any penicillin, the possibility of an allergic response, including anaphylaxis, exists, particularly in hypersensitive patients.

USAGE DURING PREGNANCY

Reproduction studies have been performed in mice and rats and have revealed no evidence of impaired fertility or harm to the fetus due to Ticarcillin. There are no well-controlled studies in pregnant women, but investigational experience does not include any positive evidence of adverse effects on the fetus. Although there is no clearly defined risk, such experience cannot exclude the possibility of infrequent or subtle damage to the fetus. Ticarcillin should be used in pregnant women only when clearly needed.

Adverse Reactions: The following adverse reactions may occur:

Hypersensitivity Reactions: Skin rashes, pruritus, urticaria, drug fever.

Gastrointestinal Disturbances: Nausea and vomiting.

Hemic and Lymphatic Systems: As with other penicillins, anemia, thrombocytopenia, leukopenia, neutropenia and eosinophilia.

Abnormalities of Blood, Hepatic and Renal Laboratory Studies: As with other semisynthetic penicillins, SGOT and SGPT elevations have been reported. To date, clinical manifestations of hepatic or renal disorders have not been observed which could be ascribed solely to Ticarcillin.

CNS: Patients, especially those with impaired renal function, may experience convulsions or neuromuscular excitability when very high doses of the drug are administered.

Other: Local reactions such as pain (rarely accompanied by induration) at the site of the injection have been reported.

Vein irritation and phlebitis can occur, particularly when undiluted solution is directly injected into the vein.

[See table on next page].

Directions For Use:

1 Gm. 3 Gm and 6 Gm Standard Vials:

Intramuscular Use: Each gram of Ticarcillin should be reconstituted with 2 ml of the desired intravenous solution listed below of 1% Lido-

Continued on next page

Beecham Laboratories—Cont.

caine Hydrochloride solution (without epinephrine). Each 2.6 ml of the resulting solution will then contain 1 Gm of Ticarcillin.
[For full product information, refer to manufacturer's package insert for Lidocaine Hydrochloride.]
As with all intramuscular preparations, TICAR (Ticarcillin Disodium) should be injected well within the body of a relatively large muscle, using usual techniques and precautions.
I.M. solutions stored at room temperature must be discarded after 24 hours or after 60 hours if stored under refrigeration.

Intravenous Use: Reconstitute each gram of Ticarcillin with 4 ml of the desired intravenous solution listed below; when dissolved, further dilute if desired. After the addition of 4 ml of diluent per gram of Ticarcillin each 1.0 ml of the resulting solution will have an approximate average concentration of 204 mg.
Direct Intravenous Injection: In order to avoid vein irritation, administer solution as slowly as possible.
Intravenous Infusion: Reconstitute the required number of vials as described above, using a suitable intravenous solution listed below, then further dilute to the desired volume. Administer by continuous or intermittent intravenous drip. Intermittent infusion should be administered over a 30 minute to 2 hour period in equally divided doses.
For the stability of TICAR in various intravenous solutions see DIRECTIONS FOR USE under Piggyback Bottles.

3 Gm Piggyback Bottles:
Direct Intravenous Injection:
The 3 gram bottle should be reconstituted with a minimum of 30 ml of the desired intravenous solution listed below.

Amount of Diluent	Concentration of Solution
100 ml	1 Gm/34 ml
60 ml	1 Gm/20 ml
30 ml	1 Gm/10 ml

In order to avoid vein irritation, the solution should be administered as slowly as possible. A dilution of approximately 1 Gm/20 ml or more

Dosage and Administration

Clinical experience indicates that in serious urinary tract and systemic infections, intravenous therapy in the higher doses should be used. Intramuscular injections should not exceed 2 grams per injection.

Adults:

Bacterial Septicemia Respiratory Tract Infections Skin and Soft-Tissue Intra-Abdominal Infections Infections of the Female Pelvis and Genital Tract	200–300 mg/kg/day by I.V. infusion in divided doses every 3, 4 or 6 hours. [Usual recommended dosage: 3 grams every 3, 4 or 6 hours, depending on weight and the severity of the infection.]
Urinary Tract Infections Complicated:	150–200 mg/kg,day by I.V. infusion in divided doses every 4 or 6 hours. [Usual recommended dosage for average (70 kg) adults: 3 grams q.i.d.]
Uncomplicated	1 gram I.M. or direct I.V. every 6 hours
Infections complicated by renal insuffiency: (1)	Initial loading dose of 3 grams I.V. followed by I.V. doses, based on creatinine clearance and type of dialysis, as indicated below:
Creatinine clearance ml/min.:	
over 60	3 grams every 4 hours
30–60	2 grams every 4 hours
10–30	2 grams every 8 hours
less than 10	2 grams every 12 hours (or 1 gram I.M. every 6 hours)
less than 10 with hepatic dysfunction	2 grams every 24 hours (or 1 gram I.M. every 12 hours)
patients on peritoneal dialysis	3 grams every 12 hours
patients on hemodialysis	2 grams every 12 hours supplemented with 3 grams after each dialysis

To calculate creatinine clearance* from a serum creatinine value use the following formula:

$$C_{cr} = \frac{(140\text{—Age})\ (\text{wt in kg})}{72 \times S_{cr}(\text{mg}/100\ \text{ml})}$$

This is the calculated creatinine clearance for adult males; for females it is 15% less.
* Cockcroft, D.W., et al, "Prediction of Creatinine Clearance from Serum Creatinine" *Nephron* 16:31–41 (1976).

(1) The half-life of Ticarcillin in patients with renal failure is approximately 13 hours.

Children: Under 40 kg (88 lbs)

The daily dose for children should not exceed the adult dosage.

Bacterial Septicemia Respiratory Tract Infections Skin and Soft-Tissue Infections Intra-Abdominal Infections Infections of the Female Pelvis and Genital Tract	200–300 mg/kg/day by I.V. infusion in divided doses every 4 or 6 hours.
Urinary Tract Infections Complicated:	150–200 mg/kg/day by I.V. infusion in divided doses every 4 to 6 hours.
Uncomplicated:	50–100 mg/kg/day I.M. or direct I.V. in divided doses every 6 or 8 hours.
Infections complicated by renal insufficiency:	Clinical data is insufficient to recommend an optimum dose.

Children weighing more than 40 kg (88 lbs) should receive adult dosages.

Neonates: In the neonate, for severe infections (sepsis) due to susceptible strains of *Pseudomonas, Proteus,* and *E. coli*, the following Ticarcillin dosages may be given I.M. or by 10–20 minutes I.V. infusion:

Infants under 2000 grams body weight:

Aged 0–7 days	75 mg/kg/12 hours (150 mg/kg/day)
Aged over 7 days	75 mg/kg/8 hours (225 mg/kg/day)

Infants over 2000 grams body weight:

Ages 0–7 days	75 mg/kg/8 hours (225 mg/kg/day)
Aged over 7 days	100 mg/kg/8 hours (300 mg/kg/day)

This dosage schedule is intended to produce peak serum concentrations of 125–150 mcg/ml one hour after a dose of Ticarcillin and trough concentrations of 25–50 mcg/ml immediately before the next dose.

NOTE: Gentamicin, tobramycin or amikacin may be used concurrently with Ticarcillin for initial therapy until results of culture and susceptibility studies are known.
Seriously ill patients should receive the higher doses. TICAR has proved to be useful in infections in which protective mechanisms are impaired, such as in acute leukemia and during therapy with immunosuppressive or oncolytic drugs.

will further reduce the incidence of vein irritation.

Intravenous Infusion: Stability studies in various intravenous solutions indicate that Ticarcillin Disodium will lose less than 10% activity at room temperature within the stated time periods at concentrations between 10 mg/ml and 50 mg/ml:

Intravenous Solution	Time Period
* Water for Injection	72 hours
Sodium Chloride Injection	72 hours
Dextrose 5% in 0.225% Sodium Chloride Solution	72 hours
Dextrose 5% in 0.45% Sodium Chloride Solution	72 hours
* Dextrose Injection 5%	72 hours
5% Alcohol, 5% Dextrose in 0.9% Sodium Chloride Solution	72 hours
* Ringer's Injection	48 hours
* Lactated Ringer's Injection	48 hours
10% Invert Sugar in Water	48 hours
5% Dextrose in Electrolyte #48 Solution	48 hours
5% Dextrose in Electrolyte #75 Solution	48 hours
5% Fructose (Levugen) in Electrolyte #75 Solution	48 hours

The above solution remain stable for 14 days if stored under refrigeration (4°C); refrigerated solutions stored longer than 72 hours should *not* be used for multidose purposes.

(*) These solutions remain stable up to 100 mg/ml concentration. After reconstitution, they can be frozen (approx. 0°F) and stored for up to 30 days without loss of potency. The stabilities of the thawed solutions are identical to the unfrozen ones listed above.

Unused solutions should be discarded after the time periods mentioned above.

It is recommended that TICAR and gentamicin sulfate, tobramycin sulfate or amikacin sulfate *not* be mixed together in the same I.V. solution due to the gradual inactivation of gentamicin sulfate, tobramycin sulfate or amikacin sulfate under these circumstances. The therapeutic effect of TICAR and these aminoglycoside drugs remains unimpaired when administered separately.

How Supplied: TICAR (Sterile Ticarcillin Disodium). Each vial contains Ticarcillin Disodium equivalent to 1 Gm, 3 Gm or 6 Gm Ticarcillin.

NDC 0029-6550-22 ....1 Gm Vial
NDC 0029-6552-26 ....3 Gm Vial
NDC 0029-6555-26 ....6 Gm Vial
NDC 0029-6552-21 ......3 Gm Piggyback Bottle

Rev. March, 1982
7182/1

TIGAN® ℞
(trimethobenzamide HCl)

Description: Tigan is an antiemetic agent. Chemically, trimethobenzamide HCl is N-[*p*-[2-(dimethylamino)-ethoxy] benzyl]-3, 4, 5-trimethoxybenzamide hydrochloride. It has a molecular weight of 424.93.

Capsules; Blue, each containing 250 mg trimethobenzamide hydrochloride; blue and white, each containing 100 mg trimethobenzamide hydrochloride.

Suppositories: (200 mg): Each suppository contains 200 mg trimethobenzamide hydrochloride and 2% benzocaine in a base compounded with polysorbate 80, white beeswax and propylene glycol monostearate.

Suppositories, Pediatric (100 mg): Each suppository contains 100 mg trimethobenzamide hydrochloride and 2% benzocaine in a base compounded with polysorbate 80, white beeswax and propylene glycol monostearate.

Ampuls: Each 2-ml ampul contains 200 mg trimethobenzamide hydrochloride compounded with 0.2% parabens (methyl and propyl) as preservatives, 1 mg sodium citrate and 0.4 mg citric acid as buffers and pH adjusted to approximately 5.0 with sodium hydroxide.

Multiple Dose Vials: Each ml contains 100 mg trimethobenzamide hydrochloride compounded with 0.45% phenol as preservative, 0.5 mg sodium citrate and 0.2 mg citric acid as buffers and pH adjusted to approximately 5.0 with sodium hydroxide.

Thera-Ject™ (Disposable Syringes): Each 2 ml contains 200 mg trimethobenzamide hydrochloride compounded with 0.45% phenol as preservative, 1 mg sodium citrate and 0.4 mg citric acid as buffers, 0.2 mg disodium edetate as stabilizer and pH adjusted to approximately 5.0 with sodium hydroxide.

Actions: The mechanism of action of Tigan as determined in animals is obscure, but may be the chemoreceptor trigger zone (CTZ), an area in the medulla oblongata through which emetic impulses are conveyed to the vomiting center; direct impulses to the vomiting center apparently are not similarly inhibited. In dogs pretreated with trimethobenzamide HCl, the emetic response to apomorphine is inhibited, while little or no protection is afforded against emesis induced by intragastric copper sulfate.

Indications: Tigan is indicated for the control of nausea and vomiting.

Contraindications: The injectable form of Tigan in children, the suppositories in premature or newborn infants, and use in patients with known hypersensitivity to trimethobenzamide are contraindicated. Since the suppositories contain benzocaine they should not be used in patients known to be sensitive to this or similar local anesthetics.

Warnings:

Caution should be exercised when administering Tigan to children for the treatment of vomiting. Antiemetics are not recommended for treatment of uncomplicated vomiting in children and their use should be limited to prolonged vomiting of known etiology. There are three principal reasons for caution:

1. There has been some suspicion that centrally acting antimetics may contribute, in combination with viral illnesses (a possible cause of vomiting in children), to development of Reye's syndrome, a potentially fatal acute childhood encephalopathy with visceral fatty degeneration, especially involving the liver. Although there is no confirmation of this suspicion, caution is nevertheless recommended.
2. The extrapyramidal symptoms which can occur secondary to Tigan may be confused with the central nervous system signs of an undiagnosed primary disease responsible for the vomiting, e.g., Reye's syndrome or other encephalopathy.
3. It has been suspected that drugs with hepatotoxic potential, such as Tigan, may unfavorably alter the course of Reye's syndrome. Such drugs should therefore be avoided in children whose signs and symptoms (vomiting) could represent Reye's syndrome. It should also be noted that salicylates and acetaminophen are hepatotoxic at large doses. Although it is not known that at usual doses they would represent a hazard in patients with the underlying hepatic disorder of Reye's syndrome, these drugs, too, should be avoided in children whose signs and symptoms could represent Reye's syndrome, unless alternative methods of controlling fever are not successful.

Tigan may produce drowsiness. Patients should not operate motor vehicles or other dangerous machinery until their individual responses have been determined.

Reye's Syndrome has been associated with the use of TIGAN and other drugs, including antiemetics, although their contribution, if any, to the cause and course of the disease hasn't been established. This syndrome is characterized by an abrupt onset shortly following a nonspecific febrile illness, with persistent, severe vomiting, lethargy, irrational behavior, progressive encephalopathy leading to coma, convulsions and death.

Usage in Pregnancy: Trimethobenzamide hydrochloride was studied in reproduction experiments in rats and rabbits and no teratogenicity was suggested. The only effects observed were an increased percentage of embryonic resorptions or stillborn pups in rats administered 20 mg and 100 mg/kg and increased resorptions in rabbits receiving 100 mg/kg. In each study these adverse effects were attributed to one or two dams. The relevance to humans is not known. Since there is no adequate experience in pregnant or lactating women who have received this drug, safety in pregnancy or in nursing mothers has not been established.

Usage with Alcohol: Concomitant use of alcohol with Tigan may result in an adverse drug interaction.

Precautions: During the course of acute febrile illness, encephalitides, gastroenteritis, dehydration and electrolyte imbalance, especially in children and the elderly or debilitated, CNS reactions such as opisthotonos, convulsions, coma and extrapyramidal symptoms have been reported with and without use of Tigan or other antiemetic agents. In such disorders caution should be exercised in administering Tigan, particularly to patients who have recently received other CNS-acting agents (phenothiazines, barbiturates, belladonna derivatives). It is recommended that severe emesis should not be treated with an antiemetic drug alone; where possible the cause of vomiting should be established. Primary emphasis should be directed toward the restoration of body fluids and electrolyte balance, the relief of fever and relief of the causative disease process. Overhydration should be avoided since it may result in cerebral edema.

The antiemetic effects of Tigan may render diagnosis more difficult in such conditions as appendicitis and obscure signs of toxicity due to overdosage of other drugs.

Adverse Reactions: There have been reports of hypersensitivity reactions and Parkinson-like symptoms. There have been instances of hypotension reported following parenteral administration to surgical patients. There have been reports of blood dyscrasias, blurring of vision, coma, convulsions, depression of mood, diarrhea, disorientation, dizziness, drowsiness, headache, jaundice, muscle cramps and opisthotonos. If these occur, the administration of the drug should be discontinued. Allergic-type skin reactions have been observed; therefore, the drug should be discontinued at the first sign of sensitization. While these symptoms will usually disappear spontaneously, symptomatic treatment may be indicated in some cases.

Dosage and Administration: (See WARNINGS and PRECAUTIONS.) Dosage should be adjusted according to the indication for therapy, severity of symptoms and the response of the patient.

Capsules, 250 mg and 100 mg

Usual Adult Dosage

One 250-mg capsule t.i.d. or q.i.d.

Usual Children's Dosage

30 to 90 lbs: One or two 100-mg capsules t.i.d. or q.i.d.

Suppositories, 200 mg (Not to be used in premature or newborn infants.)

Continued on next page

Beecham Laboratories—Cont.

Usual Adult Dosage
One suppository (200 mg) t.i.d. or q.i.d.
Usual Children's Dosage
Under 30 lbs: One-half suppository (100 mg) t.i.d. or q.i.d.
30 to 90 lbs: One-half to one suppository (100 to 200 mg) t.i.d. or q.i.d.
SUPPOSITORIES, PEDIATRIC, 100 mg (Not to be used in Premature or newborn infants).
Usual Children's Dosage
Under 30 lbs; One suppository (100 mg) t.i.d. or q.i.d.
30 to 90 lbs; One to two suppositories (100 to 200 mg) t.i.d. or q.i.d.
Injectable, 100 mg/ml (Not recommended for use in children.)
Usual Adult Dosage: 2 ml (200 mg) t.i.d. or q.i.d. intramuscularly.
Intramuscular administration may cause pain, stinging, burning, redness and swelling at the site of injection. Such effects may be minimized by deep injection into the upper outer quadrant of the gluteal region, and by avoiding the escape of solution along the route.
Note: The injectable form is intended for intramuscular administration only; it is not recommended for intravenous use.
How Supplied:

Product	Package Sizes	NDC Numbers
Capsules		
100 mg.	100's	NDC-0029-4082-30
250 mg.	100's	NDC-0029-4083-30
	500's	NDC-0029-4083-32
Suppositories		
200 mg.	10's	NDC-0029-4084-38
	50's	NDC-0029-4084-39
Suppositories Pediatric		
100 mg.	10's	NDC-0029-4088-38
Injectable Ampuls		
2 ml, 200 mg.	10's	NDC-0029-4085-22
Vials		
20 ml, 100 mg./ml	Each	NDC-0029-4086-22
Thera-Ject® (Disposable Syringe)		
2 ml, 100 mg./ml	25's	NDC-0029-4087-22

[*Shown in Product Identification Section*]

Berlex Laboratories, Inc.
WAYNE, NJ 07470

AMINODUR® (aminophylline) DURA-TABS® ℞

Description: Each Aminodur® Dura-Tab® contains 300 mg hydrous aminophylline (equivalent to 236 mg anhydrous theophylline) in a dye-free tablet matrix specially designed to provide a therapeutically effective serum level when administered every 12 hours. Aminodur minimizes the peaks and valleys of serum levels commonly found with shorter-acting theophylline products.
Aminophylline is a soluble complex containing approximately 85% anhydrous theophylline and 15% ethylenediamine.
Clinical Pharmacology: Theophylline, the active component of aminophylline, directly relaxes the smooth muscle of the bronchial airways and pulmonary blood vessels, thus acting mainly as a bronchodilator, pulmonary vasodilator and smooth muscle relaxant. The drug also possesses other actions typical of the xanthine derivatives: coronary vasodilator, diuretic, cardiac stimulant, cerebral stimulant and skeletal muscle stimulant.
No development of tolerance occurs with chronic use of theophylline.
The half-life is shortened with cigarette smoking and prolonged in alcoholism, reduced hepatic or renal function, congestive heart failure, and in patients receiving cimetidine or antibiotics such as troleandomycin, erythromycin and clindamycin. High fever for prolonged periods may decrease theophylline elimination.
The half-life of theophylline in newborn infants is prolonged (exceeding 24 hours). At about 3–6 months of age, the half-life approaches that seen in older children (3–5 hours).
Older adults with chronic obstructive pulmonary disease, patients with cor pulmonale or other causes of heart failure, and patients with liver pathology may have lower clearances with half-lives that may exceed 24 hours.
The half-life of theophylline in smokers (1 to 2 packs/day) averaged 4–5 hours among various studies, much shorter than the half-life in nonsmokers who averaged about 7–9 hours.
In a single dose study in normal adult volunteers, a dose of two Aminodur Dura-Tabs (600 mg equivalent to 472 mg anhydrous theophylline) produced a mean peak theophylline blood level of 7.6 μg/ml at 7.1 hours after administration. Aminodur Dura-Tabs were found to be equivalent in bioavailability to the reference standard Elixophyllin (theophylline) Elixir.
In a multiple dose, steady state study in normal adult volunteers, Aminodur Dura-Tabs produced relatively constant theophylline blood levels with an average difference between maximum and minimum theophylline plasma concentration of only 2.7 μg/ml.
Indications: Aminodur Dura-Tabs is indicated for relief and/or prevention of symptoms of asthma and reversible bronchospasm associated with chronic bronchitis and emphysema.
Contraindications: Hypersensitivity to any of the components.
Warnings: Since excessive theophylline doses may be associated with toxicity, periodic measurement of serum theophylline levels is recommended to assure maximal benefit without excessive risk. Incidence of toxicity increases at levels greater than 20 μg/ml. Although early signs of theophylline toxicity such as nausea and restlessness are often seen, in some cases ventricular arrhythmia or convulsions may appear without warning as the first signs of toxicity.
There is an excellent correlation between high blood levels of theophylline resulting from conventional doses and associated clinical manifestations of toxicity in (1) patients with lowered body plasma clearances (due to transient cardiac decompensation), (2) patients with liver dysfunction or chronic obstructive lung disease, (3) patients who are older than 55 years of age, particularly males.
Many patients with excessive theophylline serum levels exhibit a tachycardia.
Theophylline preparations may worsen preexisting arrhythmias.
Usage in Pregnancy: Safe use in pregnancy has not been established relative to possible adverse effects on fetal development. Therefore, use of theophylline in pregnant women should be balanced against the risk of uncontrolled asthma.
Precautions: Aminodur Dura-Tabs should not be administered concurrently with other xanthine preparations. Use with caution in patients with severe cardiac disease, severe hypoxemia, hypertension, hyperthyroidism, acute myocardial injury, cor pulmonale, liver disease, in the elderly (especially males) and in neonates. Great caution should especially be used in giving aminophylline to patients in congestive heart failure (markedly prolonged blood level curves have been observed in such patients).
Use aminophylline cautiously in patients with history of peptic ulcer.
Adverse Reactions: The most common adverse reactions are usually due to overdose and are:
Gastrointestinal: nausea, vomiting, epigastric pain, hematemesis, diarrhea;
Central nervous system: headaches, irritability, restlessness, insomnia, reflex hyperexcitability, muscle twitching, clonic and tonic generalized convulsions;
Cardiovascular: palpitation, tachycardia, extrasystoles, flushing, hypotension, circulatory failure, ventricular arrhythmias;
Respiratory: tachypnea;
Renal: albuminuria, increased excretion of renal tubular cells and red blood cells, potentiation of diuresis;
Others: hyperglycemia and inappropriate ADH (antidiuretic hormone) syndrome.
Drug Interactions: Toxic synergism with ephedrine has been documented and may occur with some other sympathomimetic bronchodilators.

Drug	Effect
Aminophylline with lithium carbonate	Increased excretion of lithium carbonate
Aminophylline with propranolol	Antagonism of propranolol effect
Theophylline with furosemide	Increased diuresis
Theophylline with hexamethonium	Decreased chronotropic effect
Theophylline with reserpine	Tachycardia
Theophylline with cimetidine	Increased theophylline blood levels
Theophylline with clindamycin, lincomycin, troleandomycin, or erythromycin	Increased theophylline blood levels

Overdosage:
Management:
A. If potential oral overdose is established and seizure has not occurred:
1. Induce vomiting;
2. Administer a cathartic,
3. Administer activated charcoal.

B. If patient is having a seizure:
1. Establish an airway;
2. Administer O_2;
3. Treat the seizure with intravenous diazepam, 0.1 to 0.3 mg/kg up to 10 mg;
4. Monitor vital signs, maintain blood pressure and provide adequate hydration.

C. Post-Seizure Coma:
1. Maintain airway and oxygenation;
2. Follow above recommendations to prevent absorption of drug, but intubation and lavage will have to be performed instead of inducing emesis, and the cathartic and charcoal will need to be introduced via a large bore gastric lavage tube;
3. Continue to provide full supportive care and adequate hydration while waiting for drug to be metabolized.

Dosage and Administration: Therapeutic serum levels associated with optimal benefit and minimal risk of toxicity are considered to be between 10 μg/ml and 20 μg/ml. Levels above 20 μg/ml may produce toxic effects. Periodic and carefully controlled monitoring of serum theophylline levels is highly recommended.
At steady-state blood levels, the following maintenance dose is recommended:
Adults: One Aminodur Dura-Tab every 12 hours* approximately 30 minutes before eating.
Not recommended for children under 12 years of age.
The average initial adult dose for a *nontheophyllinized* patient is two Aminodur Dura-Tabs, then one Aminodur Dura-Tab every 12 hours until steady-state blood levels are achieved.*
*Occasional patients may require dosing every 8 hours.

If the desired response is not achieved, dosage may be increased in approximately 25% increments at 2–3 day intervals so long as no intolerance is observed, until maximum indicated below is reached.

If gastrointestinal irritation is experienced, dosages may be taken with or after meals. Although absorption may be slowed, it is still complete.

Maximum dose without measurement of serum concentration: Not to exceed the following: (WARNING: DO NOT ATTEMPT TO MAINTAIN ANY DOSE THAT IS NOT TOLERATED.)

Age 12–16 years —	21.2 mg/kg/day †(18 mg/kg/day)
Age > 16 years—	15.2 mg/kg/day or 1100 mg/day (WHICHEVER IS LESS) *(13 mg/kg/day or 900 mg/day)

†anhydrous theophylline

NOTE: Use ideal body weight for obese patients.

Measurement of serum theophylline concentration during chronic therapy: If the above maximum doses are to be maintained or exceeded, serum theophylline measurement is recommended. This should be obtained at the approximate time of peak absorption during chronic therapy for the product used (1–2 hours for liquids and capsules that undergo rapid dissolution, 3–5 hours for sustained release preparations). It is important that the patient will have missed NO doses during the previous 48 hours and that dosing intervals will have been reasonably typical with no added doses during that period of time. DOSAGE ADJUSTMENT BASED ON SERUM THEOPHYLLINE MEASUREMENTS WHEN THESE INSTRUCTIONS HAVE NOT BEEN FOLLOWED MAY RESULT IN RECOMMENDATIONS THAT PRESENT A RISK OF TOXICITY TO THE PATIENT.

NOTE: Dosage may be titrated by breaking the tablet in half. Do not crush or chew since sustained-release properties will be lost.

How Supplied: Scored, dye-free Aminodur Dura-Tabs in bottles of:

100 Dura-Tabs ....NDC 50419-131-10
250 Dura-Tabs ....NDC 50419-131-25

Store at controlled room temperature.

DECONAMINE® Tablets ℞
DECONAMINE® Elixir ℞
DECONAMINE® SR Capsules ℞
DECONAMINE® Syrup ℞

Description:

Tablets

Each scored, white tablet contains:
chlorpheniramine maleate ....4 mg
d-pseudoephedrine hydrochloride ......60 mg

Elixir

Each 5 ml (teaspoonful) blue color liquid contains:
chlorpheniramine maleate ....2 mg
d-pseudoephedrine hydrochloride ......30 mg
alcohol 15%
in a pleasant tasting aromatic vehicle.

SR Capsules

Each sustained release, blue and yellow capsule contains:
chlorpheniramine maleate ....8 mg
d-pseudoephedrine hydrochloride ....120 mg
The capsules are designed to provide prolonged release of medication.

Syrup—No alcohol, no dye

Each 5 ml (teaspoonful) clear, colorless liquid contains:
chlorpheniramine maleate ....2 mg
d-pseudoephedrine hydrochloride ......30 mg
in a grape-flavored, aromatic vehicle

Clinical Pharmacology: Chlorpheniramine maleate antagonizes the physiological action of histamine by acting as an H_1 receptor blocking agent.

Pseudoephedrine is an orally active sympathomimetic amine and exerts a decongestant action on the nasal mucosa. It does this by vasoconstriction which results in reduction of tissue hyperemia, edema, nasal congestion and an increase in nasal airway patency. The vasoconstriction action of pseudoephedrine is similar to that of ephedrine. In the usual dose it has minimal vasopressor effects.

Indications: For relief of nasal congestion associated with the common cold, hay fever and other allergies, sinusitis, eustachian tube blockage, and vasomotor and allergic rhinitis.

Contraindications: Patients with severe hypertension, severe coronary artery disease and patients on MAO inhibitor therapy. Deconamine is also contraindicated in patients sensitive to antihistamines or sympathomimetic agents.

Warnings: Chlorpheniramine maleate should be used with extreme caution in patients with narrow angle glaucoma; stenosing peptic ulcer; pyloroduodenal obstruction; symptomatic prostatic hypertrophy; or bladder neck obstruction. Due to its mild atropine-like action, chlorpheniramine maleate should be used cautiously in patients with bronchial asthma.

Sympathomimetic amines should be used with caution in patients with hypertension, ischemic heart disease, diabetes mellitus, increased intraocular pressure, hyperthyroidism and prostatic hypertrophy. Sympathomimetics may produce central nervous system stimulation with convulsions or cardiovascular collapse with accompanying hypotension.

Precautions:

Information for patients:

Antihistamines may impair mental and physical abilities required for the performance of potentially hazardous tasks, such as driving a vehicle or operating machinery. Patients should also be warned about possible additive effects with alcohol and other central nervous system depressants (hypnotics, sedatives, tranquilizers).

Drug interactions:

Pseudoephedrine-containing drugs should not be given to patients treated with monoamine oxidase (MAO) inhibitors because of the possibility of precipitating a hypertensive crisis. MAO inhibitors also prolong and intensify the anticholinergic effects of antihistamines. Sympathomimetics may reduce the antihypertensive effect of methyldopa, reserpine, veratrum alkaloids and mecamylamine.

Alcohol and other sedative drugs will potentiate the sedative effects of chlorpheniramine.

Pregnancy:

Pregnancy Category C: Animal reproduction studies have not been conducted with Deconamine. It is also not known whether Deconamine can cause fetal harm when administered to a pregnant woman or can affect reproduction capacity. Deconamine should be given to a pregnant woman only if clearly needed.

Nursing Mothers: Due to the possible passage of pseudoephedrine and chlorpheniramine into breast milk and because of the higher than usual risk for infants from sympathomimetic amines and antihistamines, the benefit to the mother vs. the potential risk should be considered and a decision should be made whether to discontinue nursing or to discontinue the drug.

Pediatric Use: Deconamine capsules or tablets should not be given to children under 12 years of age.

Adverse Reactions:

Chlorpheniramine maleate

Slight to moderate drowsiness may occur and is the most frequent side effect. Other possible side effects of antihistamines in general include:

General: urticaria, drug rash, anaphylactic shock, photosensitivity, excessive perspiration, chills, dryness of mouth, nose and throat.

Cardiovascular: hypotension, headache, palpitation, tachycardia, extrasystoles.

Hematological: hemolytic anemia, thrombocytopenia, agranulocytosis.

CNS: sedation, dizziness, disturbed coordination, fatigue, confusion, restlessness, excitation, nervousness, tremor, irritability, insomnia, euphoria, paresthesia, blurred vision, diplopia, vertigo, tinnitus, hysteria, neuritis, convulsion.

Gastrointestinal: epigastric distress, anorexia, nausea, vomiting, diarrhea, constipation.

Genitourinary: urinary frequency, difficult urination, urinary retention, early menses.

Respiratory: thickening of bronchial secretions, tightness of chest, wheezing and nasal stuffiness.

Pseudoephedrine hydrochloride

Pseudoephedrine may cause mild central nervous system stimulation especially in those patients who are hypersensitive to sympathomimetic drugs. Nervousness, excitability, restlessness, dizziness, weakness and insomnia may also occur. Headache and drowsiness have also been reported. Large doses may cause lightheadedness, nausea and/or vomiting. Sympathomimetic drugs have also been associated with certain untoward reactions including fear, anxiety, tenseness, restlessness, tremor, weakness, pallor, respiratory difficulty, dysuria, insomnia, hallucination, convulsion, CNS depression, arrhythmias and cardiovascular collapse with hypotension.

Overdosage: Acute overdosage may produce clinical signs of CNS stimulation and variable cardiovascular effects. Pressor amines should be used with great caution in the presence of pseudoephedrine. Patients with signs of stimulation should be treated conservatively.

Dosage and Administration:

Tablets

Adults and children over 12 years, 1 tablet three or four times daily.

Children under 12 years, Deconamine Elixir or Syrup is recommended.

Elixir or Syrup

Adults and children over 12 years, 1 to 2 teaspoonfuls (5 to 10 ml) three or four times daily.

Children 6 to 12 years, ½ to 1 teaspoonful (2.5 to 5 ml) three or four times daily, not to exceed 4 teaspoonfuls in 24 hours.

Children 2 to 6 years, ½ teaspoonful (2.5 ml) three or four times daily, not to exceed 2 teaspoonfuls in 24 hours.

Children under two years, as directed by physician.

SR Capsules

Adults and children over 12 years, one capsule every 12 hours.

Children under 12 years, Deconamine Elixir or Syrup is recommended.

How Supplied:

In bottles of:

Tablets

100 ....NDC 50419-184-10
500 ....NDC 50419-184-50

Elixir

473 ml ....NDC 50419-182-16

SR Capsules

100 ....NDC 50419-181-10
500 ....NDC 50419-181-50

Syrup

473 ml ....NDC 50419-185-16

Store at controlled room temperature.

[*Shown in Product Identification Section*]

Continued on next page

Berlex—Cont.

ELIXICON® SUSPENSION ℞
(theophylline)

ELIXOPHYLLIN® CAPSULES ℞
100 mg, 200 mg
(theophylline)

ELIXOPHYLLIN® SR CAPSULES ℞
125 mg, 250 mg
(theophylline)

ELIXOPHYLLIN® ELIXIR ℞
(theophylline)

Description:

Elixicon (theophylline) Suspension
Each 5 ml (teaspoonful) contains 100 mg anhydrous theophylline in an aqueous suspension. Contains no sugar or dye. Preserved with methylparaben and propylparaben.

Elixophyllin (theophylline) Capsules
100 mg capsule—Each off-white (dye-free) soft gelatin Elixophyllin Capsule contains 100 mg anhydrous theophylline in a suspension of polyethylene glycol.
200 mg capsule—Each off-white (dye-free) soft gelatin Elixophyllin Capsule contains 200 mg anhydrous theophylline in a suspension of polyethylene glycol.

Elixophyllin (theophylline) SR Capsules
Elixophyllin SR Capsules are designed to provide a prolonged therapeutic effect.
125 mg Capsule—Each white, opaque, dye-free capsule contains 125 mg anhydrous theophylline.
250 mg Capsule—Each clear, dye-free capsule contains 250 mg anhydrous theophylline.

Elixophyllin (theophylline) Elixir
Each 15 ml (tablespoonful) of Elixophyllin Elixir contains 80 mg anhydrous theophylline and 20% alcohol in a palatable aromatic base.

Clinical Pharmacology: Theophylline directly relaxes the smooth muscle of the bronchial airways and pulmonary blood vessels, thus acting mainly as a bronchodilator, pulmonary vasodilator and smooth muscle relaxant. The drug also possesses other actions typical of the xanthine derivatives: coronary vasodilator, diuretic, cardiac stimulant, cerebral stimulant and skeletal muscle stimulant.
No development of tolerance occurs with chronic use of theophylline.
The half-life is shortened with cigarette smoking and prolonged in alcoholism, reduced hepatic or renal function, congestive heart failure, and in patients receiving cimetidine or antibiotics such as troleandomycin, erythromycin and clindamycin. High fever for prolonged periods may decrease theophylline elimination.
The half-life of theophylline in newborn infants is prolonged (exceeding 24 hours). At about 3–6 months of age, the half-life approaches that seen in older children (3–5 hours).
Older adults with chronic obstructive pulmonary disease, patients with cor pulmonale or other causes of heart failure, and patients with liver pathology may have lower clearances with half-lives that may exceed 24 hours.
The half-life of theophylline in smokers (1 to 2 packs/day) averaged 4–5 hours among various studies, much shorter than the half-life in nonsmokers who averaged about 7–9 hours.

Elixicon (theophylline) Suspension
In a single dose study in normal volunteers, a single 400 mg dose of Elixicon Suspension produced a mean peak theophylline blood level of 14.2 μg/ml at 1.5 hours after administration. Elixicon Suspension was found to be equivalent in bioavailability to the reference standard Elixophyllin (theophylline) Elixir.

Elixophyllin (theophylline) Capsules
In a single dose study in normal volunteers, a single 400 mg dose of Elixophyllin Capsules administered as two 200 mg capsules produced a mean peak theophylline blood level of 14.9 μg/ml at 1.6 hours after administration. Elixophyllin Capsules were found to be equivalent in bioavailability to the reference standard Elixophyllin (theophylline) Elixir.

Elixophyllin (theophylline) SR Capsules
In a single dose study in normal adult volunteers, a 500 mg dose of two 250 mg Elixophyllin SR Capsules produced a mean peak theophylline blood level of 7.3 μg/ml at 5.1 hours after administration. Elixophyllin SR Capsules were found to be equivalent in bioavailability to the reference standard Elixophyllin (theophylline) Elixir.
In a multiple dose, steady state study in normal adult volunteers, Elixophyllin SR Capsules produced relatively constant theophylline blood levels with an average difference between maximum and minimum theophylline plasma concentration of only 3.4 μg/ml.

Indications: For relief and/or prevention of symptoms of asthma and reversible bronchospasm associated with chronic bronchitis and emphysema.

Contraindications: Hypersensitivity to any of the components.

Warnings: Since excessive theophylline doses may be associated with toxicity, periodic measurement of serum theophylline levels is recommended to assure maximal benefit without excessive risk. Incidence of toxicity increases at levels greater than 20 μg/ml. Although early signs of theophylline toxicity such as nausea and restlessness are often seen, in some cases ventricular arrhythmia or convulsions may appear without warning as the first signs of toxicity.
There is an excellent correlation between high blood levels of theophylline resulting from conventional doses and associated clinical manifestations of toxicity in (1) patients with lowered body plasma clearances (due to transient cardiac decompensation), (2) patients with liver dysfunction or chronic obstructive lung disease, and (3) patients who are older than 55 years of age, particularly males.
Many patients with excessive theophylline serum levels exhibit a tachycardia.
Theophylline preparations may worsen preexisting arrhythmias.

Usage in Pregnancy: Safe use in pregnancy has not been established relative to possible adverse effects on fetal development; therefore, use of theophylline in pregnant women should be balanced against the risk of uncontrolled asthma.

Precautions: Theophylline should not be administered concurrently with other xanthine preparations. Use with caution in patients with severe cardiac disease, severe hypoxemia, hypertension, hyperthyroidism, acute myocardial injury, cor pulmonale, liver disease, in the elderly (especially males) and in neonates. Great caution should especially be used in giving theophylline to patients in congestive heart failure (markedly prolonged blood level curves have been observed in such patients).
Use theophylline cautiously in patients with history of peptic ulcer.

Adverse Reactions: The most common adverse reactions are usually due to overdose and are:
Gastrointestinal: nausea, vomiting, epigastric pain, hematemesis, diarrhea;
Central nervous system: headaches, irritability, restlessness, insomnia, reflex hyperexcitability, muscle twitching, clonic and tonic generalized convulsions;
Cardiovascular: palpitation, tachycardia, extrasystoles, flushing, hypotension, circulatory failure, ventricular arrhythmias;
Respiratory: tachypnea;
Renal: albuminuria, increased excretion of renal tubular cells and red blood cells, potentiation of diuresis;
Others: hyperglycemia and inappropriate ADH (antidiuretic hormone) syndrome.

Drug Interactions: Toxic synergism with ephedrine has been documented and may occur with some other sympathomimetic bronchodilators.

Drug	Effect
Theophylline with furosemide	Increased diuresis
Theophylline with hexamethonium	Decreased chronotropic effect
Theophylline with reserpine	Tachycardia
Theophylline with clindamycin, lincomycin, troleandomycin, or erythromycin	Increased theophylline blood levels
Theophylline with cimetidine	Increased theophylline blood levels

Overdosage:
Management:
A. If potential oral overdose is established and seizure has not occurred:
1) Induce vomiting;
2) Administer a cathartic,
3) Administer activated charcoal.
B. If patient is having a seizure:
1) Establish an airway;
2) Administer O_2;
3) Treat the seizure with intravenous diazepam, 0.1 to 0.3 mg/kg up to 10 mg;
4) Monitor vital signs, maintain blood pressure and provide adequate hydration.
C. Post-seizure coma:
1) Maintain airway and oxygenation;
2) Follow above recommendations to prevent absorption of drug, but intubation and lavage will have to be performed instead of inducing emesis, and the cathartic and charcoal will need to be introduced via a large bore gastric lavage tube;
3) Continue to provide full supportive care and adequate hydration while waiting for drug to be metabolized.

Dosage and Administration: Therapeutic serum levels associated with optimal benefit and minimal risk of toxicity are considered to be between 10 μg/ml and 20 μg/ml. Levels above 20 μg/ml may produce toxic effects. Periodic and carefully controlled monitoring of theophylline serum levels is highly recommended.

Elixicon (theophylline) Suspension
Average Maintenance Dosage following Theophyllinization*:

Child 6 mos. to 9 yrs. (55 lbs.):	1 teaspoonful (5 ml) q6h
Child 9–16	
(75 lbs.):	1 teaspoonful (5 ml) q6h
(110 lbs.):	1½ teaspoonfuls (7.5 ml) q6h
(145 lbs.):	2 teaspoonfuls (10 ml) q6h
Adult	
(150 lbs.):	2 teaspoonfuls (10 ml) q8h

*Dosage must be individualized. See *Individualized Dosage for Patient Population Section.*

Elixophyllin (theophylline) Capsules
Average Maintenance Dosage Following Theophyllinization*:

Adult	
(150 lbs.):	One 200 mg capsule q8h
Child 9–16	
(75 lbs.):	One 100 mg capsule q6h
Child 9–16	
(145 lbs.):	One 200 mg capsule q6h
Child <9	
(55 lbs.):	One 100 mg capsule q6h

*Dosage must be individualized. See *Individualized Dosage for Patient Population Section.*

Elixophyllin (theophylline) SR Capsules
At steady-state blood levels, the following maintenance dose is recommended:
Adults: One Elixophyllin SR Capsule 250 mg every 12 hours.*

Children ages 6 to 12: One Elixophyllin SR Capsule 125 mg every 12 hours.*

The average initial adult dose for a *nontheophyllinized* patient is two Elixophyllin SR Capsules 250 mg, then one Elixophyllin SR Capsule 250 mg every 12 hours until steady-state blood levels are achieved.*

The average initial dose for *nontheophyllinized* children ages 6 to 12 is two Elixophyllin SR Capsules 125 mg, then one Elixophyllin SR Capsule 125 mg every 12 hours until steady-state blood levels are achieved.*

* Occasional patients may require dosing every 8 hours.

If the desired response is not achieved, dosage may be increased in approximately 25% increments at 2–3 day intervals so long as no intolerance is observed, until the level indicated in the *maximum dose without measurement of serum concentration* table is reached.

Elixophyllin (theophylline) Elixir

Average Maintenance Dosage Following Theophyllinization*:

Adult (150 lbs): 2½ tablespoonfuls (37.5 ml) q8h

Child 9–16 (90 lbs.): 1½ tablespoonfuls (22.5 ml) q6h

(145 lbs): 2½ tablespoonfuls (37.5 ml) q6h

Child under 9 (45 lbs): 1 tablespoonful (15 ml) q6h

* Dosage must be individualized. See *Individualized Dosage for Patient Population Section.*

If gastrointestinal irritation is experienced, dosages may be taken with or after meals. Although absorption may be slowed, it is still complete.

Individualized Dosage for Patient Population

Acute Symptoms of Asthma Requiring Rapid Theophyllinization: (Calculations should be on basis of lean body weight.)

I. Patients not currently receiving theophylline products:

[See table above].

Group	Oral Loading Dose (Theophylline)	Maintenance Dose For Next 12 Hours (Theophylline)	Maintenance Dose Beyond 12 Hours (Theophylline)
1. Children 6 months to 9 years	6 mg/kg	4 mg/kg q4h	4 mg/kg q6h
2. Children 9–16 and young adult smokers	6 mg/kg	3 mg/kg q4h	3 mg/kg q6h
3. Otherwise healthy non-smoking adults	6 mg/kg	3 mg/kg q6h	3 mg/kg q8h
4. Older patients and patients with cor pulmonale	6 mg/kg	2 mg/kg q6h	2 mg/kg q8h
5. Patients with congestive heart failure, liver failure	6 mg/kg	2 mg/kg q8h	1–2 mg/kg q12h

II. Patients currently receiving theophylline products: Determine, where possible the time, amount, route of administration and form of the patient's last dose.

The loading dose for theophylline is based on the principle that each 0.5 mg/kg of theophylline administered as a loading dose will result in a 1 μg/ml increase in serum theophylline concentration. Ideally, then, the loading dose should be deferred if measurement of serum theophylline concentration can be rapidly obtained. If this is not possible, the clinician must exercise his judgement in selecting a dose based on the potential for benefit and risk.

Chronic Asthma: Initial Dose: 16 mg/kg/day or 400 mg/day (whichever is lower) in 3–4 divided doses at 6–8 hour intervals.

Increased Dose: The above dosage may be increased in approximately 25 percent increments at 2–3 day intervals so long as no intolerance is observed, and until the maximum indicated below is reached.

Maximum dose without measurement of serum concentration: Not to exceed the following: (WARNING: DO NOT ATTEMPT TO MAINTAIN ANY DOSE THAT IS NOT TOLERATED.)

Age <9 years—24 mg/kg/day
Age 9–12 years—20 mg/kg/day
Age 12–16 years—18 mg/kg/day
Age >16 years—13 mg/kg/day
or 900 mg/day
(WHICHEVER IS LESS)

NOTE: Use ideal body weight for obese patients.

Measurement of serum theophylline concentration during chronic therapy: If the above maximum doses are to be maintained or exceeded, serum theophylline measurement is recommended. This should be obtained at the approximate time of peak absorption during chronic therapy for the product used (1–2 hours for liquids and capsules that undergo rapid dissolution, 3–5 hours for sustained release preparations). It is important that the patient will have missed NO doses during the previous 48 hours and that dosing intervals will have been reasonably typical with no added doses during that period of time. DOSAGE ADJUSTMENT BASED ON SERUM THEOPHYLLINE MEASUREMENTS WHEN THESE INSTRUCTIONS HAVE NOT BEEN FOLLOWED MAY RESULT IN RECOMMENDATIONS THAT PRESENT RISK OF TOXICITY TO THE PATIENT.

How Supplied:

Elixicon (theophylline) Suspension

Bottles of 237 ml ....NDC 50419-112-08
NSN 6505-01-104-0397

Avoid excessive heat. Store below 30° C (86° F). Do not freeze. Shake well before using.

Elixophyllin (theophylline) Capsules

100 mg Capsules
Bottles of 100 ....NDC 50419-126-10
200 mg Capsules
Bottles of 100 ....NDC 50419-120-10
Bottles of 500 ....NDC 50419-120-50
Unit Dose Boxes
of 100 ....NDC 50419-120-11

Store at controlled room temperature.

Elixophyllin (theophylline) SR Capsules

125 mg Capsules
Bottles of 100 ....NDC 50419-129-10
NSN 6505-01-049-6812
Bottles of 500 ....NDC 50419-129-50
Unit Dose Boxes
of 100 ....NDC 50419-129-11
250 mg Capsules
Bottles of 100 ....NDC 50419-123-10
NSN 6505-01-064-9555
Bottles of 500 ....NDC 50419-123-50
Unit Dose Boxes
of 100 ....NDC 50419-123-11

Store at controlled room temperature.

Elixophyllin (theophylline) Elixir

Bottles of:
473 ml ....NDC 50419-121-16
946 ml ....NDC 50419-121-32
3785 ml ....NDC 50419-121-28

Store at controlled room temperature.

[*Shown in Product Identification Section*]

ELIXOPHYLLIN-KI® ELIXIR ℞
(theophylline/potassium iodide)

Description: Each 15 ml (tablespoonful) of Elixophyllin-KI contains 80 mg anhydrous theophylline and 130 mg potassium iodide. Alcohol 10%.

(Please refer to Elixophyllin (theophylline) Elixir for complete information on theophylline.)

Clinical Pharmacology: Potassium iodide acts as an expectorant by liquifying tenacious bronchial secretions.

Indications: For excessive tenacious mucus in chronic asthma, severe chronic and allergic bronchitis and chronic obstructive pulmonary emphysema.

Precautions: Occasionally, persons are markedly sensitive to iodides; care should be used in administering Elixophyllin-KI for the first time. Caution is recommended in patients sensitive to iodides, and in patients receiving potassium sparing diuretics or potassium supplements.

Usage in Pregnancy: Iodides readily cross the placenta and may cause thyroid enlargement in the fetus. Therefore, Elixophyllin-KI should not be used in pregnant women unless in the judgment of the physician, the potential benefits outweigh the possible hazards.

Since iodides are secreted in human milk, discontinue or decrease during breast feeding.

Adverse Reactions: Thyroid adenoma, goiter and myxedema are possible side effects of potassium iodide.

Hypersensitivity to iodides may be manifested by angioneurotic edema, cutaneous and mucosal hemorrhages, and symptoms resembling serum sickness, such as fever, arthralgia, lymph node enlargement and eosinophilia.

Iodism or chronic iodine poisoning may occur during prolonged treatment. The symptoms of iodism include a metallic taste, soreness of the mouth, increased salivation, coryza, sneezing and swelling of the eyelids. There may be severe headache, productive cough, pulmonary edema and swelling and tenderness of the salivary glands. Acneform skin lesions are seen in the seborrheic areas. Severe and sometimes fatal skin eruptions may develop. Gastric disturbance and diarrhea are common. If iodism appears, the drug should be withdrawn and the patient given appropriate supportive therapy.

Dosage and Administration Usual dose in chronic asthma. *Adults:* 30 ml (2 tablespoonfuls) t.i.d. upon arising, at 3:00 p.m. and at bedtime. *Children:* 0.2 ml per pound of body weight, t.i.d. as above. *Dosage must be individualized.*

How Supplied: Bottles of:
237 ml ....NDC 50419-124-08
3785 ml ....NDC 50419-124-28

Store at controlled room temperature.
Protect from light.

KAY CIEL® Elixir ℞
(potassium chloride)

KAY CIEL® Powder ℞
(potassium chloride)

Description: Each 15 ml (tablespoonful) contains 1.5 g (20 mEq) potassium chloride in a palatable base. Alcohol 4%. Contains no sugar. Each packet contains 1.5 g (20 mEq) potassium chloride. Contains no sugar.

Indications: Treatment and prevention of potassium deficiency occurring especially during thiazide diuretic or corticosteroid therapy,

Continued on next page

Berlex—Cont.

digitalis intoxication, low dietary intake of potassium, or as a result of excessive vomiting and diarrhea and for correction of associated hypochloremic alkalosis.
Contraindications: Impaired renal function, untreated Addison's Disease, dehydration, heat cramps and hyperkalemia.
Warnings: Do not use excessively.
Precautions: Administer with caution and adjust to the requirements of the individual patient. The patient should be checked frequently and periodic ECG recorded and/or plasma potassium levels determined. Use with caution in patients with cardiac disease. In hypokalemic states, attention should be directed toward correction of frequently associated hypochloremic alkalosis. ***PATIENTS SHOULD BE CAUTIONED TO ADHERE TO DILUTION INSTRUCTIONS TO ASSURE AGAINST GASTROINTESTINAL INJURY.***
Adverse Reactions: Potassium intoxication indicated by listlessness, mental confusion, paresthesia of the extremities, weakness of the legs, flaccid paralysis, fall in blood pressure, cardiac depression, arrhythmias, arrest and heartblock. Vomiting, nausea, abdominal discomfort and diarrhea may occur.
Dosage and Administration:
Elixir:
One tablespoonful (15 ml supplying 20 mEq) ***diluted*** in 4 ounces of cold water or fruit juice twice daily (preferably after a meal), or as directed by physician.
Powder:
Contents of 1 packet dissolved in 4 ounces of cold water or fruit juice twice daily (preferably after a meal), or as directed by physician.
Overdosage: In case of excessive use resulting in hyperkalemia or potassium intoxication, discontinue use of potassium chloride and/or take other steps to lower serum levels if indicated.
How Supplied:
Elixir: Bottles of:
118 ml..........................NDC 50419-145-04
473 ml..........................NDC 50419-145-16
3785 ml..........................NDC 50419-145-28
Powder: Boxes of:
30 packets.................. NDC 50419-144-30
NSN 6505-00-148-6984
100 packets...................NDC 50419-144-11
Store at controlled room temperature.
[*Shown in Product Identification Section*]

PYOCIDIN-OTIC® ℞
(polymyxin B-hydrocortisone)
Sterile Otic Solution

Description: Each ml contains 10,000 USP units of polymyxin B sulfate and 5 mg hydrocortisone in a vehicle containing propylene glycol and water. Sodium hydroxide or hydrochloric acid may have been added to adjust pH.
Actions: Polymyxin B sulfate is effective against the gram-negative *Pseudomonas aeruginosa*, one of the most resistant microorganisms commonly causing otitis externa. The addition of hydrocortisone to the antibiotic affords an anti-inflammatory effect and relief against allergic manifestations and reduces the possibility of sensitivity and tissue reaction.
Indications: For the treatment of superficial bacterial infections of the external auditory canal caused by organisms susceptible to the action of the antibiotic.
Contraindications: This product is contraindicated in those individuals who have shown hypersensitivity to any of its components, and in herpes simplex, vaccinia and varicella.
Warnings: As with other antibiotic preparations, prolonged treatment may result in overgrowth of nonsusceptible organisms and fungi. If the infection is not improved after one week, cultures and susceptibility tests should be repeated to verify the identity of the organism and to determine whether therapy should be changed.
Patients who prefer to warm the medication before using should be cautioned against heating the solution above body temperature, in order to avoid loss of potency.
Precautions: If sensitization or irritation occurs, medication should be discontinued promptly.
Dosage and Administration: The external auditory canal should be thoroughly cleaned and dried with a sterile cotton applicator.
For adults, 4 drops of the solution should be instilled into the affected ear 3 or 4 times daily. For infants and children, 3 drops are suggested because of the smaller capacity of the ear canal.
The patient should lie with the affected ear upward and then the drops should be instilled. This position should be maintained for 5 minutes to facilitate penetration of the drops into the ear canal. Repeat, if necessary, for the opposite ear.
If preferred, a cotton wick may be inserted into the canal and then the cotton may be saturated with the solution. This wick should be kept moist by adding further solution every four hours. The wick should be replaced at least once every 24 hours.
How Supplied: 10 ml bottle with dropper. NDC 50419-287-10.
Store at controlled room temperature.
[*Shown in Product Identification Section*]

QUINAGLUTE® ℞
(quinidine gluconate)
DURA-TABS®

Description: Each Quinaglute® Dura-Tab® contains 324 mg quinidine gluconate (equivalent to 202 mg quinidine base) in a tablet matrix specially designed for the prolonged (8 to 12 hours) release of the drug in the gastrointestinal tract. Quinaglute® Dura-Tabs® are to be administered orally.
Quinidine gluconate is the gluconate salt of quinidine (6-methoxy-α-(5-vinyl-2 quinuclidinyl)-4-quinoline-methanol), a dextrorotatory isomer of quinine. Quinidine gluconate is represented by the following structural formula:

H, CH=CH₂, H, HO, H, N, · COOH, HCOH, HOCH, HCOH, HCOH, CH₂OH, CH₃O, N

Quinidine gluconate contains 62.3% of the anhydrous quinidine alkaloid, whereas quinidine sulfate contains 82.86%. In prescribing Quinaglute® Dura-Tabs®, this factor should be considered.
Therapeutic category: Type I antiarrhythmic.
Clinical Pharmacology: The antiarrhythmic activity consists of the following basic actions:

1. In arrhythmias due to enhanced automaticity, quinidine decreases the rate of rise of slow diastolic (Phase 4) depolarization thereby depressing automaticity, particularly in ectopic foci.
2. In addition to the above, quinidine slows depolarization, repolarization and amplitude of the action potential, thus increasing its duration, leading to an increase in the refractoriness of atrial and ventricular tissue. Prolongation of the effective refractory period and an increase in conduction time may prevent the reentry phenomenon.
3. Quinidine exerts an indirect anticholinergic effect through blockade of vagal innervation. This anticholinergic effect may facilitate conduction in the atrioventricular junction.

Quinidine absorption from Quinaglute® Dura-Tabs® proceeds at a slower rate than the immediate-release products. In a single-dose pharmacokinetic study conducted in normal volunteers, the time of peak quinidine serum concentration was 1.6 hours for quinidine sulfate tablets and 3.6 hours for Quinaglute® Dura-Tabs®.
The apparent elimination half-life of quinidine ranges from 4 to 10 hours in healthy persons with a usual mean value of 6 to 7 hours. The half-life may be prolonged in elderly persons. From 60% to 80% of the dose is metabolized by the liver. Renal excretion of the intact drug comprises the remainder of the total clearance. Quinidine is approximately 75% bound to serum proteins.
In the past, plasma levels of 1.5 to 5 μg/ml have been reported as therapeutic,[1] based on non-specific assay methodology which quantitates quinidine metabolites as well as intact quinidine. The therapeutic plasma level range using newer, more specific assays has not been definitively established; however, effective reduction of premature ventricular contractions has been reported with blood levels less than 1.0 μg/ml.[2] In general, plasma quinidine levels are lower using specific assays. Clinicians requesting serum quinidine determinations should therefore also ask that the method of analysis be specified.
Due to the wide individual variation in response to quinidine therapy, the usefulness of serum quinidine levels in the planning of optimal quinidine therapy has not been clearly established. A serum quinidine concentration within the reported therapeutic range may not necessarily be the optimal concentration for some patients. In the absence of toxicity, such patients may warrant an increase in dose to achieve the desired therapeutic effect. However, for those patients in which a high blood level has been achieved without significant therapeutic response, increasing the dose to potentially toxic levels is not warranted and consideration should be given to combination or alternate therapy. In all cases, the physician should carefully consider the patient response and evidence of toxicity along with blood levels in determining optimal quinidine therapy.

[1]Koch-Weser, Arch. Int. Med. 129:763-772, 1972.
[2]Carliner et al, Am. Heart Journ. 100:483-489, 1980.

Indications and Usage: Quinaglute® Dura-Tabs® are indicated in the prevention and/or treatment of:

1. Ventricular arrhythmias
   - Premature ventricular contractions
   - Ventricular tachycardia (when not associated with complete heartblock)
2. Junctional (nodal) arrhythmias
   - A-V junctional premature complexes
   - Paroxysmal junctional tachycardia
3. Supraventricular (atrial) arrhythmias
   - Premature atrial contractions
   - Paroxysmal atrial tachycardia
   - Atrial flutter
   - Atrial fibrillation (chronic and paroxysmal)

Contraindications:

1. Idiosyncrasy or hypersensitivity to quinidine.
2. Complete A-V block.
3. Complete bundle branch block or other severe intraventricular conduction defects, especially those exhibiting a marked grade of QRS widening.
4. Digitalis intoxication manifested by A-V conduction disorders.
5. Myasthenia gravis.
6. Aberrant impulses and abnormal rhythms due to escape mechanisms.

Warnings:

1. In the treatment of atrial flutter, reversion to sinus rhythm may be preceded by a progressive reduction in the degree of A-V block to a 1:1 ratio resulting in an extremely rapid ventricular rate. This possible hazard may be reduced by digitalization prior to administration of quinidine.
2. Recent reports indicate that plasma concentrations of digoxin increase and may even double when quinidine is administered concurrently. Patients on concomitant therapy should be carefully monitored. Reduction of digoxin dosage may have to be considered.
3. Manifestations of quinidine cardiotoxicity such as excessive prolongation of the Q-T interval, widening of the QRS complex and ventricular tachyarrhythmias mandate immediate discontinuation of the drug and/or close clinical and electrocardiographic monitoring.
4. In susceptible individuals, such as those with marginally compensated cardiovascular disease, quinidine may produce clinically important depression of cardiac function such as hypotension, bradycardia, or heartblock. Quinidine therapy should be carefully monitored in such individuals.
5. Quinidine should be used with extreme caution in patients with incomplete A-V block since complete block and asystole may be produced. Quinidine may cause abnormalities of cardiac rhythm in digitalized patients and therefore should be used with caution in the presence of digitalis intoxication.
6. Quinidine should be used with caution in patients exhibiting renal, cardiac or hepatic insufficiency because of potential accumulation of quinidine in plasma leading to toxicity.
7. Patients taking quinidine occasionally have syncopal episodes which usually result from ventricular tachycardia or fibrillation. This syndrome has not been shown to be related to dose or plasma levels. Syncopal episodes frequently terminate spontaneously or in response to treatment, but sometimes are fatal.
8. A few cases of hepatotoxicity, including granulomatous hepatitis, due to quinidine hypersensitivity have been reported in patients taking quinidine. Unexplained fever and/or elevation of hepatic enzymes, particularly in the early stages of therapy, warrant consideration of possible hepatotoxicity. Monitoring liver function during the first 4–8 weeks should be considered. Cessation of quinidine in these cases usually results in the disappearance of toxicity.

Precautions: *General:* The precautions to be observed include all those applicable to quinidine. A preliminary test dose of a single tablet of quinidine sulfate may be administered to determine if the patient has an idiosyncrasy to quinidine. Hypersensitivity to quinidine, although rare, should constantly be considered, especially during the first weeks of therapy.

Hospitalization for close clinical observation, electrocardiographic monitoring, and possible determination of plasma quinidine levels is indicated when large doses are used, or with patients who present an increased risk.

Drug Interactions:

Drug	*Effect*
Quinidine with anticholinergic drugs	Additive vagolytic effect
Quinidine with cholinergic drugs	Antagonism of cholinergic effects
Quinidine with carbonic anhydrase inhibitors, sodium bicarbonate, thiazide diuretics	Alkalinization of urine resulting in decreased excretion of quinidine
Quinidine with coumarin anticoagulants	Reduction of clotting factor concentrations
Quinidine with tubocurare, succinylcholine and decamethonium	Potentiation of neuromuscular blockade
Quinidine with phenothiazines and reserpine	Additive cardiac depressive effects
Quinidine with hepatic enzyme-inducing drugs (phenobarbital, phenytoin, rifampin)	Decreased plasma half-life of quinidine
Quinidine with digoxin	Increased plasma concentrations of digoxin (See WARNINGS)

Carcinogenesis, Mutagenesis and Impairment of Fertility: Long-term studies in animals have not been performed to evaluate the carcinogenic potential of quinidine. There is currently no evidence of quinidine-induced mutagenesis or impairment of fertility.

Pregnancy: Teratogenic Effects: Pregnancy Category C. Animal reproduction studies have not been conducted with quinidine. There are no adequate and well-controlled studies in pregnant women. Quinaglute® Dura-Tabs® should be given to a pregnant woman only if clearly needed.

Nonteratogenic Effects: Like quinine, quinidine has been reported to have oxytocic properties. The significance of this property in the clinical setting has not been established.

Nursing Mothers: Caution should be exercised when Quinaglute® Dura-Tabs® are administered to a nursing woman due to passage of the drug into breast milk.

Pediatric Use: There are no adequate and well-controlled studies establishing the safety and effectiveness of Quinaglute® Dura-Tabs® in children.

Adverse Reactions: Symptoms of cinchonism, ringing in ears, headache, nausea, and/or disturbed vision may appear in sensitive patients after a single dose of the drug.

The most frequently encountered side effects to quinidine are gastrointestinal in nature. These gastrointestinal effects include nausea, vomiting, abdominal pain and diarrhea.

Less frequently encountered adverse reactions:

Cardiovascular: Widening of QRS complex, cardiac asystole, ventricular ectopic beats, idioventricular rhythms including ventricular tachycardia and fibrillation, paradoxical tachycardia, arterial embolism and hypotension.

Hematologic: Acute hemolytic anemia, hypoprothrombinemia, thrombocytopenia (purpura), agranulocytosis.

Central Nervous System: Headache, fever, vertigo, apprehension, excitement, confusion, delirium and syncope, disturbed hearing (tinnitus, decreased auditory acuity), disturbed vision (mydriasis, blurred vision, disturbed color perception, reduced vision field, photophobia, diplopia, night blindness, scotomata), optic neuritis.

Dermatologic: Rash, cutaneous flushing with intense pruritus, urticaria. Photosensitivity has also been reported.

Hypersensitivity Reactions: Angioedema, acute asthmatic episode, vascular collapse, respiratory arrest, hepatic toxicity including granulomatous hepatitis (See WARNINGS).

Although extremely rare, there have also been reports of lupus erythematosus in patients taking quinidine. A positive association with quinidine therapy has not been established.

Overdosage: If ingestion of quinidine is recent, gastric lavage, emesis and/or administration of activated charcoal may reduce absorption. Management of overdosage includes symptomatic treatment, ECG and blood pressure monitoring, cardiac pacing if indicated, and acidification of the urine. Artificial respiration and other supportive measures may be required.

IV infusion of 1/6 molar sodium lactate reportedly reduces the cardiotoxic effects of quinidine. Since marked CNS depression may occur even in the presence of convulsions, CNS depressants should not be administered. Hypotension may be treated, if necessary, with metaraminol or levarterenol after adequate fluid volume replacement. Hemodialysis has been reported to be effective in the treatment of quinidine overdosage in adults and children, but is rarely warranted.

Dosage and Administration: The dosage varies considerably depending upon the general condition and cardiovascular state of the patient. The quantity and frequency of administration of Quinaglute® Dura-Tabs® which will achieve the desired clinical results must be determined for each patient.

The ideal dosage is the minimum amount of total dose and frequency of daily administration that will prevent premature contractions, paroxysmal tachycardias and maintain normal sinus rhythm.

Prevention of premature atrial, nodal or ventricular contractions:

1 to 2 tablets every 8 or 12 hours.

Maintenance of normal sinus rhythm following conversion of paroxysmal tachycardias:

2 tablets every 12 hours or 1 ½ to 2 tablets every 8 hours are usually required.

Some patients may be maintained in normal rhythm on a dosage of 1 tablet every 8 or 12 hours; other patients may require larger doses or more frequent administration, ie, every 6 hours than the usually recommended schedule. Such increased dosage should be instituted only after careful clinical and laboratory evaluation of the patient including monitoring of plasma quinidine levels and, if possible, serial electrocardiograms.

Quinaglute® Dura-Tabs® are well tolerated with few gastrointestinal disturbances which, if they occur, may be minimized by administering the drug with food.

It is frequently desirable to determine if a patient can tolerate maintenance quinidine therapy prior to electrical conversion. Therefore, maintenance therapy may be initiated 2 to 3 days before electrical conversion is attempted. Quinaglute® Dura-Tabs® are well suited for such a program and can be administered at a maintenance dose felt necessary for a given patient as indicated above.

Note: Dosage may be titrated by breaking the tablet in half. Do not crush or chew since sustained-release properties will be lost.

How Supplied:

White to off-white round tablet imprinted with:

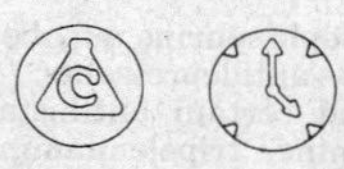

In bottles of:

100 Tablets	NDC 50419-101-10
250 Tablets	NDC 50419-101-25
500 Tablets	NDC 50419-101-50
Unit Dose Boxes of 100	NDC 50419-101-11

Store at controlled room temperature.

[*Shown in Product Identification Section*]

SUS-PHRINE® ℞
(epinephrine)
Aqueous Suspension for Subcutaneous Injection

Description: Each ml of Sus-Phrine contains 5 mg epinephrine in a sterile aqueous vehicle containing Ascorbic Acid 10 mg and Thioglycolic Acid 6.6 mg (as sodium salts), Phenol 5 mg and Glycerin (USP) 325 mg. Sodium hydroxide is added to adjust the pH. Approximately 80% of the total epinephrine is in suspension.

Continued on next page

Berlex—Cont.

Clinical Pharmacology: Sus-Phrine (epinephrine) acts at both the alpha and beta receptor sites. Beta stimulation provides bronchodilator action by relaxing bronchial muscle. Alpha stimulation increases vital capacity by relieving congestion of the bronchial mucosa and by constricting pulmonary vessels.
Sus-Phrine provides both rapid and sustained epinephrine activity. The rapid action is due to the epinephrine in solution, while the sustained activity is due to the crystalline epinephrine free base in suspension.
Indications: For the symptomatic treatment of bronchial asthma, and reversible bronchospasm associated with chronic bronchitis and emphysema.
Contraindications: Hypersensitivity to any of the components.
Narrow angle glaucoma, shock, cerebral arteriosclerosis and organic heart disease. Epinephrine is also contraindicated during general anesthesia with halogenated hydrocarbons or cyclopropane, and in local anesthesia of certain areas, e.g., fingers, toes, because of the danger of vasoconstriction producing sloughing of tissue, and in labor because the drug may delay the second stage.
Warnings: SUS-PHRINE SHOULD NOT BE EMPLOYED TO CORRECT DRUG INDUCED HYPOTENSION.
Administer with caution to elderly people; those with cardiovascular disease, diabetes, hypertension or hyperthyroidism; in psychoneurotic individuals and in pregnancy. Administer with extreme caution to patients with long-standing bronchial asthma and emphysema who have developed degenerative heart disease.
Cardiac arrhythmias may follow administration of epinephrine.
Anginal pain may be induced when coronary insufficiency is present.
Precautions: DO NOT USE IF PRODUCT IS DISCOLORED. Discoloration indicates the oxidation of epinephrine and possible loss of potency.
Use of Sus-Phrine with digitalis, mercurial diuretics or other drugs that sensitize the heart to arrhythmias is not recommended.
Sus-Phrine should not be administered concomitantly with other sympathomimetic agents, since their combined effects on the cardiovascular system may be deleterious to the patient.
The effects of epinephrine may be potentiated by tricyclic antidepressants; sodium l-thyroxine, and certain antihistamines, e.g., diphenhydramine, tripelennamine or chlorpheniramine.
Adverse Reactions: In some individuals, restlessness, anxiety, headache, tremor, weakness, dizziness, pallor, respiratory difficulties, palpitation, nausea and vomiting may occur. These reactions may be exaggerated in hyperthyroidism. Occlusion of the central retinal artery and shock have also been reported.
Also, urticaria, wheal and hemorrhage at the site of injection may occur. Repeated injections at the same site may result in necrosis from vascular constriction.
Tolerance to epinephrine may occur with prolonged use.
Overdosage: Overdosage or inadvertent intravenous injection may cause cerebrovascular hemorrhage resulting from the sharp rise in blood pressure. Fatalities may also result from pulmonary edema because of peripheral constriction and cardiac stimulation produced. Rapidly acting vasodilators such as nitrites, or alpha blocking agents may counteract the marked pressor effects. Cardiac arrhythmias may be countered by administering rapidly acting antiarrhythmic or beta blocking agents.
Dosage and Administration:
NOTE: INJECT SUBCUTANEOUSLY.
It is suggested that Sus-Phrine be administered with a tuberculin syringe and a 26 gauge, ½ inch needle.
A small initial test dose may be administered subcutaneously as a possible aid in determining patient sensitivity to epinephrine.
Site of injection should be varied to avoid necrosis at the site of injection.
Each time before withdrawing Sus-Phrine into syringe, shake vial or ampul thoroughly to disperse particles and obtain a uniform suspension. Inject promptly subcutaneously to avoid settling of suspension in the syringe.
Adults:
Adult dosage range is 0.1 to 0.3 ml depending on patient response.
Subsequent doses should be administered only when necessary and not more frequently than every six hours.
Infants 1 month to 2 years and Children 2 to 12 years:
Pediatric dose is 0.005 ml/kg (2.2 lb) body weight injected subcutaneously.
FOR CHILDREN 30 kg OR LESS MAXIMUM SINGLE DOSE IS 0.15 ml.
Subsequent doses should be administered only when necessary and not more frequently than every six hours.
Clinical Studies: Controlled studies comparing the effectiveness of Sus-Phrine and an aqueous solution of epinephrine 1:1000 were conducted in both pediatric and adult asthmatics. The studies demonstrated rapid bronchodilator acitivity following administration of either Sus-Phrine or epinephrine 1:1000; however during the 6 hour study period, a greater improvement in FEV_1 and FEF_{25-75} was observed 4 to 6 hours subsequent to Sus-Phrine administration. Improvement in WPEF was greater for Sus-Phrine than epinephrine 1:1000 3 to 8 hours following administration (10 hour study duration).
How Supplied:
In boxes of
12 × 0.3 ml ampuls ....NDC 50419-137-12
25 × 0.3 ml ampuls ....NDC 50419-137-25
5.0 ml multiple dose vial....NDC 50419-128-01
NSN 6505-01-022-2402
Store under refrigeration. Do not freeze. Do not expose to temperatures above 30° C (86°F).
[*Shown in Product Identification Section*]

Information on the Berlex products described above is based on full prescribing information in use September 1, 1982.

Beutlich, Inc.
7006 N. WESTERN AVE.
CHICAGO, IL 60645

CEO–TWO® SUPPOSITORIES

Composition: Each adult rectal suppository contains sodium bicarbonate and potassium bitartrate in a water soluble polyethylene glycol base.
Actions and Uses: The gentle pressure of the released CO_2 in the rectum stimulates peristalsis, and defecation usually results in 10 to 30 minutes. CEO-TWO® is successfully used as a bowel evacuant in spinal cord injury patients. It is gentle, effective, safe and predictable. Also used pre and post partum, pre and post operatively, or whenever the last 25cm of the lower bowel must be emptied.
Administration and Dosage: Moisten CEO-TWO® slightly with warm water before inserting. Patients should retain as long as possible.
Contraindications: As with other enemas or laxatives.
How Supplied: In packages of 10, white opaque suppositories. Keep in cool, dry place. DO NOT REFRIGERATE

HURRICAINE® TOPICAL ANESTHETIC LIQUID, GEL, and AEROSOL SPRAY

Composition: HURRICAINE® (20% Benzocaine)
Action and Indication: HURRICAINE® is a topical anesthetic for oral and mucosal application. To control pain as well as suppress the gag reflex.
Advantages: Safe, effective, 15-30 seconds, good tasting. The aerosol will not foam.
HURRICAINE® is probably the agent of choice in endoscopy since its onset is rapid, action is of short duration and virtually no systemic absorption occurs.
PATIENTS WITH A KNOWN HYPERSENSITIVITY TO BENZOCAINE SHOULD NOT USE HURRICAINE®
DO NOT USE IN EYES
NOT FOR INJECTION
KEEP OUT OF REACH OF CHILDREN
How Supplied:
AEROSOL SPRAY in 2 oz. can
LIQUID or GEL in 1 oz. bottles
LIQUID ¼cc Unit Dose

MEVANIN-C CAPSULES

Composition: Each capsule contains: Ascorbic Acid 200 mg., Hesperidin Complex 30 mg., Calcium Lactate 300 mg., Cyanocobalamin 1 mcg., Ferrous Sulfate 65 mg., Folic Acid 0.1 mg., Vitamin A 3000 USP units, Vitamin D 300 USP units, Thiamine HCl 2 mg., Riboflavin 2 mg., Pyridoxine HCl 0.5 mg., Niacin 5 mg., plus trace amounts of copper, zinc, manganese, magnesium, potassium and iodine.
Administration and Dosage: One capsule daily.
How Supplied: In bottles of 90 and 450 red and white capsules.

PERIDIN-C®

Composition: Each tablet contains Hesperidin Methyl Chalcone 50 mg., Hesperidin Complex 150 mg., Ascorbic Acid 200 mg.
Dosage: 1 tablet daily.
How Supplied: In bottles of 100 and 500 orange tablets.

Biocraft Laboratories, Inc.
92 ROUTE 46
ELMWOOD PARK, NJ 07407

NDC 0332	PRODUCT	PROD. ID. NO.
	AMITRIPTYLINE HCl TABLETS ℞	
2120	10 mg.	22
2122	25 mg.	23
2124	50 mg.	24
2126	75 mg.	25
2128	100 mg.	26
	AMOXICILLIN CAPSULES ℞	
3107	250 mg.	01
3109	500 mg.	03
	AMOXICILLIN SUSPENSION ℞	
4150	125 mg./5 ml.	
4155	250 mg./5 ml.	
	AMPICILLIN CAPSULES ℞	
3111	250 mg.	05
3113	500 mg.	06
	AMPICILLIN SUSPENSION ℞	
4129	125 mg./5 ml.	
4131	250 mg./5 ml.	
	AMPICILLIN-PROBENECID SUSPENSION ℞	
4140	1 gm. Probenecid; 3.5 gm. Amp	
	CHLOROQUINE PHOSPHATE TABLETS ℞	
2160	250 mg.	38

	CLOXACILLIN CAPSULES ℞	
3119	250 mg.	28
3121	500 mg.	30
	CLOXACILLIN SOLUTION ℞	
4159	125 mg./5 ml.	
	DICLOXACILLIN CAPSULES ℞	
3123	250 mg.	02
3125	500 mg.	04
	IMIPRAMINE HCl TABLETS ℞	
2111	10 mg.	19
2113	25 mg.	20
2117	50 mg.	21
	NEOMYCIN SULFATE TABLETS ℞	
1177	500 mg.	18
	OXACILLIN CAPSULES ℞	
3115	250 mg.	12
3117	500 mg.	14
	OXACILLIN SOLUTION ℞	
4157	250 mg./5 ml.	
	PENICILLIN G POTASSIUM SOLUTION ℞	
4115	250,000 U/5 ml.	
4117	400,000 U/5 ml.	
	PENICILLIN G POTASSIUM TABLETS ℞	
1117	200,000 Units	07
1121	250,000 Units	09
1123	400,000 Units	10
	PENICILLIN V POTASSIUM SOLUTION ℞	
4125	125 mg./5 ml.	
4127	250 mg./5 ml.	
	PENICILLIN V POTASSIUM TABLETS ℞	
1171	250 mg. ROUND	15
1172	250 mg. OVAL	16
1173	500 mg. ROUND	17
1174	500 mg. OVAL	49
	SULFAMETHOXAZOLE AND TRIMETHOPRIM TABLETS ℞	
2130	400 mg/80 mg (Single Strength)	32
2132	800 mg/160 mg (Double Strength)	33
	TRIMETHOPRIM TABLETS ℞	
2158	100 mg.	34

Bock Pharmacal Company

5435 HIGHLAND PARK DRIVE
ST. LOUIS, MO 63110

POLY-HISTINE EXPECTORANT WITH CODEINE ℞ Ⓒ

Each 5 ml. cherry flavored red syrup contains:
Codeine Phosphate ....10.0 mg.
(Warning: May be habit forming.)
Phenylpropanolamine HCl ....12.5 mg.
Brompheniramine Maleate ....2.0 mg.
Potassium Guaiacolsulfonate ....100.0 mg.
How Supplied: Bottles of 16 oz. and 1 gallon.

POLY-HISTINE EXPECTORANT PLAIN ℞

Each 5 ml. cherry flavored red syrup contains:
Phenylpropanolamine HCl .... 12.5 mg.
Brompheniramine Maleate ....2.0 mg.
Potassium Guaiacolsulfonate ....100.0 mg.
How Supplied: Bottles of 16 oz. and 1 gallon.

POLY-HISTINE-D CAPSULES ℞
Antihistamines + Decongestant

Each red-clear time release capsule imprinted BOCK contains:
Phenylpropanolamine HCl .... 50 mg.
Phenyltoloxamine Citrate .... 16 mg.
Pyrilamine Maleate .... 16 mg.
Pheniramine Maleate .... 16 mg.
How Supplied: Bottles of 100 and 1000.

POLY-HISTINE-D ELIXIR ℞
Antihistamines + Decongestant

Each 5 ml. wild cherry flavored red elixir contains:
Phenylpropanolamine HCl .... 12.5 mg.
Phenyltoloxamine Citrate .... 4.0 mg.
Pyrilamine Maleate .... 4.0 mg.
Pheniramine Maleate .... 4.0 mg.
How Supplied: Bottles of 16 oz. and 1 gallon.

POLY-HISTINE-DX CAPSULES ℞
Antihistamine + Decongestant

Each purple-clear time release capsule imprinted BOCK contains:
Pseudoephedrine HCl ....120.0 mg.
Brompheniramine Maleate ....12.0 mg.
How Supplied: Bottles of 100 and 1000.

POLY-HISTINE-DX SYRUP ℞
Antihistamine + Decongestant

Each 5 ml. grape flavored purple syrup contains:
Pseudoephedrine HCl...............................30.0 mg.
Brompheniramine Maleate ....4.0 mg.
How Supplied: Bottles of 16 oz. and 1 gallon.

PRENATE 90® ℞
Vitamin-Mineral Supplement

Each white film coated tablet contains:
Iron (Ferrous Fumarate) .... 90 mg.
Iodine (Potassium Iodine) .... 0.15 mg.
Calcium (Calcium Carbonate) .... 250 mg.
Magnesium (Magnesium Oxide) .... 20 mg.
Copper (Cupric Oxide) .... 2 mg.
Zinc (Zinc Oxide) .... 20 mg.
Folic Acid .... 1 mg.
Vitamin A (Acetate) .... 8000 I.U.
Vitamin D (Ergocalciferol) .... 400 I.U.
Vitamin E (Acetate) .... 30 I.U.
Vitamin C (Ascorbic Acid) .... 120 mg.
Vitamin B_1 (Thiamine Mononitrate) .... 3 mg.
Vitamin B_2 (Riboflavin) .... 3.4 mg.
Vitamin B_6 (Pyridoxine HCl) .... 20 mg.
Vitamin B_{12} (Cyanocobalamin) .... 12 mcg.
Niacinamide .... 20 mg.
Docusate Sodium .... 50 mg.
How Supplied: Bottles of 100's and 1000's.

THEON ELIXIR ℞

Each 5 ml. elixir contains:
Theophylline (Anhydrous) .... 50 mg.
Alcohol 10%
How Supplied: Bottles of 16 oz. and 1 gallon.

Boehringer Ingelheim Ltd.

90 EAST RIDGE
POST OFFICE BOX 368
RIDGEFIELD, CT 06877

ALUPENT® ℞
brand of metaproterenol sulfate
Bronchodilator

Tablets 10 mg	**BI-CODE 74**
Tablets 20 mg	**BI-CODE 72**
Metered Dose Inhaler 15 ml	**BI-CODE 70**
Syrup 10mg/5ml	**BI-CODE 73**
Inhalant Solution 5%	**BI-CODE 71**

Description: Chemically Alupent, brand of metaproterenol sulfate is 1-(3,5-dihydroxyphenyl)-2-isopropylaminoethanol sulfate, a white crystalline, racemic mixture of two optically active isomers. It differs from isoproterenol hydrochloride by having two hydroxyl groups attached at the meta positions on the benzene ring rather than one at the meta and one at the para position.

Clinical Pharmacology: Alupent, brand of metaproterenol sulfate, is a potent beta-adrenergic stimulator with the aerosol and inhalant solution having a rapid onset of action. It is postulated that beta-adrenergic stimulants produce many of their pharmacological effects by activation of adenyl cyclase, the enzyme which catalyzes the conversion of adenosine triphosphate to cyclic adenosine monophosphate.

Absorption, biotransformation and excretion studies following administration by inhalation have not been performed. Following oral administration in humans, an average of 40% of the drug is absorbed; it is not metabolized by catechol-O-methyltransferase or sulfatase enzymes in the gut, but is excreted primarily as glucuronic acid conjugates.

Indications and Usage: Alupent, brand of metaproterenol sulfate, is indicated as a bronchodilator for bronchial asthma, and for reversible bronchospasm which may occur in association with bronchitis and emphysema.

When administered orally or by inhalation Alupent, brand of metaproterenol sulfate, decreases reversible bronchospasm. Pulmonary function tests performed concomitantly usually show improvement following Alupent, brand of metaproterenol sulfate, administration, e.g., an increase in the one-second forced expiratory volume (FEV_1), an increase in maximum expiratory flow rate, an increase in peak expiratory flow rate, an increase in forced vital capacity, and/or a decrease in airway resistance. The resultant decrease in airway obstruction may relieve the dyspnea associated with bronchospasm.

Controlled single- and multiple-dose studies have been performed with pulmonary function monitoring. The mean duration of effect of a single dose of 20 mg of Alupent tablets or syrup, brand of metaproterenol sulfate, (i.e., the period of time during which there is a 15% or greater increase in FEV_1) was up to four hours. Four controlled multiple-dose 60-day studies, comparing the effectiveness of Alupent tablets with ephedrine tablets, have been performed. Because of difficulties in study design, only one study was available which could be analyzed in depth. This study showed a loss of efficacy with time for both Alupent tablets and ephedrine. Therefore, the physician should take this phenomenon into account in evaluating the individual patient's overall management. Further studies are in progress to adequately explain these results.

The duration of effect of a single dose of 2 to 3 inhalations of Alupent, brand of metaproterenol sulfate, (i.e., the period of time during which there is a 15% or greater increase in mean FEV_1), has varied from 1 to 5 hours. In repetitive-dosing studies (up to q.i.d.) the duration of effect for a similar dose of Alupent, brand of metaproterenol sulfate, has ranged from about one to two-and-one-half hours. Present studies are inadequate to explain the divergence in duration of the FEV_1 effect between single- and repetitive-dosing studies, respectively.

Following controlled single-dose studies with Alupent Inhalant Solution by an intermittent positive pressure breathing apparatus (IPPB) and by hand bulb nebulizers, significant improvement (15% or greater increase in FEV_1) occurred within 5 to 30 minutes and persisted for periods varying from 2 to 6 hours. In these studies the longer duration of effect occurred in the studies in which the drug was administered by IPPB, i.e., 6 hours versus 2 to 3 hours when administered by hand bulb nebulizer. In these studies the doses used were 0.3 ml by IPPB and 10 inhalations by hand bulb nebulizer.

In controlled repetitive-dosing studies by IPPB and by hand bulb nebulizer the onset of effect occurred within 5 to 30 minutes and duration ranged from 4 to 6 hours. In these studies the doses used were 0.3 ml b.i.d. or t.i.d. when given by IPPB, and 10 inhalations q.i.d. (no more often than q4h) when given by hand bulb nebulizer. As in the single-dose studies, effectiveness was measured as a sustained increase in FEV_1 of 15% or greater. In these repetitive-dosing studies there was no apparent differ-

Continued on next page

Boehringer Ingelheim—Cont.

ence in duration between the two methods of delivery.

Clinical studies were conducted in which the effectiveness of Alupent (metaproterenol sulfate) Inhalant Solution was evaluated by comparison with that of isoproterenol hydrochloride over periods of two to three months. Both drugs continued to produce significant improvement in pulmonary function throughout this period of treatment.

Contraindications: Use in patients with cardiac arrhythmias associated with tachycardia is contraindicated.

Warnings: Excessive use of adrenergic aerosols is potentially dangerous. Fatalities have been reported following excessive use of Alupent, brand of metaproterenol sulfate, as with other sympathomimetic inhalation preparations, and the exact cause is unknown. Cardiac arrest was noted in several cases.

Paradoxical bronchoconstriction with repeated excessive administration has been reported with other sympathomimetic agents. Therefore, it is possible that this phenomenon could occur with Alupent, brand of metaproterenol sulfate.

Patients should be advised to contact their physician in the event that they do not respond to their usual dose of a sympathomimetic amine aerosol.

Precautions: Because Alupent, brand of metaproterenol sulfate, is a sympathomimetic drug, it should be used with great caution in patients with hypertension, coronary artery disease, congestive heart failure, hyperthyroidism or diabetes, or when there is sensitivity to sympathomimetic amines.

Information For Patients: Extreme care must be exercised with respect to the administration of additional sympathomimetic agents. A sufficient interval of time should elapse prior to administration of another sympathomimetic agent.

Carcinogenesis: Long-term studies in mice and rats to evaluate the oral carcinogenic potential of metaproterenol sulfate have not been completed.

Pregnancy: *Teratogenic Effects: Pregnancy Category C.* Alupent, brand of metaproterenol sulfate, has been shown to be teratogenic and embryocidal in rabbits when given orally in doses 620 times the human inhalation dose and 62 times the human oral dose; the teratogenic effects included skeletal abnormalities and hydrocephalus with bone separation. Oral reproduction studies in mice, rats and rabbits showed no teratogenic or embryocidal effect at 50 mg/kg, or 310 times the human inhalation dose and 31 times the human oral dose. There are no adequate and well-controlled studies in pregnant women. Alupent, brand of metaproterenol sulfate, should be used during pregnancy only if the potential benefit justifies the potential risk to the fetus.

Nursing Mothers: It is not known whether this drug is excreted in human milk. Because many drugs are excreted in human milk, caution should be exercised when Alupent, brand of metaproterenol sulfate, is administered to a nursing woman.

Pediatric Use: Safety and effectiveness of Alupent Metered Dose Inhaler and Inhalant Solution in children below the age of 12 have not been established. The safety and efficacy of Alupent Tablets in children below the age of 6 have not been established.

Adverse Reactions: Adverse reactions are similar to those noted with other sympathomimetic agents.

The most frequent adverse reactions to Alupent, brand of metaproterenol sulfate, are nervousness, tachycardia, tremor and nausea. Less frequent adverse reactions are hypertension, palpitations, vomiting and bad taste.

Overdosage: The symptoms of overdosage are those of excessive beta adrenergic stimulation listed under **Adverse Reactions**. These reactions usually do not require treatment other than reduction of dosage and/or frequency of administration.

Dosage and Administration: ***Tablets:*** *Adults* The usual dose is 20 mg three or four times a day. *Children* Aged six to nine years or weight under 60 lbs—10 mg three or four times a day. Over nine years or weight over 60 lbs—20 mg three or four times a day.

Syrup: *Children* Aged six to nine years or weight under 60 lbs—one teaspoonful three or four times a day. Children over nine years or weight over 60 lbs—two teaspoonfuls three or four times a day. Experience in children under the age of six is limited to seventy-eight children. Of this number, forty were treated with Alupent syrup for at least one month. In this group, daily doses of approximately 1.3 to 2.6 mg/kg were well tolerated. *Adults*—two teaspoonfuls three or four times a day.

Metered Dose Inhaler: The usual single dose is two to three inhalations. With repetitive dosing, inhalation should usually not be repeated more often than about every three to four hours. Total dosage per day should not exceed 12 inhalations.

Inhalant Solution: Alupent, brand of metaproterenol sulfate, Inhalant Solution is administered by oral inhalation with the aid of a hand bulb nebulizer or an intermittent positive pressure breathing apparatus (IPPB). Usually, treatment need not be repeated more often than every four hours to relieve acute attacks of bronchospasm. As part of a total treatment program in chronic bronchospastic pulmonary diseases, Alupent, brand of metaproterenol sulfate, Inhalant Solution may be administered three to four times a day.

As with all medications, the physician should begin therapy with the lowest effective dose and then titrate the dosage according to the individual patient's requirements.

Method of Administration	Usual Single Dose	Range	Dilution
Hand bulb nebulizer	10 inhalations	5-15 inhalations	No dilution
IPPB	0.3 ml	0.2-0.3 ml	Diluted in approx. 2.5 ml of saline solution or other diluent

Alupent, brand of metaproterenol sulfate, Inhalant Solution is not recommended for use in children under 12 years of age.

How Supplied: ***Tablets:*** Alupent, brand of metaproterenol sulfate, is supplied in two dosage strengths as round, white, scored tablets in bottles of 100. Tablets of 10 mg coded Bl/74. Tablets of 20 mg coded Bl/72.

Syrup: Alupent brand of metaproterenol sulfate, is available as a cherry-flavored syrup, 10 mg per teaspoonful (5 ml), in 16 oz bottles.

Metered Dose Inhaler: Each Alupent Metered Dose Inhaler contains 225 mg of metaproterenol sulfate as a micronized powder in an inert propellant. This is sufficient medication for 300 inhalations. Each metered dose expressed from the inhaler delivers at the mouthpiece approximately 0.65 mg of metaproterenol sulfate. Alupent Metered Dose Inhaler with mouthpiece (15 ml). Alupent Metered Dose Inhaler refill (15 ml).

Inhalant Solution: Alupent, brand of metaproterenol sulfate, Inhalant Solution is supplied as a 5% solution in bottles of 10 ml with accompanying calibrated dropper. Store at room temperature; avoid excessive heat. Protect from light.

Distributed by: AL-713R-3 (5/81)

Boehringer Ingelheim Ltd.
Ridgefield, CT 06877

Under license from
Boehringer Ingelheim International GmbH
[*Shown in Product Identification Section*]

CATAPRES® ℞

brand of clonidine hydrochloride
Oral Antihypertensive

Tablets, 0.1 mg..........BI-CODE 06
Tablets, 0.2 mg..........BI-CODE 07
Tablets, 0.3 mg..........BI-CODE 11

Description: Catapres, brand of clonidine hydrochloride, an antihypertensive agent, is an imidazoline derivative and exists as a mesomeric compound. Its chemical name is 2-(2,6-dichlorophenylamino)-2-imidazoline hydrochloride.

It is an odorless, bitter, white crystalline substance soluble in water and alcohol, with a molecular weight of 266.57. The 0.1 mg tablet is equivalent to 0.087 mg of the free base.

Actions: Catapres, brand of clonidine hydrochloride, is an antihypertensive agent whose mechanism of action appears to be central alpha-adrenergic stimulation as demonstrated in animal studies. This results in the inhibition of bulbar sympathetic cardioaccelerator and sympathetic vasoconstrictor centers, thereby causing a decrease in sympathetic outflow from the brain. Initially, Catapres, brand of clonidine hydrochloride, stimulates peripheral alpha-adrenergic receptors producing transient vasoconstriction.

Catapres, brand of clonidine hydrochloride, acts relatively rapidly. The patient's blood pressure declines within 30 to 60 minutes after an oral dose, the maximum decrease occurring within 2 to 4 hours. The antihypertensive effect in humans lasts approximately 6 to 8 hours. The peak plasma level of Catapres, brand of clonidine hydrochloride, occurs in approximately 3 to 5 hours with a plasma half-life of 12 to 16 hours. Catapres, brand of clonidine hydrochloride, and its metabolites are excreted mainly in the urine. When labeled drug was administered, unchanged drug appearing in the urine accounted for about 32 percent of administered radioactivity.

Orthostatic effects are mild and infrequent since supine pressure is reduced to essentially the same extent as standing pressure. Catapres, brand of clonidine hydrochloride, does not alter normal hemodynamic responses to exercise. Acute studies with Catapres, brand of clonidine hydrochloride, in humans have demonstrated a moderate reduction (15 to 20%) of cardiac output in the supine position with no change in the peripheral resistance, while at a 45° tilt there is a smaller reduction in cardiac output and a decrease of peripheral resistance. Renal blood flow and the glomerular filtration rate remain essentially unchanged. During long-term therapy, cardiac output tends to return to control values, while peripheral resistance remains decreased. Slowing of the pulse rate has been observed in most patients given Catapres, brand of clonidine hydrochloride.

Other studies in humans have provided evidence of a reduction in plasma renin activity and in the excretion of aldosterone and catecholamines in patients treated with Catapres, brand of clonidine hydrochloride.

The exact relationship between these pharmacologic actions of Catapres, brand of clonidine hydrochloride, in humans, and its antihypertensive effect in individual patients, has not been fully elucidated at this time.

Catapres, brand of clonidine hydrochloride, has been administered together with hydralazine, guanethidine, methyldopa, reserpine, spironolactone, furosemide, chlorthalidone and thiazide diuretics without drug-to-drug interactions. The concomitant administration of a diuretic has been shown to enhance the antihypertensive efficacy of Catapres, brand of clonidine hydrochloride.

Indication: Catapres, brand of clonidine hydrochloride, is indicated in the treatment of hypertension. As an antihypertensive drug, Catapres, brand of clonidine hydrochloride, is mild to moderate in potency. It may be employed in a general treatment program with a diuretic and/or other antihypertensive agents as needed for proper patient response.

Warnings: Tolerance may develop in some patients, necessitating a reevaluation of therapy.

Use in Pregnancy: Reproduction studies have been performed with Catapres, brand of clonidine hydrochloride, in three animal species. The findings of these studies reflected no teratogenic effect but some embryotoxicity was evident at doses as low as 0.015 mg/kg (one-third the maximum recommended dose). In view of these findings, and since information on possible adverse effects in pregnant women is limited to uncontrolled clinical data, Catapres, brand of clonidine hydrochloride, is not recommended in women who are or may become pregnant unless the potential benefit outweighs the potential risk to mother and infant.

Use in Children: No clinical experience is available with the use of Catapres, brand of clonidine hydrochloride, in children. Studies are being performed to evaluate its use in the treatment of hypertension in children.

Precautions: When discontinuing Catapres, brand of clonidine hydrochloride, therapy the physician should reduce the dose gradually over 2 to 4 days to avoid a possible rapid rise in blood pressure and associated subjective symptoms such as nervousness, agitation, and headache. Patients on Catapres, brand of clonidine hydrochloride, therapy should be instructed not to discontinue therapy without consulting their physician. Rare instances of hypertensive encephalopathy and death have been recorded after abrupt cessation of Catapres, brand of clonidine hydrochloride, therapy. A causal relationship has not been established in these cases. It has been demonstrated that an excessive rise in blood pressure, should it occur, can be reversed by resumption of Catapres, brand of clonidine hydrochloride, therapy or by intravenous phentolamine.

Patients who engage in potentially hazardous activities, such as operating machinery or driving, should be advised of the sedative effect of Catapres, brand of clonidine hydrochloride. This drug may enhance the CNS-depressive effects of alcohol, barbiturates and other sedatives. Like any other antihypertensive agent, Catapres, brand of clonidine hydrochloride, should be used with caution in patients with severe coronary insufficiency, recent myocardial infarction, cerebrovascular disease or chronic renal failure.

As an integral part of their overall long-term care, patients treated with Catapres, brand of clonidine hydrochloride, should receive periodic eye examinations (see Toxicology).

Adverse Reactions: The most common reactions associated with Catapres, brand of clonidine hydrochloride, therapy are dry mouth (about 40%), drowsiness (about 35%), and sedation (about 8%). Constipation, dizziness, headache, and fatigue have been reported. Generally, these effects tend to diminish with continued therapy.

The following reactions have been associated with the drug, some of them rarely. In some instances an exact causal relationship has not been established.

Gastrointestinal: Anorexia, malaise, nausea, vomiting, parotid pain, mild transient abnormalities in liver function tests. There has been one report of possible drug-induced hepatitis without icterus and hyperbilirubinemia in a patient receiving Catapres, brand of clonidine hydrochloride, chlorthalidone and papaverine hydrochloride.

Metabolic: Weight gain, transient elevation of blood glucose or serum creatine phosphokinase, gynecomastia.

Cardiovascular: Congestive heart failure, Raynaud's phenomenon, and electrocardiographic abnormalities manifested as Wenckebach period or ventricular trigeminy.

Central Nervous System: Vivid dreams or nightmares, insomnia, other behavioral changes, nervousness, restlessness, anxiety, mental depression.

Dermatologic: Rash, angioneurotic edema, hives, urticaria, thinning of the hair, pruritus not associated with a rash.

Genitourinary: Impotence, urinary retention.

Other: Increased sensitivity to alcohol, dryness, itching or burning of the eyes, dryness of the nasal mucosa, pallor, or weakly positive Coombs' test.

Dosage and Administration: The dose of Catapres, brand of clonidine hydrochloride, must be adjusted according to the patient's individual blood pressure response. The following is a general guide to its administration.

Initial dose: One 0.1 mg tablet twice daily.

Maintenance dose: Further increments of 0.1 mg or 0.2 mg per day may be made until the desired response is achieved. The therapeutic doses most commonly employed have ranged from 0.2 mg to 0.8 mg per day given in divided doses. Studies have indicated that 2.4 mg is the maximum effective daily dose but doses as high as this have rarely been employed.

Overdosage: Profound hypotension, weakness, somnolence, diminished or absent reflexes and vomiting followed the accidental ingestion of Catapres, brand of clonidine hydrochloride, by several children from 19 months to 5 years of age. Gastric lavage and administration of an analeptic and vasopressor led to complete recovery within 24 hours. Tolazoline in intravenous doses of 10 mg at 30-minute intervals usually abolishes all effects of Catapres, brand of clonidine hydrochloride, overdosage.

Toxicology: In several studies Catapres, brand of clonidine hydrochloride, produced a dose-dependent increase in the incidence and severity of spontaneously occurring retinal degeneration in albino rats treated for six months or longer. Tissue distribution studies in dogs and monkeys revealed that Catapres, brand of clonidine hydrochloride, was concentrated in the choroid of the eye. In view of the retinal degeneration observed in rats, eye examinations were performed in 908 patients prior to the start of Catapres, brand of clonidine hydrochloride, therapy, who were then examined periodically thereafter. In 353 of these 908 patients, examinations were performed for periods of 24 months or longer. Except for some dryness of the eyes, no drug-related abnormal ophthalmologic findings were recorded and Catapres, brand of clonidine hydrochloride, did not alter retinal function as shown by specialized tests such as the electroretinogram and macular dazzle.

How Supplied: Catapres, brand of clonidine hydrochloride, is available as 0.1 mg (tan) and 0.2 mg (orange) oval, single-scored tablets in bottles of 100 and 1,000 and unit-dose packages of 100. Also available as 0.3 mg (peach) oval, single-scored tablets in bottles of 100.

98-146-073-E (7/82)

[*Shown in Product Identification Section*]

COMBIPRES® ℞

Each tablet contains:
Catapres®, brand of clonidine hydrochloride, 0.1 mg or 0.2 mg, and chlorthalidone, 15 mg
Oral Antihypertensive

Tablets 0.1 BI-CODE 08
Tablets 0.2 BI-CODE 09

WARNING

This fixed combination drug is not indicated for initial therapy of hypertension. Hypertension requires therapy titrated to the individual patient. If the fixed combination represents the dosage so determined, its use may be more convenient in patient management. The treatment of hypertension is not static, but must be reevaluated as conditions in each patient warrant.

Description: Combipres is a combination of Catapres®, brand of clonidine hydrochloride, and chlorthalidone. Catapres, an antihypertensive agent, is an imidazoline derivative and exists as a mesomeric compound. The chemical name for clonidine hydrochloride is 2-(2,6-dichlorophenylamino)-2-imidazoline hydrochloride.

It is an odorless, bitter, white crystalline substance soluble in water and alcohol, with a molecular weight of 266.57. The 0.1 mg tablet is equivalent to 0.087 mg of the free base.

Chlorthalidone is 2-chloro-5-(1-hydroxy-3-oxo-1-isoindolinyl) benzenesulfonamide.

Chlorthalidone is an oral diuretic agent indicated for the treatment of edema and hypertension. The drug has a prolonged action. It differs from other sulfonamide diuretics in that a double ring system is incorporated in its chemical structure.

Actions: Combipres:

Combipres produces a more pronounced antihypertensive response than occurs after either clonidine hydrochloride or chlorthalidone alone in equivalent doses.

Catapres (clonidine hydrochloride):

Catapres, brand of clonidine hydrochloride, is an antihypertensive agent whose mechanism of action appears to be central alpha-adrenergic stimulation as demonstrated in animal studies. This results in the inhibition of bulbar sympathetic cardioaccelerator and sympathetic vasoconstrictor centers, thereby causing a decrease in sympathetic outflow from the brain. Initially, Catapres, brand of clonidine hydrochloride, stimulates peripheral alpha-adrenergic receptors producing transient vasoconstriction.

Catapres, brand of clonidine hydrochloride, acts relatively rapidly. The patient's blood pressure declines within 30 to 60 minutes after an oral dose, the maximum decrease occurring within 2 to 4 hours. The antihypertensive effect in humans lasts approximately 6 to 8 hours. The peak plasma level of Catapres, brand of clonidine hydrochloride, occurs in approximately 3 to 5 hours with a plasma half-life of 12 to 16 hours. Catapres, brand of clonidine hydrochloride, and its metabolites are excreted mainly in the urine. When labeled drug was administered, unchanged drug appearing in the urine accounted for about 32 percent of administered radioactivity.

Orthostatic effects are mild and infrequent since supine pressure is reduced to essentially the same extent as standing pressure. Catapres, brand of clonidine hydrochloride, does not alter normal hemodynamic responses to exercise. Acute studies with Catapres, brand of clonidine hydrochloride, in humans have demonstrated a moderate reduction (15 to 20%) of cardiac output in the supine position

Continued on next page

Boehringer Ingelheim—Cont.

with no change in the peripheral resistance, while at a 45° tilt there is a smaller reduction in cardiac output and a decrease of peripheral resistance. Renal blood flow and the glomerular filtration rate remain essentially unchanged. During long-term therapy, cardiac output tends to return to control values, while peripheral resistance remains decreased. Slowing of the pulse rate has been observed in most patients given Catapres, brand of clonidine hydrochloride.

Other studies in humans have provided evidence of a reduction in plasma renin activity and in the excretion of aldosterone and catecholamines in patients treated with Catapres, brand of clonidine hydrochloride.

The exact relationship between these pharmacologic actions of Catapres, brand of clonidine hydrochloride, in humans and its antihypertensive effect in individual patients has not been fully elucidated at this time.

Catapres, brand of clonidine hydrochloride, has been administered together with hydralazine, guanethidine, methyldopa, reserpine, spironolactone, furosemide, chlorthalidone and thiazide diuretics without drug-to-drug interactions.

Chlorthalidone:

The diuretic action of chlorthalidone is thought to be due to inhibition of sodium and chloride reabsorption in the proximal tubule. It has been suggested that the initial antihypertensive action of the drug is due to a reduction of plasma volume.

Indication: Combipres is indicated in the treatment of hypertension (see box warning).

Contraindications: Combipres is contraindicated in patients with known hypersensitivity to chlorthalidone and in patients with severe renal or hepatic diseases.

Warnings: Tolerance may develop in some patients treated with Combipres. When this occurs therapy should be reevaluated.

Use in Pregnancy: No teratogenic changes have been observed following concomitant administration of chlorthalidone and Catapres, brand of clonidine hydrochloride, to pregnant rats in doses up to 0.128 mg/kg of Catapres and 32 mg/kg of chlorthalidone. However, when animals were given Catapres, brand of clonidine hydrochloride, alone in doses as low as 0.015 mg/kg (one-third the maximum recommended dose) some embryotoxicity was evident. In view of these findings and since information on possible adverse effects in pregnant women is limited to uncontrolled clinical data. Combipres is not recommended in women who are or may become pregnant unless the potential benefit outweighs the potential risk to mother and infant.

Use in Children: No clinical experience is available with the use of Combipres in children. Studies are being performed with Catapres, brand of clonidine hydrochloride, to evaluate its use in the treatment of hypertension in children.

Precautions: Catapres (clonidine hydrochloride):

When discontinuing Combipres therapy, the physician should reduce the dose gradually over 2 to 4 days to avoid a possible rapid rise in blood pressure and associated subjective symptoms such as nervousness, agitation, and headache. Patients on Combipres therapy should be instructed not to discontinue therapy without consulting their physician. Rare instances of hypertensive encephalopathy and death have been recorded after abrupt cessation of Catapres, brand of clonidine hydrochloride, therapy. A causal relationship has not been established in these cases. It has been demonstrated that an excessive rise in blood pressure, should it occur, can be reversed by resumption of Combipres therapy or by intravenous phentolamine.

Patients who engage in potentially hazardous activities, such as operating machinery or driving, should be advised of the sedative effect of the Catapres component. This drug may enhance the CNS-depressive effects of alcohol, barbiturates and other sedatives. Like any other antihypertensive agent, Combipres should be used with caution in patients with severe coronary insufficiency, recent myocardial infarction, cerebrovascular disease or chronic renal failure.

As an integral part of their overall long-term care, patients treated with Combipres should receive periodic eye examinations (see Toxicology).

Chlorthalidone:

Patients predisposed toward or affected by diabetes should be tested periodically while receiving Combipres, because of the hyperglycemic effect of chlorthalidone.

Because of the possibility of progression of renal failure, periodic determination of the BUN is indicated. If, in the physician's opinion, a rising BUN is significant, the drug should be stopped.

The chlorthalidone component of Combipres may lead to sodium and/or potassium depletion. Muscular weakness, muscle cramps, anorexia, nausea, vomiting, constipation, lethargy or mental confusion may occur. Severe dietary salt restriction is not recommended in patients receiving Combipres.

Periodic determinations of the serum potassium level will aid the physician in the detection of hypokalemia. Extra care should be given to detection of hypokalemia in patients receiving adrenal corticosteroids, ACTH or digitalis. Hypochloremic alkalosis often precedes other evidences of severe potassium deficiency. Frequently, therefore, more sensitive indicators than the potassium serum level are the serum bicarbonate and chloride concentrations. Also indicative of potassium depletion can be electrocardiographic alterations such as changes in conduction time, reduction in amplitude of the T wave, ST segment depression, prominent U wave. These abnormalities may appear with potassium depletion before the serum level of potassium decreases. To lessen the possibility of potassium deficiency, the diet, in addition to meat and vegetables, should include potassium-rich foods such as citrus fruits and bananas. If significant potassium depletion should occur during therapy, oral potassium supplements in the form of potassium chloride (3 to 4.5 g/day), fruit juice and bananas should be given.

Adverse Reactions: Combipres is generally well tolerated. The most common reactions associated with Combipres are dry mouth (about 40%), drowsiness (about 35%), and sedation (about 8%). Constipation, dizziness, headache, and fatigue have been reported. Generally, these effects tend to diminish with continued therapy.

In addition to the reactions listed above, certain adverse reactions associated with the component drugs of Combipres are shown below.

Catapres (clonidine hydrochloride):

Gastrointestinal: Anorexia, malaise, nausea, vomiting, parotid pain, mild transient abnormalities in liver function tests. One case of possible drug-induced hepatitis without icterus or hyperbilirubinemia has been reported in a patient receiving Catapres, brand of clonidine hydrochloride, chlorthalidone and papaverine hydrochloride.

Metabolic: Weight gain, transient elevation of blood glucose or serum creatine phosphokinase, gynecomastia.

Cardiovascular: Congestive heart failure, Raynaud's phenomenon, and electrocardiographic abnormalities manifested as Wenckebach period or ventricular trigeminy.

Central Nervous System: Vivid dreams or nightmares, insomnia, other behavioral changes, nervousness, restlessness, anxiety, mental depression.

Dermatologic: Rash, angioneurotic edema, hives, urticaria, thinning of the hair, pruritus not associated with a rash.

Genitourinary: Impotence, urinary retention.

Other: Increased sensitivity to alcohol, dryness, itching or burning of the eyes, dryness of the nasal mucosa, pallor, or weakly positive Coombs' test.

Chlorthalidone:

Symptoms such as nausea, gastric irritation, anorexia, constipation and cramping, weakness, dizziness, transient myopia and restlessness are occasionally observed. Headache and impotence or dysuria may occur rarely. Orthostatic hypotension has been reported and may be potentiated when chlorthalidone is combined with alcohol, barbiturates or narcotics. Skin rashes, urticaria and purpura have been reported in a few instances.

A decreased glucose tolerance evidenced by hyperglycemia and glycosuria may develop inconsistently. This condition, usually reversible on discontinuation of therapy, responds to control with antidiabetic treatment. Diabetics and those predisposed should be checked regularly.

As with other diuretic agents, hypokalemia may occur (see Precautions). Hyperuricemia may be observed on occasion and acute attacks of gout have been precipitated. In cases where prolonged and significant elevation of blood uric acid concentration is considered potentially deleterious, concomitant use of a uricosuric agent is effective in reversing hyperuricemia without loss of diuretic and/or antihypertensive activity.

Idiosyncratic drug reactions such as aplastic anemia, thrombocytopenia, leukopenia, agranulocytosis and necrotizing angiitis have occurred, but are rare.

The remote possibility of pancreatitis should be considered when epigastric pain or unexplained gastrointestinal symptoms develop after prolonged administration.

Other adverse reactions which have been reported with this general class of compounds include: jaundice, xanthopsia, paresthesia and photosensitization.

Dosage and Administration: *Dosage:* As determined by individual titration of Catapres, brand of clonidine hydrochloride, and chlorthalidone (see box warning).

The following is a general guide to the administration of the individual components of Combipres:

Catapres (clonidine hydrochloride):

Initial dose: One 0.1 mg tablet twice daily.

Maintenance dose: Further increments of 0.1 mg or 0.2 mg per day may be made until the desired response is achieved. The therapeutic doses most commonly employed have ranged from 0.2 to 0.8 mg per day, given in divided doses. Studies have indicated that 2.4 mg is the maximum effective daily dose but doses as high as this have rarely been employed.

Chlorthalidone:

The usual initial dose is 50 mg daily, which may be given in divided doses.

If the individual doses of Catapres, brand of clonidine hydrochloride, and chlorthalidone determined by titration represent the dose contained in Combipres, for convenience the patient may then be given Combipres.

Overdosage: Catapres (clonidine hydrochloride):

Profound hypotension, weakness, somnolence, diminished or absent reflexes and vomiting followed the accidental ingestion of Catapres, brand of clonidine hydrochloride, by several children from 19 months to 5 years of age. Gastric lavage and administration of an analeptic and vasopressor led to complete recovery within 24 hours. Tolazoline in intravenous doses of 10 mg at 30-minute intervals usually abolishes all effects of Catapres, brand of clonidine hydrochloride, overdosage.

Chlorthalidone:
Symptoms of overdosage include nausea, weakness, dizziness, and disturbances of electrolyte balance. There is no specific antidote, but gastric lavage is recommended, followed by supportive treatment. Where necessary, this may include intravenous dextrose and saline with potassium, administered with caution.

Toxicology: In several studies Catapres, brand of clonidine hydrochloride, produced a dose-dependent increase in the incidence and severity of spontaneously occurring retinal degeneration in albino rats treated for 6 months or longer. Tissue distribution studies in dogs and monkeys revealed that Catapres, brand of clonidine hydrochloride, was concentrated in the choroid of the eye. In view of the retinal degeneration observed in rats, eye examinations were performed in 908 patients prior to the start of Catapres, brand of clonidine hydrochloride, therapy, who were then examined periodically thereafter. In 353 of these 908 patients, examinations were performed for periods of 24 months or longer. Except for some dryness of the eyes, no drug-related abnormal ophthalmologic findings were recorded and Catapres, brand of clonidine hydrochloride, did not alter retinal function as shown by specialized tests such as the electroretinogram and macular dazzle.

How Supplied: Combipres® 0.1 (each tablet contains clonidine hydrochloride, 0.1 mg + chlorthalidone, 15 mg). It is available as pink, oval, single-scored compressed tablets in bottles of 100 and 1000.
Combipres® 0.2 (each tablet contains clonidine hydrochloride, 0.2 mg + chlorthalidone, 15 mg). It is available as blue, oval, single-scored compressed tablets in bottles of 100 and 1000.

98-146-074-C (9/81)

[*Shown in Product Identification Section*]

DULCOLAX®

brand of bisacodyl USP
Tablets of 5 mg..............................BI-CODE 12
Suppositories of 10 mg..................BI-CODE 52
Laxative

Description: Dulcolax is a contact laxative acting directly on the colonic mucosa to produce normal peristalsis throughout the large intestine. Its unique mode of action permits either oral or rectal administration, according to the requirements of the patient. Because of its gentleness and reliability of action without side effects, Dulcolax may be used whenever constipation is a problem. In preparation for surgery, proctoscopy, or radiologic examination, Dulcolax provides satisfactory cleansing of the bowel, obviating the need for an enema.
Dulcolax is a colorless, tasteless compound that is practically insoluble in water and alkaline solution. It is designated chemically bis(p-acetoxyphenyl)-2-pyridylmethane.

Actions: Dulcolax differs markedly from other laxatives in its mode of action: it is virtually nontoxic, and its laxative effect occurs on contact with the colonic mucosa, where it stimulates sensory nerve endings to produce parasympathetic reflexes resulting in increased peristaltic contractions of the colon. Administered orally, Dulcolax is absorbed to a variable degree from the small bowel but such absorption is not related to the mode of action of the compound. Dulcolax administered rectally in the form of suppositories is negligibly absorbed. The contact action of the drug is restricted to the colon, and motility of the small intestine is not appreciably influenced. Local axon reflexes, as well as segmental reflexes, are initiated in the region of contact and contribute to the widespread peristaltic activity producing evacuation. For this reason, Dulcolax may often be employed satisfactorily in patients with ganglionic blockage or spinal cord damage (paraplegia, poliomyelitis, etc.).

Indications: *Acute Constipation:* Taken at bedtime, Dulcolax tablets are almost invariably effective the following morning. When taken before breakfast, they usually produce an effect within six hours. For a prompter response and to replace enemas, the suppositories, which are usually effective in 15 minutes to one hour, can be used.

Chronic Constipation and Bowel Retraining: Dulcolax is extremely effective in the management of chronic constipation, particularly in older patients. By gradually lengthening the interval between doses as colonic tone improves, the drug has been found to be effective in redeveloping proper bowel hygiene. There is no tendency to "rebound".

Preparation for Radiography: Dulcolax tablets are excellent in eliminating fecal and gas shadows from x-rays taken of the abdominal area. For barium enemas, no food should be given following the administration of the tablets, to prevent reaccumulation of material in the cecum, and a suppository should be given one to two hours prior to examination.

Preoperative Preparation: Dulcolax tablets have been shown to be an ideal laxative in emptying the G.I. tract prior to abdominal surgery or to other surgery under general anesthesia. They may be supplemented by suppositories to replace the usual enema preparation. Dulcolax will not replace the colonic irrigations usually given patients before intracolonic surgery, but is useful in the preliminary emptying of the colon prior to these procedures.

Postoperative Care: Suppositories can be used to replace enemas, or tablets given as an oral laxative, to restore normal bowel hygiene after surgery.

Antepartum Care: Either tablets or suppositories can be used for constipation in pregnancy without danger of stimulating the uterus.

Preparation for Delivery: Suppositories can be used to replace enemas in the first stage of labor provided that they are given at least two hours before the onset of the second stage.

Postpartum Care: The same indications apply as in postoperative care, with no contraindication in nursing mothers.

Preparation for Sigmoidoscopy or Proctoscopy: For unscheduled office examinations, adequate preparation is usually obtained with a single suppository. For sigmoidoscopy scheduled in advance, however, administration of tablets the night before in addition will result in adequate preparation almost invariably.

Colostomies: Tablets the night before or a suppository inserted into the colostomy opening in the morning will frequently make irrigations unnecessary, and in other cases will expedite the procedure.

Contraindication: There is no contraindication to the use of Dulcolax, other than an acute surgical abdomen.

Precaution: Dulcolax tablets contain FD&C Yellow No. 5 (tartrazine) which may cause allergic-type reactions (including bronchial asthma) in certain susceptible individuals. Although the overall incidence of FD&C Yellow No. 5 (tartrazine) sensitivity in the general population is low, it is frequently seen in patients who also have aspirin hypersensitivity.

Adverse Reactions: As with any laxative, abdominal cramps are occasionally noted, particularly in severely constipated individuals.

Dosage:

Tablets

Tablets must be swallowed whole, not chewed or crushed, and should not be taken within one hour of antacids or milk.

Adults: Two or three (usually two) tablets suffice when an ordinary laxative effect is desired. This usually results in one or two soft, formed stools.
Up to six tablets may be safely given in preparation for special procedures when greater assurance of complete evacuation of the colon is desired. In producing such thorough emptying, these higher doses may result in several loose, unformed stools.

Children: One or two tablets, depending on age and severity of constipation, administered as above. Tablets should not be given to a child too young to swallow them whole.

Suppositories

Adults: One suppository at the time a bowel movement is required. Usually effective in 15 minutes to one hour.

Children: Half a suppository is generally effective for infants and children under two years of age. Above this age, a whole suppository is usually advisable.

Combined

In preparation for surgery, radiography and sigmoidoscopy, a combination of tablets the night before and a suppository in the morning is recommended (see Indications).

How Supplied: Dulcolax, brand of bisacodyl: Yellow, enteric-coated tablets of 5 mg in boxes of 24, bottles of 100, 1000 and unit strip packages of 100; suppositories of 10 mg in boxes of 2, 4, 8, 50 and 500.

Note: Dulcolax suppositories and tablets should be stored at temperatures not above 86°F (30°C).

Also Available: Dulcolax® Bowel Prep Kit. Each kit contains:
1 Dulcolax suppository of 10 mg bisacodyl;
4 Dulcolax tablets of 5 mg bisacodyl;
Complete patient instructions.

Clinical Applications: Dulcolax can be used in virtually any patient in whom a laxative or enema is indicated. It has no effect on the blood picture, erythrocyte sedimentation rate, urinary findings, or hepatic or renal function. It may be safely given to infants and the aged, pregnant or nursing women, debilitated patients, and may be prescribed in the presence of such conditions as cardiovascular, renal, or hepatic diseases. 026-E (5/81)

[*Shown in Product Identification Section*]

PERSANTINE® ℞

brand of dipyridamole
For Long-Term Therapy of Chronic Angina Pectoris
Tablets of 25 mg..............................BI-CODE 17
Tablets of 50 mg..............................BI-CODE 18
Tablets of 75 mg..............................BI-CODE 19

Description: Persantine, brand of dipyridamole, is classified as a coronary vasodilator. The drug is unrelated chemically to the nitrates or digitalis.

Chemistry: Persantine, brand of dipyridamole, is a homogeneous yellow crystalline powder, odorless but with a bitter taste. It is soluble in dilute acids, methanol, and chloroform. Its basic structure is a double ring of two condensed pyrimidine rings. It is designated chemically as 2,6-bis-(diethanolamino)-4,8-dipiperidino-pyrimido-(5,4-d) pyrimidine.

Actions: *Human:* Persantine, brand of dipyridamole, in therapeutic doses usually produces no significant alteration of systemic blood pressure or of blood flow in peripheral arteries; it increases coronary blood flow primarily by a selective dilation of the coronary arteries. The drug increases coronary sinus oxygen saturation without significantly altering myocardial oxygen consumption. A mild positive inotropic effect has been demonstrated in animals and man.

Animal: Experimental work in dogs subjected to artificial narrowing of one or both branches of the left coronary artery and chronically fed Persantine, brand of dipyridamole, has demonstrated an increase in intercoronary collateral circulation greater than that seen in placebo- or nitrate-treated animals exposed to identical conditions. A similar increase in collateral anastomoses over controls has been shown in healthy animals fed the drug.

Continued on next page

Boehringer Ingelheim—Cont.

In studies with heart preparations, the drug has been shown to protect against disturbances in function and fall in high-energy phosphate levels induced by hypoxia.
In animal (rat) studies using combination therapy with digitalis and dipyridamole, potentiation of digitalis toxicity occurred as measured by an augmentation of phosphorus exchange of the phosphorus-containing fractions of the myocardium. Experiments in cats, on the other hand, have shown that dipyridamole decreases the acute toxicity of digitoxin.
Studies with electron microscopy have demonstrated preservation of the anatomic structure of heart mitochondria (sarcosomes) in animals pretreated with the drug and exposed to hypoxia. Untreated animals showed dissolution of mitochondrial structure under similar conditions.

Indications: Based on a review of this drug by the National Academy of Sciences—National Research Council and/or other information, FDA has classified the indication as follows:
"Possibly" effective: For long-term therapy of chronic angina pectoris. Prolonged therapy may reduce the frequency or eliminate anginal episodes, improve exercise tolerance, and reduce nitroglycerin requirements. The drug is not intended to abort the acute anginal attack.
Final classification of the less-than-effective indications requires further investigation.

Contraindications: No specific contraindications are known.
Precautions: Since excessive doses can produce peripheral vasodilation, the drug should be used cautiously in patients with hypotension.
Persantine tablets, 25 mg, contain FD&C Yellow No. 5 (tartrazine) which may cause allergic-type reactions (including bronchial asthma) in certain susceptible individuals. Although the overall incidence of FD&C Yellow No. 5 (tartrazine) sensitivity in the general population is low, it is frequently seen in patients who also have aspirin hypersensitivity.
Adverse Reactions: Adverse reactions are minimal and transient at recommended dosages.
Instances of headache, dizziness, nausea, flushing, weakness, or syncope, mild gastrointestinal distress and skin rash have been noted during therapy. Rare cases of what appeared to be an aggravation of angina pectoris have been reported, usually at the initiation of therapy. On those uncommon occasions when adverse reactions have been persistent or intolerable to the patient, withdrawal of the medication has been followed promptly by cessation of the undesirable symptoms.
Dosage and Administration: The recommended dosage is 50 mg three times a day, taken at least one hour before meals. In some cases higher doses may be necessary but should be used with the knowledge that a significantly increased incidence of side effects is associated with increased dosage. Clinical response may not be evident before the second or third month of continuous therapy.
How Supplied:
Persantine (dipyridamole) is available as round, orange, sugar-coated tablets of 25 mg, coded 17. Bottles of 100 and 1000. Unit-dose packages of 100.
Persantine-50 (dipyridamole) is available as round, orange, sugar-coated tablets of 50 mg, coded 18. Bottles of 100 and 1000.
Persantine-75 (dipyridamole) is available as round, orange, sugar-coated tablets of 75 mg, coded 19. Bottles of 100. 98-146-510-K (7/82)
[Shown in Product Identification Section]

PRELUDIN® Ⓒ ℞

brand of phenmetrazine hydrochloride
Tablets, 25 mg USP ....BI-CODE 42
Endurets® (prolonged-action tablets), 50 mg........................BI-CODE 79
Endurets® (prolonged-action tablets), 75 mg........................BI-CODE 62

Description: Preludin, brand of phenmetrazine hydrochloride, belongs to the oxazine group of compounds and is designated chemically as 2-phenyl-3-methyltetrahydro-1,4-oxazine hydrochloride.
Phenmetrazine hydrochloride is a white, water-soluble, crystalline powder.
Actions: Preludin, brand of phenmetrazine hydrochloride, is a sympathomimetic amine with pharmacologic activity similar to the prototype drugs of this class used in obesity, the amphetamines. Actions include central nervous system stimulation and elevation of blood pressure. Tachyphylaxis and tolerance have been demonstrated with all drugs of this class in which these phenomena have been looked for.
Drugs of this class used in obesity are commonly known as "anorectics" or "anorexigenics". It has not been established, however, that the action of such drugs in treating obesity is primarily one of appetite suppression. Other central nervous system actions, or metabolic effects, may be involved, for example.
Adult obese subjects instructed in dietary management and treated with "anorectic" drugs, lose more weight on the average than those treated with placebo and diet, as determined in relatively short-term clinical trials.
The magnitude of increased weight loss of drug-treated patients over placebo-treated patients is only a fraction of a pound a week. The rate of weight loss is greatest in the first weeks of therapy for both drug and placebo subjects and tends to decrease in succeeding weeks. The possible origins of the increased weight loss due to the various drug effects are not established. The amount of weight loss associated with the use of an "anorectic" drug varies from trial to trial, and the increased weight loss appears to be related in part to variables other than the drug prescribed, such as the physician-investigator, the population treated, and the diet prescribed. Studies do not permit conclusions as to the relative importance of the drug and non-drug factors on weight loss.
The natural history of obesity is measured in years, whereas the studies cited are restricted to a few weeks' duration; thus, the total impact of drug-induced weight loss over that of diet alone must be considered clinically limited.
Preludin Endurets are formulated to release the active drug substance *in vivo* in a more gradual fashion than the standard formulation, as demonstrated by blood levels. The formulation has not been shown superior in effectiveness with respect to weight loss over the same dosage of the standard, noncontrolled-release formulations.
Indication: Preludin, brand of phenmetrazine hydrochloride, is indicated in the management of exogenous obesity as a short-term (a few weeks) adjunct in a regimen of weight reduction based on caloric restriction. The limited usefulness of agents of this class (see Actions) should be measured against possible risk factors inherent in their use such as those described below.
Contraindications: Advanced arteriosclerosis, symptomatic cardiovascular disease, moderate to severe hypertension, hyperthyroidism, known hypersensitivity or idiosyncrasy to sympathomimetic amines, glaucoma. Agitated states. Patients with a history of drug abuse. Concomitant use of CNS stimulants. During or within 14 days following the administration of monoamine oxidase inhibitors (hypertensive crises may result).
Warnings: Tolerance usually develops within a few weeks. When this occurs, the recommended dose should not be exceeded in an attempt to increase anorectic effect; rather, the drug should be discontinued.
Preludin, brand of phenmetrazine hydrochloride, may impair the ability of the patient to engage in potentially hazardous activities such as operating machinery or driving a motor vehicle; the patient should therefore be cautioned accordingly.
Drug Dependence: Preludin, brand of phenmetrazine hydrochloride, is related chemically and pharmacologically to the amphetamines. Amphetamines and related stimulant drugs have been extensively abused, and the possibility of abuse of Preludin, brand of phenmetrazine hydrochloride, should be kept in mind when evaluating the desirability of including a drug as part of a weight reduction program. Abuse of amphetamines and related drugs may be associated with intense psychological dependence and severe social dysfunction. There are reports of patients who have increased the dosage to many times that recommended. Abrupt cessation following prolonged high dosage administration results in extreme fatigue and mental depression; changes are also noted on the sleep EEG. Manifestations of chronic intoxication with anorectic drugs include severe dermatoses, marked insomnia, irritability, hyperactivity, and personality changes. The most severe manifestation of chronic intoxication is psychosis, often clinically indistinguishable from schizophrenia.
Usage in Pregnancy: Safe use in pregnancy has not been established. Animal reproductive studies demonstrated no teratogenic effects. However, the conception rate was adversely affected, as well as survival and body weight of pups at weaning. There have been clinical reports of congenital malformation associated with the use of this compound but a causal relationship has not been proved. Until more information is available, Preludin, brand of phenmetrazine hydrochloride, should not be used by women who are or may become pregnant, particularly in the first trimester, unless in the opinion of the prescribing physician the potential benefits outweigh the possible risks.
Usage in Children: Preludin, brand of phenmetrazine hydrochloride, is not recommended for use in children under 12 years of age.
Precautions: Caution should be exercised in prescribing Preludin, brand of phenmetrazine hydrochloride, for patients with even mild hypertension. Insulin requirements in diabetes mellitus may be altered in association with the use of Preludin, brand of phenmetrazine hydrochloride, and the concomitant dietary regimen. Preludin, brand of phenmetrazine hydrochloride, may decrease the hypotensive effect of guanethidine. The least amount feasible should be prescribed or dispensed at one time in order to minimize the possibility of overdosage.
Preludin Endurets, 75 mg, contain FD&C Yellow No. 5 (tartrazine) which may cause allergic-type reactions (including bronchial asthma) in certain susceptible individuals. Although the overall incidence of FD&C Yellow No. 5 (tartrazine) sensitivity in the general population is low, it is frequently seen in patients who also have aspirin hypersensitivity.
Adverse Reactions: *Cardiovascular:* Palpitation, tachycardia, elevation of blood pressure.
Central Nervous System: Overstimulation, restlessness, dizziness, insomnia, euphoria, dysphoria, tremor, headache; rarely psychotic episodes at recommended doses.
Gastrointestinal: Dryness of the mouth, unpleasant taste, diarrhea, constipation, other gastrointestinal disturbances.

Allergic: Urticaria.
Endocrine: Impotence, changes in libido.
Dosage and Administration: Preludin, brand of phenmetrazine hydrochloride, is not recommended for use in children under 12 years of age.
The maximum adult dosage is 50 to 75 mg administered as one 25-mg tablet two or three times daily, one hour before meals or as one 50-mg or 75-mg Endurets prolonged-action tablet taken daily. The scored 25-mg tablet permits adjustment of dosage to individual needs.
Since an Endurets tablet provides appetite suppression for approximately 12 hours, the time of administration should be determined by the period of the day over which the anorectic effect is desired.
Overdosage: Manifestations of acute overdosage with phenmetrazine hydrochloride include restlessness, tremor, hyperreflexia, rapid respiration, confusion, assaultiveness, hallucinations, panic states. Fatigue and depression usually follow the central stimulation. Cardiovascular effects include arrhythmias, hypertension, or hypotension and circulatory collapse. Gastrointestinal symptoms include nausea, vomiting, diarrhea and abdominal cramps. Poisoning may result in convulsions, coma, and death.
Management of acute phenmetrazine hydrochloride intoxication is largely symptomatic and includes lavage and sedation with a barbiturate. Experience with hemodialysis or peritoneal dialysis is inadequate to permit recommendation in this regard. As with the amphetamines, acidification of the urine should increase phenmetrazine hydrochloride excretion. Intravenous phentolamine has been suggested for possible acute, severe hypertension if this complicates phenmetrazine overdosage.
How Supplied: Preludin, brand of phenmetrazine hydrochloride, is available in three dosage strengths:
White, square, scored tablets of 25 mg, for b.i.d. or t.i.d. administration. Bottles of 100.
White, round Endurets prolonged-action tablets of 50 mg, for once-a-day administration. Bottles of 100.
Pink, round Endurets prolonged-action tablets of 75 mg, for once-a-day administration. Bottles of 100. 98-146-560-P (5/81)
[*Shown in Product Identification Section*]

PRELU-2® Ⓒ℞
brand of phendimetrazine tartrate
Timed Release Capsules **BI-CODE 64**
105 mg

Description: Chemical name: phendimetrazine tartrate (+) 3, 4 dimethyl-2-phenylmorpholine tartrate. Phendimetrazine tartrate is a white, odorless powder with a bitter taste. It is soluble in water, methanol and ethanol. It has a molecular weight of 341.
The capsule is manufactured in a special base which is designed for prolonged release.
Clinical Pharmacology: Phendimetrazine tartrate is a sympathomimetic amine with pharmacologic activity similar to the prototype of drugs of this class used in obesity, the amphetamines. Actions include central nervous system stimulation and elevation of blood pressure. Tachyphylaxis and tolerance have been demonstrated with all drugs of this class in which these phenomena have been looked for.
Drugs of this class used in obesity are commonly known as 'anorectics' or 'anorexigenics.' It has not been established, however, that the action of such drugs in treating obesity is primarily one of appetite suppression. Other central nervous system actions, or metabolic effects, may be involved, for example.
Adult obese subjects instructed in dietary management and treated with 'anorectic' drugs lose more weight on the average than those treated with placebo and diet, as determined in relatively short-term clinical trials.
The magnitude of increased weight loss of drug-treated patients over placebo-treated patients is only a fraction of a pound a week. The rate of weight loss is greatest in the first weeks of therapy for both drug and placebo subjects and tends to decrease in succeeding weeks. The possible origins of the increased weight loss due to the various drug effects are not established. The amount of weight loss associated with the use of an 'anorectic' drug varies from trial to trial, and the increased weight loss appears to be related in part to variables other than the drug prescribed, such as the physician-investigator, the population treated, and the diet prescribed. Studies do not permit conclusions as to the relative importance of the drug and non-drug factors on weight loss.
The natural history of obesity is measured in years, whereas the studies cited are restricted to a few weeks duration; thus, the total impact of drug-induced weight loss over that of diet alone must be considered clinically limited.
The active drug 105 mg of phendimetrazine tartrate in each capsule of this special timed release dosage form approximates the action of three 35 mg non-timed doses taken at four hour intervals.
The major route of elimination is via the kidneys where most of the drug and metabolites are excreted. Some of the drug is metabolized to phenmetrazine and also phendimetrazine-N-oxide.
The average half-life of elimination when studied under controlled conditions is about 3.7 hours for both the timed and non-timed forms. The absorption half-life of the drug from conventional non-timed 35 mg phendimetrazine tablets is appreciably more rapid than the absorption rate of the drug from the timed release formulation.
Indications and Usage: Phendimetrazine tartrate is indicated in the management of exogenous obesity as a short-term adjunct (a few weeks) in a regimen of weight reduction based on caloric restriction. The limited usefulness of agents of this class (see Clinical Pharmacology) should be measured against possible risk factors inherent in their use such as those described below.
Contraindications: Advanced arteriosclerosis, symptomatic cardiovascular disease, moderate to severe hypertension, hyperthyroidism, known hypersensitivity, or idiosyncrasy to the sympathomimetic amines, glaucoma.
Agitated states.
Patients with a history of drug abuse.
During or within 14 days following the administration of monoamine oxidase inhibitors (hypertensive crises may result).
Warnings: Tolerance to the anorectic effect usually develops within a few weeks. When this occurs, the recommended dose should not be exceeded in an attempt to increase the effect; rather, the drug should be discontinued. Phendimetrazine tartrate may impair the ability of the patient to engage in potentially hazardous activities such as operating machinery or driving a motor vehicle; the patient should therefore be cautioned accordingly.
Drug Dependence: Phendimetrazine tartrate is related chemically and pharmacologically to the amphetamines. Amphetamines and related stimulant drugs have been extensively abused, and the possibility of abuse of phendimetrazine tartrate should be kept in mind when evaluating the desirability of including a drug as part of a weight reduction program. Abuse of amphetamines and related drugs may be associated with intense psychological dependence and severe social dysfunction. There are reports of patients who have increased the dosage to many times that recommended. Abrupt cessation following prolonged high dosage administration results in extreme fatigue and mental depression; changes are also noted on the sleep EEG. Manifestations of chronic intoxication with anorectic drugs include severe dermatoses, marked insomnia, irritability, hyperactivity, and personality changes. The most severe manifestation of chronic intoxications is psychosis, often clinically indistinguishable from schizophrenia.
Usage in Pregnancy: The safety of phendimetrazine tartrate in pregnancy and lactation has not been established. Therefore phendimetrazine tartrate should not be taken by women who are or may become pregnant.
Usage in Children: Phendimetrazine tartrate is not recommended for use in children under 12 years of age.
Precautions: Caution is to be exercised in prescribing phendimetrazine tartrate for patients with even mild hypertension.
Insulin requirements in diabetes mellitus may be altered in association with the use of phendimetrazine tartrate and the concomitant dietary regimen.
Phendimetrazine tartrate may decrease the hypotensive effect of guanethidine.
The least amount feasible should be prescribed or dispensed at one time in order to minimize the possibility of overdosage.
Adverse Reactions:
Cardiovascular: Palpitation, tachycardia, elevation of blood pressure.
Central Nervous System: Overstimulation, restlessness, dizziness, insomnia, euphoria, dysphoria, tremor, headache; rarely psychotic episodes at recommended doses.
Gastrointestinal: Dryness of the mouth, unpleasant taste, diarrhea, constipation, other gastrointestinal disturbances.
Allergic: Urticaria.
Endocrine: Impotence, changes in libido.
Overdosage: Manifestations of acute overdosage with phendimetrazine tartrate include restlessness, tremor, hyperreflexia, rapid respiration, confusion, assaultiveness, hallucinations, panic states.
Fatigue and depression usually follow the central stimulation.
Cardiovascular effects include arrhythmias, hypertension or hypotension and circulatory collapse. Gastrointestinal symptoms include nausea, vomiting, diarrhea, and abdominal cramps. Fatal poisoning usually terminates in convulsions and coma. Management of acute phendimetrazine tartrate intoxication is largely symptomatic and includes lavage and sedation with a barbiturate. Experience with hemodialysis or peritoneal dialysis is inadequate to permit recommendation in this regard. Acidification of the urine increases phendimetrazine tartrate excretion. Intravenous phentolamine (Regitine) has been suggested for possible acute, severe hypertension, if this complicates phendimetrazine tartrate overdosage.
Dosage and Administration: Since this product is a timed release dosage form, limit to one timed release capsule (105 mg phendimetrazine tartrate) in the morning.
Phendimetrazine tartrate is not recommended for use in children under 12 years of age.
How Supplied: 105 mg capsules (celery and green) in bottles of 100.
Federal law prohibits dispensing without a prescription.
[*Shown in Product Identification Section*]

RESPBID® ℞
(theophylline)
Sustained release
Tablets of 250 mg and 500 mg
Oral Bronchodilator

Description: RESPBID® brand theophylline sustained release Tablets contain not less than 94.0 percent and not more than 106.0 percent of the labeled amount of $C_7H_8N_4O_2H_2O$. Theophylline, a xanthine compound, is a white, odorless, crystalline powder, having a

Continued on next page

Boehringer Ingelheim—Cont.

bitter taste. It contains one molecule of water of hydration or is anhydrous.

RESPID®, 250 mg: Each round, white, scored tablet with "BI 48" imprint contains 250 mg of theophylline, USP anhydrous in a sustained release formulation. RESPBID®, 500 mg: Each capsule-shaped, white, scored tablet with "BI 49" imprint contains 500 mg of theophylline, USP anhydrous in a sustained release formulation.

Clinical Pharmacology: Theophylline directly relaxes the smooth muscle of the bronchial airways and pulmonary blood vessels, thus acting mainly as a bronchodilator, pulmonary vasodilator and smooth muscle relaxant. The drug also possesses other actions typical of the xanthine derivatives: coronary vasodilator, diuretic, cardiac stimulant, cerebral stimulant and skeletal muscle stimulant. The actions of theophylline may be mediated through inhibition of phosphodiesterase and a resultant increase in intracellular cyclic AMP which could mediate smooth muscle relaxation. At concentrations higher than attained **in vivo**, theophylline also inhibits the release of histamine by mast cells.

In vitro, theophylline has been shown to react synergistically with beta agonists that increase intracellular cyclic AMP through the stimulation of adenyl cyclase (isoproterenol), but synergism has not been demonstrated in patient studies and more data are needed to determine if theophylline and beta agonists have clinically important additive effect **in vivo**.

Apparently, no development of tolerance occurs with chronic use of theophylline.

The half-life is shortened with cigarette smoking. The half-life is prolonged in alcoholism, reduced hepatic or renal function, congestive heart failure, and in patients receiving antibiotics such as TAO (troleandomycin), erythromycin and clindamycin. High fever for prolonged periods may decrease theophylline elimination.

Theophylline Elimination Characteristics:

	Theophylline Clearance Rates (mean ± S.D.)	Half-life Average (mean ± S.D.)
Children (over 6 months of age):	1.45 ± 0.58 ml/kg/min	3.7 ± 1.1 hrs.
Adult nonsmokers with uncomplicated asthma	0.65 ± 0.19 ml/kg/min	8.7 ± 2.2 hrs.

Newborn infants have extremely slow clearances and half-lives exceeding 24 hours which approach those seen for older children after about 3–6 months.

Older adults with chronic obstructive pulmonary disease, any patients with cor pulmonale or other causes of heart failure, and patients with liver pathology may have much lower clearances with half-lives that may exceed 24 hours.

The half-life of theophylline in smokers (1 to 2 packs/day) averaged 4–5 hours among various studies, much shorter than the half-life in nonsmokers who averaged about 7–9 hours. The increase in theophylline clearance caused by smoking is probably the result of induction of drug-metabolizing enzymes that do not readily normalize after cessation of smoking. It appears that between 3 months and 2 years may be necessary for normalization of the effect of smoking on theophylline pharmacokinetics.

RESPBID® brand theophylline has an apparent half-life of 10.7 hours. Blood levels of theophylline peak between 4 and 6 hours and the formulation is completely absorbed.

Indications: For relief of acute bronchial asthma and for reversible bronchospasm associated with chronic bronchitis and emphysema.

Contraindications: In individuals who have shown hypersensitivity to any of its components.

Warnings: Status asthmaticus is a medical emergency. Optimal therapy frequently requires additional medication including corticosteroids when the patient is not rapidly responsive to bronchodilators.

Excessive theophylline doses may be associated with toxicity and serum theophylline levels are recommended to assure maximal benefit without excessive risk. Incidence of toxicity increases at levels greater than 20 mcg/ml. Morphine, curare, and stilbamidine should be used with caution in patients with airflow obstruction since they stimulate histamine release and can induce asthmatic attacks. They may also suppress respiration leading to respiratory failure. Alternative drugs should be chosen whenever possible.

There is an excellent correlation between high blood levels of theophylline resulting from conventional doses and associated clinical manifestations of toxicity in (1) patients with lowered body plasma clearances (due to transient cardiac decompensation), (2) patients with liver dysfunction or chronic obstructive lung disease, (3) patients who are older than 55 years of age, particularly males.

There are often no early signs of less serious theophylline toxicity such as nausea and restlessness, which may appear in up to 50 percent of patients prior to onset of convulsions. Ventricular arrhythmias or seizures may be the first signs of toxicity.

Many patients who have higher theophylline serum levels exhibit a tachycardia.

Theophylline products may worsen pre-existing arrhythmias.

Usage in Pregnancy: Safe use in pregnancy has not been established relative to possible adverse effects on fetal development, but neither have adverse effects on fetal development been established. This is unfortunately true for most antiasthmatic medications. Therefore, use of theophylline in pregnant women should be balanced against the risk of uncontrolled asthma.

Precautions: Mean half-life in smokers is shorter than non-smokers; therefore smokers may require larger doses of theophylline. Theophylline should not be administered concurrently with other xanthine medications. Use with caution in patients with severe cardiac disease, severe hypoxemia, hypertension, hyperthyroidism, acute myocardial injury, cor pulmonale, congestive heart failure, liver disease, and in the elderly (especially males) and in neonates. Great caution should especially be used in giving theophylline to patients in congestive heart failure. Such patients have shown markedly prolonged theophylline blood level curves with theophylline persisting in serum for long periods following discontinuation of the drug.

Use theophylline cautiously in patients with history of peptic ulcer.

Theophylline may occasionally act as a local irritant to G.I. tract although gastrointestinal symptoms are more commonly central and associated with serum concentrations over 20 mcg/ml.

Adverse Reactions: The most consistent adverse reactions are usually due to overdose and are:

1. Gastrointestnal: nausea, vomiting, epigastric pain, hematemesis, diarrhea.
2. Central nervous system: headache, irritability, restlessness, insomnia, reflex hyperexcitability, muscle twitching, clonic and tonic generalized convulsions.
3. Cardiovascular: palpitation, tachycardia, extra systoles, flushing, hypotension, circulatory failure, life-threatening ventricular arrhythmias.
4. Respiratory: tachypnea.
5. Renal: albuminuria, increased excretion of renal tubular potentiation or diuresis, and red blood cells.
6. Others: hyperglycemia and inappropriate ADH syndrome.

Drug Interactions: Toxic synergism with ephedrine has been documented and may occur with some other sympathomimetic bronchodilators.

Drug	Effect
Aminophylline with Lithium Carbonate	Increased excretion of Lithium Carbonate
Aminophylline with Propranolol	Antagonism of Propranolol effect
Theophylline with Furosemide	Increased Diuresis of Furosemide
Theophylline with Hexamethonium	Decreased Hexamethonium-induced chromatropic effect
Theophylline with Reserpine	Reserpine-induced tachycardia
Theophylline with Chlordiazepoxide	Chlordiazepoxide-induced fatty acid mobilization
Theophylline with Cyclamycin (TAO = Triacetyloleandomycin), erythromycin, lincomycin	Increased Theophylline plasma levels

Overdosage: Management:

A. If potential oral overdose is established and seizure has not occurred:
   1) Induce vomiting.
   2) Administer a cathartic (this is particularly important if sustained release preparations have been taken).
   3) Administer activated charcoal.

B. If patient is having a seizure:
   1) Establish an airway.
   2) Administer O_2.
   3) Treat the seizure with intravenous diazepam, 0.1 to 0.3 mg/kg up to 10 mg.
   4) Monitor vital signs, maintain blood pressure and provide adequate hydration.

C. Post-Seizure Coma:
   1) Maintain airway and oxygenation.
   2) If a result of oral medication, follow above recommendations to prevent absorption of drug, but intubation and lavage will have to be performed instead of inducing emesis, and the cathartic and charcoal will need to be introduced via a large bore gastric lavage tube.
   3) Continue to provide full supportive care and adequate hydration while waiting for drug to be metabolized. In general, the drug is metabolized sufficiently rapidly so as to not warrant consideration of dialysis.

D. Animal studies suggest that phenobarbital may decrease theophylline toxicity. There is as yet, however, insufficient data to recommend pre-treatment of an overdosage with phenobarbital.

Dosage and Administration: Therapeutic serum levels associated with optimal likelihood for benefit and minimal risk of toxicity are considered to be between 10 mcg/ml and 20 mcg/ml. Levels above 20 mcg/ml may produce toxic effects. There is great variation from patient to patient in dosage needed in order to achieve a therapeutic blood level because of variable rates of elimination. Because of this wide variation from patient to patient, and the relatively narrow therapeutic blood level range, dosage must be individualized and monitoring of theophylline serum levels is highly recommended.

Dosage should be calculated on the basis of lean (ideal) body weight where mg/kg doses are stated. Theophylline does not distribute into fatty tissue.

Giving theophylline with food may prevent the rare case of stomach irritation; and though absorption may be slower, it is still complete. When rapidly absorbed products such as solutions and uncoated tablets with rapid dissolution are used, dosing to maintain "around the clock" blood levels generally requires administration every 6 hours to obtain the greatest efficacy for clinical use in children; dosing intervals up to 8 hours may be satisfactory for adults because of their slower elimination. Children, and adults requiring higher than average doses, may benefit from products with slower absorption which may allow longer dosing intervals and/or less fluctuation in serum concentration over a dosing interval during chronic therapy.

Dosage for Patient Population

Dosage schedule for Respid® brand theophylline sustained release Tablets: The calculated total daily dose of theophylline administered as Respbid® should be given in two divided daily doses, one every 12 hours. Children may require this dose to be given every 8 hours.

Acute Symptoms of Asthma Requiring Rapid Theophyllinization:

I. Not currently receiving theophylline products:

[See table above].

II. Those currently receiving theophylline products: determine, where possible, the time, amount, route of administration and form of the patient's last dose.

The loading dose for theophylline will be based on the principle that each 0.5 mg/kg of theophylline administered as a loading dose will result in a 1 mcg/ml increase in serum theophylline concentration. Ideally, then, the loading dose should be deferred if a serum theophylline concentration can be rapidly obtained. If this is not possible, the clinician must exercise his judgment in selecting a dose based on the potential for benefit and risk. When there is sufficient respiratory distress to warrant a small risk, 2.5 mg/kg of theophylline is likely to increase the serum concentration when administered as a loading dose in rapidly absorbed form by only about 5 mcg/ml. If the patient is not already experiencing theophylline toxicity, this is unlikely to result in dangerous adverse effects.

Subsequent to the modified decision regarding loading dose in this group of patients, the subsequent maintenance dosage recommendations are the same as those described above.

Comments: To achieve optimal therapeutic theophylline dosage, it is recommended to monitor serum theophylline concentrations. However, it is not always possible or practical to obtain a serum theophylline level.

Patients should be closely monitored for signs of toxicity. The present data suggest that the above dosage recommendations will achieve therapeutic serum concentrations with minimal risk of toxicity for most patients. However, some risk of toxic serum concentrations is still present.

Adverse reactions to theophylline often occur when serum theophylline levels exceed 20 mcg/ml.

Chronic Asthma:

Theophyllinization is a treatment of first choice for the management of chronic asthma (to prevent symptoms and maintain patent airways). Slow clinical titration is generally preferred to assure acceptance and safety of the medication.

Initial dose: 16 mg/kg/day or 400 mg/day (whichever is lower) in 3–4 divided doses at 6–8 hour intervals.

Increased dose: The above dosage may be increased in approximately 25 percent increments at 2–3 day intervals so long as no intolerance is observed, until the maximum indicated below is reached.

Maximum dose without measurement of serum concentration:

GROUP	ORAL LOADING DOSE (THEOPHYLLINE)	MAINTENANCE DOSE FOR NEXT 12 HOURS (THEOPHYLLINE)	MAINTENANCE DOSE BEYOND 12 HOURS (THEOPHYLLINE)
1. Children 6 months to 9 years	6 mg/kg	4 mg/kg q4hrs	4 mg/kg q6hrs
2. Children age 9–16 and young adult smokers	6 mg/kg	3 mg/kg q4h	3 mg/kg q6h
3. Otherwise healthy nonsmoking adults	6 mg/kg	3 mg/kg q6h	3 mg/kg q8h
4. Older patients and patients with cor pulmonale	6 mg/kg	2 mg/kg q6h	2 mg/kg q8h
5. Patients with congestive heart failure, liver failure	6 mg/kg	2 mg/kg q8h	1–2 mg/kg q12h

Not to exceed the following: (WARNING: DO NOT ATTEMPT TO MAINTAIN ANY DOSE THAT IS NOT TOLERATED)

Age < 9 years—24 mg/kg/day
Age 9–12 years—20 mg/kg/day
Age 12–16 years—18 mg/kg/day
Age > 16 years—13 mg/kg/day or 900 mg/day (WHICHEVER IS LESS)
NOTE: Use ideal body weight for obese patients.

Measurement of serum theophylline concentration during chronic therapy:

If the above maximum doses are to be maintained or exceeded, serum theophylline measurement is recommended. This should be obtained at the approximate time of peak absorption during chronic therapy for the product used (1–2 hours for liquids and plain uncoated tablets that undergo rapid dissolution, 3–5 hours for sustained release preparations). It is important that the patient will have missed no doses during the previous 48 hours and that dosing intervals will have been reasonably typical with no added doses during that period of time.

DOSAGE ADJUSTMENT BASED ON SERUM THEOPHYLLINE MEASUREMENTS WHEN THESE INSTRUCTIONS HAVE NOT BEEN FOLLOWED MAY RESULT IN RECOMMENDATIONS THAT PRESENT RISK OF TOXICITY TO THE PATIENT.

How Supplied:

RESPBID® brand theophylline is supplied as 250 mg white, round, scored sustained release tablets (NDC 0597-0048-01) and 500 mg white, capsule-shaped, scored sustained release tablets (NDC 0597-0049-01) in bottles of 100.

Caution: Federal law prohibits dispensing without prescription.

800172-A(6/81)

[*Shown in Product Identification Section*]

SERENTIL® ℞

brand of mesoridazine besylate

Tablets, 10 mg	**BI-CODE 20**
Tablets, 25 mg	**BI-CODE 21**
Tablets, 50 mg	**BI-CODE 22**
Tablets, 100 mg	**BI-CODE 23**
Concentrate of 25 mg/ml	**BI-CODE 25**
Ampuls of 1 ml (25 mg)	**BI-CODE 27**

Description: Serentil, brand of mesoridazine, the besylate salt of a metabolite of thioridazine, is a phenothiazine tranquilizer which is effective in the treatment of schizophrenia, organic brain disorders, alcoholism and psychoneuroses.

Serentil, brand of mesoridazine, is 10-[2(1-methyl-2-piperidyl) ethyl]-2-(methyl-sulfinyl)-phenothiazine [as the besylate].

Actions: Based upon animal studies Serentil, brand of mesoridazine, as with other phenothiazines, acts indirectly on reticular formation, whereby neuronal activity into reticular formation is reduced without affecting its intrinsic ability to activate the cerebral cortex. In addition, the phenothiazines exhibit at least part of their activities through depression of hypothalamic centers. Neurochemically, the phenothiazines are thought to exert their effects by a central adrenergic blocking action.

Indications: In clinical studies Serentil, brand of mesoridazine, has been found useful in the following disease states:

Schizophrenia: Serentil is effective in the treatment of schizophrenia. It substantially reduces the severity of emotional withdrawal, conceptual disorganization, anxiety, tension, hallucinatory behavior, suspiciousness and blunted affect in schizophrenic patients. As with other phenothiazines, patients refractory to previous medication may respond to Serentil, brand of mesoridazine.

Behavioral Problems in Mental Deficiency and Chronic Brain Syndrome: The effect of Serentil, brand of mesoridazine, was found to be excellent or good in the management of hyperactivity and uncooperativeness associated with mental deficiency and chronic brain syndrome.

Alcoholism—Acute and Chronic: Serentil, brand of mesoridazine, ameliorates anxiety, tension, depression, nausea and vomiting in both acute and chronic alcoholics without producing hepatic dysfunction or hindering the functional recovery of the impaired liver.

Psychoneurotic Manifestations: Serentil, brand of mesoridazine, reduces the symptoms of anxiety and tension, prevalent symptoms often associated with neurotic components of many disorders, and benefits personality disorders in general.

Contraindications: As with other phenothiazines, Serentil, brand of mesoridazine, is contraindicated in severe central nervous system depression or comatose states from any cause. Serentil, brand of mesoridazine, is contraindicated in individuals who have previously shown hypersensitivity to the drug.

Warnings: Where patients are participating in activities requiring complete mental alertness, (e.g., driving) it is advisable to administer the phenothiazines cautiously and to increase the dosage gradually.

Usage in Pregnancy: The safety of this drug in pregnancy has not been established; hence, it should be given only when the anticipated benefits to be derived from treatment exceed the possible risks to mother and fetus.

Usage in Children: The use of Serentil, brand of mesoridazine, in children under 12 years of age is not recommended, because safe conditions for its use have not been established.

Attention should be paid to the fact that phenothiazines are capable of potentiating central nervous system depressants (e.g., anesthetics, opiates, alcohol, etc.) as well as atropine and phosphorus insecticides.

Precautions: While ocular changes have not to date been related to Serentil, brand of mesoridazine, one should be aware that such changes have been seen with other drugs of this class.

Because of possible hypotensive effects, reserve parenteral administration for bedfast patients or for acute ambulatory cases, and keep patient lying down for at least one-half hour after injection.

Leukopenia and/or agranulocytosis have been attributed to phenothiazine therapy. A single case of transient granulocytopenia has been associated with Serentil, brand of mesorida-

Continued on next page

Boehringer Ingelheim—Cont.

zine. Since convulsive seizures have been reported, patients receiving anticonvulsant medication should be maintained on that regimen while receiving Serentil, brand of mesoridazine.

Neuroleptic drugs elevate prolactin levels; the elevation persists during chronic administration. Tissue culture experiments indicate that approximately one-third of human breast cancers are prolactin dependent in vitro, a factor of potential importance if the prescription of these drugs is contemplated in a patient with a previously detected breast cancer. Although disturbances such as galactorrhea, amenorrhea, gynecomastia, and impotence have been reported, the clinical significance of elevated serum prolactin levels is unknown for most patients. An increase in mammary neoplasms has been found in rodents after chronic administration of neuroleptic drugs. Neither clinical studies nor epidemiologic studies conducted to date, however, have shown an association between chronic administration of these drugs and mammary tumorigenesis; the available evidence is considered too limited to be conclusive at this time.

Serentil tablets contain FD&C Yellow No. 5 (tartrazine) which may cause allergic-type reactions (including bronchial asthma) in certain susceptible individuals. Although the overall incidence of FD&C Yellow No. 5 (tartrazine) sensitivity in the general population is low, it is frequently seen in patients who also have aspirin hypersensitivity.

Adverse Reactions: Drowsiness and hypotension were the most prevalent side effects encountered. Side effects tended to reach their maximum level of severity early with the exception of a few (rigidity and motoric effects) which occurred later in therapy.

With the exceptions of tremor and rigidity, adverse reactions were generally found among those patients who received relatively high doses early in treatment. Clinical data showed no tendency for the investigators to terminate treatment because of side effects.

Serentil, brand of mesoridazine, has demonstrated a remarkably low incidence of adverse reactions when compared with other phenothiazine compounds.

Central Nervous System: Drowsiness, Parkinson's syndrome, dizziness, weakness, tremor, restlessness, ataxia, dystonia, rigidity, slurring, akathisia, motoric reactions (opisthotonos) have been reported.

Autonomic Nervous System: Dry mouth, nausea and vomiting, fainting, stuffy nose, photophobia, constipation and blurred vision have occurred in some instances.

Genitourinary System: Inhibition of ejaculation, impotence, enuresis, incontinence have been reported.

Skin: Itching, rash, hypertrophic papillae of the tongue and angioneurotic edema have been reported.

Cardiovascular System: Hypotension and tachycardia have been reported. EKG changes have occurred in some instances (see Phenothiazine Derivatives: Cardiovascular Effects).

Phenothiazine Derivatives: It should be noted that efficacy, indications and untoward effects have varied with the different phenothiazines. The physician should be aware that the following have occurred with one or more phenothiazines and should be considered whenever one of these drugs is used:

Autonomic Reactions: Miosis, obstipation, anorexia, paralytic ileus.

Cutaneous Reactions: Erythema, exfoliative dermatitis, contact dermatitis.

Blood Dyscrasias: Agranulocytosis, leukopenia, eosinophilia, thrombocytopenia, anemia, aplastic anemia, pancytopenia.

Allergic Reactions: Fever, laryngeal edema, angioneurotic edema, asthma.

Hepatotoxicity: Jaundice, biliary stasis.

Cardiovascular Effects: Changes in the terminal portion of the electrocardiogram, including prolongation of the Q-T interval, lowering and inversion of the T wave and appearance of a wave tentatively identified as a bifid T or a U wave have been observed in some patients receiving the phenothiazine tranquilizers, including Serentil, brand of mesoridazine. To date, these appear to be due to altered repolarization and not related to myocardial damage. They appear to be reversible. While there is no evidence at present that these changes are in any way precursors of any significant disturbance of cardiac rhythm, it should be noted that sudden and unexpected deaths apparently due to cardiac arrest have occurred in patients previously showing characteristic electrocardiographic changes while taking the drug. The use of periodic electrocardiograms has been proposed but would appear to be of questionable value as a predictive device.

Hypotension, rarely resulting in cardiac arrest, has been noted.

Extrapyramidal Symptoms: Akathisia, agitation, motor restlessness, dystonic reactions, trismus, torticollis, opisthotonos, oculogyric crises, tremor, muscular rigidity, akinesia.

Persistent Tardive Dyskinesia: As with all antipsychotic agents, tardive dyskinesia may appear in some patients on long-term therapy or may occur after drug therapy has been discontinued. This risk seems to be greater in elderly patients on high-dose therapy, especially females. The symptoms are persistent and in some patients appear to be irreversible. The syndrome is characterized by rhythmical involuntary movements of the tongue, face, mouth or jaw (e.g., protrusion of tongue, puffing of cheeks, puckering of mouth, chewing movements). Sometimes these may be accompanied by involuntary movements of extremities.

There is no known effective treatment for tardive dyskinesia; antiparkinsonism agents usually do not alleviate the symptoms of this syndrome. It is suggested that all antipsychotic agents be discontinued if these symptoms appear.

Should it be necessary to reinstitute treatment, or increase the dosage of the agent, or switch to a different antipsychotic agent, the syndrome may be masked.

It has been reported that fine vermicular movements of the tongue may be an early sign of the syndrome and if the medication is stopped at that time, the syndrome may not develop.

Endocrine Disturbances: Menstrual irregularities, altered libido, gynecomastia, lactation, weight gain, edema. False positive pregnancy tests have been reported.

Urinary Disturbances: Retention, incontinence.

Others: Hyperpyrexia. Behavioral effects suggestive of a paradoxical reaction have been reported. These include excitement, bizarre dreams, aggravation of psychoses and toxic confusional states. More recently, a peculiar skin-eye syndrome has been recognized as a side effect following long-term treatment with phenothiazines. This reaction is marked by progressive pigmentation of areas of the skin or conjunctiva and/or accompanied by discoloration of the exposed sclera and cornea. Opacities of the anterior lens and cornea described as irregular or stellate in shape have also been reported. Systemic lupus erythematosus-like syndrome.

Dosage and Administration: The dosage of Serentil, brand of mesoridazine, as in most medications, should be adjusted to the needs of the individual. The lowest effective dosage should always be used. When maximum response is achieved, dosage may be reduced gradually to a maintenance level.

Schizophrenia: For most patients, regardless of severity, a starting dose of 50 mg. t.i.d. is recommended. The usual optimum total daily dose range is 100-400 mg per day.

Behavioral Problems in Mental Deficiency and Chronic Brain Syndrome: For most patients a starting dose of 25 mg t.i.d. is recommended. The usual optimum total daily dose range is 75-300 mg per day.

Alcoholism: For most patients the usual starting dose is 25 mg b.i.d. The usual optimum total daily dose range is 50-200 mg per day.

Psychoneurotic Manifestations: For most patients the usual starting dose is 10 mg t.i.d. The usual optimum total daily dose range is 30-150 mg per day.

Injectable Form: In those situations in which an intramuscular form of medication is indicated, Serentil, brand of mesoridazine, injectable is available. For most patients a starting dose of 25 mg is recommended. The dose may be repeated in 30 to 60 minutes, if necessary. The usual optimum total daily dose range is 25-200 mg per day.

How Supplied:

Tablets: 10 mg, 25 mg, 50 mg, and 100 mg mesoridazine (as the besylate). Bottles of 100.

Ampuls: 1 ml [25 mg mesoridazine (as the besylate)]. Inactive ingredients: disodium edetate, USP, 0.5 mg; sodium chloride, USP, 7.2 mg; carbon dioxide gas (bone dry) q.s., water for injection, USP, q.s. to 1 ml. Boxes of 20 and 100.

Concentrate: Contains 25 mg mesoridazine (as the besylate) per ml; alcohol, USP, 0.61% by volume. Immediate containers: Amber glass bottles of 4 fl oz (118 ml) packaged in cartons of 12 bottles, with an accompanying dropper graduated to deliver 10 mg, 25 mg and 50 mg of mesoridazine (as the besylate).

Storage: Below 77°F. Protect from light. Dispense in amber glass bottles only.

The concentrate may be diluted with distilled water, acidified tap water, orange juice or grape juice.

Each dose should be so diluted just prior to administration. Preparation and storage of bulk dilutions is not recommended.

Additional information available to physicians.

Pharmacology: Pharmacological studies in laboratory animals have established that Serentil, brand of mesoridazine, has a spectrum of pharmacodynamic actions typical of a major tranquilizer. In common with other tranquilizers it inhibits spontaneous motor activity in mice, prolongs thiopental and hexobarbital sleeping time in mice and produces spindles and block of arousal reaction in the EEG of rabbits. It is effective in blocking spinal reflexes in the cat and antagonizes d-amphetamine excitation and toxicity in grouped mice. It shows a moderate adrenergic blocking activity in vitro and in vivo and antagonizes 5-hydroxytryptamine in vivo. Intravenously administered, it lowers the blood pressure of anesthetized dogs. It has a weak antiacetylcholine effect in vitro.

The most outstanding activity of Serentil, brand of mesoridazine, is seen in tests developed to investigate antiemotive activity of drugs. Such tests are those in which the rat reacts to acute or chronic stress by increased defecation (emotogenic defecation) or tests in which "emotional mydriasis" is elicited in the mouse by an electric shock. In both of these tests Serentil, brand of mesoridazine, is effective in reducing emotive reactions. Its ED_{50} in inhibiting emotogenic defecation in the rat is 0.053 mg/kg (subcutaneous administration).

Serentil, brand of mesoridazine, has a potent antiemetic action. The intravenous ED_{50} against apomorphine-induced emesis in the dog is 0.64 mg/kg.

Serentil, brand of mesoridazine, in common with other phenothiazines, demonstrates antiarrhythmic activity in anesthetized dogs. Metabolic studies in the dog and rabbit with tritium labeled mesoridazine demonstrate that the compound is well absorbed from the gastrointestinal tract. The biological half-life of Serentil, brand of mesoridazine, in these studies appears to be somewhere between 24 to 48 hours. Although significant urinary excretion was observed following the administration of Serentil, brand of mesoridazine, these studies also suggest that biliary excretion is an important excretion route for mesoridazine and/or its metabolites.

Toxicity Studies

Acute LD_{50} (mg/kg):
[See table above].

Route	Mouse	Rat	Rabbit	Dog
Oral	560 ± 62.5	644 ± 48	MLD = 800	MLD = 800
I.M.	—	509M 584 F	405	—
I.V.	26 ± 0.08	—	—	—

Chronic toxicity studies were conducted in rats and dogs. Rats were administered Serentil, brand of mesoridazine, orally seven days per week for a period of seventeen months in doses up to 160 mg/kg per day. Dogs were administered Serentil, brand of mesoridazine, orally seven days per week for a period of thirteen months. The daily dosage of the drug was increased during the period of this test such that the "top-dose" group received a daily dose of 120 mg/kg of mesoridazine for the last month of the study. Untoward effects which occurred upon chronic administration of high dose-levels included:

Rats: Reduction of food intake, slowed weight gain, morphological changes in pituitary-supported endocrine organs, and melanin-like pigment deposition in renal tissues.

Dogs: Emesis, muscle tremors, decreased food intake and death associated with aspiration of oral-gastric contents into the respiratory system.

Increased intrauterine resorptions were seen with Serentil, brand of mesoridazine, in rats at 70 mg/kg and in rabbits at 125 mg/kg but not at 60 and 100 mg/kg, respectively. No drug related teratology was suggested by these reproductive studies.

Local irritation from the intramuscular injection of Serentil, brand of mesoridazine, was of the same order of magnitude as with other phenothiazines. SER-Z13 (9/80)

[*Shown in Product Identification Section*]

TORECAN® ℞
brand of thiethylperazine USP
Tablets, 10 mg ....BI-CODE 28
Suppositories, 10 mg ....BI-CODE 29
Injection, 10 mg/2 ml ampul ....BI-CODE 30
For IM use only.

Description: Torecan, brand of thiethylperazine, is a phenothiazine. Thiethylperazine is characterized by a substituted thioethyl group at position 2 in the phenothiazine nucleus, and a piperazine moiety in the side chain. The chemical designation is: 2-ethyl-mercapto-10-[3′-(1″-methyl-piperazinyl-4″)-propyl-1″] phenothiazine.

Actions: The pharmacodynamic action of Torecan, brand of thiethylperazine, in humans is unknown. However, a direct action of Torecan, brand of thiethylperazine, on both the CTZ and the vomiting center may be concluded from induced vomiting experiments in animals.

Indications: Torecan is indicated for the relief of nausea and vomiting.

Contraindications: Severe central nervous system (CNS) depression and comatose states. In patients who have demonstrated a hypersensitivity reaction (e.g., blood dyscrasias, jaundice) to phenothiazines.

Because severe hypotension has been reported after the intravenous administration of phenothiazines, this route of administration is contraindicated.

Usage in Pregnancy: Torecan, brand of thiethylperazine, is contraindicated in pregnancy.

Warnings: Phenothiazines are capable of potentiating CNS depressants (e.g., anesthetics, opiates, alcohol, etc.) as well as atropine and phosphorous insecticides.

Since Torecan, brand of thiethylperazine, may impair mental and/or physical ability required in the performance of potentially hazardous tasks such as driving a car or operating machinery, it is recommended that patients be warned accordingly.

Postoperative Nausea and Vomiting: With the use of this drug to control postoperative nausea and vomiting occurring in patients undergoing elective surgical procedures, restlessness and postoperative CNS depression during anesthesia recovery may occur. Possible postoperative complications of a severe degree of any of the known reactions of this class of drug must be considered.

Postural hypotension may occur after an initial injection, rarely with the tablet or suppository.

The administration of epinephrine should be avoided in the treatment of drug-induced hypotension in view of the fact that phenothiazines may induce a reversed epinephrine effect on occasion.

Should a vasoconstrictive agent be required, the most suitable are levarterenol and phenylephrine.

The use of this drug has not been studied following intracardiac and intracranial surgery.

Usage in Pediatrics: The safety and efficacy of Torecan, brand of thiethylperazine, in children under 12 years of age has not been established.

Nursing Mothers: Information is not available concerning the secretion of Torecan, brand of thiethylperazine, in the milk of nursing mothers. As a general rule, nursing should not be undertaken while a patient is on a drug, since many drugs are secreted in human milk.

Precautions: Abnormal movements such as extrapyramidal symptoms (EPS) (e.g., dystonia, torticollis, dysphasia, oculogyric crises, akathisia) have occurred. Convulsions have also been reported. The varied symptom complex is more likely to occur in young adults and children. Extrapyramidal effects must be treated by reduction of dosage or cessation of medication.

Torecan tablets contain FD&C Yellow No. 5 (tartrazine) which may cause allergic-type reactions (including bronchial asthma) in certain susceptible individuals. Although the overall incidence of FD&C Yellow No. 5 (tartrazine) sensitivity in the general population is low, it is frequently seen in patients who also have aspirin hypersensitivity.

Postoperative Nausea and Vomiting: When used in the treatment of the nausea and/or vomiting associated with anesthesia and surgery, it is recommended that Torecan, brand of thiethylperazine, should be administered by deep intramuscular injection at or shortly before the termination of anesthesia.

Adverse Reactions: *Central Nervous System:* Serious: Convulsions have been reported, Extrapyramidal symptoms (EPS) may occur, such as dystonia, torticollis, oculogyric crises, akathisia, and gait disturbances. Others: Occasional cases of dizziness, headache, fever and restlessness have been reported.

Drowsiness may occur on occasion, following an initial injection. Generally this effect tends to subside with continued therapy or is usually alleviated by a reduction in dosage.

Autonomic Nervous System: Dryness of the mouth and nose, blurred vision, tinnitus. An occasional case of sialorrhea together with altered gustatory sensation has been observed.

Endocrine System: Peripheral edema of the arms, hands and face.

Hepatotoxicity: An occasional case of cholestatic jaundice has been observed.

Others: An occasional case of cerebral vascular spasm and trigeminal neuralgia has been reported.

Phenothiazine Derivatives: The physician should be aware that the following have occurred with one or more phenothiazines and should be considered whenever one of these drugs is used:

Blood Dyscrasias: Serious: Agranulocytosis, leukopenia, thrombocytopenia, aplastic anemia, pancytopenia, Others: Eosinophilia, leukocytosis.

Autonomic Reactions: Miosis, obstipation, anorexia, paralytic ileus.

Cutaneous Reactions: Serious: Erythema, exfoliative dermatitis, contact dermatitis.

Hepatotoxicity: Serious: Jaundice, biliary stasis.

Cardiovascular Effects: Serious: Hypotension, rarely leading to cardiac arrest; electrocardiographic (ECG) changes.

Extrapyramidal Symptoms: Serious: Akathisia, agitation, motor restlessness, dystonic reactions, trismus, torticollis, opisthotonos, oculogyric crises, tremor, muscular rigidity, akinesia—some of which have persisted for several months or years especially in patients of advanced age with brain damage.

Endocrine Disturbances: Menstrual irregularities, altered libido, gynecomastia, weight gain. False positive pregnancy tests have been reported.

Urinary Disturbances: Retention, incontinence.

Allergic Reactions: Serious: Fever, laryngeal edema, angioneurotic edema, asthma.

Others: Hyperpyrexia. Behavioral effects suggestive of a paradoxical reaction have been reported. These include excitement, bizarre dreams, aggravation of psychoses and toxic confusional states. While there is no evidence at present that ECG changes observed in patients receiving phenothiazines are in any way precursors of any significant disturbance of cardiac rhythm, it should be noted that sudden and unexpected deaths apparently due to cardiac arrest have been reported in a few instances in hospitalized psychotic patients previously showing characteristic ECG changes. A peculiar skin-eye syndrome has also been recognized as a side effect following long-term treatment with certain phenothiazines. This reaction is marked by progressive pigmentation of areas of the skin or conjunctiva and/or accompanied by discoloration of the exposed sclera and cornea. Opacities of the anterior lens and cornea described as irregular or stellate in shape have also been reported.

Drug Interactions: Phenothiazines are capable of potentiating CNS depressants (e.g., anesthetics, opiates, alcohol, etc.) as well as atropine and phosphorous insecticides.

Phenothiazines may induce a reversed epinephrine effect on occasion.

Dosage and Administration:

Adult: Usual daily dose range is 10 mg to 30 mg.

Oral: One tablet, one to three times daily.

Intramuscular: 2 ml IM, one to three times daily. (See Precautions.)

Continued on next page

Boehringer Ingelheim—Cont.

Suppository: Insert one suppository, one to three times daily.
Children: Appropriate dosage of Torecan, brand of thiethylperazine, has not been determined in children.
How Supplied:
Tablets: Each tablet contains 10 mg thiethylperazine maleate, USP, bottles of 100.
Ampuls: Each 2 ml ampul contains in aqueous solution 10 mg thiethylperazine malate, USP; sodium metabisulfite, 0.5 mg; ascorbic acid, USP, 2.0 mg; sorbitol, NF, 40.0 mg; carbon dioxide gas q.s.; water for injection, USP, q.s. Boxes of 20 and 100.
Storage: Below 86° F; light-resistant container. Administer only if clear and colorless.
Suppositories: Each containing 10 mg thiethylperazine maleate, USP and inactive ingredient—cocoa butter, NF; packages of 12.
Storage: Below 77° F; tight container (sealed foil). TOR-Z17 (7/82)
[*Shown in Product Identification Section*]

Boots Pharmaceuticals, Inc.

6540 LINE AVENUE
SHREVEPORT, LA 71106

F–E–P CREME® ℞

Description: F-E-P Creme is a topical water soluble preparation that contains the following active ingredients:
Hydrocortisone 1.0%
Pramoxine Hydrochloride 0.5%
Clinical Pharmacology: Topical corticosteroids share anti-inflammatory, anti-pruritic and vasoconstrictive actions.
The mechanism of anti-inflammatory activity of the topical corticosteroids is unclear. Various laboratory methods, including vasoconstrictor assays, are used to compare and predict potencies and/or clinical efficacies of the topical corticosteroids. There is some evidence to suggest that a recognizable correlation exists between vasoconstrictor potency and therapeutic efficacy in man. Pramoxine Hydrochloride is a surface anesthetic agent and promptly relieves pain and itch. As it is not chemically related to the benzoate esters of the "caine" type, this compound may be used safely on the skin of those patients sensitive to the "caine" type local anesthetic.
The extent of percutaneous absorption of topical corticosteroids is determined by many factors including the vehicle, the integrity of the epidermal barrier, and the use of occlusive dressings.
Topical corticosteroids can be absorbed from normal intact skin. Inflammation and/or other disease processes in the skin increase percutaneous absorption. Occlusive dressings substantially increase the percutaneous absorption of topical corticosteroids. Thus, occlusive dressings may be a valuable therapeutic adjunct for treatment of resistant dermotoses (see–**Dosage and Administration**).
Once absorbed through the skin, hydrocortisone is handled through pharmacokinetic pathways, similar to systemically administered hydrocortisone. Hydrocortisone is more than 90% bound to plasma proteins. It is metabolized primarily in the liver and then excreted by the kidneys, mainly conjugated as glucuronides, together with a very small proportion of unchanged hydrocortisone.
Indications and Usage: F-E-P Creme is indicated for the relief of the inflammatory and pruritic manifestations of corticosteroid-responsive dermatoses.
Contraindications: F-E-P Creme is contraindicated in those patients with a history of hypersensitivity to any of the components of the preparation. It should not be used in the eye or nose.
Precautions: General. Systemic absorption of topical corticosteroids has produced reversible hypothalamic-pituitary-adrenal (HPA) axis suppression, manifestations of Cushing's syndrome, hyperglycemia, and glucosuria in some patients.
Conditions which augment systemic absorption include the application over large surface areas, prolonged use, and the addition of occlusive dressings.
As F-E-P Creme contains Pramoxine Hydrochloride, it should not be applied to extensive areas of the skin. F-E-P Creme is not intended for indefinitely prolonged use.
Children may absorb proportionally larger amounts of topical corticosteroids and thus be more susceptible to systemic toxicity (see **Precautions**–Pediatric Use).
If irritation develops, F-E-P Creme should be discontinued and appropriate therapy instituted.
In the presence of dermatological infections, the use of an appropriate antifungal or antibacterial agent should be instituted. If a favorable response does not occur promptly, the corticosteroid should be discontinued until the infection has been adequately controlled.
Information for the Patient
Patients using F-E-P Creme should receive the following information and instructions:
1. This medication is to be used as directed by the physician. It is for external use only. Avoid contact with the eyes. Do not use in the nose.
2. Patients should be advised not to use this medication for any disorder other than that for which it was prescribed.
3. The treated skin area should not be bandaged or otherwise covered or wrapped as to be occlusive unless directed by the physician.
4. Patients should report any signs of local adverse reactions, especially under occlusive dressing.
5. Parents of pediatric patients should be advised not to use tight-fitting diapers or plastic pants on a child being treated in the diaper area, as these garments may constitute occlusive dressings.
6. Discontinue the use of F-E-P Creme if redness, irritation, swelling or pain other than those from your skin disorder occur.

Laboratory Tests
The following tests may be helpful in evaluating the HPA axis suppression:
Urinary free cortisol tests
ACTH stimulation test
Carcinogenesis, Mutagenesis, and Impairment of Fertility
Long-term animal studies have not been performed to evaluate the carcinogenic potential or the effect on fertility of hydrocortisone.
Studies to determine mutagenicity with hydrocortisone have revealed negative results.
Pregnancy Category C
Corticosteroids are generally teratogenic in laboratory animals when administered systemically at relatively low dosage levels. There are no adequate and well-controlled studies in pregnant women on teratogenic effects from topically applied hydrocortisone. Therefore, F-E-P Creme should be used during pregnancy only if the potential benefit justifies the potential risk to the fetus. F-E-P Creme should not be used extensively on pregnant patients, in large amounts, or for prolonged periods of time.
Nursing Mothers
It is not known whether topically applied F-E-P Creme could result in sufficient systemic absorption to produce detectable quantities in breast milk. Systemically administered corticosteroids are secreted into breast milk in quantities not likely to have a deleterious effect on the infant. Nevertheless, caution should be exercised when F-E-P Creme is administered to a nursing woman.
Pediatric Use
Pediatric patients may demonstrate greater susceptibility to topical corticosteroid-induced HPA axis suppression and Cushing's syndrome than mature patients because of a larger skin surface area to body weight ratio.
Hypothalamic-pituitary-adrenal (HPA) axis suppression, Cushing's syndrome, and intracranial hypertension have been reported in children receiving topical corticosteroids. Manifestations of adrenal suppression in children include linear growth retardation, delayed weight gain, low plasma cortisol levels, and absence of response to ACTH stimulation. Manifestations of intracranial hypertension include bulging fortanelles, headaches, and bilateral papilledema.
Administration of F-E-P Creme to children should be limited to the least amount compatible with an effective therapeutic regimen. Chronic corticosteroid therapy may interfere with the growth and development of children.
Adverse Reactions: The following local adverse reactions are reported infrequently with topical corticosteroids, but may occur more frequently with the use of occlusive dressings. These reactions are listed in an approximately decreasing order of occurrence.
Burning, itching, irritation, dryness, folliculitis, hypertrichosis, acneiform eruptions, hypopigmentation, perioral dermatitis, allergic contact dermatitis, maceration of the skin, secondary infection, skin atrophy, striae, and miliaria. The use of Pramoxine Hydrochloride may also lead to stinging and burning.
Overdosage: Topically applied hydrocortisone can be absorbed in sufficient amounts to produce systemic effects (See **Precautions**).
Dosage and Administration: F-E-P Creme is generally applied to the affected area as a thin film from one to four times daily depending on the severity of the condition.
Occlusive dressings may be used for the management of psoriasis or recalcitrant conditions. If an infection develops, the use of occlusive dressings should be discontinued and appropriate antimicrobial therapy instituted.
How Supplied: F-E-P Creme ½ ounce (15 gm) tubes
NDC 0524-1026-51
Caution: FEDERAL LAW PROHIBITS DISPENSING WITHOUT A PRESCRIPTION.
Manufactured and Distributed By:
Boots Pharmaceuticals, Inc.
Shreveport, Louisiana 71106
Jan. 1982

LOPURIN® ℞
Allopurinol Tablets, USP

Description: LOPURIN® (Allopurinol U.S.P. in tablet form) is an orally administered xanthine oxidase inhibitor, with the chemical name 4-hydroxypyrazolo (3, 4-d) pyrimidine (HPP) (also described in U.S.P. XX as 1H-Pyrazolo (3,4-d) pyrimidin-4-ol).
Clinical Pharmacology: Allopurinol acts on purine catabolism, without disrupting the biosynthesis of vital purines, thus reducing the production of uric acid by inhibiting the biochemical reactions immediately preceding its formation. Its action differs from that of uricosuric agents, which lower the serum uric acid level by increasing urinary excretion of uric acid. Allopurinol reduces both the serum and urinary uric acid levels by inhibiting the formation of uric acid. It thereby avoids the hazard of increased hyperuricosuria in patients with gouty nephropathy or with a predisposition to the formation of uric acid stones.
Allopurinol has produced a substantial reduction in serum and urinary uric acid levels in hitherto refractory patients even in the presence of renal damage marked enough to render uricosuric drugs virtually ineffective. Salicylates may be given conjointly for their antirheumatic effect without compromising the action of Allopurinol. This is in contrast to the

nullifying effect of salicylates on uricosuric drugs.

Allopurinol is a structural analogue of the natural purine base, hypoxanthine. It is a potent inhibitor of xanthine oxidase, the enzyme responsible for the conversion of hypoxanthine to xanthine and of xanthine to uric acid, the end product of purine metabolism in man. Allopurinol is metabolized to the corresponding xanthine analogue, oxipurinol (alloxanthine), which also is an inhibitor of xanthine oxidase.

Hyperuricemia may be primary, as in gout, or secondary to diseases such as acute and chronic leukemia, polycythemia vera, multiple myeloma, and psoriasis. It may occur with the use of diuretic agents, during renal dialysis, in the presence of renal damage, during starvation or reducing diets and in the treatment of neoplastic disease where rapid resolution of tissue masses may occur.

The major disease manifestations in gout—kidney stones, tophi in soft tissues, and deposits in joints and bones—result from the deposition of urates. If progressive deposition of urates is to be arrested or reversed, it is necessary to reduce the serum uric acid to a level below the saturation point to suppress urate precipitation. Reduction may be achieved by means of uricosuric agents. Uricosurics are less effective in the presence of renal disease, and some patients develop intolerance or sensitivity to these drugs. The use of Allopurinol to block the formation of urate avoids the hazard of increased renal excretion of uric acid posed by uricosuric drugs.

The half-life of Allopurinol in the body is determined both by renal excretion and by oxidation to 4,6-dihydroxypyrazolo (3,4-d) pyrimidine (oxipurinol). The latter is also an inhibitor of xanthine oxidase, but is somewhat weaker than Allopurinol which is bound 15-fold more tightly to the enzyme than is the natural substrate, xanthine. The long half-life of oxipurinol in the plasma (18 to 30 hours), contributes significantly to the enzyme inhibition. Moreover, both Allopurinol and oxipurinol tend to inactivate xanthine oxidase, thereby further controlling the level of its activity.

Administration of Allopurinol generally results in a fall in both serum and urinary uric acid within two to three days. The magnitude of this decrease can be manipulated almost at will since it is dose-dependent. A week or more of treatment with Allopurinol may be required for the full effects of the drug to be manifest; likewise, uric acid may return to pretreatment levels slowly, usually after a period of 7 to 10 days following cessation of therapy. This reflects primarily the accumulation and slow clearance of oxipurinol. In some patients, particularly those with severe tophaceous gout and underexcretors, a dramatic fall in urinary uric acid excretion may not occur. It has been postulated that this may be due to the mobilization of urate from the tissue deposits as the serum uric acid level begins to fall.

The combined increase in hypoxanthine and xanthine excreted in the urine usually, but not always, is considerably less than the accompanying decline in urinary uric acid.

It has been shown that reutilization of both hypoxanthine and xanthine for nucleotide and nucleic acid synthesis is markedly enhanced when their oxidations are inhibited by Allopurinol. This reutilization and the normal feedback inhibition which would result from an increase in available purine nucleotides serve to regulate purine biosynthesis and, in essence, the defect of the overproducer of uric acid is thereby compensated.

Innate deficiency of xanthine oxidase, which occurs in congenital xanthinuria as an inborn error of metabolism, has been shown to be compatible with normal health. While urinary levels of oxypurines attained with full doses of Allopurinol may in exceptional cases equal those (250–600 mg per day) which in xanthinuric subjects have caused formation of urinary calculi, they usually fall in the range of 50–200 mg. Xanthine crystalluria has been reported in a few exceptional cases. Two of these had Lesch-Nyhan syndrome, which is characterized by excessive uric acid production combined with a deficiency in the enzyme, hypoxanthine-guanine phosphoribosyltransferase (HG-PRTase). This enzyme is required for the conversion of hypoxanthine and guanine to their respective nucleotides. The third case was a patient with lymphosarcoma, who produced an extremely large amount of uric acid because of rapid cell lysis during chemotherapy.

The serum concentration of oxypurines in patients receiving Allopurinol is usually in the range of 0.3 mg to 0.4 mg percent compared to a normal level of approximately 0.15 mg percent. A maximum of 0.9 mg percent was observed when the serum urate was lowered to less than 2 mg percent by high doses of the drug. In one exceptional case a value of 2.7 mg percent was reached. These are far below the saturation level at which precipitation of xanthine or hypoxanthine would be expected to occur.

The solubilities of uric acid and xanthine in the serum are similar (about 7 mg percent) while hypoxanthine is much more soluble. The finding that the renal clearance of oxypurines is at least 10 times greater than that of uric acid explains the relatively low serum oxypurine concentration at a time when the serum uric acid level has decreased markedly. At serum oxypurine levels of 0.3 mg to 0.9 mg percent, oxypurine: inulin clearance ratios were between 0.7 and 1.9. The glomerular filtration rate and urate clearance in patients receiving Allopurinol do not differ significantly from those obtained prior to therapy. The rapid renal clearance of oxypurines suggests that Allopurinol therapy should be of value in allowing a patient with gout to increase his total purine excretion.

Although the renal clearance of Allopurinol is rapid, that of oxipurinol is slow and parallels that of uric acid but is higher by a factor of about three. The clearance of oxipurinol is increased by uricosuric drugs, and as a consequence, the addition of a uricosuric agent may reduce the degree of inhibition of xanthine oxidase by oxipurinol. However, such combined therapy may be useful in achieving minimum serum uric acid levels provided the total urinary uric acid load does not exceed the competence of the patient's renal function. In some patients, where renal function is severely impaired, normal serum urate levels may not be achievable.

The danger of uric acid calculi is diminished as the uric acid excretion is reduced. The amounts of xanthine and hypoxanthine excreted in the urine generally do not exceed the solubilities of these compounds in the urine, particularly if the urine is slightly alkaline. The amounts of Allopurinol and oxipurinol excreted are likewise within the limits of their respective solubilities.

Allopurinol also inhibits the enzymatic oxidation of mercaptopurine, the sulfur-containing analogue of hypoxanthine, to 6-thiouric acid. This oxidation, which is catalyzed by xanthine oxidase, inactivates mercaptopurine. Hence, the inhibition of such oxidation by allopurinol may result in as much as 75 percent reduction in the therapeutic dose requirement of mercaptopurine when the two compounds are given together.

Indications and Use: This is not an innocuous drug and strict attention should be given to the indications for its use. Pending further investigation, its use in other hyperuricemic states is not indicated at this time.

Allopurinol is intended for:

1. treatment of gout, either primary, or secondary to the hyperuricemia associated with blood dyscrasias and their therapy;
2. treatment of primary or secondary uric acid nephropathy, with or without accompanying symptoms of gout;
3. treatment of patients with recurrent uric acid stone formation;
4. prophylactic treatment to prevent tissue urate deposition, renal calculi, or uric acid nephropathy in patients with leukemias, lymphomas and malignancies who are receiving cancer chemotherapy with its resultant elevating effect on serum uric acid levels.

Allopurinol, by promoting the resolution of tophi and urate crystals in the tissues, has relieved chronic joint pain, increased joint mobility and permitted urate sinuses to heal. The addition of Allopurinol to a uricosuric regimen has reduced the size of tophi which have been refractory to uricosuric agents alone and increased joint mobility.

Allopurinol is particularly effective in preventing the occurrence and recurrence of uric acid stones and gravel. Allopurinol is useful in therapy and prophylaxis of acute urate nephropathy in patients with neoplastic disease who are particularly susceptible to hyperuricemia and uric acid stone formation, especially after radiation therapy or the use of antineoplastic drugs.

Contraindications: Pending further investigation this drug is contraindicated for use in children with the exception of those with hyperuricemia secondary to malignancy. The drug should not be employed in nursing mothers.

Patients who have developed a severe reaction to Allopurinol should not be restarted on the drug.

Warnings: ALLOPURINOL SHOULD BE DISCONTINUED AT THE FIRST APPEARANCE OF SKIN RASH OR ANY SIGN OF ADVERSE REACTION. In some instances a skin rash may be followed by more severe hypersensitivity reactions such as exfoliative, urticarial and purpuric lesions as well as Stevens-Johnson syndrome (erythema multiforme) and very rarely a generalized vasculitis which may lead to irreversible hepatotoxicity and death.

A few cases of reversible clinical hepatotoxicity have been noted in patients taking Allopurinol and in some patients asymptomatic rises in serum alkaline phosphatase or serum transaminase have been observed. Accordingly, periodic liver function tests should be performed during the early stages of therapy, particularly in patients with pre-existing liver disease.

Due to the occasional occurrence of drowsiness, patients should be alerted to the need for due precautions when engaging in activities where alertness is mandatory.

An increase in hepatic iron concentration has been reported in rats given Allopurinol. However, laboratory experiments of several investigators show no effect of Allopurinol on iron metabolism. Nevertheless, iron salts should not be given simultaneously with Allopurinol.

This drug should not be administered to immediate relatives of patients with idiopathic hemochromatosis.

In patients receiving mercaptopurine or azathioprine the concomitant administration of 300–600 mg of allopurinol per day will require a reduction in dose to approximately one-third to one-fourth of the usual dose of mercaptopurine or azathioprine. Subsequent adjustment of doses of mercaptopurine or azathioprine should be made on the basis of therapeutic response and any toxic effects.

USAGE IN PREGNANCY AND WOMEN OF CHILDBEARING AGE: Reproduction studies showed no adverse effect of allopurinol on animal litters.

However, since the effect of xanthine oxidase inhibition on the human fetus is still unknown,

Continued on next page

Boots—Cont.

allopurinol should be used in pregnant women or women of childbearing age only if the potential benefits to the patient are weighed against the possible risk to the fetus.

Precautions: Some investigators have reported an increase in acute attacks of gout during the early stages of allopurinol administration, even when normal or subnormal serum uric acid levels have been attained. Accordingly, maintenance doses of colchicine (0.5 mg twice daily) generally should be given prophylactically when allopurinol is begun. In addition, it is recommended that the patient start with a low dose of Allopurinol (100 mg daily) and increase at weekly intervals by 100 mg until a serum uric acid level of 6 mg per 100 ml or less is attained but without exceeding the maximal recommended dose. The use of therapeutic doses of colchicine or anti-inflammatory agents may be required to suppress attacks in some cases. The attacks usually become shorter and less severe after several months of therapy. A possible explanation for these flare-ups may be the mobilization of urates from tissue deposits followed by recrystallization, due to fluctuation in the serum uric acid level. Even with adequate therapy it may require several months to deplete the uric acid pool sufficiently to achieve control of the acute episodes.

The concomitant administration of a uricosuric agent with Allopurinol may result in a decrease in urinary excretion of oxypurines as compared to their excretion with Allopurinol alone. This may possibly be due to an increased excretion of oxipurinol and a lowering of the degree of inhibition of xanthine oxidase. Such combined therapy is not contraindicated, however, and for many patients, may provide optimum control. A report by Goldfinger, et al on a patient treated with sulfinpyrazone and salicylates in addition to allopurinol showed a marked decrease in the excretion of oxypurines which they suggested was due to interference with their clearance at the renal tubular level. However, subsequent studies have indicated no interference with oxypurine clearance by salicylates. Although clinical evidence to date has not demonstrated renal precipitation of oxypurines in patients either on allopurinol alone or in combination with uricosuric agents, the possibility should be kept in mind.

It has been reported that Allopurinol prolongs the half-life of the anticoagulant, dicumarol. The clinical significance of this has not been established, but this interaction should be kept in mind when Allopurinol is given to patients already on anticoagulant therapy, and the coagulation time should be reassessed.

A fluid intake sufficient to yield a daily urinary output of at least 2 liters and the maintenance of a neutral or, preferably, slightly alkaline urine are desirable to (1) avoid the theoretic possibility of formation of xanthine calculi under the influence of allopurinol therapy and (2) help prevent renal precipitation of urates in patients receiving concomitant uricosuric agents.

A few patients with pre-existing renal disease or poor urate clearance have shown a rise in BUN during Allopurinol administration although a decrease in BUN has also been observed. Although the relationship of these observations to the drug has not been established, patients with impaired renal function require less drug and should be carefully observed during the early stages of Allopurinol administration and the drug withdrawn if increased abnormalities in renal function appear.

In patients with severely impaired renal function, or decreased urate clearance, the half-life of oxipurinol in the plasma is greatly prolonged. Therefore, a dose of 100 mg per day or 300 mg twice a week, or perhaps less, may be sufficient to maintain adequate xanthine oxidase inhibition to reduce serum urate levels. Such patients should be treated with the lowest effective dose, in order to minimize side effects.

Mild reticulocytosis has appeared in some patients, most of whom were receiving other therapeutic agents, so that significance of this observation is not known.

As with all new agents, periodic determination of liver and kidney function and complete blood counts should be performed especially during the first few months of therapy.

Adverse Reactions:

DERMATOLOGIC: Because in some instances skin rash has been followed by severe hypersensitivity reactions, it is recommended that therapy be discontinued at the first sign of rash or other adverse reaction (see WARNINGS).

Skin rash, usually maculopapular, is the adverse reaction most commonly reported.

Exfoliative, urticarial and purpuric lesions, Stevens-Johnson syndrome (erythema multiforme) and toxic epidermal necrolysis have also been reported.

A few cases of alopecia with and without accompanying dermatitis have been reported.

In some patients with a rash, restarting allopurinol therapy at lower doses has been accomplished without untoward incident.

GASTROINTESTINAL: Nausea, vomiting, diarrhea, and intermittent abdominal pain have been reported.

VASCULAR: There have been rare instances of a generalized hypersensitivity vasculitis or necrotizing angiitis which have led to irreversible hepatotoxicity and death.

HEMATOPOIETIC: Agranulocytosis, anemia, aplastic anemia, bone marrow depression, leukopenia, pancytopenia and thrombocytopenia have been reported in patients, most of whom received concomitant drugs with potential for causing these reactions. Allopurinol has been neither implicated nor excluded as a cause of these reactions.

NEUROLOGIC: There have been a few reports of peripheral neuritis occurring while patients were taking allopurinol. Drowsiness has also been reported in a few patients.

OPHTHALMIC: There have been a few reports of cataracts found in patients receiving Allopurinol. It is not known if the cataracts predated the Allopurinol therapy. "Toxic" cataracts were reported in one patient who also received an anti-inflammatory agent; again, the time of onset is unknown. In a group of patients followed by Gutman and Yu for up to five years on allopurinol therapy, no evidence of ophthalmologic effect attributable to Allopurinol was reported.

DRUG IDIOSYNCRASY: Symptoms suggestive of drug idiosyncrasy have been reported in a few patients. This was characterized by fever, chills, leukopenia or leukocytosis, eosinophilia, arthralgias, skin rash, pruritus, nausea, and vomiting.

Overdosage: Massive overdosing, or acute poisoning, by allopurinol has not been reported.

Dosage and Administration: The dosage of Allopurinol to accomplish full control of gout and to lower serum uric acid to normal or near-normal levels varies with the severity of the disease. The average is 200 to 300 mg per day for patients with mild gout and 400 to 600 mg per day for those with moderately severe tophaceous gout. The appropriate dosage may be administered in divided doses or as a single equivalent dose with the 300 mg tablet. Dosage requirements in excess of 300 mg should be supplemented in divided doses. It should also be noted that Allopurinol is generally better tolerated if taken following meals. Similar considerations govern the regulation of dosage for maintenance purposes in secondary hyperuricemia. For the prevention of uric acid nephropathy during the vigorous therapy of neoplastic disease, treatment with 600 to 800 mg daily for two to three days is advisable together with a high fluid intake. The minimal effective dosage is 100 to 200 mg daily and the maximal recommended dosage is 800 mg daily. To reduce the possibility of flare-up of acute gouty attacks, it is recommended that the patient start with a low dose of Allopurinol (100 mg daily) and increase at weekly intervals by 100 mg until a serum uric acid level of 6 mg per 100 ml or less is attained but without exceeding the maximal recommended dosage.

Normal serum urate levels are achieved in one to three weeks. The upper limit of normal is about 7 mg percent for men and postmenopausal women and 6 mg percent for premenopausal women. Too much reliance should not be placed on a single reading since, for technical reasons, estimation of uric acid may be difficult. By the selection of the appropriate dose, together with the use of uricosuric agents in certain patients, it is possible to reduce the serum uric acid level to normal and, if desired, to hold it as low as 2 to 3 mg percent indefinitely.

A fluid intake sufficient to yield a daily urinary output of at least 2 liters and the maintenance of a neutral or, preferably, slightly alkaline urine are desirable.

Since Allopurinol and its metabolites are excreted only by the kidney, accumulation of the drug can occur in renal failure, and the dose of Allopurinol should consequently be reduced. With a creatinine clearance of 20 to 10 ml/min, a daily dosage of 200 mg of allopurinol is suitable. When the creatinine clearance is less than 10 ml/min the daily dosage should not exceed 100 mg. With extreme renal impairment (creatinine clearance less than 3 ml/min) the interval between doses may also need to be lengthened.

The correct size and frequency of dosage for maintaining the serum uric acid just within the normal range is best determined by using the serum uric acid level as an index.

Children, 6 to 10 years of age, with secondary hyperuricemia associated with malignancies may be given 300 mg allopurinol daily while those under 6 years are generally given 150 mg daily. The response is evaluated after approximately 48 hours of therapy and a dosage adjustment is made if necessary.

In patients who are being treated with colchicine and/or anti-inflammatory agents, it is wise to continue this therapy while adjusting the dosage of Allopurinol, until a normal serum uric acid and freedom from acute attacks have been maintained for several months.

In transferring a patient from a uricosuric agent to Allopurinol, the dose of the uricosuric agent should be gradually reduced over a period of several weeks and the dose of allopurinol gradually increased to the required dose needed to maintain a normal serum uric acid level.

How Supplied: LOPURIN®: 100 mg (white) scored tablets, bottles of 100 and 1000; 300 mg (peach) scored tablets, bottles of 30, 100, and 500.

Animal Toxicology: In mice the LD_{50} is 160 mg/kg ip (with deaths delayed up to five days) and 700 mg/kg po (with deaths delayed up to three days). In rats the acute LD_{50} is 750 mg/kg ip >6000 mg/kg po.

In a 13 week feeding experiment in rats at a drug level of 72 mg/kg per day 2 of 10 rats died and at 225 mg/kg per day 4 of 10 died before the completion of the experiment. Both groups exhibited renal tubular damage due to the deposition of xanthine that was more extensive at the higher dose.

In chronic feeding experiments, rats showed no toxic effects at a level of 14 mg/kg per day after one year. At a level of 24 mg/kg per day for one year the rats showed very slight depression of weight gain and food intake, and 5 out of 10 of

the animals showed minor changes in the kidney tubules of the type exhibited by the rats on the higher doses described above.
Dogs survived oral doses of 30 mg/kg per day for one year with nil to minor changes in the kidney and no other significant abnormalities. At 90 mg/kg per day for one year there was some accumulation of xanthine in the kidneys with resultant chronic irritation and slight tubular changes. Occasional hemosiderin-like deposits were seen in the reticuloendothelial system. A higher dose (270 mg/kg per day) resulted in large concretions in the renal pelves, with severe destructive changes in the kidney secondary to xanthine accumulation. The deposition of xanthine appears to be a function both of the metabolic turnover of purines (which is proportionately larger in the smaller animals) and the degree of inhibition of xanthine oxidase.
Reproductive studies in rats and rabbits indicated that Allopurinol did not affect litter size, the mean weight of the progeny at birth or at three weeks postpartum, nor did it cause an increase in the number of animals born dead or with malformations.

Distributed by
Boots Pharmaceuticals, Inc.
Shreveport, Louisiana 71106
Manufactured by
Generic Pharmaceutical Corporation
Palisades Park, N.J. 07650

Licensed for Use under U.S. Patent No. 3,624,205
Rev. November 1981
[*Shown in Product Identification Section*]

RUFEN® ℞
(ibuprofen)

Description: Rufen (ibuprofen) is (±)-2-(*p*-isobutylphenyl) propionic acid. It is a white powder with a melting point of 74–77°C and is very slightly soluble in water (<1 mg/ml) and readily soluble in organic solvents such as ethanol and acetone.
Rufen is a nonsteroidal anti-inflammatory agent. It is available in 400 mg tablets for oral administration.

Clinical Pharmacology: Rufen (ibuprofen) is a nonsteroidal anti-inflammatory agent that possesses analgesic and antipyretic activities. Its mode of action, like that of other nonsteroidal anti-inflammatory agents, is not known; however, its therapeutic action is not due to pituitary-adrenal stimulation. Rufen does not alter the course of the underlying disease.
In patients treated with Rufen for rheumatoid arthritis and osteoarthritis, the anti-inflammatory action of Rufen has been shown by reduction in joint swelling, reduction in pain, reduction in duration of morning stiffness, reduction in disease activity as assessed by both the investigator and patient; and by improved functional capacity as demonstrated by an increase in grip strength, a delay in the time to onset of fatigue, and a decrease in time to walk 50 feet.
In clinical studies in patients with rheumatoid arthritis and osteoarthritis, Rufen has been shown to be comparable to aspirin in controlling the aforementioned signs and symptoms of disease activity and to be associated with a statistically significant reduction in the milder gastrointestinal side effects (see ADVERSE REACTIONS). Rufen may be well tolerated in some patients who have had gastrointestinal side effects with aspirin, but these patients when treated with Rufen should be carefully followed for signs and symptoms of gastrointestinal ulceration and bleeding.
Although it is not definitely known whether ibuprofen causes less peptic ulceration than aspirin, in one study involving 885 patients with rheumatoid arthritis treated for up to one year, there were no reports of gastric ulceration with ibuprofen whereas frank ulceration was reported in 13 patients in the aspirin group (statistically significant $p<.001$).
In clinical studies in patients with rheumatoid arthritis, Rufen has been shown to be comparable to indomethacin in controlling the aforementioned signs and symptoms of disease activity and to be associated with a statistically significant reduction of the milder gastrointestinal (see ADVERSE REACTIONS) and CNS side effects.
Rufen may be used in combination with gold salts and/or corticosteroids. When Rufen and placebo were compared in gold-treated rheumatoid arthritis patients, Rufen was consistently more effective in relieving symptoms than was placebo. However, it cannot be inferred that Rufen potentiates the effect of gold on the underlying disease. Whether or not Rufen can be used in conjunction with partially effective doses of corticosteroid for a "steroid-sparing" effect, and result in greater improvement, has not been adequately studied.
Controlled studies have demonstrated that Rufen is a more effective analgesic than propoxyphene for the relief of episiotomy pain, pain following dental extraction procedures, and for the relief of the symptoms of primary dysmenorrhea.
In patients with primary dysmenorrhea Rufen has been shown to reduce elevated levels of prostaglandin activity in the menstrual fluid and to reduce resting and active intra-uterine pressure, as well as the frequency of uterine contractions. The probable mechanism of action is to inhibit prostaglandin synthesis rather than simply to provide analgesia.
Rufen is rapidly absorbed when administered orally. Peak serum ibuprofen levels are generally attained one to two hours after administration. With single doses ranging from 200 mg to 800 mg, a dose-response relationship exists between amount of drug administered and the integrated area under the serum drug concentration vs time curve. Above 800 mg, however, the area under the curve increases less than proportional to increases in dose. There is no evidence of drug accumulation or enzyme induction.
The administration of Rufen tablets either under fasting conditions or immediately before meals and yields quite similar serum ibuprofen concentration-time profiles. When Rufen is administered immediately after a meal, there is a reduction in the rate of absorption but no appreciable decrease in the extent of absorption. The bioavailability of Rufen is minimally altered by the presence of food.
Rufen is rapidly metabolized and eliminated in the urine. The excretion of Rufen is virtually complete 24 hours after the last dose. The serum half-life of Rufen is 1.8 to 2.0 hours.
Studies have shown that following ingestion of the drug 45% to 79% of the dose was recovered in the urine within 24 hours as metabolite A (25%), (+)-2-[*p*-(2 hydroxymethylproply)phenyl] propionic acid and metabolite B(37%), (+)-2[*p*-(2 carboxy-propyl)-phenyl] propionic acid, the percentages of free and conjugated ibuprofen were approximately 1% and 14%, respectively.

Indications and Usage: Rufen (ibuprofen) is indicated for relief of the signs and symptoms of rheumatoid arthritis and osteoarthritis. It is indicated in the treatment of acute flares and in the long-term management of these diseases.
Rufen is indicated for the relief of mild to moderate pain.
Rufen is also indicated for the treatment of primary dysmenorrhea.
Since there have been no controlled trials to demonstrate whether or not there is any beneficial effect or harmful interaction with the use of Rufen in conjunction with aspirin, the combination cannot be recommended (see **Drug Interactions**).
Controlled clinical trials to establish the safety and effectiveness of Rufen in children have not been conducted.

Contraindications: Rufen (ibuprofen) should not be used in patients who have previously exhibited hypersensitivity to it, or in individuals with the syndrome of nasal polyps, angioedema and bronchospastic reactivity to aspirin or other nonsteroidal anti-inflammatory agents (see WARNINGS).

Warnings: Anaphylactoid reactions have occurred in patients with known aspirin hypersensitivity (see CONTRAINDICATIONS).
Peptic ulceration and gastrointestinal bleeding, sometimes severe, have been reported in patients receiving Rufen (ibuprofen). Peptic ulceration, perforation, or severe gastrointestinal bleeding can have a fatal outcome, and although a few such reports have been received with ibuprofen, a cause and effect relationship has not been established. Rufen should be given under close supervision to patients with a history of upper gastrointestinal tract disease, and only after consulting the ADVERSE REACTIONS section.
In patients with active peptic ulcer and active rheumatoid arthritis, attempts should be made to treat the arthritis with nonulcerogenic drugs, such as gold. If Rufen must be given, the patient should be under close supervision for signs of ulcer perforation or gastrointestinal bleeding.
As with other nonsteroidal anti-inflammatory agents, chronic studies in rats and monkeys have shown histologic evidence of mild renal toxicity as demonstrated by papillary edema and papillary necrosis, in some animals. Renal papillary necrosis has been rarely reported in humans in association with Rufen treatment.

Precautions: Blurred and/or diminished vision, scotomata, and/or changes in color vision have been reported. If a patient develops such complaints while receiving Rufen (ibuprofen), the drug should be discontinued and the patient should have an ophthalmologic examination which includes central visual fields and color vision testing.
Fluid retention and edema have been reported in association with Rufen; therefore, the drug should be used with caution in patients with a history of cardiac decompensation or hypertension.
As with other nonsteroidal anti-inflammatory drugs, borderline elevations of one or more liver tests may occur in up to 15% of patients. These abnormalities may progress, may remain essentially unchanged, or may be transient with continued therapy. The SGPT (ALT) test is probably the most sensitive indicator of liver dysfunction. Meaningful (3 times the upper limit of normal) elevations of SGPT or SGOT (AST) occurred in controlled clinical trials in less than 1% of patients. A patient with symptoms and/or signs suggesting liver dysfunction, or in whom an abnormal liver test has occurred, should be evaluated for evidence of the development of more severe hepatic reaction while on therapy with Rufen. Severe hepatic reactions, including jaundice and cases of fatal hepatitis, have been reported with ibuprofen as with other nonsteroidal anti-inflammatory drugs. Although such reactions are rare, if abnormal liver tests persist or worsen, if clinical signs and symptoms consistent with liver disease develop, or if systemic manifestations occur (e.g. eosinophilia, rash, etc.), Rufen should be discontinued.
Since Rufen is eliminated primarily by the kidneys, patients with significantly impaired renal function should be closely monitored and a reduction in dosage should be anticipated to avoid drug accumulation. Prospective studies on the safety of Rufen in patients with chronic renal failure have not been conducted.

Continued on next page

Boots—Cont.

Rufen, like other nonsteroidal anti-inflammatory agents, can inhibit platelet aggregation but the effect is quantitatively less and of shorter duration than that seen with aspirin. Ibuprofen has been shown to prolong bleeding time (but within the normal range) in normal subjects. Because this prolonged bleeding effect may be exaggerated in patients with underlying hemostatic defects, Rufen should be used with caution in persons with intrinsic coagulation defects and those on anticoagulant therapy.

Patients on Rufen should report to their physicians signs or symptoms of gastrointestinal ulceration or bleeding, blurred vision or other eye symptoms, skin rash, weight gain, or edema.

In order to avoid exacerbation of disease or adrenal insufficiency, patients who have been on prolonged corticosteroid therapy should have their therapy tapered slowly rather than discontinued abruptly when Rufen is added to the treatment program.

The antipyretic and anti-inflammatory activity of ibuprofen may reduce fever and inflammation, thus diminishing their utility as diagnostic signs in detecting complications of presumed noninfectious, noninflammatory painful conditions.

Drug-Interactions: *Coumarin-type anticoagulants.* Several short-term controlled studies failed to show that Rufen significantly affected prothrombin times or a variety of other clotting factors when administered to individuals on coumarin-type anticoagulants. However, because bleeding has been reported when Rufen and other nonsteroidal anti-inflammatory agents have been administered to patients on coumarin-type anticoagulants the physician should be cautious when administering Rufen to patients on anticoagulants.

Aspirin. Animal studies show that aspirin given with nonsteroidal anti-inflammatory agents, including Rufen, yields a net decrease in anti-inflammatory activity with lowered blood levels of the non-aspirin drug. Single dose bioavailability studies in normal volunteers have failed to show an effect of aspirin on ibuprofen blood levels. Correlative clinical studies have not been done.

Pregnancy: Reproductive studies conducted in rats and rabbits at doses somewhat less than the maximal clinical dose did not demonstrate evidence of developmental abnormalities. These data are inadequate to provide reasonable assurance that the drug will not have an adverse effect on the fetus. Rufen (ibuprofen) has been shown to inhibit prostaglandin synthesis and release. The same effect has been demonstrated by other nonsteroidal and anti-inflammatory drugs and has been associated with an increased incidence of dystocia and delayed parturition in pregnant animals when such drugs were administered late in pregnancy. Administration of Rufen is not recommended during pregnancy.

Nursing Mothers: In limited studies, an assay capable of detecting 1 mcg/ml did not demonstrate ibuprofen in the milk of lactating mothers. However, because of the limited nature of the studies and the possible adverse effects of prostaglandin inhibiting drugs on neonates. Rufen is not recommended for use in nursing mothers.

Adverse Reactions:

The most frequent type of adverse reaction occurring with Rufen (ibuprofen) is gastrointestinal. In controlled clinical trials the percentage of patients reporting one or more gastrointestinal complaints ranged from 4% to 16%.

In controlled studies when ibuprofen was compared to aspirin and indomethacin in equally effective doses, the overall incidence of gastrointestinal complaints was about half that seen in either the aspirin-, or indomethacin-treated patients.

Reactions observed during controlled clinical trials which occurred in more than 1 in 100 patients were:

Incidence greater than 1%

Gastrointestinal: nausea*, epigastric pain*, heartburn*, diarrhea, abdominal distress, nausea and vomiting, indigestion, constipation, abdominal cramps or pain, fullness of the GI tract (bloating and flatulence).

Central Nervous System: dizziness*, headache, nervousness.

Dermatologic: rash* (including maculopapular type), pruritus.

Special Senses: tinnitus.

Metabolic: decreased appetite, edema, fluid retention. Fluid retention generally responds promptly to drug discontinuation (see PRECAUTIONS).

*Reactions occurring in 3% to 9% of patients treated with Rufen. (Those reactions occurring in less than 3% of the patients are unmarked.)

Incidence less than 1%

The following adverse reactions, occurring less frequently than 1 in 100, have been reported in controlled clinical trials and from marketing experience. The probability of a causal relationship exists between Rufen and these adverse reactions:

Gastrointestinal: gastric or duodenal ulcer with bleeding and/or perforation, gastrointestinal hemorrhage, melena, gastritis, hepatitis, jaundice, abnormal liver function tests.

Dermatologic: vesiculobullous eruptions, urticaria, erythema multiforme, Stevens-Johnson syndrome and alopecia.

Central Nervous System: depression, insomnia, confusion, emotional lability, somnolence, aseptic meningitis with fever and coma.

Special Senses: hearing loss, amblyopia (blurred and/or diminished vision, scotomata and/or changes in color vision). [see PRECAUTIONS].

Hematologic: neutropenia, agranulocytosis, aplastic anemia, hemolytic anemia (sometimes Coombs' positive), thrombocytopenia with or without purpura eosinophilia, decreases in hemoglobin and hematocrit.

Cardiovascular: congestive heart failure in patients with marginal cardiac function, elevated blood pressure and palpitations.

Allergic: syndrome of abdominal pain, fever, chills, nausea and vomiting, anaphylaxis, bronchospasms (see CONTRAINDICATIONS).

Renal: acute renal failure in patients with preexisting significantly impaired renal function, decreased creatinine clearance, polyuria, azotemia, cystitis, hematuria.

Miscellaneous: dry eyes and mouth, gingival ulcers, rhinitis.

Causal relationship unknown

Other reactions have been reported but occurred under circumstances where a causal relationship could not be established. However, in these rarely reported events, the possibility cannot be excluded. Therefore these observations are being listed to serve as alerting information to the physician.

Gastrointestinal: pancreatitis

Central Nervous System: paresthesias, hallucinations, dream abnormalities, pseudotumor cerebri.

Dermatologic: toxic epidermal necrolysis, photo-allergic skin reactions.

Special Senses: conjunctivitis diplopia, optic neuritis.

Hematologic: bleeding episodes (eg., epistaxis, menorrhagia).

Allergic: serum sickness lupus erythematosus syndrome, Henoch-Schonlein vasculitis.

Endocrine: gynecomastia, hypoglycemic reaction.

Cardiovascular: arrhythmias (sinus tachycardia, sinus bradycardia).

Renal: renal papillary necrosis.

Overdosage: Approximately $1\frac{1}{2}$ hours after the reported ingestion of from 7 to 10 ibuprofen tablets (400 mg), a 19-month old child weighing 12 kg was seen in the hospital emergency room, apneic and cyanotic, responding only to painful stimuli. This type of stimulus, however, was sufficient to induce respiration. Oxygen and parenteral fluids were given, a greenish-yellow fluid was aspirated from the stomach with no evidence to indicate the presense of ibuprofen. Two hours after ingestion the child's condition seemed stable, she still responded only to painful stimuli and continued to have periods of apnea lasting from 5 to 10 seconds. She was admitted to intensive care and sodium bicarbonate was administered as well as infusions of dextrose and normal saline. By four hours postingestion she could be aroused easily, sit by herself and respond to spoken commands. Blood level of ibuprofen was 102.9 mcg/ml approximately $8\frac{1}{2}$ hours after accidental ingestion. At 12 hours she appeared to be completely recovered.

In two other reported cases where children (each weighing approximately 10 kg) had taken six tablets for an estimated acute intake of approximately 120 mg/kg, there were no signs of acute intoxication or late sequelae. Blood level in one child 90 minutes after ingestion was 700 mcg/ml about 10 times the peak levels seen in absorption-excretion studies.

A 19-year old male who had taken 8,000 mg of ibuprofen over a period of a few hours complained of dizziness, and nystagmus was noted. After hospitalization, parenteral hydration and three days bed rest, he recovered with no reported sequelae.

In cases of acute overdosage, the stomach should be emptied by vomiting or lavage, though little drug will likely be recovered if more than an hour has elapsed since ingestion. Because the drug is acidic and is excreted in the urine, it is theoretically beneficial to administer alkali and induce diuresis.

Dosage and Administration: Rheumatoid arthritis and osteoarthritis, including flareups of chronic disease.

Suggested Dosage: 400 mg t.i.d. or q.i.d. The dose of Rufen (ibuprofen) should be tailored to each patient, and may be lowered or raised from the suggested doses depending on the severity of symptoms either at time of initiating drug therapy or as the patient responds or fails to respond.

In general, patients with rheumatoid arthritis seem to require higher doses of Rufen than do patients with osteoarthritis.

The smallest dose of Rufen that yields acceptable control should be employed.

A therapeutic response to Rufen therapy is sometimes seen in a few days to a week but most often is observed by two weeks. After a satisfactory response has been achieved, the patient's dose should be reviewed and adjusted as required.

Dysmenorrhea: For the treatment of dysmenorrhea, beginning with the earliest onset of such pain, Rufen should be given in a dose of 400 mg every 4 hours as necessary.

Mild to moderate pain: 400 mg every 4 to 6 hours as necessary for the relief of pain.

In controlled analgesic clinical trials, doses of Rufen greater than 400 mg were no more effective than the 400 mg dose.

Do not exceed 2,400 mg total daily dose. If gastrointestinal complaints occur, administer Rufen with meals or milk.

How Supplied: Rufen Tablets 400 mg; round magenta sugar-coated tablets printed RUFEN 400.

Bottles of 100	NDC 0524-0039-01
Bottles of 500	NDC 0524-0039-05

Caution: Federal law prohibits dispensing without prescription.

U.S. Patent No. 3,385,886.

Manufactured for
Boots Pharmaceuticals, Inc.
Shreveport, Louisiana
By
The Boots Company PLC
Nottingham, England
Boots Pharmaceuticals, Inc.
Shreveport, Louisiana 71106

Rev. 12/81

[Shown in Product Identification Section]

RU–TUSS® EXPECTORANT ©

Description: Each fluid ounce of Ru-Tuss Expectorant contains:

Codeine Phosphate ....65.8 mg
(Warning: May Be Habit Forming)
Phenylephrine Hydrochloride ....30 mg
Pyrilamine Maleate ....20 mg
Phenylpropanolamine Hydrochloride ...20 mg
Pheniramine Maleate ....20 mg
Ammonium Chloride ....200 mg
Alcohol 5%

Ru-Tuss Expectorant is an oral antitussive, antihistaminic, nasal decongestant and expectorant preparation.

Indications and Usage: Ru-Tuss Expectorant is indicated for symptomatic relief of upper respiratory congestion associated with pharyngitis, tracheitis, bronchitis, and allergic rhinitis. Also, for the temporary relief of symptoms associated with hay fever, allergies, nasal congestion and cough due to the common cold.

Contraindications: Hypersensitivity to antihistamines. Concomitant use of an antihypertensive or antidepressant drug containing a monoamine oxidase inhibitor is contraindicated.

Ru-Tuss Expectorant is contraindicated in patients with glaucoma, bronchial asthma and in women who are pregnant.

Warnings: Ru-Tuss Expectorant contains codeine phosphate, therefore, the patient should be warned of the potential that this drug may be habit forming.

Ru-Tuss Expectorant may cause drowsiness. Patients should be warned of the possible additive effect caused by taking antihistamines with alcohol, hypnotics, sedatives and tranquilizers.

Precautions: Patients taking Ru-Tuss Expectorant should avoid driving a motor vehicle or operating dangerous machinery (See Warnings).

Caution should be taken with patients having hypertension, diabetes, hyperthyroidism and cardiovascular disease.

Caution should also be used in patients with pulmonary, hepatic or renal insufficiency.

Adverse Reactions: Ru-Tuss Expectorant may cause drowsiness, lassitude, giddiness, dryness of mucous membranes, tightness of the chest, thickening of bronchial secretions, urinary frequency and dysuria, palpitation, tachycardia, hypotension/hypertension, faintness, dizziness, tinnitus, headache, incoordination, visual disturbances, mydriasis, xerostomia, blurred vision, anorexia, nausea, vomiting, diarrhea, constipation, epigastric distress, hyperirritability, nervousness and insomnia. Overdoses may cause restlessness, excitation, delirium, tremors, euphoria, metabolic acidosis, stupor, tachycardia and even convulsions.

Dosage and Administration:

Adults: 1 or 2 teaspoonfuls, orally, every 4 hours, not to exceed 10 teaspoonfuls in any 24-hour period.

Children 6 to 12 years of age: ½ the adult dose, not to exceed 6 teaspoonfuls in any 24-hour period.

Children 2 to 6 years of age: ½ teaspoonful every 4 hours, not to exceed 3 teaspoonfuls in any 24-hour period.

Children under 2 years of age: Use as directed by a physician.

How Supplied:

Pint bottles (16 fl. oz.) NDC 0524-1010-16

Federal law prohibits dispensing without prescription.

Manufactured and Distributed by
Boots Pharmaceuticals, Inc.
Shreveport, Louisiana 71106

July 1980

RU–TUSS® WITH HYDROCODONE ©

Description: Each fluid ounce of Ru-Tuss with Hydrocodone contains:

Hydrocodone Bitartrate ....10 mg
(Warning: May Be Habit Forming)
Phenylephrine Hydrochloride ....30 mg
Phenylpropanolamine Hydrochloride ...20 mg
Pheniramine Maleate ....20 mg
Pyrilamine Maleate ....20 mg
Alcohol 5%

Ru-Tuss with Hydrocodone is an oral antitussive, antihistaminic and nasal decongestant preparation.

Indications and Usage: Ru-Tuss with Hydrocodone is indicated for the temporary relief of symptoms associated with hay fever, allergies, nasal congestion and cough due to the common cold.

Contraindications: Hypersensitivity to antihistamines. Concomitant use of an antihypertensive or antidepressant drugs containing a monoamine oxidase inhibitor is contraindicated.

Ru-Tuss with Hydrocodone is contraindicated in patients with glaucoma, bronchial asthma and in women who are pregnant.

Warnings: Patients should be warned of the potential that Ru-Tuss with Hydrocodone may be habit forming.

Ru-Tuss with Hydrocodone may cause drowsiness.

Patients should be warned of the possible additive effect caused by taking antihistamines with alcohol, hypnotics, sedatives and tranquilizers.

Precautions: Patients taking Ru-Tuss with Hydrocodone should avoid driving a motor vehicle or operating dangerous machinery (See Warnings).

Caution should be taken with patients having hypertension and cardiovascular disease.

Adverse Reactions: Ru-Tuss with Hydrocodone may cause drowsiness, lassitude, giddiness, dryness of mucous membranes, tightness of the chest, thickening of bronchial secretions, urinary frequency and dysuria, palpitation, tachycardia, hypotension/hypertension, faintness, dizziness, tinnitus, headache, incoordination, visual disturbances, mydriasis, xerostomia, blurred vision, anorexia, nausea, vomiting, diarrhea, constipation, epigastric distress, hyperirritability, nervousness and insomnia. Overdoses may cause restlessness, excitation, delirium, tremors, euphoria, stupor, tachycardia and even convulsions.

Dosage and Administration:

Adults: 2 teaspoonfuls, orally, every 4 to 6 hours.

Children 6 to 12 years of age: 1 teaspoonful every 4 to 6 hours.

Children 2 to 6 years of age: 1/2 to 1 teaspoonful ever 4 to 6 hours, according to age. Doses for children should not be repeated more than 4 times in any 24-hour period.

How Supplied:

Pint bottles (16 fl. oz) NDC 0524-1007-16

Federal law prohibits dispensing without prescription.

Manufactured and Distributed by
Boots Pharmaceuticals, Inc.
Shreveport, Louisiana 71106

Rev. 10/80

RU–TUSS® PLAIN

Description: Each fluid ounce of Ru-Tuss Plain contains:

Phenylephrine Hydrochloride ....30 mg
Phenylpropanolamine Hydrochloride ...20 mg
Pheniramine Maleate ....20 mg
Pyrilamine Maleate ....20 mg
Alcohol 5%

Ru-Tuss Plain is an oral antihistaminic and nasal decongestant preparation.

Indications and Usage: Ru-Tuss Plain is indicated for the temporary relief of symptoms associated with hay fever, allergies, and nasal congestion due to the common cold.

Contraindications: Hypersensitivity to antihistamines, concomitant use of antihypertensive or antidepressant drugs containing a monoamine oxidase (MAO) inhibitor is contraindicated. Ru-Tuss Plain is contraindicated in patients with glaucoma, bronchial asthma, and in women who are pregnant.

Warnings: Ru-Tuss Plain may cause drowsiness. Patients should be warned of the possible additive effects caused by taking antihistamines with alcohol, hypnotics, sedatives or tranquilizers.

Precautions: Patients taking Ru-Tuss Plain should avoid driving a motor vehicle or operating dangerous machinery (See Warnings). Caution should be taken with patients having hypertension and cardiovascular disease.

Adverse Reactions: Ru-Tuss Plain may cause drowsiness, lassitude, giddiness, dryness of the mucous membranes, tightness of the chest, thickening of bronchial secretions, urinary frequency and dysuria, palpitation, tachycardia, hypotension/hypertension, faintness, dizziness, tinnitus, headache, incoordination, visual disturbances, mydriasis, xerostomia, blurred vision, anorexia, nausea, vomiting, diarrhea, constipation, epigastric distress, hyperirritability, nervousness, and insomnia. Overdoses may cause restlessness, excitation, delirium, tremors and even convulsions.

Dosage and Administration:

Adults: 2 teaspoonfuls, orally, every 4 to 6 hours.

Children 6 to 12 years of age: 1 teaspoonful every 4 to 6 hours.

Children 2 to 6 years of age: ½ to 1 teaspoonful every 4 to 6 hours, according to age.

How Supplied:

Pint bottles (16 fl. oz.). NDC 0524-0009-16

Manufactured and Distributed by
Boots Pharmaceuticals, Inc.
Shreveport, Louisiana 71106

July 1980

RU–TUSS® TABLETS ℞

Description: Each prolonged action tablet contains:

Phenylephrine Hydrochloride ....25 mg
Phenylpropanolamine Hydrochloride ...50 mg
Chlorpheniramine Maleate ....8 mg
Hyoscyamine Sulfate ....0.19 mg
Atropine Sulfate ....0.04 mg
Scopolamine Hydrobromide ....0.01 mg

Ru-Tuss Tablets act continuously for 10 to 12 hours.

Ru-Tuss Tablets are an oral antihistaminic, nasal decongestant and anti-secretory preparation.

Indications and Usage: Ru-Tuss Tablets provide relief of the symptoms resulting from irritation of sinus, nasal and upper respiratory tract tissues. Phenylephrine and phenylpropanolamine combine to exert a vasoconstrictive and decongestive action while chlorpheniramine maleate decreases the symptoms of watering eyes, post nasal drip and sneezing which may be associated with an allergic-like response. The belladonna alkaloids, hyoscyamine, atropine and scopolamine further augment the anti-secretory activity of Ru-Tuss Tablets.

Contraindications: Hypersensitivity to antihistamines or sympathomimetics. Ru-Tuss Tablets are contraindicated in children under

Continued on next page

Boots—Cont.

12 years of age and in patients with glaucoma, bronchial asthma and women who are pregnant. Concomitant use of MAO inhibitors is contraindicated.
Warnings: Ru-Tuss Tablets may cause drowsiness. Patients should be warned of the possible additive effects caused by taking antihistamines with alcohol, hypnotics, sedatives or tranquilizers.
Precautions: Ru-Tuss Tablets contain belladonna alkaloids, and must be administered with care to those patients with urinary bladder neck obstruction. Caution should be exercised when Ru-Tuss Tablets are given to patients with hypertension, cardiac or peripheral vascular disease or hyperthyroidism. Patients should avoid driving a motor vehicle or operating dangerous machinery (See **Warnings:**).
Overdosage: Since the action of sustained release products may continue for as long as 12 hours, treatment of overdoses directed at reversing the effects of the drug and supporting the patient should be maintained for at least that length of time. Saline cathartics are useful for hastening evacuation of unreleased medication. In children and infants, antihistamine overdosage may produce convulsions and death.
Adverse Reactions: Hypersensitivity reactions such as rash, urticaria, leukopenia, agranulocytosis, and thrombocytopenia may occur. Other adverse reactions to Ru-Tuss Tablets may be drowsiness, lassitude, giddiness, dryness of the mucous membranes, tightness of the chest, thickening of bronchial secretions, urinary frequency and dysuria, palpitation, tachycardia, hypotension/hypertension, faintness, dizziness, tinnitus, headache, incoordination, visual disturbances, mydriasis, xerostomia, blurred vision, anorexia, nausea, vomiting, diarrhea, constipation, epigastric distress, hyperirritability, nervousness, dizziness and insomnia. Large overdoses may cause tachypnea, delirium, fever, stupor, coma and respiratory failure.
Dosage and Administration: Adults and children over 12 years of age, one tablet morning and evening. Not recommended for children under 12 years of age. Tablets are to be swallowed whole.
How Supplied:
Bottles of 100 Tablets NDC 0524-0058-01
Bottles of 500 Tablets NDC 0524-0058-05
Federal law prohibits dispensing without prescription.

Distributed by
Boots Pharmaceuticals, Inc.
Shreveport, Louisiana 71106
Manufactured by
Vitarine Company, Inc.
Springfield Gardens, New York, 11413
September 1981
[*Shown in Product Identification Section*]

TWIN-K® ℞

Description: Each 15 ml (one tablespoonful) supplies 20 mEq of potassium ions as a combination of potassium gluconate and potassium citrate in a sorbitol and saccharin solution.
Indications and Usage: For use as oral potassium therapy in the prevention or treatment of hypokalemia which may occur secondary to diuretic or corticosteroid administration. It may be used in the treatment of cardiac arrhythmias due to digitalis intoxication.
Contraindications: Severe renal impairment with oliguria or azotemia, untreated Addison's disease, adynamia episodica hereditaria, acute dehydration, heat cramps and hyperkalemia from any cause. This product should not be used in patients receiving aldosterone antagonists or triamterene.
Warnings: TWIN-K (potassium gluconate and potassium citrate) is a palatable form of oral potassium replacement. It appears that little if any potassium gluconate-citrate penetrates as far as the jejunum or ileum where enteric coated potassium chloride lesions have been noted. Excessive, undiluted doses of TWIN-K may cause a saline laxative effect.
To minimize gastrointestinal irritation, it is recommended that TWIN-K be taken with meals or diluted with water or fruit juice. A tablespoonful (15 ml) in 8 ounces of water is approximately isotonic. More than a single tablespoonful should not be taken without prior dilution.
Precautions: Potassium is a major intracellular cation which plays a significant role in body physiology. The serum level of potassium is normally 3.8–5.0 mEq/liter. While the serum or plasma level is a poor indicator of total body stores, a plasma or serum level below 3.5 mEq/liter is considered to be indicative of hypokalemia.
The most common cause of hypokalemia is excessive loss of potassium in the urine. However, hypokalemia can also occur with vomiting, gastric drainage and diarrhea.
Usually a potassium deficiency can be corrected by oral administration of potassium supplements. With normal kidney function, it is difficult to produce potassium intoxication by oral administration. However, potassium supplements must be administered with caution since, usually, the exact amount of the deficiency is not accurately known. Checks on the patient's clinical status and periodic E.K.G. and/or serum potassium levels should be made. High serum potassium levels may cause death by cardiac depression, arrhythmias or arrest.
In patients with hypokalemia who also have alkalosis and a chloride deficiency (hypokalemic hypochloremic alkalosis), there will be a requirement for chloride ions. TWIN-K is not recommended for use in these patients.
Adverse Reactions: Symptoms of potassium intoxication include paresthesias of the extremities, flaccid paralysis, listlessness, mental confusion, weakness and heaviness of the legs, fall in blood pressure, cardiac arrhythmias and heart block. Hyperkalemia may exhibit the following electrocardiographic abnormalities: disappearance of the P wave, widening and slurring of the QRS complex, changes of the ST segment and tall peaked T waves.
TWIN-K taken on an empty stomach in undiluted doses larger than 30 ml can produce gastric irritation with nausea, vomiting, diarrhea, and abdominal discomfort.
Overdosage: The administration of oral potassium supplements to persons with normal kidney function rarely causes serious hyperkalemia. However, if the renal excretory function is impaired, potentially fatal hyperkalemia can result. It is important to note that hyperkalemia is usually asymptomatic and may be manifested only by an increased serum potassium concentration with or without E.K.G. changes.
Treatment measures include:
1. Elimination of potassium containing drugs or foods.
2. Intravenous administration of 300 to 500 ml/hr of a 10% dextrose solution containing 10–20 units of crystalline insulin per 1000 milliliters.
3. Correction of acidosis.
4. Use of exchange resins or peritoneal dialysis.

In treating hyperkalemia, it should be noted that patients stabilized on digitalis can develop digitalis toxicity when the serum potassium concentration is changed too rapidly.
Dosage and Administration: The usual adult dosage is one tablespoonful (15 ml) in 8 fluid ounces of water or fruit juice, two to four times a day. This will supply 40 to 80 mEq of potassium ions. The usual preventative dose of potassium is 20 mEq per day while therapeutic doses range from 30 mEq to 100 mEq per day. Because of the potential for gastrointestinal irritation, undiluted large single doses (more than a tablespoonful or 15 ml) of TWIN-K are to be avoided.
Deviations from this schedule may be indicated, since no average total daily dose can be defined, but must be governed by close observation for clinical effects.
How Supplied:
Bottles of 1 pint (16 fl. oz.) NDC 0524-0021-16
Federal law prohibits dispensing without prescription.

Manufactured and Distributed by
Boots Pharmaceuticals, Inc.
Shreveport, Louisiana 71106
Rev. 11/81

TWIN-K-Cl® ℞

Description: Each 15 ml (one tablespoonful) supplies 15 mEq of potassium ions and 4 mEq of chloride ions as a combination of potassium gluconate, potassium citrate, and ammonium chloride, in a sorbitol and saccharin solution.
Indications: For use as oral potassium therapy in the prevention or treatment of hypokalemia which may occur secondary to diuretic or corticosteroid administration. It may be used in the treatment of cardiac arrhythmias due to digitalis intoxication.
Potassium and chloride are usually the salts of choice in the treatment of hypokalemia since chloride and potassium deficiencies are likely to be associated with each other.
Contraindications: Severe renal impairment with oliguria or azotemia, untreated Addison's disease, adynamia episodica hereditaria, acute dehydration, heat cramps and hyperkalemia from any cause. This product should not be used in patients receiving aldosterone antagonists or triamterene.
Warnings: TWIN-K-Cl is a palatable form of oral potassium replacement. Excessive, undiluted doses of TWIN-K-Cl may cause a saline laxative effect.
To minimize gastrointestinal irritation, it is recommended that TWIN-K-Cl be taken with meals or diluted with water or fruit juice. A tablespoonful (15 ml) in 8 ounces of water is approximately isotonic. More than a single tablespoonful should not be taken without prior dilution.
Precautions: Potassium is a major intracellular cation which plays a significant role in body physiology. The serum level of potassium is normally 3.8–5.0 mEq/liter. While the serum or plasma level is a poor indicator of total body stores, a plasma or serum level below 3.5 mEq/liter is considered to be indicative of hypokalemia.
The most common cause of hypokalemia is excessive loss of potassium in the urine. However, hypokalemia can also occur with vomiting, gastric drainage and diarrhea.
Usually a potassium deficiency can be corrected by oral administration of potassium supplements. With normal kidney function it is difficult to produce potassium intoxication by oral administration. However, potassium supplements must be administered with caution since, usually, the exact amount of the deficiency is not accurately known. Checks on the patient's clinical status and periodic E.K.G. and/or serum potassium levels should be made. High serum potassium levels may cause death by cardiac depression, arrhythmias or arrest.
In patients with hypokalemia who also have alkalosis and a chloride deficiency, (hypokalemic hypochloremic alkalosis) there will be a requirement for chloride ions. TWIN-K-Cl is recommended for use in these patients.
Adverse Reactions: Symptoms of potassium intoxication include paresthesias of the extremities, flaccid paralysis, listlessness, mental confusion, weakness and heaviness of the legs, fall in blood pressure, cardiac ar-

rhythmias and heart block. Hyperkalemia may exhibit the following electrocardiographic abnormalities: disappearance of the P wave, widening and slurring of the QRS complex, changes of the ST segment and tall peaked T waves.

TWIN-K-Cl taken on an empty stomach in undiluted doses larger than 30 ml can produce gastric irritation with nausea, vomiting, diarrhea, and abdominal discomfort.

Overdosage: The administration of oral potassium supplements to persons with normal kidney function rarely causes serious hyperkalemia. However, if the renal excretory function is impaired potentially fatal hyperkalemia can result. It is important to note that hyperkalemia is usually asymptomatic and may be manifested only by an increased serum potassium concentration with or without E.K.G. changes.

Treatment measures include:

1. Elimination of potassium containing drugs or foods.
2. Intravenous administration of 300 to 500 ml/hr of a 10% dextrose solution containing 10–20 units of crystalline insulin per 1000 milliliters.
3. Correction of acidosis.
4. Use of exchange resins or peritoneal dialysis.

In treating hyperkalemia, it should be noted that patients stabilized on digitalis can develop digitalis toxicity when the serum potassium concentration is changed too rapidly.

Dosage and Administration:

The usual adult dosage is one tablespoonful (15 ml) in 6–8 fluid ounces of water or fruit juice, two to four times a day. This will supply 30 to 60 mEq of potassium ions and 8 to 16 mEq of chloride ions. The usual preventative dose of potassium is 20 mEq per day while therapeutic doses range from 30 mEq to 100 mEq per day. Because of the potential for gastrointestinal irritation, undiluted large single doses (30 ml or more) of TWIN-K-Cl are to be avoided.

Deviations from this schedule may be indicated, since no average total daily dose can be defined, but must be governed by close observation for clinical effects.

How Supplied:

Bottles of 1 pint (16 fl. oz.) NDC 0524-0022-16

Federal law prohibits dispensing without prescription.

Manufactured and Distributed by
Boots Pharmaceuticals, Inc.
Shreveport, Louisiana 71106

Rev. Nov. 1980

ZORPRIN®

(Zero–Order Release Aspirin)

Description: Each capsule-shaped tablet of Zorprin contains 800 mg of acetylsalicylic acid (aspirin), formulated in a special matrix to control the release rate of aspirin after ingestion. The controlled availability of aspirin provided by Zorprin approximates zero-order release; the in vitro release of aspirin from the tablet matrix is linear and independent of the concentration of the drug.

Clinical Pharmacology: Zorprin dissolution is pH dependent. In vitro studies have shown very little aspirin to be released in acidic solutions; whereas, Zorprin releases the majority of its aspirin (90%) in a zero-order mode at a neutral to alkaline pH. It is this pH dependence of Zorprin that appears to reduce its gastrointestinal side effect potential to approximately half that of regular aspirin; the stomach and proximal duodenum are acidic while the remaining small bowel is slightly alkaline.

Bioavailability data for Zorprin have confirmed that plasma levels of salicylic acid (SA) and acetysalicylic acid (ASA) approximate zero-order release and can be measured 24 hours after a single oral dose. This substantiates a twice daily dosage regimen.

Studies of in vivo prostaglandin levels (PGE_2) have shown Zorprin plasma levels of SA and ASA to reduce PGE_2 levels 14 hours after a single oral 800 mg dose while an equivalent dose of aspirin produced a reduction of PGE_2 levels only through six hours. Zorprin's effect on other prostaglandins than PGE_2 has not been determined.

Indications and Usage: Zorprin is indicated for the treatment of rheumatoid arthritis and osteoarthritis only under the advice and supervision of a physician. The safety and efficacy of Zorprin have not been established in those rheumatoid arthritis patients who are designated by the American Rheumatism Association as Functional Class IV (incapacitated, largely or wholly bedridden, or confined to wheelchair; little or no self-care).

In patients treated with Zorprin for rheumatoid arthritis and osteoarthritis, the anti-inflammatory action of Zorprin has been shown by reduction in pain, reduction in morning stiffness and reduction in disease activity as assessed by both the investigators and patient.

In clinical studies in patients with rheumatoid arthritis and osteoarthritis, Zorprin has been shown to be comparable to regular aspirin in controlling the aforementioned signs and symptoms of disease activity and to be associated with a statistically significant reduction in the milder gastrointestinal side effects (see ADVERSE REACTIONS). Zorprin may be well tolerated in patients who have had gastrointestinal side effects with regular aspirin, but these patients when treated with Zorprin should be carefully followed for signs and symptoms of gastrointestinal bleeding and ulceration.

Since there have been no controlled trials to demonstrate whether or not there is any beneficial effect or harmful interaction with the use of Zorprin in conjunction with other nonsteroidal anti-inflammatory agents (NSAI), the combination cannot be recommended (see **Drug Interactions**).

Contraindications: Zorprin should not be used in patients known to be allergic (hypersensitive) to salicylates or in individuals with the syndrome of nasal polyps, angioedema, bronchospastic reactivity to aspirin, renal or hepatic insufficiency, hypoprothrombinemia or other bleeding disorders. Though Zorprin is not recommended for children under 5 years of age, it is contraindicated in all children with fever accompanied by dehydration.

Warnings: USE IN PREGNANCY: Aspirin interferes with maternal and infant blood clotting and lengthens the duration of pregnancy and parturition. Aspirin has produced teratogenic effects in animals and increases the incidence of stillbirths and neonatal deaths in humans. Do not take this product during the last three months of pregnancy except under the advice and supervision of a physician.

Use of this drug requires that the physician evaluate the potential benefits of the drug against any possible hazard to the mother and child and that the physician should appraise the mother of the potential hazard to the fetus.

Precautions: Appropriate precautions should be taken in prescribing Zorprin for patients who are known to be sensitive to aspirin or salicylates. Particular care should be used when prescribing this medication for patients with erosive gastritis, peptic ulcer, mild diabetes or gout. As with all salicylate drugs, caution should be urged in using Zorprin for those patients with bleeding tendencies or those on anticoagulant drug.

Large doses of salicylates should be avoided in patients with clear evidence of carditis.

In order to avoid exacerbation of disease or adrenal insufficiency, patients who have been on prolonged corticosteroid therapy should have their therapy tapered slowly rather than discontinued abruptly when Zorprin is added to the treatment program.

Drug Interactions: Aspirin may interfere with some anticoagulant and antidiabetic drugs. Uric acid-lowering drugs, which are uricosurics, are antagonized by the concomitant use of aspirin. Nonsteroidal anti-inflammatory drugs may be competitively displaced from their albumin binding sites by aspirin. This effect will ameliorate the clinical efficacy of both drugs. Also, the gastrointestinal inflammatory potential of nonsteroidal anti-inflammatory drugs may be potentiated by aspirin. Alcohol produces a synergistic effect with aspirin in causing gastrointestinal bleeding.

Pregnancy Category D. See WARNINGS Section:

Nursing Mothers: Salicylates have been detected in the breast milk of nursing mothers. Due to the slower clearance of salicylates by infants, Zorprin is not recommended for use in nursing mothers.

Adverse Reactions:

Hematologic: Aspirin interferes with blood clotting. Patients with a history of blood coagulation defects, or receiving anticoagulant drugs or with severe anemia should avoid Zorprin. Aspirin used chronically may cause a persistent iron deficiency anemia.

Gastrointestinal: Aspirin may potentiate peptic ulcer, and cause stomach distress or heartburn. Aspirin can cause an increase in occult bleeding and in some patients massive gastrointestinal bleeding. However, the greatest release of active drug from Zorprin is designed to occur in the small intestine over a period of time. This has resulted in less symptomatic gastrointestinal side effects. Patients who have had adverse G.I. reactions with other aspirin preparations have tolerated Zorprin.

Allergic: Allergic and anaphylactic reactions have been noted when hypersensitive individuals have taken aspirin. The most common allergic reaction to aspirin is the induction of bronchospasm with asthma-like symptoms. Other reactions are hives, rash, angioedema, as well as rhinitis and nasal polyposis. Fatal anaphylactic shock while not common has been reported.

Central Nervous System: Taken in overdoses, aspirin produces stimulation which may be manifested by tinnitus. Following initial stimulation, depression of the central nervous system may be noted.

Renal: Aspirin may rarely cause an increase in the severity of chronic kidney disease.

Hepatic: High doses of aspirin have been reported to produce reversible hepatic dysfunction.

Overdosage: Overdosage, if it occurs would produce the usual symptoms of salicylism: tinnitus, vertigo, headache, confusion, drowsiness, sweating, hyperventilation, vomiting or diarrhea. Plasma salicylate levels in adults may range from 50 to 80 mg/dl in the mildly intoxicated patient to 110 to 160* mg/dl in the severely intoxicated patient. An arterial blood pH of 7.1 may indicate serious poisoning. The clearance of salicylates in children is much slower than adults and should especially be kept in mind during treatment of infants; salicylate half-lives of 30 hours have been reported in infants 4–8 months old. Treatment: For mild intoxication, emptying the stomach with an emetic, or gastric lavage with 5% sodium bicarbonate. Individuals suffering from severe intoxication should, in addition, have forced diuresis by intravenous infusions of saline and sodium bicarbonate or sodium lactate, dextrose solution. In extreme cases, hemodialysis or peritoneal dialysis may be required.

[*A plasma salicylate level of 160 mg/dl in an adult is usually considered lethal.]

In order to achieve a zero-order release, the tablets of Zorprin should be swallowed whole. Breaking the tablets or disrupting

Continued on next page

Boots—Cont.

the structure will alter the release profile of the drug.

Dosage and Administration:

Adult Dosage: For mild to moderate pain associated with rheumatoid arthritis and osteoarthritis, the recommended initial dose of Zorprin is 1600 mg (2-800 mg tablets) twice a day. Because of Zorprin's prolonged release of aspirin into the bloodstream, the tablets may be taken as a b.i.d. dose. Further upward or downward adjustment of the dosage should be determined by the physician, based upon the patient's response and needs. In general, patients with rheumatoid arthritis seem to require higher doses of Zorprin than do patients with osteoarthritis.

Dosage for Juvenile Rheumatoid Arthritis: Zorprin is a zero-order release aspirin and no studies have been conducted in children with this formulation. The use of Zorprin as therapy requires that the child is able to swallow the tablet whole without chewing or crushing; consequently, Zorprin is not recommended for children below the age of 5 years.

How Supplied: Zorprin Tablets 800 mg; plain, white capsule shaped tablets.

Bottles of 100 Tablets—NDC 0524-0057-01

Manufactured and Distributed By:
Boots Pharmaceuticals, Inc.
Shreveport, Louisiana 71106
U.S. Patent No. 4,308,251

Rev 8/82

[*Shown in Product Identification Section*]

Bowman Pharmaceuticals

Division of Bowman, Inc.
5801 MAYFAIR ROAD, N.W.
NORTH CANTON, OH 44720

ACTIVATED CHARCOAL USP IN A LIQUID BASE (Bowman) OTC

12.5 gm or 25 gm

Description: The product is a mixture of activated charcoal USP, propylene glycol USP, and water. Activated charcoal is a fine black, odorless and tasteless powder which has been treated by various agents to enhance its adsorptive powers. The treatment is refered to as activation; the agents remove substances previously adsorbed on the charcoal and, in some instances, break down the granules of carbon into smaller ones having a greater total surface area, thus a greater number of adsorption sites on the charcoal molecule. Propylene glycol is a clear, colorless, viscous liquid having a slightly acid taste. Propylene glycol serves as a vehicle and a preservative.

Action: Adsorbs the toxic substances ingested by forming an effective barrier between any remaining particulate material and the gastrointestinal mucosa, thus inhibiting any gastrointestinal absorption. Testing of activated charcoal USP in a liquid base indicates that adsorption powers of the 12.5 gm size or the 25 gm size, when treated with 1 gm of an alkaloid (strychnine sulfate) adsorbs at least 99.0% of the toxin. Treatment of the product with dyes (methylene blue) produces similar results. The adsorptive properties of the activated charcoal USP in a liquid base are slightly decreased during the shelf life of the product but are still capable of adsorbing at least 99.0% of the substance tested.

Precautions: Drug/Food Interactions:

Milk, ice cream or sherbet: Should not be mixed with the product since it will decrease the adsorptive capacity of the activated charcoal.

Ipecac Syrup: When used as an antidote for oral poisoning, simultaneous administration with activated charcoal is not recommended since the ipecac is adsorbed by the charcoal. If both ipecac and activated charcoal are to be used, it is recommended that the charcoal be administered only after vomiting has been induced or completed.

Medication: The effectiveness of other medication may be decreased when used concurrently because of the adsorption by the activated charcoal.

Ineffectiveness: Activated charcoal USP in a liquid base is ineffective for mineral acids, alkalies, substances insoluble in aqueous acidic solutions. The effectiveness in the lower GI tract of the adsorbant is questionable since passage through the upper tract saturates and deactivates the agent, but drugs adsorbed in the upper tract are not desorbed in the lower intestinal tract.

Side Effects: Will color stools black which may be alarming to patient although medically insignificant.

Dosage: Many physicians and poison control centers recommend that the minimum dose should be the contents of one or two bottles (12.5–25 gm of activated charcoal). In some cases the dosage may be higher.

Administration: To be used only as directed by a physician or poison control center.

How Supplied:

12.5 gm of activated charcoal in a 2 oz. bottle with wide mouth opening for easy pouring (Bowman #0252-3636-72).

25 gm of activated charcoal in a 4 oz. squeeze bottle with a dispenser cap (Bowman #0252-3636-74).

Non-Aerosol IVY-CHEX OTC

Description: IVY-CHEX contains: SD Alcohol 40, Polyvinylpyrrolidone-vinylacetate copolymers, Methyl Salicylate, Benzalkonium Cl.

Alcohol content 89.5%. Net Contents 4 fl. oz. SDA-OHIO #1260

Indications: FOR POISON IVY, POISON OAK AND POISON SUMAC—Wash the affected area with soap and water, dry with soft towel. Spray IVY-CHEX, applying only a light coat. Relief from itching and burning is almost instantaneous. Repeat if necessary. IVY-CHEX can be easily removed with soap and water. IVY-CHEX is equally effective in reducing the swelling and itching of insect bites, from chiggers, mosquitoes, bee, wasp, etc.

Directions for Use: Hold in an upright position, approximately 6 inches from the skin, press dispenser with quick short strokes. (If nozzle clogs, pull top off pump, rinse in warm water and replace). Air dry. Warning. Flammable. Do not use near fire or while smoking. Avoid spraying near eyes.

Warning: In case of accidental ingestion seek professional assistance or contact a Poison Control Center immediately. Keep this and all drugs out of reach of children.

How Supplied: 4 oz. Non-Aerosol Spray Bottle.

IDENTIFICATION PROBLEM?

Consult PDR's

Product Identification Section

where you'll find over 900

products pictured actual size

and in full color.

Boyle & Company

13260 MOORE STREET
CERRITOS, CA 90701

CITRA® CAPSULES

Composition: Each capsule contains: Phenylephrine HCl, 10 mg., Ascorbic Acid, 50 mg., Pheniramine Maleate, 6.25 mg., Chlorpheniramine Maleate, 1 mg., Pyrilamine Maleate, 8.33 mg., Salicylamide, 227 mg., Phenacetin, 120 mg., Caffeine Alkaloid, 30 mg.

Action and Uses: Antihistaminic, Decongestant, analgesic for relief of nasal congestion, muscular aches and pains of the common cold, hay fever, and common pollen allergies.

Administration and Dosage: *Adults*—One capsule every 4 hours. *Children*—(6-12), one half adult dose.

Precautions: Patients should be advised to avoid using machinery or driving until response to antihistamines is established, and not to use longer than 10 days without consulting physician. Use with caution in patients with hypertension, cardiac disease, diabetes or hyperthyroidism.

Warning: If used in large amounts or for long periods of time may damage kidneys.

How Supplied: 100's.

CITRA® FORTE SYRUP Ⓒ ℞
CITRA® FORTE CAPSULES Ⓒ ℞

Composition:	Ea. 5cc	Ea. Cap.
Hydrocodone Bitartrate	5 mg.	5 mg.
(Warning: May be habit forming)		
Ascorbic Acid	30 mg.	50 mg.
Pheniramine Maleate	2.5 mg.	6.25 mg.
Potassium Citrate	150 mg.	
Pyrilamine Maleate	3.33 mg.	8.33 mg.
Chlorpheniramine Maleate		1 mg.
Phenylephrine HCl		10 mg.
Salicylamide		227 mg.
Caffeine Alkaloid		30 mg.
Phenacetin		120 mg.

Syrup in a palatable, alcohol 2% flavored base.

Action and Uses: *CITRA FORTE SYRUP:* Antitussive, Expectorant, Antihistaminic, Analgesic provides effective cough suppressant action, a sodium free expectorant, two antihistamines to help control allergic reactions. *CITRA FORTE CAPSULES:* Antitussive, Antihistaminic, decongestant, analgesic. Also provides cough relief and in addition three antihistamines (each in $\frac{1}{3}$ their usual dosage) for fewer side effects and broader control of the patients allergic reaction to the cough/cold process. Decongestant action shrinks mucous membranes.

Administration and Dosage: *CITRA FORTE SYRUP: Usual Adult Dose.*—One or two teaspoonfuls every 3 or 4 hours. *Children* (6-12)—one-half adult dosage. *Children under 6 years*—according to standard method of calculation. *CITRA FORTE CAPSULES: Usual Adult Dose.*—One or two capsules every 3 or 4 hours.

Precautions: Patients should be advised to avoid using machinery or driving until response to antihistamines is established. Use with caution in patients with idiosyncrasies to formula ingredients. CITRA FORTE CAPSULES should be used with caution in patients with hypertension, cardiac disease, diabetes or hyperthyroidism.

How Supplied: CITRA FORTE SYRUP in pints and gallons; CITRA FORTE CAPSULES in bottles of 50 capsules.

GLYTINIC®
(For Iron Deficiency Anemia)
Palatable Liquid or Tablets

Composition: Daily adult dose provides:
Iron (ferrous gluconate)........................100 mg.
Aminoacetic acid (Glycine)....................1.3 gm.
Vitamins B_{12} 10 mcg.; B_1 7.5 mg.; B_6 2.25 mg.; niacinamide 45 mg.; d-pantothenyl alcohol 6.5 mg.; liver, 5 gr.

Action and Uses: Ferrous Gluconate, inherently tolerable combined with amino acid, glycine, assures good toleration, assimilation, and utilization. Glycine supplies needed amino nitrogen for rapid, positive hemoglobin and hematocrit response. Patient acceptance is excellent. The liquid is surprisingly free from after-taste making it useful for all ages. Children and elderly patients will like the mild flavor and distinct freedom from gastric irritation and after-taste. Glytinic is particularly useful for patients refractory or intolerant to iron preparations.

Administration and Dosage: Liquid with or between meals: *Adults*—1 tablespoonful b.i.d.; *Children 6 to 12*—1 teaspoonful t.i.d.; 2 to 6, 1 teaspoonful b.i.d. Tablets, with or between meals: *Adults*—2 b.i.d.; *Children 6 to 12*—1 b.i.d.

How Supplied: Liquid—pints; tablets —100's.

TRIVA® COMBINATION ℞
TRIVA® DOUCHE POWDER
TRIVA® JEL ℞

Composition: TRIVA COMBINATION combines therapeutic vaginal douche and jel in a convenient and complete treatment consisting of: TRIVA POWDER containing oxyquinoline sulfate 2%; alkyl aryl sulfonate 35%; disodium edetate 0.33%; sodium sulfate 53%; dispersant (lactose) 9.67% and TRIVA JEL containing per 5 Grams oxyquinoline benzoate 7.5 mg.; alkyl aryl sulfonate 62.5 mg.; disodium edetate 2.5 mg.; aminacrine HCl 10 mg.; copper sulfate .063 mg.; sodium sulfate 6.9 mg.; in an aqueous jel base of tragacanth, Irish moss, modified lanolin, glycerin, sodium bicarbonate preserved with methyl-propyl- and butyl-parahydroxy-benzoate.

Action and Uses: TRIVA COMBINATION effectively treats Monilial and Trichomonal as well as Non-specific Vulvovaginitis. Chronic, stubborn cases as well as Monilia and Trichomonas occurring together can be successfully treated. Organisms are eradicated along with symptoms. Vaginal flora and pH return to normal spontaneously. Fungicidal, trichomonacidal, bactericidal, detergent and chelating agents are provided for a safe, simple, patient-administered 16 day treatment without need for restraints on patient's activities. Flushing and detergent action of the douche combines with the continuous action of the jel to quickly destroy the infection and stop the symptoms. Effectiveness of TRIVA COMBINATION has been demonstrated by clinical tests. Both diagnosis and cure were established by the use of special Papanicolaou smear and Sabouraud culture.

Administration and Dosage: TRIVA COMBINATION, ℞, sig: douche (1 packet in 1 qt water) at night followed immediately by one applicatorfull of JEL, continued for 15 nights followed on 16th morning by douche only. An additional course of treatment may be used if needed. Directions for complete mechanical use of product appear on each package.
TRIVA DOUCHE POWDER (individual packet dissolved in 1 qt water) alone is effective in most cases of Monilial, Trichomonal and Non-specific Vulvovaginitis. It provides rapid relief from symptoms. Particularly useful in pre- and post-operative and post-partum care. May be used adjunctively with oral treatment for Trichomonas.
TRIVA DOUCHE POWDER, sig, douche (1 packet in 1 qt water) morning and night for 12 days.
TRIVA JEL ℞, sig. one or two applicatorsful daily.
IMPORTANT: During menstruation, continue treatment as instructed.

Precautions: Occasionally, irritation occurs at the onset of treatment. In such cases it is recommended that the douche only be prescribed in one-half or less than usual strength for a day or two, then combined therapeutic treatment resumed as directed.
TRIVA COMBINATION, POWDER and JEL are spermicidal.

Side Effects: None.

Contraindications: None.

How Supplied: TRIVA COMBINATION contains 24 individual 3 Gm. packets douche powder, 1 tube 85 Gm. Jel with applicator.
TRIVA DOUCHE POWDER—Available individually, 24 individual 3 Gm. packets.
TRIVA JEL—Available individually, 1 tube 85 Gm. with applicator.

Breon Laboratories Inc.
90 PARK AVENUE
NEW YORK, NY 10016

BREOKINASE® ℞
(Urokinase For Injection)

BREOKINASE (urokinase for injection) should be used in hospitals where the recommended diagnostic and monitoring techniques are available. Thrombolytic therapy should be considered in all situations where the benefits to be achieved outweigh the risk of potentially serious hemorrhage. Although the incidence of bleeding with thrombolytic agents has been found to be no greater than with standard anticoagulation, when internal bleeding does occur, it may be more difficult to manage than that which occurs with conventional anticoagulant therapy.
Urokinase treatment should be instituted as soon as possible after the occurrence of pulmonary embolism, preferably within seven days after onset. Any delay in instituting lytic therapy to evaluate the effect of preliminary heparin therapy decreases the potential for optimal efficacy.

Description: Urokinase is an enzyme (protein) produced by the kidney and found in the urine. There are two forms differing in molecular weight but having similar effects. BREOKINASE is a sterile preparation of highly purified urokinase isolated from human urine and is predominantly the high molecular weight form (54,000 daltons). BREOKINASE is supplied as a white cake or powder in lyophilized form intended for intravenous infusion following reconstitution of each vial with 8.0 ml Sterile Water for Injection, USP. Each vial contains 250,000 I.U. of urokinase activity and approximately 0.9 millimols of sodium phosphates. Following reconstitution, a clear, practically colorless and isotonic solution of pH 7 is obtained, with 31,250 I.U. per ml.

Clinical Pharmacology: Urokinase acts on the endogenous fibrinolytic system. It converts plasminogen to the enzyme plasmin. Plasmin degrades fibrin clots as well as fibrinogen and other plasma proteins. Intravenous infusion of urokinase results in increased fibrinolytic activity. This effect disappears within a few hours after discontinuation of infusion, however an increase in thrombin time, decrease in plasma levels of fibrinogen and plasminogen, and an increase in the amount of circulating fibrin (ogen) degradation products may persist for 12–24 hours. There is a lack of correlation between embolus resolution and changes in coagulation and fibrinolytic assay results.
The efficacy of BREOKINASE in the lysis of pulmonary emboli has been established in controlled clinical studies using angiography, perfusion lung scans, and pulmonary arterial and right heart pressure measurements before and after treatment. In these studies, thrombolysis was accompanied by improved pulmonary capillary perfusion, and by reversal of the cardiopulmonary hemodynamic abnormalities towards normal.

Indications and Usage:
Pulmonary Embolism
BREOKINASE (urokinase for injection) is indicated in adults:
—for the lysis of acute massive pulmonary emboli, defined as obstruction or significant filling defects involving two or more lobar pulmonary arteries or an equivalent amount of emboli in other vessels.
—for the lysis of pulmonary emboli accompanied by unstable hemodynamics, i.e., failure to maintain blood pressure without supportive measures.

The diagnosis should be confirmed by objective means, such as pulmonary angiography using the upper extremity, or non-invasive procedures such as lung scanning. Angiographic and hemodynamic measurements and perfusion lung scans demonstrate a more rapid improvement during the first 24 hours after BREOKINASE therapy than with heparin therapy.

Contraindications: Because thrombolytic therapy increases the risk of bleeding, BREOKINASE is contraindicated in the following situations (See Warnings):
—Active internal bleeding.
—Recent (within two months) cerebrovascular accident, intracranial or intraspinal surgery.
—Intracranial neoplasm.

Warnings:
Bleeding
The aim of urokinase therapy is the production of sufficient amounts of plasmin for the lysis of intravascular deposits of fibrin; however, fibrin deposits which provide hemostasis, for example, at sites of needle punctures, will also lyse and bleeding from such sites may occur.
Intramuscular injections and non-essential handling of patients must be avoided during treatment with urokinase. Venipunctures should also be performed as carefully and infrequently as possible. Should an arterial puncture be necessary, it should be performed in an upper extremity. Pressure should be applied for at least 30 minutes followed by a pressure dressing, and the puncture site checked frequently for evidence of bleeding.
In the following conditions, the risks of thrombolytic therapy must be weighed carefully against the anticipated benefits:
—Recent (within 10 days) major surgery, obstetrical delivery, organ biopsy, previous puncture of non-compressible vessels
—Recent (within 10 days) serious gastrointestinal bleeding
—Recent trauma including cardiopulmonary resuscitation
—Severe uncontrolled arterial hypertension
—High likelihood of a left heart thrombus, e.g. mitral disease with atrial fibrillation
—Subacute bacterial endocarditis
—Hemostatic defect including those secondary to severe hepatic or renal disease
—Pregnancy
—Evidence of cerebrovascular disease
—Diabetic hemorrhagic retinopathy
—Any other condition in which bleeding constitutes a significant hazard or would be particularly difficult to manage because of its location.

If bleeding from an invasive site occurs during BREOKINASE infusion but is not severe, treatment may be continued with close clinical observation and local measures to control bleeding.

Continued on next page

Breon—Cont.

Should serious spontaneous bleeding occur, the infusion of BREOKINASE should be terminated immediately, and treatment instituted as described under ADVERSE REACTIONS.

Use of Anticoagulants

Concurrent use of anticoagulants with BREOKINASE is not recommended and may be hazardous. Before beginning BREOKINASE infusion in patients being treated with heparin, the effects of heparin should be allowed to decrease. Similarly, heparin should be withheld following BREOKINASE therapy until thrombolytic effects have diminished.

Precautions:

Use in Children

Safety and effectiveness of urokinase therapy in children have not been established; therefore, treatment of such patients is not recommended.

Pregnancy Category C

Animal reproduction studies have not been conducted with BREOKINASE. It is also not known whether BREOKINASE can cause fetal harm when administered to a pregnant woman or can affect reproduction capacity. BREOKINASE should be given to a pregnant woman only if clearly needed in the considered judgment of the treating physician.

Drug Interactions

The interaction of BREOKINASE with other drugs has not been studied. Concurrent use of drugs that may alter platelet function, e.g., aspirin, indomethacin, and phenylbutazone, should be avoided.

Patient Monitoring

Before commencing thrombolytic therapy, a thrombin time (TT), or activated partial thromboplastin time (APTT), or prothrombin time (PT) should be obtained, as well as hematocrit and platelet count. If heparin has been given, it should be discontinued and the TT or APTT should be allowed to return to less than twice the normal control value before thrombolytic therapy is started.

Opinions differ regarding monitoring of coagulation and thrombolytic status during urokinase infusion. The existence of a lytic state is usually indicated by a decrease in the fibrinogen and plasminogen levels, a prolongation of TT, APTT or PT and an increase in fibrin(ogen) degradation products. Results of coagulation and/or fibrinolytic tests, however, do not reliably predict either efficacy or risk of bleeding. Following BREOKINASE treatment, and before (re)instituting heparin, the TT or APTT should be less than twice the normal control value.

Adverse Reactions:

Bleeding

The most important side effect of BREOKINASE treatment is bleeding. However, almost all major bleeding is from sites of invasive procedures. The incidence of major bleeding complications with thrombolytic agents during recent clinical experience, based upon post-marketing surveillance, has been about 5%, and is probably not statistically different from the incidence of bleeding with conventional anticoagulants.

The types of bleeding seen with thrombolytic therapy can be placed into two broad categories:

— superficial or surface bleeding, observed mainly at invaded sites such as a venous cutdowns, arterial punctures, recent surgical sites, etc.

— internal bleeding involving the gastrointestinal tract, the genito-urinary tract, vagina, intramuscular, retroperitoneal and intracerebral sites, etc.

Several fatalities due to cerebral or retroperitoneal hemorrhage have occurred during thrombolytic treatment.

Management of Severe Bleeding

If serious bleeding occurs, urokinase therapy must be discontinued, and, if necessary, blood loss and reversal of the bleeding tendency can be effectively managed with fresh whole blood, fresh frozen plasma, or human red cell concentrates and cryoprecipitate. Dextran should not be used. Although the use of aminocaproic acid (ACA, AMICAR) in humans as an antidote for urokinase has not been documented, it may be considered in an emergency situation.

Allergic Reactions

In vitro tests with urokinase as well as intradermal tests in humans have given no evidence of induced antibody formation. Relatively mild allergic-type reactions, e.g. bronchospasm and skin rash, have been reported rarely. When such reactions occur, they usually respond to conventional therapy.

Fever

Febrile episodes have occurred in approximately 2–3% of treated patients. A cause and effect relationship to urokinase has not been established. Symptomatic treatment with acetaminophen is usually sufficient to alleviate discomfort. Aspirin is not recommended.

Dosage and Administration:

Preparation

Reconstitute BREOKINASE (urokinase for injection) by aseptically adding 8.0 ml of Sterile Water for Injection, USP, to each vial. (It is important that BREOKINASE be reconstituted *only* with Sterile Water for Injection, USP, *without* preservatives. Bacteriostatic Water for Injection or other diluents should not be used.) Swirl gently to avoid foaming. *DO NOT SHAKE.* Because BREOKINASE contains no preservatives, it should not be reconstituted until immediately before using. Any unused portion of the reconstituted material should be discarded.

Each ml of reconstituted BREOKINASE contains 31,250 I.U. of urokinase activity.

Dosing

BREOKINASE IS INTENDED FOR INTRAVENOUS INFUSION ONLY.

A priming or loading dose of 2000 I.U./lb (4400 I.U./kg) of BREOKINASE is given over a period of ten minutes. This is followed by a continuous infusion of 2000 I.U./lb/hr (4400 I.U./kg/hr) for 12 hours (see Table). A constant infusion pump independent of all other intravenous systems should be used. Do not expose reconstituted solution to excessive heat.

[See table below].

Patient Weight Lb	Kg	Total Dose I.U.*	Number Vials BREOKINASE	Total Volume BREOKINASE After Reconstitution (ml)	Loading Dose (ml/10 min)**	12 Hour Infusion Rate (ml/hr)
81–90	36.8– 40.9	2,250,000	9	72	5.5	5.5
91–100	41.4– 45.5	2,500,000	10	80	6.2	6.2
101–110	45.9– 50.0	2,750,000	11	88	6.8	6.8
111–120	50.5– 54.5	3,000,000	12	96	7.4	7.4
121–130	55.0– 59.1	3,250,000	13	104	8.0	8.0
131–140	59.5– 63.6	3,500,000	14	112	8.6	8.6
141–150	64.1– 68.2	3,750,000	15	120	9.2	9.2
151–160	68.6– 72.2	4,000,000	16	128	9.8	9.8
161–170	73.2– 77.3	4,250,000	17	136	10.5	10.5
171–180	77.7– 81.8	4,500,000	18	144	11.1	11.1
181–190	82.3– 86.4	4,750,000	19	152	11.7	11.7
191–200	86.8– 90.9	5,000,000	20	160	12.3	12.3
201–210	91.4– 95.5	5,250,000	21	168	12.9	12.9
211–220	95.9–100.0	5,500,000	22	176	13.5	13.5
221–230	100.5–104.5	5,750,000	23	184	14.2	14.2
231–240	105.0–109.1	6,000,000	24	192	14.8	14.8
241–250	109.5–113.6	6,250,000	25	200	15.4	15.4

* Loading dose plus 12 hour infusion dose

** The loading dose is administered over a ten minute period prior to the 12 hour infusion

Anticoagulation Following BREOKINASE Treatment

Following BREOKINASE infusion, treatment with heparin by continuous intravenous infusion *without a loading dose,* followed by oral anticoagulant therapy, is recommended to minimize re-thrombosis. Heparin treatment should not begin until the thrombin time has decreased to less than twice the normal control (approximately 3 to 4 hours following end of BREOKINASE infusion). Heparin treatment should then be followed by oral anticoagulant in the usual manner. See manufacturers' prescribing information for proper use of heparin and oral anticoagulants.

How Supplied: BREOKINASE is supplied as a sterile lyophilized preparation. Each vial contains 250,000 I.U. of urokinase activity and approximately 0.9 millimols sodium phosphates. The vials should be stored under refrigeration (2° to 8° C).

Code 1801 BREOKINASE 30 ml Vials

NDC 0057-1000-01

References:

1. Aoki N, Maroi M, Matsuda M, Tachiya K: The behavior of a_2-plasmin inhibitor in fibrinolytic states. *J Clin Invest 60:* 361–369, 1977.
2. Bang NU: Physiology and biochemistry of fibrinolysis. In *Thrombosis and Bleeding Disorders* (Bank NU, Beller FK, Deutsch E, Mammen EF, eds). Academic Press, 1971, pp. 292–327.
3. Bell WR: Thrombolytic Therapy: A comparison between urokinase and streptokinase. *Sem Thromb Hemost 2:*1975.
4. Bell WR: Streptokinase and urokinase in the treatment of pulmonary thromboemboli. *Thrombos Haemostas 35:*57, 1976.
5. Chesterman CN, Allington MJ, Sharp AA: Relationship of plasminogen activator to fibrin. *Nature (New Biology) 238:*15–17, 1972.
6. Collen D, Wiman B: Fact-acting plasmin inhibitor in human plasma. *Blood 51:*563, 1978.
7. Fratantoni JC, Ness P, Simon TL: Thrombolytic therapy: Current status. *N Engl J Med 293:*1073–1078, 1975.
8. Lesuk A, Terminiello L, Traver JH: Crystalline human urokinase: Some properties. *Science 147:*880, 1965.
9. Lesuk A, Terminiello L, Traver JH: Sephadex gelfiltration of human urokinase preparations. *Fed Proc 25:*194, 1966.
10. Lesuk A, Terminiello L, Traver JH, Groff JL: Biochemical and biophysical studies of human urokinase. *Thrombos Diathes Haemorrh 18:*293, 1967.
11. McNicol GP: The fibrinolytic enzyme system. *Postgrad Med J (Aug Suppl) 49:*10–12, 1973.

12. Sasahara AA, Hyers TM, Cole CM, et al: The urokinase pulmonary embolism trial. *Circulation (Suppl II) 47:*1–108, 1973.
13. Sasahara AA, Bell WR, Simon TL, Stengle JM, and Sherry S: The phase II urokinase-streptokinase pulmonary embolism trial. *Thrombos Diathes Haemorrh* (Stuttg) *33:*464–476, 1975.
14. Sherry S, Alkjaersig N, Fletcher AP: Assay of urokinase preparations with the synthetic substrate acetyl-l-lysine methyl ester. *J Lab Clin Med 64:*145, 1964.
15. Sherry S: Streptokinase, urokinase: Do they really work? *Modern Med:* 72–76, Nov. 1, 1976.
16. Urokinase pulmonary embolism trial study group: Urokinase-streptokinase embolism trial. *JAMA 229:*1606–1613, 1974.
17. Urokinase pulmonary embolism trial. *JAMA 214* (12):2163–2172, 1970.
18. Thrombolytic Therapy in Thrombosis, National Institutes of Health Consensus Development Conference, April 10–12, 1980.
19. Sharma GVRK, Burleson VA and Sasahara AA: Effect of thrombolytic therapy on pulmonary-capillary blood volume in patients with pulmonary embolism. *N Engl J Med 303:*842–845, 1980.

Supplied by:
BREON LABORATORIES INC.
New York, N.Y. 10016
Mfg. by Green Cross Corp.
Osaka, Japan
Revised February 1981 BR 884/0281

BREONESIN®
brand of guaifenesin capsules, USP

Description: Each red, oval-shaped BREONESIN capsule contains 200 mg of guaifenesin in an easy to swallow, soft gelatin capsule. BREONESIN contains no sugar or alcohol.
Indications: BREONESIN is indicated for the temporary relief of coughs. BREONESIN is an expectorant which helps to loosen phlegm (sputum) and bronchial secretions, and acts to thin mucus. Coughs due to minor throat and bronchial irritation that occur with the common cold are temporarily relieved.
Warnings: Persistent cough may indicate a serious condition. Consult your physician if cough persists for more than 1 week, recurs, or is accompanied by high fever, rash or persistent headache. Do not take this product for persistent coughs due to smoking, asthma or emphysema, or coughs accompanied by excessive secretions, except under the advice and supervision of your physician.
Dosage: Adults and Children 12 years of age and over: 1 or 2 capsules every 4 hours, not to exceed 12 capsules in a 24-hour period. Children under 12 years: as directed by your physician.
Store at controlled room temperature, between 15°C and 30°C (59°F and 86°F).
Supplied by:
BREON LABORATORIES INC.
New York, N.Y. 10016
Mfg. by R.P. Scherer Corp.
Monroe, N.C. 28110
[*Shown in Product Identification Section*]

BRONKEPHRINE® ℞
(ethylnorepinephrine hydrochloride injection, USP)
IN AQUEOUS SOLUTION

Description: BRONKEPHRINE is ethylnorepinephrine hydrochloride injection, USP. Each ml contains 2 mg ethylnorepinephrine HCl in a sterile isotonic solution of 0.7% sodium chloride with sodium acetone bisulfite 0.2% as preservative. The pH is adjusted to 2.9–4.5 with NaOH or HCl. BRONKEPHRINE is a synthetic sympathomimetic amine intended for subcutaneous or intramuscular injection. The chemical name is 1-(3, 4-dihydroxyphenyl)-2-amino-1-butanol hydrochloride.
Clinical Pharmacology: BRONKEPHRINE is primarily a beta-adrenergic agonist. Its actions are similar to those of isoproterenol, although it is less potent. Its bronchodilating properties closely simulate those of epinephrine but without significant pressor effects. It thus may be safer than epinephrine for hypertensive patients and severely ill patients in whom such effects are undesirable. It is particularly adapted for use in children because of its relative lack of adverse effects, especially central nervous system excitation. It also may be of value in diabetic asthmatics due to its lack of glycogenolytic activity.
Metabolic and pharmacokinetic data are unavailable.
Indications and Usage: BRONKEPHRINE is indicated for use as a bronchodilator for bronchial asthma and for reversible bronchospasm that may occur in association with bronchitis and emphysema.
Contraindications: BRONKEPHRINE is contraindicated in patients who are hypersensitive to any of its ingredients or with idiosyncrasy to sympathomimetic drugs.
Warnings: BRONKEPHRINE should not be administered along with epinephrine or other sympathomimetic amines because these drugs are direct cardiac stimulants and may cause excessive tachycardia.
Precautions: BRONKEPHRINE should be used with caution in persons with cardiovascular disease, a history of stroke or coronary artery disease. It is a potent drug and may cause toxic symptoms through idiosyncratic response or overdosage.
Care should be taken in anatomical selection of injection sites to avoid inadvertent intraneural or intravascular injection.
Carcinogenesis, mutagenesis, impairment of fertility: Long-term animal studies of BRONKEPHRINE to evaluate carcinogenic potential and reproduction studies in animals have not been performed. There is no evidence from human data that BRONKEPHRINE may be carcinogenic or mutagenic or that it impairs fertility.
Pregnancy Category C: Animal reproduction studies have not been conducted with BRONKEPHRINE. It is not known whether BRONKEPHRINE can cause fetal harm when administered to a pregnant woman or can affect reproduction capacity. BRONKEPHRINE should be given to a pregnant woman only if clearly needed and the potential benefits outweigh the risk.
Nursing mothers: It is not known whether BRONKEPHRINE is excreted in human milk; however, because many drugs are excreted in human milk, caution should be exercised when BRONKEPHRINE is administered to a nursing woman.
Adverse Reactions: BRONKEPHRINE is generally well tolerated. It may, however, produce changes in blood pressure (elevation or depression) or pulse rate (elevation), palpitation, headache, dizziness or nausea; as with other sympathomimetic amines.
Overdosage: The signs and symptoms of overdosage with BRONKEPHRINE are those typical of any sympathomimetic amine. Treatment should be symptomatic.
Dosage and Administration: The usual adult dose by subcutaneous or intramuscular injection is 0.5–1.0 ml. Depending on severity of the asthmatic attack, smaller doses (0.3–0.5 ml) may suffice. Dosage in children varies according to age and weight; usually 0.1 to 0.5 ml is sufficient.
How Supplied:
1 ml sterile single dose ampuls, Code #1188 (Box of 5)
NDC 0057-1001-05
1 ml sterile single dose ampuls, Code #1189 (Box of 25)
NDC 0057-1001-01
PROTECT AMPULS FROM LIGHT

BRONKODYL®S–R ℞
brand of theophylline, USP (anhydrous)
SUSTAINED RELEASE CAPSULES
300 mg

BRONKODYL® ℞
brand of theophylline, USP (anhydrous)
CAPSULES
100 mg and 200 mg
ELIXIR
80 mg per 15 ml

Description: BRONKODYL S-R—Each blue and white hard gelatin capsule contains 300 mg theophylline USP (anhydrous) in a coated bead preparation. BRONKODYL S-R capsules have been specially formulated to provide the therapeutic effect of theophylline over a prolonged period of time. Theophylline, a methylxanthine, is a white, odorless crystalline powder having a bitter taste.
BRONKODYL—Each green and white hard gelatin capsule contains theophylline USP (anhydrous) 200 mg, in a micro-pulverized form. Each brown and white hard gelatin capsule contains 100 mg. The elixir contains 80 mg theophylline per 15 ml in a 20% alcohol elixir (approximately 20 calories, 0.9 gm carbohydrate per tablespoonful).
Clinical Pharmacology: Theophylline directly relaxes smooth muscle of bronchi and pulmonary blood vessels, producing bronchodilation and pulmonary vasodilation. Other effects typical of the methylxanthines include coronary vasodilation, diuresis, and cardiac, cerebral and skeletal muscle stimulation. The actions of theophylline may be mediated through inhibition of phosphodiesterase with a resultant increase in intracellular cyclic AMP causing smooth muscle relaxation. At concentrations higher than those usually attained in vivo, theophylline also inhibits mast cell release of histamine.
In vitro, theophylline has been shown to act synergistically with beta agonists to increase intracellular cyclic AMP. However, more data are needed to determine whether there are clinically significant additive or synergistic effects **in vivo**.
Tolerance with chronic use of theophylline has not been demonstrated.
Theophylline half-life is prolonged in the presence of alcoholism, reduced hepatic or renal function, congestive heart failure, prolonged periods of high fever, and in patients receiving certain antibiotics such as troleandomycin (TAO), erythromycin and clindamycin. Half-life is shortened in cigarette smokers.
[See table above].

THEOPHYLLINE ELIMINATION

	Clearance (mean ± S.D.)	Half-life (mean ± S.D.)
Adult nonsmokers with uncomplicated asthma	0.65 ± 0.19 ml/kg/min	8.7 ± 2.2 hours
Children over six months old	1.45 ± 0.58 ml/kg/min	3.7 ± 1.1 hours

Older adults with chronic obstructive pulmonary disease, patients with cor pulmonale or other heart failure, and patients with liver

Continued on next page

Breon—Cont.

disease may have much lower clearances with half-life exceeding 24 hours.

Theophylline half-life in smokers of 1–2 packs/day averaged 4–5 hours compared with a half-life of 7–9 hours in nonsmokers. This may be due to induction of drug-metabolizing enzymes and this effect may last months to years after cessation of smoking.

Although BRONKODYL S-R is not indicated for young children or infants, it should be noted that newborns have extremely slow clearances and half-lives exceeding 24 hours. Theophylline pharmacokinetics approach those in older children after about 3–6 months of life.

In a well controlled study of normal adult volunteers, a single dose of 300 mg BRONKODYL S-R, administered as 1 capsule, resulted in a mean peak plasma concentration of 9.86 mcg/ml at 4 hours following administration. BRONKODYL S-R was found to be completely bioavailable when compared to the reference standard, theophylline elixir.

Indications: For relief and/or prevention of reversible bronchospasm associated with bronchial asthma, chronic bronchitis and emphysema.

Contraindications: BRONKODYL S-R/ BRONKODYL is contraindicated in persons with hypersensitivity to any of its components, or to other xanthines.

Warnings: All methylxanthines should be used with caution in children and in others who are currently taking bronchodilator products, especially in rectal dosage form, which may contain theophylline or related drugs.

Status asthmaticus is a medical emergency. Addition of corticosteroids and other medications to bronchodilator therapy may be required.

The incidence of toxicity increases at serum levels greater than 20 mcg/ml. There are often no early signs of theophylline toxicity, such as nausea and restlessness, which may appear in up to 50 percent of patients prior to onset of convulsions. Ventricular arrhythmias or seizures may be the first signs of toxicity. Preexisting arrhythmias may be worsened by theophylline. Tachycardia may occur in many patients who have higher theophylline serum levels.

Serum should be obtained at the time of peak drug absorption. High serum levels of theophylline may result from conventional doses in association with clinical manifestations of toxicity in certain clinical situations such as: patients with lowered body plasma clearances (due to transient cardiac decompensation), patients with liver dysfunction or chronic obstructive lung disease, patients who are more than 55 years of age, particularly males.

It is important that doses not tolerated be discontinued. In such situations if therapy is to be resumed, it should be at a lower dosage after all signs of toxicity have disappeared.

Usage in Pregnancy: Although theophylline has been used for many years, with no evidence of adverse fetal effect or teratogenicity, its safety in pregnancy has not been established. Therefore, use of BRONKODYL S-R/BRONKODYL during lactation or in women of childbearing potential requires that possible benefits of the drug be weighed against possible hazards to fetus or child.

Usage in Nursing Mothers: It has been reported that theophylline distributes readily into breast milk; therefore, the drug should not be used in nursing women.

Precautions: Smokers may require larger doses of theophylline because of a shorter half-life in these patients.

Theophylline should not be administered concurrently with other xanthines.

Caution should be observed in patients with cardiac disease, severe hypoxemia, hypertension, hyperthyroidism, acute myocardial injury, cor pulmonale, congestive heart failure, liver disease, peptic ulcer, and in the elderly and neonates. Patients with congestive heart failure in particular may have markedly prolonged serum half-lives of theophylline.

Theophylline may occasionally act as a local gastrointestinal irritant, especially in high doses and chronic use, but gastrointestinal symptoms are more commonly central and associated with serum concentrations exceeding 20 mcg/ml.

Factors known to influence the body clearance of theophylline are: cigarette smoking (increased clearance), age (decreasing clearance with increasing age), congestive heart failure (decreased clearance), liver disease (decreased clearance), pulmonary edema (decreased clearance), concurrent infection (decreased clearance), concomitant use of erythromycin, troleandomycin, clindamycin, or lincomycin (decreased clearance). In the presence of the above factors, it is advisable to monitor theophylline serum levels periodically. Any change in the patient's underlying condition may be associated with a change in theophylline clearance and therefore also requires monitoring. Other circumstances in which it is advisable to monitor serum levels include: unexplained poor control of asthmatic signs and symptoms; occurrence of toxic symptoms; addition or removal of other drugs from the therapeutic regimen which affect the metabolism of theophylline, use of unusually high doses.

Adverse Reactions: Most adverse reactions to theophylline are seen with serum levels exceeding the therapeutic range. **Gastrointestinal:** nausea, vomiting, epigastric pain, hematemesis, diarrhea. **CNS:** headache, irritability, restlessness, insomnia, reflex hyperexcitability, muscle twitching, clonic and tonic generalized convulsions. **Cardiovascular:** palpitations, tachycardia, extrasystoles, flushing, hypotension, circulatory failure, ventricular arrhythmias which may be life-threatening. **Respiratory:** tachypnea. **Renal:** diuresis, albuminuria. **Other:** hyperglycemia, inappropriate ADH secretion.

Drug Interactions: Toxic synergism with ephedrine and other sympathomimetic bronchodilators may occur.

DRUG COMBINATION	EFFECT
Aminophylline with lithium carbonate	Increased excretion of lithium carbonate
Aminophylline with propranolol	Antagonism of propranolol effect
Theophylline with furosemide	Increased diuresis
Theophylline with hexamethonium	Decreased hexamethonium-induced chronotropic effect
Theophylline with reserpine	Reserpine-induced tachycardia
Theophylline with chlordiazepoxide	Chlordiazepoxide-induced fatty acid mobilization
Theophylline with TAO (troleandomycin), erythromycin, lincomycin, clindamycin	Increased theophylline plasma levels

Dosage and Administration: Optimum therapeutic serum levels of theophylline are generally considered to lie between 10 and 20 mcg/ml. Levels above 20 mcg/ml may produce toxic effects. Because of great variation of theophylline pharmacokinetics among patients, and in the same patient at different times, dosage must be individualized and serum levels monitored as necessary. It is recommended that patients, especially those requiring immediate theophyllinization, be initially titrated on immediate release formulations, such as BRONKODYL Capsules 100 mg and 200 mg, to determine their daily dosage requirement prior to switching to a sustained release form.

BRONKODYL S-R:

Adults and Children over 12: An initial dose of 12 mg/kg/day (calculated by lean or ideal body weight) in divided doses will generally not produce excessive theophylline serum levels over 20 mcg/ml. The dose may be increased by 2 mg/kg/day every 2 days until the desired therapeutic response and blood levels are achieved if no side effects are encountered. At doses above 20 mg/kg/day, serum theophylline levels should be monitored.

The usual initial dose of BRONKODYL S-R is one 300 mg capsule every 12 hours. Some patients may require two capsules every 12 hours or individualized dosing. If the patient has been stabilized on a short-acting theophylline, therapy with BRONKODYL S-R capsules can be initiated at the same total daily dose, with half the total daily dose administered every 12 hours. If satisfactory control of symptoms is not maintaind for the full 12-hour period, or if unacceptable adverse effects occur, one-third of the total daily dosage should be administered on an every 8 hour schedule.

The **optimal maintenance dose** of theophylline is achieved by titration of blood levels. Monitoring of serum theophylline concentrations is thus recommended. For purposes of these measurements, serum should be obtained at the time of peak drug absorption (3 to 6 hours after administration of BRONKODYL S-R). In the preceding 48 hours, dosage should have been reasonably typical of the prescribed regimen and no doses should have been missed or added. Dosage adjustments based on serum theophylline measurements when these instructions have not been followed may result in dosages that present risk of toxicity to the patient.

BRONKODYL:

Rapidly absorbed theophylline preparations require administration every 6 hours, espe-

	LOADING DOSE	MAINTENANCE DOSE FOR NEXT 12 HOURS	MAINTENANCE DOSE BEYOND 12 HOURS
Children 6 months to 9 years	6 mg/kg	4 mg/kg q4h	4 mg/kg q6h
Children 9–16 years and young adults smokers	6 mg/kg	3 mg/kg q4h	3 mg/kg q6h
Otherwise healthy nonsmoking adults	6 mg/kg	3 mg/kg q6h	3 mg/kg q8h
Older patients and patients with cor pulmonale	6 mg/kg	2 mg/kg q6h	2 mg/kg q8h
Patients with congestive heart failure, liver failure	6 mg/kg	2 mg/kg q8h	1–2 mg/kg q12h

cially in children.

Rapid Theophyllinization for Patients with Acute Asthma or Bronchospasm:

For patients not currently receiving theophylline drugs:
(See table on preceding page)

For patients currently receiving theophylline drugs, the time, amount, route and form of the last dose should be determined and blood levels measured if possible before beginning treatment.

Patients should be closely monitored for signs of toxicity.

Patients with Chronic Asthma or Bronchospasm: Slow clinical titration is preferable.

Initial dose: 16 mg/kg/day or 400 mg/day (whichever is lower) in 3 to 4 divided doses at 6 to 8 hour intervals. This may be increased by about 25% at 2 to 3 day intervals if no toxicity occurs until maximum dose is reached (see below).

Maximum dose (dose not to be exceeded in absence of serum determinations)

Under 9 years of age—24 mg/kg/day
9 to 12 years of age—20 mg/kg/day
12 to 16 years of age—18 mg/kg/day
Over 16 years of age—13 mg/kg/day or 900 mg/day (whichever is lower)

During chronic therapy, periodic serum theophylline levels obtained at the time of peak absorption (1 to 2 hours after a dose of an immediate release preparation) are recommended for dosage adjustments. See Warnings and Precautions for special dosage adjustments in neonates (immediate release BRONKODYL only), the elderly, and patients with congestive heart failure, cor pulmonale, liver disease, COPD, etc.
(See table right)

Overdosage: See Adverse Reactions for signs and symptoms or theophylline overdosage.

Treatment:

A. If potential oral overdose is established and seizure has not occurred:
1) Induce vomiting.
2) Administer a cathartic.
3) Administer activated charcoal.

B. If patient is having a seizure:
1) Establish an airway.
2) Administer O_2.
3) Treat the seizure with intravenous diazepam, 0.1 to 0.3 mg/kg up to 10 mg.
4) Monitor vital signs, maintain blood pressure and provide adequate hydration.

C. Post-seizure coma:
1) Maintain airway and oxygenation.
2) If a result of oral medication, follow above recommendations to prevent absorption of drug, but intubation and lavage will have to be performed instead of inducing emesis, and the cathartic and charcoal will need to be introduced via a large bore gastric lavage tube.
3) Continue to provide full supportive care and adequate hydration while waiting for drug to be metabolized. In general, the drug is metabolized sufficiently rapidly so as to not warrant consideration of dialysis.

D. Animal studies suggest that phenobarbital may decrease theophylline toxicity. There are as yet, however, insufficient data to recommend pretreatment of an overdosage with phenobarbital.

How Supplied:

BRONKODYL S-R 300 mg **NDC** 0057-1033-10 blue and white capsules in 100's
Code 1846

BRONKODYL 100 mg **NDC** 0057-1030-10 brown and white capsules in 100's
Code 1831

BRONKODYL 200 mg **NDC** 0057-1031-10 green and white capsules in 100's
Code 1833

BRONKODYL Elixir, **NDC** 0057-1032-16 80 mg per 15 ml, in pints
Code 1835

Examples of Dosage Adjustments Based on Serum Theophylline Levels:

Peak Theophylline Level mcg/ml	Adjustment in Total Daily Dose	Comment
<5	100% increase	
5–7.5	50% increase	If patient is asymptomatic, consider trial off drug, repeat blood levels after adjustment.
8–10	20% increase	Even if patient is asymptomatic at this level an increased serum concentration may prevent symptoms during a viral URI, or heavy exposure to an inhalant allergen.
11–13	cautious 10% increase if clinically indicated	If patient is asymptomatic, no increase is necessary. If symptoms are present during URI or exercise, increase as indicated.
14–20	None	If "breakthrough" in asthmatic symptoms occurs at end of dosing interval, change to sustained-release product and repeat blood level.
	Occasional intolerance requires a 10% decrease	If side effects occur, decrease total daily dose as indicated
21–25	10% decrease	Even if side effects are absent.
26–34	25–33% decrease	Even if side effects are absent, omit next dose and decrease total daily dose as indicated. Repeat blood levels.
>35	50% decrease	Omit next two doses, decrease as indicated and repeat blood levels.

Storage: BRONKODYL S-R: Store at controlled room temperature between 15° and 30°C (59° and 86°F).

BRONKODYL S-R capsules
Mfg. by Cord Laboratories, Inc.
Broomfield, Colorado 80020
BRONKODYL capsules
Mfg. by K.V. Pharmaceutical Co.
St. Louis, Missouri 63144

[*Shown in Product Identification Section*]

BRONKOMETER® ℞
(isoetharine mesylate inhalation aerosol, USP)

Description: BRONKOMETER is a complete pocket nebulizer containing:
Isoetharine mesylate 0.61% (W/W) with saccharin, menthol, alcohol 30% (W/W), and fluorochlorohydrocarbons as gaseous propellants. Preserved with ascorbic acid 0.1% (W/W).
Isoetharine is 1-(3,4 dihydroxyphenyl)-2-isopropylamino-1-butanol. The BRONKOMETER unit delivers approximately 20 metered doses per ml of solution. Each average 56 mg delivery contains 340 mcg isoetharine.

Action: Isoetharine is a sympathomimetic amine with preferential affinity for $Beta_2$ adrenergic receptor sites of bronchial and certain arteriolar musculature, and a lower order of affinity for $Beta_1$ adrenergic receptors. Its activity in symptomatic relief of bronchospasm is rapid and of relatively long duration. By relieving bronchospasm, BRONKOMETER helps give prompt relief and significantly increases vital capacity.

Indications: BRONKOMETER is indicated for use as a bronchodilator for bronchial asthma and for reversible bronchospasm that may occur in association with bronchitis and emphysema.

Contraindications: BRONKOMETER should not be administered to patients who are hypersensitive to any of its ingredients.

Warnings: Excessive use of an adrenergic aerosol should be discouraged as it may lose its effectiveness. Occasional patients have been reported to develop severe paradoxical airway resistance with repeated excessive use of an aerosol adrenergic inhalation preparation. The cause of this refractory state is unknown. It is advisable that in such instances the use of the aerosol adrenergic be discontinued immediately and alternative therapy instituted, since in the reported cases the patients did not respond to other forms of therapy until the drug was withdrawn. Cardiac arrest has been noted in several instances.

BRONKOMETER should not be administered along with epinephrine or other sympathomimetic amines, since these drugs are direct cardiac stimulants and may cause excessive tachycardia. They may, however, be alternated if desired.

Usage in Pregnancy: Although there has been no evidence of teratogenic effects with this drug, use of any drug in pregnancy, lactation, or in women of childbearing potential requires that the potential benefit of the drug be weighed against its possible hazard to the mother or child.

Precautions: Dosage must be carefully adjusted in patients with hyperthyroidism, hypertension, acute coronary disease, cardiac asthma, limited cardiac reserve, and in individuals sensitive to sympathomimetic amines, since overdosage may result in tachycardia, palpitation, nausea, headache, or epinephrine-like side effects.

Adverse Reactions: Although BRONKOMETER is relatively free of toxic side effects, too frequent use may cause tachycardia, palpitation, nausea, headache, changes in blood pressure, anxiety, tension, restlessness, insomnia, tremor, weakness, dizziness, and excitement, as in the case with other sympathomimetic amines.

Dosage and Administration: The average adult dose is one or two inhalations. Occasionally, more may be required. It is important, however, to wait one full minute after the initial one or two inhalations in order to be certain whether another is necessary. In most cases, inhalations need not be repeated more often than every four hours, although more frequent administration may be necessary in severe cases.

How Supplied:
BRONKOMETER® 10 ml Vial with Oral Nebulizer

Continued on next page

Breon—Cont.

Code No. 1740 NDC 0057-1040-01
BRONKOMETER® 20 ml Vial with Oral Nebulizer
Code No. 1742 NDC 0057-1042-02
BRONKOMETER® 10 ml refill only
Code No. 1743 NDC 0057-1043-01
BRONKOMETER® 20 ml refill only
Code No. 1741 NDC 0057-1041-02
The bronchodilator isoetharine is also available in a convenient solution for use with conventional nebulizers, by oxygen aerosolization, and in IPPB machines as
BRONKOSOL® (isoetharine HCl) 1.0%
Bottles of 10 ml Code No. 1771
NDC 0057-1071-10
Bottles of 30 ml Code No. 1772
NDC 0057-1072-30

BRONKOSOL® ℞
(isoetharine HCl inhalation, USP, 1.0%)
BRONCHODILATOR SOLUTION FOR ORAL INHALATION

Description:
Isoetharine HCl 1.0%
in an aqueous-glycerin solution containing sodium chloride, citric acid, and sodium hydroxide, with methylparaben, propylparaben, and acetone sodium bisulfite.

BRONKOSOL® Unit Dose ℞
(isoetharine HCl inhalation, USP, 0.25%)

Description:
Isoetharine HCl 0.25%
in an aqueous-glycerine solution containing sodium chloride, citric acid and sodium hydroxide, with methylparaben, propylparaben, and acetone sodium bisulfite.

Action: Isoetharine is a sympathomimetic amine with preferential affinity for $Beta_2$ adrenergic receptor sites of bronchial and certain arteriolar musculature, and a lower order of affinity for $Beta_1$ adrenergic receptors. Its activity in symptomatic relief of bronchospasm is rapid and of relatively long duration. By relieving bronchospasm BRONKOSOL helps give prompt relief and significantly increases vital capacity.

Indications: BRONKOSOL is indicated for use as a bronchodilator for bronchial asthma and for reversible bronchospasm that may occur in association with bronchitis and emphysema.

Contraindication: BRONKOSOL should not be administered to patients who are hypersensitive to any of its ingredients.

Warnings: Excessive use of an adrenergic aerosol should be discouraged as it may lose its effectiveness. Occasional patients have been reported to develop severe paradoxical airway resistance with repeated excessive use of an aerosol adrenergic inhalation preparation. The cause of this refractory state is unknown. It is advisable that in such instances the use of the aerosol adrenergic be discontinued immediately and alternative therapy instituted, since in the reported cases the patients did not respond to other forms of therapy until the drug was withdrawn. Cardiac arrest has been noted in several instances.
BRONKOSOL should not be administered along with epinephrine or other sympathomimetic amines, since these drugs are direct cardiac stimulants and may cause excessive tachycardia. They may, however, be alternated if desired.

Usage in Pregnancy: Although there has been no evidence of teratogenic effects with this drug, use of any drug in pregnancy, lactation, or in women of childbearing potential requires that the potential benefit of the drug be weighed against its possible hazard to the mother or child.

Precautions: Dosage must be carefully adjusted in patients with hyperthyroidism, hypertension, acute coronary disease, cardiac asthma, limited cardiac reserve, and in individuals sensitive to sympathomimetic amines, since overdosage may result in tachycardia, palpitation, nausea, headache, or epinephrine-like side effects.

Adverse Reactions: Although BRONKOSOL is relatively free of toxic side effects, too frequent use may cause tachycardia, palpitation, nausea, headache, changes in blood pressure, anxiety, tension, restlessness, insomnia, tremor, weakness, dizziness, and excitement, as is the case with other sympathomimetic amines.

Dosage and Administration: BRONKOSOL can be administered by hand nebulizer, oxygen aerosolization, or intermittent positive pressure breathing (IPPB). Usually treatment need not be repeated more often than every four hours, although in severe cases more frequent administration may be necessary.

Method of Administration	Usual Dose	Range	Usual Dilution
Hand nebulizer	4 inhalations	3-7 inhalations	undiluted
Oxygen aerosolization*	½ ml	¼-½ ml	1:3 with saline or other diluent
IPPB†	½ ml	¼-1 ml	1:3 with saline or other diluent

*Administered with oxygen flow adjusted to 4 to 6 liters/minute over a period of 15 to 20 minutes.

†Usually an inspiratory flow rate of 15 liters/minute at a cycling pressure of 15 cm H_2O is recommended. It may be necessary, according to patient and type of IPPB apparatus, to adjust flow rate to 6 to 30 liters per minute, cycling pressure to 10-15 cm H_20, and further dilution according to needs of patient.

BRONKOSOL® Unit Dose—The usual adult dose is 1 BRONKOSOL Unit Dose per nebulization treatment. Usually treatment need not be repeated more often than every four hours, although in severe cases more frequent administration may be necessary.
BRONKOSOL Unit Dose can be administered by various nebulization devices, including pump-driven nebulizers and intermittent positive pressure breathing (IPPB). When administered with oxygen, adjust flow to 4 to 6 liters/-minute over a period of 15 to 20 minutes. When administered via IPPB, usually an inspiratory flow rate of 15 liters/minute at a cycling pressure of 15 cm H_2O is recommended. It may be necessary, according to patient and type of IPPB apparatus, to adjust flow rate to 6 to 30 liters per minute, cycling pressure to 10-15 cm H_2O, and to further dilute according to needs of patient.

Method of use
1. Remove BRONKOSOL Unit Dose and accompanying plunger rod from carton.
2. Screw plunger into rubber stopper at rear end of barrel.
3. Remove rubber cap from front end of barrel. To avoid contamination, do not touch open end.
4. Place open end into nebulizer cup or medication port. Depress plunger rod until barrel is empty. Discard after use.

How Supplied: BRONKOSOL for inhalation—
BRONKOSOL 1% 10 ml **NDC** 0057-1071-10
Code 1771
BRONKOSOL 1% 30 ml **NDC** 0057-1072-30
Code 1772
BRONKOSOL 2 ml
Unit Dose 10's **NDC** 0057-1003-10
Code 1773
Protect from light.
The bronchodilator isoetharine is also available in convenient, ready-to-use measured dose aerosol containers as:
Bronkometer® 10 ml Vial with Oral Nebulizer
Code 1740 **NDC** 0057-1040-01
Bronkometer® 20 ml Vial with Oral Nebulizer for desk or bedside.
Code 1742 **NDC** 0057-1042-02
Bronkometer® 10 ml Refill only
Code 1743 **NDC** 0057-1043-01
Bronkometer® 20 ml Refill only
Code 1741 **NDC** 0057-1041-02
Each contains:
Isoetharine mesylate ....0.61% W/W

BRONKOTABS®

Composition: Each tablet contains ephedrine sulfate 24 mg; guaifenesin 100 mg; theophylline 100 mg; phenobarbital 8 mg (warning: may be habit-forming).

Action and Uses: BRONKOTABS provides bronchodilatation, decongestion, promotes expectoration as well as aids in reducing local bronchial edema, and provides mild sedation—all of which actions are indicated in the treatment of bronchial asthma. For prevention or relief of the symptoms of bronchial asthma, asthmatic bronchitis, chronic bronchitis with emphysema, emphysematous bronchospasm.

Administration and Dosage: *Adults*—Patients will vary in their requirements of BRONKOTABS ; however, a dosage schedule of one tablet administered every three or four hours, four or five times daily, will usually afford symptomatic relief. *Children over six:* One-half the adult dose. *Children under six:* As directed.

Precautions: With BRONKOTABS, sympathomimetic side effects are minimal. Do not exceed the recommended dosage. Frequent or prolonged use may cause nervousness, restlessness, or sleeplessness. Use with caution if hypertension, heart disease, diabetes or hyperthyroidism is present. (Warning: Phenobarbital may be habit-forming.) This preparation may cause drowsiness. Ephedrine may cause urinary retention, especially in the presence of partial obstruction, as in prostatism.

How Supplied: Bottles of 100 and 1000 tablets.

[*Shown in Product Identification Section*]

BRONKOLIXIR®

Composition: Each 5 ml teaspoonful contains:
Ephedrine sulfate, USP ....12 mg
Guaifenesin, USP ....50 mg
Theophylline, USP ....15 mg
Phenobarbital, USP ....4 mg
(Warning: may be habit forming)
in a cherry-flavored solution containing 19% alcohol (v/v).

Action and Uses: BRONKOLIXIR is a rapidly effective cherry-flavored elixir to aid relief of symptoms of asthma and bronchitis. It promotes removal of tenacious mucus as an expectorant; relieves bronchospasm; reduces bronchial edema; serves as a mild sedative to allay anxiety-tension.

Administration and Dosage: *Adults*—Although individual requirements may vary, 2 teaspoonsful of BRONKOLIXIR every three or four hours, four times daily, usually will provide symptomatic relief. *Children over six:* One-half the adult dose. *Children under six:* As directed by physician.

Precautions: With BRONKOLIXIR, sympathomimetic side effects are minimal. Do not exceed the recommended dosage. Frequent or prolonged use may cause nervousness, restlessness, or sleeplessness. Use with caution if hypertension, heart disease, diabetes, or hyperthyroidism is present. (Warning: Phenobarbital may be habit-forming.) This preparation may cause drowsiness. Ephedrine may cause

urinary retention, especially in the presence of partial obstruction, as in prostatism.
How Supplied: Bottles of 16 oz.

CARBOCAINE® Hydrochloride ℞
brand of mepivacaine hydrochloride injection, USP

THESE SOLUTIONS ARE NOT INTENDED FOR SPINAL ANESTHESIA OR DENTAL USE.
Description: Mepivacaine hydrochloride is 1-methyl-2′, 6′-pipecoloxylidide monohydrochloride.
It is a white crystalline, odorless powder, soluble in water, but very resistant to both acid and alkaline hydrolysis. Solutions may be stored for extended periods of time without decomposition and if without vasoconstrictors may be reautoclaved when necessary.
[See table above].
Actions: Mepivacaine stabilizes the neuronal membrane and prevents the initiation and transmission of nerve impulses, thereby effecting local anesthesia.
Onset of anesthesia is rapid, the time of onset for sensory block ranging from about 3 to 20 minutes depending upon such factors as the anesthetic technique, the type of block, the concentration of the solution, and the individual patient. The degree of motor blockade produced is dependent on the concentration of the solution. A 0.5 per cent solution will be effective in small superficial nerve blocks while the 1 per cent concentration will block sensory and sympathetic conduction without loss of motor function. The 1.5 per cent solution will provide extensive and often complete motor block and the 2 per cent concentration of CARBOCAINE will produce complete sensory and motor block of any nerve group.
The duration of anesthesia also varies depending upon the technique and type of block, the concentration, and the individual. Mepivacaine will normally provide anesthesia which is adequate for 2 to 2½ hours of surgery. It has been reported that vasoconstrictors do not significantly prolong anesthesia with mepivacaine but epinephrine (1:200,000) may be added to the mepivacaine solution to promote local hemostasis and to delay systemic absorption of the anesthetic.
Mepivacaine, because of its amide structure, is not detoxified by the circulating plasma esterases. It is rapidly metabolized, with only a small percentage of the anesthetic (5 to 10 per cent) being excreted unchanged in the urine. The liver is the principal site of metabolism, with over 50 per cent of the administered dose being excreted into the bile as metabolites. Most of the metabolized mepivacaine is probably resorbed in the intestine and then excreted into the urine since only a small percentage is found in the feces. The principal route of excretion is via the kidney. Most of the anesthetic and its metabolites are eliminated within 30 hours. It has been shown that hydroxylation and N-demethylation, which are detoxification reactions, play important roles in the metabolism of the anesthetic. Three metabolites of mepivacaine have been identified from adult humans: two phenols, which are excreted almost exclusively as their glucuronide conjugates, and the N-demethylated compound (2′, 6′-pipecoloxylidide).
Mepivacaine does not ordinarily produce irritation or tissue damage.
Indications: CARBOCAINE is indicated for the production of local anesthesia by infiltration injection, peripheral nerve block, and central neural blocks by the lumbar or caudal epidural route.
Contraindications: Mepivacaine is contraindicated in patients with known hypersensitivity to the amide type of local anesthetics or to methylparaben, which is added to the multiple-dose vials.

Composition of Available Solutions

Each ml contains	Single-dose 1% vial	Multiple-dose 1% vial	Single dose 1.5% vial	Single-dose 2% vial	Multiple-dose 2% vial
Mepivacaine hydrochloride	10 mg	10 mg	15 mg	20 mg	20 mg
Sodium chloride	6.6 mg	7 mg	5.6 mg	4.6 mg	5 mg
Potassium chloride	0.3 mg	——	0.3 mg	0.3 mg	——
Calcium chloride	0.33 mg	——	0.33 mg	0.33 mg	——
Methylparaben	——	1 mg	——	——	1 mg
Water for injection	30 ml	50 ml	30 ml	20 ml	50 ml

The pH of the solutions is adjusted between 4.5 and 6.8 with sodium hydroxide or hydrochloric acid.

Warnings: RESUSCITATIVE EQUIPMENT AND DRUGS SHOULD BE IMMEDIATELY AVAILABLE WHENEVER ANY LOCAL ANESTHETIC DRUG IS USED.
Large doses of local anesthetics should not be used in patients with heart block.
Reactions resulting in fatality have occurred on rare occasions with the use of local anesthetics, even in the absence of a history of hypersensitivity.
Solutions which contain a vasoconstrictor should be used with extreme caution in patients receiving drugs known to produce alterations in blood pressure (i.e., monamine oxidase (MAO) inhibitors, tricyclic antidepressants, phenothiazines, etc.) as either severe sustained hypertension or hypotension may occur.
Usage in Children. Great care must be exercised in adhering to safe concentrations and dosages for pediatric administration (see Dosage and Administration).
Usage in Pregnancy. Safe use of mepivacaine has not been established with respect to adverse effects on fetal development. Careful consideration should be given to this fact before administering this drug to women of childbearing potential, particularly during early pregnancy. This does not exclude the use of the drug at term for obstetrical analgesia.
Vasopressor agents (administered for the treatment of hypotension related to caudal or other epidural blocks) should be used with extreme caution in the presence of oxytocic drugs as they are known to interact and may produce severe, persistent hypertension and/or rupture of cerebral blood vessels. CARBOCAINE has been used for obstetrical analgesia by the peridural and paracervical routes without evidence of adverse effects on the fetus when no more than the maximum safe dosages are used and strict adherence to technique is followed.
Local anesthetic procedures should be used with caution when there is inflammation and/or sepsis in the region of the proposed injection.
Precautions: Standard textbooks should be consulted for specific techniques and precautions for various regional anesthetic procedures.
The safety and effectiveness of a local anesthetic drug depend upon proper dosage, correct technique, adequate precautions, and readiness for emergencies.
The lowest dosage that results in effective anesthesia should be used to avoid high plasma levels and possible adverse effects. Injection of repeated doses of mepivacaine may cause significant increase in blood levels with each repeated dose due to slow accumulation of the drug or its metabolites or due to slower metabolic degradation than normal.
Tolerance varies with the status of the patient. Debilitated, elderly patients, or acutely ill patients should be given reduced doses commensurate with their weight and physical status.
Mepivacaine should be used with caution in patients with severe disturbances of cardiac rhythm, shock or heart block.

INJECTION SHOULD ALWAYS BE MADE SLOWLY AND WITH FREQUENT ASPIRATIONS TO AVOID INADVERTENT RAPID INTRAVASCULAR ADMINISTRATION WHICH CAN PRODUCE SYSTEMIC TOXICITY.
Fetal bradycardia which frequently follows paracervical block may be indicative of high fetal blood concentrations of CARBOCAINE with resultant fetal acidosis. Fetal heart rate should be monitored prior to and during paracervical block. Added risk appears to be present in prematurity, toxemia of pregnancy, and fetal distress. The physician should weigh the benefits against the risks in considering paracervical block in these conditions. Careful adherence to recommended dosage is of the utmost importance in paracervical block. Failure to achieve adequate analgesia with these doses should arouse suspicion of intravascular or fetal injection.
Case records of maternal convulsions and cardiovascular collapse following use of mepivacaine for paracervical block in early pregnancy (as anesthesia for elective abortion) suggest that systemic absorption under these circumstances may be rapid. Therefore the recommended maximum dose of 100 mg per side should not be exceeded. Injection should be made slowly and with frequent aspiration. Allow a 5-minute interval between sides.
Vasoconstrictors. Solutions containing a vasoconstrictor should be used cautiously. The decision whether or not to use a vasoconstrictor with local anesthesia depends on the physician's appraisal of the benefits as opposed to the risk, e.g., in injection of solutions containing a vasoconstrictor into areas where the blood supply is limited (e.g., ears, nose, digits) or when peripheral vascular disease is present. Furthermore, serious cardiac arrhythmias may occur if preparations containing a vasoconstrictor are employed in patients during or immediately following the administration of halothane, cyclopropane, trichloroethylene, or other related agents.
MEPIVACAINE SHOULD BE USED WITH CAUTION IN PATIENTS WITH KNOWN DRUG ALLERGIES AND SENSITIVITIES. A thorough history of the patient's prior experience with CARBOCAINE or other local anesthetics as well as concomitant or recent drug use should be taken (see Contraindications). Patients allergic to methylparaben or para-aminobenzoic acid derivatives (procaine, tetracaine, benzocaine, etc.) have not shown cross-sensitivity to agents of the amide-type such as mepivacaine. Since mepivacaine is metabolized in the liver and excreted by the kidneys, it should be used cautiously in patients with liver and renal disease.
Adverse Reactions: Systemic adverse reactions involving the central nervous system and the cardiovascular system usually result from high plasma levels due to excessive dosage,

Continued on next page

Breon—Cont.

rapid absorption, or inadvertent intravascular injection.

A small number of reactions may result from hypersensitivity, idiosyncrasy, or diminished tolerance to normal dosage.

Excitatory CNS effects commonly represent the initial signs of local anesthetic systemic toxicity. However, these reactions may be very brief or absent in some patients in which case the first manifestation of toxicity may be drowsiness merging into unconsciousness and respiratory arrest.

Cardiovascular system reactions include depression of the myocardium, hypotension (or sometimes hypertension), bradycardia, and even cardiac arrest. In obstetrics, cases of fetal bradycardia have occurred (see Precautions).

Allergic reactions are characterized by cutaneous lesions of delayed onset, or urticaria, edema, and other manifestations of allergy. The detection of sensitivity by skin testing is of limited value. As with other local anesthetics, hypersensitivity, idiosyncrasy, and anaphylactoid reactions to CARBOCAINE have occurred rarely. The reaction may be abrupt and severe, and is not usually dose related.

Sensitivity to methylparaben, a preservative added to multiple-dose vials, has been reported. Single dose vials without methylparaben are also available.

Reactions following epidural or caudal anesthesia also may include: high or total spinal block, urinary retention; fecal incontinence; loss of perineal sensation and sexual function; persistent analgesia, paresthesia, and paralysis of the lower extremities; headache and backache; and slowing of labor and consequent increased incidence of forceps delivery.

Treatment of Reactions. Toxic effects of local anesthetics require symptomatic treatment; there is no specific cure. The physician should be prepared to maintain an airway and to support ventilation with oxygen and assisted or controlled respiration as required. Supportive treatment of the cardiovascular system includes intravenous fluids and, when appropriate, vasopressors (preferably those that stimulate the myocardium, such as ephedrine). *Convulsions* may be controlled with oxygen and by the intravenous administration of diazepam or short or ultrashort-acting barbiturates. Intravenous anticonvulsant agents should only be administered by those familiar with their use and only when ventilation and oxygenation are assured. In epidural anesthesia, sympathetic blockade also occurs as a pharmacological reaction, resulting in peripheral vasodilation and often *hypotension*. The extent of the hypotension will usually depend on the number of dermatomes blocked. The blood pressure should therefore be monitored in the early phases of anesthesia. If hypotension occurs, it is readily controlled by vasoconstrictors administered either by the intramuscular or the intravenous route, the dosage of which would depend on the severity of the hypotension and the response to treatment.

Dosage and Administration: As with all local anesthetics, the dose varies and depends upon the area to be anesthetized, the vascularity of the tissues, the number of neuronal segments to be blocked, individual tolerance, and the technique of anesthesia. The lowest dose needed to provide effective anesthesia should be administered. For specific techniques and procedures, refer to standard textbooks.

The recommended single adult dose (or the total of a series of doses given in one procedure) of CARBOCAINE for unsedated, healthy, normal-sized individuals should not usually exceed 400 mg. The recommended dosage is based on requirements for the average adult and should be reduced for elderly or debilitated patients.

While maximum doses of 7 mg/kg (550 mg) have been administered without adverse effect, these are not recommended, except in exceptional circumstances and under no circumstances should the administration be repeated at intervals of less than 1½ hours. The total dose for any 24-hour period should not exceed 1000 mg because of a slow accumulation of the anesthetic or its derivatives or slower than normal metabolic degradation or detoxification with repeat administration (see Actions and Precautions).

Children tolerate the local anesthetic as well as adults. However, the pediatric dose should be carefully measured as a percentage of the total adult dose based on weight, and should not exceed 5 to 6 mg/kg (2.5 to 3 mg/lb) in children, especially those weighing less than 30 lbs. In children under 3 years of age or weighing less than 30 lbs. concentrations less than 2 per cent (e.g., 0.5 to 1.5 per cent) should be employed.

[See table below].

How Supplied:

These solutions are not intended for spinal anesthesia or dental use.

Code C-400 1% single-dose vials of 30 ml (NDC 0057-0231-01)
Code C-390 1% multiple-dose vials of 50 ml (NDC 0057-0232-01)
Code C-430 1.5% single-dose vials of 30 ml (NDC 0057-0234-01)
Code C-440 2% single-dose vials of 20 ml (NDC 0057-0236-01)
Code C-410 2% multiple-dose vials of 50 ml (NDC 0057-0237-01)

For full prescribing information on the dental use of CARBOCAINE see Cook-Waite laboratories, Inc. product listing in this publication.

Recommended Concentrations and Doses of CARBOCAINE

Procedure	Concentration	Total Dose ml	mg	Comments
Cervical, brachial, intercostal, pudendal nerve block	1%	5–40	50–400	Pudendal block; one half of total dose injected each side.
	2%	5–20	100–400	
Transvaginal block (paracervical plus pudendal)	1%	up to 30 (both sides)	up to 300 (both sides)	One half of total dose injected each side. See Precautions.
Paracervical block	1%	up to 20 (both sides)	up to 200 (both sides)	One half of total dose injected each side. This is maximum recommended dose per 90 minute period in obstetrical and non-obstetrical patients. Inject slowly, 5 minutes between sides. See Precautions.
Caudal and Epidural block	1%	15–30	150–300	Use only single dose vials which do not contain a preservative.
	1.5%	10–25	150–375	
	2%	10–20	200–400	
Infiltration	1%	up to 40	up to 400	An equivalent amount of a 0.5% solution (prepared by diluting the 1% solution with Sodium Chloride Injection, USP) may be used for large areas.
Therapeutic block	1%	1–5	10–50	
	2%	1–5	20–50	

Unused portions of solutions not containing preservatives should be discarded.

DEMEROL® APAP Ⓒ ℞
(MEPERIDINE HYDROCHLORIDE, USP) with Acetaminophen

Description: Each tablet, for oral administration, contains:

Meperidine HCl, USP ....50 mg
(WARNING: May be habit forming)
Acetaminophen, USP (APAP) ....300 mg

DEMEROL® hydrochloride, brand of meperidine hydrochloride, is a narcotic analgesic.

Meperidine hydrochloride is ethyl 1-methyl-4-phenylisonipecotate hydrochloride, a white crystalline substance with a melting point of 186° to 189° C. It is readily soluble in water and has a neutral reaction and a slightly bitter taste.

Acetaminophen is an analgesic and antipyretic.

Chemically, acetaminophen is Acetamide, N-(4-hydroxyphenyl)-4′-Hydroxyacetanilide.

Clinical Pharmacology: Meperidine hydrochloride is a narcotic analgesic with multiple actions qualitatively similar to those of morphine; the most prominent of these involve the central nervous system and organs composed of smooth muscle. The principal actions of therapeutic value are analgesia and sedation. There is some evidence which suggests that meperidine may produce less smooth muscle spasm, constipation, and depression of the cough reflex than equianalgesic doses of morphine. Meperidine, in 60 to 80 mg parenteral doses, is approximately equivalent in analgesic effect to 10 mg of morphine. The onset of action is slightly more rapid than with morphine, and the duration of action is slightly shorter. Meperidine is significantly less effective by the oral than by the parenteral route, but the exact ratio of oral to parenteral effectiveness is unknown.

Meperidine is absorbed by all routes of administration.

Meperidine is metabolized chiefly in the liver and excreted in the urine. After intravenous administration, the rapid decline of the concentration in plasma due to distribution is followed by a slower phase with a half-life of about 3 hours. In patients with cirrhosis, the half-life is increased to 6 hours. Approximately 60% of meperidine in plasma is protein bound.

Acetaminophen is a safe and effective analgesic and antipyretic.

Onset of significant analgesic and antipyretic activity of acetaminophen when administered orally occurs within 30 minutes and is maximal at approximately 2½ hours. The pharmacological mode of action of acetaminophen is unknown at this time.

Acetaminophen reduces fever by inhibiting the action of endogenous pyrogen on the hypothalamic heat regulation centers. However, the mechanisms of the antipyretic and analgesic effects of acetaminophen are uncertain.

Acetaminophen is rapidly and almost completely absorbed from the gastrointestinal tract. Peak plasma concentrations occur in 30 to 60 minutes and plasma half-life is from 1 to 3 hours.

Binding of the drug to plasma proteins is variable and dose related. 20% to 50% may be bound to plasma proteins during acute intoxication.

Acetaminophen is conjugated in the liver with glucuronic acid and to a lesser extent with sulfuric acid. Approximately 80% of acetaminophen is excreted in the urine after conjugation and about 3% is excreted unchanged. The drug is also conjugated to a lesser extent with cysteine and metabolites produced by hydroxylation and deacetylation.

DEMEROL APAP provides greater pain relief than either meperidine or acetaminophen alone.

Indications and Usage: For the relief of moderate to severe pain.

Contraindications: DEMEROL APAP should not be administered to patients who are hypersensitive to either meperidine or acetaminophen.

Meperidine is contraindicated in patients who are receiving monoamine oxidase (MAO) inhibitors or those who have received such agents within 14 days.

Therapeutic doses of meperidine have inconsistently precipitated unpredictable, severe, and occasionally fatal reactions in patients who have received such agents within 14 days. The mechanism of these reactions is unclear. Some have been characterized by coma, severe respiratory depression, cyanosis, and hypotension, and have resembled the syndrome of acute narcotic overdose. In other reactions the predominant manifestations have been hyperexcitability, convulsions, tachycardia, hyperpyrexia, and hypertension. Although it is not known that other narcotics are free of the risk of such reactions, virtually all of the reported reactions have occurred with meperidine. If a narcotic is needed in such patients, a sensitivity test should be performed in which repeated, small, incremental doses of morphine are administered over the course of several hours while the patient's condition and vital signs are under careful observation.

(Intravenous hydrocortisone or prednisolone have been used to treat severe reactions, with the addition of intravenous chlorpromazine, in those cases exhibiting hypertension and hyperpyrexia. The usefulness and safety of narcotic antagonists in the treatment of these reactions is unkown.)

Warnings:

Head Injury and Increased Intracranial Pressure: The respiratory depressant effects of meperidine and its capacity to elevate cerebrospinal fluid pressure may be markedly exaggerated in the presence of head injury, other intracranial lesions, or a preexisting increase in intracranial pressure. Furthermore, narcotics produce adverse reactions which may obscure the clinical course of patients with head injuries. In such patients, meperidine must be used with extreme caution and only if its use is deemed essential.

Precautions:

Supraventricular Tachycardias: Meperidine should be used with caution in patients with atrial flutter and other supraventricular tachycardias because of a possible vagolytic action which may produce a significant increase in the ventricular response rate.

Convulsions: Meperidine may aggravate preexisting convulsions in patients with convulsive disorders. If dosage is escalated substantially above recommended levels because of tolerance development, convulsions may occur in individuals without a history of convulsive disorders.

Acute Abdominal Conditions: The administration of meperidine or other narcotics may obscure the diagnosis or clinical course in patients with acute abdominal conditions.

Special Risk Patients: Meperidine should be given with caution and the initial dose should be reduced in certain patients such as the elderly or debilitated, and those with severe impairment of hepatic or renal function, hypothyroidism, Addison's disease, and prostatic hypertrophy or urethral stricture.

Asthma and Other Respiratory Conditions: Meperidine should be used with extreme caution in patients having an acute asthmatic attack, patients with chronic obstructive pulmonary disease or cor pulmonale, patients having a substantially decreased respiratory reserve, and patients with preexisting respiratory depression, hypoxia, or hypercapnia. In such patients, even usual therapeutic doses of narcotics may decrease respiratory drive while simultaneously increasing airway resistance to the point of apnea.

Hypotensive Effect: The administration of meperidine may result in severe hypotension in the postoperative patient or any individual whose ability to maintain blood pressure has been compromised by a depleted blood volume or the administration of drugs such as the phenothiazines or certain anesthetics.

Usage in Ambulatory Patients: Meperidine may impair the mental and/or physical abilities required for the performance of potentially hazardous tasks such as driving a car or operating machinery. The patient should be cautioned accordingly.

Meperidine, like other narcotics, may produce orthostatic hypotension in ambulatory patients.

Since acetaminophen is metabolized by the liver, the question of the safety of its use in the presence of liver disease should be considered.

Drug Interactions: Meperidine should be used with great caution and in reduced dosage in patients who are concurrently receiving other narcotic analgesics, general anesthetics, phenothiazines, other tranquilizers, sedative-hypnotics (including barbiturates), tricyclic antidepressants, and other CNS depressants (including alcohol). Respiratory depression, hypotension, and profound sedation or coma may result.

Carcinogenesis, Mutagenesis, Impairment of Fertility: Carcinogenesis, mutagenesis, and impairment of fertility studies have not been done with the combination product.

Pregnancy Category C: Meperidine has been shown to be teratogenic in hamsters. There are no adequate and well-controlled studies in pregnant women. DEMEROL should be used during pregnancy only if the potential benefit justifies potential risk to the fetus.

Labor and Delivery: When used as an obstetrical analgesic, meperidine crosses the placental barrier and can produce depression of respiration and psychophysiologic functions in the newborn. Resuscitation may be required.

Nursing Mothers: Because of the potential for serious adverse reaction in nursing infants from DEMEROL, a decision should be made whether to discontinue nursing or to discontinue the drug, taking into account the importance of the drug to the mother.

Adverse Reactions: The major hazards of DEMEROL APAP are those of meperidine.

Nervous System: Euphoria, dysphoria, weakness, headache, agitation, tremor, uncoordinated muscle movements, transient hallucinations and disorientation, visual disturbances, lightheadedness, dizziness, sedation. Inadvertent injection about a nerve trunk may result in sensory-motor paralysis which is usually, though not always, transitory.

Gastrointestinal: Dry mouth, constipation, biliary tract spasm, nausea, vomiting, and sweating.

Cardiovascular: Flushing of the face, tachycardia, bradycardia, palpitation, hypotension, syncope; to a lesser degree, circulatory depression, shock, and cardiac arrest have occurred.

Respiratory: Respiratory depression, respiratory arrest.

Genitourinary: Urinary retention.

Allergic: Pruritus, urticaria, other skin rashes.

Numerous clinical studies have shown that acetaminophen, when taken in recommended doses, is relatively free of adverse effects in most age groups, even in the presence of a variety of disease states.

A few cases of hypersensitivity to acetaminophen have been reported, as manifested by skin rashes, thrombocytopenic purpura, rarely hemolytic anemia and agranulocytosis. Occasional individuals respond to ordinary doses with nausea and vomiting or diarrhea.

Drug Abuse and Dependence: DEMEROL APAP is a Schedule II controlled substance.

No abuse pattern has been established with the combination meperidine and acetaminophen nor with acetaminophen alone.

However, psychic dependence, physical dependence, and tolerance may develop upon repeated administration of narcotics; therefore, DEMEROL APAP should be prescribed and administered with caution. However, psychic dependence is unlikely to develop when DEMEROL APAP is used for a short time for the treatment of pain. Physical dependence assumes clinically significant proportions only after several weeks of continued narcotic use, although some mild degree of physical dependence may develop after a few days of narcotic therapy. Tolerance is manifested initially by a shortened duration of analgesic effect, and subsequently by decreases in the intensity of analgesia. The rate of development of tolerance varies among patients. Withdrawal symptoms in patients dependent on DEMEROL include yawning, sweating, lacrimation, rhinorrhea, restlessness, sleeplessness, dilated pupils, gooseflesh, irritability, tremor, nausea, vomiting and diarrhea. Treatment of the abstinence syndrome is primarily symptomatic and supportive, including maintenance of proper fluid or electrolyte balance.

Overdosage:

Symptoms: The major symptoms of overdosage with DEMEROL APAP are those of overdosage with meperidine. Serious overdose with meperidine is characterized by respiratory depression (a decrease in respiratory rate and/or tidal volume, Cheyne-Stokes respiration, cyanosis), extreme somnolence progressing to stupor or coma, skeletal muscle flaccidity, cold and clammy skin, and sometimes bradycardia and hypotension. In severe overdosage, apnea, circulatory collapse, cardiac arrest, and death may occur.

In acute acetaminophen overdosage, dose-dependent, potentially fatal hepatic necrosis is the most serious adverse effect. Renal tubular necrosis, hypoglycemic coma and thrombocytopenia may also occur.

In adults, a single dose of 10 to 15 g (200 to 250 mg/kg) of acetaminophen may cause hepatotoxicity. A dose of 25 g or more is potentially fatal. The potential seriousness of the intoxica-

Continued on next page

Breon—Cont.

tion may not be evident during the first two days of acute acetaminophen poisoning. During the first 24 hours, nausea, vomiting, anorexia and abdominal pain occur. These may persist for a week or more. Liver injury may become evident the second day, initial signs being elevation of serum transaminase and lactic dehydrogenase activity, increased serum bilirubin concentration and prolongation of prothrombin time. Serum albumin concentration and alkaline phosphatase activity may remain normal. The hepatotoxicity may lead to encephalopathy, coma and death. Transient azotemia is evident in a majority of patients and acute renal failure occurs in some. There have been reports of glycosuria and impaired glucose tolerance, but hypoglycemia may also occur. Metabolic acidosis and metabolic alkalosis have been reported. Cerebral edema and nonspecific myocardial depression have also been noted. Biopsy reveals centrolobular necrosis with sparing of the periportal area. The hepatic lesions are reversible over a period of weeks or months in nonfatal cases.

The severity of the liver injury can be determined by measurement of the plasma half-life of acetaminophen during the first day of acute poisoning. If the half-life exceeds 4 hours, hepatic necrosis is likely and if the half-life is greater than 12 hours, hepatic coma will probably occur. Only minimal liver damage has developed when the serum concentration was below 120 μg/ml at 12 hours after ingestion of the drug. If serum bilirubin concentration is greater than 4 mg/100 ml during the first 5 days, encephalopathy may occur.

Treatment: Primary attention should be given to the reestablishment of adequate respiratory exchange through provision of a patent airway and institution of assisted or controlled ventilation. The narcotic antagonist, naloxone hydrochloride, is a specific antidote against respiratory depression which may result from overdosage or unusual sensitivity to narcotics, including meperidine. Therefore, an appropriate dose of this antagonist should be administered, preferably by the intravenous route, simultaneously with efforts at respiratory resuscitation.

An antagonist should not be administered in the absence of clinically significant respiratory or cardiovascular depression.

Oxygen, intravenous fluids, vasopressors, and other supportive measures should be employed as indicated.

In cases of overdosage with DEMEROL APAP tablets, the stomach should be evacuated by emesis or gastric lavage.

NOTE: In an individual physically dependent on narcotics, the administration of the usual dose of a narcotic antagonist will precipitate an acute withdrawal syndrome. The severity of this syndrome will depend on the degree of physical dependence and the dose of anatagonist administered. The use of narcotic antagonists in such individuals should be avoided if possible. If a narcotic antagonist must be used to treat serious respiratory depression in the physically dependent patient, the antagonist should be administered with extreme care and only one-fifth to one-tenth the usual initial dose administered.

There are no proven antidotes for acetaminophen and treatment of acute overdosage is purely symptomatic. Vigorous supportive therapy is required in severe intoxication. Procedures to limit the continuing absorption of the drug must be readily performed since the hepatic injury is dose dependent and occurs early in the course of intoxication. Induction of vomiting or gastric lavage, followed by oral administration of activated charcoal should be done in all cases.

If hemodialysis can be initiated within the first 12 hours, it is advocated for patients with a plasma acetaminophen concentration exceeding 120 μg/ml at 4 hours after ingestion of the drug.

Oral LD_{50} of DEMEROL in the rat: 162 mg/kg and in the mouse: 200 mg/kg.

DEMEROL is not dialysable.

Dosage and Administration:

For Relief of Pain

Dosage should be adjusted according to the severity of the pain and the response of the patient. Meperidine is less effective orally than on parenteral administration.

The usual *adult* dose is 1 or 2 tablets, repeated, if necessary, at intervals of three to four hours. Prolonged administration is not recommended. May be habit forming.

How Supplied: Code #1312 DEMEROL APAP, Pink red-mottled tablets, bottles of 100.

NDC 0057-1022-10

[*Shown in Product Identification Section*]

FERGON®
brand of ferrous gluconate
FERGON® ELIXIR

Composition: FERGON (ferrous gluconate, USP) is stabilized to maintain a minimum of ferric ions. It contains not less than 11.5 per cent iron. Each FERGON tablet contains 320 mg. FERGON Elixir 6% contains 300 mg per teaspoon.

Action and Uses: FERGON preparations produce rapid hemoglobin regeneration in patients with iron deficiency anemias. FERGON is better utilized and better tolerated than other forms of iron because of its low ionization constant and solubility in the entire pH range of the gastrointestinal tract. It does not precipitate proteins or have the astringency of more ionizable forms of iron, does not interfere with proteolytic or diastatic activities of the digestive system, and will not produce nausea, abdominal cramps, constipation or diarrhea in the great majority of patients.

FERGON preparations are indicated in anemias amenable to iron therapy: (1) hypochromic anemia of infancy and childhood; (2) idiopathic hypochromic anemia; (3) hypochromic anemia of pregnancy; and (4) anemia associated with chronic blood loss.

Administration and Dosage: Adults—one or two FERGON tablets or one or two teaspoons of FERGON Elixir three times daily. Children 6–12 years—one FERGON tablet or one teaspoon of FERGON Elixir one to three times daily, as directed by the physician. Infants—30 drops of FERGON Elixir, gradually increasing to 1 teaspoon daily.

How Supplied: FERGON, tablets of 320 mg (5 grains), bottles of 100, 500 and 1,000. FERGON Elixir 6% (5 grains per teaspoon), bottles of 1 pint.

[*Shown in Product Identification Section*]

FERGON® CAPSULES

Composition: Each FERGON Capsule contains 435 mg of ferrous gluconate, yielding 50 mg of elemental iron.

Action and Uses: FERGON preparations produce rapid hemoglobin regeneration in patients with iron deficiency anemias. FERGON is better utilized and better tolerated than other forms of iron because of its low ionization constant and solubility in the entire pH range of the gastrointestinal tract. It does not precipitate proteins or have the astringency of more ionizable forms of iron, does not interfere with proteolytic or diastatic activities of the digestive system, and will not produce nausea, abdominal cramps, constipation or diarrhea in the great majority of patients. The pellets of ferrous gluconate contained in FERGON Capsules are coated to permit maximum availability of iron in the upper small bowel, the site of maximum absorption.

FERGON preparations are indicated in anemias amenable to iron therapy: (1) hypochromic anemia of infancy and childhood; (2) idiopathic hypochromic anemia; (3) hypochromic anemia of pregnancy; and (4) anemia associated with chronic blood loss.

Administration and Dosage: 1 FERGON Capsule daily for mild to moderate iron deficiency anemia. For more severe anemia the dosage may be increased.

How Supplied: FERGON Capsules, bottles of 30.

[*Shown in Product Identification Section*]

FERGON® PLUS ℞
FOR IRON DEFICIENCY AND MACROCYTIC ANEMIAS

Description: Each sugar-coated Caplet contains:

Ferrous gluconate, USP ....500 mg
Vitamin B_{12} With Intrinsic Factor
Concentrate NF XI ....½ unit (oral)
Ascorbic acid, USP ....75 mg

Action: Vitamin B_{12} With Intrinsic Factor Concentrate as contained in 2 FERGON Plus Caplets® represents 1 NF XI oral unit of antianemia activity, that is, the amount of material which, when administered daily by mouth, produces a satisfactory hematologic and symptomatic response in patients in relapse with pernicious anemia.

Vitamin B_{12} is the principal active anti-pernicious anemia factor of liver extract and is believed to be essentially extrinsic factor. Its anti-pernicious anemia activity is approximately the same as that produced by liver extract and, like the latter, it is more effective by injection than by mouth. However, its activity on oral administration is increased by the concomitant ingestion of Intrinsic Factor Concentrate which facilitates absorption of Vitamin B_{12} from the alimentary tract.

Ferrous gluconate is better utilized and better tolerated than other forms of iron and produces rapid hemoglobin regeneration when iron deficiency is present. Vitamin C appears to play a role in the absorption of iron. Its deficiency leads to depression of bone marrow activity.

Indications: *Dietary Supplement*—FERGON Plus is useful as a dietary supplement and as a maintenance source of Vitamin B_{12}, Vitamin C and iron. However, it should be remembered that the development of the classic symptoms of pernicious anemia may in some cases be delayed by oral ingestion of Intrinsic Factor.

Therapy—FERGON Plus is indicated for all anemias amenable to iron therapy including (1) hypochromic anemia of infancy and childhood; (2) idiopathic hypochromic anemia; (3) hypochromic anemia of pregnancy; and (4) anemia associated with chronic blood loss.

FERGON Plus is also indicated for patients with anemias responding to oral Vitamin B_{12} therapy; viz., those in whom the bone marrow is in a state of megaloblastic arrest reflected in the blood stream by macrocytosis, anisocytosis and poikilocytosis, including macrocytic anemia of tropical and nontropical sprue, megaloblastic anemias of pregnancy and infancy, and pernicious anemia amenable to oral B_{12} therapy. Similarly, FERGON Plus may be given orally to patients with pernicious anemia to supplement parenterally administered Vitamin B_{12} therapy.

Note—All patients with pernicious anemia should be given periodic examinations, and laboratory studies should be performed. Some patients may not respond to orally ingested Vitamin B_{12} with Intrinsic Factor Concentrate. There is no known way to predict which patients will respond or which patients may cease to respond.

Dosage: As dietary supplement—1 Caplet daily. Therapeutic dose—1 Caplet twice daily (before the morning and evening meals).

When the condition is severe, the initial dose should be increased to 2 Caplets twice daily for one or two weeks, or specific parenteral therapy should be employed.

Caution: Federal law prohibits dispensing without prescription.

How Supplied: Bottles of 100. Code 1640 **NDC** 0057-1017-10

ISUPREL® Hydrochloride ℞

brand of isoproterenol hydrochloride injection, USP

Sterile Injection 1:5000

Description: ISUPREL hydrochloride (brand of isoproterenol hydrochloride) is 3,4-dihydroxy-α-[(isopropylamino) methyl] benzyl alcohol hydrochloride, a synthetic sympathomimetic amine that is structurally related to epinephrine but acts almost exclusively on beta receptors.

Each milliliter of the sterile 1:5000 solution contains 0.2 mg ISUPREL hydrochloride (brand of isoproterenol hydrochloride) 0.12 mg lactic acid, 1.8 mg sodium lactate, 7 mg sodium chloride, and not more than 1 mg sodium bisulfite as preservative. The pH is adjusted with hydrochloric acid. The air in the ampuls has been displaced by nitrogen gas.

Action: The primary actions of ISUPREL are on the heart and on smooth muscle of bronchi, skeletal muscle vasculature, and alimentary tract. The positive inotropic and chronotropic actions of the drug increase cardiac output. There is also an increase in venous return to the heart. With usual therapeutic doses, the increase in cardiac output is generally sufficient to maintain or increase systolic blood pressure. ISUPREL also lowers peripheral vascular resistance; the diastolic pressure, therefore, may be expected to fall in normal individuals. Thus, the mean pressure may be reduced. The rate of discharge of cardiac pacemakers is increased with isoproterenol.

ISUPREL relaxes most smooth muscle, the most pronounced effect being on bronchial and gastrointestinal smooth muscle. It produces marked relaxation in the smaller bronchi and may even dilate the trachea and main bronchi past the resting diameter.

The acute toxicity of ISUPREL in animals is much less than that of epinephrine. Excessive doses in animals or man can cause a striking drop in blood pressure, and repeated large doses in animals may result in cardiac enlargement and focal myocarditis.

Indications: Parenteral isoproterenol hydrochloride is indicated as an adjunct in the management of shock (hypoperfusion syndrome) and in the treatment of cardiac standstill or arrest; carotid sinus hypersensitivity; Adams-Stokes syndrome; and ventricular tachycardia and ventricular arrhythmias that require increased inotropic cardiac activity for therapy. It may also be used in the management of bronchospasm during anesthesia.

SHOCK (HYPOPERFUSION SYNDROME)

Shock is a complex clinical syndrome characterized by inadequate tissue perfusion, which results from one or more of the following mechanisms: loss of effective blood volume, cardiac failure, peripheral vascular failure. Rational therapy must be aimed at correcting this perfusion deficit.

Since shock is often, but by no means always, associated with lowered blood pressure, administration of vasoactive drugs that increase blood pressure without increasing blood flow may not be in the best interests of the patient. However, in cases of shock characterized chiefly by peripheral vasodilation and in shock following acute myocardial infarction, according to one group of investigators, a vasopressor such as levarterenol bitartrate injection, USP, may be indicated.[1,2]

In addition to the routine monitoring of systemic blood pressure, heart rate, urine flow, and the use of the electrocardiogram, the shock state and the response to therapy should be monitored by frequent determinations of the central venous pressure, blood pH, and blood pCO_2(or bicarbonate). Determinations of cardiac output and circulation time may also be helpful.

Adequate filling of the intravascular compartment by suitable volume expanders is of primary importance in most cases of shock, and should precede the administration of vasoactive drugs. Determination of central venous pressure is a reliable guide during volume replacement. If evidence of hypoperfusion persists after adequate volume replacement, ISUPREL may be given.

ISUPREL increases cardiac output by increasing the strength of cardiac contraction and, to a limited extent, the rate of contraction. ISUPREL also increases venous return to the heart by mobilizing blood from vascular reservoirs.[3] In addition, the peripheral and coronary vasodilating effects of the drug may aid tissue perfusion. ISUPREL may be given to patients who are fully digitalized;[4,5] in fact, ISUPREL may be particularly useful when cardiac competence cannot be restored by digitalization.

Appropriate measures should be taken to ensure adequate ventilation. Careful attention should be paid to acid-base balance and to the correction of electrolyte disturbance. In cases of shock associated with bacteremia, suitable antimicrobial therapy is, of course, imperative. In a group of 10 patients with elevated central venous pressures who were in shock from cardiac failure, isoproterenol produced increases in cardiac output of 0.33 to 4.34 liters per minute in nine of the ten.[6] Similarly, in a series of 12 patients with shock due to gram-negative bacteremia, Kardos[7] found isoproterenol to be useful in correcting the hemodynamic alterations.

Although the ultimate effect of ISUPREL on patient survival has not yet been documented, experimental studies in rats have shown that the fatal course of shock caused by transient hemorrhage was reversed by treatment with isoproterenol after replacement of blood volume.[3] In addition, clinical studies[5–15] have indicated that in a majority of patients in shock, administration of ISUPREL tends to correct the hemodynamic abnormalities.

Contraindication: Administration of ISUPREL is contraindicated in patients with tachycardia caused by digitalis intoxication.

Warning: ISUPREL infusions may produce an increase in myocardial work and oxygen consumption. These effects may be detrimental to myocardial metabolism and functioning in patients who are in cardiogenic shock secondary to coronary artery occlusion and myocardial infarction.

Precautions: ISUPREL and epinephrine should not be administered simultaneously, since both drugs are direct cardiac stimulants and their combined effects may induce serious arrhythmia. The drugs may, however, be administered alternately provided a proper interval has elapsed between doses.

Dosage of ISUPREL should be carefully adjusted particularly in patients with coronary insufficiency, diabetes, or hyperthyroidism, and in patients sensitive to sympathomimetic amines.

Hypovolemia should be corrected by suitable volume expanders before treatment with ISUPREL. Patients in shock should be closely observed during ISUPREL administration. If the heart rate exceeds 110 beats per minute, it may be advisable to decrease the infusion rate or temporarily discontinue the infusion. Doses of ISUPREL sufficient to increase the heart rate to more than 130 beats per minute may induce ventricular arrhythmia.

There has been no clinical evidence of teratogenic effects attributable to ISUPREL in more than 20 years' use of the drug. However, before administration of any drug to pregnant women or women of childbearing potential, the expected benefit of the drug should be carefully weighed against the possible risk to the mother or child.

Dosage and Administration: ISUPREL hydrochloride Solution 1:5000 should be diluted in 5 per cent Dextrose Injection, USP, before it is administered to patients in shock.

- A convenient dilution is 1 mg ISUPREL (5 ml) in 500 ml diluent (final concentration, 1:500,000).
- Concentrations up to 10 times greater have been used.[6] This may be important in patients in whom limitation of volume is essential.
- Infusion rates of 0.5 to 5 μg per minute (0.25 to 2.5 ml diluted solution 1:500,000) have been recommended.
- Rates over 30 μg per minute have been used in advanced stages of shock.

The speed of infusion should be adjusted on the basis of heart rate, central venous pressure, systemic blood pressure, and urine flow. If the heart rate exceeds 110 beats per minute, it may be advisable to decrease the infusion rate or temporarily discontinue the infusion.

CARDIAC STANDSTILL AND CARDIAC ARRHYTHMIAS

Because it has potent inotropic cardiac stimulant action with little or no pressor activity, ISUPREL hydrochloride, brand of isoproterenol hydrochloride, has been effective for the treatment of the following:

1. Adams-Stokes syndrome—atrioventricular heart block
2. Cardiac standstill (arrest)
3. Carotid sinus hypersensitivity
4. Ventricular arrhythmias, especially certain types of ventricular tachycardia and fibrillation occurring during the course of atrioventricular block.

It should be noted that in symptomatic heart block, electrical pacing is the preferred method of treatment for maintenance of an adequate ventricular rate. Moreover, in ventricular arrhythmias, especially certain types of ventricular tachycardia and fibrillation, electroshock may have to be used, and is usually the treatment of choice.

If, however, therapy with ISUPREL is elected in these conditions, intravenous administration, with constant monitoring, is preferred.

In patients with heart block and episodic ventricular tachycardia or fibrillation, ISUPREL stimulates the higher centers or nodal tissue without exciting the lower ventricular foci. In so doing, the normal idioventricular pacemaker function may take over, thereby abolishing ventricular acceleration. Epinephrine is contraindicated in patients with ventricular fibrillation because it may precipitate or prolong fibrillation by stimulation of multiple higher and lower foci. It also may further embarrass the cardiovascular system by its hypertensive action.

Intravenous administration of ISUPREL has been recommended for the management of patients with complete heart block following closure of ventricular septal defects. A 1:50,000 solution may be administered intravenously in doses ranging from 0.5 to 1.5 ml for infants and from 2 to 3 ml for adults. With such doses the heart rate accelerates and the effect often lasts for 15 or 20 minutes. Sinus rhythm sometimes occurs and persists for a variable period but often relapses again into complete block. In other cases, ISUPREL merely maintains an

Continued on next page

Breon—Cont.

acceptable heart rate somewhere above 90 to 100 beats per minute. The patient must be monitored constantly by electrocardiography.
Contraindications: Use of isoproterenol in patients with preexisting cardiac arrhythmias associated with tachycardia is generally considered contraindicated because the chronotropic effect of the drug on the heart may aggravate such disorders. Exceptions consist only of those ventricular tachycardias and ventricular arrhythmias which require increased inotropic cardiac activity for therapy.
Administration of ISUPREL is contraindicated in patients with tachycardia caused by digitalis intoxication.
Precautions: ISUPREL and epinephrine should not be administered simultaneously, since both drugs are direct cardiac stimulants and their combined effects may induce serious arrhythmia. The drugs may, however, be administered alternately provided a proper interval has elasped between doses.
Dosage of ISUPREL should be carefully adjusted in patients with coronary insufficiency, diabetes, or hyperthyroidism, and in patients sensitive to sympathomimetic amines.
If the cardiac rate increases sharply, patients with angina pectoris may experience anginal pain until the cardiac rate decreases.
There has been no clinical evidence of teratogenic effects attributable to ISUPREL in more than 20 years' use of the drug. However, before administration of any drug to pregnant women or women of childbearing potential, the expected benefit of the drug should be carefully weighed against the possible risk to the mother or child.
Adverse Reactions: Serious reactions to ISUPREL are infrequent. The following reactions, however, have been reported: flushing of the face, sweating, mild tremors, nervousness, headache, and tachycardia with palpitation manifested as a sensation of pounding in the chest. These reactions disappear quickly and usually do not require discontinuation of treatment with ISUPREL. No cumulative effects have been reported. Pulmonary edema has been reported in a patient extremely intolerant to all sympathomimetic drugs.[16]
In a few patients, presumably with organic disease of the A-V node and its branches, ISUPREL has been reported, paradoxically, to precipitate Adams-Stokes seizures during normal sinus rhythm or transient heart block.[16]
Dosage and Administration: In the treatment and prevention of cardiac standstill and cardiac arrhythmias, parenteral ISUPREL may be administered by intravenous injection, infusion, intramuscular and subcutaneous injection, and *in extremis*, by intracardiac injection.
The following table summarizes the dosage regimen suggested for various routes of administration in adults. Children may be given half the initial adult dose. In all patients, subsequent dosage and method of administration depend on the response of the ventricular rate and the rapidity with which the cardiac pacemaker can take over when the drug is gradually withdrawn.
The usual route of administration in emergency treatment of patients threatened with cardiac standstill or arrhythmia is by intravenous injection or infusion. Dosage must be regulated by monitoring of the electrocardiogram. If time is not of utmost importance, initial therapy by intramuscular or subcutaneous injection is preferred.
[See table below, left].

Dosage of ISUPREL for Cardiac Standstill and Cardiac Arrhythmias in Adults

Route of Administration	Preparation of Dilution	Initial Dose	Subsequent Dose Range
Intravenous	Dilute 1 ml of Solution 1:5000 (0.2 mg) to 10 ml with Sodium Chloride Injection, USP, or 5% Dextrose Injection, USP.	0.02 to 0.06 mg (1 to 3 ml of diluted solution 1:50,000)	0.01 to 0.2 mg (0.5 to 10 ml of diluted solution)
Intravenous infusion	Dilute 10 ml of Solution 1:5000 (2 mg) in 500 ml of 5% Dextrose Injection, USP.	5 μg/min (1.25 ml of diluted solution 1:250,000 per minute)	
Intramuscular	Use Solution 1:5000 undiluted	0.2 mg (1 ml)	0.02 to 1 mg (0.1 to 5 ml)
Subcutaneous	Use Solution 1:5000 undiluted	0.2 mg (1 ml)	0.15 to 0.2 mg (0.75 to 1 ml)
Intracardiac	Use Solution 1:5000 undiluted	0.02 mg (0.1 ml)	

BRONCHOSPASM DURING ANESTHESIA

Parenteral ISUPREL hydrochloride, brand of isoproterenol hydrochloride, has been shown under experimental and clinical conditions to be a potent bronchodilating agent. However, when given in dosages to achieve this effect, it may also have a stimulating effect on the cardiovascular system. Like epinephrine, it may produce arrhythmias in patients anesthetized with cyclopropane, and should be used with caution. ISUPREL can be used for the management of bronchospasm by helping the patient to maintain adequate ventilation and a normally functioning circulatory system.
Precautions and Adverse Reactions: See corresponding sections under "Cardiac Standstill and Cardiac Arrhythmias."
Dosage and Administration: For the management of bronchospasm during anesthesia, 1 ml of ISURPEL Solution 1:5000 is diluted to 10 ml with Sodium Chloride Injection, USP, or 5 per cent Dextrose Injection, USP. An initial dose of 0.01 to 0.02 mg (0.5 to 1 ml of the diluted solution, 1:50,000) is administered intravenously, and may be repeated when necessary.
How Supplied:
Code I-292 1 ml ampuls (0.2 mg)
UNI-NEST PAK of 25 **NDC-0057-0866-25**
Code I-330 5 ml ampuls (1 mg)
Box of 10 **NDC-0057-0867-02**
Protect from light–keep in opaque container until used.
Bibliography:

1. Gunnar, R.M., Loeb, H.S., Pietras, R.J., and Tobin, J.R., Jr.: *J.A.M.A. 202*:1124, Dec. 25, 1967.
2. Loeb, H.S., Pietras, R.J., Tobin, J.R., Jr., and Gunnar, R. M.: *Clin. Res. 15*:213, April 1967.
3. Weil, M. H. and Bradley, E.C.: *Bull. N.Y. Acad. Med. 42*:1023, Nov. 1966.
4. Cohn, J. N.: *GP 34*:78, Aug. 1966.
5. du Toit, H. J., du Plessis, J. M. E., Dommisse, J., Rorke, M. J., Theron, M. S., and de Villiers, V. P.: *Lancet 2*:143, July 16, 1966.
6. MacLean, L. D., Duff, J. H., Scott, H. M., and Peretz, D. I.: *Surg. Gynec. Obstet. 120*:1, Jan. 1965.
7. Kardos, G. G.: *New Eng. J. Med. 274*:868, April 21, 1966.
8. Duff, J. H., Scott, H. M., Peretz, D. I., Mulligan, G. W., and MacLean, L. D.: *J. Trauma 6*:145, March 1966.
9. Duff, J. H., McLean, A. P. H., Mulligan, G. W., and MacLean, L. D.: *Acad. Med. New Jersey Bull. 12*:193, Sept. 1966.
10. Duff, J. H., Peretz, D. I., Scott, H. M., Wigmore, R. A., and MacLean, L. D.: *J. Okla. Med. Ass. 59*:437, Aug. 1966.
11. Brown, R. S., Carey, J. S., Mohr, Patricia A., Monson, D. O., and Shoemaker, W. C.: *Circulation 34*:260, Aug. 1966.
12. Brown, R. S., Carey, J. S., Woodward, N. W., Mohr, Patricia A., and Shoemaker, W. C.: *Surg. Gynec. Obstet. 122*:303, Feb. 1966.
13. Wilson, J. N.: *Arch. Surg. 91*:92, July 1965.
14. Loeb, H. S., Stavrakos, C., Pietras, R. J., Tobin, J. R., Jr., and Gunnar, R. M.: *Circulation 34*:III, Oct., Suppl. 3, 1966. (abstr.)
15. Torpey, D. J.: *J.A.M.A. 202*:955, Dec. 4, 1967.
16. Schwartz, S. P. and Schwartz, L. S.: *Amer. Heart J. 57*:849, June 1959.

ISUPREL® Hydrochloride ℞

brand of isoproterenol hydrochloride, USP
MISTOMETER®

Potent Bronchodilator

Description: ISUPREL MISTOMETER is a complete nebulizing unit consisting of a plastic-coated vial of aerosol solution, detachable plastic mouthpiece with built-in nebulizer, and protective cap. The vial contains ISUPREL hydrochloride in inert propellants (dichlorodifluoromethane and dichlorotetrafluorethane) with alcohol 33 per cent (w/w) and ascorbic acid. The contents permit the delivery of not less than 300 actuations from the 16.8 g (15 ml) vial or not less than 450 actuations from the 25.2 g (22.5 ml) vial. The MISTOMETER unit delivers a measured dose of 131 μg of the bronchodilator in a fine, even mist for inhalation.
Action: ISUPREL relaxes bronchial spasm and facilitates expectoration of pulmonary secretions. It is frequently effective when epinephrine and other drugs fail, and it has a wide margin of safety. In dogs the toxic dose is 1000 times the therapeutic dose. Converted to the amount used clinically in man, this would be about 2500 times the therapeutic dose.
Indications: ISUPREL is indicated for the treatment of bronchospasm associated with acute and chronic bronchial asthma, pulmonary emphysema, bronchitis, and bronchiectasis.
Contraindication: Use of isoproterenol in patients with preexisting cardiac arrhythmias associated with tachycardia is generally considered contraindicated because the cardiac stimulant effect of the drug may aggravate such disorders.
Warnings: Excessive use of an adrenergic aerosol should be discouraged as it may lose its effectiveness.
In patients with status asthmaticus and abnormal blood gas tensions, improvement in vital capacity and in blood gas tensions may not accompany apparent relief of bronchospasm. Facilities for administering oxygen mixtures

and ventilatory assistance are necessary for such patients.

Occasional patients have been reported to develop severe paradoxical airway resistance with repeated, excessive use of isoproterenol inhalation preparations. The cause of this refractory state is unknown. It is advisable that in such instances the use of the preparation be discontinued immediately and alternative therapy instituted, since in the reported cases the patients did not respond to other forms of therapy until the drug was withdrawn.

Deaths have been reported following excessive use of isoproterenol inhalation preparations and the exact cause is unknown. Cardiac arrest was noted in several instances.

Precautions: Epinephrine should not be administered concomitantly with ISUPREL, as both drugs are direct cardiac stimulants and their combined effects may induce serious arrhythmia. If desired they may, however, be alternated, provided an interval of at least four hours has elapsed.

Isoproterenol should be used with caution in patients with cardiovascular disorders including coronary insufficiency, diabetes, or hyperthyroidism, and in persons sensitive to sympathomimetic amines.

A single treatment with the ISUPREL MISTOMETER unit is usually sufficient for controlling isolated attacks of asthma. Any patient who requires more than three aerosol treatments within a 24-hour period should be under the close supervision of his physician. Further therapy with the bronchodilator aerosol alone is inadvisable when three to five treatments within six to twelve hours produce minimal or no relief.

During the course of over 25 years of use of ISUPREL, isoproterenol, there has been no clinical evidence of teratogenic effects. However, use of any drug in pregnancy, lactation, or in women in childbearing age requires that the potential benefit of the drug be weighed against its possible hazards to the mother or child.

Adverse Reactions: The mist from the ISUPREL MISTOMETER unit contains alcohol but is generally very well tolerated. An occasional patient may experience some transient throat irritation which has been attributed to the alcohol content.

Tachycardia, palpitation, nervousness, nausea, and vomitting may occur from overdosage. Rarely do headache, flushing of the skin, tremor, dizziness, weakness, sweating, precordial distress, or anginal-type pain occur. The inhalation route is usually accompanied by a minimum of side effects. These untoward reactions disappear quickly and do not, as a rule, inconvenience the patient to the extent that the drug must be discontinued. No cumulative effects have been reported.

Dosage and Administration:

Acute Bronchial Asthma: Hold the MISTOMETER unit in an inverted position. Close lips and teeth around open end of mouthpiece. Breathe out, expelling as much air from the lungs as possible; then inhale deeply while pressing down on the bottle to activate spray mechanism. Try to hold breath for a few seconds before exhaling. Wait one full minute in order to determine the effect before considering a second inhalation. A treatment may be repeated up to 5 times daily if necessary. (See Precautions.) If carefully instructed, children quickly learn to keep the stream of mist clear of the teeth and tongue, thereby assuring inhalation into the lungs. Occlusion of the nares of very young children may be advisable to make inhalation certain.

Warm water should be run through the mouthpiece once daily to wash it and prevent clogging.

The mouthpiece may also be sanitized by immersion in alcohol.

Bronchospasm in Chronic Obstructive Lung Disease: The MISTOMETER unit provides a convenient aerosol method for delivering ISUPREL. The treatment described above for Acute Bronchial Asthma may be repeated at not less than 3 to 4 hour intervals as part of a programmed regimen of treatment of obstructive lung disease complicated by a reversible bronchospastic component. One application from the MISTOMETER unit may be regarded as equivalent in effectiveness to 5 to 7 operations of a hand-bulb nebulizer using a 1:100 solution.

Children's Dosage. In general, the technique of ISUPREL hydrochloride, brand of isoproterenol hydrochloride, aerosol solution administration to children is similar to that of adults, since children's smaller ventilatory exchange capacity automatically provides proportionally smaller aerosol intake.

How Supplied:

Isuprel Mistometer 16.8 g (15 ml)
Vial with Oral Nebulizer
Code I-350 **NDC** 0057-0878-01
Isuprel Mistometer 16.8 g (15 ml) refill only
Code I-360 **NDC** 0057-0878-02
Isuprel Mistometer 25.2 g (22.5 ml)
Vial with Oral Nebulizer
Code I-352 **NDC** 0057-0878-03
Isuprel Mistometer 25.2 g (22.5 ml) refill only
Code I-362 **NDC** 0057-0878-04

ISUPREL® Hydrochloride ℞

brand of isoproterenol hydrochloride inhalation, USP

SOLUTION 1:200
SOLUTION 1:100

Potent Bronchodilator

Description: ISUPREL hydrochloride, brand of isoproterenol hydrochloride, is available as:

Solution 1:200 in a buffered aqueous vehicle containing sodium chloride, citric acid, and glycerin with chlorobutanol 0.5 per cent and sodium bisulfite 0.3 per cent as preservatives.

Solution 1:100 in a buffered aqueous vehicle containing sodium chloride, sodium citrate, citric acid, and saccharin with chlorobutanol 0.5 per cent and sodium bisulfite 0.3 per cent as preservatives.

The air in the bottles has been displaced by nitrogen gas.

Do not use the solutions if a precipitate or brownish discoloration is observed. Although ISUPREL solutions left in nebulizers will remain clear and potent for many days, for sanitary reasons it is recommended that they be changed daily.

Action: ISUPREL relaxes bronchial spasm and facilitates expectoration of pulmonary secretions. It is frequently effective when epinephrine and other drugs fail, and it has a wide margin of safety. In dogs the toxic dose is 1000 times the therapeutic dose. Converted to the amount used clinically in man, this would be about 2500 times the therapeutic dose.

Indications: ISUPREL is indicated for the treatment of bronchospasm associated with acute and chronic bronchial asthma, pulmonary emphysema, bronchitis, and bronchiectasis.

Contraindication: Use of isoproterenol in patients with preexisting cardiac arrhythmias associated with tachycardia is generally considered contraindicated because the cardiac stimulant effect of the drug may aggravate such disorders.

Warnings: Excessive use of an adrenergic aerosol should be discouraged as it may lose its effectiveness.

In patients with status asthmaticus and abnormal blood gas tensions, improvement in vital capacity and in blood gas tensions may not accompany apparent relief of bronchospasm. Facilities for administering oxygen mixtures and ventilatory assistance are necessary for such patients.

Occasional patients have been reported to develop severe paradoxical airway resistance with repeated, excessive use of isoproterenol inhalation preparations. The cause of this refractory state is unknown. It is advisable that in such instances the use of this preparation be discontinued immediately and alternative therapy instituted, since in the reported cases the patients did not respond to other forms of therapy until the drug was withdrawn.

Deaths have been reported following excessive use of isoproterenol inhalation preparations and the exact cause is unknown. Cardiac arrest was noted in several instances.

Precautions: Epinephrine should not be administered concomitantly with ISUPREL, as both drugs are direct cardiac stimulants and their combined effects may induce serious arrhythmia. If desired they may, however, be alternated, provided an internal of at least four hours has elapsed.

Isoproterenol should be used with caution in patients with cardiovascular disorders including coronary insufficiency, diabetes, or hyperthyroidism, and in persons sensitive to sympathomimetic amines.

Any patient who requires more than three aerosol treatments within a 24-hour period should be under the close supervision of his physician. Further therapy with the bronchodilator aerosol alone is inadvisable when three to five treatments within six to twelve hours produce minimal or no relief.

During the course of over 25 years of use of ISUPREL, brand of isoproterenol, there has been no clinical evidence of teratogenic effects. However, use of any drug in pregnancy, lactation, or in women of childbearing age requires that the potential benefit of the drug be weighed against its possible hazards to the mother or child.

When compressed oxygen is employed as the aerosol propellant, the percentage of oxygen used should be determined by the patient's individual requirements to avoid depression of respiratory drive.

Adverse Reactions: Tachycardia, palpitation, nervousness, nausea, and vomiting may occur from overdosage. Rarely do headache, flushing of the skin, tremor, dizziness, weakness, sweating, precordial distress, or anginal-type pain occur. The inhalation route is usually accompanied by a minimum of side effects. These untoward reactions disappear quickly and do not, as a rule, inconvenience the patient to the extent that the drug must be discontinued. No cumulative effects have been reported.

Dosage and Administration: ISUPREL hydrochloride solutions can be administered as an aerosol mist by hand-bulb nebulizer, compressed air or oxygen operated nebulizer, or by intermittent positive pressure breathing (IPPB) devices. The method of delivery, and the treatment regimen employed in the management of the reversible bronchospastic element accompanying bronchial asthma, chronic bronchitis, and chronic obstructive lung diseases, will depend on such factors as the severity of the bronchospasm, patient age, tolerance to the medication, complicating cardiopulmonary conditions, and whether therapy is for an intermittent acute attack of bronchospasm or is part of a programmed treatment regimen for constant bronchospasm.

Acute Bronchial Asthma. *Hand-Bulb Nebulizer*—Depending on the frequency of treatment and the type of nebulizer used, a volume of ISUPREL solution, sufficient for not more than one day's treatment, should be placed in the nebulizer using the dropper provided. In time, the patient can learn to adjust the volume required. For adults and children, the 1:200 solution is administered by hand-bulb nebulization in a dosage of 5 to 15 deep inhalations (using an all glass or plastic nebulizer). In adults, the 1:100 solution may be used if a stronger solution seems to be indicated. The

Continued on next page

Breon—Cont.

dose is 3 to 7 deep inhalations. If after about 5 to 10 minutes inadequate relief is observed, these doses may be repeated one more time. If the acute attack recurs, treatments may be repeated up to 5 times daily if necessary. (See Precautions.)

Bronchospasm in Chronic Obstructive Lung Disease. *Hand-Bulb Nebulizer*—ISUPREL 1:200 or 1:100 solution may be administered daily at not less than 3 to 4 hour intervals for subacute bronchospastic attacks or as part of a programmed treatment regimen in patients with chronic obstructive lung disease with a reversible bronchospastic component. An adequate dose is usually 5 to 15 deep inhalations, using the 1:200 solution. Some patients with severe attacks of bronchospasm may require 3 to 7 deep inhalations using the ISUPREL 1:100 solution.

Nebulization by Compressed Air or Oxygen—A method often used in patients with severe chronic obstructive lung disease is to deliver the ISUPREL, brand of isoproterenol, mist in more dilute form over a longer period of time. The purpose is, not so much to increase the dose supplied, as to achieve progressively deeped bronchodilatation and thus insure that the mist achieves maximum penetration of the finer bronchioles. In this method, 0.5 ml of an ISUPREL 1:200 solution is diluted to 2 to 2.5 ml with water or isotonic saline to achieve a use concentration of 1:800 to 1:1000. If desired, 0.25 ml of the 1:100 solution may be similarly diluted to achieve the same use concentration. The diluted solution is placed in a nebulizer (e.g., DeVilbiss #640 unit) connected to either a source of compressed air or oxygen. The flow rate is regulated to suit the particular nebulizer so that the diluted ISUPREL solution will be delivered over approximately 10 to 20 minutes. A treatment may be repeated up to 5 times daily if necessary. Although the total delivered dose of ISUPREL is somewhat higher than with the treatment regimen employing the hand-bulb nebulizer, patients usually tolerate it well because of the greater dilution and longer application-time factors.

Intermittent Positive Pressure Breathing (IPPB)—Diluted solutions of ISUPREL 1:200 or 1:100 are used in a programmed regimen for the treatment of reversible bronchospasm in patients with chronic obstructive lung disease who require intermittent positive pressure breathing therapy. These devices generally have a small nebulizer, usually of 3 to 5 ml capacity, on a patient-operated side arm. The effectiveness of IPPB therapy is greatly enhanced by the simultaneous use of aerosolized bronchodilators. As with compressed air or oxygen operated nebulizers, the usual regimen is to place 0.5 ml of ISUPREL 1:200 solution diluted to 2 to 2.5 ml with water or isotonic saline in the nebulizer cup and follow the IPPB manufacturer's operating instructions. IPPB-bronchodilator treatments are usually administered over 15 to 20 minutes, up to 5 times daily if necessary.

Children's Dosage: In general, the technique of ISUPREL hydrochloride solution administration to children is similar to that of adults, since children's smaller ventilatory exchange capacity automatically provides proportionally smaller aerosol intake. However, it is generally recommended that the 1:200 solution (rather than the 1:100) be used for an acute attack of bronchospasm, and no more than 0.25 ml of the 1:200 solution should be used for each 10 to 15 minute programmed treatment in chronic bronchospastic disease.

How Supplied:

Solution 1:100
bottles of 10 ml — **NDC** 0057-0873-01

Solution 1:200
bottles of 10 ml — **NDC** 0057-0871-01
bottles of 60 ml — **NDC** 0057-0871-03

ISUPREL® Hydrochloride ℞
brand of isoproterenol hydrochloride tablets, USP
GLOSSETS®

Description: Isuprel hydrochloride (brand of isoproterenol hydrochloride) is 3,4-dihydroxy-α-[(isopropylamino)methyl]-benzyl alcohol hydrochloride, a synthetic sympathomimetic amine that is structurally related to epinephrine but acts almost exclusively on beta receptors.

Each Isuprel tablet contains 10 or 15 mg isoproterenol hydrochloride in a rapidly disintegrating base consisting of starch, lactose, sodium saccharin, and talcum with sodium bisulfite 2 mg per tablet as antioxidant.

Actions: The primary actions of Isuprel are on the heart and on smooth muscle of bronchi, skeletal muscle vasculature, and alimentary tract. The positive inotropic and chronotropic actions of the drug increase cardiac output. There is also an increase in venous return to the heart. With usual therapeutic doses, the increase in cardiac output is generally sufficient to maintain or increase systolic blood pressure. Isuprel also lowers peripheral vascular resistance; the diastolic pressure, therefore, may be expected to fall in normal individuals. Thus, the mean pressure may be reduced. The rate of discharge of cardiac pacemakers is increased with isoproterenol.

Isuprel relaxes most smooth muscle, the most pronounced effect being on bronchial and gastrointestinal smooth muscle. It produces marked relaxation in the smaller bronchi and may even dilate the trachea and main bronchi past the resting diameter.

The acute toxicity of Isuprel in animals is much less than that of epinephrine. Excessive doses in animals or man can cause a striking drop in blood pressure, and repeated large doses in animals may result in cardiac enlargement and focal myocarditis.

Indications: The sublingual or rectal dosage form of isoproterenol hydrochloride is indicated in the treatment of Adams-Stokes syndrome and atrioventricular heart block. However, the treatment of choice is electrical pacing for heart block and electroshock for emergency conditions involving ventricular arrhythmias.

This dosage form of Isuprel may also be used as a bronchodilator in the management of patients with bronchopulmonary disease.

Contraindications: Use of isoproterenol in patients with preexisting cardiac arrhythmias associated with tachycardia is generally considered contraindicated because the chronotropic effect of the drug on the heart may aggravate such disorders.

Administration of Isuprel is also contraindicated in patients with tachycardia caused by digitalis intoxication.

Warnings: In patients with status asthmaticus and abnormal blood gas tensions, improvement in vital capacity and in blood gas tensions may not accompany apparent relief of bronchospasm. Facilities for administering oxygen mixtures and ventilatory assistance are necessary for such patients.

Deaths have been reported following excessive use of isoproterenol inhalation preparations and the exact cause is unknown. Cardiac arrest was noted in several instances.

Precautions: Isuprel and epinephrine should not be administered simultaneously, since both drugs are direct cardiac stimulants and their combined effects may induce serious arrhythmia. The drugs may, however, be administered alternately provided a proper interval has elapsed between doses.

Isoproterenol should be used with caution in patients with cardiovascular disorders including coronary insufficiency, diabetes, or hyperthyroidism, and in persons sensitive to sympathomimetic amines. If precordial distress or anginal-type pain occurs, the drug should be discontinued immediately.

There has been no clinical evidence of teratogenic effects attributable to Isuprel in more than 20 years' use of the drug. However, before administration of any drug to pregnant women or women of childbearing potential, the expected benefit of the drug should be carefully weighed against the possible risk to the mother or child.

Adverse Reactions: Serious reactions to Isuprel are infrequent. The following reactions, however, have been reported: flushing of the face, sweating, mild tremors, nervousness, headache, nausea, vomiting, dizziness, weakness, and tachycardia with palpitation manifested as a sensation of pounding in the chest. These reactions generally disappear quickly and usually do not require discontinuation of treatment with Isuprel. Precordial distress or anginal-type pain occurs rarely. No cumulative effects have been reported. Pulmonary edema has been reported in a patient extremely intolerant to all sympathomimetic drugs.

In a few patients, presumably with organic disease of the A-V node and its branches, Isuprel has been reported, paradoxically, to precipitate Adams-Stokes seizures during normal sinus rhythm or transient heart block.

Dosage and Administration: *For Heart Block and Certain Ventricular Arrhythmias:* The sublingual or rectal administration of Isuprel has proven effective in the control of mild stabilized symptomatic heart block and ventricular arrhythmias. However, it should be noted that in acute symptomatic heart block, particularly in patients with post-cardiac surgery block, electrical pacing is the preferred method of treatment for maintenance of an adequate ventricular rate. Moreover, in ventricular arrhythmias, electroshock may have to be used, and is usually the treatment of choice.

If Isuprel is to be given in acute symptomatic heart block, intravenous administration, with constant monitoring, is preferred. This avoids the irregular absorption which is possible with the sublingual and rectal routes of administration. Rectal administration is more satisfactory for long-term therapy because the effect is produced within 30 minutes and lasts for two to four hours. The patient must be monitored constantly by electrocardiography. Sinus rhythm sometimes occurs and persists for a variable period but often relapses again into complete block. In other cases, Isuprel merely maintains an acceptable heart rate somewhere above 90 to 100 beats per minute.

Carotid sinus hypersensitivity with reflex cardiac standstill, induced either clinically or experimentally, can be abolished successfully by the cardiac stimulative action of Isuprel until normal automaticity returns. From 1 to 2 Isuprel Glossets administered sublingually four to six times daily may prevent heart block in patients with carotid sinus hypersensitivity.

Table 1 summarizes the dosage regimen suggested for adults.

TABLE 1
SUGGESTED DOSAGE FOR HEART BLOCK IN ADULTS

Route of Administration	Initial Dose	Subsequent Dose Range
Sublingual	10 mg	5 to 50 mg
Rectal	5 mg	5 to 15 mg

Children may be given half the initial adult dose. In all patients, subsequent dosage and method of administration depend on the response of the ventricular rate and the rapidity with which the cardiac pacemaker can take over when the drug is gradually withdrawn.

The usual route of administration of Isuprel hydrochloride in emergency treatment of patients with severe heart block is by intravenous injection or infusion. If time is not of utmost importance, initial therapy by intramuscular or subcutaneous injection is preferred. If further maintenance therapy is necessary, Isuprel Glossets may be administered sublingually. Whenever Isuprel is used for these purposes, the electrocardiogram must always be monitored.

The Glossets are particularly useful for prophylaxis and treatment of heart block since patients can administer the medication themselves.

Isuprel Glossets are usually administered sublingually; the Glossets are absorbed directly from the site of administration.

For Pulmonary Conditions with Bronchospasm: The average sublingual dose for adults is 1 tablet of 10 mg. In some cases 1 tablet of 15 mg may be required, or 2 Glossets of 10 mg, depending on the patient's response to sympathomimetic amines. However, a dosage of 15 mg four times daily or 20 mg three times daily (a total of 60 mg in one day) should not be exceeded. For children, the dose is from 5 to 10 mg (½ to 1 tablet of 10 mg), not exceeding a total of 30 mg in one day.

The Glossets are allowed to disintegrate under the tongue. Until absorption has taken place, patients are instructed not to swallow saliva. Treatment should not be repeated more often than every three or four hours, or more than three times daily.

How Supplied:
Code I-260 Isuprel Glossets 10 mg bottles of 50 NDC 0057-0875-02
Code I-270 Isuprel Glossets 15 mg bottles of 50 NDC 0057-0877-02

[Shown in Product Identification Section]

ISUPREL® ℞
Compound Elixir

Description: Each tablespoon (15 ml) of ISUPREL® Compound Elixir contains:

Phenobarbital, USP ....6 mg
Isoproterenol hydrochloride, USP ....2.5 mg
Ephedrine sulfate, USP ....12 mg
Theophylline, USP ....45 mg
Potassium iodide, USP ....150 mg
Alcohol, USP 19%

ISUPREL Compound Elixir is a balanced expectorant bronchodilator for the management of bronchial asthma, allergic coughs, and bronchitis.

Phenobarbital, 5-Ethyl-5-phenylbarbituric acid, is a barbiturate used as a sedative connective for the CNS stimulation seen with theophylline, ephedrine, and isoproterenol.

Isoproterenol hydrochloride, 3,4-Dihydroxy-α-[(isopropylamino) methyl]benzyl alcohol hydrochloride, is a synthetic sympathomimetic amine used for its beta-adrenergic bronchodilating properties.

Ephedrine sulfate, Benzenemethanol, α-[1-(methylamino) ethyl]-, Sulfate, is a non-catecholamine sympathomimetic bronchodilator.

Theophylline, 1*H*-Purine-2,6-dione, 3,7-dihydor-1,3-dimethyl-, monohydrate, is a xanthine bronchodilator.

Potassium iodide is an expectorant.

Clinical Pharmacology: ISUPREL hydrochloride (isoproterenol hydrochloride) has predominant beta sympathetic activity and ephedrine has both alpha and beta effects. Theophylline directly relaxes smooth muscle of bronchi and pulmonary blood vessels, producing bronchodilation and pulmonary vasodilation; its actions may be mediated through inhibition of phosphodiesterase with a resultant increase in intracellular cyclic AMP causing smooth muscle relaxation. The mechanism of action of potassium iodide as an expectorant is unknown. Phenobarbital is used for its mild sedative properties to allay anxiety and connect the CNS stimulation of ISUPREL (isoproterenol hydrochloride), ephedrine and theophylline.

Indications and Usage: ISUPREL Compound Elixir is indicated for the management of patients with bronchial asthma, allergic coughs, and the chronic bronchitis frequently associated with these respiratory disorders.

Contraindications: ISUPREL Compound Elixir is contraindicated in patients who are hypersensitive to any of its ingredients.

Warnings: Phenobarbital may be habit forming.

Use in pregnancy. Barbiturates can cause fetal damage when administered to a pegnant woman. Retrospective, case-controlled studies have suggested a connection between the maternal consumption of barbiturates and a higher than expected incidence of fetal abnormalities. Following oral or parenteral administration, barbiturates readily cross the placental barrier and are distributed throughout fetal tissues with highest concentrations found in the placenta, fetal liver, and brain. Fetal blood levels approach maternal blood levels following parenteral administration.

Withdrawal symptoms occur in infants born to mothers who receive barbiturates throughout the last trimester of pregnancy. If this drug is used during pregnancy or if the patient becomes pregnant while taking this drug, the patient should be apprised of the potential hazard to the fetus.

Precautions: The dosage of ISUPREL Compound Elixir must be carefully adjusted in patients with hyperthyroidism, acute coronary disease, cardiac asthma, hypertension, and limited cardiac reserve and in patients sensitive to sympathomimetic amines, since overdosage may result in tachycardia, palpitation, nausea, headache, or other epinephrine-like side effects.

Caution is also recommended in patients with prostatic hypertrophy and glaucoma.

Barbiturates may be habit forming. Tolerance and psychological and physical dependence may occur with continuing use. Barbiturates should be administered with caution, if at all, to patients who are mentally depressed, have suicidal tendencies, or a history of drug abuse. Elderly or debilitated patients may react to barbiturates with marked excitement, depression, and confusion. In some persons, barbiturates repeatedly produce excitement rather than depression.

Drug Interactions:

1. *Anticoagulants.* Phenobarbital lowers the plasma levels of dicumarol (name previously used: bishydroxycoumarin) and causes a decrease in anticoagulant activity as measured by the prothrombin time. Barbiturates can induce hepatic microsomal enzymes resulting in increased metabolism and decreased anticoagulant response of oral anticoagulants (e.g., warfarin, acenocoumarol, dicumarol, and phenprocoumon). Patients stabilized on anticoagulant therapy may require dosage adjustments if barbiturates are added to or withdrawn from their dosage regimen.

2. *Corticosteroids.* Barbiturates appar to enhance the metabolism of exogenous corticosteroids probably through the induction of hepatic microsomal enzymes. Patients stabilized on corticosteroid therapy may require dosage adjustments if barbiturates are added to or withdrawn from their dosage regimen.

3. *Griseofulvin.* Phenobarbital appears to interfere with the absorption of orally administered griseofulvin, thus decreasing its blood level. The effect of the resultant decreased blood levels of griseofulvin on therapeutic response has not been established. However, it would be preferable to avoid concomitant administration of these drugs.

4. *Doxycycline.* Phenobarbital has been shown to shorten the half-life of doxycycline for as long as 2 weeks after barbiturate therapy is discontinued. This mechanism is probably through the induction of hepatic microsomal enzymes that metabolize the antibiotic. If phenobarbital and doxycycline are administered concurrently, the clinical response to doxycycline should be monitored closely.

5. *Phenytoin, sodium valproate, valproic acid.* The effect of barbiturates on the metabolism of phenytoin appears to be variable. Some investigators report an accelerating effect, while others report no effect. Because the effect of barbiturates on the metabolism of phenytoin is not predictable, phenytoin and barbiturate blood levels should be monitored more frequently if these drugs are given concurrently. Sodium valproate and valproic acid appear to decrease barbiturate metabolism; therefore, barbiturate blood levels should be monitored and appropriate dosage adjustments made as indicated.

6. *Central nervous system depressants.* The concomitant use of other central nervous system depressants, including other sedatives or hypnotics, antihistamines, tranquilizers, or alcohol, may produce additive depressant effects.

7. *Monoamine oxidase inhibitors (MAOI).* MAOI prolong the effects of barbiturates probably because metabolism of the barbiturate is inhibited.

8. *Estradiol, estone, progesterone and other steroidal hormones.* Pretreatment with or concurrent administration of phenobarbital may decrease the effect of estradiol by increasing its metabolism. There have been reports of patients treated with antiepileptic drugs (e.g., phenobarbital) who become pregnant while taking oral contraceptives. An alternant contraceptive method might be suggested to women taking phenobarbital.

Laboratory Tests Interactions: Because of its iodide content, the Elixir may cause elevation of the protein-bound iodine.

Carcinogenesis, Mutagenesis, Impairment of Fertility: Phenobarbital sodium is carcinogenic in mice and rats after lifetime administration. In mice, it produced benign and malignant liver cell tumors. In rats, benign liver cell tumors were observed very late in life. In a 29-year epidemiological study of 9,136 patients who were treated on an anticonvulsant protocol which included phenobarbital, results indicated a higher than normal incidence of hepatic carcinoma. Previously, some of these patients were treated with thorotrast, a drug which is known to produce hepatic carcinomas. Thus, this study did not provide sufficient evidence that phenobarbital sodium is carcinogenic in humans.

A retrospective study of 84 children with brain tumors matched to 73 normal controls and 78 cancer controls (malignant disease other than brain tumors) suggested an association between exposure to barbiturates prenatally and an increased incidence of brain tumors.

Pregnancy:

1. *Teratogenic effects.* Pregnancy Category D—See WARNINGS—Use in Pregnancy above.

2. *Nonteratogenic effects.* Reports of infants suffering from long-term barbiturate exposure *in utero* included the acute withdrawal syndrome of seizures and hyperirritability from birth to a delayed onset of up to 14 days. Large doses of iodides should not be administered during pregnancy since they may cause goiter in the fetus.

Labor and delivery: Hypnotic doses of these barbiturates do not appear to significantly impair uterine activity during labor. Full anesthetic doses of barbiturates decreased the force and frequency of uterine contractions. Administration of sedative-hypnotic barbiturates to the mother during labor may result in respiratory depression in the newborn. Premature

Continued on next page

Breon—Cont.

infants are particularly susceptible to the depressant effects of barbiturates. If barbiturates are used during labor and delivery, resuscitation equipment should be available.
Data are currently not available to evaluate the effect of these barbiturates when forceps delivery or other intervention is necessary. Also, data are not available to determine the effect of these barbiturates on the later growth, development, and functional maturation of the child.
Nursing mothers: Caution should be exercised when a barbiturate is administered to a nursing woman since small amounts of barbiturates are excreted in the milk.
Adverse Reactions: Although the Elixir is generally well tolerated, symptoms of adrenergic overstimulation such as tachycardia or nervousness may occur, in which case the preparation should be temporarily discontinued and administered later at a lower dosage. Reactions to iodide include coryza, fever, acneiform eruptions, erythema of the face and chest, and painful swelling of the salivary glands. These side effects quickly subside on discontinuance of medication. Theophylline may cause gastric intolerance (nausea and vomiting).
Overdosage: The toxic dose of barbiturates varies considerably. In general, an oral dose of one gram of most barbiturates produces serious poisoning in an adult. Death commonly occurs after 2 to 10 grams of ingested barbiturate.
Overdosage of ephedrine and isoproterenol results in typical sympathomimetic signs and symptoms. Theophylline overdosage results in nausea, vomiting, convulsions, tachycardia and ventricular arrhythmias. Treatment: See standard references for treatment of overdose of barbiturates and theophylline.
Dosage and Administration:
For children from 1 to 3 years, 1 or 2 teaspoons (5 to 10 ml); **from 3 to 6 years,** 2 or 3 teaspoons (10 to 15 ml); **from 6 to 12 years,** 1 or 2 tablespoons (15 to 30 ml). The dose should be administered three times daily as needed to control symptoms.
For adults, 2 tablespoon (30 ml) three or four times daily may be given as needed. Since the severity of the disorder and the response of the patient will vary, the dose should be adjusted to individual needs, the larger doses being reserved for more severe disorders or for patients who do not respond to the smaller doses. Acute or severe attacks of bronchial asthma usually require inhalation and other therapy.
How Supplied:
Bottles of 16 fl oz,
Code 1–340 **NDC** 0057-0874-06
and Gallons, Code 1–341 **NDC** 0057-0874-08
Examine solution before using. Do not use if crystals, precipitation or cloudiness is observed.

KAYEXALATE® ℞
brand of sodium polystyrene sulfonate, USP

Cation-Exchange Resin

Description: The drug is a light brown to brown, finely ground, powdered form of sodium polystyrene sulfonate, a cation-exchange resin prepared in the sodium phase with an *in vitro* exchange capacity of approximately 3.1 mEq (*in vivo* approximately 1 mEq) of potassium per gram. The sodium content is approximately 100 mg (4.1 mEq) per gram of the drug.
Action: As the resin passes along the intestine or is retained in the colon after administration by enema, the sodium ions are partially released and are replaced by potassium ions. For the most part, this action occurs in the large intestine, which excretes potassium ions to a greater degree than does the small intestine. The efficiency of this process is limited and unpredictably variable. It commonly approximates the order of 33 per cent but the range is so large that definitive indices of electrolyte balance must be clearly monitored.
Indication: KAYEXALATE is indicated for the treatment of hyperkalemia.
Warnings: Since effective lowering of serum potassium with KAYEXALATE may take hours to days, treatment with this drug alone may be insufficient to rapidly correct severe hyperkalemia associated with states of rapid tissue breakdown (e.g., burns and renal failure) or hyperkalemia so marked as to constitute a medical emergency. Therefore, other definitive measures, including dialysis, should always be considered and may be imperative. Serious potassium efficiency can occur from KAYEXALATE therapy. The effect must be carefully controlled by frequent serum potassium determinations within each 24 hour period. Since intracellular potassium deficiency is not always reflected by serum potassium levels, the level at which treatment with KAYEXALATE should be discontinued must be determined individually for each patient. Important aids in making this determination are the patient's clinical condition and electrocardiogram. Early clinical signs of severe hypokalemia include a pattern of irritable confusion and delayed thought processes. Electrocardiographically, severe hypokalemia is often associated with a lengthened Q-T interval, widening, flattening, or inversion of the T wave, and prominent U waves. Also, cardiac arrhythmias may occur, such as premature atrial, nodal, and ventricular contractions, and supraventricular and ventricular tachycardias. The toxic effects of digitalis are likely to be exaggerated. Marked hypokalemia can also be manifested by severe muscle weakness, at times extending into frank paralysis.
Like all cation-exchange resins, KAYEXALATE is not totally selective (for potassium) in its actions, and small amounts of other cations such as magnesium and calcium can also be lost during treatment. Accordingly, patients receiving KAYEXALATE should be monitored for all applicable electrolyte disturbances. Systemic alkalosis has been reported after cation-exchange resins were administered orally in combination with nonabsorbable cation-donating antacids and laxatives such as magnesium hydroxide and aluminum carbonate. Magnesium hydroxide should not be administered with KAYEXALATE. One case of grand mal seizure has been reported in a patient with chronic hypocalcemia of renal failure who was given KAYEXALATE with magnesium hydroxide as laxative. Also, the simultaneous oral administration of KAYEXALATE with nonabsorbable cation-donating antacids and laxatives may reduce the resin's potassium exchange capability.
Precautions: Caution is advised when KAYEXALATE is administered to patients who cannot tolerate even a small increase in sodium loads (i.e., severe congestive heart failure, severe hypertension, or marked edema). In such instances compensatory restriction of sodium intake from other sources may be indicated.
If constipation occurs, patients should be treated with sorbitol (from 10 to 20 ml of 70 per cent syrup every two hours or as needed to produce one or two watery stools daily), a measure which also reduces any tendency to fecal impaction.
Adverse Reactions: KAYEXALATE may cause some degree of gastric irritation. Anorexia, nausea, vomiting, and constipation may occur especially if high doses are given. Also, hypokalemia, hypocalcemia, and significant sodium retention may occur. Occasionally diarrhea develops. Large doses in elderly individuals may cause fecal impaction (see Precautions). This effect may be obviated through usage of the resin in enemas as described under Dosage and Administration. Intestinal obstruction due to concretions of aluminum hydroxide, when used in combination with KAYEXALATE, has been reported.
Dosage and Administration: Suspensions of this drug should be freshly prepared and not stored beyond 24 hours.
The average daily adult dose of the resin is 15 to 60 g. This is best provided by administering 15 g (approximately 4 *level* teaspoons) of KAYEXALATE, brand of sodium polystyrene sulfonate, one to four times daily. One gram of KAYEXALATE contains 4.1 mEq of sodium; one level teaspoon contains approximately 3.5 g of KAYEXALATE and 15 mEq of sodium. (A heaping teaspoon may contain as much as 10 to 12 g of KAYEXALATE.) Since the *in vivo* efficiency of sodium-potassium exchange resins is approximately 33 per cent, about one third of the resin's actual sodium content is being delivered to the body.
In smaller children and infants lower doses should be employed by using as a guide a rate of 1 mEq of potassium per gram of resin as the basis for calculation.
Each dose should be given as a suspension in a small quantity of water or, for greater palatability, in syrup. The amount of fluid usually ranges from 20 to 100 ml, depending on the dose, or may be simply determined by allowing 3 to 4 ml per gram of resin. Sorbitol may be administered in order to combat constipation. The resin may be introduced into the stomach through a plastic tube and, if desired, mixed with a diet appropriate for a patient in renal failure.
The resin may also be given, although with less effective results, in a daily enema consisting (for adults) of 30 to 50 g every six hours. Each dose is administered as a warm emulsion (at body temperature) in 100 ml of aqueous vehicle, such as sorbitol. The emulsion should be agitated gently during administration. The enema should be retained as long as possible and followed by a cleansing enema.
After an initial cleansing enema, a soft, large size (French 28) rubber tube is inserted into the rectum for a distance of about 20 cm, with the tip well into the sigmoid colon, and taped in place. The resin is then suspended in the appropriate amount of aqueous vehicle at body temperature and introduced by gravity, while the particles are kept in suspension by stirring. The suspension is flushed with 50 or 100 ml of fluid, following which the tube is clamped and left in place. If back leakage occurs, the hips are elevated on pillows or a knee-chest position is taken temporarily. A somewhat thicker suspension may be used, but care should be taken that no paste is formed, because the latter has a greatly reduced exchange surface and will be particularly ineffective if deposited in the rectal ampulla. The suspension is kept in the sigmoid colon for several hours, if possible. Then, the colon is irrigated with nonsodium containing solution at body temperature in order to remove the resin. Two quarts of flushing solution may be necessary. The returns are drained constantly through a Y tube connection.
The intensity and duration of therapy depend upon the severity and resistance of hyperkalemia.
KAYEXALATE should not be heated for to do so may alter the exchange properties of the resin.
How Supplied: Jars of 1 pound (453.6 g).
Code K-450, **NDC** 0057-1075-01

LEVOPHED® Bitartrate ℞
brand of norepinephrine bitartrate injection, USP
(formerly called levarterenol bitartrate injection, USP)

Description: Levarterenol (sometimes referred to as *l-arterenol* or as *l-norepinephrine*) is a primary amine which differs from epinephrine by the absence of a methyl group on the nitrogen atom.

LEVOPHED is supplied in sterile aqueous solution in the form of the bitartrate. Each 1 ml of LEVOPHED solution contains 1 mg of LEVOPHED base, sodium chloride for isotonicity, and not more than 2 mg of sodium bisulfite as preservative. The air in the ampuls has been displaced by nitrogen gas.

Actions: LEVOPHED functions as a powerful peripheral vasoconstrictor (alpha-adrenergic action) and as a potent inotropic stimulator of the heart and dilator of coronary arteries (beta-adrenergic action). Both of these actions result in an increase in systemic blood pressure and coronary artery blood flow. Cardiac output will vary reflexly in response to systemic hypertension but is usually increased in hypotensive man when the blood pressure is raised to an optimal level. In myocardial infarction accompanied by hypotension, LEVOPHED usually increases aortic blood pressure, coronary artery blood flow, and myocardial oxygenation, thereby helping to limit the area of myocardial ischemia and infarction. Venous return is increased and the heart tends to resume a more normal rate and rhythm than in the hypotensive state.

In hypotension that persists after correction of blood volume deficits, LEVOPHED helps raise the blood pressure to an optimal level and establish a more adequate circulation.

Indications: For the restoration of blood pressure in controlling certain acute hypotensive states (e.g., pheochromocytomectomy, sympathectomy, poliomyelitis, spinal anesthesia, myocardial infarction, septicemia, blood transfusion, and drug reactions).

As an adjunct in the treatment of cardiac arrest and profound hypotension.

Contraindications: LEVOPHED should not be given to patients who are hypotensive from blood volume deficits except as an emergency measure to maintain coronary and cerebral artery perfusion until blood volume replacement therapy can be completed. If LEVOPHED is continuously administered to maintain blood pressure in the absence of blood volume replacement, the following may occur: severe peripheral and visceral vasoconstriction, decreased renal perfusion and urine output, poor systemic blood flow despite "normal" blood pressure, tissue hypoxia, and lactate acidosis.

LEVOPHED should also not be given to patients with mesenteric or peripheral vascular thrombosis (because of the risk of increasing ischemia and extending the area of infarction) unless, in the opinion of the attending physician, the administration of LEVOPHED is necessary as a life-saving procedure.

Cyclopropane and halothane anesthetics increase cardiac autonomic irritability and therefore seem to sensitize the myocardium to the action of intravenously administered epinephrine or levarterenol. Hence, the use of LEVOPHED during cyclopropane and halothane anesthesia is generally considered contraindicated because of the risk of producing ventricular tachycardia or fibrillation. The same type of cardiac arrhythmias may result from the use of LEVOPHED in patients with profound hypoxia or hypercarbia.

Warning: LEVOPHED should be used with extreme caution in patients receiving monoamine oxidase (MAO) inhibitors or antidepressants of the triptyline or imipramine types, because severe, prolonged hypertension may result.

Precautions: *Avoid Hypertension:* Because of the potency of LEVOPHED and because of varying response to pressor substances, the possibility always exists that dangerously high blood pressure may be produced with overdoses of this pressor agent. It is desirable, therefore, to record the blood pressure every two minutes from the time administration is started until the desired blood pressure is obtained, then every five minutes if administration is to be continued. The rate of flow must be watched constantly, and the patient should never be left unattended while receiving LEVOPHED. Headache may be a symptom of hypertension due to overdosage.

Site of Infusion: Whenever possible, LEVOPHED should be given into a large vein, particularly an antecubital vein because, when administered into this vein, the risk of necrosis of the overlying skin from prolonged vasoconstriction is apparently very slight. Some authors have indicated that the femoral vein is also an acceptable route of administration. A catheter tie-in technique should be avoided, if possible, since the obstruction to blood flow around the tubing may cause stasis and increased local concentration of the drug. Occlusive vascular diseases (for example, atherosclerosis, arteriosclerosis, diabetic endarteritis, Buerger's disease) are more likely to occur in the lower than in the upper extremity. Therefore, one should avoid the veins of the leg in elderly patients or in those suffering from such disorders. Gangrene has been reported in a lower extremity when LEVOPHED was given in an ankle vein.

Extravasation: The infusion site should be checked frequently for free flow. Care should be taken to avoid extravasation of LEVOPHED bitartrate, brand of levarterenol bitartrate injection, into the tissues, as local necrosis might ensue due to the vasoconstrictive action of the drug. Blanching along the course of the infused vein, sometimes without obvious extravasation, has been attributed to vasa vasorum constriction with increased permeability of the vein wall, permitting some leakage. This also may progress on rare occasions to superficial slough, particularly during infusion into leg veins in elderly patients or in those suffering from obliterative vascular disease. Hence, if blanching occurs, consideration should be given to the advisability of changing the infusion site at intervals to allow the effects of local vasoconstriction to subside.

IMPORTANT—Antidote for Extravasation Ischemia: To prevent sloughing and necrosis in areas in which extravasation has taken place, the area should be infiltrated as soon as possible with 10 to 15 ml of saline solution containing from 5 to 10 mg of **Regitine® (brand of phentolamine)**, an adrenergic blocking agent. A syringe with a fine hypodermic needle is used, and the solution is infiltrated liberally throughout the area, which is easily identified by its cold, hard, and pallid appearance. Sympathetic blockade with phentolamine causes immediate and conspicuous local hyperemic changes if the area is infiltrated within 12 hours. Therefore, phentolamine should be given as soon as possible after the extravasation is noted.

Some investigators[1] add phentolamine (5 to 10 mg) directly to the infusion flask because it is believed that the drug used in this manner is an effective antidote against sloughing should extravasation occur, whereas the systemic vasopressor activity of the LEVOPHED is not impaired.

Two investigators[2] stated that, in the treatment of patients with severe hypotension following *myocardial infarction,* thrombosis in the infused vein and perivenous reactions and necrosis may usually be prevented if 10 mg of heparin are added to each 500 ml of infusion fluid (5 per cent dextrose) containing LEVOPHED.

Sympathetic nerve block has also been suggested.

Adverse Reactions: When used as directed, LEVOPHED is more certain in action and better tolerated systemically than other pressor amines. Its therapeutic index is four times that of epinephrine. Bradycardia sometimes occurs, probably as a reflex result of a rise in blood pressure. Headache may indicate overdosage and extreme hypertension.

Overdosage with LEVOPHED may also result in severe hypertension, reflex bradycardia, marked increase in peripheral resistance, and decreased cardiac output.

Prolonged administration of any potent vasopressor may result in plasma volume depletion which should be continuously corrected by appropriate fluid and electrolyte replacement therapy. If plasma volumes are not corrected hypotension may recur when LEVOPHED is discontinued, or blood pressure may be maintained at the risk of severe peripheral vasoconstriction with diminution in blood flow and tissue perfusion.

Dosage and Administration:

Restoration of Blood Pressure in Acute Hypotensive States

Blood volume depletion should always be corrected as fully as possible before any vasopressor is administered. When, as an emergency measure, intraaortic pressures must be maintained to prevent cerebral or coronary artery ischemia, LEVOPHED bitartrate, brand of levarterenol bitartrate injection, can be administered before and concurrently with blood volume replacement.

Diluent: LEVOPHED solution should be administered in 5 per cent dextrose solution in distilled water or 5 per cent dextrose in saline solution. These fluids containing dextrose are protection against significant loss of potency due to oxidation. Administration in saline solution alone is not recommended. Whole blood or plasma, if indicated to increase blood volume, should be administered separately (for example, by use of a Y-tube and individual flasks if given simultaneously).

Average Dosage: Add 4 ml of LEVOPHED solution to 1000 ml of 5 per cent dextrose solution. Each 1 ml of this dilution contains 4 μg of LEVOPHED base. Give this dilution intravenously. Insert a plastic intravenous catheter through a suitable bore needle well advanced centrally into the vein and securely fixed with adhesive tape, avoiding, if possible, a catheter tie-in technique as this promotes stasis. A drip bulb is necessary to permit an accurate estimation of the rate of flow in drops per minute. After observing the response to an initial dose of 2 to 3 ml (from 8 to 12 μg of base) per minute, adjust the rate of flow to establish and maintain a low normal blood pressure (usually 80 to 100 mm Hg systolic) sufficient to maintain the circulation to vital organs. In previously hypertensive patients, it is recommended that the blood pressure should be raised no higher than 40 mm Hg below the preexisting systolic pressure. The average maintenance dose ranges from 0.5 to 1 ml per minute (from 2 to 4 μg of base).

High Dosage: Great individual variation occurs in the dose required to attain and maintain an adequate blood pressure. In all cases, dosage of LEVOPHED should be titrated according to the response of the patient. Occasionally much larger or even enormous daily doses (as high as 68 mg base or 17 ampuls) may be necessary if the patient remains hypotensive, but occult blood volume depletion should always be suspected and corrected when present. Central venous pressure monitoring is usually helpful in detecting and treating this situation.

Fluid Intake: The degree of dilution depends on clinical fluid volume requirements. If large volumes of fluid (dextrose) are needed at a flow rate that would involve an excessive dose of the pressor agent per unit of time, a more dilute solution than 4 μg per ml should be used. On the other hand, when large volumes of fluid

Continued on next page

Breon—Cont.

are clinically undesirable, a concentration greater than 4 μg per ml may be used.

Duration of Therapy: The infusion should be continued until adequate blood pressure and tissue perfusion are maintained without therapy. LEVOPHED infusion should be reduced gradually, avoiding abrupt withdrawal. In some of the reported cases of vascular collapse due to acute myocardial infarction, treatment was required for up to six days.

Adjunctive Treatment in Cardiac Arrest
LEVOPHED is usually administered intravenously during cardiac resuscitation to restore and maintain an adequate blood pressure after an effective heartbeat and ventilation have been established by other means. [LEVOPHED'S powerful beta-adrenergic stimulating action is also thought to increase the strength and effectiveness of systolic contractions once they occur.]

Average Dosage: To maintain systemic blood pressure during the management of cardiac arrest, LEVOPHED bitartrate, brand of levarterenol bitartrate injection, is used in the same manner as described under Restoration of Blood Pressure in Acute Hypotensive States.

How Supplied: Ampuls of 4 ml containing 4 mg LEVOPHED base, boxes of 10.

Code L-680 **NDC** 0057-1123-02

References:

1. Zucker, G. *et al.*: *Circulation 22*:935, Nov. 1960.
2. Sampson, J. and Griffith, G.: *Geriatrics 11*:60, Feb. 1956.

Regitine, trademark, CIBA Pharmaceutical Company.

MARCAINE® HYDROCHLORIDE ℞
(bupivacaine hydrochloride injection, USP)

MARCAINE® HYDROCHLORIDE WITH EPINEPHRINE 1:200,000 (AS BITARTRATE) ℞
(bupivacaine hydrochloride and epinephrine injection, USP)

Description: Bupivacaine hydrochloride is 1-butyl-2′,6′-pipecoloxylidide hydrochloride, a white crystalline powder that is freely soluble in 95 per cent ethanol, soluble in water, and slightly soluble in chloroform or acetone.

MARCAINE is available in sterile isotonic solutions with and without epinephrine (as bitartrate) 1:200,000. Solutions of MARCAINE may be reautoclaved if they do not contain epinephrine.

MARCAINE is related chemically and pharmacologically to the aminoacyl local anesthetics. It is a homologue of mepivacaine and is chemically related to lidocaine. All three of these anesthetics contain an amide linkage between the aromatic nucleus and the amino or piperidine group. They differ in this respect from the procaine-type local anesthetics, which have an ester linkage.

Actions: Parenteral administration of MARCAINE stabilizes the neuronal membrane and prevents initiation and transmission of nerve impulses, thereby effecting local anesthetic action.

The onset of action is rapid, and anesthesia may last several hours. The duration of anesthesia is significantly longer with MARCAINE than with any other commonly used local anesthetics. Anesthesia may be more prolonged with the addition of a vasoconstrictor such as epinephrine 1:200,000. It has also been noted that there is a period of analgesia that persists after the return of sensation, during which time the need for strong analgesics is reduced.

The onset of action following dental injections is usually 2 to 10 minutes and anesthesia may last two or three times longer than lidocaine and mepivacaine for dental use, in many patients up to 7 hours.

After injection of MARCAINE for caudal, epidural or peripheral nerve block in man, peak levels of MARCAINE in the blood are reached in 30 to 45 minutes, followed by a decline to insignificant levels during the next three to six hours. Because of its amide structure, MARCAINE is not detoxified by plasma esterases but is detoxified, via conjugation with glucuronic acid, in the liver. When administered in recommended doses and concentrations, MARCAINE does not ordinarily produce irritation or tissue damage, and does not cause methemoglobinemia.

Indications: Peripheral nerve block, infiltration, sympathetic block, caudal, or epidural block.

Contraindication: MARCAINE is contraindicated in patients with known hypersensitivity to it.

Warnings: RESUSCITATIVE EQUIPMENT AND DRUGS SHOULD BE READILY AVAILABLE WHEN ANY LOCAL ANESTHETIC IS USED.

Usage in Pregnancy. Reproduction studies have been performed in rats and rabbits and there is no evidence of harm to the animal fetus. The relevance to the human is not known. Safe use in pregnant women other than those in labor has not been established.

Until further clinical experience is gained, paracervical block with MARCAINE is not recommended. Fetal bradycardia frequently follows paracervical block with some amide-type local anesthetics and may be associated with fetal acidosis. Added risk appears to be present in prematurity, toxemia of pregnancy, and fetal distress.

The obstetrician is warned that severe persistent hypertension may occur after administration of certain oxytocic drugs, if vasopressors have already been used during labor (e.g., in the local anesthetic solution or to correct hypotension).

Solutions containing a vasoconstrictor, particularly epinephrine or norepinephrine, should be used with extreme caution in patients receiving monoamine oxidase (MAO) inhibitors or antidepressants of the triptyline or imipramine types, because severe, prolonged hypertension may result.

Local anesthetics which contain preservatives, i.e., those supplied in multiple dose vials, should not be used for caudal or epidural anesthesia.

Until further experience is gained in children younger than 12 years, administration of MARCAINE in this age group is not recommended.

Precautions: The safety and effectiveness of local anesthetics depend upon proper dosage, correct technique, adequate precautions, and readiness for emergencies.

The lowest dosage that gives effective anesthesia should be used in order to avoid high plasma levels and serious systemic side effects. Injection of repeated doses of MARCAINE may cause significant increase in blood levels with each additional dose, due to accumulation of the drug or its metabolites or due to slow metabolic degradation. Tolerance varies with the status of the patient. Debilitated, elderly patients and acutely ill patients should be given reduced doses commensurate with age and physical condition.

Solutions containing a vasoconstrictor should be used cautiously in areas with limited blood supply, in the presence of diseases that may adversely affect the patient's cardiovascular system, or in patients with peripheral vascular disease.

MARCAINE should be used cautiously in persons with known drugs allergies or sensitivities, particularly to the amide-type local anesthetics.

Serious dose-related cardiac arrhythmias may occur if preparations containing a vasoconstrictor such as epinephrine are employed in patients during or following the administration of chloroform, halothane, cyclopropane, trichloroethylene, or other related agents. In deciding whether to use these products concurrently in the same patient, the combined action of both agents upon the myocardium, the concentration and volume of vasoconstrictor used, and the time since injection, when applicable, should be taken into account.

Caution is advised in administration of repeat doses of MARCAINE to patients with severe liver disease.

Use in Ophthalmic Surgery: When MARCAINE 0.75% is used for retrobulbar block, complete corneal anesthesia usually precedes onset of clinically acceptable external ocular muscle akinesia. Therefore, presence of akinesia rather than anesthesia alone should determine readiness of the patient for surgery.

Use in Dentistry: Because of the long duration of anesthesia, when MARCAINE 0.5% with epinephrine is used for dental injections, patients should be cautioned about the possibility of inadvertent trauma to tongue, lips, and buccal mucosa and advised not to chew solid foods or test the anesthetized area by biting or probing.

Adverse Reactions: Reactions to MARCAINE are characteristic of those associated with other amide-type local anesthetics. A major cause of adverse reactions to this group of drugs is excessive plasma levels, which may be due to overdosage, inadvertent intravascular injection, or slow metabolic degradation.

Excessive plasma levels of the amide-type local anesthetics cause systemic reactions involving the central nervous system and the cardiovascular system. The ***central nervous system effects*** are characterized by excitation or depression. The first manifestation may be nervousness, dizziness, blurred vision, or tremors, followed by drowsiness, convulsions, unconsciousness, and possibly respiratory arrest. Since excitement may be transient or absent, the first manifestation may be drowsiness, sometimes merging into unconsciousness and respiratory arrest. Other central nervous system effects may be nausea, vomiting, chills, constriction of the pupils, or tinnitus. The ***cardiovascular manifestations*** of excessive plasma levels may include depression of the myocardium, blood pressure changes (usually hypotension), and cardiac arrest. In obstetrics, cases of fetal bradycardia have occurred (see Warnings).

Allergic reactions, which may be due to hypersensitivity, idiosyncrasy, or diminished tolerance, are characterized by cutaneous lesions (e.g., urticaria), edema, and other manifestations of allergy. Detection of sensitivity by skin testing is of doubtful value. Sensitivity to methylparaben preservatives added to multiple dose vials has been reported. Single dose vials without methylparaben are also available.

Reactions following epidural or caudal anesthesia also may include: high or total spinal block; urinary retention; fecal incontinence; loss of perineal sensation and sexual function; persistent analgesia, paresthesia, and paralysis of the lower extremities; headache and backache; and slowing of labor and increased incidence of forceps delivery.

Treatment of Reactions. Toxic effects of local anesthetics require symptomatic treatment; there is no specific cure. The physician should be prepared to maintain an airway and to support ventilation with oxygen and assisted or controlled respiration as required. Supportive treatment of the cardiovascular system includes intravenous fluids and, when appropriate, vasopressors (preferably those that stimulate the myocardium). Convulsions may be controlled with oxygen and intravenous administration, in small increments, of a barbiturate, as follows: preferably, an ultrashort-acting barbiturate such as thiopental or thiamylal; if this is not available, a short-acting barbiturate (e.g., secobarbital or pentobarbital) or diazepam. Intravenous barbiturates or anticonvulsant agents should only be administered by those familiar with their use.

Dosage and Administration: As with all local anesthetics, the dosage varies and depends upon the area to be anesthetized, the vascularity of the tissues, the number of neuronal segments to be blocked, individual tolerance, and the technique of anesthesia. The lowest dosage needed to provide effective anesthesia should be administered. For specific techniques and procedures, refer to standard textbooks.

In recommended doses, MARCAINE produces complete sensory block, but the effect on motor function differs among the three concentrations.

0.25%*—when used for caudal, epidural, or peripheral nerve block, produces incomplete motor block. Should be used for operations in which muscle relaxation is not important, or when another means of providing muscle relaxation is used concurrently. Onset of action may be slower than with the 0.5 or 0.75 per cent solutions.

0.5%*—provides motor blockade for caudal, epidural, or nerve block, but muscle relaxation may be inadequate for operations in which complete muscle relaxation is essential.

0.75%—produces complete motor block. Most useful for epidural block in abdominal operations requiring complete muscle relaxation, and for retrobulbar anesthesia.

The duration of anesthesia with MARCAINE is such that for most indications, a single dose is sufficient.

Maximum dosage limit must be individualized in each case after evaluating the size and physical status of the patient, as well as the usual rate of systemic absorption from a particular injection site. Most experience to date is with single doses of MARCAINE up to 225 mg with epinephrine 1:200,000, and 175 mg without epinephrine; more or less drug may be used depending on individualization of each case.

These doses may be repeated up to once every three hours. In clinical studies to date, total daily doses have been up to 400 mg. Until further experience is gained, this dose should not be exceeded in 24 hours. The duration of anesthetic effect may be prolonged by the addition of epinephrine.

The dosages in Table 1 have generally proved satisfactory and are recommended as a guide for use in the average adult. The dosages should be reduced for elderly or debilitated patients. Until further experience is gained, MARCAINE is not recommended for children younger than 12 years.

Use in Dentistry: The 0.5% concentration with epinephrine is recommended for infiltration and block injection in the maxillary and mandibular area when a longer duration of local anesthetic action is desired, such as for oral surgical procedures generally associated with significant postoperative pain. The average dose of 1.8 ml (9 mg) per injection site will usually suffice; an occasional second dose of 1.8 ml (9 mg) may be used if necessary to produce adequate anesthesia after making allowance for 2 to 10 minutes onset time (see ACTIONS). The lowest effective dose should be employed and time should be allowed between injections; it is recommended that the total dose for all injection sites, *spread out* over a single dental sitting, should not ordinarily exceed 90 mg for a healthy adult patient (ten 1.8 ml injections of 0.5% MARCAINE with epinephrine). Injections should be made slowly and with frequent aspirations. Until further experience is gained, MARCAINE in dentistry is not recommended for children younger than 12 years.

Unused portions of solutions not containing preservatives., i.e., those supplied in single dose ampuls, should be discarded following initial use.

Table 1. Recommended Concentrations and Doses of MARCAINE

Type of Block	Conc.	Each Dose (ml)	Each Dose (mg)	Motor Block[1]
Local infiltration	0.25%	up to max.	up to max.	______
Epidural	0.75%[2]	10–20	75–150	complete
	0.50%	10–20	50–100	moderate to complete
	0.25%	10–20	25–50	partial to moderate
Caudal	0.50%	15–30	75–150	moderate to complete
	0.25%	15–30	37.5–75	moderate
Peripheral nerves	0.50%	5 to max.	25 to max.	moderate to complete
	0.25%	5 to max.	12.5 to max.	moderate to complete
Retrobulbar	0.75%	2–4	15–30	complete
Sympathetic	0.25%	20–50	50–125	______
Dental	0.5% w/epi	1.8–3.6 per site	9–18 per site	______

[1]With continuous (intermittent) techniques, repeat doses increase the degree of motor block. The first repeat dose of 0.5% may produce complete motor block. Intercostal nerve block with 0.25% may also produce complete motor block for intraabdominal surgery.

[2]For single dose use; not for intermittent technique.

*Use only the single dose ampuls and single dose vials for caudal or epidural anesthesia; the multiple dose vials contain a preservative and therefore should not be used for these procedures.

[See table above].

How Supplied:

Store at controlled room temperature, between 15° and 30°C (59° and 86°F).

These solutions are not for spinal anesthesia.

MARCAINE hydrochloride—Sterile isotonic solutions containing sodium chloride. In multiple dose vials, each 1 ml also contains 1 mg methylparaben as antiseptic preservative. The pH of these solutions is adjusted with sodium hydroxide or hydrochloric acid. Solutions of Marcaine that do not contain epinephrine may be autoclaved. Autoclave at 15 pound pressure, 121°C (250°F) for 15 minutes.

0.25%—Contains 2.5 mg bupivacaine hydrochloride per ml

Single dose ampuls of 50 ml, boxes of 5.
Code M-601 **NDC** 0057-1212-02
M-602 Single dose vials of 10 ml, box of 10. **NDC** 0057-1212-10
M-603 Single dose vials of 30 ml, box of 10. **NDC** 0057-1212-30
Multiple dose vials of 50 ml
Code M-605 **NDC** 0057-1217-01

0.5%—Contains 5 mg bupivacaine hydrochloride per ml

Single dose ampuls of 30 ml, boxes of 5.
Code M-611 **NDC** 0057-1213-02
M-612 Single dose vials of 10 ml, box of 10. **NDC** 0057-1213-10
M-613 Single dose vials of 30 ml, box of 10. **NDC** 0057-1213-30
Multiple dose vials of 50 ml
Code M-615 **NDC** 0057-1218-01

0.75%—Contains 7.5 mg bupivacaine hydrochloride per ml

Single dose ampuls of 30 ml, boxes of 5.
Code M-621, **NDC** 0057-1214-02
M-622 Single dose vials of 10 ml, box of 10 **NDC** 0057-1214-10
M-623 Single dose vials of 30 ml, box of 10 **NDC** 0057-1214-30

MARCAINE hydrochloride with epinephrine 1:200,000 (as bitartrate)—Sterile isotonic solutions containing sodium chloride. Each 1 ml contains MARCAINE hydrochloride and 0.0091 mg epinephrine bitartrate, USP, with 0.5 mg sodium bisulfite, 0.001 ml thioglycerol, and 2 mg ascorbic acid as antioxidants, 0.0017 ml 60% sodium lactate buffer, and 0.1 mg edetate calcium disodium as stabilizer. In multiple-dose vials, each 1 ml also contains 1 mg methylparaben as antiseptic preservative. The pH of these solutions is adjusted with sodium hydroxide or hydrochloric acid. Solutions of MARCAINE that contain epinephrine should not be autoclaved and should be protected from light. Do not use if solution is discolored or contains a precipitate.

0.25% with epinephrine 1:200,000—Contains 2.5 mg bupivacaine hydrochloride per ml

Single dose ampuls of 50 ml, boxes of 5
Code M-631 **NDC** 0057-1222-02
Multiple dose vials of 50 ml, boxes of 10.
Code M-635 **NDC** 0057-1227-01

0.5% with epinephrine 1:200,000—Contains 5 mg bupivacaine hydrochloride per ml

Single dose ampuls of 30 ml, boxes of 5.
Code M-641, **NDC** 0057-1223-02
Multiple dose vials of 50 ml, boxes of 10.
Code M-645 **NDC** 0057-1228-01

0.75% with epinephrine 1:200,000—Contains 7.5 mg bupivacaine hydrochloride per ml

Single dose ampuls of 30 ml, boxes of 5.
Code M-651, **NDC** 0057-1224-02

The following table presents the solutions and packagings of MARCAINE recommended for each type of block. (An X indicates that the solution may be used for the designated block; an O indicates that it should not be used.)

[See table on next page].

MEBARAL® Ⓒ ℞

(mephobarbital tablets, USP)

Description: Mephobarbital, 5-Ethyl-1-methyl-5-phenylbarbituric acid, is a barbiturate with sedative, hypnotic and anticonvulsant properties. It occurs as a white, nearly odorless, tasteless powder and is slightly soluble in water and in alcohol.

MEBARAL is available as tablets for oral administration.

Clinical Pharmacology: Barbiturates are capable of producing all levels of CNS mood alteration from excitation to mild sedation, to hypnosis, and deep coma. Overdosage can produce death. In high enough therapeutic doses, barbiturates induce anesthesia.

Barbiturates depress the sensory cortex, decrease motor activity, alter cerebellar function, and produce drowsiness, sedation, and hypnosis.

Barbiturates are respiratory depressants. The degree of respiratory depression is dependent upon dose. With hypnotic doses, respiratory depression produced by barbiturates is similar to that which occurs during physiologic sleep with slight decrease in blood pressure and heart rate.

Studies in laboratory animals have shown that barbiturates cause reduction in the tone and contractility of the uterus, ureters, and urinary bladder. However, concentrations of the drugs required to produce this effect in hu-

Continued on next page

Breon—Cont.

mans are not reached with sedative-hypnotic doses.
Barbiturates do not impair normal hepatic function, but have been shown to induce liver microsomal enzymes, thus increasing and/or altering the metabolism of barbiturates and other drugs. (See PRECAUTIONS-DRUG INTERACTIONS below.)
MEBARAL exerts a strong sedative and anticonvulsant action but has a relatively mild hypnotic effect. It reduces the incidence of epileptic seizures in grand mal and petit mal. MEBARAL usually causes little or no drowsiness or lassitude. Hence, when it is used as a sedative or anticonvulsant, patients usually become more calm, more cheerful, and better adjusted to their surroundings without clouding of mental faculties. MEBARAL is reported to produce less sedation than does phenobarbital.
Barbiturates are weak acids that are absorbed and rapidly distributed to all tissues and fluids with high concentrations in the brain, liver, and kidneys. Lipid solubility of the barbiturates is the dominant factor in their distribution within the body. Barbiturates are bound to plasma and tissue proteins to a varying degree with the degree of binding increasing directly as a function of lipid solubility.
Approximately 50% of an oral dose of mephobarbital is absorbed from the gastrointestinal tract. Therapeutic plasma concentrations for mephobarbital have not been established nor has the half-life been determined. Following oral administration, the onset of action of the drug is 30 to 60 minutes and the duration of action is 10 to 16 hours. The primary route of mephobarbital metabolism is N-demethylation by the microsomal enzymes of the liver to form phenobarbital. Phenobarbital may be excreted in the urine unchanged or further metabolized to *p*-hydroxyphenobarbital and excreted in the urine as glucuronide or sulfate conjugates. About 75% of a single oral dose of mephobarbital is converted to phenobarbital in 24 hours. Therefore, chronic administration of mephobarbital may lead to an accumulation of phenobarbital (not mephobarbital) in plasma. It has not been determined whether mephobarbital or phenobarbital is the active agent during long-time mephobarbital therapy.

Indications and Usage: MEBARAL is indicated for use as a sedative for the relief of anxiety, tension and apprehension, and as an anticonvulsant for the treatment of grand mal and petit mal epilepsy.

Contraindications: Hypersensitivity to any barbiturate. Manifest or latent porphyria.

Warnings: 1. *Habit forming.* Barbiturates may be habit forming. Tolerance, psychological and physical dependence may occur with continued use. (See DRUG ABUSE AND DEPENDENCE below and CLINICAL PHARMACOLOGY above.) Patients who have psychological dependence on barbirurates may increase the dosage or decrease the dosage interval without consulting a physician and may subsequently develop a physical dependence on barbiturates. To minimize the possibility of overdosage or the development of dependence, the prescribing and dispensing of sedative-hypnotic barbiturates should be limited to the amount required for the interval until the next appointment. Abrupt cessation after prolonged use in the dependent person may result in withdrawal symptoms, including delirium, convulsions, and possibly death. Barbiturates should be withdrawal gradually from any patient known to be taking excessive dosage over long periods of time. (See DRUG ABUSE AND DEPENDENCE below.)
2. *Acute or chronic pain.* Caution should be exercised when barbiturates are administered to patients with acute or chronic pain, because paradoxical excitement could be induced or important symptoms could be masked. However, the use of barbiturates as sedatives in the postoperative surgical period and as adjuncts to cancer chemotherapy is well established.
3. *Use in pregnancy.* Barbiturates can cause fetal damage when administered to a pregnant woman. Retrospective, case-controlled studies have suggested a connection between the maternal consumption of barbiturates and a higher than expected incidence of fetal abnormalities. Following oral or parenteral administration, barbiturates readily cross the placental barrier and are distributed throughout fetal tissues with highest concentrations found in the placenta, fetal liver, and brain. Fetal blood levels approach maternal blood levels following parenteral administration.
Withdrawal symptoms occur in infants born to mothers who receive barbiturates throughout the last trimester of pregnancy. (See DRUG ABUSE AND DEPENDENCE below.) If this drug is used during pregnancy, or if the patient becomes pregnant while taking this drug, the patient should be apprised of the potential hazard to the fetus.
4. *Synergistic effects.* The concomitant use of alcohol or other CNS depressants may produce additive CNS depressant effects.

Precautions: *General.* Barbiturates may be habit forming. Tolerance and psychological and physical dependence may occur with continuing use. (See DRUG ABUSE AND DEPENDENCE below.) Barbiturates should be administered with caution, if at all, to patients who are mentally depressed, have suicidal tendencies, or a history of drug abuse.
Elderly or debilitated patients may react to barbiturates with marked excitement, depression, and confusion. In some persons, barbiturates repeatedly produce excitement rather than depression.
In patients with hepatic damage, barbiturates should be administered with caution and initially in reduced doses. Barbiturates should not be administered to patients showing the premonitory signs of hepatic coma.
Status epilepticus may result from the abrupt discontinuation of MEBARAL, even when administered in small daily doses in the treatment of epilepsy.
Caution and careful adjustment of dosage are required when MEBARAL is used in patients with impaired renal, cardiac or respiratory function and in patients with myasthenia gravis and myxedema. The least quantity feasible should be prescribed or dispensed at any one time in order to minimize the possibility of acute or chronic overdosage.

Vitamin D Deficiency: MEBARAL may increase vitamin D requirements, possibly by increasing vitamin D metabolism via enzyme induction. Rarely, rickets and osteomalacia have been reported following prolonged use of barbiturates.

Vitamin K: Bleeding in the early neonatal period due to coagulation defects may follow exposure to anticonvulsant drugs *in utero:* therefore, viamin K should be given to the mother before delivery or to the child at birth.
Information for the patient: Practitioners should give the following information and instructions to patients receiving barbiturates.
1. The use of barbiturates carries with it an associated risk of psychological and/or physical dependence. The patient should be warned against increasing the dose of the drug without consulting a physician.
2. Barbiturates may impair mental and/or physical abilities required for the performance of potentially hazardous tasks (e.g., driving, operating machinery, etc.).
3. Alcohol should not be consumed while taking barbiturates. Concurrent use of the barbiturates with other CNS depressants (e.g., alcohol, narcotics, tranquilizers, and antihistamines) may result in additional CNS depressant effects.

Laboratory tests. Prolonged therapy with barbiturates should be accompanied by periodic laboratory evaluation or organ systems, in-

	Infiltration	Peripheral Nerve	Retrobulbar	Caudal	Epidural	Sympathetic	Dental
0.25%							
50 ml ampul	x	x	o	x	x	x	o
10 ml vial	x	x	o	x	x	x	o
30 ml vial	x	x	o	x	x	x	o
50 ml vial (multiple dose)	x	x	o	o	o	x	o
0.25% with epinedrine 1:200,000							
50 ml ampul	x	x	o	x	x	o	o
10 ml vial	x	x	o	x	x	o	o
30 ml vial	x	x	o	x	x	o	o
50 ml vial (multiple dose)	x	x	o	o	o	o	o
0.5%							
30 ml ampul	o	x	o	x	x	o	o
10 ml vial	o	x	o	x	x	o	o
30 ml vial	o	x	o	x	x	o	o
50 ml vial (multiple dose)	o	x	o	o	o	o	o
0.5% with ephinephrine 1:200,000							
30 ml ampul	o	x	o	x	x	o	x
10 ml vial	o	x	o	x	x	o	x
30 ml vial	o	x	o	x	x	o	x
50 ml vial (multiple dose)	o	x	o	o	o	o	x
0.75%							
30 ml ampul	o	o	x	o	x	o	o
10 ml vial	o	o	x	o	x	o	o
30 ml vial	o	o	x	o	x	o	o
0.75% with epinephrine 1:200,000							
30 ml ampul	o	o	x	o	x	o	o

cluding hematopoietic, renal, and hepatic systems. (See PRECAUTIONS [*General*] above and ADVERSE REACTIONS below.)

Drug interactions. Most reports of clinically significant drug interactions occurring with the barbiturates have involved phenobarbital. However, the application of these data to other barbiturates appears valid and warrants serial blood level determinations of the relevant drugs when there are multiple therapies.

1. *Anticoagulants.* Phenobarbital lowers the plasma levels of dicumarol (name previously used: bishydroxycoumarin) and causes a decrease in anticoagulant activity as measured by the prothrombin time. Barbiturates can induce hepatic microsomal enzymes resulting in increased metabolism and decreased anticoagulant response of oral anticoagulants (e.g., warfarin, acenocoumarol, dicumarol, and phenprocoumon). Patients stablized on anticoagulant therapy may require dosage adjustments if barbiturates are added to or withdrawn from their dosage regimen.

2. *Corticosteroids.* Barbiturates appear to enhance the metabolism of exogenous corticosteroids probably through the induction of hepatic microsomal enzymes. Patients stabilized on corticosteroid therapy may require dosage adjustments if barbiturates are added to or withdrawn from their dosage regimen.

3. *Griseofulvin.* Phenobarbital appears to interfere with the absorption of orally administered griseofulvin, thus decreasing its blood level. The effect of the resultant decreased blood levels of griseofulvin on therapeutic response has not been established. However, it would be preferable to avoid concomitant administration of these drugs.

4. *Doxycycline.* Phenobarbital has been shown to shorten the half-life of doxycycline for as long as 2 weeks after barbiturate therapy is discontinued.

This mechanism is probably through the induction of hepatic microsomal enzymes that metabolize the antibiotic. If phenobarbital and doxycycline are administered concurrently, the clinical response to doxycycline should be monitored closely.

5. *Phenytoin, sodium valproate, valproic acid.* The effect of barbiturates on the metabolism of phenytoin appears to be variable. Some investigators report an accelerating effect, while others report no effect. Because the effect of barbiturates on the metabolism of phenytoin is not predictable, phenytoin and barbiturate blood levels should be monitored more frequently if these drugs are given concurrently. Sodium valproate and valproic acid appear to decrease barbiturate metabolism; therefore, barbiturate blood levels should be monitored and appropriate dosage adjustments made as indicated.

6. *Central nervous system depressants.* The concomitant use of other central nervous system depressants, including other sedatives or hypnotics, antihistamines, tranquilizers, or alcohol, may produce additive depressant effects.

7. *Monoamine oxidase inhibitors (MAOI).* MAOI prolong the effects of barbiturates probably because metabolism of the barbiturate is inhibited.

8. *Estradiol, estone, progesterone and other steroidal hormones.* Pretreatment with or concurrent administration of phenobarbital may decrease the effect of estradiol by increasing its metabolism. There have been reports of patients treated with antiepileptic drugs (e.g., phenobarbital) who become pregnant while taking oral contraceptives. An alternant contraceptive method might be suggested to women taking phenobarbital.

Carcinogenesis

1. *Animal data.* Phenobarbital sodium is carcinogenic in mice and rats after lifetime administration. In mice, it produced benign and malignant liver cell tumors. In rats, benign liver cell tumors were observed very late in life. Phenobarbital is the major metabolite of MEBARAL.

2. *Human data.* In a 29-year epidemiological study of 9,136 patients who were treated on an anticonvulsant protocol which included phenobarbital, results indicated a higher than normal incidence of hepatic carcinoma. Previously, some of these patients were treated with thorotrast, a drug which is known to produce hepatic carcinomas. Thus, this study did not provide sufficient evidence that phenobarbital sodium is carcinogenic in humans. Phenobarbital is the major metabolite of MEBARAL.

A retrospective study of 84 children with brain tumors matched to 73 normal controls and 78 cancer controls (malignant disease other than brain tumors) suggested an association between exposure to barbiturates prenatally and an increased incidence of brain tumors.

Pregnancy

1. *Teratogenic effects.* Pregnancy Category D—See WARNINGS—Use in Pregnancy above.

2. *Nonteratogenic effects.* Reports of infants suffering from long-term barbiturate exposure *in utero* included the acute withdrawal syndrome of seizures and hyperirritability from birth to a delayed onset of up to 14 days. (See DRUG ABUSE AND DEPENDENCE below.)

Labor and delivery. Hypnotic doses of these barbiturates do not appear to significantly impair uterine activity during labor. Full anesthetic doses of barbiturates decrease the force and frequency of uterine contractions. Administration of sedative-hypnotic barbiturates to the mother during labor may result in respiratory depression in the newborn. Premature infants are particularly susceptible to the depressant effects of barbiturates. If barbiturates are used during labor and delivery, resuscitation equipment should be available.

Data are currently not available to evaluate the effect of these barbiturates when forceps delivery or other intervention is necessary. Also, data are not available to determine the effect of these barbiturates on the later growth, development, and functional maturation of the child.

Nursing Mothers. Caution should be exercised when a barbiturate is administered to a nursing woman since small amounts of barbiturates are excreted in the milk.

Adverse Reactions: The following adverse reactions and their incidence were compiled from surveillance of thousands of hospitalized patients. Because such patients may be less aware of certain of the milder adverse effects of barbiturates, the incidence of these reactions may be somewhat higher in fully ambulatory patients.

More than 1 in 100 patients. The most common adverse reactions estimated to occur at a rate of 1 to 3 patients per 100 is:

Nervous system: Somnolence.

Less than 1 in 100 patients. Adverse reactions estimated to occur at a rate of less than 1 in 100 patients listed below, grouped by organ system, and by decreasing order of occurrence are:

Nervous system: Agitation, confusion, hyperkinesia, ataxia, CNS depression, nightmares, nervousness, psychiatric disturbance, hallucinations, insomnia, anxiety, dizziness, thinking abnormality.

Respiratory system: Hypoventilation, apnea.

Cardiovascular system: Bradycardia, hypotension, syncope.

Digestive system: Nausea, vomiting, constipation.

Other reported reactions: Headache, hypersensitivity reactions (angioedema, skin rashes, exfoliative dermatitis), fever, liver damage, megaloblastic anemia following chronic phenobarbital use.

Drug Abuse and Dependence: Mephobarbital is a controlled substance in Narcotic Schedule IV. Barbiturates may be habit forming. Tolerance, psychological dependence, and physical dependence may occur especially following prolonged use of high doses of barbiturates. As tolerance to barbiturates develops, the amount needed to maintain the same level of intoxication increases; tolerance to a fatal dosage, however, does not increase more than two-fold. As this occurs, the margin between an intoxicating dosage and fatal dosage becomes smaller.

Symptoms of acute intoxication with barbiturates include unsteady gait, slurred speech, and sustained nystagmus. Mental signs of chronic intoxication include confusion, poor judgment, irritability, insomnia and somatic complaints.

Symptoms of barbiturate dependence are similar to those of chronic alcoholism. If an individual appears to be intoxicated with alcohol to a degree that is radically disproportionate to the amount of alcohol in his or her blood the use of barbiturates should be suspected. The lethal dose of a barbiturate is far less if alcohol is also ingested.

The symptoms of barbiturate withdrawal can be severe and may cause death. Minor withdrawal symptoms may appear 8 to 12 hours after the last dose of a barbiturate. These symptoms usually appear in the following order: anxiety, muscle twitching, tremor of hands and fingers, progressive weakness, dizziness, distortion in visual perception, nausea, vomiting, insomnia, and orthostatic hypotension. Major withdrawal symptoms (convulsions and delirium) may occur within 16 hours and last up to 5 days after abrupt cessation of these drugs. Intensity of withdrawal symptoms gradually declines over a period of approximately 15 days. Individuals susceptible to a barbiturate abuse and dependence include alcoholics and opiate abusers, as well as other sedative-hypnotic and amphetamine abusers.

Drug dependence to barbiturates arises from repeated administration of a barbiturate or agent with barbiturate-like effect on a continuous basis, generally in amounts exceeding therapeutic dose levels. The characteristics of drug dependence to bartiturates include: (a) a strong desire or need to continue taking the drug; (b) a tendency to increase the dose; (c) a psychic dependence on the effects of the drug related to subjective and individual appreciation of those effects; and (d) a physical dependence on the effects of the drug requiring its presence for maintenance of homeostasis and resulting in a definite, characteristic, and self-limited abstinence syndrome when the drug is withdrawn.

Treatment of barbiturate dependence consists of cautious and gradual withdrawal of the drug. Barbiturate-dependent patients can be withdrawn by using a number of different withdrawal regimens. In all cases withdrawal takes an extended period of time. One method involves substituting a 30 mg dose of phenobarbital for each 100 to 200 mg dose of barbiturate that the patient has been taking. The total daily amount of phenobarbital is then administered in 3 to 4 divided doses, not to exceed 600 mg daily. Should signs of withdrawal occur on the first day of treatment, a loading dose of 100 to 200 mg of phenobarbital may be administered IM in addition to the oral dose. After stablization on phenobarbital, the total daily dose is decreased by 30 mg a day as long as withdrawal is proceeding smoothly. A modification of this regimen involves initiating treatment at the patient's regular dosage level and decreasing the daily dosage by 10% if tolerated by the patient.

Continued on next page

Breon—Cont.

Infants physically dependent on barbiturates may be given phenobarbital 3 to 10 mg/kg/day. After withdrawal symptoms (hyperactivity, disturbed sleep, tremors, hyperreflexial) are relieved, the dosage of phenobarbital should be gradually decreased and completely withdrawn over a 2-week period.

Overdosage: The toxic dose of barbiturates varies considerably. In general, an oral dose of 1 gram of most barbiturates produces serious poisoning in an adult. Death commonly occurs after 2 to 10 grams of ingested barbiturate. Barbiturate intoxication may be confused with alcoholism, bromide intoxication, and with various neurological disorders.

Acute overdosage with barbiturates is manifested by CNS and respiratory depression which may progress to Cheyne-Stokes respiration, areflexia, constriction of the pupils to a slight degree (though in severe poisoning they may show paralytic dilation), oliguria, tachycardia, hypotension, lowered body temperature and coma. Typical shock syndrome (apnea, circulatory collapse, respiratory arrest, and death) may occur.

In extreme overdose, all electrical activity in the brain may cease, in which case a "flat" EEG normally equated with clinical death cannot be accepted. This effect is fully reversible unless hypoxic damage occurs. Consideration should be given to the possibility of barbiturate intoxication even in situations that appear to involve trauma.

Complications such as pneumonia, pulmonary edema, cardiac arrhythmias, congestive heart failure, and renal failure may occur. Uremia may increase CNS sensitivity to barbiturates if renal function is impaired. Differential diagnosis should include hypoglycemia, head trauma, cerebrovascular accidents, convulsive states, and diabetic coma.

Treatment of overdosage is mainly supportive and consists of the following:

1. Maintenance of an adequate airway, with assisted respiration and oxygen administration as necessary.
2. Monitoring of vital signs and fluid balance.
3. If the patient is conscious and has not lost the gag reflex, emesis may be induced with ipecac. Care should be taken to prevent pulmonary aspiration of vomitus. After completion of vomiting, 30 grams activated charcoal in a glass of water may be administered.
4. If emesis is contraindicated, gastric lavage may be performed with a cuffed endotracheal tube in place with the patient in the face down position. Activated charcoal may be left in the emptied stomach and a saline cathartic administered.
5. Fluid therapy and other standard treatment for shock, if needed.
6. If renal function is normal, forced diuresis may aid in the elimination of the barbiturate. Alkalinization of the urine increases renal excretion of some barbiturates, including mephobarbital (which is metabolized to phenobarbital).
7. Although not recommended as a routine procedure, hemodialysis may be used in severe barbiturate intoxications or if the patient is anuric or in shock.
8. Patient should be rolled from side to side every 30 minutes.
9. Antibiotics should be given if pneumonia is suspected.
10. Appropriate nursing care to prevent hypostatic pneumonia, decubiti aspiration, and other complications of patients with altered states of consciousness.

Dosage and Administration: **Epilepsy:** Average dose for adults: 400 to 600 mg (6 to 9 grains) daily; children under 5 years: 16 to 32 mg (¼ to ½ grain) three or four times daily; children over 5 years: 32 to 64 mg (½ to 1 grain) three or four times daily. MEBARAL is best taken at bedtime if seizures generally occur at night, and during the day if attacks are diurnal.

Treatment should be started with a small dose which is gradually increased over four or five days until the optimum dosage is determined. If the patient has been taking some other antiepilptic drug, it should be tapered off as the doses of MEBARAL are increased, to guard against the temporary marked attacks that may occur when any treatment for epilepsy is changed abruptly. Similarly, when the dose is to be lowered to a maintenance level or to be discontinued, the amount should be reduced gradually over four or five days.

Special patient population. Dosage should be reduced in the elderly or debilitated because these patients may be more sensitive to barbiturates. Dosage should be reduced for patients with impaired renal function or hepatic disease.

Combination with Other Drugs: MEBARAL may be used in combination with phenobarbital, either in the form of alternating courses or concurrently. When the two drugs are used at the same time, the dose should be about one-half the amount of each used alone. The average daily dose for an adult is from 50 to 100 mg (¾ grain to 1½ grains) of phenobarbital and from 200 to 300 mg (3 to 4½ grains) of MEBARAL.

MEBARAL may also be used with phenytoin sodium; in some cases, combined therapy appears to give better results than either agent used alone, since phenytoin sodium is particularly effective for the psychomotor types of seizure but relatively ineffective for petit mal. When the drugs are employed concurrently, a reduced dose of phenytoin sodium is advisable, but the full dose of MEBARAL may be given. Satisfactory results have been obtained with an average daily dose of 230 mg (3½ grains) of phenytoin sodium plus about 600 mg (9 grains) of MEBARAL.

Sedation: Adults: 32 to 100 mg (½ to 1½ grains)—optimum dose, 50 mg (¾ grain)—three or four times daily. Children: 16 to 32 mg (¼ to ½ grain) three or four times daily.

How Supplied: **Tablets:**

32 mg (½ grain)—bottles of 250
Code M-705 ....**NDC** 0057-1231-05
32 mg (½ grain)—bottles of 1000
Code M-701 ....**NDC** 0057-1231-08
50 mg (¾ grain)—bottles of 250
Code M-715 ....**NDC** 0057-1232-05
100 mg (1½ grains)—bottles of 250
Code M-725 ....**NDC** 0057-1233-05
200 mg (3 grains)—bottles of 250
Code M-735 ....**NDC** 0057-1234-05

[*Shown in Product Identification Section*]

NOVOCAIN® ℞

brand of procaine hydrochloride injection, USP

Local Anesthetic for Major and Minor Surgery

THESE SOLUTIONS ARE NOT INTENDED FOR SPINAL OR EPIDURAL ANESTHESIA OR DENTAL USE

Description: NOVOCAIN, brand of procaine hydrochloride, is benzoic acid, 4-amino-, 2-(diethylamino)ethyl ester, monohydrochloride, the ester of diethylaminoethanol and para-aminobenzoic acid.

It is a white crystalline, odorless powder that is freely soluble in water, but less soluble in alcohol.

Composition of Available Solutions.

[See table below].

The solutions are made isotonic with sodium chloride and the pH is adjusted between 3.0 and 5.5 with sodium hydroxide and hydrochloric acid. DO NOT USE SOLUTIONS IF CRYSTALS, CLOUDINESS, OR DISCOLORATION IS OBSERVED. EXAMINE SOLUTIONS CAREFULLY BEFORE USE. REAUTOCLAVING INCREASES LIKELIHOOD OF CRYSTAL FORMATION.

Clinical Pharmacology: NOVOCAIN stabilizes the neuronal membrane and prevents the initiation and transmission of nerve impulses, thereby effecting local anesthesia. NOVOCAIN lacks surface anesthetic activity. The onset of action is rapid (2 to 5 minutes) and the duration of action is relatively short (average 1 to 1½ hours), depending upon the anesthetic technique, the type of block, the concentration, and the individual patient.

NOVOCAIN is readily absorbed following parenteral administration and is rapidly hydrolyzed by plasma cholinesterase to para-aminobenzoic acid and diethylaminoethanol.

A vasoconstrictor may be added to the NOVOCAIN solution to promote local hemostasis, delay systemic absorption, and increase duration of anesthesia.

Indications and Usage: NOVOCAIN is indicated for the production of local anesthesia by infiltration injection, nerve block, and other peripheral blocks.

Contraindication: NOVOCAIN is contraindicated in patients with a known hypersensitivity to the drug, drugs of a similar chemical configuration, or para-aminobenzoic acid or its derivatives.

Warnings: RESUSCITATIVE EQUIPMENT AND DRUGS SHOULD BE IMMEDIATELY AVAILABLE WHENEVER ANY LOCAL ANESTHETIC DRUG IS USED.

Large doses of local anesthetics should not be used in patients with heart block.

Reactions resulting in fatality have occurred on rare occasions with the use of local anesthetics, even in the absence of a history of hypersensitivity.

Solutions which contain a vasoconstrictor should be used with extreme caution in patients receiving drugs known to produce alterations in blood pressure (i.e., monoamine oxidase (MAO) inhibitors, tricyclic antidepressants, phenothiazines, etc.) as either severe or sustained hypertension or hypotension or disturbances of cardiac rhythm may occur.

Usage in Pregnancy. Safe use of NOVOCAIN has not been established with respect to adverse effects on fetal development. Careful consideration should be given to this fact before administering this drug to women of childbearing potential particularly during early pregnancy. This does not exclude the use of the drug at term for obstetrical analgesia. Vasopressor agents (administered for the treatment of hypotension or added to the anesthetic solution for vasoconstriction) should be used with extreme caution in the presence of oxytocic drugs as they may produce severe, persistent hypertension with possible rupture of a cerebral blood vessel.

Each ml contains	1% ampul	1% vial	2% vial
Procaine hydrochloride	10 mg	10 mg	20 mg
Acetone sodium bisulfite	≤ 1 mg	≤ 2 mg	≤ 2 mg
Chlorobutanol	—	≤ 2.5 mg	≤ 2.5 mg

[Acetone sodium bisulfite and chlorobutanol are added as preservatives.]

Local anesthetic procedures should be used with caution when there is inflammation and/or sepsis in the region of the proposed injection.

Precautions: Standard textbooks should be consulted for specific techniques and precautions for various regional anesthetic procedures.

The safety and effectiveness of a local anesthetic drug depend upon proper dosage, correct technique, adequate precautions, and readiness for emergencies.

Tolerance varies with the status of the patient. Debilitated, elderly patients, or acutely ill patients should be given reduced doses commensurate with their weight and physical status.

NOVOCAIN should be used with caution in patients with severe disturbances of cardiac rhythm, shock, or heart block.

INJECTION SHOULD ALWAYS BE MADE SLOWLY AND WITH FREQUENT ASPIRATIONS TO AVOID INADVERTENT RAPID INTRAVASCULAR ADMINISTRATION WHICH CAN PRODUCE SYSTEMIC TOXICITY.

Fetal bradycardia which frequently follows paracervical block may be indicative of high fetal blood concentrations of NOVOCAIN with resultant fetal acidosis. Fetal heart rate should be monitored prior to and during paracervical block. Added risk appears to be present in prematurity, toxemia of pregnancy, and fetal distress. The physician should weigh the benefits against the risks in considering paracervical block in these conditions. Careful adherence to recommended dosage is of the utmost importance in paracervical block. Failure to achieve adequate analgesia with these doses should arouse suspicion of intravascular or fetal injection.

VASOCONSTRICTORS. Solutions containing a vasoconstrictor should be used cautiously. The decision whether or not to use a vasoconstrictor with local anesthesia depends on the physician's appraisal of the benefits as opposed to the risk, e.g., in injection of solutions containing a vasoconstrictor into areas where the blood supply is limited (e.g., ears, nose, digits) or when peripheral vascular disease is present. Furthermore, serious cardiac arrhythmias may occur if preparations containing a vasoconstrictor are employed in patients during or immediately following the administration of halothane, cyclopropane, trichloroethylene, or other related agents.

NOVOVAIN SHOULD BE USED WITH CAUTION IN PATIENTS WITH KNOWN DRUG ALLERGIES AND SENSITIVITIES. A thorough history of the patient's prior experience with NOVOCAIN or other local anesthetics as well as concomitant or recent drug use should be taken (see Contraindications). NOVOCAIN should not be used in any conditions in which a sulfonamide drug is being employed since para-aminobenzoic acid inhibits the action of the sulfonamides.

Adverse Reactions: Systemic adverse reactions involving the central nervous system and the cardiovascular system usually result from high plasma levels due to excessive dosage, rapid absorption, or inadvertent intravascular injection.

A small number of reactions may result from hypersensitivity, idiosyncrasy, or diminished tolerance to normal dosage.

Excitatory CNS effects (nervousness, dizziness, blurred vision, tremors) commonly represent the initial signs of local anesthetic systemic toxicity. However, these reactions may be very brief or absent in some patients in which case the first manifestation of toxicity may be drowsiness or convulsions merging into unconsciousness and respiratory arrest.

Cardiovascular system reactions include depression of the myocardium, hypotension (or sometimes hypertension), bradycardia, and even cardiac arrest. In obstetrics, cases of fetal bradycardia have occurred (see Precautions).

Allergic reactions are characterized by cutaneous lesions of delayed onset, or urticaria, edema, and other manifestations of allergy. The detection of sensitivity by skin testing is of limited value. As with other local anesthetics, hypersensitivity, idiosyncrasy and anaphylactoid reactions have occurred rarely. The reaction may be abrupt and severe and is not usually dose related.

Treatment of Reactions. Treatment of a patient with toxic manifestations consist of assuring and maintaining a patent airway and supporting ventilation with oxygen and assisted or controlled ventilation (respiration) as required. This usually will be sufficient in the management of most reactions. Should a convulsion persist despite ventilatory therapy, small increments of anticonvulsive agents may be given intravenously, such as benzodiazepine (e.g., diazepam), or ultrashort-acting barbiturates (e.g., thiopental or thiamylal) or a short-acting barbiturate (e.g., pentobarbital or secobarbital). Cardiovascular depression may require circulatory assistance with intravenous fluids and/or vasopressors (e.g., ephedrine) as dictated by the clinical situation. Allergic reactions are rare and may occur as a result of sensitivity to the local anesthetic or methylparaben used as a preservative and are characterized by cutaneous lesions, urticaria, edema, and anaphylactoid type symptomatology. These allergic reactions should be managed by conventional means. The detection of potential sensitivity by skin testing is of limited value.

Dosage and Administration: As with all local anesthetics, the dose of NOVOCAIN varies and depends upon the area to be anesthetized, the vascularity of the tissues, the number of neuronal segments to be blocked, individual tolerance, and the technique of anesthesia. The lowest dose needed to provide effective anesthesia should be administered. For specific techniques and procedures, refer to standard textbooks.

For infiltration anesthesia, 0.25 or 0.5 percent solution; 350-600 mg is generally considered to be a single safe total dose. To prepare 60 ml of a 0.5 percent solution (5mg/ml), dilute 30 ml of the 1 percent solution with 30 ml sterile distilled water. To prepare 60 ml of a 0.25 percent solution (2.5 mg/ml), dilute 15 ml of the 1 percent solution with 45 ml sterile distilled water. 0.5 to 1 ml of epinephrine 1:1000 per 100 ml anesthetic solution may be added for vasoconstrictive effect (1:200,000 to 1:100,000) (see Warnings and Precautions).

For peripheral nerve block, 0.5 percent solution (up to 200 ml), 1 percent solution (up to 100 ml) or 2 percent solution (up to 50 ml). The use of the 2 percent solution should usually be limited to cases requiring a small volume of anesthetic solution (10-25 ml). 0.5 to 1 ml of epinephrine 1:1000 per 100 ml anesthetic solution may be added for vasoconstrictive effect (1:200,000 to 1:100,000) (see Warnings and Precautions).

THE USUAL INITIAL DOSE SHOULD NOT EXCEED 1000 MG.

Sterilization: Disinfecting agents containing heavy metals, which cause release of respective ions (mercury, zinc, copper, etc.) should not be used for skin or mucous membrane disinfection as they have been related to incidence of swelling and edema.

When chemical disinfection of multiple dose vials is desired, either pure undiluted isopropyl alcohol (91%) or 70% ethyl alcohol USP is recommended. Many commercially available brands of rubbing alcohol, as well as solutions of ethyl alcohol not of USP grade, contain denaturants which are injurious to rubber and, therefore, are not to be used. It is recommended that chemical disinfection be accomplished, by wiping the vial or ampul thoroughly with cotton or gauze that has been moistened with the recommended alcohol just prior to use.

The drug in intact ampuls and vials is sterile. The preferred method of destroying bacteria on the exterior before opening is heat sterilization (autoclaving). Immersion in antiseptic solution is not recommended.

Autoclave at 15-pound pressure, at 121°C (250°F), for 15 minutes.

How Supplied:

NOVOCAIN Solution 1 percent

Code N-162 Ampuls of 2 ml UNI-NEST PAK of 25 **NDC** 0057-1381-25

Code N-171 Ampuls of 6 ml boxes of 50 **NDC** 0057-1382-05

Code N-590 Vials of 30 ml boxes of 100 **NDC** 0057-1385-01

NOVOCAIN Solution 2 percent

Code N-190 Vials of 30 ml boxes of 100 **NDC** 0057-1386-01

Protect solutions from light.

The air in all ampuls and vials has been displaced by nitrogen gas.

NOVOCAIN® ℞

brand of procaine hydrochloride injection, USP

10% Solution for Spinal Anesthesia

Description: NOVOCAIN, brand of procaine hydrochloride, is benzoic acid, 4-amino-, 2-(diethylamino) ethyl ester, monohydrochloride, the ester of diethylaminoethanol and para-aminobenzoic acid.

It is a white crystalline, odorless powder that is freely soluble in water, but less soluble in alcohol. Each ml in the ampuls contains 100 mg procaine hydrochloride and 8 mg acetone sodium bisulfite as antioxidant. DO NOT USE SOLUTIONS IF CRYSTALS, CLOUDINESS, OR DISCOLORATION IS OBSERVED. EXAMINE SOLUTIONS CAREFULLY BEFORE USE. REAUTOCLAVING INCREASES LIKELIHOOD OF CRYSTAL FORMATION.

Clinical Pharmacology: NOVOCAIN stabilizes the neuronal membrane and prevents the initiation and transmission of nerve impulses, thereby effecting local anesthesia. NOVOCAIN lacks surface anesthetic activity. The onset of action is rapid (2 to 5 minutes) and the duration of action is relatively short (average 1 to 1½ hours), depending upon the anesthetic technique, the type of block, the concentration, and the individual patient.

NOVOCAIN is readily absorbed following parenteral administration and is rapidly hydrolyzed by plasma cholinesterase to para-aminobenzoic acid and diethylaminoethanol.

A vasoconstrictor may be added to the NOVOCAIN solution to promote local hemostasis, delay systemic absorption, and increase duration of anesthesia.

Indications and Usage: NOVOCAIN is indicated for spinal anesthesia.

Contraindications: Spinal anesthesia with NOVOCAIN is contraindicated in patients with generalized septicemia; sepsis at the proposed injection site; certain diseases of the cerebrospinal system, e.g., meningitis, syphilis; and a known hypersensitivity to the drug, drugs of a similar chemical configuration, or para-aminobenzoic acid or its derivatives.

The decision as to whether or not spinal anesthesia should be used in an individual case should be made by the physician after weighing the advantages with the risks and possible complications.

Warnings: RESUSCITATIVE EQUIPMENT AND DRUGS SHOULD BE IMMEDIATELY AVAILABLE WHENEVER ANY LOCAL ANESTHETIC DRUG IS USED. Spinal anesthesia should only be administered by those qualified to do so.

Large doses of local anesthetics should not be used in patients with heart block.

Reactions resulting in fatality have occurred on rare occasions with the use of local anes-

Continued on next page

Breon—Cont.

thetics, even in the absence of a history of hypersensitivity.

Usage in Pregnancy. Safe use of NOVOCAIN has not been established with respect to adverse effects on fetal development. Careful consideration should be given to this fact before administering this drug to women of childbearing potential particularly during early pregnancy. This does not exclude the use of the drug at term for obstetrical analgesia.

Vasopressor agents (administered for the treatment of hypotension or added to the anesthetic solution for vasoconstriction) should be used with extreme caution in the presence of oxytocic drugs as they may produce severe, persistent hypertension with possible rupture of a cerebral blood vessel.

Solutions which contain a vasoconstrictor should be used with extreme caution in patients receiving drugs known to produce alterations in blood pressure (i.e., monoamine oxidase (MAO) inhibitors, tricyclic antidepressants, phenothiazines, etc.) as either severe sustained hypertension or hypotension may occur.

Local anesthetic procedures should be used with caution when there is inflammation and/or sepsis in the region of the proposed injection.

Precautions: Standard textbooks should be consulted for specific techniques and precautions for various spinal anesthetic procedures.

The safety and effectiveness of a spinal anesthetic depend upon proper dosage, correct technique, adequate precautions, and readiness for emergencies. The lowest dosage that results in effective anesthesia should be used to avoid high plasma levels and possible adverse effects. Tolerance varies with the status of the patient. Debilitated, elderly patients, or acutely ill patients should be given reduced doses commensurate with their weight and physical status. Reduced dosages are also indicated for obstetric delivery and patients with increased intraabdominal pressure.

The decision whether or not to use spinal anesthesia in the following disease states depends on the physician's appraisal of the advantages as opposed to the risk: cardiovascular disease (i.e., shock, hypertension, anemia, etc.), pulmonary disease, renal impairment, metabolic or endocrine disorders, gastrointestinal disorders (i.e., intestinal obstruction, peritonitis, etc.), or complicated obstetrical deliveries.

NOVOCAIN SHOULD BE USED WITH CAUTION IN PATIENTS WITH KNOWN DRUG ALLERGIES AND SENSITIVITIES. A thorough history of the patient's prior experience with NOVOCAIN or other local anesthetics as well as concomitant or recent drug use should be taken (see Contraindications). NOVOCAIN should not be used in any condition in which a sulfonamide drug is being employed since para-aminobenzoic acid inhibits the action of sulfonamides.

Solutions containing a vasopressor should be used with caution in the presence of diseases which may adversely affect the cardiovascular system.

NOVOCAIN should be used with caution in patients with severe disturbances of cardiac rhythm, shock or heart block.

Adverse Reactions: Systemic adverse reactions involving the central nervous system and the cardiovascular system usually result from high plasma levels due to excessive dosage, rapid absorption, or inadvertent intravascular injection. In addition, use of inappropriate doses or techniques may result in extensive spinal blockade leading to hypotension and respiratory arrest.

A small number of reactions may result from hypersensitivity, idiosyncrasy, or diminished tolerance to normal dosage.

Excitatory CNS effect (nervousness, dizziness, blurred vision, tremors) commonly represent the initial signs of local anesthetic systemic toxicity. However, these reactions may be very brief or absent in some patients in which case the first manifestation of toxicity may be drowsiness or convulsions merging into unconsciousness and respiratory arrest.

Cardiovascular system reactions include depression of the myocardium, hypotension (or sometimes hypertension), bradycardia, and even cardic arrest.

Allergic reactions are characterized by cutaneous lesions of delayed onset, or urticaria, edema, and other manifestations of allergy. The detection of sensitivity by skin testing is of limited value. As with other local anesthetics, hypersensitivity, idiosyncrasy and anaphylactoid reactions have occurred rarely. The reaction may be abrupt and severe and is not usually dose related.

The following adverse reactions may occur with spinal anesthesia: *Central Nervous System:* post-spinal headache, meningismus, arachnoiditis, palsies, or spinal nerve paralysis. *Cardiovascular:* hypotension due to vasomotor paralysis and pooling of the blood in the venous bed. *Respiratory:* respiratory impairment or paralysis due to the level of anesthesia extending to the upper thoracic and cervical segments. *Gastrointestinal:* nausea and vomiting.

Treatment of Reactions. Toxic effects of local anesthetics require symptomatic treatment: there is no specific cure. The physician should be prepared to maintain an airway and to support ventilation with oxygen and assisted or controlled respiration as required. Supportive treatment of the cardiovascular system includes intravenous fluids and, when appropriate, vasopressors (preferably those that stimulate the myocardium, such as ephedrine). Convulsions may be controlled with oxygen and by the intravenous administration of diazepam or ultrashort-acting barbiturates or a short-acting muscle relaxant (succinylcholine). Intravenous anticonvulsant agents and muscle relaxants should only be administered by those familiar with their use and only when ventilation and oxygenation are assured. In spinal and epidural anesthesia, sympathetic blockade also occurs as a pharmacological reaction, resulting in peripheral vasodilation and often *hypotension.* The extent of the hypotension will usually depend on the number of dermatomes blocked. The blood pressure should therefore be monitored in the early phases of anesthesia.

Recommended Dosage For Spinal Anesthesia

Extent of anesthesia	NOVOCAIN 10% Solution Volume of 10% Solution (ml)	Volume of Diluent (ml)	Total Dose (mg)	Site of Injection (lumbar interspace)
Perineum	0.5	0.5	50	4th
Perineum and lower extremities	1	1	100	3rd or 4th
Up to costal margin	2	1	200	2nd, 3rd or 4th

If hypotension occurs, it is readily controlled by vasoconstrictors administered either by the intramuscular or the intravenous route, the dosage of which would depend on the severity of the hypotension and the response to treatment.

Dosage and Administration: As with all local anesthetics, the dose of NOVOCAIN varies and depends upon the area to be anesthetized, the vascularity of the tissues, the number of neuronal segments to be blocked, individual tolerance, and the technique of anesthesia. The lowest dose needed to provide effective anesthesia should be administered. For specific techniques and procedures, refer to standard textbooks.

[See table below].

THE USUAL INITIAL DOSE SHOULD NOT EXCEED 1000 MG.

The diluent may be sterile normal saline, sterile distilled water, spinal fluid; and for hyperbaric technique, sterile dextrose solution.

The usual rate of injection is 1 ml per 5 seconds. Full anesthesia and fixation usually occur in 5 minutes.

Sterilization: The drug in intact ampuls is sterile. The preferred method of destroying bacteria on the exterior of ampuls before opening is heat sterilization (autoclaving). Immersion in antiseptic solution is not recommended. **Autoclave at 15-pound pressure, at 121°C (250°F), for 15 minutes.** The diluent dextrose may show some brown discoloration due to caramelization.

How Supplied: NOVOCAIN Solution 10 percent code N-202 ampuls of 2 ml (200 mg) UNI-NEST PAK of 25 **NDC** 0057–1384–25.

Protect solutions from light.

The air in the ampuls has been displaced by nitrogen gas.

PEDIACOF® ℂ ℞

Decongestant and Soothing Cough Syrup for Children

Description: Each teaspoon (5 ml) contains:

Codeine phosphate, USP ....5.0 mg
(Warning: May be habit forming.)
Phenylephrine hydrochloride, USP .....2.5 mg
Chlorpheniramine maleate, USP ....0.75 mg
Potassium iodide, USP ....75.0 mg

with sodium benzoate 0.2% as presevative and alcohol 5%.

PEDIACOF is a pleasant-tasting, raspberry-flavored cough syrup. It contains four active ingredients in proper proportion for children.

Codeine phosphate is a white crystalline, odorless powder which is freely soluble in water. It is a narcotic analgesic.

Codeine phosphate is 7,8-Didehydro-4,5α-epoxy-3-methoxy-17 methylmorphinan-6α-ol phosphate.

Phenylephrine hydrochloride is a vasoconstrictor and pressor drug chemically related to epinephrine and ephedrine. It is a synthetic sympathomimetic agent. Chemically, phenylephrine hydrochloride is (−)-m-Hydroxy-α-[(methylamino)methyl] benzyl alcohol hydrochloride.

Chlorpheniramine maleate is an alkylamine H_1-blocking agent (antihistamine) which is chemically 2-pyridinepropanamine γ-(4-chlorophenyl)-*N, N*-dimethyl-, (Z)-2-butenedioate.

Potassium iodide is an expectorant.

Clinical Pharmacology: Codeine phosphate is an antitussive that is well recognized not only because of its efficiency and rapidity of action but also because of its relative safety in clinical use. Thus, irritating, nonproductive cough is suppressed by codeine. The codeine content of PEDIACOF is reduced to the proportion that is most suitable for children. When codeine is combined with the expectorant potassium iodide, which tends to increase bronchial secretion, coughing, although minimized, is more productive when it does occur. The continuous fatiguing effect of useless coughing is thereby avoided. Codeine is a narcotic analgesic and antitussive which resembles morphine pharmacologically. Codeine is metabolized by the liver and excreted chiefly in the urine, largely in inactive forms. A small fraction (10%) of administered codeine is demethylated to form morphine, and both free and conjugated morphine can be found in the urine after therapeutic doses of codeine. When administered subcutaneously, 120mg of codeine is approximately equivalent to 10mg of morphine. The abuse liability of codeine is generally considered to be much lower than that of morphine.

The half-life of codeine in plasma is 2.5 to 3.0 hours.

Codeine has diverse additional actions. It depresses the respiratory center, stimulates the vomiting center, depresses the cough reflex, constricts the pupils, increases the tone of the gastrointestinal and genitourinary tracts, and produces mild vasodilation.

Neo-Synephrine hydrochloride (phenylephrine hydrochloride) produces effective decongestion of the mucous membranes of the respiratory tract via its powerful postsynaptic α-receptor stimulant action. It has little effect on cardiac B-receptors. Most of its effects are due to direct action on receptors and only a small part is due to norepinephrine release. Central stimulant activity is minimal.

Chlorpheniramine maleate helps control allergic coughs and mucosal congestion. The mild anticholinergic action of chlorpheniramine maleate may aid in reducing rhinorrhea, and its mild sedative action may also be beneficial to patients whose excessive coughing has caused them to lose sleep.

Clinical experience with PEDIACOF has shown it to be a dependable medication for the relief of cough and the reduction of nasal congestion in children.

Indications and Usage: Coughs due to colds as well as coughs and congestive symptoms associated with upper respiratory tract infections such as tracheobronchitis or laryngobronchitis, croup, pharyngitis, allergic bronchitis, and infectious bronchitis, when accompanied by disturbing and fatiguing cough, have been treated successfully with PEDIACOF in children.

Contraindications: PEDIACOF is contraindicated in patients who are hypersensitive to any of its ingredients. Due to the component phenylephrine, PEDIACOF is contraindicated in patients with ventricular tachycardia or severe hypertension.

Warnings:

Respiratory Depression: Codeine produces dose-related respiratory depression by acting directly on brain stem respiratory centers. Codeine also affects centers that control respiratory rhythm, and may produce irregular and periodic breathing. If significant respiratory depression occurs, it may be antogonized by the use of naloxone hydrochloride. (See OVERDOSAGE.)

Head Injury and Increased Intracranial Pressure: The respiratory depressant effects of narcotics and their capacity to elevate cerebrospinal fluid pressure may be markedly exaggerated in the presence of head injury, other intracranial lesions, or a preexisting increase in intracranial pressure. Furthermore, narcotics can produce adverse reactions which may obscure the clinical course of patients with head injuries.

Acute Abdominal Conditions: The administration of narcotics may obscure the diagnosis or clinical course of patients with acute abdominal conditions.

Precautions: Caution should be exercised if PEDIACOF is administered to patients with cardiac disorders, other than ventricular tachycardia which is contraindicated; mild hypertension and hyperthyroidism.

Special Risk Patients:

Codeine should be used with caution in patients with impaired renal or hepatic function, hypothyroidism, Addison's disease, or urethral stricture.

In asthma, the indiscriminate use of codeine may, due to its drying action upon the mucosa of the respiratory tract, precipitate severe respiratory insufficiency resulting from increased viscosity of the bronchial secretions and suppression of the cough reflex. As with any narcotic analgesic agent, the usual precautions should be observed and the possibility of respiratory depression should be kept in mind.

Phenylephrine hydrochloride should be employed only with extreme caution in patients with hyperthyroidism, bradycardia, partial heart block, myocardial disease.

Chlorpheniramine maleate should be used with considerable caution in patients with: narrow angle glaucoma; pyloroduodenal obstruction; bladder neck obstruction. Chlorpheniramine maleate has an atropine-like action and therefore should be used with caution in patients with: a history of bronchial asthma; increased intraocular pressure; hyperthyroidism; cardiovascular disease; hypertension.

Drug Interactions:

Patients receiving other narcotic analgesics, general anesthetics, phenothiazines, tranquilizers, sedative-hypnotics, MAO inhibitors, tricyclic antidepressants, or other CNS depressants (including alcohol) concomitantly with codeine may exhibit an additive CNS depression. When such combined therapy is contemplated, the dose of one or both agents should be reduced.

Carcinogenesis, Mutagenesis, Impairment of Fertility: No long-term animal studies have been performed to evaluate PEDIACOF'S potential in these areas.

Nonteratogenic effects: Dependence has been reported in newborns whose mothers received opiates regularly during pregnancy. Withdrawal signs include irritability, excessive crying, tremors, hyperreflexia, fever, vomiting, and diarrhea. Signs usually appear during the first few days of life.

Adverse Reactions: The only significant untoward effects that have occurred are mild anorexia and an occasional tendency to constipation. However, discontinuance of PEDIACOF has seldom been required. Mild drowsiness occurs in some patients but, when cough is relieved, the quieting effect of PEDIACOF is considered beneficial in many instances. Because of its iodide content, PEDIACOF may cause elevation of the protein-bound iodine.

Adverse reactions to codeine include: *Central Nervous System:* Sedation, drowsiness, mental clouding, dizziness, lethargy, impairment of mental and physical performance, anxiety, convulsions, fear, miosis, dysphoria, psychic dependence, mood changes, and respiratory depression. *Gastrointestinal System:* Nausea, vomiting, increased pressure in the bilary tract, constipation. *Cardiovascular System:* Orthostatic hypotension, fainting, tachycardia. *Genitourinary System:* Ureteral spasm, spasm of vesical sphincters and urinary retention have been reported. *Other:* Flushing, sweating, pruritus, allergic reactions, suppressed cough reflex.

Adverse reactions to phenylephrine hydrochloride include: headache, reflex bradycardia, excitability, restlessness, and rarely arrhythmias.

Adverse reactions to chlorpheniramine maleate include: slight to moderate drowsiness. Other possible side effects common to antihistamines in general include: *General:* urticaria, drug rash, anaphylactic shock, photosensitivity, excessive perspiration, chills, dryness of mouth, nose and throat. *Cardiovascular System:* hypotension, headache, palpitations, tachycardia, extrasystoles. *Hematologic System:* hemolytic anemia, thrombocytopenia, agranulacytosis. *Nervous System:* sedation, dizziness, disturbed coordination, fatigue, confusion, restlessness, excitation, nervousness, tremor, irritability, insomnia, euphoria, paresthesias, blurred vision, diplopia, vertigo, tinnitus, acute labyrinthitis, hysteria, neuritis, convulsions. *Gastrointestinal System:* epigastric distress, anorexia, nausea, vomiting, diarrhea, constipation. *Genitourinary System:* urinary frequency, difficult urination, urinary retention, early menses. *Respiratory System:* thickening of bronchial secretions, tightness of chest and wheezing, nasal stuffiness.

Overdosage:

Codeine:

Signs and Symptoms: Overdosage with codeine is characterized by respiratory depression (a decrease in respiratory rate and/or tidal volume, Cheyne-Stokes respiration, cyanosis), pinpoint pupils, extreme somnolence progressing to stupor or coma, skeletal muscle flaccidity, cold and clammy skin, and sometimes bradycardia and hypotension. In severe overdosage, particularly by the intravenous route, apnea, circulatory collapse, cardiac arrest, and death may occur.

Treatment: Primary attention should be given to the reestablishment of adequate respiratory exchange through provision of a patent airway and institution of assisted or controlled ventilation. Naloxone hydrochloride is a specific and effective antagonist for respiratory depression which may result from overdosage. If the desired degree of counteraction and improvement in respiratory function is not obtained immediately following IV administration, it may be repeated intravenously at 2 to 3 minute intervals. Failure to obtain significant improvement after 2 or 3 doses suggests that the condition may be due partly or completely to other disease processes or non-opioid drugs. The usual initial pediatric dose is 0.01 mg/kg body weight given IV, IM, or SC. If necessary, naloxone can be diluted with Sterile Water for Injection, USP, Oxygen, intravenous fluids, vasopressors, and other supportive measures should be employed as indicated.

Oral LD_{50} in the mouse is 693 mg/kg. Codeine is not dialyzable.

Phenylephrine hydrochloride:

Signs and Symptoms: Overdosage may induce ventricular extrasystoles and short paroxysms of ventricular tachycardia, a sensation of fullness in the head and tingling of the extremities.

Treatment: Should an excessive elevation of blood pressure occur, it may be immediately relieved by an α-adrenergic blocking agent, e.g., phentolamine.

The Oral LD_{50} in the rat: is 350 mg/kg; Mouse: 120 mg/kg.

Chlorpheniramine maleate:

Signs and Symptoms: Antihistamine overdosage may vary from central nervous system depression (sedation, apnea, cardiovascular collapse) to stimulation (insomnia, hallucinations, tremors or convulsions). Other signs and symptoms may be dizziness, tinnitus, ataxia, blurred vision and hypotension. Stimulation and atropine-like signs and symptoms (dry mouth; fixed, dilated pupils; flushing; hyperthermia and gastrointestinal symptoms) are particularly likely in children.

Treatment: Emergency treatment should be started immediately. Vomiting should be induced, even if it has occurred spontaneously. Vomiting by the administration of ipecac syrup is preferred. Vomiting should *not* be induced in patients with impaired consciousness. The action of ipecac is facilitated by physical activity and by the administration of eight to twelve fluid ounces of water. If emesis does not occur within fifteen minutes, the dose of ipecac should be repeated. Precautions against aspiration must be taken, especially in infants and children. Following emesis, any drug remain-

Continued on next page

Breon—Cont.

ing in the stomach may be absorbed by activated charcoal administered as a slurry with water. If vomiting is unsuccessful, or contraindicated, gastric lavage should be performed. Isotonic and one-half isotonic saline are the lavage solutions of choice. Saline cathartics, such as milk of magnesia, draw water into the bowel by osmosis and, therefore, may be valuable for their action in rapid dilution of bowel content. After emergency treatment the patient should continue to be medically monitored. Treatment of the signs and symptoms of overdosage is symptomatic and supportive.
Stimulants (analeptic agents) should *not* be used. Vasopressors may be used to treat hypotension. Shortacting barbiturates, diazepam or paraldehyde may be administered to control seizures.
Hyperpyrexia, especially in children, may require treatment with tepid water sponge baths or a hypothermic blanket. Apnea is treated with ventilatory support.
Dosage and Administration:
PEDIACOF should be given in accordance with the needs and age of the patient. Frequency of administration may be adjusted as cough is brought under control. The following doses, to be given at 4 to 6 hour intervals, are suggested for patients under 12 years of age: **from 6 months to 1 year,** 1/4 teaspoon; **from 1 to 3 years,** 1/2 to 1 teaspoon; **from 3 to 6 years,** 1 to 2 teaspoons; and **from 6 to 12 years,** 2 teaspoons.
How Supplied:
Bottles of 16 fl oz,
Code P-915 **NDC** 0057-1509-06
Gallons, Code P-916 **NDC** 0057-1509-08
Available on prescription only.

PONTOCAINE® Hydrochloride ℞
brand of tetracaine hydrochloride, USP

Prolonged Spinal Anesthesia

Description: Tetracaine hydrochloride is 2-(dimethylamino) ethyl *p*-(butylamino) benzoate monohydrochloride. It is a white crystalline, odorless powder that is readily soluble in water, physiologic saline solution, and dextrose solution.
Tetracaine hydrochloride is a local anesthetic of the ester-linkage type, related to procaine.
PONTOCAINE hydrochloride is supplied in two forms for prolonged spinal anesthesia: Niphanoid® and 1% solution.
Niphanoid®: A sterile, instantly soluble form consisting of a network of extremely fine, highly purified particles, resembling snow.
1% solution: A sterile, isotonic, isobaric solution, each 1 ml containing 10 mg tetracaine hydrochloride, 6.7 mg sodium chloride, and not more than 2 mg acetone sodium bisulfite. The air in the ampuls has been displaced by nitrogen gas. The pH is 3.2 to 6.0.
These formulations do not contain preservatives.
Clinical Pharmacology: Parenteral administration of PONTOCAINE stabilizes the neuronal membrane and prevents initiation transmission of nerve impulses thereby effecting local anesthesia.
The onset of action is rapid, and the duration prolonged (up to two or three hours or longer of surgical anesthesia).
PONTOCAINE is detoxified by plasma esterases to para-aminobenzoic acid and diethylaminoethanol.
Indications and Usage: PONTOCAINE is indicated for the production of spinal anesthesia for procedures requiring two to three hours.
Contraindications: Spinal anesthesia with PONTOCAINE is contraindicated in patients with known hypersensitivity to tetracaine hydrochloride or to drugs of a similar chemical configuration (ester-type local anesthetics), or para-aminobenzoic acid or its derivatives; and in patients for whom spinal anesthesia as a technique is contraindicated.
The decision as to whether or not spinal anesthesia should be used for an individual patient should be made by the physician after weighing the advantages with the risks and possible complications. Contraindications to spinal anesthesia as a technique can be found in standard reference texts, and usually include generalized septicemia, infection at the site of injection, certain diseases of the cerebrospinal system, uncontrolled hypotension, etc.
Warnings: RESUSCITATIVE EQUIPMENT AND DRUGS SHOULD BE IMMEDIATELY AVAILABLE WHENEVER ANY LOCAL ANESTHETIC DRUG IS USED.
Large doses of local anesthetics should not be used in patients with heart block.
Reactions resulting in fatality have occurred on rare occasions with the use of local anesthetics, even in the absence of a history of hypersensitivity.
Precautions: The safety and effectiveness of any spinal anesthetic depend upon proper dosage, correct technique, adequate precautions, and readiness for emergencies. The lowest dosage that results in effective anesthesia should be used to avoid high plasma levels and serious systemic side effects. Tolerance varies with the status of the patient; debilitated, elderly patients or acutely ill patients should be given reduced doses commensurate with their weight, age, and physical status. Reduced doses are also indicated for obstetric patients and those with increased intraabdominal pressure.
Caution should be used in administering PONTOCAINE to patients with abnormal or reduced levels of plasma esterases.
Blood pressure should be frequently monitored during spinal anesthesia and hypotension immediately corrected.
Spinal anesthetics should be used with caution in patients with severe disturbances of cardiac rhythm, shock or heart block.
Drug Interactions: PONTOCAINE should not be used if the patient is being treated with a sulfonamide because para-aminobenzoic acid inhibits the action of sulfonamides.
Carcinogenesis, mutagenesis, impairment of fertility: Long-term animal studies to evaluate carcinogenic potential and reproduction studies in animals have not been performed. There is no evidence from human data that PONTOCAINE may be carcinogenic or that it impairs fertility.
Pregnancy Category C: Animal reproduction studies have not been conducted with PONTOCAINE. It is not known whether PONTOCAINE can cause fetal harm when administered to a pregnant woman or can affect reproduction capacity. PONTOCAINE should be given to a pregnant woman only if clearly needed and the potential benefits outweigh the risk.
Labor and delivery: Vasopressor agents administered for the treatment of hypotension resulting from spinal anesthesia may result in severe persistent hypertension and/or rupture of cerebral blood vessels if oxytocic drugs have also been administered; therefore, vasopressors should be used with extreme caution in the presence of oxytocic drugs.
PONTOCAINE has a recognized use during labor and delivery; the effect of the drug on duration of labor, incidence of forceps delivery, status of the newborn, and later growth and development of the child have not been studied.
Nursing mothers: It is not known whether PONTOCAINE is excreted in human milk; however, it is rapidly metabolized following absorption into the plasma. Because many drugs are excreted in human milk, caution should be exercised when PONTOCAINE is administered to a nursing woman.
Pediatric use: Safety and effectiveness of PONTOCAINE in children have not been established.
Adverse Reactions: Systemic adverse reactions to PONTOCAINE are characteristic of those associated with other local anesthetics and can involve the central nervous system and the cardiovascular system. Systemic reactions usually result from high plasma levels due to excessive dosage, rapid absorption, or inadvertent intravascular injection.
A small number of reactions to PONTOCAINE may result from hypersensitivity, idiosyncrasy or diminished tolerance to normal dosage.
Central nervous system effects are characterized by excitation or depression. The first manifestation may be nervousness, dizziness, blurred vision, or tremors, followed by drowsiness, convulsions, unconsciousness and possibly respiratory and cardiac arrest. Since excitement may be transient or absent, the first manifestation may be drowsiness, sometimes merging into unconsciousness and respiratory and cardiac arrest. Other central nervous system effects may be nausea, vomiting, chills, constriction of the pupils, or tinnitus.
Cardiovascular system reactions include depression of the myocardium, blood pressure changes (usually hypotension), and cardiac arrest.
Allergic reactions, which may be due to hypersensitivity, idiosyncrasy or diminished tolerance, are characterized by the cutaneous lesions (e.g., urticaria), edema, and other manifestations of allergy. Detection of sensitivity by skin testing is of limited value. Severe allergic reactions including anaphylaxis have occurred rarely and are not usually dose-related.
Reactions associated with spinal anesthesia techniques: Central nervous system: post-spinal headache, meningismus, arachnoiditis, palsies, or spinal nerve paralysis. Cardiovascular: hypotension due to vasomotor paralysis and pooling of the blood in the venous bed. Respiratory: respiratory impairment or paralysis due to the level of anesthesia extending to the upper thoracic and cervical segments. Gastrointestinal: nausea and vomiting.
Treatment of reactions: Toxic effects of local anesthetics require symptomatic treatment; there is no specific cure. **The most important measure is oxygenation of the patient by maintaining an airway and supporting ventilation.** Supportive treatment of the cardiovascular system includes intravenous fluids and, when appropriate, vasopressors (preferably those that stimulate the myocardium). Convulsions are usually controlled with adequate oxygenation alone but intravenous administration in small increments of a barbiturate (preferably an ultrashort-acting barbiturate such as thiopental and thiamylal) or diazepam can be utilized. Intravenous barbiturates or anticonvulsant agents should only be administered by those familiar with their use and only if ventilation and oxygenation have first been assured. In spinal anesthesia, sympathetic blockade also occurs as a pharmacological action, resulting in peripheral vasodilation and often hypotension. The extent of the hypotension will usually depend on the number of dermatomes blocked. The blood pressure should therefore be monitored in the early phases of anesthesia. If hypotension occurs, it is readily controlled by vasoconstrictors administered either by the intramuscular or the intravenous route, the dosage of which would depend on the severity of the hypotension and the response to treatment.
Dosage and Administration: As with all anesthetics, the dosage varies and depends upon the area to be anesthetized, the number of neuronal segments to be blocked, individual tolerance, and the technique of anesthesia. The lowest dosage needed to provide effective anesthesia should be administered. For specific

SUGGESTED DOSAGE FOR SPINAL ANESTHESIA

	Using Niphanoid		Using 1% solution		
Extent of anesthesia	Dose of Niphanoid (mg)	Volume of spinal fluid (ml)	Dose of solution (ml)	Volume of spinal fluid (ml)	Site of injection (lumbar interspace)
Perineum	5*	1	0.5 (=5 mg)*	0.5	4th
Perineum and lower extremities	10	2	1.0 (=10 mg)	1.0	3d or 4th
Up to costal margin	15 to 20†	3	1.5 to 2.0 (=15 to 20 mg)†	1.5 to 2.0	2d, 3d, or 4th

*For vaginal delivery (saddle block), from 2 to 5 mg in dextrose.
† Doses exceeding 15 mg are rarely required and should be used only in exceptional cases. Inject solution at rate of about 1 ml per 5 seconds.

techniques and procedures, refer to standard textbooks.
(See table above)
The extent and degree of spinal anesthesia depend upon dosage, specific gravity of the anesthetic solution, volume of solution used, force of the injection, level of puncture, position of the patient during and immediately after injection, etc.
When spinal fluid is added to either the Niphanoid or solution, some turbidity results, the degree depending on the pH of the spinal fluid, the temperature of the solution during mixing, as well as the amount of drug and diluent employed. This cloudiness is due to the release of the *base* from the hydrochloride. Liberation of base (which is completed within the spinal canal) is held to be essential for satisfactory results with any spinal anesthetic.
The specific gravity of spinal fluid at 25°/25°C varies under normal conditions from 1.0063 to 1.0075. A solution of the instantly soluble form (Niphanoid) in spinal fluid has only a slightly greater specific gravity. The 1% concentration in saline solution has a specific gravity of 1.0060 to 1.0074 at 25°/25°C.
A hyperbaric solution may be prepared by mixing equal volumes of the 1% solution and Dextrose Solution 10% (which is available in ampuls of 3 ml).
If the Niphanoid form is preferred, it is first dissolved in Dextrose Solution 10% in a ratio of 1 ml dextrose to 10 mg of the anesthetic. Further dilution is made with an equal volume of spinal fluid. The resulting solution now contains 5% dextrose with 5 mg of anesthetic agent per milliliter.
A hypobaric solution may be prepared by dissolving the Niphanoid in Sterile Water for Injection, USP (1 mg per milliliter). The specific gravity of this solution is essentially the same as that of water, 1.000 at 25°/25°C.
Examine ampuls carefully before use. Do not use solution if crystals, cloudiness, or discoloration is observed. Protect ampuls from light and store under refrigeration.
Sterilization of Ampuls: The drug in intact ampuls is sterile. The preferred method of destroying bacteria on the exterior of ampuls before opening is heat sterilization (autoclaving). Immersion in antiseptic solution is not recommended.
Autoclave at 15-pound pressure, at 121°C (250°F) for 15 minutes. The Niphanoid form may also be autoclaved in the same way but may lose its snowlike appearance and tend to adhere to the sides of the ampul. This may slightly decrease the rate at which the drug dissolves but does not interfere with its anesthetic potency.
Autoclaving increases likelihood of crystal formation. Unused autoclaved ampuls should be discarded. In no case should unused autoclaved ampuls be placed back in stock for later use.

How Supplied:
Niphanoid (instantly soluble) ampuls of 20 mg, boxes of 100.
Code P-841 **NDC** 0057-1577-06
1% isotonic isobaric solution: ampuls of 2 ml, UNI-NEST
PAK of 25, Code P-823 **NDC** 0057-1574-25

TRANCOPAL® ℞
brand of chlormezanone
Nonhypnotic Antianxiety Agent

Description: Trancopal (brand of chlormezanone) is [2-(p-chlorophenyl)-tetrahydro-3-methyl-4H-1, 3-thiazin-4-one 1, 1-dioxide], a white, virtually tasteless, crystalline powder with a solubility of less than 0.25 per cent w/v in water.
Clinical Pharmacology: Trancopal improves the emotional state by allaying mild anxiety, usually without impairing clarity of consciousness.
The relief of symptoms is often apparent in fifteen to thirty minutes after administration and may last up to six hours or longer.
Indications and Usage: Trancopal is indicated for the treatment of mild anxiety and tension states.
The effectiveness of chlormezanone in long-term use, that is, more than 4 months, has not been assessed by systematic clinical studies. The physician should periodically reassess the usefulness of the drug for the individual patient.
Contraindication: Contraindicated in patients with a history of a previous hypersensitivity reaction to chlormezanone.
Warnings: Should drowsiness occur, the dose should be reduced. As with other CNS-acting drugs, patients receiving chlormezanone should be warned against performing potentially hazardous tasks which require complete mental alertness, such as operating a motor vehicle or dangerous machinery. Patients should also be warned of the possible additive effects which may occur when the drug is taken with alcohol or other CNS-acting drugs.
Usage in Pregnancy. Safe use of this preparation in pregnancy or lactation has not been established, as no animal reproduction studies have been performed; therefore, use of the drug in pregnancy, lactation, or in women of childbearing age requires that the potential benefit of the drug be weighed against its possible hazards to the mother and fetus.
Adverse Reactions: Adverse effects reported to occur with Trancopal include drowsiness, drug rash, dizziness, flushing, nausea, depression, edema, inability to void, weakness, excitement, tremor, confusion and headache. Medication should be discontinued or modified as the case demands.
Jaundice, apparently of the cholestatic type, has been reported as occurring rarely during the use of chlormezanone, but was reversible on discontinuance of therapy.
Dosage and Administration: The usual **adult** dosage is 200 mg orally three or four times daily but in some patients 100 mg may suffice. The dosage for **children from 5 to 12 years** is 50 to 100 mg three or four times daily. Since the effect of CNS-acting drugs varies, treatment, particularly in children, should begin with the lowest dosage which may be increased as needed.
How Supplied:
100 mg (peach colored, scored caplets®)
bottles of 100 NDC 0057-1973-04
200 mg (green colored, scored caplets®)
bottles of 100 NDC 0057-1974-04
bottles of 1000 NDC 0057-1974-08

[*Shown in Product Identification Section*]

Bristol Laboratories
(Division of Bristol-Myers Co.)
SYRACUSE, NY 13201

AMIKIN® ℞
(amikacin sulfate)

This is the full text of the latest Official Package Circular dated August 1979 [3015 DIMO-07].

WARNINGS

Patients treated with aminoglycosides should be under close clinical observation because of the potential ototoxicity and nephrotoxicity associated with their use.
Ototoxicity, both auditory and vestibular, can occur in patients treated at higher doses or for periods longer than those recommended. The risk of amikacin-induced ototoxicity is greater in patients with renal damage. High frequency deafness usually occurs first and can be detected only by audiometric testing. Vertigo may occur and may be evidence of vestibular injury.
The ototoxicity potential of amikacin in infants is not known. Until more safety reports become available, amikacin should be used in infants only in those specific circumstances when susceptibility testing indicates that other aminoglycosides cannot be used or are otherwise contraindicated, and when the infant can be observed closely for evidence of toxicity.
Aminoglycosides are potentially nephrotoxic. Renal and eighth-nerve function should be closely monitored in patients with known or suspected renal impairment and also in those whose renal function is initially normal but who develop signs of renal dysfunction during therapy. Such impairment may be characterized by decreased creatinine clearance, the presence of cells or casts, oliguria, proteinuria, decreased urine specific gravity, or evi-

Continued on next page

Bristol—Cont.

dence of increasing nitrogen retention (increasing BUN or creatinine).
Evidence of impairment in renal, vestibular, or auditory function requires discontinuation of the drug or dosage adjustment.
Serum concentrations should be monitored when feasible, and prolonged peak concentrations above 35 mcg./ml. should be avoided. Urine should be examined for increased excretion of protein, the presence of cells and casts, and decreased specific gravity.
Concurrent and/or sequential use of topically or systemically neurotoxic or nephrotoxic antibiotics, particularly kanamycin, gentamicin, tobramycin, neomycin, streptomycin, cephaloridine, paromomycin, viomycin, polymyxin B, colistin, and vancomycin should be avoided.
AMIKIN should not be given concurrently with potent diuretics (ethacrynic acid, furosemide, meralluride sodium, sodium mercaptomerin, or mannitol). Some diuretics themselves cause ototoxicity, and intravenously administered diuretics enhance aminoglycoside toxicity by altering antibiotic concentrations in serum and tissue.

Description: Amikacin sulfate is a semisynthetic aminoglycoside antibiotic derived from kanamycin. It is $C_{22}H_{43}N_5O_{13} \cdot 2H_2SO_4$. D-Streptamine, O -3- amino -3- deoxy-α-D-glucopyranosyl- (1→6) - 0 -[6 -amino- 6 -deoxy-α-D-glucopyranosyl- (1→4)]- N^1- (4 -amino- 2 -hydroxyl- 1 -oxobutyl)- 2 deoxy-,(S)-,sulfate (1:2) (salt).
The dosage form is supplied as a sterile, colorless to light straw colored solution. The 100 mg. per 2 ml. vial contains, in addition to amikacin sulfate, 0.13% sodium bisulfite and 0.5% sodium citrate with pH adjusted to 4.5 with sulfuric acid. The 500 mg. per 2 ml. vial and the 1.0 Gm. per 4 ml. vial contain 0.66% sodium bisulfite and 2.5% sodium citrate with pH adjusted to 4.5 with sulfuric acid.

Action:

Clinical-Pharmacology

Intramuscular Administration

AMIKIN is rapidly absorbed after intramuscular administration. In normal adult volunteers, average peak serum concentrations of about 12, 16, and 21 mcg/ml are obtained 1 hour after intramuscular administration of 250-mg (3.7 mg/Kg), 375-mg (5 mg/Kg), 500-mg (7.5 mg/Kg), single doses respectively. At 10 hours, serum levels are about 0.3 mcg/ml, 1.2 mcg/ml, and 2.1 mcg/ml, respectively.
Tolerance studies in normal volunteers revealed that amikacin was well tolerated locally following repeated intramuscular dosing and, when given at maximally recommended doses, no ototoxicity or nephrotoxicity was reported. There was no evidence of drug accumulation with repeated dosing for 10 days when administered according to recommended doses.
With normal renal function about 91.9% of an intramuscular dose is excreted unchanged in the urine in the first 8 hours, and 98.2% within 24 hours. Mean urine concentrations for 6 hours are 563 mcg/ml following a 250-mg dose, 697 mcg/ml following a 375-mg dose, and 832 mcg/ml following a 500-mg dose.
Preliminary intramuscular studies in newborns of different weights (less than 1.5 Kg, 1.5 to 2.0 Kg, over 2.0 Kg) at a dose of 7.5 mg/Kg revealed that, like other aminoglycosides, serum half-life values were correlated inversely with post-natal age and renal clearances of amikacin. The volume of distribution indicates that amikacin, like other aminoglycosides, remains primarily in the extracellular fluid space of neonates. Repeated dosing every 12 hours in all the above groups did not demonstrate accumulation after 5 days.

Intravenous Administration

Single doses of 500 mg (7.5 mg/Kg) administered to normal adults as an infusion over a period of 30 minutes produced a mean peak serum concentration of 38 mcg/ml at the end of the infusion, and levels of 24 mcg/ml, 18 mcg/ml, and 0.75 mcg/ml at 30 minutes, 1 hour, and 10 hours post-infusion, respectively. Eighty-four percent of the administered dose was excreted in the urine in 9 hours and about 94% within 24 hours.
Repeat infusions of 7.5 mg/Kg every 12 hours in normal adults were well tolerated and caused no drug accumulation.

General

Pharmacokinetic studies in normal adult subjects reveal the mean serum half-life to be slightly over 2 hours with a mean total apparent volume of distribution of 24 liters (28% of the body weight). By the ultrafiltration technique, reports on serum protein binding range from 0 to 11%. The mean serum clearance rate is about 100 ml/min and the renal clearance rate is 94 ml/min in subjects with normal renal function.
Amikacin is excreted primarily by way of glomerular filtration. Patients with impaired renal function or diminished glomerular filtration pressure excrete the drug much more slowly (effectively prolonging the serum half-life). Therefore, renal function should be monitored carefully and dosage adjusted accordingly (see suggested dosage schedule under "Dosage and Administration").
Amikacin has been found in the cerebrospinal fluid, pleural fluid, and peritoneal cavity following parenteral administration.
Spinal fluid levels in normal infants are approximately 10 to 20% of the serum concentrations and may reach 50% when the meninges are inflamed. AMIKIN has been demonstrated to cross the placental barrier and yield significant concentrations in amniotic fluid. The peak fetal serum concentration is about 16% of the peak maternal serum concentration and maternal and fetal serum half-life values are about 2 and 3.7 hours, respectively.

Microbiology

Gram-negative—Amikacin is active **in vitro** against **Pseudomonas** species, **Escherichia coli, Proteus** species (indole-positive and indole-negative), **Providencia** species, **Klebsiella-Enterobacter-Serratia** species, **Acinetobacter** (formerly **Mima-Herellea**) species and **Citrobacter freundii.**
When strains of the above organisms are found to be resistant to other aminoglycosides, including gentamicin, tobramycin, and kanamycin, many are susceptible to amikacin **in vitro.**
Gram-positive—Amikacin is active **in vitro** against penicillinase and non-penicillinase-producing **Staphylococcus** species including methicillin-resistant strains. However, it has been shown to have a low order of activity against other Gram-positive organisms; viz, **Streptococcus pyogenes,** enterococci, and **Streptococcus pneumoniae** (formerly **Diplococcus pneumoniae**).
Amikacin resists degradation by most aminoglycoside inactivating enzymes known to affect gentamicin, tobramycin, and kanamycin.

Disc Susceptibility Tests

Quantitative methods that require measurement of zone diameters give the most precise estimates of antibiotic susceptibility. One such procedure* has been recommended for use with discs to test susceptibility to amikacin. Interpretation involves correlation of the diameters obtained in the disc test with MIC values for amikacin. When the causative organism is tested by the Kirby-Bauer methods of disc susceptibility, a 30-mcg amikacin disc should give a zone of 17 mm or greater to indicate susceptibility. Zone sizes of 14 mm or less indicate resistance. Zone sizes of 15 to 16 mm indicate intermediate susceptibility. With this procedure, a report from the laboratory of "susceptible" indicates that the infecting organism is likely to respond to therapy. A report of "resistant" indicates that the infecting organism is not likely to respond to therapy. A report of "intermediate susceptibility" suggests that the organism would be susceptible if the infection is confined to tissues and fluids (e.g., urine), in which high antibiotic levels are attained.

Indications and Usage: AMIKIN is indicated in the short-term treatment of serious infections due to susceptible strains of Gram-negative bacteria, including **Pseudomonas** species, **Escherichia coli,** species of indole-positive and indole-negative **Proteus, Providencia** species, **Klebsiella-Enterobacter-Serratia** species, and **Acinetobacter (Mima-Herellea)** species.
Clinical studies have shown AMIKIN to be effective in bacteremia and septicemia (including neonatal sepsis); in serious infections of the respiratory tract, bones and joints, central nervous system (including meningitis) and skin and soft tissue; intra-abdominal infections (including peritonitis); and in burns and post-operative infections (including post-vascular surgery). Clinical studies have shown AMIKIN also to be effective in serious complicated and recurrent urinary tract infections due to these organisms. Aminoglycosides, including AMIKIN injectable, are not indicated in uncomplicated initial episodes of urinary tract infections unless the causative organisms are not susceptible to antibiotics having less potential toxicity.
Bacteriologic studies should be performed to identify causative organisms and their susceptibilities to amikacin. AMIKIN may be considered as initial therapy in suspected Gram-negative infections and therapy may be instituted before obtaining the results of susceptibility testing. Clinical trials demonstrated that AMIKIN was effective in infections caused by gentamicin and/or tobramycin resistant strains of Gram-negative organisms, particularly **Proteus rettgeri, Providencia stuartii, Serratia marcescens,** and **Pseudomonas aeruginosa.** The decision to continue therapy with the drug should be based on results of the susceptibility tests, the severity of the infection, the response of the patient, and the important additional considerations contained in the "Warning" box above.
AMIKIN has also been shown to be effective in staphylococcal infections and may be considered as initial therapy under certain conditions in the treatment of known or suspected staphylococcal disease such as, severe infections where the causative organism may be either a Gram-negative bacterium or a staphylococcus, infections due to susceptible strains of staphylococci in patients allergic to other antibiotics, and in mixed staphylococcal/-Gram-negative infections.
Amikacin may be indicated in the treatment of neonatal sepsis when susceptibility testing indicates that other aminoglycosides cannot be used. In certain severe infections such as neonatal sepsis, concomitant therapy with a penicillin-type drug may be indicated because of the possibility of infections due to Gram-positive organisms such as streptococci or pneumococci.

Contraindications: A history of hypersensitivity to amikacin is a contraindication for its use.

Warning: See "Warning" box above.

Precautions: AMIKIN is potentially nephrotoxic, ototoxic, and neurotoxic. The concurrent or serial use of other ototoxic or nephrotoxic agents should be avoided either systemically or topically because of the potential for additive effects. Such agents include antibacterial drugs such as kanamycin, gentamicin, tobramycin, neomycin, streptomycin, cephaloridine, paromomycin, viomycin, polymyxin B, colistin, and vancomycin as well as certain diuretic agents such as ethacrynic acid or furosemide.

Ototoxicity

See "Warning" box.

Nephrotoxicity

Since AMIKIN is present in high concentrations in the renal excretory system, patients should be well hydrated to minimize chemical irritation of the renal tubules. Kidney function should be assessed by the usual methods prior to starting therapy and daily during the course of treatment.

If signs of renal irritation appear (casts, white or red cells or albumin), hydration should be increased. A reduction in dosage (see "Dosage and Administration") may be desirable if other evidence of renal dysfunction occurs such as decreased creatinine clearance, decreased urine specific gravity, increased BUN, creatinine, or oliguria. If azotemia increases or if a progressive decrease in urinary output occurs, treatment should be stopped.

Note: When patients are well hydrated and kidney function is normal the risk of nephrotoxic reactions with amikacin is low if the dosage recommendations (see "Dosage and Administration") are not exceeded.

Neurotoxicity

Neuromuscular blockade and muscular paralysis have been demonstrated in the cat with high doses of amikacin (188 mg/Kg). The possibility of neuromuscular blockade and respiratory paralysis should be considered when amikacin is administered concomitantly with anesthetic or neuromuscular blocking drugs. If blockade occurs, calcium salts may reverse this phenomenon.

Other

Cross-allergenicity among aminoglycosides has been demonstrated. As with other antibiotics the use of amikacin may result in overgrowth of nonsusceptible organisms. If this occurs, appropriate therapy should be instituted.

Pregnancy

Reproduction studies have been performed in rats and mice and have revealed no evidence of impaired fertility or harm to the fetus due to amikacin. There are no well-controlled studies in pregnant women but investigational experience does not include any positive evidence of adverse effects on the fetus. Although there is no clearly defined risk, such experience cannot exclude the possibility of infrequent or subtle damage to the fetus. AMIKIN should be used in pregnant women only when clearly needed. It is not known whether this drug is excreted in human milk. As a general rule, nursing should not be undertaken while a patient is on a drug since many drugs are excreted in human milk.

Adverse Reactions:

Ototoxicity

See "Warning" box.

Nephrotoxocity

Albuminuria, presence of red and white cells, casts, azotemia, and oliguria have been reported.

Other

In addition to those described above, other adverse reactions which have been reported on rare occasions are skin rash, drug fever, headache, paresthesia, tremor, nausea and vomiting, eosinophilia, arthralgia, anemia, hypotension.

Overdosage

In the event of overdosage or toxic reaction, peritoneal dialysis or hemodialysis will aid in the removal of amikacin from the blood.

Dosage and Administration: The patient's pretreatment body weight should be obtained for calculation of correct dosage. AMIKIN may be given intramuscularly or intravenously.

Intramuscular Administration for Patients with Normal Renal Function

The recommended dosage for adults, children, and older infants (see Box "Warning") with normal renal function is 15 mg/Kg/day divided into 2 or 3 equal doses administered at equally-divided intervals, i.e., 7.5 mg/Kg q.12h. or 5 mg/Kg q.8h. Treatment of patients in the heavier weight classes shall not exceed 1.5 Gm/day.

When amikacin is indicated in newborns (see Box "Warning"), it is recommended that a loading dose of 10 mg/Kg be administered initially to be followed with 7.5 mg/Kg every 12 hours.

The usual duration of treatment is 7 to 10 days. The total daily dose by all routes of administration should not exceed 15 mg/Kg/day. In the unusual circumstances where treatment beyond 10 days is considered, the use of AMIKIN should be reevaluated and, if continued, renal and auditory functions should be monitored daily.

At the recommended dosage level, uncomplicated infections due to amikacin-sensitive organisms should respond in 24 to 48 hours. If definite clinical response does not occur within 3 to 5 days, therapy should be stopped and the antibiotic sensitivity pattern of the invading organism should be rechecked. Failure of the infection to respond may be due to resistance of the organism or to the presence of septic foci requiring surgical drainage.

When AMIKIN is indicated in uncomplicated urinary tract infections, a dose of 250 mg twice daily may be used.

Intramuscular Administration for Patients with Impaired Renal Function

Whenever possible, serum amikacin concentrations should be monitored by appropriate assay procedures. Doses may be adjusted in patients with impaired renal function either by administering normal doses at prolonged intervals or by administering reduced doses at a fixed interval.

Both methods are based on the patient's creatinine clearance or serum creatinine values since these have been found to correlate with aminoglycoside half-lives in patients with diminished renal function. These dosage schedules must be used in conjunction with careful clinical and laboratory observations of the patient and should be modified as necessary. Neither method should be used when dialysis is being performed.

Normal Dosage at Prolonged Intervals

If the creatinine clearance rate is not available and the patient's condition is stable, a dosage interval in hours for the normal dose can be calculated by multiplying the patient's serum creatinine by nine, e.g., if the serum creatinine concentration is 2 mg/100 ml the recommended single dose (7.5 mg/Kg) should be administered every 18 hours.

Reduced Dosage at Fixed Time Intervals

When renal function is impaired and it is desirable to administer AMIKIN at a fixed time interval, dosage must be reduced. In these patients serum AMIKIN concentrations should be measured to assure accurate administration of AMIKIN and to avoid concentrations above 35 mcg/ml. If serum assay determinations are not available and the patient's condition is stable, serum creatinine and creatinine clearance values are the most readily available indicators of the degree of renal impairment to use as a guide for dosage.

First, initiate therapy by administering a normal dose, 7.5 mg/Kg, as a loading dose. This loading dose is the same as the normally recommended dose which would be calculated for a patient with a normal renal function as described above.

To determine the size of maintenance doses administered every 12 hours, the loading dose should be reduced in proportion to the reduction in the patient's creatinine clearance rate:

$$\text{Maintenance Dose Every 12 Hours} = \frac{\text{observed CC in ml/min}}{\text{normal CC in ml/min}} \times \text{calculated loading dose in mg}$$

(CC—creatinine clearance rate)

An alternate rough guide for determining reduced dosage at twelve-hour intervals (for patients whose steady state serum creatinine values are known) is to divide the normally recommended dose by the patient's serum creatinine.

The above dosage schedules are not intended to be rigid recommendations but are provided as guides to dosage when the measurement of amikacin serum levels is not feasible.

Intravenous Administration

The individual dose, the total daily dose, and the total cumulative dose of AMIKIN are identical to the dose recommended for intramuscular administration. The solution for intravenous use is prepared by adding the contents of a 500-mg vial to 100 or 200 ml of sterile diluent such as normal saline or 5% Dextrose in Water or any other compatible solution.

The solution is administered to adults over a 30- to 60-minute period. The total daily dose should not exceed 15 mg/Kg/day and may be divided into either 2 or 3 equally-divided doses at equally-divided intervals.

In pediatric patients the amount of fluid used will depend on the amount ordered for the patient. It should be a sufficient amount to infuse the amikacin over a 30- to 60-minute period. Infants should receive a 1- to 2-hour infusion. Amikacin should not be physically premixed with other drugs but should be administered separately according to the recommended dose and route.

Stability in IV Fluids

Amikin is stable for 24 hours at room temperature, at concentrations of 0.25 and 5.0 mg/ml in the following solutions:

5% Dextrose Injection, U.S.P.

5% Dextrose and 0.2% Sodium Chloride Injection, U.S.P.

5% Dextrose and 0.45% Sodium Chloride Injection, U.S.P.

0.9% Sodium Chloride Injection, U.S.P.

Lactated Ringer's Injection, U.S.P.

Normosol®M in 5% Dextrose Injection, U.S.P. (or Plasma-Lyte 56 Injection in 5% Dextrose in Water)

Normosol®R in 5% Dextrose Injection, U.S.P. (or Plasma-Lyte 148 Injection in 5% Dextrose in Water)

Supply: AMIKIN is supplied as a colorless solution which requires no refrigeration. It is stable at room temperature for at least two years. At times the solution may become a very pale yellow; this does not indicate a decrease in potency.

AMIKIN (amikacin sulfate injection)

NDC 0015-3015-20—100 mg per 2 ml

NDC 0015-3020-20—500 mg per 2 ml

NDC 0015-3020-21—Disposable Syringe (500 mg per 2 ml)

NDC 0015-3023-20—1.0 gm per 4 ml

For information on package sizes available, refer to the current price schedule.

---

*Bauer, A. W., Kirby, W. M. M., Sherris, J. C., and Turck, M.: Antibiotic Testing by a Standardized Single Disc Method, Am. J. Clin. Pathol., 45:493, 1966; Standardized Disc Susceptibility Test, FEDERAL REGISTER, 37:20527-29, 1972.

AZOTREX® Capsules ℞

(tetracycline phosphate complex with sulfonamide and analgesic)

This is the full text of the latest Official Package Circular dated May 1972 [4325 DIRO-05].

Description: Each capsule contains:

Tetrex® (tetracycline phosphate complex) equivalent to ....125 mg. tetracycline HCl activity

Continued on next page

Bristol—Cont.

Sulfamethizole ....250 mg.
Phenazopyridine HCl .... 50 mg.

This formula provides comprehensive treatment of common urinary tract infections, since the organisms causing the vast majority of such infections are sensitive to one or more of its antibacterial components.

Tetracycline phosphate complex has the same actions and uses as the parent antibiotic, tetracycline, or its hydrochloride salt. However, the phosphate complex is more rapidly and completely absorbed from the gastrointestinal tract than is the free base or its salts and therefore produces somewhat higher blood levels after oral administration. Tetracycline is excreted primarily by the kidneys.

Laboratory and clinical studies have shown that tetracycline is effective against **D. pneumoniae,** alpha- and beta-hemolytic streptococci, many strains of staphylococci, **N. gonorrhoeae, N. meningitidis, E. coli,** certain clostridia, **H. influenzae, Klebsiella pneumoniae,** Shigella, **Enterobacter aerogenes** and some strains of Salmonella. Tetracycline is also effective against **Entamoeba histolytica,** certain Rickettsia and viruses of the lymphogranuloma-psittacosis-trachoma group.

Sulfamethizole, the sulfonamide component of these capsules, is absorbed rapidly and almost completely from the intestinal tract into the blood stream. It is excreted rapidly by way of the kidneys, with the result that a high concentration is established in the urinary tract 1 to 2 hours after ingestion. The lower degree of acetylation of sulfamethizole assures greater effectiveness with minimum renal toxicity. It may be administered to patients sensitive to other sulfonamides, since there is little cross-sensitization.

Phenazopyridine HCl has a long clinical history of successful use as a urinary analgesic that provides prompt relief of pain and alleviates dysuria, frequency, and urgency.

Indications:
Based on a review of this drug by the National Academy of Sciences—National Research Council and/or other information, FDA has classified the indications as follows:
Lacking substantial evidence of effectiveness for the labeled indications.
Final classification for the less-than-effective indications requires further investigation.
This drug provides systemic and local antibacterial action in acute and chronic urinary tract infections due to organisms sensitive to tetracycline and sulfamethizole. It may be used in mixed infections where the invading organisms are more sensitive to the combination than to either antibacterial agent alone and is not intended for the treatment of infections where complete response to either component might be expected.
It is indicated in the treatment of cystitis, urethritis, pyelonephritis, ureteritis, and prostatitis due to bacterial infection, prior to and following genitourinary surgery and instrumentation, prophylactically in patients with urethrostomies and cord bladders.
In geriatrics this drug is particularly useful when exacerbations of infection occur in such conditions as cystocele, prostatitis, and nonspecific urethritis.
Infections caused by beta-hemolytic streptococci should be treated for at least 10 days to help prevent the occurrence of rheumatic fever or acute glomerulonephritis.

Contraindications: The drug should not be used in patients with a history of sensitivity to one of the components; or in prematures, neonates, pregnant females at term; or in patients with chronic glomerulonephritis, uremia, severe hepatitis, hepatic or renal failure, or severe pyelitis of pregnancy.

Warnings: Certain hypersensitive individuals may develop a photodynamic reaction precipitated by direct exposure to natural or artificial sunlight during the use of tetracycline. This reaction is usually of the photoallergic type which may also be produced by other tetracycline derivatives. Individuals with a history of photosensitivity reactions should be instructed to avoid direct exposure to natural or artificial sunlight while under treatment with this or other tetracycline drugs, and treatment should be discontinued at first evidence of skin discomfort.

n.b. The incidence of photodynamic reactions varies markedly among various drugs of the tetracycline family. Many of these reactions have been reported in the literature from demethylchlortetracycline. Occasional cases from chlortetracycline, a few cases from oxytetracycline, and rare cases from tetracycline, tetracycline hydrochloride, and tetracycline phosphate complex have been reported.

If renal impairment exists, even usual oral or parenteral doses may lead to excessive systemic accumulation of the tetracycline and possible liver toxicity. Under such conditions, lower than usual doses are indicated, and if therapy is prolonged, tetracycline serum level determinations may be advisable.

Severe blood dyscrasias (including granulocytopenia and pancytopenia) have been associated with sulfonamide administration. Deposition of crystals within the kidney can result in oliguria or anuria. Monitoring renal, hepatic, and hematopoietic function is advisable when therapy is prolonged or repetitious.

This drug should be used only after critical appraisal in patients with liver damage, renal damage, urinary obstructions, or blood dyscrasias. Deaths have been reported from hypersensitivity reactions, agranulocytosis, aplastic anemia and other blood dyscrasias associated with sulfonamide administration.

When used intermittently or for a prolonged period, blood counts and liver and kidney function tests should be performed.

Precautions: Patients should be informed that the azo dye will impart an orange-red color to the urine.

Prolonged use of these capsules may lead to renal toxicity or to superinfection with resistant organisms (yeasts, Pseudomonas, antibiotic-resistant Staphylococci). If superinfection occurs, appropriate therapy should be instituted.

Infants may occasionally exhibit signs of increased cerebrospinal fluid pressure with bulging fontanels when on full therapeutic doses. Signs and symptoms disappear on cessation of tetracycline therapy.

In the treatment of gonorrhea, patients with a suspected lesion of syphilis should have darkfield examinations before receiving tetracycline and monthly serologic tests for a minimum of four months.

Tetracycline may form a stable calcium complex in any bone-forming tissue with no serious harmful effects reported thus far in humans. However, use of tetracycline during tooth development (last trimester of pregnancy, neonatal period, and early childhood) may cause discoloration of the teeth (yellow-grey-brownish). This effect occurs mostly during long-term use of the drug, but it has also been observed in usual short treatment courses.

Care should be taken to assure adequate fluid intake and urinary output.

This drug should be used with caution in persons having significant allergies and/or asthma.

Adverse Reactions: As in all sulfonamide therapy, the following reactions may occur: nausea, vomiting, diarrhea, hepatitis, pancreatitis, blood dyscrasias, neuropathy, drug fever, skin rash, injection of the conjunctiva and sclera, petechiae, purpura, hematuria and crystalluria. The side effects found with tetracycline therapy, namely glossitis, stomatitis, proctitis and vaginitis may occur. The dosage should be decreased or the drug withdrawn depending upon the severity of the reaction.

Dosage: Adult: One or two capsules 4 times a day. Patients with severe urinary tract infections or those who respond slowly to therapy may require higher doses.

In acute uncomplicated urinary tract infections, therapy should be continued until urine specimens become sterile, i.e., 7 to 14 days.

The medication should be given on an empty stomach. Calcium, in particular, interferes with the absorption of tetracycline.

Supply: AZOTREX Capsules (Tetracycline Phosphate Complex with Sulfonamide and Analgesic).

NDC 0015-4325

For information on package sizes available, refer to the current price schedule.

BETAPEN®-VK ℞

(penicillin V potassium)
Tablets (Film Coated) and Oral Solution

This is the full text of the latest Official Package Circular dated August 1980 [7506 DIR-07].

Description: Betapen-VK is the potassium salt of penicillin V. The oral solutions contain in each 5 ml. (teaspoonful) 125 mg. or 250 mg. of penicillin V activity respectively.

Clinical Pharmacology: Penicillin V exerts a bactericidal action against penicillin-susceptible microorganisms during the stage of active multiplication. It acts through the inhibition of biosynthesis of cell wall mucopeptide. It is not active against the penicillinase-producing bacteria, which include many strains of staphylococci. The drug exerts high **in vitro** activity against staphylococci (except penicillinase-producing strains), streptococci (Groups A, C, G, H, L, and M) and pneumococci. Other organisms susceptible **in vitro** to penicillin V are **Corynebacterium diphtheriae, Bacillus anthracis,** Clostridia, **Actinomyces bovis, Streptobacillus moniliformis, Listeria monocytogenes,** Leptospira and **Neisseria gonorrhoeae. Treponema pallidum** is extremely susceptible.

Penicillin V has the distinct advantage over penicillin G in resistance to inactivation by gastric acid. It may be given with meals; however, blood levels are slightly higher when the drug is given on an empty stomach. Average blood levels are two to five times higher than the levels following the same dose of oral penicillin G and also show much less individual variation.

Once absorbed, penicillin V is about 80% bound to serum protein. Tissue levels are highest in the kidney, with lesser amounts in the liver, skin, and intestines. Small amounts are found in all other body tissues and the cerebrospinal fluid. The drug is excreted as rapidly as it is absorbed in individuals with normal renal function; however, recovery of the drug from the urine indicates that only about 25% of the dose is absorbed. In neonates, young infants, and individuals with impaired renal function, excretion is considerably delayed.

Indications and Usage: Betapen-VK is indicated in the treatment of mild to moderately severe infections due to penicillin G-susceptible microorganisms. Therapy should be guided by bacteriological studies (including susceptibility tests) and by clinical response.

Note: Severe pneumonia, empyema, bacteremia, pericarditis, meningitis, and arthritis should not be treated with oral penicillins during the acute stage.

Indicated surgical procedures should be performed.

The following infections will usually respond to adequate doses of penicillin V: Streptococcal Infections (without bacteremia). Mild to moderate infections of the upper respiratory tract, scarlet fever, and mild erysipelas.

Note: Streptococci in Groups A, C, G, H, L, and M are very susceptible to penicillin. Other groups, including Group D (enterococcus) are resistant.

Pneumococcal Infections—Mild to moderately severe infections of the respiratory tract.

Staphylococcal Infections—penicillin G-susceptible. Mild infections of the skin and soft tissue.

Note: Reports indicate an increasing number of strains of staphylococci resistant to penicillin G, emphasizing the need for culture and susceptibility studies in treating suspected staphylococcal infections.

Fusospirochetosis (Vincent's gingivitis and pharyngitis)—Mild to moderately severe infections of the oropharynx usually respond to therapy with oral penicillin.

Note: Necessary dental care should be accomplished in infections involving gum tissue.

Medical conditions in which oral penicillin therapy is indicated as prophylaxis: For the prevention of recurrence following rheumatic fever and/or chorea. Prophylaxis with oral penicillin on a continuing basis has proven effective in preventing recurrence of these conditions.

Although no controlled clinical efficacy studies have been conducted penicillin V has been suggested by the American Heart Association and the American Dental Association for use as part of a parenteral-oral regimen and as an alternative oral regimen for prophylaxis against bacterial endocarditis in patients with congenital heart disease or rheumatic or other acquired valvular heart disease when they undergo dental procedures and surgical procedures of the respiratory tract.[1] Since it may happen that **alpha**-hemolytic streptococci, relatively resistant to penicillin, may be found when patients are receiving continuous oral penicillin for secondary prevention of rheumatic fever, prophylactic agents other than penicillin may be chosen for these patients and prescribed in addition to their continuous rheumatic fever prophylactic regimen. Oral penicillin should not be used as adjunctive prophylaxis for genitourinary instrumentation or surgery, lower intestinal tract surgery, sigmoidoscopy, and childbirth.

Note: When selecting antibiotics for the prevention of bacterial endocarditis the physician or dentist should read the full joint statement of the American Heart Association and the American Dental Association.[1]

Contraindications: A previous hypersensitivity reaction to any penicillin is a contraindication.

Warning: Serious and occasionally fatal hypersensitivity (anaphylactoid) reactions have been reported in patients on penicillin therapy. Although anaphylaxis is more frequent following parenteral therapy, it has occurred in patients on oral penicillins. These reactions are more apt to occur in individuals with a history of sensitivity to multiple allergens.

There have been well documented reports of individuals with a history of penicillin hypersensitivity reactions who experienced severe hypersensitivity reactions when treated with cephalosporins. Before therapy with a penicillin, careful inquiry should be made concerning previous hypersensitivity reactions to penicillins, cephalosporins, and other allergens. If an allergic reaction occurs, the drug should be discontinued and the patient treated with the usual agents, e.g., antihistamines, pressor amines, corticosteroids.

Precautions: Penicillins should be used with caution in individuals with a history of significant allergies and/or asthma.

The oral route of administration should not be relied upon in patients with severe illness, or with nausea, vomiting, gastric dilatation, cardiospasm or intestinal hypermotility.

Occasional patients will not absorb therapeutic amounts of orally administered penicillins.

In streptococcal infections, therapy must be sufficient to eliminate the organism (10 days minimum); otherwise the sequelae of streptococcal disease may occur. Cultures should be taken following completion of treatment to determine whether streptococci have been eradicated.

Prolonged use of antibiotics may promote the overgrowth of nonsusceptible organisms, including fungi. Should superinfection occur, appropriate measures should be taken.

Adverse Reactions: Although the incidence of reactions to oral penicillins has been reported with much less frequency than following parenteral therapy, it should be remembered that all degrees of hypersensitivity, including fatal anaphylaxis, have been reported with oral penicillin.

The most common reactions to oral penicillin are nausea, vomiting, epigastric distress, diarrhea, and black hairy tongue. The hypersensitivity reactions reported are skin eruptions (maculopapular to exfoliative dermatitis), urticaria and other serum sickness reactions, laryngeal edema and anaphylaxis. Fever and eosinophilia may frequently be the only reaction observed. Hemolytic anemia, leukopenia, thrombocytopenia, neuropathy, and nephropathy are infrequent reactions and usually associated with high doses of parenteral penicillin.

Administration and Dosage: The dosage of Betapen-VK should be determined according to the susceptibility of the causative organism and the severity of infection, and adjusted to the clinical response of the patient.

The usual dosage recommendations for adults and children 12 years and over are as follows:

Streptococcal Infections—mild to moderately severe—of the upper respiratory tract and including scarlet fever and erysipelas: 125 to 250 mg. (200,000 to 400,000 units) every 6 to 8 hours for 10 days.

Pneumococcal Infections—mild to moderately severe—of the respiratory tract, including otitis media: 250 mg. (400,000 units) every 6 hours until the patient has been afebrile for at least 2 days.

Staphylococcal Infections—mild infections of skin and soft tissue (culture and sensitivity tests should be performed): 250 mg. (400,000 units) every 6 to 8 hours.

Fusospirochetosis (Vincent's Infection) of the oropharynx—mild to moderately severe infections: 250 mg. (400,000 units) every 6 to 8 hours.

For the prevention of recurrence following rheumatic fever and/or chorea: 125 mg. (200,000 units) twice daily on a continuing basis.

For prophylaxis against bacterial endocarditis[1] in patients with congenital heart disease or rheumatic or other acquired valvular heart disease when undergoing dental procedures or surgical procedures of the upper respiratory tract, 1 of 2 regimens may be selected:

(1) For the oral regimen, give 2 grams of penicillin V (1 gram for children under 60 lbs) ½ to 1 hour before the procedure, and then, 500 mg (250 mg for children under 60 lbs) every 6 hours for 8 doses; or

(2) For the combined parenteral-oral regimen, give 1 million units of aqueous crystalline penicillin G (30,000 units/kg in children) intramuscularly mixed with 600,000 units procaine penicillin G (600,000 units for children) ½ to 1 hour before the procedure, and then, oral penicillin V, 500 mg for adults or 250 mg for children less than 60 lbs, every 6 hours for 8 doses. Doses for children should not exceed recommendations for adults for a single dose or for a 24-hour period.

Directions for Dispensing Oral Solutions: Prepare this formulation at the time of dispensing. For ease in preparation, add water to the bottle in two portions and shake well after each addition. Add the total amount of water as directed on the labeling of the package being dispensed. The reconstituted solutions are stable for 14 days under refrigeration.

How Supplied: BETAPEN-VK (penicillin V potassium) for Oral Solution. Each 5 ml. of reconstituted solution contains penicillin V potassium equivalent to 125 or 250 mg. penicillin V.

NDC 0015-7506—125 mg
NDC 0015-7507—250 mg

BETAPEN-VK (penicillin V potassium) Tablets (Film Coated). Each tablet contains penicillin V potassium equivalent to 250 or 500 mg. penicillin V.

NDC 0015-7508-250 mg.
NDC 0015-7509-500 mg.

For information on package sizes available, refer to the current price schedule.

Reference:

1. American Heart Association. 1977. Prevention of bacterial endocarditis. Circulation. 56:139A-143A.

[*Shown in Product Identification Section*]

BiCNU® ℞

(carmustine [BCNU])

This is the full text of the latest Official Package Circular dated November 1981 [3012 DIM-07].

WARNING

BiCNU should be administered preferably by individuals experienced in antineoplastic therapy. Since delayed bone marrow toxicity is the major toxicity, complete blood counts should be monitored frequently for at least 6 weeks after a dose. Repeat doses of BiCNU should not be given more frequently than every 6 weeks. The bone marrow toxicity of BiCNU is cumulative, and therefore dosage adjustment must be considered on the basis of nadir blood counts from prior dose (see dosage adjustment table under **Dosage**).

It is recommended that liver function, pulmonary function, and renal function tests also be monitored.

Description: BiCNU (1,3-bis (2-chloroethyl)-1-nitrosourea) is one of the nitrosoureas. It is a white lyophilized powder with a molecular weight of 214.06. It is highly soluble in alcohol and poorly soluble in water. It is also highly soluble in lipids.

Action: BiCNU alkylates DNA and RNA and has also been shown to inhibit several enzymes by carbamoylation of amino acids in proteins.

Intravenously administered BiCNU is rapidly degraded, with no intact drug detectable after 15 minutes. However, in studies with C^{14} labeled drug, prolonged levels of the isotope were observed in the plasma and tissue, probably representing radioactive fragments of the parent compound.

It is thought that the antineoplastic and toxic activities of BiCNU may be due to metabolites. Approximately 60 to 70% of a total dose is excreted in the urine in 96 hours and about 10% as respiratory CO_2. The fate of the remainder is undetermined.

Because of the high lipid solubility and the relative lack of ionization at a physiological pH, BiCNU crosses the blood brain barrier quite effectively. Levels of radioactivity in the CSF are 50% or greater than those measured concurrently in plasma.

Indications: BiCNU is indicated as palliative therapy as a single agent or in established combination therapy with other approved chemotherapeutic agents in the following:

Continued on next page

Bristol—Cont.

1. **Brain tumors**—glioblastoma, brainstem glioma, medulloblastoma, astrocytoma, ependymoma, and metastatic brain tumors.
2. **Multiple myeloma**—in combination with prednisone.
3. **Hodgkin's Disease**—as secondary therapy in combination with other approved drugs in patients who relapse while being treated with primary therapy, or who fail to respond to primary therapy.
4. **Non-Hodgkin's lymphomas**—as secondary therapy in combination with other approved drugs for patients who relapse while being treated with primary therapy, or who fail to respond to primary therapy.

Contraindications: BiCNU should not be given to individuals who have demonstrated a previous hypersensitivity to it.

BiCNU should not be given to individuals with decreased circulating platelets, leukocytes, or erythrocytes either from previous chemotherapy or other causes.

Warnings: Safe use in pregnancy has not been established. BiCNU is embryotoxic and teratogenic in rats and embryotoxic in rabbits at dose levels equivalent to the human dose. BiCNU also affects fertility in male rats at doses somewhat higher than the human dose. BiCNU is carcinogenic in rats and mice, producing a marked increase in tumor incidence in doses approximating those employed clinically.

Nitrosourea therapy does have carcinogenic potential. The occurrence of acute leukemia and bone marrow dysplasias have been reported in patients following nitrosourea therapy.

Precautions: BiCNU should be administered preferably by individuals experienced in antineoplastic therapy. Since delayed bone marrow toxicity is the major toxicity, complete blood counts should be monitored frequently for at least 6 weeks after a dose. Repeat doses of BiCNU should not be given more frequently than every 6 weeks. The bone marrow toxicity of BiCNU is cumulative, and therefore dosage adjustment must be considered on the basis of nadir blood counts from prior dose (see Dosage Adjustment Table under DOSAGE).

It is recommended that liver function tests also be monitored.

Safe Use in Pregnancy has not been established. Therefore, the benefit to risk of toxicity must be carefully weighed.

See "Warnings" section for information on carcinogenesis.

Adverse Reactions:

Hematopoietic

The most frequent and most serious toxicity of BiCNU is delayed myelosuppression. It usually occurs 4 to 6 weeks after drug administration and is dose-related. Platelet nadirs occur at 4 to 5 weeks; leukocyte nadirs occur at 5 to 6 weeks post therapy. Thrombocytopenia is generally more severe than leukopenia. However both may be dose limiting toxicities. Anemia also occurs, but is generally less severe.

Gastrointestinal

Nausea and vomiting after IV administration of BiCNU are noted frequently. This toxicity appears within 2 hours of dosing, usually lasting 4 to 6 hours, and is dose-related. Prior administration of antiemetics is effective in diminishing and sometimes preventing this side effect.

Hepatic

When high doses of BiCNU have been employed, a reversible type of hepatic toxicity, manifested by increased transaminase, alkaline phosphatase and bilirubin levels, has been reported in a small percentage of patients.

Pulmonary—Pulmonary toxicity characterized by pulmonary infiltrate and/or fibrosis have been reported in some patients receiving prolonged therapy with BiCNU.

Renal—Renal abnormalities consisting of decrease in kidney size, progressive azotemia and renal failure have been reported in patients who received large cumulative doses after prolonged therapy with BiCNU and related nitrosoureas. Kidney damage has also been reported occasionally in patients receiving lower total doses.

Local

Burning at the site of injection is common but true thrombosis is rare.

Other

Rapid IV infusion of BiCNU may produce intensive flushing of the skin and suffusion of the conjunctiva within 2 hours, lasting about 4 hours.

Accidental contact of reconstituted BiCNU with the skin has caused burning and hyperpigmentation of the affected areas.

Dosage: The recommended dose of BiCNU as single agent in previously untreated patients is 200 mg/m^2 intravenously every 6 weeks. This may be given as a single dose or divided into daily injections such as 100 mg/m^2 on 2 successive days. When BiCNU is used in combination with other myelosuppressive drugs or in patients in whom bone marrow reserve is depleted, the doses should be adjusted accordingly.

A repeat course of BiCNU should not be given until circulating blood elements have returned to acceptable levels (platelets above 100,000/mm^3; leukocytes above 4,000/mm^3), and this is usually in 6 weeks. Blood counts should be monitored frequently and repeat courses should not be given before 6 weeks because of delayed toxicity.

Doses subsequent to the initial dose should be adjusted according to the hematologic response of the patient to the preceding dose. The following schedule is suggested as a guide to dosage adjustment:

Nadir After Prior Dose		Percentage of Prior Dose to be Given
Leukocytes	Platelets	
>4000 -	>100,000 -	100%
3000-3999	75,000-99,999	100%
2000-2999	25,000-74,999	70%
<2000 -	<25,000 -	50%

Preparation of Intravenous Solutions: Dissolve BiCNU with 3 ml of the supplied sterile diluent and then aseptically add 27 ml of Sterile Water for Injection, U.S.P., to the alcohol solution. Each ml of the resulting solution will contain 3.3 mg of BiCNU in 10% ethanol having a pH of 5.6 to 6.0. Accidental contact of reconstituted BiCNU with the skin has caused transient hyperpigmentation of the affected areas.

Reconstitution as recommended results in a clear, colorless solution which may be further diluted with Sodium Chloride for Injection, U.S.P., or 5% Dextrose for Injection, U.S.P.

The reconstituted solution should be used intravenously only and should be administered by IV drip over a 1 to 2 hour period. Injection of BiCNU over shorter periods of time may produce intense pain and burning at the site of injection.

Important Note: The lyophilized dosage formulation contains no preservatives and is not intended as a multiple dose vial.

Stability: Unopened vials of the dry powder must be stored in a refrigerator (2°C to 8°C). The recommended storage of unopened vials prevents significant decomposition for at least 2 years.

After reconstitution as recommended, decomposition of BiCNU at room temperature is linear with time. After 3 hours, appoximately 6% of the solution has decomposed and after 6 hours, approximately 8%.

Refrigeration (4°C) of the reconstituted BiCNU significantly increases the stability of the solution. After 24 hours, when protected from light, there is only 4% decomposition. Further dilution of the reconstituted solution with 500 ml. of Sodium Chloride for Injection, U.S.P., or 5% Dextrose for Injection, U.S.P., results in a solution which is stable for 48 hours when protected from light and refrigerated.

Important Note: BiCNU has a low melting point (approximately 30.5°C–32.0°C). Exposure of the drug to this temperature or above will cause the drug to liquify and appear as an oil film in the bottom of the vials. This is a sign of decomposition and vials should be discarded.

Supply: BiCNU (Carmustine [BCNU]). Each package contains a vial containing 100 mg. carmustine and a vial containing 3 ml. sterile diluent.

NDC 0015-3012

For information on package sizes available, refer to the current price schedule.

BLENOXANE® ℞

(sterile bleomycin sulfate)

This is the full text of the latest Official Package Circular dated February 1982 [3010 DIR-12].

WARNING

It is recommended that Blenoxane be administered under the supervision of a qualified physician experienced in the use of cancer chemotherapeutic agents.

Appropriate management of therapy and complications is possible only when adequate diagnostic and treatment facilities are readily available.

Pulmonary fibrosis is the most severe toxicity associated with Blenoxane. The most frequent presentation is pneumonitis occasionally progressing to pulmonary fibrosis. Its occurrence is higher in elderly patients and in those receiving greater than 400 units total dose, but pulmonary toxicity has been observed in young patients and those treated with low doses.

A severe idiosyncratic reaction consisting of hypotension, mental confusion, fever, chills, and wheezing has been reported in approximately 1% of lymphoma patients treated with Blenoxane.

Description: Blenoxane (sterile bleomycin sulfate) is a mixture of cytotoxic glycopeptide antibiotics isolated from a strain of **Streptomyces verticillus.** It is freely soluble in water.

Note: A unit of bleomycin is equal to the formerly used milligram activity. The term milligram activity is a misnomer and was changed to units to be more precise.

Action: Although the exact mechanism of action of Blenoxane is unknown, available evidence would seem to indicate that the main mode of action is the inhibition of DNA synthesis with some evidence of lesser inhibition of RNA and protein synthesis.

In mice, high concentrations of Blenoxane are found in the skin, lungs, kidneys, peritoneum, and lymphatics. Tumor cells of the skin and lungs have been found to have high concentrations of Blenoxane in contrast to the low concentrations found in hematopoietic tissue. The low concentrations of Blenoxane found in bone marrow may be related to high levels of Blenoxane degradative enzymes found in that tissue.

In patients with a creatinine clearance of >35 ml. per minute, the serum or plasma terminal elimination half-life of bleomycin is approximately 115 minutes. In patients with a creatinine clearance of <35 ml. per minute, the plasma or serum terminal elimination half-life increases exponentially as the creatinine clearance decreases. In humans, 60 to 70% of an administered dose is recovered in the urine as active bleomycin.

Indications: Blenoxane should be considered a palliative treatment. It has been shown to be useful in the management of the following neoplasms either as a single agent or in proven combinations with other approved chemotherapeutic agents:

Squamous Cell Carcinoma—Head and neck including mouth, tongue, tonsil, nasopharynx, oropharynx, sinus, palate, lip, buccal mucosa, gingiva, epiglottis, skin, larynx, penis, cervix, and vulva. The response to Blenoxane is poorer in patients with head and neck cancer previously irradiated.

Lymphomas—Hodgkin's, reticulum cell sarcoma, lymphosarcoma.

Testicular Carcinoma—Embryonal cell, choriocarcinoma, and teratocarcinoma.

Contraindications: Blenoxane is contraindicated in patients who have demonstrated a hypersensitive or an idiosyncratic reaction to it.

Warnings: Patients receiving Blenoxane must be observed carefully and frequently during and after therapy. It should be used with extreme caution in patients with significant impairment of renal function or compromised pulmonary function.

Pulmonary toxicities occur in 10% of treated patients. In approximately 1%, the nonspecific pneumonitis induced by Blenoxane progresses to pulmonary fibrosis, and death. Although this is age and dose related, the toxicity is unpredictable. Frequent roentgenograms are recommended.

Idiosyncratic reactions similar to anaphylaxis have been reported in 1% of lymphoma patients treated with Blenoxane. Since these usually occur after the first or second dose, careful monitoring is essential after these doses.

Renal or hepatic toxicity, beginning as a deterioration in renal or liver function tests, have been reported, infrequently. These toxicities may occur, however, at any time after initiation of therapy.

Usage in Pregnancy: Safe use of Blenoxane in pregnant women has not been established.

Adverse Reactions:

Pulmonary—This is potentially the most serious side effect, occurring in approximately 10% of treated patients. The most frequent presentation is pneumonitis occasionally progressing to pulmonary fibrosis. Approximately 1% of patients treated have died of pulmonary fibrosis. Pulmonary toxicity is both dose and age-related, being more common in patients over 70 years of age and in those receiving over 400 units total dose. This toxicity, however, is unpredictable and has been seen occasionally in young patients receiving low doses.

Because of lack of specificity of the clinical syndrome, the identification of patients with pulmonary toxicity due to Blenoxane has been extremely difficult. The earliest symptom associated with Blenoxane pulmonary toxicity is dyspnea. The earliest sign is fine rales.

Radiographically, Blenoxane-induced pneumonitis produces nonspecific patchy opacities, usually of the lower lung fields. The most common changes in pulmonary function tests are a decrease in total lung volume and a decrease in vital capacity. However, these changes are not predictive of the development of pulmonary fibrosis.

The microscopic tissue changes due to Blenoxane toxicity include bronchiolar squamous metaplasia, reactive macrophages, atypical alveolar epithelial cells, fibrinous edema, and interstitial fibrosis. The acute stage may involve capillary changes and subsequent fibrinous exudation into alveoli producing a change similar to hyaline membrane formation and progressing to a diffuse interstitial fibrosis resembling the Hamman-Rich syndrome. These microscopic findings are nonspecific, e.g., similar changes are seen in radiation pneumonitis, pneumocystic pneumonitis.

To monitor the onset of pulmonary toxicity, roentgenograms of the chest should be taken every 1 to 2 weeks. If pulmonary changes are noted, treatment should be discontinued until it can be determined if they are drug related. Recent studies have suggested that sequential measurement of the pulmonary diffusion capacity for carbon monoxide (DL_{co}) during treatment with Blenoxane may be an indicator of subclinical pulmonary toxicity. It is recommended that the DL_{co} be monitored monthly if it is to be employed to detect pulmonary toxicities, and thus the drug should be discontinued when the DL_{co} falls below 30 to 35% of the pretreatment value.

Idiosyncratic Reactions—In approximately 1% of the lymphoma patients treated with Blenoxane an idiosyncratic reaction, similar to anaphylaxis clinically, has been reported. The reaction may be immediate or delayed for several hours, and usually occurs after the first or second dose. It consists of hypotension, mental confusion, fever, chills, and wheezing. Treatment is symptomatic including volume expansion, pressor agents, antihistamines, and corticosteroids.

Integument and Mucus Membranes—These are the most frequent side effects, being reported in approximately 50% of treated patients. These consist of erythema, rash, striae, vesiculation, hyperpigmentation, and tenderness of the skin. Hyperkeratosis, nail changes, alopecia, pruritus, and stomatitis have also been reported. It was necessary to discontinue Blenoxane therapy in 2% of treated patients because of these toxicities.

Skin toxicity is a relatively late manifestation usually developing in the 2nd and 3rd week of treatment after 150 to 200 units of Blenoxane have been administered and appears to be related to the cumulative dose.

Other—Fever, chills, and vomiting were frequently reported side effects. Anorexia and weight loss are common and may persist long after termination of this medication. Pain at tumor site, phlebitis, and other local reactions were reported infrequently.

There are isolated reports of Raynaud's phenomenon occurring in patients with testicular carcinomas treated with a combination of Blenoxane and Velban®. It is currently unknown if the cause for the Raynaud's phenomenon in these cases is the disease, Blenoxane, Velban, or a combination of any or all of these.

Dosage: **Because of the possibility of an anaphylactoid reaction, lymphoma patients should be treated with 2 units or less for the first 2 doses. If no acute reaction occurs, then the regular dosage schedule may be followed.**

The following dose schedule is recommended:

Squamous cell carcinoma, lymphosarcoma, reticulum cell sarcoma, testicular carcinoma—0.25 to 0.50 units/Kg. (10 to 20 units/M.^{2}) given intravenously, intramuscularly, or subcutaneously weekly or twice weekly.

Hodgkin's Disease—0.25 to 0.50 units/Kg. (10 to 20 units/M.^{2}) given intravenously, intramuscularly, or subcutaneously weekly or twice weekly. After a 50% response, a maintenance dose of 1 unit daily or 5 units weekly intravenously or intramuscularly should be given.

Pulmonary toxicity of Blenoxane appears to be dose-related with a striking increase when the total dose is over 400 units. Total doses over 400 units should be given with great caution.

Note: When Blenoxane is used in combination with other antineoplastic agents, pulmonary toxicities may occur at lower doses.

Improvement of Hodgkin's Disease and testicular tumors is prompt and noted within two weeks. If no improvement is seen by this time, improvement is unlikely. Squamous cell cancers respond more slowly, sometimes requiring as long as three weeks before any improvement is noted.

Administration: Blenoxane may be given by the intramuscular, intravenous, or subcutaneous routes.

Intramuscular or Subcutaneous—Dissolve the contents of a Blenoxane vial in 1 to 5 ml. of Sterile Water for Injection, U.S.P., Sodium Chloride for Injection, U.S.P., 5% Dextrose Injection, U.S.P., or Bacteriostatic Water for Injection, U.S.P.

Intravenous—Dissolve the contents of the vial in 5 ml. or more of a solution suitable for injection, e.g., physiologic saline or glucose, and administer slowly over a period of ten minutes.

Stability: The sterile powder is stable for a period of 24 months and should not be used after the expiration date is reached.

Blenoxane is stable for 24 hours at room temperature in Sodium Chloride or 5% Dextrose Solution.

Blenoxane is stable for 24 hours in 5% Dextrose containing heparin 100 units per ml. or 1000 units per ml.

Supply: Each vial contains 15 units of Blenoxane as sterile bleomycin sulfate.

NDC 0015-3010-20

For information on package sizes available, refer to the current price sheet.

BRISTAGEN™ ℞

(gentamicin sulfate injection)
40 mg per ml
Each ml contains gentamicin sulfate equivalent to 40 mg gentamicin
For Parenteral Administration

This is the full text of the latest Official Package Circular dated August 1980 [3300DIM-01].

WARNINGS

Because of the potential toxicity associated with their use, patients treated with aminoglycosides should be under close clinical observation.

BRISTAGEN Injectable, like other aminoglycosides, is potentially nephrotoxic. The risk is greater in patients with impaired renal function and in those receiving high dosage or prolonged therapy.

Neurotoxicity manifested by ototoxicity, both auditory and vestibular, can occur in patients treated with BRISTAGEN Injectable, primarily in those with preexisting renal damage and in patients with normal renal function treated for longer periods than recommended and/or with higher doses. Other manifestations of neurotoxicity may include convulsions, muscle twitching, numbness and skin tingling.

Renal and eighth cranial nerve function should be closely monitored, particularly in patients with known or suspected reduced renal function at onset of therapy and also in those whose renal function is initially normal but who later develop signs of renal dysfunction during therapy. Urine should be examined for increased excretion of protein, the presence of cells or casts, and decreased specific gravity. BUN, serum creatinine, or creatinine clearance should be determined periodically. When feasible, in patients old enough to be tested, particularly high-risk patients, it is recommended that serial audiograms be obtained. Evidence of ototoxicity (vertigo, dizziness, tinnitus, roaring in the ears or hearing loss) or nephrotoxicity requires dosage adjustment or discontinuance of the drug. As is true with other aminoglycosides, on rare occasions changes in renal and eighth cranial nerve function may not become manifest until soon after completion of therapy.

When feasible, serum concentrations of aminoglycosides should be monitored to assure adequate levels and to avoid poten-

Continued on next page

Bristol—Cont.

tially toxic levels. When monitoring gentamicin peak concentrations, dosage should be adjusted so that prolonged levels above 12 mcg/ml are avoided. Dosage should also be adjusted so that trough levels above 2 mcg/ml are avoided. Excessive peak and /or trough serum concentrations of aminoglycosides may increase the risk of renal and eighth cranial nerve toxicity. If overdose or toxic reactions should occur, hemodialysis or peritoneal dialysis will aid in removal of gentamicin from the blood.
Avoid concurrent and/or sequential systemic or topical use of other potentially neurotoxic and/or nephrotoxic drugs, such as colistin, paromomycin, polymyxin B, cisplatin, streptomycin, kanamycin, neomycin, cephaloridine, amikacin, viomycin, vancomycin and tobramycin. Other factors which may increase patient risk of toxicity are advanced age and dehydration.
Avoid concurrent use of gentamicin with potent diuretics, such as ethacrynic acid or furosemide, since certain diuretics by themselves may cause ototoxicity. When administered intravenously, diuretics may enhance aminoglycoside toxicity by altering the antibiotic concentration in serum and tissue.

Description: Gentamicin sulfate, a water-soluble antibiotic of the aminoglycoside group, is derived from **Micromonospora purpurea**, an actinomycete. BRISTAGEN Injectable is a sterile, aqueous solution for parenteral administration. Each ml contains gentamicin sulfate, equivalent to 40 mg gentamicin base, 1.8 mg methylparaben and 0.2 mg propylparaben as preservatives; 3.2 mg sodium bisulfite; and 0.1 mg edetate disodium.
Clinical Pharmacology: Peak serum concentrations usually occur between 30 and 60 minutes after intramuscular administration of BRISTAGEN Injectable. Serum levels are measurable for 6 to 8 hours. Administration by intravenous infusion over a 2-hour period results in serum concentrations similar to those obtained by intramuscular administration.
In patients with normal renal function, peak serum concentrations of gentamicin (mcg/ml) are usually up to 4 times the single intramuscular dose (mg/kg); i.e., a 1-mg/kg injection in adults may be expected to result in a peak serum concentration up to 4 mcg/ml; a 1.5 mg/kg dose may produce peaks up to 6 mcg/ml. While some variation is to be expected due to a number of variables such as age, body temperature, surface area and physiologic differences, the individual patient given the same dose tends to have similar levels on repeated determinations. Administered at 1 mg/kg every 8 hours for the usual 7- to 10-day treatment period to patients with normal renal function, gentamicin does not accumulate in the serum. Gentamicin, like all aminoglycosides, may accumulate in the serum and tissues of patients treated with higher doses and for prolonged periods. This is particularly true in the presence of impaired renal function. In adult patients, treatment with gentamicin dosages of 4 mg/kg/day or higher for 7 to 10 days may result in a slight, progressive rise in both peak and trough concentrations. In patients with impaired renal function, gentamicin is cleared from the body more slowly than in those with normal renal function. The severer the impairment, the slower the clearance. (Dosage must be adjusted.)
Peak serum concentrations may be lower than usual in adult patients who have a large volume of this fluid since gentamicin is distributed in extracellular fluid. Serum concentrations of gentamicin in febrile patients may be lower than those in afebrile patients given the same dose. As body temperature returns to normal, serum concentrations of the drug may rise. A shorter than usual serum half-life may be associated with febrile and anemic states. (Dosage adjustment is usually not necessary.) In severely burned patients, the half-life may be significantly decreased and result in serum concentrations lower than anticipated from the mg/kg dose.
Protein binding studies have indicated that the degree of gentamicin binding is low. Depending upon the methods used for testing, this may be between 0 and 30%.
In patients with normal renal function, after initial administration, generally 70% or more of the gentamicin dose is recoverable in the urine in 24 hours. Concentrations in urine above 100 mcg/ml may be achieved. The drug is excreted principally by glomerular filtration. Little, if any, metabolic transformation occurs. After several days of treatment, the amount excreted in the urine approaches the daily dose administered. As with other aminoglycosides, a small amount of the gentamicin dose may be retained in the tissues, especially in the kidneys. Weeks after drug administration was discontinued, minute quantities of aminoglycosides have been detected in the urine. Renal clearance of gentamicin is similar to that of endogenous creatinine.
There is decreased concentration of aminoglycosides in urine and in their penetration into defective renal parenchyma in patients with marked impairment of renal function. This decreased drug excretion, together with the potential nephrotoxicity of aminoglycosides, should be considered when treating such patients who have urinary tract infections.
Probenecid has no affect on the renal tubular transport of gentamicin.
The serum creatinine and endogenous creatinine clearance rate level have a high correlation with the half-life of gentamicin in serum. Results of these tests may serve as guides for adjusting dosage in patients with renal functional impairment (see **DOSAGE AND ADMINISTRATION**).
Gentamicin can be detected in serum, lymph, tissues, sputum, and in pleural, synovial and peritoneal fluids following parenteral administration. Concentrations in renal cortex sometimes may be 8 times higher than the usual serum levels. Concentrations in bile, in general, are low and suggest minimal biliary excretion. Gentamicin crosses the peritoneal as well as the placental membranes. Aminoglycosides diffuse poorly into the subarachnoid space after parenteral administration. Concentrations of gentamicin in cerebrospinal fluid are often low and dependent upon dose, rate of penetration, and degree of meningeal inflammation. Following intramuscular or intravenous administration, there is minimal penetration of gentamicin into occular tissues.
Microbiology: Tests **in vitro** have demonstrated that gentamicin is a bactericidal antibiotic which acts by inhibiting normal protein synthesis in susceptible microorganisms. Gentamicin is active against a wide variety of pathogenic bacteria including **Escherichia coli, Proteus** species, (indole-positive and indole-negative), **Pseudomonas aeruginosa,** species of the Klebsiella-Enterobacter-Serratia group, **Citrobacter** species and **Staphylococcus** species (including penicillin- and methicillin-resistant strains). It is also active **in vitro** against species of Salmonella and Shigella. The following bacteria are usually resistant to aminoglycosides: **Streptococcus pneumoniae,** most species of streptococci, particularly group D, and anaerobic organisms, such as **Bacteroides** species or **Clostridium** species.
In vitro studies have shown that an aminoglycoside combined with an antibiotic interfering with cell wall synthesis may act synergistically against some group D streptococcal strains. The combination of gentamicin and penicillin G has a synergistic bactericidal effect against virtually all strains of **Streptococcus faecalis** and its varieties (**S. faecalis** var. **liquifaciens, S. faecalis** var. **zymogenes**), **S. faecium** and **S. durans. In vitro,** an enhanced killing effect against many of these strains has also been shown with combinations of gentamicin and ampicillin, carbenicillin, nafcillin, or oxacillin.
The combined effect of gentamicin and carbenicillin is synergistic for many strains of **Pseudomonas aeruginosa.** Synergism against other gram-negative organisms has been shown **in vitro** with combinations of gentamicin and cephalosporins. Gentamicin may be active against clinical isolates of bacteria resistant to other aminoglycosides. Bacterial resistance to gentamicin generally developes slowly.
Susceptibility Testing: Using the method described by Bauer **et. al.** (**Am J Clin Path** 45:493, 1966; **Federal Register** 37:20527–20529, 1972), a disc containing 10 mcg of gentamicin should give a zone of inhibition of 13 mm or more to indicate susceptibility of the infecting organism. A zone of 12 mm or less indicates that the infecting organism is likely to be resistant. It may be desirable, in certain conditions, to do additional susceptibility testing by the tube or agar dilution method; gentamicin substance is available for this purpose.
Indications and Usage: BRISTAGEN Injectable is indicated in the treatment of serious infections caused by susceptible strains of the following microorganisms: **Pseudomonas aeruginosa, Proteus** species (indole-positive and indole-negative), **Escherichia coli,** Klebsiella-Enterobacter-Serratia species, **Citrobacter** species and **Staphylococcus** species (coagulase-positive and coagulase-negative).
BRISTAGEN Injectable has been shown by clinical studies to be effective in bacterial neonatal sepsis; bacterial septicemia; and serious bacterial infections of the central nervous system (meningitis), urinary tract, respiratory tract, gastrointestinal tract (including peritonitis), skin, bone and soft tissue (including burns). The aminoglycosides, including gentamicin, are not indicated in uncomplicated first episodes of urinary tract infections unless the causative organisms are susceptible to these antibiotics and are not susceptible to antibiotics having less potential for toxicity.
Specimens for bacterial culture should be obtained to identify causative organisms and to determine their susceptibility to gentamicin.
BRISTAGEN may be considered as initial therapy in suspected or confirmed gram-negative infections. Therapy may be instituted before obtaining results of susceptibility testing. The decision to continue therapy with this drug should be based on the results of susceptibility tests, the severity of the infection, and the important concepts contained in the "WARNINGS Box" above. If the causative organisms are resistant to gentamicin, other appropriate therapy should be instituted.
In serious infections when the causative organisms are unknown, BRISTAGEN may be administered as initial therapy in conjunction with a penicillin-type or cephalosporin-type of drug before the results of susceptibility testing are known. If anaerobic organisms are suspected as etiologic agents, consideration should be given to other suitable antimicrobial therapy in conjunction with gentamicin. Appropriate antibiotic therapy should then be continued following identification of the organism and its susceptibility.
BRISTAGEN has been used effectively in combination with carbenicillin for the treatment of life-threatening infections caused by **Pseudomonas aeruginosa.** Effectiveness, when used in conjunction with a penicillin-type drug for the treatment of endocarditis caused by group D streptococci, has been demonstrated.
BRISTAGEN Injectable has also been shown to be effective in the treatment of serious

DOSAGE SCHEDULE I
DOSAGE SCHEDULE FOR ADULTS WITH NORMAL RENAL FUNCTION
(Dose at 8-Hour Intervals)
40 mg per ml

Patient's Weight* lb	(Kg)	Usual Dosage for Serious Infections 1 mg/kg q8h (3 mg/kg/day) mg/dose q8h	ml/dose	Dosage for Life-Threatening Infections (Reduce As Soon As Clinically Indicated) 1.7 mg/kg q8h** (5 mg/kg/day) mg/dose q8h	ml/dose
88	(40)	40	1.0	66	1.6
99	(45)	45	1.1	75	1.9
110	(50)	50	1.25	83	2.1
121	(55)	55	1.4	91	2.25
132	(60)	60	1.5	100	2.5
143	(65)	65	1.6	108	2.7
154	(70)	70	1.75	116	2.9
165	(75)	75	1.9	125	3.1
176	(80)	80	2.0	133	3.3
187	(85)	85	2.1	141	3.5
198	(90)	90	2.25	150	3.75
209	(95)	95	2.4	158	4.0
220	(100)	100	2.5	166	4.2

* The dose of aminoglycosides in obese patients should be based on an estimate of the lean body mass.

** For q6h schedules, dose should be recalculated.

staphylococcal infections. While not considered the antibiotic of first choice, BRISTAGEN Injectable may be used when penicillins or other less potentially toxic drugs are contraindicated and bacterial susceptibility tests and clinical judgment indicate its use. Its use may also be considered in mixed infections caused by susceptible strains of staphylococci and gram-negative organisms.

In the neonate with suspected bacterial sepsis or staphylococcal pneumonia, a penicillin-type drug is also usually indicated as concomitant therapy with gentamicin.

Contraindications: Hypersensitivity to gentamicin is a contraindication to its use. Because of the known cross-sensitivity of patients to drugs in this class, a history of hypersensitivity or serious toxic reactions to other aminoglycosides may contraindicate use of gentamicin.

Warnings: See "WARNINGS Box" above.

Precautions: Neurotoxic and nephrotoxic antibiotics may be absorbed in significant quantities from body surfaces after local irrigation or application. This potential toxic effect of antibiotics administered in this fashion should be considered.

Increased nephrotoxicity has been reported following concomitant administration of aminoglycoside antibiotics and cephalosporins.

Neuromuscular blockade and respiratory paralysis have been reported in the cat receiving high doses (40 mg/kg) of gentamicin. These phenomena possibly occurring in man should be considered if aminoglycosides are administered by any route to patients receiving anesthetics, or to patients receiving neuromuscular-blocking agents, such as tubocurarine, succinylcholine, or decamethonium, or in patients receiving massive transfusions of citrate-anticoagulated blood. Administration of calcium salts may reverse the neuromuscular blockade.

Aminoglycosides should be used with caution in patients with neuromuscular disorders such as myasthenia gravis or parkinsonism. These drugs may aggravate muscle weakness due to their potential curare-like effects on the neuromuscular junction.

Elderly patients may have reduced renal function. This may not be evident in the results of routine screening tests, such as BUN or serum creatinine. A creatinine clearance determination may be more useful. Monitoring of renal function during treatment with gentamicin is particularly important in such patients.

Cross-allergenicity among aminoglycosides has been demonstrated.

Patients should be well hydrated during treatment.

The **in vitro** mixing of gentamicin and carbenicillin results in a rapid and significant inactivation of gentamicin. This interaction has not been demonstrated in patients with normal renal function who received both drugs by different routes of administration. A reduction in gentamicin serum half-life has been reported in patients with severe renal dysfunction receiving carbenicillin concomitantly with gentamicin.

Treatment with gentamicin may result in overgrowth of nonsusceptible organisms. If this occurs, appropriate therapy is indicated.

See "WARNINGS Box" regarding concurrent and/or sequential use of other neurotoxic and /or nephrotoxic antibiotics, concurrent use of potent diuretics, and for other essential information.

Usage in Pregnancy

Safety for use in pregnancy has not been established.

Adverse Reactions:

Nephrotoxicity

Adverse renal effects, demonstrated by the presence of casts, cells, or protein in the urine or by rising BUN, NPN, serum creatinine or oliguria, have been reported. They occur more often in patients with a history of renal impairment and in patients treated for longer periods or with larger dosage than recommended.

Note: The risk of toxic reactions is low in patients with normal renal function if they do not receive BRISTAGEN Injectable at higher doses or for longer periods of time than recommended.

Neurotoxicity

Serious adverse effects on both auditory and vestibular branches of the eighth nerve have been reported. These occur primarily in patients with renal impairment and in patients on high doses and/or prolonged therapy. Symptoms include dizziness, vertigo, tinnitus, roaring in the ears and hearing loss which may be irreversible. Hearing loss is likely to be manifested initially by diminution of high-tone acuity. Other factors which may increase the risk of toxicity include previous exposure to other ototoxic drugs, excessive dosage and dehydration.

Convulsions, muscle twitching, numbness and skin tingling have also been reported.

Other reported adverse reactions possibly related to gentamicin include vomiting, nausea, weight loss, decreased appetite, increased salivation, fever, headache, stomatitis, alopecia, urticaria, itching, rash, generalized burning, visual disturbances, laryngeal edema, purpura, joint pain, lethargy, anaphylactoid reactions, hypertension, hypotension, acute organic brain syndrome, pseudotumor cerebri, splenomegaly, pulmonary fibrosis, respiratory depression, transient hepatomegaly, and depression.

Laboratory abnormalities possibly related to gentamicin include potassium, magnesium, sodium, bilirubin, serum LDH, increased and decreased reticulocyte counts, decreased serum calcium, increased levels of serum transaminase (SGPT, SGOT), anemia, thrombocytopenia, transient agranulocytosis, leukopenia, granulocytosis and eosinophilia.

Although local tolerance of BRISTAGEN Injectable is generally excellent, there has been an occasional report of pain at the injection site. Subcutaneous atrophy or fat necrosis suggesting local irritation has been reported rarely.

Overdosage: Should overdose or toxic reactions occur, hemodialysis or peritoneal dialysis will aid in the removal of gentamicin from the blood.

Dosage and Administration: BRISTAGEN Injectable may be given intravenously or intramuscularly. Pretreatment body weight should be obtained for calculation of correct dosage. The dosage in obese patients should be based on an estimate of the lean body mass. It is desirable to limit the duration of treatment with aminoglycosides to short term.

Patients with Normal Renal Function

Adults: The recommended dosage of BRISTAGEN Injectable for patients with serious infections and normal renal function is 3 mg/kg/day, administered in 3 equal doses every 8 hours (Schedule I).

For patients with life-threatening infections, dosages up to 5 mg/kg/day may be administered in 3 or 4 equal doses. This dosage should be reduced to 3 mg/kg/day as soon as clinically indicated (Schedule I).

To determine the adequacy and safety of the dosage, it is desirable to measure both peak and trough serum concentrations of gentamicin. When such measurements are feasible, they should be carried out periodically during therapy to assure adequate but not excessive drug levels. For example, the peak concentration (at 30 to 60 minutes after intramuscular injection) is expected to be in the range of 4 to 6 mcg/ml. When monitoring peak concentrations after parenteral administration, dosage should be adjusted so that prolonged levels above 12 mcg/ml are avoided. When monitoring trough concentrations (just prior to the next dose), dosage should be adjusted so that levels above 2 mcg/ml are avoided. The adequacy of a serum level for a particular patient must take into consideration the susceptibility of the causative organism, the severity of the infection, and the status of the patient's host-defense mechanisms.

In patients with extensive burns, altered pharmacokinetics can result in reduced serum concentrations of aminoglycosides. In such patients treated with gentamicin, measurement of serum concentrations is recommended as a basis for ongoing dosage adjustment.

[See table above].

The usual duration of treatment for all patients is 7 to 10 days. A longer course of therapy may be necessary in difficult and complicated infections. In these cases, monitoring of

Continued on next page

Bristol—Cont.

renal, auditory, and vestibular functions is recommended since toxicity is more likely to occur when treatment is extended for more than 10 days. Dosage should be reduced if clinically indicated.

For Intravenous Administration

The intravenous administration of gentamicin may be particularly useful for patients with bacterial septicemia or those in shock. It may also be the preferred route for some patients with congestive heart failure, hematologic disorders, severe burns, or those with reduced muscle mass. For intermittent intravenous administration in adults, a single dose of BRISTAGEN Injectable may be diluted in 50 to 200 ml of Sterile Isotonic Saline Solution or in a sterile solution of 5% Dextrose in Water. The solution may be infused over a period of ½ to 2 hours.

For Intramuscular Administration

The recommended dosage for intramuscular and intravenous administration is identical.

BRISTAGEN Injectable should not be physically premixed with other drugs. Its administration is separate in accordance with the recommended route of administration and dosage schedule.

Patients with Impaired Renal Function

Dosage must be adjusted in patients with impaired renal function. Whenever possible serum concentrations of gentamicin should be monitored. One method of dosage adjustment is to increase the interval between doses. The serum creatinine concentration has a high correlation with the serum half-life of gentamicin. This test may provide guidance for adjustment of the interval between doses. The interval between doses (in hours) may be approximated by multiplying the serum creatinine level (mg/100 ml) by 8. For example, a patient weighing 70 kg with a serum creatinine level of 3 mg/100 ml could be given 70 mg (1 mg/kg) every 24 hours (3 × 8).

In patients having serious systemic infections and renal impairment, it may be desirable to administer the antibiotic more frequently but in reduced dosage. In these patients, serum concentrations of gentamicin should be measured so that adequate but not excessive levels result. Intermittent peak and trough concentration measured during therapy will provide optimal guidance for adjusting dosage. After the usual initial dose, a rough guide for determining reduced dosage at 8-hour intervals is to divide the normally recommended dose by the serum creatinine level (Schedule II). For example, after an initial dose of 70 mg (1 mg/kg), a patient weighing 70 kg with a serum creatinine level of 2 mg/100 ml could be given 35 mg every 8 hours (70÷2). It should be noted that the status of renal function may be changing over the course of the infectious process and that deteriorating renal function may require a greater reduction in dosage than that specified in the above guidelines for patients with stable renal impairment.

(See table below)

In adults with renal failure undergoing hemodialysis, the amount of gentamicin removed from the blood may vary depending upon several factors including the dialysis method used. An 8-hour hemodialysis may reduce serum concentrations by approximately 50%. The recommended dosage at the end of each dialysis period is 1 to 1.7 mg/kg depending upon the severity of infection.

The above dosage schedules are not intended as rigid recommendations but are provided as guides to dosage when measurement of gentamicin serum levels is not feasible.

A variety of methods are available to measure gentamicin concentrations in body fluids; these include microbiologic, enzymatic and radioimmunoassay techniques.

How Supplied: BRISTAGEN Injectable, 40 mg per ml, for parenteral administration.

NDC 0015-3300-20—2 ml vial, 40 mg/ml (80 mg)

NDC 0015-3300-18—2 ml disposable syringe, 40 mg/ml (80 mg) 1¼″ × 22 gauge staked needle

NDC 0015-3301-18—1.5 ml disposable syringe, 40 mg/ml (60 mg) 1¼″ × 22 gauge staked needle.

For information on package sizes available, refer to the current price schedule. BRISTAGEN Injectable is a clear, stable solution that requires no refrigeration.

DOSAGE SCHEDULE II
DOSAGE ADJUSTMENT FOR PATIENTS WITH IMPAIRED RENAL FUNCTION
(Dose at 8-Hour Intervals After the Usual Initial Dose)

Serum Creatinine (mg%)	Approximate Creatinine Clearance Rate (ml/min/1.73M2)	Percent of Usual Dose Shown in Schedule I
≤1.0	>100	100
1.1–1.3	70–100	80
1.4–1.6	55– 70	65
1.7–1.9	45– 55	55
2.0–2.2	40– 45	50
2.3–2.5	35– 40	40
2.6–3.0	30– 35	35
3.1–3.5	25– 30	30
3.6–4.0	20– 25	25
4.1–5.1	15– 20	20
5.2–6.6	10– 15	15
6.7–8.0	< 10	10

BRISTAMYCIN® ℞

(erythromycin stearate)
Tablets
Film Coated
250 mg.

This is the full text of the latest Official Package Circular dated September, 1980 [8367DIR-06].

Description: Bristamycin (erythromycin stearate) is produced by a strain of **Streptomyces erythraeus** and belongs to the macrolide group of antibiotics. It is basic and readily forms salts with acids. The base, the stearate salt, and the esters are poorly soluble in water and are suitable for oral administration.

Actions: The mode of action of erythromycin is inhibition of protein synthesis without affecting nucleic acid synthesis. Resistance to erythromycin of some strains of **Haemophilus influenzae** and staphylococci has been demonstrated. Culture and susceptibility testing should be done. If the Kirby-Bauer method of disc susceptibility is used, a 15-mcg erythromycin disc should give a zone diameter of at least 18 mm when tested against an erythromycin susceptible organism.

A single oral 250-mg dose of Bristamycin given to a fasting adult produces in 2 hours a serum level of from 0.4 mcg/ml to 1.3 mcg/ml. The peak serum level rises with repeated administration.

Orally administered Bristamycin is readily absorbed by most patients, especially on an empty stomach, but patient variation is observed.

After absorption, Bristamycin diffuses readily into most body fluids. In the absence of meningeal inflammation, low concentrations are normally achieved in the spinal fluid but passage of the drug across the blood-brain barrier increases in meningitis. In the presence of normal hepatic function, Bristamycin is concentrated in the liver and excreted in the bile; the effect of hepatic dysfunction on excretion of Bristamycin by the liver into the bile is not known. After oral administration, less than 5 percent of the activity of the administered dose can be recovered in the urine.

Bristamycin crosses the placental barrier but fetal plasma levels are low.

Indications and Usage: Although no controlled clinical efficacy trials have been conducted, oral erythromycin has been suggested by the American Heart Association and American Dental Association for use in a regimen for prophylaxis against bacterial endocarditis in patients hypersensitive to penicillin who have congenital heart disease or rheumatic or other acquired valvular heart disease when they undergo dental procedures and surgical procedures of the upper respiratory tract.[1] Erythromycin is not suitable prior to genitourinary or gastrointestinal tract surgery.

Note: When selecting antibiotics for the prevention of bacterial endocarditis the physician or dentist should read the full joint statement of the American Heart Association and the American Dental Association.[1]

Streptococcus pyogenes (Group A beta-hemolytic streptococci): Upper and lower respiratory tract, skin, and soft tissue infections of mild to moderate severity.

Injectable penicillin G benzathine is considered by the American Heart Association to be the drug of choice in the treatment and prevention of streptococcal pharyngitis and in long-term prophylaxis of rheumatic fever.

When oral medication is preferred for treatment of streptococcal pharyngitis, penicillin G, V, or erythromycin are alternate drugs of choice.

When oral medication is given, the importance of strict adherence by the patient to the prescribed dosage regimen must be stressed.

A therapeutic dose should be administered for at least 10 days.

Staphylococcus aureus:

Acute infections of skin and soft tissue of mild to moderate severity. Resistance may develop during treatment.

Streptococcus pneumoniae: (formerly **Diplococcus pneumoniae)**

Upper respiratory tract infections (e.g. otitis media, pharyngitis) and lower respiratory tract infections (e.g. pneumonia) of mild to moderate degree.

Mycoplasma pneumoniae (Eaton agent, PPLO):

In the treatment of primary atypical pneumonia, when due to this organism.

Hemophilus influenzae:

For upper respiratory tract infections of mild to moderate severity when used concomitantly with adequate doses of sulfonamides. Not all strains of this organism are susceptible at the erythromycin concentrations ordinarily achieved (see appropriate sulfonamide labeling for prescribing information).

Treponema pallidum:

Bristamycin is an alternate choice of treatment for primary syphilis in patients allergic to the penicillins. In treatment of primary syphilis, spinal fluid examinations should be

done before treatment and as part of follow up after therapy.
Corynebacterium diphtheriae and **Corynebacterium minutissimum:**
As an adjunct to antitoxin, to prevent establishment of carriers, and to eradicate the organism in carriers.
In the treatment of erythrasma.
Entamoeba histolytica:
In the treatment of intestinal amebiasis only. Extra-enteric amebiasis requires treatment with other agents.
Listeria monocytogenes:
Infections due to this organism.
Neisseria gonorrheae:
Erythromycin lactobionate for injection in conjunction with erythromycin stearate or base orally, as an alternative drug in treatment of acute pelvic inflammatory disease caused by **N. gonorrhoeae** in female patients with a history of sensitivity to penicillin. Before treatment of gonorrhea, patients who are suspected of also having syphilis should have a microscopic examination for **T. pallidum** (by immunofluorescence or darkfield) before receiving erythromycin, and monthly serologic tests for a minimum of 4 months.
Legionnaires' disease:
Although no controlled clinical efficacy studies have been conducted, **in vitro** and limited preliminary clinical data suggest that erythromycin may be effective in treating Legionnaires' disease.
Contraindications: Bristamycin is contraindicated in patients with known hypersensitivity to this antibiotic.
Warnings: Usage in Pregnancy: Safety for use in pregnancy has not been established.
Precautions: Erythromycin is principally excreted by the liver. Caution should be exercised in administering the antibiotic to patients with impaired hepatic function. There have been reports of hepatic dysfunction, with or without jaundice, occurring in patients receiving oral erythromycin products.
Recent data from studies of erythromycin reveal that its use in patients who are receiving high doses of theophylline may be associated with an increase of serum theophylline levels and potential theophylline toxicity. In case of theophylline toxicity and/or elevated serum theophylline levels, the dose of theophylline should be reduced while the patient is receiving concomitant erythromycin therapy.
Surgical procedures should be performed when indicated.
Adverse Reactions: The most frequent side effects of erythromycin preparations are gastrointestinal, such as abdominal cramping and discomfort, and are dose-related. Nausea, vomiting, and diarrhea occur infrequently with usual oral doses.
During prolonged or repeated therapy, there is a possibility of overgrowth of nonsusceptible bacteria or fungi. If such infections occur, the drug should be discontinued and appropriate therapy instituted.
Mild allergic reactions such as urticaria and other skin rashes have occurred. Serious allergic reactions, including anaphylaxis, have been reported.
Dosage and Administration: Optimum blood levels are obtained when doses are given on an empty stomach.
Adults: 250 mg every 6 hours is the usual dose. Dosage may be increased up to 4 or more Grams per day according to the severity of the infection.
Children: Age, weight, and severity of the infection are important factors in determining the proper dosage. 30 to 50 mg/Kg/day (15 to 25 mg/lb/day) in divided doses, is the usual dose. For more severe infections this dose may be doubled.
If dosage is desired on a twice-a-day schedule in either adults or children, one-half of the total daily dose may be given every 12 hours, 1 hour before meals.
In the treatment of streptococcal infections, a therapeutic dosage of erythromycin should be administered for at least 10 days. In continuous **prophylaxis** of streptococcal infections in persons with a history of rheumatic heart disease, the dose is 250 mg twice a day.
For treatment of primary syphilis: 30 to 40 Grams given in divided doses over a period of 10 to 15 days.
For dysenteric amebiasis: 250 mg 4 times daily for 10 to 14 days, for adults; 30 to 50 mg/Kg/day in divided doses for 10 to 14 days, for children.
For treatment of Legionnaires' disease: Although optimal doses have not been established, doses utilized in reported clinical data were those recommended above (1 to 4 Grams erythromycin stearate, daily in divided doses).
For prophylaxis against bacterial endocarditis[1] in patients with congenital heart disease or rheumatic or other acquired valvular heart disease when undergoing dental procedures or surgical procedures of the upper respiratory tract, give 1 Gram (20 mg/Kg for children) orally 1½ to 2 hours before the procedure, and then 500 mg (10 mg/Kg for children) orally every 6 hours for 8 doses.
How Supplied: Bristamycin (erythromycin stearate) Tablets, Film Coated. Erythromycin stearate equivalent to 250 mg erythromycin per tablet.
NDC 0015-8367—250 mg mg
For information on package sizes available, refer to the current price schedule.
Reference:
1. American Heart Association. 1977. Prevention of bacterial endocarditis. Circulation **56**:139A-143A.

[*Shown in Product Identification Section*]

BRISTOJECT®

The following products are available in prefilled, disposable Bristoject® syringes:

NDC-0015	PRODUCT
	ATROPINE SULFATE ℞
9410-87	0.5 mg in 5 ml, 22 ga × 1½″
9411-87	1 mg in 10 ml, 22 ga × 1½″
	CALCIUM CHLORIDE ℞
9422-78	1 gram in 10 ml (10%), 22 ga × 1½″
9422-75	1 gram in 10 ml (10%), 18 ga × 3½″
	DIPHENHYDRAMINE HCl
9085-87	50 mg in 5 ml, 22 ga × 1½″
	DEXTROSE ℞
9424-87	50% (25 grams in 50 ml), 18 ga × 1½″
	EPINEPHRINE ℞
9423-77	1 mg in 10 ml (1:10,000), 22 ga × 1½″
9423-87	1 mg in 10 ml (1:10,000), 18 ga × 3½″
	LIDOCAINE HCl ℞
9149-87	50 mg in 5 ml (1%), 22 ga × 1½″
9151-87	100 mg in 5 ml (2%), 22 ga × 1½″
9161-87	100 mg in 10 ml (1%), 22 ga × 1½″
9179-87	1 gram in 25 ml (4%), Inject-all™ Syringe
9140-90	2 grams in 50 ml (4%), Inject-all™ Syringe
9142-87	1 gram in 5 ml (20%) Inject-all™ Syringe Safety Vial™
9143-87	2 grams in 10 ml (20%) Inject-all™ Syringe Safety Vial™
	MAGNESIUM SULFATE ℞
9266-87	50% (5 grams in 10 ml), 20 ga × 2½″
	METARAMINOL BITARTRATE ℞
9440-90	100 mg in 10 ml (1%), Inject-all™ Syringe
	SODIUM BICARBONATE ℞
9121-87	44.6 mEq in 50 ml (7.5%), 18 ga × 1½″
9124-87	50 mEq in 50 ml (8.4%), 18 ga × 1½″
9125-87	(Ped) 10 mEq in 10 ml (8.4%), 22 ga × 1½″
9115-87	(Infant) 5 mEq in 10 ml (4.2%) 22 ga × 1½″

BUFFERIN® WITH CODEINE NO. 3 TABLETS ©III

This is the full text of the latest Official Package Circular dated June 1981 [5711DIR-01].
Description: Each tablet contains 325 mg aspirin (acetylsalicylic acid), buffered with Di-Alminate.® Bristol-Myer's brand of aluminum glycinate (¾ gr) 48.6 mg, and magnesium carbonate (1½ gr) 97.2 mg, and (½ gr) 30 mg codeine phosphate (warning: may be habit forming).
Clinical Pharmacology: Aspirin is a non-narcotic analgesic which alleviates pain both centrally and peripherally. It also has both antipyretic and anti-inflammatory effects. Di-Alminate helps prevent the stomach upset often caused by plain aspirin. Codeine is a narcotic analgesic and antitussive.
Indications: For the relief of mild to moderate pain.
Contraindications: Hypersensitivity to any of the components.
Warnings:
Drug dependence: Codeine can produce drug dependence of the morphine type and, therefore, has the potential for being abused. Psychic dependence, physical dependence and tolerance may develop upon repeated administration of this drug, and it should be prescribed and administered with the same degree of caution appropriate to the use of other oral, narcotic-containing medications. Like other narcotic-containing medications, the drug is subject to the Federal Controlled Substances Act.
Use in ambulatory patients: Codeine may impair the mental and/or physical abilities required for the performance of potentially hazardous tasks such as driving a car or operating machinery. The patient using this drug should be cautioned accordingly.
Interaction with other central nervous system (CNS) depressants: Patients receiving other narcotic analgesics, general anesthetics, phenothiazines, other tranquilizers, sedative-hypnotics, or other CNS depressants (including alcohol) concomitantly with this drug may exhibit an additive CNS depression. When such combined therapy is contemplated, the dose of one or both agents should be reduced.
Use in pregnancy: Safe use in pregnancy has not been established relative to possible adverse effects on fetal development. Therefore, this drug should not be used in pregnant women unless, in the judgment of the physician, the potential benefits outweigh the possible hazards.
Precautions:
Head injury and increased intracranial pressure: The respiratory depressant effects of narcotics and their capacity to elevate cerebrospinal fluid pressure may be markedly exaggerated in the presence of head injury, other intracranial lesions or a pre-existing increase in intracranial pressure. Furthermore, narcotics produce adverse reactions which may ob-

Continued on next page

Bristol—Cont.

scure the clinical course of patients with head injuries.

Acute abdominal conditions: The administration of this drug or other narcotics may obscure the diagnosis or clinical course in patients with acute abdominal conditions.

Allergic: Precautions should be taken in administering salicylates to persons with known allergies: patients with nasal polyps are more likely to be hypersensitive to aspirin.

Special risk patients: This drug should be given with caution to certain patients such as the elderly or debilitated, and those with severe impairment of hepatic or renal function, hypothyroidism, Addison's disease, prostatic hypertrophy or urethral stricture, peptic ulcer or coagulation disorders.

Adverse Reactions: The most frequently observed adverse reactions to codeine include light-headedness, dizziness, sedation, nausea and vomiting. These effects seem to be more prominent in ambulatory than in nonambulatory patients, and some of these adverse reactions may be alleviated if the patient lies down. Other adverse reactions include euphoria, dysphoria, constipation and pruritis.

The most frequently observed adverse reactions to aspirin include headache, vertigo, ringing in the ears, mental confusion, drowsiness, sweating, thirst, nausea and vomiting. Occasional patients experience gastric irritation and bleeding with aspirin. Some patients are unable to take salicylates without developing nausea and vomiting. The Di-Alminate buffering agent in this product helps prevent the stomach upset often caused by plain aspirin. Hypersensitivity may be manifested by a skin rash or even an anaphylactic reaction. With these exceptions, most of the side-effects occur after repeated administration of large doses.

Dosage and Administration: Dosage should be adjusted according to the severity of the pain and the response of the patient. It may occasionally be necessary to exceed the usual dosage recommended below in cases of more severe pain or in those patients who have become tolerant to the analgesic effect of narcotics.

BUFFERIN with Codeine #3 tablets are given orally. The usual adult dose in one or two tablets every four hours as required.

Drug Interactions: The CNS depressant effects of this drug may be additive with that of other CNS depressants. See "WARNINGS."

Overdosage: Signs and symptoms: Serious overdose of this drug is characterized by respiratory depression (a decrease in respiratory rate and/or tidal volume, Cheyne-Stokes respiration, cyanosis), extreme somnolence progressing to stupor or coma, skeletal muscle flaccidity, cold and clammy skin and sometimes bradycardia and hypotension. In severe overdose, apnea, circulatory collapse, cardiac arrest and death may occur.

Treatment: Treatment consists primarily of management of codeine intoxication and acid base imbalance due to salicylism. Primary attention should be given to the establishment of adequate respiratory exchange through provision of a patent airway and the institution of assisted or controlled ventilation. The narcotic antagonist naloxone is a specific antidote for respiratory depression which may result from overdose or unusual sensitivity to narcotics. Therefore, an appropriate dose of an antagonist should be administered, preferably by the intravenous route, simultaneously with efforts at respiratory resuscitation. Since the duration of action of this drug may exceed that of the antagonist, the patient should be kept under continued surveillance and repeated doses of the antagonist should be administered as needed to maintain adequate respiration.

An antagonist should not be administered in the absence of clinically-significant respiratory or cardiovascular depression. Oxygen, intravenous fluids, vasopressors and other supportive measures should be employed as indicated.

Gastric emptying may be useful in removing unabsorbed drug.

How Supplied: BUFFERIN® with Codeine No. 3—White, round tablets, available as follows:

NDC 0015-5711-60—bottles of 100 tablets

CeeNU® ℞
(lomustine [CCNU])

This is the full text of the latest Official Package Circular dated November 1981 [3030 DIM-09].

WARNING

CeeNU should be administered by individuals experienced in the use of antineoplastic therapy.

Since the major toxicity is delayed bone marrow suppression, blood counts should be monitored weekly for at least 6 weeks after a dose. (See "Adverse Reactions.") At the recommended dosage, courses of CeeNU should not be given more frequently than 6 weeks.

Caution should be used in administering CeeNU to patients with decreased circulating platelets, leukocytes, or erythrocytes. (See "Dosage and Administration.")

Liver function should be monitored periodically. (See "Adverse Reactions.")

Description: CeeNU 1-(2-chloroethyl)-3 cyclohexyl-1-nitrosoureais is one of a group of nitrosoureas. It is a yellow powder with the empirical formula of $C_9H_{16}ClN_3O_2$ and a molecular weight of 233.71. CeeNU is soluble in 10% ethanol (0.05 mg. per ml.) and in absolute alcohol (70 mg. per ml.). CeeNU is relatively insoluble in water (<0.05 mg. per ml.). It is relatively unionized at a physiological pH.

Action: It is generally agreed that CeeNU acts as an alkylating agent but, as with other nitrosoureas, it may also inhibit several key enzymatic processes.

CeeNU may be given orally. Following oral administration of radioactive CeeNU at doses ranging from 30 mg/M^2 to 100 mg/M^2, about half of the radioactivity given was excreted within 24 hours. The serum half-life of the drug and/or metabolites ranges from 16 hours to 2 days. Tissue levels are comparable to plasma levels at 15 minutes after intravenous administration.

Because of the high lipid solubility and the relative lack of ionization at a physiological pH, CeeNU crosses the blood brain barrier quite effectively. Levels of radioactivity in the CSF are 50% or greater than those measured concurrently in plasma.

Indications: CeeNU is indicated as palliative therapy to be employed in addition to other modalities, or in established combination therapy with other approved chemotherapeutic agents in the following:

Brain tumors—both primary and metastatic, in patients who have already received appropriate surgical and/or radiotherapeutic procedures;

Hodgkin's Disease—as a secondary therapy.

Contraindications: CeeNU should not be given to individuals who have demonstrated a previous hypersensitivity to it.

Warnings: Safe use in pregnancy has not been established. CeeNU is embryotoxic and teratogenic in rats and embryotoxic in rabbits at dose levels equivalent to the human dose. CeeNU also affects fertility in male rats at doses somewhat higher than the human dose. CeeNU is carcinogenic in rats and mice, producing a marked increase in tumor incidence in doses approximating those employed clinically.

Nitrosourea therapy does have carcinogenic potential. The occurrence of acute leukemia and bone marrow dysplasias have been reported in patients following nitrosourea therapy.

Precautions: CeeNU should be administered by individuals experienced in the use of antineoplastic therapy.

Since the major toxicity is delayed bone marrow suppression blood counts should be monitored weekly for at least 6 weeks after a dose. (See "Adverse Reactions".)

At the recommended dosage, courses of CeeNU should not be given more frequently than every 6 weeks.

Caution should be used in administering CeeNU to patients with decreased circulating platelets, leukocytes, or erythrocytes. (See "Dosage and Administration".)

Liver function should be monitored periodically. (See "Adverse Reactions".)

See "Warnings" section for information on carcinogenesis.

Adverse Reactions: Nausea and vomiting may occur 3 to 6 hours after an oral dose and usually last less than 24 hours. The frequency and duration may be reduced by the use of antiemetics prior to dosing and by the administration of CeeNU to fasting patients.

Thrombocytopenia occurs at about 4 weeks after a dose of CeeNU and persists for 1 to 2 weeks.

Leukopenia occurs at about 6 weeks after a dose of CeeNU and persists for 1 to 2 weeks. Approximately 65% of patients develop white blood counts below 5000 wbc/mm^3 and 36% develop white blood counts below 3000 wbc/mm^3.

CeeNU may produce cumulative myelosuppression, manifested by more depressed indices or longer duration of suppression after repeated doses.

Other toxicities: Stomatitis, alopecia, anemia, and hepatic toxicity, manifested by transient reversible elevation of liver function tests, have been reported infrequently.

Neurological reactions such as disorientation, lethargy, ataxia, and dysarthria have been noted in some patients receiving CeeNU. However, the relationship to medication in these patients is unclear.

Renal abnormalities consisting of decrease in kidney size, progressive azotemia and renal failure have been reported in patients who received large cumulative doses after prolonged therapy with CeeNU and related nitrosoureas. Kidney damage has also been reported occasionally in patients receiving lower total doses.

Dosage and Administration: The recommended dose of CeeNU in adults and children is 130 mg/M^2 as a single dose by mouth every 6 weeks.

In individuals with compromised bone marrow function, the dose should be reduced to 100 mg/M^2 every 6 weeks.

A repeat course of CeeNU should not be given until circulating blood elements have returned to acceptable levels (platelets above 100,000/mm^3; leukocytes above 4,000/mm^3). Blood counts should be monitored weekly and repeat courses should not be given before 6 weeks because the hematologic toxicity is delayed and cumulative.

Doses subsequent to the initial dose should be adjusted according to the hematologic response of the patient to the preceding dose. The following schedule is suggested as a guide to dosage adjustment:

Nadir After Prior Dose		Percentage of Prior Dose to be Given
Leukocytes	Platelets	
> 4000	> 100,000	100%
3000-3999	75,000-99,999	100%
2000-2999	25,000-74,999	70%
< 2000	< 25,000	50%

When CeeNU is used in combination with myelosuppressive drugs, the doses should be adjusted accordingly.

Stability: CeeNU capsules are stable for at least 2 years when stored at room temperature in well closed containers. Avoid excessive heat (over 40°C).

Supply: This dose pack of CeeNU (Lomustine [CCNU]) Capsules contains;

NDC 0015-3032-13—2—100 mg capsules (Green/Green)

NDC 0015-3031-13—2—40 mg capsules (Purple/Green)

NDC 0015-3030-13—2—10 mg capsules (Purple/Purple)

Directions to the Pharmacist

The capsules are to provide enough medication for a single dose. The total dose prescribed by the physician can be obtained (to within 10 mg) by determining the appropriate combination of the enclosed capsule strengths.

The appropriate number of capsules of each size should be placed in a single vial to which the patient information label (gummed label provided) explaining the differences in the appearance of the capsules is affixed.

Example: A patient dose of 240 mg can be obtained by combining two 100 mg capsules and one 40 mg capsule. The remaining capsules (if any) should be discarded.

A patient information sticker, to be placed on dispensing container, is enclosed.

Also Available: Individual bottles of 20 capsules each.

NDC 0015-3032-20—20—100 mg. capsules (Green/Green)

NDC 0015-3031-20—20—40 mg. capsules (Purple/Green)

NDC 0015-3030-20—20—10 mg. capsules (Purple/Purple)

[*Shown in Product Identification Section*]

CEFADYL® ℞

(sterile cephapirin sodium)

This is the full text of the latest Official Package Circular dated November 1981. [7628DIR-23].

Description: Cefadyl (sterile cephapirin sodium) is a cephalosporin antibiotic intended for intramuscular or intravenous administration only. Each 500 mg contains 1.18 milliequivalents of sodium.

Cefadyl is the sodium salt of 7-α-(4-pyridylthio)-acetamido-cephalosporanic acid and has the following structural formula.

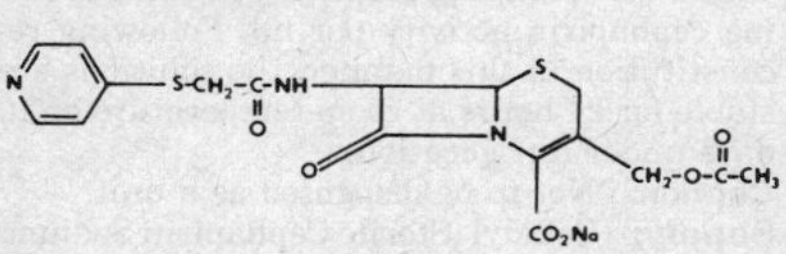

Clinical Pharmacology:

Human Pharmacology

Following intramuscular administration of single 500-mg and 1-gram doses to normal volunteers, average peak serum levels of 9.0 and 16.4 mcg/ml, respectively, were attained at 30 minutes, declining to 0.7 and 1.0 mcg/ml, respectively, at 4 hours and 0.2 and 0.3 mcg/ml, respectively, at 6 hours.

Cefadyl and its metabolites were excreted primarily by the kidneys. Antibiotic activity in the urine was equivalent to 35% of a 500-mg dose 6 hours after I.M. injection, and to 65% of a 500-mg dose 12 hours after injection. Following an I.M. dose of 500 mg, peak urine levels averaged 900 mcg/ml within the first 6 hours.

Following rapid intravenous administration of single 500-mg, 1-gram, and 2-gram doses, peak serum levels of 35, 67, and 129 mcg/ml, respectively, were attained at 5 minutes, declining to 6.7, 14.0, and 31.7 mcg/ml, respectively, at 30 minutes and 0.27, 0.61, and 1.11 mcg/ml, respectively, at 3 hours.

Seventy percent of the administered dose was recovered in the urine within 6 hours.

Repetitive intravenous administration of 1-gram doses over 6-hour periods produced serum levels between 4.5 and 5.5 mcg/ml.

At therapeutic drug levels, normal human serum binds Cefadyl to the extent of 44 to 50%.

The average serum half-life of Cefadyl in patients with normal renal function is approximately 36 minutes.

The major metabolite of cephapirin is desacetyl cephapirin which has been shown to contribute to antibacterial activity.

Controlled studies in normal adult volunteers revealed that Cefadyl was well tolerated intramuscularly. In controlled studies of volunteers and of patients receiving I.V. Cefadyl, the incidence of venous irritation was low.

Microbiology

In vitro tests demonstrate that the action of cephalosporins results from inhibition of cell-wall synthesis. Cefadyl is active against the following organisms **in vitro:**

- Beta-hemolytic streptococci and other streptococci.
- (Many strains of enterococci, e.g. **S. faecalis**, are relatively resistant.)
- **Staphylococcus aureus** (penicillinase and nonpenicillinase-producing).
- **Staphylococcus epidermidis** (methicillin-susceptible strains).
- **Streptococcus pneumoniae** (formerly **Diplococcus pneumoniae)**
- **Haemophilus influenzae**
- Klebsiella species
- **Proteus mirabilis**
- **Escherichia coli**

Most strains of Enterobacter and indole-positive Proteus **(P. vulgaris, P. morganii, P. rettgeri)** are resistant to Cefadyl. Methicillin-resistant staphylococci, Serratia, Pseudomonas, Mima, and Herellea species are almost uniformly resistant to Cefadyl.

Disc Susceptibility Tests. — Quantitative methods that require measurement of zone diameters give the most precise estimates of antibiotic susceptibility. One such procedure* has been recommended for use with discs for testing susceptibility to cephalosporin class antibiotics. Interpretations correlate diameters of the disc test with MIC values for Cefadyl. With this procedure, a report from the laboratory of "susceptible" indicates that the infecting organism is likely to respond to therapy. A report of "resistant" indicates that the infecting organism is not likely to respond to therapy. A report of "intermediate susceptibility" suggests that the organism would be susceptible if high dosage is used, or if the infection is confined to tissues and fluid (e.g., urine), in which high antibiotic levels are attained.

Indications: Cefadyl is indicated in the treatment of infections caused by susceptible strains of the designated microorganisms in the diseases listed below. Culture and susceptibility studies should be performed. Therapy may be instituted before results of susceptibility studies are obtained.

Respiratory tract infections caused by **S. pneumoniae** (formerly **D. pneumoniae**); **Staphylococcus aureus** (penicillinase and nonpenicillinase-producing), Klebsiella species, **H. influenzae** and Group A beta-hemolytic streptococci.

Skin and skin structure infections caused by **Staphylococcus aureus** (penicillinase and nonpenicillinase-producing), **Staphylococcus epidermidis** (methicillin-susceptible strains), **E. coli, P. mirabilis,** Klebsiella species, and Group A beta-hemolytic streptococci.

Urinary tract infections caused by **Staphylococcus aureus** (penicillinase and nonpenicillinase-producing), **E. coli, P. mirabilis,** and Klebsiella species.

Septicemia caused by **Staphylococcus aureus** (penicillinase and nonpenicillinase-producing), **S. viridans, E. coli,** Klebsiella species and Group A beta-hemolytic streptococci.

Endocarditis caused by **Streptococcus viridans** and **Staphylococcus aureus** (penicillinase and nonpenicillinase-producing).

Osteomyelitis caused by **Staphylococcus aureus** (penicillinase and nonpenicillinase-producing), Klebsiella species, **P. mirabilis,** and Group A beta-hemolytic streptococci.

Perioperative Prophylaxis —The prophylactic administration of Cefadyl preoperatively and postoperatively may reduce the incidence of certain postoperative infections in patients undergoing surgical procedures which are classified as contaminated or potentially contaminated, e.g., vaginal hysterectomy.

The perioperative use of Cefadyl may also be effective in surgical patients in whom infection at the operative site would present a serious risk, e.g., during open-heart surgery and prosthetic arthroplasty.

The prophylactic administration of Cefadyl should be discontinued within a 24 hour period after the surgical procedure in surgery where the occurrence of infection may be particularly devastating, e.g., open-heart surgery and prosthetic arthroplasty. The prophylactic administration of Cefadyl may be continued for 3 to 5 days following completion of surgery. If there are signs of infection, specimens for culture should be obtained for the identification of the causative organism so that appropriate therapy may be instituted (See Dosage and Administration.)

Note: If the susceptibility tests show that the causative organism is resistant to Cefadyl, other appropriate therapy should be instituted.

Contraindications: Cefadyl is contraindicated in persons who have shown hypersensitivity to cephalosporin antibiotics.

Warnings: IN PENICILLIN-ALLERGIC PATIENTS, CEPHALOSPORINS SHOULD BE USED WITH GREAT CAUTION. THERE IS CLINICAL AND LABORATORY EVIDENCE OF PARTIAL CROSS-ALLERGENICITY OF THE PENICILLINS AND THE CEPHALOSPORINS, AND THERE ARE INSTANCES OF PATIENTS WHO HAVE HAD REACTIONS TO BOTH DRUGS (INCLUDING FATAL ANAPHYLAXIS AFTER PARENTERAL USE).

Any patient who has demonstrated some form of allergy, particularly to drugs, should receive antibiotics cautiously and then only when absolutely necessary. No exceptions should be made with regard to Cefadyl.

SERIOUS ANAPHYLACTOID REACTIONS REQUIRE IMMEDIATE EMERGENCY TREATMENT WITH EPINEPHRINE, OXYGEN, INTRAVENOUS STEROIDS, AND AIRWAY MANAGEMENT, INCLUDING INTUBATION, SHOULD ALSO BE ADMINISTERED AS INDICATED.

Precautions: Usage in Pregnancy—Pregnancy Category B. Reproduction studies have been performed in rats and mice and have revealed no evidence of impaired fertility or harm to the fetus due to Cefadyl. There are however no well controlled studies in pregnant women. Because animal studies are not always predictive of human response, this drug should be used during pregnancy only if clearly indicated.

Nursing Mothers—Cefadyl may be present in human milk in small amounts. Caution should be exercised when Cefadyl is administered to a nursing woman.

The renal status of the patients should be determined prior to and during Cefadyl therapy, since in patients with impaired renal function, a reduced dose may be appropriate (see Dosage, Adults). When Cefadyl was given to patients with marked reduction in renal function and to

Continued on next page

Bristol—Cont.

renal transplant patients, no adverse effects were reported.

Prolonged use of Cefadyl may result in the overgrowth of nonsusceptible organisms. Careful observation of the patient is essential. If superinfection occurs during therapy, appropriate measures should be taken.

With high urine concentrations of cephapirin, false-positive glucose reactions may occur if Clinitest, Benedict's Solution, or Fehling's Solution are used. Therefore, it is recommended that glucose tests based on enzymatic glucose oxidase reactions (such as Clinistix or Tes-Tape) be used.

Increased nephrotoxicity has been reported following concomitant administration of cephalosporins and aminoglycoside antibiotics.

Adverse Reactions:

Hypersensitivity—Cephalosporins were reported to produce the following reactions: maculopapular rash, urticaria, reactions resembling serum sickness, and anaphylaxis. Eosinophilia and drug fever have been observed to be associated with other allergic reactions. These reactions are most likely to occur in patients with a history of allergy, particularly to penicillin.

Blood—During large scale clinical trials, rare instances of neutropenia, leukopenia, and anemia were reported. Some individuals, particularly those with azotemia, have developed positive direct Coombs' test during therapy with other cephalosporins.

Liver—Elevations in SGPT or SGOT, alkaline phosphatase, and bilirubin have been reported.

Kidney—Rises in BUN have been observed; their frequency increases in patients over 50 years old.

Dosage and Administration:

Adults—The usual dose is 500 mg to 1 gram every 4 to 6 hours intramuscularly or intravenously. The lower dose of 500 mg is adequate for certain infections, such as skin and skin structure and most urinary tract infections. However, the higher dose is recommended for more serious infections.

Very serious or life-threatening infections may require doses up to 12 grams daily. The intravenous route is preferable when high doses are indicated.

Depending upon the causative organism and the severity of infection, patients with reduced renal function (moderately severe oliguria or serum creatinine above 5.0 mg/100 ml) may be treated adequately with a lower dose 7.5 to 15 mg/Kg of cephapirin every 12 hours. Patients with severely reduced renal function and who are to be dialyzed should receive the same dose just prior to dialysis and every 12 hours thereafter.

Perioperative Prophylactic Use—To prevent postoperative infection in contaminated or potentially contaminated surgery. Recommended doses are:

a. 1 to 2 grams IM or IV administered ½ hour to 1 hour prior to the start of surgery.
b. 1 to 2 grams during surgery (administration modified depending on the duration of the operative procedure).
c. 1 to 2 grams IV or IM every 6 hours for 24 hours postoperatively.

It is important (1) the preoperative dose be given just prior to the start of surgery (½ to 1 hour) so that adequate antibiotic levels are present in the serum and tissues at the time of initial surgical incision, and (2) Cefadyl be administered, if necessary, at appropriate intervals during surgery to provide sufficient levels of the antibiotic at the anticipated moments of greatest exposure to infective organisms.

In surgery where the occurrence of infection may be particularly devastating, e.g., open-heart surgery and prosthetic arthroplasty, the prophylactic administration of Cefadyl may be continued for 3 to 5 days following completion of surgery.

Children—The dosage is in accordance with age, weight, and severity of infection. The recommended total daily dose is 40 to 80 mg/Kg (20 to 40 mg/lb) administered in four equally divided doses.

The drug has not been extensively studied in infants, therefore, in the treatment of children under the age of three months the relative benefit/risk should be considered.

Therapy in beta-hemolytic streptococcal infections should continue for at least 10 days.

Where indicated surgical procedures should be performed in conjunction with antibiotic therapy.

Intramuscular Injection

The 500-mg and 1-gram vials should be reconstituted with 1 or 2 ml of Sterile Water for Injection, U.S.P., or Bacteriostatic Water for Injection, U.S.P., respectively. Each 1.2 ml contains 500 mg of cephapirin. All injections should be deep in the muscle mass.

Intravenous Injection

The intravenous route may be preferable for patients with bacteremia, septicemia, or other severe or life-threatening infections who may be poor risks because of lowered resistance resulting from such debilitating conditions as malnutrition, trauma, surgery, diabetes, heart failure, or malignancy, particularly if shock is present or impending. If patient has impaired renal function, a reduced dose may be indicated (see Dosage, Adults). In conditions such as septicemia, 6 to 8 grams per day may be given intravenously for several days at the beginning of therapy; then, depending on the clinical response and laboratory findings, the dosage may gradually be reduced.

When the infection has been refractory to previous forms of treatment and multiple sites have been involved, daily doses up to 12 grams have been used.

Intermittent Intravenous Injection

The contents of the 500-mg, 1-gram or 2-gram vial should be diluted with 10 ml or more of the specified diluent and administered slowly over a 3- to 5-minute period or may be given with intravenous infusions.

Intermittent Intravenous Infusion with Y-Tube

Intermittent intravenous infusion with a Y-type administration set can also be accomplished while bulk intravenous solutions are being infused. However, during infusion of the solution containing Cefadyl it is desirable to discontinue the other solution. When this technique is employed, careful attention should be paid to the volume of the solution containing Cefadyl so that the calculated dose will be infused. When a Y-tube hookup is used, the contents of the 4-gram vial of cephapirin should be diluted by addition of 40 ml of Bacteriostatic Water for Injection, U.S.P., Dextrose Injection, U.S.P., or Sodium Chloride Injection, U.S.P.

STABILITY

Utility Time For Cefadyl In Various Diluents At Concentrations Ranging From 20 to 400 mg/ml

Diluent	Approximate Concentration (mg/ml)	Utility Time 25°C	Utility Time 4°C
Water for Injection	50 to 400	12 hours	10 days
Bacteriostatic Water for Injection with Benzyl Alcohol or Parabens	250 to 400	48 hours	10 days
Normal Saline	20 to 100	24 hours	10 days
5% Dextrose in Water	20 to 100	24 hours	10 days

All of the above solutions can be frozen immediately after reconstitution and stored at −15°C for 60 days before use. After thawing at room temperature (25°C), all of the solutions are stable for at least 12 hours at room temperature or 10 days under refrigeration (4°C).

The pH of the resultant solution ranges from 6.5 to 8.5. During these storage conditions, no precipitation occurs. A change in solution color during this storage time does not affect the potency.

Compatibility with the Infusion Solution

Cefadyl is stable and compatible for 24 hours at room temperature at concentrations between 2 mg/ml and 30 mg/ml in the following solutions.

- Sodium Chloride Injection, U.S.P.
- 5% W/V Dextrose in Water, U.S.P.
- Sodium Lactate Injection, U.S.P.
- 5% Dextrose in Normal Saline, U.S.P.
- 10% Invert Sugar in Normal Saline
- 10% Invert Sugar in Water
- 5% Dextrose + 0.2% Sodium Chloride Injection, U.S.P.
- Lactated Ringer's Injection, U.S.P.
- Lactated Ringer's with 5% Dextrose
- 5% Dextrose + 0.45% Sodium Chloride Injection, U.S.P.
- Ringer's Injection, U.S.P.
- 10% Dextrose Injection, U.S.P.
- Sterile Water for Injection, U.S.P.
- 20% Dextrose Injection, U.S.P.
- 5% Sodium Chloride in Water
- 5% Dextrose in Ringer's Injection
- Normosol® R
- Normosol® R in 5% Dextrose Injection
- Ionosol® D-CM
- Ionosol® G in 10% Dextrose Injection

In addition, Cefadyl, at a concentration of 4 mg/ml, is stable and compatible for 10 days under refrigeration (4°C) or 14 days in the frozen state (−15°C) followed by 24 hours at room temperature (25°C) in all of the intravenous solutions listed above.

"Piggyback" I.V. Package:

This glass vial contains the labeled quantity of Cefadyl and is intended for intravenous administration. The diluent and volume are specified on the label.

Hospital Bulk Package:

This glass vial contains 20 grams Cefadyl and is designed for use in the pharmacy in preparing I.V. additives. Add 67 ml of Sodium Chloride Injection, U.S.P., or Dextrose Injection, U.S.P. The resulting solution will contain 250 mg cephapirin activity per ml. Following reconstitution in this manner, the solutions are stable for 24 hours at room temperature or 10 days under refrigeration.

Caution: Not to be dispensed as a unit.

Supply: Cefadyl (Sterile Cephapirin Sodium) for I.M. or I.V. Injection. Cephapirin sodium equivalent to 500 mg, 1 gram, 2 grams, 4 grams, or 20 grams cephapirin.

NDC 0015-7627-28—500-mg vial
NDC 0015-7628-28—1-gram vial
NDC 0015-7629-30—2-gram vial
NDC 0015-7628-22—1-gram "piggyback" vial
NDC 0015-7629-28—2-gram "piggyback" vial
NDC 0015-7630-20—4-gram "piggyback" vial
NDC 0015-7613-20—20-gram Hospital Bulk Package

For information on package sizes available, refer to the current price schedule.

---

*Bauer, A. W., Kirby, W. M. M., Sherris, J. C. and Turck, M.: Antibiotic Testing by a Standardized Single Disc Method, Am. J. Clin. Pathol., 45:493, 1966; Standardized Disc Susceptibility Test, FEDERAL REGISTER 37:20527–29, 1972.

DYNAPEN® ℞
(dicloxacillin sodium)
Capsules-125 mg., 250 mg. and 500 mg.
Dicloxacillin sodium
For Oral Suspension
62.5 mg./5 ml.

This is the full text of the latest Official Package Circular dated February 1978 [7856 DIR-09].

Description: DYNAPEN (dicloxacillin sodium monohydrate) is an antibacterial agent of the isoxazolyl penicillin series. It is the monohydrate sodium salt of 3-(2, 6-dichlorophenyl)-5-methyl-4-isoxazolyl penicillin. The drug resists destruction by the enzyme penicillinase (beta-lactamase). It has been demonstrated to be especially efficacious in the treatment of penicillinase-producing staphylococcal infections and effective in the treatment of other commonly encountered Gram-positive coccal infections.

Pharmacology: DYNAPEN (dicloxacillin sodium) is resistant to destruction by acid and is exceptionally well absorbed from the gastrointestinal tract. Oral administration of dicloxacillin gives blood levels considerably in excess of those attained with equivalent doses of any other presently available oral penicillin. The levels are comparable to those achieved with intramuscular administration of similar doses of penicillin G. Studies[1] with an oral dose of 125 mg. gave average serum levels at 60 minutes of 4.74 mcg./ml. At four hours, average levels were 0.62 mcg./ml. The 125 mg. dose gave peak blood levels 5 times higher than those of 250 mg. of penicillin G and 2 to 4 times higher than those of 250 mg. of Penicillin V Potassium. Serum levels after oral administration are directly proportional to dosage at unit doses of 125, 250, 500, and 1000 mg.[1,2,3] as measured at the two-hour level.

Actions (Microbiology): DYNAPEN (dicloxacillin sodium) is active against most Gram-positive cocci including beta-hemolytic streptococci, pneumococci, and susceptible staphylococci. Because of its resistance to the enzyme penicillinase, it is active against penicillinase-producing staphylococci.

The average Minimal Inhibitory Concentrations (M.I.C.'s) of DYNAPEN (dicloxacillin sodium) for these organisms are as follows:

	Average M.I.C. (mcg./ml.)
Group A beta-hemolytic streptococcus	0.05
Diplococcus pneumoniae	0.10
Staphylococcus (nonpenicillinase-producing)	0.20
Staphylococcus (penicillinase-producing)	0.30

Disc Susceptibility Tests

Quantitative methods that require measurement of zone diameters give the most precise estimates of antibiotic susceptibility. One such procedure* has been recommended for use with discs for testing susceptibility to methicillin class antibiotics. Interpretations correlate diameters on the disc test with MIC values for methicillin. With this procedure, a report from the laboratory of "susceptible" indicates that the infecting organism is likely to respond to therapy. A report of "resistant" indicates that the infecting organism is not likely to respond to therapy. A report of "intermediate susceptibility" suggests that the organism would be susceptible if high dosage is used, or if the infection is confined to tissues and fluids (e.g., urine), in which high antibiotic levels are attained.

Indications: Although the principal indication for dicloxacillin sodium is in the treatment of infections due to penicillinase-producing staphylococci, it may be used to initiate therapy in such patients in whom a staphylococcal infection is suspected. (See Important Note below.)

Bacteriologic studies to determine the causative organisms and their susceptibility to dicloxacillin sodium should be performed.

In serious, life-threatening infections, oral preparations of the penicillinase-resistant penicillins should not be relied on for initial therapy.

Important Note: When it is judged necessary that treatment be initiated before definitive culture and susceptibility results are known, the choice of dicloxacillin sodium should take into consideration the fact that it has been shown to be effective only in the treatment of infections caused by pneumococci, Group A beta-hemolytic streptococci, and penicillin G-resistant and penicillin G-susceptible staphylococci. If the bacteriology report later indicates the infection is due to an organism other than a penicillin G-resistant staphylococcus susceptible to dicloxacillin sodium, the physician is advised to continue therapy with a drug other than dicloxacillin sodium or any other penicillinase-resistant semi-synthetic penicillin.

Recent studies have reported that the percentage of staphylococcal isolates resistant to penicillin G outside the hospital is increasing, approximating the high percentage of resistant staphylococcal isolates found in the hospital. For this reason, it is recommended that a penicillinase-resistant penicillin be used as initial therapy for any suspected staphylococcal infection until culture and susceptibility results are known.

Dicloxacillin sodium is a compound that acts through a mechanism similar to that of methicillin against penicillin G-resistant staphylococci. Strains of staphylococci resistant to methicillin have existed in nature and it is known that the number of these strains reported has been increasing. Such strains of staphylococci have been capable of producing serious disease, in some instances resulting in fatality. Because of this, there is concern that widespread use of the penicillinase-resistant penicillins may result in the appearance of an increasing number of staphylococcal strains which are resistant to these penicillins.

Methicillin-resistant strains are almost always resistant to all other penicillinase-resistant penicillins (cross resistance with cephalosporin derivatives also occurs frequently). Resistance to any penicillinase-resistant penicillin should be interpreted as evidence of clinical resistance to all, in spite of the fact that minor variations in **in vitro** susceptibility may be encountered when more than one penicillinase-resistant penicillin is tested against the same strain of staphylococcus.

Contraindications: A history of allergic reactions to penicillins or cephalosporins should be considered a contraindication.

Precautions: As with any penicillin, a careful inquiry about sensitivity or allergic reactions to penicillins, cephalosporins, or other allergens should be made before the drug is prescribed. Allergic reactions are more likely to occur in hypersensitive individuals. Should an allergic reaction occur during therapy, the drug should be discontinued and the patient treated with the usual agents (epinephrine, corticosteroids, antihistamines).

As with other agents capable of altering flora, the possibility of superinfection with mycotic organisms or other pathogens exists during the periods of use of this drug. Should superinfection occur, appropriate treatment should be initiated and discontinuation of dicloxacillin therapy should be considered.

As with any potent drug, periodic assessment of organ system function, including renal, hepatic, and hematopoietic systems, is strongly recommended.

Experience in the neonatal period is limited. Therefore, a dose for the newborn is not recommended at this time.

Safety for use in pregnancy has not been established.

Adverse Reactions: Gastrointestinal disturbances such as nausea, vomiting, epigastric discomfort, flatulence, and loose stools have been noted in some patients receiving DYNAPEN (dicloxacillin sodium). Pruritus, urticaria, skin rashes, and allergic symptoms have been occasionally encountered, as with all penicillins. Mildly elevated SGOT levels (less than 100 units) have been reported in a few patients for whom pretherapeutic determinations were not made. Minor changes in the results of cephalin flocculation tests have been noted without other evidence of hepatic dysfunction. Eosinophilia, with or without overt allergic manifestations, has been noted in some patients during therapy.

Dosage: For mild-to-moderate upper respiratory and localized skin and soft tissue infections due to susceptible organisms:

Adults and children weighing 40 Kg. (88 lbs.) or more: 125 mg. q.6h.

Children weighing less than 40 Kg. (88 lbs.): 12.5 mg./Kg./day in equally-divided doses q.6h.

For more severe infections such as those of the lower respiratory tract or disseminated infections:

Adults and children weighing 40 Kg. (88 lbs.) or more: 250 mg. q.6h. or higher.

Children weighing less than 40 Kg. (88 lbs.): 25 mg./Kg./day or higher in equally-divided doses q.6h.

Experience in the neonatal period is limited. Therefore, a dose for the newborn is not recommended at this time.

Studies indicate that this material is best absorbed when taken on an empty stomach, preferably one to two hours before meals.

N.B. INFECTIONS CAUSED BY GROUP A BETA-HEMOLYTIC STREPTOCOCCI SHOULD BE TREATED FOR AT LEAST 10 DAYS TO HELP PREVENT THE OCCURRENCE OF ACUTE RHEUMATIC FEVER OR ACUTE GLOMERULONEPHRITIS.

Directions for Dispensing Oral Suspension: Prepare these formulations at the time of dispensing. For ease in preparation, add water to the bottle in two portions and shake well after each addition. Add the total amount of water as directed on the labeling of the package being dispensed. The reconstituted formulation is stable for 14 days under refrigeration.

References:

1. Data on file at Bristol Laboratories.
2. Bennett, J.V., Gravenkemper, C.F., Brodie, J.L., and Kirby, W.M.M., "Dicloxacillin, a New Antibiotic: Clinical Studies and Laboratory Comparisons with Oxacillin and Cloxacillin." Antimicrobial Agents and Chemotherapy, 1964, pp. 257-262.
3. Naumann, P. and Kempf, E., "Dicloxacillin, a New Acid and Penicillinase Stable Oral Penicillin." Arzneimittel-Forschung, **15**, pp. 139-145, 1965.

Supply: DYNAPEN (dicloxacillin sodium) for Oral Suspension, 62.5 mg per 5 ml.

NDC 0015-7856—80 ml, 100 ml and 200 ml bottles

DYNAPEN (dicloxacillin sodium) Capsules. Each capsule contains dicloxacillin sodium equivalent to 125, 250, or 500 mg dicloxacillin.

NDC 0015-7892-125 mg
NDC 0015-7893-250 mg
NDC 0015-7658-500 mg

For information on package sizes available, refer to the current price schedule.

[*Shown in Product Identification Section*]

*Bauer, A. W., Kirby, W. M. M., Sherris J. C. and Turck, M.: Antibiotic Testing by a Standardized Single Disc Method, Am. J. Clin. Pathol., 45:493, 1966; Standardized Disc Susceptibility Test, FEDERAL REGISTER 37:20527–29, 1972.

Continued on next page

Bristol—Cont.

KANTREX® CAPSULES ℞
(kanamycin sulfate)
Not for Systemic Use

This is the full text of the latest Official Package Circular dated January 1978 [3506 DIRO-08]

Description: Kanamycin sulfate is a water soluble aminoglycoside antibiotic derived from **Streptomyces kanamyceticus.** It is supplied in oral formulation for topical effect within the gastrointestinal tract, because it is absorbed only very slightly when administered orally, and is excreted unchanged in the feces.

Actions: Kanamycin is poorly absorbed from the normal gastrointestinal tract. The small absorbed fraction is rapidly excreted with normal kidney function. The unabsorbed portion of the drug is eliminated unchanged in the feces.

Most intestinal bacteria are eliminated rapidly following oral administration of kanamycin, with bacterial suppression persisting for 48 to 72 hours.

Indications:

Suppression of Intestinal Bacteria—Kanamycin is indicated when supression of the normal bacterial flora of the bowel is desirable for short-term adjunctive therapy.

Hepatic Coma—Prolonged administration has been shown to be effective adjunctive therapy in **Hepatic Coma** by reduction of the ammonia-forming bacteria in the intestinal tract. The subsequent reduction in blood ammonia has resulted in neurologic improvement.

Contraindications: This drug is contraindicated in the presence of intestinal obstruction and in individuals with a history of hypersensitivity to the drug.

Warnings: Although negligible amounts of kanamycin are absorbed through intact intestinal mucosa (approximately 1 percent), the possibility of increased absorption from ulcerated or denuded areas should be considered. If renal insufficiency develops during treatment, the dosage should be reduced or the antibiotic discontinued. Urine and blood examinations and audiometric tests should be given prior to and during extended therapy in individuals with hepatic and/or renal disease.

Usage in Pregnancy: Safety for use in pregnancy has not been established.

Precautions: Caution should be taken in concurrent use of other ototoxic and/or nephrotoxic antimicrobial drugs while kanamycin is administered orally. These include streptomycin, neomycin, polymyxin B, colistin, viomycin, gentamicin, and cephaloridine.

The concurrent use of potent diuretics (e.g. ethacrynic acid, furosemide, and mannitol, particularly when the diuretics are given intravenously) should be avoided. They may cause cumulative adverse effects of the kanamycin on the kidney and auditory nerve.

Prolonged use of oral kanamycin may result in overgrowth of nonsusceptible organisms, particularly fungi. If this occurs, appropriate therapy should be instituted.

Adverse Reactions: The most common adverse reactions to oral kanamycin are nausea, vomiting, and diarrhea. The "Malabsorption Syndrome" characterized by increased fecal fat, decreased serum carotene, and fall in xylose absorption has been reported with prolonged therapy. Nephrotoxicity and ototoxicity have been reported following prolonged and high dosage therapy in hepatic coma.

Dosage and Administration For Oral Use Only:

Suppression of Intestinal Bacteria:

1. As an adjunct in therapy of Hepatic Coma for extended therapy: 8 to 12 Gm. per day in divided doses.
2. As an adjunct to mechanical cleansing of the large bowel in short term therapy: 1.0 Gm. (2 capsules) every hour for 4 hours followed by 1.0 Gm. (2 capsules) every 6 hours for 36 to 72 hours.

Duration of therapy within this range depends on the condition of the patient, the type and amount of concurrent mechanical cleansing (catharsis and enemas), and the customary medical routine.

Supply: KANTREX (kanamycin sulfate) Capsules. Kanamycin sulfate equivalent to 500 mg kanamycin per capsule.

NDC 0015-3506—500mg

For information on package sizes available, refer to the current price schedule.

[*Shown in Product Identification Section*]

KANTREX® INJECTION ℞
(kanamycin sulfate injection)
500 mg. per 2 ml.; 1.0 Gm. per 3 ml.

KANTREX® PEDIATRIC INJECTION ℞
(kanamycin sulfate injection)
75 mg. per 2 ml.

This is the full text of the latest Official Package Circular dated November 1978 [3502DIM-09].

WARNING

Patients treated with aminoglycosides by any route should be under close clinical observation because of the potential toxicity associated with their use. As with other aminoglycosides, the major toxic effects of kanamycin sulfate are its action on the auditory and vestibular branches of the eighth nerve and the renal tubules. Loss of high frequency perception usually occurs before clinical hearing loss and can be detected by audiometric testing. There may not be clinical symptoms to warn of developing cochlear damage. Vertigo may occur and may be evidence of vestibular injury. Renal impairment may be characterized by decreased creatinine clearance, the presence of cells or casts, oliguria, proteinuria, decreased urine specific gravity, or evidence of increasing nitrogen retention (increasing BUN, NPN or serum creatinine).

In patients with impaired kidney function, the risks of severe ototoxic and nephrotoxic reactions are sharply increased. In such cases, either the total daily dosage should be reduced, or the interval between doses lengthened, or both. Assessment of renal function and audiograms should be obtained before treatment if possible and monitored frequently during the course of therapy (see "Precautions"). If there is evidence of progressive renal dysfunction (increasing NPN, BUN, serum creatinine or oliguria) during therapy, audiometric tests are advised and discontinuation of the drug should be considered.

Elderly patients, patients with preexisting tinnitus or vertigo or known subclinical deafness, those having received prior ototoxic drugs, and patients receiving a total dose of more than 15 g of kanamycin sulfate should be carefully observed for signs of eighth nerve damage. Loss of hearing may occur in such patients even with normal renal function.

Neuromuscular blockade with respiratory paralysis may occur when kanamycin sulfate is administered intraperitoneally concomitantly with anesthesia and muscle-relaxing drugs. Although there have been isolated reports of respiratory depression following intraperitoneal instillation of kanamycin, there is no conclusive proof that this side effect can be produced with recommended doses of the drug.

The concurrent and or sequential systemic or topical use of kanamycin and other potentially ototoxic, nephrotoxic, and/or neurotoxic drugs, particularly streptomycin, polymyxin B, colistin, neomycin, gentamicin, cephaloradine, paromomycin, tobramycin, amikacin, vancomycin and viomycin should be avoided because the toxicity may be additive.

Kanamycin sulfate should not be given concurrently with potent diuretics (ethacrynic acid, furosemide, meralluride sodium, sodium mercaptomerin, or mannitol). Some diuretics themselves cause ototoxicity, and intravenously administered diuretics may enhance aminoglycoside toxicity by altering antibiotic concentrations in serum and tissue.

Description: Kanamycin sulfate is an aminoglycoside antibiotic produced by **Streptomyces kanamyceticus.** It is $C_{18}H_{36}N_4O_{11} \cdot 2H_2SO_4$ · D - Streptomine, 0 - 3-amino-3-deoxy-α-D- glucopyranosyl— (1→6) - 0 - [6 - amino - 6-deoxy-α-D-glucopyranosyl-(1→4)]- 2-deoxy, sulfate 1:2 (salt). It consists of two amino sugars glycosidically linked to deoxystreptamine.

Kanamycin sulfate injection, sterile solution for parenteral administration, contains respectively: kanamycin sulfate 75 mg, 500 mg, and 1 g; sodium bisulfite, an antioxidant, 0.099%, 0.66%, and 0.45%, and sodium citrate, 0.33%, 2.2%, and 2.2% with pH of each dosage form adjusted to 4.5 with sulfuric acid.

Action:

Clinical Pharmacology

The drug is rapidly absorbed after intramuscular injection and peak serum levels are generally reached within approximately one hour. Doses of 7.5 mg/Kg give mean peak levels of 22 mcg/ml. At 8 hours following a 7.5 mg/Kg dose, mean serum levels are 3.2 mcg/ml. Intravenous administration of kanamycin over a period of one hour resulted in serum concentrations similar to those obtained by intramuscular administration.

Kanamycin diffuses rapidly into most body fluids including synovial and peritoneal fluids and bile. Significant levels of the drug appear in cord blood and amniotic fluid following intramuscular administration to pregnant patients. Spinal fluid concentrations in normal infants are approximately 10 to 20 percent of serum levels and may reach 50 percent when the meninges are inflamed.

Studies in normal adult patients have shown only trace levels of kanamycin in spinal fluid. No data are available on adults with meningitis.

The drug is excreted almost entirely by glomerular filtration and is not reabsorbed by the renal tubules. Hence, high concentrations are attained in the nephron, and the urine may contain levels 10 to 20 times higher than those in serum. Renal excretion is extremely rapid. In patients with normal renal function, approximately one-half of the administered dose is cleared within 4 hours and excretion is complete within 24 to 48 hours. Patients with impaired renal function or with diminished glomerular filtration pressure excrete kanamycin more slowly. Such patients may build up excessively high blood levels which greatly increase the risk of ototoxic reactions.

Microbiology

Kanamycin sulfate is a bactericidal antibiotic which acts by inhibiting the synthesis of protein in susceptible microorganisms. Kanamycin sulfate is active **in vitro** against many strains of **Staphylococcus aureus** (including penicillinase and nonpenicillinase-producing strains). **Staphylococcus epidermidis, N. gonorrhoeae, H. influenzae, E. coli, Enterobacter aerogenes,** Shigella, Salmonella, **K. pneumoniae, Serratia marcescens, Acinetobacter,** and many strains of both indole-positive and indole-negative **Proteus** that are frequently resistant to other antibiotics. Bacterial resistance to kanamycin develops slowly in most susceptible organisms. **In vitro** studies have demonstrated that an aminoglycoside combined with an antibiotic which interferes with cell wall synthesis (i.e., penicillins or cephalosporins) acts synergistically against some strains of Gram-negative organisms and enterococci (**Streptococcus faecalis**).

Susceptibility testing: The infecting organism should be cultured and its susceptibility demonstrated as a guide to therapy. If the Kirby-Bauer method of disc susceptibility is used, a 30-mcg kanamycin disc should give a zone of inhibition of 17 mm or more when tested against a kanamycin-susceptible bacterial strain. A zone of 16 mm or less indicates that the infecting organism is likely to be resistant. In certain conditions, it may be desirable to do additional susceptibility testing by the tube or Agar dilution method. Kanamycin reference standard is available for this purpose.

Indications and Usage: Kanamycin is indicated in the treatment of serious infections caused by susceptible strains of microorganisms. Bacteriological studies to identify the causative organisms and to determine their susceptibility to kanamycin should be performed. Therapy may be instituted prior to obtaining the results of susceptibility testing. Kanamycin may be considered as initial therapy in the treatment of infections where one or more of the following are the known or suspected pathogens: **E. coli, Proteus** species (both indole-positive and indole-negative), **Enterobacter aerogenes, Klebsiella pneumoniae, Serratia marcescens, Acinetobacter.** The decision to continue therapy with the drug should be based on results of the susceptibility tests, the response of the infection to therapy, and the important additional concepts contained in the "Warning" box above.

In serious infections when the causative organisms are unknown, Kantrex may be administered as initial therapy in conjunction with a penicillin- or cephalosporin-type drug before obtaining results of susceptibility testing. If anerobic organisms are suspected, consideration should be given to using other suitable antimicrobial therapy in conjunction with kanamycin.

Although kanamycin is not the drug of choice for staphylococcal infections, it may be indicated under certain conditions for the treatment of known or suspected staphylococcal disease. These situations include the initial therapy of severe infections where the organism is thought to be either a Gram-negative bacterium or a staphylococcus, infections due to susceptible strains of staphylococci in patients allergic to other antibiotics, and mixed staphylococcal/Gram-negative infections.

Contraindications: A history of hypersensitivity or toxic reaction to one aminoglycoside may also contraindicate the use of any other aminoglycoside, because of the known cross-sensitivity and cumulative effects of drugs in this category.

THIS DRUG IS NOT INDICATED IN LONG-TERM THERAPY (e.g. Tuberculosis) BECAUSE OF THE TOXIC HAZARD ASSOCIATED WITH EXTENDED ADMINISTRATION.

Warning: See "Warning" box above.

Precautions:

Ototoxicity: In patients with renal dysfunction an audiogram should be obtained before treatment and repeated frequently during therapy. Therapy should be stopped if tinnitus or subjective hearing loss develops, or if follow-up audiograms show loss of high frequency perception.

It should be emphasized that since renal function may alter appreciably during therapy, the serum creatinine should be checked daily or more frequently. Changes in the concentration would, of course, necessitate changes in the dosage frequency.

Nephrotoxicity: Because of the high concentration of kanamycin sulfate in the urinary excretory system, patients should be well-hydrated to prevent chemical irritation of the renal tubules. Kidney function should be assessed by the usual methods, e.g., urinalysis, BUN, serum creatinine, prior to starting therapy and periodically during the course of treatment. If signs of renal irritation appear, such as casts, white or red cells, and albumin, hydration should be increased and a reduction in dosage may be desirable (see "Dosage and Administration"). These signs usually disappear when treatment is completed. However, if azotemia or a progressive decrease in urine output occurs, treatment should be stopped.

The possibility of neuromuscular blockade with respiratory paralysis should be considered if aminoglycosides are administered by any route in patients receiving anesthetics, in patients receiving neuromuscular-blocking agents such as tubocurarine, succinylcholine, decamethonium or in patients receiving massive transfusions of citrate-anticoagulated blood. In all cases, patients should be observed carefully for signs of respiratory depression. If blockade occurs, calcium salts or neostigmine may reverse this phenomenon.

NOTE: The risk of toxic reactions is low in well-hydrated patients with normal kidney function, who receive a total dose of 15 g of kanamycin or less.

Because of the possibility of additive effects of other potentially ototoxic, neurotoxic, and/or nephrotoxic drugs, the concurrent or sequential administration of these drugs with kanamycin sulfate should be avoided (see "Warning" box).

Increased nephrotoxicity has been reported following concomitant parenteral administration of aminoglycoside antibiotics and cephalothin.

Since kanamycin sulfate and methicillin inactivate each other in vitro, they should not be physically mixed together in the same solution intended for parenteral administration. However, this inactivation has not been demonstrated in patients who receive both drugs by different routes of administration. (See "Dosage and Administration.")

Elderly patients may have reduced renal function which may not be evident in the results of routine screening tests, such as BUN or serum creatinine. A creatinine clearance determination may be more helpful. Monitoring of renal function during treatment is particularly important in such patients.

Aminoglycosides should be used with caution in patients with myasthenia gravis since these drugs may aggravate muscle weakness because of their curare-like effect on the neuromuscular function.

Kanamycin sulfate should not be given concurrently with potent diuretics (see "Warning" box).

Neurotoxic and nephrotoxic antibiotics may be absorbed from body surfaces after local irrigation or application. The potential toxic effect of aminoglycosides administered in this fashion should be considered (see "Warning" box).

Cross-allergenicity among aminoglycosides has been demonstrated.

As with other antibiotics, kanamycin sulfate administration may result in overgrowth of nonsusceptible organisms, including fungi. If superinfection occurs, appropriate therapy should be instituted.

Pregnancy:

Reproduction studies have been performed in rats and rabbits and have revealed no evidence of impaired fertility or teratogenic effects. Dosages of 200 mg/Kg/day in pregnant rats and pregnant guinea pigs led to hearing impairment in the offspring. There are no well-controlled studies in pregnant women but clinical experience does not include any positive evidence of adverse effects on the fetus. Although there is no clearly defined risk, such experience cannot exclude the possibility of infrequent or subtle damage to the fetus. Kantrex should be used in pregnant women only when clearly needed.

Adverse Reactions:

Nephrotoxicity—Albuminuria, presence of red and white cells, and granular casts; azotemia and oliguria have been reported.

Ototoxicity—Tinnitus, vertigo, and partial reversible to irreversible hearing loss have been reported, usually associated with higher than recommended dosage. Rapid development of hearing loss has been reported in patients with poor kidney function treated concurrently with kanamycin and one of the rapid-acting diuretic agents given intravenously. These have included ethacrynic acid, furosemide, and mannitol.

Other—Some local irritation or pain may follow intramuscular injection. Other adverse reactions of the drug reported on rare occasions are skin rash, drug fever, headache, and paresthesia.

Overdosage: In the event of overdosage or toxic reaction, hemodialysis or peritoneal dialysis will aid in the removal of kanamycin from the blood. In the newborn infant, exchange transfusions may also be considered.

Dosage and Administration:

Intramuscular Route: Inject deeply into the upper outer quadrant of the gluteal muscle. The recommended dose for adults or children is 15 mg/Kg/day in two equally divided dosages administered at equally divided intervals, i.e. 7.5 mg/Kg q12h. If continuously high blood levels are desired, the daily dose of 15 mg/Kg may be given in equally divided doses every 6 or 8 hours. Treatment of patients in the heavier weight classes, i.e. >100 Kg, should not exceed 1.5 g/day.

In patients with impaired renal function, it is desirable to follow therapy by appropriate serum assays. If this is not feasible, a suggested method is to reduce the frequency of administration in patients with renal dysfunction. The interval between doses may be calculated with the following formula:

Serum creatinine (mg/100 ml) $\times$ 9 = Dosage Interval (in hours): e.g., if the serum creatinine is 2 mg, the recommended dose (7.5 mg/Kg) should be administered every 18 hours. Changes in creatinine concentration during therapy would, of course, necessitate changes in the dosage frequency.

The usual duration of treatment is 7 to 10 days. The total daily dose by all routes of administration should not exceed 1.5 g/day.

At the recommended dosage level, uncomplicated infections due to kanamycin-susceptible organisms should respond to therapy in 24 to 48 hours. If definite clinical response does not occur within 3 to 5 days, therapy should be stopped and the antibiotic susceptibility pattern of the invading organism should be rechecked. Failure of the infection to respond may be due to resistance of the organism or to the presence of septic foci requiring surgical drainage.

Intravenous Administration: The dose should not exceed 15 mg/Kg per day and must be administered slowly. The solution for intravenous use is prepared by adding the contents of a 500-mg vial to 100 to 200 ml of sterile diluent such as Normal Saline or 5% Dextrose in Water, or the contents of a 1 g vial to 200 to 400 ml of sterile diluent. The appropriate dose is administered over a 30- to 60-minute period. The total daily dose should be divided into two or three equally divided doses.

In pediatric patients the amount of diluent used should be sufficient to infuse the kanamycin sulfate over a 30- to 60-minute period.

Kanamycin sulfate injection should not be physically mixed with other antibacterial agents but each should be administered separately in accordance with its recommended route of administration and dosage schedule.

Intraperitoneal Use: (following exploration for established peritonitis or after peritoneal

Continued on next page

Bristol—Cont.

contamination due to fecal spill during surgery.)

Adults: 500 mg diluted in 20 ml sterile distilled water may be instilled through a polyethylene catheter sutured into the wound at closure. If possible, instillation should be postponed until the patient has fully recovered from the effects of anesthesia and muscle-relaxing drugs (see "Warning" box).

Aerosol Treatment: 250 mg two to four times a day. Withdraw 250 mg (1 ml) from 500-mg vial and dilute it with 3 ml Physiological Saline and nebulize.

Other Routes of Administration: Kantrex Injection in concentrations of 0.25 percent (2.5 mg/ml) has been used as an irrigating solution in abscess cavities, pleural space, peritoneal and ventricular cavities. Possible absorption of Kantrex by such routes must be taken into account and dosage adjustments should be arranged so that a maximum total dose of 1.5 g/day by all routes of administration is not exceeded.

PEDIATRIC DOSAGE GUIDE FOR KANTREX PEDIATRIC INJECTION, 75 mg/2 ml— AMOUNT PER 24 HOURS TO BE GIVEN IN DIVIDED DOSES

Weight in Pounds	Weight in Kilograms	Daily Dosage in Milligrams	Daily Dosage in Milliliters
2.2	1.00	15.0	0.4
2.8	1.25	18.8	0.5
3.3	1.50	22.5	0.6
3.9	1.75	26.2	0.7
4.4	2.00	30.0	0.8
5.0	2.25	33.8	0.9
5.5	2.50	37.5	1.0
6.0	2.75	41.2	1.1
6.6	3.00	45.0	1.2
7.7	3.50	52.5	1.4
8.8	4.00	60.0	1.6
9.9	4.50	67.5	1.8
11.0	5.00	75.0	2.0

Stability: Occasionally, some vials may darken during the shelf-life of the product, but this does not indicate a loss of potency.

How Supplied: KANTREX INJECTION (kanamycin sulfate injection)

NDC 0015-3502-20—500 mg per 2 ml

NDC 0015-3502-24—Disposable Syringe (500 mg per 2 ml)

NDC 0015-3503-20—1 g per 3 ml

KANTREX PEDIATRIC INJECTION (kanamycin sulfate injection)

NDC 0015-3512-20—75 mg per 2 ml (activity assayed as kanamycin base)

KETAJECT® ℞
(ketamine hydrochloride injection)

This is the full text of the latest Official Package Circular dated June 1980 [8340 DIMO-08].

SPECIAL NOTE

EMERGENCE REACTIONS HAVE OCCURRED IN APPROXIMATELY 12 PERCENT OF PATIENTS.

THE PSYCHOLOGICAL MANIFESTATIONS VARY IN SEVERITY BETWEEN PLEASANT DREAM-LIKE STATES, VIVID IMAGERY, HALLUCINATIONS, AND EMERGENCE DELIRIUM. IN SOME CASES THESE STATES HAVE BEEN ACCOMPANIED BY CONFUSION, EXCITEMENT, AND IRRATIONAL BEHAVIOR WHICH A FEW PATIENTS RECALL AS AN UNPLEASANT EXPERIENCE. THE DURATION ORDINARILY LASTS NO MORE THAN A FEW HOURS; IN A FEW CASES, HOWEVER, RECURRENCES HAVE TAKEN PLACE UP TO 24 HOURS POSTOPERATIVELY. NO RESIDUAL PSYCHOLOGICAL EFFECTS ARE KNOWN TO HAVE RESULTED FROM USE OF KETAJECT.

THE INCIDENCE OF THESE EMERGENCE PHENOMENA IS LEAST IN THE YOUNG (15 YEARS OF AGE OR LESS) AND ELDERLY (OVER 65 YEARS OF AGE) PATIENT. ALSO, THEY ARE LESS FREQUENT WHEN THE DRUG IS GIVEN INTRAMUSCULARLY.

THESE REACTIONS MAY BE REDUCED IF VERBAL, TACTILE, AND VISUAL STIMULATION OF THE PATIENT IS MINIMIZED DURING THE RECOVERY PERIOD. THIS DOES NOT PRECLUDE THE MONITORING OF VITAL SIGNS. IN ADDITION, THE USE OF A SMALL HYPNOTIC-DOSE OF A SHORT-ACTING OR ULTRASHORT-ACTING BARBITURATE MAY BE REQUIRED TO TERMINATE A SEVERE EMERGENCE REACTION. THE INCIDENCE OF EMERGENCE REACTIONS IS REDUCED AS EXPERIENCE WITH THE DRUG IS GAINED.

WHEN KETAJECT IS USED ON AN OUTPATIENT BASIS, THE PATIENT SHOULD NOT BE RELEASED UNTIL RECOVERY FROM ANESTHESIA IS COMPLETE AND THEN SHOULD BE ACCOMPANIED BY A RESPONSIBLE ADULT.

Description: Ketaject is a nonbarbiturate anesthetic chemically designated *dl* 2-(o-chlorophenyl)-2-(methylamino) cyclohexanone hydrochloride. It is formulated as a slightly acid (pH 3.5 to 5.5) solution for intravenous or intramuscular injection in concentrations containing the equivalent of either 10, 50, or 100 mg. ketamine base per milliliter and contains not more than 0.1 mg./ml. Phemerol® (benzethonium chloride) as a preservative. The 10 mg./ml. solution has been made isotonic with sodium chloride.

Action: Ketaject is a rapid-acting general anesthetic producing an anesthetic state characterized by profound analgesia, normal pharyngeal-laryngeal reflexes, normal or slightly enhanced skeletal muscle tone, cardiovascular and respiratory stimulation; and occasionally a transient and minimal respiratory depression.

A patent airway is maintained partly by virtue of unimpaired pharyngeal and laryngeal reflexes. (See Warnings and Precautions.)

The anesthetic state produced by Ketaject has been termed "dissociative anesthesia" in that it appears to selectively interrupt association pathways of the brain before producing somesthetic sensory blockade. It may selectively depress the thalamoneocortical system before significantly obtunding the more ancient cerebral centers and pathways (reticular-activating and limbic systems).

Elevation of blood pressure begins shortly after injection, reaches a maximum within a few minutes, and usually returns to preanesthetic values within 15 minutes after injection. The median peak rise has ranged from 20 to 25% of preanesthetic values.

Ketamine has a wide margin of safety; several instances of unintentional administration of overdoses of Ketaject (up to ten times that usually required) have been followed by prolonged but complete recovery.

Indications:

Ketaject is recommended:

1. as the sole anesthetic agent for diagnostic and surgical procedures that do not require skeletal muscle relaxation. Ketaject is best suited for short procedures but it can be used, with additional doses, for longer procedures.
2. for the induction of anesthesia prior to the administration of other general anesthetic agents.
3. to supplement low-potency agents, such as nitrous oxide.

Specific areas of application are described in the section Clinical Studies.

Contraindications: Ketamine hydrochloride is contraindicated in those in whom a significant elevation of blood pressure would constitute a serious hazard and in those who have shown hypersensitivity to the drug.

Warnings:

1. Ketaject should be used by or under the direction of physicians experienced in administering general anesthetics and in maintenance of an airway and in the control of respiration.
2. Cardiac function should be continually monitored during the procedure in patients found to have hypertension or cardiac decompensation.
3. Barbiturates and Ketaject, being chemically incompatible because of precipitate formation, should not be injected from the same syringe.
4. Prolonged recovery time may occur if barbiturates and/or narcotics are used concurrently with Ketaject.
5. Postoperative confusional states may occur during the recovery period.
6. Respiratory depression may occur with overdosage or too rapid a rate of administration of Ketaject, in which case supportive ventilation should be employed. Mechanical support of respiration is preferred to administration of analeptics.

Usage in Pregnancy: Since the safe use in pregnancy, including obstetrics (either vaginal or abdominal delivery), has not been established, such use is not recommended (see Animal Reproduction).

Precautions:

1. Because pharyngeal and laryngeal reflexes are usually active, Ketaject should not be used alone in surgery or diagnostic procedures of the pharynx, larynx, or bronchial tree. Mechanical stimulation of the pharynx should be avoided, whenever possible, if Ketaject is used alone. Muscle relaxants, with proper attention to respiration, may be required in both of these instances.
2. Resuscitative equipment should be ready for use.
3. **The incidence of emergence reactions may be reduced** if verbal and tactile stimulation of the patient is minimized during the recovery period. This does not preclude the monitoring of vital signs (see Special Note).
4. The intravenous dose should be administered over a period of 60 seconds. More rapid administration may result in respiratory depression or apnea and enhanced pressor response.
5. In surgical procedures involving visceral pain pathways, Ketaject should be supplemented with an agent which obtunds visceral pain.
6. Use with caution in the chronic alcoholic and the acutely alcohol-intoxicated patients.
7. An increase in cerebrospinal fluid pressure has been reported following administration of ketamine hydrochloride. Use with extreme caution in patients with preanesthetic elevated cerebrospinal fluid pressure.

Adverse Reactions:

Cardiovascular: Blood pressure and pulse rate are frequently elevated following administration of Ketaject. However, hypotension and bradycardia have been observed. Arrhythmia has also occurred.

Respiration: Although respiration is frequently stimulated, severe depression of respiration or apnea may occur following rapid intravenous administration of high doses of Ketaject. Laryngospasms and other forms of airway obstruction have occurred during Ketaject anesthesia.

Eye: Diplopia and nystagmus have been noted following Ketaject administration. It also may cause a slight elevation in intraocular pressure measurement.

Psychological: (See Special Note.)
Neurological: In some patients, enhanced skeletal muscle tone may be manifested by tonic and clonic movements sometimes resembling seizures (see Dosage and Administration).
Gastrointestinal: Anorexia, nausea, and vomiting have been observed; however, this is not usually severe and allows the great majority of patients to take liquids by mouth shortly after regaining consciousness (see Dosage and Administration).
General: Local pain and exanthema at the injection site have infrequently been reported. Transient erythema and/or morbilliform rash have also been reported.

Dosage and Administration:

Preoperative Preparations:

1. While vomiting has been reported following Ketaject administration, airway protection is usually afforded because of active laryngeal-pharyngeal reflexes. However, since these reflexes may also be diminished by supplementary anesthetics or muscle relaxants, the possibility of aspiration must be considered. Ketaject is recommended for use in the patient whose stomach is not empty when, in the judgment of the practitioner, the benefits of the drug outweigh the possible risks.
2. Atropine, scopolamine, or other drying agents should be given at an appropriate interval prior to induction.

Dosage: As with other general anesthetic agents, the individual response to Ketaject is somewhat varied depending on the dose, route of administration, and age of patients, so that dosage recommendation cannot be absolutely fixed. The drug should be titrated against the patient's requirements.
Onset and Duration: Because of rapid induction following the initial intravenous injection, the patient should be in a supported position during administration.
The onset of action of Ketaject is rapid; an intravenous dose of 2 mg./Kg. (1 mg./lb.) of body weight usually produces surgical anesthesia within 30 seconds after injection, with the anesthetic effect usually lasting five to ten minutes. If a longer effect is desired, additional increments can be administered intravenously or intramuscularly to maintain anesthesia without producing significant cumulative effects.
Intramuscular doses, from experience primarily in children, in a range of 9 to 13 mg./Kg. (4 to 6 mg./lb.) usually produce surgical anesthesia within 3 to 4 minutes following injection, with the anesthetic effect usually lasting 12 to 25 minutes.

Induction:

Intravenous Route: The initial dose of Ketaject administered intravenously may range from 1 mg./Kg. to 4.5 mg./Kg. (0.5 to 2 mg./lb.). The average amount required to produce five to ten minutes of surgical anesthesia has been 2 mg./Kg. (1 mg./lb.).
NOTE: The 100 mg./ml. concentration of Ketaject should not be injected intravenously without proper dilution. It is recommended the drug be diluted with an equal volume of either Sterile Water for Injection, U.S.P., Normal Saline, or 5% Dextrose in Water.
Rate of Administration: It is recommended that Ketaject be administered slowly (over a period of 60 seconds). More rapid administration may result in respiratory depression and enhanced pressor response.
Intramuscular Route: The initial dose of Ketaject administered intramuscularly may range from 6.5 to 13 mg./Kg. (3 to 6 mg./lb.). A dose of 10 mg./Kg. (5 mg./lb.) will usually produce 12 to 25 minutes of surgical anesthesia.
Maintenance of Anesthesia: Increments of one-half to the full induction dose may be repeated as needed for maintenance of anesthesia. However, it should be noted that purposeless and tonic-clonic movements of extremities may occur during the course of anesthesia. These movements do not imply a light plane and are not indicative of the need for additional doses of the anesthetic.
It should be recognized that the larger the total dose of Ketaject administered the longer will be the time to complete recovery.
Supplementary Agents: Ketaject is clinically compatible with the commonly used general and local anesthetic agents when an adequate respiratory exchange is maintained.

Animal Pharmacology and Toxicology:

Toxicity: The acute toxicity of Ketaject has been studied in several species. In mature mice and rats, the intraperitoneal LD_{50} values are approximately 100 times the average human intravenous dose and approximately 20 times the average human intramuscular dose. A slightly higher acute toxicity observed in neonatal rats was not sufficiently elevated to suggest an increased hazard when used in children. Daily intravenous injections in rats of five times the average human intravenous dose and intramuscular injections in dogs at four times the average human intramuscular dose demonstrated excellent tolerance for as long as six weeks. Similarly, twice weekly anesthetic sessions of one, three, or six hours duration in monkeys over a four-to-six week period were well tolerated.
Interaction With Other Drugs Commonly Used for Preanesthetic Medication: Large doses (three or more times the equivalent effective human dose) of morphine, meperidine, and atropine increased the depth and prolonged the duration of anesthesia produced by a standard anesthetizing dose of Ketaject in Rhesus monkeys. The prolonged duration was not of sufficient magnitude to contraindicate the use of these drugs for preanesthetic medication in human clinical trials.
Blood Pressure: Blood pressure responses to Ketaject vary with the laboratory species and experimental conditions. Blood pressure is increased in normotensive and renal hypertensive rats with and without adrenalectomy and under pentobarbital anesthesia.
Intravenous Ketaject produces a fall in arterial blood pressure in the Rhesus monkey and a rise in arterial blood pressure in the dog. In this respect the dog mimics the cardiovascular effect observed in man. The pressor response to Ketaject injected into intact, unanesthetized dogs is accompanied by a tachycardia, rise in cardiac output, and a fall in total peripheral resistance. It causes a fall in perfusion pressure following a large dose injected into an artificially perfused vascular bed (dog hindquarters), and it has little or no potentiating effect upon vasoconstriction responses of epinephrine or norepinephrine. The pressor response to Ketaject is reduced or blocked by chlorpromazine (central depressant and peripheral α-adrenergic blockade), by β-adrenergic blockade, and by ganglionic blockade. The tachycardia and increase in myocardial contractile force seen in intact animals does not appear in isolated hearts (Langendorff) at a concentration of 0.1 mg. of Ketaject nor in Starling dog heart-lung preparations at a Ketaject concentration of 50 mg./Kg. of HLP. These observations support the hypothesis that the hypertension produced by Ketaject is due to selective activation of central cardiac stimulating mechanisms leading to an increase in cardiac output. The dog myocardium is not sensitized to epinephrine and Ketaject appears to have a weak antiarrhythmic activity.
Metabolic Disposition: Ketaject is rapidly absorbed following parenteral administration. Animal experiments indicated that Ketaject was rapidly distributed in body tissues, with relatively high concentrations appearing in body fat, liver, lung, and brain; lower concentrations were found in the heart, skeletal muscle, and blood plasma. Placental transfer of the drug was found to occur in pregnant dogs and monkeys. No significant degree of binding to serum albumin was found with Ketaject.
Balance studies in rats, dogs, and monkeys resulted in the recovery of 85 to 95% of the dose in the urine, mainly in the form of degradation products. Small amounts of drug were also excreted in the bile and feces. Balance studies with tritium-labeled Ketaject in human subjects (1 mg./lb. given intravenously) resulted in the mean recovery of 91% of the dose in the urine and 3% in the feces. Peak plasma levels averaged about 0.75 μg./ml., and CSF levels were about 0.2 μg./ml., one hour after dosing.
Ketaject undergoes N-demethylation and hydroxylation of the cyclohexanone ring, with the formation of water-soluble conjugates which are excreted in the urine. Further oxidation also occurs with the formation of a cyclohexenone derivative. The unconjugated N-demethylated metabolite was found to be less than one sixth as potent as Ketaject. The unconjugated demethyl cyclohexenone derivative was found to be less than one tenth as potent as Ketaject. Repeated doses of Ketaject administered to animals did not produce any detectable increase in microsomal enzyme activity.
Reproduction: Male and female rats, when given five times the average human intravenous dose of Ketaject for three consecutive days about one week before mating had a reproductive performance equivalent to that of saline-injected controls. When given to pregnant rats and rabbits intramuscularly at twice the average human intramuscular dose during the respective periods of organogenesis, the litter characteristics were equivalent to those of saline-injected controls. A small group of rabbits was given a single large dose (six times the average human dose) of Ketaject on Day 6 of pregnancy to simulate the effect of an excessive clinical dose around the period of nidation. The outcome of pregnancy was equivalent in control and treated groups.
To determine the effect of Ketaject on the perinatal and postnatal period, pregnant rats were given twice the average human intramuscular dose during Days 18 to 21 of pregnancy. Litter characteristics at birth and through the weaning period were equivalent to those of the control animals. There was a slight increase in incidence of delayed parturition by one day in treated dams of this group. Three groups each of mated beagle bitches were given 2.5 times the average human intramuscular dose twice weekly for the three weeks of the first, second, and third trimesters of pregnancy, respectively, without the development of adverse effects in the pups.
Clinical Studies: Ketaject was initially studied in over 12,000 operative and diagnostic procedures, involving over 10,000 patients from 105 separate studies. During the course of these studies Ketaject was administered as the sole agent, as induction for other general agents, or to supplement low-potency agents. Specific areas of application have included the following:

1. debridement, painful dressings, and skin grafting in burn patients, as well as other superficial surgical procedures.
2. neurodiagnostic procedures such as pneumoencephalograms, ventriculograms, myelograms, and lumbar punctures.
3. diagnostic and operative procedures of the eye, ear, nose, and mouth, including dental extractions.
4. diagnostic and operative procedures of the pharynx, larynx, or bronchial tree. NOTE: Muscle relaxants, with proper attention to respiration, may be required (see Precautions).
5. sigmoidoscopy and minor surgery of the anus and rectum, and circumcision.

Continued on next page

Bristol—Cont.

6. extraperitoneal procedures used in gynecology such as dilatation and curettage.
7. orthopedic procedures such as closed reductions, manipulations, femoral pinning, amputations, and biopsies.
8. as an anesthetic in poor-risk patients with depression of vital functions.
9. in procedures where the intramuscular route of administration is preferred.
10. in cardiac catheterization procedures.

In these studies, the anesthesia was rated either "excellent" or "good" by the anesthesiologist and the surgeon at 90 and 93%, respectively; rated "fair" at 6 and 4%, respectively; and rated "poor" at 4 and 3%, respectively. In a second method of evaluation, the anesthesia was rated "adequate" in at least 90%, and "inadequate" in 10% or less of the procedures.

How Supplied: Ketaject is supplied as the hydrochloride in concentrations equivalent to ketamine base.

NDC 0015-8340-27—Each 50-ml. vial contains 10 mg./ml.

NDC 0015-8341-10—Each 10-ml. vial contains 50 mg./ml.

NDC 0015-8343-05—Each 5-ml. vial contains 100 mg./ml.

LYSODREN® ℞
(mitotane)

This is the full text of the latest Official Package Circular dated August 1978 [3080DIM-01].

> Treatment should be instituted in the hospital until a stable dosage regimen is achieved. Lysodren should be temporarily discontinued immediately following shock or severe trauma since adrenal suppression is its prime action. Exogenous steroids should also be administered in such circumstances, since the depressed adrenal may not immediately start to secrete steroids.

LYSODREN (mitotane) is an oral chemotherapeutic agent.

Description: LYSODREN (mitotane) is best known by its trivial name, o,p'-DDD, and is chemically, 1.1 dichloro-2 (o-chlorophenyl)-2-(p-chlorophenyl) ethane.

LYSODREN is a white granular solid composed of clear colorless crystals.

LYSODREN is tasteless and has a slight pleasant aromatic odor.

Action: LYSODREN (mitotane) can best be described as an adrenal cytotoxic agent, although it can cause adrenal inhibition, apparently without cellular destruction. Its biochemical mechanism of action is unknown. Data are available to suggest that the drug modifies the peripheral metabolism of steroids as well as directly suppressing the adrenal cortex. The administration of LYSODREN alters the extra-adrenal metabolism of cortisol in man, leading to a reduction in measurable 17-hydroxy corticosteroids, even though plasma levels of corticosteroids do not fall. The drug apparently causes increased formation of 6-β-hydroxy cortisol.

Indications: LYSODREN is indicated only in the treatment of inoperable adrenal cortical carcinoma of both functional and non-functional types.

Contraindications: The only contraindication for LYSODREN is known hypersensitivity to the drug.

Warnings: Lysodren should be temporarily discontinued immediately following shock or severe trauma, since adrenal suppression is its prime action. Exogenous steroids should also be administered in such circumstances, since the depressed adrenal may not immediately start to secrete steroids.

LYSODREN should be administered with care to patients with liver disease other than metastatic lesions from the adrenal cortex, since the metabolism of LYSODREN may be interfered with and the drug may accumulate.

All possible tumor tissue should be surgically removed from large metastatic masses before LYSODREN administration is instituted. This is necessary to minimize the possibility of infarction and hemorrhage in the tumor due to a rapid positive effect of the drug.

Long-term continuous administration of high doses of LYSODREN may lead to brain damage and impairment of function. Behavioral and neurological assessments should be made at regular intervals when continuous LYSODREN treatment exceeds two years.

Uses in Pregnancy and Lactation: The safety of LYSODREN in pregnancy or lactation has not been established. Treatment of women who are, or who may become pregnant, should be undertaken only after consideration of the benefits versus the possibility of harm to mother and child.

Precautions: Adrenal insufficiency may develop in patients treated with LYSODREN, and adrenal steroid replacement should be considered for these patients.

Since sedation, lethargy, vertigo, and other CNS side effects can occur, ambulatory patients should be cautioned about driving, operating machinery, and other hazardous pursuits requiring mental and physical alertness.

Adverse Reactions: A very high percentage of patients treated with LYSODREN have shown at least one type of side effect. The main types of adverse reactions consist of the following:

1. Gastrointestinal disturbances, which consisted of anorexia, nausea or vomiting, and in some cases diarrhea, occurred in about 80% of the patients.
2. Central nervous system side effects occurred in 40% of the patients. These consisted primarily of depression as manifested by lethargy and somnolence (25%), and dizziness or vertigo (15%).
3. Skin toxicity was observed in about 15% of the cases. In some instances, however, this side effect subsided while the patients were maintained on drug.

Infrequently occurring side effects involve the eye (visual blurring, diplopia, lens opacity, toxic retinopathy); the genitourinary system (hematuria, hemorrhagic cystitis, and albuminuria); cardiovascular system (hypertension, orthostatic hypotension, and flushing); and some miscellaneous complaints including generalized aching, hyperpyrexia, and lowered PBI.

Dosage and Administration: The recommended treatment schedule is to start the patient at 9-10 grams of LYSODREN per day in divided doses, either q.i.d. or t.i.d. If severe side effects appear, the dose should be reduced until the maximum tolerated dose is achieved. If the patient can tolerate higher doses and improved clinical response appears possible, the dose should be increased until adverse reactions interfere. Experience has shown that the maximum tolerated dose (MTD) will vary from 2-16 grams per day, but has usually been 8-10 grams per day. The highest doses used in the studies to date were 18-19 grams per day.

Treatment should be instituted in the hospital until a stable dosage regimen is achieved.

Treatment should be continued as long as clinical benefits are observed. Maintenance of clinical status or slowing of growth of metastatic lesions can be considered clinical benefits if they can clearly be shown to have occurred.

If no clinical benefits are observed after three months at the maximum tolerated dose, the case may be considered a clinical failure. However, 10% of the patients who showed a measurable response required more than three months at the MTD. Early diagnosis and prompt institution of treatment improve the probability of a positive clinical response.

How Supplied: LYSODREN is available as a 500 mg. scored tablet in bottles of 100.

Animal Studies: Dogs were used for much of the experimental work with LYSODREN (1). Doses as low as 4 mg/kg/day may produce some effects upon the canine adrenals. However, most of the data suggest that toxicity occurs between 80-200 mg/kg/day, primarily as a result of LYSODREN'S effect upon the adrenals. At doses of 100 mg/kg/day and higher of LYSODREN, deaths occurred in some of the dogs after two to four weeks of administration. The primary action of LYSODREN is upon the adrenal cortex. The toxicity observed in animals appears to result from suppression of the activity of the adrenal cortex. The production of adrenal steroids has been shown to be reduced in most of the studies.

A toxicity study was conducted in rats at doses as high as 300 mg/kg/day for 28 days. There were no deaths nor was there any evidence of organ changes in these animals. In this study even the adrenal cortex showed no evidence of change, indicating that the rodent appears to be highly resistant to LYSODREN.

In both dogs and rats, there was a dose-related rise in alkaline phosphatase. In dogs, there were signs of histological changes in the liver at the high doses (50-100 mg/kg/day).

A dose of 300 mg/kg/day administered to guinea pigs resulted in death in one of three animals and reduction in cortisol levels. Death was probably due to adrenal insufficiency (2).

Metabolic Studies of LYSODREN in Man: One study (3) with adrenal carcinoma patients indicated that about 40% of oral LYSODREN was absorbed, and approximately 10% was recovered in the urine as a water-soluble metabolite. A small amount was excreted in the bile and the balance was apparently stored in the tissues. When administered parenterally, approximately 25% of the dose was found in the urine as a water-soluble metabolite.

Blood levels were determined during and following administration of LYSODREN. Both unchanged drug and metabolite were measured. The levels in patients receiving doses from 5-15 grams per day varied from 7-90 micrograms/ml of unchanged LYSODREN and 29-54 micrograms/ml of the metabolite. These studies indicated no relationship between blood levels and therapeutic and/or toxic effects.

Following discontinuation of the drug, LYSODREN blood levels fell, but persisted for several weeks. In most patients blood levels became undetectable after six to nine weeks. In one patient who had received a total of 1900 grams of LYSODREN, high blood levels were found ten weeks after stopping the drug. Autopsy data have provided evidence that LYSODREN is found in most tissues of the body. Fat tissues were the primary site of storage. In one patient a very large number of tissues were examined and the drug was found in essentially every tissue. LYSODREN appears to be converted, in part, to a water-soluble metabolite. This material has not been characterized, but is only found in the urine and blood of patients receiving LYSODREN. Examination of bile was made and found to contain no unchanged LYSODREN. There was metabolite in the bile, and this would indicate that biliary excretion is a significant route of removal of this metabolite from the body.

Clinical Studies: Hutter and Kayhoe (4) reported on the clinical features and the results of LYSODREN treatment of 138 patients with adrenal cortical carcinoma, and compared their findings with 48 treated patients previously reported in the literature. Subsequent to their report, 115 patients given drug were studied. There is no evidence of a cure as a consequence of the administration of LYSODREN. A number of patients have been treated intermittently, treatment being restarted when severe symptoms reappeared. Patients often do not respond after the third or fourth such course. Experience accumulated to date suggests that continuous treatment with the maximum possible dosage of LYSODREN would be the best approach.

A substantial percentage of the patients treated showed signs of adrenal insufficiency. It therefore appears necessary to watch for and institute steroid replacement in those patients. It has been shown that the metabolism of exogenous steroids is modified and consequently somewhat higher doses than just replacement therapy may be required.

There was significant reduction in tumor mass following LYSODREN administration in about 50%, and a significant reduction in elevated steroid excretion in about 80% of the evaluable patients studied to date (4). Clinical effectiveness can be shown by reduction in tumor mass, reduction in pain, weakness or anorexia, and reduction of steroid symptoms.

Bibliography:

1. a) Nelson, A A, Woodward, G: *Archives of Pathology,* 48:387, 1949.
   b) Nichols, J: Studies on an Adrenal Cortical Inhibitor, in *The Adrenal Cortex,* Scranton, Pa., Harper and Row, 1961, p 83.
2. Kupfer, D, *et al: Life Sciences,* 3:959, 1964.
3. Moy, R H: *J Lab Clin Med,* 58:296, 1961.
4. Hutter, A M, Kahoe, D E: *Am J Med,* 41:572, 581, 1966.

Manufactured by Anabolic, Inc.
Irvine, California 92664
[*Shown in Product Identification Section*]

MEXATE™ ℞
(methotrexate sodium for injection)

This is the full text of the latest Official Package Circular dated November, 1980 [3050DIM-07].

WARNING

METHOTREXATE MUST BE USED ONLY BY PHYSICIANS EXPERIENCED IN ANTIMETABOLITE CHEMOTHERAPY.

BECAUSE OF THE POSSIBILITY OF FATAL OR SEVERE TOXIC REACTIONS THE PATIENT SHOULD BE FULLY INFORMED BY THE PHYSICIAN OF THE RISK INVOLVED AND SHOULD BE UNDER HIS CONSTANT SUPERVISION.

DEATHS HAVE BEEN REPORTED WITH THE USE OF METHOTREXATE IN THE TREATMENT OF PSORIASIS, IN THE TREATMENT OF PSORIASIS METHOTREXATE SHOULD BE RESTRICTED TO SEVERE, RECALCITRANT, DISABLING PSORIASIS WHICH IS NOT ADEQUATELY RESPONSIVE TO OTHER FORMS OF THERAPY, BUT ONLY WHEN THE DIAGNOSIS HAS BEEN ESTABLISHED AS BY BIOPSY AND/OR AFTER DERMATOLOGIC CONSULTATION.

1. Methotrexate may produce marked depression of bone marrow, anemia, leukopenia, thrombocytopenia and bleeding.
2. Methotrexate may be hepatotoxic, particularly at high dosage or with prolonged therapy. Liver atrophy, necrosis, cirrhosis, fatty changes, and periportal fibrosis have been reported. Since changes may occur without previous signs of gastrointestinal or hematologic toxicity, it is imperative that hepatic function be determined prior to initiation of treatment and monitored regularly throughout therapy. Special caution is indicated in the presence of preexisting liver damage or impaired hepatic function. Concomitant use of other drugs with hepatotoxic potential (including alcohol) should be avoided.
3. Methotrexate has caused fetal death and/or congenital anomalies, therefore, it is not recommended in women of childbearing potential unless there is appropriate medical evidence that the benefits can be expected to outweigh the considered risks. Pregnant psoriatic patients should not receive Methotrexate.
4. Impaired renal function is usually a contraindication.
5. Diarrhea and ulcerative stomatitis are frequent toxic effects and require interruption of therapy; otherwise hemorrhagic enteritis and death from intestinal perforation may occur.

METHOTREXATE HAS BEEN ADMINISTERED IN VERY HIGH DOSAGE FOLLOWED BY LEUCOVORIN RESCUE IN EXPERIMENTAL TREATMENT OF CERTAIN NEOPLASTIC DISEASES. THIS PROCEDURE IS INVESTIGATIONAL AND HAZARDOUS.

Description: Methotrexate is an antimetabolite used in the treatment of certain neoplastic diseases.

Methotrexate Sodium Parenteral is available in 20, 50, and 100 mg strengths, each available as lyophilized powder in vials, containing no preservatives, for single use only.

Each 20 mg vial contains Methotrexate, 20 mg, prepared as the sodium salt; sodium hydroxide to adjust pH to about 8.5.

Each 50 mg vial contains Methotrexate, 50 mg, prepared as the sodium salt; sodium hydroxide to adjust pH to about 8.5.

Each 100 mg vial contains Methotrexate, 100 mg, prepared as the sodium salt; sodium hydroxide to adjust pH to about 8.5.

Each 250 mg vial contains methotrexate 250 mg prepared as the sodium salt; sodium hydroxide to adjust pH to about 8.5.

Action: Methotrexate has as its principle mechanism of action the competitive inhibition of the enzyme folic acid reductase. Folic acid must be reduced to tetrahydrofolic acid by this enzyme in the process of DNA synthesis and cellular replication.

Methotrexate inhibits the reduction of folic acid and interferes with tissue-cell reproduction.

Actively proliferating tissues such as malignant cells, bone marrow, fetal cells, dermal epithelium, buccal and intestinal mucosa and cells of the urinary bladder are in general more sensitive to this effect of Methotrexate. Cellular proliferation in malignant tissue is greater than in most normal tissue and thus Methotrexate may impair malignant growth without irreversible damage to normal tissues.

After parenteral injection, peak serum levels are seen in about 30 to 60 minutes. Approximately one half the absorbed Methotrexate is reversibly bound to serum protein, but exchanges with body fluids easily and diffuses into the body tissue cells.

Excretion of single daily doses occurs through the kidneys in amounts from 55% to 88% or higher within 24 hours. Repeated doses daily result in more sustained serum levels and some retention of Methotrexate over each 24-hour period which may result in accumulation of the drug within the tissues. The liver cells appear to retain certain amounts of the drug for prolonged periods even after a single therapeutic dose. Methotrexate is retained in the presence of impaired renal function and may increase rapidly in the serum and in the tissue cells under such conditions. Methotrexate does not penetrate the blood cerebrospinal fluid barrier in therapeutic amounts when given parenterally. High concentrations of the drug when needed may be attained by direct intrathecal administration. In psoriasis, the rate of production of epithelial cells in the skin is greatly increased over normal skin. This differential in reproductive rates is the basis for use of Methotrexate to control the psoriatic process.

Indications:

Anti-neoplastic Chemotherapy

Methotrexate is indicated for the treatment of gestational choriocarcinoma, and in patients with chorioadenoma destruens and hydatidiform mole.

Methotrexate is indicated for the palliation of acute lymphocytic leukemia. It is also indicated in the treatment and prophylaxis of meningeal leukemia. Greatest effect has been observed in palliation of acute lymphoblastic (stem-cell) leukemias in children. In combination with other anticancer drugs or suitable agents Methotrexate may be used for induction of remission, but it is most commonly used, as described in the literature, in the maintenance of induced remissions.

Methotrexate is also effective in the treatment of the advanced stages (III and IV, Peters Staging System) of lymphosarcoma, particularly in those cases in children, and in advanced cases of mycosis fungoides.

Psoriasis Chemotherapy (See box warnings.)

Because of high risk attending its use. Methotrexate is only indicated in the symptomatic control of severe, recalcitrant, disabling psoriasis which is not adequately responsive to other forms of therapy, **but only when the diagnosis has been established, as by biopsy and/or after dermatologic consultation.**

Contraindications: Pregnant psoriatic patients should not receive Methotrexate. Psoriatic patients with severe renal or hepatic disorders should not receive Methotrexate. Psoriatic patients with preexisting blood dyscrasias, such as bone marrow hypoplasia, leukopenia, thrombocytopenia or anemia, should not receive Methotrexate.

Warnings: See box warnings.

Precautions: Methotrexate has a high potential toxicity, usually dose-related. The physician should be familiar with the various characteristics of the drug and its established clinical usage. Patients undergoing therapy should be subject to appropriate supervision so that signs or symptoms of possible toxic effects or adverse reactions may be detected and evaluated with minimal delay. Pretreatment and periodic hematologic studies are essential to the use of Methotrexate in chemotherapy because of its common effect of hematopoietic suppression. This may occur abruptly and on apparent safe dosage, and any profound drop in blood-cell count indicates immediate stopping of the drug and appropriate therapy. In patients with malignant disease who have preexisting bone marrow aplasia, leukopenia, thrombocytopenia or anemia, the drug should be used with caution, if at all.

Methotrexate is excreted principally by the kidneys. Its use in the presence of impaired renal function may result in accumulation of toxic amounts or even additional renal damage. The patient's renal status should be determined prior to and during Methotrexate therapy and proper caution exercised should significant renal impairment be disclosed. Drug dosage should be reduced or discontinued until renal function is improved or restored.

In general, the following laboratory tests are recommended as part of essential clinical evaluation and appropriate monitoring of patients chosen for or receiving Methotrexate therapy; complete hemogram; hematocrit; urinalysis; renal function tests; and liver function tests. A chest x-ray is also recommended. The purpose is to determine any existing organ dysfunction or system impairment. The tests should be performed prior to therapy, at appropriate periods during therapy and after termination of therapy. It may be useful or important to perform liver biopsy or bone marrow aspiration studies

Continued on next page

Bristol—Cont.

where high dose or long-term therapy is being followed.

Methotrexate is bound in part to serum albumin after absorption and toxicity may be increased because of displacement by certain drugs such as salicylates, sulfonamides, diphenylhydantoin, phenylbutazone, and some antibacterials as tetracycline, chloramphenicol and para-amino-benzoic acid. These drugs, especially salicylates, phenylbutazone, and sulfonamides, whether antibacterial, hypoglycemic or diuretic, should not be given concurrently until the significance of these findings is established.

Vitamin preparations containing folic acid or its derivatives may alter responses to Methotrexate.

Methotrexate should be used with extreme caution in the presence of infection, peptic ulcer, ulcerative colitis, debility and in extreme youth or old age.

If profound leukopenia occurs during therapy, bacterial infection may occur or become a threat. Cessation of the drug and appropriate antibiotic therapy is usually indicated. In severe bone marrow depression, blood or platelet transfusions may be necessary.

Since it is reported that Methotrexate may have an immunosuppressive action, this factor must be taken into consideration in evaluating the use of the drug where immune responses in a patient may be important or essential.

In all instances where the use of Methotrexate is considered for chemotherapy, the physician must evaluate the need and usefulness of the drug against the risks of toxic effects or adverse reaction. Most such adverse reactions are reversible if detected early. When such effects or reactions do occur, the drug should be reduced in dosage or discontinued and appropriate corrective measures should be taken, according to the clinical judgment of the physician. Reinstitution of Methotrexate therapy should be carried out with caution, with adequate consideration of further need for the drug and alertness as to possible recurrence of toxicity.

Adverse Reactions: The most common adverse reactions include ulcerative stomatitis, leukopenia, nausea and abdominal distress. Others reported are malaise, undue fatigue, chills and fever, dizziness and decreased resistance to infection. In general, the incidence and severity of side effects are considered to be dose-related. Adverse reactions as reported for the various systems are as follows:

Skin: erythematous rashes, pruritus, urticaria, photosensitivity, depigmentation, alopecia, ecchymosis, telangiectasia, acne, furunculosis. Lesions of psoriasis may be aggravated by concomitant exposure to ultraviolet radiation.

Blood: bone marrow depression, leukopenia, thrombocytopenia, anemia, hypogammaglobulinemia, hemorrhage from various sites, septicemia.

Alimentary System: gingivitis, pharyngitis, stomatitis, anorexia, vomiting, diarrhea, hematemesis, melena, gastrointestinal ulceration and bleeding, enteritis, hepatic toxicity resulting in acute liver atrophy, necrosis, fatty metamorphosis, periportal fibrosis, or hepatic cirrhosis.

Urogenital System: renal failure, azotemia, cystitis, hematuria; defective oogenesis or spermatogenesis, transient oligospermia, menstrual dysfunction; infertility, abortion, fetal defects, severe nephropathy.

Central Nervous System: headaches, drowsiness, blurred vision. Aphasia, hemiparesis, paresis and convulsions have also occurred following administration of Methrotrexate.

There have been reports of leucoencephalopathy following intravenous administration of Methotrexate to patients who have had craniospinal irradiation.

After the intrathecal use of Methotrexate, the central nervous system toxicity which may occur can be classified as follows: (1) chemical arachnoiditis manifested by such symptoms as headache, back pain, vomiting, nuchal rigidity, and fever, (2) paresis, usually transient, manifested by paraplegia associated with involvement with one or more spinal nerve roots, (3) leucoencephalopathy manifested by confusion, irritability, somnolence, ataxia, dementia, and occasionally major convulsions and coma.

Other reactions related to or attributed to the use of Methotrexate, such as pneumonitis, metabolic changes, precipitating diabetes, osteoporotic effects, abnormal tissue cell changes, and even sudden death have been reported.

Dosage and Administration:

Anti-neoplastic chemotherapy

Methotrexate sodium parenteral may be given by intramuscular, intravenous, intraarterial or intrathecal route. Initial treatment is usually undertaken with the patient under hospital care.

*For conversion of mg/kg b.w. to mg/M^2 of body surface or the reverse, a ratio of 1:30 is given as a guideline. The conversion factor varies between 1:20 and 1:40 depending on age and body build.

Choriocarcinoma and similar trophoblastic diseases: Methotrexate is administered intramuscularly in doses of 15 to 30 mg daily for a 5 day course. Such courses are usually repeated for 3 to 5 times as required, with rest periods of one or more weeks interposed between courses, until any manifesting toxic symptoms subside. The effectiveness of therapy is ordinarily evaluated by 24 hour quantitative analysis of urinary chorionic gonadotropin hormone (CGH), which should return to normal or less than 50 IU/24 hr usually after the 3rd or 4th course and usually be followed by a complete resolution of measurable lesions in 4 to 6 weeks. One to two courses of Methotrexate after normalization of CGH is usually recommended.

Before each course of the drug careful clinical assessment is essential. Cyclic combination therapy of Methotrexate with other antitumor drugs has been reported as being useful.

Since hydatidiform mole may precede choriocarcinoma, prophylactic chemotherapy with Methotrexate has been recommended. Chorioadenoma destruens is considered to be an invasive form of hydatidiform mole. Methotrexate is administered in these disease states in doses similar to those recommended for choriocarcinoma.

Leukemia: Acute lymphatic (lymphoblastic) leukemia in children and young adolescents is the most responsive to present day chemotherapy. In young adults and older patients, clinical remission is more difficult to obtain and early relapse is more common. In chronic lymphatic leukemia, the prognosis for adequate response is less encouraging.

Methotrexate alone or in combination with steroids was used initially for induction of remission of lymphoblastic leukemias. More recently corticosteroid therapy in combination with other antileukemic drugs or in cyclic combinations with Methotrexate included appear to produce rapid and effective remissions. When used for induction, Methotrexate in doses of 3.3 mg/M^2 in combination with prednisone 60 mg/M^2, given daily, produced remission in 50% of patients treated, usually within a period of 4 to 6 weeks. Methotrexate alone or in combination with other agents appears to be the drug of choice for securing maintenance of drug-induced remissions. When remission is achieved and supportive care has produced general clinical improvement, maintenance therapy is initiated, as follows: Methotrexate is administered 2 times weekly intramuscularly in doses of 30 mg/M^2. It has also been given in doses of 2.5 mg/kg intravenously every 14 days. If and when relapse does occur, reinduction of remission can again usually be obtained by repeating the initial induction regimen. Various experts have recently introduced a variety of dosage schedules for both induction and maintenance of remission with various combinations of alkylating and antifolic agents. Multiple drug therapy with several agents, including Methotrexate, given concomitantly is gaining increasing support in both the acute and chronic forms of leukemia. The physician should familiarize himself with the new advances in antileukemic therapy.

Acute granulocytic leukemia is rare in children but common in adults. This form of leukemia responds poorly to chemotherapy and remissions are short with relapses common, and resistance to therapy develops rapidly.

Meningeal leukemia: Patients with leukemia are subject to leukemic invasion of the central nervous system. This may manifest characteristic signs or symptoms or may remain silent and be diagnosed only by examination of the cerebrospinal fluid which contains leukemic cells in such cases. Therefore, the CSF should be examined in all leukemic patients. Since passage of Methotrexate from blood serum to the cerebrospinal fluid is minimal, for adequate therapy the drug is administered intrathecally. It is now common practice because of the noted increased frequency of meningeal leukemia to administer Methotrexate intrathecally as prophylaxis in all cases of lymphocytic leukemia.

By intrathecal injection, the sodium salt of Methotrexate is administered in solution in doses of 12 mg per square meter of body surface or in an empirical dose of 15 mg. The solution is made in a strength of 1 mg per ml with an appropriate, sterile, preservative-free medium such as Sodium Chloride Injection, U.S.P.

For the treatment of meningeal leukemia. Methotrexate is given at intervals of 2 to 5 days. Methotrexate is administered until the cell count of the cerebrospinal fluid returns to normal. At this point one additional dose is advisable.

For prophylaxis against meningeal leukemia, the dosage is the same as for treatment except for the intervals of administration. On this subject, it is advisable for the physician to consult the medical literature.

Large doses may cause convulsions. Untoward side effects may occur with any given intrathecal injection and are commonly neurological in character. Methotrexate given by intrathecal route appears significantly in the systemic circulation and may cause systemic Methotrexate toxicity. Therefore systemic antileukemic therapy with the drug should be appropriately adjusted, reduced or discontinued. Focal leukemic involvement of the central nervous system may not respond to intrathecal chemotherapy and is best treated with radiotherapy.

Lymphomas: In Burkitt's Tumor, Stages III, Methotrexate has produced prolonged remissions in some cases. In Stage III Methotrexate is commonly given concomitantly with other antitumor agents. Treatment in all stages usually consists of several courses of the drug interposed with 7 to 10 day rest periods. Lymphosarcomas in Stage III may respond to combined drug therapy with Methotrexate given in doses of 0.625 mg to 2.5 mg/kg daily.

Mycosis fungoides: Therapy with Methotrexate appears to produce clinical remissions in about one half of the cases treated. Dosage is usually daily by mouth for weeks or months. Dose levels of drug and adjustment of dose regimen by reduction or cessation of drug are guided by patient response and hematologic monitoring. Methotrexate has also been given intramuscularly in doses of 50 mg once weekly or 25 mg 2 times weekly.

Psoriasis Chemotherapy

The patient should be fully informed of the risks involved and should be under constant supervision of the physician.

Assessment of renal function, liver function, and blood elements should be made by history, physical examination, and laboratory tests (such as CBC, urinalysis, serum creatinine, liver function studies, and liver biopsy if indicated) before beginning Methotrexate, periodically during Methotrexate therapy, and before reinstituting Methotrexate therapy after a rest period. Appropriate steps should be taken to avoid conception during and for at least eight weeks following Methotrexate therapy.

There are three commonly used general types of dosage schedules:

1. weekly oral or parenteral intermittent large doses
2. divided dose intermittent oral schedule over a 36-hour period
3. daily oral with a rest period

All schedules should be continually tailored to the individual patient. Dose schedules cited below pertain to an average 70 Kg adult. An initial test dose one week prior to initiation of therapy is recommended to detect any idiosyncrasy. A suggested dose range is 5 to 10 mg parenterally.

Recommended starting dose schedule:

Weekly single IM or IV dose schedule:

10 to 25 mg per week until adequate response is achieved. With this dosage schedule, 50 mg per week should ordinarily not be exceeded.

Special Note: Available data suggests that schedule 3 (daily oral with a rest period) may carry an increased risk of serious liver pathology.

Dosages may be gradually adjusted to achieve optimal clinical response, but not to exceed the maximum stated in the schedule.

Once optimal clinical response has been achieved, the dosage schedule should be reduced to the lowest possible amount of drug and to the longest possible rest period. The use of Methotrexate may permit the return to conventional topical therapy, which should be encouraged.

Antidote for Overdosage

Leucovorin (citrovorum factor) is a potent agent for neutralizing the immediate toxic effects of Methotrexate on the hematopoietic system. Where large doses or overdoses are given, Calcium Leucovorin may be administered by intravenous infusion in doses up to 75 mg within 12 hours, followed by 12 mg intramuscularly every 6 hours for 4 doses. Where average doses of Methotrexate appear to have an adverse effect, 2 to 4 ml (6 to 12 mg) of Calcium Leucovorin may be given intramuscularly every 6 hours for 4 doses. In general, where overdosage is suspected, the dose of Leucovorin should be equal to or higher than the offending dose of Methotrexate and should best be administered within the first hour. Use of Calcium Leucovorin after an hour delay is much less effective.

Caution:

Pharmacist: Because of its potential to cause severe toxicity, Methotrexate therapy requires close supervision of the patient by the physician. Pharmacists should dispense no more than a seven (7) day supply of the drug at one time. Refill of such prescriptions should be by direct order (written or oral) of the physician only.

Directions for Use: Reconstitute immediately prior to use with 2 to 10 ml. depending on route of administration, of an appropriate preservative-free medium such as Sodium Chloride Injection, U.S.P.

Note: Store dry powder and reconstituted solution at room temperature protected from light.

Supply: Mexate (Methotrexate Sodium) for Injection.

NDC 0015-3050-20—20 mg vial
NDC 0015-3051-20—50 mg vial
NDC 0015-3052-20—100 mg vial
NDC 0015-3053-20—250 mg vial

MUTAMYCIN® ℞
(mitomycin for injection)

This is the full text of the latest Official Package Circular dated December 1978 [3001DIR-12].

WARNING

Mutamycin should be administered under the supervision of a qualified physician experienced in the use of cancer chemotherapeutic agents. Appropriate management of therapy and complications is possible only when adequate diagnostic and treatment facilities are readily available. Bone marrow suppression, notably thrombocytopenia and leukopenia, which may contribute to overwhelming infections in an already compromised patient, is the most common and severe of the toxic effects of Mutamycin (see "Warnings" and "Adverse Reactions" sections).

Description: Mutamycin (also known as mitomycin and/or mitomycin-C) is an antibiotic isolated from the broth of **Streptomyces caespitosus** which has been shown to have antitumor activity. The compound is heat stable, has a high melting point, and is freely soluble in organic solvents.

Action: Mutamycin selectively inhibits the synthesis of deoxyribonucleic acid (DNA). The guanine and cytosine content correlates with the degree of Mutamycin-induced cross-linking. At high concentrations of the drug, cellular RNA and protein synthesis are also suppressed.

In humans, Mutamycin is rapidly cleared from the serum after intravenous administration. Time required to reduce the serum concentration by 50% after a 30 mg. bolus injection is 17 minutes. After injection of 30 mg., 20 mg., or 10 mg. I.V., the maximal serum concentrations were 2.4 mcg./ml., 1.7 mcg./ml., and 0.52 mcg./ml., respectively. Clearance is effected primarily by metabolism in the liver, but metabolism occurs in other tissues as well. The rate of clearance is inversely proportional to the maximal serum concentration because, it is thought, of saturation of the degradative pathways.

Approximately 10% of a dose of Mutamycin is excreted unchanged in the urine. Since metabolic pathways are saturated at relatively low doses, the percent of a dose excreted in urine increases with increasing dose. In children, excretion of intravenously administered Mutamycin is similar.

Animal Toxicology—Mutamycin has been found to be carcinogenic in rats and mice. At doses approximating the recommended clinical dose in man, it produces a greater than 100 percent increase in tumor incidence in male Sprague-Dawley rats, and a greater than 50 percent increase in tumor incidence in female Swiss mice.

Indications: Mutamycin is not recommended as single-agent, primary therapy. It has been shown to be useful in the therapy of disseminated adenocarcinoma of the stomach or pancreas in proven combinations with other approved chemotherapeutic agents and as palliative treatment when other modalities have failed. Mutamycin is not recommended to replace appropriate surgery and/or radiotherapy.

Contraindications: Mutamycin is contraindicated in patients who have demonstrated a hypersensitive or idiosyncratic reaction to it in the past.

Mutamycin is contraindicated in patients with thrombocytopenia, coagulation disorder, or an increase in bleeding tendency due to other causes.

Warnings: Patients being treated with Mutamycin must be observed carefully and frequently during and after therapy.

The use of Mutamycin results in a high incidence of bone marrow suppression, particularly thrombocytopenia and leukopenia. Therefore, the following studies should be obtained repeatedly during therapy and for at least 7 weeks following therapy: platelet count, white blood cell count, differential, and hemoglobin. The occurrence of a platelet count below 150,000, or a WBC below 4,000, or a progressive decline in either is an indication for interruption of therapy.

Patients should be advised of the potential toxicity of this drug, particularly bone marrow suppression. Deaths have been reported due to septicemia as a result of leukopenia due to the drug.

Patients receiving Mutamycin should be observed for evidence of renal toxicity. Mutamycin should not be given to patients with a serum creatinine greater than 1.7 mg. percent.

Usage in Pregnancy—Safe use of Mutamycin in pregnant women has not been established. Teratological changes have been noted in animal studies. The effect of Mutamycin on fertility is unknown.

Adverse Reactions: **Bone Marrow Toxicity**— This was the most common and most serious toxicity, occurring in 605 of 937 patients (64.4%). Thrombocytopenia and/or leukopenia may occur anytime within 8 weeks after onset of therapy with an average time of 4 weeks. Recovery after cessation of therapy was within 10 weeks. About 25% of the leukopenic or thrombocytopenic episodes did not recover. Mutamycin produces cumulative myelosuppression.

Integument and Mucus Membrane Toxicity—This has occurred in approximately 4% of patients treated with Mutamycin. Cellulitis at the injection site has been reported and is occasionally severe. Stomatitis and alopecia also occurred frequently.

Renal Toxicity—2% of 1,281 patients demonstrated a statistically significant rise in creatinine. There appeared to be no correlation between total dose administered or duration of therapy and the degree of renal impairment.

Pulmonary Toxicity—This has occurred infrequently but can be severe. Dyspnea with a nonproductive cough and radiographic evidence of pulmonary infiltrates may be indicative of Mutamycin-induced pulmonary toxicity. If other etiologies are eliminated, Mutamycin therapy should be discontinued. Steroids have been employed as treatment of this toxicity, but the therapeutic value has not been determined.

Acute Side Effects Due to Mutamycin were fever, anorexia, nausea, and vomiting. They occurred in about 14% of 1,281 patients.

Other Undesirable Side Effects that have been reported during Mutamycin therapy have been headache, blurring of vision, confusion, drowsiness, syncope, fatigue, edema, thrombophlebitis, hematemesis, diarrhea, and pain. These did not appear to be dose related and were not unequivocally drug related. They may have been due to the primary or metastatic disease processes.

Dosage and Administration: Mutamycin should be given intravenously only, using care to avoid extravasation of the compound. If extravasation occurs, cellulitis, ulceration, and slough may result.

Each vial contains either mitomycin 5 mg. and mannitol 10 mg. or mitomycin 20 mg. and mannitol 40 mg. To administer, add Sterile Water for Injection, 10 ml. or 40 ml. respectively. Shake to dissolve. If product does not dissolve immediately, allow to stand at room temperature until solution is obtained.

After full hematological recovery (see guide to dosage adjustment) from any previous chemotherapy, either of the following dosage schedules may be used at 6 to 8 week intervals.

Continued on next page

Bristol—Cont.

Because of cumulative myelosuppression, patients should be fully reevaluated after each course of Mutamycin, and the dose reduced if the patient has experienced any toxicities. Doses greater than 20 mg./M.^{2} have not been shown to be more effective, and are more toxic than lower doses.

(1) 20 mg./M.^{2} intravenously as a single dose via a functioning intravenous catheter.

(2) 2 mg./M.^{2}/day intravenously for 5 days. After a drug-free interval of 2 days, 2 mg./M.^{2}/day for 5 days, thus making the total initial dose 20 mg./M.^{2} given over 10 days. The following schedule is suggested as a guide to dosage adjustment:

Nadir After Prior Dose		Percentage of Prior Dose to be Given
Leukocytes	Platelets	
>4000	>100,000	100%
3000–3999	75,000–99,999	100%
2000–2999	25,000–74,999	70%
<2000	<25,000	50%

No repeat dosage should be given until leukocyte count has returned to 3000 and platelet count to 75,000.

When Mutamycin is used in combination with other myelosuppressive agents, the doses should be adjusted accordingly. If the disease continues to progress after two courses of Mutamycin, the drug should be stopped since chances of response are minimal.

Stability:

1. **Unreconstituted** Mutamycin is stable for at least 2 years at room temperature. Avoid excessive heat (over 40°C).
2. **Reconstituted** with Sterile Water for Injection to a concentration of 0.5 mg. per ml., Mutamycin is stable for 14 days refrigerated or 7 days at room temperature.
3. **Diluted** in various IV fluids at room temperature, to a concentration of 20 to 40 micrograms per ml:

IV Fluid	Stability
5% Dextrose Injection	3 hours
0.9% Sodium Chloride Injection	12 hours
Sodium Lactate Injection	24 hours

4. **The combination** of Mutamycin (5 mg. to 15 mg.) and heparin (1,000 units to 10,000 units) in 30 ml. of 0.9% Sodium Chloride Injection is stable for 48 hours at room temperature.

Supply:

Mutamycin (mitomycin) for Injection.

NDC 0015-3001-20—Each vial contains 5 mg. mitomycin.

NDC 0015-3002-20—Each vial contains 20 mg. mitomycin.

NAFCIL™ ℞

(nafcillin sodium for injection)
For Intramuscular or Intravenous Injection

This is the full text of the latest Official Package Circular dated May 1979 [7224DIR-07].

Description: NAFCIL (nafcillin sodium as the monohydrate) is 6-(2-ethoxy-1-nophthamido)-penicillanic acid, a penicillinase-resistant semisynthetic penicillin.

Microbiology: NAFCIL is a bactericidal penicillin which has shown activity **in vitro** against both penicillin G-susceptible and penicillin G-resistant strains of **Staphylococcus aureus** as well as against pneumococcus, beta-hemolytic streptococcus, and alpha streptococcus (veridans).

In experimental mouse infections induced with pneumococci, beta-hemolytic streptococci, and both penicillin G-susceptible and penicillin G-resistant strains of **Staphylococcus aureus**, nafcillin sodium was compared with methicillin and oxacillin. Regardless of the route of drug administration (intramuscular or oral) nafcillin sodium was consistently and significantly more effective than the other two penicillins.

The fate of a penicillin G-resistant strain of **Staphylococcus aureus** was determined in the kidneys of mice treated with penicillin G, methicillin, and nafcillin sodium. Animals injected with the nafcillin sodium showed negative cultures after the fourteenth day, whereas positive kidney cultures were obtained during the entire 28-day period from mice treated with penicillin G and methicillin.

Disc Susceptibility Tests

Quantitative methods that require measurement of zone diameters give the most precise estimates of antibiotic susceptibility. One such procedure* has been recommended for use with discs for testing susceptibility to methicillin class antibiotics. Interpretations correlate diameters on the disc test with MIC values for methicillin. With this procedure, a report from the laboratory of "susceptible" indicates that the infecting organism is likely to respond to therapy. A report of "resistant" indicates that the infecting organism is not likely to respond to therapy. A report of "intermediate susceptibility" suggests that the organism would be susceptible if high dosage is used, or if the infection is confined to tissues and fluids (e.g., urine), in which high antibiotic levels are attained.

Pharmacology: NAFCIL is relatively nontoxic for animals. The acute LD^{50} of this product by oral administration in rats and mice was greater than 5 g./Kg.; by intramuscular administration in rats 2800 mg./Kg.; by intraperitoneal administration in rats 1240 mg./Kg.; and by intravenous administration in mice 1140 mg./Kg. The intraperitoneal LD^{50} in dogs is 600 mg./Kg. Animal studies indicated that local tissue responses following intramuscular administration of 25% solutions were minimal and resembled those of penicillin G rather than methicillin.

Animal studies indicate that antibacterial amounts are concentrated in the bile, kidney, lung, heart, spleen, and liver. Eighty-four percent of an intravenously administered dose can be recovered by biliary cannulation and 13 percent by renal excretion in 24 hours. High and prolonged tissue levels can be demonstrated by both biological activity assays and C^{14} distribution patterns.

At comparable dosage intramuscular absorption of this product is nearly equivalent to that of intramuscular methicillin, and oral absorption to that of oral oxacillin. Blood concentrations may be tripled by the concurrent use of probenecid. Clinical studies with nafcillin sodium in infants under three days of age and prematures have revealed higher blood levels and slower rates of urinary excretion than in older children and adults.

Studies of the effect of this product on reproduction in rats and rabbits have been completed and reveal no fetal or maternal abnormalities. These studies include the observation of the effects of administration of the drug before conception and continuously through weaning (one generation).

Indications: Although the principal indication for nafcillin sodium is in the treatment of infections due to penicillinase-producing staphylococci, it may be used to initiate therapy in such patients in whom a staphylococcal infection is suspected. (See Important Note following.)

Bacteriologic studies to determine the causative organisms and their susceptibility to nafcillin sodium should be performed.

Important Note: When it is judged necessary that treatment be initiated before definitive culture and susceptibility results are known, the choice of nafcillin sodium should take into consideration the fact that it has been shown to be effective only in the treatment of infections caused by pneumococci, Group A beta-hemolytic streptococci and penicillin G-resistant and penicillin G-susceptible staphylococci. If the bacteriology report later indicates the infection is due to an organism other than a penicillin G-resistant staphylococcus susceptible to nafcillin sodium, the physician is advised to continue therapy with a drug other than nafcillin sodium or any other penicillinase-resistant semisynthetic penicillin.

Recent studies have reported that the percentage of staphylococcal isolates resistant to penicillin G outside the hospital is increasing, approximating the high percentage of resistant staphylococcal isolates found in the hospital. For this reason, it is recommended that a penicillinase-resistant penicillin be used as initial therapy for any suspected staphylococcal infection until culture and susceptibility results are known.

Nafcillin sodium is a compound that acts through a mechanism similar to that of methicillin against penicillin G-resistant staphylococci. Strains of staphylococci resistant to methicillin have existed in nature and it is known that the number of these strains reported has been increasing. Such strains of staphylococci have been capable of producing serious disease, in some instances resulting in fatality. Because of this, there is concern that widespread use of the penicllinase-resistant penicillins may result in the appearance of an increasing number of staphylococcal strains which are resistant to these penicillins.

Methicillin-resistant strains are almost always resistant to all other penicillinase-resistant penicillins (cross resistance with cephalosporin derivatives also occurs frequently). Resistance to any penicillinase-resistant penicillin should be interpreted as evidence of clinical resistance to all, in spite of the fact that minor variations in **in vitro** susceptibility may be encountered when more than one penicillinase-resistant penicillin is tested against the same strain of staphylococcus.

Contraindications: A history of allergic reaction to any of the penicillins is a contraindication.

Warnings:

Warning: Serious and occasionally fatal hypersensitivity (anaphylactoid) reactions have been reported in patients on penicillin therapy. Although anaphylaxis is more frequent following parenteral therapy it has occurred in patients on oral penicillins. These reactions are more apt to occur in individuals with a history of sensitivity to multiple allergens.

There have been reports of individuals with a history of penicillin hypersensitivity reactions who have experienced severe hypersensitivity reactions when treated with a cephalosporin. Before therapy with a penicillin, careful inquiry should be made concerning previous hypersensitivity reactions to penicillins, cephalosporins, and other allergens. If an allergic reaction occurs, appropriate therapy should be instituted, and discontinuation of nafcillin therapy considered. The usual agents (antihistamines, pressor amines, corticosteroids) should be readily available.

Precautions: As with any potent drug, periodic assessment of organ system function, including renal, hepatic and hematopoietic, should be made during prolonged therapy.

The possibility of bacterial and fungal overgrowth should be kept in mind during long-term therapy. If overgrowth of resistant organisms occurs, appropriate measures should be taken.

The oral route of administration should not be relied upon in patients with severe illness, or

with nausea, vomiting, gastric dilatation, cardiospasm, or intestinal hypermotility.
Safety for use in pregnancy has not been established.
Particular care should be taken with intravenous administration because of the possibility of thrombophlebitis.
Adverse Reactions: Reactions to nafcillin sodium have been infrequent and mild in nature. As with other penicillins, the possibility of an anaphylactic reaction or serum sickness-like reactions should be considered. A careful history should be taken. Patients with histories of hay fever, asthma, urticaria, or previous sensitivity to penicillin are more likely to react adversely.
The few reactions associated with the intramuscular use of nafcillin sodium have been skin rash, pruritus, and possible drug fever. As with other penicillins, reactions from oral use of the drug have included nausea, vomiting, diarrhea, urticaria, and pruritus.
Dosage and Administration: It is recommended that parenteral therapy be used initially in severe infections. The patient should be placed on oral therapy with this product as soon as the clinical condition warrants.
Intravenous Route: 500 mg. every 4 hours; double the dose if necessary in very severe infections. The required amount of drug should be diluted in 15 to 30 ml. of Sterile Water for Injection, U.S.P. or Sodium Chloride Injection, U.S.P. and injected over a 5 to 10 minute period. This may be accomplished through the tubing of an intravenous infusion if desirable.
Stability studies on nafcillin sodium at concentrations of 2 mg./ml. and 30 mg./ml. in the following intravenous solutions indicate the drug will lose less than 10% activity at room temperature (70°F) during the time period stipulated:

Isotonic sodium chloride	24 hours
5% dextrose in water	24 hours
5% dextrose in 0.4% sodium chloride solution	24 hours
Ringer's solution	24 hours
M/6 sodium lactate solution (conc. of 30 mg./ml.)	24 hours

Discard any unused portions of intravenous solutions after 24 hours. Only those solutions listed above should be used for the intravenous infusion of NAFCIL (nafcillin sodium). The concentration of the antibiotic should fall within the range of 2 to 30 mg./ml. The drug concentrate and the rate and volume of the infusion should be adjusted so that the total dose of nafcillin is administered before the drug loses its stability in the solution in use.
There is no clinical experience available on the use of this agent in neonates or infants for this route of administration.
This route of administration should be used for relatively short-term therapy (24 to 48 hours) because of the occasional occurrence of thrombophlebitis particularly in elderly patients.
Intramuscular Route: 500 mg. every 6 hours in adults; decrease the interval to 4 hours if necessary in severe infections. In infants and children a dose of 25 mg. per Kg. (about 12 mg. per pound) twice daily is usually adequate.
For neonates 10 mg. per Kg. is recommended twice daily.
Reconstitute with Sterile Water for Injection, U.S.P., 0.9% Sodium Chloride Injection, U.S.P. or Bacteriostatic water for Injection, U.S.P. (with benzyl alcohol or parabens); add 1.8 ml to the 500 mg vial for 2 ml resulting solution; 3.4 ml to the 1 g vial for 4 ml resulting solution; 6.6 ml to the 2 g vial for 8 ml resulting solution. All reconstituted vials have a concentration of 250 mg per ml.
The clear solution should be administered by deep intragluteal injection immediately after reconstitution.
INFECTIONS CAUSED BY GROUP A BETA-HEMOLYTIC STREPTOCOCCI SHOULD BE TREATED FOR AT LEAST 10 DAYS TO HELP PREVENT THE OCCURRENCE OF ACUTE RHEUMATIC FEVER OR ACUTE GLOMERULONEPHRITIS.
"Piggyback"I.V. Package: This glass vial contains the labeled quantity of Nafcillin and is intended for intravenous administration. The diluent and volume are specified on the label of each package.
Reconstituted Stability: Reconstitute with the required amount of Sterile Water for Injection, U.S.P., 0.9% Sodium Chloride Injection, U.S.P. or Bacteriostatic Water for Injection. U.S.P. (with benzyl alcohol or parabens). The resulting solutions are stable for 3 days at room temperature or 7 days under refrigeration and frozen.
When the "piggyback" vial is reconstituted with either Sterile Water for Injection, U.S.P. or 0.9% Sodium Chloride Injection, U.S.P. and the resulting solutions are in a concentration of 10 to 200 mg/ml, the solutions are stable for 24 hours at room temperature or 7 days under refrigeration.
Hospital Bulk Package: This glass vial contains 10 grams Nafcil and is designed for use in the pharmacy in preparing I.V. additives. Add 93 ml Sterile Water for Injection, U.S.P. or 0.9% Sodium Chloride Injection, U.S.P. The resulting solution will contain 100 milligrams nafcillin activity per ml. Solutions in a concentration of 10 mg to 200 mg per ml are stable for 24 hours at room temperature or seven days under refrigeration. Solutions in a concentration of 250 mg per ml are stable for three days at room temperature or seven days under refrigeration and frozen.
Caution: NOT TO BE DISPENSED AS A UNIT.
Supply: NAFCIL (nafcillin sodium) for injection. Nafcillin sodium equivalent to 500 mg., 1.0 Gm., 2.0 Gm., or 10 Gm. nafcillin per vial.
NDC 0015-7224-20—500 mg. vial
NDC 0015-7225-20—1.0-Gm. vial
NDC 0015-7226-20—2.0-Gm. vial
NDC 0015-7225-28—1.0-Gm. "piggyback" vial.
NDC 0015-7226-28—2.0-Gm. "piggyback" vial.
NDC 0015-7101-28—10 gram Hospital Bulk Package
For information on package sizes available, refer to the current price schedule.

*Bauer, A. W., Kirby, W. M. M., Sherris, J. C. and Turck, M.: Antibiotic Testing by a Standardized Single Disc Method, Am. J. Clin. Pathol., 45:493, 1966; Standardized Disc Susceptibility Test, FEDERAL REGISTER 37:20527-29, 1972.

	For immediate action	For delayed action	Total contents
Each sustained-action tablet contains:			
Phenylpropanolamine hydrochloride	20.0 mg	20.0 mg	40.0 mg
Phenylephrine hydrochloride	5.0 mg	5.0 mg	10.0 mg
Phenyltoloxamine citrate	7.5 mg	7.5 mg	15.0 mg
Chlorpheniramine maleate	2.5 mg	2.5 mg	5.0 mg
Each teaspoonful (5 ml) of syrup contains:			
Phenylpropanolamine hydrochloride			20.0 mg
Phenylephrine hydrochloride			5.0 mg
Phenyltoloxamine citrate			7.5 mg
Chlorpheniramine maleate			2.5 mg

Each pediatric formulation contains the following ingredients:	Pediatric Syrup each 5-ml contains:	Pediatric Drops each 1-ml dropper contains:
Phenylpropanolamine hydrochloride	5.0 mg	5.0 mg
Phenylephrine hydrochloride	1.25 mg	1.25 mg
Phenyltoloxamine citrate	2.0 mg	2.0 mg
Chlorpheniramine maleate	0.5 mg	0.5 mg

NALDECON® ℞

Tablets, Syrup, Pediatric Drops and Pediatric Syrup For Oral Use Only

This is the full text of the latest Official Package Circular dated October 1981 [5600DIR-14].
Description:
Naldecon is a preparation containing:
[See table above].
Clinical Pharmacology:
Phenylpropanolamine Hydrochloride
The drug may directly stimulate adrenergic receptors but probably indirectly stimulates both alpha (α) and beta (β) adrenergic receptors by releasing norepinephrine from its storage sites. Phenylpropanolamine increases heart rate, force of contraction and cardiac output, and excitability. It acts on α receptors in the mucosa of the respiratory tract, producing vasoconstriction which results in shrinkage of swollen mucous membranes, reduction of tissue, hyperemia, edema and nasal congestion, and an increase in nasal airway patency. Phenylpropanolamine causes CNS stimulation and reportedly has an anorexigenic effect.
Phenylephrine Hydrochloride
Phenylephrine acts predominantly by a direct action on alpha (α) adrenergic receptors. In therapeutic doses, the drug has no significant stimulant effect on the beta (β) adrenergic receptors of the heart. Following oral administration, constriction of blood vessels in the nasal mucosa may relieve nasal congestion. In therapeutic doses the drug causes little, if any, central nervous system stimulation.
Phenyltoloxamine Citrate
Phenyltoloxamine is an H_1 blocking agent which interferes with the action of histamine primarily in capillaries surrounding mucous tissues and sensory nerves of nasal and adjacent areas. It has the ability to interfere with certain actions of acetylcholine-inhibiting secretions in the nose, mouth and pharynx. It commonly causes CNS depression.
Chlorpheniramine Maleate
Chlorpheniramine competitively antagonizes most of the smooth muscle stimulating actions of histamine on the H_1 receptors of the GI tract, uterus, large blood vessels and bronchial muscle. It also antagonizes the action of histamine that results in increased capillary permeability and the formation of edema.
Indications and Usage: For the relief of nasal congestion and eustachian tube congestion associated with the common cold, sinusitis and acute upper respiratory infections. Also indicated symptomatic relief of perennial and seasonal allergic rhinitis, vasomotor rhinitis. Decongestants in combination with antihistamines have been used to relieve eustachian

Continued on next page

Bristol—Cont.

tube congestion associated with acute eustachian salpingitis, aerotitis and serous otitis media.
Contraindications: Patients with severe hypertension, severe coronary artery disease, patients on MAO inhibitor therapy; patients with narrow angle glaucoma, urinary retention, peptic ulcer and during an asthmatic attack. Also contraindicated in patients with hypersensitivity or idiosyncrasy to sympathomimetic amines or antihistamines.
Warnings: Sympathomimetic amines should be used judiciously and sparingly in patients with hypertension, diabetes mellitus, ischemic heart disease, increased intraocular pressure, hyperthyroidism or prostatic hypertrophy. See, however, CONTRAINDICATIONS. Sympathomimetics may produce central nervous system stimulation with convulsions or cardiovascular collapse with accompanying hypotension.
Antihistamines may impair mental and physical abilities required for the performance of potentially hazardous tasks, such as driving a vehicle or operating machinery, and may impair mental alertness in children. Chlorpheniramine and phenyltoloxamine have an atropine-like action and should be used with caution in patients with increased intraocular pressure, cardiovascular disease, hypertension or in patients with a history of bronchial asthma. See, however, CONTRAINDICATIONS.
Do not exceed recommended dosage.
Precautions: Patients with diabetes, hypertension, cardiovascular disease and hyperreactivity to ephedrine. The antihistaminics may cause drowsiness and ambulatory patients who operate machinery or motor vehicles should be cautioned accordingly.
Drug Interactions: MAO inhibitors and beta adrenergic blockers increase the effect of sympathomimetics. Sympathomimetics may reduce the antihypertensive effects of methyldopa, mecamylamine, reserpine and veratrum alkaloids. Concomitant use of antihistamines with alcohol, tricyclic antidepressants, barbiturates and other CNS depressants may have an additive effect.
Pregnancy Category C: Animal reproduction studies have not been conducted with Naldecon. It is also not known whether Naldecon can cause fetal harm when administered to a pregnant woman or can effect reproductive capacity. Naldecon should be given to a pregnant woman only if clearly needed.
Nursing Mothers: Caution should be exercised when this drug is given to nursing mothers due to the higher than usual risk of the sympathomimetic amines in infants.
Adverse Reactions: Hyperreactive individuals may display ephedrine-like reactions such as tachycardia, palpitations, headache, dizziness or nausea. Patients sensitive to antihistamines may experience mild sedation. Sympathomimetics have been associated with certain untoward reactions including restlessness, tremor, weakness, pallor, respiratory difficulty, dysuria, insomnia, hallucinations, convulsions, CNS depression, arrhythmias and cardiovascular collapse with hypotension. Possible side effects of antihistamines are drowsiness, restlessness, dizziness, weakness, dry mouth, anorexia, nausea, vomiting, headache, nervousness, blurring of vision, polyuria, heartburn, dysuria and, very rarely, dermatitis.
Dosage and Administration: This chart represents single dosages for the products listed below. Usual dosage schedule for Naldecon Pediatric Drops, Naldecon Pediatric Syrup and Naldecon Syrup is every 3 to 4 hours, not to exceed four doses in a 24-hour period. For sustained-action Naldecon Tablets, doses should be administered on arising, in midafternoon, and at bedtime.
[See table below].
How Supplied:
NDC 0015-5600—Naldecon Tablets
NDC 0015-5601—Naldecon Syrup
NDC 0015-5615—Naldecon Pediatric Drops
NDC 0015-5616—Naldecon Pediatric Syrup
For information on package sizes available, refer to the current price schedule.
[*Shown in Product Identification Section*]

Single Dosage for ...	Naldecon Pediatric Drops	Naldecon Pediatric Syrup	Naldecon Syrup	Naldecon Tablets
3 to 6 months (10–20 lbs)	¼ dropperful (0.25 ml)			
6 to 12 months (20–30 lbs)	½ dropperful (0.5 ml)	½ teaspoonful		
1 to 6 years (30–50 lbs)	1 dropperful (1.0 ml)	1 teaspoonful		
6 to 12 years (over 50 lbs)		2 teaspoonfuls	½ teaspoonful	½ tablet
over 12 years			1 teaspoonful	1 tablet

NALDECON-CX® SUSPENSION Ⓒ
Decongestant/Expectorant/Antitussive

Description: Each teaspoonful (5 ml) of Naldecon-CX Suspension contains:
Phenylpropanolamine HC1 ....18 mg
Guaifenesin ....200 mg
Codeine Phosphate
(Warning: May be Habit Forming) ...10 mg
Indications: Provide prompt relief from cough and nasal congestion due to the common cold, bronchitis, nasopharyngitis, and influenza. Codeine temporarily quiets non-productive coughing by its antitussive action while guaifenesin's expectorant action helps loosen phlegm and bronchial secretions. Phenylpropanolamine reduces swelling of nasal passages and shrinks swollen membranes. This combination production is antihistamine and alcohol free.
Contraindications: Hypersensitivity to guaifenesin, codeine or sympathomimetic amines.
Warnings: Nervousness, dizziness or sleeplessness may occur if recommended dosage is exceeded. Do not give this product to a child with high blood pressure, heart disease, diabetes or thyroid disease except under the advice and supervision of a physician. Do not give this product to a child presently taking a prescription drug containing a monamine oxidase inhibitor except under the advice and supervision of a physician. Do not administer this product for persistent or chronic cough associated with asthma or emphysema or when cough is accompanied by excessive secretions, except under the care and advice of a physician. A persistent cough may be a sign of a serious condition. If cough persists for more than 1 week, tends to recur, or is accompanied by high fever, rash or persistent headaches, consult a physician.
Dosage and Administration: Children 2 to 6 years—½ teaspoon 4 times daily. 6 to 12 years—1 teaspoon 4 times daily. Over 12 years—2 teaspoons 4 times daily.
How Supplied: Naldecon-CX Suspension—4 oz. and pint bottles.
(1) 5/81

NALDECON-DX® PEDIATRIC SYRUP OTC

Description: Each teaspoonful (5 ml.) of Naldecon-DX Syrup contains:
dextromethorphan hydrobromide ....7.5 mg
phenylpropanolamine hydrochloride ......9 mg
guaifenesin ....100 mg
alcohol 5%
Indications: Provide prompt relief from cough and nasal congestion due to the common cold, bronchitis, nasopharyngitis and recurrent bronchial coughing. Dextromethorphan temporarily quiets non-productive coughing by its antitussive action while guaifenesin's expectorant action helps loosen phlegm and bronchial secretions. Phenylpropanolamine reduces swelling of nasal passages; shrinks swollen membranes. This combination product is antihistamine-free.
Contraindications: Hypersensitivity to guaifenesin, dextromethorphan or sympathomimetic amines.
Warnings: Nervousness, dizziness or sleeplessness may occur if recommended dosage is exceeded. Do not give this product to a child with high blood pressure, heart disease, diabetes or thyroid disease except under the advice and supervision of a physician. Do not give this product to a child presently taking a prescription drug containing a monamine oxidase inhibitor except under the advice and supervision of a physician. Do not administer this product for persistent or chronic cough such as occurs with asthma or emphysema or when cough is accompanied by excessive secretions except under the care and advice of a physician. A persistent cough may be a sign of a serious condition. If cough persists for more than 1 week, tends to recur, or is accompanied by high fever, rash or persistent headaches, consult a physician.
Dosage and Administration: Children 2 to 6 years—1 teaspoonful 4 times daily. Over 6 years—2 teaspoons 4 times daily.
How Supplied: Naldecon-DX Syrup in 4 oz. and pint bottles.
(1) 8/80

NALDECON-EX PEDIATRIC DROPS OTC

Description: Each 1 ml. dropper of Naldecon-EX contains:
phenylpropanolamine hydrochloride ......9 mg
guaifenesin ....30 mg
alcohol 0.6%
Indications: Combined decongestant/expectorant designed specifically to promptly reduce the swelling of nasal membranes and to help loosen phlegm and bronchial secretions through productive coughing. This dual action is of particular value in infants with common cold, acute bronchitis, bronchiolitis, tracheobronchitis, nasopharyngitis and croup. This combination product is antihistamine-free.
Contraindications: Hypersensitivity to guaifenesin or sympathomimetic amines.
Warnings: Nervousness, dizziness or sleeplessness may occur if recommended dosage is exceeded. Do not give this product to a child with high blood pressure, heart disease, diabetes or thyroid disease except under the advice and supervision of a physician. Do not give this product to a child presently taking a prescription drug containing a monamine oxidase inhibitor except under the advice and supervi-

sion of a physician. Do not administer this product for persistent or chronic cough such as occurs with asthma or emphysema or when cough is accompanied by excessive secretions except under the care and advice of a physician. A persistent cough may be a sign of a serious condition. If cough persists for more than 1 week, tends to recur, or is accompanied by high fever, rash or persistent headaches, consult a physician.

Dosage and Administration: Dose should be adjusted to age or weight and be given 4 times a day (see calibrations on dropper). Administer by mouth only.

1-3 Months: (8-12 lbs.)	¼ ml
4-6 Months: (13-17 lbs.)	½ ml
7-9 Months: (18-20 lbs.)	¾ ml
10 Months or over (21 lbs. or more)	1 ml

Bottle label dosage reads as follows: children under 2 years of age: use only as directed by a physician.

How Supplied: Naldecon-EX Pediatric Drops in 30 ml. bottles with calibrated dropper.

(1) 8/80

PALLACE™ ℞
(megestrol acetate)

This is the full text of the latest Official Package Circular dated September 1981 [3601DIR-01].

THE USE OF PROGESTATIONAL AGENTS DURING THE FIRST FOUR MONTHS OF PREGNANCY IS NOT RECOMMENDED.

Progestational agents have been used beginning with the first trimester of pregnancy in an attempt to prevent habitual abortion or treat threatened abortion. There is no adequate evidence that such use is effective and there is evidence of potential harm to the fetus when such drugs are given during the first four months of pregnancy.

Furthermore, in the vast majority of women, the cause of abortion is a defective ovum, which progestational agents could not be expected to influence. In addition, the use of progestational agents, with their uterine-relaxant properties, in patients with fertilized defective ova may cause a delay in spontaneous abortion. Therefore, the use of such drugs during the first four months of pregnancy is not recommended.

Several reports suggest an association between intrauterine exposure to female sex hormones and congenital anomalies, including congenital heart defects and limb reduction defects.[1–5] One study[4] estimated a 4.7-fold increased risk of limb reduction defects in infants exposed in utero to sex hormones (oral contraceptives, hormone withdrawal tests for pregnancy, or attempted treatment for threatened abortion).

Some of these exposures were very short and involved only a few days of treatment. The data suggest that the risk of limb reduction defects in exposed fetuses is somewhat less than 1 in 1,000.

If the patient is exposed to Pallace during the first four months of pregnancy or if she becomes pregnant while taking this drug, she should be apprised of the potential risks to the fetus.

Description: Megestrol acetate is a white, crystalline solid chemically described as 17α-acetoxy-6-methyl-pregna-4,6-diene-3,20-dione. Its molecular weight is 384.5. The empirical formula is $C_{24}H_{32}O_4$.

Actions: While the precise mechanism by which Pallace (megestrol acetate) produces its antineoplastic effects against endometrial carcinoma is unknown at the present time, an antiluteinizing effect mediated via the pituitary has been postulated. There is also evidence to suggest a local effect as a result of the marked changes brought about by the direct instillation of progestational agents into the endometrial cavity. Likewise, the antineoplastic action of Pallace (megestrol acetate) on carcinoma of the breast is unclear.

Indications: Pallace (megestrol acetate) is indicated for the palliative treatment of advanced carcinoma of the breast or endometrium (i.e., recurrent, inoperable, or metastatic disease). It should not be used in lieu of currently accepted procedures such as surgery, radiation, or chemotherapy.

Contraindications: As a diagnostic test for pregnancy.

Warnings: Administration for up to 7 years of megestrol acetate to female dogs is associated with an increased incidence of both benign and malignant tumors of the breast. Comparable studies in rats and ongoing studies in monkeys are not associated with an increased incidence of tumors. The relationship of the dog tumors to humans is unknown but should be considered in assessing the benefit-to-risk ratio when prescribing Pallace and in surveillance of patients on therapy.

The use of Pallace (megestrol acetate) in other types of neoplastic disease is not recommended.

Precautions: There are no specific precautions identified for the use of Pallace (megestrol acetate) when used as recommended. Close, customary surveillance is indicated for any patient being treated for recurrent or metastatic cancer. Use with caution in patients with a history of thrombophlebitis.

Adverse Reactions: No untoward effects have been ascribed to Pallace (megestrol acetate) therapy. Reports have been received of patients developing carpal tunnel syndrome, deep vein thrombophlebitis and alopecia while taking megestrol acetate.

Overdosage: No serious side effects have resulted from studies involving Pallace (megestrol acetate) administered in dosages as high as 800 mg/day.

Dosage and Administration: Breast cancer: 160 mg/day (40 q.i.d.).

Endometrial carcinoma: 40-320 mg/day in divided doses.

At least two months of continuous treatment is considered an adequate period for determining the efficacy of Pallace (megestrol acetate).

How Supplied: Pallace is available as white, scored tablets containing 20 mg or 40 mg megestrol acetate in bottles of 100 tablets each.

NDC 0015-3601-60, 20 mg tablets, Bottles of 100

NDC 0015-3602-60, 40 mg tablets, Bottles of 100

References:

1. Gal I. Kirman B and Stern J: "Hormonal Pregnancy Tests and Congenital Malformation," Nature 216:83, 1967.
2. Levy EP, Cohen A and Fraser FC: "Hormone Treatment During Pregnancy and Congenital Heart Defects," Lancet 1:611, 1973.
3. Nora J and Nora A: "Birth Defects and Oral Contraceptives," Lancet 1:941, 1973.
4. Janench DT, Piper JM and Glebatis DM: "Oral Contraceptives and Congenital Limb-Reduction Defects," N Eng J Med, 291:697, 1974.
5. Heinonen OP, Slone D, Monson RR, Hook EB and Shapiro S: "Cardiovascular Birth Defects and Antenatal Exposure to Female Sex Hormones," N Eng J Med, 296:67, 1977.

Patient Labeling For Pallace™

Warning For Women

There is an increased risk of birth defects in children whose mothers take this drug during the first four months of pregnancy.

Pallace is similar to the progesterone hormones naturally produced by the body. Progesterone and progesterone-like drugs are used to treat menstrual disorders, to test if the body is producing certain hormones, and to treat some forms of cancer in women.

They have been used as a test for pregnancy but such use is no longer considered safe because of possible damage to a developing baby. Also, more rapid methods for testing for pregnancy are now available.

These drugs have also been used to prevent miscarriage in the first few months of pregnancy. No adequate evidence is available to show that they are effective for this purpose and there is evidence of an increased risk of birth defects, such as heart or limb defects, if these drugs are taken during the first four months of pregnancy. Furthermore, most cases of early miscarriage are due to causes which could not be helped by these drugs.

The exact risk of taking this drug early in pregnancy and having a baby with a birth defect is not known. However, one study found that babies born to women who had taken sex hormones (such as progesterone-like drugs) during the first three months of pregnancy were 4 to 5 times more likely to have abnormalities of the arms or legs than if their mothers had not taken such drugs. Some of these women had taken these drugs for only a few days. The chance that an infant whose mother had taken this drug will have this type of defect is about 1 in 1,000.

If you take Pallace and later find you were pregnant when you took it, be sure to discuss this with your doctor as soon as possible.

PLATINOL® ℞
(cisplatin for injection)

This is the full text of the latest Official Package Circular dated April 1982 [3070DIM-16].

WARNING

Platinol (cisplatin) should be administered under the supervision of a qualified physician experienced in the use of cancer chemotherapeutic agents. Appropriate management of therapy and complications is possible only when adequate diagnostic and treatment facilities are readily available.

Cumulative renal toxicity associated with Platinol is severe. Other major dose-related toxicities are myelosuppression and nausea and vomiting.

Ototoxicity, which may be more pronounced in children, and is manifested by tinnitus, and/or loss of high frequency hearing and occasionally deafness, is significant.

Anaphylactic-like reactions to Platinol have been reported. Facial edema, bronchoconstriction, tachycardia, and hypotension may occur within minutes of Platinol administration. Epinephrine, corticosteroids, and antihistamines have been effectively employed to alleviate symptoms (see "Warnings" and "Adverse Reactions" sections).

Description: Platinol (cisplatin) (cis-diamminedichloroplatinum) is a heavy metal complex containing a central atom of platinum surrounded by two chloride atoms and two ammonia molecules in the cis position. It is a white lyophylized powder with the molecular formula $Pt\,Cl_2H_6N_2$, and a molecular weight of 300.1. It is soluble in water or saline at 1 mg/ml and in dimethylformamide at 24 mg/ml. It has a melting point of 207°C.

Action: Platinol has biochemical properties similar to that of bifunctional alkylating agents producing interstrand and intrastrand

Continued on next page

Bristol—Cont.

crosslinks in DNA. It is apparently cell-cycle non-specific. Following a single I.V. dose, Platinol concentrates in liver, kidneys, and large and small intestines in animals and humans. Platinol apparently has poor penetration into the CNS.
Plasma levels of radioactivity decay in a biphasic manner after an I.V. bolus dose of radioactive Platinol to patients. The initial plasma half-life is 25 to 49 minutes, and the post-distribution plasma half-life is 58 to 73 hours. During the post-distribution phase, greater than 90% of the radioactivity in the blood is protein bound. Platinol is excreted primarily in the urine. However, urinary excretion is incomplete with only 27 to 43% of the radioactivity being excreted within the first 5 days post-dose in human beings. There are insufficient data to determine whether biliary or intestinal excretion occurs.
Indications: Platinol is indicated as palliative therapy to be employed as follows:
Metastatic Testicular Tumors—in established combination therapy with other approved chemotherapeutic agents in patients with metastatic testicular tumors who have already received appropriate surgical and/or radiotherapeutic procedures. An established combination therapy consists of Platinol, Blenoxane (Bleomycin Sulfate) and Velban (Vinblastine Sulfate).
Metastatic Ovarian Tumors—in established combination therapy with other approved chemotherapeutic agents in patients with metastatic ovarian tumors who have already received appropriate surgical and/or radiotherapeutic procedures. An established combination consists of Platinol and Adriamycin (Doxorubicin Hydrochloride). Platinol, as a single agent, is indicated as secondary therapy in patients with metastatic ovarian tumors refractory to standard chemotherapy who have not previously received Platinol therapy.
Advanced Bladder Cancer—Platinol is indicated as a single agent for patients with transitional cell bladder cancer which is no longer amenable to local treatments such as surgery and/or radiotherapy.
Contraindications: Platinol is contraindicated in patients with preexisting renal impairment. Platinal should not be employed in myelosuppressed patients, or patients with hearing impairment.
Platinol is contraindicated in patients with a history of allergic reactions to Platinol or other platinum-containing compounds.
Warnings: Platinol produces cumulative nephrotoxicity which may be potentiated by aminoglycoside antibiotics. The serum creatinine, BUN, creatinine clearance and magnesium, potassium and calcium levels should be measured prior to initiating therapy, and prior to each subsequent course. At the recommended dosage, Platinol should not be given more frequently than once every 3 to 4 weeks (see "Adverse Reactions").
Anaphylactic-like reactions to Platinol have been reported. These reactions have occurred within minutes of administration to patients with prior exposure to Platinol, and have been alleviated by administration of epinephrine, corticosteroids and antihistamines.
Since ototoxicity of Platinol is cumulative, audiometric testing should be performed prior to initiating therapy and prior to each subsequent dose of drug (see "Adverse Reactions").
Safe use in human pregnancy has not been established. Platinol is mutagenic in bacteria and produces chromosome aberrations in animal cells in tissue culture. In mice Platinol is teratogenic and embryotoxic.
Platinol has not been studied for its carcinogenic potential but compounds with similar mechanisms of action and mutagenicity have been reported to be carcinogenic.
Precautions: Peripheral blood counts should be monitored weekly. Liver function should be monitored periodically. Neurologic examination should also be performed regularly (see "Adverse Reactions").
Adverse Reactions:
Nephrotoxicity
Dose-related and cumulative renal insufficiency is the major dose-limiting toxicity of Platinol. Renal toxicity has been noted in 28 to 36% of patients treated with a single dose of 50 mg/M^2. It is first noted during the second week after a dose and is manifested by elevations in BUN and creatinine, serum uric acid and/or a decrease in creatinine clearance. **Renal toxicity becomes more prolonged and severe with repeated courses of the drug. Renal function must return to normal before another dose of Platinol can be given.**
Impairment of renal function has been associated with renal tubular damage. The administration of Platinol using a 6- to 8-hour infusion with intravenous hydration, and mannitol has been used to reduce nephrotoxicity. However, renal toxicity still can occur after utilization of these procedures.
Ototoxicity
Ototoxicity has been observed in up to 31% of patients treated with a single dose of Platinol 50 mg/M^2, and is manifested by tinnitus and/or hearing loss in the high frequency range (4,000 to 8,000 Hz). Decreased ability to hear normal conversational tones may occur occasionally. Ototoxic effects may be more severe in children receiving Platinol. Hearing loss can be unilateral or bilateral and tends to become more frequent and severe with repeated doses. It is unclear whether Platinol-induced ototoxicity is reversible. Careful monitoring of audiometry should be performed prior to initiation of therapy and prior to subsequent doses of Platinol.
Hematologic
Myelosuppression occurs in 25 to 30% of patients treated with Platinol. The nadirs in circulating platelets and leukocytes occur between days 18 to 23 (range 7.5 to 45) with most patients recovering by day 39 (range 13 to 62). Leukopenia and thrombocytopenia are more pronounced at higher doses (>50 mg/M^2). Anemia (decrease of >2 g hemoglobin/100 ml) occurs at approximately the same frequency and with the same timing as leukopenia and thrombocytopenia.
Gastrointestinal
Marked nausea and vomiting occur in almost all patients treated with Platinol, and are occasionally so severe that the drug must be discontinued. Nausea and vomiting usually begin within one to four hours after treatment and last up to 24 hours. Various degrees of nausea and anorexia may persist for up to one week after treatment.
Other Toxicities:
Serum Electrolyte Disturbances
Hypomagnesemia, hypocalcemia, hypokalemia and hypophosphatemia have been reported to occur in patients treated with Platinol and are probably related to renal tubular damage. Tetany has occasionally been reported in those patients with hypocalcemia and hypomagnesemia. Generally, normal serum electrolyte levels are restored by administering supplemental electrolytes and discontinuing Platinol.
Hyperuricemia
Hyperuricemia has been reported to occur at approximately the same frequency as the increases in BUN and serum creatinine. It is more pronounced after doses greater than 50 mg/M^2, and peak levels of uric acid generally occur between 3 to 5 days after the dose. Allopurinol therapy for hyperuricemia effectively reduces uric acid levels.
Neurotoxicity
Neurotoxicity, usually characterized by peripheral neuropathies, has occurred in some patients. Loss of taste and seizures have also been reported. Neuropathies resulting from Platinol treatment may occur after prolonged therapy (4 to 7 months); however, neurologic symptoms have been reported to occur after a single dose.
Platinol therapy should be discontinued when the symptoms are first observed. Preliminary evidence suggests peripheral neuropathy may be irreversible in some patients.
Anaphylactic-like Reactions
Anaphylactic-like reactions have been occasionally reported in patients previously exposed to Platinol. The reactions consist of facial edema, wheezing, tachycardia and hypotension within a few minutes of drug administration. Reactions may be controlled by intravenous epinephrine, corticosteroids or antihistamines. Patients receiving Platinol should be observed carefully for possible anaphylactic-like reactions and supportive equipment and medication should be available to treat such a complication.
Other toxicities reported to occur infrequently are cardiac abnormalities, anorexia and elevated SGOT.
Dosage and Administration:
Note: Needles or intravenous sets containing aluminum parts that may come in contact with Platinol should not be used for preparation or administration. Aluminum reacts with Platinol, causing precipitate formation and a loss of potency.
Metastatic Testicular Tumors—An effective combination for the treatment of patients with metastatic testicular carcinomas includes Platinol, Blenoxane (Bleomycin Sulfate) and Velban (Vinblastine Sulfate). Remission induction therapy consists of Platinol, Blenoxane (Bleomycin Sulfate) and Velban (Vinblastine Sulfate) in the following doses:

PLATINOL—20 mg/M^2 I.V. daily for 5 days (days 1–5) every three weeks for three courses.

BLENOXANE® (Bleomycin Sulfate)—30 units I.V. weekly (Day 2 of each week) for 12 consecutive doses.

VELBAN® (Vinblastine Sulfate)—0.15 to 0.2 mg/Kg I.V. twice weekly (Days 1 and 2) every three weeks for four courses (a total of eight doses).

Maintenance therapy for patients who respond to the above regimen consists of Velban (Vinblastine Sulfate) 0.3 mg/Kg I.V. every 4 weeks for a total of 2 years.
For directions for the administration of Blenoxane (Bleomycin Sulfate) and Velban (Vinblastine Sulfate), refer to their respective package insert.
Metastatic Ovarian Tumors—An effective combination for the treatment of patients with metastatic ovarian tumors includes Platinol and Adriamycin (Doxorubicin Hydrochloride) in the following doses:

PLATINOL—50 mg/M^2 I.V. once every 3 weeks (Day 1).

ADRIAMYCIN™ (Doxorubicin Hydrochloride)—50 mg/M^2 I.V. once every 3 weeks (Day 1).

For directions for the administration of Adriamycin (Doxorubicin Hydrochloride), refer to the Adriamycin (Doxorubicin Hydrochloride) package insert.
In combination therapy, Platinol and Adrilamycin (Doxorubicin Hydrochloride) are administered sequentially.
As a single agent, Platinol should be administered at a dose of 100 mg/M^2 I.V. once every 4 weeks.
Advanced Bladder Cancer—Platinol should be administered as a single agent at a dose of 50–70 mg/m^2 I.V. once every 3 to 4 weeks depending on the extent of prior exposure to radiation therapy and/or prior chemotherapy. For heavily pretreated patients an initial dose of 50

mg/m^2 repeated every 4 weeks is recommended.
Pretreatment hydration with 1 to 2 liters of fluid infused for 8 to 12 hours prior to a Platinol dose is recommended. The drug is then diluted in 2 liters of 5% Dextrose in ½ or ⅓N Saline containing 37.5 g of mannitol, and infused over a 6- to 8-hour period. Adequate hydration and urinary output must be maintained during the following 24 hours.
A repeat course of Platinol should not be given until the serum creatinine is below 1.5 mg/100 ml, and/or the BUN is below 25 mg/100 ml. A repeat course should not be given until circulating blood elements are at an acceptable level (platelets $\geq$100,000/mm^3, WBC $\geq$4,000/mm^3). Subsequent doses of Platinol should not be given until an audiometric analysis indicates that auditory acuity is within normal limits.
As with other potentially toxic compounds, caution should be exercised in handling the powder and preparing the solution of cisplatin. Skin reactions associated with accidental exposure to cisplatin may occur. The use of gloves is recommended. If cisplatin powder or solution contact skin or mucosae, immediately wash the skin or mucosae thoroughly with soap and water.
Preparation of Intravenous Solutions: The 10 mg and 50 mg vials should be reconstituted with 10 ml or 50 ml of Sterile Water for Injection, U.S.P., respectively. Each ml of the resulting solution will contain 1 mg of Platinol.
Reconstitution as recommended results in a clear, colorless solution.
The reconstituted solution should be used intravenously only and should be administered by I.V. infusion over a 6- to 8-hour period. (See Dosage and Administration.)
Stability: Unopened vials of the dry powder must be stored in a refrigerator (2°C to 8°C). The recommended storage of unopened vials provides a stable product for 2 years.
The reconstituted solution is stable for 20 hours at room temperature (27°C).
Important Note: Once reconstituted, the solution should be kept at room temperature (27°C). If the reconstituted solution is refrigerated a precipitate will form.
Supply: PLATINOL (cisplatin) for Injection
NDC 0015-3070-20—Each amber vial contains 10 mg of cisplatin.
NDC 0015-3072-20—Each amber vial contains 50 mg of cisplatin.

POLYCILLIN® ℞
(ampicillin)
CAPSULES
250 mg. and 500 mg.
For Oral Suspension
125 mg. per 5 ml., 250 mg. per 5 ml., 500 mg. per 5 ml.
Pediatric Drops
100 mg. per ml.

POLYCILLIN-N®
(sterile ampicillin sodium)
For Intramuscular or Intravenous Injection

This is the full text of the latest Combined Official Package Circulars dated October 1977 [7988DIRO-16 Polycillin] *and May 1979* [7401DIRO-24 Polycillin-N]. (S 9/78)
Description: Polycillin (ampicillin) is a synthetic penicillin with a broad spectrum of bactericidal activity against both penicillin-susceptible Gram-positive organisms and many common Gram-negative pathogens.
Polycillin-N (sterile ampicillin sodium) contains 2.9 milliequivalents of sodium per 1 gram of drug.
Actions:
Pharmacology
Polycillin is stable in the presence of gastric acid and is well-absorbed from the gastrointestinal tract. It diffuses readily into most body tissues and fluids. However, penetration into the cerebrospinal fluid and brain occurs only when the meninges are inflamed. Ampicillin is excreted largely unchanged in the urine and its excretion can be delayed by concurrent administration of probenecid. The active form appears in the bile in higher concentrations than those found in serum. Ampicillin is the least serum-bound of all the penicillins, averaging about 20% compared to approximately 60 to 90% for other penicillins. Polycillin is well-tolerated by most patients and has been given in doses of 2 grams daily for many weeks without adverse reactions.
Microbiology
The following bacteria have been shown in **in vitro** studies to be susceptible to Polycillin:
GRAM-POSITIVE ORGANISMS: Hemolytic and nonhemolytic streptococci, **D. pneumoniae,** non-penicillinase-producing staphylococci, Clostridia spp., **B. anthracis, Listeria monocytogenes,** and most strains of enterococci.
GRAM-NEGATIVE ORGANISMS: H. influenzae, N. gonorrhoeae, N. meningitidis, Proteus mirabilis, and many strains of Salmonella, Shigella, and **E. coli.**
Polycillin does not resist destruction by penicillinase. Polycillin Susceptibility Test Discs, 10 mcg. should be used to estimate the **in vitro** susceptibility of bacteria to Polycillin.
Indications: Polycillin is indicated for the treatment of infections due to susceptible Gram-positive organisms including streptococci, pneumococci, penicillin G-susceptible staphylococci, and enterococci, and susceptible strains of Gram-negative bacteria including **H. influenzae, E. coli, Proteus mirabilis, N. gonorrhoeae, N. meningitidis,** Shigella, **S. typhosa** and other Salmonella.
Bacteriology studies to determine the causative organisms and their susceptibility to ampicillin should be performed. Therapy may be instituted prior to obtaining results of susceptibility testing.
It is advisable to reserve the parenteral form of this drug for moderately severe and severe infections and for patients who are unable to take the oral forms. A change to oral Polycillin (ampicillin) may be made as soon as appropriate.
Indicated surgical procedures should be performed.
Contraindications: A history of a previous hypersensitivity reaction to any of the penicillins is a contraindication.
Warning: Serious and occasionally fatal hypersensitivity (anaphylactoid) reactions have been reported in patients on penicillin therapy. Although anaphylaxis is more frequent following parenteral therapy, it has occurred in patients on oral penicillins. These reactions are more apt to occur in individuals with a history of sensitivity to multiple allergens.
There have been well-documented reports of individuals with a history of penicillin hypersensitivity reactions who have experienced severe hypersensitivity reactions when treated with a cephalosporin. Before therapy with a penicillin, careful inquiry should be made concerning previous hypersensitivity reactions to penicillins, cephalosporins, and other allergens.
Serious anaphylactoid reactions require immediate emergency treatment with epinephrine. Oxygen, intravenous steroids, and airway management, including intubation, should also be administered as indicated.
USAGE IN PREGNANCY: Safety for use in pregnancy has not been established.
Precautions: The possibility of superinfections with mycotic organisms or bacterial pathogens should be kept in mind during therapy. In such cases, discontinue the drug and substitute appropriate treatment.
As with any potent drug, periodic assessment of organ system function, including renal, hepatic, and hematopoietic, should be made during prolonged therapy.
With high urine concentrations of ampicillin, false-positive glucose reactions may occur if Clinitest, Benedict's Solution, or Fehling's Solution are used. Therefore, it is recommended that glucose tests based on enzymatic glucose oxidase reactions (such as Clinistix or Tes-Tape) be used.
Adverse Reactions: As with other penicillins, it may be expected that untoward reactions will be essentially limited to sensitivity phenomena. They are more likely to occur in individuals who have previously demonstrated hypersensitivity to penicillins and in those with a history of allergy, asthma, hay fever, or urticaria.
The following adverse reactions have been reported as associated with the use of ampicillin:
Gastrointestinal—Glossitis, stomatitis, black "hairy" tongue, nausea, vomiting, enterocolitis, pseudomembranous colitis, and diarrhea. (These reactions are usually associated with oral dosage forms.)
Hypersensitivity reactions—Skin rashes and urticaria have been reported frequently. A few cases of exfoliative dermatitis and erythema multiforme have been reported. Anaphylaxis is the most serious reaction experienced and has usually been associated with the parenteral dosage form.
Note: Urticaria, other skin rashes, and serum sickness-like reactions may be controlled with antihistamines and, if necessary, systemic corticosteroids. Whenever such reactions occur, ampicillin should be discontinued, unless, in the opinion of the physician, the condition being treated is life threatening and amenable only to ampicillin therapy. Serious anaphylactic reactions require the immediate use of epinephrine, oxygen, and intravenous steroids.
Liver—A moderate rise in serum glutamic oxaloacetic transaminase (SGOT) has been noted, particularly in infants, but the significance of this finding is unknown. Mild transitory SGOT elevations have been observed in individuals receiving larger (two to four times) than usual and oft-repeated intramuscular injections. Evidence indicates that glutamic oxaloacetic transaminase (GOT) is released at the site of intramuscular injection of ampicillin sodium and that the presence of increased amounts of this enzyme in the blood does not necessarily indicate liver involvement.
Hemic and Lymphatic Systems—Anemia, thrombocytopenia, thrombocytopenic purpura, eosinophilia, leukopenia, and agranulocytosis have been reported during therapy with the penicillins. These reactions are usually reversible on discontinuation of therapy and are believed to be hypersensitivity phenomena.
Other—Since infectious mononucleosis is viral in origin, ampicillin should not be used in the treatment. A high percentage of patients with mononucleosis who received ampicillin developed a skin rash.
Dosage:
Infections of the respiratory tract and soft tissues:
Oral: Patients weighing 20 Kg. (44 lbs.) or more: 250 mg. every 6 hours.
Patients weighing less than 20 Kg. (44 lbs.): 50 mg./Kg./day in equally divided doses at 6-to 8-hour intervals.
Parenteral: Patients weighing 40 Kg. (88 lbs.) or more: 250 to 500 mg. every 6 hours.
Patients weighing less than 40 Kg. (88 lbs.): 25 to 50 mg./Kg./day in equally divided doses at 6-to 8-hour intervals.
Infections of the gastrointestinal and genitourinary tracts:
Oral: Patients weighing 20 Kg. (44 lbs.) or more: 500 mg. every 6 hours.

Continued on next page

Bristol—Cont.

Patients weighing less than 20 Kg. (44 lbs.): 100 mg./Kg./day in equally divided doses at 6-to 8-hour intervals.
Infections of the gastrointestinal and genitourinary tracts (including those caused by Neisseria gonorrhoeae in females).
Parenteral: Patients weighing 40 Kg. (88 lbs.) or more: 500 mg. every 6 hours.
Patients weighing less than 40 Kg. (88 lbs.): 50 mg./Kg./day in equally divided doses at 6-to 8-hour intervals.
In the treatment of chronic urinary tract and intestinal infections, frequent bacteriological and clinical appraisal is necessary. Smaller doses than those recommended above should not be used. Higher doses should be used for stubborn or severe infections. In stubborn infections, therapy may be required for several weeks. It may be necessary to continue clinical and/or bacteriological follow-up for several months after cessation of therapy.
Urethritis in males or females due to N. gonorrhoeae:
Oral: 3.5 Grams, with 1.0 Gram probenecid, administered simultaneously.
Urethritis in males due to N. gonorrhoeae:
Parenteral: Adult: Two doses of 500 mg. each at an interval of 8 to 12 hours. Treatment may be repeated if necessary or extended if required.
In the treatment of complications of gonorrheal urethritis, such as prostatitis and epididymitis, prolonged and intensive therapy is recommended. Cases of gonorrhea with a suspected primary lesion of syphilis should have darkfield examinations before receiving treatment. In all other cases where concomitant syphilis is suspected, monthly serological tests should be made for a minimum of four months. The parenteral doses for the preceding infections may be given by either the intramuscular or intravenous route. A change to oral Polycillin (ampicillin) may be made when appropriate.
Bacterial Meningitis
Parenteral ONLY: Adults and Children: 150 to 200 mg./Kg./day in equally divided doses every 3 to 4 hours. (Treatment may be initiated with intravenous drip therapy and continued with intramuscular injections.) The doses for other infections may be given by either the intravenous or intramuscular route.
Septicemia
Parenteral ONLY: Adults and Children: 150 to 200 mg./Kg./day. Start with intravenous administration for at least three days and continue with the intramuscular route every 3 to 4 hours.
Treatment of all infections should be continued for a minimum of 48 to 72 hours beyond the time that the patient becomes asymptomatic or evidence of bacterial eradication has been obtained. A minimum of 10-days treatment is recommended for any infection caused by Group A beta-hemolytic streptococci to help prevent the occurrence of acute rheumatic fever or acute glomerulonephritis.
The following Dosage chart may be useful as a guide to therapy with the Pediatric Drops.
[See table below].
Note: For ease in administration, the dropper assembly is calibrated at the 62.5–mg. level (½ dropperful), at the 94–mg. level (¾ dropperful), and at the 125–mg. level (1 dropperful). Children over 10 Kg. (22 pounds) would generally be dosed with Polycillin for Oral Suspension.

Polycillin-N—Reconstitution Volumes

NDC 0015	Label Claim	Recommended Amount of Diluent	Withdrawable Volume	Concentration (in mg/ml)
7401-20	125 mg.	1.2 ml.	1.0 ml.	125 mg.
7402-20	250 mg.	1.0 ml.	1.0 ml.	250 mg.
7403-20	500 mg.	1.8 ml.	2.0 ml.	250 mg.
7404-20	1.0 gram	3.5 ml.	4.0 ml.	250 mg.
7405-20	2.0 gram	6.8 ml.	8.0 ml.	250 mg.

Directions for Dispensing Oral Suspension and Pediatric Drops: Prepare these formulations at the time of dispensing. For ease in preparation, add water to the bottle in two portions and shake well after each addition. Add the total amount of water as directed on the labeling of the package being dispensed. The reconstituted formulation is stable for 14 days under refrigeration.
Parenteral—Directions For Use: Use only freshly prepared solutions. Intramuscular and intravenous injections should be administered within one hour after preparation, since the potency may decrease significantly after this period.
For Intramuscular Use: Dissolve contents of a vial with the amount of Sterile Water for Injection, U.S.P. or Bacteriostatic Water for Injection, U.S.P., listed in the table below.
[See table above].
While Polycillin-N, 1.0 g. and 2.0 g., are primarily for intravenous use, they may be administered intramuscularly when the 250-mg. or 500-mg. vials are unavailable. In such instances, dissolve in 3.5 or 6.8 ml. Sterile Water for Injection, U.S.P. or Bacteriostatic Water for Injection, U.S.P., respectively. The resulting solution will provide a concentration of 250 mg. per ml.
Polycillin-N, 125 mg., is intended primarily for pediatric use. It also serves as a convenient dosage form when small parenteral doses of the antibiotic are required.
For Direct Intravenous Use: Add 5 ml. Sterile Water for Injection, U.S.P. or Bacteriostatic Water for Injection, U.S.P. to the 125-, 250-, and 500- mg. vials and administer slowly over a 3- to 5- minute period. Polycillin-N, 1.0 Gm. or 2.0 Gm., may also be given by direct intravenous administration. Dissolve in 7.4 or 14.8 ml. Sterile Water for Injection, U.S.P., or Bacteriostatic Water for Injection, U.S.P. respectively, and administer slowly over at least 10 to 15 minutes. CAUTION: More rapid administration may result in convulsive seizures.
For Administration by Intravenous Drip: Reconstitute as directed above (For Direct Intravenous Use) prior to diluting with Intravenous Solution. Stability studies on ampicillin sodium at several concentrations in various intravenous solutions indicate the drug will lose less than 10% activity at the temperatures noted for the time periods stated:
[See table on next page].
Only those solutions listed above should be used for the intravenous infusion of Polycillin-N. The concentrations should fall within the range specified. The drug concentration and the rate and volume of the infusion should be adjusted so that the total dose of ampicillin is administered before the drug loses its stability in the solution in use.
"Piggyback" I.V. Package: These glass vials contain the labeled quantity of POLYCILLIN-N and are intended for intravenous administration. The diluent and volume are specified on the label of each package.
Hospital Bulk Package: This glass vial contains 10 grams ampicillin and is designed for use in the pharmacy in preparing I.V. additives. Add 94 ml Sterile Water for Injection, U.S.P. The resulting solution will contain 100 milligrams ampicillin activity per ml, and is stable up to one hour at room temperature. Diluting further within one hour to 5 mg to 10 mg per ml, the resulting solution will remain stable for 8 hours at room temperature or 72 hours under refrigeration.
Caution: NOT TO BE DISPENSED AS A UNIT.
Supply: Polycillin (ampicillin) for Oral Suspension. Each 5 ml. of reconstituted suspension contains ampicillin trihydrate equivalent to 125, 250, or 500 mg. ampicillin.
NDC 0015-7988—125 mg., 80 ml., 100 ml., 150 ml. and 200 ml. bottles
NDC 0015-7998—250 mg., 80 ml., 100 ml., 150 ml. and 200 ml. bottle
NDC 0015-7884—500 mg., 100 ml. bottle
Polycillin (ampicillin) Capsules. Ampicillin trihydrate equivalent to 250 or 500 mg. ampicillin per capsule.
NDC 0015-7992—250 mg.
NDC 0015-7993—500 mg.
[*Shown in Product Identification Section*]
Polycillin (ampicillin) for oral suspension. Each ml. of reconstituted pediatric drops contains ampicillin trihydrate equivalent to 100 mg. ampicillin.
NDC 0015-7884—100 mg., 20 ml. bottles.
Polycillin-N (sterile ampicillin sodium) for I.M. or I.V. Injection. Ampicillin sodium equivalent to 125, 250, 500 mg., 1 g or 2 g ampicillin per vial.
NDC 0015-7401-20—125–mg. vial.
NDC 0015-7402-20—250–mg. vial.
NDC 0015-7403-20—500–mg. vial.
NDC 0015-7404-20—1.0–Gm. vial.
NDC 0015-7405-20—2.0 Gm. vial.
NDC 0015-7403-94—500 mg. "piggyback" vial.
NDC 0015-7404-94—1.0 gram "piggyback" vial.
NDC 0015-7405-95—2.0 gram "piggyback" vial.
NDC 0015-7100-98—10 gram Hospital Bulk Package
For information on package sizes available, refer to the current price sheets.

Pediatric Drops—Dosage Chart

Weight		Infection	
Kg.	Lb.	Respiratory	GU/GI
Up to 5	Up to 11	62.5 mg. q. 6h. (½ dropperful q. 6h.)	125 mg. q. 6h. (1 dropperful q. 6h.)
5 to 7.5	11 to 16.5	94 mg. q. 6h. (¾ dropperful q. 6h.)	188 mg. q. 6h. (1½ dropperfuls q. 6h.)
7.6 to 10	16.6 to 22	125 mg. q. 6h. (1 dropperful q. 6h.)	250 mg. q. 6h. (2 dropperfuls q. 6h.)

POLYCILLIN-PRB® ℞
(ampicillin-probenecid)
For Oral Suspension
Ampicillin Trihydrate equivalent to 3.5 Grams ampicillin with 1.0 Gram probenecid

This is the full text of the latest Official Package Circular dated October 1977 [7607 DIRO-06].
Description: Polycillin-PRB (ampicillin-probenecid) is a semisynthetic penicillin in combination with probenecid.
Actions:
Pharmacology
Ampicillin is stable in the presence of gastric acid and is well-absorbed from the gastrointes-

tinal tract. It diffuses readily into most body tissues and fluids. However, penetration into the cerebrospinal fluid and brain occurs only when the meninges are inflamed. Ampicillin is excreted largely unchanged in the urine and its excretion can be delayed by concurrent administration of probenecid. The active form appears in the bile in higher concentrations than those found in serum. Ampicillin is the least serum-bound of all the penicillins, averaging about 20% compared to approximately 60 to 90% for other penicillins. Probenecid inhibits the renal tubular secretion of penicillins causing an increased serum level of the antibiotic.

Microbiology

Neisseria gonorrhoeae has been shown in **in vitro** studies to be susceptible to ampicillin.

Indications: Ampicillin-probenecid is indicated for the treatment of uncomplicated infections (urethral, endocervical, or rectal) due to **N. gonorrhoeae** in males and females.

Susceptibility studies should be performed with recurrent infections or when resistant strains are encountered. Therapy may be instituted prior to obtaining results of susceptibility testing.

Contraindications:

Ampicillin

A history of previous hypersensitivity reactions to any of the penicillins is a contraindication.

Probenecid

Polycillin-PRB should not be given to individuals with a known hypersensitivity to probenecid. It is not recommended for patients with known blood dyscrasias, uric acid kidney stones or during an acute attack of gout.

Warnings: Serious and occasionally fatal hypersensitivity reactions have been reported in patients on penicillin therapy. Although anaphylaxis is more frequent following parenteral therapy, it has occurred in patients on oral penicillins. These reactions are more apt to occur in individuals with a history of sensitivity to multiple allergens.

There have been well-documented reports of individuals with a history of penicillin hypersensitivity reactions who have experienced severe hypersensitivity reactions when treated with a cephalosporin. Before therapy with a penicillin, careful inquiry should be made concerning previous hypersensitivity reactions to penicillins, cephalosporins, and other allergens. If an allergic reaction occurs, the patient should be treated with the usual agents, e.g., pressor amines, antihistamines, and corticosteroids. Serious anaphylactoid reactions require emergency treatment with epinephrine. Oxygen, intravenous steroids, and airway management, including intubation, should also be administered as indicated.

USAGE IN PREGNANCY: Safety for use in pregnancy has not been established.

Precautions: Cases of gonococcal infection with a suspected lesion of syphilis should have darkfield examinations ruling out syphilis before receiving ampicillin. Patients who do not have suspected lesions of syphilis and are treated with ampicillin should have a follow-up serologic test for syphilis each month for four months to detect syphilis that may have been masked by treatment for gonorrhea. Patients with gonorrhea who also have syphilis should be given additional appropriate parenteral penicillin treatment.

Adverse Reactions: As with other penicillins, it may be expected that untoward reactions to ampicillin will be essentially limited to sensitivity phenomena. They are more likely to occur in individuals who have previously demonstrated hypersensitivity to penicillins and in those with a history of allergy, asthma, hay fever, or urticaria.

The following adverse reactions have been reported as associated with the use of ampicillin:

Gastrointestinal—Glossitis, stomatitis, black "hairy" tongue, nausea, vomiting, enterocolitis, pseudomembranous colitis, and diarrhea. (These reactions are usually associated with oral dosage forms.)

Polycillin-N IV Stability

Room Temperature (25°C.)

Diluent	Concentrations	Stability Periods
Sterile Water for Injection	up to 30 mg./ml.	8 hours
Isotonic Sodium Chloride	up to 30 mg./ml.	8 hours
M/6 Sodium Lactate Solution	up to 30 mg./ml.	8 hours
5% Dextrose in Water	10 to 20 mg./ml.	2 hours
5% Dextrose in Water	up to 2 mg./ml.	4 hours
5% Dextrose in 0.45% NaCl	up to 2 mg./ml.	4 hours
10% Invert Sugar in Water	up to 2 mg./ml.	4 hours
Lactated Ringer's Solution	up to 30 mg./ml.	8 hours
Refrigerated (4°C.)		
Sterile Water for Injection	30 mg./ml.	48 hours
Sterile Water for Injection	up to 20 mg./ml.	72 hours
Isotonic Sodium Chloride	30 mg./ml.	48 hours
Isotonic Sodium Chloride	up to 20 mg./ml.	72 hours
Lactated Ringer's Solution	up to 30 mg./ml.	24 hours
M/6 Sodium Lactate	up to 30 mg./ml.	8 hours
5% Dextrose in Water	up to 20 mg./ml.	4 hours
5% Dextrose in 0.45% NaCl	up to 10 mg./ml.	4 hours
10% Invert Sugar	up to 20 mg./ml.	3 hours

Hypersensitivity reactions—Skin rashes and urticaria have been reported frequently. A few cases of exfoliative dermatitis and erythema multiforme have been reported. Anaphylaxis is the most serious reaction experienced and has usually been associated with the parenteral form.

Serious acute hypersensitivity reactions may require the use of epinephrine, oxygen, and airway management, which may include endotracheal intubation, intravenous steroids, and repletion of plasma volume.

Liver—A moderate rise in serum glutamic oxaloacetic transaminase (SGOT) has been noted, but the significance of this finding is unknown.

Hemic and Lymphatic Systems—Anemia, thrombocytopenia, thrombocytopenic purpura, eosinophilia, leukopenia, and agranulocytosis have been reported during therapy with the penicillins. These reactions are usually reversible on discontinuation of therapy and are believed to be hypersensitivity phenomena.

Dosage: Acute N. gonorrhoeae infections in adult males and females.

3.5 Grams ampicillin, with 1.0 Gram probenecid, administered simultaneously. One bottle contains enough of each drug for the required single dose.

It is desirable that follow-up cultures be obtained from the original site(s) of infection 7 to 14 days after therapy.

In women, it is also desirable to obtain culture test-of-cure from both the endocervical and anal canal.

Directions For Dispensing Oral Suspension: Prepare this formulation at the time of dispensing. For ease in preparation, add water to the bottle in two portions and shake well after each addition. Add the total amount of water as directed on the labeling of the package being dispensed. The reconstituted formulation is stable for 24 hours at room temperature.

Supply: POLYCILLIN-PRB (Ampicillin-Probenecid) for Oral Suspension. Ampicillin Trihydrate equivalent to 3.5 Grams ampicillin with 1.0 Gram probenecid, single-dose bottle. **NDC** 0015-7607

POLYMOX® ℞

(amoxicillin)

CAPSULES

250 mg. and 500 mg.

FOR ORAL SUSPENSION

125 mg. per 5 ml., 250 mg. per 5 ml.

PEDIATRIC DROPS

50 mg. per ml.

This is the full text of the latest Official Package Circular dated May 1976 [7276DIRO-07].

Description: Polymox® (amoxicillin) is a semisynthetic penicillin, an analogue of ampicillin, with a broad spectrum of bactericidal activity against Gram-positive organisms and many Gram-negative pathogens.

Actions:

Pharmacology

Polymox® is stable in the presence of gastric acid and is well absorbed from the gastrointestinal tract and may be given with no regard to food. It diffuses readily into most body tissues and fluids, with the exception of brain and spinal fluid, except when meninges are inflamed. The half-life of amoxicillin is 61.3 minutes. Most of the amoxicillin is excreted unchanged in the urine; its excretion can be delayed by concurrent administration of probenecid. Amoxicillin is not highly protein-bound. In blood serum, amoxicillin is approximately 20% protein-bound as compared to 60% for penicillin-G.

Orally administered doses of 250 mg. and 500 mg. amoxicillin capsules result in average peak blood levels one to two hours after administration in the range of 3.5 mcg./ml. to 5.0 mcg./ml. and 5.5 mcg./ml. to 7.5 mcg./ml. respectively.

Orally administered doses of amoxicillin suspension 125 mg./5 ml., and 250 mg./5 ml., result in average peak blood levels one to two hours after administration in the range of 1.5 mcg./ml. to 3.0 mcg./ml. and 3.5 mcg./ml. to 5.0 mcg./ml. respectively.

Detectable serum levels are observed up to 8 hours after an orally administered dose of amoxicillin. Approximately 60 percent of an orally administered dose of amoxicillin is excreted in the urine within six to eight hours.

Microbiology

Polymox® (amoxicillin) is similar to ampicillin in its bactericidal action against susceptible organisms during the stage of active multiplication. It acts through the inhibition of biosynthesis of cell wall mucopeptides. **In vitro** studies have demonstrated the susceptibility of most strains of the following Gram-positive bacteria: alpha- and beta-hemolytic streptococci, **Diplococcus pneumoniae,** nonpenicillinase-producing staphylococci, and **Streptococcus faecalis.** It is active **in vitro** against many strains of **Haemophilus influenzae, Neisseria gonorrhoeae, Escherichia coli** and **Proteus mirabilis.** Because it does not resist destruction by penicillinase, it is **not** effective against penicillinase-producing bacteria, particularly resistant staphylococci. All strains of Pseudomonas and most strains of Klebsiella and Enterobacter are resistant.

Disc Susceptibility Tests

Quantitative methods that require measurement of zone diameters give the most precise

Continued on next page

Bristol—Cont.

estimates of antibiotic susceptibility. One such procedure* has been recommended for use with discs for testing susceptibility to ampicillin-class antibiotics. Interpretations correlate diameters on the disc test with MIC values for amoxicillin. With this procedure, a report from the laboratory of "susceptible" indicates that the infecting organism is likely to respond to therapy. A report of "resistant" indicates that the infecting organism is not likely to respond to therapy. A report of "intermediate susceptibility" suggests that the organism would be susceptible if high dosage is used, or if the infection is confined to tissues and fluids (e.g., urine), in which high antibiotic levels are attained.

Indications: Polymox® (amoxicillin) is indicated in the treatment of infections due to susceptible strains of the following:

GRAM-NEGATIVE ORGANISMS—**H. influenzae, E. coli, P. mirabilis** and **N. gonorrhoeae.**

GRAM-POSITIVE ORGANISMS—Streptococci (including **Streptococcus faecalis**), **D. pneumoniae,** and nonpenicillinase-producing staphylococci.

Therapy may be instituted prior to obtaining results from bacteriological and susceptibility studies to determine the causative organisms and their susceptibility to amoxicillin.

Indicated surgical procedures should be performed.

Contraindications: A history of a previous hypersensitivity reaction to any of the penicillins is a contraindication.

Warning: Serious and occasionally fatal hypersensitivity (anaphylactoid) reactions have been reported in patients on penicillin therapy. Although anaphylaxis is more frequent following parenteral therapy, it has occurred in patients on oral penicillins. These reactions are more apt to occur in individuals with a history of sensitivity to multiple allergens.

There have been well-documented reports of individuals with a history of penicillin hypersensitivity reactions who have experienced severe hypersensitivity reactions when treated with a cephalosporin. Before therapy with a penicillin, careful inquiry should be made concerning previous hypersensitivity reactions to penicillins, cephalosporins, and other allergens.

SERIOUS ANAPHYLACTOID REACTIONS REQUIRE IMMEDIATE EMERGENCY TREATMENT WITH EPINEPHRINE. OXYGEN, INTRAVENOUS STEROIDS, AND AIRWAY MANAGEMENT, INCLUDING INTUBATION, SHOULD ALSO BE ADMINISTERED AS INDICATED.

Usage In Pregnancy: Safety for use in pregnancy has not been established.

Precautions: The possibility of superinfections with mycotic organisms or bacterial pathogens should be kept in mind during therapy. In such cases, discontinue the drug and substitute appropriate treatment.

As with any potent drug, periodic assessment of organ system function, including renal, hepatic, and hematopoietic, should be made during prolonged therapy.

Adverse Reactions: As with other penicillins, it may be expected that untoward reactions will be essentially limited to sensitivity phenomena. They are more likely to occur in individuals who have previously demonstrated hypersensitivity to penicillins and in those with a history of allergy, asthma, hay fever, or urticaria.

The following adverse reactions have been reported as associated with the use of penicillin:

Gastrointestinal—Glossitis, stomatitis, black "hairy" tongue, nausea, vomiting, and diarrhea. (These reactions are usually associated with oral dosage forms.)

Hypersensitivity Reactions—Skin rashes and urticaria have been reported frequently. A few cases of exfoliative dermatitis and erythema multiforme have been reported. Anaphylaxis is the most serious reaction experienced and has usually been associated with the parenteral dosage form.

Note: Urticaria, other skin rashes, and serum sickness-like reactions may be controlled with antihistamines and, if necessary, systemic corticosteroids. Whenever such reactions occur, penicillin should be discontinued unless, in the opinion of the physician, the condition being treated is life threatening and amenable only to penicillin therapy. Serious anaphylactic reactions require the immediate use of epinephrine, oxygen, and intravenous steroids.

Liver—A moderate rise in serum glutamic oxaloacetic transaminase (SGOT) has been noted, particularly in infants, but the significance of this finding is unknown.

Hemic and Lymphatic Systems—Anemia, thrombocytopenia, thrombocytopenic purpura, eosinophilia, leukopenia, and agranulocytosis have been reported during therapy with the penicillins. These reactions are usually reversible on discontinuation of therapy and are believed to be hypersensitivity phenomena.

Dosage and Administration: Infections of the ear, nose, and throat due to streptococci, pneumococci, nonpenicillinase-producing staphylococci and **H. influenzae;**

Infections of the genitourinary tract due to **E. coli, Proteus mirabilis,** and **Streptococcus faecalis;**

Infections of the skin and soft-tissues due to streptococci, susceptible staphylococci, and **E. coli:**

Usual Dosage: Adults: 250 mg. every 8 hours.
Children: 20 mg./Kg./day in divided doses every 8 hours.

Children weighing 20 Kg. or more should be dosed according to the adult recommendations.

In severe infections or those caused by less susceptible organisms: 500 mg. every 8 hours for adults, and 40 mg./Kg./day in divided doses every 8 hours for children may be needed.

Infections of the lower respiratory tract, due to streptococci, pneumococci, nonpenicillinase-producing staphylococci, and **H. influenzae:**

Usual Dosage: Adults: 500 mg. every 8 hours.
Children: 40 mg./Kg./day in divided doses every 8 hours.

Children weighing 20 Kg. or more should be dosed according to the adult recommendations.

Larger doses may be required for stubborn or severe infections.

The children's dosage is intended for individuals whose weight will not cause a dosage to be calculated greater than that recommended for adults.

Gonorrhea, acute uncomplicated ano-genital and urethral infections due to **N. gonorrhoeae:** (males and females) 3 grams as a single oral dose.

Cases of gonorrhea with a suspected lesion of syphilis should have dark-field examinations before receiving amoxicillin, and monthly serological tests for a minimum of four months. It should be recognized that in the treatment of chronic urinary tract infections, frequent bacteriological and clinical appraisals are necessary. Smaller doses than those recommended above should not be used. Even higher doses may be needed at times. In stubborn infections, therapy may be required for several weeks. It may be necessary to continue clinical and/or bacteriological follow-up for several months after cessation of therapy. Except for gonorrhea, treatment should be continued for a minimum of 48 to 72 hours beyond the time that the patient becomes asymptomatic or evidence of bacterial eradication has been obtained. It is recommended that there be at least 10 days treatment for any infection caused by hemolytic streptococci to prevent the occurrence of acute rheumatic fever or glomerulonephritis.

Dosage and Administration of Pediatric Drops: Usual dosage for all indications except infections of the lower respiratory tract:

Under 6 Kg. (13 lbs.): 0.5 ml. every 8 hours.
6-8 Kg. (13 to 18 lbs.): 1 ml. every 8 hours.
Infections of the lower respiratory tract:
Under 6 Kg. (13 lbs.): 1 ml. every 8 hours.
6-8 Kg. (13 to 18 lbs.): 2 ml. every 8 hours.

Children weighing more than 8 Kg. (18 lbs.) should receive the appropriate dose of the Oral Suspension 125 mg. or 250 mg./5 ml.

After reconstitution, the required amount of suspension should be placed directly on the child's tongue for swallowing. Alternate means of administration are to add the required amount of suspension to formula, milk, fruit juice, water, ginger ale, or cold drinks. These preparations should then be taken immediately. To be certain the child is receiving full dosage, such preparations should be consumed in entirety.

Directions For Dispensing Oral Suspension and Pediatric Drops:

Prepare these formulations at the time of dispensing. For ease in preparation, add water to the bottle in two portions and shake well after each addition. Add the total amount of water as directed on the labeling of the package being dispensed.

The reconstituted formulation is stable for 14 days at either room temperature or refrigeration.

How Supplied:

Polymox (amoxicillin) Capsules. Each capsule contains amoxicillin trihydrate equivalent to 250 or 500 mg. amoxicillin.

NDC 0015-7278—250 mg., bottles of 100 and 500.

NDC 0015-7279—500 mg., bottles of 50 and 100.

[*Shown in Product Identification Section*]

Polymox (amoxicillin) for Oral Suspension. Each 5 ml. of reconstituted suspension contains amoxicillin trihydrate equivalent to 125 or 250 mg. amoxicillin.

NDC 0015-7276—125 mg., 80 ml., 100 ml. and 150 ml. bottles.

NDC 0015-7277—250 mg., 80 ml., 100 ml. and 150 ml. bottles.

Polymox (amoxicillin) for Oral Suspension. Each ml. of reconstituted pediatric drops contains amoxicillin trihydrate equivalent to 50 mg. amoxicillin.

NDC 0015-7277—50 mg.

For information on package sizes available, refer to the current price sheets.

---

*Bauer, A.W., Kirby, W.M.M., Sherris, J.C., and Turck, M.: Antibiotic Testing by a Standardized Single Disc Method, Am. J. Clin. Pathol., 45:493, 1966; Standardized Disc Susceptibility Test, FEDERAL REGISTER 37:20527–29, 1972.

PROSTAPHLIN® ℞
(oxacillin sodium)
Capsules, Oral Solution, I.M. or I.V.

This is the full text of the latest Combined Official Package Circulars dated May 1978 [7977DIRO-09 Prostaphlin Capsules and Oral Solution *May 1978*] [7979DIR-22 Prostaphlin Injectable]. October 1981 (16) 7/82

Description: PROSTAPHLIN (oxacillin sodium monohydrate) is sodium 5-methyl-3-phenyl-4-isoxazolyl penicillin, a penicillinase-resistant, acid-resistant, semi-synthetic penicillin. Each gram of PROSTAPHLIN For Injection contains approximately 2.8 mEq. of sodium and is buffered with 40 mg. dibasic sodium phosphate.

Actions and Pharmacology: Prostaphlin is active against staphylococci (both penicillin

G-susceptible and resistant), pneumococci, and streptococci.

It is resistant to destruction by acid and is well-absorbed from the gastrointestinal tract. Distribution studies in man indicate that oxacillin can be detected in bile, amniotic fluid, cord serum and human milk and in trace amounts in normal cerebrospinal fluid.

The drug is well tolerated. Oral doses of 500 mg. to 2.0 Gm. every 6 hours for a period of one month produced no side effects in 40 normal adult volunteers. Intramuscular doses of 250 to 1000 mg. 4 times daily for 30 days produced no side effects in 40 normal adult volunteers. Laboratory and physical examinations showed no significant changes from control levels in the test subjects.

A single 250-mg. oral dose gives a 1-hour peak serum level of 1.65 mcg./ml. A 500-mg. dose peaks at about 2.6 mcg./ml. Peak serum levels with the oral solution occur somewhat earlier, about one-half hour after dosing. A single dose of 250-mg. oral solution gives a peak serum level of 1.9 mcg./ml.; of 500-mg., 4.8 mcg./ml. Intramuscular injections give peak serum levels 30 minutes after injection. A 250-mg. dose gives a level of 5.3 mcg./ml. while a 500-mg. dose peaks at 10.9 mcg./ml. Intravenous injection gives a peak about 5 minutes after the injection is completed. Slow I.V. dosing with 500 mg. gives a 5-minute peak of 43 mcg./ml. with a half-life of 20 to 30 minutes.

PROSTAPHLIN is active against most Gram-positive cocci including beta-hemolytic streptococci, pneumococci and nonpenicillinase-producing staphylococci. Because of its resistance to the enzyme penicillinase, it is also active against penicillinase-producing staphylococci.

Disc Susceptibility Tests: Quantitative methods that require measurement of zone diameters give the most precise estimates of antibiotic susceptibility. One such procedure* has been recommended for use with discs for testing susceptibility to methicillin class antibiotics. Interpretations correlate diameters on the disc test with MIC values for methicillin. With this procedure, a report from the laboratory of "susceptible" indicates that the infecting organism is likely to respond to therapy. A report of "resistant" indicates that the infecting organism is not likely to respond to therapy. A report of "intermediate susceptibility" suggests that the organism would be susceptible if high dosage is used, or if the infection is confined to tissues and fluids (e.g., urine), in which high antibiotic levels are attained.

Indications: Although the principal indication for oxacillin sodium is in the treatment of infections due to penicillinase-producing staphylococci, it may be used to initiate therapy in such patients in whom a staphylococcal infection is suspected. (See Important Note below.)

Bacteriologic studies to determine the causative organisms and their susceptibility to oxacillin sodium should be performed.

In serious life-threatening infections, oral preparations of the penicillinase-resistant penicillins should not be relied on for initial therapy.

Important Note: When it is judged necessary that treatment be initiated before definitive culture and susceptibility results are known, the choice of oxacillin sodium should take into consideration the fact that it has been shown to be effective only in the treatment of infections caused by pneumococci, Group A beta-hemolytic streptococci, and penicillin G-resistant and penicillin G-susceptible staphylococci. If the bacteriology report later indicates the infection is due to an organism other than a penicillin G-resistant staphylococcus susceptible to oxacillin sodium, the physician is advised to continue therapy with a drug other than oxacillin sodium or any other penicillinase-resistant semisynthetic penicillin.

Recent studies have reported that the percentage of staphylococcal isolates resistant to penicillin G outside the hospital is increasing, approximating the high percentage of resistant staphylococcal isolates found in the hospital. For this reason, it is recommended that a penicillinase-resistant penicillin be used as initial therapy for any suspected staphylococcal infection until culture and susceptibility results are known.

Oxacillin sodium is a compound that acts through a mechanism similar to that of methicillin against penicillin G-resistant staphylococci. Strains of staphylococci resistant to methicillin have existed in nature and it is known that the number of these strains reported has been increasing. Such strains of staphylococci have been capable of producing serious disease, in some instances resulting in fatality. Because of this, there is concern that widespread use of the penicillinase-resistant penicillins may result in the appearance of an increasing number of staphylococcal strains which are resistant to these penicillins.

Methicillin-resistant strains are almost always resistant to all other penicillinase-resistant penicillins (cross resistance with cephalosporin derivatives also occurs frequently). Resistance to any penicillinase-resistant penicillin should be interpreted as evidence of clinical resistance to all, in spite of the fact that minor variations in **in vitro** susceptibility may be encountered when more than one penicillinase-resistant penicillin is tested against the same strain of staphylococcus.

Contraindications: A previous hypersensitivity reaction to any penicillin is a contraindication.

Warnings: Serious and occasionally fatal hypersensitivity (anaphylactoid) reactions have been reported in patients on penicillin therapy. Although anaphylaxis is more frequent following parenteral therapy, it has occurred in patients on oral penicillins. These reactions are more apt to occur in individuals with a history of sensitivity to multiple allergens.

There have been well documented reports of individuals with a history of penicillin hypersensitivity reactions who have experienced severe hypersensitivity reactions when treated with a cephalosporin. Before therapy with a penicillin, careful inquiry should be made concerning previous hypersensitivity reactions to penicillins, cephalosporins, and other allergens. If an allergic reaction occurs, the drug should be discontinued and the patient treated with the usual agents e.g., pressor amines, antihistamines, and corticosteroids.

Precautions: Penicillin should be used with caution in individuals with histories of significant allergies and/or asthma.

The oral route of administration should not be relied upon in patients with severe illness, or with nausea, vomiting, gastric dilatation, cardiospasm, or intestinal hypermotility.

Occasional patients will not absorb therapeutic amounts of orally administered penicillin.

The possibility of bacterial and/or fungal overgrowth should be kept in mind during long-term therapy. If overgrowth of resistant organisms occurs, appropriate measures should be taken.

As with any potent drug, periodic assessment of organ system function, including renal, hepatic and hematopoietic, should be made during long-term therapy.

Experience in premature and newborn infants is limited. Caution should be exercised in administration of the drug to such patients and frequent evaluation of organ system function is recommended.

Safety for use in pregnancy has not been established.

Adverse Reactions: The hypersensitivity reactions reported are skin rashes, urticaria, serum sickness and anaphylactic reactions. Symptomatic and asymptomatic elevations of S.G.O.T. and S.G.P.T. have been reported following I.V./I.M. and oral use of oxacillin. Hypersensitivity has been considered to be the cause in most instances which are reversible. Pathological study has shown either a cholestatic or nonspecific hepatitis. Oral lesions such as glossitis and stomatitis have been reported. Fever, eosinophilia, oral and rectal moniliasis have also been reported. Hemolytic anemia, transient neutropenia with evidence of granulocytopenia or thrombocytopenia, neuropathy, and nephrotoxicity (oliguria, albuminuria, hematuria, pyuria, and/or cylindruria) are infrequent and usually associated with high doses of parenteral penicillin. Thrombophlebitis has occurred in a small percentage of patients after intravenous therapy.

In some newborns and infants receiving high doses of oxacillin sodium (150 to 175 mg./Kg./day), transient hematuria, albuminuria and azotemia have been encountered. Although the causal relationship is not entirely clear, infants and newborns treated with high doses of the drug should be observed closely for signs of renal impairment.

Administration and Dosage:

ORAL

Usual Adult Dose: For mild to moderate infections of the skin, soft tissue or upper respiratory tract—500 mg. every 4 to 6 hours for a minimum of 5 days.

Pediatric Dose: Children weighing more than 40 Kg. (88 lbs.) should receive adult dosage. Children weighing less than 40 Kg. (88 lbs.): For mild to moderately severe infections of the skin, soft tissue or upper respiratory tract—50 mg./Kg./day (25 mg./lb./day) in equally-divided doses at 6-hour intervals for at least 5 days.

Note: In serious or life-threatening infections, such as staphylococcal septicemia or other deep-seated severe infections, oral preparations of the penicillinase-resistant penicillins should not be relied upon for initial therapy. Oral absorption may be unreliable. Infections caused by Group A beta-hemolytic streptococci: The use of penicillin G, penicillin V, or phenethicillin is the preferred treatment, because of their greater activity against this agent. PROSTAPHLIN parenteral or parenteral methicillin sodium is advisable for initial treatment of these conditions.

Following initial control of the infections with the parenteral preparations, oral PROSTAPHLIN may be given for follow-up therapy in the following doses:

Adults: 1.0 Gm. every 4 to 6 hours.
Children: 100 mg/Kg./day (50 mg./lb./day) or greater in equally-divided doses at 4 to 6 hours intervals.

In serious systemic infection, therapy should be continued for at least 1 to 2 weeks after the patient is afebrile and cultures are sterile. Treatment of osteomyelitis may require several months of intensive therapy. The best use for this oral medication is in the prolonged follow-up therapy following successful initial treatment with parenterally administered penicillinase-resistant penicillin.

This medication is best taken on an empty stomach, preferably 1 to 2 hours before meals.

Directions for Dispensing Oral Solution

Prepare these formulations at the time of dispensing. For ease in preparation, add water to the bottle in two portions and shake well after each addition. Add the total amount of water as directed on the labeling of the package being dispensed. The reconstituted formulation is stable for 3 days at room temperature or 14 days under refrigeration.

PARENTERAL

The parenteral form of this drug should be considered for patients who are unable to take the oral form. The route of administration, however, should be changed to the oral form when parenteral therapy is no longer necessary.

For mild-to-moderate upper respiratory and localized skin and soft tissue infections:

Continued on next page

Bristol—Cont.

Adults and children weighing 40 Kg. (88 lbs.) or more: 250 mg. to 500 mg. every 4 to 6 hours.

Children weighing less than 40 Kg. (88 lbs.): 50 mg./Kg./day (25 mg./lb./day) in equally-divided doses every 6 hours.

Note: Absorption and excretion data indicate that doses of 25 mg./Kg./day (12.5 mg./lb./day) in prematures and neonates provide adequate therapeutic levels.

For more severe infections such as those of the lower respiratory tract or disseminated infections:

Adults and children weighing 40 Kg. (88 lbs.) or more: 1 Gm. or higher every 4 to 6 hours.

Children weighing less than 40 Kg. (88 lbs.): 100 mg./Kg./day (50 mg./lb./day) or higher in equally-divided doses every 4 to 6 hours.

Very severe infections may require very high doses and prolonged therapy.

INFECTIONS CAUSED BY GROUP A BETA-HEMOLYTIC STREPTOCOCCI SHOULD BE TREATED FOR AT LEAST 10 DAYS TO HELP PREVENT THE OCCURRENCE OF ACUTE RHEUMATIC FEVER OR ACUTE GLOMERULONEPHRITIS.

Directions For Use:

For Intramuscular Use: Use Sterile Water for Injection, U.S.P. Add 1.4 ml. to the 250-mg. vial, 2.7 ml. to the 500-mg. vial, 5.7 ml. to the 1.0-gram vial, 11.5 ml. to the 2.0-Gm. vial and 23 ml. to the 4.0-Gm. vial. Shake well until a clear solution is obtained. After reconstitution, vials will contain 250 mg. of active drug per 1.5 ml. of solution. The reconstituted solution is stable for 3 days at 70°F. or for one week under refrigeration (40°F.).

For Direct Intravenous Use: Use Sterile Water for Injection, U.S.P. or Sodium Chloride Injection, U.S.P. Add 5 ml. to the 250-mg. and 500-mg. vials, 10 ml. to the 1.0-gram vial, 20 ml. to the 2.0-gram vial, and 40 ml. to the 4.0-gram vial. Withdraw the entire contents and administer slowly over a period of approximately 10 minutes.

For Administration by Intravenous Drip: Reconstitute as directed above (For Direct Intravenous Use) prior to diluting with intravenous Solution. Stability studies on oxacillin sodium at concentrations of 0.5 mg./ml. and 2 mg./ml. in the intravenous solutions listed below indicate that the drug will lose less than 10% activity at room temperature (70°F.) during a six-hour period:

I.V. Solution
Normal Saline Solution
5% Dextrose in Water
5% Dextrose in Normal Saline
10% D-Fructose in Water
10% D-Fructose in Normal Saline
Lactated Ringer's Solution
Lactated Potassic Saline Injection
10% Invert Sugar in Water
10% Invert Sugar in Normal Saline
10% Invert Sugar plus 0.3% Potassium Chloride in Water
Travert 10% Electrolyte #1
Travert 10% Electrolyte #2
Travert 10% Electrolyte #3

Only those solutions listed above should be used for the intravenous infusion of PROSTAPHLIN. The concentration of the antibiotic should fall within the range of 0.5 to 2.0 mg./ml. The drug concentration and the rate and volume of the infusion should be adjusted so that the total dose of oxacillin is administered before the drug loses its stability in the solution in use.

"Piggyback" I.V. Package: This glass vial contains the labeled quantity of Prostaphlin and is intended for intravenous administration. The diluent and volume are specified on the label of each package.

Following reconstitution, the solution is stable for 24 hours at room temperature.

Hospital Bulk Package: This glass vial contains 10 grams Prostaphlin and is designed for use in the pharmacy in preparing I.V. additives. Add 93 ml of Sterile Water for Injection, U.S.P. The resulting solution will contain 100 mg oxacillin activity per ml. Following reconstitution in this manner, the solutions are stable for 24 hours at room temperature.

CAUTION. NOT TO BE DISPENSED AS A UNIT.

Supply: PROSTAPHLIN (oxacillin sodium) Capsules. Each capsule contains oxacillin sodium equivalent to 250 or 500 mg. oxacillin.
NDC-0015-7977—250 mg.
NDC-0015-7982—500 mg.

[*Shown in Product Identification Section*]

PROSTAPHLIN (oxacillin sodium) for Oral Solution. Each 5 ml. of reconstituted solution contains oxacillin sodium equivalent to 250 mg. oxacillin.
NDC-0015-7985—250 mg., 100 ml. bottles.

PROSTAPHLIN (oxacillin sodium) for Injection. Oxacillin sodium equivalent to 250, 500 mg., 1, 2, 4 or 10 grams oxacillin per vial.
NDC 0015-7978—250 mg. vial
NDC 0015-7979—500 mg. vial
NDC 0015-7981—1.0 Gm. vial
NDC 0015-7970—2.0 Gm. vial
NDC 0015-7300—4.0 Gm. vial
NDC 0015-7981—1.0-Gm. "Piggyback" vial.
NDC 0015-7970—2.0-Gm. "Piggyback" vial.
NDC 0015-7300—4.0-Gm. "Piggyback" vial.
NDC 0015-7103-28—10 gram—Hospital Bulk Package

For information on package sizes available, refer to the current price sheets.

---

*Bauer, A.W., Kirby, W.M.M., Sherris, J.C. and Turck, M.: Antibiotic Testing by a Standardized Single Disc Method, Am. J. Clin. Pathol., 45:493, 1966; Standardized Disc Susceptibility Test, FEDERAL REGISTER 37:20527–29, 1972.

SALURON® ℞
(hydroflumethiazide)

This is the full text of the latest Official Package Circular dated December 1976 [5410DIRO-10].

Description: Saluron (hydroflumethiazide) is a potent oral diuretic-antihypertensive agent of low toxicity developed by Bristol Laboratories.

Action: The mechanism of action results in an interference with the renal tubular mechanism of electrolyte reabsorption. At maximal therapeutic dosage all thiazides are approximately equal in their diuretic potency. The mechanism whereby thiazides function in the control of hypertension is unknown.

Indications: Saluron is indicated as adjunctive therapy in edema associated with congestive heart failure, hepatic cirrhosis, and corticosteroid and estrogen therapy.

Saluron has also been found useful in edema due to various forms of renal dysfunction such as nephrotic syndrome, acute glomerulonephritis, and chronic renal failure.

Saluron is indicated in the management of hypertension either as the sole therapeutic agent or to enhance the effectiveness of other antihypertensive drugs in the more severe forms of hypertension.

Usage in Pregnancy: The routine use of diuretics in an otherwise healthy woman is inappropriate and exposes mother and fetus to unnecessary hazard. Diuretics do not prevent development of toxemia of pregnancy, and there is no satisfactory evidence that they are useful in the treatment of developed toxemia.

Edema during pregnancy may arise from pathological causes or from the physiologic and mechanical consequences of pregnancy. Thiazides are indicated in pregnancy when edema is due to pathologic causes, just as they are in the absence of pregnancy (however, see Warnings, below). Dependent edema in pregnancy, resulting from restriction of venous return by the expanded uterus, is properly treated through elevation of the lower extremities and use of support hose; use of diuretics to lower intravascular volume in this case is illogical and unnecessary. There is hypervolemia during normal pregnancy which is harmful to neither the fetus nor the mother (in the absence of cardiovascular disease), but which is associated with edema, including generalized edema, in the majority of pregnant women. If this edema produces discomfort, increased recumbency will often provide relief. In rare instances, this edema may cause extreme discomfort which is not relieved by rest. In these cases, a short course of diuretics may provide relief and may be appropriate.

Contraindications: Patients with anuria or hypersensitivity to this or other sulfonamide derived drugs.

Warnings: Saluron should be used with caution in severe renal disease. In patients with renal disease, thiazides may precipitate azotemia. Cumulative effects of the drug may develop in patients with impaired renal function.

Thiazides should be used with caution in patients with impaired hepatic function or progressive liver disease, since minor alterations of fluid and electrolyte balance may precipitate hepatic coma.

Thiazides may be additive or potentiative of the action of other antihypertensive drugs. Potentiation occurs with ganglionic or peripheral adrenergic blocking drugs.

Sensitivity reactions may occur in patients with a history of allergy or bronchial asthma.

The possibility of exacerbation or activation of systemic lupus erythematosus has been reported.

Usage in Pregnancy: Thiazides cross the placental barrier and appear in cord blood. The use of thiazides in pregnant women requires that the anticipated benefit be weighed against possible hazards to the fetus. These hazards include fetal or neonatal jaundice, thrombocytopenia, and possibly other adverse reactions which have occurred in the adult.

Nursing Mothers: Thiazides appear in breast milk. If use of the drug is deemed essential, the patient should stop nursing.

Precautions: Periodic determination of serum electrolytes to detect possible electrolyte imbalance should be performed at appropriate intervals.

All patients receiving thiazide therapy should be observed for clinical signs of fluid or electrolyte imbalance; namely, hyponatremia, hypochloremic alkalosis, and hypokalemia. Serum and urine electrolyte determinations are particularly important when the patient is vomiting excessively or receiving parenteral fluids. Medication such as digitalis may also influence serum electrolytes. Warning signs, irrespective of cause, are: Dryness of mouth, thirst, weakness, lethargy, drowsiness, restlessness, muscle pains or cramps, muscular fatigue, hypotension, oliguria, tachycardia, and gastrointestinal disturbances such as nausea and vomiting.

Hypokalemia may develop with thiazides as with any other potent diuretic, especially with brisk diuresis, when severe cirrhosis is present, or during concomitant use of corticosteroids or ACTH.

Interference with adequate oral electrolyte intake will also contribute to hypokalemia. Digitalis therapy may exaggerate metabolic effects of hypokalemia especially with reference to myocardial activity.

Any chloride deficit is generally mild and usually does not require specific treatment except under extraordinary circumstances (as in liver disease or renal disease). Dilutional hyponatremia may occur in edematous patients in hot

weather; appropriate therapy is water restriction, rather than administration of salt except in rare instances when the hyponatremia is life-threatening. In actual salt depletion, appropriate replacement is the therapy of choice.
Hyperuricemia may occur or frank gout may be precipitated in certain patients receiving thiazide therapy.
Insulin requirements in diabetic patients may be increased, decreased, or unchanged. Latent diabetes mellitus may become manifested during thiazide administration.
Thiazide drugs may increase the responsiveness to tubocurarine.
The antihypertensive effects of the drug may be enhanced in the postsympathectomy patient.
Thiazides may decrease arterial responsiveness to norepinephrine. This diminution is not sufficient to preclude effectiveness of the pressor agent for therapeutic use.
If progressive renal impairment becomes evident, as indicated by a rising nonprotein nitrogen or blood urea nitrogen, a careful reappraisal of therapy is necessary with consideration given to withholding or discontinuing diuretic therapy.
Thiazides may decrease serum PBI levels without signs of thyroid disturbance.

Adverse Reactions:

A. Gastrointestinal system reactions: Anorexia, gastric irritation, nausea, vomiting, cramping, diarrhea, constipation, jaundice (intrahepatic cholestatic jaundice), pancreatitis.
B. Central nervous system reactions: Dizziness, vertigo, parasthesias, headache, xanthopsia.
C. Hematologic reactions: Leukopenia, agranulocytosis, thrombocytopenia, aplastic anemia.
D. Dermatologic-Hypersensitivity reactions: Purpura, photo-sensitivity, rash, urticaria, necrotizing angiitis (vasculitis) (cutaneous vasculitis).
E. Cardiovascular reaction: Orthostatic hypotension may occur and may be aggravated by alcohol, barbiturates, or narcotics.
F. Other: Hyperglycemia, glycosuria, hyperuricemia, muscle spasm, weakness, restlessness.

Whenever adverse reactions are moderate or severe, thiazide dosage should be reduced or therapy withdrawn.

Dosage and Administration: The average adult diuretic dose is 25 to 200 mg. per day. The average adult antihypertensive dose is 50 to 100 mg. per day.
Therapy should be individualized according to patient response. This therapy should be titrated to gain maximal therapeutic response as well as the minimal dose possible to maintain that therapeutic response.

How Supplied: NDC 0015-5410—Saluron Tablets, scored, 50 mg., bottles of 100.
[*Shown in Product Identification Section*]

SALUTENSIN®
SALUTENSIN–Demi™ ℞
(hydroflumethiazide, reserpine Antihypertensive Formulation)

This is the full text of the latest Official Package Circular dated March 1977 [5436 DIMO-07].

WARNING
This fixed combination drug is not indicated for initial therapy of hypertension. Hypertension requires therapy titrated to the individual patient. If the fixed combination represents the dosage so determined, its use may be more convenient in patient management. The treatment of hypertension is not static, but must be reevaluated as conditions in each patient warrant.

Description: Salutensin combines two antihypertensive agents: Saluron® (hydroflumethiazide) and reserpine. The chemical name for hydroflumethiazide is 3,4-dihydro-7-sulfamyl-6-trifluoromethyl-2H-1,2,4-benzothiadiazine-1, 1-dioxide. Reserpine (3,4,5-trimethoxybenzoyl methyl reserpate) is a crystalline alkaloid derived from Rauwolfia serpentina.

Each Salutensin tablet contains:
Saluron (hydroflumethiazide).... 50 mg
Reserpine .... 0.125 mg
Each Salutensin-Demi tablet contains:
Saluron (hydroflumethiazide).... 25 mg
Reserpine .... 0.125 mg

Actions: Hydroflumethiazide is an oral diuretic-antihypertensive agent. It exerts its effect by inhibiting renal tubular reabsorption, inducing increased excretion of sodium and chloride and water with variable concomitant loss of potassium and bicarbonate as well. When used alone as an antihypertensive agent, hydroflumethiazide usually induces a gradual but sustained decrease in abnormally elevated blood pressure—both systolic and diastolic.
Hypertensive patients who have been maintained on chlorothiazide or hydrochlorothiazide may also be maintained on hydroflumethiazide.
The component, reserpine, probably produces its antihypertensive effects through depletion of tissue stores of catecholamines (epinephrine and norepinephrine) from peripheral sites. By contrast, its sedative and tranquilizing properties are thought to be related by depletion of 5-hydroxytryptamine from the brain.
Reserpine is characterized by slow onset of action and sustained effect. Both its cardiovascular and central nervous system effects may persist following withdrawal of the drug.
Careful observation for changes in blood pressure must be made when Salutensin is used with other antihypertensive drugs. The dosage of other agents must be reduced by at least 50 percent as soon as Salutensin is added to the regimen to prevent excessive drop in blood pressure. As the blood pressure falls under the potentiating effect of Salutensin, a further reduction in dosage or even discontinuation of other antihypertensive drugs may be necessary.
Hypertension therapy requires therapy titrated to the individual patient. If a fixed combination represents the dosage so determined its use may be more convenient in patient management.

Indications: Hypertension (see box warning).

Contraindications: Salutensin is contraindicated in patients who have previously demonstrated hypersensitivity to its components. Patients with anuria or oliguria should not be given this medication. The presence of an active peptic ulcer, ulcerative colitis, or severe depression contraindicates the use of reserpine. It is also contraindicated in patients receiving electroconvulsive therapy.

Warnings: Azotemia may be precipitated or increased by hydroflumethiazide. Special caution is necessary in patients with impaired renal function to avoid cumulative or toxic effects.
Since in hepatic cirrhosis, minor alterations of fluid and electrolyte balance may precipitate coma, hydroflumethiazide should be given with caution.
The possibility of sensitivity reactions should be considered in patients with a history of allergy or bronchial asthma.
Hydroflumethiazide potentiates the action of other antihypertensive drugs. Therefore, the dosage of these agents, especially the ganglion blockers, must be reduced by at least 50 percent as soon as hydroflumethiazide is added to the regimen.
The possibility of exacerbation or activation of systemic lupus erythematosus has been reported for sulfonamide derivatives (including thiazides) and reserpine.
The occurrence of mental depression due to reserpine in doses of 0.25 mg daily or less is unusual. In any event, Salutensin should be discontinued at the first sign of depression.
There have been several reports, published and unpublished, concerning nonspecific small bowel lesions consisting of stenosis with or without ulceration, associated with the administration of enteric coated thiazides with potassium salts. These lesions may occur with enteric coated potassium tablets alone or when they are used with nonenteric coated thiazides, or certain other oral diuretics.
These small bowel lesions have caused obstruction, hemorrhage, and perforation. Surgery was frequently required and deaths have occurred.
Available information tends to implicate enteric coated potassium salts, although lesions of this type also occur spontaneously. CAUTION: Coated potassium-containing formulations should be administered only when indicated, and should be discontinued immediately if abdominal pain, distention, nausea, vomiting, or gastrointestinal bleeding occurs.
Coated potassium tablets should be used only when adequate dietary supplementation is not practical.

Usage in Pregnancy and the Child-Bearing Age
Since thiazides and reserpine appear in breast milk, Salutensin is contraindicated in nursing mothers. If use of the drug is deemed essential, the patient should stop nursing. Reserpine has been demonstrated to cross the placental barrier in guinea pigs with depression of adrenal catecholamine stores in the newborn. There is some evidence that side effects such as nasal congestion, lethargy, depressed Moro reflex, and bradycardia may appear in infants born of reserpine-treated mothers. Thiazides cross the placental barrier and appear in cord blood. When Salutensin is used in women of child-bearing age, the potential benefits of the drug should be weighed against the possible hazards to the fetus. These hazards include fetal or neonatal jaundice, thrombocytopenia, and possibly other adverse reactions which have occurred in the adult.

Precautions:

Hydroflumethiazide
Careful check should be kept for signs of fluid and electrolyte imbalance. Serum and urine electrolyte determinations are particularly important when the patient is vomiting excessively or receiving parenteral fluids. Warning signs, irrespective of cause, are: dryness of mouth, thirst, weakness, lethargy, drowsiness, restlessness, muscle pains or cramps, muscular fatigue, hypotension, oliguria, tachycardia, and gastrointestinal disturbances.
Potassium excretion is usually minimal. However, hypokalemia may develop with hydroflumethiazide as with any other potent diuretic, especially with brisk diuresis, when severe cirrhosis is present, or during concomitant use of steroids or ACTH. Interference with adequate electrolyte intake will contribute to hypokalemia. Digitalis therapy may exaggerate metabolic effects of hypokalemia especially with reference to myocardial activity. If dietary salt is unduly restricted, especially during hot weather, in severely edematous patients with congestive failure or renal disease, a low salt syndrome may complicate therapy with thiazides.
Hypokalemia may be avoided or treated by use of potassium chloride or giving foods with a high potassium content. Any chloride deficit may similarly be corrected by use of ammonium chloride (excepting patients with hepatic disease) and largely prevented by a near normal salt intake.
Thiazide drugs may increase the responsiveness to tubocurarine. The antihypertensive effect of the drug may be enhanced in the post-

Continued on next page

Bristol—Cont.

sympathectomy patient. Hydroflumethiazide decreases arterial responsiveness to norepinephrine, as do other thiazides, necessitating due care in surgical patients. It is recommended that thiazides be discontinued 48 hours before elective surgery. Orthostatic hypotension may occur and may be potentiated by alcohol, barbiturates, or narcotics.
Pathological changes in the parathyroid glands with hypercalcemia and hypophosphatemia have been observed in a few patients on prolonged thiazide therapy. The common complications of hyperparathyroidism such as renal lithiasis, bone resorption, and peptic ulceration have not been seen. The effect of discontinuance of thiazide therapy on serum calcium and phosphorus levels may be helpful in assessing the need for parathyroid surgery in such patients. Parathyroidectomy has been followed by subjective clinical improvement in most patients, but is without effect on the hypertension. Following surgery, thiazide therapy may be resumed.
Caution is necessary in patients with hyperuricemia or a history of gout, since gout may be precipitated. Insulin requirements in diabetic patients may be increased, decreased, or unchanged. In latent diabetics, hydroflumethiazide, in common with other benzothiadiazines, may cause hyperglycemia and glycosuria.

Reserpine

Since reserpine may increase gastric secretion and motility, it should be used cautiously in patients with a history of peptic ulcer, ulcerative colitis, or other gastrointestinal disorder. This compound may precipitate biliary colic in patients with gallstones, or bronchial asthma in susceptible persons.
Reserpine may cause hypotension including orthostatic hypotension. In hypertensive patients on reserpine therapy significant hypotension and bradycardia may develop during surgical anesthesia. Therefore, the drug should be discontinued two weeks before giving anesthesia. For emergency surgical procedures, it may be necessary to give vagal blocking agents parenterally to prevent or reverse hypotension and/or bradycardia.
Anxiety or depression, as well as psychosis, may develop during reserpine therapy. If depression is present when therapy is begun, it may be aggravated. Mental depression is unusual with reserpine doses of 0.25 mg daily or less. In any case, Salutensin should be discontinued at the first sign of depression. Extreme caution should be used in treating patients with a history of mental depression, and the possibility of suicide should be kept in mind.
As with most antihypertensive therapy, caution should be exercised when treating hypertensive patients with renal insufficiency, since they adjust poorly to lowered blood pressure levels. Use reserpine cautiously with digitalis and quinidine; cardiac arrhythmias have occurred with reserpine preparations. Thiazides may decrease serum P.B.I. levels without signs of thyroid disturbance.

Adverse Reactions:

Hydroflumethiazide

A. Gastrointestinal System Reactions: Anorexia, gastric irritation, nausea, vomiting, cramping, diarrhea, constipation, jaundice (intrahepatic cholestatic jaundice), pancreatitis, hyperglycemia, and glycosuria.
B. Central Nervous System Reactions: dizziness, vertigo, parasthesias, headache, and xanthopsia.
C. Hematologic Reactions: leukopenia, thrombocytopenia, agranulocytosis, and aplastic anemia.
D. Dermatologic-Hypersensitivity Reactions: purpura, photosensitivity, rash, urticaria, and necrotizing angiitis (vasculitis) (cutaneous vasculitis).
E. Cardiovascular Reaction: orthostatic hypotension may occur and may be aggravated by alcohol, barbiturates or narcotics.
F. Miscellaneous: muscle spasm, weakness, and restlessness.

Whenever adverse reactions are moderate or severe, thiazide dosage should be reduced or therapy withdrawn.

Reserpine

Side effects due to reserpine often disappear with continued use and most can be controlled by reducing the dosage. Rarely, it may be necessary to discontinue therapy. The reactions most often reported include: excessive sedation, nightmares, nasal congestion, conjunctival injection, enhanced susceptibility to colds, muscular aches, headache, dizziness, dyspnea, anorexia, nausea, increased intestinal motility, diarrhea, weight gain, dryness of the mouth, blurred vision, flushing of the skin and pruritus. Skin rash, dysuria, syncope, nonpuerperal lactation, impotence or decreased libido, increased salivation, vomiting, bradycardia, mental depression, nervousness, paradoxical anxiety, epistaxis, purpura due to thrombocytopenia, angina pectoris and other direct cardiac effects (e.g., premature ventricular contractions, fluid retention, congestive failure), and central nervous system sensitization manifested by dull sensorium, deafness, glaucoma, uveitis, and optic atrophy also have been noted. In some patients reserpine has produced a syndrome similar to Parkinson's disease, though this effect usually is reversible with decreased dosage or discontinuation of therapy. Salutensin should be given with caution to hypertensive patients who also have coronary artery disease to avoid a precipitous drop in blood pressure.

Dosage: As determined by individual titration (see box warning).
The usual adult dose of Salutensin is one tablet once or twice daily. If a smaller amount of thiazide diuretic is desired, Salutensin-Demi, one tablet once or twice daily, can be given. Most patients will respond to this dosage level. In refractory cases, the physician may carefully increase the dose to three or four tablets per day in divided doses providing the proper precautions are observed—careful attention to serum uric acid, fasting blood sugar, BUN or NPN, and serum electrolyte levels. (See sections on Precautions and Warnings above.)
When the desired blood pressure reduction has been achieved, the dose should be reduced to the minimum effective dose for the individual patient.
Careful observation for changes in blood pressure must be made when Salutensin is used with other antihypertensive drugs. The dosage of other agents must be reduced by at least 50 percent as soon as Salutensin is added to the regimen to prevent excessive drop in blood pressure. As the blood pressure falls under the potentiating effect of Salutensin, a further reduction in dosage or even discontinuation of other antihypertensive drugs may be necessary.

Supply:
Salutensin Tablets—**NDC** 0015-5436
Salutensin-Demi Tablets—**NDC** 0015-5455
For information on package sizes available, refer to the current price schedule.

[*Shown in Product Identification Section*]

STADOL® ℞
(butorphanol tartrate)

This is the full text of the latest Official Package Circular dated October 1979 [5644DIM-04].

Description: Stadol (butorphanol tartrate), sterile, parenteral, narcotic agonist-antagonist, analgesic, is a member of the phenanthrene series. The chemical name is levo-N-cyclobutylmethyl-6, 10aβ-dihydroxy-1,2,3,9,10, 10a-hexahydro- (4H) - 10, 4a-iminoethanophenanthrene tartrate. It is a white crystalline substance soluble in aqueous solution. The dose is expressed as the salt. One milligram of tartrate salt is equivalent to 0.68 milligram of base. In addition to Stadol (butorphanol tartrate), each ml contains 3.3 mg citric acid, 6.4 mg sodium citrate and 6.4 mg sodium chloride. The molecular weight is 477.56 and the molecular formula is $C_{21}H_{29}NO_2 \cdot C_4H_6O_6$

Clinical Pharmacology: Stadol is a potent analgesic. The duration of analgesia is generally 3 to 4 hours and is approximately equivalent to that of morphine. The onset time for analgesia is within 10 minutes following intramuscular injection and very rapidly following intravenous administration. Peak analgesic activity is obtained at 30 to 60 minutes following intramuscular injection and more rapidly following intravenous administration.

Narcotic Antagonist Activity

Stadol has narcotic antagonist activity which is approximately equivalent to that of nalorphine, 30 times that of pentazocine and 1/40 that of naloxone (Narcan®) as measured by the antagonism of morphine analgesia in the rat tail flick test.

Mechanism of Analgesic Action

The exact mechanism of action of Stadol is unknown. It is felt that the class of narcotic antagonist analgesics exert their analgesic effect via a central nervous system mechanism. Currently, it is believed the site of action of centrally acting analgesics is subcortical, possibly in the limbic system.

Effect on Respiration

At the analgesic dose of 2 mg, Stadol depresses respiration to a degree equal to 10 mg morphine. The magnitude of respiratory depression with Stadol is not appreciably increased at doses of 4 mg. In contrast to the magnitude of respiratory depression, the duration of respiratory depression with Stadol is dose-related. Any respiratory depression produced by Stadol is reversible by naloxone which is a specific antagonist.

Cardiovascular Effects

The hemodynamic changes after the intravenous administration of Stadol are similar to the reported hemodynamic changes after pentazocine. The changes include increased pulmonary artery pressure, pulmonary wedge pressure, left ventricular end-diastolic pressure, systemic arterial pressure, and pulmonary vascular resistance. Although smaller than those following pentazocine, these changes are nevertheless in a direction which increases the work of the heart, especially in the pulmonary circuit.

Indications and Usage: Stadol is recommended for the relief of moderate to severe pain. Stadol can also be used for preoperative or preanesthetic medication, as a supplement to balanced anesthesia, and for the relief of prepartum pain.

Contraindications: Stadol should not be administered to patients who have been shown to be hypersensitive to it.

Warnings:

Patients Physically Dependent on Narcotics

Because of its antagonist properties, Stadol is not recommended for patients physically dependent on narcotics. Detoxification in such patients is required prior to use.
Due to the difficulty in assessing addiction in patients who have recently received substantial amounts of narcotic medication, caution should be used in the administration of Stadol. Detoxification of such patients prior to usage should be carefully considered.

Drug Dependence

Special care should be exercised in administering Stadol to emotionally unstable patients and to those with a history of drug misuse. When long-term therapy is contemplated, such patients should be closely supervised. Even though Stadol has a low physical dependence liability, care should be taken that individuals who may be prone to drug abuse are closely supervised. It is important to avoid increases in dose and frequency of injections by the patient and to prevent the use of the drug in anticipation of pain rather than for the relief of pain.

Head Injury and Increased Intracranial Pressure

Although there is no clinical experience in patients with head injury, it can be assumed that Stadol, like other potent analgesics, elevates cerebrospinal fluid pressure. Therefore the use of Stadol in cases of head injury can produce effects (e.g., miosis) which may obscure the clinical course of patients with head injuries. In such patients Stadol must be used with extreme caution and only if its use is deemed essential.

Cardiovascular Effects

Because Stadol increases the work of the heart, especially the pulmonary circuit, (see Clinical Pharmacology), the use of this drug in acute myocardial infarction or in cardiac patients with ventricular dysfunction or coronary insufficiency should be limited to those who are hypersensitive to morphine sulfate or meperidine.

Precautions:

Certain Respiratory Conditions

Because Stadol causes some respiratory depression, it should be administered only with caution and low dosage to patients with respiratory depression (e.g., from other medication, uremia, or severe infection), severely limited respiratory reserve, bronchial asthma, obstructive respiratory conditions, or cyanosis.

Impaired Renal or Hepatic Function

Although laboratory tests have not indicated that Stadol causes or increases renal or hepatic impairment, the drug should be administered with caution to patients with such impairment. Extensive liver disease may predispose to greater side effects and greater activity from the usual clinical dose, possibly the result of decreased metabolism of the drug by the liver.

Biliary Surgery

Clinical studies have not been done to establish the safety of Stadol administration to patients about to undergo surgery of the biliary tract.

Usage as a Pre-Operative or Pre-Anesthetic Medication

Slight increases in systolic blood pressure may occur, therefore caution should be employed when Stadol is used in the hypertensive patient.

Usage in Balanced Anesthesia

The use of pancuronium in combination with Stadol may cause an increase in conjunctival changes.

Usage in Pregnancy

The safety of Stadol for use in pregnancy prior to the labor period has not been established; therefore, this drug should be used in pregnant patients only when in the judgment of the physician its use is deemed essential to the welfare of the patient.

Reproduction studies have been performed in rats, mice, and rabbits and have revealed no evidence of impaired fertility or harm to the fetus due to Stadol at about 2.5 to 5 times the human dose.

Usage in Labor and Delivery

Safety to the mother and fetus following the administration of Stadol during labor has been established. Patients receiving Stadol during labor have experienced no adverse effects other than those observed with commonly used analgesics. Stadol should be used with caution in women delivering premature infants.

Usage in Nursing Mothers

The use of Stadol in lactating mothers who are nursing their infants is not recommended, since it is not known whether this drug is excreted in milk. Stadol has been used safely for labor pain in mothers who subsequently nursed their infants.

Usage in Children

Safety and efficacy in children below age 18 years have not been established at present.

Adverse Reactions: The most frequent adverse reactions in 1250 patients treated with Stadol are: sedation (503, 40%), nausea (82, 6%), clammy/sweating (76, 6%).

Less frequent reactions are: headache (35, 3%), vertigo (33, 3%), floating feeling (33, 3%), dizziness (23, 2%), lethargy (19, 2%), confusion (15, 1%), lightheadedness (12, 1%).

Other adverse reactions which may occur (reported incidence of less than 1%) are:

CNS: nervousness, unusual dreams, agitation, euphoria, hallucinations

Autonomic: flushing and warmth, dry mouth, sensitivity to cold

Cardiovascular: palpitation, increase or decrease of blood pressure

Gastrointestinal: vomiting

Respiratory: slowing of respiration, shallow breathing

Dermatological: rash or hives

Eye: diplopia or blurred vision

Overdosage:

Manifestations

Although there have been no experiences of overdosage with Stadol during clinical trials, this may occur due to accidental or intentional misuse as well as therapeutic use. Based on the pharmacology of Stadol, overdosage could produce some degree of respiratory depression and variable cardiovascular and central nervous system effects.

Treatment

The immediate treatment of suspected Stadol overdosage is intravenous naloxone. The respiratory and cardiac status of the patient should be evaluated constantly and appropriate supportive measures instituted, such as oxygen, intravenous fluids, vasopressors, and assisted or controlled respiration.

Dosage and Administration:

Adults:

Intramuscular—The usual recommended single dose is 2 mg. This may be repeated every three to four hours, as necessary. The effective dosage range, depending on the severity of pain, is 1 to 4 mg repeated every three to four hours. At this time, there is insufficient clinical data to recommend single doses beyond 4 mg.

Intravenous—The usual recommended single dose for intravenous administration is 1 mg repeated every three to four hours as necessary. The effective dosage range, depending on the severity of pain, is 0.5 to 2 mg repeated every three to four hours.

Concomitant Use with Tranquilizers

According to accepted procedure, the dose of Stadol should be reduced when administered concomitantly with phenothiazines and other tranquilizers which may potentiate the action of Stadol.

Children:

Since there is no clinical experience in children under 18 years, Stadol is not recommended in this age group.

Storage Conditions

Store at room temperature.

Supply: Stadol (butorphanol tartrate) Injection for I.M. or I.V. use, is available as follows:

NDC 0015-5644-20—2 mg per ml, 2-ml vial
NDC 0015-5645-20—1 mg per ml, 1-ml vial
NDC 0015-5646-20—2 mg per ml, 1-ml vial
NDC 0015-5646-23—2 mg per ml, 1-ml Disposable Syringe
NDC 0015-5648-20—2 mg per ml, 10-ml multi-dose vial

For information on package sizes available, refer to the current price schedule.

STAPHCILLIN® ℞

(methicillin sodium for Injection)
Buffered
For I.M. Or I.V. Use

This is the full text of the latest Official Package Circular dated October 1981 [7961DIR-16].

Description: Staphcillin (methicillin sodium monohydrate) is a semisynthetic penicillin: 2,6-dimethoxyphenyl penicillin. It is supplied as the sodium salt in a parenteral dosage form. Each Gm. of Staphcillin is equivalent to 900 mg. methicillin activity and is buffered with 50 mg. sodium citrate.

Actions and Pharmacology: Staphcillin is a bactericidal penicillin, highly resistant to staphylococcal penicillinase and equally active against penicillin-susceptible and penicillinase-producing strains of Staphylococcus aureus. Methicillin is considerably less active than penicillin G against streptococci and pneumococci. It is not acid-resistant and must be administered by intramuscular or intravenous injection. A 1-Gram intramuscular dose gives a peak blood level of approximately 12 mcg./ml. which drops off to about 1 mcg./ml. within a 4-hour period. Methicillin is rapidly excreted unchanged in the urine in individuals with normal kidney function. Impairment in kidney function results in elevated blood levels which may require adjustment of dosage and treatment intervals. Protein binding of methicillin is approximately 40%. The drug penetrates body tissues well, and diffuses readily into pleural, pericardial, and synovial fluids. As with all penicillins, absorption into spinal fluids is poor under normal conditions. However, higher concentrations may be attained in the presence of meningeal inflammation.

Disc Susceptibility Tests

Quantitative methods that require measurement of zone diameters give the most precise estimates of antibiotic susceptibility. One such procedure* has been recommended for use with discs for testing susceptibility to methicillin class antibiotics. Interpretations correlate diameters on the disc test with MIC values for methicillin. With this procedure, a report from the laboratory of "susceptible" indicates that the infecting organism is likely to respond to therapy. A report of "resistant" indicates that the infecting organism is not likely to respond to therapy. A report of "intermediate susceptibility" suggests that the organism would be susceptible if high dosage is used, or if the infection is confined to tissues and fluids (e.g., urine), in which high antibiotic levels are attained.

*Bauer, A. W., Kirby, W. M. M., Sherris, J. C. and Turck, M.: Antibiotic Testing by a Standard Single Disc Method, Am. J. Clin. Pathol., 45:493, 1966; Standardized Disc Susceptibility Test, FEDERAL REGISTER 37:20527-29, 1972.

Indications: Although the principal indication for methicillin sodium is in the treatment of infections due to penicillinase-producing staphylococci, it may be used to initiate therapy in such patients in whom a staphylococcal infection is suspected. (See Important Note below.)

Bacteriologic studies to determine the causative organisms and their susceptibility to methicillin sodium should be performed.

Important Note: When it is judged necessary that treatment be initiated before definitive culture and susceptibility results are known, the choice of methicillin sodium should take into consideration the fact that it has been shown to be effective only in the treatment of infections caused by pneumococci, Group A beta-hemolytic streptococci, and penicillin G-resistant and penicillin G-susceptible staphylococci. If the bacteriology report later indicates the infection is due to an organism other than a penicillin G-resistant staphylococcus susceptible to methicillin sodium, the physician is advised to continue therapy with a drug other than methicillin sodium or any other penicillinase-resistant semisynthetic penicillin.

Recent studies have reported that the percentage of staphylococcal isolates resistant to penicillin G outside the hospital is increasing, ap-

Continued on next page

Bristol—Cont.

proximating the high percentage of resistant staphylococcal isolates found in the hospital. For this reason, it is recommended that a penicillinase-resistant penicillin be used as initial therapy for any suspected staphylococcal infection until culture and susceptibility results are known.

Strains of staphylococci resistant to methicillin have existed in nature and it is known that the number of these strains reported has been increasing. Such strains of staphylococci have been capable of producing serious disease, in some instances resulting in fatality. Because of this, there is concern that widespread use of the penicillinase-resistant penicillins may result in the appearance of an increasing number of staphylococcal strains which are resistant to these penicillins.

Methicillin-resistant strains are almost always resistant to all other penicillinase-resistant penicillins (cross-resistance with cephalosporin derivatives also occurs frequently). Resistance to any penicillinase-resistant penicillin should be interpreted as evidence of clinical resistance to all, in spite of the fact that minor variations in **in vitro** susceptibility may be encountered when more than one penicillinase-resistant penicillin is tested against the same strain of staphylococcus.

Contraindications: A previous hypersensitivity reaction to any penicillin is a contraindication.

Warning: Serious and occasionally fatal hypersensitivity (anaphylactoid) reactions have been reported in patients on penicillin therapy. Although anaphylaxis is more frequent following parenteral therapy, it has occurred in patients on oral penicillins. These reactions are more apt to occur in individuals with a history of sensitivity to multiple allergens.

There have been well documented reports of individuals with a history of penicillin hypersensitivity reactions who have experienced severe hypersensitivity reactions when treated with a cephalosporin. Before therapy with a penicillin, careful inquiry should be made concerning previous hypersensitivity reactions to penicillins, cephalosporins, and other allergens. If an allergic reaction occurs, the drug should be discontinued and the patient treated with the usual agents e.g., pressor amines, antihistamines, and corticosteroids.

Precautions: Penicillin should be used with caution in individuals with histories of significant allergies and/or asthma.

As with any potent drug, periodic assessment of organ system functions, including renal, hepatic, and hematopoietic, should be made during prolonged therapy.

The possibility of bacterial and/or fungal overgrowth should be kept in mind during long-term therapy. If overgrowth of resistant organisms occurs, appropriate measures should be taken.

Safety for use in pregnancy has not been established.

Because of incompletely developed renal function in infants, methicillin may not be completely excreted, with abnormally high blood levels resulting. Frequent blood levels are advisable in this age group with dosage adjustments when necessary.

Adverse Reactions: The hypersensitivity reactions reported are skin rashes, urticaria, serum sickness, and anaphylactic reactions. Oral lesions such as glossitis and stomatitis have been reported. Fever, eosinophilia, oral and rectal moniliasis have also been reported. Hemolytic anemia, transient neutropenia with evidence of granulocytopenia or thrombocytopenia, neuropathy, and nephrotoxicity (oliguria, albuminuria, hematuria, pyuria, and/or cylindruria) are infrequent and usually associated with high doses of parenteral penicillin.

Dosage and Administration: The drug is well tolerated when given by deep intragluteal or intravenous injection. As is the case with other antibiotics, the duration of therapy should be determined by the clinical and bacteriological response of the patient. Therapy should be continued for at least 48 hours after the patient has become afebrile, asymptomatic, and cultures are negative. In serious systemic infection, therapy should be continued for at least 1 to 2 weeks after the patient is afebrile and cultures are sterile.

Treatment of osteomyelitis may require several months of intensive therapy.

Oral penicillinase-resistant penicillins may be of special value in follow-up therapy because of the difficulty of maintaining prolonged parenteral treatment.

Intramuscular Route: The usual adult dose is 1 Gm. every 4 or 6 hours. Infants' and children's dosage is 25 mg./Kg. (approximately 12 mg./lb.) every 6 hours.

Intravenous Route: The usual adult dose is 1 Gm. every 6 hours using 50 ml. of Sodium Chloride Injection, U.S.P. at the rate of 10 ml. per minute.

The number of instances in which the drug was administered intravenously to infants and children is not large enough to permit specific intravenous dosage recommendations.

Directions For Use:

For Intramuscular Use: Use Sterile Water for Injection, U.S.P. or Sodium Chloride Injection U.S.P. Add 1.5 ml. to the 1.0-Gm. vial, 5.7 ml. to the 4.0-Gm. vial, and 8.6 ml. to the 6.0-Gm. vial, and withdraw the entire contents. Each 1.0 ml. will contain approximately 500 mg. of Staphcillin. The solutions are stable for 24 hours at room temperature and 4 days under refrigeration.

For Direct Intravenous Use: Further dilute each 1.0 ml. of solution, reconstituted as above, with 25 ml. of Sodium Chloride Injection, U.S.P. and inject at the rate of 10 ml. per minute.

For Administration by Intravenous Drip: Reconstitute as directed above (For Intramuscular Use) prior to diluting with Intravenous Solution. Stability studies on Staphcillin at concentrations of 2 mg./ml., 10 mg./ml., and 20 mg./ml. in various intravenous solutions indicate the drug will lose less than 10% activity at room temperature (70°F.) during an 8-hour period.

I.V. Solution

Isotonic Sodium Chloride
5% Dextrose in Water
5% Dextrose in Normal Saline
10% D-Fructose in Water
10% D-Fructose in Normal Saline
M/6 Sodium r-Lactate Solution
Lactated Ringer's Injection
Lactated Potassic Saline Injection
5% Plasma Hydrolysate in Water
10% Invert Sugar in Water
*10% Invert Sugar in Normal Saline
10% Invert Sugar plus 0.3% Potassium Chloride in Water
Travert 10% Electrolyte #1
Travert 10% Electrolyte #2
Travert 10% Electrolyte #3

*At a concentration of 2 mg./ml., Staphcillin is stable for only 4 hours in this solution. Concentrations between 10 mg./ml. and 30 mg./ml. are stable for 8 hours.

Only those solutions listed above should be used for the intravenous infusion of Staphcillin. The concentration of the antibiotic should fall within the range specified. The drug concentration and the rate and volume of the infusion should be adjusted so that the total dose of methicillin is administered before the drug loses its stability in the solution in use.

If another agent is used in conjunction with methicillin therapy, **it should not be physically mixed** with methicillin but should be administered separately.

"Piggyback" I.V. Package: This glass vial contains the labeled quantity of Staphcillin and is intended for intravenous administration. The diluent and volume are specified on the label of each package.

Discard solution after 24 hours at room temperature.

Hospital Bulk Package: This glass vial contains 10 grams Staphcillin and is designed for use in the pharmacy in preparing I.V. additives. Add 94 ml Sterile Water for Injection, U.S.P. or Sodium Chloride Injection, U.S.P. The resulting solution will contain 100 mg methicillin sodium per ml, which is equivalent to 90 mg per ml methicillin activity.

Following reconstitution in this manner, the resulting solutions are stable for 24 hours at room temperature.

Caution: NOT TO BE DISPENSED AS A UNIT.

Supply:

STAPHCILLIN (methicillin sodium for Injection) buffered.

NDC 0015-7961-20—1.0-gram vial.
NDC 0015-7964-20—4.0-gram vial.
NDC 0015-7965-20—6.0-gram vial.
NDC 0015-7961-28—1.0-gram "piggyback" vial.
NDC 0015-7964-28—4.0-gram "piggyback" vial.
NDC 0015-7012-28—10-gram Hospital Bulk Package.

For information on package sizes available, refer to the current price schedule.

TEGOPEN® ℞
(cloxacillin sodium)
For Oral Solution
Capsules

This is the full text of the latest Official Package Circular dated January 1978 [7935DIRO-10].

Description: Tegopen (cloxacillin sodium monohydrate) is a member of the Bristol family of synthetic penicillins. It has been demonstrated to be especially efficacious in the treatment of penicillinase-producing staphylococcal infections and effective in the treatment of other commonly encountered Gram-positive coccal infections.

Actions:

Pharmacology

Cloxacillin is resistant to destruction by acid and is well-absorbed from the gastrointestinal tract.

Microbiology

Cloxacillin is active against most Gram-positive cocci including beta-hemolytic streptococci, pneumococci, and nonpenicillinase-producing staphylococci. Because of its resistance to the enzyme penicillinase, it is also active against penicillinase-producing staphylococci.

Disc Susceptibility Tests

Quantitative methods that require measurement of zone diameters give the most precise estimates of antibiotic susceptibility. One such procedure* has been recommended for use with discs for testing susceptibility to methicillin class antibiotics. Interpretations correlate diameters on the disc test with MIC values for methicillin. With this procedure, a report from the laboratory of "susceptible" indicates that the infecting organism is likely to respond to therapy. A report of "resistant" indicates that the infecting organism is not likely to respond to therapy. A report of "intermediate susceptibility" suggests that the organism would be susceptible if high dosage is used, or if the infection is confined to tissues and fluids (e.g. urine), in which high antibiotic levels are attained.

Indications: Although the principal indication for cloxacillin sodium is in the treatment of infections due to penicillinase-producing staphylococci, it may be used to initiate therapy in such patients in whom a staphylococcal infection is suspected. (See Important Note below.)

Bacteriologic studies to determine the causative organisms and their susceptibility to cloxacillin sodium should be performed.

In serious, life-threatening infections, oral preparations of the penicillinase-resistant penicillins should not be relied on for initial therapy.

Important Note: When it is judged necessary that treatment be initiated before definitive culture and susceptibility results are known, the choice of cloxacillin sodium should take into consideration the fact that it has been shown to be effective only in the treatment of infections caused by pneumococci, Group A beta-hemolytic streptococci, and penicillin G-resistant and penicillin G-susceptible staphylococci. If the bacteriology report later indicates the infection is due to an organism other than a penicillin G-resistant staphylococcus susceptible to cloxacillin sodium, the physician is advised to continue therapy with a drug other than cloxacillin sodium or any other penicillinase-resistant semi-synthetic penicillin.

Recent studies have reported that the percentage of staphylococcal isolates resistant to penicillin G outside the hospital is increasing, approximating the high percentage of resistant staphylococcal isolates found in the hospital. For this reason, it is recommended that a penicillinase-resistant penicillin be used as initial therapy for any suspected staphylococcal infection until culture and susceptibility results are known.

Cloxacillin sodium is a compound that acts through a mechanism similar to that of methicillin against penicillin G-resistant staphylococci. Strains of staphylococci resistant to methicillin have existed in nature and it is known that the number of these strains reported has been increasing. Such strains of staphylococci have been capable of producing serious disease, in some instances resulting in fatality. Because of this, there is concern that widespread use of the penicillinase-resistant penicillins may result in the appearance of an increasing number of staphylococcal strains which are resistant to these penicillins.

Methicillin-resistant strains are almost always resistant to all other penicillinase-resistant penicillins (cross resistance with cephalosporin derivatives also occurs frequently). Resistance to any penicillinase-resistant penicillin should be interpreted as evidence of clinical resistance to all, in spite of the fact that minor variations in **in vitro** susceptibility may be encountered when more than one penicillinase-resistant penicillin is tested against the same strain of staphylococcus.

Contraindications: A history of a previous hypersensitivity reaction to any of the penicillins is a contraindication.

Warning: Serious and occasionally fatal hypersensitivity (anaphylactoid) reactions have been reported in patients on penicillin therapy. Although anaphylaxis is more frequent following parenteral therapy, it has occurred in patients on oral penicillins. These reactions are more apt to occur in individuals with a history of sensitivity to multiple allergens.

There have been well documented reports of individuals with a history of penicillin hypersensitivity reactions who have experienced severe hypersensitivity reactions when treated with a cephalosporin. Before therapy with a penicillin, careful inquiry should be made concerning previous hypersensitivity reactions to penicillins, cephalosporins, and other allergens. If an allergic reaction occurs, the drug should be discontinued and the patient treated with the usual agents e.g., pressor amines, antihistamines, and corticosteroids.

Usage in Pregnancy

Safety for use in pregnancy has not been established.

Precautions: The possibility of the occurrence of superinfections with mycotic organisms or other pathogens should be kept in mind when using this compound, as with other antibiotics. If superinfection occurs during therapy, appropriate measures should be taken.

As with any potent drug, periodic assessment of organ system function, including renal, hepatic, and hematopoietic, should be made during long-term therapy.

Adverse Reactions: Gastrointestinal disturbances, such as nausea, epigastric discomfort, flatulence, and loose stools, have been noted by some patients. Mildly elevated SGOT levels (less than 100 units) have been reported in a few patients for whom pretherapeutic determinations were not made. Skin rashes and allergic symptoms, including wheezing and sneezing, have occasionally been encountered. Eosinophilia, with or without overt allergic manifestations, has been noted in some patients during therapy.

Dosage: For mild-to-moderate upper respiratory and localized skin and soft tissue infections due to susceptible organisms:

Adults and children weighing 20 Kg. (44 lbs.) or more: 250 mg. q. 6h.

Children weighing less than 20 Kg. (44 lbs.): 50 mg./Kg./day in equally-divided doses q. 6h.

For more severe infections such as those of the lower respiratory tract or disseminated infections:

Adults and children weighing 20 Kg. (44 lbs.) or more: 500 mg. or higher q. 6h.

Children weighing less than 20 Kg. (44 lbs.): 100 mg./Kg./day or higher in equally-divided doses q. 6h.

Studies indicate that this material is best absorbed when taken on an empty stomach, preferably one to two hours before meals.

N.B.: INFECTIONS CAUSED BY GROUP A BETA-HEMOLYTIC STREPTOCOCCI SHOULD BE TREATED FOR AT LEAST 10 DAYS TO HELP PREVENT THE OCCURRENCE OF ACUTE RHEUMATIC FEVER OR ACUTE GLOMERULONEPHRITIS.

Directions For Dispensing Oral Solution: Prepare solution at the time of dispensing. For ease in preparation, add the water in two portions, shaking well after each addition. Add the total amount of water as directed on the labeling of the package being dispensed. Refrigerated, the solution is stable for 14 days.

Supply:

TEGOPEN (cloxacillin sodium) Capsules. Each capsule contains cloxacillin sodium equivalent to 250 mg. or 500 mg. cloxacillin.

NDC 0015-7935—250 mg.
NDC 0015-7496—500 mg.

[*Shown in Product Identification Section*]

TEGOPEN (cloxacillin sodium) for Oral Solution. Each 5 ml. of reconstituted solution contains cloxacillin sodium equivalent to 125 mg. cloxacillin.

NDC 0015-7941—125 mg., 100 ml. and 200 ml. bottles

For information on package sizes available, refer to the current price schedule.

---

*Bauer, A. W., Kirby, W. M. M., Sherris, J. C. and Turck, M.: Antibiotic Testing by a Standardized Single Disc Method, Am. J. Clin. Pathol., 45:493, 1966; Standardized Disc Susceptibility Test, FEDERAL REGISTER 37:20527-29, 1972.

TETREX® ℞

(tetracycline phosphate complex)
Capsules 250 mg.
bidCAPS® 500 mg.

This is the full text of the latest Official Package Circular dated January 1978 [4322DIRO-14].

Description:

Each capsule contains:

Tetrex (tetracycline phosphate complex equivalent to tetracycline HCl activity) .....250 mg.

bidCaps (tetracycline phosphate complex equivalent to tetracycline HCl activity) ...500 mg.

Actions and Pharmacology: The tetracyclines are primarily bacteriostatic and are thought to exert their antimicrobial effect by inhibition of protein synthesis. Tetracyclines are active against a wide range of Gram-negative and Gram-positive organisms.

The drugs in the tetracycline class have closely similar antimicrobial spectra, and cross-resistance among them appears complete. Microorganisms may be considered highly sensitive if the M.I.C. (minimum inhibitory concentration) is not more than 4.0 mcg./ml. and intermediate if the M.I.C. is 4.0 to 12.5 mcg./ml.

Susceptibility plate testing: A tetracycline disc may be used to determine microbial susceptibility to drugs in the tetracycline class. If the Kirby-Bauer method of disc sensitivity is used, a 30-mcg. tetracycline disc should give a zone of over 18 mm. when tested against a tetracycline-sensitive bacterial strain.

Tetracyclines are readily absorbed and are bound to plasma proteins in varying degree. They are concentrated by the liver in the bile and excreted in the urine and feces at high concentrations and in a biologically active form.

Tetrex has the same actions and uses as the parent antibiotic, tetracycline, or its hydrochloride salt. However, the phosphate complex is more rapidly and more completely absorbed from the gastrointestinal tract than is the free base or its salts and therefore produces somewhat higher blood levels after oral administration.

Indications:

Tetracycline is indicated in infections caused by the following microorganisms:

Rickettsiae: Rocky Mountain spotted fever, typhus fever and the typhus group, Q fever, rickettsialpox, tick fevers,

Mycoplasma pneumoniae (PPLO, Eaton agent),

Agents of psittacosis and ornithosis,

Agents of lymphogranuloma venereum and granuloma inguinale,

The spirochetal agent of relapsing fever **(Borrelia recurrentis).**

The following Gram-negative organisms:

Haemophilus ducreyi (chancroid),

Pasteurella pestis and **Pasteurella tularensis,**

Bartonella bacilliformis,

Bacteroides species,

Vibrio comma and **Vibrio fetus,**

Brucella species (in conjunction with streptomycin).

Because many strains of the following groups of microorganisms have been shown to be resistant to tetracyclines, culture and susceptibility testing are recommended.

Tetracycline is indicated for treatment of infections caused by the following Gram-negative microorganisms, when bacteriologic testing indicates appropriate susceptibility to the drug.

Escherichia coli,

Enterobacter aerogenes (formerly **Aerobacter aerogenes),**

Shigella species,

Mima species and **Herellea** species,

Haemophilus influenzae (respiratory infections),

Klebsiella species (respiratory and urinary infections).

The following Gram-positive organisms when bacteriologic testing indicates appropriate susceptibility to the drug:

Streptococcus species:

Up to 44 percent of strains of **Streptococcus pyogenes** and 74 percent of **Streptococcus faecalis** have been found to be resistant to tetracycline drugs. Therefore, tetracycline should not be used for streptococcal disease unless the organism has been demonstrated to be sensitive.

Continued on next page

Bristol—Cont.

For upper respiratory infections due to Group A beta-hemolytic streptococci, penicillin is the usual drug of choice, including prophylaxis of rheumatic fever.

Diplococcus pneumoniae,
Staphylococcus aureus, skin and soft tissue infections. Tetracyclines are not the drugs of choice in the treatment of any type of staphylococcal infections.

When penicillin is contraindicated, tetracyclines are alternative drugs in the treatment of infections due to:

Neisseria gonorrhoeae,
Treponema pallidum and **Treponema pertenue** (syphilis and yaws),
Listeria monocytogenes,
Clostridium species,
Bacillus anthracis,
Fusobacterium fusiforme (Vincent's infection),
Actinomyces species.

In acute intestinal amebiasis, the tetracyclines may be a useful adjunct to amebicides.

In severe acne, the tetracyclines may be useful adjunctive therapy.

Tetracyclines are indicated in the treatment of trachoma, although the infectious agent is not always eliminated, as judged by immunofluorescence.

Inclusion conjunctivitis may be treated with oral tetracyclines or with a combination of oral and topical agents.

Contraindications: This drug is contraindicated in persons who have shown hypersensitivity to any of the tetracyclines.

Warnings: THE USE OF DRUGS OF THE TETRACYCLINE CLASS DURING TOOTH DEVELOPMENT (LAST HALF OF PREGNANCY, INFANCY, AND CHILDHOOD TO THE AGE OF 8 YEARS) MAY CAUSE PERMANENT DISCOLORATION OF THE TEETH (YELLOW-GRAY-BROWN.)

This adverse reaction is more common during long-term use of the drugs but has been observed following repeated short-term courses. Enamel hypoplasia has also been reported. TETRACYCLINES, THEREFORE, SHOULD NOT BE USED IN THIS AGE GROUP UNLESS OTHER DRUGS ARE NOT LIKELY TO BE EFFECTIVE OR ARE CONTRAINDICATED.

If renal impairment exists, even usual oral or parenteral doses may lead to excessive systemic accumulation of the drug and possible liver toxicity. Under such conditions, lower than the usual doses are indicated and if therapy is prolonged, serum level determinations of the drug may be advisable.

Photosensitivity manifested by exaggerated sunburn reaction has been observed in some individuals taking tetracyclines. Patients apt to be exposed to direct sunlight or ultraviolet light should be advised that this reaction can occur with tetracycline drugs and treatment should be discontinued at the first evidence of skin erythema.

The anti-anabolic action of the tetracyclines may cause an increase in BUN. While this is not a problem in those with normal renal function, in patients with significantly impaired function, higher serum levels of tetracycline may lead to azotemia, hyperphosphatemia, and acidosis.

Usage in Pregnancy: (See above "Warnings" about use during tooth development.)

Results of animal studies indicate that tetracyclines cross the placenta, are found in fetal tissues, and can have toxic effects on the developing fetus (often related to retardation of skeletal development). Evidence of embryotoxicity has also been noted in animals treated early in pregnancy.

Usage in Newborns, Infants, and Children: (See above "Warning" about use during tooth development.)

All tetracyclines form a stable calcium complex in any bone forming tissue. A decrease in the fibula growth rate has been observed in prematures given oral tetracycline in doses of 25 mg./Kg. every 6 hours. This reaction was shown to be reversible when the drug was discontinued.

Tetracyclines are present in the milk of lactating women who are taking a drug in this class.

Precautions: As with other antibiotics, use of this drug may result in overgrowth of nonsusceptible organisms, including fungi. If superinfection occurs, appropriate therapy should be instituted.

When used in the treatment of gonorrhea, a darkfield examination should be made of any lesions suggestive of syphilis before treatment is started and serologic tests for syphilis should be made monthly for at least 4 months afterwards.

Because the tetracyclines have been shown to depress plasma prothrombin activity, patients who are on anticoagulant therapy may require downward adjustment of their anticoagulant dosage.

In long-term therapy, periodic laboratory evaluation of organ systems, including hematopoietic, renal, and hepatic studies should be performed.

INFECTIONS DUE TO GROUP A BETA-HEMOLYTIC STREPTOCOCCI SHOULD BE TREATED FOR A MINIMUM OF 10 DAYS.

Since bacteriostatic drugs may interfere with the bactericidal action of penicillin, it is advisable to avoid giving tetracyclines in conjunction with penicillin.

Adverse Reactions:

Gastrointestinal: Anorexia, nausea, vomiting, diarrhea, glossitis, dysphagia, enterocolitis, and inflammatory lesions (with monilial overgrowth) in the anogenital region. These reactions have been caused by both oral and parenteral administration of tetracyclines.

Skin: Maculopapular and erythematous rashes. Exfoliative dermatitis has been reported but is uncommon. Photosensitivity is discussed above. (See "Warnings".)

Renal Toxicity: Rise in BUN has been reported and is apparently dose related. (See "Warnings".)

Hypersensitivity reactions: Urticaria, angioneurotic edema, anaphylaxis, anaphylactoid purpura, pericarditis, and exacerbation of systemic lupus erythematosus.

Bulging fontanels have been reported in young infants following therapeutic dosage. This sign disappeared rapidly when the drug was discontinued.

Blood: Hemolytic anemia, thrombocytopenia, neutropenia, and eosinophilia have been reported.

When given over prolonged periods, tetracyclines have been reported to produce brown-black microscopic discoloration of thyroid glands. No abnormalities of thyroid function studies are known to occur.

Administration and Dosage:

Capsules

Adults: The usual dose is 1 Gram per day in 4 divided doses of 250 mg. each. Severe infections require higher doses.

For children above eight years of age: The usual dose is 25 mg./Kg./day (12.5 mg./lb./day) in 4 divided doses. Children weighing more than 40 Kg. (88 lbs.) should be given the adult doses.

bidCAPS

Adults: The usual dose is 500 mg. b.i.d. Severe infections require higher doses.

For treatment of brucellosis, 500 mg. tetracycline four times daily for 3 weeks should be accompanied by streptomycin, 1 Gram intramuscularly twice daily the first week and once daily the second week.

For treatment of syphilis, a total of 30 to 40 Grams in equally divided doses over a period of 10 to 15 days should be given. Close follow-up including laboratory tests is recommended.

For treatment of pustular acne, the dosage may be reduced as soon as pustular element is controlled.

Treatment of uncomplicated gonorrhea, when penicillin is contraindicated, tetracycline may be used for the treatment of both males and females in the following divided dosage schedule: 1.5 Grams initially followed by 0.5 Grams q.i.d. for a total of 9.0 Grams.

Concomitant therapy: Iron salts and antacids containing aluminum, calcium, or magnesium impair absorption and should not be given to patients taking oral tetracycline.

Foods and some dairy products also interfere with absorption. Oral forms of tetracycline should be given 1 hour before or 2 hours after meals. Pediatric oral dosage forms should not be given with milk formulas and should be given at least 1 hour prior to feeding.

Therapy should be continued for at least 24 to 48 hours after symptoms and fever have subsided.

In patients with renal impairment: (See "Warnings".) Total dosage should be decreased by reduction of recommended individual doses and/or by extending time intervals between doses.

In the treatment of streptococcal infections, a therapeutic dose of tetracycline should be administered for at least 10 days.

Supply:

TETREX (tetracycline phosphate complex) Capsules equivalent to 250 mg. tetracycline HCl activity.

NDC 0015-4322—250 mg.

[Shown in Product Identification Section]

TETREX bidCaps (tetracycline phosphate complex) Capsules equivalent to 500 mg. tetracycline HCl activity.

NDC 0015-4330—500 mg.

[Shown in Product Identification Section]

ULTRACEF™ ℞
cefadroxil
CAPSULES, TABLETS AND ORAL SUSPENSION

This is the full text of the latest Office Package Circular dated November, 1981 [7271DIR-09].

Description: ULTRACEF (cefadroxil) is a semisynthetic cephalosporin antibiotic intended for oral administration. It is a white to yellowish-white crystalline powder. It is soluble in water and it is acid-stable. It is chemically designated as 7-[[D-2-amino-2-(4-hydroxyphenyl) acetyl]amino]-3-methyl-8-oxo-5-thia-1-azabicyclo [4.2.0]oct-2-ene-2-carboxylic acid monohydrate.

Clinical Pharmacology: ULTRACEF (cefadroxil) is rapidly absorbed after oral administration. Following single doses of 500 and 1000 mg, average peak serum concentrations were approximately 16 and 28 mcg/ml, respectively. Measurable levels were present 12 hours after administration. Over 90 percent of the drug is excreted unchanged in the urine within 24 hours. Peak urine concentrations are approximately 1800 mcg/ml during the period following a single 500-mg oral dose. Increases in dosage generally produce a proportionate increase in ULTRACEF urinary concentration. The urine antibiotic concentration, following a 1-gram dose, was maintained well above the MIC of susceptible urinary pathogens for 20 to 22 hours.

Microbiology: **In vitro** tests demonstrate that the cephalosporins are bactericidal because of their inhibition of cell-wall synthesis. ULTRACEF is active against the following organisms **in vitro:**

Beta-hemolytic streptococci
Staphylococci, including coagulase-positive, coagulase-negative, and penicillinase-producing strains

Streptococcus (Diplococcus) pneumoniae
Escherichia coli
Proteus mirabilis
Klebsiella species

Note: Most strains of Enterococci (**Streptococcus faecalis** and **S. faecium**) are resistant to ULTRACEF. It is not active against most strains of **Enterobacter** species. **P. Morganii**, and **P. vulgaris**. It has no activity against **Pseudomonas** species and **Acinetobacter calcoaceticus** (formerly **Mima** and **Herellea** species).

Disc Susceptibility Tests—Quantitative methods that require measurement of zone diameters give the most precise estimates of antibiotic susceptibility. One recommended procedure (CFR Section 460.1) uses a cephalosporin-class disc for testing susceptibility; interpretations correlate zone diameters of this disc test with MIC values for ULTRACEF. With this procedure, a report from the laboratory of "resistant" indicates that the infecting organism is not likely to respond to therapy. A report of "intermediate susceptibility" suggests that the organism would be susceptible if the infection is confined to the urinary tract, as ULTRACEF produces high antibiotic levels in the urine.

Indications: ULTRACEF (cefadroxil) is indicated for the treatment of the following infections when caused by susceptible strains of the designated microorganisms:

Urinary tract infections caused by **E. coli, P. mirabilis,** and **Klebsiella** species.

Skin and skin structure infections caused by staphylococci and/or streptococci.

Pharyngitis and tonsillitis caused by Group A beta-hemolytic streptococci. (Penicillin is the usual drug of choice in the treatment and prevention of streptococcal infections, including the prophylaxis of rheumatic fever. ULTRACEF is generally effective in the eradication of streptococci from the nasopharynx; however substantial data establishing the efficacy of ULTRACEF in the subsequent prevention of rheumatic fever are not available at present.)

Note: Culture and susceptibility tests should be initiated prior to and during therapy. Renal function studies should be performed when indicated.

Contraindications: ULTRACEF (cefadroxil) is contraindicated in patients with known allergy to the cephalosporin group of antibiotics.

Warning:

IN PENICILLIN-ALLERGIC PATIENTS, CEPHALOSPORIN ANTIBIOTICS SHOULD BE USED WITH GREAT CAUTION. THERE IS CLINICAL AND LABORATORY EVIDENCE OF PARTIAL CROSS-ALLERGENICITY OF THE PENICILLINS AND THE CEPHALOSPORINS, AND THERE ARE INSTANCES OF PATIENTS WHO HAVE HAD REACTIONS TO BOTH DRUGS (INCLUDING FATAL ANAPHYLAXIS AFTER PARENTERAL USE).

Any patient who had demonstrated a history of some form of allergy, particularly to drugs, should receive antibiotics cautiously and then only when absolutely necessary. No exception should be made with regard to ULTRACEF (cefadroxil).

Pseudomembranous colitis has been reported with the use of cephalosporins (and other broad spectrum antibiotics); therefore, it is important to consider its diagnosis in patients who develop diarrhea in association with antibiotic use.

Treatment with broad spectrum antibiotics alters normal flora of the colon and may permit overgrowth of clostridia. Studies indicate a toxin produced by **Clostridium difficile** is one primary cause of antibiotic-associated colitis. Cholestyramine and colestipol resins have been shown to bind the toxin **in vitro**.

Mild cases of colitis may respond to drug discontinuance alone.

Moderate to severe cases should be managed with fluid, electrolyte and protein supplementation as indicated.

When the colitis is not relieved by drug discontinuance or when it is severe, oral vancomycin is the treatment of choice for antibiotic-associated pseudomembranous colitis produced by **C. difficile**. Other causes of colitis should also be considered.

Precautions: Patients should be followed carefully so that any side effects or unusual manifestations of drug idiosyncrasy may be detected. If a hypersensitivity reaction occurs, the drug should be discontinued and the patient treated with the usual agents (e.g., epinephrine or other pressor amines, antihistamines, or corticosteroids).

ULTRACEF (cefadroxil) should be used with caution in the presence of markedly impaired renal function (creatinine clearance rate of less than 50 ml/min/1.73M^2). (See DOSAGE AND ADMINISTRATION.) In patients with known or suspected renal impairment, careful clinical observation and appropriate laboratory studies should be made prior to and during therapy.

Prolonged use of ULTRACEF may result in the overgrowth of nonsusceptible organisms. Careful observation of the patient is essential. If superinfection occurs during therapy, appropriate measures should be taken.

Positive direct Coombs' tests have been reported during treatment with the cephalosporin antibiotics. In hematologic studies or in transfusion cross-matching procedures when antiglobulin tests are performed on the minor side or in Coombs' testing of newborns whose mothers have received cephalosporin antibiotics before parturition, it should be recognized that a positive Coombs' test may be due to the drug.

ULTRACEF should be prescribed with caution in individuals with a history of gastrointestinal disease, particularly colitis.

Usage in Pregnancy: Pregnancy Category B: Reproduction studies have been performed in mice and rats at doses up to 11 times the human dose and have revealed no evidence of impaired fertility or harm to the fetus due to cefadroxil. There are, however, no adequate and well controlled studies in pregnant women. Because animal reproduction studies are not always predictive of human response, this drug should be used during pregnancy only if clearly needed.

Nursing Mothers: Caution should be exercised when cefadroxil is administered to a nursing mother.

Adverse Reactions:

Gastrointestinal — Symptoms of pseudomembranous colitis can appear during antibiotic treatment. Nausea and vomiting have been reported rarely. Administration with food decreases nausea and does not decrease absorption. Diarrhea and dysuria have also occurred.

Hypersensitivity — Allergies (in the form of rash, urticaria, and angioedema) have been observed. These reactions usually subsided upon discontinuation of the drug.

Other reactions have included genital pruritus, genital moniliasis, vaginitis, and moderate transient neutropenia.

Dosage and Administration: ULTRACEF (cefadroxil) is acid stable and may be administered orally without regard to meals. Administration with food may be helpful in diminishing potential gastrointestinal complaints occasionally associated with oral cephalosporin therapy.

Adults

Urinary Tract Infections — for uncomplicated lower urinary tract infections (i.e. cystitis) the usual dosage is 1 or 2 grams per day in single (q.d.) or divided doses (b.i.d.).

For all other urinary tract infections the usual dosage is 2 grams per day in divided doses (b.i.d.).

Skin and Skin Structure Infections — For skin and skin structure infections the usual dosage is 1 gram per day in single (q.d.) or divided doses (b.i.d.).

Pharyngitis and Tonsillitis — Treatment of Group A beta-hemolytic streptococcal pharyngitis and tonsillitis — 1 gram per day in divided doses (b.i.d.) for 10 days.

Children — The recommended daily dosage for children is 30 mg/kg/day in divided doses every 12 hours as indicated:

Child's Weight		Ultracef Oral Suspension	
lbs	Kg	125 mg/5 ml	250 mg/5 ml
10	4.5	½ tsp. b.i.d.	
20	9.1	1 tsp. b.i.d.	½ tsp. b.i.d.
30	13.6	1 ½ tsp. b.i.d.	¾ tsp. b.i.d.
40	18.2	2 tsp. b.i.d.	1 tsp. b.i.d.
50	22.7	2 ½ tsp. b.i.d.	1 ¼ tsp. b.i.d.

In the treatment of beta-hemolytic, streptococcal infections, a therapeutic dosage of Ultracef should be administered for at least ten days.

In patients with renal impairment, the dosage of cefadroxil should be adjusted according to creatinine clearance rates to prevent drug accumulation. The following schedule is suggested. In adults, the initial dose is 1000 mg of ULTRACEF (cefadroxil) and the maintenance dose (based on the creatinine clearance rate [ml/min/1.73M^2]) is 500 mg at the time intervals listed below.

Creatinine Clearances	Dosage Interval
0-10 ml/min	36 hours
10-25 ml/min	24 hours
25-50 ml/min	12 hours

Patients with creatinine clearance rates over 50 ml/min may be treated as if they were patients having normal renal function.

How Supplied: ULTRACEF (cefadroxil) tablets. Each tablet contains cefadroxil monohydrate equivalent to 1 gram cefadroxil.

NDC 0015-7286—1 gram

ULTRACEF (cefadroxil) capsules. Each capsule contains cefadroxil monohydrate equivalent to 500 mg cefadroxil.

NDC 0015-7271—500 mg

ULTRACEF (cefadroxil) for oral suspension. Each 5 ml of reconstituted suspension contains cefadroxil monohydrate equivalent to 125 mg or 250 mg cefadroxil.

NDC 0015-7283—125 mg
NDC 0015-7284—250 mg

Directions for mixing are included on the label. Shake well before using. Keep container tightly closed.

Store reconstituted suspension in refrigerator, discard unused portion after 14 days.

For information on package sizes available, refer to the current price schedule.

[*Shown in Product Identification Section*]

VERSAPEN®-K CAPSULES

(hetacillin potassium)

VERSAPEN® ℞

(hetacillin)

Oral Suspension, Pediatric Drops

This is the full text of the latest Official Package Circular dated April 1979 [7805DIR-15].

Description: Versapen (hetacillin) is a semisynthetic antibiotic derived from the penicillin nucleus, 6-aminopenicillanic acid. **The antibiotic activity of hetacillin is provided by its rapid conversion to ampicillin.**

Actions:

Pharmacology

Oral preparations of hetacillin are acid stable and, therefore, well absorbed. Food retards absorption. In the conversion of hetacillin to ampicillin at a pH of 7.1, the hetacillin half-life is 20 minutes. Oral formulations of hetacillin and hetacillin potassium equivalent to 225 mg.

Continued on next page

Bristol—Cont.

and 450 mg. of ampicillin activity provide peak blood levels in the range of 1.7 to 2.1 mcg./ml. and 2.5 to 2.7 mcg./ml., respectively.
Ampicillin diffuses readily into most body tissues and fluids. However, penetration into the cerebrospinal fluid and brain occurs only when the meninges are inflamed. Ampicillin is excreted largely unchanged in the urine and its excretion can be delayed by concurrent administration of probenecid. The active form appears in the bile in higher concentrations than those found in the serum. Ampicillin is the least serum-bound of all the penicillins, averaging about 20% compared to approximately 60 to 90% for other penicillins.

Microbiology
No antibacterial activity has been demonstrated for the hetacillin moiety itself. Hetacillin, upon conversion to the active drug, ampicillin, is similar to benzyl penicillin in its bactericidal action against susceptible organisms during the stage of active multiplication.
The following bacteria have been shown in **in vitro** studies to be susceptible to ampicillin.
Gram-Positive Organisms—Hemolytic and nonhemolytic streptococci, **D. pneumoniae,** non-penicillinase-producing staphylococci, Clostridia spp., **B. anthracis, Listeria monocytogenes,** and most strains of enterococci.
Gram-Negative Organisms—H. influenzae, N. gonorrhoeae, N. meningitidis, Proteus mirabilis, and many strains of Salmonella, Shigella, and **E. coli.**
The drug does not resist destruction by penicillinase and hence is not effective against penicillin G-resistant staphylococci. Ampicillin Susceptibility Test Discs, 10 micrograms, should be used to estimate the **in vitro** susceptibility of bacteria to hetacillin.
Indications: Versapen is indicated in the treatment of susceptible strains of the following organisms in the diseases listed. Bacteriology studies to determine the causative organisms and their susceptibility should be performed. Therapy may be instituted prior to obtaining results of susceptibility testing.
Group A beta-hemolytic streptococcus: Tonsillitis, pharyngitis, otitis media, skin and soft tissue infections. (Injectable benzathine penicillin is considered to be the drug of choice in treatment and prevention of streptococcal pharyngitis and in long-term prophylaxis of rheumatic fever. Versapen is effective in the eradication of streptococci from the nasopharynx; however, data establishing the efficacy of orally administered Versapen in the subsequent prevention of rheumatic fever are not available at present.)
Diplococcus pneumoniae: Broncho- and lobar pneumonia, otitis media.
Non-penicillinase-producing **Staphylococcus aureus:** Skin and soft tissue infections, otitis media.
Haemophilus influenzae: Bronchitis, bronchopneumonia, otitis media.
Escherichia coli: Cystitis, pyelonephritis, prostatitis/urethritis, skin and soft tissue infections.
Proteus mirabilis: Cystitis, pyelonephritis, skin and soft tissue infections.
Enterococcus (Streptococcus faecalis): Cystitis, pyelonephritis, prostatitis/urethritis.
Shigella species: Shigellosis.
Indicated surgical procedures should be performed.
Contraindications: A history of a previous hypersensitivity reaction to any of the penicillins is a contraindication.
Warnings: Serious and occasionally fatal hypersensitivity (anaphylactic) reactions have been reported in patients on penicillin therapy. Although anaphylaxis is more frequent following parenteral therapy, it has occurred in patients on oral penicillins. These reactions are more apt to occur in individuals with a history of sensitivity to multiple allergens.
There have been reports of individuals with a history of penicillin hypersensitivity reactions who experienced severe hypersensitivity reactions when treated with cephalosporins. Before therapy with a penicillin, careful inquiry should be made concerning previous hypersensitivity reactions to penicillins, cephalosporins, and other allergens.
Serious anaphylactoid reactions require immediate emergency treatment with epinephrine. Oxygen, intravenous steroids, and airway management, including intubation, should also be administered as indicated.
Usage in Pregnancy: Safety for use in pregnancy has not been established.
Precautions: The possibility of superinfection with mycotic or bacterial pathogens should be kept in mind during therapy. In such cases, discontinue the drug and substitute appropriate treatment.
As with any potent drug, periodic assessment of renal, hepatic, and hematopoietic function should be made during prolonged therapy.
This oral preparation should not be relied upon in patients with severe illness or with nausea, vomiting, gastric dilatation, cardiospasm, or intestinal hypermotility.
Adverse Reactions: As with other penicillins, it may be expected that untoward reactions will be essentially limited to sensitivity phenomena. They are more likely to occur in individuals who have previously demonstrated hypersensitivity to penicillins and in those with a history of allergy, asthma, hay fever, or urticaria.
The following adverse reactions have been reported:
Gastrointestinal: Glossitis, stomatitis, black "hairy" tongue, nausea, vomiting, enterocolitis, pseudomembranous colitis, and diarrhea. (These reactions are usually associated with oral dosage forms.)
Hypersensitivity reactions: Skin rashes and urticaria have been reported frequently. A few cases of exfoliative dermatitis and erythema multiforme have been reported. Anaphylaxis is the most serious reaction experienced and has usually been associated with the parenteral dosage form.
Note: Urticaria, other skin rashes, and serum sickness-like reactions may be controlled with antihistamines and, if necessary, systemic corticosteroids. Whenever such reactions occur, the drug should be discontinued, unless, in the opinion of the physician, the condition being treated is life threatening and amenable only to this therapy.
Liver: A moderate rise in serum glutamic oxaloacetic transaminase (SGOT) has been noted, particularly in infants, but the significance of this finding is unknown.
Hemic and Lymphatic Systems: Anemia, thrombocytopenia, thrombocytopenic purpura, eosinophilia, leukopenia, and agranulocytosis have been reported during therapy with the penicillins. These reactions are usually reversible on discontinuation of therapy and are believed to be hypersensitivity phenomena.
Other: Since infectious mononucleosis is viral in origin, hetacillin should not be used in the treatment. A high percentage of patients with mononucleosis who received ampicillin developed a skin rash.
Dosage: Infections of the upper and lower respiratory tracts; those of the skin and soft tissue; and infections of the gastrointestinal and genitourinary tracts due to susceptible organisms:
Patients weighing 88 lbs. (40 Kg.) or more: 225 to 450 mg. q.i.d., depending on the severity of the infection.
Patients weighing less than 88 lbs. (40 Kg.): 22.5 to 45 mg./Kg./day or 10 to 20 mg./lb./day, depending on the severity of the infection.
Urinary and gastrointestinal tract infections may require prolonged and intensive therapy at doses higher than those recommended above. It may be necessary to maintain therapy for several weeks and to continue bacteriologic and/or clinical follow-up for several months after cessation of therapy.
The oral drug should be administered in a fasting state to insure maximum absorption.
For very severe infections in adults or children, treatment should be initiated with parenteral ampicillin.
INFECTIONS DUE TO GROUP A BETA-HEMOLYTIC STREPTOCOCCI SHOULD BE TREATED FOR A MINIMUM OF TEN DAYS.

Directions for Dispensing Oral Suspension and Pediatric Drops

Prepare these formulations at the time of dispensing. For ease in preparation, add water to the bottle in two portions and shake well after each addition. Add the total amount of water as directed on the labeling of the package being dispensed. The reconstituted formulation is stable 14 days under refrigeration.
Supply: VERSAPEN-K (hetacillin potassium) Capsules. Hetacillin potassium equivalent to 225 or 450 mg. ampicillin per capsule.
NDC 0015-7805—225 mg.
NDC 0015-7806—450 mg.
[*Shown in Product Identification Section*]
VERSAPEN (hetacillin) for Oral Suspension. Each 5 ml. of reconstituted oral suspension contains hetacillin equivalent to 112.5 or 225 mg. ampicillin.
NDC 0015-7808—112.5 mg., 100 ml. bottle
NDC 0015-7809—225 mg., 100 ml. bottle
VERSAPEN (hetacillin) Pediatric Drops. Each ml. of reconstituted pediatric drops contains hetacillin equivalent to 112.5 mg. ampicillin.
NDC 0015-7807—112.5 mg.
For informtion on package sizes available, refer to the current price schedule.

Bristol-Myers Products
(Div. of Bristol-Myers Co.)
345 PARK AVENUE
NEW YORK, NY 10154

ARTHRITIS STRENGTH BUFFERIN®
Analgesic

Composition: Aspirin $7\frac{1}{2}$ gr. (486 mg.) in a formulation buffered with Di-Alminate,® Bristol-Myers' brand of Aluminum Glycinate 1.125 gr. (72.9 mg.) and Magnesium Carbonate 2.25 gr. (145.8 mg.).
Action and Uses: ARTHRITIS STRENGTH BUFFERIN is specially formulated to give temporary relief from the minor aches and pains, stiffness, swelling and inflammation of arthritis and rheumatism. ARTHRITIS STRENGTH BUFFERIN also reduces pain and fever of colds and "flu" and provides fast, effective pain relief for: simple headache, lower back muscular aches from fatigue, sinusitis, neuralgia, neuritis, tooth extraction, muscle strain, athletic soreness, painful distress associated with normal menstrual periods. The leading aspirin substitute acetaminophen cannot provide relief from inflammation.
ARTHRITIS STRENGTH BUFFERIN PROVIDES INGREDIENTS FOR STOMACH PROTECTION JUST LIKE REGULAR BUFFERIN WHICH HELP PREVENT THE STOMACH UPSET ASPIRIN OFTEN CAUSES.
Contraindications: Hypersensitivity to salicylates.
Caution: If pain persists for more than 10 days or redness is present or in Arthritic or Rheumatic conditions affecting children under 12, consult physician immediately. Do not take without consulting physician if under medical care, pregnant or nursing a baby. WARNING: Keep this and all medicines out of children's

reach. In case of accidental overdose, contact a physician immediately.
Administration and Dosage: Two tablets with water. Repeat after four hours if necessary. Do not exceed 8 tablets in any 24 hour period. If dizziness, impaired hearing or ringing in ear occurs, discontinue use. Not recommended for children.
Overdose: (Symptoms and Treatment) Typical of aspirin.
How Supplied: Tablets in bottles of 40 and 100. Samples available upon request.
Product Identification: White elongated tablet.
Literature Available: Upon request.

BUFFERIN® Analgesic

Composition: Aspirin 5 gr. (324 mg.) in a formulation buffered with Di-Alminate®, Bristol-Myers's brand of Aluminum Glycinate ¾ gr. (48.6 mg.), and Magnesium Carbonate 1½ gr. (97.2 mg.).
Action and Uses: Bufferin® is for relief of simple headache; and for temporary relief of: minor arthritic pain, the painful discomforts and fever of colds and "flu", menstrual cramps, muscular aches from fatigue and toothache. Bufferin® helps prevent the stomach upset often caused by plain aspirin.
Contraindications: Hypersensitivity to salicylates.
Caution: If pain persists for more than 10 days or redness is present or, in Arthritic or Rheumatic conditions affecting children under 12, consult physician immediately. Do not take without consulting physician if under medical care, pregnant or nursing a baby. Consult a dentist for toothache promptly.
Warning: Keep this and all medicines out of children's reach. In case of accidental overdose, consult a physician immediately.
Dosage: 2 tablets every four hours as needed. Do not exceed 12 tablets in 24 hours, unless directed by a physician. For children 6-12, one-half dose. Under 6, consult physician.
Overdose: (Symptoms and treatment) Typical of aspirin.
How Supplied: Tablets in bottles of 12, 36, 60, 100, 165, 225, and 375. For hospital and clinical use: bottle—1,000; boxed 200x2 tablet foil packets. Samples available on request.
Product Identification Mark: White tablet with letter "B" on one surface.
Literature Available: Upon request.

EXTRA–STRENGTH BUFFERIN®

Composition: Each tablet and capsule contains aspirin 500 mg. in a formulation buffered with Di-Alminate®, Bristol-Myers' brand of Aluminum Glycinate 75 mg. and Magnesium Carbonate 150 mg.
Action and Uses: Extra-Strength BUFFERIN provides fast extra-strength pain relief, and is gentler on the stomach than plain aspirin. Each 2 tablet/capsule dose contains 1000 mg. of aspirin, the maximum quantity recommended without a prescription. Extra-Strength BUFFERIN is formulated to help prevent the stomach upset that plain aspirin can cause. Provides relief of headaches, menstrual cramps, toothache, muscular aches painful discomforts and fever of colds or flu, and temporary relief from the minor aches, pain and inflammation of arthritis and rheumatism.
Contraindications: Hypersensitivity to salicylates.
Caution: If pain persists for more than 10 days, or redness is present, or in arthritic or rheumatic conditions affecting children under 12, consult a physician immediately. Do not take without consulting a physician if under medical care, pregnant or nursing a baby. Consult a dentist for toothache promptly.
Warning: KEEP THIS AND ALL MEDICINES OUT OF CHILDREN'S REACH. IN CASE OF ACCIDENTAL OVERDOSE, CONSULT A PHYSICIAN IMMEDIATELY.
Administration and Dosage: Tablets—2 tablets every 4 hours as needed. Do not exceed 8 tablets in 24 hours, or give to children 12 or under, unless directed by a physician. Capsules—2 capsules every 4 hours as needed. Do not exceed 8 capsules in 24 hours, or give to childen 12 or under, unless directed by a physician.
How Supplied: Bottles of 30, 60 and 100 tablets. Capsules in bottles of 24's, 50's and 75's. All sizes packaged in child resistant closures except 60's (for tablets); 50's (for capsules) which are sizes not recommended for households with young children.
Product Identification Mark: White, elongated tablets with "ESB" imprinted on one side. White and blue capsules with "EXTRA-STRENGTH BUFFERIN" imprinted on 3 sides.

	COMTREX Tablets	COMTREX Liquid	COMTREX Capsules
Acetaminophen	325 mg.	650 mg.	325 mg.
Phenylpropanolamine HCl:	12 ½ mg.	25 mg.	12 ½ mg.
Chlorpheniramine Maleate:	1 mg.	2 mg.	1 mg.
Dextromethorphan HBr	10 mg.	20 mg.	10 mg.
Alcohol:	—	20% by Volume	—

COMTREX®
Multi-Symptom Cold Reliever

Composition: Each tablet, fluid ounce (30 ml.), and capsule contains:
[See table above].
Action and Uses: COMTREX® contains safe and effective fast acting ingredients including a non-aspirin analgesic, a decongestant, an antihistamine and a cough reliever. COMTREX relieves these major cold symptoms: nasal and sinus congestion, runny nose, sneezing, post nasal drip, watery eyes, coughing, fever, minor sore throat pain (systemically), headache, body aches and pain.
Contraindications: Hypersensitivity to acetaminophen or antihistamines.
Caution: Do not take without consulting a physician if under medical care, pregnant or nursing a baby. Do not drive a car or operate machinery while taking this cold remedy as it may cause drowsiness.
Warning: Keep this and all medicine out of children's reach. In case of accidental overdose, consult a physician immediately. Persistent cough may indicate the presence of a serious condition. Persons with a high fever or persistent cough, or with high blood pressure, diabetes, heart or thyroid disease should not use this preparation unless directed by a physician. Do not use for more than 10 days unless directed by a physician.
Administration and Dosage:
Tablets—Adults: 2 tablets every 4 hours as needed not to exceed 12 tablets in 24 hours. Children 6-12 years: ½ the adult dose. Under 6, consult a physician.
Liquid—Adults: 1 fluid ounce (30 ml.) every 4 hours as needed, not to exceed 6 fluid ounces (180 ml.) in 24 hours. Children 6-12 years: ½ the adult dose. Under 6, consult a physician.
Capsules—Adults 2 capsules every 4 hours as needed not to exceed 12 capsules in 24 hours. Children 6–12 years: ½ the adult dose. Under 6, consult a physician.
Overdose: The signs and symptoms observed would be those produced by the acetaminophen, which may cause hepatotoxicity in some patients. Since clinical and laboratory evidence may be delayed up to 1 week, close clinical monitoring and serial hepatic enzyme determinations are recommended.
How Supplied: Tablets in bottles of 12's, 24's, 50's, 100's. Capsules in bottles of 16's and 36's. Liquid in 6 oz. and 10 oz. plastic bottles. Samples available on request.
Product Identification Mark: Yellow tablet with letter "C" on one surface. Orange and Yellow capsules with "Bristol-Myers" and "Comtrex" on one side.
Literature Available: Upon request.

CONGESPIRIN®
Chewable Cold Tablets for Children

Composition: Each tablet contains aspirin 81 mg. (1¼ grains) phenylephrine hydrochloride (1¼ mg.).
Action and Uses: For the temporary relief of nasal congestion, fever, aches and pains of the common cold or "flu". Plus an effective nasal decongestant to help relieve stuffiness, runny nose and sneezing from colds.
Dosage and Administration:
Under Age 2 consult your physician.

2–3 YRS.	2 TABLETS
4–5 YRS.	3 TABLETS
6–8 YRS.	4 TABLETS
9–10 YRS.	5 TABLETS
11 YRS.	6 TABLETS
12+ YRS.	8 TABLETS

Repeat dose in four hours if necessary. Do not give more than four doses per day unless prescribed by your physician.
Caution: If child is under medical care, do not administer without consulting physician. Do not exceed recommended dosage. Consult your physician if symptoms persist or if high fever, high blood pressure, heart disease, diabetes or thyroid disease is present. Do not administer for more than 10 days unless directed by your physician.
Warning: KEEP THIS AND ALL MEDICINES OUT OF CHILDREN'S REACH. IN CASE OF ACCIDENTAL OVERDOSAGE, CONTACT A PHYSICIAN IMMEDIATELY.
How Supplied: Tablets in bottles of 36.
Product Identification Mark: Two layer (orange/white) circular tablet with letter "C" imprinted on the orange side.

CONGESPRIN®
Liquid Cold Medicine

Composition: Each 5 ml. teaspoon contains Acetaminophen 130 mg., Phenylpropanolamine Hydrochloride 6 ¼ mg., Alcohol 10% by volume.
Action and Uses: Reduces fever and relieves aches and pains associated with colds and "flu". Contains an effective decongestant for the temporary relief of nasal congestion due to the common cold, hay fever or other respiratory allergies. Reduces swelling of nasal passages, shrinks swollen membranes, restores freer breathing.
Dosage and Administration:
Children 3–5, 1 teaspoon every 3–4 hours.
Children 6–12, 2 teaspoons every 3–4 hours.
Children under 3 years use only as directed by your physician.
Do not give more than 4 doses a day unless directed by your physician.
Caution: If child is under medical care, do not administer without consulting physician. Do not exceed recommended dosage. Consult your physician if symptoms persist or if high fever, high blood pressure, heart disease, diabetes or thyroid disease is present. Do not administer for more than 10 days unless directed by your physician.
Warning: KEEP THIS AND ALL MEDICINES OUT OF CHILDREN'S REACH. IN

Continued on next page

Bristol-Myers—Cont.

CASE OF ACCIDENTAL OVERDOSAGE, CONTACT A PHYSICIAN IMMEDIATELY.
How Supplied: In 3 oz. plastic, unbreakable bottles.

DATRIL® Analgesic

Composition: Each tablet contains acetaminophen 5 gr. (325 mg.)
Actions and Uses: The **DATRIL** formula contains a safe, effective, non-aspirin analgesic that relieves pain fast, without causing the gastric bleeding that aspirin tablets can cause. DATRIL is also less likely to cause the nausea and stomach upset that plain aspirin tablets can cause. DATRIL provides relief from the pain of: • Headache • Colds or "flu" • Bursitis • Menstrual discomfort • Sinusitis • Muscular aches due to fatigue or overexertion • Muscular backache • Neuralgia. **DATRIL** also helps reduce fever of colds or "flu" and provides temporary relief from toothache and minor arthritic or rheumatic aches and pain. For most persons with peptic ulcer **DATRIL** may be used safely and comfortably when taken as directed for recommended conditions.
Contraindications: There have been rare reports of skin rash or glossitis attributed to acetaminophen. Discontinue use if a sensitivity reaction occurs. However, acetaminophen is usually well tolerated by aspirin-sensitive patients.
Caution: If pain persists for more than 10 days or redness is present or in arthritic or rheumatic conditions affecting children under 12, consult physician immediately. Do not take without consulting a physician if under medical care, pregnant or nursing a baby. Consult a dentist for toothache promptly.
Warning: Do not give to children under 6 or use for more than 10 days unless directed by a physician. Keep this and all medicines out of reach of children. In case of accidental overdose contact a physician promptly.
Dosage: 2 tablets every four hours, 1 to 4 times daily as needed, or as directed by a physician. For children 6–12 years of age use half the adult dose.
Overdose: A massive overdose of acetaminophen may cause hepatotoxicity in some patients. Since clinical and laboratory evidence may be delayed up to 1 week, close clinical monitoring and serial hepatic enzyme determinations are recommended.
How Supplied: Tablets in bottles of 24 and 100. Samples available on request.
Product Identification Mark: White tablet with name "Datril" on one surface.
Literature Available: Upon request.

EXTRA-STRENGTH DATRIL™

Composition: Each tablet contains acetaminophen, 500 mg.
Actions and Uses: Extra-Strength DATRIL has been specially developed to provide fast, extra-strength pain relief. It contains a non-aspirin ingredient (acetaminophen) which is less likely to irritate the stomach than plain aspirin. Extra-Strength DATRIL is fast-acting. Extra-Strength DATRIL tablets are for the temporary relief of minor aches, pains, headaches and fever. For most persons with peptic ulcer Extra-Strength DATRIL may be used when taken as directed for recommended conditions.
Contraindictions: There have been rare reports of skin rash or glossitis attributed to acetaminophen. Discontinue use if a sensitivity reaction occurs. However, acetaminophen is usually well tolerated by aspirin-sensitive patients.
Caution: Severe or recurrent pain or high or continued fever may be indicative of serious illness. Under these conditions consult a physician.
Warning: Do not give to children 12 and under or use for more than 10 days unless directed by a physician. Do not take without consulting a physician if under medical care, pregnant or nursing a baby. Keep this and all medicines out of reach of children. In case of accidental overdose contact a physician immediately.
Dosage: Adults: Two tablets. May be repeated in 4 hours if needed. Do not exceed 8 tablets in any 24 hour period.
Overdose: A massive overdose of acetaminophen may cause hepatotoxicity in some patients. Since clinical and laboratory evidence may be delayed up to 1 week, close clinical monitoring and serial hepatic enzyme determinations are recommended.
How Supplied: Tablets in bottles of 24's, 50's and 72's. Samples available on request.
Product Identification Mark: White tablet with DATRIL 500 on one surface.
Literature Available: Upon request.

EXCEDRIN® Analgesic

Composition: Each tablet and capsule contains Acetaminophen 250 mg.; Aspirin 250 mg.; and Caffeine 65 mg.
Action and Uses: Extra-Strength Excedrin provides fast, effective relief from pain of: headache, sinusitis, colds or 'flu', muscular aches and menstrual discomfort. Also recommended for temporary relief of toothaches and minor arthritic pains.
Contraindications: Hypersensitivity to salicylates or acetaminophen.
Caution: If sinus or arthritis pain persists (say for a week), or if skin redness is present, or in arthritic conditions affecting children under 12, consult physician immediately. Consult dentist for toothache promptly. Do not take without consulting physician if under medical care, pregnant or nursing a baby.
Warning: Do not exceed 8 tablets/capsules in 24 hours or use for more than 10 days unless directed, or give to children under 12. Keep this and all medicines out of children's reach. In case of accidental overdose, contact a physician immediately.
Administration and Dosage: Tablets—Individuals 12 and over, take 2 tablets every 4 hours as needed. Capsules—Individuals 12 and over, take 2 capsules every 4 hours as needed.
How Supplied: Bottles of 12, 36, 60, 100, 165, 225, and 375 tablets. Capsules in bottles of 24's, 40's and 60's. A metal tin of 12 tablets. All sizes packaged in child resistant closures except 100's (for tablets); 60's (for capsules) which are sizes not recommended for households with young children.
Product Identification Mark: White, circular tablet with letter "E" imprinted on both sides. Red capsules with "EXCEDRIN" printed on 2 sides.
Literature Available: Upon request.

EXCEDRIN P.M.® Nighttime Analgesic

Composition: Each tablet contains Acetaminophen 500 mg. and Pyrilamine Maleate 25 mg.
Action and Uses: Excedrin P.M. has a special formula that provides prompt relief of nighttime pain and aids sleep for people with headache, bursitis, colds or "flu", sinusitis, muscle aches and menstrual discomfort. Also recommended for temporary relief of toothaches and minor arthritic pain.
Contraindications: Hypersensitivity to acetaminophen.
Caution: If sinus or arthritis pain persists (say for a week) or if skin redness is present, or in arthritic conditions affecting children under 12 consult physician immediately. Do not drive a car or operate machinery after use. Consult dentist for toothache promptly. Do not take without consulting physician if under medical care, pregnant or nursing a baby.
Warning: Do not exceed 2 tablets in 24 hours, or give to children under 12 or use for more than 10 days unless directed by physician. KEEP THIS AND ALL MEDICINES OUT OF CHILDREN'S REACH. IN CASE OF ACCIDENTAL OVERDOSE, CONTACT A PHYSICIAN IMMEDIATELY. If sleeplessness persists for more than two weeks, consult your physician. Insomnia may be a symptom of serious underlying medical ailments. Take this product with caution if alcohol is being consumed. DO NOT TAKE THIS PRODUCT IF YOU HAVE ASTHMA, GLAUCOMA OR ENLARGEMENT OF THE PROSTATE GLAND EXCEPT UNDER THE ADVICE AND SUPERVISION OF A PHYSICIAN.
Administration and Dosage: Adults take two tablets at bedtime to help relieve pain and aid sleep.
How Supplied: Bottles of 10, 30, 50, and 80 tablets. All sizes packaged in child resistant closures except 50's, which is a size not recommended for households with young children.
Product Identification Mark: Blue/green circular tablet with letters "PM" imprinted on one side.

4-WAY® Cold Tablets

Composition: Each tablet contains aspirin 324 mg., phenylpropanolamine HCl 12 ½ mg., and chlorpheniramine maleate 2 mg.
Action and Uses: For temporary relief of minor aches and pains, fever, nasal congestion and runny nose as may occur in the common cold.
Dosage and Administration:
Adults—2 tablets every 4 hours, if needed. Do not exceed 6 tablets in 24 hours. Children 6–12 years—1 tablet every 4 hours. Do not exceed 4 tablets in 24 hours. Under age 6, consult a physician.
Warning: Do not take without consulting a physician if under medical care, pregnant or nursing a baby.
Caution: This preparation may cause drowsiness. Do not drive or operate machinery while taking this medication. Individuals with high blood pressure, heart disease, diabetes, or thyroid disease should use only as directed by physician. Do not exceed recommended dosage. KEEP THIS AND ALL MEDICINES OUT OF CHILDREN'S REACH. IN CASE OF ACCIDENTAL OVERDOSE, CONTACT PHYSICIAN IMMEDIATELY.
How Supplied: Carded 15's and bottles of 36's and 60's.
Product Identification Mark: Pink and White tablet with number "4" on one surface.

4-WAY® Nasal Spray

Composition: Phenylephrine hydrochloride 0.5%, naphazoline hydrochloride 0.05%, pyrilamine maleate 0.2%, in a buffered isotonic aqueous solution with thimerosal 0.005% added as a preservative. Also available in a mentholated formula.
Action and Uses: For relief of nasal congestion, runny nose, sneezing, itching nose, and watery eyes which may be symptoms of the common cold, sinusitis, nasal allergies, or hay fever.
Dosage and Administration: With head in a normal upright position, put atomizer tip into nostril. Squeeze atomizer with firm, quick pressure while inhaling. Adults-spray twice into each nostril. Children 6-12-spray once. Under 6-consult physician. Repeat in three hours, if needed.
Warning: Overdosage in young children may cause marked sedation. Do not exceed recommended dosage. Follow directions carefully. If symptoms persist, consult physician. The use of this dispenser by more than one person may spread infection. Keep out of children's reach.

How Supplied: Atomizers of ½ fluid ounce and 1 fluid ounce.

4-WAY® Long Acting Nasal Spray

Composition: Xylometazoline Hydrochloride 0.1% in a buffered isotonic aqueous solution. Thimerosal, 0.005% added as a preservative. Also available in a mentholated formula.
Action and Uses: Provides temporary relief of nasal congestion due to the common cold, sinusitis, hayfever or other upper respiratory allergies.
Dosage and Administration: With head in a normal upright position, put atomizer tip into nostril. Squeeze atomizer with firm, quick pressure while inhaling. Adults: Spray 2 or 3 times in each nostril every 8 to 10 hours. For children under 12, consult physician.
Warning: For adult use only. Do not give this product to children under 12 years except under the advice and supervision of a physician. Do not exceed recommended dosage because symptoms may occur such as burning, stinging, sneezing, or an increase of nasal discharge. Do not use this product for more than 3 days. If symptoms persist, consult a physician. The use of this dispenser by more than one person may spread infection.
KEEP OUT OF CHILDREN'S REACH.
How Supplied: Atomizers of ½ fluid ounce.

NO DOZ® TABLETS

Composition: Each tablet contains 100 mg. Caffeine. No Doz is non-habit forming.
Action and Uses: Helps restore mental alertness.
Dosage and Administration:
For Adults: 2 tablets initially, thereafter, 1 tablet every three hours should be sufficient.
Caution: Do not take without consulting physician if under medical care, pregnant or nursing a baby. No stimulant should be substituted for normal sleep in activities requiring physical alertness.
KEEP THIS AND ALL MEDICINES OUT OF THE REACH OF CHILDREN.
How Supplied: Carded 15's and 36's and bottles of 60's.
Product Identification Mark: A white tablet with No Doz on one side.

PAZO® HEMORRHOID OINTMENT/SUPPOSITORIES

Composition: Triolyte®, Bristol-Myers brand of the combination of benzocaine (0.8%) and ephedrine sulphate (0.24%); zinc oxide (4.0%); camphor (2.18%), in an emollient base.
Action and Uses: Pazo helps shrink swelling of inflamed hemorrhoid tissue. Provides prompt, temporary relief of burning itch and pain in many cases.
Administration:
Ointment—Apply stainless Pazo well up in rectum night and morning, and after each bowel movement. Repeat as often during the day as may be necessary to maintain comfort. Continue for one week after symptoms subside. When applicator is used, lubricate applicator first with Pazo. Insert slowly, then simply press tube.
Suppositories—Remove foil and insert one Pazo suppository night and morning, and after each bowel movement. Repeat as often during the day as may be necessary to maintain comfort. Continue for one week after symptoms subside.
Warning: If the underlying condition persists or recurs frequently, despite treatment, or if any bleeding or hard irreducible swelling is present, consult your physician.
Keep out of children's reach. Keep in a cool place.
How Supplied:
Ointment—1-ounce and 2-ounce tubes with plastic applicator.
Suppositories—Boxes of 12 and 24 wrapped in silver foil.
Literature Available: Yes.

The Brown Pharmaceutical Company, Inc.

2500 WEST SIXTH STREET
P.O. BOX 57925
LOS ANGELES, CA 90057

ANDROID®-5 ℞
Methyltestosterone U.S.P. 5 mg. (Buccal Tablets)

ANDROID®-10 ℞
Methyltestosterone U.S.P. 10 mg.

ANDROID®-25 ℞
Methyltestosterone U.S.P. 25 mg.

Description: Methyltestosterone is an androgenic steroid which occurs as white or creamy white crystals or crystalline powder.
Action: The actions of anabolic steroids are similar to those of male sex hormones.
As methyltestosterone is a 17-methylated steroid it is protected to a certain extent from the liver. Consequently, oral administration does not result in rapid destruction of the preparation by its passage through the hepatic system.
Indications:
In the Male:
1. Eunuchoidism and eunuchism.
2. Climacteric symptoms when these are secondary to androgen deficiency.
3. Impotence due to androgen deficiency.
4. Postpuberal cryptorchidism with evidence of hypogonadism.

In the Female:
1. Prevention of postpartum breast pain and engorgement. There is no satisfactory evidence that this drug prevents or suppresses lactation.
2. Palliation of androgen-responsive, advancing, inoperable mammary cancer in women who are more than 1 year, but less than 5 years postmenopausal or who have been proven to have a hormone-dependent tumor as shown by previous beneficial response to castration.

Contraindications: Carcinoma of the male breast; known or suspected carcinoma of the prostate; cardiac, hepatic, or renal decompensation; hypercalcemia; impaired liver function; prepuberal males; patients easily stimulated; pregnancy; and breast feeding.
Warnings: Hypercalcemia may occur in immobilized patients and in breast cancer patients. In patients with cancer, hypercalcemia may indicate progression of bony metastasis, in which case the drug should be discontinued. Watch female patients closely for signs of virilization. Some effects such as voice changes may not be reversible even when the drug is stopped.
Discontinue the drug if cholestatic hepatitis with jaundice appears or liver function tests become abnormal.
Precautions: Patients with cardiac, renal or hepatic derangement may retain sodium and water with resulting edema formation.
Males, especially the elderly, may become overly stimulated.
Priapism or excessive sexual stimulation may develop.
Oligospermia and reduced ejaculatory volume may occur after prolonged administration or excessive dosage.
Hypersensitivity and gynecomastia may occur.
Alterations in liver function tests (e.g. increased BSP retention and SGOT levels) and rarely jaundice have been reported and appear to be directly related to the dose of the drug. When any of these effects appear, the androgen should be stopped; if restarted, a lower dosage should be utilized.
Use cautiously in young boys to avoid possible premature epiphyseal closure or precocious sexual development.
The PBI may decrease during androgen therapy without clinical significance.
Adverse Reactions: Hypersensitivity, including skin manifestations and anaphylactoid reactions; acne; decreased ejaculatory volume; oligospermia; gynecomastia; edema; priapism; hypercalcemia; especially in immobile patients and those with metastatic breast carcinoma; virilization in females; cholestatic jaundice. There have been rare reports of hepatocellular neoplasms and peliosis hepatis in patients who have received androgenic-anabolic steroids, usually over prolonged periods of time.
Dosage and Administration: Dosage must be strictly individualized. Daily requirements are best administered in divided doses. The following chart is suggested as an average daily dosage guide. Duration of therapy will depend upon the response of the condition being treated and the appearance of adverse reactions.
Note: Buccal tablets have approximately twice the potency of the orally ingested hormone.
Indications:

	Average Daily Dosage Buccal	Tablet
In the Male:		
Eunuchism and eunuchoidism	5 to 20 mg.	10 to 40 mg.
Male climacteric and male impotency	5 to 20 mg.	10 to 40 mg.
Cryptorchidism-postpuberal	15 mg.	30 mg.
In the female:		
Postpartum breast pain & engorgement (3 to 5 days)	40 mg.	80 mg.
Breast cancer	100 mg.	200 mg.

Administration of Buccal Tablets: Buccal tablets should not be swallowed since the hormone is meant to be absorbed through the mucous membranes. Place buccal tablet in the upper or lower buccal pouch between the gum and cheek. Avoid eating, drinking, chewing, or smoking while the buccal tablet is in place. Proper oral hygienic measures are particularly important after the use of buccal tablets.
How Supplied: Tablets of 10 mg. and 25 mg. concentrations and buccal tablets of 5 mg. concentration.
[*Shown in Product Identification Section*]

ANDROID-F® ℞
Fluoxymesterone 10 mg.

Composition:
Android-F—10 mg. NDC 0248-6998-01
Each white scored tablet contains:
Fluoxymesterone ....10 mg.
Administration and Dosage: See Insert.
How Supplied: Available in bottles of 60 and 250.
[*Shown in Product Identification Section*]

LIPO-NICIN®/100 mg. Tablets ℞
LIPO-NICIN®/250 mg. Tablets
LIPO-NICIN®/300 mg. Timed Caps

Composition:
LIPO-NICIN®/100 mg.
Each blue tablet contains:
Nicotinic Acid ....100 mg.
Niacinamide .... 75 mg.
Ascorbic Acid ....150 mg.
Thiamine HCl (B-1) .... 25 mg.
Riboflavin (B-2) .... 2 mg.
Pyridoxine HCl (B-6) .... 10 mg.

Continued on next page

Brown—Cont.

LIPO-NICIN /250 mg.
Each yellow tablet contains:
Nicotinic Acid .... 250 mg.
Niacinamide .... 75 mg.
Ascorbic Acid .... 150 mg.
Thiamine HCl (B-1) .... 25 mg.
Riboflavin (B-2) .... 2 mg.
Pyridoxine HCl (B-6) .... 10 mg.
LIPO-NICIN®/300 mg. Timed Caps
Each red capsule contains:
Nicotinic Acid .... 300 mg.
Vitamin C (Ascorbic Acid) .... 150 mg.
Vitamin B_1 (Thiamine HCl) .... 25 mg.
Vitamin B_2 (Riboflavin) .... 2 mg.
Pyridoxine HCl (B_6) .... 10 mg.
In a special base so prepared that the active ingredients are released over a period of 6 to 8 hours.

Action and Uses: For use as a vasodilator in the symptoms of cold feet, leg cramps, dizziness, memory loss or tinnitus when associated with impaired peripheral circulation. Also provides concomitant administration of the listed vitamins.
The warm tingling flush which may follow each dose is one of the therapeutic effects that often produce psychologic benefits to the patient.

Side Effects: Flushing with heat and itching, in some cases followed by sweating, nausea and abdominal cramps. This reaction is usually transient. Nausea caused by high acidity can be relieved by nonabsorbable antacid.

Caution: Federal law prohibits dispensing without prescription.

Administration and Dosage:
LIPO-NICIN /100 mg.—1 to 5 tablets daily.
LIPO-NICIN /250 mg.—1 to 3 tablets daily.
LIPO-NICIN® /300 mg Timed— 1 to 2 capsules daily.

Available: Bottles of 100, 500.

Literature Available: Samples.

Burroughs Wellcome Co.

3030 CORNWALLIS ROAD
RESEARCH TRIANGLE PARK,
NC 27709

LITERATURE AVAILABLE: Folders, circulars, file cards, films, slides, lecture guides and monographs.

ACTIFED® TABLETS and SYRUP

(See PDR For Nonprescription Drugs)

ACTIFED-C® EXPECTORANT ℞ ©

Description: Each 5 ml (1 teaspoonful) contains: codeine phosphate 10 mg (Warning —may be habit-forming), Actidil® (Triprolidine Hydrochloride) 2 mg, Sudafed® (Pseudoephedrine Hydrochloride) 30 mg, Guaifenesin 100 mg.
Preservatives: methylparaben 0.1%, sodium benzoate 0.1%.

Action: Actifed-C Expectorant is useful in both "wet" and "dry" coughs, and is effective whether the etiology is infectious or allergic. The etiology of cough is such that drug therapy designed to produce relief may be called upon to provide several therapeutic actions simultaneously. The ingredients of Actifed-C Expectorant were selected because they produce the following desirable effects:

Antitussive: For many years codeine has been universally accepted as one of the most consistently effective cough suppressants. As used in Actified-C Expectorant, codeine provides welcome reduction of excessive cough without productive expectoration.

Expectorant: Guaifenesin (glyceryl guaiacolate) reduces the viscosity of secretions, thereby increasing the efficiency of the cough reflex and of ciliary action in removing accumulated secretions from the trachea and bronchi. Unlike many other expectorants, guaifenesin (glyceryl guaiacolate) rarely causes gastric irritation.

Decongestant: Some degree of mucosal congestion is usually present along with all coughs. The decongestant effect of Sudafed (Pseudoephedrine Hydrochloride) provides gratifying relief to many patients so affected. In cases complicated by upper respiratory congestion, it also helps keep the nasal passages clear and the sinus ostia and eustachian tubes patent.

Antihistaminic: The frequent association of allergy with cough makes antihistaminic action desirable. The antihistamine, Actidil (Triprolidine Hydrochloride) when combined with the sympathomimetic amine, pseudoephedrine hydrochloride, often provides a greater degree of relief from allergy than either drug used alone.

> **Indications:** Based on a review of this drug by the National Academy of Sciences—National Research Council and/or other information, FDA has classified the indications as follows:
> "Lacking substantial evidence of effectiveness as a fixed combination": For the symptomatic relief of cough in conditions such as: the common cold, acute bronchitis, allergic asthma, bronchiolitis, croup, emphysema, tracheobronchitis.
> Final classificaion of the less-than-effective indications requires further investigation.

Contraindications:
Use in Newborn or Premature Infants: This drug should *not* be used in newborn or premature infants.
Use in Nursing Mothers: Because of the higher risk of antihistamines, codeine and sympathomimetic amines for infants generally and for newborn and premature in particular, Actifed-C Expectorant therapy is contraindicated in nursing mothers.
***Use in Lower Respiratory Disease:* Antihistamines *should NOT* be used to treat lower respiratory tract symptoms including asthma.**
Actifed-C Expectorant is also contraindicated in the following conditions:
Hypersensitivity to: 1) Triprolidine Hydrochloride and other antihistamines of similar chemical structure; 2) sympathomimetic amines including pseudoephedrine; and/or 3) any of the other ingredients.
Monoamine oxidase inhibitor therapy (see Drug Interaction Section)

Warnings: Actifed-C Expectorant should be used with considerable caution in patients with:
Increased intraocular pressure (Narrow angle glaucoma)
Stenosing peptic ulcer
Pyloroduodenal obstruction
Symptomatic prostatic hypertrophy
Bladder neck obstruction
Hypertension
Diabetes mellitus
Ischemic heart disease
Hyperthyroidism

Sympathomimetics may produce central nervous stimulation with convulsions or cardiovascular collapse with accompanying hypotension. Codeine can produce drug dependence of the morphine type, and therefore has the potential of being abused.
Use in Children: As in adults, the combination of an antihistamine and sympathomimetic amine can elicit either mild stimulation or mild sedation in children. While it is difficult to predict the result of an *overdosage* of a combination of triprolidine, pseudoephedrine, and codeine the following is known about the individual components:
In infants and children especially, antihistamine in overdosage may cause hallucination, convulsion or death. Large doses of pseudoephedrine are known to cause weakness, lightheadedness, nausea and/or vomiting. An overdosage of codeine may cause CNS depression with muscular twitching and convulsion, weakness, disturbed vision, dyspnea, respiratory depression, collapse and coma.
Use in Pregnancy: Experience with this drug in pregnant women is inadequate to determine whether there exists a potential for harm to the developing fetus.
Use with CNS Depressants: Triprolidine and codeine phosphate have additive effects with alcohol and other CNS depressants (hypnotics, sedatives, tranquilizers, etc.)
Use in Activities Requiring Mental Alertness: Patients should be warned about engaging in activities requiring mental alertness as driving a car or operating appliances, machinery, etc.
Use in the Elderly (approximately 60 years or older): Antihistamines are more likely to cause dizziness, sedation and hypotension in elderly patients. Overdosages of sympathomimetics in this age group may cause hallucinations, convulsions, CNS depression, and death.

Precautions: Actifed-C Expectorant should be used with caution in patients with:
history of bronchial asthma, increased intraocular pressure, hyperthyroidism, cardiovascular disease, hypertension.

Drug Interactions: MAO inhibitors prolong and intensify the anticholinergic (drying) effects of antihistamines and overall effects of sympathomimetics. Sympathomimetics may reduce the antihypertensive effects of methyldopa, decamylamine, reserpine, and veratrum alkaloids.
The CNS depressant effect of triprolidine hydrochloride and codeine phosphate may be additive with that of other CNS depressants.

Adverse Reactions:
1. *General:* Urticaria, drug rash, anaphylactic shock, photosensitivity, excessive perspiration, chills, dryness of mouth, nose and throat.
2. *Cardiovascular System:* Hypotension, headache, palpitations, tachycardia, extrasystoles.
3. *Haemotologic System:* Hemolytic anemia, thrombocytopenia, agranulocytosis.
4. *Nervous System:* Sedation, sleepiness, dizziness, disturbed coordination, fatigue, confusion, restlessness, excitation, nervousness, tremor, irritability, insomnia, euphoria, paresthesias, blurred vision, diplopia, vertigo, tinnitus, acute labyrinthitis, hysteria, neuritis, convulsions, CNS depression, hallucination.
5. *G.I. System:* Epigastric distress, anorexia, nausea, vomiting, diarrhea, constipation.
6. *G.U. System:* Urinary frequency, difficult urination, urinary retention, early menses.
7. *Respiratory System:* Thickening of bronchial secretions, tightness of chest and wheezing, nasal stuffiness.

Note: Guaifenesin has been shown to produce a color interference with certain clinical laboratory determinations of 5-hydroxyindoleacetic acid (5-HIAA) and vanillymandelic acid (VMA).

Overdosage: Actifed-C Expectorant overdosage reactions may vary from central nervous system depression to stimulation. Stimulation is particularly likely in children. Atropine-like signs and symptoms: dry mouth; fixed, dilated pupils; flushing; and gastrointestinal symptoms may also occur.
If Vomiting Has Not Occurred Spontaneously the patient should be induced to vomit. This is best done by having him use syrup of ipecac. Precautions against aspiration must be taken, especially in infants and children.

If Attempts to Induce Vomiting Are Unsuccessful gastric lavage is indicated. Isotonic and ½ isotonic saline is the lavage solution of choice.
Saline cathartics, are valuable for their action in rapid dilution of bowel content.
Stimulants should *not* be used.
Vasopressors may be used to treat hypotension.
Naloxone may be used to treat codeine toxicity.

Dosage and Administration:
DOSAGE SHOULD BE INDIVIDUALIZED ACCORDING TO THE NEEDS AND RESPONSE OF THE PATIENT.
Usual Dose:

	Teaspoonfuls (5 ml)	
Adults and children 12 years and older	2	
Children 6 to 12 years	1	3–4 times
Children 4 to 6 years	¾	a day
Children 2 to 4 years	½	

How Supplied: Bottles of 1 pint, 1 gallon and 4 oz Unit of Use Bottle with Child Resistant Cap.

AEROSPORIN® ℞
brand Polymyxin B Sulfate
Sterile Powder
Polymyxin B Sulfate for Parenteral and/or Ophthalmic Administration

WARNING
CAUTION: **WHEN THIS DRUG IS GIVEN INTRAMUSCULARLY AND/OR INTRATHECALLY, IT SHOULD BE GIVEN ONLY TO HOSPITALIZED PATIENTS, SO AS TO PROVIDE CONSTANT SUPERVISION BY A PHYSICIAN.**
RENAL FUNCTION SHOULD BE CAREFULLY DETERMINED AND PATIENTS WITH RENAL DAMAGE AND NITROGEN RETENTION SHOULD HAVE REDUCED DOSAGE. PATIENTS WITH NEPHROTOXICITY DUE TO POLYMYXIN B SULFATE USUALLY SHOW ALBUMINURIA, CELLULAR CASTS, AND AZOTEMIA. DIMINISHING URINE OUTPUT AND A RISING BUN ARE INDICATIONS FOR DISCONTINUING THERAPY WITH THIS DRUG.
NEUROTOXIC REACTIONS MAY BE MANIFESTED BY IRRITABILITY, WEAKNESS, DROWSINESS, ATAXIA, PERIORAL PARESTHESIA, NUMBNESS OF THE EXTREMITIES, AND BLURRING OF VISION. THESE ARE USUALLY ASSOCIATED WITH HIGH SERUM LEVELS FOUND IN PATIENTS WITH IMPAIRED RENAL FUNCTION AND/OR NEPHROTOXICITY. THE CONCURRENT USE OF OTHER NEPHROTOXIC AND NEUROTOXIC DRUGS, PARTICULARLY KANAMYCIN, STREPTOMYCIN, CEPHALORIDINE, PAROMOMYCIN, TOBRAMYCIN, POLYMYXIN E (COLISTIN), NEOMYCIN, GENTAMICIN, AND VIOMYCIN, SHOULD BE AVOIDED.
THE NEUROTOXICITY OF POLYMYXIN B SULFATE CAN RESULT IN RESPIRATORY PARALYSIS FROM NEUROMUSCULAR BLOCKADE, ESPECIALLY WHEN THE DRUG IS GIVEN SOON AFTER ANESTHESIA AND/OR MUSCLE RELAXANTS.
USAGE IN PREGNANCY: THE SAFETY OF THIS DRUG IN HUMAN PREGNANCY HAS NOT BEEN ESTABLISHED.

Description: Polymyxin B sulfate is one of a group of basic polypeptide antibiotics derived from *B polymyxa (B aerosporous).*
Aerosporin brand Sterile Polymyxin B Sulfate is in powder form suitable for preparation of sterile solutions for intramuscular, intravenous drip, intrathecal, or ophthalmic use.
In the medical literature, dosages have frequently been given in terms of equivalent weight of pure polymyxin B base. Each milligram of pure polymyxin B base is equivalent to 10,000 units of polymyxin B and each microgram of pure polymyxin B base is equivalent to 10 units of polymyxin B.
Aqueous solutions of Aerosporin brand Polymyxin B Sulfate may be stored up to 12 months without significant loss of potency if kept under refrigeration. In the interest of safety, solutions for parenteral use should be stored under refrigeration and any unused portion should be discarded after 72 hours. Polymyxin B sulfate should not be stored in alkaline solutions since they are less stable.

Actions: Aerosporin brand Polymyxin B Sulfate has a bactericidal action against almost all gram-negative bacilli except the *Proteus* group. Polymyxins increase the permeability of bacterial cell wall membranes. All gram-positive bacteria, fungi, and the gram-negative cocci, *N gonorrhoeae* and *N meningitidis*, are resistant.
Susceptibility plate testing: If the Kirby-Bauer method of disc susceptibility testing is used, a 300-unit polymyxin B disc should give a zone of over 11 mm when tested against a polymyxin B-susceptible bacterial strain.
Polymyxin B sulfate is not absorbed from the normal alimentary tract. Since the drug loses 50 percent of its activity in the presence of serum, active blood levels are low. Repeated injections may give a cumulative effect. Levels tend to be higher in infants and children. The drug is excreted slowly by the kidneys. Tissue diffusion is poor and the drug does not pass the blood brain barrier into the cerebrospinal fluid. In therapeutic dosage, polymyxin B sulfate causes some nephrotoxicity with tubule damage to a slight degree.

Indications: Acute Infections Caused by Susceptible Strains of *Pseudomonas aeruginosa.*
Polymyxin B sulfate is a drug of choice in the treatment of infections of the urinary tract, meninges, and bloodstream caused by susceptible strains of *Ps aeruginosa.* It may also be used topically and subconjunctivally in the treatment of infections of the eye caused by susceptible strains of *Ps aeruginosa.*
It may be indicated in serious infections caused by susceptible strains of the following organisms, when less potentially toxic drugs are ineffective or contraindicated:
H. influenzae, specifically meningeal infections.
Escherichia coli, specifically urinary tract infections.
Aerobacter aerogenes, specifically bacteremia.
Klebsiella pneumoniae, specifically bacteremia.
Note. In Meningeal Infections, Polymyxin B Sulfate Should Be Administered Only by the Intrathecal Route.

Contraindications: This drug is contraindicated in persons with a prior history of hypersensitivity reactions to the polymyxins.

Precautions: See "Warning" box.
Baseline renal function should be done prior to therapy, with frequent monitoring of renal function and blood levels of the drug during parenteral therapy.
Avoid concurrent use of a curariform muscle relaxant and other neurotoxic drugs (ether, tubocurarine, succinylcholine, gallamine, decamethonium and sodium citrate) which may precipitate respiratory depression. If signs of respiratory paralysis appear, respiration should be assisted as required, and the drug discontinued.
As with other antibiotics, use of this drug may result in overgrowth of nonsusceptible organisms, including fungi. If superinfection occurs, appropriate therapy should be instituted.

Adverse Reactions: See "Warning" box.
Nephrotoxic reactions: Albuminuria, cylinduria, azotemia, and rising blood levels without any increase in dosage.
Neurotoxic reactions: Facial flushing, dizziness progressing to ataxia, drowsiness, peripheral paresthesias (circumoral and stocking-glove), apnea due to concurrent use of curariform muscle relaxants and other neurotoxic drugs or inadvertent overdosage, and signs of meningeal irritation with intrathecal administration, e.g., fever, headache, stiff neck and increased cell count and protein cerebrospinal fluid.
Other reactions occasionally reported: Drug fever, urticarial rash, pain (severe) at intramuscular injection sites, and thrombophlebitis at intravenous injection sites.

Dosage and Administration:
PARENTERAL:
Intravenous. Dissolve 500,000 units polymyxin B sulfate in 300-500 cc of 5 percent dextrose in water for continuous intravenous drip.
Adults and children. 15,000-25,000 units/kg body weight/day in individuals with normal kidney function. This amount should be reduced from 15,000 units/kg downward for individuals with kidney impairment. Infusions may be given every 12 hours; however, the total daily dose must not exceed 25,000 units/kg/day.
Infants. Infants with normal kidney function may receive up to 40,000 units/kg/day without adverse effects.
Intramuscular. Not recommended routinely because of severe pain at injection sites, particularly in infants and children. Dissolve 500,000 units polymyxin B sulfate in 2 cc sterile distilled water (Water for Injection, U.S.P.) or sterile physiologic saline (Sodium Chloride Injection, U.S.P.) or 1 percent procaine hydrochloride solution.
Adults and children. 25,000-30,000 units/kg/day. This should be reduced in the presence of renal impairment. The dosage may be divided and given at either 4- or 6-hour intervals.
Infants. Infants with normal kidney function may receive up to 40,000 units/kg/day without adverse effects.
Note. Doses as high as 45,000 units/kg/day have been used in limited clinical studies in treating prematures and newborn infants for sepsis caused by *Ps aeruginosa.*
Intrathecal. A treatment of choice for *Ps aeruginosa* meningitis. Dissolve 500,000 units polymyxin B sulfate in 10 cc of sterile physiologic saline (Sodium Chloride Injection, U.S.P.) for 50,000 units per ml dosage unit.
Adults and children over 2 years of age. Dosage is 50,000 units once daily intrathecally for 3-4 days, then 50,000 units once every other day for at least 2 weeks after cultures of the cerebrospinal fluid are negative and sugar content has returned to normal.
Children under 2 years of age. 20,000 units once daily, intrathecally for 3-4 days or 25,000 units once every other day. Continue with a dose of 25,000 units once every other day for at least 2 weeks after cultures of the cerebrospinal fluid are negative and sugar content has returned to normal.
IN THE INTEREST OF SAFETY, SOLUTIONS FOR PARENTERAL USE SHOULD BE STORED UNDER REFRIGERATION, AND ANY UNUSED PORTIONS SHOULD BE DISCARDED AFTER 72 HOURS.

TOPICAL:
Ophthalmic. Dissolve 500,000 units polymyxin B sulfate in 20-50 cc sterile distilled water (Water for Injection, U.S.P.) or sterile physiologic saline (Sodium Chloride Injection U.S.P.) for a 10,000-25,000 units per cc concentration.
For the treatment of *Ps aeruginosa* infections of the eye, a concentration of 0.1 percent to 0.25 percent (10,000 units to 25,000 units per cc) is administered 1-3 drops every hour, increasing the intervals as response indicates.
Subconjunctival injection of up to 10,000 units/day may be used for the treatment of *Ps aeruginosa* infections of the cornea and conjunctiva.
Note. Avoid total systemic and ophthalmic instillation over 25,000 units/kg/day.

Continued on next page

Burroughs Wellcome—Cont.

AVAILABLE DOSAGE FORM
500,000 units.
Rubber-stoppered vial with flip off cap.
Vial—VA NSN 6505-00-913-3124

ALKERAN® ℞
(Melphalan)
2 mg Scored Tablets

> **WARNING:** *There are many reports of patients with multiple myeloma who have developed acute, non-lymphatic leukemia following therapy with alkylating agents (including melphalan). Evaluation of published reports strongly suggests that melphalan is leukemogenic in patients with multiple myeloma.*
> *There is a greatly increased incidence of acute, non-lymphatic leukemia in women with ovarian carcinoma treated with alkylating agents (including melphalan).*
> *Melphalan is a carcinogen in animals and must be presumed to be so in humans. Although the palliation to be anticipated from the use of melphalan in multiple myeloma and ovarian carcinoma is generally felt to greatly outweigh the possible induction of a second neoplasm, the potential benefits and the potential risk of carcinogenesis must be evaluated on an individual basis.*
> *Melphalan has been observed to produce chromosomal aberrations in human cells* in vitro *and* in vivo. *Melphalan is potentially mutagenic and teratogenic in humans, although the extent of the risk is unknown.*

Description: Alkeran (melphalan), also known as L-phenylalanine mustard, phenylalanine mustard, L-PAM, or L-sarcolysin, is a phenylalanine derivative of nitrogen mustard. Chemically, it is *p*-di(2-chloroethyl)amino-L-phenylalanine.
Alkeran (melphalan) is the active L-isomer of the compound and was first synthesized in 1953 by Bergel and Stock; the D-isomer, known as medphalan, is less active against certain animal tumors, and the dose needed to produce effects on chromosomes is larger than that required with the L-isomer. The racemic (DL—) form is known as merphalan or sarcolysin.

Clinical Pharmacology:

***In Vitro* Studies:**

a. **Stability.** Melphalan is a highly reactive, bifunctional alkylating agent. It is a nitrogen mustard derivative. In water at 37° C it undergoes rapid, first-order hydrolysis with a rate constant of 0.83 hr^{-1}. In protein-containing solutions hydrolysis is retarded; in human plasma at 37° C *in vitro* the rate constant varies between 0.31 and 0.45 hr^{-1}.[1]
b. **Protein Binding and Dialysis.** After incubating ^{14}C-melphalan in human plasma at 37° C for eight hours, Chang *et al* found that only 70% of the carbon-14 label was removed by methanol extraction.[1] Almost none of the methanol-extractable ^{14}C-melphalan was in the form of parent drug at that time. Equilibrium dialysis of ^{14}C-melphalan in human plasma at 37° C (30μg of melphalan per ml plasma) against 0.05 M phosphate buffer, pH 7.4, demonstrated that 30% of the carbon-14 remained undialyzable after equilibrium had been reached at eight hours. These observations may indicate alkylation of plasma proteins by melphalan.[1]

***In Vivo* Studies:**
Alberts *et al*[2] found that plasma melphalan levels are highly variable after oral dosing, both with respect to the time of the first appearance of melphalan in plasma and to the peak concentrations achieved. Whether this results from incomplete gastrointestinal absorption or a variable "first pass" hepatic metabolism is unknown. Five patients were studied after both oral and intravenous dosing with 0.6 mg/kg as a single bolus dose by each route. The areas under the plasma concentration-time curves after oral administration averaged 61 ± 26% (± standard deviation; range 25 to 89%) of those following intravenous administration. In ten patients given a single, oral dose of 0.6 mg/kg of melphalan, the terminal plasma half-disappearance time of parent drug was 101 ± 63 minutes. the 24-hour urinary excretion of parent drug in these patients was 10 ± 6%, suggesting that renal clearance is not a major route of elimination of parent drug.
Tattersall *et al*[3], using universally labeled ^{14}C-melphalan, found substantially less radioactivity in the urine of patients given the drug by mouth (30% of administered dose in nine days) than in the urine of those given it intravenously (35 to 65% in seven days). Following either oral or intravenous administration, the pattern of label recovery was similar, with the majority being recovered in the first 24 hours. Following oral administration, peak radioactivity occurred in plasma at two hours and then disappeared with a half-life of approximately 160 hours. in one patient where parent drug (rather than just radiolabel) was determined, the melphalan half-disappearance time was 67 minutes.[3]

Indications: Alkeran (melphalan) is indicated for the palliative treatment of multiple myeloma and for the palliation of non-resectable epithelial carcinoma of the ovary.

Contraindications: Melphalan should not be used in patients whose disease has demonstrated a prior resistance to this agent. Patients who have demonstrated hypersensitivity to melphalan should not be given the drug. There may be cross-sensitivity (skin rash) between melphalan and chlorambucil (Leukeran®).

Warnings: As with other nitrogen mustard drugs, excessive dosage will produce marked bone marrow depression. Frequent blood counts are essential to determine optimal dosage and to avoid toxicity. The drug should be discontinued or the dosage reduced upon evidence of depression of the bone marrow.
USAGE IN PREGNANCY: Safe use of melphalan has not been established with respect to adverse effects on fetal development. Therefore, it should be used in women of child-bearing potential and particularly during early pregnancy only when, in the judgment of the physician, the potential benefits outweigh the possible hazards.

Precautions: Melphalan should be used with extreme caution in patients whose bone marrow reserve may have been compromised by prior irradiation or chemotherapy, or whose marrow function is recovering from previous cytotoxic therapy.
A recommendation as to whether or not dosage reduction should be made routinely in patients with impaired creatinine clearance cannot be made because:

(a) there is considerable inherent patient-to-patient variability in the systemic availability of melphalan in patients with normal renal function, and
(b) there is only a small amount of the administered dose that appears as parent drug in the urine of patients with normal renal function.

Patients with azotemia should be closely observed, however, in order to make dosage reductions, if required, at the earliest possible time.
If the leukocyte count falls below 3,000 cells/μl, or the platelet count below 100,000/μl, the drug should be discontinued until the peripheral blood cell counts have recovered.

Adverse Reactions: Nausea and vomiting have followed the use of high doses of Alkeran (melphalan). Dose-related bone marrow depression produces anemia, neutropenia and thrombocytopenia. Skin rashes, both maculopapular and urticarial, have been reported. Rare instances of bronchopulmonary dysplasia and pulmonary fibrosis have been reported.[4]

Dosage and Administration:
Multiple Myeloma: The usual oral dose is 6 mg (3 tablets) daily. The entire daily dose may be given at one time. It is adjusted, as required, on the basis of blood counts done at approximately weekly intervals. After two to three weeks of treatment, the drug should be discontinued for up to four weeks during which time the blood count should be followed carefully. When the white blood cell and platelet counts are rising, a maintenance dose of 2 mg daily may be instituted. Because of the patient-to-patient variation in melphalan plasma levels following oral administration of the drug, several investigators have recommended that melphalan dosage be cautiously escalated until some myelosuppression is observed, in order to assure that potentially therapeutic levels of the drug have been reached.[2,3]
Other dosage regimens have been used by various investigators. Osserman and Takatsuki[5,6] have used an initial course of 10 mg/day for seven to ten days. They report the maximal suppression of the leukocyte and platelet counts occurs within three to five weeks and recovery within four to eight weeks. Continuous maintenance therapy with 2 mg/day is instituted when the white blood cell count is greater than 4,000 and the platelet count is greater than 100,000. Dosage is adjusted to between 1 and 3 mg/day depending upon the hematological response. It is desirable to try to maintain a significant degree of bone marrow depression so as to keep the leukocyte count in the range of 3,000 to 3,500 cells/μl.
Hoogstraten *et al*[7] have started treatment with 0.15 mg/kg/day for seven days. This is followed by a rest period of at least 14 days, but it may be as long as five to six weeks. Maintenance therapy is started when the white blood cell and platelet counts are rising. The maintenance dose is 0.05 mg/kg per day or less and is adjusted according to the blood count.
Available evidence suggests that about one third to one half of the patients with multiple myeloma show a favorable response to oral administration of the drug.
One study by Alexanian *et al*[8] has shown that the use of melphalan in combination with prednisone significantly improves the percentage of patients with multiple myeloma who achieve palliation. One regimen has been to administer courses of melphalan at 0.25 mg/kg/day for four consecutive days (or, 0.20 mg/kg/day for five consecutive days) for a total dose of 1 mg/kg per course. These four- to five-day courses are then repeated every four to six weeks if the granulocyte count and the platelet count have returned to normal levels.
Melphalan has been used with other cytotoxic agents in an attempt to increase the response rate. It is not known at present whether the addition of other cytotoxic agents to a combination of melphalan and prednisone significantly increases either the response rate or the duration of survival.
It is to be emphasized that response may be very gradual over many months; it is important that repeated courses or continuous therapy be given since improvement may continue slowly over many months and the maximum benefit may be missed if treatment is abandoned too soon.
Epithelial Ovarian Cancer: One commonly employed regimen for the treatment of ovarian carcinoma has been to administer melphalan at a dose of 0.2 mg/kg daily for five days as a single course. Courses are repeated every four to five weeks depending upon hematologic tolerance.[9,10]

How Supplied: White, scored 2 mg tablets imprinted with "WELLCOME" and "A2A"; bottle of 50.

References:

1. Chang SY, Alberts DS, Farquhar D, *et al:* Hydrolysis and protein binding of melphalan. J. Pharm. Sci., *67:*682, 1978.
2. Alberts DS, Chang SY, Chen H-S, *et al:* Oral melphalan kinetics, Clin. Pharm. Ther., *26:*737, 1979.
3. Tattersall MHN, Jarman M, Newlands ES, *et al:* Pharmaco-Kinetics of melphalan following oral or intravenous administration in patients with malignant disease. Eur. J. Cancer, *14:*507, 1978.
4. Taetle R, Dickman PS, Feldman PS: Pulmonary histopathologic changes associated with melphalan therapy. Cancer, *42:*1239, 1978.
5. Osserman EF: Therapy of plasma cell myeloma with melphalan (1-phenylalanine mustard). Proc. Am. Assoc. Cancer Res, *4:*50, 1963.
6. Osserman EF, Takatsuki, K: Plasma cell myeloma: gamma globulin synthesis and structure. Medicine, *42:*357, 1963.
7. Hoogstraten B, Sheehe PR, Cuttner J: Melphalan in multiple myeloma. Blood, *30:*74, 1967.
8. Alexanian R, Haut A, Kahn AU, *et al:* Treatment for multiple myeloma. Combination chemotherapy with different melphalan dose regimens. JAMA, *208:*1680, 1969.
9. Smith JP and Rutledge FN: Chemotherapy in advanced ovarian cancer, Natl. Cancer Inst. Monogr., *42:*141, 1975
10. Young RC, Chabner BA, Hubbard SP, *et al:* Advanced ovarian adenocarcinoma. A prospective clinical trial of melphalan (L-PAM) versus combination chemotherapy. N. Eng. J. Med., *299:*1261, 1978.

[*Shown in Product Identification Section*]

ANECTINE® ℞
(Succinylcholine Chloride)
Injection, USP

ANECTINE® ℞
(Succinylcholine Chloride)
Sterile Powder Flo-Pack®

This drug should be used only by individuals familiar with its actions, characteristics and hazards.

Description: Anectine (succinylcholine chloride) is an ultra short-acting depolarizing-type, skeletal muscle relaxant for intravenous administration. Succinylcholine chloride is a white, odorless, slightly bitter powder and very soluble in water. The drug is unstable in alkaline solutions but relatively stable in acid solutions, depending upon the concentration of the solution and the storage temperature. Solutions of succinylcholine chloride should be stored under refrigeration to preserve potency. Anectine Injection is a sterile solution for intravenous injection, containing 20 mg succinylcholine chloride in each ml and made isotonic with sodium chloride. The pH is adjusted to 3.5 with hydrochloric acid. Methylparaben (0.1%) is added as a preservative. Anectine® Flo-Pack is a sterile powder, containing either 500 mg or 1000 mg of succinylcholine chloride in each vial.

The chemical name for succinylcholine chloride is 2,2′-[(1,4-dioxo-1,4-butanediyl) bis(oxy)]-bis [*N,N,N*-trimethylethanaminium] dichloride.

Clinical Pharmacology: Succinylcholine is a depolarizing skeletal muscle relaxant. As does acetylcholine, it combines with the cholinergic receptors of the motor end plate to produce depolarization. This depolarization may be observed as fasciculations. Subsequent neuromuscular transmission is inhibited so long as adequate concentration of succinylcholine remains at the receptor site. Onset of flaccid paralysis is rapid (less than one minute after intravenous administration), and with single administration lasts approximately 4–6 minutes.

Succinylcholine is rapidly hydrolyzed by plasma pseudocholinesterase to succinylmonocholine (which possesses nondepolarizing muscle relaxant properties) and then more slowly to succinic acid and choline. About 10% of the drug is excreted unchanged in the urine. The paralysis following administration of succinylcholine is selective, initially involving consecutively the levator muscles of the face, muscles of the glottis and finally the intercostals and the diaphragm and all other skeletal muscles. Succinylcholine has no direct action on the uterus or other smooth muscle structures. Because it is highly ionized and has low fat solubility, it does not readily cross the placenta.

Tachyphylaxis occurs with repeated administration.

When succinylcholine is given over a prolonged period of time, the characteristic depolarizing neuromuscular block (Phase 1 block) may change to a block with characteristics superficially resembling a non-depolarizing block (Phase II block). This may be associated with prolonged respiratory depression or apnea in patients who manifest the transition to Phase II block. When this diagnosis is confirmed by peripheral nerve stimulation, it may be reversed with anticholinesterase drugs such as neostigmine (See Precautions).

While succinylcholine has no direct effect on the myocardium, changes in rhythm may result from vagal stimulation, such as may result from surgical procedures (particularly in children) or from potassium-mediated alterations in electrical conductivity. These effects are enhanced by cyclopropane and halogenated anesthetics.

Succinylcholine causes a slight, transient increase in intraocular pressure immediately after its injection and during the fasciculation phase, and slight increases may persist after onset of complete paralysis. This suggests that the drug should not be used in the presence of open eye injuries.

Succinylcholine has no effect on consciousness, pain threshold or cerebration. It should be used only with adequate anesthesia.

Indications and Usage: Succinylcholine chloride is indicated as an adjunct to general anesthesia, to facilitate endotracheal intubation, and to provide skeletal muscle relaxation during surgery or mechanical ventilation.

Contraindications: Succinylcholine is contraindicated for persons with genetically determined disorders of plasma pseudocholinesterase, personal or familial history of malignant hyperthermia, myopathies associated with elevated creatine phosphokinase (CPK) values, known hypersensitivity to the drug, acute narrow angle glaucoma, and penetrating eye injuries.

Warnings: Succinylcholine should be used only by those skilled in the management of artificial respiration and only when facilities are instantly available for endotracheal intubation and for providing adequate ventilation of the patient, including the administration of oxygen under positive pressure and the elimination of carbon dioxide. The clinician must be prepared to assist or control respiration.

Succinylcholine should not be mixed with short-acting barbiturates in the same syringe or administered simultaneously during intravenous infusion through the same needle. Solutions of succinylcholine have an acid pH, whereas those of barbiturates are alkaline. Depending upon the resultant pH of a mixture of solutions of these drugs, either free barbituric acid may be precipitated or succinylcholine hydrolyzed.

Succinylcholine administration has been associated with acute onset of fulminant hypermetabolism of skeletal muscle known as malignant hyperthermic crisis. This frequently presents as intractable spasm of the jaw muscles which may progress to generalized rigidity, increased oxygen demand, tachycardia, tachypnea and profound hyperpyrexia. Successful outcome depends on recognition of early signs, such as jaw muscle spasm, lack of laryngeal relaxation or generalized rigidity to initial administration of succinylcholine for endotracheal intubation, or failure of tachycardia to respond to deepening anesthesia. Skin mottling, rising temperature and coagulopathies occur late in the course of the hypermetabolic process. Recognition of the syndrome is a signal for discontinuance of anesthesia, attention to increased oxygen consumption, correction of metabolic acidosis, support of circulation, assurance of adequate urinary output and institution of measures to control rising temperature. Dantrolene sodium, intravenously, is recommended as an adjunct to supportive measures in the management of this problem. Consult literature references or the dantrolene prescribing information for additional information about the management of malignant hyperthermic crisis. Routine, continuous monitoring of temperature is recommended as an aid to early recognition of malignant hyperthermia.

Precautions:

General: Low levels or abnormal variants of pseudocholinesterase may be associated with prolonged respiratory depression or apnea following the use of succinylcholine. Low levels of pseudocholinesterase may occur in patients with the following conditions: burns, severe liver disease or cirrhosis, cancer, severe anemia, pregnancy, malnutrition, severe dehydration, collagen diseases, myxedema, and abnormal body temperature. Also, exposure to neurotoxic insecticides, antimalarial or anti-cancer drugs, monoamine oxidase inhibitors, contraceptive pills, pancuronium, chlorpromazine, ecothiopate iodide, or neostigmine may result in low levels of pseudocholinesterase. Succinylcholine should be administered with extreme care to such patients. If low pseudocholinesterase activity is suspected, a small test dose of from 5 to 10 mg of succinylcholine may be administered, or relaxation may be produced by the cautious administration of a 0.1% solution of the drug by intravenous drip. Apnea or prolonged muscle paralysis should be treated with controlled respiration.

Succinylcholine should be administered with great caution to patients recovering from severe trauma, those suffering from electrolyte imbalance, those receiving quinidine, and those who have been digitalized recently or who may have digitalis toxicity, because in these circumstances it may induce serious cardiac arrhythmias or cardiac arrest. Great caution should be observed also in patients with pre-existing hyperkalemia, those who are paraplegic, or have suffered extensive or severe burns, extensive denervation of skeletal muscle due to disease or injury of the central nervous system, or have degenerative or dystrophic neuromuscular disease, because such patients tend to become severely hyperkalemic when given succinylcholine.

When succinylcholine is given over a prolonged period of time, the characteristic depolarization block of the myoneural junction (Phase I block) may change to a block with characteristics superficially resembling a nondepolarizing block (Phase II block). Prolonged respiratory depression or apnea may be observed in patients manifesting this transition to Phase II block. The transition from Phase I to Phase II block has been reported in 7 of 7 patients studied under halothane anesthesia after an accumulated dose of 2 to 4 mg/kg succinylcholine (administered in repeated, di-

Continued on next page

Burroughs Wellcome—Cont.

vided doses). The onset of Phase II block coincided with the onset of tachyphylaxis and prolongation of spontaneous recovery. In another study, using balanced anesthesia (N_2O/O_2/-narcotic-thiopental) and succinylcholine infusion, the transition was less abrupt, with great individual variability in the dose of succinylcholine required to produce Phase II block. Of 32 patients studied, 24 developed Phase II block. Tachyphylaxis was not associated with the transition to Phase II block, and 50% of the patients who developed Phase II block experienced prolonged recovery.

When Phase II block is suspected in cases of prolonged neuromuscular blockage, positive diagnosis should be made by peripheral nerve stimulation, prior to administration of any anticholinesterase drug. Reversal of Phase II block is a medical decision which must be made upon the basis of the individual clinical pharmacology and the experience and judgment of the physician. The presence of Phase II block is indicated by fade of responses to successive stimuli (preferably "train of four"). The use of anticholinesterase drugs to reverse Phase II block should be accompanied by appropriate doses of atropine to prevent disturbances of cardiac rhythm. After adequate reversal of Phase II block with an anticholinesterase agent, the patient should be continually observed for at least 1 hour for signs of return of muscle relaxation. Reversal should not be attempted unless: (1) a peripheral nerve stimulator is used to determine the presence of Phase II block (since anti-cholinesterase agents will potentiate succinylcholine-induced Phase I block), and (2) spontaneous recovery of muscle twitch has been observed for at least 20 minutes and has reached a plateau with further recovery proceeding slowly; this delay is to ensure complete hydrolysis of succinylcholine by pseudocholinesterase prior to administration of the anticholinesterase agent. Should the type of block be misdiagnosed, depolarization of the type initially induced by succinylcholine, that is depolarizing block, will be prolonged by an anticholinesterase agent.

Succinylcholine should be used with caution, if at all, during ocular surgery and in patients with glaucoma. The drug should be employed with caution in patients with fractures or muscle spasm because the initial muscle fasciculations may cause additional trauma.

Neuromuscular blockade may be prolonged in patients with hypokalemia or hypocalcemia.

Drug Interactions: Drugs which may enhance the neuromuscular blocking action of succinylcholine include: phenelzine, promazine, oxytocin, aprotinin, certain nonpenicillin antibiotics, quinidine, β-adrenergic blockers, procainamide, lidocaine, trimethaphen, lithium carbonate, magnesium salts, quinine, chloroquin, propanidid, diethylether, and isoflurane.

If other relaxants are to be used during the same procedure, the possibility of a synergistic or antagonistic effect should be considered.

Pregnancy: **Teratogenic Effects:** Pregnancy Category C.

Animal reproduction studies have not been conducted with succinylcholine chloride. It is also not known whether succinylcholine can cause fetal harm when administered to a pregnant woman or can affect reproduction capacity. Succinylcholine should be given to a pregnant woman only if clearly needed.

Nonteratogenic Effects: Pseudocholinesterase levels are decreased by approximately 24% during pregnancy and for several days postpartum. Therefore, a higher proportion of patients may be expected to show sensitivity (prolonged apnea) to succinylcholine when pregnant than when nonpregnant.

Labor and Delivery: Succinylcholine is commonly used to provide muscle relaxation during delivery by caesarean section. While small amounts of succinylcholine are known to cross the placental barrier, under normal conditions the quantity of drug that enters fetal circulation after a single dose of 1 mg/kg to the mother will not endanger the fetus. However, since the amount of drug that crosses the placental barrier is dependent on the concentration gradient between the maternal and fetal circulations, residual neuromuscular blockade (apnea and flaccidity) may occur in the neonate after repeated high doses to, or in the presence of, atypical pseudocholinesterase in the mother.

Adverse Reactions: Adverse reactions consist primarily of an extension of the drug's pharmacological actions. It causes profound muscle relaxation resulting in respiratory depression to the point of apnea; this effect may be prolonged. Hypersensitivity to the drug may exist in rare instances. The following additional adverse reactions have been reported: cardiac arrest, malignant hyperthermia, arrhythmias, bradycardia, tachycardia, hypertension, hypotension, hyperkalemia, prolonged respiratory depression or apnea, increased intraocular pressure, muscle fasciculation, postoperative muscle pain, myoglobinemia, excessive salivation, and rash.

Dosage and Administration: The dosage of succinylcholine is essentially individualized and its administration should always be determined by the clinician after careful assessment of the patient. To avoid distress to the patient, succinylcholine should not be administered before unconsciousness has been induced. Succinylcholine should not be mixed with short-acting barbiturates in the same syringe or administered simultaneously during intravenous infusion through the same needle.

For Short Surgical Procedures: The average dose for relaxation of short duration is 0.6 mg/kg (~2.0 ml) Anectine (succinylcholine chloride) Injection given intravenously. The optimum dose will vary among individuals and may be from 0.3 to 1.1 mg/kg for adults (1.0 to 4.0 ml). Following administration of doses in this range, relaxation develops in about 1 minute; maximum muscular paralysis may persist for about 2 minutes, after which recovery takes place within 4 to 6 minutes. However, very large doses may result in more prolonged apnea. An initial test dose of 0.1 mg/kg (~0.5 ml) may be used to determine the sensitivity of the patient and the individual recovery time.

For Long Surgical Procedures: The dosage of succinylcholine administered by infusion depends upon the duration of the surgical procedure and the need for muscle relaxation. The average rate for an adult ranges between 2.5 and 4.3 mg per minute.

Solutions containing from 0.1% to 0.2% (1 to 2 mg per ml) succinylcholine have commonly been used for continuous intravenous drip. Solutions of 0.1% or 0.2% may conveniently be prepared by adding 1 g succinylcholine (the contents of one Anectine Sterile Powder Flo-Pack unit containing 1 g succinylcholine chloride) respectively to 1,000 or 500 ml of sterile solution, such as sterile 5% dextrose solution or sterile isotonic saline solution. The more dilute solution (0.1% or 1 mg per ml) is probably preferable from the standpoint of ease of control of the rate of administration of the drug and, hence, of relaxation. This intravenous drip solution containing 1 mg per ml may be administered at a rate of 0.5 mg (0.5 ml) to 10 mg (10 ml) per minute to obtain the required amount of relaxation. The amount required per minute will depend upon the individual response as well as the degree of relaxation required. The 0.2% solution may be especially useful in those cases where it is desired to avoid overburdening the circulation with a large volume of fluid. It is recommended that neuromuscular function be carefully monitored with a peripheral nerve stimulator when using succinylcholine by infusion in order to avoid overdose, detect development of Phase II block, follow its rate of recovery, and assess the effects of reversing agents.

Solutions of succinylcholine must be used within 24 hours after preparation. Discard unused solutions.

Intermittent intravenous injections of succinylcholine may also be used to provide muscle relaxation for long procedures. An intravenous injection of 0.3 to 1.1 mg/kg may be given initially, followed, at appropriate intervals, by further injections of 0.04 to 0.07 mg/kg to maintain the degree of relaxation required.

The intravenous dose of succinylcholine is 2 mg/kg for infants and small children. For older children and adolescents the dose is 1 mg/kg.

Intramuscular Use: If necessary, succinylcholine may be given intramuscularly to infants, older children or adults when a suitable vein is inaccessible. A dose of up to 3 to 4 mg/kg may be given, but not more than 150 mg total dose should be administered by this route. The onset of effect of succinylcholine given intramuscularly is usually observed in about 2 to 3 minutes.

How Supplied: For immediate injection of single doses for short procedures:

Anectine® Injection, 20 mg succinylcholine chloride in each ml.

Multiple-dose vials of 10 ml.

Box of 12 vials, NDC-0081-0071-95.

DOD NSN 6505-00-133-4309

Store in refrigerator at 2°-8°C (36°-46°F). The multi-dose vials are stable for up to 14 days at room temperature without significant loss of potency.

For preparation of intravenous drip solutions only:

Anectine® Flo-Pack®, 500 mg sterile succinylcholine chloride powder.

Box of 12 vials, NDC-0081-0085-15.

Anectine® Flo-Pack®, 1000 mg sterile succinylcholine chloride powder.

Box of 12 vials, NDC-0081-0086-15.

DOD NSN 6505-01-028-2260

Anectine Flo-Pack does not require refrigeration. Solutions of succinylcholine must be used within 24 hours after preparation. Discard unused solutions.

TABLE I

Dosage Form	Contains	Equivalency in Terms of Piperazine Hexahydrate
Syrup	Piperazine Citrate Anhydrous 550 mg per 5 cc (1 teaspoonful)	500 mg per teaspoonful
Scored Tablet	Piperazine Citrate Anhydrous 550 mg per tablet	500 mg per tablet

ANTEPAR® ℞
brand Piperazine
Syrup/Tablet

Description: (See Table I left).

Piperazine hexahydrate is a white, crystalline substance.

Actions: Clinical investigations in man have demonstrated its activity against the human

pinworm, *Enterobius vermicularis*, and against the "common roundworm," *Ascaris lumbricoides.*
Piperazine produces a paralysis of ascaris muscle with resultant expulsion of the worm through intestinal peristalsis.
Systemic absorption of piperazine is variable and the drug is excreted essentially unchanged.
Indications: For the treatment of ascariasis ("common roundworm" infection) and enterobiasis (pinworm infection).
Contraindications: This product is contraindicated in patients with impaired renal or hepatic function, convulsive disorders, or a history of hypersensitivity reactions from piperazine and its salt.
Warnings: Because of potential neurotoxicity of this drug, especially in children, prolonged or repeated treatment in excess of that recommended should be avoided.
Usage in Pregnancy: Safety of this drug for use during pregnancy has not been established.
Precautions: If CNS, significant gastrointestinal, or hypersensitivity reactions occur, the drug should be discontinued.
In patients with severe malnutrition, or anemia, appropriate caution should be exercised.
Adverse Reactions: The following reactions have been reported, usually due to excessive dosage:
Gastrointestinal—nausea, vomiting, abdominal cramps, and diarrhea.
Central nervous system—headache, vertigo, ataxia, tremors, choreiform movement, muscular weakness, hyporeflexia, paresthesia, blurring of vision, paralytic strabismus, convulsion, EEG abnormalities, sense of detachment, and memory defect.
Hypersensitivity—urticaria, erythema multiforme, purpura, fever, and arthralgia.
Dosage and Administration: *For ascariasis ("common roundworm" infection):*
Adults—a single daily dose of 3.5 g (hexahydrate equivalent) for 2 consecutive days.
Children—a single daily dose of 75 mg (hexahydrate equivalent)/kg of body weight/day for 2 consecutive days, with maximum daily dose of 3.5 g. See Table II above.

TABLE II

Patient's Weight	ANTEPAR (For Roundworms) Daily Dose for Two Consecutive Days	
15 lbs	1 tablet or teaspoonful	(0.5 g)
30 lbs	2 tablets or teaspoonfuls	(1.0 g)
45 lbs	3 tablets or teaspoonfuls	(1.5 g)
60 lbs	4 tablets or teaspoonfuls	(2.0 g)
75 lbs	5 tablets or teaspoonfuls	(2.5 g)
90 lbs	6 tablets or teaspoonfuls	(3.0 g)
105 lbs or over	7 tablets or teaspoonfuls (maximum daily dose)	(3.5 g)

In severe infections, the treatment course may be repeated after a *one* week interval. In circumstances where it is desired to apply mass therapy of ascariasis as a public health measure and where repeated therapy is not practicable, one single dose of 70 mg per pound of body weight, up to a maximum dose of 3 g, may be used, as described by Swartzwelder and Goodwin.* This procedure is successful in removing ascarids in the great majority of cases. However, the maximum cure rate is usually obtained with the multiple-dose regimen.

***References:**

Swartzwelder C, Miller JH, Sappenfield RW: Treatment of ascariasis in children with a single dose of piperazine citrate. Pediatrics 16(1):115, 1955
Goodwin LG, Standen OD: Treatment of roundworm with piperazine citrate (Antepar). Brit MJ 2:1332, 1954

For enterobiasis (pinworm infection): Adults and children—a single daily dose of 65 mg (hexahydrate equivalent)/kg of body weight/day, with a maximum daily dose of 2.5 g, for 7 consecutive days. See Table III below.

TABLE III

Patient's Weight	ANTEPAR (For Pinworms) Daily Dose For Seven Consecutive Days	
17 lbs	1 tablet or teaspoonful	(0.5 g)
34 lbs	2 tablets or teaspoonfuls	(1.0 g)
51 lbs	3 tablets or teaspoonfuls	(1.5 g)
68 lbs	4 tablets or teaspoonfuls	(2.0 g)
85 lbs and over	5 tablets or teaspoonfuls (maximum daily dose)	(2.5 g)

In severe infections, the treatment course may be repeated after a *one* week interval.
Use of laxatives or enema and dietary restriction are not necessary.
To prevent reinfection practice of personal and environmental hygiene should be recommended.
How Supplied:
ANTEPAR® brand Piperazine Citrate SYRUP 550 mg per 5 cc (equivalent to 500 mg piperazine hexahydrate). Bottle of 1 pint.
ANTEPAR® brand Piperazine Citrate TABLETS 550 mg scored (equivalent to 500 mg piperazine hexahydrate). Bottles of 100. Imprinted Y4A for identification.
Antepar Syrup
Pint DoD NSN 6505-00-598-8561
[*Shown in Product Identification Section*]

A.P.C. with Codeine Tablets ℞ Ⓒ
TABLOID® BRAND

Description: Tabloid A.P.C. with Codeine is supplied in tablet form for oral administration. Each tablet contains aspirin (acetylsalicylic acid) 227 mg, phenacetin 162 mg, and caffeine 32 mg, plus codeine phosphate in one of the following strengths: No. 2–15 mg, No. 3–30 mg, and No. 4–60 mg. (Warning—may be habit-forming.)
Tabloid A.P.C. with Codeine has analgesic, antipyretic and anti-inflammatory effects.
Clinical Pharmacology:
Aspirin: The analgesic, anti-inflammatory and antipyretic effects of aspirin are believed to result from inhibition of the synthesis of certain prostaglandins. Aspirin interferes with clotting mechanisms primarily by diminishing platelet aggregation; at high doses prothrombin synthesis can be inhibited.
Aspirin in solution is rapidly absorbed from the stomach and from the upper small intestine. About 50 percent of an oral dose is absorbed in 30 minutes and peak plasma concentrations are reached in about 40 minutes. Higher than normal stomach pH or the presence of food slightly delays absorption.
Once absorbed, aspirin is mainly hydrolyzed to salicylic acid and distributed to all body tissues and fluids, including fetal tissue, breast milk and the central nervous system (CNS). Highest concentrations are found in plasma, liver, renal cortex, heart and lung.
From 50 to 80 percent of the salicylic acid and its metabolites in plasma are loosely bound to plasma proteins. The plasma half-life of total salicylate is about 30 hours, with a 650 mg dose. Higher doses of aspirin cause increases in plasma salicylate half-life. Metabolism occurs primarily in the hepatocytes. The major metabolites are salicyluric acid (75%), the phenolic and acyl glucuronides of salicylate (15%), and gentisic and gentisuric acid (<1%).
Almost all of a therapeutic dose of aspirin is excreted through the kidneys, either as salicylic acid or the above-mentioned metabolic products. Renal clearance of salicylates is greatly augmented by an alkaline urine, as is produced by concurrent administration of sodium bicarbonate or potassium citrate.
Toxic salicylate blood levels are usually above 30 mg/100 ml. The single lethal dose of aspirin in normal adults is approximately 25–30 g, but patients have recovered from much larger doses with appropriate treatment.
Phenacetin: The mechanism through which phenacetin relieves pain is uncertain.
Phenacetin is rapidly absorbed from the gastrointestinal tract and reaches peak plasma concentrations in one-half to two hours. The physiologic half-life of phenacetin varies from about one-half to one and one-half hours: the drug is almost completely cleared from the body five hours after ingestion. About 30 to 40 percent of phenacetin is bound to plasma protein. Phenacetin and its pharmacologically active metabolite, acetaminophen, are distributed throughout the body tissues and fluids, including fetal tissue, breast milk and the CNS. Their concentration in body fluids, including milk, is relatively uniform, but the extent to which phenacetin and acetaminophen are taken up by various body tissues has not been established. About 75 to 80 percent of phenacetin is rapidly de-ethylated in liver to acetaminophen, which reaches peak plasma concentration in one to two hours and has a half-life of one to three hours. The therapeutic plasma concentration of acetaminophen is reported to be 0.5–2.0 mg/100 ml and the lethal concentration is 150 mg/100 ml. About 80 percent of the derived acetaminophen is excreted in urine after conjugation, primarily as the glucuronide; 3 percent is excreted unchanged. Other metabolites are formed by deacetylation and hydroxylation.
Phenacetin is metabolized by deacetylation (to para-phenetidin) and hydroxylation to a number of breakdown products; traces of phenacetin are eliminated unchanged. Toxic effects (sedation, dizziness) have been seen with single doses of 2 g. The minimum lethal dose has been estimated to be 5–20 g, but adults have recovered completely from acute overdoses of 50–60 g.
Caffeine: In ordinary doses, caffeine stimulates the CNS to elevate mood, decrease fatigue, promote alertness and improve motor skills. Caffeine also reduces susceptibility to fatigue by increasing the strength of skeletal muscle contractions. At higher doses or in the presence of medullary depressants, caffeine has been shown to stimulate respiration.
Caffeine exerts central and peripheral effects on heart rate that tend to offset each other except at high doses, when its direct positive chronotropic action predominates and an increased heart rate results. Caffeine also causes

Continued on next page

Burroughs Wellcome—Cont.

a moderate increase in myocardial contractility. While the balance between its central and peripheral effects on blood vessels generally favors vasodilation, caffeine causes vasoconstriction in the cerebral circulation. This effect is thought to explain its efficacy in relieving headache. In addition, caffeine has mild diuretic and smooth-muscle relaxant properties.
Like most xanthines, caffeine is rapidly absorbed and distributed in all body tissues and fluids, including the CNS, fetal tissues and breast milk. About 90 percent of an administered dose is metabolized in the liver to approximately equal amounts of 1-methyl-xanthine and 1-methyluric acid; the remainder is excreted unchanged in the urine.
Caffeine achieves its peak effect in about 2 hours; the plasma half-life is about 1.5 hours. The dose level at which toxicity occurs is about 1 g. The single lethal dose is estimated to be over 10 g.
Codeine: Codeine probably exerts its analgesic effect through actions on opiate receptors in the CNS.
Codeine is readily absorbed from the gastrointestinal tract, and a therapeutic dose reaches peak analgesic effectiveness in about 2 hours and persists for 4 to 6 hours. Oral codeine (60 mg) given to healthy males has been shown to achieve peak blood levels of 0.016 mg/100 ml at approximately one hour post-dose. The codeine plasma half-life for a 60 mg oral dose is about 2.9 hours. Blood levels causing CNS depression begin at 0.05–0.19 mg/100 ml. The single lethal dose of codeine in adults is estimated to be approximately 0.5–1.0 g.
Codeine is rapidly distributed from blood to body tissues and taken up preferentially by parenchymatous organs such as liver, spleen and kidney. It passes the blood-brain barrier and is found in fetal tissue and breast milk.
The drug is not bound by plasma protein nor is it accumulated in body tissues. Codeine is metabolized in the liver to morphine and norcodeine, each representing about 10 percent of the administered dose of codeine. About 90 percent of the dose is excreted within 24 hours, primarily through the kidneys. Urinary excretion products are free and glucuronide-conjugated codeine (about 70%), free and conjugated norcodeine (about 10%), free and conjugated morphine (about 10%), normorphine (under 4%) and hydrocodone (<1%). The remainder of the dose appears in the feces.
Indications and Usage: Tabloid A.P.C. with Codeine is indicated for the relief of mild, moderate, and moderate to severe pain.
Contraindications: Tabloid A.P.C. with Codeine is contraindicated under the following conditions:
(1) hypersensitivity or intolerance to aspirin, phenacetin, caffeine or codeine.
(2) severe bleeding, disorders of coagulation or primary hemostasis, including hemophilia, hypoprothrombinemia, von Willebrand's disease, the thrombocytopenias, thrombasthenia and other ill-defined hereditary platelet dysfunctions, as well as such associated conditions as severe vitamin K deficiency and severe liver damage.
(3) anticoagulant therapy, and
(4) peptic ulcer, or other serious gastrointestinal lesions.

Warnings: Therapeutic doses of aspirin can cause anaphylactic shock and other severe allergic reactions. A history of allergy is often lacking.
Significant bleeding can result from aspirin therapy in patients with peptic ulcer or other gastrointestinal lesions, and in patients with bleeding disorders. Aspirin administered preoperatively may prolong the bleeding time.
Nephrotoxicity (renal papillary necrosis), frequently accompanied by urinary tract infection, has been reported in a small percentage of individuals consuming analgesic mixtures regularly in large amounts for long periods. Carcinoma of the renal pelvis and urinary bladder has been associated with chronic abuse of analgesic mixtures.
In the presence of head injury or other intracranial lesions, the respiratory depressant effects of codeine and other narcotics may be markedly enhanced, as well as their capacity for elevating cerebrospinal fluid pressure. Narcotics also produce other CNS depressant effects, such as drowsiness, that may further obscure the clinical course of patients with head injuries.
Codeine or other narcotics may obscure signs on which to judge the diagnosis or clinical course of patients with acute abdominal conditions.

Precautions:
General: Tabloid A.P.C. with Codeine should be prescribed with caution for certain special-risk patients such as the elderly or debilitated, and for those with severe impairment of renal or hepatic function, gallbladder disease or gallstones, respiratory impairment, cardiac arrhythmias, inflammatory disorders of the gastrointestinal tract, hypothyroidism. Addison's disease, prostatic hypertrophy or urethral stricture, coagulation disorders, head injuries, acute abdominal conditions and patients known to be taking other analgesic-antipyretic medications. Patients' self-medication habits should be investigated to determine their use of such medications. Tabloid A.P.C. with Codeine should not be prescribed for long-term therapy unless specifically indicated.
Precautions should be taken when administering salicylates to persons with known allergies. Hypersensitivity to aspirin is particularly likely in patients with nasal polyps, and relatively common in those with asthma.
In persons with glucose-6-phosphate dehydrogenase deficiency, phenacetin can cause acute hemolytic anemia.
In persons with renal insufficiency, a typically mild but progressive hemolytic anemia can occur with long-term use of phenacetin. Patients with renal insufficiency appear to be especially susceptible to renal inflammatory lesions characteristic of so-called analgesic nephropathy associated with chronic abuse of analgesic medications.
Patients with severe heart disease should not receive high doses of caffeine, since it can cause tachycardia or extrasystoles and thus precipitate cardiac failure.
Palpitations that may be caused by caffeine are usually of significance only in patients with severe heart disease. Caffeine may cause gastrointestinal irritation and, in susceptible persons, overstimulation, "jitters" or insomnia.
Information for Patients: Tabloid A.P.C. with Codeine may impair the mental and/or physical abilities required for performance of potentially dangerous tasks such as driving a car or operating machinery. Such tasks should be avoided while taking Tabloid A.P.C. with Codeine.
Alcohol and other CNS depressants may produce an additive CNS depression when taken with Tabloid A.P.C. with Codeine, and should be avoided.
Patients with severe heart disease should be advised to reduce their total intake of caffeine. Codeine may be habit-forming when used over long periods or in high doses. Chronic use of Tabloid A.P.C. with Codeine at high doses for long periods of time may result in kidney or liver damage. Patients should take this drug only for as long as prescribed, in the amounts prescribed, and no more frequently than prescribed.
Laboratory Tests: Hypersensitivity to aspirin cannot be detected by skin testing or radioimmunoassay procedures.
The primary screening tests for detecting a bleeding tendency are platelet count, bleeding time, activated partial thromboplastin time and prothrombin time.
In patients with severe hepatic or renal disease, effects of therapy should be monitored with serial liver and/or renal function tests.
Drug Interactions: Tabloid A.P.C. with Codeine may *enhance* the effects of:
(1) monoamine oxidase (MAO) inhibitors,
(2) oral anticoagulants, causing bleeding by inhibiting prothrombin formation in the liver and displacing anticoagulants from plasma protein binding sites,
(3) oral antidiabetic agents and insulin, causing hypoglycemia by contributing an additive effect, and by displacing the oral antidiabetic agents from secondary binding sites,
(4) 6-mercaptopurine and methotrexate, causing bone marrow toxicity and blood dyscrasias by displacing these drugs from secondary binding sites,
(5) penicillins and sulfonamides, increasing their blood levels by displacing these drugs from protein binding sites,
(6) non-steroidal anti-inflammatory agents, increasing the risk of peptic ulceration and bleeding by contributing additive effects,
(7) other narcotic analgesics, alcohol, general anesthetics, tranquilizers such as chlordiazepoxide, sedative-hypnotics, or other CNS depressants, causing increased CNS depression,
(8) corticosteroids, potentiating steroid anti-inflammatory effects by displacing steroids from protein binding sites. Aspirin intoxication may occur with corticosteroid withdrawal because steroids promote renal clearance of salicylates.

Tabloid A.P.C. with Codeine may *diminish* the effects of:
(1) uricosuric agents such as probenecid and sulfinpyrazone, reducing their effectiveness in the treatment of gout. Aspirin competes with these agents for protein binding sites.

Aspirin and its metabolites may be caused to accumulate in the body, perhaps to toxic levels, by para-amino-salicylic acid, furosemide, and vitamin C. Phenobarbital decreases the effects of phenacetin by accelerating its excretion. Sorbitol and polysorbate accelerate the absorption of phenacetin. High doses of caffeine can cause a potentially lethal hypertensive reaction in the presence of MAO inhibitors. Caffeine and stimulants such as amphetamines may combine to cause excessive excitation or "nervousness".
Drug/Laboratory Test Interactions:
Aspirin: Aspirin may interfere with the following laboratory determinations in blood: serum amylase, fasting blood glucose, carbon dioxide, cholesterol, protein, protein bound iodine, uric acid, prothrombin time, bleeding time, and spectrophotometric detection of barbiturates. Aspirin may interfere with the following laboratory determinations in urine: glucose, 5-hydroxyindoleacetic acid, Gerhardt ketone, vanillylmandelic acid (VMA), protein, uric acid, and diacetic acid.
Phenacetin: Phenacetin may interfere with laboratory determinations of 5-hydroxyindoleacetic acid and glucose in urine.
Caffeine: Caffeine may interfere with laboratory determinations of bilirubin, fasting blood glucose, and uric acid in blood, and catecholamines and 5-hydroxyindoleacetic acid in urine.
Codeine: Codeine may increase serum amylase levels.
Carcinogenesis, Mutagenesis, Impairment of Fertility: No adequate long-term studies have been conducted in animals to determine whether codeine has a potential for carcinogenesis, mutagenesis, or impairment of fertility.
Adequate long-term studies have been conducted in mice and rats with aspirin, phenace-

tin and caffeine given alone or in combination. No evidence of carcinogenesis was seen in these studies. No adequate animal studies have been conducted with aspirin, phenacetin or caffeine to determine whether they have a potential for mutagenesis or impairment of fertility.

***Pregnancy:* Teratogenic Effects:** Pregnancy Category C. Animal reproduction studies have not been conducted with Tabloid A.P.C. with Codeine. It is also not known whether Tabloid A.P.C. with Codeine can cause fetal harm when administered to a pregnant woman or can affect reproduction capacity. Tabloid A.P.C. with Codeine should be given to a pregnant woman only if clearly needed.

Reproductive studies in rats and mice have shown aspirin to be teratogenic and embryocidal at four to six times the human therapeutic dose. Studies in pregnant women, however, have not shown that aspirin increases the risk of abnormalities when administered during the first trimester of pregnancy. In controlled studies involving 41,337 pregnant women and their offspring, there was no evidence that aspirin taken during pregnancy caused stillbirth, neonatal death or reduced birthweight. In controlled studies of 50,282 pregnant women and their offspring, aspirin administration in moderate and heavy doses during the first four lunar months of pregnancy showed no teratogenic effect.

Reproduction studies have been performed in rats and mice at doses up to 10 times the human dose and have revealed no evidence of impaired fertility or harm to the fetus due to caffeine.

Reproduction studies have been performed in rabbits and rats at doses up to 150 times the human dose and have revealed no evidence of impaired fertility or harm to the fetus due to codeine.

Nonteratogenic Effects: Therapeutic doses of aspirin in pregnant women close to term may cause bleeding in mother, fetus, or neonate. During the last six months of pregnancy, regular use of aspirin in high doses may prolong pregnancy and delivery.

The risk of methemoglobinemia or hemolytic anemia occurring in the fetus may be increased by: (1) regular ingestion of high doses of phenacetin during pregnancy, (2) renal insufficiency in the mother and/or fetus, (3) glucose-6-phosphate dehydrogenase deficiency, or (4) a genetically acquired abnormality in phenacetin metabolism.

Labor and Delivery: Ingestion of aspirin prior to delivery may prolong delivery or lead to bleeding in the mother or neonate. Ingestion of phenacetin may cause methemoglobinemia or hemolytic anemia. Use of codeine during labor may lead to respiratory depression in the neonate.

Nursing Mothers: All components of Tabloid A.P.C. with Codeine are excreted in breast milk in small amounts, but the significance of their effects on nursing infants is not known. Because of the potential for serious adverse reactions in nursing infants from Tabloid A.P.C. with Codeine, a decision should be made whether to discontinue nursing or to discontinue the drug, taking into account the importance of the drug to the mother.

Adverse Reactions:

Codeine: The most frequently observed adverse reactions to codeine include light-headedness, dizziness, drowsiness, nausea, vomiting, constipation and depression of respiration. Less common reactions to codeine include euphoria, dysphoria, pruritus and skin rashes.

Aspirin: Mild intoxication (salicylism) can occur in response to chronic use of large doses. Manifestations include nausea, vomiting, hearing impairment, tinnitus, diminished vision, headache, dizziness, drowsiness, metal confusion, hyperpnea, hyperventilation, tachycardia, sweating and thirst.

Therapeutic doses of aspirin can induce mild or severe allergic reactions manifested by skin rashes, urticaria, angioedema, rhinorrhea, asthma, abdominal pain, nausea, vomiting, or anaphylactic shock. A history of allergy is often lacking, and allergic reactions may occur in patients who have previously taken aspirin without any ill effects. Allergic reactions to aspirin are most likely to occur in patients with a history of allergic disease, especially in patients with nasal polyps or asthma.

Some patients are unable to take aspirin or other salicylates without developing nausea or vomiting. Occasional patients respond to aspirin (usually in large doses) with dyspepsia or heartburn, which may be accompanied by occult bleeding. Excessive bruising or bleeding is sometimes seen in patients with mild disorders of primary hemostasis who regularly use low doses of aspirin.

Prolonged use of aspirin can cause painless erosion of gastric mucosa, occult bleeding and, infrequently, iron-deficiency anemia. High doses of aspirin can exacerbate symptoms of peptic ulcer and, occasionally cause extensive bleeding.

Excessive bleeding can follow injury or surgery in patients with or without known bleeding disorders who have taken therapeutic doses of aspirin within the preceding 10 days.

Hepatotoxicity has been reported in association with prolonged use of large doses of aspirin in patients with lupus erythematosus, rheumatoid arthritis, or rheumatic disease.

Bone-marrow depression, manifested by weakness, fatigue, or abnormal bruising or bleeding, has occasionally been reported.

In patients with glucose-6-phosphate dehydrogenase deficiency, aspirin can cause a mild degree of hemolytic anemia.

In hyperuricemic persons, low doses of aspirin may reduce the effectiveness of uricosuric therapy or precipitate an attack of gout.

Phenacetin: In therapeutic doses, side effects of phenacetin are generally limited to occasional sedation, skin rashes or, uncommonly, drug fever.

Adverse reactions to phenacetin are usually the result of acute overdosage or chronic abuse of analgesic mixtures containing phenacetin. Toxic doses can cause dizziness, drowsiness or stimulation, methemoglobinemia and sulfhemoglobinemia (cyanosis, fatigue), and, rarely, hepatic necrosis (gastrointestinal symptoms possibly followed by general obtundation) or nephropathy (cloudy urine due to cells, casts, organism, sloughed tissue, edema of lower legs).

Caffeine: Usual doses of caffeine may cause gastric disturbances in some persons. Side effects are usually due to hyperresponsiveness or overdosage, actue or chronic. Toxic doses can cause nervousness, excitement, insomnia, muscle tenderness or tremors, tinnitus, scintillating scotomas, headache on withdrawal of the drug, diuresis, tachycardia and extrasystoles.

Drug Abuse and Dependence: Like other medications containing a narcotic analgesic, Tabloid A.P.C. with Codeine is controlled by the Drug Enforcement Administration and is classified under Schedule III.

Tabloid A.P.C. with Codeine can produce drug dependence of the morphine type; therefore, it has the potential for being abused. Psychic dependence, physical dependence and tolerance may develop on repeated administration. The dependence liability of codeine has been found to be too small to permit a full definition of its characteristics. Studies indicate that addiction to codeine is extremely uncommon and requires very high parenteral doses.

When dependence on codeine occurs at therapeutic doses, it appears to require from one to two months to develop, and withdrawal symptoms are mild. Most patients on long-term oral codeine therapy show no signs of physical dependence upon abrupt withdrawal.

Overdosage: Severe intoxication, caused by overdose of Tabloid A.P.C. with Codeine may produce: skin eruptions, dyspnea, vertigo, double vision, delusions, hallucinations, garbled speech, excitability, restlessness, delirium, constricted pupils, a positive Babinski sign, respiratory depression (slow and shallow breathing, Cheyne-Stokes respiration), cyanosis, clammy skin, muscle flaccidity, circulatory collapse, stupor and coma. In children, difficulty in hearing, tinnitus, dim vision, headache, dizziness, drowsiness, confusion, rapid breathing, sweating, thirst, nausea, vomiting, hyperpyrexia, dehydration and convulsions are prominent signs. The most severe manifestations from A.P.C. result from cardiovascular and respiratory insufficiency secondary to aspirin-induced acid-base and electrolyte disturbances, complicated by hyperthermia and dehydration. The most severe manifestations from codeine are associated with respiratory depression.

Respiratory alkalosis is characteristic of the early phase of intoxication with aspirin while hyperventilation is occurring, and is quickly followed by metabolic acidosis in most people with severe intoxication. This occurs more readily in children. Hypoglycemia may occur in children who have taken large overdoses. Other laboratory findings associated with aspirin intoxication include ketonuria, hyponatremia, hypokalemia, and occasionally proteinuria. A slight rise in lactic dehydrogenase and hydroxybutyric dehydrogenase may occur.

Hemolytic anemia due to phenacetin is possible and should be monitored by periodic laboratory tests.

Methemoglobin and sulfhemoglobin formation are seldom clinically significant in adults but may contribute to general toxicity. When prominent, they appear as a grayish cyanosis seen most clearly in the lips and nailbeds. Definitive diagnosis is made by spectroscopic analysis of a water-diluted (1:100) blood specimen, which shows an abnormal band at 630 m for methemoglobin and at 618 m for sulfhemoglobin.

Concentrations of aspirin in plasma above 30 mg/100 ml are associated with toxicity. (See Clinical Pharmacology section for information on factors influencing aspirin blood levels.)

The single lethal dose of aspirin in adults is probably about 25–30 g, but is not known with certainty.

Toxic and lethal concentrations of phenacetin in human fluids are not known with certainty. Patient response per phenacetin dose may be greater than usual in infants, in patients with renal insufficiency or hepatic insufficiency and in those with a glucose-6-phosphate dehydrogenase deficiency or a decreased ability to convert phenacetin to acetaminophen. Toxic effects (e.g. sedation) have been seen with single doses of 2 g. The minimum lethal dose has been estimated to be 5–20 g, but adults have recovered from acute overdoses of 50–60 g.

Toxic and lethal concentrations of caffeine in human fluids are not known with certainty. Patient response per dose is increased in the presence of renal or hepatic insufficiency. Toxic manifestations may appear with a caffeine dose of 1 g. The single lethal dose in man is generally estimated to be over 10 g, but the lowest reported lethal dose was 3.2 g or 57 mg/kg.

The toxic plasma concentration of codeine is not known with certainty. Experimental production of mild to moderate CNS depression in healthy, nontolerant subjects occurred at plasma concentrations of 0.05–0.19 mg/100 ml when codeine was given by intravenous infusion. The single lethal dose of codeine in adults is estimated to be from 0.5–1.0 g. It is also estimated that 5 mg/kg could be fatal in children.

Continued on next page

Burroughs Wellcome—Cont.

Hemodialysis and peritoneal dialysis can be performed to reduce the body aspirin content. Phenacetin is dialyzable, but dialysis of the drug and its major metabolite, acetaminophen, has not yet been established as an effective means of altering the consequences of acute phenacetin overdosage. Caffeine and codeine are theoretically dialyzable but the procedure has not been clinically established for either.
Treatment of overdosage consists primarily of support of vital functions, management of codeine-induced respiratory depression, increasing salicylate elimination, and correcting the acid-base imbalance due primarily to salicylism.
In a comatose patient, primary attention should be given to establishment of adequate respiratory exchange through provision of a patent airway and the institution of assisted or controlled ventilation. The narcotic antagonist naloxone is a specific antidote for respiratory depression which may result from overdosage or unusual sensitivity to narcotics. Therefore, an appropriate dose of an antagonist should be administered, preferably by the intravenous route, simultaneously with efforts at respiratory resuscitation. Since the duration of action of Tabloid A.P.C. with Codeine may exceed that of the antagonist, the patient should be kept under continued surveillance and repeated doses of the antagonist should be administered as needed to maintain adequate respiration.
A narcotic antagonist should not be administered in absence of clinically significant respiratory or cardiovascular depression.
Gastric emptying (Syrup of Ipecac) and/or lavage is recommended as soon as possible after ingestion, even if the patient has vomited spontaneously. (Apomorphine should not be used as an emetic for Tabloid A.P.C. with Codeine, since it may potentiate hypotension and respiratory depression.) Administration of activated charcoal as a slurry is beneficial after lavage and/or emesis, if less than three hours have passed since ingestion. Charcoal adsorption should *not* be employed prior to emesis or lavage.
Severity of aspirin intoxication is determined by measuring the blood salicylate level. Acid-base status should be closely followed with serial blood gas and serum pH measurements. Fluid and electrolyte balance should also be regularly monitored.
A serum salicylate level of 30 mg/100 ml or higher indicates a need for enhanced salicylate excretion that can be achieved through body-fluid supplementation and urine alkalinization if renal function is normal. In mild intoxication, urine flow can be increased by forcing oral fluids and giving potassium citrate capsules. (DO NOT GIVE BICARBONATE BY MOUTH SINCE IT INCREASES THE RATE OF SALICYLATE ABSORPTION.)
In severe cases, hyperthermia and hypovolemia as well as respiratory depression are the major immediate threats to life. Children should be sponged with tepid water. Replacement fluid should be administered intravenously in adequate amount and augmented with sufficient bicarbonate to correct acidosis, with monitoring of plasma electrolytes and pH, to promote alkaline diuresis of salicylate if renal function is normal. Complete control may also require infusion of glucose to control hypoglycemia.
Potassium deficiency may also be corrected through the infusion, once adequate urinary output is assured. Plasma or plasma expanders may be needed if fluid replacement is insufficient to maintain normal blood pressure or adequate urinary output.
In patients with renal insufficiency or in cases of life-threatening intoxication, dialysis is usually required. Peritoneal dialysis or exchange transfusion is indicated in infants and young children, and hemodialysis in older patients. Oxygen, intravenous fluids, vasopressors and other supportive measures should be employed as needed.

Dosage and Administration: Dosage is adjusted according to the severity of pain and the response of the patient. It may occasionally be necessary to exceed the usual dosage recommended below when pain is severe or the patient has become tolerant to the analgesic effect of codeine. Tabloid A.P.C. with Codeine is given orally. The usual adult dose for Tabloid A.P.C. with Codeine No. 2 and No. 3 is one or two tablets every four hours as required. The usual adult dose for Tabloid A.P.C. with Codeine No. 4 is one tablet every four hours as required.
Tabloid A.P.C. with Codeine should be taken with food or a full glass of milk or water to lessen gastric irritation.

How Supplied:
Tabloid A.P.C. with Codeine No. 2: (white tablet embossed with "TABLOID BRAND" and "2")

Bottle of 100	NDC 0081-0343-55
Bottle of 500	NDC 0081-0343-70
Bottle of 1000	NDC 0081-0343-75

Tabloid A.P.C. with Codeine No. 3: (white tablet embossed with "TABLOID BRAND" and "3")

Bottle of 100	NDC 0081-0356-55
Bottle of 500	NDC 0081-0356-70
Bottle of 1000	NDC 0081-0356-75

Tabloid A.P.C. with Codeine No. 4: (white tablet embossed with "TABLOID BRAND" and "4")

Bottle of 100	NDC 0081-0369-55
Bottle of 500	NDC 0081-0369-70
Bottle of 1000	NDC 0081-0369-75

Store at 15°–30°C (59°–86°F) in a dry place and protect from light.
[*Shown in Product Identification Section*]

CARDILATE® TABLETS ℞
(Erythrityl Tetranitrate)

Description: Cardilate (erythrityl tetranitrate) is an antianginal drug that belongs to the organic nitrate class of pharmaceutical agents. Erythrityl tetranitrate is soluble in alcohol, ether and glycerol, but insoluble in water. It has the empirical formula $C_4H_6N_4O_{12}$, molecular weight of 302.12 and melting point of 61°C.
Erythrityl tetranitrate is known chemically as *(R*S*)*-1,2,3,4-butanetetrol tetranitrate and has the following structural formula:

```
        CH2ONO2
        |
   H---C---ONO2
        |
   H---C---ONO2
        |
        CH2ONO2
```

In the pure state, erythrityl tetranitrate will explode upon percussion, but properly diluted with lactose, as in Cardilate tablets, it is nonexplosive. Since it is a low melting solid, erythrityl tetranitrate does not evaporate from the Cardilate tablets.
Cardilate Oral/Sublingual Tablets contain either 5, 10 or 15 mg erythrityl tetranitrate dispersed in lactose, with disintegration characteristics that permit sublingual or oral (swallowed) administration. Cardilate Chewable Tablets contain 10 mg erythrityl tetranitrate and lactose, with wintergreen flavoring to enhance patient acceptance.

Clinical Pharmacology: Cardilate exerts its effects by relaxation of vascular smooth muscle.[1] The action is maximal on the post-capillary vessels, including the large veins. Venodilatation results in peripheral blood pooling, which decreases venous return to the heart, central venous pressure and pulmonary capillary wedge pressure (preload reduction).[2] Pulmonary arteriolar dilatation causes a reduction in pulmonary vascular resistance.[2] A decrease in systemic arterial pressure (afterload reduction) can also occur, but is usually less pronounced. Augmentation of cardiac output generally occurs in those patients with increased filling pressures and high resting systemic vascular resistance.[2]

Mechanism of Action: The inadequate myocardial oxygenation that precipitates angina can be corrected by: (1) increasing the supply of oxygen to ischemic myocardium through direct dilatation of the large coronary conductance vessels or (2) decreasing the myocardial oxygen demand secondary to a reduction of cardiac work (preload and afterload reduction).[3] The beneficial effect of Cardilate probably involves both mechanisms.

Pharmacokinetics and Metabolism: Cardilate is readily absorbed from the sublingual, buccal and gastrointestinal mucosae. The peak effect from a swallowed dose is diminished but of longer duration when compared to the sublingual route.[4] The biotransformation of Cardilate is thought to occur by reductive hydrolysis catalyzed by the hepatic enzyme glutathione-organic nitrate reductase.[3] Differences in response among various nitrates may relate to both intrinsic potency at cardiovascular sites, as well as factors related to pharmacokinetics and biotransformation.[5]
Time to onset of effect is approximately 5 minutes for the sublingual and chewable routes and 15 to 30 minutes for swallowed tablets, with peak effect in 15 minutes and 60 minutes, respectively. Duration of action will vary, but vasodilatory effects have been demonstrated for up to 3 hours after sublingual and chewable administration[4,6] and for 6 hours after the oral (swallowed) route.[4]

Indications and Usage: Cardilate (Erythrityl Tetranitrate) is intended for the prophylaxis and long-term treatment of patients with frequent or recurrent anginal pain and reduced exercise tolerance associated with angina pectoris, rather than for the treatment of the acute attack of angina pectoris, since its onset is somewhat slower than that of nitroglycerin.

Contraindications: Cardilate should not be administered to individuals with a known hypersensitivity or idiosyncratic reaction to organic nitrates.

Warnings: The use of nitrates in acute myocardial infarction or congestive heart failure should be undertaken only under close clinical observation and/or in conjunction with hemodynamic monitoring.

Precautions:
General: Cardilate should be used with caution in patients with severe liver or renal disease. Development of tolerance and cross-tolerance to the effects of erythrityl tetranitrate and other organic nitrates may occur. However, recent studies in patients with chronic heart failure[1] indicate that nitrates produce sustained beneficial hemodynamic effects.
Carcinogenesis, Mutagenesis, Impairment of Fertility: No long-term studies in animals have been performed.
Pregnancy: Teratogenic Effects. Pregnancy Category C. Animal reproduction studies have not been conducted with Cardilate. It is also not known whether Cardilate can cause fetal harm when administered to a pregnant woman or can affect reproduction capacity. Cardilate should be given to a pregnant woman only if clearly needed.
Nursing Mothers: It is not known whether this drug is excreted in human milk. Because many drugs are excreted in human milk, caution should be exercised when Cardilate is administered to a nursing woman.
Pediatric Use: Safety and effectiveness in children have not been established.

Adverse Reactions: The most frequent adverse reaction in patients treated with Cardilate is headache. Lowering the dose and the use of analgesics will help control headaches, which usually diminish or disappear as therapy is continued. Other adverse reactions occurring are the following: cutaneous vasodilatation with flushing, and transient episodes of dizziness and weakness, plus other signs of cerebral ischemia associated with postural hypotension. Occasional individuals exhibit marked sensitivity to the hypotensive effects of organic nitrates, and severe responses (e.g., nausea, vomiting, weakness, restlessness, pallor, perspiration and collapse) can occur even with the usual therapeutic dose. Alcohol may enhance this effect. Drug rash and/or exfoliative dermatitis may occasionally occur.

Overdosage: Accidental overdosage of Cardilate may result in severe hypotension and reflex tachycardia, which can be treated by laying the patient down and elevating the legs. If further treatment is required, the administration of intravenous fluids or other means of treating hypotension should be considered.

Dosage and Administration:

Oral/Sublingual Tablets: The Cardilate Oral/Sublingual Tablet can be placed under the tongue or swallowed. Sublingual therapy may be initiated with a dose of 5 to 10 mg prior to each anticipated physical or emotional stress, and at bedtime for patients subject to nocturnal attacks of angina. The dose may be increased as needed.

If the patient is to swallow the tablet, therapy may be initiated with 10 mg before each meal, as well as mid-morning and mid-afternoon if needed, and at bedtime for patients subject to nocturnal attacks. The dose may be increased or decreased as needed.

Dosage titration up to 100 mg daily has been well tolerated, but temporary headache is more apt to occur with increasing doses. When headache occurs, the dose should be reduced for a few days. If headache is troublesome during adjustment of dosage, it may be effectively relieved with an analgesic.

Chewable Tablets: Cardilate Chewable Tablets offer the advantages of the sublingual tablet in a wintergreen-flavored tablet. Dosage, time of onset and maximum effect are the same as for the sublingual tablet, if the tablet is thoroughly chewed and kept in the mouth for as long as possible.

How Supplied:

CARDILATE (Erythrityl Tetranitrate) ORAL/SUBLINGUAL TABLETS (scored).

5 mg: Bottles of 100 (NDC-0081-0166-55), Imprint "CARDILATE P2B" (round, white).

10 mg: Bottles of 100 (NDC-0081-0168-55) and 1000 (NDC-0081-0168-75). Imprint "CARDILATE X7A" (square, white).

CARDILATE (Erythrityl Tetranitrate) CHEWABLE TABLETS (scored),

10 mg: Bottles of 100 (NDC-0081-0161-55). Imprint "CARDILATE X7A" (round, white).

All tablets should be stored at 15°–25°C (59°–77°F) in a dry place and dispensed in glass.

References:

1. Chatterjee K, Parmley WW: Vasodilator Therapy for Chronic Heart Failure. *Ann Rev Pharmacol Toxicol, 20*:475–512, 1980.
2. Goldberg S. Mann T, Grossman W: Nitrate Therapy of Heart Failure in Valvular Heart Disease. *Am J Med, 66*:161–66, 1978.
3. Needleman P, Johnson EM: Vasodilators and the Treatment of Angina. In: AG Gilman, LS Goodman, A Gilman, eds. The Pharmacological Basis of Therapeutics, 6th Edition, New York: Macmillan Publishing Co., Inc. 819–33, 1980.
4. Hannemann RE, Erb RJ, Stoltman WP, Bronson EC, Williams EJ, Long RA, Hull JH, Starbuck RR: Digital Plethysmograph for Assessing Erythrityl Tetranitrate Bioavailability. *Clin Pharmacol Ther, 29*:35–9, 1981.
5. Wastila WB, Namm DH, Maxwell RA: Comparison of the Vascular Effects of Several Organic Nitrates in Anesthetized Rats and Dogs after Intravenous and Intraportal Administration. Vascular Neuroeffector Mechanisms. 2nd Int. Symp., Odense. Basel: Karger Publishing Co. 216–25, 1975.
6. Haffty GB, Nakamura Y, Spodick DH, Long RA, Hull JH: Bioavailability of Organic Nitrates: a Comparison of Methods for Evaluating Plethysmographic Responses. *J Clin Pharmacol. 22*:117–124, 1982.

[*Shown in Product Identification Section*]

CORTISPORIN® CREAM ℞

Polymyxin B—Neomycin—Gramicidin—Hydrocortisone

Description: Each gram contains: Aerosporin® brand Polymyxin B Sulfate 10,000 units; neomycin sulfate 5 mg (equivalent to 3.5 mg neomycin base); gramicidin 0.25 mg; hydrocortisone acetate 5 mg (0.5%).

Preservative: methylparaben 0.25%

The base contains the inactive ingredients liquid petrolatum, white petrolatum, propylene glycol, polyoxyethylene polyoxypropylene compound, emulsifying wax and purified water.

The base is a smooth vanishing cream with a pH of approximately 5.0. The acid pH helps restore normal cutaneous acidity. The cream is cosmetically acceptable and may be easily removed with water. Owing to its excellent spreading and penetrating properties, the cream facilitates treatment of hairy and intertriginous areas. It may also be of value in selective cases where the lesions are moist. The antibiotics diffuse readily from the base into fluids of the skin or tissues.

Action: The cream is useful wherever the anti-inflammatory and antipruritic action of hydrocortisone is indicated in conjunction with the bactericidal action of polymyxin B, neomycin, and gramicidin. For anti-inflammatory action, the acetate salt of the naturally-occurring adrenal corticosteroid hydrocortisone is used. Wide range antibacterial action, approaching the ideal, is provided by the overlapping spectra of polymyxin B, neomycin, and gramicidin. The range of action of this combination includes virtually all pathogenic bacteria found topically, and the three antibacterials are bactericidal, rather than bacteriostatic. The index of allergenicity of this combination has been shown over the years to be low and the rarity of topical irritation has been well demonstrated.

Polymyxin B is one of a group of closely related substances produced by various strains of *Bacillus polymyxa*. Its activity is sharply restricted to gram-negative bacteria, including many strains of *Pseudomonas aeruginosa*.

Neomycin, isolated from *Streptomyces fradiae*, has antibacterial activity *in vitro* against a wide range of gram-negative and gram-positive organisms, with effectiveness against many strains of *Proteus*.

Gramicidin has particular action *in vitro* against certain gram-positive bacteria.

Indications: Based on a review of this drug by the National Academy of Sciences—National Research Council and/or other information, FDA has classified the indications as follows:

"Possibly" effective: General: The cream is indicated in the treatment of topical bacterial infections caused by organisms sensitive to the antibiotic ingredients, and when the anti-inflammatory and/or anti-allergic action of the hydrocortisone is indicated as in burns, wounds, and skin grafts; otitis externa; also following surgical procedures. Dermatologic: Atopic, contact, stasis and infectious eczematoid dermatitis; neurodermatitis; eczema; anogenital pruritus. It may also be useful as an adjunct in certain pyodermas, such as impetigo, during specific systemic antibiotic therapy for these infections.

Final classification of the less-than-effective indications requires further investigation.

Contraindications: Not for use in the eyes or in the external ear canal if the eardrum is perforated. This drug is contraindicated in tuberculous, fungal or viral lesions of the skin (herpes simplex, vaccinia and varicella). This product is contraindicated in those individuals who have shown hypersensitivity to any of its components.

Warning: Because of the potential hazard of nephrotoxicity and ototoxicity due to neomycin, care should be exercised when using this product in treating extensive burns, trophic ulceration and other extensive conditions where absorption of neomycin is possible. In burns where more than 20 percent of the body surface is affected, especially if the patient has impaired renal function or is receiving other aminoglycoside antibiotics concurrently, not more than one application a day is recommended.

When using neomycin-containing products to control secondary infection in the chronic dermatoses, such as chronic otitis externa or stasis dermatitis, it should be borne in mind that the skin in these conditions is more liable than is normal skin to become sensitized to many substances, including neomycin. The manifestation of sensitization to neomycin is usually a low grade reddening with swelling, dry scaling and itching; it may be manifest simply as a failure to heal. During long-term use of neomycin-containing products, periodic examination for such signs is advisable and the patient should be told to discontinue the product if they are observed. These symptoms regress quickly on withdrawing the medication. Neomycin-containing applications should be avoided for that patient thereafter.

Precautions: As with other antibacterial preparations, prolonged use may result in overgrowth of nonsusceptible organisms, including fungi. Appropriate measures should be taken if this occurs. Use of steroids on infected areas should be supervised with care as anti-inflammatory steroids may encourage spread of infection. If this occurs steroid therapy should be stopped and appropriate antibacterial drugs used. Generalized dermatological conditions may require systemic corticosteroid therapy. As the safety of topical steroid preparations during pregnancy has not been fully established, they should not be used unnecessarily, on extended areas, in large amounts, or for prolonged periods of time, in pregnancy.

Adverse Reactions: When steroid preparations are used for long periods of time in intertriginous areas or over extensive body areas, with or without occlusive non-permeable dressings, striae may occur; also there exists the possibility of systemic side effects when steroid preparations are used over larger areas or for a long period of time.

Neomycin is a not uncommon cutaneous sensitizer. Articles in the current literature indicate an increase in the prevalence of persons allergic to neomycin. Ototoxicity and nephrotoxicity have been reported (see Warning section).

Dosage and Administration: A small quantity of the cream should be applied 2 to 4 times daily, as required. The cream should, if conditions permit, be gently rubbed into the affected areas. In chronic conditions, withdrawal of treatment is carried out by decreasing the frequency of application, until the cream finally is applied as infrequently as once a week.

How Supplied: Tube of 7.5 g.

Continued on next page

Burroughs Wellcome—Cont.

CORTISPORIN® OINTMENT ℞
Polymyxin B-Bacitracin-Neomycin-Hydrocortisone

Description: Each gram contains: Aerosporin® brand Polymyxin B Sulfate 5,000 units; bacitracin zinc 400 units; neomycin sulfate 5 mg (equivalent to 3.5 mg neomycin base); hydrocortisone 10 mg (1%); special white petrolatum qs.

Indications: Based on a review of this drug by the National Academy of Sciences—National Research Council and/or other information, FDA has classified the indications as follows:
"Possibly" effective: General: The ointment is indicated in the treatment of topical bacterial infections caused by organisms sensitive to the antibiotic ingredients, and when the anti-inflammatory and/or anti-allergic action of the hydrocortisone is indicated, e.g., such conditions as burns, wounds, skin grafts; otitis externa; and plastic, proctologic, gynecologic, or general surgical procedures. Dermatologic: Atopic, contact, stasis and infectious eczematoid dermatitis; neurodermatitis; eczema; anogenital pruritus. It may also be useful as an adjunct in certain pyodermas, such as impetigo, during specific systemic antibiotic therapy for these infections.
Final classification of the less-than-effective indications requires further investigation.

Contraindications: This product is contraindicated in those individuals who have shown hypersensitivity to any of its components. Do not use in the external ear canal if the eardrum is perforated.
Warning: Because of the potential hazard of nephrotoxicity and ototoxicity due to neomycin, care should be exercised when using this product in treating extensive burns, trophic ulceration and other extensive conditions where absorption of neomycin is possible. In burns where more than 20 percent of the body surface is affected, especially if the patient has impaired renal function or is receiving other aminoglycoside antibiotics concurrently, not more than one application a day is recommended.
When using neomycin-containing products to control secondary infection in the chronic dermatoses, such as chronic otitis externa or stasis dermatitis, it should be borne in mind that the skin in these conditions is more liable than is normal skin to become sensitized to many substances, including neomycin. The manifestation of sensitization to neomycin is usually a low grade reddening with swelling, dry scaling and itching; it may be manifest simply as a failure to heal. During long-term use of neomycin-containing products, periodic examination for such signs is advisable and the patient should be told to discontinue the product if they are observed. These symptoms regress quickly on withdrawing the medication. Neomycin-containing applications should be avoided for that patient thereafter.
Precautions: As with any antibiotic preparation, prolonged use may result in the overgrowth of nonsusceptible organisms, including fungi. Appropriate measures should be taken if this occurs. Use of steroids on infected areas should be supervised with care as anti-inflammatory steroids may encourage spread of infection. If this occurs steroid therapy should be stopped and appropriate antibacterial drugs used. Generalized dermatological conditions may require systemic corticosteroid therapy. As the safety of topical steroid preparations during pregnancy has not been fully established, they should not be used unnecessarily, on extended areas, in large amounts, or for prolonged periods of time, in pregnancy.
Adverse Reactions: When steroid preparations are used for long periods of time in intertriginous areas or over extensive body areas, with or without occlusive nonpermeable dressings, striae may occur; also there exists the possibility of systemic side effects when steroid preparations are used over larger areas or for a long period of time.
Neomycin is a not uncommon cutaneous sensitizer. Articles in the current literature indicate an increase in the prevalence of persons allergic to neomycin. Ototoxicity and nephrotoxicity have been reported (see Warning section).
Dosage and Administration: A thin film is applied 2 to 4 times daily. In chronic conditions, withdrawal of treatment is carried out by decreasing the frequency of application, until the ointment is applied as infrequently as once a week.
How Supplied: Tube of ½ oz with applicator tip.

CORTISPORIN® OPHTHALMIC OINTMENT Sterile ℞
(POLYMYXIN B–BACITRACIN–NEOMYCIN–HYDROCORTISONE)

Description: Cortisporin® Ophthalmic Ointment (polymyxin B-bacitracin-neomycin-hydrocortisone) is a sterile antimicrobial ointment for ophthalmic use. Each gram contains Aerosporin® (polymyxin B sulfate) 10,000 units, bacitracin zinc 400 units, neomycin sulfate 5 mg (equivalent to 3.5 mg neomycin base), hydrocortisone 10 mg (1%) and special white petrolatum, qs.
Polymyxin B sulfate is the sulfate salt of polymyxin B_1 and B_2 which are produced by the growth of *Bacillus polymyxa* (Prazmowski) Migula (Fam. Bacillaceae). It has a potency of not less than 6,000 Polymyxin B units per mg, calculated on an anhydrous basis.
Bacitracin zinc is the zinc salt of bacitracin, a mixture of related cyclic polypeptides (mainly bacitracin A) produced by the growth of an organism of the *licheniformis* group of *Bacillus subtilis* (Fam. Bacillaceae). It has a potency of not less than 40 bacitracin units per mg. The precise structural formula is not known. Neomycin sulfate is the sulfate salt of neomycin B and C which are produced by the growth of *Streptomyces fradiae* Waksman (Fam. Streptomycetaceae). It has a potency equivalent of not less than 600 μg of neomycin standard per mg, calculated on an anhydrous basis.
Hydrocortisone, 11β, 17, 21-Trihydroxy-4-pregnene-3, 20-dione, is an anti-inflammatory hormone.
Clinical Pharmacology: Corticoids suppress the inflammatory response to a variety of agents and they probably delay or slow healing. Since corticoids may inhibit the body's defense mechanism against infection, a concomitant antimicrobial drug may be used when this inhibition is considered to be clinically significant in a particular case.
The anti-infective component in the combination is included to provide action against specific organisms susceptible to it. Polymyxin B is considered active against the following microorganisms: gram-negative bacilli (excepting *Proteus*), including virtually all strains of *Pseudomonas aeruginosa* and *H. influenza* (Koch-Weeks bacillus).
Neomycin sulfate is considered active against the following microorganisms: many strains of gram-positive and gram-negative organisms, including many strains of *Proteus vulgaris* and *Staphylococcus aureus* but not streptococci. Bacitracin is considered active against the following microorganisms: gram-positive bacilli and cocci, and extends the spectrum to include hemolytic streptococci.
When a decision to administer both a corticoid and antimicrobials is made, the administration of such drugs in combination has the advantage of greater patient compliance and convenience, with the added assurance that the appropriate dosage of both drugs is administered, plus assured compatibility of ingredients when both types of drug are in the same formulation and, particularly, that the correct volume of drug is delivered and retained.
The relative potency of corticosteroids depends on the molecular structure, concentration, and release from the vehicle.
Indications and Usage: For steroid-responsive inflammatory ocular conditions for which a corticosteroid is indicated and where bacterial infection or a risk of bacterial ocular infection exists.
Ocular steroids are indicated in inflammatory conditions of the palpebral and bulbar conjunctiva, cornea and anterior segment of the globe where the inherent risk of steroid use in certain infective conjunctivitides is accepted to obtain a diminution in edema and inflammation. They are also indicated in chronic anterior uveitis and corneal injury from chemical, radiation, or thermal burns, or penetration of foreign bodies.
The use of a combination drug with an anti-infective component is indicated where the risk of infection is high or where there is an expectation that potentially dangerous numbers of bacteria will be present in the eye.
The particular anti-infective drugs in this product are active against the following common bacterial eye pathogens: *Staphylococcus aureus*, Streptococci, including *Streptococcus pneumoniae*, *Escherichia coli*, *Haemophilus influenzae*, *Klebsiella/Enterobacter* species, *Neisseria* species and *Pseudomonas aeruginosa*.
The product does not provide adequate coverage against: *Serratia marcescens*.
Contraindications: Epithelial herpes simplex keratitis (dendritic keratitis), vaccinia, varicella, and many other viral diseases of the cornea and conjunctiva. Mycobacterial infection of the eye. Fungal diseases of ocular structures. Hypersensitivity to a component of the medication. (Hypersensitivity to the antibiotic component occurs at a higher rate than for other components.)
The use of these combinations is contraindicated after uncomplicated removal of a corneal foreign body.
Warnings: Prolonged use may result in glaucoma, with damage to the optic nerve, defects in visual acuity and fields of vision, and posterior subcapsular cataract formation. Prolonged use may suppress the host response and thus increase the hazard of secondary ocular infections. In those diseases causing thinning of the cornea or sclera, perforations have been known to occur with the use of topical steroids. In acute purulent conditions of the eye, steroids may mask infection or enhance existing infection. If these products are used for 10 days or longer, intraocular pressure should be routinely monitored even though it may be difficult in children and uncooperative patients.
Employment of steroid medication in the treatment of herpes simplex requires great caution.
Neomycin sulfate may cause cutaneous sensitization. A precise incidence of hypersensitivity reactions (primarily skin rash) due to topical neomycin is not known.
Precautions: The initial prescription and renewal of the medication order beyond 8 grams should be made by a physician only after examination of the patient with the aid of magnification, such as slit lamp biomicroscopy and, where appropriate, fluorescein staining.
The possibility of persistent fungal infections of the cornea should be considered after prolonged steroid dosing.
Adverse Reactions: Adverse reactions have occurred with steroid/anti-infective combination drugs which can be attributed to the steroid component, the anti-infective component,

or the combination. Exact incidence figures are not available since no denominator of treated patients is available.
Reactions occurring most often from the presence of the anti-infective ingredient are allergic sensitizations. The reactions due to the steroid component in decreasing order of frequency are elevation of intraocular pressure (IOP) with possible development of glaucoma, and infrequent optic nerve damage, posterior subcapsular cataract formation; and delayed wound healing.
Secondary Infection: The development of secondary infection has occurred after use of combinations containing steroids and antimicrobials. Fungal infections of the cornea are particularly prone to develop coincidentally with long-term applications of steroid. The possibility of fungal invasion must be considered in any persistent corneal ulceration where steroid treatment has been used.
Secondary bacterial ocular infection following suppression of host responses also occurs.
Dosage and Administration: Apply the ointment in the affected eye every 3 or 4 hours, depending on the severity of the infection. In chronic conditions, withdrawal of treatment is carried out by decreasing the frequency of application, until the ointment is applied as infrequently as once a week.
Not more than 8 grams should be prescribed initially and the prescription should not be refilled without further evaluation as outlined in Precautions above.
How Supplied: Tube of ⅛ oz with ophthalmic tip (**NDC**-0081-0197-86). Store at 15°–30°C (59°–86°F).
DOD NSN 6505-01-102-4303

CORTISPORIN® OPHTHALMIC SUSPENSION Sterile ℞

(Polymyxin B-Neomycin-Hydrocortisone)

Description: Cortisporin® Ophthalmic Suspension (Polymyxin B-Neomycin-Hydrocortisone) is a sterile antimicrobial suspension for ophthalmic use. Each ml contains: Aerospórin® (Polymyxin B sulfate) 10,000 units, neomycin sulfate (equivalent to 3.5 mg neomycin base) 5 mg and hydrocortisone, 10 mg (1%). The vehicle contains the inactive ingredients cetyl alcohol, glyceryl monostearate, mineral oil, polyoxyl 40 stearate, propylene gylcol, water for injection, and thimerosal (preservative) 0.001%.
Polymyxin B Sulfate is the sulfate salt of polymyxin B_1 and B_2 which are produced by the growth of *Bacillus polymyxa* (Prazmowski) migula (Fam. Bacillaceae). It has a potency of not less than 6,000 Polymyxin B units per mg, calculated on an anhydrous basis.
Clinical Pharmacology: Corticoids suppress the inflammatory response to a variety of agents and they probably delay or slow healing. Since corticoids may inhibit the body's defense mechanism against infections, a concomitant antimicrobial drug may be used when this inhibition is considered to be clinically significant in a particular case.
The anti-infective component in the combination is included to provide action against specific organisms susceptible to it. Polymyxin B is considered active against the following microorganisms: gram-negative bacilli (excepting *Proteus*), including virtually all strains of *Pseudomonas aeruginosa* and *H. influenza* (Koch-Weeks bacillus). Neomycin B sulfate is considered active against the following microorganisms: many strains of gram-positive and gram-negative organisms, including many strains of *Proteus vulgaris* and *Staphylococcus aureus*, but not streptococci.
When a decision to administer both a corticoid and antimicrobials is made, the administration of such drugs in combination has the advantage of greater patient compliance and convenience, with the added assurance that the appropriate dosage of both drugs is administered, plus assured compatibility of ingredients when both types of drug are in the same formulation and, particularly, that the correct volume of drug is delivered and retained.
The relative potency of corticosteroids depends on the molecular structure, concentration, and release from the vehicle.
Indications and Usage: For steroid-responsive inflammatory ocular conditions for which a corticosteroid is indicated and where bacterial infection or a risk of bacterial ocular infection exists.
Ocular steroids are indicated in inflammatory conditions of the palpebral and bulbar conjunctiva, cornea and anterior segment of the globe where the inherent risk of steroid use in certain infective conjunctivitides is accepted to obtain a diminution in edema and inflammation. They are also indicated in chronic anterior uveitis and corneal injury from chemical, radiation, or thermal burns, or penetration of foreign bodies.
The use of a combination drug with an anti-infective component is indicated where the risk of infection is high or where there is an expectation that potentially dangerous numbers of bacteria will be present in the eye.
The particular anti-infective drugs in this product are active against the following common bacterial eye pathogens: *Staphylococcus aureus, Escherichia coli, Haemophilus influenzae, Klebsiella-Enterobacter* species, *Neisseria* species, and *Pseudommonas aeruginosa.*
The product does not provide adequate coverage against: *Serratia marcescens* and Streptococci, including *Streptococcus pneumoniae.*
Contraindications: Epithelial herpes simplex keratitis (dendritic keratitis), vaccinia, varicella, and many other viral diseases of the cornea and conjunctiva. Mycobacterial infection of the eye. Fungal diseases of ocular structures. Hypersensitivity to a component of the medication. (Hypersensitivity to the antibiotic component occurs at a higher rate than for other components.)
The use of these combinations is always contraindicated after uncomplicated removal of a corneal foreign body.
Warnings: Prolonged use may result in glaucoma, with damage to the optic nerve, defects in visual acuity and fields of vision, and posterior subcapsular cataract formation. Prolonged use may suppress the host response and thus increase the hazard of secondary ocular infections. In those diseases causing thinning of the cornea or sclera, perforations have been known to occur with the use of topical steroids. In acute purulent conditions of the eye, steroids may mask infection or enhance existing infection. If these products are used for 10 days or longer, intraocular pressure should be routinely monitored even though it may be difficult in children and uncooperative patients.
Employment of steroid medication in the treatment of herpes simplex requires great caution.
Neomycin sulfate may cause cutaneous sensitization. A precise incidence of hypersensitivity reactions (primarily skin rash) due to topical neomycin is not known.
Precautions: The initial prescription and renewal of the medication order beyond 20 milliliters should be made by a physician only after examination of the patient with the aid of magnification, such as slit lamp biomicroscopy and, where appropriate, fluorescein staining.
The possibility of persistent fungal infections of the cornea should be considered after prolonged steroid dosing.
Adverse Reactions: Adverse reactions have occurred with steroid/anti-infective combination drugs which can be attributed to the steroid component, the anti-infective component, or the combination. Exact incidence figures are not available since no denominator of treated patients is available.
Reactions occurring most often from the presence of the anti-infective ingredient are allergic sensitizations. The reactions due to the steroid component in decreasing order of frequency are: elevation of intraocular pressure (IOP) with possible development of glaucoma, and infrequent optic nerve damage; posterior subcapsular cataract formation; and delayed wound healing.
Secondary Infection: The development of secondary infection has occurred after use of combinations containing steroids and antimicrobials. Fungal infections of the cornea are particularly prone to develop coincidentally with long-term applications of steroid. The possibility of fungal invasion must be considered in any persistent corneal ulceration where steroid treatment has been used.
Secondary bacterial ocular infection following suppression of host responses also occurs.
Dosage and Administration: One or two drops in the affected eye every three or four hours, depending on the severity of the condition. The suspension may be used more frequently if necessary. The patient should be instructed to avoid contaminating the dropper with material from the eye, fingers, or other sources. This caution is necessary if the sterility of the suspension is to be preserved.
SHAKE WELL BEFORE USING.
Not more than 20 milliliters should be prescribed initially and the prescription should not be refilled without further evaluation as outlined in Precautions above.
How Supplied: Bottle of 5 ml with Sterile Dropper (NDC-0081-0193-84). Store at 15°–25°C (59°–77°F).
DOD NSN 6505-00-764-9042

CORTISPORIN® OTIC SOLUTION Sterile ℞

Polymyxin B-Neomycin-Hydrocortisone

Description: Each cc contains:
Aerosporin® brand Polymyxin B Sulfate ....10,000 Units
Neomycin sulfate ....5 mg
(equivalent to 3.5 mg neomycin base)
Hydrocortisone ....10 mg (1%)
The vehicle contains the inactive ingredients cupric sulfate, glycerin, hydrochloric acid, propylene glycol, water for injection and potassium metabisulfite (preservative) 0.1%.
Action: Hydrocortisone, the naturally occurring adrenal corticosteroid, affords antiallergic, antipruritic and anti-inflammatory activity.
Polymyxin B is one of a group of closely related substances produced by various strains of *Bacillus polymyxa.* Its activity is sharply restricted to gram-negative bacteria, including many strains of *Pseudomonas aeruginosa.*
Neomycin, isolated from *Streptomyces fradiae,* has antibacterial activity *in vitro* against a wide range of gram-negative and gram-positive organisms, with effectiveness against many strains of *Proteus.*
Indications: For the treatment of superficial bacterial infections of the external auditory canal caused by organisms susceptible to the action of the antibiotics.
Contraindications: This product is contraindicated in those individuals who have shown hypersensitivity to any of its components, and in herpes simplex, vaccinia and varicella.
Warnings: As with other antibiotic preparations, prolonged treatment may result in overgrowth of nonsusceptible organisms and fungi. If the infection is not improved after one week, cultures and susceptibility tests should be repeated to verify the identity of the organism and to determine whether therapy should be changed.
When using neomycin-containing products to control secondary infection in the chronic dermatoses, such as chronic otitis externa, it should be borne in mind that the skin in these conditions is more liable than is normal skin to

Continued on next page

Burroughs Wellcome—Cont.

become sensitized to many substances, including neomycin. The manifestation of sensitization to neomycin is usually a low grade reddening with swelling, dry scaling and itching; it may be manifest simply as a failure to heal. During long-term use of neomycin-containing products, periodic examination for such signs is advisable and the patient should be told to discontinue the product if they are observed. These symptoms regress quickly on withdrawing the medication. Neomycin-containing applications should be avoided for that patient thereafter.

Precautions: If sensitization or irritation occurs, medication should be discontinued promptly.

This drug should be used with care when the integrity of the tympanic membrane is in question because of the possibility of ototoxicity caused by neomycin.

Patients who prefer to warm the medication before using should be cautioned against heating the solution above body temperature, in order to avoid loss of potency.

Treatment should not be continued for longer than ten days.

Allergic cross-reactions may occur which could prevent the use of any or all of the following antibiotics for the treatment of future infections: kanamycin, paromomycin, streptomycin, and possibly gentamicin.

Adverse Reactions: Neomycin is a not uncommon cutaneous sensitizer. There are articles in the current literature that indicate an increase in the prevalence of persons sensitive to neomycin.

Stinging and burning have been reported when this drug has gained access to the middle ear.

Dosage and Administration: The external auditory canal should be thoroughly cleansed and dried with a sterile cotton applicator.

For adults, 4 drops of the solution should be instilled into the affected ear 3 or 4 times daily. For infants and children, 3 drops are suggested because of the smaller capacity of the ear canal.

The patient should lie with the affected ear upward and then the drops should be instilled. This position should be maintained for 5 minutes to facilitate penetration of the drops into the ear canal. Repeat, if necessary, for the opposite ear.

If preferred, a cotton wick may be inserted into the canal and then the cotton may be saturated with the solution. This wick should be kept moist by adding further solution every four hours. The wick should be replaced at least once every 24 hours.

The patient should be instructed to avoid contaminating the dropper with material from the ear, fingers, or other source. This caution is necessary if the sterility of the drops is to be preserved.

How Supplied: Bottle of 10 cc with sterile dropper.

10 cc—DoD **NSN 6505-01-014-1378**
10 cc—VA **NSN 6505-01-023-4751**

CORTISPORIN® OTIC SUSPENSION ℞
Sterile
Polymyxin B-Neomycin-Hydrocortisone

Description: Each cc contains: Aerosporin® brand Polymyxin B Sulfate 10,000 units; neomycin sulfate 5 mg (equivalent to 3.5 mg neomycin base); hydrocortisone 10 mg (1%).

The vehicle contains the inactive ingredients cetyl alcohol, propylene glycol, polysorbate 80, water for injection and thimerosal (preservative) 0.01%.

Action: Hydrocortisone, the naturally occurring adrenal corticosteroid, affords antiallergic, antipruritic and anti-inflammatory activity.

Polymyxin B is one of a group of closely related substances produced by various strains of *Bacillus polymyxa.* Its activity is sharply restricted to gram-negative bacteria, including many strains of *Pseudomonas aeruginosa.*

Neomycin, isolated from *Streptomyces fradiae,* has antibacterial activity *in vitro* against a wide range of gram-negative and gram-positive organisms, with effectiveness against many strains of *Proteus.*

Indications: For the treatment of superficial bacterial infections of the external auditory canal caused by organisms susceptible to the action of the antibiotics, and for the treatment of infections of mastoidectomy and fenestration cavities caused by organisms susceptible to the antibiotics.

Contraindications: This product is contraindicated in those individuals who have shown hypersensitivity to any of its components, and in herpes simplex, vaccinia and varicella.

Warnings: As with other antibiotic preparations, prolonged treatment may result in overgrowth of nonsusceptible organisms and fungi. If the infection is not improved after one week, cultures and susceptibility tests should be repeated to verify the identity of the organism and to determine whether therapy should be changed.

When using neomycin-containing products to control secondary infection in the chronic dermatoses, such as chronic otitis externa, it should be borne in mind that the skin in these conditions is more liable than is normal skin to become sensitized to many substances, including neomycin. The manifestation of sensitization to neomycin is usually a low grade reddening with swelling, dry scaling and itching; it may be manifest simply as a failure to heal. During long-term use of neomycin-containing products, periodic examination for such signs is advisable and the patient should be told to discontinue the product if they are observed. These symptoms regress quickly on withdrawing the medication. Neomycin-containing applications should be avoided for that patient thereafter.

Precautions: If sensitization or irritation occurs, medication should be discontinued promptly.

This drug should be used with care in cases of perforated eardrum and in longstanding cases of chronic otitis media because of the possibility of ototoxicity caused by neomycin.

Patients who prefer to warm the medication before using should be cautioned against heating the solution above body temperature, in order to avoid loss of potency.

Treatment should not be continued for longer than ten days.

Allergic cross-reactions may occur which could prevent the use of any or all of the following antibiotics for the treatment of future infections: kanamycin, paromomycin, streptomycin, and possibly gentamicin.

Adverse Reactions: Neomycin is a not uncommon cutaneous sensitizer. There are articles in the current literature that indicate an increase in the prevalence of persons sensitive to neomycin.

Dosage and Administration: The external auditory canal should be thoroughly cleansed and dried with a sterile cotton applicator.

For adults, 4 drops of the suspension should be instilled into the affected ear 3 or 4 times daily. For infants and children, 3 drops are suggested because of the smaller capacity of the ear canal.

The patient should lie with the affected ear upward and then the drops should be instilled. This position should be maintained for 5 minutes to facilitate penetration of the drops into the ear canal. Repeat, if necessary, for the opposite ear.

If preferred, a cotton wick may be inserted into the canal and then the cotton may be saturated with the suspension. This wick should be kept moist by adding further suspension every four hours. The wick should be replaced at least once every 24 hours.

The patient should be instructed to avoid contaminating the dropper with material from the ear, fingers, or other source. This caution is necessary if the sterility of the drops is to be preserved. SHAKE WELL BEFORE USING.

How Supplied: Bottle of 10 cc with sterile dropper.

10cc DoD **NSN 6505-01-043-0230**
10cc VA **NSN 6505-00-932-3247**

DARAPRIM® ℞
brand Pyrimethamine

Description: Each scored tablet contains 25 mg Daraprim brand Pyrimethamine (2, 4- diamino-5-p-chlorophenyl-6-ethylpyrimidine).

Actions and Benefits: Daraprim is a folic acid antagonist, and the rationale for its therapeutic action is based on the differential requirement between host and parasite for nucleic acid precursors involved in growth. This activity is highly selective against plasmodia and *Toxoplasma gondii.* Daraprim does not destroy gametocytes, but arrests sporogony in the mosquito.

Indications: Daraprim brand Pyrimethamine is indicated for the chemoprophylaxis of malaria due to susceptible strains of plasmodia. Fast-acting schizonticides (chloroquine, amodiaquin, quinacrine or quinine) are indicated and preferable for the treatment of acute attacks. However, conjoint use of Daraprim will initiate *transmission control* and *suppressive cure.*

Daraprim is also indicated for the treatment of toxoplasmosis. For this purpose the drug should be used conjointly with a sulfonamide since synergism exists with this combination.

Warnings: The dosage of pyrimethamine required for the treatment of toxoplasmosis is 10 to 20 times the recommended antimalarial dosage and approaches the toxic level. If signs of folic or folinic acid deficiency develop (see Adverse Reactions) reduce the dosage or discontinue the drug according to the response of the patient. Folinic acid (leucovorin) may be administered in a dosage of 3 to 9 mg intramuscularly daily for 3 days, or as required to produce a return of depressed platelet or white blood cell counts to safe levels.

Patients should be warned to keep Daraprim out of the reach of children since accidental ingestion has led to fatality.

Use in Pregnancy: Pyrimethamine, like other folic acid antagonists, may, in large doses, produce teratogenic effects in laboratory animals. The large doses required to treat toxoplasmosis should be used only after a definitive diagnosis of acute toxoplasmosis has been made, and the possibility of teratogenic effects from the drug has been carefully weighed against the possible risks of permanent damage to the fetus from the infection.

Concurrent administration of folinic acid is recommended when pyrimethamine is used for treatment of toxoplasmosis during pregnancy.

Precautions: The recommended dosage for malaria suppression should not be exceeded. In patients receiving high dosage, as for the treatment of toxoplasmosis, semi-weekly blood counts, including platelet counts, should be made. In patients with convulsive disorders a small "starting" dose (for toxoplasmosis) is recommended to avoid the potential nervous system toxicity of pyrimethamine.

Adverse Reactions: With large doses, anorexia and vomiting may occur. Vomiting may be minimized by giving the medication with meals; it usually disappears promptly upon reduction of dosage. Also, large doses as used in toxoplasmosis may produce megaloblastic anemia, leukopenia, thrombocytopenia, pancytopenia and atrophic glossitis. Acute intoxication may follow the ingestion of an excessive amount of pyrimethamine; this may involve central nervous system stimulation including convulsions. In such cases a parenteral barbiturate may be indicated followed by folinic acid (leucovorin).

Dosage and Administration:

For Chemoprophylaxis of Malaria: Adults and children over 10 years—25 mg (1 tablet) once weekly.

Children 4 through 10 years—12.5 mg (½ tablet) once weekly.

Infants and children under 4 years—6.25 mg (¼ tablet) once weekly.

Regimens planned to include *suppressive cure* should be extended through any characteristic periods of early recrudescence and late relapse for at least 10 weeks in each case.

For Treatment of Acute Attacks: Daraprim is recommended in areas where only susceptible plasmodia exist. The drug is not recommended alone in the treatment of acute attacks of malaria in non-immune persons. Fast-acting schizonticides (chloroquine, amodiaquin, quinacrine or quinine) are indicated for treatment of acute attacks. However, conjoint Daraprim dosage of 25 mg daily for two days will initiate *transmission control* and *suppressive cure.* Should circumstances arise wherein Daraprim must be used alone in semi-immune persons, the adult dosage for an acute attack is 50 mg daily for 2 days; children 4 through 10 years old may be given 25 mg daily for 2 days. In any event, clinical cure should be followed by the once-weekly regimen described above.

For Toxoplasmosis: The dosage of Daraprim brand Pyrimethamine in the treatment of toxoplasmosis must be carefully adjusted so as to provide maximum therapeutic effect and a minimum of side effects. At the high dosage required, there is a marked variation in the tolerance to the drug. Young patients may tolerate higher doses than older individuals.

The adult *starting* dose is 50 to 75 mg of the drug daily, together with 1 to 4 g daily of a sulfonamide drug of the sulfapyrimidine type, e.g., sulfadiazine, triple-sulfa. This dosage is ordinarily continued for 1 to 3 weeks, depending on the response of the patient and his tolerance of the therapy. The dosage may then be reduced to about one-half that previously given for each drug and continued for an additional 4 or 5 weeks.

The pediatric dosage of Daraprim is 1 mg/kg per day divided into 2 equal daily doses; after 2 to 4 days this dose may be reduced to one-half and continued for approximately one month. The usual pediatric sulfonamide dosage is used in conjunction with Daraprim.

Supplied: Tablets, scored, 25 mg, bottles of 100. Tablets bear identification, A3A.

100—DoD NSN 6505-00-926-4765

[*Shown in Product Identification Section*]

EMPIRIN
ASPIRIN TABLETS
ASPIRIN—325 mg (5 grs)

(See PDR for Nonprescription Drugs)

EMPIRIN® with Codeine Tablets ℞ Ⓒ

Description: Empirin with Codeine is supplied in tablet form for oral administration. Each tablet contains aspirin (acetylsalicylic acid) 325 mg plus codeine phosphate in one of the following strengths: No. 2–15 mg, No. 3–30 mg, and No. 4–60 mg. (Warning—may be habit-forming.)

Empirin with Codeine has analgesic, antipyretic and anti-inflammatory effects.

Clinical Pharmacology:

Aspirin: The analgesic, anti-inflammatory and antipyretic effects of aspirin are believed to result from inhibition of the synthesis of certain prostaglandins. Aspirin interferes with clotting mechanisms primarily by diminishing platelet aggregation; at high doses prothrombin synthesis can be inhibited.

Aspirin in solution is rapidly absorbed from the stomach and from the upper small intestine. About 50 percent of an oral dose is absorbed in 30 minutes and peak plasma concentrations are reached in about 40 minutes. Higher than normal stomach pH or the presence of food slightly delays absorption.

Once absorbed, aspirin is mainly hydrolyzed to salicylic acid and distributed to all body tissues and fluids, including fetal tissue, breast milk and the central nervous system (CNS). Highest concentrations are found in plasma, liver, renal cortex, heart and lung.

From 50 to 80 percent of the salicylic acid and its metabolites in plasma are loosely bound to proteins. The plasma half-life of total salicylate is about 3.0 hours, with a 650 mg dose. Higher doses of aspirin cause increases in plasma salicylate half-life. Metabolism occurs primarily in the hepatocytes. The major metabolites are salicyluric acid (75%), the phenolic and acyl glucuronides of salicylate (15%), and gentisic and gentisuric acid (<1%).

Almost all of a therapeutic dose of aspirin is excreted through the kidneys, either as salicylic acid or the above mentioned metabolic products. Renal clearance of salicylates is greatly augmented by an alkaline urine, as is produced by concurrent administration of sodium bicarbonate or potassium citrate.

Toxic salicylate blood levels are usually above 30 mg/100 ml. The single lethal dose of aspirin in normal adults is approximately 25–30 g, but patients have recovered from much larger doses with appropriate treatment.

Codeine: Codeine probably exerts its analgesic effect through actions on opiate receptors in the CNS.

Codeine is readily absorbed from the gastrointestinal tract, and a therapeutic dose reaches peak analgesic effectiveness in about 2 hours and persists for 4 to 6 hours. Oral codeine (60 mg) given to healthy males has been shown to achieve peak blood levels of 0.016 mg/100 ml at approximately one hour post-dose. The codeine plasma half-life for a 60 mg oral dose is about 2.9 hours. Blood levels causing CNS depression begin at 0.05–0.19 mg/100 ml. The single lethal dose of codeine in adults is estimated to be approximately 0.5–1.0 g.

Codeine is rapidly distributed from blood to body tissues and taken up preferentially by parenchymatous organs such as liver, spleen and kidney. It passes the blood-brain barrier and is found in fetal tissue and breast milk. The drug is not bound by plasma proteins nor is it accumulated in body tissues. Codeine is metabolized in liver to morphine and norcodeine, each representing about 10 percent of the administered dose of codeine. About 90 percent of the dose is excreted within 24 hours, primarily through the kidneys. Urinary excretion products are free and glucuronide-conjugated codeine (about 70%), free and conjugated norcodeine (about 10%), free and conjugated morphine (about 10%), normorphine (under 4%) and hydrocodone (<1%). The remainder of the dose appears in the feces.

Indications and Usage: Empirin® with Codeine is indicated for the relief of mild, moderate, and moderate to severe pain.

Contraindications: Emprin with Codeine is contraindicated under the following conditions:

(1) hypersensitivity or intolerance to aspirin or codeine,
(2) severe bleeding, disorders of coagulation or primary hemostasis, including hemophilia, hypoprothrombinemia, von Willebrand's disease, the thrombocytopenias, thrombasthenia and other ill-defined hereditary platelet dysfunctions, and well as such associated conditions as severe vitamin K deficiency and severe liver damage,
(3) anticoagulant therapy, and
(4) peptic ulcer, or other serious gastrointestinal lesions.

Warnings: Therapeutic doses of aspirin can cause analphylactic shock and other severe allergic reactions. A history of allergy is often lacking.

Significant bleeding can result from aspirin therapy in patients with peptic ulcer or other gastrointestinal lesions, and in patients with bleeding disorders. Aspirin administered preoperatively may prolong the bleeding time.

In the presence of head injury or other intracranial lesions, the respiratory depressant effects of codeine and other narcotics may be markedly enhanced, as well as their capacity for elevating cerebrospinal fluid pressure. Narcotics also produce other CNS depressant effects, such as drowsiness, that may further obscure the clinical course of patients with head injuries.

Codeine or other narcotics may obscure signs on which to judge the diagnosis or clinical course of patients with acute abdominal conditions.

Precautions:

General: Empirin® with Codeine should be prescribed with caution for certain special-risk patients such as the elderly or debilitated, and those with severe impairment of renal or hepatic function, gallbladder disease or gallstones, respiratory impairment, cardiac arrhythmias, inflammatory disorders of the gastrointestinal tract, hypothyroidism, Addison's disease, prostatic hypertrophy or urethral stricture, coagulation disorders, head injuries, or acute abdominal conditions. Empirin® with Codeine should not be prescribed for long-term therapy unless specifically indicated.

Precautions should be taken when administering salicylates to persons with known allergies. Hypersensitivity to aspirin is particularly likely in patients with nasal polyps, and relatively common in those with asthma.

Information for Patients: Empirin with Codeine may impair the mental and/or physical abilities required for the performance of potentially hazardous tasks such as driving a car or operating machinery. Such tasks should be avoided while taking Empirin with Codeine.

Alcohol and other CNS depressants may produce an additive CNS depression when taken with Empirin with Codeine, and should be avoided.

Codeine may be habit-forming when used over long periods or in high doses. Patients should take the drug only for as long as it is prescribed, in the amounts prescribed, and no more frequently than prescribed.

Laboratory Tests: Hypersensitivity to aspirin cannot be detected by skin testing or radioimmunoassay procedures.

The primary screening tests for detecting a bleeding tendency are platelet count, bleeding time, activated partial thromboplastin time and prothrombin time.

In patients with severe hepatic or renal disease, effects of therapy should be monitored with serial liver and/or renal function tests.

Drug Interactions: Empirin® with Codeine may *enhance* the effects of:

(1) monoamine oxidase (MAO) inhibitors,
(2) oral anticoagulants, causing bleeding by inhibiting prothrombin formation in the liver and displacing anticoagulants from plasma protein binding sites,
(3) oral antidiabetic agents and insulin, causing hypoglycemia by contributing an additive effect, and by displacing the oral antidiabetic agents from secondary binding sites,
(4) 6-mercaptopurine and methotrexate, causing bone marrow toxicity and blood dyscrasias by displacing these drugs from secondary binding sites,
(5) penicillins and sulfonamides, increasing their blood levels by displacing these drugs from protein binding sites,

Continued on next page

Burroughs Wellcome—Cont.

(6) non-steroidal anti-inflammatory agents, increasing the risk of peptic ulceration and bleeding by contributing additive effects.
(7) other narcotic analgesics, alcohol, general anesthetics, tranquilizers such as chlordiazepoxide, sedative-hypnotics, or other CNS depressants, causing increased CNS depression,
(8) corticosteroids, potentiating steroid anti-inflammatory effects by displacing steroids from protein binding sites. Aspirin intoxication may occur with corticosteroid withdrawal because steroids promote renal clearance of salicylates.

Empirin® with Codeine may *diminish* the effects of:
(1) uricosuric agents such as probenecid and sulfinpyrazone, reducing their effectiveness in the treatment of gout. Aspirin competes with these agents for protein binding sites.

Aspirin and its metabolites may be caused to accumulate in the body, perhaps to toxic levels, by para-aminosalicylic acid, furosemide, and vitamin C.

Drug/Laboratory Test Interactions:
Aspirin: Aspirin may interfere with the following laboratory determinations in blood: serum amylase, fasting blood glucose, carbon dioxide, cholesterol, protein, protein bound iodine, uric acid, prothrombin time, bleeding time, and spectrophotometric detection of barbiturates. Aspirin may interfere with the following laboratory determinations in urine: glucose, 5-hydroxyindoleacetic acid, Gerhardt ketone, vanillylmandelic acid (VMA), protein, uric acid, and diacetic acid.
Codeine: Codeine may increase serum amylase levels.
Carcinogenesis, Mutagenesis, Impairment of Fertility: No adequate long-term studies have been conducted in animals to determine whether codeine has a potential for carcinogenesis, mutagenesis, or impairment of fertility.
Adequate long-term studies have been conducted in mice and rats with aspirin, alone or in combination with other drugs, in which no evidence of carcinogenesis was seen. No adequate studies have been conducted in animals to determine whether aspirin has a potential for mutagenesis or impairment of fertility.
Pregnancy: **Teratogenic Effects:** Pregnancy Category C. Animal reproduction studies have not been conducted with Empirin® with Codeine. It is also not known whether Empirin with Codeine can cause fetal harm when administered to a pregnant woman or can affect reproduction capacity. Empirin with Codeine should be given to a pregnant woman only if clearly needed.
Reproductive studies in rats and mice have shown aspirin to be teratogenic and embryocidal at four to six times the human therapeutic dose. Studies in pregnant women, however, have not shown that aspirin increases the risk of abnormalities when administered during the first trimester of pregnancy. In controlled studies involving 41,337 pregnant women and their offspring, there was no evidence that aspirin taken during pregnancy caused stillbirth, neonatal death or reduced birthweight. In controlled studies of 50,282 pregnant women and their offspring, aspirin administration in moderate and heavy doses during the first four lunar months of pregnancy showed no teratogenic effect.
Reproduction studies have been performed in rabbits and rats at doses up to 150 times the human dose and have revealed no evidence of impaired fertility or harm to the fetus due to codeine.
Nonteratogenic Effects: Therapeutic doses of aspirin in pregnant women close to term may cause bleeding in mother, fetus, or neonate. During the last six months of pregnancy, regular use of aspirin in high doses may prolong pregnancy and delivery.
Labor and Delivery: Ingestion of aspirin prior to delivery may prolong delivery or lead to bleeding in the mother or neonate. Use of codeine during labor may lead to respiratory depression in the neonate.
Nursing Mothers: Aspirin and codeine are excreted in breast milk in small amounts, but the significance of their effects on nursing infants is not known. Because of the potential for serious adverse reactions in nursing infants from Empirin® with Codeine, a decision should be made whether to discontinue nursing or to discontinue the drug, taking into account the importance of the drug to the mother.

Adverse Reactions:
Codeine: The most frequently observed adverse reactions to codeine include light-headedness, dizziness, drowsiness, nausea, vomiting, constipation and depression of respiration. Less common reactions to codeine include euphoria, dysphoria, pruritis and skin rashes.
Aspirin: Mild aspirin intoxication (salicylism) can occur in response to chronic use of large doses. Manifestations include nausea, vomiting, hearing impairment, tinnitus, diminished vision, headache, dizziness, drowsiness, mental confusion, hyperpnea, hyperventilation, tachycardia, sweating and thirst.
Therapeutic doses of aspirin can induce mild or severe allergic reactions manifested by skin rashes, urticaria, angioedema, rhinorrhea, asthma, abdominal pain, nausea, vomiting, or anaphylactic shock. A history of allergy is often lacking, and allergic reactions may occur even in patients who have previously taken aspirin without any ill effects. Allergic reactions to aspirin are most likely to occur in patients with a history of allergic disease, especially in patients with nasal polyps or asthma. Some patients are unable to take aspirin or other salicylates without developing nausea or vomiting. Occasional patients respond to aspirin (usually in large doses) with dyspepsia or heartburn, which may be accompanied by occult bleeding. Excessive bruising or bleeding is sometimes seen in patients with mild disorders of primary hemostasis who regularly use low doses of aspirin.
Prolonged use of aspirin can cause painless erosion of gastric mucosa, occult bleeding and, infrequently, iron-deficiency anemia. High doses of aspirin can exacerbate symptoms of peptic ulcer and, occasionally, cause extensive bleeding.
Excessive bleeding can follow injury or surgery in patients with or without known bleeding disorders who have taken therapeutic doses of aspirin within the preceding 10 days.
Hepatotoxicity has been reported in association with prolonged use of large doses of aspirin in patients with lupus erythematosus, rheumatoid arthritis and rheumatic disease.
Bone marrow depression, manifested by weakness, fatigue, or abnormal bruising or bleeding, has occasionally been reported.
In patients with glucose-6-phosphate dehydrogenase deficiency, aspirin can cause a mild degree of hemolytic anemia.
In hyperuricemic persons, low doses of aspirin may reduce the effectiveness of uricosuric therapy or precipitate an attack of gout.
Drug Abuse and Dependence: Like other medications containing a narcotic analgesic, Empirin® with Codeine is controlled by the Drug Enforcement Administration and is classified under Schedule III.
Empirin with Codeine can produce drug dependence of the morphine type; therefore, it has a potential for being abused. Psychic dependence, physical dependence and tolerance may develop on repeated administration.
The dependence liability of codeine has been found to be too small to permit a full definition of its characteristics. Studies indicate that addiction to codeine is extremely uncommon and requires very high parenteral doses.
When dependence on codeine occurs at therapeutic doses, it appears to require from one to two months to develop, and withdrawal symptoms are mild. Most patients on long-term oral codeine therapy show no signs of physical dependence upon abrupt withdrawal.
Overdosage: Severe intoxication, caused by overdose of Empirin® with Codeine may produce: skin eruptions, dyspnea, vertigo, double vision, delusions, hallucinations, garbled speech, excitability, restlessness, delirium, constricted pupils, a positive Babinski sign, respiratory depression (slow and shallow breathing; Cheyne-Stokes respiration), cyanosis, clammy skin, muscle flaccidity, circulatory collapse, stupor and coma. In children, difficulty in hearing, tinnitus, dim vision, headache, dizziness, drowsiness, confusion, rapid breathing, sweating, thirst, nausea, vomiting, hyperpyrexia, dehydration and convulsions are prominent signs. The most severe manifestations from aspirin result from cardiovascular and respiratory insufficiency secondary to acid-base and electrolyte disturbances, complicated by hyperthermia and dehydration. The most severe manifestations from codeine are associated with respiratory depression.
Respiratory alkalosis is characteristic of the early phase of intoxication with aspirin while hyperventilation is occurring, but is quickly followed by metabolic acidosis in most people with severe intoxication. This occurs more readily in children. Hypoglycemia may occur in children who have taken large overdoses. Other laboratory findings associated with aspirin intoxication include ketonuria, hyponatremia, hypokalemia, and occasionally proteinuria. A slight rise in lactic dehydrogenase and hydroxybutyric dehydrogenase may occur.
Concentrations of aspirin in plasma above 30 mg/100 ml are associated with toxicity. (See Clinical Pharmacology Section for information on factors influencing aspirin blood levels.) The single lethal dose of aspirin in adults is probably about 25–30 g, but is not known with certainty.
The toxic plasma concentration of codeine is not known with certainty. Experimental production of mild to moderate CNS depression in healthy, nontolerant subjects occurred at plasma concentrations of 0.05–0.19 mg/100 ml when codeine was given by intravenous infusion. The single lethal dose of codeine in adults is estimated to be from 0.5–1.0 g. It is also estimated that 5 mg/kg could be fatal in children.
Hemodialysis and peritoneal dialysis can be performed to reduce the body aspirin content. Codeine is theoretically dialyzable but the procedure has not been clinically established.
Treatment of overdosage consists primarily of support of vital functions, management of codeine-induced respiratory depression, increasing salicylate elimination, and correcting the acid-base imbalance due primarily to salicylism.
In a comatose patient, primary attention should be given to establishment of adequate respiratory exchange through provisions of a patent airway and the institution of assisted or controlled ventilation. The narcotic antagonist naloxone is a specific antidote for respiratory depression which may result from overdose or unusual sensitivity to narcotics. Therefore, an appropriate dose of an antagonist should be administered, preferably by the intravenous route, simultaneously with efforts at respiratory resuscitation. Since the duration of action of Empirin® with Codeine may exceed that of the antagonist, the patient should be kept under continued surveillance and repeated doses of the antagonist should be administered as needed to maintain adequate respiration.
A narcotic antagonist should not be administered in the absence of clinically significant respiratory or cardiovascular depression.

Gastric emptying (Syrup of Ipecac) and/or lavage is recommended as soon as possible after ingestion, even if the patient has vomited spontaneously. (Apomorphine should not be used as an emetic for Empirin® with Codeine, since it may potentiate hypotension and respiratory depression.) Administration of activated charcoal as a slurry is beneficial after lavage and/or emesis, if less than three hours have passed since ingestion. Charcoal adsorption should *not* be employed prior to emesis or lavage.
Severity of aspirin intoxication is determined by measuring the blood salicylate level. Acid-base status should be closely followed with serial blood gas and serum pH measurements. Fluid and electrolyte balance should also be regularly monitored.
A serum salicylate level of 30 mg/100 ml or higher indicates a need for enhanced salicylate excretion that can be achieved through body-fluid supplementation and urine alkalinization if renal function is normal. In mild intoxication, urine flow can be increased by forcing oral fluids and giving potassium citrate capsules. (DO NOT GIVE BICARBONATE BY MOUTH SINCE IT INCREASES THE RATE OF SALICYLATE ABSORPTION.)
In severe cases, hyperthermia and hypovolemia, as well as respiratory depression are the major immediate threats to life. Children should be sponged with tepid water. Replacement fluid should be administered intravenously and augmented with sufficient bicarbonate to correct acidosis, with monitoring of plasma electrolytes and pH, to promote alkaline diuresis of salicylate if renal function is normal. Complete control may also require infusion of glucose to control hypoglycemia.
Potassium deficiency may also be corrected through the infusion, once adequate urinary output is assured. Plasma or plasma expanders may be needed if fluid replacement is insufficient to maintain normal blood pressure or adequate urinary output.
In patients with renal insufficiency or in cases of life-threatening intoxication, dialysis is usually required. Peritoneal dialysis or exchange transfusion is indicated in infants and young children, and hemodialysis in older patients.
Oxygen, intravenous fluids, vasopressors and other supportive measures should be employed as needed.

Dosage and Administration: Dosage is adjusted according to the severity of pain and the response of the patient. It may occasionally be necessary to exceed the usual dosage recommended below when pain is severe or the patient has become tolerant to the analgesic effect of codeine. Empirin® with Codeine is given orally. The usual adult dose for Empirin with Codeine No. 2 and No. 3 is one or two tablets every four hours as required. The usual adult dose for Empirin with Codeine No. 4 is one tablet every four hours as required.
Empirin® with Codeine should be taken with food or a full glass of milk or water to lessen gastric irritation.

How Supplied:
Empirin with Codeine 15 mg No. 2: (white tablet imprinted with "EMPIRIN" and "2")

Bottle of 100	NDC 0081-0215-55
Bottle of 1000	NDC 0081-0215-75
Dispenserpak® of 25	NDC 0081-0215-25

Empirin with Codeine 30 mg No. 3: (white tablet imprinted with "EMPIRIN" and "3")

Bottle of 100	NDC 0081-0220-55
Bottle of 500	NDC 0081-0220-70
Bottle of 1000	NDC 0081-0220-75
Dispenserpak® of 25	NDC 0081-0220-25

Empirin with Codeine 60 mg No. 4: (white tablet imprinted with "EMPIRIN" and "4")

Bottle of 100	NDC 0081-0225-55
Bottle of 500	NDC 0081-0225-70
Bottle of 1000	NDC 0081-0225-75
Dispenserpak® of 25	NDC 0081-0225-25

Store at 15°–30°C (59°–86°F) in a dry place and protect from light.
[Shown in Product Identification Section]

EMPRACET® with Codeine Phosphate ℞ Ⓒ 30 mg, No. 3; 60 mg, No. 4

Description: Each Empracet with Codeine Phosphate tablet contains codeine phosphate* 30 mg in No. 3 and 60 mg in No. 4 (**WARNING:** May be habit-forming) and acetaminophen 300 mg.
Acetaminophen occurs as a white, odorless crystalline powder, possessing a slightly bitter taste. Codeine is an alkaloid, obtained from opium or prepared from morphine by methylation. Codeine occurs as colorless or white crystals, effloresces slowly in dry air and is affected by light.

Actions: Acetaminophen is a nonopiate, non-salicylate analgesic and antipyretic. Codeine is an opiate analgesic and antitussive. Codeine retains at least one-half of its analgesic activity when administered orally.

Indications: No. 3—for relief of mild to moderate pain; No. 4—for the relief of moderate to moderately severe pain.

Contraindications: Hypersensitivity to acetaminophen or codeine.

Warnings:

Drug Dependence: Codeine can produce drug dependence of the morphine type, and therefore has the potential for being abused. Psychic dependence, physical dependence and tolerance may develop upon repeated administration of this drug and it should be prescribed and administered with the same degree of caution appropriate to the use of other oral narcotic medications. This acetaminophen and codeine dosage form is subject to the Federal Controlled Substances Act (Schedule III).

Precautions:

General:

Head injury and increased intracranial pressure: The respiratory depressant effects of narcotics and their capacity to elevate cerebrospinal fluid pressure may be markedly exaggerated in the presence of head injury, other intracranial lesions or a pre-existing increase in intracranial pressure. Furthermore, narcotics, produce adverse reactions which may obscure the clinical course of patients with head injuries.

Acute abdominal conditions: The administration of products containing codeine or other narcotics may obscure the diagnosis or clinical course in patients with acute abdominal conditions.

Special risk patients: Acetaminophen with codeine should be given with caution to certain patients, such as the elderly or debilitated, and those with severe impairment of hepatic or renal function, hypothyroidism, Addison's disease, and prostatic hypertrophy or urethral stricture.

Information for Patients: Codeine may impair the mental and/or physical abilities required for the performance of potentially hazardous tasks such as driving a car or operating machinery. The patient taking this drug should be cautioned accordingly.

Drug Interactions: Patients receiving other narcotic analgesics, antipsychotics, antianxiety, or other CNS depressants (including alcohol) concomitantly with acetaminophen and codeine may exhibit additive CNS depression due to the codeine component. When such therapy is contemplated, the dose of one or both agents should be reduced.
The use of MAO inhibitors or tricyclic antidepressants with codeine preparations may increase the effect of either the antidepressant or codeine.
The concurrent use of anticholinergics with codeine may produce paralytic ileus.

Usage in Pregnancy: Safe use in pregnancy has not been established relative to possible adverse effects on fetal development. Therefore, acetaminophen and codeine should not be used in pregnant women unless, in the judgment of the physician, the potential benefits outweigh the possible hazards.

Nursing Mothers: It is not known whether the components of this drug are excreted in human milk. Because many drugs are excreted in human milk, caution should be exercised when acetaminophen and codeine is administered to a nursing woman.

Adverse Reactions: The most frequently observed adverse reactions include light-headedness, dizziness, sedation, shortness of breath, nausea and vomiting. These effects seem to be more prominent in ambulatory than in non-ambulatory patients, and some of these adverse reactions may be alleviated if the patient lies down.
Other adverse reactions include euphoria, dysphoria, constipation and pruritus. At higher doses, codeine has most of the disadvantages of morphine, including respiratory depression.

Overdosage:

Acetaminophen:

Signs and Symptoms: Acetaminophen in massive overdosage may cause hepatic toxicity in some patients. In all cases of suspected overdose, immediately call your regional poison center or the Rocky Mountain Poison Center's toll-free number (800-525-6115) for assistance in diagnosis and for directions in the use of N-acetylcysteine as an antidote, a use currently restricted to investigational status.
In adults, hepatic toxicity has rarely been reported with acute overdoses of less than 10 grams and fatalities with less than 15 grams. Importantly, young children seem to be more resistant than adults to the hepatotoxic effect of an acetaminophen overdose. Despite this, the measures outlined below should be initiated in any adult or child suspected of having ingested an acetaminophen overdose.
Early symptoms following a potentially hepatotoxic overdose may include: nausea, vomiting, diaphoresis and general malaise. Clinical and laboratory evidence of hepatic toxicity may not be apparent until 48 to 72 hours post-ingestion.

Treatment: The stomach should be emptied promptly by lavage or by induction of emesis with syrup of ipecac. Patients' estimates of the quantity of a drug ingested are notoriously unreliable. Therefore, if an acetaminophen overdose is suspected, a serum acetaminophen assay should be obtained as early as possible, but no sooner than four hours following ingestion. Liver function studies should be obtained initially and repeated at 24-hour intervals.
The antidote, N-acetylcysteine, should be administered as early as possible, and within 16 hours of the overdose ingestion for optimal results. Following recovery, there are no residual, structural or functional hepatic abnormalities.

Codeine:

Signs and Symptoms: Serious overdose with codeine is characterized by respiratory depression (a decrease in respiratory rate and/or tidal volume. Cheyne-Stokes respiration, cyanosis), extreme somnolence progressing to stupor or coma, skeletal muscle flaccidity, cold and clammy skin, and sometimes bradycardia and hypotension. In severe overdosage, apnea, circulatory collapse, cardiac arrest, and death may occur.

Treatment: Primary attention should be given to the reestablishment of adequate respiratory exchange through provision of a patent airway and the institution of assisted or controlled ventilation. The narcotic antagonist naloxone is a specific antidote against respiratory depression which may result from over-

Continued on next page

Burroughs Wellcome—Cont.

dosage or unusual sensitivity to narcotics, including codeine. Therefore, an appropriate dose of naloxone (see package insert) should be administered preferably by the intravenous route, and simultaneously with efforts at respiratory resuscitation. Since the duration of action of codeine may exceed that of the antagonist, the patient should be kept under continued surveillance and repeated doses of the antagonist should be administered as needed to maintain adequate respiration.

An antagonist should not be administered in the absence of clinically significant respiratory or cardiovascular depression. Oxygen, intravenous fluids, vasopressors and other supportive measures should be employed as indicated.

Gastric emptying may be useful in removing unabsorbed drug.

Dosage and Administration: Dosage should be adjusted according to severity of pain and response of the patient. However, it should be kept in mind that tolerance to codeine can develop with continued use and that the incidence of untoward effects is dose related. This product is inappropriate even in high doses for severe or intractable pain. Adult doses of codeine higher than 60 mg fail to give commensurate relief of pain, but merely prolong analgesia and are associated with an appreciably increased incidence of undesirable side effects. Equivalently high doses in children would have similar effects.

The usual adult dose is one tablet every four hours, as required.

How Supplied: Empracet® with Codeine phosphate 30 mg. No. 3 is available in tablets (peach) coded with "Empracet 3" and "K9B." Bottles of 100, (NDC-0081-0315-55) 500 (NDC-0081-0315-70) and Dispenserpak® of 25 (NDC-0081-0315-25). Empracet® with Codeine Phosphate 60 mg, No. 4, is available in tablets (peach), coded with "EMPRACET 4" and "L9B." Bottles of 100 (NDC-0081-0327-55) and 500 (NDC-0081-0327-70).

[*Shown in Product Identification Section*]

EMPRAZIL® TABLETS ℞

Description: Emprazil® Tablets are intended for oral administration. Each tablet contains Sudafed® (pseudoephedrine hydrochloride) 20 mg, aspirin (acetylsalicylic acid) 200 mg, phenacetin 150 mg, and caffeine 30 mg.

Emprazil has analgesic, antipyretic, anti-inflammatory, and nasal decongestant effects.

Clinical Pharmacology:

Pseudoephedrine: Pseudoephedrine acts as an indirect sympathomimetic agent by stimulating sympathetic (adrenergic) nerve endings to release norepinephrine. Norepinephrine in turn stimulates alpha and beta receptors throughout the body. The action of pseudoephedrine hydrochloride is apparently more specific on the blood vessels of the upper respiratory tract and less specific for the blood vessels of the systemic circulation. The vasoconstriction elicited at these sites results in the shrinkage of swollen tissues in the sinuses and nasal passages.

Pseudoephedrine is rapidly and almost completely absorbed from the gastrointestinal tract. After a 60 mg dose (tablet), peak plasma concentrations are reached in from ½ to 2 hours. Within the normal urine pH ranges, mean plasma half-life is 6 to 7 hours. However, considerable variation in half-life has been observed (from about 4½ to 10 hours) which is attributed to individual differences in absorption and excretion. Excretion rates are also altered by urine pH, increasing with acidification and decreasing with alkalinization. As a result, mean half-life falls to about 4 hours at pH 5 and increases to 12 to 13 hours at pH 8.

After administration of a 60 mg tablet, 87 to 96% of the pseudoephedrine is cleared from the body within 24 hours. The drug is distributed to body tissues and fluids, including fetal tissue, breast milk and the CNS. About 55 to 75% of an administered dose is excreted unchanged in the urine; the remainder is apparently metabolized in the liver to inactive compounds by N-demethylation, parahydroxylation and oxidative deamination.

Aspirin: The analgesic, anti-inflammatory and antipyretic effects of aspirin are believed to result from inhibition of the synthesis of certain prostaglandins. Aspirin interferes with clotting mechanisms primarily by diminishing platelet aggregation; at high doses prothrombin synthesis can be inhibited.

Aspirin in solution is rapidly absorbed from the stomach and from the upper small intestine. About 50 percent of an oral dose is absorbed in 30 minutes and peak plasma concentrations are reached in about 40 minutes. Higher than normal stomach pH or the presence of food slightly delays absorption.

Once absorbed, aspirin is mainly hydrolyzed to salicylic acid and distributed to all body tissues and fluids, including fetal tissue, breast milk and the central nervous system (CNS). Highest concentrations are found in plasma, liver, renal cortex, heart and lung.

From 50 to 80 percent of the salicylic acid and its metabolites in plasma are loosely bound to plasma proteins. The plasma half-life of total salicylate is about 3.0 hours, with a 650 mg dose. Higher doses of aspirin cause increases in plasma salicylate half-life. Metabolism occurs primarily in the hepatocytes. The major metabolites are salicyluric acid (75%), the phenolic and acyl glucuronides of salicylate (15%), and gentisic and gentisuric acid (<1%).

Almost all of a therapeutic dose of aspirin is excreted through the kidneys, either as salicylic acid or the above-mentioned metabolic products. Renal clearance of salicylates is greatly augmented by an alkaline urine, as is produced by concurrent administration of sodium bicarbonate or potassium citrate.

Toxic salicylate blood levels are usually above 30 mg/100 ml. The single lethal dose of aspirin in normal adults is approximately 25–30 g, but patients have recovered from much larger doses with appropriate treatment.

Phenacetin: The mechanism through which phenacetin relieves pain is uncertain.

Phenacetin is rapidly absorbed from the gastrointestinal tract and reaches peak plasma concentrations in one-half to two hours. The physiologic half-life of phenacetin varies from about one-half to one and one-half hours; the drug is almost completely cleared from the body five hours after ingestion. About 30 to 40 percent of phenacetin is bound to plasma protein. Phenacetin and its pharmacologically active metabolite, acetaminophen, are distributed throughout the body tissues and fluids, including fetal tissue, breast milk and the CNS. Their concentration in body fluids, including milk, is relatively uniform, but the extent to which phenacetin and acetaminophen are taken up by various body tissues has not been established. About 75 to 80 percent of phenacetin is rapidly de-ethylated in liver to acetaminophen, which reaches peak plasma concentration in one to two hours and has a half-life of one to three hours. The therapeutic plasma concentration of acetaminophen is reported to be 0.5–2.0 mg/100 ml and the lethal concentration is 150 mg/100 ml. About 80 percent of the derived acetaminophen is excreted in urine after conjugation, primarily as the glucuronide; 3 percent is excreted unchanged. Other metabolites are formed by deacetylation and hydroxylation.

Phenacetin is metabolized by deacetylation (to para-phenetidin) and hydroxylation to a number of breakdown products; traces of phenacetin are eliminated unchanged. Toxic effects (sedation, dizziness) have been seen with single doses of 2 g. The minimum lethal dose has been estimated to be 5–20 g, but adults have recovered completely from acute overdoses of 50–60 g.

Caffeine: In ordinary doses, caffeine stimulates the CNS to elevate mood, decrease fatigue, promote alertness and improve motor skills. Caffeine also reduces susceptibility to fatigue by increasing the strength of skeletal muscle contractions. At higher doses or in the presence of medullary depressants, caffeine has been shown to stimulate respiration.

Caffeine exerts central and peripheral effects on heart rate that tend to offset each other except at high doses, when its direct positive chronotropic action predominates and an increased heart rate results.

Caffeine also causes a moderate increase in myocardial contractility. While the balance between its central and peripheral effects on blood vessels generally favors vasodilation, caffeine causes vasoconstriction in the cerebral circulation. This effect is thought to explain its efficacy in relieving headache. In addition, caffeine has mild diuretic and smooth-muscle relaxant properties.

Like most xanthines, caffeine is rapidly absorbed and distributed to all body tissues and fluids, including the CNS, fetal tissues and breast milk. About 90 percent of an administered dose is metabolized in the liver to approximately equal amounts of 1-methyl-xanthine and 1-methyluric acid; the remainder is excreted unchanged in the urine.

Caffeine achieves its peak effect in about 2 hours; the plasma half-life is about 1.5 hours. The dose level at which toxicity occurs is about 1 g. The single lethal dose is estimated to be over 10 g.

Indications and Usage: Emprazil Tablets are a combination of analgesic, antipyretic and decongestant agents for the relief of symptoms associated with upper respiratory tract infections.

Contraindications: Emprazil is contraindicated under the following conditions:

(1) hypersensitivity or intolerance to pseudoephedrine, aspirin, phenacetin, or caffeine,
(2) severe hypertension, severe coronary artery disease and in patients on MAO inhibitor therapy,
(3) severe bleeding, disorders of coagulation or primary hemostasis, including hemophilia, hypoprothrombinemia, von Willebrand's disease, the thrombocytopenias, thrombasthenia and other ill-defined hereditary platelet dysfunctions, as well as such associated conditions as severe vitamin K deficiency and severe liver damage.
(4) anticoagulant therapy, and
(5) peptic ulcer, or other serious gastrointestinal lesions.

Warnings: Therapeutic doses of aspirin can cause anaphylactic shock and other severe allergic reactions. A history of allergy is often lacking.

Significant bleeding can result from aspirin therapy in patients with peptic ulcer or other gastrointestinal lesions, and in patients with bleeding disorders. Aspirin administered preoperatively may prolong the bleeding time.

Nephrotoxicity (renal papillary necrosis), frequently accompanied by urinary tract infection, has been reported in a small percentage of individuals consuming analgesic mixtures regularly in large amounts for long periods. Carcinoma of the renal pelvis and urinary bladder has been associated with chronic abuse of analgesic mixtures.

Pseudoephedrine should be used judiciously and sparingly in patients with hypertension, diabetes mellitus, ischemic heart disease, increased intraocular pressure, hyperthyroidism, and prostatic hypertrophy.

Use in Elderly: The elderly (approximately 60 years or older) are more likely to have adverse reactions to sympathomimetics.

Precautions:

General: Emprazil should be prescribed with caution for certain special-risk patients such as the elderly or debilitated, and for those with severe impairment of renal or hepatic function, cardiac arrhythmias, inflammatory disorders of the gastrointestinal tract, coagulation disorders, and patients known to be taking other analgesic-antipyretic-decongestant medications. Patients' self-medication habits should be investigated to determine their use of such medications. Emprazil should not be prescribed for long-term therapy unless specifically indicated.

Precautions should be taken when administering salicylates to persons with known allergies. Hypersensitivity to aspirin is particularly likely in patients with nasal polyps, and relatively common in those with asthma.

In persons with glucose-6-phosphate dehydrogenase deficiency, phenacetin can cause acute hemolytic anemia.

In persons with renal insufficiency, a typically mild but progressive hemolytic anemia can occur with long-term use of phenacetin. Patients with renal insufficiency appear to be especially susceptible to renal inflammatory lesions characteristic of so-called analgesic nephropathy associated with chronic abuse of analgesic medications.

Patients with severe heart disease should not receive high doses of caffeine, since it can cause tachycardia or extrasystoles and thus precipitate cardiac failure. Palpitations that may be caused by caffeine are usually of significance only in patients with severe heart disease. Caffeine may cause gastrointestinal irritation and, in susceptible persons, over-stimulation, "jitters" or insomnia.

Information for Patients: Emprazil should not be used by persons intolerant to sympathomimetics used for the relief of nasal or sinus congestion. Such drugs include ephedrine, epinephrine, and phenylephrine. Symptoms of intolerance include dizziness, weakness, difficulty in breathing, tenseness, muscle tremors or palpitations.

Patients with severe heart disease should be advised to reduce their total intake of caffeine. Chronic use of Emprazil at high doses for long periods of time may result in kidney or liver damage. Patients should take this drug only for as long as it is prescribed, in the amounts prescribed, and no more frequently than prescribed.

Laboratory Tests: Hypersensitivity to aspirin cannot be detected by skin testing or radioimmunoassay procedures.

The primary screening tests for detecting a bleeding tendency are platelet count, bleeding time, activated partial thromboplastin time and prothrombin time.

In patients with severe hepatic or renal disease, effects of therapy should be monitored with serial liver and/or renal function tests.

Drug Interactions: Emprazil may *enhance* the effects of:

(1) monoamine oxidase (MAO) inhibitors,
(2) oral anticoagulants, causing bleeding by inhibiting prothrombin formation in the liver and displacing anticoagulants from plasma protein binding sites,
(3) oral antidiabetic agents and insulin, causing hypoglycemia by contributing an additive effect, and by displacing the oral antidiabetic agents from secondary binding sites,
(4) 6-mercaptopurine and methotrexate, causing bone marrow toxicity and blood dyscrasias by displacing these drugs from secondary binding sites,
(5) penicillins and sulfonamides, increasing their blood levels by displacing these drugs from protein binding sites,
(6) non-steroidal anti-inflammatory agents, increasing the risk of peptic ulceration and bleeding by contributing additive effects.
(7) corticosteroids, potentiating steroid anti-inflammatory effects by displacing steroids from protein binding sites.
Aspirin intoxication may occur with corticosteroid withdrawal because steroids promote renal clearance of salicylates.

Emprazil may *diminish* the effects of:

(1) the antihypertensive effects of guanethidine, bethanidine, methyldopa, and reserpine;
(2) uricosuric agents such as probenecid and sulfinpyrazone, reducing their effectiveness in the treatment of gout. Aspirin competes with these agents for protein binding sites.

Aspirin and its metabolites may be caused to accumulate in the body, perhaps to toxic levels, by para-amino-salicylic acid, furosemide, and vitamin C. Phenobarbital decreases the effects of phenacetin by accelerating its excretion. Sorbitol and polysorbate accelerate the absorption of phenacetin. High doses of caffeine can cause a potentially lethal hypertensive reaction in the presence of MAO inhibitors. High doses of caffeine and propoxyphene can cause fatal convulsions by additive CNS stimulation. Caffeine and stimulants such as amphetamines may combine to cause excessive excitation or "nervousness".

Drug/Laboratory Test Interactions:

Aspirin: Aspirin may interfere with the following laboratory determinations in blood: serum amylase, fasting blood glucose, carbon dioxide, cholesterol, protein, protein bound iodine, uric acid, prothrombin time, bleeding time, and spectrophotometric detection of barbiturates. Aspirin may interfere with the following laboratory determinations in urine: glucose, 5-hydroxyindoleacetic acid, Gerhardt ketone, vanillylmandelic acid (VMA), protein, uric acid, and diacetic acid.

Phenacetin: Phenacetin may interfere with laboratory determinations of 5-hydroxyindoleacetic acid and glucose in urine.

Caffeine: Caffeine may interfere with laboratory determinations of bilirubin, fasting blood glucose, and uric acid in blood, and catecholamines and 5-hydroxyindoleacetic acid in urine.

Carcinogenesis, Mutagenesis, Impairment of Fertility: No adequate long-term studies have been conducted in animals to determine whether pseudoephedrine has a potential for carcinogenesis, mutagenesis, or impairment of fertility.

Adequate long-term studies have been conducted in mice and rats with aspirin, phenacetin and caffeine given alone or in combination. No evidence of carcinogenesis was seen in these studies. No adequate animal studies have been conducted with aspirin, phenacetin or caffeine to determine whether they have a potential for mutagenesis or impairment of fertility.

Pregnancy: **Teratogenic Effects:** Pregnancy Category C. Animal reproduction studies have not been conducted with Emprazil. It is also not known whether EMPRAZIL can cause fetal harm when administered to a pregnant woman or can affect reproduction capacity. Emprazil should be given to a pregnant woman only if clearly needed.

Teratology studies have been performed in rats at doses up to 150 times the human dose and have revealed no evidence of teratogenic harm to the fetus due to pseudoephedrine. However, overt signs of toxicity were observed in the dams which was reflected in reduced average weight, length and rate of skeletal ossification in their fetuses.

Reproductive studies in rats and mice have shown aspirin to be teratogenic and embryocidal at four to six times the human therapeutic dose. Studies in pregnant women, however, have not shown that aspirin increases the risk of abnormalities when administered during the first trimester of pregnancy. In controlled studies involving 41,337 pregnant women and their offspring, there was no evidence that aspirin taken during pregnancy caused stillbirth, neonatal death or reduced birthweight. In controlled studies of 50,282 pregnant women and their offspring, aspirin administration in moderate and heavy doses during the first four lunar months of pregnancy showed no teratogenic effect.

Reproduction studies have been performed in rats and mice at doses up to 10 times the human dose and have revealed no evidence of impaired fertility or harm to the fetus due to caffeine.

Nonteratogenic Effects: Therapeutic doses of aspirin in pregnant women close to term may cause bleeding in mother, fetus, or neonate. During the last six months of pregnancy, regular use of aspirin in high doses may prolong pregnancy and delivery.

The risk of methemoglobinemia or hemolytic anemia occurring in the fetus may be increased by: (1) regular ingestion of high doses of phenacetin during pregnancy, (2) renal insufficiency in the mother and/or fetus, (3) glucose-6-phosphate dehydrogenase deficiency, or (4) a genetically acquired abnormality in phenacetin metabolism.

Labor and Delivery: Ingestion of aspirin prior to delivery may prolong delivery or lead to bleeding in the mother or neonate. Ingestion of phenacetin may cause methemoglobinemia or hemolytic anemia.

Nursing Mothers: All components of Emprazil are excreted in breast milk in small amounts, but the significance of their effects on nursing infants is not known. Because of the potential for serious adverse reactions in nursing infants from Emprazil, a decision should be made whether to discontinue nursing or to discontinue the drug, taking into account the importance of the drug to the mother.

Adverse Reactions:

Pseudoephedrine: Hyperactive individuals may display ephedrine-like reactions such as tachycardia, palpitations, headache, dizziness or nausea. Sympathomimetic drugs have been associated with certain untoward reactions including fear, anxiety, tenseness, restlessness, tremor, weakness, pallor, respiratory difficulty, dysuria, insomnia, hallucinations, CNS depression, arrhythmias, and anorexia.

Aspirin: Mild aspirin intoxication (salicylism) can occur in response to chronic use of large doses. Manifestations include nausea, vomiting, hearing impairment, tinnitus, diminished vision, headache, dizziness, drowsiness, mental confusion, hyperpnea, hyperventilation, tachycardia, sweating and thirst.

Therapeutic doses of aspirin can induce mild or severe allergic reactions manifested by skin rashes, urticaria, angioedema, rhinorrhea, asthma, abdominal pain, nausea, vomiting, or anaphylactic shock. A history of allergy is often lacking, and allergic reactions may occur in patients who have previously taken aspirin without any ill effects. Allergic reactions to aspirin are most likely to occur in patients with a history of allergic disease, especially in patients with nasal polyps or asthma.

Some patients are unable to take aspirin or other salicylates without developing nausea or vomiting. Occasional patients respond to aspirin (usually in large doses) with dyspepsia or heartburn, which may be accompanied by occult bleeding. Excessive bruising or bleeding is sometimes seen in patients with mild disorders of primary hemostasis who regularly use low doses of aspirin.

Prolonged use of aspirin can cause painless erosion of gastric mucosa, occult bleeding and, infrequently, iron-deficiency anemia. High doses of aspirin can exacerbate symptoms of peptic ulcer and, occasionally, cause extensive bleeding.

Excessive bleeding can follow injury or surgery in patients with or without known bleed-

Continued on next page

Burroughs Wellcome—Cont.

ing disorders who have taken therapeutic doses of aspirin within the preceding 10 days.
Hepatotoxicity has been reported in association with prolonged use of large doses of aspirin in patients with lupus erythematosus, rheumatoid arthritis, or rheumatic disease.
Bone-marrow depression, manifested by weakness, fatigue, or abnormal bruising or bleeding, has occasionally been reported.
In patients with glucose-6-phosphate dehydrogenase deficiency aspirin can cause a mild degree of hemolytic anemia.
In hyperuricemic persons, low doses of aspirin may reduce the effectiveness of uricosuric therapy or precipitate an attack of gout.
Phenacetin: In therapeutic doses, side effects of phenacetin are generally limited to occasional sedation, skin rashes or, uncommonly, drug fever.
Adverse reactions to phenacetin are usually the result of acute overdosage or chronic abuse of analgesic mixtures containing phenacetin. Toxic doses can cause dizziness, drowsiness or stimulation, methemoglobinemia and sulfhemoglobinemia (cyanosis, fatigue), and, rarely, hepatic necrosis (gastrointestinal symptoms possibly followed by general obtundation) or nephropathy (cloudy urine due to cells, casts, organisms, sloughed tissue; edema of lower legs).
Caffeine: Usual doses of caffeine may cause gastric disturbances in some persons. Side effects are usually due to hyperresponsiveness or overdosage, acute or chronic. Toxic doses can cause nervousness, excitement, insomnia, muscle tenderness or tremors, tinnitus, scintillating scotomas, headache on withdrawal of the drug, diuresis, tachycardia and extrasystoles.
Overdosage: Severe intoxication, caused by overdose of EMPRAZIL may produce skin eruptions, dyspnea, vertigo, double vision, delusions, hallucinations, garbled speech, excitability, restlessness, delirium, fixed pupils, a positive Babinski sign, cyanosis, circulatory collapse, stupor and coma. In children, difficulty in hearing, tinnitus, dim vision, headache, dizziness, drowsiness, confusion, rapid breathing, sweating, thirst, nausea, vomiting, hyperpyrexia, dehydration and convulsions are prominent signs.
The most severe manifestations from aspirin result from cardiovascular and respiratory insufficiency secondary to acid-base and electrolyte disturbances, complicated by hyperthermia and dehydration.
Respiratory alkalosis is characteristic of the early phase of intoxication with aspirin while hyperventilation is occurring, and is quickly followed by metabolic acidosis with severe intoxication. This occurs more readily in children. Hypoglycemia may occur in children who have taken large overdoses. Other laboratory findings associated with aspirin intoxication include ketonuria, hyponatremia, hypokalemia, and occasionally proteinuria. A slight rise in lactic dehydrogenase and hydroxybutyric dehydrogenase may occur.
Hemolytic anemia due to phenacetin is possible and should be monitored by periodic laboratory tests.
Methemoglobin and sulfhemoglobin formation are seldom clinically significant in adults but may contribute to general toxicity. When prominent, they appear as a grayish cyanosis seen most clearly in the lips and nailbeds. Definitive diagnosis is made by spectroscopic analysis of a water-diluted (1:100) blood specimen, which shows an abnormal band at 630 m for methemoglobin and at 618 m for sulfhemoglobin.
Concentrations of aspirin in plasma above 30 mg/100 ml are associated with toxicity. (See Clinical Pharmacology section for information on factors influencing aspirin blood levels).
The single lethal dose of aspirin in adults is probably about 25–30 g, but is not known with certainty.
Toxic and lethal concentrations of phenacetin in human fluids are not known with certainty.
Patient response per phenacetin dose may be greater than usual in infants, in patients with renal insufficiency or hepatic insufficiency and in those with a glucose-6-phosphate dehydrogenase deficiency or a decreased ability to convert phenacetin to acetaminophen. Toxic effects (e.g., sedation) have been seen with single doses of 2 g. The minimum lethal dose has been estimated to be 5–20 g, but adults have recovered from acute overdoses of 50–60 g.
Toxic and lethal concentrations of caffeine in human fluids are not known with certainty.
Patient response per dose is increased in the presence of renal or hepatic insufficiency.
Toxic manifestations may appear with a caffeine dose of 1 g. The single lethal dose in man is generally estimated to be over 10 g, but the lowest reported lethal dose was 3.2 g or 57 mg/kg.
Hemodialysis and peritoneal dialysis can be performed to reduce the body aspirin content. Phenacetin is dialyzable, but dialysis of the drug and its major metabolite, acetaminophen, has not yet been established as an effective means of altering the consequence of acute phenacetin overdosage. Pseudoephedrine and caffeine are theoretically dialyzable but the procedure has not been clinically established.
Overdosage with pseudoephedrine can cause excessive CNS stimulation associated with such manifestations as excitement, nervousness or anxiety, restlessness and insomnia. Other manifestations include tachycardia, hypertension, unusually intense pallor, mydriasis, hyperglycemia and urinary retention.
Severe overdosage with sympathomimetic agents may cause greater CNS stimulation (tachypnea or hyperpnea, hallucinations, convulsions) or CNS depression (stupor, respiratory depression), arrhythmias, bradycardia, hypotension and circulatory collapse. No laboratory findings are of specific diagnostic value. No organ damage or significant metabolic derangement is associated with pseudoephedrine overdosage.
The mean LD_{50} (single oral dose) of pseudoephedrine is 726 mg/kg in the mouse, 2206 mg/kg in the rat, and 1177 mg/kg in the rabbit. The toxic and lethal concentrations in human biologic fluids are not known. Excretion rates increase with urine acidification and decrease with alkalinization.
Insufficient data are available to estimate toxic and lethal doses in man. Few reports of toxicity due to pseudoephedrine have been published, and no cases of fatal overdosage are known.
There is no specific antidote for pseudoephedrine. If instituted within one hour of overdosage, therapy is initially aimed at reducing further drug absorption by use of emetics and gastric lavage. If renal function is adequate, forced osmotic diuresis and acidification of urine with ammonium chloride will accelerate excretion of the drug.
Treatment of overdosage consists primarily of support of vital functions, increasing salicylate elimination, and correcting the acid-base imbalance due primarily to salicylism.
In a comatose patient, primary attention should be given to establishment of adequate respiratory exchange through provisions of a patent airway and the institution of assisted or controlled ventilation.
Gastric emptying (Syrup of Ipecac) and/or lavage is recommended as soon as possible after ingestion, even if the patient has vomited spontaneously. Administration of activated charcoal as a slurry is beneficial after lavage and/or emesis, if less than three hours have passed since ingestion. Charcoal absorption should *not* be employed prior to emesis or lavage.
Severity of aspirin intoxication is determined by measuring the blood salicylate level. Acid-base status should be closely followed with serial blood gas and serum pH measurements. Fluid and electrolyte balance should also be regularly monitored.
A serum salicylate level of 30 mg/100 ml or higher indicates a need for enhanced salicylate excretion that can be achieved through body-fluid supplementation and urine alkalinization if renal function is normal. In mild intoxication, urine flow can be increased by forcing oral fluids and giving potassium citrate capsules. (DO NOT GIVE BICARBONATE BY MOUTH SINCE IT INCREASES THE RATE OF SALICYLATE ABSORPTION.)
In severe cases, hyperthermia and hypovolemia as well as respiratory depression are the major immediate threats to life. Children should be sponged with tepid water. Replacement fluid should be administered intravenously in adequate amount and augmented with sufficient bicarbonate to correct acidosis, with monitoring of plasma electrolytes and pH, to promote alkaline diuresis of salicylate if renal function is normal. Complete control may also require infusion of glucose to control hypoglycemia.
Potassium deficiency may also be corrected through the infusion, once adequate urinary output is assured. Plasma or plasma expanders may be needed if fluid replacement is insufficient to maintain normal blood pressure or adequate urinary output.
In patients with renal insufficiency or in cases of life-threatening intoxication, dialysis is usually required. Peritoneal dialysis or exchange transfusion is indicated in infants and young children, and hemodialysis in older patients.
Oxygen, intravenous fluids, vasopressors and other supportive measures should be employed as needed.
Dosage and Administration: The recommended dosage for adults and children over 12 years of age is one or two tablets three times daily, as required. Dosage for children 6 through 12 years of age is one tablet three times daily, as required.
Emprazil should be taken with food or a full glass of milk or water to lessen gastric irritation.
How Supplied: Orange and white tablet embossed with "TABLOID BRAND."
Bottle of 100 NDC # 0081-0300-55
Store at 15°–30°C (59°–86°F) in a dry place and protect from light.
[*Shown in Product Identification Section*]

EMPRAZIL-C® TABLETS ℞ Ⓒ

Description: EMPRAZIL-C® Tablets are intended for oral administration. Each tablet contains SUDAFED® (pseudoephedrine hydrochloride) 20 mg, aspirin (acetylsalicyclic acid) 200 mg, phenacetin 150 mg, caffeine 30 mg, and codeine phosphate 15 mg. (Warning—may be habit-forming.)
EMPRAZIL-C® has antitussive, analgesic, antipyretic, anti-inflammatory and nasal decongestant effects.
Clinical Pharmacology:
Pseudoephedrine: Pseudoephedrine acts as an indirect sympathomimetic agent by stimulating sympathetic (adrenergic) nerve endings to release norepinephrine. Norepinephrine in turn stimulates alpha and beta receptors throughout the body. The action of pseudoephedrine hydrochloride is apparently more specific on the blood vessels of the upper respiratory tract and less specific for the blood vessels of the systemic circulation. The vasoconstriction elicited at these sites results in the shrinkage of swollen tissues in the sinuses and nasal passages.
Pseudoephedrine is rapidly and almost completely absorbed from the gastrointestinal tract. After a 60 mg dose (tablet), peak plasma concentrations are reached in from ½ to 2

hours. Within the normal urine pH ranges, mean plasma half-life is 6 to 7 hours. However, considerable variation in half-life has been observed (from about 4½ to 10 hours) which is attributed to individual differences in absorption and excretion. Excretion rates are also altered by urine pH, increasing with acidification and decreasing with alkalinization. As a result, mean half-life falls to about 4 hours at pH 5 and increases to 12 to 13 hours at pH 8. After administration of a 60 mg tablet, 87 to 96% of the pseudoephedrine is cleared from the body within 24 hours. The drug is distributed to body tissues and fluids, including fetal tissue, breast milk and the CNS. About 55 to 75% of an administered dose is excreted unchanged in the urine; the remainder is apparently metabolized in the liver to inactive compounds by N-demethylation, parahydroxylation and oxidative deamination.

Aspirin: The analgesic, anti-inflammatory and antipyretic effects of aspirin are believed to result from inhibition of the synthesis of certain prostaglandins. It interferes with clotting mechanisms primarily by diminishing platelet aggregation; at high doses prothrombin synthesis can be inhibited.

Aspirin in solution is rapidly absorbed from the stomach and from the upper small intestine. About 50 percent of an oral dose is absorbed in 30 minutes and peak plasma concentrations are reached in about 40 minutes. Higher than normal stomach pH or the presence of food slightly delays absorption.

Once absorbed, aspirin is mainly hydrolyzed to salicylic acid and distributed to all body tissues and fluids, including fetal tissue, breast milk and the central nervous system (CNS). Highest concentrations are found in plasma, liver, renal cortex, heart and lung.

From 50 to 80 percent of the salicylic acid and its metabolites in plasma are loosely bound to plasma proteins. The plasma half-life of total salicylate is about 3.0 hours with a 650 mg dose. Higher doses of aspirin cause increases in plasma salicylate half-life. Metabolism occurs primarily in the hepatocytes. The major metabolites are salicyluric acid (75%), the phenolic and acyl glucuronides of salicylate (15%), and gentisic and gentisuric acid (<1%).

Almost all of a therapeutic dose of aspirin is excreted through the kidneys, either as salicylic acid or the above-mentioned metabolic products. Renal clearance of salicylates is greatly augmented by an alkaline urine, as is produced by concurrent administration of sodium bicarbonate or potassium citrate.

Toxic salicylate blood levels are usually above 30 mg/100 ml. The single lethal dose of aspirin in normal adults is approximately 25-30 g, but patients have recovered from much larger doses with appropriate treatment.

Phenacetin: The mechanism through which phenacetin relieves pain is uncertain.

Phenacetin is rapidly absorbed from the gastrointestinal tract and reaches peak plasma concentrations in one-half to two hours. The physiologic half-life of phenacetin varies from about one-half to one and one-half hours; the drug is almost completely cleared from the body five hours after ingestion. About 30 to 40 percent of phenacetin is bound to plasma protein. Phenacetin and its pharmacologically active metabolite, acetaminophen, are distributed throughout the body tissues and fluids, including fetal tissue, breast milk and the CNS. Their concentration in body fluids, including milk, is relatively uniform, but the extent to which phenacetin and acetaminophen are taken up by various body tissues has not been established. About 75 to 80 percent of phenacetin is rapidly de-ethylated in liver to acetaminophen, which reaches peak plasma concentration in one to two hours and has a half-life of one to three hours. The therapeutic plasma concentration of acetaminophen is reported to be 0.5-2.0 mg/100 ml and the lethal concentration is 150 mg/100 ml. About 80 percent of the derived acetaminophen is excreted in urine after conjugation, primarily as the glucuronide; 3 percent is excreted unchanged. Other metabolites are formed by deacetylation and hydroxylation.

Phenacetin is metabolized by deacetylation (to para-phenetidin) and hydroxylation to a number of breakdown products; traces of phenacetin are eliminated unchanged. Toxic effects (sedation, dizziness) have been seen with single doses of 2 g. The minimum lethal dose has been estimated to be 5-20 g, but adults have recovered completely from acute overdoses of 50-60 g.

Caffeine: In ordinary doses, caffeine stimulates the CNS to elevate mood, decrease fatigue, promote alertness and improve motor skills. Caffeine also reduces susceptibility to fatigue by increasing the strength of skeletal muscle contractions. At higher doses or in the presence of medullary depressants, caffeine has been shown to stimulate respiration.

Caffeine exerts central and peripheral effects on heart rate that tend to offset each other except at high doses, when its direct positive chronotropic action predominates and an increased heart rate results.

Caffeine also causes a moderate increase in myocardial contractility. While the balance between its central and peripheral effects on blood vessels generally favors vasodilation, caffeine causes vasoconstriction in the cerebral circulation. This effect is thought to explain its efficacy in relieving headache. In addition, caffeine has mild diuretic and smooth-muscle relaxant properties.

Like most xanthines, caffeine is rapidly absorbed and distributed to all body tissues and fluids, including the CNS, fetal tissues and breast milk. About 90 percent of an administered dose is metabolized in the liver to approximately equal amounts of 1-methylxanthine and 1-methyluric acid; the remainder is excreted unchanged in the urine.

Caffeine achieves its peak effect in about 2 hours; the plasma half-life is about 1.5 hours. The dose level at which toxicity occurs is about 1 g. The single lethal dose is estimated to be over 10 g.

Codeine: Codeine probably exerts its analgesic effect through actions on opiate receptors in the CNS. Its antitussive activity supposedly arises from its ability to depress the medullary (brain) cough center thereby raising its threshold for incoming cough impulses.

Codeine is readily absorbed from the gastrointestinal tract, and a therapeutic dose reaches peak analgesic effectiveness in about 2 hours and persists for 4 to 6 hours. Oral codeine (60 mg) given to healthy males has been shown to achieve peak blood levels of 0.016 mg/100 ml at approximately one hour post-dose. The codeine plasma half-life for a 60 mg oral dose is about 2.9 hours.

Blood levels causing CNS depression begin at 0.05-0.19 mg/100 ml. The single lethal dose of codeine in adults is estimated to be approximately 0.5-1.0 g.

Codeine is rapidly distributed from blood to body tissues and taken up preferentially by parenchymatous organs such as liver, spleen and kidney. It passes the blood brain barrier and is found in fetal tissue and breast milk.

The drug is not bound by plasma proteins nor is it accumulated in body tissues. Codeine is metabolized in liver to morphine and norcodeine, each representing about 10 percent of the administered dose of codeine. About 90 percent of the dose is excreted within 24 hours, primarily through the kidneys. Urinary excretion products are free and glucuronide-conjugated codeine (about 70%), free and conjugated norcodeine (about 10%), free and conjugated morphine (about 10%), normorphine (under 4%) and hydrocodone (<1%). The remainder of the dose appears in the feces.

Indications and Usage: EMPRAZIL-C Tablets are a combination of antitussive, analgesic, antipyretic and decongestant agents for the relief of symptoms associated with upper respiratory tract infections.

Contraindications: EMPRAZIL-C is contraindicated under the following conditions:

(1) hypersensitivity or intolerance to pseudoephedrine, aspirin, phenacetin, caffeine or codeine;
(2) severe hypertension, severe coronary artery disease and in patients on MAO inhibitor therapy;
(3) severe bleeding, disorders of coagulation or primary hemostasis, including hemophilia, hypoprothrombinemia, von Willebrand's disease, the thrombocytopenias, thrombasthenia and other ill-defined hereditary platelet dysfunctions, as well as such associated conditions as severe vitamin K deficiency and severe liver damage;
(4) anticoagulant therapy; and
(5) peptic ulcer or other serious gastrointestinal lesions.

Warnings: Therapeutic doses of aspirin can cause anaphylactic shock and other severe allergic reactions. A history of allergy is often lacking.

Significant bleeding can result from aspirin therapy in patients with peptic ulcer or other gastrointestinal lesions, and in patients with bleeding disorders. Aspirin administered preoperatively may prolong the bleeding time.

Nephrotoxicity (renal papillary necrosis), frequently accompanied by urinary tract infection, has been reported in a small percentage of individuals consuming analgesic mixtures regularly in large amounts for long periods. Carcinoma of the renal pelvis and urinary bladder has been associated with chronic abuse of analgesic mixtures.

Pseudoephedrine should be used judiciously and sparingly in patients with hypertension, diabetes mellitus, ischemic heart disease, increased intraocular pressure, hyperthyroidism, and prostatic hypertrophy.

Use in Elderly: The elderly (approximately 60 years or older) are more likely to have adverse reactions to sympathomimetics.

In the presence of head injury or other intracranial lesions, the respiratory depressant effects of codeine and other narcotics may be markedly enhanced, as well as their capacity for elevating cerebrospinal fluid pressure. Narcotics also produce other CNS depressant effects, such as drowsiness, that may further obscure the clinical course of patients with head injuries.

Codeine or other narcotics may obscure signs on which to judge the diagnosis or clinical course of patients with acute abdominal conditions.

Precautions:

General: EMPRAZIL-C should be prescribed with caution for certain special-risk patients such as the elderly or debilitated, and for those with severe impairment of renal or hepatic function, gall-bladder disease or gallstones, respiratory impairment, cardiac arrhythmias, inflammatory disorders of the gastrointestinal tract, hypothyroidism, Addison's disease, urethral stricture, coagulation disorders, head injuries, acute abdominal conditions and patients known to be taking other antitussive, analgesic-antipyretic-decongestant medications. Patients' self-medication habits should be investigated to determine their use of such medications. EMPRAZIL-C should not be prescribed for long-term therapy unless specifically indicated.

Precautions should be taken when administering salicylates to persons with known allergies. Hypersensitivity to aspirin is particularly likely in patients with nasal polyps, and relatively common in those with asthma.

Continued on next page

Burroughs Wellcome—Cont.

In persons with glucose-6-phosphate dehydrogenase deficiency, phenacetin can cause acute hemolytic anemia.
In persons with renal insufficiency, a typically mild but progressive hemolytic anemia can occur with long-term use of phenacetin. Patients with renal insufficiency appear to be especially susceptible to renal inflammatory lesions characteristic of so-called analgesic nephropathy associated with chronic abuse of analgesic medications.
Patients with severe heart disease should not receive high doses of caffeine, since it can cause tachycardia or extrasystoles and thus precipitate cardiac failure. Palpitations that may be caused by caffeine are usually of significance only in patients with severe heart disease. Caffeine may cause gastrointestinal irritation and, in susceptible persons, over-stimulation, "jitters" or insomnia.
Information for Patients: EMPRAZIL-C may impair the mental and/or physical abilities required for performance of potentially hazardous tasks such as driving a car or operating machinery. Such tasks should be avoided while taking EMPRAZIL-C.
EMPRAZIL-C should not be used by persons intolerant to sympathomimetics used for the relief of nasal or sinus congestion. Such drugs include ephedrine, epinephrine, and phenylephrine. Symptoms of intolerance include dizziness, weakness, difficulty in breathing, tenseness, muscle tremors or palpitations.
Alcohol and other CNS depressants may produce an additive CNS depression when taken with EMPRAZIL-C, and should be avoided.
Patients with severe heart disease should be advised to reduce their total intake of caffeine. Codeine may be habit-forming when used over long periods or in high doses. Chronic use of EMPRAZIL-C at high doses for long periods of time may result in kidney or liver damage. Patients should take the drug only for as long as it is prescribed, in the amounts prescribed, and no more frequently than prescribed.
Laboratory Tests: Hypersensitivity to aspirin cannot be detected by skin testing or radioimmunoassay procedures.
The primary screening tests for detecting a bleeding tendency are platelet count, bleeding time, activated partial thromboplastin time and prothrombin time.
In patients with severe hepatic or renal disease, effects of therapy should be monitored with serial liver and/or renal function tests.
Drug Interactions: EMPRAZIL-C may enhance the effects of:
(1) monoamine oxidase (MAO) inhibitors;
(2) oral anticoagulants, causing bleeding by inhibiting prothrombin formation in the liver and displacing anticoagulants from plasma protein binding sites;
(3) oral antidiabetic agents and insulin, causing hypoglycemia by contributing an additive effect, and by displacing the oral antidiabetic agents from secondary binding sites;
(4) 6-mercaptopurine and methotrexate, causing bone marrow toxicity and blood dyscrasias by displacing these drugs from secondary binding sites;
(5) penicillins and sulfonamides, increasing their blood levels by displacing these drugs from protein binding sites;
(6) non-steroidal anti-inflammatory agents, increasing the risk of peptic ulceration and bleeding by contributing additive effects;
(7) other narcotic analgesics, alcohol, general anesthetics, tranquilizers such as chlordiazepoxide, sedative-hypnotics, or other CNS depressants, causing increased CNS depression;
(8) corticosteroids, potentiating steroid anti-inflammatory effects by displacing steroids from protein binding sites. Aspirin intoxication may occur with corticosteroid withdrawal because steriods promote renal clearance of salicylates.

EMPRAZIL-C may *diminish* the effects of:
(1) the antihypertensive effects of guanethidine, bethanidine, methyldopa, and reserpine;
(2) uricosuric agents such as probenecid and sulfinpyrazone, reducing their effectiveness in the treatment of gout. Aspirin competes with these agents for protein binding sites.

Aspirin and its metabolites may be caused to accumulate in the body, perhaps to toxic levels, by para-amino-salicylic acid, furosemide, and vitamin C. Phenobarbital decreases the effects of phenacetin by accelerating its excretion. Sorbitol and polysorbate accelerate the absorption of phenacetin. High doses of caffeine can cause a potentially lethal hypertensive reaction in the presence of MAO inhibitors. High doses of caffeine and propoxyphene can cause fetal convulsions by additive CNS stimulation. Caffeine and stimulants such as amphetamines may combine to cause excessive excitation or "nervousness".
Drug/Laboratory Test Interactions:
Aspirin: Aspirin may interfere with the following laboratory determinations in blood: serum amylase, fasting blood glucose, carbon dioxide, cholesterol, protein bound iodine, uric acid, prothrombin time, bleeding time, and spectrophotometric detection of barbiturates. Aspirin may interfere with the following laboratory determinations in urine: glucose, 5-hydroxyindoleacetic acid, Gerhardt ketone, vanillylmandelic acid (VMA), protein, uric acid, and diacetic acid.
Phenacetin: Phenacetin may interfere with laboratory determinations of 5-hydroxyindoleacetic acid and glucose in urine.
Caffeine: Caffeine may interfere with laboratory determinations of bilirubin, fasting blood glucose, and uric acid in blood, and catecholamines and 5-hydroxyindoleacetic acid in urine.
Codeine: Codeine may increase serum amylase levels.
Carcinogenesis, Mutagenesis, Impairment of Fertility: No adequate long-term studies have been conducted in animals to determine whether codeine and pseudoephedrine have a potential for carcinogenesis, mutagenesis, or impairment of fertility.
Adequate long-term studies have been conducted in mice and rats with aspirin, phenacetin and caffeine given alone or in combination. No evidence of carcinogenesis was seen in these studies. No adequate animal studies have been conducted with aspirin, phenacetin or caffeine to determine whether they have a potential for mutagenesis or impairment of fertility.
Pregnancy: **Teratogenic Effects:** Pregnancy Category C. Animal reproduction studies have not been conducted with EMPRAZIL-C. It is also not known whether EMPRAZIL-C can cause fetal harm when administered to a pregnant woman or can affect reproduction capacity. EMPRAZIL-C should be given to a pregnant woman only if clearly needed.
Teratology studies have been performed in rats at doses up to 150 times the human dose and have revealed no evidence of teratogenic harm to the fetus due to pseudoephedrine. However, overt signs of toxicity were observed in the dams which was reflected in reduced average weight, length and rate of skeletal ossification in their fetuses.
Reproductive studies in rats and mice have shown aspirin to be teratogenic and embryocidal at four to six times the human therapeutic dose. Studies in pregnant women, however, have not shown that aspirin increases the risk of abnormalities when administered during the first trimester of pregnancy. In controlled studies involving 41,337 pregnant women and their offspring, there was no evidence that aspirin taken during pregnancy caused stillbirth, neonatal death or reduced birthweight. In controlled studies of 50,282 pregnant women and their offspring, aspirin administration in moderate and heavy doses during the first four lunar months of pregnancy showed no teratogenic effect.
Reproduction studies have been performed in rats and mice at doses up to 10 times the human dose and have revealed no evidence of impaired fertility or harm to the fetus due to caffeine.
Reproduction studies have been performed in rabbits and rats at doses up to 150 times the human dose and have revealed no evidence of impaired fertility or harm to the fetus due to codeine.
Nonteratogenic Effects: Therapeutic doses of aspirin in pregnant women close to term may cause bleeding in mother, fetus, or neonate. During the last six months of pregnancy, regular use of aspirin in high doses may prolong pregnancy and delivery.
The risk of methemoglobinemia or hemolytic anemia occurring in the fetus may be increased by: (1) regular ingestion of high doses of phenacetin during pregnancy. (2) renal insufficiency in the mother and/or fetus, (3) glucose-6-phosphate dehydrogenase deficiency, or (4) a genetically acquired abnormality in phenacetin metabolism.
Labor and Delivery: Ingestion of aspirin prior to delivery may prolong delivery or lead to bleeding in the mother or neonate. Ingestion of phenacetin may cause methemoglobinemia or hemolytic anemia. Use of codeine during labor may lead to respiratory depression in the neonate.
Nursing Mothers: All components of EMPRAZIL-C are excreted in breast milk in small amounts, but the significance of their effects on nursing infants is not known. Because of the potential for serious adverse reactions in nursing infants from EMPRAZIL-C, a decision should be made whether to discontinue nursing or to discontinue the drug, taking into account the importance of the drug to the mother.

Adverse Reactions:
Codeine: The most frequently observed adverse reactions to codeine include light-headedness, dizziness, drowsiness, nausea, vomiting, constipation and depression of respiration. Less common reactions to codeine include euphoria, dysphoria, pruritus and skin rashes.
Pseudoephedrine: Hyperactive individuals may display ephedrine-like reactions such as tachycardia, palpitations, headache, dizziness or nausea. Sympathomimetic drugs have been associated with certain untoward reactions including fear, anxiety, tenseness, restlessness, tremor, weakness, pallor, respiratory difficulty, dysuria, insomnia, hallucinations, CNS depression, arrhythmias, and anorexia.
Aspirin: Mild aspirin intoxication (salicylism) can occur in response to chronic use of large doses. Manifestations include nausea, vomiting, hearing impairment, tinnitus, diminished vision, headache, dizziness, drowsiness, mental confusion, hyperpnea, hyperventilation, tachycardia, sweating and thirst.
Therapeutic doses of aspirin can induce mild or severe allergic reactions manifested by skin rashes, urticaria, angioedema, rhinorrhea, asthma, abdominal pain, nausea, vomiting, or anaphylactic shock. A history of allergy is often lacking, and allergic reactions may occur in patients who have previously taken aspirin without any ill effects. Allergic reactions to aspirin are most likely to occur in patients with a history of allergic disease, especially in patients with nasal polyps or asthma.
Some patients are unable to take aspirin or other salicylates without developing nausea or vomiting. Occasional patients respond to aspirin (usually in large doses) with dyspepsia or heartburn, which may be accompanied by occult bleeding. Excessive bruising or bleeding is

sometimes seen in patients with mild disorders of primary hemostasis who regularly use low doses of aspirin.

Prolonged use of aspirin can cause painless erosion of gastric mucosa, occult bleeding and, infrequently, iron-deficiency anemia. High doses of aspirin can exacerbate symptoms of peptic ulcer and, occasionally, cause extensive bleeding.

Excessive bleeding can follow injury or surgery in patients with or without known bleeding disorders who have taken therapeutic doses of aspirin within the preceding 10 days.

Hepatotoxicity has been reported in association with prolonged use of large doses of aspirin in patients with lupus erythematosus, rheumatoid arthritis, or rheumatic disease.

Bone-marrow depression, manifested by weakness, fatigue, or abnormal bruising or bleeding, has occasionally been reported.

In patients with glucose-6-phosphate dehydrogenase deficiency, aspirin can cause a mild degree of hemolytic anemia.

In hyperuricemic persons, low doses of aspirin may reduce the effectiveness of uricosuric therapy or precipitate an attack of gout.

Phenacetin: In therapeutic doses, side effects of phenacetin are generally limited to occasional sedation, skin rashes or, uncommonly, drug fever.

Adverse reactions to phenacetin are usually the result of acute overdosage or chronic abuse of analgesic mixtures containing phenacetin. Toxic doses can cause dizziness, drowsiness or stimulation, methemoglobinemia and sulfhemoglobinemia (cyanosis, fatigue), and, rarely, hepatic necrosis (gastrointestinal symptoms possibly followed by general obtundation) or nephropathy (cloudy urine due to cells, casts, organisms, sloughed tissue; edema of lower legs).

Caffeine: Usual doses of caffeine may cause gastric disturbances in some persons. Side effects are usually due to hyperresponsiveness or overdosage, acute or chronic. Toxic doses can cause nervousness, excitement, insomnia, muscle tenderness or tremors, tinnitus, scintillating scotomas, headache on withdrawal of the drug, diuresis, tachycardia and extrasystoles.

Drug Abuse and Dependence: Like other medications containing a narcotic analgesic, EMPRAZIL-C is controlled by the Drug Enforcement Administration and is classified under Schedule III.

EMPRAZIL-C can produce drug dependence of the morphine type, and therefore it has a potential for being abused. Psychic dependence, physical dependence and tolerance may develop on repeated administration.

The dependence liability of codeine has been found to be too small to permit a full definition of its characteristics. Studies indicate that addiction to codeine is extremely uncommon and requires very high parenteral doses.

When dependence on codeine occurs at therapeutic doses, it appears to require from one to two months to develop, and withdrawal symptoms are mild. Most patients on long-term oral codeine therapy show no signs of physical dependence upon abrupt withdrawal.

Overdosage: Severe intoxication, caused by overdose of EMPRAZIL-C may produce skin eruptions, dyspnea, vertigo, double vision, delusions, hallucinations, garbled speech, excitability, restlessness, delirium, constricted pupils, a positive Babinski sign, respiratory depression (slow and shallow breathing; Cheyne-Stokes respiration), cyanosis, clammy skin, muscle flaccidity, circulatory collapse, stupor and coma. In children, difficulty in hearing, tinnitus, dim vision, headache, dizziness, drowsiness, confusion, rapid breathing, sweating, thirst, nausea, vomiting, hyperpyrexia, dehydration and convulsions are prominent signs. The most severe manifestations from aspirin result from cardiovascular and respiratory insufficiency secondary to acid-base and electrolyte disturbances, complicated by hyperthermia and dehydration. The most severe manifestations from codeine are associated with respiratory depression.

Respiratory alkalosis is characteristic of the early phase of intoxication with aspirin while hyperventilation is occurring but is quickly followed by metabolic acidosis in most people with severe intoxication. This occurs more readily in children. Hypoglycemia may occur in children who have taken large overdoses. Other laboratory findings associated with aspirin intoxication include ketonuria, hyponatremia, hypokalemia, and occasionally proteinuria. A slight rise in lactic dehydrogenase and hydroxybutyric dehydrogenase may occur.

Hemolytic anemia due to phenacetin is possible and should be monitored by periodic laboratory tests.

Methemoglobin and sulfhemoglobin formation are seldom clinically significant in adults but may contribute to general toxicity. When prominent, they appear as a grayish cyanosis seen most clearly in the lips and nailbeds. Definitive diagnosis is made by spectroscopic analysis of a water-diluted (1:100) blood specimen, which shows an abnormal band at 630 m for methemoglobin and 618 m for sulfhemoglobin.

Concentrations of aspirin in plasma above 30 mg/100 ml are associated with toxicity. (See Clinical Pharmacology section for information on factors influencing aspirin blood levels.) The single lethal dose of aspirin in adults is probably about 25-30 g, but it is not known with certainty.

Toxic and lethal concentrations of phenacetin in human fluids are not known with certainty. Patient response per phenacetin dose may be greater than usual in infants, in patients with renal insufficiency or hepatic insufficiency and in those with a glucose-6-phosphate dehydrogenase deficiency or a decreased ability to convert phenacetin to acetaminophen. Toxic effects (e.g., sedation) have been seen with single doses of 2 g. The minimum lethal dose has been estimated to be 5-20 g, but adults have recovered from acute overdoses of 50-60 g.

Toxic and lethal concentrations of caffeine in human fluids are not known with certainty. Patient response per dose is increased in the presence of renal or hepatic insufficiency. Toxic manifestations may appear with a caffeine dose of 1 g. The single lethal dose in man is generally estimated to be over 10 g, but the lowest reported lethal dose was 3.2 g or 57 mg/kg.

The toxic plasma concentration of codeine is not known with certainty. Experimental production of mild to moderate CNS depression in healthy, nontolerant subjects occurred at plasma concentrations of 0.05-0.19 mg/100 ml when codeine was given by intravenous infusion. The single lethal dose of codeine in adults is estimated to be from 0.5-1.0 g. It is also estimated that 5 mg/kg could be fatal in children.

Hemodialysis and peritoneal dialysis can be performed to reduce the body aspirin content. Phenacetin is dialyzable, but dialysis of the drug and its major metabolite, acetaminophen, has not yet been established as an effective means of altering the consequence of acute phenacetin overdosage. Pseudoephedrine, caffeine and codeine are theoretically dialyzable, but the procedures have not been clinically established.

Overdosage with pseudoephedrine can cause excessive CNS stimulation associated with such manifestations as excitement, nervousness or anxiety, restlessness and insomnia. Other manifestations include tachycardia, hypertension, unusually intense pallor, mydriasis, hyperglycemia and urinary retention. Severe overdosage with sympathomimetic agents may cause greater CNS stimulation (tachypnea or hyperpnea, hallucinations, convulsions) or CNS depression (stupor, respiratory depression), arrhythmias, bradycardia, hypotension and circulatory collapse. No laboratory findings are of specific diagnostic value. No organ damage or significant metabolic derangement is associated with pseudoephedrine overdosage.

The mean LD_{50} (single oral dose) of pseudoephedrine is 726 mg/kg in the mouse, 2206 mg/kg in the rat, and 1177 mg/kg in the rabbit. The toxic and lethal concentrations in human biologic fluids are not known. Excretion rates increase with urine acidification and decrease with alkalinization.

Insufficient data are available to estimate toxic and lethal doses in man. Few reports of toxicity due to pseudoephedrine have been published, and no cases of fatal overdosage are known.

There is no specific antidote for pseudoephedrine. If instituted within one hour of overdosage, therapy is initially aimed at reducing further drug absorption by use of emetics and gastric lavage. If renal function is adequate, forced osmotic diuresis and acidification of urine with ammonium chloride will accelerate excretion of the drug.

Treatment of overdosage consists primarily of support of vital functions, management of codeine-induced respiratory depression, increasing salicylate elimination, and correcting the acid-base imbalance due primarily to salicylism.

In a comatose patient, primary attention should be given to establishment of adequate respiratory exchange through provisions of a patent airway and the institution of assisted or controlled ventilation. The narcotic antagonist naloxone is a specific antidote for respiratory depression which may result from overdose or unusual sensitivity to narcotics. Therefore, an appropriate dose of an antagonist should be administered preferably by the intravenous route, simultaneously with efforts at respiratory resuscitation. Since the duration of action of EMPRAZIL-C may exceed that of the antagonist, the patient should be kept under continued surveillance and repeated doses of the antagonist should be administered as needed to maintain adequate respiration.

A narcotic antagonist should not be administered in the absence of clinically significant respiratory or cardiovascular depression.

Gastric emptying (Syrup of Ipecac) and/or lavage is recommended as soon as possible after ingestion, even if the patient has vomited spontaneously. (Apomorphine should not be used as an emetic for EMPRAZIL-C, since it may potentiate hypotension and respiratory depression.) Administration of activated charcoal as a slurry is beneficial after lavage and/or emesis, if less than three hours have passed since ingestion. Charcoal adsorption should *not* be employed prior to emesis or lavage.

Severity of aspirin intoxication is determined by measuring the blood salicylate level. Acid-base status should be closely followed with serial blood gas and serum pH measurements. Fluid and electrolyte balance should also be regularly monitored.

A serum salicylate level of 30 mg/100 ml or higher indicates a need for enhanced salicylate excretion that can be achieved through body-fluid supplementation and urine alkalinization if renal function is normal. In mild intoxication, urine flow can be increased by forcing oral fluids and giving potassium citrate capsules. (DO NOT GIVE BICARBONATE BY MOUTH SINCE IT INCREASES THE RATE OF SALICYLATE ABSORPTION.)

In severe cases, hyperthermia and hypovolemia as well as respiratory depression, are the major immediate threats to life. Children should be sponged with tepid water. Replacement fluid should be administered intravenously and augmented with sufficient bicarbonate to correct acidosis and with monitoring

Continued on next page

Burroughs Wellcome—Cont.

of plasma electrolytes and pH, to promote alkaline diuresis of salicylate if renal function is normal. Complete control may also require infusion of glucose to control hypoglycemia.
Potassium deficiency may also be corrected through the infusion, once adequate urinary output is assured. Plasma or plasma expanders may be needed if fluid replacement is insufficient to maintain normal blood pressure or adequate urinary output.
In patients with renal insufficiency or in cases of life-threatening intoxication, dialysis is usually required. Peritoneal dialysis or exchange transfusion is indicated in infants and young children, and hemodialysis in older patients.
Oxygen, intravenous fluids, vasopressors and other supportive measures should be employed as needed.

Dosage and Administration: The recommended dosage for adults and children over 12 years of age is one or two tablets three times daily, as required. Dosage for children 6 through 12 years of age is one tablet three times daily, as required.
EMPRAZIL-C should be taken with food or a full glass of milk or water to lessen gastric distress.

How Supplied: White tablet with orange core imprinted "BW&CO."
Bottle of 100 NDC #0081-0303-55
Store at 15°-30°C (59°-86°F) in a dry place and protect from light.
[*Shown in Product Identification Section*]

FEDRAZIL® TABLETS

(See PDR for Nonprescription Drugs).

IMURAN® ℞

brand
Azathioprine Injection
(as the sodium salt)
equivalent to
100 mg azathioprine
sterile lyophilized material

An adjunct for the prevention of rejection in renal homotransplantation.

Caution: Imuran brand Azathioprine is a potent drug. In view of its hematopoietic toxicity, complete blood counts, including platelets, should be performed frequently. See below under WARNINGS.

Description: Imuran brand Azathioprine is an imidazolyl derivative of mercaptopurine and its action is similar to the latter drug. Chemically azathioprine is 6-[(1-methyl-4-nitro imidazol-5-yl)thio]purine. As the Sodium Salt of Imuran brand Azathioprine the drug is sufficiently soluble in water to make a 1.0 percent solution. Such a solution is stable for approximately two weeks when stored at temperatures between 59° and 86° F after which it undergoes increasing hydrolysis to form mercaptopurine. The compound is also split into mercaptopurine by sulfhydryl compounds such as cysteine, glutathione and hydrogen sulfide.

Action:

Metabolism: Following the intravenous administration of therapeutic doses of the Sodium Salt of Imuran to man (equivalent to 150–300 mg per day of azathioprine) the drug quickly leaves the circulation and very little unchanged drug is recovered in the urine. Azathioprine is split extensively to mercaptopurine, which is then subject to catabolic destruction to form a variety of oxidized and methylated derivatives, among which 6-thiouric acid predominates. The latter is formed by the oxidation of mercaptopurine by xanthine oxidase. The proportions of the different metabolites vary from individual to individual depending upon the relative amounts of the catabolic enzymes available. After eight hours there is little or no unchanged drug or mercaptopurine in the urine. A small portion (about 10 percent) of azathioprine is split *in vivo* between the sulfur and the purine ring to give 1-methyl-4-nitro-5-thioimidazole in which the sulfur is derived from the original molecule. Although elimination of azathioprine is mainly by metabolic destruction, small amounts of unchanged drug and mercaptopurine are eliminated by the kidney, and the biological effectiveness and toxicity may, therefore, be increased as much as twofold in the anuric patient. Imuran brand Azathioprine and mercaptopurine show moderate binding (about 30 percent) to serum proteins, but both the unchanged drug and its metabolic products appear to be dialyzable.
Blood levels of Imuran and of the mercaptopurine derived from it are extremely low (below 1 μg/ml) at therapeutic doses, as determined by studies with radio-active material. In any event, blood levels are of little or no predictive value, since the magnitude and duration of the clinical response cannot be predicted from the blood levels. The effects of this drug and its active metabolite, mercaptopurine, may appear long after clearance is complete.

Please see IMURAN® brand Azathioprine Tablets monograph for information on: Immunosuppressive Properties, Human Homotransplantation, Indications, Contraindications, Warnings, Precautions and Adverse Reactions.

Dosage: The intravenous administration of sodium salt of azathioprine has a particular advantage during the first 24–96 hours post-renal homotransplantation, during which time the patient may be unable to receive Imuran orally. As soon as the patient recovers sufficiently from the operation a transfer should be made to oral medication. The dosage of the Sodium Salt of Imuran brand Azathioprine which will be tolerated or will be effective will vary from patient to patient and, therefore, careful management is necessary to obtain the optimum therapeutic effect without incurring toxicity. Caution must be exercised to avoid toxicity, the chief manifestation of which is depression of the bone marrow, resulting most commonly in leukopenia and less often in thrombocytopenia and bleeding. SINCE THIS DRUG MAY HAVE A DELAYED ACTION, IT IS IMPORTANT TO REDUCE DOSAGE OR WITHDRAW THE MEDICATION TEMPORARILY AT THE FIRST SIGN OF AN ABNORMALLY LARGE FALL IN THE LEUKOCYTE COUNT AND/OR OTHER EVIDENCE OF PERSISTENT DEPRESSION OF THE BONE MARROW. The effect of renal failure on tolerance to azathioprine appears to be somewhat variable. Patients with impaired renal function may have slower elimination of the drug and its metabolites, with a consequent cumulative effect; therefore, the dosage may need to be appropriately reduced.
The usual initial post-renal transplantation dose is approximately 3–5 mg/kg per day of azathioprine administered intravenously. Adjunct therapy of various types has generally been used in suppressing rejection of renal homografts and this may add to the toxic potential of the regimen. Dosage must be adjusted to attempt to provide satisfactory maintenance of the homograft without producing toxic effects; it may be possible to reduce maintenance dosage to 1 to 2 mg/kg per day.

Preparation of Solution: Inject into the vial 10 ml sterile water for injection. Swirl the vial until solution results. The resultant solution should be used within 24 hours. It has an approximate pH of 9.6 and is for intravenous use only. For infusion, a further dilution may be made with sterile saline or glucose saline by withdrawing the appropriate dosage from the vial and transferring it aseptically to the infusion solution.

How Supplied: 20 ml vial (contains the equivalent of 100 mg azathioprine). Also available: Imuran® brand Azathioprine Tablets, 50 mg scored.

IMURAN® ℞

(Azathioprine)
50 mg Scored Tablets

20 ml vial (as the sodium salt) for I.V. injection, equivalent to 100 mg Azathioprine sterile lyophilized material.

> **Warning:** Chronic immunosuppression with this purine antimetabolite increases *risk of neoplasia* in humans. Physicians using this drug should be very familiar with this risk as well as with the mutagenic potential to both men and women and with possible hematologic toxicities. See below under WARNINGS.

Description: Azathioprine is chemically 6-[(1-methyl-4-nitro-imidazol-5-yl)thio] purine. It is an imidazolyl derivative of 6-mercaptopurine (Purinethol®) and many of its biological effects are similar to those of the parent compound.
Azathioprine is insoluble in water, but may be dissolved with addition of one molar equivalent of alkali. The sodium salt of azathioprine is sufficiently soluble to make a 10 mg/ml water solution which is stable for 24 hours at 59° to 86°F (15° to 30° C). Azathioprine is stable in solution at neutral or acid pH but hydrolysis to mercaptopurine occurs in excess sodium hydroxide (0.1N), especially on warming. Conversion to mercaptopurine also occurs in the presence of sulfhydryl compounds such as cysteine, glutathione and hydrogen sulfide.

Clinical Pharmacology and Actions

Metabolism[1]**:** Azathioprine is well absorbed following oral administration. Maximum serum radioactivity occurs at one to two hours after oral ^{35}S-azathioprine and decays with a half-life of five hours. This is not an estimate of the half-life of azathioprine itself but is the decay rate for all ^{35}S-containing metabolites of the drug. Because of extensive metabolism, only a fraction of the radioactivity is present as azathioprine. Usual doses produce blood levels of azathioprine, and of mercaptopurine derived from it, which are low (<1 mcg/ml). Blood levels are of little predictive value for therapy since the magnitude and duration of clinical effects correlate with thiopurine nucleotide levels in tissues rather than with plasma drug levels. Azathioprine and mercaptopurine are moderately bound to serum proteins (30%) and are partially dialyzable.
Azathioprine is cleaved *in vivo* to mercaptopurine. Both compounds are rapidly eliminated from blood and are oxidized or methylated in erythrocytes and liver, no azathioprine or mercaptopurine is detectable in urine after eight hours. Conversion to inactive 6-thiouric acid by xanthine oxidase is an important degradative pathway, and the inhibition of this pathway in patients receiving allopurinol (Zyloprim®) is the basis for the azathioprine dosage reduction required in these patients (see DOSAGE AND ADMINISTRATION). Proportions of metabolites are different in individual patients, and this presumably accounts for variable magnitude and duration of drug effects. Renal clearance is probably not important in predicting biological effectiveness or toxicities, although dose reduction is practiced in patients with poor renal function.

Homograft Survival[1,2]**:** Summary information from transplant centers and registries indicates relatively universal use of Imuran® with or without other immunosuppressive agents.[3,4,5] Although the use of azathioprine for inhibition of renal homograft rejection is well established, the mechanism(s) for this action are somewhat obscure. The drug suppresses hypersensitivities of the cell-mediated type and causes variable alterations in antibody production. Suppression of T-cell effects, including ablation of T-cell suppression, is dependent on the temporal relationship to antigenic stimulus or engraftment. This agent has little effect on established graft rejections or secondary responses.

Alterations in specific immune responses or immunologic functions in transplant recipients are difficult to relate specifically to immunosuppression by azathioprine. These patients have subnormal responses to vaccines, low numbers of T-cells, and abnormal phagocytosis by peripheral blood cells, but their mitogenic responses, serum immunoglobulins and secondary antibody responses are usually normal. Transplant recipients on azathioprine also receive corticosteroids and may be given antilymphocyte globulin; there are no known hazards or toxicities due to interactions of these agents.

Immunoinflammatory Response: Azathioprine suppresses disease manifestations as well as underlying pathology in animal models of auto-immune disease. For example, the severity of adjuvant arthritis is reduced by azathioprine.

The mechanisms whereby azathioprine affects auto-immune diseases are not known. Azathioprine is immunosuppressive, delayed hypersensitivity and cellular cytotoxicity tests being suppressed to a greater degree than are antibody responses. In the rat model of adjuvant arthritis, azathioprine has been shown to inhibit the lymph node hyperplasia which precedes the onset of the signs of the disease. Both the immunosuppressive and therapeutic effects in animal models are dose-related. Azathioprine is considered a slow acting drug and effects may persist after the drug has been discontinued.

Indications and Usage: Imuran® is indicated as an adjunct for the prevention of rejection in renal homotransplantation. It is also indicated for the management of severe, active rheumatoid arthritis unresponsive to rest, aspirin or other nonsteroidal anti-inflammatory drugs, or to agents in the class of which gold is an example.

Renal Homotransplantation: Imuran is indicated as an adjunct for the prevention of rejection in renal homotransplantation. Experience with over 16,000 transplants shows a five-year patient survival of 35% to 55%, but this is dependent on donor, match for HLA antigens, anti-donor or anti B-cell alloantigen antibody and other variables. The effect of Imuran on these variables has not been tested in controlled trials.

Rheumatoid Arthritis[6,7]: Imuran is indicated only in adult patients meeting criteria for classic or definite rheumatoid arthritis as specified by the American Rheumatism Association[8]. Imuran should be restricted to patients with severe, active and erosive disease not responsive to conventional management including rest, aspirin or other non-steroidal drugs or to agents in the class of which gold is an example. Rest, physiotherapy and salicylates should be continued while Imuran is given, but it may be possible to reduce the dose of corticosteroids in patients on Imuran. The combined use of Imuran with gold, antimalarials or penicillamine has not been studied for either added benefit or unexpected adverse effects. The use of Imuran with these agents cannot be recommended.

Contraindications: Imuran should not be given to patients who have shown hypersensitivity to the drug.

Imuran should not be used for treating rheumatoid arthritis in pregnant women.

Patients with rheumatoid arthritis previously treated with alkylating agents (cyclophosphamide, chlorambucil, melphalan or others) may have a prohibitive risk of neoplasia if treated with Imuran.

Warnings: Severe *leukopenia and/or thrombocytopenia* may occur in patients on Imuran. Macrocytic anemia and severe bone marrow depression may also occur. Hematologic toxicities are dose related and may be more severe in renal transplant patients whose homograft is undergoing rejection. It is suggested that patients on Imuran have complete blood counts, including platelet counts, weekly during the first month, twice monthly for the second and third months of treatment, then monthly or more frequently if dosage alterations or other therapy changes are necessary. Delayed hematologic suppression may occur. Prompt reduction in dosage or temporary withdrawal of the drug may be necessary if there is a rapid fall in, or persistently low leukocyte count or other evidence of bone marrow depression. Leukopenia does not correlate with therapeutic effect, therefore the dose should not be increased intentionally to lower the white blood cell count.

Serious infections are a constant hazard for patients on chronic immunosuppression, especially for homograft recipients. Fungal, viral, bacterial and protozoal infections may be fatal and should be treated vigorously. Reduction of azathioprine dosage and/or use of other drugs should be considered.

Imuran® is mutagenic in animals and humans, carcinogenic in animals, and may increase the patient's *risk of neoplasia.* Renal transplant patients are known to have an increased risk of malignancy, predominantly skin cancer and reticulum cell or lymphomatous tumors.[9] Information is available on the spontaneous neoplasia risk in Rheumatoid Arthritis[11], and on neoplasia following immunosuppressive therapy of other autoimmune diseases[12]. It has not been possible to define the precise risk of neoplasia due to Imuran[10], but the risk is lower for patients with rheumatoid arthritis than for transplant recipients. However, acute myelogenous leukemia as well as solid tumors have been reported in patients with rheumatoid arthritis who have received azathioprine. Data on neoplasia in patients receiving Imuran can be found under Adverse Reactions.

Pregnancy Warning[13]: Imuran should not be given during pregnancy without careful weighing of risk versus benefit. Whenever possible, use of Imuran in pregnant patients should be avoided.

Imuran has been shown to be mutagenic in both male and female animals. Chromosomal abnormalities have also been documented in patients, however, the abnormalities in humans were reversed upon discontinuance of the drug.[14]

Imuran is teratogenic in rodents. Transplacental transmission of azathioprine and its metabolites has been reported in man.[15] Limited immunologic and other abnormalities have occurred in some infants born of renal homograft recipients on Imuran. Benefit versus risk must be weighed carefully before use of Imuran in patients of reproductive potential. This drug should not be used for treating rheumatoid arthritis in pregnant women.

Precautions: Patient information: Patients being started on Imuran should be informed of the necessity of periodic blood counts while they are receiving the drug and should be encouraged to report any unusual bleeding or bruising to their physician. They should be advised of the danger of infection while receiving Imuran and encouraged to report signs and symptoms of infection to their physician. Careful dosage instructions should be given to the patient, especially when Imuran is being administered in the presence of impaired renal function or concomitantly with allopurinol (see DOSAGE AND ADMINISTRATION). Patients should be advised of the potential risks of the use of Imuran during pregnancy and during the nursing period. The increased risk of neoplasia following Imuran therapy should be explained to the patient.

Adverse Reactions: The principal and potentially serious toxic effects of Imuran® are hematologic and gastrointestinal. The risks of secondary infection and neoplasia are also important. The frequency and severity of adverse reactions depend on the dose and duration of Imuran as well as on the patient's underlying disease or concomitant therapies. The incidence of hematologic toxicities and neoplasia encountered in groups of renal homograft recipients is significantly higher than that in studies employing Imuran for rheumatoid arthritis. The relative incidences in clinical studies are summarized below:

Toxicity	*Renal Homograft*	*Rheumatoid Arthritis*
Leukopenia		
Any Degree	< 50%	28 %
$< 2500/mm^3$	16%	5.3%
Neoplasia		
Lymphoma	0.5%	
Others	2.8%	

*18 reported cases; denominator unknown.

Hematologic: Leukopenia and/or thrombocytopenia are dose dependent and may occur late in the course of Imuran therapy. Dose reduction or temporary withdrawal allows reversal of these toxicities. Infection may occur as a secondary manifestation of bone marrow suppression or leukopenia, but the incidence of infection in renal homotransplantation is 30 to 60 times that in rheumatoid arthritis. Macrocytic anemia and/or bleeding have been reported in two patients on Imuran.

Gastrointestinal: Nausea and vomiting may occur within the first few months of Imuran therapy, and occurred in approximately 12% of 676 rheumatoid arthritis patients. The frequency of gastric disturbance can be reduced by administration of the drug in divided doses and/or after meals. Vomiting with abdominal pain may occur rarely with a hypersensitivity pancreatitis. Hepatotoxicity with elevated serum alkaline phosphatase and bilirubin is known to occur with thiopurines including Imuran and 6-mercaptopurine (Purinethol®). This toxic hepatitis with biliary stasis is known to occur in homograft recipients and has been generally reversible after interruption of Imuran. Hepatotoxicity has been uncommon in rheumatoid arthritis patients on Imuran (less than 1%).

Others: Additional side effects of low frequency have been reported. These include skin rashes (approximately 2%), alopecia, fever, arthralgias, diarrhea, steatorrhea and negative nitrogen balance (all less than 1%).

Dosage and Administration: Renal Homotransplantation: The dose of Imuran® required to prevent rejection and minimize toxicity will vary with individual patients; this necessitates careful management. Initial dose is usually 3 to 5 mg/kg daily, beginning at the time of transplant. Imuran is usually given as a single daily dose on the day of, and in a minority of cases one to three days before, transplantation. Imuran is often initiated with the intravenous administration of the sodium salt, with subsequent use of tablets (at the same dose level) after the post-operative period. Intravenous administration of the sodium salt is indicated only in patients unable to tolerate oral medications. Dose reduction to maintenance levels of 1 to 3 mg/kg daily is usually possible. The dose of Imuran should not be increased to toxic levels because of threatened rejection. Discontinuation may be necessary for severe hematologic or other toxicity, even if rejection of the homograft may be a consequence of drug withdrawal.

Rheumatoid Arthritis: Imuran is usually given on a daily basis. The initial dose should be approximately 1.0 mg/kg (50 to 100 mg) given as a single dose or on a twice daily schedule. The dose may be increased, beginning at six to eight weeks and thereafter by steps at four-week intervals, if there are no serious toxicities and if initial response is unsatisfactory. Dose increments should be 0.5 mg/kg daily, up to a

Continued on next page

Burroughs Wellcome—Cont.

maximum dose of 2.5 mg/kg/day. Therapeutic response occurs after several weeks of treatment, usually six to eight; an adequate trial should be a minimum of 12 weeks. Patients not improved after twelve weeks can be considered refractory. Imuran may be continued long-term in patients with clinical response, but patients should be monitored carefully, and gradual dosage reduction should be attempted to reduce risk of toxicities. Maintenance therapy should be at the lowest effective dose, and the dose given can be lowered incrementally with changes of 0.5 mg/kg or approximately 25 mg daily every four weeks while other therapy is kept constant. The optimum duration of maintenance Imuran has not been determined. Imuran can be discontinued abruptly, but delayed effects are possible.

Use in Renal Dysfunction: Relatively oliguric patients, especially those with tubular necrosis in the immediate post-cadaveric transplant period, may have delayed clearance of Imuran or its metabolites, may be particularly sensitive to this drug and may require lower doses.

Use with Allopurinol (Zyloprim®): The principal pathway for detoxification of Imuran is inhibited by allopurinol (Zyloprim). Patients receiving Imuran and Zyloprim concomitantly should have a dose reduction of Imuran, to approximately 1/3 to 1/4 the usual dose.

Parenteral Administration: Add 10 ml of sterile Water for Injection, and swirl until a clear solution results. This solution is for intravenous use only; it has a pH of approximately 9.6, and it should be used within twenty-four hours. Further dilution into sterile saline or dextrose is usually made for infusion; the final volume depends on time for the infusion, usually 30-60 minutes but as short as 5 minutes and as long as 8 hours for the daily dose.

How Supplied: 50 mg yellow, scored tablets imprinted with "IMURAN" and "K7A" on each tablet; bottle of 100.

20 ml vial containing the equivalent of 100 mg azathioprine (as the sodium salt). The sterile, lyophilized sodium salt is yellow, and should be dissolved in sterile Water for Injection (see Parenteral Administration under DOSAGE AND ADMINISTRATION).

References:

1. Elion, G.B. and G.H. Hitchings, "Azathioprine" in *Handbook of Experimental Pharmacology,* Vol. 38, ed. by Sartorelli and Johns, Springer Verlag, New York, 1975.
2. McIntosh, J., P. Hansen *et al.,* "Defective Immune and Phagocytic Functions in Uremia and Renal Transplantation," *Int. Arch. Allergy Appl. Immunol.,* 51:544–559, 1976.
3. Advisory Committee, Renal Transplant Registry, "The 12th Report of the Human Renal Transplant Registry," *JAMA,* 233:787–796, 1975.
4. McGeown, M., "Immunosuppression for Kidney Transplantation," *Lancet,* ii:310—312, 1973.
5. Simmons, R.L., E.J. Thompson *et al.,* "115 Patients with First Cadaver Kidney Transplants Followed Two to Seven and a Half Years," *Am. J. Med.,* 62:234–242, 1977.
6. Fye, K. and N. Talal, "Cytotoxic Drugs in the Treatment of Rheumatoid Arthritis," *Ration. Drug Ther., 9*(4): 1–5, 1975.
7. Davis, J.D., H.B. Muss, and R.A. Turner, "Cytotoxic Agents in the Treatment of Rheumatoid Arthritis," *South. Med. J., 71* (1): 58–64, 1978.
8. McEwen, C., "The Diagnosis and Differential Diagnosis of Rheumatoid Arthritis," *Arthritis and Allied Conditions,* Philadelphia, Lea and Febiger, pp. 403–418, 1972.
9. Hoover, R. and J.F. Fraumeni, "Risk of Cancer in Renal Transplant Recipients," *Lancet,* 2:55–57, 1973.
10. Sieber, S.M. and R.H. Adamson, "Toxicity of Antineoplastic Agents in Man," *Adv. Cancer Res.,* 22:57–155, 1975.
11. Lewis, R.B., C.W. Castor, R.E. Knisley, and G.C. Bole, "Frequency of Neoplasia in Systemic Lupus Erythematosus and Rheumatoid Arthritis," *Arthritis Rheum., 19*(6): 1256–1260, 1976.
12. Louie, S. and R.S. Schwartz, "Immunodeficiency and the Pathogenesis of Lymphoma and Leukemia," *Semin. Hematol., 15*(2): 117–138, 1978.
13. Tagatz, G.E. and R.L. Simmons, "Pregnancy After Renal Transplantation," *Ann. Intern. Med.,* 82:113–114, 1975 (Editorial).
14. Hunter, T., M.B. Urowitz, D.A. Gordon, H.A. Smythe and M.A. Ogryzlo, Azathioprine in Rheumatoid Arthritis. A Long-Term Follow-Up Study, Arthritis Rheum., *18*(1): 15–20, 1975.
15. Saarikoski, S. and M. Sepalla, Immunosuppressive During Pregnancy: Transmission of Azathioprine and its Metabolites from the Mother to the Fetus, Am. J. Obstet. Gynecol., *115*(8): 1100–1106, 1973.

[*Shown in Product Identification Section*]

KEMADRIN® ℞
brand Procyclidine Hydrochloride

Description: 1-cyclohexyl-1-phenyl-3-pyrrolidinopropan-1-ol hydrochloride. Developed in The Wellcome Research Laboratories.

Indications: Kemadrin brand Procyclidine Hydrochloride is indicated for the treatment of parkinsonism including the postencephalitic, arteriosclerotic and idiopathic types. Partial control of the parkinsonism symptoms is the usual therapeutic accomplishment. Procyclidine hydrochloride is usually more efficacious in the relief of rigidity than tremor; but tremor, fatigue, weakness and sluggishness are frequently beneficially influenced. It can be substituted for all previous medications in mild and moderate cases. For the control of more severe cases other drugs may be added to procyclidine therapy as indications warrant.

Clinical reports indicate that procyclidine often successfully relieves the symptoms of extrapyramidal dysfunction (dystonia, dyskinesia, akathisia and parkinsonism) which accompany the therapy of mental disorders with phenothiazine and rauwolfia compounds. In addition to minimizing the symptoms induced by tranquilizing drugs, the drug effectively controls sialorrhea resulting from neuroleptic medication. At the same time freedom from the side effects induced by tranquilizer drugs, as provided by the administration of procyclidine, permits a more sustained treatment of the patient's mental disorder.

Clinical results in the treatment of parkinsonism indicate that most patients experience subjective improvement characterized by a feeling of well-being and increased alertness, together with diminished salivation and a marked improvement in muscular coordination as demonstrated by objective tests of manual dexterity and by increased ability to carry out ordinary self-care activities. While the drug exerts a mild atropine-like action and therefore causes mydriasis, this may be kept minimal by careful adjustment of the daily dosage.

Contraindications: Procyclidine hydrochloride should not be used in angle-closure glaucoma although simple type glaucomas do not appear to be adversely affected.

Warnings:

Use in Children

Safety and efficacy have not been established in the pediatric age group; therefore, the use of procyclidine hydrochloride in this age group requires that the potential benefits be weighed against the possible hazards to the child.

Pregnancy Warning

The safe use of this drug in pregnancy has not been established; therefore, the use of procyclidine hydrochloride in pregnancy, lactation or in women of childbearing age requires that the potential benefits be weighed against the possible hazards to the mother and child.

Precautions: Conditions in which inhibition of the parasympathetic nervous system is undesirable such as tachycardia and urinary retention (such as may occur with marked prostatic hypertrophy) require special care in the administration of the drug. Hypotensive patients who receive the drug should be observed closely. Occasionally, particularly in older patients, mental confusion and disorientation may occur with the development of agitation, hallucinations and psychotic-like symptoms.

Patients with mental disorders occasionally experience a precipitation of a psychotic episode when the dosage of antiparkinsonism drugs is increased to treat the extrapyramidal side effects of phenothiazine and rauwolfia derivatives.

Adverse Reactions: Anticholinergic effects can be produced by therapeutic doses although these can frequently be minimized or eliminated by careful dosage. They include: dryness of the mouth, mydriasis, blurring of vision, giddiness, light headedness and gastrointestinal disturbances such as nausea, vomiting, epigastric distress and constipation. Occasionally an allergic reaction such as a skin rash may be encountered. Feelings of muscular weakness may occur. Acute suppurative parotitis as a complication of dry mouth has been reported.

Dosage and Administration:

For Parkinsonism

The dosage of the drug for the treatment of parkinsonism depends upon the age of the patient, the etiology of the disease, and individual responsiveness. Therefore, the dosage must remain flexible to permit adjustment to the individual tolerance and requirements of each patient. In general, younger and postencephalitic patients require and tolerate a somewhat higher dosage than older patients and those with arteriosclerosis.

For Patients Who Have Received No Other Therapy

The usual dose of procyclidine hydrochloride for initial treatment is 2 to 2.5 mg administered three times daily after meals. If well tolerated, this dose may be gradually increased to 4 to 5 mg three times a day and occasionally 4 to 5 mg given before retiring. In some cases smaller doses may be employed with good therapeutic results.

Occasionally a patient is encountered who cannot tolerate a bedtime dose of the drug. In such cases it may be desirable to adjust dosage so that the bedtime dose is omitted and the total daily requirement is administered in three equal daytime doses. It is best administered during or after meals to minimize the development of side reactions.

To Transfer Patients to Kemadrin brand Procyclidine Hydrochloride from Other Therapy

Patients who have been receiving other drugs may be transferred to procyclidine hydrochloride. This is accomplished gradually by substituting 2 to 2.5 mg three times a day for all or part of the original drug. The dose of procyclidine is then increased as required while that of the other drug is correspondingly omitted or decreased until complete replacement is achieved. The total daily dosage may then be adjusted to the level which produces maximum benefit.

For Drug-Induced Extrapyramidal Symptoms

For treatment of symptoms of extrapyramidal dysfunction induced by tranquilizer drugs during the therapy of mental disorders, the dosage of procyclidine hydrochloride will depend on the severity of side effects associated with tranquilizer administration. In general the larger the dosage of the tranquilizer the more severe will be the associated symptoms, including rigidity and tremors. Accordingly, the drug dosage should be adjusted to suit the needs of the individual patient and to provide maximum relief of the induced symptoms. A convenient method to establish the daily dosage of procyclidine is to begin with the administration of 2 to 2.5 mg three times daily. This may be increased by 2 to 2.5 mg daily increments until the patient obtains relief of symptoms. In most cases excellent results will be obtained with 10 to 20 mg daily.

How Supplied: Scored tablets of 2 mg and 5 mg, bottles of 100. 2 mg tablet bears Wellcome I.D. code imprint, F4B.

[*Shown in Product Identification Section*]

LANOXICAPS® ℞

(Digoxin Solution in Capsules)
50 μg (0.05 mg) I.D. Imprint A2C (red)
100 μg (0.1 mg) I.D. Imprint B2C (yellow)
200 μg (0.2 mg) I.D. Imprint C2C (green)

Description: Digoxin is one of the cardiac (or digitalis) glycosides, a closely related group of drugs having in common specific effects on the myocardium. These drugs are found in a number of plants. Digoxin is extracted from the leaves of *Digitalis lanata*. The term "digitalis" is used to designate the whole group. The glycosides are composed of two portions: a sugar and a cardenolide (hence "glycosides").

Digoxin has the empirical formula $C_{41}H_{64}O_{14}$, a molecular weight of 780.96 and melting and decomposition points above 235°C. The drug is practically insoluble in water and in ether; slightly soluble in diluted (50%) alcohol and in chloroform; and freely soluble in pyridine. Digoxin powder is composed of odorless white crystals.

Digoxin has the chemical name: 3β-[(0-2.6-dideoxy-β-D-ribo-hexopyranosyl-(1→4)-0-2,6-dideoxy-β-D-ribo-hexopyranosyl-(1→4)-2,6-dideoxy-β-D-ribo-hexopyranosyl)oxy]-12β, 14-dihydroxy-5β-card-20(22)-enolide, and the structure shown:

Lanoxicaps is a stable solution of digoxin enclosed within a soft gelatin capsule for oral use. Each capsule contains the labeled amount of digoxin USP dissolved in a solvent comprised of polyethylene glycol 400 USP, 8 percent ethyl alcohol, propylene glycol USP and purified water USP.

Clinical Pharmacology:

Mechanism of Action: The influence of digitalis glycosides on the myocardium is dose-related, and involves both a direct action on cardiac muscle and the specialized conduction system, and indirect actions on the cardiovascular system mediated by the autonomic nervous system. The indirect actions mediated by the autonomic nervous system involve a vagomimetic action, which is responsible for the effects of digitalis on the sino-atrial (SA) and atrioventricular (AV) nodes; and also a baroreceptor sensitization which results in increased carotid sinus nerve activity and enhanced sympathetic withdrawal for any given increment in mean arterial pressure. The pharmacologic consequences of these direct and indirect effects are: 1) an increase in the force and velocity of myocardial systolic contraction (positive inotropic action); 2) a slowing of heart rate (negative chronotropic effect); and 3) decreased conduction velocity through the AV node. In higher doses, digitalis increases sympathetic outflow from the central nervous system (CNS) to both cardiac and peripheral sympathetic nerves. This increase in sympathetic activity may be an important factor in digitalis cardiac toxicity. Most of the extracardiac manifestations of digitalis toxicity are also mediated by the CNS.

PRODUCT	BIOAVAILABILITY	EQUIVALENT DOSES (IN MG)*		
Lanoxin® Tablet	60–80%	0.125	0.25	0.5
Lanoxin Elixir	70–85%	0.125	0.25	0.5
Lanoxin Injection/IM	70–85%	0.125	0.25	0.5
Lanoxin Injection/IV	100%	0.1	0.2	0.4
Lanoxicaps Capsules	90–100%	0.1	0.2	0.4

*1 mg = 1000 μg

Pharmacokinetics:

Absorption—Gastrointestinal absorption of digoxin is a passive process. Absorption of digoxin from Lanoxicaps capsules has been demonstrated to be 90 to 100% complete compared to an identical intravenous dose of digoxin. Conventional digoxin tablets are absorbed 60 to 80%. The enhanced absorption from Lanoxicaps compared to digoxin tablets and elixir is associated with reduced between-patient and within-patient variability in steady-state serum concentrations. The peak serum concentrations are higher than those observed after tablets. When digoxin tablets or capsules are taken after meals, the rate of absorption is slowed, but the total amount of digoxin absorbed is usually unchanged. When taken with meals high in bran fiber, however, the amount absorbed from an oral dose may be reduced. Comparisons of the systemic availability and equivalent doses for digoxin preparations are shown in the following table:

[See table above].

Distribution—Following drug administration, a 6 to 8 hour distribution phase is observed. This is followed by a much more gradual serum concentration decline, which is dependent on digoxin elimination from the body. The peak height and slope of the early portion (absorption/distribution phases) of the serum concentration-time curve are dependent upon the route of administration and the absorption characteristics of the formulation. Clinical evidence indicates that the early high serum concentrations (particularly high for digoxin capsules) do not reflect the concentration of digoxin at its site of action, but that with chronic use, the steady-state post-distribution serum levels are in equilibrium with tissue levels and correlate with pharmacologic effects. In individual patients, these post-distribution serum concentrations are linearly related to maintenance dosage and may be useful in evaluating therapeutic and toxic effects (see Serum Digoxin Concentrations in DOSAGE AND ADMINISTRATION section).

Digoxin is concentrated in tissues and therefore has a large apparent volume of distribution. Digoxin crosses both the blood-brain barrier and the placenta. At delivery, serum digoxin concentration in the newborn is similar to the serum level in the mother. Approximately 20 to 25% of plasma digoxin is bound to protein. Serum digoxin concentrations are not significantly altered by large changes in fat tissue weight, so that its distribution space correlates best with lean (ideal) body weight, not total body weight.

Pharmacologic Response—The approximate times to onset of effect and to peak effect of all the Lanoxin and Lanoxicaps preparations are given in the following table:

[See table below].

Excretion—Elimination of digoxin follows first-order kinetics (that is, the quantity of digoxin eliminated at any time is proportional to the total body content). Following intravenous administration to normal subjects, 50 to 70% of a digoxin dose is excreted unchanged in the urine. Renal excretion of digoxin is proportional to glomerular filtration rate and is largely independent of urine flow. In subjects with normal renal function, digoxin has a half-life of 1.5 to 2.0 days. The half-life in anuric patients is prolonged to 4 to 6 days. Digoxin is not effectively removed from the body by dialysis, exchange transfusion or during cardiopulmonary by-pass because most of the drug is in tissue rather than circulating in the blood.

Indications and Usage:

Heart Failure: The increased cardiac output resulting from the inotropic action of digoxin ameliorates the disturbances characteristic of heart failure (venous congestion, edema, dyspnea, orthopnea and cardiac asthma).

Digoxin is more effective in "low output" (pump) failure than in "high output" heart failure secondary to arteriovenous fistula, anemia, infection or hyperthyroidism.

Digoxin is usually continued after failure is controlled, unless some known precipitating factor is corrected. Studies have shown, however, that even though hemodynamic effects can be demonstrated in almost all patients, corresponding improvement in the signs and symptoms of heart failure is not necessarily apparent. Therefore, in patients in whom digoxin may be difficult to regulate, or in whom the risk of toxicity may be great (e.g., patients with unstable renal function or whose potassium levels tend to fluctuate) a cautious withdrawal of digoxin may be considered. If digoxin is discontinued, the patient should be regularly monitored by clinical evidence of recurrent heart failure.

Atrial Fibrillation: Digoxin reduces ventricular rate and thereby improves hemodynamics. Palpitation, precordial distress or weakness are relieved and concomitant congestive failure ameliorated. Digoxin should be continued in doses necessary to maintain the desired ventricular rate.

Atrial Flutter: Digoxin slows the heart and regular sinus rhythm may appear. Frequently the flutter is converted to atrial fibrillation with a controlled ventricular response. Digoxin treatment should be maintained if atrial fibrillation persists. (Electrical cardioversion is

PRODUCT	TIME TO ONSET OF EFFECT*	TIME TO PEAK EFFECT*
Lanoxin® Tablet	0.5–2 hours	2–6 hours
Lanoxin Elixir	0.5–2 hours	2–6 hours
Lanoxin Injection/IM	0.5–2 hours	2–6 hours
Lanoxin Injection/IV	5–30 minutes†	1–4 hours
Lanoxicaps Capsules	0.5–2 hours	2–6 hours

*Documented for ventricular response rate in atrial fibrillation, inotropic effect and electrocardiographic changes.
†Depending upon rate of infusion.

Continued on next page

Burroughs Wellcome—Cont.

often the treatment of choice for atrial flutter. See discussion of cardioversion in PRECAUTIONS section.)

Paroxysmal Atrial Tachycardia (PAT): Digoxin may convert PAT to sinus rhythm by slowing conduction through the AV node. If heart failure has ensued or paroxysms recur frequently, digoxin should be continued. In infants, digoxin is usually continued for 3 to 6 months after a single episode of PAT to prevent recurrence.

Contraindications: Digitalis glycosides are contraindicated in ventricular fibrillation.

In a given patient, an untoward effect requiring permanent discontinuation of other digitalis preparations usually constitutes a contraindication to digoxin. Hypersensitivity to digoxin itself is a contraindication to its use. Allergy to digoxin, though rare, does occur. It may not extend to all such preparations, and another digitalis glycoside may be tried with caution.

Warnings: Digitalis alone or with other drugs has been used in the treatment of obesity. This use of digoxin or other digitalis glycosides is unwarranted. Moreover, since they may cause potentially fatal arrhythmias or other adverse effects, the use of these drugs solely for the treatment of obesity is dangerous.

It is recommended that digoxin in soft capsules be administered in divided daily doses to minimize any potential adverse reactions, since peak serum digoxin concentrations resulting from the capsules are approximately twice those after bioequivalent tablet doses (400 μg of Lanoxicaps are bioequivalent to 500 μg of tablets). Studies are underway to determine if there are any increased risks associated with the higher peaks that occur with single daily dosing of soft gelatin capsules.

Anorexia, nausea, vomiting and arrhythmias may accompany heart failure or may be indications of digitalis intoxication. Clinical evaluation of the cause of these symptoms should be attempted before further digitalis administration. In such circumstances determination of the serum digoxin concentration may be an aid in deciding whether or not digitalis toxicity is likely to be present. If the possibility of digitalis intoxication cannot be excluded, cardiac glycosides should be temporarily withheld, if permitted by the clinical situation.

Patients with renal insufficiency require smaller than usual maintenance doses of digoxin (see DOSAGE AND ADMINISTRATION section).

Heart failure accompanying acute glomerulonephritis requires extreme care in digitalization. Relatively low loading and maintenance doses and concomitant use of antihypertensive drugs may be necessary and careful monitoring is essential. Digoxin should be discontinued as soon as possible.

Patients with severe carditis, such as carditis associated with rheumatic fever or viral myocarditis, are especially sensitive to digoxin-induced disturbances of rhythm.

Newborn infants display considerable variability in their tolerance to digoxin. Premature and immature infants are particularly sensitive, and dosage must not only be reduced but must be individualized according to their degree of maturity.

Note: Digitalis glycosides are an important cause of accidental poisoning in children.

Precautions:

General: Digoxin toxicity develops more frequently and lasts longer in patients with renal impairment because of the decreased excretion of digoxin. Therefore, it should be anticipated that dosage requirements will be decreased in patients with moderate to severe renal disease (see DOSAGE AND ADMINISTRATION section). Because of the prolonged half-life, a longer period of time is required to achieve an initial or new steady-state concentration in patients with renal impairment than in patients with normal renal function.

In patients with hypokalemia, toxicity may occur despite serum digoxin concentrations within the "normal range", because potassium depletion sensitizes the myocardium to digoxin. Therefore, it is desirable to maintain normal serum potassium levels in patients being treated with digoxin. Hypokalemia may result from diuretic, amphotericin B or corticosteroid therapy, and from dialysis or mechanical suction of gastrointestinal secretions. It may also accompany malnutrition, diarrhea, prolonged vomiting, old age and long-standing heart failure. In general, rapid changes in serum potassium or other electrolytes should be avoided, and intravenous treatment with potassium should be reserved for special circumstances as described below (see TREATMENT OF ARRHYTHMIAS PRODUCED BY OVERDOSAGE section).

Calcium, particularly when administered rapidly by the intravenous route, may produce serious arrhythmias in digitalized patients. Hypercalcemia from any cause predisposes the patient to digitalis toxicity. On the other hand, hypocalcemia can nullify the effects of digoxin in man; thus, digoxin may be ineffective until serum calcium is restored to normal. These interactions are related to the fact that calcium affects contractility and excitability of the heart in a manner similar to digoxin.

Hypomagnesemia may predispose to digitalis toxicity. If low magnesium levels are detected in a patient on digoxin, replacement therapy should be instituted.

Quinidine causes a rise in serum digoxin concentration, with the implication that digitalis intoxication may result. This rise appears to be proportional to the quinidine dose. Interestingly, both the digoxin clearance and the volume of distribution are reduced, so that the serum half-life may not change. Because of the considerable variability of this interaction, digoxin dosage should be carefully individualized.

Patients with acute myocardial infarction or severe pulmonary disease may be unusually sensitive to digoxin-induced disturbances of rhythm.

Atrial arrhythmias associated with hypermetabolic states (e.g. hyperthyroidism) are particularly resistant to digoxin treatment. Large doses of digoxin are not recommended as the only treatment of these arrhythmias and care must be taken to avoid toxicity if large doses of digoxin are required. In hypothyroidism, the digoxin requirements are reduced. Digoxin responses in patients with compensated thyroid disease are normal.

Reduction of digoxin dosage may be desirable prior to electrical cardioversion to avoid induction of ventricular arrhythmias, but the physician must consider the consequences of rapid increase in ventricular response to atrial fibrillation if digoxin is withheld 1 to 2 days prior to cardioversion. If there is a suspicion that digitalis toxicity exists, elective cardioversion should be delayed. If it is not prudent to delay cardioversion, the energy level selected should be minimal at first and carefully increased in an attempt to avoid precipitating ventricular arrhythmias.

Incomplete AV block, especially in patients with Stokes-Adams attacks, may progress to advanced or complete heart block if digoxin is given.

In some patients with sinus node disease (i.e. Sick Sinus Syndrome), digoxin may worsen sinus bradycardia or sino-atrial block.

In patients with Wolff-Parkinson-White Syndrome and atrial fibrillation, digoxin can enhance transmission of impulses through the accessory pathway. This effect may result in extremely rapid ventricular rates and even ventricular fibrillation.

Digoxin may worsen the outflow obstruction in patients with idiopathic hypertrophic subaortic stenosis (IHSS). Unless cardiac failure is severe, it is doubtful whether digoxin should be employed.

Patients with chronic constrictive pericarditis may fail to respond to digoxin. In addition, slowing of the heart rate by digoxin in some patients may further decrease cardiac output.

Patients with heart failure from amyloid heart disease or constrictive cardiomyopathies respond poorly to treatment with digoxin.

Digoxin is not indicated for the treatment of sinus tachycardia unless it is associated with heart failure.

Intramuscular injection of digoxin is extremely painful and offers no advantages unless other routes of administration are contraindicated.

Laboratory Tests: Patients receiving digoxin should have their serum electrolytes and renal function (BUN and/or serum creatinine) assessed periodically; the frequency of assessments will depend on the clinical setting. For discussion of serum digoxin concentrations, see DOSAGE AND ADMINISTRATION section.

Drug Interactions: Potassium-depleting *corticosteroids* and *diuretics* may be major contributing factors to digitalis toxicity. *Calcium*, particularly if administered rapidly by the intravenous route, may produce serious arrhythmias in digitalized patients. *Quinidine* causes a rise in serum digoxin concentration, with the implication that digitalis intoxication may result. *Antacids, kaolin-pectin, sulfasalazine, neomycin* and *cholestyramine* may interfere with intestinal digoxin absorption, resulting in unexpectedly low serum concentrations. *Thyroid* administration to a digitalized, hypothyroid patient may increase the dose requirement of digoxin. Concomitant use of digoxin and *sympathomimetics* increases the risk of cardiac arrhythmias, because both enhance ectopic pacemaker activity. *Succinylcholine* may cause a sudden extrusion of potassium from muscle cells, and may thereby cause arrhythmias in digitalized patients. Although *propranolol* and digoxin may be useful in combination to control atrial fibrillation, their additive effects on AV node conduction can result in complete heart block.

Carcinogenesis, Mutagenesis, Impairment of Fertility: There have been no long-term studies performed in animals to evaluate carcinogenic potential.

Pregnancy: Pregnancy Category C. Animal reproduction studies have not been conducted with digoxin. It is also not known whether digoxin can cause fetal harm when administered to a pregnant woman or can affect reproduction capacity. Digoxin should be given to a pregnant woman only if clearly needed.

Nursing Mothers: Studies have shown that digoxin concentrations in the mother's serum and milk are similar. However, the estimated daily dose to a nursing infant will be far below the usual infant maintenance dose. Therefore, this amount should have no pharmacologic effect upon the infant. Nevertheless, caution should be exercised when digoxin is administered to a nursing woman.

Adverse Reactions: The frequency and severity of adverse reactions to digoxin depend on the dose and route of administration, as well as on the patient's underlying disease or concomitant therapies (see PRECAUTIONS section). The overall incidence of adverse reactions has been reported as 5 to 20%, with 15 to 20% of them being considered serious (one to four percent of patients receiving digoxin). Evidence suggests that the incidence of toxicity has decreased since the introduction of the serum digoxin assay and improved standardization of digoxin tablets. Cardiac toxicity accounts for about one-half, gastrointestinal disturbances for about one-fourth, and CNS and other toxicity for about one-fourth of these adverse reactions.

Adults:

Cardiac—Unifocal or multiform ventricular premature contractions, especially in bigeminal or trigeminal patterns, are the most common arrhythmias associated with digoxin toxicity in adults with heart disease. Ventricular tachycardia may result from digitalis toxicity. Atrioventricular (AV) dissociation, accelerated junctional (nodal) rhythm and atrial tachycardia with block are also common arrhythmias caused by digoxin overdosage.

Excessive slowing of the pulse is a clinical sign of digoxin overdosage. AV block (Wenckebach) of increasing degree may proceed to complete heart block.

Note: The electrocardiogram is fundamental in determining the presence and nature of these cardiac disturbances. Digoxin may also induce other changes in the ECG (e.g. PR prolongation, ST depression), which represent digoxin effect and may or may not be associated with digitalis toxicity.

Gastrointestinal—Anorexia, nausea, vomiting and less commonly diarrhea are common early symptoms of overdosage. However, uncontrolled heart failure may also produce such symptoms.

CNS—Visual disturbances (blurred or yellow vision), headache, weakness, apathy and psychosis can occur.

Other—Gynecomastia is occasionally observed.

Infants and Children: Toxicity differs from the adult in a number of respects. Anorexia, nausea, vomiting, diarrhea and CNS disturbances may be present but are rare as initial symptoms in infants. Cardiac arrhythmias are more reliable signs of toxicity. Digoxin in children may produce any arrhythmia. The most commonly encountered are conduction disturbances or supraventricular tachyarrhythmias, such as atrial tachycardia with or without block, and junctional (nodal) tachycardia. Ventricular arrhythmias are less common. Sinus bradycardia may also be a sign of impending digoxin intoxication, especially in infants, even in the absence of first degree heart block. Any arrhythmia or alteration in cardiac conduction that develops in a child taking digoxin should initially be assumed to be a consequence of digoxin intoxication.

Treatment of Arrhythmias Produced By Overdosage:

Adults: Digoxin should be discontinued until all signs of toxicity are gone. Discontinuation may be all that is necessary if toxic manifestations are not severe and appear only near the expected time for maximum effect of the drug. Potassium salts are commonly used, particularly if hypokalemia is present. Potassium chloride in divided oral doses totaling 3 to 6 grams of the salt (40 to 80 mEq K +) for adults may be given provided renal function is adequate (see below for potassium recommendations in Infants and Children).

When correction of the arrhythmia is urgent and the serum potassium concentration is low or normal, potassium should be administered intravenously in 5% dextrose injection. For adults, a total of 40 to 80 mEq (diluted to a concentration of 40 mEq per 500 ml) may be given at a rate not exceeding 20 mEq per hour, or slower if limited by pain due to local irritation. Additional amounts may be given if the arrhythmia is uncontrolled and potassium well-tolerated. ECG monitoring should be performed to watch for any evidence of potassium toxicity (e.g. peaking of T waves) and to observe the effect on the arrhythmia. The infusion may be stopped when the desired effect is achieved.

Note: Potassium should not be used and may be dangerous in heart block due to digoxin, unless primarily related to supraventricular tachycardia. Other agents that have been used for the treatment of digoxin intoxication include lidocaine, procainamide, propranolol and phenytoin, although use of the latter must be considered experimental. In advanced heart block, temporary ventricular pacing may be beneficial.

Infants and Children: See Adult section for general recommendations for the treatment of arrhythmias produced by overdosage and for cautions regarding the use of potassium.

If a potassium preparation is used to treat toxicity, it may be given orally in divided doses totaling 1 to 1.5 mEq K + per kilogram (kg) body weight (1 gram of potassium chloride contains 13.4 mEq K +).

When correction of the arrhythmia with potassium is urgent, approximately 0.5 mEq/kg of potassium per hour may be given intravenously, with careful ECG monitoring. The intravenous solution of potassium should be dilute enough to avoid local irritation; however, especially in infants, care must be taken to avoid intravenous fluid overload.

Dosage and Administration: Recommended dosages are average values that may require considerable modification because of individual sensitivity or associated conditions. Diminished renal function is the most important factor requiring modification of recommended doses.

Due to the more complete absorption of digoxin from soft capsules, recommended oral doses are only 80 percent of those for Tablets, Elixir and I.M. Injection.

Because the significance of the higher peak serum concentrations associated with once daily capsules is not established, divided daily dosing is presently recommended for:

1. Infants and children under 10 years of age,
2. Patients requiring a daily dose of 300 μg (0.3 mg) or greater;
3. Patients with a previous history of digitalis toxicity;
4. Patients considered likely to become toxic;
5. Patients in whom compliance is not a problem.

Where compliance is considered a problem, single daily dosing may be appropriate.

In deciding the dose of digoxin, several factors must be considered:

1. The disease being treated Atrial arrhythmias may require larger doses than heart failure.
2. The body weight of the patient. Doses should be calculated based upon lean or ideal body weight.
3. The patient's renal function, preferably evaluated on the basis of creatinine clearance.
4. Age is an important factor in infants and children.
5. Concomitant disease states, drugs or other factors likely to alter the expected clinical response to digoxin (see PRECAUTIONS and Drug Interactions sections).

Digitalization may be accomplished by either of two general approaches that vary in dosage and frequency of administration, but reach the same endpoint in terms of total amount of digoxin accumulated in the body.

1. Rapid digitalization may be achieved by administering a loading dose based upon projected body digoxin stores, then calculating the maintenance dose as a percentage of the loading dose.
2. More gradual digitalization may be obtained by beginning an appropriate maintenance dose, thus allowing digoxin body stores to accumulate slowly. Steady-state serum digoxin concentrations will be achieved in approximately 5 half-lives of the drug for the individual patient. Depending upon the patient's renal function, this will take between one and three weeks.

Adults:

Adults—Rapid Digitalization with a Loading Dose: Peak body digoxin stores of 8 to 12 μg/kg should provide therapeutic effect with minimum risk of toxicity in most patients with heart failure and normal sinus rhythm. Larger stores (10 to 15 μg/kg) are ofter required for adequate control of ventricular rate in patients with atrial flutter or fibrillation. Because of altered digoxin distribution and elimination, projected peak body stores for patients with renal insufficiency should be conservative (i.e. 6 to 10 μg/kg) [see PRECAUTIONS section].

The loading dose should be based on the projected peak body stores and administered in several portions, with roughly half the total given as the first dose. Additional fractions of this planned total dose may be given at 6 to 8 hour intervals, **with careful assessment of clinical response before each additional dose.** If the patient's clinical response necessitates a change from the calculated dose of digoxin, then calculation of the maintenance dose should be based upon the amount actually given.

In previously undigitalized patients, a single initial Lanoxicaps dose of 400 to 600 μg (0.4 to 0.6 mg) usually produces a detectable effect in 0.5 to 2 hours that becomes maximal in 2 to 6 hours. Additional doses of 100 to 300 μg (0.1 to 0.3 mg) may be given cautiously at 6 to 8 hour intervals until clinical evidence of an adequate effect is noted. The usual amount of Lanoxicaps that a 70 kg patient required to achieve 8 to 15 μg/kg peak body stores is 600 to 1000 μg (0.6 to 1.0 mg).

Although peak body stores are mathematically related to loading doses and are utilized to calculate maintenance doses, they do not correlate with measured serum concentrations. This discrepancy is caused by digoxin distribution within the body during the first 6 to 8 hours following a dose. Serum concentrations drawn during this time are usually not interpretable.

The maintenance dose should be based upon the percentage of the peak body stores lost each day through elimination. The following formula has had wide clinical use:

$$\text{Maintenance Dose} = \text{Peak Body Stores (i.e. Loading Dose} \times \frac{\text{\% Daily Loss}}{100}$$

$$\text{Where: \% Daily Loss} = 14 + \text{Ccr}/5$$

Ccr is creatinine clearance, corrected to 70 kg body weight or 1.73 m^2 body surface area. **For adults,** if only serum creatinine concentrations (Scr) are available, a Ccr (corrected to 70 kg body weight) may be estimated in men as (140—Age)/Scr. For women, this result should be multiplied by 0.85.

Note: This equation cannot be used for estimating creatinine clearance in infants or children.

A common practice involves the use of Lanoxin® Injection to achieve rapid digitalization, with conversion to Lanoxicaps or Lanoxin Tablets for maintenance therapy. If patients are switched from IV to oral digoxin formulations, allowances must be made for differences in bioavailability when calculating maintenance dosages (see table, CLINICAL PHARMACOLOGY section).

Adults—Gradual Digitalization with a Maintenance Dose: The following table provides average Lanoxicaps daily maintenance dose requirements for patients with heart failure based upon lean body weight and renal function:

[See table on bottom next page].

Example—based on the above table, a patient in heart failure with an estimated lean body weight of 70 kg and a Ccr of 60 ml/min, should be given 200 μg (0.2 mg) of Lanoxicaps per day, usually taken as a 100 μg (0.1 mg) capsule after the morning and evening meals. Steady-state serum concentrations should not be anticipated before 11 days.

Infants and Children: Digitalization must be individualized. Divided daily dosing is recommended for infants and young children. In

Continued on next page

Burroughs Wellcome—Cont.

these patients, where dosage adjustment is frequent and outside the fixed dosages available, Lanoxicaps may not be the formulation of choice. Children over 10 years of age require adult dosages in proportion to their body weight.

In the newborn period, renal clearance of digoxin is diminished and suitable dosage adjustments must be observed. This is especially pronounced in the premature infant. Beyond the immediate newborn period, children generally require proportionally larger doses than adults on the basis of body weight or body surface area.

Lanoxin® Injection Pediatric can be used to achieve rapid digitalization, with conversion to an oral Lanoxin formulation for maintenance therapy. If patients are switched from IV to oral digoxin tablets or elixir, allowances must be made for differences in bioavailability when calculating maintenance dosages (see bioavailability table in CLINICAL PHARMACOLOGY section and dosing table below).

Intramuscular injection of digoxin is extremely painful and offers no advantages unless other routes of administration are contraindicated.

Digitalizing and daily maintenance doses for each age group are given below and should provide therapeutic effect with minimum risk of toxicity in most patients with heart failure and normal sinus rhythm. Larger doses are often required for adequate control of ventricular rate in patients with atrial flutter or fibrillation.

The loading dose should be administered in several portions, with roughly half the total given as the first dose. Additional fractions of this planned total dose may be given at 6 to 8 hour intervals, **with careful assessment of clinical response before each additional dose.** If the patient's clinical response necessitates a change from the calculated dose of digoxin, then calculation of the maintenance dose should be based upon the amount actually given.

[See table above].

More gradual digitalization can also be accomplished by beginning an appropriate maintenance dose. The range of percentages provided above can be used in calculating this dose for patients with normal renal function. In children with renal disease, digoxin dosing must be carefully titrated based upon desired clinical response.

Long-term use of digoxin is indicated in many children who have been digitalized for acute heart failure, unless the cause is transient. Children with severe congenital heart disease, even after surgery, may require digoxin for prolonged periods.

It cannot be overemphasized that both the adult and pediatric dosage guidelines provided are based upon average patient response and substantial individual variation can be expected. Accordingly, ultimate dosage selection must be based upon clinical assessment of the patient.

Usual Digitalizing and Maintenance Dosages for Lanoxicaps in Children with **Normal Renal Function Based on Lean Body Weight**

Age	Digitalizing* Dose (μg/kg)	**Daily** † Maintenance Dose (μg/kg)
2–5 Years	25–35	25–35% of the oral or IV loading dose ‡
5–10 Years	15–30	
Over 10 years	8–12	

*IV digitalizing doses are the same as Lanoxicaps digitalizing doses.
†Divided daily dosing is recommended for children under 10 years of age.
‡Projected or actual digitalizing dose providing desired clinical response.

Serum Digoxin Concentrations: Measurement of serum digoxin concentrations can be helpful to the clinician in determining the state of digitalization and in assigning certain probabilities to the likelihood of digoxin intoxication. Studies in adults considered adequately digitalized (without evidence of toxicity) show that about two-thirds of such patients have serum digoxin levels ranging from 0.8 to 2.0 ng/ml. Patients with atrial fibrillation or atrial flutter require and appear to tolerate higher levels than do patients with other indications. On the other hand, in adult patients with clinical evidence of digoxin toxicity, about two-thirds will have serum digoxin levels greater than 2.0 ng/ml. Thus, whereas levels less than 0.8 ng/ml are infrequently associated with toxicity, levels greater than 2.0 ng/ml are often associated with toxicity. Values in between are not very helpful in deciding whether a certain sign or symptom is more likely caused by digoxin toxicity or by something else. There are rare patients who are unable to tolerate digoxin even at serum concentrations below 0.8 ng/ml. Some researchers suggest that infants and young children tolerate slightly higher serum concentrations than do adults.

To allow adequate time for equilibration of digoxin between serum and tissue, **sampling of serum concentrations for clinical use should be at least 6 to 8 hours after the last dose,** regardless of the route of administration or formulation used. On a twice daily dosing schedule, there will be only minor differences in serum digoxin concentrations whether sampling is done at 8 or 12 hours after a dose. After a single daily dose, the concentration will be 10 to 25% lower when sampled at 24 versus 8 hours, depending upon the patient's renal function. Ideally, sampling for assessment of steady-state concentrations should be done just before the next dose.

If a discrepancy exists between the reported serum concentration and the observed clinical response, the clinician should consider the following possibilities:

1. Analytical problems in the assay procedure.
2. Inappropriate serum sampling time.
3. Administration of a digitalis glycoside other than digoxin.
4. Conditions (described in WARNINGS and PRECAUTIONS sections) causing an alteration in the sensitivity of the patient to digoxin.
5. The patient falls outside the norm in his response to or handling of digoxin. This decision should only be reached after exclusion of the other possibilities and generally should be confirmed by additional correlations of clinical observations with serum digoxin concentrations.

The serum concentration data should always be interpreted in the overall clinical context and an isolated serum concentration value should not be used alone as a basis for increasing or decreasing digoxin dosage.

Adjustment of Maintenance Dose in Previously Digitalized Patients: Lanoxicaps maintenance doses in individual patients on steady-state digoxin can be adjusted upward or downward in proportion to the ratio of the desired versus the measured serum concentration. For example, a patient at steady-state on 100 μg (0.1 mg) of Lanoxicaps per day with a measured serum concentration of 0.7 ng/ml, should have the dose increased to 200 μg (0.2 mg) per day to achieve a steady-state serum concentration of 1.4 ng/ml, **assuming the serum digoxin concentration measurement is correct, renal function remains stable during this time and the needed adjustment is not the result of a problem with compliance.**

Dosage Adjustment When Changing Preparations: The absolute bioavailability of the capsule formulation is greater than that of the standard tablets and very near that of the intravenous dosage form. As a result the doses recommended for Lanoxicaps capsules are the same as those for Lanoxin® Injection (see CLINICAL PHARMACOLOGY section). Adjustments in dosage will seldom be necessary when converting a patient from intravenous to Lanoxicaps formulation. The differences in bioavailability between Lanoxin Injection or Lanoxicaps, and Lanoxin Elixir Pediatric or Lanoxin Tablets must be considered when changing patients from one dosage form to another.

Lanoxin Injection and Lanoxicaps doses of 100 μg (0.1 mg) and 200 μg (0.2 mg) are approximately equivalent to 125 μg (0.125 mg) and 250 μg (0.25 mg) doses of Lanoxin Tablets and Elixir Pediatric (see table in CLINICAL PHARMACOLOGY section). Intramuscular injection of digoxin is extremely painful and offers no advantages unless other routes of administration are contraindicated.

How Supplied:

LANOXICAPS (DIGOXIN SOLUTION IN CAPSULES), 50 μg (0.05 mg): bottles of 100, Imprint A2C (red), NDC-0081-0270-55

LANOXICAPS (DIGOXIN SOLUTION IN CAPSULES), 100 μg (0.1 mg)* bottles of 100, Imprint B2C (yellow), NDC 0081-0272-55

LANOXICAPS (DIGOXIN SOLUTION IN CAPSULES), 200 μg (0.2 mg)* bottles of 100, Imprint C2C (green), NDC-0081-0274-55

Store at 15°–30°C (59°–86°F) in a dry place and protect from light.

Usual Lanoxicaps Daily Maintenance Dose Requirements (μg) for Estimated Peak Body Stores of 10 μg/kg

		Lean Body Weight (kg/lbs)							
		50/110	60/132	70/154	80/176	90/198	100/220		
Corrected Ccr (ml/min per 70 kg)	0	50	100	100	100	150	150	22	Number of Days Before Steady-State Achieved
	10	100	100	100	150	150	150	19	
	20	100	100	150	150	150	200	16	
	30	100	150	150	150	200	200	14	
	40	100	150	150	200	200	250	13	
	50	150	150	200	200	250	250	12	
	60	150	150	200	200	250	300	11	
	70	150	200	200	250	250	300	10	
	80	150	200	200	250	300	300	9	
	90	150	200	250	250	300	350	8	
	100	200	200	250	300	300	350	7	

Also Available:
LANOXIN® (DIGOXIN) TABLETS, Scored 125 µg (0.125 mg): Bottles of 100 and 1000: Unit Dose Pack of 1000; Unit of Use Bottles of 30. Imprinted with LANOXIN and Y3B (yellow).
LANOXIN (DIGOXIN) TABLETS, Scored 250 µg (0.25 mg): Bottles of 100, 1000 and 5000; Unit Dose Pack of 100; Unit of Use bottles of 30 and 100. Imprinted with LANOXIN and X3A (white).
LANOXIN (DIGOXIN) TABLETS Scored 500 µg (0.5 mg): Bottles of 100. Imprinted with LANOXIN and T9A (Green)
LANOXIN (DIGOXIN) ELIXIR PEDIATRIC, 50 µg (0.05 mg) per ml; bottle of 60 ml with calibrated dropper.
LANOXIN (DIGOXIN) INJECTION, 500 µg (0.5 mg) in 2 ml (250 µg [0.25 mg] per ml); boxes of 12 and 100 ampuls.
LANOXIN (DIGOXIN) INJECTION PEDIATRIC, 100 µg (0.1 mg) in 1 ml; box of 50 ampuls.
*U.S. Patent No. 4088750

LANOXIN® ℞
(Digoxin)
Tablets/Injections/Elixir Pediatric

Description: Digoxin is one of the cardiac (or digitalis) glycosides, a closely related group of drugs having in common specific effects on the myocardium. These drugs are found in a number of plants. Digoxin is extracted from the leaves of *Digitalis lanata*. The term "digitalis" is used to designate the whole group. The glycosides are composed of two portions: a sugar and a cardenolide (hence "glycosides").

Digoxin has the empirical formula $C_{41}H_{64}O_{14}$, a molecular weight of 780.96 and melting and decomposition points above 235°C. The drug is practically insoluble in water and in ether, slightly soluble in diluted (50%) alcohol and in chloroform; and freely soluble in pyridine. Digoxin powder is composed of odorless white crystals.

Digoxin has the chemical name: 3β-[(0-2,6-dideoxy-β - D - ribo-hexopyranosyl - (1→4)-0-2,6-dideoxy -β-D-ribo-hexopyranosyl - (1→4)-2,6 - dideoxy -β- D - ribo - hexopyranosyl) oxy] - 12β,14-dihydroxy-5β-card-20(22)-enolide.

Lanoxin Tablets with 125µg (0.125 mg), 250 µg (0.25 mg) or 500 µg (0.5 mg) digoxin USP are intended for oral use. Each tablet contains the labeled amount of digoxin USP dispersed in lactose and other inert ingredients.

Lanoxin brand Digoxin Injection and Injection Pediatric are sterile solutions of digoxin for intravenous or intramuscular injection. The vehicle contains 40% propylene glycol and 10% alcohol. The injection is buffered to a pH of 6.8 to 7.2 with 0.3 percent sodium phosphate and 0.08 percent anhydrous citric acid. Each 2 cc ampul of Lanoxin Injection contains 500 µg (0.5 mg) digoxin [250 µg (0.25 mg) per cc]. Each 1 cc ampul of Lanoxin Injection Pediatric contains 100 µg (0.1 mg) digoxin. Dilution is not required.

Lanoxin Elixir Pediatric is a stable solution of digoxin specially formulated for oral use in infants and children. Each cc contains 50 µg (0.05 mg) digoxin USP. The lime-flavored elixir contains 10% alcohol. Each package is supplied with a specially calibrated dropper to facilitate the administration of accurate dosage even in premature infants. This 1 cc dropper is marked in divisions of 0.1 cc, each corresponding to 5 µg (0.005 mg) digoxin.

PRODUCT	ABSOLUTE BIOAVAILABILITY	EQUIVALENT DOSES (IN MG*)		
Lanoxin Tablet	60–80%	0.125	0.25	0.5
Lanoxin Elixir	70–85%	0.125	0.25	0.5
Lanoxin Injection/IM	70–85%	0.125	0.25	0.5
Lanoxin Injection/IV	100%	0.1	0.2	0.4

*1 mg = 1000 µg

Clinical Pharmacology:

Mechanism of Action:
The influence of digitalis glycosides on the myocardium is dose-related, and involves both a direct action on cardiac muscle and the specialized conduction system, and indirect actions on the cardiovascular system mediated by the autonomic nervous system. The indirect actions mediated by the autonomic nervous system involve a vagomimetic action, which is responsible for the effects of digitalis on the sino-atrial (SA) and atrioventricular (AV) nodes; and also a baroreceptor sensitization which results in increased carotid sinus nerve activity and enhanced sympathetic withdrawal for any given increment in mean arterial pressure. The pharmacologic consequences of these direct and indirect effects are: 1) an increase in the force and velocity of myocardial systolic contraction (positive inotropic action); 2) a slowing of heart rate (negative chronotropic effect); and 3) decreased conduction velocity through the AV node. In higher doses, digitalis increases sympathetic outflow from the central nervous system (CNS) to both cardiac and peripheral sympathetic nerves. This increase in sympathetic activity may be an important factor in digitalis cardiac toxicity. Most of the extracardiac manifestations of digitalis toxicity are also mediated by the CNS.

Pharmacokinetics:
Note: The following data are from studies performed in adults, unless otherwise stated.

Absorption—Gastrointestinal absorption of digoxin is a passive process. Absorption of digoxin from the Lanoxin® tablet formulation has been demonstrated to be 60 to 80% complete and absorption of digoxin from the Lanoxin® Elixir Pediatric formulation, 70 to 85% complete compared to an identical intravenous dose of digoxin (absolute bioavailability). When digoxin elixir or tablets are taken after meals, the rate of absorption is slowed, but the total amount of digoxin absorbed is usually unchanged. When taken with meals high in bran fiber, however, the amount absorbed from an oral dose may be reduced. Comparison of the systemic availability and equivalent doses for digoxin preparations are shown in the following table.
[See table above].

Distribution—Following drug administration, a 6 to 8 hour distribution phase is observed. This is followed by a much more gradual serum concentration decline, which is dependent on digoxin elimination from the body. The peak height and slope of the early portion (absorption/distribution phases) of the serum concentration-time curve are dependent upon the route of administration and the absorption characteristics of the formulation. Clinical evidence indicates that the early high serum concentrations do not reflect the concentration of digoxin at its site of action, but that with chronic use, the steady-state post-distribution serum levels are in equilibrium with tissue levels and correlate with pharmacologic effects. In individual patients, these post-distribution serum concentrations are linearly related to maintenance dosage and may be useful in evaluating therapeutic and toxic effects (see Serum Digoxin Concentrations in DOSAGE AND ADMINISTRATION section).

Digoxin is concentrated in tissues and therefore has a large apparent volume of distribution. Digoxin crosses both the blood-brain barrier and the placenta. At delivery, serum digoxin concentration in the newborn is similar to the serum level in the mother. Approximately 20 to 25% of plasma digoxin is bound to protein. Serum digoxin concentrations are not significantly altered by large changes in fat tissue weight, so that its distribution space correlates best with lean (ideal) body weight, not total body weight.

Pharmacologic Response—The approximate times to onset of effect and to peak effect of all the Lanoxin® preparations are given in the following table:
[See table below].

Excretion—Elimination of digoxin follows first-order kinetics (that is, the quantity of digoxin eliminated at any time is proportional to the total body content). Following intravenous administration to normal subjects, 50 to 70% of a digoxin dose is excreted unchanged in the urine. Renal excretion of digoxin is proportional to glomerular filtration rate and is largely independent of urine flow. In subjects with normal renal function, digoxin has a half-life of 1.5 to 2.0 days. The half-life in anuric patients is prolonged to 4 to 6 days. Digoxin is not effectively removed from the body by dialysis, exchange transfusion or during cardiopulmonary by-pass because most of the drug is in tissue rather than circulating in the blood.

Indications and Usage:

Heart Failure:
The increased cardiac output resulting from the inotropic action of digoxin ameliorates the disturbances characteristic of heart failure (venous congestion, edema, dyspnea, orthopnea and cardiac asthma).

Digoxin is more effective in "low output" (pump) failure than in "high output" heart failure secondary to arteriovenous fistula, anemia, infection or hyperthyroidism.

Digoxin should usually be continued after failure is controlled unless some known precipitating factor has been corrected. If digoxin is discontinued the patient should be evaluated periodically for clinical evidence of recurrent heart failure.

Atrial Fibrillation:
Digoxin reduces ventricular rate and thereby improves hemodynamics. Palpitation, precordial distress or weakness are relieved and concomitant congestive failure ameliorated. Digoxin should be continued in doses necessary to maintain the desired ventricular rate.

Atrial Flutter:
Digoxin slows the heart and regular sinus rhythm may appear. Frequently the flutter is converted to atrial fibrillation with a controlled ventricular response. Digoxin treatment should be maintained if atrial fibrillation

Continued on next page

PRODUCT	TIME TO ONSET OF EFFECT*	TIME TO PEAK EFFECT*
Lanoxin Tablet	0.5–2 hours	2–6 hours
Lanoxin Elixir	0.5–2 hours	2–6 hours
Lanoxin Injection/IM	0.5–2 hours	2–6 hours
Lanoxin Injection/IV	5–30 minutes†	1–4 hours

*Documented for ventricular response rate in atrial fibrillation, inotropic effect and electrocardiographic changes.
†Depending upon rate of infusion.

Burroughs Wellcome—Cont.

persists. (Electrical cardioversion is often the treatment of choice for atrial flutter. See discussion of cardioversion in PRECAUTIONS section.)

Paroxysmal Atrial Tachycardia (PAT):
Digoxin may convert PAT to sinus rhythm by slowing conduction through the AV node. If heart failure has ensued or paroxysms recur frequently, digoxin should be continued. In infants, digoxin is usually continued for 3 to 6 months after a single episode of PAT to prevent recurrence.

Contraindications: Digitalis glycosides are contraindicated in ventricular fibrillation.
In a given patient, an untoward effect requiring discontinuation of other digitalis preparations usually constitutes a contraindication to digoxin. Hypersensitivity to digoxin itself is a contraindication to its use. Allergy to digoxin, though rare, does occur. It may not extend to all such preparations, and another digitalis glycoside may be tried with caution.

Warnings: Digitalis alone or with other drugs has been used in the treatment of obesity. This use of digoxin or other digitalis glycosides is unwarranted. Moreover, since they may cause potentially fatal arrhythmias or other adverse effects, the use of these drugs solely for the treatment of obesity is dangerous.
Anorexia, nausea, vomiting and arrhythmias may accompany heart failure or may be indications of digitalis intoxication. Clinical evaluation of the cause of these symptoms should be attempted before further digitalis administration. In such circumstances determination of the serum digoxin concentration may be an aid in deciding whether or not digitalis toxicity is likely to be present. If the possibility of digitalis intoxication cannot be excluded, cardiac glycosides should be temporarily withheld, if permitted by the clinical situation.
Patients with renal insufficiency require smaller than usual maintenance doses of digoxin (see DOSAGE AND ADMINISTRATION section).
Heart failure accompanying acute glomerulonephritis requires extreme care in digitalization. Relatively low loading and maintenance doses and concomitant use of antihypertensive drugs may be necessary and careful monitoring is essential. Digoxin should be discontinued as soon as possible.
Patients with severe carditis, such as carditis associated with rheumatic fever or viral myocarditis, are especially sensitive to digoxin-induced disturbances of rhythm.
Newborn infants display considerable variability in their tolerance to digoxin. Premature and immature infants are particularly sensitive, and dosage must not only be reduced but must be individualized according to their degree of maturity.
Note: Digitalis glycosides are an important cause of accidental poisoning in children.

Precautions:

General:
Digoxin toxicity develops more frequently and lasts longer in patients with renal impairment because of the decreased excretion of digoxin. Therefore, it should be anticipated that dosage requirements will be decreased in patients with moderate to severe renal disease (see DOSAGE AND ADMINISTRATION section).
Because of the prolonged half-life, a longer period of time is required to achieve an initial or new steady-state concentration in patients with renal impairment than in patients with normal renal function.
In patients with hypokalemia, toxicity may occur despite serum digoxin concentrations within the "normal range", because potassium depletion sensitizes the myocardium to digoxin. Therefore, it is desirable to maintain normal serum potassium levels in patients being treated with digoxin. Hypokalemia may result from diuretic, amphotericin B or corticosteroid therapy, and from dialysis or mechanical suction of gastrointestinal secretions. It may also accompany malnutrition, diarrhea, prolonged vomiting, old age and long-standing heart failure. In general, rapid changes in serum potassium or other electrolytes should be avoided, and intravenous treatment with potassium should be reserved for special circumstances as described below (see TREATMENT OF ARRHYTHMIAS PRODUCED BY OVERDOSAGE section).
Calcium, particularly when administered rapidly by the intravenous route, may produce serious arrhythmias in digitalized patients. Hypercalcemia from any cause predisposes the patient to digitalis toxicity. On the other hand, hypocalcemia can nullify the effects of digoxin in man; thus, digoxin may be ineffective until serum calcium is restored to normal. These interactions are related to the fact that calcium affects contractility and excitability of the heart in a manner similar to digoxin.
Hypomagnesemia may predispose to digitalis toxicity. If low magnesium levels are detected in a patient on digoxin, replacement therapy should be instituted.
Quinidine causes a rise in serum digoxin concentration, with the implication that digitalis intoxication may result. This rise appears to be proportional to the quinidine dose. Interestingly, both the digoxin clearance and the volume of distribution are reduced, so that the serum half-life may not change. Because of the considerable variability of this interaction, digoxin dosage should be carefully individualized.
Patients with acute myocardial infarction or severe pulmonary disease may be unusually sensitive to digoxin-induced disturbances of rhythm.
Atrial arrhythmias associated with hypermetabolic states (e.g. hyperthyroidism) are particularly resistant to digoxin treatment. Large doses of digoxin are not recommended as the only treatment of these arrhythmias and care must be taken to avoid toxicity if large doses of digoxin are required. In hypothyroidism, the digoxin requirements are reduced. Digoxin responses in patients with compensated thyroid disease are normal.
Reduction of digoxin dosage may be desirable prior to electrical cardioversion to avoid induction of ventricular arrhythmias, but the physician must consider the consequences of rapid increase in ventricular response to atrial fibrillation if digoxin is withheld 1 to 2 days prior to cardioversion. If there is a suspicion that digitalis toxicity exists, elective cardioversion should be delayed. If it is not prudent to delay cardioversion, the energy level selected should be minimal at first and carefully increased in an attempt to avoid precipitating ventricular arrhythmias.
Incomplete AV block, especially in patients with Stokes-Adams attacks, may progress to advanced or complete heart block if digoxin is given.
In some patients with sinus node disease (i.e. Sick Sinus Syndrome), digoxin may worsen sinus bradycardia or sino-atrial block.
In patients with Wolff-Parkinson-White Syndrome and atrial fibrillation, digoxin can enhance transmission of impulses through the accessory pathway. This effect may result in extremely rapid ventricular rates and even ventricular fibrillation.
Digoxin may worsen the outflow obstruction in patients with idiopathic hypertrophic subaortic stenosis (IHSS). Unless cardiac failure is severe, it is doubtful whether digoxin should be employed.
Patients with chronic constrictive pericarditis may fail to respond to digoxin. In addition, slowing of the heart rate by digoxin in some patients may further decrease cardiac output. Patients with heart failure from amyloid heart disease or constrictive cardiomyopathies respond poorly to treatment with digoxin.
Digoxin is not indicated for the treatment of sinus tachycardia unless it is associated with heart failure.
Intramuscular injection of digoxin is extremely painful and offers no advantages unless other routes of administration are contraindicated.

Laboratory Tests:
Patients receiving digoxin should have their serum electrolytes and renal function (BUN and/or serum creatinine) assessed periodically; the frequency of assessments will depend on the clinical setting. For discussion of serum digoxin concentrations, see DOSAGE AND ADMINISTRATION section.

Drug Interactions:
Potassium-depleting *corticosteroids* and *diuretics* may be major contributing factors to digitalis toxicity. *Calcium*, particularly if administered rapidly by the intravenous route, may produce serious arrhythmias in digitalized patients. *Quinidine* causes a rise in serum digoxin concentration, with the implication that digitalis may result. *Antacids, kaolin-pectin, sulfasalazine, neomycin* and *cholestyramine* may interfere with intestinal digoxin absorption, resulting in unexpectedly low serum concentrations. *Thyroid* administration to a digitalized, hypothyroid patient may increase the dose requirement of digoxin. Concomitant use of digoxin and *sympathomimetics* increases the risk of cardiac arrhythmias because both enhance ectopic pacemaker activity. *Succinylcholine* may cause a sudden extrusion of potassium from muscle cells, and may therefore cause arrhythmias in digitalized patients. Although *propranolol* and digoxin may be useful in combination to control atrial fibrillation, their additive effects on AV node conduction can result in complete heart block.

Carcinogenesis, Mutagenesis, Impairment of Fertility:
There have been no long-term studies in animals to evaluate carcinogenic potential.

Pregnancy:
Pregnancy Category A. Studies in pregnant women have not shown that digoxin increases the risk of fetal abnormalities during all trimesters of pregnancy. If this drug is used during pregnancy, the possibility of fetal harm appears remote. Because studies cannot rule out the possibility of harm, however, digoxin should be used during pregnancy only if clearly needed.

Nursing Mothers:
Studies have shown that digoxin concentrations in the mother's serum and milk are similar. However, the estimated daily dose to a nursing infant will be far below the usual infant maintenance dose. Therefore, this amount should have no pharmacologic effect upon the infant. Nevertheless, caution should be exercised when digoxin is administered to a nursing woman.

Adverse Reactions: The frequency and severity of adverse reactions to digoxin depend on the dose and route of administration, as well as on the patient's underlying disease or concomitant therapies (see PRECAUTIONS section). The overall incidence of adverse reactions has been reported as 5 to 20%, with 15 to 20% of them being considered serious (one to four percent of patients receiving digoxin). Evidence suggests that the incidence of toxicity has decreased since the introduction of the serum digoxin assay and improved standardization of digoxin tablets. Cardiac toxicity accounts for about one-half, gastrointestinal disturbances for about one-fourth, and CNS and other toxicity for about one-fourth of these adverse reactions.

Adults:
Cardiac—Unifocal or multiform ventricular premature contractions, especially in bigeminal or trigeminal patterns, are the most com-

mon arrhythmias associated with digoxin toxicity in adults with heart disease. Ventricular tachycardia may result from digitalis toxicity. Atrioventricular (AV) dissociation, accelerated junctional (nodal) rhythm and atrial tachycardia with block are also common arrhythmias caused by digoxin overdosage.

Excessive slowing of the pulse is a clinical sign of digoxin overdosage. AV block (Wenckebach) of increasing degree may proceed to complete heart block.

Note: The electrocardiogram is fundamental in determining the presence and nature of these cardiac disturbances. Digoxin may also induce other changes in the ECG (e.g. PR prolongation, ST depression), which represent digoxin effect and may or may not be associated with digitalis toxicity.

Gastrointestinal—Anorexia, nausea, vomiting and less commonly diarrhea are common early symptoms of overdosage. However, uncontrolled heart failure may also produce such symptoms.

CNS—Visual disturbances (blurred or yellow vision), headache, weakness, apathy and psychosis can occur.

Other—Gynecomastia is occasionally observed.

Infants and Children:

Toxicity differs from the adult in a number of respects. Anorexia, nausea, vomiting, diarrhea and CNS disturbances may be present but are rare as initial symptoms in infants. Cardiac arrhythmias are more reliable signs of toxicity. Digoxin in children may produce any arrhythmia.

Cardiac—Conduction disturbances or supraventricular tachyarrhythmias, such as atrioventricular (AV) block (Wenckebach), atrial tachycardia with or without block and junctional (nodal) tachycardia are the most common arrhythmias associated with digoxin toxicity in children. Ventricular arrhythmias, such as unifocal or multiform ventricular premature contractions, especially in bigeminal or trigeminal patterns, are less common. Ventricular tachycardia may result from digitalis toxicity. Sinus bradycardia may also be a sign of impending digoxin intoxication, especially in infants, even in the absence of first degree heart block. Any arrhythmias or alteration in cardiac conduction that develops in a child taking digoxin should initially be assumed to be a consequence of digoxin intoxication.

Note: The electrocardiogram is fundamental in determining the presence and nature of these cardiac disturbances. Digoxin may also induce other changes in the ECG (e.g. PR prolongation ST depression), which represent digoxin effect and may or may not be associated with digitalis toxicity.

Gastrointestinal—Anorexia, nausea, vomiting and diarrhea may be early symptoms of overdosage. However, uncontrolled heart failure may also produce such symptoms.

CNS—Visual disturbances (blurred or yellow vision), headache, weakness, apathy and psychosis can occur. These may be difficult to recognize in infants and children.

Other—Gynecomastia is occasionally observed.

Treatment of Arrhythmias Produced by Overdosage:

Adults:

Digoxin should be discontinued until all signs of toxicity are gone. Discontinuation may be all that is necessary if toxic manifestations are not severe.

Potassium salts are commonly used, particularly if hypokalemia is present. Potassium chloride in divided oral doses totaling 3 to 6 grams of the salt (40 to 80 mEq K+) for adults may be given provided renal function is adequate (see below for potassium recommendations in Infants and Children).

When correction of the arrhythmia is urgent and the serum potassium concentration is low or normal, potassium should be administered intravenously in 5% dextrose injection. For adults, a total of 40 to 80 mEq (diluted to a concentration of 40 mEq per 500 ml) may be given at a rate not exceeding 20 mEq per hour, or slower if limited by pain due to local irritation. Additional amounts may be given if the arrhythmia is uncontrolled and potassium well-tolerated. ECG monitoring should be performed to watch for any evidence of potassium toxicity (e.g. peaking of T waves) and to observe the effect on the arrhythmia. The infusion may be stopped when the desired effect is achieved.

Note: Potassium should not be used and may be dangerous in heart block due to digoxin, unless primarily related to supraventricular tachycardia.

Other agents that have been used for the treatment of digoxin intoxication include lidocaine, procainamide, propranolol and phenytoin, although use of the latter must be considered experimental. In advanced heart block, temporary ventricular pacing may be beneficial.

Infants and Children:

See Adult section for general recommendations for the treatment of arrhythmias produced by overdosage and for cautions regarding the use of potassium.

If a potassium preparation is used to treat toxicity, it may be given orally in divided doses totaling 1 to 1.5 mEq K+ per kilogram (kg) body weight (1 gram of potassium chloride contains 13.4 mEq K+).

When correction of the arrhythmia with potassium is urgent, approximately 0.5 mEq/kg of potassium per hour may be given intravenously, with careful ECG monitoring. The intravenous solution of potassium should be dilute enough to avoid local irritation; however, especially in infants, care must be taken to avoid intravenous fluid overload.

Dosage and Administration: *Recommended dosages are average values that may require considerable modification because of individual sensitivity or associated conditions.* Diminished renal function is the most important factor requiring modification of recommended doses.

Parenteral administration of digoxin should be used only when the need for rapid digitalization is urgent or when the drug cannot be taken orally. Intramuscular injection can lead to severe pain at the injection site, thus intravenous administration is preferred. If the drug must be administered by the intramuscular route, it should be injected deep into the muscle followed by massage. No more than 500 μg (2 cc) of Lanoxin Injection or 200 μg (2 cc) of Lanoxin Injection Pediatric should be injected into a single site.

Lanoxin® Injection and Injection Pediatric can be administered undiluted or diluted with a 4-fold or greater volume of sterile water for injection, 0.9% sodium chloride injection or 5% dextrose injection. The use of less than a 4-fold volume of diluent could lead to precipitation of the digoxin. Immediate use of the diluted product is recommended.

If tuberculin syringes are used to measure very small doses, one must be aware of the problem of inadvertent overadministration of digoxin. The syringe should *not* be flushed with the parenteral solution after its contents are expelled into an indwelling vascular catheter.

Slow infusion of Lanoxin® Injection or Injection Pediatric is preferable to bolus administration. Rapid infusion of digitalis glycosides has been shown to cause systemic and coronary arteriolar constriction, which may be clinically undesirable. Caution is thus advised: Lanoxin Injection or Injection Pediatric should probably be administered over a period of 5 minutes or longer. Mixing of Lanoxin Injections with other drugs in the same container or simultaneous administration in the same intravenous line is not recommended.

In deciding the dose of digoxin, several factors must be considered:

1. The disease being treated. Atrial arrhythmias may require larger doses than heart failure.
2. The body weight of the patient. Doses should be calculated based upon lean or ideal body weight.
3. The patient's renal function, preferably evaluated on the basis of creatinine clearance.
4. Age is an important factor in infants and children.
5. Concomitant disease states, drugs or other factors likely to alter the expected clinical response to digoxin (see PRECAUTIONS and Drug Interactions sections).

Digitalization may be accomplished by either of two general approaches that vary in dosage and frequency of administration, but reach the same endpoint in terms of total amount of digoxin accumulated in the body.

1. Rapid digitalization may be achieved by administering a loading dose based upon projected peak body digoxin stores, then calculating the maintenance dose as a percentage of the loading dose.
2. More gradual digitalization may be obtained by beginning an appropriate maintenance dose, thus allowing digoxin body stores to accumulate slowly. Steady-state serum digoxin concentration will be achieved in approximately 5 half-lives of the drug for the individual patient. Depending upon the patient's renal function, this will take between one and three weeks.

Adults:

Adults—Rapid Digitalization with a Loading Dose. Peak body digoxin stores of 8 to 12 μg/kg should provide therapeutic effect with minimum risk of toxicity in most patients with heart failure and normal sinus rhythm. Larger stores (10 to 15 μg/kg) are often required for adequate control of ventricular rate in patients with atrial flutter or fibrillation. Because of altered digoxin distribution and elimination, projected peak body stores for patients with renal insufficiency should be conservative (i.e. 6 to 10 μg/kg) [see PRECAUTIONS section].

The loading dose should be based on the projected peak body stores and administered in several portions, with roughly half the total given as the first dose. Additional fractions of this planned total dose may be given at 4 to 8 hour intervals IV or 6 to 8 hour intervals orally, with *careful assessment of clinical response before each additional dose.*

If the patient's clinical response necessitates a change from the calculated dose of digoxin, then calculation of the maintenance dose should be based upon the amount actually given.

In previously undigitalized patients, a single initial intravenous Lanoxin® Injection dose of 400 to 600 μg (0.4 to 0.6 mg) usually produces a detectable effect in 5 to 30 minutes that becomes maximal in 1 to 4 hours. Additional doses of 100 to 300 μg (0.1 to 0.3 mg) may be given cautiously at 4 to 8 hour intervals until clinical evidence of an adequate effect is noted. The usual amount of Lanoxin Injection that a 70 kg patient requires to achieve 8 to 15 μg/kg peak body stores is 600 to 1000 μg (0.6 to 1.0 mg).

A single initial Lanoxin® Tablet or Elixir Pediatric dose of 500 to 750 μg (0.5 to 0.75 mg) usually produces a detectable effect in 0.5 to 2 hours that becomes maximal in 2 to 6 hours. Additional doses of 125 to 375 μg (0.125 to 0.375 mg) may be given cautiously at 6 to 8 hour intervals until clinical evidence of an adequate effect is noted. The usual amount of Lanoxin Tablets or Elixir that a 70 kg patient requires to achieve 8 to 15 μg peak body stores is 750 to 1250 μg (0.75 to 1.25 mg).

Continued on next page

Burroughs Wellcome—Cont.

Usual Lanoxin Daily Maintenance Dose Requirements (μg)
For Estimated Peak Body Stores of 10 $\mu g/kg$

		Lean Body Weight (kg/lbs)						
		50/110	**60/132**	**70/154**	**80/176**	**90/198**	**100/200**	Number of Days Before Steady-State Achieved
Corrected Ccr (ml/min per 70 kg)	0	63*†	125	125	125	188††	188	22
	10	125	125	125	188	188	188	19
	20	125	125	188	188	188	250	16
	30	125	188	188	188	250	250	14
	40	125	188	188	250	250	250	13
	50	188	188	250	250	250	250	12
	60	188	188	250	250	250	375	11
	70	188	250	250	250	250	375	10
	80	188	250	250	250	375	375	9
	90	188	250	250	250	375	500	8
	100	250	250	250	375	375	500	7

* 63 μg = 0.063 mg
† ½ of 125 μg tablet or 125 μg every other day
†† 1½ of 125 μg tablet.

Example—based on the above table, a patient in heart failure with an estimated lean body weight of 70 kg and a Ccr of 60 ml/min, should be given a 250 μg (0.25 mg) Lanoxin® Tablet each day, usually taken after the morning meal. Steady-state serum concentrations should not be anticipated before 11 days.

Although peak body stores are mathematically related to loading doses and are utilized to calculate maintenance doses, they do not correlate with measured serum concentrations. This discrepancy is caused by digoxin distribution within the body during the first 6 to 8 hours following a dose. Serum concentrations drawn during this time are usually not interpretable. The maintenance dose should be based upon the percentage of the peak body stores lost each day through elimination. The following formula has had wide clinical use:

[See table below].

Ccr is creatinine clearance, corrected to 70 kg body weight or 1.73 m^2 body surface area. *For adults,* if only serum creatinine concentrations (Scr) are available, a Ccr (corrected to 70 kg body weight) may be estimated in men as (140–Age)/Scr. For women, this result should be multiplied by 0.85.

Note: This equation cannot be used for estimating creatinine clearance in infants or children.

A common practice involves the use of Lanoxin® Injection to achieve rapid digitalization, with conversion to Lanoxin Tablets for maintenance therapy. If patients are switched from IV to oral digoxin formulations, allowances must be made for differences in bioavailability when calculating maintenance dosages (see table, CLINICAL PHARMACOLOGY section).

Adults—Gradual Digitalization with a Maintenance Dose: The following table provides average Lanoxin Tablet daily maintenance dose requirements for patients with heart failure based upon lean body weight and renal function:

[See table above].

Infants and Children:

Digitalization must be individualized. Divided daily dosing is recommended for infants and young children. Children over 10 years of age require adult dosages in proportion to their body weight.

In the newborn period, renal clearance of digoxin is diminished and suitable dosage adjustments must be observed. This is especially pronounced in the premature infant. Beyond the immediate newborn period, children generally require proportionally larger doses than adults on the basis of body weight or body surface area.

Infants and Children—Rapid Digitalization with a Loading Dose: Lanoxin Injection Pediatric can be used to achieve rapid digitalization, with conversion to an oral Lanoxin formulation for maintenance therapy. If patients are switched from IV to oral digoxin tablets or elixir, allowances must be made for differences in bioavailability when calculating maintenance dosages (see bioavailability table in CLINICAL PHARMACOLOGY section and dosing tables below).

Intramuscular injection of digoxin is extremely painful and offers no advantages unless other routes of administration are contraindicated.

Digitalizing and daily maintenance doses for each age group are given below and should provide therapeutic effect with minimum risk of toxicity in most patients with heart failure and normal sinus rhythm. Larger doses are often required for adequate control of ventricular rate in patients with atrial flutter or fibrillation.

The loading dose should be administered in several portions, with roughly half the total given as the first dose. Additional fractions of this planned total dose may be given at 6 to 8 hour intervals with Lanoxin Tablets or Elixir or at 4 to 8 hour intervals with Lanoxin Injection or Injection Pediatric *with careful assessment of clinical response before each additional dose.* If the patient's clinical response necessitates a change from the calculated dose of digoxin, then calculation of the maintenance dose should be based upon the amount actually given.

[See table on next page].

Infants and Children—Gradual Digitalization With A Maintenance Dose: More gradual digitalization can also be accomplished by beginning an appropriate maintenance dose. The range of percentages provided above can be used in calculating this dose for patients with normal renal function. In children with renal disease, digoxin dosing must be carefully titrated based upon desired clinical response.

Long-term use of digoxin is indicated in many children who have been digitalized for acute heart failure, unless the cause is transient. Children with severe congenital heart disease, even after surgery, may require digoxin for prolonged periods.

It cannot be overemphasized that both the adult and pediatric dosage guidelines provided are based upon average patient response and substantial individual variation can be expected. Accordingly, ultimate dosage selection must be based upon clinical assessment of the patient.

Serum Digoxin Concentrations:

Measurement of serum digoxin concentrations can be helpful to the clinician in determining the state of digitalization and in assigning certain probabilities to the likelihood of digoxin intoxication. Studies in adults considered adequately digitalized (without evidence of toxicity) show that about two-thirds of such patients have serum digoxin levels ranging from 0.8 to 2.0 ng/ml. Patients with atrial fibrillation or atrial flutter require and appear to tolerate higher levels than do patients with other indications. On the other hand, in adult patients with clinical evidence of digoxin toxicity, about two-thirds will have serum digoxin levels greater than 2.0 ng/ml. Thus, whereas levels less than 0.8 ng/ml are infrequently associated with toxicity, levels greater than 2.0 ng/ml are often associated with toxicity. Values in between are not very helpful in deciding whether a certain sign or symptom is more likely caused by digoxin toxicity or by something else. There are rare patients who are unable to tolerate digoxin even at serum concentrations below 0.8 ng/ml. Some researchers suggest that infants and young children tolerate slightly higher serum concentrations than do adults.

To allow adequate time for equilibration of digoxin between serum and tissue, *sampling of serum concentrations for clinical use should be at least 6 to 8 hours after the last dose,* regardless of the route of administration or formulation used. On a twice daily dosing schedule, there will be only minor differences in serum digoxin concentrations whether sampling is done at 8 or 12 hours after a dose. After a single daily dose, the concentration will be 10 to 25% lower when sampled at 24 versus 8 hours, depending upon the patient's renal function. Ideally, sampling for assessment of steady-state concentrations should be done just before the next dose.

If a discrepancy exists between the reported serum concentration and the observed clinical response, the clinician should consider the following possibilities:

1. Analytical problems in the assay procedure.
2. Inappropriate serum sampling time.
3. Administration of a digitalis glycoside other than digoxin.
4. Conditions (described in WARNINGS and PRECAUTIONS sections) causing an alteration in the sensitivity of the patient to digoxin.
5. The patient falls outside the norm in his response to or handling of digoxin. This decision should only be reached after exclusion of the other possibilities and generally should be confirmed by additional correlations of clinical observations with serum digoxin concentrations.

The serum concentration data should always be interpreted in the overall clinical context and an isolated serum concentration value should not be used alone as a basis for increasing or decreasing digoxin dosage.

Adjustment of Maintenance Dose in Previously Digitalized Patients:

Maintenance doses in individual patients on steady-state digoxin can be adjusted upward or downward in proportion to the ratio of the desired versus the measured serum concentration. For example, a patient at steady-state on 125 μg (0.125 mg) of Lanoxin Tablets per day with a measured serum concentration of 0.7 ng/ml, should have the dose increased to 250 μg (0.25 mg) per day to achieve a steady-state serum concentration of 1.4 ng/ml, *assuming the serum digoxin concentration measurement is correct, renal function remains stable during this time and the needed adjustment is not the result of a problem with compliance.*

Dosage Adjustment When Changing Preparations:

$$\text{Maintenance Dose} = \text{Peak Body Stores (i.e. Loading Dose)} \times \frac{\%\ \text{Daily Loss}}{100}$$

$$\text{Where: } \%\ \text{Daily Loss} = 14 + \text{Ccr}/5$$

The differences in bioavailability between injectable Lanoxin and Lanoxin Elixir Pediatric or Lanoxin Tablets must be considered when changing patients from one dosage form to another.

Lanoxin Injection doses of 100 µg (0.1 mg) and 200 µg (0.2 mg) are approximately equivalent to 125 µg (0.125 mg) and 250 µg (0.25 mg) doses of Lanoxin Tablets and Elixir Pediatric (see table in CLINICAL PHARMACOLOGY section). Intramuscular injection of digoxin is extremely painful and offers no advantages unless other routes of administration are contraindicated.

How Supplied:

LANOXIN® (DIGOXIN) TABLETS, Scored 125 µg (0.125 mg): Bottles of 100 (NDC-0081-0242-55) and 1000 (NDC-0081-0242-75); Unit dose pack of 1000 (200 x 5's) (NDC-0081-0242-72); Unit of Use bottles of 30 (NDC-0081-0242-30). Imprinted with LANOXIN and Y3B (yellow). Store at 15°–30°C (59°–86°F) in a dry place and protect from light.

LANOXIN (DIGOXIN) TABLETS, Scored 250 µg (0.25 mg): Bottles of 100 (NDC-0081-0249-55), 500 (NDC-0081-0249-70), 1000 (NDC-0081-0249-75) and 5000 (NDC-0081-0249-80); Unit dose pack of 100 (10 x 10) (NDC-0081-0249-77); Unit of Use bottles of 30 (NDC-0081-0249-30) and 100 (NDC-0081-0249-17). Imprinted with LANOXIN and X3A (white). Store at 15°–30°C (59°–86°F) in a dry place.

LANOXIN (DIGOXIN) TABLETS, Scored 500 µg (0.5 mg): Bottles of 100 (NDC-0081-0253-55). Imprinted with LANOXIN and T9A (green). Store at 15°–30°C (59°–86°F) in a dry place and protect from light.

LANOXIN (DIGOXIN) INJECTION, 500 µg (0.5 mg) in 2 cc [250 µg (0.25 mg) per cc]; boxes of 12 (NDC-0081-0260-15) and 100 ampuls (NDC-0081-0260-55). Store at 15°–30°C (59°–86°F) and protect from light.

LANOXIN (DIGOXIN) INJECTION PEDIATRIC, 100 µg (0.1 mg) in 1 cc; box of 50 ampuls (NDC-0081-0262-35). Store at 15°–30°C (59°–86°F) and protect from light.

LANOXIN (DIGOXIN) ELIXIR PEDIATRIC, 50 µg (0.05 mg) per ml; bottle of 60 ml with calibrated dropper (NDC-0081-0264-81). Store at 15°–30°C (59°–86°F) and protect from light.

[*Tablets Shown in Product Identification Section*]

Usual Digitalizing and Maintenance Dosages for **Lanoxin® Tablets or Lanoxin® Elixir Pediatric** in Children with *Normal Renal Function Based on Lean Body Weight*

Age	Digitalizing* Dose (µg/kg)	*Daily* † Oral Maintenance Dose (µg/kg)
Premature	20–30	20–30% of *oral* loading dose††
Full-Term	25–35	
1–24 Months	35–60	
2–5 Years	30–40	25–35% of *oral* loading dose
5–10 Years	20–35	
Over 10 years	10–15	

Usual Digitalizing and Maintenance Dosages for **Lanoxin® Injection or Lanoxin® Injection Pediatric** in Children with *Normal Renal Function Based on Lean Body Weight*

Age	Digitalizing* Dose (µg/kg)	*Daily* † IV Maintenance Dose (µg/kg)
Premature	15–25	20–30% of the IV loading dose††
Full-Term	20–30	
1–24 Months	30–50	
2–5 Years	25–35	25–35% of the IV loading dose
5–10 Years	15–30	
Over 10 Years	8–12	

* IV digitalizing doses are 80% of oral digitalizing doses.
† Divided daily dosing is recommended for children under 10 years of age.
†† Projected or actual digitalizing dose providing desired clinical response.

LEUKERAN® ℞
(Chlorambucil)
2 mg Sugar-coated Tablets

> **WARNING:** LEUKERAN (CHLORAMBUCIL) CAN SEVERELY SUPPRESS BONE MARROW FUNCTION.
> CHLORAMBUCIL IS A CARCINOGEN IN MICE AND MUST BE PRESUMED TO BE SO IN HUMANS.
> CHLORAMBUCIL IS PROBABLY MUTAGENIC AND TERATOGENIC IN HUMANS.
> CHLORAMBUCIL AFFECTS HUMAN FERTILITY.
> SEE "WARNINGS" AND "PRECAUTIONS" SECTIONS.

Description: Leukeran® (chlorambucil), a bifunctional alkylating agent of the nitrogen mustard type, was first synthesized by Everett *et al.*[1] It is known chemically as *p*-(di-2-chlorethyl) aminophenylbutyric acid.

Haddow[2,3] discovered that chlorambucil was a powerful inhibitor of the transplanted Walker rat tumor 256 and had the pharmacologic effects of nitrogen mustard compounds. Subsequent clinical investigation showed that the drug was of value in producing remissions in chronic lymphocytic leukemia and in the treatment of malignant lymphomas and Hodgkin's disease.

Pharmacology and Toxicity: Pharmacologic studies,[2,3,4,5] in rats showed that oral absorption is good, being slightly less than intraperitoneal absorption. A single dose of 12.5 mg/kg intraperitoneally produces typical nitrogen mustard effects. These include loss of weight the first three days, atrophy of intestinal mucosa and of lymphoid organs, severe lymphopenia becoming maximal in four days, transient mild anemia lasting ten days, and thrombocytopenia. Rapid recovery occurs, commonly within 72 hours, and the animal appears normal in about one week, although the bone marrow and blood may not become completely normal for about three weeks. An intraperitoneal dose of 18.5 mg/kg kills about 50 per cent of the rats, with the development of convulsions. As much as 50 mg/kg has been given orally to rats as a single dose with recovery. Chlorambucil is only partially radiomimetic, producing chiefly the lymphoid effects of x-radiation as contrasted with Myleran® (busulfan) which produces mainly the myeloid effects.[4,5]

In humans, single oral doses of 20 mg or more may produce nausea and vomiting. In therapeutic doses the depressant effect on the bone marrow is only moderate and rapidly reversible. Patients with lymphomas are more sensitive to the drug and smaller doses are indicated and are therapeutically useful. With excessive doses or prolonged therapy amounting to a total accumulated dosage approaching 6.5 mg/kg (about 450 mg for a patient) there may develop pancytopenia with possible irreversible bone marrow damage. Patients will usually respond to considerably less total dosage of drug than this if they are to respond at all.

Indications: Leukeran® (chlorambucil) is indicated in the treatment of chronic lymphatic (lymphocytic) leukemia, malignant lymphomas including lymphosarcoma, giant follicular lymphoma and Hodgkin's disease. It is not curative in any of these disorders but may produce clinically useful palliation.

Contraindications: Chlorambucil should not be used in patients whose disease has demonstrated a prior resistance to the agent. Patients who have demonstrated hypersensitivity to chlorambucil should not be given the drug. There may be cross-hypersensitivity (skin rash) between chlorambucil and melphalan.

Warnings: Because of the carcinogenic, mutagenic and teratogenic potential, the use of chlorambucil to treat non-malignant conditions should be considered only after careful assessment of the benefit-to-risk ratio as it applies to the individual patient.

Carcinogenesis and Leukemogenesis: Three cases of acute myelogenous leukemia occurred in thirteen women who received daily chlorambucil for more than five years as adjuvant therapy for carcinoma of the breast.[6,7]

There are many additional reports of acute leukemia arising in patients with both malignant[8] and non-malignant[9] diseases following chlorambucil treatment. In many instances, these patients also received other chemotherapeutic agents or some form of radiation therapy. The quantitation of the risk of chlorambucil-induction of leukemia or carcinoma in humans is not possible. Evaluation of published reports of leukemia developing in patients who have received chlorambucil (and other alkylating agents) suggests that the risk of leukemogenesis increases with both chronicity of treatment and large cumulative doses. However, it has proved impossible to define a cumulative dose below which there is no risk of the induction of secondary malignancy. The potential benefits from chlorambucil therapy must be weighed on an individual basis against the possible risk of the induction of a secondary malignancy.

Use in Pregnancy: Safe use of chlorambucil has not been established with respect to adverse effects on fetal development. The problem of whether to use cancer chemotherapeutic agents in the treatment of leukemia during pregnancy has been reviewed by Smith *et al.*[10] and by Sokal and Lessmann.[11] Whenever possible, it seems best to defer use of these drugs until after the first trimester. Women of childbearing potential should be counseled about the mutagenic and teratogenic potential of alkylating agents.

Precautions: Patients must be followed carefully to avoid life-endangering damage to the bone marrow during treatment. Weekly examination of the blood should be made to determine hemoglobin levels, total and differential leukocyte counts, and quantitative platelet counts. Also, during the first 3 to 6 weeks of therapy, it is recommended that

Continued on next page

Burroughs Wellcome—Cont.

white blood cell counts be made 3 or 4 days after each of the weekly complete blood counts. Galton *et al.*[12] have suggested that in following patients it is helpful to plot the blood counts on a chart at the same time that body weight, temperature, spleen size, etc. are recorded. It is considered dangerous to allow a patient to go more than two weeks without hematological and clinical examination during treatment.

Many patients develop a slowly progressive lymphopenia during treatment. The lymphocyte count usually rapidly returns to normal levels upon completion of drug therapy. Most patients have some neutropenia after the third week of treatment and this may continue for up to ten days after the last dose. Subsequently, the neutrophil count usually rapidly returns to normal. Severe neutropenia appears to be related to dosage and usually occurs only in patients who have received a total dosage of 6.5 mg/kg or more in one course. About one-quarter of all patients receiving this dosage, and one-third of those receiving this dosage in eight weeks or less may be expected to develop severe neutropenia.[12]

While it is not necessary to discontinue chlorambucil at the first evidence of a fall in neutrophil count, it must be remembered that the fall may continue for ten days after the last dose and that as the total dose approaches 6.5 mg/kg there is real risk of causing irreversible bone marrow damage. Galton *et al.*[12] reported that most patients who received benefit from chlorambucil required a smaller dosage than this amount. The dosage should be decreased if leukocyte or platelet counts fall below normal values and should be discontinued for more severe depression.

Chlorambucil should not be given at full dosages before four weeks after a full course of radiation therapy or chemotherapy because of the vulnerability of the bone marrow to damage under these conditions. If the pretherapy leukocyte or platelet counts are depressed from bone marrow disease process prior to institution of therapy, the treatment should be instituted at a reduced dosage.

Persistently low neutrophil and platelet counts or peripheral lymphocytosis suggest bone marrow infiltration. If confirmed by bone marrow examination, the daily dosage of chlorambucil should not exceed 0.1 mg/kg. Chlorambucil appears to be relatively free from gastrointestinal side effects or other evidence of toxicity apart from the bone marrow depressant action.

Adverse Reactions: Apart from the depressant action on the bone marrow, side effects rarely occur with therapeutic doses. Gastric discomfort may occasionally be observed, especially with large dosage. Occasional drug fever and skin rashes (sometimes urticarial) have been reported.

Chlorambucil may be capable of producing a syndrome of bronchopulmonary dysplasia and pulmonary fibrosis similar to that seen with busulfan and cyclophosphamide.[13]

A high incidence of sterility has been documented when chlorambucil is administered to prepubertal and pubertal males.[14] Prolonged or permanent azoospermia has also been observed in adult males.[15] While most reports of gonadal dysfunction secondary to chlorambucil have related to males, the induction of amenorrhea in females with alkylating agents is well documented and chlorambucil is capable of producing amenorrhea.

Rare instances of hepatotoxicity with jaundice have been attributed to chlorambucil.[16,17]

Seizures have been observed in children following accidental overdose[18], during investigational therapy of nephrotic syndrome[19], and in an adult following repeated challenges with chlorambucil.[20]

Dosage and Administration: The usual oral dosage is 0.1 to 0.2 mg/kg body weight daily for three to six weeks as required. This usually amounts to 4 to 10 mg a day for the average patient. The entire daily dose may be given at one time. These dosages are for initiation of therapy or for short courses of treatment. The dosage must be carefully adjusted according to the response of the patient and must be reduced as soon as there is an abrupt fall in the white blood cell count. Patients with Hodgkin's disease usually require 0.2 mg/kg daily whereas patients with other lymphomas or chronic lymphocytic leukemia usually require only 0.1 mg/kg daily. When lymphocytic infiltration of the bone marrow is present, or when the bone marrow is hypoplastic, the daily dose should not exceed 0.1 mg/kg (about 6 mg for the average patient).

An alternate schedule for the treatment of chronic lymphocytic leukemia employing intermittent, bi-weekly, pulse doses of chlorambucil has been reported by Knospe *et al.*[21] Chlorambucil was administered orally with an initial single dose of 0.4 mg/kg. Doses were repeated every two weeks and increased by 0.1 mg/kg until control of lymphocytosis or toxicity was observed. Subsequent doses were modified up or down to produce mild hematologic toxicity. It was felt that the response rate of chronic lymphocytic leukemia to this bi-weekly schedule of chlorambucil administration was similar to that previously reported with daily administration and that hematologic toxicity was less than that encountered in studies using daily chlorambucil.

Radiation and cytotoxic drugs render the bone marrow more vulnerable to damage and chlorambucil should be used with particular caution within four weeks of a full course of radiation therapy or chemotherapy. However, small doses of palliative radiation over isolated foci remote from the bone marrow will not usually depress the neutrophil and platelet count. In these cases chlorambucil may be given in the customary dosage.

It is presently felt that short courses of treatment are safer than continuous maintenance therapy although both methods have been effective. It must be recognized that continuous therapy may give the appearance of "maintenance" in patients who are actually in remission and have no immediate need for further drug. If maintenance dosage is used, it should not exceed 0.1 mg/kg daily and may well be as low as 0.03 mg/kg daily. A typical maintenance dose is 2 mg to 4 mg daily, or less, depending on the status of the blood counts. It may, therefore, be desirable to withdraw the drug after maximal control has been achieved since intermittent therapy reinstituted at time of relapse may be as effective as continuous treatment.

How Supplied: White sugar-coated tablet containing 2 mg chlorambucil; in bottles of 50. **(NDC**-0081-0635-35.)

Store at 15°–30°C (59°–86°F) in a dry place.

References:

1. Everett, J.L., Roberts, J.R., and Ross, W.C.J.: Aryl-2-halogen-oalkylamines. Part XII. Some Carboxylic Derivatives of NN-Di-2-chloroethylaniline. J. Chem. Soc., p. 2386, 1953.
2. Haddow, A.: New Cytotoxic and Radiomimetic Agents. Annual Report Brit. Emp. Cancer Campaign, *30*:25, 1952.
3. Haddow, A.: Mode of Action of Carcinogenic Agents on Cells. Acta Unio internat contra cancrum, *9*:675, 1953.
4. Elson, L.A.: Comparison of the Physiological Response to Radiation and to Radiomimetic Chemicals. Radiobiology Symposium: pp. 235–242, London (Butterworth) 1954.
5. Elson, L.A.: A Comparison of the Effects of Radiation and Radiomimetic Chemicals on the Blood. Brit. J. Haematol., *1*:104, 1955.
6. Lerner, H.: Acute Myelogenous Leukemia in Patients Receiving Chlorambucil as Long-Term Therapy for Stage II Breast Cancer. Cancer Treat. Reports. *62*:1135, 1978.
7. Lerner, H.: Second Malignancies Diagnosed in Breast Cancer Patients While Receiving Adjuvant Chemotherapy at the Pennsylvania Hospital. Proc. Amer. Assoc. Cancer Res. and Amer. Soc. Clin. Oncol., *18*:340 (Abstract C-295), 1977.
8. Zarrabi, M.H. *et al.*: Chronic Lymphocytic Leukemia Terminating in Acute Leukemia. Arch. Intern. Med., *137(8)*: 1059, 1977.
9. Cameron, S.: Chlorambucil and Leukemia. N. Eng. J. Med., *296*:1065, 1977.
10. Smith, R.B.W., Sheehy, T.W., and Rothberg, H.: Hodgkin's Disease and Pregnancy. A.M.A. Arch. Int. Med., *102*:777, 1958.
11. Sokal, J.E., and Lessmann, E.M.: Effects of Cancer Chemotherapeutic Agents on the Human Fetus. JAMA, *172*:1765, 1960.
12. Galton, D.A.G., Israels, L.G., Nabarro, J.D.N., and Till, M.: Clinical Trials of p-(Di-2-chloroethylamino)-phenylbutyric Acid (CB 1348) in Malignant Lymphoma. Brit. M.J., *2*:1172, 1955.
13. Cole, S.R., Myers, T.J., and Klatsky, A.V.: Pulmonary Disease With Chlorambucil Therapy. Cancer, *41*:455, 1978.
14. Guesry, P., Lenoir, G., and Broyer, M.: Gonadal Effects of Chlorambucil Given to Prepubertal and Pubertal Boys for Nephrotic Syndrome. J. Pediatr., *92*:299, 1978.
15. Richter, P., *et al.*: Effect of Chlorambucil on Spermatogenesis in the Human with Malignant Lymphoma. Cancer, *25*:1026, 1970.
16. Koler, R.D. and Forsgren, A.L.: Hepatotoxicity Due to Chlorambucil, JAMA, *167*:316, 1958.
17. Amromin, G.D., Deliman, R.M., Shanbrom, E.: Liver Damage After Chemotherapy for Leukemia and Lymphoma. Gastroenterol. *42*:401, 1962.
18. Wolfson, S. and Olney, M.B.: Accidental Ingestion of a Toxic Dose of Chlorambucil. JAMA, *165*:239, 1957.
19. Williams, S.A., Makker, S.P., and Grupe, W.E.: Seizures: A Significant Side Effect of Chlorambucil Therapy in Children. J. Pediatr., *93*:516, 1978.
20. Naysmith, A. and Robson, R.H.: Focal Fits During Chlorambucil Therapy. Postgrad. Med. J., *55*:806, 1979.
21. Knospe, W.H., *et al.*: Bi-Weekly Chlorambucil Treatment of Chronic Lymphocytic Leukemia. Cancer. *33*:555, 1974.

[*Shown in Product Identification Section*]

MANTADIL® CREAM ℞

Description: Mantadil® Cream contains the antihistamine chlorcyclizine hydrochloride 2% and the corticosteroid hydrocortisone acetate 0.5%, preserved with methylparaben 0.25% in a vanishing cream base. The inactive ingredients are liquid and white petrolatum, emulsifying wax and purified water.

Mantadil Cream is an ANTIPRURITIC-ANTI-INFLAMMATORY-ANESTHETIC for topical administration.

Chlorcyclizine hydrochloride is known chemically as 1-[(4-Chlorophenyl) phenylmethyl]-4-methylpiperazine monohydrochloride.

Hydrocortisone acetate is the acetate ester of cortisol, known chemically as 17-hydroxycorticosterone 21-acetate.

The pH of this product is approximately 4.5.

Clinical Pharmacology: Chlorcyclizine hydrochloride is an H_1 histamine-receptor antagonist that will occupy receptor sites in effector cells to the exclusion of histamine. It blocks most of the effects of histamine mediated by H_1

receptors, including contraction of smooth muscle and increased capillary permeability. Absorption of chlorcyclizine hydrochloride into the skin is rapid following topical application, whereas systemic absorption from the skin is minimal. Chlorcyclizine hydrochloride prevents local edema and provides local anesthetic and antipruritic action in the skin. Hydrocortisone acetate administered topically suppresses most inflammatory and allergic responses in the skin. Following topical application, it is absorbed rapidly into the skin, where it reduces local heat, redness, swelling, and tenderness. A small part of the dose applied to broken skin is absorbed systemically and metabolized by the liver.

Indications and Usage: Mantadil Cream is indicated for the treatment of pruritic skin eruptions and other dermatoses including: eczema (allergic, nuchal and nummular); dermatitis (atopic, lichenoid and seborrheic); contact dermatitis including poison ivy, poison oak and poison sumac; localized neurodermatitis; insect bites; sunburn; intertrigo; and anogenital pruritus.

Contraindications: This preparation is contraindicated in patients who are hypersensitive to any of its components; in tuberculosis of the skin, vaccinia, varicella, and herpes simplex. As with other topical products containing hydrocortisone, the cream should not be used in bacterial infections of the skin unless antibacterial therapy is concomitant.

Not for ophthalmic use.

Warnings: Oral chlorcyclizine is teratogenic in animals. Long-term reproduction studies of topical chlorcyclizine have not been conducted in humans.

Precautions:

General: If signs of irritation develop with use of this cream, treatment should be discontinued and appropriate therapy instituted.

Any of the side effects reported following systemic use of corticosteroids, including adrenal suppression, may also occur following their topical use, especially in infants and children. Systemic absorption of topically applied steroids will be increased if extensive body surface areas are treated or if the occlusive technique is used. Under these circumstances, suitable precautions should be taken when long-term use is anticipated, particularly in infants and children.

Carcinogenesis, Mutagenesis, Impairment of Fertility:

Oral chlorcyclizine is teratogenic in animals. Long-term reproduction studies of topical chlorcyclizine have not been conducted. It is poorly absorbed percutaneously.

Pregnancy: **Teratogenic Effects:**

Pregnancy Category C. Animal reproduction studies have not been conducted with Mantadil Cream. It is also not known whether Mantadil Cream can cause fetal harm when administered to a pregnant woman or can affect reproduction capacity. Mantadil Cream should be given to a pregnant woman only if clearly needed.

Nursing Mothers: Hydrocortisone acetate appears in human milk following oral administration of the drug.

Caution should be exercised when hydrocortisone acetate is administered to a nursing woman.

It is not known whether chlorcyclizine hydrochloride is excreted in human milk. Because many drugs are excreted in human milk, caution should be exercised when chlorcyclizine hydrochloride is administered to a nursing woman.

Adverse Reactions: Allergic contact dermatitis may occur with topical application of chlorcyclizine hydrochloride. Systemic side effects have been reported after topical application of antihistamines to large areas of skin. The following local adverse reactions have been reported with topical corticosteroids, especially under occlusive dressings: irritation, folliculitis, hypertrichosis, acneiform eruptions, hypopigmentation, allergic contact dermatitis, secondary infection, skin atrophy, striae and miliaria.

Overdosage: With continued application of topical corticosteroid on large areas of damaged skin and under occlusion, there is a remote possibility that sufficient absorption could occur to produce Cushing's syndrome. This is more likely in children.

Systemic toxicity following application of chlorcyclizine has never been reported.

The oral LD_{50} of chlorcyclizine hydrochloride in the mouse is 300 mg/kg.

The intraperitoneal LD_{50} of hydrocortisone acetate in the mouse is 2300 mg/kg.

Dosage and Administration: Apply to the skin two to five times daily. If the condition of the skin will permit, the cream should be well rubbed in.

How Supplied: Mantadil Cream (Chlorcyclizine hydrochloride 2% and hydrocortisone acetate 0.5%) is available in 15 gram tubes (**NDC**-0081-0650-94).

Store at 15°-30°C (59°-86°F).

Compatibility Table
Marezine brand Cyclizine Lactate Injection

Forms a clear solution with: (i.e., can be mixed with)	Is not compatible with: (requires separate injection)
Atropine sulfate	Oxytetracycline hydrochloride
Meperidine hydrochloride (Demerol)	Chlortetracycline hydrochloride
Morphine sulfate	Penicillin
Tetracycline hydrochloride	Any solution with pH of 6.8 or higher (this includes Pentothal sodium and other soluble barbiturates)
Streptomycin sulfate	
Pyridoxine hydrochloride*	
Codeine phosphate and sulfate	
Alphaprodine HCl (Nisentil)	
Scopolamine hydrobromide*	
Pantopon (Hydrochlorides of opium alkaloids)*	
Hydromorphone (Dilaudid)*	*Administer within 4–10 minutes

MAREZINE® ℞
brand Cyclizine Lactate Injection
50 mg in 1 cc

Description: Chemically, cyclizine is N-benzhydryl-N′ methylpiperazine, and has a molecular weight of 266.4.

It is a white crystalline solid having a bitter taste, and is soluble in water and isotonic saline.

Marezine brand Cyclizine Lactate Injection is a sterile solution for INTRAMUSCULAR INJECTION ONLY.

Action: Marezine brand Cyclizine has antiemetic, anticholinergic and antihistaminic properties. It also reduces the sensitivity of the labyrinthine apparatus. The exact mechanism of action is unknown. In dogs the drug prevents emesis from intravenous threshold doses of apomorphine, but it is much less effective in blocking emesis from orally administered copper sulfate. These data suggest that the action is mediated through the chemoreceptive trigger zone.

Indications: For the treatment of nausea and vomiting of motion sickness when the oral route cannot be used.

Contraindications: Marezine is contraindicated in individuals who have shown a previous hypersensitivity to the drug.

Warnings: Patients may become drowsy while taking Marezine and should be cautioned against engaging in activities requiring mental alertness, e.g., driving a car or operating heavy machinery or appliances.

Use in Children: Clinical studies establishing safety and efficacy in children have not been done; therefore, usage in this age group and nursing mothers cannot be recommended.

Use with CNS Depressants: May have additive effects with alcohol and other CNS depressants (hypnotics, sedatives, tranquilizers, antianxiety agents, etc.).

Precautions: Because of its anticholinergic action, Marezine should be used with caution and appropriate monitoring in patients with glaucoma, obstructive disease of the gastrointestinal or genitourinary tract, and in elderly males with possible prostatic hypertrophy. Incipient glaucoma may be precipitated by anticholinergic drugs such as Marezine. The drug may have a hypotensive action. This may be confusing or dangerous in postoperative patients and should influence the decision on using the drug postoperatively.

Adverse Reactions: Urticaria, drug rash, dryness of mouth, nose and throat, drowsiness, restlessness, excitation, nervousness, insomnia, euphoria, anorexia, nausea, vomiting, diarrhea, constipation, hypotension, blurred vision, diplopia, vertigo, tinnitus, palpitation, tachycardia, urinary frequency, difficult urination, urinary retention, auditory and visual hallucinations have been reported, particularly when dosage recommendations are exceeded. Cholestatic jaundice has occurred in association with the use of Marezine.

Dosage and Administration: Marezine brand Cyclizine Lactate Injection is administered INTRAMUSCULARLY. The usual dose is 1 cc (50 mg) every 4 to 6 hours as necessary.

Overdosage:

Symptoms of Overdosage: Moderate overdosage may cause hyperexcitability alternating with drowsiness. Massive overdosage may cause convulsions; hallucinations; respiratory paralysis.

Treatment: Appropriate supportive and symptomatic treatment. Consider dialysis.

Caution: Do not use morphine or other respiratory depressants.

[See table above].

How Supplied:

MAREZINE® brand CYCLIZINE LACTATE INJECTION
50 mg in 1 cc
Boxes of 100 ampuls

The injection should be stored in a cold place. It may develop a slight yellow tint if stored at room temperature for several months; however, it retains full potency.

Also Available:

MAREZINE® brand CYCLIZINE HYDROCHLORIDE
50 mg Scored TABLETS
Boxes of 12
Bottles of 100 and 1000

[*Shown in Product Identification Section*]

Continued on next page

Burroughs Wellcome—Cont.

MYLERAN® ℞
(Busulfan)
2 mg Scored Tablets

Warnings: Myleran® (busulfan) is a potent drug. It should not be used unless a diagnosis of chronic myelogenous leukemia has been adequately established and the responsible physician is knowledgeable in assessing response to chemotherapy.
Myleran (busulfan) can induce severe bone marrow hypoplasia. Reduce or discontinue the dosage immediately at the first sign of any unusual depression of bone marrow function as reflected by an abnormal decrease in any of the formed elements of the blood. A bone marrow examination should be performed if the bone marrow status is uncertain.
SEE "WARNINGS" SECTION FOR INFORMATION REGARDING BUSULFAN-INDUCED LEUKEMOGENESIS IN HUMANS.

Description: Myleran (busulfan) (1,4-butanediol dimethanesulfonate) is a bifunctional alkylating agent. It is the most clinically useful member of a series of sulfonic acid esters of dihydric, straight chain, aliphatic alcohols synthesized by Haddow and Timmis at the Chester Beatty Research Institute.[1] It is the tetramethylene member (n = 4) of the series $CH_3SO_2O\text{-}(\text{-}CH_2\text{-})_n\ OSO_2CH_3$. It is *not* a structural analog of the nitrogen mustards.
The activity of busulfan in chronic myelogenous leukemia was first reported by D.A.G. Galton in 1953.[2]
Clinical Pharmacology: No analytical method has been found which permits the quantitation of non-radiolabeled busulfan or its metabolites in biological tissues or plasma. All studies of the pharmacokinetics of busulfan in humans have employed radiolabeled drug using either sulfur-35 (labeling the "carrier" portion of the molecule) or carbon-14 or tritium in the alkane portion of the 4-carbon chain (labels in the "alkylating" portion of the molecule).
Studies with ^{35}S-busulfan.[3] Following the intravenous administration of a single therapeutic dose of ^{35}S-busulfan, there was rapid disappearance of radioactivity from the blood; 90 to 95% of the ^{35}S-label disappeared within three to five minutes after injection. Thereafter, a constant, low level of radioactivity (1 to 3% of the injected dose) was maintained during the subsequent forty-eight hour period of observation. Following the oral administration of ^{35}S-busulfan, there was a lag period of one-half to two hours prior to the detection of radioactivity in the blood. However, at four hours the (low) level of circulating radioactivity was comparable to that obtained following intravenous administration.
After either oral or intravenous administration of ^{35}S-busulfan to humans, 45 to 60% of the radioactivity was recovered in the urine in the forty-eight hours after administration; the majority of the total urinary excretion occurred in the first twenty-four hours. In man, over 95% of the urinary sulfur-35 occurs as ^{35}S-methanesulfonic acid.
The fact that urinary recovery of sulfur-35 was equivalent, irrespective of whether the drug was given intravenously or orally, suggests virtually complete absorption by the oral route.
Studies with ^{14}C-busulfan.[3] Oral and intravenous administration of 1,4-^{14}C-busulfan showed the same rapid initial disappearance of plasma radioactivity with a subsequent low-level plateau as observed following the administration of ^{35}S-labeled drug. Cumulative radioactivity in the urine after forty-eight hours was 25 to 30% of the administered dose (contrasting with 45 to 60% for ^{35}S-busulfan) and suggests a slower excretion of the alkylating portion of the molecule and its metabolites than for the sulfonoxymethyl moieties. Regardless of the route of administration, 1,4-^{14}C-busulfan yielded a complex mixture of at least 12 radiolabeled metabolites in urine; the main metabolite being 3-hydroxytetrahydrothiophene-1, 1-dioxide.
Studies with ^{3}H-busulfan.[4] Human pharmacokinetic studies have been conducted employing busulfan labeled with tritium on the tetramethylene chain. These experiments confirmed a rapid initial clearance of the radioactivity from plasma, irrespective of whether the drug was given orally or intravenously, and showed a gradual accumulation of radioactivity in the plasma after repeated doses. Urinary excretion of less than 50% of the total dose given suggested a slow elimination of the metabolic products from the body.
There is no experience with the use of dialysis in an attempt to modify the clinical toxicity of busulfan. One technical difficulty would derive from the extremely poor water solubility of busulfan. Additionally, all studies of the metabolism of busulfan employing radiolabeled materials indicate rapid chemical reactivity of the parent compound with prolonged retention of some of the metabolites (particularly the metabolites arising from the "alkylating" portion of the molecule). The effectiveness of dialysis at removing significant quantities of unreacted drug would be expected to be minimal in such a situation.
No information is available regarding the penetration of busulfan into brain or cerebrospinal fluid.
Biochemical Pharmacology: In aqueous media, busulfan undergoes a wide range of nucleophilic substitution reactions. While this chemical reactivity is relatively non-specific, alkylation of the DNA is felt to be an important biological mechanism for its cytotoxic effect.[3] Coliphage T7 exposed to busulfan was found to have the DNA crosslinked by intrastrand crosslinkages, but no interstrand linkages were found.
The metabolic fate of busulfan has been studied in rats and humans using ^{14}C- and ^{35}S-labeled materials.[3,6,7] In man,[3] as in the rat,[7] almost all of the radioactivity in ^{35}S-labeled busulfan is excreted in the urine in the form of ^{35}S-methanesulfonic acid. No unchanged drug was found in human urine,[3] although a small amount has been reported in rat urine.[7] Roberts and Warwick demonstrated that the formation of methanesulfonic acid *in vivo* in the rat is not due to a simple hydrolysis of busulfan to 1,4-butanediol, since only about 4% of 2,3-^{14}C-busulfan was excreted as carbon dioxide whereas 2,3-^{14}C-1,4-butanediol was converted almost exclusively to carbon dioxide.[6] The predominant reaction of busulfan in the rat is the alkylation of sulfhydryl groups (particularly cysteine and cysteine-containing compounds) to produce a cyclic sulfonium compound which is the precursor of the major urinary metabolite of the 4-carbon portion of the molecule, 3-hydroxytetrahydrothiophene-1, 1-dioxide.[6] This has been termed a "sulfur-stripping" action of busulfan and it may modify the function of certain sulfur-containing amino acids, polypeptides, and proteins; whether this action makes an important contribution to the cytotoxicity of busulfan is unknown.
The biochemical basis for acquired resistance to busulfan is largely a matter of speculation. Although altered transport of busulfan into the cell is one possibility, increased intracellular inactivation of the drug before it reaches the DNA is also possible. Experiments with other alkylating agents have shown that resistance to this class of compounds may reflect an acquired ability of the resistant cell to repair alkylation damage more effectively.[5]
Indications and Usage: Myleran® (busulfan) is indicated for the palliative treatment of chronic myelogenous (myeloid, myelocytic, granulocytic) leukemia. Although not curative, busulfan reduces the total granulocyte mass, relieves symptoms of the disease, and improves the clinical state of the patient. Approximately 90% of adults with previously untreated chronic myelogenous leukemia will obtain hematologic remission with regression or stabilization of organomegaly following the use of busulfan. It has been shown to be superior to splenic irradiation with respect to survival times and maintenance of hemoglobin levels, and to be equivalent to irradiation at controlling splenomegaly.[8]
It is not clear whether busulfan unequivocally prolongs the survival of responding patients beyond the 31 months experienced by an untreated group of historical controls.[9] Median survival figures of 31–42 months have been reported for several groups of patients treated with busulfan, but concurrent control groups of comparable, untreated patients are not available.[8,10,11,12] The median survival figures reported from different studies will be influenced by the percentage of "poor risk" patients initially entered into the particular study. Patients who are alive two years following the diagnosis of chronic myelogenous leukemia, and who have been treated during that period with busulfan, are estimated to have a mean annual mortality rate during the second to fifth year which is approximately two-thirds that of patients who received either no treatment, conventional x-ray or ^{32}P-irradiation, or chemotherapy with minimally active drugs.[13]
Busulfan is clearly less effective in patients with chronic myelogenous leukemia who lack the Philadelphia (Ph^1) chromosome.[14] Also, the so-called "juvenile" type of chronic myelogenous leukemia, typically occurring in young children and associated with the absence of a Philadelphia chromosome, responds poorly to busulfan.[15] The drug is of no benefit in patients whose chronic myelogenous leukemia has entered a "blastic" phase.
Contraindications: Myleran® (busulfan) should not be used unless a diagnosis of chronic myelogenous leukemia has been adequately established and the responsible physician is knowledgeable in assessing response to chemotherapy.
Myleran should not be used in patients whose chronic myelogenous leukemia has demonstrated prior resistance to this drug.
Myleran is of no value in chronic lymphocytic leukemia, acute leukemia, or in the "blastic crisis" of chronic myelogenous leukemia.
Warnings: The most frequent, serious side effect of treatment with busulfan is the induction of bone marrow failure (which may or may not be anatomically hypoplastic) resulting in severe pancytopenia. The pancytopenia caused by busulfan may be more prolonged than that induced with other alkylating agents. It is generally felt that the usual cause of busulfan-induced pancytopenia is the failure to stop administration of the drug soon enough; individual idiosyncrasy to the drug does not seem to be an important factor. *Myleran should be used with extreme caution and exceptional vigilance in patients whose bone marrow reserve may have been compromised by prior irradiation or chemotherapy, or whose marrow function is recovering from previous cytotoxic therapy.* Although recovery from busulfan-induced pancytopenia may take from one month to two years, this complication is potentially reversible and the patient should be vigorously supported through any period of severe pancytopenia.[16]
A rare, important complication of busulfan therapy is the development of bronchopulmonary dysplasia with pulmonary fibrosis.[17] Symptoms have been reported to occur within eight months to ten years after initiation of

therapy—the average duration of therapy being four years. The histologic findings associated with "busulfan lung" mimic those seen following pulmonary irradiation. Clinically, patients have reported the insidious onset of cough, dyspnea, and low-grade fever. Pulmonary function studies have revealed diminished diffusion capacity and decreased pulmonary compliance. It is important to exclude more common conditions (such as opportunistic infections or leukemic infiltration of the lungs) with appropriate diagnostic techniques. If measures such as sputum cultures, virologic studies, and exfoliative cytology fail to establish an etiology for the pulmonary infiltrates, lung biopsy may be necessary to establish the diagnosis. Treatment of established busulfan-induced pulmonary fibrosis is unsatisfactory; in most cases the patients have died within six months after the diagnosis was established. There is no specific therapy for this complication other than the immediate discontinuation of busulfan. The administration of corticosteroids has been suggested, but the results have not been impressive or uniformly successful.

Busulfan may cause cellular dysplasia in many organs in addition to the lung. Cytologic abnormalities characterized by giant, hyperchromatic nuclei have been reported in lymph nodes, pancreas, thyroid, adrenal glands, liver, and bone marrow. This cytologic dysplasia may be severe enough to cause difficulty in interpretation of exfoliative cytologic examinations from the lung, bladder, breast, and the uterine cervix.

In addition to the widespread epithelial dysplasia that has been observed during busulfan therapy, chromosome aberrations have been reported in cells from patients receiving busulfan.

Busulfan is mutagenic in mice and, possibly, in man.

A number of malignant tumors have been reported in patients on busulfan therapy and this drug may be a human carcinogen. Four cases of acute leukemia occurred among 243 patients treated with busulfan as adjuvant chemotherapy following surgical resection of bronchogenic carcinoma. All four cases were from a subgroup of 19 of these 243 patients who developed pancytopenia while taking busulfan five to eight years before leukemia became clinically apparent. These findings suggest that busulfan is leukemogenic, although its mode of action is uncertain.[18]

Busulfan may cause fetal harm when administered to a pregnant woman. Although there have been a number of cases reported where apparently normal children have been born after busulfan treatment during pregnancy.[19] one case has been cited where a malformed baby was delivered by a mother treated with busulfan. During the pregnancy that resulted in the malformed infant, the mother received x-ray therapy early in the first trimester, mercaptopurine until the third month, then busulfan until delivery.[20] In pregnant rats, busulfan produces sterility in both male and female offspring due to the absence of germinal cells in testes and ovaries.[21] Germinal cell aplasia or sterility in offspring of mothers receiving busulfan during pregnancy has not been reported in humans. If this drug is used during pregnancy or if the patient becomes pregnant while taking this drug, the patient should be apprised of the potential hazard to the fetus.

Ovarian suppression and amenorrhea with menopausal symptoms commonly occur during busulfan therapy in premenopausal patients. Busulfan interferes with spermatogenesis in experimental animals, and there have been clinical reports of sterility, azoospermia and testicular atrophy in male patients.

Precautions: General: The most consistent, dose-related toxicity is bone marrow suppression. This may be manifest by anemia, leukopenia, thrombocytopenia, or any combination of these. It is imperative that patients be instructed to report promptly the development of fever, sore throat, signs of local infection, bleeding from any site, or symptoms suggestive of anemia. Any one of these findings may indicate busulfan toxicity; however, they may also indicate transformation of the disease to an acute "blastic" form. Since busulfan may have a delayed effect, it is important to withdraw the medication temporarily at the first sign of an abnormally large or exceptionally rapid fall in any of the formed elements of the blood. *Patients should never be allowed to take the drug without close medical supervision.*

Laboratory Tests: It is recommended that evaluation of the hemoglobin or hematocrit, total white blood cell count and differential count, and quantitative platelet count be obtained weekly while the patient is on busulfan therapy. In cases where the cause of fluctuation in the formed elements of the peripheral blood is obscure, bone marrow examination may be useful for evaluation of marrow status. A decision to increase, decrease, continue, or discontinue a given dose of busulfan must be based not only on the absolute hematologic values, but also on the rapidity with which changes are occurring. The dosage of busulfan may need to be reduced if this agent is combined with other drugs whose primary toxicity is myelosuppression. Occasional patients may be unusually sensitive to busulfan administered at standard dosage and suffer neutropenia or thrombocytopenia after a relatively short exposure to the drug. Busulfan should not be used where facilities for complete blood counts, including quantitative platelet counts, are not available at weekly (or more frequent) intervals.

Carcinogenesis, Mutagenesis, Impairment of Fertility: See "WARNINGS" section.

Pregnancy: ***Teratogenic effects:*** Pregnancy Category D. See "WARNINGS" section.

Non-Teratogenic effects: There have been reports in the literature of small infants being born after the mothers received busulfan during pregnancy, in particular, during the third trimester.[22] One case was reported where an infant had mild anemia and neutropenia at birth after busulfan was administered to the mother from the eighth week of pregnancy to term.[19]

Nursing Mothers: It is not known whether this drug is excreted in human milk. Because of the potential for tumorigenicity shown for Myleran (bulsulfan) in animal and human studies, a decision should be made whether to discontinue nursing or to discontinue the drug, taking into account the importance of the drug to the mother.

Adverse Reactions:

Hematological Effects: The most frequent, serious, toxic effect of busulfan is myelosuppression resulting in leukopenia, thrombocytopenia, and anemia. Myelosuppression is most frequently the result of a failure to discontinue dosage in the face of an undetected decrease in leukocyte or platelet counts.[16]

Pulmonary: Interstitial pulmonary fibrosis has been reported rarely, but it is a clinically significant adverse effect when observed and calls for immediate discontinuation of further administration of the drug. The role of corticosteroids in arresting or reversing the fibrosis has been reported to be beneficial in some cases and without effect in others.[17]

Cardiac: One case of endocardial fibrosis has been reported in a 79-year-old woman who received a total dose of 7,200 mg of busulfan over a period of nine years for the management of chronic myelogenous leukemia.[23] At autopsy, she was found to have endocardial fibrosis of the left ventricle in addition to interstitial pulmonary fibrosis.

Ocular: Busulfan is capable of inducing cataracts in rats and there have been several reports indicating that this is a rare complication in humans. In the few cases reported in humans, cataracts have occurred only after prolonged administration of busulfan.[24]

Dermatologic: Hyperpigmentation is the most common adverse skin reaction and occurs in 5–10% of patients, particularly those with a dark complexion.

Metabolic: In a few cases, a clinical syndrome closely resembling adrenal insufficiency and characterized by weakness, severe fatigue, anorexia, weight loss, nausea and vomiting, and melanoderma has developed after prolonged busulfan therapy. The symptoms have sometimes been reversible when busulfan was withdrawn. Adrenal responsiveness to exogenously administered ACTH has usually been normal. However, pituitary function testing with metyrapone revealed a blunted urinary 17-hydroxycorticosteroid excretion in two patients.[25] Following the discontinuation of busulfan (which was associated with clinical improvement), rechallenge with metyrapone revealed normal pituitary-adrenal function.

Hyperuricemia and/or hyperuricosuria are not uncommon in patients with chronic myelogenous leukemia. Additional rapid destruction of granulocytes may accompany the initiation of chemotherapy and increase the urate pool. Adverse effects can be minimized by increased hydration, urine alkalinization, and the prophylactic administration of a xanthine oxidase inhibitor such as Zyloprim® (allopurinol).

Miscellaneous: Other reported adverse reactions include; urticaria, erythema multiforme, erythema nodosum, alopecia, porphyria cutanea tarda, excessive dryness and fragility of the skin with anhidrosis, dryness of the oral mucous membranes and cheilosis, gynecomastia, cholestatic jaundice, and myasthenia gravis. Most of these are single case reports, and in many a clear cause and effect relationship with busulfan has not been demonstrated.

Overdosage: There is no known antidote to busulfan. The principal toxic effect is on the bone marrow. Survival after a single 140 mg dose has been reported in an 18 kg, 4 year old child,[26] but hematologic toxicity is likely to be more profound with chronic overdosage. The hematologic status should be closely monitored and vigorous supportive measures instituted if necessary.

Dosage and Administration: Busulfan is administered orally. The usual adult dose for *remission induction* is four to eight mg. total dose, daily. Dosing on a weight basis (mg/kg) is the same for both children and adults, approximately 60 μg per kg of body weight or 1.8 mg per square meter of body surface, daily. Since the rate of fall of the leukocyte count is dose related, daily doses exceeding four mg per day should be reserved for patients with the most compelling symptoms; the greater the total daily dose, the greater is the possibility of inducing bone marrow aplasia.

A decrease in the leukocyte count is not usually seen during the first ten to fifteen days of treatment; the leukocyte count may actually increase during this period and it should not be interpreted as resistance to the drug, nor should the dose be increased.[27] Since the leukocyte count may continue to fall for more than one month after discontinuing the drug, it is important that busulfan be discontinued *prior* to the total leukocyte count falling into the normal range. When the total leukocyte count has declined to approximately 15,000/μl the drug should be withheld.

With a constant dose of busulfan, the total leukocyte count declines exponentially; a weekly plot of the leukocyte count on semilogarithmic graph paper aids in predicting the time when therapy should be discontinued.[28] With the recommended dose of busulfan, a normal leukocyte count is usually achieved in twelve to twenty weeks.

Continued on next page

Burroughs Wellcome—Cont.

During remission, the patient is examined at monthly intervals and treatment resumed with the induction dosage when the total leukocyte count reaches approximately 50,000/µl. When remission is shorter than three months, maintenance therapy of 1 to 3 mg daily may be advisable in order to keep the hematological status under control and prevent rapid relapse.

How Supplied: White, scored tablets containing 2 mg busulfan, imprinted with "WELLCOME" and "K2A" on each tablet; in bottle of 25.

References:

1. Haddow, A., and Timmis, G.M.: Myleran in Chronic Myeloid Leukaemia; Chemical Constitution and Biological Action. Lancet *1*: 207–208, 1953.
2. Galton, D.A.G.: Myleran in Chronic Myeloid Leukaemia, Lancet *1*: 208–213, 1953.
3. Nadkarni, M.V., Trams, E.G., and Smith, P.K.: Preliminary Studies on the Distribution and Fate of TEM, TEPA, and Myleran in the Human. Cancer Res. *19*: 713–718, 1959.
4. Vodopick, H., Hamilton, H.E., Jackson, H.L., Peng, C.T., and Sheets, R.F.: Metabolic Fate of Tritiated Busulfan in Man. J. Lab. & Clin. Med. *73*: 266–276, 1969.
5. Fox, B.W.: Mechanism of Action of Methanesulfonates. In, *Antineoplastic and Immunosuppressive Agents,* Part II. (Edited by A.C. Sartorelli and D.G. Johns) Berlin, Springer-Verlag, 35–46, 1975.
6. Roberts, J.J., and Warwick, G.P.: The Mode of Action of Alkylating Agents—III. The Formation of 3-hydroxytetrahydrothiophene-1:1-dioxide from 1:4-dimethanesulphonyloxybutane (Myleran), S-β-L-alanyltetrahydrothiophenium mesylate, tetrahydrothiophene and tetrahydrothiophene-1:1-dioxide in the Rat, Rabbit and Mouse, Biochem. Pharmacol. *6*: 217–227, 1961.
7. Peng, C.T.: Distribution and Metabolic Fate of S^{35} Labeled Myleran (Bulsulfan) in Normal and Tumor Bearing Rats. J. Pharmac. Exp. Therap. *120*: 229–238, 1957.
8. Medical Research Council's Working Party for Therapeutic Trials in Leukemia: Chronic Granulocytic Leukaemia: Comparison of Radiotherapy and Bulsulphan Therapy, Brit. Med. J. *1*: 201–208, 1968.
9. Minot, G.R., Buckman, T.E., and Isaacs, R.: Chronic Myelogenous Leukemia: Age Incidence, Duration, and Benefit Derived From Irradiation, JAMA *82*: 1489–1494, 1924.
10. Haut, A., Abbott, W.S., Wintrobe, M.M., and Cartwright, G.E.: Busulfan in the Treatment of Chronic Myelocytic Leukemia. The Effect of Long Term Intermittent Therapy. Blood *17*: 1–19, 1961.
11. Monfardini, S., Gee, T., Fried J. and Clarkson, B.: Survival in Chronic Myelogenous Leukemia: Influence of Treatment and Extent of Disease at Diagnosis. Cancer *31*: 492–501, 1973.
12. Conrad, F.G.: Survival in Chronic Granulocytic Leukemia. Arch. Intern. Med. *131*: 684–685, 1973.
13. Sokal, J.E.: Evaluation of Survival Data for Chronic Myelocytic Leukemia. Am. J. Hematol. *1*: 493–500, 1976.
14. Ezdinli, E.Z., Sokal, J.E., Crosswhite, L., and Sandberg, A.A.: Philadelphia-Chromosome-Positive and -Negative Chronic Myelocytic Leukemia. Ann. Intern. Med. *72*: 175–182, 1970.
15. Smith, K.L., and Johnson, W.: Classification of Chronic Myelocytic Leukemia in Children. Cancer *34*: 670–679, 1974.
16. Stuart, J.J., Crocker, D.L., and Roberts, H.R.: Treatment of Busulfan-Induced Pancytopenia. Arch. Intern. Med. *136*: 1181–1183, 1976.
17. Sostman, H.D., Matthay, R.A., and Putman, C.E.: Cytotoxic Drug-Induced Lung Disease. Am. J. Med. *62*: 608–615, 1977.
18. Stott, H., Fox, W., Girling, D.J., Stephens, R.J., and Galton, D.A.G.: Acute Leukemia After Busulphan. Brit. Med. J. *2*: 1513–1517, 1977.
19. Dugdale, M. and Fort, A.T.: Busulfan Treatment of Leukemia During Pregnancy. Case Report and Review of the Literature. JAMA *199*: 131–133, 1967.
20. Diamond, I., Anderson, M.M. and McCreadie, S.R.: Transplacental Transmission of Busulfan (Myleran®) in a Mother with Leukemia. Pediatrics *25*: 85–90, 1960.
21. Bollag, W.: Cytostatica in der Schwangershaft, Schweiz. Med. Wochenschr. *84*: 393–395, 1954.
22. Boros, S.J. and Reynolds, J.W.: Intrauterine Growth Retardation Following Third-Trimester-Exposure to Busulfan. Am. J. Obstet. Gynecol. *129*: 111–112, 1977.
23. Weinberger, A., Pinkhas, J., Sandbank, U., Shaklai, M., and Vries, A. de: Endocardial Fibrosis Following Busulfan Treatment. JAMA *231*: 495, 1975.
24. Ravindranathan, M.P., Paul, V.J., and Kuriakose, E.T.: Cataract after Busulphan Treatment. Brit. Med. J. *1*: 218–219, 1972.
25. Vivacqua, R.J., Haurani, F.I., and Erslev, A.J.: "Selective", Pituitary Insufficiency Secondary to Busulfan. Ann. Intern. Med. *67*: 380–387, 1967.
26. Oliveira, H.P. de, Cruz, E., Fonseca, A. de S., and Medeiros, M.: Accidental Ingestion of a Toxic Dose of Myleran by a Child. Acta Haemat. (Basel) *29*: 249–255, 1963.
27. Stryckmans, P.A.: Current Concepts in Chronic Myelogenous Leukemia. Semin. Hematol. *11*: 101–139, 1974.
28. Galton, D.A.G.: Chemotherapy of Chronic Myelocytic Leukaemia. Semin. Hematol. *6*: 323–343, 1969.

[*Shown in Product Identification Section*]

NEOSPORIN® AEROSOL ℞

Polymyxin B—Bacitracin—Neomycin Powder For Topical Use Only (Not Sterile)

Description: Each aerosol spray packing of 90 g contains: Aerosporin® brand Polymyxin B Sulfate 100,000 units; bacitracin zinc 8,000 units; neomycin sulfate 100 mg (equivalent to 70 mg neomycin base).
Inert propellant: dichlorodifluoromethane and trichloromonofluoromethane.
Approximate spraying time of the container is 100 seconds.

Action: The combination of Aerosporin brand Polymyxin B Sulfate with neomycin and bacitracin was selected because it most nearly meets the criteria for an ideal topical antibacterial preparation. The spectrum of action encompasses most pathogenic bacteria found topically, and the three antibiotics are bactericidal rather than bacteriostatic. When used topically, polymyxin B, neomycin and bacitracin are rarely irritating, and absorption from skin or mucous membrane is insignificant. The index of allergenicity of this combination has been shown over the years to be low. And finally, since these antibiotics are seldom used systemically, the patient is spared sensitization to those antibiotics which might later be required systemically.
Polymyxin B is one of a group of closely related substances produced by various strains of *Bacillus polymyxa.* Its activity is sharply restricted to gram-negative bacteria, including many strains of *Pseudomonas aeruginosa.*
Neomycin, isolated from *Streptomyces fradiae,* has antibacterial activity *in vitro* against a wide range of gram-negative and gram-positive organisms, with effectiveness against many strains of *Proteus.*
Bacitracin, an antibiotic substance derived from cultures of *Bacillus subtilis* (Tracy), exerts antibacterial action *in vitro* against a variety of gram-positive and a few gram-negative organisms.

Indications: Based on a review of this drug by the National Academy of Sciences-National Research Council and/or other information, FDA has classified the indications as follows:
"Possibly" effective: For topical administration for the treatment of the listed localized infections or for suppressive therapy in such conditions:

Biopsy sites	Abrasions
Vascular ulcers	Cuts
Decubitus ulcers	Lacerations
Burns	Infected eczemas
Dermabrasion	Infected dermatoses
	Skin grafts and donor sites

Final classification of the less-than-effective indications requires further investigation.

Contraindications: This product is contraindicated in those individuals who have shown hypersensitivity to any of its components.

Warning: Because of the potential hazard of nephrotoxicity and ototoxicity due to neomycin, care should be exercised when using this product in treating extensive burns, trophic ulceration and other extensive conditions where absorption of neomycin is possible. In burns where more than 20 percent of the body surface is affected, especially if the patient has impaired renal function or is receiving other aminoglycoside antibiotics concurrently, not more than one application a day is recommended.
When using neomycin-containing products to control secondary infection in the chronic dermatoses, such as chronic otitis externa or stasis dermatitis, it should be borne in mind that the skin in these conditions is more liable than is normal skin to become sensitized to many substances, including neomycin. The manifestation of sensitization to neomycin is usually a low grade reddening with swelling, dry scaling and itching; it may be manifest simply as failure to heal. During long-term use of neomycin-containing products, periodic examination for such signs is advisable and the patient should be told to discontinue the product if they are observed. These symptoms regress quickly on withdrawing the medication. Neomycin-containing applications should be avoided for that patient thereafter.

Precautions: As with other antibiotic preparations, prolonged use may result in overgrowth of nonsusceptible organisms including fungi. Appropriate measures should be taken if this occurs. Do not spray in the eyes. Contents are under pressure, but are not flammable. Do not puncture or incinerate container.

Adverse Reactions: Neomycin is a not uncommon cutaneous sensitizer. Articles in the current literature indicate an increase in the prevalence of persons allergic to neomycin. Ototoxicity and nephrotoxicity have been reported (see Warning section).

Dosage and Administration: SHAKE WELL before each spraying. Remove cap, twist off tamper-proof seal and press button to spray affected area. Container will operate in either upright or inverted position. Use one-second intermittent sprays from a distance of about 8 inches. Prolonged spraying is unnecessary and wastes medication.

How Supplied: Aerosol spray can of 90 g.

NEOSPORIN®-G CREAM ℞

Polymyxin B—Neomycin—Gramicidin

Description: Each gram contains:
Aerosporin® brand Polymyxin B Sulfate 10,000 units; neomycin sulfate 5 mg (equiva-

lent to 3.5 mg neomycin base); gramicidin 0.25 mg.
Inactive ingredients: liquid petrolatum, white petrolatum, purified water, propylene glycol, polyoxyethylene polyoxypropylene compound, emulsifying wax, and 0.25% methylparaben as preservative.

Indications: Based on a review of this drug by the National Academy of Sciences—National Research Council and/or other information, FDA has classified the indications as follows:
"Possibly" effective: For topical administration for the treatment of the listed localized infections or for suppressive therapy in such conditions: primary pyodermas (impetigo, ecthyma, sycosis vulgaris, paronychia); secondary infected dermatoses (eczema, herpes and seborrheic dermatitis); traumatic lesions (inflamed or suppurating as a result of bacterial infection).
Final classification of the less-than-effective indications requires further investigation.

Contraindications: Not for use in the eyes or in the external ear canal if the eardrum is perforated. This product is contraindicated in those individuals who have shown hypersensitivity to any of its components.
Warning: Because of the potential hazard of nephrotoxicity and ototoxicity due to neomycin, care should be exercised when using this product in treating extensive burns, trophic ulceration and other extensive conditions where absorption of neomycin is possible. In burns where more than 20 percent of the body surface is affected, especially if the patient has impaired renal function or is receiving other aminoglycoside antibiotics concurrently, not more than one application a day is recommended.
When using neomycin-containing products to control secondary infection in the chronic dermatoses, such as chronic otitis externa or stasis dermatitis, it should be borne in mind that the skin in these conditions is more liable than is normal skin to become sensitized to many substances, including neomycin. The manifestation of sensitization to neomycin is usually a low grade reddening with swelling, dry scaling and itching; it may be manifest simply as a failure to heal. During long-term use of neomycin-containing products, periodic examination for such signs is advisable and the patient should be told to discontinue the product if they are observed. These symptoms regress quickly on withdrawing the medication. Neomycin-containing applications should be avoided for that patient thereafter.
Precautions: As with other antibacterial preparations, prolonged use may result in overgrowth of nonsusceptible organisms, including fungi. Appropriate measures should be taken if this occurs.
Adverse Reactions: Neomycin is a not uncommon cutaneous sensitizer. Articles in the current literature indicate an increase in the prevalence of persons allergic to neomycin. Ototoxicity and nephrotoxicity have been reported (see Warning section).
Dosage and Administration: A small quantity of the cream should be applied 2 to 5 times daily, as required. The cream should, if conditions permit, be gently rubbed into the affected areas.
How Supplied: Tube of 15 g.
15 g—DoD & VA NSN 6505-00-926-2159

NEOSPORIN® G.U. IRRIGANT ℞

brand Neomycin Sulfate—Polymyxin B Sulfate G.U. Irrigant, Sterile. A Concentrated Antibiotic Solution To Be Diluted For Urinary Bladder Irrigation. NOT FOR INJECTION.

Description: Each cc contains neomycin sulfate equivalent to neomycin base 40 mg, polymyxin B sulfate 200,000 units, water for injection qs. Multiple-dose vial contains methylparaben 1 mg (0.1%) as preservative.
Action: Polymyxin B sulfate is bactericidal to most gram-negative bacilli, including clinically isolated strains of *Pseudomonas aeruginosa (B pyocyaneus).* This organism is conspicuously absent from the spectra of most other antibiotic agents, but it is highly susceptible to polymyxin B sulfate, which is acknowledged to be an effective agent for the treatment and prophylaxis of *Pseudomonas* infections.
Neomycin sulfate is bactericidal against a wide range of gram-negative and gram-positive organisms. It is particularly effective against many strains of *Proteus.*
When used topically, polymyxin B sulfate and neomycin are rarely irritating. Since these antibiotics are seldom used systemically, the patient is spared sensitization to those antibiotics which might later be required systemically.
Indications: To be used as a continuous irrigant or rinse for short-term use *(up to 10 days)* in the urinary bladder of abacteriuric patients to help prevent bacteriuria and gram-negative rod bacteremia, associated with the use of indwelling catheters.
Contraindications: This product is contraindicated in those individuals who have shown hypersensitivity to any of its components.
Precautions: As with other antibiotic preparations, prolonged use may result in overgrowth of nonsusceptible organisms, including fungi. Appropriate measures should be taken if this occurs. The safety and effectiveness of this preparation for use in the care of patients with recent lower urinary tract surgery have not been established.
Neomycin toxicity: Neomycin is nephrotoxic and ototoxic, particularly when given parenterally in higher than recommended doses. Cases of nephrotoxicity and/or ototoxicity have been reported following its use in treatment of extensive burns and irrigation of wounds. Although the possibility of these reactions is remote with the use of the minimal amount in bladder irrigations, such may occur if these bladder irrigations are continued over the recommended time of "under 10 days"; caution should be observed.
Adverse Reactions: Hypersensitivity reactions: According to current medical literature there has been an increase in the prevalence of neomycin hypersensitivity, however, topical application to mucous membrane rarely results in local or systemic reactions.
Dosage and Administration: This preparation is specifically designed for use with "three-way" catheters or with other catheter systems permitting *continuous* irrigation of the urinary bladder.
Using sterile precautions, one (1) cc of Neosporin G.U. Irrigant should be added to a 1,000 cc container of isotonic saline solution. This container should then be connected to the inflow lumen of the "three-way" catheter which has been inserted with full aseptic precautions; use of a sterile lubricant is recommended during insertion of the catheter. The outflow lumen should be connected, via a sterile disposable plastic tube, to a disposable plastic collection bag.
Inflow rate, for most patients, of the 1,000 cc saline solution of neomycin and polymyxin B, should be adjusted to a slow drip to deliver about 1,000 cc every twenty-four hours. If the patient's urine output exceeds 2 liters per day it is recommended that the inflow rate should be adjusted to deliver 2,000 cc of the solution in a twenty-four hour period.
It is important that the rinse of the bladder be *continuous:* the inflow or rinse solution should not be interrupted for more than a few minutes.
Clinical Background: Extremely high rates of infection of the urinary tract following indwelling catheterization have been reported. The serious sequelae of urinary tract infections, such as hypertension, pregnancy toxemia, premature labor, perinatal mortality, azotemia and renal failure have been substantiated. Recently the seriousness and increasing incidence of gram-negative rod bacteremia have been appreciated—and clear recognition of its close association with indwelling catheterization noted.
Clinical and experimental evidence has demonstrated that organisms gain entrance to the bladder by way of, through, and around the catheter. Significant bacteriuria is then induced by bacterial multiplication in the bladder urine, in the mucoid film often present between catheter and urethra and in other sites. Although recently acquired bacteriuria may or may not have clinical significance, Kass has demonstrated that the hallmark of urinary tract infection is the repeated presence in the urine of large numbers of pathogenic bacteria, usually over 100,000 organisms/ml.
The use of closed systems with indwelling catheters has been shown to reduce the risk of infection. However, evidence has been presented[1] that disconnections of the junctions in the closed system, whether irrigated or not, were associated with a doubling of the infection rates. Therefore, stringent procedures, such as taping the inflow and outflow junctions at the catheter, should be observed to insure the junctional integrity of the system.
The effectiveness of a three-way catheter and a continuous neomycin-polymyxin B bladder rinse in preventing bacteriuria after indwelling catheterization was first reported by Martin and Bookrajian: "The selection of neomycin and polymyxin as the active components of a continuous bladder rinse solution was based on the evidence that both compounds are bactericidal in low concentration, that few potential urinary tract pathogens are resistant to both, and that the use of 2 drugs against a pathogen sensitive to both will reduce the probability of acquisition of resistance to either."
In a controlled study of the efficacy of the three-way catheter system with constant neomycin-polymyxin B bladder rinse, Meyers et al demonstrated that the cumulative rates of acquisition of bacteriuria were only 4, 6 and 10 percent after 5, 10 and 15 days of catheterization, respectively.
Elimination of the standard indwelling catheter and institution of routine hospitalwide use of the three-way catheter with continuous neomycin-polymyxin B bladder rinse has been reported to cause a marked reduction in the incidence of both fatal and nonfatal gram-negative rod bacteremia.
How Supplied: Ampul of 1 cc, boxes of 12 and 100 ampuls. 20 cc multiple-dose vials.

1. Warren, J.W., Platt, R., Thomas, R.J., Rosner, B. and Kass, E.H., Antibiotic Irrigation and Catheter-Associated Urinary Tract Infections. New Eng. J. Med., 299:570, 1978.

NEOSPORIN® OINTMENT

Polymyxin B-Bacitracin-Neomycin

Description: Each gram contains: Aerosporin® brand Polymyxin B Sulfate 5,000 units; bacitracin zinc 400 units; neomycin sulfate 5 mg (equivalent to 3.5 mg neomycin base); special white petrolatum qs.
Action: The overlapping spectra of the antibiotics provide effective antibacterial action

Continued on next page

Burroughs Wellcome—Cont.

against most commonly occurring bacteria known to be topical invaders. The range of antibacterial activity encompasses many bacteria which are, or have become, resistant to other antibiotics or chemicals—notably *Pseudomonas* and *Staphylococcus*. In susceptible organisms, resistance rarely develops, even on repeated or prolonged use.

Indications: *Therapeutically*, (as an adjunct to systemic therapy when indicated), for topical infections, primary or secondary, due to susceptible organisms, as in: infected burns, skin grafts, surgical incisions, otitis externa; primary pyodermas (impetigo, ecthyma, sycosis vulgaris, paronychia); secondarily infected dermatoses (eczema, herpes, and seborrheic dermatitis); traumatic lesions, inflamed or suppurating as a result of bacterial infection. *Prophylactically*, the ointment may be used to prevent bacterial contamination in burns, skin grafts, incisions, and other clean lesions. For abrasions, minor cuts and wounds accidentally incurred, its use may prevent the development of infection and permit wound healing.

Contraindications: Not for use in the eyes or external ear canal if the eardrum is perforated. This product is contraindicated in those individuals who have shown hypersensitivity to any of its components.

Warning: Because of the potential hazard of nephrotoxicity and ototoxicity due to neomycin, care should be exercised when using this product in treating extensive burns, trophic ulceration and other extensive conditions where absorption of neomycin is possible. In burns where more than 20 percent of the body surface is affected, especially if the patient has impaired renal function or is receiving other aminoglycoside antibiotics concurrently, not more than one application a day is recommended.

When using neomycin-containing products to control secondary infection in the chronic dermatoses, such as chronic otitis externa or stasis dermatitis, it should be borne in mind that the skin in these conditions is more liable than is normal skin to become sensitized to many substances, including neomycin. The manifestation of sensitization to neomycin is usually a low grade reddening with swelling, dry scaling and itching; it may be manifest simply as a failure to heal. During long term use of neomycin-containing products, periodic examination for such signs is advisable and the patient should be told to discontinue the product if they are observed. These symptoms regress quickly on withdrawing the medication. Neomycin-containing applications should be avoided for that patient thereafter.

Precautions: As with other antibacterial products, prolonged use may result in overgrowth of nonsusceptible organisms, including fungi. Appropriate measures should be taken if this occurs.

Adverse Reactions: Neomycin is a not uncommon cutaneous sensitizer. Articles in the current literature indicate an increase in the prevalence of persons allergic to neomycin. Ototoxicity and nephrotoxicity have been reported (see Warning section).

Dosage and Administration: Apply a small quantity to the affected area 2 to 5 times daily, depending on the severity of the condition. May be left exposed or covered with a dressing, as indicated.

How Supplied: Tubes of 1 oz and ½ oz and foil packet of 1/32 oz (approx.) in box of 144 for topical use only.

NEOSPORIN® OINTMENT ℞
Polymyxin B-Bacitracin-Neomycin
OPHTHALMIC
Sterile

Description: Each gram contains: Aerosporin® brand Polymyxin B Sulfate 10,000 units; bacitracin zinc 400 units; neomycin sulfate 5 mg (equivalent to 3.5 mg. neomycin base); special white petrolatum qs.

Actions: Polymyxin B is one of a group of closely related substances produced by various strains of *Bacillus polymyxa*. Its activity is sharply restricted to gram-negative bacteria, including many strains of *Pseudomonas aeruginosa*.

Neomycin, isolated from *Streptomyces fradiae*, has antibacterial activity *in vitro* against a wide range of gram-negative and gram-positive organisms, with effectiveness against many strains of *Proteus*.

Bacitracin, an antibiotic substance derived from cultures of *Bacillus subtilis* (Tracy), exerts antibacterial action *in vitro* against a variety of gram-positive and a few gram-negative organisms.

Indications: This product is indicated in the short-term treatment of superficial external ocular infections caused by organisms susceptible to one or more of the antibiotics contained therein.

Contraindications: This product is contraindicated in those persons who have shown sensitivity to any of its components.

Warnings: Prolonged use may result in overgrowth of nonsusceptible organisms. Ophthalmic ointment may retard corneal healing.

Precautions: Culture and susceptibility testing should be performed during treatment.

Allergic cross-reactions may occur which could prevent the use of any or all of the following antibiotics for the treatment of future infections: kanamycin, paromomycin, streptomycin, and possibly gentamicin.

Adverse Reactions: Neomycin is a not uncommon cutaneous sensitizer. Articles in the current literature indicate an increase in the prevalence of persons allergic to neomycin.

Dosage and Administration: Apply the ointment every 3 or 4 hours, depending on the severity of the infection.

How Supplied: Tube of ⅛ oz with ophthalmic tip.

⅛ oz. × 12—DoD NSN 6505-00-530-6469

NEOSPORIN® OPHTHALMIC SOLUTION Sterile ℞
Polymyxin B-Neomycin-Gramicidin

Description: Each ml contains: Aerosporin® brand Polymyxin B Sulfate 10,000 units; neomycin sulfate 2.5 mg (equivalent to 1.75 mg neomycin base); gramicidin 0.025 mg. Vehicle contains alcohol 0.5%, thimerosal (preservative) 0.001% and the inactive ingredients propylene glycol, polyoxyethylene polyoxypropylene compound, sodium chloride and water for injection.

Indications: This product is indicated in the short-term treatment of superficial external ocular infections caused by organisms susceptible to one or more of the antibiotics contained therein.

Contraindications: This product is contraindicated in those persons who have shown sensitivity to any of its components.

Warnings: Prolonged use may result in overgrowth of nonsusceptible organisms.

Precautions: Culture and susceptibility testing should be performed during treatment.

Allergic cross-reactions may occur which could prevent the use of any or all of the following antibiotics for the treatment of future infections: kanamycin, paromomycin, streptomycin, and possibly gentamicin.

Adverse Reactions: Neomycin is a not uncommon cutaneous sensitizer. Articles in the current literature indicate an increase in the prevalence of persons allergic to neomycin.

Dosage and Administration: The suggested dosage is one or two drops in the affected eye, two to four times daily, or more frequently, as required. In acute infections initiate therapy with one or two drops every 15 to 30 minutes, reducing the frequency of instillation gradually as the infection is controlled.

The patient should be instructed to avoid contaminating the applicator tip with material from an infected eye or other source. This is best done by preventing the tip from touching the eyelid or surrounding areas. This caution is necessary in order to keep the sterile solution as free from contaminating organisms as possible.

How Supplied: 10 cc Drop Dose® (plastic dispenser bottle).

10 cc—DoD NSN 6505-00-890-1299
10 cc—VA NSN 6505-01-012-2906

NEOSPORIN® POWDER ℞
Polymyxin B—Bacitracin—Neomycin
For Topical Use Only (Not Sterile)

Description: Each gram contains: Aerosporin® brand Polymyxin B Sulfate 5,000 units; bacitracin zinc 400 units; neomycin sulfate 5 mg (equivalent to 3.5 mg neomycin base); in a special lactose base.

Indications: Based on a review of this drug by the National Academy of Sciences—National Research Council and/or other information, FDA has classified the indications as follows:

"Possibly" effective: For topical administration for the treatment of the listed localized infections or for suppressive therapy in such conditions:

Prophylactic:
Postoperative and traumatic surface wounds
Biopsy sites
Skin grafts and donor sites
Dermabrasion
Therapeutic (when infected by susceptible organisms):
Vascular ulcers
Decubitus ulcers
Pyodermas
Infected eczemas
Infected dermatoses

Final classification of the less-than-effective indications requires further investigation.

Contraindications: This product is contraindicated in those individuals who have shown hypersensitivity to any of its components.

Warning: Because of the potential hazard of nephrotoxicity and ototoxicity due to neomycin, care should be exercised when using this product in treating extensive burns, trophic ulceration and other extensive conditions where absorption of neomycin is possible. In burns where more than 20 percent of the body surface is affected, especially if the patient has impaired renal function or is receiving other aminoglycoside antibiotics concurrently, not more than one application a day is recommended.

When using neomycin-containing products to control secondary infection in the chronic dermatoses, such as chronic otitis externa or stasis dermatitis, it should be borne in mind that the skin in these conditions is more liable than is normal skin to become sensitized to many substances, including neomycin. The manifestation of sensitization to neomycin is usually a low grade reddening with swelling, dry scaling and itching; it may be manifest simply as a failure to heal. During long term use of neomycin-containing products, periodic examination for such signs is advisable and the patient should be told to discontinue the product if

they are observed. These symptoms regress quickly on withdrawing the medication. Neomycin-containing applications should be avoided for that patient thereafter.
Precautions: As with other antibiotic preparations, prolonged use may result in overgrowth of nonsusceptible organisms, including fungi. Appropriate measures should be taken if this occurs. It is to be noted that the powder is not intended for sterile use in surgical procedures such as those involving abdominal or thoracic body cavities.
Adverse Reactions: Neomycin is a not uncommon cutaneous sensitizer. Articles in the current literature indicate an increase in the prevalence of persons allergic to neomycin. Ototoxicity and nephrotoxicity have been reported (see Warning section).
Dosage and Administration: Apply lightly to the area to be treated as often as needed; treated area may be covered with a dressing or left exposed, as desired. In biopsy sites, dermabraded areas, etc., the powder may be mixed with a little powdered gelatin foam to provide concurrent hemostasis.
How Supplied: Shaker-top vial of 10 g.

POLYSPORIN® OINTMENT
Polymyxin B-Bacitracin

Description: Each gram contains: Aerosporin brand Polymyxin B Sulfate 10,000 units; bacitracin zinc 500 units in a special white petrolatum qs.
Action: Combined antibiotic action against gram-negative and gram-positive organisms.
Indications: *Therapeutically,* (as an adjunct to systemic therapy when indicated), for topical infections, primary or secondary, due to susceptible organisms, as in: infected burns, skin grafts, surgical incisions, otitis externa; primary pyodermas (impetigo, ecthyma, sycosis vulgaris, paronychia); secondarily infected dermatoses (eczema, herpes, and seborrheic dermatitis); traumatic lesions, inflamed or suppurating as a result of bacterial infection. *Prophylactically,* the ointment may be used to prevent bacterial contamination in burns, skin grafts, incisions, and other clean lesions. For abrasions, minor cuts and wounds accidentally incurred, its use may prevent the development of infection and permit wound healing.
Contraindication: This product is contraindicated in those individuals who have shown hypersensitivity to any of its components.
Precaution: As with other antibiotic products, prolonged use may result in overgrowth of nonsusceptible organisms including fungi. Appropriate measures should be taken if this occurs.
Dosage and Administration: Apply 2 to 5 times daily, depending on the severity of the infection.
How Supplied: Tubes of ½ oz, 1 oz and 1/32 oz (approx.) foil packet in box of 144.
1 oz.—VA NSN 6505-00-579-9110

POLYSPORIN® OPHTHALMIC OINTMENT ℞
Polymyxin B—Bacitracin
Sterile

Description: Each gram contains: Aerosporin® brand Polymyxin B Sulfate 10,000 units; bacitracin zinc 500 units; special white petrolatum qs.
Action: Polymyxin B attacks gram-negative bacilli, including virtually all strains of *Pseudomonas aeruginosa* and *H influenzae* species. Bacitracin is active against most gram-positive bacilli and cocci, including hemolytic streptococci.
Indications: For the treatment of superficial ocular infections involving the conjunctiva and/or cornea caused by organisms susceptible to polymyxin B sulfate and bacitracin zinc.
Contraindications: This product is contraindicated in those individuals who have shown hypersensitivity to any of its components.
Warnings: Ophthalmic ointments may retard corneal healing.
Precautions: As with other antibiotic preparations, prolonged use may result in overgrowth of nonsusceptible organisms, including fungi. Appropriate measures should be taken if this occurs.
Dosage and Administration: Apply the ointment every 3 or 4 hours, depending on the severity of the infection.
How Supplied: Tube of ⅛ oz with ophthalmic tip.

PROLOPRIM® ℞
(Trimethoprim)
100 mg Scored Tablets

Description: Proloprim® (trimethoprim)* is a synthetic antibacterial, available in scored white tablets, each containing 100 mg trimethoprim. Trimethoprim is 2, 4-diamino-5-(3,4,5,-trimethoxybenzyl) pyrimidine. It is a white to light yellow, odorless, bitter compound with a molecular weight of 290.3.
Clinical Pharmacology: Trimethoprim is rapidly absorbed following oral administration. Mean peak serum levels of approximately 1.0 mcg/ml occur 1 to 4 hours after oral administration of a single 100 mg dose. A single 200 mg dose will result in serum levels approximately twice as high. The half-life of trimethoprim is 8 to 10 hours.
Trimethoprim exists in the blood as free, protein-bound and metabolized forms. Approximately 44% of trimethoprim is protein-bound in the blood. The free form is considered to be the therapeutically active form. Excretion of trimethoprim is chiefly by the kidneys through glomerular filtration and tubular secretion. Urine concentrations of trimethoprim are considerably higher than are the concentrations in the blood.
Trimethoprim urine levels, after a single oral dose of 100 mg, ranged from 30 to 160 mcg/ml during the 0 to 4 hour period and declined to approximately 18 to 91 mcg/ml during the 8 to 24 hour period. After oral administration, 50% to 60% of trimethoprim is excreted in the urine within 24 hours, approximately 80% of this being unmetabolized trimethoprim.
Microbiology: Proloprim blocks the production of tetrahydrofolic acid from dihydrofolic acid by binding to and reversibly inhibiting the enzyme dihydrofolate reductase. This binding is very much stronger for the bacterial enzyme than for the corresponding mammalian enzyme. Thus, Proloprim selectively interferes with bacterial biosynthesis of nucleic acids and proteins.
In vitro serial dilution tests have shown that the spectrum of antibacterial activity of Proloprim includes the common urinary tract pathogens with the exception of *Pseudomonas aeruginosa.*

REPRESENTATIVE MINIMUM INHIBITORY CONCENTRATIONS FOR TRIMETHOPRIM-SUSCEPTIBLE ORGANISMS

Bacteria	Trimethoprim MIC—mcg/ml (Range)
Escherichia coli	0.05–1.5
Proteus mirabilis	0.5 –1.5
Klebsiella pneumoniae	0.5 –5.0
Enterobacter species	0.5 –5.0
Staphylococcus species, coagulase-negative	0.15–5.0

The recommended quantitative disc susceptibility method[1,2] may be used for estimating the susceptibility of bacteria to Proloprim.
Reports from the laboratory giving results of the standardized test using the 5 mcg trimethoprim disc should be interpreted according to the following criteria:
Organisms producing zones of 16 mm or greater are classified as susceptible whereas those producing zones of 11 to 15 mm are classified as having intermediate susceptibility. A report from the laboratory of "Susceptible" to trimethoprim or "Intermediate" susceptibility to trimethoprim indicates that the infection is likely to respond when, as in uncomplicated urinary tract infections, effective therapy is dependent upon the urine concentration of trimethoprim.
Organisms producing zones of 10 mm or less are reported as resistant, indicating that other therapy should be selected.
Dilution methods for determining susceptibility are also used, and results are reported as the minimum drug concentration inhibiting microbial growth (MIC)[3].
If the MIC is 8 mcg per ml or less, the microorganism is considered "susceptible". If the MIC is 16 mcg per ml or greater the microorganism is considered "resistant".
Normal vaginal and fecal flora are the source of most pathogens causing urinary tract infections. It is therefore relevant to consider the suppressive effect of trimethoprim in these sites.
Concentrations of trimethoprim in vaginal secretions are consistently greater than those found simultaneously in the serum, being typically 1.6 times the concentration of simultaneously obtained serum samples. Sufficient trimethoprim is excreted in the feces to markedly reduce or eliminate trimethoprim susceptible organisms from the fecal flora.
The dominant fecal organisms *(non-Enterobacteriaceae), Bacteroides* spp. and *Lactobacillus* spp., are not susceptible to trimethoprim levels obtained with the recommended dosage.
Indications and Usage: For the treatment of initial episodes of uncomplicated urinary tract infections due to susceptible strains of the following organisms: *Escherichia coli, Proteus mirabilis, Klebsiella pneumoniae* and *Enterobacter* species and coagulase-negative *Staphylococcus* species, including *S. saprophyticus.* Cultures and susceptibility tests should be performed to determine the susceptibility of the bacteria to trimethoprim. Therapy may be initiated prior to obtaining the results of these tests.
Contraindications: Proloprim is contraindicated in individuals hypersensitive to trimethoprim and in those with documented megaloblastic anemia due to folate deficiency.
Warnings: Experience with trimethoprim alone is limited, but it has been reported rarely to interfere with hematopoiesis, especially when administered in large doses and/or for prolonged periods.
The presence of clinical signs such as sore throat, fever, pallor or purpura may be early indications of serious blood disorders. Complete blood counts should be obtained if any of these signs are noted in a patient receiving trimethoprim and the drug discontinued if a significant reduction in the count of any formed blood element is found.
Precautions:
General: Trimethoprim should be given with caution to patients with possible folate deficiency. Folates may be administered concomitantly without interfering with the antibacterial action of trimethoprim. Trimethoprim should also be given with caution to patients with impaired renal or hepatic function.
Pregnancy: Teratogenic Effects: Pregnancy Category C. Trimethoprim has been shown to be teratogenic in the rat when given in doses 40 times the human dose. In some rabbit studies, an overall increase in fetal loss (dead and resorbed and malformed conceptuses) was associated with doses 6 times the human therapeutic dose. While there are no large well-controlled studies on the use of trimethoprim in pregnant

Continued on next page

Burroughs Wellcome—Cont.

women, Brumfitt and Pursell[4] reported the outcome of 186 pregnancies during which the mother received either placebo or trimethoprim in combination with sulfamethoxazole. The incidence of congenital abnormalities was 4.5% (3 of 66) in those who received placebo and 3.3% (4 of 120) in those receiving trimethoprim plus sulfamethoxazole. There were no abnormalities in the 10 children whose mothers received the drug during the first trimester. In a separate survey, Brumfitt and Pursell also found no congenital abnormalities in 35 children whose mothers had received trimethoprim plus sulfamethoxazole at the time of conception or shortly thereafter.

Because trimethoprim may interfere with folic acid metabolism, Proloprim should be used during pregnancy only if the potential benefit justifies the potential risk to the fetus.

Nursing Mothers: Trimethoprim is excreted in human milk. Because trimethoprim may interfere with folic acid metabolism, caution should be exercised when Proloprim is administered to a nursing mother.

Pediatric Use: The safety of trimethoprim in infants under 2 months has not been demonstrated. The effectiveness of trimethoprim has not been established in children under 12 years of age.

Adverse Reactions: The adverse effects encountered most often with trimethoprim are rash and pruritus. Other adverse effects reported involved the gastrointestinal and hematopoietic systems.

Dermatologic Reactions: Rash, pruritus and exfoliative dermatitis. At the recommended dosage regimens of 100 mg b.i.d. or 200 mg q.d., the incidence of rash is 2.9% to 6.7%. In clinical studies which employed high doses of Proloprim, an elevated incidence of rash was noted. These rashes were maculopapular, morbilliform, pruritic and generally mild to moderate, appearing 7 to 14 days after the initiation of therapy.

Gastrointestinal Reactions: Epigastric distress, nausea, vomiting, and glossitis.

Hematologic Reactions: Thrombocytopenia, leukopenia, neutropenia, megaloblastic anemia, and methemoglobinemia.

Miscellaneous Reactions: Fever, elevation of serum transaminases and bilirubin, and increases in BUN and serum creatinine levels.

Overdosage:

Acute: Signs of acute overdosage with trimethoprim may appear following ingestion of 1 gram or more of the drug and include nausea, vomiting, dizziness, headaches, mental depression, confusion and bone marrow depression (SEE CHRONIC OVERDOSAGE). Treatment consists of gastric lavage and general supportive measures. Acidification of the urine will increase renal elimination of trimethoprim. Peritoneal dialysis is not effective and hemodialysis only moderately effective in eliminating the drug.

Chronic: Use of trimethoprim at high doses and/or for extended periods of time may cause bone marrow depression manifested as thrombocytopenia, leukopenia and/or megaloblastic anemia. If signs of bone marrow depression occur, trimethoprim should be discontinued and the patient should be given leucovorin, 3 to 6 mg intramuscularly daily for three days, or as required to restore normal hematopoiesis.

Dosage and Administration: The usual oral adult dosage is 100 mg of Proloprim every 12 hours or 200 mg of Proloprim every 24 hours, each for 10 days.

The use of trimethoprim in patients with a creatinine clearance of less than 15 ml/min is not recommended. For patients with a creatinine clearance of 15 to 30 ml/min, the dose should be 50 mg every 12 hours. The effectiveness of trimethoprim has not been established in children under 12 years of age.

How Supplied: 100 mg (white) scored tablets, imprinted with "PROLOPRIM 09A"—bottle of 100 (NDC-0081-0820-55) and unit dose pack of 100 (NDC-0081-0820-56). Store at 15°–30°C (59°–86°F) in a dry place.

References:

1. Bauer AW, Kirby WMM, Sherris JC, Turck M: Antibiotic Susceptibility Testing by Standardized Single Disk Method. Am J Clin Path *45*: 493–496, 1966.
2. Approved Standard ASM-2 Performance Standards for Antimicrobial Disc Susceptibility Test: National Committee for Clinical Laboratory Standards, 771 East Lancaster Avenue, Villanova, Pennsylvania 19085.
3. Ericsson HM and Sherris JC: Antibiotic Sensitivity Testing. Report of an International Collaborative Study. Acta Pathologica et Microbiologica Scandinavica, Section B, Suppl. 217, 1971, pp. 1–90.
4. Brumfitt W and Pursell R: Trimethoprim/Sulfamethoxazole in the Treatment of Bacteriuria in Women. J Inf Dis Suppl *128*: S657–S663, 1973.

*Mfd. under Pat. #3,956,327.

[*Shown in Product Identification Section*]

PURINETHOL® ℞

(Mercaptopurine)
50 mg Scored Tablets

Caution: Purinethol® (mercaptopurine) is a potent drug. It should not be used unless a diagnosis of acute leukemia or chronic myelogenous leukemia has been adequately established and the responsible physician is knowledgeable in assessing response to chemotherapy.

Description: Purinethol® (mercaptopurine) (6-mercaptopurine) was synthesized and developed by Hitchings, Elion, and associates at the Wellcome Research Laboratories.[1] It is one of a large series of purine analogues which interfere with nucleic acid biosynthesis. Mercaptopurine is an analogue of the purine bases adenine and hypoxanthine:

Biochemical Pharmacology: Mercaptopurine competes with hypoxanthine and guanine for the enzyme hypoxanthine-guanine phosphoribosyltransferase (HGPRTase) and is itself converted to thioinosinic acid (TIMP). This intracellular nucleotide inhibits several reactions involving inosinic acid (IMP), including the conversion of IMP to xanthylic acid (XMP) and the conversion of IMP to adenylic acid (AMP) via adenylosuccinate (SAMP). In addition, 6-methylthioinosinate (MTIMP) is formed by the methylation of TIMP. Both TIMP and MTIMP have been reported to inhibit glutamine-5-phosphoribosylpyrophosphate amidotransferase, the first enzyme unique to the *de novo* pathway for purine ribonucleotide synthesis.[2]

Experiments indicate that radiolabeled mercaptopurine may be recovered from the DNA in the form of deoxythioguanosine.[3] Some mercaptopurine is converted to nucleotide derivatives of 6-thioguanine (6-TG) by the sequential actions of inosinate (IMP) dehydrogenase and xanthylate (XMP) aminase, converting TIMP to thioguanylic acid (TGMP).

Animal tumors that are resistant to mercaptopurine have lost the ability to convert mercaptopurine to TIMP. However, it is clear that resistance to mercaptopurine may be acquired by other means as well, particularly in human leukemias.

It is not known exactly which of any one or more of the biochemical effects of mercaptopurine and its metabolites are directly or predominantly responsible for cell death.[4]

The catabolism of mercaptopurine and its metabolites is complex. In man, after oral administration of ^{35}S-6-mercaptopurine, urine contains intact mercaptopurine, thiouric acid (formed by direct oxidation by xanthine oxidase, probably via 6-mercapto-8-hydroxypurine) and a number of 6-methylated thiopurines. The methylthiopurines yield appreciable amounts of inorganic sulfate.[2] The importance of the metabolism by xanthine oxidase relates to the fact that Zyloprim® (allopurinol) inhibits this enzyme and retards the catabolism of mercaptopurine and its active metabolites. A significant reduction in mercaptopurine dosage is mandatory if a potent xanthine oxidase inhibitor and Purinethol (mercaptopurine) are used simultaneously in a patient (see "WARNINGS").

Clinical Pharmacology: Clinical studies have shown that the absorption of an oral dose of mercaptopurine in man is incomplete and variable, averaging approximately 50% of the administered dose.[5] The factors influencing absorption are unknown. Intravenous administration of an investigational preparation of mercaptopurine revealed a plasma half-disappearance time of 21 minutes in children and 47 minutes in adults. The volume of distribution usually exceeded that of the total body water.[5]

Following the oral administration of ^{35}S-6-mercaptopurine in one subject, a total of 46% of the dose could be accounted for in the urine (as parent drug and metabolites) in the first 24 hours. Metabolites of mercaptopurine were found in urine within the first 2 hours after administration. Radioactivity (in the form of sulfate) could be found in the urine for weeks afterwards.[2]

There is negligible entry of mercaptopurine into cerebrospinal fluid.

Plasma protein binding averages 19% over the concentration range 10 to 50 micrograms per milliliter (a concentration only achieved by intravenous administration of mercaptopurine at doses exceeding 5 to 10 mg/kg).[5]

Monitoring plasma levels of mercaptopurine during therapy is of questionable value.[2] It is technically difficult to determine plasma concentrations which are seldom greater than 1 to 2 micrograms per milliliter after a therapeutic oral dose. More significantly, mercaptopurine enters rapidly into the anabolic and catabolic pathways for purines and the active intracellular metabolites have appreciably longer half-lives than the parent drug. The biochemical effects of a single dose of mercaptopurine are evident long after the parent drug has disappeared from plasma. Because of this rapid metabolism of mercaptopurine to active intracellular derivatives, hemodialysis would not be expected to appreciably reduce toxicity of the drug. There is no known pharmacologic antagonist to the biochemical actions of mercaptopurine *in vivo.*

Indications and Usage: Purinethol (mercaptopurine) is indicated for remission induction, remission consolidation, and maintenance therapy of the acute leukemias. The response to this agent depends upon the particular sub-classification of the acute leukemia (lymphatic, myelogenous, undifferentiated, etc.) and the age of the patient (child or adult). Purinethol (mercaptopurine) is also indicated for the palliative treatment of chronic myelogenous (granulocytic) leukemia.

a) **Acute Lymphatic (Lymphocytic, Lymphoblastic) Leukemia:** Acute lymphatic leukemia occurring in children responds, in general, more favorably to mercaptopurine than the same disorder occuring in adults. Given as a single agent for remission induction, mercaptopurine induces complete remission in approximately 25% of children and 10% of adults. These results can be improved upon considerably by using multiple, carefully selected agents in combination. Reliance upon mercaptopurine alone is seldom justified. The duration of complete remission induced in children with acute lymphatic leukemia is so brief without the use of maintenance therapy that some form of drug therapy is considered essential following remission induction. Mercaptopurine, as a single agent, is capable of significantly prolonging complete remission duration in children; however, combination therapy with multiple agents has produced results superior to that achieved with mercaptopurine alone. The effectiveness of mercaptopurine in maintenance programs in adult acute lymphatic leukemia has not been established.

b) **Acute Myelogenous (and Acute Myelomonocytic) Leukemia:** As a single agent, mercaptopurine will induce complete remission in approximately 10% of children and adults with acute myelogenous leukemia or its sub-classifications. These results are inferior to those achieved with combination chemotherapy employing optimum treatment schedules.

c) **Chronic Myelogenous (Granulocytic) Leukemia:** Mercaptopurine is one of several agents with demonstrated efficacy in the treatment of chronic myelogenous leukemia. Approximately 30 to 50% of patients with chronic myelogenous leukemia obtain an objective response to mercaptopurine. This is less than the 90% objective responses with busulfan, and, of these two agents, Myleran® (busulfan) is usually regarded as the preferred drug for initial therapy.

d) **Central Nervous System Leukemia:** Mercaptopurine is not effective for prophylaxis or treatment of central nervous system leukemia.

e) **Other Neoplasms:** Purinethol (mercaptopurine) is not effective in chronic lymphatic leukemia, the lymphomas (including Hodgkin's Disease), or solid tumors.

Contraindications: Purinethol (mercaptopurine) should not be used unless a diagnosis of acute leukemia or chronic myelogenous leukemia has been adequately established and the responsible physician is knowledgeable in assessing response to chemotherapy.

Mercaptopurine should not be used in patients whose disease has demonstrated prior resistance to this drug. In animals and man there is usually complete cross-resistance between Purinethol (mercaptopurine) and Tabloid® brand thioguanine.

Warnings:

a) **Bone Marrow Toxicity:** The most consistent, dose-related toxicity is bone marrow suppression. This may be manifest by anemia, leukopenia, thrombocytopenia, or any combination of these. Any of these findings may also indicate progression of the underlying disease. It is imperative that patients be instructed to report promptly the development of fever, sore throat, signs of local infection, bleeding from any site, or symptoms suggestive of anemia. Since mercaptopurine may have a delayed effect, it is important to withdraw the medication temporarily at the first sign of an abnormally large fall in any of the formed elements of the blood.

b) **Hepatotoxicity:**[5] Purinethol (mercaptopurine) is hepatotoxic in animals and man; deaths have been reported from hepatic necrosis. Hepatic injury can occur with any dosage, but seems to occur with greatest frequency when doses of 2.5 mg/kg/day are exceeded. The histologic pattern of mercaptopurine hepatotoxicity includes features of both intrahepatic cholestasis and parenchymal cell necrosis, either of which may predominate. It is not clear how much of the hepatic damage is due to direct toxicity from the drug and how much may be due to a hypersensitivity reaction. In some patients jaundice has cleared following withdrawal of mercaptopurine and reappeared with its reintroduction.

Published reports have cited widely varying incidences of overt hepatotoxicity; several reports have indicated that as many as 10 to 40% of patients with acute leukemia develop jaundice while receiving treatment with mercaptopurine. Usually, clinically detectable jaundice appears early in the course of treatment (one to two months). However, jaundice has been reported as early as one week and as late as eight years after the start of treatment with mercaptopurine.

Monitoring of serum transaminase levels, alkaline phosphatase, and bilirubin levels may allow early detection of hepatotoxicity. It is advisable to monitor these liver function tests at weekly intervals when first beginning therapy and at monthly intervals thereafter. Liver function tests may be advisable more frequently in patients who are receiving mercaptopurine with other hepatotoxic drugs or with known pre-existing liver disease.

The concomitant administration of mercaptopurine with other hepatotoxic agents requires especially careful clinical and biochemical monitoring of hepatic function. Combination therapy involving mercaptopurine with other drugs not felt to be hepatotoxic should nevertheless be approached with caution. The combination of mercaptopurine with doxorubicin (Adriamycin®) was reported to be hepatotoxic in 19 of 20 patients undergoing remission-induction therapy for leukemia resistant to previous therapy.

The hepatotoxicity has been associated in some cases with anorexia, diarrhea, jaundice, and ascites. Hepatic encephalopathy has occurred.

The onset of clinical jaundice, hepatomegaly, or anorexia with tenderness in the right hypochondrium are immediate indications for withholding mercaptopurine until the exact etiology can be identified. Likewise, any evidence of deterioration in liver function studies, toxic hepatitis, or biliary stasis should prompt discontinuation of the drug and lead to a search for an etiology of the hepatotoxicity.

c) **Interaction with Zyloprim® (Allopurinol): When allopurinol and mercaptopurine are administered concomitantly, it is imperative that the dose of mercaptopurine be reduced to one-third to one-quarter of the usual dose. Failure to observe this dosage reduction will result in a delayed catabolism of mercaptopurine and the strong likelihood of inducing severe toxicity.**

d) **Immunosuppression:** Mercaptopurine recipients may manifest decreased cellular hypersensitivities and impaired allograft rejection. Induction of immunity to infectious agents or vaccines will be subnormal in these patients; the degree of immunosuppression will depend on antigen dose and temporal relationship to drug. This drug effect is similar to that of Imuran® (azathioprine) and should be carefully considered with regard to intercurrent infections and risk of subsequent neoplasia.

e) **Mutagenesis and Carcinogenesis:** Purinethol (mercaptopurine) causes chromosomal aberrations in animals and man and induces dominant-lethal mutations in male mice. Carcinogenic potential exists in man, but the extent of the risk is unknown.

f) **Teratogenesis:** Mercaptopurine has embryopathic effects in rats. Women receiving mercaptopurine in the first trimester of pregnancy have an increased incidence of abortion; the risk of malformation in offspring surviving first trimester exposure is not accurately known. In a series of twenty-eight women receiving mercaptopurine after the first trimester of pregnancy, three mothers died undelivered, one delivered a stillborn child, and one aborted; there were no cases of macroscopically abnormal fetuses. Since such experience cannot exclude the possibility of fetal damage, mercaptopurine should be used during pregnancy only if the benefit clearly justifies the possible risk to the fetus, and particular caution should be given to the use of mercaptopurine in the first trimester of pregnancy.

g) **Effects on Fertility:** The effect of mercaptopurine on human fertility is unknown for either males or females.

Precautions: The safe and effective use of Purinethol demands a thorough knowledge of the natural history of the condition being treated. For example, remission induction of adult acute leukemia virtually always necessitates the production of moderate to severe bone marrow hypoplasia. The degree of myelosuppression acceptable in this disease would not be desirable in the management of chronic granulocytic leukemia. After selection of an initial dosage schedule, therapy will frequently need to be modified depending upon the patient's response and manifestations of toxicity.

The most frequent, serious, toxic effect of mercaptopurine is myelosuppression resulting in leukopenia, thrombocytopenia, and anemia. These toxic effects are often unavoidable during the induction phase of adult acute leukemia if remission induction is to be successful. Whether or not these manifestations demand modification or cessation of dosage depends both upon the response of the underlying disease and a careful consideration of supportive facilities (granulocyte and platelet transfusions) which may be available. Life-threatening infections and bleeding have been observed as a consequence of mercaptopurine induced granulocytopenia and thrombocytopenia. Severe hematologic toxicity may require supportive therapy with platelet transfusions for bleeding, and antibiotics and granulocyte transfusions if sepsis is documented.

If it is not the intent to intentionally induce bone marrow hypoplasia, it is important to discontinue the drug temporarily at the first evidence of an abnormally large fall in white blood cell count, platelet count, or hemoglobin concentration. In many patients with severe depression of the formed elements of the blood due to mercaptopurine, the bone marrow appears hypoplastic on aspiration or biopsy, whereas in other cases it may appear normocellular. The qualitative changes in the erythroid elements toward the megaloblastic series, characteristically seen with the folic acid antagonists and some other antimetabolites, are not seen with this drug.

It is recommended that evaluation of the hemoglobin or hematocrit, total white blood cell count and differential count, and quantitative platelet count be obtained weekly while the patient is on mercaptopurine therapy. In cases where the cause of fluctuations in the formed elements in the peripheral blood is obscure, bone marrow examination may be useful for the evaluation of marrow status. The decision to increase, decrease, continue, or discontinue a given dosage of mercaptopurine must be based not only on the absolute hematologic values, but also upon the rapidity with which changes are occurring. In many instances, particularly during the induction phase of acute leukemia, complete blood counts will need to be done more frequently than once weekly in order to evaluate the effect of the therapy. The dosage of mercaptopurine may need to be reduced when this agent is combined with other drugs whose primary toxicity is myelosuppression.

It is probably advisable to start with smaller dosages in patients with impaired renal function, since the latter might result in slower elimination of the drug and a greater cumulative effect.

Continued on next page

Burroughs Wellcome—Cont.

See "WARNINGS" section for information on immunosuppression, mutagenesis and carcinogenesis, teratogenesis, and effects on fertility.

Adverse Reactions: Intestinal ulceration has been reported.[8] Nausea, vomiting and anorexia are uncommon during initial administration, but they may occur during toxicity. Mild diarrhea and sprue-like symptoms have been noted occasionally, but it is difficult at present to attribute these to the medication. Oral lesions are rarely seen, and when they occur they resemble thrush rather than antifolic ulcerations.

Hyperuricemia frequently occurs in patients receiving mercaptopurine as a consequence of rapid cell lysis accompanying the antineoplastic effect. Adverse effects can be minimized by increased hydration, urine alkalinization, and the prophylactic administration of a xanthine oxidase inhibitor such as Zyloprim® (allopurinol). The dosage of mercaptopurine should be reduced to one-third to one-quarter of the usual dose if Zyloprim® (allopurinol) is given concurrently.

Drug fever has been very rarely reported with mercaptopurine. Before attributing fever to mercaptopurine, every attempt should be made to exclude more common causes of pyrexia, such as sepsis, in patients with acute leukemia.

Overdosage: There is no known pharmacologic antagonist of mercaptopurine. The drug should be discontinued immediately if unintended toxicity occurs during treatment. If a patient is seen immediately following an accidental overdosage of the drug, induced emesis may be useful. Hemodialysis is thought to be of marginal use due to the rapid intracellular incorporation of mercaptopurine into active metabolites with long persistence.

Dosage and Administration:

a) **Induction and Consolidation Therapy:** Purinethol (mercaptopurine) is administered orally. The dosage which will be tolerated or will be effective varies from patient-to-patient, and therefore careful titration is necessary to obtain the optimum therapeutic effect without incurring excessive, unintended toxicity. The usual initial dosage for children and adults is 2.5 mg/kg of body weight per day (100 to 200 mg in the average adult and 50 mg in an average 5 year old child). Children with acute leukemia have tolerated this dose without difficulty in most cases; it may be continued daily for several weeks or more in some patients. If, after four weeks at this dosage, there is no clinical improvement and no definite evidence of leukocyte or platelet depression, the dosage may be increased up to 5 mg/kg daily.

A dosage of 2.5 mg/kg per day may result in a rapid fall in leukocyte count within 1 to 2 weeks in some adults with acute leukemia and high total leukocyte counts, as well as in certain adults with chronic myelocytic leukemia.

The total daily dosage may be given at one time. It is calculated to the nearest multiple of 25 mg. The dosage of mercaptopurine should be reduced to one-third to one-quarter of the usual dose if Zyloprim® (allopurinol) is given concurrently. Since the drug may have a delayed action, it should be discontinued at the first sign of an abnormally large or rapid fall in the leukocyte or platelet count. If subsequently the leukocyte count or platelet count remains constant for two or three days, or rises, treatment may be resumed.

b) **Maintenance Therapy:** If a complete hematologic remission is obtained with mercaptopurine, either alone or in combination with other agents, maintenance therapy should be considered. This is indicated in children with acute lymphatic leukemia. The use of mercaptopurine in maintenance schedules for adults with acute leukemia has not been established to be effective. If remission is achieved, maintenance doses will vary from patient to patient. A usual daily maintenance dose of mercaptopurine is 1.5 to 2.5 mg/kg/day as a single dose. It is to be emphasized that in children with acute lymphatic leukemia in remission, superior results have been obtained when mercaptopurine has been combined with other agents (most frequently with methotrexate) for remission maintenance. Mercaptopurine should rarely be relied upon as a single agent for the maintenance of remissions induced in acute leukemia.

How Supplied: Cream-colored, scored tablets containing 50 mg mercaptopurine, imprinted with "WELLCOME" and "04A" on each tablet; bottles of 25 and 250.

References:

1. New York Academy of Sciences: 6-mercaptopurine. ANN NY ACAD SCI *60:* 359–507 (1954).
2. Elion GB: Biochemistry and pharmacology of purine analogues. FED PROC *26:* 898–904 (1967).
3. Scannell JP, Hitchings GH: Thioguanine in deoxyribonucleic acid from tumors of 6-mercaptopurine-treated mice. PROC SOC EXP BIOL MED *122:* 627–629 (1966).
4. Paterson ARP, Tidd DM: 6-thiopurines. pp. 384–403. In: Sartorelli AC, Johns DG, ed. Antineoplastic and Immunosuppressive Agents, Part II, Berlin, Springer-Verlag, 1975.
5. Loo TL, Luce JK, Sullivan MP, Frei E: Clinical pharmacologic observations on 6-mercaptopurine and 6-methylthiopurine ribonucleoside. CLIN PHARMACOL THER *9:* 180–194 (1968).
6. Schein PS, Winokur SH: Immunosuppressive and cytotoxic chemotherapy: long-term complications. ANN INTERN MED *82:* 84–95 (1975).
7. Stern MH, Minow MD, Casey MD: Hepatotoxicity in patients treated with adriamycin and 6-mercaptopurine for refractory leukemia. AM J CLIN PATHOL *63:* 758–759 (1975).
8. Clark PA, Hsia YE, Huntsman RG: Toxic complications of treatment with 6-mercaptopurine. BR MED J *1:* 393–395 (1960).

[*Shown in Product Identification Section*]

SEPTRA® ℞
I.V. INFUSION

Description: Septra I.V. Infusion, a sterile solution for intravenous infusion only, is a synthetic antibacterial combination product. Each 5 ml ampul contains 80 mg trimethoprim* (16 mg/ml) and 400 mg sulfamethoxazole (80 mg/ml) compounded with 40% propylene glycol, 10% ethyl alcohol and 0.3% diethanolamine; 1% benzyl alcohol and 0.1% sodium metabisulfite as preservatives, water for injection, and pH adjusted to approximately 10 with sodium hydroxide.

Trimethoprim is 2,4-diamino-5-(3,4,5-trimethoxybenzyl)pyrimidine. It is a white to light yellow, odorless, bitter compound with a molecular weight of 290.3.

Sulfamethoxazole is N^1-(5-methyl-3-isoxazolyl)sulfanilamide. It is an almost white in color, odorless, tasteless compound with a molecular weight of 253.28.

Clinical Pharmacology: Following a one-hour intravenous infusion of a single dose of 160 mg trimethoprim plus 800 mg sulfamethoxazole to 11 patients whose weight ranged from 105 lbs. to 165 lbs. (mean, 143 lbs.), the mean peak plasma concentrations of trimethoprim and sulfamethoxazole were 3.4 ± 0.3 μg/ml and 46.3 ± 2.7 μg/ml, respectively. Following repeated intravenous administration of the same dose at eight-hour intervals, the mean plasma concentrations just prior to and immediately after each infusion at steady state were 5.6 ± 0.6 μg/ml and 8.8 ± 0.9 μg/ml for trimethoprim and 70.6 ± 7.3 μg/ml and 105.6 ± 10.9 μg/ml for sulfamethoxazole. The mean plasma half-life was 11.3 ± 0.7 hours for trimethoprim and 12.8 ± 1.8 hours for sulfamethoxazole. All of these 11 patients had normal renal function and their age ranged from 17 to 78 years (median, 60 years)[1].

Pharmacokinetic studies in children and adults suggest an age dependent half-life of trimethoprim as indicated in the following table.[2]

Age (yrs.)	No. of Patients	Mean TMP Half-life (hours)
<1	2	7.67
1–10	9	5.49
10–20	5	8.19
20–63	6	12.82

Sulfamethoxazole exists in the blood as free, conjugated and protein-bound forms; trimethoprim is present as free and protein-bound and metabolized forms. The free forms are considered to be the therapeutically active forms. Approximately 44 percent of trimethoprim and 70 percent of sulfamethoxazole are protein-bound in blood. The presence of 10 mg percent sulfamethoxazole in plasma decreases the protein binding of trimethoprim to an insignificant degree; trimethoprim does not influence the protein binding of sulfamethoxazole.

Excretion of Septra is chiefly by the kidneys through both glomerular filtration and tubular secretion. Urine concentrations of both sulfamethoxazole and trimethoprim are considerably higher than are the concentrations in the blood. When administered together as in Septra, neither sulfamethoxazole nor trimethoprim affects the urinary excretion pattern of the other.

Microbiology: Sulfamethoxazole inhibits bacterial synthesis of dihydrofolic acid by competing with *para*-aminobenzoic acid. Trimethoprim blocks the production of tetrahydrofolic acid from dihydrofolic acid by binding to and reversibly inhibiting the required enzyme, dihydrofolate reductase. Thus, Septra blocks two consecutive steps in the biosynthesis of nucleic acids and proteins essential to many bacteria.

In vitro studies have shown that bacterial resistance develops more slowly with Septra than with trimethoprim or sulfamethoxazole alone.

In vitro serial dilution tests have shown that the spectrum of antibacterial activity of Septra includes common bacterial pathogens with the exception of *Pseudomonas aeruginosa.* The following organisms are usually susceptible: *Escherichia coli, Klebsiella-Enterobacter, Proteus mirabilis,* indole-positive *Proteus* species, *Haemophilus influenzae (including ampicillin-resistant strains), Streptococcus, pneumoniae, Shigella flexneri* and *Shigella sonnei.* It should be noted, however, that there are little clinical data on the use of Septra I.V. infusion in serious systemic infections due to *Haemophilus influenzae* and *Streptococcus pneumoniae.*

[See table on next page].

The recommended quantitative disc susceptibility method may be used for estimating the susceptibility of bacteria to Septra.[3,4] With this procedure, a report from the laboratory of "Susceptible to trimethoprim-sulfamethoxazole" indicates that the infection is likely to respond to therapy with Septra. If the infection is confined to the urine, a report of "Intermediate susceptibility to trimethoprim-sulfamethoxazole" also indicates that the infection is likely to respond. A report of "Resistant to trimethoprim-sulfamethoxazole" indicates that the infection is unlikely to respond to therapy with Septra.

Indications and Usage:

PNEUMOCYSTIS CARINII PNEUMONITIS: Septra I.V. Infusion is indicated in the treatment of *Pneumocystis carinii* pneumonitis in children and adults.

SHIGELLOSIS: Septra I.V. Infusion is indicated in the treatment of enteritis caused by susceptible strains of *Shigella flexneri* and *Shigella sonnei* in children and adults.

URINARY TRACT INFECTIONS: Septra I.V. Infusion is indicated in the treatment of severe or complicated urinary tract infections due to susceptible strains of *Escherichia coli, Klebsiella-Enterobacter* and *Proteus* sp. when oral administration of Septra is not feasible and when the organism is not suceptible to single agent antibacterials effective in the urinary tract.

Cultures and susceptibility tests should be performed to determine the susceptibility of the bacteria to Septra. Therapy may be initiated prior to obtaining the results of these tests.

Contraindications: Hypersensitivity to trimethoprim or sulfonamides. Patients with documented megaloblastic anemia due to folate deficiency. Pregnancy at term and during the nursing period, because sulfonamides pass the placenta and are excreted in the milk and may cause kernicterus.

Infants less than two months of age.

Warnings: SEPTRA I.V. INFUSION SHOULD NOT BE USED IN THE TREATMENT OF STREPTOCOCCAL PHARYNGITIS. Clinical studies have documented that patients with Group A, β-hemolytic streptococcal tonsillopharyngitis have a greater incidence of bacteriologic failure when treated with Septra than do those patients treated with penicillin as evidenced by failure to eradicate this organism from the tonsillopharyngeal area.

Deaths associated with the administration of sulfonamides have been reported from hypersensitivity reactions, agranulocytosis, aplastic anemia and other blood dyscrasias. Experience with trimethoprim alone is much more limited, but it has been reported to interfere with hematopoiesis in occasional patients. In elderly patients concurrently receiving certain diuretics, primarily thiazides, as increased incidence of thrombopenia with purpura has been reported.

The presence of clinical signs such as sore throat, fever, pallor, purpura or jaundice may be early indications of serious blood disorders.

Precautions:

General: Septra should be given with caution to patients with impaired renal or hepatic function, to those with possible folate deficiency and to those with severe allergy or bronchial asthma. In glucose-6-phosphate dehydrogenase-deficient individuals, hemolysis may occur. This reaction is frequently dose-related. Adequate fluid intake must be maintained in order to prevent crystalluria and stone formation.

Local irritation and inflammation due to extravascular infiltration of the infusion has been observed with Septra I.V. Infusion. If this occurs the infusion should be discontinued and restarted at another site.

Laboratory Tests: Appropriate culture and susceptibility studies should be performed before and throughout treatment. Complete blood counts should be done frequently in patients receiving Septra; if a significant reduction in the count of any formed blood element is noted, Septra should be discontinued. Urinalyses with careful microscopic examination and renal function tests should be performed during therapy, particularly for those patients with impaired renal function.

Drug Interactions: It has been reported that Septra may prolong the prothrombin time in patients who are receivng the anticoagulant warfarin. This interaction should be kept in mind when Septra is given to patients already on anticoagulant therapy, and the coagulation time should be reassessed.

REPRESENTATIVE MINIMUM INHIBITORY CONCENTRATION VALUES FOR SEPTRA SUSCEPTIBLE ORGANISMS (MIC-mcg/ml)

Bacteria	TMP Alone	SMX Alone	TMP/SMX (1:19) TMP	SMX
Escherichia coli	0.05–1.5	1.0–245	0.05–0.5	0.95–9.5
Proteus species (indole positive)	0.5–5.0	7.35–300	0.05–1.5	0.95–28.5
Proteus mirabilis	0.5–1.5	7.35–30	0.05–0.15	0.95–2.85
Klebsiella-Enterobacter	0.15–5.0	2.45–245	0.05–1.5	0.95–28.5
Haemophilus influenzae	0.15–1.5	2.85–95	0.015–0.15	0.285–2.85
Streptococcus pneumoniae	0.15–1.5	7.35–24.5	0.05–0.15	0.95–2.85
Shigella flexneri †	<0.01–0.04	<0.16–>320	<0.002–0.03	0.04–0.625
Shigella sonnei †	0.02–0.08	0.625–>320	0.004–0.06	0.08–1.25

TMP = Trimethoprim
SMX = Sulfamethoxazole

†Rudoy, R.C., Nelson, J.D., Haltalin, K.C. Antimicrobial Agents and Chemotherapy 5:439-43, 1974.

Carcinogenesis, Mutagenesis, Impairment of Fertility:

Carcinogenesis: Long-term studies in animals to evaluate carcinogenic potential have not been conducted with Septra I.V. Infusion.

Mutagenesis: Bacterial mutagenic studies have not been performed with sulfamethoxazole and trimethoprim in combination. Trimethoprim was demonstrated to be non-mutagenic in the Ames assay. No chromosomal damage was observed in human leukocytes cultured *in vitro* with sulfamethoxazole and trimethoprim alone or in combination; the concentrations used exceeded blood levels of these compounds following therapy with Septra. Observations of leukocytes obtained from patients treated with Septra revealed no chromosomal abnormalities.

Impairment of Fertility: Septra I.V. Infusion has not been studied in animals for evidence of impairment of fertility. However, studies in rats at oral dosages as high as 70 mg/kg trimethoprim plus 350 mg/kg sulfamethoxazole daily showed no adverse effects on fertility or general reproductive performance.

Pregnancy: Teratogenic Effects: Pregnancy Category C. In rats, oral doses of 533 mg/kg sulfamethoxazole or 200 mg/kg trimethoprim produced teratological effects manifested mainly as cleft palates.

The highest dose which did not cause cleft palates in rats was 512 mg/kg sulfamethoxazole or 192 mg/kg trimethoprim when administered separately. In two studies in rats, no teratology was observed when 512 mg/kg of sulfamethoxazole was used in combination with 128 mg/kg of trimethoprim. In one study, however, cleft palates were observed in one litter out of 9 when 355 mg/kg, of sulfamethoxazole was used in combination with 88 mg/kg of trimethoprim.

In some rabbit studies, an overall increase in fetal loss (dead and resorbed and malformed conceptuses) was associated with doses of trimethoprim 6 times the human therapeutic dose.

While there are no large, well-controlled studies on the use of trimethoprim plus sulfamethoxazole in pregnant women. Brumfitt and Pursell[5] reported the outcome of 186 pregnancies during which the mother received either placebo or oral trimethoprim in combination with sulfamethoxazole. The incidence of congenital abnormalities was 4.5% (3 of 66) in those who received placebo and 3.3% (4 of 120) in those receiving trimethoprim plus sulfamethoxazole. There were no abnormalities in the 10 children whose mothers received the drug during the first trimester. In a separate survey, Brumfitt and Pursell also found no congenital abnormalities in 35 children whose mothers had received oral trimethoprim plus sulfamethoxazole at the time of conception or shortly thereafter.

Because trimethoprim plus sulfamethoxazole may interfere with folic acid metabolism, Septra I.V. Infusion should be used during pregnancy only if the potential benefit justifies the potential risk to the fetus.

Nonteratogenic Effects: See "CONTRAINDICATIONS" section.

Nursing Mothers: See "CONTRAINDICATIONS" section.

Adverse Reactions: The most frequent adverse reactions reported for Septra I.V. Infusion are nausea and vomiting, thrombocytopenia, and rash. These occurred in less than one in twenty patients. Local reaction, pain and slight irritation on I.V. administration are infrequent. Thrombophlebitis has rarely been observed. For completeness, all major reactions to sulfonamides and to trimethoprim are included below, even though they may not have been reported with Septra I.V. Infusion.

Allergic Reactions: Generalized skin eruptions, pruritus, urticaria, erythema multiforme, Stevens-Johnson syndrome, epidermal necrolysis, serum sickness, exfoliative dermatitis, anaphylactoid reactions, periorbital edema, conjunctival and scleral injection, photosensitization, arthralgia and allergic myocarditis.

Blood Dyscrasias: Megaloblastic anemia, hemolytic anemia, purpura, thrombopenia, leukopenia, agranulocytosis, aplastic anemia, hypoprothrombinemia and methemoglobinemia.

Gastrointestinal Reactions: Glossitis, stomatitis, nausea, emesis, abdominal pains, hepatitis, diarrhea, pseudomembranous colitis and pancreatitis.

C.N.S. Reactions: Headache, peripheral neuritis, mental depression, ataxia, convulsions, hallucinations, tinnitus, vertigo, insomnia, apathy, fatigue, muscle weakness and nervousness.

Miscellaneous Reactions: Drug fever, chills, and toxic nephrosis with oliguria and anuria. Periarteritis nodosa and L. E. phenomenon have occurred.

The sulfonamides bear certain chemical similarities to some goitrogens, diuretics (acetazolamide and the thiazides) and oral hypoglycemic agents. Cross-sensitivity may exist with these agents. Diuresis and hypoglycemia have occurred rarely in patients receiving sulfonamides.

Continued on next page

Burroughs Wellcome—Cont.

Overdosage: Since there has been no extensive experience in humans with single doses of Septra I.V. Infusion in excess of 25 ml (400 mg trimethoprim and 2000 mg sulfamethoxazole), the maximum tolerated dose in humans is unknown.

Use of Septra I.V. Infusion at high doses and/or for extended periods of time may cause bone marrow depression manifested as thrombopenia, leukopenia, and/or megaloblastic anemia. If signs of bone marrow depression occur, the patient should be given leucovorin 3 to 6 mg intramuscularly daily for three days, or as required to restore normal hematopoiesis.

Peritoneal dialysis is not effective and hemodialysis only moderately effective in eliminating trimethoprim and sulfamethoxazole.

The LD_{50} of Septra I.V. Infusion in mice is 700 mg/kg or 7.3 ml/kg; in rats and rabbits the LD_{50} is >500 mg/kg or >5.2 ml/kg. The vehicle produced the same LD_{50} in each of these species as the active drug.

The signs and symptoms noted in mice, rats and rabbits with Septra I.V. Infusion or its vehicle at the high I.V. doses used in acute toxicity studies included ataxia, decreased motor activity, loss of righting reflex, tremors or convulsions, and/or respiratory depression.

Dosage and Administration: [CONTRAINDICATED IN INFANTS LESS THAN TWO MONTHS OF AGE.] CAUTION—SEPTRA I.V. INFUSION MUST BE DILUTED IN 5% DEXTROSE IN WATER SOLUTION PRIOR TO ADMINISTRATION. DO NOT MIX SEPTRA I.V. INFUSION WITH OTHER DRUGS OR SOLUTIONS. RAPID OR BOLUS INJECTION MUST BE AVOIDED.

Children and Adults:

PNEUMOCYSTIS CARINII PNEUMONITIS: Total daily dose is 15 to 20 mg/kg (based on the trimethoprim component) given in three to four equally divided doses every 6 or 8 hours for up to 14 days. One investigator noted that a total daily dose of 10 to 15 mg/kg was sufficient in 10 adult patients with normal renal function.[6]

SEVERE URINARY TRACT INFECTIONS AND SHIGELLOSIS: Total daily dose is 8 to 10 mg/kg (based on the trimethoprim component) given in two to four equally divided doses every 6, 8 or 12 hours for up to 14 days for severe urinary tract infections and 5 days for shigellosis.

For Patients with Impaired Renal Function: When renal function is impaired, a reduced dosage should be employed using the following table:

Creatinine Clearance (ml/min)	Recommended Dosage Regimen
Above 30	Use Standard Regimen
15–30	½ the Usual Regimen
Below 15	Use Not Recommended

Method of Preparation: Septra I.V. Infusion must be diluted. EACH 5 ml AMPUL SHOULD BE ADDED TO 125 ml OF 5% DEXTROSE IN WATER. After diluting with 5% dextrose in water the solution should not be refrigerated and should be used within 6 hours. If upon visual inspection there is cloudiness or evidence of crystallization after mixing, the solution should be discarded and a fresh solution prepared.

The following infusion sets have been tested and found satisfactory: unit-dose glass containers (McGaw Laboratories, Cutter Laboratories, Inc., and Abbott Laboratories); unit-dose plastic containers (Viaflex™ from Travenol Laboratories and Accumed™ from McGaw Laboratories). No other systems have been tested and therefore no others can be recommended.

NOTE: In those instances where fluid restriction is desirable, each ampul may be added to 75 ml of 5% dextrose in water. Under these circumstances the solution should be mixed just prior to use and should be administered within two (2) hours. If upon visual inspection there is cloudiness or evidence of crystallization after mixing, the solution should be discarded and a fresh solution prepared.

Administration: The solution should be given by intravenous infusion over a period of 60 to 90 minutes. Rapid infusion or bolus injections must be avoided. Septra I.V. Infusion should not be given intramuscularly.

How Supplied: 5 ml ampuls, containing 80 mg trimethoprim (16 mg/ml) and 400 mg sulfamethoxazole (80 mg/ml) for infusion with 5% dextrose in water. Boxes of 10 (NDC-0081-0856-10)

STORE AT ROOM TEMPERATURE 15°–30°C (59°–86°F). DO NOT REFRIGERATE.

Also available in tablets containing 80 mg trimethoprim and 400 mg sulfamethoxazole (bottles of 40, 100, 500 and 1000 tablets; unit dose pack of 100); oral suspension containing 40 mg trimethoprim and 200 mg sulfamethoxazole in each 5 ml (bottle of 473 ml; Unit of Use: bottle of 100 ml with child-resistant cap) and double strength, oval-shaped, pink, scored tablets containing 160 mg trimethoprim and 800 mg sulfamethoxazole (bottle of 100, unit dose pack of 100, and Compliance™ Pak of 20).

References:

1. Grose WE, Bodey GP, Loo TL: Clinical Pharmacology of Intravenously Administered Trimethoprim-Sulfamethoxazole. Antimicrob Agents Chemother *15:* 447, 1979.
2. Siber GR, Gorham C, Durbin W, Lesko L, Levin MJ: Pharmacology of Intravenous Trimethoprim-Sulfamethoxazole in Children and Adults. Current Chemotherapy and Infectious Diseases, American Society for Microbiology, Washington, D.C., 1980, Vol. 1, pp. 691–692.
3. Bauer AW, Kirby WMM, Sherris JC, Turck M: Antibiotic Susceptibility Testing by Standardized Single Disk Method. Am J Clin Path *45:* 493, 1966.
4. Approved Standard ASM-2 Performance Standards for Antimicrobial Disc Susceptibility Test: National Committee for Clinical Laboratory Standards, 771 East Lancaster Avenue, Villanova, Pennsylvania 19085.
5. Brumfitt W and Pursell R: Trimethoprim/-Sulfamethoxazole in the Treatment of Bacteriuria in Women. J Inf Dis Suppl *128:*S657, 1973.
6. Winston DJ, Lau WK, Gale RP, Young LS: Trimethoprim-Sulfamethoxazole for the Treatment of *Pneumocystis carinii* pneumonia. Ann Int Med *92:* 762–769, 1980.

*Mfd. under Pat. 3,956,327

SEPTRA® TABLETS and SUSPENSION ℞
SEPTRA ® DS TABLETS Double Strength

Description: Septra is a synthetic antibacterial combination product, available in scored pink tablets, each containing 80 mg trimethoprim* and 400 mg sulfamethoxazole and in double strength, pink, scored tablets, each containing 160 mg trimethoprim and 800 mg sulfamethoxazole.

*Mfd. under Pat. 3,956,327

Also available as a pink, cherry flavored oral suspension, each teaspoonful (5 ml) containing the equivalent of 40 mg trimethoprim and 200 mg sulfamethoxazole compounded with 0.26% alcohol.

Trimethoprim is 2,4-diamino-5-(3,4,5-trimethoxybenzl) pyrimidine. It is a white to light yellow, odorless, bitter compound with a molecular weight of 290.3.

Sulfamethoxazole is N^1-(5-methyl-3-isoxazolyl) sulfanilamide. It is an almost white in color, odorless, tasteless compound with a molecular weight of 253.28.

Clinical Pharmacology:

Septra is rapidly absorbed following oral administration. The blood levels of trimethoprim and sulfamethoxazole are similar to those achieved when each component is given alone. Peak blood levels for the individual components occur one to four hours after oral administration. The half-lives of sulfamethoxazole and trimethoprim, 10 and 8 to 10 hours respectively, are relatively the same regardless of whether these compounds are administered as individual components or as Septra. Detectable amounts of trimethoprim and sulfamethoxazole are present in the blood 24 hours after drug administration. Free sulfamethoxazole and trimethoprim blood levels are proportionately dose-dependent. On repeated administration, the steady-state ratio of trimethoprim to sulfamethoxazole levels in the blood is about 1:20.

Sulfamethoxazole exists in the blood as free, conjugated and protein-bound forms; trimethoprim is present as free, protein-bound and metabolized forms. The free forms are considered to be the therapeutically active forms. Approximately 44 percent of trimethoprim and 70 percent of sulfamethoxazole are protein-bound in the blood. The presence of 10 mg percent sulfamethoxazole in plasma decreases the protein binding of trimethoprim to an insignificant degree; trimethoprim does not influence the protein binding of sulfamethoxazole.

Excretion of Septra is chiefly by the kidneys through both glomerular filtration and tubular secretion. Urine concentrations of both sulfamethoxazole and trimethoprim are considerably higher than are the concentrations in the blood. When administered together as in Septra, neither sulfamethoxazole nor trimethoprim affects the urinary excretion pattern of the other.

Microbiology: Sulfamethoxazole inhibits bacterial synthesis of dihydrofolic acid by competing with *para*-aminobenzoic acid. Trimethoprim blocks the production of tetrahydrofolic acid from dihydrofolic acid by binding to and reversibly inhibiting the required enzyme, dihydrofolate reductase. Thus, Septra blocks two consecutive steps in the biosynthesis of nucleic acids and proteins essential to many bacteria.

In vitro studies have shown that bacterial resistance develops more slowly with Septra than with trimethoprim or sulfamethoxazole alone.

In vitro serial dilution tests have shown that the spectrum of antibacterial activity of Septra includes the common urinary tract pathogens with the exception of *Pseudomonas aeruginosa.* The following organisms are usually susceptible: *Escherichia coli, Klebsiella-Enterobacter, Proteus mirabilis* and indole-positive *Proteus* species.

In addition, the usual spectrum of antimicrobial activity of Septra includes the following bacterial pathogens isolated from middle ear exudate and bronchial secretions: *Haemophilus influenzae,* including ampicillin resistant strains, and *Streptococcus pneumoniae. Shigella flexneri* and *Shigella sonnei* are also usually susceptible.

[See table on next page].

The recommended quantitative disc susceptibility method (Federal Register *37*:20527–29, 1972; Bauer AW, Kirby WMM, Sherris JC, Turck M: Antibiotic susceptibility testing by a standarized single disk method, Am J Clin Path *45*:493, 1966) may be used for estimating the susceptibility of bacteria to Septra. With this procedure, a report from the laboratory of "Susceptible to trimethoprim-sulfamethoxazole" indicates that the infection is likely to respond to therapy with Septra. If the infection is confined to the urine, a report of "Intermediate susceptibility to trimethoprim-sulfamethoxazole" also indicates that the infection is likely to respond. A report of "Resistant to trimethoprim-sulfamethoxazole" indicates that the infection is unlikely to respond to therapy with Septra.

Indications and Usage:
URINARY TRACT INFECTIONS: **For the treatment of urinary tract infections due to susceptible strains of the following organisms:** *Escherichia coli, Klebsiella-Enterobacter, Proteus mirabilis, Proteus vulgaris, Proteus morganii.* **It is recommended that initial episodes of uncomplicated urinary tract infections be treated with a single effective antibacterial agent rather than the combination.**
Note: Currently, the increasing frequency of resistant organisms is a limitation of the usefulness of all antibacterial agents, especially in the treatment of these urinary tract infections.
ACUTE OTITIS MEDIA: **For the treatment of acute otitis media in children due to susceptible strains of** *Haemophilus influenzae* **or** *Streptococcus pneumoniae* **when in the judgment of the physician Septra offers some advantage over the use of other antimicrobial agents. To date, there are limited data on the safety of repeated use of Septra in children under two years of age. Septra is not indicated for prophylactic or prolonged administration in otitis media at any age.**
ACUTE EXACERBATIONS OF CHRONIC BRONCHITIS IN ADULTS: **For the treatment of acute exacerbations of chronic bronchitis due to susceptible strains of** *Haemophilus influenzae* **or** *Streptococcus pneumoniae,* **when in the judgment of the physician, Septra offers some advantage over the use of a single antimicrobial agent.**
SHIGELLOSIS: **For the treatment of enteritis caused by susceptible strains of** *Shigella flexneri* **and** *Shigella sonnei* **when antibacterial therapy is indicated.**
PNEUMOCYSTIS CARINII **PNEUMONITIS: Septra is also indicated in the treatment of documented** *Pneumocystis carinii* **pneumonitis.**

Contraindications: Hypersensitivity to trimethoprim or sulfonamides. Patients with documented megaloblastic anemia due to folate deficiency. Pregnancy at term and during the nursing period, because sulfonamides pass the placenta and are excreted in the milk and may cause kernicterus. Infants less than two months of age.

Warnings: SEPTRA SHOULD NOT BE USED IN THE TREATMENT OF STREPTOCOCCAL PHARYNGITIS. Clinical studies have documented that patients with Group A β-hemolytic streptococcal tonsillopharyngitis have a greater incidence of bacteriologic failure when treated with Septra than do those patients treated with penicillin as evidenced by failure to eradicate this organism from the tonsillopharyngeal area.
Deaths associated with the administration of sulfonamides have been reported from hypersensitivity reactions, agranulocytosis, aplastic anemia and other blood dyscrasias. Experience with trimethoprim alone is much more limited, but it has been reported to interfere with hematopoiesis in occasional patients. In elderly patients concurrently receiving certain diuretics, primarily thiazides, an increased incidence of thrombopenia with purpura has been reported.
The presence of clinical signs such as sore throat, fever, pallor, purpura or jaundice may be early indications of serious blood disorders. Complete blood counts should be done frequently in patients receiving Septra. If a significant reduction in the count of any formed blood element is noted, Septra should be discontinued.

Precautions: *General:* Septra should be given with caution to patients with impaired renal or hepatic function, to those with possible folate deficiency and to those with severe allergy or bronchial asthma. In glucose-6-phosphate dehydrogenase-deficient individuals, hemolysis may occur. This reaction is frequently dose-related. Adequate fluid intake must be maintained in order to prevent crystalluria and stone formation. Urinalyses with careful microscopic examination and renal function tests should be performed during therapy, particularly for those patients with impaired renal function.

REPRESENTATIVE MINIMUM INHIBITORY CONCENTRATION VALUES FOR SEPTRA SUSCEPTIBLE ORGANISMS (MIC-mcg/ml)

Bacteria	TMP Alone	SMX Alone	TMP/SMX (1:19) TMP	TMP/SMX (1:19) SMX
Escherichia coli	0.05–1.5	1.0 –245	0.05 –0.5	0.95 – 9.5
Proteus species (indole positive)	0.5 –5.0	7.35 –300	0.05 –1.5	0.95 –28.5
Proteus mirabilis	0.5 –1.5	7.35 – 30	0.05 –0.15	0.95 – 2.85
Klebsiella-Enterobacter	0.15–5.0	2.45 –245	0.05 –1.5	0.95 –28.5
Haemophilus influenzae	0.15–1.5	2.85 – 95	0.015 –0.15	0.285 – 2.85
Streptococcus pneumoniae	0.15–1.5	7.35 – 24.5	0.05 –0.15	0.95 – 2.85
Shigella flexneri†	<0.01–0.04	<0.16 –> 320	<0.002 –0.03	0.04 –0.625
Shigella sonnei†	0.02–0.08	0.625 –> 320	0.004 –0.06	0.08 –1.25

TMP = Trimethoprim SMX = Sulfamethoxazole
†Rudoy, R.C., Nelson, J.D., Haltalin, K.C. *Antimicrobial Agents and Chemotherapy 5:*439–43, 1974.

It has been reported that Septra may prolong the prothrombin time of patients who are receiving the anticoagulant warfarin. This interaction should be kept in mind when Septra is given to patients already on anticoagulant therapy, and the coagulation time should be reassessed.
Pregnancy: Teratogenic Effects: Pregnancy Category C. In rats, doses of 533 mg/kg sulfamethoxazole or 200 mg/kg trimethoprim produced teratological effects manifested mainly as cleft palates. The highest dose which did not cause cleft palates in rats was 512 mg/kg sulfamethoxazole or 192 mg/kg trimethoprim when administered separately. In two studies in rats, no teratology was observed when 512 mg/kg of sulfamethoxazole was used in combination with 128 mg/kg of trimethoprim. In one study, however, cleft palates were observed in one litter out of 9 when 355 mg/kg of sulfamethoxazole was used in combination with 88 mg/kg of trimethoprim.
In some rabbit studies, an overall increase in fetal loss (dead and resorbed and malformed conceptuses) was associated with doses of trimethoprim 6 times the human therapeutic dose.
While there are no large well-controlled studies on the use of trimethoprim plus sulfamethoxazole in pregnant women, Brumfitt and Pursell (Trimethoprim/Sulfamethoxazole in the Treatment of Bacteriuria in Women. J Inf Dis Suppl 128:S657-S663, 1973.) reported the outcome of 186 pregnancies during which the mother received either placebo or trimethoprim in combination with sulfamethoxazole. The incidence of congenital abnormalities was 4.5% (3 of 66) in those who received placebo and 3.3% (4 of 120) in those receiving trimethoprim plus sulfamethoxazole. There were no abnormalities in the 10 children whose mothers received the drug during the first trimester. In a separate survey, Brumfitt and Pursell also found no congenital abnormalities in 35 children whose mothers had received trimethoprim plus sulfamethoxazole at the time of conception or shortly thereafter.
Because trimethoprim plus sulfamethoxazole may interfere with folic acid metabolism, Septra should be used during pregnancy only if the potential benefit justifies the potential risk to the fetus.
Nonteratogenic Effects: See "CONTRAINDICATIONS" section.
Nursing Mothers: See "CONTRAINDICATIONS" section.

Adverse Reactions: For completeness, all major reactions to sulfonamides and to trimethoprim are included below even though they may not have been with Septra.
Blood Dyscrasias: Agranulocytosis, aplastic anemia, megaloblastic anemia, thrombopenia, leukopenia, hemolytic anemia, purpura, hypoprothrombinemia and methemoglobinemia.
Allergic Reactions: Erythema multiforme, Stevens-Johnson syndrome, generalized skin eruptions, epidermal necrolysis, urticaria, serum sickness, pruritus, exfoliative dermatitis, anaphylactoid reactions, periorbital edema, conjuctival and scleral injection, photosensitization, arthralgia and allergic myocarditis.
Gastrointestinal Reactions: Glossitis, stomatitis, nausea, emesis, abdominal pains, hepatitis, diarrhea, pseudomembraneous colitis and pancreatitis.
C.N.S. Reactions: Headache, peripheral neuritis, mental depression, convulsions, ataxia, hallucinations, tinnitus, vertigo, insomnia, apathy, fatigue, muscle weakness and nervousness.
Miscellaneous Reactions: Drug fever, chills, and toxic nephrosis with oliguria and anuria. Periarteritis nodosa and L.E. phenomenon have occurred.
The sulfonamides bear certain chemical similarities to some goitrogens, diuretics (acetazolamide and the thiazides) and oral hypoglycemic agents. Goiter production, diuresis and hypoglycemia have occurred rarely in patients receiving sulfonamides. Cross-sensitivity may exist with these agents. Rats appear to be especially susceptible to the goitrogenic effects of sulfonamides, and long-term administration has produced thyroid malignancies in the species.

Dosage and Administration: Not recommended for use in infants less than two months of age.
URINARY TRACT INFECTIONS AND SHIGELLOSIS IN ADULTS AND CHILDREN. ACUTE OTITIS MEDIA IN CHILDREN.
Adults: The usual adult dosage for the treatment of urinary tract infections is one Septra DS Tablet or two Septra Tablets or four tea-

Continued on next page

Burroughs Wellcome—Cont.

spoonfuls (20 ml) Septra Suspension every 12 hours for 10 to 14 days. An identical daily dosage is used for 5 days in the treatment of shigellosis.

Children: The recommended dose for children with urinary tract infections or acute otitis media is 8 mg/kg trimethoprim and 40 mg/kg sulfamethoxazole per 24 hours, given in two divided doses every 12 hours for 10 days. In children weighing 88 lbs (40 kg) or more, the dosage is one Septra DS Tablet or two Septra Tablets every 12 hours for 10 days. An identical daily dosage is used for 5 days in the treatment of shigellosis. The following table is a guideline for the attainment of this dosage using Septra Tablets or Suspension.

Children: Two months of age or older

Weight		Dose—every 12 hours	
lb	kg	Teaspoonfuls	Tablets
22	10	1 (5 ml)	
44	20	2 (10 ml)	1
66	30	3 (15 ml)	1 ½
88	40	4 (20 ml)	2 (or 1 DS Tablet)

For patients with renal impairment:

Creatinine Clearance (ml/min)	Recommended Dosage Regimen
Above 30	Usual Standard Regimen
15–30	Half of the usual dosage regimen
Below 15	Use Not Recommended

Acute Exacerbations of Chronic Bronchitis in Adults: The usual adult dosage in the treatment of acute exacerbations of chronic bronchitis is one Septra DS tablet or two Septra tablets or four teaspoonfuls (20 ml) of Septra Suspension every 12 hours for 14 days.

PNEUMOCYSTIS CARINII **PNEUMONITIS:** The recommended dosage for patients with documented *Pneumocystis carinii* pneumonitis is 20 mg/kg trimethoprim and 100 mg/kg sulfamethoxazole per 24 hours given in equally divided doses every 6 hours for 14 days. The following table is a guideline for the attainment of this dosage in children.

Weight		Dose—every 6 hours	
lb	kg	Teaspoonfuls	Tablets
18	8	1 (5 ml)	½
35	16	2 (10 ml)	1
53	24	3 (15 ml)	1 ½
70	32	4 (20 ml)	2 (or 1 DS Tablet)

How Supplied: TABLETS, containing 80 mg trimethoprim and 400 mg sulfamethoxazole—bottles of 100, 500 and 1000 tablets; unit dose pack of 100. Regular strength tablets bear identification, SEPTRA Y2B.

ORAL SUSPENSION, containing the equivalent of 40 mg trimethoprim and 200 mg sulfamethoxazole in each teaspoonful (5 ml), cherry flavored—bottles of 100 ml and 473 ml.

Also available in double strength, oval-shaped, pink, scored tablets containing 160 mg trimethoprim and 800 mg sulfamethoxazole—Compliance™ Pak of 20, bottles of 100 and 250 and unit dose pack of 100. Double strength tablets bear identification, SEPTRA DS O2C.

[*Shown in Product Identification Section*]

SUDAFED® COUGH SYRUP
Decongestant/Cough Suppressant/Expectorant

(See PDR for Nonprescription Drugs)

SUDAFED® PLUS SYRUP/TABLETS

(See PDR for Nonprescription Drugs)

TABLOID® BRAND THIOGUANINE ℞
40 mg Scored Tablets

CAUTION: Tabloid® brand thioguanine is a potent drug. It should not be used unless a diagnosis of acute leukemia or chronic myelogenous leukemia has been adequately established and the responsible physician is knowledgeable in assessing response to chemotherapy.

Description: Tabloid brand thioguanine (6-thioguanine; 2-amino-6-thiopurine; 2-amino-6-mercaptopurine) was synthesized and developed by Hitchings, Elion, and associates at the Wellcome Research Laboratories. It is one of a large series of purine analogues which interfere with nucleic acid biosynthesis.[1]

Thioguanine is an analogue of the nucleic acid constituent guanine, and is closely related structurally and functionally to Purinethol® brand mercaptopurine (6-mercaptopurine).

1. Thioguanine competes with hypoxanthine and guanine for the enzyme hypoxanthine-guanine phosphoribosyltransferase (HGPRTase) and is itself converted to 6-thioguanylic acid (TGMP). This nucleotide reaches high intracellular concentrations at therapeutic doses. TGMP interferes at several points with the synthesis of guanine nucleotides. It inhibits *de novo* purine biosynthesis by pseudo-feedback inhibition of glutamine-5-phosphoribosylpyrophosphate amidotransferase—the first enzyme unique to the *de novo* pathway for purine ribonucleotide synthesis. TGMP also inhibits the conversion of inosinic acid (IMP) to xanthylic acid (XMP) by competition for the enzyme inosinic acid (IMP) dehydrogenase. At one time TGMP was felt to be a significant inhibitor of ATP:GMP phosphotransferase (guanylate kinase)[2], but recent results have shown this not to be so.[3]
2. Thioguanylic acid is further converted to the di- and tri-phosphates, thioguanosine diphosphate (TGDP) and thioguanosine triphosphate (TGTP) (as well as their 2′-deoxyribosyl analogues), by the same enzymes which metabolize guanine nucleotides.[4] Thioguanine nucleotides are incorporated into both the RNA and the DNA by phosphodiester linkages[5] and it has been argued that incorporation of such fraudulent bases contributes to the cytotoxicity of thioguanine.
3. Thus, thioguanine has multiple metabolic effects and, at present, it is not possible to designate one major site of action. Its tumor inhibitory properties may be due to one or more of its effects on (a) feedback inhibition of *de novo* purine synthesis; (b) inhibition of purine nucleotide interconversions; or (c) incorporation into the DNA and the RNA. The net consequence of its actions is a sequential blockade of the synthesis and utilization of the purine nucleotides.[2,4,6]
4. The catabolism of thioguanine and its metabolites is complex and shows significant differences between man and the mouse.[5,7] In both humans and mice, after oral administration of ^{35}S-6-thioguanine, urine contains virtually no detectable intact thioguanine. While deamination and subsequent oxidation to thiouric acid occurs only to a small extent in man, it is the main pathway in mice. The product of deamination by guanase, 6-thioxanthine, is inactive, having negligible antitumor activity. This pathway of thioguanine inactivation is not dependent on the action of xanthine oxidase and an inhibitor of that enzyme (such as Zyloprim® brand allopurinol) will not block the detoxification of thioguanine even though the inactive 6-thioxanthine is normally further oxidized by xanthine oxidase to thiouric acid before it is eliminated. In man, methylation of thioguanine is much more extensive than in the mouse. The product of methylation, 2-amino-6-methylthiopurine, is also substantially less active and less toxic than thioguanine and its formation is likewise unaffected by the presence of allopurinol. Appreciable amounts of inorganic sulfate are also found in both murine and human urine, presumably arising from further metabolism of the methylated derivatives.
5. In some animal tumors, resistance to the effect of thioguanine correlates with the loss of HGPRTase activity and the resulting inability to convert thioguanine to thioguanylic acid. However, other resistance mechanisms, such as increased catabolism of TGMP by a nonspecific phosphatase, may be operative. Although not invariable, it is usual to find cross-resistance between thioguanine and its close analogue, mercaptopurine.

Clinical Pharmacology:

1. Clinical studies have shown that the absorption of an oral dose of thioguanine in man is incomplete and variable, averaging approximately 30% of the administered dose (range: 14–46%).[5,7] Following oral administration of ^{35}S-6-thioguanine, total plasma radioactivity reached a maximum at eight hours and declined slowly thereafter. Parent drug represented only a very small fraction of the total plasma radioactivity at any time, being virtually undetectable throughout the period of measurements.
2. The oral administration of radiolabeled thioguanine revealed only trace quantities of parent drug in the urine. However, a methylated metabolite, 2-amino-6-methylthiopurine (MTG), appeared very early, rose to a maximum six to eight hours after drug administration, and was still being excreted after 12 to 22 hours. Radiolabeled sulfate appeared somewhat later than MTG but was the principal metabolite after eight hours. Thiouric acid and some unidentified products were found in the urine in small amounts.[7]
3. Intravenous administration of ^{35}S-6-thioguanine disclosed a median plasma half-disappearance time of 80 minutes (range: 25–240 minutes) when the compound was given in single doses of 65 to 300 mg/m^2. Although initial plasma levels of thioguanine did correlate with the dose level, there was no correlation between the plasma half-disappearance time and the dose.[5]
4. Thioguanine is incorporated into the DNA and the RNA of human bone marrow cells. Studies with intravenous ^{35}S-6-thioguanine have shown that the amount of thioguanine incorporated into nucleic acids is more than 100 times higher after five daily doses than after a single dose. With the 5-dose schedule, from one-half to virtually all of the guanine in the residual DNA was replaced by thioguanine.[5]
5. Tissue distribution studies of ^{35}S-6-thioguanine in mice showed only traces of radioactivity in brain after oral administration. No measurements have been made of thioguanine concentrations in human cerebrospinal fluid, but observations on tissue distribution in animals, together with the lack of CNS penetration by the closely related compound, mercaptopurine, suggests that thioguanine does not reach therapeutic concentrations in the CSF.
6. Monitoring of plasma levels of thioguanine during therapy is of questionable value.[7] There is technical difficulty in determining

plasma concentrations which are seldom greater than 1 to 2 micrograms per ml after a therapeutic oral dose. More significantly, thioguanine enters rapidly into the anabolic acid and catabolic pathways for purines and the active intracellular metabolites have appreciably longer half-lifes than the parent drug. The biochemical effects of a single dose of thioguanine are evident long after the parent drug has disappeared from plasma. Because of this rapid metabolism of thioguanine to active intracellular derivatives, hemodialysis would not be expected to appreciably reduce toxicity of the drug.

Indications:

The Acute Leukemias: Tabloid brand thioguanine is indicated for remission induction, remission consolidation, and maintenance therapy of the acute leukemias. The response to this agent depends upon the particular subclassification of the acute leukemia (lymphatic, myelogenous, undifferentiated, etc.), the age of the patient (child or adult), and whether or not thioguanine is used in previously treated or previously untreated patients. Thioguanine induces complete remissions in approximately 50% of previously untreated children with acute leukemia when the drug is used as a single agent. These results can be improved upon considerably, however, by using multiple carefully selected agents in combination. Reliance upon thioguanine alone is seldom justified for initial remission induction in children with acute leukemia. The duration of complete remission induced in children with acute leukemia is so brief without the use of maintenance therapy that some form of drug therapy is essential following successful remission induction.

In adults, thioguanine has been most frequently employed in combination with other agents (particularly with cytosine arabinoside) for the treatment of acute myelogenous (granulocytic) leukemia and acute lymphatic (lymphocytic, lymphoblastic) leukemia. The incidence of complete remission induction has varied widely, depending upon the particular combination of agents used, the classification of the leukemia (lymphatic, in general, responding better than myelogenous), the age of the patient (younger patients faring better than older), and whether the results are reported by a single institution or a large cooperative group.

Because of the brief duration of "unmaintained" complete remissions following successful remission induction, most therapy for adult acute leukemia currently employs some form of maintenance chemotherapy.

Thioguanine is not effective for prophylaxis or treatment of central nervous system leukemia.

Chronic Myelogenous (Granulocytic) Leukemia: Thioguanine is one of several agents with demonstrated efficacy in the treatment of chronic myelogenous leukemia. Approximately 50% of patients with chronic myelogenous leukemia have an objective response to thioguanine. This is less than the 90% objective responses with busulfan and, of these two agents, Myleran® brand busulfan is usually regarded as the preferred drug for initial therapy.

Other Neoplasms: Tabloid brand thioguanine is not effective in chronic lymphatic leukemia, the lymphomas (including Hodgkin's Disease), multiple myeloma, or solid tumors.

Contraindications: Thioguanine should not be used in patients whose disease has demonstrated prior resistance to this drug. In animals and man, there is usually complete cross-resistance between Purinethol brand mercaptopurine and Tabloid brand thioguanine.

Warnings: While thioguanine may be used in patients with anemia, thrombocytopenia, and granulocytopenia secondary to leukemia, these same abnormalities may be produced as a result of a direct, myelotoxic effect of the drug.

The safe and effective use of thioguanine demands a thorough knowledge of the natural history of the condition being treated. For example, remission induction of acute leukemia in adults virtually always necessitates the production of moderate to severe bone marrow hypoplasia. The degree of myelosuppression acceptable in this disease would not be desirable in the management of chronic granulocytic leukemia. After selection of an initial dosage schedule, therapy will frequently need to be modified depending upon the patient's response and manifestations of toxicity.

Evaluation of response to thioguanine therapy requires frequent examination of the peripheral blood for changes in the formed elements. Bone marrow examination (aspiration and/or biopsy) may be helpful in distinguishing between resistance to therapy, progression of leukemia, and marrow hypoplasia induced by therapy.

The most consistent, dose-related toxicity is bone marrow suppression. This may be manifest by anemia, leukopenia, thrombocytopenia, or any combination of these. Any one of these findings may also reflect progression of the underlying disease. It is imperative that patients be instructed to report promptly the development of fever, sore throat, signs of local infection, bleeding from any site, or symptoms suggestive of anemia. Since thioguanine may have a delayed effect, it is important to withdraw the medication temporarily at the first sign of an abnormally large fall in any of the formed elements of the blood.

It is recommended that evaluation of the hemoglobin concentration or hematocrit, total white blood cell count and differential count, and quantitative platelet count be obtained weekly while the patient is on thioguanine therapy. In cases where the cause of fluctuations in the formed elements in the peripheral blood is obscure, bone marrow examination may be useful for the evaluation of marrow status. The decision to increase, decrease, continue or discontinue a given dosage of thioguanine must be based not only on the absolute hematologic values, but also upon the rapidity with which changes are occurring. In many instances, particularly during the induction phase of acute leukemia, complete blood counts will need to be done more frequently than once weekly in order to evaluate the effect of the therapy. The dosage of thioguanine may need to be reduced when this agent is combined with other drugs whose primary toxicity is myelosuppression.

Although the effect usually occurs slowly over a period of two to four weeks, occasionally there may be a rapid fall in leukocyte count within one to two weeks. This may occur in some adults with acute leukemia and high total leukocyte counts as well as in certain adults with chronic granulocytic leukemia. For this reason, it is important to observe such patients carefully. Since the drug may have a delayed action, it should be discontinued at the first sign of an abnormally large fall in the leukocyte or platelet count. If, subsequently, the leukocyte or platelet count remains constant for two or three days, or rises, treatment may be resumed.

Myelosuppression is often unavoidable during the induction phase of adult acute leukemia if remission induction is to be successful. Whether or not this demands modification or cessation of dosage depends both upon the response of the underlying disease and a careful consideration of supportive facilities (granulocyte and platelet transfusions) which may be available. Life-threatening infections and bleeding have been observed as a consequence of thioguanine induced granulocytopenia and thrombocytopenia.

If it is not the intent to intentionally induce bone marrow hypoplasia, it is important to discontinue the drug temporarily at the first evidence of abnormally large, or excessively rapid, fall in white blood cell count, platelet count, or hemoglobin concentration. In many patients with severe depression of the formed elements of the blood due to thioguanine, the bone marrow appears hypoplastic on aspiration or biopsy, whereas in other cases it may appear normocellular. The qualitative changes in the erythroid elements toward the megaloblastic series, characteristically seen with the folic acid antagonist and some other antimetabolites, are not seen with this drug. Carcinogenic potential exists in man, but the extent of the risk is unknown.

The effect of thioguanine on the immunocompetence of patients is unknown.

Drugs such as thioguanine are potential mutagens and teratogens. Because of the possibility of fetal damage, thioguanine should be used during pregnancy only if the benefit clearly justifies the potential risk to the fetus; whenever possible, use of the drug should be deferred until after the first trimester of pregnancy. The effects of thioguanine upon fertility, both in males and females, together with potential hazards to the fetus are unknown when the drug is employed either as a single agent or is used in combination chemotherapeutic regimens.

Two cases have been reported in which fathers have sired children with congenital abnormalities after chemotherapy with multiple antineoplastic agents (including thioguanine) was stopped.[8]

Precautions: A few cases of jaundice have been reported in patients with leukemia receiving thioguanine. It has been reported that two adult male patients and four children, all with acute myelogenous leukemia, developed veno-occlusive hepatic disease while receiving chemotherapy for their leukemia.[9] All six patients had received cytosine arabinoside prior to treatment with thioguanine and some were receiving other chemotherapy in addition to thioguanine when they became symptomatic. While veno-occlusive hepatic disease has not been reported in patients treated with thioguanine alone, it is recommended that thioguanine be withheld if there is evidence of toxic hepatitis or biliary stasis, and that appropriate clinical and laboratory investigations be initiated to establish the etiology of the hepatic dysfunction.

It is advisable to monitor liver function tests (serum transaminases, alkaline phosphatase, bilirubin) at weekly intervals when first beginning therapy and at monthly intervals thereafter. Liver function tests may be advisable more frequently in patients who are receiving thioguanine with known pre-existing liver disease or with other hepatotoxic drugs. Patients should be instructed to discontinue thioguanine immediately if clinical jaundice is detected.

Deterioration in liver function studies while receiving thioguanine should prompt discontinuation of treatment and a search for an explanation of the hepatotoxicity.

See **WARNINGS** section for information on immunosuppression, carcinogenesis, mutagenesis, and impairment of fertility.

Adverse Reactions:

Gastrointestinal Symptoms: Nausea, vomiting, anorexia, and stomatitis may occur, particularly with overdosage. While no significant clinical differences between thioguanine and mercaptopurine have been noted with respect to action or side effects, it has been observed that occasional patients may experience better gastrointestinal tolerance to one or the other drug. The onset of clinical jaundice, hepatomegaly, or anorexia with tenderness in the right hypochondrium are immediate indications for withholding thioguanine until the exact etiology can be identified.

Continued on next page

Burroughs Wellcome—Cont.

Other: Hyperuricemia frequently occurs in patients receiving thioguanine as a consequence of rapid cell lysis accompanying the antineoplastic effect. Adverse effects can be minimized by increased hydration, urine alkalinization, and the prophylactic administration of a xanthine oxidase inhibitor such as Zyloprim brand allopurinol. Unlike Purinethol brand mercaptopurine and Imuran® brand azathioprine, thioguanine may be continued in the usual dosage when allopurinol is used conjointly to inhibit uric acid formation.

Overdosage: There is no known pharmacologic antagonist of thioguanine. The drug should be discontinued immediately if unintended toxicity occurs during treatment. Severe hematologic toxicity may require supportive therapy with platelet transfusions for bleeding, and granulocyte transfusions and antibiotics if sepsis is documented. If a patient is seen immediately following an accidental overdosage of the drug, induced emesis may be useful. Hemodialysis is thought to be of marginal use due to the rapid intracellular incorporation of thioguanine into active metabolites with long persistence.

Dosage and Administration: Tabloid brand thioguanine is administered orally. The dosage which will be tolerated or which will be effective varies from patient-to-patient and careful dose titration is necessary to obtain the optimum therapeutic effect without incurring excessive, unintended toxicity. The usual initial dosage for children and adults is approximately 2 mg/kg of body weight per day. If, after four weeks on this dosage, there is no clinical improvement and no leukocyte or platelet depression, the dosage may be cautiously increased to 3 mg/kg per day. The total daily dose may be given at one time. It is usually calculated to the closest multiple of 20 mg.

The dosage of thioguanine used does not depend on whether or not the patient is receiving Zyloprim brand allopurinol; *this is in contradistinction to the dosage reduction which is mandatory when mercaptopurine or azathioprine is used simultaneously with allopurinol.*

If a complete hematologic remission is obtained with thioguanine, either alone or in combination with other agents, maintenance therapy should be instituted. If remission is achieved, maintenance doses and schedules incorporating thioguanine will vary from patient-to-patient depending upon the regimen being used.

How Supplied: Greenish-yellow, scored tablets containing 40 mg thioguanine, imprinted with "WELLCOME" and "U3B" on each tablet; in bottle of 25.

References:

1. Hitchings, G.H., and Elion, G.B: The Chemistry and Biochemistry of Purine Analogs. Ann. N.Y. Acad. Sci. *60:*195–199, 1954.
2. Miech, R.P., Parks, R.E., Jr., Anderson, J.H., Jr., and Sartorelli, A.C.: An Hypothesis on the Mechanism of Action of 6-Thioguanine. Biochem. Pharmacol. *16:*2222–2227, 1967.
3. Miller, R.L., Adamczyk, D.L., and Spector, T.: Reassessment of the Interactions of Guanylate Kinase and 6-Thioguanosine 5′-Phosphate. Proc. Am. Assoc. Cancer Res. *18:*6, 1977. *Abstract.*
4. Paterson, A.R.P., and Tidd, D.N.: 6-Thiopurines. In: *Antineoplastic and Immunosuppressive Agents,* Part II. (Edited by A.C. Sartorelli and D.G. Johns.) Berlin, Springer-Verlag, 384–403, 1975.
5. LePage, G.A., and Whitecar, J.P., Jr.: Pharmacology of 6-Thioguanine in Man. Cancer Res. *31:*1627–1631, 1971.
6. Nelson, J.A., Carpenter, J.W., Rose, L.N., and Adamson, D.J.: Mechanisms of Action of 6-Thioguanine, 6-Mercaptopurine, and 8-Azaguanine. Cancer Res. *35:*2872–2878, 1975.
7. Elion, G.B.: Biochemistry and Pharmacology of Purine Analogues. Fed. Proc. *26:*898–904, 1967.
8. Russell, J.A., Powle, R.L., and Oliver, R.T.D.: Conception and Congenital Abnormalities After Chemotherapy of Acute Myelogenous Leukaemia in Two Men. Brit. Med. J. *1:*1508, 1976.
9. Griner, P.F., Elbadawi, A., and Packman, C.H.: Veno-Occlusive Disease of the Liver After Chemotherapy of Acute Leukemia. Ann. Inter. Med. *85:*578–582, 1976.

[Shown in Product Identification Section]

VASOXYL® ℞
(Methoxamine Hydrochloride)
INJECTION
20 mg in 1 ml

Description: Vasoxyl (Methoxamine Hydrochloride) Injection is a sterile solution for intramuscular or intravenous injection, made isotonic with sodium chloride. Each ml contains 20 mg methoxamine hydrochloride. Citric acid anhydrous 0.3% and sodium citrate 0.3% are added as buffers and potassium metabisulfite 0.1% is added as an antioxidant.

Methoxamine is a sympathomimetic amine. Chemically, methoxamine is α-(1-aminoethyl)-2,5-dimethoxybenzenemethanol hydrochloride. It is available as the hydrochloride in sterile aqueous solution for parenteral use.

The structural formula is as follows:

CH_3O / ring —CH(OH)—CH(NH_2)—CH_3 · HCl / OCH_3

Actions: Vasoxyl (Methoxamine Hydrochloride) Injection is a vasopressor agent which produces a prompt and prolonged rise in blood pressure following parenteral administration. It is especially useful for maintaining blood pressure during operations under spinal anesthesia; it may also safely be used during general anesthesia.

The outstanding characteristic is potent, prolonged pressor action following parenteral administration. Unlike most pressor amines, there is no increase in cardiac rate but rather on occasions a decrease in rate develops as the blood pressure increases. This bradycardia is apparently caused by a carotid sinus reflex mediated over the vagus nerve. It is abolished by atropine.

The pressor action appears to be due primarily to peripheral vasoconstriction. Dripps has pointed out that evidence for direct action on blood vessels is provided by the observation of intense constriction along the course of a vein into which methoxamine has been injected. Taube and Fassett have shown that methoxamine increases central venous pressure. Methoxamine hydrochloride has the distinct advantage of being free of central stimulating action. This has been demonstrated by de Beer in laboratory studies as well as by Fassett in electroencephalogram tracings of patients receiving the drug. Pressor action without central stimulation may be especially desirable in patients undergoing surgery under spinal anesthesia.

Of special significance is the conclusion of Stutzman, Pettinga and Fruggiero that "Methoxamine does not increase the irritability of the cyclopropane-sensitized heart. It is a safe pressor agent for use during cyclopropane anesthesia." It has already been noted that it tends to slow the ventricular rate; large doses may produce bradycardia, but do not cause ventricular tachycardia, fibrillation, or an increased sinoauricular rate.

Finally, tachyphylaxis does not appear to be a factor clinically; Dripps states that he has never observed true tachyphylaxis to methoxamine.

Indications: For supporting, restoring or maintaining blood pressure during anesthesia (including cyclopropane anesthesia).

For terminating some episodes of paroxysmal supraventricular tachycardia.

Contraindications: Methoxamine is contraindicated as a combination with local anesthetics to prolong their action at local sites.

Precautions: The use of Vasoxyl (Methoxamine Hydrochloride) Injection is not a substitute for the replacement of blood, plasma, fluids and electrolytes which should promptly be restored when loss has occurred.

Caution should be observed when used closely following the parenteral injection of ergot alkaloids, to prevent an excessive rise in blood pressure. Caution should be exercised to avoid overdosage so that undesirably high blood pressure or excessive bradycardia will not occur. (Bradycardia may be abolished with atropine.) While 20 mg Vasoxyl (Methoxamine Hydrochloride) Injection intramuscularly has been used by some anesthesiologists, with favorable results, most studies indicate that 10 to 15 mg intramuscularly is adequate to give a satisfactory pressor response. A second dose should not be given until the previous one has had time to act (about 15 minutes). The intravenous route should be reserved for emergencies where a strong immediate pressor response is imperative, in which case not more than 5 mg may be given slowly.

Vasoxyl (Methoxamine Hydrochloride) Injection, like other vasopressor agents, should be used with care in patients with hyperthyroidism or severe hypertension. It is to be noted, however, that patients with hypertension may suffer greater or more serious fall in blood pressure than those with normal blood pressure when under spinal anesthesia, hence a pressor drug may be especially valuable properly used under these circumstances.

The possibility exists that the increase in peripheral resistance produced by methoxamine may produce or exacerbate heart failure associated with a diseased myocardium, due to the production of an increased workload.

Adverse Reactions: Methoxamine may on occasion produce sustained excessive blood pressure elevations with severe headache, pilomotor response, a desire to void and projectile vomiting, particularly with high dosage.

Dosage: (Methoxamine Hydrochloride) Injection is administered by either intramuscular or intravenous administration.

The usual intravenous dose of methoxamine for emergencies is 3 to 5 mg, injected slowly. Intravenous injection may be supplemented by intramuscular injections to provide a more prolonged effect. The usual intramuscular dose is 10 to 15 mg. This may be given shortly before or at the time of administering spinal anesthesia to prevent a fall in blood pressure. The tendency for the blood pressure to fall is greater with higher levels of spinal anesthesia, hence the dosage may be adjusted accordingly; 10 mg may be adequate at lower spinal levels while 15 to 20 mg may be required at high levels of spinal anesthesia. Repeated doses may be given if necessary but time should be allowed for the previous dose to act (see Precautions).

For purposes of correcting a fall in blood pressure an intramuscular injection of 10 to 15 mg methoxamine hydrochloride may be given depending upon the degree of fall. In cases where the systolic pressure falls to 60 mm or less, or whenever an emergency exists, an intravenous injection of 3 to 5 mg Vasoxyl (Methoxamine Hydrochloride) Injection is indicated. This may be accompanied by 10 to 15 mg intramuscularly to provide more prolonged effect.

For preoperative and postoperative use in cases of only moderate hypotension 5 to 10 mg intramuscularly may be adequate. In paroxysmal supraventricular tachycardia the average dose is 10 mg intravenously injected slowly.

How Supplied: Vasoxyl (Methoxamine Hydrochloride) Injection 20 mg in 1 ml: 1 ml ampuls; boxes of 12.

VIROPTIC® OPHTHALMIC SOLUTION, 1% ℞
(trifluridine) Sterile

Description: VIROPTIC® is the brand name for trifluridine (also known as trifluorothymidine, F_3TdR, F_3T), an antiviral drug for topical treatment of epithelial keratitis caused by Herpes simplex virus. The chemical name of trifluridine is 5-trifluoromethyl-2′-deoxyuridine.

VIROPTIC sterile ophthalmic solution contains 1% trifluridine in an aqueous solution with acetic acid and sodium acetate (buffers), sodium chloride, and thimerosal 0.001% (added as a preservative).

Clinical Pharmacology: Trifluridine is a fluorinated pyrimidine nucleoside with *in vitro* and *in vivo* activity against Herpes simplex virus, types 1 and 2 and vacciniavirus. Some strains of Adenovirus are also inhibited *in vitro.*

Trifluridine interferes with DNA synthesis in cultured mammalian cells. However, its antiviral mechanism of action is not completely known.

In vitro perfusion studies on excised rabbit corneas have shown that trifluridine penetrates the intact cornea as evidenced by recovery of parental drug and its major metabolite, 5-carboxy-2′-deoxyuridine, on the endothelial side of the cornea. Absence of the corneal epithelium enhances the penetration of trifluridine approximately two-fold.

Intraocular penetration of trifluridine occurs after topical instillation of VIROPTIC into human eyes. Decreased corneal integrity or stromal or uveal inflammation may enhance the penetration of trifluridine into the aqueous humor. Unlike the results of ocular penetration of trifluridine *in vitro,* 5-carboxy-2′-deoxyuridine was not found in detectable concentrations within the aqueous humor of the human eye.

Systemic absorption of trifluridine following therapeutic dosing with VIROPTIC appears to be negligible. No detectable concentrations of trifluridine or 5-carboxy-2′-deoxyuridine were found in the sera of adult healthy normal subjects who had VIROPTIC instilled into their eyes seven times daily for 14 consecutive days.

Indications and Usage: VIROPTIC brand Trifluridine Ophthalmic Solution, 1% is indicated for the treatment of primary keratoconjunctivitis and recurrent epithelial keratitis due to Herpes simplex virus, types 1 and 2. VIROPTIC is also effective in the treatment of epithelial keratitis that has not responded clinically to the topical administration of idoxuridine or when ocular toxicity or hypersensitivity to idoxuridine has occurred. In a smaller number of patients found to be resistant to topical vidarabine, VIROPTIC was also effective.

The clinical efficacy of VIROPTIC in the treatment of stromal keratitis and efficacy due to Herpes simplex virus or ophthalmic infections caused by vacciniavirus and Adenovirus has not been established by well-controlled clinical trials. VIROPTIC has not been shown to be effective in the prophylaxis of Herpes simplex virus keratoconjunctivitis and epithelial keratitis by well-controlled clinical trials. VIROPTIC is not effective against bacterial, fungal or chlamydial infections of the cornea or nonviral trophic lesions.

During controlled multicenter clinical trials, 92 of 97 (95%) patients (78 of 81 with dendritic and 14 of 16 with geographic ulcers) responded to VIROPTIC therapy as evidenced by complete corneal re-epithelialization within the 14 day therapy period. In these controlled studies, 56 of 75 (75%) patients (49 of 58 with dendritic and 7 of 17 with geographic ulcers) responded to idoxuridine therapy. The mean time to corneal re-epithelialization of dendritic ulcers (6 days) and geographic ulcers (7 days) was similar for both therapies. In other clinical studies, VIROPTIC was evaluated in the treatment of Herpes simplex virus keratitis in patients who were unresponsive or intolerant to the topical administration of idoxuridine or vidarabine. VIROPTIC was effective in 138 of 150 (92%) patients (109 of 114 with dendritic and 29 of 36 with geographic ulcers) as evidenced by corneal re-epithelialization. The mean time to corneal re-epithelialization was 6 days for patients with dendritic ulcers and 12 days for patients with geographic ulcers.

Contraindications: VIROPTIC brand Trifluridine Ophthalmic Solution, 1%, is contraindicated for patients who develop hypersensitivity reactions or chemical intolerance to trifluridine.

Warnings:
The recommended dosage and frequency of administration should not be exceeded (see Dosage and Administration).

Precautions:
General: VIROPTIC brand Trifluridine Ophthalmic Solution, 1% should be prescribed only for patients who have a clinical diagnosis of herpetic keratitis.

VIROPTIC may cause mild local irritation of the conjunctiva and cornea when instilled but these effects are usually transient.

Although documented *in vitro* viral resistance to trifluridine has not been reported following multiple exposure to VIROPTIC, the possibility exists of viral resistance development.

Drug Interactions: The following drugs have been administered topically to the eye and concurrently with VIROPTIC in a limited number of patients without apparent evidence of adverse interaction; antibiotics—chloramphenicol, erythromycin, polymyxin B sulfate, bacitracin, gentamicin sulfate, tetracycline HCl, sodium sulfacetamide, neomycin sulfate; steroids—dexamethasone, dexamethasone sodium phosphate, prednisolone acetate, prednisolone sodium phosphate, hydrocortisone, fluorometholone; and other ophthalmic drugs—atropine sulfate, scopolamine hydrobromide, naphazoline hydrochloride, cyclopentolate hydrochloride, homatropine hydrobromide, pilocarpine, 1-epinephrine hydrochloride, sodium chloride.

Carcinogenesis, Mutagenesis, Impairment of Fertility: Mutagenic Potential. Trifluridine has been shown to exert mutagenic, DNA damaging and cell transforming activities in various standard *in vitro* test systems, and clastogenic activity in *Vicia faba* cells.

Although the significance of these test results is not clear or fully understood, there exists the possibility that mutagenic agents may cause genetic damage in humans.

Oncogenic Potential. The oncogenic potential of trifluridine is unknown at this time. The oncogenic potential of trifluridine in rodents is being evaluated.

Pregnancy: The drug should not be prescribed for pregnant women unless the potential benefits outweigh the potential risks.

Teratogenic Potential. Kury and Crosby[1] found that trifluridine was teratogenic when injected directly into the yolk sac of developing chick embryos. Itoi *et al.*[2] found that topical application of 1% trifluridine ophthalmic solution to the eyes of rabbits on days 6–18 of pregnancy produced no teratogenic effects. Trifluridine was not teratogenic when given subcutaneously to rats at doses up to 5.0 mg/kg/day although drug induced fetal toxicity (delayed ossification of portions of the skeletal system) was observed at the 2.5 mg/kg/day dose level. Trifluridine was not teratogenic when given subcutaneously to rabbits at doses up to 5.0 mg/kg/day. Drug induced fetal toxicity (delayed ossification of portions of the skeletal system) was observed at the 2.5 mg/kg/day dose level. A 1.0 mg/kg/day dose was considered to be a no effect level in both rats and rabbits. Based upon these findings in animals, it is unlikely that VIROPTIC would cause embryonic or fetal damage if given in the recommended ophthalmic dosage to pregnant women. A safe dose, however, has not been established for the human embryo or fetus.

Nursing Mothers: It is unlikely that trifluridine is excreted in human milk after ophthalmic instillation of VIROPTIC because of the relatively small dosage (<5.0 mg/day), its dilution in body fluids and its extremely short half-life (approximately 12 minutes). The drug should not be prescribed for nursing mothers unless the potential benefits outweigh the potential risks.

Adverse Reactions: The most frequent adverse reactions reported during controlled clinical trials were mild, transient burning or stinging upon instillation (4.6%) and palpebral edema (2.8%). Other adverse reactions in decreasing order of reported frequency were superficial punctate keratopathy, epithelial keratopathy, hypersensitivity reaction, stromal edema, irritation, keratitis sicca, hyperemia, and increased intraocular pressure.

Overdosage: Overdosage by ocular instillation is unlikely because any excess solution should be quickly expelled from the conjunctival sac.

Acute overdosage by accidental oral ingestion of VIROPTIC has not occurred. However, should such ingestion occur, the 75 mg dosage of trifluridine in a 7.5 ml bottle of VIROPTIC is not likely to produce adverse effects. Single intravenous doses of 15–30 mg/kg/day in children and adults with neoplastic disease produce reversible bone marrow depression as the only potentially serious toxic effect and only after 3–5 courses of therapy.[3] The acute oral LD_{50} in the mouse and rat was 4379 mg/kg or higher.

Dosage and Administration: Instill one drop of VIROPTIC Ophthalmic Solution, 1% onto the cornea of the affected eye every two hours while awake for a maximum daily dosage of nine drops until the corneal ulcer has completely re-epithelialized. Following re-epithelialization, treatment for an additional seven days of one drop every four hours while awake for a minimum daily dosage of five drops is recommended.

If there are no signs of improvement after seven days of therapy or complete re-epithelialization has not occurred after 14 days of therapy, other forms of therapy should be considered. Continuous administration of VIROPTIC for periods exceeding 21 days should be avoided because of potential ocular toxicity.

How Supplied: VIROPTIC Opthalmic Solution, 1% is supplied as a sterile ophthalmic solution in a plastic Drop-Dose® dispenser bottle of 7.5 ml. (NDC-0081-0968-02)

Store under refrigeration 2° to 8°C (36° to 46°F)

Animal Pharmacology and Animal Toxicology: Corneal wound healing studies in rabbits showed that VIROPTIC did not significantly retard closure of epithelial wounds. However, mild toxic changes such as intracellular edema of the basal cell layer, mild thinning of the overlying epithelium and reduced strength of stromal wounds were observed.

Whereas instillation of VIROPTIC into rabbit eyes during a subchronic toxicity study produced some degree of corneal epithelial thinning, a 12-month chronic toxicity study in rabbits in which VIROPTIC was instilled into eyes in intermittent, multiple, full-therapy courses showed no drug related changes in the cornea.

References:

1. Kury, G. and R.J. Crosby—The teratogenic effect of 5-trifluoromethyl-2′-deoxyuridine

Continued on next page

Burroughs Wellcome—Cont.

in chicken embryos. *Toxicol. Appl. Pharmacol.* 11(1):72–80, 1967.
2. Itoi, M., J.W. Gefter, N. Kaneko, Y. Ishii, R.M. Ramer and A.R. Gasset—Teratogenicities of ophthalmic drugs. I. Antiviral ophthalmic drugs. *Arch. Ophthalmol.* 93(1):46–51, 1975.
3. Ansfield, F.J. and G. Ramirez—Phase I and II Studies of 2′-deoxy-5-(trifluoromethyl)-uridine (NSC-75520). *Cancer Chemother. Rep.* (Pt. 1) 55(2):205–208, 1971.

U.S. Patent No. 3,201,387

ZOVIRAX® (Acyclovir) ℞
Ointment 5%

Description: Zovirax is the brand name for acyclovir, an antiviral drug against herpes viruses. Zovirax Ointment 5% is a formulation for topical administration. Each gram of Zovirax Ointment 5% contains 50 mg of acyclovir in a polyethylene glycol (PEG) base.
The chemical name of acyclovir is 9-[(2-hydroxyethoxy)methyl]guanine.
Acyclovir is a white, crystalline powder with a molecular weight of 225 Daltons, and a maximum solubility in water of 1.3 mg/ml.

Clinical Pharmacology: Acyclovir is a synthetic acyclic purine nucleoside analogue with *in vitro* inhibitory activity against Herpes simplex types 1 and 2 (HSV-1 and HSV-2), varicella-zoster, Epstein-Barr and cytomegalovirus. In cell cultures, the inhibitory activity of acyclovir for Herpes simplex virus is highly selective. Cellular thymidine kinase does not effectively utilize acyclovir as a substrate. Herpes simplex virus-coded thymidine kinase, however, converts acyclovir into acyclovir monophosphate, a nucleotide. The monophosphate is further converted into diphosphate by cellular guanylate kinase and into triphosphate by a number of cellular enzymes.[1] Acyclovir triphosphate interferes with Herpes simplex virus DNA polymerase and inhibits viral DNA replication. Acyclovir triphosphate also inhibits cellular α-DNA polymerase but to a lesser degree. *In vitro*, acyclovir triphosphate can be incorporated into growing chains of DNA by viral DNA polymerase and to a much smaller extent by cellular α-DNA polymerase.[2] When incorporation occurs, the DNA chain is terminated.[3] Acyclovir is preferentially taken up and selectively converted to the active triphosphate form by herpesvirus-infected cells. Thus, acyclovir is much less toxic *in vitro* for normal uninfected cells because: 1) less is taken up; 2) less is converted to the active form; 3) cellular α-DNA polymerase is less sensitive to the effects of the active form.
The relationship between *in vitro* susceptibility of Herpes simplex virus to antiviral drugs and clinical response has not been established. The techniques and cell culture types used for determining *in vitro* susceptibility may influence the results obtained. Using a quantitative assay to determine the acyclovir concentration producing 50% inhibition of viral cytopathic effect (ID_{50}), 28 HSV-1 clinical isolates had a mean ID_{50} of 0.17 μg/ml and 32 HSV-2 clinical isolates had a mean ID_{50} of 0.46 μg/ml.* Results from other studies using different assays have yielded mean ID_{50} values for clinical HSV-1 isolates of 0.018, 0.03 and 0.043 μg/ml and for clinical HSV-2 isolates of 0.027, 0.36 and 0.03 μg/ml, respectively.[4,5,6]
Two clinical pharmacology studies were performed with Zovirax Ointment 5% in adult immunocompromised patients, at risk of developing mucocutaneous Herpes simplex virus infections or with localized varicella-zoster infections. These studies were designed to evaluate the dermal tolerance, systemic toxicity and percutaneous absorption of acyclovir. In one of these studies, which included 16 inpatients, the complete ointment or its vehicle were randomly administered in a dose of 1 cm strips (25 mg acyclovir) four times a day for seven days to an intact skin surface area of 4.5 square inches. No local intolerance, systemic toxicity or contact dermatitis were observed. In addition, no drug was detected in blood and urine by radioimmunoassay (sensitivity, 0.01 μg/ml).
The other study included eleven patients with localized varicella-zoster. In this uncontrolled study, acyclovir was detected in the blood of 9 patients and in the urine of all patients tested. Acyclovir levels in plasma ranged from <0.01 to 0.28 μg/ml in eight patients with normal renal function, and from <0.01 to 0.78 μg/ml in one patient with impaired renal function. Acyclovir excreted in the urine ranged from <0.02 to 9.4 percent of the daily dose. Therefore, systemic absorption of acyclovir after topical application is minimal.

Indications And Usage: Zovirax (Acyclovir) Ointment 5% is indicated in the management of initial herpes genitalis and in limited non-life-threatening mucocutaneous Herpes simplex virus infections in immunocompromised patients. In clinical trials of initial herpes genitalis, Zovirax Ointment 5% has shown a decrease in healing time and in some cases a decrease in duration of viral shedding and duration of pain. In studies in immunocompromised patients with mainly herpes labialis, there was a decrease in duration of viral shedding and a slight decrease in duration of pain.
By contrast, in studies of recurrent herpes genitalis and of herpes labialis in nonimmunocompromised patients; there was no evidence of clinical benefit; there was some decrease in duration of viral shedding.
Diagnosis: Whereas cutaneous lesions associated with Herpes simplex infections are often characteristic, the finding of multinucleated giant cells in smears prepared from lesion exudate or scrapings may assist in the diagnosis.[7] Positive cultures for Herpes simplex virus offer a reliable means for confirmation of the diagnosis. In genital herpes, appropriate examinations should be performed to rule out other sexually transmitted diseases.

Contraindications: Zovirax Ointment 5% is contraindicated for patients who develop hypersensitivity or chemical intolerance to the components of the formulation.

Warnings: Zovirax Ointment 5% is intended for cutaneous use only and should not be used in the eye.

Precautions:
General: The recommended dosage, frequency of applications, and length of treatment should not be exceeded (see DOSAGE AND ADMINISTRATION). There exist no data which demonstrate that the use of Zovirax Ointment 5% will either prevent transmission of infection to other persons or prevent recurrent infections when applied in the absence of signs and symptoms. Zovirax Ointment 5% should not be used for the prevention of recurrent HSV infections. Although clinically significant viral resistance associated with the use of Zovirax Ointment 5% has not been observed, this possibility exists.
Drug Interactions: Clinical experience has identified no interactions resulting from topical or systemic administration of other drugs concomitantly with Zovirax Ointment 5%.
Carcinogenesis, Mutagenesis, Impairment of Fertility: Acyclovir was tested in lifetime bioassays in rats and mice at single daily doses of 50, 150 and 450 mg/kg/day given by gavage. These studies showed no statistically significant difference in the incidence of benign and malignant tumors produced in drug-treated as compared to control animals, nor did acyclovir induce the occurrence of tumors earlier in drug-treated animals as compared to controls. In 2 *in vitro* cell transformation assays, used to provide preliminary assessment of potential oncogenicity in advance of these more definitive lifetime bioassays in rodents, conflicting results were obtained. Acyclovir was positive at the highest dose used in one system and the resulting morphologically transformed cells formed tumors when inoculated into immunosuppressed, syngeneic, weanling mice. Acyclovir was negative in another transformation system.
No chromosome damage was observed at maximum tolerated parenteral doses of 100 mg/kg acyclovir in rats or Chinese hamsters; higher doses of 500 and 1000 mg/kg were clastogenic in Chinese hamsters. In addition, no activity was found in a dominant lethal study in mice. In 9 of 11 microbial and mammalian cell assays, no evidence of mutagenicity was observed. In 2 mammalian cell assays (human lymphocytes and L5178Y mouse lymphoma cells *in vitro*), positive response for mutagenicity and chromosomal damage occurred, but only at concentrations at least 1000 times the plasma levels achieved in man following topical application.
Acyclovir does not impair fertility or reproduction in mice at oral doses up to 450 mg/kg/day or in rats at subcutaneous doses up to 25 mg/kg/day. In rabbits given a high dose of acyclovir (50 mg/kg/day, s.c.), there was a statistically significant decrease in implantation efficiency.
Pregnancy: ***Teratogenic Effects. Pregnancy Category C.*** Acyclovir has been known to cause a statistically significant decrease in implantation efficiency in rabbits, when given at subcutaneous doses providing mean plasma levels of drug 2.2 times those expected from use in patients with normal renal function.
Reproduction studies were negative for impairment of fertility or harm to the fetus in mice given oral doses, and in rats given subcutaneous doses providing mean plasma levels of drug 84 times and 4 times (respectively) greater than those expected from use in patients with normal renal function.
Acyclovir was not teratogenic after subcutaneous administration of up to 50 mg/kg/day during the period of organogenesis in rats and rabbits; doses up to 450 mg/kg given daily by gavage to mice were not teratogenic. There are, however, no adequate and well-controlled studies in pregnant women. Acyclovir should be used during pregnancy only if the potential benefit justifies the potential risk to the fetus.
Nursing Mothers: It is not known whether this drug is excreted in human milk. Because many drugs are excreted in human milk, caution should be exercised when Zovirax is administered to a nursing woman.

Adverse Reactions: Because ulcerated genital lesions are characteristically tender and sensitive to any contact or manipulation, patients may experience discomfort upon application of ointment. In the controlled clinical trials, mild pain (including transient burning and stinging) was reported by 103 (28.3%) of 364 patients treated with acyclovir and by 115 (31.1%) of 370 patients treated with placebo; treatment was discontinued in 2 of these patients. Other local reactions among acyclovir-treated patients included pruritis in 15 (4.1%), rash in 1 (0.3%) and vulvitis in 1 (0.3%).
Among the placebo-treated patients, pruritus was reported by 17 (4.6%) and rash by 1 (0.3%).
In all studies, there was no significant difference between the drug and placebo group in the rate or type of reported adverse reactions nor were there any differences in abnormal clinical laboratory findings.

Overdosage: Overdosage by topical application of Zovirax Ointment 5% is unlikely because of limited transcutaneous absorption (see Clinical Pharmacology).

Dosage And Administration: Apply sufficient quantity to adequately cover all lesions every 3 hours 6 times per day for 7 days. The dose size per application will vary depending upon the total lesion area but should approximate a one-half inch ribbon of ointment per 4 square inches of surface area. A finger cot or rubber glove should be used when applying Zovirax to prevent autoinoculation of other body sites and transmission of infection to other persons. **Therapy should be initiated as early as possible following onset of signs and symptoms.**

How Supplied: Zovirax Ointment 5% is supplied in 15 g tubes (NDC 0081-0993-94). Each gram contains 50 mg acyclovir in a polyethylene glycol base. Store at 15°–25°C (59°–78°F) in a dry place.

Animal Pharmacology And Animal Toxicology: Topical treatment of guinea pigs with 10% acyclovir in polyethylene glycol ointment for three weeks did not result in cutaneous irritation or systemic toxicity. Also, a wide variety of animal tests by parenteral routes demonstrated that acyclovir has a low order of toxicity. Acyclovir did not cause dermal sensitization in guinea pigs.

References

1. Miller WH and Miller RL J Biol Chem *255*(15):7204–7207, 1980.
2. Furman PA et al. J Virol *32*(1):72–77, 1979.
3. Derse D et al. J Biol Chem *256*(22): 11447–11451, 1981.
4. Collins P and Bauer DJ. J Antimicrob Chemother *5*:431–436, 1979.
5. Crumpacker CS et al. Antimicrob Agents Chemother *15*:642–645, 1979.
6. De Clercq E et al. J Infect Dis *141*:563–574, 1980.
7. Naib ZM et al. Cancer Res *33*1452–1463, 1973.

*Data on file at Burroughs Wellcome Co.

U.S. Patent No. 4199574

ZOVIRAX® Sterile Powder ℞
(Acyclovir Sodium)
FOR INTRAVENOUS INFUSION ONLY

Description: Zovirax is the brand name for acyclovir, an antiviral drug active against herpesviruses. Zovirax Sterile Powder is a formulation for intravenous administration. Each vial of Zovirax Sterile Powder contains 549 mg of sterile lyophilized acyclovir sodium equivalent to 500 mg of acyclovir.

The chemical name of acyclovir sodium is 9-[(2-hydroxyethoxy)methyl]guanine sodium; it has the following structural formula:

[structural formula: acyclovir sodium, $CH_2OCH_2CH_2OH$ side chain, H_2N, Na^+]

Acyclovir sodium is a white, crystalline powder with a molecular weight of 247 daltons, and a solubility in water exceeding 100 mg/ml. Recommended reconstitution with 10 ml diluent per vial yields 50 mg/ml acyclovir (pH approximately 11). Further dilution in any appropriate intravenous solution must be performed before infusion (see Method of Preparation). At physiologic pH, acyclovir exists as the un-ionized form with a molecular weight of 225 daltons and a maximum solubility of 2.5 mg/ml at 37°C.

Clinical Pharmacology: Acyclovir is a synthetic acyclic purine nucleoside analogue with *in vitro* and *in vivo* inhibitory activity against Herpes simplex, varicella-zoster, Epstein-Barr and cytomegalovirus. In cell cultures, the inhibitory activity of acyclovir for Herpes simplex is highly selective. Cellular thymidine kinase does not effectively utilize acyclovir as a substrate. Herpes simplex virus-coded thymidine kinase, however, converts acyclovir into acyclovir monophosphate, a nucleotide analogue. The monophosphate is further converted into diphosphate by cellular guanylate kinase and into triphosphate by a number of cellular enzymes.[1] Acyclovir triphosphate interferes with Herpes simplex virus DNA polymerase and inhibits viral DNA replication. Acyclovir triphosphate also inhibits cellular α-DNA polymerase but to a lesser degree. *In vitro*, acyclovir triphosphate can be incorporated into growing chains of DNA by viral DNA polymerase and to a much smaller extent by cellular α-DNA polymerase.[2] When incorporation occurs, the DNA chain is terminated.[3] Acyclovir is preferentially taken up and selectively converted to the active triphosphate form by herpesvirus-infected cells. Thus, acyclovir is much less toxic *in vitro* for normal uninfected cells because: 1) less is taken up; 2) less is converted to the active form; 3) cellular α-DNA polymerase is less sensitive to the effects of the active form.

The relationship between *in vitro* susceptibility of Herpes simplex virus to antiviral drugs and clinical response has not been established. The techniques and cell types used for determining *in vitro* susceptibility may influence the results obtained. With a quantitative assay to determine the acyclovir concentration producing 50% inhibition of viral cytopathic effect (ID_{50}), 28 HSV-1 clinical isolates had a mean ID_{50} of 0.17 μg/ml and 32 HSV-2 clinical isolates had a mean ID_{50} of 0.46 μg/ml. Results from other studies using different assays have yielded mean ID_{50} values for clinical HSV-1 isolates of 0.018, 0.03 and 0.43 μg/ml and for clinical HSV-2 isolates of 0.027, 0.36 and 0.03 μg/ml, respectively.[4,5,6]

Pharmacokinetics: The pharmacokinetics of acyclovir has been evaluated in 95 patients (9 studies). Results were obtained in adult patients with normal renal function during Phase I/II studies after single doses ranging from 0.5 to 15 mg/kg and after multiple doses ranging from 2.5 to 15 mg/kg every 8 hours. Pharmacokinetics was also determined in pediatric patients with normal renal function ranging in age from 1 to 17 years at doses of 250 mg/M^2 or 500 mg/M^2 every 8 hours. In these studies, dose-independent pharmacokinetics is observed in the range of 0.5 to 15 mg/kg. Proportionality between dose and plasma levels is seen after single doses or at steady state after multiple dosing.[7] When Zovirax was administered to adults at 5 mg/kg (approximately 250 mg/M^2) by 1-hr infusions every 8 hours, mean steady-state peak and trough concentrations of 9.8 μg/ml (5.5 to 13.8 μg/ml) and 0.7 μg/ml (0.2 to 1.0 μg/ml), respectively, were achieved. Similar concentrations are achieved in children over 1 year of age when doses of 250 mg/M^2 are given every 8 hours. Concentrations achieved in the cerebrospinal fluid are approximately 50% of plasma values. Plasma protein binding is relatively low (9% to 33%) and drug interactions involving binding site displacement are not anticipated.[7]

Renal excretion of unchanged drug by glomerular filtration and tubular secretion is the major route of acyclovir elimination accounting for 62 to 91% of the dose as determined by ^{14}C-labelled drug. The only major urinary metabolite detected is 9-carboxymethoxymethylguanine. This may account for up to 14.1% of the dose in patients with normal renal function. An insignificant amount of drug is recovered in feces and expired CO_2 and there is no evidence to suggest tissue retention.[7] However, postmortem examinations have shown that acyclovir is widely distributed in tissues and body fluids including brain, kidney, lung, liver, muscle, spleen, uterus, vaginal mucosa, vaginal secretions, cerebrospinal fluid and herpetic vesicular fluid.

In a Phase I study in 3 adult volunteers, 1 g of probenecid was administered orally prior to a single 1-hour 5 mg/kg intravenous infusion of acyclovir. The acyclovir half-life and area under the plasma concentration-time curve increased by 18 and 40%, respectively, compared to a control infusion of acyclovir without probenecid. The mean urinary excretion of acyclovir decreased from 79% to 69% of the dose indicating that probenecid can influence the renal excretion of acyclovir.[6]

The half-life and total body clearance of acyclovir is dependent on renal function as shown below.[7]

Creatinine Clearance (ml/min/1.73M^2)	Half-Life (hr)	Total Body Clearance (ml/min/1.73M^2)
>80	2.5	327
50–80	3.0	248
15–50	3.5	190
0 (Anuric)	19.5	29

Zoviraz was administered at a dose of 2.5 mg/kg to 6 adult patients with severe renal failure. The peak and trough plasma levels during the 47 hours preceding hemodialysis were 8.5 μg/ml and 0.7 μg/ml, respectively. Consult DOSAGE AND ADMINISTRATION section for recommended adjustments in dosing based upon creatinine clearance.

The half-life and total body clearance of acyclovir in pediatric patients over 1 year of age is similar to those in adults with normal renal function (see DOSAGE AND ADMINISTRATION).

Indications and Usage: Zovirax Sterile Powder is indicated for the treatment of initial and recurrent mucosal and cutaneous Herpes simplex (HSV-1 and HSV-2) infections in immunocompromised adults and children. It is also indicated for severe initial clinical episodes of herpes genitalis in patients who are not immunocompromised.

These indications are based on the results of several double-blind, placebo-controlled studies which evaluated the drug's effect on virus excretion, complete healing of lesions, and relief of pain.

Herpes Simplex Infections in Immunocompromised Patients

A multicenter trial of Zovirax Sterile Powder at a dose of 250 mg/M^2 every 8 hours (750 mg/M^2/day) for 7 days was conducted in 97 immunocompromised patients with oro-facial, esophageal, genital and other localized infections (50 treated with Zovirax and 47 with placebo). Zoviraz significantly decreased virus excretion, reduced pain, and promoted scabbing and rapid healing of lesions.[9,10,11]

Initial Episodes of Herpes Genitalis

A controlled trial was conducted in 28 patients with severe initial episodes of herpes genitalis with a Zovirax dosage of 5 mg/kg every 8 hours for 5 days (12 patients treated with Zovirax and 16 with placebo). Significant treatment effects were seen in elimination of virus from lesions and in reduction of healing times.[12]

In a similar study, 15 patients with initial episodes of genital herpes were treated with Zovirax 5 mg/kg every 8 hours for 5 days and 15 with placebo. Zovirax decreased the duration of viral excretion, new lesion formation, duration of vesicles and promoted more rapid healing of all lesions.[13]

Diagnosis

The use of appropriate laboratory diagnostic procedures will help to establish the etiologic diagnosis. Positive cultures for Herpes simplex virus offer a reliable means for confirmation of the diagnosis. In initial episodes of genital herpes, appropriate examinations should be performed to rule out other sexually transmitted diseases. Whereas cutaneous lesions associated with Herpes simplex infections are often characteristic, the finding of multinucleated giant cells in smears prepared from lesions exudate or scrapings may assist in the diagnosis.[14]

Contraindications: Zovirax Sterile Powder is contraindicated for patients who develop hypersensitivity to the drug.

Continued on next page

Burroughs Wellcome—Cont.

Warnings: Zovirax Sterile Powder is intended for intravenous infusion only, and should not be administered topically, intramuscularly, orally, subcutaneously, or in the eye. Intravenous infusions must be given over a period of at least 1 (one) hour to prevent renal tubular damage (see PRECAUTIONS and DOSAGE AND ADMINISTRATION).

Precautions:

General: The recommended dosage, frequency and length of treatment should not be exceeded (see DOSAGE AND ADMINISTRATION).

Although the aqueous solubility of acyclovir sodium (for infusion) is > 100 mg/ml, precipitation of acyclovir crystals in renal tubules can occur if the maximum solubility of free acyclovir (2.5 mg/ml at 37°C in water) is exceeded or if the drug is administered by bolus injection. This complication causes a rise in serum creatinine and blood urea nitrogen (BUN), and a decrease in renal creatinine clearance. Ensuing renal tubular damage can produce acute renal failure.

Abnormal renal function (decreased creatinine clearance) can occur as a result of acyclovir administration and depends on the state of the patient's hydration, other treatments, and the rate of drug administration. Bolus administration of the drug leads to a 10% incidence of renal dysfunction, while in controlled studies, infusion of 5 mg/kg (250 mg/M^2) over an hour was associated with a lower frequency—4.6%. Concomitant use of other nephrotoxic drugs, pre-existing renal disease, and dehydration make further renal impairment with acyclovir more likely. In most instances, alterations of renal function were transient and resolved spontaneously or with improvement of water and electrolyte balance, drug dosage adjustment or discontinuation of drug administration. However, in some instances, these changes may progress to acute renal failure.

Administration of Zovirax by intravenous infusion must be accompanied by adequate hydration. Since maximum urine concentration occurs within the first 2 hours following infusion, particular attention should be given to establishing sufficient urine flow during that period in order to prevent precipitation in renal tubules.

When dosage adjustments are required they should be based on estimated creatinine clearance (See DOSAGE AND ADMINISTRATION).

Approximately 1% of patients receiving intravenous acyclovir have manifested encephalopathic changes characterized by either lethargy, obtundation, tremors, confusion, hallucinations, agitation, seizures or coma. Zovirax should be used with caution in those patients who have underlying neurologic abnormalities and those with serious renal, hepatic, or electrolyte abnormalities or significant hypoxia. It should also be used with caution in patients who have manifested prior neurologic reactions to cytotoxic drugs or those receiving concomitant intrathecal methotrexate or interferon.

Exposure of HSV isolates to acyclovir *in vitro* can lead to the emergence of less sensitive viruses. These viruses usually are deficient in thymidine kinase (required for acyclovir activation) and are less pathogenic in animals. Similar isolates have been observed in 6 severely immunocompromised patients during the course of controlled and uncontrolled studies of intravenously administered Zovirax. These occurred in patients with congenital severe combined immunodeficiencies or following bone marrow transplantation. The presence of these viruses was not associated with a worsening of clinical illness and, in some instances, the virus disappeared spontaneously. The possibility of the appearance of less sensitive viruses must be borne in mind when treating such patients. The relationship between the *in vitro* sensitivity of herpesviruses to acyclovir and clinical response to therapy has yet to be established.

Drug Interactions: Co-administration of probenecid with acyclovir has been shown to increase the mean half-life and the area under the concentration-time curve. Urinary excretion and renal clearance were correspondingly reduced. Clinical experience has identified no other significant interactions resulting from administration of other drugs concomitantly with Zovirax Sterile Powder.

Carcinogenesis, Mutagenesis, Impairment of Fertility: Acyclovir was tested in lifetime bioassays in rats and mice at single daily doses of 50, 150 and 450 mg/kg given by gavage. There was no statiscally significant difference in the incidence of tumors between treated and control animals, nor did acyclovir appear to shorten the latency of tumors. In 2 *in vitro* cell transformation assays, used to provide preliminary assessment of potential oncogenicity in advance of these more definitive lifetime bioassays in rodents, conflicting results were obtained. Acyclovir was positive at the highest dose used in one system and the resulting morphologically transformed cells formed tumors when inoculated into immunosuppressed, syngeneic, weanling mice. Acyclovir was negative in another transformation system.

No chromosome damage was observed at maximum tolerated parenteral doses of 100 mg/kg acyclovir in rats or Chinese hamsters; higher doses of 500 and 100 mg/kg were clastogenic in Chinese hamsters. In addition, no activity was found in a dominant lethal study in mice. In 9 of 11 microbial and mammalian cell assays, no evidence of mutagenicity was observed. In 2 mammalian cell assays (human lymphocytes and L5178Y mouse lymphoma cells *in vitro*), positive responses for mutagenicity and chromosomal damage occurred, but only at concentrations at least 25 times the acyclovir plasma levels achieved in man.

Acyclovir does not impair fertility or reproduction in mice at oral doses up to 450 mg/kg/day. In female rabbits treated subcutaneously with acyclovir subsequent to mating, there was a statistically significant decrease in implantation efficiency but no concomitant decrease in litter size at a dose of 50 mg/kg/day.

Pregnancy: Teratogenic Effects. Pregnancy Category C. Acyclovir was not teratogenic in the mouse (450 mg/kg/day, p.o.), rabbit (50 mg/kg/day, s.c.) or rat (50 mg/kg/day, s.c.).

Although maximum tolerated doses were tested in the teratology studies, the plasma levels obtained did not exaggerate maximum plasma levels that might occur with clinical use of intravenous acyclovir.

There have been no adequate and well-controlled studies in pregnant women. Acyclovir should be used during pregnancy only if the potential benefit justifies the potential risk to the fetus.

Nursing Mothers: It is not known whether this drug is excreted in human milk. Because many drugs are excreted in human milk, caution should be exercised when Zovirax is administered to a nursing woman.

Adverse Reactions: The most frequent adverse reactions reported during controlled clinical trials of Zovirax in 64 patients were inflammation or phlebitis at the injection site following infiltration of the I.V. fluid in 9 (14.0%), transient elevations of serum creatinine in 3 (4.7%), and rash or hives in 3 (4.7%). Less frequent adverse reactions were diaphoresis, hematuria, hypotension, headache and nausea, each of which occurred in 1 patient (1.6%). Of the 63 patients receiving placebo, 3 (4.8%) experienced inflammation/phlebitis and 3 (4.8%) experienced rash or itching. Hematuria and nausea were experienced by placebo recipients at the same frequency.

Among 51 immunocompromised patients, one, a bone marrow transplant recipient with pneumonitis, developed seizures, cerebral edema, coma and expired with changes consistent with cerebral anoxia on postmortem biopsy; another immunocompromised patient exhibited coarse tremor and clonus.

Additional adverse reactions were reported in uncontrolled trials. The most frequent adverse reaction was elevated serum creatinine. This occurred in 9.8 percent of patients, usually following rapid (less than 10 minutes) intranvenous infusion. Less frequent adverse experiences were thrombocytosis and jitters, each in 0.4% of patients.

Approximately 1% of patients receiving intravenous acyclovir have manifested encephalopathic changes characterized by either lethargy, obtundation, tremors, confusion, hallucinations, agitation, seizures or coma (see PRECAUTIONS).

Overdosage: No acute massive overdosage of the intravenous form has been reported.

Doses administered to humans have been as high as 1200 mg/M^2 (28 mg/kg) three times daily for up to two weeks. Peak plasma concentrations have reached 80 μg/ml. Precipitation of free acyclovir in renal tubules may occur when the solubility in the intratubular fluid is exceeded (see PRECAUTIONS). Acyclovir is dialyzable. In the event of acute renal failure and anuria, the patient may benefit from hemodialysis until renal function is restored (see DOSAGE AND ADMINISTRATION).

Dosage and Administration: CAUTION—RAPID OR BOLUS INTRAVENOUS AND INTRAMUSCULAR OR SUBCUTANEOUS INJECTION MUST BE AVOIDED.

Dosage: ***MUCOSAL AND CUTANEOUS HERPES SIMPLEX (HSV-1 and HSV-2) INFECTIONS IN IMMUNOCOMPROMISED PATIENTS***—5 mg/kg infused at a constant rate over 1 hour, every 8 hours (15 mg/kg/day) for 7 days in adult patients with normal renal function. In children under 12 years of age, more accurate dosing can be attained by infusing 250 mg/M^2 at a constant rate over 1 hour, every 8 hours (750 mg/M^2/day) for 7 days.

SEVERE INITIAL CLINICAL EPISODES OF HERPES GENITALIS—The same dose given above—administered for 5 days.

Therapy should be initiated as early as possible following onset of signs and symptoms.

PATIENTS WITH ACUTE OR CHRONIC RENAL IMPAIRMENT: Refer to DOSAGE AND ADMINISTRATION section for recommended doses, and adjust the dosing interval as indicated in the table below.

Creatinine Clearance (ml/min/1.73M^2)	Dose (mg/kg)	Dosing Interval (hours)
>50	5	8
25–50	5	12
10–25	5	24
0–10	2.5	24

Hemodialysis: For patients who require dialysis, the mean plasma half-life of acyclovir during hemodialysis is approximately 5 hours. This results in a 60% decrease in plasma concentrations following a 6 hour dialysis period. Therefore, the patient's dosing schedule should be adjusted so that a dose is administered after each dialysis.

Method of Preparation: Each 10 ml vial contains acyclovir sodium equivalent to 500 mg of acyclovir. The contents of the vial should be dissolved in 10 ml of sterile water for injection yielding a final concentration of 50 mg/ml of acyclovir (pH approximately 11). Shake the vial well to assure complete dissolution before measuring and transferring each individual dose.

Administration: The calculated dose should then be removed and added to any appropriate intravenous solution at a volume selected for administration during each 1 hour infusion. Infusion concentrations of approximately 7 mg/ml or lower are recommended. In clinical studies, the average 70 kg adult received approximately 60 ml of fluid per dose. Higher concentrations (e.g., 10 mg/ml) may produce phlebitis or inflammation at the injection site upon inadvertent extravasation. Standard, commercially available electrolyte and glucose solutions are suitable for intravenous administration; biologic or colloidal fluids (e.g., blood products, protein solutions, etc.) are not recommended.

Once in solution in the vial at a concentration of 50 mg/ml, the drug should be used within 12 hours. Once diluted for administration, each dose should be used within 24 hours. Refrigeration of reconstituted solutions may result in formation of a precipitate which will redissolve at room temperature.

How Supplied: ZOVIRAX Sterile Powder is supplied in 10 ml sterile vials, each containing acyclovir sodium equivalent to 500 mg of acyclovir, carton of 25 (NDC 0081-0995-95). Store at 15°-30°C (59°-86°F).

Also available: ZOVIRAX Ointment, 5% in 15 g tubes. Each gram contains 50 mg acyclovir in a polyethylene glycol base.

References

1. W.H. Miller and R.L. Miller, J. Biol. Chem. *225*(15): 7204–7207, 1980.
2. P.A. Furman, *et al.*, J. Virol. *32*(1): 72–77, 1979.
3. D. Derse, *et al.*, J. Biol. Chem. *256*(22): 11447–11451, 1981.
4. P. Collins and D.J. Bauer. J. Antimicrob. Chemother. *5*:431–436, 1979.
5. C.S. Crumpacker, *et al.*, Antimicrob. Agents Chemother. *15*:642–645, 1979.
6. E. De Clercq. *et al.*, J. Infect. Dis. *141*563–574, 1980.
7. M.R. Blum, *et al.*, Am. J. Med. *73*(1A): 186–192, Jul. 20, 1982.
8. O.L. Laskin, *et al.*, Antimicrob. Agents Chemother. *21*(5): 804–807, May 1982.
9. C.D. Mitchell, *et al.*, Lancet *1*(8235): 1389–1392, Jun. 27, 1981.
10. J.C. Wade, *et al.*, Ann. Intern. Med. *96*(3): 265–269, Mar. 1982.
11. J.D. Meyers, *et al.*, Am. J. Med. *73*(1A): 229–235, Jul. 20, 1982.
12. Data on file, Burroughs Wellcome Co.
13. A. Mindel, *et al.*, Lancet *1*(8274): 697–700, Mar. 27, 1982.
14. Z.M. Naib, *et al.*, Cancer Res. *33*:1452–1463, 1973.

ZYLOPRIM ® ℞

brand Allopurinol*
100 mg Scored Tablets and
300 mg Scored Tablets

Description: Allopurinol is a xanthine oxidase inhibitor with the chemical name 4-hydroxypyrazolo (3,4-d) pyrimidine (HPP).

Clinical Pharmacology: Zyloprim (Allopurinol) acts on purine catabolism, without disrupting the biosynthesis of vital purines, thus reducing the production of uric acid by inhibiting the biochemical reactions immediately preceding its formation. Its action differs from that of uricosuric agents, which lower the serum uric acid level by increasing urinary excretion of uric acid. Zyloprim reduces both the serum and urinary uric acid levels by inhibiting the formation of uric acid. It thereby avoids the hazard of increased hyperuricosuria in patients with gouty nephropathy or with a predisposition to the formation of uric acid stones.

Zyloprim has produced a substantial reduction in serum and urinary uric acid levels in hitherto refractory patients even in the presence of renal damage marked enough to render uricosuric drugs virtually ineffective. Salicylates may be given conjointly for their antirheumatic effect without compromising the action of allopurinol. This is in contrast to the nullifying effect of salicylates on uricosuric drugs.

Zyloprim is a structural analogue of the natural purine base, hypoxanthine. It is a potent inhibitor of xanthine oxidase, the enzyme responsible for the conversion of hypoxanthine to xanthine and of xanthine to uric acid, the end product of purine metabolism in man. Zyloprim is metabolized to the corresponding xanthine analogue, oxipurinol (alloxanthine), which also is an inhibitor of xanthine oxidase.

Hyperuricemia may be primary, as in gout, or secondary to diseases such as acute and chronic leukemia, polycythemia vera, multiple myeloma, and psoriasis. It may occur with the use of diuretic agents, during renal dialysis, in the presence of renal damage, during starvation or reducing diets and in the treatment of neoplastic disease where rapid resolution of tissue masses may occur.

The major disease manifestations in gout—kidney stones, tophi in soft tissues, and deposits in joints and bones—result from the deposition of urates. If progressive deposition of urates is to be arrested or reversed, it is necessary to reduce the serum uric acid to a level below the saturation point to suppress urate precipitation. Reduction may be achieved by means of uricosuric agents. Uricosurics are less effective in the presence of renal disease, and some patients develop intolerance or sensitivity to these drugs. The use of allopurinol to block the formation of urate avoids the hazard of increased renal excretion of uric acid posed by uricosuric drugs.

The half-life of Zyloprim in the body is determined both by renal excretion and by oxidation to 4,6-dihydroxypyrazolo (3,4-d) pyrimidine (oxipurinol). The latter is also an inhibitor of xanthine oxidase, but is somewhat weaker than allopurinol which is bound 15-fold more tightly to the enzyme than is the natural substrate, xanthine. The long half-life of oxipurinol in the plasma (18 to 30 hours), contributes significantly to the enzyme inhibition. Moreover, both allopurinol and oxipurinol tend to inactivate xanthine oxidase, thereby further controlling the level of its activity.

Administration of Zyloprim generally results in a fall in both serum and urinary uric acid within two to three days. The magnitude of this decrease can be manipulated almost at will since it is dose-dependent. A week or more of treatment with allopurinol may be required for the full effects of the drug to be manifest; likewise, uric acid may return to pretreatment levels slowly, usually after a period of seven to 10 days following cessation of therapy. This reflects primarily the accumulation and slow clearance of oxipurinol. In some patients, particularly those with severe tophaceous gout and underexcretors, a dramatic fall in urinary uric acid excretion may not occur. It has been postulated that this may be due to the mobilization of urate from the tissue deposits as the serum uric acid level begins to fall.

The combined increase in hypoxanthine and xanthine excreted in the urine usually, but not always, is considerably less than the accompanying decline in urinary uric acid.

It has been shown that reutilization of both hypoxanthine and xanthine for nucleotide and nucleic acid synthesis is markedly enhanced when their oxidations are inhibited by allopurinol. This reutilization and the normal feedback inhibition which would result from an increase in available purine nucleotides serve to regulate purine biosynthesis and, in essence, the defect of the overproducer of uric acid is thereby compensated.

Innate deficiency of xanthine oxidase, which occurs in congenital xanthinuria as an inborn error of metabolism, has been shown to be compatible with normal health. While urinary levels of oxypurines attained with full doses of allopurinol may in exceptional cases equal those (250–600 mg per day) which in xanthinuric subjects have caused formation of urinary calculi, they usually fall in the range of 50–200 mg. Xanthine crystalluria has been reported in a few exceptional cases. Two of these had Lesch-Nyhan syndrome, which is characterized by excessive uric acid production combined with a deficiency in the enzyme, hypoxanthine-guanine phosphoribosyltransferase (HG-PRTase). This enzyme is required for the conversion of hypoxanthine and guanine to their respective nucleotides. The third case was a patient with lymphosarcoma, who produced an extremely large amount of uric acid because of rapid cell lysis during chemotherapy.

The serum concentration of oxypurines in patients receiving allopurinol is usually in the range of 0.3 mg to 0.4 mg percent compared to a normal level of approximately 0.15 mg percent. A maximum of 0.9 mg percent was observed when the serum urate was lowered to less than 2 mg percent by high doses of the drug. In one exceptional case a value of 2.7 mg percent was reached. These are far below the saturation level at which precipitation of xanthine or hypoxanthine would be expected to occur.

The solubilities of uric acid and xanthine in the serum are similar (about 7 mg percent) while hypoxanthine is much more soluble. The finding that the renal clearance of oxypurines is at least 10 times greater than that of uric acid explains the relatively low serum oxypurine concentration at a time when the serum uric acid level has decreased markedly. At serum oxypurine levels of 0.3 mg to 0.9 mg percent, oxypurine: inulin clearance ratios were between 0.7 and 1.9. The glomerular filtration rate and urate clearance in patients receiving allopurinol do not differ significantly from those obtained prior to therapy. The rapid renal clearance of oxypurines suggests that allopurinol therapy should be of value in allowing a patient with gout to increase his total purine excretion.

Although the renal clearance of allopurinol is rapid, that of oxipurinol is slow and parallels that of uric acid but is higher by a factor of about three. The clearance of oxipurinol is increased by uricosuric drugs, and as a consequence, the addition of a uricosuric agent may reduce the degree of inhibition of xanthine oxidase by oxipurinol. However, such combined therapy may be useful in achieving minimum serum uric acid levels provided the total urinary uric acid load does not exceed the competence of the patient's renal function. In some patients, where renal function is severely impaired, normal serum urate levels may not be achievable.

The danger of uric acid calculi is diminished as the uric acid excretion is reduced. The amounts of xanthine and hypoxanthine excreted in the urine generally do not exceed the solubilities of these compounds in the urine, particularly if the urine is slightly alkaline. The amounts of allopurinol and oxipurinol excreted are likewise within the limits of their respective solubilities.

Zyloprim also inhibits the enzymatic oxidation of mercaptopurine, the sulfur-containing analogue of hypoxanthine, to 6-thiouric acid. This oxidation, which is catalyzed by xanthine oxidase, inactivates mercaptopurine. Hence, the inhibition of such oxidation by allopurinol may result in as much as 75 percent reduction in the therapeutic dose requirement of mercaptopurine when the two compounds are given together.

Indications and Use: This is not an innocuous drug and strict attention should be given to the indications for its use. Pending further investigation, its use in other hyperuricemic states is not indicated at this time.

Continued on next page

Burroughs Wellcome—Cont.

Zyloprim® (allopurinol) is intended for:

1. treatment of gout, either primary, or secondary to the hyperuricemia associated with blood dyscrasias and their therapy;
2. treatment of primary or secondary uric acid nephropathy, with or without accompanying symptoms of gout;
3. treatment of patients with recurrent uric acid stone formation;
4. prophylactic treatment to prevent tissue urate deposition, renal calculi, or uric acid nephropathy in patients with leukemias, lymphomas and malignancies who are receiving cancer chemotherapy with its resultant elevating effect on serum uric acid levels.

Allopurinol, by promoting the resolution of tophi and urate crystals in the tissues, has relieved chronic joint pain, increased joint mobility and permitted urate sinuses to heal. The addition of allopurinol to a uricosuric regimen has reduced the size of tophi which have been refractory to uricosuric agents alone and increased joint mobility.

Zyloprim is particularly effective in preventing the occurrence and recurrence of uric acid stones and gravel. Zyloprim is useful in therapy and prophylaxis of acute urate nephropathy in patients with neoplastic disease who are particularly susceptible to hyperuricemia and uric acid stone formation, especially after radiation therapy or the use of antineoplastic drugs.

Contraindications: Pending further investigation this drug is contraindicated for use in children with the exception of those with hyperuricemia secondary to malignancy. The drug should not be employed in nursing mothers.

Patients who have developed a severe reaction to Zyloprim should not be restarted on the drug.

Warnings: ZYLOPRIM SHOULD BE DISCONTINUED AT THE FIRST APPEARANCE OF SKIN RASH OR ANY SIGN OF ADVERSE REACTION. In some instances a skin rash may be followed by more severe hypersensitivity reactions such as exfoliative, urticarial and purpuric lesions as well as Stevens-Johnson syndrome (erythema multiforme) and very rarely a generalized vasculitis which may lead to irreversible hepatotoxicity and death.

A few cases of reversible clinical hepatotoxicity have been noted in patients taking Zyloprim and in some patients asymptomatic rises in serum alkaline phosphatase or serum transaminase have been observed. Accordingly, periodic liver function tests should be performed during the early stages of therapy, particularly in patients with pre-existing liver disease.

Due to the occasional occurrence of drowsiness, patients should be alerted to the need for due precautions when engaging in activities where alertness is mandatory.

Occasional cases of hypersensitivity have been reported in patients with renal compromise receiving thiazides and Zyloprim concurrently. For this reason, in this clinical setting, such combination should be administered with caution.

In patients receiving Purinethol® (mercaptopurine) or Imuran® (azathioprine), the concomitant administration of 300–600 mg of Zyloprim per day will require a reduction in dose to approximately one-third to one-fourth of the usual dose of mercaptopurine or azathioprine. Subsequent adjustment of doses of Purinethol or Imuran should be made on the basis of therapeutic response and any toxic effects.

Usage in Pregnancy and Women of Childbearing Age: Reproductive studies showed no adverse effect of Zyloprim on animal litters. However, since the effect of xanthine oxidase inhibition on the human fetus is still unknown, Zyloprim should be used in pregnant women or women of childbearing age only if the potential benefits to the patient are weighed against the possible risk to the fetus.

Precautions: Some investigators have reported an increase in acute attacks of gout during the early stages of allopurinol administration, even when normal or subnormal serum uric acid levels have been attained. Accordingly, maintenance doses of colchicine (0.5 mg twice daily) generally should be given prophylactically when allopurinol is begun. In addition, it is recommended that the patient start with a low dose of allopurinol (100 mg daily) and increase at weekly intervals by 100 mg until a serum uric acid level of 6 mg per 100 ml or less is attained but without exceeding the maximal recommended dose. The use of therapeutic doses of colchicine or anti-inflammatory agents may be required to suppress attacks in some cases. The attacks usually become shorter and less severe after several months of therapy. A possible explanation for these flare-ups may be the mobilization of urates from tissue deposits followed by recrystallization, due to fluctuation in the serum uric acid level. Even with adequate therapy it may require several months to deplete the uric acid pool sufficiently to achieve control of the acute episodes.

The concomitant administration of a uricosuric agent with Zyloprim may result in a decrease in urinary excretion of oxypurines as compared to their excretion with allopurinol alone. This may possibly be due to an increased excretion of oxipurinol and a lowering of the degree of inhibition of xanthine oxidase. Such combined therapy is not contraindicated, however, and for many patients, may provide optimum control. A report by Goldfinger, et al on a patient treated with sulfinpyrazone and salicylates in addition to allopurinol showed a marked decrease in the excretion of oxypurines which they suggested was due to interference with their clearance at the renal tubular level. However, subsequent studies in our laboratories have indicated no interference with oxypurine clearance by salicylates. Although clinical evidence to date has not demonstrated renal precipitation of oxypurines in patients either on Zyloprim alone or in combination with uricosuric agents, the possiblity should be kept in mind.

It has been reported that allopurinol prolongs the half-life of the anticoagulant, dicumarol. The clinical significance of this has not been established, but this interaction should be kept in mind when allopurinol is given to patients already on anticoagulant therapy, and the coagulation time should be reassessed.

A fluid intake sufficient to yield a daily urinary output of at least 2 liters and the maintenance of a neutral or, preferably, slightly alkaline urine are desirable to (1) avoid the theoretic possibility of formation of xanthine calculi under the influence of Zyloprim therapy and (2) help prevent renal precipitation of urates in patients receiving concomitant uricosuric agents.

A few patients with preexisting renal disease or poor urate clearance have shown a rise in BUN during Zyloprim administration although a decrease in BUN has also been observed. Although the relationship of these observations to the drug has not been established, patients with impaired renal function require less drug and should be carefully observed during the early stages of Zyloprim administration and the drug withdrawn if increased abnormalities in renal function appear.

In patients with severely impaired renal function, or decreased urate clearance, the half-life of oxipurinol in the plasma is greatly prolonged. Therefore, a dose of 100 mg per day or 300 mg twice a week, or perhaps less, may be sufficient to maintain adequate xanthine oxidase inhibition to reduce serum urate levels. Such patients should be treated with the lowest effective dose, in order to minimize side effects.

Mild reticulocytosis has appeared in some patients, most of whom were receiving other therapeutic agents, so that the significance of this observation is not known.

Periodic determination of liver and kidney function and complete blood counts should be performed especially during the first few months of therapy.

Adverse Reactions:

Dermatologic: Because in some instances skin rash has been followed by severe hypersensitivity reactions, it is recommended that therapy be discontinued at the first sign of rash or other adverse reaction (see WARNINGS). Skin rash, usually maculopapular, is the adverse reaction most commonly reported. The incidence of skin rash may be increased in the presence of renal disorders.

Exfoliative, urticarial and purpuric lesions, Stevens-Johnson syndrome (erythema multiforme) and toxic epidermal necrolysis have also been reported.

A few cases of alopecia with and without accompanying dermatitis have been reported. In some patients with a rash, restarting Zyloprim therapy at lower doses has been accomplished without untoward incident.

Gastrointestinal: Nausea, vomiting, diarrhea, and intermittent abdominal pain have been reported.

Hepatic: Rare cases of granulomatous hepatitis and hepatic necrosis have been reported.

Vascular: There have been rare instances of a generalized hypersensitivity vasculitis or necrotizing angiitis which have led to irreversible hepatotoxicity and death.

Hematopoietic: Agranulocytosis, anemia, aplastic anemia, bone marrow depression, leukopenia, pancytopenia and thrombocytopenia have been reported in patients, most of whom received concomitant drugs with potential for causing these reactions. Zyloprim has been neither implicated nor excluded as a cause of these reactions.

Renal: Rare cases of renal failure have been reported in hypertensive patients who received thiazides and Zyloprim concurrently. Some patients had evidence of hypersensitivity to allopurinol.

Neurologic: There have been a few reports of peripheral neuritis occurring while patients were taking Zyloprim.

Drowsiness has also been reported in a few patients.

Ophthalmic: There have been a few reports of cataracts found in patients receiving Zyloprim. It is not known if the cataracts predated the Zyloprim therapy. "Toxic" cataracts were reported in one patient who also received an anti-inflammatory agent; again, the time of onset is unknown. In a group of patients followed by Gutman and Yu for up to five years on Zyloprim therapy, no evidence of ophthalmologic effect attributable to Zyloprim was reported.

Drug Idiosyncrasy: Symptoms suggestive of drug idiosyncrasy have been reported in a few patients. This was characterized by fever, chills, leukopenia or leukocytosis, eosinophilia, arthralgias, skin rash, pruritus, nausea and vomiting.

Overdosage: Massive overdosing, or acute poisoning, by Zyloprim has not been reported.

Dosage and Administration: The dosage of Zyloprim brand Allopurinol to accomplish full control of gout and to lower serum uric acid to normal or near-normal levels varies with the severity of the disease. The average is 200 to 300 mg per day for patients with mild gout and 400 to 600 mg per day for those with moderately severe tophaceous gout. The appropriate dosage may be administered in divided doses or as a single equivalent dose with the 300 mg tablet. Dosage requirements in excess of 300 mg should be supplemented in divided doses. It should also be noted that allopurinol is generally better tolerated if taken following meals. Similar considerations govern the regulation of dosage for maintenance purposes in secondary hyperuricemia. For the prevention of uric acid nephropathy during the vigorous therapy of neoplastic disease, treatment with 600 to 800 mg daily for two or three days is advisable together with a high fluid intake. The minimal effective dosage is 100 to 200 mg daily and the maximal recommended dosage is 800 mg daily. To reduce the possiblity of flare-up of acute gouty attacks, it is recommended that the patient start with a low dose of allopurinol (100 mg daily) and increase at weekly intervals by 100 mg until a serum uric acid level of 6 mg per 100 ml or less is attained but without exceeding the maximal recommended dosage.

Normal serum urate levels are achieved in one to three weeks. The upper limit of normal is about 7 mg percent for men and postmenopausal women and 6 mg percent for premenopausal women. Too much reliance should not be placed on a single reading since, for technical reasons, estimation of uric acid may be difficult. By the selection of the appropriate dose, together with the use of uricosuric agents in certain patients, it is possible to reduce the serum uric acid level to normal and, if desired, to hold it as low as 2 to 3 mg percent indefinitely.

A fluid intake sufficient to yield a daily urinary output of at least 2 liters and the maintenance of a neutral or, preferably, slightly alkaline urine are desirable.

Since allopurinol and its metabolites are excreted only by the kidney, accumulation of the drug can occur in renal failure, and the dose of allopurinol should consequently be reduced. With a creatinine clearance of 20 to 10 ml/min, a daily dosage of 200 mg of Zyloprim is suitable. When the creatinine clearance is less than 10 ml/min the daily dosage should not exceed 100 mg. With extreme renal impairment (creatinine clearance less than 3 ml/min) the interval between doses may also need to be lengthened.

The correct size and frequency of dosage for maintaining the serum uric acid just within the normal range is best determined by using the serum uric acid level as an index.

Children, 6 to 10 years of age, with secondary hyperuricemia associated with malignancies may be given 300 mg allopurinol daily while those under 6 years are generally given 150 mg daily. The response is evaluated after approximately 48 hours of therapy and a dosage adjustment is made if necessary.

In patients who are being treated with colchicine and/or anti-inflammatory agents, it is wise to continue this therapy while adjusting the dosage of Zyloprim, until a normal serum uric acid and freedom from acute attacks have been maintained for several months.

In transferring a patient from a uricosuric agent to Zyloprim, the dose of the uricosuric agent should be gradually reduced over a period of several weeks and the dose of allopurinol gradually increased to the required dose needed to maintain a normal serum uric acid level.

How Supplied: 100 mg (white) scored tablets, bottles of 100 and 1000; unit dose pack of 1000. Tablets bear identification, ZYLOPRIM U4A. 300 mg (peach) scored tablets, bottles of 30, 100, 500 and unit dose pack of 1000. Tablets bear identification, ZYLOPRIM C9B.

100 mg × 100—DoD & VA
NSN 6505-00-998-4381

300 mg × 30—VA
NSN 6505-01-006-5974

300 mg × 100—VA
NSN 6505-01-004-3952

300 mg × 100—DoD
NSN 6505-00-149-1438

Animal Toxicology: In mice the LD_{50} is 160 mg/kg ip (with deaths delayed up to five days) and 700 mg/kg po (with deaths delayed up to three days). In rats the acute LD_{50} is 750 mg/kg ip > 6000 mg/kg po.

In a 13 week feeding experiment in rats at a drug level of 72 mg/kg per day 2 of 10 rats died and at 225 mg/kg per day 4 of 10 died before the completion of the experiment. Both groups exhibited renal tubular damage due to the deposition of xanthine that was more extensive at the higher dose.

In chronic feeding experiments, rats showed no toxic effects at a level of 14 mg/kg per day after one year. At a level of 24 mg/kg per day for one year the rats showed very slight depression of weight gain and food intake, and 5 out of 10 of the animals showed minor changes in the kidney tubules of the type exhibited by the rats on the higher doses described above.

Dogs survived oral doses of 30 mg/kg per day for one year with nil to minor changes in the kidney and no other significant abnormalities. At 90 mg/kg per day for one year there was some accumulation of xanthine in the kidneys with resultant chronic irritation and slight tubular changes. Occasional hemosiderin-like deposits were seen in the reticuloendothelial system. A higher dose (270 mg/kg per day) resulted in large concretions in the renal pelves, with severe destructive changes in the kidney secondary to xanthine accumulation. The deposition of xanthine appears to be a function both of the metabolic turnover of purines (which is proportionately larger in the smaller animals) and the degree of inhibition of xanthine oxidase.

Reproductive studies in rats and rabbits indicated that Zyloprim did not affect litter size, the mean weight of the progeny at birth or at three weeks postpartum, nor did it cause an increase in the number of animals born dead or with malformations.

*3,624,205 (Use Patent)
[*Shown in Product Identification Section*]

Burton, Parsons & Company

A Division of Alcon Laboratories, Inc.
6201 SOUTH FREEWAY
FORT WORTH, TX 76134

KONSYL®

Plantago Ovata Coating
Brand of Psyllium Hydrophilic Mucilloid

Composition: Konsyl contains 100% highly refined mucilloid of the blond psyllium seed. It forms moist, smooth bulk which disperses intimately with the contents of the intestine to promote natural elimination.

Action and Uses: Konsyl provides nonirritating bulk for the treatment of chronic constipation, spastic constipation, nonspecific diarrhea, irritable colon, following anorectal surgery, rectal disorders, and wherever intensive bulk producing therapy is indicated.

Administration and Dosage: A rounded teaspoonful one to three times each day. Reduce dosage for children according to age. In cases of constipation, each dose should be taken with a full glass of fluid. In cases of diarrhea, each dose should be taken in one-third of a glass of fluid. The patient should be instructed to stir Konsyl into a glass of water, fruit juice, or milk, and drink promptly. Dosage and/or its frequency can be reduced as symptoms disappear.

Side Effects: None.

Precautions: None.

Contraindications: Where obstruction of the bowel exists as the result of growths, adhesions or other causes, Konsyl may, by its bulk, cause difficulty.

How Supplied: Powder, containers of 6, 12 and 18 ounces.

L. A. FORMULA®

Plantago Ovata Coating
Brand of Psyllium Hydrophilic Mucilloid

Composition: L. A. Formula contains 50% Plantago Ovata Coating (blond psyllium) dispersed in an equal amount of dextrose. It forms moist, smooth bulk which disperses intimately with the contents of the intestine to provide natural elimination. Each dose contains approximately 22 calories and a negligible amount of sodium.

Action and Uses: L. A. Formula is prepared by an ultra-fine pulverization process which permits quick dispersion, yet delays gel formation. Its high degree of palatability provides good patient acceptance.

L. A. Formula provides nonirritating bulk for the treatment of chronic constipation, spastic constipation, nonspecific diarrhea, irritable colon, following anorectal surgery, rectal disorders, and wherever intensive bulk producing therapy is indicated.

Administration and Dosage: A rounded teaspoonful one to three times each day. Reduce dosage for children according to age. In cases of constipation, each dose should be taken with a full glass of fluid. In cases of diarrhea, each dose should be taken in one-third glass of fluid. The patient should be instructed to stir L. A. Formula into a glass of water, fruit juice, or milk, and drink promptly. Dosage and/or its frequency can be reduced as the symptoms disappear.

Side Effects: None.

Precautions: None.

Contraindications: Where obstruction of the bowel exists as the result of growths, adhesions or other causes, L. A. Formula may, by its bulk, cause difficulty.

How Supplied: Powder, containers of 7, 14 and 21 ounces.

C & M Pharmacal, Inc.

1519 E. EIGHT MILE ROAD
HAZEL PARK, MI 48030-2696

VERR–CANTH–C&M ℞

for the removal of benign epithelial growths

Description: Cantharidin 0.7% in an adherent-film-forming base of ethylcellulose, cellosolve, collodion, castor oil, penederm (octylphenylpolyethylene glycol), acetone.

Note: Cap tightly immediately after use. Keep away from heat and flame. If Verr-Canth thickens (loss of solvent by evaporation) add minimum amount of acetone needed to obtain original consistency, mixing well.

Action: The well-known vesicating and macerating effect of cantharidin is enhanced by the adherency of the film and by the penederm which facilitates its release from the film.

Indications: Verr-Canth is to be used topically for the removal of benign epithelial growths such as verruca vulgaris or molluscum contagiosum. For unusually resistant warts see Verrusol-C&M.

Cautions: Verr-Canth is a potent vesicant and is to be used (applied) only by the doctor. It is recommended that care be used in the selection of patients to be treated with Verr-Canth and method used, the doctor developing his own experience and technique. Care should be used in selection of site of application since residual pigmentation may occur (rarely). It is recommended that patients be advised of effect and possible results of treatment. Do not use on mucosal tissue. Do not use if growth or sur-

Continued on next page

C & M Pharmacal—Cont.

rounding tissue is inflamed or irritated. Do not use for diabetics, or people with poor blood-circulation, nor for moles, birthmarks, or unusual warts with hair growing from them.
If any Verr-Canth contacts eye or mucosal tissue or normal skin, flush immediately with water for 15 minutes, removing the film precipitated by the water.
Method: Using the thin-tipped applicator provided, apply Verr-Canth to the growth, one drop at a time, covering it completely. Allow a few minutes to dry. Cover with a nonporous adhesive bandage making sure that none of the medicinal is able to escape. (Prior to the application of the Verr-Canth some of the growth's surface may be removed, if deemed advisable, by paring or by gentle abrasion with a coarse cloth or emery board. Bleeding is to be avoided.) Tape should be left on as long as possible up to 24 hours for warts, up to 6 hours for molluscum. If any Verr-Canth film is still present it should be covered with a Band-aid or similar covering. When treating palpebral warts great care must be used in applying Verr-Canth making certain that film is thoroughly dry and warning patient not to touch the eyelid.
Removal of necrotic material should be done by the doctor. Growth is usually removed with the tape or it may be pared out. If necessary, repeat applications of Verr-Canth can be made when area is free of irritation or inflammation. After the removal of the growth, the use of a mild antibacterial until area heals is advisable.
How Supplied: 7.5 cc bottle with thin-tipped applicator attached to inside of cap. NDC 0398-0085-75.

VERREX–C&M ℞

for the removal of benign epithelial growths such as common warts

Description: Salicylic acid 30.0%, podophyllin 10.0%, penederm 0.5% (octylphenylpolyethylene glycol) in an adherent-film-forming vehicle of ethylcellulose, cellosolve, collodion, castor oil, acetone.
Caution: Federal law prohibits dispensing without prescription.
Action: The well-known keratolytic salicylic acid and roentgomimetic, antimetasticizing podophyllin are present at maximum levels; the surfactant penederm facilitates release from the film and penetration.
Indications: Verrex is to be used topically for the removal of benign epithelial growths such as common warts.
Cautions: Verrex is an extremely potent medicinal and it is recommended that care be used in the selection of patients to use Verrex, as well as location of warts to be treated. Do not use near eyes or on mucosal tissue (genital, anal). Do not use if wart or surrounding skin is inflamed or irritated. Large areas should not be treated at one time since discomfort may be excessive and systemic absorption may result. It is recommended that Verrex not be used for pregnant women, diabetics, or people with poor blood-circulation; nor on moles, birthmarks, or unusual warts with hair growing from them. Care should be used in selection of site of application since residual pigmentation may occur. It is recommended that the patient be advised of effect and possible results of treatment. Verrex is very flammable: keep away from fire or flame. Cap tightly immediately after use. Store at room temperature away from heat.
If any Verrex contacts eyes or mucosal tissue flush with water for 15 minutes, removing film precipitated by the water.
KEEP OUT OF REACH OF CHILDREN
Method: Wash affected area and soak in warm water for 5 minutes, then dry. Apply one or two drops of Verrex to growth allowing each drop to dry completely. Do not allow Verrex to contact normal skin. Cover with appropriate adhesive bandage which will cover but not adhere to the wart itself making sure that none of the Verrex film escapes. Use once daily for two days to a week, as required. After the removal of the growth the use of a mild anti-bacterial agent until area heals is advisable.
Note: When Verrex is applied by the doctor some of the growth's surface may be removed by rubbing gently with a coarse cloth or emery board after soaking with warm water and drying just prior to initial application. Bleeding is to be avoided.
How Supplied: 7.5 cc bottle with thin-tipped applicator attached to inside of cap. NDC 0398-0080-75.

VERRUSOL–C&M ℞

for the removal of benign epithelial growths such as common warts

Description: Salicylic acid 30.0%, podophyllin 5.0%, cantharidin 1.0%, penederm 0.5% (octylphenylpolyethylene glycol) in an adherent-film-forming vehicle of ethylcellulose, cellosolve, collodion, castor oil, acetone.
Note: If Verrusol thickens (loss of solvent by evaporation) add minimum amount of acetone needed to obtain original consistency, mixing well.
Action: Verrusol provides a convenient combination in a single vehicle of well-known wart-removing agents. Salicylic acid and cantharidin, both at maximum levels, serve as keratolytic and vesicating agents, respectively; podophyllin provides roentgomimetic and antimetasticizing effects and the surfactant penederm facilitates release from the film and penetration.
Indications: Verrusol is to be used by the doctor (see below) topically for the removal of warts.
Cautions: **Verrusol is an extremely potent medicinal and is to be used (applied) only by the doctor.** Do not use near eyes or on mucosal tissue (genital, anal). Do not use if wart or surrounding skin is inflamed or irritated. Large areas should not be treated at one time since discomfort may be excessive and systemic absorption may result. Care and caution should be used in selection of patients to be treated with Verrusol and method used, the doctor developing his own experience and technique. It is recommended that Verrusol not be used for pregnant women, diabetics, or people with poor blood-circulation; nor on moles, birthmarks, or unusual warts with hair growing from them. Care should be used in selection of site of application since residual pigmentation may occur. It is recommended that the patient be advised of effect and possible results of treatment.
Verrusol is very flammable: keep away from fire or flame. Cap tightly immediately after use. Store at room temperature away from heat. If any Verrusol contacts eyes or mucosal tissue flush with warm water for 15 minutes, removing film precipitated by the water.
Method: Using the thin-tipped applicator provided, apply Verrusol to the wart one drop at a time until it is covered: allow each drop to dry before adding the next. When dry, cover with a non-porous, slightly elastic tape making sure none of the dried Verrusol is able to escape. Blister forms within 24 hours. It is often painful and inflamed. (Aspirin with codeine or other analgesics may be needed during this period.) Tape should be left on as long as possible up to 24 hours. Growth is usually removed with the tape; or it is pared out after tape is removed. The use of a mild antibacterial agent until area heals is recommended.
Verrusol has been in active use since 1962—with very gratifying results.
How Supplied: 7.5 cc bottle with thin-tipped applicator attached to inside of cap. NDC 0398-0081-75.

Campbell Laboratories, Inc.

300 EAST 51st STREET
P.O. BOX 812, F.D.R. STATION
NEW YORK, NY 10022

HERPECIN-L® Cold Sore Lip Balm OTC

Composition: A soothing, emollient, cosmetically pleasant lip balm incorporating pyridoxine HCl; allantoin; the sunscreen, octyl p-(dimethylamino)-benzoate (Padimate O); and titanium dioxide in a balanced, acidic lipid system. (All ingredients appear on the package. Does not contain any "caines", antibiotics, phenol or camphor.) (NDC 38083-777-31)
Actions and Uses: HERPECIN-L® relieves dryness and chapping by providing a lipid barrier to help restore normal moisture balance to labial tissues. The sunscreen is effective in 2900-3200 AU range while titanium dioxide blocks, scatters and reflects the sun's rays. Pyridoxine is reputed to act as a co-enzyme in the metabolism of amino acids.
Administration: (1) *Recurrent "cold sores, sun and fever blisters":* Simply put, users report the sooner and more often applied, the better the results. Frequent sufferers report that with *prophylactic* use (B.I.D./P.R.N.), their attacks are fewer and less severe. Most recurrent herpes labialis patients are aware of the *prodromal* symptoms: tingling, itching, burning. At this stage, or if the lesion has already developed, HERPECIN-L should be applied liberally as often as convenient—at least *every hour* (qq. hor.). The prodrome will often persist and remind the patient to continue to reapply HERPECIN-L. (2) *Outdoor sun/winter protection:* Apply during and after exposure (and after swimming) and again at bedtime (h.s.). (3) *Dry, chapped lips:* Apply as needed.
Note: HERPECIN-L is for peri-oral use only; not for "canker sores" (aphthous stomatitis). Primary attacks, usually in children and young adults, are normally intra-oral and accompanied by foul breath, pain and fever. Lasting up to six weeks, they are most resistant to treatment. Adjunctive therapy for pain, fever and secondary infection may be indicated. "Mouth breathing" is often causative of excessive chapping. Malocclusion (narrowed bite) may be suspected in angular chelosis.
Adverse Reactions: A few, rare instances of topical sensitivity to pyridoxine HCl (Vitamin B_6) have been reported. Discontinue use if allergic reaction develops.
Contraindications: HERPECIN-L does not contain any steroids; oral or topical corticosteroids are normally contraindicated in *herpes* infections.
How Supplied: 2.8 gm. swivel tubes. O.T.C.
Samples Available: Yes.

The Carlton Corporation

83 N. SUMMIT STREET
TENAFLY, NJ 07670

CALPHOSAN® ℞

(calcium glycerophosphate/calcium lactate)
calcium/phosphorus solution in metabolic disorders involving low calcium

Composition: CALPHOSAN is a specially processed solution containing calcium glycerophosphate and calcium lactate. CALPHOSAN is isotonic, with a pH of about 7 or above. (Other calcium solutions are usually quite acid, with pH values of 4.5 to 5.5) Each 10 ml. CALPHOSAN contains calcium glycerophosphate 50 mg. and calcium lactate 50 mg. in a physiological solution of sodium chloride, with 0.25% phenol as a preservative.
Advantages: Intramuscular injections of CALPHOSAN raise blood serum calcium levels, do not raise the calcium levels above normal.

Usually intramuscular injections of CALPHOSAN are without pain, inflammatory reactions or sloughing.

Indications: Conditions associated with hypocalcemia: tetany, hypoparathyroidism (postoperative and idiopathic).

Administration: One or two 10 ml. injections of CALPHOSAN each week for the first four or five weeks, and on a when-needed basis thereafter, is usually sufficient to raise blood calcium levels.

Contraindications: Hypercalcemia; and in view of the fact that hypercalcemia is associated with sarcoidosis and bone metastasis of neoplastic processes, it should not be used in those conditions. As there is a similarity in the actions of calcium and digitalis on the contractility and excitability of the heart muscle, CALPHOSAN is contraindicated in fully digitalized patients. **Do not use intramuscularly in infants and young children.**

Availability: 10 ml. ampuls in boxes of 10s and 100s; and 60 ml. multiple dose vials.

Also Available: CALPHOSAN B-12: Calphosan plus 300 mcg. vitamin B_{12} per 10 ml.

Carnrick Laboratories, Inc.

65 HORSE HILL ROAD
CEDAR KNOLLS, NJ 07927

AMEN® ℞

(medroxyprogesterone acetate tablet U.S.P. 10 mg)

Caution: Federal Law Prohibits Dispensing Without Prescription

Warning:

The Use of Progestational Agents During the First Four Months of Pregnancy is Not Recommended.

Progestational agents have been used beginning with the first trimester of pregnancy in an attempt to prevent habitual abortion or treat threatened abortion. There is no adequate evidence that such use is effective and there is evidence of potential harm to the fetus when such drugs are given during the first four months of pregnancy. Furthermore, in the vast majority of women, the cause of abortion is a defective ovum, which progestational agents could not be expected to influence. In addition, the use of progestational agents, with their uterine-relaxant properties, in patients with fertilized defective ova may cause a delay in spontaneous abortion. Therefore, the use of such drugs during the first four months of pregnancy is not recommended.

Several reports suggest an association between intrauterine exposure to female sex hormones and congenital anomalies, including congenital heart defects and limb reduction defects (Refs. 1-5). One study (Ref. 4) estimated a 4.7-fold increased risk of limb reduction defects in infants exposed in utero to sex hormones (oral contraceptives, hormone withdrawal test for pregnancy, or attempted treatment for threatened abortion). Some of these exposures were very short and involved only a few days of treatment. The data suggest that the risk of limb reduction defects in exposed fetuses is somewhat less than 1 in 1,000.

If the patient is exposed to Amen® during the first four months of pregnancy or if she becomes pregnant while taking this drug, she should be apprised of the potential risks to the fetus.

Description: Amen® (medroxyprogesterone acetate U.S.P.) is a derivative of progesterone. It is a white to off-white, odorless crystalline powder, stable in air, melting between 200° and 210° C. It is freely soluble in chloroform, soluble in acetone and in dioxane, sparingly soluble in alcohol and in methanol, slightly soluble in ether, and insoluble in water.

The chemical name for medroxyprogesterone acetate is Pregn-4-ene-3,20-dione, 17-(acetyloxy)-6-methyl-, (6α)-. The structural formula is:

Actions: Amen® (medroxyprogesterone acetate), administered orally in the recommended dose to women with adequate endogenous estrogen, transforms proliferative endometrium into secretory endometrium. Androgenic and anabolic effects have been noted, but the drug is apparently devoid of significant estrogenic activity.

Indications: Amen® (medroxyprogesterone acetate) is indicated in secondary amenorrhea and abnormal uterine bleeding due to hormonal imbalance in the absence of organic pathology, such as submucous fibroids or uterine cancer.

Contraindications: **1.** Thrombophlebitis, thromboembolic disorders, cerebral apoplexy or patients with a past history of these conditions. **2.** Liver dysfunction or disease. **3.** Known or suspected malignancy of breast or genital organs. **4.** Undiagnosed vaginal bleeding. **5.** Missed abortion. **6.** As a diagnostic test for pregnancy. **7.** Known sensitivity to medroxyprogesterone acetate.

Warnings: **1.** The physician should be alert to the earliest manifestations of thrombotic disorders (thrombophlebitis, cerebrovascular disorders, pulmonary embolism, and retinal thrombosis). Should any of these occur or be suspected, the drug should be discontinued immediately.

2. Beagle dogs treated with medroxyprogesterone acetate developed mammary nodules, some of which were malignant. Although nodules occasionally appeared in control animals, they were intermittent in nature, whereas the nodules in the drug treated animals were larger, more numerous, persistent, and there were some breast malignancies with metastases, their significance with respect to humans has not been established.

3. Discontinue medication pending examination if there is sudden partial or complete loss of vision, or if there is sudden onset of proptosis, diplopia or migraine. If examination reveals papilledema, or retinal vascular lesions, medication should be withdrawn.

Detectable amounts of progestin have been identified in the milk of mothers receiving the drug. The effect of this on the nursing infant has not been determined. Masculinization of the female fetus has occurred when progestins have been used in pregnant women.

4. Retrospective studies of morbidity and mortality in Great Britain and studies of morbidity in the United States have shown a statistically significant association between thrombophlebitis, pulmonary embolism, and cerebral thrombosis and embolism and the use of oral contraceptives. There have been three principal studies in Great Britain[6–8] leading to this conclusion and one[9] in this country. The estimate of the relative risk of thromboembolism in the study by Vessey and Doll[8] was about sevenfold, while Sartwell and Associates[9] in the United States found a relative risk of 4.4, meaning that the users are several times as likely to undergo thromboembolic disease without evident cause as non-users. The American study also indicated that the risk did not persist after discontinuation of administration, and that it was not enhanced by long continued administration. The American study was not designed to evaluate a difference between products.

Precautions: **1.** The pretreatment physical examination should include special reference to breast and pelvic organs, as well as Papanicolaou smear.

2. Because this drug may cause some degree of fluid retention, conditions which might be influenced by this factor, such as epilepsy, migraine, asthma, cardiac or renal dysfunction require careful observation.

3. In cases of breakthrough bleeding, as in all cases of irregular bleeding per vaginum, nonfunctional causes should be borne in mind. In cases of undiagnosed vaginal bleeding adequate diagnostic measures are indicated.

4. Patients who have a history of psychic depression should be carefully observed and the drug discontinued if the depression recurs to a serious degree.

5. Any possible influence of prolonged progestin therapy on pituitary, ovarian, adrenal, hepatic or uterine functions awaits further study.

6. A decrease in glucose tolerance has been observed in a small percentage of patients on estrogen-progestin combination drugs. The mechanism of this decrease is obscure. For this reason, diabetic patients should be carefully observed while receiving progestin therapy.

7. The age of the patient constitutes no absolute limiting factor although treatment with progestins may mask the onset of the climacteric.

8. The pathologist should be advised of progestin therapy when relevant specimens are submitted.

9. Because of the occasional occurence of thrombotic disorders, (thrombophlebitis, pulmonary embolism, retinal thrombosis, and cerebrovascular disorders) in patients taking estrogen-progestin combinations and since the mechanism is obscure, the physician should be alert to the earliest manifestation of these disorders.

10. Information for the patient. See text of Patient Package Insert which is printed below.

Patient Labeling for Amen®—Warning for Women

There is an increased risk of birth defects in children whose mothers take this drug during the first four months of pregnancy.

Amen® is similar to the progesterone hormones naturally produced by the body. Progesterone and progesterone-like drugs are used to treat menstrual disorders, to test if the body is producing certain hormones, and to treat some forms of cancer in women.

They have been used as a test for pregnancy but such use is no longer considered safe because of possible damage to a developing baby. Also, more rapid methods for testing for pregnancy are now available. These drugs have also been used to prevent miscarriage in the first few months of pregnancy. No adequate evidence is available to show that they are effective for this purpose and there is evidence of an increased risk of birth defects, such as heart or limb defects, if these drugs are taken during the first four months of pregnancy. Furthermore, most cases of early miscarriage are due to causes which could not be helped by these drugs.

The exact risk of taking this drug early in pregnancy and having a baby with a birth defect is not known. However, one study found that babies born to women who had taken sex hormones (such as progesterone-like drugs) during the first three months of pregnancy were 4 to 5 times more likely to have abnormalities of the arms or legs than if their mothers had not taken such drugs. Some of these women had taken these drugs for only a few days. The

Continued on next page

Carnrick—Cont.

chance that an infant whose mother had taken this drug will have this type of defect is about 1 in 1,000.
If you take Amen® and later find you were pregnant when you took it, be sure to discuss this with your doctor as soon as possible.

Adverse Reactions: The following adverse reactions have been associated with the use of medroxyprogesterone acetate.
Breast: In a few instances, breast tenderness or galactorrhea have occurred.
Pregnancy: A few cases of clitoral hypertrophy have been reported in new born females, whose mothers received medroxyprogesterone acetate during pregnancy. Prolonged postpartum bleeding, postabortal bleeding and missed abortion have been reported.
Psychic: An occasional patient has experienced nervousness, insomnia, somnolence, fatigue or dizziness.
Thromboembolic phenomena: Thromboembolic phenomena including thrombophlebitis and pulmonary embolism have been reported.
Skin and mucous membranes: Sensitivity reactions ranging from pruritus, urticaria, angioneurotic edema to generalized rash and anaphylaxis have occasionally been reported. Acne, alopecia, or hirsutism have been reported in a few cases.
Gastrointestinal: Rarely, nausea has been reported. Jaundice, including neonatal jaundice, has been noted in a few instances.
Miscellaneous: Rare cases of headache and hyperpyrexia have been reported. The following adverse reactions have been observed in women taking progestins including medroxyprogesterone acetate: breakthrough bleeding; spotting; change in menstrual flow; amenorrhea; edema; change in weight (increase or decrease); changes in cervical erosion and cervical secretions; cholestatic jaundice; rash (allergic) with and without pruritus; melasma or chloasma; mental depression.
A statistically significant association has been demonstrated between use of estrogen-progestin combination drugs and the following serious adverse reactions; thrombophlebitis, pulmonary embolism and cerebral thrombosis and embolism. For this reason patients on progestin therapy should be carefully observed.
Although available evidence is suggestive of an association, such a relationship has been neither confirmed nor refuted for the following serious adverse reactions: neuro-ocular lesions, e.g., retinal thrombosis and optic neuritis.
The following adverse reactions have been observed in patients receiving estrogen-progestin combination drugs; rise in blood pressure in susceptible individuals; premenstrual-like syndrome; changes in libido; changes in appetite; cystitis-like syndrome; headache; nervousness; dizziness; fatigue; backache; hirsutism; loss of scalp hair; erythema multiforme; erythema nodosum; hemorrhagic eruption; itching.
In view of these observations, patients on progestin therapy should be carefully observed.
Female fetal masculinization has been observed in patients receiving progestins. The following laboratory results may be altered by the use of estrogen-progestin combination drugs: Increased sulfobromophthalein and other hepatic function tests; Coagulation tests: increase in prothrombin factors VII, VIII, IX and X; Metyrapone test; Pregnanediol determination.
Dosage and Administration: Secondary Amenorrhea—Amen® (medroxyprogesterone acetate) may be employed in doses ranging from 5 to 10 mg. daily depending upon the degree of endometrial stimulation desired. The dose should be given daily for 5 to 10 days beginning on the assumed 16th to 21st day of the cycle. In patients with poorly developed endometria, conventional estrogen therapy should be given in conjunction with Amen®. Following therapy with the preceding doses of Amen®, withdrawal bleeding usually occurs within three days. **Abnormal uterine bleeding, (due to hormonal imbalance in the absence of organic pathology, such as submucous fibroids or uterine cancers)**—Amen® may be given in doses ranging from 5 to 10 mg. for 5 to 10 days beginning on the assumed or calculated 16th to 21st day of the cycle. (Hamblen, E.C. et al, Brook Lodge Symposium on Progesterone, page 201, Brook Lodge Press, Augusta, Michigan, 1961).
When bleeding is due to a deficiency of both ovarian hormones, as indicated by a poorly developed proliferative endometrium, estrogens should be used in conjunction with Amen®. If bleeding is controlled satisfactorily, two subsequent cycles of treatment should be given.

References: 1. Gal, I., B. Kirman, and J. Stern, "Hormonal Pregnancy Tests and Congenital Malformation," Nature, 216:83, 1967.
2. Levy, E. P., A. Cohen, and F. C. Fraser, "Hormone Treatment During Pregnancy and Congenital Heart Defects," Lancet, 1:611, 1973.
3. Nora, J. and A. Nora, "Birth Defects and Oral Contraceptives," Lancet, 1:941, 1973.
4. Janerich, D. T., J. M. Piper, and D. M. Glebatis, "Oral Contraceptives and Congenital Limb-Reduction Defects," New England Journal of Medicine, 291:697, 1974.
5. Heinonen, 0. P., D. Slone, R. R. Monson, E. B. Hook, and S. Shapiro, "Cardiovascular Birth Defects and Antenatal Exposure to Female Sex Hormones," New England Journal of Medicine, 296:67, 1977.
6. Royal College of General Practitioners; Oral Contraception and Thromboembolic Disease. J. Coll. Gen. Prac., 13:267–279, 1967.
7. Inman, W. H. W. and Vessey, M. P.: Investigation of Deaths From Pulmonary Coronary and Cerebral Thrombosis and Embolism in Women in Child-Bearing Age, Brit. Med. J., 2:193–199, 1968.
8. Vessey, M. P. and Doll, R.: Investigation of Relation Between Use of Oral Contraceptives and Thromboembolic Disease. A Further Report, Brit. Med. J., 2:651–657, 1969.
9. Sartwell, P. E., Masi, A. T., Arthes, G. R., Greene, R. R., and Smith, H. E.: Thromboembolism and Oral Contraceptives: An Epidemiological Case-Control Study, Am. J. Epidem., 90: 365–380, (Nov.) 1969.

How Supplied: Amen® is a scored tablet containing 10 mg. of medroxyprogesterone acetate USP and is available in bottles of 50 (NDC 0086-0049-05) and 1000 (NDC 0086-0049-90).
The most recent revision of this labeling is January 1982.
Manufactured for Carnrick Laboratories, Inc.
[Shown in Product Identification Section]

BONTRIL® PDM Ⓒ
(brand of phendimetrazine tartrate 35 mg. tablets)

Dosage and Administration: Usual Adult Dosage: Dosage should be individualized to obtain an adequate response with the lowest effective dose. In some cases 17½ mg. per dose may be adequate. 1 tablet (35 mg.) b.i.d. or t.i.d. one hour before meals. Dosage should not exceed 2 tablets t.i.d.
How Supplied: Three layered green, white and yellow tablets with 8648 on the scored side and the letter "C" on the other. Bottles of 100, NDC 0086-0048-10. Bottles of 1,000, NDC 0086-0048-90.
Caution: Federal law prohibits dispensing without prescription.
Manufactured for Carnrick Laboratories, Inc.
[Shown in Product Identification Section]

BONTRIL® SLOW-RELEASE Ⓒ
(brand of phendimetrazine tartrate slow-release capsules 105 mg

Description: Phendimetrazine tartrate, as the dextro isomer, has the chemical name of (+)-3,4-Dimethyl-2-phenylmorpholine Tartrate.
The structural formula is as follows:

M.W. 341

Phendimetrazine tartrate is a white, odorless powder with a bitter taste. It is soluble in water, methanol and ethanol.
Actions: Phendimetrazine tartrate is a sympathomimetic amine with pharmacological activity similar to the prototype drugs of this class used in obesity, the amphetamines. Actions include central nervous system stimulation and elevation of blood pressure. Tachyphylaxis and tolerance have been demonstrated with all drugs of this class in which these phenomena have been looked for.
Drugs of this class used in obesity are commonly known as "anorectics" or "anorexigenics". It has not been established, however, that the action of such drugs in treating obesity is primarily one of appetite suppression. Other central nervous system actions or metabolic effects may be involved.
Adult obese subjects instructed in dietary management and treated with anorectic drugs lose more weight on the average than those treated with placebo and diet, as determined in relatively short term clinical trials.
The magnitude of increased weight loss of drug-treated patients over placebo-treated patients is only a fraction of a pound a week. The rate of weight loss is greatest in the first weeks of therapy for both drug and placebo subjects and tends to decrease in succeeding weeks. The possible origin of the increased weight loss due to the various drug effects is not established. The amount of weight loss associated with the use of an anorectic drug varies from trial to trial, and the increased weight loss appears to be related in part to variables other than the drug prescribed, such as the physician investigator, the population treated, and the diet prescribed. Studies do not permit conclusions as to the relative importance of the drug and non-drug factors on weight loss.
The natural history of obesity is measured in years, whereas the studies cited are restricted to a few weeks duration; thus, the total impact of drug-induced weight loss over that of diet alone must be considered clinically limited.
The active drug 105 mg of phendimetrazine tartrate in each capsule of this special slow-release dosage form approximates the action of three 35 mg non-time release doses taken at 4 hours intervals.
The major route of elimination is via the kidneys where most of the drug and metabolites are excreted. Some of the drug is metabolized to phenmetrazine and also phendimetrazine-N-oxide.
The average half-life of elimination when studied under controlled conditions is about 1.9 hours for the non-time and 9.8 hours for the slow-release dosage form. The absorption half-life of the drug from conventional non-time 35 mg phendimetrazine tablets is approximately the same. These data indicate that the slow-release product has a similar onset of action to the conventional non-time-release product and, in addition, has a prolonged therapeutic effect.
Indications: Phendimetrazine tartrate is indicated in the managment of exogenous obesity as a short term adjunct (a few weeks) in a regimen of weight reduction based on caloric

restriction. The limited usefulness of agents of this class (see ACTIONS) should be measured against possible risk factors inherent in their use such as those described below.

Contraindications: Advanced arteriosclerosis, symptomatic cardiovascular disease, moderate and severe hypertension, hyperthyroidism, known hypersensitivity, or idiosyncrasy to the sympathomimetic amines. Agitated states. Patients with a history of drug abuse. Use in Patients taking other CNS stimulants including monoamine oxidase inhibitors.

Warnings: Tolerance to the anorectic effect usually develops within a few weeks. When this occurs, the recommended dose should not be exceeded in an attempt to increase the effect; rather, the drug should be discontinued. Use of phendimetrazine within 14 days following the administration of monoamine oxidase inhibitors may result in a hypertensive crisis. Abrupt cessation of administration following prolonged high dosage results in extreme fatigue and depression. Because of the effect on the central nervous system phendimetrazine tartrate may impair the ability of the patient to engage in potentially hazardous activities such as operating machinery or driving a motor vehicle; the patient should therefore be cautioned accordingly.

Precautions: Caution is to be exercised in prescribing phendimetrazine for patients with even mild hypertension.
Insulin requirements in diabetes mellitus may be altered in association with the use of phendimetrazine and the concomitant dietary regimen.
Phendimetrazine may decrease the hypotensive effect of guanethidine.
The least amount feasible should be prescribed or dispensed at one time in order to minimize the possibility of overdosage.

Usage in Pregnancy: Safe use in pregnancy has not been established. Until more information is available, phendimetrazine tartrate should not be taken by women who are or may become pregnant unless, in the opinion of the physician, the potential benefits outweigh the possible hazards.

Usage in Children: Phendimetrazine tartrate is not recommended for use in children under 12 years of age.

Adverse Reactions: **Cardiovascular:** Palpitation, tachycardia, elevation of blood pressure.
Central Nervous System: Overstimulation, restlessness, dizziness, insomnia, tremor, headache, rarely psychotic episodes at recommended doses, agitation, flushing, sweating, blurring of vision.
Gastrointestinal: Dryness of the mouth, diarrhea, constipation, nausea, stomach pain.
Genitourinary: Changes in libido, urinary frequency, dysuria.

Drug Abuse and Dependence:
Controlled Substance: Phendimetrazine is a Schedule III controlled substance.
Dependence: Phendimetrazine Tartrate is related chemically and pharmacologically to the amphetamines. Amphetamines and related stimulant drugs have been extensively abused, and the possibility of abuse of phendimetrazine should be kept in mind when evaluating the desirability of including a drug as part of a weight reduction program. Abuse of amphetamines and related drugs may be associated with intense psychological dependence and severe social dysfunction. There are reports of patients who have increased the dosage to many times that recommended. Abrupt cessation following prolonged high dosage administration results in extreme fatigue and mental depression; changes are also noted on the sleep EEG. Manifestations of chronic intoxication with anorectic drugs include severe dermatoses, marked insomnia, irritability, hyperactivity and personality changes. The most severe manifestation of chronic intoxications is psychosis, often clinically indistinguishable from schizophrenia.

Overdosage: Manifestations of acute overdosage may include restlessness, tremor, hyperreflexia, rapid respiration, confusion, assaultiveness, hallucinations, panic states.
Fatigue and depression usually follow the central stimulation.
Cardiovascular effects include arrhythmias, hypertension, or hypotension and circulatory collapse. Gastrointestinal symptoms include nausea, vomiting, diarrhea, and abdominal cramps. Poisoning may result in convulsions, coma, and death.
Management of acute intoxication is largely symptomatic and includes lavage and sedation with a barbiturate. Experience with hemodialysis or peritoneal dialysis is inadequate to permit recommendation in this regard.
Acidification of the urine increases phendimentrazine tartrate excretion.
Intravenous phentolamaine (Regitine) has been suggested for possible acute, severe hypotension, if this complicates overdosage.

Dosage and Administration: One Slow-Release Capsule (105 mg) in the morning, taken 30-60 minutes before the morning meal. Phendimetrazine Tartrate is not recommended for use in children under twelve years of age.

How Supplied: Phendimetrazine Slow-Release Capsules 105 mg is supplied in bottles of 100 opaque green and clear yellow capsules, imprinted with the letter "C" and 8647. NDC # 0086-0047-10.
Store at controlled room temperature, 15°–30°C(59°–86°F).

Caution: Federal law prohibits dispensing without prescription.
Manufactured For: Carnrick Laboratories, Inc.
[*Shown in Product Identification Section*]

CAPITAL® with CODEINE
(acetaminophen with codeine)
Tablets Ⓒ **Suspension** Ⓒ

Caution: Federal law prohibits dispensing without prescription.

Description:
Each CAPITAL® with CODEINE tablet contains:

Codeine Phosphate*	30 mg
***WARNING:** May be habit forming	
Acetaminophen	325 mg

CAPITAL® with CODEINE suspension contains (in each 5ml):

Codeine Phosphate*	12 mg
***WARNING:** May be habit forming	
Acetaminophen	120 mg

Acetaminophen occurs as a white, odorless crystalline powder, possessing a slightly bitter taste. Codeine is an alkaloid, obtained from opium or prepared from morphine by methylation. Codeine occurs as colorless or white crystals, efforesces slowly in dry air and is affected by light.

Actions: Acetaminophen is a nonopiate, non-salicylate analgesic and antipyretic. Codeine is an opiate analgesic and antitussive. Codeine retains at least one-half of its analgesic activity when administered orally.

Indications: CAPITAL® with CODEINE tablets are indicated for the relief of mild to moderately severe pain. CAPITAL® with CODEINE suspension is indicated for the relief of mild to moderate pain.

Contraindications: Hypersensitivity to acetaminophen or codeine.

Warnings:
Drug Dependence: Codeine can produce drug dependence of the morphine type, and therefore, has the potential for being abused. Psychic dependence, physical dependence and tolerance may develop upon repeated administration of this drug and it should be prescribed and administered with the same degree of caution appropriate to the use of other oral narcotic medications.
CAPITAL® with CODEINE tablets is subject to the Federal Controlled Substances Act (Schedule III). CAPITAL® with CODEINE suspension is subject to the Federal Controlled Substances Act (Schedule V).

Precautions:

1. **General:**
   Head Injury and increased intracranial pressure: The respiratory depressant effects of narcotics and their capacity to elevate cerebrospinal fluid pressure may be markedly exaggerated in the presence of head injury, other intracranial lesions or a pre-existing increase in intracranial pressure. Furthermore, narcotics produce adverse reactions which may obscure the clinical course of patients with head injuries.
   Acute abdominal conditions: The administration of products containing codeine or other narcotics may obscure the diagnosis or clinical course in patients with acute abdominal conditions.
   Special risk patients: Acetaminophen with codeine should be given with caution to certain patients such as elderly or debilitated, and those with severe impairment of hepatic or renal funcion, hypothyroidism, Addison's disease, and prostatic hypertrophy or urethral stricture.
2. **Information for Patients:**
   Codeine may impair the mental and/or physical abilities required for the performance of potentially hazardous tasks such as driving a car or operating machinery. The patient taking this drug should be cautioned accordingly.
3. **Drug Interactions:**
   Patients receiving other narcotic analgesics, antipsychotics, antianxiety, or other CNS depressants (including alcohol) concomitantly with acetaminophen and codeine may exhibit additive CNS depression due to the codeine component. When such therapy is contemplated, the dose of one or both agents should be reduced. The use of MAO inhibitors or tricyclic antidepressants with codeine preparations may increase the effect of either the antidepressant or codeine.
   The concurrent use of anticholinergics with codeine may produce paralytic ileus.
4. **Usage in Pregancy:**
   Safe use in pregnancy has not been established relative to possible adverse effects on fetal development. Therefore, acetaminophen and codeine should not be used in pregnant women unless, in the judgment of the physician, the potential benefits outweigh the possible hazards.
5. **Nursing Mothers:**
   Problems in humans have not been documented; however, risk-benefit must be considered since acetaminophen (in very low concentrations) and codeine are excreted in breast milk.
6. **Pediatric Use:**
   Safety and effectiveness of the suspension in children below the age of 3 have not been established. Tablets should not be administered to children under 12.

Adverse Reactions: The most frequently observed adverse reactions include light-headedness, dizziness, sedation, shortness of breath, nausea, and vomiting. These effects seem to be more prominent in ambulatory than in non-ambulatory patients, and some of these adverse reactions may be alleviated if the patient lies down.
Other adverse reactions include euphoria, dysphoria, constipation and pruritus. At higher doses codeine has most of the disadvantages of morphine including respiratory depression.

Continued on next page

Carnrick—Cont.

Overdosage:

Acetaminophen:

Signs and Symptoms: Acetaminophen in massive overdosage may cause hepatic toxicity in some patients. In all cases of suspected overdose, immediately call your regional poison center or the Rocky Mountain Poison Center's toll-free number (800 525-6115) for assistance in diagnosis and for directions in the use of N-acetylcysteine as an antidote, a use currently restricted to investigational status. In adults, hepatic toxicity has rarely been reported with acute overdoses of less than 10 grams and fatalities with less than 15 grams. Importantly, young children seem to be more resistant than adults to the hepatotoxic effect of an acetaminophen overdose. Despite this, the measures outlined below should be initiated in any adult or child suspected of having ingested an acetaminophen overdose.

Early symptoms following a potentially hepatotoxic overdose may include: nausea, vomiting, diaphoresis and general malaise. Clinical and laboratory evidence of hepatic toxicity may not be apparent until 48 to 72 hours post-ingestion.

Treatment: The stomach should be emptied promptly by lavage or by induction of emesis with syrup of ipecac. Patients' estimates of the quantity of a drug ingested are notoriously unreliable. Therefore, if an acetaminophen overdose is suspected, a serum acetaminophen assay should be obtained as early as possible, but no sooner than four hours following ingestion. Liver function studies should be obtained initially and repeated at 24-hour intervals.

The antidote, N-acetylcysteine, should be administered as early as possible, and within 16 hours of the overdose ingestion for optimal results. Following recovery, there are no residual, structural or functional hepatic abnormalities.

Codeine:

Signs and Symptoms: Serious overdose with codeine is characterized by respiratory depression (a decrease in respiratory rate and/or tidal volume, Cheyne-Stokes respiration, cyanosis), extreme somnolence progressing to stupor or coma, skeletal muscle flaccidity, cold and clammy skin, and sometimes bradycardia and hypotension. In severe overdosage, apnea, circulatory collapse, cardiac arrest and death may occur.

Treatment: Primary attention should be given to the reestablishment of adequate respiratory exchange through provision of a patent airway and the institution of assisted or controlled ventilation. The narcotic antagonist naloxone is a specific antidote against respiratory depression which may result from overdosage or unusual sensitivity to narcotics, including codeine. Therefore, an appropriate dose of naloxone (see package insert) should be administered, preferably by the intravenous route, and simultaneously with efforts at respiratory resuscitation. Since the duration of acion of codeine may exceed that of the antagonist, the patient should be kept under continued surveillance and repeated doses of the antagonist should be administered as needed to maintain adequate respiration.

An antagonist should not be administered in the absence of clinically significant respiratory or cardiovascular depression. Oxygen, intravenous fluids, vasopressors and other supportive measures should be employed as indicated.

Gastric emptying may be useful in removing unabsorbed drug.

Dosage and Administration: Dosage should be adjusted according to severity of pain and response of the patient. However, it should be kept in mind that tolerance to codeine can develop with continued use and that the incidence of untoward effects is dose related. This product is inappropriate even in high doses for severe or intractable pain. Adult doses of codeine higher than 60 mg. fail to give commensurate relief of pain but merely prolong analgesia and are associated with an appreciably increased incidence of undesirable side effects. Equivalently high doses in children would have similar effects.

CAPITAL® with CODEINE tablets are given orally. Adults: One tablet for mild to moderate pain. Two tablets for moderate to moderately severe pain. Doses can be repeated up to every 4 hours as required.

CAPITAL® with CODEINE suspension is given orally. The usual doses are: Children (3 to 6 years): One teaspoonful (5 ml) 3 or 4 times daily. (7 to 12 years): Two teaspoonfuls (10 ml) 3 or 4 times daily. Adults: One tablespoonful (15 ml) every 4 hours as needed.

SHAKE WELL BEFORE USING

How Supplied: CAPITAL® with CODEINE tablets: Pale blue scored tablet imprinted with 8644 and a sunburst on the scored side and the letter "C" on the other. Bottles of 100 tablets, NDC 0086-0044-10. Bottles of 1000 tablets, NDC 0086-0044-90. Store at Controlled Room Temperature 15°–30°C (59°–86°F) in a dry place.

CAPTIAL® with CODEINE suspension: a pink, pleasantly flavored suspension—16 oz. bottles, NDC 0086-0046-16. Store at Controlled Room Temperature 15°-30°C (59°–86°F)

The most recent revision of this labeling is May 1982

Manufactured for: Carnrick Laboratories, Inc.

[*Shown in Product Identification Section*]

MIDRIN™ ℞

Caution: Federal law prohibits dispensing without prescription.

Description: Each red capsule with pink band contains Isometheptene Mucate 65 mg., Dichloralphenazone 100 mg., and Acetaminophen 325 mg.

Isometheptene Mucate is a white crystalline powder having a characteristic aromatic odor and bitter taste. It is an unsaturated aliphatic amine with sympathomimetic properties.

Dichloralphenazone is a white, microcrystalline powder, with slight odor and tastes saline at first, becoming acrid. It is a mild sedative.

Acetaminophen, a non-salycylate, occurs as a white, odorless, crystalline powder possessing a slightly bitter taste.

Actions: Isometheptene Mucate, a sympathomimetic amine, acts by constricting dilated cranial and cerebral arterioles, thus reducing the stimuli that lead to vascular headaches. Dichloralphenazone, a mild sedative, reduces the patient's emotional reaction to the pain of both vascular and tension headaches. Acetaminophen raises the threshold to painful stimuli, thus exerting an analgesic effect against all types of headaches.

Indications: For relief of tension and vascular headaches.*

* Based on a review of this drug (isometheptene mucate) by the National Academy of Sciences-National Research Council and/or other information, FDA has classified the other indication as "Possibly" effective in the treatment of migraine headache. Final classification of the less-than-effective indication requires further investigation.

Contraindications: Midrin is contraindicated in glaucoma and/or severe cases of renal disease, hypertension, organic heart disease, hepatic disease and in those patients who are on monoamine-oxidase (MAO) inhibitor therapy.

Precautions: Caution should be observed in hypertension, peripheral vascular disease and after recent cardiovascular attacks.

Adverse Reactions: Transient dizziness and skin rash may appear in hypersensitive patients. This can usually be eliminated by reducing the dose.

Dosage and Administration: FOR RELIEF OF MIGRAINE HEADACHE: The usual adult dosage is two capsules at once, followed by one capsule every hour until relieved, up to 5 capsules within a twelve hour period.

FOR RELIEF OF TENSION HEADACHE: The usual adult dosage is one or two capsules every four hours up to 8 capsules a day.

How Supplied: Red capsules imprinted with pink band, the letter "C" and 86120. Bottles of 50 capsules, NDC 0086-0120-05. Bottles of 100 capsules, NDC 0086-0120-10. Store at controlled room temperature 15–30°C (59–86°F) in a dry place.

The most recent revision of this labeling is Jan. 1982.

Manufactured for Carnrick Laboratories, Inc.

[*Shown in Product Identification Section*]

NOLAHIST™

(phenindamine tartrate)

Description: Each tablet contains:

Phenindamine Tartrate .... 25 mg

Indications: For temporary relief of running nose, sneezing, itching of the nose or throat and itchy and watery eyes as may occur in allergic rhinitis (such as hay fever).

Dosage: Adult oral dosage is one tablet every 4 to 6 hours not to exceed six tablets in 24 hours. Children 6 to under 12 years oral dosage is one-half tablet every 4 to 6 hours not to exceed 3 tablets in 24 hours. For children under 6 years, there is no recommended dosage except under the advice and supervision of a physician.

Warnings: May cause drowsiness. May cause excitability espcially in children. Do not take this product if you have asthma, glaucoma or difficulty in urination due to enlargement of the prostate gland except under the advice and supervision of a physician. Do not give this product to children under 6 years except under the advise and supervision of a physician. As with any drug, if you are pregnant or nursing a baby, seek professional advice before using this product. Keep this and all medication out of the reach of children. In case of accidental overdose, seek professional assistance or contact a Poison Control Center immediately.

Cautions: May cause nervousness and insomnia in some individuals. Avoid driving a motor vehicle or operating heavy machinery. Avoid alcoholic beverages while taking this product.

How Supplied: White, capsule-shaped, scored tablet inscribed with 8652 on one side and the letter C on the other side in bottles of 100. Each tablet contains phenindamine tartrate 25 mg. (NDC 0086-0052-10)

Keep tightly closed away from light.

Manufactured for Carnrick Laboratories, Inc.

[*Shown in Product Identification Section*]

NOLAMINE® ℞

Description:

Each timed release tablet contains:

Phenindamine tartrate .... 24 mg

Chlorpheniramine maleate .... 4 mg

Phenylpropanolamine hydrochloride .. 50 mg

Formulated to provide 8 to 12 hours of continuous relief.

Caution: Federal law prohibits dispensing without prescription.

Indications: As a nasal decongestant associated with the common cold, sinusitis, hay fever and other allergies.

Contraindications: Hypersensitivity to any of the components. Contraindicated in concurrent MAO inhibitor therapy.
Side Effects: Nervousness, insomnia, tremors, dizziness and drowsiness may occur occasionally.
Precautions: Antihistamines may cause drowsiness and should be used with caution in patients who operate motor vehicles or dangerous machinery. Use with caution in patients with hypertension, cardiovascular disease, diabetes or hyperthyroidism. Ths product should be used with caution in patients with prostatic hypertrophy or glaucoma.
Dosage: Usual adult dose: Orally, one tablet every 8 hours. In mild cases, one tablet every 10 to 12 hours.
How Supplied: Pink, timed release tablets coded C 86204 in bottles of 100 (NDC 0086-0204-10) and 250 (NDC 0086-0204-25). Store at room temperature.
Manufactured for Carnrick Laboratories, Inc.
[*Shown in Product Identification Section*]

PHRENILIN® and PHRENILIN® FORTE ℞

Caution: Federal Law Prohibits Dispensing Without Prescription

Description: PHRENILIN®: Each PHRENILIN® tablet, an analgesic-sedative combination for oral administration contains: butalbital, USP 50 mg., (Warning—May be habit forming); acetaminophen, USP 325 mg.
PHRENILIN® FORTE: Each PHRENILIN® FORTE capsule, an analgesic-sedative combination for oral administration, contains: butalbital, USP 50 mg., (Warning—May be habit forming); acetaminophen, USP 650 mg.

$CH_2{=}CHCH_2$ / $(CH_3)_2CHCH_2$ — O, H, O, NH, O

Butalbital

Butalbital, 5-allyl-5-isobutyl-barbituric acid, a white odorless crystalline powder, is a short to intermediate acting barbiturate.

HO—⟨benzene⟩—NHCOCH$_3$

Acetaminophen

Acetaminophen, N-acetyl-p-amino-phenol, occurs as a white, odorless, crystalline powder, possessing a slightly bitter taste. Acetaminophen is a non-salicylate, non-narcotic analgesic, and antipyretic.
Clinical Pharmacology: Pharmacologically, Butalbital-Acetaminophen combines the analgesic properties of acetaminophen with the anxiolytic and muscle relaxant properties of butalbital.
Butalbital is a short to intermediate acting barbiturate which produces mild sedation. Barbiturates are capable of producing all levels of CNS mood alteration from excitation to mild sedation, to hypnosis, and deep coma. Overdosage can produce death.
Barbiturates depress the sensory cortex, decrease motor activity, alter cerebellar function, and produce drowsiness, sedation, and hypnosis. Barbiturates are respiratory depressants. The degree of respiratory depression is dependent on dose.
Barbiturates do not impair normal hepatic function, but have been shown to induce liver microsomal enzymes, thus increasing and/or altering the metabolism of barbiturates and other drugs.
Acetaminophen is a non-narcotic analgesic and antipyretic. Acetaminophen produces analgesia by elevation of the pain threshold and antipyresis through action on the hypothalamic heat-regulating center.

Pharmacokinetics: The onset and duration of action, which is related to the rate at which the barbiturates are redistributed throughout the body, varies among persons and in the same person from time to time. Butalbital has a duration of action from 3 to 6 hours.
Barbiturates are weak acids that are absorbed and rapidly distributed to all tissues and fluids with high concentrations in the brain, liver, and kidneys. The more lipid soluble the barbiturate, the more rapidly it penetrates all tissues of the body. Barbiturates are bound to plasma and tissue proteins to a varying degree with the degree of binding increasing directly as a function of lipid solubility.
Barbiturates are metabolized primarily by the hepatic microsomal enzyme system and the metabolic products are excreted in the urine, and less commonly, in the feces. The inactive metabolites of the barbiturates are excreted as conjugates of glucoronic acid.
Acetaminophen is rapidly and almost completely absorbed from the gastrointestinal tract, producing maximum serum concentrations within 30 minutes to one hour. The plasma half-life varies from one to three hours. Acetaminophen is relatively uniformly distributed throughout most body fluids and is approximately 25% protein bound. Approximately 90 to 95% of a dose is metabolized in the liver, primarily by conjugation with glucuronic acid, sulfuric acid, and cysteine. Excretion is renal; primarily as conjugates. About 3% of a dose may be excreted unchanged.
Indications and Usage: PHRENILIN® and PHRENILIN® FORTE are indicated for the relief of the symptom complex of tension (or muscle contraction) headache.
Contraindications: Hypersensitivity to any of the components. Patients with porphyria.
Warnings: Acetaminophen in massive overdosage may cause hepatotoxicity in some patients. (See OVERDOSAGE.)
Habit Forming: Barbiturates may be habit forming. Tolerance, psychological and physical dependence may occur with continued use. (See DRUG ABUSE AND DEPENDENCE.) Abrupt cessation after prolonged use in the dependent person may result in withdrawal symptoms, including delirium, convulsions, and possibly death. Barbiturates should be withdrawn gradually from any patient known to be taking excessive dosage over long periods of time.
Acute or Chronic Pain: Caution should be exercised when barbiturates are administered to patients with acute or chronic pain, because paradoxical excitement could be induced or important symptoms could be masked.
Use in Pregnancy: (See PRECAUTIONS section.)
Synergistic Effects: The concomitant use of alcohol or other CNS depressants may produce additive CNS depressant effects.
Precautions:
General: Barbiturates may be habit forming. Tolerance and psychological and physical dependence may occur with continuing use. (See DRUG ABUSE AND DEPENDENCE.) Barbiturates should be administered with caution, if at all, to patients who are mentally depressed, have suicidal tendencies, or a history of drug abuse.
Elderly or debilitated patients may react to barbiturates with marked excitement, depression, and confusion. In some persons, barbiturates repeatedly produce excitement rather than depression.
In patients with hepatic damage, barbiturates should be administered with caution and initially in reduced doses. Barbiturates should not be administered to patients showing the premonitory signs of hepatic coma.
Use with caution in patients with severe renal function impairment.
Do not exceed recommended dosage. Excessive or prolonged use should be avoided.

Information for Patients: Practitioners should give the following information and instructions to patients receiving barbiturates.
1. The use of barbiturates carries with it an associated risk of psychological and/or physical dependence. The patient should be warned against increasing the dose of the drug without consulting a physician.
2. Barbiturates may impair mental and/or physical abilities required for the performance of potentially hazardous tasks (e.g., driving, operating machinery, etc.)
3. Alcohol should not be consumed while taking barbiturates. Concurrent use of the barbiturates with other CNS depressants (e.g., alcohol, narcotics, tranquilizers, and antihistamines) may result in additional CNS depressant effects.

Drug Interactions: The concomitant use of other central nervous system depressants, including other sedatives or hypnotics, antihistamines, tranquilizers, or alcohol, may produce additive depressant effects. When such combined therapy is necessary, the dose of one or more agents may need to be reduced.
The presence of barbiturates decreases the effects of oral anticoagulants, griseofulvin, doxycycline, corticosteroids, and possibly phenytoin. Monoamine oxidase inhibitors (MAOI) prolong the effects of barbiturates.
Use in Pregnancy: Animal reproduction studies have not been conducted with PHRENILIN® or PHRENILIN® FORTE. It is also not known whether PHRENILIN® or PHRENILIN® FORTE can cause fetal harm when administered to a pregnant woman or can affect reproduction capacity.
BUTALBITAL:
First trimester: The teratogenic potential of butalbital has not been studied in either animals or humans. Although teratogenic effects with this combination medication have not been reported clinically, risk-benefit must be considered since other barbiturates have been shown to increase the risk of fetal abnormalities in humans. If this drug is used during pregnancy, or if the patient becomes pregnant while taking this drug, the patient should be apprised of the potential hazard to the fetus.
Third trimester: Use of barbiturates throughout the last trimester of pregnancy may cause physical dependence with resulting withdrawal symptoms (convulsions and hyperirritability) in the neonate. These withdrawal symptoms may occur up to 14 days after birth. (See DRUG ABUSE AND DEPENDENCE.)
Also, one study in humans has shown that prenatal exposure to barbiturates may be associated with an increased incidence of brain tumors. In addition, use of barbiturates during pregnancy may be associated with neonatal hemorrhage due to reduction in levels of vitamin K-dependent clotting factors in the neonate.
Labor and delivery: Use of barbiturates just prior to or during delivery may cause respiratory depression in the neonate, especially the premature neonate, because of immature hepatic function.
ACETAMINOPHEN:
Problems in humans have not been documented; however, controlled studies have not been done. Risk-benefit must be considered since acetaminophen crosses the placenta.
Nursing Mothers:
BUTALBITAL—
Barbiturates are excreted in breast milk; use by nursing mothers may cause CNS depression, bradycardia, or respiratory depression in the infant.
ACETAMINOPHEN:
Problems in humans have not been documented; however, risk-benefit must be considered. Although peak concentrations of 10 to 15 mcg per ml have been measured in breast milk

Continued on next page

Carnrick—Cont.

1 to 2 hours following maternal ingestion of a single 650-mg dose, neither acetaminophen nor its metabolites were detected in the urine of the nursing infants. The half-life in breast milk is 1.35 to 3.5 hours.
Caution should be exercised when PHRENILIN® or PHRENILIN® FORTE is administered to a nursing woman.
Pediatric Use: Safety and effectiveness in children below the age of 12 have not been established.
Adverse Reactions: Drowsiness, dizziness, nausea, vomiting, constipation and skin rash may occur.
Drug Abuse and Dependence: Barbiturates may be habit forming. Tolerance, psychological dependence, and physical dependence may occur especially following prolonged use of high doses of barbiturates.
The average daily dose for the barbiturate addict is usually about 1.5 grams. As tolerance to barbiturates develops, the amount needed to maintain the same level of intoxication increases; tolerance to a fatal dosage, however, does not increase more than two-fold. As this occurs, the margin between an intoxicating dosage and fatal dosage becomes smaller.
Symptoms of acute intoxication with barbiturates include unsteady gait, slurred speech, and sustained nystagmus. Mental signs of chronic intoxication include confusion, poor judgment, irritability, insomnia, and somatic complaints.
Symptoms of barbiturate dependence are similar to those of chronic alcoholism. If an individual appears to be intoxicated with alcohol to a degree that is radically disproportionate to the amount of alcohol in his or her blood the use of barbiturates should be suspected. The lethal dose of a barbiturate is far less if alcohol is also ingested.
The symptoms of barbiturate withdrawal can be severe and may cause death. Major withdrawal symptoms (convulsions and delirium) may occur within 16 hours and last up to 5 days after abrupt cessation of these drugs. Intensity of withdrawal symptoms gradually declines over a period of approximately 15 days. Individuals susceptible to barbiturate abuse and dependence include alcoholics and opiate abusers, as well as other sedative-hypnotic and amphetamine abusers.
Treatment of barbiturate dependence consists of cautious and gradual withdrawal of the drug. Barbiturate-dependent patients can be withdrawn by using a number of different withdrawal regimens. One method involves initiating treatment at the patient's regular dosage level and decreasing the daily dosage by 10 percent if tolerated by the patient.
Overdosage:
BARBITURATES:
Signs and Symptoms: The toxic dose of barbiturates varies considerably. In general, an oral dose of 1 gram of most barbiturates produces serious poisoning in an adult. Death commonly occurs after 2 to 10 grams of ingested barbiturate. Barbiturate intoxication may be confused with alcoholism, bromide intoxication, and with various neurological disorders.
Acute overdosage with barbiturates is manifested by CNS and respiratory depression which may progress to Cheyne-Stokes respiration, areflexia, constriction of the pupils to a slight degree (though in severe poisoning they may show paralytic dilation), oliguria, tachycardia, hypotension, lowered body temperature, and coma. Typical shock syndrome (apnea, circulatory collapse, respiratory arrest, and death) may occur.
In extreme overdose, all electrical activity in the brain may cease, in which case a "flat" EEG normally equated with clinical death cannot be accepted. This effect is fully reversible unless hypoxic damage occurs. Consideration should be given to the possibility of barbiturate intoxication even in situations that appear to involve trauma.
Complications such as pneumonia, pulmonary edema, cardiac arrhythmias, congestive heart failure, and renal failure may occur. Uremia may increase CNS sensitivity to barbiturates if renal function is impaired. Differential diagnosis should include hypoglycemia, head trauma, cerebrovascular accidents, convulsive states, and diabetic coma.
Treatment: Treatment of barbiturate overdosage is mainly supportive and consists of the following:
1. Maintenance of an adequate airway, with assisted respiration and oxygen administration as necessary. 2. Monitoring of vital signs and fluid balance. 3. If the patient is conscious and has not lost the gag reflex, emesis may be induced with ipecac. Care should be taken to prevent pulmonary aspiration of vomitus. After completion of vomiting, 30 grams activated charcoal in a glass of water may be administered. 4. If emesis is contraindicated, gastric lavage may be performed with a cuffed endotracheal tube in place with the patient in the face down position. Activated charcoal may be left in the emptied stomach and a saline cathartic administered. 5. Fluid therapy and other standard treatment for shock, if needed. 6. If renal function is normal, forced diuresis may aid in the elimination of the barbiturate. Alkalinization of the urine increases renal excretion of some barbiturates. 7. Although not recommended as a routine procedure, hemodialysis may be used in severe barbiturate intoxications or if the patient is anuric or in shock. 8. Patient should be rolled from side to side every 30 minutes. 9. Antibiotics should be given if pneumonia is suspected. 10. Appropriate nursing care to prevent hypostatic pneumonia, decubiti, aspiration, and other complications of patients with altered states of consciousness.
ACETAMINOPHEN:
Signs and Symptoms: Acetaminophen in massive overdosage may cause hepatic toxicity in some patients. In all cases of suspected overdose, immediately call your regional poison center or the Rocky Mountain Poison Center's toll-free number (800-525-6115) for assistance in diagnosis and for directions in the use of N-acetylcysteine as an antidote, a use currently restricted to investigational status.
In adults, hepatic toxicity has rarely been reported with acute overdoses of less than 10 grams and fatalities with less than 15 grams. Importantly, young children seem to be more resistant than adults to the hepatotoxic effect of an acetaminophen overdose. Despite this, the measures outlined below should be initiated in any adult or child suspected of having ingested an acetaminophen overdose.
Early symptoms following a potentially hepatotoxic overdose may include: nausea, vomiting, diaphoresis, and general malaise. Clinical and laboratory evidence of hepatic toxicity may not be apparent until 48 to 72 hours post-ingestion.
Treatment: The stomach should be emptied promptly by lavage or by induction of emesis with syrup of ipecac. Patients' estimates of the quantity of a drug ingested are notoriously unreliable. Therefore, if an acetaminophen overdose is suspected, a serum acetaminophen assay should be obtained as early as possible, but no sooner than four hours following ingestion. Liver function studies should be obtained initially and repeated at 24-hour intervals.
The antidote, N-acetylcysteine, should be administered as early as possible, and within 16 hours of the overdose ingestion for optimal results. Following recovery, there are no residual, structural or functional hepatic abnormalities.
Dosage and Administration:
PHRENILIN®: One or two tablets every four hours. Total daily dosage should not exceed six tablets.
PHRENILIN® FORTE: One capsule every 4-6 hours. Total daily dosage should not exceed three capsules.
How Supplied:
PHRENILIN®: Pale violet scored tablets with the letter 'C' on one side and 8650 on the other, in bottles of 100 (NDC 0086-0050-10).
PHRENILIN® FORTE: Amethyst, opaque capsules imprinted with the letter 'C' and 8656, in bottles of 100 (NDC 0086-0056-10).
Manufactured for Carnrick Laboratories, Inc.
(11/82)
[*Shown in Product Identification Section*]

PROPAGEST™ and PROGAGEST™ SYRUP
(Phenylpropanolamine HCl)

Description:
PROPAGEST™—Each tablet contains:
Phenylpropanolamine HCl .... 25 mg.
PROPAGEST™ SYRUP —Each 5 ml. (one teaspoonful) contains:
Phenylpropanolamine HCl .... 12.5 mg.
Indications: For the temporary relief of nasal congestion associated with the common cold, sinusitis, hay fever or other upper respiratory allergies.
Dosage:
PROPAGEST™
Adult oral dosage is one tablet every 4 hours not to exceed 6 tablets in 24 hours. Children 6 to under 12 years oral dosage is one-half tablet every 4 hours not to exceed 3 tablets in 24 hours. Children 2 to under 6 years, use PROPAGEST™ SYRUP.
PROPAGEST™ SYRUP
Indicated dosage may be given every 4 hours. Do not exceed 6 doses in 24 hours.
Adult oral dosage ....2 teaspoonfuls
Children 6 to under 12 years
oral dosage ....1 teaspoonful
Children 2 to under 6 years
oral dosage ....½ teaspoonful
For children under 2 years, there is no recommended dosage except under the advice and supervision of a physician.
Warnings: Do not exceed recommended dosage because at higher doses nervousness, dizziness, sleeplessness, rapid pulse or high blood pressure may occur.
If symptoms do not improve within 7 days or are accompanied by high fever, consult a physician before continuing use. Do not take this product if you have high blood pressure, heart disease, diabetes or thyroid disease except under the advice and supervision of a physician.
DRUG INTERACTION PRECAUTION: Do not take this product if you are presently taking a prescription antihypertensive or antidepressant drug containing a monoamine oxidase inhibitor except under the advice and supervision of a physician.
Consult your physician if pregnant or nursing or taking other medication.
Our labeling states:
KEEP THIS AND ALL MEDICATION OUT OF THE REACH OF CHILDREN.
In case of accidental overdose, seek professional assistance or contact a Poison Control Center immediately.
Keep tightly closed away from light and store at room temperature.
How Supplied: PROPAGEST™—White, oval scored tablets containing 25 mg. phenylpropanolamine HCl in bottles of 100. (NDC 0086-0051-10)
PROPAGEST™ SYRUP —Orange-flavored, colorless, syrup containing 12.5 mg. phenylpropanolamine HCl per 5 ml. in bottles of 16 fluid ounces (NDC 0086-0053-16) and in bottles of 4 fluid ounces (NDC 0086-0053-04).
Manufactured for Carnrick Laboratories, Inc.
[*Shown in Product Identification Section*]

SINULIN®

Description: Each tablet contains: phenylpropanolamine HCl 37.5 mg., chlorpheniramine maleate 2 mg., acetaminophen 325 mg., salicylamide 250 mg., homatropine methylbromide 0.75 mg.
Indications: For relief of sinus congestion and headache.
Warning: Not to be used by persons with high blood pressure, diabetes, heart or thyroid disease, glaucoma or excessive pressure within the eye. Elderly persons and children under 12 use only as directed by a physician. As with any drug, if you are pregnant or nursing a baby, seek professional advice before using this product.
Precaution: If drowsiness occurs, do not drive a car or operate machinery. Discontinue use if rapid pulse, dizziness or blurring of vision occurs. If dryness of mouth occurs reduce dosage. Not for frequent or prolonged use. If eye pain occurs, discontinue and see your physician immediately as this can indicate glaucoma.
Overdosage: In case of accidental overdose, seek professional assistance or contact a poison control center immediately.
Dosage: Adults: 1 tablet every 4 hours. Not more than 4 tablets daily. If symptoms persist for more than 10 days consult physician.
How Supplied: Peach color, scored tablets inscribed with 8625 on one side and C logo on the other. Bottles of 20 (NDC 0086-0250-02), 7 boxes of 24 blisters (NDC 0086-0250-24) and Bottles of 100 (NDC 0086-0250-10).
Manufactured for Carnrick Laboratories, Inc.
[*Shown in Product Identification Section*]

Center Laboratories
Division of EM Industries, Inc.
35 CHANNEL DRIVE
PORT WASHINGTON, NY 11050

EPIPEN® ℞
Epinephrine Auto-Injector

Description: EpiPen provides epinephrine for intramuscular auto-injection in a sterile solution prepared from epinephrine with the aid of hydrochloric acid in pyrogen-free water. The EpiPen Auto-Injector contains 2 ml Epinephrine Injection 1:1,000, and is designed to deliver a dose of 0.3 ml. Each ml contains: Active: 1.00 mg epinephrine. Inactive: 6.00 mg sodium chloride, 1.67 mg sodium bisulfite, and hydrochloric acid to adjust pH.
Actions: Epinephrine is a sympathomimetic drug, acting on both alpha and beta receptors. It is the drug of choice for the emergency treatment of severe allergic reactions such as the sting of Hymenoptera insects: bees, wasps, hornets, and yellow jackets. The strong vasoconstrictor action of epinephrine acts quickly to counter vasodilation and resulting increased capillary permeability. By its effect on smooth muscle, epinephrine relaxes the bronchioles, thereby relieving wheezing and dyspnea. Its action also relieves angioedema or hives.
Indications: Epinephrine is indicated in the emergency treatment of anaphylactic reactions to insect stings. The EpiPen Auto-Injector is intended for immediate self-administration by individuals with a history of hypersensitivity to insect stings. It is designed as emergency supportive therapy only and is not a replacement or substitute for subsequent medical or hospital care, nor is it intended to supplant conventional insect venom hyposensitization.
Contraindications: Epinephrine is contraindicated in individuals with organic brain damage.
Warnings: Epinephrine is sensitive to light and heat. Store in a cool dark place. Before using, check EpiPen to make sure solution in Auto-Injector is not brown in color. If it is discolored or contains a precipitate, do not use. Every effort should be made to avoid possible inadvertent intravascular administration through appropriate selection of an injection site such as the thigh or deltoid. Do not inject into buttock.
Large doses or accidental intravenous injection of epinephrine may result in cerebral hemorrhage due to sharp rise in blood pressure. Rapidly acting vasodilators can counteract the marked pressor effects of epinephrine. Epinephrine should be administered with extreme caution to patients who have developed degenerative heart disease. Use of epinephrine with drugs that sensitize the heart to arrhythmias is not recommended. Anginal pain may be induced by epinephrine in patients with coronary insufficiency.
Precautions: The effects of epinephrine may be potentiated by tricyclic antidepressants; certain antihistamines, e.g., diphenhydramine, tripelennamine, d-chlorpheniramine; and sodium 1-thyroxine.
Administer with caution to hyperthyroid individuals; psychoneurotic individuals, individuals with cardiovascular disease, hypertension, or diabetes, elderly individuals, pregnant women, and children under 6 years of age.
Adverse Reactions: Transient and minor side effects of epinephrine include palpitation, respiratory difficulty, pallor, dizziness, weakness, tremor, headache, throbbing, restlessness, tenseness, anxiety and fear.
Ventricular arrhythmias may follow administration of epinephrine.
Dosage and Administration: A physician who prescribes EpiPen should take appropriate steps to insure that his patient understands the indications and use of this device thoroughly. The physician should review with the patient, in detail, the package insert and operation of the EpiPen Auto-Injector. Inject the delivered dose of the EpiPen Auto-Injector (0.3ml Epinephrine Injection, 1:1,000) intramuscularly into the anteriolateral aspect of the thigh or the deltoid region of the arm.
Caution: Federal (U.S.A.) law prohibits dispensing without a prescription.

Central Pharmaceuticals, Inc.
SEYMOUR, IN 47274

CODICLEAR DH Syrup Ⓒ ℞

A clear, colorless, sweet-tasting syrup for oral administration, which is alcohol-free, sugar-free and dye-free.
Each teaspoonful (5 ml.) contains:
Hydrocodone bitartrate ....5 mg.
(Warning - May be habit forming)
Potassium guaiacolsulfonate ....300 mg.
Indications: For the temporary relief of dry, nonproductive cough due to colds, pertussis or influenza.
Contraindications: Hypersensitivity to any of the ingredients.
Warnings: Hydrocodone can produce drug dependence and therefore has the potential for being abused. Codiclear DH should be prescribed and administered with the degree of caution appropriate for this type product.
Precautions:
General: The hydrocodone in this product may exhibit additive effects with other CNS depressants, including alcohol. Respiratory depression can be a real hazard so caution should be used, especially in patients with chronic obstructive pulmonary disease.
Information for Patients: The hydrocodone may cause drowsiness and ambulatory patients who operate machinery or motor vehicles should be cautioned accordingly.
Drug Interactions: Concommitant use of hydrocodone with alcohol and/or other CNS depressants may have an additive effect.
Pregnancy: The safety of use of this product in pregnancy has not been established.
Adverse Reactions: Adverse reactions include drowsiness, lassitude, nausea, giddiness, constipation, respiratory depression and addiction.
Overdosage: Symptoms of overdosage include respiratory depression, extreme somnolence progressing to stupor or coma, skeletal muscle flaccidity, cold and clammy skin and other symptoms common with narcotic overdosage.
Primary treatment consists of insuring adequate respiration through provision of a patent airway and the institution of assisted or controlled ventilation. Naloxone hydrochloride should be administered in small intravenous doses (consult specific product labeling before use). In addition, oxygen, intravenous fluids, vasopressors and other supportive measures should be employed as indicated. Gastric emptying may be useful in removing unabsorbed drug. Activated charcoal may also be of benefit.
Dosage and Administration: Adults and older children–1 to 1½ teaspoonfuls; children, 6 to 12 years of age–½ to 1 teaspoonful; children, 3 to 6 years of age–¼ to ½ teaspoonful. These doses may be given four times daily as needed. Not recommended for children under 3 years of age.
How Supplied:
Bottles of 4 fl. oz.–NDC 0131-5034-64
Bottles of 1 pint–NDC 0131-5034-70

CODIMAL® DH Ⓒ ℞
CODIMAL® DM
CODIMAL® PH Ⓒ
CODIMAL® EXPECTORANT

Composition: Each teaspoonful (5 ml) of CODIMAL DH contains: Hydrocodone Bitartrate 1.66 mg. (Warning—May be habit forming); Phenylephrine Hydrochloride 5.0 mg.; Pyrilamine Maleate 8.33 mg.
Each teaspoonful (5 ml) of CODIMAL DM contains: Dextromethorphan hydrobromide 10 mg.; Phenylephrine hydrochloride 5 mg.; Pyrilamine maleate 8.33 mg.; Alcohol 4%. Sugar-free.
Each teaspoonful (5 ml) of CODIMAL PH contains: Codeine Phosphate 10 mg. (Warning —May be habit forming); Phenylephrine Hydrochloride 5 mg.; Pyrilamine Maleate 8.33 mg.
Each teaspoonful (5 ml) of CODIMAL EXPECTORANT contains: Phenylpropanolamine Hydrochloride 25 mg.; Guaifenesin 100 mg.
Indications: For temporary relief of cough due to the common cold or other upper respiratory infection or irritation.
Contraindications: In persons with a known hypersensitivity to any of the ingredients.
Precautions: Should be administered with extreme caution to patients with hypertension, heart disease, diabetes, thyroid disease or vascular disease, or those receiving MAO inhibitors. Codeine and its derivative, Hydrocodone Bitartrate, are narcotic agents and the usual precautions in their use should be observed, particularly in infants and elderly patients.
Side Effects: Occasional drowsiness, blurred vision, palpitation, flushing, nervousness or gastrointestinal upsets.
Warnings: Patients should be instructed not to drive or operate machinery while taking the medication; and not to administer it to patients with a high fever or persistent cough unless so directed by a physician.
Administration and Dosage: Codimal DH, Codimal DM and Codimal PH: Adults and older children—1 to 2 teaspoonfuls; children 6 to 12—1 teaspoonful; children 2 to 6—½ teaspoonful. These doses may be taken every 4

Continued on next page

Central—Cont.

hours. Children 6 months to 2 years—¼ teaspoonful every 6 hours.
Codimal Expectorant: Adults and older children—1 teaspoonful; children, 6 to 12 years—½ teaspoonful; children, 2 to 6—¼ teaspoonful. This dose may be taken every four hours.
How Supplied: Bottles of 4 ounces, pints and gallons.

CODIMAL®-L.A. CENULES® ℞

Description: Each Cenule® (Timed Release Capsule) contains:
Chlorpheniramine maleate .... 8 mg.
Pseudoephedrine hydrochloride .... 120 mg.
in a specially prepared base to provide prolonged action.
Indications: For the temporary relief of symptoms of the common cold, allergic rhinitis (hay fever) and sinusitis.
Contraindications: Hypersensitivity to any of the ingredients. Also contraindicated in patients with severe hypertension, severe coronary artery disease, patients on MAO inhibitor therapy, patients with narrow-angle glaucoma, urinary retention, peptic ulcer and during an asthmatic attack.
Should not be used in children under 12 years or in nursing mothers.
Warnings: Considerable caution should be exercised in patients with hypertension, diabetes mellitus, ischemic heart disease, hyperthyroidism, increased intraocular pressure and prostatic hypertrophy. The elderly (60 years or older) are more likely to exhibit adverse reactions.
Antihistamines may cause excitability, especially in children. At dosages higher than the recommended dose, nervousness, dizziness or sleeplessness may occur.
Precautions:
General: Caution should be exercised in patients with high blood pressure, heart disease, diabetes or thyroid disease. The antihistamine in this product may exhibit additive effects with other CNS depressants, including alcohol.
Information for Patients: Antihistamine may cause drowsiness and ambulatory patients who operate machinery or motor vehicles should be cautioned accordingly.
Drug Interactions: MAO inhibitors and beta adrenergic blockers increase the effects of sympathomimetics. Sympathomimetics may reduce the antihypertensive effects of methyldopa, mecamylamine, reserpine and veratrum alkaloids. Concomitant use of antihistamines with alcohol and other CNS depressants may have an additive effect.
Pregnancy: The safety of use of this product in pregnancy has not been established.
Adverse Reactions: Adverse reactions include drowsiness, lassitude, nausea, giddiness, dryness of mouth, blurred vision, cardiac palpitations, flushing, increased irritability or excitement (especially in children).
Dosage and Administration: Adults and children over 12 years of age—1 capsule orally every 12 hours.
How Supplied:
Bottle of 100 Cenules® NDC 0131-4213-37
Bottle of 1000 Cenules® NDC 0131-4213-43
[*Shown in Product Identification Section*]

CO-XAN® SYRUP Ⓒ ℞

Each tablespoonful (15 ml) contains:
Theophylline .... 165 mg.
(as 330 mg. theophylline sodium glycinate)
Codeine phosphate .... 15 mg.
(WARNING—May be habit forming)
Ephedrine hydrochloride .... 25 mg.
Guaifenesin .... 100 mg.
Alcohol 10 %

How Supplied:
Pint NDC 0131-5145-70
Gallon NDC 0131-5145-72

DI-GESIC™ Ⓒ ℞

Each tablet contains:
Hydrocodone bitartrate .... 5 mg.
(WARNING—May be habit forming)
Aspirin .... 230 mg.
Acetaminophen .... 150 mg.
Caffeine .... 30 mg.
Indications: For the relief of moderate to moderately severe pain.
Contraindications: Hypersensitivity to any of the ingredients; intracranial lesion associated with increased intracranial pressure; status asthmaticus; liver disease.
Warnings: At high doses or in sensitive patients, hydrocodone may produce dose-related respiratory depression and/or elevated cerebrospinal fluid pressure. Extreme care should be used in the presence of head injury or other intracranial lesions. The administration of narcotics may obscure the diagnosis or clinical course of patients with acute abdominal conditions.
Ambulatory patients: hydrocodone, like other narcotics, may impair the mental and/or physical abilities required for the performance of potentially hazardous tasks, such as driving a car or operating machinery; patients should be cautioned accordingly.
Precautions: General: As with any narcotic, analgesic agent, DI-GESIC should be used with caution in elderly or debilitated patients and those with conditions where the respiratory depression or CNS depression will cause additional risks. Examples are severe impairment of hepatic or renal function, hypothyroidism and pulmonary disease. Salicylates should be used with extreme caution in the presence of peptic ulcer or coagulation abnormalities.
Pregnancy: Safe use in pregnancy has not been established relative to potential adverse effects on fetal development. Therefore, this product should not be used in pregnant women, unless in the judgment of the physician, the potential benefits outweigh the possible hazards.
Nursing Mothers: As a general rule, nursing should not be undertaken when a patient is receiving this product, since it may be present in the milk of the nursing mothers.
Pediatric Use: Safety and effectiveness in children have not been established.
Adverse Reactions: Adverse reactions include light headedness, dizziness, sedation, nausea and vomiting, euphoria, dysphoria, constipation, skin rash and pruritus.
Drug Abuse and Dependence: This product is a Schedule III Controlled Substance. Because of the hydrocodone content, some abuse might be expected. Psychic dependence, physical dependence and tolerance may develop upon repeated administration. It should be prescribed and administered with caution. However, psychic dependence is unlikely to develop when DI-GESIC tablets are used for a short time for the treatment of pain. Physical dependence, the condition in which continued administration of the drug is required to prevent the appearance of a withdrawal syndrome, assumes clinically significant proportions only after several weeks of continued narcotic use, although some mild degree of physical dependence may develop after a few days of narcotic therapy.
Overdosage: Serious overdose with hydrocodone is characterized by respiratory depression (a decrease in respiratory rate and/or tidal volume, cheyne-stokes respiration, cyanosis), extreme somnolence progressing to stupor or coma, skeletal muscle flaccidity, cold and clammy skin, and sometimes, bradycardia and hypotension. In severe overdosage, apnea, circulatory collapse, cardiac arrest and death may occur.
Treatment: Primary attention should be given to the reestablishment of adequate respiratory exchange through provision of a patent airway and the institution of assisted or controlled ventilation. The narcotic antagonist, naloxone, is the treatment of choice against respiratory depression. Therefore, an appropriate dose of naloxone (see package insert) should be administered, preferably by the intravenous route, and simultaneously with efforts at respiratory resuscitation. Since the duration of action of hydrocodone may exceed that of the antagonist, the patient should be kept under continued surveillance and repeated doses of the antagonist should be administered as needed to maintain adequate respiration.
An antagonist should not be administered in the absence of clinically significant respiratory or cardiovascular depression. Oxygen, intravenous fluids, vasopressors and other supportive measures should be employed as indicated.
Gastric emptying may be useful in removing unabsorbed drug.
Dosage and Administration: Adults—One or two tablets every four to six hours as needed for pain. Dosage should be adjusted according to the severity of the pain and the response of the patient. Total dosage should be limited to eight tablets in 24 hours.
How Supplied: Flat, truncated oval, bisected white tablets inscribed with the Central logo on one side and the number 31 and the score on the other side.
Bottles of 100 tablets—NDC 0131-2310-37
Bottles of 1000 tablets—NDC 0131-2310-43
[*Shown in Product Identification Section*]

NEOLAX® TABLETS ℞

Description: Each NEOLAX Tablet contains: Dehydrocholic Acid 240 mg. and Docusate sodium 50 mg.
Clinical Pharmacology: The actions of NEOLAX are the result of the combination of complementary activities of its ingredients. Dehydrocholic acid, the oxidation product of cholic acid, is a potent hydrocholeretic. It is a mild laxative that has shown very low toxicity in both experimental animals and in clinical use. The mechanism by which dehydrocholic acid increases the frequency of bowel movements is unknown. Docusate sodium affects the surface tension and increases the water content of the stool, making it softer and, therefore, easier to pass. This softening, combined with the laxative effect of dehydrocholic acid, alleviates both of these symptoms of constipation.
Indications: A mild laxative and fecal softener as an aid in the treatment of chronic functional constipation, particularly in the elderly.
Contraindications: Biliary tract obstruction, acute hepatitis, or sensitivity to any of its ingredients.
Precautions: Patients should be examined periodically to prevent fluid and electrolyte deficiencies due to excessive laxative effects or inadequate intake.
Administration and Dosage: One or two tablets three times daily with meals. This dosage should be reduced as the condition is relieved.
How Supplied:
Bottles of 100 NDC 0131-2187-37
Bottles of 1000 NDC 0131-2187-43
Unit Dose Pkg. of 100 NDC 0131-2187-86

NIFEREX® Tablets/Elixir
NIFEREX®-150 Capsules
NIFEREX® with Vitamin C Tablets
(polysaccharide-iron complex)

Composition: NIFEREX is a highly water-soluble complex of iron and a low molecular weight polysaccharide. Each NIFEREX-150

Capsule contains 150 mg. elemental iron. Each NIFEREX Film Coated Tablet and each NIFEREX with Vitamin C Chewable Tablet contains 50 mg. elemental iron. In addition, each NIFEREX with Vitamin C tablet contains Ascorbic acid, U.S.P., 100 mg. and Sodium ascorbate, 168.75 mg. Each 5 ml. (teaspoonful) NIFEREX Elixir contains 100 mg. elemental iron, alcohol 10% (sugar free).

Action and Uses: NIFEREX is an easily assimilated source of iron for treatment of uncomplicated iron deficiency anemia. Because NIFEREX is a polysaccharide bound iron complex, it is relatively nontoxic and there are relatively few, if any, of the gastrointestinal side effects associated with iron therapy, thus permitting full therapeutic dosage (150 to 300 mg. elemental iron daily) in a single dose if desirable. There is no staining of teeth and no metallic aftertaste.

Indications: For treatment of uncomplicated iron deficiency anemia.

Contraindications: In patients with hemochromatosis and hemosiderosis, and in those with a known hypersensitivity to any of the ingredients.

Administration and Dosage: ADULTS: One or two NIFEREX-150 Capsules daily, or one or two NIFEREX or NIFEREX with Vitamin C Tablets twice daily, *or* one or two teaspoonfuls NIFEREX Elixir daily. CHILDREN 6 to 12 years of age: One or two NIFEREX *or* one NIFEREX with Vitamin C Tablet daily, or one teaspoonful NIFEREX Elixir daily; Children 2 to 6 years of age: ½ teaspoonful NIFEREX Elixir daily. Children under 2 years: ¼ teaspoonful daily.

How Supplied: NIFEREX-150 Capsules: Bottles of 100 and 1,000. NIFEREX Elixir: Bottles of 8 ounces and one gallon. NIFEREX Tablets: Bottles of 100 and 1,000. NIFEREX with Vitamin C Chewable Tablets: Bottles of 50.

[*Shown in Product Identification Section*]

NIFEREX®-150 FORTE Capsules ℞
NIFEREX® FORTE Elixir ℞

Each capsule Niferex®-150 Forte contains:
Iron (Elemental) ....150 mg.
(as polysaccharide-iron complex)
Folic Acid ....1 mg.
Vitamin B_{12}....................25 mcg.

Each teaspoon (5 ml) Niferex® Forte Elixir contains:
Iron (Elemental) ....100 mg.
(as polysaccharide-iron complex)
Folic Acid ....1 mg.
Vitamin B_{12}....................25 mcg.
Alcohol 10%
Sugar-Free

Indications: Iron deficiency anemia and/or nutritional megaloblastic anemias due to inadequate diet.

Warnings: Folic acid alone is improper therapy in the treatment of pernicious anemia and other megaloblastic anemias where vitamin B_{12} is deficient.

Precaution: Folic acid, especially in doses above 0.1 mg. daily, may obscure pernicious anemia, in that hematologic remission may occur while neurological manifestations remain progressive.

Adverse Reactions: Allergic sensitization has been reported following both oral and parenteral administration of folic acid.

Dosage And Administration: Adults: One capsule or one teaspoonful daily. Children: 6 to 12 yrs.—1 teaspoonful daily; 2 to 6 yrs.—½ teaspoonful daily; under 2 yrs.—¼ teaspoonful daily.

How Supplied:
NIFEREX-150 FORTE CAPSULES

Bottle of 100	NDC 0131-4330-37
Bottle of 1000	NDC 0131-4330-43

NIFEREX FORTE ELIXIR

Bottle of 4 fl. oz.	NDC 0131-5065-64

[*Capsules Shown in Product Identification Section*]

NIFEREX®—PN TABLETS ℞
(MODIFIED FORMULA)

Description: Each film-coated tablet for oral administration contains:
Iron (Elemental) ....60 mg.
(as polysaccharide-iron complex)
Folic acid ....1 mg.
Ascorbic acid ....50 mg.
(as sodium ascorbate)
Cyanocobalamin (Vitamin B_{12}) ....3 mcg.
Vitamin A ....4000 I.U.
Vitamin D_2....................400 I.U.
Thiamine mononitrate ....3 mg.
Riboflavin ....3 mg.
Pyridoxine hydrochloride ....2 mg.
Niacinamide ....10 mg.
Calcium carbonate ....312 mg.
Zinc sulfate USP ....80 mg.
(as 50 mg. dried zinc sulfate)

Indications: For the prevention and/or treatment of dietary vitamin and mineral deficiencies associated with pregnancy and lactation.

Contraindications: Hypersensitivity to any of the ingredients.

Warnings: Folic acid alone is improper therapy in the treatment of pernicious anemia and other megaloblastic anemias where vitamin B_{12} is deficient.

Precautions: Folic acid, especially in doses above 0.1 mg. daily may obscure pernicious anemia, in that hematologic remission may occur while neurological manifestations remain progressive.

Adverse Reactions: Allergic sensitization has been reported following both oral and parenteral administration of folic acid.

Dosage and Administration: One tablet daily or as prescribed by a physician.

How Supplied:
Bottles of 100 tablets–NDC 0131-2209-37
Bottles of 1000 tablets–NDC 0131-2209-43

[*Shown in Product Identification Section*]

SYNOPHYLATE® Tablets/Elixir ℞
(theophylline sodium glycinate)
SYNOPHYLATE®-GG Tablets/Syrup ℞
(theophylline sodium glycinate and guaifenesin)

SYNOPHYLATE (theophylline sodium glycinate) Elixir or Tablets contain per tbsp. (15 ml.) or per tablet: theophylline sodium glycinate, 330 mg. (equivalent to 165 mg. theophylline). (Alcohol 20% in the elixir).

SYNOPHYLATE-GG Syrup or Tablets contain per tbsp. (15 ml.) or per tablet: theophylline sodium glycinate, 300 mg. (equivalent to 150 mg. theophylline); guaifenesin 100 mg. (Alcohol 10% in the syrup).

How Supplied:

SYNOPHYLATE TABLETS	
100	**NDC** 0131-2251-37
1000	**NDC** 0131-2251-43
SYNOPHYLATE ELIXIR	
Pint	**NDC** 0131-5089-70
Gallon	**NDC** 0131-5089-72
SYNOPHYLATE-GG TABLETS	
100	**NDC** 0131-2253-37
1000	**NDC** 0131-2253-43
SYNOPHYLATE-GG SYRUP	
Pint	**NDC** 0131-5092-70
Gallon	**NDC** 0131-5092-72

THEOCLEAR® L.A.-130 CENULES® ℞
THEOCLEAR® L.A.-260 CENULES® ℞
THEOCLEAR®-80 Syrup ℞
(theophylline anhydrous)

Description: THEOCLEAR L.A. 130 and THEOCLEAR L.A.-260: Each Cenule® contains 130 mg. or 260 mg. of theophylline anhydrous in a sustained release bead formulation. **THEOCLEAR-80:** Each 15 ml. (1 tablespoonful) contains 80 mg. Anhydrous Theophylline as the active ingredient. Other ingredients are saccharin sodium; tartaric acid; benzoic acid; citric acid; sorbitol; glycerin; propylene glycol; artificial flavor and purified water q.s. This formulation provides an alcohol-free, dye-free, and sugar-free vehicle containing no corn byproducts.

Indications: For relief and/or prevention of symptoms from asthma and reversible bronchospasm associated with chronic bronchitis and emphysema.

Contraindications: In individuals who have shown hypersensitivity to any of its components.

Warnings: Status asthmaticus is a medical emergency. Optimal therapy frequently requires additional medication including corticosteroids when the patient is not rapidly responsive to bronchodilators.

Excessive theophylline doses may be associated with toxicity thus serum theophylline levels are recommended to assure maximal benefit without excessive risk. Incidence of toxicity increases at levels greater than 20 mcg/ml. Morphine, curare, and stilbamidine should be used with caution in patients with airflow obstruction since they stimulate histamine release and can induce asthmatic attacks. They may also suppress respiration leading to respiratory failure. Alternative drugs should be chosen whenever possible.

There is an excellent correlation between high blood levels of theophylline resulting from conventional doses and associated clinical manifestations of toxicity in (1) patients with lowered body plasma clearances (due to transient cardiac decomposition), (2) patients with liver dysfunction or chronic obstructive lung disease, (3) patients who are older than 55 years of age, particularly males.

There are often no early signs of less serious theophylline toxicity such as nausea and restlessness, which may appear in up to 50 percent of patients prior to onset of convulsions. Ventricular arrhythmias or seizures may be the first signs of toxicity.

Many patients who have higher theophylline serum levels exhibit a tachycardia.

Theophylline products may worsen pre-existing arrhythmias.

Usage in Pregnancy: Safe use in pregnancy has not been established relative to possible adverse effects on fetal development, but neither have adverse effects on fetal development been established. This is, unfortunately, true for most antiasthmatic medications. Therefore, use of theophylline in pregnant women should be balanced against the risk of uncontrolled asthma.

Precautions: Mean half-life in smokers is shorter than non-smokers, therefore, smokers may require larger doses of theophylline. Theophylline should not be administered concurrently with other xanthine medications. Use with caution in patients with severe cardiac disease, severe hypoxemia, hypertension, hyperthyroidism, acute myocardial injury, cor pulmonale, congestive heart failure, liver disease, and in the elderly (especially males) and in neonates. Great caution should especially be used in giving theophylline to patients in congestive heart failure. Such patients have shown markedly prolonged theophylline blood level curves with theophylline persisting in serum for long periods following discontinuation of the drug.

Use theophylline cautiously in patients with history of peptic ulcer. Theophylline may occasionally act as a local irritant to G.I. tract although gastrointestinal symptoms are more commonly central and associated with serum concentrations over 20 mcg/ml.

Adverse Reactions: The most consistent adverse reactions are usually due to overdose and are:

1. Gastrointestinal: nausea, vomiting, epigastric pain, hematemesis, diarrhea.

Continued on next page

Central—Cont.

2. Central nervous system: headaches, irritability, restlessness, insomnia, reflex hyperexcitability, muscle twitching, clonic and tonic generalized convulsions.
3. Cardiovascular: palpitation, tachycardia, extra systoles, flushing, hypotension, circulatory failure, life threatening ventricular arrhythmias.
4. Respiratory: tachypnea.
5. Renal: albuminuria, increased excretion of renal tubular cells and red blood cells; potentiation of diuresis.
6. Others: hyperglycemia and inappropriate ADH syndrome.

Dosage and Administration: Therapeutic serum levels associated with optimal likelihood for benefit and minimal risk of toxicity are considered to be between 10 mcg/ml and 20 mcg/ml. Levels above 20 mcg/ml may produce toxic effects. There is great variation from patient to patient in dosage needed in order to achieve a therapeutic blood level because of variable rates of elimination. Because of this wide variation from patient to patient, and the relatively narrow therapeutic blood level range, dosage must be individualized and monitoring of theophylline serum levels is highly recommended.

Dosage should be calculated on the basis of lean (ideal) body weight where mg/kg doses are stated. Theophylline does not distribute into fatty tissue.

Giving theophylline with food may prevent the rare case of stomach irritation; and though absorption may be slower, it is still complete. When rapidly absorbed products such as solutions are used, dosing to maintain "around the clock" blood levels generally requires administration every 6 hours to obtain the greatest efficacy for clinical use in children; dosing intervals up to 8 hours may be satisfactory for adults because of their slower elimination. Children, and adults requiring higher than average doses, may benefit from products with slower absorption which may allow longer dosing intervals and/or less fluctuation in serum concentration over a dosing interval during chronic therapy.

[See table below].

The loading dose for theophylline will be based on the principle that each .5 mg/kg of theophylline administered as a loading dose will result in a 1 mcg/ml increase in serum theophylline concentration. Ideally, then, the loading dose should be deferred if a serum theophylline concentration can be rapidly obtained. If this is not possible, the clinician must exercise his judgment in selecting a dose based on the potential for benefit and risk. When there is sufficient respiratory distress to warrant a small risk, 2.5 mg/kg of theophylline is likely to increase the serum concentration when administered as a loading dose in rapidly absorbed form by only about 5 mcg/ml. If the patient is not already experiencing theophylline toxicity, this is unlikely to result in dangerous adverse effects.

Subsequent to the modified decision regarding loading dose in this group of patients, the subsequent maintenance dosage recommendations are the same as those described above.

Comments: To achieve optimal therapeutic theophylline dosage, it is recommended to monitor serum theophylline concentrations. However, it is not always possible or practical to obtain a serum theophylline level.

Patients should be closely monitored for signs of toxicity. The present data suggest that the above dosage recommendations will achieve therapeutic serum concentrations with minimal risk of toxicity for most patients. However, some risk of toxic serum concentrations is still present.

Adverse reactions to theophylline often occur when serum theophylline levels exceed 20 mcg/ml.

Chronic Asthma:

Theophyllinization is a treatment of first choice for the management of chronic asthma (to prevent symptoms and maintain patent airways). Slow clinical titration is generally preferred to assure acceptance and safety of the medication.

Initial dose: 16 mg/kg/day or 400 mg/day (whichever is lower) in 3–4 divided doses at 6–8 hour intervals. (520 mg/day in 1–2 divided doses at 12 hour intervals for sustained release formulations.)

Increased dose: The above dosage may be increased in approximately 25 percent increments at 2–3 day intervals so long as no intolerance is observed, until the maximum indicated below is reached.

Maximum dose without measurement of serum concentrations:

Not to exceed the following: (WARNING: DO NOT ATTEMPT TO MAINTAIN ANY DOSE THAT IS NOT TOLERATED)

Age < 9 years - 24 mg/kg/day
Age 9–12 years - 20 mg/kg/day
Age 12–16 years - 18 mg/kg/day
Age > 16 years - 13 mg/kg/day or 900 mg/day (WHICHEVER IS LESS)

Note: Use ideal body weight for obese patients.

Measurement of serum theophylline concentration during chronic therapy:

If the above maximum doses are to be maintained or exceeded, serum theophylline measurement is recommended. This should be obtained at the approximate time of peak absorption during chronic therapy for the product used (1–2 hours for liquids, 3–5 hours for sustained release preparations). It is important that the patient will have missed no doses during the previous 48 hours and that dosing intervals will have been reasonably typical with no added doses during that period of time. DOSAGE ADJUSTMENT BASED ON SERUM THEOPHYLLINE MEASUREMENTS WHEN THESE INSTRUCTIONS HAVE NOT BEEN FOLLOWED MAY RESULT IN RECOMMENDATIONS THAT PRESENT RISK OF TOXICITY TO THE PATIENT.

How Supplied:

THEOCLEAR L.A.-260 CENULES
Bottle of 100 NDC 0131-4248-37
Bottle of 1000 NDC 0131-4248-43
THEOCLEAR L.A.-130 CENULES
Bottle of 100 NDC 0131-4247-37
Bottle of 1000 NDC 0131-4247-43
THEOCLEAR-80 SYRUP
One Pint NDC 0131-5098-70
One Gallon NDC 0131-5098-72

[*Shown in Product Identification Section*]

DOSAGE FOR PATIENT POPULATION
Acute Symptoms of Asthma Requiring Rapid Theophyllinization:
I. Not currently receiving theophylline products

GROUP	ORAL LOADING DOSE (THEOPHYLLINE)	MAINTENANCE DOSE FOR NEXT 12 HOURS (THEOPHYLLINE)	MAINTENANCE DOSE BEYOND 12 HOURS (THEOPHYLLINE)
1. Children 6 months to 9 years	6 mg/kg	4 mg/kg q4h	4 mg/kg q6h
2. Children age 9-16 and smoking young adults	6 mg/kg	3 mg/kg q4h	3 mg/kg q6h
3. Otherwise healthy nonsmoking adults	6 mg/kg	3 mg/kg q6h	3 mg/kg q8h
4. Older adults and patients with cor pulmonale	6 mg/kg	2 mg/kg q6h	2 mg/kg q8h
5. Patients with congestive heart failure, liver failure	6 mg/kg	2 mg/kg q8h	1-2 mg/kg q12h

II. Those currently receiving theophylline products: Determine, where possible, the time, amount, route of administration and form of the patient's last dose.

Cetylite Industries, Inc.

P.O. BOX CN6
9051 RIVER ROAD
PENNSAUKEN, NJ 08110

CETACAINE® ℞
TOPICAL ANESTHETIC

A BRAND OF
Benzocaine 14.0%
Butyl Aminobenzoate 2.0%
Tetracaine Hydrochloride 2.0%
Benzalkonium Chloride 0.5%
Cetyl Dimethyl Ethyl Ammonium Bromide 0.005%
In a bland water soluble base.

Action: Cetacaine produces anesthesia rapidly in approximately 30 seconds.

Indications: Cetacaine is a topical anesthetic indicated for the production of anesthesia of accessible mucous membrane.

Cetacaine Spray is indicated for use to control pain or gagging. Cetacaine in all forms is indicated for use to control pain.

Dosage and Administration: Cetacaine Spray should be applied for approximately one second or less for normal anesthesia. Only limited quantity of Cetacaine is required for anesthesia and a spray in excess of 2 seconds is contraindicated. Average expulsion rate of residue from spray, at normal temperatures, is 200 mg. per second.

Tissue need not be dried prior to application of Cetacaine.

Cetacaine should be applied directly to the site where pain control is required.

Cetacaine Liquid or Cetacaine Ointment may be applied with a cotton pledget or directly to tissue. Cotton pledget should not be held in position for extended periods of time, since local reactions to benzoate topical anesthetics are related to the length of time of application.

Adverse Reactions: Although systemic reactions to Cetacaine have not been reported, local reactions to benzoate topical anesthetics may be associated with the condition of the mucous membrane treated and the length of time of application. Dehydration of the epithehum or a slight escharotic effect may result from prolonged contact. Allergic reactions are known to occur in some patients with preparations containing benzocaine.

Usage in Pregnancy: Safe use of Cetacaine has not been established with respect to possible adverse effects upon fetal development. Therefore Cetacaine should not be used during early pregnancy, unless in the judgment of a physician the potential benefits outweigh the unknown hazards.

Routine precaution for the use of any topical anesthetic should be observed when Cetacaine is used.

Contraindications:
Cetacaine is not for injection.
Do not use in the eyes.
To avoid excessive systemic absorption, Cetacaine should not be applied to large areas of denuded or inflamed tissue.
Cetacaine should not be administered to patients who are hypersensitive to any of its ingredients.
Individual dosage of tetracaine hydrochloride in excess of 20 mg. is contraindicated. Cetacaine should not be used under dentures or cotton rolls, as retention of the active ingredients under a denture or cotton roll could possibly cause a slight escharotic effect.
Jetco Cannula: The Jetco cannula for Cetacaine Spray is specially designed for accessibility and application of Cetacaine, at the required site of pain control.
The Jetco cannula is supplied in various sizes and shapes.
The Jetco cannula is inserted firmly onto the protruding plastic tubing on each bottle of Cetacaine Spray.
The Jetco cannula may be removed and reinserted as many times as required for cleansing or sterilization.
Packaging Available:
Aerosol Spray 56 gm., including propellant.
Liquid 56 gm. bottle.
Ointment, flavored, 37 gram jar.
Hospital Gel, 29 grams in polyethylene tube.
Caution: Federal law prohibits dispensing Cetacaine without prescription.
Keep out of reach of children.

CETYLCIDE® SOLUTION

Composition:

Cetyl Dimethyl Ethyl Ammonium Bromide	6.5%
Benzalkonium Chloride U.S.P.	6.5%
Isopropyl Alcohol	13.0%
Inert Ingredients	74.0%

Formulation contains Sodium Nitrite
Indications and Uses: Cetylcide is for use in the chemical disinfection of dental and surgical instruments. Cetylcide, when diluted, is a potent germicidal solution combining high bactericidal and bacteriostatic action against most kinds of pathogenic bacteria.
Germicides containing a Quarternary Ammonium derivative should not be relied upon to destroy spore bearing organisms, mycobacterium tuberculosis or the etiologic agent of viral hepatitis. Thus, instruments suspected of such contamination should be sterilized by heat. Needles, hypodermic syringes, corroded instruments or those with deep narrow crevices, as well as hinged or defective plated instruments, should be sterilized by heat. To maintain disinfection they may then be immersed in Cetylcide Solution.
How Supplied: 10 cc ampules, 32 ounce bottles, and 16 ounce bottles.

Important Notice

Before prescribing or administering any product described in PHYSICIANS' DESK REFERENCE always consult the PDR Supplement for possible new or revised information.

CIBA Pharmaceutical Company

Division of CIBA-GEIGY Corporation
SUMMIT, NJ 07901

To provide a convenient and accurate means of identifying CIBA solid dosage form products, a code number has been imprinted on all tablets and capsules. To help you quickly identify a CIBA Tablet or Capsule by its code number, a numerical listing of codes (with corresponding product names) and an alphabetical listing of products (with corresponding codes and list numbers) have been compiled below.

CIBA Code #	ALPHABETICAL LISTING	List Number
	Antrenyl® bromide	
	(oxyphenonium bromide)	
15	TABLETS, 5 mg (white, scored)	
	100s	2410
	Anturane®	
	(sulfinpyrazone USP)	
41	TABLETS (white, single-scored) each containing 100 mg sulfinpyrazone USP	
	100s	1910
168	CAPSULES (green) each containing 200 mg sulfinpyrazone USP	
	100s	1920
	Apresazide®	
	(hydralazine HCl and hydrochlorothiazide)	
139	CAPSULES 25/25 (light blue and white opaque), each containing 25 mg hydralazine HCl and 25 mg hydrochlorothiazide	
	100s	3131
149	CAPSULES 50/50 (pink and white opaque), each containing 50 mg hydralazine HCl and 50 mg hydrochlorothiazide	
	100s	3132
159	CAPSULES 100/50 (pink flesh and white opaque), each containing 100 mg hydralazine HCl and 50 mg hydrochlorothiazide	
	100s	3133
	Apresoline® hydrochloride	
	(hydralazine hydrochloride USP)	
37	TABLETS, 10 mg (pale yellow, dry-coated)	
	100s	2629
	1000s	2627
	Consumer Pack 100s	2603
39	TABLETS, 25 mg (deep blue, dry-coated)	
	100s	2611
	500s	2613
	1000s	2615
	Accu-Pak® 100s	2647
	Consumer Pack 100s	2606
73	TABLETS, 50 mg (light blue, dry-coated	
	100s	2619
	500s	2621
	1000s	2623
	Accu-Pak® 100s	2648
	Consumer Pack 100s	2643
101	TABLETS, 100 mg (peach, dry-coated)	
	100s	2638
	Apresoline®-Esidrix®	
	(hydralazine hydrochloride and hydrochlorothiazide)	
129	TABLETS (orange, dry-coated), each containing 25 mg hydralazine hydrochloride and 15 mg hydrochlorothiazide	
	100s	3120
	Cytadren®	
	(aminoglutethamide)	
24	TABLETS-250 mg (white, round, scored into quarters)	
	100s	2120
	Esidrix®	
	(hydrochlorothiazide USP)	
22	TABLETS, 25 mg (pink, scored)	
	100s	4310
	1000s	4313
	Accu-Pak® 100s	4312
	Consumer Pack 100s	4325
46	TABLETS, 50 mg (yellow, scored)	
	100s	4315
	1000s	4318
	Accu-Pak® 100s	4317
	Consumer Pack 30s	4328
	60s	4331
	100s	4330
192	TABLETS, 100 mg (blue, scored)	
	100s	4340
	Esimil®	
47	TABLETS (white, scored), each containing 10 mg guanethidine monosulfate and 25 mg hydrochlorothiazide	
	100s	4503
	Consumer Pack 100s	4512
	Ismelin® sulfate	
	(guanethidine monosulfate)	
49	TABLETS, 10 mg (pale yellow, scored)	
	100s	5010
	1000s	5012
	Consumer Pack 100s	5003
103	TABLETS, 25 mg (white, scored)	
	100s	5020
	1000s	5022
	Consumer Pack 100s	5026
	Lithobid®	
	(lithium carbonate)	
65	TABLETS, 300 mg (peach colored)	
	100s	0210
	1000s	0220
	Accu-Pak® 100s	0230
	Ludiomil®	
	(maprotiline hydrochloride)	
110	TABLETS, 25 mg (oval, dark orange, coated)	
	100s	1710
	Accu-Pak® 100s	1714
26	TABLETS, 50 mg (round, dark orange, coated)	
	100s	1720
	Accu-Pak® 100s	1721
135	TABLETS, 75 mg (oval, white, coated)	
	100s	1730
	Accu-Pak® 100s	1732
	Metandren®	
	(methyltestosterone USP)	
30	TABLETS, 10 mg (white, scored)	
	100s	1414
32	TABLETS, 25 mg (pale yellow, scored)	
	100s	1418
51	LINGUETS®, 5 mg (white)	
	100s	1432
64	LINGUETS®, 10 mg (yellow)	
	100s	1438
	Metopirone®	
	(metyrapone USP)	
130	TABLETS, 250 mg (white, scored)	
	18s	5403

Continued on next page

The full prescribing information for each CIBA drug is contained herein and is that in effect as of October 1, 1982.

CIBA—Cont.

Regitine® hydrochloride
(phentolamine hydrochloride USP)
152 TABLETS, 50 mg (white, scored)
100s 6814

Rimactane®
(rifampin USP)
154 CAPSULES, 300 mg (opaque scarlet and caramel)
30s 8903
60s 8904
100s 8901

Rimactane®/INH Dual Pack
(rifampin USP) (isoniazid USP)
8912 Each Dual Pack contains two Rimactane 300-mg CAPSULES and one INH 300-mg TABLET 8912

Ritalin® hydrochloride ©
(methylphenidate hydrochloride USP)
07 TABLETS, 5 mg (yellow)
100s 7410
500s 7412
1000s 7414
03 TABLETS, 10 mg (pale green, scored)
100s 7416
500s 7418
1000s 7420
Accu-Pak® 100s 7415
34 TABLETS, 20 mg (pale yellow, scored)
100s 7422
1000s 7426

Ritalin-SR®©
(methylphenidate hydrochloride) sustained-release tablets
16 TABLETS, 20 mg (round, white, scored)
100s 7442

Ser-Ap-Es®
71 TABLETS (light salmon pink, dry-coated), each containing 0.1 mg reserpine, 25 mg hydralazine hydrochloride and 15 mg hydrochlorothiazide
100s 6610
1000s 6612
Accu-Pak® 100s 6605
Consumer Pack
100s 6617

Serpasil®
(reserpine USP)
35 TABLETS, 0.1 mg (white)
100s 7610
1000s 7614
36 TABLETS, 0.25 mg (white, scored)
100s 7616
500s 7618
1000s 7620
Consumer Pack
100s 7607

Serpasil®-Apresoline®
(reserpine and hydralazine hydrochloride)
40 TABLETS #1 (yellow, dry-coated), each containing 0.1 mg reserpine and 25 mg hydralazine hydrochloride
100s 7721
104 TABLETS #2 (yellow, dry-coated), each containing 0.2 mg reserpine and 50 mg hydralazine hydrochloride
100s 7709

Serpasil®-Esidrix®
(reserpine and hydrochlorothiazide)
13 TABLETS #1 (light orange), each containing 0.1 mg reserpine and 25 mg hydrochlorothiazide
100s 7010
1000s 7012
97 TABLETS #2 (light orange), each containing 0.1 mg reserpine and 50 mg hydrochlorothiazide
100s 7020
1000s 7022

Slow-K®
(potassium chloride)
165 TABLETS (pale orange, sugar-coated), each containing 8 mEq (600 mg) potassium chloride
100s 2807
1000s 2811
Accu-Pak®
100s 2817
Consumer Pack
100s 2815

CIBA Code # NUMERICAL LISTING

Ritalin® hydrochloride ©
(methylphenidate hydrochloride USP)
03 TABLETS, 10 mg (pale green, scored)
07 TABLETS, 5 mg (yellow)

Serpasil®-Esidrix®
(reserpine and hydrochlorothiazide)
13 TABLETS #1 (light orange), each containing 0.1 mg reserpine and 25 mg hydrochlorothiazide

Antrenyl® bromide
(oxyphenonium bromide)
15 TABLETS, 5 mg (white, scored)

Ritalin-SR®
(methylphenidate hydrochloride) sustained-release tablets
16 TABLETS, 20 mg (round, white, scored)

Esidrix®
(hydrochlorothiazide USP)
22 TABLETS, 25 mg (pink, scored)

Cytadren®
(aminoglutethamide)
24 TABLETS, 250 mg (white, round, scored into quarters)

Ludiomil®
(maprotiline hydrochloride)
26 TABLETS, 50 mg (round, dark orange, coated)

Metandren®
(methyltestosterone USP)
30 TABLETS, 10 mg (white, scored)

Metandren®
(methyltestosterone USP)
32 TABLETS, 25 mg (pale yellow, scored)

Ritalin® hydrochloride ©
(methylphenidate hydrochloride USP)
34 TABLETS, 20 mg (pale yellow, scored)

Serpasil®
(reserpine USP)
35 TABLETS, 0.1 mg (white)
36 TABLETS, 0.25 mg (white, scored)

Apresoline® hydrochloride
(hydralazine hydrochloride USP)
37 TABLETS, 10 mg (pale yellow, dry-coated)
39 TABLETS, 25 mg (deep blue, dry-coated)

Serpasil®-Apresoline®
(reserpine and hydralazine hydrochloride)
40 TABLETS #1 (yellow, dry-coated), each containing 0.1 mg reserpine and 25 mg hydralazine hydrochloride

Anturane®
(sulfinpyrazone USP)
41 TABLETS (white, single-scored) each containing 100 mg sulfinpyrazone USP

Esidrix®
(hydrochlorothiazide USP)
46 TABLETS, 50 mg (yellow, scored)

Esimil®
47 TABLETS (white, scored), each containing 10 mg guanethidine monosulfate and 25 mg hydrochlorothiazide

Ismelin® sulfate
(guanethidine monosulfate)
49 TABLETS, 10 mg (pale yellow, scored)

Metandren®
(methyltestosterone USP)
51 LINGUETS®, 5 mg (white)

Metandren®
(methyltestosterone USP)
64 LINGUETS®, 10 mg (yellow)

Lithobid®
(lithium carbonate)
65 TABLETS, 300 mg (peach colored)

Ser-Ap-Es®
71 TABLETS (light salmon pink, dry-coated), each containing 0.1 mg reserpine, 25 mg hydralazine hydrochloride and 15 mg hydrochlorothiazide

Apresoline® hydrochloride
(hydralazine hydrochloride USP)
73 TABLETS, 50 mg (light blue, dry-coated)

Serpasil®-Esidrix®
(reserpine and hydrochlorothiazide)
97 TABLETS #2 (light orange), each containing 0.1 mg reserpine and 50 mg hydrochlorothiazide

Apresoline® hydrochloride
(hydralazine hydrochloride USP)
101 TABLETS, 100 mg (peach, dry-coated)

Ismelin® sulfate
(guanethidine monosulfate)
103 TABLETS, 25 mg (white, scored)

Serpasil®-Apresoline®
(reserpine and hydralazine hydrochloride)
104 TABLETS #2 (yellow, dry-coated), each containing 0.2 mg reserpine and 50 mg hydralazine hydrochloride

Ludiomil®
(maprotiline hydrochloride)
110 TABLETS, 25 mg (oval, dark orange coated)

Apresoline®-Esidrix®
(hydralazine hydrochloride and hydrochlorothiazide)
129 TABLETS (orange, dry-coated), each containing 25 mg hydralazine hydrochloride and 15 mg hydrochlorothiazide

Metopirone®
(metyrapone USP)
130 TABLETS, 250 mg (white, scored)

Apresazide®
(hydralazine HCl and hydrochlorothiazide)

Ludiomil®
(maprotiline hydrochloride)
135 TABLETS, 75 mg (oval, white, coated)
139 CAPSULES 25/25 (light blue and white opaque), each containing 25 mg hydralazine hydrochloride and 25 mg hydrochlorothiazide
149 CAPSULES 50/50 (pink and white opaque), each containing 50 mg hydralazine hydrochloride and 50 mg hydrochlorothiazide

Regitine® hydrochloride
(phentolamine hydrochloride USP)
152 TABLETS, 50 mg (white, scored)

Rimactane®
(rifampin USP)
154 CAPSULES, 300 mg (opaque scarlet and caramel)

Rimactane®/INH Dual Pack
(rifampin USP) (isoniazid USP)
8912 Each Dual Pack contains two Rimactane 300-mg CAPSULES and one INH 300-mg TABLET

Apresazide®
(hydralazine HCl and hydrochlorothiazide)
159 CAPSULES 100/50 (pink flesh and white opaque), each containing 100 mg hydralazine hydrochloride and 50 mg hydrochlorothiazide
Slow-K®
(potassium chloride)
165 TABLETS (pale orange, sugar-coated), each containing 8 mEq (600 mg) potassium chloride
Anturane®
(sulfinpyrazone USP)
168 CAPSULES (green) each containing 200 mg sulfinpyrazone USP
Esidrix®
(hydrochlorothiazide USP)
192 TABLETS, 100 mg (blue, scored)

ANTRENYL® bromide ℞
(oxyphenonium bromide)

Indications: Peptic Ulcer, as adjunctive therapy.
Contraindications: Glaucoma; obstructive uropathy (for example, bladder neck obstruction due to prostatic hypertrophy); obstructive disease of the gastrointestinal tract (as in achalasia, paralytic ileus, pyloroduodenal stenosis, etc.); intestinal atony of the elderly or debilitated patient; unstable cardiovascular status in acute hemorrhage; severe ulcerative colitis; toxic megacolon complicating ulcerative colitis; myasthenia gravis; hypersensitivity.
Warnings: In the presence of a high environmental temperature, heat prostration can occur with drug use (fever and heat stroke due to decreased sweating).
Diarrhea may be an early symptom of incomplete intestinal obstruction, especially in patients with ileostomy or colostomy. In this instance, treatment with Antrenyl would be inappropriate and possibly harmful.
Anticholinergics may produce drowsiness or blurred vision. Therefore, patients should be warned not to engage in activities requiring mental alertness (such as operating a motor vehicle or other machinery) or perform hazardous work while taking Antrenyl.
Usage in Pregnancy
The safe use of this drug in pregnant women or during lactation has not been established. Therefore, the benefits must be weighed against the potential hazards.
Precautions: Give cautiously to patients with autonomic neuropathy; hepatic or renal disease; early evidence of ileus (as in peritonitis); ulcerative colitis (large doses may suppress intestinal motility to the point of producing a paralytic ileus and the use of anticholinergics may precipitate or aggravate the serious complication of toxic megacolon); hyperthyroidism; coronary heart disease; congestive heart failure; cardiac arrhythmias; hypertension; nonobstructing prostatic hypertrophy; hiatal hernia associated with reflux esophagitis, since anticholinergic drugs may aggravate this condition.
It should be noted that the use of anticholinergic drugs in the treatment of gastric ulcer may produce a delay in gastric emptying time and may complicate such therapy (antral stasis). Do not rely on the use of Antrenyl in the presence of biliary tract disease. Investigate any tachycardia before giving anticholinergic (atropine-like) drugs, since they may increase the heart rate.
With overdosage, a curare-like action may occur.
Use cautiously in debilitated patients with chronic lung disease, because reduction in bronchial secretions can lead to inspissation and formation of bronchial plugs. All anticholinergic agents should be used with caution in patients over 40 years of age because of the increased incidence of glaucoma in this age group.
Adverse Reactions: Anticholinergics produce certain effects which may be physiologic or toxic, depending upon the individual patient's response. The physician must delineate these. Adverse reactions may include xerostomia; urinary hesitancy and retention; blurred vision; tachycardia; palpitations; mydriasis; dilatation of the pupil; cycloplegia; increased ocular tension; loss of taste; headaches; nervousness; drowsiness; weakness; dizziness; insomnia; nausea; vomiting; impotence; suppression of lactation; constipation; bloated feeling; severe allergic reaction or drug idiosyncrasies, including anaphylaxis, urticaria, and other dermal manifestation; some degree of mental confusion and/or excitement, especially in elderly persons.
Decreased sweating is another adverse reaction that may occur. It should be noted that adrenergic innervation of the eccrine sweat glands on the palms and soles make complete control of sweating impossible. An end point of complete anhidrosis cannot occur because large doses of drug would be required, and this would produce severe side effects from parasympathetic paralysis.
Dosage and Administration: Average adult dosage is 10 mg (2 tablets) 4 times daily for several days. Dosage may then be reduced, depending on patient's response.
Not for use in children.
Overdosage: Treatment is the same as for atropine overdosage. Gastric lavage or, in the absence of coma, an emetic should be given, and activated charcoal slurry instilled into the stomach. If central nervous system excitation occurs, a short-acting barbiturate may be used. Avoid long-acting sedatives; the central depressive action of these agents may coincide with depression produced by oxyphenonium in later stages. Fever may be combated with ice bags, alcohol sponges, and other appropriate measures.
How Supplied: *Tablets,* 5 mg (white, scored); bottles of 100. C77-16 Rev. 3/77
[*Shown in Product Identification Section*]

ANTURANE® ℞
(sulfinpyrazone USP)
Tablets Capsules

Indications: Anturane is indicated for the treatment of:
1. Chronic gouty arthritis
2. Intermittent gouty arthritis

Contraindications: Patients with an active peptic ulcer or symptoms of gastrointestinal inflammation or ulceration should not receive the drug.
The drug is contraindicated in patients with a history or the presence of:
1. Hypersensitivity to phenylbutazone or other pyrazoles
2. Blood dyscrasias

Warnings: Studies on the teratogenicity of pyrazole compounds in animals have yielded inconclusive results. Up to the present time, however, there have been no reported cases of human congenital malformation proved to be due to the use of the drug.
It is suggested that Anturane be used with caution in pregnant women, weighing the potential risks against the possible benefits.
Precautions: As with all pyrazole compounds, patients receiving Anturane should be kept under close medical supervision and periodic blood counts are recommended. It may be administered with care to patients with a history of healed peptic ulcer.
Recent reports have indicated that Anturane potentiates the action of certain sulfonamides, such as sulfadiazine and sulfisoxazole. In addition, other pyrazole compounds (phenylbutazone) have been observed to potentiate the hypoglycemic sulfonylurea agents, as well as insulin. In view of these observations, it is suggested that Anturane be used with caution in conjunction with sulfa drugs, the sulfonylurea hypoglycemic agents and insulin.
Because Anturane is a potent uricosuric agent, it may precipitate urolithiasis and renal colic, especially in the initial stages of therapy. For this reason, an adequate fluid intake and alkalinization of the urine are recommended. In cases with significant renal impairment, periodic assessment of renal function is indicated. Occasional cases of renal failure have been reported; but a cause-and-effect relationship has not always been clearly established.
Salicylates antagonize the uricosuric action of Anturane and for this reason their concomitant use is contraindicated in gouty arthritis.
Anturane may accentuate the action of coumarin-type anticoagulants and further depress prothrombin activity when these medications are employed simultaneously.
Note: Anturane has minimal anti-inflammatory effect and is not intended for the relief of an acute attack of gout.
In the initial stages of therapy, because of the marked ability of Anturane to mobilize urates, acute attacks of gouty arthritis may be precipitated.
Adverse Reactions: The most frequently reported adverse reactions with Anturane have been upper gastrointestinal disturbances. In these patients it is advisable to administer the drug with food, milk, or antacids. Despite this precaution, Anturane may aggravate or reactivate peptic ulcer.
Rash has been reported. In most instances, this reaction did not necessitate discontinuance of therapy. In general, Anturane has not been observed to affect electrolyte balance.
Blood dyscrasias (anemia, leukopenia, agranulocytosis, thrombocytopenia and aplastic anemia) have rarely been reported. There has also been a published report associating Anturane, administered concomitantly with other drugs including colchicine, with leukemia following long-term treatment of patients with gout. However, the circumstances involved in the two cases reported are such that a cause-and-effect relationship to Anturane has not been clearly established.
Overdosage:
Symptoms: Nausea, vomiting, diarrhea, epigastric pain, ataxia, labored respiration, convulsions, coma. Possible symptoms, seen after overdosage with other pyrazolone derivatives: anemia, jaundice, ulceration.
Treatment: No specific antidote. Induce emesis; gastric lavage; supportive treatment (intravenous glucose infusions, analeptics).
Dosage and Administration:
Initial: 200–400 mg daily in two divided doses, with meals or milk, gradually increasing when necessary to full maintenance dosage in one week.
Maintenance:
400 mg daily, given in two divided doses, as above. This dosage may be increased to 800 mg daily, if necessary, and may sometimes be reduced to as low as 200 mg daily after the blood urate level has been controlled. Treatment should be continued without interruption even in the presence of acute exacerbations, which can be concomitantly treated with phenylbutazone or colchicine. Patients previously controlled with other uricosuric therapy may be transferred to Anturane at full maintenance dosage.
How Supplied: White, single-scored tablets of 100 mg, bottles of 100 (NDC 0083-0041-30). Green capsules of 200 mg, bottles of 100 (NDC 0083-0168-30).
Dispense in tight container (USP).
C80-24 (1/81)
[*Shown in Product Identification Section*]

The full prescribing information for each CIBA drug is contained herein and is that in effect as of October 1, 1982.

Continued on next page

CIBA—Cont.

APRESAZIDE® ℞
(hydralazine HCl and hydrochlorothiazide)
25/25 Capsules
50/50 Capsules
100/50 Capsules

> **Warning**
> This fixed combination drug is not indicated for initial therapy of hypertension. Hypertension requires therapy titrated to the individual patient. If the fixed combination represents the dosage so determined, its use may be more convenient in patient management. The treatment of hypertension is not static, but must be reevaluated as conditions in each patient warrant.

Indications
Hypertension. (See box warning.)

Contraindications
Hydralazine
Hypersensitivity to hydralazine; coronary artery disease; and mitral valvular rheumatic heart disease.
Hydrochlorothiazide
Anuria; hypersensitivity to this or other sulfonamide-derived drugs.

Warnings
Hydralazine
Hydralazine may produce in a few patients a clinical picture simulating systemic lupus erythematosus. In such patients hydralazine should be discontinued unless the benefit-to-risk determination requires continued antihypertensive therapy with this drug. Symptoms and signs usually regress when the drug is discontinued but residua have been detected many years later. Long-term treatment with steroids may be necessary.
Complete blood counts, L.E. cell preparations, and antinuclear antibody titer determinations are indicated before and periodically during prolonged therapy with hydralazine even though the patient is asymptomatic. These studies are also indicated if the patient develops arthralgia, fever, chest pain, continued malaise or other unexplained signs or symptoms.
A positive antinuclear antibody titer and/or positive L.E. cell reaction requires that the physician carefully weigh the implications of the test results against the benefits to be derived from antihypertensive therapy with hydralazine.
Use MAO inhibitors with caution in patients receiving hydralazine.
When other potent parenteral antihypertensive drugs, such as diazoxide, are used in combination with hydralazine, patients should be continuously observed for several hours for any excessive fall in blood pressure. Profound hypotensive episodes may occur when diazoxide injection and hydralazine are used concomitantly.

Hydrochlorothiazide
Use with caution in severe renal disease. In patients with renal disease, thiazides may precipitate azotemia. Cumulative effects of the drug may develop in patients with impaired renal function.
Thiazides should be used with caution in patients with impaired hepatic function or progressive liver disease, since minor alterations of fluid and electrolyte imbalance may precipitate hepatic coma.
Thiazides may add to or potentiate the action of other antihypertensive drugs. Potentiation occurs with ganglionic or peripheral adrenergic blocking drugs.
Sensitivity reactions are more likely to occur in patients with a history of allergy or bronchial asthma.
The possibility of exacerbation or activation of systemic lupus erythematosus has been reported.

Usage in Pregnancy
Hydralazine
Animal studies indicate that hydralazine is teratogenic in mice, possibly in rabbits, and not in rats. Teratogenic effects observed were cleft palate and malformations of facial and cranial bones. Although clinical experience does not include any positive evidence of adverse effects on the human fetus, hydralazine should not be used during pregnancy unless the expected benefit clearly justifies the potential risk to the fetus.
Hydrochlorothiazide
Thiazides cross the placental barrier and appear in cord blood. The use of thiazides in pregnant women requires that the anticipated benefit be weighed against possible hazards to the fetus. These hazards include fetal or neonatal jaundice, thrombocytopenia, and possibly other adverse reactions which have occurred in the adult.
Nursing Mothers: Thiazides appear in breast milk. If the use of the drug is deemed essential, the patient should stop nursing.

Precautions
Hydralazine
Myocardial stimulation produced by hydralazine can cause anginal attacks and ECG changes of myocardial ischemia. The drug has been implicated in the production of myocardial infarction. It must, therefore, be used with caution in patients with suspected coronary artery disease.
The "hyperdynamic" circulation caused by hydralazine may accentuate specific cardiovascular inadequacies. An example is that hydralazine may increase pulmonary artery pressure in patients with mitral valvular disease. The drug may reduce the pressor responses to epinephrine. Postural hypotension may result from hydralazine but is less common than with ganglionic blocking agents. Use with caution in patients with cerebral vascular accidents.
In hypertensive patients with normal kidneys who are treated with hydralazine, there is evidence of increased renal blood flow and a maintenance of glomerular filtration rate. In some instances improved renal function has been noted where control values were below normal prior to hydralazine administration. However, as with any antihypertensive agent, hydralazine should be used with caution in patients with advanced renal damage.
Peripheral neuritis, evidenced by paresthesias, numbness, and tingling, has been observed. Published evidence suggests an antipyridoxine effect and the addition of pyridoxine to the regimen if symptoms develop.
Blood dyscrasias, consisting of reduction in hemoglobin and red cell count, leukopenia, agranulocytosis, and purpura, have been reported. If such abnormalities develop, discontinue therapy. Periodic blood counts are advised during prolonged therapy.
Hydrochlorothiazide
Periodic determination of serum electrolytes to detect possible electrolyte imbalance should be performed at appropriate intervals. All patients receiving thaizide therapy should be observed for clinical signs of fluid or electrolyte imbalance; namely, hyponatremia, hypochloremic alkalosis, and hypokalemia. Serum and urine electrolyte determinations are particularly important when the patient is vomiting excessively or receiving parenteral fluids. Medication such as digitalis may also influence serum electrolytes. Warning signs are dryness of mouth, thirst, weakness, lethargy, drowsiness, restlessness, muscle pains or cramps, muscular fatigue, hypotension, oliguria, tachycardia, and gastrointestinal disturbance such as nausea or vomiting.
Hypokalemia may develop, especially with brisk diuresis, when severe cirrhosis is present, or during concomitant use of steroids or ACTH. Interference with adequate oral intake of electrolytes will also contribute to hypokalemia. Hypokalemia can sensitize or exaggerate the response of the heart to the toxic effects of digitalis (*eg*, increased ventricular irritability).
Any chloride deficit is generally mild and usually does not require specific treatment except under extraordinary circumstances (as in liver disease or renal disease). Dilutional hyponatremia may occur in edematous patients in hot weather; appropriate therapy is water restriction rather than administration of salt, except in rare instances when the hyponatremia is life-threatening. In actual salt depletion, appropriate replacement is the therapy of choice.
Hyperuricemia may occur or frank gout may be precipitated in certain patients receiving thiazide therapy.
Insulin requirements in diabetic patients may be increased, decreased, or unchanged. Latent diabetes may become manifest during thiazide administration.
Thiazide drugs may increase the responsiveness to tubocurarine.
The antihypertensive effects of the drug may be enhanced in the postsympathectomy patient. Thiazides may decrease arterial responsiveness to norepinephrine. This diminution is not sufficient to preclude effectiveness of the pressor agent for therapeutic use.
If progressive renal impairment becomes evident, withholding or discontinuing diuretic therapy should be considered.
Thiazides may decrease serum PBI levels without signs of thyroid disturbance.
Calcium excretion is decreased by thiazides. Pathological changes in the parathyroid gland with hypercalcemia and hypophosphatemia have been observed in a few patients on prolonged thiazide therapy. The common complications of hyperparathyroidism such as renal lithiasis, bone resorption, and peptic ulceration have not been seen. Thiazides should be discontinued before carrying out tests for parathyroid function.
The Apresazide capsules (100/50) contain FD&C Yellow No. 5 (tartrazine) which may cause allergic-type reactions (including bronchial asthma) in certain susceptible individuals. Although the overall incidence of FD&C Yellow No. 5 (tartrazine) sensitivity in the general population is low, it is frequently seen in patients who also have aspirin hypersensitivity.

Adverse Reactions
Hydralazine
Adverse reactions with hydralazine are usually reversible when dosage is reduced. However, in some cases it may be necessary to discontinue the drug.
Common: Headache; palpitations; anorexia; nausea; vomiting; diarrhea; tachycardia; angina pectoris.
Less frequent: Nasal congestion; flushing; lacrimation; conjunctivitis; peripheral neuritis, evidenced by paresthesias, numbness, and tingling; edema; dizziness; tremors; muscle cramps; psychotic reactions characterized by depression, disorientation, or anxiety; hypersensitivity (including rash, urticaria, pruritus, fever, chills, arthralgia, eosinophilia, and, rarely, hepatitis); constipation; difficulty in micturition; dyspnea; paralytic ileus; lymphadenopathy; splenomegaly; blood dyscrasias, consisting of reduction in hemoglobin and red cell count, leukopenia, agranulocytosis and purpura; hypotension; paradoxical pressor response.
Hydrochlorothiazide
Gastrointestinal: Anorexia, gastric irritation, nausea, vomiting, cramping, diarrhea, constipation, jaundice (intrahepatic cholestatic), pancreatitis, sialadenitis.

Central Nervous System: Dizziness, vertigo, paresthesias, headache, xanthopsia.
Hematologic: Leukopenia, thrombocytopenia, agranulocytosis, aplastic anemia.
Cardiovascular: Orthostatic hypotension (may be potentiated by alcohol, barbiturates, or narcotics).
Hypersensitivity: Purpura, photosensitivity, rash, urticaria, necrotizing angiitis, Stevens-Johnson syndrome, and other hypersensitivity reactions.
Other: Hyperglycemia, glycosuria, hyperuricemia, muscle spasm, weakness, restlessness.
When adverse reactions are moderate or severe, thiazide dosage should be reduced or therapy withdrawn.

Dosage and Administration: As determined by individual titration (see box warning).
Usual dosage is one Apresazide Capsule twice daily, the strength depending upon individual requirement following titration. For maintenance, adjust dosage to lowest effective level. When necessary, other antihypertensives such as sympathetic inhibitors may be added gradually in reduced dosages; watch effects carefully.

How Supplied: *25/25 Capsules* (light blue and white opaque), each containing 25 mg hydralazine hydrochloride and 25 mg hydrochlorothiazide; bottles of 100.
50/50 Capsules (pink and white opaque), each containing 50 mg hydralazine hydrochloride and 50 mg hydrochlorothiazide; bottles of 100.
100/50 Capsules (pink flesh and white opaque), each containing 100 mg hydralazine hydrochloride and 50 mg hydrochlorothiazide; bottles of 100.
Dispense in tight, light-resistant container (USP).

C80-11 (1/80)

[*Shown in Product Identification Section*]

APRESOLINE® hydrochloride (hydralazine hydrochloride USP) Tablets ℞

Listed in USP, a Medicare designated compendium.

Indications: Essential hypertension, alone or as an adjunct.

Contraindications: Hypersensitivity to hydralazine; coronary artery disease; and mitral valvular rheumatic heart disease.

Warnings: Hydralazine may produce in a few patients a clinical picture simulating systemic lupus erythematosus. In such patients hydralazine should be discontinued unless the benefit-to-risk determination requires continued antihypertensive therapy with this drug. Symptoms and signs usually regress when the drug is discontinued but residua have been detected many years later. Long-term treatment with steroids may be necessary.
Complete blood counts, L. E. cell preparations, and antinuclear antibody titer determinations are indicated before and periodically during prolonged therapy with hydralazine even though the patient is asymptomatic. These studies are also indicated if the patient develops arthralgia, fever, chest pain, continued malaise or other unexplained signs or symptoms.
A positive antinuclear antibody titer and/or positive L.E. cell reaction requires that the physician carefully weigh the implications of the test results against the benefits to be derived from antihypertensive therapy with hydralazine.
Use MAO inhibitors with caution in patients receiving hydralazine.
When other potent parenteral antihypertensive drugs, such as diazoxide, are used in combination with hydralazine, patients should be continuously observed for several hours for any excessive fall in blood pressure. Profound hypotensive episodes may occur when diazoxide injection and Apresoline (hydralazine hydrochloride) are used concomitantly.

Usage in Pregnancy: Animal studies indicate that hydralazine is teratogenic in mice, possibly in rabbits, and not in rats. Teratogenic effects observed were cleft palate and malformations of facial and cranial bones. Although clinical experience does not include any positive evidence of adverse effects on the human fetus, hydralazine should not be used during pregnancy unless the expected benefit clearly justifies the potential risk to the fetus.

Precautions: Myocardial stimulation produced by Apresoline can cause anginal attacks and ECG changes of myocardial ischemia. The drug has been implicated in the production of myocardial infarction. It must, therefore, be used with caution in patients with suspected coronary artery disease.
The "hyperdynamic" circulation caused by Apresoline may accentuate specific cardiovascular inadequacies. An example is that Apresoline may increase pulmonary artery pressure in patients with mitral valvular disease. The drug may reduce the pressor responses to epinephrine. Postural hypotension may result from Apresoline, but is less common than with ganglionic blocking agents. Use with caution in patients with cerebral vascular accidents.
In hypertensive patients with normal kidneys who are treated with Apresoline, there is evidence of increased renal blood flow and a maintenance of glomerular filtration rate. In some instances improved renal function has been noted where control values were below normal prior to Apresoline administration. However, as with any antihypertensive agent, Apresoline should be used with caution in patients with advanced renal damage.
Peripheral neuritis, evidenced by paresthesias, numbness, and tingling, has been observed. Published evidence suggests an antipyridoxine effect and the addition of pyridoxine to the regimen if symptoms develop.
Blood dyscrasias, consisting of reduction in hemoglobin and red cell count, leukopenia, agranulocytosis, and purpura, have been reported. If such abnormalities develop, discontinue therapy. Periodic blood counts are advised during prolonged therapy.
The Apresoline tablets (10 and 100 mg) contain FD&C Yellow No. 5 (tartrazine) which may cause allergic-type reactions (including bronchial asthma) in certain susceptible individuals. Although the overall incidence of FD&C Yellow No. 5 (tartrazine) sensitivity in the general population is low, it is frequently seen in patients who also have aspirin hypersensitivity.

Adverse Reactions: Adverse reactions with Apresoline are usually reversible when dosage is reduced. However, in some cases it may be necessary to discontinue the drug.
Common: Headache; palpitations; anorexia; nausea; vomiting; diarrhea; tachycardia; angina pectoris.
Less Frequent: Nasal congestion; flushing; lacrimation; conjunctivitis; peripheral neuritis, evidenced by paresthesias, numbness, and tingling; edema; dizziness; tremors; muscle cramps; psychotic reactions characterized by depression, disorientation, or anxiety; hypersensitivity (including rash, urticaria, pruritus, fever, chills, arthralgia, eosinophilia, and, rarely, hepatitis); constipation; difficulty in micturition; dyspnea; paralytic ileus; lymphadenopathy; splenomegaly; blood dyscrasias, consisting of reduction in hemoglobin and red cell count, leukopenia, agranulocytosis, and purpura; hypotension; paradoxical pressor response.

Dosage and Administration
Initiate therapy in gradually increasing dosages; adjust according to individual response. Start with 10 mg 4 times daily for the first 2 to 4 days, increase to 25 mg 4 times daily for balance of first week. For second and subsequent weeks, increase dosage to 50 mg 4 times daily. For maintenance, adjust dosage to lowest effective levels.
The incidence of toxic reactions, particularly the L. E. cell syndrome, is high in the group of patients receiving large doses of Apresoline.
In a few resistant patients, up to 300 mg Apresoline daily may be required for a significant antihypertensive effect. In such cases, a lower dosage of Apresoline combined with a thiazide, reserpine, or both may be considered. However, when combining therapy, individual titration is essential to insure the lowest possible therapeutic dose of each drug.

Overdosage
Signs and Symptoms
Hypotension, tachycardia, headache and generalized skin flushing are to be expected. Myocardial ischemia and cardiac arrhythmia can develop; profound shock can occur in severe overdosage.
Treatment
Evacuate gastric contents, taking adequate precautions against aspiration and for protection of the airway; instill activated charcoal slurry, if general conditions permit. These manipulations may have to be omitted or carried out after cardiovascular status has been stabilized, since they might precipitate cardiac arrhythmias or increase the depth of shock.
Support of the cardiovascular system is of primary importance. Shock should be treated with volume expanders without resorting to use of vasopressors, if possible. If a vasopressor is required, use one that is least likely to precipitate or aggravate cardiac arrhythmia. Digitalization may be necessary. Renal function must be monitored and supported as required. No experience has been reported with extracorporeal or peritoneal dialysis.

How Supplied: *Tablets,* 10 mg (pale yellow, dry-coated); bottles of 100 and 1000. *Tablets,* 25 mg (deep blue, dry-coated) and 50 mg (light blue, dry-coated); bottles of 100, 500, 1000 and Accu-Pak® blister units of 100. *Tablets,* 100 mg (peach, dry-coated); bottles of 100.
Dispense in tight, light-resistant container (USP).

C80-15 (1/80)

[*Shown in Product Identification Section*]

APRESOLINE® hydrochloride (hydralazine hydrochloride USP) Parenteral ℞

Listed in USP, a Medicare designated compendium.

Indications
Severe essential hypertension when the drug cannot be given orally or when there is an urgent need to lower blood pressure.

Contraindications: Hypersensitivity to hydralazine; coronary artery disease; and mitral valvular rheumatic heart disease.

Warnings: Hydralazine may produce in a few patients a clinical picture simulating systemic lupus erythematosus. In such patients hydralazine should be discontinued unless the benefit-to-risk determination requires continued antihypertensive therapy with this drug. Symptoms and signs usually regress when the drug is discontinued but residua have been detected many years later. Long-term treatment with steroids may be necessary.
Complete blood counts, L. E. cell preparations, and antinuclear antibody titer determinations are indicated before and periodically during prolonged therapy with hydralazine even though the patient is asymptomatic. These studies are also indicated if the patient develops arthralgia, fever, chest pain, continued

Continued on next page

The full prescribing information for each CIBA drug is contained herein and is that in effect as of October 1, 1982.

CIBA—Cont.

malaise, or other unexplained signs or symptoms.

A positive antinuclear antibody titer and/or positive L.E. cell reaction requires that the physician carefully weigh the implications of the test results against the benefits to be derived from antihypertensive therapy with hydralazine.

Use MAO inhibitors with caution in patients receiving hydralazine.

When other potent parenteral antihypertensive drugs, such as diazoxide, are used in combination with hydralazine, patients should be continuously observed for several hours for any excessive fall in blood pressure. Profound hypotensive episodes may occur when diazoxide injection and Apresoline (hydralazine hydrochloride) are used concomitantly.

Usage in Pregnancy

Animal studies indicate that hydralazine is teratogenic in mice, possibly in rabbits, and not in rats. Teratogenic effects observed were cleft palate and malformations of facial and cranial bones. Although clinical experience does not include any positive evidence of adverse effects on the human fetus, hydralazine should not be used during pregnancy unless the expected benefit clearly justifies the potential risk to the fetus.

Precautions: Myocardial stimulation produced by Apresoline can cause anginal attacks and ECG changes of myocardial ischemia. The drug has been implicated in the production of myocardial infarction. It must, therefore, be used with caution in patients with suspected coronary artery disease.

The "hyperdynamic" circulation caused by Apresoline may accentuate specific cardiovascular inadequacies. An example is that Apresoline may increase pulmonary artery pressure in patients with mitral valvular disease. The drug may reduce the pressor responses to epinephrine. Postural hypotension may result from Apresoline, but is less common than with ganglionic blocking agents. Use with caution in patients with cerebral vascular accidents.

In hypertensive patients with normal kidneys who are treated with Apresoline, there is evidence of increased renal blood flow and a maintenance of glomerular filtration rate. In some instances improved renal function has been noted where control values were below normal prior to Apresoline administration. However, as with any antihypertensive agent, Apresoline should be used with caution in patients with advanced renal damage.

Peripheral neuritis, evidenced by paresthesias, numbness, and tingling, has been observed. Published evidence suggests an antipyridoxine effect and the addition of pyridoxine to the regimen if symptoms develop.

Blood dyscrasias, consisting of reduction in hemoglobin and red cell count, leukopenia, agranulocytosis, and purpura, have been reported. If such abnormalities develop, discontinue therapy. Periodic blood counts are advised during prolonged therapy.

Adverse Reactions: Adverse reactions with Apresoline are usually reversible when dosage is reduced. However, in some cases it may be necessary to discontinue the drug.

Common: Headache; palpitations; anorexia; nausea; vomiting; diarrhea; tachycardia; angina pectoris.

Less Frequent: Nasal congestion; flushing; lacrimation; conjunctivitis; peripheral neuritis, evidenced by paresthesias, numbness, and tingling; edema; dizziness; tremors; muscle cramps; psychotic reactions characterized by depression, disorientation, or anxiety; hypersensitivity (including rash, urticaria, pruritus, fever, chills, arthralgia, eosinophilia, and, rarely, hepatitis); constipation; difficulty in micturition; dyspnea; paralytic ileus; lymphadenopathy; splenomegaly; blood dyscrasias, consisting of reduction in hemoglobin and red cell count, leukopenia, agranulocytosis, and purpura; hypotension; paradoxical pressor response.

Dosage and Administration: When there is urgent need, therapy in the hospitalized patient may be initiated intravenously or intramuscularly. Use parenteral Apresoline only when the drug cannot be given orally. Usual dose is 20 to 40 mg, repeated as necessary. Certain patients (especially those with marked renal damage) may require a lower dose. Check blood pressure frequently. It may begin to fall within a few minutes after injection, with an average maximal decrease occurring in 10 to 80 minutes. In cases where there is a previously existing increased intracranial pressure, lowering the blood pressure may increase cerebral ischemia. Most patients can be transferred to oral Apresoline within 24 to 48 hours.

Overdosage

Signs and Symptoms

Hypotension, tachycardia, headache and generalized skin flushing are to be expected. Myocardial ischemia and cardiac arrhythmia can develop; profound shock can occur in severe overdosage.

Treatment

Support of the cardiovascular system is of primary importance. Shock should be treated with volume expanders without resorting to use of vasopressors, if possible. If a vasopressor is required, use one that is least likely to precipitate or aggravate cardiac arrhythmia. Digitalization may be necessary. Renal function must be monitored and supported as required. No experience has been reported with extracorporeal or peritoneal dialysis.

How Supplied: *Ampuls,* 1 ml, each ml containing 20 mg hydralazine hydrochloride, 0.1 ml propylene glycol with 0.065% methyl-*p*-hydroxybenzoate and 0.035% propyl-*p*-hydroxybenzoate as preservatives in water; cartons of 5. C80-42 (5/80)

APRESOLINE®-ESIDRIX® ℞

(hydralazine hydrochloride and hydrochlorothiazide)

> **Warning**
> This fixed combination drug is not indicated for initial therapy of hypertension. Hypertension requires therapy titrated to the individual patient. If the fixed combination represents the dosage so determined, its use may be more convenient in patient management. The treatment of hypertension is not static, but must be reevaluated as conditions in each patient warrant.

Indications

Hypertension. (See box warning.)

Contraindications

Hydralazine

Hypersensitivity to hydralazine; coronary artery disease; and mitral valvular rheumatic heart disease.

Hydrochlorothiazide

Anuria; hypersensitivity to this or other sulfonamide-derived drugs.

Warnings

Hydralazine

Hydralazine may produce in a few patients a clinical picture simulating systemic lupus erythematosus. In such patients hydralazine should be discontinued unless the benefit-to-risk determination requires continued antihypertensive therapy with this drug. Symptoms and signs usually regress when the drug is discontinued but residua have been detected many years later. Long-term treatment with steroids may be necessary.

Complete blood counts, L. E. cell preparations, and antinuclear antibody titer determinations are indicated before and periodically during prolonged therapy with hydralazine even though the patient is asymptomatic. These studies are also indicated if the patient develops arthralgia, fever, chest pain, continued malaise or other unexplained signs or symptoms.

A positive antinuclear antibody titer and/or positive L. E. cell reaction requires that the physician carefully weigh the implications of the test results against the benefits to be derived from antihypertensive therapy with hydralazine.

Use MAO inhibitors with caution in patients receiving hydralazine.

When other potent parenteral antihypertensive drugs, such as diazoxide, are used in combination with hydralazine, patients should be continuously observed for several hours for any excessive fall in blood pressure. Profound hypotensive episodes may occur when diazoxide injection and Apresoline (hydralazine hydrochloride) are used concomitantly.

Hydrochlorothiazide

Use with caution in severe renal disease. In patients with renal disease, thiazides may precipitate azotemia. Cumulative effects of the drug may develop in patients with impaired renal function.

Thiazides should be used with caution in patients with impaired hepatic function or progressive liver disease, since minor alterations of fluid and electrolyte imbalance may precipitate hepatic coma.

Thiazides may add to or potentiate the action of other antihypertensive drugs. Potentiation occurs with ganglionic or peripheral adrenergic blocking drugs.

Sensitivity reactions are more likely to occur in patients with a history of allergy or bronchial asthma.

The possibility of exacerbation or activation of systemic lupus erythematosus has been reported.

Usage in Pregnancy

Hydralazine

Animal studies indicate that hydralazine is teratogenic in mice, possibly in rabbits, and not in rats. Teratogenic effects observed were cleft palate and malformations of facial and cranial bones. Although clinical experience does not include any positive evidence of adverse effects on the human fetus, hydralazine should not be used during pregnancy unless the expected benefit clearly justifies the potential risk to the fetus.

Hydrochlorothiazide

Thiazides cross the placental barrier and appear in cord blood. The use of thiazides in pregnant women requires that the anticipated benefit be weighed against possible hazards to the fetus. These hazards include fetal or neonatal jaundice, thrombocytopenia, and possibly other adverse reactions which have occurred in the adult.

Nursing Mothers: Thiazides appear in breast milk. If the use of the drug is deemed essential, the patient should stop nursing.

Precautions

Hydralazine

Myocardial stimulation produced by hydralazine can cause anginal attacks and ECG changes of myocardial ischemia. The drug has been implicated in the production of myocardial infarction. It must, therefore, be used with caution in patients with suspected coronary artery disease.

The "hyperdynamic" circulation caused by hydralazine may accentuate specific cardiovascular inadequacies. An example is that hydralazine may increase pulmonary artery pressure in patients with mitral valvular disease. The drug may reduce the pressor responses to epinephrine. Postural hypotension may result from hydralazine but is less common than with ganglionic blocking agents. Use with caution in patients with cerebral vascular accidents.

In hypertensive patients with normal kidneys who are treated with hydralazine, there is evidence of increased renal blood flow and a maintenance of glomerular filtration rate. In some instances improved renal function has been noted where control values were below normal prior to hydralazine administration. However, as with any antihypertensive agent, hydralazine should be used with caution in patients with advanced renal damage.

Peripheral neuritis, evidenced by paresthesias, numbness, and tingling, has been observed. Published evidence suggests an antipyridoxine effect and the addition of pyridoxine to the regimen if symptoms develop.

Blood dyscrasias, consisting of reduction in hemoglobin and red cell count, leukopenia, agranulocytosis, and purpura, have been reported. If such abnormalities develop, discontinue therapy. Periodic blood counts are advised during prolonged therapy.

Hydrochlorothiazide

Periodic determination of serum electrolytes to detect possible electrolyte imbalance should be performed at appropriate intervals. All patients receiving thiazide therapy should be observed for clinical signs of fluid or electrolyte imbalance; namely, hyponatremia, hypochloremic alkalosis, and hypokalemia. Serum and urine electrolyte determinations are particularly important when the patient is vomiting excessively or receiving parenteral fluids. Medication such as digitalis may also influence serum electrolytes. Warning signs are dryness of mouth, thirst, weakness, lethargy, drowsiness, restlessness, muscle pains or cramps, muscular fatigue, hypotension, oliguria, tachycardia, and gastrointestinal disturbance such as nausea or vomiting.

Hypokalemia may develop, especially with brisk diuresis, when severe cirrhosis is present, or during concomitant use of steroids or ACTH. Interference with adequate oral intake of electrolytes will also contribute to hypokalemia. Hypokalemia can sensitize or exaggerate the response of the heart to the toxic effects of digitalis (*eg*, increased ventricular irritability).

Any chloride deficit is generally mild and usually does not require specific treatment except under extraordinary circumstances (as in liver disease or renal disease). Dilutional hyponatremia may occur in edematous patients in hot weather; appropriate therapy is water restriction rather than administration of salt, except in rare instances when the hyponatremia is life-threatening. In actual salt depletion, appropriate replacement is the therapy of choice.

Hyperuricemia may occur or frank gout may be precipitated in certain patients receiving thiazide therapy.

Insulin requirements in diabetic patients may be increased, decreased, or unchanged. Latent diabetes may become manifest during thiazide administration.

Thiazide drugs may increase the responsiveness to tubocurarine.

The antihypertensive effects of the drug may be enhanced in the postsympathectomy patient. Thiazides may decrease arterial responsiveness to norepinephrine. This diminution is not sufficient to preclude effectiveness of the pressor agent for therapeutic use.

If progressive renal impairment becomes evident, withholding or discontinuing diuretic therapy should be considered.

Thiazides may decrease serum PBI levels without signs of thyroid disturbance.

Calcium excretion is decreased by thiazides. Pathological changes in the parathyroid gland with hypercalcemia and hypophosphatemia have been observed in a few patients on prolonged thiazide therapy. The common complications of hyperparathyroidism such as renal lithiasis, bone resorption, and peptic ulceration have not been seen. Thiazides should be discontinued before carrying out tests for parathyroid function.

Adverse Reactions

Hydralazine

Adverse reactions with hydralazine are usually reversible when dosage is reduced. However, in some cases it may be necessary to discontinue the drug.

Common: Headache; palpitations; anorexia; nausea; vomiting; diarrhea; tachycardia; angina pectoris.

Less frequent: Nasal congestion; flushing; lacrimation; conjunctivitis; peripheral neuritis, evidenced by paresthesias, numbness, and tingling; edema; dizziness; tremors; muscle cramps; psychotic reactions characterized by depression, disorientation, or anxiety; hypersensitivity (including rash, urticaria, pruritus, fever, chills, arthralgia, eosinophilia, and, rarely, hepatitis); constipation; difficulty in micturition; dyspnea; paralytic ileus; lymphadenopathy; splenomegaly; blood dyscrasias, consisting of reduction in hemoglobin and red cell count, leukopenia, agranulocytosis and purpura; hypotension; paradoxical pressor response.

Hydrochlorothiazide

Gastrointestinal: Anorexia, gastric irritation, nausea, vomiting, cramping, diarrhea, constipation, jaundice (intrahepatic cholestatic), pancreatitis, sialadenitis.

Central Nervous System: Dizziness, vertigo, paresthesias, headache, xanthopsia.

Hematologic: Leukopenia, thrombocytopenia, agranulocytosis, aplastic anemia.

Cardiovascular: Orthostatic hypotension (may be potentiated by alcohol, barbiturates, or narcotics).

Hypersensitivity: Purpura, photosensitivity, rash, urticaria, necrotizing angiitis, Stevens-Johnson syndrome, and other hypersensitivity reactions.

Other: Hyperglycemia, glycosuria, hyperuricemia, muscle spasm, weakness, restlessness.

When adverse reactions are moderate or severe, thiazide dosage should be reduced or therapy withdrawn.

Dosage and Administration: As determined by individual titration (see box warning).

Usual dosage is 1 tablet t.i.d. (maximal dosage is 2 tablets t.i.d.). For maintenance, adjust dosage to lowest effective level.

When necessary, other antihypertensives may be added gradually in reduced dosages. When the drug is given in conjunction with ganglionic blocking agents, dosage must be reduced by at least 50% and effects should be watched carefully.

Overdosage

Hydralazine

Signs and Symptoms

Hypotension, tachycardia, headache and generalized skin flushing are to be expected. Myocardial ischemia and cardiac arrhythmia can develop; profound shock can occur in severe overdosage.

Treatment

Evacuate gastric contents, taking adequate precautions against aspiration and for protection of the airway; instill activated charcoal slurry, if general conditions permit. These manipulations may have to be omitted or carried out after cardiovascular status has been stabilized, since they might precipitate cardiac arrhythmias or increase the depth of shock.

Support of the cardiovascular system is of primary importance. Shock should be treated with volume expanders without resorting to use of vasopressors, if possible. If a vasopressor is required, use one that is least likely to precipitate or aggravate cardiac arrhythmia. Digitalization may be necessary. Renal function must be monitored and supported as required. No experience has been reported with extracorporeal or peritoneal dialysis.

Hydrochlorothiazide

Signs and Symptoms

Diuresis is to be expected; lethargy of varying degree may appear and may progress to coma within a few hours, with minimal depression of respiration and cardiovascular function and without significant serum electrolyte changes or dehydration. The mechanism of CNS depression with thiazide overdosage is unknown. GI irritation and hypermotility may occur; temporary elevation of BUN has been reported and serum electrolyte changes could occur, especially in patients with impairment of renal function.

Treatment

Evacuate gastric contents but take care to prevent aspiration, especially in the stuporous or comatose patient. GI effects are usually of short duration, but may require symptomatic treatment.

Monitor serum electrolyte levels and renal function; institute supportive measures as required individually to maintain hydration, electrolyte balance, respiration and cardiovascular-renal function.

How Supplied: *Tablets* (orange, dry-coated), each containing 25 mg hydralazine hydrochloride and 15 mg hydrochlorothiazide; bottles of 100. C78-52 (1/79)

[*Shown in Product Identification Section*]

CORAMINE® ℞

(nikethamide)
Solution
Ampuls

Description: Coramine, nikethamide, is a central nervous system (CNS) stimulant, available as an aqueous solution (25% w/w) for oral administration and in 1.5-ml ampuls for parenteral administration. Nikethamide is N,N-diethyl-3-pyridinecarboxamide.

Nikethamide is a clear, colorless to pale yellow, somewhat viscous liquid that crystallizes in the cold and melts again as the temperature rises. It has a faint, characteristic, aromatic odor and a peculiar, bitter taste. Its solutions are clear and nearly colorless and have a faint amine-like odor. Nikethamide is miscible with water, with alcohol, and with ether. Its molecular weight is 178.24.

Clinical Pharmacology: The mechanism of action of Coramine is unknown. Coramine stimulates the CNS at all levels of the cerebrospinal axis; it also acts as a respiratory and circulatory stimulant.

Coramine is generally given by the intravenous or intramuscular route, but it is absorbed from all routes of administration. Nikethamide is converted to nicotinamide and then excreted as n-methylnicotinamide.

Pharmacokinetic data in humans are not available.

Indications and Usage: Coramine is indicated for the treatment of CNS depression, respiratory depression, and circulatory failure, particularly when these are due to the effects of CNS depressant drugs.

Combined with electroshock therapy, Coramine helps restore respiration more quickly and may reduce the number of treatments required in cases of psychotic excitement.

Contraindications: Coramine is contraindicated in patients with hypersensitivity to nikethamide or related compounds.

Warnings: Coramine should not be injected intra-arterially, as arterial spasm and thrombosis may result.

Precautions:

Carcinogenesis, Mutagenesis, Impairment of Fertility

Long-term carcinogenicity studies in animals have not been conducted with Coramine.

Pregnancy Category C

Animal reproduction studies have not been conducted with Coramine. It is also not known

Continued on next page

The full prescribing information for each CIBA drug is contained herein and is that in effect as of October 1, 1982.

CIBA—Cont.

whether Coramine can cause fetal harm when administered to a pregnant woman or can affect reproduction capacity. Coramine should be given to a pregnant woman only if clearly needed.

Labor and Delivery
The effect of Coramine on labor and delivery or on the newborn is unknown.

Nursing Mothers
It is not known whether this drug is excreted in human milk. Because many drugs are excreted in human milk, caution should be exercised when Coramine is administered to a nursing woman.

Pediatric Use
Safety and effectiveness in children have not been established.

Adverse Reactions: The difference between the clinically effective dose and that producing side effects varies but is often small. The following side effects that have been reported may, in fact, be the result of overdosage.
The most common side effect is an unpleasant feeling or burning or itching, especially at the back of the nose. Occasionally, flushing or a subjective feeling of warmth, sneezing, coughing, sweating, nausea, vomiting, generalized restlessness, fearfulness, changing depth and frequency of respiration, tachycardia, elevated blood pressure, tics (especially facial), and convulsions have also been reported.

Overdosage:

Acute Toxicity
The highest known doses survived are 6,250 mg orally (17-year-old woman) and 375 mg intramuscularly (3-year-old girl).
Intravenous LD_{50} in rats: 152 mg/kg.

Signs and Symptoms
Coughing, sneezing, hyperpnea, and muscle tremors can occur. Heart rate and blood pressure may increase, although probably not markedly. With severe overdosage, as may occur with injection, generalized muscle spasm and convulsive seizures can occur.

Treatment
Treatment is usually not required, except in severe overdosage. In such cases, a short-acting barbiturate is effective in controlling the generalized muscle spasm and convulsions that may be present.
Since the oral solution is rapidly absorbed, attempts to induce emesis or to perform gastric lavage are of little value and, in the presence of paroxysmal coughing or sneezing, could result in complications from aspiration.

Dosage and Administration: Although Coramine is readily absorbed after oral, subcutaneous, or intramuscular administration, it is most effective by the intravenous route.

Parenteral

Anesthetic Overdosage. *To Shorten Narcosis:* 4 ml intravenously or intramuscularly.
To Increase Amplitude of Respiration: 2-5 ml intravenously.
To Overcome Respiratory Depression: 5-10 ml intravenously, repeated as necessary.
To Combat Respiratory Paralysis: 15 ml intravenously as the minimal initial dose, repeated as required. Other methods of resuscitation, including artificial respiration, should also be employed as indicated. If cardiac arrest is also present, 0.5-1.0 ml administered intracardially may be of some benefit.

Narcotic, Hypnotic, and Carbon Monoxide Poisoning. The initial dose is 5-10 ml intravenously, followed by 5 ml every 5 minutes for the first hour, depending on the response. Thereafter, 5-ml booster doses may be given every hour if needed or, in more serious cases, as often as every half hour. Artificial respiration, gastric lavage, oxygen, and other means of stimulation should also be employed.

Cardiac Decompensation and Coronary Occlusion. In emergencies 5-10 ml intravenously or intramuscularly may be given.

Shock. The primary treatment of shock requires oxygen and adequate solutions, including blood or plasma, for volume replacement. Given in doses of 10-15 ml intravenously or intramuscularly initially and repeated as indicated by the response, Coramine may be of value in compensating peripheral circulation until blood or plasma is available.

Acute Alcoholism. The initial dose is 5-20 ml intravenously to overcome CNS depression, repeated as necessary.

Electroshock Therapy. The recommended dose is 5 ml of Coramine diluted with an equal volume of sterile, distilled water in a 10-ml syringe and injected rapidly into an antecubital vein. The electrical stimulus is applied when the patient's face flushes and the respiratory rate increases noticeably, usually within 1 minute after injection.

Oral
For maintenance therapy, 3-5 ml of the oral solution may be given every 4-6 hours, when indicated.

HOW SUPPLIED
Available as 25% (by weight) aqueous solution.

Ampuls 1.5 ml
Cartons of 20 ....NDC 0083-3234-61

Oral Solution
Bottles of 3 fluid ounces (approx. 90 ml) NDC 0083-3234-61

Dispense in tight, light-resistant container (USP).

C82-22 (8/82)

CYTADREN® ℞
(aminoglutethimide)

Description: Cytadren is available as 250-mg tablets of aminoglutethimide for oral administration. It acts as an inhibitor of adrenal cortical steroid synthesis. The chemical name is α-(p-aminophenyl)-α-ethylglutarimide.
Empirical formula: $C_{13}H_{16}N_2O_2$. Molecular weight: 232.28. Melting point: 149°–150°C. It is very slightly soluble in water but is readily soluble in most organic solvents.

Clinical Pharmacology: Cytadren inhibits the exzymatic conversion of cholesterol to Δ^5-pregnenolone, thereby reducing the synthesis of adrenal glucocorticoids, mineralocorticoids and other steroids. Evidence suggests that aminoglutethimide acts by binding to the hemoprotein, cytochrome P_{450}, and that it may also affect other steps in the synthesis and metabolism of steroids.
In human volunteers the major portion of aminoglutethimide is excreted unchanged in the urine within 24 hours. The N-acetyl derivative of aminoglutethimide also has been found in the urine of subjects receiving the parent drug. The half-life of the drug in man is not known.
Aminoglutethimide was marketed previously as an anticonvulsant but was withdrawn from marketing for that indication in 1966 because of the effects on the adrenal gland.

Indications and Usage: Cytadren is indicated for the suppression of adrenal function in selected patients with Cushing's syndrome. Plasma cortisol levels (morning) in patients with adrenal carcinoma and ectopic ACTH-producing tumors were reduced on the average to about one-half the pretreatment levels, and in patients with adrenal hyperplasia to about two-thirds of the pretreatment levels during one to three months on Cytadren. Data available from the few patients with adrenal adenoma who were treated suggest similar reductions in plasma cortisol levels. Measurements of plasma cortisol showed reductions to at least 50% of baseline or to normal levels in one-third or more of patients studied, depending on diagnostic groups and time of measurement.
Because aminoglutethimide does not affect the underlying disease process, it has been used primarily during clinical investigations either as an interim measure until more definitive therapy such as surgery can be undertaken, or in cases where such therapy is not appropriate. Only small numbers of patients have been treated for longer than 3 months. A decreased effect or escape from a favorable effect seems to occur more frequently in pituitary dependent Cushing's syndrome, probably because of increasing ACTH levels in response to decreasing glucocorticoid levels.
Cytadren should be used only in those patients who are demonstrated to respond to it.

Contraindications: Cytadren is contraindicated in those patients with serious forms and/or more severe manifestations of hypersensitivity to glutethimide or aminoglutethimide.

Warnings: Cytadren may cause adrenal cortical hypofunction, especially under conditions of stress such as surgery, trauma, or acute illness. Patients should be carefully monitored and given hydrocortisone and mineralocorticoid supplements as indicated. Dexamethasone should not be used. (See Drug Interactions.)
Cytadren also may suppress aldosterone production by the adrenal cortex and may cause orthostatic or persistent hypotension. The blood pressure should be followed in all patients at appropriate intervals. Patients should be advised of the possible occurrence of weakness and dizziness as symptoms of hypotension, and of measures to be taken should they occur.
Cytadren can cause fetal harm when administered to a pregnant woman. In about 5000 patients in the earlier experience with the drug, two cases of pseudohermaphroditism were reported in female infants whose mothers took Cytadren and concomitant anticonvulsants. Normal pregnancies have also occurred during the administration of Cytadren. When administered to rats at doses ½ and 1¼ times the maximum human dose Cytadren caused a decrease in fetal implantation, increase in fetal deaths and a variety of teratogenic effects. The compound also caused pseudohermaphroditism in rats treated with approximately three times the highest recommended human dose. If this drug must be used during pregnancy, or if the patient becomes pregnant while taking the drug, the patient should be apprised of the potential hazard to the fetus.

Precautions:

1. *General:* This drug should be administered only by physicians familiar with its use and hazards. Therapy should be initiated in a hospital. See Dosage and Administration.
2. *Information for Patients:* Patients should be warned that drowsiness may occur and that in its presence they should not drive, operate potentially dangerous machinery, or engage in other activities with possibly harmful effects.
   Patients should also be warned of the possibility of hypotension and its symptoms (see Warnings).
3. *Laboratory Tests:* Hypothyroidism may occur in association with aminoglutethimide; hence, appropriate clinical observations should be made and laboratory studies of thyroid function performed as indicated. Supplementary thyroid hormone may be required.
   Hematologic abnormalities in patients receiving Cytadren have been reported (see Adverse Reactions). Therefore, baseline hematologic studies should be followed by periodic hematologic checks.
   Since elevations in SGOT, alkaline phosphatase, and bilirubin have been reported, appropriate clinical observations and regular laboratory studies should be performed before and during therapy.
   Serum electrolytes should be determined periodically.
4. *Drug Interactions:* Cytadren accelerates the metabolism of dexamethasone; therefore, if glucocorticoid replacement is needed, hydrocortisone should be prescribed.

5. *Carcinogenesis, Mutagenesis, Impairment of Fertility:* No mutagenesis studies or animal carcinogenicity studies have been performed. Cytadren affects fertility in female rats. (See Warnings.) Whether it does so in humans has not been determined.
6. *Pregnancy:* Pregnancy category D. See Warnings section.
7. *Pediatric Use:* Safety and effectiveness have not been established by adequate and well-controlled studies in children. See Clinical Studies section for additional information.

Adverse Reactions: Untoward effects have been reported in about two out of three patients treated with Cytadren as the only adrenal cortical suppressant for four or more weeks in Cushing's syndrome. The most frequent and reversible side effects such as drowsiness (approximately one in three), morbilliform skin rash (one in six), nausea and anorexia (each approximately one in eight) often disappear spontaneously within one or two weeks of continued therapy.

Other effects observed are:

Hematologic abnormalities: In four of 27 patients with adrenal carcinoma who were treated with Cytadren for at least four weeks, there were single occurrences of neutropenia, leukopenia (patient received o,p'DDD concomitantly), pancytopenia (5-fluorouracil also administered), and agranulocytosis. The latter two were considered by the investigators not to be related to the administration of Cytadren. One patient with adrenal hyperplasia showed decreased hemoglobin and hematocrit during the course of treatment with Cytadren. In 1214 non-Cushingoid patients, transient leukopenia, the only hematological effect, was reported once. Coombs-negative hemolytic anemia was reported in one patient. In approximately 300 patients with nonadrenal malignancy, 10 to 12 cases showed some degree of anemia and two developed pancytopenia while taking Cytadren.

Endocrine effects: Adrenal insufficiency occurred during four or more weeks of Cytadren therapy in one of thirty patients with Cushing's syndrome. This may involve the glucocorticoids as well as the mineralocorticoids. Hypothyroidism, occasionally associated with thyroid enlargement, may be detected early or confirmed by measuring the plasma levels of the thyroid hormones. Masculinization and hirsutism have occasionally occurred in females as has precocious sex development in males.

CNS effects: Headache and dizziness, possibly caused by lowered vascular resistance or orthostasis have occurred in about one in twenty patients.

Cardiovascular effects: Hypotension, occasionally orthostatic, occurred in one of thirty patients receiving Cytadren, and tachycardia in one of forty.

Gastrointestinal and liver: Vomiting occurred in one of thirty cases. Isolated instances of abnormal liver function tests have been reported. Suspected hepatotoxicity occurred in less than one in a thousand.

Skin: In addition to a rash (one in six cases and often reversible on continued therapy), pruritus was reported in one of twenty cases. These may be allergic or hypersensitivity reactions. Urticaria has occurred rarely.

Miscellaneous: Fever, possibly related to therapy, has been reported in several patients on Cytadren therapy for less than four weeks in duration and with the administration of other drugs. Myalgia occurred in one of 30 patients.

Overdosage: Intentional overdosage with aminoglutethimide has caused ataxia, sedation, and deep coma with hyperventilation and hypotension. No reports of death have been found following doses estimated to have been as high as 7 grams. Gastric lavage and unspecified supportive treatment have been employed. Full consciousness following deep coma was regained forty hours or less after ingestion of three or four grams without lavage. No evidence of hematologic, renal, or hepatic effects were subsequently found. Dialysis may be considered in severe intoxication.

Extreme weakness has been reported with divided doses of 3 grams/day in patients.

A parenteral glucocorticoid, preferably hydrocortisone, and/or a mineralocorticoid, such as fludrocortisone, may be indicated in the event of extreme prostration due to adrenocortical hypofunction.

Dosage and Administration:

Adults: Treatment should be instituted in a hospital until a stable dosage regimen is achieved. Therapy should be initiated with 250 mg orally q.i.d., preferably at 6-hour intervals. Adrenal cortical response should be followed by careful monitoring of plasma cortisol until the desired level of suppression is achieved. If cortisol suppression is inadequate, the dosage may be increased in increments of 250 mg daily at intervals of one to two weeks to a total daily dose of 2 grams. Dose reduction or temporary discontinuation may be required in the event of adverse responses, including extreme drowsiness, severe skin rash, or excessively low cortisol levels. If a skin rash persists for longer than five to eight days, or becomes severe, the drug should be discontinued. It may be possible to reinstate therapy at a lower dosage following the disappearance of a mild or moderate rash.

Mineralocorticoid replacement therapy (e.g., fludrocortisone) may be necessary. If glucocorticoid replacement therapy is needed, 20–30 mg of hydrocortisone orally in the morning will replace endogenous secretion.

How Supplied: Tablets 250 mg (white, round and scored into quarters) bottles of 100 (NDC 0083-0024-30).

Clinical Studies: Clinical investigations included 9 patients in the age range 2½ to 16 years; 4 of these were aged 10 or less. However, of the 9, seven received other therapies (drugs or irradiation) either concomitantly or within a short period prior to Cytadren. Diagnoses included 5 with adrenal carcinoma, 3 with adrenal hyperplasia, and one with ectopic ACTH-producing tumor. Treatment duration in this group ranged from 3 days to 6½ months. Dosages ranged from 0.375 gm daily to 1.5 gm daily. In general, smaller doses were used for younger patients; for example, a 2½-year-old received 0.5–0.75 gm/day, a 3⁸⁄₁₂-year-old received 0.5 gm/day, and all of the others over 10 years of age were given 0.75–1.5 gm daily. Results are difficult to evaluate because of the concomitant therapy, duration of therapy, or inadequate laboratory documentation. Most did show decreases of plasma or urinary steroids at some time during treatment, but these may have been due to other therapeutic modalities or their combinations.

Dispense in tight, light-resistant container (USP).

C80-36 (11/80)

[*Shown in Product Identification Section*]

DESFERAL® mesylate (deferoxamine mesylate USP) ℞

Description: Desferal is available as the mesylate salt of deferoxamine. Its solubility in water is greater than 25%; 500 mg will dissolve in 2 ml distilled water.

Chemically, it is N-[5-[3-[(5-Aminopentyl) hydroxycarbamoyl] propionamido] pentyl] - 3 - [[5-(N-hydroxyacetamido) pentyl] carbamoyl] propionohydroxamic acid monomethanesulfonate (salt).

Actions: Desferal is a compound with a specific ability to chelate iron, forming a stable complex which prevents the iron from entering into further chemical reactions. This chelate is readily soluble in water and passes easily through the kidney, giving the urine a characteristic reddish color. Some is also excreted in the feces via the bile. Theoretically, 100 parts by weight of Desferal are capable of binding approximately 8.5 parts by weight of ferric iron. In studies thus far in man and animals, Desferal does not cause any demonstrable increase in the excretion of electrolytes and trace metals.

Indications: To facilitate the removal of iron in the treatment of acute iron intoxication and in chronic iron overload due to transfusion-dependent anemias.

ACUTE IRON INTOXICATION

Desferal is an adjunct to, and not a substitute for, standard measures generally used in treating acute iron intoxication which may include the following:

1. Induction of emesis with syrup of ipecac.
2. Gastric lavage.
3. Suction and maintenance of clear airway.
4. Control of shock with intravenous fluids, blood, oxygen, and vasopressors.
5. Correction of acidosis.

CHRONIC IRON OVERLOAD

Desferal can promote iron excretion in patients who have secondary iron overload from multiple transfusions (such as occur in some chronic anemias including thalassemia). One controlled study has found that long-term therapy with Desferal slows accumulation of hepatic iron and retards or eliminates progression of hepatic fibrosis.

Iron mobilization by Desferal is relatively poor in patients under the age of three with relatively small degrees of iron overload. The drug should ordinarily be withheld in such patients unless a demonstration of significant iron mobilization (eg, one mg of iron per day or more) can be demonstrated.

Desferal is not indicated for the treatment of primary hemochromatosis, since phlebotomy is the method of choice for removing excess iron in this indication.

Contraindications: Desferal is contraindicated in patients with severe renal disease or anuria, since the drug and the chelate which it forms with iron are excreted primarily by the kidney.

Warnings: Rarely, cataracts have been observed in patients who received the drug over prolonged periods in the treatment of chronic iron storage diseases. Slit-lamp examinations performed in patients treated with Desferal for acute iron intoxication have not revealed cataracts. Slit-lamp examinations are recommended periodically in patients treated for chronic iron overload.

Usage in Pregnancy

Skeletal anomalies were noted in the fetuses of two animal species at doses just above those recommended for humans. Therefore, Desferal should not be administered to women of childbearing potential, particularly during early pregnancy, except when in the judgment of the physician the potential benefits outweigh the possible hazards.

Precautions: Flushing of the skin, urticaria, hypotension, and even shock have occurred in a few patients when Desferal has been administered by rapid intravenous injection. To avoid these reactions, DESFERAL SHOULD BE GIVEN INTRAMUSCULARLY, OR BY SLOW SUBCUTANEOUS OR INTRAVENOUS INFUSION.

Adverse Reactions: Occasionally, pain and induration at the site of injection have been reported. Side effects reported in patients treated for acute iron intoxication include generalized erythema, urticaria, and hypotension, which occurred with rapid intravenous injec-

Continued on next page

The full prescribing information for each CIBA drug is contained herein and is that in effect as of October 1, 1982.

CIBA—Cont.

tion. Adverse effects reported in patients receiving long-term therapy for chronic iron storage diseases include allergic-type reactions (cutaneous wheal formation, generalized itching, rash, anaphylactic reaction), blurring of vision, dysuria, abdominal discomfort, diarrhea, leg cramps, tachycardia, and fever. Adverse effects reported in patients receiving subcutaneous therapy include localized pain, pruritus, erythema, skin irritation and swelling. These reactions might also occur in an occasional patient treated for acute iron intoxication.

Dosage and Administration: Since little of the drug is absorbed when administered orally, it is necessary to administer Desferal parenterally to chelate the iron that has been absorbed.

ACUTE IRON INTOXICATION

Intramuscular Administration

Intramuscular administration is preferred and should be used for ALL PATIENTS NOT IN SHOCK.

Dose: One gm should be administered initially. This may be followed by 0.5 gm every four hours for two doses. Depending upon the clinical response, subsequent doses of 0.5 gm may be administered every four to twelve hours. The total amount administered should not exceed 6 gm in twenty-four hours.

Preparation of Solution for Intramuscular Administration: Dissolve the Desferal by adding 2 ml sterile water for injection to each vial. Make sure that the drug is completely dissolved and then withdraw the drug and administer intramuscularly.

Intravenous Administration

This route should be used ONLY FOR PATIENTS IN A STATE OF CARDIOVASCULAR COLLAPSE and then ONLY BY SLOW INFUSION. THE RATE OF INFUSION SHOULD NOT EXCEED 15 mg/kg/hour.

Dose: An initial dose of 1 gm should be administered at a rate NOT TO EXCEED 15 mg/kg/hour. This may be followed by 0.5 gm every four hours for two doses. Depending upon the clinical response, subsequent doses of 0.5 gm may be administered every four to twelve hours. The total amount administered should not exceed 6 gm in twenty-four hours. As soon as the clinical condition of the patient permits, intravenous administration should be discontinued and the drug administered intramuscularly.

Preparation of Solution for Intravenous Administration: Dissolve the Desferal by adding 2 ml sterile water for injection to each vial. Make sure that the drug is completely dissolved and then withdraw the drug and add to physiologic saline, glucose in water, or Ringer's lactate solution and administer at a rate NOT TO EXCEED 15 mg/kg/hour.

CHRONIC IRON OVERLOAD

The more effective of the following two routes of administration must be individualized for each patient.

Intramuscular Administration: 0.5 to 1.0 gm daily administered intramuscularly. In addition, 2.0 gm should be administered intravenously with each unit of blood transfused. However, Desferal should be administered separately from blood. The rate of intravenous infusion must not exceed 15 mg/kg/hour.

Subcutaneous Administration: 1.0 gm to 2.0 gm (20–40 mg/kg/day) administered daily over 8 to 24 hours utilizing a small portable pump capable of providing continuous mini-infusion. The duration of infusion must be individualized. In some patients iron excretion will be as great after a short infusion of 8 to 12 hours as it is if the same dose is given over a 24-hour period.

Preparation of Solution for Subcutaneous Administration: Dissolve the Desferal by adding 2.0 ml sterile water to each vial. Make sure that the drug is completely dissolved and then withdraw the drug in syringe to be used for administration.

Note: Desferal reconstituted with sterile water may be stored under sterile conditions and protected from light at room temperature for not longer than one week.

How Supplied: *Vials,* each containing 500 mg lyophilized deferoxamine mesylate sterile, for INTRAMUSCULAR, SUBCUTANEOUS, OR INTRAVENOUS administration; cartons of 4.

C80-22 (1/80)

ESIDRIX® ℞
(hydrochlorothiazide USP)

Listed in USP, a Medicare designated compendium.

Indications:

Hypertension: In the management of hypertension either as the sole therapeutic agent or to enhance the effect of other antihypertensive drugs in the more severe forms of hypertension.

Edema: As adjunctive therapy in edema associated with congestive heart failure, hepatic cirrhosis, and corticosteroid and estrogen therapy.

Esidrix has also been found useful in edema due to various forms of renal dysfunction, such as the nephrotic syndrome, acute glomerulonephritis, and chronic renal failure.

Usage in Pregnancy: The routine use of diuretics in an otherwise healthy woman is inappropriate and exposes mother and fetus to unnecessary hazard. Diuretics do not prevent development of toxemia of pregnancy, and there is no satisfactory evidence that they are useful in the treatment of developed toxemia. Edema during pregnancy may arise from pathological causes or from the physiologic and mechanical consequences of pregnancy. Thiazides are indicated in pregnancy when edema is due to pathologic causes, just as they are in the absence of pregnancy (however, see WARNINGS). Dependent edema in pregnancy, resulting from restriction of venous return by the expanded uterus, is properly treated through elevation of the lower extremities and use of support hose; use of diuretics to lower intravascular volume in this case is illogical and unnecessary. There is hypervolemia during normal pregnancy which is not harmful to either the fetus or the mother (in the absence of cardiovascular disease) but which is associated with edema, including generalized edema, in the majority of pregnant women. If this edema produces discomfort, increased recumbency will often provide relief. In rare instances, this edema may cause extreme discomfort which is not relieved by rest. In these cases, a short course of diuretics may provide relief and may be appropriate.

Contraindications: Anuria; hypersensitivity to this or other sulfonamide-derived drugs.

Warnings: Use with caution in severe renal disease. In patients with renal disease, thiazides may precipitate azotemia. Cumulative effects of the drug may develop in patients with impaired renal function.

Thiazides should be used with caution in patients with impaired hepatic function or progressive liver disease, since minor alterations of fluid and electrolyte imbalance may precipitate hepatic coma.

Thiazides may add to or potentiate the action of other antihypertensive drugs. Potentiation occurs with ganglionic or peripheral adrenergic blocking drugs.

Sensitivity reactions are more likely to occur in patients with a history of allergy or bronchial asthma.

The possibility of exacerbation or activation of systemic lupus erythematosus has been reported.

Usage in Pregnancy

Thiazides cross the placental barrier and appear in cord blood. The use of thiazides in pregnant women requires that the anticipated benefit be weighed against possible hazards to the fetus. These hazards include fetal or neonatal jaundice, thrombocytopenia, and possibly other adverse reactions which have occurred in the adult.

Nursing Mothers: Thiazides appear in breast milk. If the use of the drug is deemed essential, the patient should stop nursing.

Precautions: Periodic determination of serum electrolytes to detect possible electrolyte imbalance should be performed at appropriate intervals. All patients receiving thiazide therapy should be observed for clinical signs of fluid or electrolyte imbalance: namely, hyponatremia, hypochloremic alkalosis, and hypokalemia. Serum and urine electrolyte determinations are particularly important when the patient is vomiting excessively or receiving parenteral fluids. Medication such as digitalis may also influence serum electrolytes. Warning signs are dryness of mouth, thirst, weakness, lethargy, drowsiness, restlessness, muscle pains or cramps, muscular fatigue, hypotension, oliguria, tachycardia, and gastrointestinal disturbance such as nausea or vomiting.

Hypokalemia may develop, especially with brisk diuresis, when severe cirrhosis is present, or during concomitant use of steroids or ACTH. Interference with adequate oral intake of electrolytes will also contribute to hypokalemia. Hypokalemia can sensitize or exaggerate the response of the heart to the toxic effects of digitalis (eg, increased ventricular irritability).

Any chloride deficit is generally mild and usually does not require specific treatment except under extraordinary circumstances (as in liver disease or renal disease). Dilutional hyponatremia may occur in edematous patients in hot weather; appropriate therapy is water restriction, rather than administration of salt except in rare instances when the hyponatremia is life-threatening. In actual salt depletion, appropriate replacement is the therapy of choice.

Hyperuricemia may occur or frank gout may be precipitated in certain patients receiving thiazide therapy.

Insulin requirements in diabetic patients may be increased, decreased, or unchanged. Latent diabetes may become manifest during thiazide administration.

Thiazide drugs may increase the responsiveness to tubocurarine.

The antihypertensive effects of the drug may be enhanced in the postsympathectomy patient. Thiazides may decrease arterial responsiveness to norepinephrine. This diminution is not sufficient to preclude effectiveness of the pressor agent for therapeutic use.

If progressive renal impairment becomes evident, withholding or discontinuing diuretic therapy should be considered.

Thiazides may decrease serum PBI levels without signs of thyroid disturbance.

Calcium excretion is decreased by thiazides. Pathological changes in the parathyroid gland with hypercalcemia and hypophosphatemia have been observed in a few patients on prolonged thiazide therapy. The common complications of hyperparathyroidism such as renal lithiasis, bone resorption, and peptic ulceration have not been seen. Thiazides should be discontinued before carrying out tests for parathyroid function.

Adverse Reactions:

Gastrointestinal: Anorexia, gastric irritation, nausea, vomiting, cramping, diarrhea, constipation, jaundice (intrahepatic cholestatic), pancreatitis, sialadenitis

Central Nervous System: Dizziness, vertigo, paresthesias, headache, xanthopsia

Hematologic: Leukopenia, agranulocytosis, thrombocytopenia, aplastic anemia

Cardiovascular: Orthostatic hypotension (may be potentiated by alcohol, barbiturates, or narcotics)

Hypersensitivity: Purpura, photosensitivity, rash, urticaria, necrotizing angiitis, Stevens-Johnson syndrome, and other hypersensitivity reactions

Other: Hyperglycemia, glycosuria, hyperuricemia, muscle spasm, weakness, restlessness

Whenever adverse reactions are moderate or severe, thiazide dosage should be reduced or therapy withdrawn.

Dosage and Administration: Therapy should be individualized according to patient response. Dosage should be titrated to gain maximal therapeutic response as well as the minimal dose possible to maintain that therapeutic response.

Adults

Hypertension

To Initiate Therapy: Usual dose is 75 mg daily. May be given as a single dose every morning.

Maintenance: After a week dosage may be adjusted downward to as little as 25 mg a day, or upward to as much as 100 mg daily.

Combined Therapy: When necessary, other antihypertensive agents may be added cautiously. Since this drug potentiates the antihypertensive effect of other agents, such additions should be gradual. Dosages of ganglionic blockers in particular should be halved initially.

Edema

To Initiate Diuresis: 25 to 200 mg daily for several days, or until dry weight is attained.

Maintenance: 25 to 100 mg daily or intermittently depending on patient's response. A few refractory patients may require up to 200 mg daily.

Infants and Children

The usual pediatric dosage is administered twice daily.

The total daily dosage for infants up to 2 years of age: 12.5 to 37.5 mg; for children 2 to 12 years of age: 37.5 to 100 mg. Dosage should be based on body weight at the rate of 1 mg per pound, but infants below 6 months of age may require 1.5 mg per pound.

Overdosage

Signs and Symptoms

Diuresis is to be expected; lethargy of varying degree may appear and may progress to coma within a few hours, with minimal depression of respiration and cardiovascular function and without significant serum electrolyte changes or dehydration. The mechanism of CNS depression with thiazide overdosage is unknown. GI irritation and hypermotility may occur; temporary elevation of BUN has been reported and serum electrolyte changes could occur, especially in patients with impairment of renal function.

Treatment

Evacuate gastric contents but take care to prevent aspiration, especially in the stuporous or comatose patient. GI effects are usually of short duration, but may require symptomatic treatment.

Monitor serum electrolyte levels and renal function; institute supportive measures as required individually to maintain hydration, electrolyte balance, respiration and cardiovascular-renal function.

How Supplied: *Tablets,* 100 mg (blue, scored); bottles of 100. *Tablets,* 50 mg (yellow, scored); bottles of 30, 60, 100, 1000, 5000 and Accu-Pak® blister units of 100.

Tablets, 25 mg (pink, scored); bottles of 100, 1000 and 5000. C78-1 Rev. 1/78

[*Shown in Product Identification Section*]

ESIMIL® ℞

guanethidine monosulfate 10 mg
hydrochlorothiazide 25 mg

> **Warning**
> This fixed combination drug is not indicated for initial therapy of hypertension. Hypertension requires therapy titrated to the individual patient. If the fixed combination represents the dosage so determined, its use may be more convenient in patient management. The treatment of hypertension is not static, but must be reevaluated as conditions in each patient warrant.

Indications

Hypertension. (See box warning.)

Contraindications

Guanethidine

Known or suspected pheochromocytoma; hypersensitivity; frank congestive heart failure not due to hypertension; use of MAO inhibitors.

Hydrochlorothiazide

Anuria; hypersensitivity to this or other sulfonamide-derived drugs.

Warnings: Guanethidine and hydrochlorothiazide are potent drugs and their use can lead to disturbing and serious clinical problems. Physicians should be familiar with both drugs and their combination before prescribing, and patients should be warned not to deviate from instructions.

Guanethidine

> Orthostatic hypotension can occur frequently and patients should be properly instructed about this potential hazard. Fainting spells may occur unless the patient is forewarned to sit or lie down with the onset of dizziness or weakness. Postural hypotension is most marked in the morning and is accentuated by hot weather, alcohol, or exercise. Dizziness or weakness may be particularly bothersome during the initial period of dosage adjustment and with postural changes, such as arising in the morning. The potential occurrence of these symptoms may require alteration of previous daily activity. The patient should be cautioned to avoid sudden or prolonged standing or exercise while taking the drug.

Concurrent use of guanethidine and rauwolfia derivatives may cause excessive postural hypotension, bradycardia, and mental depression.

If possible, withdraw therapy two weeks prior to surgery to reduce the possibility of vascular collapse and cardiac arrest during anesthesia. If emergency surgery is indicated, preanesthetic and anesthetic agents should be administered cautiously in reduced dosage. Oxygen, atropine, vasopressors, and adequate solutions for volume replacement should be ready for immediate use to counteract vascular collapse in the surgical patient. Vasopressors should be used only with extreme caution, since guanethidine augments the responsiveness to exogenously administered norepinephrine and vasopressors with respect to blood pressure and their propensity for the production of cardiac arrhythmias.

Dosage requirements may be reduced in the presence of fever.

Exercise special care when treating patients with a history of bronchial asthma; asthmatics are more apt to be hypersensitive to catecholamine depletion and their condition may be aggravated.

Hydrochlorothiazide

Use with caution in severe renal disease. In patients with renal disease, thiazides may precipitate azotemia. Cumulative effects of the drug may develop in patients with impaired renal function.

Thiazides should be used with caution in patients with impaired hepatic function or progressive liver disease, since minor alterations of fluid and electrolyte imbalance may precipitate hepatic coma.

Thiazides may add to or potentiate the action of other antihypertensive drugs. Potentiation occurs with ganglionic or peripheral adrenergic blocking drugs.

Sensitivity reactions are more likely to occur in patients with a history of allergy or bronchial asthma.

The possibility of exacerbation or activation of systemic lupus erythematosus has been reported.

Usage in Pregnancy

Guanethidine

The safety of guanethidine for use in pregnancy has not been established; therefore, this drug should be used in pregnant patients only when, in the judgment of the physician, its use is deemed essential to the welfare of the patient.

Hydrochlorothiazide

Thiazides cross the placental barrier and appear in cord blood. The use of thiazides in pregnant women requires that the anticipated benefit be weighed against possible hazards to the fetus. These hazards include fetal or neonatal jaundice, thrombocytopenia, and possibly other adverse reactions which have occurred in the adult.

Nursing Mothers: Thiazides appear in breast milk. If the use of the drug is deemed essential, the patient should stop nursing.

Precautions

Guanethidine

The effects of guanethidine are cumulative over long periods; initial doses should be small and increased gradually in small increments.

Use very cautiously in hypertensive patients with: renal disease and nitrogen retention or rising BUN levels, since decreased blood pressure may further compromise renal function; coronary disease with insufficiency or recent myocardial infarction; cerebral vascular disease, especially with encephalopathy.

Do not give to patients with severe cardiac failure except with extreme caution since guanethidine may interfere with the compensatory role of the adrenergic system in producing circulatory adjustment in patients with congestive heart failure.

In patients with incipient cardiac decompensation, watch for weight gain or edema, which may be averted by the concomitant administration of a thiazide.

Remember that both digitalis and guanethidine slow the heart rate.

Use cautiously in patients with a history of peptic ulcer or other chronic disorders which may be aggravated by a relative increase in parasympathetic tone.

Amphetamine-like compounds, stimulants (*eg,* ephedrine, methylphenidate), tricyclic antidepressants (*eg,* amitriptyline, imipramine, desipramine) and other psychopharmacologic agents (*eg,* phenothiazines and related compounds), and oral contraceptives may reduce the hypotensive effect of guanethidine.

MAO inhibitors should be discontinued for at least one week before starting therapy with guanethidine.

Hydrochlorothiazide

Periodic determination of serum electrolytes to detect possible electrolyte imbalance should be performed at appropriate intervals. All patients receiving thiazide therapy should be

Continued on next page

The full prescribing information for each CIBA drug is contained herein and is that in effect as of October 1, 1982.

CIBA—Cont.

observed for clinical signs of fluid or electrolyte imbalance; namely, hyponatremia, hypochloremic alkalosis, and hypokalemia. Serum and urine electrolyte determinations are particularly important when the patient is vomiting excessively or receiving parenteral fluids. Medication such as digitalis may also influence serum electrolytes. Warning signs are dryness of mouth, thirst, weakness, lethargy, drowsiness, restlessness, muscle pains or cramps, muscular fatigue, hypotension, oliguria, tachycardia, and gastrointestinal disturbance such as nausea or vomiting.
Hypokalemia may develop, especially with brisk diuresis, when severe cirrhosis is present, or during concomitant use of steroids or ACTH. Interference with adequate oral intake of electrolytes will also contribute to hypokalemia. Hypokalemia can sensitize or exaggerate the response of the heart to the toxic effects of digitalis (*eg,* increased ventricular irritability).
Any chloride deficit is generally mild and usually does not require specific treatment except under extraordinary circumstances (as in liver disease or renal disease). Dilutional hyponatremia may occur in edematous patients in hot weather; appropriate therapy is water restriction rather than administration of salt, except in rare instances when the hyponatremia is life-threatening. In actual salt depletion, appropriate replacement is the therapy of choice.
Hyperuricemia may occur or frank gout may be precipitated in certain patients receiving thiazide therapy.
Insulin requirements in diabetic patients may be increased, decreased, or unchanged. Latent diabetes may become manifest during thiazide administration.
Thiazide drugs may increase the responsiveness to tubocurarine.
The antihypertensive effects of the drug may be enhanced in the postsympathectomy patient. Thiazides may decrease arterial responsiveness to norepinephrine. This diminution is not sufficient to preclude effectiveness of the pressor agent for therapeutic use.
If progressive renal impairment becomes evident, withholding or discontinuing diuretic therapy should be considered.
Thiazides may decrease serum PBI levels without signs of thyroid disturbance.
Calcium excretion is decreased by thiazides. Pathological changes in the parathyroid gland with hypercalcemia and hypophosphatemia have been observed in a few patients on prolonged thiazide therapy. The common complications of hyperparathyroidism such as renal lithiasis, bone resorption, and peptic ulceration have not been seen. Thiazides should be discontinued before carrying out tests for parathyroid function.

Adverse Reactions

Guanethidine

Frequent reactions due to sympathetic blockade: dizziness, weakness, lassitude, and syncope resulting from either postural or exertional hypotension.
Frequent reactions due to unopposed parasympathetic activity: bradycardia, increase in bowel movements, and diarrhea. Diarrhea may be severe at times and necessitate discontinuance of the medication.
Other common reactions: inhibition of ejaculation, a tendency toward fluid retention and edema with occasional development of congestive heart failure.
Other less common reactions: dyspnea, fatigue, nausea, vomiting, nocturia, urinary incontinence, dermatitis, scalp hair loss, dry mouth, rise in BUN, ptosis of the lids, blurring of vision, parotid tenderness, myalgia, muscle tremor, mental depression, chest pains (angina), chest paresthesias, nasal congestion, weight gain, and asthma in susceptible individuals. Although a causal relationship has not been established, a few instances of blood dyscrasias (anemia, thrombocytopenia, and leukopenia) and of priapism have been reported.

Hydrochlorothiazide

Gastrointestinal: Anorexia, gastric irritation, nausea, vomiting, cramping, diarrhea, constipation, jaundice (intrahepatic cholestatic), pancreatitis, sialadenitis
Central Nervous System: Dizziness, vertigo, paresthesias, headache, xanthopsia
Hematologic: Leukopenia, thrombocytopenia, agranulocytosis, aplastic anemia
Cardiovascular: Orthostatic hypotension (may be potentiated by alcohol, barbiturates, or narcotics)
Hypersensitivity: Purpura, photosensitivity, rash, urticaria, necrotizing angiitis, Stevens-Johnson syndrome, and other hypersensitivity reactions
Other: Hyperglycemia, glycosuria, hyperuricemia, muscle spasm, weakness, restlessness
Whenever adverse reactions are moderate or severe, thiazide dosage should be reduced or therapy withdrawn.

Dosage and Administration: As determined by individual titration (see box warning).
The usual dosage of Esimil is 2 tablets daily. As with any antihypertensive, dosage should be individually titrated for the patient. Depending upon the degree of hypertension, the patient should be started on the lowest possible dose (usually 1 tablet daily) and then gradually increased at weekly intervals until the desired response is obtained. Blood pressure should be recorded with the patient in the supine position and again after 10 minutes of standing. Dosage should be increased only if the standing blood pressure has not been reduced to desired levels. Dosage adjustment should be made at not less than weekly intervals; maximal dosage should not exceed 4 tablets daily. If additional effect is desirable, supplement individually with guanethidine tablets.
Do not give MAO inhibitors with Esimil. Stop ganglionic blockers before instituting therapy with Esimil. Wait at least one week after one drug is discontinued before starting Esimil.
When Esimil is to be substituted for other antihypertensive agents, the change should be made gradually. In general, dosage of the agent to be discontinued should be discontinued by one-half, and Esimil should be started at 1 tablet daily. Follow this schedule for at least one week; then, dosage of the previous therapy may be halved again and dosage of Esimil increased to 2 tablets daily. At the next week interval, the previously used drugs can generally be discontinued. Titrate dosage of Esimil at weekly intervals as mentioned above.
Patients receiving more than 75 mg guanethidine alone may do well on a smaller dose if also given hydrochlorothiazide. Because of the ratio of the combination, they are probably not candidates for Esimil.

Overdosage

Guanethidine

Signs and Symptoms

Postural hypotension [with dizziness, blurring of vision, etc., possibly progressing to syncope when standing] and bradycardia are most likely to occur; diarrhea, possibly severe, also may occur. Unconsciousness is unlikely if adequate blood pressure and cerebral perfusion can be maintained by appropriate positioning [supine] and by other treatment as required.

Treatment

In previously normotensive patients, treatment has consisted essentially of restoring blood pressure and heart rate to normal by keeping patient in supine position. Normal homeostatic control usually returns gradually over a 72-hour period in these patients.
In previously hypertensive patients, particularly those with impaired cardiac reserve or other cardiovascular-renal disease, intensive treatment may be required to support vital functions and/or to control cardiac irregularities that might be present. Supine position must be maintained; if vasopressors are required, it must be remembered that guanethidine may increase responsiveness as to blood pressure rise and occurrence of cardiac arrhythmias.
Diarrhea, if severe or persistent, should be treated symptomatically to reduce intestinal hypermotility, with due attention to maintenance of hydration and electrolyte balance.

Hydrochlorothiazide

Signs and Symptoms

Diuresis is to be expected; lethargy of varying degree may appear and may progress to coma within a few hours, with minimal depression of respiration and cardiovascular function and without significant serum electrolyte changes or dehydration. The mechanism of CNS depression with thiazide overdosage is unknown. GI irritation and hypermotility may occur; temporary elevation of BUN has been reported and serum electrolyte changes could occur, especially in patients with impairment of renal function.

Treatment

Evacuate gastric contents but take care to prevent aspiration, especially in the stuporous or comatose patient. GI effects are usually of short duration, but may require symptomatic treatment.
Monitor serum electrolyte levels and renal function; institute supportive measures as required individually to maintain hydration, electrolyte balance, respiration and cardiovascular-renal function.

How Supplied:

Tablets—round, white, scored (imprinted CIBA 47)
10 mg guanethidine monosulfate
25 mg hydrochlorothiazide
Bottles of 100 ....NDC 0083-0047-30
Consumer Pack—One Unit
12 bottles—
100 tablets each ....NDC 0083-0047-65
Dispense in tight container (USP) C82-15 (7/82)
[*Shown in Product Identification Section*]

INH (isoniazid USP) ℞
Tablets

Warning:
Severe and sometimes fatal hepatitis associated with isoniazid therapy may occur and may develop even after many months of treatment. The risk of developing hepatitis is age related. Approximate case rates by age are: 0 per 1,000 for persons under 20 years of age, 3 per 1,000 for persons in the 20–34 year age group, 12 per 1,000 for persons in the 35–49 year age group, 23 per 1,000 for persons in the 50–64 year age group, and 8 per 1,000 for persons over 65 years of age. The risk of hepatitis is increased with daily consumption of alcohol. Precise data to provide a fatality rate for isoniazid-related hepatitis is not available; however, in a U.S. Public Health Service Surveillance Study of 13,838 persons taking isoniazid, there were 8 deaths among 174 cases of hepatitis.
Therefore, patients given isoniazid should be carefully monitored and interviewed at monthly intervals. Serum transaminase concentration becomes elevated in about 10–20 percent of patients, usually during the first few months of therapy but it can occur at any time. Usually enzyme levels return to normal despite continuance of drug but in some cases progressive liver dysfunction occurs. Patients should be instructed to report immediately any of the prodromal symptoms of hepatitis, such as fatigue, weakness, malaise, anorexia, nausea, or vomiting. If these symptoms appear or if signs suggestive of hepatic damage are detected, isoniazid should be

discontinued promptly, since continued use of the drug in these cases has been reported to cause a more severe form of liver damage.
Patients with tuberculosis should be given appropriate treatment with alternative drugs. If isoniazid must be reinstituted, it should be reinstituted only after symptoms and laboratory abnormalities have cleared. The drug should be restarted in very small and gradually increasing doses and should be withdrawn immediately if there is any indication of recurrent liver involvement.
Preventive treatment should be deferred in persons with acute hepatic diseases.

Indications: For all forms of tuberculosis in which organisms are susceptible.
For preventive therapy for the following groups, in order of priority:
1. Household members and other close associates of persons with recently diagnosed tuberculous disease.
2. Positive tuberculin skin test reactors with findings on the chest roentgenogram consistent with nonprogressive tuberculous disease, in whom there are neither positive bacteriologic findings nor a history of adequate chemotherapy.
3. Newly infected persons.
4. Positive tuberculin skin test reactors in the following special clinical situations: prolonged therapy with adrenocorticosteroids; immunosuppressive therapy; some hematologic and reticuloendothelial diseases, such as leukemia or Hodgkin's disease; diabetes mellitus; silicosis; after gastrectomy.
5. Other positive tuberculin reactors under 35 years of age.
The risk of hepatitis must be weighed against the risk of tuberculosis in positive tuberculin reactors over the age of 35. However, the use of isoniazid is recommended for those with the additional risk factors listed above (1–4) and on an individual basis in situations where there is likelihood of serious consequences to contacts who may become infected.
Contraindications: Isoniazid is contraindicated in patients who develop severe hypersensitivity reactions, including drug-induced hepatitis. Previous isoniazid-associated hepatic injury: severe adverse reactions to isoniazid, such as drug fever, chills, and arthritis; acute liver disease of any etiology.
Warnings: See the boxed warning.
Ophthalmologic examinations (including ophthalmoscopy) should be done *before* INH is started and periodically thereafter, even without occurrence of visual symptoms.
Carcinogenesis
Isoniazid has been reported to induce pulmonary tumors in a number of strains of mice.
Usage in Pregnancy and Lactation
It has been reported that in both rats and rabbits, isoniazid may exert an embryocidal effect when administered orally during pregnancy, although no isoniazid-related congenital anomalies have been found in reproduction studies in mammalian species (mice, rats, and rabbits). Isoniazid should be prescribed during pregnancy only when therapeutically necessary. The benefit of preventive therapy should be weighed against a possible risk to the fetus. Preventive treatment generally should be started after delivery because of the increased risk of tuberculosis for new mothers.
Since isoniazid is known to cross the placental barrier and to pass into maternal breast milk, neonates and breast-fed infants of isoniazid treated mothers should be carefully observed for any evidence of adverse effects.
Precautions: Use of isoniazid should be carefully monitored in the following:
1. Patients who are receiving phenytoin concurrently. Isoniazid may decrease the excretion of phenytoin or may enhance its effects. To avoid phenytoin intoxication, appropriate adjustment of the anticonvulsant should be made.
2. Daily users of alcohol. Daily ingestion of alcohol may be associated with a higher incidence of isoniazid hepatitis.
3. Patients with current chronic liver disease or severe renal dysfunction.
Adverse Reactions: The most frequent reactions are those affecting the nervous system and the liver.
Nervous system reactions: Peripheral neuropathy is the most common toxic effect. It is dose-related, occurs most often in the malnourished and in those predisposed to neuritis (*eg,* alcoholics and diabetics), and is usually preceded by paresthesias of the feet and hands. The incidence is higher in "slow inactivators".
Other neurotoxic effects, which are uncommon with conventional doses, are convulsions, toxic encephalopathy, optic neuritis and atrophy, memory impairment, and toxic psychosis.
Gastrointestinal reactions: Nausea, vomiting, epigastric distress.
Hepatic reactions: Elevated serum transaminases (SGOT; SGPT), bilirubinemia, bilirubinuria, jaundice and occasionally severe and sometimes fatal hepatitis. The common prodromal symptoms are anorexia, nausea, vomiting, fatigue, malaise, and weakness. Mild and transient elevation of serum transaminase levels, occurs in 10 to 20 percent of persons taking isoniazid. The abnormality usually occurs in the first 4 to 6 months of treatment but can occur at any time during therapy. In most instances, enzyme levels return to normal with no necessity to discontinue medication. In occasional instances, progressive liver damage occurs, with accompanying symptoms. In these cases, the drug should be discontinued immediately. The frequency of progressive liver damage increases with age. It is rare in persons under 20, but occurs in up to 2.3 percent of those over 50 years of age.
Hematologic reactions: Agranulocytosis; hemolytic, sideroblastic, or aplastic anemia; thrombocytopenia; and eosinophilia.
Hypersensitivity reactions: Fever, skin eruptions (morbilliform, maculopapular, purpuric, or exfoliative), lymphadenopathy and vasculitis.
Metabolic and endocrine reactions: Pyridoxine deficiency, pellagra, hyperglycemia, metabolic acidosis, and gynecomastia
Miscellaneous reactions: Rheumatic syndrome and systemic lupus erythematosus-like syndrome.
Overdosage:
Signs and Symptoms
Isoniazid overdosage produces signs and symptoms within 30 minutes to 3 hours after ingestion. Nausea, vomiting, dizziness, slurring of speech, blurring of vision, and visual hallucinations (including bright colors and strange designs), are among the early manifestations. With marked overdosage, respiratory distress and CNS depression, progressing rapidly from stupor to profound coma, are to be expected, along with severe, intractable seizures. Severe metabolic acidosis, acetonuria, and hyperglycemia are typical laboratory findings.
Treatment
Untreated or inadequately treated cases of gross isoniazid overdosage can terminate fatally, but good response has been reported in most patients brought under adequate treatment within the first few hours after drug ingestion.
Secure the airway and establish adequate respiratory exchange. Gastric lavage within the first 2 to 3 hours is advised, but should not be attempted until convulsions are under control. To control convulsions administer I.V. short-acting barbiturates and I.V. pyridoxine (usually 1 mg/1mg isoniazid ingested).
Obtain blood samples for immediate determination of gases, electrolytes, BUN, glucose, etc.; type and crossmatch blood in preparation for possible hemodialysis.
Rapid control of metabolic acidosis is fundamental to management. Give I.V. sodium bicarbonate at once and repeat as needed, adjusting subsequent dosage on the basis of laboratory findings (*ie,* serum sodium, pH, etc.).
Forced osmotic diuresis must be started early and should be continued for some hours after clinical improvement to hasten renal clearance of drug and help prevent relapse; monitor fluid intake and output.
Hemodialysis is advised for severe cases; if this is not available, peritoneal dialysis can be used along with forced diuresis.
Along with measures based on initial and repeated determination of blood gases and other laboratory tests as needed, utilize meticulous respiratory and other intensive care to protect against hypoxia, hypotension, aspiration pneumonitis, etc.
Dosage and Administration (See also indications):
NOTE—For preventive therapy of tuberculous infection it is recommended that physicians be familiar with the joint recommendations of the American Thoracic Society, American Lung Association, and the Center for Disease Control, as published in the American Review of Respiratory Diseases Vol. 110, No. 3, September 1974, or CDC's Morbidity and Mortality Weekly Report, Vol. 24, No. 8, February 22, 1975.
For treatment of active tuberculosis: Isoniazid is used in conjunction with other effective antituberculous agents.
If the bacilli become resistant, therapy must be changed to agents to which the bacilli are susceptible.
Usual oral dosage
Adults: 5 mg/kg up to 300 mg daily in a single dose.
Infants and children: 10–20 mg/kg depending on severity of infection, (up to 300–500 mg daily) in a single dose.
For preventive therapy
Adults: 300 mg/day in a single dose.
Infants and children: 10 mg/kg (up to 300 mg daily) in a single dose.
Continuous administration of isoniazid for a sufficient period is an essential part of the regimen because relapse rates are higher if chemotherapy is stopped prematurely. In the treatment of tuberculosis, resistant organisms may multiply and the emergence of resistant organisms during the treatment may necessitate a change in the regimen.
Concomitant administration of pyridoxine (B_6) is recommended in the malnourished and in those predisposed to neuropathy (*eg,* alcoholics and diabetics).
How Supplied: *Tablets,* 300 mg (white, scored); available as Rimactane® (rifampin USP) /INH Dual Pack containing 30 INH Tablets and 60 Rimactane 300-mg Capsules.
C78-15 Rev. 3/78

ISMELIN® sulfate ℞
(guanethidine monosulfate)

Listed in USP, a Medicare designated compendium.

Indications: *Moderate and severe hypertension* either alone or as an adjunct.
Renal hypertension, including that secondary to pyelonephritis, renal amyloidosis, and renal artery stenosis.
Contraindications: Known or suspected pheochromocytoma; hypersensitivity; frank con-

Continued on next page

The full prescribing information for each CIBA drug is contained herein and is that in effect as of October 1, 1982.

CIBA—Cont.

gestive heart failure not due to hypertension; use of MAO inhibitors.

Warnings: Ismelin is a potent drug and can lead to disturbing and serious clinical problems. Before prescribing, physicians should familiarize themselves with the details of its use and warn patients not to deviate from instructions.

> Orthostatic hypotension can occur frequently and patients should be properly instructed about this potential hazard. Fainting spells may occur unless the patient is forewarned to sit or lie down with the onset of dizziness or weakness. Postural hypotension is most marked in the morning and is accentuated by hot weather, alcohol, or exercise. Dizziness or weakness may be particularly bothersome during the initial period of dosage adjustment and with postural changes, such as arising in the morning. The potential occurrence of these symptoms may require alteration of previous daily activity. The patient should be cautioned to avoid sudden or prolonged standing or exercise while taking the drug.

Concurrent use of Ismelin and rauwolfia derivatives may cause excessive postural hypotension, bradycardia, and mental depression.

If possible, withdraw therapy two weeks prior to surgery to reduce the possibility of vascular collapse and cardiac arrest during anesthesia. If emergency surgery is indicated, preanesthetic and anesthetic agents should be administered cautiously in reduced dosage. Oxygen, atropine, vasopressors, and adequate solutions for volume replacement should be ready for immediate use to counteract vascular collapse in the surgical patient. Vasopressors should be used only with extreme caution, since Ismelin augments the responsiveness to exogenously administered norepinephrine and vasopressors with respect to blood pressure and their propensity for the production of cardiac arrhythmias.

Dosage requirements may be reduced in the presence of fever.

Exercise special care when treating patients with a history of bronchial asthma; asthmatics are more apt to be hypersensitive to catecholamine depletion and their condition may be aggravated.

Usage in Pregnancy

The safety of Ismelin for use in pregnancy has not been established; therefore this drug should be used in pregnant patients only when, in the judgment of the physician, its use is deemed essential to the welfare of the patient.

Precautions: The effects of guanethidine are cumulative over long periods; initial doses should be small and increased gradually in small increments.

Use very cautiously in hypertensive patients with: renal disease and nitrogen retention or rising BUN levels, since decreased blood pressure may further compromise renal function; coronary disease with insufficiency or recent myocardial infarction; cerebral vascular disease, especially with encephalopathy.

Do not give to patients with severe cardiac failure except with extreme caution since Ismelin may interfere with the compensatory role of the adrenergic system in producing circulatory adjustment in patients with congestive heart failure.

In patients with incipient cardiac decompensation, watch for weight gain or edema, which may be averted by the concomitant administration of a thiazide.

Remember that both digitalis and Ismelin slow the heart rate.

Use cautiously in patients with a history of peptic ulcer or other chronic disorders which may be aggravated by a relative increase in parasympathetic tone.

Amphetamine-like compounds, stimulants (*eg*, ephedrine, methylphenidate), tricyclic antidepressants (*eg*, amitriptyline, imipramine, desipramine) and other psychopharmacologic agents (*eg*, phenothiazines and related compounds), and oral contraceptives may reduce the hypotensive effect of guanethidine.

MAO inhibitors should be discontinued for at least one week before starting therapy with Ismelin.

Adverse Reactions:

Frequent reactions due to sympathetic blockade: dizziness, weakness, lassitude, and syncope resulting from either postural or exertional hypotension.

Frequent reactions due to unopposed parasympathetic activity: bradycardia, increase in bowel movements, and diarrhea. Diarrhea may be severe at times and necessitate discontinuance of the medication.

Other common reactions: inhibition of ejaculation, a tendency toward fluid retention and edema with occasional development of congestive heart failure.

Other less common reactions: dyspnea, fatigue, nausea, vomiting, nocturia, urinary incontinence, dermatitis, scalp hair loss, dry mouth, rise in BUN, ptosis of the lids, blurring of vision, parotid tenderness, myalgia, muscle tremor, mental depression, chest pains (angina), chest paresthesias, nasal congestion, weight gain, and asthma in susceptible individuals. Although a causal relationship has not been established, a few instances of blood dyscrasias (anemia, thrombocytopenia, and leukopenia) and of priapism have been reported.

Dosage and Administration: Better control may be obtained, especially in the initial phases of treatment, if the patient can have his blood pressure recorded regularly at home.

Ambulatory Patients. Begin treatment with small doses (10 mg). Increase gradually, depending upon the patient's response. Ismelin has a long duration of action; therefore, dosage increases should not be made more often than every 5 to 7 days, unless the patient is hospitalized.

Take blood pressure in the supine position, after standing for ten minutes, and immediately after exercise if feasible. Increase dosage only if there has been *no* decrease in standing blood pressure from the previous levels. The average daily dose is 25 to 50 mg; only 1 dose a day is usually required.

Dosage Chart for Ambulatory Patients

Visits at Intervals of 5 to 7 Days	*Daily Dose*
Visit No. 1 (Start with 10-mg tablets)	10 mg
Visit No. 2	20 mg
Visit No. 3 (Patient can be changed to 25-mg tablets whenever convenient)	30 mg (three 10-mg tablets) or 37.5 mg (one and one-half 25-mg tablets)
Visit No. 4	50 mg

Visit No. 5 (and subsequent). Dosage may be increased by 12.5 mg or 25 mg if necessary.

Reduce dosage in any of the following 3 situations:

1. *Normal supine pressure*
2. *Excessive orthostatic fall in pressure*
3. *Severe diarrhea*

Hospitalized Patients. Initial oral dose is 25 to 50 mg, increased by 25 or 50 mg daily or every other day as indicated. This higher dosage is possible because hospitalized patients can be watched carefully. Unless absolutely impossible, take the standing blood pressure regularly. Patients should not be discharged from the hospital until the effect of the drug on the standing blood pressure is known. *Patients should be told about the possibility of orthostatic hypotension and warned not to get out of bed without help during the period of dosage adjustment.*

Combination Therapy. Ismelin may be added gradually to thiazides and/or hydralazine. Thiazide diuretics enhance the effectiveness of Ismelin and may reduce the incidence of edema. When thiazide diuretics are added to the regimen in patients on Ismelin, it is usually necessary to reduce the dosage of Ismelin. After control is established, reduce dosage of all drugs to the lowest effective level.

When replacing MAO inhibitors, at least one week should elapse before commencing treatment with Ismelin.

In many cases ganglionic blockers will have been stopped before Ismelin is started. It may be advisable, however, to withdraw the blocker gradually to prevent a spiking blood pressure response during the transfer period.

Overdosage

Signs and Symptoms

Postural hypotension [with dizziness, blurring of vision, etc., possibly progressing to syncope when standing] and bradycardia are most likely to occur; diarrhea, possibly severe, also may occur. Unconsciousness is unlikely if adequate blood pressure and cerebral perfusion can be maintained by appropriate positioning [supine] and by other treatment as required.

Treatment

In previously normotensive patients, treatment has consisted essentially of restoring blood pressure and heart rate to normal by keeping patient in supine position. Normal homeostatic control usually returns gradually over a 72-hour period in these patients.

In previously hypertensive patients, particularly those with impaired cardiac reserve or other cardiovascular-renal disease, intensive treatment may be required to support vital functions and/or to control cardiac irregularities that might be present. Supine position must be maintained; if vasopressors are required, it must be remembered that Ismelin may increase responsiveness as to blood pressure rise and occurrence of cardiac arrhythmias.

Diarrhea, if severe or persistent, should be treated symptomatically to reduce intestinal hypermotility, with due attention to maintenance of hydration and electrolyte balance.

Tablets 10 mg — pale yellow, scored (imprinted 49 CIBA)

Bottles of 100 ....NDC 0083-0049-30
Bottles of 1000 ....NDC 0083-0049-40
Consumer Pack—One Unit
(12 bottles - 100 tablets each) ....NDC 0083-0049-65
Accu-Pak® Unit Dose (blister pack)
Box of 100 (strips of 10) .NDC 0083-0049-32

Tablets 25 mg — white, scored (imprinted 103 CIBA)

Bottles of 100 ....NDC 0083-0103-30
Bottles of 1000 ....NDC 0083-0103-40
Consumer Pack—One Unit
(12 bottles-100 tablets each) ....NDC 0083-0103-65
Accu-Pak® Unit Dose (blister pack)
Box of 100 (strips of 10) .NDC 0083-0103-32

Dispense in tight container (USP)

C81-20 (6/81)

[*Shown in Product Identification Section*]

LITHOBID® ℞
(lithium carbonate)
slow-release tablets (not USP)

CIBALITH-S™ Syrup ℞
(lithium citrate)

> **WARNING**
> Lithium toxicity is closely related to serum lithium levels, and can occur at doses close to therapeutic levels. Facilities for prompt and accurate serum lithium

determinations should be available before initiating therapy.

Description:

Lithobid: Each film-coated slow-release tablet contains 300 mg of lithium carbonate, 40 mg of sodium chloride, equivalent to 15.7 mg of sodium. This slowly dissolving film-coated tablet is designed to give postadministration serum lithium peaks lower than obtained with conventional oral lithium dosage forms.

Cibalith-S: Each 5 ml of this lithium citrate syrup contains 8 mEq of lithium ion (Li^+), equivalent to the amount of lithium in 300 mg of lithium carbonate.

Lithium carbonate is a white, light alkaline powder with molecular formula Li_2CO_3 and molecular weight 73.89. Lithium is an element of the alkali-metal group with atomic number 3, atomic weight 6.94 and an emission line at 671 nm on the flame photometer.

Lithium citrate is prepared in solution from lithium hydroxide and citric acid in a ratio approximating di-lithium citrate.

Indications: Lithium is indicated in the treatment of manic episodes of manic-depressive illness. Maintenance therapy prevents or diminishes the intensity of subsequent episodes in those manic-depressive patients with a history of mania.

Typical symptoms of mania include pressure of speech, motor hyperactivity, reduced need for sleep, flight of ideas, grandiosity, elation, poor judgment, aggressiveness, and possibly hostility. When given to a patient experiencing a manic episode, lithium may produce a normalization of symptomatology within 1 to 3 weeks.

Warnings: Lithium should generally not be given to patients with significant renal or cardiovascular disease, severe debilitation or dehydration, or sodium depletion, and to patients receiving diuretics, since the risk of lithium toxicity is very high in such patients. If the psychiatric indication is life-threatening, and if such a patient fails to respond to other measures, lithium treatment may be undertaken with extreme caution, including daily serum lithium determinations and adjustment to the usually low doses ordinarily tolerated by these individuals. In such instances, hospitalization is a necessity.

Lithium toxicity is closely related to serum lithium levels, and can occur at doses close to therapeutic levels (see DOSAGE AND ADMINISTRATION).

Lithium therapy has been reported in some cases to be associated with morphologic changes in the kidneys. The relationship between such changes and renal function has not been established.

Outpatients and their families should be warned that the patient must discontinue lithium therapy and contact his physician if such clinical signs of lithium toxicity as diarrhea, vomiting, tremor, mild ataxia, drowsiness, or muscular weakness occur.

Lithium may prolong the effects of neuromuscular blocking agents. Therefore, neuromuscular blocking agents should be given with caution to patients receiving lithium.

Lithium may impair mental and/or physical abilities. Caution patients about activities requiring alertness (*e.g.,* operating vehicles or machinery).

Combined use of haloperidol and lithium: An encephalopathic syndrome (characterized by weakness, lethargy, fever, tremulousness and confusion, extrapyramidal symptoms, leucocytosis, elevated serum enzymes, BUN and FBS) followed by irreversible brain damage has occurred in a few patients treated with lithium plus haloperidol. A causal relationship between these events and the concomitant administration of lithium and haloperidol has not been established; however, patients receiving such combined therapy should be monitored closely for early evidence of neurological toxicity and treatment discontinued promptly if such signs appear. The possibility of similar adverse interactions with other antipsychotic medications exists.

Usage in Pregnancy

Adverse effects on nidation in rats, embryo viability in mice, and metabolism *in vitro* of rat testis and human spermatozoa have been attributed to lithium, as have teratogenicity in submammalian species and cleft palates in mice. Studies in rats, rabbits and monkeys have shown no evidence of lithium-induced teratology.

There are lithium birth registries in the United States and elsewhere; however there are at the present time insufficient data to determine the effects of lithium on human fetuses. Therefore, at this point, lithium should not be used in pregnancy, especially the first trimester, unless in the opinion of the physician, the potential benefits outweigh the possible hazards.

Usage in Nursing Mothers

Lithium is excreted in human milk. Nursing should not be undertaken during lithium therapy except in rare and unusual circumstances where, in the view of the physician, the potential benefits to the mother outweigh possible hazards to the child.

Usage in Children

Since information regarding the safety and effectiveness of lithium in children under 12 years of age is not available, its use in such patients is not recommended at this time.

Precautions: The ability to tolerate lithium is greater during the acute manic phase and decreases when manic symptoms subside (see DOSAGE AND ADMINISTRATION).

The distribution space of lithium approximates that of total body water. Lithium is primarily excreted in urine with insignificant excretion in feces. Renal excretion of lithium is proportional to its plasma concentration. The half-elimination time of lithium is approximately 24 hours. Lithium decreases sodium reabsorption by the renal tubules which could lead to sodium depletion. Therefore, it is essential for the patient to maintain a normal diet, including salt, and an adequate fluid intake (2500–3000 ml) at least during the initial stabilization period. Decreased tolerance to lithium has been reported to ensue from protracted sweating or diarrhea and, if such occur, supplemental fluid and salt should be administered.

In addition to sweating and diarrhea, concomitant infection with elevated temperatures may also necessitate a temporary reduction or cessation of medication.

Previously existing underlying disorders do not necessarily constitute a contraindication to lithium treatment; where hypothyroidism exists, careful monitoring of thyroid function during lithium stabilization and maintenance allows for correction of changing thyroid parameters, if any, where hypothroidism occurs during lithium stabilization and maintenance, supplemental thyroid treatment may be used.

Indomethacin (50 mg t.i.d.) has been reported to increase steady-state plasma lithium levels from 30 to 59 percent. There is also some evidence that other nonsteroidal, anti-inflammatory agents may have a similar effect. When such combinations are used, increased plasma lithium level monitoring is recommended.

Adverse Reactions: Adverse reactions are seldom encountered at serum lithium levels below 1.5 mEq/l, except in the occasional patient sensitive to lithium. Mild-to-moderate toxic reactions may occur at levels from 1.5–2.5 mEq/l, and moderate-to-severe reactions may be seen at levels from 2.0–2.5 mEq/l, depending upon individual response to the drug.

Fine hand tremor, polyuria and mild thirst may occur during initial therapy for the acute manic phase, and may persist throughout treatment. Transient and mild nausea and general discomfort may also appear during the first few days of lithium administration. These side effects are an inconvenience rather than a disabling condition, and usually subside with continued treatment or a temporary reduction or cessation of dosage. If persistent, a cessation of dosage is indicated.

Diarrhea, vomiting, drowsiness, muscular weakness and lack of coordination may be early signs of lithium intoxication, and can occur at lithium levels below 2.0 mEq/l. At higher levels, giddiness, ataxia, blurred vision, tinnitus and a large output of dilute urine may be seen. Serum lithium levels above 3.0 mEq/l may produce a complex clinical picture involving multiple organs and organ systems. Serum lithium levels should not be permitted to exceed 2.0 mEq/l during the acute treatment phase.

The following toxic reactions have been reported and appear to be related to serum lithium levels, including levels within the therapeutic range.

Neuromuscular: tremor, muscle hyperirritability (fasciculations, twitching, clonic movements of whole limbs), ataxia, choreoathetotic movements, hyperactive deep tendon reflexes.

Central Nervous System: blackout spells, epileptiform seizures, slurred speech, dizziness, vertigo, incontinence of urine or feces, somnolence, psychomotor retardation, restlessness, confusion, stupor, coma.

Cardiovascular: cardiac arrhythmia, hypotension, peripheral circulatory collapse.

Gastrointestinal: anorexia, nausea, vomiting, diarrhea.

Genitourinary: albuminuria, oliguria, polyuria, glycosuria.

Dermatologic: drying and thinning of hair, anesthesia of skin, chronic folliculitis, xerosis cutis, alopecia, exacerbation of psoriasis.

Autonomic Nervous System: blurred vision, dry mouth.

Miscellaneous: fatigue, lethargy, tendency to sleep, dehydration, weight loss, transient scotomata.

Thyroid Abnormalities: euthyroid goiter and/or hypothyroidism (including myxedema) accompanied by lower T_3 and $T_4.I_{131}$ iodine uptake may be elevated (See Precautions). Paradoxically, rare cases of hyperthyroidism have been reported.

EEG Changes: diffuse slowing, widening of frequency spectrum, potentiation and disorganization of background rhythm.

EKG Changes: reversible flattening, isoelectricity or inversion of T-waves.

Miscellaneous reactions unrelated to dosage are: transient electroencephalographic and electrocardiographic changes, leucocytosis, headache, diffuse nontoxic goiter with or without hypothyroidism, transient hyperglycemia, generalized pruritus with or without rash, cutaneous ulcers, albuminuria, worsening of organic brain syndromes, excessive weight gain, edematous swelling of ankles or wrists, and thirst or polyuria, sometimes resembling diabetes insipidus and metallic taste.

A single report has been received of the development of painful discoloration of fingers and toes and coldness of the extremities within one day of the starting of treatment of lithium. The mechanism through which these symptoms (resembling Raynaud's Syndrome) developed is not known. Recovery followed discontinuance.

Dosage and Administration:

Acute Mania: Optimal patient response can usually be established and maintained with

Continued on next page

The full prescribing information for each CIBA drug is contained herein and is that in effect as of October 1, 1982.

CIBA—Cont.

the following dosages:

Lithobid ....900 mg b.i.d. or 600 mg t.i.d. (1800 mg per day)

Cibalith-S ....10 ml (2 teaspoons) (16 mEq of lithium) t.i.d.

Such doses will normally produce an effective serum lithium level ranging between 1.0 and 1.5 mEq/l. Dosage must be individualized according to serum levels and clinical response. Regular monitoring of the patient's clinical state and of serum lithium levels is necessary. Serum levels should be determined twice per week during the acute phase, and until the serum level and clinical condition of the patient have been stabilized.

Long-Term Control: The desirable serum lithium levels are 0.6 to 1.2 mEq/l. Dosage will vary from one individual to another, but usually the following dosages will maintain this level:

Lithobid ....900 mg to 1200 mg per day given in two or three divided doses.

Cibalith-S ....5 ml (1 teaspoon) (8 mEq of lithium) t.i.d. or q.i.d.

Serum lithium levels in uncomplicated cases receiving maintenance therapy during remission should be monitored at least every two months. Patients abnormally sensitive to lithium may exhibit toxic signs at serum levels of 1.0 to 1.5 mEq/l. Elderly patients often respond to reduced dosage, and may exhibit signs of toxicity at serum levels ordinarily tolerated by other patients.

N.B.: Blood samples for serum lithium determinations should be drawn immediately prior to the next dose when lithium concentrations are relatively stable (i.e., 8–12 hours after previous dose). Total reliance must not be placed on serum levels alone. Accurate patient evaluation requires both clinical and laboratory analysis.

Overdosage: The toxic levels for lithium are close to the therapeutic levels. It is therefore important that patients and their families be cautioned to watch for early toxic symptoms and to discontinue the drug and inform the physician should they occur. Toxic symptoms are listed in detail under ADVERSE REACTIONS.

Treatment: No specific antidote for lithium poisoning is known. Early symptoms of lithium toxicity can usually be treated by reduction or cessation of dosage of the drug and resumption of the treatment at a lower dose after 24 to 48 hours. In severe cases of lithium poisoning, the first and foremost goal of treatment consists of elimination of this ion from the patient.

Treatment is essentially the same as that used in barbiturate poisoning: 1) gastric lavage 2) correction of fluid and electrolyte imbalance and 3) regulation of kidney functioning. Urea, mannitol, and aminophylline all produce significant increases in lithium excretion. Hemodialysis is an effective and rapid means of removing the ion from the severely toxic patient. Infection prophylaxis, regular chest x-rays, and preservation of adequate respiration are essential.

How Supplied:

Lithobid, lithium carbonate 300 mg, peach-colored, slow-release tablets are supplied in bottles of 100's & 1000's and in unit-dose boxes of 100's.

[*Shown in Product Identification Section*]

Cibalith-S, lithium citrate syrup, 8 mEq of lithium ion per 5 ml (1 teaspoon) is supplied as a sugar-free, raspberry-flavored syrup in bottles of 480 ml.

C81-70 (1/82)

Dist. by: CIBA Pharmaceutical Company
Div. of CIBA-GEIGY Corporation
Summit, NJ 07901

LOCORTEN® ℞

(flumethasone pivalate USP)
Cream

Description: Locorten, flumethasone pivalate USP, is a topical anti-inflammatory, antipruritic corticosteroid, available as a cream containing 0.03% flumethasone pivalate USP in a water-washable base of cetyl alcohol NF, sodium lauryl sulfate NF, propylene glycol USP, methylparaben NF, propylparaben NF, and purified water USP.

Flumethasone pivalate is 6α, 9-difluoro-11β,17,21-trihydroxy-16α-methylpregna-1,4-diene-3,20-dione 21-trimethylacetate.

Flumethasone pivalate USP is a white to off-white, crystalline powder with a molecular weight of 494.57. It is insoluble in water, slightly soluble in methanol, and very slightly soluble in chloroform and in methylene chloride.

Clinical Pharamcology: Topical corticosteroids have anti-inflammatory, antipruritic, and vasoconstrictive actions.

The mechanism of anti-inflammatory activity of the topical corticosteroids is unclear. Various laboratory methods, including vasoconstrictor assays, are used to compare and predict potencies and clinical efficacies of the topical corticosteroids. There is some evidence to suggest that a recognizable correlation exists between vasoconstrictor potency and therapeutic efficacy in man. Vasoconstriction assays indicate that Locorten penetrates to the dermis and blanching is maximal after approximately 10 hours.

Pharmacokinetics

The extent of percutaneous absorption of topical corticosteroids is determined by many factors, including the vehicle, the integrity of the epidermal barrier, and the use of occulsive dressings.

Topical corticosteroids can be absorbed from normal intact skin. Inflammation and other disease processes in the skin increase percutaneous absorption. Occlusive dressings substantially increase the percutaneous absorption of topical corticosteroids. Thus, occlusive dressings may be a valuable therapeutic adjunct for treatment of resistant dermatoses. (See **Dosage and Administration.**)

Once absorbed through the skin, topical corticosteroids are handled through pharmacokinetic pathways similar to systemically administered corticosteroids. Corticosteroids are bound to plasma proteins in varying degrees. Corticosteroids are metabolized primarily in the liver and are then excreted by the kidneys. Some of the topical corticosteroids and their metabolites are also excreted into the bile.

Indications and Usage: Locorten is indicated for the relief of the inflammatory and pruritic manifestations of corticosteroids-responsive dermatoses.

Contraindications: Locorten is contraindicated in those patients with a history of hypersensitivity to any of the components of the preparation.

Precautions:

General

Systemic absorption of topical corticosteroids has produced reversible hypothalamic-pituitary-adrenal (HPA) axis suppression, manifestations of Cushing's syndrome, hyperglycemia, and glucosuria in some patients.

Conditions that augment systemic absorption include the application of the more potent steroids, use over large surface areas, prolonged use, and the addition of occlusive dressings.

Therefore, patients receiving a large dose of a potent topical steroid applied to a large surface area or under an occlusive dressing should be evaluated periodically for evidence of HPA axis suppression by using the urinary free cortisol and ACTH stimulation tests. If HPA axis suppression is noted, an attempt should be made to withdraw the drug, to reduce the frequency of application, or to substitute a less potent steroid.

Recovery of HPA axis function is generally prompt and complete upon discontinuation of the drug. Infrequently, signs and symptoms of steroid withdrawal may occur, requiring supplemental systemic corticosteroids.

Children may absorb proportionally larger amounts of topical corticosteroids and thus be more susceptible to systemic toxicity. (See **Precautions, Pediatric use.**)

If irritation develops, topical corticosteroids should be discontinued and appropriate therapy instituted.

In the presence of dermatological infections, the use of an appropriate antifungal or antibacterial agent should be instituted. If a favorable response does not occur promptly, the corticosteroids should be discontinued until the infection has been adequarely controlled.

Information for Patients

Patients using topical corticosteroids should receive the following information and instructions:

1. This medication is to be used as directed by the physician. It is for external use only. Avoid contact with the eyes.
2. This medication should not be used for any disorder other than that for which it was prescribed.
3. The treated skin area should not be bandaged or otherwise covered or wrapped as to be occlusive unless directed by the physician.
4. Any signs of local adverse reactions, especially under occlusive dressing, should be reported to the physician.
5. Tight-fitting diapers or plastic pants should not be used on a child being treated in the diaper area, as these garments may constitute occlusive dressings.

Laboratory Tests

The urinary free cortisol and ACTH stimulation tests may be helpful in evaluating the HPA axis suppression.

Carcinogenesis, Mutagenesis, Impairment of Fertility

Long-term animal studies have not been performed to evaluate the carcinogenic potential or the effect on fertility of topical corticosteroids.

Studies to determine mutagenicity with prednisolone and hydrocortisone have revealed negative results.

Pregnancy Category C

Corticosteroids are generally teratogenic in laboratory animals when administered systemically at relatively low dosage levels. The more potent corticosteroids have been shown to be teratogenic after dermal application in laboratory animals. There are no adequate and well-controlled studies in pregnant women on teratogenic effects from topically applied corticosteroids. Therefore, topical corticosteroids should be used during pregnancy only if the potential benefit justifies the potential risk to the fetus. Drugs of this class should not be used extensively on pregnant patients, in large amounts, or for prolonged periods of time.

Nursing Mothers

It is not known whether topical administration of corticosteroids could result in sufficient systemic absorption to produce detectable quantities in breast milk. Systemically administered corticosteroids are secreted into breast milk in quantities *not* likely to have a deleterious effect on the infant. Nevertheless, caution should be exercised when topical corticosteroids are administered to a nursing woman.

Pediatric Use

Pediatric patients may demonstrate greater susceptibility to topical corticosteroid-induced HPA axis suppression and Cushing's syndrome than mature patients because of a larger skin-surface-area to body-weight ratio.

HPA axis suppression, Cushing's syndrome, and intracranial hypertension have been reported in children receiving topical corticosteroids. Manifestations of adrenal suppression in

children include linear growth retardation, delayed weight gain, low plasma cortisol levels, and absence of response to ACTH stimulation. Manifestations of intracranial hypertension include bulging fontanelles, headaches, and bilateral papilledema.
Administration of topical corticosteroids to children should be limited to the least amount compatible with an effective therapeutic regimen. Chronic corticosteroid therapy may interfere with the growth and development of children.

Adverse Reactions: The following local adverse reactions are reported infrequently with topical corticosteroids but may occur more frequently with the use of occlusive dressings. These reactions are listed in an approximate decreasing order of occurrence: burning, itching, irritation, dryness, folliculitis, hypertrichosis, acneiform eruptions, hypopigmentation, perioral dermatitis, allergic contact dermatitis, maceration of the skin, secondary infection, skin atrophy, striae, miliaria.

Overdosage: Topically applied corticosteroids can be absorbed in sufficient amounts to produce systemic effects. (See **Precautions**).

Dosage and Administration: A small amount of Locorten should be applied to affected areas three or four times daily; the cream should be gently rubbed in until it disappears. Treatment should be continued for a few days after the lesions clear.

Occlusive Dressings

Occlusive dressings may be used for the management of psoriasis or recalcitrant conditions, such as chronic neurodermatitis, lichen planus, or lichen simplex chronicus.
Locorten should be gently rubbed in until it disappears. Then an additional thin coating of cream is applied and the entire area covered with a pliable plastic film. If the lesions are dry, the dressing should be airtight and watertight. Moist lesions need not be completely sealed. Dressing changes should be determined on an individual basis. This may be as frequent as once or twice daily or every 3 or 4 days. Reapplication of Locorten is required at each dressing change. Usually, the longer the patient is treated with occlusive dressings the more rapid is the rate of response.

Note: Sensitivity to occlusive dressings or adhesive may occur. In these cases, hypoallergenic materials should be substituted. Some plastic films may be flammable; care should be exercised in their use. Infection may develop when occlusive dressings are used; lesions should be carefully inspected between dressings.

How Supplied:

Cream water-washable base

Tubes of 15 g ....NDC 0083-5301-83
Tubes of 60 g ....NDC 0083-5301-86

Do not store above 86°F (30°C)

C82-38 (11/82)
665253

LUDIOMIL® ℞

(maprotiline hydrochloride)
Tablets

Description: Ludiomil®, maprotiline hydrochloride, is an antidepressant for oral administration which belongs to a new chemical series, dibenzo-bicyclo-octadienes. Its molecular weight is 315.5, and its empirical formula is $C_{20}H_{24}Cl\ N$.
Ludiomil is a white, odorless, stable, crystalline powder which is slightly soluble in water. It melts at 236–246°C.

Clinical Pharmacology: The mechanism of action of Ludiomil is not precisely known. It does not act primarily by stimulation of the central nervous system and is not a monoamine oxidase inhibitor. The postulated mechanism of Ludiomil is that it acts primarily by potentiation of central adrenergic synapses by blocking reuptake of norepinephrine at nerve endings. This pharmacologic action is thought to be responsible for the drug's antidepressant and anxiolytic effects.
The mean time to peak is 12 hours.[1] The half-life of elimination averages 51 hours.[1,2]
Steady-state levels measured prior to the morning dose on a one-dosage regimen are summarized as follows:[2]

Regimen	Average Minimum Concentration ng/ml	95% Confidence Limits ng/ml
50 mg x 3 daily	238	181–295

Indications and Usage: Ludiomil is indicated for the treatment of depressive illness in patients with depressive neurosis (dysthymic disorder) and manic-depressive illness, depressed type (major depressive disorder). Ludiomil is also effective for the relief of anxiety associated with depression.

Contraindications: Ludiomil is contraindicated in patients hypersensitive to Ludiomil and in patients with known or suspected seizure disorders. It should not be given concomitantly with monoamine oxidase (MAO) inhibitors. A minimum of 14 days should be allowed to elapse after discontinuation of MAO inhibitors before treatment with Ludiomil is initiated. Effects should be monitored with gradual increase in dosage until optimum response is achieved. The drug is not recommended for use during the acute phase of myocardial infarction.

Warnings: Extreme caution should be used when this drug is given to:
—patients with a history of myocardial infarction;
—patients with a history or presence of cardiovascular disease because of the possibility of conduction defects, arrhythmias, myocardial infarction, strokes and tachycardia.

Precautions:

General: The possibility of suicide in seriously depressed patients is inherent in their illness and may persist until significant remission occurs. Therefore, patients must be carefully supervised during all phases of treatment with Ludiomil, and prescriptions should be written for the smallest number of tablets consistent with good patient management.
Seizures have been reported in patients treated with Ludiomil. These have occurred in patients both with and without a past history of seizures. While it must be noted that a cause-and-effect relationship has not been established, the risk of seizures may be reduced by initiating therapy at low dosage. Because of the long half-life of Ludiomil (average 51 hours) initial dosage should be maintained for two weeks before being raised gradually in small increments (see **Dosage and Administration**).
Hypomanic or manic episodes have been known to occur in some patients taking tricyclic antidepressant drugs, particularly in patients with cyclic disorders. Such occurrences have also been noted, rarely, with Ludiomil.
Prior to elective surgery, Ludiomil should be discontinued for as long as clinically feasible, since little is known about the interaction between Ludiomil and general anesthetics.
Ludiomil should be administered with caution in patients with increased intraocular pressure, history of urinary retention, or history of narrow-angle glaucoma because of the drug's anticholinergic properties.

Information for Patients: Warn patients to exercise caution about potentially hazardous tasks, or operating automobiles or machinery since the drug may impair mental and/or physical abilities.
Ludiomil may enhance the response to alcohol, barbiturates, and other CNS depressants, requiring appropriate caution of administration.

Laboratory Tests: Although not observed with Ludiomil, the drug should be discontinued if there is evidence of pathologic neutrophil depression. Leukocyte and differential counts should be performed in patients who develop fever and sore throat during therapy.

Drug Interactions: Close supervision and careful adjustment of dosage are required when administering Ludiomil concomitantly with anticholinergic or sympathomimetic drugs because of the possibility of additive atropine-like effects.
Concurrent administration of Ludiomil with electroshock therapy should be avoided because of the lack of experience in this area.
Caution should be exercised when administering Ludiomil to hyperthyroid patients or those on thyroid medication because of the possibility of enhanced potential for cardiovascular toxicity of Ludiomil.
Ludiomil should be used with caution in patients receiving guanethidine or similar agents since it may block the pharmacologic effects of these drugs.
(See "Information for Patients")

Carcinogenesis, Mutagenesis, Impairment of Fertility: Carcinogenicity and chronic toxicity studies have been conducted in laboratory rats and dogs. No drug- or dose-related occurrence of carcinogenesis was evident in rats receiving daily oral doses up to 60 mg/kg of Ludiomil for eighteen months or in dogs receiving daily oral doses up to 30 mg/kg of Ludiomil for one year. In addition, no evidence of mutagenic activity was found in offspring of female mice mated with males treated with up to 60 times the maximum daily human dose.

Pregnancy Category B: Reproduction studies have been performed in female laboratory rabbits, mice, and rats at doses up to 1.3, 7, and 9 times the maximum daily human dose respectively and have revealed no evidence of impaired fertility or harm to the fetus due to Ludiomil. There are, however, no adequate and well-controlled studies in pregnant women. Because animal reproduction studies are not always predictive of human response, this drug should be used during pregnancy only if clearly needed.

Labor and Delivery: Although the effect of Ludiomil on labor and delivery is unknown, caution should be exercised as with any drug with CNS depressant action.

Nursing Mothers: Ludiomil is excreted in breast milk. At steady state, the concentrations in milk correspond closely to the concentrations in whole blood. Caution should be exercised when Ludiomil is administered to a nursing woman.

Pediatric Use: Safety and effectiveness in children below the age of 18 have not been established.

Adverse Reactions: The following adverse reactions have been noted with Ludiomil and are generally similar to those observed with tricyclic antidepressants.

Cardiovascular: Rare occurrences of hypotension, hypertension, tachycardia, palpitation, arrhythmia, heart block, and syncope have been reported with Ludiomil.

Psychiatric: Nervousness (6%), anxiety (3%), insomnia (2%), and agitation (2%); rarely, confusional states (especially in the elderly), hallucinations, disorientation, delusions, restlessness, nightmares, hypomania, mania, exacerbation of psychosis, decrease in memory, and feelings of unreality.

Neurological: Drowsiness (16%), dizziness (8%), tremor (3%), and, rarely, numbness, tingling, motor hyperactivity, akathisia, seizures, EEG alterations, tinnitus, extrapyramidal symptoms, ataxia, and dysarthria.

Anticholinergic: Dry mouth (22%), constipation (6%), and blurred vision (4%); rarely, ac-

Continued on next page

The full prescribing information for each CIBA drug is contained herein and is that in effect as of October 1, 1982.

CIBA—Cont.

commodation disturbances, mydriasis, urinary retention, and delayed micturition.

Allergic: Rare instances of skin rash, petechiae, itching, photosensitization, edema, and drug fever.

Gastrointestinal: Nausea (2%) and, rarely, vomiting, epigastric distress, diarrhea, bitter taste, abdominal cramps and dysphagia.

Endocrine: Rare instances of increased or decreased libido, impotence, and elevation or depression of blood sugar levels.

Other: Weakness and fatigue (4%) and headache (4%); rarely, altered liver function, jaundice, weight loss or gain, excessive perspiration, flushing, urinary frequency, increased salivation, and nasal congestion.

Note: Although the following adverse reactions have not been reported with Ludiomil, its pharmacologic similarity to tricyclic antidepressants requires that each reaction be considered when administering Ludiomil.

—Bone marrow depression, including agranulocytosis, eosinophilia, purpura, and thrombocytopenia, myocardial infarction, stroke, peripheral neuropathy, sublingual adenitis, black tongue, stomatitis, paralytic ileus, gynecomastia in the male, breast enlargement and galactorrhea in the female, and testicular swelling.

Overdosage:

Animal Oral LD_{50}: The oral LD_{50} of Ludiomil is 600-750 mg/kg in mice, 760-900 mg/kg in rats, > 1000 mg/kg in rabbits, > 300 mg/kg in cats, and > 30 mg/kg in dogs.

Signs and Symptoms: Data dealing with overdosage in humans are limited with only a few cases on record. Symptoms are drowsiness, tachycardia, ataxia, vomiting, cyanosis, hypotension, shock, restlessness, agitation, hyperpyrexia, muscle rigidity, athetoid movements, mydriasis, cardiac arrhythmias, impaired cardiac condition. In severe cases, loss of consciousness and generalized convulsions may occur. Since congestive heart failure has been seen with overdosages of tricyclic antidepressants, it should be considered with Ludiomil overdosage.

Treatment: There is no specific antidote. Induced emesis and gastric lavage are recommended. It may be helpful to leave the tube in the stomach with irrigation and continual aspiration of stomach contents possibly promoting more rapid elimination of the drug from the body. The room should be darkened, allowing only minimal external stimulation to reduce the tendency to convulsions.

1. The intravenous administration of 1 to 3 mg of physostigmine has been reported to reverse the signs and symptoms of overdosage with tricyclic antidepressants. Repeat doses at intervals of 30 to 60 minutes may be necessary.
2. Hyperirritability and convulsions may be treated with carefully titrated parenteral barbiturates. Barbiturates should not be employed, however, if drugs that inhibit monoamine oxidase have also been taken by the patient in overdosage or in recent therapy. Similarly, barbiturates may induce respiratory depression, particularly in children. It is therefore advisable to have equipment available for artificial ventilation and resuscitation when barbiturates are employed. Paraldehyde may be used effectively in some children to counteract muscular hypertonus and convulsions with less likelihood of causing respiratory depression.
3. Shock (circulatory collapse) should be treated with supportive measures such as intravenous fluids, oxygen, and corticosteroids.
4. Hyperpyrexia should be controlled by whatever means available, including ice packs if necessary.
5. Signs of congestive heart failure may be satisfactorily treated by rapid digitalization.
6. Dialysis is of little value because of the low plasma concentration of this drug.

Dosage and Administration: A single daily dose is an alternative to divided daily doses. Therapeutic effects are sometimes seen within 3 to 7 days, although as long as 2 to 3 weeks are usually necessary.

Initial Adult Dosage: An initial dosage of 75 mg daily is suggested for outpatients with mild-to-moderate depression. However, in some patients, particularly the elderly, an initial dosage of 25 mg daily may be used. Because of the long half-life of Ludiomil, the initial dosage should be maintained for two weeks. The dosage may then be increased gradually in 25 mg increments as required and tolerated. Most patients respond to a dose of 150 mg daily, but daily dosage as high as 225 mg may be required in some cases.

More severely depressed, hospitalized patients should be given an initial daily dose of 100 mg to 150 mg which may be gradually increased as required and tolerated. Most hospitalized patients with moderate-to-severe depression respond to a daily dosage of 150 mg to 225 mg, although dosages as high as 300 mg may be required in some cases. Daily dosage of 300 mg should not be exceeded.

Elderly Patients: In general, lower dosages are recommended for patients over 60 years of age. Dosages of 50 mg to 75 mg daily are usually satisfactory as maintenance therapy for elderly patients who do not tolerate higher amounts.

Maintenance: Dosage during prolonged maintenance therapy should be kept at the lowest effective level. Dosage may be reduced to levels of 75 mg to 150 mg daily during such periods, with subsequent adjustment depending on therapeutic response.

How Supplied:

Tablets 25 mg—oval, dark orange, coated (imprinted CIBA 110)
Bottle of 100—NDC 0083-0110-30
Accu-Pak® Unit Dose (blister pack)
Box of 100 (strips of 10)—NDC 0083-0110-32

Tablets 50 mg—round, dark orange, coated (imprinted CIBA 26)
Bottle of 100—NDC 0083-0026-30
Accu-Pak® Unit Dose (blister pack)
Box of 100 (strips of 10)—NDC 0083-0026-32

Tablets 75 mg—oval, white, coated (imprinted CIBA 135)
Bottles of 100—NDC 0083-0135-30
Accu-Pak® Unit Dose (blister pack)
Box of 100 (strips of 10)—NDC 0083-0135-32

Dispense in tight container (USP).

1. Alkalay D, et al. Bioavailability and kinetics of maprotiline. *Clin Pharmacol Ther* 1980; **27** (5): 697–703.
2. Riess W, et al. The pharmacokinetic properties of maprotiline (Ludiomil®) in man. *J Int Med Res* 1975; **3** (2): 16–41.

C82-57 (10/82)

[*Shown in Product Identification Section*]

METANDREN® ℞
(methyltestosterone USP)
Linguets® and Tablets

Listed in USP, a Medicare designated compendium.

Indications

In the Male

1. Eunuchoidism and eunuchism.
2. Climacteric symptoms when these are secondary to androgen deficiency.
3. Impotence due to androgen deficiency.
4. Postpuberal cryptorchidism with evidence of hypogonadism.

In the Female

1. Prevention of postpartum breast pain and engorgement. There is no satisfactory evidence that this drug prevents or suppresses lactation.
2. Palliation of androgen-responsive, advancing, inoperable mammary cancer, in women who are more than 1 year, but less than 5 years postmenopausal or who have been proven to have a hormone-dependent tumor as shown by previous beneficial response to castration.

Contraindications: Carcinoma of the male breast; known or suspected carcinoma of the prostate; cardiac, hepatic, or renal decompensation; hypercalcemia; impaired liver function; prepuberal males; patients easily stimulated; pregnancy; and breast feeding.

Warnings: Hypercalcemia may occur in immobilized patients and in breast cancer patients. In patients with cancer hypercalcemia may indicate progression of bony metastasis, in which case the drug should be discontinued. Watch female patients closely for signs of virilization. Some effects such as voice changes may not be reversible even when the drug is stopped.

Discontinue the drug if cholestatic hepatitis with jaundice appears or liver function tests become abnormal.

Precautions: Patients with cardiac, renal, or hepatic derangement may retain sodium and water with resulting edema formation.

Males, especially the elderly, may become overly stimulated.

Priapism or excessive sexual stimulation may develop.

Oligospermia and reduced ejaculatory volume may occur after prolonged administration or excessive dosage.

Hypersensitivity and gynecomastia may occur.

Alterations in liver function tests (*eg,* increased BSP retention and SGOT levels) and rarely jaundice have been reported and appear to be directly related to the dose of the drug. When any of these effects appear, the androgen should be stopped; if restarted, a lower dosage should be utilized.

Use cautiously in young boys to avoid possible premature epiphyseal closure or precocious sexual development.

The PBI may decrease during androgen therapy without clinical significance.

The Metandren Linguets® (10 mg) and tablets (25 mg) contain FD&C Yellow No. 5 (tartrazine) which may cause allergic-type reactions (including bronchial asthma) in certain susceptible individuals. Although the overall incidence of FD&C Yellow No. 5 (tartrazine) sensitivity in the general population is low, it is frequently seen in patients who also have aspirin hypersensitivity.

Adverse Reactions: Hypersensitivity, including skin manifestations and anaphylactoid reactions; acne; decreased ejaculatory volume; oligospermia; gynecomastia; edema; priapism; hypercalcemia, especially in immobile patients and those with metastatic breast carcinoma; virilization in females; cholestatic jaundice. There have been rare reports of hepatocellular neoplasms and peliosis hepatis in association with long-term androgenic-anabolic steroid therapy.

Dosage and Administration: Dosage must be strictly individualized. Daily requirements are best administered in divided doses. The following chart is suggested as an average daily dosage guide. Duration of therapy will depend upon the response of the condition being treated and the appearance of adverse reactions.

NOTE: Linguets have approximately twice the potency of the orally ingested hormone.

INDICATIONS	AVERAGE DAILY DOSAGE *Linguets*	*Tablets*
In the Male		
Eunuchism and eunuchoidism	5 to 20 mg	10 to 40 mg

Male climacteric and male impotence ....5 to 20 mg 10 to 40 mg
Cryptorchidism—postpuberal ....15 mg 30 mg

In the Female

Postpartum breast pain and engorgement (3 to 5 days) ....40 mg 80 mg
Breast cancer.................. 100 mg 200 mg

Administration of Linguets
Linguets should not be swallowed since the hormone is meant to be absorbed through the mucous membranes. Place Linguet in the upper or lower buccal pouch between the gum and cheek. Avoid eating, drinking, chewing, or smoking while the Linguet is in place. Proper oral hygienic measures are particularly important after the use of Linguets.

How Supplied: *Linguets,* 5 mg (white); bottles of 100. *Linguets,* 10 mg (yellow); bottles of 100. *Tablets,* 10 mg (white, scored) and 25 mg (pale yellow, scored); bottles of 100.
LINGUETS® (tablets for mucosal absorption CIBA)
Dispense in tight, light-resistant container (USP).

C80-18 (1/80)

[*Shown in Product Identification Section*]

METOPIRONE® ℞

(metyrapone USP)
Tablets
Diagnostic Test of Pituitary Function

Description: A synthetic compound prepared in the CIBA Research Laboratories, Metopirone is 2-Methyl-1,2-di-3-pyridyl-1-propanone (USP).

Actions: Immediate effect of reducing cortisol production by inhibition of adrenal 11-β-hydroxylation. In the normal person, a compensatory increase in ACTH release follows and the secretion of 11-desoxycortisol and 11-desoxycorticosterone, "17-hydroxycorticoids," are markedly accelerated.

Indications: A diagnostic test drug for hypothalamico-pituitary function.

Contraindications: Adrenal cortical insufficiency, hypersensitivity.

Warnings: Usage in Pregnancy: The safety of metyrapone in pregnant women has not been established.

Precautions: All corticosteroid therapy must be discontinued prior to and during metyrapone testing.
Ability of adrenals to respond to exogenous ACTH should be demonstrated before metyrapone is employed as a test.
Drug may induce acute adrenal insufficiency in patients with reduced adrenal secretory capacity.
Erroneous results in pituitary function as determined by the metyrapone test may occur in patients taking diphenylhydantoin for as long as two weeks following cessation of therapy. A subnormal response may also occur in pregnant women and in patients on estrogen therapy.

Adverse Reactions: Nausea, abdominal discomfort, dizziness, headache, sedation, and allergic rash have been reported.

Dosage and Administration:

Day 1: Control period—Collect 24-hour urine with measurement of 17-hydroxycorticosteroids (17-OHCS) or 17-ketogenic steroids (17-KGS).

Day 2: ACTH test—Standard ACTH test such as administering 50 units ACTH by infusion over 8 hours and measurement of 24 hours urinary steroids.

Days 3-4: Rest period.

Day 5: Metyrapone administration:
Adults—750 mg orally, every 4 hours for 6 doses. A single dose is approximately equivalent to 15 mg/kg.
Children—15 mg/kg orally, every 4 hours for 6 doses. A minimal single dose of 250 mg is recommended.

Day 6: Post-oral metyrapone measurement—24-hour steroid determination for effect.

Interpretation

ACTH
The normal 24-hour urinary excretion of 17-OHCS ranges from 3 to 12 mg. Following continuous intravenous infusion of 50 units ACTH over a period of 8 hours, the 17-OHCS excretion is increased to 15 to 45 mg per 24 hours.

Metyrapone

a. **Normal response:** In patients with a normally functioning pituitary, the administration of metyrapone is followed by a two- to four-fold increase of 17-OHCS excretion or doubling of 17-KGS excretion.

b. **Subnormal response:** Subnormal response in patients without adrenal insufficiency is indicative of some degree of impairment of pituitary function, either panhypopituitarism or partial hypopituitarism (limited pituitary reserve).
   1. *Panhypopituitarism* is readily diagnosed by the classical clinical and chemical evidences of hypogonadism, hypothyroidism, and hypoadrenocorticism. These patients usually have subnormal basal urinary steroid levels. Depending upon the duration of the disease and degree of adrenal atrophy, they may fail to respond to exogenous ACTH in the normal manner. Metyrapone administration is not essential in the diagnosis, but if given, it will not induce an appreciable increase in urinary steroids.
   2. *Partial hypopituitarism* or limited pituitary reserve is the more difficult diagnosis as these patients do not present the classical signs and symptoms of hypopituitarism. Measurements of target organ functions often are normal under basal conditions. The response to exogenous ACTH is usually normal, producing the expected rise of urinary steroids (17-OHCS or 17-KGS). The response, however, to metyrapone is *subnormal;* that is, no significant increase in 17-OHCS or 17-KGS excretion occurs.
   This failure to respond to metyrapone may be interpreted as evidence of impaired pituitary-adrenal reserve. In view of the normal response to exogenous ACTH, the failure to respond to metyrapone is inferred to be related to a defect in the CNS-pituitary mechanisms which normally regulate ACTH secretions. Presumably the ACTH secreting mechanisms of these individuals are already working at their maximal rates to meet everyday conditions and possess limited "reserve" capacities to secrete additional ACTH either in response to stress or to decreased cortisol levels occurring as a result of metyrapone administration.

c. **Excessive response:** An excessive excretion of 17-OHCS or 17-KGS above the normal range after metyrapone administration is suggestive of Cushing's syndrome associated with adrenal hyperplasia. These patients have an elevated excretion of urinary corticosteroids under basal conditions and will often, but not invariably, show a "supernormal" response to ACTH and also to metyrapone, excreting more than 35 mg per 24 hours of either 17-OHCS or 17-KGS.

How Supplied: *Tablets,* 250 mg (white, scored); bottles of 18.
Dispense in tight, light-resistant container (USP).

C79-13 (7/79)

[*Shown in Product Identification Section*]

NUPERCAINAL®

Anesthetic Ointment
Pain-Relief Cream

> **Caution:**
> **Nupercainal** products are not for prolonged or extensive use and should never be applied in or near the eyes.
> **Consult labels before using.**
> **Keep this and all medications out of reach of children.**
> NUPERCAINAL SHOULD NOT BE SWALLOWED. SWALLOWING OR USE OF A LARGE QUANTITY IS HAZARDOUS, PARTICULARLY TO CHILDREN. CONSULT A PHYSICIAN OR POISON CONTROL CENTER IMMEDIATELY.

Indications: Nupercainal Ointment and Cream are fast-acting, long-lasting pain relievers that you can use for a number of painful skin conditions. **Nupercainal Anesthetic Ointment** is for hemorrhoids and for general use. **Nupercainal Pain-Relief Cream** is for general use only. The **Cream** is half as strong as the **Ointment.**

How to use Nupercainal Anesthetic Ointment (for general use). This soothing Ointment helps lubricate dry, inflamed skin and gives fast, temporary relief of pain and itching. It is recommended for sunburn, nonpoisonous insect bites, minor burns, cuts, and scratches. **DO NOT USE THIS PRODUCT IN OR NEAR YOUR EYES.**
Apply to affected areas gently. If necessary, cover with a light dressing for protection. Do not use more than 1 ounce of Ointment in a 24-hour period for an adult, do not use more than one-quarter of an ounce in a 24-hour period for a child. If irritation develops, discontinue use and consult your doctor.

How to use Nupercainal Anesthetic Ointment for fast, temporary relief of pain and itching due to hemorrhoids (also known as piles). Remove cap from tube and set it aside. Attach the white plastic applicator to the tube. Squeeze the tube until you see the Ointment begin to come through the little holes in the applicator. Using your finger, lubricate the applicator with the Ointment. Now insert the entire applicator gently into the rectum. Give the tube a good squeeze to get enough Ointment into the rectum for comfort and lubrication. Remove applicator from rectum and wipe it clean. Apply additional Ointment to anal tissues to help relieve pain, burning, and itching. For best results use Ointment morning and night and after each bowel movement. After each use detach applicator, and wash it off with soap and water. Put cap back on tube before storing. In case of rectal bleeding, discontinue use and consult your doctor.

Pain-Relief Cream for general use. This Cream is particularly effective for fast, temporary relief of pain and itching associated with sunburn, cuts, scratches, minor burns and nonpoisonous insect bites. **DO NOT USE THIS PRODUCT IN OR NEAR YOUR EYES.** Apply liberally to affected area and rub in gently. This Cream is water-washable, so be sure to reapply after bathing, swimming or sweating. If irritation develops, discontinue use and consult your doctor.

Nupercainal Anesthetic Ointment contains 1% (one percent) dibucaine USP in a lubricant base. Available in tubes of 1 and 2 ounces. **Nupercainal Pain-Relief Cream** contains 0.5% (one-half of one percent) dibucaine USP in a

Continued on next page

The full prescribing information for each CIBA drug is contained herein and is that in effect as of October 1, 1982.

CIBA—Cont.

water-soluble base. Available in 1 1/2 ounce tubes.

Dibucaine USP is officially classified as a "topical anesthetic" and is one of the strongest and longest lasting of all pain relievers. It is not a narcotic.

C81-17 (5/81)

NUPERCAINAL™ Suppositories

Caution:
Nupercainal Suppositories are not for prolonged or extensive use. Contact with the eyes should be avoided.
Consult labels before using.
Keep this and all medications out of reach of children.
NUPERCAINAL SUPPOSITORIES SHOULD NOT BE SWALLOWED. SWALLOWING CAN BE HAZARDOUS, PARTICULARLY TO CHILDREN. IN THE EVENT OF ACCIDENTAL SWALLOWING CONSULT A PHYSICIAN OR POISON CONTROL CENTER IMMEDIATELY.

Indications: Nupercainal Suppositories are for the temporary relief from itching, burning, and discomfort due to hemorrhoids or other anorectal disorders.

How to use Nupercainal Suppositories for hemorrhoids (also known as piles) or other anorectal disorders.
Tear off one suppository along the perforated line. Remove foil wrapper. Insert the suppository, rounded end first, well into the anus until you can feel it moving into your rectum. For best results, use one suppository after each bowel movement and as needed, but not to exceed 6 in a 24-hour period. Each suppository is sealed in its own foil packet to reduce danger of leakage when carried in pocket or purse. **To prevent melting, do not store above 86°F (30°C).**

Nupercainal Suppositories contain 2.4 gram cocoa butter, .25 gram zinc oxide, .1 gram bismuth subgallate, and acetone sodium bisulfite as preservative.

Dist. by:
CIBA Pharmaceutical Company
Division of CIBA-GEIGY Corporation
Summit, New Jersey 07901

C82-56 (12/82)

NUPERCAINE® hydrochloride ℞ (dibucaine hydrochloride USP) 1:200 (0.5%)

Listed in USP, a Medicare designated compendium.

Specially Prepared for Isobaric Spinal Anesthesia According to the Method of Keyes and McLellan*

*Keyes, E. L., and McLellan, A. M.: *Amer J Surg 9:*1 (July) 1930. Not to be confused with the method of Howard Jones wherein the technique is somewhat different and the dibucaine hydrochloride solution is much weaker (1:1500) or with the Heavy Solution Nupercaine® hydrochloride (dibucaine hydrochloride).

Principle: A small volume of this concentrated solution of dibucaine hydrochloride is mixed with cerebrospinal fluid and injected in a final concentration of 1:1000.

Solution: Nupercaine hydrochloride 1:200 is an isobaric, isotonic, phosphate-buffered solution.

Specific Gravity
1.0062 (15.5°C) 1.0060 (20.0°C) 1.0059 (37.0°C)

Equipment

Syringe: Luer-Lok all-glass syringe, capacity 10 ml.

Needles: One needle of convenient size to transfer solution from the ampul into the syringe. One spinal needle with an accurately fitted stylet. It is suggested that a needle no larger than No. 22 be used. Larger sizes, permitting loss of spinal fluid, contribute to postinjection headache.

The bevel of the needle is important. It should be short with an angle of no less than 45° to decrease the possibility that part of the dibucaine hydrochloride solution might escape into the extradural space during the injection.

Because dibucaine hydrochloride is precipitated by minute amounts of alkali, syringes and needles should be rinsed with acidified distilled water to remove traces of alkaline salts and small foreign particles.

Ampuls: As part of the meticulous technique for administration of any spinal anesthetic agent, ampuls should be prepared as follows: Autoclave sterilization, considered by several authorities to be the best method. Dibucaine hydrochloride 1:200 solution (method of Keyes and McLellan) is stable as to pH, color and chemical assay when subjected to 3 repeated sterilizations at 121°C for 30 minutes.

Preparation of the Patient: Food and liquid, unless otherwise contraindicated, may be given freely up to the night before surgery. Enemas may be given.

It is recommended that a mild hypnotic be given the night before the operation. One-half to one hour before the patient is brought into the operating room, ¼ grain (15 mg) of morphine sulfate [with 1/200 gr (0.33 mg) of scopolamine hydrobromide as recommended by Keyes and McLellan] is administered. If necessary, ⅙ gr (10 mg) of morphine is given shortly before spinal puncture.

Position of the Patient: The sitting position facilitates injection. If necessary, the lateral position may be employed; care must be taken so that the vertebral column is straight and without lateral curvature.

Insertion of the Spinal Needle: The patient sits bending well forward, and the puncture is made at the L_3-L_4 interspace. (If he is in the lateral position he should be fully flexed.) The D_{12}-L_1 interspace can be the site of injection for upper abdominal operations and L_1-L_2 for gynecological surgery.

When the spinal needle is in the correct position, the stylet is removed and about 2 ml cerebrospinal fluid is allowed to escape. The stylet is replaced. If the tapped fluid is bloody after 2 ml have flowed or if there is radiating pain, there has been incorrect placement of the needle. It should be withdrawn and inserted at another interspace.

Once the needle is correctly inserted, it is very important to avoid displacing it from the subdural space.

Suggested Dosages

Surgical Area	*Dose (mg)*	*Volume (ml)*
Perineum and lower limbs	2.5 to 5	0.5 to 1
Lower abdomen	5 to 7.5	1 to 1.5
Upper abdomen	10	2

The size of the individual, the degree of anesthesia desired and particularly the experience of the physician may modify these recommended dosages.

Note: The maximum dose should never be more than 10 mg (2 ml).

Injection: The desired amount of Nupercaine hydrochloride (dibucaine hydrochloride) 1:200 is drawn up into the syringe by the "transfer" needle. With the stylet removed from the positioned spinal needle, the syringe is attached. If the patient is in the upright position, cerebrospinal fluid pressure usually will force the fluid out into the syringe to mix with the dibucaine hydrochloride 1:200 solution. If fluid does not flow easily, gentle aspiration may be used. The appropriate volume of cerebrospinal fluid (4 times the volume of the dibucaine hydrochloride 1:200 solution) is withdrawn and allowed to mix with the dibucaine hydrochloride. [See table 1 below.].

About one-third of the mixture is then injected, after which spinal fluid is again aspirated. Following this, one-half of the remaining contents of the syringe is injected. Another aspiration is then followed by injection of the remainder of the mixture.

The whole injection should be carried out very slowly.

Regulation of Anesthesia: When injection is complete, the needle is removed, the skin swabbed with antiseptic, sterile gauze fixed, and the patient is placed in Trendelenburg position.

Immediately after dibucaine hydrochloride is injected subdurally, it is advisable to inject ¾ to 1½ gr (50 to 100 mg) ephedrine intramuscularly. This usually prevents a fall in blood pressure in case the anesthetic solution ascends higher than desired.

For operations on the abdominal viscera a 20° Trendelenburg position is used; with surgery on the lower abdomen, perineum and lower limbs, the tilt may be decreased to 10° to 15°. The level of anesthesia should be determined after 1 or 2 minutes so that the tilt of the table can be adjusted for the desired level of anesthesia.

With correct technique and dosage, anesthesia with Nupercaine hydrochloride (dibucaine hydrochloride) should be sufficiently developed after 10 to 15 minutes. Failure of this to occur suggests either:

(1) Separation of dibucaine hydrochloride because of alkalinity of the syringe or needle.
(2) Extradural injection of the anesthetic solution.

Anesthesia lasts, on the average, up to six hours. This is followed by a period of slowly returning sensibility during which the patient is free from postoperative discomfort.

General Contraindications

Absolute

1. Disease of the cerebrospinal system, such as meningitis, cranial hemorrhage, tumors, poliomyelitis.
2. Moribund patients.
3. Blood stream infection.
4. Pernicious anemia with cord symptoms.
5. Arthritis, spondylitis, and other diseases of the spinal column rendering spinal puncture impossible. The presence of tuberculosis or metastatic lesions in the column is also a contraindication.
6. Pyogenic infection of the skin at or adjacent to the site of puncture.

Table 1

Dilution of Dibucaine Hydrochloride 1:200 by Cerebrospinal Fluid

Ml Dibucaine Hydrochloride 1:200	*Ml Cerebrospinal Fluid*	*Final Concentration Dibucaine Hydrochloride*	*Mg Dibucaine Hydrochloride Per Dose*
0.5	2	1:1000	2.5
1	4	1:1000	5
1.5	6	1:1000	7.5
2	8	1:1000	10

Relative

1. **Hysteria or excessive nervous tension.** This difficulty may frequently be overcome by the preoperative administration of morphine sulfate ⅙ to ¼ gr (10 to 15 mg), scopolamine 1/150 to 1/100 gr (0.43 to 0.65 mg), or a sedative.
2. **Chronic backache.** The patient may blame any exacerbation of symptoms, either immediate or late, on the spinal anesthesia.
3. **Preoperative headache of long duration or history of migraine.** Exacerbation of symptoms may follow spinal injection.
4. **Hypersensitivity to drugs.** This drug may be used frequently in patients who have shown a sensitivity to procaine. However, in all patients in whom drug sensitivity is suspected, a skin test should be performed by injecting intradermally a small amount (0.1 ml) of dibucaine hydrochloride and at the same time injecting intradermally a small amount (0.1 ml) of physiologic salt solution as a control. Reaction may be local (redness), or systemic (dyspnea, agitation). Use of the drug is absolutely contraindicated in the presence of local reaction if there is a history of drug idiosyncrasy.
5. **Possibility of severe hemorrhage during operation.** Judgment in this case must include consideration of the amount of possible hemorrhage, the height of anesthesia to be induced, and the facilities available to control shock.
6. **Shock.** All forms of anesthesia are poorly borne by patients in shock. Systolic blood pressure should be raised to at least 105 mm Hg before operation is contemplated.
7. **Hypotension.** In cases not due to Addison's disease or associated with severe shock, this has become of relatively little importance because of the effectiveness of ephedrine in restoring pressure to normal (see *Complications:* Hypotension).
8. **Hemorrhagic spinal fluid.** Where clear spinal fluid cannot be obtained, the needle should be withdrawn and puncture made at another interspace. This is important in order to avoid the possibility of intravenous injection of the drug.
9. **Cardiac decompensation, massive pleural effusions, and markedly increased intra-abdominal pressure** as in massive ascites and tumors.

Warnings

1. An extremely potent anesthetic agent and therefore is to be used in much smaller concentrations than other local anesthetics.
2. As is true for any spinal anesthetic agent, the anesthetist should remain in constant attendance. Ephedrine and oxygen should be held in readiness in order to effectively combat a sudden fall in blood pressure should such occur. Likewise, a quick-acting barbiturate should be readily available so that any evidence of toxicity, as manifested by excitement, may be treated promptly.
3. Persons with known drug sensitivity should be pretested before using any of the local anesthetic agents.

Cautions: Authorities agree that spinal anesthesia should not be induced unless the anesthetist is: (1) equipped to provide a rigidly aseptic technique; (2) prepared to remain in constant attendance; (3) equipped to deal with complications or side effects that may arise; (4) familiar with the contraindications to spinal anesthesia.

Complications and Side Effects

1. **Respiratory.** Cessation of respiration may occur from spread of the anesthetic into the cervical region. This is absolutely prevented by following the technique described. It may also occur because of medullary anoxia which follows the circulatory collapse incident to severe hypotension.
   Treatment: Intubation to assure an adequate airway; artificial respiration; oxygen; respiratory stimulant repeated as necessary.
2. **Hypotension.** The fall of blood pressure produced by spinal anesthesia is due to a number of factors, most important of which are: (1) sudden vasodilatation incident to paralysis of sympathetic vasomotor fibers and (2) loss of muscle tone with decrease in venous pressure, venous return, and cardiac output. The degree of fall therefore depends upon the number of segments involved, being greatest in high spinal anesthesia and practically nonexistent when the effect is confined to the perineal area alone.
   There have been several reports indicating that Nupercaine hydrochloride (dibucaine hydrochloride) has less effect upon blood pressure than does a comparable degree of anesthesia produced by procaine.
   Treatment: The prophylactic use of 25 mg ephedrine given intramuscularly before the anesthetic is injected is advised by many authorities. It may be omitted in low spinals. An additional dose of 25 mg should be given *intravenously* if a fall below 100 mm Hg occurs. This dose may be repeated; total should not exceed 100 mg. Fluids, plasma, or whole blood should be administered intravenously when severe fall of blood pressure occurs. In *obstetrical patients,* raising the legs to the vertical position is the most effective initial procedure to increase blood pressure.
3. **Postanesthetic Headache.** Since this is usually due to leakage of spinal fluid, incidence will decrease as technique improves.
   Prophylaxis: A needle of small caliber (not over 20 or 22 gauge) should be used. Some authorities recommend special needles, one of 20 gauge to penetrate the skin and fascia and an inner needle of 24 gauge to pierce the dura. It has also been recommended that the needle be introduced with the bevel held laterally so as to cut fewer fibers of the dura. The needle should remain in place for several seconds after injection to allow time for equalization of pressure.
   Treatment: Tight abdominal binder. Hydration of the patient with either oral or intravenous fluids. One ml surgical pituitrin or 100 mg ephedrine. Rapid relief has been reported after intraspinal or caudal injection of 30 ml sterile saline.
4. **Nausea and Vomiting.** These may occur from psychic causes, drop in blood pressure, or intra-abdominal manipulation.
   Treatment: When caused by hypotension, inhalations of 100 percent oxygen in conjunction with a vasopressor may be found effective. Light cyclopropane or an intravenous barbiturate will control that which is due to intra-abdominal manipulation.
5. **Palsies.** Transient nerve palsies, usually involving the abducens, have occasionally been reported. This very uncommon complication generally occurs during the second week and clears up by the third or fourth week. Temporary or permanent transverse myelitis may follow the use of spinal anesthetic agents (see *Warnings*).
6. **Meningitis.** An aseptic technique should practically preclude the occurrence of this complication. Aseptic meningitis or meningismus, usually of rapid and benign course, has occurred after spinal anesthesia as it has also in cases where no spinal puncture has been carried out. Lundy has called attention to the fact that meningitides following spinal anesthesia may occur without relation to the method but due to pathologically proved metastases from distant foci. However, even the remote possibility of this complication reinforces the necessity for an absolutely sterile technique.
7. **Drug Idiosyncrasy.** The use of this drug is exceptionally free of this hazard. Patients giving a history of hypersensitivity to drugs, however, should be skin tested (see *Contraindications*).
   Treatment: The occurrence of motor excitement requires the anticonvulsant action of an intravenous barbiturate.

How Supplied: *Ampuls,* for spinal anesthesia, 2 ml, 1:200 (method of Keyes and McLellan), each ampul containing 10 mg dibucaine hydrochloride, 10 mg sodium chloride, 4 mg sodium phosphate monobasic, 0.9 mg sodium phosphate dibasic, and water q.s.; cartons of 10.
C80-50 (7/80)

NUPERCAINE® hydrochloride ℞
(dibucaine hydrochloride USP)
1:1500

Listed in USP, a Medicare designated compendium.

Specially Prepared for Hypobaric Spinal Anesthesia According to the Method of Howard Jones*

*Not to be confused with the method of Keyes and McLellan wherein the technique is completely different and the dibucaine hydrochloride solution is much more concentrated.

Principle: A relatively large volume of this solution of dibucaine hydrochloride with a specific gravity *less* than that of the cerebrospinal fluid (hypobaric) is injected without previous removal of fluid.

Solution: Nupercaine hydrochloride 1:1500 in saline. Specific Gravity: 1.0038 (15.5°C), 1.0036 (37°C).

Equipment

Syringe: Luer-Lok syringe with a capacity of 20 ml, accurately gauged, made of neutral glass.

Needles: Rustless needles, 20 gauge and 3½ inches in length; short bevels.

Large needles inflict unnecessary trauma; their use is apt to be followed by postinjection backache and headache, presumably due to trauma and leakage of spinal fluid. With a needle as slender as 22 gauge or more, longer than 3½ inches, bending is apt to occur when the needle is held by the hub and attempt made to puncture the skin; on the other hand, needles less than 3½ inches long may be too short for obese patients. The bevel of the needle is of importance; if it is less than 45 degrees, the chance of having a portion of the lumen outside the dura is increased, although the tip lies in the subdural space; the result being that a part or all of the anesthetic solution escapes extradurally when the attempt is made to inject it. The spinal puncture needle should be furnished with an accurately fitting stylet. The needle should be carefully examined and tested by bending before sterilization.

Syringes and needles are sterilized, preferably in an autoclave, then rinsed in slightly acidulated distilled water or 95% alcohol (2 to 3 drops of dilute hydrochloric acid to the liter), and covered with a sterile towel. This procedure is of importance, both for removing any small foreign particles and also to neutralize any alkalinity.

Ampuls: As part of the meticulous technique for administration of any spinal anesthetic agent, ampuls should be prepared as follows:

Continued on next page

The full prescribing information for each CIBA drug is contained herein and is that in effect as of October 1, 1982.

CIBA—Cont.

Autoclave sterilization, considered by several authorities to be the best method. Dibucaine hydrochloride 1:1500 solution (method of Howard Jones) is stable as to pH, color and chemical assay when subjected to 3 repeated sterilizations at 121°C for 30 minutes.

Preoperative Procedure: The patient's confidence should be gained. Food and liquids, unless contraindicated, may be given freely up to the night preceding surgery; enemas may be given.

A mild hypnotic is indicated in order to provide sleep the night preceding the operation; 1/4 gr morphine sulfate is administered 1/2 to 1 hour before the patient is brought to the operating room. If necessary, 1/6 gr morphine may be given shortly before puncture.

Administration: The patient is placed in the right lateral position, after his back has been painted with tincture of iodine over an area extending a palm's breadth below the scapular angle to the gluteal cleft, washed with 70% alcohol and draped with sterile cloth or towels. It is important to have the patient in a lateral position when making the subdural injection, because the solution with the specific gravity lighter than the one of the spinal fluid (usually 1.005 to 1.007) will ascend rapidly in the canal, with possible involvement of the medullary centers, if the sitting position is adopted.

The lumbar puncture is made between the 2nd and 3rd vertebrae or between the 3rd and 4th, according to the level of the operation. The needle, inserted in the proper interspace, is pushed 1 mm further after the first appearance of cerebrospinal fluid, and a few drops are allowed to escape. The syringe is then attached, care being taken not to displace the needle. The injection is made very slowly and should be discontinued for 3 to 4 seconds when an increasing resistance is encountered. The needle is, under these circumstances, maintained strictly in the position adopted to minimize leakage. No efforts should be made to decrease the resistance by moving the needle, but pauses are made after the injection of each succeeding 2 ml of the solution.

While barbotage is practiced in the administration of the buffered (1:200) solution of Nupercaine hydrochloride (dibucaine hydrochloride), it should *never* be employed with the hypobaric (1:1500) concentration.

Upon the completion of the injection, that is, the selected volume of the solution (see dosage), the needle is allowed to remain in place for 1 or 2 minutes to permit increased subdural pressure to return to normal.

Position Following Injection: The needle withdrawn, the patient is immediately turned flat in the prone position for 5 to 10 minutes to enable the light solution to impregnate the posterior roots. If there is a pronounced degree of dorsal curvature, the table may be tilted, fastened down with the head-piece flexed to bring the head below the level of the dorsal region. The patient is then turned on his back in a slight Trendelenburg position (head 2 inches below feet), which is maintained throughout the operation.

Dosage: For anesthesia of the lower extremities as high as the pelvis, 4 mg (6 ml solution, 1:1500) are usually sufficient. 7.5 to 10 mg (11 to 15 ml) will be required for most abdominal operations.

Usually, dosage above 15 ml is not necessary. The volume of solution to pass the level of D_5 is roughly calculated by subtracting from the number of inches given by the measurement of the distance from the spine C_7 to the interiliac line (4 for males and 6 for females). For caudal block, 6 ml is usually sufficient; 10 ml for the level D_{10}, 12 ml for D_7-D_8. For operations of longer duration on the stomach or duodenum, up to 20 ml may be required (16 ml for a 5-foot woman, 17 ml for a 5-foot man with 1 ml added for every 3 inches over 5 feet—to a maximum of 20 ml). For anesthesia in the lower part of the abdomen, divide 100 by the number of the uppermost thoracic nerve segment which is to be anesthetized. The result is the amount (in ml) of Nupercaine hydrochloride (dibucaine hydrochloride) solution to be used.

Approximate Dosage

Dosage for:	Concentration	Amount
Upper Abdominal	1:1500	15 to 18 ml
Lower Abdominal	1:1500	10 to 15 ml
Simple Caudal Block	1:1500	6 ml

Obstetrical Contraindications To Spinal Anesthesia: (1) Pelvic disproportion, (2) placenta praevia, (3) abruptio placenta, (4) unengaged head, and (5) necessity for intrauterine manipulations such as podalic version.

General Contraindications

Absolute

1. Disease of the cerebrospinal system, such as meningitis, cranial hemorrhage, tumors, poliomyelitis.
2. Moribund patients.
3. Blood stream infection.
4. Pernicious anemia with cord symptoms.
5. Arthritis, spondylitis, and other diseases of the spinal column rendering spinal puncture impossible. The presence of tuberculosis or metastatic lesions in the column is also a contraindication.
6. Pyogenic infection of the skin at or adjacent to the site of puncture.

Relative

1. **Hysteria or excessive nervous tension.** This difficulty may frequently be overcome by the preoperative administration of morphine sulfate 1/6 to 1/4 gr (10 to 15 mg), scopolamine 1/150 to 1/100 gr (0.43 to 0.65 mg), or a sedative.
2. **Chronic backache.** The patient may blame any exacerbation of symptoms, either immediate or late, on the spinal anesthesia.
3. **Preoperative headache of long duration or history of migraine.** Exacerbation of symptoms may follow spinal injection.
4. **Hypersensitivity to drugs.** This drug may be used frequently in patients who have shown a sensitivity to procaine. However, in all patients in whom drug sensitivity is suspected, a skin test should be performed by injecting intradermally a small amount (0.1 ml) of dibucaine hydrochloride and at the same time injecting intradermally a small amount (0.1 ml) of physiologic salt solution as a control. Reaction may be local (redness), or systemic (dyspnea, agitation). Use of the drug is absolutely contraindicated in the presence of local reaction if there is a history of drug idiosyncrasy.
5. **Possibility of severe hemorrhage during operation.** Judgment in this case must include consideration of the amount of possible hemorrhage, the height of anesthesia to be induced, and the facilities available to control shock.
6. **Shock.** All forms of anesthesia are poorly borne by patients in shock. Systolic blood pressure should be raised to at least 105 mm Hg before operation is contemplated.
7. **Hypotension.** In cases not due to Addison's disease or associated with severe shock, this has become of relatively little importance because of the effectiveness of ephedrine in restoring pressure to normal (see *Complications:* Hypotension).
8. **Hemorrhagic spinal fluid.** Where clear spinal fluid cannot be obtained, the needle should be withdrawn and puncture made at another interspace. This is important in order to avoid the possibility of intravenous injection of the drug.
9. **Cardiac decompensation, massive pleural effusions, and markedly increased intra-abdominal pressure** as in massive ascites and tumors.

Warnings

1. An extremely potent anesthetic agent and therefore is to be used in much smaller concentrations than other local anesthetics.
2. As is true for any spinal anesthetic agent, the anesthetist should remain in constant attendance. Ephedrine and oxygen should be held in readiness in order to effectively combat a sudden fall in blood pressure should such occur. Likewise, a quick-acting barbiturate should be readily available so that any evidence of toxicity, as manifested by excitement, may be treated promptly.
3. Persons with known drug sensitivity should be pretested before using any of the local anesthetic agents.

Cautions: Authorities agree that spinal anesthesia should not be induced unless the anesthetist is: (1) equipped to provide a rigidly aseptic technique; (2) prepared to remain in constant attendance; (3) equipped to deal with complications or side effects that may arise; (4) familiar with the contraindications to spinal anesthesia.

Complications and Side Effects

1. **Respiratory.** Cessation of respiration may occur from spread of the anesthetic into the cervical region. This is absolutely prevented by following the technique described. It may also occur because of medullary anoxia which follows the circulatory collapse incident to severe hypotension.

   Treatment: Intubation to assure an adequate airway; artificial respiration; oxygen; respiratory stimulant repeated as necessary.

2. **Hypotension.** The fall of blood pressure produced by spinal anesthesia is due to a number of factors, most important of which are: (1) sudden vasodilatation incident to paralysis of sympathetic vasomotor fibers and (2) loss of muscle tone with decrease in venous pressure, venous return, and cardiac output. The degree of fall therefore depends upon the number of segments involved, being greatest in high spinal anesthesia and practically nonexistent when the effect is confined to the perineal area alone.

   There have been several reports indicating that Nupercaine hydrochloride (dibucaine hydrochloride) has less effect upon blood pressure than does a comparable degree of anesthesia produced by procaine.

   Treatment: The prophylactic use of 25 mg ephedrine given intramuscularly before the anesthetic is injected is advised by many authorities. It may be omitted in low spinals. An additional dose of 25 mg should be given *intravenously* if a fall below 100 mm Hg occurs. This dose may be repeated; total should not exceed 100 mg. Fluids, plasma, or whole blood should be administered intravenously when severe fall of blood pressure occurs. In *obstetrical patients,* raising the legs to the vertical position is the most effective initial procedure to increase blood pressure.

3. **Postanesthetic Headache.** Since this is usually due to leakage of spinal fluid, incidence will decrease as technique improves.

   Prophylaxis: A needle of small caliber (not over 20 or 22 gauge) should be used. Some authorities recommend special needles, one of 20 gauge to penetrate the skin and fascia and an inner needle of 24 gauge to pierce the dura. It has also been recommended that the needle be introduced with the bevel held laterally so as to cut fewer fibers of the dura. The needle should remain in place for several seconds after injection to allow time for equalization of pressure.

Treatment: Tight abdominal binder. Hydration of the patient with either oral or intravenous fluids. One ml surgical pituitrin or 100 mg ephedrine. Rapid relief has been reported after intraspinal or caudal injection of 30 ml sterile saline.

4. **Nausea and Vomiting.** These may occur from psychic causes, drop in blood pressure, or intra-abdominal manipulation.
   Treatment: When caused by hypotension, inhalations of 100 percent oxygen in conjunction with a vasopressor may be found effective. Light cyclopropane or an intravenous barbiturate will control that which is due to intra-abdominal manipulation.
5. **Palsies.** Transient nerve palsies, usually involving the abducens, have occasionally been reported. This very uncommon complication generally occurs during the second week and clears up by the third or fourth week. Temporary or permanent transverse myelitis may follow the use of spinal anesthetic agents (see *Warnings*).
6. **Meningitis.** An aseptic technique should practically preclude the occurrence of this complication. Aseptic meningitis or meningismus, usually of rapid and benign course, has occurred after spinal anesthesia as it has also in cases where no spinal puncture has been carried out. Lundy has called attention to the fact that meningitides following spinal anesthesia may occur without relation to the method but due to pathologically proved metastases from distant foci. However, even the remote possibility of this complication reinforces the necessity for an absolutely sterile technique.
7. **Drug Idiosyncrasy.** The use of this drug is exceptionally free of this hazard. Patients giving a history of hypersensitivity to drugs, however, should be skin tested (see *Contraindications*).
   Treatment: The occurrence of motor excitement requires the anticonvulsant action of an intravenous barbiturate.

How Supplied: *Ampuls*, for spinal anesthesia, 20 ml, 1:1500 (method of Howard Jones), each ml containing 0.667 mg dibucaine hydrochloride, 5 mg sodium chloride, and water q.s.; cartons of 12. C80-54 (7/80)

HEAVY SOLUTION NUPERCAINE® hydrochloride (dibucaine hydrochloride) with Dextrose 5% For Spinal Anesthesia ℞

Indications: Heavy Solution Nupercaine hydrochloride is indicated for the production of low spinal anesthesia.

Contraindications: Shock, hypovolemia due to hemorrhage, and severe anemia; septicemia; pernicious anemia with evidence of spinal cord involvement; infection of the skin or subcutaneous tissue at or near the puncture site; tuberculosis or metastatic lesions in the lumbar spine; history of hypersensitivity to dibucaine or related compounds; in obstetrics: abruptio placenta, placenta praevia with significant bleeding, and early stages of labor (see Dosage and Administration); diseases, syndromes, or situations causing increased intra-abdominal pressure, such as ascites, tumors, or advanced pregnancy (unless in preparation for vaginal delivery).

Warnings: Nupercaine hydrochloride is a highly potent agent and therefore is to be used in lower concentration and lower total dosage than certain other local anesthetic drugs.

Pooling of a concentrated solution of Nupercaine hydrochloride or any other anesthetic agent in the conus may cause irreversible nerve damage. Therefore, the patient must not be kept in the sitting position for more than one minute following injection of the drug.

Do not inject Nupercaine during uterine contractions since spinal fluid currents may carry the drug further cephalad than desired.

The possibility of severe bleeding during planned surgery and the facilities available to manage the resulting complications must be considered in the selection of anesthesia.

To avoid intravascular injection, do not administer spinal anesthesia in the presence of blood noted in attempting lumbar puncture. If the fluid does not clear after entering the dural space, repeat lumbar puncture is recommended; use of another interspace should be considered.

Low spinal anesthesia of the type provided by Heavy Nupercaine is not recommended for delivery involving abdominal operation, nor does it provide the uterine relaxation necessary for obstetrical manipulations such as internal podalic version.

Precautions: Spinal anesthesia should not be undertaken unless the anesthesiologist is familiar with techniques of and contraindications to spinal anesthesia, equipped to provide a rigidly aseptic technique, prepared to remain in constant attendance, monitoring patient's condition continuously, and equipped to deal with any complications that may arise.

Impairment of respiration may result from spread of the anesthetic above the desired level; this can be minimized by following the administration techniques described. It can also occur because of medullary hypoxia associated with circulatory collapse incident to severe hypotension, requiring intensive supportive treatment.

Hypotension during spinal anesthesia may be related to a number of factors, most important of which are sudden vasodilation incident to paralysis of sympathetic vasomotor fibers and loss of muscle tone with decrease in venous pressure, venous return, and cardiac output. The degree of hypotension relates to the number of vasoconstrictor fibers blocked, being greater in a higher level of spinal anesthesia. If the operative conditions permit, it may be possible to restore blood pressure to an acceptable level without drugs by repositioning the patient and administering intravenous fluids. In obstetrics, lateral displacement of the uterus to the left may raise the blood pressure by improving venous return to the heart. If a vasopressor is necessary, one having both central and peripheral actions (*eg*, ephedrine) should be administered as needed. Plasma expanders or whole blood may also be required; adequate respiratory exchange must be maintained.

The use of spinal anesthesia in patients with cardiac disease depends upon the practitioner's evaluation of the type and severity of the physiological disturbance weighed against the possible pharmacological changes resulting from the anesthesia, and upon his ability to manage any possible complications.

In the presence of neurological disease (*eg*, meningitis, spinal block, hemorrhage, poliomyelitis, migraine, headache of long duration) or conditions involving the back (*eg*, arthritis, spondylitis, chronic backache), the decision to use spinal anesthesia will depend upon the practitioner's evaluation of the disease process and its possible implications. In these circumstances, the patient may ascribe signs and symptoms of previously existing disease or exacerbations of chronic backache to the spinal anesthetic.

Selection of another form of anesthesia should be considered if the patient is uncooperative, hysterical, or excessively nervous or apprehensive. Use of spinal anesthesia in such cases will depend upon the practitioner's ability to evaluate and to manage the individual situation.

Adverse Reactions

Postanesthetic Headache. This can be minimized by use of small caliber needles (24 to 26 gauge) specially designed to prevent spinal fluid leakage and by keeping patient flat on back, without a pillow, for appropriate period after delivery or operation.

Nausea and Vomiting. These may result from psychic causes, fall in blood pressure, intra-abdominal manipulation, or concomitant medication.

Palsies. Nerve palsies, involving extra-ocular muscles, legs, vesical and anal sphincters, have occasionally been reported. These usually are transient and clear completely, but in rare instances a permanent residual has been reported.

Meningitis, Myelitis. Careful selection of patients, use of strictest aseptic techniques, and scrupulous care to avoid injury to meninges and cord during anesthetic drug injection should prevent infectious and traumatic complications almost entirely. Instances of aseptic meningitis or myelitis have occurred, occasionally with permanent residual and fatal termination. Aseptic meningitis or myelitis also have been reported in rare instances following diagnostic lumbar puncture without spinal anesthesia, following various operations for which spinal anesthesia was not used and spinal tap was done, and following pregnancy and delivery without use of spinal anesthesia or spinal tap.

Meningismus also has been reported, evidently without infection, and usually clears promptly.

Dosage and Administration: Heavy Solution Nupercaine hydrochloride has a specific gravity greater than that of spinal fluid. When introduced into the spinal subarachnoid space, it will gravitate toward the lowest point; with the patient in sitting position, it settles toward the conus.

If injection is made with patient recumbent and the Trendelenburg position is immediately assumed, flow of anesthetic will be cephalad. Extent of upward spread will depend upon rate, force and volume of fluid injected, and length of time the Trendelenburg position is maintained. **Level of anesthesia and extent of involvement must be precisely regulated by careful attention to the various techniques described herein.**

Syringe should be filled with required amount of solution prior to lumbar puncture in order to reduce possibility of dislodgment of needle. Injection is made as rapidly as gentle pressure will permit, with needle held firmly to prevent dislodgment. The latter detail is of utmost importance, because failure to obtain anesthesia after an apparently satisfactory lumbar puncture may be due to dislodgment of needle during injection of solution. Needle should be kept in place for a few seconds after injection to permit equalization of pressure.

Directions for amount of solution, rapidity of injection, and positioning of patient following injection must be followed precisely to obtain desired level of anesthesia and to minimize complications.

Inasmuch as Nupercaine hydrochloride is readily precipitated by even the slightest amount of alkali, needles and syringes must be thoroughly rinsed in distilled water prior to autoclaving. As part of the meticulous technique for administration of any spinal anesthetic agent, ampuls should be autoclaved to assure sterility of exterior surface. Heavy Solution Nupercaine hydrochloride can be resterilized once at 121° C for 30 minutes; repeated autoclaving produces progressive lowering of pH and darkening of color, probably from caramelization of the dextrose contained. Any

Continued on next page

The full prescribing information for each CIBA drug is contained herein and is that in effect as of October 1, 1982.

CIBA—Cont.

ampul showing discoloration after resterilization must be discarded.

Heavy Solution Nupercaine hydrochloride should be used only in accordance with the following techniques:

Obstetric Analgesia Not Involving Abdominal Operation

Dose: 1 ml Heavy Solution Nupercaine hydrochloride is the amount most frequently used. However, greater duration of anesthesia will result from the use of 2 ml.

Time of Injection: Low spinal anesthesia is not intended to relieve the pains of early labor; these can be controlled adequately by other methods. There is general agreement that the injection should not be made until the cervix is well effaced, the head fixed in the pelvis, and the labor progressing satisfactorily. Parmley and Adriani advise injection after the cervix is 5 to 6 cm dilated and 60 to 80 percent effaced. Injection must not be made during uterine contractions, since currents in the spinal fluid may carry solution cephalad.

Position of Patient at Injection: Sitting with legs over side of bed or delivery table, supported by an attendant. Downward pressure on the head to increase flexion should be avoided.

Injection: Draw Heavy Solution Nupercaine into syringe before lumbar puncture. After introduction of needle into subarachnoid space, make injection to count of 1-and-2-and-3 (approximately 2 to 3 seconds). Keep patient sitting for exactly 30 seconds, then place her flat, with head supported by two pillows, or in Fowler's position of 5 degrees.

Under no circumstances is patient allowed to remain in sitting position for more than one minute after injection of the hyperbaric solution, since pooling in the conus can produce irreversible nerve damage.

Saddle Block Anesthesia in Rectal and Urologic Surgery Not Involving Abdominal Surgery

Position of Patient at Injection: *Sitting.* Under no circumstances should the patient be allowed to remain in the sitting position for longer than one minute after injection of the hyperbaric solution since pooling of the anesthetic in the conus can produce irreversible nerve damage.

Dose: For anesthesia of the perineum, rectum, lower scrotum, and penis, inject 1 ml Heavy Solution Nupercaine hydrochloride and allow the patient to sit upright for only 60 seconds. For anesthesia of fundus of the uterus, dome of the bladder, and other pelvic structures, in addition to the areas previously mentioned, inject 2 ml Heavy Solution Nupercaine hydrochloride and allow patient to sit upright for 0 to 5 seconds.

Position Following Injection: Place patient down immediately at expiration of the required number of seconds, with head supported by two pillows and table placed in Fowler's position at an angle of 5 degrees. After allowing at least 10 minutes for fixation of the anesthetic level, determining by sensory testing (as by pin-prick) that the level has ceased to rise, place patient in desired position for operation.

How Supplied: *Ampuls,* 2 ml, each ampul containing 5 mg Nupercaine hydrochloride (0.25%) and 100 mg dextrose in water.

Cartons of 10 ....NDC 0083-5662-10

C80-44 (7/80)

OCUSERT® ℞

(pilocarpine)

Pilo-20/Pilo-40 Ocular Therapeutic System

For full prescribing information, including placement and removal instructions, consult the Physicians' Desk Reference for Ophthalmology.

PERCORTEN® acetate ℞

(desoxycorticosterone acetate pellets USP)

Pellets

Listed in USP, a Medicare designated compendium.

Indications: As partial replacement therapy for primary and secondary adrenocortical insufficiency in Addison's disease and for the treatment of salt-losing adrenogenital syndrome.

Contraindications: Hypersensitivity to desoxycorticosterone acetate; hypertension; congestive heart failure.

Warnings: Mineralocorticoids should be accompanied by adequate glucocorticoid therapy in adrenal insufficiency or the salt-losing form of the adrenogenital syndrome.

Usage in Pregnancy

If it is necessary to give steroids during pregnancy, the newborn infant should be watched closely for signs of hypoadrenalism and appropriate therapy instituted if such signs are present.

Precautions: All patients receiving Percorten should be watched for evidence of intercurrent infection. Should infection occur, appropriate anti-infective therapy should be initiated.

If edema occurs, dietary sodium restriction may be required. Frequent blood electrolyte determinations should be performed; potassium supplementation may be necessary.

Adverse Reactions: Generalized edema; frontal or occipital headaches; hypertension and cardiac enlargement, especially if hypertension was present before the onset of adrenal insufficiency; arthralgia and tendon contractures; extreme weakness of extremities with ascending paralysis secondary to low serum potassium; cardiac arrhythmias; hypersensitivity reactions; rarely, irritation at site of pellet implantation.

Dosage and Administration: Mineralocorticoid therapy may not be necessary if the patient can be controlled with an adequate salt intake and glucocorticoid therapy.

If mineralocorticoid therapy is necessary, dosage must be individualized according to the severity of the disease and the response of the patient and should be accompanied by adequate amounts of glucocorticoid.

Percorten pellets should be implanted only after the optimal daily maintenance dose of Percorten acetate in Oil has been carefully determined. Any attempt to implant a number of pellets not exactly calculated on the basis of the optimal daily maintenance dose by injection may lead to irreparable damage.

For the determination of the ultimate optimal maintenance dose, several weeks are required. It is advisable, therefore, in order to eliminate the possibility of overdosage, that the patient be maintained on Percorten acetate in Oil for at least 2 to 3 months prior to pellet implantation.

Calculation of Pellet Requirement

One pellet is implanted for each 0.5 mg of the daily injected maintenance dose of Percorten acetate in Oil. For example, an addisonian patient whose optimal maintenance requirement is 5 mg Percorten acetate in Oil should receive a maximum of 10 pellets.

Technique of Pellet Implantation

Pellets should be implanted only in a fully equipped operating room. Aseptic precautions and careful hemostasis are primary requirements for successful implantation.

The infrascapular region has been selected as the most suitable site for the implantation. Strict asepsis is observed. The operative field is prepared with iodine and alcohol, and the site of incision is anesthetized. A 2- to 4-cm transverse incision is made a few centimeters below the inferior angle of the scapula. A number of small pockets, according to the number of pellets to be implanted, are prepared in the subcutaneous tissue by blunt dissection, radiating from the incision. The pellets, which have been removed previously from the vial under sterile conditions and kept close at hand on a sterile towel, are placed in the pockets with forceps. The use of a nasal dilator, introduced into the opening of the pocket, has been found helpful, as it permits the placing of the pellet sufficiently far away from the incision. If the pellet is not placed at least 2 cm away from the incision, the chances are greatly increased that it may be extruded later. No pellet should be extruded spontaneously if implanted aseptically, sufficiently far away from the incision, and if careful hemostasis is observed. It is a matter of technique and experience whether each single pellet pocket should be closed with an individual suture, or whether the skin incision only should be closed with subcuticular sutures of fine black silk. It is possible to insert as many as 15 pellets through a single incision by this technique.

Observation After Implantation

On the average, the pellets last for a period of 8 to 12 months. In case of infection, disease, or other stress, supplementary Percorten acetate in Oil injections may be necessary until the patient has returned to the condition established when the pellets were implanted.

In a few instances, it has been necessary to remove pellets, although the maintenance dose was adequately determined prior to implantation. The occurrence of edema, excessive gain in weight, and rise in blood pressure are signs of overdosage.

Reimplantation of Pellets

The effect of the implanted pellets fades after approximately 8 to 12 months. A gradual decrease in *blood pressure* and *weight,* increased fatigue, and loss of appetite are usually the first indications of this decrease in hormonal supply, and the patient must be carefully watched. It may be necessary to resume daily injections of Percorten acetate in Oil with slowly increasing doses. During a period of from 4 to 6 weeks, it is possible to ascertain anew the maintenance requirement of Percorten acetate in Oil; from this dosage the number of new pellets to be implanted can be calculated. Under no circumstances should pellets be arbitrarily implanted on the basis of the initial assay, as the condition of the patient may have undergone a definite change in hormone requirement during the year.

How Supplied: *Pellets,* each containing approximately 125 mg desoxycorticosterone acetate; cartons of 1. C80-61 (2/81)

PERCORTEN® pivalate ℞

(desoxycorticosterone pivalate)

Not USP, differs in pH range (5.0-8.5)

INTRAMUSCULAR REPOSITORY

Indications: As partial replacement therapy for primary and secondary adrenocortical insufficiency in Addison's disease and for treatment of salt-losing adrenogenital syndrome.

Contraindications: Hypersensitivity to Percorten pivalate suspension or any of its ingredients. Patients with hypertension or cardiac disease.

Warnings: Since Percorten pivalate is potent and long-acting, do not administer more frequently than once per month.

Usage in Pregnancy

The safe use of this drug in pregnant women or during lactation has not been established. Therefore, the benefits must be weighed against the potential hazards.

Precautions: Patients with Addison's disease are more sensitive to the action of the hormone and may exhibit side effects in an exaggerated degree.

Since Percorten pivalate is a potent adrenocortical preparation which may produce side effects, patients should be closely watched. Treatment should be stopped in the event of a significant increase in weight or blood pres-

sure, or the development of edema or cardiac enlargement.
Sodium retention and the loss of potassium are accelerated by a high intake of sodium. Hence, it may be necessary to restrict intake of sodium and increase that of potassium.
Only if absolutely necessary should a glucose tolerance test (particularly intravenous) be performed, as addisonian patients with or without desoxycorticosterone therapy have the tendency to react with severe hypoglycemia within 3 hours.
Adverse Reactions: Like other adrenocortical hormones, Percorten pivalate may cause severe side effects if dosage is too high or prolonged. It may cause increased blood volume, edema, elevation of blood pressure, and enlargement of the heart shadow. In patients with essential hypertension or a tendency toward its development, a marked rise in blood pressure may follow administration of this drug.
Headache, arthralgia, weakness, ascending paralysis, low potassium syndrome, and hypersensitivity may occur.
On rare occasions, irritation at the site of injection has been reported.
Dosage and Administration: In treating Addison's disease, Percorten pivalate should be used only in conjunction with other supplemental measures (*eg,* other hormonal agents, electrolytes, control of infection).
At initiation of treatment, the daily requirement for maintenance therapy should be determined with desoxycorticosterone acetate in oil. For each mg of desoxycorticosterone acetate in oil, 1 ml (25 mg) Percorten pivalate suspension is to be injected intramuscularly through a 20-gauge needle into the upper outer quadrant of one or both buttocks.
The average dose is 25 to 100 mg every 4 weeks.
How Supplied: *Multiple-Dose Vials,* 4 ml, each ml containing 25 mg desoxycorticosterone pivalate, 10.5 mg methylcellulose, 3 mg sodium carboxymethylcellulose, 1 mg polysorbate 80, and 8 mg sodium chloride with 0.002% thimerosal added as preservative in aqueous suspension.
Cartons of 1 ....NDC 0083-2222-01
For intramuscular use only.
Shake well before using.
C81-12 (2/81)

PRISCOLINE® hydrochloride ℞
(tolazoline hydrochloride USP)
Parenteral/Intra-Arterial

Listed in USP, a Medicare designated compendium.

Indications
Based on a review of this drug by the National Academy of Sciences-National Research Council and/or other information, FDA has classified the indications as follows:
"Possibly" effective: Spastic peripheral vascular disorders associated with acrocyanosis, acroparesthesia, arteriosclerosis obliterans, Buerger's disease, causalgia, diabetic arteriosclerosis, gangrene, endarteritis, frostbite (sequelae), post-thrombotic conditions (thrombophlebitis), Raynaud's disease, and scleroderma.
Final classification of the less-than-effective indications requires further investigation.

Contraindications: Priscoline is contraindicated following a cerebrovascular accident; known or suspected coronary artery disease; hypersensitivity to tolazoline.
Warnings: Priscoline stimulates gastric secretion and may activate peptic ulcers. Use cautiously in patients with gastritis or known or suspected peptic ulcer.
In patients with mitral stenosis, parenterally administered Priscoline may produce either a fall or a rise in pulmonary artery pressure and total pulmonary resistance, hence must be used with caution in known or suspected mitral stenosis.
Usage in Pregnancy
The safe use of this drug in pregnant women or during lactation has not been established. Therefore, the benefits must be weighed against the potential hazards.
Precautions: Because of the risks involved, intra-arterial administration should be used only by those thoroughly familiar with the procedure and, preferably, only in the hospital or a clinic facility (see Dosage and Administration).
Adverse Reactions: Although side effects are generally mild and may decrease progressively during continued therapy, cardiac arrhythmias, anginal pain, and marked hypertension have been reported. Exacerbations of peptic ulcer have also occurred.
Other side effects include nausea, vomiting, diarrhea, epigastric discomfort, tachycardia, flushing, slight rise or fall in blood pressure, increased pilomotor activity with tingling or chilliness, rash and edema.
Thrombocytopenia, leukopenia, psychiatric reactions characterized by confusion or hallucinations, hepatitis, oliguria and hematuria have been reported rarely.
Intra-arterial administration, in addition to the above, may also produce a feeling of warmth or a "burning sensation" in the injected extremity, transient weakness, transient postural vertigo, palpitations, formication, and apprehension. Rarely, a paradoxical response (further decrease in an already impaired blood supply) may occur in a seriously damaged limb with incipient or established gangrene. This usually disappears with continued treatment and may usually be prevented by prior administration of histamine.
Dosage and Administration: Dosage should be individualized according to the condition being treated and the response of the patient.
Subcutaneous, Intramuscular, or *Intravenous:* 10 to 50 mg 4 times daily. Start with low doses, increasing with patient under close observation until optimal dosage (as determined by appearance of flushing) is established. Keeping patient warm will often increase effectiveness of drug.
Intra-arterial: This approach should not be used except in carefully selected cases and only after it has been determined that maximal benefit has been achieved with other forms of parenteral administration.
Caution: Because of the risks involved, and because of the special technique and strict aseptic precautions required with intra-arterial injection, this approach should be used only by those thoroughly familiar with the procedure and, preferably, only in the hospital or a clinic facility.
Initially, 25 mg (1 ml) is given slowly as a test dose to determine the response. Subsequently, the average single dose may be 50 to 75 mg (2 to 3 ml) per injection, depending on the observed response.
One or 2 injections daily are usually required initially to achieve maximum response. For maintenance, 2 or 3 injections weekly may be enough to sustain improved circulation, but more may be needed.
Overdosage
Signs and Symptoms: Increased pilomotor activity, peripheral vasodilatation and skin flushing, and, in rare instances, hypotension to shock levels.
Treatment: In treating hypotension, placement of the patient in the head-low position and the administration of intravenous fluids is most important. If a vasopressor is necessary, one having both central and peripheral action (*eg,* ephedrine) may be administered as needed. Do not use epinephrine or norepinephrine, since large doses of Priscoline may cause "epinephrine reversal" (further reduction in blood pressure followed by an exaggerated rebound).
How Supplied: *Multiple-dose Vials,* 10 ml, each ml containing 25 mg tolazoline hydrochloride, 0.65% sodium citrate, 0.65% tartaric acid, and 0.5% chlorobutanol as preservative in water; cartons of 1. C82-5 (3/82)

PRIVINE®
0.05% Nasal Solution
0.05% Nasal Spray

Caution: Do not use Privine if you have glaucoma. Privine is an effective nasal decongestant when you use it in the recommended dosage. If you use too much, too long, or too often, Privine may be harmful to your nasal mucous membranes and cause burning, stinging, sneezing or an increased runny nose.
Do not use Privine by mouth.
Keep this and all medications out of the reach of children. Do not use Privine with children under 6 years of age, except with the advice and supervision of a doctor.
OVERDOSAGE IN YOUNG CHILDREN MAY CAUSE MARKED SEDATION AND IF SEVERE, EMERGENCY TREATMENT MAY BE NECESSARY.
IF NASAL STUFFINESS PERSISTS AFTER 3 DAYS OF TREATMENT, DISCONTINUE USE AND CONSULT A DOCTOR.
Privine is a nasal decongestant that comes in two forms: Nasal Solution (in a bottle with a dropper) and Nasal Spray (in a plastic squeeze bottle). Both are for prompt, and prolonged relief of nasal congestion due to common colds, sinusitis, hay fever, etc.
How to use Nasal Solution: Squeeze rubber bulb to fill dropper with proper amount of medication. For best results, tilt head as far back as possible and put two drops of solution into your right nostril. Then lean head forward, inhaling and turning your head to the left. Refill dropper by squeezing bulb. Now tilt head as far back as possible and put two drops of solution into your left nostril. Then lean head forward, inhaling, and turning your head to the right. Use only 2 drops in each nostril. Do not repeat this dosage more than every 3 hours.
The Privine dropper bottle is designed to make administration of the proper dosage easy and to prevent accidental overdosage. Privine will not cause sleeplessness, so you may use it before going to bed.
Important: After use, be sure to rinse the dropper with very hot water. This helps prevent contamination of the bottle with bacteria from nasal secretions. Use of the dispenser by more than one person may spread infection.
Note: Privine Nasal Solution may be used on contact with glass, plastic, stainless steel and specially treated metals used in atomizers. Do not let the solution come in contact with reactive metals, especially aluminum. If solution becomes discolored, it should be discarded.
How to use Nasal Spray: For best results do not shake the plastic squeeze bottle.
Remove cap. With head held upright, spray twice into each nostril. Squeeze the bottle sharply and firmly while sniffing through the nose.
For best results use every 4 to 6 hours. Do not use more often than every 3 hours.
Avoid overdosage. Follow directions for use carefully.
Privine Nasal Solution contains 0.05% naphazoline hydrochloride USP with benzalkonium chloride as a preservative. Available in bottles of .66 fl. oz. (20 ml) with dropper, and bottles of 16 fl. oz. (473 ml). Privine Nasal Spray contains

Continued on next page

The full prescribing information for each CIBA drug is contained herein and is that in effect as of October 1, 1982.

CIBA—Cont.

0.05% naphazoline hydrochloride USP with benzalkonium chloride as a preservative. Available in plastic squeeze bottles of ½ fl. oz. (15 ml).

C80-5 (1/80)

REGITINE® ℞
(phentolamine USP)

Listed in USP a Medicare designated compendia.

Indications
Oral and Parenteral Regitine
Prevention or control of hypertensive episodes that may occur in a patient with pheochromocytoma as a result of stress or manipulation during preoperative preparation and surgical excision.
Parenteral Regitine
Prevention and treatment of dermal necrosis and sloughing following intravenous administration or extravasation of norepinephrine.
Diagnosis of pheochromocytoma—Regitine blocking test.
Contraindications: Myocardial infarction, history of myocardial infarction, coronary insufficiency, angina or other evidence suggestive of coronary artery disease. Hypersensitivity to phentolamine or related compounds.
Warnings: Myocardial infarction, cerebrovascular spasm, and cerebrovascular occlusion have been reported to occur following the administration of phentolamine, usually in association with marked hypotensive episodes with shock-like states which occasionally follow parenteral administration.
For screening tests in patients with hypertension, the generally available urinary assay of catecholamines or other biochemical assays have largely supplanted the Regitine and other pharmacological tests for reasons of accuracy and safety. None of the chemical or pharmacological tests is infallible in the diagnosis of pheochromocytoma. The Regitine test is not the procedure of choice and should be reserved for cases in which additional confirmatory evidence is necessary, and the relative risks involved in conducting the test have been considered.
Usage in Pregnancy: The safe use of this drug in pregnant women or during lactation has not been established. Therefore, the benefits must be weighed against the potential hazards.
Precautions: Tachycardia and cardiac arrhythmias may occur with the use of Regitine or other alpha adrenergic blocking agents. When possible, defer administration of cardiac glycosides until cardiac rhythm returns to normal.
Adverse Reactions: Acute and prolonged hypotensive episodes, tachycardia, and cardiac arrhythmias have been reported, most frequently after parenteral administration. In addition, weakness, dizziness, flushing, orthostatic hypotension, nasal stuffiness, nausea, vomiting, and diarrhea may occur.
Dosage and Administration
1. Prevention or control of hypertensive episodes in the patient with pheochromocytoma.
To control and prevent paroxysmal attacks prior to surgery, the usual adult dosage is 50 mg (1 tablet) of Regitine hydrochloride orally 4 to 6 times daily. In certain severe cases, higher doses may be required. In children, smaller doses generally suffice; 25 mg (½ tablet) orally 4 to 6 times daily is suggested initially.
For use in preoperative reduction of elevated blood pressure, inject 5 mg of Regitine mesylate (1 mg for children) intravenously or intramuscularly 1 or 2 hours before surgery (and repeat if necessary).
During surgery administer Regitine mesylate (5 mg for adults, 1 mg for children) intravenously as indicated to help prevent or control paroxysms of hypertension, tachycardia, respiratory depression, convulsions, or other effects of epinephrine intoxication. (Postoperatively, norepinephrine may be given to control the hypotension which commonly follows complete removal of a pheochromocytoma.)
2. Prevention and treatment of dermal necrosis and sloughing following intravenous administration or extravasation of norepinephrine.
For prevention, add 10 mg Regitine mesylate to each liter of solution containing norepinephrine. The pressor effect of norepinephrine is not affected.
For treatment, inject Regitine mesylate (5 to 10 mg in 10 ml saline) into the area of extravasation within 12 hours.
3. Diagnosis of pheochromocytoma—Regitine blocking test.

a. **Intravenous**

Preparation.
Review the *Contraindications, Warnings,* and *Precautions.* Withhold sedatives, analgesics, and all other medication not deemed essential (such as digitalis and insulin) for at least 24 hours (preferably 48 to 72 hours) prior to the test. Withhold antihypertensive drugs until blood pressure returns to the untreated, hypertensive level. Do not perform test on a patient who is normotensive.

Procedure.

1. Keep patient at rest in the supine position throughout the test, preferably in a quiet, darkened room. Delay Regitine injection until blood pressure is stabilized, as evidenced by blood pressure readings taken every 10 minutes for at least one-half hour.
2. Dissolve 5 mg Regitine mesylate in 1 ml Sterile Water for Injection. Dose for adults is 5 mg; for children, 1 mg.
3. Insert the syringe needle into vein, delay injection until pressor response to venipuncture has subsided.
4. Inject Regitine rapidly. Record blood pressure immediately after injection, at 30-second intervals for the first 3 minutes, and at 60-second intervals for the next 7 minutes.

Interpreting the Test
Positive response, suggestive of pheochromocytoma, is indicated by a drop in blood pressure of more than 35 mm Hg systolic and 25 mm Hg diastolic pressure. A typical positive response may be a drop of 60 mm Hg systolic and 25 mm Hg diastolic. Maximal depressor pressure effect usually is evident within 2 minutes after injection. Return to pre-injection pressure commonly occurs within 15 to 30 minutes, but may return more rapidly.
If blood pressure falls to a dangerous level, treat patient as outlined under "Overdosage."
A positive response should always be confirmed by other diagnostic procedures, preferably the measurement of urinary catecholamines or their metabolites.
Negative response is indicated when the blood pressure is unchanged, elevated, or is reduced less than 35 mm Hg systolic and 25 mm Hg diastolic after injection of Regitine. A negative response to this test does not exclude the diagnosis of pheochromocytoma, especially in patients with paroxysmal hypertension in whom the incidence of false negative responses is high.

b. **Intramuscular**

If the intramuscular test for pheochromocytoma is preferred, preparation is the same as for the intravenous test. Then dissolve 5 mg Regitine mesylate in 1 ml Sterile Water for Injection. Dose for adults is 5 mg intramuscularly; for children, 3 mg. Record blood pressure every 5 minutes for 30 to 45 minutes following intramuscular injection. Positive response is indicated by a drop in blood pressure of 35 mm Hg systolic and 25 mm Hg diastolic or greater within 20 minutes following injection.

c. **Reliability**

The test is most reliable in detecting pheochromocytoma in patients with sustained hypertension, and least reliable in those with paroxysmal hypertension. False positive tests may occur in patients with hypertension without pheochromocytoma.

Overdosage: In the event of a drop in blood pressure to dangerous level or other evidence of shock-like conditions, treat vigorously and promptly. Include intravenous infusion of norepinephrine, titrated to maintain blood pressure to normotensive level, and all available supportive measures. Do not use epinephrine since it may cause a paradoxical fall in blood pressure.
How Supplied
Vials, each containing 5 mg phentolamine mesylate USP and 25 mg mannitol in lyophilized form and accompanied by ampul containing 1 ml Sterile Water for Injection; cartons of 1.
The reconstituted solution should be used upon preparation and should not be stored.
Tablets (white, scored), each containing 50 mg phentolamine hydrochloride USP; bottles of 100.

C81-11 (1/81)

[*Shown in Product Identification Section*]

RIMACTANE® ℞
(rifampin USP)

Indications
Pulmonary Tuberculosis
In the initial treatment and in the retreatment of pulmonary tuberculosis, Rimactane must be used in conjunction with at least one other antituberculous drug.
Frequently used regimens have been the following:
isoniazid and Rimactane
ethambutol and Rimactane
isoniazid, ethambutol, and Rimactane
Neisseria Meningitidis Carriers
Rimactane is indicated for the treatment of asymptomatic carriers of *N. meningitidis* to eliminate meningococci from the nasopharynx.
Rimactane is not indicated for the treatment of meningococcal infection.
To avoid the indiscriminate use of Rimactane, diagnostic laboratory procedures, including serotyping and susceptibility testing, should be performed to establish the carrier state and the correct treatment. In order to preserve the usefulness of Rimactane in the treatment of asymptomatic meningococcal carriers, it is recommended that the drug be reserved for situations in which the risk of meningococcal meningitis is high.
Both in the treatment of tuberculosis and in the treatment of meningococcal carriers, small numbers of resistant cells, present within large populations of susceptible cells, can rapidly become the predominating type. Since rapid emergence of resistance can occur, culture and susceptibility tests should be performed in the event of persistent positive cultures.
Contraindications: A history of previous hypersensitivity reaction to any of the rifamycins.
Warnings: Rifampin has been shown to produce liver dysfunction. There have been fatalities associated with jaundice in patients with liver disease or receiving rifampin concomitantly with other hepatotoxic agents. Since an increased risk may exist for individuals with liver disease, benefits must be weighed carefully against the risk of further liver damage. Periodic liver function monitoring is mandatory.
The possibility of rapid emergence of resistant meningococci restricts the use of Rimactane to short-term treatment of the asymptomatic carrier state. Rimactane is not to be used for the treatment of meningococcal disease.

Several studies of tumorigenicity potential have been done in rodents. In one strain of mice known to be particularly susceptible to the spontaneous development of hepatomas, rifampin given at a level 2–10 times the maximum dosage used clinically, resulted in a significant increase in the occurrence of hepatomas in female mice of this strain after one year of administration. There was no evidence of tumorigenicity in the males of this strain, in males or females of another mouse strain, or rats.

Usage in Pregnancy: Although rifampin has been reported to cross the placental barrier and appear in cord blood, the effect of Rimactane, alone or in combination with other antituberculous drugs, on the human fetus is not known. An increase in congenital malformations, primarily spina bifida and cleft palate, has been reported in the offspring of rodents given oral doses of 150-250 mg/kg/day of rifampin during pregnancy.

The possible teratogenic potential in women capable of bearing children should be carefully weighed against the benefits of therapy.

Precautions: Rimactane is not recommended for intermittent therapy; the patient should be cautioned against intentional or accidental interruption of the daily dosage regimen since rare renal hypersensitivity reactions have been reported when therapy was resumed in such cases.

Rifampin has been observed to increase the requirements for anticoagulant drugs of the coumarin type. The cause of this phenomenon is unknown. In patients receiving anticoagulants and rifampin concurrently, it is recommended that the prothrombin time be performed daily or as frequently as necessary to establish and maintain the required dose of anticoagulant.

Urine, feces, saliva, sputum, sweat, and tears may be colored red-orange by rifampin and its metabolites. Soft contact lenses may be permanently stained. Individuals to be treated should be made aware of these possibilities.

It has been reported that the reliability of oral contraceptives may be affected in some patients being treated for tuberculosis with rifampin in combination with at least one other antituberculous drug. In such cases, alternative contraceptive measures may need to be considered.

Rifampin has been reported to diminish the effects of concurrently administered methadone, oral hypoglycemics, corticosteroids, dapsone, and digitalis preparations; appropriate dosage adjustments may be necessary if indicated by the patient's clinical condition.

When rifampin is taken in combination with PAS, decreased rifampin serum levels may result. Therefore, the drugs should be given at least 4 hours apart.

Therapeutic levels of rifampin have been shown to inhibit standard assays for serum folate and vitamin B_{12}. Alternative methods must be considered when determining folate and vitamin B_{12} concentrations in the presence of rifampin.

Since rifampin has been reported to cross the placental barrier and appear in cord blood, neonates of rifampin-treated mothers should be carefully observed for any evidence of adverse effects. Rifampin is excreted in breast milk.

Adverse Reactions: Gastrointestinal disturbances such as heartburn, epigastric distress, anorexia, nausea, vomiting, gas, cramps, and diarrhea have been noted in some patients. Headache, drowsiness, fatigue, ataxia, dizziness, inability to concentrate, mental confusion, visual disturbances, muscular weakness, fever, pains in extremities, generalized numbness, and menstrual disturbances have also been noted.

Hypersensitivity reactions have been reported. Encountered occasionally have been pruritus, urticaria, rash, pemphigoid reaction, eosinophilia, sore mouth, sore tongue, and exudative conjunctivitis. Rarely, hepatitis or a shock-like syndrome with hepatic involvement and abnormal liver function tests have been reported. Transient abnormalities in liver function tests (*eg*, elevations in serum bilirubin, BSP, alkaline phosphatase, serum transaminases) have also been observed. The BSP test should be performed prior to the morning dose of rifampin to avoid false-positive results.

Thrombocytopenia, transient leukopenia, hemolytic anemia, and decreased hemoglobin have been observed. Thrombocytopenia has occurred when rifampin and ethambutol were administered concomitantly according to an intermittent dose schedule twice weekly and in high doses.

Elevations in BUN and serum uric acid have occurred. Rarely, hemolysis, hemoglobinuria, hematuria, renal insufficiency or acute renal failure have been reported and are generally considered to be hypersensitivity reactions. These have usually occurred during intermittent therapy or when treatment was resumed following intentional or accidental interruption of a daily dosage regimen and were reversible when rifampin was discontinued and appropriate therapy instituted.

Although rifampin has been reported to have an immunosuppressive effect in some animal experiments, available human data indicate that this has no clinical significance.

Dosage and Administration: It is recommended that Rimactane be administered once daily, either one hour before or two hours after a meal.

Data are not available for determination of dosage for children under 5.

Pulmonary Tuberculosis

Adults: 600 mg (two 300-mg Capsules) in a single daily administration.

Children: 10 to 20 mg/kg, not to exceed 600 mg/day.

In the treatment of pulmonary tuberculosis, Rimactane must be used in conjunction with at least one other antituberculous agent. In general, therapy should be continued until bacterial conversion and maximal improvement have occurred.

Meningococcal Carriers

It is recommended that Rimactane be administered once daily for four consecutive days in the following doses:

Adults: 600 mg (two 300-mg Capsules) in a single daily administration.

Children: 10 to 20 mg/kg, not to exceed 600 mg/day.

Susceptibility Testing

Pulmonary Tuberculosis: Rifampin susceptibility powders are available for both direct and indirect methods of determining the susceptibility of strains of mycobacteria. The MIC's of susceptible clinical isolates when determined in 7H10 or other non-egg-containing media have ranged from 0.1 to 2 mcg/ml.

Meningococcal Carriers: Susceptibility discs containing 5 mcg rifampin are available for susceptibility testing of *N. meningitidis*.

Quantitative methods that require measurement of zone diameters give the most precise estimates of antibiotic susceptibility. One such procedure[1] has been recommended for use with discs for testing susceptibility to rifampin. Interpretations correlate zone diameters from the disc test with MIC (minimal inhibitory concentration) values for rifampin. A range of MIC's from 0.1 to 1 mcg/ml has been found *in vitro* for susceptible strains of *N. meningitidis*. With this procedure, a report from the laboratory of "resistant" indicates that the organism is not likely to be eradicated from the nasopharynx of asymptomatic carriers.

How Supplied: *Capsules,* 300 mg (opaque scarlet and caramel); bottles of 30, 60, and 100. Also available, Rimactane®/INH (isoniazid USP) Dual Pack containing 60 Rimactane Capsules and 30 INH 300-mg Tablets.

Reference:

1. Bauer, A. W., Kirby, W. M. M., Sherris, J. C., and Turck, M. Antibiotic susceptibility testing by a standardized single disk method. Am. J. Clin. Path. 45:493-496, 1966.

C79-20 (9/79)

[*Shown in Product Identification Section*]

RITALIN® hydrochloride Ⓒ
(methylphenidate hydrochloride USP)
tablets

RITALIN-SR® Ⓒ
(methylphenidate hydrochloride)
sustained-release tablets

Description: Ritalin is a white, odorless, fine crystalline powder, solutions of which are acid to litmus. It is freely soluble in water.

Clinical Pharmacology: Ritalin is a mild central nervous system stimulant.

The mode of action in man is not completely understood, but Ritalin presumably activates the brain stem arousal system and cortex to produce its stimulant effect.

There is neither specific evidence which clearly establishes the mechanism whereby Ritalin produces its mental and behavioral effects in children, nor conclusive evidence regarding how these effects relate to the condition of the central nervous system.

Ritalin in the SR tablets is more slowly but as extensively absorbed as in the regular tablets. Relative bioavailability of the SR tablet compared to the Ritalin tablet, measured by the urinary excretion of Ritalin major metabolite (α-phenyl-2-piperidine acetic acid) was 105% (49–168%) in children and 101% (85–152%) in adults. The time to peak rate in children was 4.7 hours (1.3–8.2 hours) for the SR tablets and 1.9 hours (0.3–4.4 hours) for the tablets. An average of 67% of SR tablet dose was excreted in children as compared to 86% in adults.

Indications

Based on a review of this drug by the National Academy of Sciences-National Research Council and/or other information, FDA has classified the indications as follows:

Effective: Attention Deficit Disorders (previously known as Minimal Brain Dysfunction in Children). Other terms being used to describe the behavioral syndrome below include: Hyperkinetic Child Syndrome, Minimal Brain Damage, Minimal Cerebral Dysfunction, Minor Cerebral Dysfunction.

Ritalin is indicated as an integral part of a total treatment program which typically includes other remedial measures (psychological, educational, social) for a stabilizing effect in children with a behavioral syndrome characterized by the following group of developmentally inappropriate symptoms: moderate-to-severe distractibility, short attention span, hyperactivity, emotional lability, and impulsivity. The diagnosis of this syndrome should not be made with finality when these symptoms are only of comparatively recent origin. Nonlocalizing (soft) neurological signs, learning disability, and abnormal EEG may or may not be present, and a diagnosis of central nervous system dysfunction may or may not be warranted.

Special Diagnostic Considerations

Specific etiology of this syndrome is unknown, and there is no single diagnostic test. Adequate diagnosis requires the use

Continued on next page

The full prescribing information for each CIBA drug is contained herein and is that in effect as of October 1, 1982.

CIBA—Cont.

not only of medical but of special psychological, educational, and social resources. Characteristics commonly reported include: chronic history of short attention span, distractibility, emotional lability, impulsivity, and moderate-to-severe hyperactivity; minor neurological signs and abnormal EEG. Learning may or may not be impaired. The diagnosis must be based upon a complete history and evaluation of the child and not solely on the presence of one of one or more of these characteristics. Drug treatment is not indicated for all children with this syndrome. Stimulants are not intended for use in the child who exhibits symptoms secondary to environmental factors and/or primary psychiatric disorders, including psychosis. Appropriate educational placement is essential and psychosocial intervention is generally necessary. When remedial measures alone are insufficient, the decision to prescribe stimulant medication will depend upon the physician's assessment of the chronicity and severity of the child's symptoms.

Effective: Narcolepsy

"Possibly" effective: Mild depression; Apathetic or Withdrawn Senile Behavior

Final classification of the less-than-effective indications requires further investigation.

Contraindications: Marked anxiety, tension, and agitation are contraindications to Ritalin, since the drug may aggravate these symptoms. Ritalin is contraindicated also in patients known to be hypersensitive to the drug, in patients with glaucoma, and in patients with motor tics or with a family history or diagnosis of Tourette's syndrome.

Warnings: Ritalin should not be used in children under six years, since safety and efficacy in this age group have not been established.

Sufficient data on safety and efficacy of long-term use of Ritalin in children are not yet available. Although a causal relationship has not been established, suppression of growth (*ie*, weight gain, and/or height) has been reported with the long-term use of stimulants in children. Therefore, patients requiring long-term therapy should be carefully monitored.

Ritalin should not be used for severe depression of either exogenous or endogenous origin. Clinical experience suggests that in psychotic children, administration of Ritalin may exacerbate symptoms of behavior disturbance and thought disorder.

Ritalin should not be used for the prevention or treatment of normal fatigue states.

There is some clinical evidence that Ritalin may lower the convulsive threshold in patients with prior history of seizures, with prior EEG abnormalities in absence of seizures, and, very rarely, in absence of history of seizures and no prior EEG evidence of seizures. Safe concomitant use of anticonvulsants and Ritalin has not been established. In the presence of seizures, the drug should be discontinued.

Use cautiously in patients with hypertension. Blood pressure should be monitored at appropriate intervals in all patients taking Ritalin, especially those with hypertension.

Symptoms of visual disturbances have been encountered in rare cases. Difficulties with accommodation and blurring of vision have been reported.

Drug Interactions

Ritalin may decrease the hypotensive effect of guanethidine. Use cautiously with pressor agents and MAO inhibitors.

Human pharmacologic studies have shown that Ritalin may inhibit the metabolism of coumarin anticoagulants, anticonvulsants (phenobarbital, diphenylhydantoin, primidone), phenylbutazone, and tricyclic antidepressants (imipramine, desipramine). Downward dosage adjustments of these drugs may be required when given concomitantly with Ritalin.

Usage in Pregnancy

Adequate animal reproduction studies to establish safe use of Ritalin during pregnancy have not been conducted. Therefore, until more information is available, Ritalin should not be prescribed for women of childbearing age unless, in the opinion of the physician, the potential benefits outweigh the possible risks.

Drug Dependence

Ritalin should be given cautiously to emotionally unstable patients, such as those with a history of drug dependence or alcoholism, because such patients may increase dosage on their own initiative.

Chronically abusive use can lead to marked tolerance and psychic dependence with varying degrees of abnormal behavior. Frank psychotic episodes can occur, especially with parenteral abuse. Careful supervision is required during drug withdrawal, since severe depression as well as the effects of chronic overactivity can be unmasked. Long-term follow-up may be required because of the patient's basic personality disturbances.

Precautions: Patients with an element of agitation may react adversely; discontinue therapy if necessary.

Periodic CBC, differential, and platelet counts are advised during prolonged therapy.

Drug treatment is not indicated in all cases of this behavioral syndrome and should be considered only in light of the complete history and evaluation of the child. The decision to prescribe Ritalin should depend on the physician's assessment of the chronicity and severity of the child's symptoms and their appropriateness for his/her age. Prescription should not depend solely on the presence of one or more of the behavioral characteristics.

When these symptoms are associated with acute stress reactions, treatment with Ritalin is usually not indicated.

Long-term effects of Ritalin in children have not been well established.

Adverse Reactions: Nervousness and insomnia are the most common adverse reactions but are usually controlled by reducing dosage and omitting the drug in the afternoon or evening. Other reactions include hypersensitivity (including skin rash, urticaria, fever, arthralgia, exfoliative dermatitis, erythema multiforme with histopathological findings of necrotizing vasculitis, and thrombocytopenic purpura); anorexia; nausea; dizziness; palpitations; headache; dyskinesia; drowsiness; blood pressure and pulse changes, both up and down; tachycardia; angina; cardiac arrhythmia; abdominal pain; weight loss during prolonged therapy. There have been rare reports of Tourette's syndrome. Toxic psychosis has been reported. Although a definite causal relationship has not been established, the following have been reported in patients taking this drug: leukopenia and/or anemia; a few instances of scalp hair loss.

In children, loss of appetite, abdominal pain, weight loss during prolonged therapy, insomnia, and tachycardia may occur more frequently; however, any of the other adverse reactions listed above may also occur.

Dosage and Administration: Dosage should be individualized according to the needs and responses of the patient.

Adults

Tablets: Administer in divided doses 2 or 3 times daily, preferably 30 to 45 minutes before meals. Average dosage is 20 to 30 mg daily. Some patients may require 40 to 60 mg daily. In others, 10 to 15 mg daily will be adequate. Patients who are unable to sleep if medication is taken late in the day should take the last dose before 6 p.m.

SR Tablets: Ritalin SR Tablets have a duration of action of approximately 8 hours. Therefore, Ritalin SR tablets may be used in place of Ritalin tablets when the 8 hour dosage of Ritalin SR corresponds to the titrated 8 hour dosage of Ritalin.

Children (6 years and over)

Ritalin should be initiated in small doses, with gradual weekly increments. Daily dosage above 60 mg is not recommended.

If improvement is not observed after appropriate dosage adjustments over a one-month period, the drug should be discontinued.

Tablets: Start with 5 mg twice daily (before breakfast and lunch) with gradual increments of 5 to 10 mg weekly.

SR Tablets: Ritalin SR tablets have a duration of action of approximately 8 hours. Therefore, Ritalin SR tablets may be used in place of Ritalin tablets when the 8 hour dosage of Ritalin SR corresponds to the titrated 8 hour dosage of Ritalin.

If paradoxical aggravation of symptoms or other adverse effects occur, reduce dosage, or, if necessary, discontinue the drug.

Ritalin should be periodically discontinued to assess the child's condition. Improvement may be sustained when the drug is either temporarily or permanently discontinued.

Drug treatment should not and need not be indefinite and usually may be discontinued after puberty.

Overdosage: Signs and symptoms of acute overdosage, resulting principally from overstimulation of the central nervous system and from excessive sympathomimetic effects, may include the following: vomiting, agitation, tremors, hyperreflexia, muscle twitching, convulsions (may be followed by coma), euphoria, confusion; hallucinations, delirium, sweating, flushing, headache, hyperpyrexia, tachycardia, palpitations, cardiac arrhythmias, hypertension, mydriasis, and dryness of mucous membranes.

Treatment consists of appropriate supportive measures. The patient must be protected against self-injury and against external stimuli that would aggravate overstimulation already present. If signs and symptoms are not too severe and the patient is conscious, gastric contents may be evacuated by induction of emesis or gastric lavage. In the presence of severe intoxication, use a carefully titrated dosage of a *short-acting* barbiturate *before* performing gastric lavage.

Intensive care must be provided to maintain adequate circulation and respiratory exchange; external cooling procedures may be required for hyperpyrexia.

Efficacy of peritoneal dialysis or extracorporeal hemodialysis for Ritalin overdosage has not been established.

How Supplied:

Tablets 20 mg—round, pale yellow, scored (imprinted CIBA 34)

Bottles of 100 ....NDC 0083-0034-30
Bottles of 1000 ....NDC 0083-0034-40

Tablets 10 mg —round, pale green, scored (imprinted CIBA 3)

Bottles of 100 ....NDC 0083-0003-30
Bottles of 500 ....NDC 0083-0003-35
Bottles of 1000 ....NDC 0083-0003-40
Accu-Pak® Unit Dose (blister pack)
Box of 100 (strips of 10) NDC 0083-0003-32

Tablets 5 mg—round, yellow (imprinted CIBA 7)

Bottles of 100 ....NDC 0083-0007-30
Bottles of 500 ....NDC 0083-0007-35
Bottles of 1000 ....NDC 0083-0007-40

SR Tablets 20 mg—round, white, coated (imprinted CIBA 16)

Bottles of 100 ....NDC 0083-0016-30

Note: SR Tablets are color-additive free.

Do not store above 86°F (30°C). Protect from moisture.

Dispense in tight, light-resistant container (USP).

C82-63 (Rev. 1/83)

SER-AP-ES® ℞
reserpine 0.1 mg
hydralazine hydrochloride 25 mg
hydrochlorothiazide 15 mg
Combination Tablets

Warning
This fixed combination drug is not indicated for initial therapy of hypertension. Hypertension requires therapy titrated to the individual patient. If the fixed combination represents the dosage so determined, its use may be more convenient in patient management. The treatment of hypertension is not static, but must be reevaluated as conditions in each patient warrant.

Indications
Hypertension. (See box warning.)

Contraindications

Reserpine
Known hypersensitivity, mental depression (especially with suicidal tendencies), active peptic ulcer, ulcerative colitis, and patients receiving electroconvulsive therapy.

Hydralazine
Hypersensitivity to hydralazine; coronary artery disease; and mitral valvular rheumatic heart disease.

Hydrochlorothiazide
Anuria; hypersensitivity to this or other sulfonamide-derived drugs.

Warnings

Reserpine
Extreme caution should be exercised in treating patients with a history of mental depression. Discontinue the drug at first sign of despondency, early morning insomnia, loss of appetite, impotence, or self-deprecation. Drug-induced depression may persist for several months after drug withdrawal and may be severe enough to result in suicide.
MAO inhibitors should be avoided or used with extreme caution.

Hydralazine
Hydralazine may produce in a few patients a clinical picture simulating systemic lupus erythematosus. In such patients hydralazine should be discontinued unless the benefit-to-risk determination requires continued antihypertensive therapy with this drug. Symptoms and signs usually regress when the drug is discontinued but residua have been detected many years later. Long-term treatment with steroids may be necessary.
Complete blood counts, L. E. cell preparations, and antinuclear antibody titer determinations are indicated before and periodically during prolonged therapy with hydralazine, even though the patient is asymptomatic. These studies are also indicated if the patient develops arthralgia, fever, chest pain, continued malaise or other unexplained signs or symptoms.
A positive antinuclear antibody titer and/or positive L. E. cell reaction requires that the physician carefully weigh the implications of the test results against the benefits to be derived from antihypertensive therapy with hydralazine.
Use MAO inhibitors with caution in patients receiving hydralazine.
When other potent parenteral antihypertensive drugs, such as diazoxide, are used in combination with hydralazine, patients should be continuously observed for several hours for any excessive fall in blood presssure. Profound hypotensive episodes may occur when diazoxide injection and hydralazine are used concomitantly.

Hydrochlorothiazide
Use with caution in severe renal disease. In patients with renal disease, thiazides may precipitate azotemia. Cumulative effects of the drug may develop in patients with impaired renal function.
Thiazides should be used with caution in patients with impaired hepatic function or progressive liver disease, since minor alterations of fluid and electrolyte imbalance may precipitate hepatic coma.
Thiazides may add to or potentiate the action of other antihypertensive drugs. Potentiation occurs with ganglionic or peripheral adrenergic blocking drugs.
Sensitivity reactions are more likely to occur in patients with a history of allergy or bronchial asthma.
The possibility of exacerbation or activation of systemic lupus erythematosus has been reported.

Usage in Pregnancy

Reserpine
The safety of reserpine for use during pregnancy or lactation has not been established; therefore, the drug should be used in pregnant patients or in women of childbearing potential only when, in the judgment of the physician, it is essential to the welfare of the patient. Increased respiratory tract secretions, nasal congestion, cyanosis, and anorexia may occur in neonates and breast-fed infants of reserpine-treated mothers since reserpine crosses the placental barrier and appears in maternal breast milk.

Hydralazine
Animal studies indicate that hydralazine is teratogenic in mice, possibly in rabbits, and not in rats. Teratogenic effects observed were cleft palate and malformations of facial and cranial bones. Although clinical experience does not include any positive evidence of adverse effects on the human fetus, hydralazine should not be used during pregnancy unless the expected benefit clearly justifies the potential risk to the fetus.

Hydrochlorothiazide
Thiazides cross the placental barrier and appear in cord blood. The use of thiazides in pregnant women requires that the anticipated benefit be weighed against possible hazards to the fetus. These hazards include fetal or neonatal jaundice, thrombocytopenia, and possibly other adverse reactions which have occurred in the adult.
Nursing Mothers: Thiazides appear in breast milk. If the use of the drug is deemed essential, the patient should stop nursing.

Precautions

Reserpine
Since reserpine increases gastrointestinal motility and secretion, it should be used cautiously in patients with a history of peptic ulcer, ulcerative colitis, or gallstones (biliary colic may be precipitated).
Caution should be exercised when treating hypertensive patients with renal insufficiency since they adjust poorly to lowered blood pressure levels.
Use reserpine cautiously with digitalis and quinidine, since cardiac arrhythmias have occurred with rauwolfia preparations.
Preoperative withdrawal of reserpine does not assure that circulatory instability will not occur. It is important that the anesthesiologist be aware of the patient's drug intake and consider this in the overall management, since hypotension has occurred in patients receiving rauwolfia preparations. Anticholinergic and/or adrenergic drugs (*eg,* metaraminol, norepinephrine) have been employed to treat adverse vagocirculatory effects.

Hydralazine
Myocardial stimulation produced by hydralazine can cause anginal attacks and ECG changes of myocardial ischemia. The drug has been implicated in the production of myocardial infarction. It must, therefore, be used with caution in patients with suspected coronary artery disease.
The "hyperdynamic" circulation caused by hydralazine may accentuate specific cardiovascular inadequacies. An example is that hydralazine may increase pulmonary artery pressure in patients with mitral valvular disease. The drug may reduce the pressor responses to epinephrine. Postural hypotension may result from hydralazine but is less common than with ganglionic blocking agents. Use with caution in patients with cerebral vascular accidents.
In hypertensive patients with normal kidneys who are treated with hydralazine, there is evidence of increased renal blood flow and a maintenance of glomerular filtration rate. In some instances improved renal function has been noted where control values were below normal prior to hydralazine administration. However, as with any antihypertensive agent, hydralazine should be used with caution in patients with advanced renal damage.
Peripheral neuritis, evidenced by paresthesias, numbness, and tingling, has been observed. Published evidence suggests an antipyridoxine effect and the addition of pyridoxine to the regimen if symptoms develop.
Blood dyscrasias, consisting of reduction in hemoglobin and red cell count, leukopenia, agranulocytosis, and purpura, have been reported. If such abnormalities develop, discontinue therapy. Periodic blood counts are advised during prolonged therapy.

Hydrochlorothiazide
Periodic determination of serum electrolytes to detect possible electrolyte imbalance should be performed at appropriate intervals. All patients receiving thiazide therapy should be observed for clinical signs of fluid or electrolyte imbalance; namely, hyponatremia, hypochloremic alkalosis, and hypokalemia. Serum and urine electrolyte determinations are particularly important when the patient is vomiting excessively or receiving parenteral fluids. Medication such as digitalis may also influence serum electrolytes. Warning signs are dryness of mouth, thirst, weakness, lethargy, drowsiness, restlessness, muscle pains or cramps, muscular fatigue, hypotension, oliguria, tachycardia, and gastrointestinal disturbance such as nausea or vomiting.
Hypokalemia may develop, especially with brisk diuresis, when severe cirrhosis is present, or during concomitant use of steroids or ACTH. Interference with adequate oral intake of electrolytes will also contribute to hypokalemia. Hypokalemia can sensitize or exaggerate the response of the heart to the toxic effects of digitalis (*eg,* increased ventricular irritability).
Any chloride deficit is generally mild and usually does not require specific treatment except under extraordinary circumstances (as in liver disease or renal disease). Dilutional hyponatremia may occur in edematous patients in hot weather; appropriate therapy is water restriction rather than administration of salt, except in rare instances when the hyponatremia is life-threatening. In actual salt depletion, appropriate replacement is the therapy of choice.
Hyperuricemia may occur or frank gout may be precipitated in certain patients receiving thiazide therapy.
Insulin requirements in diabetic patients may be increased, decreased, or unchanged. Latent diabetes may become manifest during thiazide administration.
Thiazide drugs may increase the responsiveness to tubocurarine.
The antihypertensive effects of the drug may be enhanced in the postsympathectomy pa-

Continued on next page

The full prescribing information for each CIBA drug is contained herein and is that in effect as of October 1, 1982.

CIBA—Cont.

tient. Thiazides may decrease arterial responsiveness to norepinephrine. This diminution is not sufficient to preclude effectiveness of the pressor agent for therapeutic use.
If progressive renal impairment becomes evident, withholding or discontinuing diuretic therapy should be considered.
Thiazides may decrease serum PBI levels without signs of thyroid disturbance.
Calcium excretion is decreased by thiazides. Pathological changes in the parathyroid gland with hypercalcemia and hypophosphatemia have been observed in a few patients on prolonged thiazide therapy. The common complications of hyperparathyroidism such as renal lithiasis, bone resorption, and peptic ulceration have not been seen. Thiazides should be discontinued before carrying out tests for parathyroid function.

Adverse Reactions

Reserpine

Rauwolfia preparations have caused gastrointestinal reactions including hypersecretion, nausea, vomiting, anorexia, and diarrhea; cardiovascular reactions including angina-like symptoms, arrhythmias (particularly when used concurrently with digitalis or quinidine), and bradycardia; central nervous system reactions including drowsiness, depression, nervousness, paradoxical anxiety, nightmares, rare parkinsonian syndrome and other extrapyramidal tract symptoms, and CNS sensitization manifested by dull sensorium, deafness, glaucoma, uveitis, and optic atrophy. Nasal congestion is a frequent occurrence. Pruritus, rash, dryness of mouth, dizziness, headache, dyspnea, syncope, epistaxis, purpura and other hematologic reactions, impotence or decreased libido, dysuria, muscular aches, conjunctival injection, weight gain, breast engorgement, pseudolactation, and gynecomastia have been reported. These reactions are usually reversible and disappear after the drug is discontinued.
Water retention with edema in patients with hypertensive vascular disease may occur rarely, but the condition generally clears with cessation of therapy or with the administration of a diuretic agent.

Hydralazine

Adverse reactions with hydralazine are usually reversible when dosage is reduced. However, in some cases it may be necessary to discontinue the drug.
Common: Headache; palpitations; anorexia; nausea; vomiting; diarrhea; tachycardia; angina pectoris.
Less Frequent: Nasal congestion; flushing; lacrimation; conjunctivitis; peripheral neuritis, evidenced by paresthesias, numbness, and tingling; edema; dizziness; tremors; muscle cramps; psychotic reactions characterized by depression, disorientation, or anxiety; hypersensitivity (including rash, urticaria, pruritus, fever, chills, arthralgia, eosinophilia, and, rarely, hepatitis); constipation; difficulty in micturition; dyspnea; paralytic ileus; lymphadenopathy; splenomegaly; blood dyscrasias, consisting of reduction in hemoglobin and red cell count, leukopenia, agranulocytosis, and purpura; hypotension; paradoxical pressor response.

Hydrochlorothiazide

Gastrointestinal: Anorexia, gastric irritation, nausea, vomiting, cramping, diarrhea, constipation, jaundice (intrahepatic cholestatic), pancreatitis, sialadenitis
Central Nervous System: Dizziness, vertigo, paresthesias, headache, xanthopsia
Hematologic: Leukopenia, thrombocytopenia, agranulocytosis, aplastic anemia
Cardiovascular: Orthostatic hypotension (may be potentiated by alcohol, barbiturates, or narcotics)
Hypersensitivity: Purpura, photosensitivity, rash, urticaria, necrotizing angiitis, Stevens-Johnson syndrome, and other hypersensitivity reactions
Other: Hyperglycemia, glycosuria, hyperuricemia, muscle spasm, weakness, restlessness
Whenever adverse reactions are moderate or severe, thiazide dosage should be reduced or therapy withdrawn.

Dosage and Administration: As determined by individual titration (see box warning). Usual dosage is 1 to 2 tablets t.i.d.
Since the antihypertensive effects of reserpine are not immediately apparent, maximal reduction in blood pressure from a given dosage may not occur for 2 weeks. For maintenance, adjust dosage to lowest patient requirement.
When necessary, more potent antihypertensives may be added gradually in dosages reduced by at least 50 percent. Watch effects carefully.

Overdosage

Reserpine

Signs and Symptoms

Impairment of consciousness may occur and may range from drowsiness to coma, depending upon the severity of overdosage. Flushing of the skin, conjunctival injection, and pupillary constriction are to be expected. Hypotension, hypothermia, central respiratory depression, and bradycardia may develop in cases of severe overdosage. Diarrhea may also occur.

Treatment

Evacuate stomach contents, taking adequate precautions against aspiration and for the protection of the airway; instill activated charcoal slurry.
Treat the effect of reserpine overdosage symptomatically. If hypotension is severe enough to require treatment with a vasopressor, use one having a direct action upon vascular smooth muscle (*eg* phenylephrine, levarterenol, metaraminol). Since reserpine is long-acting, observe the patient carefully for at least 72 hours, administering treatment as required.

Hydralazine

Signs and Symptoms

Hypotension, tachycardia, headache and generalized skin flushing are to be expected. Myocardial ischemia and cardiac arrhythmia can develop; profound shock can occur in severe overdosage.

Treatment

Evacuate gastric contents, taking adequate precautions against aspiration and for protection of the airway; instill activated charcoal slurry, if general conditions permit. These manipulations may have to be omitted or carried out after cardiovascular status has been stabilized, since they might precipitate cardiac arrhythmias or increase the depth of shock.
Support of the cardiovascular system is of primary importance. Shock should be treated with volume expanders without resorting to use of vasopressors, if possible. If a vasopressor is required, use one that is least likely to precipitate or aggravate cardiac arrhythmia. Digitalization may be necessary. Renal function must be monitored and supported as required.
No experience has been reported with extracorporeal or peritoneal dialysis.

Hydrochlorothiazide

Signs and Symptoms

Diuresis is to be expected; lethargy of varying degree may appear and may progress to coma within a few hours, with minimal depression of respiration and cardiovascular function and without significant serum electrolyte changes or dehydration. The mechanism of CNS depression with thiazide overdosage is unknown. GI irritation and hypermotility may occur; temporary elevation of BUN has been reported and serum electrolyte changes could occur, especially in patients with impairment of renal function.

Treatment

Evacuate gastric contents but take care to prevent aspiration, especially in the stuporous or comatose patient. GI effects are usually of short duration, but may require symptomatic treatment.
Monitor serum electrolyte levels and renal function; institute supportive measures as required individually to maintain hydration, electrolyte balance, respiration and cardiovascular-renal function.

How Supplied: *Tablets* (light salmon pink, dry-coated), each containing 0.1 mg reserpine, 25 mg hydralazine hydrochloride, and 15 mg hydrochlorothiazide; bottles of 100, 1000 and Accu-Pak® blister units of 100.

C78-53 (1/79)

[*Shown in Product Identification Section*]

SERPASIL® ℞
(reserpine USP)
Tablets

Listed in USP, a Medicare designated compendium.

Indications

Mild essential hypertension; also useful as adjunctive therapy with other antihypertensive agents in the more severe forms of hypertension; relief of symptoms in agitated psychotic states (*eg*, schizophrenia), primarily in those individuals unable to tolerate phenothiazine derivatives or those who also require antihypertensive medication.

Contraindications: Known hypersensitivity, mental depression (especially with suicidal tendencies), active peptic ulcer, ulcerative colitis, and patients receiving electroconvulsive therapy.

Warnings: Extreme caution should be exercised in treating patients with a history of mental depression. Discontinue the drug at first sign of despondency, early morning insomnia, loss of appetite, impotence, or self-deprecation. Drug-induced depression may persist for several months after drug withdrawal and may be severe enough to result in suicide.
MAO inhibitors should be avoided or used with extreme caution.

Usage in Pregnancy

The safety of reserpine for use during pregnancy or lactation has not been established; therefore, the drug should be used in pregnant patients or in women of childbearing potential only when, in the judgment of the physician, it is essential to the welfare of the patient. Increased respiratory tract secretions, nasal congestion, cyanosis, and anorexia may occur in neonates and breast-fed infants of reserpine-treated mothers since reserpine crosses the placental barrier and also appears in maternal breast milk.

Precautions: Since Serpasil increases gastrointestinal motility and secretion, it should be used cautiously in patients with a history of peptic ulcer, ulcerative colitis, or gallstones (biliary colic may be precipitated).
Caution should be exercised when treating hypertensive patients with renal insufficiency since they adjust poorly to lowered blood pressure levels.
Use Serpasil cautiously with digitalis and quinidine since cardiac arrhythmias have occurred with rauwolfia preparations.
Preoperative withdrawal of reserpine does not assure that circulatory instability will not occur. It is important that the anesthesiologist be aware of the patient's drug intake and consider this in the overall management, since hypotension has occurred in patients receiving rauwolfia preparations. Anticholinergic and/or adrenergic drugs (*eg*, metaraminol, norepinephrine) have been employed to treat adverse vagocirculatory effects.

Adverse Reactions: Rauwolfia preparations have caused gastrointestinal reactions including hypersecretion, nausea, vomiting, anorexia, and diarrhea; cardiovascular reactions including angina-like symptoms, arrhythmias (particularly when used concurrently with digitalis or quinidine), bradycardia; central nervous system reactions including drowsiness, depression, nervousness, paradoxical anxiety, nightmares, rare parkinsonian syndrome and other extrapyramidal tract symptoms, and CNS sensitization manifested by dull sensorium, deafness, glaucoma, uveitis, and optic atrophy. Nasal congestion is a frequent occurrence. Pruritus, rash, dryness of mouth, dizziness, headache, dyspnea, syncope, epistaxis, purpura and other hematologic reactions, impotence or decreased libido, dysuria, muscular aches, conjunctival injection, weight gain, breast engorgement, pseudolactation, and gynecomastia have been reported. These reactions are usually reversible and usually disappear after the drug is discontinued.

Water retention with edema in patients with hypertensive vascular disease may occur rarely, but the condition generally clears with cessation of therapy or with the administration of a diuretic agent.

Dosage and Administration

For Hypertension: In the average patient not receiving other antihypertensive agents, the usual initial dose is 0.5 mg daily for 1 or 2 weeks. For maintenance, reduce to 0.1 mg to 0.25 mg daily. Higher doses should be used cautiously, because serious mental depression and other side effects may be increased considerably.

For Psychiatric Disorders: The usual initial dose is 0.5 mg, with a range of 0.1 mg to 1.0 mg. Adjust dosage upward or downward according to the patient's response.

Concomitant use of Serpasil with ganglionic blocking agents, guanethidine, veratrum, hydralazine, methyldopa, chlorthalidone, or thiazides necessitates careful titration of dosage with each agent.

Overdosage

Signs and Symptoms

Impairment of consciousness may occur and may range from drowsiness to coma, depending upon the severity of overdosage. Flushing of the skin, conjunctival injection, and pupillary constriction are to be expected. Hypotension, hypothermia, central respiratory depression, and bradycardia may develop in cases of severe overdosage. Diarrhea may also occur.

Treatment

Evacuate stomach contents, taking adequate precautions against aspiration and for the protection of the airway; instill activated charcoal slurry.

Treat the effects of reserpine overdosage symptomatically. If hypotension is severe enough to require treatment with a vasopressor, use one having a direct action upon vascular smooth muscle (*eg,* phenylephrine, levarterenol, metaraminol). Since reserpine is long-acting, observe the patient carefully for at least 72 hours, administering treatment as required.

How Supplied

Tablets 0.1 mg — white (imprinted 35 CIBA)
Bottles of 100 ....NDC 0083-0035-30
Bottles of 1000 ....NDC 0083-0035-40

Tablets 0.25 mg — white, scored (imprinted 36 CIBA)
Bottles of 100 ....NDC 0083-0036-30
Bottles of 500 ....NDC 0083-0036-35
Bottles of 1000 ....NDC 0083-0036-40
Consumer Pack — One Unit
(12 bottles — 100 tablets each) ....NDC 0083-0036-65

Dispense in tight, light-resistant container (USP).

C81-15 (5/81)

[*Shown in Product Identification Section*]

SERPASIL® ℞
(reserpine USP)
Parenteral Solution

Listed in USP, a Medicare designated compendium.

Indications: Hypertensive emergencies, such as acute hypertensive encephalopathy, in which it is desired to reduce blood pressure rapidly; psychiatric conditions only to initiate treatment in those patients unable to accept oral medication or to control symptoms of extreme agitation.

Contraindications: Known hypersensitivity, mental depression (especially with suicidal tendencies), active peptic ulcer, ulcerative colitis, and patients receiving electroconvulsive therapy.

Warnings: Extreme caution should be exercised in treating patients with a history of mental depression. Discontinue the drug at first sign of despondency, early morning insomnia, loss of appetite, impotence, or self-deprecation. Drug-induced depression may persist for several months after drug withdrawal and may be severe enough to result in suicide.

MAO inhibitors should be avoided or used with extreme caution.

Usage in Pregnancy

The safety of reserpine for use during pregnancy or lactation has not been established; therefore, the drug should be used in pregnant patients or in women of childbearing potential only when, in the judgment of the physician, it is essential to the welfare of the patient. Increased respiratory tract secretions, nasal congestion, cyanosis, and anorexia may occur in neonates and breast-fed infants of reserpine-treated mothers since reserpine crosses the placental barrier and also appears in maternal breast milk.

Precautions: Since Serpasil increases gastrointestinal motility and secretion, it should be used cautiously in patients with a history of peptic ulcer, ulcerative colitis, or gallstones (biliary colic may be precipitated).

Caution should be exercised when treating hypertensive patients with renal insufficiency since they adjust poorly to lowered blood pressure levels.

Use Serpasil cautiously with digitalis and quinidine since cardiac arrhythmias have occurred with rauwolfia preparations.

Preoperative withdrawal of reserpine does not assure that circulatory instability will not occur. It is important that the anesthesiologist be aware of the patient's drug intake and consider this in the overall management, since hypotension has occurred in patients receiving rauwolfia preparations. Anticholinergic and/or adrenergic drugs (*eg,* metaraminol, norepinephrine) have been employed to treat adverse vagocirculatory effects.

Adverse Reactions: Rauwolfia preparations have caused gastrointestinal reactions including hypersecretion, nausea, vomiting, anorexia, and diarrhea; cardiovascular reactions including angina-like symptoms, arrhythmias (particularly when used concurrently with digitalis or quinidine), bradycardia; central nervous system reactions including drowsiness, depression, nervousness, paradoxical anxiety, nightmares, rare parkinsonian syndrome and other extrapyramidal tract symptoms, and CNS sensitization manifested by dull sensorium, deafness, glaucoma, uveitis, and optic atrophy. Nasal congestion is a frequent occurrence. Pruritus, rash, dryness of mouth, dizziness, headache, dyspnea, syncope, epistaxis, purpura and other hematologic reactions, impotence or decreased libido, dysuria, muscular aches, conjunctival injection, weight gain, breast engorgement, pseudolactation, and gynecomastia have been reported. These reactions are usually reversible and usually disappear after the drug is discontinued.

Water retention with edema in patients with hypertensive vascular disease may occur rarely, but the condition generally clears with cessation of therapy or with the administration of a diuretic agent.

Dosage and Administration: Serpasil may be administered intramuscularly in the short-term treatment of hypertensive crises. Because of the varying responsiveness, a titration procedure should be used. An initial dose of 0.5 to 1 mg intramuscularly is followed at intervals of 3 hours, if necessary, by doses of 2 and 4 mg until the blood pressure falls to the desired level. If the 4-mg dose is ineffective, other antihypertensive agents should be used. An initial dose larger than 0.5 mg may induce severe hypotension, particularly in patients with cerebral hemorrhage.

Serpasil may be administered intramuscularly in psychiatric emergencies to initiate treatment in those patients unable to accept oral medication or to control extreme agitation. The usual dose is from 2.5 mg to 5.0 mg, following a small initial dose to test patient responsiveness.

Concomitant use of Serpasil with ganglionic blocking agents, guanethidine, veratrum, hydralazine, methyldopa, chlorthalidone, or thiazides necessitates careful titration of dosage with each agent.

Overdosage

Signs and Symptoms

Impairment of consciousness may occur and may range from drowsiness to coma, depending upon the severity of overdosage. Flushing of the skin, conjunctival injection, and pupillary constriction are to be expected. Hypotension, hypothermia, central respiratory depression, and bradycardia may develop in cases of severe overdosage. Diarrhea may also occur.

Treatment

Hypotension is likely to require major therapeutic attention. If a vasopressor is necessary, use one having a direct action upon vascular smooth muscle (*eg,* phenylephrine, levarterenol, metaraminol).

If bradycardia becomes marked, especially with cardiac arrhythmia, consider use of vagal blocking agents along with other appropriate measures.

Treat other effects of reserpine overdosage symptomatically. Since reserpine is long-acting, observe the patient carefully for at least 72 hours, administering treatment as required.

How Supplied

Parenteral Solution: Each ml contains 2.5 mg reserpine, 0.1 ml dimethylacetamide, 10 mg adipic acid, 0.1 mg versene, 0.01 ml benzyl alcohol, 0.05 ml polyethylene glycol, 0.5 mg ascorbic acid, and 0.1 mg sodium sulfite in water. *Ampuls,* 2 ml; cartons of 5.

C78-61 (3/79)

SERPASIL®-APRESOLINE® ℞
hydrochloride
(reserpine and hydralazine hydrochloride)
Combination Tablets

Warning

This fixed combination drug is not indicated for initial therapy of hypertension. Hypertension requires therapy titrated to the individual patient. If the fixed combination represents the dosage so determined, its use may be more convenient in patient management. The treatment of hypertension is not static, but must be reevaluated as conditions in each patient warrant.

Continued on next page

The full prescribing information for each CIBA drug is contained herein and is that in effect as of October 1, 1982.

CIBA—Cont.

Indications

Hypertension. (See box warning.)

Contraindications

Reserpine

Known hypersensitivity, mental depression (especially with suicidal tendencies), active peptic ulcer, ulcerative colitis, and patients receiving electroconvulsive therapy.

Hydralazine

Hypersensitivity to hydralazine; coronary artery disease; and mitral valvular rheumatic heart disease.

Warnings

Reserpine

Extreme caution should be exercised in treating patients with a history of mental depression. Discontinue the drug at first sign of despondency, early morning insomnia, loss of appetite, impotence, or self-deprecation. Drug-induced depression may persist for several months after drug withdrawal and may be severe enough to result in suicide.

MAO inhibitors should be avoided or used with extreme caution.

Hydralazine

Hydralazine may produce in a few patients a clinical picture simulating systemic lupus erythematosus. In such patients hydralazine should be discontinued unless the benefit-to-risk determination requires continued antihypertensive therapy with this drug. Symptoms and signs usually regress when the drug is discontinued but residua have been detected many years later. Long-term treatment with steroids may be necessary.

Complete blood counts, L. E. cell preparations, and antinuclear antibody titer determinations are indicated before and periodically during prolonged therapy with hydralazine, even though the patient is asymptomatic. These studies are also indicated if the patient develops arthralgia, fever, chest pain, continued malaise, or other unexplained signs or symptoms.

A positive antinuclear antibody titer and/or positive L. E. cell reaction requires that the physician carefully weigh the implications of the test results against the benefits to be derived from antihypertensive therapy with hydralazine.

Use MAO inhibitors with caution in patients receiving hydralazine.

When other potent parenteral antihypertensive drugs, such as diazoxide, are used in combination with hydralazine, patients should be continuously observed for several hours for any excessive fall in blood pressure. Profound hypotensive episodes may occur when diazoxide injection and Apresoline (hydralazine hydrochloride) are used concomitantly.

Usage in Pregnancy

Reserpine

The safety of reserpine for use during pregnancy or lactation has not been established; therefore, the drug should be used in pregnant patients or in women of childbearing potential only when, in the judgment of the physician, it is essential to the welfare of the patient. Increased respiratory tract secretions, nasal congestion, cyanosis, and anorexia may occur in neonates and breast-fed infants of reserpine-treated mothers since reserpine crosses the placental barrier and appears in maternal breast milk.

Hydralazine

Animal studies indicate that hydralazine is teratogenic in mice, possibly in rabbits, and not in rats. Teratogenic effects observed were cleft palate and malformations of facial and cranial bones. Although clinical experience does not include any positive evidence of adverse effects on the human fetus, hydralazine should not be used during pregnancy unless the expected benefit clearly justifies the potential risk to the fetus.

Precautions

Reserpine

Since reserpine increases gastrointestinal motility and secretion, it should be used cautiously in patients with a history of peptic ulcer, ulcerative colitis, or gallstones (biliary colic may be precipitated).

Caution should be exercised when treating hypertensive patients with renal insufficiency, since they adjust poorly to lowered blood pressure levels.

Use reserpine cautiously with digitalis and quinidine since cardiac arrhythmias have occurred with rauwolfia preparations.

Preoperative withdrawal of reserpine does not assure that circulatory instability will not occur. It is important that the anesthesiologist be aware of the patient's drug intake and consider this in the overall management, since hypotension has occurred in patients receiving rauwolfia preparations. Anticholinergic and/or adrenergic drugs (*eg*, metaraminol, norepinephrine) have been employed to treat adverse vagocirculatory effects.

Hydralazine

Myocardial stimulation produced by hydralazine can cause anginal attacks and ECG changes of myocardial ischemia. The drug has been implicated in the production of myocardial infarction. It must, therefore, be used with caution in patients with suspected coronary artery disease.

The "hyperdynamic" circulation caused by hydralazine may accentuate specific cardiovascular inadequacies. An example is that hydralazine may increase pulmonary artery pressure in patients with mitral valvular disease. The drug may reduce the pressor responses to epinephrine. Postural hypotension may result from hydralazine but is less common than with ganglionic blocking agents. Use with caution in patients with cerebral vascular accidents.

In hypertensive patients with normal kidneys who are treated with hydralazine, there is evidence of increased renal blood flow and a maintenance of glomerular filtration rate. In some instances improved renal function has been noted where control values were below normal prior to hydralazine administration. However, as with any antihypertensive agent, hydralazine should be used with caution in patients with advanced renal damage.

Peripheral neuritis, evidenced by paresthesias, numbness, and tingling, has been observed. Published evidence suggests an antipyridoxine effect and the addition of pyridoxine to the regimen if symptoms develop.

Blood dyscrasias, consisting of reduction in hemoglobin and red cell count, leukopenia, agranulocytosis, and purpura, have been reported. If such abnormalities develop, discontinue therapy. Periodic blood counts are advised during prolonged therapy.

The Serpasil-Apresoline tablets (#1 and #2) contain FD&C Yellow No. 5 (tartrazine) which may cause allergic-type reactions (including bronchial asthma) in certain susceptible individuals. Although the overall incidence of FD&C Yellow No. 5 (tartrazine) sensitivity in the general population is low, it is frequently seen in patients who also have aspirin hypersensitivity.

Adverse Reactions

Reserpine

Rauwolfia preparations have caused gastrointestinal reactions including hypersecretion, nausea, vomiting, anorexia, and diarrhea; cardiovascular reactions including angina-like symptoms, arrhythmias (particularly when used concurrently with digitalis or quinidine), and bradycardia; central nervous system reactions including drowsiness, depression, nervousness, paradoxical anxiety, nightmares, rare parkinsonian syndrome and other extrapyramidal tract symptoms, and CNS sensitization manifested by dull sensorium, deafness, glaucoma, uveitis, and optic atrophy. Nasal congestion is a frequent occurrence. Pruritus, rash, dryness of mouth, dizziness, headache, dyspnea, syncope, epistaxis, purpura and other hematologic reactions, impotence or decreased libido, dysuria, muscular aches, conjunctival injection, weight gain, breast engorgement, pseudolactation, and gynecomastia have been reported. These reactions are usually reversible and disappear after the drug is discontinued.

Water retention with edema in patients with hypertensive vascular disease may occur rarely, but the condition generally clears with cessation of therapy or with the administration of a diuretic agent.

Hydralazine

Adverse reactions with hydralazine are usually reversible when dosage is reduced. However, in some cases it may be necessary to discontinue the drug.

Common: Headache; palpitations; anorexia; nausea; vomiting; diarrhea; tachycardia; angina pectoris.

Less Frequent: Nasal congestion; flushing; lacrimation; conjunctivitis; peripheral neuritis, evidenced by paresthesias, numbness, and tingling; edema; dizziness; tremors; muscle cramps; psychotic reactions characterized by depression, disorientation, or anxiety; hypersensitivity (including rash, urticaria, pruritus, fever, chills, arthralgia, eosinophilia, and, rarely, hepatitis); constipation; difficulty in micturition; dyspnea; paralytic ileus; lymphadenopathy; splenomegaly; blood dyscrasias, consisting of reduction in hemoglobin and red cell count, leukopenia, agranulocytosis, and purpura; hypotension; paradoxical pressor response.

Dosage and Administration: As determined by individual titration (see box warning).

Step 1: a. Start with reserpine alone. Average dosage: 0.5 mg daily.

b. Continue for at least one week. If results prove satisfactory—as they will in many cases—no other medication is required. For maintenance, reduce dosage to 0.25 mg or less daily.

Step 2: a. Should more than the therapeutic action of reserpine be indicated, therapy with *Tablet #2* (reserpine 0.2 mg/hydralazine hydrochloride 50 mg) should be initiated—one tablet 4 times a day.

b. When reduction of dosage is indicated, *Tablet #1* (reserpine 0.1 mg/hydralazine hydrochloride 25 mg) should be used—one tablet 4 times a day.

Side effects associated with hydralazine (headache, tachycardia, palpitation) are seldom encountered when the patient has been "primed" with reserpine before combination therapy is begun. Should side effects appear, however, reduction of dosage to one *Tablet #1* two to four times a day for a few days will usually alleviate them.

In cases where further individualization of dosage is necessary, the adjustment may be made by increasing or decreasing the dosage of reserpine and/or hydralazine.

For maintenance, daily dosage of hydralazine should probably not exceed 200 mg, nor should the dosage of reserpine exceed 1 mg.

For Patients on Hydralazine.

Patients already on this drug may be given a combination tablet as required. With the addition of reserpine, it is usually possible to reduce the dose of hydralazine.

Overdosage

Reserpine

Signs and Symptoms

Impairment of consciousness may occur and may range from drowsiness to coma, depending upon the severity of overdosage. Flushing of the skin, conjunctival injection, and pupillary constriction are to be expected. Hypotension, hypothermia, central respiratory depression, and bradycardia may develop in cases of severe overdosage. Diarrhea may also occur.

Treatment

Evacuate stomach contents, taking adequate precautions against aspiration and for the protection of the airway; instill activated charcoal slurry.

Treat the effects of reserpine overdosage symptomatically. If hypotension is severe enough to require treatment with a vasopressor, use one having a direct action upon vascular smooth muscle (*eg*, phenylephrine, levarterenol, metaraminol). Since reserpine is long-acting, observe the patient carefully for at least 72 hours, administering treatment as required.

Hydralazine

Signs and Symptoms

Hypotension, tachycardia, headache and generalized skin flushing are to be expected. Myocardial ischemia and cardiac arrhythmia can develop; profound shock can occur in severe overdosage.

Treatment

Evacuate gastric contents, taking adequate precautions against aspiration and for protection of the airway; instill activated charcoal slurry, if general conditions permit. These manipulations may have to be omitted or carried out after cardiovascular status has been stabilized, since they might precipitate cardiac arrhythmias or increase the depth of shock.

Support of the cardiovascular system is of primary importance. Shock should be treated with volume expanders without resorting to use of vasopressors, if possible. If a vasopressor is required, use one that is least likely to precipitate or aggravate cardiac arrhythmia. Digitalization may be necessary. Renal function must be monitored and supported as required.

No experience has been reported with extracorporeal or peritoneal dialysis.

How Supplied

Tablets #2 (yellow, dry-coated), each containing 0.2 mg reserpine and 50 mg hydralazine hydrochloride; bottles of 100.

Tablets #1 (yellow, dry-coated), each containing 0.1 mg reserpine and 25 mg hydralazine hydrochloride; bottles of 100.

Dispense in tight, light-resistant container (USP).

C80-19 (1/80)

[*Shown in Product Identification Section*]

SERPASIL®-ESIDRIX® ℞

(reserpine and hydrochlorothiazide)
Combination Tablets

> **Warning**
> This fixed combination drug is not indicated for initial therapy of hypertension. Hypertension requires therapy titrated to the individual patient. If the fixed combination represents the dosage so determined, its use may be more convenient in patient management. The treatment of hypertension is not static, but must be reevaluated as conditions in each patient warrant.

Indications

Hypertension. (See box warning.)

Contraindications

Reserpine

Known hypersensitivity, mental depression (especially with suicidal tendencies), active peptic ulcer, ulcerative colitis, and patients receiving electroconvulsive therapy.

Hydrochlorothiazide

Anuria; hypersensitivity to this or other sulfonamide-derived drugs.

Warnings

Reserpine

Extreme caution should be exercised in treating patients with a history of mental depression. Discontinue the drug at first sign of despondency, early morning insomnia, loss of appetite, impotence, or self-deprecation. Drug-induced depression may persist for several months after drug withdrawal and may be severe enough to result in suicide.

MAO inhibitors should be avoided or used with extreme caution.

Hydrochlorothiazide

Use with caution in severe renal disease. In patients with renal disease, thiazides may precipitate azotemia. Cumulative effects of the drug may develop in patients with impaired renal function.

Thiazides should be used with caution in patients with impaired hepatic function or progressive liver disease, since minor alterations of fluid and electrolyte imbalance may precipitate hepatic coma.

Thiazides may add to or potentiate the action of other antihypertensive drugs. Potentiation occurs with ganglionic or peripheral adrenergic blocking drugs.

Sensitivity reactions are more likely to occur in patients with a history of allergy or bronchial asthma.

The possibility of exacerbation or activation of systemic lupus erythematosus has been reported.

Usage in Pregnancy

Reserpine

The safety of reserpine for use during pregnancy or lactation has not been established; therefore, the drug should be used in pregnant patients or in women of childbearing potential only when, in the judgment of the physician, it is essential to the welfare of the patient. Increased respiratory tract secretions, nasal congestion, cyanosis, and anorexia may occur in neonates and breast-fed infants of reserpine-treated mothers, since reserpine crosses the placental barrier and appears in maternal breast milk.

Hydrochlorothiazide

Thiazides cross the placental barrier and appear in cord blood. The use of thiazides in pregnant women requires that the anticipated benefit be weighed against possible hazards to the fetus. These hazards include fetal or neonatal jaundice, thrombocytopenia, and possibly other adverse reactions which have occurred in the adult.

Nursing Mothers: Thiazides appear in breast milk. If the use of the drug is deemed essential, the patient should stop nursing.

Precautions

Reserpine

Since reserpine increases gastrointestinal motility and secretion, it should be used cautiously in patients with a history of peptic ulcer, ulcerative colitis, or gallstones (biliary colic may be precipitated).

Caution should be exercised when treating hypertensive patients with renal insufficiency since they adjust poorly to lowered blood pressure levels.

Use reserpine cautiously with digitalis and quinidine since cardiac arrhythmias have occurred with rauwolfia preparations.

Preoperative withdrawal of reserpine does not assure that circulatory instability will not occur. It is important that the anesthesiologist be aware of the patient's drug intake and consider this in the overall management, since hypotension has occurred in patients receiving rauwolfia preparations. Anticholinergic and/or adrenergic drugs (*eg*, metaraminol, norepinephrine) have been employed to treat adverse vagocirculatory effects.

Hydrochlorothiazide

Periodic determination of serum electrolytes to detect possible electrolyte imbalance should be performed at appropriate intervals. All patients receiving thiazide therapy should be observed for clinical signs of fluid or electrolyte imbalance; namely, hyponatremia, hypochloremic alkalosis, and hypokalemia. Serum and urine electrolyte determinations are particularly important when the patient is vomiting excessively or receiving parenteral fluids. Medication such as digitalis may also influence serum electrolytes. Warning signs are dryness of mouth, thirst, weakness, lethargy, drowsiness, restlessness, muscle pains or cramps, muscular fatigue, hypotension, oliguria, tachycardia, and gastrointestinal disturbance such as nausea or vomiting.

Hypokalemia may develop, especially with brisk diuresis, when severe cirrhosis is present, or during concomitant use of steroids or ACTH. Interference with adequate oral intake of electrolytes will also contribute to hypokalemia. Hypokalemia can sensitize or exaggerate the response of the heart to the toxic effects of digitalis (*eg*, increased ventricular irritability).

Any chloride deficit is generally mild and usually does not require specific treatment except under extraordinary circumstances (as in liver disease or renal disease). Dilutional hyponatremia may occur in edematous patients in hot weather; appropriate therapy is water restriction rather than administration of salt, except in rare instances when the hyponatremia is life-threatening. In actual salt depletion, appropriate replacement is the therapy of choice.

Hyperuricemia may occur or frank gout may be precipitated in certain patients receiving thiazide therapy.

Insulin requirements in diabetic patients may be increased, decreased, or unchanged. Latent diabetes may become manifest during thiazide administration.

Thiazide drugs may increase the responsiveness to tubocurarine.

The antihypertensive effects of the drug may be enhanced in the postsympathectomy patient. Thiazides may decrease arterial responsiveness to norepinephrine. This diminution is not sufficient to preclude effectiveness of the pressor agent for therapeutic use.

If progressive renal impairment becomes evident, withholding or discontinuing diuretic therapy should be considered.

Thiazides may decrease serum PBI levels without signs of thyroid disturbance.

Calcium excretion is decreased by thiazides. Pathological changes in the parathyroid gland with hypercalcemia and hypophosphatemia have been observed in a few patients on prolonged thiazide therapy. The common complications of hyperparathyroidism such as renal lithiasis, bone resorption, and peptic ulceration have not been seen. Thiazides should be discontinued before carrying out tests for parathyroid function.

The Serpasil-Esidrix tablets (#1 and #2) contain FD&C Yellow No. 5 (tartrazine) which may cause allergic-type reactions (including bronchial asthma) in certain susceptible individuals. Although the overall incidence of FD&C Yellow No. 5 (tartrazine) sensitivity in the general population is low, it is frequently seen in patients who also have aspirin hypersensitivity

Adverse Reactions

Reserpine

Rauwolfia preparations have caused gastrointestinal reactions including hypersecretion, nausea, vomiting, anorexia, and diarrhea; cardiovascular reactions including angina-like symptoms, arrhythmias (particularly when used concurrently with digitalis or quinidine), and bradycardia; central nervous system reactions including drowsiness, depression, nervousness, paradoxical anxiety, nightmares, rare parkinsonian syndrome and other extrapyramidal tract symptoms, and CNS sensitization manifested by dull sensorium, deafness, glaucoma, uveitis, and optic atrophy. Nasal

Continued on next page

The full prescribing information for each CIBA drug is contained herein and is that in effect as of October 1, 1982.

CIBA—Cont.

congestion is a frequent occurrence. Pruritus, rash, dryness of mouth, dizziness, headache, dyspnea, syncope, epistaxis, purpura and other hematologic reactions, impotence or decreased libido, dysuria, muscular aches, conjunctival injection, weight gain, breast engorgement, pseudolactation, and gynecomastia have been reported. These reactions are usually reversible and disappear after the drug is discontinued.

Water retention with edema in patients with hypertensive vascular disease may occur rarely, but the condition generally clears with cessation of therapy or with the administration of a diuretic agent.

Hydrochlorothiazide

Gastrointestinal: Anorexia, gastric irritation, nausea, vomiting, cramping, diarrhea, constipation, jaundice (intrahepatic cholestatic), pancreatitis, sialadenitis

Central Nervous System: Dizziness, vertigo, paresthesias, headache, xanthopsia

Hematologic: Leukopenia, thrombocytopenia, agranulocytosis, aplastic anemia

Cardiovascular: Orthostatic hypotension (may be potentiated by alcohol, barbiturates, or narcotics)

Hypersensitivity: Purpura, photosensitivity, rash, urticaria, necrotizing angiitis, Stevens-Johnson syndrome, and other hypersensitivity reactions

Other: Hyperglycemia, glycosuria, hyperuricemia, muscle spasm, weakness, restlessness

Whenever adverse reactions are moderate or severe, thiazide dosage should be reduced or therapy withdrawn.

Dosage and Administration: As determined by individual titration (see box warning).

Usual dosage is 2 Tablets #2 daily in single or divided doses. For patients requiring less hydrochlorothiazide, substitute Tablets #1.

Since antihypertensive effects of reserpine are not immediately apparent, maximal reduction in blood pressure from a given dosage may not occur for 2 weeks. For maintenance, reduce dosage to lowest effective level; as little as 1 tablet daily may suffice.

When necessary, more potent antihypertensive agents may be added gradually in reduced dosages. Watch effects carefully.

Overdosage

Reserpine

Signs and Symptoms

Impairment of consciousness may occur and may range from drowsiness to coma, depending upon the severity of overdosage. Flushing of the skin, conjunctival injection, and pupillary constriction are to be expected. Hypotension, hypothermia, central respiratory depression, and bradycardia may develop in cases of severe overdosage. Diarrhea may also occur.

Treatment

Evacuate stomach contents, taking adequate precautions against aspiration and for the protection of the airway; instill activated charcoal slurry.

Treat the effects of reserpine overdosage symptomatically. If hypotension is severe enough to require treatment with a vasopressor, use one having a direct action upon vascular smooth muscle (*eg,* phenylephrine, levarterenol, metaraminol). Since reserpine is long-acting, observe the patient carefully for at least 72 hours, administering treatment as required.

Hydrochlorothiazide

Signs and Symptoms

Diuresis is to be expected; lethargy of varying degree may appear and may progress to coma within a few hours, with minimal depression of respiration and cardiovascular function and without significant serum electrolyte changes or dehydration. The mechanism of CNS depression with thiazide overdosage is unknown. GI irritation and hypermotility may occur; temporary elevation of BUN has been reported and serum electrolyte changes could occur, especially in patients with impairment of renal function.

Treatment

Evacuate gastric contents but take care to prevent aspiration, especially in the stuporous or comatose patient. GI effects are usually of short duration, but may require symptomatic treatment.

Monitor serum electrolyte levels and renal function; institute supportive measures as required individually to maintain hydration, electrolyte balance, respiration and cardiovascular-renal function.

How Supplied: *Tablets #1* (light orange), each containing 0.1 mg reserpine and 25 mg hydrochlorothiazide; bottles of 100 and 1000.

Tablets #2 (light orange), each containing 0.1 mg reserpine and 50 mg hydrochlorothiazide; bottles of 100 and 1000.

Dispense in tight, light-resistant container (USP).

C80-20 (1/80)

[Shown in Product Identification Section]

SLOW-K® ℞

(potassium chloride)
slow-release tablets

Description: Slow-K is a sugar-coated (not enteric-coated) tablet containing 600 mg potassium chloride (equivalent to 8 mEq) in a wax matrix. This formulation is intended to provide a controlled release of potassium from the matrix to minimize the likelihood of producing high localized concentrations of potassium within the gastrointestinal tract.

Actions: Potassium ion is the principal intracellular cation of most body tissues. Potassium ions participate in a number of essential physiological processes, including the maintenance of intracellular tonicity, the transmission of nerve impulses, the contraction of cardiac, skeletal, and smooth muscle and the maintenance of normal renal function.

Potassium depletion may occur whenever the rate of potassium loss through renal excretion and/or loss from the gastrointestinal tract exceeds the rate of potassium intake. Such depletion usually develops slowly as a consequence of prolonged therapy with oral diuretics, primary or secondary hyperaldosteronism, diabetic ketoacidosis, severe diarrhea, or inadequate replacement of potassium in patients on prolonged parenteral nutrition. Potassium depletion due to these causes is usually accompanied by a concomitant deficiency of chloride and is manifested by hypokalemia and metabolic alkalosis. Potassium depletion may produce weakness, fatigue, disturbances of cardiac rhythm (primarily ectopic beats), prominent U-waves in the electrocardiogram, and in advanced cases flaccid paralysis and/or impaired ability to concentrate urine.

Potassium depletion associated with metabolic alkalosis is managed by correcting the fundamental causes of the deficiency whenever possible and administering supplemental potassium chloride, in the form of high potassium food or potassium chloride solution or tablets. In rare circumstances (*eg,* patients with renal tubular acidosis) potassium depletion may be associated with metabolic acidosis and hyperchloremia. In such patients potassium replacement should be accomplished with potassium salts other than the chloride, such as potassium bicarbonate, potassium citrate, or potassium acetate.

Indications: BECAUSE OF REPORTS OF INTESTINAL AND GASTRIC ULCERATION AND BLEEDING WITH SLOW-RELEASE POTASSIUM CHLORIDE PREPARATIONS, THESE DRUGS SHOULD BE RESERVED FOR THOSE PATIENTS WHO CANNOT TOLERATE OR REFUSE TO TAKE LIQUID OR EFFERVESCENT POTASSIUM PREPARATIONS OR FOR PATIENTS IN WHOM THERE IS A PROBLEM OF COMPLIANCE WITH THESE PREPARATIONS.

1. For therapeutic use in patients with hypokalemia with or without metabolic alkalosis; in digitalis intoxication and in patients with hypokalemic familial periodic paralysis.
2. For prevention of potassium depletion when the dietary intake of potassium is inadequate in the following conditions: Patients receiving digitalis and diuretics for congestive heart failure; hepatic cirrhosis with ascites; states of aldosterone excess with normal renal function; potassium-losing nephropathy, and certain diarrheal states.
3. The use of potassium salts in patients receiving diuretics for uncomplicated essential hypertension is often unnecessary when such patients have a normal dietary pattern. Serum potassium should be checked periodically, however, and, if hypokalemia occurs, dietary supplementation with potassium-containing foods may be adequate to control milder cases. In more severe cases supplementation with potassium salts may be indicated.

Contraindications: Potassium supplements are contraindicated in patients with hyperkalemia since a further increase in serum potassium concentration in such patients can produce cardiac arrest. Hyperkalemia may complicate any of the following conditions: chronic renal failure, systemic acidosis such as diabetic acidosis, acute dehydration, extensive tissue breakdown as in severe burns, adrenal insufficiency, or the administration of a potassium-sparing diuretic (*eg,* spironolactone, triamterene).

Wax-matrix potassium chloride preparations have produced esophageal ulceration in certain cardiac patients with esophageal compression due to an enlarged left atrium.

All solid dosage forms of potassium supplements are contraindicated in any patient in whom there is cause for arrest or delay in tablet passage through the gastrointestinal tract. In these instances, potassium supplementation should be with a liquid preparation.

Warnings:

Hyperkalemia

In patients with impaired mechanisms for excreting potassium, the administration of potassium salts can produce hyperkalemia and cardiac arrest. This occurs most commonly in patients given potassium by the intravenous route but may also occur in patients given potassium orally. Potentially fatal hyperkalemia can develop rapidly and be asymptomatic.

The use of potassium salts in patients with chronic renal disease, or any other condition which impairs potassium excretion, requires particularly careful monitoring of the serum potassium concentration and appropriate dosage adjustment.

Interaction with Potassium-Sparing Diuretics

Hypokalemia should not be treated by the concomitant administration of potassium salts and a potassium-sparing diuretic (*eg,* spironolactone or triamterene), since the simultaneous administration of these agents can produce severe hyperkalemia.

Gastrointestinal lesions

Potassium chloride tablets have produced stenotic and/or ulcerative lesions of the small bowel and deaths. These lesions are caused by a high localized concentration of potassium ion in the region of a rapidly dissolving tablet, which injures the bowel wall and thereby produces obstruction, hemorrhage, or perforation. Slow-K is a wax-matrix tablet formulated to provide a controlled rate of release of potassium chloride and thus to minimize the possibility of a high local concentration of potassium ion near the bowel wall. While the reported frequency of small-bowel lesions is much less with wax-matrix tablets (less than one per 100,000 patient-years) than with enteric-coated potassium chloride tablets (40–50 per

100,000 patient-years) cases associated with wax-matrix tablets have been reported both in foreign countries and in the United States. In addition, perhaps because the wax-matrix preparations are not enteric-coated and release potassium in the stomach, there have been reports of upper gastrointestinal bleeding associated with these products. The total number of gastrointestinal lesions remains approximately one per 100,000 patient-years. Slow-K should be discontinued immediately and the possibility of bowel obstruction or perforation considered if severe vomiting, abdominal pain, distention, or gastrointestinal bleeding occurs.

Metabolic acidosis

Hypokalemia in patients with metabolic *acidosis* should be treated with an alkalinizing potassium salt such as potassium bicarbonate, potassium citrate, or potassium acetate.

Precautions: The diagnosis of potassium depletion is ordinarily made by demonstrating hypokalemia in a patient with a clinical history suggesting some cause for potassium depletion. In interpreting the serum potassium level, the physician should bear in mind that acute alkalosis *per se* can produce hypokalemia in the absence of a deficit in total body potassium, while acute acidosis *per se* can increase the serum potassium concentration into the normal range even in the presence of a reduced total body potassium. The treatment of potassium depletion, particularly in the presence of cardiac disease, renal disease, or acidosis, requires careful attention to acid-base balance and appropriate monitoring of serum electrolytes, the electrocardiogram, and the clinical status of the patient.

Adverse Reactions: The most common adverse reactions to oral potassium salts are nausea, vomiting, abdominal discomfort, and diarrhea. These symptoms are due to irritation of the gastrointestinal tract and are best managed by diluting the preparation further, taking the dose with meals, or reducing the dose. One of the most severe adverse effects is hyperkalemia (see Contraindications, Warnings and Overdosage). There also have been reports of upper and lower gastrointestinal conditions including obstruction, bleeding, ulceration and perforation (see Contraindications and Warnings); other factors known to be associated with such conditions were present in many of these patients.

Skin rash has been reported rarely.

Overdosage: The administration of oral potassium salts to persons with normal excretory mechanisms for potassium rarely causes serious hyperkalemia. However, if excretory mechanisms are impaired or if potassium is administered too rapidly intravenously, potentially fatal hyperkalemia can result (see Contraindications and Warnings). It is important to recognize that hyperkalemia is usually asymptomatic and may be manifested only by an increased serum potassium concentration and characteristic electrocardiographic changes (peaking of T-waves, loss of P-wave, depression of S-T segment, and prolongation of the QT interval). Late manifestations include muscle paralysis and cardiovascular collapse from cardiac arrest.

Treatment measures for hyperkalemia include the following: (1) elimination of foods and medications containing potassium and of potassium-sparing diuretics; (2) intravenous administration of 300 to 500 ml/hr of 10% dextrose solution containing 10–20 units of insulin per 1,000 ml; (3) correction of acidosis, if present, with intravenous sodium bicarbonate; (4) use of exchange resins, hemodialysis, or peritoneal dialysis.

In treating hyperkalemia, it should be recalled that in patients who have been stabilized on digitalis, too rapid a lowering of the serum potassium concentration can produce digitalis toxicity.

Dosage and Administration: The usual dietary intake of potassium by the average adult is 40 to 80 mEq per day. Potassium depletion sufficient to cause hypokalemia usually requires the loss of 200 or more mEq of potassium from the total body store. Dosage must be adjusted to the individual needs of each patient but is typically in the range of 20 mEq per day for the prevention of hypokalemia to 40–100 mEq per day or more for the treatment of potassium depletion.

Note: Slow-K slow-release tablets must be swallowed whole and never crushed or chewed.

How Supplied:

Tablets 600 mg potassium chloride (equiv. to 8 mEq) —round, buff colored, sugar-coated (imprinted CIBA 165)

Bottles of 100 ....NDC 0083-0165-30
Bottles of 1000 ....NDC 0083-0165-40
Consumer Pack—One Unit
(12 Bottles—100 tablets each) ....NDC 0083-0165-65
Accu-Pak® Unit Dose (Blister pack)
Box of 100 (strips of 10) ..NDC 0083-0165-32

Protect from moisture. Protect from light. Do not store above 86°F (30°C).

Dispense in tight, light-resistant container (USP).

C82-58 (Rev. 1/83)

[*Shown in Product Identification Section*]

TRANSDERM®-NITRO ℞

(nitroglycerin)

Transdermal Therapeutic System

Description: Transderm-Nitro (nitroglycerin) transdermal therapeutic system is a flat unit designed to provide controlled release of nitroglycerin through a semipermeable membrane continuously for 24 hours following application to intact skin. Nitroglycerin (glyceryl trinitrate) is a prompt-acting vasodilator for the relief and prevention of anginal attacks. Systems are rated to release *in vivo* 5 and 10 mg nitroglycerin over 24 hours and are in sizes of 10 and 20 cm^2 respectively.

One-fifth of the total nitroglycerin in the system is delivered transdermally to the patient over 24 hours; the remainder serves as the thermodynamic energy source to release the drug and remains in the system. The rated release of drug is dependent upon the area of the system; 0.5 mg nitroglycerin is delivered *in vivo* for every cm^2 of system size.

The Transderm-Nitro system comprises four layers as shown below. Proceeding from the visible surface towards the surface attached to the skin, these layers are: 1) a tan-colored backing layer (aluminized plastic) that is impermeable to nitroglycerin; 2) a drug reservoir containing nitroglycerin adsorbed on lactose, colloidal silicon dioxide, and silicone medical fluid; 3) an ethylene/vinyl acetate copolymer membrane that is permeable to nitroglycerin; and 4) a layer of hypoallergenic silicone adhesive. Prior to use, a protective peel strip is removed from the adhesive surface.

Cross section of the system:

Backing
Drug Reservoir
Semipermeable Membrane
Adhesive
Protective Peel Strip

Actions: When the Transderm-Nitro system is applied to the skin, nitroglycerin is absorbed continuously through the skin into the systemic circulation. This results in active drug reaching the target organs (heart, extremities) before being inactivated by the liver. Nitroglycerin is a smooth muscle relaxant with vascular effects manifested predominantly by venous dilatation and pooling. The major beneficial effect of nitroglycerin in angina pectoris is a reduction in myocardial oxygen consumption secondary to vascular smooth muscle relaxation and consequent reduced cardiac preload and afterload. In recent years there has been an increasing recognition of a direct vasodilator effect of nitroglycerin on the coronary vessels.

In clinical studies transdermal absorption of nitroglycerin from a nitroglycerin system occurred in a continuous and well-controlled manner, for a minimum of 24 hours. Therapeutic effect can be anticipated 30 minutes after application steps 1 the system and to be maintained for 30 minutes after its removal.

Indications and Usage: Transderm-Nitro system is indicated for the prevention and treatment of angina pectoris due to coronary artery disease.

Contraindications: Intolerance of organic nitrate drugs, marked anemia, increased intraocular pressure or increased intracranial pressure.

Warnings: In patients with acute myocardial infarction or congestive heart failure, Transderm-Nitro system should be used under careful clinical and/or hemodynamic monitoring.

In terminating treatment of anginal patients, both the dosage and frequency of application must be gradually reduced over a period of 4 to 6 weeks to prevent sudden withdrawal reactions, which are characteristic of all vasodilators in the nitroglycerin class.

Precautions: Symptoms of hypotension, such as faintness, weakness or dizziness, particularly orthostatic hypotension may be due to overdosage. When these symptoms occur, the dosage should be reduced or use of the product discontinued.

Transderm-Nitro system is not intended for immediate relief of anginal attacks. For this purpose occasional use of the sublingual preparations may be necessary.

Adverse Reactions: Transient headaches are the most common side effect, especially when higher doses of the drug are used. These headaches should be treated with mild analgesics while Transderm-Nitro therapy is continued. When such headaches are unresponsive to treatment, the nitroglycerin dosage should be reduced or use of the product discontinued.

Adverse reactions reported less frequently include hypotension, increased heart rate, faintness, flushing, dizziness, nausea, vomiting, and dermatitis. These symptoms are attributable to the known pharmacologic effects of nitroglycerin, but may be symptoms of overdosage. When they persist the dose should be reduced or use of the product discontinued.

Dosage and Administration: Therapy should be initiated with application of one Transderm-Nitro 5 system to the desired area of skin. Many patients prefer the chest; if hair is likely to interfere with system adhesion or removal, it can be clipped prior to placement of the system. Each system is designed to remain in place for 24 hours, and each successive application should be to a different skin area. Transderm-Nitro system should not be applied to the distal parts of the extremities.

The usual dosage is one Transderm-Nitro 5 system every 24 hours. Some patients, however, may require the Transderm-Nitro 10 system. If a single Transderm-Nitro 5 system fails to provide adequate clinical response, the patient should be instructed to remove it and apply either two Transderm-Nitro 5 systems or one Transderm-Nitro 10 system. More systems may be added as indicated by continued careful monitoring of clinical response.

The optimal dosage should be selected based upon the clinical response, side effects, and the effects of therapy upon blood pressure. The greatest attainable decrease in resting blood

Continued on next page

The full prescribing information for each CIBA drug is contained herein and is that in effect as of October 1, 1982.

CIBA—Cont.

pressure that is not associated with clinical symptoms of hypotension especially during orthostasis indicates the optimal dosage. To decrease adverse reactions, the size and/or number of systems should be tailored to the individual patient's needs.
Do not store above 86°F (30°C).

Patient Instructions For Applications: A patient leaflet is supplied with the systems.

How Supplied:
[See Table 1 below].

Dist. by **CIBA Pharmaceutical Company**
Division of CIBA-GEIGY Corporation
Summit, New Jersey 07901
C82-16 (3/82)

PATIENT INSTRUCTION SHEET
How to use

Transderm®-Nitro
nitroglycerin
Transdermal Therapeutic System

The usual starting dose is one Transderm-Nitro 5 system. The dose may vary, however, depending on your individual response to the system. For instance, your doctor may decide to increase or decrease the size of the system, or prescribe a combination of systems, to suit your particular needs.

Where to place Transderm-Nitro
Select any area of skin on the body, **EXCEPT** the extremities below the knee or elbow. The chest is the preferred site, but the back is an excellent alternative because it is usually free of hair, skin folds, and excessive muscular movement. The area should be clean, dry, and hairless. If hair is likely to interfere with system adhesion or removal, clip the hair prior to applying the system. Do not shave. Take care to avoid areas with cuts or irritations. Do **NOT** apply the system immediately after showering or bathing. It is best to wait until you are certain the skin is completely dry.

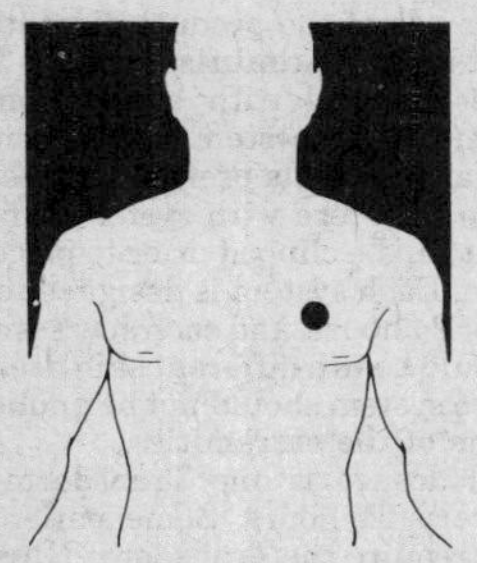

How to apply Transderm-Nitro

1. Open the package containing the system by tearing at the indicated indentations: then remove the system from the package *(Figure A)*.

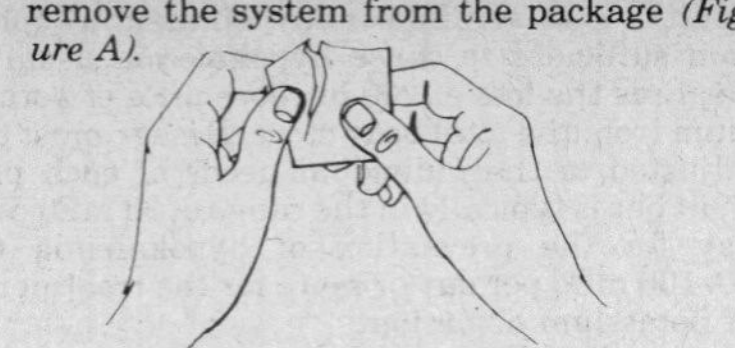

Figure A

2. Carefully pick up the system lengthwise with the tab up *(Figure B)*.

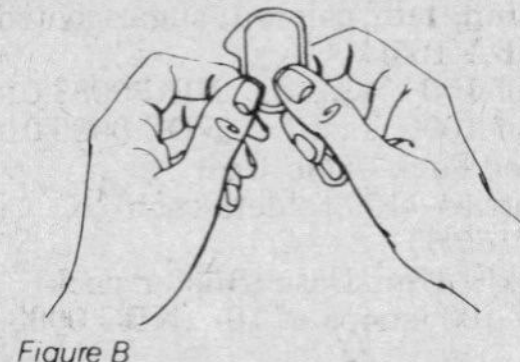

Figure B

3. With your thumbs, begin to remove the protective backing from the system at the tab *(Figure C)*. Do not touch the inside of the exposed system, because the adhesive covers the entire surface.

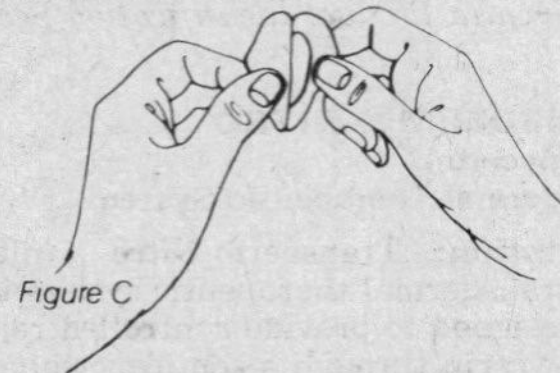

Figure C

4. Continue to remove the backing *slowly* along the length of the system, allowing the system to rest on the outside of your fingers *(Figure D)*.

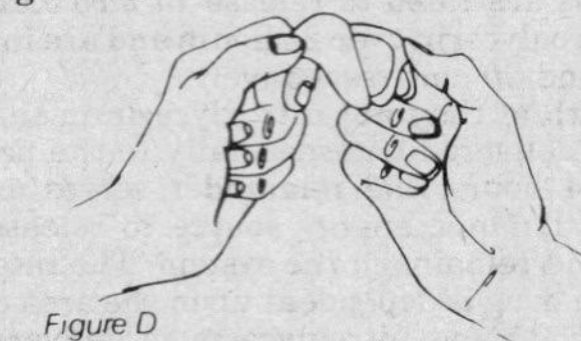

Figure D

5. Place the exposed, adhesive side of the system on the chosen skin site. It is extremely important to *press firmly* in place with the palm of your hand, and maintain the pressure for *10–15 seconds (Figure E)*.

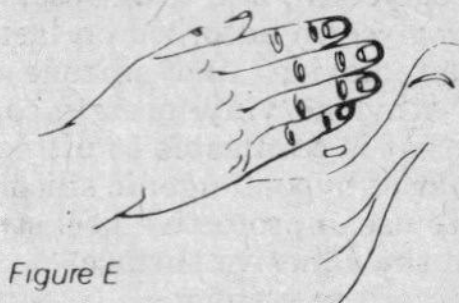

Figure E

6. Circle the outside edge of the system with one or two fingers *(Figure F)*. This, along with step 5, will insure optimum adhesion. Once the system is in place, *do not* test the adhesion by pulling on it. For your information, the adhesive in the Transderm-Nitro system will not feel as sticky as that on an adhesive bandage.

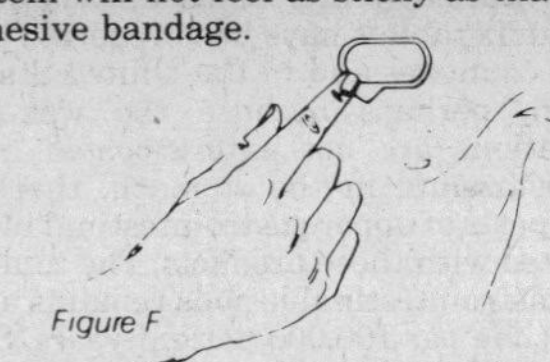

Figure F

7. Remove and discard the system after 24 hours. Dispose of the system by conventional means, such as in a trash container. Place a new system on a different skin site, following steps 1–6.

Please note:
Contact with water, as in bathing, swimming, or showering will not affect the system. In the unlikely event that a system falls off, discard it and put a new one on a different skin site.

Precautions: The most common side effect that is encountered is transient headaches. These often decrease as therapy is continued, but may require treatment with a mild analgesic. Although uncommon, faintness, flushing, and dizziness may occur, especially when suddenly rising from the recumbent (lying horizontal) position. If these latter symptoms do occur, the system should be removed from the skin and your physician should be notified. For changes in dosage and frequency of application, consult your physician.
Keep these systems and all drugs out of the reach of children.

DO NOT STORE ABOVE 86°F (30°C).

Dist. by:
CIBA Pharmaceutical Company
Division of CIBA-GEIGY Corporation
Summit, New Jersey 07901
C82-55 (9/82)

[*Shown in Product Identification Section*]

Table 1

Transderm-Nitro System Rated Release *in vivo*	Total Nitroglycerin in System	System Size	Carton Size
5 mg/24 hr	25 mg	10 cm^2	30 Systems (NDC 0083-2105-26)
5 mg/24 hr	25 mg	10 cm^2	7 Systems (NDC 0083-2105-07)
10 mg/24 hr	50 mg	20 cm^2	30 Systems (NDC 0083-2110-26)

TRANSDERM®-SCŌP ℞
scopolamine
(formerly Transderm -V)

Transdermal Therapeutic System

Programmed delivery *in vivo* of 0.5 mg scopolamine over 3 days

Description: The Transderm-Scōp scopolamine system is a circular flat unit designed for continuous release of scopolamine following application to an area of intact skin on the head, behind the ear. Clinical evaluation has demonstrated that the system provides effective antiemetic and antinauseant actions when tested against motion-sickness stimuli in adults.
The Transderm-Scōp system is a 0.2-mm thick film with four layers. Proceeding from the visible surface towards the surface attached to the skin, these layers are: 1) a backing layer of tan-colored, aluminized polyester film; 2) a drug reservoir of scopolamine, mineral oil, and polyisobutylene; 3) a microporous polypropylene membrane that controls the rate of delivery of scopolamine from the system to the skin surface; and 4) an adhesive formulation of mineral oil, polyisobutylene, and scopolamine. Prior to use, a protective peel strip of siliconized polyester which covers layer 4 is removed.
The mineral oil (12.4 mg) and polyisobutylene (11.4 mg) inactive components are not released from the system.
Release-Rate Concept: The Transderm-Scōp system, 2.5 cm^2 in area, contains 1.5 mg scopolamine. The system is programmed to deliver 0.5 mg scopolamine, at an approximately constant rate to the systemic circulation, over the 3-day lifetime of the system. An initial priming dose of scopolamine, released from the adhesive layer of the system, saturates the skin binding sites for scopolamine and rapidly brings the plasma concentration to the required steady-state level. The continuous con-

trolled release of scopolamine that flows from the drug reservoir through the rate-controlling membrane then maintains the plasma level constant.

Clinical Pharmacology: The formulation of the Transderm-Scōp system contains as its sole active agent the drug scopolamine, a belladonna alkaloid with well-known pharmacological properties. The drug has a long history of oral and parenteral use for central anticholinergic activity, including prophylaxis of motion sickness. This formulation provides for a gradual release of scopolamine from an adhesive matrix of mineral oil and polyisobutylene applied to the postauricular skin.

Clinical Results: The Transderm-Scōp system provides antiemetic protection within several hours following application of the system behind the ear. In 195 adult subjects of different racial origins who participated in clinical efficacy studies at sea or in a controlled motion environment, there was a 75% reduction in the incidence of motion-induced nausea and vomiting. The Transderm-Scōp system provided significantly greater protection than that obtained with oral dimenhydrinate.

Indications and Usage: The Transderm-Scōp system is indicated for prevention of nausea and vomiting associated with motion sickness in adults. The system should be applied only to skin in the postauricular area.

Contraindications: The Transderm-Scōp system should not be used in patients with known hypersensitivity to scopolamine or any of the components of the adhesive matrix making up the therapeutic system.

Warnings: The Transderm-Scōp system should not be used in children and should be used with special caution in the elderly.

Since drowsiness, disorientation, and confusion may occur with the use of scopolamine, patients should be warned of the possibility and cautioned against engaging in activities that require mental alertness, such as driving a motor vehicle or operating dangerous machinery.

Potentially alarming idiosyncratic reactions may occur with ordinary therapeutic doses of scopolamine.

Precautions: Scopolamine should be used with caution in patients with glaucoma, pyloric obstruction, or urinary bladder neck obstruction. Caution should be exercised when administering an antiemetic or antimuscarinic drug to patients suspected of having intestinal obstruction.

The Transderm-Scōp system should be used with special caution in the elderly or in individuals with impaired metabolic, liver, or kidney functions, because of the increased likelihood of central nervous system effects.

Information for Patients: Since scopolamine can cause temporary dilation of the pupils and blurred vision if it comes in contact with the eyes, the patient should be strongly advised to wash the hands thoroughly with soap and water immediately after handling the unit.

Patients should be warned against driving a motor vehicle or operating dangerous machinery.

Pregnancy: Fertility studies were performed in female rats and revealed no evidence of impaired fertility or harm to the fetus due to scopolamine hydrobromide administered by daily subcutaneous injection. In the highest-dose group (plasma level approximately 500 times the level achieved in humans using a transdermal system), reduced maternal body weights were observed. Teratogenic studies were performed in pregnant rats and rabbits with scopolamine hydrobromide by daily intravenous injection. No adverse effects were recorded in rats. In rabbits, the highest dose (plasma level approximately 100 times the level achieved in humans using a transdermal system) of drug administered had a marginal embryotoxic effect. Transderm-Scōp should be used during pregnancy only if the anticipated benefit justifies the potential risk to the fetus.

Nursing Mothers: It is not known whether scopolamine is excreted in human milk. As a general rule, nursing should not be undertaken while a patient is on a drug, since many drugs are excreted in human milk.

Usage in Children: Children are particularly susceptible to the side effects of belladonna alkaloids. The Transderm-Scōp system should not be used in children because it is not known whether this system will release an amount of scopolamine that could produce serious adverse effects in children.

Adverse Reactions: The most frequent adverse reaction to the Transderm-Scōp system is dryness of the mouth. This occurs in about two thirds of the people. A less frequent adverse reaction is drowsiness, which occurs in less than one sixth of the people. Transient impairment of eye accommodation, including blurred vision and dilation of the pupils, is also observed. The following adverse reactions have also been reported on infrequent occasions during use of the Transderm-Scōp system: disorientation; memory disturbances; dizziness; restlessness; giddiness; hallucinations; confusion; difficulty urinating; rashes and erythema; and dry, itchy, or red eyes.

Overdosage: Overdosage with scopolamine may cause disorientation, memory disturbances, restlessness, giddiness, hallucinations or confusion. Should these symptoms occur, the Transderm-Scōp system should be immediately removed. Appropriate parasympathomimetic therapy should be initiated if these symptoms are severe.

Dosage and Administration: *Adults: Initiation of Therapy:* One Transderm-Scōp system (unit), programmed to deliver 0.5 mg scopolamine over three days, should be applied to the hairless area behind one ear at least 4 hours before the antiemetic effect is required.

Handling: After applying the system on dry skin behind the ear, the hands should be washed thoroughly with soap and water and dried. Upon removal of the system, it should be discarded, and the hands and application site washed thoroughly with soap and water and dried, to prevent any traces of scopolamine from coming into direct contact with the eyes. A patient brochure is available.

Continuation of Therapy: Should a system become displaced, it should be discarded, and a fresh system placed on the hairless area behind the other ear. If therapy is required for longer than 72 hours, the first system should be discarded, and a fresh system placed on the hairless area behind the other ear.

Children: Children are particularly susceptible to the side effects of belladonna alkaloids. The Transderm-Scōp system should not be used in children because it is not known whether this system will release an amount of scopolamine that could produce serious adverse effects in children.

How Supplied: Transderm-Scōp systems are available in 2-unit blister packs—NDC **17314-4345-1.**

Storage and Handling: The system should be stored at room temperature.

71 4342-0-2 665941 (5/82)

Mfd. by:
ALZA Corporation
Palo Alto, CA 94304
Dist. by:
CIBA Pharmaceutical Co.
Div. of CIBA-GEIGY Corp.
Summit, NJ 07901

Information for the Patient About—

TRANSDERM®-SCŌP
Generic Name—scopolamine, pronounced skoe-POL-a-meen
(formerly Transderm -V)
Transdermal Therapeutic System

The Transderm-Scōp system helps to prevent the nausea and vomiting of motion sickness up to 72 hours. It is an adhesive unit that you place behind your ear several hours before you travel.

Be sure to wash your hands thoroughly with soap and water immediately after handling the system (unit), so that any drug that might get on your hands will not come into contact with your eyes.

Also, be careful about driving or operating any machinery while using the system because the drug may make you drowsy.

THE TRANSDERM-SCŌP SYSTEM SHOULD NOT BE USED IN CHILDREN AND SHOULD BE USED WITH SPECIAL CAUTION IN THE ELDERLY.

How the Transderm-Scōp System Works

A group of nerve fibers deep inside the ear helps people keep their balance. For some people, the motion of ships, airplanes, trains, automobiles, and buses increases the activity of these nerve fibers. This increased activity causes the *dizziness, nausea, and vomiting* of motion sickness. People may have one, some, or all of these symptoms.

Transderm-Scōp contains the drug scopolamine, which helps reduce the activity of the nerve fibers in the inner ear. When the Transderm-Scōp system is placed on the skin behind one of the ears, scopolamine passes through the skin and into the bloodstream. One system may be kept in place for 72 hours if needed.

Precautions: Before using Transderm-Scōp be sure to tell your doctor if you—

- Are pregnant or nursing (or planning to become pregnant)
- Have glaucoma (increased pressure in the eyeball)
- Have (or have had) any metabolic, liver, or kidney disease
- Have any obstructions of the stomach or intestine
- Have trouble urinating or any bladder obstruction
- Have any skin allergy or have had a skin reaction such as a rash or redness to any drug, especially scopolamine, or chemical or food substance.

Any of these conditions could make the Transderm-Scōp system unsuitable for you. Also tell your doctor if you are taking any other medicines.

The Transderm-Scōp system should not be used in children. The safety of its use in children has not been determined. Children and the elderly may be particularly sensitive to the effects of scopolamine.

Side Effects: The most common side effect experienced by people using the Transderm-Scōp system is dryness of the mouth. This occurs in about two thirds of the people. A less frequent side effect is drowsiness, which occurs in less than one sixth of the people. Temporary blurring of vision and dilation (widening) of the pupils may occur, especially if the drug is on your hands and comes in contact with the eyes. On infrequent occasions, disorientation; memory disturbances; dizziness; restlessness; giddiness; hallucinations; confusion; difficulty urinating; skin rashes or redness; and dry, itchy, or red eyes have been reported. If these effects do occur, remove the system and call your doctor. Since drowsiness, disorientation, and confusion may occur with use of scopolamine, be careful driving or operating any dangerous machinery, especially when you first start using the drug system.

How to Use the Transderm-Scōp System

Transderm-Scōp may be kept at room temperature until use.

Continued on next page

The full prescribing information for each CIBA drug is contained herein and is that in effect as of October 1, 1982.

CIBA—Cont.

1. Plan to apply one Transderm-Scōp system (unit) at least 4 hours before you need it.
2. Select a hairless area of skin behind one ear, taking care to avoid any cuts or irritations. Wipe the area with a clean, dry tissue.
3. Peel the package open and remove the system (Figure 1).

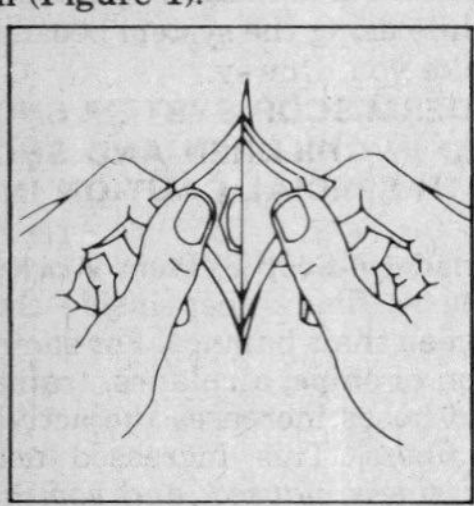

(Figure 1)

4. Remove the clear plastic six-sided backing from the round system. Try not to touch the adhesive surface on the drug system with your hands (Figure 2).

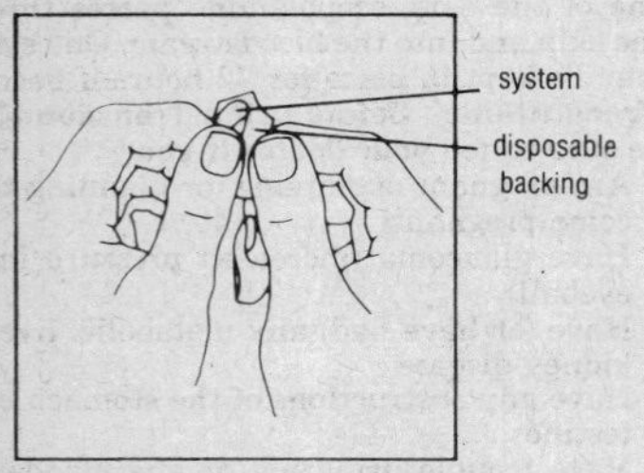

(Figure 2)

5. Firmly apply the adhesive surface (metallic side) to the dry area of skin behind the ear so that the tan-colored side is showing (Figure 3). Make good contact, especially around the edge. Once you have placed the system behind your ear, do not move it for as long as you want to use it (up to 3 days).

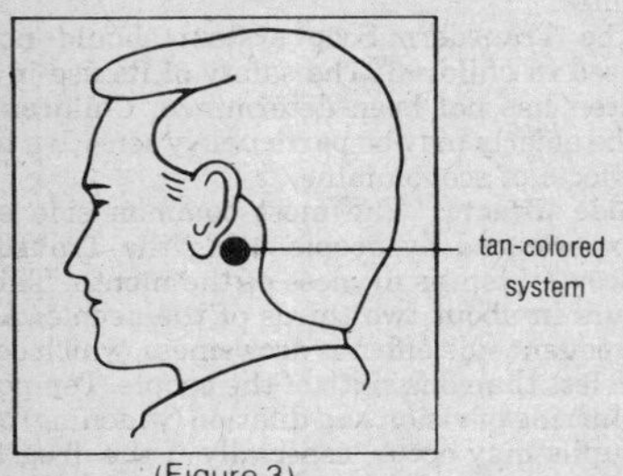

(Figure 3)

6. ***Important:*** **After the system is in place, be sure to wash your hands thoroughly with soap and water to remove any scopolamine. If this drug were to contact your eyes, it could cause temporary blurring of vision and dilation (widening) of the pupils (the dark circles in the center of your eyes). This is not serious, and your pupils should return to normal.**
7. Remove the system after 3 days and throw it away. (You may remove it sooner if you are no longer concerned about motion sickness.) After removing the system, be sure to wash your hands and the area behind your ear thoroughly with soap and water.
8. If you wish to control nausea for longer than 3 days, remove the first system after 3 days and place a new one behind the other ear, repeating instructions 2 to 7.
9. Keep the system dry, if possible, to prevent it from falling off. Limited contact with water, however, as in bathing or swimming, will not affect the system. In the unlikely event that the system falls off, throw it away and put a new one behind the other ear.

This leaflet presents a summary of information about Transderm-Scōp. If you would like more information, or if you have any questions, ask your doctor or pharmacist. There is also a more technical leaflet available, written for your doctor. If you would like to read the leaflet, ask your pharmacist to let you see a copy. You may need the help of your doctor or pharmacist to understand some of the information.

Mfd. by:
ALZA Corporation
Palo Alto, CA 94304
Dist. by:
CIBA Pharmaceutical Co.
Division of CIBA-GEIGY Corp.
Summit, NJ 07901
72-4342-0-2 665951 (5/82)

VIOFORM®
(iodochlorhydroxyquin USP)

Listed in USP, a Medicare designated compendium.

Indications and Directions For Use:
A soothing antifungal and antibacterial preparation for the treatment of inflamed conditions of the skin, such as eczema, athlete's foot and other fungal infections.
Apply to the affected area 2 or 3 times a day or use as directed by physician.
Caution: May prove irritating to sensitized skin in rare cases. If this should occur, discontinue treatment and consult physician. May stain.
KEEP OUT OF REACH OF CHILDREN.
How Supplied:
Ointment, 3% iodochlorhydroxyquin in a petrolatum base; tubes of 1 ounce.
Cream, 3% iodochlorhydroxyquin in a water-washable base; tubes of 1 ounce.
(7/80)

VIOFORM®-HYDROCORTISONE ℞
(iodochlorhydroxyquin and hydrocortisone)

Indications
Based on a review of this drug by the National Academy of Sciences-National Research Council and/or other information, FDA has classified the indications as follows:
"Possibly" effective: Contact or atopic dermatitis; impetiginized eczema; nummular eczema; infantile eczema; endogenous chronic infectious dermatitis; stasis dermatitis; pyoderma; nuchal eczema and chronic eczematoid otitis externa; acne urticata; localized or disseminated neurodermatitis; lichen simplex chronicus; anogenital pruritus (vulvae, scroti, ani); folliculitis; bacterial dermatoses; mycotic dermatoses such as tinea (capitis, cruris, corporis, pedis); moniliasis; intertrigo.
Final classification of the less-than-effective indications requires further investigation.

Contraindications: Hypersensitivity to Vioform-Hydrocortisone, or any of its ingredients or related compounds; lesions of the eye; tuberculosis of the skin; most viral skin lesions (including herpes simplex, vaccinia, and varicella).
Warnings: *This product is not for ophthalmic use.*
In the presence of systemic infections, appropriate systemic antibiotics should be used.
Usage in Pregnancy: Although topical steroids have not been reported to have an adverse effect on pregnancy, the safety of their use in pregnant women has not been absolutely established. In laboratory animals, increases in incidence of fetal abnormalities have been associated with exposure of gestating females to topical corticosteroids, in some cases at rather low dosage levels. Therefore, drugs of this class should not be used extensively on pregnant patients in large amounts or for prolonged periods of time.
Precautions: May prove irritating to sensitized skin in rare cases. If irritation occurs, discontinue therapy. Staining of skin and fabrics may occur. Additionally, there are rare reports of discoloration of hair and nails.
Signs and symptoms of systemic toxicity, electrolyte imbalance, or adrenal suppression have not been reported with Vioform-Hydrocortisone. Nevertheless, the possibility of suppression of the pituitary-adrenal axis during therapy should be kept in mind, especially when the drug is used under occlusive dressings, for a prolonged period, or for treating extensive cutaneous areas since significant absorption of corticosteroid may occur under these conditions, particularly in children and infants.
Vioform may be absorbed through the skin and interfere with thyroid function tests. If such tests are contemplated, wait at least one month between discontinuation of therapy and performance of these tests. The ferric chloride test for phenylketonuria (PKU) can yield a false-positive result if Vioform is present in the diaper or urine.
Prolonged use may result in overgrowth of nonsusceptible organisms requiring appropriate therapy.
Adverse Reactions: There have been a few reports of rash and hypersensitivity.
The following local adverse reactions have been reported with topical corticosteroids, especially under occlusive dressings: burning; itching; irritation; dryness; folliculitis; hypertrichosis; acneiform eruptions; hypopigmentation; perioral dermatitis; allergic contact dermatitis; maceration of the skin; secondary infection; skin atrophy; striae; miliaria. Discontinue therapy if any untoward reaction occurs.
Dosage and Administration: Apply a thin layer to the affected parts 3 or 4 times daily. The *Cream,* because of its slight drying effect, is primarily useful for moist, weeping lesions; the *Lotion* is particularly suitable for application behind the ears and in intertriginous areas of the body; the *Ointment* is best used for dry lesions accompanied by thickening and scaling of the skin.
The *Mild Cream* and *Mild Ointment* should be used when treating lesions involving extensive body areas or less severe dermatoses.
How Supplied: *Cream,* 3% iodochlorhydroxyquin and 1% hydrocortisone in a water-washable base containing stearyl alcohol, cetyl alcohol, stearic acid, petrolatum, sodium lauryl sulfate, and glycerin in water; tubes of 5 and 20 Gm.
Ointment, 3% iodochlorhydroxyquin and 1% hydrocortisone in a petrolatum base; tubes of 20 Gm.
Lotion, 3% iodochlorhydroxyquin and 1% hydrocortisone in a water-washable base containing stearic acid, cetyl alcohol, lanolin, propylene glycol, sorbitan trioleate, polysorbate 60, triethanolamine, methylparaben, propylparaben, and perfume Flora in water; plastic squeeze bottles of 15 ml.
Mild Cream, 3% iodochlorhydroxyquin and 0.5% hydrocortisone in a water-washable base containing stearyl alcohol, cetyl alcohol, stearic acid, petrolatum, sodium lauryl sulfate, and glycerin in water; tubes of ½ and 1 ounce.
Mild Ointment, 3% iodochlorohydroxyquin and 0.5% hydrocortisone in a petrolatum base; tubes of 1 ounce. C79-1 (5/79)

Circle Pharmaceuticals, Inc.

10377 HAGUE ROAD
INDIANAPOLIS, IN 46256

TUSQUELIN ℞

Composition: Each teaspoonful (5 ml.) contains: Dextromethorphan HBr, 15 mg.; Chlorpheniramine Maleate, 2 mg.; Phenylpropanolamine HCl, 5 mg.; Phenylephrine HCl, 5 mg.; Alcohol, 5%.
Action and Uses: Tusquelin is a very palatable antitussive with antihistamine, bronchodilating, and nasal decongestant action, suitable for all ages.
Administration and Dosage: *Adults*—One or two teaspoonfuls four times a day, or more, as indicated. *Children*—½ to 1 teaspoonful three or four times a day, as indicated.
Side Effects: If side effects are encountered, dosage should be reduced or medication withdrawn. Professional care in supervising dosage for the very young is essential.
Precautions: This preparation may cause drowsiness. Do not drive or operate machinery while taking this medication. Do not give to children under six years of age or exceed the recommended dosage unless directed by physician. Individuals with high blood pressure, heart disease, diabetes or thyroid disease should use only as directed by physician.
Contraindications: Sensitivity to any of the components.
How Supplied: Syrup, pints. (In a pleasant vanilla-citrus syrup base.)

Connaught Laboratories, Inc.

SWIFTWATER, PA 18370

Distributed in the Continental U.S.A. by:
Elkins-Sinn, Inc.,
A subsidiary of A.H. Robins Co.
2 Esterbrook Lane
Cherry Hill, NJ 08034

The following is a product listing only. Full product and prescribing information is contained in the package insert.

DIPHTHERIA ANTITOXIN, USP ℞
(Purified, Concentrated Globulin—EQUINE)

Expiration Dating—60 Months
How Supplied: 20,000 unit vial.

DIPHTHERIA AND TETANUS TOXOIDS AND PERTUSSIS VACCINE ADSORBED USP ℞
(For Pediatric Use)

Expiration Dating—18 Months
How Supplied: 7.5 ml vial.

FLUZONE® ℞
(Influenza Virus Vaccine USP)
(Zonal Purified, Whole Virion)
and
(Zonal Purified, Subvirion)
(Formula consistent with current USPHS requirements)

Expiration Dating—June 30 of following year.
How Supplied: 5 ml vial (10 doses, 0.5 ml each).

MENOMUNE®-A/C/Y/W-135 ℞
(Meningococcal Polysaccharide Vaccine, Groups A,C,Y and W-135 Combined)
(Freeze-Dried)

Expiration Dating—24 Months
How Supplied: 10 dose vial with 6 ml diluent (needle and syringe administration); 50 dose vial with 27.5 ml diluent (jet injector administration only).

MENOMUNE®- A/C ℞
(Meningococcal Polysaccharide Vaccine, Groups A and C Combined)
(Freeze-Dried)

Expiration Dating—24 Months
How Supplied: 10 dose vial with 6 ml diluent (needle and syringe administration); 50 dose vial with 27.5 ml diluent (jet injector administration only).
Also available as single entity vaccines, Group A or Group C. Contact Elkins-Sinn/A.H. Robins for information.

TETANUS AND DIPHTHERIA TOXOIDS ADSORBED USP ℞
(For Adult Use)

Expiration Dating—24 Months
How Supplied: 5 ml vial.

TETANUS TOXOID ADSORBED USP ℞

Expiration Dating—24 Months
How Supplied: 5 ml vial.

TETANUS TOXOID USP ℞
("Fluid" or "Plain")

Expiration Dating—24 Months
How Supplied: 7.5 ml vial

YF-VAX™ (Yellow Fever Vaccine) ℞
(Live, 17D Virus, Avian Leukosis-Free, Stabilized)
(Freeze-Dried)

Expiration Dating—12 Months
How Supplied: 1 dose vial with 0.6 ml diluent; 5 dose vial with 3 ml diluent; 20 dose vial with 12 ml diluent.

Connaught Laboratories, Ltd.

1755 STEELES AVENUE WEST
WILLOWDALE, ONTARIO M2R3T4, CANADA

Distributed in the Continental U.S.A. by:
Elkins-Sinn, Inc.,
A subsidiary of A.H. Robins Co.
2 Esterbrook Lane
Cherry Hill, NJ 08034

POLIOMYELITIS VACCINE (PURIFIED) ℞
(For the Prevention of Poliomyelitis [Inactivated, Salk Type])

Expiration Dating—12 Months
How Supplied: 1 ml ampul, package of 5; 10 ml vial.

TUBERCULIN PURIFIED PROTEIN DERIVATIVE ℞
(Concentrated Solution in 50% Glycerine for Multiple Puncture Test [Heaf])

Expiration Dating—24 Months
How Supplied: 1 ml vial.

TUBERSOL® ℞
Tuberculin Purified Protein Derivative (Mantoux)

Expiration Dating—24 Months
How Supplied: 1 U.S. Unit (TU) per test dose (0.1 ml), package of 10 vials; 5 U.S. Units (TU) per test dose (0.1 ml), package of 10 vials and 50 vials; 250 U.S. Units (TU) per test dose (0.1 ml), package of 10 vials.

Cook-Waite Laboratories, Inc.

90 PARK AVENUE
NEW YORK, NEW YORK 10016

CARBOCAINE® ℞
hydrochloride 3% Injection
(mepivacaine hydrochloride injection, USP)
CARBOCAINE® ℞
hydrochloride 2%
with NEO–COBEFRIN®
1:20,000 Injection
(mepivacaine hydrochloride and levonordefrin injection, USP)

THESE SOLUTIONS ARE INTENDED FOR DENTAL USE ONLY.

Description: Mepivacaine hydrochloride is 1-methyl-2′, 6′-pipecoloxylidide monohydrochloride.
It is a white, crystalline, odorless powder soluble in water, but very resistant to both acid and alkaline hydrolysis.
Levonordefrin is (−)-α-(1-Aminoethyl)-3, 4-dihydroxybenzyl alcohol.
It is a white or buff-colored crystalline solid, freely soluble in aqueous solutions of mineral acids, but practically insoluble in water.
DENTAL CARTRIDGES MAY NOT BE AUTOCLAVED.

COMPOSITION	CARTRIDGE	
Each ml contains:	2%	3%
mepivacaine hydrochloride	20.0 mg	30.0 mg
levonordefrin	0.05 mg	—
sodium chloride	4.0 mg	3.0 mg
acetone sodium bisulfite not more than	2.0 mg	—
water for injection qs ad	1.0 ml	1.0 ml

The pH of the 2% cartridge solution is adjusted between 3.3 and 5.5 with NaOH or HCl.
The pH of the 3% cartridge solution is adjusted between 4.5 and 6.8 with NaOH or HCl.
Clinical Pharmacology: Carbocaine stabilizes the neuronal membrane and prevents the initiation and transmission of nerve impulses, thereby effecting local anesthesia.
CARBOCAINE is rapidly metabolized, with only a small percentage of the anesthetic (5 to 10 per cent) being excreted unchanged in the urine. CARBOCAINE, because of its amide structure, is not detoxified by the circulating plasma esterases. The liver is the principal site of metabolism, with over 50 per cent of the administered dose being excreted into the bile as metabolites. Most of the metabolized mepivacaine is probably resorbed in the intestine and then excreted into the urine since only a small percentage is found in the feces. The principal route of excretion is via the kidney. Most of the anesthetic and its metabolites are eliminated within 30 hours. It has been shown that hydroxylation and N-demethylation, which are detoxification reactions, play important roles in the metabolism of the anesthetic. Three metabolites of mepivacaine have been identified from adult humans: two phenols, which are excreted almost exclusively as their glucuronide conjugates, and the N-demethylated compound (2′,6′-pipecoloxylidide).
The onset of action is rapid (30 to 120 seconds in the upper jaw; 1 to 4 minutes in the lower jaw) and CARBOCAINE Hydrochloride 3% without vasoconstrictor will ordinarily provide operating anesthesia of 20 minutes in the upper jaw and 40 minutes in the lower jaw.
CARBOCAINE hydrochloride 2% with Neo-Cobefrin 1:20,000 (brand of mepivacaine hydrochloride and levonordefrin injection) provides anesthesia of longer duration for more prolonged procedures, 1 hour to 2.5 hours in

Continued on next page

Cook-Waite—Cont.

the upper jaw and 2.5 hours to 5.5 hours in the lower jaw.

CARBOCAINE does not ordinarily produce irritation or tissue damage.

Neo-Cobefrin (brand of levonordefrin) is a sympathomimetic amine used as a vasoconstrictor in local anesthetic solutions. It has pharmacologic activity similar to that of epinephrine but it is more stable than epinephrine. In equal concentrations, Neo-Cobefrin is less potent than epinephrine in raising blood pressure, and as a vasoconstrictor.

Indications: Carbocaine is indicated for the production of local anesthesia for dental procedures by infiltration injection or nerve block.

Contraindications: Mepivacaine is contraindicated in patients with a known hypersensitivity to amide type local anesthetics.

Warnings: RESUSCITATIVE EQUIPMENT AND DRUGS SHOULD BE IMMEDIATELY AVAILABLE. (See Adverse Reactions).

Reactions resulting in fatality have occurred on rare occasions with the use of local anesthetics, even in the absence of a history of hypersensitivity.

The solution which contains a vasoconstrictor should be used with extreme caution for patients whose medical history and physical evaluation suggest the existence of hypertension, arteriosclerotic heart disease, cerebral vascular insufficiency, heart block, thyrotoxicosis and diabetes, etc. The solution which contains a vasoconstrictor, should also be used with extreme caution in patients receiving drugs known to produce blood pressure alterations (i.e., MAO inhibitors, tricyclic anti-depressants, phenothiazines, etc.) as either sustained hypotension or hypertension may occur.

Usage in Children. Great care must be exercised in adhering to safe concentrations and dosages for pedodontic administration (see Dosage and Administration).

Usage in Pregnancy. Safe use of mepivacaine has not been established with respect to adverse effects on fetal development. Careful consideration should be given to this fact before administration during pregnancy.

Local anesthetic procedures should be used with caution when there is inflammation and/or sepsis in the region of the proposed injection.

Precautions: The safety and effectiveness of mepivacaine depend upon proper dosage, correct technique, adequate precautions, and readiness for emergencies.

The lowest dose that results in effective anesthesia should be used to avoid high plasma levels and possible adverse effects. Injection of repeated doses of mepivacaine may cause significant increase in blood levels with each repeated dose due to slow accumulation of the drug or its metabolites, or due to slower metabolic degradation than normal.

Tolerance varies with the status of the patient. Debilitated, elderly patients, acutely ill patients, and children should be given reduced doses commensurate with their weight and physical status.

Mepivacaine should be used with caution in patients with a history of severe disturbances of cardiac rhythm or heart block.

INJECTIONS SHOULD ALWAYS BE MADE SLOWLY WITH ASPIRATION TO AVOID INTRAVASCULAR INJECTION AND THEREFORE SYSTEMIC REACTION TO BOTH LOCAL ANESTHETIC AND VASOCONSTRICTOR.

If sedatives are employed to reduce patient apprehension, use reduced doses, since local anesthetic agents, like sedatives, are central nervous system depressants which in combination may have an additive effect. Young children should be given minimal doses of each agent.

Changes in sensorium such as excitation, disorientation, drowsiness, may be early indications of a high blood level of the drug and may occur following inadvertent intravascular administration or rapid absorption of mepivacaine.

Solutions containing a vasoconstrictor should be used cautiously in the presence of diseases which may adversely affect the patient's cardiovascular system. Serious cardiac arrhythmias may occur if preparations containing a vasoconstrictor are employed in patients during or following the administration of chloroform, halothane, cyclopropane, trichloroethylene, or other related agents.

Mepivacaine SHOULD BE USED WITH CAUTION IN PATIENTS WITH KNOWN DRUG ALLERGIES AND SENSITIVITIES. A thorough history of the patient's prior experience with mepivacaine or other local anesthetics as well as concomitant or recent drug use should be taken (see Contraindications). Patients allergic to methylparaben or para-aminobenzoic acid derivatives (procaine, tetracaine, benzocaine, etc.) have not shown cross-sensitivity to agents of the amide type such as mepivacaine.

Since mepivacaine is metabolized in the liver and excreted by the kidneys, it should be used cautiously in patients with liver and renal disease.

Adverse Reactions: Systemic adverse reactions involving the central nervous system and the cardiovascular system usually result from high plasma levels due to excessive dosage, rapid absorption, or inadvertent intravascular injection.

A small number of reactions may result from hypersensitivity, idiosyncrasy or diminished tolerance to normal dosage on the part of the patient.

Reactions involving the *central nervous system* are characterized by excitation and/or depression. Nervousness, dizziness, blurred vision, or tremors may occur followed by drowsiness, convulsions, unconsciousness, and possibly respiratory arrest. Since excitement may be transient or absent, the first manifestations may be drowsiness merging into unconsciousness and respiratory arrest.

Reactions involving the *cardiovascular system* include depression of the myocardium, hypotension, bradycardia, and even cardiac arrest.

Allergic reactions are rare and may occur as a result of sensitivity to the local anesthetic and are characterized by cutaneous lesions of delayed onset or urticaria, edema and other manifestations of allergy. The detection of sensitivity by skin testing is of limited value. As with other local anesthetics, anaphylactoid reactions to CARBOCAINE have occurred rarely. The reaction may be abrupt and severe and is not usually dose related.

Treatment of a patient with toxic manifestations consists of assuring and maintaining a patent airway and supporting ventilation (respiration) as required. This usually will be sufficient in the management of most reactions. Should a convulsion persist despite ventilatory therapy, small increments of anticonvulsive agents may be given intravenously, such as benzodiazepine (e.g., diazepam) or ultra-short acting barbiturates (e.g., thiopental or thiamylal) or short-acting barbiturate (e.g., pentobarbital or secobarbital). Cardiovascular depression may require circulatory assistance with intravenous fluids and/or vasopressor (e.g., ephedrine) as dictated by the clinical situation. Allergic reactions should be managed by conventional means.

Dosage and Administration: As with all local anesthetics, the dose varies and depends upon the area to be anesthetized, the vascularity of the tissues, individual tolerance and the technique of anesthesia. The lowest dose needed to provide effective anesthesia should be administered. For specific techniques and procedures refer to standard dental manuals and textbooks.

For infiltration and block injections in the upper or lower jaw, the average dose of 1 cartridge will usually suffice.

Each cartridge contains 1.8 ml. (36 mg. of 2% or 54 mg. of 3%).

Five cartridges (180 mg. of the 2% solution or 270 mg. of the 3% solution) are usually adequate to effect anesthesia of the entire oral cavity. Whenever a larger dose seems to be necessary for an extensive procedure, the maximum dose should be calculated according to that patient's weight. A dose of up to 3 mg. per pound of body weight may be administered. At any single dental sitting the total dose for all injected sites should not exceed 400 mg. in adults.

The maximum pediatric dose should be *carefully calculated* and should not exceed 5 cartridges (180 mg. of the 2% solution and 270 mg. of the 3% solution). The maximum pediatric dose should be calculated as:

$$\text{Maximum Dose for Children} = \frac{\text{Child's Weight (lbs.)}}{150} \times \text{Maximum Recommended Dose for Adults (400 mg.)}$$

When using CARBOCAINE for infiltration or regional block anesthesia, injection should always be made slowly and with frequent aspiration.

Any unused portion of a cartridge should be discarded.

Disinfection of Cartridges: As in the case of any cartridge, the diaphragm should be disinfected before needle puncture. The diaphragm should be thoroughly swabbed with either pure 91% isopropyl alcohol or 70% ethyl alcohol, USP just prior to use. Many commercially available alcohol solutions contain ingredients which are injurious to container components, and therefore, should not be used. Cartridges should not be immersed in any solution.

How Supplied: Both formulas are available in 1.8 ml. cartridges, containers of 50, to fit the Carpule® Aspirator.

The 2% solution should be stored at controlled room temperature, between 15° and 30° C (59° and 86° F).

Marketed by:
COOK-WAITE LABORATORIES, INC.
Mfg. by Sterling Drug Inc.
New York, N.Y. 10016
Carbocaine and Neo-Cobefrin
are the registered trademarks
of Sterling Drug Inc.
Revised March 1982 CO 160/0382

For full prescribing information on the medical use of Carbocaine, see Breon Laboratories product listing in this publication.

CooperCare, Inc.
DERMATOLOGY PRODUCTS
3145 PORTER DRIVE
PALO ALTO, CA 94304

AVEENO® BATH
REGULAR FORMULA AND OILATED FOR DRY SKIN

AVEENO® BATHS contain Colloidal Oatmeal, a natural oat derivative developed specially for soothing and cleansing itchy, sore, sensitive skin.

AVEENO® BATHS contain no soaps or synthetic detergents that may be harmful to the skin. They cleanse naturally because of their unique adsorptive properties.

Infants and children with sensitive skin will also benefit from soothing, calming AVEENO® Colloidal Oatmeal baths.

Aveeno®bar
Regular for normal to oily skin

Aveeno®bar Regular is made especially for sensitive skin that is irritated by ordinary soaps.
More than 50% of this mild skin cleanser is colloidal oatmeal, noted for its soothing and protective qualities.
Aveeno®bar Regular is completely soapfree. It leaves no harsh alkaline film to irritate delicate skin. . . it leaves it feeling soft and comfortable.
Ingredients: Aveeno® Colloidal Oatmeal, 50%; specially selected lanolin derivative; in a sudsing soapfree base containing a mild surfactant.

Aveenobar®
MEDICATED FOR ACNE
(FORMERLY ACNAVEEN®)

Aveeno®bar Medicated is a special soapfree cleansing bar for acne. It contains colloidal oatmeal, 2% sulfur, and 2% salicylic acid, to help cleanse and soothe irritated skin.
Ingredients: Aveeno® Colloidal Oatmeal, 50%; sulfur, 2%; salicylic acid, 2%; in a sudsing soapfree base containing a mild surfactant.

Aveenobar®
OILATED FOR DRY SKIN
(FORMERLY EMULAVE®)

Aveeno®bar Oilated is a unique, soapfree cleanser for dry, sensitive skin that is irritated by ordinary soaps. Aveeno®bar Oilated contains over 29% skin-softening emollients to help replace natural skin oils and 30% colloidal oatmeal, recommended for its soothing and protective qualities.
Ingredients: A combination of vegetable oils, specially selected lanolin derivative and glycerine 29%, Aveeno® Colloidal Oatmeal, 30%; in a sudsing soapfree base containing a mild surfactant.

BENISONE® ℞
(Betamethasone Benzoate Gel, USP)
Gel 0.025%

BENISONE® ℞
(Betamethasone Benzoate)
Cream 0.025%

BENISONE® ℞
(Betamethasone Benzoate)
Ointment 0.025%

BENISONE® ℞
(Betamethasone Benzoate)
Lotion 0.025%

For external use only
Caution: Federal law prohibits dispensing without prescription.
Description: Benisone Gel/Cream/Ointment/Lotion contains the active fluorinated corticosteroid compound betamethasone benzoate, the 17-benzoate ester of betamethasone, having the chemical formula of 9-fluoro-11β-methylpregna-1, 4-diene-3, 20-dione benzoate. Its chemical structure is:

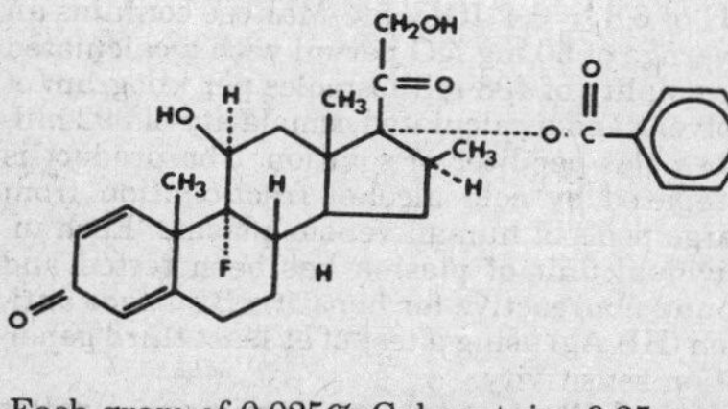

CH₂OH, C=O, HO, H, CH₃, O, C, CH₃, H, CH₃, H, F, H, O

Each gram of 0.025% Gel contains 0.25 mg of betamethasone benzoate in a specially formulated gel base consisting of 13.8% (w/w) alcohol, carboxyvinyl polymer, propylene glycol, disodium edetate, diisopropanolamine and purified water. The gel is self-liquefying, clear, greaseless and nonstaining. The active ingredient is completely solubilized and remains in the clear film without crystallization after evaporation of volatile substances.
Each gram of 0.025% Cream contains 0.25 mg of betamethasone benzoate in a water-washable emollient cream base consisting of cetyl alcohol, glyceryl stearate, light mineral oil, propylene glycol, disodium monooleamidosulfosuccinate, citric acid and purified water.
Each gram of 0.025% Ointment contains 0.25 mg of betamethasone benzoate in an emollient ointment base of light mineral oil, glyceryl stearate, food starch-modified and polyethylene. In this formulation the active ingredient is micronized to provide uniform distribution and optimal activity.
Each gram of 0.025% Lotion contains 0.25 mg of betamethasone benzoate in a water miscible, oil- and fat-free vehicle consisting of cetyl alcohol, stearyl alcohol, propylene glycol, sodium lauryl sulfate, purified water, and propyl-, butyl-, and methylparabens as preservatives.
Clinical Pharmacology: Topical corticosteroids share antiinflammatory, antipruritic and vasoconstrictive actions.
The mechanism of antiinflammatory activity of the topical corticosteroids is unclear. Various laboratory methods, including vasoconstrictor assays, are used to compare and predict potencies and/or clinical efficacies of the topical corticosteroids. There is some evidence to suggest that a recognizable correlation exists between vasoconstrictor potency and therapeutic efficacy in man.
Pharmacokinetics
The extent of percutaneous absorption of topical corticosteroids is determined by many factors including the vehicle, the integrity of the epidermal barrier, and the use of occlusive dressings.
Topical corticosteroids can be absorbed from normal intact skin. Inflammation and/or other disease processes in the skin increase percutaneous absorption. Occlusive dressings substantially increase the percutaneous absorption of topical corticosteroids. Thus, occlusive dressings may be a valuable therapeutic adjunct for treatment of resistant dermatoses. (See *DOSAGE AND ADMINISTRATION.*)
Once absorbed through the skin, topical corticosteroids are handled through pharmacokinetic pathways similar to systemically administered corticosteroids. Corticosteroids are bound to plasma proteins in varying degrees. Corticosteroids are metabolized primarily in the liver and are then excreted by the kidneys. Some of the topical corticosteroids and their metabolites are also excreted into the bile.
Indications and Usage: Topical corticosteroids are indicated for the relief of the inflammatory and pruritic manifestations of corticosteroid-responsive dermatoses.

Contraindications: Topical corticosteroids are contraindicated in those patients with a history of hypersensitivity to any of the components of the preparation.

Precautions:
General
Systemic absorption of topical corticosteroids has produced reversible hypothalamic-pituitary-adrenal (HPA) axis suppression, manifestations of Cushing's syndrome, hyperglycemia and glucosuria in some patients. Conditions which augment systemic absorption include the application of the more potent steroids, use over large surface areas, prolonged use, and the addition of occlusive dressings.
Therefore, patients receiving a large dose of a potent topical steroid applied to a large surface area or under an occlusive dressing should be evaluated periodically for evidence of HPA axis suppression by using the urinary free cortisol and ACTH stimulation tests. If HPA axis suppression is noted, an attempt should be made to withdraw the drug, to reduce the frequency of application, or to substitute a less potent steroid.
Recovery of HPA axis function is generally prompt and complete upon discontinuation of the drug. Infrequently, signs and symptoms of steroid withdrawal may occur, requiring supplemental systemic corticosteroids.
Children may absorb proportionally larger amounts of topical corticosteroids and thus be more susceptible to systemic toxicity (See *PRECAUTIONS—Pediatric Use*).
If irritation develops, topical corticosteroids should be discontinued and appropriate therapy instituted.
In the presence of dermatological infections, the use of an appropriate antifungal or antibacterial agent should be instituted. If a favorable response does not occur promptly, the corticosteroid should be discontinued until the infection has been adequately controlled.
Information for the Patient
Patients using topical corticosteroids should receive the following information and instructions:
1. This medication is to be used as directed by the physician. It is for external use only. Avoid contact with the eyes.
2. Patients should be advised not to use this medication for any disorder other than for which it was prescribed.
3. The treated skin area should not be bandaged or otherwise covered or wrapped as to be occlusive unless directed by the physician.
4. Patients should report any signs of local adverse reactions especially under occlusive dressing.
5. Parents of pediatric patients should be advised not to use tight-fitting diapers or plastic pants on a child being treated in the diaper area, as these garments may constitute occlusive dressings.
Laboratory Tests
The following tests may be helpful in evaluating the HPA axis suppression:
Urinary free cortisol test
ACTH stimulation test
Carcinogenesis, Mutagenesis, and Impairment of Fertility
Long-term animal studies have not been performed to evaluate the carcinogenic potential or the effect on fertility of topical corticosteroids.
Studies to determine mutagenicity with prednisolone and hydrocortisone have revealed negative results.
Pregnancy Category C
Corticosteroids are generally teratogenic in laboratory animals when administered systemically at relatively low dosage levels. The more potent corticosteroids have been shown to be teratogenic after dermal application in laboratory animals. There are no adequate and well-controlled studies in pregnant women or teratogenic effects from topically applied corticosteroids. Therefore, topical corticosteroids should be used during pregnancy only if the potential benefit justifies the potential risk to the fetus. Drugs of this class should not be used extensively on pregnant patients, in large amounts, or for prolonged periods of time.
Nursing Mothers
It is not known whether topical administration of corticosteroids could result in sufficient systemic absorption to produce detectable quantities in breast milk. Systemically administered corticosteroids are secreted into breast milk in quantities *not* likely to have a deleterious effect on the infant. Nevertheless, caution should be exercised when topical corticosteroids are administered to a nursing woman.
Pediatric Use
Pediatric patients may demonstrate greater susceptibility to topical corticosteroid-induced HPA axis suppression and Cushing's syndrome than

Continued on next page

CooperCare—Cont.

mature patients because of a larger skin surface area to body weight ratio.
Hypothalamic-pituitary-adrenal (HPA) axis suppression, Cushing's syndrome, and intracranial hypertension have been reported in children receiving topical corticosteroids. Manifestations of adrenal suppression in children include linear growth retardation, delayed weight gain, low plasma cortisol levels, and absence of response to ACTH stimulation. Manifestations of intracranial hypertension include bulging fontanelles, headaches, and bilateral papilledema.
Administration of topical corticosteroids to children should be limited to the least amount compatible with an effective therapeutic regimen. Chronic corticosteroid therapy may interfere with the growth and development of children. Benisone (betamethasone benzoate) Gel/Cream/Ointment/Lotion are not for Ophthalmic use.
Adverse Reactions: The following local adverse reactions are reported infrequently with topical corticosteroids, but may occur more frequently with the use of occlusive dressings. These reactions are listed in an approximate decreasing order of occurence:

- Burning
- Itching
- Irritation
- Dryness
- Folliculitis
- Hypertrichosis
- Acneiform eruptions
- Hypopigmentation
- Perioral dermatitis
- Allergic contact dermatitis
- Maceration of the skin
- Secondary infection
- Skin atrophy
- Striae
- Miliaria

Overdosage: Topically applied corticosteroids can be absorbed in sufficient amounts to produce systemic effects (See *PRECAUTIONS*).
Dosage and Administration: Topical corticosteroids are generally applied to the affected area as a thin film from two to four times daily depending on the severity of the condition.
Occlusive dressings may be used for the management of psoriasis or recalcitrant conditions. If an infection develops, the use of occlusive dressings should be discontinued and appropriate antimicrobial therapy instituted.

How Supplied:
Benisone Gel 0.025% is supplied in 15 gram (N 0041-0280-15) and 60 gram (N 0041-0280-60) tubes.
Benisone Cream 0.025% is supplied in 15 gram (N 0041-0281-15) and 60 gram (N 0041-0281-60) tubes.
Benisone Ointment 0.025% is supplied in 15 gram (N 0041-0283-15) and 60 gram (N 0041-0283-60) tubes.
Benisone Lotion 0.025% is supplied in 15 ml (N 0041-0284-15) and 60 ml (N 0041-0284-60) plastic bottles.
Store between 59°–86° F.
US Patent 3,529,060
US Patent 3,749,773
January, 1982
Distributed by
Cooper Care, Inc.
DERMATOLOGY PRODUCTS
Palo Alto, Ca 94304
Manufactured by

PARKE-DAVIS
Div of Warner-Lambert Co
Morris Plains, NJ 07950

0280G030

PENTRAX®
Tar Shampoo with Fractar®

Description: Pentrax Tar Shampoo contains 8.75% Fractar® (which is equal to 4.3% crude coal tar), a standardized tax extract, a blend of highly concentrated detergents, and conditioning agents. Spectrophotometric standardization, based on hydrocarbon analysis assures uniform tar content from batch to batch. Pentrax Tar Shampoo does not contain hexachlorophene, parabens or other preservatives.
Action and Indications: Coal tar helps correct abnormalities of keratinization by decreasing epidermal proliferation and dermal infiltration. Pentrax Tar Shampoo is indicated for the adjunctive, topical management of dandruff, seborrheic dermatitis, psoriasis and subacute and chronic eczematous dermatoses of the scalp.
Advantages: Pentrax Tar Shampoo contains all the desirable crude coal tar fractions without undesirable pitch. It has excellent lathering qualities and leaves hair clean and manageable.
Contraindications: Pentrax Tar Shampoo is contraindicated in patients with a history of hypersensitivity to tar and other components of the formulation.
Precautions: Not for ophthalmic use. Minor dematologic side effects have been reported from the use of topical tar preparations. These include irritation, folliculitis from long-term use, allergic contact dermatitis and phototoxicity. May stain dyed or colored hair. Keep of the reach of children.
Directions: Apply Pentrax® Tar Shampoo to wet hair; massage, adding water liberally to produce lather. Rinse. Reapply. Second lather may be allowed to remain up to 10 minutes. Rinse. Shampoo twice weekly.
Packaging:
4 fluid ounce plastic bottles.
NDC 0041-3916-04
8 fluid ounce plastic bottles.
NDC 0041-3916-08

TEXACORT® Scalp Lotion ℞

Caution: Federal law prohibits dispensing without prescription.
Texacort Scalp Lotion contains hydrocortisone in a concentration of 1% (10 mg per gram). Hydrocortisone (cortisol) has the chemical formula of pregn-4-ene-3,20-dione, 11,17,21-trihydroxy, (11β)-. The vehicle contains: 33% alcohol, propylene glycol, polysorbate 20, benzalkonium chloride, and purified water. Texacort Scalp Lotion is lipid-free and paraben-free.
Actions: Topical steroids are primarily effective because of their antiinflammatory, antipruritic and vasoconstrictive actions.
Indications: For relief of the inflammatory manifestations of corticosteroid responsive dermatoses.
Contraindications: Topical steroids are contraindicated in those patients with a history of hypersensitivity to any components of the preparation.
Precautions: If irritation develops, Texacort Scalp Lotion should be discontinued and appropriate therapy instituted.
In the presence of an infection the use of an appropriate antifungal or antibacterial agent should be instituted. If a favorable response does not occur promptly, the corticosteroid should be discontinued until the infection has been adequately controlled.
If extensive areas are treated or if the occlusive technique is used there will be increased systemic absorption of the corticosteroid and suitable precautions should be taken, particularly in children and infants.
Although topical steroids have not been reported to have an adverse effect on human pregnancy, the safety of their use in pregnant women has not been absolutely established. In laboratory animals, increases in incidence of fetal abnormalities have been associated with exposure of gestating females to topical corticosteroids, in some cases at rather low dosage levels. Therefore, drugs of this class should not be used extensively on pregnant patients, in large amounts, or for prolonged periods of time.
Texacort Scalp Lotion is not for ophthalmic use.
Adverse Reactions: The following local adverse reactions have been reported with topical corticosteroids, especially under occlusive dressings: burning, itching, irritation, dryness, folliculitis, hypertrichosis, acneform eruptions, hypopigmentation, perioral dermatitis, allergic contact dermatitis, maceration of the skin, secondary infection, skin atrophy, striae and miliaria.
Dosage and Administration: Apply to affected areas 2 or 4 times daily. When a favorable response is obtained, gradually reduce dosage and eventually discontinue.
How Supplied: Texacort Scalp Lotion is supplied in 1 fl oz bottles with dropper (N 0064-3912-01).
Store between 59°–86° F [15°–30° C].

CooperVision Pharmaceuticals Inc.
SAN GERMAN, PUERTO RICO 00753

OPHTHALMIC PRODUCTS

For information on CooperVision Pharmaceuticals Inc. prescription and OTC ophthalmic products, consult the Physicians' Desk Reference For Ophthalmology. For literature, service items or sample material, contact your CooperVision Pharmaceuticals Inc. representative. See a complete listing of products in the Manufacturers' Index section of this book.

Cutter Biological
DIV. CUTTER LABORATORIES, INC.
2200 POWELL STREET
EMERYVILLE, CA 94608

GAMASTAN® ℞
(Immune Serum Globulin—Human U.S.P.)
2 ml., 10 ml. vials

GAMIMUNE® ℞
IMMUNE GLOBULIN INTRAVENOUS, 5%
(In 10% Maltose)

Description: Immune Globulin Intravenous, 5% in 10% Maltose (IGIV,5%-Maltose)-Gamimune®—is a sterile 5 $\pm$ 1% solution of human protein stabilized with 0.1 $\pm$ 0.015 M glycine and 10 $\pm$ 2% maltose; it contains no preservatives. The immunoglobulin is selectively reduced under controlled conditions using dithiothreitol and alkylated with iodoacetamide to render it suitable for intravenous administration. The preparation contains not less than 90% immunoglobulin and has a pH of 6.8 $\pm$ 0.4. IGIV,5%-Maltose contains an average of 50 mg lgG per ml with a calculated osmolality of 438 milliosmoles per kilogram of solvent and a calculated osmolarity of 392 milliosmoles per liter of solution. The product is prepared by cold alcohol fractionation from large pools of human venous plasma. Each individual unit of plasma has been tested and found nonreactive for hepatitis B surface antigen (HB_sAg) using a test of at least third-generation sensitivity.
Clinical Pharmacology: Gamimune supplies IgG antibodies for prevention or attenuation of infectious diseases. The half-life of Gamimune is approximately three weeks but individual patient variation in half-life has been ob-

served. Thus, this variable as well as the amount of immunoglobulin administered per dose is important in determining the frequency of administration of the drug for each patient. Maltose is added to the solution in a 10% concentration for stabilization of the protein. A comparative clinical study of IGIV with and without maltose showed the incidence of adverse effects was significantly less with the maltose-containing preparation.

The intravenous administration of solutions of maltose have been studied by several investigators. Healthy subjects tolerated the infusions well and no adverse effects were observed at a rate of 0.25 g maltose/kg per hour. In safety studies conducted by Cutter Laboratories, infusions of 10% maltose administered at 0.27 to 0.62 g maltose/kg per hour to normal subjects produced either mild side effects (e.g., headache) or no adverse reaction. Following intravenous infusions of maltose, maltose was detected in the peripheral blood, there was a dose dependent excretion of maltose and glucose in the urine and a mild diuretic effect. These alterations were tolerated without significant adverse effects.

Since one milliliter of IGIV,5%-Maltose contains 0.1 g of maltose, the recommended dose of 0.1 to 0.2 g IGIV,5%-Maltose per kilogram body weight (see Dosage and Administration) would result in the patient receiving a total of 0.2 g to 0.4 g maltose per kilogram body weight given over 2 to 4 hours. These amounts are within those levels tolerated in the Cutter safety studies cited above.

Indications and Usage: Immune Globulin Intravenous,5% in 10% Maltose (IGIV,5%-Maltose)-Gamimune® is indicated for the maintenance treatment of patients who are unable to produce sufficient amounts of IgG antibodies. Usage of Gamimune may be preferred to that of intramuscular immunoglobulin preparations especially in patients who require an immediate increase in intravascular immunoglobulin levels, in patients with a small muscle mass, and in patients with bleeding tendencies in whom intramuscular injections are contraindicated. It may be used in disease states such as congenital agammaglobulinemia (e.g., x-linked agammaglobulinemia), common variable hypogammaglobulinemia, x-linked immunodeficiency with hyper IgM, and combined immunodeficiency.[5,7,9,18,19]

In a cooperative comparative study of Immune Globulin Intravenous, 10% (IGIV, 10%) and Immune Serum Globulin (Human)-Gamastan® in hypogammaglobulinemic patients, the same doses of IGIV,10% and Gamastan were equally effective in the prevention of severe acute infections.

Contraindications: IGIV,5%-Maltose is contraindicated in individuals who are known to have had an anaphylactic or severe systemic response to Immune Serum Globulin (Human). Individuals with selective IgA deficiencies should not receive IGIV,5%-Maltose or any immune globulin preparation.

Warnings: IGIV,5%-Maltose should only be administered intravenously as the intramuscular route has not yet been evaluated.

IGIV,5%-Maltose can, on occasion, cause a precipitous fall in blood pressure and the clinical picture of anaphylaxis even when the patient is not known to be sensitive to immune globulin preparations. These reactions appear to be related to the rate of infusion. Accordingly, the infusion rate given under "Dosage and Administration" should be closely followed, at least until the physician has had sufficient experience with a given patient. The patient's vital signs should be monitored continuously and careful observation made for any symptoms throughout the entire infusion. Epinephrine should be available for treatment of any acute anaphylactoid reaction.

Precautions:

Drug Interactions

Although Gamimune may be diluted with 5% dextrose, no other drug interactions or compatibilities have been evaluated. It is recommended that the infusion of Gamimune be given via separate line, by itself, without mixing with other intravenous fluids or medications the patient might be receiving.

Pregnancy Category C

Animal reproduction studies have not been conducted with Gamimune. It is also not known whether Gamimune can cause fetal harm when administered to a pregnant woman or can affect reproduction capacity. Gamimune should be given to a pregnant woman only if clearly needed.

Adverse Reactions: In an investigation of the incidence of side effects to IGIV,5%-Maltose, only 10% of the patients exhibited any side effects. Those reported were mild back pain in one patient during the infusion, nausea in another patient, and flushing in a third.[11]

True anaphylactic reactions to IGIV,5%-Maltose would be expected to occur only in recipients with documented prior histories of severe allergic reactions to intramuscular immune serum globulin.

Dosage and Administration: The usual dose of Immune Globulin Intravenous,5% in 10% Maltose (IGIV,5%-Maltose)-Gamimune® for prophylaxis in immunodeficiency syndromes is 100 mg/kg of body weight (i.e., 2 ml/kg body weight) administered once a month by intravenous infusion. If the clinical response is inadequate or the level of IgG achieved in the circulation is felt to be insufficient, the dosage may be increased to 200 mg/kg body weight (i.e., 4 ml/kg body weight) or the infusion may be repeated more frequently than once a month. However, controlled studies have not yet been undertaken to determine whether any increase in efficacy can be obtained with the larger dose or more frequent administration.

Recent investigations confirm that Gamimune is well tolerated and not likely to produce side effects when infused at the indicated rate.[11] It is recommended that Gamimune be infused, by itself, at a rate of 0.01 to 0.02 ml/kg body weight per minute for thirty minutes. If the patient does not experience any discomfort, the rate may be increased to between 0.02 and 0.04 ml/kg body weight per minute. If side effects occur, the rate should be reduced or the infusion interrupted until the symptoms subside. The infusion may then be resumed at a rate which is tolerated by the patient.

Caution: U.S. Federal law prohibits dispensing without a prescription.

Storage: Store at 2 to 8°C (35 to 46°F). Solution that has been frozen should not be used. Any vial that has been entered should be used promptly. Partially used vials should be discarded. Do not use after expiration date. Do not use if turbid.

How Supplied: Gamimune is supplied as 50 to 100 ml single dose vials.

14-7617-201
(Rev Apr 1981)

HYPERAB® ℞

(Rabies Immune Globulin—Human)

2 ml. (300 IU) pediatric vial
10 ml. (1500 IU) adult vial

HYPERHEP® ℞

(Hepatitis B Immune Globulin—Human)

1 ml., 5 ml. vials

HYPER-TET® ℞

(Tetanus Immune Globulin—Human U.S.P.)

250 units vial or prefilled disposable syringe

HYPERTUSSIS® ℞

(Pertussis Immune Globulin—Human, U.S.P.)

1.25 ml. vial

HypRho®-D ℞

Rh_o(D) Immune Globulin (Human)

Description: Rh_o(D) Immune Globulin (Human)—HypRho®-D is a sterile solution of immune globulin containing antibodies to Rh_o(D) prepared from human venous plasma collected from carefully screened donors. It contains $16.5 \pm 1.5\%$ protein stabilized with 0.3 M glycine and preserved with 1:10,000 thimerosal (a mercury derivative). The pH is adjusted with sodium carbonate. HypRho-D has been titered against and the potency found equal to or greater than that of the U.S. Food and Drug Administration Reference Rh_o(D) Immune Globulin (Human). One vial or syringe has been shown to effectively suppress the immunizing potential of 15 ml of Rh_o(D) positive or D^u positive packed red blood cells.

This product has been prepared from large pools of human venous plasma. Each individual unit of plasma has been found nonreactive for hepatitis B surface antigen (HBsAg) using a U.S. Federally approved test of at least third-generation sensitivity.

Clinical Pharmacology: HypRho-D is used to prevent isoimmunization in the Rh_o(D) negative, D^u negative individual exposed to Rh_o(D) positive or D^U positive blood as the result of a fetomaternal hemorrhage occuring during a delivery of a Rh_o(D) positive or D^U positive infant, abortion (either spontaneous or induced), or following amniocentesis. Similarly, immunization resulting in the production of anti-Rh_o(D) following transfusion of Rh positive red cells to a Rh_o(D) negative recipient may be prevented by administering Rh_o(D) immune globulin.

Rh hemolytic disease of the newborn is the result of the active immunization of a Rh_o(D) negative, D^u negative mother by Rh_o(D) positive or D^u positive red cells entering the maternal circulation during a previous delivery, abortion or amniocentesis or as a result of red cell transfusion. HypRho-D acts by suppressing the specific immune response of Rh_o(D) negative individuals to Rh_o(D) positive red blood cells.

The administration of Rh_o(D) Immune Globulin within 72 hours of a full-term delivery of an infant to a Rh_o(D) negative, D^u negative mother at risk reduced the incidence of Rh isoimmunization from 12–13% reduces 1–2%. The 1–2% treatment failures are probably due to isoimmunization occurring during the latter part of pregnancy or following delivery. Bowman, et al, have reported that the incidence of isoimmunization can be further reduced from approximately 1.6% to less than 0.1% by administering Rh_o(D) Immune Globulin in two doses, one antenatal at 28 weeks gestation and another following delivery.

Indications and Usage:

Pregnancy and Other Obstetric Conditions

HypRho-D is recommended for the prevention of Rh hemolytic disease of the newborn by its administration to the Rh_o(D) negative, D^u negative mother within 72 hours after birth of a Rh_o(D) positive or D^u positive infant, providing the following criteria are met:

1. The mother must be Rh_o(D) negative, D^u negative and must not already be sensitized to the Rh_o(D) factor.
2. Her child must be Rh_o(D) positive or D^u positive, and should have a negative direct Coombs test. A positive direct Coombs test may be caused by antibodies other than Rh_o(D) and

Continued on next page

Cutter—Cont.

while this does not contraindicate therapy with HypRho-D, it should be investigated. A positive direct Coombs test due to anti-Rh_o(D) is a contraindication to the use of HypRho-D. Even though Rh hemolytic disease of the newborn is less frequent when there is ABO incompatibility between the Rh_o(D) negative mother and the Rh_o(D) positive fetus, protection against Rh_o(D) sensitization may be incomplete, and treatment of the mother with HypRho-D is indicated in such cases.

If Rh_o(D) Immune Globulin (Human)—HypRho®-D is administered antepartum, it is essential that the mother receive another dose of HypRho-D after delivery of a Rh_o(D) positive or D^u positive infant.

HypRho-D should be administered within 72 hours to all nonimmunized Rh_o(D) negative, D^u negative women who have undergone spontaneous or induced abortion, following ruptured tubal pregnancy or following amniocentesis unless the blood type of the fetus or the father is known to be Rh_o(D) negative, R^u negative. If the fetal blood type is unknown, one must assume that it is Rh_o(D) positive, and HypRho-D should be administered to the mother.

Transfusion

HypRho-D may be used to prevent isoimmunization in Rh_o(D) negative, D^u negative individuals who have been transfused with Rh_o(D) positive or D^u positive red blood cells or blood components containing red blood cells.

Contraindications: HypRho-D is contraindicated for use in:

1. A Rh_o(D) positive or D^u positive individual.
2. A Rh_o(D) negative or D^u negative individual previously sensitized to the Rh_o(D) or D^u antigen.

Warnings:

1. Solutions which have been frozen should not be used.
2. Partially used vials or syringes must be discarded.
3. Babies born of women given Rh immune globulin antepartum may have a weakly positive direct Coomb's test at birth.

Precautions: NEVER ADMINISTER **HypRho-D** INTRAVENOUSLY. NEVER ADMINISTER TO THE NEONATE.

The presence of fetal cells in a maternal blood sample, or passive antibody given to the mother antepartum can affect the interpretation of laboratory tests to identify and monitor the patient for HypRho-D. If in doubt as to the patient's Rh type or immune status, HypRho-D should be administered.

Adverse Reactions: Reactions to Rh_o(D) Immune Globulin (Human) are infrequent in Rh_o(D) negative, D^u negative individuals and consist primarily of slight soreness at the site of injection and slight temperature elevation. While sensitization to repeated injections of human immune globulin is extremely rare, it has occurred. Elevated bilirubin levels have been reported in some individuals receiving multiple doses of Rh_o(D) Immune Globulin (Human) following mismatched tranfusions. This is believed to be due to a relatively rapid rate of foreign red cell destruction.

No instances of transmission of hepatitis have been reported from the use of human immune globulin prepared by the fractionation methods employed at Cutter Laboratories, Inc.

Dosage and Administration:

Pregnancy and Other Obstetric Conditions

1. For postpartum prophylaxis, administer one vial or syringe of HypRho-D intramuscularly, preferably within 72 hours of delivery. Although a lesser degree of protection is afforded if Rh antibody is administered beyond the 72-hour period, HypRho-D may still be given. However, full-term deliveries can vary in their dosage requirements depending on the magnitude of the fetomaternal hemorrhage. One vial or syringe of HypRho-D provides sufficient antibody to prevent Rh sensitization if the **packed red blood cell** volume that has entered the circulation is 15 ml or less. In instances where a large (greater than 30 ml of whole blood or 15 ml **packed red blood cells**) fetomaternal hemorrhage is suspected, a fetal red cell count by an approved laboratory technique (e.g. Modified Kleihauer-Betke acid elution stain technique) should be performed to determine the dosage of immune globulin required. The **packed red blood cell** volume of the calculated fetomaternal hemorrhage is divided by 15 ml to obtain the number of vials or syringes of HypRho-D for administration.

2. For antenatal prophylaxis, one vial or syringe of Rh_o(D) Immune Globulin (Human)—HypRho®D is administered intramuscularly at approximately 28 weeks. This must be followed by another full dose (one vial or one syringe), preferably within 72 hours following delivery, if the infant is Rh positive.

3. Following miscarriage, abortion, or ectopic pregnancy, it is recommended that one vial or syringe of HypRho-D be given. If more than 15 ml of packed red cells is suspected, due to fetomaternal hemorrhage, the same dose modification in #1 above applies.

Transfusion

In the case of a transfusion of Rh_o(D) positive or D^u positive red cells to a Rh_o(D) negative, D^u negative recipient, the volume of Rh positive whole blood administered is multiplied by the hematocrit of the donor unit giving the volume of **packed red blood cells** transfused. The volume of **packed red blood cells** is divided by 15 ml which provides the number of vials or syringes of HypRho-D to be administered.

If the dose calculated results in a fraction, the next whole number of vials or syringes should be administered (e.g., if 1.4, give 2 vials or 2 syringes). HypRho-D should be administered within 72 hours after the red cell transfusion, but preferably as soon as possible.

Injection Procedure

DO NOT INJECT INTRAVENOUSLY. DO NOT INJECT NEONATE.

A. Single Vial or Syringe Dose
   INJECT ENTIRE CONTENTS OF THE VIAL OR SYRINGE INTO THE INDIVIDUAL INTRAMUSCULARLY.

B. Multiple Vial or Syringe Dose
   1. Calculate the number of vials or syringes of HypRho-D to be given (See Dosage section).
   2. The total volume of HypRho-D can be given in divided doses at different sites at one time or the total dose may be divided and injected at intervals, provided the total dosage is given within 72 hours of the fetomaternal hemorrhage or transfusion. USING STERILE TECHNIQUE, INJECT THE ENTIRE CONTENTS OF THE CALCULATED NUMBER OF VIALS OR SYRINGES INTRAMUSCULARLY INTO THE PATIENT.

Storage: Store at 2–8°C (35–46°F). Do not freeze. Do not use after expiration date. Do not store after entry.

How Supplied: HypRho-D is available in vials and syringes as follows:

Product Code	Contents
621-10	Ten single dose vials of HypRho-D Package insert giving directions for use and patient identification cards.
621-22	Ten single dose syringes of HypRho-D. Package insert giving directions for use and patient identification cards.

Caution: U.S. Federal law prohibits dispensing without a prescription.

14-7621-102
(Rev May 1982)

KOĀTE® ℞
(Antihemophilic Factor—Human—Factor VIII, AHF, AHG)

250 AHF units, approx., with 10 ml. Sterile Water for Injection, U.S.P., and sterile filter needle.
500 AHF units, approx., with 20 ml. Sterile Water for Injection, U.S.P., and sterile filter needle.
1000 AHF units, approx., with 40 ml. Sterile Water for Injection, U.S.P., and sterile filter needle.
1500 AHF units, approx., with 40 ml. Sterile Water for Injection, U.S.P., and sterile filter needle.

KONŸNE® ℞
(Factor IX Complex—Human—Factors II, VII, IX and X)

500 unit vial, approx., with 20 ml. Sterile Water for Injection, U.S.P., and sterile filter needle.
1000 unit vial, approx., with 40 ml. Sterile Water for Injection, U.S.P., and sterile filter needle.

PLAGUE VACCINE, U.S.P. ℞
20 ml. vials

Dalin Pharmaceuticals, Inc.
74-80 MARINE STREET
FARMINGDALE, NY 11735

CELLUZYME™
Chewable Digestive Enzyme Tablets with Simethicone

Description: Green, spearmint-flavored, chewable, palatable tablets. Each tablet contains Cellulase 9 mg., Amylase 30 mg., Protease 6 mg., Lipase 20 mg., Simethicone 25 mg.
Action and Uses: To relieve the discomfort of: Intestinal Gas • Vegetable Bezoars • Functional Gastrointestinal Disorders • Pancreatic Insufficiency • Dyspepsia • Flatulence • Bloating.
Contraindications: A known sensitivity to any ingredient.
Dosage: Chew or swallow 1 or 2 tablets with meals and at bedtime.
How Supplied: 100 tablets. Hospital Unit Dose Available.
Remarks: DOES NOT CONTAIN PANCREATIN.

DALIDYNE™
Lotion
Effective Treatment for the Oral Cavity

Composition: Methylbenzethonium Chloride, Benzocaine, Tannic Acid, Camphor, Chlorothymol, Menthol, Benzyl Alcohol in a Specially Prepared Aromatized Base. Alcohol 61%.
Action and Uses: A cooling, soothing, quick-drying lotion possessing germicidal, fungicidal, anesthetic, astringent and healing properties used in the treatment of: Aphthous Stomatitis • Teething Pains • Herpes Simplex • Denture Irritations • Trench Mouth • Cheilosis, Avitaminosis • Thrush • Gingivitis • Throat Irritations (as mouth wash or gargle).
Administration and Dosage: Topical Application: Dry area and apply several times a day with cotton applicator. As Gargle or Mouth Wash: ½ teaspoonful in ½ glass of warm water several times a day.
How Supplied: 1 fl. oz.

SORBUTUSS®
Sugar Free for the Diabetic Cough Patient
Alcohol Free for the Alcoholic Patient

Composition: Each teaspoonful (5 cc.) contains d-methorphan hydrobromide 10 mg., glycerol guaiacolate 100 mg., potassium citrate

85 mg., citric acid 35 mg., in a palatable, mint-flavored, glycerin-sorbitol vehicle.

Action and Uses: Effective sugar-free and alcohol-free antitussive and expectorant with mucolytic properties for relief of coughs and coughs due to colds.

No
- Sugar
- Alcohol
- Antihistamines
- Decongestants
- Sodium

Recommended for all patients including diabetic, cardiac, hypertensive, geriatric and alcoholic. Soothing for coughs due to smoking.

Administration and Dosage: *Adults*—2 teaspoonfuls every 3 to 4 hours. *Children*—in proportion.

How Supplied: Bottles of 4 fl. oz., pints and gallons.

Remarks: SUGAR-FREE and SODIUM-FREE, NON-NARCOTIC and NON-ALCOHOLIC.

Danbury Pharmacal, Inc.

131 WEST STREET
P.O. BOX 296
DANBURY, CT 06810

PRODUCT IDENTIFICATION CODE

Danbury Prescription Capsules and Tablets are identified with a symbol DAN and the NDC Product Number.

Controlled Substance Products are identified with the Danbury NDC Number 591- followed by a letter identifying the product.

To quickly identify a product, a compilation of most of Danbury's products is listed below in alphabetical order with corresponding product codes.

NDC# 0591-	PRODUCT	IMPRINT
5370	Bethanechol Chloride Tablets, 5 mg.	U: DAN L: 5370
5369	Bethanechol Chloride Tablets, 10 mg.	U: DAN L: 5369
5402	Bethanechol Chloride Tablets, 25 mg.	U: DAN L: 5402
5515	Bethanechol Chloride Tablets, 50 mg.	U: DAN L: 5515
5541	Carisoprodol Compound Tablets	U: DAN L: 5541
5513	Carisoprodol Tablets, 350 mg.	U: DAN L: 5513
5548	Chloroquine Phosphate Tablets, 250 mg.	U: DAN L: 5548
5549	Chloroquine Phosphate Tablets, 500 mg.	U: DAN L: 5549
5444	Chlorothiazide Tablets, 250 mg.	U: DAN L: 5444
5016	Chlorpheniramine Maleate T.D. Capsules, 8 mg.	DAN/ 5016
5017	Chlorpheniramine Maleate T.D. Capsules, 12 mg.	DAN/ 5017
5336	Chlorpheniramine Maleate T.D. Tablets, 8 mg.	U: DAN L: 5336
5332	Chlorpheniramine Maleate T.D. Tablets, 12 mg.	U: DAN L: 5332
5507	Chlorthalidone Tablets, 25 mg.	U: DAN L: 5507
5518	Chlorthalidone Tablets, 50 mg.	U: DAN L: 5518
5495	Chlorzoxazone Tablets, 250 mg.	U: DAN L: 5495
5509	Chlorzoxazone with APAP Tablets, 250 mg.	U: DAN L: 5509
0944	Colchicine Tablets, 0.6 mg.	U: DAN L: 944
5325	Col-Probenecid Tablets, 0.5 mg./500 mg.	U: DAN L: 5325
5484	Cyproheptadine HCl. Tablets, 4 mg.	U: DAN L: 5484
5309	Dicyclomine HCl. Capsules, 10 mg.	DAN/ 5309
5383	Dicyclomine HCl. Tablets, 20 mg.	U: DAN L: 5383
5002	Diphenhydramine HCl. Capsules, 25 mg.	DAN/ 5002
5003	Diphenhydramine HCl. Capsules, 50 mg.	DAN/ 5003
5510	Dipyridamole Tablets, 25 mg.	DAN/ 5510
5376	Disulfiram Tablets, 250 mg.	U: DAN L: 5376
5368	Disulfiram Tablets, 500 mg.	U: DAN L: 5368
5535	Doxycycline Hyclate Capsules (Equivalent to 50 mg. Doxycycline)	DAN/ 5535
5440	Doxycycline Hyclate Capsules (Equivalent to 100 mg. Doxycycline)	DAN/ 5440
5504	Ergoloid Mesylates Oral Tablets 1.0 mg.	U: DAN L: 5504
5502	Ergoloid Mesylates Sublingual Tablets, 0.5 mg.	U: DAN L: 5502
5501	Ergoloid Mesylates Sublingual Tablets, 1.0 mg.	U: DAN L: 5501
5479	Erythromycin Estolate Capsules, 250 mg.	DAN/ 5479
5216	Folic Acid Tablets, 1.0 mg.	U: DAN L: 5216
5493	Glycopyrrolate Tablets, 1 mg.	U: DAN L: 5493
5494	Glycopyrrolate Tablets, 2 mg.	U: DAN L: 5494
5050	Hydralazine HCl. Tablets, 25 mg.	U: DAN L: 5050
5055	Hydralazine HCl. Tablets, 50 mg.	U: DAN L: 5055
5428	Hydrochlorothiazide, Hydralazine HCl., Reserpine Tablets, 15 mg., 25 mg. 0.1 mg.	U: DAN L: 5428
5406	Hydrochlorothiazide/Reserpine Tablets, 25 mg./0.125 mg.	U: DAN L: 5406
5407	Hydrochlorothiazide/Reserpine Tablets 50 mg./0.125 mg.	U: DAN L: 5407
5345	Hydrochlorothiazide Tablets, 50 mg.	U: DAN L: 5345
5183	Hydrocortisone Tablets, 20 mg.	U: DAN L: 5183
5532	Hydroxyzine Pamoate Capsules (Equivalent to 50 mg. Hydroxyzine HCl.)	DAN/ 5532
5537	Hydroxyzine Pamoate Capsules (Equivalent to 100 mg. Hydroxyzine HCl.)	DAN/ 5537
0528	Isoniazid Tablets, 50 mg.	U: DAN L: 528
0525	Isoniazid Tablets, 100 mg.	U: DAN L: 525
0526	Isoniazid Tablets, 300 mg.	U: DAN L: 526
5374	Isosorbide Dinitrate Oral Tablets, 5 mg.	U: DAN L: 5374
5373	Isosorbide Dinitrate Oral Tablets, 10 mg.	U: DAN L: 5373
5387	Isosorbide Dinitrate Sublingual Tablets, 2.5 mg.	U: DAN L: 5387
5385	Isosorbide Dinitrate Sublingual Tablets, 5 mg.	U: DAN L: 5385
5400	Isoxsuprine HCl. Tablets, 10 mg.	U: 10 L: DAN/ 5400
5401	Isoxsuprine HCl. Tablets, 20 mg.	U: 20 L: DAN/ 5401
5381	Methocarbamol Tablets, 500 mg.	U: DAN L: 5381
5382	Methocarbamol Tablets, 750 mg.	U: DAN L: 5382
5540	Metronidazole Tablets, 250 mg.	U: DAN L: 5540
5552	Metronidazole Tablets, 500 mg.	U: DAN L: 5552
5342	Nylidrin HCl. Tablets, 6 mg.	U: DAN L: 5342
5390	Nylidrin HCl. Tablets, 12 mg.	U: DAN L: 5390
0938	Papaverine HCl. Tablets, 100 mg.	U: DAN L: 938
5196	Papaverine HCl. T.D. Capsules, 150 mg.	DAN/ 5196
5521	Phenylbutazone Tablets, 100 mg.	U: DAN L: 5521
5059	Prednisolone Tablets, 5 mg.	U: DAN L: 5059
5052	Prednisone Tablets, 5 mg.	U: DAN L: 5052
5442	Prednisone Tablets, 10 mg.	U: DAN L: 5442
5443	Prednisone Tablets, 20 mg.	U: DAN L: 5443
5490	Prednisone Tablets, 50 mg.	U: DAN L: 5490
5321	Primidone Tablets, 250 mg.	U: DAN L: 5321
5347	Probenecid Tablets, 500 mg.	U: DAN L: 5347
5026	Procainamide HCl. Capsules, 250 mg.	DAN/ 5026
5350	Procainamide HCl. Capsules, 375 mg.	DAN/ 5350
5333	Procainamide HCl. Capsules, 500 mg.	DAN/ 5333
5257	Propantheline Bromide Tablets, 15 mg.	DAN/ 5257
5204	Pseudoephedrine HCl. Tablets, 60 mg.	U: DAN L: 5204
5516	Quindan Tablets (Quinine Sulfate Tablets, 260 mg.)	U: DAN L: 5516
5538	Quinidine Gluconate Sustained Action Tablets, 324 mg.	U: DAN L: 5538
5453	Quinidine Sulfate Tablets, 100 mg.	U: DAN L: 5453
5438	Quinidine Sulfate Tablets, 200 mg.	U: DAN L: 5438
5454	Quinidine Sulfate Tablets, 300 mg.	U: DAN L: 5454
5496	Spironolactone/Hydrochlorothiazide Tablets	U: DAN L: 5496
5503	Sulfasalazine Tablets, 500 mg.	DAN/ 5503
5514	Sulfinpyrazone Tablets, 100 mg.	U: DAN L: 5514
5162	Tetracycline HCl. Capsules, 250 mg.	DAN/ 5162
5520	Tetracycline HCl. Capsules, 500 mg.	DAN/ 5520
5481	Theofedral Tablets	U: DAN L: 5481
5508	Tolbutamide Tablets, 500 mg.	U: DAN L: 5508
5388	Triamcinolone Tablets, 4 mg.	U: DAN L: 5388
5335	Trihexyphenidyl HCl. Tablets, 2 mg.	U: DAN L: 5335
5337	Trihexyphenidyl HCl. Tablets, 5 mg.	U: DAN L: 5337
5058	Tripelennamine HCl. Tablets, 50 mg.	U: DAN L: 5058
5434	Tripodrine Tablets	U: DAN L: 5434

CONTROLLED SUBSTANCE PRODUCTS

NDC#	SCHEDULE#	PRODUCT	IMPRINT
5238	C-IV	Meprobamate Tablets, 400 mg.	591-A
5239	C-IV	Meprobamate Tablets, 200 mg.	591-B
5069	C-IV	Phenobarbital Tablets, 1/4 gr.	591-C
5180	C-IV	Phenobarbital Tablets, 1/2 gr.	591-D
5073	C-IV	Phenobarbital Tablets, 1/8 gr.	591-E
5519	C-III	Butalbital with Acetaminophen Tablets	591-F

Continued on next page

Danbury—Cont.

5366	C-III	Glutethimide Tablets, 500 mg.	591-J
5346	C-IV	Phenobarbital Tablets, $1\frac{1}{2}$ gr.	591-O
5476	C-IV	Phenobarbital Tablets, 30 mg.	591-T
5478	C-IV	Phenobarbital Tablets, 60 mg.	591-V

Delmont Laboratories, Inc.

P.O. BOX AA
SWARTHMORE, PA 19081

STAPHAGE LYSATE (SPL)™
BACTERIAL ANTIGEN MADE FROM STAPHYLOCOCCUS

Description: STAPHAGE LYSATE (SPL)™ is a whole culture vaccine, in solution, of two strains of lysed *Staphylococcus aureus,* Serologic Types I & III, specially selected for their broad antigenic spectrum.
How Supplied: 1-ml ampules, boxes of 10 (NDC 48532-0299-2), for subcutaneous and aerosol use; 10-ml multiple-dose vials (NDC 48532-0299-1) for aerosol, topical, and oral use.
For complete prescribing information and literature, please write, or call (215) 543-3365.

Dermik Laboratories, Inc.

1777 WALTON ROAD
DUBLIN HALL
BLUE BELL, PA 19422

ANTHRA-DERM® Ointment ℞
(anthralin) 1%, ½%, ¼%, $\frac{1}{10}$%
FOR TOPICAL USE ONLY

Description: Each gram of Anthra-Derm® (anthralin) Ointment 0.1%, 0.25%, 0.5% and 1.0% contains 1 mg, 2.5 mg, 5 mg and 10 mg, respectively of anthralin in a base consisting of mineral oil and white petrolatum. Anthralin is an anti-psoriatic agent with cytostatic, irritant and weak antimicrobial properties.
Clinical Pharmacology: Although the exact mechanism of anthralin's activity is unknown, there is experimental evidence that anthralin binds DNA, inhibiting synthesis of nucleic protein, and thus reduces mitotic activity.
Absorption in man has not been determined. However, based on a study in piglets it would appear to be quite low.
Indications and Usage: For the topical treatment of psoriasis.
Contraindications: Anthra-Derm® (anthralin) Ointment is contraindicated in patients with acute psoriasis or where inflammation is present, and in those patients with a history of hypersensitivity to any of the ingredients.
Warnings: Although no renal, hepatic or hematologic abnormalities have been reported as a result of topical application of Anthra-Derm® (anthralin) Ointment, caution is advised in patients with renal disease. Patients with renal disease and those having extensive and prolonged applications should have periodic urine tests for albuminuria. Discontinue use if sensitivity reactions occur.
Precautions: General: When redness is observed on adjacent normal skin, reduce frequency of application. For external use only. Do not apply to face, genitalia or intertriginous areas. Wash area thoroughly and carefully after using. Keep out of the reach of children. Anthralin is a tumor-promoting agent in 2-stage carcinogenesis on mouse skin. However, there have not been any reports of such effects in humans at the usual dosages.
Pregnancy: Pregnancy Category C. Animal reproduction studies have not been conducted with anthralin. It is also not known whether anthralin can cause fetal harm when administered to a pregnant woman or can affect reproduction capacity. Anthra-Derm® Ointment should be given to a pregnant woman only if clearly needed.
Nursing mothers: It is not known whether this drug is excreted in human milk. Because many drugs are excreted in milk and because of the potential for tumorigenicity shown for anthralin in animal studies, a decision should be made whether to discontinue nursing or to discontinue the drug, taking into account the importance of the drug to the mother.
Pediatric use: Safety and effectiveness in children have not been established.
Adverse Reactions: Irritation of normal skin is the most frequently reported adverse reaction. Anthra-Derm® may, temporarily, stain skin and hair.
Dosage and Administration: The usual dosage regimen begins with the lowest concentration (0.1%) and is gradually increased until the desired effect is obtained. Apply in a thin layer to affected areas once or twice daily, or as directed by a physician.
How Supplied: Anthra-Derm® (anthralin) Ointment 0.1%, 0.25%, 0.5% and 1.0% is available in 1.5 oz (42.5 g) tubes.
Caution: Federal law prohibits dispensing without a prescription.

5 BENZAGEL® MICROGEL™
(5% benzoyl peroxide) and
10 BENZAGEL® FORMULA
(10% benzoyl peroxide)
Acne Gels

Description: Each gram of 5 Benzagel® and 10 Benzagel® contains 50 mg and 100 mg respectively, of benzoyl peroxide in a gel vehicle of purified water, carbomer 940, sodium hydroxide, dioctyl sodium sulfosuccinate, alkyl polyglycol ether, fragrance and alcohol 14%. Benzoyl peroxide is an antibacterial and keratolytic agent.
Clinical Pharmacology: Benzoyl peroxide is an antibacterial agent which has been shown to be effective against *Propionibacterium* acnes. This action is believed to be responsible for its usefulness in acne. One study in the rhesus monkey demonstrated a percutaneous absorption of about 1.8 μg per cm² of benzoyl peroxide or 45% of the applied dose in a 24-hour period. The absorbed benzoyl peroxide was completely converted in the skin to benzoic acid.
Indication and Usage: 5 & 10 Benzagel® may be used alone topically for mild to moderate acne and as an adjunct in acne treatment regimens which might include retinoic acid products, systemic antibiotics, and/or sulfur and salicylic acid containing preparations. The active ingredient, benzoyl peroxide, exerts a desquamative and antibacterial action. It provides mild peeling and keratolytic activity.
Contraindications: Benzagel® should not be used by patients having known sensitivity to benzoyl peroxide or any of its components.
Warnings: If itching, redness, burning, swelling or undue dryness occurs, discontinue use.
Precautions: For external use only. Not for ophthalmic use. Keep away from eyes and mucosae. Very fair individuals should begin with a single application at bedtime allowing overnight medication. May bleach colored fabrics. Keep this and all medications out of the reach of children.
Carcinogenesis, Mutagenesis and Impairment of Fertility—Long-term studies in animals have not been performed to evaluate carcinogenic potential.
Pregnancy Category C—Animal reproduction studies have not been conducted with benzoyl peroxide. It is also not known whether benzoyl peroxide can cause fetal harm when administered to a pregnant woman or can affect reproduction capacity. Benzoyl peroxide should be given to a pregnant woman only if clearly needed.
Nursing Mothers—It is not known whether this drug is excreted in human milk. Because many drugs are excreted in human milk, caution should be exercised when benzoyl peroxide is administered to a nursing woman.
Pediatric Use: Safety and effectiveness in children under the age of 12 have not been established.
Adverse Reactions: Irritation and contact dermatitis are the most frequent side reactions to benzoyl peroxide.
Dosage and Administration: Wash and dry affected areas prior to application. Apply sparingly one or more times daily.
How Supplied: 5 & 10 Benzagel® are available in 1.5 oz (42.5 g) and 3 oz (85 g) plastic tubes; 5 Benzagel® contains 50 mg benzoyl peroxide per gram and 10 Benzagel® contains 100 mg benzoyl peroxide per gram.
Caution: Federal law prohibits dispensing without prescription.

HYTONE® Cream, Lotion and Ointment ℞
(hydrocortisone)

Description: *Cream*—Each gram of 1% and 2½% Cream contains 10 mg or 25 mg, respectively, of hydrocortisone in a water-washable base of purified water, propylene glycol, glyceryl monostearate SE, cholesterol and related sterols, isopropyl myristate, polysorbate 60, cetyl alcohol, sorbitan monostearate, polyoxyl 40 stearate and sorbic acid.
Lotion—Each ml of 1% and 2½% Lotion contains 10 mg or 25 mg, respectively, of hydrocortisone in a vehicle consisting of carbomer 940, propylene glycol, polysorbate 40, propylene glycol stearate, cholesterol and related sterols, isopropyl myristate, sorbitan palmitate, cetyl alcohol, triethanolamine, sorbic acid, simethicone and purified water.
Ointment—Each gram of 1% and 2½% contains 10 mg or 25 mg, respectively, of hydrocortisone in a topical emollient base of mineral oil, white petrolatum and sorbitan sesquioleate.
Chemically, hydrocortisone is 11, 17, 21-trihydroxypregn-4-ene 3, 20-dione ($C_{21}H_{30}O_5$) and is represented by the following structural formula:

Its molecular weight is 362.47 and its CAS Registry Number is 50-23-7. The topical corticosteroids including hydrocortisone, constitute a class of primarily synthetic steroids used as anti-inflammatory and antipruritic agents.
Clinical Pharmacology: Topical corticosteroids share anti-inflammatory, antipruritic and vasoconstrictive actions. The mechanism of anti-inflammatory activity of the topical corticosteroids is unclear. Various laboratory methods, including vasoconstrictor assays, are used to compare and predict potencies and/or clinical efficacies of the topical corticosteroids. There is some evidence to suggest that a recognizable correlation exists between vasoconstrictor potency and therapeutic efficacy in man.

Pharmacokinetics

The extent of percutaneous absorption of topical corticosteroids is determined by many factors including the vehicle, the integrity of the epidermal barrier, and the use of occlusive dressings.
Topical corticosteroids can be absorbed from normal intact skin. Inflammation and/or other disease processes in the skin increase

percutaneous absorption. Occlusive dressings substantially increase the percutaneous absorption of topical corticosteroids. Thus, occlusive dressings may be a valuable therapeutic adjunct for treatment of resistant dermatoses. (See *DOSAGE AND ADMINISTRATION.*)

Once absorbed through the skin, topical corticosteroids are handled through pharmacokinetic pathways similar to systemically administered corticosteroids. Corticosteroids are bound to plasma proteins in varying degrees. Corticosteroids are metabolized primarily in the liver and are then excreted by the kidneys. Some of the topical corticosteroids and their metabolites are also excreted into the bile.

Indications and Usage: Topical corticosteroids are indicated for the relief of the inflammatory and pruritic manifestations of corticosteroid-responsive dermatoses.

Contraindications: Topical corticosteroids are contraindicated in those patients with a history of hypersensitivity to any of the components of the preparation.

Precautions:

General—Systemic absorption of topical corticosteroids has produced reversible hypothalamic-pituitary-adrenal (HPA) axis suppression, manifestations of Cushing's syndrome, hyperglycemia, and glucosuria in some patients.

Conditions which augment systemic absorption include the application of the more potent steroids, use over large surface areas, prolonged use, and the addition of occlusive dressings.

Therefore, patients receiving a large dose of a potent topical steroid applied to a large surface area or under an occlusive dressing should be evaluated periodically for evidence of HPA axis suppression by using the urinary free cortisol and ACTH stimulation tests. If HPA axis suppression is noted, an attempt should be made to withdraw the drug, to reduce the frequency of application, or to substitute a less potent steroid.

Recovery of HPA axis function is generally prompt and complete upon discontinuation of the drug. Infrequently, signs and symptoms of steroid withdrawal may occur, requiring supplemental systemic corticosteroids.

Children may absorb proportionally larger amounts of topical corticosteroids and thus be more susceptible to systemic toxicity (See PRECAUTIONS—Pediatric Use).

If irritation develops, topical corticosteroids should be discontinued and appropriate therapy instituted.

In the presence of dermatological infections, the use of an appropriate antifungal or antibacterial agent should be instituted. If a favorable response does not occur promptly, the corticosteroid should be discontinued until the infection has been adequately controlled.

Information for the Patient—Patients using topical corticosteroids should receive the following information and instructions:

1. This medication is to be used as directed by the physician. It is for external use only. Avoid contact with the eyes.
2. Patients should be advised not to use this medication for any disorder other than for which it was prescribed.
3. The treated skin area should not be bandaged or otherwise covered or wrapped as to be occlusive unless directed by the physician.
4. Patients should report any signs of local adverse reactions, especially under occlusive dressing.
5. Parents of pediatric patients should be advised not to use tight-fitting diapers or plastic pants on a child being treated in the diaper area, as these garments may constitute occlusive dressings.

Laboratory Tests—The following tests may be helpful in evaluating the HPA axis suppression:

Urinary free cortisol test
ACTH stimulation test

Carcinogenesis, Mutagenesis, and Impairment of Fertility—Long-term animal studies have not been performed to evaluate the carcinogenic potential or the effect on fertility of topical corticosteroids.

Studies to determine mutagenicity with prednisolone and hydrocortisone have revealed negative results.

Pregnancy Category C—Corticosteroids are generally teratogenic in laboratory animals when administered systemically at relatively low dosage levels. The more potent corticosteroids have been shown to be teratogenic after dermal application in laboratory animals. There are no adequate and well-controlled studies in pregnant women on teratogenic effects from topically applied corticosteroids. Therefore, topical corticosteroids should be used during pregnancy only if the potential benefit justifies the potential risk to the fetus. Drugs of this class should not be used extensively on pregnant patients, in large amounts, or for prolonged periods of time.

Nursing Mothers—It is not known whether topical administration of corticosteroids could result in sufficient systemic absorption to produce detectable quantities in breast milk. Systemically administered corticosteroids are secreted into breast milk in quantities *not* likely to have a deleterious effect on the infant. Nevertheless, caution should be exercised when topical corticosteroids are administered to a nursing woman.

Pediatric Use—**Pediatric patients may demonstrate greater susceptibility to topical corticosteroid-induced HPA axis suppression and Cushing's syndrome than mature patients because of a larger skin surface area to body weight ratio.**

Hypothalamic-pituitary-adrenal (HPA) axis suppression, Cushing's syndrome, and intracranial hypertension have been reported in children receiving topical corticosteroids. Manifestations of adrenal suppression in children include linear growth retardation, delayed weight gain, low plasma cortisol levels, and absence of response to ACTH stimulation. Manifestations of intracranial hypertension include bulging fontanelles, headaches, and bilateral papilledema.

Administration of topical corticosteroids to children should be limited to the least amount compatible with an effective therapeutic regimen. Chronic corticosteroid therapy may interfere with the growth and development of children.

Adverse Reactions: The following local adverse reactions are reported infrequently with topical corticosteroids, but may occur more frequently with the use of occlusive dressings. These reactions are listed in an approximate decreasing order of occurrence:

Burning	Perioral dermatitis
Itching	Allergic contact dermatitis
Irritation	Maceration of the skin
Dryness	Secondary infection
Folliculitis	Skin atrophy
Hypertrichosis	Striae
Acneiform eruptions	Miliaria
Hypopigmentation	

Overdosage: Topically applied corticosteroids can be absorbed in sufficient amounts to produce systemic effects (See PRECAUTIONS).

Dosage and Administration: Topical corticosteroids are generally applied to the affected area as a thin film from two to four times daily depending on the severity of the condition. Occlusive dressings may be used for the management of psoriasis or recalcitrant conditions.

If an infection develops, the use of occlusive dressings should be discontinued and appropriate antimicrobial therapy instituted.

How Supplied: *Cream*—2½% - tube 1 oz NDC 0066-0095-01; 1% - tube 1 oz NDC 0066-0083-01 and jar 4 oz NDC 0066-0083-04; ½% - jar 4 oz NDC 0066-0082-04 and tube 1 oz (OTC) NDC 0066-0082-01.

Lotion—2½% - bottle 2 oz NDC 0066-0098-02; 1% - bottle 4 oz NDC 0066-0090-04.

Ointment—2 ½% - tube 1 oz NDC 0066-0085-01; 1% - tube 1 oz NDC 0066-0087-01 and jar 4 oz NDC 0066-0087-04; ½% (OTC) - tube 1 oz NDC 0066-0086-01.

Caution: Federal law prohibits dispensing without prescription

SULFACET-R® Acne Lotion ℞
(sodium sulfacetamide 10% and sulfur 5%)

Description: Each gram of Sulfacet-R® Acne Lotion (sodium sulfacetamide 10% and sulfur 5%) as dispensed, contains 100 mg of sodium sulfacetamide and 50 mg of sulfur in a flesh-tinted lotion of purified water, alkylaryl sulfonic acid salts, hydroxyethylcellulose, propylene glycol, xanthan gum, lauric myristic diethanolamide, polyoxyethylene laurate, butylparaben, methylparaben, silicone emulsion, talc, zinc oxide, titanium dioxide, attapulgite, iron oxides, pH buffers and 2-bromo-2-nitropropane-1, 3 diol.

Sodium sulfacetamide is a sulfonamide with antibacterial activity while sulfur acts as a keratolytic agent. Chemically sodium sulfacetamide is N'-[(4-aminophenyl)sulfonyl]-acetamide, monosodium salt, monohydrate.

Clinical Pharmacology: The most widely accepted mechanism of action of sulfonamides is the Woods-Fildes theory which is based on the fact that sulfonamides act as competitive antagonists to para-aminobenzoic acid (PABA), an essential component for bacterial growth. While absorption through intact skin has not been determined, sodium sulfacetamide is readily absorbed from the gastrointestinal tract when taken orally and excreted in the urine, largely unchanged. The biological half-life has variously been reported as 7 to 12.8 hours.

The exact mode of action of sulfur in the treatment of acne is unknown, but it has been reported that it inhibits the growth of p. acnes and the formation of free fatty acids.

Indications: Sulfacet-R® is indicated in the topical control of acne vulgaris, acne rosacea and seborrheic dermatitis.

Contraindications: Sulfacet-R® Acne Lotion is contraindicated for use by patients having known hypersensitivity to sulfonamides, sulfur, or any other component of this preparation. Sulfacet-R® Acne Lotion is not to be used by patients with kidney disease.

Warnings: Although rare, sensitivity to sodium sulfacetamide may occur. Therefore, caution and careful supervision should be observed when prescribing this drug for patients who may be prone to hypersensitivity to topical sulfonamides. Systemic toxic reactions such as agranulocytosis, acute hemolytic anemia, purpura hemorrhagica, drug fever, jaundice, and contact dermatitis indicate hypersensitivity to sulfonamides. Particular caution should be employed if areas of denuded or abraded skin are involved.

Precautions: General—if irritation develops, use of the product should be discontinued and appropriate therapy instituted. For external use only. Keep away from eyes. Patients should be carefully observed for possible local irritation or sensitization during long-term therapy. The object of this therapy is to achieve desquamation without irritation, but sodium sulfacetamide and sulfur can cause reddening and scaling of epidermis. These side effects are not unusual in the treatment of acne vulgaris, but patients should be cautioned about the possibility. Keep out of the reach of children.

Continued on next page

Dermik—Cont.

Carcinogenesis, Mutagenesis and Impairment of Fertility—Long-term studies in animals have not been performed to evaluate carcinogenic potential.
Pregnancy—Pregnancy Category C. Animal reproduction studies have not been conducted with Sulfacet-R® Acne Lotion. It is also not known whether Sulfacet-R® Acne Lotion can cause fetal harm when administered to a pregnant woman or can affect reproduction capacity. Sulfacet-R® Acne Lotion should be given to a pregnant woman only if clearly needed.
Nursing Mothers—It is not known whether sodium sulfacetamide is excreted in the human milk following topical use of Sulfacet-R® Acne Lotion. However, small amounts of orally administered sulfonamides have been reported to be eliminated in human milk. In view of this and because many drugs are excreted in human milk, caution should be exercised when Sulfacet-R® Acne Lotion is administered to a nursing woman.
Pediatric Use—Safety and effectiveness in children under the age of 12 have not been established.
Adverse Reactions: Although rare, sodium sulfacetamide may cause local irritation.
Dosage and Administration: Shake well before using. Apply a thin film to affected areas with light massaging to blend in each application 1 to 3 times daily. Each package contains a Dermik Color Blender™ which enables the patient to alter the basic shade of the lotion so that it matches the skin color exactly.
(Important to the Pharmacist—At the time of dispensing, add contents of vial* to the bottle. Shake well and/or stir with a glass rod to insure uniform dispersion. Place expiration date of four (4) months on bottle label.)
*Sulfa-Pak™ vial contains 2.4 grams of sodium sulfacetamide.
How Supplied: 1 oz (28.35 g) bottles
Caution: Federal law prohibits dispensing without prescription.

VANOXIDE-HC® Acne Lotion ℞
(Clear)
LOROXIDE-HC® Acne Lotion ℞
(Flesh-Tinted)

Description: Each gram of Vanoxide-HC® Lotion contains, as dispensed, 50 mg benzoyl peroxide, and 5 mg hydrocortisone. Each gram of Loroxide-HC® Lotion contains as dispensed, 55 mg benzoyl peroxide, and 5 mg hydrocortisone. Each is incorporated in a water washable lotion of purified water, calcium phosphate, propylene glycol, caprylic/capric triglyceride, propylene glycol monostearate, laneth-10 acetate, decyl oleate, polysorbate 20, cetyl alcohol, mineral oil, lanolin alcohol, sodium phosphate, sodium biphosphate, stearyl heptanoate, hydroxyethylcellulose, tetrasodium EDTA, cyclohexanediamine tetraacetic acid, propylparaben, methylparaben, vegetable oil, monoglyceride citrate, simethicone, BHT, sodium hydroxide, BHA, propyl gallate, FD&C colors. Loroxide-HC® Lotion contains a caramel color in place of FD&C color and in addition to the foregoing, its lotion contains kaolin, talc and titanium dioxide.
Clinical Pharmacology: Benzoyl peroxide is an antibacterial agent which has been shown to be effective against *Propionibacterium acnes.* This action is believed to be largely responsible for its usefulness. In addition, benzoyl peroxide exerts a desquamative and keratolytic action. One study in the rhesus monkey demonstrated a percutaneous absorption of about 1.8 μg per cm^2 of benzoyl peroxide or 45% of the applied dose in a 24-hour period. The absorbed benzoyl peroxide was completely converted in the skin to benzoic acid.
Topical steroids are primarily effective because of their anti-inflammatory, antipruritic and vasoconstrictive actions.
Indications and Usage: Treatment of acne vulgaris and oily skin.
Contraindications: Vanoxide-HC® Lotion and Loroxide-HC® Lotion are contraindicated in individuals having known sensitivity to benzoyl peroxide, hydrocortisone or any of the components of the product. Topical steroids are contraindicated in viral diseases of the skin, such as varicella or vaccinia.
Warnings: If itching, redness, swelling or undue dryness occurs, discontinue use.
Precautions: For external use only. Keep away from the eyes and mucosae. Very fair individuals should begin with a single application at bedtime allowing overnight medication. May bleach colored fabrics.
Carcinogenesis, Mutagenesis, Impairment of Fertility—Long-term studies in animals have not been performed to evaluate carcinogenic potential.
Pregnancy, Category C—Animal reproduction studies have not been conducted with either Vanoxide-HC® Lotion or Loroxide-HC® Lotion. It is not known whether Vanoxide-HC® Lotion or Loroxide-HC® can cause fetal harm when administered to a pregnant woman or can affect reproduction capacity. Vanoxide-HC® Lotion and Loroxide-HC® Lotion should be given to a pregnant woman only if clearly needed.
Nursing Mothers—It is not known whether these drugs are excreted in human milk. Because many drugs are excreted in human milk, caution should be exercised when Vanoxide-HC® Lotion and Loroxide-HC® Lotion are administered to a nursing woman.
Pediatric Use—Safety and effectiveness in children under the age of 12 have not been established.
Adverse Reactions: Irritation and contact dermatitis are the most frequent side reactions to benzoyl peroxide. Although 0.5% hydrocortisone is considered safe, the following adverse reactions have been reported with topical corticosteroids, especially under occlusive dressings: burning, itching, irritation, dryness, folliculitis, hypertrichosis, acneform eruptions, hypopigmentation, perioral dermatitis, allergic contact dermatitis, maceration of the skin, secondary infection, skin atrophy, striae, miliaria.
Dosage and Administration: Shake well before using. Apply a thin film 1 to 3 times daily with gentle massaging to blend with skin, or as directed by physician.
How Supplied: Bottles, 25 grams net weight as dispensed. Package contains a bottle of lotion base and a Benzie-Pak™ vial containing a mixture of benzoyl peroxide, 35%, and calcium phosphate, 65%. Net weight of vial is 3.8 grams. A Dermik Color Blender™ is also provided with Loroxide-HC® Lotion which enables the patient to alter the basic shade of the lotion to match the skin color.
To the Pharmacist—At the time of dispensing, add contents of Benzie-Pak™ to the lotion in the bottle. Shake well and/or stir with glass rod to ensure uniform dispersion. Place expiration date of three (3) months on bottle label.
Caution: Federal law prohibits dispensing without prescription.

VLEMASQUE®
(6% sulfurated lime solution)

Description: Contains sulfurated lime solution 6%, S.D. alcohol 7% in a drying clay mask.
Indication: For the treatment of acne.
Directions: Daily, apply generous layer over entire face and neck, or as directed by physician. Avoid eyes, nostrils and lips. Leave on for 20-25 minutes. Remove with lukewarm water, using a gentle circular motion. Pat dry.
Warnings: Keep away from eyes. In case of contact, flush eyes thoroughly. For external use only. If any irritation appears, stop treatment immediately and consult physician.
How Supplied: 4 oz. jars

VYTONE® CREAM
(hydrocortisone-iodoquinol)

Description: Each gram of Vytone® Cream 0.5% and 1% contains 5 mg or 10 mg of hydrocortisone, respectively, and 10 mg of iodoquinol in a greaseless base of purified water, propylene glycol, glyceryl monostearate SE, cholesterol and related sterols, isopropyl myristate, polysorbate 60, cetyl alcohol, sorbitan monostearate, polyoxyl 40 stearate, sorbic acid, and polysorbate 20.
Chemically, hydrocortisone is 11, 17, 21-trihydroxypregn-4-ene-3, 20-dione ($C_{21}H_{30}O_5$) and is represented by the following structural formula:

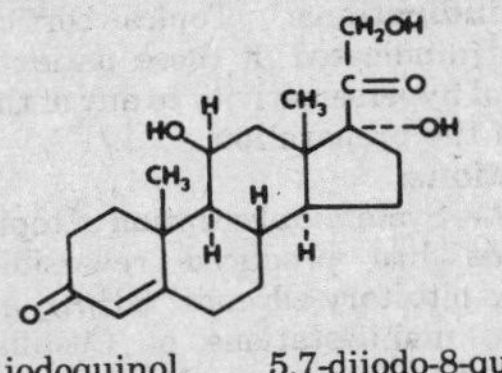

and iodoquinol, 5,7-diiodo-8-quinolinol ($C_9H_5I_2NO$) is represented by the following structure.

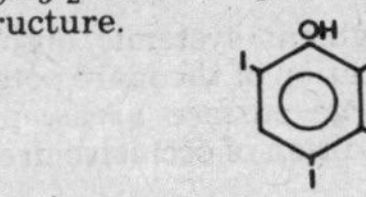

Hydrocortisone is an anti-inflammatory and antipruritic agent, while iodoquinol is an antifungal and antibacterial agent.
Clinical Pharmacology: Hydrocortisone has anti-inflammatory, antipruritic and vasoconstrictor properties. The mechanism of anti-inflammatory activity is unclear. There is some evidence to suggest that a recognizable correlation exists between vasoconstrictor potency and therapeutic efficacy in man.
Iodoquinol has both antifungal and antibacterial properties.
Pharmacokinetics
The extent of percutaneous absorption of topical corticosteroids is determined by many factors including vehicle, the integrity of the epidermal barrier, and the use of occlusive dressings.
Hydrocortisone can be absorbed from normal intact skin. Inflammation and/or other inflammatory disease processes in the skin increase percutaneous absorption. Occlusive dressings substantially increase the percutaneous absorption of topical corticosteroids.
Once absorbed through the skin, hydrocortisone is metabolized in the liver and most body tissues to hydrogenated and degraded forms such as tetrahydrocortisone and tetrahydrocortisol. These are excreted in the urine, mainly conjugated as glucuronides, together with a very small proportion of unchanged hydrocortisone.
There are no data available regarding the percutaneous absorption of iodoquinol; however, following oral administration, 3–5% of the dose was recovered in the urine as a glucuronide.

Indications and Usage: Based on a review of a related drug by the National Research Council and subsequent FDA classification for that drug, the indications are as follows:
"Possibly" Effective: Contact or atopic dermatitis; impetiginized eczema; nummular eczema; infantile eczema; endogenous chronic infectious dermatitis; stasis dermatitis; pyoderma; nuchal eczema and chronic eczematoid otitis externa; acne urticata; localized or disseminated neurodermatitis; lichen simplex chronicus; ano-

genital pruritus (vulvae, scroti, ani); folliculitis, bacterial dermatoses; mycotic dermatoses such as tinea (capitis, cruris, corporis, pedis); moniliasis, intertrigo. Final classification of the less-than-effective indications requires further investigation.

Contraindications: Vytone® Cream is contraindicated in those patients with a history of hypersensitivity to hydrocortisone, iodoquinol or any other components of the preparation.
Warnings and Precautions: For external use only. Keep away from eyes. If irritation develops, the use of Vytone® Cream should be discontinued and appropriate therapy instituted. Staining of the skin and fabrics may occur. If extensive areas are treated or if the occlusive technique is used, the possibility exists of increased systemic absorption of the corticosteroid, and suitable precautions should be taken. Children may absorb proportionally larger amounts of topical corticosteroids and thus be more susceptible to systemic toxicity. Parents of pediatric patients should be advised not to use tight-fitting diapers or plastic pants on a child being treated in the diaper area, as these garments may constitute occlusive dressings. Iodoquinol may be absorbed through the skin and interfere with thyroid function tests. If such tests are contemplated, wait at least one month after discontinuance of therapy to perform these tests. The ferric chloride test for phenylketonuria (PKU) can yield a false positive result if iodoquinol is present in the diaper or urine.
Prolonged use may result in overgrowth of non-susceptible organisms requiring appropriate therapy. Keep out of reach of children.
Carcinogenesis, Mutagenesis and Impairment of Fertility: Long-term animal studies have not been performed to evaluate the carcinogenic potential or the effect on fertility of hydrocortisone or iodoquinol.
In vitro studies to determine mutagenicity with hydrocortisone have revealed negative results. Mutagenicity studies have not been conducted with iodoquinol.
Pregnancy Category C: Animal reproductive studies have not been conducted with Vytone® Cream. It is not known whether Vytone® Cream can cause fetal harm when administered to a pregnant woman or can affect reproductive capacity. Vytone® Cream should be given to a pregnant woman only if clearly needed.
Nursing Mothers: It is not known whether this drug is excreted in human milk. Because many drugs are excreted in human milk, caution should be exercised when Vytone® Cream is administered to a nursing woman.
Pediatric Use: Safety and effectiveness in children under the age of 12 have not been established.
Adverse Reactions: The following local adverse reactions are reported infrequently with topical corticosteroids. These reactions are listed in an approximate decreasing order of occurrence.

Burning	Perioral dermatitis
Itching	Allergic contact dermatitis
Irritation	Maceration of the skin
Dryness	Secondary infection
Folliculitis	Skin atrophy
Hypertrichosis	Striae
Acneiform eruptions	Miliaria
Hypopigmentation	

Dosage and Administration: Apply to affected area 3 to 4 times daily in accordance with physician's directions.
How Supplied:
½%-Tube 1 oz NDC 0066-0049-01,
1%-Tube 1 oz NDC 0066-0051-01
Caution: Federal law prohibits dispensing without prescription.

ZETAR® EMULSION (Coal Tar) ℞

Description: Zetar® Emulsion, coal tar, is a liquid for topical application, following dilution in aqueous media. Each ml contains 300 mg whole coal tar in polysorbates. It is a topical anti-eczematic. The complete chemical composition of coal tar has not been ascertained; components are grouped into six categories: aromatic hydrocarbons, acidic phenolic compounds, cyclic nitrogen compounds, organic sulfur compounds, nonacidic phenolics and nonbasic nitrogen compounds.
Clinical Pharmacology: There is no confirmed scientific evidence as to the clinical pharmacologic effects of coal tar. Its actions in humans have been reported in the literature as antiseptic, antipruritic, antiparasitic, antifungal, antibacterial, keratoplastic and antiacanthotic. Vasoconstrictive activity of coal tar has also been reported.
Indications and Usage: Zetar® Emulsion is indicated for the relief of symptoms associated with generalized, persistent dermatoses such as psoriasis, eczema, atopic dermatitis and seborrheic dermatitis.
Contraindications: Not to be used on open or infected lesions.
Warnings: Application of coal tar may elicit a pustular eruption or a cyst (epidermal) like reaction.
Patients who have previously exhibited sensitivity to tars must be under careful and continuous supervision by the physician.
Precautions: For external (topical) use only. Keep away from the eyes. When used in the bath, add lukewarm water (not hot water). For 72 hours following treatment with coal tar, patients should avoid exposure to either direct sunlight or sunlamps (ultra-violet A and/or B) unless directed by physician, as this drug may photoactivate the skin. Prior to exposure to sunlight, completely remove all tar from skin. Sensitization or dermatitis may occur after prolonged use. If irritation develops or increases, discontinue use and consult physician. Keep out of the reach of children.
While no known drug interactions have been reported pertaining to the clinical use of this drug in patients, the concomitant use of drugs with phototoxic and/or photoactivating potential is not recommended (i.e. tetracyclines, psoralens, topical retinoic acid).
Carcinogenesis—Coal tar applied to the skin of mice resulted in an increase in epidermal carcinomas. Painting rabbit ears with coal tar appears to increase self-limiting keratoacanthomas. To date, existing reports do not suggest an increased incidence of skin cancer in psoriatics treated with coal tar.
Pregnancy Category C—Animal reproduction studies have not been conducted with Zetar® Emulsion (coal tar). It is also not known whether Zetar® Emulsion can cause fetal harm when administered to a pregnant woman or can affect reproduction capacity. Zetar® Emulsion should be given to a pregnant woman only if clearly needed.
Nursing Mothers—It is not known whether this drug is excreted in human milk. Because of the tumorigenicity shown for coal tar in animal studies, a decision should be made whether to discontinue nursing or to discontinue the drug, taking into account the importance of the drug to the mother.
Adverse Reactions: Application of coal tar may result in superficial folliculitis. Patients hypersensitive to coal tar may exhibit a pustular or keratocystic response.
Dosage and Administration: Add 3 to 5 teaspoonfuls of Zetar® Emulsion to a bath of lukewarm water. This is mixed throughout the bath. The patient immerses in the bath for 15 to 20 minutes. The interval recommended between dosing is from once-a-day to once every third day, and usual duration of treatment is 30 to 45 days.
If the physician decides to administer supplemental ultraviolet irradiation (Goeckerman treatment) to the patient (ultraviolet B; A or A/B), this may be accomplished between 2 and 72 hours. A determination of minimal erythemal dosage (MED) should be made for each patient; initial irradiation should be suberythemal, not to exceed MED.
Compounding: Zetar® Emulsion (coal tar) may be utilized in compounding prescriptions in aqueous based vehicles requiring coal tar. Each ml of Zetar® Emulsion contains 300 mg whole coal tar.
How Supplied: Zetar® Emulsion (coal tar) is available in 6 fl oz (177 ml) plastic bottles. The strength of the preparation is 300 mg coal tar/ml.
SHAKE WELL before each use. No special handling or storage conditions are required.
Caution: Federal law prohibits dispensing without prescription.

ZETAR® SHAMPOO

Description: WHOLE Coal Tar (as Zetar®) 1.0% in a golden foam shampoo which produces soft, fluffy abundant lather.
Actions and Indications: Antiseptic, antibacterial, antiseborrheic. Loosens and softens scales and crusts. Indicated in psoriasis, seborrhea, dandruff, cradle-cap and other oily, itchy conditions of the body and scalp.
Contraindications: Acute inflammation, open or infected lesions.
Precautions: If undue skin irritation develops or increases, discontinue use and consult physician. In rare instances, temporary discoloration of blond, bleached, or tinted hair may occur. Avoid contact with eyes.
Dosage and Administration: Massage into moistened scalp. Rinse. Repeat; leave on 5 minutes. Rinse thoroughly.
How Supplied: 6 oz. Plastic Bottles.

Dista Products Company

Division of Eli Lilly and Company
307 EAST McCARTY STREET
INDIANAPOLIS, IN 46285

LEGEND

Hyporets®—*Disposable Syringes, Dista*
Identi-Code®—*Formula Identification Code, Dista*
Identi-Dose®—*Unit Dose Medication, Dista*
Pulvules®—*Filled Gelatin Capsules, Dista*
℞Pak—*Prescription Package, Dista*
Traypak™—*Multivial Carton, Dista*

IDENTI-CODE® Index

Illustrations of examples of products bearing Identi-Code® appear in the Product Identification Section.

Identi-Code® Product Name

CO3-C22 (Coated Tablets)

CO3 Ilotycin®
Composition (Each Enteric-Coated Tablet): Erythromycin, USP, 250 mg

C19 Mi-Cebrin®
Composition (Each Coated Tablet): Thiamine (vitamin B_1), 10 mg; riboflavin (vitamin B_2), 5 mg; pyridoxine (vitamin B_6), 1.7 mg; pantothenic acid, 10 mg; niacinamide, 30 mg; vitamin B_{12}

Continued on next page

Dista—Cont.

(activity equivalent), 3 mcg; ascorbic acid (vitamin C), 100 mg; *dl*-alpha tocopheryl acetate (vitamin E), 5.5 IU (5.5 mg); vitamin A, 10,000 IU (3 mg); vitamin D, 400 IU (10 mcg); contains also (approximately): iron (as ferrous sulfate), 15 mg; copper (as the sulfate), 1 mg; iodine (as potassium iodide), 0.15 mg; manganese (as the glycerophosphate), 1 mg; magnesium (as the hydroxide), 5 mg; zinc (as the chloride), 1.5 mg

C20 Mi-Cebrin T®
Composition (Each Coated Tablet): Thiamine mononitrate (vitamin B_1), 15 mg; riboflavin (vitamin B_2), 10 mg; pyridoxine hydrochloride (vitamin B_6), 2 mg; pantothenic acid (as calcium pantothenate), 10 mg; niacinamide, 100 mg; vitamin B_{12} (activity equivalent), 7.5 mcg; ascorbic acid (vitamin C), 150 mg; *dl*-alpha tocopheryl acetate (vitamin E), 5.5 IU (5.5 mg); vitamin A, 10,000 IU (3 mg); vitamin D, 400 IU (10 mcg); contains also (approximately): iron (as ferrous sulfate), 15 mg; copper (as the sulfate), 1 mg; iodine (as potassium iodide), 0.15 mg; manganese (as the glycerophosphate), 1 mg; magnesium (as the hydroxide), 5 mg; zinc (as the chloride), 1.5 mg

C22 Becotin®-T
Composition (Each Coated Tablet): Thiamine mononitrate (vitamin B_1), 15 mg; riboflavin (vitamin B_2), 10 mg; pyridoxine hydrochloride (vitamin B_6), 5 mg; niacinamide, 100 mg; pantothenic acid (as calcium pantothenate), 20 mg; vitamin B_{12} (activity equivalent), 4 mcg; ascorbic acid (vitamin C) (as sodium ascorbate), 300 mg

F62-H77 (Pulvules®)

F62 Becotin®
Composition (Each Pulvule®): Thiamine hydrochloride (vitamin B_1), 10 mg; riboflavin (vitamin B_2), 10 mg; pyridoxine (vitamin B_6), 4.1 mg; niacinamide, 50 mg; pantothenic acid, 25 mg; vitamin B_{12} (activity equivalent), 1 mcg

F77 Becotin® with Vitamin C
Composition (Each Pulvule®): Thiamine hydrochloride (vitamin B_1), 10 mg; riboflavin (vitamin B_2), 10 mg; pyridoxine (vitamin B_6), 4.1 mg; niacinamide, 50 mg; pantothenic acid, 25 mg; vitamin B_{12} (activity equivalent), 1 mcg; ascorbic acid (vitamin C), 150 mg

3042 Co-Pyronil®, Pediatric
Composition (Each Pulvule®): pyrrobutamine phosphate, 7.5 mg; cyclopentamine hydrochloride, 6.25 mg

3043 Co-Pyronil®
Composition (Each Pulvule®): pyrrobutamine phosphate, 15 mg; cyclopentamine hydrochloride, 12.5 mg

3055 Cinobac®
Composition (Each Pulvule®): Cinoxacin, USP, 250 mg

3056 Cinobac®
Composition (Each Pulvule®): Cinoxacin, USP, 500 mg

H07 Ilosone®
Composition (Each Pulvule®): Erythromycin Estolate, USP, 125 mg (equiv. to erythromycin)

H09 Ilosone®
Composition (Each Pulvule®): Erythromycin Estolate, USP, 250 mg (equiv. to erythromycin)

H69 Keflex®
Composition (Each Pulvule®): Cephalexin, USP, 250 mg

H71 Keflex®
Composition (Each Pulvule®): Cephalexin, USP, 500 mg

©H74 Valmid®
Composition (Each Pulvule®): Ethinamate, USP, 500 mg

H76 Nalfon®
Composition (Each Pulvule®): Fenoprofen Calcium, USP, 200 mg (equiv. to fenoprofen)

H77 Nalfon®
Composition (Each Pulvule®): Fenoprofen Calcium, USP, 300 mg (equiv. to fenoprofen)

U05-U59 (Compressed Tablets)

U05 Ilosone® Chewable
Composition (Each Compressed Tablet): Erythromycin Estolate, USP, 125 mg (equiv. to erythromycin)

U25 Ilosone® Chewable
Composition (Each Compressed Tablet): Erythromycin Estolate, USP, 250 mg (equiv. to erythromycin)

U26 Ilosone®
Composition (Each Compressed Tablet): Erythromycin Estolate, USP, 500 mg (equiv. to erythromycin)

U59 Nalfon®
Composition (Each Compressed Tablet): Fenoprofen Calcium, USP, 600 mg (equiv. to fenoprofen)

U60 Keflex®
Composition (Each Compressed Tablet): Cephalexin, 1 g

W03-W68 (Miscellaneous)

W03 Ilosone®, for Oral Suspension
Composition (When Mixed as Directed): Each 5 ml contain erythromycin estolate equivalent to 125 mg erythromycin (USP).

W14 Cordran® Tape
Composition: Flurandrenolide, USP, 4 mcg/sq cm

W15 Ilosone® Liquid, Oral Suspension
Composition: Each 5 ml contain erythromycin estolate equivalent to 125 mg erythromycin (USP).

W17 Ilosone® Liquid, Oral Suspension
Composition: Each 5 ml contain erythromycin estolate equivalent to 250 mg erythromycin (USP).

W18 Ilosone® Ready-Mixed Drops
Composition: Each ml contains erythromycin estolate equivalent to 100 mg erythromycin (USP).

W21 For Oral Suspension, Keflex®
Composition (When Mixed as Directed): Each 5 ml contain 125 mg cephalexin (USP).

W22 For Pediatric Drops, Keflex®
Composition (When Mixed as Directed): Each ml contains 100 mg cephalexin (USP).

W68 For Oral Suspension, Keflex®
Composition (When Mixed as Directed): Each 5 ml contain 250 mg cephalexin (USP).

UNIT-DOSE PACKAGING

Identi-Dose® (unit dose medication, Dista)
Closed-circuit control of medication from pharmacy to nurse to patient and return. Simplifies counting and dispensing whether in single-unit or prescription-size quantities. Fits into any dispensing system for ready identification and legibility, better inventory control, protection from contamination, easier handling and recording under Medicare, prevention of drug loss through pilferage or spilling, better control of Federal Controlled Substances, and less chance of medication errors.
The following products are available through normal channels of supply:

Identi-Dose®
Pulvules®
No.
325 Becotin® with Vitamin C
402 Keflex®, 250 mg
403 Keflex®, 500 mg
375 Ilosone®, 250 mg
3043 Co-Pyronil®
Tablets
No.
23 Ilotycin®, 250 mg
1790 Mi-Cebrin®
1807 Mi-Cebrin T®
1810 Becotin®-T
1863 Ilosone®, 500 mg
1896 Keflex®, 1 g
Miscellaneous
No.
M-201 Keflex®, for Oral Suspension, 125 mg/5 ml
M-202 Keflex®, for Oral Suspension, 250 mg/5 ml

BECOTIN® OTC
(vitamin B complex)

Description: Each Pulvule® contains—
Thiamine Hydrochloride (Vitamin B_1) .... 10 mg
Riboflavin (Vitamin B_2) .... 10 mg
Pyridoxine (Vitamin B_6) .... 4.1 mg
Niacinamide .... 50 mg
Pantothenic Acid .... 25 mg
Vitamin B_{12} (Activity Equivalent) .... 1 mcg

Indications: Prophylaxis or treatment of vitamin B complex deficiencies. Acute B complex deficiencies may be precipitated by concurrent diseases or by surgical procedures, particularly of the gastrointestinal tract. The following symptoms of vitamin B complex deficiencies have been described: loss of appetite, nausea, burning tongue, vomiting, headache, general uneasiness or indisposition, nervousness, apprehensive mental depression, hypersensitivity to noise, mental confusion, fatigue, burning sensation of the skin, sore mouth and tongue, and burning and itching of the eyes.

Dosage: *Prophylaxis*—1 Pulvule a day. *Treatment*—2 or 3 Pulvules a day, or as directed by the physician.

How Supplied: *Pulvules No. 300, Becotin® (vitamin B complex, Dista), F62** (No. 0, Dark-Blue), in bottles of 100. [050180]

*Identi-Code® symbol.

BECOTIN®-T OTC
(vitamin B complex with vitamin C, therapeutic)

Description: Becotin-T is an easy-to-swallow, cinnamon-brown tablet which provides therapeutic quantities of vitamin B complex and vitamin C.
Each tablet contains—
Thiamine Mononitrate (Vitamin B_1) ...... 15 mg
Riboflavin (Vitamin B_2) .... 10 mg
Pyridoxine Hydrochloride (Vitamin B_6) .... 5 mg
Niacinamide .... 100 mg
Pantothenic Acid (as Calcium Pantothenate) .... 20 mg
Vitamin B_{12} (Activity Equivalent) .... 4 mcg

Ascorbic Acid (Vitamin C)
(as Sodium Ascorbate) ....300 mg

Becotin-T is especially useful as an adjunct to specific therapy in medical or surgical aftercare. By restoring normal tissue levels of these easily depleted water-soluble vitamins, Becotin-T reduces morbidity—helps shorten convalescence.

Indications: For the prevention or treatment of concurrent vitamin B complex and vitamin C deficiencies.

Dosage: 1 or 2 tablets a day, or as directed by the physician.

How Supplied: *Tablets No. 1810, Becotin®-T (vitamin B complex with vitamin C, therapeutic, Dista), C22,** Coated, Cinnamon Brown, in bottles of 100 and 1000 and in 10 strips of 10 individually labeled blisters each containing 1 tablet (ID100). [050180]

*Identi-Code® symbol.

BECOTIN® WITH VITAMIN C OTC
(vitamin B complex with vitamin C)

Description: Each Pulvule® contains—

Thiamine Hydrochloride
(Vitamin B_1)..10 mg
Riboflavin
(Vitamin B_2)..10 mg
Pyridoxine
(Vitamin B_6)..4.1 mg
Niacinamide..50 mg
Pantothenic Acid..25 mg
Vitamin B_{12} (Activity Equivalent)..........1 mcg
Ascorbic Acid
(Vitamin C)..150 mg

Indications: For the prevention or treatment of concurrent vitamin B complex and vitamin C deficiencies. *See also under* Becotin®.

Dosage: *Prophylaxis*—1 Pulvule a day. *Treatment*—2 or 3 Pulvules a day, or as directed by the physician.

How Supplied: *Pulvules No. 325, Becotin® with Vitamin C (vitamin B complex with vitamin C, Dista), F77** (No. 0, Green Body, Dark-Blue Cap), in bottles of 100, 500, and 1000 and in 10 strips of 10 individually labeled blisters each containing 1 Pulvule (ID100). [050180]

*Identi-Code® symbol.

CINOBAC® ℞
(cinoxacin)

Description: Cinobac® (cinoxacin, Dista) is a synthetic antimicrobial agent for oral administration. It is 1-ethyl-1,4-dihydro-4-oxo-[1,3]dioxolo[4,5-g]cinnoline-3-carboxylic acid and occurs as white or very light-yellow needle-shaped crystals. Cinobac is available as 250 and 500-mg Pulvules®. Examples of other antibacterial drugs in this class are nalidixic acid and oxolinic acid.

Clinical Pharmacology: Cinoxacin is rapidly absorbed after oral administration. A 500-mg dose produced a peak serum concentration of 15 mcg per ml, which declined to approximately 1 to 2 mcg per ml 6 hours after administration, as determined by fluorometric assay. A 500-mg dose produced an average urine concentration of approximately 300 mcg per ml during the first 4 hours and approximately 100 mcg per ml during the second 4-hour period. These urine concentrations are many times greater than the minimum inhibitory concentration (MIC) of cinoxacin for most gram-negative organisms commonly found in urinary tract infections.

Ninety-seven percent of a 500-mg oral dose of radiolabeled cinoxacin was recovered in the urine within 24 hours, 60% of which was present as unaltered cinoxacin and the remainder as inactive metabolic products.

The presence of food did not affect the total absorption of cinoxacin. Peak serum concentrations were reduced, but the 24-hour urinary recovery of antibacterial activity was unaltered. The mean serum half-life is 1.5 hours.

Microbiology—Cinoxacin has in vitro activity against a wide variety of aerobic gram-negative bacilli, particularly strains of *Enterobacteriaceae.* In vitro tests demonstrate that cinoxacin is bactericidal. The mode of action has been shown to be inhibition of bacterial DNA replication. It is active within the range of urinary pH.

Cinoxacin is active against most strains of the following organisms: *Escherichia coli, Klebsiella* species, *Enterobacter* species (including *E. aerogenes, E. cloacae,* and *E. hafniae), Proteus mirabilis,* and *P. vulgaris.*

Cinoxacin is not active against *Pseudomonas,* enterococci, or staphylococci. Cross-resistance with drugs in this class (nalidixic acid and oxolinic acid) has been demonstrated. Bacterial resistance to cinoxacin has been reported in less than 4% of patients treated with recommended doses; however, bacterial resistance to cinoxacin has not been shown to be transferable via R-factor.

Susceptibility Tests—Quantitative methods give the most precise estimates of susceptibility to antibacterial drugs. For purposes of judging susceptibility of bacterial isolates to cinoxacin, minimum inhibitory concentration and disc test breakpoints were established on the basis of (1) human drug bioavailability studies and (2) test results obtained with normally susceptible strains compared with results from resistant strains. The breakpoints have been verified by comparison with results of the clinical trials with cinoxacin.

One quantitative method, a standardized disc test, has been recommended.* Reports from the laboratory giving results of the standardized test using the 100-mcg cinoxacin disc should be interpreted according to the following criteria:

Organisms producing zones of 19 mm or greater are classified as susceptible, whereas those producing zones of 15 to 18 mm are classified as having intermediate susceptibility. Organisms in either of these categories are likely to respond to therapy if the infection is confined to the urinary tract.

Organisms producing zones of 14 mm or less are reported as resistant, indicating that other therapy should be selected.

Certain strains of *Enterobacteriaceae* exhibit heterogeneity of resistance to cinoxacin. These strains produce isolated colonies within the inhibition zone. When such strains are encountered, the clear inhibition zone should be measured *within* the isolated colonies.

Dilution methods for determining susceptibility are also used, and results are reported as the minimum drug concentration inhibiting microbial growth (MIC).

If the MIC is 16 mcg per ml or less, the microorganism is considered "susceptible"; if greater than 16 mcg per ml and less than 64 mcg per ml, it is "intermediate"; and it is "resistant" if the MIC is 64 mcg per ml or greater.

*Approved Standard ASM-2 Performance Standards for Antimicrobial Disc Susceptibility Tests; National Committee for Clinical Laboratory Standards, 771 East Lancaster Avenue, Villanova, Pennsylvania 19085.

Indications and Usage: Cinobac® (cinoxacin, Dista) is indicated for the treatment of initial and recurrent urinary tract infections in adults caused by the following susceptible microorganisms: *E. coli, P. mirabilis, P. vulgaris, Klebsiella pneumoniae* and *Klebsiella* species, and *Enterobacter* species.

In vitro susceptibility testing should be performed prior to administration of the drug and, when clinically indicated, during treatment.

Contraindication: Cinobac® (cinoxacin, Dista) is contraindicated in patients with a history of hypersensitivity to cinoxacin.

Warnings: The use of cinoxacin in prepubertal children and during pregnancy is not recommended. The oral administration of a single 250-mg-per-kg dose of cinoxacin caused lameness in immature dogs. Histologic examination of the weight-bearing joints of these dogs revealed permanent lesions of the cartilage. Related drugs (e.g., nalidixic acid, oxolinic acid) also produce erosions of the cartilage in weight-bearing joints and other signs of arthropathy in immature animals of various species.

Precautions: *General*—Since Cinobac® (cinoxacin, Dista) is eliminated primarily by the kidney, the usual dosage should be lower in patients with reduced renal function (*see* Dosage and Administration). Administration of Cinobac is not recommended for anuric patients.

Cinobac should be used with caution in patients with a history of hepatic disease.

Pregnancy—Pregnancy Category B—Reproduction studies have been performed in rats and rabbits at doses up to 10 times the daily human dose and have revealed no evidence of impaired fertility or harm to the fetus due to cinoxacin. There are, however, no adequate and well-controlled studies in pregnant women. **Since cinoxacin, like other drugs in its class, causes arthropathy in immature animals, its use during pregnancy is not recommended (*see* Warnings).**

Nursing Mothers—It is not known whether cinoxacin is excreted in human milk. Because other drugs in this class are excreted in human milk and because of the potential for serious adverse reactions from cinoxacin in nursing infants, a decision should be made to discontinue nursing or to discontinue the drug, taking into account the importance of the drug to the mother.

Pediatric Use—Cinoxacin is not recommended for use in prepubertal children (*see* Warnings).

Adverse Reactions: In clinical studies in 1118 patients, the following adverse effects were considered related to cinoxacin therapy:

Gastrointestinal—Nausea was reported most commonly and occurred in less than 3 in 100 patients. Other side effects, occurring less frequently (1 in 100), were anorexia, vomiting, abdominal cramps, and diarrhea.

Central Nervous System—The most frequent side effects were headache and dizziness, reported by 1 in 100 patients. Other adverse reactions possibly related to Cinobac® (cinoxacin, Dista) include insomnia, tingling sensation, perineal burning, photophobia, and tinnitus, and these were reported by less than 1 in 100 patients.

Hypersensitivity—Rash, urticaria, pruritus, and edema were reported by less than 3 in 100 patients.

Laboratory values that were reported to be abnormal were, in order of frequency, BUN (1 in 100) and SGOT, SGPT, serum creatinine, and alkaline phosphatase (each less than 1 in 100).

Although not observed in the 1118 patients treated with cinoxacin, the following side effects have been reported for other drugs in the same pharmacologically active and chemically related class: restlessness, nervousness, overbrightness of lights, change in color perception, difficulty in focusing, decrease in visual acuity, double vision, abdominal pain, weakness, constipation, angioedema, erythema and bullae, feelings of disorientation or agitation or acute anxiety, palpitation, soreness of the gums, drowsiness, joint stiffness, swelling of the extremities, metallic taste, toxic psychosis or convulsions (rare), reduction in hematocrit/hemoglobin, and eosinophilia.

Continued on next page

Dista—Cont.

All adverse reactions observed with drugs in this class were reversible.

Dosage and Administration: The usual adult dosage for the treatment of urinary tract infections is 1 g daily, administered orally in 2 or 4 divided doses (500 mg b.i.d. or 250 mg q.i.d.) for 7 to 14 days. Although susceptible organisms may be eradicated within a few days after therapy has begun, the full treatment course is recommended.

Impaired Renal Function—When renal function is impaired, a reduced dosage must be employed. After an initial dose of 500 mg, a maintenance dosage schedule should be used (*see* table).

MAINTENANCE DOSAGE GUIDE FOR PATIENTS WITH RENAL IMPAIRMENT

Creatinine Clearance (ml/min/1.73 m^2)	Renal Function	Dosage
>80	Normal	500 mg b.i.d.
80–50	Mild Impairment	250 mg t.i.d.
<50–20	Moderate Impairment	250 mg b.i.d.
<20	Marked Impairment	250 mg q.d.

Administration of Cinobac® (cinoxacin, Dista) to anuric patients is not recommended.

When only serum creatinine is available, the following formula (based on sex, weight, and age of the patient) may be used to convert this value into creatinine clearance. The serum creatinine should represent a steady state of renal function.

Males: $\frac{\text{Weight (kg)} \times (146-\text{age})}{72 \times \text{serum creatinine}}$

Females: 0.9 x male value

How Supplied: Pulvules:
250 mg, orange and green (No. 3055)—40
500 mg, orange and green (No. 3056)—50

Animal Pharmacology: Crystalluria, sometimes associated with secondary urinary tract pathology, occurs in laboratory animals treated orally with cinoxacin. In the rhesus monkey, crystalluria (without urinary tract pathology) has been noted at doses as low as 50 mg/kg/day (lowest dose tested). Cinoxacin-related crystalluria has not been observed in humans receiving twice the recommended daily dosage.

Cinoxacin and related drugs have been shown to cause arthropathy in immature animals of most species tested (*see* Warnings).

Some drugs of this class have been shown to have oculotoxic potential. Cinoxacin administered to cats at high dosages (200 mg/kg/day) resulted in retinal degeneration and other ocular changes. The dog appeared to be somewhat resistant to these effects, but high dosages (500 mg/kg/day) resulted in mild retinal atrophy. No cinoxacin-related ocular changes were noted in the rabbit, rat, or monkey or in human studies. (In one of the studies in the monkey, cinoxacin was administered for 1 year at 10 times the recommended clinical dose.)

[091080]

[*Shown in Product Identification Section*]

CO-PYRONIL® ℞
(pyrrobutamine compound)

Description: Each Pulvule® Co-Pyronil® (pyrrobutamine compound, Dista) contains—
Pyronil® (pyrrobutamine phosphate, Dista)............15 mg
Clopane® Hydrochloride (cyclopentamine hydrochloride, Dista)............12.5 mg

Each Pulvule Co-Pyronil, Pediatric, contains—
Pyronil® (pyrrobutamine phosphate, Dista)............7.5 mg
Clopane® Hydrochloride (cyclopentamine hydrochloride, Dista)............6.25 mg

Each 5 ml (approximately 1 teaspoonful) of Suspension Co-Pyronil contain—
Pyrrobutamine naphthalene disulfonate............6.73 mg
(Equivalent to 7.5 mg Pyronil)
Cyclopentamine hydroxybenzoyl benzoate............13.49 mg
(Equivalent to 6.25 mg Clopane Hydrochloride)

Pyronil is an antihistamine. It is soluble in warm water to the extent of 10 percent.

Clopane Hydrochloride is the hydrochloride of 1-cyclopentyl-2-methylaminopropane.

The formula of Co-Pyronil formerly included methapyrilene hydrochloride. The salts used in preparing the Pulvules are different from those in the suspension; the active ingredients are the same.

Actions: Pyronil® (pyrrobutamine phosphate, Dista) is an antihistamine. Side effects of antihistamines include sedation and some anticholinergic (drying) effects.

Pyronil is effective for approximately nine to 11 hours.

Clopane® Hydrochloride (cyclopentamine hydrochloride, Dista) is an ephedrine-like drug that is orally effective as a sympathomimetic and is present in the mixture to provide a constricting effect on the dilated blood vessels of the allergic person's swollen mucous membranes. It results in less central-nervous-system stimulation than ephedrine and, therefore, in fewer side effects, such as tension and insomnia. It also has a more prolonged action than ephedrine.

Indications: Co-Pyronil is indicated in seasonal and perennial allergic rhinitis and in vasomotor rhinitis.

Contraindications: *In Newborn or Premature Infants*—Antihistamines should *not* be used in newborn or premature infants.

In Nursing Mothers—Since antihistamines are hazardous for all infants, especially newborns and prematures, they are contraindicated in nursing mothers.

In Lower Respiratory Disease—Antihistamines should not be used to treat lower respiratory tract symptoms, including asthma.

Co-Pyronil should not be used in patients with hypersensitivity to Pyronil® (pyrrobutamine phosphate, Dista), to other antihistamines of similar chemical structure, or to Clopane® Hydrochloride (cyclopentamine hydrochloride, Dista).

Pyronil is contraindicated in patients receiving monoamine oxidase (MAO) inhibitors (*see* Drug Interactions) and in those with narrow-angle glaucoma, stenosing peptic ulcer, symptomatic prostatic hypertrophy, bladder neck obstruction, or pyloroduodenal obstruction.

Warnings: *Use in Children*—In infants and children especially, *overdosage* of antihistamines may cause hallucinations, convulsions, and death.

As in adults, antihistamines may diminish mental alertness in children. In the young child particularly, they may produce excitation.

Use in Pregnancy—Adequate reproduction studies have not been performed in animals. There is insufficient information as to whether this drug may reduce fertility in men or women or have teratogenic or other adverse effects on the fetus.

Use with C.N.S. Depressants—Pyronil® (pyrrobutamine phosphate, Dista) may add to the depressant effects of alcohol and other C.N.S. depressants (hypnotics, sedatives, tranquilizers, antianxiety agents, etc.).

Use When Activities Require Mental Alertness—Patients should be warned against engaging in activities requiring mental alertness, such as driving a car or operating appliances, machinery, etc.

Precautions: Like other antihistamines, Pyronil® (pyrrobutamine phosphate, Dista) has some action similar to that of atropine and, therefore, should be used with caution in patients with a history of bronchial asthma, increased intraocular pressure, hyperthyroidism, cardiovascular-renal disease, hypertension, or diabetes.

In the presence of prostatism, the administration of sympathomimetic drugs may cause urinary retention.

Adverse Reactions: *The most frequent adverse reactions to antihistamines:* sedation; sleepiness; dryness of mouth, nose, and throat; thickening of bronchial secretions; dizziness; epigastric distress; and disturbed coordination.

Other adverse reactions that occur with antihistamines: fatigue, confusion, restlessness, excitation, nervousness, insomnia, euphoria, anorexia, nausea, vomiting, diarrhea, constipation, hypotension, tightness of chest and wheezing, urticaria, drug rash, anaphylactic shock, blurred vision, diplopia, vertigo, tinnitus, headache, palpitation, tachycardia, nasal stuffiness, urinary frequency, difficult urination, urinary retention, photosensitivity, hemolytic anemia, leukopenia, and agranulocytosis.

Persons hypersensitive to sympathomimetics may report nervousness and insomnia. Clopane® Hydrochloride (cyclopentamine hydrochloride, Dista) causes less central-nervous-system stimulation than do other sympathomimetic drugs commonly employed.

The side effects of antihistamines and Clopane Hydrochloride tend to be counteracted by the combined administration of these medications. In most instances, Clopane Hydrochloride, a sympathomimetic, will prevent the drowsiness produced by Pyronil® (pyrrobutamine phosphate, Dista).

Administration and Dosage: Dosage of Co-Pyronil should be adjusted to the requirements and response of the patient.

Pulvules and Suspension
Usual Adult Dosage
Mild symptoms—1 Pulvule or 2 teaspoonfuls q. 12 h.
Moderate symptoms—1 Pulvule or 2 teaspoonfuls q. 8 h.
Severe symptoms—2 Pulvules or 4 teaspoonfuls q. 8 h. or 1 Pulvule or 2 teaspoonfuls q. 4 h.

Pediatric Pulvules and Suspension
Usual Dosage for Children—40 to 60 Pounds
Mild symptoms—1 Pulvule or 1 teaspoonful q. 12 h.
Moderate symptoms—1 Pulvule or 1 teaspoonful q. 8 h.
Severe symptoms—2 Pulvules or 2 teaspoonfuls q. 8 h.

Suspension
Usual Dosage for Children—20 to 40 Pounds
Mild symptoms—½ teaspoonful q. 12 h.
Moderate symptoms—½ teaspoonful q. 8 h.
Severe symptoms—½ to 1 teaspoonful q. 8 h.

The maximum dosages recommended for severe symptoms should not be exceeded. Side effects will increase with larger doses, but there will be no greater clinical efficacy.

Drug Interactions: MAO inhibitors prolong and intensify the anticholinergic (drying) effects of antihistamines.

Management of Overdosage: Reactions from overdosage of antihistamines may range from central-nervous-system depression to stimulation, especially in children. Also, signs and symptoms similar to those from atropine—dry mouth; fixed, dilated pupils; flushing; etc.—as well as gastrointestinal symptoms may appear.

If vomiting has not occurred spontaneously, the patient should be induced to vomit unless an excessive time has elapsed. Precautions must be taken against aspiration, especially in infants and children.

If vomiting is unsuccessful, gastric lavage is indicated within three hours after ingestion and even later if large amounts of milk or cream were taken beforehand. Isotonic or one-

half isotonic saline is the solution of choice for lavage.
Saline cathartics, such as milk of magnesia, draw water into the bowel by osmosis and, therefore, are valuable for their action in the rapid dilution of bowel contents.
Stimulants should *not* be used.
Levarterenol Bitartrate, USP, may be used for hypotension—1 ml of a 0.2 percent solution (0.1 percent base) in 250 ml of diluent. Drip at 0.5 ml/minute to give 2 mcg of base/minute or 2 mcg/m^2/minute intravenously. The dose should be titrated with blood pressure.
CAUTION: Slough results from extravascular leakage. The extravasated area should be treated quickly by infiltrating Phentolamine Mesylate, USP, or Phentolamine Hydrochloride, USP, 5 to 10 mg in 15 ml of saline solution.

How Supplied: (℞) *Pulvules No. 3043, Co-Pyronil® (pyrrobutamine compound, Dista), 3043** (No. 3, Yellow Opaque Body, Green Opaque Cap), in bottles of 100 (NDC 0777-3043-02) and 1000 (NDC 0777-3043-04) and in 10 strips of 10 individually labeled blisters each containing 1 Pulvule (ID100) (NDC 0777-3043-33).
(℞) *Pulvules, Pediatric, No. 3042, Co-Pyronil® (pyrrobutamine compound, Dista), 3042** (No. 4, Dark-Red), in bottles of 100 (NDC 0777-3042-02).
(℞) *Suspension No. M-5047, Co-Pyronil® (pyrrobutamine compound, Dista),* in 16-fl-oz bottles (NDC 0777-5047-05). *Avoid freezing.*
[062282]

*Identi-Code® symbol.

CORDRAN® and CORDRAN® SP ℞
(flurandrenolide) USP

Description: Cordran® (Flurandrenolide, USP, Dista) is a potent corticosteroid intended for topical use. It occurs as white to off-white, fluffy, crystalline powder and is odorless. Cordran is practically insoluble in water and in ether. One g dissolves in 72 ml of alcohol and in 10 ml of chloroform. The molecular weight of Cordran is 436.52.
The chemical name of Cordran is 6α-fluoro-16α-hydroxyhydrocortisone-16, 17-acetonide; its empirical formula is $C_{24}H_{33}FO_6$.
Each g of Cream Cordran® SP (Flurandrenolide Cream, USP, Dista) contains 0.5 mg (0.05 percent) or 0.25 mg (0.025 percent) flurandrenolide in an emulsified base composed of cetyl alcohol, citric acid, mineral oil, polyoxyl 40 stearate, propylene glycol, sodium citrate, stearic acid, and purified water.
Each g of Ointment Cordran® (Flurandrenolide Ointment, USP, Dista) contains 0.5 mg (0.05 percent) or 0.25 mg (0.025 percent) flurandrenolide in a base composed of white wax, cetyl alcohol, sorbitan sesquioleate, and white petrolatum.
Each ml of Lotion Cordran® (Flurandrenolide Lotion, USP, Dista) contains 0.5 mg (0.05 percent) flurandrenolide in an oil-in-water emulsion base composed of glycerin, cetyl alcohol, stearic acid, glyceryl monostearate, mineral oil, polyoxyl 40 stearate, menthol, benzyl alcohol, and purified water.

Clinical Pharmacology: Cordran® (flurandrenolide, Dista) is primarily effective because of its anti-inflammatory, antipruritic, and vasoconstrictive actions.
The mechanism of the anti-inflammatory effect of topical corticosteroids is not completely understood. Various laboratory methods, including vasoconstrictor assays, are used to compare and predict potencies and/or clinical efficacies of the topical corticosteroids. There is some evidence to suggest that a recognizable correlation exists between vasoconstrictor potency and therapeutic efficacy in man. Corticosteroids with anti-inflammatory activity may stabilize cellular and lysosomal membranes. There is also the suggestion that the effect on the membranes of lysosomes prevents the release of proteolytic enzymes and, thus, plays a part in reducing inflammation.
Evaporation of water from the lotion vehicle produces a cooling effect which is often desirable in the treatment of acutely inflamed or weeping lesions.
Pharmacokinetics—The extent of percutaneous absorption of topical corticosteroids is determined by many factors, including the vehicle, the integrity of the epidermal barrier, and the use of occlusive dressings.
Topical corticosteroids can be absorbed from normal intact skin. Inflammation and/or other disease processes in the skin increase percutaneous absorption. Occlusive dressings substantially increase the percutaneous absorption of topical corticosteroids. Thus, occlusive dressings may be a valuable therapeutic adjunct for treatment of resistant dermatoses. *See* Dosage and Administration.
Once absorbed through the skin, topical corticosteroids are handled through pharmacokinetic pathways similar to those of systemically administered corticosteroids. Corticosteroids are bound to plasma proteins in varying degrees. Corticosteroids are metabolized primarily in the liver and then excreted in the kidneys. Some of the topical corticosteroids and their metabolites are also excreted into the bile.

Indications and Usage: Cordran® (flurandrenolide, Dista) is indicated for the relief of the inflammatory and pruritic manifestations of corticosteroid-responsive dermatoses.

Contraindications: Topical corticosteroids are contraindicated in patients with a history of hypersensitivity to any of the components of these preparations.

Precautions: *General Precautions*—Systemic absorption of topical corticosteroids has produced reversible hypothalamic-pituitary-adrenal (HPA) axis suppression, manifestations of Cushing's syndrome, hyperglycemia, and glucosuria in some patients.
Conditions which augment systemic absorption include application of the more potent steroids, use over large surface areas, prolonged use, and the addition of occlusive dressings.
Therefore, patients receiving a large dose of a potent topical steroid applied to a large surface area or under an occlusive dressing should be evaluated periodically for evidence of HPA axis suppression by using urinary-free cortisol and ACTH stimulation tests. If HPA axis suppression is noted, an attempt should be made to withdraw the drug, to reduce the frequency of application, or to substitute a less potent steroid.
Recovery of HPA axis function is generally prompt and complete upon discontinuation of the drug. Infrequently, signs and symptoms of steroid withdrawal may occur, so that supplemental systemic corticosteroids are required.
Children may absorb proportionately larger amounts of topical corticosteroids and thus be more susceptible to systemic toxicity *See* Precautions—Usage in Children.
If irritation develops, topical corticosteroids should be discontinued and appropriate therapy instituted.
In the presence of dermatologic infections, the use of an appropriate antifungal or antibacterial agent should be instituted. If a favorable response does not occur promptly, Cordran should be discontinued until the infection has been adequately controlled.
Information for the Patient—Patients using topical corticosteroids should receive the following information and instructions.

1. This medication is to be used as directed by the physician. It is for external use only. Avoid contact with the eyes.
2. Patients should be advised not to use this medication for any disorder other than that for which it was prescribed.
3. The treated skin area should not be bandaged or otherwise covered or wrapped in order to be occlusive unless the patient is directed to do so by the physician.
4. Patients should report any signs of local adverse reactions, especially under occlusive dressing.
5. Parents of pediatric patients should be advised not to use tightfitting diapers or plastic pants on a child being treated in the diaper area, because these garments may constitute occlusive dressings.

Laboratory Tests—The following tests may be helpful in evaluating the HPA axis suppression:

Urinary-free cortisol test
ACTH stimulation test

Carcinogenesis, Mutagenesis, and Impairment of Fertility—Long-term animal studies have not been performed to evaluate the carcinogenic potential or the effect on fertility of topical corticosteroids.
Studies to determine mutagenicity with prednisolone and hydrocortisone have revealed negative results.
Usage in Pregnancy—Pregnancy Category C—Corticosteroids are generally teratogenic in laboratory animals when administered systemically at relatively low dosage levels. The more potent corticosteroids have been shown to be teratogenic after dermal application in laboratory animals. There are no adequate and well-controlled studies in pregnant women on teratogenic effects from topically applied corticosteroids. Therefore, topical corticosteroids should be used during pregnancy only if the potential benefit justifies the potential risk to the fetus. Drugs of this class should not be used extensively on pregnant patients or in large amounts or for prolonged periods of time.
Nursing Mothers—It is not known whether topical administration of corticosteroids could result in sufficient systemic absorption to produce detectable quantities in breast milk. Systemically administered corticosteroids are secreted into breast milk in quantities *not* likely to have a deleterious effect on the infant. Nevertheless, caution should be exercised when topical corticosteroids are administered to a nursing woman.
Usage in Children—Pediatric patients may demonstrate greater susceptibility to topical corticosteroid-induced HPA axis suppression and Cushing's syndrome than do mature patients because of a larger skin surface area to body weight ratio.
Hypothalamic-pituitary-adrenal (HPA) axis suppression, Cushing's syndrome, and intracranial hypertension have been reported in children receiving topical corticosteroids. Manifestations of adrenal suppression in children include linear growth retardation, delayed weight gain, low plasma cortisol levels, and absence of response to ACTH stimulation. Manifestations of intracranial hypertension include bulging fontanelles, headaches, and bilateral papilledema.
Administration of topical corticosteroids to children should be limited to the least amount compatible with an effective therapeutic regimen. Chronic corticosteroid therapy may interfere with the growth and development of children.

Adverse Reactions: The following local adverse reactions are reported infrequently with topical corticosteroids but may occur more frequently with the use of occlusive dressings. These reactions are listed in an approximate decreasing order of occurrence:
Burning
Itching
Irritation

Continued on next page

Dista—Cont.

Dryness
Folliculitis
Hypertrichosis
Acneiform eruptions
Hypopigmentation
Perioral dermatitis
Allergic contact dermatitis
Maceration of the skin
Secondary infection
Skin atrophy
Striae
Miliaria

Overdosage: Topically applied corticosteroids can be absorbed in sufficient amounts to produce systemic effects (*See* Precautions).

Dosage and Administration: Topical corticosteroids are generally applied to the affected area as a thin film one to four times daily, depending on the severity of the condition.

Occlusive dressings may be used for the management of psoriasis or recalcitrant conditions. If an infection develops, the use of occlusive dressings should be discontinued and appropriate antimicrobial therapy instituted.

For moist lesions, a small quantity of the cream or lotion should be rubbed gently into the affected areas two or three times a day. For dry, scaly lesions, the ointment is applied as a thin film to affected areas two or three times daily.

Use with Occlusive Dressings

The technique of occlusive dressings (for management of psoriasis and other persistent dermatoses) is as follows:

1. Remove as much as possible of the superficial scaling before applying Cream Cordran® SP (flurandrenolide, Dista) or Ointment or Lotion Cordran. Soaking in a bath will help soften the scales and permit easier removal by brushing, picking, or rubbing.
2. Rub Cream Cordran SP or Ointment or Lotion Cordran thoroughly into the affected areas.
3. Cover with an occlusive plastic film such as polyethylene, Saran Wrap™, or Handi-Wrap®. (When Cream Cordran SP or Lotion Cordran is used, added moisture may be provided by placing a slightly dampened cloth or gauze over the lesion before the plastic film is applied.)
4. Seal the edges to adjacent normal skin with tape or hold in place by a gauze wrapping.
5. For convenience, the patient may remove the dressing during the day. The dressing should then be reapplied each night.
6. For daytime therapy, the condition may be treated by rubbing Cream Cordran SP or Ointment or Lotion Cordran sparingly into the affected areas.
7. In more resistant cases, leaving the dressing in place for three to four days at a time may result in a better response.
8. Thin polyethylene gloves are suitable for treatment of the hands and fingers; plastic garment bags may be utilized for treating lesions on the trunk or buttocks. A tight shower cap is useful in treating lesions on the scalp.

Occlusive Dressings Have the Following Advantages—1. Percutaneous penetration of the corticosteroid is enhanced.

2. Medication is concentrated on the areas of skin where it is most needed.

3. This method of administration frequently is more effective in very resistant dermatoses than is the conventional application of Cordran® (flurandrenolide, Dista).

Precautions to Be Observed in Therapy with Occlusive Dressings—Treatment should be continued for at least a few days after clearing of the lesions. If it is stopped too soon, a relapse may occur. Reinstitution of treatment frequently will cause remission.

Because of the increased hazard of secondary infection from resistant strains of staphylococci among hospitalized patients, it is suggested that the use of occlusive plastic films for corticosteroid therapy in such cases be restricted.

Generally, occlusive dressings should not be used on weeping, or exudative, lesions.

When large areas of the body are covered, thermal homeostasis may be impaired. If elevation of body temperature occurs, use of the occlusive dressing should be discontinued.

Rarely, a patient may develop miliaria, folliculitis, or a sensitivity to either the particular dressing material or a combination of Cordran® (flurandrenolide, Dista) and the occlusive dressing. If miliaria or folliculitis occurs, use of the occlusive dressing should be discontinued. Treatment by inunction with a corticosteroid such as Cordran may be continued. If the sensitivity is caused by the particular material of the dressing, substitution of a different material may be tried.

Warnings—Some plastic films are readily flammable. Patients should be cautioned against the use of any such material.

When plastic films are used on infants and children, the persons caring for the patients must be reminded of the danger of suffocation if the plastic material accidentally covers the face.

How Supplied:

(℞) *Cordran® (Flurandrenolide, USP), 0.05%, Lotion No. M-128,* in 15-ml (NDC 0777-2352-47) and 60-ml (NDC 0777-2352-97) plastic squeeze bottles. *Avoid freezing.*

(℞) *Cordran® (Flurandrenolide, USP), 0.025%, Ointment No. 79,* in 30-g (NDC 0777-1824-67) and 60-g (NDC 0777-1824-97) tubes and in 225-g (NDC 0777-1824-88) jars.

(℞) *Cordran® (Flurandrenolide, USP), 0.05%, Ointment No. 85,* in 15-g (NDC 0777-1826-47), 30-g (NDC 0777-1826-67), and 60-g (NDC 0777-1826-97) tubes and in 225-g (NDC 0777-1826-88) jars.

(℞) *Cordran® SP (Flurandrenolide, USP), 0.025%, Cream No. 9,* in 30-g (NDC 0777-6034-67) and 60-g (NDC 0777-6034-97) tubes and in 225-g (NDC 0777-6034-88) jars.

(℞) *Cordran® SP (Flurandrenolide, USP), 0.05%, Cream No. 11,* in 15-g (NDC 0777-6035-47), 30-g (NDC 0777-6035-67), and 60-g (NDC 0777-6035-97) tubes and in 225-g (NDC 0777-6035-88) jars.

Cream No. 11, 0.05%—15 g—6505-00-890-1554A; 60 g—6505-00-728-2623A; 225 g—6505-00-728-2624

Lotion No. M-128, 0.05%—15 ml—6505-00-926-9110

Ointment No. 85, 0.05%—15 g—6505-00-728-2626 [052682A]

CORDRAN®-N ℞

(flurandrenolide with neomycin sulfate)

Description: Cordran® (Flurandrenolide, USP, Dista) is a potent corticosteroid intended for topical use. The chemical formula of Cordran is 6α-fluoro-16α-hydroxyhydrocortisone 16,17-acetonide.

Each g of Cordran-N cream contains 0.5 mg (0.05 percent) flurandrenolide and 5 mg neomycin sulfate (equivalent to 3.5 mg neomycin base) in a base composed of stearic acid, cetyl alcohol, mineral oil, polyoxyl 40 stearate, ethylparaben, glycerin, and purified water.

Each g of Cordran-N ointment contains 0.5 mg (0.05 percent) flurandrenolide and 5 mg neomycin sulfate (equivalent to 3.5 mg neomycin base) in a base composed of white wax, cetyl alcohol, sorbitan sesquioleate, and white petrolatum.

Actions: Cordran® (flurandrenolide, Dista) is primarily effective because of its anti-inflammatory, antipruritic, and vasoconstrictive actions.

The addition of neomycin broadens the usefulness of Cordran so that dermatoses complicated by actual skin infections may be treated more effectively and with safety.

Indications: On the basis of a review of this drug by the National Academy of Sciences—National Research Council and/ or other information, FDA has classified the following indications as "possibly" effective.

For relief of the inflammatory manifestations of corticosteroid-responsive dermatoses complicated by bacterial infections.

Final classification of the less-than-effective indications requires further investigation.

Contraindications: Topical corticosteroids are contraindicated in patients with a history of hypersensitivity to any of the components of these preparations.

Warning: Because of the potential hazard of nephrotoxicity and ototoxicity, prolonged use or use of large amounts of this product should be avoided in the treatment of skin infections following extensive burns, trophic ulceration, and other conditions in which absorption of neomycin is possible.

Precautions: If irritation develops, the product should be discontinued and appropriate therapy instituted.

Patients with superficial fungus or yeast infections should be treated with additional appropriate methods and observed frequently.

Prolonged use of neomycin preparations may result in the overgrowth of nonsusceptible organisms. If this occurs, appropriate measures should be taken.

There are articles in the current medical literature that indicate an increase in the prevalence of persons who are sensitive to neomycin.

If extensive areas are treated or if the occlusive technique is used, there will be increased systemic absorption of the corticosteroid, and suitable precautions should be taken, particularly in children and infants.

Although topical corticosteroids have not been reported to have an adverse effect on human pregnancy, the safety of their use on pregnant women has not been absolutely established. In laboratory animals, increases in incidence of fetal abnormalities have been associated with exposure of gestating females to topical corticosteroids, in some cases at rather low dosage levels. Therefore, drugs of this class should not be used extensively, in large amounts, or for prolonged periods of time on pregnant patients.

These products are not for ophthalmic use.

Adverse Reactions: The following local adverse reactions have been reported with topical corticosteroid formulations:

Acneform eruptions
Allergic contact dermatitis
Burning
Dryness
Folliculitis
Hypertrichosis
Hypopigmentation
Irritation
Itching
Perioral dermatitis

The following may occur more frequently with occlusive dressings:

Maceration of the skin
Miliaria
Secondary infection
Skin atrophy
Striae

Topical neomycin has been reported to cause allergic contact dermatitis, ototoxicity, and nephrotoxicity.

Administration and Dosage: For moist lesions, a small quantity of the cream should be rubbed gently into the affected areas two or three times a day. For dry, scaly lesions, the ointment is applied as a thin film to affected areas two or three times daily.

Use with Occlusive Dressings—See under Cordran and Cordran SP.

How Supplied: (℞) *Cordran®-N (flurandrenolide with neomycin sulfate, Dista), Cream No. 12,* in 15, 30, and 60-g tubes.
(℞) *Cordran®-N (flurandrenolide with neomycin sulfate, Dista), Ointment No. 86,* in 15, 30, and 60-g tubes.
[081880]

CORDRAN® TAPE ℞
(flurandrenolide tape)
USP

Description: Cordran Tape is a transparent, inconspicuous, plastic surgical tape, impervious to moisture. It contains Cordran® (flurandrenolide, Dista), a potent corticosteroid. *See also under* Cordran® and Cordran SP.
Each square centimeter contains 4 mcg of flurandrenolide uniformly distributed in the adhesive layer. The tape is made of a thin, matte-finish polyethylene film which is slightly elastic and highly flexible.
The adhesive is a synthetic copolymer of acrylate ester and acrylic acid which is free from substances of plant origin. The pressure-sensitive adhesive surface is covered with a protective paper liner to permit handling and trimming before application.
Clinical Pharmacology: Cordran® (flurandrenolide, Dista) is primarily effective because of its anti-inflammatory, antipruritic, and vasoconstrictive actions.
See also under Cordran and Cordran SP.
The tape serves as both a vehicle and an occlusive dressing. Retention of insensible perspiration by the tape results in hydration of the stratum corneum and improved diffusion of the medication. The skin is protected from scratching, rubbing, desiccation, and chemical irritation. The tape acts as a mechanical splint to fissured skin. Since it prevents removal of the medication by washing or the rubbing action of clothing, the tape formulation provides a sustained action.
Pharmacokinetics—See under Cordran and Cordran SP.
Indications and Usage: For relief of the inflammatory and pruritic manifestations of corticosteroid-responsive dermatoses, particularly dry, scaling localized lesions.
Contraindications: Topical corticosteroids are contraindicated in patients with a history of hypersensitivity to any of the components of this preparation.
Use of Cordran® Tape (flurandrenolide tape, Dista) is not recommended for lesions exuding serum or in intertriginous areas.
Precautions: *See under* Cordran and Cordran SP.
Adverse Reactions: *See under* Cordran and Cordran SP.
Dosage and Administration: Occlusive dressings may be used for the management of psoriasis or recalcitrant conditions.
If an infection develops, the use of occlusive dressings should be discontinued and appropriate antimicrobial therapy instituted.
Replacement of the tape every 12 hours produces the lowest incidence of adverse reactions, but it may be left in place for 24 hours if it is well tolerated and adheres satisfactorily.
When necessary, the tape may be used at night only and removed during the day.
If ends of the tape loosen prematurely, they may be trimmed off and replaced with fresh tape.
The directions given below are included on a separate package insert for the patient to follow unless otherwise instructed by the physician.

Application of Cordran Tape

> IMPORTANT: Skin should be clean and dry before tape is applied. Tape should always be cut, never torn.

DIRECTIONS FOR USE:
1. Prepare skin as directed by your physician or as follows: Gently clean the area to be covered to remove scales, crusts, dried exudates, and any previously used ointments or creams. A germicidal soap or cleanser should be used to prevent the development of odor under the tape. Shave or clip the hair in the treatment area to allow good contact with the skin and comfortable removal. If shower or tub baths are to be taken, they should be completed before the tape is applied. The skin should be dry before application of the tape.
2. Remove tape from package and cut a piece slightly larger than area to be covered. Round off corners.
3. Pull white paper from transparent tape. Be careful that tape does not stick to itself.
4. Apply tape, keeping skin smooth; press tape into place.

REPLACEMENT OF TAPE:
Unless instructed otherwise by your physician, replace tape after 12 hours. Cleanse skin and allow it to dry for one hour before applying new tape.
IF IRRITATION OR INFECTION DEVELOPS, REMOVE TAPE AND CONSULT PHYSICIAN.

How Supplied: (℞) *Cordran® Tape (Flurandrenolide Tape, USP), M-170, W14,** 4 mcg flurandrenolide/sq cm, in Small Rolls 24 inches long and 3 inches wide (60 cm x 7.5 cm) (NDC 0777-2314-24) and in Large Rolls 80 inches long and 3 inches wide (200 cm x 7.5 cm) (NDC 0777-2314-28), in single packages.
Directions for the patient are included in each package. [062182]
Cordran Tape is manufactured by Minnesota Mining and Mfg. Co., St. Paul, Minnesota 55101, for Dista Products Company.

*Identi-Code® symbol.

ILOSONE® ℞
(erythromycin estolate)
USP

> **WARNING**
> Hepatic dysfunction with or without jaundice has occurred, chiefly in adults, in association with erythromycin estolate administration. It may be accompanied by malaise, nausea, vomiting, abdominal colic, and fever. In some instances, severe abdominal pain may simulate an abdominal surgical emergency.
> If the above findings occur, discontinue Ilosone® (erythromycin estolate, Dista) promptly.
> Ilosone is contraindicated for patients with a known history of sensitivity to this drug and for those with preexisting liver disease.

Description: Erythromycin is produced by a strain of *Streptomyces erythraeus* and belongs to the macrolide group of antibiotics. It is basic and readily forms salts with acids. The base, the stearate salt, and the esters are poorly soluble in water and are suitable for oral administration.
Ilosone® (erythromycin estolate, Dista) is the lauryl sulfate salt of the propionyl ester of erythromycin.
Actions: Erythromycin inhibits protein synthesis without affecting nucleic acid synthesis. Some strains of *Haemophilus influenzae* and staphylococci have demonstrated resistance to erythromycin. Culture and susceptibility testing should be done. If the Bauer-Kirby method of disc susceptibility testing is used, a 15-mcg erythromycin disc should give a zone diameter of at least 18 mm when tested against an erythromycin-susceptible organism.
Orally administered erythromycin estolate is readily and reliably absorbed. Because of acid stability, serum levels are comparable whether the estolate is taken in the fasting state or after food. After a single 250-mg dose, blood concentrations average 0.29, 1.2, and 1.2 mcg/ml respectively at two, four, and six hours. Following a 500-mg dose, blood concentrations average 3, 1.9, and 0.7 mcg/ml respectively at two, six, and 12 hours.
After oral administration, serum antibiotic levels consist of erythromycin base and propionyl erythromycin ester. The propionyl ester continuously hydrolyzes to the base form of erythromycin to maintain an equilibrium ratio of approximately 20 percent base and 80 percent ester in the serum.
After absorption, erythromycin diffuses readily into most body fluids. In the absence of meningeal inflammation, low concentrations are normally achieved in the spinal fluid, but passage of the drug across the blood-brain barrier increases in meningitis. In the presence of normal hepatic function, erythromycin is concentrated in the liver and excreted in the bile; the effect of hepatic dysfunction on excretion of erythromycin by the liver into the bile is not known. After oral administration, less than 5 percent of the administered dose can be recovered as the active form in the urine.
Erythromycin crosses the placental barrier, but fetal plasma levels are low.
Indications: *Streptococcus pyogenes* (Group A Beta-Hemolytic)—Upper and lower respiratory tract, skin, and soft-tissue infections of mild to moderate severity.
Injectable penicillin G benzathine is considered by the American Heart Association to be the drug of choice in the treatment and prevention of streptococcal pharyngitis and in long-term prophylaxis of rheumatic fever.
When oral medication is preferred for treating the above-mentioned conditions, penicillin G or V or erythromycin is the alternate drug of choice.
The importance of the patient's strict adherence to the prescribed dosage regimen must be stressed when oral medication is given. A therapeutic dose should be administered for at least ten days.
Alpha-Hemolytic Streptococci (Viridans Group)—Although no controlled clinical efficacy trials have been conducted, oral erythromycin has been suggested by the American Heart Association and American Dental Association for use in a regimen for prophylaxis against bacterial endocarditis in patients hypersensitive to penicillin who have congenital and/or rheumatic or other acquired valvular heart disease when they undergo dental procedures and surgical procedures of the upper respiratory tract.[1] Erythromycin is not suitable for such prophylaxis prior to genitourinary or gastrointestinal tract surgery.
Note: When selecting antibiotics for the prevention of bacterial endocarditis, the physician or dentist should read the full joint statement of the American Heart Association and the American Dental Association.[1]
Staphylococcus aureus—Acute infections of skin and soft tissue which are mild to moderately severe. Resistance may develop during treatment.
S. (Diplococcus) pneumoniae—Infections of the upper respiratory tract (e.g., otitis media, pharyngitis) and lower respiratory tract (e.g., pneumonia) of mild to moderate severity.

Continued on next page

Dista—Cont.

Mycoplasma pneumoniae (Eaton Agent, PPLO) —In the treatment of respiratory tract infections due to this organism.

H. influenzae—May be used concomitantly with adequate doses of sulfonamides in treating upper respiratory tract infections of mild to moderate severity. Not all strains of this organism are susceptible at the erythromycin concentrations ordinarily achieved (see appropriate sulfonamide labeling for prescribing information).

Treponema pallidum—Erythromycin is an alternate choice of treatment for primary syphilis in penicillin-allergic patients. In primary syphilis, spinal-fluid examinations should be done before treatment and as part of follow-up after therapy.

Corynebacterium diphtheriae—As an adjunct to antitoxin, to prevent establishment of carriers, and to eradicate the organism in carriers.

C. minutissimum—In the treatment of erythrasma.

Entamoeba histolytica—In the treatment of intestinal amebiasis only. Extraenteric amebiasis requires treatment with other agents.

Listeria monocytogenes—Infections due to this organism.

Legionnaires' Disease—Although no controlled clinical efficacy studies have been conducted, in vitro and limited preliminary clinical data suggest that erythromycin may be effective in treating Legionnaires' disease.

Contraindication: Erythromycin is contraindicated in patients with known hypersensitivity to this antibiotic.

Warnings: (*See* Warning box above.) The administration of erythromycin estolate has been associated with the infrequent occurrence of cholestatic hepatitis. Laboratory findings have been characterized by abnormal hepatic function test values, peripheral eosinophilia, and leukocytosis. Symptoms may include malaise, nausea, vomiting, abdominal cramps, and fever. Jaundice may or may not be present. In some instances, severe abdominal pain may simulate the pain of biliary colic, pancreatitis, perforated ulcer, or an acute abdominal surgical problem. In other instances, clinical symptoms and results of liver function tests have resembled findings in extrahepatic obstructive jaundice.

Initial symptoms have developed in some cases after a few days of treatment but generally have followed one or two weeks of continuous therapy. Symptoms reappear promptly, usually within 48 hours after the drug is readministered to sensitive patients. The syndrome seems to result from a form of sensitization, occurs chiefly in adults, and has been reversible when medication is discontinued.

Usage in Pregnancy—Safety of this drug for use during pregnancy has not been established.

Precautions: Since erythromycin is excreted principally by the liver, caution should be exercised in administering the antibiotic to patients with impaired hepatic function.

Recent data from studies of erythromycin reveal that its use in patients who are receiving high doses of theophylline may be associated with an increase in serum theophylline levels and potential theophylline toxicity. In case of theophylline toxicity and/or elevated serum theophylline levels, the dose of theophylline should be reduced while the patient is receiving concomitant erythromycin therapy.

Surgical procedures should be performed when indicated.

Adverse Reactions: The most frequent side effects of erythromycin preparations are gastrointestinal (e.g., abdominal cramping and discomfort) and are dose related. Nausea, vomiting, and diarrhea occur infrequently with usual oral doses.

During prolonged or repeated therapy, there is a possibility of overgrowth of nonsusceptible bacteria or fungi. If such infections arise, the drug should be discontinued and appropriate therapy instituted.

Mild allergic reactions, such as urticaria and other skin rashes, have occurred. Serious allergic reactions, including anaphylaxis, have been reported.

Administration and Dosage: *Adults*—The usual dosage is 250 mg every six hours. This may be increased up to 4 g or more/day according to the severity of the infection.

Children—Age, weight, and severity of the infection are important factors in determining the proper dosage. The usual regimen is 30 to 50 mg/kg/day in divided doses. For more severe infections, this dosage may be doubled.

If administration is desired on a twice-a-day schedule in either adults or children, one-half of the total daily dose may be given every 12 hours.

Streptococcal Infections—For the treatment of streptococcal pharyngitis and tonsillitis, the usual dosage range is 20 to 50 mg/kg/day in divided doses.

Body Weight	Total Daily Dose
10 kg or less (less than 25 lb)	250 mg
11–18 kg (25–40 lb)	375 mg
18–25 kg (40–55 lb)	500 mg
25–36 kg (55–80 lb)	750 mg
36 kg or more (more than 80 lb)	1000 mg (adult dose)

In the treatment of group A beta-hemolytic streptococcal infections, a therapeutic dosage of erythromycin should be administered for at least ten days. In continuous prophylaxis of streptococcal infections in persons with a history of rheumatic heart disease, the dosage is 250 mg twice a day.

For prophylaxis against bacterial endocarditis[1] in patients with rheumatic, congenital, or other acquired valvular heart disease when undergoing dental procedures or surgical procedures of the upper respiratory tract, the dosage schedule for adults is 1 g (20 mg/kg for children) orally one and one-half to two hours before the procedure and then 500 mg (10 mg/kg for children) orally every six hours for eight doses.

Primary Syphilis—A regimen of 20 g of erythromycin estolate in divided doses over a period of ten days has been shown to be effective in the treatment of primary syphilis.

Dysenteric Amebiasis—Dosage for adults is 250 mg four times daily for 10 to 14 days; for children, 30 to 50 mg/kg/day in divided doses for 10 to 14 days.

Legionnaires' Disease—Although optimum doses have not been established, doses utilized in reported clinical data were those recommended above (1 to 4 g erythromycin estolate daily in divided doses).

Reference: 1. American Heart Association: Prevention of Bacterial Endocarditis, Circulation, *56*:139A, 1977.

How Supplied: (℞) *Pulvules® Ilosone® (Erythromycin Estolate Capsules, USP): No. 374, H07,** 125 mg (equivalent to erythromycin) (No. 2, Ivory Opaque Body, Red Opaque Cap), in bottles of 24 (NDC 0777-0807-24) and 100 (NDC 0777-0807-02); *No. 375, H09,** 250 mg (equivalent to erythromycin) (No. 0, Ivory Opaque Body, Red Opaque Cap), in bottles of 24 (NDC 0777-0809-24) and 100 (NDC 0777-0809-02) and in 10 strips of 10 individually labeled blisters each containing 1 Pulvule (ID100) (NDC 0777-0809-33).

[*Shown in Product Identification Section*]

(℞) *Tablets Ilosone® (Erythromycin Estolate Tablets, USP), No. 1863, U26,** 500 mg (equivalent to erythromycin), Specially Coated, Light-Pink (capsule-shaped, scored), in bottles of 50 (NDC 0777-2126-50) and in 10 strips of 10 individually labeled blisters each containing 1 tablet (ID100) (NDC 0777-2126-33).

(℞) *Tablets Ilosone® Chewable (Erythromycin Estolate Tablets, USP), No. 1834, U05,** 125 mg (equivalent to erythromycin), Light-Pink, in bottles of 50 (NDC 0777-2105-50); *No. 1865, U25,** 250 mg (equivalent to erythromycin), Light-Pink, in bottles of 50 (NDC 0777-2125-50).

(℞) *Ilosone® Liquid (Erythromycin Estolate Oral Suspension, USP), M-148, W15,** in 100-ml (NDC 0777-2315-48) and 16-fl-oz (NDC 0777-2315-05) bottles.

Each 5 ml contain erythromycin estolate equivalent to 125 mg erythromycin in an orange-flavored vehicle. *Shake well before using. Refrigerate to maintain optimum taste.*

(℞) *Ilosone® Liquid (Erythromycin Estolate Oral Suspension, USP), M-153, W17,** in 100-ml (NDC 0777-2317-48) and 16-fl-oz (NDC 0777-2317-05) bottles.

Each 5 ml contain erythromycin estolate equivalent to 250 mg erythromycin in a cherry-flavored vehicle. *Shake well before using. Refrigerate to maintain optimum taste.*

(℞) *Ilosone® (Erythromycin Estolate for Oral Suspension, USP), M-104, W03,** in 60 (NDC 0777-2303-97) and 150-ml-size (NDC 0777-2303-68) packages.

Each 60-ml-size package consists of a bottle containing erythromycin estolate equivalent to 1.5 g erythromycin. At the time of dispensing, 48 ml of water are added to provide 60 ml of an oral suspension.

Each 150-ml-size package consists of a bottle containing erythromycin estolate equivalent to 3.75 g erythromycin. At the time of dispensing, 120 ml of water are added to provide 150 ml of an oral suspension.

When mixed as directed, each 5 ml (approximately 1 teaspoonful) will contain erythromycin estolate equivalent to 125 mg erythromycin. After being mixed, the suspension may be kept at room temperature for 14 days without significant loss of potency. *Shake well before using. Keep tightly closed.*

(℞) *Ilosone® Ready-Mixed Drops (Erythromycin Estolate Oral Suspension, USP), M-159, W18,** in 10-ml bottles (NDC 0777-2318-37).

Each package consists of a bottle containing erythromycin estolate equivalent to 1 g erythromycin in a pleasantly flavored vehicle and a special dropper calibrated at approximately 25 mg and 50 mg.

Each ml contains erythromycin estolate equivalent to 100 mg erythromycin. *Shake well before using. Refrigerate to maintain optimum taste.* [061682]

Pulvules No. 375, 250 mg—100's—6505-00-890-1388A

*Identi-Code® symbol.

ILOTYCIN® ℞
(erythromycin)
Ointment, USP

Description: Ilotycin® (erythromycin, Dista) is a wide-range antibiotic discovered in the research laboratories of Eli Lilly and Company and produced from a strain of *Streptomyces erythraeus.*

Indications: On the basis of a review of this drug by the National Academy of Sciences—National Research Council and/or other information, FDA has classified the following indications as "possibly" effective.

Ilotycin® (erythromycin, Dista) ointment is possibly effective in the treatment of superficial topical infections due to organisms sensitive to its action. The therapeutic spectrum of Ilotycin includes streptococci, staphylococci, pneumococci, and other gram-positive bacteria. In addition,

Ilotycin is effective against some gram-negative organisms, *Neisseria, Haemophilus,* corynebacteria, clostridia, and certain parasitic (e.g., *Entamoeba histolytica*), rickettsial, and large-virus infections.
Final classification of the less-than-effective indications requires further investigation.

Contraindication: This drug is contraindicated in patients with a history of sensitivity to erythromycin.
Precautions and Adverse Reactions: The use of antimicrobial agents may be associated with the overgrowth of antibiotic-resistant organisms; in such a case, antibiotic administration should be stopped and appropriate measures taken.
As with any other medicament intended for topical use, there is always the possibility that sensitivity reactions will occur in certain individuals.
Administration: Ointment Ilotycin® (erythromycin, Dista) should be applied to the affected areas three or four times daily.
How Supplied: (℞) *Ointment No. 90, Ilotycin® (Erythromycin Ointment, USP),* 10 mg per g, in ½-oz and 1-oz tubes and in 16-oz jars. Contains mineral oil and white petrolatum. *Store at controlled room temperature, 15° to 30° C (59° to 86° F).*

[010880]

ILOTYCIN® ℞
(erythromycin)
Ophthalmic Ointment, USP

Description: Ilotycin® (erythromycin, Dista) is a wide-range antibiotic discovered in the research laboratories of Eli Lilly and Company and produced from a strain of *Streptomyces erythraeus.* The special sterile ophthalmic ointment base, containing mineral oil and white petrolatum, flows freely over the conjunctiva.
Indications: For the treatment of superficial ocular infections involving the conjunctiva and/or cornea caused by organisms susceptible to Ilotycin® (erythromycin, Dista).
For prophylaxis of ophthalmia neonatorum due to *Neisseria gonorrhoeae* or *Chlamydia trachomatis.* The Center for Disease Control (U.S.P.H.S.) and the Committee on Drugs, the Committee on Fetus and Newborn, and the Committee on Infectious Diseases of the American Academy of Pediatrics recommend 1 percent silver nitrate solution in single-dose ampoules or single-use tubes of an ophthalmic ointment containing 0.5 percent erythromycin or 1 percent tetracycline as "effective and acceptable regimens for prophylaxis of gonococcal ophthalmia neonatorum."[1] (For infants born to mothers with clinically apparent gonorrhea, intravenous or intramuscular injections of aqueous crystalline penicillin G should be given: a single dose of 50,000 units for term infants or 20,000 units for infants of low birth weight. Topical prophylaxis alone is inadequate for these infants.[1]) Ophthalmic Ointment Ilotycin also has been effective for prevention of neonatal conjunctivitis due to *C. trachomatis,*[2] a condition that may develop one to several weeks after delivery in infants of mothers whose birth canals harbor the organism.
Contraindication: This drug is contraindicated in patients with a history of hypersensitivity to erythromycin.
Precautions: The use of antimicrobial agents may be associated with the overgrowth of antibiotic-resistant organisms; in such a case, antibiotic administration should be stopped and appropriate measures taken.
Adverse Reactions: As with any other medicament intended for topical use, there is always the possibility that sensitivity reactions will occur in certain individuals. If such reactions develop, the medication should be discontinued.
Dosage and Administration: In the treatment of external ocular infections, Ophthalmic Ointment Ilotycin® (erythromycin, Dista) should be applied directly to the infected structure one or more times daily, depending on the severity of the infection.
For prophylaxis of neonatal gonococcal or chlamydial conjunctivitis, a ribbon of ointment approximately 0.5 to 1 cm in length should be instilled into each conjunctival sac. The ointment should not be flushed from the eye following instillation. A new tube should be used for each infant. Infants born by cesarean section as well as those delivered by the vaginal route should receive prophylaxis.

References: 1. American Academy of Pediatrics: Prophylaxis and Treatment of Neonatal Gonococcal Infections, Pediatrics, *65:*1047, 1980.
2. Hammerschlag, M. R., *et al.:* Erythromycin Ointment for Ocular Prophylaxis of Neonatal Chlamydial Infection, J.A.M.A., *244:*2291, 1980.

How Supplied: (℞) *Sterile Ophthalmic Ointment No. 52, Ilotycin® (Erythromycin Ophthalmic Ointment, USP),* 5 mg per g, in ⅛-oz tamperproof tubes (NDC 0777-1863-17). *Store at controlled room temperature, 15° to 30° C (59° to 86° F).*

[020381]

ILOTYCIN® ℞
(erythromycin)
Tablets, USP
(Enteric-Coated)

Description: Erythromycin is produced by a strain of *Streptomyces erythraeus* and belongs to the macrolide group of antibiotics. It is basic and readily forms salts with acids. The base, the stearate salt, and the esters are poorly soluble in water and are suitable for oral administration.
Tablets Ilotycin® (erythromycin, Dista) are specially coated to protect the contents from the inactivating effect of gastric acid and to permit efficient absorption of the antibiotic in the small intestine.
Each enteric-coated tablet contains 250 mg erythromycin.
Actions: Erythromycin inhibits protein synthesis without affecting nucleic acid synthesis. Some strains of *Haemophilus influenzae* and staphylococci have demonstrated resistance to erythromycin. Some strains of *H. influenzae* that are resistant in vitro to erythromycin alone are susceptible to erythromycin and sulfonamides used concomitantly. Culture and susceptibility testing should be done. If the Bauer-Kirby method of disc susceptibility testing is used, a 15-mcg erythromycin disc should give a zone diameter of at least 18 mm when tested against an erythromycin-susceptible organism.
Tablets Ilotycin® (erythromycin, Dista) are well absorbed and may be given without regard to meals.
After absorption, erythromycin diffuses readily into most body fluids. In the absence of meningeal inflammation, low concentrations are normally achieved in the spinal fluid, but passage of the drug across the blood-brain barrier increases in meningitis. In the presence of normal hepatic function, erythromycin is concentrated in the liver and excreted in the bile; the effect of hepatic dysfunction on excretion of erythromycin by the liver into the bile is not known. After oral administration, less than 5 percent of the administered dose can be recovered as the active form in the urine.
Erythromycin crosses the placental barrier, but fetal plasma levels are low.
Indications: *Streptococcus pyogenes* (Group A Beta-Hemolytic)—Upper and lower respiratory tract, skin, and soft-tissue infections of mild to moderate severity.
Injectable penicillin G benzathine is considered by the American Heart Association to be the drug of choice in the treatment and prevention of streptococcal pharyngitis and in long-term prophylaxis of rheumatic fever.
When oral medication is preferred for treating the above-mentioned conditions, penicillin G or V or erythromycin is the alternate drug of choice.
The importance of the patient's strict adherence to the prescribed dosage regimen must be stressed when oral medication is given. A therapeutic dose should be administered for at least ten days.
Alpha-Hemolytic Streptococci (Viridans Group)—Although no controlled clinical efficacy trials have been conducted, oral erythromycin has been suggested by the American Heart Association and American Dental Association for use in a regimen for prophylaxis against bacterial endocarditis in patients hypersensitive to penicillin who have congenital and/or rheumatic or other acquired valvular heart disease when they undergo dental procedures and surgical procedures of the upper respiratory tract.[1] Erythromycin is not suitable for such prophylaxis prior to genitourinary or gastrointestinal tract surgery.
Note: When selecting antibiotics for the prevention of bacterial endocarditis, the physician or dentist should read the full joint statement of the American Heart Association and the American Dental Association.[1]
Staphylococcus aureus—Acute infections of skin and soft tissue which are mild to moderately severe. Resistance may develop during treatment.
S. (Diplococcus) pneumoniae—Infections of the upper respiratory tract (e.g., otitis media, pharyngitis) and lower respiratory tract (e.g., pneumonia) of mild to moderate severity.
Mycoplasma pneumoniae (Eaton Agent, PPLO)—In the treatment of respiratory tract infections due to this organism.
H. influenzae—May be used concomitantly with adequate doses of sulfonamides in treating upper respiratory tract infections of mild to moderate severity. Not all strains of this organism are susceptible at the erythromycin concentrations ordinarily achieved (see appropriate sulfonamide labeling for prescribing information).
Treponema pallidum—Erythromycin is an alternate choice of treatment for primary syphilis in penicillin-allergic patients. In primary syphilis, spinal-fluid examinations should be done before treatment and as part of follow-up after therapy.
Corynebacterium diphtheriae—As an adjunct to antitoxin, to prevent establishment of carriers, and to eradicate the organism in carriers.
C. minutissimum—In the treatment of erythrasma.
Entamoeba histolytica—In the treatment of intestinal amebiasis only. Extraenteric amebiasis requires treatment with other agents.
Listeria monocytogenes—Infections due to this organism.
Neisseria gonorrhoeae—In female patients with a history of sensitivity to penicillin, a parenteral erythromycin (such as the gluceptate) may be administered in conjunction with an oral erythromycin as alternate therapy in acute pelvic inflammatory disease caused by *N. gonorrhoeae.* In the treatment of gonorrhea, patients suspected of having concomitant syphilis should have microscopic examinations (by immunofluorescence or darkfield) before receiving erythromycin and monthly serologic tests for a minimum of four months.
Bordetella pertussis—Erythromycin is effective in eliminating the organism from the nasopharynx of infected individuals and in rendering them noninfectious. Some clinical studies suggest that erythromycin may be helpful

Continued on next page

Dista—Cont.

in the prophylaxis of pertussis in exposed susceptible individuals.
Legionnaires' Disease—Although no controlled clinical efficacy studies have been conducted, in vitro and limited preliminary clinical data suggest that erythromycin may be effective in treating Legionnaires' disease.
Contraindication: Erythromycin is contraindicated in patients with known hypersensitivity to this antibiotic.
Warning: *Usage in Pregnancy*—Safety of this drug for use during pregnancy has not been established.
Precautions: Since erythromycin is excreted principally by the liver, caution should be exercised in administering the antibiotic to patients with impaired hepatic function. There have been reports of hepatic dysfunction, with or without jaundice, occurring in patients taking oral erythromycin products.
Recent data from studies of erythromycin reveal that its use in patients who are receiving high doses of theophylline may be associated with an increase in serum theophylline levels and potential theophylline toxicity. In case of theophylline toxicity and/or elevated serum theophylline levels, the dose of theophylline should be reduced while the patient is receiving concomitant erythromycin therapy.
Surgical procedures should be performed when indicated.
Adverse Reactions: The most frequent side effects of erythromycin preparations are gastrointestinal (e.g., abdominal cramping and discomfort) and are dose related. Nausea, vomiting, and diarrhea occur infrequently with usual oral doses.
During prolonged or repeated therapy, there is a possibility of overgrowth of nonsusceptible bacteria or fungi. If such infections arise, the drug should be discontinued and appropriate therapy instituted.
Mild allergic reactions, such as urticaria and other skin rashes, have occurred. Serious allergic reactions, including anaphylaxis, have been reported.
Administration and Dosage: Tablets Ilotycin® (erythromycin, Dista) are well absorbed whether given immediately after meals or between meals on an empty stomach.
Adults—The usual dosage is 250 mg every six hours. This may be increased up to 4 g or more per day according to the severity of the infection.
Children—Age, weight, and severity of the infection are important factors in determining the proper dosage. The usual regimen is 30 to 50 mg per kg per day in divided doses. For more severe infections, this dosage may be doubled. If administration is desired on a twice-a-day schedule in either adults or children, one-half of the total daily dose may be given every 12 hours.
Streptococcal Infections—In the treatment of group A beta-hemolytic streptococcal infections, a therapeutic dosage of erythromycin should be administered for at least ten days. In continuous prophylaxis of streptococcal infections in persons with a history of rheumatic heart disease, the dosage is 250 mg twice a day. For prophylaxis against bacterial endocarditis[1] in patients with rheumatic, congenital, or other acquired valvular heart disease when undergoing dental procedures or surgical procedures of the upper respiratory tract, the dosage schedule for adults is 1 g (20 mg/kg for children) orally one and one-half to two hours before the procedure and then 500 mg (10 mg/kg for children) orally every six hours for eight doses.
Primary Syphilis—30 to 40 g given in divided doses over a period of 10 to 15 days.
Acute Pelvic Inflammatory Disease Caused by N. gonorrhoeae—Ilotycin® Gluceptate (Sterile Erythromycin Gluceptate, USP, Dista), 500 mg intravenously every six hours for at least three days, followed by Ilotycin, 250 mg every six hours for seven days.
Dysenteric Amebiasis—250 mg four times daily for 10 to 14 days for adults; 30 to 50 mg per kg per day in divided doses for 10 to 14 days for children.
Pertussis—Although optimum dosage and duration of treatment have not been established, the dosage of erythromycin utilized in reported clinical studies was 40 to 50 mg per kg per day, given in divided doses for five to 14 days.
Legionnaires' Disease—Although optimum doses have not been established, doses utilized in reported clinical data were those recommended above (1 to 4 g erythromycin base daily in divided doses).
Reference: 1. American Heart Association: Prevention of Bacterial Endocarditis, Circulation, *56:* 139A, 1977.
How Supplied: (℞) *Tablets No. 23, Ilotycin® (Erythromycin Tablets, USP) (Enteric-Coated), C03,** 250 mg, Orange, in bottles of 24, 100, and 500 and in 20 strips of 5 individually labeled blisters each containing 1 tablet (ID100).
[032081]

---

*Identi-Code® symbol.

ILOTYCIN® GLUCEPTATE ℞
(erythromycin gluceptate)
Sterile, USP
IntraVenous

Description: Erythromycin is produced by a strain of *Streptomyces erythraeus* and belongs to the macrolide group of antibiotics. It is basic and readily forms salts with acids.
Actions: Erythromycin inhibits protein synthesis without affecting nucleic acid synthesis. Some strains of *Haemophilus influenzae* and staphylococci have demonstrated resistance to erythromycin. Culture and susceptibility testing should be done. If the Bauer-Kirby method of disc susceptibility testing is used, a 15-mcg erythromycin disc should give a zone diameter of at least 18 mm when tested against an erythromycin-susceptible organism.
Intravenous injection of 200 mg of erythromycin produces peak serum levels of 3 to 4 mcg per ml at one hour and 0.5 mcg per ml at six hours.
Erythromycin diffuses readily into the body fluids. Only low concentrations are normally achieved in the spinal fluid, but passage of the drug across the blood-brain barrier increases in meningitis. In the presence of normal hepatic function, erythromycin is concentrated in the liver and excreted in the bile; the effect of hepatic dysfunction on excretion of erythromycin by the liver into the bile is not known. From 12 to 15 percent of intravenously administered erythromycin is excreted in active form in the urine.
Erythromycin crosses the placental barrier, but fetal plasma levels are low.
Indications: *Streptococcus pyogenes* (Group A Beta-Hemolytic)—Upper and lower respiratory tract, skin, and soft-tissue infections of mild to moderate severity.
Injectable penicillin G benzathine is considered by the American Heart Association to be the drug of choice in the treatment and prevention of streptococcal pharyngitis and in long-term prophylaxis of rheumatic fever.
Staphylococcus aureus—Acute infections of skin and soft tissue which are mild to moderately severe. Resistance may develop during treatment.
S. (Diplococcus) pneumoniae—Infections of the upper respiratory tract (e.g., otitis media, pharyngitis) and lower respiratory tract (e.g., pneumonia) of mild to moderate severity.
Mycoplasma pneumoniae (Eaton Agent, PPLO)—In the treatment of respiratory tract infections due to this organism.
H. influenzae—May be used concomitantly with adequate doses of sulfonamides in treating upper respiratory tract infections of mild to moderate severity. Not all strains of this organism are susceptible at the erythromycin concentrations ordinarily achieved (see appropriate sulfonamide labeling for prescribing information).
Corynebacterium diphtheriae—As an adjunct to antitoxin.
Listeria monocytogenes—Infections due to this organism.
Neisseria gonorrhoeae—In female patients with a history of sensitivity to penicillin, a parenteral erythromycin (such as the gluceptate) may be administered in conjunction with an oral erythromycin as alternate therapy in acute pelvic inflammatory disease caused by *N. gonorrhoeae*. In the treatment of gonorrhea, patients suspected of having concomitant syphilis should have microscopic examinations (by immunofluorescence or darkfield) before receiving erythromycin and monthly serologic tests for a minimum of four months.
Legionnaires' Disease—Although no controlled clinical efficacy studies have been conducted, in vitro and limited preliminary clinical data suggest that erythromycin may be effective in treating Legionnaires' disease.
Contraindication: Intravenous erythromycin is contraindicated in patients with known hypersensitivity to this antibiotic.
Warning: *Usage in Pregnancy*—Safety of this drug for use during pregnancy has not been established.
Precautions: Side effects following the use of intravenous erythromycin are rare. Occasional venous irritation has been encountered, but if the injection is given slowly, in dilute solution, preferably by continuous intravenous infusion over 20 to 60 minutes, pain and vessel trauma are minimized.
Since erythromycin is excreted principally by the liver, caution should be exercised in administering the antibiotic to patients with impaired hepatic function.
Recent data from studies of erythromycin reveal that its use in patients who are receiving high doses of theophylline may be associated with an increase in serum theophylline levels and potential theophylline toxicity. In case of theophylline toxicity and/or elevated serum theophylline levels, the dose of theophylline should be reduced while the patient is receiving concomitant erythromycin therapy.
Surgical procedures should be performed when indicated.
Adverse Reactions: Allergic reactions, ranging from urticaria and mild skin eruptions to anaphylaxis, have occurred with intravenously administered erythromycin.
During prolonged or repeated therapy, there is a possibility of overgrowth of nonsusceptible bacteria or fungi. If such infections arise, the drug should be discontinued and appropriate therapy instituted.
Variations in liver function have been observed following daily doses at high levels or after prolonged therapy. Hepatic function tests should be performed when such therapy is given.
Reversible hearing loss associated with the intravenous infusion of 4 g or more per day of erythromycin has been reported rarely.
Administration and Dosage: Prepare the initial solution of Ilotycin® Gluceptate (erythromycin gluceptate, Dista) by (1) adding at least 10 ml of Sterile Water for Injection to the 250 or 500-mg vial or at least 20 ml of Sterile Water for Injection to the 1-g vial of Ilotycin Gluceptate and (2) shaking the vial until all of the drug is dissolved.
It is important that the product be diluted only *with Sterile Water for Injection without preservatives.*
After reconstitution, the sterile solutions should be stored in a refrigerator and used within seven days.

When all of the drug is dissolved, the solution may then be added to 0.9% Sodium Chloride Injection or to 5% Dextrose in Water to give 1 g per liter for slow, continuous infusion. I.V. fluid admixtures with a pH below 5.5 tend to lose potency rapidly. Therefore, such solutions should be administered completely within four hours after dilution.

If the period of administration is prolonged, the pH of the infusion fluid should be buffered to neutrality with a sterile agent such as Neut® (Sodium Bicarbonate 4% Additive Solution, Abbott) or Buff™ (Phosphate-Carbonate Buffer, Travenol). For administration of the antibiotic ir 500 or 1000 ml of 5% Dextrose in Water, add one ampoule full-strength Buff or 5 ml of Neut; for administration of the antibiotic in the same volumes of 0.9% Sodium Chloride Injection, add one ampoule half-strength Buff or 5 ml of Neut. These solutions should be completely administered within 24 hours after dilution.

If the medication is to be given in 100 to 250 ml of fluid by a volume control set such as Metriset® (McGaw), Volu-Trole® "B" (Cutter), Soluset® (Abbott), or Buretrol® (Baxter-Travenol), the I.V. fluid should be buffered in its primary container before being added to the volumetric administration set.

If the medication is to be given by intermittent injection, one-fourth of the total daily dose can be given in 20 to 60 minutes by slow intravenous injection of 250 to 500 mg in 100 to 250 ml of 0.9% Sodium Chloride Injection or 5% Dextrose in Water. Injection should be sufficiently slow to avoid pain along the vein.

The recommended I.V. dosage for severe infections in adults and children is 15 to 20 mg/kg of body weight/day. Higher doses (up to 4 g/day) may be given in very severe infections. Continuous infusion is preferable, but administration in divided doses at intervals of no more than every six hours is also effective.

For treatment of acute pelvic inflammatory disease caused by *N. gonorrhoeae*, administer 500 mg Ilotycin Gluceptate intravenously every six hours for at least three days, followed by 250 mg Ilotycin® (Erythromycin Tablets, USP, Dista) every six hours for seven days.

Patients receiving intravenous erythromycin should be changed to the oral dosage form as soon as possible.

For Treatment of Legionnaires' Disease—Although optimum doses have not been established, doses utilized in reported clinical data were those recommended above (1 to 4 g daily in divided doses).

How Supplied: (℞) *Vials Ilotycin® Gluceptate (Sterile Erythromycin Gluceptate, USP), I.V.,* rubber-stoppered (Dry Powder): *No. 524,* 250 mg (equivalent to erythromycin), 30-ml size (NDC 0777-1404-01); *No. 538,* 500 mg (equivalent to erythromycin), 30-ml size (NDC 0777-1409-01); and *No. 646,* 1 g (equivalent to erythromycin), 30-ml size (NDC 0777-1441-01), in singles (10 per carton).

[020582]

KEFLEX® (cephalexin) USP ℞

Description: Keflex® (cephalexin, Dista) is a semisynthetic cephalosporin antibiotic intended for oral administration. It is 7-(D-α-amino-α-phenylacetamido) - 3 - methyl - 3 - cephem - 4 - carboxylic acid, monohydrate.

The nucleus of cephalexin is related to that of other cephalosporin antibiotics. The compound is a zwitterion; i.e., the molecule contains both a basic and an acidic group. The isoelectric point of cephalexin in water is approximately 4.5 to 5.

The crystalline form of cephalexin which is available is a monohydrate. It is a white crystalline solid having a bitter taste. Solubility in water is low at room temperature; 1 or 2 mg/ml may be dissolved readily, but higher concentrations are obtained with increasing difficulty.

The cephalosporins differ from penicillins in the structure of the bicyclic ring system. Cephalexin has a *D*-phenylglycyl group as substituent at the 7-amino position and an unsubstituted methyl group at the 3-position.

Clinical Pharmacology: *Human Pharmacology*—Keflex® (cephalexin, Dista) is acid stable and may be given without regard to meals. It is rapidly absorbed after oral administration. Following doses of 250 mg, 500 mg, and 1 g, average peak serum levels of approximately 9, 18, and 32 mcg/ml respectively were obtained at one hour. Measurable levels were present six hours after administration. Cephalexin is excreted in the urine by glomerular filtration and tubular secretion. Studies showed that over 90 percent of the drug was excreted unchanged in the urine within eight hours. During this period, peak urine concentrations following the 250-mg, 500-mg, and 1-g doses were approximately 1000, 2200, and 5000 mcg/ml respectively.

Microbiology—In vitro tests demonstrate that the cephalosporins are bactericidal because of their inhibition of cell-wall synthesis. Keflex is active against the following organisms in vitro:

- Beta-hemolytic streptococci
- Staphylococci, including coagulase-positive, coagulase-negative, and penicillinase-producing strains
- *Streptococcus (Diplococcus) pneumoniae*
- *Escherichia coli*
- *Proteus mirabilis*
- *Klebsiella* sp.
- *Haemophilus influenzae*
- *Neisseria catarrhalis*

Note—Most strains of enterococci *(S. faecalis)* and a few strains of staphylococci are resistant to Keflex. It is not active against most strains of *Enterobacter* sp., *P. morganii,* and *P. vulgaris.* It has no activity against *Pseudomonas* or *Herellea* species. When tested by in vitro methods, staphylococci exhibit cross-resistance between Keflex and methicillin-type antibiotics.

Disc Susceptibility Tests—Quantitative methods that require measurement of zone diameters give the most precise estimates of antibiotic susceptibility. One such procedure (*Am. J. Clin. Pathol., 45:*493, 1966; *Federal Register, 39:*19182–19184, 1974) has been recommended for use with discs for testing susceptibility to cephalothin. Interpretations correlate zone diameters of the disc test with MIC values for Keflex. With this procedure, a report from the laboratory of "resistant" indicates that the infecting organism is not likely to respond to therapy. A report of "intermediate susceptibility" suggests that the organism would be susceptible if the infection is confined to the urine, in which high antibiotic levels can be obtained, or if high dosage is used in other types of infection.

Indications and Usage: Keflex® (cephalexin, Dista) is indicated for the treatment of the following infections when caused by susceptible strains of the designated microorganisms:

- Respiratory tract infections caused by *S. pneumoniae* and group A beta-hemolytic streptococci (Penicillin is the usual drug of choice in the treatment and prevention of streptococcal infections, including the prophylaxis of rheumatic fever. Keflex is generally effective in the eradication of streptococci from the nasopharynx; however, substantial data establishing the efficacy of Keflex in the subsequent prevention of rheumatic fever are not available at present.)
- Otitis media due to *S. pneumoniae, H. influenzae,* staphylococci, streptococci, and *N. catarrhalis*
- Skin and skin-structure infections caused by staphylococci and/or streptococci
- Bone infections caused by staphylococci and/or *P. mirabilis*
- Genitourinary tract infections, including acute prostatitis, caused by *E. coli, P. mirabilis,* and *Klebsiella* sp.

Note—Culture and susceptibility tests should be initiated prior to and during therapy. Renal function studies should be performed when indicated.

Contraindication: Keflex® (cephalexin, Dista) is contraindicated in patients with known allergy to the cephalosporin group of antibiotics.

Warnings: BEFORE CEPHALEXIN THERAPY IS INSTITUTED, CAREFUL INQUIRY SHOULD BE MADE CONCERNING PREVIOUS HYPERSENSITIVITY REACTIONS TO CEPHALOSPORINS AND PENICILLIN. CEPHALOSPORIN C DERIVATIVES SHOULD BE GIVEN CAUTIOUSLY TO PENICILLIN-SENSITIVE PATIENTS.

SERIOUS ACUTE HYPERSENSITIVITY REACTIONS MAY REQUIRE EPINEPHRINE AND OTHER EMERGENCY MEASURES.

There is some clinical and laboratory evidence of partial cross-allergenicity of the penicillins and the cephalosporins. Patients have been reported to have had severe reactions (including anaphylaxis) to both drugs.

Any patient who has demonstrated some form of allergy, particularly to drugs, should receive antibiotics cautiously. No exception should be made with regard to Keflex® (cephalexin, Dista).

Pseudomembranous colitis has been reported with virtually all broad-spectrum antibiotics (including macrolides, semisynthetic penicillins, and cephalosporins); therefore, it is important to consider its diagnosis in patients who develop diarrhea in association with the use of antibiotics. Such colitis may range in severity from mild to life-threatening.

Treatment with broad-spectrum antibiotics alters the normal flora of the colon and may permit overgrowth of clostridia. Studies indicate that a toxin produced by *Clostridium difficile* is one primary cause of antibiotic-associated colitis.

Mild cases of pseudomembranous colitis usually respond to drug discontinuance alone. In moderate to severe cases, management should include sigmoidoscopy, appropriate bacteriologic studies, and fluid, electrolyte, and protein supplementation. When the colitis does not improve after the drug has been discontinued, or when it is severe, oral vancomycin is the drug of choice for antibiotic-associated pseudomembranous colitis produced by *C. difficile.* Other causes of colitis should be ruled out.

Usage in Pregnancy—Safety of this product for use during pregnancy has not been established.

Precautions: *General Precautions*—Patients should be followed carefully so that any side effects or unusual manifestations of drug idiosyncrasy may be detected. If an allergic reaction to Keflex® (cephalexin, Dista) occurs, the drug should be discontinued and the patient treated with the usual agents (e.g., epinephrine or other pressor amines, antihistamines, or corticosteroids).

Prolonged use of Keflex may result in the overgrowth of nonsusceptible organisms. Careful observation of the patient is essential. If superinfection occurs during therapy, appropriate measures should be taken.

Positive direct Coombs' tests have been reported during treatment with the cephalosporin antibiotics. In hematologic studies or in transfusion cross-matching procedures when antiglobulin tests are performed on the minor side or in Coombs' testing of newborns whose mothers have received cephalosporin antibiotics before parturition, it should be recognized that a positive Coombs' test may be due to the drug.

Keflex should be administered with caution in the presence of markedly impaired renal function. Under such conditions, careful clinical

Continued on next page

Dista—Cont.

observation and laboratory studies should be made because safe dosage may be lower than that usually recommended.
Indicated surgical procedures should be performed in conjunction with antibiotic therapy.
As a result of administration of Keflex, a false-positive reaction for glucose in the urine may occur. This has been observed with Benedict's and Fehling's solutions and also with Clinitest® tablets but not with Tes-Tape® (Glucose Enzymatic Test Strip, USP, Lilly).
Broad-spectrum antibiotics should be prescribed with caution in individuals with a history of gastrointestinal disease, particularly colitis.
Usage in Pregnancy—Pregnancy Category B—The daily oral administration of cephalexin to rats in doses of 250 or 500 mg/kg prior to and during pregnancy, or to rats and mice during the period of organogenesis only, had no adverse effect on fertility, fetal viability, fetal weight, or litter size. Note that the safety of cephalexin during pregnancy in humans has not been established.
Cephalexin showed no enhanced toxicity in weanling and newborn rats as compared with adult animals. Nevertheless, because the studies in humans cannot rule out the possibility of harm, Keflex should be used during pregnancy only if clearly needed.
Nursing Mothers—The excretion of cephalexin in the milk increased up to four hours after a 500-mg dose; the drug reached a maximum level of 4 mcg/ml, then decreased gradually, and had disappeared eight hours after administration. Caution should be exercised when Keflex is administered to a nursing woman.
Adverse Reactions: *Gastrointestinal*—Symptoms of pseudomembranous colitis may appear either during or after antibiotic treatment. Nausea and vomiting have been reported rarely. The most frequent side effect has been diarrhea. It was very rarely severe enough to warrant cessation of therapy. Dyspepsia and abdominal pain have also occurred.
Hypersensitivity—Allergies (in the form of rash, urticaria, and angioedema) have been observed. These reactions usually subsided upon discontinuation of the drug. Anaphylaxis has also been reported.
Other reactions have included genital and anal pruritus, genital moniliasis, vaginitis and vaginal discharge, dizziness, fatigue, and headache.
Eosinophilia, neutropenia, and slight elevations in SGOT and SGPT have been reported.
Dosage and Administration: Keflex® (cephalexin, Dista) is administered orally.
Adults—The adult dosage ranges from 1 to 4 g daily in divided doses. The usual adult dose is 250 mg q. 6 h. For skin and skin-structure infections, a dosage of 500 mg may be administered q. 12 h. For more severe infections or those caused by less susceptible organisms, larger doses may be needed. If daily doses of Keflex greater than 4 g are required, parenteral cephalosporins, in appropriate doses, should be considered.
Children—The usual recommended daily dosage for children is 25 to 50 mg/kg in divided doses. For skin and skin-structure infections, the total daily dose may be divided and administered q. 12 h.
[See table below].
In severe infections, the dosage may be doubled.
In the therapy of otitis media, clinical studies have shown that a dosage of 75 to 100 mg/kg/day in four divided doses is required.
In the treatment of beta-hemolytic streptococcal infections, a therapeutic dosage of Keflex should be administered for at least ten days.
How Supplied: (℞) *For Oral Suspension, Keflex® (Cephalexin for Oral Suspension, USP), M-201, W21,** in 60 (NDC 0777-2321-97), 100 (NDC 0777-2321-48), and 200-ml-size (NDC 0777-2321-89) packages and in unit-dose bottles of 100 (ID100) (NDC 0777-2321-33).
Each 60-ml-size package contains 1.5 g cephalexin in a dry, pleasantly flavored mixture. At the time of dispensing, add 36 ml of water to the dry mixture in the bottle in *two* portions. Shake well after each addition.
Each 100-ml-size package contains 2.5 g cephalexin in a dry, pleasantly flavored mixture. At the time of dispensing, add 60 ml of water in *two* portions to the dry mixture in the bottle. Shake well after each addition.
Each 200-ml-size package contains 5 g cephalexin in a dry, pleasantly flavored mixture. At the time of dispensing, add 120 ml of water in *two* portions to the dry mixture in the bottle. Shake well after each addition.
When mixed as directed, each 5 ml (approximately 1 teaspoonful) will contain 125 mg cephalexin. After mixing, store in a refrigerator. The mixture may be kept for 14 days without significant loss of potency. *Shake well before using. Keep tightly closed.*
(℞) *For Oral Suspension, Keflex® (Cephalexin for Oral Suspension, USP), M-202, W68,** in 100 (NDC 0777-2368-48) and 200-ml-size (NDC 0777-2368-89) packages and in unit-dose bottles of 100 (ID100) (NDC 0777-2368-33).
Each 100-ml-size package contains 5 g cephalexin in a dry, pleasantly flavored mixture. At the time of dispensing, add 60 ml of water in *two* portions to the dry mixture in the bottle. Shake well after each addition.
Each 200-ml-size package contains 10 g cephalexin in a dry, pleasantly flavored mixture. At the time of dispensing, add 124 ml of water in *two* portions to the dry mixture in the bottle. Shake well after each addition.
When mixed as directed, each 5 ml (approximately 1 teaspoonful) will contain 250 mg cephalexin. After mixing, store in a refrigerator. The mixture may be kept for 14 days without significant loss of potency. *Shake well before using. Keep tightly closed.*
(℞) *For Pediatric Drops, Keflex® (Cephalexin for Oral Suspension, USP), M-204, W22,** in 10-ml-size packages (NDC 0777-2322-37).
This package contains 1 g cephalexin in a dry, pleasantly flavored mixture and a special dropper calibrated at approximately 25 and 50 mg. At the time of dispensing, add 5.5 ml of water to the dry mixture in the bottle. Close with original bottle cap and shake promptly until all of the powder is in suspension. Remove detachable portion of bottle label but leave white tab affixed.
When mixed as directed, each ml will contain 100 mg cephalexin. After being mixed, the suspension may be kept in a refrigerator for 14 days without significant loss of potency. *Shake well before using. Keep tightly closed.*
(℞) *Pulvules® Keflex® (Cephalexin Capsules, USP): No. 402, H69,** 250 mg (No. 0, White Opaque Body, Dark-Green Opaque Cap), and *No. 403, H71,** 500 mg (No. 0, Light-Green Opaque Body, Dark-Green Opaque Cap), in bottles of 20 (NDC 0777-0869-20 and 0871-20) and 100 (NDC 0777-0869-02 and 0871-02) and in 10 strips of 10 individually labeled blisters each containing 1 Pulvule (ID100) (NDC 0777-0869-33 and 0871-33).
(℞) *Tablets No. 1896, Keflex® (Cephalexin Tablets, USP), U60,** 1 g, Green (capsule-shaped), in bottles of 24 (NDC 0777-2160-24) and in 10 strips of 10 individually labeled blisters each containing 1 tablet (ID100) (NDC 0777-2160-33). [060882]
[*Shown in Product Identification Section*]
Pulvules No. 402, 250 mg—100's—6505-00-165-6545(A); ID100's—6505-00-197-9200(A)
Pulvules No. 403, 500 mg—100's—6505-00-183-8543A; ID100's—6505-00-171-1213(A)
M-201—For Oral Suspension—100-ml size —6505-00-009-1833

* Identi-Code® symbol.

Keflex Suspension

Child's Weight	125 mg/5 ml	250 mg/5 ml
10 kg (22 lb)	½ to 1 tsp q.i.d.	¼ to ½ tsp q.i.d.
20 kg (44 lb)	1 to 2 tsp q.i.d.	½ to 1 tsp q.i.d.
40 kg (88 lb)	2 to 4 tsp q.i.d.	1 to 2 tsp q.i.d.

or

Child's Weight	125 mg/5 ml	250 mg/5 ml
10 kg (22 lb)	1 to 2 tsp b.i.d.*	½ to 1 tsp. b.i.d.*
20 kg (44 lb)	2 to 4 tsp b.i.d.	1 to 2 tsp b.i.d.
40 kg (88 lb)	4 to 8 tsp b.i.d.	2 to 4 tsp b.i.d.

* Note: The b.i.d. dosage is indicated only for skin and skin-structure infections.

MI-CEBRIN® OTC
(vitamins-minerals)

Description: Each tablet contains—

Thiamine (Vitamin B_1)	10 mg
Riboflavin (Vitamin B_2)	5 mg
Pyridoxine (Vitamin B_6)	1.7 mg
Pantothenic Acid	10 mg
Niacinamide	30 mg
Vitamin B_{12} (Activity Equivalent)	3 mcg
Ascorbic Acid (Vitamin C)	100 mg
dl-Alpha Tocopheryl Acetate (Vitamin E)	5.5 IU (5.5 mg)
Vitamin A	10,000 IU (3 mg)
Vitamin D	400 IU (10 mcg)
Contains also—	approximately
Iron (as Ferrous Sulfate)	15 mg
Copper (as the Sulfate)	1 mg
Iodine (as Potassium Iodide)	0.15 mg
Manganese (as the Glycerophosphate)	1 mg
Magnesium (as the Hydroxide)	5 mg
Zinc (as the Chloride)	1.5 mg

Mi-Cebrin offers a comprehensive vitamin-mineral formula in a yellow tablet of convenient size. The use of synthetic vitamins A and D eliminates any unpleasant fish-liver-oil odor or taste.
Indications: For the prevention or treatment of multiple vitamin and mineral deficiencies and in states of subnutrition. Both vitamins and minerals are essential components of vital physiologic mechanisms, including many enzyme systems. Although trace elements are known constituents of foodstuffs, their exact role in nutrition has not been defined. Studies have shown that foodstuffs may be lacking in these elements when grown in soil notably deprived of its normal constituents.
Dosage: 1 tablet a day, or as directed by the physician.
How Supplied: *Tablets No. 1790, Mi-Cebrin® (vitamins-minerals, Dista), C19,** Coated, Yellow, in bottles of 60, 100, and 1000 and in 10 strips of 10 individually labeled blisters each containing 1 tablet (ID100). [050180]

*Identi-Code® symbol.

MI-CEBRIN T® OTC
(vitamin-minerals therapeutic)

Description: Each tablet contains—

Thiamine Mononitrate (Vitamin B_1)	15 mg

Riboflavin (Vitamin B_2) ....10 mg
Pyridoxine Hydrochloride (Vitamin B_6) ....2 mg
Pantothenic Acid (as Calcium Pantothenate) ....10 mg
Niacinamide ....100 mg
Vitamin B_{12} (Activity Equivalent) ....7.5 mcg
Ascorbic Acid (Vitamin C) ....150 mg
dl-Alpha Tocopheryl Acetate (Vitamin E) ....5.5 IU (5.5 mg)
Vitamin A ....10,000 IU (3 mg)
Vitamin D ....400 IU (10 mcg)
Contains also— approximately
Iron (as Ferrous Sulfate) ....15 mg
Copper (as the Sulfate) ....1 mg
Iodine (as Potassium Iodide) ....0.15 mg
Manganese (as the Glycerophosphate) ....1 mg
Magnesium (as the Hydroxide) ....5 mg
Zinc (as the Chloride) ....1.5 mg

Mi-Cebrin T is an extended-range therapeutic vitamin-mineral tablet formulated to aid patient recovery. Each tablet contains ten vitamins and six minerals and is specially coated to protect the full potency of the ingredients.

Indications: For the therapeutic management of surgical patients and patients with burns or injuries, febrile diseases, or poor dietary intake.

Precaution: Rarely, vitamins A and D in large doses daily for several months or longer cause toxicity.

Dosage: 1 tablet a day, or as directed by the physician.

How Supplied: *Tablets No. 1807, Mi-Cebrin T® (vitamin-minerals therapeutic, Dista), C20,** Coated, Orange, in bottles of 30, 100, and 1000 and in 10 strips of 10 individually labeled blisters each containing 1 tablet (ID100).

[050180]

*Identi-Code® symbol.

NALFON®
NALFON® 200
(fenoprofen calcium) USP

℞

Description: Nalfon® (fenoprofen calcium, Dista) is a nonsteroidal, anti-inflammatory, antiarthritic drug. Pulvules® and Tablets Nalfon contain fenoprofen calcium as the dihydrate in an amount equivalent to 200 mg or 300 mg (Pulvules) or 600 mg (Tablets) of fenoprofen. Chemically, Nalfon is an arylacetic acid derivative.

Nalfon is a white crystalline powder, soluble in alcohol (95%) to the extent of approximately 15 mg/ml at 25°C, slightly soluble in water, and insoluble in benzene.

The pK_a of Nalfon is 4.5 at 25°C.

Clinical Pharmacology: Nalfon® (fenoprofen calcium, Dista) is a nonsteroidal, anti-inflammatory, antiarthritic drug that also prossesses analgesic and antipyretic activities. Its exact mode of action is unknown, but it is thought that prostaglandin synthetase inhibition is involved. Nalfon has been shown to inhibit prostaglandin synthetase isolated from bovine seminal vesicles. Reproduction studies in rats have shown Nalfon to be associated with prolonged labor and difficult parturition when given during late pregnancy. Evidence suggests that this may be due to decreased uterine contractility resulting from the inhibition of prostaglandin synthesis. Its action is not mediated through the adrenal gland.

Fenoprofen shows anti-inflammatory effects in rodents by inhibiting the development of redness and edema in acute inflammatory conditions and by reducing soft-tissue swelling and bone damage associated with chronic inflammation. It exhibits analgesic activity in rodents by inhibiting the writhing response caused by the introduction of an irritant into the peritoneal cavities of mice and by elevating pain thresholds to pressure in edematous hindpaws of rats. In rats made febrile by the subcutaneous administration of brewer's yeast, fenoprofen produces antipyretic action. These effects are characteristic of nonsteroidal, anti-inflammatory, antipyretic, analgesic drugs.

The results in humans confirmed the anti-inflammatory and analgesic actions found in animals. The emergence and degree of erythemic response were measured in adult male volunteers exposed to ultraviolet irradiation. The effects of Nalfon, aspirin, and indomethacin were compared separately with those of a placebo. All three drugs demonstrated antierythemic activity.

In patients with rheumatoid arthritis, the anti-inflammatory action of Nalfon has been evidenced by relief of pain; by increase in grip strength; by reductions in joint swelling, duration of morning stiffness, and disease activity (as assessed by both the investigator and the patient); and by increased mobility (a decrease in the number of joints having limited motion).

The use of Nalfon® (fenoprofen calcium, Dista) in combination with gold salts or corticosteroids has been studied in patients with rheumatoid arthritis. The studies, however, were inadequate in demonstrating whether further improvement is obtained by adding Nalfon to maintenance therapy with gold salts or steroids. Whether or not Nalfon, used in conjunction with partially effective doses of a corticosteroid, has a "steroid-sparing" effect is unknown.

In patients with osteoarthritis, the anti-inflammatory and analgesic effects of Nalfon have been demonstrated by reduction in tenderness on pressure; relief of pain with motion and at rest; reductions in night pain, stiffness, swelling, and overall disease activity (as assessed by both the patient and the investigator); and increased range of motion in involved joints.

In patients with rheumatoid arthritis and osteoarthritis, clinical studies have shown Nalfon to be comparable to aspirin in controlling the aforementioned measures of disease activity, but mild gastrointestinal adverse reactions (nausea, dyspepsia) and tinnitus occurred less frequently than in aspirin-treated patients. It is not known whether Nalfon causes less peptic ulceration than does aspirin.

In patients with pain, the analgesic action of Nalfon has produced a reduction in pain intensity, an increase in pain relief, improvement in total analgesia scores, and a sustained analgesic effect.

Under fasting conditions, Nalfon is rapidly absorbed, and peak plasma levels of 50 mcg/ml are achieved within two hours after oral administration of 600-mg doses. Good dose proportionality was observed between 200-mg and 600-mg doses in fasting male volunteers. The plasma half-life is approximately three hours. About 90% of a single oral dose is eliminated within 24 hours as fenoprofen glucuronide and 4′-hydroxyfenoprofen glucuronide, the major urinary metabolites of fenoprofen. Fenoprofen is highly bound (99%) to albumin.

The concomitant administration of antacid (containing both aluminum and magnesium hydroxide) does not interfere with absorption of Nalfon.

There is less suppression of collagen-induced platelet aggregation with single doses of Nalfon than there is with aspirin.

Indications and Usage: Nalfon® (fenoprofen calcium, Dista) is indicated for relief of the signs and symptoms of rheumatoid arthritis and osteoarthritis. It is recommended for the treatment of acute flares and exacerbations and for the long-term management of these diseases.

Nalfon is also indicated for the relief of mild to moderate pain.

Controlled trials are currently in progress to establish the safety and efficacy of Nalfon in children.

Contraindications: Nalfon® (fenoprofen calcium, Dista) is contraindicated in patients who have shown hypersensitivity to it.

The drug should not be administered to patients with a history of significantly impaired renal function.

Nalfon should not be given to patients in whom aspirin and other nonsteroidal anti-inflammatory drugs induce the symptoms of asthma, rhinitis, or urticaria, because cross-sensitivity to these drugs occurs in a high proportion of such patients.

Warnings: Nalfon® (fenoprofen calcium, Dista) should be given under close supervision to patients with a history of upper gastrointestinal tract disease and only after the Adverse Reactions section has been consulted. Gastrointestinal bleeding, sometimes severe (with fatalities having been reported), may occur in patients receiving Nalfon as with other nonsteroidal anti-inflammatory drugs.

If Nalfon must be given to patients with an active peptic ulcer, the patient should be on a vigorous anti-ulcer treatment regimen and under close supervision for signs of ulcer perforation or severe gastrointestinal bleeding.

Since Nalfon has been marketed, there have been reports of genitourinary tract problems in patients taking it. The most frequently reported problems have been episodes of dysuria, cystitis, hematuria, interstitial nephritis, and the nephrotic syndrome. This syndrome may be preceded by the appearance of fever, rash, arthralgia, oliguria, and azotemia and may progress to anuria. There may also be substantial proteinuria, and, on renal biopsy, electron microscopy has shown foot process fusion and T-lymphocyte infiltration in the renal interstitium. Early recognition of the syndrome and withdrawal of the drug have been followed by rapid recovery. Administration of steroids and the use of dialysis have also been included in the treatment. Because syndrome with some of these characteristics has also been reported with other nonsteroidal anti-inflammatory drugs, it is recommended that patients who have had these reactions with other such drugs not be treated with Nalfon. In patients with possibly compromised renal function, periodic renal function examinations should be done.

Precautions: In chronic studies in rats, high doses of Nalfon®(fenoprofen calcium, Dista) caused elevation of serum transaminase and hepatocellular hypertrophy. In clinical trials, some patients developed elevation of serum transaminase, LDH, and alkaline phosphatase that persisted for some months and usually, but not always, declined despite continuation of the drug. The significance of this is unknown. It is recommended, therefore, that Nalfon be discontinued if any significant liver abnormalities occur.

As with other nonsteroidal anti-inflammatory drugs, borderline elevations of one or more liver tests may occur in up to 15 percent of patients. These abnormalities may progress, may remain essentially unchanged, or may be transient with continued therapy. The SGPT (ALT) test is probably the most sensitive indicator of liver dysfunction. Meaningful (three times the upper limit of normal) elevations of SGPT or SGOT (AST) occurred in controlled clinical trials in less than 1 percent of patients. A patient with symptoms and/or signs suggesting liver dysfunction, or in whom an abnormal liver test has occurred, should be elavulated for evidence of the development of more severe hepatic reaction while on therapy with Nalfon. Severe hepatic reactions, including jaundice and cases of fatal hepatitis, have been reported with Nalfon as with other nonsteroidal anti-inflammatory drugs. Although such reactions are rare, if abnormal liver tests persist or worsen, if clinical signs and symptoms consistent with liver disease develop, or if systemic

Continued on next page

Dista—Cont.

manifestations occur (e.g., eosinophilia, rash, etc.), Nalfon should be discontinued.
Safe use of Nalfon during pregnancy and lactation has not been established; therefore, administration to pregnant patients and nursing mothers is not recommended. Reproduction studies have been performed in rats and rabbits. When fenoprofen was given to rats during pregnancy and continued to the time of labor, parturition was prolonged. Similar results have been found with other nonsteroidal anti-inflammatory drugs that inhibit prostaglandin synthetase.
In patients receiving Nalfon and a steroid concomitantly, any reduction in steroid dosage should be gradual in order to avoid the possible complications of sudden steroid withdrawal.
Patients with initial low hemoglobin values who are receiving long-term therapy with Nalfon should have a hemoglobin determination at reasonable intervals.
Peripheral edema has been observed in some patients taking Nalfon; therefore, Nalfon should be used with caution in patients with compromised cardiac function or hypertension. The possibility of renal involvement should be considered.
Studies to date have not shown changes in the eyes attributable to the administration of Nalfon. However, adverse ocular effects have been observed with other anti-inflammatory drugs. Eye examinations, therefore, should be performed if visual disturbances occur in patients taking Nalfon.
Caution should be exercised by patients whose activities require alertness if they experience central-nervous-system side effects from Nalfon.
Since the safety of Nalfon has not been established in patients with impaired hearing, these patients should have periodic tests of auditory function during chronic therapy with Nalfon.
Nalfon decreases platelet aggregation and may prolong bleeding time. Patients who may be adversely affected by prolongation of the bleeding time should be carefully observed when Nalfon is administered.
Drug Interactions: The coadministration of aspirin decreases the biologic half-life of fenoprofen because of an increase in metabolic clearance that results in a greater amount of hydroxylated fenoprofen in the urine. Although the mechanism of interaction between fenoprofen and aspirin is not totally known, enzyme induction and displacement of fenoprofen from plasma albumin binding sites are possibilities. Because Nalfon® (fenoprofen calcium, Dista) has not been shown to produce any additional effect beyond that obtained with aspirin alone and because aspirin increases the rate of excretion of Nalfon, the concomitant use of Nalfon and salicylates is not recommended.
Chronic administration of phenobarbital, a known enzyme inducer, may be associated with a decrease in the plasma half-life of fenoprofen. When phenobarbital is added or withdrawn, dosage adjustment of Nalfon may be required.
In vitro studies have shown that fenoprofen, because of its affinity for albumin, may displace from their binding sites other drugs which are also albumin bound, and this may lead to drug interaction. Theoretically, fenoprofen could likewise be displaced. Patients receiving hydantoin, sulfonamides, or sulfonylureas should be observed for increased activity of these drugs and, therefore, signs of toxicity to these drugs. In patients receiving coumarin-type anticoagulants, the addition of Nalfon to therapy could prolong the prothrombin time. Patients receiving both drugs should be under careful observation.
Adverse Reactions: During clinical studies for rheumatoid arthritis or osteoarthritis, complaints were compiled from a checklist of potential adverse reactions, from which the following data emerged. These encompass observations in 3391 patients, including 188 observed for at least 52 weeks. During short-term studies for analgesia, the incidence of adverse reactions was markedly lower than that seen in longer-term studies.
INCIDENCE GREATER THAN 1%
Probable Causal Relationship
Digestive System—During clinical trials with Nalfon® (fenoprofen calcium, Dista), the most common adverse reactions were gastrointestinal in nature and occurred in about 14% of patients. In decending order of frequency, these reactions included dyspepsia,* constipation,* nausea,* vomiting,* abdominal pain, anorexia, occult blood in the stool, diarrhea, flatulence, and dry mouth.
The drug was discontinued because of adverse gastrointestinal reactions in less than 2% of patients.
Nervous System—The most frequent adverse neurologic reactions were headache and somnolence, which occurred in about 15% of patients. Dizziness,* tremor, confusion, and insomnia were noted less frequently.
Nalfon was discontinued in less than 0.5% of patients because of these side effects.
Skin and Appendages—Pruritus,* rash, increased sweating, and urticaria.
Nalfon was discontinued in about 1% of patients because of an adverse effect related to the skin.
Special Senses—Tinnitus, blurred vision, and decreased hearing.
Nalfon was discontinued in less than 0.5% of patients because of adverse effects related to the special senses.
Cardiovascular—Palpitations* and tachycardia.
Nalfon was discontinued in about 0.5% of patients because of adverse cardiovascular reactions.
Miscellaneous—Nervousness,* asthenia,* dyspnea, fatigue, and malaise.

* Reactions in 3% to 9% of patients treated with Nalfon. (Those reactions occurring in less than 3% of the patients are unmarked.)

INCIDENCE LESS THAN 1%
Probable Causal Relationship
The following adverse reactions, occurring in less than 1% of patients, were reported in controlled clinical trials and through voluntary reports since Nalfon® (fenoprofen calcium, Dista) was initially marketed. The probability of a causal relationship exists between Nalfon and these adverse reactions:
Digestive System—Gastritis, peptic ulcer with/without perforation, and/or gastrointestinal hemorrhage. Increases in alkaline phosphatase, LDH, and SGOT, jaundice, and cholestatic hepatitis were observed (*see* Precautions).
Genitourinary Tract—Dysuria, cystitis, hematuria, oliguria, azotemia, anuria, interstitial nephritis, nephrosis, and papillary necrosis (*see* Warnings).
Hematologic—Purpura, bruising, hemorrhage, thrombocytopenia, hemolytic anemia, agranulocytosis, and pancytopenia.
Miscellaneous—Peripheral edema and anaphylaxis.
INCIDENCE LESS THAN 1%
Causal Relationship Unknown
Other reactions have been reported but occurred in circumstances in which a causal relationship could not be established. However, with these rarely reported reactions, the possibility of such a relationship cannot be excluded. Therefore, these observations are listed to alert the physician.
Skin and Appendages—Stevens-Johnson syndrome, angioneurotic edema, exfoliative dermatitis, and alopecia.
Digestive System—Aphthous ulcerations of the buccal mucosa, metallic taste, and pancreatitis.
Cardiovascular—Atrial fibrillation, pulmonary edema, electrocardiographic changes, and supraventricular tachycardia.
Nervous System—Depression, disorientation, seizures, and trigeminal neuralgia.
Special Senses—Burning tongue, diplopia, and optic neuritis.
Hematologic—Aplastic anemia.
Miscellaneous—Personality change, lymphadenopathy, mastodynia, and fever.
Overdosage: No specific information is available on the treatment of overdosage with Nalfon® (fenoprofen calcium, Dista). If it should occur, standard procedures to evacuate gastric contents and to support vital functions should be employed. Since Nalfon is acidic and is excreted in the urine, it may be beneficial to administer alkali and charcoal and induce diuresis. Furosemide did not lower blood levels.
Dosage and Administration: *Analgesia*—For the treatment of mild to moderate pain, the recommended dosage is 200 mg every four to six hours, as needed.
Rheumatoid Arthritis and Osteoarthritis—The suggested dosage is 300 to 600 mg three or four times a day. The dose should be tailored to the needs of the patient and may be increased or decreased depending on the severity of the symptoms. Dosage adjustments may be made after initiation of drug therapy or during exacerbations of the disease. Total daily dosage should not exceed 3200 mg.
If gastrointestinal complaints occur, Nalfon® (fenoprofen calcium, Dista) may be administered with meals or with milk. Although the total amount absorbed is not affected, peak blood levels are delayed and diminished.
Patients with rheumatoid arthritis generally seem to require larger doses of Nalfon than do those with osteoarthritis. The smallest dose that yields acceptable control should be employed.
Although improvement may be seen in a few days in many patients, an additional two to three weeks may be required to gauge the full benefits of therapy.
How Supplied: (℞) *Pulvules Nalfon® 200 (Fenoprofen Calcium, Capsules, USP): No. 415, H76,** 200 mg (equivalent to fenoprofen) (No. 1, White Opaque Body, Ocher Opaque Cap), in an ℞Pak of 100 (NDC 0777-0876-02).
*Pulvules Nalfon, No. 416, H77,** 300 mg (equivalent to fenoprofen) (No. 0, Yellow Opaque Body, Ocher Opaque Cap), in an ℞Pak of 100 (NDC 0777-0877-02) and in bottles of 500 (NDC 0777-0877-03).
(℞) *Tablets Nalfon® (Fenoprofen Calcium Tablets, USP), No. 1900, U59,** 600 mg (equivalent to fenoprofen), Yellow (paracapsule-shaped, scored), in an ℞Pak of 100 (NDC 0777-2159-02) and in bottles of 500 (NDC 0777-2159-03).
[070182]
[*Shown in Product Identification Section*]

* Identi-Code® symbol.

NEBCIN® ℞
(tobramycin sulfate)
Injection, USP

WARNINGS
Patients treated with Nebcin® (Tobramycin Sulfate Injection, USP, Dista) and other aminoglycosides should be under close clinical observation, because these drugs have an inherent potential for causing ototoxicity and nephrotoxicity.
Neurotoxicity, manifested as both auditory and vestibular ototoxicity, can occur. The auditory changes are irreversible, are usually bilateral, and may be partial or total. Eighth-nerve impairment and nephrotoxicity may develop, primarily in pa-

tients having preexisting renal damage and in those with normal renal function to whom aminoglycosides are administered for longer periods or in higher doses than those recommended. Other manifestations of neurotoxicity may include numbness, skin tingling, muscle twitching, and convulsions. The risk of aminoglycoside-induced hearing loss increases with the degree of exposure to either high peak or high trough serum concentrations. Patients who develop cochlear damage may not have symptoms during therapy to warn them of eighth-nerve toxicity, and partial or total irreversible bilateral deafness may continue to develop after the drug has been discontinued. Rarely, nephrotoxicity may not become manifest until the first few days after cessation of therapy. Aminoglycoside-induced nephrotoxicity usually is reversible.

Renal and eighth-nerve function should be closely monitored in patients with known or suspected renal impairment and also in those whose renal function is initially normal but who develop signs of renal dysfunction during therapy. Peak and trough serum concentrations of aminoglycosides should be monitored periodically during therapy to assure adequate levels and to avoid potentially toxic levels. Prolonged serum concentrations above 12 mcg/ml should be avoided. Rising trough levels (above 2 mcg/ml) may indicate tissue accumulation. Such accumulation, excessive peak concentrations, advanced age, and cumulative dose may contribute to ototoxicity and nephrotoxicity (*see* Precautions). Urine should be examined for decreased specific gravity and increased excretion of protein, cells, and casts. Blood urea nitrogen, serum creatinine, and creatinine clearance should be measured periodically. When feasible, it is recommended that serial audiograms be obtained in patients old enough to be tested, particularly high-risk patients. Evidence of impairment of renal, vestibular, or auditory function requires discontinuation of the drug or dosage adjustment.

Nebcin should be used with caution in premature and neonatal infants because of their renal immaturity and the resulting prolongation of serum half-life of the drug. Concurrent and sequential use of other neurotoxic and/or nephrotoxic antibiotics, particularly other aminoglycosides (e.g., amikacin, streptomycin, neomycin, kanamycin, gentamicin, and paromomycin), cephaloridine, viomycin, polymyxin B, colistin, cisplatin, and vancomycin, should be avoided. Other factors that may increase patient risk are advanced age and dehydration.

Aminoglycosides should not be given concurrently with potent diuretics, such as ethacrynic acid and furosemide. Some diuretics themselves cause ototoxicity, and intravenously administered diuretics enhance aminoglycoside toxicity by altering antibiotic concentrations in serum and tissue.

Aminoglycosides can cause fetal harm when administered to a pregnant woman (*see* Precautions).

Description: Tobramycin sulfate, a water-soluble antibiotic of the aminoglycoside group, is derived from the actinomycete *Streptomyces tenebrarius.* Nebcin® (tobramycin sulfate, Dista), Injection, is a clear and colorless sterile aqueous solution for parenteral administration.

Each ml also contains 5 mg phenol as a preservative, 3.2 mg sodium bisulfite, 0.1 mg edetate disodium, and water for injection, q.s. Sulfuric acid and/or sodium hydroxide may have been added to adjust the *p*H. Tobramycin is 4-0-[2,6-diamino-2, 3, 6-trideoxy-α-D-glucopyranosyl]-6-0- [3-amino-3-deoxy-α-D-glucopyranosyl] -2- deoxystreptamine.

Clinical Pharmacology: Tobramycin is rapidly absorbed following intramuscular administration. Peak serum concentrations of tobramycin occur between 30 and 90 minutes after intramuscular administration. Following an intramuscular dose of 1 mg/kg of body weight, maximum serum concentrations reach about 4 mcg/ml, and measurable levels persist for as long as eight hours. Therapeutic serum levels are generally considered to range from 4 to 6 mcg/ml. When Nebcin® (tobramycin sulfate, Dista) is administered by intravenous infusion over a one-hour period, the serum concentrations are similar to those obtained by intramuscular administration. Nebcin is poorly absorbed from the gastrointestinal tract.

In patients with normal renal function, except neonates, Nebcin administered every eight hours does not accumulate in the serum. However, in those with reduced renal function and in neonates, the serum concentration of the antibiotic is usually higher and can be measured for longer periods of time than in normal adults. Dosage for such patients must, therefore, be adjusted accordingly (*see* Dosage and Administration).

Following parenteral administration, little, if any, metabolic transformation occurs, and tobramycin is eliminated almost exclusively by glomerular filtration. Renal clearance is similar to that of endogenous creatinine. Ultrafiltration studies demonstrate that practically no serum protein binding occurs. In patients with normal renal function, up to 84 percent of the dose is recoverable from the urine in eight hours and up to 93 percent in 24 hours.

Peak urine concentrations ranging from 75 to 100 mcg/ml have been observed following the intramuscular injection of a single dose of 1 mg/kg. After several days of treatment, the amount of tobramycin excreted in the urine approaches the daily dose administered. When renal function is impaired, excretion of Nebcin is slowed, and accumulation of the drug may cause toxic blood levels.

The serum half-life in normal individuals is two hours. An inverse relationship exists between serum half-life and creatinine clearance, and the dosage schedule should be adjusted according to the degree of renal impairment (*see* Dosage and Administration). In patients undergoing dialysis, 25 to 70 percent of the administered dose may be removed, depending on the duration and type of dialysis.

Tobramycin can be detected in tissues and body fluids after parenteral administration. Concentrations in bile and stools ordinarily have been low, which suggests minimum biliary excretion. Tobramycin has appeared in low concentration in the cerebrospinal fluid following parenteral administration, and concentrations are dependent on dose, rate of penetration, and degree of meningeal inflammation. It has also been found in sputum, peritoneal fluid, synovial fluid, and abscess fluids, and it crosses the placental membranes. Concentrations in the renal cortex are several times higher than the usual serum levels.

Probenecid does not affect the renal tubular transport of tobramycin.

Microbiology—In vitro tests demonstrate that tobramycin is bactericidal and that it acts by inhibiting the synthesis of protein in bacterial cells.

Tobramycin is usually active against most strains of the following organisms in vitro and in clinical infections:

Pseudomonas aeruginosa
Proteus species (indole-positive and indole-negative), including *Proteus mirabilis, P. morganii, P. rettgeri,* and *P. vulgaris*
Escherichia coli
Klebsiella-Enterobacter-Serratia group
Citrobacter species
Providencia species
Staphylococci, including *Staphylococcus aureus* (coagulase-positive and coagulase-negative)

Aminoglycosides have a low order of activity against most gram-positive organisms, including *Streptococcus pyogenes, S. pneumoniae,* and enterococci.

Although most strains of group D streptococci demonstrate in vitro resistance, some strains in this group are susceptible. In vitro studies have shown that an aminoglycoside combined with an antibiotic which interferes with cell-wall synthesis affects some group D streptococcal strains synergistically. The combination of penicillin G and tobramycin results in a synergistic bactericidal effect in vitro against certain strains of *S. faecalis.* However, this combination is not synergistic against other closely related organisms, e.g., *S. faecium.* Speciation of group D streptococci alone cannot be used to predict susceptibility. Susceptibility testing and tests for antibiotic synergism are emphasized.

Cross-resistance between aminoglycosides occurs and depends largely on inactivation by bacterial enzymes.

Susceptibility Tests—If the FDA Standardized Disc Test method (formerly the Bauer-Kirby-Sherris-Turck method) of disc susceptibility testing is used, a disc containing 10 mcg tobramycin should give a zone of at least 15 mm when tested against a tobramycin-susceptible bacterial strain, a zone of 13 to 14 mm against strains of intermediate susceptibility, and a zone of 12 mm or less against resistant organisms. The minimum inhibitory concentration correlates are $\leq$ 4 mcg/ml for susceptibility and $\geq$ 8 mcg/ml for resistance.

Indications and Usage: Nebcin® (tobramycin sulfate, Dista) is indicated for the treatment of serious bacterial infections caused by susceptible strains of the designated microorganisms in the diseases listed below:

Septicemia in the neonate, child, and adult caused by *P. aeruginosa, E. coli,* and *Klebsiella* species

Lower respiratory tract infections caused by *P. aeruginosa, Klebsiella* species, *Enterobacter* species, *Serratia* species, *E. coli,* and *S. aureus* (penicillinase and non-penicillinase-producing strains)

Serious central-nervous-system infections (meningitis) caused by susceptible organisms

Intra-abdominal infections, including peritonitis, caused by *E. coli, Klebsiella* species, and *Enterobacter* species.

Skin, bone, and skin-structure infections caused by *P. aeruginosa, Proteus* species, *E. coli, Klebsiella* species, *Enterobacter* species, and *S. aureus*

Complicated and recurrent urinary tract infections caused by *P. aeruginosa, Proteus* species (indole-positive and indole-negative), *E. coli, Klebsiella* species, *Enterobacter* species, *Serratia* species, *S. aureus, Providencia* species, and *Citrobacter* species

Aminoglycosides, including Nebcin, are not indicated in uncomplicated initial episodes of urinary tract infections unless the causative organisms are not susceptible to antibiotics having less potential toxicity. Nebcin may be considered in serious staphylococcal infections when penicillin or other potentially less toxic drugs are contraindicated and when bacterial susceptibility testing and clinical judgment indicate its use.

Bacterial cultures should be obtained prior to and during treatment to isolate and identify etiologic organisms and to test their susceptibility to tobramycin. If susceptibility tests show that the causative organisms are resist-

Continued on next page

Dista—Cont.

ant to tobramycin, other appropriate therapy should be instituted. In patients in whom a serious life-threatening gram-negative infection is suspected, including those in whom concurrent therapy with a penicillin or cephalosporin and an aminoglycoside may be indicated, treatment with Nebcin may be initiated before the results of susceptibility studies are obtained. The decision to continue therapy with Nebcin® (tobramycin sulfate, Dista) should be based on the results of susceptibility studies, the severity of the infection, and the important additional concepts discussed in the WARNINGS box above.

Contraindications: A hypersensitivity to any aminoglycoside is a contraindication to the use of tobramycin. A history of hypersensitivity or serious toxic reactions to aminoglycosides may also contraindicate the use of any other aminoglycoside because of the known cross-sensitivity of patients to drugs in this class.

Warnings: *See* WARNINGS box above.

Precautions: Serum and urine specimens for examination should be collected during therapy, as recommended in the WARNINGS box. Serum calcium, magnesium, and sodium should be monitored.

Peak and trough serum levels should be measured periodically during therapy. Prolonged concentrations above 12 mcg/ml should be avoided. Rising trough levels (above 2 mcg/ml) may indicate tissue accumulation. Such accumulation, advanced age, and cumulative dosage may contribute to ototoxicity and nephrotoxicity. It is particularly important to monitor serum levels closely in patients with known renal impairment.

A useful guideline would be to perform serum level assays after two or three doses, so that the dosage could be adjusted if necessary, and also at three to four-day intervals during therapy. In the event of changing renal function, more frequent serum levels should be obtained and the dosage or dosage interval adjusted according to the guidelines provided in the Dosage and Administration section.

In order to measure the peak level, a serum sample should be drawn about 30 minutes following intravenous infusion or one hour after an intramuscular injection. Trough levels are measured by obtaining serum samples at eight hours or just prior to the next dose of Nebcin®(tobramycin sulfate, Dista). These suggested time intervals are intended only as guidelines and may vary according to institutional practices. It is important, however, that there be consistency within the individual patient program unless computerized pharmacokinetic dosing programs are available in the institution. These serum-level assays may be especially useful for monitoring the treatment of severely ill patients with changing renal function or of those infected with less sensitive organisms or those receiving maximum dosage.

Neuromuscular blockade and respiratory paralysis have been reported in cats receiving very high doses of tobramycin (40 mg/kg). The possibility that prolonged or secondary apnea may occur should be considered if tobramycin is administered to anesthetized patients who are also receiving neuromuscular blocking agents, such as succinylcholine, tubocurarine, or decamethonium, or in patients receiving massive transfusions of citrated blood. If neuromuscular blockade occurs, it may be reversed by the administration of calcium salts.

Cross-allergenicity among aminoglycosides has been demonstrated.

In patients with extensive burns, altered pharmacokinetics may result in reduced serum concentrations of aminoglycosides. In such patients treated with Nebcin, measurement of serum concentration is especially recommended as a basis for determination of appropriate dosage.

Elderly patients may have reduced renal function that may not be evident in the results of routine screening tests, such an BUN or serum creatinine. A creatinine clearance determination may be more useful. Monitoring of renal function during treatment with aminoglycosides is particularly important in such patients.

An increased incidence of nephrotoxicity has been reported following concomitant administration of aminoglycoside antibiotics and cephalosporins.

Aminoglycosides should be used with caution in patients with muscular disorders, such as myasthenia gravis or parkinsonism, since these drugs may aggravate muscle weakness because of their potential curare-like effect on neuromuscular function.

Aminoglycosides may be absorbed in significant quantities from body surfaces after local irrigation or application and may cause neurotoxicity and nephrotoxicity.

See WARNINGS box regarding concurrent use of potent diuretics and concurrent and sequential use of other neurotoxic or nephrotoxic drugs.

The inactivation of tobramycin and other aminoglycosides by beta-lactam-type antibiotics (penicillins or cephalosporins) has been demonstrated in vitro and in patients with severe renal impairment. Such inactivation has not been found in patients with normal renal function who have been given the drugs by separate routes of administration.

Therapy with tobramycin may result in overgrowth of nonsusceptible organisms. If overgrowth of nonsusceptible organisms occurs, appropriate therapy should be initiated.

Pregnancy Category D—Aminoglycosides can cause fetal harm when administered to a pregnant woman. Aminoglycoside antibiotics cross the placenta, and there have been several reports of total irreversible bilateral congenital deafness in children whose mothers received streptomycin during pregnancy. Serious side effects to mother, fetus, or newborn have not been reported in the treatment of pregnant women with other aminoglycosides. If tobramycin is used during pregnancy or if the patient becomes pregnant while taking tobramycin, she should be apprised of the potential hazard to the fetus.

Usage in Children—See Indications and Usage and Dosage and Administration.

Adverse Reactions: *Neurotoxicity*—Adverse effects on both the vestibular and auditory branches of the eighth nerve have been noted, especially in patients receiving high doses or prolonged therapy, in those given previous courses of therapy with an ototoxin, and in cases of dehydration. Symptoms include dizziness, vertigo, tinnitus, roaring in the ears, and hearing loss. Hearing loss is usually irreversible and is manifested initially by diminution of high-tone acuity. Tobramycin and gentamicin sulfates closely parallel each other in regard to ototoxic potential.

Nephrotoxicity—Renal function changes, as shown by rising BUN, NPN, and serum creatinine and by oliguria, cylindruria, and increased proteinuria, have been reported, especially in patients with a history of renal impairment who are treated for longer periods or with higher doses than those recommended. Adverse renal effects can occur in patients with initially normal renal function.

Clinical studies and studies in experimental animals have been conducted to compare the nephrotoxic potential of tobramycin and gentamicin. In some of the clinical studies and in the animal studies, tobramycin caused nephrotoxicity significantly less frequently than gentamicin. In some other clinical studies, no significant difference in the incidence of nephrotoxicity between tobramycin and gentamicin was found.

Other reported adverse reactions possibly related to Nebcin® (tobramycin sulfate, Dista) include anemia, granulocytopenia, and thrombocytopenia; and fever, rash, itching, urticaria, nausea, vomiting, headache, lethargy, pain at the injection site, mental confusion, and disorientation. Laboratory abnormalities possibly related to Nebcin include increased serum transaminases (SGOT, SGPT); increased serum LDH and bilirubin; decreased serum calcium, magnesium, sodium, and potassium; and leukopenia, leukocytosis, and eosinophilia.

Overdosage: In the event of overdosage or toxic reaction, hemodialysis or peritoneal dialysis will reduce serum levels. Hemodialysis is preferable because it is more efficient in reducing serum levels.

Dosage and Administration: Nebcin® (tobramycin sulfate, Dista) may be given intramuscularly or intravenously. Recommended dosages are the same for both routes. The patient's pretreatment body weight should be obtained for calculation of correct dosage. It is desirable to measure both peak and trough serum concentrations (*see* WARNINGS box and Precautions).

Administration for Patients with Normal Renal Function—Adults with Serious Infections: 3 mg/kg/day in three equal doses every eight hours (*see* Table 1).

Adults with Life-Threatening Infections: Up to 5 mg/kg/day may be administered in three or four equal doses (*see* Table 1). The dosage should be reduced to 3 mg/kg/day as soon as clinically indicated. To prevent increased toxicity due to excessive blood levels, dosage should not exceed 5 mg/kg/day unless serum levels are monitored.

[See table on next page].

Children: 6 to 7.5 mg/kg/day in three or four equally divided doses (2 to 2.5 mg/kg every eight hours or 1.5 to 1.89 mg/kg every six hours).

Premature or Full-Term Neonates One Week of Age or Less: Up to 4 mg/kg/day may be administered in two equal doses every 12 hours. It is desirable to limit treatment to a short term. The usual duration of treatment is seven to ten days. A longer course of therapy may be necessary in difficult and complicated infections. In such cases, monitoring of renal, auditory, and vestibular functions is advised, because neurotoxicity is more likely to occur when treatment is extended longer than ten days.

Administration for Patients with Impaired Renal Function—Whenever possible, serum tobramycin concentrations should be monitored during therapy.

Following a loading dose of 1 mg/kg, subsequent dosage in these patients must be adjusted, either with reduced doses administered at eight-hour intervals or with normal doses given at prolonged intervals. Both of these methods are suggested as guides to be used when serum levels of tobramycin cannot be measured directly. They are based on either the creatinine clearance or the serum creatinine of the patient, because these values correlate with the half-life of tobramycin. The dosage schedules derived from either method should be used in conjunction with careful clinical and laboratory observations of the patient and should be modified as necessary. Neither method should be used when dialysis is being performed.

Reduced dosage at eight-hour intervals: When the creatinine clearance rate is 70 ml or less per minute or when the serum creatinine value is known, the amount of the reduced dose can be determined by multiplying the normal dose from Table 1 by the percent of normal dose from the accompanying nomogram.

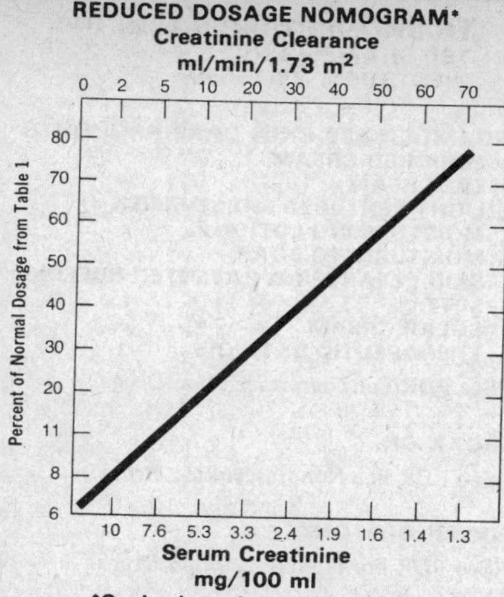

*Scales have been adjusted to facilitate dosage calculations.

An alternate rough guide for determining reduced dosage at eight-hour intervals (for patients whose steady-state serum creatinine values are known) is to divide the normally recommended dose by the patient's serum creatinine.

Normal dosage at prolonged intervals: If the creatinine clearance rate is not available and the patient's condition is stable, a dosage frequency *in hours* for the dosage given in Table 1 can be determined by multiplying the patient's serum creatinine by six.

Dosage in Obese Patients—The appropriate dose may be calculated by using the patient's estimated lean body weight plus 40 percent of the excess as the basic weight on which to figure mg/kg.

Intramuscular Administration—Nebcin may be administered by withdrawing the appropriate dose directly from a vial or by using a prefilled Hyporet® (disposable syringe, Dista).

Intravenous Administration—For intravenous administration, the usual volume of diluent (0.9% Sodium Chloride Injection or 5% Dextrose Injection) is 50 to 100 ml for adult doses. For children, the volume of diluent should be proportionately less than for adults. The diluted solution usually should be infused over a period of 20 to 60 minutes. Infusion periods of less than 20 minutes are not recommended, because peak serum levels may exceed 12 mcg/ml (*see* WARNINGS box).

Nebcin® (tobramycin sulfate, Dista) should not be physically premixed with other drugs but should be administered separately according to the recommended dose and route.

How Supplied: (℞) *Vials (Multiple Dose) Nebcin® (Tobramycin Sulfate Injection, USP): No. 781,* 80 mg (equivalent to tobramycin) per 2 ml, 2 ml, rubber-stoppered, in singles (10 per carton (NDC 0777-1499-01) and in Traypak™ (multivial carton, Dista) of 25 (NDC 0777-1499-25); *No. 7090,* 40 mg (equivalent to tobramycin) per ml, 1.2 g per 30 ml (Pharmacy Bulk Package), rubber-stoppered, in Traypak of 6 (NDC 0777-7090-16).

(℞) *Vials (Multiple Dose) No. 782, Nebcin® (Tobramycin Sulfate Injection, USP), Pediatric,* 20 mg (equivalent to tobramycin) per 2 ml, 2 ml, rubber-stoppered, in singles (10 per carton) (NDC 0777-0501-01).

(℞) *Hyporets® (disposable syringes, Dista) Nebcin® (Tobramycin Sulfate Injection, USP): No. 55,* 60 mg (equivalent to tobramycin) per 1.5 ml, 1.5 ml, in packages of 24 (NDC 0777-0509-24), and *No. 42,* 80 mg (equivalent to tobramycin) per 2 ml, 2 ml, in packages of 24 (NDC 0777-0503-24). Each Hyporet is scored with a 10-mg (0.25-ml) fractional dose scale. [050582]

TABLE 1. DOSAGE SCHEDULE GUIDE FOR NEBCIN® (TOBRAMYCIN SULFATE) IN ADULTS WITH NORMAL RENAL FUNCTION
(Dosage at Eight-Hour Intervals)

For Patient Weighing		Usual Dose for Serious Infections 1 mg/kg q. 8 h. (Total, 3 mg/kg/day)		Maximum Dose for Life-Threatening Infections (Reduce as soon as possible) 1.66 mg/kg q. 8 h. (Total, 5 mg/kg/day)	
kg	lb	mg/dose q. 8 h.	ml/dose*	mg/dose q. 8 h.	ml/dose*
120	264	120 mg	3 ml	200 mg	5 ml
115	253	115 mg	2.9 ml	191 mg	4.75 ml
110	242	110 mg	2.75 ml	183 mg	4.5 ml
105	231	105 mg	2.6 ml	175 mg	4.4 ml
100	220	100 mg	2.5 ml	166 mg	4.2 ml
95	209	95 mg	2.4 ml	158 mg	4 ml
90	198	90 mg	2.25 ml	150 mg	3.75 ml
85	187	85 mg	2.1 ml	141 mg	3.5 ml
80	176	80 mg	2 ml	133 mg	3.3 ml
75	165	75 mg	1.9 ml	125 mg	3.1 ml
70	154	70 mg	1.75 ml	116 mg	2.9 ml
65	143	65 mg	1.6 ml	108 mg	2.7 ml
60	132	60 mg	1.5 ml	100 mg	2.5 ml
55	121	55 mg	1.4 ml	91 mg	2.25 ml
50	110	50 mg	1.25 ml	83 mg	2.1 ml
45	99	45 mg	1.1 ml	75 mg	1.9 ml
40	88	40 mg	1 ml	66 mg	1.6 ml

*Applicable to all product forms except Nebcin, Pediatric, Injection (*see* How Supplied).

NEBCIN® ℞

(tobramycin sulfate)
Sterile

This vial is intended for use by the hospital pharmacist in the extemporaneous preparation of I.V. solutions.

Warnings: *See under* Nebcin, Injection, USP.

Description: Tobramycin sulfate, a water-soluble antibiotic of the aminoglycoside group, is derived from the actinomycete *Streptomyces tenebrarius.* Nebcin® (tobramycin sulfate, Dista), Sterile, is supplied as a sterile dry powder and is intended for solution in Sterile Water for Injection, USP. Sulfuric acid and/or sodium hydroxide may have been added during manufacture to adjust the *p*H. Each vial contains 1200 mg of tobramycin activity. After dilution, the solution will contain 40 mg of tobramycin per ml. The product contains no preservative. *See also under* Nebcin, Injection, USP.

Clinical Pharmacology, Indications and Usage, Contraindications, Warnings, Precautions, Adverse Reactions, and **Overdosage:** *See under* Nebcin, Injection, USP.

Dosage and Administration: The patient's pretreatment body weight should be obtained for calculation of correct dosage. It is desirable to measure both peak and trough serum concentrations (*see* WARNINGS box and Precautions).

Administration for Patients with Normal Renal Function—Adults with Serious Infections: 3 mg/kg/day in three equal doses every eight hours (*see* Table 1 under Nebcin, Injection, USP).

Adults with Life-Threatening Infections: Up to 5 mg/kg/day may be administered in three or four equal doses (*see* Table 1). The dosage should be reduced to 3 mg/kg/day as soon as clinically indicated. To prevent increased toxicity due to excessive blood levels, dosage should not exceed 5 mg/kg/day unless serum levels are monitored.

Children: 6 to 7.5 mg/kg/day in three or four equally divided doses (2 to 2.5 mg/kg every eight hours or 1.5 to 1.89 mg/kg every six hours).

Premature or Full-Term Neonates One Week of Age or Less: Up to 4 mg/kg/day may be administered in two equal doses every 12 hours.

It is desirable to limit treatment to a short term. The usual duration of treatment is seven to ten days. A longer course of therapy may be necessary in difficult and complicated infections. In such cases, monitoring of renal, auditory, and vestibular functions is advised, because neurotoxicity is more likely to occur when treatment is extended longer than ten days.

Administration for Patients with Impaired Renal Function—Whenever possible, serum tobramycin concentrations should be monitored during therapy.

Following a loading dose of 1 mg/kg, subsequent dosage in these patients must be adjusted, either with reduced doses administered at eight-hour intervals or with normal doses given at prolonged intervals. Both of these methods are suggested as guides to be used when serum levels of tobramycin cannot be measured directly. They are based on either the creatinine clearance or the serum creatinine of the patient, because these values correlate with the half-life of tobramycin. The dosage schedules derived from either method should be used in conjunction with careful clinical and laboratory observations of the patient and should be modified as necessary. Neither method should be used when dialysis is being performed.

Reduced dosage at eight-hour intervals: When the creatinine clearance rate is 70 ml or less per minute or when the serum creatinine value is known, the amount of the reduced dose can be determined by multiplying the normal dose from Table 1 by the percent of normal dose from the nomogram *under* Nebcin, Injection, USP.

An alternate rough guide for determining reduced dosage at eight-hour intervals (for patients whose steady-state serum creatinine values are known) is to divide the normally recommended dose by the patient's serum creatinine.

Normal dosage at prolonged intervals: If the creatinine clearance rate is not available and the patient's condition is stable, a dosage frequency *in hours* for the dosage given in Table 1 can be determined by multiplying the patient's serum creatinine by six.

Continued on next page

Dista—Cont.

Dosage in Obese Patients—The appropriate dose may be calculated by using the patient's estimated lean body weight plus 40 percent of the excess as the basic weight on which to figure mg/kg.
Intravenous Administration—For intravenous administration, the usual volume of diluent (0.9% Sodium Chloride Injection or 5% Dextrose Injection) is 50 to 100 ml for adult doses. For children, the volume of diluent should be proportionately less than for adults. The diluted solution usually should be infused over a period of 20 to 60 minutes. Infusion periods of less than 20 minutes are not recommended, because peak serum levels may exceed 12 mcg/ml (*see* WARNINGS box).
Nebcin® (tobramycin sulfate, Dista) should not be physically premixed with other drugs but should be administered separately according to the recommended dose and route.
Preparation and Storage of Solution: Nebcin, Sterile, is supplied as a dry powder. The contents of the vial (No. 7040) should be diluted with 30 ml of Sterile Water for Injection, USP, to provide a solution containing 40 mg of tobramycin per ml. Prior to reconstitution, the vial should be stored at controlled room temperature, 59° to 86°F (15° to 30°C). After reconstitution, the solution should be kept in a refrigerator and used within 96 hours. If kept at room temperature, the solution must be used within 24 hours.
How Supplied: (℞) *Vials No. 7040, Nebcin® (tobramycin sulfate, Dista), Sterile,* 1.2 g (equivalent to tobramycin), 40-ml size, rubber-stoppered (Dry Powder), in a Traypak™ (multivial carton, Dista) of 6 (NDC 0777-7040-16).
[050682]

VALMID® Ⓒ
(ethinamate)
Capsules, USP

Description: Valmid® (ethinamate, Dista) is 1-ethinyl-cyclohexyl-carbamate. It is a nonirritating, colorless, faintly bitter, stable crystalline powder with a melting point of 96°-98° C. Valmid is relatively insoluble in water but quite soluble in many alcohols and oils.
Action: Valmid® (ethinamate, Dista) is a hypnotic agent for oral administration. Its site and mechanism of action are unknown.
Clinical Pharmacology: Valmid® (ethinamate, Dista) is rapidly absorbed after oral administration. Following a single oral dose of 1 g, peak plasma levels are reached in approximately 36 minutes and decline to negligible values over the next eight hours. Approximately 36 percent of the administered dose appears in the urine within 24 hours. The effect of multiple doses and prolonged administration on pharmacodynamics and pharmacokinetics is not known.
Indications and Usage: Valmid® (ethinamate, Dista) is a short-acting hypnotic. It has not been sufficiently well studied with currently available sleep laboratory techniques to delimit its value in specific types of insomnia. Valmid is best used for limited periods. Should insomnia persist, drug-free intervals of one week or more should elapse before re-treatment is considered. Attempts should be made to find alternative nondrug therapy for chronic insomnia. The prolonged administration of Valmid is not recommended, since it has not been shown to be effective for a period of more than seven days.
Contraindication: Valmid® (ethinamate, Dista) is contraindicated in patients with known hypersensitivity to the drug.
Warnings: Patients receiving Valmid® (ethinamate, Dista) should be cautioned about possible additive effects when it is taken in combination with alcohol or other CNS depressants. Patients should be cautioned against becoming involved in hazardous occupations requiring complete mental alertness, such as operating machines or driving a motor vehicle, shortly after ingestion of the drug.
Precautions: *Drug Interactions*—If Valmid is to be administered in combination with other drugs known to have a hypnotic or CNS-depressant effect, consideration should be given to the potential additive effects.
Carcinogenesis—Long-term studies in animals have *not* been performed to evaluate carcinogenic potential.
Usage in Pregnancy—Pregnancy Category C—Animal reproduction studies have not been conducted with Valmid. It is also not known whether the drug can cause fetal harm when administered to a pregnant woman or can affect reproduction capacity. Valmid should be given to a pregnant woman only if clearly needed.
Nursing Mothers—It is not known whether this drug is excreted in human milk. Because many drugs are excreted in human milk, caution should be exercised when Valmid is administered to a nursing woman.
Usage in Children—Safety and effectiveness in children below the age of 15 years have not been established.
Adverse Reactions: Rare cases of thrombocytopenic purpura and drug idiosyncrasy with fever have been reported. Paradoxical excitement in children, mild gastrointestinal symptoms, and skin rashes have occurred after the use of Valmid® (ethinamate, Dista).
Drug Abuse and Dependence: *Controlled Substance*—Valmid® (ethinamate, Dista) is a Schedule IV drug.
Dependence—Drug dependence characterized by both a psychologic and a physical dependence has occurred when Valmid has been taken at higher than recommended doses for prolonged intervals. It is, therefore, desirable to exercise caution in administering Valmid to individuals who are addiction-prone and to those whose history suggests that they may increase dosage on their own initiative. It is advisable to limit repeated prescriptions without adequate medical supervision.
In the event that an individual has established dependence on Valmid, withdrawal must be accomplished with extreme care. Abrupt withdrawal may cause a typical abstinence syndrome accompanied by convulsions. Withdrawal may be accomplished by hospitalizing the patient and reducing the addictive daily dose at a rate of 500 to 1000 mg every two or three days. Psychiatric follow-up is indicated.
Overdosage: In suicidal overdosage, CNS and respiratory depression should be treated in the same manner as barbiturate intoxication. Valmid® (ethinamate, Dista) is dialyzable.
Dosage and Administration: For insomnia, 1 or 2 Pulvules (500 mg or 1 g) of Valmid® (ethinamate, Dista) should be taken 20 minutes before retiring.
Special Patient Population—Since the risk of oversedation, dizziness, confusion, and/or ataxia substantially increases with the administration of large doses of sedatives and hypnotics in the elderly and debilitated, it is recommended that a single 500-mg Pulvule be the dose given to such individuals. Should this dose prove to be ineffective, clinical judgment must weigh the risk of increasing the dosage against the potential hazards mentioned above.
How Supplied: (Ⓒ) *Pulvules No. 399, Valmid® (Ethinamate Capsules, USP), H74,** 500 mg (No. 0, Light-Blue Opaque Body, Blue Opaque Cap), in bottles of 100 (NDC 0777-0874-02).
[051982]
[*Shown in Product Identification Section*]

*Identi-Code® symbol.

Doak Pharmacal Co., Inc.
700 SHAMES DRIVE
WESTBURY, NY 11590

FORMULA 405 SKIN CARE PRODUCTS
ENRICHED CREAM
EYE CREAM
LIGHT TEXTURED MOISTURIZER
MOISTURIZING LOTION
MOISTURIZING SOAP
SKIN CLEANSER & PATENTED BUFFING MITT
SOLAR CREAM
THERAPEUTIC BATH OIL

(See PDR For Nonprescription Drugs)

DOAK OIL
(See PDR For Nonprescription Drugs)

DOAK OIL FORTE
(See PDR For Nonprescription Drugs)

DOAK TAR LOTION
(See PDR For Nonprescription Drugs)

DOAK TAR SHAMPOO
(See PDR For Nonprescription Drugs)

LAVATAR TAR BATH
(See PDR For Nonprescription Drugs)

TARPASTE
(See PDR For Nonprescription Drugs)

TERSASEPTIC HYGIENIC SKIN CLEANSER
(See PDR For Nonprescription Drugs)

Dorsey Laboratories
Division of Sandoz, Inc.
LINCOLN, NE 68501

ACID MANTLE® CREME AND LOTION

Description: A greaseless, water-miscible preparation containing buffered aluminum acetate.
Indications: Provides relief from mild skin irritation due to exposure to soaps, detergents, chemicals, alkalis. Aids in the treatment of diaper rash, acne, eczema and dry, rough, scaly skin from varied causes.
Application: Apply several times daily, especially after wet work.
Caution: Limited compatibility and stability with Vitamin A, neomycin and water-soluble antibiotics. For external use only. Not for ophthalmic use.
How Supplied: Creme: 1 oz tubes; 4 oz and 1 lb jars. Lotion: 4 oz.

CAMA® INLAY-TABS®

Description: Each CAMA INLAY-TAB contains: aspirin, USP, 600 mg. (10 grains); magnesium hydroxide, USP, 150 mg.; aluminum hydroxide dried gel, USP, 150 mg.
Indications: An analgesic in arthritis and rheumatism.
Contraindications: Hypersensitivity to salicylates.
Warnings: The antipyretic effect of salicylates may mask the diagnostic importance of persistent fever.
Precautions: The occasional occurrence of mild salicylism may require adjustment of dosage.
Adverse Reactions: Overdosage of salicylates will cause tinnitus, nausea, vomiting and gastrointestinal upsets and bleeding.

Dosage and Administration: Adults—one tablet every four hours. Physicians may increase the dosage as required to provide satisfactory relief of symptoms. Usually, a dose of one to two tablets four times daily is adequate.
How Supplied: Cama Inlay-Tabs (white with salmon inlay) in bottles of 100 and 250.

DORCOL® PEDIATRIC COUGH SYRUP

Description: Each teaspoonful (5 ml) of DORCOL Pediatric Cough Syrup contains: phenylpropanolamine hydrochloride 6.25 mg, guaifenesin 50 mg, dextromethorphan hydrobromide 5 mg, alcohol 5%.
Indications: Provides prompt relief of cough and nasal congestion due to the common cold. The expectorant component helps loosen bronchial secretions. The decongestant, expectorant and antitussive are provided in an antihistamine-free formula.
Contraindications: DORCOL Pediatric Cough Syrup is contraindicated in the presence of hypersensitivity to any of the ingredients. The use of pressor amines such as phenylpropanolamine hydrochloride is contraindicated in those patients taking monoamine oxidase inhibitors for antihypertensive or antidepressant indications.
Precautions: Exercise prescribing caution in patients with persistent or chronic cough such as occurs with chronic bronchitis, bronchial asthma, or emphysema. Use with caution in patients with hypertension, hyperthyroidism cardiovascular disease or diabetes mellitus.
Adverse Reactions: Occasional blurred vision, cardiac palpitations, flushing, gastrointestinal upsets, nervousness, dizziness, or sleeplessness may occur.
Dosage and Administration: Children 6–12 years—2 teaspoonfuls every 4 hours. Children 2–6 years—1 teaspoonful every 4 hours. The suggested dosage in pediatric patients 3 months to 2 years of age is 3 drops per kilogram of body weight administered every four hours. For nighttime cough relief, give the last dose at bedtime.
How Supplied: DORCOL Pediatric Cough Syrup (grape-colored) in 4 fl oz and 8 fl oz bottles.

KANULASE® TABLETS

Description: Each KANULASE TABLET contains: Dorase® (cellulase) standardized to 9 mg.; pancreatin, N.F., 500 mg.; glutamic acid hydrochloride 200 mg.; ox bile extract 100 mg.; pepsin 150 mg.
Indications: Kanulase is designed to diminish intestinal gas in healthy persons and in those patients having digestive disorders. Cellulase disintegrates the cell walls of plant foods, releasing starch for digestion in the upper intestinal tract, and thus reducing gas formation in the colon. Kanulase further reduces gas formation by aiding in the digestion of fats, proteins and starches.
Precautions: Kanulase contains glutamic acid hydrochloride which is not usually given to patients with peptic ulcer.
Dosage and Administration: Adults—1 or 2 tablets, swallowed whole, at mealtimes. If looseness of stools occurs decrease the dosage.
How Supplied: Kanulase Tablets (pink) in bottles of 50.

PABIRIN® BUFFERED TABLETS

Description: Each BUFFERED PABIRIN TABLET contains: aspirin 300 mg., aminobenzoic acid 300 mg., dried aluminum hydroxide gel 100 mg.
Indications: An analgesic for temporary relief from minor aches and pains associated with arthritis and rheumatism.
Contraindications: Sensitivity to salicylates.
Precautions: When administered concurrently, aminobenzoic acid inhibits bacteriostatic action of sulfonamides.
Dosage and Administration: Adults: 2 tablets every four hours, 4 to 6 times daily.
How Supplied: Buffered Pabirin Tablets (dark pink) in bottles of 100.

TRIAMINIC® EXPECTORANT

Description: Each teaspoonful (5 ml) of TRIAMINIC Expectorant contains: phenylpropanolamine hydrochloride 12.5 mg, guaifenesin 100 mg, alcohol 5%.
Indications: Provides prompt relief of cough and nasal congestion due to the common cold. The expectorant component helps loosen bronchial secretions. The decongestant and expectorant are provided in an antihistamine-free formula.
Contraindications: TRIAMINIC Expectorant is contraindicated in the presence of hypersensitivity to any of the ingredients. The use of pressor amines such as phenylpropanolamine hydrochloride is contraindicated in those patients taking monoamine oxidase inhibitors for antihypertensive or antidepressant indications.
Precautions: Exercise prescribing caution in patients with persistent or chronic cough such as occurs with chronic bronchitis, bronchial asthma, or emphysema. Use with caution in patients with hypertension, hyperthyroidism, cardiovascular disease or diabetes mellitus.
Adverse Reactions: Occasional blurred vision, cardiac palpitations, flushing, gastrointestinal upsets, nervousness, dizziness, or sleeplessness may occur.
Dosage and Administration: Adults—2 teaspoonfuls every 4 hours. Children 6–12 years—1 teaspoonful every 4 hours. Children 2–6—½ teaspoonful every 4 hours. The suggested dosage in pediatric patients 3 months to 2 years of age is 4 to 5 drops per kilogram of body weight administered every four hours.
How Supplied: TRIAMINIC Expectorant (yellow) in 4 fl oz, 8 fl oz and pint bottles.

TRIAMINIC® SYRUP

Description: Each teaspoonful (5 ml) of TRIAMINIC Syrup contains: phenylpropanolamine hydrochloride 12.5 mg and chlorpheniramine maleate 2 mg in a nonalcoholic vehicle.
Indications: For the temporary relief of nasal congestion, sneezing, and itchy watery eyes that may occur in hay fever or other upper respiratory allergies, the common cold and sinusitis.
Contraindications: TRIAMINIC Syrup is contraindicated in the presence of hypersensitivity to any of the ingredients. The use of pressor amines such as phenylpropanolamine hydrochloride is contraindicated in those patients taking monoamine oxidase inhibitors for antihypertensive or antidepressant indications.
Precautions: Caution should be observed in operating a motor vehicle or performing potentially hazardous tasks requiring mental alertness. Alcoholic beverages and other CNS depressants may potentiate the sedative effects of antihistamines. Caution should be observed in the presence of hypertension, hyperthyroidism, cardiovascular disease or diabetes mellitus. Because of anticholinergic action of antihistamines they should be administered with caution to patients with bronchial asthma, narrow angle glaucoma, stenosing peptic ulcer, pyloroduodenal obstruction, prostatic hypertrophy or other bladder neck obstruction.
Adverse Reactions: Drowsiness, blurred vision, palpitations, flushing, gastrointestinal upsets, nervousness, dizziness, or sleeplessness may occur. May cause excitability especially in children.
Dosage and Administration: Adults—two teaspoonfuls every 4 hours. Children 6–12 years—1 teaspoonful every 4 hours, children 2–6—½ teaspoonful every 4 hours. The suggested dosage in pediatric patients 3 months to 2 years of age is 4 to 5 drops per kilogram of body weight administered every four hours.
How Supplied: TRIAMINIC Syrup (orange), in 4 fl oz, 8 fl oz and pint bottles.

TRIAMINIC-DM® COUGH FORMULA

Description: Each teaspoonful (5 ml) of TRIAMINIC-DM Cough Formula contains: phenylpropanolamine hydrochloride 12.5 mg and dextromethorphan hydrobromide 10 mg in a nonalcoholic vehicle.
Indications: Provides prompt, temporary relief of cough and nasal congestion due to the common cold. The decongestant and antitussive are provided in an antihistamine free formula.
Contraindications: TRIAMINIC-DM Cough Formula is contraindicated in the presence of hypersensitivity to any of the ingredients. The use of pressor amines such as phenylpropanolamine hydrochloride is contraindicated in those patients taking monoamine oxidase inhibitors for antihypertensive or antidepressant indications.
Precautions: Exercise prescribing caution in patients with persistent or chronic cough such as occurs with chronic bronchitis, bronchial asthma, or emphysema. Use with caution in patients with hypertension, hyperthyroidism, cardiovascular disease or diabetes mellitus.
Adverse Reactions: Occasional blurred vision, cardiac palpitations, flushing, gastrointestinal upsets, nervousness, dizziness, or sleeplessness may occur.
Dosage and Administration: Adults—2 teaspoonfuls every 4 hours. Children 6–12 years—1 teaspoonful every 4 hours. Children 2–6 years—½ teaspoonful every 4 hours. The suggested dosage in pediatric patients 3 months to 2 years of age is 1½ drops per kilogram of body weight administered every 4 hours.
How Supplied: TRIAMINIC-DM Cough Formula (dark red) in 4 fl oz and 8 fl oz bottles.

TRIAMINIC-12™ Sustained-Release Tablets

Each tablet contains: phenylpropanolamine hydrochloride 75 mg and chlorpheniramine maleate 12 mg. TRIAMINIC-12 Tablets contain the nasal decongestant phenylpropanolamine and the antihistamine chlorpheniramine, in a formulation providing 12 hours of symptomatic relief.
Indications: For the temporary relief of nasal congestion due to the common cold, hay fever or other upper respiratory allergies and associated with sinusitis. Helps decongest sinus openings, sinus passages; promotes nasal and/or sinus drainage; temporarily restores freer breathing through the nose.
For temporary relief of running nose, sneezing, itching of the nose or throat and itchy and watery eyes as may occur in allergic rhinitis (such as hay fever).
Dosage: Adults and children over 12 years of age—1 tablet swallowed whole every 12 hours.
NOTE: The nonactive portion of the tablet that supplies the active ingredients may occasionally appear in the stool as a soft mass.
Warnings: This product is not recommended for use in children under 12 years of age. Use with caution in patients with high blood pressure, heart disease, diabetes, thyroid disease, asthma, glaucoma or difficulty in urination due to enlargement of the prostate gland. Do

Continued on next page

Dorsey Labs.—Cont.

not exceed the recommended dosage because at higher doses nervousness, dizziness, or sleeplessness may occur. This preparation may cause drowsiness; this preparation may cause excitability, especially in children.
Caution: Patients should be advised to avoid driving a motor vehicle or operating heavy machinery. Patients should also be advised to avoid alcoholic beverages while taking this product. Use with caution in pregnant and nursing mothers.
Drug Interaction Precaution: Use with caution in patients presently taking a prescription antihypertensive or antidepressant drug containing a monamine oxidase inhibitor.
How Supplied: TRIAMINIC-12 Tablets (orange), imprinted "Dorsey" on one side, in blister packs of 10 and 20.

TRIAMINICIN® TABLETS

(See PDR For Nonprescription Drugs)

TRIAMINICOL® DECONGESTANT COUGH SYRUP

Description: Each teaspoonful (5 ml.) of TRIAMINICOL COUGH SYRUP contains: phenylpropanolamine hydrochloride 12.5 mg., pheniramine maleate 6.25 mg., pyrilamine maleate 6.25 mg.; dextromethorphan hydrobromide 15 mg.; ammonium chloride 90 mg., in a palatable vehicle.
Indications: For relief of coughs, especially when accompanied by stuffed and runny noses, due to the common cold. It combines the effective, nonnarcotic, antitussive action of dextromethorphan hydrobromide with a proven nasal decongestant.
Precautions: Patients should be advised not to drive a car or operate dangerous machinery if drowsiness occurs. Use with caution in the presence of hypertension, hyperthyroidism, cardiovascular disease or diabetes.
Adverse Reactions: Occasional drowsiness, blurred vision, cardiac palpitations, flushing, dizziness, nervousness or gastrointestinal upsets.
Dosage and Administration: Adults—2 teaspoonfuls every 4 hours; children 6 to 12—1 teaspoonful every 4 hours; children 2 to 6—½ teaspoonful every 4 to 6 hours. For nighttime cough relief, give the last dose at bedtime.
How Supplied: Triaminicol Decongestant Cough Syrup (dark red) in 4 fl. oz. and 8 fl. oz. bottles.

TUSSAGESIC® TABLETS/SUSPENSION

(See PDR For Nonprescription Drugs)

URSINUS® INLAY-TABS®

(See PDR For Nonprescription Drugs)

Dorsey Pharmaceuticals

Division of Sandoz, Inc.
E. HANOVER, NJ 07936

ASBRON G® ELIXIR and ASBRON G® INLAY-TABS® ℞

Description: Each ASBRON G INLAY-TAB and tablespoonful (15 ml) of ASBRON G Elixir contains: theophylline sodium glycinate 300 mg (equivalent to 150 mg theophylline), guaifenesin 100 mg. The elixir supplies the active ingredients in a solution containing 15% alcohol. ASBRON G contains a bronchodilator and an expectorant.
Theophylline sodium glycinate, a methylxanthine, is a white crystalline powder that is freely soluble in water, has a slight ammoniacal odor and a bitter taste. It is an equimolar mixture of theophylline sodium and glycine buffered by an additional mole of the essential amino acid, glycine.
The expectorant component is guaifenesin (formerly called glyceryl guaiacolate) which helps loosen and thus clear the bronchial passageways of bothersome, thickened mucus. Guaifenesin, 3-(o-methoxyphenoxy)-1,2-propanediol, occurs as a fine, white powder having a bitter, aromatic taste and a slight odor of guaiacol. The powder tends to become lumpy on storage. It is freely soluble in alcohol and soluble in water.
Clinical Pharmacology: Theophylline sodium glycinate is more stable in the presence of hydrochloric acid due to the buffering action of glycine with subsequent reduction of the chance of theophylline precipitation in the stomach. This and the high solubility of the product are suggested as the reasons why this product has better gastric tolerance than aminophylline.
Theophylline, the active ingredient of theophylline sodium glycinate, accounts for 50% of the weight of this compound. Theophylline sodium glycinate is highly effective in relaxing the smooth muscle of the bronchioles and the pulmonary blood vessels, thus acting primarily as a bronchodilator, pulmonary vasodilator and smooth muscle relaxant. Like other xanthines, theophylline sodium glycinate is a coronary vasodilator, a diuretic, a cerebral, cardiac and skeletal muscle stimulant.
Theophylline acts by inhibiting phosphodiesterase which causes an increase in intracellular cyclic AMP. This action produces smooth muscle relaxation and inhibits the release of histamine and other bronchoconstricting mediators from mast cells.
In vitro, using human white blood cells, theophylline has been shown to react synergistically with beta agonists to increase intracellular cyclic AMP. More data is required to clearly establish if theophylline and the beta agonists are synergistic or additive in vivo.
Even after prolonged therapy, it has not been possible to demonstrate the development of tolerance to theophylline sodium glycinate.
The half-life of theophylline varies from individual to individual. Since effective bronchodilatation depends upon maintaining serum theophylline levels between 10-20 mg/dl (10-20 mcg/ml), the determination of serum theophylline can be of value.

The half-life of theophylline is prolonged in alcoholism, in patients with reduced hepatic or renal function, congestive heart failure and in patients receiving antibiotics such as triacetyloleandomycin, erythromycin, clindamycin and lincomycin. Fever can also prolong theophylline half-life.
Cigarette smoking (1-2 packs per day) enhances theophylline elimination. The half-life of theophylline is shortened with cigarette smoking. This effect is probably related to the induction of enzymes and requires between three months and two years to normalize after stopping tobacco usage.
By increasing respiratory tract fluid, guaifenesin reduces the viscosity of tenacious secretions and acts as an expectorant. The drug is effective in productive as well as nonproductive cough, but is of particular value in dry, nonproductive cough which tends to injure the mucous membranes of the air passages.
[See table below].

THEOPHYLLINE ELIMINATION CHARACTERISTICS

Group	Theophylline Renal Clearance Rates	Half-Life Average
1. Children	1.4 ml/kg/min	3.5 hours
2. Adults with uncomplicated asthma	1.2 ml/kg/min	7 hours
3. Older adults with chronic obstructive pulmonary disease	0.6 ml/kg/min	up to 24 hours
4. Adults with chronic obstructive pulmonary disease and cor pulmonale or other causes of heart failure and liver pathology	0.6 ml/kg/min and less	may exceed 24 hours
5. Young smokers	Not available	4.3 hours

Indications and Usage: For relief of acute bronchial asthma and for reversible bronchospasm associated with chronic bronchitis and emphysema.
Contraindications: ASBRON G INLAY-TABS and ASBRON G Elixir are contraindicated in individuals who have shown hypersensitivity to any of the components.
Warnings: There is an excellent correlation between high theophylline blood levels and the clinical manifestations of toxicity in (1) patients with lowered body plasma clearances (due to transient cardiac decomposition), (2) chronic obstructive lung disease or patients with liver dysfunction, (3) patients who are older than 55 years of age, particularly males. There are often no early signs of theophylline toxicity such as nausea and restlessness which may appear in up to 50% of patients. Convulsions or ventricular arrhythmias may be the first signs of toxicity.
Excessive doses of theophylline sodium glycinate may be expected to be toxic and serum theophylline levels are recommended to monitor therapy. The incidence of toxicity increases significantly at levels greater than 20 mcg/ml. Many patients who have higher theophylline serum levels exhibit tachycardia. Theophylline products often worsen preexisting arrhythmias.
ASBRON G INLAY-TABS, ASBRON G Elixir and other oral theophylline compounds should never be used to treat status asthma.
Precautions:
General: Theophylline should be used with caution in patients with severe cardiovascular disease, severe hypoxemia, hypertension, hyperthyroidism, acute myocardial injury, obstructive lung disease, liver disease, in the elderly and in neonates.
Great caution should be used in giving theophylline to patients in congestive heart failure. Such patients have markedly prolonged theophylline blood levels which have persisted for long periods after discontinuation of the drug. Smokers have a shorter mean half-life of theophylline than nonsmokers and may require larger doses of theophylline.
Theophylline sodium glycinate should not be administered concurrently with other theophylline containing products.
Theophylline should be given with caution to patients with a history of peptic ulcer. Theophylline may act as a local irritant in the gastrointestinal tract.
Information for Patients: The importance of adherence to the prescribed dosage regimen should be stressed. Patients should be informed of symptoms associated with theophylline toxicity such as nausea and restlessness.
Laboratory Tests: There is great patient-to-patient variation in the serum half-life of theophylline. Therefore, when possible, serum theophylline levels should be measured to assist in titration of dosage.

Drug Interactions: The use of theophylline sodium glycinate with ephedrine and other sympathomimetic bronchodilators may result in a significant increase in side effects.

Drug	Effect
Aminophylline with Lithium Carbonate	Increased excretion of Lithium Carbonate
Aminophylline with Propranolol	Antagonism of Propranolol effect
Theophylline with Furosemide	Increased Diuresis of Furosemide
Theophylline with Reserpine	Reserpine-induced Tachycardia
Theophylline with Chlordiazepoxide	Chlordiazepoxide-induced fatty acid mobilization
Theophylline with Cyclamycin (TAO = Triacetyloleandomycin): erythromycin lincomycin	Increased Theophylline plasma levels

Drug/Laboratory Test Interactions

Theophylline has been shown to increase the urinary excretion of catecholamines. The VMA test for catechols may be falsely elevated by guaifenesin. Theophylline may increase the apparent serum uric acid in certain manual or automated chemical procedures by being treated as if it were uric acid. Guaifenesin may increase renal clearance for urate and thereby lower the serum uric acid. It may also falsely elevate the level of urinary 5H1AA in certain serotonin metabolite chemical tests.

Carcinogenesis, Mutagenesis, Impairment of Fertility: No data are available on the long-term potential for carcinogenicity, mutagenicity or impairment of fertility in animals or humans.

Pregnancy: *Pregnancy Category C*—Animal reproduction studies have not been conducted with ASBRON-G. Safe use in pregnancy has not been established relative to possible adverse effects on fetal development. Therefore, theophylline should not be used in pregnant patients unless, in the judgment of the physician, the potential benefits outweigh possible hazards.

Nursing Mothers: It is not known whether this drug is excreted in human milk. Because many drugs are excreted in human milk, caution should be observed when ASBRON G INLAY-TABS or ASBRON-G Elixir is administered to a nursing mother.

Pediatric Use: See Dosage and Administration Section for mg/kg dosage in pediatric patients.

Adverse Reactions: Included in this listing which follows are adverse reactions, some of which may have been reported with theophylline sodium glycinate. However, pharmacological similarities among the xanthine drugs require that each of the reactions be considered when theophylline is administered. The most consistent adverse reactions are usually due to overdosage of theophylline sodium glycinate and are:

1. Gastrointestinal: nausea, vomiting, epigastric pain, hematemesis, diarrhea.
2. Central Nervous System: headaches, irritability, restlessness, insomnia, reflex hyperexcitability, muscle twitching, clonic and tonic generalized convulsions.
3. Cardiovascular: palpitation, tachycardia, extrasystoles, flushing hypotension, circulatory failure, life-threatening ventricular arrhythmias.
4. Respiratory: tachypnea.
5. Renal: albuminuria, increased excretion of renal tubular cells and red blood cells; potentiation of diuresis.
6. Others: hyperglycemia and inappropriate ADH syndrome.

Overdosage (Management):

A. If potential oral overdose is established and seizure has not occurred: (1) induce vomiting and resort to gastric lavage if the patient fails to vomit within 20-30 minutes; (2) administer a cathartic (this is particularly important if sustained-release preparations have been taken) and activated charcoal after successful vomiting has been induced or adequate gastric lavage performed.
B. If patient is having a seizure: (1) establish an airway; (2) administer O_2; (3) treat the seizure with intravenous diazepam 0.1 to 0.3 mg/kg up to 10 mg; (4) monitor vital signs, maintain blood pressure and provide adequate hydration.
C. Postseizure Coma: (1) maintain airway and oxygenation; (2) if a result of oral medication, follow above recommendations to prevent absorption of drug, but tracheal intubation and lavage will have to be performed instead of inducing emesis, and the cathartic and charcoal will need to be introduced via a large bore gastric lavage tube; (3) continue to provide full supportive care and adequate hydration while waiting for drug to be metabolized. In general, the drug is metabolized sufficiently rapidly so as to not warrant consideration of dialysis.

Dosage and Administration: Therapeutic serum levels associated with optimal likelihood for benefit and minimal risk of toxicity are between 10-20 mcg/ml. There is great variation from patient to patient in the dosage of theophylline needed to achieve a therapeutic blood level because of variable rates of elimination. Because of this and because of the relatively narrow therapeutic blood level range associated with optimal results, the monitoring of serum theophylline levels is highly recommended. (See Laboratory Tests)

Usual Dosage: Adults—1 or 2 tablets or tablespoonfuls (15-30 ml), 3 or 4 times daily. Children 6 to 12—2 or 3 teaspoonfuls (10-15 ml), 3 or 4 times daily. Children 3 to 6—1 to 1½ teaspoonfuls (5-7.5 ml), 3 or 4 times daily. Children 1 to 3—½ to 1 teaspoonful (2.5-5 ml), 3 or 4 times daily.

Dosage Titration:

A. FOR PATIENTS NOT CURRENTLY RECEIVING THEOPHYLLINE PRODUCTS: [See table above].

	Oral Loading Dose (Theophylline Sodium Glycinate	Maintenance Dose For Next 12 Hours (Theophylline Sodium Glycinate)	Maintenance Dose Beyond 12 Hours (Theophylline Sodium Glycinate)
1. Infants	8 mg/kg *(4 mg/kg)	3-8 mg/kg q6h *(1.5-4.0 mg/kg q6h)	4-6 mg/kg q6h *(2-3 mg/kg q6h)**
2. Children 6 months to 9 years	12 mg/kg *(6 mg/kg)	8 mg/kg q4h *(4 mg/kg q4h)	8 mg/kg q6h *(4 mg/kg q6h)
3. Children age 9-16 and young adult Smokers	12 mg/kg *(6 mg/kg)	6 mg/kg q4h *(3 mg/kg q4h)	6 mg/kg q6h *(3 mg/kg q6h)
4. Otherwise healthy nonsmoking adults	12 mg/kg *(6 mg/kg)	6 mg/kg q6h *(3 mg/kg q6h)	6 mg/kg q8h *(3 mg/kg q8h)
5. Older patients and patients with cor pulmonale	12 mg/kg *(6 mg/kg)	4 mg/kg q6h *(2 mg/kg q6h)	4 mg/kg q8h *(2 mg/kg q8h)
6. Patients with congestive heart failure, liver failure	12 mg/kg *(6 mg/kg)	4 mg/kg q8h *(2 mg/kg q8h)	2-4 mg/kg q12h *(1-2 mg/kg q12h)

Equivalent theophylline dosage indicated in parenthesis and marked with an asterisk (*).
** PEDIATRICS, Vol. 55, No. 5, May 1975.

B. FOR PATIENTS CURRENTLY RECEIVING THEOPHYLLINE PRODUCTS: Determine, where possible, the time, amount, route of administration and form of the patient's last dose of theophylline.

The loading dose of theophylline will be based on the principle that each 0.5 mg/kg of theophylline administered as a loading dose will result in a 1 mcg/ml increase in serum theophylline concentration. Ideally, then, the loading dose should be deferred if a serum theophylline concentration can be rapidly obtained. If this is not possible, the clinician must exercise his judgment in selecting a dose based on the potential for benefit and risk. When there is sufficient respiratory distress to warrant a small risk, 2.5 mg/kg of theophylline is likely to increase the serum concentration when administered as a loading dose in rapidly absorbed form by only about 5 mcg/ml. If the patient is not already experiencing theophylline toxicity, this is unlikely to result in dangerous adverse effects.

Measurement of serum theophylline concentration during chronic therapy:

Blood for peak theophylline determinations should be obtained 1-2 hours after a dose of theophylline sodium glycinate. When determining theophylline serum concentrations in patients who have received chronic therapy, it is essential to establish that no doses were omitted in the 48 hours prior to the determination. Missed doses could result in recommendations of future doses that would cause serious toxicity due to overdosage.

DOSAGE ADJUSTMENT BASED ON SERUM THEOPHYLLINE MEASUREMENTS WHEN THESE INSTRUCTIONS HAVE NOT BEEN FOLLOWED MAY RESULT IN RECOMMENDATIONS THAT PRESENT RISK OF TOXICITY TO THE PATIENT.

PATIENTS SHOULD NEVER BE MAINTAINED ON A DOSAGE OF THEOPHYLLINE THAT IS NOT WELL TOLERATED. Patients experiencing toxic side effects should be instructed to skip the next regular dose and to resume theophylline therapy at a lower dosage when all side effects have disappeared.

Maximum Dose Without Measurement of Serum Concentration: Not to exceed the following: (WARNING: DO NOT ATTEMPT TO MAINTAIN ANY DOSAGE THAT IS NOT WELL TOLERATED.)

[See table on next page].

Use ideal (lean) body weight for obese patients in computing dosage.

Dosage should always be calculated on the basis of ideal (lean) body weight when mg/kg doses are stated. Theophylline does not distribute into fatty tissues. NEVER ATTEMPT TO MAINTAIN A DOSAGE THAT IS NOT WELL TOLERATED BY THE PATIENT.

How Supplied: ASBRON G INLAY-TABS (green with white inlay) in bottles of 100. ASBRON G Elixir (green) in pint bottles.

Caution: Federal law prohibits dispensing without prescription.

[*Shown in Product Identification Section*]

Continued on next page

Dorsey Pharm.—Cont.

BELLERGAL® Tablets and BELLERGAL-S® Tablets ℞

Description: Each BELLERGAL Tablet contains: phenobarbital, USP, central sedative (Warning: May be habit forming), 20.0 mg; Gynergen® (ergotamine tartrate, USP) sympathetic inhibitor, 0.3 mg; Bellafoline® (levorotatory alkaloids of belladonna, as malates) parasympathetic inhibitor, 0.1 mg. Each BELLERGAL-S Tablet contains: phenobarbital, USP, central sedative (Warning: May be habit forming), 40.0 mg; Gynergen (ergotamine tartrate, USP) sympathetic inhibitor, 0.6 mg; Bellafoline (levorotatory alkaloids of belladonna, as malates) parasympathetic inhibitor, 0.2 mg.

Clinical Pharmacology: Based on the concept that functional disorders frequently involve hyperactivity of both the sympathetic and parasympathetic nervous systems, the ingredients in BELLERGAL are combined to provide a balanced preparation designed to correct imbalance of the autonomic nervous system. The integrated action of BELLERGAL is effected through the combined administration of ergotamine and the levorotatory alkaloids of belladonna, specific inhibitors of the sympathetic and parasympathetic respectively, reinforced by the synergistic action of phenobarbital in dampening the cortical centers. It should be noted that on a weight basis the levorotatory alkaloids of belladonna have approximately twice the pharmacological effect as do the usual racemic mixtures.

Indications and Usage: BELLERGAL is employed in the management of disorders characterized by nervous tension and exaggerated autonomic response: *Menopausal disorders* with hot flushes, sweats, restlessness and insomnia. *Cardiovascular disorders* with palpitation, tachycardia, chest oppression and vasomotor disturbances. *Gastrointestinal disorders* with hypermotility, hypersecretion, "nervous stomach," and alternately diarrhea and constipation.

Genitourinary—uterine cramps, etc.

Premenstrual tension.

Interval treatment of *recurrent, throbbing headache.*

Contraindications: Peripheral vascular disease, coronary heart disease, hypertension, impaired hepatic or renal function, sepsis, pregnancy, nursing mothers and glaucoma. The concomitant administration of ergotamine and dopamine should be avoided, due to the increased potential for ischemic vasoconstriction. Phenobarbital is contraindicated in patients with a history of manifest or latent porphyria. Phenobarbital is contraindicated in those patients in whom the drug produces restlessness and/or excitement. BELLERGAL is contraindicated in patients with a demonstrated hypersensitivity to any of the components.

Warnings: Total weekly dosage of ergotamine tartrate should not exceed 10 mg. (This dosage corresponds to 33 BELLERGAL Tablets or 16 BELLERGAL-S Tablets). Due to presence of a barbituate, may be habit forming.

Precautions: Even though the ergotamine tartrate content of this product is low and untoward effects have been rare and of minor significance, caution should be exercised if large or prolonged dosage is contemplated, and physicians should be alert to possible peripheral vascular complications in patients sensitive to ergot. Due to the presence of the anticholinergic agent, special caution should be excerised in the use of this drug in patients with bronchial asthma or obstructive uropathy.

BELLERGAL-S contains FD&C Yellow No. 5 (tartrazine) which may cause allergic-type reactions (including bronchial asthma) in certain susceptible individuals. Although the overall incidence of FD&C Yellow No. 5 (tartrazine) sensitivity in the general population is low, it is frequently seen in patients who also have aspirin hypersensitivity.

Information for patients: Patients on large or prolonged dosage should be asked to report numbness or tingling of extremities, claudication or other symptoms of peripheral vasoconstriction.

Drug Interactions:

1. Oral Anticoagulants: Phenobarbital may lower the plasma levels of dicumarol (name previously used: bishydroxycoumarin) and may cause a decrease in anticoagulant activity as measured by the prothrombin time. More frequent monitoring of prothrombin time responses is indicated whenever phenobarbital is initiated or discontinued, and the dosage of anticoagulants should be adjusted accordingly.
2. CNS depressants: Combined administration of phenobarbital and CNS depressants such as alcohol, tricyclic antidepressants, phenothiazines and narcotic analgesics may result in a potentiation of the depressant action.
3. Beta adrenergic blocking agents: Although proof is lacking, several reports in the literature suggest a possible interaction between ergot alkaloids and beta adrenergic blocking agents. This interaction may result in excessive vasoconstriction. Although many patients can apparently take propranolol and ergot alkaloids without ill effects, there is enough evidence of an interaction to dictate closer surveillance of patients so treated.
4. Hepatic metabolism: Through the mechanism of enzyme induction caused by phenobarbital, a number of substances have been shown to be metabolized at an increased rate. In these cases, clinical responses should be closely monitored and appropriate dosage adjustments made. Included are such substances as griseofulvin, quinidine, doxycycline and estrogen. Although the meaning of published reports regarding the effects of phenobarbital on estrogen metabolism are unclear at this time, if avoidance of pregnancy is critical, consideration should be given to alternative methods of contraception.
5. Phenytoin, sodium valproate, valproic acid: The effect of barbiturates on the metabolism of phenytoin appears to be variable. Some investigators report an accelerating effect, while others report no effect. Because the effect of barbiturates on the metabolism of phenytoin is not predictable, phenytoin and barbiturate blood levels should be monitored more frequently if these drugs are given concurrently. Sodium valproate and valproic acid appear to decrease barbiturate metabolism; therefore, barbiturate blood levels should be monitored and appropriate dosage adjustments made as indicated.
6. Tricyclic antidepressants: Due to the presence of levorotatory alkaloids of belladonna, concomitant administration of tricyclic antidepressants may result in additive anticholinergic effects.

Carcinogenesis: No data are available on the long-term potential for carcinogenicity in animals or humans.

Pregnancy: *Pregnancy Category X*—due to the potential uterotonic effects of the ergot alkaloids, the use of BELLERGAL during pregnancy is contraindicated. See "Contraindications" section.

Nursing Mothers: A number of ergot alkaloids inhibit the secretion of prolactin. Therefore, BELLERGAL is contraindicated in nursing mothers. See "Contraindications" section.

Pediatric Use: Safety and effectiveness in children have not been established.

Adverse Reactions: Tingling and other paresthesias of the extremities, blurred vision, palpitations, dry mouth, decreased sweating, decreased gastrointestinal motility, urinary retention, tachycardia, flushing, drowsiness occur rarely.

Drug Abuse and Dependence: Barbiturates may be habit-forming. Tolerance, psychological dependence, and physical dependence may occur especially following prolonged use of high doses. Daily administration in excess of 400 mg of pentobarbital or secobarbital for approximately 90 days is likely to produce some degree of physical dependence. By way of comparison, the phenobarbital component of BELLERGAL and BELLERGAL-S at the highest recommended daily dosage amounts to 120 mg and 80 mg respectively.

Overdosage:

Management of Overdosage: While severe symptoms of overdosage with BELLERGAL have not been reported, theoretically they could occur. It is imperative to note that overdosage symptoms with BELLERGAL may be attributable to any one or more of the three active ingredients. Which toxic manifestations might predominate in any individual case would be impossible to predict but one should be alert to the various possibilities. When anticholinergic/antispasmodic drugs are taken in sufficient overdose to produce such severe symptoms, prompt treatment should be instituted. Gastric lavage and other measures to limit intestinal absorption should be initiated without delay.

Cholinesterase inhibitors administered parenterally may be necessary for treatment of the serious manifestations of anticholinergic overdosage. Additionally, symptomatic therapy, including oxygen, sedatives and control of hyperthermia may be necessary.

Acute barbiturate overdosage symptoms with BELLERGAL, while possible, have not been reported. While the usual procedures for handling barbiturate poisoning should be employed, keep in mind the possibility of anticholinergic overdosing effects.

Acute ergot overdosage symptoms with BELLERGAL, while possible, have not been reported. The usual procedures for handling ergot overdosage include the administration of a peripheral vasodilator to counteract the vasospasm.

Dosage and Administration: BELLERGAL Tablets: Four tablets daily (one in the morning, one at noon and two at bedtime) is the dose usually employed. In more resistant cases begin with six tablets daily, then gradually reduce dosage at weekly intervals according to response. Where required, continue with the smallest effective dose to maintain the improved status of the patient. BELLERGAL-S Tablets: One in the morning and one in the evening.

How Supplied: BELLERGAL Tablets (flesh pink, sugar-coated) in bottles of 100 and 1000.

Age	Theophylline Sodium Glycinate	Equivalent Theophylline
Under 9 years	48 mg/kg/day	24 mg/kg/day
9-12 years	40 mg/kg/day	20 mg/kg/day
12-16 years	36 mg/kg/day	18/mg/kg/day
Over 16 years	26 mg/kg/day or 1800 mg/day (WHICHEVER IS LESS)	13 mg/kg/day or 900 mg/day (WHICHEVER IS LESS)

BELLERGAL-S Tablets (compressed, scored tablets of tricolored pattern: dark green, orange and light lemon yellow) in bottles of 100.

[*Shown in Product Identification Section*]

GRIS–PEG® ℞
(griseofulvin ultramicrosize)
Tablets, USP 125 and 250 mg

Description: Gris-PEG Tablets contain ultramicrosize crystals of griseofulvin, an antibiotic derived from a species of *Penicillium*. Each Gris-PEG Tablet contains 125 mg or 250 mg griseofulvin ultramicrosize.

Action: *Microbiology*—Griseofulvin is fungistatic with *in vitro* activity against various species of *Microsporum, Epidermophyton* and *Trichophyton*. It has no effect on bacteria or other genera of fungi.

Human Pharmacology—Following oral administration, griseofulvin is deposited in the keratin precursor cells and has a greater affinity for diseased tissue. The drug is tightly bound to the new keratin which becomes highly resistant to fungal invasions.

Controlled bioavailability studies of Gris-PEG have demonstrated blood levels regarded as adequate.

Thus, the efficiency of gastrointestinal absorption of the ultramicrocrystalline formulation of Gris-PEG is approximately twice that of conventional microsized griseofulvin. This factor permits the oral intake of half as much griseofulvin per tablet but there is no evidence, at this time, that this confers any significant clinical differences in regard to safety and efficacy.

Indications: Gris-PEG (griseofulvin ultramicrosize) is indicated for the treatment of the following ringworm infections: *Tinea corporis* (ringworm of the body), *Tinea pedis* (athlete's foot), *Tinea cruris* (ringworm of the thigh), *Tinea barbae* (barber's itch), *Tinea capitis* (ringworm of the scalp), and *Tinea unguium* (onychomycosis, ringworm of the nails), when caused by one or more of the following genera of fungi: *Trichophyton rubrum, Trichophyton tonsurans, Trichophyton mentagrophytes, Trichophyton interdigitalis, Trichophyton verrucosum, Trichophyton megnini, Trichophyton gallinae, Trichophyton crateriform, Trichophyton sulphureum, Trichophyton schoenleini, Microsporum audiouini, Microsporum canis, Microsporum gypseum* and *Epidermophyton floccosum*. NOTE: Prior to therapy, the type of fungi responsible for the infection should be identified. The use of the drug is not justified in minor or trivial infections which will respond to topical agents alone. Griseofulvin is *not* effective in the following: Bacterial infections, Candidiasis (Moniliasis), Histoplasmosis, Actinomycosis, Sporotrichosis, Chromoblastomycosis, Coccidioidomycosis, North American Blastomycosis, Cryptococcosis (Torulosis), *Tinea versicolor* and Nocardiosis.

Contraindications: This drug is contraindicated in patients with porphyria, hepatocellular failure, and in individuals with a history of sensitivity to griseofulvin.

Warnings: *Prophylactic Usage*—Safety and Efficacy of Griseofulvin for Prophylaxis of Fungal Infections Has Not Been Established. *Animal Toxicology*—Chronic feeding of griseofulvin, at levels ranging from 0.5 to 2.5% of the diet, resulted in the development of liver tumors in several strains of mice, particularly in males. Smaller particle sizes result in an enhanced effect. Lower oral dosage levels have not been tested. Subcutaneous administration of relatively small doses of griseofulvin, once a week, during the first three weeks of life has also been reported to induce hepatomata in mice. Although studies in other animal species have not yielded evidence of tumorigenicity, these studies were not of adequate design to form a basis for conclusions in this regard. In subacute toxicity studies, orally administered griseofulvin produced hepatocellular necrosis in mice, but this has not been seen in other species. Disturbances in porphyrin metabolism have been reported in griseofulvin treated laboratory animals. Griseofulvin has been reported to have a colchicine-like effect on mitosis and cocarcinogenicity with methylcholanthrene in cutaneous tumor induction in laboratory animals. *Usage in Pregnancy*—The safety of this drug during pregnancy has not been established. *Animal Reproduction Studies*—It has been reported in the literature that griseofulvin was found to be embryotoxic and teratogenic on oral administration to pregnant rats. Pups with abnormalities have been reported in the litters of a few bitches treated with griseofulvin. Additional animal reproduction studies are in progress. Suppression of spermatogenesis has been reported to occur in rats, but investigation in man failed to confirm this.

Precautions: Patients on prolonged therapy with any potent medication should be under close observation. Periodic monitoring of organ system function, including renal, hepatic and hematopoietic, should be done. Since griseofulvin is derived from species of *Penicillium*, the possibility of cross sensitivity with penicillin exists; however, known penicillin-sensitive patients have been treated without difficulty. Since a photosensitivity reaction is occasionally associated with griseofulvin therapy, patients should be warned to avoid exposure to intense natural or artificial sunlight. Should a photosensitivity reaction occur, lupus erythematosus may be aggravated. Griseofulvin decreases the activity of warfarin-type anticoagulants so that patients receiving these drugs concomitantly may require dosage adjustment of the anticoagulant during and after griseofulvin therapy. Barbiturates usually depress griseofulvin activity and concomitant administration may require a dosage adjustment of the antifungal agent.

Adverse Reactions: When adverse reactions occur, they are most commonly of the hypersensitivity type such as skin rashes, urticaria, and rarely, angioneurotic edema, and may necessitate withdrawal of therapy and appropriate countermeasures. Paresthesias of the hands and feet have been reported rarely after extended therapy. Other side effects reported occasionally are oral thrush, nausea, vomiting, epigastric distress, diarrhea, headache, fatigue, dizziness, insomnia, mental confusion, and impairment of performance of routine activities. Proteinuria and leukopenia have been reported rarely. Administration of the drug should be discontinued if granulocytopenia occurs. When rare, serious reactions occur with griseofulvin, they are usually associated with high dosages, long periods of therapy, or both.

Dosage and Administration: Accurate diagnosis of the infecting organism is essential. Identification should be made either by direct microscopic examination of a mounting of infected tissue in a solution of potassium hydroxide or by culture on an appropriate medium. Medication must be continued until the infecting organism is completely eradicated as indicated by appropriate clinical or laboratory examination. Representative treatment periods are *tinea capitis*, 4 to 6 weeks; *tinea corporis* 2 to 4 weeks; *tinea pedis*, 4 to 8 weeks; *tinea unguium*—depending on rate of growth—fingernails, at least 4 months; toenails, at least 6 months.

General measures in regard to hygiene should be observed to control sources of infection or reinfection. Concomitant use of appropriate topical agents is usually required, particularly in treatment of *tinea pedis*. In some forms of athlete's foot, yeasts and bacteria may be involved as well as fungi. Griseofulvin will not eradicate the bacterial or monilial infection.

Adults: Daily administration of 250 mg (as a single dose or in divided amounts) will give a satisfactory response in most patients with *tinea corporis, tinea cruris,* and *tinea capitis.*

For those fungus infections more difficult to eradicate, such as *tinea pedis* and *tinea unguium*, a divided daily dosage of 500 mg is recommended. In all cases, the dosage should be individualized.

Children: Approximately 2.5 mg per pound of body weight per day is an effective dose for most children. On this basis, the following dosage schedule is suggested: Children weighing 30 to 50 pounds—62.5 mg to 125 mg daily. Children weighing over 50 pounds—125 mg to 250 mg daily.

Children 2 years of age and younger—dosage has not been established.

Dosage should be individualized, as is done for adults. Clinical experience with griseofulvin in children with *tinea capitis* indicates that a single daily dose is effective. Clinical relapse will occur if the medication is not continued until the infecting organism is eradicated.

How Supplied: Gris-PEG (griseofulvin ultramicrosize) Tablets, 125 mg (white, elliptical-shaped) and Gris-PEG (griseofulvin ultramicrosize) Tablets, 250 mg (white, capsule-shaped embossed "Gris-PEG" on one side). The 125 mg strength is available in bottles of 100 and 500; the 250 mg strength is available in bottles of 100. Both strengths are scored and film-coated.

HYDERGINE® ℞
(ergoloid mesylates) tablets, USP (ORAL)
(ergoloid mesylates) tablets, USP (SUBLINGUAL)
(ergoloid mesylates) liquid

Caution: Federal law prohibits dispensing without a prescription.

Description:

Hydergine tablet 1 mg and Hydergine sublingual tablet 1 mg, each contains ergoloid mesylates USP as follows: dihydroergocornine mesylate 0.333 mg, dihydroergocristine mesylate 0.333 mg, and dihydroergocryptine (dihydro-alpha-ergocryptine and dihydro-beta-ergocryptine in the proportion of 2:1) mesylate, representing a total of 1 mg.

Hydergine sublingual tablet 0.5 mg, each contains ergoloid mesylates USP as follows: dihydroergocornine mesylate 0.167 mg, dihydroergocristine mesylate 0.167 mg, and dihydroergocryptine (dihydro-alpha-ergocryptine and dihydro-beta-ergocryptine in the proportion of 2:1) mesylate, representing a total of 0.5 mg.

Hydergine liquid 1mg/ml, each ml contains ergoloid mesylates USP as follows: dihydroergocornine mesylate 0.333 mg, dihydroergocristine mesylate 0.333 mg, and dihydroergocryptine (dihydro-alpha-ergocryptine and dihydro-beta-ergocryptine in the proportion of 2:1) mesylate, representing a total of 1 mg; alcohol, USP, 30% by volume.

Pharmacokinetic Properties

Bioequivalence studies were performed in which Hydergine® (ergoloid mesylates) tablets were administered orally and Hydergine sublingual tablets were administered sublingually to human subjects. Hydergine tablets are rapidly but incompletely absorbed from the gastrointestinal tract. Following administration, the oral tablets resulted in slightly higher peak levels when compared to the sublingual dosage form. Hydergine substance undergoes a rapid first pass liver metabolism and less than 50% of the therapeutic moiety reaches the systemic circulation. The peak plasma levels of single, orally administered doses are achieved within one hour and by 24 hours the plasma levels are not detectable.

Actions: There is no specific evidence which clearly establishes the mechanism by which Hydergine tablets, sublingual tablets, and liquid produce mental effects, nor is there conclusive evidence that the drug particularly affects cerebral arteriosclerosis or cerebrovascular insufficiency.

Continued on next page

Dorsey Pharm.—Cont.

Indications: A proportion of individuals over sixty who manifest signs and symptoms of an idiopathic decline in mental capacity (i.e., cognitive and interpersonal skills, mood, self-care, apparent motivation) can experience some symptomatic relief upon treatment with Hydergine preparations. The identity of the specific trait(s) or condition(s), if any, which would usefully predict a response to Hydergine therapy is not known. It appears, however, that those individuals who do respond come from groups of patients who would be considered clinically to suffer from some ill-defined process related to aging or to have some underlying dementing condition (i.e., primary progressive dementia, Alzheimer's dementia, senile onset, multi-infarct dementia).

Before prescribing Hydergine® (ergoloid mesylates) therapy, the physician should exclude the possibility that the patient's signs and symptoms arise from a potentially reversible and treatable condition. Particular care should be taken to exclude delirium and dementiform illness secondary to systemic disease, primary neurological disease, or primary disturbance of mood.

Hydergine preparations are not indicated in the treatment of acute or chronic psychosis, regardless of etiology (see CONTRAINDICATIONS section).

The decision to use Hydergine therapy in the treatment of an individual with a symptomatic decline in mental capacity of unknown etiology should be continually reviewed since the presenting clinical picture may subsequently evolve sufficiently to allow a specific diagnosis and a specific alternative treatment. In addition, continued clinical evaluation is required to determine whether any initial benefit conferred by Hydergine therapy persists with time.

The efficacy of Hydergine therapy was evaluated using a special rating scale known as the SCAG (Sandoz-Clinical Assessment Geriatric). The specific items on this scale on which modest but statistically significant changes were observed at the end of twelve weeks include: mental alertness, confusion, recent memory, orientation, emotional lability, self-care, depression, anxiety/fears, cooperation, sociability, appetite, dizziness, fatigue, bothersome (ness), and an overall impression of clinical status.

Contraindications: Hydergine® (ergoloid mesylates) tablets, sublingual tablets, and liquid are contraindicated in individuals who have previously shown hypersensitivity to the drug. Hydergine preparations are also contraindicated in patients who have psychosis, acute or chronic, regardless of etiology.

Precautions: *Practitioners are advised that because the target symptoms are of unknown etiology careful diagnosis should be attempted before prescribing Hydergine tablets, sublingual tablets, and liquid.*

Adverse Reactions: Hydergine tablets, sublingual tablets, and liquid have not been found to produce serious side effects. Some sublingual irritation, transient nausea, and gastric disturbances have been reported. Hydergine tablets, sublingual tablets, and liquid do not possess the vasoconstrictor properties of the natural ergot alkaloids.

Dosage and Administration: 1 mg three times daily.

Alleviation of symptoms is usually gradual and results may not be observed for 3-4 weeks.

How Supplied:

Hydergine tablets (for oral use):
1 mg, round, white, embossed "HYDERGINE 1" on one side, triangle (S) other side. Packages of 100 and 500.

Hydergine sublingual tablets:
1 mg, oval, white, embossed "HYDERGINE" on one side, "78-77" other side. Packages of 100 and 1000.
0.5 mg, round, white, embossed "HYDERGINE 0.5" on one side, triangle (S) other side. Packages of 100 and 1000.

[*Shown in Product Identification Section*]

Hydergine liquid:
1 mg/ml. Bottles of 100 ml with an accompanying dropper graduated to deliver 1 mg.

© 1982 Sandoz, Inc.

KLORVESS® EFFERVESCENT GRANULES, TABLETS and KLORVESS® (potassium chloride) 10% LIQUID ℞

Description: Klorvess Effervescent Granules: Each packet (2.8 g) contains 20 mEq each of potassium and chloride supplied by potassium chloride 1.125 g, potassium bicarbonate 0.5 g, L-lysine monohydrochloride 0.913 g in a sodium-, sugar- and carbohydrate-free effervescent formulation. Dissolution of the packet contents in water provides the potassium and chloride available for oral ingestion as potassium chloride, potassium bicarbonate, potassium citrate and L-lysine monohydrochloride.

Klorvess Effervescent Tablets: Each dry, sodium- and sugar-free effervescent tablet contains 20 mEq each of potassium and chloride supplied by potassium chloride 1.125 g, potassium bicarbonate 0.5 g, L-lysine mono- hydrochloride 0.913 g. Dissolution of the tablet in water provides the potassium and chloride available for oral ingestion as potassium chloride, potassium bicarbonate, potassium citrate and L-lysine monohydrochloride.

Klorvess (potassium chloride) 10% Liquid: Each tablespoonful (15 ml) contains 20 mEq of potassium chloride (provided by potassium chloride 1.5 g) in a palatable, cherry-with-pit flavored vehicle, alcohol 1%.

Indications: For the prevention and treatment of potassium depletion and hypokalemic-hypochloremic alkalosis. Deficits of body potassium and chloride can occur as a consequence of therapy with potent diuretic agents and adrenal corticosteroids.

Contraindications: Severe renal impairment characterized by azotemia or oliguria, untreated Addison's disease, Familial Periodic Paralysis, acute dehydration, heat cramps, patients receiving aldosterone-inhibiting or potassium-sparing diuretic agents, or hyperkalemia from any cause.

Precautions: In response to a rise in the concentration of body potassium, renal excretion of the ion is increased. In the presence of normal renal function and hydration, it is difficult to produce potassium intoxication by oral potassium salt supplements.

Since the extent of potassium deficiency cannot be accurately determined, it is prudent to proceed cautiously in undertaking potassium replacement. Periodic evaluations of the patient's clinical status, serum electrolytes and the EKG should be carried out when replacement therapy is undertaken. This is particularly important in patients with cardiac disease and those patients receiving digitalis.

High serum concentrations of potassium may cause death through cardiac depression, arrhythmia or cardiac arrest.

To minimize gastrointestinal irritation associated with potassium chloride preparations, patients should dissolve the packet contents of Klorvess Effervescent Granules or each Klorvess Effervescent Tablet in 3 to 4 ounces of water or fruit juice, or dilute each tablespoonful of Klorvess (potassium chloride) 10% Liquid in 3 to 4 ounces of water. Both of these solutions should be ingested slowly with or immediately after meals.

Adverse Reactions: Abdominal discomfort, diarrhea, nausea and vomiting may occur with the use of potassium salts.

The symptoms and signs of potassium intoxication include paresthesias, heaviness, muscle weakness and flaccid paralysis of the extremities. Potassium intoxication can produce listlessness, mental confusion, a fall in blood pressure, shock, cardiac arrhythmias, heart block and cardiac arrest.

The EKG picture of hyperkalemia is characterized by the early appearance of tall, peaked T waves. The R wave is decreased in amplitude and the S wave deepens; the QRS complex widens progressively. The P wave widens and decreases in amplitude until it disappears. Occasionally, an apparent elevation of the RS-T junction and a cove plane RS-T segment and T wave will be noted in AVL.

Dosage and Administration: Klorvess Effervescent Granules and Tablets: Adults—Contents of one packet or one tablet (20 mEq each of potassium and chloride) completely dissolved in 3 to 4 ounces of cold water, fruit juice or other liquid 2 to 4 times daily depending upon the requirements of the patient.

Klorvess (potassium chloride) 10% Liquid: Adults—One tablespoonful (15 ml) of Klorvess Liquid (20 mEq of potassium chloride) completely diluted in 3 to 4 ounces of water 2 to 4 times daily depending upon the requirements of the patient.

Both of these solutions should be ingested slowly with meals or immediately after eating. Deviations from these recommended dosages may be indicated in certain cases of hypokalemia based upon the patient's status. The average total daily dosage must be governed by the patient's response as determined by frequent evaluation of serum electrolytes, EKG and clinical status.

Overdosage: Potassium intoxication may result from overdosage of potassium or from therapeutic dosage in conditions stated under "Contraindications." Hyperkalemia, when detected, must be treated immediately because lethal levels can be reached in a few hours.

Treatment of Hyperkalemia:

1. Dextrose solution, 10 or 25% containing 10 units of crystalline insulin per 20 g dextrose, given IV in a dose of 300 to 500 ml in an hour.
2. Adsorption and exchange of potassium using sodium or ammonium cycle cation exchange resins, orally and as retention enema. (Caution: Ammonium compounds should not be used in patients with hepatic cirrhosis.)
3. Hemodialysis and peritoneal dialysis.
4. The use of potassium-containing foods or medicaments must be eliminated.

In digitalized patients too rapid a lowering of plasma potassium concentration can cause digitalis toxicity.

How Supplied: Klorvess Effervescent Granules—packages of 30 packets (2.8 g each). Klorvess Effervescent Tablets (white) – 60 tablets (2 units of 30 effervescent tablets each). Each tablet is individually foil wrapped. Klorvess (potassium chloride) 10% Liquid (dark red) – as a cherry-with-pit flavored liquid in pint and gallon bottles. Klorvess Tablets and Liquid are also available in institutional packaging as follows: Klorvess Tablets – 30 and 1000 tablets; Klorvess Liquid – 36 (3 × 12) × 4 oz Unit-of-Use bottles and 100 (4 × 25) × 15 ml Unit-Dose bottles. ℞

[*Shown in Product Identification Section*]

METAPREL® ℞
(metaproterenol sulfate)
METERED DOSE INHALER, SYRUP and TABLETS

Each Metered Dose Inhaler contains: metaproterenol sulfate 225 mg as a micronized powder in an inert propellant. Each teaspoonful (5 ml) of syrup contains: metaproterenol sulfate 10 mg. Tablets contain: metaproterenol sulfate 10 and 20 mg.

Description: Chemically, Metaprel (metaproterenol sulfate) is 1-(3, 5-dihydroxyphenyl)-2-isopropylaminoethanol sulfate, a white, crystalline, racemic mixture of two optically active isomers. It differs from isoproterenol hydrochloride by having two hydroxyl groups attached at the meta positions on the benzene ring rather than one at the meta and one at the para position.

Actions: Metaprel (metaproterenol sulfate) is a potent beta-adrenergic stimulator with the metered dose inhaler having a rapid onset of action. It is postulated that beta-adrenergic stimulants produce many of their pharmacological effects by activation of adenyl cyclase, the enzyme which catalyzes the conversion of adenosine triphosphate to cyclic adenosine monophosphate.

Absorption, biotransformation and excretion studies following administration by inhalation have not been performed. Following oral administration in humans, an average of 40 percent of the drug is absorbed; it is not metabolized by catechol-O-methyltransferase or sulfatase enzymes in the gut but is excreted primarily as glucuronic acid conjugates.

Metered Dose Inhaler: When administered by oral inhalation, Metaprel (metaproterenol sulfate) decreases reversible bronchospasm. Pulmonary function tests performed concomitantly usually show improvement following aerosol Metaprel (metaproterenol sulfate) administration, e.g., an increase in the one-second forced expiratory volume (FEV_1), an increase in maximum expiratory flow rate, an increase in forced vital capacity, and/or a decrease in airway resistance. The resultant decrease in airway obstruction may relieve the dyspnea associated with bronchospasm.

Controlled single- and multiple-dose studies have been performed with pulmonary function monitoring. The duration of effect of a *single dose* of two to three inhalations of Metaprel (metaproterenol sulfate) (that is, the period of time during which there is a 20 percent or greater increase in FEV_1) has varied from one to five hours.

In repetitive-dosing studies (up to q.i.d.) the duration of effect for a similar dose of Metaprel (metaproterenol sulfate) has ranged from about one to two-and-one-half hours. Present studies are inadequate to explain the divergence in duration of the FEV_1 effect between single- and repetitive-dosing studies, respectively.

Syrup: When administered orally, Metaprel (metaproterenol sulfate) decreases reversible bronchospasm. Pulmonary function tests performed after the administration of Metaprel (metaproterenol sulfate) usually show improvement, e.g., an increase in the one-second forced expiratory volume (FEV_1), an increase in maximum expiratory flow rate, an increase in peak expiratory flow rate, an increase in forced vital capacity, and/or a decrease in airway resistance. The decrease in airway obstruction may relieve the dyspnea associated with bronchospasm.

Pulmonary function has been monitored in controlled single- and multiple-dose studies. The duration of effect of a single dose of Metaprel (metaproterenol sulfate) Syrup (that is, the period of time during which there is a 15 percent or greater increase in mean FEV_1) was up to four hours.

Tablets: When administered orally, Metaprel (metaproterenol sulfate) decreases reversible bronchospasm. Pulmonary function tests performed concomitantly usually show improvement following Metaprel (metaproterenol sulfate) administration, e.g., an increase in the one-second forced expiratory volume (FEV_1), an increase in maximum expiratory flow rate, an increase in forced vital capacity, and/or a decrease in airway resistance. The resultant decrease in airway obstruction may relieve the dyspnea associated with bronchospasm.

Controlled single- and multiple-dose studies have been performed with pulmonary function monitoring. The mean duration of effect of a single dose of 20 mg of Metaprel (metaproterenol sulfate) (that is, the period of time during which there is a 15 percent or greater increase in FEV_1) was up to four hours. Four controlled multiple-dose 60-day studies, comparing the effectiveness of metaproterenol sulfate tablets with ephedrine tablets, have been performed. Because of difficulties in study design, only one study was available which could be analyzed in depth. This study showed a loss of efficacy with time for both metaproterenol sulfate and ephedrine. Therefore, the physician should take this phenomenon into account in evaluating the individual patient's overall management. Further studies are in progress to adequately explain these results.

Indications: Metaprel (metaproterenol sulfate) is indicated as a bronchodilator for bronchial asthma, and for reversible bronchospasm which may occur in association with bronchitis and emphysema.

Contraindications: Use in patients with cardiac arrhythmias associated with tachycardia is contraindicated.

Warnings: Excessive use of adrenergic aerosols is potentially dangerous. Fatalities have been reported following excessive use of metaproterenol sulfate as with other sympathomimetic inhalation preparations, and the exact cause is unknown. Cardiac arrest was noted in several cases.

Paradoxical bronchoconstriction with repeated excessive administration has been reported with other sympathomimetic agents. Therefore, it is possible that this phenomenon could occur with Metaprel (metaproterenol sulfate).

Patients should be advised to contact their physician in the event that they do not respond to their *usual dose* of a sympathomimetic amine aerosol.

Precautions: Extreme care must be exercised with respect to the administration of additional sympathomimetic agents. A sufficient interval of time should elapse prior to administration of another sympathomimetic agent.

Because metaproterenol sulfate is a sympathomimetic drug, it should be used with great caution in patients with hypertension, coronary artery disease, congestive heart failure, hyperthyroidism and diabetes, or when there is sensitivity to sympathomimetic amines.

Usage in Pregnancy: Safety in pregnancy has not been established. Metaproterenol should not be used except with caution during pregnancy, weighing the drug's benefit to the patient against potential risk to the fetus. Studies of metaproterenol in mice, rats and rabbits have revealed no significant teratogenic effects at oral doses up to 50 mg/kg (310 times the recommended daily human inhalational dose or 31 times the recommended daily human oral dose). In rabbits, fetal loss and teratogenic effects have been observed at and above oral doses of 50 and 100 mg/kg, respectively.

Adverse Reactions: Adverse reactions such as tachycardia, hypertension, palpitations, nervousness, tremor, nausea and vomiting have been reported. These reactions are similar to those noted with other sympathomimetic agents.

Dosage and Administration: Metered Dose Inhaler: The usual single dose is two to three inhalations. With repetitive dosing, inhalation should usually not be repeated more often than about every three to four hours. Total dosage per day should not exceed 12 inhalations.

Metaprel (metaproterenol sulfate) Metered Dose Inhaler is not recommended for children under 12 years of age because there is not sufficient data on administration of the dosage form in this age group.

Syrup: Children aged 6–9 years or weight under 60 lbs—one teaspoonful three or four times a day. Children over 9 years or weight over 60 lbs—two teaspoonfuls three or four times a day. Experience in children under the age of six is limited to seventy-eight children. Of this number, forty were treated with metaproterenol sulfate syrup for at least one month. In this group, daily doses of approximately 1.3 to 2.6 mg/kg were well tolerated. Adults—two teaspoonfuls three or four times a day.

Tablets: The usual adult dose is one 20 mg tablet three or four times a day. Children aged 6–9 years or weight under 60 lbs—10 mg three or four times a day. Over 9 years or weight over 60 lbs—20 mg three or four times a day. Metaprel tablets are not recommended for use in children under 6 years at this time. (Please refer to the Actions section for further information on clinical experience with this product.)

If Metaprel (metaproterenol sulfate) is administered before or after other sympathomimetic bronchodilators, caution should be exercised with respect to possible potentiation of adrenergic effects.

Symptoms of Overdosage: The symptoms of overdosage are those of excessive beta-adrenergic stimulation listed under Adverse Reactions.

How Supplied: Metered Dose Inhaler: Each Metaprel (metaproterenol sulfate) Metered Dose Inhaler contains 225 mg of metaproterenol sulfate as a micronized powder in an inert propellant. This is sufficient medication for 300 inhalations. Each metered dose expressed from the inhaler delivers at the mouthpiece approximately 0.65 mg of metaproterenol sulfate.

Metaprel Metered Dose Inhaler with mouthpiece (15 cc)

Metaprel Metered Dose Inhaler refill (15 cc)

Syrup: Metaprel (metaproterenol sulfate) (red) is available as a cherry-flavored syrup, 10 mg per teaspoonful (5 ml), in pint bottles.

Tablets: Round, scored, white 10 and 20 mg tablets in bottles of 100.

[*Tablets Shown in Product Identification Section*]

METAPREL® ℞

(metaproterenol sulfate)
Inhalant Solution 5%

Description: METAPREL (metaproterenol sulfate) Inhalant Solution is a bronchodilator administered by oral inhalation with the aid of a hand bulb nebulizer or an intermittent positive pressure breathing apparatus (IPPB). It contains METAPREL 5% in a pH adjusted aqueous solution containing disodium edetate and sodium metabisulfite as preservatives.

Chemically, METAPREL (metaproterenol sulfate) is 1-(3,5 dihydroxyphenyl)-2-isopropylaminoethanol sulfate, a white crystalline, racemic mixture of two optically active isomers. It differs from isoproterenol hydrochloride by having two hydroxyl groups attached at the meta positions on the benzene ring rather than one at the meta and one at the para position.

Clinical Pharmacology: METAPREL (metaproterenol sulfate) is a potent beta-adrenergic stimulator with a rapid onset of action. It is postulated that beta-adrenergic stimulants produce many of their pharmacological effects by activation of adenyl cyclase, the enzyme which catalyzes the conversion of adenosine triphosphate to cyclic adenosine monophosphate.

Absorption, biotransformation and excretion studies following administration by inhalation have not been performed. Following oral administration in humans, an average of 40% of the drug is absorbed; it is not metabolized by catechol-O-methyltransferase but is excreted primarily as glucuronic acid conjugates.

Continued on next page

Dorsey Pharm.—Cont.

Indications and Usage: METAPREL (metaproterenol sulfate) Inhalant Solution is indicated as a bronchodilator for bronchial asthma and for reversible bronchospasm which may occur in association with bronchitis and emphysema.

Following controlled single-dose studies by an intermittent positive pressure breathing apparatus (IPPB) and by hand bulb nebulizers, significant improvement (15% or greater increase in FEV_1) occurred within 5 to 30 minutes and persisted for periods varying from 2 to 6 hours. In these studies, the longer duration of effect occurred in the studies in which the drug was administered by IPPB, i.e., 6 hours versus 2 to 3 hours when administered by hand bulb nebulizer. In these studies the doses used were 0.3 ml by IPPB and 10 inhalations by hand bulb nebulizer.

In controlled repetitive-dosing studies by IPPB and by hand bulb nebulizer the onset of effect occurred within 5 to 30 minutes and duration ranged from 4 to 6 hours. In these studies the doses used were 0.3 ml bid or tid when given by IPPB, and 10 inhalations qid (no more often than q4h) when given by hand bulb nebulizer. As in the single-dose studies, effectiveness was measured as a sustained increase in FEV_1 of 15% or greater. In these repetitive-dosing studies there was no apparent difference in duration between the two methods of delivery.

Clinical studies were conducted in which the effectiveness of METAPREL (metaproterenol sulfate) Inhalant Solution was evaluated by comparison with that of isoproterenol hydrochloride over periods of two to three months. Both drugs continued to produce significant improvement in pulmonary function throughout this period of treatment.

Contraindications: Use in patients with cardiac arrhythmias associated with tachycardia is contraindicated.

Warnings: Excessive use of adrenergic aerosols is potentially dangerous. Fatalities have been reported following excessive use of METAPREL (metaproterenol sulfate) as with other sympathomimetic inhalation preparations, and the exact cause is unknown. Cardiac arrest was noted in several cases.

Paradoxical bronchoconstriction with repeated excessive administration has been reported with sympathomimetic agents.

Patients should be advised to contact their physician in the event that they do not respond to their usual dose of sympathomimetic amine aerosol.

Precautions: Because METAPREL (metaproterenol sulfate) Inhalant Solution is a sympathomimetic drug, it should be used with great caution in patients with hypertension, coronary artery disease, congestive heart failure, hyperthyroidism or diabetes, or when there is sensitivity to sympathomimetic amines.

Information For Patients: Extreme care must be exercised with respect to the administration of additional sympathomimetic agents. A sufficient interval of time should elapse prior to administration of another sympathomimetic agent.

Carcinogenesis: Long-term studies in mice and rats to evaluate the oral carcinogenic potential of metaproterenol sulfate have not been completed.

Pregnancy: *Teratogenic Effects: Pregnancy Category C.* METAPREL has been shown to be teratogenic and embryocidal in rabbits when given orally in doses 620 times the human inhalational dose; the teratogenic effects included skeletal abnormalities and hydrocephalus with bone separation. Oral reproduction studies in mice, rats and rabbits showed no teratogenic or embryocidal effect at 50 mg/kg, or 310 times the human inhalational dose. There are no adequate and well-controlled studies in pregnant women. Metaprel Inhalant Solution should be used during pregnancy only if the potential benefit justifies the potential risk to the fetus.

Nursing Mothers: It is not known whether this drug is excreted in human milk. Because many drugs are excreted in human milk, caution should be exercised when METAPREL (metaproterenol sulfate) is administered to a nursing woman.

Pediatric Use: Safety and effectiveness in children below the age of 12 have not been established.

Adverse Reactions: Adverse reactions are similar to those noted with other sympathomimetic agents.

The most frequent adverse reactions to METAPREL (metaproterenol sulfate) are nervousness, tachycardia, tremor and nausea. Less frequent adverse reactions are hypertension, palpitations, vomiting and bad taste.

Overdosage: The symptoms of overdosage are those of excessive beta-adrenergic stimulation listed under ADVERSE REACTIONS. These reactions usually do not require treatment other than reduction of dosage and/or frequency of administration.

Dosage and Administration: METAPREL (metaproterenol sulfate) Inhalant Solution is administered by oral inhalation with the aid of a hand bulb nebulizer or an intermittent positive pressure breathing apparatus (IPPB).

Usually, treatment need not be repeated more often than every four hours to relieve acute attacks of bronchospasm. As part of a total treatment program in chronic bronchospastic pulmonary diseases, METAPREL (metaproterenol sulfate) Inhalant Solution may be administered three to four times a day.

As with all medications, the physician should begin therapy with the lowest effective dose and then titrate the dosage according to the individual patient's requirements.

[See table below].

METAPREL (metaproterenol sulfate) Inhalant Solution is not recommended for use in children under 12 years of age.

How Supplied: METAPREL (metaproterenol sulfate) Inhalant Solution is supplied as a 5% solution in bottles of 10 ml with accompanying calibrated dropper.

Method of Administration	Usual Single Dose	Range	Dilution
Hand nebulizer	10 inhalations	5–15 inhalations	No dilution
IPPB	0.3 ml	0.2–0.3 ml	Dilute in approx. 2.5 ml of saline solution or other diluent

NEO-CALGLUCON® SYRUP
(glubionate calcium)
Palatable and Readily Absorbable Calcium Supplement.

Description: Each teaspoonful (5 ml) of NEO-CALGLUCON (glubionate calcium) Syrup contains: glubionate calcium 1.8 g (calcium content 115 mg—providing the same amount as 1.2 g calcium gluconate), benzoic acid (as preservative) 5.0 mg.

Adequate calcium intake is particularly important during periods of bone growth in childhood and adolescence, during pregnancy and lactation. An adequate supply of calcium is considered necessary in adults, especially those over 40, to prevent a negative calcium balance which may contribute to the development of osteoporosis. The following are the US Government Recommended Daily Allowances (US RDA) of calcium.

Age Period	Calcium Requirements
Infants	0.6 g
Children under 4 years	0.8 g
Adults and children over 4	1.0 g
Pregnant and lactating women	1.3 g

Eight ounces of whole milk provide approximately 267 mg of calcium. One tablespoonful (15 ml) of NEO-CALGLUCON Syrup contains 345 mg of calcium.

Indications:

1. As a *dietary supplement* where calcium intake may be inadequate:
   a. childhood and adolescence
   b. pregnancy
   c. lactation
   d. postmenopausal females and in the aged
2. In the *treatment* of calcium deficiency states which may occur in diseases such as:
   a. tetany of the newborn*
   b. hypoparathyroidism, acute* and chronic
   c. pseudohypoparathyroidism
   d. postmenopausal and senile osteoporosis
   e. rickets and osteomalacia

   *As a supplement to parenterally administered calcium.

Contraindications: Patients with renal calculi.

Warnings: Certain dietary substances interfere with the absorption of calcium. These include oxalic acid (found in large quantities in rhubarb and spinach), phytic acid (bran and whole cereals) and phosphorus (milk and other dairy products).

Administration of corticosteroids may interfere with calcium absorption.

Precautions: When calcium is administered in therapeutic amounts for prolonged periods, hypercalcemia and hypercalciuria may result. This is most likely to occur in patients with hypoparathyroidism who are receiving high doses of Vitamin D. It can be avoided by frequent checks of plasma and urine calcium levels. Urine calcium levels may rise before plasma calcium levels. The former may be checked by determining 24-hour calcium excretion or by the Sulkowitch test.

Adverse Reactions: NEO-CALGLUCON (glubionate calcium) Syrup is exceptionally well tolerated. Gastrointestinal disturbances are exceedingly rare. A fatal case of hypercalcemia associated with an overdose of NEO-CALGLUCON Syrup has been reported in a two pound neonate. Symptoms of hypercalcemia include anorexia, nausea, vomiting, constipation, abdominal pain, dryness of the mouth, thirst and polyuria.

Dosage and Administration: NEO-CALGLUCON (glubionate calcium) Syrup should be administered before meals to enhance absorption.

[See table on next page].

How Supplied: NEO-CALGLUCON Syrup (straw yellow) in pint bottles.

TAVIST-1® (clemastine fumarate) ℞
TABLETS 1.34 mg
TAVIST® (clemastine fumarate)
TABLETS 2.68 mg

Description: TAVIST (clemastine fumarate) belongs to the benzhydryl ether group of antihistaminic compounds. The chemical name is (+)-2-[2-[(p-chloro-α-methyl-α-phenyl benzyl) oxy]ethyl]-1-methylpyrrolidine* hydrogen fumarate.

*U.S. Patent No. 3,097,212.

Actions: TAVIST is an antihistamine with anticholinergic (drying) and sedative side effects. Antihistamines appear to compete with histamine for cell receptor sites on effector cells. The inherently long duration of antihistaminic effects of TAVIST has been demonstrated in wheal and flare studies. In normal

	Grams of Supplemental Calcium Provided Daily	Percentage of US Recommended Daily Allowance (US RDA)
I. As a Dietary Supplement: Adults and children 4 or more years of age—1 tablespoonful 3 times daily.	1.0 g	104
Pregnant or lactating women—1 tablespoonful 4 times daily.	1.4 g	106
Children under 4 years of age—2 teaspoonfuls 3 times daily.	0.7 g	86
Infants—1 teaspoonful 5 times daily (may be taken undiluted, mixed with infant's formula or fruit juice). (Part of need is supplied by diet)	0.6 g	96

	Grams of Supplemental Ca Provided Daily
II. In the treatment of Calcium Deficiency States: *Tetany of the Newborn* (Tetany of the newborn appears to be a transient physiologic hypoparathyroidism related to the maturation of the parathyroid glands. Adequate parathyroid gland function usually occurs within one week after birth.) Serum calcium should be determined before therapy is instituted. Hypocalcemia is defined as a serum calcium below 8 mg/100 ml or 4 mEq/liter. It is advisable to lower the solute and phosphorus loads in the feeding as well as to provide extra calcium. Intravenous administration of calcium solutions may be necessary for prompt relief of symptoms.	
Dose: Infants with confirmed hypocalcemia may be benefited by the oral administration of calcium salts so as to provide ELEMENTAL CALCIUM in a dosage of 50 to 150 mg/kg/day divided into three or more doses. (NEO-CALGLUCON contains 115 mg ELEMENTAL CALCIUM per 5 ml teaspoon.) The lower dosage range should be employed if calcium is also being provided by the parenteral route. Whole milk formulas which are high in phosphorus should be eliminated in order to increase the calcium/phosphorus ratio. Supplemental oral calcium should be gradually reduced over a period of two or three weeks after the condition has completely stabilized.	See left-hand column
Hypoparathyroidism	
Acute	
Intravenous administration of calcium solutions may be necessary for prompt correction of hypocalcemia. Supplementary calcium should be given orally as soon as possible.	
Dose: 1–3 tablespoonfuls 3 times daily	1.0–3.1
Chronic	
Dose: 1–3 tablespoonfuls daily	0.3–1.0
Pseudohypoparathyroidism	
Dose: 1–3 tablespoonfuls daily	0.3–1.0
Osteoporosis, postmenopausal and senile	
Dose: 1–2 tablespoonfuls 3 times daily	1.0–2.1

Rickets and Osteomalacia

Treatment of these disorders consists of the administration of Vitamin D orally. The addition of calcium to the therapeutic regimen may be desirable to provide calcium needed for remineralization and to avoid hypocalcemia which occurs not infrequently in the early days of treatment. Dosages should be those recommended above under Dietary Supplement.

human subjects who received histamine injections over a 24-hour period, the antihistaminic activity of TAVIST reached a peak at 5–7 hours, persisted for 10–12 hours and, in some cases, for as long as 24 hours. Pharmacokinetic studies in man utilizing ^{3}H and ^{14}C labeled compound demonstrate that: TAVIST (clemastine fumarate) is rapidly and nearly completely absorbed from the gastrointestinal tract, peak plasma concentrations are attained in 2–4 hours, and urinary excretion is the major mode of elimination.

Indications: TAVIST-1 Tablets 1.34 mg are indicated for the relief of symptoms associated with allergic rhinitis such as sneezing, rhinorrhea, pruritus and lacrimation.

TAVIST Tablets 2.68 mg are indicated for the relief of symptoms associated with allergic rhinitis such as sneezing, rhinorrhea, pruritus, and lacrimation. TAVIST Tablets 2.68 mg are also indicated for the relief of mild, uncomplicated allergic skin manifestations of urticaria and angioedema.

It should be noted that TAVIST (clemastine fumarate) is indicated for the dermatologic indications at the 2.68 mg dosage level only.

Contraindications: *Use in Nursing Mothers:* Because of the higher risk of antihistamines for infants generally and for newborns and prematures in particular, antihistamine therapy is contraindicated in nursing mothers.

Use in Lower Respiratory Disease: Antihistamines should not be used to treat lower respiratory tract symptoms including asthma.

Antihistamines are also contraindicated in the following conditions:

Hypersensitivity to TAVIST (clemastine fumarate) or other antihistamines of similar chemical structure.

Monamine oxidase inhibitor therapy (see Drug Interaction Section).

Warnings: Antihistamines should be used with considerable caution in patients with: narrow angle glaucoma, stenosing peptic ulcer, pyloroduodenal obstruction, symptomatic prostatic hypertrophy, and bladder neck obstruction.

Use in Children: Safety and efficacy of TAVIST have not been established in children under the age of 12.

Use in Pregnancy: Experience with this drug in pregnant women is inadequate to determine whether there exists a potential for harm to the developing fetus.

Use with CNS Depressants: TAVIST has additive effects with alcohol and other CNS depressants (hypnotics, sedatives, tranquilizers, etc.)

Use in Activities Requiring Mental Alertness: Patients should be warned about engaging in activities requiring mental alertness such as driving a car or operating appliances, machinery, etc.

Use in the Elderly (approximately 60 years or older): Antihistamines are more likely to cause dizziness, sedation, and hypotension in elderly patients.

Precautions: TAVIST (clemastine fumarate) should be used with caution in patients with: history of bronchial asthma, increased intraocular pressure, hyperthyroidism, cardiovascular disease, and hypertension.

Drug Interactions: MAO inhibitors prolong and intensify the anticholinergic (drying) effects of antihistamines.

Adverse Reactions: Transient drowsiness, the most common adverse reaction associated with TAVIST (clemastine fumarate), occurs relatively frequently and may require discontinuation of therapy in some instances.

Antihistaminic Compounds: It should been noted that the following reactions have occurred with one or more antihistamines and, therefore, should be kept in mind when prescribing drugs belonging to this class, including TAVIST. The most frequent adverse reactions are underlined.

1. *General:* Urticaria, drug rash, anaphylactic shock, photosensitivity, excessive perspiration, chills, dryness of mouth, nose, and throat.
2. *Cardiovascular System:* Hypotension, headache, palpitations, tachycardia, extrasystoles.
3. *Hematologic System:* Hemolytic anemia, thrombocytopenia, agranulocytosis.
4. *Nervous System:* Sedation, sleepiness, dizziness, disturbed coordination, fatigue, confusion, restlessness, excitation, nervousness, tremor, irritability, insomnia, euphoria, paresthesias, blurred vision, diplopia, vertigo, tinnitus, acute labyrinthitis, hysteria, neuritis, convulsions.
5. *GI System:* Epigastric distress, anorexia, nausea, vomiting, diarrhea, constipation.
6. *GU System:* Urinary frequency, difficult urination, urinary retention, early menses.
7. *Respiratory System:* Thickening of bronchial secretions, tightness of chest and wheezing, nasal stuffiness.

Continued on next page

Dorsey Pharm.—Cont.

Overdosage: Antihistamine overdosage reactions may vary from central nervous system depression to stimulation. Stimulation is particularly likely in children. Atropine-like signs and symptoms: dry mouth; fixed, dilated pupils; flushing; and gastrointestinal symptoms may also occur.

If vomiting has not occurred spontaneously the conscious patient should be induced to vomit. This is best done by having him drink a glass of water or milk after which he should be made to gag. Precautions against aspiration must be taken, especially in infants and children.

If vomiting is unsuccessful gastric lavage is indicated within 3 hours after ingestion and even later if large amounts of milk or cream were given beforehand. Isotonic and ½ isotonic saline is the lavage solution of choice.

Saline cathartics, such as milk of magnesia, by osmosis draw water into the bowel and therefore, are valuable for their action in rapid dilution of bowel content.

Stimulants should *not* be used.

Vasopressors may be used to treat hypotension.

Dosage and Administration: DOSAGE SHOULD BE INDIVIDUALIZED ACCORDING TO THE NEEDS AND RESPONSE OF THE PATIENT.

TAVIST-1 Tablets 1.34 mg: The recommended starting dose is one tablet twice daily. Dosage may be increased as required, but not to exceed six tablets daily.

TAVIST Tablets 2.68 mg: The maximum recommended dosage is one tablet three times daily. Many patients respond favorably to a single dose which may be repeated as required, but not to exceed three tablets daily.

How Supplied: TAVIST-1 Tablets: 1.34 mg clemastine fumarate. White, oval compressed, scored tablet, embossed "43" bisect "80" on one side, "TAVIST" on the other. Packages of 100.

TAVIST Tablets: 2.68 mg clemastine fumarate. White, round compressed tablet, embossed "43" over "70" and scored on one side, "TAVIST" on the other. Packages of 100.

[*Shown in Product Identification Section*]

TRIAMINIC® ©
Expectorant with Codeine

Description: Each teaspoonful (5 ml) of TRIAMINIC Expectorant with Codeine contains: codeine phosphate 10 mg (Warning: May be habit forming), phenylpropanolamine hydrochloride 12.5 mg, guaifenesin 100 mg, alcohol 5%.

Indications: For use in providing temporary relief of coughs and nasal congestion due to the common cold, when the antitussive properties of codeine are desired. The expectorant component helps loosen bronchial secretions. The ingredients are provided in an antihistamine-free formula.

Contraindications: TRIAMINIC Expectorant with Codeine is contraindicated in the presence of hypersensitivity to any of the ingredients. The use of pressor amines such as phenylpropanolamine hydrochloride is contraindicated in those patients taking monoamine oxidase inhibitors for antihypertensive or antidepressant indications. Continuous dosage over an extended period is generally contraindicated since codeine phosphate may cause addiction.

Precautions: Exercise prescribing caution in patients with persistent or chronic cough such as occurs with chronic bronchitis, bronchial asthma, or emphysema. Use with caution in patients with hypertension, hyperthyroidism, cardiovascular disease, diabetes mellitus, chronic pulmonary disease or shortness of breath. Exercise caution in prescribing this product to children taking other drugs.

Adverse Reactions: Occasional blurred vision, cardiac palpitations, flushing, gastrointestinal upsets, nervousness, dizziness, sleeplessness and drowsiness. May cause or aggravate constipation.

Dosage and Administration: Adults—2 teaspoonfuls every 4 hours. Children 6 to 12 years—1 teaspoonful every 4 hours. Children 2 to 6 years—½ teaspoonful every 4 hours. The suggested dosage in pediatric patients 3 months to 2 years of age is 2 drops per kilogram of body weight administered every four hours.

How Supplied: TRIAMINIC Expectorant with Codeine (green) in 4 fl oz and pint bottles. TRIAMINIC Expectorant with Codeine is a Schedule V controlled substance.

TRIAMINIC JUVELETS® ℞
(Timed Release)
TRIAMINIC® TABLETS (Timed Release) ℞

Description: TRIAMINIC JUVELETS (Timed Release): Each tablet contains phenylpropanolamine hydrochloride 25 mg, pheniramine maleate 12.5 mg, pyrilamine maleate 12.5 mg.

TRIAMINIC Tablets (Timed Release): Each tablet contains phenylpropanolamine hydrochloride 50 mg, pheniramine maleate 25 mg, pyrilamine maleate 25 mg.

These products combine the nasal decongestant properties of phenylpropanolamine hydrochloride with the antihistaminic activities of pheniramine maleate and pyrilamine maleate.

Phenylpropanolamine hydrochloride, a sympathomimetic drug, is structurally related to ephedrine and amphetamine. Pheniramine maleate is an antihistamine of the alkylamine class while pyrilamine maleate belongs to the ethylenediamine class.

Clinical Pharmacology: Phenylpropanolamine presumably acts on α-adrenergic receptors in the mucosa of the respiratory tract producing vasoconstriction which results in shrinkage of swollen mucous membranes, reduction of tissue hyperemia, edema and nasal congestion, and an increase in nasal airway patency. Its pharmacologic properties are analogous to those of ephedrine. Antihistamines competitively act as H_1 receptor antagonists of histamine. They exhibit anticholinergic (drying) and sedative side effects. There are several classes of antihistamines which vary with respect to potency, dosage and the relative incidence of side effects. Antihistamines inhibit the effects of histamine on capillary permeability and on vascular, bronchial and many other types of smooth muscle. This accounts for the predominant use of antihistamines in hypersensitivity states.

Indications and Usage: For relief from such symptoms as nasal congestion, and postnasal drip associated with colds, allergies, sinusitis and rhinitis. Also for the relief of symptoms associated with allergic rhinitis such as sneezing, rhinorrhea, pruritus and lacrimation.

Contraindications: These formulas are contraindicated in patients exhibiting hypersensitivity to any of the components. Antihistamines are contraindicated in patients receiving monamine oxidase inhibitors since these agents prolong and intensify the anticholinergic effects of antihistamines (see Drug Interactions). Antihistamines <u>should</u> <u>not</u> be used to treat lower respiratory tract symptoms. Sympathomimetic preparations are contraindicated in patients with severe hypertension, severe coronary artery disease and in patients receiving MAO inhibitor therapy due to potentiation of the pressor effects of phenylpropanolamine.

Nursing Mothers: Because of the higher risk of antihistamines for newborns and prematures in particular, antihistamine therapy is contraindicated in nursing mothers.

Warnings: Sympathomimetics should be used with caution in patients with hypertension, hyperthyroidism, diabetes mellitus and cardiovascular disease. Antihistamines should be used with caution in patients with narrow angle glaucoma, stenosing peptic ulcer, pyloroduodenal obstruction, symptomatic prostatic hypertrophy and bladder neck obstruction. Antihistamines have additive effects with alcohol and other CNS depressants (hypnotics, sedatives, tranquilizers, etc.). Patients should be warned about engaging in activities requiring mental alertness such as driving a car or operating machinery.

Use In The Elderly (approximately 60 years or older): Antihistamines are more likely to cause dizziness, sedation and hypotension in elderly patients. Overdosages of sympathomimetics in this age group may cause hallucinations, convulsions, CNS depression and death in elderly patients.

Precautions:

General: Use with caution in patients with hypertension, hyperthyroidism, diabetes mellitus, cardiovascular disease, bronchial asthma, increased intraocular pressure (see WARNINGS).

Information For Patients: Patients should be informed of the potential for sedation or drowsiness and warned about driving or operating machinery. The concomitant consumption of alcoholic beverages or other sedative drugs should be avoided.

Drug Interactions:

(1) Monamine oxidase inhibitors: MAO inhibitors prolong and intensify the anticholinergic effects of antihistamines and potentiate the pressor effects of sympathomimetics.
(2) Alcohol and CNS depressants: These agents potentiate the sedative effects of antihistamines.
(3) Certain antihypertensives: Sympathomimetics may reduce the antihypertensive effects of methyldopa, mecamylamine, reserpine and veratrum alkaloids.

Carcinogenesis, Mutagenesis, Impairment Of Fertility: No data are available on the long-term potential for carcinogenicity, mutagenicity or impairment of fertility in animals or humans.

Pregnancy: *Pregnancy Category C*—Animal reproduction studies have not been conducted. Safe use in pregnancy has not been established relative to possible adverse effects on fetal development. Therefore, TRIAMINIC should not be used in pregnant patients unless, in the judgment of the physician, the potential benefits outweigh possible hazards.

Nursing Mothers: see CONTRAINDICATIONS.

Pediatric Use: TRIAMINIC JUVELETS are intended for administration to children 6 to 12 years of age (see DOSAGE AND ADMINISTRATION). It is important to note the variability of response infants and small children exhibit to antihistamines and sympathomimetics. As in adults, the combination of an antihistamine and sympathomimetic can elicit either mild stimulation or mild sedation in children. In the young child, mild stimulation is the response most frequently seen. In infants and children, overdosage of antihistamines may cause hallucinations, convulsions or death.

Adverse Reactions: The most frequent adverse reactions are underlined.

(1) *General:* Urticaria, drug rash, anaphylactic shock, photosensitivity, excessive perspiration, chills, dryness of mouth, nose and throat.
(2) *Cardiovascular System:* Hypotension, headache, palpitations, tachycardia, extrasystoles.
(3) *Hematologic System:* Hemolytic anemia, thrombocytopenia, agranulocytosis.
(4) *Nervous System:* <u>Sedation, sleepiness, dizziness, disturbed coordination,</u> fatigue, confusion, <u>restlessness, excitation, nervousness,</u> tremor, irritability, <u>insomnia,</u> euphoria, paresthesias, blurred vi-

sion, diplopia, vertigo, tinnitus, acute labyrinthitis, hysteria, neuritis, convulsions, CNS depression, hallucinations.
(5) *GI System:* Epigastic distress, anorexia, nausea, vomiting, diarrhea, constipation.
(6) *GU System:* Urinary frequency, difficult urination, urinary retention, early menses.
(7) *Respiratory System:* Thickening of bronchial secretions, tightness of chest and wheezing, nasal stuffiness.

Overdosage: TRIAMINIC product overdosage reactions may vary from central nervous system depression to stimulation. Stimulation is particularly likely in children. Atropine-like signs and symptoms: dry mouth; fixed, dilated pupils; flushing; and gastrointestinal symptoms may also occur.

If vomiting has not occurred spontaneously, the conscious patient should be induced to vomit. This is best done by having the patient drink a glass of water or milk after which they should be made to gag. Precautions against aspiration must be taken, especially in infants and children.

If vomiting is unsuccessful gastric lavage is indicated within three hours after ingestion and even later if large amounts of milk or cream were given beforehand. Isotonic and ½ isotonic saline is the lavage solution of choice.

Saline cathartics, such as milk of magnesia, by osmosis draw water into the bowel and therefore, are valuable for their action in rapid dilution of bowel content.

Stimulants should *not* be used. Vasopressors may be used to treat hypotension.

Dosage and Administration: TRIAMINIC JUVELETS (Timed Release): Children 6 to 12—1 tablet, swallowed whole, in the morning, midafternoon and before retiring. Adults—2 tablets on same dosage schedule.

TRIAMINIC Tablets (Timed Release): Adults and children over 12 years—1 tablet swallowed whole, in the morning, midafternoon and before retiring.

How Supplied: TRIAMINIC Tablets (Timed Release) (yellow, round, film-coated, imprinted "Dorsey" on one side) in bottles of 100 and 250. TRIAMINIC JUVELETS (Timed Release) (pink, round, film-coated, imprinted "Dorsey" on one side) in bottles of 50.

[*Shown in Product Identification Section*]

TRIAMINIC® ORAL INFANT DROPS ℞

Description: TRIAMINIC Oral Infant Drops: Each ml contains phenylpropanolamine hydrochloride 20 mg, pheniramine maleate 10 mg, pyrilamine maleate 10 mg.

This product combines the nasal decongestant properties of phenylpropanolamine hydrochloride with the antihistaminic activities of pheniramine maleate and pyrilamine maleate.

Phenylpropanolamine hydrochloride, a sympathomimetic drug, is structurally related to ephedrine and amphetamine. Pheniramine maleate is an antihistamine of the alkylamine class while pyrilamine maleate belongs to the ethylenediamine class.

Clinical Pharmacology: Phenylpropanolamine presumably acts on α-adrenergic receptors in the mucosa of the respiratory tract producing vasoconstriction which results in shrinkage of swollen mucous membranes, reduction of tissue hyperemia, edema and nasal congestion, and an increase in nasal airway patency. Its pharmacologic properties are analogous to those of ephedrine. Antihistamines competitively act as H_1 receptor antagonists of histamine. They exhibit anticholinergic (drying) and sedative side effects. There are several classes of antihistamines which vary with respect to potency, dosage and the relative incidence of side effects. Antihistamines inhibit the effects of histamine on capillary permeability and on vascular, bronchial and many other types of smooth muscle. This accounts for the predominant use of antihistamines in hypersensitivity states.

Indications and Usage: For relief from such symptoms as nasal congestion, and postnasal drip associated with colds, allergies, sinusitis and rhinitis. Also for the relief of symptoms associated with allergic rhinitis such as sneezing, rhinorrhea, pruritus and lacrimation.

Contraindications: TRIAMINIC Oral Infant Drops are contraindicated in patients exhibiting hypersensitivity to any of the components. Antihistamines are contraindicated in patients receiving monamine oxidase inhibitors since these agents prolong and intensify the anticholinergic effects of antihistamines (see Drug Interactions). Antihistamines should not be used to treat lower respiratory tract symptoms. Sympathomimetic preparations are contraindicated in patients with severe hypertension, severe coronary artery disease and in patients receiving MAO inhibitor therapy due to potentiation of the pressor effects of phenylpropanolamine.

Warnings: Sympathomimetics should be used with caution in patients with hypertension, hyperthyroidism, diabetes mellitus and cardiovascular disease. Antihistamines should be used with caution in patients with narrow angle glaucoma, stenosing peptic ulcer, pyloroduodenal obstruction, symptomatic prostatic hypertrophy and bladder neck obstruction. Antihistamines have additive effects with other CNS depressants (hypnotics, sedatives, tranquilizers, alcohol, etc.). Warn mothers that drowsiness may occur. When prescribing antihistamine preparations, patients should be cautioned against mechanical activity requiring alertness.

Precautions:

General: Use with caution in patients with hypertension, hyperthyroidism, diabetes mellitus, cardiovascular disease, bronchial asthma, increased intraocular pressure (see WARNINGS).

Information For Patients: Mothers should be informed of the potential for sedation or drowsiness.

Drug Interactions

(1) Monamine oxidase inhibitors: MAO inhibitors prolong and intensify the anticholinergic effects of antihistamines and potentiate the pressor effects of sympathomimetics.
(2) Alcohol and CNS depressants: These agents potentiate the sedative effects of antihistamines.
(3) Certain antihypertensives: Sympathomimetics may reduce the antihypertensive effects of methyldopa, mecamylamine, reserpine and veratrum alkaloids.

Carcinogenesis, Mutagenesis, Impairment Of Fertility: No data are available on the long-term potential for carcinogenicity, mutagenicity or impairment of fertility in animals or humans.

Pediatric Use: TRIAMINIC Oral Infant Drops have been formulated to provide safe and effective symptomatic relief for infants and small children. Precise dosage (on a body weight basis) is facilitated through the use of the plastic squeeze bottle with attached dropper tip (see DOSAGE AND ADMINISTRATION). It is important to note the variability of response infants and small children exhibit to antihistamines and sympathomimetics. As in adults, the combination of an antihistamine and sympathomimetic can elicit either mild stimulation or mild sedation in children. In the young child, mild stimulation is the response most frequently seen. In infants and children, overdosage of antihistamines may cause hallucinations, convulsions or death.

Adverse Reactions: The most frequent adverse reactions are underlined.

(1) *General:* Urticaria, drug rash, anaphylactic shock, photosensitivity, excessive perspiration, chills, dryness of mouth, nose, and throat.
(2) *Cardiovascular System:* Hypotension, headache, palpitations, tachycardia, extrasystoles.
(3) *Hematologic System:* Hemolytic anemia, thrombocytopenia, agranulocytosis.
(4) *Nervous System:* Sedation, sleepiness, dizziness, disturbed coordination, fatigue, confusion, restlessness, excitation, nervousness, tremor, irritability, insomnia, euphoria, paresthesias, blurred vision, diplopia, vertigo, tinnitus, acute labyrinthitis, hysteria, neuritis, convulsions, CNS depression, hallucinations.
(5) *GI System:* Epigastic distress, anorexia, nausea, vomiting, diarrhea, constipation.
(6) *GU System:* Urinary frequency, difficult urination, urinary retention.
(7) *Respiratory System:* Thickening of bronchial secretions, tightness of chest and wheezing, nasal stuffiness.

Overdosage: TRIAMINIC product overdosage reactions may vary from central nervous system depression to stimulation. Stimulation is particularly likely in children. Atropine-like signs and symptoms: dry mouth; fixed, dilated pupils; flushing; and gastrointestinal symptoms may also occur.

If vomiting has not occurred spontaneously the conscious patient should be induced to vomit. This is best done by having the patient drink a glass of water or milk after which they should be made to gag. Precautions against aspiration must be taken, especially in infants and children.

If vomiting is unsuccessful gastric lavage is indicated within three hours after ingestion and even later if large amounts of milk or cream were given beforehand. Isotonic and 1/2 isotonic saline is the lavage solution of choice.

Saline cathartics such as milk of magnesia, by osmosis draw water into the bowel and therefore, are valuable for their action in rapid dilution of bowel content.

Stimulants should *not* be used. Vasopressors may be used to treat hypotension.

Dosage and Administration: TRIAMINIC Oral Infant Drops: 1 drop per 2 pounds of body weight administered orally four times daily. The prescribed number of drops may be put directly into child's mouth or on a spoon for administration.

How Supplied: TRIAMINIC Oral Infant Drops in 15 ml plastic squeeze bottles which deliver approximately 24 drops per ml. Store TRIAMINIC Oral Infant Drops at room temperature.

Drug Industries Co., Inc.
3237 HILTON ROAD
FERNDALE, MI 48220

AL-VITE ℞
(high potency vitamin formula with intrinsic factor + Vitamin D_3)

Composition: Each capsule shaped tablet contains: Vitamin A Palmitate, 10,000 USP Units, Vitamin D_3 (activ. 7-Dehydrocholesterol), 400 USP Units, Vitamin E (from D-Alpha Tocopheryl Acetate Concentrate), 25 int. Units, Vitamin C (Ascorbic Acid), 200 mg., Vitamin B_1 (Thiamine Mononitrate), 20 mg., Vitamin B_2 (Riboflavin), 10 mg., Vitamin B_6 (pyridoxine Hydrochloride), 6 mg., Calcium Pantothenate, 20 mg., Niacinamide, 100 mg., Vitamin B_{12} with Intrinsic Factor Concentrate, ½ N.F. Unit (oral).

Action and Uses: Provides Vitamins A, D, C and B Complex factors in therapeutic amounts. For use in multiple vitamin deficiencies.

Administration and Dosage: One or two tablets daily or as directed by the physician.

Side Effects: None known when taken as directed.

Continued on next page

Drug Industries—Cont.

Caution: This preparation is not a reliable substitute for parenterally administered cyanocobalamin (vitamin B_{12}) in the management of pernicious anemia. Periodic examinations and laboratory studies of pernicious anemia patients are essential.
Contraindications: Idiosyncrasy to any component.
How Supplied: Bottles of 100 and 500 light orange capsule shaped tablets.

BILAX CAPSULES™ ℞

Composition: Each Bilax Capsule contains:
Dehydrocholic Acid ....50 mg.
Dioctyl Sodium Sulfosuccinate ....100 mg.
Action and Uses: The actions of Bilax are the result of the combination of complementary activities of its ingredients. Dioctyl Sodium Sulfosuccinate effects the surface tension and increases the water content of the stool, making it softer and therefore, easier to pass. The softening, combined with the laxative effect of Dehydrocholic Acid, alleviates symptoms of constipation.
Indications: A mild laxative and fecal softener designed as an aid in the treatment of functional constipation, particularly in the elderly.
Contraindications: Biliary tract obstruction, acute hepatitis, or sensitivity to any of its ingredients.
Precautions: Patients should be examined periodically to prevent fluid and electrolyte deficiencies due to excessive laxative effects or inadequate intake.
Administration and Dosage: One or two capsules three times daily with meals. This dosage should be reduced as the condition is relieved.
How Supplied: Bottles of 100.
Bottles of 500.
NDC 261-0157-01

HEMO-VITE ℞
(hematinic with vitamins and intrinsic factor)

Composition: Each tablet contains: Ferrous Fumarate, 240.0 mg., Copper Sulfate, 1.0 mg., Vitamin C (ascorbic acid) 150.0 mg., Vitamin B_1(Thiamine Hydrochloride) 5.0 mg., Vitamin B_2(Riboflavin), 5.0 mg., Vitamin B_6(Pyridoxine Hydrochloride), 1.0 mg., Calcium Pantothenate, 10.0 mg., Niacinamide, 50.0 mg., Folic Acid, .2 mg., Vitamin B_{12}(Crystalline with Intrinsic Factor Concentrate), ½ N.F. Unit (oral)
Action and Uses: For the treatment and prevention of iron deficiency anemias. Contains the well tolerated effective fumarate salt of iron.
Administration and Dosage: One or two tablets daily after meals or as directed by the physician.
Precautions: If any symptoms of intolerance appear, the medication should be discontinued. Prolonged administration requires closer medical supervision. Folic acid may obscure the symptoms of pernicious anemia while neurological destruction is progressive. Patients with pernicious anemia should be treated with parenteral B_{12}
HEMO-VITE should not be used in cases of serious folic acid deficiency where therapeutic amounts of folic acid are needed.
Side Effects: None known when used as directed.
Contraindications: Idiosyncrasy to any component.
How Supplied: Bottles of 100 and 500 black capsule shaped tablets.
Also available in Hemo-Vite Liquid—pint bottles.

SINOVAN TIMED™ ℞

Composition: Each black and clear timed capsule contains 8 mg. Chlorpheniramine Maleate, 20 mg. of Phenylephrine Hydrochloride, and 2.5 mg. of Methscopolamine Nitrate in a special base that provides a prolonged therapeutic effect of from about 10 to 12 hours.
Action and Uses: Provides temporary relief of the distressing symptoms accompanying the common cold, hay fever, and similar allergic conditions.
Contraindications: Pyloric obstruction, prostatic hypertrophy, intolerance to anticholinergic or antisecretory drugs, glaucoma, hepatitis, asthma, and toxemia of pregnancy.
Administration and Dosage: One capsule in the morning and at bedtime.
How Supplied: In bottles of 100 and 1000.

TRILAX™ ℞
(laxative, fecal softener, choleretic)

Composition: Each blue and white capsule contains:
Dioctyl Sodium Sulfosuccinate ....200 mg.
Yellow Phenolphthalein ....30 mg.
Dehydrocholic Acid ....20 mg.
Action and Uses: Provides softening of the feces, homogenization, and laxative action without the discomfort of bowel distention, pain, cramping, or interference of vitamin absorption. For use in geriatric, obstetric, cardiac and surgical patients, and in those with hepatic or biliary disease or other conditions causing biliary stasis without complete mechanical obstruction of the common duct where increase in volume of fluid bile is desired.
Contraindications: TRILAX is contraindicated in patients with biliary tract obstruction and severe acute hepatitis.
Administration and Dosage: One or two capsules at bedtime for 2 or 3 days. Dosage may then be adjusted to meet individual needs.
How Supplied: Bottles of 100.
Bottles of 500.
NDC 261-0103-01

Dura Pharmaceuticals, Inc.
P.O. BOX 28331
SAN DIEGO, CA 92128

DURA-TAP/PD™ ℞
Antihistamine/Decongestant

Description: Each timed release capsule contains:
Brompheniramine maleate ....6 mg.
Phenylephrine hydrochloride ....10 mg.
Phenylpropanolamine hydrochloride ...10 mg.
in specially prepared base to provide prolonged action.
This product contains ingredients of the following therapeutic classes: antihistamine and decongestant.
Clinical Pharmacology: Brompheniramine maleate is an alkylamine type antihistamine. This group of antihistamines are among the most active histamine antagonists and are generally effective in relatively low doses. The drugs are not so prone to produce drowsiness and are among the most suitable agents for daytime use; but again, a significant proportion of patients do experience this effect. Phenylpropanolamine hydrochloride and phenylephrine hydrochloride are sympathomimetics which act predominantly on alpha receptors and have little action on beta receptors. They, therefore, function as oral nasal decongestants with minimal CNS stimulation.
Indications: For the temporary relief of symptoms of the common cold, allergic rhinitis (hay fever) and sinusitis.
Contraindications: Hypersensitivity to any of the ingredients. Also contraindicated in patients with severe hypertension, severe coronary artery disease, patients on MAO inhibitor therapy, patients with narrow-angle glaucoma, urinary retention, peptic ulcer and during an asthmatic attack.
Should not be used in nursing mothers.
Warnings: Considerable caution should be exercised in patients with hypertension, diabetes mellitus, ischemic heart disease, hyperthyroidism, increased intraocular pressure and prostatic hypertrophy. The elderly (60 years or older) are more likely to exhibit adverse reactions.
Antihistamines may cause excitability, especially in children. At dosages higher than the recommended dose, nervousness, dizziness or sleeplessness may occur.
Precautions:
General: Caution should be exercised in patients with high blood pressure, heart disease, diabetes or thyroid disease. The antihistamine in this product may exhibit additive effects with other CNS depressants, including alcohol.
Information for Patients: Antihistamines may cause drowsiness and ambulatory patients who operate machinery or motor vehicles should be cautioned accordingly.
Drug Interactions: MAO inhibitors and beta adrenergic blockers increase the effects of sympathomimetics. Sympathomimetics may reduce the antihypertensive effects of methyldopa, mecamylamine, reserpine and veratrum alkaloids. Concommitant use of antihistamines with alcohol and other CNS depressants may have an additive effect.
Pregnancy: The safety of use of this product in pregnancy has not been established.
Adverse Reactions: Adverse reactions include drowsiness, lassitude, nausea, giddiness, dryness of mouth, blurred vision, cardiac palpitations, flushing, increased irritability or excitement (especially in children).
Dosage and Administration: Children over 6 years of age—1 capsule orally every 12 hours.
How Supplied: DURA-TAP/PD™ capsules are supplied in bottles of 100 NDC #'s 51479-004-01.
Caution: FEDERAL LAW PROHIBITS DISPENSING WITHOUT A PRESCRIPTION.
DISPENSE IN TIGHT CONTAINERS AS DEFINED IN USP/NF.
STORE BETWEEN 15°-30°C (59°-86°F).
DISPENSE IN CHILD RESISTANT CONTAINERS.
Manufactured by Central Pharmaceuticals, Inc., Seymour, Indiana 47274.
Manufactured for Dura Pharmaceuticals, Inc., San Diego, California 92128.
Issued 7/82.

DURA-VENT™ ℞
Decongestant/Expectorant

Description: Each continuous release blue and clear capsule imprinted "Dura-Vent™" contains:
Phenylpropanolamine Hydrochloride 75 mg
Guaifenesin ....400 mg
in a special base to provide a prolonged therapeutic effect.
Clinical Pharmacology: Phenylpropanolamine hydrochloride is an effective vasocontrictor that decongest swollen mucus membranes of the entire respiratory tract. Guaifenesin enhances the flow of respiratory tract fluid, promoting ciliary action and facilitating removal of viscid, inspissated mucous.
Indications and Usage: Dura-Vent™ is indicated for the relief of symptoms associated with bronchitis, bronchial asthma, pulmonary emphysema, sinusitis and related conditions. Symptoms include an increase of respiratory tract fluids and relief of congestion in the treatment of acute or chronic pulmonary disorders where tenacious mucous plugs and congestion complicate the problem.
Contraindications: Dura-Vent™ is contraindicated in individuals with known hypersen-

sitivity to sympathomimetics, severe hypertension or in patients receiving MAO inhibitors.

Precautions: Dura-Vent™ should be used with caution in the presence of hypertension, hyperthyroidism, diabetes or heart disease and in those patients who may be sensitive to sympathomimetics.

Pregnancy: Animal reproduction studies have not been conducted with Dura-Vent™. It is also not known whether Dura-Vent™ can cause fetal harm when administered to a pregnant woman or can affect reproduction capacity. Dura-Vent™ should be given to a pregnant woman only if clearly needed.

Nursing Mothers: It is not known whether this drug is excreted in human milk. Because many drugs are excreted in human milk, caution should be exercised when Dura-Vent™ is administered to a nursing woman.

Adverse Reactions: Central nervous system stimulation may occur with overdosage. May cause urinary retention in patients with benign prostatic hypertrophy.

Overdosage: Central nervous system stimulation may occur with overdosage. Since the effects of Dura-Vent™ may last up to 12 hours, treatment of overdosage directed toward supporting the patient and reversing the effects of the drug should be continued for at least that length of time. Saline cathartics may be useful in hastening the evacuation of unreleased medication.

Dosage and Administration: Adults and children over 12 years, orally one capsule every 12 hours, not to exceed two capsules every 24 hours.

How Supplied: Capsules of Dura-Vent™ are supplied in bottles of 100. Keep in tight, light-resistant containers.
NDC 51479-001-01

Warning: Federal law prohibits dispensing without prescription.

DURA-VENT™/A ℞

Decongestant/Antihistamine

Description: Each continuous release clear capsule imprinted "Dura-Vent™/A contains:

Phenylpropanotamine Hydrochlorde . 75 mg
Chlorpheniramine Maleate .... 10 mg

Clinical Pharmacology: Dura-Vent™/A is a combination of an orally effective nasal decongestant together with a highly effective antihistamine, prepared in continuous release form to provide comprehensive relief of nasal congestion and inflammation associated with colds, allergies and upper respiratory infection.

Phenylpropanolamine Hydrochloride—The drug may directly stimulate adrenergic receptors but probably indirectly stimulates both alpha (a) and beta (B) adrenergic receptors by releasing norepinephrine from its storage sites. Phenylpropanolamine increases heart rate, force of contraction and cardiac output, and excitability. It acts on (a) receptors in the mucosa of the respiratory tract, producing vasoconstriction which results in shrinkage of swollen mucous membranes, reduction of tissue, hyperemia, edema and nasal airway patency. Phenylpropanolamine causes CNS stimulation and reportedly has an anorexigenic effect.

Chlorpheniramine Maleate—Chlorpheniramine competitively antagonizes most of the smooth muscle stimulating actions of histamine on the H_1 receptors of the gastrointestinal tract, uterus, large blood vessels and bronchial muscle. It also antagonizes the action of histamine that results in increased capillary permeability and the formation of edema.

Indications and Usage: For the relief of nasal congestion and eustacian tube congestion associated with the common cold, sinusitis and acute upper respiratory infections. Also indicated symptomatic relief of perennial and seasonal allergic rhinitis, vasomotor rhinitis. Decongestants in combination with antihistamines have been used to relieve eustacian tube congestion associated with acute eustachian salpingitis, aerotitis and serous otitis media. N.B.: A final determination has not been made on the effectiveness of this drug combination in accordance with efficacy requirements of the 1962 Amendments to the Food, Drug and Cosmetic Act.

Contraindications: Patients with severe hypertension, severe coronary artery disease, patients on MAO inhibitor therapy; patients with narrow angle glaucoma, urinary retention, peptic ulcer and during an asthmatic attack. Also contraindicated in patients with hypersensitivity or idiosyncrasy to sympathomimetic amines or antihistamines.

Warnings: Sympathomimetic amines should be used judiciously and sparingly in patients with hypertension, diabetes mellitus, ischemic heart disease, increased intraocular pressure, hyperthyroidism or prostatic hypertrophy. See CONTRAINDICATIONS. Sympathomimetics may produce central nervous system stimulation with convulsions or cardiovascular collapse with accompanying hypotension.

Antihistamines may impair mental and physical abilities required for the performance of potentially hazardous tasks, such as driving a vehicle or operating machinery and may impair mental alertness in children. Chlorpheniramine has an atropine-like action and should be used with caution in patients with increased intraocular pressure, cardiovascular disease, hypertension or in patients with a history of bronchial asthma. See CONTRAINDICATIONS.

Do not exceed recommended dosage.

Precautions: Patients with diabetes, hypertension and cardiovascular disease. The antihistamines may cause drowsiness, and ambulatory patients who operate machinery or motor vehicles should be cautioned accordingly.

Drug Interactions: MAO inhibitors and beta adrenergic blockers increase the effect of sympathomimetics. Sympathomimetics may reduce the antihypertensive effects of methyldopa, mecamylamine, reserpine and veratrum alkaloids. Concomitant use of antihistamines with alcohol, tricyclic antidepressants, barbiturates and other CNS depressants may have an additive effect.

Use in Pregnancy: Animal reproduction studies have not been conducted with Dura-Vent™/A. It is also not known whether Dura-Vent™/A can cause fetal harm when administered to a pregnant woman or can affect reproductive capacity. Dura-Vent™/A should be given to a pregnant woman only if clearly needed.

Nursing Mothers: Caution should be exercised when this drug is given to nursing mothers due to the higher than usual risk of the sympathomimetic amines in infants.

Pediatric Usage: Safety and effectiveness in children have not been established.

Overdosage: Symptoms may vary from central nervous system depression to stimulation. Also, atropine-like signs and symptoms (dry mouth, fixed, dilated pupils, flushing, etc.) as well as gastrointestinal symptoms may occur. Marked cerebral irritation resulting in jerking of muscles and possible convulsions may be followed by deep stupor and respiratory failure.

Treatment of Overdosage: Immediate evacuation of the stomach should be induced by emesis and gastric lavage. Since much of the capsule medication is coated for gradual release, saline cathartics should be administered to hasten evacuation of pellets that have not already released medication.

Respiratory depression should be treated promptly with oxygen. Do not treat respiratory or CNS depression with analeptics that might precipitate convulsions; if convulsions or marked CNS excitement occurs, only short-acting barbiturates or chloral hydrate should be used.

Adverse Reactions: Patients sensitive to antihistamines may experience mild sedation. Sympathomimetics have been associated with certain untoward reactions including restlessness, tremor, weakness, pallor, respiratory difficulty, dysuria, insomnia, hallucinations, convulsions, CNS depression, arrhythmias and cardiovascular collapse with hypotension. Possible side effects of antihistamines are drowsiness, restlessness, dizziness, weakness, dry mouth, anorexia, nausea, vomiting, headache, nervousness, blurring of vision, polyuria, heartburn, dysuria and, very rarely, dermatitis.

Dosage and Administration: Adults and children over 12 years of age, one capsule every 12 hours.

How Supplied: Dura-Vent™/A capsules are supplied in bottles of 100.
NDC 51479-002-01

Warning: Federal law prohibits dispensing without prescription.

DURA-VENT™/DA ℞

Antihistamine/Decongestant/Anticholinergic

Description: Each brown and clear capsule contains:

Chlorpheniramine maleate .... 8 mg.
Phenylephrine hydrochloride .... 20 mg.
Methscopolamine nitrate .... 2.5 mg.

in a specially prepared base to provide prolonged action.

This product contains ingredients in the following therapeutic classes; antihistamine, decongestant and anticholinergic.

Clinical Pharmacology: Chlorpheniramine maleate is an alkylamine-type antihistamine. This group of antihistamines are among the most active histamine antagonists and are generally effective in relatively low doses. The drugs are not so prone to produce drowsiness and are among the most suitable agents for daytime use; but again, a significant proportion of patients do experience this effect. Phenylephrine HCl is a sympathomimetic which acts predominantly on alpha receptors and has little action on beta receptors. It therefore functions as an oral nasal decongestant with minimal CNS stimulation. Methscopolamine nitrate is a quaternary ammonium derivative of scopolamine, which posseses the peripheral actions of the belladonna alkaloids, but does not exhibit the central actions because of its lack of ability to cross the blood-brain barrier. In this formulaion, it is used because of its antisecretory effects on the respiratory system.

Indications: For the temporary relief of symptoms of the common cold, allergic rhinitis (hay-fever) and sinusitis.

Contraindications: Hypersensitivity to any of the ingredients. Also contraindicated in patients with severe hypertension, severe coronary artery disease, patients on MAO inhibitor therapy, patients with narrow-angle glaucoma, urinary retention, peptic ulcer and during as asthmatic attack.

Should not be used in children under 12 years or in nursing mothers.

Warnings: Considerable caution shold be exercised in patients with hypertension, diabetes mellitus, ischemic heart disease, hyperthyroidism, increased intraocular pressure and prostatic hypertrophy. The elderly (60 years or older) are more likely to exhibit adverse reactions.

Antihistamines may cause excitability, especially in children. At dosages higher than the recommended dose, nervousness, dizziness or sleeplessness may occur.

Continued on next page

Dura—Cont.

Precautions: General: Caution should be exercised in patients with high blood pressure, heart disease, diabetes or thyroid disease. The antihistamine in this produce may exhibit additive effects with other CNS depressants, including alcohol.
Information for Patients: Antihistamine may cause drowsiness and ambulatory patients who operate machinery or motor vehicles should be cautioned accordingly.
Drug Interactions: MAO inhibitors and beta adrenergic blockers increase the effects of sympathomimetics. Sympathomimetics may reduce the antihypertensive effects of methyldopa, mecamylamine, reserpine and veratrum alkaloids. Concomitant use of antihistamines with alcohol and other CNS depressants may have an additive effect.
Pregnancy: The safety of use of this product in pregnancy has not been established.
Adverse Reactions: Adverse reactions include drowsiness, lassitude, nausea, giddiness, dryness of mouth, blurred vision, cardiac palpitations, flushing, increased irritability or excitement (especially in children).
Dosage and Administration: Adults and children over 12 years of age–1 capsule orally every 12 hours.
STORE AND DISPENSE IN TIGHT CONTAINERS AS DEFINED IN USP/NF. STORE BETWEEN 59°–86°F. DISPENSE IN CHILD-RESISTANT CONTAINERS.
How Supplied: Dura-Vent™/DA capsules are supplied in bottles of 100.
NDC: 51470-003-01
Warning: Federal Law Prohibits Dispensing Without Prescription.

Eaton Laboratories

See NORWICH EATON PHARMACEUTICALS, INC. Professional Products Group

Edwards Pharmacal, Inc.

100 EAST HALE
OSCEOLA, AR 72370

BLANEX® Capsules ℞

Description: Each capsule contains:
Chlorzoxazone ....250 mg.
Acetaminophen ....300 mg.
How Supplied: Capsules in bottles of 100 (NDC 0485-0031-01). Dispense in tight, light-resistant container.

C-SPAN Capsules

(See PDR For Nonprescription Drugs)

DOUBLE-A ℞

Description: Each enteric coated tablet contains:
Acetaminophen ....5 grains
Aspirin ....5 grains
How Supplied: Double-A is an oval shaped tablet with Double-A imprinted in red, supplied in bottles of 100 (NDC 0485-0034-01).

ECEE PLUS Tablets

(See PDR For Nonprescription Drugs)

NICO-VERT® Capsules ℞

Description: Each capsule contains:
Niacin ....50 mg.
Dimenhydrinate ....25 mg.
How Supplied: Bottles of 100 orange and black imprinted capsules (NDC 0485-0025-01). Dispense in tight, light-resistant container.

RYMED® Capsules ℞

Description: Each maroon and white capsule contains:
Phenylephrine HCl ....5 mg.
Phenylpropanolamine HCl ....45 mg.
Guaifenesin ....200 mg.
How Supplied: Maroon and white capsule monogrammed "RYMED", supplied in bottles of 100 capsules. Keep in tight, light-resistant container. (NDC 0485-0028-01)

RYMED®-JR. Capsules ℞

Description: Each capsule contains:
Guaifenesin ....100 mg.
Phenylpropanolamine HCL ....22.5 mg.
Phenylephrine HCL ....2.5 mg.
How Supplied: Bottles of 100 (NDC 0485-0030-01).

RYMED® Liquid ℞

Description: Each 5 cc contains:
Guaifenesin ....100 mg.
Phenylpropanolamine HCl ....20 mg.
Phenylephrine HCl ....5 mg.
Alcohol 5%
How Supplied: Rymed Liquid is supplied in pints (NDC 0485-0027-16).

RYMED®-TR Capsules ℞

Description: Each capsule contains:
Guaifenesin ....300 mg.
Phenylpropanolamine HCL ....75 mg.
Phenylephrine HCL ....10 mg.
How Supplied: Bottles of 100 (NDC 0485-0032-01).

SLYN-LL Ⓒ ℞

Description: Each capsule contains:
Phendimetrazine Tartrate ....105 mg.
How Supplied: Slyn-LL is a brown and clear capsule supplied in bottles of 100 (NDC 0485-0033-01).

UROGESIC® Tablets ℞

Description: Each tablet contains:
Phenazopyridine HCl ....100 mg.
Hyoscymine Hydrobromide ....0.12 mg.
Atropine Sulfate ....0.08 mg.
Scopolamine Hydrobromide ....0.0003 mg.
How Supplied: UROGESIC, a red, sugar-coated tablet is packaged in bottles of 100 and 500 (NDC 04875-0008-01).

IDENTIFICATION PROBLEM?

Consult PDR's

Product Identification Section

where you'll find over 900

products pictured actual size

and in full color.

Elder Pharmaceuticals Inc.

705 E. MULBERRY ST.
BRYAN, OH 43506

BENOQUIN® ℞
(Monobenzone Cream)

Contains: Monobenzone, USP, 20% in a water-washable base consisting of water, cetyl alcohol, propylene glycol, sodium lauryl sulfate, and white wax.
Action: Potent Depigmenting Agent.
Indications: For final depigmentation in extensive vitiligo.
BENOQUIN is not recommended for freckling, hyperpigmentation due to photosensitization following use of certain perfumes (berlock dermatitis), melasma (chloasma) of pregnancy, and hyperpigmentation following inflammation of the skin. BENOQUIN is of no value in the treatment of cafe-au-lait spots, pigmented nevi, malignant melanoma, or pigment resulting from pigments other than melanin, including, bile, silver, and artificial pigments.
Warning: BENOQUIN is a potent depigmenting agent, not a mild cosmetic bleach. Do not use except for final depigmentation in extensive vitiligo.
Federal (U.S.A.) law prohibits dispensing without prescription.
Adverse Reactions: Discontinue use if irritation, burning sensation, or dermatitis occurs.
Dosage and Administration: Apply and rub into the pigmented areas to be treated, two or three times daily.
Note: Depigmentation is usually observed after one to four months of therapy. If satisfactory results have not been obtained within four months, treatment should be discontinued.
How Supplied: BENOQUIN Cream, 20% in 1¼ oz. tubes (NDC 0163-0380-34).

ELAQUA® XX

Composition: Urea 20%, water, mineral oil, white petrolatum, microcrystalline cellulose, polyethylene glycol 400, cetyl alcohol, cetearyl alcohol and ceteareth 20, imidazolidinyl urea, p-hydroxybenzoic acid esters.
Actions and Uses: ELAQUA XX contains 20% urea, which increases the water binding capacity of the stratum corneum. The urea is combined with an emollient base that helps retain existing skin moisture and maintains the skin in a soft and supple condition.
Indications: ELAQUA XX is a therapeutic strength moisturizing cream for use in diseases where severe dry skin is a problem such as: atopic dermatitis, psoriasis, xerosis, and other hyperkeratotic conditions.
Administration: ELAQUA XX should be applied two or three times a day or as needed. The moisturizing action of ELAQUA XX will be most effective if it is applied when the skin is still moist after washing or bathing.
Caution: FOR EXTERNAL USE ONLY. Do not use near eyes. Discontinue use if irritation or rash occurs. Keep out of the reach of children.
How Supplied: Cream—1½ ounce (NDC 0163-0367-39)—in a beige plastic squeeze tube.

ELDER PSORALITE®

The Elder Psoralite is a full-body ultraviolet phototherapy medical device possessing a special interior elliptical shape to ensure uniform body irradiation. Series 53000-UVA (44 UVA lamps) and Series 56000-UVA/UVB (36 UVA lamps and 8 UVB lamps) are equipped with a Joulee® Control System wherein a microprocessor and two recessed remote sensors insure administration of the desired joules as well as an independent timer that functions as a regulating monitor on the joule dosimeter. Series 43000-UVB is available with either 8, 12, or 24 UVB lamps. A Gralab timer provides excellent control of the time of exposure.

ELDOPAQUE Forte® Cream ℞
Hydroquinone 4% Skin Bleaching Agent

CAUTION: FEDERAL LAW (U.S.A.) PROHIBITS DISPENSING WITHOUT A PRESCRIPTION.
FOR EXTERNAL USE ONLY

Description: Each gram of Eldopaque Forte contains 40 mg of hydroquinone in an opaque sunblocking base of water, stearic acid, talc, polyethylene glycol stearates, propylene glycol, glyceryl stearate, iron oxides, mineral oil, squalane, disodium EDTA, sodium metabisulfite, and potassium sorbate.

Clinical Pharmacology: Topical application of hydroquinone produces a reversible depigmentation of the skin by inhibition of the enzymatic oxidation of tyrosine to 3, 4-dihydroxyphenylalanine (dopa) and suppression of other melanocyte metabolic processes. Exposure to sunlight or ultraviolet light will cause repigmentation which may be prevented by the sunblocking agents contained in Eldopaque Forte.

Indications and Usage: Eldopaque Forte is indicated for the gradual bleaching of hyperpigmented skin conditions such as chloasma, melasma, freckles, senile lentigines, and other unwanted areas of melanin hyperpigmentation.

Contraindications: Prior history of sensitivity or allergic reaction to this product or any of its ingredients. The safety of topical hydroquinone use during pregnancy or in children (12 years and under) has not been established.

Warnings:

A. CAUTION: Hydroquinone is a skin bleaching agent which may produce unwanted cosmetic effects if not used as directed. The physician should be familiar with the contents of this insert before prescribing or dispensing this medication.

B. Test for skin sensitivity before using Eldopaque Forte by applying a small amount to an unbroken patch of skin and check in 24 hours. Minor redness is not a contraindication, but where there is itching or vesicle formation or excessive inflammatory response, further treatment is not advised. Close patient supervision is recommended. Contact with the eyes should be avoided. If no bleaching or lightening effect is noted after 2 months of treatment use, Eldopaque Forte should be discontinued. Eldopaque Forte is formulated for use as a skin bleaching agent and should not be used for the prevention of sunburn.

C. Sunscreen use is an essential aspect of hydroquinone therapy because even minimal sunlight exposure sustains melanocytic activity. The sunscreens in Eldopaque Forte provide the necessary sun protection during skin bleaching therapy. After clearing and during maintenance therapy, sun exposure should be avoided on bleached skin by application of a sunscreen or sunblock agent, or protective clothing to prevent repigmentation.

D. Keep this and all medications out of the reach of children. In case of accidental ingestion, call a physician or a poison control center immediately.

Precautions: SEE WARNINGS.

A. Pregnancy Category C. Animal reproduction studies have not been conducted with topical hydroquinone. It is also not known whether hydroquinone can cause fetal harm when used topically on a pregnant woman or affect reproductive capacity. It is not known to what degree, if any, topical hydroquinone is absorbed systemically. Topical hydroquinone should be used in women only when clearly indicated.

B. Nursing mothers. It is not known whether topical hydroquinone is absorbed or excreted in human milk. Caution is advised when topical hydroquinone is used by a nursing mother.

C. Pediatric usage. Safety and effectiveness in children below the age of 12 years have not been established.

Adverse Reactions: No systemic adverse reactions have been reported. Occasional hypersensitivity (localized contact dermatitis) may occur in which case the medication should be discontinued and the physician notified immediately.

Overdosage: There have been no systemic reactions from the use of topical hydroquinone or the sunblockers in Eldopaque Forte. However, treatment should be limited to relatively small areas of the body at one time since some patients experience a transient skin reddening and a mild burning sensation which does not preclude treatment.

Drug Dosage and Administration: A thin application of Eldopaque Forte should be applied to the affected area twice daily or as directed by a physician. Do not rub in. There is no recommendation for children under 12 years of age except under the advice and supervision of a physician.

How Supplied: Eldopaque Forte is available as follows:

Size	NDC Number
0.5 ounce tube	0163-0395-35
1.0 ounce tube	0163-0395-31

Available without prescription for maintenance therapy: Eldopaque® (2% Hydroquinone) in ½ ounce (NDC 0163-0518-35) and 1 ounce (NDC 0163-0518-31) tubes.

ELDOQUIN Forte® Cream ℞
Hydroquinone 4% Skin Bleaching Agent

CAUTION: FEDERAL LAW (U.S.A.) PROHIBITS DISPENSING WITHOUT A PRESCRIPTION.
FOR EXTERNAL USE ONLY

Description: Each gram of Eldoquin Forte contains 40 mg of hydroquinone in a vanishing cream base of water, stearic acid, propylene glycol, polyethylene glycol-40 stearate, propylene glycol-25 stearate, glyceryl stearate, mineral oil, squalane, propylparaben, and sodium metabisulfite.

Clinical Pharmacology: Topical application of hydroquinone produces a reversible depigmentation of the skin by inhibition of the enzymatic oxidation of tyrosine to 3, 4-dihydroxyphenylalanine (dopa) and suppression of the other melanocyte metabolic processes. Exposure to sunlight or ultraviolet light will cause repigmentation of the bleached areas. Eldoquin Forte is indicated for the gradual bleaching of hyperpigmented skin conditions such as chloasma, melasma, freckles, senile lentigines, and other unwanted areas of melanin hyperpigmentation. It is intended for night-time use only since it contains no sunblocking agents. For daytime usage, Solaquin Forte™ or Eldopaque Forte® should be prescribed.

Contraindications: Prior history of sensitivity or allergic reaction to this product or any of its ingredients. The safety of topical hydroquinone use during pregnancy or in children (12 years and under) has not been established.

Warnings:

A. CAUTION: Hydroquinone is a skin bleaching agent which may produce unwanted cosmetic effects if not used as directed. The physician should be familiar with the contents of this insert before prescribing or dispensing this medication.

B. Test for skin sensitivity before using Eldoquin Forte by applying a small amount to an unbroken patch of skin and check in 24 hours. Minor redness is not a contraindication, but where there is itching or vesicle formation or excessive inflammatory response, further treatment is not advised. Close patient supervision is recommended. Contact with the eyes should be avoided. If no bleaching or lightening effect is noted after 2 months of treatment, the medication should be discontinued.

C. There are no sunblocking or sunscreening agents in Eldoquin Forte and since minimal sunlight exposure may reverse the bleaching effect of this preparation, it should be used only at night or on areas of the body covered by protective clothing. During the daytime, sunblocking or broad spectrum sunscreen preparations or protective clothing should be used to prevent the bleached areas from repigmentation. For daytime bleaching of unwanted pigmented areas, the use of Solaquin Forte™ or Eldopaque Forte® should be considered.

D. Keep this and all medication out of the reach of children. In case of accidental ingestion, call a physician or a poison control center immediately.

Precautions: SEE WARNINGS.

A. Pregnancy Category C. Animal reproduction studies have not been conducted with topical hydroquinone. It is also not known whether hydroquinone can cause fetal harm when used topically on a pregnant woman or affect reproductive capacity. It is not known to what degree, if any, topical hydroquinone is absorbed systemically. Topical hydroquinone should be used in women only when clearly indicated.

B. Nursing mothers. It is not known whether topical hydroquinone is absorbed or excreted in human milk. Caution is advised when topical hydroquinone is used by a nursing mother.

C. Pediatric usage. Safety and effectiveness in children below the age of 12 years have not been established.

Adverse Reactions: No systemic adverse reactions have been reported. Occasional hypersensitivity (localized contact dermatitis) may occur in which case the medication should be discontinued and the physician notified immediately.

Overdosage: There have been no systemic reactions from the use of topical hydroquinone in Eldoquin Forte. However, treatment should be limited to relatively small areas of the body at one time since some patients experience a transient skin reddening and a mild burning sensation which does not preclude treatment.

Drug Dosage and Administration: Eldoquin Forte should be applied to the affected area and rubbed in well twice daily or as directed by a physician. There is no recommended dosage for children under 12 years of age except under the advice and supervision of a physician.

How Supplied: ELDOQUIN FORTE is available as follows:

Size	NDC Number
0.5 ounce tube	0163-0394-35
1.0 ounce tube	0163-0394-31

Available without prescription for maintenance therapy: Eldoquin® (2% Hydroquinone) in ½ ounce (NDC 0163-0382-35) and 1 ounce tubes (NDC 0163-0382-31); Eldoquin Lotion (2% Hydroquinone) in ½ ounce bottles (NDC 0163-0423-35).

FOTOTAR® Cream ℞
Therapeutic Coal Tar Cream
FOR EXTERNAL USE ONLY

Caution: FEDERAL (U.S.A.) LAW PROHIBITS DISPENSING WITHOUT A PRESCRIPTION.

Description: Each gram of Fototar Cream contains 20 mg. of Coal Tar extract (equivalent to 16 mg. of Coal Tar, USP) in an emollient moisturizing cream base containing purified water, white petrolatum, mineral oil, microcrystalline cellulose, PEG 8, stearyl alcohol, glyceryl stearate PEG 100 stearate blend, coceth 6, imidazolidinyl urea, methylparaben, and propylparaben.

Continued on next page

Elder—Cont.

Clinical Pharmacology: The mechanism of action of coal tar products is largely unknown. Coal tars have antiseptic qualities, because they contain many substituted phenols. Coal tars also act as mild irritants and have a keratoplastic and antipruritic action. Coal tars have a photosensitizing effect and have been used for years with sunlight or ultraviolet (UV) radiation (Goeckerman Therapy) for the treatment of psoriasis. Coal tars have been successfully used in the treatment of seborrhea, eczema, psoriasis, lichen simplex chronicus, and other chronic skin diseases with lichenification. Refinement of the crude coal tars has not lessened their therapeutic effectiveness and has increased patient acceptability.

Indications: Fototar is indicated in chronic skin disorders that are responsive to coal tars such as psoriasis, infantile and atopic eczema, seborrhea, lichen simplex chronicus, and other chronic skin disorders exhibiting lichenification. Fototar is useful in the Goeckerman program (tars plus UV radiation) in the treatment of psoriasis or other conditions responding to this combined therapy.

Contraindications:

A. Fototar is contraindicated in patients with a history of sensitivity to this product or with a history of sensitivity to coal tar products.

B. Fototar should not be used on patients who have a disease characterized by photosensitivity such as lupus erythematosus or allergy to sunlight.

Warnings:

A. Fototar should not be applied to inflamed or broken skin except on the advice of a physician.

B. Since Fototar is photosensitizing, care must be exercised in exposing the areas of application to excessive UV or sunlight for 24 hours. In the Goeckerman treatment of psoriasis or other skin conditions, care must be taken against overexposure of the areas of application during therapeutic UV radiation or subsequent to such treatment because serious burns may result. Sunscreening or sunblocking agents or protective clothing for at least 24 hours after treatment is recommended to protect the treated areas against additional UV exposure from sunlight.

C. Fototar contains a coal tar derivative. Coal tar preparations should not be used in patients with an exacerbation of psoriasis since this may precipitate total body exfoliation.

D. In psoriatic patients receiving Goeckerman therapy, care should be taken that Fototar application and/or subsequent sunlight exposure be avoided over normal skin since this may cause the appearance of new psoriatic lesions in areas of skin trauma (Koebner Phenomenon).

E. Contact with the eyes should be avoided.

F. Staining of clothing may occur which is normally removed by standard laundry methods. Use on the scalp may cause temporary staining of light colored hair.

Precautions:

A. Patients should be advised of the photosensitizing effect of Fototar.

B. Laboratory tests—none required.

C. Carcinogenesis. Skin cancer following the use of Fototar has not been seen. The use of crude coal tar combined with UV radiation in the production of skin cancer has been studied with conflicting results. Stern, et al, 1980, estimated an increased risk for such cancer in patients with high exposure to tar and ultraviolet radiation compared with those lacking high exposure. They recommended continued surveillance for tumors among psoriatic patients who receive long-term tar and/or UV radiation therapy. However, Pittelkow, et al, 1981, did a 25 year follow-up study on patients receiving combined crude coal tar and UV radiation for psoriasis at the Mayo Clinic and found the incidence of skin cancer not appreciably increased above the expected incidence for the general population, and concluded that this combined regimen (Goeckerman) could be used with minimal risk for skin cancer in the treatment of psoriasis.

D. Pregnancy Category C. Animal reproduction studies have not been conducted with Fototar. It is not known whether Fototar can cause fetal harm when administered to a pregnant woman or can affect reproductive capacity. Fototar should be given to a pregnant woman only if clearly indicated.

E. Nursing Mothers. The absorption of Fototar in nursing mothers has not been studied and caution should be exercised when Fototar is administered to a nursing woman.

F. Pediatric Use. Safety and effectiveness of Fototar in children have not been established.

Adverse Reactions:

A. SEE WARNINGS

B. Chemical folliculitis has been observed in areas of skin which have received long term coal tar applications. This phenomenon has not been observed with the use of Fototar, but its possibility should be borne in mind. This reaction normally clears if coal tar is discontinued or frequency of application reduced.

Overdosage:

A. SEE WARNINGS about use on normal skin.

B. If Fototar is accidentally ingested, call a physician or a poison control center for instructions.

Dosage and Administration: Fototar should be rubbed in the desired area well prior to UV radiation. After several minutes, the excess cream remaining on the skin can be patted with paper tissues to remove the excess.

How Supplied: Fototar (NDC 0163-0373-03) is supplied in 3.0 ounce plastic tubes.

OXSORALEN® CAPSULES ℞

(Methoxsalen, 10 mg)

CAUTION: FEDERAL LAW PROHIBITS DISPENSING WITHOUT PRESCRIPTION.
CAUTION: METHOXSALEN IS A POTENT DRUG. READ ENTIRE BROCHURE BEFORE PRESCRIBING OR DISPENSING THIS MEDICATION.

> Methoxsalen with UV radiation should be used only by physicians who have special competence in the diagnosis and treatment of psoriasis and vitiligo and who have special training and experience in photochemotherapy. Psoralen and ultraviolet radiation therapy should be under constant supervision of such a physician. For the treatment of patients with psoriasis, photochemotherapy should be restricted to patients with severe, recalcitrant, disabling psoriasis which is not adequately responsive to other forms of therapy, and only when the diagnosis has been supported by biopsy. Because of the possibilities of ocular damage, aging of the skin, and skin cancer (including melanoma), the patient should be fully informed by the physician of the risks inherent in this therapy.

Description: Oxsoralen (Methoxsalen, 8-Methoxypsoralen) Capsules, 10 mg. Methoxsalen is a naturally occuring photoactive substance found in the seeds of the Ammi majus (Umbelliferae) plant. It belongs to a group of compounds known as psoralens, or furocoumarins. The chemical name of methoxsalen is 9-methoxy-7H-furo[3,2-g][1]-benzopyran-7-one.

Clinical Pharmacology: The combination treatment regimen of psoralen (P) and ultraviolet radiation of 320-400 nm wavelength commonly referred to as UVA is known by the acronym, PUVA. Skin reactivity to UVA (320-400 nm) radiation is markedly enhanced by the ingestion of methoxsalen. The drug reaches its maximum bioavailability 1½-3 hours after oral administration and may last for up to 8 hours (Pathak et al, 1974). Methoxsalen is reversibly bound to serum albumen and is also preferentially taken up by epidermal cells (Artuc et al, 1979). At a dose which is six times larger than that used in humans, it induces mixed function oxidases in the liver of mice (Mandula et al, 1978). In both mice and man, methoxsalen is rapidly metabolized. Approximately 95% of the drug is excreted as a series of metabolites in the urine within 24 hours (Pathak et al, 1977).

The exact mechanism of action of methoxsalen with the epidermal melanocytes and keratinocytes is not known. The best known biochemical reaction of methoxsalen is with DNA. Methoxsalen, upon photoactivation, conjugates and forms covalent bonds with DNA which leads to the formation of both monofunctional (addition to a single strand of DNA) and bifunctional adducts (crosslinking of psoralen to both strands of DNA)(Dall'Acqua et al, 1971; Cole, 1970; Musajo et al, 1974; Dall'Acqua et al, 1979). Reactions with proteins have also been described (Yoshikawa et al, 1979).

Methoxsalen acts as a photosensitizer. Administration of the drug and subsequent exposure to UVA can lead to cell injury. Orally administered methoxsalen reaches the skin via the blood and UVA penetrates well into the skin. If sufficient cell injury occurs in the skin, an inflammatory reaction occurs. The most obvious manifestation of this reaction is delayed erythema, which may not begin for several hours and peaks at 48-72 hours. The inflammation is followed, over several days to weeks, by repair which is manifested by increased melanization of the epidermis and thickening of the stratum corneum. The mechanisms of therapy are not known. In the treatment of vitiligo, it has been suggested that melanocytes in the hair follicle are stimulated to move up the follicle and to repopulate the epidermis (Ortonne et al, 1979). In the treatment of psoriasis, the mechanism is most often assumed to be DNA photodamage and resulting decrease in cell proliferation but other vascular, leukocyte, or cell regulatory mechanisms may also be playing some role. Psoriasis is a hyperproliferative disorder and other agents known to be therapeutic for psoriasis are known to inhibit DNA synthesis.

Indications and Usage:

A. Photochemotherapy (methoxsalen with long wave UVA radiation) is indicated for the symptomatic control of severe, recalcitrant, disabling psoriasis not adequately responsive to other forms of therapy and when the diagnosis has been supported by biopsy. Photochemotherapy is intended to be administered only in conjunction with a schedule of controlled doses of long wave ultraviolet radiation.

B. Photochemotherapy (methoxsalen with long wave ultraviolet radiation) is indicated for the repigmentation of idiopathic vitiligo.

Contraindications:

A. Patients exhibiting idiosyncratic reactions to psoralen compounds.

B. Patients possessing a specific history of light sensitive disease states should not initiate methoxsalen therapy. Diseases associated with photosensitivity include lupus erythematosus, porphyria cutanea tarda, erythropoietic protoporphyria, variegate porphyria, xeroderma pigmentosum, and albinism.

C. Patients exhibiting melanoma or possessing a history of melanoma.

D. Patients exhibiting invasive squamous cell carcinomas.

E. Patients with aphakia, because of the significantly increased risk of retinal damage due to the absence of lenses.

Warnings—General:

A. Skin Burning: Serious burns from either UVA or sunlight (even through window glass) can result if the recommended dosage of the drug and/or exposure schedules are not maintained.

B. Carcinogenicity.

1. ANIMAL STUDIES: Topical or intraperitoneal methoxsalen has been reported to be a potent photocarcinogen in albino mice and hairless mice. However, methoxsalen given by the oral route to albino mice or by any route in pigmented mice is considerably less phototoxic or carcinogenic (Hakim et al, 1960; Pathak et al, 1959).

2. HUMAN STUDIES: A prospective study of 1380 patients over 5 years revealed an approximately nine-fold increase in risks of squamous cell carcinoma among PUVA treated patients. (Stern et al, 1979 and Stern et al, 1980) This increase in risk appears greatest among patients who are fair skinned or had pre-PUVA exposure to 1) prolonged tar and UVB treatment, 2) ionizing radiation, or 3) arsenic.

In addition, an approximately two-fold increase in the risk of basal cell carcinoma was noted in this study. Roenigk et al, 1980 studied 690 patients for up to 4 years and found no increase in the risk of non-melanoma skin cancer. However, patients in this cohort had significantly less exposure to PUVA than in the Stern et al study. After 5 years, two of 1380 patients in the Stern et al PUVA study have developed malignant melanoma. In addition, more than 1/5 of patients in this cohort have developed macular pigmented lesions on the buttocks. While there is no evidence that an increased risk of melanoma exists in PUVA treated patients, these observations indicate the need for continued evaluation of melanoma risk in PUVA treated patients.

In a study in Indian patients treated for 4 years for vitiligo, 12 percent developed keratoses, but not cancer, in the depigmented, vitiliginous areas (Mosher, 1980). Clinically, the keratoses were keratotic papules, actinic keratosis-like macules, nonscaling dome-shaped papules, and lichenoid porokeratotic-like papules.

C. Cataractogenicity:

1. ANIMAL STUDIES: Exposure to large doses of UVA causes cataracts in animals, and this effect is enhanced by the administration of methoxsalen (Cloud et al, 1960; Cloud et al, 1961; Freeman et al, 1969).

2. HUMAN STUDIES: It has been found that the concentration of methoxsalen in the lens is proportional to the serum level. If the lens is exposed to UVA during the time methoxsalen is present in the lens, photochemical action may lead to irreversible binding of methoxsalen to proteins and the DNA components of the lens (Lerman et al, 1980). However, if the lens is shielded from UVA, the methoxsalen will diffuse out of the lens in a 24 hour period. Patients should be told emphatically to wear UVA-absorbing, wrap-around sunglasses for the twenty-four (24) hour period following ingestion of methoxsalen, whether exposed to direct or indirect sunlight in the open or through a window glass.

Among patients using proper eye protection, there is no evidence for a significantly increased risk of cataracts in association with PUVA therapy. Thirty-five of 1380 patients have developed cataracts in the five years since their first PUVA treatment. This incidence is comparable to that expected in a population of this size and age distribution. No relationship between PUVA dose and cataract risk in this group has been noted.

D. Actinic Degeneration: Exposure to sunlight and/or ultraviolet radiation may result in "premature aging" of the skin.

E. Basal Cell Carcinomas: Patients exhibiting multiple basal cell carcinomas or having a history of basal cell carcinomas should be diligently observed and treated.

F. Radiation Therapy: Patients having a history of previous x-ray therapy or grenz ray therapy should be diligently observed for signs of carcinoma.

G. Arsenic Therapy: Patients having a history of previous arsenic therapy should be diligently observed for signs of carcinoma.

H. Hepatic Diseases: Patients with hepatic insufficiency should be treated with caution since hepatic biotransformation is necessary for drug urinary excretion.

I. Cardiac Diseases: Patients with cardiac diseases or others who may be unable to tolerate prolonged standing or exposure to heat stress should not be treated in a vertical UVA chamber.

J. Total Dosage: The total cumulative dose of UVA that can be given over long periods of time with safety has not as yet been established.

K. Concomitant Therapy: Special care should be exercised in treating patients who are receiving concomitant therapy (either topically or systemically) with known photosensitizing agents such as anthralin, coal tar or coal tar derivatives, griseofulvin, phenothiazines, nalidixic acid, halogenated salicylanilides (bacteriostatic soaps), sulfonamides, tetracyclines, thiazides and certain organic staining dyes such as methylene blue, toluidine blue, rose bengal, and methyl orange.

Precautions:

A. General-Applicable To Both Vitiligo and Psoriasis Treatment

1. BEFORE METHOXSALEN INGESTION

Patients must not sunbathe during the 24 hours prior to methoxsalen ingestion and UV exposure. The presence of a sunburn may prevent an accurate evaluation of the patient's response to photochemotherapy.

2. AFTER METHOXSALEN INGESTION

a. UVA-absorbing wrap-around sunglasses should be worn during daylight for 24 hours after methoxsalen ingestion. The protective eyewear must be designed to prevent entry of stray radiation to the eyes, including that which may enter from the sides of the eyewear. The protective eyewear is used to prevent the irreversible binding of methoxsalen to the proteins and DNA components of the lens. Cataracts form when enough of the binding occurs. Visual discrimination should be permitted by the eyewear for patient well-being and comfort.

b. Patients must avoid sun exposure, even through window glass or cloud cover, for at least 8 hours after methoxsalen ingestion. If sun exposure cannot be avoided, the patient should wear protective devices such as a hat and gloves, and/or apply sunscreens which contain ingredients that filter out UVA radiation (e.g. sunscreens containing benzophenone and/or PABA esters which exhibit a sun protective factor equal to or greater than 15). These chemical sunscreens should be applied to all areas that might be exposed to the sun (including lips). Sunscreens should not be applied to areas affected by psoriasis until after the patient has been treated in the UVA chamber.

3. DURING PUVA THERAPY

a. Total UVA-absorbing/blocking goggles mechanically designed to give maximal ocular protection must be worn. Failure to do so may increase the risk of cataract formation. A reliable radiometer can be used to verify elimination of UVA transmission through the goggles.

b. Abdominal skin, breasts, genitalia, and other sensitive areas should be protected for approximately 1/3 of the initial exposure time until tanning occurs.

c. Unless affected by disease, male genitalia should be shielded.

4. AFTER COMBINED METHOXSALEN/UVA THERAPY

a. UVA-absorbing wrap-around sunglasses should be worn during the daylight for 24 hours after combined methoxsalen /UVA therapy.

b. Patients should not sunbathe for 48 hours after therapy. Erythema and/or burning due to photochemotherapy and sunburn due to sun exposure are additive.

5. VITILIGO THERAPY

a. The dosage of methoxsalen should not be increased above 0.6 mg/kg since overdosage may result in serious burning of the skin.

b. Eye and skin sun protection as described in the Precautions-General section should be observed.

B. Information For Patients: See Patient Package Insert.

C. Laboratory Tests:

1. Patients should have an ophthalmologic examination prior to start of therapy, and thence yearly.

2. Patients should have the following tests prior to the start of therapy and should be retested 6-12 months subsequently. Additional tests at more extended time periods should be conducted as clinically indicated.

a. Complete Blood Count (Hemoglobin or Hematocrit; White Blood Count-if abnormal, a differential count).

b. Anti-nuclear Antibodies.

c. Liver Function Tests.

d. Renal Function Tests (Creatinine or Blood Urea Nitrogen).

D. Drug Interactions: See Warnings Section.

E. Carcinogenesis: See Warnings Section.

F. Pregnancy:

Pregnancy Category C. Animal reproduction studies have not been conducted with methoxsalen. It is also not known whether methoxsalen can cause fetal harm when administered to a pregnant woman or can affect reproduction capacity. Methoxsalen should be given to a woman only if clearly needed.

G. Nursing Mothers:

It is not known whether this drug is excreted in human milk. Because many drugs are excreted in human milk, caution should be exercised when methoxsalen is administered to a nursing woman.

H. Pediatric Use:

Safety in children has not been established. Potential hazards of long-term therapy include the possibilities of carcinogenicity and cataractogenicity as described in the Warnings Section as well as the probability of actinic degeneration which is also described in the Warnings Section.

Adverse Reactions:

A. Methoxsalen

The most commonly reported side effect of methoxsalen alone is nausea, which occurs with approximately 10% of all patients. This effect may be minimized or avoided by instructing the patient to take methoxsalen with milk or food, or to divide the dose into two portions, taken approximately one-half hour apart. Other effects include nervousness, insomnia, and psychological depression.

B. Combined Methoxsalen/UVA Therapy

1. PRURITUS: This adverse reaction occurs with approximately 10% of all patients. In most cases, pruritus can be alleviated with frequent application of bland emollients or other topical agents; severe pruritus may require systemic treatment. If pruritus is unresponsive to these measures, shield pruritic areas from further UVA exposure until

Continued on next page

Elder—Cont.

the condition resolves. If intractable pruritus is generalized, UVA treatment should be discontinued until the pruritus disappears.

2. ERYTHEMA: Mild, transient erythema at 24-48 hours after PUVA therapy is an expected reaction and indicates that a therapeutic interaction between methoxsalen and UVA occurred. Any area showing moderate erythema (greater than Grade 2—See Table 1 for grades of erythema) should be shielded during subsequent UVA exposures until the erythema has resolved. Erythema greater than Grade 2 which appears within 24 hours after UVA treatment may signal a potentially severe burn. Erythema may become progressively worse over the next 24 hours, since the peak erythemal reaction characteristically occurs 48 hours or later after methoxsalen ingestion. The patient should be protected from further UVA exposures and sunlight, and should be monitored closely.

3. IMPORTANT DIFFERENCES BETWEEN PUVA ERYTHEMA AND SUNBURN: PUVA-induced inflammation differs from sunburn or UVB phototherapy in several ways. The *in situ* depth of photochemistry is deeper within the tissue because UVA is transmitted further into the skin. The DNA lesions induced by PUVA are very different from UV-induced thymine dimers and may lead to a DNA crosslink. This DNA lesion may be more problematic to the cell because crosslinks are more lethal and psoralen-DNA photoproducts may be "new" or unfamiliar substrates for DNA repair enzymes. DNA synthesis is also suppressed longer after PUVA. The time course of delayed erythema is different with PUVA and may not involve the usual mediators seen in sunburn. PUVA-induced redness may be just beginning at 24 hours, when UVB erythema has already passed its peak. The erythema dose-response curve is also steeper for PUVA. Compared to equally erythemogenic doses of UVB, the histologic alterations induced by PUVA show more dermal vessel damage and longer duration of epidermal and dermal abnormalities.

4. OTHER ADVERSE REACTIONS: Those reported include edema, dizziness, headache, malaise, depression, hypopigmentation, vesiculation and bullae formation, non-specific rash, herpes simplex, miliaria, urticaria, folliculitis, gastrointestinal disturbances, cutaneous tenderness, leg cramps, hypotension, and extension of psoriasis.

Overdosage: In the event of methoxsalen overdosage, induce emesis and keep the patient in a darkened room for at least 24 hours. Emesis is beneficial only within the first 2 to 3 hours after ingestion of methoxsalen, since maximum blood levels are reached by this time.

Drug Dosage & Administration:

A. Vitiligo Therapy

1. DRUG DOSAGE: Two capsules (10 mg each) in one dose taken with milk or in food two to four hours before ultraviolet light exposure.

2. LIGHT EXPOSURE: The exposure time to sunlight should comply with the following guide:

	Basic Skin Color		
	Light	Medium	Dark
Initial Exposure	15 min	20 min	25 min
Second Exposure	20 min	25 min	30 min
Third Exposure	25 min	30 min	35 min
Fourth Exposure	30 min	35 min	40 min

Subsequent Exposure: Gradually increase exposure based on erythema and tenderness of the amelanotic skin.

Therapy should be on alternate days and never two consecutive days.

B. Psoriasis Therapy

1. DRUG DOSAGE-INITIAL THERAPY: The methoxsalen capsules should be taken two hours before UVA exposure with some food or milk according to the following table:

Patient's Weight (kg.)	(lbs.)	Dose (mg.)
<30	<65	10
30-50	65-100	20
51-65	101-145	30
66-80	146-175	40
81-90	176-200	50
91-115	201-250	60
>115	>250	70

Additional drug dosage directions are as follows:

a. Weight Change: In the event that the weight of a patient changes during treatment such that he/she falls into an adjacent weight range/dose category, no change in the dose of methoxsalen is usually required. If, in the physician's opinion, however, a weight change is sufficiently great to modify the drug dose, then an adjustment in the time of exposure to UVA should be made.

b. Dose/Week: The number of doses per week of methoxsalen capsules will be determined by the patient's schedule of UVA exposures. In no case should treatments be given more often than once every other day because the full extent of phototoxic reactions may not be evident until 48 hours after each exposure.

c. Dosage Increase: Dosage may be increased by 10 mg. after the fifteenth treatment under the conditions outlined in the section titled PUVA Treatment Protocol, part B)4)b).

UVA Radiation Source Specifications & Information:

A. Irradiance Uniformity

The following specifications should be met with the window of the detector held in a vertical plane:

1. Vertical variation: For readings taken at any point along the vertical center axis of the chamber (to within 15 cm from the top and bottom), the lowest reading should not be less than 70 percent of the highest reading.

2. Horizontal variation: Throughout any specific horizontal plane, the lowest reading must be at least 80 percent of the highest reading, excluding the peripheral 3 cm of the patient treatment space.

B. Patient Safety Features

The following safety features should be present: (1) Protection from electrical hazard: All units should be grounded and conform to applicable electrical codes. The patient or operator should not be able to touch any live electrical parts. There should be ground fault protection. (2) Protective shielding of lamps: The patient should not be able to come in contact with the bare lamps. In the event of lamp breakage, the patient should not be exposed to broken lamp components. (3) Hand rails and hand holds: Appropriate supports should be available to the patient. (4) Patient viewing window: A window which blocks UV should be provided for viewing the patient during treatment. (5) Door and latches: Patients should be able to open the door from the inside with only slight pressure to the door. (6) Non-skid floor: The floor should be of a non-skid nature. (7) Thermoregulation: Sufficient air flow should be provided for patient safety and comfort, limiting temperature within the UVA radiator cabinet to approximately less than 100°F. (8) Timer: The irradiator should be equipped with an automatic timer which terminates the exposure at the conclusion of a pre-set time interval. (9) Patient alarm device: An alarm device within the UVA irradiator chamber should be accessible to the patient for emergency activation. (10) Danger label: The unit should have a label prominently displayed which reads as follows: Danger-Ultraviolet radiation-Follow your physicians instructions-Failure to use protective eyewear may result in eye injury.

C. UVA Exposure Dosimetry Measurements:

The maximum radiant exposure or irradiance (within ± 15 percent) of UVA (320-400 nm) delivered to the patient should be determined by using an appropriate radiometer calibrated to be read in Joules/cm^2 or mW/cm^2. In the absence of a standard measuring technique approved by the National Bureau of Standards, the system should use a detector corrected to a cosine spatial response. The use and recalibration frequency of such a radiometer for a specific UVA irradiator chamber should be specified by the manufacturer because the UVA dose (exposure) is determined by the design of the irradiator, the number of lamps, and the age of the lamps. If irradiance is measured, the radiometer reading in mW/cm^2 is used to calculate the exposure time in minutes to deliver the required UVA dose in Joules/cm^2 to a patient in the UVA irradiator cabinet. The equation is:

$$\text{Exposure Time in Minutes} = \frac{\text{Desired UVA Dose (J/cm}^2)}{0.06 \times \text{Irradiance (mW/cm}^2)}$$

Overexposure due to human error should be minimized by using an accurate automatic timing device, which is set by the operator and controlled by energizing and de-energizing the UVA irradiator lamp. The timing device calibration interval should be specified by the manufacturer. Safety systems should be included to minimize the possibility of delivering a UVA exposure which exceeds the prescribed dose, in the event that the timer of radiometer should malfunction.

D. UVA Spectral Output Distribution

The spectral distributions of the lamps should meet the following specifications:

Wavelength band (nanometers)	Output[1]
<310	<1
310 to 320	1 to 3
320 to 330	4 to 8
330 to 340	11 to 17
340 to 350	18 to 25
350 to 360	19 to 28
360 to 370	15 to 23
370 to 380	8 to 12
380 to 390	3 to 7
390 to 400	1 to 3

[1]As a percentage of total irradiance between 320 and 400 nanometers.

PUVA Treatment Protocol:

A. Initial Exposure: The initial UVA exposure radiation level and corresponding time of exposure is determined by the patient's skin characteristics for sun burning and tanning as follows:

[See table on top next page].

B. Clearing Phase: Specific recommendations for patient treatment are as follows:

1. SKIN TYPES I, II, and III. Patients with skin types I, II, and III may be treated 2 or 3 times per week. UVA exposure may be held constant or increased by up to 1.0 Joule/cm^2 at each treatment, according to the patient's response. If erythema occurs, however, do not increase exposure time until erythema resolves. The severity and extent of the patient's erythema may be used to determine whether the next exposure should be shortened, omitted, or maintained at the previous dosage. See Adverse Reactions section for additional information.

2. SKIN TYPES IV, V, and VI. Patients with skin types IV, V, and VI may be treated 2 or 3 times per week. UVA exposure may be held constant or increased by up to 1.5 Joules/cm^2 at each treatment unless erythema occurs. If erythema occurs, follow instructions outlined above in the procedures for patients with skin types I, II, and III.

3. ERYTHRODERMIC PSORIASIS. Patients with erythrodermic psoriasis should

be treated with special attention because pre-existing erythema may obscure observations of possible treatment-related phototoxic erythema. These patients may be treated 2 or 3 times per week, as a Type I patient.

4. MISCELLANEOUS SITUATIONS:

a. If there is no response after a total of 10 treatments, the exposure of UVA energy may be increased by an additional 0.5-1.0 Joules/cm^2 above the prior incremental increases for each treatment. (Example: a patient whose exposure dosage is being increased by 1.0 Joule/cm^2 may now have all subsequent doses increased by 1.5-2.0 Joules/cm^2.)

b. If there is no response, or only minimal response, after 15 treatments, the dosage of methoxsalen may be increased by 10 mg. (a one-time increase in dosage). This increased dosage may be continued for the remainder of the course of treatment but should not be exceeded.

c. If a patient misses a treatment, the UVA exposure time of the next treatment should not be increased. If more than one treatment is missed, reduce the exposure by 0.5 Joule/cm^2 for each treatment missed.

d. If the lower extremities are not responding as well as the rest of the body and do not show erythema, cover all other body areas and give 25 percent of the present exposure dose as an additional exposure to the lower extremities. This additional exposure to the lower extremities should be terminated if erythema develops on these areas.

e. Non-responsive psoriasis: If a patient's generalized psoriasis is not responding, or if the condition appears to be worsening during treatment, the possibility of a generalized phototoxic reaction should be considered. This may be confirmed by the improvement of the condition following temporary discontinuance of this therapy for two weeks. If no improvement occurs during the interruption of treatment, this patient may be considered a treatment failure.

Skin Type	History	Recommended Joules/cm^2
I	Always burn, never tan (Patients with erythrodermic psoriasis are to be classed as Type I for determination of UVA dosage.)	0.5 J/cm^2
II	Always burn, but sometimes tan	1.0 J/cm^2
III	Sometimes burn, but always tan	1.5 J/cm^2
IV	Never burn, always tan	2.0 J/cm^2
	Physician Examination	
V*	Moderately pigmented	2.5 J/cm^2
VI*	Blacks	3.0 J/cm^2

[*Patients with natural pigmentation of these types should be classified into a lower skin type category if the sunburning history so indicates.]

C. Alternative Exposure Schedule:

As an alternative to increasing the UVA exposure at each treatment, the following schedule may be followed; this schedule may reduce the total number of Joules/cm^2 received by the patient over the entire course of therapy.

1. Incremental increases in UVA exposure for all patients may range from 0.5 to 1.5 Joules/cm^2, according to the patient's response to therapy.
2. Once Grade 2 clearing (see Table 2) has been reached and the patient is progressing adequately, UVA dosage is held constant. The dosage is maintained until Grade 4 clearing is reached.
3. If the rate of clearing significantly decreases, exposure dosage may be increased at each treatment (0.1-1.5 Joules/cm^2) until Grade 3 clearing and a satisfactory progress rate is attained. The UVA exposure will be held constant again until Grade 4 clearing is attained. These increases may be used also if the rate of clearing significantly decreases between Grade 3 and Grade 4 response. However, the possibility of a phototoxic reaction should be considered; see Non-responsive Psoriasis, above.
4. In summary, this schedule raises slightly the increments (Joules/cm^2) of UVA dosage, but limits these increases to those periods when the patient is not responding adequately. Otherwise, the UVA exposure is held at the lowest effective dose.

D. Maintenance Phase:

The goal of maintenance treatment is to keep the patient symptom-free as possible with the least amount of UVA exposure.

1. SCHEDULE OF EXPOSURES: When patients have achieved 95 percent clearing, or Grade 4 response (Table 2), they may be placed on the following maintenance schedules (M_1-M_4), in sequence. It is recommended that each maintenance schedule be adhered to for at least 2 treatments (unless erythema or psoriatic flare occurs, in which case see (2a) and (2b) below).

Maintenance Schedules

M_1–once/week
M_2–once/2 weeks
M_3–once/3 weeks
M_4–p.r.n. (i.e. for flares)

2. LENGTH OF EXPOSURE: The UVA exposure for the first maintenance treatment of any schedule (except M_4 as noted below) is the same as that of the patient's last treatment under the previous schedule. For skin types I-IV, however, it is recommended that the maximum UVA dosage during maintenance treatments not exceed the following:

Skin Type	Joules/cm^2/treatment
I	12
II	14
III	18
IV	22

If the patient develops erythema or new lesions of psoriasis, proceed as follows:

a. Erythema: During maintenance therapy, the patient's tan and threshold dose for erythema may gradually decrease. If maintenance treatments produce significant erythema, the exposure to UVA should be decreased by 25 percent until further treatments no longer produce erythema.

b. Psoriasis: If the patient develops new areas of psoriasis during maintenance therapy (but still is classified as having a Grade 4 response), the exposure to UVA may be increased by 0.5-1.5 Joules/cm^2 at each treatment; this is appropriate for all types of patients. These increases are continued until the psoriasis is brought under control and the patient is again clear. The exposure being administered when this clearing is reached should be used for further maintenance treatment.

3. FLARES DURING MAINTENANCE: If the patient flares during maintenance treatment (i.e., develops psoriasis on more than 5 percent of the originally involved areas of the body) his maintenance treatment schedule may be changed to the preceding maintenance or clearing schedule. The patient may be kept on his schedule until again 95 percent clear. If the original maintenance treatment schedule is unable to control the psoriasis, the schedule may be changed to a more frequent regimen. If a flare occurs less than 6 weeks after the last treatment, 25 percent of the maximum exposure received during the clearing phase may be used and proceed with the clearing schedule previously followed for this patient. (At 95 percent clearing follow regular maintenance until the optimum maintenance schedule is determined for the patient.) If more than 6 weeks have elapsed since the last treatment was given, treat patients as if they were beginning therapy insofar as exposure dosages are concerned, since their threshold for erythema may have decreased.

Table 1.—Grades of Erythema

Grade	Erythema Level
0	No erythema
1	Minimally perceptible erythema—faint pink
2	Marked erythema but with no edema
3	Fiery erythema with edema
4	Fiery erythema with edema and blistering

[See table below].

How Supplied: Oxsoralen Capsules, each containing 10 mg. of methoxsalen (8-methoxypsoralen) packaged in amber glass bottles are available as follows:

Unit Count	NDC Number
30	NDC 0163-0600-30
100	NDC 0163-0600-01

[*Shown in Product Identification Section*]

Also Available: OXSORALEN Lotion (Methoxsalen 1%) in 1 ounce bottles (NDC 0163-0402-31) For Topical Use.

Oxsoralen lotion should never be dispensed to a patient for home application.

Table 2.—Response to Therapy

Grade	Criteria	Percent Improvement (compared to original extent of disease)
−1	Psoriasis worse	0
0	No change	0
1	Minimal improvement—slightly less scale and/or erythema	5-20
2	Definite improvement—partial flattening of all plagues—less scaling and less erythema	20-50
3	Considerable improvement—nearly complete flattening of all plagues but borders of plagues still palpable	50-95
4	Clearing; complete flattening of plagues including borders; plagues may be outlined by pigmentation	95

OXSORALEN® LOTION 1% ℞
(methoxsalen 1%)

CAUTION: FEDERAL LAW PROHIBITS DISPENSING WITHOUT A PRESCRIPTION.
CAUTION: METHOXSALEN LOTION IS A POTENT DRUG. READ ENTIRE BROCHURE BEFORE PRESCRIBING OR USING THIS MEDICATION.
WARNING: METHOXSALEN LOTION IS A POTENT DRUG CAPABLE OF PRODUCING SEVERE BURNS IF IMPROPERLY USED. IT SHOULD BE APPLIED ONLY BY A PHYSICIAN UNDER CONTROLLED CONDITIONS

Continued on next page

Elder—Cont.

FOR LIGHT EXPOSURE AND SUBSEQUENT LIGHT SHIELDING. THIS PREPARATION SHOULD NEVER BE DISPENSED TO A PATIENT.

Description: Each ml. of Oxsoralen Lotion contains 10 mg. in an inert vehicle containing alcohol, propylene glycol, acetone, and water. Methoxsalen is a naturally occurring substance found in the seeds of the Ammi majus (Umbelliferae) plant; it belongs to a group of compounds known as psoralens or furocoumarins. The chemical name of methoxsalen is 9-methoxy-7H-furo(3, 2g) (1)-benzopyran-7-one. It has the following structure:

Clinical Pharmacology: The exact mechanism of action of methoxsalen with the epidermal melanocytes and keratinocytes is not known. Psoralens given orally are preferentially taken up by epidermal cells (Artuc et al, 1979). The best known biochemical reaction of methoxsalen is with DNA. Methoxsalen, upon photoactivation, conjugates and forms covalent bonds with DNA which leads to the formation of both monofunctional (addition to a single strand of DNA) and bifunctional adducts (crosslinking of psoralen to both strands of DNA) (Dall'Acqua et al, 1971). Reactions with proteins have also been described (Yoshikawa et al, 1979).

Methoxsalen acts as a photosensitizer. Topical application of this drug and subsequent exposure to UVA, whether artificial or sunlight, can cause cell injury. If sufficient cell injury occurs in the skin an inflammatory reaction will result. The most obvious manifestation of this reaction is delayed erythema which may not begin for several hours and may not peak for 2 to 3 days or longer. It is crucial to realize that the length of time the skin remains sensitized or when the maximum erythema will occur is quite variable from person to person. The erythematous reaction is followed over several days or weeks by repair which is manifested by increased melanization of the epidermis and thickening of the stratum corneum. The exact mechanics are unknown but it has been suggested melanocytes in the hair follicles are stimulated to move up the follicle and to repopulate the epidermis. (Ortonne, et al, 1979)

Indications and Usage: As a topical repigmenting agent in vitiligo in conjunction with controlled doses of ultraviolet A (320–400 nm) or sunlight.

Contraindications:

A. Patients exhibiting idiosyncratic reactions to psoralen compounds or a history of sensitivity reactions to them.
B. Patients exhibiting melanoma or with a history of melanoma.
C. Patients exhibiting invasive skin carcinoma generally.
D. Patients with photosensitivity diseases such as porphyria, acute lupus erythematosus, xeroderma pigmentosum, etc.
E. Children under 12 since clinical studies to determine the efficacy and safety of treatment in this age group have not been done.

Warnings:

A. **Skin Burns**

Serious skin burns from either UVA or sunlight (even through window glass) can result if recommended exposure schedule is exceeded and/or protective covering or sunscreens are not used. The blistering of the skin sometimes encountered after UV exposure generally heals without complication or scarring. (Farrington Daniels, Jr, M.D., personal communication). Suitable covering of the area of application or a topical sunblock should follow the therapeutic UVA exposure.

B. **Carcinogenicity**

1. Animal Studies. Topical methoxsalen has been reported to be a potent photocarcinogen in certain strains of mice. (Pathak et al 1959).
2. Human Studies. None of our clinical investigators reported skin cancers as a complication of topical treatment for vitiligo. However, it is recommended that caution be exercised when the patient is fair-skinned or has a history of prior coal tar UV treatment, or has had ionizing radiation or taken arsenical compounds. Such patients who subsequently have oral psoralen—UVA treatment (PUVA) are at increased risk for developing skin cancer.

C. **Concomitant Therapy**

Special care should be exercised in treating patients who are receiving concomitant therapy (either topically or systemically) with known photosensitizing agents such as anthralin, coal tar or coal tar derivatives, griseofulvin, phenothiazines, nalidixic acid, halogenated salicylanilides (bacteriostatic soaps), sulfonamides, tetracyclines, thiazides and certain organic staining dyes such as methylene blue, toluidine blue, rose bengal, and methyl orange.

Precautions:

A. This product should be applied only in small well defined lesions and preferably on lesions which can be protected by clothing or a sunscreen from subsequent exposure to radiant UVA. If this product is used to treat vitiligo of face or hands, be very emphatic when instructing patient to keep the treated areas protected from light by use of protective clothing or sunscreening agents. The area of application may be highly photosensitive for several days and may result in severe burn injury if exposed to additional UV or sunlight.
B. CARCINOGENESIS: See Warning Section
C. Pregnancy Category C. Animal reproduction studies have not been conducted with topical methoxsalen. It is also not known whether methoxsalen can cause fetal harm when used topically on a pregnant woman or affect reproductive capacity. It is not known to what degree, if any, topical methoxsalen is absorbed systemically. Topical methoxsalen should be used in women only when clearly indicated.
D. Nursing Mothers. It is not known whether topical methoxsalen is absorbed or excreted in human milk. Caution is advised when topical methoxsalen is used in a nursing mother.
E. Pediatric Usage. Safety and effectiveness in children below the age of 12 years have not been established.

Adverse Reactions: Systemic adverse reactions have not been reported. The most common adverse reaction is severe burns of the treated area from overexposure to UVA, including sunlight. TREATMENT MUST BE INDIVIDUALIZED. Minor blistering of the skin is not a contraindication to further treatment and generally heals without incident. Treatment would be the standard for burn therapy. Since 1953, many studies have demonstrated the safety and effectiveness of topical methoxsalen and UVA for the treatment of vitiligo when used as directed. (Lerner, A.B., et al, 1953) (Fitzpatrick, T.B., et al, 1966) (Fulton, James F. et al, 1969)

Overdosage: This does not apply to topical usage. In the unlikely event that the lotion is ingested, standard procedures for poisoning should be followed, including gastric lavage. Protection from UVA or daylight for hours or days would also be necessary and the patient kept in a darkened room.

Administration: The OXSORALEN® Lotion is applied to a well-defined area of vitiligo by the physician and the area is then exposed to a suitable source of UVA. Initial exposure time should be conservative and not exceed that which is predicted to be one-half the minimal erythema dose. Treatment intervals should be regulated by the erythema response and once a week is recommended or less often depending on the results. The hands and fingers of the person applying the medication should be protected by gloves or finger cots to avoid photosensitization and possible burns.

Pigmentation may begin after a few weeks but significant repigmentation may require up to 6 to 9 months of treatment. Periodic re-treatment may be necessary to retain all of the new pigment. Idiopathic vitiligo is reversible but not equally reversible in every patient. Treatment must be individualized. Repigmentation will vary in completeness, time of onset, and duration. Repigmentation occurs more rapidly in fleshy areas such as face, abdomen, and buttocks and less rapidly over less fleshy areas such as the dorsum of the hands or feet.

How Supplied: Oxsoralen Lotion containing 1% methoxsalen (8-methoxypsoralen) packaged in 1 ounce amber glass bottles (NDC 0163-0402-31).

RVP®
(Red Petrolatum-ELDER)

Composition: Red petrolatum, paraben and lanolin-free sunscreen. Now improved with 2.5% surfactants for easier application and easier removal with soap and water.

Action and Use: Topical sunscreen. Absorbs erythemal spectrum through 340 nanometers, but allows the tanning rays to pass. RVP gives sun protection and sun tanning when applied before sun exposure in the thinnest possible film.

Resists water and perspiration; safe around the eyes and on the lips.

How Supplied: 2 ounce tube (NDC 0163-0384-02).

RVPaba® LIP STICK
5% ParaAminobenzoic Acid (PABA) + Red Petrolatum (RVP)

Actions and Uses: RVPaba LIP STICK is a topical sunscreen and protectant for lips and small areas of exposed dermis. ParaAminobenzoic Acid (Paba) in Red Petrolatum (RVP) absorbs burning UV in a wide spectrum. Protects against sunburn, windburn and chapping winter or summer. RVPaba LIP STICK contains no perfumes or colors.

Dosage and Administration: Apply to lips and other sensitive areas of the face and hands before exposure to the sun. Reapply as needed.

Caution: Individuals sensitive to Paba should not use RVPaba LIP STICK.

Supply: 1/7 oz. lipstick tubes (NDC 0163-0505-41).

Military—Cold Climate Stock #6508-00-116-1479. Hot Climate Stock #6508-00-116-1473.

RVPaque® (Physical Sunscreen)

Composition: Red petrolatum, zinc oxide, and 2-ethoxyethyl p-methoxycinnamate in a greaseless, water-resistant base.

Actions and Uses: Unlike chemical sunscreens, RVPaque functions by reflecting instead of absorbing incident solar radiation. It therefore provides a significant barrier to a wide range of solar wavelengths including visible light. Tinted to blend with most skin tones.

Indications: RVPaque provides extra sun protection in any condition in which ultraviolet and visible light are contraindicated. It may be used adjunctively with depigmenting and skin bleaching agents.

To Use: Apply in a uniformly thin film which is visible to areas requiring exclusion of light. Reapply if removed by abrasion.

Contraindications: None reported; discontinue use if reaction develops.

How Supplied: ½ ounce (NDC 0163-0397-35) and 1¼ ounce tubes (NDC 0163-0397-34).

SOLAQUIN Forte™ Cream ℞
Hydroquinone 4% Skin Bleaching Agent
CAUTION: FEDERAL (U.S.A.) LAW PROHIBITS DISPENSING WITHOUT PRESCRIPTION.
FOR EXTERNAL USE ONLY.

Description: Each gram of Solaquin Forte contains 40 mg hydroquinone, 50 mg ethyl dihydroxypropyl PABA, 30 mg dioxybenzone and 20 mg oxybenzone in a bland emollient cream of water, glyceryl stearate, octyldodecyl stearoyl stearate, glyceryl dilaurate, quaternium-26, coceth-6, stearyl alcohol, diethylaminoethyl stearate, dimethicone, polysorbate-80, lactic acid, ascorbic acid, hydroxyethylcellulose, quaternium-14, myristylkonium chloride, disodium EDTA, and sodium metabisulfite.

Clinical Pharmacology: Topical application of hydroquinone produces a reversible depigmentation of the skin by inhibition of the enzymatic oxidation of tyrosine to 3, 4-dihydroxyphenylalanine (dopa) and suppression of other melanocyte metabolic processes. Exposure to sunlight or ultraviolet light will cause repigmentation which may be prevented by the broad spectrum sunscreen agents contained in Solaquin Forte.

Indications and Usage: Solaquin Forte is indicated for the gradual bleaching of hyperpigmented skin conditions such as chloasma, melasma, freckles, senile lentigines, and other unwanted areas of melanin hyperpigmentation.

Contraindications: Prior history of sensitivity or allergic reaction to this product or any of its ingredients. The safety of topical hydroquinone use during pregnancy or in children (12 years and under) has not been established.

Warnings:

A. CAUTION: Hydroquinone is a skin bleaching agent which may produce unwanted cosmetic effects if not used as directed. The physician should be familiar with the contents of this insert before prescribing or dispensing this medication.
B. Test for skin sensitivity before using Solaquin Forte by applying a small amount to an unbroken patch of skin and check in 24 hours. Minor redness is not a contraindication, but where there is itching or vesicle formation or excessive inflammatory response further treatment is not advised. Close patient supervision is recommended. Contact with the eyes should be avoided. If no bleaching or lightening effect is noted after 2 months of treatment use, Solaquin Forte should be discontinued. Solaquin Forte is formulated for use as a skin bleaching agent and should not be used for the prevention of sunburn.
C. Sunscreen use is an essential aspect of hydroquinone therapy because even minimal sunlight exposure sustains melanocytic activity. The sunscreens in Solaquin Forte provide the necessary sun protection during skin bleaching therapy. After clearing and during maintenance therapy, sun exposure should be avoided on bleached skin by application of a sunscreen or sunblock agent or protective clothing to prevent repigmentation.
D. Keep this and all medication out of the reach of children. In case of accidental ingestion, call a physician or a poison control center immediately.

Precautions: SEE WARNINGS.

A. Pregnancy Category C. Animal reproduction studies have not been conducted with topical hydroquinone. It is also not known whether hydroquinone can cause fetal harm when used topically on a pregnant woman or affect reproductive capacity. It is not known to what degree, if any, topical hydroquinone is absorbed systemically. Topical hydroquinone should be used in women only when clearly indicated.
B. Nursing mothers. It is not known whether topical hydroquinone is absorbed or excreted in human milk. Caution is advised when topical hydroquinone is used by a nursing mother.
C. Pediatric usage. Safety and effectiveness in children below the age of 12 years have not been established.

Adverse Reactions: No systemic adverse reactions have been reported. Occasional hypersensitivity (localized contact dermatitis) may occur in which case the medication should be discontinued and the physician notified immediately.

Overdosage: No systemic reactions from the topical use of Solaquin Forte have been noted. However, treatment should be limited to relatively small areas of the body at one time since some patients experience a transient skin reddening and a mild burning sensation which does not preclude treatment.

Drug Dosage and Administration: Solaquin Forte should be applied to the affected area and rubbed in well twice daily or as directed by a physician. There is no recommended dosage for children under 12 years of age except under the advice and supervision of a physician.

How Supplied: SOLAQUIN FORTE is available as follows:

Size	NDC Number
0.5 ounce tube	0163-0396-35
1.0 ounce tube	0163-0396-31

Available without prescription for maintenance therapy: Solaquin (2% Hydroquinone) in 1 ounce tubes (NDC 0163-0372-31).

TRISORALEN® ℞
(Trioxsalen) Elder

To facilitate repigmentation in vitiligo, increase tolerance to solar exposure and enhance pigmentation.

Caution: *THIS IS A POTENT DRUG.*

Caution: Federal (U.S.A.) law prohibits dispensing without prescription.

Description: Trisoralen Tablets 5 mg.
TRISORALEN is the first synthetic psoralen compound made available to the medical profession. It possesses greater activity than Methoxsalen, yet the LD 50 is six times that of Methoxsalen.
Contains color additives including FD&C Yellow No. 5 (Tartrazine).

Actions: Pigment formation with TRISORALEN.
The normal pigmentation of the skin is due to melanin which is produced in the cytoplasm of the melanocytes located in the basal layers of the epidermis at its junction with the dermis. Melanin is formed by the oxidation of tyrosine to DOPA (Dihydroxyphenylalanine) with tyrosinase as catalyst. This enzymatic reaction, however, must be activated by radiant energy in the form of ultraviolet light, preferably between 2900 and 3800 angstroms (black light). The exact mechanism of the action of psoralens in the process of melanogenesis is not known. One group of investigators feel that the psoralens have a specific effect on the epidermis or, more specifically, on the melanocytes. Another group feels that the primary response to the psoralens is an inflammatory one and that the process of melanogenesis is secondary.

Indications: TRISORALEN taken approximately two hours before measured periods of exposure to ultraviolet facilitates:

1. Repigmentation of idiopathic vitiligo. Repigmentation, not equally reversible in every patient, will vary in completeness, time of onset, and duration. The rate of completeness of pigmentation with respect to locations of lesions, occurs more rapidly on fleshy regions, such as the face, abdomen, and buttocks, and less rapidly over bony areas such as the dorsum of the hands and feet. Repigmentation may begin after a few weeks; however, significant results may take as long as six to nine months, and repigmentation, at the optimum level, may, in some cases, require maintenance dosage to retain the new pigment. If follicular repigmentation is not apparent after three months of daily treatment, treatment should be discontinued as a failure.
2. Increasing tolerance to sunlight. In blond persons and those with fair complexions who suffer painful reactions when exposed to sunlight, TRISORALEN aids in increasing resistance to solar damage. Certain persons who are allergic to sunlight or exhibit sun sensitivity may be benefited by the protective action of TRISORALEN. In albinism, TRISORALEN will increase the tolerance of the skin to sunlight, although no pigment is formed. This protective action seems to be related to the thickening of the horny layer and retention of melanin which produces a thickened melanized stratum corneum and formation of a stratum lucidum.
3. Enhancing pigmentation. The use of TRISORALEN accelerates pigmentation only when the administration of the drug is followed by exposure of the skin to sunlight or ultraviolet irradiation. The increase in pigmentation is not immediate but occurs gradually within a few days of repeated exposure and may become equivalent in a degree to that achieved by a full summer of sun exposure. Since sufficient pigment will have been formed within two weeks of continuous therapy, the use of TRISORALEN should not be continued beyond this period. Pigmentation can be maintained by periodic exposure to sunlight.

Contraindications: In those diseases associated with photosensitivity, such as porphyria, acute lupus erythematosus, or leukoderma of infectious origin. To date, the safety of this drug in young persons (12 and under), has not been established and is, therefore contraindicated. No preparation with any photosensitizing capacity, internal or external should be used concomitantly with TRISORALEN therapy.

Warnings: *TRISORALEN IS A POTENT DRUG.*
Read entire brochure before prescribing or dispensing this medication. The dosage of this medication should not be increased.
The dosage of TRISORALEN and exposure time should not be increased. Overdosage and/or overexposure may result in serious burning and blistering. When used to increase tolerance to sunlight or accelerate tanning, TRISORALEN total dosage should not exceed 28 tablets, taken in daily single doses of two tablets on a continuous or interrupted regimen. To prevent harmful effects, the physician should carefully instruct the patient to adhere to the prescribed dosage schedule and procedure.

Precautions: Accidental Overdosage:
If an overdose of TRISORALEN or ultraviolet light has been taken, emesis should be encouraged. The individual should be kept in a darkened room for eight hours or until cutaneous reactions subside. The treatment for severe reactions resulting from overdosage or overexposure should follow accepted procedures for treatment of severe burns. There have not been any clinical reports or tests to verify that more severe reactions may result from the concomitant ingestion of furocoumarin-containing food while on TRISORALEN therapy; but the physician should warn the patient that taking limes, figs, parsley, parsnips, mustard, carrots and celery, might be dangerous.
This product contains FD&C Yellow No. 5 (Tartrazine) which may cause allergic-type reactions (including bronchial asthma) in certain susceptible individuals. Although the overall incidence of FD&C Yellow No. 5 (Tartrazine)

Continued on next page

Elder—Cont.

sensitivity is low, it is frequently seen in patients who also have aspirin hypersensitivity.
Adverse Reactions and Side Effects: Severe burns can result from excessive sunlight or sun lamp ultraviolet exposure.
Occasionally, there may occur gastric discomfort; to minimize this gastric effect, the tablets may be taken with milk or after a meal. Some patients who are unable to tolerate 10 mg. will tolerate 5 mg. This dosage produces the same therapeutic effect but more slowly.
Dosage: (Adults and children over 12 years of age)
VITILIGO: Two tablets daily, taken two to four hours before measured periods of ultraviolet exposure or fluorescent black light. (See suggested sun exposure guide.)
To increase tolerance to sunlight and/or enhance pigmentation: Two tablets daily, taken two hours before measured periods of exposure to sun or ultraviolet irradiation. Not to be continued for longer than 14 days. The dosage should NOT be increased, as severe burning may occur. (See suggested sun exposure guide.)

SUGGESTED SUN EXPOSURE GUIDE
The exposure time to sunlight should be limited according to the following plan:

	Basic Skin Color	
	Light	Medium
Initial Exposure	15 min.	20 min.
Second Exposure	20 min.	25 min.
Third Exposure	25 min.	30 min.
Fourth Exposure	30 min.	35 min.
Subsequent Exposure:	Gradually increase exposure based on erythema and tenderness.	

Sunglasses should be worn during exposure and the lips protected with a light-screening lipstick.

SUN-LAMP EXPOSURE: Should be initiated according to directions of the sun-lamp manufacturer.

How Supplied: TRISORALEN Tablets 5 mg. in bottles of 28 (NDC 0163-0303-28) and 100 (NDC 0163-0303-01).
Military—TRIOXSALEN Tablets 5 mg. stock # 6505-00-560-7022.
[*Shown in Product Identification Section*]

VITADYE®
(Cosmetic Cover for hypopigmented skin)

Composition: Certified dyes and dihydroxyacetone in a special solvent base.
Use: To cover light colored or white patches of skin. For external use only.
Administration: Apply Vitadye to hypopigmented areas with the applicator provided and let it dry for ten to fifteen minutes. To obtain a darker shade, additional applications may be made. Allow each application to dry before reapplying. After the desired shade is achieved, allow three hours before washing or rubbing the area. The artificial color will normally last two to four days. Use Vitadye to maintain the desired color.
Concomitant Therapy: Vitadye transmits most UVA radiation so it can be used concurrently with psoralens in vitiligo therapy.
Precaution: If rash or irritation of the skin develops, discontinue use and contact a physician.
Caution: Vitadye when wet will stain clothing.
Warning: Keep this and all drugs out of the reach of children. In case of accidental ingestion, seek professional assistance or contact a poison control center immediately. Avoid open flame.
How Supplied: Vitadye is available in ½ fluid ounce (NDC 0163-0413-35) and 2 fluid ounce (NDC 0163-0413-02) packages.

Elkins-Sinn, Inc.
A subsidiary of A. H. Robins Company
2 ESTERBROOK LANE
P.O. BOX 5483
CHERRY HILL, NJ 08034

Elkins-Sinn's DOSETTE® line offers a broad spectrum of injectable products in a variety of single-dose containers—DOSETTE vials, DOSETTE ampuls, and DOSETTE syringes. Easily adaptable to any hospital pharmacy set-up, the DOSETTE system combines easily identifiable, clearly printed product labeling with space-conserving packaging. Each DOSETTE single-dose container is characterized by product name and strength in large, bold-faced type, important usage and storage data, lot identification number, and expiration date. Elkins-Sinn also produces a vast number of multiple dose vials. Listed below are some major ESI products. Additional syringe products are currently being marketed. For a complete catalog and price list, direct inquiries to Customer Service. For specific product information, direct inquiries to the Professional Services Department.

DOSETTE® SYRINGES

Dexamethasone Sodium Phosphate Injection, USP
4 mg/1 ml
10 mg/1ml
Gentamicin Sulfate Injection, USP
60 mg/1.5 ml
80 mg/2 ml
Hydroxyzine Hydrochloride Intramuscular Injection
25 mg/1 ml
50 mg/1 ml
100 mg/2 ml

DOSETTE® VIALS

Aminophylline Injection, USP
250 mg/10 ml
500 mg/20 ml
Atropine Sulfate Injection, USP
400 mcg/1ml (0.4 mg, 1/150 gr)
1.0 mg/1 ml
1.2 mg/1 ml
Codeine Phosphate Injection, USP
30 mg/1 ml
60 mg/1 ml
Cyanocobalamin Injection, USP (Vit. B-12)
1 mg/1 ml (1000 mcg)
Dexamethasone Sodium Phosphate Injection, USP
4 mg/1 ml
10 mg/1 ml
Dexpanthenol Injection
500 mg/2 ml
Dextrose Injection, USP
50%-50 ml
Diphenhydramine Hydrochloride Injection, USP
50 mg/1 ml
Dopamine HCl Injection
200 mg/5 ml
400 mg/5 ml
Furosemide Injection, USP
20 mg/2 ml
40 mg/4 ml
100 mg/10 ml
Gentamicin Sulfate Injection, USP
20 mg/2 ml (Pediatric)
80 mg/2 ml
Hep-Lock® (Heparin Sodium for IV Flush)
10 USP units/1 ml
100 USP units/1 ml
Heparin Sodium Injection, USP
1000 USP units/1 ml
5000 USP units/1 ml
10,000 USP units/1 ml
Hydromorphone Hydrochloride Injection, USP
2 mg/1 ml
Hydroxyzine Hydrochloride Intramuscular Injection
25 mg/1 ml
50 mg/1ml
75 mg/1.5 ml
100 mg/2 ml
Lidocaine Hydrochloride Injection, USP
1%-2 ml
2%/2 ml
Lidocaine Hydrochloride Injection for Intravenous Use in Cardiac Arrhythmias
50 mg/5 ml
100 mg/5 ml
1 gram/25 ml
2 grams/50 ml
Meperidine Hydrochloride Injection, USP
25 mg/1 ml
50 mg/1 ml
75 mg/1 ml
100 mg/1 ml
Mineral Oil, Sterile Light
10 ml
30 ml
Morphine Sulfate Injection, USP
8 mg/1 ml (1/8 gr)
10 mg/1 ml (1/6 gr)
15 mg/1 ml (1/4 gr)
Pentobarbital Sodium Injection, USP
100 mg/2 ml
Phenobarbital Sodium Injection, USP
65 mg/1 ml
130 mg/1 ml
Phenytoin Sodium Injection
(formerly Sodium Diphenylhydantoin)
100 mg/2 ml
250 mg/5 ml
Scopolamine Hydrobromide Injection, USP
400 mcg/1 ml (0.4 mg, 1/150 gr)
Sodium Nitroprusside Injection, USP
50 mg
Thiamine Hydrochloride Injection, USP
100 mg/1 ml
Vials, Sterile Empty
2 ml

DOSETTE® AMPULS

Aminophylline Injection, USP
250 mg/10 ml
500 mg/20 ml
Atropine Sulfate Injection, USP
400 mcg/1 ml (0.4 mg, 1/150 gr)
400 mcg/0.5 ml (0.4 mg, 1/150 gr)
Calcium Chloride Injection, USP,
1 gram/10 ml (10%)
Calcium Gluconate Injection, USP,
1 gram/10 ml (10%)
Chlorpromazine Hydrochloride Injection, USP
25 mg/1 ml
50 mg/2 ml
Cyanocobalamin Injection, USP (Vit. B-12)
1 mg/1 ml (1000 mcg)
Digoxin Injection, USP
0.5 mg/2 ml
Dopamine HCl Injection
200 mg/5 ml
400 mg/5 ml
Epinephrine Injection, USP,
1 mg/1 ml (1:1000)
Furosemide Injection, USP
20 mg/2 ml
40 mg/4 ml
100 mg/10 ml
Isoproterenol Hydrochloride Injection, USP
1 mg/5 ml (1:5000)
Magnesium Sulfate Injection, USP,
1 gram/2 ml (50%)
Meperidine Hydrochloride Injection, USP
25 mg/1 ml
50 mg/1 ml
75 mg/1 ml
100 mg/1 ml
Methylene Blue Injection, USP,
1%-10 ml

Morphine Sulfate Injection, USP
8 mg/1 ml (1/8 gr)
10 mg/1 ml (1/6 gr)
15 mg/1 ml (1/4 gr)
Paraldehyde Sterile, USP
5 ml
Phenytoin Sodium Injection
(formerly Sodium Diphenylhydantoin)
100 mg/2 ml
250 mg/5 ml
Potassium Chloride Injection, USP
20 mEq/10 ml
40 mEq/20 ml
Prochlorperazine Edisylate Injection, USP
10 mg/2 ml
Promethazine Hydrochloride Injection, USP
25 mg/1 ml
50 mg/1 ml
Sodium Chloride Injection, USP,
0.9%-5 ml
0.9%-10 ml
Sotradecol® (Sodium Tetradecyl Sulfate)
1%-2 ml
3%-2 ml
Water for Injection, USP
5 ml
10 ml

MULTIPLE DOSE VIAL

Aminocaproic Acid Injection, USP
250 mg/ml-20 ml
Atropine Sulfate Injection, USP
400 mcg/ml (0.4 mg, 1/150 gr)-20 ml
Chlorpromazine Hydrochloride Injection, USP
25 mg/ml-10 ml
Cyanocobalamin Injection, USP (Vit. B-12)
1 mg/ml (1000 mcg)-10 ml, 30 ml
Dexamethasone Sodium Phosphate Injection, USP
4 mg/ml-5 ml, 25 ml
10 mg/ml-10 ml
Gentamicin Sulfate Injection, USP
40 mg/ml-20 ml
Hep-Lock® (Heparin Sodium for IV Flush)
10 USP units/ml-10 ml, 30 ml
100 USP units/ml-10 ml, 30 ml
Heparin Sodium Injection, USP
1000 USP units/ml-10 ml, 30 ml
5000 USP units/ml-10 ml
10,000 USP units/ml-4 ml
Hydrocortisone Sodium Succinate For Injection, USP
100 mg
250 mg
500 mg
1000 mg (1 gram)
Hydroxyzine Hydrochloride Intramuscular Injection
50 mg/ml
Lidocaine Hydrochloride Injection, USP
1%-30 ml, 50 ml
2%-30 ml, 50 ml
Lidocaine Hydrochloride and Epinephrine 1:100,000 Injection, USP
1%-30 ml
2%-30 ml
Metaraminol Bitartrate Injection, USP
10 mg/ml (1%)-10 ml
Methylprednisolone Sodium Succinate for Injection, USP
40 mg
125 mg
500 mg
1000 mg (1 gram)
Neostigmine Methylsulfate Injection, USP
1 mg/ml (1:1000)-10 ml
Potassium Chloride Injection, USP
2 mEq/ml-30 ml
Procaine Hydrochloride Injection, USP
1%-30 ml
2%-30 ml
Sodium Chloride Injection, USP
0.9%-30 ml
Vials, Sterile Empty
5 ml
10 ml
30 ml

Water for Injection, USP
30 ml

SOTRADECOL® ℞

(Sodium Tetradecyl Sulfate)
For Intravenous Use Only

Description: Sotradecol (sodium tetradecyl sulfate) Injection is a sterile solution containing in each ml sodium tetradecyl sulfate 10 mg (1%) or 30 mg (3%) in Water for Injection with 0.02 ml benzyl alcohol and buffered with dibasic sodium phosphate. pH is adjusted to 7–8.1 with monobasic sodium phosphate or sodium hydroxide.

Actions: The product is a mild sclerosing agent which acts by irritation of the vein intimal endothelium.

Indications: Indicated in the treatment of small uncomplicated varicose veins of the lower extremities.

The benefit-to-risk ratio should be considered in selected patients who are great surgical risks due to conditions such as old age.

Contraindications: Contraindicated in acute superficial thrombophlebitis; underlying arterial disease; varicosities caused by abdominal and pelvic tumors, uncontrolled diabetes mellitus, thyrotoxicosis, tuberculosis, neoplasms, asthma, sepsis, blood dyscrasias, acute respiratory or skin diseases; and any condition which causes the patient to be bedridden. Do not use if precipitated.

Warnings: Sotradecol (sodium tetradecyl sulfate) should be used in pregnant women only when clearly needed. See Precautions.

Precautions: For varicosities, sclerotherapy should not be undertaken if tests such as the Trendelenberg and Perthes, and angiography show significant valvular or deep venous incompetence. The physician should bear in mind the fact that injection necrosis may result from direct injection of sclerosing agents. The drug should be administered by physicians who are familiar with an acceptable injection technique. Because of the danger of extension of thrombosis into the deep venous system, thorough pre-injection evaluation for valvular competency should be carried out, and slow injections with a small amount (not over 2 ml) of the preparation should be injected into the varicosity. In particular, deep venous patency must be determined by angiography and/or the Perthes test before sclerotherapy is undertaken.

No well controlled studies have been performed on patients taking anti-ovulatory agents. The physician must use judgment and evaluate any patient taking anti-ovulatory drugs prior to initiating treatment with Sotradecol (sodium tetradecyl sulfate). See Adverse Reactions.

Pregnancy category C. Adequate reproduction studies have not been performed in animals to determine whether this drug affects fertility in males or females, has teratogenic potential, or has other adverse effects on the fetus. There are no well-controlled studies in pregnant women, but investigational and marketing experience does not include any positive evidence of adverse effects on the fetus. Although there is no clearly defined risk, such experience cannot exclude the possibility of infrequent or subtle damage to the human fetus.

Adverse Reactions: Post-operative complication of sloughing may occur. A permanent discoloration, usually small and hardly noticeable may occur at the site of injection, and may be objectionable from a cosmetic viewpoint. Allergic reactions have been reported. Therefore, as a precaution against anaphylactic shock, it is recommended that an injection of 0.5 ml of the product into a varicosity be followed by observance of the patient for several hours before a larger injection is administered. The possibility of an anaphylactic reaction should always be kept in mind, and the physician should be prepared to treat it appropriately. In extreme emergencies, 0.25 ml of a 1:1000 solution of epinephrine (0.25 mg) intravenously should be used and side reactions controlled with antihistamines.

One death has been reported in a patient who received Sotradecol (sodium tetradecyl sulfate) and who had been receiving an anti-ovulatory agent. Another death (fatal pulmonary embolism) has been reported in a 36-year-old female treated with sodium tetradecyl acetate and who was not taking oral contraceptives.

Dosage and Administration: For intravenous use only. Do not use if precipitated. The strength of solution required depends on the size and degree of varicosity. In general, the 3% solution will be found most useful, with the 1% solution preferred for small varicosities. The dosage should be kept small, using 0.5 to 2 ml for each injection, and the maximum single treatment should not exceed 10 ml.

Literature describing various current techniques of administration is available upon request from the Professional Services Department.

How Supplied:
1% — 2 ml Dosette® Ampuls, 5's — #1514-34 (NDC 0641-1514-34)
3% — 2 ml Dosette® Ampuls, 5's — #1516-34 (NDC 0641-1516-34)

Endo Laboratories, Inc.

Subsidiary of the DuPont Company
ONE RODNEY SQUARE
WILMINGTON, DE 19898

Endo Inc.

MANATI, PUERTO RICO 00701
Subsidiary of Endo Laboratories, Inc.
Subsidiary of the DuPont Company

Endo Pharmaceuticals, Inc.

MANATI, PUERTO RICO 00701
Subsidiary of Endo Laboratories, Inc.
Subsidiary of the DuPont Company

Products indicated by a dagger are products of Endo Inc.

PRODUCT IDENTIFICATION CODES

The Endo Logo and a code number is imprinted on all Endo tablets and a code number appears on the following capsules. This identifies each specific Endo product. Below is an alphabetical listing of each Endo product with the corresponding identification number.

PRODUCT	IDENT. NO.
COUMADIN® crystalline warfarin sodium Tablets	
2 mg	170
2½ mg	171
5 mg	172
7½ mg	173
10 mg	174
ENDECON® (decongestant, analgesic, antipyretic) Tablets	030
HYCODAN® (hydrocodone bitartrate/homatropine methylbromide combination) Tablets Ⓒ	042
HYCOMINE® COMPOUND (hydrocodone bitartrate/chlorpheniramine maleate/phenylephrine hydrochloride/APAP/caffeine) Tablets Ⓒ	048

Continued on next page

Endo—Cont.

MOBAN® (molindone hydrochloride) Tablets	
5 mg	072
10 mg	073
25 mg	074
50 mg	076
100 mg	077
†**PERCOCET® 5** (oxycodone/APAP combination) Tablets Ⓒ	127
†**PERCODAN®** (oxycodone/aspirin combination) Tablets Ⓒ	135
†**PERCODAN®-DEMI** (oxycodone/aspirin combination) Tablets Ⓒ	136
PERCOGESIC® with CODEINE (analgesic with codeine) Tablets Ⓒ	133
REMSED® promethazine hydrochloride Tablets 50 mg	051
SYMMETREL® amantadine hydrochloride Capsules 100 mg	105
VALPIN® 50 anisotropine methylbromide Tablets 50 mg	161
VALPIN® 50-PB (anisotropine methylbromide with phenobarbital) Tablets	162

COUMADIN® ℞
(crystalline warfarin sodium, U.S.P.)*

Description: COUMADIN (crystalline warfarin sodium), a prothrombinopenic anticoagulant, is chemically crystalline sodium warfarin isopropanol clathrate. The crystallization of warfarin sodium virtually eliminates trace impurities present in amorphous warfarin sodium, thus achieving a crystalline product of the highest purity. Warfarin* is the coined generic name for 3-(α-Acetonylbenzyl)-4-hydroxycoumarin. On a dose-for-dose basis, COUMADIN (crystalline warfarin sodium) is therapeutically equivalent to amorphous warfarin sodium.

Actions: COUMADIN and other coumarin anticoagulants act by depressing synthesis in the liver of several factors which are known to be active in the coagulation mechanisms in a variety of diseases characterized by thromboembolic phenomena. The resultant **in vivo** effect is a sequential depression of Factors VII, IX, X and II. The degree of depression is dependent upon the dosage administered. Anticoagulants have no direct effect on an established thrombus, nor do they reverse ischemic tissue damage. However, once a thrombosis has occurred, anticoagulant treatment aims to prevent further extension of the formed clot and prevents secondary thromboembolic complications which may result in serious and possible fatal sequelae.

After oral administration, absorption is essentially complete, and maximal plasma concentrations are reached in 1 to 9 hours. Approximately 97% is bound to albumin within the plasma. COUMADIN usually induces hypoprothrombinemia in 36 to 72 hours, and its duration of action may persist for 4 to 5 days, thus producing a smooth, long lasting response curve. Little is known of the metabolic pathways involved in the biotransformation of oral anticoagulants in man. However, their metabolites appear to be eliminated principally in the urine.

Indications: Based on a review of this drug by the National Academy of Sciences—National Research Council and/or other information, FDA has classified the indications as follows:

Effective: COUMADIN is indicated for the prophylaxis and treatment of venous thrombosis and its extension, the treatment of atrial fibrillation with embolization, the prophylaxis and treatment of pulmonary embolism, and as an adjunct in the treatment of coronary occlusion.

"Possibly" effective: as an adjunct in the treatment of transient cerebral ischemic attacks.

Final classification of the less-than-effective indication requires further investigation.

Contraindications: Anticoagulation is contraindicated in any localized or general physical condition or personal circumstance in which the hazard of hemorrhage might be greater than its potential clinical benefits, such as:

Pregnancy—COUMADIN is contraindicated in pregnancy because the drug passes through the placental barrier and may cause fatal hemorrhage to the fetus in utero. Furthermore, there have been reports of birth malformations in children born to mothers who have been treated with warfarin during pregnancy. Women of childbearing potential who are candidates for anticoagulant therapy should be carefully evaluated and the indications critically reviewed with the patient. If the patient becomes pregnant while taking this drug, she should be apprised of the potential risks to the fetus, and the possibility of termination of the pregnancy should be discussed in light of those risks.

Hemorrhagic tendencies or blood dyscrasias.

Recent or contemplated surgery of: (1) central nervous system; (2) eye; (3) traumatic surgery resulting in large open surfaces.

Bleeding tendencies associated with active ulceration or overt bleeding of: (1) gastrointestinal, genitourinary or respiratory tracts; (2) cerebrovascular hemorrhage; (3) aneurysms—cerebral, dissecting aorta; (4) pericarditis and pericardial effusions; (5) subacute bacterial endocarditis.

Threatened abortion, eclampsia and preeclampsia.

Inadequate laboratory facilities or unsupervised senility, alcoholism, psychosis; or lack of patient cooperation.

Spinal puncture and other diagnostic or therapeutic procedures with potential for uncontrollable bleeding.

Miscellaneous: major regional, lumbar block anesthesia and malignant hypertension.

Warnings: Warfarin sodium is a potent drug with a half-life of 2½ days; therefore its effects may become more pronounced as daily maintenance doses overlap. It cannot be emphasized too strongly that treatment of each patient is a highly individualized matter. Dosage should be controlled by periodic determinations of prothrombin time or other suitable coagulation tests. Determinations of whole blood clotting and bleeding times are not effective measures for control of therapy. Heparin prolongs the one-stage prothrombin time. Therefore, to obtain a valid prothrombin time when heparin and COUMADIN (crystalline warfarin sodium) are given together, a period of at least 5 hours should elapse after the last intravenous dose and 24 hours after the last subcutaneous dose of heparin, before blood is drawn.

Caution should be observed when warfarin sodium is administered in any situation or physical condition where added risk of hemorrhage is present.

Administration of anticoagulants in the following conditions will be based upon clinical judgment in which the risks of anticoagulant therapy are weighed against the risk of thrombosis or embolization in untreated cases. The following may be associated with these increased risks:

Lactation—coumarins may pass into the milk of mothers and cause a prothrombinopenic state in the nursing infant.

Severe to moderate hepatic or renal insufficiency.

Infectious diseases or disturbances of intestinal flora—sprue, antibiotic therapy.

Trauma which may result in internal bleeding.

Surgery or trauma resulting in large exposed raw surfaces.

Indwelling catheters.

Severe to moderate hypertension.

Miscellaneous: polycythemia vera, vasculitis, severe diabetes, severe allergic and anaphylactic disorders.

Patients with congestive heart failure may become more sensitive to COUMADIN, thereby requiring more frequent laboratory monitoring, and reduced doses of COUMADIN.

Concurrent use of anticoagulants with streptokinase or urokinase is not recommended and may be hazardous. (Please note recommendations accompanying these preparations.)

Abrupt cessation of anticoagulant therapy is not generally recommended; taper dose gradually over three to four weeks.

Precautions: Periodic determination of prothrombin time or other suitable coagulation test is essential.

Numerous factors, alone or in combination, including travel, changes in diet, environment, physical state and medication may influence response of the patient to anticoagulants. It is generally good practice to monitor the patient's response with additional prothrombin time determinations in the period immediately after discharge from the hospital, and whenever other medications are initiated, discontinued or taken haphazardly. The following factors are listed for your reference; however, other factors may also affect the prothrombin response.

The following factors, alone or in combination, may be responsible for increased prothrombin time response:

ENDOGENOUS FACTORS: Carcinoma; collagen disease; congestive heart failure; diarrhea; elevated temperature; hepatic disorders—infectious hepatitis, hyperthyroidism; jaundice; poor nutritional state; vitamin K deficiency—steatorrhea.

EXOGENOUS FACTORS: Alcohol†; allopurinol; aminosalicylic acid; anabolic steroids; antibiotics; bromelains; chloral hydrate†; chlorpropamide; chymotrypsin; cimetidine; cinchophen; clofibrate; COUMADIN overdosage; dextran; dextrothyroxine; diazoxide; dietary deficiencies; diuretics†; disulfiram; drugs affecting blood elements; ethacrynic acid; fenoprofen; glucagon; hepatotoxic drugs; ibuprofen; indomethacin; inhalation anesthetics; mefenamic acid; methyldopa; methylphenidate; metronidazole; monoamine oxidase inhibitors; nalidixic acid: naproxen; oxolinic acid; oxyphenbutazone; pyrazolones; phenylbutazone; phenyramidol; phenytoin; prolonged hot weather; prolonged narcotics; quinidine; quinine; salicylates; sulfinpyrazone; sulfonamides, long acting; sulindac; thyroid drugs; tolbutamide; triclofos sodium; trimethoprim/-sulfamethoxazole; unreliable prothrombin time determinations.

†Increased and decreased prothrombin time responses have been reported.

The following factors, alone or in combination, may be responsible for decreased prothrombin time response:

ENDOGENOUS FACTORS: Edema; hereditary resistance to coumarin therapy; hyperlipemia; hypothyroidism.

EXOGENOUS FACTORS: Adrenocortical steroids; alcohol†; antacids; antihistamines; barbiturates; carbamazepine; chloral hydrate†; chlordiazepoxide; cholestyramine; COUMADIN underdosage; diet high in vitamin K; diuretics†; ethchorvynol; glutethimide; griseofulvin; haloperidol; meprobamate; oral contraceptives; paraldehyde; primidone; rifampin; unreliable prothrombin time determinations; vitamin C.

† Increased and decreased prothrombin time responses have been reported.

A patient may be exposed to a combination of the above factors, some of which may increase and some decrease his sensitivity to COUMADIN (crystalline warfarin sodium). Because the net effect on his prothrombin time response may be unpredictable under these circumstances, more frequent laboratory monitoring is advisable.

Drugs not yet shown to interact or not to interact with coumarins are best regarded with suspicion, and when their administration is started or stopped, the prothrombin time should be determined more often than usual. Coumarins also affect the action of other drugs. Hypoglycemic agents (chlorpropamide and tolbutamide) and anticonvulsants (phenytoin and phenobarbital) may accumulate in the body as a result of interference with either their metabolism or excretion.

Adverse Reactions: Potential side effects of COUMADIN (crystalline warfarin sodium) include:

1. Minor or major hemorrhage from any tissue or organ—which is an extension of the physiologic activity of prothrombinopenia. The signs and symptoms will vary according to the location and degree or extent of the bleeding. Therefore the possibility of hemorrhage should be considered in evaluating the condition of any anticoagulated patient with complaints which do not indicate an obvious diagnosis. Bleeding during anticoagulant therapy does not always correlate with prothrombin activity. (See TREATMENT FOR OVERDOSAGE.) Bleeding which occurs when the prothrombin time is within the therapeutic range warrants diagnostic investigation since it may unmask a previously unsuspected lesion, e.g., tumor, ulcer etc.
2. Side effects other than hemorrhage are infrequent and consist of alopecia, urticaria, dermatitis, fever, nausea, diarrhea, abdominal cramping, a syndrome called "purple toes," hypersensitivity reactions and a reaction consisting of hemorrhagic infarction and necrosis of the skin.
3. Priapism has been associated with anticoagulant administration, however, a causal relationship has not been established.

Dosage and Laboratory Control: The aim of anticoagulant therapy is to impede the coagulation or clotting mechanism to such an extent that thrombosis will not occur, but at the same time avoiding such extensive impairment as might produce spontaneous bleeding. Effective therapeutic levels with minimal complications can best be achieved in cooperative and well-instructed patients, who keep the doctor informed of their status between visits. COUMADIN patient aids are available to physicians on request.

The administration and dosage of COUMADIN must be individualized for each patient according to the particular patient's sensitivity to the drug as indicated by the prothrombin time. The prothrombin time reflects the depression of vitamin K dependent Factors VII, X and II. These factors, in addition to Factor IX, are affected by coumarin anticoagulants. There are several modifications of the Quick one-stage prothrombin time and the physician should become familiar with the specific method used in his laboratory.

Administration of COUMADIN should be gauged according to prothrombin time determinations by a suitable method. The blood prothrombin time should usually be determined daily after the administration of the initial dose until prothrombin time results stabilize in the therapeutic range. Intervals between subsequent prothrombin time determinations should be based upon the physician's judgment of the patient's reliability and response to warfarin in order to maintain the individual within the therapeutic range. Acceptable intervals for prothrombin time determinations have usually fallen within the range of one to four weeks. Satisfactory levels for maintenance of therapeutic anticoagulation are 1½ to 2½ times the normal prothrombin time (e.g. 18 to 30 seconds, with a control of 12 seconds).

Induction—Induction may be initiated with 10 to 15 mg daily and thereafter (usually 2 or 3 days) adjusted according to prothrombin time response. The basis for this no-loading dose regimen is that the depression of Factors II, IX, and X is not accelerated by the administration of a loading dose. Avoidance of a large priming dose may minimize the possibility of excessive increases in prothrombin time.

Alternatively, 40 to 60 mg for average adult or 20 to 30 mg for elderly and/or debilitated patients for one dose only administered orally, intravenously, or intramuscularly.

Maintenance—Most patients are satisfactorily maintained at a dose of 2 to 10 mg daily. Flexibility of dosage is provided by breaking scored tablets in half. The individual dose and interval should be gauged by the patient's prothrombin response.

Duration of therapy—The duration of therapy in each patient should be individualized. In general, anticoagulant therapy should be continued until the danger of thrombosis and embolism has passed.

Treatment during dentistry and surgery—The management of patients who undergo dental and surgical procedures requires close liaison between attending physicians, surgeons and dentists. Interruption of anticoagulant therapy may precipitate thromboembolism, and conversely, if anticoagulants are maintained at full doses, some patients may hemorrhage excessively. If it is elected to administer anticoagulants prior to, during, or immediately following dental or surgical procedures, it is recommended that the dosage of COUMADIN (crystalline warfarin sodium) be adjusted to maintain the prothrombin time at approximately 1½ to 2½ times the control level. The operative site should be sufficiently limited to permit the effective use of local procedures for hemostasis including absorbable hemostatic agents, sutures, and pressure dressings if necessary. Under these conditions dental and surgical procedures may be performed without undue risk of hemorrhage.

COUMADIN with Heparin—Since a delay intervenes between the administration of the initial dose and the therapeutic prolongation of prothrombin time, it may be advisable in emergency situations to administer sodium heparin initially along with COUMADIN. The initial dose of heparin and injectable COUMADIN may be administered together in the same syringe.

It should be noted that heparin may affect the prothrombin time, and therefore, when patients are receiving both heparin and COUMADIN, the blood sample for prothrombin time determination should be drawn just prior to the next heparin dosage, at least 5 hours after the last intravenous injection or 24 hours after the last subcutaneous injection.

Treatment For Overdosage: Excessive prothrombinopenia, with or without bleeding, is readily controlled by discontinuing COUMADIN (crystalline warfarin sodium), and if necessary, the oral or parenteral administration of vitamin K_1. The appearance of microscopic hematuria, excessive menstrual bleeding, melena, petechiae or oozing from nicks made while shaving are early manifestations of hypoprothrombinemia beyond a safe and satisfactory level.

In excessive prothrombinopenia with mild or no bleeding, omission of one or more doses of COUMADIN may suffice; and if necessary, small doses of vitamin K_1 orally, 2.5 to 10 mg will usually correct the problem.

If minor bleeding persists, or progresses to frank bleeding, vitamin K_1 in doses of 5 to 25 mg may be given parenterally. (Please note recommendations accompanying vitamin K preparations prior to use.)

Fresh whole blood transfusions should be considered in cases of severe bleeding or prothrombinopenic states unresponsive to vitamin K_1. Resumption of COUMADIN administration reverses the effect of vitamin K_1, and a therapeutic hypoprothrombinemia level can again be obtained.

Supplied: **Tablets:** COUMADIN (crystalline warfarin sodium, USP). For oral use, single scored, imprinted numerically in bottles with potencies and colors as follows:

100's and 1000's:	100's:
2 mg lavender	7½ mg yellow
2½ mg orange	10 mg white
5 mg peach	

Also available in Hospital Unit-dose blister package of 100.

Injection: Available as single injection units of amorphous warfarin sodium lyophilized for intravenous or intramuscular use in a box of 6 units for use immediately after reconstitution. 50 mg: Unit consists of 1 vial, 50 mg; sodium chloride, 10 mg; thimerosal, 0.2 mg. pH is adjusted with sodium hydroxide, accompanied by a 2 ml ampul Sterile Water for Injection. Sterile Water for Injection contains no antimicrobial or other substance, and it is not suitable for intravascular injection without first having been made approximately isotonic by the addition of a suitable solute. Use only for reconstitution of the lyophilized product.

---

* Present as crystalline sodium warfarin isopropanol clathrate.

Injection manufactured by Lypho-Med, Inc., Chicago, Illinois 60651 for Endo Laboratories, Inc.

COUMADIN® is a registered U.S. trademark of Endo Laboratories, Inc.

6037-19

[*Shown in Product Identification Section*]

HYCODAN® ©
Tablets and Syrup

Description: Each HYCODAN® Tablet or teaspoonful (5 ml) contains:

Hydrocodone bitartrate........................ 5 mg
WARNING: May be habit forming
Homatropine methylbromide.............. 1.5 mg

Hydrocodone is 7, 8-dihydrocodeinone, a derivative of codeine.

Actions: Hydrocodone is a centrally acting narcotic antitussive providing cough relief for up to 6 hours.

Indications: Based on a review of this drug by the National Academy of Sciences-National Research Council and/or other information, FDA has classified HYCODAN® Tablets and Syrup as follows:

"Probably" effective: for the symptomatic relief of cough.

Final classification of this "probably" effective indication requires further investigation.

Contraindications: HYCODAN® should not be used in patients with glaucoma or hypersensitivity to hydrocodone or homatropine methylbromide.

Warnings: HYCODAN® should be prescribed and administered with the same degree of caution appropriate for the use of other oral narcotic-containing medications since it can produce drug dependence and, therefore, has the potential for abuse. Patients should be warned not to drive a car or operate machinery if they become drowsy or show impaired mental and/or physical abilities while taking HYCODAN®. Patients receiving narcotic analgesics, phenothiazines, other tranquilizers, sedative-hypnotics or other central nervous

Continued on next page

Endo—Cont.

system depressants (including alcohol) concomitantly with HYCODAN® may exhibit an additive central nervous system depression. When such combined therapy is contemplated, the dose of one or both agents should be reduced.

Precautions: Before prescribing medication to suppress or modify cough, it is important to ascertain that the underlying cause of cough is identified, that modification of cough does not increase the risk of clinical or physiologic complications, and that appropriate therapy for the primary disease is provided.

Adverse Reactions: Adverse reactions when they occur include sedation, nausea, vomiting and constipation.

Dosage and Administration: HYCODAN® should be taken after meals and at bedtime, not less than 4 hours apart. Treatment should be started with the suggested initial dose and subsequent doses adjusted if required.
[See table below].

Drug Interactions: The central nervous system depressant effects of HYCODAN® may be additive with that of other central nervous system depressants. See WARNINGS.

Management of Overdosage:

Signs and Symptoms: Serious overdose with HYCODAN® may be characterized by respiratory depression, extreme somnolence progressing to stupor or coma, skeletal muscle flaccidity, cold and clammy skin, and sometimes bradycardia and hypotension. In severe overdosage, apnea, circulatory collapse, cardiac arrest and death may occur. The ingestion of very large amounts of HYCODAN® may, in addition, result in acute homatropine intoxication.

Treatment: Primary attention should be given to the reestablishment of adequate respiratory exchange through provision of a patent airway and the institution of assisted or controlled ventilation. The narcotic antagonist naloxone hydrochloride (NARCAN®) is a specific antidote against respiratory depression which may result from overdosage or unusual sensitivity to narcotics including hydrocodone. Therefore, an appropriate dose of naloxone hydrochloride should be administered, (usual initial adult dose: 0.4 mg) preferably by the intravenous route and simultaneously with efforts at respiratory resuscitation. Since the duration of action of hydrocodone may exceed that of the antagonist, the patient should be kept under continued surveillance and repeated doses of the antagonist should be administered as needed to maintain adequate respiration. Oxygen, intravenous fluids, vasopressors and other supportive measures should be employed as indicated, including treatment for anticholinergic drug intoxication. Gastric emptying may be useful in removing unabsorbed drug. Activated charcoal may be of benefit.

How Supplied: As white, scored tablets in bottles of 100 and 500 or as a red-colored, wild cherry flavored syrup in bottles of one pint and one gallon.

Oral prescription where permitted by State law.

HYCODAN® is a registered trademark of Endo Laboratories, Inc. NARCAN® is a registered U.S. trademark of Endo Pharmaceuticals, Inc.
6014-10

HYCODAN® DOSAGE AND ADMINISTRATION

Usual Dosage

	TABLETS Initial dose	TABLETS Maximum single dose	SYRUP teaspoonful (5 ml) Initial dose	SYRUP teaspoonful (5 ml) Maximum single dose
Adults	1	3	1 tsp.	3 tsps.
Children				
over 12 years	1	2	1 tsp.	2 tsps.
2 to 12 years	½	1	½ tsp.	1 tsp.
under 2 years	¼	¼	¼ tsp.	¼ tsp.

HYCOMINE® Ⓒ

Pediatric Syrup

Description: HYCOMINE Pediatric Syrup contains hydrocodone (dihydrocodeinone) bitartrate, a semi-synthetic centrally-acting narcotic antitussive and phenylpropanolamine hydrochloride, a sympathomimetic amine decongestant for oral administration.

Each teaspoonful (5 ml) contains:
Hydrocodone bitartrate .... 2.5 mg
Warning: May be habit forming
Phenylpropanolamine
hydrochloride .... 12.5 mg

Clinical Pharmacology: Clinical trials have proven hydrocodone bitartrate to be an effective antitussive agent which is pharmacologically 2 to 8 times as potent as codeine. At equi-effective doses, its sedative action is greater than codeine. The precise mechanism of action of hydrocodone and other opiates is not known, however, hydrocodone is believed to act by directly depressing the cough center. In excessive doses hydrocodone, like other opium derivatives, will depress respiration. The effect of hydrocodone in therapeutic doses on the cardiovascular system is insignificant. The constipation effects of hydrocodone are much weaker than that of morphine and no stronger than that of codeine. Hydrocodone can produce miosis, euphoria, physical and psychological dependence. At therapeutic antitussive doses, it does exert analgesic effects. Following a 10 mg oral dose of hydrocodone administered to five adult male human subjects, the mean peak concentration was 23.6 ± 5.2 ng/ml. Maximum serum levels were achieved at 1.3 ± 0.3 hours and the half-life was determined to be 3.8 ± 0.3 hours. Hydrocodone exhibits a complex pattern of metabolism including O-demethylation, N-demethylation and 6-keto reduction to the corresponding 6-α- and 6-β-hydroxymetabolites.

Phenylpropanolamine effects its vasoconstrictor activity by releasing noradrenaline from sympathetic nerve endings, and from direct stimulation of α-adrenoreceptors in blood vessels.

Indications and Usage: HYCOMINE Pediatric Syrup is indicated for the symptomatic relief of cough and nasal congestion.

Contraindications: HYCOMINE Pediatric Syrup is contraindicated in patients hypersensitive to hydrocodone or phenylpropanolamine and concurrent MAO inhibitor therapy. Patients known to be hypersensitive to other opioids or sympathomimetic amines may exhibit cross sensitivity to HYCOMINE Pediatric Syrup. Phenylpropanolamine is contraindicated in patients with heart disease, hypertension, diabetes or hyperthyroidism. Hydrocodone is contraindicated in the presence of an intracranial lesion associated with increased intracranial pressure; and whenever ventilatory function is depressed.

Warnings: May be habit forming. Hydrocodone can produce drug dependence of the morphine type and therefore has the potential for being abused. Psychic dependence, physical dependence and tolerance may develop upon repeated administration of HYCOMINE Pediatric Syrup and it should be prescribed and administered with the same degree of caution appropriate to the use of other narcotic drugs (See DRUG ABUSE AND DEPENDENCE).

Respiratory Depression: HYCOMINE Pediatric Syrup produces dose-related respiratory depression by directly acting on brain stem respiratory centers. If respiratory depression occurs, it may be antagonized by the use of NARCAN® (naloxone hydrochloride) and other supportive measures when indicated.

Head Injury and Increased Intracranial Pressure: The respiratory depressant properties of narcotics and their capacity to elevate cerebrospinal fluid pressure may be markedly exaggerated in the presence of head injury, other intracranial lesions or a pre-existing increase in intracranial pressure. Furthermore, narcotics produce adverse reactions which may obscure the clinical course of patients with head injuries.

Acute Abdominal Conditions: The administration of HYCOMINE Pediatric Syrup or other narcotics may obscure the diagnosis or clinical course of patients with actue abdominal conditions.

Phenylpropanolamine: Hypertensive crises can occur with concurrent use of phenylpropanolamine and monoamine oxidase (MAO) inhibitors, indomethacin or with beta-blockers and methyldopa.

If a hypertensive crisis occurs these drugs should be discontinued immediately and therapy to lower blood pressure should be instituted immediately. Fever should be managed by means of external cooling.

Precautions: Before prescribing medication to suppress or modify cough, it is important to ascertain that the underlying cause of cough is identified, that modification of cough does not increase the risk of clinical or physiologic complications, and that appropriate therapy for the primary disease is provided.

Usage in Ambulatory Patients: Hydrocodone, like all narcotics, may impair the mental and/ or physical abilities required for the performance of potentially hazardous tasks such as operating recreational vehicles or machinery; phenylpropanolamine may produce a rapid pulse, dizziness or palpitations; patients should be cautioned accordingly.

Drug Interactions: Patients receiving other narcotic analgesics, general anesthetics, phenothiazines, other tranquilizers, sedative-hypnotics or other CNS depressants (including alcohol) concomitantly with hydrocodone may exhibit an additive CNS depression. When such combined therapy is contemplated, the dose of one or both agents should be reduced. The use of phenylpropanolamine with other sympathomimetic amines and MAO inhibitors may produce an additive elevation blood pressure. (See WARNINGS).

Carcinogenesis, mutagenesis, impairment of fertility: Carcinogenicity, mutagenicity and reproduction studies have not been conducted with HYCOMINE Pediatric Syrup.

Usage in Pregnancy: Pregnancy Category C. Animal reproduction studies have not been conducted with HYCOMINE Pediatric Syrup. It is also not known whether HYCOMINE Pediatric Syrup can cause fetal harm when administered to a pregnant woman or can affect reproductive capacity. HYCOMINE Pediatric Syrup should be given to a pregnant woman only if clearly needed.

Nonteratogenic effects: Babies born to mothers who have been taking opioids regularly prior to delivery will be physically dependent. The withdrawal signs include irritability and excessive crying, tremors, hyperactive reflexes, increased respiratory rate, increased stools, sneezing, yawning, vomiting and fever. The intensity of the syndrome does not always correlate with the duration of maternal opioid use or dose. There is no consensus on the best method of managing withdrawal. Chlorpromazine 0.7–1.0 mg/kg q 6 h, phenobarbital 2 mg/kg q 6 h, and paregoric 2–4 drops/kg q 4 h, have been used to treat withdrawal symptoms in infants. The duration of therapy is 4 to 28 days, with the dosages decreased as tolerated.

Nursing mothers: It is not known whether this drug is excreted in human milk. Because many drugs are excreted in human milk and because of the potential for serious adverse reactions in nursing infants from HYCOMINE Pediatric Syrup, a decision should be made whether to discontinue nursing or discontinue the drug, taking into account the importance of the drug to the mother.

Pediatric use: Safety and effectiveness in children below the age of 6 years have not been established.

Adverse Reactions:

Respiratory System: Hydrocodone produces dose-related respiratory depression by acting directly on brain stem respiratory centers.

Cardiovascular System: Hypertension, postural hypotension, tachycardia and palpitations.

Genitourinary System: Ureteral spasm, spasm of vesical sphincters and urinary retention have been reported with opiates.

Central Nervous System: Sedation, drowsiness, mental clouding, lethargy, impairment of mental and physical performance, anxiety, fear, dysphoria, dizziness, psychic dependence, mood changes, and blurred vision.

Gastrointestinal System: Nausea and vomiting occur more frequently in ambulatory than in recumbent patients.

Drug Abuse and Dependence: Special care should be exercised in prescribing hydrocodone for emotionally unstable patients and for those with a history of drug misuse. Such patients should be closely supervised when long-term therapy is contemplated.

HYCOMINE Pediatric Syrup is a Schedule III narcotic. Psychic dependence, physical dependence, and tolerance may develop upon repeated administration of narcotics; therefore, HYCOMINE Pediatric Syrup should always be prescribed and administered with caution.

Physical dependence is the condition in which continued administration of the drug is required to prevent the appearance of a withdrawal syndrome.

Patients physically dependent on opioids will develop an abstinence syndrome upon abrupt discontinuation of the opioid or following the administration of a narcotic antagonist. The character and severity of the withdrawal symptoms are related to the degree of physical dependence. Manifestations of opioid withdrawal are similar to but milder than that of morphine and include lacrimation, rhinorrhea, yawning, sweating, restlessness, dilated pupils, anorexia, gooseflesh, irritability and tremor. In more severe forms, nausea, vomiting, intestinal spasm and diarrhea, increased heart rate and blood pressure, chills, and pains in bones and muscles of the back and extremities may occur. Peak effects will usually be apparent at 48 to 72 hours.

Treatment of withdrawal is usually managed by providing sufficient quantities of an opioid to suppress **severe** withdrawal symptoms and then gradually reducing the dose of opioid over a period of several days.

Overdosage:

Signs and Symptoms: Serious overdosage with HYCOMINE Pediatric Syrup is characterized by respiratory depression (a decrease in respiratory rate and/or tidal volume, Cheyne-Stokes respiration, cyanosis), extreme somnolence progressing to stupor or coma, skeletal muscle flaccidity, cold and clammy skin, and sometimes bradycardia and hypotension. In severe overdosage apnea, circulatory collapse, cardiac arrest, and death may occur.

The signs and symptoms of overdosage of the individual components of HYCOMINE Pediatric Syrup may be modified in varying degrees by the presence of other active ingredients. Overdosage with phenylpropanolamine alone may result in tremor, restlessness, increased motor activity, agitation and hallucinations.

Treatment: Primary attention should be given to the reestablishment of adequate respiratory exchange through provision of a patent airway and the institution of assisted or controlled ventilation. The narcotic antagonist naloxone hydrochloride (NARCAN®) is a specific antidote against respiratory depression which may result from overdosage or unusual sensitivity to narcotics including hydrocodone. Therefore, an appropriate dose of naloxone hydrochloride should be administered (usual initial child dose; 0.01 mg/kg body weight. For further information see NARCAN® full prescribing information) preferably by the intravenous route, simultaneously with efforts at respiratory resuscitation. Since the duration of action of hydrocodone may exceed that of the antagonist, the patient should be kept under continued surveillance and repeated doses of the antagonist should be administered as needed to maintain adequate respiration. Oxygen, intravenous fluids, vasopressors and other supportive measures should be employed as indicated.

Gastric emptying may be useful in removing unabsorbed drug. Activated charcoal may be of benefit.

Dosage and Administration:

Usual Dosage: (age 6–12 years) One teaspoonful (5 ml) after meals and at bedtime, not less than 4 hours apart (not to exceed 6 teaspoonsful in a 24 hour period).

How Supplied: HYCOMINE Pediatric Syrup is available as a green-colored, fruit flavored syrup in bottles as follows:

One pint: NDC 0056-0247-16

Store at controlled room temperature (59°–86° F, 15°–30° C).

HYCOMINE® is a Registered Trademark of Endo Laboratories, Inc. NARCAN® is a Registered U.S. Trademark of Endo Pharmaceuticals, Inc.

6130-2

HYCOMINE® ©

Syrup

Description: HYCOMINE Syrup contains hydrocodone (dihydrocodeinone) bitartrate, a semi-synthetic centrally-acting narcotic antitussive and phenylpropanolamine hydrochloride, a sympathomimetic amine decongestant for oral administration.

Each teaspoonful (5 ml) contains:

Hydrocodone bitartrate .... 5 mg

Warning: May be habit forming

Phenylpropanolamine hydrochloride .. 25 mg

Clinical Pharmacology: Clinical trials have proven hydrocodone bitartrate to be an effective antitussive agent which is pharmacologically 2 to 8 times as potent as codeine. At equi-effective doses, its sedative action is greater than codeine. The precise mechanism of action of hydrocodone and other opiates is not known, however, hydrocodone is believed to act by directly depressing the cough center, in excessive doses hydrocodone, like other opium derivatives, will depress respiration. The effects of hydrocodone in therapeutic doses on the cardiovascular system is insignificant. The constipation effects of hydrocodone are much weaker than that of morphine and no stronger than that of codeine. Hydrocodone can produce miosis, euphoria, physical and psychological dependence. At therapeutic antitussive doses, it does exert analgesic effects. Following a 10 mg oral dose of hydrocodone administered to five adult male human subjects, the mean peak concentration was 23.6 ± 5.2 ng/ml. Maximum serum levels were achieved at 1.3 ± 0.3 hours and the half-life was determined to be 3.8 ± 0.3 hours. Hydrocodone exhibits a complex pattern of metabolism including O-demethylation, N-demethylation and 6-keto reduction to the corresponding 6-α- and 6-β-hydroxymetabolites.

Phenylpropanolamine effects its vasoconstrictor activity by releasing noradrenaline from sympathetic nerve endings, and from direct stimulation of α-adrenoreceptors in blood vessels.

Indications and Usage: HYCOMINE Syrup is indicated for the symptomatic relief of cough and nasal congestion.

Contraindications: HYCOMINE is contraindicated in patients hypersensitive to hydrocodone or phenylpropanolamine, and concurrent MAO inhibitor therapy. Patients known to be hypersensitive to other opioids or sympathomimetic amines may exhibit cross sensitivity to HYCOMINE. Phenylpropanolamine is contraindicated in patients with heart disease, hypertension, diabetes or hyperthyroidism. Hydrocodone is contraindicated in the presence of an intracranial lesion associated with increased intracranial pressure; and whenever ventilatory function is depressed.

Warnings: May be habit forming. Hydrocodone can produce drug dependence of the morphine type and therefore has the potential for being abused. Psychic dependence, physical dependence and tolerance may develop upon repeated administration of HYCOMINE and it should be prescribed and administered with the same degree of caution appropriate to the use of other narcotic drugs (See DRUG ABUSE AND DEPENDENCE).

Respiratory Depression: HYCOMINE produces dose-related respiratory depression by directly acting on brain stem respiratory centers. If respiratory depression occurs, it may be antagonized by the use of NARCAN® (naloxone hydrochloride) and other supportive measures when indicated.

Head Injury and Increased Intracranial Pressure: The respiratory depression properties of narcotics and their capacity to elevate cerebrospinal fluid pressure may be markedly exaggerated in the presence of head injury, other intracranial lesions or a pre-existing increase in intracranial pressure. Furthermore, narcotics produce adverse reactions which may obscure the clinical course of patients with head injuries.

Acute abdominal conditions: The administration of HYCOMINE or other narcotics may obscure the diagnosis or clinical course of patients with acute abdominal conditions.

Phenylpropanolamine: Hypertensive crises can occur with concurrent use of phenylpropanolamine and monoamine oxidase (MAO) inhibitors, indomethacin or with beta-blockers and methyldopa.

If a hypertensive crisis occurs these drugs should be discontinued immediately and therapy to lower blood pressure should be instituted immediately. Fever should be managed by means of external cooling.

Precautions: Before prescribing medication to suppress or modify cough, it is important to ascertain that the underlying cause of cough is identified, that modification of cough does not increase the risk of clinical or physiologic complications, and that appropriate therapy for the primary disease is provided.

Usage in Ambulatory Patients: Hydrocodone, like all narcotics, may impair the mental and /or physical abilities required for the performance of potentially hazardous tasks such as driving a car or operating machinery; phenylpropanolamine may produce a rapid pulse, dizziness or palpitations; patients should be cautioned accordingly.

Drug Interactions: Patients receiving other narcotic analgesics, general anesthetics, phenothiazines, other tranquilizers, sedative-hyp-

Continued on next page

Endo—Cont.

notics or other CNS depressants (including alcohol) concomitantly with hydrocodone may exhibit an additive CNS depression. When such combined therapy is contemplated, the dose of one or both agents should be reduced. The use of phenylpropanolamine with other sympathomimetic amines and MAO inhibitors may produce an additive elevation of blood pressure (See WARNINGS).

Carcinogenesis, mutagenesis, Impairment of fertility: Carcinogenicity, mutagenicity and reproduction studies have not been conducted with HYCOMINE.

Usage in Pregnancy: Pregnancy Category C. Animal reproduction studies have not been conducted with HYCOMINE. It is also not known whether HYCOMINE can cause fetal harm when administered to a pregnant woman or can affect reproductive capacity. HYCOMINE should be given to a pregnant woman only if clearly needed.

Nonteratogenic effects: Babies born to mothers who have been taking opioids regularly prior to delivery will be physically dependent. The withdrawal signs include irritability and excessive crying, tremors, hyperactive reflexes, increased respiratory rate, increased stools, sneezing, yawning, vomiting and fever. The intensity of the syndrome does not always correlate with the duration of maternal opioid use or dose. There is no consensus on the best method of managing withdrawal. Chlorpromazine 0.7–1.0 mg/kg q 6 h, phenobarbital 2 mg/kg q 6 h, and paregoric 1–4 drops/kg q 4 h, have been used to treat withdrawal symptoms in infants. The duration of therapy is 4 to 28 days, with the dosages decreased as tolerated.

Nursing mothers: It is not known whether this drug is excreted in human milk. Because many drugs are excreted in human milk and because of the potential for serious adverse reactions in nursing infants from HYCOMINE, a decision should be made whether to discontinue nursing or discontinue the drug, taking into account the importance of the drug to the mother.

Pediatric use: HYCOMINE Syrup should not be used in children.

Adverse Reactions:

Respiratory System: Hydrocodone produces dose-related respiratory depression by acting directly on brain stem respiratory centers.

Cardiovascular System: Hypertension, postural hypotension, tachycardia and palpitations.

Genitourinary System: Ureteral spasm, spasm of vesical sphincters and urinary retention have been reported with opiates.

Central Nervous Systems: Sedation, drowsiness, mental clouding, lethargy, impairment of mental and physical performance, anxiety, fear, dysphoria, dizziness, psychic dependence, mood changes and blurred vision.

Gastrointestinal System: Nausea and vomiting occur more frequently in ambulatory than in recumbent patients.

Drug Abuse and Dependence: Special care should be exercised in prescribing hydrocodone for emotionally unstable patients and for those with a history of drug misuse. Such patients should be closely supervised when long-term therapy is contemplated.

HYCOMINE Syrup is a Schedule III narcotic. Psychic dependence, physical dependence, and tolerance may develop upon repeated administration of narcotics; therefore, HYCOMINE Syrup should always he prescribed and administered with caution. Physical dependence is the condition in which continued administration of the drug is required to prevent the appearance of a withdrawal syndrome.

Patients physically dependent on opioids will develop an abstinence syndrome upon abrupt discontinuation of the opioid or following the administration of a narcotic antagonist. The character and severity of the withdrawal symptoms are related to the degree of physical dependence. Manifestations of opioid withdrawal are similar to but milder than that of morphine and include lacrimation, rhinorrhea, yawning, sweating, restlessness, dilated pupils, anorexia, gooseflesh, irritability and tremor. In more severe forms, nausea, vomiting, intestinal spasm and diarrhea, increased heart rate and blood pressure, chills, and pains in bones and muscles of the back and extremities may occur. Peak effects will usually be apparent at 48 to 72 hours.

Treatment of withdrawal is usually managed by providing sufficient quantities of an opioid to suppress severe withdrawal symptoms and then gradually reducing the dose of opioid over a period of several days.

Overdosage:

Signs and Symptoms: Serious overdosage with HYCOMINE is characterized by respiratory depression (a decrease in respiratory rate and/or tidal volume, Cheyne-Stokes respiration, cyanosis), extreme somnolence progressing to stupor or coma, skeletal muscle flaccidity, cold and clammy skin, and sometimes bradycardia and hypotension. In severe overdosage apnea, circulatory collapse, cardiac arrest, and death may occur.

The signs and symptoms of overdosage of the individual components of HYCOMINE Syrup may be modified in varying degrees by the presence of other active ingredients. Overdosage with phenylpropanolamine alone may result in tremor, restlessness, increased motor activity, agitation and hallucinations.

Treatment: Primary attention should be given to the reestablishment of adequate respiratory exchange through provision of a patent airway and the institution of assisted or controlled ventilation. The narcotic antagonist naloxone hydrochloride (NARCAN®) is a specific antidote against respiratory depression which may result from overdosage or unusual sensitivity to narcotics including hydrocodone. Therefore, an appropriate dose of naloxone hydrochloride should be administered (usual initial adult dose 0.4 mg. For further information see NARCAN® full prescribing information) preferably by the intravenous route, simultaneously with efforts at respiratory resuscitation. Since the duration of action of hydrocodone may exceed that of the antagonist, the patient should be kept under continued surveillance and repeated doses of the antagonist should be administered as needed to maintain adequate respiration. Oxygen, intravenous fluids, vasopressors and other supportive measures should be employed as indicated.

Gastric emptying may be useful in removing unabsorbed drug. Activated charcoal may be of benefit.

Dosage and Administration: Usual Adult Dose: One teaspoonful (5 ml) after meals and at bedtime, not less than 4 hours apart (not to exceed 6 teaspoonful in a 24 hour period).

How Supplied: HYCOMINE® Syrup is available as an orange-colored, fruit-flavored syrup in bottles as follows:

One pint:	NDC 0056-0246-16
One gallon:	NDC 0056-0246-82

Store at controlled room temperature (59°–86°F, 15°–30°C).

HYCOMINE® is an Endo Registered Trademark. NARCAN® is an Endo Registered U.S. Trademark of Endo Pharmaceuticals, Inc.

6129-1

HYCOMINE® COMPOUND ©

Description: HYCOMINE Compound tablets contain hydrocodone (dihydrocodeinone) bitartrate, a semi-synthetic centrally-acting narcotic antitussive; chlorpheniramine maleate, an antihistamine; phenylephrine hydrochloride, a sympathomimetic amine decongestant; acetaminophen, an analgesic/antipyretic; and caffeine, a centrally-acting stimulant; for oral administration.

Each HYCOMINE Compound tablet contains:

Hydrocodone bitartrate	5 mg
WARNING: May be habit forming	
Chlorpheniramine maleate	2 mg
Phenylephrine hydrochloride	10 mg
Acetaminophen	250 mg
Caffeine	30 mg

Clinical Pharmacology: Clinical trials have proven hydrocodone bitartrate to be an effective antitussive agent which is pharmacologically 2 to 8 times as potent as codeine. At equi-effective doses, its sedative action is greater than codeine. The precise mechanism of action of hydrocodone and other opiates is not known, however, hydrocodone is believed to act by directly depressing the cough center. In excessive doses hydrocodone, like other opium derivatives, will depress respiration. The effects of hydrocodone in therapeutic doses on the cardiovascular system is insignificant. The constipation effects of hydrocodone are much weaker than that of morphine and no stronger than that of codeine. Hydrocodone can produce miosis, euphoria, physical and psychological dependence. At therapeutic antitussive doses, it does exert analgesic effects. Following a 10 mg oral dose of hydrocodone administered to five adult male human subjects, the mean peak concentration was 23.6 ± 5.2 ng/ml. Maximum serum levels were achieved at 1.3 ± 0.3 hours and the half-life was determined to be 3.8 ± hours. Hydrocodone exhibits a complex pattern of metabolism including O-demethylation, N-demethylation and 6-keto reduction to the corresponding 6-α- and 6-β-hydroxymetabolites.

Chlorpheniramine maleate is a competitive H_1-receptor histamine blocking drug, thereby counteracting the effects of histamine release associated with allergic manifestations of upper respiratory tract inflammatory disorders. H_1-blocking drugs inhibit the actions of histamine on smooth muscle, capillary permeability, and can both stimulate and depress the central nervous system. Phenylephrine hydrochloride effects its vasoconstrictor activity by releasing noradrenaline from sympathetic nerve endings, and from direct stimulation of α-adreno-receptors in blood vessels. Acetaminophen is an antipyretic and peripherally acting analgesic. Caffeine is a central nervous system stimulant.

Indications and Usage: HYCOMINE Compound is indicated for the symptomatic relief of cough, nasal congestion, and discomfort associated with upper respiratory tract infections.

Contraindications: HYCOMINE Compound is contraindicated in patients hypersensitive to any component of the drug, and concurrent MAO inhibitor therapy. Patients known to be hypersensitive to other opioids, antihistamines, or sympathomimetic amines may exhibit cross sensitivity with HYCOMINE Compound. Phenylephrine is contraindicated in patients with heart disease, hypertension, diabetes or hyperthyroidism. Hydrocodone is contraindicated in the presence of an intracranial lesion associated with increased intracranial pressure; and whenever ventilatory function is depressed.

Warnings: May be habit forming. Hydrocodone can produce drug dependence of the morphine type and therefore has the potential for being abused. Psychic dependence, physical dependence and tolerance may develop upon repeated administration of HYCOMINE Compound and it should be prescribed and administered with the same degree of caution appropriate to the use of other narcotic drugs. (See DRUG ABUSE AND DEPENDENCE).

Respiratory Depression: HYCOMINE Compound produces dose-related respiratory depression by directly acting on brain stem respiratory centers. If respiratory depression occurs, it may be antagonized by the use of NAR-

CAN® (naloxone hydrochloride) and other supportive measures when indicated.

Head Injury and Increased Intracranial Pressure: The respiratory depressant properties of narcotics and their capacity to elevate cerebrospinal fluid pressure may be markedly exaggerated in the presence of head injury, other intracranial lesions or a pre-existing increase in intracranial pressure. Furthermore, narcotics produce adverse reactions which may obscure the clinical course of patients with head injuries.

Acute abdominal conditions: The administration of HYCOMINE Compound or other narcotics may obscure the diagnosis or clinical course of patients with acute abdominal conditions.

Phenylephrine: Hypersensitive crises can occur with concurrent use of phenylephrine and monoamine oxidase (MAO) inhibitors, indomethacin or with beta-blockers and methyldopa.

If a hypertensive crisis occurs these drugs should be discontinued immediately and therapy to lower blood pressure should be instituted immediately. Fever should be managed by means of external cooling.

Chlorpheniramine: Antihistamines may produce drowsiness or excitation, particularly in children and elderly patients.

Precautions: Before prescribing medication to suppress or modify cough, it is important to ascertain that the underlying cause of cough is identified, that modification of cough does not increase the risk of clinical or physiologic complications, and that appropriate therapy for the primary disease is provided.

Usage in Ambulatory Patients: Hydrocodone, like all narcotics, and antihistamines such as chlorpheniramine maleate, may impair the mental and/or physical abilities required for the performance of potentially hazardous tasks such as driving a car or operating machinery; phenylephrine may produce a rapid pulse, dizziness or palpitations; patients should be cautioned accordingly.

Drug Interactions: Patients receiving other narcotic analgesics, general anesthetics, phenothiazines, other tranquilizers, sedative-hypnotics or other CNS depressants (including alcohol) concomitantly with hydrocodone may exhibit an additive CNS depression. When such combined therapy is contemplated, the dose of one or both agents should be reduced. The use of phenylephrine with other sympathomimetic amines and MAO inhibitors may produce an additive elevation of blood pressure. MAO inhibitors may prolong the anticholinergic effects of antihistamines. (See WARNINGS).

Carcinogenesis, mutagenesis, impairment of fertility: Carcinogenicity, mutagenicity, and reproduction studies have not been conducted with HYCOMINE Compound.

Usage in Pregnancy: Pregnancy Category C. Animal reproduction studies have not been conducted with HYCOMINE Compound. It is also not known whether HYCOMINE Compound can cause fetal harm when administered to a pregnant woman or can affect reproductive capacity. HYCOMINE Compound should be given to a pregnant woman only if clearly needed.

Nonteratogenic effects: Babies born to mothers who have been taking opioids regularly prior to delivery will be physically dependent. The withdrawal signs include irritability and excessive crying, tremors, hyperactive reflexes, increased respiratory rate, increased stools, sneezing, yawning, vomiting and fever. The intensity of the syndrome does not always correlate with the duration of maternal opioid use or dose. Chlorpromazine 0.7–1.0 mg/kg q 6 h, phenobarbital 2 mg/kg q 6 h, and paregoric 2–4 drops/kg q 4 h, have been used to treat withdrawal symptoms in infants. The duration of therapy is 4 to 28 days, with the dosages decreased as tolerated.

Nursing mothers: It is not known whether this drug is excreted in human milk. Because many drugs are excreted in human milk and because of the potential for serious adverse reactions in nursing infants from HYCOMINE Compound, a decision should be made whether to discontinue nursing or discontinue the drug, taking into account the importance of the drug to the mother.

Pediatric use: Safety and effectiveness in children below the age of 2 years have not been established.

Adverse Reactions:

Respiratory System: Hydrocodone produces dose-related respiratory depression by acting directly on brain stem respiratory centers.

Cardiovascular System: Hypertension, postural hypotension, tachycardia and palpitations.

Genitourinary System: Ureteral spasm, spasm of vesical sphincters and urinary retention have been reported with opiates.

Central Nervous System: Sedation, drowsiness, mental clouding, lethargy, impairment of mental and physical performance, anxiety, fear, dysphoria, dizziness, psychic dependence, mood changes, and blurred vision.

Gastrointestinal System: Nausea and vomiting occur more frequently in ambulatory than in recumbent patients.

Drug Abuse and Dependence: Special care should be exercised in prescribing hydrocodone for emotionally unstable patients and for those with a history of drug misuse. Such patients should be closely supervised when long-term therapy is contemplated.

HYCOMINE Compound is a Schedule III narcotic. Psychic dependence, physical dependence, and tolerance may develop upon repeated administration of narcotics; therefore, HYCOMINE Compound should always be prescribed and administered with caution. Physical dependence is the condition in which continued administration of the drug is required to prevent the appearance of a withdrawal syndrome.

Patients physically dependent on opioids will develop an abstinence syndrome upon abrupt discontinuation of the opioid or following the administration of a narcotic antagonist. The character and severity of the withdrawal symptoms are related to the degree of physical dependence. Manifestations of opioid withdrawal are similar to but milder than that of morphine and include lacrimation, rhinorrhea, yawning, sweating, restlessness, dilated pupils, anorexia, gooseflesh, irritability and tremor. In more severe forms, nausea, vomiting, intestinal spasms and diarrhea, increased heart rate and blood pressure, chills, and pains in bones and muscles of the back and extremities may occur. Peak effects will usually be apparent at 48 to 72 hours.

Treatment of withdrawal is usually managed by providing sufficient quantities of an opioid to suppress **severe** withdrawal symptoms and then gradually reducing the dose of opioid over a period of several days.

Overdosage: The signs and symptoms of overdosage of the individual components of HYCOMINE Compound may be modified in varying degrees by the presence of other active ingredients.

Signs and Symptoms: Serious overdosage with hydrocodone is characterized by respiratory depression (a decrease in respiratory rate and/or tidal volume. Cheyne-Stokes respiration, cyanosis), extreme somnolence progressing to stupor or coma, skeletal muscle flaccidity, cold and clammy skin, and sometimes bradycardia and hypotension. In severe overdosage apnea, circulatory collapse, cardiac arrest, and death may occur. The ingestion of large amounts of acetaminophen may produce hepatic toxicity.

The signs and symptoms of overdosage of the individual components of HYCOMINE Compound may be modified in varying degrees by the presence of other active ingredients. Overdosage with phenylephrine alone may result in tremor, restlessness, increased motor activity, agitation and hallucinations.

Treatment: Primary attention should be given to the reestablishment of adequate respiratory exchange through provision of a patent airway and the institution of assisted or controlled ventilation. The narcotic antagonist naloxone hydrochloride (NARCAN®) is a specific antidote against respiratory depression which may result from overdosage or unusual sensitivity to narcotics including hydrocodone. Therefore, an appropriate dose of naloxone hydrochloride should be administered (usual initial adult dose: 0.4 mg; usual initial child dose is 0.01 mg/kg body weight. For further information see NARCAN® full prescribing information) preferably by the intravenous route, simultaneously with efforts at respiratory resuscitation. Since the duration of action of hydrocodone may exceed that of the antagonist, the patient should be kept under continued surveillance and repeated doses of the antagonist should be administered as needed to maintain adequate respiration. Oxygen, intravenous fluids, vasopressors and other supportive measures should be employed as indicated. Gastric emptying may be useful in removing unabsorbed drug. Activated charcoal may be of benefit.

Treatment of acute acetaminophen overdosage is purely symptomatic.

Dosage and Administration: Usual dosage, not less than 4 hours apart:

Adults: 1 tablet 4 times a day
Children: 6 to 12 years: ½ tablet 4 times a day
Children: 2 to 6 years: ½ tablet twice daily

How Supplied: HYCOMINE® Compound is available as a coral pink, scored tablet in bottles as follows:

Bottles of 100 NDC 0056-0048-70
Bottles of 500 NDC 0056-0048-85

Store at controlled room temperature (59°–86° F, 15°–30° C)

HYCOMINE® is a Registered Trademark of Endo Laboratories, Inc.
NARCAN® is a Registered U.S. Trademark of Endo Laboratories, Inc.
6015-7

[*Shown in Product Identification Section*]

HYCOTUSS® ©
Expectorant

Description: HYCOTUSS Expectorant Syrup contains hydrocodone (dihydrocodeinone) bitartrate, a semi-synthetic centrally-acting narcotic, antitussive and guaifenesin, an expectorant for oral administration.

Each teaspoonful (5 ml) contains:
Hydrocodone bitartrate .... 5 mg
Warning: May be habit forming
Guaifenesin .... 100 mg
Alcohol U.S.P. 10% v/v

Clinical Pharmacology: Clinical trials have proven hydrocodone bitartrate to be an effective antitussive agent which is pharmacologically 2 to 8 times as potent as codeine. At equi-effective doses, its sedative action is greater than codeine. The precise mechanism of action of hydrocodone and other opiates is not known, however, hydrocodone is believed to act by directly depressing the cough center. In excessive doses hydrocodone, like other opium derivatives, can depress respiration. The effects of hydrocodone in therapeutic doses on the cardiovascular system is insignificant. The constipation effects of hydrocodone are much weaker than that of morphine and no stronger than that of codeine. Hydrocodone can produce miosis, euphoria, physical and psychological dependence. At therapeutic antitussive doses, it does exert analgesic effects. Following a 10 mg oral dose of hydrocodone administered to five male human subjects, the

Continued on next page

Endo—Cont.

mean peak concentration was 23.6 ± 5.2 ng/ml. Maximum serum levels were achieved at 1.3 ± 0.3 hours and half-life was determined to be 3.8 ± 0.3 hours. Hydrocodone exhibits a complex pattern of metabolism including O-demethylation, N-demethylation and 6-keto reduction to the corresponding 6-α- and 6-β-hydroxymetabolites.

The exact mechanism of action is not established but guaifenesin is believed to act by stimulating receptors in the gastric mucosa that initiates a reflex secretion of respiratory tract fluid, thereby increasing the volume and decreasing the viscosity of bronchial secretions. Studies with guaifenesin indicate that it is rapidly absorbed from the gastrointestinal tract and has a half-life of one hour.

Indications and Usage: HYCOTUSS Expectorant is indicated for the symptomatic relief of irritating non-productive cough associated with upper and lower respiratory tract congestion.

Contraindications: HYCOTUSS Expectorant is contraindicated in patients hypersensitive to hydrocodone or guaifenesin. Patients known to be hypersensitive to other opioids may exhibit cross sensitivity to HYCOTUSS Expectorant. Hydrocodone is contraindicated in the presence of an intracranial lesion associated with increased intracranial pressure; and whenever ventilatory function is depressed.

Warnings: May be habit forming. Hydrocodone can produce drug dependence of the morphine type and therefore has the potential for being abused. Psychic dependence, physical dependence and tolerance may develop upon repeated administration of HYCOTUSS Expectorant and it should be prescribed and administered with the same degree of caution appropriate to the use of other narcotic drugs (See DRUG ABUSE AND DEPENDENCE).

Respiratory Depression: HYCOTUSS Expectorant produces dose-related respiratory depression by directly acting on the brain stem respiratory centers. If respiratory depression occurs, it may be antagonized by the use of NARCAN® (naloxone hydrochloride) and other supportive measures when indicated.

Head Injury and Increased Intracranial Pressure: The respiratory depressant properties of narcotics and their capacity to elevate cerebrospinal fluid pressure may be markedly exaggerated in the presence of head injury, other intracranial lesions or a pre-existing increase in intracranial pressure. Furthermore, narcotics produce adverse reactions which may obscure the clinical course of patients with head injuries.

Acute Abdominal Conditions: The administration of HYCOTUSS Expectorant or other opioids may obscure the diagnosis or clinical course of patients with acute abdominal conditions.

Precautions: Before prescribing medication to suppress or modify cough, it is important to ascertain that the underlying cause of cough is identified, that modification of cough does not increase the risk of clinical or physiologic complications, and that appropriate therapy for the primary disease is provided.

Usage in Ambulatory Patients: Hydrocodone, like all narcotics, may impair the mental and/or physical abilities required for the performance of potentially hazardous tasks such as driving a car or operating machinery, and patients should be warned accordingly.

Drug Interactions: Patients receiving other narcotic analgesics, general anesthetics, phenothiazines, other tranquilizers, sedative hypnotics or other CNS depressants (including alcohol) concomitantly with hydrocodone may exhibit an additive CNS depression. When such combined therapy is contemplated, the dose of one or both agents should be reduced. (See WARNINGS).

Laboratory Interactions: The metabolite of guaifenesin has been found to produce an apparent increase in urinary 5-hydroxyindoleacetic acid, and guaifenesin therefore may interfere with the interpretation of this test for the diagnosis of carcinoid syndrome. Guaifenesin administration should be discontinued 24 hours prior to the collection of urine specimens for the determination of 5-hydroxyindoleacetic acid.

Carcinogenesis, mutagenesis, impairment of fertility: Carcinogenicity, mutagenicity and reproduction studies have not been conducted with HYCOTUSS Expectorant.

Usage in Pregnancy: Pregnancy Category C. Animal reproduction studies have not been conducted with HYCOTUSS Expectorant. It is also not known whether HYCOTUSS Expectorant can cause fetal harm when administered to a pregnant woman or can affect reproductive capacity. HYCOTUSS Expectorant should be given to a pregnant woman only if clearly needed.

Nonteratogenic effects: Babies born to mothers who have been taking opioids regularly prior to delivery will be physically dependent. The withdrawal signs include irritability and excessive crying, tremors, hyperactive reflexes, increased respiratory rate, increased stools, sneezing, yawning, vomiting and fever. The intensity of the syndrome does not always correlate with the duration of maternal opioid use or dose. There is no consensus on the best method of managing withdrawal. Chlorpromazine 0.7–1.0 mg/kg q 6 h, phenobarbital 2 mg/kg q 6 h, and paregoric 2–4 drops/kg q 4 h, have been used to treat withdrawal symptoms in infants. The duration of therapy is 4 to 28 days, with the dosages decreased as tolerated.

Nursing mothers: It is not known whether this drug is excreted in human milk. Because many drugs are excreted in human milk and because of the potential for serious adverse reactions in nursing infants from HYCOTUSS Expectorant, a decision should be made whether to discontinue nursing or discontinue the drug, taking into account the importance of the drug to the mother.

Adverse Reactions:

Respiratory System: Hydrocodone produces dose-related respiratory depression by acting directly on brain stem respiratory centers.

Cardiovascular System: Hypertension, postural hypotension and palpitations.

Genitourinary System: Ureteral spasm, spasm of vesical sphincters and urinary retention have been reported with opiates.

Central Nervous System: Sedation, drowsiness, mental clouding, lethargy, impairment of mental and physical performance, anxiety, fear, dysphoria, dizziness, psychic dependence, mood changes and blurred vision.

Gastrointestinal System: Nausea and vomiting occur more frequently in ambulatory than in recumbent patients.

Drug Abuse and Dependence: Special care should be exercised in prescribing hydrocodone for emotionally unstable patients and for those with a history of drug misuse. Such patients should be closely supervised when long-term therapy is contemplated.

HYCOTUSS Expectorant is a Schedule III narcotic. Psychic dependence, physical dependence and tolerance may develop upon repeated administration of narcotics; therefore, HYCOTUSS Expectorant should always be prescribed and administered with caution. Physical dependence is the condition in which continued administration of the drug is required to prevent the appearance of a withdrawal syndrome.

Patients physically dependent on opioids will develop an abstinence syndrome upon abrupt discontinuation of the opioid or following the administration of a narcotic antagonist. The character and severity of the withdrawal symptoms are related to the degree of physical dependence. Manifestations of opioid withdrawal are similar to but milder than that of morphine and include lacrimation, rhinorrhea, yawning, sweating, restlessness, dilated pupils, anorexia, gooseflesh, irritability and tremor. In more severe forms, nausea, vomiting, intestinal spasm and diarrhea, increased heart rate and blood pressure, chills, and pains in bones and muscles of the back and extremities may occur. Peak effects will usually be apparent at 48 to 72 hours.

Treatment of withdrawal is usually managed by providing sufficient quantities of an opioid to suppress **severe** withdrawal symptoms and then gradually reducing the dose of opioid over a period of several days.

Overdosage:

Signs and Symptoms: Serious overdosage with HYCOTUSS Expectorant is characterized by respiratory depression (a decrease in respiratory rate and/or tidal volume, Cheyne-Stokes respiration, cyanosis), extreme somnolence progressing to stupor or coma, skeletal muscle flaccidity, cold and clammy skin, and sometimes bradycardia and hypotension. In severe overdosage apnea, circulatory collapse, cardiac arrest, and death may occur.

Treatment: Primary attention should be given to the reestablishment of adequate respiratory exchange through provision of a patent airway and the institution of assisted or controlled ventilation. The narcotic antagonist naloxone hydrochloride (NARCAN®) is a specific antidote against respiratory depression which may result from overdosage or unusual sensitivity to narcotics including hydrocodone. Therefore, an appropriate dose of naloxone hydrochloride should be administered (usual initial adult dose: 0.4 mg. For further information see NARCAN® full prescribing information) preferably by the intravenous route, simultaneously with efforts at respiratory resuscitation. Since the duration of action of hydrocodone may exceed that of the antagonist, the patient should be kept under continued surveillance and repeated doses of the antagonist should be administered as needed to maintain adequate respiration. Oxygen, intravenous fluids, vasopressors and other supportive measures should be employed as indicated.

Gastric emptying may be useful in removing unabsorbed drug. Activated charcoal may be of benefit.

Dosage and Administration:

Usual Adult Dose: One teaspoonful (5 ml) after meals and at bedtime, not less than 4 hours apart (not to exceed 6 teaspoonsful in a 24 hour period). Treatment should be initiated with one teaspoonful and subsequent doses, up to a maximum single dose of 3 teaspoonsful, adjusted if required.

Usual Children's Dose:

Over 12 years: Initial dose 1 teaspoonful; maximum single dose, 2 teaspoonsful.

2 to 12 years: Initial dose ½ teaspoonful; maximum single dose, 1 teaspoonful.

Under 2 years: Dosage should be calculated as Hydrocodone, 0.3 mg/kg/24 hours, divided into four equal doses.

How Supplied: HYCOTUSS Expectorant is available as an orange-colored, butterscotch flavored syrup in bottles as follows:

One pint: NDC 0056-0235-16

Store at controlled room temperature (59°–86° F, 15°–30° C).

HYCOTUSS ® is a Registered Trademark of Endo Laboratories, Inc. NARCAN® is a Registered U.S. Trademark of Endo Pharmaceuticals, Inc.

6131-1

MOBAN® ℞
(molindone hydrochloride)
Tablets and Concentrate

Description: MOBAN® (molindone hydrochloride) is a dihydroindolone compound which is not structurally related to the phenothiazines, the butyrophenones or the thioxanthenes.

MOBAN® is 3-ethyl-6, 7-dihydro-2-methyl-5-(morpholinomethyl) indol-4(5H)-one hydrochloride. It is a white crystalline powder, freely soluble in water and alcohol and has a molecular weight of 312.67.

Actions: MOBAN® (molindone hydrochloride) has a pharmacological profile in laboratory animals which predominantly resembles that of major tranquilizers causing reduction of spontaneous locomotion and aggressiveness, suppression of a conditioned response and antagonism of the bizarre stereotyped behavior and hyperactivity induced by amphetamines. In addition, MOBAN® antagonizes the depression caused by the tranquilizing agent tetrabenazine.

In human clinical studies tranquilization is achieved in the absence of muscle relaxing or incoordinating effects. Based on EEG studies, MOBAN® exerts its effect on the ascending reticular activating system.

Human metabolic studies show MOBAN® (molindone hydrochloride) to be rapidly absorbed and metabolized when given orally. Unmetabolized drug reached a peak blood level at 1.5 hours. Pharmacological effect from a single oral dose persists for 24–36 hours. There are 36 recognized metabolites with less than 2–3% unmetabolized MOBAN® being excreted in urine and feces.

Indications: MOBAN® (molindone hydrochloride) is indicated in the management of the manifestations of schizophrenia.

Contraindications: MOBAN® (molindone hydrochloride) is contraindicated in severe central nervous system depression (alcohol, barbiturates, narcotics, etc.) or comatose states, and in patients with known hypersensitivity to the drug.

Warnings:

Usage in Pregnancy: Studies in pregnant patients have not been carried out. Reproduction studies have been performed in the following animals:

Pregnant Rats oral dose— 20 mg/kg/day —10 days
no adverse effect
40 mg/kg/day —10 days
no adverse effect

Pregnant Mice oral dose— 20 mg/kg/day —10 days
slight increase resorptions
40 mg/kg/day —10 days
slight increase resorptions

Pregnant Rabbits oral dose—5 mg/kg/day —12 days
no adverse effect
10 mg/kg/day —12 days
no adverse effect
20 mg/kg/day —12 days
no adverse effect

Animal reproductive studies have not demonstrated a teratogenic potential. The anticipated benefits must be weighed against the unknown risks to the fetus if used in pregnant patients.

Nursing Mothers: Data are not available on the content of MOBAN® (molindone hydrochloride) in the milk of nursing mothers.

Usage in Children: Use of MOBAN® (molindone hydrochloride) in children below the age of twelve years is not recommended because safe and effective conditions for its usage have not been established.

Moban® has not been shown effective in the management of behavorial complications in patients with mental retardation.

Precautions: Some patients receiving MOBAN® (molindone hydrochloride) may note drowsiness initially and they should be advised against activities requiring mental alertness until their response to the drug has been established.

Increased activity has been noted in patients receiving MOBAN®. Caution should be exercised where increased activity may be harmful.

MOBAN® does not lower the seizure threshold in experimental animals to the degree noted with more sedating antipsychotic drugs. However, in humans convulsive seizures have been reported in a few instances.

The physician should be aware that this tablet preparation contains calcium sulfate as an excipient and that calcium ions may interfere with the absorption of preparations containing phenytoin sodium and tetracyclines.

MOBAN® has an antiemetic effect in animals. A similar effect may occur in humans and may obscure signs of intestinal obstruction or brain tumor.

Neuroleptic drugs elevate prolactin levels; the elevation persists during chronic administration. Tissue culture experiments indicate that approximately one-third of human breast cancers are prolactin dependent in vitro, a factor of potential importance if the prescription of these drugs is contemplated in a patient with a previously detected breast cancer. Although disturbances such as galactorrhea, amenorrhea, gynecomastia, and impotence have been reported, the clinical significance of elevated serum prolactin levels is unknown for most patients. An increase in mammary neoplasms has been found in rodents after chronic administration of neuroleptic drugs. Neither clinical studies nor epidemiologic studies conducted to date however, have shown an association between chronic administration of these drugs and mammary tumorigenesis; the available evidence is considered too limited to be conclusive at this time.

Adverse Reactions:

CNS Effects

The most frequently occurring effect is initial drowsiness that generally subsides with continued usage of the drug or lowering of the dose.

Noted less frequently were depression, hyperactivity and euphoria.

Neurological

Extrapyramidal Reactions

Extrapyramidal reactions noted below may occur in susceptible individuals and are usually reversible with appropriate management.

Akathisia

Motor restlessness may occur early.

Parkinson Syndrome

Akinesia, characterized by rigidity, immobility and reduction of voluntary movements and tremor, have been observed. Occurrence is less frequent than akathisia.

Dystonic Syndrome

Prolonged abnormal contractions of muscle groups occur infrequently. These symptoms may be managed by the addition of a synthetic antiparkinson agent (other than L-dopa), small doses of sedative drugs, and/or reduction in dosage.

Tardive Dyskinesia

Neuroleptic drugs are known to cause a syndrome of dyskinetic movements commonly referred to as tardive dyskinesia. The movements may appear during treatment or upon withdrawal of treatment and may be either reversible or irreversible (i.e., persistent) upon cessation of further neuroleptic administration. Reports of reversible tardive dyskinesia in association with MOBAN® therapy have been received. Reports of the irreversible variety have not been received, but this cannot be used to predict that MOBAN® cannot cause an irreversible dyskinetic syndrome.

The syndrome is known to have a variable latency for development and the duration of the latency cannot be determined reliably. It is thus wise to assume that any neuroleptic agent has the capacity to induce the syndrome and act accordingly until sufficient data has been collected to settle the issue definitely for a specific drug product. In the case of neuroleptics known to produce the irreversible syndrome, the following has been observed:

Tardive dyskinesia associated with other agents has appeared in some patients on long-term therapy and has also appeared after drug therapy has been discontinued. The risk appears to be greater in elderly patients on high-dose therapy, especially females. The symptoms are persistent and in some patients appear to be irreversible. The syndrome is characterized by rhythmical involuntary movements of the tongue, face, mouth or jaw (e.g., protrusion of tongue, puffing of cheeks, puckering of mouth, chewing movements). There may be involuntary movements of extremities.

There is no known effective treatment of tardive dyskinesia; antiparkinsonism agents usually do not alleviate the symptoms of this syndrome. It is suggested that all antipsychotic agents be discontinued if these symptoms appear. Should it be necessary to reinstitute treatment, or increase the dosage of the agent, or switch to a different antipsychotic agent, the syndrome may be masked. It has been reported that fine vermicular movements of the tongue may be an early sign of the syndrome and if the medication is stopped at that time the syndrome may not develop.

Autonomic Nervous System

Occasionally blurring of vision, tachycardia, nausea, dry mouth and salivation have been reported. Urinary retention and constipation may occur particularly if anticholinergic drugs are used to treat extrapyramidal symptoms.

Hematological

There have been rare reports of leucopenia and leucocytosis. If such reactions occur, treatment with MOBAN® may continue if clinical symptoms are absent. Alterations of blood glucose, liver function tests, B.U.N., and red blood cells have not been considered clinically significant.

Metabolic and Endocrine Effects

Alteration of thyroid function has not been significant. Amenorrhea has been reported infrequently. Resumption of menses in previously amenorrheic women has been reported. Initially heavy menses may occur. Galactorrhea and gynecomastia have been reported infrequently. Increase in libido has been noted in some patients. Although both weight gain and weight loss have been in the direction of normal or ideal weight, excessive weight gain has not occurred with MOBAN®.

Cardiovascular

Rare, transient, non-specific T wave changes have been reported on E.K.G. Association with a clinical syndrome has not been established. Rarely has significant hypotension been reported.

Ophthalmological

Lens opacities and pigmentary retinopathy have not been reported where patients have received MOBAN® (molindone hydrochloride). In some patients, phenothiazine induced lenticular opacities have resolved following discontinuation of the phenothiazine while continuing therapy with MOBAN®.

Skin

Early, non-specific skin rash, probably of allergic origin, has occasionally been reported. Skin pigmentation has not been seen with MOBAN® usage alone.

MOBAN® (molindone hydrochloride) has certain pharmacological similarities to other antipsychotic agents. Because adverse reactions are often extensions of the pharmacological activity of a drug, all of the known pharmacological effects associated with other antipsychotic drugs should be kept in mind when MOBAN® is used. Upon abrupt withdrawal after prolonged high dosage an abstinence syndrome has not been noted.

Continued on next page

Endo—Cont.

Dosage and Administration: Initial and maintenance doses of MOBAN® (molindone hydrochloride) should be individualized.
Initial Dosage Schedule: The usual starting dosage is 50–75 mg/day.
—Increase to 100 mg/day in 3 or 4 days.
—Based on severity of symptomatology, dosage may be titrated up or down depending on individual patient response.
—An increase to 225 mg/day may be required in patients with severe symptomatology.

Elderly and debilitated patients should be started on lower dosage.
Maintenance Dosage Schedule:
1. Mild—5 mg–15 mg three or four times a day.
2. Moderate—10 mg–25 mg three or four times a day.
3. Severe—225 mg/day may be required.

Drug Interactions: Potentiation of drugs administered concurrently with MOBAN® (molindone hydrochloride) has not been reported. Additionally, animal studies have not shown increased toxicity when MOBAN® is given concurrently with representative members of three classes of drugs (i.e., barbiturates, chloral hydrate and antiparkinson drugs).
Management of Overdosage: Symptomatic, supportive therapy should be the rule.
Gastric lavage is indicated for the reduction of absorption of MOBAN® (molindone hydrochloride) which is freely soluble in water.
Since the adsorption of MOBAN® (molindone hydrochloride) by activated charcoal has not been determined, the use of this antidote must be considered of theoretical value.
Emesis in a comatose patient is contraindicated. Additionally, while the emetic effect of apomorphine is blocked by MOBAN® in animals, this blocking effect has not been determined in humans.
A significant increase in the rate of removal of unmetabolized MOBAN® from the body by forced diuresis, peritoneal or renal dialysis would not be expected. (Only 2% of a single ingested dose of MOBAN® is excreted unmetabolized in the urine.) However, poor response of the patient may justify use of these procedures.
While the use of laxatives or enemas might be based on general principles, the amount of unmetabolized MOBAN® in feces is less than 1%. Extrapyramidal symptoms have responded to the use of diphenhydramine (Benadryl*) and the synthetic anticholinergic antiparkinson agents (i.e., Artane*, Cogentin*, Akineton*).
How Supplied: As tablets in bottles of 100's with potencies and colors as follows:

5 mg orange
10 mg lavender
25 mg light green
50 mg blue
100 mg tan

As a concentrate containing 20 mg molindone hydrochloride per ml in 4 oz. (120 ml) bottles.

*Benadryl—Trademark, Parke-Davis and Co.
*Artane—Trademark, Lederle Laboratories
*Cogentin—Trademark, Merck Sharp & Dohme
*Akineton—Trademark, Knoll Pharmaceutical Co.
6102-9
MOBAN is an Endo registered U.S. trademark.
[*Shown in Product Identification Section*]

NARCAN® INJECTION ℞
NARCAN® NEONATAL INJECTION ℞
(naloxone hydrochloride)
Narcotic Antagonist

Description: NARCAN (naloxone hydrochloride), a narcotic antagonist, is a synthetic congener of oxymorphone. In structure it differs from oxymorphone in that the methyl group on the nitrogen atom is replaced by an allyl group.
Naloxone hydrochloride occurs as a white to slightly off-white powder, and is soluble in water, in dilute acids, and in strong alkali; slightly soluble in alcohol; practically insoluble in ether and in chloroform.
NARCAN injection is available as a sterile solution for intravenous, intramuscular and subcutaneous administration in two concentrations, 0.02 mg and 0.4 mg of naloxone hydrochloride per ml. Each ml of either strength contains 8.6 mg of sodium chloride; and 2.0 mg of methylparaben and propylparaben as preservatives in a ratio of 9 to 1. pH is adjusted to 3.5 ± 0.5 with hydrochloric acid.
Clinical Pharmacology: NARCAN (naloxone hydrochloride) prevents or reverses the effects of opioids including respiratory depression, sedation and hypotension. Also, it can reverse the psychotomimetic and dysphoric effects of agonist-antagonist such as pentazocine.
NARCAN (naloxone hydrochloride) is an essentially pure narcotic antagonist, i.e., it does not possess the "agonistic" or morphine-like properties characteristic of other narcotic antagonists; NARCAN does not produce respiratory depression, psychotomimetic effects or pupillary constriction. In the absence of narcotics or agonistic effects of other narcotic antagonists it exhibits essentially no pharmacologic activity.
NARCAN has not been shown to produce tolerance nor to cause physical or psychological dependence.
In the presence of physical dependence on narcotics NARCAN will produce withdrawal symptoms.
Mechanisms of Action: While the mechanism of action of NARCAN is not fully understood, the preponderance of evidence suggests that NARCAN antagonizes the opioid effects by competing for the same receptor sites.
When NARCAN is administered intravenously the onset of action is generally apparent within two minutes; the onset of action is only slightly less rapid when it is administered subcutaneously or intramuscularly. The duration of action is dependent upon the dose and route of administration of NARCAN. Intramuscular administration produces a more prolonged effect than intravenous administration. The requirement for repeat doses of NARCAN, however, will also be dependent upon the amount, type and route of administration of the narcotic being antagonized.
Following parenteral administration NARCAN is rapidly distributed in the body. It is metabolized in the liver, primarily by glucuronide conjugation and excreted in urine. In one study the serum half-life in adults ranged from 30 to 81 minutes (mean 64 ± 12 minutes). In a neonatal study the mean plasma half-life was observed to be 3.1 ± 0.5 hours.
Indications and Usage: NARCAN is indicated for the complete or partial reversal of narcotic depression, including respiratory depression, induced by opioids including natural and synthetic narcotics, propoxyphene, methadone and the narcotic-antagonist analgesics: nalbuphine, pentazocine and butorphanol. NARCAN is also indicated for the diagnosis of suspected acute opioid overdosage.
Contraindications: NARCAN is contraindicated in patients known to be hypersensitive to it.
Warnings: NARCAN should be administered cautiously to persons including newborns of mothers who are known or suspected to be physically dependent on opioids. In such cases an abrupt and complete reversal of narcotic effects may precipitate an acute abstinence syndrome.
The patient who has satisfactorily responded to NARCAN should be kept under continued surveillance and repeated doses of NARCAN should be administered, as necessary, since the duration of action of some narcotics may exceed that of NARCAN.
NARCAN is not effective against respiratory depression due to non-opioid drugs.
Precautions: In addition to NARCAN, other resuscitative measures such as maintenance of a free airway, artificial ventilation, cardiac massage, and vasopressor agents should be available and employed when necessary to counteract acute narcotic poisoning.
Several instances of hypotension, hypertension, ventricular tachycardia and fibrillation, and pulmonary edema have been reported. These have occurred in postoperative patients most of whom had pre-existing cardiovascular disorders or received other drugs which may have similar adverse cardiovascular effects. Although a direct cause and effect relationship has not been established, NARCAN should be used with caution in patients with pre-existing cardiac disease or patients who have received potentially cardiotoxic drugs.
Carcinogenesis, Mutagenesis, Impairment of Fertility: Carcinogenicity and mutagenicity studies have not been performed with NARCAN. Reproductive studies in mice and rats demonstrated no impairment of fertility.
Use in Pregnancy: Pregnancy Catagory B: Reproduction studies performed in mice and rats at doses up to 1,000 times the human dose, revealed no evidence of impaired fertility or harm to the fetus due to NARCAN. There are, however, no adequate and well controlled studies in pregnant women. Because animal reproduction studies are not always predictive of human response, NARCAN should be used during pregnancy only if clearly needed.
Nursing Mothers: It is not known whether NARCAN is excreted in human milk. Because many drugs are excreted in human milk, caution should be exercised when NARCAN is administered to a nursing woman.
Adverse Reactions: Abrupt reversal of narcotic depression may result in nausea, vomiting, sweating, tachycardia, increased blood pressure, and tremulousness. In postoperative patients, larger than necessary dosage of NARCAN may result in significant reversal of analgesia, and in excitement. Hypotension, hypertension, ventricular tachycardia and fibrillation, and pulmonary edema have been associated with the use of NARCAN postoperatively (see PRECAUTIONS & USAGE IN ADULTS-POSTOPERATIVE NARCOTIC DEPRESSION). Seizures have beer reported to occur infrequently after the administration of naloxone; however, a causal relationship has not been established.
Overdosage: There is no clinical experience with NARCAN overdosage in humans.
In the mouse and rat the intravenous LD_{50} is 150 ± 5 mg/kg and 109 ± 4 mg/kg respectively. In acute subcutaneous toxicity studies in newborn rats the LD_{50} (95% CL) is 260 (228-296) mg/kg. Subcutaneous injection of 100 mg/kg/day in rats for 3 weeks produced only transient salivation and partial ptosis following injection: no toxic effects were seen at 10 mg/kg/day for 3 weeks.
Dosage and Administration: NARCAN (naloxone hydrochloride) may be administered intravenously, intramuscularly, or subcutaneously. The most rapid onset of action is achieved by intravenous administration and it is recommended in emergency situations.
Since the duration of action of some narcotics may exceed that of NARCAN the patient should be kept under continued surveillance and repeated doses of NARCAN should be administered, as necessary.
Intravenous Infusion: NARCAN may be diluted for intravenous infusion in normal saline or 5% dextrose solutions. The addition of 2 mg of NARCAN in 500 ml of either solution provides a concentration of 0.004 mg/ml. Mixtures should be used within 24 hours. After 24

hours, the remaining unused solution must be discarded. The rate of administration should be titrated in accordance with the patient's response.

Parenteral drug products should be inspected visually for particulate matter and discoloration prior to administration whenever solution and container permit. NARCAN should not be mixed with preparations containing bisulfite, metabisulfite, long-chain or high molecular weight anions, or any solution having an alkaline pH. No drug or chemical agent should be added to NARCAN unless its effect on the chemical and physical stability of the solution has first been established.

Usage in Adults:

Narcotic Overdose—Known or Suspected: An initial dose of 0.4 mg to 2 mg of NARCAN may be administered intravenously. If the desired degree of counteraction and improvement in respiratory functions is not obtained, it may be repeated at 2 to 3 minute intervals. If no response is observed after 10 mg of NARCAN have been administered, the diagnosis of narcotic induced or partial narcotic induced toxicity should be questioned. Intramuscular or subcutaneous administration may be necessary if the intravenous route is not available.

Postoperative Narcotic Depression: For the partial reversal of narcotic depression following the use of narcotics during surgery, smaller doses of NARCAN are usually sufficient. The dose of NARCAN should be titrated according to the patient's response. For the initial reversal of respiratory depression, NARCAN should be injected in increments of 0.1 to 0.2 mg intravenously at two to three minute intervals to the desired degree of reversal i.e. adequate ventilation and alertness without significant pain or discomfort. Larger than necessary dosage of NARCAN may result in significant reversal of analgesia and increase in blood pressure. Similarly, too rapid reversal may induce nausea, vomiting, sweating or circulatory stress.

Repeat doses of NARCAN may be required within one to two hour intervals depending upon the amount, type (i.e., short or long acting) and time interval since last administration of narcotic. Supplemental intramuscular doses have been shown to produce a longer lasting effect.

Usage in Children:

Narcotic Overdose—Known or Suspected: The usual initial dose in children is 0.01 mg/kg body weight given I.V. If this dose does not result in the desired degree of clinical improvement, a subsequent dose of 0.1 mg/kg body weight may be administered. If an I.V. route of administration is not available, NARCAN may be administered I.M. or S.C. in divided doses. If necessary, NARCAN can be diluted with sterile water for injection.

Postoperative Narcotic Depression: Follow the recommendations and cautions under **Adult Postoperative Depression.** For the initial reversal of respiratory depression NARCAN should be injected in increments of 0.005 mg to 0.01 mg intravenously at two to three minute intervals to the desired degree of reversal.

Usage in Neonates:

Narcotic-Induced Depression: The usual initial dose is 0.01 mg/kg body weight administered I.V., I.M., or S.C. This dose may be repeated in accordance with adult administration guidelines for postoperative narcotic depression.

HOW SUPPLIED: 0.4 mg/ml of NARCAN® (naloxone hydrochloride) for intravenous, intramuscular and subcutaneous administration. Available as follows:

1 ml ampuls in
boxes of 10 NDC 0590-0365-10
1 ml disposable prefilled syringes.
boxes of 10 NDC 0590-0365-15
boxes of 25 NDC 0590-0365-25
10 ml vials NDC 0590-0365-05

0.02 mg/ml of NARCAN® (naloxone hydrochloride) NEONATAL INJECTION for intravenous, intramuscular and subcutaneous administration. Available as:

2 ml ampuls in
boxes of 10 NDC 0590-0367-10

Endo Pharmaceuticals, Inc.
Manati, Puerto Rico 00701
Subsidiary of Endo Laboratories, Inc.
Subsidiary of the Du Pont Company
NARCAN® is a Registered Trademark of Endo Pharmaceuticals, Inc.
6108-2/Rev. Apr., 1982

[*Shown in Product Identification Section*]

NUBAIN® ℞
(nalbuphine hydrochloride)

Description: NUBAIN (nalbuphine hydrochloride) is a synthetic narcotic agonist-antagonist analgesic of the phenanthrene series. It is chemically related to both the widely used narcotic antagonist, naloxone, and the potent narcotic analgesic, oxymorphone.

Nalbuphine hydrochloride is (-)-17-(cyclobutylmethyl)-4, 5α-epoxy-morphinan-3,6α, 14-triol, hydrochloride.

Each ml of the injectable aqueous solution of NUBAIN contains 10 mg of nalbuphine hydrochloride.

Actions: NUBAIN is a potent analgesic. Its analgesic potency is essentially equivalent to that of morphine on a milligram basis.

Its onset of action occurs within 2 to 3 minutes after intravenous administration, and in less than 15 minutes following subcutaneous or intramuscular injection. The plasma half-life of nalbuphine is 5 hours and in clinical studies the duration of analgesic activity has been reported to range from 3 to 6 hours.

The narcotic antagonist activity of NUBAIN is one-fourth as potent as nalorphine and 10 times that of pentazocine.

Indications: For the relief of moderate to severe pain. NUBAIN can also be used for preoperative analgesia, as a supplement to surgical anesthesia, and for obstetrical analgesia during labor.

Contraindications: NUBAIN should not be administered to patients who are hypersensitive to it.

Warnings:

Drug Dependence NUBAIN has been shown to have a low abuse potential which is approximate to that of pentazocine. When compared with drugs which are not mixed agonist-antagonists, it has been reported that nalbuphine's potential for abuse would be less than that of codeine and propoxyphene. Psychological and physical dependence and tolerance may follow the abuse or misuse of nalbuphine. Therefore, caution should be observed in prescribing it for emotionally unstable patients, or for individuals with a history of narcotic abuse. Such patients should be closely supervised when long-term therapy is contemplated.

Care should be taken to avoid increases in dosage or frequency of administration which in susceptible individuals might result in physical dependence.

Abrupt discontinuation of NUBAIN following prolonged use has been followed by symptoms of narcotic withdrawal, i.e., abdominal cramps, nausea and vomiting, rhinorrhea, lacrimation, restlessness, anxiety, elevated temperature and piloerection.

Use in Ambulatory Patients NUBAIN may impair the mental or physical abilities required for the performance of potentially dangerous tasks such as driving a car or operating machinery. Therefore, NUBAIN should be administered with caution to ambulatory patients who should be warned to avoid such hazards.

Use in Emergency Procedures Maintain patient under observation until recovered from NUBAIN effects that would affect driving or other potentially dangerous tasks.

Use in Children Clinical experience to support administration to patients under 18 years is not available at present.

Use in Pregnancy (other than labor) Safe use of NUBAIN in pregnancy has not been established. Although animal reproductive studies have not revealed teratogenic or embryotoxic effects, nalbuphine should only be administered to pregnant women when, in the judgment of the physician, the potential benefits outweigh the possible hazards.

Use During Labor and Delivery NUBAIN can produce respiratory depression in the neonate. It should be used with caution in women delivering premature infants.

Head Injury and Increased Intracranial Pressure The possible respiratory depressant effects and the potential of potent analgesics to elevate cerebrospinal fluid pressure (resulting from vasodilation following CO_2 retention) may be markedly exaggerated in the presence of head injury, intracranial lesions or a preexisting increase in intracranial pressure. Furthermore, potent analgesics can produce effects which may obscure the clinical course of patients with head injuries. Therefore, NUBAIN should be used in these circumstances only when essential, and then should be administered with extreme caution.

Interaction With Other Central Nervous System Depressants Although NUBAIN possesses narcotic antagonist activity, there is evidence that in nondependent patients it will not antagonize a narcotic analgesic administered just before, concurrently, or just after an injection of NUBAIN. Therefore, patients receiving a narcotic analgesic, general anesthetics, phenothiazines, or other tranquilizers, sedatives, hypnotics, or other CNS depressants (including alcohol) concomitantly with NUBAIN may exhibit an additive effect. When such combined therapy is contemplated, the dose of one or both agents should be reduced.

Precautions:

Impaired Respiration At the usual adult dose of 10 mg/70 kg, NUBAIN causes some respiratory depression approximately equal to that produced by equal doses of morphine. However, in contrast to morphine, respiratory depression is not appreciably increased with higher doses of NUBAIN. Respiratory depression induced by NUBAIN can be reversed by NARCAN® (naloxone hydrochloride) when indicated. NUBAIN should be administered with caution at low doses to patients with impaired respiration (e.g., from other medication, uremia, bronchial asthma, severe infection, cyanosis or respiratory obstructions).

Impaired Renal or Hepatic Function Because NUBAIN is metabolized in the liver and excreted by the kidneys, patients with renal or liver dysfunction may over-react to customary doses. Therefore, in these individuals, NUBAIN should be used with caution and administered in reduced amounts.

Myocardial Infarction As with all potent analgesics, NUBAIN should be used with caution in patients with myocardial infarction who have nausea or vomiting.

Biliary Tract Surgery As with all narcotic analgesics, NUBAIN should be used with caution in patients about to undergo surgery of the biliary tract since it may cause spasm of the sphincter of Oddi.

Adverse Reactions: The most frequent adverse reaction in 1066 patients treated with NUBAIN is sedation 381(36%).

Less frequent reactions are: sweaty/clammy 99(9%), nausea/vomiting 68(6%), dizziness/vertigo 58(5%), dry mouth 44(4%), and headache 27(3%).

Other adverse reactions which may occur (reported incidence of 1% or less) are:

Continued on next page

Endo—Cont.

CNS Effects nervousness, depression, restlessness, crying, euphoria, floating, hostility, unusual dreams, confusion, faintness, hallucinations, dysphoria, feeling of heaviness, numbness, tingling, unreality. The incidence of psychotomimetic effects, such as unreality, depersonalization, delusions, dysphoria and hallucinations has been shown to be less than that which occurs with pentazocine.

Cardiovascular Hypertension, hypotension, bradycardia, tachycardia.

Gastrointestinal Cramps, dyspepsia, bitter taste.

Respiration Depression, dyspnea, asthma.

Dermatological Itching, burning, urticaria.

Miscellaneous Speech difficulty, urinary urgency, blurred vision, flushing and warmth.

Dosage and Administration: The usual recommended adult dose is 10 mg for a 70 kg individual, administered subcutaneously, intramuscularly or intravenously; this dose may be repeated every 3 to 6 hours as necessary. Dosage should be adjusted according to the severity of the pain, physical status of the patient, and other medications which the patient may be receiving. (See Interaction with Other Central Nervous System Depressants under WARNINGS). In non-tolerant individuals, the recommended single maximum dose is 20 mg, with a maximum total daily dose of 160 mg.

Patients Dependent on Narcotics Patients who have been taking narcotics chronically may experience withdrawal symptoms upon the administration of NUBAIN. If unduly troublesome, narcotic withdrawal symptoms can be controlled by the slow intravenous administration of small increments of morphine, until relief occurs. If the previous analgesic was morphine, meperidine, codeine, or other narcotic with similar duration of activity, one-fourth of the anticipated dose of NUBAIN can be administered initially and the patient observed for signs of withdrawal, i.e., abdominal cramps, nausea and vomiting, lacrimation, rhinorrhea, anxiety, restlessness, elevation of temperature or piloerection. If untoward symptoms do not occur, progressively larger doses may be tried at appropriate intervals until the desired level of analgesia is obtained with NUBAIN.

Management of Overdosage The immediate intravenous administration of NARCAN® (naloxone hydrochloride) is a specific antidote. Oxygen, intravenous fluids, vasopressors and other supportive measures should be used as indicated.

The administration of single doses of 72 mg of NUBAIN subcutaneously to eight normal subjects has been reported to have resulted primarily in symptoms of sleepiness and mild dysphoria.

How Supplied: NUBAIN® (nalbuphine hydrochloride) injection for intramuscular, subcutaneous, or intravenous use (10 mg/ml) is available in:

NDC #0590-0385 10 mg/ml, 1 ml ampuls (box of 10)

NDC #0590-0384 10 mg/ml, 2 ml ampuls (box of 10)

NDC #0590-0386 10 mg/ml, 10 ml vials

Each ml contains 10 mg nalbuphine hydrochloride, 0.1% sodium chloride, 0.94% sodium citrate, 1.26% citric acid anhydrous, 0.1% sodium metabisulfite, and 0.2% of a 9:1 mixture of methylparaben and propylparaben as preservative; pH is adjusted with hydrochloric acid.

NUBAIN® is a Registered Trademark of Endo Pharmaceuticals, Inc.

NARCAN® is a Registered Trademark of Endo Pharmaceuticals, Inc.

6109

[*Shown in Product Identification Section*]

NUMORPHAN® Ⓒ
(oxymorphone hydrochloride)
injection

Description: NUMORPHAN (oxymorphone hydrochloride), a semisynthetic narcotic substitute for morphine, is a potent analgesic.

NUMORPHAN is 4,5α-Epoxy-3, 14-dihydroxy-17-methylmorphinan-6-one hydrochloride.

Oxymorphone hydrochloride occurs as a white or slightly off-white, odorless powder, sparingly soluble in alcohol and ether, but freely soluble in water.

NUMORPHAN injection is available in two concentrations, 1.0 mg and 1.5 mg of oxymorphone hydrochloride per ml. Both strengths contain sodium chloride 0.8%; with methylparaben 0.18%, propylparaben 0.02% and sodium dithionite 0.1%, as preservatives. pH is adjusted with sodium hydroxide.

Actions: NUMORPHAN (oxymorphone hydrochloride) is a potent narcotic analgesic. Administered parenterally, one mg of NUMORPHAN is approximately equivalent in analgesic activity to 10 mg of morphine sulfate.

The onset of action is rapid; initial effects are usually perceived within 5 to 10 minutes. Its duration of action is approximately 3 to 6 hours.

NUMORPHAN produces mild sedation and causes little depression of the cough reflex. These properties make it particularly useful in postoperative patients.

Indications: NUMORPHAN (oxymorphone hydrochloride) is indicated for the relief of moderate to severe pain. This drug is also indicated parenterally for preoperative medication, for support of anesthesia, for obstetrical analgesia, and for relief of anxiety in patients with dyspnea associated with acute left ventricular failure and pulmonary edema.

Contraindications: Safe use of NUMORPHAN (oxymorphone hydrochloride) in children under 12 years of age has not been established. This drug should not be used in patients known to be hypersensitive to morphine analogs.

Warnings: *May be habit forming.* As with other narcotic drugs, tolerance and addiction may develop. The addicting potential of the drug appears to be about the same as for morphine. Like other narcotic-containing medications, NUMORPHAN is subject to the Federal Controlled Substances Act.

Interaction with other central nervous system depressants: Patients receiving other narcotic analgesics, general anesthetics, phenothiazines, other tranquilizers, sedatives, hypnotics or other CNS depressants (including alcohol) concomitantly with NUMORPHAN may exhibit an additive CNS depression. When such combined therapy is contemplated, the dose of one or both agents should be reduced.

Safe use in pregnancy has not been established (relative to possible adverse effects on fetal development). As with other analgesics, the use of NUMORPHAN (oxymorphone hydrochloride) in pregnancy, in nursing mothers, or in women of child-bearing potential requires that the possible benefits of the drug be weighed against the possible hazards to the mother and the child.

Precautions: The same care and caution should be taken when administering NUMORPHAN (oxymorphone hydrochloride) as when other potent narcotic analgesics are used. It should be borne in mind that some respiratory depression may occur as with all potent narcotics especially when other analgesic and/or anesthetic drugs with depressant action have been given shortly before administration of NUMORPHAN.

The respiratory depressant effects of narcotics and their capacity to elevate cerebrospinal fluid pressure may be markedly exaggerated in the presence of head injury, other intracranial lesions or a pre-existing increase in intracranial pressure. Furthermore narcotics produce adverse reactions which may obscure the clinical course of patients with head injuries.

As with other analgesics, caution must also be exercised in elderly and debilitated patients and in patients who are known to be sensitive to central nervous system depressants, such as those with cardiovascular, pulmonary, or hepatic disease, in hypothyroidism (myxedema), acute alcoholism, delirium tremens, convulsive disorders, bronchial asthma and kyphoscoliosis. Debilitated and elderly patients and those with severe liver diseases should receive smaller doses of NUMORPHAN.

Adverse Reactions: As with all potent narcotic analgesics, possible side effects include drowsiness, nausea, vomiting, miosis, itching, dysphoria, light-headedness, and headache. Respiratory depression may occur with oxymorphone as with other narcotics.

Dosage and Administration: Usual Adult Dosage of NUMORPHAN (oxymorphone hydrochloride) Injection: Subcutaneous or intramuscular administration: initially 1 mg to 1.5 mg, repeated every 4 to 6 hours as needed. Intravenous: 0.5 mg initially. In nondebilitated patients the dose can be cautiously increased until satisfactory pain relief is obtained. For analgesia during labor 0.5 mg to 1 mg intramuscularly is recommended.

Management of Overdosage: *Signs and Symptoms:* Serious overdosage with NUMORPHAN is characterized by respiratory depression (a decrease in respiratory rate and/or tidal volume, Cheyne-Stokes respiration, cyanosis), extreme somnolence progressing to stupor or coma, skeletal muscle flaccidity, cold and clammy skin, and sometimes bradycardia and hypotension. In severe overdosage, apnea, circulatory collapse, cardiac arrest and death may occur.

Treatment: Primary attention should be given to the reestablishment of adequate respiratory exchange through provision of a patent airway and the institution of assisted or controlled ventilation. The narcotic antagonist naloxone hydrochloride (NARCAN®) is a specific antidote against respiratory depression which may result from overdosage or unusual sensitivity to narcotics including oxymorphone. Therefore, an appropriate dose of naloxone hydrochloride should be administered (usual initial adult dose: 0.4 mg) preferably by the intravenous route and simultaneously with efforts at respiratory resuscitation. Since the duration of action of oxymorphone may exceed that of the antagonist, the patient should be kept under continued surveillance and repeated doses of the antagonist should be administered as needed to maintain adequate respiration.

Oxygen, intravenous fluids, vasopressors and other supportive measures should be employed as indicated.

How Supplied:

For Injection: DEA Order Form Required

1 mg/ml	1 ml ampuls, boxes of 10 and 100
1.5 mg/ml	1 ml ampuls, boxes of 10 and 100
	10 ml multiple dose vial, individual box

NUMORPHAN® is a Registered Trademark of Endo Pharmaceuticals, Inc.

NARCAN® is a Registered Trademark of Endo Pharmaceuticals, Inc.

6110

†PERCOCET®-5 Ⓒ

Description:

Each tablet of PERCOCET®-5 contains:

Oxycodone hydrochloride ....5 mg

WARNING: May be habit forming

Acetaminophen (APAP) ....325 mg

The oxycodone component is 14-hydroxydihydrocodeinone, a white, odorless crystalline powder which is derived from the opium alkaloid, thebaine.

Actions: The principal analgesic ingredient, oxycodone, is a semisynthetic narcotic with multiple actions qualitatively similar to those of morphine; the most prominent of these involve the central nervous system and organs composed of smooth muscle. The principal actions of therapeutic value of the oxycodone in PERCOCET®-5 are analgesia and sedation.
Oxycodone is similar to codeine and methadone in that it retains at least one half of its analgesic activity when administered orally.
PERCOCET®-5 also contains the non-narcotic antipyretic-analgesic acetaminophen.
Indications: For the relief of moderate to moderately severe pain.
Contraindications: Hypersensitivity to oxycodone or acetaminophen.
Warnings:
Drug Dependence: Oxycodone can produce drug dependence of the morphine type and, therefore, has the potential for being abused. Psychic dependence, physical dependence and tolerance may develop upon repeated administration of PERCOCET®-5, and it should be prescribed and administered with the same degree of caution appropriate to the use of other oral narcotic-containing medications. Like other narcotic-containing medications, PERCOCET®-5 is subject to the Federal Controlled Substances Act.
Usage in ambulatory patients: Oxycodone may impair the mental and/or physical abilities required for the performance of potentially hazardous tasks such as driving a car or operating machinery. The patient using PERCOCET®-5 should be cautioned accordingly.
Interaction with other central nervous system depressants: Patients receiving other narcotic analgesics, general anesthetics, phenothiazines, other tranquilizers, sedative-hypnotics or other CNS depressants (including alcohol) concomitantly with PERCOCET®-5 may exhibit an additive CNS depression. When such combined therapy is contemplated, the dose of one or both agents should be reduced.
Usage in pregnancy: Safe use in pregnancy has not been established relative to possible adverse effects on fetal development. Therefore, PERCOCET®-5 should not be used in pregnant women unless, in the judgment of the physician, the potential benefits outweigh the possible hazards.
Usage in children: PERCOCET®-5 should not be administered to children.
Precautions:
Head injury and increased intracranial pressure: The respiratory depressant effects of narcotics and their capacity to elevate cerebrospinal fluid pressure may be markedly exaggerated in the presence of head injury, other intracranial lesions or a pre-existing increase in intracranial pressure. Furthermore, narcotics produce adverse reactions which may obscure the clinical course of patients with head injuries.
Acute abdominal conditions: The administration of PERCOCET®-5 or other narcotics may obscure the diagnosis or clinical course in patients with acute abdominal conditions.
Special risk patients: PERCOCET®-5 should be given with caution to certain patients such as the elderly or debilitated, and those with severe impairment of hepatic or renal function, hypothyroidism, Addison's disease, and prostatic hypertrophy or urethral stricture.
Adverse Reactions: The most frequently observed adverse reactions include light headedness, dizziness, sedation, nausea and vomiting. These effects seem to be more prominent in ambulatory than in nonambulatory patients, and some of these adverse reactions may be alleviated if the patient lies down.
Other adverse reactions include euphoria, dysphoria, constipation, skin rash and pruritus.
Dosage and Administration: Dosage should be adjusted according to the severity of the pain and the response of the patient. It may occasionally be necessary to exceed the usual dosage recommended below in cases of more severe pain or in those patients who have become tolerant to the analgesic effect of narcotics. PERCOCET®-5 is given orally. The usual adult dose is one tablet every 6 hours as needed for pain.
Drug Interactions: The CNS depressant effects of PERCOCET®-5 may be additive with that of other CNS depressants. See WARNINGS.
Management of Overdosage:
Signs and Symptoms: Serious overdose with PERCOCET®-5 is characterized by respiratory depression (a decrease in respiratory rate and/or tidal volume, Cheyne-Stokes respiration, cyanosis), extreme somnolence progressing to stupor or coma, skeletal muscle flaccidity, cold and clammy skin, and sometimes bradycardia and hypotension. In severe overdosage, apnea, circulatory collapse, cardiac arrest and death may occur. The ingestion of very large amounts of PERCOCET®-5 may, in addition, result in acute hepatic toxicity.
Treatment: Primary attention should be given to the reestablishment of adequate respiratory exchange through provision of a patent airway and the institution of assisted or controlled ventilation. The narcotic antagonist naloxone hydrochloride (NARCAN®) is a specific antidote against respiratory depression which may result from overdosage or unusual sensitivity to narcotics including oxycodone. Therefore, an appropriate dose of naloxone hydrochloride should be administered (usual adult dose: 0.4 mg) preferably by the intravenous route, simultaneously with efforts at respiratory resuscitation. Since the duration of action of oxycodone may exceed that of the antagonist, the patient should be kept under continued surveillance and repeated doses of the antagonist should be administered as needed to maintain adequate respiration.
Oxygen, intravenous fluids, vasopressors and other supportive measures should be employed as indicated.
Gastric emptying may be useful in removing unabsorbed drug.
Acetaminophen in massive overdosage may cause hepatotoxicity in some patients. Clinical and laboratory evidence of hepatotoxicity may be delayed for up to one week. Close clinical monitoring and serial hepatic enzyme determinations are therefore recommended.
Treatment of acute acetaminophen overdosage is purely symptomatic.
How Supplied: White, scored tablets in bottles of 100 and 500; Hospital blister pack of 25 tablets in units of 250 and 1,000 tablets.
DEA Order Form Required
PERCOCET® is a registered Trademark of Endo, Inc. NARCAN® is a Registered U.S. Trademark of Endo Pharmaceuticals, Inc.
6090-2

†Product of Endo Inc.
[*Shown in Product Identification Section*]

†PERCODAN® Ⓒ
†PERCODAN®-DEMI
Tablets

Description:
Each tablet of PERCODAN® contains:
Oxycodone hydrochloride ....4.50 mg
WARNING: May be habit forming
Oxycodone terephthalate ....0.38 mg
WARNING: May be habit forming
Aspirin ....325 mg
Each tablet of PERCODAN®-Demi contains:
Oxycodone hydrochloride ....2.25 mg
WARNING: May be habit forming
Oxycodone terephthalate ....0.19 mg
WARNING: May be habit forming
Aspirin ....325 mg
The oxycodone component is 14-hydroxydihydrocodeinone, a white odorless crystalline powder which is derived from the opium alkaloid, thebaine.
Actions: The principal ingredient, oxycodone, is a semisynthetic narcotic analgesic with multiple actions qualitatively similar to those of morphine; the most prominent of these involve the central nervous system and organs composed of smooth muscle. The principal actions of therapeutic value of the oxycodone in PERCODAN® and PERCODAN®-Demi are analgesia and sedation.
Oxycodone is similar to codeine and methadone in that it retains at least one half of its analgesic activity when administered orally.
PERCODAN® and PERCODAN®-Demi also contain the non-narcotic antipyretic-analgesic, aspirin.
Indications: For the relief of moderate to moderately severe pain.
Contraindications: Hypersensitivity to oxycodone or aspirin.
Warnings:
Drug Dependence: Oxycodone can produce drug dependence of the morphine type and, therefore, has the potential for being abused. Psychic dependence, physical dependence and tolerance may develop upon repeated administration of PERCODAN® and PERCODAN®-Demi, and it should be prescribed and administered with the same degree of caution appropriate to the use of other oral narcotic-containing medications. Like other narcotic-containing medications, PERCODAN® and PERCODAN®-Demi are subject to the Federal Controlled Substances Act.
Usage in ambulatory patients: Oxycodone may impair the mental and/or physical abilities required for the performance of potentially hazardous tasks such as driving a car or operating machinery. The patient using PERCODAN® and PERCODAN®-Demi should be cautioned accordingly.
Interaction with other central nervous system depressants: Patients receiving other narcotic analgesics, general anesthetics, phenothiazines, other tranquilizers, sedative-hypnotics or other CNS depressants (including alcohol) concomitantly with PERCODAN® and PERCODAN®-Demi may exhibit an additive CNS depression. When such combined therapy is contemplated, the dose of one or both agents should be reduced.
Usage in pregnancy: Safe use in pregnancy has not been established relative to possible adverse effects on fetal development. Therefore, PERCODAN® and PERCODAN®-Demi should not be used in pregnant women unless, in the judgment of the physician, the potential benefits outweigh the possible hazards.
Usage in children: PERCODAN® should not be administered to children. PERCODAN®-Demi, containing half the amount of oxycodone, can be considered. (See Dosage and Administration for PERCODAN®-Demi).
Salicylates should be used with caution in the presence of peptic ulcer or coagulation abnormalities.
Precautions:
Head injury and increased intracranial pressure: The respiratory depressant effects of narcotics and their capacity to elevate cerebrospinal fluid pressure may be markedly exaggerated in the presence of head injury, other intracranial lesions or a pre-existing increase in intracranial pressure. Furthermore, narcotics produce adverse reactions which may obscure the clinical course of patients with head injuries.
Acute abdominal conditions: The administration of PERCODAN® and PERCODAN®-Demi or other narcotics may obscure the diagnosis or clinical course in patients with acute abdominal conditions.
Special risk patients: PERCODAN® and PERCODAN®-Demi should be given with cau-

Continued on next page

Endo—Cont.

tion to certain patients such as the elderly or debilitated, and those with severe impairment of hepatic or renal function, hypothyroidism, Addison's disease, and prostatic hypertrophy or urethral stricture.

Adverse Reactions: The most frequently observed adverse reactions include light headedness, dizziness, sedation, nausea and vomiting. These effects seem to be more prominent in ambulatory than in nonambulatory patients, and some of these adverse reactions may be alleviated if the patient lies down.

Other adverse reactions include euphoria, dysphoria, constipation and pruritus.

Dosage and Administration: Dosage should be adjusted according to the severity of the pain and the response of the patient. It may occasionally be necessary to exceed the usual dosage recommended below in cases of more severe pain or in those patients who have become tolerant to the analgesic effect of narcotics. PERCODAN® and PERCODAN®-Demi are given orally.

PERCODAN®: The usual adult dose is one tablet every 6 hours as needed for pain.

PERCODAN®-Demi: Adults—One or two tablets every six hours. Children 12 years and older—One-half tablet every six hours. Children 6 to 12 years—One-quarter tablet every six hours. PERCODAN®-Demi is not indicated for children under 6 years of age.

Drug Interactions: The CNS depressant effects of PERCODAN® and PERCODAN®-Demi may be additive with that of other CNS depressants. See WARNINGS.

Aspirin may enhance the effect of anticoagulants and inhibit the uricosuric effects of uricosuric agents.

Management of Overdosage:

Signs and Symptoms: Serious overdose with PERCODAN® or PERCODAN®-Demi is characterized by respiratory depression (a decrease in respiratory rate and/or tidal volume, Cheyne-Stokes respiration, cyanosis), extreme somnolence progressing to stupor or coma, skeletal muscle flaccidity, cold and clammy skin, and sometimes bradycardia and hypotension. In severe overdosage, apnea, circulatory collapse, cardiac arrest and death may occur. The ingestion of very large amounts of PERCODAN® or PERCODAN®-Demi may, in addition, result in acute salicylate intoxication.

Treatment: Primary attention should be given to the reestablishment of adequate respiratory exchange through provision of a patent airway and the institution of assisted or controlled ventilation. The narcotic antagonist naloxone hydrochloride (NARCAN®) is a specific antidote against respiratory depression which may result from overdosage or unusual sensitivity to narcotics, including oxycodone. Therefore, an appropriate dose of naloxone hydrochloride should be administered (usual adult dose: 0.4 mg) preferably by the intravenous route, simultaneously with efforts at respiratory resuscitation. Since the duration of action of oxycodone may exceed that of the antagonist, the patient should be kept under continued surveillance and repeated doses of the antagonist should be administered as needed to maintain adequate respiration.

Oxygen, intravenous fluids, vasopressors and other supportive measures should be employed as indicated.

Gastric emptying may be useful in removing unabsorbed drug.

How Supplied:

PERCODAN®—Yellow, scored tablets in bottles of 100, 500 and 1,000; Hospital blister pack of 25 tablets in units of 250 and 1,000 tablets.

PERCODAN®-Demi—Pink, scored tablets in bottles of 100 and 500.

[Shown in Product Identification Section]
DEA Order Form Required.

PERCODAN is a registered U.S. trademark of Endo Inc.

†Products of Endo Inc.
6117-1/6118-1

NARCAN is a Registered U.S. Trademark of Endo Pharmaceuticals, Inc.

PERCOGESIC® with Codeine Ⓒ

Description: PERCOGESIC with Codeine tablets contain a peripherally-acting analgesic, antipyretic acetaminophen; an antihistamine, phenyltoloxamine citrate; and a centrally-acting narcotic analgesic codeine phosphate for oral administration.

Each PERCOGESIC with Codeine tablet contains:

Codeine phosphate .... 32.4 mg
 Warning: May be habit forming
Acetaminophen .... 325 mg
Phenyltoloxamine citrate .... 30 mg

Clinical Pharmacology: Codeine phosphate is an analgesic which acts centrally. It is rapidly absorbed following oral administration and the plasma half-life is about 2.5 to 3 hours. Codeine is metabolized in the liver and excreted chiefly in the urine as conjugated products; however, a portion (approximately 10%) is demethylated to form morphine. Codeine depresses the cough reflex and can produce constipation, miosis, euphoria, physical and psychological dependence. At therapeutic analgesic doses it has antitussive action. In excessive doses, it can produce respiratory depression.

Acetaminophen is a non-narcotic peripherally acting analgesic and antipyretic agent. It is absorbed rapidly from the gastrointestinal tract and metabolized in the liver. The plasma half-life is 1 to 4 hours after therapeutic doses. It is excreted in the urine.

Phenyltoloxamine citrate is a competitive H_1-receptor histamine blocking drug which inhibits the action of histamine. It can both stimulate and depress the central nervous system. In addition, H_1-blocking drugs inhibit the actions of histamine on smooth muscle and capillary permeability. In combination with acetaminophen, it enhances the analgesic action of acetaminophen.

Indications and Usage: PERCOGESIC with Codeine is indicated for the relief of mild to moderate pain.

Contraindications: PERCOGESIC with Codeine is contraindicated in patients hypersensitive to any component of the drug and concurrent MAO inhibitor therapy. Patients known to be hypersensitive to other opioids or antihistamines may exhibit cross sensitivity to PERCOGESIC with Codeine. Codeine is contraindicated in the presence of an intracranial lesion associated with increased intracranial pressure and whenever ventilatory function is depressed.

Warnings: May be habit forming. Codeine can produce drug dependence of the morphine type and therefore has the potential for being abused. Psychic dependence, physical dependence and tolerance may develop upon repeated administration of PERCOGESIC with Codeine, and it should be prescribed and administered with the same degree of caution appropriate to the use of other narcotic drugs (See DRUG ABUSE AND DEPENDENCE).

Respiratory Depression: PERCOGESIC with Codeine produces dose-related respiratory depression by directly acting on brain stem respiratory centers. If respiratory depression occurs, it may be antagonized by the use of NARCAN® (naloxone hydrochloride) and other supportive measures when indicated.

Head Injury and Increased Intracranial Pressure: The respiratory depressant properties of narcotics and their capacity to elevate cerebrospinal fluid pressure may be markedly exaggerated in the presence of head injury, other intracranial lesions or a pre-existing increase in intracranial pressure. Furthermore, narcotics produce adverse reactions which may obscure the clinical course of patients with head injuries.

Acute abdominal conditions: The administration of PERCOGESIC with Codeine or other narcotics may obscure the diagnosis or clinical course of patients with acute abdominal conditions.

Antihistamines may produce drowsiness or excitation, particularly in children and elderly patients.

Precautions: As with all narcotic medication, care should be exercised in prescribing PERCOGESIC with Codeine in view of the possibility of unwanted suppression of productive cough.

Usage in Ambulatory Patients: Codeine, like all narcotics, and antihistamines such as phenyltoloxamine, may impair the mental and/or physical abilities required for the performance of potentially hazardous tasks, such as driving a car or operating machinery, and patients should be warned accordingly.

Drug Interactions: Patients receiving other narcotic analgesics, general anesthetics, phenothiazines, other tranquilizers, sedative-hypnotics or other CNS depressants (including alcohol) concomitantly with codeine may exhibit an additive CNS depression. When such combined therapy is contemplated, the dose of one or both agents should be reduced. MAO inhibitors may prolong the anticholinergic effects of antihistamines.

Carcinogenesis, mutagenesis, impairment of fertility: Carcinogenicity, mutagenicity and reproduction studies have not been conducted with PERCOGESIC with Codeine.

Usage in Pregnancy: Pregnancy Category C. Animal reproduction studies have not been conducted with PERCOGESIC with Codeine. It is also not known whether PERCOGESIC with Codeine can cause fetal harm when administered to a pregnant woman or can affect reproductive capacity. PERCOGESIC with Codeine should be given to a pregnant woman only if clearly needed.

Nonteratogenic effects: Babies born to mothers who have been taking opioids regularly prior to delivery will be physically dependent. The withdrawal signs include irritability and excessive crying, tremors, hyperactive reflexes, increased respiratory rate, increased stools, sneezing, yawning, vomiting and fever. The intensity of the syndrome does not always correlate with the duration of maternal opioid use or dose. There is no consensus on the best method of managing withdrawal. Chlorpromazine 0.7–1.0 mg/kg q 6 h, phenobarbital 2 mg/kg q 6 h, and paregoric 2–4 drops/kg q 4 h, have been used to treat withdrawal symptoms in infants. The duration of therapy is 4 to 28 days, with the dosage decreased as tolerated.

Nursing mothers: It is not known whether this drug is excreted in human milk. Because many drugs are excreted in human milk and because of the potential for serious adverse reactions in nursing infants from PERCOGESIC with Codeine, a decision should be made whether to discontinue nursing or discontinue the drug, taking into account the importance of the drug to the mother.

Pediatric use: Safety and effectiveness in children below the age of 5 years have not been established.

Adverse Reactions:

Respiratory System: Codeine produces dose-related respiratory depression by acting directly on brain stem respiratory centers.

Cardiovascular System: Hypertension, postural hypotension, tachycardia and palpitations.

Genitourinary System: Ureteral spasm, spasm of vesical sphincters, urinary retention have been reported with opiates.

Central Nervous System: Sedation, drowsiness, mental clouding, lethargy, impairment of mental and physical performance, anxiety, fear, dysphoria, dizziness, psychic dependence, mood changes and blurred vision.

Gastrointestinal System: Nausea and vomiting occur more frequently in ambulatory than in recumbent patients.

Drug Abuse and Dependence: Special care should be exercised in prescribing codeine for emotionally unstable patients and for those with a history of drug misuse. Such patients should be closely supervised when long-term therapy is contemplated.

PERCOGESIC with Codeine is a Schedule III narcotic. Psychic dependence, physical dependence, and tolerance may develop upon repeated administration of narcotics; therefore, PERCOGESIC with Codeine should be prescribed and administered with caution. Physical dependence is the condition in which continued administration of the drug is required to prevent the appearance of a withdrawal syndrome.

Patients physically dependent on opioids will develop an abstinence syndrome upon abrupt discontinuation of the opioid or following the administration of a narcotic antagonist. The character and severity of the withdrawal symptoms are related to the degree of physical dependence. Manifestations of opioid withdrawal are similar to but milder than that of morphine and include lacrimation, rhinorrhea, yawning, sweating, restlessness, dilated pupils, anorexia, gooseflesh, irritability and tremor. In more severe forms, nausea, vomiting, intestinal spasm and diarrhea, increased heart rate and blood pressure, chills, and pains in bones and muscles of the back and extremities may occur. Peak effects will usually be apparent at 48 to 72 hours.

Treatment of withdrawal is usually managed by providing sufficient quantities of an opioid to suppress **severe** withdrawal symptoms and then gradually reducing the dose of opioid over a period of several days.

Overdosage: The signs and symptoms of overdosage of the individual components of PERCOGESIC with Codeine may be modified in varying degrees by the presence of other active ingredients.

Signs and Symptoms: Serious overdosage with codeine is characterized by respiratory depression (a decrease in respiratory rate and/or tidal volume, Cheyne-Stokes respiration, cyanosis), extreme somnolence progressing to stupor coma, skeletal muscle flaccidity, cold and clammy skin, and sometimes bradycardia and hypertension. In severe overdosage apnea, circulatory collapse, cardiac arrest, and death may occur. The ingestion of a large amount of acetaminophen may produce hepatic toxicity.

Treatment: Primary attention should be given to the reestablishment of adequate respiratory exchange through provision of a patent airway and institution of assisted or controlled ventilation. The narcotic antagonist naloxone hydrochloride (NARCAN®) is a specific antidote against respiratory depression which may result from overdosage or unusual sensitivity to narcotics including codeine. Therefore, an appropriate dose of naloxone hydrochloride should be administered (usual initial adult dose: 0.4 mg; usual initial child dose is 0.01 mg/kg body weight; for further information see NARCAN® full prescribing information), preferably by the intravenous route, simultaneously with efforts at respiratory resuscitation. Since the duration of action of codeine may exceed that of the antagonist, the patient should be kept under continued surveillance and repeated doses of the antagonist should be administered as needed to maintain adequate respiration. Oxygen, intravenous fluids, vasopressors and other supportive measures should be employed as indicated.

Gastric emptying may be useful in removing unabsorbed drug. Activated charcoal may be of benefit.

Treatment of acute acetaminophen overdosage is purely symptomatic.

Dosage and Administration:

Adults: One to two tablets every 4 hours as needed for pain.

Children: 5 to 12 years: ½ to 1 tablet every four hours as needed for pain.

How Supplied: PERCOGESIC with Codeine is available as a white scored tablet in bottles as follows:

Bottles of 100	NDC 0056-0133-70
Bottles of 1000	NDC 0056-0133-90

Store at controlled room temperature (59°–86°F, 15°–30°C).

PERCOGESIC® is a Registered Trademark of Endo Laboratories, Inc.

NARCAN® is a Registered Trademark of Endo Pharmaceuticals, Inc.

6024-8/Rev. Sept. 1981

REMSED® TABLETS ℞
(promethazine hydrochloride)

Description: REMSED (promethazine hydrochloride) is a phenothiazine derivative.

Actions: REMSED, a phenothiazine, possesses antihistaminic, sedative, anti-motion, antiemetic and anticholinergic effects. The duration of action is generally from 4 to 6 hours. As an antihistamine it acts by competitive antagonism, but does not block the release of histamine. It antagonizes in varying degrees most, but not all, of the pharmacological effects of histamine.

Indications: REMSED (promethazine hydrochloride) is indicated for the production of light sleep from which the patient can be easily aroused.

In addition, REMSED can provide:

a) sedation in both children and adults.
b) relief of apprehension
c) preoperative, postoperative, and obstetric sedation.

REMSED can also be of clinical use as follows:

a) adjunctive therapy with meperidine or other analgesics for control of postoperative pain.
b) for prevention and control of nausea and vomiting associated with anesthesia and surgery.
c) as an antiemetic in postoperative patients.
d) for active and prophylactic treatment of motion sickness.

Contraindications: REMSED is contraindicated in comatose patients. It is also contraindicated in patients receiving monoamine oxidase inhibitors and in patients who have received large amounts of central nervous system depressants (alcohol, barbiturates, narcotics, etc.). Additionally, the drug is contraindicated in patients who have demonstrated an idiosyncrasy or hypersensitivity to REMSED or to other phenothiazines.

REMSED is contraindicated in patients with bone marrow depression, narrow-angle glaucoma, bladder neck obstruction, prostatic hypertrophy, pyloroduodenal obstruction and stenosing peptic ulcer. The drug should not be used in patients during asthmatic attacks or to treat lower respiratory tract symptoms.

REMSED is contraindicated in newborn or premature infants. It should not be used in acutely ill or dehydrated children because there is an increased susceptibility to dystonias.

Warnings: REMSED may impair the mental and/or physical abilities required for the performance of potentially hazardous tasks such as driving a vehicle or operating machinery. Similarly, it may impair mental alertness in children. The concomitant use of alcohol or other central nervous system depressants may have an additive effect. Patients should be warned accordingly.

Usage in Pregnancy: The safe use of REMSED has not been established with respect to the possible adverse effects upon fetal development. Therefore, it should not be used in women of childbearing potential, particularly during early pregnancy, or in lactating women unless in the judgment of the physician the potential benefits outweigh the possible risks. There are reports of jaundice and prolonged extrapyramidal symptoms in infants whose mothers received phenothiazines during pregnancy. Therefore, the use of this drug during early pregnancy, or in lactating women, should be undertaken only after weighing possible risks against potential benefit. REMSED may interfere with the accuracy of diagnostic tests for pregnancy.

Caution should be exercised when administering REMSED to children for the treatment of vomiting. Antiemetics are not recommended for treatment of uncomplicated vomiting in children and their use should be limited to prolonged vomiting of known etiology. There are three principal reasons for caution:

1. There has been some suspicion that centrally acting antiemetics may contribute, in combination with viral illnesses (a possible cause of vomiting in children), to development of Reye's syndrome, a potentially fatal acute childhood encephalopathy with visceral fatty degeneration, especially involving the liver. Although there is no confirmation of this suspicion, caution is nevertheless recommended.
2. The extrapyramidal symptoms which can occur secondary to REMSED may be confused with the central nervous system signs of an undiagnosed primary disease responsible for the vomiting, e.g., Reye's syndrome or other encephalopathy.
3. It has been suspected that drugs with hepatotoxic potential, such as REMSED, may unfavorably alter the course of Reye's syndrome. Such drugs should therefore be avoided in children whose signs and symptoms (vomiting) could represent Reye's syndrome.

It should also be noted that salicylates and acetaminophen are hepatotoxic at large doses. Although it is not known that at usual doses they would represent a hazard in patients with the underlying hepatic disorder of Reye's syndrome, these drugs, too, should be avoided in children whose signs and symptoms could represent Reye's syndrome, unless alternative methods of controlling fever are not successful.

Precautions: REMSED (promethazine hydrochloride) may significantly affect the actions of other drugs. It may increase, prolong or intensify the sedative action of central nervous system depressants such as anesthetics, barbiturates or alcohol. The dose of a narcotic or barbiturate may be reduced to ¼ or ½ the usual amount when REMSED is administered concomitantly. Excessive amounts of REMSED, relative to a narcotic, may lead to restlessness and motor hyperactivity in the patient with pain.

REMSED can block and even reverse some of the actions of epinephrine.

The drug should also be used cautiously in persons with acute or chronic respiratory impairment, particularly children, because of possible suppression of the cough reflex.

REMSED should be used cautiously in persons with cardiovascular disease, impairment of liver function or a history of ulcer disease.

Because of its antiemetic effect, REMSED may mask signs of overdosage of toxic drugs or may obscure conditions such as brain tumor or intestinal obstruction.

Continued on next page

Endo—Cont.

Neuroleptic drugs elevate prolactin levels; the elevation persists during chronic administration. Tissue culture experiments indicate that approximately one-third of human breast cancers are prolactin dependent in vitro, a factor of potential importance if the prescription of these drugs is contemplated in a patient with a previously detected breast cancer. Although disturbances such as galactorrhea, amenorrhea, gynecomastia, and impotence have been reported, the clinical significance of elevated serum prolactin levels is unknown for most patients. An increase in mammary neoplasms has been found in rodents after chronic administration of neuroleptic drugs. Neither clinical studies nor epidemiologic studies conducted to date, however, have shown an association between chronic administration of these drugs and mammary tumorigenesis; the available evidence is considered too limited to be conclusive at this time.

Adverse Reactions:
Note: Not all of the following adverse reactions have been reported with this specific drug; however, pharmacological similarities among phenothiazine derivatives require that each be considered when REMSED is administered. There have been occasional reports of sudden death in patients receiving phenothiazine derivatives chronically.

CNS Effects: Drowsiness is the most prominent CNS effect of this drug. Extrapyramidal reactions occur, particularly with high dosages. Hyperreflexia has been reported in the newborn when a phenothiazine was used during pregnancy. Other reported reactions include blurred vision, diplopia, dizziness, euphoria, fatigue, grand mal seizures, incoordination, insomnia, lassitude, nervousness, tinnitus and tremors.

Cardiovascular Effects: Postural hypotension is the most common cardiovascular effect of REMSED. Reflex tachycardia may be seen. Bradycardia, faintness, dizziness and cardiac arrest have been reported. EKG changes, including blunting of T waves and prolongation of the Q-T interval, may be seen.

Gastrointestinal: Anorexia, constipation, dry mouth, epigastric distress, nausea and vomiting may occur.

Genitourinary: Urinary frequency and dysuria may occur.

Allergic Reactions: These include anaphylactoid reactions, angioedema, asthma, dermatitis, laryngeal edema and urticaria.

The following adverse reactions have been reported with all phenothiazines but are less common with REMSED: agranulocytosis, leukopenia, jaundice and extrapyramidal reactions.

Dosage and Administration: The usual adult daytime dose is 12.5 mg to 25 mg, 3 to 4 times daily. The usual adult bedtime dose is 50 mg. The dose for preoperative, postoperative and obstetrical sedation is 25 mg to 50 mg; 50 mg will provide sedation and relief of apprehension in early stages of labor.

Pediatric and geriatric doses may be adjusted according to age and weight.

When used prophylactically for motion sickness, the usual adult dose is 12.5 mg to 25 mg, 3 or 4 times daily. An initial dose of 25 mg should be taken ½ to 1 hour before anticipated travel.

Overdosage: Signs of overdosage include excitation, ataxia, incoordination, athetosis, convulsion and coma. Common signs in children are fixed, dilated pupils, fever and a flushed face. The treatment is symptomatic and supportive.

Drug Interactions: Phenothiazine medications include a large number of related molecular structures with many pharmacologic actions, including antihistaminic, antinauseant, antihypertensive, sedative and tranquilizing properties. As a result, they may interact with other medications, potentiating those drugs having similar pharmacologic effects, and antagonizing others having the opposite actions. Whenever REMSED is used concomitantly with other medications, the patient should be observed carefully for drug interactions.

How Supplied: REMSED is available as: Tablets—50 mg (light blue, scored) in bottles of 100.

REMSED® is an Endo Registered U.S. Trademark.
6048-3-4

SYMMETREL® ℞
(amantadine hydrochloride)

Description SYMMETREL is designated generically as amantadine hydrochloride and chemically as 1-adamantanamine hydrochloride.

Amantadine hydrochloride is a stable white or nearly white crystalline powder, freely soluble in water and soluble in alcohol and in chloroform.

Amantadine hydrochloride has pharmacological actions as both an anti-Parkinson and an antiviral drug.

SYMMETREL is available in capsules and syrup.

Clinical Pharmacology: SYMMETREL is readily absorbed, is not metabolized, and is excreted unchanged in the urine.

After oral administration of a single dose of 100 mg. maximum blood levels are reached, based on the mean time of the peak urinary excretion rate, in approximately 4 hours; the peak excretion rate is approximately 5 mg/hr; the mean half-life of the excretion rate approximates 15 hours.

The mechanism of action of SYMMETREL in the treatment of Parkinson's disease and drug-induced extrapyramidal reactions is not known. It has been shown to cause an increase in dopamine release in the animal brain. The drug does not possess anticholinergic activity in animal tests at doses similar to those used clinically. The antiviral activity of SYMMETREL against influenza A virus is not completely understood. The mode of action of SYMMETREL appears to be the prevention of the release of infectious viral nucleic acid into the host cell. SYMMETREL does not appear to interfere with the immunogenicity of inactivated influenza A virus vaccine.

Indications and Usage: **Parkinson's Disease/Syndrome and Drug-Induced Extrapyramidal Reactions:** SYMMETREL is indicated in the treatment of idiopathic Parkinson's disease (Paralysis Agitans), postencephalitic parkinsonism, drug-induced extrapyramidal reactions, and symptomatic parkinsonism which may follow injury to the nervous system by carbon monoxide intoxication. It is indicated in those elderly patients believed to develop parkinsonism in association with cerebral arteriosclerosis. In the treatment of Parkinson's disease, SYMMETREL is less effective than levodopa, (1)-3-(3, 4-dihydroxyphenyl)-L-alanine, and its efficacy in comparison with the anticholinergic antiparkinson drugs has not yet been established. Although anticholinergic type side effects have been noted with SYMMETREL when used in patients with drug-induced extrapyramidal reactions, there is a lower incidence of these side effects than that observed with anticholinergic antiparkinson drugs.

Influenza A Virus Respiratory Tract Illness: SYMMETREL (amantadine hydrochloride) is indicated in the prevention and treatment of respiratory tract illness caused by influenza A virus strains. SYMMETREL should be considered especially for high risk patients, close household or hospital ward contacts of index cases and patients with severe influenza A virus illness. In the prophylaxis of influenza due to A virus strains, early immunization as periodically recommended by the Public Health Service Advisory Committee on Immunization Practices is the method of choice. When early immunization is not feasible, or when the vaccine is contraindicated or not available. SYMMETREL can be used for chemoprophylaxis against influenza A virus illness. Because SYMMETREL does not appear to suppress antibody response, it can be used chemoprophylactically in conjunction with inactivated influenza A virus vaccine until protective antibody responses develop. There is no clinical evidence that this drug has efficacy in the prophylaxis or treatment of viral respiratory tract illnesses other than those caused by influenza A virus strains.

Contraindications: SYMMETREL in contraindicated in patients with known hypersensitivity to the drug.

Warnings: Patients with a history of epilepsy or other "seizures" should be observed closely for possible increased seizure activity.

Patients with a history of congestive heart failure or peripheral edema should be followed closely as there are patients who developed congestive heart failure while receiving SYMMETREL.

Patients with Parkinson's disease improving on SYMMETREL should resume normal activities gradually and cautiously, consistent with other medical considerations, such as the presence of osteoporosis or phlebothrombosis.

Patients receiving SYMMETREL who note central nervous system effects or blurring of visions should be cautioned against driving or working in situations where alertness is important.

Precautions: SYMMETREL (amantadine hydrochloride) should not be discontinued abruptly since a few patients with Parkinson's disease experienced a parkinsonian crisis, i.e., a sudden marked clinical deterioration, when this medication was suddenly stopped. The dose of anticholinergic drugs or of SYMMETREL should be reduced if atropine-like effects appear when these drugs are used concurrently.

The dose of SYMMETREL may need careful adjustment in patients with renal impairment, congestive heart failure, peripheral edema, or orthostatic hypotension. Since SYMMETREL is not metabolized and is mainly excreted in the urine, it may accumulate when renal function is inadequate.

Care should be exercised when administering SYMMETREL to patients with liver disease, a history of recurrent eczematoid rash, or to patients with psychosis or severe psychoneurosis not controlled by chemotherapeutic agents. Careful observation is required when SYMMETREL is administered concurrently with central nervous system stimulants.

No long-term studies in animals have been performed to evaluate the carcinogenic potential of SYMMETREL.

The mutagenic potential of the drug has not yet been determined in experimental systems.

Pregnancy Category C: SYMMETREL (amantadine hydrochloride) has been shown to be embryotoxic and teratogenic in rats at 50 mg/kg/day, about 12 times the recommended human dose, but not at 37 mg/kg/day. Embryotoxic and teratogenic drug effects were not seen in rabbits which received up to 25 times the recommended human dose. There are no adequate and well-controlled studies in pregnant women.

SYMMETREL should be used during pregnancy only if the potential benefit justifies the potential risk to the embryo or the fetus.

Nursing Mothers: SYMMETREL is excreted in human milk. Caution should be exercised when SYMMETREL is administered to a nursing woman.

Pediatric Use: The safety and efficacy of SYMMETREL in newborn infants, and infants below the age of 1 year have not been established.

Adverse Reactions: The most frequently occurring serious adverse reactions are depression, congestive heart failure, orthostatic hypotensive episodes, psychosis, and urinary retention. Rarely convulsions, leukopenia, and neutropenia have been reported.
Other adverse reactions of a less serious nature which have been observed are the following: hallucinations, confusion, anxiety and irritability, anorexia, nausea, and constipation; ataxia and dizziness (lightheadedness); livedo reticularis and peripheral edema. Adverse reactions observed less frequently are the following: vomiting; dry mouth; headache; dyspnea; fatigue, insomnia, and a sense of weakness. Infrequently, skin rash, slurred speech, and visual disturbances have been observed. Rarely eczematoid dermatitis and oculogyric episodes have been reported.
Overdosage: There is no specific antidote. However, slowly administered intravenous physostigmine in 1 and 2 mg doses in an adult[1] at 1 to 2 hour intervals and 0.5 mg doses in a child[2] at 5 to 10 minute intervals up to a maximum of 2 mg/hour have been reported to be effective in the control of central nervous system toxicity caused by amantadine hydrochloride. For acute overdosing, general supportive measures should be employed along with immediate gastric lavage or induction of emesis. Fluids should be forced, and if necessary, given intravenously. The pH of the urine has been reported to influence the excretion rate of SYMMETREL. Since the excretion rate of SYMMETREL increases rapidly when the urine is acidic, the administration of urine acidifying drugs may increase the elimination of the drug from the body. The blood pressure, pulse, respiration and temperature should be monitored. The patient should be observed for hyperactivity and convulsions; if required, sedation, and anticonvulsant therapy should be administered. The patient should be observed for the possible development of arrhythmias and hypotension, if required, appropriate antiarrhythmic and antihypotensive therapy should be given. The blood electrolytes, urine pH and urinary output should be monitored. If there is no record of recent voiding, catheterization should be done. The possibility of multiple drug ingestion by the patient should be considered.
[1]D.F. Casey, N. Engl. J. Med. 298:516, 1978.
[2]C.D. Berkowitz, J. Pediatr. 95:144, 1979.
Dosage and Administration:
Dosage for Parkinsonism:
Adult: The usual dose of SYMMETREL (amantadine hydrochloride) is 100 mg twice a day when used alone. SYMMETREL has an onset of action usually within 48 hours.
The initial dose of SYMMETREL is 100 mg daily for patients with serious associated medical illnesses or who are receiving high doses of other antiparkinson drugs. After one to several weeks at 100 mg once daily, the dose may be increased to 100 mg twice daily, if necessary. Occasionally, patients whose responses are not optimal with SYMMETREL at 200 mg daily may benefit from an increase up to 400 mg daily in divided doses. However, such patients should be supervised closely by their physicians.
Patients initially deriving benefit from SYMMETREL not uncommonly experience a fall-off of effectiveness after a few months. Benefit may be regained by increasing the dose to 300 mg daily. Alternatively, temporary discontinuation of SYMMETREL for several weeks, followed by reinitiation of the drug, may result in regaining benefit in some patients. A decision to use other antiparkinson drugs may be necessary.
Dosage for Concomitant Therapy
Some patients who do not respond to anticholinergic antiparkinson drugs may respond to SYMMETREL. When SYMMETREL or anticholinergic antiparkinson drugs are each used with marginal benefit, concomitant use may produce additional benefit.
When SYMMETREL and levodopa are initiated concurrently, the patient can exhibit rapid therapeutic benefits. SYMMETREL should be held constant at 100 mg daily or twice daily while the daily dose of levodopa is gradually increased to optimal benefit.
When SYMMETREL is added to optimal well-tolerated doses of levodopa, additional benefit may result, including smoothing out the fluctuations in improvement which sometimes occur in patients on levodopa alone. Patients who require a reduction in their usual dose of levodopa because of development of side effects may possibly regain lost benefit with the addition of SYMMETREL.
Dosage for Drug-induced Extrapyramidal Reactions:
Adult: The usual dose of SYMMETREL (amantadine hydrochloride) is 100 mg twice a day. Occasionally, patients whose responses are not optimal with SYMMETREL at 200 mg daily may benefit from an increase up to 300 mg daily in divided doses.
Dosage for Prophylaxis and Treatment of Influenza A
Virus Respiratory Tract Illness:
Adult: The adult daily dosage of SYMMETREL (amantadine hydrochloride) is 200 mg; two 100 mg capsules (or four teaspoonfuls of syrup) as a single daily dose, or the daily dosage may be split into one capsule of 100 mg (or two teaspoonfuls of syrup) twice a day. If central nervous system effects develop on once-a-day dosage, a split dosage schedule may reduce such complaints.
Children: 1 yr.–9 yrs. of age: The total daily dose should be calculated on the basis of 2 to 4 mg/lb/day (4.4 to 8.8 mg/kg/day), but not to exceed 150 mg per day.
9 yrs.–12 yrs. of age: The total daily dose is 200 mg given as one capsule of 100 mg (or two teaspoonfuls of syrup) twice a day.
Prophylactic dosing should be started in anticipation of contact or as soon as possible after contact with individuals with influenza A virus respiratory illness. SYMMETREL should be continued daily for at least 10 days following a known exposure. If SYMMETREL is used chemoprophylactically in conjunction with inactivated influenza A virus vaccine until protective antibody responses develop, then it should be administered for 2 to 3 weeks after the vaccine has been given. When inactivated influenza A virus vaccine is unavailable or contraindicated, SYMMETREL should be administered for up to 90 days in case of possible repeated and unknown exposures. Treatment of influenza A virus illness should be started as soon as possible after onset of symptoms and should be continued for 24 to 48 hours after the disappearance of symptoms.
How Supplied: SYMMETREL (amantadine hydrochloride).
Capsules: (bottles of 100 and 500)–each red, soft gelatin capsule contains 100 mg amantadine hydrochloride.
Syrup: (1 pint)–each 5 ml (1 teaspoonful) of syrup contains 50 mg amantadine hydrochloride.
SYMMETREL is a DuPont Registered U.S. Trademark
Capsules manufactured by
R.P. Scherer-North America,
St. Petersburg, Florida 33702
For Endo Laboratories, Inc.
6043-11
[*Shown in Product Identification Section*]

TESSALON® ℞
(benzonatate NF)

Description: TESSALON®, a nonnarcotic antitussive agent, is 2, 5, 8, 11, 14, 17, 20, 23, 26-nonaoxaoctacosan-28-yl p-(butylamino) benzoate.
Actions: TESSALON® acts peripherally by anesthetizing the stretch receptors located in the respiratory passages, lungs, and pleura by dampening their activity and thereby reducing the cough reflex at its source. It begins to act within 15 to 20 minutes and its effect lasts for 3 to 8 hours. TESSALON® has no inhibitory effect on the respiratory center in recommended dosage.
Indications: Symptomatic relief of cough.
Contraindications: Hypersensitivity to benzonatate or related compounds.
Warnings: **Usage in Pregnancy:** The safe use of this drug in pregnant women or during lactation has not been established. Therefore, the benefits must be weighed against the potential hazards.
Precautions: Release of TESSALON® from the perle in the mouth can produce a temporary local anesthesia of the oral mucosa. Therefore, the perles should be swallowed without chewing.
Adverse Reactions: Sedation, headache, mild dizziness, pruritus and skin eruptions, nasal congestion, constipation, nausea, gastrointestinal upset, sensation of burning in the eyes, a vague "chilly" sensation, numbness in the chest, and hypersensitivity have been reported.
Dosage and Administration: *Adults and Children over 10:* Usual dose is one 100 mg perle t.i.d. as required. If necessary, up to 6 perles daily may be given.
Overdosage: No clinically significant cases have been reported, to our knowledge. The drug is chemically related to tetracaine and other topical anesthetics and shares various aspects of their pharmacology and toxicology. Drugs of this type are generally well absorbed after ingestion.
Signs and Symptoms
If perles are chewed or dissolved in the mouth, oropharyngeal anesthesia will develop rapidly. CNS stimulation may cause restlessness and tremors which may proceed to clonic convulsions followed by profound CNS depression.
Treatment
Evacuate gastric contents and administer copious amounts of activated charcoal slurry. Even in the conscious patient, cough and gag reflexes may be so depressed as to necessitate special attention to protection against aspiration of gastric contents and orally administered materials.
Convulsions should be treated with a *short-acting* barbiturate given intravenously and carefully titrated for the smallest effective dosage.
Intensive support of respiration and cardiovascular-renal function is an essential feature of the treatment of severe intoxication from overdosage.
Do not use CNS stimulants.
How Supplied: Perles, 100 mg (yellow); bottles of 100.
6075-7
TESSALON is manufactured by R.P. Scherer-North America, St. Petersburg, Florida 33702 for Endo Laboratories, Inc.
[*Shown in Product Identification Section*]

VALPIN® 50 ℞
anisotropine methylbromide 50 mg

Description: VALPIN® 50 is anisotropine methylbromide, a quaternary ammonium salt which differs chemically from atropine and most other anticholinergics in the substitution of an aliphatic for an aromatic side chain in the acid moiety of the ester.
Chemically, VALPIN® 50 is 2-propyl pentanoyl tropinium methylbromide. Its stability both to acid and alkaline hydrolysis minimizes inactivation.

Continued on next page

Endo—Cont.

Actions: VALPIN® 50 inhibits gastric acid secretion and reduces gastrointestinal motility.

Indications: For use as adjunctive therapy in the treatment of peptic ulcer.

AS WITH ALL ANTICHOLINERGICS, IT SHOULD BE NOTED THAT AT THE PRESENT TIME THERE IS LACK OF CONCURRENCE AS TO THEIR VALUE IN THE TREATMENT OF GASTRIC ULCER. IT HAS NOT BEEN SHOWN CONCLUSIVELY WHETHER ANTICHOLINERGIC DRUGS AID IN THE HEALING OF A PEPTIC ULCER, DECREASE THE RATE OF RECURRENCES OR PREVENT COMPLICATION.

Contraindications: Glaucoma; obstructive uropathy (for example, bladder neck obstruction due to prostatic hypertrophy); obstructive disease of the gastrointestinal tract (as in achalasia, pyloroduodenal stenosis, etc.); paralytic ileus, intestinal atony of the elderly or debilitated patient; unstable cardiovascular status in acute hemorrhage; severe ulcerative colitis; toxic megacolon complicating ulcerative colitis; myasthenia gravis.

Warnings:

Use in Pregnancy Since the safety of these preparations in pregnancy, lactation or in women of child-bearing age has not been established, use of the drugs in such patients requires that the potential benefits of the drug be weighed against possible hazards to the mother and child.

In the presence of a high environmental temperature, heat prostration can occur with drug use (fever and heat stroke due to decreased sweating).

Diarrhea may be an early symptom of incomplete intestinal obstruction, especially in patients with ileostomy or colostomy. In this instance treatment with this drug would be inappropriate and possibly harmful.

VALPIN® 50 may produce drowsiness or blurred vision. In this event, the patient should be warned not to engage in activities requiring mental alertness such as operating a motor vehicle or other machinery or perform hazardous work while taking this drug.

Precautions:

Use with caution in patients with:

—Autonomic neuropathy.

—Hepatic or renal disease.

—Ulcerative colitis—large doses may suppress intestinal motility to the point of producing a paralytic ileus and the use of this drug may precipitate or aggravate the serious complication of toxic megacolon.

—Hyperthyroidism, coronary heart disease, congestive heart failure, cardiac arrhythmias, hypertension and non-obstructing prostatic hypertrophy.

—Hiatal hernia associated with reflux esophagitis since anticholinergic drugs may aggravate this condition.

It should be noted that the use of anticholinergic drugs in the treatment of gastric ulcer may produce a delay in gastric emptying time and may complicate such therapy (antral stasis).

Do not rely on the use of the drug in the presence of complication of biliary tract disease.

Investigate any tachycardia before giving anticholinergic (atropine-like) drugs since they may increase the heart rate.

With overdosage, a curare-like action may occur.

Adverse Reactions: Anticholinergic drugs produce certain effects which may be physiologic or toxic depending upon the individual patient's response. The physician must delineate these.

Adverse reactions may include xerostomia; urinary hesitancy and retention; blurred vision and tachycardia; palpitations; mydriasis; cycloplegia; increased ocular tension; loss of taste; headaches; nervousness; drowsiness; weakness; dizziness; insomnia; nausea; vomiting; impotence; suppression of lactation; constipation; bloated feeling; severe allergic reaction or drug idiosyncrasies including anaphylaxis; urticaria and other dermal manifestations; some degree of mental confusion and/or excitement especially in elderly persons. Decreased sweating is another adverse reaction that may occur.

Dosage and Administration: To be effective dosage must be titrated to individual patient needs. Usual adult dosage—VALPIN® 50 mg tablet; one tablet 3 times daily.

Management of Overdosage: While overdosage intoxication with anisotropine methylbromide has not been reported, theoretically it could occur since anisotropine methylbromide is an anticholinergic drug. When anticholinergic drugs are taken in sufficient overdose to produce severe symptoms, prompt treatment should be instituted. If the drug has been taken orally, gastric lavage and other measures to limit intestinal absorption should be initiated without delay. Physostigmine administered parenterally may be necessary for treatment of the serious manifestations of intoxication. Additionally, symptomatic therapy, including oxygen, sedatives, and control of hyperthermia may be necessary.

How Supplied: VALPIN® 50: 50 mg anisotropine methylbromide in each scored, beige tablet.

Bottles of 100 tablets.

Animal Pharmacology and Toxicology: VALPIN® 50 (anisotropine methylbromide) is a relatively non-toxic drug. In dogs, mice, rats and guinea pigs both acute toxic and chronic toxic dose-levels are at many times in excess of the clinically useful range.

Both **in vitro** and oral **in vivo** data in mice and rats indicate that VALPIN® 50 (anisotropine methylbromide) is at least 2 or 3 times as potent as homatropine methylbromide in antispasmodic action while it is less than two-thirds as active in mydriatic effect. It has less than one-fiftieth of the mydriatic activity of atropine sulfate. In inhibition of salivary flow, VALPIN® 50 (anisotropine methylbromide) is one-fifth as active as homatropine methylbromide and only one-hundredth as active as atropine sulfate. This pharmacologic profile is consistent with relative specificity of action of the gastrointestinal smooth muscle and the lesser tendency to produce side effects.

VALPIN® is an Endo registered U.S. trademark

6083-5

VALPIN® 50-PB ℞

(anisotropine methylbromide 50 mg with phenobarbital 15 mg)

Description: VALPIN® 50-PB is anisotropine methylbromide with phenobarbital. Anisotropine methylbromide differs chemically from atropine and most other anticholinergics/ antispasmodics in the substitution of an aliphatic for an aromatic side chain in the acid moiety of the ester.

Chemically, anisotropine methylbromide is 2-propyl pentanoyl tropinium methylbromide. Its stability both to acid and alkaline hydrolysis minimizes inactivation.

Actions: VALPIN® 50-PB (anisotropine methylbromide with phenobarbital), like other anticholinergic/antispasmodic drugs, effectively produces visceral smooth muscle relaxation. Consequently, VALPIN® 50-PB may provide effective control of smooth muscle spasm seen in motility disorders of the gastrointestinal tract, such as spastic colon and functional gastrointestinal disorders.

Indications: AS WITH ALL ANTICHOLINERGICS/ANTISPASMODICS, IT SHOULD BE NOTED THAT AT THE PRESENT TIME THERE IS LACK OF CONCURRENCE AS TO THEIR VALUE IN THE TREATMENT OF GASTRIC ULCER. IT HAS NOT BEEN SHOWN CONCLUSIVELY WHETHER ANTICHOLINERGIC/ANTISPASMODIC DRUGS AID IN THE HEALING OF A PEPTIC ULCER, DECREASE THE RATE OF RECURRENCES OR PREVENT COMPLICATION.

Based on a review of this drug by the National Academy of Sciences—National Research Council and/or other information, FDA has classified the following indications as "possibly" effective.

Indicated for use as adjunctive therapy in the treatment of peptic ulcer; irritable bowel syndrome (irritable colon, spastic colon, mucous colitis, acute enterocolitis, and functional gastrointestinal disorders); and in neurogenic bowel disturbances (including the splenic flexure syndrome and neurogenic colon).

THESE FUNCTIONAL DISORDERS ARE OFTEN RELIEVED BY VARYING COMBINATIONS OF SEDATIVE, REASSURANCE, PHYSICIAN INTEREST, AMELIORATION OF ENVIRONMENTAL FACTORS.

Final classification of the less-than-effective indications requires further investigation.

Contraindications: Glaucoma; obstructive uropathy (for example, bladder neck obstruction due to prostatic hypertrophy); obstructive disease of the gastrointestinal tract (as in achalasia, pyloroduodenal stenosis, etc.); paralytic ileus, intestinal atony of the elderly or debilitated patient; unstable cardiovascular status in acute hemorrhage; severe ulcerative colitis; toxic megacolon complicating ulcerative colitis; myasthenia gravis.

Phenobarbital is contraindicated in acute intermittent porphyria. VALPIN® 50-PB is contraindicated in those patients in whom phenobarbital produces restlessness and/or excitement.

Warnings:

Use in Pregnancy: Since the safety of these preparations in pregnancy, lactation or in women of child-bearing age has not been established, use of the drugs in such patients requires that the potential benefits of the drug be weighed against possible hazards to the mother and child.

In the presence of a high environmental temperature, heat prostration can occur with drug use (fever and heat stroke due to decreased sweating).

Diarrhea may be an early symptom of incomplete intestinal obstruction, especially in patients with ileostomy or colostomy. In this instance treatment with this drug would be inappropriate and possibly harmful.

VALPIN® 50-PB may produce drowsiness or blurred vision. In this event, the patient should be warned not to engage in activities requiring mental alertness such as operating a motor vehicle or other machinery or perform hazardous work while taking this drug.

Phenobarbital: Phenobarbital may decrease the prothrombin time response to oral anticoagulants. More frequent monitoring of prothrombin time responses is indicated whenever phenobarbital is initiated or discontinued, and the dosage of anticoagulants should be adjusted accordingly.

Phenobarbital may be habit forming and should not be administered to individuals known to be addiction prone or to those with a history of physical and/or psychological dependence upon habit forming drugs.

Precautions: Use with caution in patients with:

—Autonomic neuropathy.
—Hepatic or renal disease.
—Ulcerative colitis—large doses may suppress intestinal motility to the point of producing a paralytic ileus and the use of this drug may precipitate or aggravate the serious complication of toxic megacolon.
—Hyperthyroidism, coronary heart disease, congestive heart failure, cardiac arrhythmias, hypertension and non-obstructing prostatic hypertrophy.
—Hiatal hernia associated with reflux esophagitis since anticholinergic/antispasmodic drugs may aggravate this condition.

It should be noted that the use of anticholinergic/antispasmodic drugs in the treatment of gastric ulcer may produce a delay in gastric emptying time and may complicate such therapy (antral stasis).

Do not rely on the use of the drug in the presence of complication of biliary tract disease.

Investigate any tachycardia before giving anticholinergic/antispasmodic (atropine-like) drugs since they may increase the heart rate.

With overdosage, a curare-like action may occur.

Adverse Reactions: Anticholinergic/antispasmodic drugs produce certain effects which may be physiologic or toxic depending upon the individual patient's response. The physician must delineate these.

Adverse reactions may include xerostomia; urinary hesitancy and retention; blurred vision and tachycardia; palpitations; mydriasis; cycloplegia; increased ocular tension; loss of taste; headaches; nervousness; drowsiness; weakness; dizziness; insomnia; nausea; vomiting; impotence; suppression of lactation; constipation; bloated feeling; severe allergic reaction or drug idiosyncrasies including anaphylaxis; urticaria and other dermal manifestations; some degree of mental confusion and/or excitement especially in elderly persons. Decreased sweating is another adverse reaction that may occur.

Phenobarbital: In some patients phenobarbital may produce excitement rather than a sedative effect, as well as musculoskeletal pain. Some patients may acquire a sensitivity to barbiturates.

Dosage and Administration: To be effective, the dosage must be titrated to the individual patient's needs. Usual adult dosage—VALPIN® 50-PB: one tablet 3 times daily.

Management of Overdosage: While overdosage intoxication with anisotropine methylbromide with phenobarbital has not been reported, theoretically it could occur since anisotropine methylbromide is an anticholinergic/antispasmodic drug. When anticholinergic/antispasmodic drugs are taken in sufficient overdose to produce severe symptoms, prompt treatment should be instituted. If the drug has been taken orally, gastric lavage and other measures to limit intestinal absorption should be initiated without delay. Physostigmine administered parenterally may be necessary for treatment of the serious manifestations of intoxication. Additionally, symptomatic therapy, including oxygen, sedatives, and control of hyperthermia may be necessary.

Acute barbiturate intoxication with VALPIN® 50-PB, while possible, has not been reported. While the usual procedures for handling barbiturate poisoning should be employed, keep in mind the possibility of anticholinergic overdosing effects.

How Supplied: VALPIN® 50-PB: 50 mg anisotropine methylbromide and 15 mg of phenobarbital (*Warning:* May be habit forming) in each scored, white tablet.

Bottles of 100 tablets.

Animal Pharmacology and Toxicology: Anisotropine methylbromide is a relatively non-toxic drug. In dogs, mice, rats and guinea pigs both acute toxic and chronic toxic dose-levels are at many times in excess of the clinically useful range.

Both in vitro and oral in vivo data in mice and rats indicate that anisotropine methylbromide is at least 2 or 3 times as potent as homatropine methylbromide in antispasmodic action while it is less than two-thirds as active in mydriatic effect. It has less than one-fiftieth of the mydriatic activity of atropine sulfate. In inhibition of salivary flow, anisotropine methylbromide is one-fifth as active as homatropine methylbromide and only one-hundredth as active as atropine sulfate. This pharmacologic profile is consistent with relative specificity of action of the gastrointestinal smooth muscle and the lesser tendency to produce side effects.

VALPIN is an Endo registered U.S. trademark

6084-3

Everett Laboratories, Inc.

76 FRANKLIN STREET
EAST ORANGE, NEW JERSEY 07017

ANAFED Capsules and Syrup ℞

Antihistamine-Decongestant

Each timed release capsule contains: Chlorpheniramine Maleate 8 mg., Pseudoephedrine HCl. 120 mg.

Each tsp. contains: Chlorpheniramine Maleate 2 mg., Pseudoephedrine HCl. 30 mg.

Supplied: Bottles of 100 yellow/clear capsules; Pints, pineapple flavor.

FLORVITE Chewable Tablets ℞

Children's Vitamins + Fluoride

Supplied: Multiflavored chewable tablets in bottles of 100 and 1000.

FLORVITE Drops ℞

Children's Vitamins + Fluoride

Supplied: Bottles of 50 ml.

FLORVITE + IRON Chewable Tablets ℞

Children's Vitamins + Iron + Fluoride

Supplied: Grape flavored chewable tablets in bottles of 100.

FLORVITE + IRON Drops ℞

Children's Vitamins-Iron-Fluoride

Supplied: Bottles of 50 ml.

LIBIDINAL Soft Gel Capsules OTC

Each capsule contains: Zinc Gluconate 150 mg., Vitamin E 400 I.U.

Supplied: Bottles of 60 sugar and salt free capsules.

PAVATYM Capsules ℞

Each timed release capsule contains: Papaverine HCl. 150 mg.

Supplied: Bottles of 100 and 1000 capsules and Unit Dose packs of 100. Capsules imprinted EVERETT.

REPAN Tablets ℞

Each tablet contains: Butalbital 50 mg. (Warning: May be habit forming.), Caffeine (Anhydrus) 40 mg., Acetaminophen 325 mg.

Supplied: Bottles of 100 tablets imprinted EVERETT and 162.

VITAFOL Tablets ℞

Vitamins, Minerals, Iron, Folic Acid Supplement

Supplied: Bottles of 100 and 1000 pink film coated tablets.

Ferndale Laboratories, Inc.

780 W. EIGHT MILE ROAD
FERNDALE, MI 48220

AQUAPHYLLIN SYRUP ℞

(Theophylline, anhydrous 80 mg/15 ml)
Dye-Free, Alcohol-free and saccharin-free.

AQUAPHYLLIN SUGARBEADS 50 mg. CAPSULES

(Theophylline, anhydrous USP)
Dye-free

Actions and Uses: Theophylline is most effective in relaxing smooth muscles of bronchi, particularly if there is bronchial constriction, as in asthma. AQUAPHYLLIN is indicated for relief of acute bronchial asthma and for reversible bronchospasm associated with chronic asthma, bronchitis and emphysema.

Dosage and Administration:

AQUAPHYLLIN SYRUP:

Severe Asthma Attack: Adults—75 ml (5 tablespoonfuls). Children—One ml per kg. body weight, Do not repeat within six hours.

Maintenance 24-Hour Therapy: Adults for first six doses—45 ml (3 tablespoonfuls) upon every 6–8 hours, then 30 ml (2 tablespoonfuls) doses every 6–8 hours.

Children 3 to 5 mg. of theophylline per kg. body weight every 6–8 hours. It is recommended that dosage increases be based on serum theophylline determinations, particularly when exceeding the usual dosage range.

AQUAPHYLLIN SUGARBEADS 50 mg CAPSULES:

Maintenance 24-hour Therapy: Adults for first six doses—5 capsules upon every 6–8 hours, then 3 capsules every 6–8 hours. Children—3 to 5 mg of theophylline per kg. body weight every 6–8 hours. It is recommended that dosage increases be based on serum theophylline determination, particularly when exceeding the usual dosage range. To administer in small children, mix the content of capsule in favorite semi-solid food or dessert (e.g. apple sauce).

Adverse Effects: Nausea, vomiting, epigastric or substernal pain, palpitation, headache, dizziness may occur.

How Supplied:

Liquid: Pints, gallons and unit dose vials.

Capsules: Bottles of 100 and 1000.

KRONOFED–A–JR KRONOCAPS* ℞

Dye-Free, Sustained Release

Each capsule contains:
Pseudoephedrine HCl ....60 mg.
Chlorpheniramine Maleate ....4 mg.

How Supplied: Bottles of 100 and 500 capsules.

*Detailed information is available upon request.

KRONOFED–A KRONOCAPS* ℞

Dye-Free, Sustained Release

Each capsule contains:
Pseudoephedrine HCl ....120 mg.
Chlorpheniramine maleate ....8 mg.

How Supplied: Bottles of 100 and 500 capsules.

* Detailed information is available upon request.

KRONOHIST KRONOCAPS* ℞

Timed Disintegration Capsules.

Each Capsule contains:
Chlorpheniramine Maleate ....4 mg.
Pyrilamine Maleate ....25 mg.
Phenylpropanolamine HCl ....50 mg.

How Supplied: Bottles of 100 and 1000 capsules.

* Detailed information is available upon request.

Continued on next page

Ferndale—Cont.

LIQUI-DOSS*

Contains: Dioctyl Sodium Sulfosuccinate and mineral oil in a self-emulsifying, pleasantly flavored base.
How Supplied: Pints and unit dose vials.
* Detailed information is available upon request.

PRAMOSONE CREAM, LOTION AND OINTMENT ℞

Description: Pramosone Cream: Contains Hydrocortisone acetate 0.5% or 1% and Pramoxine HCl 1% in a hydrophilic base containing stearic acid, cetyl alcohol, aquaphor, isopropyl palmitate, polyoxyl 40 stearate, propylene glycol, potassium sorbate 0.1%, sorbic acid 0.1%, triethanolamine lauryl sulfate and water.
Pramosone Lotion: Contains Hydrocortisone acetate 0.5%, 1% or 2.5% and Pramoxine HCl 1% in a base containing forlan-L, cetyl alcohol, stearic acid, di-isopropyl adipate, polyoxyl 40 stearate, silicon, triethanolamine, glycerine, polyvinylpyrolidone, potassium sorbate 0.1%, sorbic acid 0.1% and water.
Pramosone Ointment: Contains Hydrocortisone acetate 1% and Pramoxine HCl 1% in an emollient ointment base containing Sorbitan sesquioleate, Water, Aquaphor and White petrolatum.
Actions: Hydrocortisone acetate is a corticosteroid. Topically, it is primarily effective because of its anti-inflammatory, anti-pruritic and vaso-constrictive actions. Pramoxine hydrochloride is a topical anesthetic which provides temporary relief from itching and pain.
Indications: For relief of the inflammatory manifestations of corticosteroid responsive dermatoses.
Contraindications: Topical steroids are contraindicated in viral diseases of the skin, such as varicella and vaccinia. Topical steroids are contraindicated in those patients with a history of hypersensitivity to any of the components of the preparation. Topical steroids should not be used when circulation is markedly impaired.
Precautions: If irritation develops, the product should be discontinued and appropriate therapy instituted. In the presence of an infection, the use of appropriate antifungal or antibacterial agents should be instituted. If a favorable response does not occur promptly, the corticosteroid should be discontinued until the infection has been adequately controlled. If extensive areas are treated or if the occlusive technique is used, the possibility exists of increased systemic absorption of the corticosteroid and suitable precautions should be taken. The product is not for opthalmic use.
Warnings: USAGE IN PREGNANCY: Although topical steroids have not been reported to have an adverse effect on the fetus, the safety of their use in pregnant females has not absolutely been established. Therefore, they should not be used extensively on pregnant patients, or in large amounts, or for prolonged periods of time.
Caution: Federal law prohibits despensing without prescription.
Adverse Reactions: The following local adverse reactions have been reported with topical corticosteroids, especially under occlusive dressings.
Burning, Itching, Irritation, Dryness, Folliculitis, Hypertrichosis, Acneiform eruptions, Hypopigmentation, Perioral dermatitis, Allergic Contact Dermatitis, Maceration of the skin, Secondary infection, Skin atrophy, Striae, and Miliaria.
Dosage and Administration: Apply to affected area 3 or 4 times daily.
How Supplied: CREAM: ½% or 1% in 1 oz. tube and lb. jar. LOTION: ½% or 1% in 1¼ fl. oz., 4 fl. oz., and 8 fl. oz., and HIGH POTENCY: 2½% in 2 fl. oz. plastic dispenser bottles. OINTMENT: 1 oz. tubes, 4 oz. jars and lb jars.

PRAX LOTION*
(Pramoxine HCl 1% in a hydrophilic lotion base)

Available: 15 ml and 120 ml dispenser bottle.
* Additional information available upon request.

Fisons Corporation
Pharmaceutical Division
TWO PRESTON COURT
BEDFORD, MA 01730

In addition to the products described in this section, Fisons also distributes the following products. On these and all Fisons products, information may be obtained by addressing Fisons Corporation, 2 Preston Court, Bedford, MA 01730.

BACID® CAPSULES OTC
lactobacillus acidophilus

ERGOMAR® ℞
ergotamine tartrate
2.0 mg sublingual tablet

KONDREMUL® OTC
KONDREMUL® with CASCARA
KONDREMUL® with PHENOLPHTHALEIN
mineral oil microemulsion

NEO-CULTOL® OTC
refined mineral oil, jelly, chocolate flavored

PERSISTIN® OTC
salicylsalicylic acid - 7 ½ gr.
aspirin - 2 ½ gr.

PROFERDEX™ ℞
iron dextran injection, USP
complex of ferric hydroxide
and dextran in a 0.9% sodium
chloride solution.

TUSSCAPINE® COUGH SUSPENSION and TABLETS OTC
noscapine

VAPO-ISO® ℞
isoproterenol HCl
solution 0.5% (1:200)

VAPONEFRIN® SOLUTION OTC
(racepinephrine)

VITRON-C® OTC
ferrous fumarate - 200 mg
ascorbic acid - 125 mg

VITRON-C PLUS® OTC
ferrous fumarate - 400 mg
ascorbic acid - 250 mg

INTAL® Nebulizer Solution ℞
(cromolyn sodium, USP)
For Inhalation Use Only—Not for Injection

Description: Each ampule of Intal (cromolyn sodium, USP) Nebulizer Solution contains 20 mg cromolyn sodium in 2 ml of purified water for inhalation. Chemically, cromolyn sodium is the disodium salt of 1,3-bis (2-carboxychromon-5-yloxy)-2-hydroxypropane. Intal Nebulizer Solution is clear, colorless, sterile and has a pH of 4.0-7.0.
The molecular structure is:

Pharmacological Category: Mast cell stabilizer/anti-allergic.
Therapeutic Category: Anti-asthmatic.
Clinical Pharmacology: *In vitro* and *in vivo* animal studies have shown that cromolyn sodium inhibits the degranulation of sensitized mast cells which occurs after exposure to specific antigens. Cromolyn sodium inhibits the release of histamine and SRS-A (the slow-reacting substance of anaphylaxis). Bronchial asthma induced by the inhalation of specific antigens can be inhibited to varying degrees by pretreatment with cromolyn sodium.
Another activity demonstrated *in vitro* is the capacity of cromolyn sodium to inhibit the degranulation of non-sensitized rat mast cells by phospholipase A and the subsequent release of chemical mediators. An additional *in vitro* study showed that cromolyn sodium did not inhibit the enzymatic activity of released phospholipase A on its specific substrate.
Cromolyn sodium has no intrinsic bronchodilator, antihistaminic or anti-inflammatory activity. Because of its prophylactic mechanism of action, Intal Nebulizer Solution has no role in the treatment of an acute attack of asthma.
Cromolyn sodium is poorly absorbed from the gastrointestinal tract. After inhalation of Intal capsules, about 8 percent of the total dose administered is deposited in the lung, absorbed, and rapidly excreted unchanged in the bile and urine. The remainder of the dose is either exhaled or deposited in the oropharynx, swallowed and excreted via the alimentary tract.
Indications and Usage: Intal Nebulizer Solution is indicated in the management of patients with bronchial asthma in whom the frequency, intensity and predictability of episodes indicate the use of a continuing program of symptomatic medication. Such patients must have a significant bronchodilator-reversible component to their airway obstruction as demonstrated by a generally accepted pulmonary function test of airway mechanics.
If improvement occurs, it will ordinarily occur within the first 4 weeks of administration as manifested by a decrease in the severity of clinical symptoms of asthma, or in the need for concomitant therapy, or both.
A decision to continue the administration of Intal Nebulizer Solution on a long term basis is justified if introduction of the drug into the patient's regime:
- produces a significant reduction in the severity of the symptoms of asthma, or
- permits a significant reduction in or elimination of steroids, or
- permits better management of patients who have intolerable side effects to sympathomimetic agents or methylxanthines.

Contraindications: Intal Nebulizer Solution is contraindicated in those patients who have shown hypersensitivity to cromolyn sodium.
Warnings: Intal (cromolyn sodium, USP) Nebulizer Solution has no role in the treatment of an acute attack of asthma, especially status asthmaticus.
The prophylactic effect of cromolyn sodium is usually evident after several weeks of treatment, although some patients show an almost immediate response.
In some animal toxicity studies, a previously unreported proliferative arterial lesion found predominantly in the kidneys occurred in both treated and untreated macaque monkeys. The incidence of the lesion was approximately equal in the treated and untreated animals. The relevance of these data to man is unknown. In considering the long-term administration of Intal Nebulizer Solution to a patient, the physician should take into consideration the possible risk as well as the degree of efficacy achieved in the individual patient.
Precautions:
General: In view of the biliary and renal routes of excretion for cromolyn sodium, consideration should be given to decreasing the dosage or discontinuing the administration of

the drug in patients with impaired renal or hepatic function.

If eosinophilic pneumonia (pulmonary infiltrates with eosinophilia) occurs during the course of Intal Nebulizer Solution therapy, the drug should be discontinued.

Occasionally patients may experience cough and/or bronchospasm following cromolyn sodium inhalation. At times, patients with cromolyn sodium induced bronchospasm may not be able to continue its administration despite prior bronchodilator administration. Rarely very severe bronchospasm has been encountered.

Symptoms of asthma may recur if Intal® Nebulizer Solution is reduced below the recommended dosage, or discontinued.

Carcinogenesis, Mutagenesis, Impairment of Fertility: Long-term studies have been conducted in mice (12 months and 18 months), rats (18 months), and in hamsters (24 months) using cromolyn sodium. The drug had no effect on the incidence of neoplasia in these studies.

No evidence of chromosomal damage or cytotoxic activity was obtained in various mutagenicity studies.

Reproduction studies performed in rabbits, rats, and mice at doses up to 600 times the human dose have revealed no evidence of impaired fertility or harm to the fetus due to cromolyn sodium.

Pregnancy: Teratogenic Effects: Pregnancy Category B. There are no adequate and well-controlled studies in pregnant women. Because animal reproduction studies are not always predictive of human response, this drug should be used during pregnancy only if clearly needed.

Reproduction studies with parenterally administered cromolyn sodium have been performed in rabbits, rats and mice. Adverse fetal effects (increased resorptions and decreased fetal weight) were noticed only at very high parenteral doses that produced maternal toxicity. The relevance to the human is not known.

Nursing Mothers: It is not known whether this drug is excreted in human milk. Because many drugs are excreted in human milk, caution should be exercised when Intal Nebulizer Solution is administered to a nursing woman.

Pediatric Use: Safety and effectiveness in children below the age of 2 years have not been established.

Adverse Reactions: The adverse reactions which have been observed in clinical trials with Intal Nebulizer Solution are noted as follows:

Cough
Nasal congestion
Nausea
Sneezing
Wheezing

Other reactions have been reported in clinical trails; however, a causal relationship could not be established:

Drowsiness
Nasal itching
Nose bleed
Nose burning
Serum sickness
Stomach ache

In addition, adverse reactions have been reported with Intal (cromolyn sodium) 20 mg Capsules. The most frequently reported adverse reactions attributed to Intal capsules (on the basis of reoccurrence following readministration) involve the respiratory tract and include:

Bronchospasm
Cough
Laryngeal edema (rare)
Nasal congestion
Pharyngeal irritation
Wheezing

Other adverse reactions which have also been attributed to Intal capsules (on the basis of reoccurrence following readministration) are:

Angioedema
Dizziness
Dysuria and urinary frequency
Joint swelling and pain
Lacrimation
Nausea and headache
Rash
Swollen parotid gland
Urticaria

In addition, the following adverse reactions have been reported as rare events and it is unclear whether these are attributable to Intal capsules:

Anaphylaxis
Anemia
Exfoliative dermatitis
Hemoptysis
Hoarseness
Myalgia
Nephrosis
Periarteritic vasculitis
Pericarditis
Peripheral neuritis
Photodermatitis
Polymyositis
Pulmonary infiltratis with eosinophilia
Vertigo

Dosage and Administration: The usual starting dosage for adults and children 2 years of age and over is the contents of one ampule administered by nebulization four times a day. One ampule contains 20 mg cromolyn sodium. Intal Nebulizer Solution should be administered from a power-operated nebulizer having an adequate flow rate, equipped with a suitable face mask. Hand operated nebulizers are not suitable for the administration of Intal Nebulizer Solution. Patients should be advised that the effect of Intal Nebulizer Solution therapy is dependent upon its administration at regular intervals, as directed. Intal Nebulizer Solution should be introduced into the patient's therapeutic regimen when the acute episode has been controlled, the airway cleared and the patient is able to inhale adequately.

Once a patient is stabilized on Intal® Nebulizer Solution, if there is no need for steroids, the frequency of administration may be titrated downward to the least frequent level consistent with the desired effect. The usual decrease is from four to three Intal Nebulizer Solution ampules per day. It is important that the dosage be reduced slowly, maintaining close supervision of the patient, to avoid exacerbation of asthma. It should be emphasized that in patients who have been titrated to less than four ampules per day, an increase in dosage may be needed if the patient's clinical condition worsens.

Corticosteroid Treatment and Its Relation to Intal Nebulizer Solution Use: An attempt to decrease corticosteroid administration and particularly to institute an alternate day regimen should be made in asthmatic patients receiving corticosteroids. Concomitant corticosteroids, as well as bronchodilators, should be continued following the introduction of Intal Nebulizer Solution. If the patient improves, an attempt to decrease corticosteroids should be made. Even if the steroid-dependent patient fails to improve following Intal Nebulizer Solution administration, gradual tapering of steroid dosage may nonetheless be attempted. It is important that the dose be reduced slowly, maintaining close supervision of the patient to avoid an exacerbation of asthma.

It should be borne in mind that prolonged corticosteroid therapy frequently causes a reduction in the activity and size of the adrenal cortex. Relative adrenocortical insufficiency upon discontinuation of therapy may be avoided by gradual reduction of dosage.

However, a potentially critical degree of insufficiency may persist asymptomatically for some time even after gradual discontinuation of adrenocortical steroids. Therefore, if a patient is subjected to significant stress, such as a severe asthmatic attack, surgery, trauma or severe illness while being treated or within one year (occasionally up to two years) after corticosteroid treatment has been terminated, consideration should be given to reinstituting corticosteroid therapy. When the inhalation of Intal Nebulizer Solution is impaired, as may occur in severe exacerbation of asthma, a temporary increase in the amount of corticosteroids and/or other medications may be required.

It is particularly important that great care be exercised if for any reason Intal Nebulizer Solution is withdrawn in cases where its use has permitted a reduction in the maintenance dose of steroids. In such cases, continued close supervision of the patient is essential since there may be sudden reappearance of severe manifestations of asthma which will require immediate therapy and possible reintroduction of corticosteroids.

Clinical Usage: A number of variables must be considered in evaluating the patient response to a drug used in the treatment of bronchial asthma—for example, concomitant treatment with other drugs, the fact that part of the trial may be conducted during the pollen season, the age of the patient, the duration and severity of disease, etc. In most studies of Intal® (cromolyn sodium) 20 mg Capsules, the drug was evaluated as part of the total care program for asthmatic patients, and the role of each of these factors could not be evaluated. It is emphasized that at the initiation of cromolyn sodium therapy, it is being added to a total care program and that patients may continue to require sympathomimetic amines, methylxanthines, and corticosteroids and antibiotics when indicated.

In clinical studies utilizing Intal Nebulizer Solution, physicians were able to reduce or eliminate the use of concomitant asthma medications, particularly methylxanthines.

Many clinical studies have been performed with Intal Capsules in patients with bronchial asthma. Controlled evaluations of the drug in comparison with a placebo have usually been of a crossover design with treatment periods lasting 4 to 6 weeks. In most of these studies, the investigator has concluded that cromolyn sodium is efficacious in comparison with the placebo. The proportion of patients responding to cromolyn sodium is usually reported to be in the majority, and an occasional patient is said to have a dramatic response. Significant improvement in pulmonary function tests is rarely reported, with the exception of one study in children in which approximately one-third of the patients showed an increase in Forced Expiratory Volume at 0.75 seconds ($FEV_{0.75}$) after three months therapy with cromolyn sodium.

One collaborative study of Intal capsules involving over 250 patients was sufficiently large to permit multivariate statistical analysis of the results. In this study, patients' symptom scores were measured according to the following scale: 0 (no symptoms), 1 (trivial), 2 (mild), 3 (annoying), 4 (moderate), 5 (severe), and 6 (incapacitating). The indices that were measured included day wheezing, night wheezing, day breathlessness, night breathlessness, day cough, night cough, etc. The study was crossover in design and patients were treated with cromolyn sodium and with placebo for a period of four weeks each. The study as a whole included a large number of patients whose mean baseline symptom scores were less than 2. Changes in mean symptom scores as a result of cromolyn sodium treatment were, for the group as a whole, usually less than one unit. Little clinical benefit was manifested in this group with trivial to mild symptoms. In patients who were most symptomatic (i.e., those whose baseline symptom scores ranged from 2 to 6) changes in mean symptom scores due to cromolyn sodium were greater than one unit. Pulmonary function studies in the total group showed no essential changes attributable to cromolyn sodium. It is inferred from this study that a clinically significant response to cromolyn sodium is most likely in patients with severe perennial asthma who are highly symptomatic (see Indications).

Another group of studies has been performed to determine whether the administration of Intal capsules has a corticosteroid-sparing effect. These studies have shown that a number of steroid dependent patients who have had several unsuccessful attempts to reduce or omit corticosteroids may do so after the administration of cromolyn sodium (see special section in Dosage and Administration).

Continued on next page

Fisons—Cont.

Long-term controlled studies relating specifically to the issue of tolerance are not available, but uncontrolled observations have not to this point revealed evidence of resistance or tolerance to the drug. Because the degree of response in an individual patient cannot be predicted, long-term therapy with cromolyn sodium is indicated only in patients who show a significant initial clinical response (see Indications).

How Supplied: Intal Nebulizer Solution is supplied in a double ended glass ampule containing 20 mg cromolyn sodium in 2 ml purified water.

NDC 0585-0673-01 48 ampules × 2 ml

Intal Nebulizer Solution should be stored below 30°C (86°F) and protected from direct light.

Caution: Federal law prohibits dispensing without prescription.

Also available as:

INTAL® ℞
(cromolyn sodium)
20 mg Capsules
For Inhalation Only
For Use With The SPINHALER®
TURBO-INHALER

Description: Chemically, cromolyn sodium is the disodium salt of 1,3-bis (2-carboxychromon-5-yloxy)-2-hydroxypropane.

It is soluble in water. Each capsule contains 20 mg cromolyn sodium in micronized form together with 20 mg of lactose powder added to improve the flow properties of the material. The contents of the capsule are intended for inhalation only, with the SPINHALER® turbo-inhaler.

Please see package insert for complete instructions.

SOMOPHYLLIN® Oral Liquid ℞
SOMOPHYLLIN®-DF Oral Liquid ℞
(aminophylline, USP)
SOMOPHYLLIN® Rectal Solution ℞
(aminophylline enema, USP)
SOMOPHYLLIN®-T Capsules ℞
(anhydrous theophylline, USP)
SOMOPHYLLIN®-CRT Capsules ℞
(anhydrous theophylline, USP)

Description: **Somophyllin Oral Liquid** contains anhydrous aminophylline (USP) equal to not less than 85.0 percent and not more than 86.5 percent of anhydrous theophylline and not less than 13.5 percent and not more than 15.0 percent of ethylenediamine, an inactive ingredient. Aminophylline is white or slightly yellowish granules, having a slight ammoniacal odor and a bitter taste. **Somophyllin® Oral Liquid** is a red raspberry flavored solution. **Somophyllin®-DF Oral Liquid** is a dye free colorless to light straw colored raspberry flavored solution. For both products, each 5 ml (teaspoonful) contains anhydrous aminophylline 105 mg (equivalent to 90 mg anhydrous theophylline) in a palatable, aqueous vehicle. Each 15 ml (tablespoonful) contains anhydrous aminophylline 315 mg (equivalent to 270 mg anhydrous theophylline).

Theophylline is the active ingredient.

Somophyllin Rectal Solution contains anhydrous aminophylline (USP) equal to not less than 85.0 percent and not more than 86.5 percent of anhydrous theophylline and not less than 13.5 percent and not more than 15.0 percent of ethylenediamine, an inactive ingredient. Aminophylline is white or slightly yellowish granules, having a slight ammoniacal odor and a bitter taste. **Somophyllin Rectal Solution** is a concentrated aqueous solution for rectal administration with the Rectal Ject syringe. Each 5 ml contains anhydrous aminophylline 300 mg (equivalent to 255 mg anhydrous theophylline).

Theophylline is the active ingredient.

Somophyllin-T Capsules (anhydrous theophylline, USP) contain not less than 94.0 percent and not more than 106.0 percent of the labeled amount of anhydrous theophylline. Theophylline is a white, odorless, crystalline powder, having a bitter taste.

Somophyllin-T Capsules are white, soft gelatin, liquid-filled capsules. They are supplied in four strengths: 50 mg, 100 mg, 200 mg, and 250 mg.

Each **Somophyllin-CRT** capsule contains anhydrous theophylline (USP) in a formulation to provide a prolonged therapeutic effect. **Somophyllin-CRT Capsules** contain not less than 90.0 percent and not more than 110.0 percent of the labelled amount of anhydrous theophylline. Theophylline, a xanthine compound, is a white, odorless, crystalline powder having a bitter taste.

Somophyllin-CRT Capsules are supplied in 50 mg, 100 mg and 250 mg strengths.

Clinical Pharmacology: Theophylline directly relaxes the smooth muscle of the bronchial airways and pulmonary blood vessels, thus acting mainly as a bronchodilator, pulmonary vasodilator and smooth muscle relaxant. The drug also possesses other actions typical of the xanthine derivatives: coronary vasodilation; diuresis; cardiac, cerebral and skeletal muscle stimulation. The actions of theophylline may be mediated through inhibition of phosphodiesterase and a resultant increase in intracellular cyclic AMP which could mediate smooth muscle relaxation. At concentrations higher than those attained *in vivo,* theophylline also inhibits the release of histamine by mast cells.

In vitro, theophylline has been shown to act synergistically with beta agonists (isoproterenol) that increase intracellular cyclic AMP through the stimulation of adenyl cyclase, but synergism has not been demonstrated in patient studies. More data are needed to determine if theophylline and beta agonists have a clinically important additive effect *in vivo.* Apparently, no development of tolerance occurs with chronic use of theophylline.

The half-life of theophylline is shortened with cigarette smoking. It is prolonged in alcoholism, reduced hepatic or renal function, congestive heart failure, and in patients receiving antibiotics such as TAO (troleandomycin), erythromycin and clindamycin. High fever for prolonged periods may reduce the rate of theophylline elimination.

Theophylline Elimination Characteristics:

	Theophylline Clearance Rates (mean ± S.D.)	Half-life Average (mean ± S.D.)
Children (over 6 months of age)	1.45 ± 0.58 ml/kg/min	3.7 ± 1.1 hrs.
Adult non-smokers with uncomplicated asthma	0.65 ± 0.19 ml/kg/min	8.7 ± 2.2 hrs.

Newborn infants have extremely slow theophylline clearance rates. The theophylline half-life in newborn infants may exceed 24 hours. Not until 3–6 months of age do these rates approach those seen in older children.

Older adults with chronic obstructive pulmonary disease, any patients with cor pulmonale or other causes of heart failure, and patients with liver pathology may have much slower clearance rates with a half-life that may exceed 24 hours.

The half-life of theophylline in smokers (1 to 2 packs/day) averaged 4–5 hours among various studies, much shorter than the half-life in nonsmokers which averaged about 7–9 hours. The increase in theophylline clearance caused by smoking is probably the result of induction of drug-metabolizing enzymes that do not readily normalize after cessation of smoking. It appears that between 3 months and 2 years may be necessary for normalization of the effect of smoking on theophylline pharmacokinetics.

Indications: ***For relief and/or prevention of symptoms from asthma and reversible bronchospasm associated with chronic bronchitis and emphysema.***

Contraindications: These products are contraindicated in individuals who have shown hypersensitivity to their components.

Warnings: ***Status asthmaticus is a medical emergency. Optimal therapy frequently requires additional medication including corticosteroids when the patient is not rapidly responsive to bronchodilators.***

Excessive theophylline doses may be associated with toxicity. The determination of serum theophylline levels is recommended to assure maximal benefit without excessive risk. Incidence of toxicity increases at serum theophylline levels greater than 20 mcg/ml. Morphine, curare, and stilbamidine should be used with caution in patients with airflow obstruction because they stimulate histamine release and they can induce asthmatic attacks. These drugs may also suppress respiration leading to respiratory failure. Alternative drugs should be chosen whenever possible.

There is an excellent correlation between high blood levels of theophylline resulting from conventional doses and associated clinical manifestations of toxicity in (1) patients with lowered body plasma clearances (due to transient cardiac decompensation), (2) patients with liver dysfunction or chronic obstructive lung disease, (3) patients who are older than 55 years of age, particularly males.

Less serious signs of theophylline toxicity such as nausea and restlessness may appear in up to 50 percent of patients. However, serious side effects such as ventricular arrhythmias and convulsions may appear without warning as the first signs of toxicity.

Many patients who have higher theophylline serum levels exhibit tachycardia.

Theophylline products may worsen preexisting arrhythmias.

Usage in Pregnancy: Safe use in pregnancy has not been established relative to possible adverse effects on fetal development, but neither have adverse effects on fetal development been established. This is true for most antiasthmatic medications. Use of theophylline in pregnant women should be balanced against the risk of uncontrolled asthma.

Precautions: Mean half-life in smokers is shorter than nonsmokers, therefore smokers may require larger doses of theophylline. Theophylline should not be administered concurrently with other xanthine medications. Use with caution in patients with severe cardiac disease, severe hypoxemia, hypertension, hyperthyroidism, acute myocardial injury, cor pulmonale, congestive heart failure, liver disease, in the elderly (especially males) and in neonates. In particular, great caution should be used in giving theophylline to patients with congestive heart failure. Frequently, such patients have markedly prolonged theophylline serum levels with theophylline persisting in serum for long periods following discontinuation of the drug.

Use theophylline cautiously in patients with history of peptic ulcer. Theophylline may occasionally act as a local irritant to G.I. tract although gastrointestinal symptoms are more commonly centrally mediated and associated with serum drug concentrations over 20 mcg/ml.

Adverse Reactions: The most consistent adverse reactions are usually due to overdose and are:

1. Gastrointestinal: nausea, vomiting, epigastric pain, hematemesis, diarrhea.
2. Central nervous system: headaches, irritability, restlessness, insomnia, reflex hyperexcitability, muscle twitching, clonic and tonic generalized convulsions.

3. Cardiovascular: palpitation, tachycardia, extra systoles, flushing, hypotension, circulatory failure, life threatening ventricular arrhythmias.
4. Respiratory: tachypnea.
5. Renal: albuminuria, increased excretion of renal tubular and red blood cells, potentiates diuresis.
6. Others: hyperglycemia and inappropriate ADH syndrome; rash (*ethylenediamine*).

Drug Interactions: Toxic synergism with ephedrine has been documented and may occur with some other sympathomimetic bronchodilators.

Drug	Effect
Aminophylline with lithium carbonate	Increased excretion of lithium carbonate
Aminophylline with propranolol	Antagonism of propranolol effect
Theophylline with clindamycin, troleandomycin, erythromycin, lincomycin, cimetidine	Increased theophylline plasma levels

Overdosage:

Management:

A. If potential oral overdose is established and seizure has not occurred:
1. Induce vomiting.
2. Administer a cathartic (this is particularly important if sustained release preparations have been taken).
3. Administer activated charcoal.

B. If patient is having a seizure:
1. Establish an airway.
2. Administer oxygen.
3. Treat the seizure with intravenous diazepam, 0.1 to 0.3 mg/kg up to 10 mg.
4. Monitor vital signs, maintain blood pressure and provide adequate hydration.

C. Post-seizure coma:
1. Maintain airway and oxygenation.
2. If a result of oral medication, follow above recommendations to prevent absorption of drug, but intubation and lavage will have to be performed instead of inducing emesis, and the cathartic and charcoal will need to be introduced via a large bore gastric lavage tube.
3. Continue to provide full supportive care and adequate hydration while waiting for drug to be metabolized. In general, the drug is metabolized sufficiently rapidly so as not to warrant consideration of dialysis.

D. Animal studies suggest that phenobarbital may decrease theophylline toxicity. There is as yet, however, insufficient data to recommend pretreatment of an overdosage with phenobarbital.

E. For overdosage of **Somophyllin Rectal Solution:**

Discontinue drug:
1. Treatment is symptomatic.
2. Use appropriate supportive measures.
3. Prudent use of sympathomimetics.

Dosage and Administration: Therapeutic serum levels associated with optimal likelihood for benefit and minimal risk of toxicity are considered to be between 10 mcg/ml and 20 mcg/ml. Levels above 20 mcg/ml may produce toxic effects. There is great variation from patient to patient in dosage needed in order to achieve a therapeutic blood level because of variable rates of elimination. Because of this wide interpatient variation and the relatively narrow therapeutic blood level range, dosage must be individualized. Monitoring of theophylline serum levels is highly recommended. Dosage should be calculated on the basis of lean (ideal) body weight where mg/kg doses are stated. Theophylline does not distribute into fatty tissue.

Giving theophylline with food may prevent the rare case of stomach irritation; and though absorption may be slower, it is still complete.

	Loading Dose Aminophylline/ Theophylline	Maintenance Dose for Next 12 Hours Aminophylline/ Theophylline	Maintenance Dose Beyond 12 Hours Aminophylline/ Theophylline
1. Children 6 months to 9 years	7 mg/kg *(6 mg/kg)	4.7 mg/kg q4 hrs. *(4 mg/kg q4 hrs)	4.7 mg/kg q6 hrs *(4 mg/kg q6 hrs)
2. Children age 9–16 and young adult smokers	7 mg/kg *(6 mg/kg)	3.5 mg/kg q4 hrs *(3 mg/kg q4 hrs)	3.8 mg/kg q6 hrs *(3 mg/kg q6 hrs)
3. Otherwise healthy nonsmoking adults	7 mg/kg *(6 mg/kg)	3.5 mg/kg q6 hrs *(3 mg/kg q6 hrs)	3.5 mg/kg q8 hrs *(3 mg/kg q8 hrs)
4. Older patients and patients with cor pulmonale	7 mg/kg *(6 mg/kg)	2.4 mg/kg q6 hrs *(2 mg/kg q6 hrs)	2.4 mg/kg q8 hrs *(2 mg/kg q8 hrs)
5. Patients with congestive heart failure, liver failure	7 mg/kg *(6 mg/kg)	2.4 mg/kg q8 hrs *(2 mg/kg q8 hrs)	1.2-2.4 mg/kg q12 hrs *(1-2 mg/kg q12 hrs)

When rapidly absorbed products such as **Somophyllin® Oral Liquid, Somophyllin-DF Oral Liquid,** or **Somophyllin-T Capsules** are used, dosing to maintain "around-the-clock" blood levels generally requires administration every 6 hours to obtain the greatest efficacy for clinical use in children; dosing intervals up to 8 hours may be satisfactory for adults because they eliminate theophylline more slowly. Children, and adults requiring higher than average doses, may benefit from products with slower absorption which may allow longer dosing intervals and/or less fluctuation in serum concentration over a dosing interval during chronic therapy.

Due to the marked variation in theophylline metabolism in infants under 6 months of age, these drugs are not recommended for infants under 6 months of age.

Dosage for Patient Population

Acute Symptoms of Asthma Requiring Rapid Theophyllinization:

Anhydrous theophylline indicated in *( )

I. Not currently receiving theophylline products:

[See table above].

II. Those currently receiving theophylline products: Determine, where possible, the time, amount, route of administration and form of the patient's last dose.

The loading dose for theophylline will be based on the principle that each 0.5 mg/kg of theophylline administered as a loading dose will result in a 1.0 mcg/ml increase in serum theophylline concentration. Ideally, then, the loading dose should be deferred if a serum theophylline concentration can be obtained rapidly. If this is not possible, the clinician must exercise his judgment in selecting a dose based on the potential for benefit and risk. When there is sufficient respiratory distress to warrant a small risk, 2.5 mg/kg of theophylline is likely to increase the serum concentration when administered as a loading dose in rapidly absorbed form by approximately 5 mcg/ml. If the patient is not experiencing theophylline toxicity, this is unlikely to result in dangerous adverse effects.

Subsequent to the decision regarding modification of the loading dose for this group of patients, the maintenance dosage recommendations are the same as those described above.

Comments: It is recommended that serum theophylline concentrations be monitored in order to obtain optimal therapeutic theophylline dosage. However, it is not always possible or practical to obtain a serum theophylline level. Therefore, patients should be closely monitored for signs of toxicity. The present data suggest that the above dosage recommendations will achieve therapeutic serum concentrations with minimal risk of toxicity for most patients. However, some risk of toxic serum concentrations is still present.

Adverse reactions to theophylline often occur when serum theophylline levels exceed 20 mcg/ml.

Chronic Asthma: Theophylline administration is a treatment of first choice for the management of chronic asthma (to prevent symptoms and maintain patent airways). Slow clinical titration is generally preferred to assure acceptance and safety of the medications.

Initial Dose: 16 mg/kg/day or 400 mg/day (whichever is lower) in 3–4 divided doses at 6–8 hour intervals.

Increased Dose: The above dosage may be increased in approximately 25 percent increments at 2–3 day intervals so long as no intolerance is observed, until the maximum dose indicated below is reached.

NOTE: Somophyllin–CRT Capsules are designed to release theophylline slowly but completely. It is recommended that the daily dosage requirement first be established by monitoring serum theophylline levels while the patient has been receiving an immediately available oral liquid such as **Somophyllin® Oral Liquid** for several days. Thereafter, conversion to **Somophyllin–CRT Capsules** can be accomplished by administering one half of the total daily theophylline requirement every 12 hours. Rapid theophyllinization should not be attempted using controlled release formulations.

Maximum dose where the serum concentration is not measured:

(Warning: *Do Not Attempt to Maintain Any Dose That is Not Tolerated)*

Not to exceed the following:

Age <9 years	28.2 mg/kg/day *(24 mg/kg/day)
Age 9–12 years	23.5 mg/kg/day *(20 mg/kg/day)
Age 12–16 years	21.2 mg/kg/day *(18 mg/kg/day)
Age >16 years	15.2 mg/kg/day or 1100 mg/day (WHICHEVER IS LESS) *(13 mg/kg/day or 900 mg/day) (WHICHEVER IS LESS)

NOTE: Use ideal body weight for obese patients.
Anhydrous theophylline indicated in *( ).

Measurement of serum theophylline concentration during chronic therapy:

If the above maximum doses are to be maintained or exceeded, serum theophylline measurement is recommended. This should be obtained at the approximate time of peak absorption (1-2 hours for immediate release products and 4-6 hours for sustained release products) during chronic therapy. It is important that the patient will have missed *no* doses during the previous 48 hours and that dosing intervals will have been reasonably typical with no added doses during that period of time. *Dosage Adjustment Based on Serum Theophylline Measurements When These Instructions Have Not Been Followed May Result in Recommenda-*

Continued on next page

Fisons—Cont.

tions That Present Risk of Toxicity to the Patient.

Final adjustment of dosage: See Table I.

Caution should be exercised for younger children who cannot complain of minor side effects. Older adults, those with cor pulmonale, congestive heart failure, and/or liver disease, may have unusually low dosage requirements and thus may experience toxicity at the maximal dosage recommended above.

It is important that no patient be maintained on any dosage that is not tolerated. In instructing patients to increase dosage according to the schedule above, they should be instructed not to take a subsequent dose if apparent side effects occur and to resume therapy at a lower dose once adverse effects have disappeared. (See table below)

How Supplied:

Somophyllin® Oral Liquid
NDC 0585-2218-80 8 Fl. oz. bottle
NDC 0585-2218-82 32 Fl. oz. bottle

Somophyllin®-DF Oral Liquid
NDC 0585-0218-84 8 Fl. oz. bottle

Somophyllin Rectal Solution is available in nonbreakable bottles of 3 fl. oz. solution and 5 fl. oz. solution with accompanying Rectal Ject syringe, plastic applicator tips and patient instructions.
NDC 0585-1218-20 3 fl. oz. bottle
NDC 0585-1218-25 5 fl. oz. bottle

Caution: Protect from cold. If crystals appear, redissolve by immersing bottle in warm water. Wash syringe after application.

Somophyllin-T Capsules, 50 mg, 100 mg, 200 mg, and 250 mg, in white, imprinted, soft gelatin capsules — bottles of 100.
NDC 0585-9318-35 50 mg capsules
NDC 0585-3318-40 100 mg capsules
NDC 0585-4318-50 200 mg capsules
NDC 0585-5318-60 250 mg capsules

Somophyllin-CRT Capsules, 50 mg, 100 mg and 250 mg, in white and clear, imprinted gelatin capsules—bottles of 100.
NDC 0585-8218-30 50 mg capsules—imprinted S-CRT 50
NDC 0585-6218-70 100 mg capsules—imprinted S-CRT 100
NDC 0585-7218-75 250 mg capsules—imprinted S-CRT 250

Caution: Federal law prohibits dispensing without a prescription. Keep tightly closed and out of reach of children.

TABLE I

Peak Theophylline Serum Level mcg/ml	Adjustment in Total Daily Dose	Comment
<5	100% increase	If patient is asymptomatic, consider trial off drug; repeat blood levels after adjustment.
5–7.5	50% increase	
8–10	20% increase	Even if patient is asymptomatic at this level, an increased serum concentration may prevent symptoms during a viral URI, or heavy exposure to an inhalent allergen.
11–13	Cautious 10% increase if clinically indicated	If patient is asymptomatic, no increase is necesary. If symptoms present during URI or exercise, increase as indicated.
14–20	None	If "breakthrough" in asthmatic symptoms present at end of dosing interval, change to sustained-release product and repeat blood level.
	Occasional intolerance requires a 10% decrease	If side effects present, decrease total daily dose as indicated.
21–25	10% decrease	Even if side effects are absent.
26–34	25–33% decrease	Even if side effects are absent, omit next dose and decrease total daily dose as indicated. Repeat blood levels.
≥ 35	Omit next two doses. 50% decrease	Resume at 50% of previous dose and repeat blood levels.

C. B. Fleet Co., Inc.
4615 MURRAY PL.
LYNCHBURG, VA. 24506

FLEET® BABYLAX

Active Ingredient: Glycerin (USP)
Indications: For temporary relief of constipation in infants and young children.
Actions: The exact mode of action of glycerin administered rectally as a laxative is not known. It has been suggested that glycerin causes dehydration of exposed tissues to produce an irritant effect which results in a laxative response.
Warning: For rectal use only. Glycerin administered rectally may produce rectal discomfort in some individuals. Frequent or prolonged use of laxatives may result in dependence. Do not use when nausea, vomiting or abdominal pain is present. If use results in unusual pain or side effects, consult a physician. Keep this and all drugs out of the reach of children. If a sudden change in bowel habits persists over two weeks, consult a physician before using a laxative. This product should not be used longer than one week except under a physician's advice.
Dosage and Administration: Children under 6 years of age: 1 rectal applicator containing 4 ml. of glycerin as needed or as directed by physician. Hold unit upright. Remove protective shield and discard. With steady pressure, gently insert stem with tip pointing toward navel. Squeeze unit until nearly all liquid is expelled. Remove tip from rectum. Note: A small amount of liquid will remain in unit. Usually produces a bowel movement within 30 minutes. Store and use at room temperature.
How Supplied: Six 4 ml. rectal applicators per package.
Is This Product O.T.C.: Yes.
Literature Available: Yes.

FLEET® BRAND BISACODYL ENEMA
(bisacodyl U.S.P.)

Composition: Each 30 ml (delivered dose) contains 10 mg. of bisacodyl, U.S.P. suspended in an aqueous medium. The FLEET® Bisacodyl Enema unit, with a 2-inch prelubricated Comfortip®, contains 1¼ fl. oz. of enema suspension in a ready-to-use plastic squeeze bottle. Designed for quick, convenient administration by nurse or patient according to instructions. Disposable after single use.
Action and Uses: FLEET® Bisacodyl Enema is a contact laxative acting directly on the colonic mucosa to produce peristalsis. FLEET® Bisacodyl Enema actually produces peristalsis and evacuation of the large intestine by stimulating sensory nerve endings in the colonic mucosa to produce parasympathetic reflexes. FLEET® Bisacodyl Enema is very effective usually producing an evacuation within 5 to 20 minutes. FLEET® Bisacodyl Enema may be used whenever a laxative or enema is indicated. It is useful as a laxative for relief of constipation, in bowel cleansing before X-ray and endoscopic examination.
Warning: Frequent or prolonged use of any laxative may result in dependence. Do not use when nausea, vomiting or abdominal pain is present. If use results in unusual pain or other side effects, contact a physician. Keep this and all medication out of the reach of children. In case of accidental overdose or ingestion, contact the nearest poison control center.
Precautions: Do not administer to children under two years of age.
Dosage and Administration: Adults—one unit or as directed by a physician. This dosage is not recommended for children under two years of age. Administration: Preferred position—Lying on left side with left knee slightly bent and the right leg drawn up, or knee-chest position. Rubber diaphragm at base of tube prevents accidental leakage and assures controlled flow of the enema solution. May be used at room temperature.
How Supplied: FLEET® Bisacodyl Enema is supplied in 1¼ fl. oz. ready-to-use squeeze bottle.
Is this Product OTC: Yes.
Literature Available: Professional literature mailed on request.

FLEET® BRAND ENEMA

Composition: Each 118 ml (delivered dose) contains 19 g. sodium biphosphate and 7 g. sodium phosphate. The FLEET Enema unit, with a 2-inch, prelubricated Comfortip™, contains 4½ fl. oz. of enema solution in a hand-size plastic squeeze bottle. Designed for quick, convenient administration by nurse or patient according to instructions. Disposable after single use.
Action and Uses: FLEET Enema is useful as a laxative in the relief of constipation, and as a bowel evacuant for a variety of diagnostic, surgical, and therapeutic indications. FLEET Enema provides thorough yet safe cleansing action and induces complete emptying of the left colon usually within 2 to 5 minutes without pain or spasm. FLEET Enema may be used for the relief of constipation; as a routine enema; preparation for rectal examination; during pregnancy and pre- and postnatally; preoperative cleansing and general postoperative care; to help relieve fecal or barium impaction.
Contraindications: Do not use when nausea, vomiting, or abdominal pain is present.
Warnings: Frequent or prolonged use of enemas may result in dependence. Do not use in patients with megacolon, as hypernatremic dehydration may occur. Use with caution in

patients with impaired renal function as hyperphosphatemia and hypocalcemia may occur.
Precautions: Do not administer to children under two years of age unless directed by a physician.
Administration and Dosage: Preferred position: Lying on left side with left knee slightly bent and the right leg drawn up, or knee-chest position. Dosage: Adults, 4 fl. oz.; Children two years or older, 2 fl. oz., or as directed by physician. Rubber diaphragm at base of tube prevents accidental leakage and assures controlled flow of the enema solution. May be used at room temperature. Each 118 ml. (delivered dose) contains 4.4 g. sodium.
How Supplied: FLEET Enema is supplied in 4½ fl. oz. ready-to-use squeeze bottle. Pediatric size, 2¼ fl. oz.
Is This Product O.T.C.: Yes.
Literature Available: Professional literature mailed on request.

FLEET® BRAND MINERAL OIL ENEMA

Composition: The FLEET Mineral Oil Enema unit, with a 2-inch, prelubricated Comfortip™, contains 4½ fl.oz. (133 ml.) mineral oil USP in a hand-size plastic squeeze bottle.
Action and Uses: Serves to soften and lubricate hard stools, easing their passage without irritating the mucosa. Results approximate a normal bowel movement in that only the rectum, sigmoid, and part or all of the descending colon are evacuated. Indicated for relief of fecal impaction; valuable in relief of constipation when straining must be avoided (in hypertension, coronary occlusion, proctologic procedures, postoperative care); for removal of barium sulfate residues from the colon after barium administration for GI series or outlining the left atrium; to obtain the laxative benefits of mineral oil while avoiding possible untoward effects of oral administration such as (1) interference with intestinal absorption of fat-soluble vitamins A, D, E and K and other nutrients (2) danger of systemic absorption (3) possible risk of lipid pneumonia due to aspiration.
Contraindications: Do not use when nausea, vomiting, or abdominal pain is present.
Warnings: Frequent or prolonged use of enemas may result in dependence. Take only when needed or when prescribed by a physician.
Precautions: Do not administer to children under two years of age unless directed by a physician.
Administration and Dosage: For rectal administration only. Ready-to-use unit permits easy, rapid administration by physician, nurse, or patient; disposable after single use. *Adults,* 4 fl.oz. *Children two years or older,* one quarter to one half the adult dose, or as directed by physician.
How Supplied: FLEET Mineral Oil Enema is supplied in 4½ fl.oz. ready-to-use squeeze bottle.
Is This Product O.T.C.: Yes.
Literature Available: Professional literature available on request.

FLEET® BRAND
Buffered Laxative
PHOSPHO®-SODA

Composition: Each 100 ml. of regular or flavored PHOSPHO-SODA contains 48 g. sodium biphosphate and 18 g. sodium phosphate in a stable, buffered aqueous solution.
Action and Uses: Versatile in action as a gentle laxative or purgative, according to dosage. Usually works within one hour when taken before meals, or overnight when taken at bedtime. Virtually free from likelihood of GI discomfort and irritation, PHOSPHO-SODA is pleasant to take, safe for all age groups. Useful before diagnostic examinations or bowel surgery.
Contraindications: Do not use when nausea, vomiting, or abdominal pain is present.
Warnings: Frequent or prolonged use of this preparation may result in dependence on laxatives. Do not use in patients with megacolon, as hypernatremic dehydration may occur. Use with caution in patients with impaired renal function as hyperphosphatemia and hypocalcemia may occur.
Administration and Dosage: Mix required dose with one-half glass cold clear liquid and follow with a full glass of water, preferably on arising or at least 30 minutes before a meal, or at bedtime for overnight action.
As a laxative: 4 teaspoonfuls, diluted as directed.
As a purgative: 8 teaspoonfuls, diluted as directed.
Children: One half the adult dose for children 10 years old or older; one quarter the adult dose for children between 5 and 10 years of age. Each recommended dose (4 teaspoonfuls) contains 96.4 meq. sodium.
How Supplied: Regular or Flavored, in bottles of 3 and 8 fl. oz.; 1½ fl. oz. size for hospitals.
Is This Product O.T.C.: Yes.
Literature Available: Professional literature on request.

FLEET® BRAND PREP KITS
Bowel Evacuant

Description: FLEET® Prep Kit No. 1 contains:
1. FLEET® Phospho®-Soda—1½ oz. Ingredients: Each teaspoonful (5 ml) contains : Active Ingredients: Sodium Biphosphate 2.4 Gm. and Sodium Phosphate 0.9 Gm.
2. FLEET® Bisacodyl—4 laxative tablets. Ingredients: Each enteric-coated tablet contains Bisacodyl, NF, 5 mg.
3. FLEET® Bisacodyl—1 laxative suppository. Ingredients: Bisacodyl, NF, 10 mg.
4. 1 Patient Instruction Sheet.

FLEET® Prep Kit No. 2 contains:
1. FLEET® Phospho®-Soda—1½ oz.
2. FLEET® Bisacodyl—4 tablets.
3. FLEET® Bagenema—1. Ingredients: Liquid castile soap ⅔ fl. oz.
4. 1 Patient Instruction Sheet.

FLEET® Prep Kit No. 3 contains:
1. FLEET® Phospho®-Soda—1½ oz.
2. FLEET® Bisacodyl—4 tablets.
3. FLEET® Bisacodyl Enema—1 laxative enema. Ingredients: 1–30 ml. dose containing 10 mg. of Bisacodyl.
4. 1 Patient Instruction Sheet.

FLEET® Prep Kit No. 4 contains:
1. FLEET® Flavored Castor Oil Emulsion-1½ oz.
Ingredients: Each tablespoonful (15 ml.) contains: Active Ingredients: Castor Oil U.S.P. 10 ml.
2. FLEET® Bisacodyl—4 tablets.
3. FLEET® Bisacodyl—1 suppository.
4. 1 Patient Instruction Sheet.

FLEET® Prep Kit No. 5 contains:
1. FLEET® Flavored Castor Oil Emulsion-1½ oz.
2. FLEET® Bisacodyl—4 tablets.
3. FLEET® Bagenema—1.
4. 1 Patient Instruction Sheet.

FLEET® Prep Kit No. 6 contains:
1. FLEET® Flavored Castor Oil Emulsion-1½ oz.
2. FLEET® Bisacodyl—4 tablets.
3. FLEET® Bisacodyl Enema—30 ml.
4. 1 Patient Instruction Sheet.

Actions: Bowel Evacuant.
Indications: Preparation of the colon for radiology (prior to barium enemas or I.V.P.'s), surgery, and many proctologic and colonoscopic procedures.
Warnings: Each recommended dose ((1½ oz.) (45ml)) of Phospho®-Soda contains 216.9 milli-equivalents (mEq) of Sodium. Persons on a low salt diet should consult a health professional before use.
Do not use in patients with megacolon, as hypernatremic dehydration may occur. Use with caution in patients with impaired renal function as hyperphosphatemia and hypocalcemia may occur. Castor Oil affects the small intestine, and regular use may cause excessive loss of water and body salts which can have debilitating effects.
General Warnings: Do not use when nausea, vomiting, or abdominal pain is present. Frequent or prolonged use may result in a dependence on laxatives.
These Kits should not be used by patients under 6 years of age.
Dosage and Administration: See Patient Instruction Sheet for 12, 18 and 24 hour preparation schedule in each kit.
How Supplied:

FLEET® Prep Kit No. 1 contains:
1. 1½ oz. FLEET® Phospho®-Soda
2. 4 tablets—FLEET® Bisacodyl
3. 1 suppository—FLEET® Bisacodyl
4. 1 Patient Instruction Sheet

FLEET® Prep Kit No. 2 contains:
1. 1½ oz. FLEET® Phospho®-Soda
2. 4 tablets—FLEET® Bisacodyl
3. 1 FLEET® Bagenema
4. 1 Patient Instruction Sheet

FLEET® Prep Kit No. 3 contains:
1. 1½ oz. FLEET® Phospho®-Soda.
2. 4 tablets FLEET® Bisacodyl.
3. 1 FLEET® Bisacodyl Enema.
4. 1 Patient Instruction Sheet.

FLEET® Prep Kit No. 4 contains:
1. 1½ oz. FLEET® Flavored Castor Oil Emulsion.
2. 4 tablets FLEET® Bisacodyl.
3. 1 suppository FLEET Bisacodyl.
4. 1 Patient Instruction Sheet.

FLEET® Prep Kit No. 5 contains:
1. 1½ oz. FLEET® Flavored Castor Oil Emulsion.
2. 4 tablets FLEET® Bisacodyl.
3. 1 FLEET® Bagenema.
4. 1 Patient Instruction Sheet.

FLEET® Prep Kit No. 6 contains:
1. 1½ oz. FLEET® Flavored Castor Oil Emulsion.
2. 4 tablets FLEET® Bisacodyl.
3. 1 FLEET Bisacodyl Enema.
4. 1 Patient Instruction Sheet.

Shipping Unit: 48 FLEET® Prep Kits per carton.
For full prescribing information on specific products, see individual listings (FLEET® Phospho®-Soda, FLEET® Bisacodyl Enema and FLEET® Flavored Castor Oil Emulsion).
Is this Product O.T.C.: Yes.
Literature Available: Yes.

FLEET® FLAVORED CASTOR OIL EMULSION

Ingredients: Each tablespoonful (15 ml.) contains:
Active Ingredients: Castor oil U.S.P. 10 ml.
Inactive Ingredients: Water, flavoring, emulsifying agents, propylene glycol, sodium benzoate, citric acid and sodium saccharin.
Indications: For the treatment of isolated bouts of constipation and preparation of the colon for x-ray and endoscopic examination. (See FLEET® Prep Kit listings.)
Actions: Works directly on the small intestine to promote bowel movement.
Dosage and Administration: Adults: 3 tablespoonfuls (45 ml.) Children 2 to 6 years: 1 tablespoonful (15 ml.) Children up to 2 years: 1 teaspoonful (5 ml.) For best results, take on an empty stomach. Follow with one full glass of cool water.
General Warnings: Do not use when nausea, vomiting or abdominal pain is present.

Continued on next page

Fleet—Cont.

Frequent or prolonged use may result in a dependence on laxatives. Not to be used on a daily basis, except under the direction of a physician. If you have noticed a sudden change in bowel habits that persists over a period of two weeks, consult a physician before using a laxative. If the recommended use of this product for one week has had no effect, discontinue use and consult a physician. Castor oil affects the small intestine and regular use may cause excessive loss of water and body salts, which can have a debilitating effect. Keep this and all drugs out of the reach of children. In case of accidental overdose, consult a physician immediately.
How Supplied: Bottles of 1½ oz. and 3 fl. oz.
Is This Product O.T.C.: Yes.
Literature Available: Yes.

SUMMER'S EVE®
MEDICATED DOUCHE

Active Ingredient: Potassium Sorbate 1%
Indications: For temporary relief of minor vaginal itching and irritation.
Actions: Potassium Sorbate has been proven effective for minor vaginal irritation and itching. It is clear and colorless, and leaves no stain or messiness on the skin or clothing.
Warning: Douching does not prevent pregnancy. Do not use during pregnancy except with the approval of a physician. If douching results in pain, soreness, itching, excessive dryness, or irritation, stop douching. If symptoms persist after 10 days, consult a physician. Keep out of reach of children.
Dosage and Administration: 4½ ounces of sanitized solution in a unique one-piece, one-time use disposable unit. Remove the sanitary overwrap. Pull up the flexible nozzle until it clicks and locks, and Summer's Eve® Medicated Douche is ready to use. After use, the unit is discarded.
How Supplied: 4½ oz. single pack or twin pack containing two 4½ oz. units.
Is This Product O.T.C.: Yes.
Literature Available: Yes.

SUMMER'S EVE®
MEDICATED VAGINAL SUPPOSITORIES

Active Ingredient: Potassium Sorbate 3%
Indications: For temporary relief of minor vaginal irritation and itching.
Actions: Potassium Sorbate has been proved effective for minor vaginal irritation and itching. It is clear and colorless, and leaves no stain or messiness on the skin or clothing.
Warning: This product does not prevent pregnancy. Do not use during pregnancy except with the approval of a physician. If usage results in pain, soreness, excessive dryness or irritation, discontinue use. If original symptoms persist after 10 days, consult a physician. Keep out of the reach of children.
Dosage and Administration: Remove foil wrap. Place suppository into applicator. Gently insert applicator and suppository into the vagina. Push plunger to deposit suppository. Use whenever symptoms are present, but for no more than 10 days or as directed by a physician. Store and use at room temperature. Cleanse applicator afer each use.
How Supplied: 10 suppositories with plastic applicator per package.
Is This Product O.T.C.: Yes.
Literature Available: Yes.

Products are cross-indexed by

generic and chemical names in the

YELLOW SECTION

Fleming & Company
1600 FENPARK DR.
FENTON, MO 63026

AEROLATE SR & JR & III Capsules ℞
(theophylline, anhydrous T.D.)

AEROLATE LIQUID
(theophylline, anhydrous)

Composition: Contains theophylline 4 grs. (260 mg) as SR, 2 grs (130 mg) as JR, 1 gr. as III (65 mg), in red/clear capsules. Liquid has 160 mg theophyllin/15cc in a non-sugar, non-alcoholic, non-saccharin tangerine flavored base.
Action and Uses: Timed action pellets bypass stomach to prevent gastric upset. Bronchodilation is achieved through bowel absorption only. Liquid is for the acute attack primarily.
Administration and Dosage: One capsule every 12 hours. Every 8 hours in severe attacks. Liquid—adults—40 ml (2.5 tablespoonfuls) for acute attack. Children—0.25 ml/lb. Maintainance therapy—adults—for the first 6 doses, 25 ml (1.5 tablespoonfuls) before breakfast, at 3 p.m., at bedtime. Then 15 ml doses at above times. Children—0.15ml/lb. at these times, then 0.1ml/lb per dose.
Side Effects: Nausea, vomiting, epigastric or substernal pain, palpitation, headache, dizziness may occur.
How Supplied: Capsules in bottles of 100 and 1000.
Liquid in pints and gallons.

CONGESS SR & JR Capsules ℞
Expectorant/Decongestant T.D.

Composition: Contains guaifenesin 250 mgs/pseudoephedrine 120 mgs as SR; guaifenesin 125 mgs/pseudoephedrine 60 mgs as JR in blue/pink capsules.
Action and Uses: To loosen mucus plugs in upper respiratory tract and congestion in acute pulmonary disorders, and in coughing. Nasal decongestion and alleviation of bronchospasm is also achieved up to 12 hrs. that accompany most coughs, especially during the nocturnal period.
Indications: Nasal congestion, sinusitis, acute aerotitis media, bronchial asthma, serous otitis media, and symptoms of the common cold.
Dosage: Adults and children over 12 yrs. one SR capsule every 12 hrs. Under 12 yrs. one JR capsule as prescribed by physician.
Precaution and Side Effects: Use with care in severe hypertension, heart disease, hyperthyroidism, diabetes. Low grade sensitivity to drugs may be experienced.
Contraindications: Glaucoma, prostatic hypertrophy, patients receiving MAO inhibitors.
How Supplied: Plastic bottles of 100 and 1000 capsules.

EXTENDRYL ℞
T.D. Capsules SR & JR, Syrup and Tablets

Each timed action SR capsule contains phenylepherine HCl 20 mg; methscopolamine nitrate 2.5 mg; chlorpheniramine maleate 8 mg. The JR potency is exactly half-strength. Green/red color for both. Each 5 cc of root beer flavored syrup and tablet contains: phenylephrine HCl 10 mg; methscopolamine nitrate 1.25 mg; chlorpheniramine maleate 2 mg.
Action and Uses: Antihistaminic-decongestant for relief of respiratory congestion; allergic rhinitis; allergic skin reactions of urticaria and angioedema.
Administration and Dosage: Capsules—one every 12 hrs of the SR for adults; one JR every 12 hrs for children 6–12 yrs. Syrup-two teaspoonfuls every 4 hrs for adults; children 1 teaspoonful every 4 hrs. Tablets—adults two and children one every 4 hrs. Do not exceed 4 doses in 24 hrs.
Children under 6 yrs. as recommended by a physician.
Precautions: Withdraw therapy if drowsiness occurs. Patients are cautioned against driving or operating mechanical devices.
Contraindications: Glaucoma, cardiac disease, hyperthyroidism and hypertension.
How Supplied: Capsules and tablets in bottles of 100 and 1000. Syrup in pints and gallons.

MARBLEN
Suspensions and Tablet

(See PDR For Nonprescription Drugs)

NEPHROX SUSPENSION
(aluminum hydroxide)
Antacid Suspension

(See PDR For Nonprescription Drugs)

NICOTINEX Elixir
nicotinic acid

(See PDR For Nonprescription Drugs)

OCEAN MIST
(buffered saline)

(See PDR For Nonprescription Drugs)

PIMA Syrup ℞
(potassium iodide)

Composition: Contains KI 5 grs./tsp., in a black raspberry flavored base.
Action and Uses: An expectorant in the symptomatic treatment of chronic pulmonary diseases where tenacious mucus complicates the problem, including bronchial asthma, bronchitis and pulmonary emphysema.
Administration and Dosage: Children—one half to one tsp. and adults one or two tsp. every 4-6 hours.
Side Effects: May include gastrointestinal upset, metallic taste, minor skin eruptions, nausea, vomiting and epigastric pain. Therapy should be withdrawn.
Precautions: In patients sensitive to iodides, in hyperthyroidism, and in rare cases iodine-induced goiter may occur.
How Supplied: Plastic pints and gallons.

PURGE
(flavored castor oil)

(See PDR For Nonprescription Drugs)

RUM-K ℞
(potassium chloride 15% conc.)

Description: Each 10 ml. contains 1.5 Gm. potassium chloride (20 mEq) in a butter/rum synthetic flavored base that is alcohol and sugar free.
Indications: Hypokalemic-hypochloremic alkalosis; digitalis toxicity; hypokalemia prevention secondary to corticosteroid or diuretic administration.
Contraindications: Impaired renal function, untreated Addison's Disease, acute dehydration, heat cramps, hyperkalemia.
Precautions: Do not use in patients with low urinary output or renal decompensation. Potassium replacements vary and should be individualized. Patients should be checked frequently, ECG and plasma K+ levels should be made. High serum concentrations of K+ cause death thru cardiac depression, arrhythmias or arrest. Use with caution in cardiac disease.
Adverse Reactions: Vomiting, nausea, abdominal discomfort, diarrhea may occur. Symptoms and signs of potassium overdose include paresthesias of extremities, flaccid paralysis, listlessness, fall in blood pressure, weakness and heaviness of the legs, cardiac

arrhythmias and heart block. Hyperkalemia may cause ECG changes as disappearance of the P wave, widening and slurring of QRS complex, changes of the S-T segment, tall peaked T waves.

Dosage and Administration: Adults—two teaspoonsful (10ml) in 4–6 oz water 2 to 4 times daily after meals to supply 40–80 mEq of elemental potassium and chloride. Larger doses may be required and administered under close supervision due to possible potassium intoxication or saline laxative effect.

How Supplied: 2 oz; 4 oz; pints and gallons.

S-P-T ℞
(Pork thyroid "liquid" capsules USP)

Composition: S-P-T is prepared by special process from cleaned, fresh pork thyroid glands, deprived of connective tissue, defatted and suspended in soy bean oil and encapsulated in gelatin for greater oral absorption. The active hormones (T4 and T3) are available in their natural state in a ratio of approximately 2.5:1, as in humans, to insure therapeutic availability. Capsules are standardized by USP method for iodine content and also biologically to insure 100% metabolic potency.

Action: To increase metabolic rate of body tissues. S-P-T is replacement therapy for diminished or absent thyroid function. Effect develops slowly and is fully reached in 10—14 days per grain increase in most instances.

Indications: As replacement therapy in hypothyroidism, cretinism, myxedema, and after surgery following complete thyroidectomy.

Contraindications: In thyrotoxicosis, angina pectoris, myocardial infarction and hypertension unless complicated by hypothyroidism, and uncorrected adrenal insufficiency.

Precaution and Side Effects: Overdosage may cause tachycardia, angina pectoris, diarrhea, nervousness, sweating, headache and increased pulse action. In most cases, reduction of dosage overcomes side effects.

Dosage and Administration: Patients should be titrated starting at lower levels and increasing by 1 gr every 2 weeks until mild thyromimetic effects are noted. Then lower the dose to the level at which the patient felt best, as patients vary widely as to thyroid need.

Warnings: Drugs with thyroid hormone activity, alone or together with other therapeutic agents, have been used for the treatment of obesity. In euthyroid patients, doses within the range of daily hormonal requirements are ineffective for weight reduction. Larger doses may produce serious or even life-threatening manifestations of toxicity, particularly when given in association with sympathomimetic amines such as those used for their anorectic effects.

How Supplied: As 1 gr (green); 2 gr (brown); 3 gr (red); 5 gr (black) gelatin sealed capsules in bottles of 100 and 1000.

Important Notice

Before prescribing or administering any product described in PHYSICIANS' DESK REFERENCE always consult the PDR Supplement for possible new or revised information.

Flint Laboratories
(Division of Travenol Laboratories, Inc.)
DEERFIELD, IL 60015

CHOLOXIN® ℞
(Dextrothyroxine Sodium Tablets, USP) Flint

Description: CHOLOXIN (dextrothyroxine sodium) is the sodium salt of the dextrorotatory isomer of thyroxine. It is chemically described as D-3,5,3′,5′-tetraiodothyronine sodium salt.

Clinical Pharmacology: The predominant effect of CHOLOXIN (dextrothyroxine sodium) is the reduction of serum cholesterol levels in hyperlipidemic patients. Beta lipoprotein and triglyceride fractions may also be reduced from previously elevated levels.

Available evidence indicates that CHOLOXIN (dextrothyroxine sodium) stimulates the liver to increase catabolism and excretion of cholesterol and its degradation products via the biliary route into the feces. Cholesterol synthesis is not inhibited and abnormal metabolic endproducts do not accumulate in the blood.

Indication and Usage: For treatment of hyperlipidemia in patients with no known heart disease.

This is not an innocuous drug. Strict attention should be paid to the indications and contraindications.

CHOLOXIN (dextrothyroxine sodium) is an antilipidemic agent used as an adjunct to diet and other measures for the reduction of elevated serum cholesterol (low density lipoproteins) in euthyroid patients with no known evidence of organic heart disease.

It has not been clearly established whether the drug-induced lowering of serum cholesterol or lipid levels has a detrimental, beneficial, or no effect on the morbidity or mortality due to atherosclerosis or coronary heart disease. Several years will be required before current investigations will yield an answer to this question.

Contraindications: The administration of CHOLOXIN (dextrothyroxine sodium) to euthyroid patients with one or more of the following conditions is contraindicated:

1. Known organic heart disease, including angina pectoris; history of myocardial infarction; cardiac arrhythmia or tachycardia, either active or in patients with demonstrated propensity for arrhythmias; rheumatic heart disease; history of congestive heart failure; and decompensated or borderline compensated cardiac status.
2. Hypertensive states (other than mild, labile systolic hypertension).
3. Advanced liver or kidney disease.
4. Pregnancy.
5. Nursing mothers.
6. History of iodism.

Warnings:

Drugs with thyroid hormone activity, alone or together with other therapeutic agents, have been used for the treatment of obesity. In euthyroid patients, doses within the range of daily hormonal requirements are ineffective for weight reduction. Larger doses may produce serious or even life threatening manifestations of toxicity, particularly when given in association with sympathomimetic amines such as those used for their anorectic effects.

CHOLOXIN (dextrothyroxine sodium) may potentiate the effects of anticoagulants on prothrombin time. Reductions of anticoagulant dosage by as much as 30% have been required in some patients. Consequently, the dosage of anticoagulants should be reduced by one-third upon initiation of CHOLOXIN (dextrothyroxine sodium) therapy and the dosage subsequently readjusted on the basis of prothrombin time. The prothrombin time of patients receiving anticoagulant therapy concomitantly with CHOLOXIN (dextrothyroxine sodium) therapy should be observed as frequently as necessary, at least weekly during the first few weeks of treatment.

In the surgical patient, it is wise to consider withdrawal of the drug two weeks prior to surgery if the use of anticoagulants during surgery is contemplated.

Special consideration must be given to the dosage of other thyroid medications used concomitantly with CHOLOXIN (dextrothyroxine sodium). As with all thyroactive drugs, hypothyroid patients are more sensitive than euthyroid patients to a given dose of dextrothyroxine sodium.

The injection of epinephrine into patients with coronary artery disease may precipitate an episode of coronary insufficiency. This condition may be enhanced in patients receiving thyroid analogues. These phenomena should be kept in mind when catecholamine injections are required in dextrothyroxine sodium-treated patients with coronary artery disease.

Since the possibility of precipitating cardiac arrhythmias during surgery may be greater in patients treated with thyroid hormones, it may be wise to discontinue CHOLOXIN (dextrothyroxine sodium) in euthyroid patients at least two weeks prior to an elective operation. During emergency surgery in euthyroid patients, the patients should be carefully observed.

There are reports that dextrothyroxine sodium in diabetic patients is capable of increasing blood sugar levels with a resultant increase in requirements of insulin or oral hypoglycemic agents. Special attention should be paid to parameters necessary for good control of the diabetic state in dextrothyroxine sodium-treated subjects and to dosage requirements of insulin or other antidiabetic drugs. If dextrothyroxine sodium is later withdrawn from patients who had required a dosage increase of insulin or oral hypoglycemic agents during its administration, the dosage of antidiabetic drugs should be reduced and adjusted to maintain good control of the diabetic state.

When impaired liver and/or kidney function are present, the advantages of CHOLOXIN (dextrothyroxine sodium) therapy must be weighed against the possibility of deleterious results.

Precautions: It is expected that patients on CHOLOXIN (dextrothyroxine sodium) therapy will show increased serum thyroxine levels. These increased serum thyroxine values are evidence of absorption and transport of the drug, and should NOT be interpreted as evidence of hypermetabolism; therefore, they may not be used to determine the effective dose of dextrothyroxine sodium. Thyroxine values in the range of 10 to 25 mcg% in dextrothyroxine sodium-treated patients are common.

If signs or symptoms of iodism develop during dextrothyroxine sodium therapy, the drug should be discontinued.

A few children with familial hypercholesterolemia have been treated with CHOLOXIN (dextrothyroxine sodium) for periods of one year or longer with no adverse effects on growth. However, it is recommended that the drug be continued in patients in this age group only if a significant serum cholesterol-lowering effect is observed.

The 2 mg and 6 mg tablets of CHOLOXIN (dextrothyroxine sodium) contain FD&C Yellow No. 5 (tartrazine) which may cause allergic-type reactions (including bronchial asthma) in certain susceptible individuals. Although the overall incidence of FD&C Yellow No. 5 (tartrazine) sensitivity in the general population is low, it is frequently seen in patients who also have aspirin hypersensitivity.

Continued on next page

Flint—Cont.

Usage in Women of Childbearing Age: Women of childbearing age with familial hypercholesterolemia or hyperlipemia should not be deprived of the use of this drug; it can be given to those patients exercising strict birth control procedures. Since pregnancy may occur despite the use of birth control procedures, administration of CHOLOXIN (dextrothyroxine sodium) to women of this age group should be undertaken only after weighing the possible risk to the fetus against the possible benefits to the mother. Teratogenic studies in two animal species have resulted in no abnormalities in the offspring.

Adverse Reactions: The side effects attributed to CHOLOXIN (dextrothyroxine sodium) therapy are, for the most part, due to increased metabolism, and may be minimized by following the recommended dosage schedule. Adverse effects are least commonly seen in euthyroid patients with no signs or symptoms of organic heart disease.

In the absence of known organic heart disease, some cardiac changes may be precipitated during dextrothyroxine sodium therapy. Angina pectoris, extrasystoles, ectopic beats, supraventricular tachycardia, ECG evidence of ischemic myocardial changes and increase in heart size have all been observed. Myocardial infarctions, both fatal and nonfatal, have occurred, but these are not unexpected in untreated patients in the age groups studied. It is not known whether any of these infarcts were drug related.

Changes in clinical status that may be related to the metabolic action of the drug include the development of insomnia, nervousness, palpitations, tremors, loss of weight, lid lag, sweating, flushing, hyperthermia, hair loss, diuresis, and menstrual irregularities. Gastrointestinal complaints during therapy have included dyspepsia, nausea and vomiting, constipation, diarrhea, and decrease in appetite.

Other side effects reported to be associated with dextrothyroxine sodium therapy include the development of headache, changes in libido (increase or decrease), hoarseness, tinnitus, dizziness, peripheral edema, malaise, tiredness, visual disturbances, psychic changes, paresthesia, muscle pain, and various bizarre subjective complaints. Skin rashes, including a few which appeared to be due to iodism, and itching have been attributed to dextrothyroxine sodium by some investigators. Gallstones have been discovered in occasional dextrothyroxine sodium-treated patients and cholestatic jaundice has occurred in one patient, although its relationship to dextrothyroxine sodium therapy was not established.

In several instances, the previously existing conditions of the patient appeared to continue or progress during the administration of dextrothyroxine sodium. A worsening of peripheral vascular disease, sensorium, exophthalmos and retinopathy have been reported.

Dextrothyroxine sodium potentiates the effects of anticoagulants on prothrombin time, thus indicating a decrease in the dosage requirements of the anticoagulants. On the other hand, dosage requirements of antidiabetic drugs have been reported to be increased during dextrothyroxine sodium therapy (see WARNINGS section).

Dosage and Administration: For **adult** euthyroid hypercholesterolemic patients, the recommended maintenance dose of CHOLOXIN (dextrothyroxine sodium) is 4 to 8 mg per day. The initial dose should be 1 to 2 mg daily, to be increased in 1 to 2 mg increments at intervals of not less than one month to a maximal level of 4 to 8 mg daily.

For **pediatric** hypercholesterolemic patients, the recommended maintenance dose of CHOLOXIN (dextrothyroxine sodium) is approximately 0.1 mg (100 mcg) per kilogram. The initial dosage should be approximately 0.05 mg (50 mcg) per kilogram daily, increased at not more than 0.05 mg (50 mcg) per kilogram increments at monthly intervals. The recommended maximal dose is 4 mg daily.

If signs or symptoms of cardiac disease develop during the treatment period, the drug should be withdrawn.

How Supplied: CHOLOXIN (dextrothyroxine sodium) Tablets are supplied as scored, color-coded tablets in 4 concentrations: 1 mg-orange... 2 mg-yellow... 4 mg-white... 6 mg-green.

Literature Available: Upon request.

[*Shown in Product Identification Section*]

SILVER SULFADIAZINE CREAM ℞

Description: 1% Silver Sulfadiazine Cream is a topical antibacterial preparation which has as its active antimicrobial ingredient silver sulfadiazine. The active moiety is contained within an opaque, white, water-miscible cream base.

Each 1000 grams of 1% Silver Sulfadiazine Cream contains 10 grams of silver sulfadiazine. The cream base contains White Petrolatum, USP; Stearyl Alcohol, NF; Isopropyl Myristate, NF; Sorbitan Monooleate, NF; Polyoxyl 40 Stearate, NF; Propylene Glycol, USP; and Purified Water, USP; with 0.3% Methylparaben, NF, as a preservative.

Silver sulfadiazine has an empirical formula of $C_{10}H_9AgN_4O_2S$, molecular weight of 357.14, and structural formula as shown:

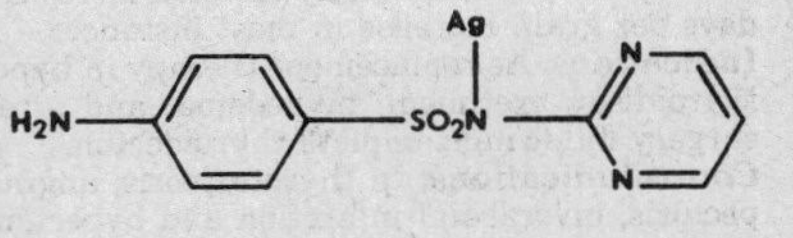

Clinical Pharmacology: 1% Silver Sulfadiazine Cream has demonstrated *in vitro* antimicrobial activity against actual clinical burn wound isolates. Representative organisms included numerous strains of gram-negative and gram-positive bacteria and yeasts. *In vitro* test results evaluating the antimicrobial effectiveness of silver sulfadiazine are summarized in Table 1. All microorganisms analyzed for susceptibility are isolates from burn patients obtained nationwide.

[See table bottom left].

1% Silver Sulfadiazine Cream exerts its principal antimicrobial effect at the level of the cell membrane and cell wall. The mechanism and site of action differ from sodium sulfadiazine and silver nitrate. *In vitro* analysis has demonstrated that the bactericidal activity exerted by 1% Silver Sulfadiazine Cream is superior to sulfadiazine alone.

1% Silver Sulfadiazine Cream may be especially applicable to the treatment of pediatric burn patients, because it is not a carbonic anhydrase inhibitor. There have been no reports of acidosis attributable to treatment with 1% Silver Sulfadiazine Cream.

Indications and Usage: 1% Silver Sulfadiazine Cream is a topical antibacterial preparation which is indicated as an adjunct to currently accepted principles of burn wound care, for the prevention and treatment of burn wound sepsis in patients with partial and full thickness burns.

Contraindications: Since sulfonamide derivatives are known to increase the possibility of kernicterus[1], 1% Silver Sulfadiazine Cream should not be used in pregnant women approaching or at term, premature infants, or neonates less than two months of age.

Warnings: 1% Silver Sulfadiazine Cream should be administered with caution to patients with a history of hypersensitivity to silver sulfadiazine. It is not known whether prior sensitivity to other sulfonamides will precipitate an allergic response to 1% Silver Sulfadiazine Cream.

Should manifestation of allergic response to 1% Silver Sulfadiaz'ne Cream be observed, continuation of therapy must be weighed

TABLE 1
NUMBER OF SENSITIVE BURN ISOLATED STRAINS/
TOTAL BURN ISOLATED STRAINS TESTED

	CONCENTRATION OF SILVER SULFADIAZINE	
Genus & Species	**62.5 mcg/ml**	**125 mcg/ml**
Pseudomonas aeruginosa	46/54	50/54
Pseudomonas cepacia	2/3	2/3
Pseudomonas species	2/3	2/3
Enterobacter cloacae	6/14	6/14
Enterobacter aerogenes	4/6	4/6
Enterobacter agglomerans	1/1	1/1
Klebsiella pneumoniae	4/4	4/4
Klebsiella species	1/3	1/3
Escherichia coli	11/15	11/15
Serratia liquifaciens	3/3	3/3
Serratia marcescens	6/6	6/6
Serratia rubidae	2/2	2/2
Serratia species	0/1	1/1
Proteus mirabilis	8/8	8/8
Proteus morganii	8/9	8/9
Proteus rettgeri	1/1	1/1
Proteus vulgaris	3/4	4/4
Providencia species	3/3	3/3
Citrobacter diversus	0/2	0/2
Shigella species	1/2	1/2
Acinetobacter anitratum	2/2	2/2
Aeromonas hydrophilia	3/3	3/3
Arizona hinshawii	1/1	1/1
Alcaligenes faecalis	2/2	2/2
Staphylococcus aureus	7/7	7/7
Streptococcus Group D (including *Enterococcus*)	17/18	18/18
Bacillus species	0/1	1/1
Candida albicans	1/3	3/3
Candida species	0/1	1/1

against the potential hazards of the particular allergic reaction.
While 1% Silver Sulfadiazine Cream is exerting a bacteriostatic effect on the burn wound, fungal proliferation in and below the eschar may occur. However, the incidence of clincially reported fungal superinfection is low.
1% Silver Sulfadiazine Cream should be used with caution in patients with a history of glucose-6-phosphate dehydrogenase deficiency, as hemolysis may occur.
When treatment with 1% Silver Sulfadiazine Cream involves prolonged administration and /or large burn surfaces, considerable amounts of silver sulfadiazine are absorbed. Serum sulfa concentrations may approach adult therapeutic levels (8-12 mg%).
In extensively burned patients, serum sulfa concentrations and renal function should be closely monitored, and urine should be analyzed for presence of sulfa crystals.

Precautions: Following administration of 1% Silver Sulfadiazine Cream, absorption of sulfadiazine has been reported. In addition, small amounts of silver are absorbed over the course of repeated application of 1% Silver Sulfadiazine Cream. Impairment of hepatic and renal functions which results in diminished excretion of drug constituents may lead to accumulation of silver and sulfadiazine moieties. In the presence of hepatic and/or renal dysfunction, the therapeutic benefits of continued silver sulfadiazine administration must be assessed in light of the possibility of accumulation of by-products.
When utilizing topical enzymatic preparations for debridement of partial and full thickness burn wounds, concomitant or alternating topical antimicrobial therapy must be employed.
Pregnancy Category C. Animal reproduction studies have not been conducted with 1% Silver Sulfadiazine Cream. It is also not known whether 1% Silver Sulfadiazine Cream can cause fetal harm when administered to a pregnant woman or can affect reproduction capacity. 1% Silver Sulfadiazine Cream should be given to a pregnant woman only if clearly needed. To date, there are no reports in the medical literature which associate 1% Silver Sulfadiazine Cream therapy with adverse effects on the fetus or reproductive capacity.
1% Silver Sulfadiazine Cream should be administered to pregnant women only when the physician decides that the potentially life-saving benefits of silver sulfadiazine therapy in the larger burn (extent greater than 20% body surface area) outweigh possible hazard to the fetus.
There is no evidence that topical application of 1% Silver Sulfadiazine Cream results in excretion of any of its constituents in human milk. However, since all sulfonamide derivatives are known to increase the possibility of kernicterus, caution should be exercised when 1% Silver Sulfadiazine Cream is administered to nursing women.

Adverse Reactions: Several cases of transient leukopenia have been reported in patients receiving silver sulfadiazine therapy. Leukopenia associated with silver sulfadiazine administration is primarily characterized by decreased neutrophil count. Maximal white blood cell depression occurs within two to four days of initiation of therapy. Rebound to normal leukocyte levels follows onset within two to three days. Recovery is not influenced by continuation of silver sulfadiazine therapy. This reaction has been reported to occur in approximately one in twenty patients.[6,7]
A low incidence of other adverse reactions has been reported. These include burning sensation, rashes and pruritus, and rarely, interstitial nephritis.
It is often difficult to differentiate topical reactions which are precipitated by 1% Silver Sulfadiazine Cream from those resulting from routine burn wound effects, or caused by hypersensitivity to other therapeutic agents being administered concurrently to the patient. During the treatment of burns over large body surfaces (greater than 20% body surface area), significant amounts of silver sulfadiazine are systemically absorbed. Therefore, it is possible that any adverse reactions associated with sulfonamides may occur.

Dosage and Administration: In the patients with a major burn, evaluation of airway and fluid replacement needs should precede treatment of the burn wound. After appropriate resuscitative measures are instituted, the burn wound is evaluated for extent and depth, and an appropriate treatment regimen is instituted.
1% Silver Sulfadiazine Cream should be applied to a thickness of at least 1/16 inch, to selected burned surfaces once or twice daily.
It is recommended that a protocol for management of the burn wound using accepted principles and techniques of debridement be followed. 1% Silver Sulfadiazine Cream should be applied with sterile gloves.
1% Silver Sulfadiazine Cream will provide antimicrobial protection when used with either open treatment or occlusive dressing regimens. When treating patients utilizing the open method, care must be taken to promptly reapply 1% Silver Sulfadiazine Cream whenever it is removed by patient movement.
Daily hydrotherapy facilitates debridement of loosened eschar and removal of accumulated debris. 1% Silver Sulfadiazine Cream should be reapplied immediately after hydrotherapy.
Treatment of burns with topical antimicrobial agents has been reported to allow spontaneous healing of deep partial thickness burn wounds, by preventing bacterial proliferation which could otherwise cause conversion to full thickness loss. However, delayed separation of eschar associated with the use of topical antimicrobial agents such as 1% Silver Sulfadiazine Cream may require definitive surgical treatment of the eschar.
1% Silver Sulfadiazine Cream should be applied continually until either spontaneous healing or grafting of the burn wound is achieved.
In order to avoid the possibility of infection, 1% Silver Sulfadiazine Cream should not be withdrawn from the therapeutic regimen until definitive wound closure is accomplished, unless there is a significant adverse reaction to the drug.

How Supplied: 1% Silver Sulfadiazine Cream is supplied in plastic jars containing 50 and 400 grams.
Store between 15°–30° C (59°–86° F).

References:

1. **AMA Drug Evaluations,** Fourth Edition: Chapter 77, Sulfonamides and related compounds. 1980, p 1309.
2. Delaveau P, Friedrich-Noue P: Cutaneous absorption and urinary elimination of silver sulfadiazine compounds used in the treatment of burns. **Therapy 32**:563-572, 1977.
3. Dimick AR: Experience with the use of proteolytic enzyme (Travase®) in burn patients. **J Trauma 17**:948-955, 1977.
4. Fox CL Jr: Silver Sulfadiazine - A new topical therapy for Pseudomonas in burns. Therapy of Pseudomonas infection in burns. **Arch Surg 96**:184-188, 1968.
5. Fox CL, Modak SM: Mechanism of silver sulfadiazine action of burn wound infections. **Antimicrobial Agents for Chemotherapy 5**:582-588, 1974.
6. Harrison HN: Pharmacology of sulfadiazine silver - its attachment to burned human and rat skin and studies of gastrointestinal absorption and extension. **Arch Surg 114**:281-285, 1979.
7. Jarret F, Ellerbe S, Demling R: Acute leukopenia during topical burn therapy with silver sulfadiazine. **Amer J Surg 135**:818-819, 1978.
8. Kiker RG, Carvajal HF, Mlcak RP, Larson DL: A controlled study of the effects of silver sulfadiazine on white blood cell counts in burned children. **J Trauma 17**:835-836, 1977.
9. Krizek TJ: Emergency nonsurgical escharotomy in the burned extremity. **Ortho Rev,** July 1975, p 53-55.
10. Pennisi BR, Abril F, Cappozzi A: The combined efficacy of Travase and silver sulfadiazine in the acute burn. **Burns 2**:169-172, 1976.
11. Rodeheaver G: Proteolytic enzymes as adjuncts to antimicrobial prophylaxis of contaminated wounds. **Amer J Surg 129**:537-544, 1975.

Literature Available: Upon request.
[*Shown in Product Identification Section*]

SYNTHROID® ℞

(Levothyroxine Sodium, USP) Flint
Synthroid Tablets—for oral administration
Synthroid Injection—for parenteral administration after reconstitution

Description: SYNTHROID (levothyroxine sodium) **Tablets** and SYNTHROID for **Injection** contain synthetic crystalline levothyroxine sodium (L-thyroxine). L-thyroxine is the principal hormone secreted by the normal thyroid gland.

Pharmacologic Category: SYNTHROID (levothyroxine sodium) **Tablets,** taken orally, provide hormone that is absorbed readily from the gastrointestinal tract. SYNTHROID **Injection** is effective by any parenteral route. Following absorption, the synthetic L-thyroxine provided by SYNTHROID (levothyroxine sodium) products cannot be distinguished from L-thyroxine that is secreted endogenously. Each is bound to the same serum proteins and each exhibits a six to seven day circulating half-life in the euthyroid individual.
Both SYNTHROID (levothyroxine sodium) products will provide L- thyroxine (T_4) as a substrate for physiologic deiodination to L-triiodothyronine (T_3). Therefore, patients taking SYNTHROID (levothyroxine sodium) products will demonstrate normal blood levels of L-triiodothyronine even when the thyroid gland has been removed surgically or destroyed by radioiodine. Administration of levothyroxine sodium alone will result in complete physiologic thyroid replacement.

Indications and Usage: SYNTHROID (levothyroxine sodium) products serve as specific replacement therapy for reduced or absent thyroid function of any etiology. SYNTHROID (levothyroxine sodium) **Injection** can be used intravenously whenever a rapid onset of effect is critical, and either intravenously or intramuscularly in hypothyroid patients whenever the oral route is precluded for long periods of time.

Contraindications: There are no absolute contraindications to SYNTHROID (levothyroxine sodium) therapy. Relative contraindications include acute myocardial infarction, uncorrected adrenal insufficiency and thyrotoxicosis (see WARNINGS).

Warnings:

> Drugs with thyroid hormone activity, alone or together with other therapeutic agents, have been used for the treatment of obesity. In euthyroid patients, doses within the range of daily hormonal requirements are ineffective for weight reduction. Larger doses may produce serious or even life threatening manifestations of toxicity, particularly when given in association with sympathomimetic amines such as those used for their anorectic effects.

Continued on next page

Flint—Cont.

Patients with cardiovascular diseases warrant particularly close attention during the restoration of normal thyroid function by any thyroid drug. In such cases, low initial dosage increased slowly by small increments is indicated. Occasionally, the cardiovascular capacity of the patient is so compromised that the metabolic demands of the normal thyroid state cannot be met. Clinical judgment will then dictate a less-than-complete restoration of thyroid status.
Endocrine disorders such as diabetes mellitus, adrenal insufficiency (Addison's disease), hypopituitarism and diabetes insipidus are characterized by signs and symptoms which may be diminished in severity or obscured by hypothyroidism. SYNTHROID (levothyroxine sodium) therapy for such patients may aggravate the intensity of previously obscured symptoms and require appropriate adjustment of therapeutic measures directed at these concomitant disorders.
Thyroid replacement may potentiate the effects of anticoagulants. Patients on anticoagulant therapy should have frequent prothrombin determinations when instituting thyroid replacement to gauge the need to reduce anticoagulant dosage.
Precautions: Overdosage with any thyroid drug may produce the signs and symptoms of thyrotoxicosis, but resistance to such factitious thyrotoxicosis is the general rule. With SYNTHROID (levothyroxine sodium) **Tablets**, the relatively slow onset of action minimizes the risk of overdose but close observation in the weeks following institution of a dosage regimen is advised. Treatment of thyroid hyperactivity induced by oral medication is confined to interruption of therapy for a week, followed by reinstitution of daily therapy at an appropriately reduced dosage.
Close observation of the patient following the administration of SYNTHROID (levothyroxine sodium) **Injection** is advised, and appropriate adjustment of repeated dosage is recommended.
The 100 mcg (0.1 mg) and 300 mcg (0.3 mg) tablets of SYNTHROID (levothyroxine sodium) contain FD&C Yellow No. 5 (tartrazine) which may cause allergic-type reactions (including bronchial asthma) in certain susceptible individuals. Although the overall incidence of FD&C Yellow No. 5 (tartrazine) sensitivity in the general population is low, it is frequently seen in patients who also have aspirin hypersensitivity.
Adverse Reactions: Adverse reactions are due to overdose and are those of induced hyperthyroidism.
Dosage and Administration: For most adults, a final dosage of 100 mcg. (0.1 mg.) to 200 mcg. (0.2 mg.) of SYNTHROID (levothyroxine sodium) **Tablets** daily will provide adequate thyroid replacement, and only occasionally will patients require larger doses. Failure to respond adequately to a daily oral intake of 400 mcg. (0.4 mg.) or more is rare and should prompt reconsideration of the diagnosis of hypothyroidism, special investigation of the patient in terms of malabsorption of L-thyroxine from the gastrointestinal tract or evaluation of patient compliance to therapy.
The concomitant appearance of other diseases, especially cardiovascular diseases, usually dictates a replacement regimen with initial doses smaller than 100 mcg. (0.1 mg.) per day. In otherwise healthy adults with relatively recent onset of hypothyroidism, full replacement doses of 150 mcg. (0.15 mg.) or 200 mcg. (0.2 mg.) have been instituted immediately without untoward effect and with good therapeutic response. General experience, however, favors a more cautious approach in view of the possible presence of subclinical disorders of the cardiovascular system or other endocrinopathies.
The age and general physicial condition of the patient and the severity and duration of hypothyroid symptoms determine the starting dosage and the rate of incremental dosage increase leading to a final maintenance dosage. In the elderly patient with long standing disease, evidence of myxedematous infiltration and symptomatic, functional or electrocardiographic evidence of cardiovascular dysfunction, the starting dose may be as little as 25 mcg. (0.025 mg.) per day. Further incremental increases of 25 mcg. (0.025 mg.) per day may be instituted at three to four week intervals depending on patient response. Conversely, otherwise healthy adults may be started at higher daily doses and raised to a full replacement dose in two to three weeks. Clearly it is the physician's judgment of the severity of the disease and close observation of patient response which determine the rate and extent of dosage increase.
Appropriate laboratory tests are beneficial in monitoring thyroid replacement therapy. Although measurements of normal blood levels of thyroxine in patients on oral replacement regimens frequently coincide with clinical impressions of normal thyroid status, higher than normal levels occur occasionally and should not be considered evidence of overdosage per se. In all cases, clinical impressions of the well-being of the patient take precedence over laboratory determinations of appropriate individual dosage.
In infants and children, there is a great urgency to achieve full thyroid replacement because of the critical importance of thyroid hormone in sustaining growth and maturation. Despite the smaller body size, the dosage needed to sustain a full rate of growth, development and general thriving is higher in the child than in the adult.
The recommended daily replacement dosage of levothyroxine sodium in childhood is: 0-1 years: 9 mcg/kg; 1-5 years: 6 mcg/kg; 6-10 years: 4 mcg/kg; 11-20 years: 3 mcg/kg. Dose is administered once daily only. Optimal maintenance levels should be adjusted individually to obtain both normal serum free T_4 estimates (i.e., free T_4 index) and Thyroid Stimulating Hormone (TSH) values after several weeks of therapy for hypothyroidism. An exception may be seen in congenital hypothyroidism where elevated serum TSH values may persist for the first 2-3 years of life despite normalization of free T_4 measurements. In such cases, it generally is recommended that maintenance of normal serum free T_4 values alone should be considered therapeutically sufficient.
In myxedema coma or stupor, without concomitant severe heart disease, 200 to 500 mcg. of SYNTHROID (levothyroxine sodium) **Injection** may be administered intravenously as a solution containing 100 mcg./ml. DO NOT ADD TO OTHER INTRAVENOUS FLUIDS. Although the patient may show evidence of increased responsivity within six to eight hours, full therapeutic effect may not be evident until the following day. An additional 100 to 300 mcg. or more may be given on the second day if evidence of significant and progressive improvement has not occurred. Like the oral dosage form, SYNTHROID (levothyroxine sodium) **Injection** produces a predictable increase in the circulating level of hormone with a long half-time. This usually precludes the need for multiple injections but continued daily administration of lesser amounts parenterally should be maintained until the patient is fully capable of accepting a daily oral dose. A daily maintenance dose of 50 to 100 mcg parenterally should suffice to maintain a euthyroid state.
In the presence of concomitant heart disease, the sudden administration of such large doses of L-thyroxine intravenously is clearly not without its cardiovascular risks. Under such circumstances, intravenous therapy should not be undertaken without weighing the alternative risks of the myxedema coma and the cardiovascular disease. Clinical judgment in this situation may dictate smaller intravenous doses of SYNTHROID (levothyroxine sodium) **Injection.**
SYNTHROID (levothyroxine sodium) **Injection** by intravenous or intramuscular routes can be substituted for the oral dosage form when ingestion of SYNTHROID (levothyroxine sodium) **Tablets** is precluded for long periods of time. The initial parenteral dosage should be approximately one half of the previously established oral dosage of levothyroxine sodium tablets. Close observation of the patient, with increase in dosage as needed, is recommended.
How Supplied: SYNTHROID (levothyroxine sodium) **Tablets** are supplied as scored, color-coded potency-marked tablets in 6 concentrations: 25 mcg. (0.025 mg.)—orange . . . 50 mcg. (0.05 mg.)—white . . . 100 mcg. (0.1 mg.)—yellow . . . 150 mcg. (0.15 mg.)—blue . . . 200 mcg. (0.2 mg.)—pink . . . 300 mcg. (0.3 mg.)—green.
SYNTHROID (levothyroxine sodium) **Injection** is lyophilized in the final container with 10 mg Mannitol, USP and 0.7 mg tribasic sodium phosphate anhydrous. pH may be adjusted with sodium hydroxide. It is supplied in color-coded 10 ml vials in 3 concentrations: 100 mcg — blue. . . 200 mcg—gray. . . 500 mcg—yellow.
Directions for Reconstitution: Reconstitute the lyophilized levothyroxine sodium by aseptically adding 5 ml. of 0.9% Sodium Chloride Injection, USP or Bacteriostatic Sodium Chloride Injection, USP with Benzyl Alcohol, only. Shake vial to insure complete mixing. **Use immediately** after reconstitution. Do not add to other intravenous fluids. Discard any unused portion.
Literature Available: Upon request.
[*Shown in Product Identification Section*]

TRAVASE® OINTMENT ℞
(Sutilains Ointment, USP)

Description: TRAVASE Ointment (Sutilains Ointment, USP) is a sterile preparation of proteolytic enzymes, elaborated by **Bacillus subtilis,** in a hydrophobic ointment base consisting of 95% white petrolatum and 5% polyethylene. One gram of ointment contains approximately 82,000 casein units* of proteolytic activity.
*A casein unit is the amount of enzyme required to produce the same optical density at 275 mμ as that of a solution of 1.5 mcg. tyrosine/ml. after the enzyme has been incubated with 35 mg. of casein at 37° C. for one minute.
Action: TRAVASE Ointment selectively digests necrotic soft tissues by proteolytic action. It dissolves and facilitates the removal of necrotic tissues and purulent exudates that otherwise impair formation of granulation tissue and delay wound healing.
At body temperatures these proteolytic enzymes have optimal activity in the pH range from 6.0 to 6.8.
Indications: For wound debridement—TRAVASE Ointment is indicated as an adjunct to established methods of wound care for biochemical debridement of the following lesions:

- Second and third degree burns,
- Decubitus ulcers,
- Incisional, traumatic, and pyogenic wounds,
- Ulcers secondary to peripheral vascular disease.

Contraindications: Application of TRAVASE Ointment is contraindicated in the following conditions:

- Wounds communicating with major body cavities,
- Wounds containing exposed major nerves or nervous tissue,
- Fungating neoplastic ulcers,
- Wounds in women of child-bearing potential—because of lack of laboratory evi-

dence of effects of TRAVASE Ointment upon the developing fetus.

Warning: Do not permit TRAVASE Ointment to come into contact with the eyes. In treatment of burns or lesions about the head or neck, should the ointment inadvertently come into contact with the eyes, the eyes should be immediately rinsed with copious amounts of water, preferably sterile.

Precautions: A moist environment is essential to optimal activity of the enzyme. Enzyme activity may also be impaired by certain agents. **In vitro**, several detergents and antiseptics (benzalkonium chloride, hexachlorophene, iodine, and nitrofurazone) may render the substrate indifferent to the action of the enzyme. Compounds such as thimerosal, containing metallic ions, interfere directly with enzyme activity to a slight degree, whereas neomycin, sulfamylon, streptomycin, and penicillin do not affect enzyme activity. In cases where adjunctive topical therapy has been used and no dissolution of slough occurs after treatment with TRAVASE Ointment for 24 to 48 hours, further application, because of interference by the adjunctive agents, is unlikely to be rewarding.

In cases where there is existent or threatening invasive infection, appropriate systemic antibiotic therapy should be instituted concurrently.

Although there have been no reports of systemic allergic reaction to TRAVASE Ointment in humans, studies have shown that there may be an antibody response in humans to absorbed enzyme material.

Adverse Reactions: Adverse reactions consist of mild, transient pain, paresthesias, bleeding and transient dermatitis. Pain usually can be controlled by administration of mild analgesics. Side effects severe enough to warrant discontinuation of therapy occasionally have occurred.

If bleeding or dermatitis occurs as a result of the application of TRAVASE Ointment, therapy should be discontinued. No systemic toxicity has been observed as a result of the topical application of TRAVASE Ointment.

Dosage and Administration:

STRICT ADHERENCE TO THE FOLLOWING IS REQUIRED FOR EFFECTIVE RESULTS OF TREATMENT

1. Thoroughly cleanse and irrigate wound area with sodium chloride or water solutions. Wound MUST be cleansed of antiseptics or heavy-metal antibacterials which may denature enzyme or alter substrate characteristics (e.g., hexachlorophene, silver nitrate, benzalkonium chloride, nitrofurazone).
2. Thoroughly moisten wound area either through tubbing, showering, or wet soaks (e.g., sodium chloride or water solutions).
3. Apply TRAVASE Ointment in a thin layer assuring intimate contact with necrotic tissue and complete wound coverage extending to ¼ to ½ inch beyond the area to be debrided.
4. Apply loose moist dressings.
5. Repeat entire procedure 3 to 4 times per day for best results.

How Supplied: TRAVASE Ointment (Sutilains Ointment, USP) is supplied sterile in one-half ounce (14.2 g) tubes. Each gram contains 82,000 casein units of proteolytic activity in a hydrophobic ointment base.

The ointment must be refrigerated at 2° to 8° C (35° to 46° F).

[*Shown in Product Identification Section*]

Products are cross-indexed by generic and chemical names in the

YELLOW SECTION

Fluoritab Corporation

P.O. BOX 381
FLINT, MICHIGAN 48501

FLUORITAB® ℞
sodium fluoride (Active Ingredient)

Composition:

Sodium fluoride	2.2 mg.
Inert organic filler	75.8 mg.

Each tablet contains 1 mg. of fluorine (as fluoride ion)

Action and Uses: FLUORITAB dietary fluoride products are straight fluoride and contain no other active ingredients. They are to provide optimum fluoride where water supplies are deficient in fluorine. Dietary fluoride is beneficial in providing teeth that are more resistant to decay. Fluorine combines with calcium to form the apatite molecule of teeth and bone to form fluorapatite crystals.

Administration and Dosage: FLUORITAB dietary fluoride can be given in baby formulas, or in any liquid. They can be swallowed quickly, or permitted to remain in the mouth to dissolve, which may provide surface benefit to tooth enamel. Fluoride must be taken on a continued basis throughout the period of tooth formation to be fully effective.

Dosage should provide the child with ½ mg. per day from birth to 3 years of age and 1 mg. per day from 3 years of age up.

Water supplies with 0.2 parts per million or less require supplementing with ½ mg. and 1 mg. dosage per day for children under and over 3, respectively. Water supplies with 0.2 to 0.6 parts per million require ¼ mg. and ½ mg. dosage per day for children under 3 and over 3 respectively.

Side Effects: Excess fluoride is to be avoided, as it may cause dental fluorosis (mottling of the teeth).

Precautions: Where water with 0.7 P.P.M. of fluoride is used, dietary fluoride ought not be used.

Contraindications: None.

Overdosage: (*Symptoms and Treatment*): The total contents of our safety limited packages can be taken without any effect.

How Supplied: FLUORITAB TABLETS are supplied in bottles of 100, scored, easily divided 1.2 grain tablets, 1 mg. fluorine per tablet. FLUORITAB LIQUID is supplied in 19 cc. (480 drop) (.25 mg. fluorine per drop) polyethelene squeeze type dropper bottles.

Product Identification Mark(s): FLUORITAB products have the "FLUORITAB" name on all packages.

Remarks: FLUORITAB dietary fluoride was the first dietary fluoride product given A.D.A. acceptance (July, 1958). We adhere rigidly to their recommendation of restricting our package size to their safety admonition: *Never* to sell packages containing more than 264 mg. of sodium fluoride.

Literature Available: Reprints, educational folders and prescription instructions will be sent free, on request.

IDENTIFICATION PROBLEM?

Consult PDR's

Product Identification Section

where you'll find over 900

products pictured actual size

and in full color.

Forest Laboratories, Inc.

919 THIRD AVENUE
NEW YORK, NEW YORK 10022

BROCON® C.R.* Tablets ℞

Description: Each tablet contains:

Brompheniramine Maleate	12 mg
Phenylephrine Hydrochloride	15 mg
Phenylpropanolamine Hydrochloride	15 mg

Actions: Brocon C.R. reduces excessive nasopharyngeal secretion and diminishes inflammatory mucosal edema and congestion in the upper respiratory tract. The antihistaminic action of brompheniramine maleate reduces or abolishes the allergic response of nasal tissue. It is complemented by the mild vasoconstrictor action of phenylephrine hydrochloride and phenylpropanolamine hydrochloride, which provides a nasal decongestant effect.

Indications: Based on a review of this drug by the National Academy of Sciences-National Research Council and/or other information, FDA has classified the indication(s) as follows: "Possibly" effective for the symptomatic treatment of seasonal and perennial allergic rhinitis and vasomotor rhinitis; and for treatment of urticaria and pruritus due to allergens of drugs; and allergic conjunctivitis.

Final classification of the less-than-effective indication requires further investigation.

Contraindications: Hypersensitivity to any of the ingredients. Brompheniramine is contraindicated during pregnancy and in patients who are receiving concurrent MAO inhibitors. Because of its drying and thickening effect on the lower respiratory secretions, it is not recommended in the treatment of bronchial asthma.

Warnings: In infants and children particularly, over-dosage of antihistamines may produce convulsions and death.

Precautions: Administer with caution to patients with cardiac or peripheral vascular disease or hypertension. Until the patient's response has been determined, he should be warned against engaging in operations requiring alertness, such as driving an automobile, operating machinery, etc. Patients receiving antihistamines should be warned against possible additive effects with CNS depressants such as alcohol, hypnotics, sedatives, tranquilizers, etc.

Adverse Reactions: Hypersensitivity reactions such as rash, leukopenia, urticaria, agranulocytosis and thrombocytopenia, drowsiness, lassitude, giddiness, dryness of the mucous membranes, tightness of the chest, thickening of bronchial secretions, palpitation, hypotension/hypertension, urinary frequency and dysuria, headache, faintness, dizziness, tinnitus, incoordination, visual disturbances, mydriasis, CNS-depressant and stimulant effect, anorexia, nausea, vomiting, diarrhea, constipation and epigastric distress.

Dosage and Administration: Adults and children over 12 years of age: One tablet morning and evening. If indicated, one tablet every 8 hours may be given.

How Supplied: Bottles of 100, 500 and 1000.

Caution: Federal law prohibits dispensing without prescription.

---

*Synchron™ System, a special base to provide a controlled release—U.S. Patent 3,870,790—Other U.S. Patents Pending.

GEIGY Pharmaceuticals

Division of CIBA-GEIGY Corporation
ARDSLEY, NY 10502

GY-CODE® INDEX

GEIGY Pharmaceuticals has established a Drug Identity Code System entitled GY-CODE. This system affords a convenient and accurate means of uniquely identifying each Geigy solid dosage form on which the GY-CODE number and the name "Geigy" appear. The GY-CODE number also appears as part of the National Drug Code number.

GY-CODE NUMBER	PROD. DESCRIPTION	NATIONAL DRUG CODE
11 Tofranil® Tablets		
	imipramine hydrochloride USP 25 mg.	
	Coral-colored (black Geigy imprint) coated tablets	
	100's	0028-0011-01
	1000's	0028-0011-10
	100's Unit Dose Pkg.	0028-0011-61
	Gy-Pak® 100's	
	One unit (12 × 100)	0028-0011-65
	Six units (72 × 100)	0028-0011-65
14 Butazolidin® Tablets		
	phenylbutazone USP 100 mg.	
	Red, film-coated tablets	
	100's	0028-0014-01
	1000's	0028-0014-10
	100's Unit Dose Pkg.	0028-0014-61
20 Tofranil-PM® Capsules		
	imipramine pamoate 75 mg.	
	Coral-colored capsules	
	30's	0028-0020-26
	100's	0028-0020-01
	1000's	0028-0020-10
	100's Unit Dose Pkg.	0028-0020-61
21 Tofranil® Tablets		
	imipramine hydrochloride USP 10 mg.	
	Triangular, coral-colored, coated tablets	
	100's	0028-0021-01
	1000's	0028-0021-10
22 Tofranil-PM® Capsules		
	imipramine pamoate 150 mg.	
	Coral-colored capsules	
	30's	0028-0022-26
	100's	0028-0022-01
	100's Unit Dose Pkg.	0028-0022-61
23 Lioresal® Tablets		
	baclofen 10 mg.	
	White, oval, scored tablets	
	100's	0028-0023-01
	100's Unit Dose Pkg.	0028-0023-61
24 Tandearil® Tablets		
	oxyphenbutazone USP 100 mg.	
	Tan, coated tablets	
	100's	0028-0024-01
	1000's	0028-0024-10
	100's Unit Dose Pkg.	0028-0024-61
33 Lioresal® Tablets		
	baclofen 20 mg.	
	White, capsule shaped, scored tablets	
	100's	0028-0033-01
	100's Unit Dose Pkg.	0028-0033-61
40 Tofranil-PM® Capsules		
	imipramine pamoate 100 mg.	
	Dark yellow/coral-colored capsules	
	30's	0028-0040-26
	100's	0028-0040-01
42 Constant-T™ Tablets		
	theophylline (anhydrous) 200 mg.	
	Light pink, oval, scored tablets	
	100's	0028-0042-01
	100's Unit Dose Pkg.	0028-0042-61
	Gy-Pak® 60's	
	One Unit (12 × 60)	0028-0042-73
	Six Units (72 × 60)	0028-0042-73
43 PBZ® Tablets		
	tripelennamine hydrochloride USP 50 mg.	
	Light blue, scored tablets	
	100's	0028-0043-01
	1000's	0028-0043-10
44 Butazolidin® Capsules		
	phenylbutazone USP 100 mg.	
	Orange/white capsules	
	100's	0028-0044-01
	1000's	0028-0044-10
	100's Unit Dose Pkg.	0028-0044-61
	Gy-Pak® 100's	
	One Unit (12 × 100)	0028-0044-65
	Six Units (72 × 100)	0028-0044-65
45 Tofranil-PM® Capsules		
	imipramine pamoate 125 mg.	
	Light yellow/coral-colored capsules	
	30's	0028-0045-26
	100's	0028-0045-01
47 Tegretol® Chewable Tablets		
	carbamazepine USP	
	Round, red-speckled, pink, single-scored tablets	
	100's	0028-0047-01
	100's Unit Dose Pkg.	0028-0047-61
48 PBZ-SR® Tablets		
	tripelennamine hydrochloride 100 mg.	
	Lavender-colored tablets	
	100's	0028-0048-01
51 Lopressor® Tablets		
	metoprolol tartrate 50 mg.	
	Light red, capsule-shaped, scored tablets	
	100's	0028-0051-01
	1000's	0028-0051-10
	100's Unit Dose Pkg.	0028-0051-61
	Gy-Pak® 60's	
	One Unit (12x60)	0028-0051-73
	Six Units (72x60)	0028-0051-73
	Gy-Pak® 100's	
	One Unit (12 × 100)	0028-0051-65
	Six Units (72 × 100)	0028-0051-65
57 Constant-T™ Tablets		
	theophylline (anhydrous) 300 mg.	
	Light blue, oval, scored tablets	
	100's	0028-0057-01
	100's Unit Dose Pkg.	0028-0057-61
	Gy-Pak® 60's	
	One Unit (12 × 60)	0028-0057-73
	Six Units (72 × 60)	0028-0057-73
60 PBZ® Lontabs® Tablets		
	tripelennamine hydrochloride 50 mg.	
	Light green Lontabs® tablets	
	100's	0028-0060-01
67 Tegretol® Tablets		
	carbamazepine USP 200 mg.	
	White, single-scored tablets	
	100's	0028-0067-01
	1000's	0028-0067-10
	100's Unit Dose Pkg.	0028-0067-61
	Gy-Pak® 100's	
	One Unit (12 × 100)	0028-0067-65
	Six Units (72 × 100)	0028-0067-65
71 Lopressor® Tablets		
	metoprolol tartrate 100 mg.	
	Light blue, capsule-shaped, scored tablets	
	100's	0028-0071-01
	1000's	0028-0071-10
	100's Unit Dose Pkg.	0028-0071-61
	Gy-Pak® 60's	
	One Unit (12 × 60)	0028-0071-73
	Six Units (72 × 60)	0028-0071-73
	Gy-Pak® 100's	
	One Unit (12 × 100)	0028-0071-65
	Six Units (72 × 100)	0028-0071-65
72 Brethine® Tablets		
	terbutaline sulfate USP 2.5 mg.	
	Oval, white, scored tablets	
	100's	0028-0072-01
	1000's	0028-0072-10
	100's Unit Dose Pkg.	0028-0072-61
	Gy-Pak® 90's	
	One Unit (12 × 90)	0028-0072-90
	Six Units (72 × 90)	0028-0072-90
	Gy-Pak® 100's	
	One Unit (12 × 100)	0028-0072-65
	Six Units (72 × 100)	0028-0072-65
74 Tofranil® Tablets		
	imipramine hydrochloride USP 50 mg.	
	Coral-colored (white Geigy imprint) coated tablets	
	100's	0028-0074-01
	1000's	0028-0074-10
	100's Unit Dose Pkg.	0028-0074-61
	Gy-Pak® 100's	
	One unit (12 × 100)	0028-0074-65
	Six units (72 × 100)	0028-0074-65
95 PBZ® Tablets		
	tripelennamine hydrochloride USP 25 mg.	
	Green, sugar-coated tablets	
	100's	0028-0095-01
105 Brethine® Tablets		
	terbutaline sulfate USP 5 mg.	
	Round, scored, white tablets	
	100's	0028-0105-01
	1000's	0028-0105-10
	100's Unit Dose Pkg.	0028-0105-61
	Gy-Pak® 90's	
	One Unit (12 × 90)	0028-0105-90
	Six Units (72 × 90)	0028-0105-90
	Gy-Pak® 100's	
	One unit (12 × 100)	0028-0105-65
	Six units (72 × 100)	0028-0105-65
134 PBZ® Tablets with Ephedrine		
	tripelennamine hydrochloride	
	Per Tablet:	
	tripelennamine hydrochloride 25 mg.	
	ephedrine sulfate 12 mg.	
	White, dry-coated tablets	
	100's	0028-0134-01
6114 Otrivin® Nasal Drops (0.1%)		
	xylometazoline hydrochloride USP	
	20 ml.	0028-6114-58
6116 Otrivin® Pediatric (0.05%)		
	xylometazoline hydrochloride USP	
	20 ml.	0028-6116-58
6118 Otrivin® Spray (0.1%)		
	xylometazoline hydrochloride USP	
	15 ml.	0028-6118-57
6925 PBZ® Elixir		
	Per 5-ml. teaspoon:	
	tripelennamine citrate USP 37.5 mg.	
	(equivalent to 25 mg. tripelennamine hydrochloride)	
	473 ml.	0028-6925-16
6946 PBZ® Antihistamine Cream		
	tripelennamine hydrochloride	
	Cream 2% (water-washable base)	
	1 oz.	0028-6946-76

BRETHINE® ℞

terbutaline sulfate USP
Tablets of 5 mg **GY-CODE 105**
Tablets of 2.5 mg **GY-CODE 72**

Description: Brethine, a synthetic sympathomimetic amine, may be chemically described as α-[(*tert*-Butylamino) methyl] -3,5- dihydroxybenzyl alcohol sulfate.

Brethine, terbutaline sulfate, is a water soluble, colorless, crystalline solid. Tablets containing terbutaline sulfate should be stored at controlled room temperature.

Each scored, white tablet contains 5 mg (equivalent to 4.1 mg of free base) or 2.5 mg (equivalent to 2.05 mg of free base) of terbutaline sulfate.

Actions: Brethine is a β-adrenergic receptor agonist which has been shown by *in vitro* and *in vivo* pharmacological studies in animals to exert a preferential effect on β_2-adrenergic receptors such as those located in bronchial smooth muscle. Controlled clinical studies in patients who were administered the drug orally have revealed proportionally greater changes in pulmonary function parameters than in heart rate or blood pressure. While this *suggests* a relative preference for the β_2 receptor in man, the usual cardiovascular effects commonly associated with sympathomimetic agents were also observed with Brethine.

Brethine has been shown in controlled clinical studies to relieve bronchospasm in chronic obstructive pulmonary disease.

This action is manifested by a clinically significant increase in pulmonary function as demonstrated by an increase of 15% or more in FEV_1 and in $FEF_{25\text{-}75\%}$. Following administration of Brethine tablets, a measurable change in flow rate is usually observed in 30 minutes, and a clinically significant improvement in pulmonary function occurs at 60–120 minutes. The maximum effect usually occurs within 120-180 minutes. Brethine also produces a clinically significant decrease in airway and pulmonary resistance which persists for at least four hours or longer. Significant bronchodilator action, as measured by various pulmonary function determinations (airway resistance, $FEF_{25\text{-}75\%}$, or PEFR), has been demonstrated in some studies for periods up to eight hours.

Clinical studies were conducted in which the effectiveness of Brethine was evaluated in comparison with ephedrine over periods up to three months. Both drugs continued to produce significant improvement in pulmonary function throughout this period of treatment.

Indications: Brethine is indicated as a bronchodilator for bronchial asthma and for reversible bronchospasm which may occur in association with bronchitis and emphysema.

Contraindications: Brethine is contraindicated when there is known hypersensitivity to sympathomimetic amines.

Warnings: *Usage in Pregnancy:* Animal reproductive studies have been negative with respect to adverse effects on fetal development. The safe use of Brethine has not, however, been established in human pregnancy. As with any medication, the use of the drug in pregnancy, lactation, or women of childbearing potential requires that the expected therapeutic benefit of the drug be weighed against its possible hazards to the mother or child.

Usage in Pediatrics: Brethine tablets are not presently recommended for children below the age of 12 years due to insufficient clinical data in this pediatric group.

Precautions: Brethine should be used with caution in patients with diabetes, hypertension, hyperthyroidism, and a history of seizures.

As with other sympathomimetic bronchodilator agents, Brethine should be administered cautiously to cardiac patients, especially those with associated arrhythmias.

The concomitant use of Brethine with other sympathomimetic agents is not recommended, since their combined effect on the cardiovascular system may be deleterious to the patient. However, this does not preclude the use of an aerosol bronchodilator of the adrenergic stimulant type for the relief of an acute bronchospasm in patients receiving chronic oral Brethine therapy.

Adverse Reactions: Commonly observed side effects include nervousness and tremor. Other reported reactions include headache, increased heart rate, palpitations, drowsiness, nausea, vomiting, sweating, and muscle cramps. These reactions are generally transient in nature and usually do not require treatment. The frequency of these side effects appears to diminish with continued therapy. In general, all the side effects observed are characteristic of those commonly seen with sympathomimetic amines.

Dosage and Administration: The usual oral dose of Brethine for adults is 5 mg administered at approximately six-hour intervals, three times daily, during the hours the patient is usually awake. If side effects are particularly disturbing, the dose may be reduced to 2.5 mg three times daily, and still provide a clinically significant improvement in pulmonary function. A dose of 2.5 mg, three times daily, also is recommended for children in the 12- to 15-year group. Brethine is not recommended at present for use in children below the age of 12 years. In adults, a total dose of 15 mg should not be exceeded in a 24-hour period. In children, a total dose of 7.5 mg should not be exceeded in a 24-hour period.

Overdosage: Overdosage experience is limited. Excessive beta-adrenergic receptor stimulation may augment the signs or symptoms listed under **Adverse Reactions** and they may be accompanied by other adrenergic effects. Treat the alert patient who has taken excessive oral medication by emptying the stomach by means of induced emesis, followed by gastric lavage. In the unconscious patient, secure the airway with a cuffed endotracheal tube before beginning lavage (do not induce emesis). Instillation of activated charcoal slurry may help reduce absorption of terbutaline sulfate. Maintain adequate respiratory exchange. Provide cardiac and respiratory support as needed. Continue observation until symptom-free.

How Supplied: Round, scored, white tablets of 5 mg are supplied in bottles of 100 and 1,000 and Unit Dose Packages of 100; and oval, scored, white tablets of 2.5 mg are supplied in bottles of 100 and 1,000 and Unit Dose Packages of 100.

C80-57 (12/80)

[*Shown in Product Identification Section*]

BRETHINE® ℞

terbutaline sulfate USP GY-CODE 7507
Ampuls
A sterile aqueous solution for subcutaneous injection.

Description: Brethine, α-[(*tert*-Butylamino) methyl]- 3,5-dihydroxybenzyl alcohol sulfate is a synthetic sympathomimetic amine.

Brethine is a water soluble colorless crystalline solid. Solutions are sensitive to excessive heat and light, and ampuls should therefore be stored at controlled room temperature with protection from light by storage in their original carton until dispensed. Solutions should not be used if discolored.

Each milliliter of sterile isotonic solution contains 1.0 mg of terbutaline sulfate (equivalent to 0.82 mg of free base), 8.9 mg of sodium chloride, and hydrochloric acid to adjust the pH to 3.0–5.0.

Actions: Brethine is a β-adrenergic receptor agonist which has been shown by *in vitro* and *in vivo* pharmacological studies in animals to exert a preferential effect on β_2-adrenergic receptors such as those located in bronchial smooth muscle.

However, controlled clinical studies in patients who were administered the drug subcutaneously have not revealed a preferential β_2 adrenergic effect.

Brethine has been shown in controlled clinical studies to relieve acute bronchospasm in acute and chronic obstructive pulmonary disease, resulting in a clinically significant increase in pulmonary flow rates, e.g., an increase of 15% or greater in FEV_1. Following administration of 0.25 mg of subcutaneous Brethine, a measurable change in flow rate is usually observed within five minutes, and a clinically significant increase in FEV_1 occurs by 15 minutes following the injection. The maximum effect usually occurs within 30–60 minutes and clinically significant bronchodilator activity has been observed to persist for 90 minutes to four hours. The duration of clinically significant improvement is comparable to that found with equimilligram doses of epinephrine.

Indications: Brethine is indicated as a bronchodilator for bronchial asthma and for reversible bronchospasm which may occur in association with bronchitis and emphysema.

Contraindications: Brethine is contraindicated when there is known hypersensitivity to sympathomimetic amines.

Warnings: *Usage in Pregnancy:* Animal reproductive studies have been negative with respect to adverse effects on fetal development. The safe use of Brethine has not, however, been established in human pregnancy. As with any medication, the use of the drug in pregnancy, lactation, or women of childbearing potential requires that the expected therapeutic benefit of the drug be weighed against its possible hazards to the mother or child.

Usage in Pediatrics: Studies are in progress to define the safe and effective dose of Brethine in children. Therefore, until such studies are completed and evaluated, Brethine is not recommended for use in pediatrics.

Precautions: Brethine should be used with caution in patients with diabetes, hypertension, hyperthyroidism, and a history of seizures.

As with other sympathomimetic bronchodilator agents, Brethine should be administered cautiously to cardiac patients, especially those with associated arrhythmias.

The concomitant use of Brethine with other sympathomimetic agents is not recommended, since their combined effect on the cardiovascular system may be deleterious to the patient.

Preparation of Other Dosage Forms: Use of the subcutaneous injection for preparation of other dosage forms, i.e., I.V. infusion, is inappropriate. Sterility and accurate dosing cannot be assured if the ampuls are not used in accordance with **Dosage and Administration.**

Carcinogenesis, Mutagenesis, Impairment of Fertility: An 18-month oral (feeding) carcinogenicity study of terbutaline (5, 50, and 200 mg/kg, corresponding to 500x, 5000x, and 20,000x the clinical subcutaneous dose) in NMRI strain mice revealed no drug-related tumorigenicity. Mutagenicity and fertility studies were not performed.

Pregnancy Category B: Reproduction studies have been performed in mice and rats at doses up to 1,000 times the human dose and have revealed no evidence of impaired fertility or harm to the fetus due to terbutaline. There are, however, no adequate and well-controlled studies in pregnant women. Because animal reproduction studies are not always predictive of human response, this drug should be used during pregnancy only if clearly needed.

Usage in Labor and Delivery: Serious adverse reactions have been reported following administration of terbutaline sulfate to women in labor. These reports have included transient hypokalemia, pulmonary edema and hypoglycemia in the mother and hypoglycemia in the neonatal children of women treated with terbutaline parenterally.

Pediatric Use: Studies are in progress to define the safe and effective dose of Brethine in children. Therefore, until such studies are completed and evaluated, Brethine is not recommended for use in pediatrics.

Adverse Reactions: Commonly observed side effects include increases in heart rate, nervousness, tremor, palpitations and dizziness. These occur more frequently at doses in excess of 0.25 mg. Other reported reactions include headache, nausea, vomiting, anxiety, and muscle cramps. These reactions are transient in nature and usually do not require treatment. In general, all side effects are characteristic of those commonly seen with sympathomimetic amines such as epinephrine.

Dosage and Administration: The usual subcutaneous dose of Brethine is 0.25 mg injected into the lateral deltoid area. If significant clinical improvement does not occur by 15–30 minutes, a second dose of 0.25 mg may be administered. A total dose of 0.5 mg should not be exceeded within a four-hour period. If a patient fails to respond to a second 0.25-mg dose of Brethine within 15–30 minutes, other therapeutic measures should be considered.

Continued on next page

The full prescribing information for each GEIGY drug is contained herein and is that in effect as of October 1, 1982.

Geigy—Cont.

Overdosage: Overdosage experience is limited. Excessive beta-adrenergic receptor stimulation may augment the signs or symptoms listed under **Adverse Reactions** and they may be accompanied by other adrenergic effects. In the case of subcutaneous injectable terbutaline overdosage, the patient should be treated symptomatically under guidelines for sympathomimetic overdosage.

How Supplied:
Ampuls 1-mg/ml (2-ml size ampul, expiration-dated)

Box of 10	NDC 0028-7507-23
Box of 100	NDC 0028-7507-01

Protect from light by storing ampuls in original carton until dispensed.
Keep at controlled room temperature (59°–86°F) 15°-30°C. Do not use if solution is discolored.

C81-31 (3/82)

BUTAZOLIDIN® ℞
phenylbutazone USP GY-CODE 14
Tablets
Capsules
Nonhormonal Antiarthritic
Anti-Inflammatory Agent

Important Note: Butazolidin cannot be considered a simple analgesic and should never be administered casually. Each patient should be carefully evaluated before treatment is started and should remain constantly under the close supervision of the physician. The following cautions should be observed:

1. Therapy should not be initiated until a careful detailed history and complete physical and laboratory examination, including a complete hemogram and urinalysis, etc., of the patient have been made. These examinations should be made at regular, frequent intervals throughout the duration of this drug therapy.
2. Patients should be carefully selected, avoiding those in whom it is contraindicated as well as those who will respond to ordinary therapeutic measures, or those who cannot be observed at frequent intervals.
3. Patients taking this drug should be warned not to exceed the recommended dosage, since this may lead to toxic effects, and should discontinue the drug and report to the physician immediately any sign of:
   a. Fever, sore throat, lesions in the mouth (symptoms of blood dyscrasia).
   b. Dyspepsia, epigastric pain, symptoms of anemia, unusual bleeding, unusual bruising, black or tarry stools or other evidence of intestinal ulceration.
   c. Skin rashes.
   d. Significant weight gain or edema.
4. A trial period of one week of therapy is considered adequate to determine the therapeutic effect of the drug. In the absence of a favorable response, therapy should be discontinued.
   a. In the elderly (sixty years and over) the drug should be restricted to short-term treatment periods only—if possible, *one week* maximum.
5. **Before prescribing Butazolidin for an individual patient, read thoroughly the information contained under each heading which follows:**

Description: Butazolidin should not be considered as a simple analgesic that can be prescribed for indiscriminate use. Butazolidin is closely related chemically and pharmacologically, including toxic effects, to the well-known pyrazolines (pyrazole compounds) amidopyrine and antipyrine.
Butazolidin is 4-Butyl-1,2-diphenyl-3,5-pyrazolidinedione, with a molecular weight of 308.38.
It is very slightly soluble in water; freely soluble in acetone and in ether; soluble in alcohol.

Clinical Pharmacology: Butazolidin is a nonsalicylate, nonsteroidal, anti-inflammatory drug. It has anti-inflammatory, antipyretic, analgesic and mild uricosuric properties that produce symptomatic relief but do not alter the disease process.
The exact mechanism of the anti-inflammatory effects of Butazolidin has not been elucidated, but clinical pharmacology studies have shown that Butazolidin inhibits certain factors believed to be involved in the inflammatory process. These processes are (1) prostaglandin synthesis; (2) leucocyte migration; (3) release and/or activity of lysosomal enzymes.
Phenylbutazone is rapidly absorbed after oral administration of Butazolidin. Tests conducted in 18 healthy adult male volunteers indicated that a peak plasma concentration of 43.3 ($\pm$3.1) mg/l was attained within 2.5 ($\pm$1.4) hours after the ingestion of three 100-mg tablets. In these same volunteers, the apparent elimination half-life was 84 ($\pm$23) hours. About 98% of the drug is bound to human serum albumin.
Twenty-one days after oral administration of ^{14}C-labelled drug, 61% was recovered from the urine and 27% from the feces. However, only about 1% of total urinary radioactivity represents unchanged drug. The sum of nonconjugated urinary metabolites (oxyphenbutazone, γ-hydroxyphenylbutazone, p,γ-dihydroxyphenylbutazone), and phenylbutazone itself amounted to only about 10%. About 40% of the total urinary radioactivity was excreted as the C(4)-glucuronide of phenylbutazone and an additional 12% was identified as the C(4)-glucuronide of γ-hydroxyphenylbutazone.
The major metabolite of phenylbutazone in human plasma is oxyphenbutazone; steady-state plasma levels about 50% of those of phenylbutazone. Less than 2% of the dose of phenylbutazone appears in the urine as oxyphenbutazone.

Indications: The indications for Butazolidin are:
Acute Gouty Arthritis
Active Rheumatoid Arthritis
Active Ankylosing Spondylitis
Short-term treatment of acute attacks of degenerative joint disease of the hips and knees not responsive to other treatment.
Painful Shoulder (peritendinitis, capsulitis, bursitis, and acute arthritis of that joint)

Contraindications:
1. *Age:* Butazolidin is contraindicated in children 14 years of age or younger since controlled clinical trials in patients of this age group have not been conducted.
2. *Other Medical Conditions.* Butazolidin is contraindicated in patients with incipient cardiac failure, blood dyscrasias, pancreatitis, parotitis, stomatitis, polymyalgia rheumatica, temporal arteritis, senility, drug allergy, and in the presence of severe renal, cardiac and hepatic disease, and in patients with a history of peptic ulcer disease, or symptoms of gastrointestinal inflammation or active ulceration because serious adverse reactions or aggravation of existing medical problems can occur.
3. *Concomitant Medications:* Butazolidin should not be used in combination with other drugs which accentuate or share a potential for similar toxicity.

It is also inadvisable to administer Butazolidin in combination with other potent drugs because of the possibility of increased toxic reactions from Butazolidin and other agents. (see also *Drug Interactions.*)
Butazolidin is contraindicated in patients with a history or suggestion of prior toxicity, sensitivity, or idiosyncrasy to phenylbutazone or oxyphenbutazone.

Warnings: Based on reports of clinical experience with phenylbutazone and related compounds, the following warnings should be considered by the physician prior to prescribing the drug:
1. *Gastrointestinal:* Upper G.I. diagnostic tests should be performed in patients with persistent or severe dyspepsia. Peptic ulceration, reactivation of latent peptic ulcer, perforation and gastrointestinal bleeding, sometimes severe, have been reported. As with other nonsteroidal anti-inflammatory drugs, borderline elevations of values measured by one or more liver tests may occur in up to 15% of patients. These abnormalities may progress, may remain essentially unchanged, or may be transient with continued therapy. The SGPT (ALT) test is probably the most sensitive indicator of liver dysfunction. Meaningful elevations (three times the upper limit of normal) of SGPT or SGOT (AST) have occurred in controlled clinical trials in less than 1% of patients. A patient with symptoms and/or signs suggesting liver dysfunction, or in whom an abnormal liver test has occurred, should be evaluated for evidence of the development of more severe hepatic reactions while on therapy with Butazolidin. Severe hepatic reactions, including jaundice and cases of fatal hepatitis, have been reported with Butazolidin as with other nonsteroidal anti-inflammatory drugs. Although such reactions are rare, if abnormal liver tests persist or worsen, if clinical signs and symptoms consistent with liver disease develop, or if systemic manifestations (e.g., eosinophilia, rash, etc.) occur, therapy with Butazolidin be discontinued.
2. *Hematologic: Frequent and regular hematologic evaluations should be performed on patients receiving the drug for periods over one week.* Any significant change in the total white count, relative decrease in granulocytes, appearance of immature forms or fall in hematocrit should be a signal for immediate cessation of therapy and a complete hematologic investigation. Serious, sometimes fatal blood dyscrasias, including aplastic anemia have been reported to occur. Hematologic toxicity may occur suddenly or many days or weeks after cessation of treatment as manifest by the appearance of anemia, leukopenia, thrombocytopenia or clinically significant hemorrhagic diathesis. There have been published reports associating phenylbutazone with leukemia. However, the circumstances involved in these reports are such that a cause-and-effect relationship to the drug has not been clearly established.
3. *Pregnancy:* Reproductive studies in animals, although inconclusive, exhibited evidence of possible embryotoxicity. It is, therefore, recommended that this drug should be used with caution during pregnancy. The benefits should be weighed against the potential risk to the fetus.
4. *Nursing Mothers:* Caution is also advised in prescribing Butazolidin in nursing mothers since the drug may appear in cord blood and breast milk.
5. Patients reporting visual disturbances while receiving the drug should discontinue treatment and have an ophthalmologic examination because ophthalmologic adverse reactions have been reported (see **Adverse Reactions:** *Special Senses*)
6. In the aging (forty years and over), there appears to be an increase in the possibility of adverse reactions. Butazolidin should be used with commensurately greater care in the elderly and should be avoided altogether in the senile patient.
7. Like other drugs with prostaglandin synthetase inhibition activity, Butazolidin may precipitate acute episodes of asthmatic attacks in patients with asthma.
8. Butazolidin increases sodium retention. Evidence of fluid retention in patients in whom there is danger of cardiac decompen-

sation is an indication to discontinue the drug.

Precautions: Because of potential serious adverse reactions to Butazolidin, the following precautions should be observed in the use of the drug:

—A careful diagnostic physical examination and history should be performed on all patients at regular intervals while the patient is receiving the drug.

—Butazolidin is not recommended for chronic use in the elderly.

—Hematologic evaluation should be performed at frequent and regular intervals and additional laboratory examinations performed as indicated.

—Patients should be instructed to report immediately the occurrence of high fever, severe sore throat, stomatitis, salivary gland enlargement, tarry stools, unusual bleeding or bruising, sudden weight gain, or edema.

—The drug reduces iodine uptake by the thyroid and may interfere with laboratory tests of thyroid function (see **Adverse Reactions:** *Endocrine-Metabolic*)

—The patient should be cautioned regarding participation in activities requiring alertness and coordination and that the concomitant ingestion of alcohol with Butazolidin may further impair psychomotor skills.

Drug Interactions: Butazolidin is highly bound to serum proteins. If its affinity for protein binding is higher than other concurrently administered drugs, the actions and toxicity of the other drug may be increased.

Butazolidin accentuates the prothrombin depression produced by coumarin-type anticoagulants. When administered alone, it does not affect prothrombin activity.

The pharmacologic action of insulin, antidiabetic, and sulfonamide drugs may be potentiated by the simultaneous administration of Butazolidin.

Concomitant administration of phenylbutazone and phenytoin may result in increased serum levels of phenytoin which could lead to increased phenytoin toxicity.

Adverse Reactions: Based upon reports of clinical experience with phenylbutazone and related compounds, the following adverse reactions have been reported.

The adverse reactions listed in the following table have been arranged into three groups: (1) incidence greater than 1%, (2) incidence less than 1% and (3) causal relationship unknown. The incidence for group (1) was obtained from sixty-eight (68) clinical trials reported in the literature (5369 patients). The incidence for group (2) was based on reports in clinical trials, in the literature, and on voluntary reports since marketing. The reactions in group (3) have been reported but occurred under circumstances where a causal relationship could not be established. In some patients the reported reactions may have been unrelated to the administration of Butazolidin. However, in these reported events, the possibility cannot be excluded. Therefore these observations are being listed to serve as alerting information to physicians. Before prescribing this drug for an individual patient, the physician should be familiar with the following:

(1) Incidence greater than 1%	(2) Incidence less than 1%
*GASTROINTESTINAL (See **Warnings**)*	
nausea dyspepsia/including indigestion and heartburn abdominal discomfort/distress *(See Note)*	vomiting abdominal distention with flatulence constipation diarrhea esophagitis gastritis salivary gland enlargement stomatitis, sometimes with ulceration ulceration and perforation of the intestinal tract including acute and reactivated peptic ulcer with perforation, hemorrhage and hematemesis anemia due to gastrointestinal bleeding which may be occult hepatitis, both fatal and nonfatal, sometimes associated with evidence of cholestasis
*HEMATOLOGICAL (See **Warnings**)*	
None	anemia leukopenia thrombocytopenia with associated purpura, petechiae, and hemorrhage pancytopenia aplastic anemia bone marrow depression agranulocytosis and agranulocytic anginal syndrome hemolytic anemia
HYPERSENSITIVITY	
None	urticaria anaphylactic shock arthralgia, drug fever hypersensitivity angiitis (polyarteritis) and vasculitis Lyell's syndrome serum sickness Stevens-Johnson syndrome activation of systemic lupus erythematosus aggravation of temporal arteritis in patients with polymyalgia rheumatica
DERMATOLOGIC	
rash	pruritus erythema nodosum erythema multiforme nonthrombocytopenic purpura
CARDIOVASCULAR, FLUID AND ELECTROLYTE	
edema/water retention *(See Note)*	sodium and chloride retention fluid retention and plasma dilution cardiac decompensation (congestive heart failure) with edema and dyspnea metabolic acidosis respiratory alkalosis hypertension pericarditis interstitial myocarditis with muscle necrosis and perivascular granulomata
RENAL	
None	hematuria proteinuria ureteral obstruction with uric acid crystals anuria glomerulonephritis acute tubular necrosis cortical necrosis renal stones nephrotic syndrome impaired renal function and renal failure associated with azotemia
CENTRAL NERVOUS SYSTEM	
None	headache drowsiness agitation confusional states and lethargy tremors numbness weakness
*ENDOCRINE-METABOLIC (See **Precautions**)*	
None	hyperglycemia
*SPECIAL SENSES (See **Warnings**)*	
Ocular: None Otic: None	 hearing loss tinnitus

(3) Causal relationship unknown—incidence less than 1%: *Hematological* (see **Warnings**) —Leukemia (There have been reports associating phenylbutazone with leukemia. However, the circumstances involved in these reports are such that a cause-and-effect relationship to the drug has not been clearly established.) *Endocrine—Metabolic* (see **Precautions**)—Thyroid hyperplasia; goiters associated with hyperthyroidism and hypothyroidism; pancreatitis. *Special Senses* (see **Warnings**)—Blurred vision; optic neuritis; toxic amblyopia; scotomata; retinal detachment; retinal hemorrhage; oculomotor palsy.

Overdosage: *Signs and Symptoms:* Include any of the following: nausea, vomiting, epigastric pain, excessive perspiration, euphoria, psychosis, headaches, giddiness, vertigo, hyperventilation, insomnia, tinnitus, difficulty in hearing, edema (sodium retention), hypertension, cyanosis, respiratory depression, agitation, hallucinations, stupor, convulsions, coma, hematuria, and oliguria. Hepatomegaly, jaundice, and ulceration of the buccal or gastrointestinal mucosa have been reported as late manifestations of massive overdosage.

Reported laboratory abnormalities following overdosage include: respiratory or metabolic acidosis, impaired hepatic or renal function, and abnormalities of formed blood elements.

Treatment: In the alert patient, empty the stomach promptly by induced emesis followed by lavage. In the obtunded patient, secure the airway with a cuffed endotracheal tube before beginning lavage (do not induce emesis). Maintain adequate respiratory exchange, do not use respiratory stimulants. Treat shock with appropriate supportive measures. Control seizures with intravenous diazepam or short-acting barbiturates. Dialysis may be helpful if renal function is impaired.

Dosage and Administration: Butazolidin should be used at the smallest effective dosage to afford rapid relief of severe symptoms. It is contraindicated in children under 14 years of age and in senile patients.

If a favorable symptomatic response to treatment is not obtained after one week, the drug should be discontinued. When a favorable therapeutic response has been obtained, the dosage should be reduced and then discontinued as soon as possible.

In elderly patients (sixty years and over) every effort must be made to discontinue therapy on, or as soon as possible after, the seventh day,

Continued on next page

The full prescribing information for each GEIGY drug is contained herein and is that in effect as of October 1, 1982.

Geigy—Cont.

because of the exceedingly high risk of severe fatal toxic reactions in this age group.
To minimize gastric upset, the drug should be taken with milk or with meals.
In selecting the appropriate dosage in any specific case, consideration should be given to the patient's age, weight, general health, and any other factors that may influence his response to the drug.
Rheumatoid Arthritis, Ankylosing Spondylitis, Acute Attacks of Degenerative Joint Disease, and Painful Shoulder: Initial Dosage: The initial daily dose in adult patients is 300 to 600 mg as 3 to 4 divided doses. Maximum therapeutic response is usually obtained at a total daily dose of 400 mg. A trial period of one week of therapy is considered adequate to determine the therapeutic effect of the drug. In the absence of a favorable response, therapy should be discontinued.
Maintenance Dosage: When improvement is obtained, dosage should be promptly decreased to the minimum effective level necessary to maintain relief, not exceeding 400 mg daily because of the possibility of cumulative toxicity. A satisfactory clinical response may be obtained with daily doses as low as 100 to 200 mg daily.
Acute Gouty Arthritis: Satisfactory results are obtained after an initial dose of 400 mg followed by 100 mg every 4 hours. The articular inflammation usually subsides within 4 days and treatment should not be continued longer than one week.
How Supplied:
Tablets 100 mg—round, red, film-coated (imprinted GEIGY 14)
Bottles of 100 ....NDC 0028-0014-01
Bottles of 1000 ....NDC 0028-0014-10
Unit Dose (blister pack)
Box of 100 (strips of 10) .....NDC 0028-0014-61
Capsules 100 mg—orange and white (imprinted GEIGY 44)
Bottles of 100 ....NDC 0028-0044-01
Bottles of 1000 ....NDC 0028-0044-10
Gy-Pak® — One Unit
(12 bottles — 100
capsules each) ....NDC 0028-0044-65
Unit Dose (blister pack)
Box of 100 (strips of 10) .....NDC 0028-0044-61
Dispense in tight, light-resistant container (USP).
NOTE: Reactions occurring in 3% to 9% of patients treated with phenylbutazone (those reactions occurring in less than 3% of the patients are unmarked).
C82-34 (8/82)
[*Shown in Product Identification Section*]

CONSTANT-T™ ℞

theophylline (anhydrous)
Sustained-Action Tablets
Tablets
200 mg
300 mg

Description: Constant-T Sustained-Action Tablets contain anhydrous theophylline. Constant-T is available in two strengths: 200-mg and 300-mg oval, scored tablets. Theophylline, a xanthine compound, is a white, odorless crystalline powder, having a bitter taste.
Actions: The pharmacologic actions of Constant-T are as a bronchodilator, pulmonary vasodilator and smooth muscle relaxant, since the drug directly relaxes the smooth muscle of the bronchial airways and pulmonary blood vessels. Theophylline also possesses other actions typical of the xanthine derivatives: coronary vasodilator, diuretic, cardiac stimulant, cerebral stimulant and skeletal muscle stimulant. The actions of theophylline may be mediated through inhibition of phosphodiesterase and a resultant increase in intracellular cyclic AMP which could mediate smooth muscle relaxation. No development of tolerance appears to occur with chronic use of theophylline.
The half-life is shortened with cigarette smoking and prolonged in alcoholism, reduced hepatic or renal function, congestive heart failure, and in patients receiving certain antibiotics (see **Drug Interactions**). High fever for prolonged periods may decrease theophylline elimination. Children over six months of age have rapid clearances with average half-lives of approximately 3–5 hours. Newborn infants have extremely slow clearances and half-lives exceeding 24 hours. Older adults with chronic obstructive pulmonary disease, any patients with cor pulmonale or other causes of heart failure, and patients with liver pathology may have much lower clearances with half-lives that exceed 24 hours. The half-life of theophylline in smokers (1–2 packs per day) averages 4–5 hours; the half-life in nonsmokers averages 7–9 hours.
In single-dose studies, adjusting the data to dosing equivalent to 8 mg/kg body weight, Constant-T produced mean peak theophylline blood levels of 9.1 ± 0.7 μg/ml at 5.0 ± 1.2 hours with the 200-mg dosage form, and 9.8 ± 0.9 μg/ml at 4.6 ± 0.9 hours with the 300-mg dosage form. In a multidose, steady-state, 5-day study, Constant-T achieved constant intrasubject theophylline levels with an average peak-trough difference of only 3.4 μg/ml. This is indicative of smooth and stable maintenance therapeutic theophylline levels throughout a 12-hour dosing interval.
Indications: Symptomatic relief and/or prevention of asthma and reversible bronchospasm associated with chronic bronchitis and emphysema.
Contraindications: Constant-T is contraindicated in individuals who have shown hypersensitivity to any of its components or to xanthine derivatives.
Warnings: Excessive theophylline doses may be associated with toxicity; serum theophylline levels should be monitored to assure maximum benefit with minimum risk. Incidence of toxicity increases at serum levels greater than 20 μg/ml. High blood levels of theophylline resulting from conventional doses are correlated with clinical manifestations of toxicity in: patients with lowered body plasma clearances; patients with liver dysfunction or chronic obstructive lung disease, and patients who are older than 55 years of age, particularly males. There are often no early signs of less serious theophylline toxicity such as nausea and restlessness, which may appear in up to 50% of patients prior to onset of convulsions. Ventricular arrhythmias or seizures may be the first signs of toxicity. Many patients who have higher theophylline serum levels exhibit a tachycardia. Theophylline products may worsen preexisting arrhythmias.
Usage in Pregnancy: Safe use in pregnancy has not been established relative to possible adverse effects on fetal development, but neither have adverse effects on fetal development been established. This is, unfortunately, true for most antiasthmatic medications. Therefore, use of theophylline in pregnant women should be balanced against the risk of uncontrolled asthma.
Precautions: CONSTANT-T TABLETS SHOULD NOT BE CHEWED OR CRUSHED.
Theophyllines should not be administered concurrently with other xanthine medications. It should be used with caution in patients with severe cardiac disease, severe hypoxemia, hypertension, hyperthyroidism, acute myocardial injury, cor pulmonale, congestive heart failure, liver disease and in the elderly, particularly males, and in neonates. Great caution should be used in giving theophylline to patients in congestive heart failure since these patients show markedly prolonged theophylline blood level curves. Use theophylline cautiously in patients with history of peptic ulcer. Theophylline may occasionally act as a local irritant to GI tract although gastrointestinal symptoms are more commonly central and associated with high serum concentrations above 20 μg/ml.
Adverse Reactions: The most consistent adverse reactions are usually due to overdose and are:
Gastrointestinal: Nausea, vomiting, epigastric pain, hematemesis, diarrhea.
Central Nervous System: Headaches, irritability, restlessness, insomnia, reflex hyperexcitability, muscle twitching, clonic and tonic generalized convulsions.
Cardiovascular: Palpitation, tachycardia, extrasystoles, flushing, hypotension, circulatory failure, life-threatening ventricular arrhythmias.
Respiratory: Tachypnea.
Renal: Albuminuria, increased excretion of renal tubular cells and red blood cells; potentiation of diuresis.
Others: Hyperglycemia and inappropriate ADH syndrome.
Drug Interactions:

Drug	*Effect*
Theophylline with Furosemide	Increased Diuresis
Theophylline with Hexamethonium	Decreased Chronotropic Effect
Theophylline with Reserpine	Tachycardia
Theophylline with Cyclamycin (TAO), Erythromycin, or Lincomycin	Increased Theophylline Blood Levels

Overdosage
Management:
A. If potential oral overdose is established and seizure has not occurred:
  1) Induce vomiting.
  2) Administer a cathartic (this is particularly important if sustained-release preparations have been taken).
  3) Administer activated charcoal.
B. If patient is having a seizure:
  1) Establish an airway.
  2) Administer 0_2.
  3) Treat the seizure with intravenous diazepam, 0.1 to 0.3 mg/kg up to 10 mg.
  4) Monitor vital signs, maintain blood pressure and provide adequate hydration.
C. Postseizure coma:
  1) Maintain airway and oxygenation.
  2) If a result of oral medication, follow above recommendations to prevent absorption of the drug, but intubation and lavage will have to be performed instead of inducing emesis, and the cathartic and charcoal will need to be introduced via a large-bore gastric lavage tube.
  3) Continue to provide full supportive care and adequate hydration while waiting for drug to be metabolized. In general, the drug is metabolized sufficiently rapidly so as to not warrant consideration of dialysis.

Dosage and Administration: Therapeutic serum levels associated with optimal likelihood for benefit and minimal risk of toxicity are considered to be between 10 and 20 μg/ml. There is a great variation from patient to patient in dosage needed in order to achieve a therapeutic blood level due to variable rates of elimination. Because of this wide variation from patient to patient, and the relatively narrow therapeutic range, dosage must be individualized.
THE AVERAGE INITIAL CHILDREN'S (15 to 20 kg) DOSE IS ONE-HALF OF A CONSTANT-T 200-mg TABLET q12h.
THE AVERAGE INITIAL CHILDREN'S (20 to 25 kg) DOSE IS ONE-HALF (150 mg) OF A CONSTANT-T 300-mg TABLET q12h.
THE AVERAGE INITIAL ADULT AND CHILDREN'S (OVER 25 kg) DOSE IS ONE CONSTANT-T 200-mg TABLET q12h.

If the desired response is not achieved with the above AVERAGE INITIAL DOSAGE recommendations, and there are no adverse reactions, the dose may be increased, after 3 days, to the following MAXIMUM DOSE WITHOUT MEASUREMENT OF SERUM CONCENTRATION.

MAXIMUM DOSE WITHOUT MEASUREMENT OF SERUM CONCENTRATION

	Dose Per Interval
Children (15–20 kg)	150 mg q12h
Children (20–25 kg)	200 mg q12h
Children (25–35 kg)	250 mg q12h
Adults and Children (over 35 kg)	300 mg q12h

If increased dose is not tolerated because of headaches or stomach upset (nausea, vomiting, diarrhea, etc.), decrease dose to AVERAGE INITIAL DOSE. If tolerated, the dose may be increased, after 3 days, to the following MINIMUM DOSE REQUIRING MEASUREMENT OF SERUM CONCENTRATION.

MINIMUM DOSE REQUIRING MEASUREMENT OF SERUM CONCENTRATION

	Dose Per Interval
Children (15–20 kg)	200 mg q12h
Children (20–30 kg)	250 mg q12h
Children (30–35 kg)	300 mg q12h
Children (35–40 kg)	350 mg q12h
Adults and Children (over 40 kg)	400 mg q12h

CHECK SERUM CONCENTRATION BETWEEN 3 AND 8 HOURS AFTER A DOSE WHEN NONE HAVE BEEN MISSED OR ADDED FOR AT LEAST 3 DAYS.

If serum theophylline concentration is between 10 and 20 μg/ml, maintain dose, if tolerated. RECHECK SERUM THEOPHYLLINE CONCENTRATION AT 6- TO 12-MONTH INTERVALS.*

* Finer adjustments in dosage may be needed for some patients.

Take the following action if the serum theophylline concentration is too high.

20 to 25 μg/ml—Decrease dose by 50 mg q12h.

25 to 30 μg/ml—Skip next dose and decrease subsequent doses by 25% to the nearest 50 mg q12h.

Over 30 μg/ml—Skip next 2 doses and decrease subsequent doses by 50% to nearest 50 mg q12h. RECHECK SERUM THEOPHYLLINE CONCENTRATION.

Take the following action if the serum theophylline concentration is too low.

7.5 to 10 μg/ml—Increase dose by 25% to the nearest 50 mg.†

5 to 7.5 μg/ml—Increase dose by 25% to the nearest 50 mg and RECHECK SERUM THEOPHYLLIINE FOR GUIDANCE IN FURTHER DOSAGE ADJUSTMENT.

† Dividing the daily dosage into 3 doses administered at 8-hour intervals may be indicated if symptoms occur repeatedly at the end of a dosing interval.

DOSAGE ADJUSTMENT, BASED ON SERUM THEOPHYLLINE CONCENTRATION MEASUREMENTS WHEN THESE INSTRUCTIONS HAVE NOT BEEN FOLLOWED. MAY RESULT IN RECOMMENDATIONS THAT PRESENT RISK OF TOXICITY TO THE PATIENT.

How Supplied:

Sustained-Action Tablets 200 mg—
light pink, oval, scored (imprinted Geigy 42)
Bottles of 100 ....NDC 0028-0042-01
Gy-Pak®—One Unit
12 bottles—
60 tablets each ....NDC 0028-0042-73
Unit Dose (blister pack)
Box of 100 (strips of 10) .NDC 0028-0042-61
Sustained-Action Tablets 300 mg—
light blue, oval, scored (imprinted Geigy 57)
Bottles of 100 ....NDC 0028-0057-01
Gy-Pak®—One Unit
12 bottles—
60 tablets each ....NDC 0028-0057-73
Unit Dose (blister pack)
Box of 100
(strips of 10) ....NDC 0028-0057-61

Storage Conditions:
Do not store above 86°F. Protect from moisture. *Dispense in tight, light-resistant container (USP).*

C82-19 (6/82)

Dist. by:
GEIGY Pharmaceuticals
Div. of CIBA-GEIGY Corp.
Ardsley, New York 10502
[*Shown in Product Identification Section*]

LIORESAL® 10 mg ℞
baclofen
Muscle Relaxant, Antispastic 20 mg ℞

Description: Lioresal is 4-amino-3-(*p*-chlorophenyl) butyric acid, a white to off-white crystalline substance.

It is slightly soluble in water and poorly soluble in organic solvents. Molecular weight: 213.67.

Actions: The precise mechanism of action of Lioresal is not fully known. Lioresal is capable of inhibiting both monosynaptic and polysynaptic reflexes at the spinal level, possibly by hyperpolarization of afferent terminals, although actions at supraspinal sites may also occur and contribute to its clinical effect. Although Lioresal is an analog of the putative inhibitory neurotransmitter gamma-aminobutyric acid (GABA), there is no conclusive evidence that actions on GABA systems are involved in the production of its clinical effects. In studies with animals, Lioresal has been shown to have general CNS depressant properties as indicated by the production of sedation with tolerance, somnolence, ataxia, and respiratory and cardiovascular depression. Lioresal is rapidly and extensively absorbed and eliminated. Absorption may be dose-dependent, being reduced with increasing doses. Lioresal is excreted primarily by the kidney in unchanged form and there is relatively large intersubject variation in absorption and/or elimination.

Indications: Lioresal is useful for the alleviation of signs and symptoms of spasticity resulting from multiple sclerosis, particularly for the relief of flexor spasms and concomitant pain, clonus, and muscular rigidity.

Patients should have reversible spasticity so that Lioresal treatment will aid in restoring residual function.

Lioresal may also be of some value in patients with spinal cord injuries and other spinal cord diseases.

Lioresal is not indicated in the treatment of skeletal muscle spasm resulting from rheumatic disorders.

The efficacy of Lioresal in stroke, cerebral palsy, and Parkinson's disease has not been established and, therefore, it is not recommended for these conditions.

Contraindications: Hypersensitivity to baclofen.

Warnings:

a. *Abrupt Drug Withdrawal:* Hallucinations and seizures have occurred on abrupt withdrawal of Lioresal. Therefore, except for serious adverse reactions, the dose should be reduced slowly when the drug is discontinued.

b. *Impaired Renal Function:* Because Lioresal is primarily excreted unchanged through the kidneys, it should be given with caution, and it may be necessary to reduce the dosage.

c. *Stroke:* Lioresal has not significantly benefited patients with stroke. These patients have also shown poor tolerability to the drug.

d. *Pregnancy:* Lioresal has been shown to increase the incidence of omphaloceles (ventral hernias) in fetuses of rats given approximately 13 times the maximum dose recommended for human use, at a dose which caused significant reductions in food intake and weight gain in dams. This abnormality was not seen in mice or rabbits. There was also an increased incidence of incomplete sternebral ossification in fetuses of rats given approximately 13 times the maximum recommended human dose, and an increased incidence of unossified phalangeal nuclei of forelimbs and hindlimbs in fetuses of rabbits given approximately 7 times the maximum recommended human dose. In mice, no teratogenic effects were observed, although reductions in mean fetal weight with consequent delays in skeletal ossification were present when dams were given 17 or 34 times the human daily dose. There are no studies in pregnant women. Lioresal should be used during pregnancy only if the benefit clearly justifies the potential risk to the fetus.

Precautions: Safe use of Lioresal in children under age 12 has not been established, and it is, therefore, not recommended for use in children.

Because of the possibility of sedation, patients should be cautioned regarding the operation of automobiles or other dangerous machinery, and activities made hazardous by decreased alertness. Patients should also be cautioned that the central nervous system effects of Lioresal may be additive to those of alcohol and other CNS depressants.

Lioresal should be used with caution where spasticity is utilized to sustain upright posture and balance in locomotion or whenever spasticity is utilized to obtain increased function.

In patients with epilepsy, the clinical state and electroencephalogram should be monitored at regular intervals, since deterioration in seizure control and EEG have been reported occasionally in patients taking Lioresal.

It is not known whether this drug is excreted in human milk. As a general rule, nursing should not be undertaken while a patient is on a drug since many drugs are excreted in human milk.

A dose-related increase in incidence of ovarian cysts and a less marked increase in enlarged and/or hemorrhagic adrenal glands was observed in female rats treated chronically with Lioresal. The relevance of these findings to humans is not known.

Adverse Reactions: The most common is transient drowsiness (10–63%). In one controlled study of 175 patients, transient drowsiness was observed in 63% of those receiving Lioresal compared to 36% of those in the placebo group. Other common adverse reactions are dizziness (5–15%), weakness (5–15%) and fatigue (2–4%). Others reported:

Neuropsychiatric: Confusion (1–11%), headache (4–8%), insomnia (2–7%); and, rarely, euphoria, excitement, depression, hallucinations, paresthesia, muscle pain, tinnitus, slurred speech, coordination disorder, tremor, rigidity, dystonia, ataxia, blurred vision, nystagmus, strabismus, miosis, mydriasis, diplopia, dysarthria, epileptic seizure.

Cardiovascular: Hypotension (0–9%). Rare instances of dyspnea, palpitation, chest pain, syncope.

Gastrointestinal: Nausea (4–12%), constipation (2–6%); and, rarely, dry mouth, anorexia, taste disorder, abdominal pain, vomiting, diarrhea, and positive test for occult blood in stool.

Genitourinary: Urinary frequency (2–6%); and, rarely, enuresis, urinary retention, dysuria, impotence, inability to ejaculate, nocturia, hematuria.

Other: Instances of rash, pruritus, ankle edema, excessive perspiration, weight gain, nasal congestion.

Continued on next page

The full prescribing information for each GEIGY drug is contained herein and is that in effect as of October 1, 1982.

Geigy—Cont.

Some of the CNS and genitourinary symptoms may be related to the underlying disease rather than to drug therapy.
The following laboratory tests have been found to be abnormal in a few patients receiving Lioresal: increased SGOT, elevated alkaline phosphatase, and elevation of blood sugar.
Overdosage: *Signs and Symptoms:* Vomiting, muscular hypotonia, drowsiness, accommodation disorders, coma, respiratory depression, and seizures.
Treatment: In the alert patient, empty the stomach promptly by induced emesis followed by lavage. In the obtunded patient, secure the airway with a cuffed endotracheal tube before beginning lavage (do not induce emesis). Maintain adequate respiratory exchange, do not use respiratory stimulants.
Dosage and Administration: The determination of optimal dosage requires individual titration. Start therapy at a low dosage and increase gradually until optimum effect is achieved (usually between 40–80 mg daily).
The following dosage titration schedule is suggested:
5 mg t.i.d. for 3 days
10 mg t.i.d. for 3 days
15 mg t.i.d. for 3 days
20 mg t.i.d. for 3 days
Thereafter additional increases may be necessary but the total daily dose should not exceed a maximum of 80 mg daily (20 mg q.i.d.).
The lowest dose compatible with an optimal response is recommended. If benefits are not evident after a reasonable trial period, patients should be slowly withdrawn from the drug (see **Warnings** *Abrupt Drug Withdrawal*).
How Supplied:
Tablets 10 mg—white, oval, single scored (imprinted 23 Geigy)
Bottles of 100 ....NDC 0028-0023-01
Unit Dose (blister pack)
Box of 100 (strips of 10) .NDC 0028-0023-61
Tablets 20 mg—white, capsule shaped, scored (imprinted 33 Geigy)
Bottles of 100 ....NDC 0028-0033-01
Unit Dose (blister pack)
Box of 100 (strips of 10) NDC 0028-0033-61
Dispense in tight container (USP).
C82-66 (Rev. 2/83)
[*Shown in Product Identification Section*]

LOPRESSOR® ℞
metoprolol tartrate
Tablets of 50 mg GY-CODE 51
Tablets of 100 mg GY-CODE 71
An antihypertensive beta-blocking agent

Description: Lopressor, a synthetic selective beta$_1$-adrenoreceptor blocking agent, may be chemically described as 1-isopropylamino-3-[p-(2-methoxyethyl)-phenoxy]-2-propanol *dextro*-tartrate.
Lopressor is a water-soluble, white, crystalline solid. It is supplied for oral administration.
Clinical Pharmacology: Lopressor is a beta-adrenergic receptor blocking agent. *In vitro* and *in vivo* animal studies show it has a preferential effect on beta$_1$ adrenoreceptors, chiefly located in cardiac muscle. This preferential effect is not absolute, however, and at higher doses, metoprolol inhibits beta$_2$ adrenoreceptors, chiefly located in the bronchial and vascular musculature.
Clinical pharmacology studies have confirmed the beta-blocking activity as shown by (1) reduction in heart rate and cardiac output at rest and on exercise, (2) reduction of systolic blood pressure on exercise, (3) inhibition of isoproterenol-induced tachycardia, and (4) reduction of reflex orthostatic tachycardia.
Beta$_1$ selectivity has been confirmed: (1) In normal subjects by the inability of Lopressor to reverse the beta$_2$-mediated vasodilating effects of epinephrine. This contrasts with the effect of nonselective (beta$_1$ plus beta$_2$) beta blockers, such as propranolol, which completely reverse the vasodilating effects of epinephrine. (2) In asthmatic patients, Lopressor reduces FEV$_1$ and FVC significantly less than propranolol in equivalent beta$_1$-receptor blocking doses.
Metoprolol has no intrinsic sympathomimetic activity and only weak membrane-stabilizing activity. Metoprolol crosses the blood-brain barrier and has been reported in the CSF in a concentration 78% of the simultaneous plasma concentration. Animal and human experiments indicate that metoprolol slows the sinus rate and decreases AV nodal conduction.
Lopressor has been shown in controlled clinical studies to be an effective antihypertensive agent when used as monotherapy, or as concomitant therapy with thiazide-type diuretics. In hypertension, dosages in the range of 100 to 450 mg daily have been shown to be effective. In controlled, comparative, clinical studies, Lopressor was shown to be as effective an antihypertensive agent as propranolol, methyldopa, and thiazide-type diuretics. It was equally effective in supine and standing positions.
The mechanism of the antihypertensive effects of beta-blocking agents has not been elucidated. However, several possible mechanisms have been proposed and include (1) competitive antagonism of catecholamines at peripheral (especially cardiac) adrenergic neuron sites, leading to decreased cardiac output, (2) a central effect leading to reduced sympathetic outflow to the periphery, and (3) suppression of renin activity.
In man, absorption of Lopressor is rapid and complete. Plasma levels following oral administration, however, approximate 50% of levels following intravenous administration, indicating about 50% first-pass metabolism. Plasma levels achieved are highly variable. Only a small fraction of the drug (about 12 percent) is bound to human serum albumin. Elimination is mainly by biotransformation in the liver and the plasma half-life is three to four hours. Significant beta-blocking effect (as measured by reduction of exercise heart rate) occurs within one hour after oral administration. The duration of pharmacologic effect as measured by reduction of exercise heart rate is dose-related. For example, the time for a 50-percent reduction of the maximum registered effect after single oral doses of 20, 50, and 100 mg was 3.3, 5.0, and 6.4 hours respectively in normal subjects.
Following repeated oral doses of 100 mg twice daily, a significant reduction in exercise systolic blood pressure was evident at 12 hours. Because of variable plasma levels attained with a given dose and the lack of a consistent relationship of antihypertensive activity to dose, selection of proper dosage requires individual titration.
There is a linear relationship between plasma levels and reduction of exercise heart rate. However, antihypertensive activity does not appear to be related to plasma levels.
Indications: Lopressor is indicated in the management of hypertension. It may be used alone or in combination with other antihypertensive agents, especially thiazide-type diuretics.
Contraindications: Lopressor is contraindicated in sinus bradycardia, heart block greater than first degree, cardiogenic shock, and overt cardiac failure (see **Warnings**).
Warnings: ***Cardiac Failure:*** Sympathetic stimulation is a vital component supporting circulatory function in congestive heart failure, and beta blockade carries the potential hazard of further depressing myocardial contractility and precipitating more severe failure. In hypertensive patients who have congestive heart failure controlled by digitalis and diuretics, Lopressor should be administered cautiously. Both digitalis and metoprolol slow AV conduction.
In Patients Without a History of Cardiac Failure continued depression of the myocardium with beta-blocking agents over a period of time can, in some cases, lead to cardiac failure. At the first sign or symptom of impending cardiac failure, patients should be fully digitalized and/or be given a diuretic, and the response observed closely. If cardiac failure continues, despite adequate digitalization and diuretic, Lopressor therapy should be withdrawn.
Ischemic Heart Disease: Following abrupt cessation of therapy with certain beta-blocking agents, exacerbations of angina pectoris and, in some cases, myocardial infarction have been reported. Even in the absence of overt angina pectoris, when discontinuing therapy, Lopressor should not be withdrawn abruptly, and patients should be cautioned against interruption of therapy without the physician's advice.
Bronchospastic Diseases: **PATIENTS WITH BRONCHOSPASTIC DISEASES SHOULD IN GENERAL NOT RECEIVE BETA BLOCKERS. Because of its relative beta$_1$ selectivity, however, Lopressor may be used with caution in patients with bronchospastic disease who do not respond to, or cannot tolerate, other antihypertensive treatment. Since beta$_1$ selectivity is not absolute, a beta$_2$-stimulating agent should be administered concomitantly and the lowest possible dose of metoprolol should be used. It may be prudent initially to administer metoprolol in smaller doses three times daily, instead of larger doses two times daily, to avoid the higher plasma levels associated with the longer dosing interval. (See Dosage and Administration.)**
Major Surgery: The necessity or desirability of withdrawal of beta-blocking therapy prior to major surgery is controversial. It should be noted, however, that the impaired ability of the heart to respond to reflex adrenergic stimuli may augment the risks of general anesthesia and surgical procedures.
Metoprolol, like other beta blockers, is a competitive inhibitor of beta-receptor agonists and its effects can be reversed by administration of such agents, e.g., dobutamine or isoproterenol. However, such patients may be subject to protracted severe hypotension. Difficulty in restarting and maintaining the heart beat has also been reported with beta blockers.
Diabetes Mellitus: Beta-adrenergic blockade may mask symptoms of hypoglycemia (e.g., tachycardia) and may potentiate insulin-induced hypoglycemia. Lopressor should therefore be used with caution in diabetic patients, especially those with labile diabetes.
Thyrotoxicosis: Beta-adrenergic blockade may mask certain clinical signs (e.g., tachycardia) of hyperthyroidism. Patients suspected of developing thyrotoxicosis should be managed carefully to avoid abrupt withdrawal of beta blockade which might precipitate a thyroid storm.
Precautions: ***Impaired Hepatic or Renal Function:*** The drug should be used with caution in patients with impaired hepatic or renal function.
Drug Interactions: Catecholamine-depleting drugs (e.g., reserpine) may have an additive effect when given with beta-blocking agents. Patients treated with Lopressor plus a catecholamine depletor should therefore be closely observed for evidence of hypotension and/or marked bradycardia which may produce vertigo, syncope, or postural hypotension.
Long-Term Animal Studies: Long-term studies in animals have been conducted to evaluate toxic effects and carcinogenic potential. In a one-year study in dogs, there was no evidence of drug-induced toxicity at or below oral doses of 105 mg/kg per day. Two-year studies in rats at three oral dosage levels of up to 800 mg/kg per day did not indicate an increase in the development of spontaneously occurring benign or malignant neoplasms of any type. The only

histologic changes which appeared to be drug-related were an increased incidence of generally mild focal accumulation of foamy macrophages in pulmonary alveoli and a slight increase in biliary hyperplasia. Neither finding represents symptoms of a known disease entity in man. In a 21-month study in mice at three oral dose levels of up to 750 mg/kg per day, benign lung tumors (small adenomas) occurred more frequently in female mice receiving the highest dose than in untreated control animals. There was no increase in malignant lung tumors or total (benign plus malignant) lung tumors. The overall incidence of tumors or malignant tumors was also unaffected by metoprolol administration.

Usage in Pregnancy: Reproduction studies in animals did not reveal any evidence of impaired fertility or of teratogenic potential. There was evidence in the rat of increased post-implantation loss and decreased neonatal survival (threshold between 50 and 500 mg/kg). Distribution studies in mice confirm exposure of the fetus when metoprolol is administered to the pregnant animal. There are no well-controlled studies in pregnant women. Lopressor should be used in pregnant women only when clearly needed.

Nursing Mothers: It is not known whether this drug is excreted in human milk. Since most drugs are excreted in human milk, nursing should not be undertaken by mothers receiving metoprolol.

Usage in Children: Safety and effectiveness in children have not been established.

Adverse Reactions: Most adverse effects have been mild and transient.

Central Nervous System: Tiredness and dizziness have occurred in about 10 of 100 patients. Depression was reported in about 5 of 100 patients. Headache, nightmares, and insomnia have also been reported but drug relationship is not clear.

Cardiovascular: Shortness of breath and bradycardia have occurred in approximately 3 of 100 patients. Cold extremities; arterial insufficiency, usually of the Raynaud type; palpitations and congestive heart failure have been reported. See **Contraindications, Warnings,** and **Precautions.**

Respiratory: Wheezing (bronchospasm) has been reported in less than 1 of 100 patients. See **Warnings.**

Gastrointestinal: Diarrhea has occurred in about 5 of 100 patients. Nausea, gastric pain, constipation, flatulence, and heartburn have been reported in 1 of 100 or less.

Allergic: Pruritus has occurred in less than 1 of 100 patients.

Miscellaneous: Peyronie's disease has been reported in less than 1 of 100,000 patients.

The oculomucocutaneous syndrome associated with the beta blocker practolol has not been reported with Lopressor during investigational use and foreign marketing experience.

Potential Adverse Effects: In addition, a variety of adverse effects not listed above have been reported with other beta-adrenergic blocking agents, and should be considered potential adverse effects of metoprolol.

Central Nervous System: Reversible mental depression progressing to catatonia; visual disturbances; hallucinations; an acute reversible syndrome characterized by disorientation for time and place, short-term memory loss, emotional lability, slightly clouded sensorium, and decreased performance on neuropsychometrics.

Cardiovascular: Intensification of AV block (See **Contraindications**).

Hematologic: Agranulocytosis, nonthrombocytopenic purpura, thrombocytopenic purpura.

Allergic: Erythematous rash, fever combined with aching and sore throat, laryngospasm and respiratory distress.

Miscellaneous: Reversible alopecia.

Clinical Laboratory Test Findings: Elevated blood urea levels in patients with severe heart disease, elevated serum transaminase, alkaline phosphatase, lactate dehydrogenase.

Overdosage: To date, only one case of extreme overdosage has been reported. A 19-year-old man ingested 200 50-mg tablets (160 mg/kg) and on hospital admission was conscious with peripheral cyanosis, weak heart sounds and an unmeasurable blood pressure. Only the femoral pulse was palpable. EKG showed sinus rhythm 60-70/minute with normal AV conduction, ST segments and T-waves. Blood analysis revealed excess base (−5 mEq/L), pH 7.41 pCO_2 29 mmHg and bicarbonate 20 mEq/L. Treatment consisted of gastric lavage, 2L Ringer's solution, metaraminol 10 mg, glucagon 6 mg, 150 mmol sodium bicarbonate. Fluid retention noted during the first 6 hours was treated with furosemide. Two hours after admission, blood levels of Lopressor of 12,200 ng/g of plasma were recorded (normal maximum values after 100 mg orally is about 100/ng/g plasma). Complete recovery occurred within 12 hours without signs of cardiovascular depression.[1]

No specific information on emergency treatment of overdosage is available. Therefore, on the basis of the pharmacologic actions of Lopressor, the following general measures should be employed:

Gastric Lavage.

Bradycardia: Administer atropine. If there is no response to vagal blockade administer isoproterenol cautiously.

Hypotension: Administer vasopressors, e.g., epinephrine or levarterenol.

Bronchospasm: Administer a $beta_2$-stimulating agent and/or a theophylline derivative.

Cardiac Failure: Administer a digitalis glycoside and diuretic. In shock resulting from inadequate cardiac contractility, the administration of dobutamine may be considered.

Dosage and Administration: Dosage of Lopressor should be individualized. The usual initial dose is 50 mg twice daily whether used alone or added to a diuretic. The dosage may be increased at weekly (or longer) intervals until optimum blood pressure reduction is achieved. In general, the maximum effect of any given dosage level will be apparent after one week of therapy. Usual maintenance dosage is approximately 100 mg twice a day, with a range of 100 to 450 mg per day. Dosages above 450 mg per day have not been studied. While twice-daily dosing is effective and can maintain a reduction in blood pressure throughout the day, some patients, especially when lower dosages are used, will experience a modest rise in blood pressure toward the end of the 12-hour dosing interval. This can be evaluated by measuring blood pressure near the end of the dosing interval to determine whether satisfactory control is being maintained throughout the day. If control is not adequate, a larger dose, or three times daily therapy, may achieve better control. $Beta_1$ selectivity diminishes as dosage of Lopressor is increased.

This drug should be stored at controlled room temperature and protected from moisture.

How Supplied: Tablets of 50 mg (capsule-shaped, scored, light red, film-coated) and 100 mg (capsule-shaped, scored, light blue, film-coated) are supplied in bottles of 100 and 1,000 and Unit Dose Packages of 100.

Store at controlled room temperature and protect from moisture.

Dispense in tight, light-resistant container (USP).

[1]Moller, B HS: Massive intoxication with metoprolol. Br Med J *1* (6003):222 (Jan. 24) 1976.

C80-82 (12/80)

[*Shown in Product Identification Section*]

OTRIVIN®

xylometazoline hydrochloride USP
Adult Nasal Spray and Drops 0.1%
Pediatric Nasal Drops 0.05%

Description: Otrivin, xylometazoline HCl, a sympathomimetic amine, is a white, odorless, crystalline powder which is soluble in water and freely soluble in alcohol. Chemically, it is 2-(4-*tert*-butyl-2,6-dimethylbenzyl)-2-imidazoline monohydrochloride.

This preparation is available in 0.1% solution for adults and 0.05% solution for children under 12.

Nasal Spray contains 0.1% and *Nasal Drops* contain 0.1% or 0.05% xylometazoline hydrochloride NF, potassium phosphate monobasic, potassium chloride, sodium phosphate dibasic, sodium chloride, and benzalkonium chloride 1:5,000 as preservative in water.

Actions: Its sympathomimetic (adrenergic) action constricts the smaller arterioles of the nasal passages, effecting a decongesting action. This vasoconstriction results from alpha adrenergic receptor stimulation of vascular smooth muscle.

Indications: For decongestion of the nasal mucosa.

Contraindications: Narrow-angle glaucoma. Concurrent MAO inhibitor therapy. Tricyclic antidepressant therapy. Hypersensitivity to any component of this preparation.

Sensitivity to even small doses of adrenergic substances as manifested by sleeplessness, dizziness, lightheadedness, weakness, tremulousness, or cardiac arrhythmias.

Warnings: Systemic effects from the use of topical decongestants may occur due to rapid absorption through the nasal mucous membrane and from gastrointestinal absorption if given in excess so that the solution is swallowed. Such reactions are most likely to occur in infants and the elderly.

Because of the possibility of generalized vasoconstriction and tachycardia, nose drops (as all sympathomimetic amines) should be used very cautiously in patients with hypertension, heart disease, including angina, hyperthyroidism and advanced arteriosclerotic conditions.

Overdosage may produce profound CNS depression in children, possibly requiring intensive supportive treatment.

Usage in Pregnancy: Clinical data are inadequate to establish conditions for safe use of nose drops in pregnancy.

Directions:

Nasal Spray 0.1%—Spray 2 or 3 times into each nostril every 8–10 hours. With head upright, squeeze sharply and firmly while inhaling (sniffing) through the nose.

Nasal Drops 0.1%—For adults and children 12 years and older. Put 2 or 3 drops into each nostril every 8 to 10 hours. Tilt head as far back as possible. Immediately bend head forward toward knees, hold a few seconds, then return to upright position.

Pediatric Nasal Drops 0.05%—For children 2 to 12 years of age. Put 2 or 3 drops into each nostril every 8 to 10 hours. Tilt head as far back as possible. Immediately bend head forward toward knees, hold a few seconds, then return to upright position.

How Supplied: *Otrivin Nasal Spray/Nasal Drops* are available in unbreakable plastic spray packages of ½ fl oz (15 ml) and in plastic dropper bottles of .66 fl oz (20 ml).

Otrivin Pediatric Nasal Drops Available in plastic dropper bottles of .66 fl oz (20 ml).

(8/80)

Continued on next page

The full prescribing information for each GEIGY drug is contained herein and is that in effect as of October 1, 1982.

Geigy—Cont.

PBZ-SR® GY-CODE 48 ℞
tripelennaminne HCl
sustained-release tablets
Tablets of 100 mg

Description: PBZ-SR Tablets are available as the hydrochloride salt of tripelennamine, 2-[benzyl[2-(dimethylamino)ethyl]-amino]pyridine, in a wax matrix. This formulation is intended to provide a gradual and prolonged release of tripelennamine from the matrix. Tripelennamine hydrochloride is an antihistamine occurring as a white, crystalline powder that slowly darkens on exposure to light and is freely soluble in water and alcohol.
Actions: Antihistamines are competitive antagonists of histamine, which also produce central nervous system effects (both stimulant and depressant) and peripheral anticholinergic, atropine-like effects (e.g., drying).
Indications: Perennial and seasonal allergic rhinitis; vasomotor rhinitis; allergic conjunctivitis due to inhalant allergens and foods; mild, uncomplicated allergic skin manifestations of urticaria and angioedema; amelioration of allergic reactions to blood or plasma; dermographism; anaphylactic reactions as adjunctive therapy to epinephrine and other standard measures after the acute manifestations have been controlled.
Contraindications: PBZ-SR should not be used in premature infants, neonates, or nursing mothers; patients receiving MAO inhibitors; patients with narrow-angle glaucoma, stenosing peptic ulcer, symptomatic prostatic hypertrophy, bladder neck obstruction, pyloroduodenal obstruction, lower respiratory tract symptoms (including asthma), or hypersensitivity to tripelennamine or related compounds.
Warnings: Antihistamines often produce drowsiness and may reduce mental alertness in children and adults. Patients should be warned about engaging in activities requiring mental alertness (e.g., driving a car, operating machinery or hazardous appliances). In elderly patients, approximately 60 years or older, antihistamines are more likely to cause dizziness, sedation and hypotension.
Patients should be warned that the central nervous system effects of PBZ-SR may be additive with those of alcohol and other CNS depressants (e.g., hypnotics, sedatives, tranquilizers, antianxiety agents).
Antihistamines may produce excitation, particularly in children.
Usage in Pregnancy
Although no tripelennamine-related teratogenic potential or other adverse effects on the fetus have been observed in limited animal reproduction studies, the safe use of this drug in pregnancy or during lactation has not been established. Therefore, the drug should not be used during pregnancy or lactation unless, in the judgment of the physician, the expected benefits outweigh the potential hazards.
Usage in Children
In infants and children particularly, antihistamines in overdosage may produce hallucinations, convulsions and/or death.
Precautions: PBZ-SR, like other antihistamines, has atropine-like, anticholinergic activity and should be used with caution in patients with increased intraocular pressure, hyperthyroidism, cardiovascular disease, hypertension, or history of bronchial asthma.
Adverse Reactions: The most frequent adverse reactions to antihistamines are sedation or drowsiness; sleepiness; dryness of the mouth, nose, and throat; thickening of bronchial secretions; dizziness; disturbed coordination; epigastric distress.
Other adverse reactions which may occur are: fatigue; chills; confusion; restlessness; excitation; hysteria; nervousness; irritability; insomnia; euphoria; anorexia; nausea; vomiting; diarrhea; constipation; hypotension; tightness in the chest; wheezing; blurred vision; diplopia; vertigo; tinnitus; convulsions; headache; palpitations; tachycardia; extrasystoles; nasal stuffiness; urinary frequency; difficult urination; urinary retention; leukopenia; hemolytic anemia; thrombocytopenia; agranulocytosis; aplastic anemia; allergic or hypersensitivity reactions, including drug rash, urticaria, anaphylactic shock, and photosensitivity. Although the following may have been reported to occur in association with some antihistamines, they have not been known to result from the use of PBZ-SR: excessive perspiration, tremor, paresthesias, acute labyrinthitis, neuritis and early menses.
Dosage and Administration: Dosage should be individualized according to the needs and response of the patient.
Adults: One 100-mg PBZ-SR Tablet in the morning and one in the evening is generally adequate. In difficult cases, one 100-mg PBZ-SR Tablet every 8 hours may be required.
Children: PBZ-SR Tablets are not intended for use in children.
Overdosage:
Signs and Symptoms
The greatest danger from acute overdosage with antihistamines is their central nervous system effects which produce depression and/or stimulation.
In children, stimulation predominates initially in a syndrome which may include excitement, hallucinations, ataxia, incoordination, athetosis, and convulsions followed by postictal depression. Dry mouth, fixed dilated pupils, flushing of the face, and fever are common and resemble the syndrome of atropine poisoning.
In adults, CNS depression (i.e., drowsiness, coma) is more common. CNS stimulation is rare; fever and flushing are uncommon.
In both children and adults, there can be a terminal deepening of coma and cardiovascular collapse; death can occur, especially in infants and children.
Treatment
There is no specific therapy for acute overdosage with antihistamines. General symptomatic and supportive measures should be instituted promptly and maintained for as long as necessary.
In the conscious patient, vomiting should be induced even though it may have occurred spontaneously. If vomiting cannot be induced, gastric lavage is indicated. Adequate precautions must be taken to protect against aspiration, especially in infants and children. Charcoal slurry or other suitable agent should be instilled into the stomach after vomiting or lavage. Saline cathartics or milk of magnesia may be of additional benefit.
In the unconscious patient, the airway should be secured with a cuffed endotracheal tube before attempting to evacuate the gastric contents. Intensive supportive and nursing care is indicated, as for any comatose patient.
If breathing is significantly impaired, maintenance of an adequate airway and mechanical support of respiration is the safest and most effective means of providing for adequate oxygenation of tissues to prevent hypoxia (especially brain hypoxia during convulsions).
Hypotension is an early sign of impending cardiovascular collapse and should be treated vigorously. Although general supportive measures are important, specific treatment with intravenous infusion of a vasopressor (e.g., levarterenol bitartrate) titrated to maintain adequate blood pressure is also necessary.
Do *not* use CNS stimulants.
Convulsions should be controlled by careful titration of a short-acting barbiturate, repeated as necessary.
Ice packs and cooling sponge baths can aid in reducing the fever commonly seen in children.
How Supplied: *PBZ-SR Tablets,* 100 mg (lavender), each containing 100 mg tripelennamine hydrochloride; bottles of 100.
Dispense in tight container (USP).

C78-44 (12/78)

[*Shown in Product Identification Section*]

PBZ® ℞
tripelennamine
Tablets GY-CODE 95
Elixir GY-CODE 6925
Listed in USP, a Medicare designated compendium.

Description: PBZ Tablets are available as the hydrochloride salt and PBZ Elixir as the citrate salt of 2-[benzyl[2-(dimethylamino) ethyl]-amino]pyridine. Tripelennamine hydrochloride is an antihistamine occurring as a white, crystalline powder that slowly darkens on exposure to light and is freely soluble in water and alcohol.
Actions: Antihistamines are competitive antagonists of histamine, which also produce central nervous system effects (both stimulant and depressant) and peripheral anticholinergic, atropine-like effects (e.g., drying).
Indications: Perennial and seasonal allergic rhinitis; vasomotor rhinitis; allergic conjunctivitis due to inhalant allergens and foods; mild, uncomplicated allergic skin manifestations of urticaria and angioedema; amelioration of allergic reactions to blood or plasma; dermographism; anaphylactic reactions as adjunctive therapy to epinephrine and other standard measures after the acute manifestations have been controlled.
Contraindications: PBZ should not be used in premature infants, neonates, or nursing mothers; patients receiving MAO inhibitors; patients with narrow-angle glaucoma, stenosing peptic ulcer, symptomatic prostatic hypertrophy, bladder neck obstruction, pyloroduodenal obstruction, lower respiratory tract symptoms (including asthma), or hypersensitivity to tripelennamine or related compounds.
Warnings: Antihistamines often produce drowsiness and may reduce mental alertness in children and adults. Patients should be warned about engaging in activities requiring mental alertness (e.g., driving a car, operating machinery or hazardous appliances). In elderly patients, approximately 60 years or older, antihistamines are more likely to cause dizziness, sedation and hypotension.
Patients should be warned that the central nervous system effects of PBZ may be additive with those of alcohol and other CNS depressants (e.g., hypnotics, sedatives, tranquilizers, antianxiety agents).
Antihistamines may produce excitation, particularly in children.
Usage in Pregnancy
Although no tripelennamine-related teratogenic potential or other adverse effects on the fetus have been observed in limited animal reproduction studies, the safe use of this drug in pregnancy or during lactation has not been established. Therefore, the drug should not be used during pregnancy or lactation unless, in the judgment of the physician, the expected benefits outweigh the potential hazards.
Usage in Children
In infants and children particularly, antihistamines in overdosage may produce hallucinations, convulsions and/or death.
Precautions: PBZ, like other antihistamines, has atropine-like, anticholinergic activity and should be used with caution in patients with increased intraocular pressure, hyperthyroidism, cardiovascular disease, hypertension, or history of bronchial asthma.
The PBZ tablets (25 mg) contain FD&C Yellow No. 5 (tartrazine) which may cause allergic-type reactions (including bronchial asthma) in certain susceptible individuals. Although the overall incidence of FD&C Yellow No. 5 (tartrazine) sensitivity in the general population is low, it is frequently seen in patients who also have aspirin hypersensitivity.

Adverse Reactions: The most frequent adverse reactions to antihistamines are sedation or drowsiness; sleepiness; dryness of the mouth, nose, and throat; thickening of bronchial secretions; dizziness; disturbed coordination; epigastric distress.

Other adverse reactions which may occur are: fatigue; chills; confusion; restlessness; excitation; hysteria; nervousness; irritability; insomnia; euphoria; anorexia; nausea; vomiting; diarrhea; constipation; hypotension; tightness in the chest; wheezing; blurred vision; diplopia; vertigo; tinnitus; convulsions; headache; palpitations; tachycardia; extrasystoles; nasal stuffiness; urinary frequency; difficult urination; urinary retention; leukopenia; hemolytic anemia; thrombocytopenia; agranulocytosis; aplastic anemia; allergic or hypersensitivity reactions, including drug rash, urticaria, anaphylactic shock, and photosensitivity. Although the following may have been reported to occur in association with some antihistamines, they have not been known to result from the use of PBZ: excessive perspiration, tremor, paresthesias, acute labyrinthitis, neuritis and early menses.

Dosage and Administration: Dosage should be individualized.

Usual Adult Dose: 25 to 50 mg every four to six hours. As little as 25 mg may control symptoms, but as much as 600 mg daily may be given in divided doses, if necessary.

Children and Infants: 5 mg/kg/24 hours or 150 mg/m^2/24 hours divided into four to six doses. Do not exceed maximum total dose of 300 mg/24 hours.

Note: Recommended dosages are based on the hydrochloride salt; each ml of Elixir (tripelennamine citrate) is equivalent to 5 mg tripelennamine hydrochloride.

Overdosage

Signs and Symptoms

The greatest danger from acute overdosage with antihistamines is their central nervous system effects which produce depression and/or stimulation.

In children, stimulation predominates initially in a syndrome which may include excitement, hallucinations, ataxia, incoordination, athetosis, and convulsions followed by postictal depression. Dry mouth, fixed dilated pupils, flushing of the face, and fever are common and resemble the syndrome of atropine poisoning.

In adults, CNS depression (i.e., drowsiness, coma) is more common. CNS stimulation is rare; fever and flushing are uncommon.

In both children and adults, there can be a terminal deepening of coma and cardiovascular collapse; death can occur, especially in infants and children.

Treatment

There is no specific therapy for acute overdosage with antihistamines. General symptomatic and supportive measures should be instituted promptly and maintained for as long as necessary.

In the conscious patient, vomiting should be induced even though it may have occurred spontaneously. If vomiting cannot be induced, gastric lavage is indicated. Adequate precautions must be taken to protect against aspiration, especially in infants and children. Charcoal slurry or other suitable agent should be instilled into the stomach after vomiting or lavage. Saline cathartics or milk of magnesia may be of additional benefit.

In the unconscious patient, the airway should be secured with a cuffed endotracheal tube before attempting to evacuate the gastric contents. Intensive supportive and nursing care is indicated, as for any comatose patient.

If breathing is significantly impaired, maintenance of an adequate airway and mechanical support of respiration is the safest and most effective means of providing for adequate oxygenation of tissues to prevent hypoxia (especially brain hypoxia during convulsions).

Hypotension is an early sign of impending cardiovascular collapse and should be treated vigorously. Although general supportive measures are important, specific treatment with intravenous infusion of a vasopressor (e.g., levarterenol bitartrate) titrated to maintain adequate blood pressure may be necessary.

Do *not* use CNS stimulants.

Convulsions should be controlled by careful titration of a short-acting barbiturate, repeated as necessary.

Ice packs and cooling sponge baths can aid in reducing the fever commonly seen in children.

How Supplied:

Tablets (light blue, scored), containing 50 mg PBZ® hydrochloride (tripelennamine hydrochloride USP); bottles of 100 and 1000.

Tablets (green, sugar-coated), containing 25 mg tripelennamine hydrochloride; bottles of 100.

Elixir (green, cinnamon-flavored), containing 37.5 mg PBZ® citrate (tripelennamine citrate USP) per 5 ml (equivalent to 25 mg tripelennamine hydrochloride); bottles of 473 ml (approx. 1 pint).

Dispense in tight, light-resistant container (USP).

C80-12 (1/80)

[*Shown in Product Identification Section*]

PBZ® Lontabs® GY-CODE 60 ℞
tripelennamine
Tablets of 50 mg

Description: PBZ Lontabs (long-acting tablets) are available as the hydrochloride salt of 2-[benzyl[2-(dimethylamino)ethyl]-amino]pyridine. Tripelennamine hydrochloride is an antihistamine occurring as a white, crystalline powder that slowly darkens on exposure to light and is freely soluble in water and alcohol.

Actions: Antihistamines are competitive antagonists of histamine, which also produce central nervous system effects (both stimulant and depressant) and peripheral anticholinergic, atropine-like effects (e.g., drying).

Indications: Perennial and seasonal allergic rhinitis; vasomotor rhinitis; allergic conjunctivitis due to inhalant allergens and foods; mild, uncomplicated allergic skin manifestations of urticaria and angioedema; amelioration of allergic reactions to blood or plasma; dermographism; anaphylactic reactions as adjunctive therapy to epinephrine and other standard measures after the acute manifestations have been controlled.

Contraindications: PBZ should not be used in premature infants, neonates, or nursing mothers; patients receiving MAO inhibitors; patients with narrow-angle glaucoma, stenosing peptic ulcer, symptomatic prostatic hypertrophy, bladder neck obstruction, pyloroduodenal obstruction, lower respiratory tract symptoms (including asthma), or hypersensitivity to tripelennamine or related compounds.

Warnings: Antihistamines often produce drowsiness and may reduce mental alertness in children and adults. Patients should be warned about engaging in activities requiring mental alertness (e.g., driving a car, operating machinery or hazardous appliances). In elderly patients, approximately 60 years or older, antihistamines are more likely to cause dizziness, sedation and hypotension.

Patients should be warned that the central nervous system effects of tripelennamine may be additive with those of alcohol and other CNS depressants (e.g., hypnotics, sedatives, tranquilizers, antianxiety agents).

Antihistamines may produce excitation, particularly in children.

Usage in Pregnancy

Although no tripelennamine-related teratogenic potential or other adverse effects on the fetus have been observed in limited animal reproduction studies, the safe use of this drug in pregnancy or during lactation has not been established. Therefore, the drug should not be used during pregnancy or lactation unless, in the judgment of the physician, the expected benefits outweigh the potential hazards.

Usage in Children

In infants and children particularly, antihistamines in overdosage may produce hallucinations, convulsions and/or death.

Precautions: PBZ, like other antihistamines, has atropine-like, anticholinergic activity and should be used with caution in patients with increased intraocular pressure, hyperthyroidism, cardiovascular disease, hypertension, or history of bronchial asthma.

PBZ Lontab® tablets (50 mg) contain FD&C Yellow No. 5 (tartrazine) which may cause allergic-type reactions (including bronchial asthma) in certain susceptible individuals. Although the overall incidence of FD&C Yellow No. 5 (tartrazine) sensitivity in the general population is low, it is frequently seen in patients who also have aspirin hypersensitivity.

Adverse Reactions: The most frequent adverse reactions to antihistamines are sedation or drowsiness; sleepiness; dryness of the mouth, nose, and throat; thickening of bronchial secretions; dizziness; disturbed coordination; epigastric distress.

Other adverse reactions which may occur are fatigue; chills; confusion; restlessness; excitation; hysteria; nervousness; irritability; insomnia; euphoria; anorexia; nausea; vomiting; diarrhea; constipation; hypotension; tightness in the chest; wheezing; blurred vision; diplopia; vertigo; tinnitus; convulsions; headache; palpitations; tachycardia; extrasystoles; nasal stuffiness; urinary frequency; difficult urination; urinary retention; leukopenia; hemolytic anemia; thrombocytopenia; agranulocytosis; aplastic anemia; allergic or hypersensitivity reactions, including drug rash, urticaria, anaphylactic shock, and photosensitivity. Although the following may have been reported to occur in association with some antihistamines, they have not been known to result from the use of PBZ: excessive perspiration, tremor, paresthesias, acute labyrinthitis, neuritis and early menses.

Dosage and Administration: Dosage should be individualized according to the needs and response of the patient.

The effects of PBZ Lontabs begin within 15 to 30 minutes and generally last up to 8 hours.

Adults: 100 mg in the morning and 100 mg in the evening is generally adequate for "around-the-clock" allergic protection. In difficult cases, 100 mg every 8 hours may be required.

Children Over 5: One 50-mg Lontab in the morning and one in the evening is usually sufficient, but some children may require one every 8 hours.

Overdosage:

Signs and Symptoms

The greatest danger from acute overdosage with antihistamines is their central nervous system effects which produce depression and/or stimulation.

In children, stimulation predominates initially in a syndrome which may include excitement, hallucinations, ataxia, incoordination, athetosis, and convulsions followed by postictal depression. Dry mouth, fixed dilated pupils, flushing of the face, and fever are common and resemble the syndrome of atropine poisoning.

In adults, CNS depression (i.e., drowsiness, coma) is more common. CNS stimulation is rare; fever and flushing are uncommon.

In both children and adults, there can be a terminal deepening of coma and cardiovascular collapse; death can occur, especially in infants and children.

Continued on next page

The full prescribing information for each GEIGY drug is contained herein and is that in effect as of October 1, 1982.

Geigy—Cont.

Treatment

There is no specific therapy for acute overdosage with antihistamines. General symptomatic and supportive measures should be instituted promptly and maintained for as long as necessary.

In the conscious patient, vomiting should be induced even though it may have occurred spontaneously. If vomiting cannot be induced, gastric lavage is indicated. Adequate precautions must be taken to protect against aspiration, especially in infants and children. Charcoal slurry or other suitable agent should be instilled into the stomach after vomiting or lavage. Saline cathartics or milk of magnesia may be of additional benefit.

In the unconscious patient, the airway should be secured with a cuffed endotracheal tube before attempting to evacuate the gastric contents. Intensive supportive and nursing care is indicated, as for any comatose patient.

If breathing is significantly impaired, maintenance of an adequate airway and mechanical support of respiration is the safest and most effective means of providing for adequate oxygenation of tissues to prevent hypoxia (especially brain hypoxia during convulsions).

Hypotension is an early sign of impending cardiovascular collapse and should be treated vigorously. Although general supportive measures are important, specific treatment with intravenous infusion of a vasopressor (e.g., levarterenol bitartrate) titrated to maintain adequate blood pressure is also necessary.

Do *not* use CNS stimulants.

Convulsions should be controlled by careful titration of a short-acting barbiturate, repeated as necessary.

Ice packs and cooling sponge baths can aid in reducing the fever commonly seen in children.

How Supplied:

LONTABS® 50 mg—round, light green (imprinted GEIGY 60)

Bottles of 100 ....NDC 0028-0060-01

LONTABS® (Long-acting tablets)

Dispense in tight, light-resistant container (USP).

C82-43 (11/82)

PBZ® tripelennamine GY-CODE 134 ℞
Tablets with Ephedrine

Description: PBZ Tablets with Ephedrine contain 25 mg tripelennamine hydrochloride and 12 mg ephedrine sulfate. PBZ hydrochloride is an antihistamine occurring as a white, crystalline powder that darkens slowly on exposure to light and is freely soluble in water and alcohol; chemically, it is 2-[benzyl[2-(dimethylamino)ethyl]-amino]pyridine hydrochloride.

Actions:

Tripelennamine

Antihistamines are competitive antagonists of histamine, which also produce central nervous system effects (both stimulant and depressant) and peripheral anticholinergic, atropine-like effects (e.g., drying).

Ephedrine

Ephedrine differs from epinephrine mainly in its efficacy after oral administration, its much longer duration of action, its more pronounced central actions, and its much lower potency. Bronchial muscle relaxation is less prominent but more sustained with ephedrine than with epinephrine.

Indications

Based on a review of this drug by the National Academy of Sciences-National Research Council and/or other information, FDA has classified the indications as follows:

"Probably" Effective: For the symptomatic treatment of seasonal and perennial allergic rhinitis and vasomotor rhinitis.

Final classification of the less-than-effective indications requires further investigation.

Contraindications: PBZ Tablets with Ephedrine should not be used in premature infants, neonates, or nursing mothers; patients receiving MAO inhibitors; patients with narrow-angle glaucoma, stenosing peptic ulcer, symptomatic prostatic hypertrophy, bladder neck obstruction, pyloroduodenal obstruction, lower respiratory tract symptoms (including asthma), or hypersensitivity to tripelennamine, ephedrine or related compounds.

Warnings:

Tripelennamine

Antihistamines often produce drowsiness and may reduce mental alertness in children and adults. Patients should be warned about engaging in activities requiring mental alertness (e.g., driving a car, operating machinery or hazardous appliances). In elderly patients, approximately 60 years or older, antihistamines are more likely to cause dizziness, sedation and hypotension.

Patients should be warned that the central nervous system effects of PBZ may be additive with those of alcohol and other CNS depressants (e.g., hypnotics, sedatives, tranquilizers, anti-anxiety agents).

Antihistamines may produce excitation, particularly in children.

Ephedrine

Use cautiously in patients with degenerative heart disease (anginal pain may be induced in patients with angina pectoris) and in hyperthyroid and hypertensive individuals, who are particularly susceptible to the untoward and pressor responses to ephedrine.

Usage in Pregnancy

Although no tripelennamine-related teratogenic potential or other adverse effects on the fetus have been observed in limited animal reproduction studies, the safe use of this drug in pregnancy or during lactation has not been established. Therefore, the drug should not be used during pregnancy or lactation unless, in the judgment of the physician, the expected benefits outweigh the potential hazards.

Usage in Children

In infants and children particularly, antihistamines in overdosage may produce hallucinations, convulsions and/or death.

Precautions: PBZ, like other antihistamines, has atropine-like, anticholinergic activity and should be used with caution in patients with increased intraocular pressure, hyperthyroidism, cardiovascular disease, hypertension, or history of bronchial asthma.

Adverse Reactions:

Tripelennamine

The most frequent adverse reactions to antihistamines are sedation or drowsiness; sleepiness; dryness of the mouth, nose, and throat; thickening of bronchial secretions; dizziness; disturbed coordination; epigastric distress.

Other adverse reactions which may occur are: fatigue; chills; confusion; restlessness; excitation; hysteria; nervousness; irritability; insomnia; euphoria; anorexia; nausea; vomiting; diarrhea; constipation; hypotension; tightness in the chest; wheezing; blurred vision; diplopia; vertigo; tinnitus; convulsions; headache; palpitations; tachycardia; extrasystoles; nasal stuffiness; urinary frequency; difficult urination; urinary retention; leukopenia; hemolytic anemia; thrombocytopenia; agranulocytosis; aplastic anemia; allergic or hypersensitivity reactions, including drug rash, urticaria, anaphylactic shock, and photosensitivity. Although the following may have been reported to occur in association with some antihistamines, they have not been known to result from the use of PBZ: excessive perspiration, tremor, paresthesias, acute labyrinthitis, neuritis and early menses.

Ephedrine

Occasionally peripheral vasoconstriction, irritability, palpitations, tremors, insomnia, in some cases anxiety, or other side effects which may be encountered with the sympathomimetic drugs. Psychotic symptoms with paranoid delusions have been described following chronic overdosage (self-medication).

Dosage and Administration: Dosage should be individualized according to the needs and the response of the patient.

Adults: 1 or 2 tablets every 4 hours.

Older Children: 1 tablet 4 times a day.

Overdosage:

Tripelennamine

Signs and Symptoms

The greatest danger from acute overdosage with antihistamines is their central nervous system effects which produce depression and/or stimulation.

In children, stimulation predominates in a syndrome which may include excitement, hallucinations, ataxia, incoordination, athetosis, and convulsions followed by postictal depression. Dry mouth, fixed dilated pupils, flushed face, and fever are common and resemble the syndrome of atropine poisoning.

In adults, CNS depression (i.e., drowsiness, coma) is more common. CNS stimulation is rare; fever and flushing are uncommon.

In both children and adults, there can be a terminal deepening of coma and cardiovascular collapse; death can occur, especially in infants and children.

Treatment

There is no specific therapy for acute overdosage with antihistamines. General symptomatic and supportive measures should be instituted promptly and maintained for as long as necessary.

In the conscious patient, vomiting should be induced even though it may have occurred spontaneously. If vomiting cannot be induced, gastric lavage is indicated. Adequate precautions must be taken to protect against aspiration, especially in infants and children. Charcoal slurry or other suitable agent should be instilled into the stomach after vomiting or lavage. Saline cathartics or milk of magnesia may be of additional benefit.

In the unconscious patient, the airway should be secured with a cuffed endotracheal tube before attempting to evacuate the gastric contents. Intensive supportive and nursing care is indicated, as for any comatose patient.

If breathing is significantly impaired, maintenance of an adequate airway and mechanical support of respiration is the safest and most effective means of providing for adequate oxygenation of tissues to prevent hypoxia (especially brain hypoxia during convulsions).

Hypotension is an early sign of impending cardiovascular collapse and should be treated vigorously. Although general supportive measures are important, specific treatment with intravenous infusion of a vasopressor (e.g., levarterenol bitartrate) titrated to maintain adequate blood pressure is also necessary.

Do *not* use CNS stimulants.

Convulsions should be controlled by careful titration of a short-acting barbiturate, repeated as necessary.

Ice packs and alcohol sponge baths can aid in reducing the fever commonly seen in children.

How Supplied: *Tablets with Ephedrine* (white, dry-coated), each containing 25 mg tripelennamine hydrochloride and 12 mg ephedrine sulfate; bottles of 100.

Dispense in tight container (USP).

C78-46 (12/78)

PBZ® hydrochloride
tripelennamine hydrochloride
Cream **GY-CODE 6946**
Antihistamine

Indications: For the temporary relief of itching due to minor skin disorders, ivy and oak poisoning, hives, sunburn, insect bites (nonpoisonous), and stings.
Directions: Apply gently to the affected area 3 or 4 times daily or according to physician's directions.
Caution: If the condition persists or irritation develops, discontinue use and consult physician. Do not use in eyes.
KEEP OUT OF REACH OF CHILDREN.
How Supplied:
Cream, 2% tripelennamine hydrochloride in a water-washable base; tubes of 1 ounce.
(1/80)

TANDEARIL® ℞
oxyphenbutazone USP
A Potent Anti-Inflammatory Agent
Tablets of 100 mg **GY-CODE 24**

Important Note: Tandearil cannot be considered a simple analgesic and should never be administered casually. Each patient should be carefully evaluated before treatment is started and should remain constantly under the close supervision of the physician. The following cautions should be observed:

1. Therapy should not be initiated until a careful detailed history and complete physical and laboratory examination, including a complete hemogram and urinalysis, etc., of the patient have been made. These examinations should be made at regular, frequent intervals throughout the duration of this drug therapy.
2. Patients should be carefully selected, avoiding those in whom it is contraindicated as well as those who will respond to ordinary therapeutic measures, or those who cannot be observed at frequent intervals.
3. Patients taking this drug should be warned not to exceed the recommended dosage, since this may lead to toxic effects, and should discontinue the drug and report to the physician immediately any sign of:
   a. Fever, sore throat, lesions in the mouth (symptoms of blood dyscrasia).
   b. Dyspepsia, epigastric pain, symptoms of anemia, unusual bleeding, unusual bruising, black or tarry stools or other evidence of intestinal ulceration.
   c. Skin rashes.
   d. Significant weight gain or edema.
4. A trial period of one week of therapy is considered adequate to determine the therapeutic effect of the drug. In the absence of a favorable response, therapy should be discontinued.
   a. In the elderly (sixty years and over) the drug should be restricted to short-term treatment periods only—if possible, *one week* maximum.
5. **Before prescribing Tandearil for an individual patient, read thoroughly the information contained under each heading which follows:**

Description: Tandearil should not be considered as a simple analgesic that can be prescribed for indiscriminate use. Tandearil is closely related chemically and pharmacologically, including toxic effects, to the well-known pyrazolines (pyrazole compounds) amidopyrine and antipyrine.
Chemically, Tandearil is 4-Butyl-1-(p-hydroxyphenyl) 2-phenyl-3,5-pyrazolidinedione monohydrate, the parahydroxy analog of Butazolidin®, brand of phenylbutazone USP.
It has anti-inflammatory and antipyretic action as well as analgesic and mild uricosuric properties resulting in symptomatic relief only. **The disease process itself is unaltered by this drug.**
Clinical Pharmacology: In man, oxyphenbutazone is completely absorbed after oral administration of Tandearil. After ingestion of three 100-mg tablets, peak plasma concentration of oxyphenbutazone has been measured at 34.9 (± 5.3) mg/l within six hours. After therapeutic doses, about 98 percent of the drug is bound to human serum albumin. Elimination is mainly by biotransformation in the liver, and the plasma half-life has been measured as 72 (± 15 hours). Urinary excretion consists mostly of metabolites.
Indications: The indications for Tandearil are:
Acute Gouty Arthritis
Active Rheumatoid Arthritis
Active Ankylosing Spondylitis
Short-term treatment of acute attacks of degenerative joint disease of the hips and knees not responsive to other treatment.
Painful Shoulder (peritendinitis, capsulitis, bursitis, and acute arthritis of that joint)
Contraindications:

1. *Age:* Tandearil is contraindicated in children 14 years of age or younger since controlled clinical trials in patients of this age group have not been conducted.
2. *Other Medical Conditions:* Tandearil is contraindicated in patients with incipient cardiac failure, blood dyscrasias, pancreatitis, parotitis, stomatitis, polymyalgia rheumatica, temporal arteritis, senility, drug allergy, and in the presence of severe renal, cardiac and hepatic disease, and in patients with a history of peptic ulcer disease, or symptoms of gastrointestinal inflammation or active ulceration because serious adverse reactions or aggravation of existing medical problems can occur.
3. *Concomitant Medications:* Tandearil should not be used in combination with other drugs which accentuate or share a potential for similar toxicity.
   It is also inadvisable to administer Tandearil in combination with other potent drugs because of the possibility of increased toxic reactions from Tandearil and other agents. (See also *Drug Interactions.*)
   Tandearil is contraindicated in patients with a history or suggestion of prior toxicity, sensitivity, or idiosyncrasy to phenylbutazone or oxyphenbutazone.

Warnings: Based on reports of clinical experience with oxyphenbutazone and related compounds, the following warnings should be considered by the physician prior to prescribing the drug:

1. *Gastrointestinal:* Upper G.I. diagnostic tests should be performed in patients with persistent or severe dyspepsia. Peptic ulceration, reactivation of latent peptic ulcer, perforation and gastrointestinal bleeding, sometimes severe, have been reported.
   As with other nonsteroidal anti-inflammatory drugs, borderline elevations of values measured by one or more liver tests may occur in up to 15% of patients. These abnormalities may progress, may remain essentially unchanged, or may be transient with continued therapy. The SGPT (ALT) test is probably the most sensitive indicator of liver dysfunction. Meaningful elevations (three times the upper limit of normal) of SGPT or SGOT (AST) have occurred in controlled clinical trials in less than 1% of patients. A patient with symptoms and/or signs suggesting liver dysfunction, or in whom an abnormal liver test has occurred, should be evaluated for evidence of the development of more severe hepatic reactions while on therapy with Tandearil. Severe hepatic reactions, including jaundice and cases of fatal hepatitis, have been reported with Tandearil as with other nonsteroidal anti-inflammatory drugs. Although such reactions are rare, if abnormal liver tests persist or worsen, if clinical signs and symptoms consistent with liver disease develop, or if systemic manifestations (e.g., eosinophilia, rash, etc.) occur, therapy with Tandearil should be discontinued.
2. *Hematologic: Frequent and regular hematologic evaluations should be performed on patients receiving the drug for periods over one week.* Any significant change in the total white count, relative decrease in granulocytes, appearance of immature forms, or fall in hematocrit should be a signal for immediate cessation of therapy and a complete hematologic investigation. Serious, sometimes fatal blood dyscrasias, including aplastic anemia have been reported to occur. Hematologic toxicity may occur suddenly or many days or weeks after cessation of treatment as manifest by the appearance of anemia, leukopenia, thrombocytopenia or clinically significant hemorrhagic diathesis. There have been published reports associating oxyphenbutazone with leukemia. However, the circumstances involved in these reports are such that a cause-and-effect relationship to the drug has not been clearly established.
3. *Pregnancy:* Reproductive studies in animals, although inconclusive, exhibited evidence of possible embryotoxicity. It is, therefore, recommended that this drug should be used with caution during pregnancy. The benefits should be weighed against the potential risk to the fetus.
4. *Nursing Mothers:* Caution is also advised in prescribing Tandearil in nursing mothers since the drug may appear in cord blood and breast milk.
5. Patients reporting visual disturbances while receiving the drug should discontinue treatment and have an ophthalmologic examination because ophthalmologic adverse reactions have been reported (see **Adverse Reactions:** *Special Senses*).
6. In the aging (forty years and over), there appears to be an increase in the possibility of adverse reactions. Tandearil should be used with commensurately greater care in the elderly and should be avoided altogether in the senile patient.
7. Like other drugs with prostaglandin synthetase inhibition activity, Tandearil may precipitate acute episodes of asthmatic attacks in patients with asthma.
8. Tandearil increases sodium retention. Evidence of fluid retention in patients in whom there is danger of cardiac decompensation is an indication to discontinue the drug.

Precautions: Because of potential serious adverse reactions to Tandearil, the following precautions should be observed in the use of the drug:
—A careful diagnostic physical examination and history should be performed on all patients at regular intervals while the patient is receiving the drug.
—Tandearil is not recommended for chronic use in the elderly.
—Hematologic evaluation should be performed at frequent and regular intervals and additional laboratory examinations performed as indicated.
—Patients should be instructed to report immediately the occurrence of high fever, severe sore throat, stomatitis, salivary

Continued on next page

The full prescribing information for each GEIGY drug is contained herein and is that in effect as of October 1, 1982.

Geigy—Cont.

gland enlargement, tarry stools, unusual bleeding or bruising, sudden weight gain, or edema.

—The drug reduces iodine uptake by the thyroid and may interfere with laboratory tests of thyroid function (see **Adverse Reactions**: *Endocrine-Metabolic*).

—The patient should be cautioned regarding participation in activities requiring alertness and coordination, and that the concomitant ingestion of alcohol with Tandearil may further impair psychomotor skills.

Drug Interactions: Tandearil is highly bound to serum proteins. If its affinity for protein binding is higher than other concurrently administered drugs, the actions and toxicity of the other drug may be increased.

Tandearil accentuates the prothrombin depression produced by coumarin-type anticoagulants. When administered alone, it does not affect prothrombin activity.

The pharmacologic action of insulin, antidiabetic, and sulfonamide drugs may be potentiated by the simultaneous administration of Tandearil.

Concomitant administration of oxyphenbutazone and phenytoin may result in increased serum levels of phenytoin which could lead to increased phenytoin toxicity.

Adverse Reactions: Based upon reports of clinical experience with oxyphenbutazone and related compounds, the following adverse reactions have been reported.

The adverse reactions listed in the following table have been arranged into three groups: (1) incidence greater than 1%, (2) incidence less than 1% and (3) causal relationship unknown. The incidence for group (1) was obtained from fifty-seven (57) clinical trials reported in the literature (3713 patients). The incidence for group (2) was based on reports in clinical trials, in the literature, and on voluntary reports since marketing. The reactions in group (3) have been reported but occurred under circumstances where a causal relationship could not be established. In some patients the reported reactions may have been unrelated to the administration of Tandearil. However, in these reported events, the possibility cannot be excluded. Therefore these observations are being listed to serve as alerting information to physicians. Before prescribing this drug for an individual patient, the physician should be familiar with the following:

(1) Incidence greater than 1%	**(2) Incidence less than 1%**
GASTROINTESTINAL (See Warnings)	
gastrointestinal upset	nausea dyspepsia/including indigestion and heartburn abdominal and epigastric distress vomiting abdominal distention with flatulence constipation diarrhea esophagitis gastritis salivary gland enlargement stomatitis, sometimes with ulceration ulceration and perforation of the intestinal tract including acute and reactivated peptic ulcer with perforation, hemorrhage and hematemesis anemia due to gastrointestinal bleeding which may be occult hepatitis, both fatal and nonfatal, sometimes associated with evidence of cholestasis
HEMATOLOGICAL (See Warnings)	
None	anemia leukopenia thrombocytopenia with associated purpura, petechiae, and hemorrhage pancytopenia aplastic anemia bone marrow depression agranulocytosis and agranulocytic anginal syndrome hemolytic anemia
HYPERSENSITIVITY	
None	urticaria anaphylactic shock arthralgia, drug fever hypersensitivity angiitis (polyarteritis) and vasculitis Lyell's syndrome serum sickness Stevens-Johnson syndrome activation of systemic lupus erythematosus aggravation of temporal arteritis in patients with polymyalgia rheumatica
DERMATOLOGIC	
None	pruritus drug rashes erythema nodosum erythema multiforme nonthrombocytopenic purpura
CARDIOVASCULAR, FLUID AND ELECTROLYTE	
None	sodium and chloride retention fluid retention and plasma dilution cardiac decompensation (congestive heart failure) with edema and dyspnea metabolic acidosis respiratory alkalosis hypertension pericarditis interstitial myocarditis with muscle necrosis and perivascular granulomata
RENAL	
None	hematuria proteinuria ureteral obstruction with uric acid crystals anuria glomerulonephritis acute tubular necrosis cortical necrosis renal stones nephrotic syndrome impaired renal function and renal failure associated with azotemia
CENTRAL NERVOUS SYSTEM	
None	headache drowsiness agitation confusional states and lethargy tremors numbness weakness
ENDOCRINE-METABOLIC (See Precautions)	
None	None
SPECIAL SENSES (See Warnings)	
Ocular:	
None	None
Otic:	
None	hearing loss tinnitus

(3) Causal relationship unknown—Incidence less than 1%: *Hematological* (see **Warnings**)—Leukemia (There have been reports associating oxyphenbutazone with leukemia. However, the circumstances involved in these reports are such that a cause-and-effect relationship to the drug has not been clearly established) *Endocrine—Metabolic* (see **Precautions**)— Thyroid hyperplasia; goiters associated with hyperthyroidism and hypothyroidism; pancreatitis; hyperglycemia. *Special Senses* (see **Warnings**)—Blurred vision; optic neuritis; toxic amblyopia; scotomata; retinal detachment; retinal hemorrhage; oculomotor palsy.

Overdosage: *Signs and Symptoms:* Include any of the following: nausea, vomiting, epigastric pain, excessive perspiration, euphoria, psychosis, headaches, giddiness, vertigo, hyperventilation, insomnia, tinnitus, difficulty in hearing, edema (sodium retention), hypertension, cyanosis, respiratory depression, agitation, hallucinations, stupor, convulsions, coma, hematuria, and oliguria. Hepatomegaly, jaundice, and ulceration of the buccal or gastrointestinal mucosa have been reported as late manifestations of massive overdosage.

Reported laboratory abnormalities following overdosage include: respiratory or metabolic acidosis, impaired hepatic or renal function, and abnormalities of formed blood elements.

Treatment: In the alert patient, empty the stomach promptly by induced emesis followed by lavage. In the obtunded patient, secure the airway with a cuffed endotracheal tube before beginning lavage (do not induce emesis). Maintain adequate respiratory exchange, do not use respiratory stimulants. Treat shock with appropriate supportive measures. Control seizures with intravenous diazepam or short-acting barbiturates. Dialysis may be helpful if renal function is impaired.

Dosage and Administration: Tandearil should be used at the smallest effective dosage to afford rapid relief of severe symptoms. It is contraindicated in children under 14 years of age and in senile patients.

If a favorable symptomatic response to treatment is not obtained after one week, the drug should be discontinued. When a favorable therapeutic response has been obtained, the dosage should be reduced and then discontinued as soon as possible.

In elderly patients (sixty years and over) every effort must be made to discontinue therapy on, or as soon as possible after, the seventh day, because of the exceedingly high risk of severe fatal toxic reactions in this age group.

To minimize gastric upset, the drug should be taken with milk or with meals.

In selecting the appropriate dosage in any specific case, consideration should be given to the patient's age, weight, general health, and any other factors that may influence his response to the drug.

Rheumatoid Arthritis, Ankylosing Spondylitis, Acute Attacks of Degenerative Joint Disease, and Painful Shoulder: Initial Dosage: The initial daily dose in adult patients is 300 to 600 mg as 3 to 4 divided doses. Maximum therapeutic response is usually obtained at a total daily dose of 400 mg. A trial period of one week of therapy is considered adequate to determine the therapeutic effect of the drug. In the absence of a favorable response, therapy should be discontinued.

Maintenance Dosage: When improvement is obtained, dosage should be promptly decreased to the minimum effective level necessary to maintain relief, not exceeding 400 mg daily because of the possibility of cumulative toxicity. A satisfactory clinical response may be obtained with daily doses as low as 100 to 200 mg daily.

Acute Gouty Arthritis: Satisfactory results are obtained after an initial dose of 400 mg followed by 100 mg every 4 hours. The articular inflammation usually subsides within 4 days and treatment should not be continued longer than one week.

How Supplied:

Tablets 100 mg—round, tan, sugar-coated (imprinted Geigy 24)

Bottle of 100 ....NDC 0028-0024-01
Bottle of 1000 ....NDC 0028-0024-10
Unit Dose Packages—Blister–Packed
Box of 100 ....NDC 0028-0024-61

Dispense in tight container (USP).

C82-41 (8/82)

[*Shown in Product Identification Section*]

TEGRETOL® ℞

carbamazepine USP

Chewable Tablets of 100 mg—red-speckled, pink GY-CODE 47

Tablets of 200 mg—white GY-CODE 67

WARNING
SERIOUS AND SOMETIMES FATAL ABNORMALITIES OF BLOOD CELLS (APLASTIC ANEMIA, AGRANULOCYTOSIS, THROMBOCYTOPENIA, AND LEUKOPENIA) HAVE BEEN REPORTED FOLLOWING TREATMENT WITH TEGRETOL, CARBAMAZEPINE. EARLY DETECTION OF HEMATOLOGIC CHANGE IS IMPORTANT SINCE, IN SOME PATIENTS, APLASTIC ANEMIA IS REVERSIBLE.
COMPLETE PRETREATMENT BLOOD COUNTS, INCLUDING PLATELET AND POSSIBLY RETICULOCYTE AND SERUM IRON, SHOULD BE OBTAINED. ANY SIGNIFICANT ABNORMALITIES SHOULD RULE OUT USE OF THE DRUG. THESE SAME TESTS SHOULD BE REPEATED AT FREQUENT INTERVALS, POSSIBLY WEEKLY DURING THE FIRST THREE MONTHS OF THERAPY AND MONTHLY THEREAFTER FOR AT LEAST TWO TO THREE YEARS. THE DRUG SHOULD BE STOPPED IF ANY EVIDENCE OF BONE MARROW DEPRESSION DEVELOPS.
PATIENTS SHOULD BE MADE AWARE OF THE EARLY TOXIC SIGNS AND SYMPTOMS OF A POTENTIAL HEMATOLOGIC PROBLEM, SUCH AS FEVER, SORE THROAT, ULCERS IN THE MOUTH, EASY BRUISING, PETECHIAL OR PURPURIC HEMORRHAGE, AND SHOULD BE ADVISED TO DISCONTINUE THE DRUG AND TO REPORT TO THE PHYSICIAN IMMEDIATELY IF ANY SUCH SIGNS OR SYMPTOMS APPEAR.

This drug is not a simple analgesic and should not be used for the relief of trivial aches or pains. Treatment of epilepsy should be restricted to those classifications listed under "INDICATIONS AND USAGE."

Before prescribing Tegretol, the physician should be thoroughly familiar with the details of this prescribing information, particularly regarding use with other drugs, especially those which accentuate toxicity potential.

Description: Tegretol, carbamazepine USP, is an anticonvulsant and specific analgesic for trigeminal neuralgia, available as chewable tablets of 100 mg and tablets of 200 mg for oral administration. Its chemical name is 5H-dibenz[b,f]azepine-5-carboxamide.

Carbamazepine USP is a white to off-white powder, practically insoluble in water and soluble in alcohol and in acetone.

Clinical Pharmacology: In controlled clinical trials, Tegretol has been shown to be effective in the treatment of psychomotor and grand mal seizures, as well as trigeminal neuralgia.

It has demonstrated anticonvulsant properties in rats and mice with electrically and chemically induced seizures. It appears to act by reducing polysynaptic response and blocking the posttetanic potentiation. Tegretol greatly reduces or abolishes pain induced by stimulation of the infraorbital nerve in cats and rats. It depresses thalamic potential and bulbar and polysynaptic reflexes, including the linguomandibular reflex in cats. Tegretol is chemically unrelated to other anticonvulsants or other drugs used to control the pain of trigeminal neuralgia. The mechanism of action remains unknown.

Tegretol tablets are adequately absorbed after oral administration at a slower rate than a solution, thus avoiding undesirably high peak concentrations. Tegretol in blood is 76% bound to plasma proteins. Plasma levels of Tegretol are variable and may range from 0.5-25 μg/ml, with no apparent relationship to the daily intake of the drug. Usual adult therapeutic levels are between 4 and 12 μg/ml. Following oral administration, serum levels peak at 4 to 5 hours. The CSF/serum ratio is 0.22, similar to the 22% unbound Tegretol in serum. Because Tegretol may induce its own metabolism, the half-life is also variable. Initial half-life values range from 25-65 hours, with 12-17 hours on repeated doses. Tegretol is metabolized in the liver. After oral administration of ^{14}C-carbamazepine, 72% of the administered radioactivity was found in the urine and 28% in the feces. This urinary radioactivity was composed largely of hydroxylated and conjugated metabolites, with only 3% of unchanged Tegretol. Transplacental passage of Tegretol is rapid (30 to 60 minutes), and the drug is accumulated in fetal tissues, with higher levels found in liver and kidney than in brain and lungs.

Indications and Usage:

Epilepsy: Tegretol is indicated for the following conditions in patients who have not responded satisfactorily to treatment with other agents such as phenytoin, phenobarbital, or primidone:

1. Partial seizures with complex symptomatology (psychomotor, temporal lobe). Patients with these seizures appear to show greater improvement than those with other types.
2. Generalized tonic-clonic seizures (grand mal).
3. Mixed seizure patterns which include the above, or other partial or generalized seizures.

Absence seizures (petit mal) do not appear to be controlled by Tegretol.

Because of the necessity for frequent laboratory evaluation for potentially serious side effects, Tegretol is not recommended as the drug of first choice in seizure disorders. It should be reserved for patients whose seizures are difficult to control or patients experiencing marked side effects (e.g., excessive sedation).

Trigeminal Neuralgia: Tegretol is indicated in the treatment of the pain associated with true trigeminal neuralgia.

Beneficial results have also been reported in glossopharyngeal neuralgia.

Contraindications: Tegretol should not be used in patients with a history of previous bone marrow depression, hypersensitivity to the drug, or known sensitivity to any of the tricyclic compounds, such as amitriptyline, desipramine, imipramine, protriptyline, nortriptyline, etc. Likewise, on theoretical grounds its use with monoamine oxidase inhibitors is not recommended. Before administration of Tegretol, MAO inhibitors should be discontinued for a minimum of fourteen days, or longer if the clinical situation permits.

Warnings: The drug should be discontinued if evidence of significant bone marrow depression occurs, as follows:

1) Erythrocytes	less than 4,000,000/cu mm
Hematocrit	less than 32%
Hemoglobin	less than 11 gm/100 ml
2) Leukocytes	less than 4000/cu mm
3) Platelets	less than 100,000/cu mm
4) Reticulocytes	less than 0.3% (20,000/cu mm)

5) Serum iron greater than 150 μg/100 ml

Patients with a history of adverse hematologic reaction to any drug may be particularly at risk.

Tegretol has shown mild anticholinergic activity; therefore, patients with increased intraocular pressure should be closely observed during therapy.

Because of the relationship of the drug to other tricyclic compounds, the possibility of activation of a latent psychosis and, in elderly patients, of confusion or agitation should be borne in mind.

Precautions:

General: Before initiating therapy, a detailed history and physical examination should be made.

Therapy should be prescribed only after critical benefit-to-risk appraisal in patients with a history of cardiac, hepatic or renal damage, adverse hematologic reaction to other drugs, or interrupted courses of therapy with Tegretol.

Information for Patients: Since dizziness and drowsiness may occur, patients should be cautioned about the hazards of operating machinery or automobiles or engaging in other potentially dangerous tasks.

Laboratory Tests: Complete pretreatment blood counts, including platelets and possibly reticulocytes and serum iron, should be obtained. Any significant abnormalities should rule out use of the drug. These same tests should be repeated at frequent intervals, possibly weekly, during the first three months of therapy and monthly thereafter for at least two to three years.

Baseline and periodic evaluations of liver function, particularly in patients with a history of liver disease, must be performed during treatment with this drug since liver damage may occur. The drug should be discontinued immediately in cases of aggravated liver dysfunction or active liver disease.

Baseline and periodic eye examinations, including slit-lamp, funduscopy and tonometry, are recommended since many phenothiazines and related drugs have been shown to cause eye changes.

Baseline and periodic complete urinalysis and BUN determinations are recommended for patients treated with this agent because of observed renal dysfunction.

Monitoring of blood levels (see **CLINICAL PHARMACOLOGY**) has increased the efficacy and safety of anticonvulsants. This monitoring may be particularly useful in cases of dramatic increase in seizure frequency and for verification of compliance. In addition, measurement of drug serum levels may aid in determining the cause of toxicity when more than one medication is being used.

Continued on next page

The full prescribing information for each GEIGY drug is contained herein and is that in effect as of October 1, 1982.

Geigy—Cont.

Thyroid function tests have been reported to show decreased values with Tegretol administered alone.

Drug Interactions: The simultaneous administration of phenobarbital, phenytoin, or primidone, or a combination of two, produces a marked lowering of serum levels of Tegretol. The half-lives of phenytoin, warfarin, doxycycline were significantly shortened when administered concurrently with Tegretol. The doses of these drugs may therefore have to be increased when Tegretol is added to the therapeutic regime.

Concomitant administration of Tegretol and erythromycin has been reported to result in elevated plasma levels of carbamazepine resulting in toxicity in some cases.

Alterations of thyroid function have been reported in combination therapy with other anticonvulsant medications.

Breakthrough bleeding has been reported among patients receiving concomitant oral contraceptives and their reliability may be adversely affected.

Carcinogenicity, Mutagenesis, Impairment of Fertility: Carbamazepine, when administered to Sprague-Dawley rats for two years in the diet at doses of 25, 75, and 250 mg/kg/day, resulted in a dose-related increase in the incidence of hepatocellular tumors in females and of benign interstitial cell adenomas in the testes of males.

Carbamazepine must, therefore, be considered to be carcinogenic in Sprague-Dawley rats. Bacterial and mammalian mutagenicity studies using carbamazepine produced negative results. The significance of these findings relative to the use of carbamazepine in humans is, at present, unknown.

Pregnancy Category C: Tegretol has been shown to have adverse effect in reproduction studies in rats when given orally in dosages 10–25 times the maximum human daily dosage of 1200 mg. In rat teratology studies, 2 of 135 offspring showed kinked ribs at 250 mg/kg and 4 of 119 offspring at 650 mg/kg showed other anomalies (cleft palate, 1; talipes, 1; anophthalmos, 2). In reproduction studies in rats, nursing offspring demonstrated a lack of weight gain and an unkempt appearance at a maternal dosage level of 200 mg/kg.

There are no adequate and well-controlled studies in pregnant women. Tegretol should be used during pregnancy only if the potential benefit justifies the potential risk to the fetus. It is important to note that anticonvulsant drugs should not be discontinued in patients in whom the drug is administered to prevent major seizures because of the strong possibility of precipitating status epilepticus with attendant hypoxia and threat to life. In individual cases where the severity and frequency of the seizure disorder are such that removal of medication does not pose a serious threat to the patient, discontinuation of the drug may be considered prior to and during pregnancy, although it cannot be said with any confidence that even minor seizures do not pose some hazard to the developing embryo or fetus.

Labor and Delivery: The effect of Tegretol on human labor and delivery is unknown.

Nursing Mothers: During lactation, concentration of Tegretol in milk is approximately 60% of the maternal plasma concentration.

Because of the potential for serious adverse reactions in nursing infants from carbamazepine, a decision should be made whether to discontinue nursing or to discontinue the drug, taking into account the importance of the drug to the mother.

Pediatric Use: Safety and effectiveness in children below the age of 6 years have not been established.

Adverse Reactions: If adverse reactions are of such severity that the drug must be discontinued, the physician must be aware that abrupt discontinuation of any anticonvulsant drug in a responsive epileptic patient may lead to seizures or even status epilepticus with its life-threatening hazards.

The most severe adverse reactions have been observed in the hemopoietic system (see boxed WARNING), the skin and the cardiovascular system.

The most frequently observed adverse reactions, particularly during the initial phases of therapy, are dizziness, drowsiness, unsteadiness, nausea, and vomiting. To minimize the possibility of such reactions, therapy should be initiated at the low dosage recommended.

The following additional adverse reactions have been reported:

Hemopoietic System: Aplastic anemia, agranulocytosis, thrombocytopenia, leukopenia, leukocytosis, eosinophilia.

Skin: Pruritic and erythematous rashes, urticaria, Stevens-Johnson syndrome, photosensitivity reactions, alterations in skin pigmentation, exfoliative dermatitis, erythema multiforme and nodosum, purpura, aggravation of disseminated lupus erythematosus, alopecia, and diaphoresis. In certain cases, discontinuation of therapy may be necessary.

Cardiovascular System: Congestive heart failure, edema, aggravation of hypertension, hypotension, syncope and collapse, aggravation of coronary artery disease, arrhythmias and A-V block, primary thrombophlebitis, recurrence of thrombophlebitis, and adenopathy or lymphadenopathy.

Some of these cardiovascular complications have resulted in fatalities. Myocardial infarction has been associated with other tricyclic compounds.

Liver: Abnormalities in liver function tests, cholestatic and hepatocellular jaundice, hepatitis.

Respiratory System: Pulmonary hypersensitivity characterized by fever, dyspnea, pneumonitis or pneumonia.

Genitourinary System: Urinary frequency, acute urinary retention, oliguria with elevated blood pressure, azotemia, renal failure, and impotence. Albuminuria, glycosuria, elevated BUN and microscopic deposits in the urine have also been reported.

Testicular atrophy occurred in rats receiving Tegretol orally from 4 to 52 weeks at dosage levels of 50 to 400 mg/kg/day. Additionally, rats receiving Tegretol in the diet for two years at dosage levels of 25, 75, and 250 mg/kg/day had a dose-related incidence of testicular atrophy and aspermatogenesis. In dogs, it produced a brownish discoloration, presumably a metabolite, in the urinary bladder at dosage levels of 50 mg/kg and higher. Relevance of these findings to humans is unknown.

Nervous System: Dizziness, drowsiness, disturbances of coordination, confusion, headache, fatigue, blurred vision, visual hallucinations, transient diplopia, oculomotor disturbances, nystagmus, speech disturbances, abnormal involuntary movements, peripheral neuritis and paresthesias, depression with agitation, talkativeness, tinnitus, and hyperacusis.

There have been reports of associated paralysis and other symptoms of cerebral arterial insufficiency, but the exact relationship of these reactions to the drug has not been established.

Digestive System: Nausea, vomiting, gastric distress and abdominal pain, diarrhea, constipation, anorexia, and dryness of the mouth and pharynx, including glossitis and stomatitis.

Eyes: Scattered, punctate, cortical lens opacities, as well as conjunctivitis have been reported. Although a direct causal relationship has not been established, many phenothiazines and related drugs have been shown to cause eye changes.

Musculoskeletal System: Aching joints and muscles and leg cramps.

Metabolism: Fever and chills. Inappropriate antidiuretic hormone syndrome has been reported.

Drug Abuse and Dependence: No evidence of abuse potential has been associated with Tegretol, nor is there evidence of psychological or physical dependence in humans.

Overdosage:

Acute Toxicity

Lowest known lethal dose: adults, >60 g (39-year-old man). Highest known doses survived: adults, 30 g (31-year-old woman); children, 10 g (6-year-old boy); small children, 5 g (3-year-old girl).

Oral LD_{50} in animals (mg/kg); mice, 1100-3750; rats, 3850-4025; rabbits, 1500-2680; guinea pigs, 920.

Signs and Symptoms

The first signs and symptoms appear after 1-3 hours. Neuromuscular disturbances are the most prominent. Cardiovascular disorders are generally milder, and severe cardiac complications occur only when very high doses (>60 g) have been ingested.

Respiration: Irregular breathing, respiratory depression.

Cardiovascular System: Tachycardia, hypotension or hypertension, shock, conduction disorders.

Nervous System and Muscles: Impairment of consciousness ranging in severity to deep coma. Convulsions, especially in small children. Motor restlessness, muscular twitching, tremor, athetoid movements, opisthotonos, ataxia, drowsiness, dizziness, mydriasis, nystagmus, adiadochokinesia, ballism, psychomotor disturbances, dysmetria. Initial hyperreflexia, followed by hyporeflexia.

Gastrointestinal Tract: Nausea, vomiting.

Kidneys and Bladder: Anuria or oliguria, urinary retention.

Laboratory Findings: Isolated instances of overdosage have included leukocytosis, reduced leukocyte count, glycosuria and acetonuria. EEG may show dysrhythmias.

Combined Poisoning: When alcohol, tricyclic antidepressants, barbiturates or hydantoins are taken at the same time, the signs and symptoms of acute poisoning with Tegretol may be aggravated or modified.

Treatment

The prognosis in cases of severe poisoning is critically dependent upon prompt elimination of the drug, which may be achieved by inducing vomiting, irrigating the stomach, and by taking appropriate steps to diminish absorption. If these measures cannot be implemented without risk on the spot, the patient should be transferred at once to a hospital, while ensuring that vital functions are safeguarded. There is no specific antidote.

Elimination of the Drug: Induction of vomiting.

Gastric lavage. Even when more than 4 hours have elapsed following ingestion of the drug, the stomach should be repeatedly irrigated, especially if the patient has also consumed alcohol.

Measures to Reduce Absorption: Activated charcoal, laxatives.

Measures to Accelerate Elimination:

Forced diuresis.

Dialysis is indicated only in severe poisoning associated with renal failure. Replacement transfusion is indicated in severe poisoning in small children.

Respiratory Depression: Keep the airways free; resort, if necessary, to endotracheal intubation, artificial respiration, and administration of oxygen.

Hypotension, Shock: Keep the patient's legs raised and administer a plasma expander. If blood pressure fails to rise despite measures taken to increase plasma volume, use of vasoactive substances should be considered.

Convulsions: Diazepam or barbiturates.

Warning: Diazepam or barbiturates may aggravate respiratory depression (especially in children), hypotension, and coma. However, barbiturates should not be used if drugs that inhibit monoamine oxidase have also been taken by the patient either in overdosage or in recent therapy (within one week).

Surveillance: Respiration, cardiac function (ECG monitoring), blood pressure, body temperature, pupillary reflexes, and kidney and bladder function should be monitored for several days.

Treatment of Blood Count Abnormalities: If evidence of bone marrow depression develops, the following recommendations are suggested: 1) stop the drug, (2) perform daily CBC, platelet and reticulocyte counts, (3) do a bone marrow aspiration and trephine biopsy immediately and repeat with sufficient frequency to monitor recovery.

Special periodic studies might be helpful as follows: (1) white cell and platelet antibodies, (2) ^{59}Fe—ferrokinetic studies, (3) peripheral blood cell typing, (4) cytogenetic studies on marrow and peripheral blood, (5) bone marrow culture studies for colony-forming units, (6) hemoglobin electrophoresis for A_2 and F hemoglobin, and (7) serum folic acid and B_{12}levels.

A fully developed aplastic anemia will require appropriate, intensive monitoring and therapy, for which specialized consultation should be sought.

Dosage and Administration: Monitoring of blood levels has increased the efficacy and safety of anticonvulsants (see **PRECAUTIONS Laboratory Tests**). Dosage should be adjusted to the needs of the individual patient. A low initial daily dosage with a gradual increase is advised. As soon as adequate control is achieved, the dosage may be reduced very gradually to the minimum effective level. Tablets should be taken with meals.

Epilepsy (see **INDICATIONS AND USAGE**)

Adults and children over 12 years of age—Initial: 200 mg b.i.d. on the first day. Increase gradually by adding up to 200 mg per day using a t.i.d. or q.i.d. regimen until the best response is obtained. Dosage should generally not exceed 1000 mg daily in children 12 to 15 years of age, and 1200 mg daily in patients above 15 years of age. Doses up to 1600 mg daily have been used in adults in rare instances. ***Maintenance:*** Adjust dosage to the minimum effective level, usually 800-1200 mg daily.

Children 6-12 years of age—Initial: 100 mg b.i.d. on the first day. Increase gradually by adding 100 mg per day using a t.i.d. or q.i.d. regimen until the best response is obtained. Dosage should generally not exceed 1000 mg. ***Maintenance:*** Adjust dosage to the minimum effective level, usually 400–800 mg daily.

Combination Therapy: Tegretol may be used alone or with other anticonvulsants. When added to existing anticonvulsant therapy, the drug should be added gradually while the other anticonvulsants are maintained or gradually decreased, except phenytoin, which may have to be increased. (see **PRECAUTIONS Drug Interactions**).

Trigeminal Neuralgia (see **INDICATIONS AND USAGE**)

Initial: 100 mg b.i.d. on the first day for a total daily dose of 200 mg. This daily dose may be increased by up to 200 mg a day using increments of 100 mg every 12 hours only as needed to achieve freedom from pain. Do not exceed 1200 mg daily.

Maintenance: Control of pain can be maintained in most patients with 400 mg to 800 mg daily. However, some patients may be maintained on as little as 200 mg daily, while others may require as much as 1200 mg daily. At least once every 3 months throughout the treatment period, attempts should be made to reduce the dose to the minimum effective level or even to discontinue the drug.

How Supplied:

Chewable Tablets 100 mg—round, red-speckled, pink, single-scored (imprinted Geigy 47)

Bottles of 100 .... NDC 0028-0047-01

Unit Dose (blister pack)
Box of 100
(strips of 10) .... NDC 0028-0047-61

Tablets 200 mg—round, white, single-scored (imprinted Geigy 67)

Bottles of 100 .... NDC 0028-0067-01
Bottles of 1000 .... NDC 0028-0067-10

Gy-Pak®—One Unit
12 bottles—100 tablets each ....
.... NDC 0028-0067-65

Unit Dose (blister pack)
Box of 100
(strips of 10) .... NDC 0028-0067-61

Protect from moisture.

Dispense in tight container (USP).

C82-48 (1/83)

[*Shown in Product Identification Section*]

TOFRANIL® ℞

imipramine hydrochloride USP

Tablets of 10 mg	**GY-CODE 21**
Tablets of 25 mg	**GY-CODE 11**
Tablets of 50 mg	**GY-CODE 74**

For oral administration

Ampuls, 2 cc

For intramuscular administration

Each 2 cc ampul contains: imipramine hydrochloride USP, 25 mg; ascorbic acid, 2 mg; sodium bisulfite, 1 mg; sodium sulfite, anhydrous, 1 mg

Description: Tofranil, the original tricyclic antidepressant, is a member of the dibenzazepine group of compounds. It is designated 5-[3-(Dimethylamino)propyl] - 10, 11 - dihydro - 5H-dibenz[b,f]azepine Monohydrochloride. Its molecular weight is 316.9 and its empirical formula is $C_{19}H_{25}N_2Cl$.

Tofranil is a white, crystalline substance that turns yellowish or reddish on long exposure to light. It is easily soluble in water, fairly soluble in acetone or alcohol, but almost insoluble in ether. It melts at 170–174° C.

Clinical Pharmacology: The mechanism of action of Tofranil is not definitely known. However, it does not act primarily by stimulation of the central nervous system. The clinical effect is hypothesized as being due to potentiation of adrenergic synapses by blocking uptake of norepinephrine at nerve endings. The mode of action of the drug in controlling childhood enuresis is thought to be apart from its antidepressant effect.

Indications: *Depression:* For the relief of symptoms of depression. Endogenous depression is more likely to be alleviated than other depressive states. One to three weeks of treatment may be needed before optimal therapeutic effects are evident.

Childhood Enuresis: May be useful as temporary adjunctive therapy in reducing enuresis in children aged 6 years and older, after possible organic causes have been excluded by appropriate tests. In patients having daytime symptoms of frequency and urgency, examination should include voiding cystourethrography and cystoscopy, as necessary. The effectiveness of treatment may decrease with continued drug administration.

Contraindications: The concomitant use of monoamine oxidase inhibiting compounds is contraindicated. Hyperpyretic crises or severe convulsive seizures may occur in patients receiving such combinations. The potentiation of adverse effects can be serious, or even fatal. When it is desired to substitute Tofranil in patients receiving a monoamine oxidase inhibitor, as long an interval should elapse as the clinical situation will allow, with a minimum of 14 days. Initial dosage should be low and increases should be gradual and cautiously prescribed.

The drug is contraindicated during the acute recovery period after a myocardial infarction. Patients with a known hypersensitivity to this compound should not be given the drug. The possibility of cross-sensitivity to other dibenzazepine compounds should be kept in mind.

Warnings:

Children: A dose of 2.5 mg/kg/day of imipramine hydrochloride should not be exceeded in childhood. ECG changes of unknown significance have been reported in pediatric patients with doses twice this amount.

Extreme caution should be used when this drug is given to:

- patients with cardiovascular disease because of the possibility of conduction defects, arrhythmias, congestive heart failure, myocardial infarction, strokes and tachycardia. These patients require cardiac surveillance at all dosage levels of the drug;
- patients with increased intraocular pressure, history of urinary retention, or history of narrow-angle glaucoma because of the drug's anticholinergic properties;
- hyperthyroid patients or those on thyroid medication because of the possibility of cardiovascular toxicity;
- patients with a history of seizure disorder because this drug has been shown to lower the seizure threshold;
- patients receiving guanethidine, clonidine, or similar agents, since imipramine hydrochloride may block the pharmacologic effects of these drugs;
- patients receiving methylphenidate hydrochloride. Since methylphenidate hydrochloride may inhibit the metabolism of imipramine hydrochloride, downward dosage adjustment of imipramine hydrochloride may be required when given concomitantly with methylphenidate hydrochloride.

Tofranil may enhance the CNS depressant effects of alcohol. Therefore, it should be borne in mind that the dangers inherent in a suicide attempt or accidental overdosage with the drug may be increased for the patient who uses excessive amounts of alcohol. (See **Precautions.**)

Since imipramine hydrochloride may impair the mental and/or physical abilities required for the performance of potentially hazardous tasks, such as operating an automobile or machinery, the patient should be cautioned accordingly.

Precautions: An ECG recording should be taken prior to the initiation of larger-than-usual doses of imipramine hydrochloride and at appropriate intervals thereafter until steady state is achieved. (Patients with any evidence of cardiovascular disease require cardiac surveillance at all dosage levels of the drug. See **Warnings.**) Elderly patients and patients with cardiac disease or a prior history of cardiac disease are at special risk of developing the cardiac abnormalities associated with the use of imipramine hydrochloride.

It should be kept in mind that the possibility of suicide in seriously depressed patients is inherent in the illness and may persist until significant remission occurs. Such patients should be carefully supervised during the early phase of treatment with imipramine hydrochloride, and may require hospitalization. Prescriptions should be written for the smallest amount feasible.

Hypomanic or manic episodes may occur, particularly in patients with cyclic disorders. Such reactions may necessitate discontinuation of the drug. If needed, imipramine hydrochloride may be resumed in lower dosage when these episodes are relieved. Administration of a tranquilizer may be useful in controlling such episodes.

Continued on next page

The full prescribing information for each GEIGY drug is contained herein and is that in effect as of October 1, 1982.

Geigy—Cont.

An activation of the psychosis may occasionally be observed in schizophrenic patients and may require reduction of dosage and the addition of a phenothiazine.
Concurrent administration of imipramine hydrochloride with electroshock therapy may increase the hazards; such treatment should be limited to those patients for whom it is essential, since there is limited clinical experience.

Usage During Pregnancy and Lactation:

Animal reproduction studies have yielded inconclusive results. (See also **Animal Pharmacology & Toxicology.**)

There have been no well-controlled studies conducted with pregnant women to determine the effect of imipramine hydrochloride on the fetus. However, there have been clinical reports of congenital malformations associated with the use of the drug. Although a causal relationship between these effects and the drug could not be established, the possibility of fetal risk from the maternal ingestion of imipramine hydrochloride cannot be excluded. Therefore, imipramine hydrochloride should be used in women who are or might become pregnant only if the clinical condition clearly justifies potential risk to the fetus.

Limited data suggest that imipramine hydrochloride is likely to be excreted in human breast milk. As a general rule, a women taking a drug should not nurse since the possibility exists that the drug may be excreted in breast milk and be harmful to the child.

Usage in Children: The effectiveness of the drug in children for conditions other than nocturnal enuresis has not been established.

The safety and effectiveness of the drug as temporary adjunctive therapy for nocturnal enuresis in children less than 6 years of age has not been established.

The safety of the drug for long-term, chronic use as adjunctive therapy for nocturnal enuresis in children 6 years of age or older has not been established; consideration should be given to instituting a drug-free period following an adequate therapeutic trial with a favorable response.

A dose of 2.5 mg/kg/day should not be exceeded in childhood. ECG changes of unknown significance have been reported in pediatric patients with doses twice this amount.

Patients should be warned that imipramine hydrochloride may enhance the CNS depressant effects of alcohol. (See **Warnings.**)
Imipramine hydrochloride should be used with caution in patients with significantly impaired renal or hepatic function.
Patients who develop a fever and a sore throat during therapy with imipramine hydrochloride should have leukocyte and differential blood counts performed. Imipramine hydrochloride should be discontinued if there is evidence of pathological neutrophil depression.
Prior to elective surgery, imipramine hydrochloride should be discontinued for as long as the clinical situation will allow.
In occasional susceptible patients or in those receiving anticholinergic drugs (including antiparkinsonism agents) in addition, the atropine-like effects may become more pronounced (e.g., paralytic ileus). Close supervision and careful adjustment of dosage is required when imipramine hydrochloride is administered concomitantly with anticholinergic drugs.
Avoid the use of preparations, such as decongestants and local anesthetics, which contain any sympathomimetic amine (e.g., epinephrine, norepinephrine), since it has been reported that tricyclic antidepressants can potentiate the effects of catecholamines.
Caution should be exercised when imipramine hydrochloride is used with agents that lower blood pressure.
Imipramine hydrochloride may potentiate the effects of CNS depressant drugs.
Patients taking imipramine hydrochloride should avoid excessive exposure to sunlight since there have been reports of photosensitization.
Both elevation and lowering of blood sugar levels have been reported with imipramine hydrochloride use.
The Tofranil tablets (10, 25, 50 mg) contain FD&C Yellow No. 5 (tartrazine) which may cause allergic-type reactions (including bronchial asthma) in certain susceptible individuals. Although the overall incidence of FD&C Yellow No. 5 (tartrazine) sensitivity in the general population is low, it is frequently seen in patients who also have aspirin hypersensitivity.

Adverse Reactions: Note: Although the listing which follows includes a few adverse reactions which have not been reported with this specific drug, the pharmacological similarities among the tricyclic antidepressant drugs require that each of the reactions be considered when imipramine is administered.
Cardiovascular: Orthostatic hypotension, hypertension, tachycardia, palpitation, myocardial infarction, arrhythmias, heart block, ECG changes, precipitation of congestive heart failure, stroke.
Psychiatric: Confusional states (especially in the elderly) with hallucinations, disorientation, delusions; anxiety, restlessness, agitation; insomnia and nightmares; hypomania; exacerbation of psychosis.
Neurological: Numbness, tingling, paresthesias of extremities; incoordination, ataxia, tremors; peripheral neuropathy; extrapyramidal symptoms; seizures, alterations in EEG patterns; tinnitus.
Anticholinergic: Dry mouth, and, rarely, associated sublingual adenitis; blurred vision, disturbances of accommodation, mydriasis; constipation, paralytic ileus; urinary retention, delayed micturition, dilation of the urinary tract.
Allergic: Skin rash, petechiae, urticaria, itching, photosensitization; edema (general or of face and tongue); drug fever; cross-sensitivity with desipramine.
Hematologic: Bone marrow depression including agranulocytosis; eosinophilia; purpura; thrombocytopenia.
Gastrointestinal: Nausea and vomiting, anorexia, epigastric distress, diarrhea; peculiar taste, stomatitis, abdominal cramps, black tongue.
Endocrine: Gynecomastia in the male; breast enlargement and galactorrhea in the female; increased or decreased libido, impotence; testicular swelling; elevation or depression of blood sugar levels.
Other: Jaundice (simulating obstructive); altered liver function; weight gain or loss; perspiration; flushing; urinary frequency; drowsiness; dizziness, weakness and fatigue; headache; parotid swelling; alopecia; proneness to falling.
Withdrawal Symptoms: Though not indicative of addiction, abrupt cessation of treatment after prolonged therapy may produce nausea, headache and malaise.
Note: In enuretic children treated with Tofranil the most common adverse reactions have been nervousness, sleep disorders, tiredness, and mild gastrointestinal disturbances. These usually disappear during continued drug administration or when dosage is decreased. Other reactions which have been reported include constipation, convulsions, anxiety, emotional instability, syncope, and collapse. All of the adverse effects reported with adult use should be considered.

Dosage and Administration:
Depression: Lower dosages are recommended for elderly patients and adolescents. Lower dosages are also recommended for outpatients as compared to hospitalized patients who will be under close supervision. Dosage should be initiated at a low level and increased gradually, noting carefully the clinical response and any evidence of intolerance. Following remission, maintenance medication may be required for a longer period of time, at the lowest dose that will maintain remission.
Parenteral administration should be used only for starting therapy in patients unable or unwilling to use oral medication. The oral form should supplant the injectable as soon as possible.
Oral:—Usual Adult Dose: Hospitalized patients—Initially, 100 mg/day in divided doses gradually increased to 200 mg/day as required. If no response after two weeks, increase to 250-300 mg/day.
Outpatients—Initially, 75 mg/day increased to 150 mg/day. Dosages over 200 mg/day are not recommended. Maintenance, 50-150 mg/day.
Adolescent and geriatric patients—Initially, 30–40 mg/day; it is generally not necessary to exceed 100 mg/day.
Parenteral: Initially, up to 100 mg/day intramuscularly in divided doses.
Childhood Enuresis: Initially, an oral dose of 25 mg/day should be tried in children aged 6 and older. Medication should be given one hour before bedtime. If a satisfactory response does not occur within one week, increase the dose to 50 mg nightly in children under 12 years; children over 12 may receive up to 75 mg nightly. A daily dose greater than 75 mg does not enhance efficacy and tends to increase side effects. Evidence suggests that in early night bedwetters, the drug is more effective given earlier and in divided amounts, i.e., 25 mg in midafternoon, repeated at bedtime. Consideration should be given to instituting a drug-free period following an adequate therapeutic trial with a favorable response. Dosage should be tapered off gradually rather than abruptly discontinued; this may reduce the tendency to relapse. Children who relapse when the drug is discontinued do not always respond to a subsequent course of treatment.
A dose of 2.5 mg/kg/day should not be exceeded. ECG changes of unknown significance have been reported in pediatric patients with doses twice this amount.
The safety and effectiveness of Tofranil as temporary adjunctive therapy for nocturnal enuresis in children less than 6 years of age has not been established.

Overdosage: Children have been reported to be more sensitive than adults to an acute overdosage of imipramine hydrochloride. An acute overdose of any amount in infants or young children, especially, must be considered serious and potentially fatal.
Signs and Symptoms: These may vary in severity depending upon factors such as the amount of drug absorbed, the age of the patient, and the interval between drug ingestion and the start of treatment. Blood and urine levels of imipramine may not reflect the severity of poisoning; they have chiefly a qualitative rather than quantitative value, and are unreliable indicators in the clinical management of the patient.
CNS abnormalities may include drowsiness, stupor, coma, ataxia, restlessness, agitation, hyperactive reflexes, muscle rigidity, athetoid and choreiform movements, and convulsions.
Cardiac abnormalities may include arrhythmia, tachycardia, ECG evidence of impaired conduction, and signs of congestive failure.
Respiratory depression, cyanosis, hypotension, shock, vomiting, hyperpyrexia, mydriasis, and diaphoresis may also be present.
Treatment: Because CNS involvement, respiratory depression and cardiac arrhythmia can occur suddenly, hospitalization and close ob-

servation are necessary, even when the amount ingested is thought to be small or the initial degree of intoxication appears slight or moderate. All patients with ECG abnormalities should have continuous cardiac monitoring for at least 72 hours and be closely observed until well after cardiac status has returned to normal; relapses may occur after apparent recovery.

The *slow* intravenous administration of physostigmine salicylate has been reported to reverse most of the cardiovascular and CNS effects of overdosage with tricyclic antidepressants. In adults, 1 to 3 mg has been reported to be effective. In children, start with 0.5 mg and repeat at 5-minute intervals to determine the minimum effective dose; do not exceed 2 mg. Because of the short duration of action of physostigmine, repeat the effective dose at 30- to 60-minute intervals, as necessary. Avoid rapid injection to reduce the possibility of physostigmine-induced convulsions.

In the alert patient, empty the stomach promptly by induced emesis followed by lavage. In the obtunded patient, secure the airway with a cuffed endotracheal tube before beginning lavage (do not induce emesis). Continue lavage for 24 hours or longer, depending on the apparent severity of intoxication. Use normal or half-normal saline to avoid water intoxication, especially in children. Instillation of activated charcoal slurry may help reduce absorption of imipramine.

Minimize external stimulation to reduce the tendency to convulsions. If anticonvulsants are necessary, diazepam, short-acting barbiturates, paraldehyde or methocarbamol may be useful. Do not use barbiturates if MAO inhibitors have been taken recently.

Maintain adequate respiratory exchange. Do not use respiratory stimulants.

Shock should be treated with supportive measures, such as intravenous fluids, oxygen and corticosteroids. Digitalis may increase conduction abnormalities and further irritate an already sensitized myocardium. If congestive heart failure necessitates rapid digitalization, particular care must be exercised.

Hyperpyrexia should be controlled by whatever external means are available, including ice packs and cooling sponge baths, if necessary.

Hemodialysis, peritoneal dialysis, exchange transfusions and forced diuresis have been generally reported as ineffective because of the rapid fixation of imipramine in tissues. Blood and urine levels of imipramine may not correlate with the degree of intoxication, and are unreliable indicators in the clinical management of the patient.

How Supplied: Triangular, sugar-coated, coral-colored tablets of 10 mg in bottles of 100 and 1000; round, sugar-coated, coral-colored (black Geigy imprint) tablets of 25 mg in bottles of 100, 1000 and 5000 and unit strip packages of 100; round, sugar-coated, coral-colored (white Geigy imprint) tablets of 50 mg in bottles of 100, 1000 and 5000 and unit strip packages of 100; ampuls for intramuscular administration only, each containing 25 mg in 2 cc of solution (1.25%), in boxes of 10.

Note: On storage, very minute crystals may form in some ampuls. This has no influence on the therapeutic efficacy of the preparation, and the crystals redissolve when the affected ampuls are immersed in hot tap water for one minute.

Animal Pharmacology & Toxicology:

A. *Acute:* Oral LD_{50} ranges are as follows:

Rat	355 to 682 mg/kg
Dog	100 to 215 mg/kg

Depending on the dosage in both species, toxic signs proceeded progressively from depression, irregular respiration and ataxia to convulsions and death.

B. *Reproduction/Teratogenic:* The overall evaluation may be summed up in the following manner:

Oral: Independent studies in three species (rat, mouse and rabbit) revealed that when Tofranil is administered orally in doses up to approximately 2½ times the maximum human dose in the first 2 species and up to 25 times the maximum human dose in the third species, the drug is essentially free from teratogenic potential. In the three species studied, only one instance of fetal abnormality occurred (in the rabbit) and in that study there was likewise an abnormality in the control group. However, evidence does exist from the rat studies that some systemic and embryotoxic potential is demonstrable. This is manifested by reduced litter size, a slight increase in the stillborn rate and a reduction in the mean birth weight.

Parenteral: In contradistinction to the oral data, Tofranil does exhibit a slight but definite teratogenic potential when administered by the subcutaneous route. Drug effects on both the mother and fetus in the rabbit are manifested in higher resorption rates and decrease in mean fetal birth weights, while teratogenic findings occurred at a level of 5 times the maximum human dose. In the mouse, teratogenicity occurred at 1½ and 6½ times the maximum human dose, but no teratogenic effects were seen at levels 3 times the maximum human dose. Thus, in the mouse, the findings are equivocal.

Dispense in tight container (USP).

C80-3 (1/80)

[*Shown in Product Identification Section*]

For full prescribing information on Enuresis, please refer to Tofranil® imipramine hydrochloride USP, on page 973.

TOFRANIL-PM® ℞

imipramine pamoate

Capsules of 75 mg	**GY-CODE 20**
Capsules of 100 mg	**GY-CODE 40**
Capsules of 125 mg	**GY-CODE 45**
Capsules of 150 mg	**GY-CODE 22**

For oral administration

Each 75-mg capsule contains imipramine pamoate equivalent to 75 mg of imipramine hydrochloride.

Each 100-mg capsule contains imipramine pamoate equivalent to 100 mg of imipramine hydrochloride.

Each 125-mg capsule contains imipramine pamoate equivalent to 125 mg of imipramine hydrochloride.

Each 150-mg capsule contains imipramine pamoate equivalent to 150 mg of imipramine hydrochloride.

Description: Tofranil-PM is the pamoate salt of imipramine. It is designated bis 5-[3-(Dimethylamino)propyl] - 10, 11 - dihydro - 5H-dibenz[b,f]azepine compound (2:1) with 4,4-methylene-bis- [3-hydroxy-2-naphthoic acid] with the empirical formula $C_{61}H_{64}N_4O_6$.

Tofranil-PM is a fine, yellow, tasteless and odorless powder. It is soluble in ethyl alcohol, acetone, ethyl ether, chloroform and carbon tetrachloride. It is insoluble in water.

Clinical Pharmacology: The mechanism of action of imipramine is not definitely known. However, it does not act primarily by stimulation of the central nervous system. The clinical effect is hypothesized as being due to potentiation of adrenergic synapses by blocking uptake of norepinephrine at nerve endings.

Indications: For the relief of symptoms of depression. Endogenous depression is more likely to be alleviated than other depressive states. One to three weeks of treatment may be needed before optimal therapeutic effects are evident.

Contraindications: The concomitant use of monoamine oxidase inhibiting compounds is contraindicated. Hyperpyretic crises or severe convulsive seizures may occur in patients receiving such combinations. The potentiation of adverse effects can be serious, or even fatal. When it is desired to substitute Tofranil-PM in patients receiving a monoamine oxidase inhibitor, as long an interval should elapse as the clinical situation will allow, with a minimum of 14 days. Initial dosage should be low and increases should be gradual and cautiously prescribed.

The drug is contraindicated during the acute recovery period after a myocardial infarction. Patients with a known hypersensitivity to this compound should not be given the drug. The possibility of cross-sensitivity to other dibenzazepine compounds should be kept in mind.

Warnings: Extreme caution should be used when this drug is given to:

- patients with cardiovascular disease because of the possibility of conduction defects, arrhythmias, congestive heart failure, myocardial infarction, strokes and tachycardia. These patients require cardiac surveillance at all dosage levels of the drug;
- patients with increased intraocular pressure, history of urinary retention, or history of narrow-angle glaucoma because of the drug's anticholinergic properties;
- hyperthyroid patients or those on thyroid medication because of the possibility of cardiovascular toxicity;
- patients with a history of seizure disorder because this drug has been shown to lower the seizure threshold;
- patients receiving guanethidine, clonidine, or similar agents, since imipramine pamoate may block the pharmacologic effects of these drugs;
- patients receiving methylphenidate hydrochloride. Since methylphenidate hydrochloride may inhibit the metabolism of imipramine pamoate, downward dosage adjustment of imipramine pamoate may be required when given concomitantly with methylphenidate hydrochloride.

Since imipramine pamoate may impair the mental and/or physical abilities required for the performance of potentially hazardous tasks, such as operating an automobile or machinery, the patient should be cautioned accordingly.

Tofranil-PM may enhance the CNS depressant effects of alcohol. Therefore, it should be borne in mind that the dangers inherent in a suicide attempt or accidental overdosage with the drug may be increased for the patient who uses excessive amounts of alcohol. (See **Precautions.**)

Usage in Children: Tofranil-PM should not be used in children of any age because of the increased potential for acute overdosage due to the high unit potency (75 mg, 100 mg, 125 mg and 150 mg). Each capsule contains imipra-

Continued on next page

The full prescribing information for each GEIGY drug is contained herein and is that in effect as of October 1, 1982.

Geigy—Cont.

mine pamoate equivalent to 75 mg, 100 mg, 125 mg or 150 mg imipramine hydrochloride.

Precautions: An ECG recording should be taken prior to the initiation of larger-than-usual doses of imipramine pamoate and at appropriate intervals thereafter until steady state is achieved. (Patients with any evidence of cardiovascular disease require cardiac surveillance at all dosage levels of the drug. See **Warnings.**) Elderly patients and patients with cardiac disease or a prior history of cardiac disease are at special risk of developing the cardiac abnormalities associated with the use of imipramine pamoate. It should be kept in mind that the possibility of suicide in seriously depressed patients is inherent in the illness and may persist until significant remission occurs. Such patients should be carefully supervised during the early phase of treatment with imipramine pamoate and may require hospitalization. Prescriptions should be written for the smallest amount feasible.

Hypomanic or manic episodes may occur, particularly in patients with cyclic disorders. Such reactions may necessitate discontinuation of the drug. If needed, imipramine pamoate may be resumed in lower dosage when these episodes are relieved. Administration of a tranquilizer may be useful in controlling such episodes.

An activation of the psychosis may occasionally be observed in schizophrenic patients and may require reduction of dosage and the addition of a phenothiazine.

Concurrent administration of imipramine pamoate with electroshock therapy may increase the hazards; such treatment should be limited to those patients for whom it is essential, since there is limited clinical experience.

Usage During Pregnancy and Lactation:

Animal reproduction studies have yielded inconclusive results. (See also **Animal Pharmacology & Toxicology.**)

There have been no well-controlled studies conducted with pregnant women to determine the effect of imipramine on the fetus. However, there have been clinical reports of congenital malformations associated with the use of the drug. Although a causal relationship between these effects and the drug could not be established, the possibility of fetal risk from the maternal ingestion of imipramine cannot be excluded. Therefore, imipramine should be used in women who are or might become pregnant only if the clinical condition clearly justifies potential risk to the fetus.

Limited data suggest that imipramine is likely to be excreted in human breast milk. As a general rule, a woman taking a drug should not nurse since the possibility exists that the drug may be excreted in breast milk and be harmful to the child.

Patients should be warned that imipramine pamoate may enhance the CNS depressant effects of alcohol. (See **Warnings.**)

Imipramine pamoate should be used with caution in patients with significantly impaired renal or hepatic function.

Patients who develop a fever and a sore throat during therapy with imipramine pamoate should have leukocyte and differential blood counts performed. Imipramine pamoate should be discontinued if there is evidence of pathological neutrophil depression.

Prior to elective surgery, imipramine pamoate should be discontinued for as long as the clinical situation will allow.

In occasional susceptible patients or in those receiving anticholinergic drugs (including antiparkinsonism agents) in addition, the atropine-like effects may become more pronounced (e.g., paralytic ileus). Close supervision and careful adjustment of dosage is required when imipramine pamoate is administered concomitantly with anticholinergic drugs.

Avoid the use of preparations, such as decongestants and local anesthetics, which contain any sympathomimetic amine (e.g., epinephrine, norepinephrine), since it has been reported that tricyclic antidepressants can potentiate the effects of catecholamines.

Caution should be exercised when imipramine pamoate is used with agents that lower blood pressure.

Imipramine pamoate may potentiate the effects of CNS depressant drugs.

Patients taking imipramine pamoate should avoid excessive exposure to sunlight since there have been reports of photosensitization.

Both elevation and lowering of blood sugar levels have been reported with imipramine pamoate use.

The Tofranil-PM capsules (100 and 125 mg) contain FD&C Yellow No. 5 (tartrazine) which may cause allergic-type reactions (including bronchial asthma) in certain susceptible individuals. Although the overall incidence of FD&C Yellow No. 5 (tartrazine) sensitivity in the general population is low, it is frequently seen in patients who also have aspirin hypersensitivity.

Adverse Reactions: Note: Although the listing which follows includes a few adverse reactions which have not been reported with this specific drug, the pharmacological similarities among the tricyclic antidepressant drugs require that each of the reactions be considered when imipramine is administered.

Cardiovascular: Orthostatic hypotension, hypertension, tachycardia, palpitation, myocardial infarction, arrhythmias, heart block, ECG changes, precipitation of congestive heart failure, stroke.

Psychiatric: Confusional states (especially in the elderly) with hallucinations, disorientation, delusions; anxiety, restlessness, agitation; insomnia and nightmares; hypomania; exacerbation of psychosis.

Neurological: Numbness, tingling, paresthesias of extremities; incoordination, ataxia, tremors; peripheral neuropathy; extrapyramidal symptoms; seizures, alterations in EEG patterns; tinnitus.

Anticholinergic: Dry mouth, and, rarely, associated sublingual adenitis; blurred vision, disturbances of accommodation, mydriasis; constipation, paralytic ileus; urinary retention, delayed micturition, dilation of the urinary tract.

Allergic: Skin rash, petechiae, urticaria, itching, photosensitization; edema (general or of face and tongue); drug fever; cross-sensitivity with desipramine.

Hematologic: Bone marrow depression including agranulocytosis; eosinophilia; purpura; thrombocytopenia.

Gastrointestinal: Nausea and vomiting, anorexia, epigastric distress, diarrhea; peculiar taste, stomatitis, abdominal cramps, black tongue.

Endocrine: Gynecomastia in the male; breast enlargement and galactorrhea in the female; increased or decreased libido, impotence; testicular swelling; elevation or depression of blood sugar levels.

Other: Jaundice (simulating obstructive); altered liver function; weight gain or loss; perspiration; flushing; urinary frequency; drowsiness, dizziness, weakness and fatigue; headache; parotid swelling; alopecia; proneness to falling.

Withdrawal Symptoms: Though not indicative of addiction, abrupt cessation of treatment after prolonged therapy may produce nausea, headache and malaise.

Dosage and Administration: The following recommended dosages for Tofranil-PM should be modified as necessary by the clinical response and any evidence of intolerance.

Initial Adult Dosage:

Outpatients—Therapy should be initiated at 75 mg/day. Dosage may be increased to 150 mg/day which is the dose level at which optimum response is usually obtained. If necessary, dosage may be increased to 200 mg/day. Dosage higher than 75 mg/day may also be administered on a once-a-day basis after the optimum dosage and tolerance have been determined. The daily dosage may be given at bedtime. In some patients it may be necessary to employ a divided-dose schedule.

As with all tricyclics, the antidepressant effect of imipramine may not be evident for one to three weeks in some patients.

Hospitalized Patients—Therapy should be initiated at 100–150 mg/day and may be increased to 200 mg/day. If there is no response after two weeks, dosage should be increased to 250–300 mg/day.

Dosage higher than 150 mg/day may also be administered on a once-a-day basis after the optimum dosage and tolerance have been determined. The daily dosage may be given at bedtime. In some patients it may be necessary to employ a divided-dose schedule.

As with all tricyclics, the antidepressant effect of imipramine may not be evident for one to three weeks in some patients.

Adult Maintenance Dosage: Following remission, maintenance medication may be required for a longer period of time at the lowest dose that will maintain remission after which the dosage should gradually be decreased.

The usual maintenance dosage is 75–150 mg/day. The total daily dosage can be administered on a once-a-day basis, preferably at bedtime. In some patients it may be necessary to employ a divided-dose schedule.

In cases of relapse due to premature withdrawal of the drug, the effective dosage of imipramine should be reinstituted.

Adolescent and Geriatric Patients: Therapy in these age groups should be initiated with Tofranil®, brand of imipramine hydrochloride, tablets at a total daily dosage of 25–50 mg, since Tofranil-PM capsules are not available in these strengths. Dosage may be increased according to response and tolerance, but it is generally unnecessary to exceed 100 mg/day in these patients. Tofranil-PM capsules may be used when total daily dosage is established at 75 mg or higher.

The total daily dosage can be administered on a once-a-day basis, preferably at bedtime. In some patients it may be necessary to employ a divided-dose schedule.

As with all tricyclics, the antidepressant effect of imipramine may not be evident for one to three weeks in some patients.

Adolescent and geriatric patients can usually be maintained at lower dosage. Following remission, maintenance medication may be required for a longer period of time at the lowest dose that will maintain remission after which the dosage should gradually be decreased.

The total daily maintenance dosage can be administered on a once-a-day basis, preferably at bedtime. In some patients it may be necessary to employ a divided-dose schedule.

In cases of relapse due to premature withdrawal of the drug, the effective dosage of imipramine should be reinstituted.

Overdosage: Children have been reported to be more sensitive than adults to an acute overdosage of imipramine pamoate. An acute overdose of any amount in infants or young children, especially, must be considered serious and potentially fatal.

Signs and Symptoms: These may vary in severity depending upon factors such as the amount of drug absorbed, the age of the patient, and the interval between drug ingestion and the start of treatment. Blood and urine levels of imipramine may not reflect the severity of poisoning; they have chiefly a qualitative rather than quantitative value, and are unreliable indicators in the clinical management of the patient.

CNS abnormalities may include drowsiness, stupor, coma, ataxia, restlessness, agitation, hyperactive reflexes, muscle rigidity, athetoid and choreiform movements, and convulsions.

Cardiac abnormalities may include arrhythmia, tachycardia, ECG evidence of impaired conduction, and signs of congestive failure.

Respiratory depression, cyanosis, hypotension, shock, vomiting, hyperpyrexia, mydriasis, and diaphoresis may also be present.

Treatment: Because CNS involvement, respiratory depression and cardiac arrhythmia can occur suddenly, hospitalization and close observation are necessary, even when the amount ingested is thought to be small or the initial degree of intoxication appears slight or moderate. All patients with ECG abnormalities should have continuous cardiac monitoring for at least 72 hours and be closely observed until well after cardiac status has returned to normal; relapses may occur after apparent recovery.

The *slow* intravenous administration of physostigmine salicylate has been reported to reverse most of the cardiovascular and CNS effects of overdosage with tricyclic antidepressants. In adults, 1 to 3 mg has been reported to be effective. In children, start with 0.5 mg and repeat at 5-minute intervals to determine the minimum effective dose; do not exceed 2 mg. Because of the short duration of action of physostigmine, repeat the effective dose at 30- to 60-minute intervals, as necessary. Avoid rapid injection to reduce the possibility of physostigmine-induced convulsions.

In the alert patient, empty the stomach promptly by induced emesis followed by lavage. In the obtunded patient, secure the airway with a cuffed endotracheal tube before beginning lavage (do not induce emesis). Continue lavage for 24 hours or longer, depending on the apparent severity of intoxication. Use normal or half-normal saline to avoid water intoxication, especially in children. Instillation of activated charcoal slurry may help reduce absorption of imipramine.

Minimize external stimulation to reduce the tendency to convulsions. If anticonvulsants are necessary, diazepam, short-acting barbiturates, paraldehyde or methocarbamol may be useful. Do not use barbiturates if MAO inhibitors have been taken recently.

Maintain adequate respiratory exchange. Do not use respiratory stimulants.

Shock should be treated with supportive measures, such as intravenous fluids, oxygen and corticosteroids. Digitalis may increase conduction abnormalities and further irritate an already sensitized myocardium. If congestive heart failure necessitates rapid digitalization, particular care must be exercised.

Hyperpyrexia should be controlled by whatever external means are available, including ice packs and cooling sponge baths, if necessary.

Hemodialysis, peritoneal dialysis, exchange transfusions and forced diuresis have been generally reported as ineffective because of the rapid fixation of imipramine in tissues. Blood and urine levels of imipramine may not correlate with the degree of intoxication, and are unreliable indicators in the clinical management of the patient.

How Supplied: Tofranil-PM is available as follows:

75-mg, coral-colored capsules equivalent to 75 mg imipramine hydrochloride in bottles of 30, 100 and 1,000 capsules, and unit strip packages of 100.

100-mg, dark yellow/coral-colored capsules equivalent to 100 mg imipramine hydrochloride in bottles of 30, 100 and 1,000 capsules.

125-mg, light yellow/coral-colored capsules equivalent to 125 mg imipramine hydrochloride in bottles of 30, 100 and 1,000 capsules.

150-mg, coral-colored capsules equivalent to 150 mg imipramine hydrochloride in bottles of 30, 100 and 1,000 capsules, and unit strip packages of 100.

Animal Pharmacology & Toxicology

A. *Acute:* Oral LD_{50}:

Mouse	2185 mg/kg
Rat (F)	1142 mg/kg
(M)	1807 mg/kg
Rabbit	1016 mg/kg
Dog	693 mg/kg (Emesis ED_{50})

B. *Subacute:*

Two three-month studies in dogs gave evidence of an adverse drug effect on the testes, but only at the highest dose level employed, i.e., 90 mg/kg (10 times the maximum human dose). Depending on the histological section of the testes examined, the findings consisted of a range of degenerative changes up to and including complete atrophy of the seminiferous tubules, with spermatogenesis usually arrested.

Human studies show no definitive effect on sperm count, sperm motility, sperm morphology or volume of ejaculate.

Rat

One three-month study was done in rats at dosage levels comparable to those of the dog studies. No adverse drug effect on the testes was noted in this study, as confirmed by histological examination.

C. *Reproduction/Teratogenic:*

Oral: Imipramine pamoate was fed to male and female albino rats for 28 weeks through two breeding cycles at dose levels of 15 mg/kg/day and 40 mg/kg/day (equivalent to 2½ and 7 times the maximum human dose). No abnormalities which could be related to drug administration were noted in gross inspection. Autopsies performed on pups from the second breeding likewise revealed no pathological changes in organs or tissues; however, a decrease in mean litter size from both matings was noted in the drug-treated groups and significant growth suppression occurred in the nursing pups of both sexes in the high group as well as in the females of the low-level group. Finally, the lactation index (pups weaned divided by number left to nurse) was significantly lower in the second litter of the high-level group.

Dispense in tight container (USP).

C80-9 (1/80)

[*Shown in Product Identification Section*]

Geneva Generics

2599 W. MIDWAY BLVD.
BROOMFIELD, CO 80020

NDC 0781	PRODUCT	
	APAP w/CODEINE TABLETS	℞ Ⓒ
1752-01	½ gr., 100's	
1654-01	1 gr., 100's	
	AMINOPHYLLINE TABLETS	℞
1214-01	1 ½ gr., 100's	
1318-01	3 gr., 100's	
	AMITRIPTYLINE HCl. TABLETS	℞
1486-01	10mg., 100's	
1487-01	25mg., 100's	
1488-01	50mg., 100's	
1489-01	75mg., 100's	
1490-01	100mg., 100's	
1491-01	150mg., 100's	
7210-70	**ANTIBIOTIC EAR DROPS** 10 cc	℞
	ASPIRIN (325mg.) w/CODEINE TABLETS	℞ Ⓒ
1660-01	30mg. (½ gr.), 100's	
1875-01	60mg. (1 gr.), 100's	
1225-01	**AZO-SULFISOXAZOLE TABLETS** 100's	℞
7023-01	**BISACODYL SUPPOSITORIES** 10mg., 100's	OTC
1307-01	**CALTRO TABLETS** (Vitamin D-2, Calcium—from Oyster Shell Powder, with Trace Minerals from Oyster Shell), 100's	OTC
1050-01	**CARISOPRODOL TABLETS** 100's	℞
1055-01	**CARISOPRODOL COMPOUND TABLETS** (Carisoprodol, Phenacetin, Caffeine), 100's	℞
2235-01	**CHLORAL HYDRATE CAPSULES** 500mg., 100's	℞ Ⓒ
	CHLORDIAZEPOXIDE CAPSULES	℞ Ⓒ
2080-01	5mg., 100's	
2082-01	10mg., 100's	
2084-01	25 mg., 100's	
	CHLOROTHIAZIDE TABLETS	℞
1944-01	250mg., 100's	
1940-01	500mg., 100's	
1970-01	**CHLOROTHIAZIDE (250mg.) w/RESERPINE TABLETS** 0.125mg., 100's	℞
	CHLORPHENIRAMINE MALEATE T.D. CAPSULES	℞
2602-01	8mg., 100's	
2699-01	12mg., 100's	
	CHLORPROMAZINE HCl. TABLETS	℞
1715-01	10mg., 100's	
1716-01	25mg., 100's	
1717-01	50mg., 100's	
1718-01	100mg., 100's	
1719-01	200mg., 100's	
4009-08	**CHLORPROMAZINE CONCENTRATE SYRUP** 100mg./cc., 8 oz.	℞
1698-01	**CHLORZOXAZONE (250mg.) w/APAP TABLETS** 300mg., 100's	℞
	CONJUGATED ESTROGENS TABLETS	℞
1135-01	0.625mg., 100's	
1835-01	1.25mg., 100's	
1625-01	2.5mg., 100's	
	CYCLANDELATE CAPSULES	℞
2668-01	200mg., 100's	
2670-01	400mg., 100's	
1125-01	**CYPROHEPTADINE HCl. TABLETS** 4mg., 100's	℞
6315-04	**DEPROIST EXPECTORANT w/CODEINE** (Codeine Phosphate, Phenylpropanolamine, Guaifenesin, Alcohol) 4 oz.	℞ Ⓒ
	DIPHENHYDRAMINE CAPSULES	℞
2458-01	25mg., 100's	
2498-01	50mg., 100's	
	DIPYRIDAMOLE TABLETS	℞
1890-01	25mg., 100's	
1678-01	50 mg., 100's	
1478-01	75mg., 100's	
1600-01	**DISOBROM TABLETS** (Dexbrompheniramine Maleate, d-isoephedrine Sulfate,) 100's	℞
1060-01	**DISULFIRAM TABLETS** 250 mg., 100's	℞
	DSS CAPSULES	OTC
2408-01	100mg., 100's	
2795-01	250mg., 100's	
6804-16	**DSS SYRUP** 20mg.,/5ml., 16 oz.	OTC
2653-01	**DSS w/CASANTHRANOL CAPSULES** 30mg., 100's	OTC
	ERGOLOID MESYLATES TABLETS	℞
1990-01	0.5 mg., 100's (Sublingual)	
1255-01	1.0 mg., 100's (Sublingual)	
	FUROSEMIDE TABLETS	℞
1818-01	20mg., 100's	
1966-01	40mg., 100's	

Continued on next page

Geneva—Cont.

1827-01 **GLUTETHIMIDE TABLETS** ℞ C
500mg., 100's

HYDRALAZINE HCl. TABLETS ℞
1732-01 10mg., 100's
1733-01 25mg., 100's
1734-01 50mg., 100's

HYDROCHLOROTHIAZIDE TABLETS ℞
1480-01 25mg., 100's
1481-01 50mg., 100's
1735-01 100mg., 100's

1010-01 **HYDROCHLOROTHIAZIDE 25 w/RESERPINE TABLETS** ℞
0.125mg., 100's

1011-01 **HYDROCHLOROTHIAZIDE 50 w/RESERPINE TABLETS** ℞
0.125mg., 100's

HYDROXYZINE TABLETS ℞
133201 10mg., 100's
133401 25mg., 100's
133601 50mg., 100's

IMIPRAMINE TABLETS ℞
1762-01 10mg., 100's
1764-01 25mg., 100's
1766-01 50mg., 100's

ISOSORBIDE DINITRATE TABLETS ℞
1635-01 5mg., 100's (Oral)
1565-01 5mg., 100's (Sublingual)
1556-01 10mg., 100's (Oral)
1695-01 20mg., 100's

2520-01 **ISOSORBIDE DINITRATE T.D. CAPSULES** ℞
40mg., 100's

1417-01 **ISOSORBIDE DINITRATE T.D. TABLETS** ℞
40mg., 100's

ISOXSUPRINE TABLETS ℞
1840-01 10mg., 100's
1842-01 20mg., 100's

1262-01 **LONOX TABLETS** ℞ C
(Diphenoxylate HCl., Atropine Sulfate), 100's

MECLIZINE HCl. TABLETS OTC
1345-01 12.5mg., 100's
1375-01 25mg., 100's

1410-01 **MEPROBAMATE TABLETS** ℞ C
400mg., 100's

METHOCARBAMOL TABLETS ℞
1760-01 500mg., 100's
1750-01 750mg., 100's

1740-01 **METRONIDAZOLE TABLETS** ℞
250 mg., 100's

6532-42 **MYGEL SUSPENSION** OTC
(Aluminum Hydroxide, Magnesium Hydroxide, Simethicone), 1–11

NITROFURANTOIN CAPSULES ℞
2160-01 50mg., 100's
2162-01 100mg., 100's

NITROFURANTOIN TABLETS ℞
1139-01 50mg., 100's
1282-01 100mg., 100's

NITROGLYCERIN T.D. CAPSULES ℞
2718-60 2.5mg., 60's
2786-01 6.5mg., 100's

NYLIDRIN TABLETS ℞
1406-01 6mg., 100's
1413-01 12mg., 100's

1370-01 **P.E.T.N. S.R. TABLETS** ℞
80mg., 100's

2000-01 **PAPAVERINE T.D. CAPSULES** ℞
150mg., 100's

2440-01 **PHENYLBUTAZONE CAPSULES** ℞
100 mg., 100's

1440-01 **PHENYLBUTAZONE TABLETS** ℞
100mg., 100's

6003-52 **POLYVITE WITH FLUORIDE DROPS**
(Vitamin A, Vitamin D, Vitamin E, Vitamin C, Thiamine, Riboflavin, Niacin, Vitamin B-6, Vitamin B-12, Fluoride), 50ml.

POTASSIUM CHLORIDE ELIXIR ℞
6040-16 10% Sugar Free, 16 oz.
6790-16 20% Sugar Free, 16 oz.

6846-16 **POTASSIUM GLUCONATE ELIXIR (K-G ELIXIR)** ℞
20mEq/15ml., 16 oz.

1540-01 **PREDNISOLONE TABLETS** ℞
5mg., 100's

PREDNISONE TABLETS ℞
1495-01 5mg., 100's
1500-01 10mg., 100's
1485-01 20mg., 100's
1450-01 50mg., 100's

1040-01 **PRIMIDONE TABLETS** ℞
250mg. 100's

1021-01 **PROBENECID TABLETS** ℞
0.5gm., 100's

1023-01 **PROBENECID & COLCHICINE TABLETS** ℞
0.5gm., 100's

2315-01 **PROCAINAMIDE CAPSULES** ℞
500mg., 100's

PROCHLORPERAZINE TABLETS ℞
1120-01 5mg., 100's
1122-01 10mg., 100's
1124-01 25mg., 100's

2060-01 **PRO-ISO CAPSULES** ℞
(Prochlorperazine as the Maleate, Isopropamide as the Iodide), 100's

6035-16 **PROMETHAZINE DM (Ped) EXPECTORANT** ℞
16 oz.

6598-16 **PROMETHAZINE EXPECTORANT PLAIN** ℞
16 oz.

6960-16 **PROMETHAZINE w/CODEINE EXPECTORANT** ℞ C
16 oz.

6685-16 **PROMETHAZINE VC EXPECTORANT** ℞
16 oz.

6997-16 **PROMETHAZINE VC w/CODEINE EXPECTORANT** ℞ C
16 oz.

1855-01 **PROPANTHELINE BROMIDE TABLETS** ℞
15mg., 100's

2140-01 **PROPOXYPHENE HCl. CAPSULES** ℞ C
65mg., 100's

2365-01 **PROPOXYPHENE COMPOUND 65 CAPSULES** ℞ C
100's

1378-01 **PROPOX 65 w/APAP TABLETS** ℞ C
650mg., 100's

2360-01 **PSEUDOEPHEDRINE S.R. CAPSULES** ℞
120 mg., 100's

1535-01 **PSEUDOEPHEDRINE TABLETS** ℞
60mg., 100's

1804-01 **QUINIDINE GLUCONATE S.R. TABLETS** ℞
324 mg., 100's

1900-01 **QUINIDINE SULFATE TABLETS** ℞
3 gr., 100's

2995-01 **QUININE CAPSULES** ℞
200 mg., 100's

2997-01 **QUININE SULFATE TABLETS** OTC
5 gr., 100's

1925-01 **QUIPHILE TABLETS** ℞
(Quinine Sulfate, Aminophylline-as dihydrate), 100's

2426-01 **RESAID T.D. CAPSULES** ℞
(Phenylpropanolamine HCl., Chlorpheniramine Maleate, Isopropamide) 100's

2846-01 **RESCAPS-D T.D. CAPSULES** ℞
(Caramiphen Edisylate, Chlorpheniramine Maleate, Phenylpropanolamine HCl., Atropine Sulfate), 100's

1598-01 **SPIRONOLACTONE TABLETS** ℞
25mg., 100's

1150-01 **SPIRONOLACTONE (25mg.) w/HYDRO-CHLOROTHIAZIDE TABLETS** ℞
25mg., 100's

1261-01 **SULFAMETHOXAZOLE TABLETS** ℞
500mg., 100's

1045-01 **SULFASALAZINE TABLETS** ℞
500mg., 100's

1015-01 **SULFISOXAZOLE TABLETS** ℞
500mg., 100's

1988-01 **T.E.H. TABLETS** ℞
(Ephedrine Sulfate, Theophylline, Hydroxyzine HCl.), 100's

1325-01 **T.E.P. TABLETS** OTC
(Theophylline Anhydrous, Ephedrine HCl., Phenobarbital), 100's

6710-16 **TAMINE ELIXIR** ℞
16 oz.

6785-16 **TAMINE EXPECTORANT** ℞
16 oz.

6275-16 **TAMINE EXPECTORANT DC** ℞
16 oz.

115301 **TAMINE S.R. TABLETS** ℞
(Brompheniramine Maleate, Phenylephrine Hydrochloride, Phenylpropanolamine Hydrochloride), 100's

6600-16 **THEOPHYLLINE ELIXIR** ℞
16 oz.

1704-01 **TOLBUTAMIDE TABLETS** ℞
0.5g., 100's

1670-01 **TRIAMCINOLONE TABLETS** ℞
4mg., 100's

1180-01 **TRICHLORMETHIAZIDE TABLETS** ℞
4mg., 100's

1663-01 **TRIFED TABLETS** ℞
(Triprolidine HCl., Pseudoephedrine HCl.), 100's

6510-16 **TRIFED SYRUP** ℞
16 oz.

6520-16 **TRIFED-C SYRUP** ℞ C
16 oz.

TRIFLUOPERAZINE TABLETS ℞
1030-01 1 mg., 100's
1032-01 2 mg., 100's
1034-01 5 mg., 100's
1036-01 10 mg., 100's

6005-52 **TRIPLEVITE WITH FLUORIDE DROPS** ℞
(Vitamin A, Vitamin D, Vitamin C, Fluoride), 1-50cc.

1340-01 **UROBLUE TABLETS** ℞
(Atropine Sulfate, Hyoscyamine, Methenamine, Methylene Blue, Phenyl Salicylate, Benzoic Acid), 100's

Gerber Products Company
FREMONT, MI 49412

MBF* (Meat Base Formula) Liquid Hypoallergenic Infant feeding Formula, Gerber

Composition: Hypoallergenic liquid formula made from water, beef hearts, sugar, sesame oil, modified tapioca starch, tricalcium phosphate, calcium citrate, potassium chloride, magnesium chloride, iodized salt, sodium ascorbate, ferrous sulfate, tocopheryl acetate, thiamin hydrochloride, vitamin A palmitate, calcium pantothenate, pyridoxine hydrochloride, vitamin D, cupric sulfate, phytonadione (vitamin K_1), folic acid, potassium iodide and biotin.

Nutrient Content: 1:1 dilution contains 20 cal/fl.oz., 12.2% solids, 2.2% protein, 3.2% fat and 6.0% carbohydrate with a Ca/P ratio of 1.5. Vitamin and mineral content per 15 fl. oz. can is:

Vitamin A	1600.0	I.U.
Vitamin D	360.0	I.U.
Vitamin K	24.0	mcg
Vitamin E	6.6	I.U.
Vitamin C	54.0	mg
Vitamin B_1 (Thiamin)	0.54	mg
Vitamin B_2 (Riboflavin)	0.90	mg
Vitamin B_6 (Pyridoxine)	0.78	mg

Vitamin B_{12}	7.8	mcg
Niacin	3.6	mg
Folic Acid	24.0	mcg
Pantothenic Acid	1.8	mg
Biotin	9.0	mcg
Choline	90.0	mg
Inositol	150.0	mg
Calcium	900.0	mg
Phosphorus	600.0	mg
Magnesium	36.0	mg
Iron	12.0	mg
Iodine	30.0	mcg
Zinc	3.0	mg
Copper	0.36	mg
Manganese	30.0	mcg
Sodium	246.0	mg
Potassium	486.0	mg
Chloride	438.0	mg

Action and Uses: A nutritionally adequate formula for infants and children intolerant to cow's and goat's milk whose symptoms may be diarrhea, colic, eczema, upper respiratory, etc. Useful in the management of galactosemia and milk induced steatorrhea.
Administration and Dosage: Provides 20 cal/fl.oz. when diluted 1:1; similar to other milk-based and soy-based infant formulas. Concentrated liquid added to previously boiled (not hot) water is to be divided among prescribed number of bottles, easily fed thru cross-cut nipples.
MBF's content of essential nutrients conforms to the infant formula standard established by the U.S. Food and Drug Administration in 1971 and the 1980 American Academy of Pediatrics infant formula recommendations.
Side Effects: None.
Precautions: None.
Contraindications: None.
How Supplied: Concentrated Liquid, 15 fl. oz. cans.
Literature Available: Yes.
*Trademark

Geriatric Pharm. Corp.
397 JERICHO TURNPIKE
FLORAL PARK, NY 11001

B-C-BID CAPSULES
B Complex with Vitamin C
SUSTAINED RELEASE
BY MICRODIALYSIS DIFFUSION

Composition: Each capsule contains: Vitamin B-1 15 mg., Vitamin B-2 10 mg., Vitamin B-6 5 mg., Niacinamide 50 mg., Calcium Pantothenate 10 mg., Vitamin C 300 mg., and Vitamin B-12 (Cyanocobalamin) 5 mcg.
Medication is released at a smooth, continuous, predictable rate dependent only upon the presence of fluid in the G.I. tract, and not dependent on pH and other variables. *No regurgitation; no after-taste.*
On b.i.d. dosage, this smooth, continuous release of B-C-BID's essential vitamins frees your patient from the "peak and valley" effect of ordinary capsules or tablets.
Dosage: For continuous 24 hour therapy, one capsule after breakfast and one after supper.

CEVI-BID Capsules (500 mg. Vitamin C)
SUSTAINED RELEASE
BY MICRO-DIALYSIS DIFFUSION

Composition: Each CEVI-BID capsule contains 500 mg. Vitamin C.
Action and Uses: For treatment of Vitamin C deficiency. CEVI-BID maintains optimal blood levels of Vitamin C around the clock on b.i.d. dosage, and avoids "peak and valley" effects of ordinary Vitamin C tablets. Medication is released at a smooth, continuous, predictable rate dependent only upon the presence of fluid in the G.I. tract and independent of pH or other variables.
Dosage: For continuous 24 hour therapy, one capsule after breakfast and one after supper.

GER-O-FOAM™ Analgesic Anesthetic Foam

Composition: Aerosol foam containing methyl salicylate 30% and benzocaine 3% in a specially-processed oil emulsion.
Action and Uses: For topical application in alleviating minor pains of musculoskeletal conditions such as osteoarthritis, rheumatoid arthritis and low back pain. GER-O-FOAM permits increased range of motion by decreasing pain.
Administration and Dosage: Massage into affected area 2 or 3 times daily.
Precautions: If a rash or irritation occurs, discontinue. Avoid application in or near eyes, mucous membranes or open wounds.
How Supplied: 4 oz. Aerosol cans.

GUSTASE®
Gastrointestinal Enzyme Tablets

Composition: Each GUSTASE tablet contains GERILASE (standardized amylolytic enzyme) 30 mg., GERIPROTASE (standardized proteolytic enzyme) 6 mg., GERICELLULASE (standardized cellulolytic enzyme) 2 mg.
Action and Uses: GUSTASE is indicated in dyspepsia, colitis, flatulence, diverticulitis, abdominal distension, etc. GUSTASE is effective in a broad pH spectrum (3–10), and is not enteric coated.
Administration and Dosage: One tablet during or immediately after meals.

ISO-BID® CAPSULES 40 mg. ℞
SUSTAINED RELEASE BY
MICRO-DIALYSIS DIFFUSION

Composition: Each ISO-BID SUSTAINED-MEDICATION CAPSULE contains 40 mg. Isosorbide Dinitrate. Medication is released at a smooth, continuous, predictable rate dependent only upon the presence of fluid in the G.I. tract; not dependent on the variable digestive processes.
Mode of Action: The mechanism of action of ISO-BID, like all nitrates, is the relaxation of smooth muscle. The relationship between this and its clinical usefulness is obscure, since the exact cause of anginal pain is presently unknown. ISO-BID is intended to decrease the frequency and severity of anginal attacks, and thus effect a decrease in the need for nitroglycerin. These should be the criteria for the success of ISO-BID therapy, since there is a wide variation in symptomatic response to treatment. Isosorbide Dinitrate is widely accepted as a safe and useful therapeutic agent in the treatment of angina pectoris.

Indications: Based on a review of this drug by the National Academy of Sciences—National Research Council and/or other information, FDA has classified the indications as follows:
"*Possibly*" *effective:* When taken orally ISO-BID SUSTAINED MEDICATION CAPSULES are indicated for the relief of angina pectoris (pain of coronary artery disease). ISO-BID SUSTAINED RELEASE CAPSULES are not intended to abort the acute anginal episode, but are widely regarded as useful in the prophylactic treatment of angina pectoris. Final classification of the less-than-effective indication requires further investigation.

Contraindication: Idiosyncrasy to this drug.
Warnings: Data supporting the use of nitrites during the early days of the acute phase of myocardial infarction (the period during which clinical and laboratory findings are unstable) are insufficient to establish safety.
Precautions: Use with caution in patients with glaucoma. Tolerance to this drug, and cross-tolerance to other nitrites and nitrates may occur.
Patients with gastric hypermotility for any reason, where the duration of passage through the gastrointestinal tract may be less than normal, should take sublingual nitroglycerin rather than sustained release medications.
Adverse Reactions: Cutaneous vasodilation with flushing. Headache may commonly occur, and may be both severe and persistent. Transient dizziness and weakness, in addition to other signs of cerebral ischemia associated with postural hypotension may occasionally be seen. ISO-BID can act as a physiological antagonist to norepinephrine, histamine, acetylcholine and many other medications. An occasional patient may show marked sensitivity to the hypotensive effects of nitrite; severe responses (nausea, vomiting, weakness, restlessness, pallor, excessive sweating and collapse) can occur, even with the usual therapeutic dosage. Alcohol may enhance this effect. A drug rash and/or exfoliative dermatitis is occasionally seen.
Dosage: One 40mg. ISO-BID CAPSULE every 12 hours on an empty stomach according to need, for continuous 24-hour therapy. This dosage schedule is particularly convenient in the management of nocturnal angina. Some patients may require higher dosage levels. In these patients, dosage should be titrated, and may require two ISO-BID CAPSULES b.i.d.

Gilbert Laboratories
31 FAIRMOUNT AVENUE
CHESTER, NEW JERSEY 07930

ESGIC® ℞
Tablets and Capsules

Description: Each ESGIC tablet or capsule, an analgesic sedative combination, for oral administration contains: isobutylallylbarbituric acid, (butalbital, U.S.P.), 50 mg., (WARNING: may be habit forming); caffeine, U.S.P., 40 mg.; and acetaminophen, U.S.P., 325 mg.
Clinical Pharmacology: Pharmacologically, ESGIC employs the analgesic properties of acetaminophen with the sedative and muscle relaxant properties of isobutylallylbarbituric acid. Many clinicians report that nervous tension and anxiety underlie stress (muscle contraction) headache. ESGIC was formulated to be an effective means of treating the target symptoms of the stress headache syndrome. These include headache pain, nervous tension and contraction of muscles of the head, neck and shoulder region. Acetaminophen may be used safely by most persons sensitive to aspirin.
Isobutylallylbarbuturic acid is an intermediate-acting barbiturate which produces mild sedation. Barbiturates are capable of producing all levels of CNS mood alteration from excitation to mild sedation, to hypnosis, and deep coma. Overdosage can produce death.
Barbiturates depress the sensory cortex, decrease motor activity, alter cerebellar function, and produce drowsiness, sedation, and hypnosis. Barbiturates are respiratory depressants. The degree of respiratory depression is dependent on dose.
Barbiturates do not impair normal hepatic function, but have been shown to induce liver microsomal enzymes, thus increasing and/or altering the metabolism of barbiturates and other drugs.
The analgesic action of acetaminophen involves peripheral and central influences, but the specific mechanism is as yet undetermined. Antipyretic activity is medicated through hypothalmic heat regulating centers. Acetami-

Continued on next page

Gilbert—Cont.

nophen inhibits prostaglandin synthetase. Therapeutic doses of acetaminophen have negligible effects on the cardiovascular or respiratory systems; however, toxic doses may cause circulatory failure and rapid, shallow breathing.

PHARMACOKINETICS. The onset and duration of action, which is related to the rate at which the barbiturates are redistributed throughout the body varies among persons and in the same person from time to time. Isobutylallylbarbituric acid has a duration of action from 3 to 6 hours.

Barbiturates are weak acids that are absorbed and rapidly distributed to all tissues and fluids with high concentrations in the brain, liver, and kidneys. The more lipid soluble the barbiturate, the more rapidly it penetrates all tissues of the body. Barbiturates are bound to plasma and tissue proteins to a varying degree with degree of binding increasing directly as a function of lipid solubility.

Barbiturates are metabolized primarily by the hepatic microsomal enzyme system and the metabolic products are excreted in the urine, and less commonly, in the feces. The inactive metabolites of the barbiturates are excreted as conjugates of glucuronic acid.

Acetaminophen is rapidly and almost completely absorbed from the gastrointestinal tract, producing maximum serum concentrations within 30 minutes to one hour. The plasma half-life in adults and children ranges from 0.90 hours to 3.25 hours with an average of approximately 2 hours. The drug distributes uniformly in most body fluids and is approximately 25% protein bound. Acetaminophen is conjugated in the liver, with less than 3% of the dose excreted unchanged in 24 hours. The primary metabolic pathway is conjugation to sulfate and glucuronide by-products. A minor oxidative pathway forms cysteine and mercapturic acid. These compounds are subsequently excreted by the kidneys into the urine.

Indications: ESGIC is indicated for the relief of the symptom complex of stress or muscle contraction headache.

Contraindications: Hypersensitivity to acetaminophen, caffeine, or barbiturates. Patients with prophyria.

Warnings: Acetaminophen in massive overdosage may cause hepatotoxicity in some patients (see OVERDOSAGE).

Habit Forming: Barbiturates may be habit forming. Tolerance, psychological and physical dependence may occur with continued use. (See DRUG ABUSE AND DEPENDENCE). Abrupt cessation after prolonged use in the dependent person may result in withdrawal symptoms, including delirium, convulsions, and possibly death. Barbiturates should be withdrawn gradually from any patient known to be taking excessive dosage over long periods of time.

Use in Pregnancy: Barbiturates can cause fetal damage when administered to a pregnant woman. Retrospective, case-controlled studies have suggested a connection between the maternal consumption of barbiturates and a higher than expected incidence of fetal abnormalities. Following oral or parenteral administration, barbiturates readily cross the placental barrier and are distributed throughout fetal tissues with highest concentrations found in the placenta, fetal liver, and brain. Fetal blood levels approach maternal blood levels following parenteral administration.

Withdrawal symptoms occur in infants born to mothers who receive barbiturates throughout the last trimester of pregnancy. (See DRUG ABUSE AND DEPENDENCE). If this drug is used during pregnancy, or if the patient becomes pregnant while taking this drug, the patient should be apprised of the potential hazards to the fetus.

Synergistic Effects: The concomitant use of alcohol or other CNS depressants may produce additive CNS depressant effects.

Precautions: *General:* Barbiturates may be habit forming. Tolerance and psychological and physical dependence may occur with continuing use. (See DRUG ABUSE AND DEPENDENCE). Barbiturates should be administered with caution, if at all, to patients who are mentally depressed, have suicidal tendencies, or a history of drug abuse.

Elderly or debilitated patients may react to barbiturates with marked excitement, depression, and confusion. In some persons, barbiturates repeatedly produce excitement rather than depression.

In patients with hepatic damage, barbiturates should be administered with caution and initially in reduced doses. Barbiturates should not be administered to patients showing the premonitory signs of hepatic coma.

Information For Patients: Practitioners should give the following information and instructions to patients receiving barbiturates.

1. The use of barbiturates carries with it an associated risk of psychological and/or physical dependence. The patient should be warned against increasing the dose of the drug without consulting a physician.
2. Barbiturates may impair mental and/or physical abilities required for the performance of potentially hazardous tasks (e.g., driving, operating machinery, etc.).
3. Alcohol should not be consumed while taking barbiturates. Concurrent use of the barbiturates with other CNS depressants (e.g., alcohol, narcotics, tranquilizers, and antihistamines) may result in additional CNS depressant effects.

Drug Interactions: The concomitant use of other central nervous system depressants, including other sedatives or hypnotics, antihistamines, tranquilizers, or alcohol, may produce additive depressant effects. When such combined therapy is necessary, the dose of one or more agents may need to be reduced.

The presence of barbiturates decreases the effects of oral anticoagulants, griseofulvin, doxycycline, corticosteroids and possibly phenytoin. Monoamine oxidase inhibitors (MAOI) prolong the effects of barbiturates.

Pregnancy Category D: (See WARNINGS section). Barbiturates can cause fetal harm when administered to pregnant women. If ESGIC is used during pregnancy, or if the patient becomes pregnant while taking ESGIC, the patient should be apprised of the potential hazard to the fetus.

Nursing Mothers: The effects of ESGIC on infants of nursing mothers are not known. Barbiturates are excreted in the breast milk of nursing mothers. Caution should be exercised when ESGIC is administered to a nursing woman.

Pediatric Use: Safety and effectiveness in children below the age of 12 have not been established.

Adverse Reactions: The most frequent adverse reactions are drowsiness and dizziness. Less frequent adverse reactions are lightheadedness, nausea and skin rash.

Drug Abuse and Dependence:

Barbiturates may be habit forming: Tolerance, psychological dependence, and physical dependence may occur especially following prolonged use of high doses of barbiturates. The average daily dose for the barbiturate addict is usually about 1,500 mg. As tolerance to barbiturates develops, the amount needed to maintain the same level of intoxication increases; tolerance to a fatal dosage, however, does not increase more than two-fold. As this occurs, the margin between an intoxication dosage and fatal dosage becomes smaller. The lethal dose of a barbiturate is far less if alcohol is also ingested. Major withdrawal symptoms (convulsions and delirium) may occur within 16 hours and last up to 5 days after abrupt cessation of these drugs. Intensity of withdrawal symptoms gradually declines over a period of approximately 15 days.

Treatment of barbiturate dependence consists of cautious and gradual withdrawal of the drug. Barbiturate-dependent patients can be withdrawn by using a number of different withdrawal regimens. One method involves initiating treatment at the patient's regular dosage level and decreasing the daily dosage by 10 percent if tolerated by the patient.

Overdosage: The toxic effects of acute overdosage of ESGIC are attributable mainly to its barbiturate component. The toxic effects of acetaminophen which may be masked by the barbiturate, may also occur and should not be overlooked. Because toxic effects of caffeine occur in very high dosages only, the possibility of significant caffeine toxicity from ESGIC overdosage is unlikely.

Barbiturates: The toxic dose of barbiturates varies considerably. In general, an oral dose of 1 gram of most barbiturates produces serious poisoning in an adult. Death commonly occurs after 2 to 10 grams of ingested barbiturate. Barbiturate intoxication may be confused with alcoholism, bromide intoxication, and with various neurological disorders.

Acute overdosage with barbiturates is manifested by CNS and respiratory depression which may progress to Cheyne-Stokes respiration, aroflexia, constriction of the pupils to a slight degree (though in severe poisoning they may show paralytic dilation), oliguria, tachycardia, hypotension, lowered body temperature, and coma. Typical shock syndrome (apena, circulatory collapse, respiratory arrest, and death) may occur.

In extreme overdose, all electrical activity in the brain may cease, in which case a "flat" EEG normally equated with clinical death cannot be accepted. This effect is fully reversible unless hypoxic damage occurs. Consideration should be given to the possibility of barbiturate intoxication even in situations that appear to involve trauma.

Complications such as pneumonia, pulmonary edema, cardiac arrhythmias, congestive heart failure, and renal failure may occur. Uremia may increase CNS sensitivity to barbiturates if renal function is impaired. Differential diagnosis should include hypoglycemia, head trauma, cerebrovascular accidents, convulsive states, and diabetic coma.

Treatment of overdosage is mainly supportive and consists of the following:

1. Maintenance of an adequate airway, with assisted respiration and oxygen administration as necessary.
2. Monitoring of vital signs and fluid balance.
3. If the patient is conscious and has not lost the gag reflex, emesis may be induced with ipecac. Care should be taken to prevent pulmonary aspiration of vomitus. After completion of vomiting, 30 grams activated charcoal in a glass of water may be administered.
4. If emesis is contraindicated, gastric lavage may be performed with a cuffed endotracheal tube in place with the patient in the face down position. Activated charcoal may be left in the emptied stomach and a salin cathartic administered.
5. Fluid therapy and other standard treatment for shock, if needed.
6. If renal function is normal, forced diuresis may aid in the elimination of the barbiturate. Alkalinization of the urine increases renal excretion of some barbiturates.
7. Although not recommended as a routine procedure, hemodialysis may be used in severe barbiturate intoxications or if the patient is anuric or in shock.
8. Patient should be rolled from side to side every 30 minutes.

9. Antibiotics should be given if pneumonia is suspected.
10. Appropriate nursing care to prevent hypostatic pneumonia, decubiti, aspiration, and other complications of patients with altered states of consciousness.

Acetaminophen: Acetaminophen in massive overdosage may cause hepatic toxicity in some patients. In adults, hepatic toxicity has rarely been reported with less than 10 grams and fatalities with less than 15 grams, taken as single, massive overdoses. Importantly, for reasons not fully understood, young children seem to be more resistant than adults to the hepatotoxic effect of an acetaminophen overdose.

Early symptoms following a potentially hepatotoxic overdose may include: nausea, vomiting, diaphoresis and general malaise. Clinical and laboratory evidence of hepatic toxicity usually are not apparent until 48 to 72 hours postingestion. Following recovery there are no residual, structural or functional hepatic abnormalities.

Since patients' estimates of the quantity of a drug ingested are notoriously unreliable, if an acetaminophen overdose is suspected a serum acetaminophen assay should be obtained as early as possible, but no sooner than four hours following ingestion. Liver function studies should be obtained initially and repeated at 24 hour intervals.

Antidotal therapy with N-acetylcysteine appears effective in preventing and/or minimizing the toxic effects of acetaminophen. For optimal results, the antidote should be administered within 16 hours of ingestion of the overdose.

The Rocky Mountain Poison Center (303-629-1123) should be contacted for assistance in interpreting plasma levels and for directions on the administration of N-acetylcysteine as an antidote, a use currently restricted to investigational status.

Dosage and Administration: One or two tablets or capsules taken orally every four hours. Total daily dose should not exceed six tablets or capsules.

How Supplied: *ESGIC tablets:* White, round, compressed tablet. Supplied in bottles of 100 tablets. NDC #0535-0011-01. Tablets imprinted with Gilbert Laboratories logo on one side and 535-11 on the opposite side.

ESGIC capsules: White, opaque capsules imprinted with Gilbert Laboratories Logo and 535-12 in black print. Supplied in bottles of 100 capsules. NDC #0535-0012-01.

Revised 12/80

[*Shown in Product Identification Section*]

Glaxo Inc.

1900 WEST COMMERCIAL BLVD.
FT. LAUDERDALE, FL 33309

B C G Vaccine, USP ℞

For Intradermal Use
Freeze–Dried

Description: BCG Vaccine, USP, is a standardized preparation of living BCG bacillus in the dry form for use in immunization against tuberculosis. It is prepared from a Glaxo culture of the Danish substrain of BCG bacillus. The organisms are harvested, suspended in a medium consisting of suitable concentrations of dextran, glucose, and Triton WR 1339, and then freeze-dried. This vaccine, when reconstituted as directed, contains not less than 8 million and not more than 26 million colony-forming units per ml.

Indications: BCG Vaccine induces active immunity to tuberculosis. The Advisory Committee on Immunization Practices of the U.S. Public Health Service has made the following specific recommendations[1] for the use of BCG Vaccine.

1. BCG vaccination should be seriously considered for persons who have negative tuberculin skin tests and repeated exposure to persistently untreated or ineffectively treated sputum-positive cases of pulmonary tuberculosis.
2. BCG vaccination should be considered for well-defined communities or groups if an excessive rate of new infections can be demonstrated and the usual surveillance and treatment programs have failed or have been shown not to be applicable.

Contraindications: BCG Vaccine is contraindicated in tuberculin-positive individuals, subjects with fresh smallpox vaccinations, and burn patients. In addition, BCG Vaccine should not be given to individuals being given prolonged treatment with corticosteroids or other immunosuppressive therapy or to those with hypogammaglobulinemia or any other disorder in which the natural immunologic capacity of the host may be altered. Although chronic diseases involving the skin are not contraindications, individuals with such conditions should be vaccinated in a healthy area of skin. BCG Vaccine will not be effective if given during isoniazid (INH) administration, because INH inhibits multiplication of BCG.

Precautions: BCG vaccination is not normally undertaken without prior determination that the patient is nonreactive to a tuberculin skin test. The individual to be vaccinated should first be tuberculin-tested by a suitable method. A Mantoux test with 5 T.U. of Tuberculin P.P.D. (Purified Protein Derivative) is suitable. If this test is negative, the person may be vaccinated immediately. The test should be performed within the 6-week period preceding vaccination. The protection from tuberculosis afforded by BCG vaccination is only relative and is not permanent or entirely predictable. If the tuberculin test again becomes negative and the risk of infection continues, BCG vaccination may need to be repeated. Although no harmful effects on the fetus have been observed with BCG Vaccine, it is prudent to refrain from vaccination during pregnancy unless there is excessive risk of unavoidable exposure to infectious tuberculosis.

Interpretation of Tuberculin Test—After BCG vaccination, it is usually not possible to distinguish between a tuberculin reaction caused by virulent supra-infection and a reaction resulting from persistent postvaccination sensitivity. Therefore, caution is advised in attributing a positive skin test to BCG (except in the immediate postvaccination period), especially if the vaccinee has recently been exposed to infective tuberculosis.

Tuberculosis in Vaccinated Persons—Since full, lasting protection from BCG vaccination cannot be assured, tuberculosis should be included in the differential diagnosis of any tuberculosis-like illness in a BCG vaccinee.

Method of Use: Using appropriate aseptic technique, add 1 ml of Sterile Water for Injection to each 1-ml-size multiple-dose ampoule of vaccine. Allow to stand for approximately 1 minute. Avoid shaking, since this results in foaming. The process of withdrawing the solution from the ampoule will yield a homogeneous suspension.

Dosage and Administration: After the vaccine has been prepared, the immunizing dose of 0.1 ml is given by **intradermal** injection. A 0.05-ml dose may be given to infants under 28 days of age. Following reconstitution, the ampoule should be used immediately, and any material remaining in the ampoule should be discarded.

Before use, the product should be stored at a uniform temperature between 2° and 8°C (36° and 46°F), preferably at the lower limit. Do not expose vaccine to light.

The Normal Local Reaction: After proper intradermal injection of the immunizing dose, the initial skin lesion usually appears within 7 to 10 days. The normal lesion consists of a small red papule at the site of injection: it reaches its maximum diameter of approximately 8 mm after about 5 weeks. The top of the papule scales, ulcerates, and dries, and the whole lesion gradually shrinks to a smooth or scaly pink or bluish scar approximately 3 months after vaccination and becomes a smooth or pitted white scar in approximately 6 months.

A postvaccinal tuberculin test should be conducted 2 to 3 months after vaccination. If the test is negative, the vaccination should be repeated.

Other Reactions: The Glaxo BCG strain used has proved to be associated with a very low incidence of untoward reactions. However, BCG vaccination has been associated with adverse reactions, including severe or prolonged ulceration at the vaccination site, lymphadenitis, osteomyelitis, disseminated BCG infection, and death. The reported frequency of complications, mostly from other countries, has varied greatly, depending on the substrain of BCG used and on the extent of the surveillance effort. For example the occurrence of ulceration and lymphadenitis has been reported to range from 1 to 10%, depending on the vaccine, the dosage, and the age of vaccinees. Osteomyelitis has been noted in 1 per 1,000,000 vaccinees, although recent information indicates that the rate may be as high as 5 per 100,000 in newborns. Disseminated BCG infection and death are very rare; they range from 1 to 10 per 10,000,000 vaccinees and occur almost exclusively in children with impaired immune response. Autoinoculation ulcers are seen occasionally. Abscesses in the skin at the site of inoculation may occur from secondary infection. Rarely, abscesses may develop in the regional lymph nodes draining the site of the BCG vaccination.

Granulomas, appearing approximately 4 to 6 weeks following the vaccination, have been reported at the site of the injection. They may result from application of irritating dressings to a normal BCG reaction or may occur occasionally as an idiosyncrasy. Such granulomas may persist for variable periods of time and may have a keloid scar after final healing. Rarely, persistent lupus reactions of the skin that required treatment have been reported. For these, isoniazid in a daily dose of 4 mg per kg of body weight has been recommended. One case of histiocytoma at the vaccination site required excision.[2] Transient urticaria of the limbs and trunk has been observed following BCG vaccination, and one instance of erythema nodosum occurred in a large series of vaccinees in England.

How Supplied: BCG Vaccine, USP is supplied in a 1-ml-size package (NDC 0173-0339-65)

References:

1. U.S. Department of Health, Education, and Welfare: BCG Vaccines, Morbidity and Mortality Weekly Report, *28*:21, 1979.
2. Hartson, W.: Uncommon Skin Reactions after BCG Vaccination, Tubercle, *40*:265, 1959.

BECLOVENT® INHALER ℞

(beclomethasone dipropionate)
For oral inhalation only

Description: Beclomethasone dipropionate, the active component of BECLOVENT® (beclomethasone dipropionate) Inhaler, is an anti-inflammatory steroid having the chemical name 9 - Chloro - 11β, 17, 21 - trihydroxy - 16β-methylpregna- 1, 4 - diene - 3, 20 - dione 17, 21 - dipropionate.

BECLOVENT® Inhaler is a metered-dose aerosol unit containing a microcrystalline suspension of beclomethasone dipropionate-trichloromonofluoromethane clathrate in a mixture of propellants (trichloromonofluoromethane and dichlorodifluoromethane) with oleic

Continued on next page

Glaxo—Cont.

acid. Each canister contains beclomethasone dipropionate – trichloromonofluoromethane clathrate having a molecular proportion of beclomethasone dipropionate to trichloromonofluoromethane between 3:1 and 3:2. Each actuation delivers from the mouthpiece a quantity of clathrate equivalent to 42 mcg. of beclomethasone dipropionate. The contents of one canister provide at least 200 oral inhalations.

Clinical Pharmacology: Beclomethasone 17, 21-dipropionate is a diester of beclomethasone, a synthetic corticosteroid which is chemically related to prednisolone. Beclomethasone differs from prednisolone only in having a chlorine at the 9-alpha and a methyl group at the 16-beta position in place of hydrogen. Animal studies showed that beclomethasone dipropionate has potent anti-inflammatory activity. When administered systemically to mice, the anti-inflammatory activity was accompanied by other typical features of glucocorticoid action including thymic involution, liver glycogen deposition, and pituitary-adrenal suppression. However, after systemic administration to rats, the anti-inflammatory action was associated with little or no effect on other tests of glucocorticoid activity.

Beclomethasone dipropionate is sparingly soluble and is poorly mobilized from subcutaneous or intramuscular injection sites. However, systemic absorption occurs after all routes of administration. When given to animals in the form of an aerosolized suspension of the trichloromonofluoromethane clathrate, the drug is deposited in the mouth and nasal passages, the trachea and principal bronchi, and in the lung; a considerable portion of the drug is also swallowed. Absorption occurs rapidly from all respiratory and gastrointestinal tissues, as indicated by the rapid clearance of radioactively labeled drug from local tissues and appearance of tracer in the circulation. There is no evidence of tissue storage of beclomethasone dipropionate or its metabolites. Lung slices can metabolize beclomethasone dipropionate rapidly to beclomethasone 17-monopropionate and more slowly to free beclomethasone (which has very weak anti-inflammatory activity). However, irrespective of the route of administration (injection, oral, or aerosol), the principal route of excretion of the drug and its metabolites is the feces. Less than 10% of the drug and its metabolites is excreted in the urine. In humans, 12% to 15% of an orally administered dose of beclomethasone dipropionate was excreted in the urine as both conjugated and free metabolites of the drug.

The mechanisms responsible for the anti-inflammatory action of beclomethasone dipropionate are unknown. The precise mechanism of the aerosolized drug's action in the lung is also unknown.

Indications: BECLOVENT® (beclomethasone dipropionate) Inhaler is indicated only for patients who require chronic treatment with corticosteroids for control of the symptoms of bronchial asthma. Such patients would include those already receiving systemic corticosteroids, and selected patients who are inadequately controlled on a non-steroid regimen and in whom steroid therapy has been withheld because of concern over potential adverse effects.

BECLOVENT® Inhaler is NOT indicated:

1. For relief of asthma which can be controlled by bronchodilators and other non-steroid medications.
2. In patients who require systemic corticosteroid treatment infrequently.
3. In the treatment of non-asthmatic bronchitis.

Contraindications: BECLOVENT® Inhaler is contraindicated in the primary treatment of status asthmaticus or other acute episodes of asthma where intensive measures are required.

Hypersensitivity to any of the ingredients of this preparation contraindicates its use.

Warnings:
Particular care is needed in patients who are transferred from systemically active corticosteroids to BECLOVENT® Inhaler because deaths due to adrenal insufficiency have occurred in asthmatic patients during and after transfer from systemic corticosteroids to aerosol beclomethasone dipropionate. After withdrawal from systemic corticosteroids, a number of months are required for recovery of hypothalamic-pituitary-adrenal (HPA) function. During this period of HPA suppression, patients may exhibit signs and symptoms of adrenal insufficiency when exposed to trauma, surgery or infections, particularly gastroenteritis. Although BECLOVENT® Inhaler may provide control of asthmatic symptoms during these episodes, it does NOT provide the systemic steroid which is necessary for coping with these emergencies.

During periods of stress or a severe asthmatic attack, patients who have been withdrawn from systemic corticosteroids should be instructed to resume systemic steroids (in large doses) immediately and to contact their physician for further instruction. These patients should also be instructed to carry a warning card indicating that they may need supplementary systemic steroids during periods of stress or a severe asthma attack. To assess the risk of adrenal insufficiency in emergency situations, routine tests of adrenal cortical function, including measurement of early morning resting cortisol levels, should be performed periodically in all patients. An early morning resting cortisol level may be accepted as normal only if it falls at or near the normal mean level.

Localized infections with *Candida albicans* or *Aspergillus niger* have occurred frequently in the mouth and pharynx and occasionally in the larynx. Positive cultures for oral *Candida* may be present in up to 75% of patients. Although the frequency of clinically apparent infection is considerably lower, these infections may require treatment with appropriate antifungal therapy or discontinuance of treatment with BECLOVENT® Inhaler.

BECLOVENT® Inhaler is not to be regarded as a bronchodilator and is not indicated for rapid relief of bronchospasm.

Patients should be instructed to contact their physician immediately when episodes of asthma which are not responsive to bronchodilators occur during the course of treatment with BECLOVENT® (beclomethasone dipropionate). During such episodes, patients may require therapy with systemic corticosteroids.

There is no evidence that control of asthma can be achieved by the administration of BECLOVENT® in amounts greater than the recommended doses.

Transfer of patients from systemic steroid therapy to BECLOVENT® Inhaler may unmask allergic conditions previously suppressed by the systemic steroid therapy, e.g., rhinitis, conjunctivitis, and eczema.

Precautions: During withdrawal from oral steroids, some patients may experience symptoms of systemically active steroid withdrawal, e.g., joint and/or muscular pain, lassitude and depression, despite maintenance or even improvement of respiratory function (See DOSAGE AND ADMINISTRATION for details).

In responsive patients, beclomethasone dipropionate may permit control of asthmatic symptoms without suppression of HPA function, as discussed below (See CLINICAL STUDIES). Since beclomethasone dipropionate is absorbed into the circulation and can be systemically active, the beneficial effects of BECLOVENT® Inhaler in minimizing or preventing HPA dysfunction may be expected only when recommended dosages are not exceeded.

The long-term effects of beclomethasone dipropionate in human subjects are still unknown. In particular, the local effects of the agent on developmental or immunologic processes in the mouth, pharynx, trachea, and lung are unknown. There is also no information about the possible long-term systemic effects of the agent.

The potential effects of BECLOVENT® on acute, recurrent, or chronic pulmonary infections, including active or quiescent tuberculosis, are not known. Similarly, the potential effects of long-term administration of the drug on lung or other tissues are unknown.

Pulmonary infiltrates with eosinophilia may occur in patients on BECLOVENT® Inhaler therapy. Although it is possible that in some patients this state may become manifest because of systemic steroid withdrawal when inhalational steroids are administered, a causative role for beclomethasone dipropionate and/or its vehicle cannot be ruled out.

Use in Pregnancy: Glucocorticoids are known teratogens in rodent species and beclomethasone dipropionate is no exception.

Teratology studies were done in rats, mice, and rabbits treated with subcutaneous beclomethasone dipropionate. Beclomethasone dipropionate was found to produce fetal resorption, cleft palate, agnathia, microstomia, absence of tongue, delayed ossification and partial agenesis of the thymus. Well-controlled trials relating to fetal risk in humans are not available. Glucocorticoids are secreted in human milk. It is not known whether beclomethasone dipropionate would be secreted in human milk but it is safe to assume that it is likely. The use of beclomethasone dipropionate in pregnancy, nursing mothers, or women of childbearing potential requires that the possible benefits of the drug be weighed against the potential hazards to the mother, embryo, or fetus. Infants born of mothers who have received substantial doses of corticosteroids during pregnancy should be carefully observed for hypoadrenalism.

Adverse Reactions: Deaths due to adrenal insufficiency have occurred in asthmatic patients during and after transfer from systemic corticosteroids to aerosol beclomethasone dipropionate (See WARNINGS).

Suppression of HPA function (reduction of early morning plasma cortisol levels) has been reported in adult patients who received 1600 mcg. daily doses of BECLOVENT® (beclomethasone dipropionate) for one month. A few patients on BECLOVENT® have complained of hoarseness or dry mouth. Bronchospasm and rash have been reported rarely.

Dosage and Administration: Adults: The usual dosage is two inhalations (84 mcg.) given three or four times a day. In patients with severe asthma, it is advisable to start with 12 to 16 inhalations a day and adjust the dosage downward according to the response of the patient. The maximal daily intake should not exceed 20 inhalations, 840 mcg. (0.84 mg.), in adults.

Children 6 to 12 years of age: The usual dosage is one or two inhalations (42 to 84 mcg.) given three or four times a day according to the response of the patient. The maximal daily intake should not exceed ten inhalations, 420 mcg. (0.42 mg.), in children 6 to 12 years of age. Insufficient clinical data exist with respect to the administration of BECLOVENT® Inhaler in children below the age of 6.

Rinsing the mouth after inhalation is advised. Patients receiving bronchodilators by inhalation should be advised to use the bronchodilator before BECLOVENT® Inhaler in order to enhance penetration of beclomethasone dipropionate into the bronchial tree. After use of an aerosol bronchodilator several minutes should elapse before use of the BECLOVENT® Inhaler to reduce the potential toxicity from the inhaled fluorocarbon propellants in the two aerosols.

Different considerations must be given to the following groups of patients in order to obtain the full therapeutic benefit of BECLOVENT® Inhaler.

Patients not receiving systemic steroids: The use of BECLOVENT® Inhaler is straightforward in patients who are inadequately controlled with non-steroid medications but in whom systemic steroid therapy has been withheld because of concern over potential adverse reactions. In patients who respond to BECLOVENT®, an improvement in pulmonary function is usually apparent within one to four weeks after the start of BECLOVENT® Inhaler.

Patients receiving systemic steroids: In those patients dependent on systemic steroids, transfer to BECLOVENT® and subsequent management may be more difficult because recovery from impaired adrenal function is usually slow. Such suppression has been known to last for up to 12 months. Clinical studies, however, have demonstrated that BECLOVENT® may be effective in the management of these asthmatic patients and may permit replacement or significant reduction in the dosage of systemic corticosteroids.

The patient's asthma should be reasonably stable before treatment with BECLOVENT® Inhaler is started. Initially, the aerosol should be used concurrently with the patient's usual maintenance dose of systemic steroid. After approximately one week, gradual withdrawal of the systemic steroid is started by reducing the daily or alternate daily dose. The next reduction is made after an interval of one or two weeks, depending on the response of the patient. Generally, these decrements should not exceed 2.5 mg. of prednisone or its equivalent. A slow rate of withdrawal cannot be overemphasized. During withdrawal, some patients may experience symptoms of systemically active steroid withdrawal, e.g., joint and/or muscular pain, lassitude and depression, despite maintenance or even improvement of respiratory function. Such patients should be encouraged to continue with the Inhaler but should be watched carefully for objective signs of adrenal insufficiency, such as hypotension and weight loss. If evidence of adrenal insufficiency occurs, the systemic steroid dose should be boosted temporarily and thereafter further withdrawal should continue more slowly.

During periods of stress or a severe asthma attack, transfer patients will require supplementary treatment with systemic steroids. Exacerbations of asthma which occur during the course of treatment with BECLOVENT® (beclomethasone dipropionate) Inhaler should be treated with a short course of systemic steroid which is gradually tapered as these symptoms subside. There is no evidence that control of asthma can be achieved by administration of BECLOVENT® in amounts greater than the recommended doses.

Directions for Use: Illustrated patient instructions for proper use accompany each package of BECLOVENT® Inhaler.

CONTENTS UNDER PRESSURE. Do not puncture. Do not use or store near heat or open flame. Exposure to temperatures above 120°F may cause bursting. Never throw container into fire or incinerator. Keep out of reach of children.

How Supplied: BECLOVENT® Inhaler 16.8 g canister with oral adapter and patient's instructions (NDC 0173-0312-88) and Beclovent Inhaler Refill 16.8 g canister only with patient's instructions (NDC 0173-0312-98).

[*Shown in Product Identification Section*]

BECONASE® Nasal Inhaler ℞
brand of beclomethasone dipropionate, USP
For Nasal Inhalation Only

Description: Beclomethasone dipropionate, USP, the active component of BECONASE Nasal Inhaler, is an anti-inflammatory steroid having the chemical name, 9-Chloro-11β, 17, 21-trihydroxy-16β-methylpregna-1, 4-diene-3, 20-dione 17,21-dipropionate.

Beclomethasone dipropionate is a white to creamy-white, odorless powder with a molecular weight of 521.25. It is very slightly soluble in water; very soluble in chloroform; and freely soluble in acetone and in alcohol.

BECONASE Nasal Inhaler is a metered-dose aerosol unit containing a microcrystalline suspension of beclomethasone dipropionate-trichloromonofluoromethane clathrate in a mixture of propellants (trichloromonofluoromethane and dichlorodifluoromethane) with oleic acid. Each canister contains beclomethasone dipropionate-trichloromonofluoromethane clathrate having a molecular proportion of beclomethasone dipropionate to trichloromonofluoromethane between 3:1 and 3:2. Each actuation delivers from the nasal adapter a quantity of clathrate equivalent to 42 mcg of beclomethasone dipropionate, USP. The contents of one canister provide at least 200 metered doses.

Clinical Pharmacology: Beclomethasone 17,21-dipropionate is a diester of beclomethasone, a synthetic corticosteroid which is chemically related to dexamethasone. Beclomethasone differs from dexamethasone only in having a chlorine at the 9-alpha position in place of a fluorine. Animal studies showed that beclomethasone dipropionate has potent glucocorticoid and weak mineralocorticoid activity. The mechanisms for the anti-inflammatory action of beclomethasone dipropionate are unknown. The precise mechanism of the aerosolized drug's action in the nose is also unknown. Biopsies of nasal mucosa obtained during clinical studies showed no histopathologic changes when beclomethasone dipropionate was administered intranasally.

The effects of beclomethasone dipropionate on hypothalamic-pituitary-adrenal (HPA) function have been evaluated in adult volunteers by other routes of administration. Studies are currently being undertaken with beclomethasone dipropionate by the intranasal route, which may demonstrate that there is more or that there is less absorption by this route of administration. There was no suppression of early morning plasma cortisol concentrations when beclomethasone dipropionate was administered in a dose of 1000 mcg/day for one month as an oral aerosol or for three days by intramuscular injection. However, partial suppression of plasma cortisol concentration was observed when beclomethasone dipropionate was administered in doses of 2000 mcg/day either by oral aerosol or intramuscularly. Immediate suppression of plasma cortisol concentrations was observed after single doses of 4000 mcg of beclomethasone dipropionate. Suppression of HPA function (reduction of early morning plasma cortisol levels) has been reported in adult patients who received 1600 mcg daily doses of oral beclomethasone dipropionate for one month. In clinical studies using beclomethasone dipropionate intranasally, there was no evidence of adrenal insufficiency.

Beclomethasone dipropionate is sparingly soluble. When given by nasal inhalation in the form of an aerosolized suspension, the drug is deposited primarily in the nasal passages. A portion of the drug is swallowed. Absorption occurs rapidly from all respiratory and gastrointestinal tissues. There is no evidence of tissue storage of beclomethasone dipropionate or its metabolites. *In vitro* studies, have shown that tissue other than the liver (lung slices) can rapidly metabolize beclomethasone dipropionate to beclomethasone 17-monopropionate and more slowly to free beclomethasone (which has very weak anti-inflammatory activity). However, irrespective of the route of entry the principal route of excretion of the drug and its metabolites is the feces. In humans, 12% to 15% of an orally administered dose of beclomethasone dipropionate is excreted in the urine as both conjugated and free metabolites of the drug. The half-life of beclomethasone dipropionate in humans is approximately 15 hours.

Studies have shown that the degree of binding to plasma proteins is 87%.

Indications and Usage: BECONASE Nasal Inhaler is indicated for the relief of the symptoms of seasonal or perennial rhinitis in those cases poorly responsive to conventional treatment.

Clinical studies have shown that improvement is usually apparent within a few days. However, symptomatic relief may not occur in some patients for as long as 2 weeks. Although systemic effects are minimal at recommended doses, BECONASE should not be continued beyond 3 weeks in the absence of significant symptomatic improvement. BECONASE should not be used in the presence of untreated localized infection involving the nasal mucosa.

Contraindications: Hypersensitivity to any of the ingredients of this preparation contraindicates its use.

Warnings: The replacement of a systemic corticosteroid with BECONASE Nasal Inhaler can be accompanied by signs of adrenal insufficiency.

When transfered to BECONASE Nasal Inhaler, careful attention must be given to patients previously treated for prolonged periods with systemic corticosteroids. This is particularly important in those patients who have associated asthma or other clinical conditions, where too rapid a decrease in systemic corticosteroids may cause a severe exacerbation of their symptoms.

Studies have shown that the combined administration of alternate-day prednisone systemic treatment and orally inhaled beclomethasone increase the likelihood of HPA suppression compared to a therapeutic dose of either one alone. Therefore, BECONASE treatment should be used with caution in patients already on alternate day prednisone regimens for any disease.

Precautions: General: During withdrawal from oral steroids, some patients may experience symptoms of withdrawal, e.g., joint and /or muscular pain, lassitude, and depression.

In clinical studies with beclomethasone dipropionate administered intranasally, the development of localized infections of the nose and pharynx with *Candida albicans* has occurred only rarely. When such an infection develops, it may require treatment with appropriate local therapy or discontinuance of treatment with BECONASE Nasal Inhaler.

Beclomethasone dipropionate is absorbed into the circulation. Use of excessive doses of BECONASE Nasal Inhaler may suppress HPA function.

BECONASE should be used with caution, if at all, in patients with active or quiescent tuberculous infections of the respiratory tract, or in untreated fungal, bacterial, systemic viral infections or ocular herpes simplex.

Because of the inhibitory effect of corticosteroids on wound healing, patients who have experienced recent nasal septal ulcers, nasal surgery, or trauma should not use a nasal corticosteroid until healing has occurred.

Although, systemic effects have been minimal with recommended doses, this potential increases with excessive doses. Therefore, larger than recommended doses should be avoided.

Information for Patients: Patients should use BECONASE Nasal Inhaler at regular intervals since its effectiveness depends on its regu-

Continued on next page

Glaxo—Cont.

lar use. The patient should take the medication as directed. It is not acutely effective and the prescribed dosage should not be increased. Instead nasal vasoconstrictors or oral antihistamines may be needed until the effects of BECONASE Nasal Inhaler are fully manifested. One to two weeks may pass before full relief is obtained. The patient should contact the doctor if symptoms do not improve, or if the condition worsens, or if sneezing or nasal irritation occurs. For the proper use of this unit and to attain maximum improvement, the patient should read and follow the accompanying Patient's Instructions carefully.

Carcinogenesis, Mutagenesis, Impairment of Fertility: Treatment of rats for a total of 95 weeks, 13 weeks by inhalation and 82 weeks by the oral route, resulted in no evidence of carcinogenic activity. Mutagenic studies have not been performed.

Impairment of fertility, as evidenced by inhibition of the estrous cycle in dogs, was observed following treatment by the oral route. No inhibition of the estrous cycle in dogs was seen following treatment with beclomethasone dipropionate by the inhalation route.

Pregnancy Category C: Like other corticoids, parenteral (subcutaneous) beclomethasone dipropionate has been shown to be teratogenic and embryocidal in the mouse and rabbit when given in doses approximately ten times the human dose. In these studies, beclomethasone was found to produce fetal resorption, cleft palate, agnathia, microstomia, absence of tongue, delayed ossification, and agenesis of the thymus. No teratogenic or embryocidal effects have been seen in the rat when beclomethasone dipropionate was administered by inhalation at 10 times the human dose or orally at 1000 times the human dose. There are no adequate and well-controlled studies in pregnant women. Beclomethasone dipropionate should be used during pregnancy only if the potential benefit justifies the potential risk to the fetus.

Nonteratogenic Effects: Hypoadrenalism may occur in infants born of mothers receiving corticosteroids during pregnancy. Such infants should be carefully observed.

Nursing Mothers: It is not known whether beclomethasone dipropionate is excreted in human milk. Because other corticosteroids are excreted in human milk, caution should be exercised when BECONASE Nasal Inhaler is administered to nursing women.

Pediatric Use: Safety and effectiveness in children below the age of 12 years have not been established.

Adverse Reactions: In general, side effects in clinical studies have been primarily associated with the nasal mucous membranes.

Adverse reactions reported in controlled clinical trials and long term open studies in patients treated with BECONASE are described below.

Sensations of irritation and burning in the nose (11 per 100 patients) following the use of BECONASE Nasal Inhaler have been reported. Also, occasional sneezing attacks (10 per 100 patients) have occurred immediately following the use of the intranasal inhaler.

Localized infections of the nose and pharynx with *Candida albicans* have occurred rarely. (See PRECAUTIONS).

Less than 2 per 100 patients reported transient episodes of bloody discharge from the nose.

Ulceration of the nasal mucosa has been reported rarely. Systemic corticosteroid side effects were not reported during the controlled clinical trials. If recommended doses are exceeded, however, or if individuals are particularly sensitive, symptoms of hypercorticism, i.e., Cushing's syndrome, could occur.

Dosage and Administration: *Adults and Children 12 years of age and over:* the usual dosage is one inhalation (42 mcg) in each nostril two to four times a day (total dose 168–336 mcg/day). Patients can often be maintained on a maximum dose of one inhalation in each nostril three times a day (252 mcg/day).

In patients who respond to BECONASE Nasal Inhaler, an improvement of the symptoms of seasonal or perennial rhinitis usually becomes apparent within a few days after the start of BECONASE Inhaler therapy.

The therapeutic effects of corticosteroids, unlike those of decongestants are not immediate. This should be explained to the patient in advance in order to ensure cooperation and continuation of treatment with the prescribed dosage regimen.

BECONASE Nasal Inhaler is *not* recommended for children below 12 years of age.

In the presence of excessive nasal mucus secretion or edema of the nasal mucosa, the drug may fail to reach the site of intended action. In such cases it is advisable to use a nasal vasoconstrictor during the first two to three days of BECONASE Nasal Inhaler therapy.

Directions for Use: Illustrated patient instructions for proper use accompany each package of BECONASE Nasal Inhaler.

CONTENTS UNDER PRESSURE. Do not puncture. Do not use or store near heat or open flame. Exposure to temperatures above 120°F may cause bursting. Never throw container into fire or incinerator. Keep out of reach of children.

Overdosage: When used at excessive doses, systemic corticosteroid effects such as hypercorticism and adrenal suppression may appear. If such symptoms appear, the dosage should be decreased. The oral LD_{50} of beclomethasone dipropionate is greater than 1 g/kg. One canister of BECONASE contains 8.4 mg. of beclomethasone dipropionate, therefore acute overdosage is unlikely.

How Supplied: BECONASE Nasal Inhaler, 16.8 g canister; box of one. Supplied with nasal adapter and patient's instructions; (0173-0336-88).

Store between 2° and 30°C (36° and 86°F).

[*Shown in Product Identification Section*]

CORTICAINE® Cream ℞

Description: Corticaine Cream contains hydrocortisone 0.5% and dibucaine 0.5% in a washable, non-greasy, mentholated, cream base composed of esters of mixed saturated fatty acids, stearyl alcohol, glycerin, polysorbate 40 and purified water with methylparaben and propylparaben as preservatives. Corticaine Cream is an anti-inflammatory and local anesthetic cream for topical and intrarectal use.

Clinical Pharmacology: Hydrocortisone is a corticosteroid that acts to reduce swelling, itching, hyperemia and other manifestations of inflammation regardless of the cause. Dibucaine, an amide-type local anesthetic, provides relief from pain, itching and burning by reversibly blocking nerve conduction when applied topically. Because dibucaine is an amide, it can often be used in patients sensitive to ester-type local anesthetics such as procaine and tetracaine. The base has a soothing, lubricant action.

Indications and Usage: Corticaine Cream is indicated for the relief of the inflammatory manifestations of corticosteroid-responsive dermatosis. When combined with other recognized therapeutic measures, it is recommended for the symptomatic relief of itching, pain and irritation of certain anorectal, anogenital and dermatological conditions. On the skin, it offers symptomatic relief in atopic dermatitis, sumac or ivy dermatitis, mild sunburn, minor burns, insect bites, prickly heat, eczema, postanal surgery, diaper rash and intertrigo. When introduced into the rectum, it helps to relieve the itching, pain and inflammation of internal hemorrhoids, as well as the anorectal discomfort of associated conditions such as proctitis, papillitis and cryptitis. When applied perianally, it can provide symptomatic relief from pruritus ani and external hemorrhoids.

Contraindications: Local tuberculosis, fungal and viral infections. Topical steroids and local anesthetics are contraindicated in those patients with a history of hypersensitivity to any of the components of the preparation. Not recommended for use in such diseases as pemphigus and discoid lupus erythematosus.

Precautions: GENERAL: Avoid use in the eyes. Do not apply to extensive areas for prolonged periods or with occlusive dressings as there may be increased systemic absorption of the ingredients. If irritation develops, the product should be discontinued and appropriate therapy instituted. In the presence of a secondary bacterial infection, the use of an appropriate antibacterial agent should be instituted; if a favorable response does not occur promptly, this preparation should be discontinued until the infection has been adequately controlled. Should not be used rectally without adequate proctologic examination. Not to be used with anorectal fistulas and abscesses.

USAGE IN PREGNANCY: Although topical steroids have not been reported to have an adverse effect on human pregnancy, the safety of their use in pregnant women has not been absolutely established. In laboratory animals, increases in incidence of fetal abnormalities have been associated with exposure of gestating females to topical corticosteroids—in some cases, at rather low dosage levels. Therefore, drugs of this class should not be used extensively on pregnant patients, in large amounts, or for prolonged periods of time.

Adverse Reactions: The following local adverse reactions have been reported with topical corticosteroids, especially under occlusive dressings: burning sensations, itching, irritation, dryness, folliculitis, hypertrichosis, acneform eruptions, hypopigmentation, perioral dermatitis, allergic contact dermatitis, maceration of the skin, secondary infection, skin atrophy, striae and miliaria.

Dosage and Administration: FOR RECTAL USE—Cleanse the rectal area and dry thoroughly before use. Attach plastic applicator to tube, and squeeze tube lightly to fill applicator with cream. Lubricate applicator with cream, then gently insert into rectum and squeeze tube again lightly to extrude a similar applicator dose of cream into the rectum. Can also be applied topically to irritated anorectal tissues. Use morning and evening and after each bowel movement. Recommended duration of treatment: 2 to 6 days.

FOR TOPICAL USE—Apply to affected areas of the skin 2 to 4 times daily. Recommended duration of treatment: 2 weeks.

How Supplied: Corticaine Cream (hydrocortisone 0.5% and dibucaine 0.5%) is supplied in a 1 oz tube with a rectal applicator (NDC 0173-0320-72). Keep container well-closed and store betwen 59° and 86° F. (15° and 30° C.).

[*Shown in Product Identification Section*]

CORTICAINE® SUPPOSITORIES ℞

Rectal Suppositories with Hydrocortisone

Description: CORTICAINE SUPPOSITORIES contain hydrocortisone acetate, 10 mg, in a hydrogenated vegetable oil base with zinc oxide and menthol. CORTICAINE SUPPOSITORIES are an anti-inflammatory for rectal use.

Clinical Pharmacology: Hydrocortisone is a corticosteroid that acts directly on the anorectal tissues to reduce swelling, itching, hyperemia and other manifestations of the tissue response to acute inflammation, regardless of the cause. The combination of hydrocortisone and the soothing ingredients of the base tends to reduce inflammation and edema.

Indications and Usage: When introduced into the rectum, CORTICAINE SUPPOSITORIES help to relieve the symptoms of internal hemorrhoids and serve as an adjunct in the treatment of the discomfort associated with proctitis, papillitis, cryptitis and other inflammatory conditions of the anorectum.

Contraindications: CORTICAINE SUPPOSITORIES are contraindicated in patients with local tuberculosis and viral infections and in those individuals with a history of hypersensitivity to any of the components of the preparation.

Precautions:

General—If irritation develops, the product should be discontinued and appropriate therapy instituted. In the presence of a secondary bacterial infection, the use of an appropriate antibacterial should be instituted; if a favorable response does not occur promptly, this preparation should be discontinued until the infection has been adequately controlled. Should not be used without adequate proctologic examination. Not to be used with anorectal fistulas and abscesses.

Use in Pregnancy—Although topical steroids have not been reported to have an adverse effect on human pregnancy, the safety of their use in pregnant women has not been absolutely established. In laboratory animals, increases in the incidence of fetal abnormalities have been associated with exposure of gestating females to topical steroids; in some cases at rather low dosage levels. Therefore, drugs of this class should not be used extensively on pregnant patients, in large amounts or for prolonged periods of time.

Pediatric Use—Safety and effectiveness in children have not been established.

Adverse Reactions: The following local adverse reactions have been reported with corticosteroid suppositories: burning, itching, irritation, dryness, folliculitis, hypopigmentation, allergic contact dermatitis and secondary infection.

Dosage and Administration: Insert one suppository in the rectum twice daily, morning and evening. Recommended duration of treatment, two to six days.

How Supplied: CORTICAINE SUPPOSITORIES (hydrocortisone acetate, 10 mg) are supplied in blue plastic containers of 12 (NDC 0173-0333-00). Keep at room temperature 59°–86°F. May be refrigerated. Dispense in original plastic container.

[*Shown in Product Identification Section*]

ETHATAB® Tablets ℞
(Ethaverine Hydrochloride)

Description: Each yellow Ethatab tablet contains Ethaverine Hydrochloride 100 mg.

Action: Ethatab acts directly on the smooth muscle cells, without involving the autonomic nervous system or its receptors. It produces smooth muscle relaxation, particularly where spasm exists, affecting the larger blood vessels, especially systemic, peripheral and pulmonary vessels, smooth muscle of the intestines, biliary tree, and ureters.

Indications: In peripheral and cerebral vascular insufficiency associated with arterial spasm; also useful as a smooth muscle spasmolytic in spastic conditions of the gastrointestinal and genitourinary tracts.

Contraindications: The use of Ethatab is contraindicated in the presence of complete atrioventricular dissociation.

Precautions: As with vasodilators, Ethatab should be administered with caution to patients with glaucoma. The safety of ethaverine hydrochloride during pregnancy or lactation has not been established; therefore it should not be used in pregnant women or in women of childbearing age unless, in the judgement of the physician, its use is deemed essential to the welfare of the patient.

Side Effects: Even though the incidence of side effects as reported in the literature is very low, it is possible for a patient to evidence nausea, anorexia, abdominal distress, dryness of the throat, hypotension, malaise, lassitude, drowsiness, flushing, sweating, vertigo, respiratory depression, cardiac depression, cardiac arrhythmia and headache. If these side effects occur, reduce dosage or discontinue medication.

Dosage and Administration: In mild or moderate disease, the usual dose for adults is one tablet three times a day. In more difficult cases, dosage may be increased to two tablets three times a day. It is most effective given early in the course of the vascular disorder. Because of the chronic nature of the disease, long-term therapy is required.

Supplied: Ethatab Tablets. Bottles of 100 and 500 tablets. Also available in unit dose packages of 100's.

[*Shown in Product Identification Section*]

HISTABID® ℞
DURACAP®
Timed Action Capsules

Description: Each HISTABID® DURACAP® timed-action capsule for oral administration contains:

Chlorpheniramine Maleate ....8 mg.
Phenylpropanolamine
Hydrochloride ....75 mg.

Clinical Pharmacology: The antihistamine component of HISTABID®, chlorpheniramine maleate, appears to act by competing with histamine for H-1 receptors on effector cells. It reduces or abolishes the allergic response to histamine of most tissues and smooth muscles. The decongestant component, phenylpropanolamine hydrochloride, provides vasoconstriction mediated by its action on the autonomic nervous system to produce a physiologic antagonism of the chemical mediators of allergy. HISTABID® reduces nasal congestion and secretions, and the ophthalmic and bronchial manifestations of the allergic response.

Indications: HISTABID® is indicated in conditions in which nasal decongestion is desired concurrently with the action of an antihistamine. Indicated for the symptomatic relief of upper respiratory allergic reactions (Hay Fever), perennial and seasonal allergic rhinitis, vasomotor rhinitis, allergic conjunctivitis due to inhalant allergies and foods, and mild, uncomplicated allergic skin manifestations of urticaria and angioedema.

Contraindications: HISTABID® should not be used in patients taking MAO inhibitors nor in those hypersensitive to any of the components.

Precautions:

General—HISTABID® should be used with considerable caution in patients with narrow angle glaucoma, stenosing peptic ulcer, pyloroduodenal obstruction, symptomatic prostatic hypertrophy, bladder neck obstruction, hypertension, thyroid disease, diabetes and heart disease. The risk of antihistamine-induced dizziness, sedation and hypotension is greater in elderly patients (over 60 years).

Information for Patients—Patients should be warned about engaging in activities requiring mental alertness, such as driving a car or operating appliances, machinery, etc.

Drug Interactions—HISTABID® should not be used in patients taking MAO inhibitors. Antihistamines have additive effects with alcohol and other CNS depressants (hypnotics, sedatives, tranquilizers, etc.).

Usage in Pregnancy—Pregnancy Category C. Animal reproduction studies have not been conducted with HISTABID®. It is also not known whether HISTABID® can cause fetal harm when administered to a pregnant woman or can affect reproduction capacity. HISTABID® should be given to pregnant women only if clearly needed.

Nursing Mothers—it is not known whether this drug is excreted in human milk. Because many drugs are excreted in human milk caution should be exercised when HISTABID® is administered to a nursing woman.

Pediatric Use—Safety and effectiveness of HISTABID® in children below the age of 6 have not been established.

Adverse Reactions:

General—Urticaria, drug rash, anaphylactic shock, photosensitivity, excessive perspiration, chills, dryness of mouth, nose and throat.

Cardiovascular System—Hypotension, hypertension, headache, palpitaions tachycarida, extrasystoles and angina pain.

Hematologic System—Hemolytic anemia, thrombocytopenia, agranulocytosis.

Nervous System—Sedation, dizziness, disturbed coordination, fatigue, confusion, restlessness, excitation, nervousness, tremor, irritability, insomnia, euphoria, paresthesias, blurred vision, diplopia, vertigo, tinnitus, acute labyrinthitis, hysteria, neuritis and convulsions.

Gastrointestinal System—Epigastric distress, anorexia, nausea, vomiting, diarrhea, constipation.

Genitourinary System—Urinary frequency, difficult urination, urinary retention, early menses.

Respiratory System—Thickening of bronchial secretions, tightness of chest and wheezing, nasal stuffiness.

Overdosage:

Symptoms—Overdosage symptoms may vary from central nervous system depression to stimulation. Peripheral atropine-like signs and symptoms as well as grastrointestinal symptoms may occur. Marked cerebral irritation resulting in jerking of muscles and possible convulsions may be followed by deep stupor and respiratory failure. Acute hypertension or cardiovascular collapse with accompanying hypotension may occur.

Treatment—If spontaneous vomiting has not occurred, immediate evacuation of the stomach should be induced by emesis or gastric lavage. Saline cathartics, as milk of magnesia, by osmosis draw water into the bowel and, therefore, are valuable for their action in rapid dilution of bowel content. Respiratory depression should be treated promptly with oxygen. Do not treat CNS depression with analeptics which might precipitate convulsions. If convulsions or marked CNS excitement occur, use only shortacting depressants.

Dosage and Administration: Adults and children over 6 years, one capsule on arising and one capsule 12 hours later. The DURACAP® form provides for prolonged therapeutic effect providing effect throughout the day, and if taken at bedtime, relief is made possible throughout the night.

How Supplied: HISTABID® DURACAP® capsules, pink and clear beadfilled capsules imprinted with "Glaxo", are supplied in bottles of 100 (NDC 0173-0309-13) and 500 (NDC 0173-0309-14) each.

[*Shown in Product Identification Section*]

THEOBID® & THEOBID® JR. ℞
DURACAP®
(Sustained Action Capsules)

Description: Two strengths of anhydrous theophylline sustained action capsules for oral administration are available. Each blue and clear THEOBID DURACAP capsule contains:

Theophylline, Anhydrous ....260 mg.

Each two-toned blue THEOBID JR. DURACAP capsule contains:

Theophylline, Anhydrous ....130 mg.

THEOBID and THEOBID JR. DURACAP capsules are bronchodilators.

Clinical Pharmacology: Theophylline directly relaxes the smooth muscle of the bron-

Continued on next page

Glaxo—Cont.

chial airways and pulmonary blood vessels, thus acting mainly as a bronchodilator, pulmonary vasodilator and smooth muscle relaxant. The drug also possesses other actions typical of the xanthine derivatives, such as coronary vasodilator, diuretic, cardiac stimulant, cerebral stimulant and skeletal muscle stimulant effects. The actions of theophylline may be mediated through inhibition of phosphodiesterase with a resultant increase in intracellular cyclic AMP which could mediate smooth muscle relaxation. At concentrations higher than attained *in vivo,* theophylline also inhibits the release of histamine by mast cells.

In vitro, theophylline has been shown to react synergistically with beta agonists (e.g. isoproterenol) that increase intracellular cyclic AMP through the stimulation of adenyl cyclase, but synergism has not been demonstrated in patient studies and more data is needed to determine if theophylline and beta agonists have clinically important additive effects *in vivo.*

Apparently no development of tolerance occurs with chronic use of theophylline.

The half life of theophylline is shortened with cigarette smoking and is prolonged in alcoholism, reduced hepatic or renal function, congestive heart failure and in patients receiving antibiotics such as TAO (troleandomycin), erythromycin and clindamycin. High fever for prolonged periods may decrease theophylline elimination.

THEOPHYLLINE ELIMINATION CHARACTERISTICS

Theophylline Elimination Characteristics—Children (over 6 months of age) have theophylline clearance rates of 1.45 ± 0.58 ml/kg/min (mean ± S.D.) with half-life of 3.7 ± 1.1 hours (mean ± S.D.). Adult nonsmokers, with uncomplicated asthma, have theophylline clearance rates of 0.65 ± 0.19 ml/kg/min (mean ± S.D.) with half-life of 8.7 ± 2.2 hours (mean ± S.D.).

Newborn infants have extremely slow clearances and half-lives exceeding 24 hours which approach those seen for older children after about 3–6 months.

Older adults with chronic obstructive pulmonary disease, any patients with corpulmonale or other causes of heart failure, and patients with liver pathology may have much lower clearances with half-lives that may exceed 24 hours.

The half-life of theophylline in smokers (1 to 2 packs/day) averaged 4–5 hours among various studies, much shorter than the half-life in nonsmokers who averaged about 7–9 hours. The increase in theophylline clearance caused by smoking is probably the result of induction of drug-metabolizing enzymes that do not readily normalize after cessation of smoking. It appears that between 3 months and 2 years may be necessary for normalization of the effect of smoking on theophylline pharmacokinetics.

Indications and Usage: For relief of acute bronchial asthma and for reversible bronchial spasm associated with chronic bronchitis and emphysema.

Contraindications: In individuals who have shown hypersensitivity to any of its components or xanthine derivatives.

Warnings: Excessive theophylline doses may be associated with toxicity and measurement of serum theophylline levels are recommended to assure maximal benefit without excessive risk. Incidence of toxicity increases at levels greater than 20 mcg/ml. Morphine, curare and stilbamidine should be used with caution in patients with airflow obstruction since they stimulate histamine release and can induce asthmatic attacks. They may also suppress respiration leading to respiratory failure. Alternative drugs should be chosen whenever possible.

There is an excellent correlation between high blood levels of theophylline resulting from conventional doses and associated clinical manifestations of toxicity in (1) patients with lowered body plasma clearances, (2) patients with liver dysfunction or chronic obstructive lung disease, (3) patients who are older than 55 years of age, particularly males.

There are often no early signs of less serious theophylline toxicity such as nausea and restlessness, which may appear in up to 50 percent of patients prior to onset of convulsions. Ventricular arrhythmias or seizures may be the first signs of toxicity.

Many patients who have high theophylline serum levels exhibit a tachycardia. Theophylline products may worsen preexisting arrhythmias.

Precautions:

General: Theophylline should not be administered concurrently with other xanthine medications. Use with caution in patients with severe cardiac disease, severe hypoxemia, hypertension, hyperthyroidism, acute myocardial injury, corpulmonale, congestive heart failure, liver disease, and in the elderly (especially males) and in neonates. Great caution should especially be used in giving theophylline to patients in congestive heart failure. Such patients have shown markedly prolonged theophylline blood level curves with theophylline persisting in serum for long periods following discontinuation of the drug.

Use theophylline cautiously in patients with a history of peptic ulcers. Theophylline may occasionally act as a local irritant to G.I. tract although gastrointestinal symptoms are more commonly central and associated with serum concentrations over 20 mcg/ml.

Drug Interactions: Theophylline antagonizes the action of propranolol. Theophylline increases diuresis of furosemide. Theophylline decreases hexamethonium-induced chronotropic effect. Theophylline potentiates reserpine-induced tachycardia. Troleandomycin (TAO), erythromycin, lincomycin and clindamycin increases theophylline plasma levels.

Usage in Pregnancy: Safe use in pregnancy has not been established relative to possible adverse effects on fetal development, but neither have adverse effects on fetal development been established. This is, unfortunately, true for most antiasthmatic medications. Therefore, use of theophylline in pregnant women should be balanced against the risk of uncontrolled asthma.

Nursing Mothers:

Cautions should be exercised when theophylline is administered to a nursing woman.

Adverse Reactions: The most consistent adverse reactions are usually due to overdose and are :

1. Gastrointestinal: nausea, vomiting, epigastric pain, hematemesis, diarrhea.
2. Central nervous system: headaches, irritability, restlessness, insomnia, reflex hyperexcitability, muscle twitching, clonic and tonic generalized convulsions.
3. Cardiovascular: palpitations, tachycardia, extra systoles, flushing, hypotension, circulatory failure, life threatening ventricular arrhythmias.
4. Respiratory: tachypnea.
5. Renal: albuminuria, increased excretion of renal tubular cells and red blood cells, potentiation of diuresis.
6. Others: hyperglycemia and inappropriate ADH syndrome.

Overdosage:

Management—

A. If potential oral overdose is established and seizure has not occurred:
   1. Induce vomiting.
   2. Administer a cathartic (this is particularly important if sustained preparations have been taken),
   3. Administer activated charcoal.

B. If patient is having a seizure:
   1. Establish an airway.
   2. Administer O_2,
   3. Treat the seizure with intravenous diazepam, 0.1 to 0.3 mg/kg up to 10 mg.
   4. Monitor vital signs, maintain blood pressure and provide adequate hydration.

C. Post-seizure coma:
   1. Maintain airway and oxygenation,
   2. If a result of oral medication, follow above recommendations to prevent absorption of drug, but intubation and lavage will have to be performed instead of inducing emesis, and the cathartic and charcoal will need to be introduced via a large bore gastric lavage tube,
   3. Continue to provide full supportive care and adequate hydration while waiting for drug to be metabolized. In general, the drug is metabolized sufficiently rapidly so as to not warrant consideration of dialysis.

Dosage and Administration: Therapeutic serum levels associated with optimal likelihood for benefit and minimal risk of toxicity are considered to be between 10 mcg/ml and 20 mcg/ml. Levels above 20 mcg/ml may produce toxic effects. There is great variation from patient to patient in dosage needed in order to achieve a therapeutic blood level because of variable rates of elimination. Because of this wide variation from patient to patient, and the relatively narrow therapeutic blood level range, dosage must be individualized and monitoring of theophylline serum levels is highly recommended.

Initial Dosage—The initial dosage of Theobid is approximately 8 mg/kg/12 hr or 260 mg every 12 hr, whichever is less. This dosage can be provided as Theobid Jr. 130 mg capsules, Theobid 260 mg capsules, or a combination of the 130 mg and 260 mg capsules. The initial dosage is conservative and will provide the assurance that serum theophylline levels will not exceed 20 mcg/ml.

Dosage Adjustment—The Theobid dosage should be increased by 130 or 260 mg/day at three day intervals so long as the drug is tolerated and there is no nausea, vomiting, diarrhea or headache. Minor side effects such irritability, nervousness and insomnia may occur, but most patients become tolerant to such side effects within a few days. The dosage, if tolerated, should be increased to, but not exceed:

12 mg/kg/12 hr for patients under 9 years*
10 mg/kg/12 hr for patients 9–12 years
9 mg/kg/12 hr for patients 12–16 years
6.5 mg/kg/12 hr for patients over 16 years or 900 mg/day, whichever is less

If any increase in dose is associated with adverse effects, i.e., nausea, vomiting, diarrhea or headache, the next dose should be skipped and subsequent doses should be reduced to the previously tolerated dose. If higher doses than those listed above are required, it is recommended that such dosage adjustments be monitored by serum theophylline levels.

*Rapid theophylline clearance rates in some patients may require 8 mg/kg administered at 8 hr intervals.

How Supplied: Theobid Duracap capsules, blue and clear capsules imprinted with "Glaxo", are supplied in bottles of 60 (NDC #0173-0268-12) and 500 capsules (NDC #0173-0268-14) as well as Unit Dose packs of 100 capsules (NDC #0173-0268-17).

The two-tone blue Theobid Jr. Duracap 130 mg capsules are supplied in bottles of 60 (NDC #0173-0295-12) and 500 capsules (NDC #0173-0295-14). Each capsule is imprinted with "Glaxo."

[*Shown in Product Identification Section*]

TRI–CONE® Capsules

Composition: Each white and black capsule contains:

Amylase ....10 mg
Prolase ....10 mg
Lipase ....10 mg
Simethicone ....40 mg

Actions and Uses: Tri-cone is indicated for the symptomatic relief of functional digestive disorders characterized by functional gastric bloating, dyspepsia, and flatulence resulting from failure to chew food properly, inadequate digestive competency due to disease or age, or faulty dietary habits. Tri-Cone is also indicated as a supplement to normal enzyme activity of the body in absorptive and assimilative defects associated with surgery on the stomach, small bowel, or pancreas and associated with chronic pancreatitis and pancreatic insufficiency.

Simethicone acts to relieve or alleviate the pain and other symptoms of gaseousness produced by bacterial fermentation and aerophagia.

The enzymes, particularly the proteolytic enzyme, do not require acid conditions to be activated which may be of special benefit in aiding digestion in geriatric patients with insufficient gastric acidity due to hypochlorhydria.

Contraindications: Known allergy to an ingredient.

Dosage: Two or three capsules after meals as required to relieve the symptoms of gas and aid digestion of fats, starches and proteins.

How Supplied: Bottles of 60 and 500 capsules.

[*Shown in Product Identification Section*]

TRI–CONE® PLUS Capsules ℞

Description: Each TRI-CONE® PLUS capsule for oral administration contains:

Amylase ....10 mg.
Prolase ....10 mg.
Lipase ....10 mg.
Simethicone ....40 mg.
Hyoscyamine Sulfate ....0.025 mg.

TRI-CONE® PLUS Capsules are a digestant, antiflatulent and intestinal antispasmodic.

Indications and Usage: TRI-CONE® PLUS is indicated for the symptomatic relief of functional digestive disorders characterized by functional gastric bloating, dyspepsia, and flatulence resulting from failure to chew food properly, inadequate digestive competency due to disease or age, or faulty dietary habits. TRI-CONE® PLUS is also indicated as a supplement to normal enzyme activity of the body in absorptive and assimilative defects associated with surgery on the stomach, small bowel, or pancreas and associated with chronic pancreatitis and pancreatic insufficiency. Simethicone acts to relieve or alleviate the pain and other symptoms of gaseousness produced by bacterial fermentation and aerophagia. The enzymes, particularly the proteolytic enzyme, do not require acid conditions to be activated which may be of special benefit in aiding digestion in geriatric patients with insufficient gastric acidity due to hypochlorhydria.

Hyoscyamine is added to TRI-CONE® PLUS capsules for its spasmolytic effect in the alimentary tract, which aids in the relief of pain due to spasm of the gastrointestinal musculature.

Contraindications: Acute glaucoma, advanced renal or hepatic disease, biliary or gastrointestinal tract obstruction or a hypersensitivity to any ingredient.

Precautions: General—Administer with caution to patients with incipient glaucoma, prostatic hypertrophy and known sensitivity to pork or enzymes.

Use in Pregnancy—Pregnancy Category C. Animal reproduction studies have not been conducted with TRI-CONE® PLUS. It is also not known whether TRI-CONE® PLUS can cause fetal harm when administered to a pregnant woman or can affect reproduction capacity. TRI-CONE® PLUS should be given to a pregnant woman only if clearly needed.

Use in Nursing Mothers—It is not known whether this drug is excreted in human milk. Because many drugs are excreted in human milk, caution should be exercised when TRI-CONE® PLUS is administered to a nursing woman.

Pediatric Use—Safety and effectiveness in children below the age of 12 have not been established.

Adverse Reactions: Mild dryness of the mouth, blurring of vision and difficult urination may occur at higher dosage levels.

Dosage and Administration: Usual adult dose, two or three capsules with or after meals.

How Supplied: TRI-CONE® PLUS capsules, two-tone green capsules imprinted with "Glaxo," are supplied in bottles of 60 (NDC 0173-0315-22) and 500 (NDC 0173-0315-24) capsules each.

[*Shown in Product Identification Section*]

TRINSICON® ℞
Hematinic Concentrate With Intrinsic Factor

A highly potent oral antianemia preparation

Description: Each capsule contains—

Special Liver-Stomach Concentrate (containing Intrinsic Factor) ....240 mg.
Cobalamin Concentrate, USP, equivalent to Cobalamin ....7.5 mcg.
(The total vitamin B_{12} activity in the Special Liver-Stomach Concentrate and the Cobalamin Concentrate, USP, is 15 micrograms.)
Iron, Elemental ....110 mg.
(as Ferrous Fumarate)
Ascorbic Acid (Vitamin C) ....75 mg.
Folic Acid ....0.5 mg.

Clinical Pharmacology: *Vitamin B_{12} with* Intrinsic Factor—When secretion of intrinsic factor in gastric juice is inadequate or absent (e.g., in Addisonian pernicious anemia or after gastrectomy), vitamin B_{12} in physiologic doses is absorbed poorly, if at all. The resulting deficiency of vitamin B_{12} leads to the clinical manifestations of pernicious anemia. Similar megaloblastic anemias may develop in fish tapeworm *(Diphyllobothrium latum)* infection or after a surgically created small-bowel blind loop; in these situations, treatment requires freeing the host of the parasites or bacteria which appear to compete for the available vitamin B_{12}. Strict vegetarianism and malabsorption syndromes may also lead to vitamin B_{12} deficiency. In the latter case, parenteral therapy, or oral therapy with so-called massive doses of vitamin B_{12}, may be necessary for adequate treatment of the patient.

Potency of intrinsic factor concentrates is determined physiologically, i.e., by their use in patients with pernicious anemia. The liver-stomach concentrate with intrinsic factor and the vitamin B_{12} contained in 2 Trinsicon capsules provide 1½ times the minimum amount of therapeutic agent which, when given daily in an uncomplicated case of pernicious anemia, will produce a satisfactory reticulocyte response and relief of anemia and symptoms.

Concentrates of intrinsic factor derived from hog gastric, pyloric, and duodenal mucosa have been used successfully in patients who lack intrinsic factor. For example, Fouts *et al.* maintained patients with pernicious anemia in clinical remission with oral therapy (liver extracts or intrinsic factor concentrate with vitamin B_{12}) for as long as 29 years.

After total gastrectomy, Ficarra found multifactor preparations taken orally to be "just as effective in maintaining blood levels as any medication that has to be administered parenterally." His study was based on 24 patients who had survived for 5 years after total gastrectomy for cancer and who had been taking 2 Trinsicon capsules daily.

Folic Acid—Folic acid deficiency is the immediate cause of most, if not all, cases of nutritional megaloblastic anemia and of the megaloblastic anemias of pregnancy and infancy; usually, it is also at least partially responsible for the megaloblastic anemias of malabsorption syndromes, e.g., tropical and nontropical sprue.

It is apparent that in vitamin B_{12} deficiency (e.g., pernicious anemia), lack of this vitamin results in impaired utilization of folic acid. There are other evidences of the close folic acid-vitamin B_{12} interrelationship: (1) B_{12} influences the storage, absorption, and utilization of folic acid, and (2), as a deficiency of B_{12} progresses, the requirement for folic acid increases. However, folic acid does not change the requirement for vitamin B_{12}.

Iron—A very common anemia is that due to iron deficiency. In most cases, the response to iron salts is prompt, safe, and predictable. Within limits, the response is quicker and more certain to large doses of iron than to small doses.

Each Trinsicon capsule furnishes 110 mg. of elemental iron (as ferrous fumarate) to provide a maximum response.

Ascorbic Acid—Vitamin C plays a role in anemia therapy. It augments the conversion of folic acid to its active form, folinic acid. In addition, ascorbic acid promotes the reduction of ferric iron in food to the more readily absorbed ferrous form. Severe and prolonged vitamin C deficiency is associated with an anemia which is usually hypochromic but occasionally megaloblastic in type.

Indications and Usage: Trinsicon® (hematinic concentrate with intrinsic factor) is a multifactor preparation effective in the treatment of anemias that respond to oral hematinics, including pernicious anemia and other megaloblastic anemias and also iron-deficiency anemia. Therapeutic quantities of hematopoietic factors that are known to be important are present in the recommended daily dose.

Contraindications: Hemochromatosis and hemosiderosis are contraindications to iron therapy.

Precautions:

General Precautions—Anemia is a manifestation that requires appropriate investigation to determine its cause or causes.

Folic acid *alone* is unwarranted in the treatment of pure vitamin B_{12} deficiency states, such as pernicious anemia. Folic acid may obscure pernicious anemia in that the blood picture may revert to normal while neurological manifestations remain progressive.

As with all preparations containing intrinsic factor, resistance may develop in some cases of pernicious anemia to the potentiation of absorption of physiologic doses of vitamin B_{12}. If resistance occurs, parenteral therapy, or oral therapy with so-called massive doses of vitamin B_{12} may be necessary for adequate treatment of the patient. No single regimen fits all cases, and the status of the patient observed in follow-up is the final criterion for adequacy of therapy. Periodic clinical and laboratory studies are considered essential and are recommended.

Usage in Pregnancy—Pregnancy Category C—Animal reproduction studies have not been conducted with Trinsicon. It is also not known whether Trinsicon can cause fetal harm when administered to a pregnant woman or can affect reproduction capacity. Trinsicon should be given to a pregnant women only if clearly needed.

Nursing Mothers—It is not known whether this drug is excreted in human milk. Because many drugs are excreted in human milk, caution should be exercised when Trinsicon is administered to a nursing woman.

Continued on next page

Glaxo—Cont.

Usage in Children—Safety and effectiveness in children below the age of 10 have not been established.

Adverse Reactions: Rarely, iron in therapeutic doses produces gastrointestinal reactions, such as diarrhea or constipation. Reducing the dose and administering it with meals will minimize these effects in the iron-sensitive patient.

In extremely rare instances, skin rash suggesting allergy has been noted following the oral administration of liver-stomach material. Allergic sensitization has been reported following both oral and parenteral administration of folic acid.

Overdosage:

Symptoms—Those of iron intoxication, which may include pallor and cyanosis, vomiting, hematemesis, diarrhea, melena, shock, drowsiness, and coma.

Treatment—For specific therapy, exchange transfusion and chelating agents. For general management, gastric and rectal lavage with sodium bicarbonate solution or milk, administration of intravenous fluids and electrolytes, and use of oxygen.

Dosage: One capsule twice a day. (Two capsules daily produce a standard response in the average uncomplicated case of pernicious anemia.)

How Supplied: Capsules, dark pink and dark red (No. 2). Bottles of 60 (NDC 0173-0337-22), bottles of 500 (NDC 0173-0337-24), and Unit Dose Packs of 100 capsules (NDC 0173-0337-27).

VENTOLIN® Inhaler ℞
(albuterol)
Bronchodilator Aerosol
FOR ORAL INHALATION ONLY

Description: The active component of VENTOLIN Inhaler is albuterol (α'-[(*tert*-butylamino)methyl]-4-hydroxy-*m*-xylene-α, α'-diol), a relatively selective beta$_2$-adrenergic bronchodilator.

Albuterol is the official generic name in the United States. The international generic name for the drug is salbutamol. The molecular weight of albuterol is 239.3.

VENTOLIN Inhaler is a metered-dose aerosol unit for oral inhalation. It contains a microcrystalline suspension of albuterol in propellants (trichloromonofluoromethane and dichlorodifluoromethane) with oleic acid. Each actuation delivers from the mouthpiece 90 mcg of albuterol. Each canister provides at least 200 inhalations.

Clinical Pharmacology: The prime action of beta-adrenergic drugs is to stimulate adenyl cyclase, the enzyme which catalyzes the formation of cyclic-3′, 5′-adenosine monophosphate (cyclic AMP) from adenosine triphosphate (ATP). The cyclic AMP thus formed mediates the cellular responses. By virtue of its relatively selective action on beta$_2$-adrenoceptors, albuterol relaxes smooth muscle of the bronchi, uterus, and vascular supply to skeletal muscle, but may have less cardiac stimulant effects than does isoproterenol.

Albuterol is longer acting than isoproterenol by any route of administration in most patients because it is not a substrate for the cellular uptake processes for catecholamines nor for catechol-O-methyl transferase.

Because of its gradual absorption from the bronchi, systemic levels of albuterol are low after inhalation of recommended doses. Studies undertaken with four subjects administered tritiated albuterol, resulted in maximum plasma concentrations occurring within two to four hours. Due to the sensitivity of the assay method, the metabolic rate and half-life of elimination of albuterol in plasma could not be determined. However, urinary excretion provided data indicating that albuterol has an elimination half-life of 3.8 hours. Approximately 72 percent of the inhaled dose is excreted within 24 hours in the urine, and consists of 28 percent of unchanged drug and 44 percent as metabolite.

Results of animal studies show that albuterol does not pass the blood-brain barrier.

The effects of rising doses of albuterol and isoproterenol aerosols were studied in volunteers and asthmatic patients. Results in normal volunteers indicated that albuterol is ½ to ¼ as active as isoproterenol in producing increases in heart rate. In asthmatic patients similar cardiovascular differentiation between the two drugs was also seen.

Indications and Usage: VENTOLIN Inhaler is indicated for the relief of bronchospasm in patients with reversible obstructive airway disease.

In controlled clinical trials the onset of improvement in pulmonary function was within 15 minutes, as determined by both maximal midexpiratory flow rate (MMEF) and FEV$_1$. MMEF measurements also showed that near maximum improvement in pulmonary function generally occurs within 60 to 90 minutes following 2 inhalations of albuterol and that clinically significant improvement generally continues for 3 to 4 hours in most patients. In clinical trials, some patients with asthma showed a therapeutic response (defined by maintaining FEV$_1$ values 15 percent or more above base line) which was still apparent at 6 hours. Continued effectiveness of albuterol was demonstrated over a 13-week period in these same trials.

Contraindications: VENTOLIN Inhaler is contraindicated in patients with a history of hypersensitivity to any of its components.

Warnings: As with other adrenergic aerosols, the potential for paradoxical bronchospasm should be kept in mind. If it occurs, the preparation should be discontinued immediately and alternative therapy instituted.

Fatalities have been reported in association with excessive use of inhaled sympathomimetic drugs. The exact cause of death is unknown, but cardiac arrest following the unexpected development of a severe acute asthmatic crisis and subsequent hypoxia is suspected.

The contents of VENTOLIN Inhaler are under pressure. Do not puncture. Do not use or store near heat or open flame. Exposure to temperatures above 120°F may cause bursting. Never throw container into fire or incinerator. Keep out of reach of children.

Precautions: Although it has less effect on the cardiovascular system than isoproterenol at recommended dosages, albuterol is a sympathomimetic amine and as such should be used with caution in patients with cardiovascular disorders, including coronary insufficiency and hypertension, in patients with hyperthyroidism or diabetes mellitus, and in patients who are unusually responsive to sympathomimetic amines.

Large doses of intravenous albuterol have been reported to aggravate preexisting diabetes and ketoacidosis. The relevance of this observation to the use of VENTOLIN Inhaler is unknown, since the aerosol dose is much lower than the doses given intravenously.

Although there have been no reports concerning the use of VENTOLIN Inhaler during labor and delivery, it has been reported that high doses of albuterol administered intravenously inhibit uterine contractions. Although this effect is extremely unlikely as a consequence of aerosol use, it should be kept in mind.

Information For Patients: The action of VENTOLIN Inhaler may last up to six hours and therefore it should not be used more frequently than recommended. Do not increase the number or frequency of doses without medical consultation. If symptoms get worse, medical consultation should be sought promptly. While taking VENTOLIN Inhaler, other inhaled medicines should not be used unless prescribed.

See Illustrated Patient Instructions For Use.

Drug Interactions: Other sympathomimetic aerosol bronchodilators or epinephrine should not be used concomitantly with albuterol.

Albuterol should be administered with caution to patients being treated with monoamine oxidase inhibitors or tricyclic antidepressants, since the action of albuterol on the vascular system may be potentiated.

Beta-receptor blocking agents and albuterol inhibit the effect of each other.

Carcinogenesis, Mutagenesis, and Impairment of Fertility: In a 2 year study in the rat, albuterol sulfate caused a significant dose-related increase in the incidence of benign leiomyomatas of the mesovarium at doses corresponding to 111, 555, and 2,800 times the maximum human inhalational dose. The relevance of these findings to humans is not known. An 18-month study in mice revealed no evidence of tumorigenicity. Studies with albuterol revealed no evidence of mutagenesis. Reproduction studies in rats revealed no evidence of impaired fertility.

Teratogenic Effects—Pregnancy Category C: Albuterol has been shown to be teratogenic in mice when given in doses corresponding to 14 times the human dose. There are no adequate and well-controlled studies in pregnant women. Albuterol should be used during pregnancy only if the potential benefit justifies the potential risk to the fetus. A reproduction study in CD-1 mice with albuterol (0.025, 0.25, and 2.5 mg/kg, corresponding to 1.4, 14, and 140 times the maximum human inhalational dose) showed a cleft palate formation in 5 of 111 (4.5 percent) fetuses at 0.25 mg/kg and in 10 or 108 (9.3 percent) fetuses at 2.5 mg/kg. None were observed at 0.025 mg/kg. Cleft palate also occurred in 22 of 72 (30.5 percent) fetuses treated with 2.5 mg/kg isoproterenol (positive control). A reproduction study in Stride Dutch rabbits revealed cranioschisis in 7 of 19 (37 percent) fetuses at 50 mg/kg, corresponding to 2,800 times the maximum human inhalational dose.

Nursing Mothers: It is not known whether this drug is excreted in human milk. Because of the potential for tumorigenicity shown for albuterol in animal studies, a decision should be made whether to discontinue nursing or to discontinue the drug, taking into account the importance of the drug to the mother.

Pediatric Use: Safety and effectiveness in children below the age of 12 years have not been established.

Adverse Reactions: The adverse reactions of albuterol are similar in nature to those of other sympathomimetic agents, although the incidence of certain cardiovascular effects is less with albuterol. A 13-week double-blind study compared albuterol and isoproterenol aerosols in 147 asthmatic patients. The results of this study showed that the incidence of cardiovascular effects was: palpitations, less than 10 per 100 with albuterol and less than 15 per 100 with isoproterenol. The incidences of tachycardia and increased blood pressure were 10 per 100 and less than 5 per 100, respectively, with both drugs. In the same study, both drugs caused tremor or nausea in less than 15 patients per 100; dizziness or heartburn in less than 5 per 100 patients. Nervousness occurred in less than 10 per 100 patients receiving albuterol and in less than 15 per 100 patients receiving isoproterenol.

In addition, albuterol, like other sympathomimetic agents, can cause adverse reactions such as hypertension, angina, vomiting, vertigo, central stimulation, insomnia, headache, unusual taste, and drying or irritation of the oropharynx.

Overdosage: Exaggeration of the effects listed in ADVERSE REACTIONS can occur. Anginal pain and hypertension may result.

The oral LD_{50} in male and female rats and mice was greater than 2,000 mg/kg. The aerosol LD_{50} could not be determined.
Dialysis is not appropriate treatment for overdosage of VENTOLIN Inhaler. The judicious use of a cardioselective beta-receptor blocker, such as metoprolol tartrate, is suggested, bearing in mind the danger of inducing an asthmatic attack.
Dosage and Administration: The usual dosage for adults and children 12 years and older is 2 inhalations repeated every 4 to 6 hours; in some patients, 1 inhalation every 4 hours may be sufficient. More frequent administration of a larger number of inhalations is not recommended. The use of VENTOLIN Inhaler can be continued as medically indicated to control recurring bouts of bronchospasm. During this time most patients gain optimal benefit from regular use of the inhaler. Safe usage for periods extending over several years has been documented.
If a previously effective dosage regimen fails to provide the usual relief, medical advice should be sought immediately as this is often a sign of seriously worsening asthma which would require reassessment of therapy.
How Supplied: VENTOLIN Inhaler, 17.0 g canister; box of one. Each actuation delivers 90 mcg of albuterol from the mouthpiece. It is supplied with an oral adapter and patient's instructions: (NDC 0173-0321-88). Also available, VENTOLIN Inhaler Refill, 17.0 g canister only with patient's instructions (NDC 0173-0321-98).
Store between 15° and 30°C (59° to 86°F).
[*Shown in Product Identification Section*]

VENTOLIN® Tablets ℞
(albuterol)

Description: VENTOLIN Tablets contain albuterol sulfate, a relatively selective $beta_2$-adrenergic bronchodilator. Albuterol sulfate has the chemical name α^1-[(*tert*-Butylamino)-methyl]-4-hydroxy-*m*-xylene-α,α-diol sulfate (2:1)(salt).
Albuterol sulfate has a molecular weight of 576.7 and the empirical formula $(C_{13}H_{21}NO_3)_2 \cdot H_2SO_4$. Albuterol sulfate is a white crystalline powder, soluble in water and slightly soluble in ethanol.
The international generic name for albuterol base is salbutamol.
Each VENTOLIN Tablet contains 2 or 4 mg of albuterol as 2.4 and 4.8 mg of albuterol sulfate, respectively.
Clinical Pharmacology: The prime action of beta-adrenergic drugs is to stimulate adenyl cyclase, the enzyme which catalyzes the formation of cyclic-3',5'-adenosine monophosphate (cyclic AMP) from adenosine triphosphate (ATP). The cyclic AMP thus formed mediates the cellular responses. Based on pharmacologic studies in animals, albuterol appears to exert direct and preferential action on $beta_2$-adrenoceptors including those of the bronchial tree and uterus, and may have less cardiac stimulant effect than isoproterenol, when given in the usual recommended dose.
Albuterol is longer acting than isoproterenol in most patients by any route of administration because it is not a substrate for the cellular uptake processes for catecholamines nor for catechol-O-methyl transferase.
In three normal volunteers given tablets containing 6 mg tritiated albuterol sulfate, the maximum plasma concentrations of albuterol occurred within 2.5 hours. In other studies, the analysis of peak plasma samples indicated that the metabolite of albuterol represented 80% of the radioactivity present. Albuterol was shown to have a plasma half-life ranging from 2.7 to 5.0 hours when administered orally. Analysis of urine samples showed that 76% of the dose was excreted over 3 days, with the majority of the dose being excreted within the first 24 hours. Sixty percent of this radioactivity was shown to be the metabolite. Feces collected over this period contained 4% of the administered dose.
Animal studies show that albuterol does not pass the blood-brain barrier.
Indications and Usage: VENTOLIN Tablets are indicated for the relief of bronchospasm in patients with reversible obstructive airway disease.
In controlled clinical trials in patients with asthma, the onset of improvement in pulmonary function, as measured by maximal midexpiratory flow rate, MMEF, *was noted* within 30 minutes after a dose of VENTOLIN Tablets with peak improvement occurring between 2 to 3 hours. In controlled clinical trials in which measurements were conducted for 6 hours, significant clinical improvement in pulmonary function (defined as maintaining a 15% or more increase in FEV, and a 20% or more increase in MMEF over baseline values) was observed in 60% of patients at 4 hours and in 40% at 6 hours. No decrease in the effectiveness of VENTOLIN Tablets has been reported in patients who received long-term treatment with the drug in uncontrolled studies for periods up to 6 months.
Contraindications: VENTOLIN Tablets are contraindicated in patients with a history of hypersensitivity to any of its components.
Precautions: General: Although albuterol usually has minimal effects on the $beta_1$-adrenoceptors of the cardiovascular system at the recommended dosage, occassionally the usual cardiovascular and CNS stimulatory effects common to all sympathomimetic agents have been seen with patients treated with albuterol necessitating discontinuation. Therefore, albuterol should be used with caution in patients with cardiovascular disorders, including coronary insufficiency and hypertension, in patients with hyperthyroidism or diabetes mellitus, and in patients who are unusually responsive to sympathomimetic amines.
Large doses of intravenous albuterol have been reported to aggravate preexisting diabetes mellitus and ketoacidosis. The relevance of this observation to the use of VENTOLIN Tablets is unknown.
Although there have been no reports concerning the use of VENTOLIN Tablets during labor and delivery, high doses of albuterol administered intravenously are reported to inhibit uterine contractions. Although this effect is extremely unlikely as a consequence of oral use, it should be kept in mind.
Information for Patients: The action of VENTOLIN Tablets may last for six hours or longer and therefore it should not be taken more frequently than recommended. Do not increase the dose or frequency of medication without medical consultation. If symptoms get worse, medical consultation should be sought promptly.
Drug Interactions: The concomitant use of VENTOLIN Tablets and other oral sympathomimetic agents is not recommended since such combined use may lead to deleterious cardiovascular effects. This recommendation does not preclude the judicious use of an aerosol bronchodilator of the adrenergic stimulant type in patients receiving VENTOLIN Tablets. Such concomitant use, however, should be individualized and not given on a routine basis. If regular co-administration is required, then alternative therapy should be considered.
Albuterol should be administered with extreme caution to patients being treated with monoamine oxidase inhibitors or tricyclic antidepressants, since the action of albuterol on the vascular system may be potentiated.
Beta-receptor blocking agents and albuterol inhibit the effect of each other.
Carcinogenesis, Mutagenesis, and Impairment of Fertility: Albuterol sulfate, like other agents in its class, caused a significant dose-related increase in the incidence of benign leiomyomas of the mesovarium in a 2-year study in the rat, at doses corresponding to 3, 16, and 78 times the maximum human oral dose. In another study this effect was blocked by the co-administration of propranolol. The relevance of these findings to humans is not known. An 18-month study in mice and a lifetime study in hamsters revealed no evidence of tumorigenicity. Studies with albuterol revealed no evidence of mutagenesis. Reproduction studies in rats revealed no evidence of impaired fertility.
Teratogenic Effects-Pregnancy Category C: Albuterol has been shown to be teratogenic in mice when given subcutaneously in doses corresponding to 0.4 times the maximum human oral dose.
There are no adequate and well-controlled studies in pregnant women. Albuterol should be used during pregnancy only if the potential benefit justifies the potential risk to the fetus.
A reproduction study in CD-1 mice with albuterol showed cleft palate formation in 5 of 111 (4.5%) fetuses at 0.25 mg/kg and in 10 of 108 (9.3%) fetuses at 2.5 mg/kg, none were observed at 0.025 mg/kg. Cleft palate also occurred in 22 of 72 (30.5%) fetuses treated with 2.5 mg/kg isoproterenol (positive control). A reproduction study in Stride Dutch rabbits revealed cranioschisis in 7 of 19 (37%) fetuses at 50 mg/kg, corresponding to 78 times the maximum human oral dose of albuterol.
Nursing Mothers: It it not known whether this drug is excreted in human milk. Because of the potential for tumorigenicity shown for albuterol in animal studies, a decision should be made whether to discontinue nursing or to discontinue the drug, taking into account the importance of the drug to the mother.
Pediatric Use: Safety and effectiveness in children below the age of 12 years have not been established.
Adverse Reactions: The adverse reactions to albuterol are similar in nature to those of other sympathomimetic agents. The most frequent adverse reactions to VENTOLIN Tablets were nervousness and tremor, with each occurring in approximately 20 of 100 patients. Other reported reactions were headache, 7 of 100 patients; tachycardia and palpitations, 5 of 100 patients; muscle cramps, 3 of 100 patients; insomnia, nausea, weakness, and dizziness, each occurred in 2 of 100 patients. Drowsiness, flushing, restlessness, irritability, chest discomfort, and difficulty in micturition each occurred in less than 1 of 100 patients.
In addition, albuterol, like other sympathomimetic agents, can cause adverse reactions such as hypertension, angina, vomiting, vertigo, central stimulation, unusual taste, and drying or irritation of the oropharynx.
The reactions are generally transient in nature, and it is usually not necessary to discontinue treatment with VENTOLIN Tablets. In selected cases, however, dosage may be reduced temporarily; after the reaction has subsided, dosage should be increased in small increments to the optimal dosage.
Overdosage: Manifestations of overdosage include anginal pain, hypertension and exaggeration of the effects listed in **ADVERSE REACTIONS.**
The oral LD_{50} in rats and mice was greater than 2,000 mg/kg.
Dialysis is not appropriate treatment for overdosage of VENTOLIN Tablets. The judicious use of a cardioselective beta-receptor blocker, such as metoprolol tartrate, is suggested, bearing in mind the danger of inducing an asthmatic attack.
Dosage and Administration: The following dosages of VENTOLIN Tablets are expressed in terms of albuterol base.
Usual Dose: The usual starting dosage for adults and children 12 years and over is 2 mg or 4 mg three or four times a day.

Continued on next page

Glaxo—Cont.

Dosage Adjustment: Doses above 4 mg, four times a day should be used only when the patient fails to respond. If a favorable response does not occur with the 4 mg initial dosage, it should be cautiously increased step wise up to a maximum of 8 mg four times a day as tolerated.

Elderly Patients and Those Sensitive to Beta-Adrenergic Stimulators: An initial dosage of 2 mg three or four times a day is recommended for elderly patients and for those with a history of unusual sensitivity to beta-adrenergic stimulators. If adequate bronchodilatation is not obtained, dosage may be increased gradually to as much as 8 mg three or four times a day.

The total daily dose should not exceed 32 mg in adults and children 12 years and over.

How Supplied: VENTOLIN Tablets, 2 mg albuterol as the sulfate, white, round, compressed tablets, impressed with the product name (VENTOLIN) and the number 2 on one side, and scored on the other with "GLAXO" impressed on each side of the score; bottles of 100 (NDC 0173-0341-43).

VENTOLIN Tablets, 4 mg albuterol as the sulfate, white, round, compressed tablets, impressed with the product name (VENTOLIN) and the number 4 on one side, and scored on the other with "GLAXO" impressed on each side of the score; bottles of 100 (NDC 0173-0342-43).

Store between 2° and 30°C (36° and 86°F).

[Shown in Product Identification Section]

VICON-C® Capsules
(Therapeutic Vitamins and Minerals)

Composition: Each yellow and orange capsule contains:

Ascorbic Acid .... 300 mg.
Niacinamide .... 100 mg.
Thiamine Mononitrate .... 20 mg.
d-Calcium Pantothenate .... 20 mg.
Riboflavin .... 10 mg.
Pyridoxine Hydrochloride .... 5 mg.
Magnesium Sulfate USP* .... 70 mg.
Zinc Sulfate USP** .... 80 mg.

* As 50 mg. of dried Magnesium Sulfate
** As 50 mg. of dried Zinc Sulfate.

Actions and Uses: VICON-C® is indicated in the treatment of patients with deficiencies of, or increased requirements for Vitamin C, B-Complex vitamins, zinc and/or magnesium. The components of Vicon-C® have important roles in nutrition, tissue growth and repair, and the prevention of hemorrhage. Tissue injury resulting from trauma, burns or surgery may rapidly deplete the body stores of Vitamin C, the B-Complex vitamins and zinc. Patients maintained on parenteral fluids for extended periods or patients with burns, wounds or diarrhea often develop deficiencies of Vitamin C, the B-Complex vitamins and zinc.

VICON-C® is recommended for deficiencies or the prevention of deficiencies of Vitamin C, the B-Complex vitamins, magnesium and/or zinc in conditions such as febrile diseases, chronic or acute infections, burns fractures, surgery, toxic conditions, physiologic stress, alcoholism, pregnancy, lactation, geriatrics, gastritis, peptic ulcer, colitis and in conditions involving special diets and weight-reduction diets. It is also recommended in dentistry for these deficiencies in conditions such as herpetic stomatitis, aphthous stomatitis, cheilosis, herpangina, gingivitis and states involving oral surgery.

Administration and Dosage: One capsule 2 or 3 times daily or as directed by a physician for treatment of deficiencies.

How Supplied: Bottles of 60 and 500 Capsules and Unit Dose Pack of 100 Capsules.

[Shown in Product Identification Section]

VICON®-PLUS Capsules
(Therapeutic Vitamins and Minerals)

Composition: Each red and beige capsule contains:

Vitamin A .... 4,000 I.U.
Vitamin E .... 50 I.U.
Ascorbic Acid .... 150 mg.
Zinc Sulfate USP* .... 80 mg.
Magnesium Sulfate USP** .... 70 mg.
Niacinamide .... 25 mg.
Thiamine Mononitrate .... 10 mg.
d-Calcium Pantothenate .... 10 mg.
Riboflavin .... 5 mg.
Manganese Chloride .... 4 mg.
Pyridoxine HCl .... 2 mg.

* As 50 mg. of Dried Zinc Sulfate
** As 50 mg. of Dried Magnesium Sulfate

Vicon-Plus is an extended range vitamin-mineral supplement formulated to aid patient recovery by helping to meet increased nutritional demands.

Indications: For nutritional supplementation of the patient undergoing physiologic stress due to surgery, burns, trauma, febrile illnesses, or poor nutrition.

Dosage: 1 capsule twice daily or as prescribed by a physician for treatment of deficiencies. Dosage should not exceed 8 capsules daily due to the possible toxicity of large dosages of vitamin A.

How Supplied: In bottles of 60 capsules and 500 capsules.

[Shown in Product Identification Section]

VICON FORTE® Capsules ℞
(Therapeutic Vitamins-Minerals)

Description: Each black and orange capsule for oral administration contains:

Vitamin A .... 8,000 I.U.
Vitamin E .... 50 I.U.
Ascorbic Acid .... 150 mg.
Zinc Sulfate USP* .... 80 mg.
Magnesium Sulfate USP** .... 70 mg.
Niacinamide .... 25 mg.
Thiamine Mononitrate .... 10 mg.
d-Calcium Pantothenate .... 10 mg.
Riboflavin .... 5 mg.
Manganese Chloride .... 4 mg.
Pyridoxine Hydrochloride .... 2 mg.
Folic Acid .... 1 mg.
Vitamin B_{12}(Cyanocobalamin) .... 10 mcg.

* As 50 mg. of Dried Zinc Sulfate
** As 50 mg. of Dried Magnesium Sulfate

VICON FORTE® is a therapeutic vitamin-mineral preparation.

Indications and Usage: VICON FORTE® is indicated for the treatment and/or prevention of vitamin and mineral deficiencies associated with restricted diets, improper food intake, alcoholism, and decreased absorption. VICON FORTE® is also indicated in patients with increased requirements for vitamins and minerals due to chronic disease, infection, and burns and in persons using alcohol to excess. Pre- and post-operative use of VICON FORTE® can provide the increased amounts of vitamins and minerals necessary for optimal recovery from the stress of surgery.

Contraindications: None known.

Precautions: General—Folic acid in doses above 0.1 mg daily may obscure pernicious anemia in that hematologic remission can occur while neurological manifestations remain progressive.

Dosage and Administration: One capsule daily or as directed by the physician.

How Supplied: Capsules, orange and black imprinted with "Glaxo," and "316" in bottles of 60 (NDC 0173-0316-22) and 500 (NDC 0173-0316-24) capsules each and in unit dose packs of 100 (NDC 0173-0316-27) capsules.

[Shown in Product Identification Section]

VI-ZAC® Capsules
(Therapeutic Vitamin-Mineral)

Composition: Each orange capsule contains:

Vitamin A .... 5000 I.U.
Ascorbic Acid .... 500 mg
Vitamin E .... 50 I.U.
Zinc Sulfate USP .... 80 mg

* as 50 mg Dried Zinc Sulfate.

Actions and Uses: VI-ZAC is indicated in the treatment of patients with deficiencies of, or increased requirements for, Vitamins A, C and E and zinc. The VI-ZAC formulation is a limited vitamin-mineral formulation designed to meet special needs. It is particularly indicated where there is no requirement for supplemental amounts of the B-Complex vitamins and their attendant appetite stimulation. The formulation is also designed for patients who cannot tolerate magnesium supplements but do need supplemental amounts of zinc.

Precautions: Although rarely encountered, vitamin A in large doses daily for several months or longer may cause toxicity.

Dosage: One or two capsules daily or as directed by the physician for the treatment of deficiencies.

How Supplied: In bottles of 60 and 500 capsules.

[Shown in Product Identification Section]

Glenbrook Laboratories
Division of Sterling Drug Inc.
90 PARK AVENUE
NEW YORK, NY 10016

BAYER ASPIRIN AND BAYER CHILDREN'S CHEWABLE ASPIRIN
Aspirin (Acetylsalicylic Acid)

Composition: Bayer Aspirin—Aspirin 5 grains. (325 mg.) contains a thin, inert, methylcellulose coating for easier swallowing. This is not an enteric coating and does not alter the onset of action of Bayer Aspirin.

Bayer Children's Chewable Aspirin—Aspirin 1¼ grains (81 mg.) per orange flavored chewable tablet.

Actions and Uses: Analgesic, antipyretic, anti-inflammatory, antiplatelet. For relief of headache; painful discomfort and fever of colds and flu; sore throats; muscular aches and pains; temporary relief of minor pains of arthritis, rheumatism, bursitis, lumbago, sciatica; toothache, teething pains, and pain following dental procedures; neuralgia and neuritic pain; functional menstrual pain; sleeplessness when caused by minor painful discomforts; painful discomfort and fever accompanying immunizations.

For antiplatelet use: In recurrent transient ischemic attacks or stroke in men. See below.

Administration and Dosage: The following dosages are those provided in the packaging, as appropriate for self-medication. Larger or more frequent dosage may be necessary as appropriate to the condition or needs of the patient.

The methyl-cellulose coating makes Bayer Aspirin particularly appropriate for those who must take frequent doses of aspirin and for those who have difficulty in swallowing uncoated tablets.

Bayer Aspirin—5 grain (325 mg.) tablets

Usual Adult Dose: One or two tablets with water. May be repeated every four hours as necessary up to 12 tablets a day.

Children's Dose: To be administered only under adult supervision.

Under 2 years .... per physician
2 to under 4 years .... ½ tablet
4 to under 6 years .... ¾ tablet
6 to under 9 years .... 1 tablet
9 to under 11 years .... 1¼ tablets

11 to under 12 years........................$1\frac{1}{2}$ tablets
Over 12 years..............................same as adult
Indicated dosage may be repeated every 4 hours, up to but not more than five times a day.
For Antiplatelet Use: In recurrent TIA's or stroke in men. See below.
Larger dosage may be prescribed per physician.
Bayer Children's Chewable Aspirin—$1\frac{1}{4}$ grain (81mg.) tablets.

Dosage

To be administered only under adult supervision. For children under 2 consult physician.

Age (years)	Weight (lbs.)	Dosage
2 up to 4	27 to 35	2 tablets
4 up to 6	36 to 45	3 tablets
6 up to 9	46 to 65	4 tablets
9 up to 11	66 to 76	5 tablets
11 up to 12	77 to 83	6 tablets
12 and over	84 and over	8 tablets

Indicated dosage may be repeated every 4 hours, up to but not more than five times a day.
Larger dosage may be prescribed per physician.
For Antiplatelet Use: In recurrent TIA's and stroke in men.
Indication: There is evidence that aspirin is safe and effective for reducing the risk of recurrent transient ischemic attacks or stroke in men who have had transient ischemia of the brain due to fibrin platelet emboli.
There is no evidence that aspirin is effective in reducing TIA's in women, or is of benefit in the treatment of completed strokes in men or women.
Patients presenting with signs and symptoms of TIA's should have a complete medical and neurologic evaluation. Consideration should be given to other disorders which resemble TIA's. It is important to evaluate and treat, if appropriate, other diseases associated with TIA's and stroke, such as hypertension and diabetes.
Dosage: The recommended dosage for this new indication is 1,300 mg/day (650 mg twice/day or 325 mg four times a day).
Precaution: A complete medical and neurologic examination should be performed on the male individual with recurrent TIA or stroke prior to instituting antiplatelet therapy with aspirin. The differential diagnosis should include consideration of disorders that resemble TIA's. An assessment of the presence and need for treatment of other diseases associated with TIA's or stroke, such as diabetes and hypertension, should be made.
The landmark studies which showed the effectiveness of aspirin in men with recurrent TIA's or stroke used a standard unbuffered aspirin preparation. It has been reported that concurrent administration of unabsorbable antacids may alter the available aspirin in plasma by decreasing the aspirin/salicylate ratio; the significance of this finding on recurrent TIA's has not been assessed clinically.
How Supplied:
Bayer Aspirin 5 grains (325 mg.)—
NDC-12843-101-10, packs of 12 tablets
NDC-12843-101-11, bottles of 24 tablets
NDC-12843-101-17, bottles of 50 tablets
NDC-12843-101-12, bottles of 100 tablets
NDC-12843-101-20, bottles of 200 tablets
NDC-12843-101-13, bottles of 300 tablets
Child-resistant safety closures on 12s, 24s, 50s, 200s, 300s. Bottle of 100s available without safety closure for households without small children.
Bayer Children's Chewable Aspirin $1\frac{1}{4}$ grains (81 mg.)—
NDC-12843-131-05, bottle of 36 tablets with child-resistant safety closure.
Samples available on request.

BAYER® CHILDREN'S COLD TABLETS

Composition: Each tablet contains phenylpropanolamine HCl 3.125 mg., aspirin $1\frac{1}{4}$ gr. (81 mg.); the tablets are orange flavored and chewable.
Action and Uses: Bayer Children's Cold Tablets combine two effective ingredients: a gentle decongestant to relieve nasal congestion and ease breathing, and genuine Bayer Aspirin to reduce fever and relieve minor aches and pains of colds and flu.
Administration and Dosage: The following dosage is provided in the packaging.
Under 3 years - consult physician
3 years - 1 tablet
4 to 5 years - 2 tablets
6 to 12 years - 4 tablets
Indicated dosage may be repeated every four hours up to but not more than four times a day.
Larger or more frequent dosage may be necessary as appropriate to the condition or needs of the patient.
Contraindications: Side effects at higher doses may include nervousness, dizziness, sleeplessness. To be used with caution in presence of high blood pressure, heart disease, diabetes, asthma, or thyroid disease.
How Supplied: NDC-12843-181-01, bottles of 30 tablets with child-resistant safety closure. Samples available on request.

BAYER® COUGH SYRUP FOR CHILDREN

Composition: Each 5 ml. (1 tsp.) contains phenylpropanolamine HCl 9 mg. and dextromethorphan hydrobromide 7.5 mg., alcohol 5% Cherry flavored.
Action and Uses: Bayer Cough Syrup for Children combines two effective ingredients in a syrup with a very appealing cherry flavor: a gentle nasal decongestant and a cough suppressant.
Administration and Dosage: The following dosage is provided on the packaging.
Under 2 years ....per physician
2–5 years: 1 teaspoon every 4 hours, not to exceed 4 teaspoons every 24 hours.
6–12 years: 2 teaspoons every 4 hours, not to exceed 8 teaspoons every 24 hours.
Contraindications and Precautions: To be used with caution in presence of high blood pressure, heart disease, diabetes, asthma, or thyroid disease.
How Supplied: NDC–12843-401-02, 3.0 oz. bottles. Samples available on request.

BAYER® TIMED-RELEASE ASPIRIN (aspirin)

Description: Each oblong white scored tablet contains 10 grains (650 mg.) of aspirin in microencapsulation form.
Indications: Bayer Timed-Release Aspirin is indicated for the temporary relief of low grade pain amenable to relief with salicylates, such as in rheumatoid arthritis, osteoarthritis, spondylitis, bursitis and other forms of rheumatism, as well as in many common musculoskeletal disorders. It possesses the same advantages for other types of prolonged aches and pains, such as minor injuries, dental pain and dysmenorrhea. Its long-lasting effectiveness should also make it valuable as an analgesic in simple headache, colds, grippe, flu and other similar conditions in which aspirin is indicated for symptomatic relief, either by itself or as an adjunct to specific therapy.
Dosage: Two Bayer Timed-Release Aspirin tablets q. 8 h. provide effective long-lasting pain relief. This two-tablet (20 grain or 1300 mg.) dose of timed-release aspirin promptly produces salicylate blood levels greater than those achieved by a 10-grain (650 mg.) dose of regular aspirin, and in the second 4 hour period produces a salicylate blood level curve which approximates that of two successive 10-grain doses of regular aspirin at 4 hour intervals. The 10-grain scored Bayer Timed-Release Aspirin tablets permit administration of aspirin in multiples of 5 grains (325 mg.), allowing individualization of dosage to meet the specific needs of the patient.
For the convenience of patients on a regular aspirin dosage schedule, two 10-grain Bayer Timed-Release Aspirin tablets may be administered with water every 8 hours. Whenever necessary, two tablets (20 grains) may be given before retiring to provide effective analgesic and anti-inflammatory action—for relief of pain throughout the night and lessening of stiffness upon arising. Do not exceed 6 tablets in 24 hours. Bayer Timed-Release Aspirin has been made in a special capsule-shaped tablet to permit easy swallowing. However, for patients who do have difficulty, Bayer Timed-Release Aspirin tablets may be gently crumbled in the mouth and swallowed with water without loss of timed-release effect. There is no bitter "aspirin" taste. For children under 12, per physician.
Side Effects: Side effects encountered with regular aspirin may be encountered with Bayer Timed-Release Aspirin. Tinnitus and dizziness are the ones most frequently encountered.
Contraindications and Precautions: Bayer Timed-Release Aspirin is contraindicated in patients with marked aspirin hypersensitivity, and should be given with extreme caution to any patient with a history of adverse reaction to salicylates. It may cautiously be tried in patients intolerant to aspirin because of gastric irritation, but the usual precautions for any form of aspirin should be observed in patients with gastric ulcers, bleeding tendencies, asthma, or hypoprothrombinemia.
Supplied:

Tablets in Bottle of 30's	NDC-12843-191-72
Tablets in Bottle of 72's	NDC-12843-191-74
Tablets in Bottle of 125's	NDC-12843-191-76

All sizes packaged in child-resistant safety closure except 72's which is a size recommended for households without young children.
Samples available upon request.

MIDOL®

Composition: Each Caplet® contains Aspirin 454 mg (7 grains); Cinnamedrine Hydrochloride 14.9 mg; Caffeine 32.4 mg.
Action and Uses: Analgesic, antispasmodic. For fast relief of functional menstrual pain, cramps, irritability; headache, aches from swelling, and the irritability associated with premenstrual tension; headache, and low backache associated with menstruation.
Usage Adult Dosage: Two Caplets with water. Repeat two Caplets every four hours as needed, up to eight Caplets per day.
How Supplied: White, capsule-shaped Caplets.
NDC-12843-151-29, professional dispenser, 250 2-Caplet Packets
NDC-12843-151-02, sample size of 6 Caplets
NDC-12843-151-34, strip packs of 12 Caplets
NDC-12843-151-36, bottles of 30 Caplets
NDC-12843-151-38, bottles of 60 Caplets
Child-resistant safety closures on bottles of 30 and 60 Caplets.
Samples Supplied: Available upon request.

PHILLIPS' MILK OF MAGNESIA

Composition: A suspension of magnesium hydroxide, meeting all USP specifications.
Action and Uses: Phillips' Milk of Magnesia is a mild saline laxative and is indicated for the relief of constipation especially in patients with hemorrhoids, obstetric patients, cardiacs, and in geriatric patients where straining at stool is contraindicated. Phillips' also acts as an antacid, and is effective for the relief of symptoms associated with gastric hyperacidity.
Administration and Dosage: As a laxative, adults 2 to 4 tbsp. followed by a glass of water.

Continued on next page

Glenbrook—Cont.

Children-infants 1 tsp.; over one year 1/4 to 1/2 adult dose, depending on age. As a antacid, 1 to 3 tsps. with a little water, up to four times a day. Children-1 to 12 years: 1/4 to 1/2 adult dose up to four times a day.
Contraindications: Abdominal pain, nausea, vomiting or other symptoms of appendicitis.
How Supplied: Phillips' Milk of Magnesia is available in regular and mint in bottles of:

Regular	
4 fl. oz.	NDC-12843-353-01
12 fl. oz.	NDC-12843-353-02
26 fl. oz.	NDC-12843-353-03
Mint	
4 fl oz.	NDC-12843-363-04
12 fl. oz.	NDC-12843-363-05
26 fl. oz.	NDC-12843-363-06

Also available in tablet form.

VANQUISH®

Composition: Each Caplet contains aspirin 227 mg., acetaminophen 194 mg., caffeine 33 mg., dried aluminum hydroxide gel 25 mg.; magnesium hydroxide 50 mg.
Action and Uses: A buffered analgesic, antipyretic for relief of headache; muscular aches and pains; neuralgia and neuritic pain; pain following dental procedures; for painful discomforts and fever of colds and flu; functional menstrual pain, headache and pain due to cramps; temporary relief from minor pains of arthritis, rheumatism, bursitis, lumbago, sciatica.
Usual Adult Dosage: Two caplets with water. May be repeated every four hours if necessary up to 12 tablets per day. Larger or more frequent doses may be prescribed by physician if necessary.
Contraindications: Hypersensitivity to salicylates.
(To be used with caution during anticoagulant therapy or in asthmatic patients.)
How Supplied: White, capsule-shaped Caplets in bottles of:
15 Caplets NDC 12843-171-42
30 Caplets NDC 12843-171-44
60 Caplets NDC 12843-171-46
100 Caplets NDC 12843-171-48

Glenwood, Inc.
83 N. SUMMIT STREET
TENAFLY, NJ 07670

MYOTONACHOL™ ℞
Bethanechol Chloride—Oral

Description: Bethanechol chloride is an ester of a choline-like compound.
Actions: Bethanechol chloride is a synthetic choline ester with postganglionic parasympathomimetic actions mediated via direct stimulation of cholinergic receptors. Its actions are similar to those of acetylcholine—the natural neurohormonal mediator of postganglionic parasympathetic receptors and of certain sympathetic nerves (sweat glands and some blood vessels)—which usually produce smooth muscle stimulation. However, unlike acetylcholine, bethanechol chloride is not inactivated by cholinesterases and therefore has more prolonged effects. Bethanechol chloride's principal effects are due predominately to its muscarinic action, i.e., stimulating micturition and gastrointestinal peristalsis while its nicotinic action is slight. Its cardiovascular effects when administered orally, are ordinarily inconspicious and constitute a slight transient fall in diastolic pressure with a minor reflex tachycardia. Other effects of bethanechol chloride's parasympathetic stimulating actions include contracted pupils, salivation, constricted bronchi, and dilated splanchnic vessels. The pharmacological actions of bethanechol chloride are more efficaciously produced following subcutaneous than with oral administration.
Indications: Acute postoperative and postpartum nonobstructive (functional) urinary retention, and neurogenic atony of the urinary bladder with retention.
Contraindications: Bethanechol chloride is contraindicated in the presence of mechanical obstruction of the gastrointestinal or urinary tracts and hollow viscera, or in conditions where the integrity of the gastrointestinal or bladder wall is questionable. Also, it is contraindicated in spastic, including peptic ulcer or acute in flammatory conditions of the gastrointestinal tract, or peritonitis.
Other major contraindications to the use of bethanechol chloride are latent or active asthma, hyperthyroidism, and coronary occlusion. Additional contraindications are bradycardia, atrio-ventricular conduction defects, vasomotor instability, hypotention, hypertention, coronary artery disease, epilepsy and parkinsonism.
Precautions: Special care and consideration are required when bethanechol chloride is administered to patients concomitantly being treated with other drugs with which pharmacologic interactions may occur. Examples of drugs with potentials for such interactions are: quinidine and procainamide, which may antagonize cholinergic effects; cholinergic drugs, particularly cholinesterase inhibitors, where additive effects may occur. When administered to patients receiving ganglionic blocking compounds a critical fall in blood pressure may occur which usually is preceeded by severe abdominal symptoms.
Adverse Reactions: Untoward effects are usually due to overdosage but occur infrequently with the oral administration of bethanechol chloride. Abdominal discomfort, salivation, flushing of the skin ("hot feeling"), sweating, nausea and vomiting are early signs of overdosage. Asthmatic attacks, especially in asthmatic individuals may be precipitated. Substernal pressure or pain may occur, however, it is uncertain whether this is due to bronchoconstriction, or spasm of the esophagus. Myocardial hypoxia must be considered if a marked fall in blood pressure occurs.
Transient syncope with cardiac arrest, transient complete heart block, dyspnea, and orthostatic hypotention may be associated with large doses. Patients with hypertention may react to the drug with a precipitious fall in blood pressure. Short periods of atrial fibrillation have been observed in hyperthyroid individuals following the administration of cholinergic drugs. Also, involuntary defecation and urinary urgency may occur after large doses.
Atropine sulfate is a specific antidote. A dose of 0.5 mg.—1.0 mg. (1/100 grain–1/50 grain), for intramuscular or intravenous administration, should be readily available to counteract severe toxic cardiovascular or bronchoconstrictor responses to bethanechol chloride.
Dosage and Administration: The usual adult oral dose is administered with 5, 10 or 25 mg. tablets, three or four times daily. The minimum effective dose is determined by giving 5 or 10 mg. initially and repeating in the same amounts at one or two hour intervals, to a maximum of 30 mg., until the desired response is obtained. The drug's effects appear within 60 to 90 minutes and persist for an hour.
How Supplied: Myotonachol.
10 mg. tablets, flat, NDC 0516-0021-01 in bottles of 100s.
25 mg. tablets, flat, NDC 0516-0022-01 in bottles of 100s.
[*Shown in Product Identification Section*]

POTABA® ℞
Potassium p-Aminobenzoate, Glenwood
Systemic ANTIFIBROSIS THERAPY

Formula: POTABA is chemically a pure potassium p-aminobenzoate, KPAB.

> **Indications:** Based on a review of this drug by the National Academy of Sciences-National Research Council and/or other information, FDA has classified the indications as follows:
> "Possibly" effective: Potassium aminobenzoate is possibly effective in the treatment of scleroderma, dermatomyositis, morphea, linear scleroderma, pemphigus, and Peyronie's disease.
> Final classification of the less-than-effective indications requires further investigation.

Advantages: POTABA offers a means of treatment of serious and often chronic entities involving fibrosis and nonsuppurative inflammation.
Pharmacology: P-Aminobenzoate is considered a member of the vitamin B complex. Small amounts are found in cereal, eggs, milk and meats. Detectable amounts are normally present in human blood, spinal fluid, urine, and sweat. PABA is a component of several biologically important systems, and it participates in a number of fundamental biological processes. It has been suggested that the antifibrosis action of POTABA is due to its mediation of increased oxygen uptake at the tissue level. Fibrosis is believed to occur from either too much serotonin or too little monoamine oxidase activity over a period of time. Monoamine oxidase requires an adequate supply of oxygen to function properly. By increasing oxygen supply at the tissue level POTABA may enhance MAO activity and prevent or bring about regression of fibrosis.
Clinical Uses:
PEYRONIE'S DISEASE: 21 patients with Peyronie's disease were placed on POTABA therapy for periods ranging from 3 months to 2 years. Pain disappeared from 16 of 16 cases in which it had been present. There was objective improvement in penile deformity in 10 of 17 patients, and decrease in plaque size in 16 of 21. The authors suggest that this medication offers no hazard of further local injury as may result from other therapy. There were no significant untoward effects encountered on long term POTABA therapy.
SCLERODERMA: Of 135 patients with diffuse systemic sclerosis treated with POTABA every patient but one has shown softening of the involved skin if treatment has been continued for 3 months or longer. The responses have been reported in a number of publications. The treatment program consists of systemic antifibrosis therapy with POTABA, physical therapy, including deep breathing exercises and dynamic traction splints where indicated, and bethanechol chloride (MYOCHOLINE, Glenwood) for relief of dysphagia as well as small doses of reserpine for amelioration of Raynaud's phenomena.
DERMATOMYOSITIS: Five patients with scleroderma and 2 with dermatomyositis were treated with POTABA. There was striking clinical improvement in each patient. Doses of 15-20 grams per day were well tolerated, and patients were easily able to take these doses.
MORPHEA and LINEAR SCLERODERMA: All 14 patients with localized forms of scleroderma placed on long-term Potaba treatment showed softening of the sclerotic component of their disorder. Treatment is particularly indicated in patients where persistent compressive sclerosis may contribute even greater disfigurement or functional embarrassment from secondary pressure atrophy.

Dosage and Administration: The average adult daily dose of POTABA is 12 grams, usually given in four to six divided doses. Tablets and capsules 0.5 gram are given at the rate of 4 tablets or capsules 6 times daily, or 6 given four times daily, usually with meals, and at bedtime with a snack. Tablets must be dissolved in an adequate amount of liquid to prevent gastrointestinal upset.
POTABA Envules contain 2 grams pure drug each, and constitute the individual average dose. 6 Envules are given for a total of 12 grams POTABA daily.
POTABA Powder is used to prepare solutions, which are kept refrigerated, but for no longer than one week. 100 grams POTABA powder make 1 quart of 10% solution when dissolved in potable tap water. Children are given 1 gram POTABA daily in divided doses for each 10 lbs. of body weight.
Side Effects: Anorexia, nausea, fever and rash have occurred infrequently and subside with omission of the drug. Desensitization can be accomplished and treatment resumed.
Precautions: Should anorexia or nausea occur, therapy is interrupted until the patient is eating normally again. This permits prompt subsidence of symptoms and also avoids the possible development of hypoglycemia. Give cautiously to patients with renal disease. If a hypersensitivity reaction should occur, Potaba should be stopped.
Contraindications: POTABA should not be administered to patients taking sulfonamides.
How Supplied: POTABA Capsules 0.5 gm. in 250's and 1,000's; POTABA Envules 2.0 gm. in boxes of 50's; POTABA Powder, pure, in 100 gm. and 1 lb.; POTABA Tablets 0.5 gm. in 100's and 1,000's.
[Shown in Product Identification Section]

YODOXIN ℞
(iodoquinol Tablets, U.S.P.)
210 mg. and 650 mg. Tablets

Composition: Each tablet contains: Iodoquinol, U.S.P. 210 mg. or 650 mg.
Description: Iodoquinol is of a light yellowish to tan color, nearly odorless and stable in air. The compound is practically insoluble in water, and sparingly soluble in most other solvents. It contains 64 per cent organically bound iodine.
Action: Iodoquinol is amebicidal against Entamoeba histolytica and is considered effective against the trophozoite and cyst forms.
Indications: Iodoquinol is used in the treatment of intestinal amebiasis.
Contraindications: Known hypersensitivity to iodine and 8-hydroxyquinolines. Contraindicated in patients with hepatic damage.
Warnings: Optic neuritis, optic atrophy, and peripheral neuropathy have been reported following prolonged high dosage theraphy with halogenated 8-hydroxyquinolines. Long term use of this drug should be avoided.
Use in Pregnancy: Safety for use in pregnancy or during lactation has not been established.
Precautions: Iodoquinol should be used with caution in patients with thyroid disease.
Protein-bound serum iodine levels may be increased during treatment with iodoquinol and therefore interfere with certain thyroid function tests. These effects may persist for as long as six months after discontinuation of therapy. Discontinue the drug if hypersensitivity reactions occur.
Adverse Reactions: Skin: various forms of skin eruptions (acneiform papular and pustular; ballae; vegetating of tuberous iododerma), urticaria and pruritus. Gastrointestinal: nausea, vomiting, abdominal cramps, diarrhea, and pruritus ani.
Fever, chills, headache, vertigo and enlargement of thyroid have been reported. Optic neuritis, optic atrophy and peripheral neuropathy have been reported in association with prolonged high-dosage 8-hydroxyquinoline therapy.
Dosage and Administration: Usual adult dose: (210 mgm. each) 3 tablets three times daily, after meals for 20 days. Children 6 to 12 years: (210 mgm. each) 2 tablets, t.i.d. Children under 6: (210 mgm. each) one tablet per 15 pounds of body weight. Usual adult dose: (650 mgm. each) One tablet three times a day for twenty days, to be taken after meals. Children (650 mgm. each): For twenty days, 40 mg. per Kg. of body weight daily divided into 3 doses.
How Supplied: 210 mgm. NDC-00516-0092-01 bottle of 100 tablets and NDC-00516-0092-10 bottle of 1,000 tablets. 650 mgm. NDC-00516-0093-01 bottle of 100 tablets and NDC-00516-0093-10 bottle of 1,000 tablets.
Storage: Store at Controlled Room Temperature 15-30° C. (59-86°F.)
Caution: Federal law prohibits dispensing without prescription.

Mfg. for:
GLENWOOD INC.
Tenafly, New Jersey 07670
by VITARINE CO., Springfield Gardens, N.Y. 11413
5/82
[Shown in Product Identification Section]

Gray Pharmaceutical Co.
100 CONNECTICUT AVENUE
NORWALK, CT 06856

X-PREP® LIQUID
(standardized extract of senna fruit)

Action and Uses: An easy-to-administer, palatable, highly effective bowel evacuant for the preparation of the intestinal tract prior to G.I. and urological radiography as well as colonoscopy, sigmoidoscopy and other diagnostic bowel procedures. In addition, X-Prep Liquid may be used for preparation of the bowel prior to elective colon surgery. Permits excellent visualization without residual oil droplets. X-PREP Liquid is fully prepared in a single dose container—all the patient has to do is drink the contents of one small bottle (2½ fl. oz.). Good patient cooperation is ensured because of highly pleasant taste. Predictable effectiveness helps reduce or eliminate the need for enemas prior to radiography.
Contraindications: Acute surgical abdomen.
Caution: In diabetic patients, the physician should be aware of the sugar content of X-PREP Liquid (50 grams per 2½ fl. oz. dose).
Adverse Reactions: As with all potent purgatives, some patients may experience abdominal discomfort and nausea; vomiting is rare.
Administration and Dosage: For adults: X-PREP Liquid: entire contents of bottle should be taken between 2:00 and 4:00 p.m. on the day prior to diagnostic procedure or elective colon surgery. Patients should be advised to expect a thorough, strong bowel action to begin approximately six hours later. After X-PREP Liquid is taken, diet should be confined to clear fluids.
X-PREP Liquid has proved to be effective following the above regimen. However, at physician's discretion, X-PREP Liquid may be given in divided doses, particularly to elderly or debilitated patients. The following split dosage regimens are equally effective: (1) One-half (½) of the contents of the bottle is taken at bedtime two days prior to diagnostic procedure. On day prior to examination, remaining contents of bottle is taken, also at bedtime. OR (2) On the day prior to examination, one-half (½) contents of bottle is taken at noon and the remaining one-half (½) at 4:00 p.m.
Some physicians prefer the hydration method, with 24-hour liquid diet and consumption of several extra glasses of water during this period, prior to the administration of X-PREP Liquid. Morning enema is optional. X-PREP Liquid may be successfully combined with adjunctive laxative suppositories or citrate of magnesia
How Supplied: 2½ fl. oz. bottles (alcohol 7% by volume), each providing a single, complete adult dose.
Now Available—Two X-PREP® Bowel Evacuant Kits.
Kit #1 contains: Two SENOKOT-S® Tablets (standardized senna concentrate and docusate sodium), one bottle of X-PREP Liquid 2½ fl. oz., and one RECTOLAX® Suppository (bisacodyl 10 mg), plus easy-to-follow patient instructions for hydration, clear liquid diet, and the correct time-sequence for administering the above laxatives.
Kit #2 contains: One dose CITRALAX™ Granules 1.06 oz. (effervescent citrate/sulfate of magnesia), one bottle of X-PREP Liquid 2½ fl. oz., and one RECTOLAX® Suppository (bisacodyl 10 mg), plus easy-to-follow patient instructions.

Guardian Chemical
a division of United-Guardian, Inc.
P.O. Box 2500
SMITHTOWN, N.Y. 11787

CLORPACTIN® WCS-90
(brand of sodium oxychlorosene)

Composition: Stabilized organic derivative of hypochlorous acid. A white, water soluble powder with a characteristic smell of hypochlorous acid. Active chlorine derived from calcium hypochlorite: 3–4%.
Action and Uses: For use as a topical antiseptic for treating localized infections, particularly when resistant organisms are present. Complete spectrum (bacteria, fungi, viruses, mold, yeast and spores); effective in cases of antibiotic resistance; nontoxic and non-allergenic in use concentrations.
Administration and Dosage: Applied by irrigation, instillations, spray, soaks or wet compresses, preferably thoroughly cleansing with gravity flow irrigation or syringe to provide copious quantities of fresh solution to remove the organic wastes and debris from the site of the involvement. Also for preoperative skin preparation and postoperative protection. Generally applied as the 0.4% solution in water, or isotonic saline, but as the 0.1% to 0.2% in Urology and Ophthalmology.
Contraindications: The use of this product is contraindicated where the site of the infection is not exposed to the direct contact with the solution. Not for systemic use.
How Supplied: In boxes containing 5 x 2 gram bottles.

LUBRASEPTIC® JELLY

Composition: Active ingredients: Aryl phenols, as phenyl phenol 0.1%, Alkyl phenols, as amyl phenol 0.02%, in water miscible form as an acid complex. Phenyl mercuric nitrate 0.007%.
Uses: For urethral instillation, prior to insertion of cystoscopes or sounds; for urethral dilations in the case of strictures. For proctologic use, in cases of hemorrhoids, or for post-hemorrhoidectomies, to provide increased comfort between and during the passage of stools. For endotracheal intubation. For use whenever a sterile water soluble lubricant is required: on cystoscopes and proctoscopes, in urological, rectal, and vaginal examinations or for use as a sterile dressing on burns, abrasions, and decubitus ulcers (bedsores).
Precautions and Side Effects: No serious side effects or contraindications are known. Urethral instillation, in some individuals, may cause a temporary burning or stinging sensa-

Continued on next page

Guardian—Cont.

tion but this usually disappears in several minutes. Excessive pressure should be avoided when instilling where strictures may exist.
How Supplied: In boxes containing 24 sterile packets each with a 10 gram "bellows" shaped tube of jelly and a urethral Disposatip.

pHos-pHaid® ℞
(brand of urinary acidifier)

Composition: Each 0.5 Gm. tablet contains ammonium biphosphate, 190 mg., sodium biphosphate, 200 mg., and sodium acid pyrophosphate, 110 mg. pH: approximately 4.5. Sodium content: less than one grain per tablet.
Action and Uses: pHos-pHaid is a highly effective urinary acidifier which, in conjunction with an acid ash diet, can decrease the urinary pH to a 5–5.5 level. Useful in increasing the solubility of calcium in the urine to assist in preventing formation of calculi in the urinary tract.
Administration and Dosage: In conjunction with an acidifying diet, the recommended dosage is two 0.5 Gm. tablets, followed by a glass of water, t.i.d. Occasionally, higher dosage is required and may be employed when necessary.
Side Effects: Occasional hyperacidity, particularly where gastritis or ulceration exists, and/or occasional nausea have been observed in some patients on a high dosage level. This may be decreased or eliminated by the use of the Enteric-Coated tablets. Excessive doses may also act as a saline cathartic and cause diarrhea. In such cases dosage should be decreased until the symptoms disappear. In cases of severe or extensive renal damage, pHos-pHaid should be administered with caution.
How Supplied: In color-coded tablets, either regular or Enteric- Coated.

Size	*Type*	*Packaged*	*Color*
0.5 Gm.	Reg.	90 & 500	Blue
0.5 Gm.	Ent.-Coat	90 & 500	Orange
0.25 Gm.	Reg.	150	Pink
0.25 Gm.	Ent.-Coat	150	Green

Literature Available: Literature on pHos-pHaid and Acid Ash Diet Sheets are available to physicians on request.

RENACIDIN® ℞

Composition: Active Ingredients (in a 300 gram bottle): Citric acid, anhydrous, 156–171 grams; D-gluconic acid (primarily as the lactone), 21–30 grams. Inert Ingredients: Purified magnesium hydroxycarbonate, 75–87 grams; Magnesium Acid Citrate ($MgHC_6H_5O_7$), 9–15 grams; Calcium (as the carbonate), 2–6 grams; Water, combined and free, 17–21 grams.
Action and Uses: For use in preparing solutions for irrigating indwelling urethral catheters and the urinary bladder in order to dissolve or prevent formation of calcifications.
Administration and Dosage: As a 10% solution (sterile) in distilled water. Irrigation is carried out with 1-2 ounces, b.i.d. or t.i.d. by means of a small, sterile, rubber syringe.
Side Effects: Only occasionally will a patient complain of some temporary pain or burning sensation from this procedure, in which case use of the solution should be discontinued.
Contraindications: It is contraindicated for therapy or preventive therapy above the ureteral-vesical junction; therefore it is contraindicated for ureteral catheters, nephrostomy or pyelostomy tubes or renal lavage for dissolving calculi. Contraindicated for biliary calculi.
How Supplied: In bottles containing 300 grams; also in boxes containing six 25 gram bottles.

W. E. Hauck, Inc.
P.O. BOX 1065
ROSWELL, GA 30075

BESTA® CAPSULES OTC
(Therapeutic Vitamins and Minerals)

Supplied: Bottles of 100.

CANTRI VAGINAL CREAM ℞

Composition: Sulfisoxazole 10%; Aminacrine HCl 0.2%; Allantoin 2.0%.
Supplied: 90 Gm. tube with reusable applicator.

CHLORAFED H.S. TIMECELLES* ℞

Composition: Chlorpheniramine Maleate 4 mg.; Pseudoephedrine HCl 60 mg.
* In special time release beads.
Supplied: Bottles of 100.

CHLORAFED LIQUID OTC
(Corn, Dye, Alcohol, Sugar Free)

Composition: Each 5 ml. of liquid contains: Chlorpheniramine Maleate 2 mg.; Pseudoephedrine HCl 30 mg.
Supplied: 4 oz. and pints.

CHLORAFED TIMECELLES* ℞

Composition: Chlorpheniramine Maleate 8 mg.; Pseudoephedrine HCl-120 mg.;
*In special time release beads.
Supplied: Bottles of 100 and 500

ENTUSS TABLETS and LIQUID Ⓒ ℞
(Sugar, Alcohol, Corn, Tartrazine Free)

Composition: Each tablet contains: Hydrocodone Bitartrate 5 mg., Guaifenesin 300 mg. Each 5 ml. of liquid contains: Hydrocodone Bitartrate 5 mg. Potassium Guaiacolsulfonate 300 mg.
Supplied: Tablets—bottles of 100. Liquid—pints.

G–1® CAPSULES ℞
G–2® CAPSULES Ⓒ ℞
G–3® CAPSULES Ⓒ ℞

Composition: Each G-1 Capsule contains: Acetaminophen 500 mg., Butalbital 50 mg., Caffeine 40 mg. Each G-2 Capsule contains: Acetamionphen 500 mg., Butalbital 50 mg., Codeine PO_4 15 mg. Each G-3 Capsule contains: Acetamionphen 500 mg., Butalbital 50 mg., Codeine PO_4 30 mg.
Supplied: Bottles of 100.

GERAVITE ELIXIR ℞

Each 15 ml. contains: Lysine 150 mg.; Thiamine HCl 1 mg.; Riboflavin 1.2 mg.; Niacinamide 100 mg.; Cyanocobalamin 10 mcg.; Alcohol 15%
Supplied: Pints and gallons.

HISTOR–D® TIMECELLES* ℞

Composition: Chlorpheniramine Maleate 8 mg.; Phenylephrine 20 mg.; Methscopolamine Nitrate 2.5 mg.
*In special time release beads.
Supplied: Bottles of 100 and 500.

ISOTRATE TIMECELLES ℞
(Isosorbide Dinitrate)

Composition: Each Timecelle contains: 40 mg. Isosorbide Dinitrate in a microdialysis release base which lasts for 12 hours. Orange and clear capsules imprinted Isotrate T.C.
Supplied: Bottles of 100 and 500.

OTIC–H.C. EAR DROPS ℞

Composition: Each ml. contains: Chloroxylenol 1 mg., Hydrocortisone 10 mg., Pramoxine 10 mg., in a non-aqueous Propylene Glycol vehicle with Acetic Acid and Benzalkonium Chloride.
Supplied: 10 ml. dropper tip bottle.

WEHLESS–105 TIMECELLES Ⓒ ℞

Composition: Each capsule contains: Phendimetrazine Tartrate 105 mg. in a sustained release base which lasts for 10 hours. Black and clear capsule imprinted WEHLESS T.C. 105 mg.
Supplied: Bottles of 100.

Hawaii Diet Plan, Inc.
737 BISHOP STREET
SUITE 2990
HONOLULU, HI 96813

THE HAWAII DIET

(See PDR For Nonprescription Drugs)

Health Care Products Division of Consolidated Chemical, Inc.
3224 SOUTH KINGSHIGHWAY BLVD.
ST. LOUIS, MO 63139

FORMULA MAGIC®
Lubricating Body Talc

Composition: Talc, Magnesium Carbonate, Mineral Oil, Fragrance, DMDM Hydantoin.
HPD 1895-202
Action: U.S.P. Talc based body powder and nursing lubricant. Aids in preventing excoriation and friction chafing. Aids in controlling odor.
Precautions: Non-irritating to skin. Practically non-toxic. Slight eye irritant. In case of eye contact flush with water.
Dosage and Administration: Apply liberally to patient's body. Provides a protective barrier against chafing.
How Supplied: 4 oz., 12 oz.

PERINEAL/OSTOMY SPRAY CLEANER™

Composition: Water, Cocamidopropylamine Oxide, Witch Hazel, Coco Betaine, DMDM Hydantoin, Fragrance, FD&C Red #33, FD&C Blue #1.
HPD 1895-117
Action: A gentle, effective spray cleaner for cleaning, refreshing, and deodorizing the perineal area, stoma sites, and stoma appliances.
Precautions: Non-irritating to skin. Practically non-toxic. May cause slight eye discomfort. In case of eye contact flush with water.
Dosage and Administration: Spray directly on entire perineal area, or peristomal skin or in stoma appliance for quick odor control and thorough cleaning. See label for full instructions.
How Supplied: 8 oz., 1 gallon.

SATIN®

Composition: Water, Ammonium Laureth Sulfate, Cocamide DEA, PEG-8, Glycol Stearate, Sodium Cocoyl Sarcosinate, Chloroxylenol, Tetrasodium EDTA, Lanolin Oil, Citric Acid, Fragrance, D&C Yellow #10.
HPD 1895-101
Action: Skin cleanser and shampoo for daily use. Aids in reducing odor.
Precautions: Non-irritating to skin. Practically non-toxic. Moderate eye irritant. In case of eye contact flush with water.

Dosage and Administration: Apply directly to skin or hair or to dampened washcloth. Wash in normal manner. Rinse thoroughly.
How Supplied: 8 oz., 16 oz., 1 gallon.

SKIN MAGIC™

Composition: Water, Stearic Acid, Mineral Oil, Propylene Glycol, Isostearyl Alcohol, Glycol Stearate, Stearamide DEA, Triethanolamine, Cetyl Alcohol, Myristyl Propionate, Lanolin Oil, Fragrance, Propylparaben, DMDM Hydantoin, Methylparaben, Carbomer 934, Sodium Borate.
HPD 1895-201
Action: Emollient body rub and skin lotion. Soothes and moisturizes dry irritated skin. Aids in reducing odor.
Precautions: Non-irritating to skin. Practically non-toxic. Slight eye irritant. In case of eye contact flush with water.
Dosage and Administration: Apply liberally and massage into skin.
How Supplied: 4 oz., 8 oz., 1 gallon.

Herbert Laboratories

Dermatology Division of Allergan Pharmaceuticals, Inc.
2525 DUPONT DRIVE
IRVINE, CA 92713

AEROSEB-DEX® ℞

(dexamethasone)
Topical aerosol spray

Description: The topical corticosteroids constitute a class of primarily synthetic steroids used as anti-inflammatory and anti-pruritic agents.
Chemical Name: Pregna-1, 4-diene-3, 20-dione, 9-fluoro-11, 17, 21-trihydroxy-16-methyl-, (11β, 16α)-.
Contains:
dexamethasone 0.01%
alcohol 68.5%
with: isopropyl myristate and propellant (butane).
Each 1 second of spray dispenses approximately 0.02 mg of dexamethasone.
Clinical Pharmacology: Topical corticosteroids share anti-inflammatory, anti-pruritic and vasoconstrictive actions.
The mechanism of anti-inflammatory activity of the topical corticosteroids is unclear. Various laboratory methods, including vasoconstrictor assays, are used to compare and predict potencies and/or clinical efficacies of the topical corticosteroids. There is some evidence to suggest that a recognizable correlation exists between vasoconstrictor potency and therapeutic efficacy in man.
Pharmacokinetics: The extent of percutaneous absorption of topical corticosteroids is determined by many factors including the vehicle, the integrity of the epidermal barrier and the use of occlusive dressings.
Topical corticosteroids can be absorbed from normal intact skin. Inflammation and/or other disease processes in the skin increase percutaneous absorption. Occlusive dressings substantially increase the percutaneous absorption of topical corticosteroids. Thus, occlusive dressings may be a valuable therapeutic adjunct for treatment of resistant dermatoses (see DOSAGE AND ADMINISTRATION).
Once absorbed through the skin, topical corticosteroids are handled through pharmacokinetic pathways similar to systemically administered corticosteroids. Corticosteroids are bound to plasma proteins in varying degrees. Corticosteroids are metabolized primarily in the liver and are then excreted by the kidneys. Some of the topical corticosteroids and their metabolites are also excreted into the bile.

Indications and Usage: Topical corticosteroids are indicated for the relief of the inflammatory and pruritic manifestations of corticosteroid-responsive dermatoses. Aeroseb-Dex is particularly useful in treating conditions of the scalp such as seborrheic dermatitis.
Contraindications: Topical corticosteroids are contraindicated in those patients with a history of hypersensitivity to any of the components of the preparation.
Precautions:
General: Systemic absorption of topical corticosteroids has produced reversible hypothalamic-pituitary-adrenal (HPA) axis suppression, manifestations of Cushing's syndrome, hyperglycemia and glucosuria in some patients.
Conditions which augment systemic absorption include the application of more potent steroids, use over large surface areas, prolonged use and the addition of occlusive dressings.
Therefore, patients receiving a large dose of a potent topical steroid applied to a large surface area or under an occlusive dressing should be evaluated periodically for evidence of HPA axis suppression by using the urinary free cortisol and ACTH stimulation tests. If HPA axis suppression is noted, an attempt should be made to withdraw the drug, to reduce the frequency of application, or to substitute a less potent steroid.
Recovery of HPA axis function is generally prompt and complete upon discontinuation of the drug. Infrequently, signs and symptoms of steroid withdrawal may occur, requiring supplemental systemic corticosteroids.
Children may absorb proportionally larger amounts of topical corticosteroids and thus be more susceptible to systemic toxicity (see PRECAUTIONS—Pediatric Use).
This medication contains alcohol. It may produce irritation or burning sensations in open lesions. If irritation develops, topical corticosteroids should be discontinued and appropriate therapy instituted.
In the presence of dermatological infections, the use of an appropriate antifungal or antibacterial agent should be instituted. If a favorable response does not occur promptly, the corticosteroid should be discontinued until the infection has been adequately controlled.
Information for the Patient: Patients using topical corticosteroids should receive the following information and instructions:

1. This medication is to be used as directed by the physician. It is for external use only. Avoid contact with the eyes. When used about the face, the eyes should be covered and inhalation of the spray should be avoided.
2. Patients should be advised not to use this medication for any disorder other than for which it was prescribed.
3. The treated skin area should not be bandaged or otherwise covered or wrapped as to be occlusive unless directed by the physician.
4. Patients should report any signs of local adverse reactions especially under occlusive dressing.
5. Parents of pediatric patients should be advised not to use tight-fitting diapers or plastic pants on a child being treated in the diaper area, as these garments may constitute occlusive dressings.

Laboratory Tests. The urinary free cortisol test and the ACTH stimulation test may be helpful in evaluating the HPA axis suppression.
Carcinogenesis, mutagenesis, impairment of fertility: Long-term animal studies have not been performed to evaluate the carcinogenic potential or the effect of topical corticosteroids on fertility.
Studies to determine mutagenicity with prednisolone and hydrocortisone have revealed negative results.

Pregnancy Category C: Corticosteroids are generally teratogenic in laboratory animals when administered systemically at relatively low dosage levels. The more potent corticosteroids have been shown to be teratogenic after dermal application in laboratory animals. There are no adequate and well-controlled studies in pregnant women on teratogenic effects from topically applied corticosteroids. Therefore, topical corticosteroids should be used during pregnancy only if the potential benefit justifies the potential risk to the fetus. Drugs of this class should not be used extensively on pregnant patients, in large amounts, or for prolonged periods of time.
Nursing Mothers: It is not known whether topical administration of corticosteroids could result in sufficient systemic absorption to produce detectable quantities in breast milk. Systemically administered corticosteroids are secreted into breast milk in quantities not likely to have a deleterious effect on the infant. Nevertheless, caution should be exercised when topical corticosteroids are administered to a nursing woman.
Pediatric Use: Pediatric patients may demonstrate greater susceptibility to topical corticosteroid-induced HPA axis suppression and Cushing's syndrome than mature patients because of a larger skin surface area to body weight ratio.
Hypothalamic-pituitary-adrenal (HPA) axis suppression, Cushing's syndrome and intracranial hypertension have been reported in children receiving topical corticosteroids. Manifestations of adrenal suppression in children include linear growth retardation, delayed weight gain, low plasma cortisol levels and absence of response to ACTH stimulation. Manifestations of intracranial hypertension include bulging fontanelles, headaches and bilateral papilledema.
Administration of topical corticosteroids to children should be limited to the least amount compatible with an effective therapeutic regimen. Chronic corticosteroid therapy may interfere with the growth and development of children.
Adverse Reactions: The following local adverse reactions are reported infrequently with topical corticosteroids, but may occur more frequently with the use of occlusive dressings. These reactions are listed in an approximate decreasing order of occurrence:
Burning
Itching
Irritation
Dryness
Folliculitis
Hypertrichosis
Acneiform eruptions
Hypopigmentation
Perioral dermatitis
Allergic contact dermatitis
Maceration of the skin
Secondary infection
Skin atrophy
Striae
Miliaria
Overdosage: Topically applied corticosteroids can be absorbed in sufficient amounts to produce systemic effects (see PRECAUTIONS).
Dosage and Administration: Aeroseb-Dex® should be applied to the affected area two or three times daily depending on the severity of the condition.
Occlusive dressings may be used for management of psoriasis or recalcitrant conditions.
If an infection develops, the use of occlusive dressings should be discontinued and appropriate antimicrobial therapy instituted.
For use on the scalp: Apply to dry scalp after shampoo. Shake well before spraying.

1. Hold aerosol upright. Slide applicator tube under the hair so that it touches scalp.

Continued on next page

Herbert—Cont.

Spray while moving tube to all affected areas, keeping tube under hair and in contact with scalp throughout treatment. Spraying should take 1 to 2 seconds.
2. If some areas of the scalp are not covered adequately, they may be "spot" sprayed by sliding applicator tube through hair to touch scalp—press and immediately release spray button.
3. It is unnecessary to massage medication into the scalp.
4. Be sure that the tip of the applicator tube stops at the hairline so that forehead and eyes are not sprayed.

For other dermatoses: Remove applicator tube. Shake well before spraying. Hold the can upright, approximately six inches from the area to be treated. Spray each four-inch square of affected area for one or two seconds, two or three times a day.
Note: For best results and to avoid wasting medication, it is important to follow the application instructions carefully (application instructions appear on the carton; however, it is preferable that the physician demonstrate the proper application method to the patient).
Caution: Flammable. Do not spray near flame or heated surfaces. If medication accidentally gets in the eyes, wash thoroughly with water and contact physician immediately. Keep out of the reach of children. Contents under pressure. Do not puncture, incinerate, or expose to temperatures above 120°F.
How Supplied: In a 58 gm aerosol with applicator tube.* On prescription only.
*U.S. Patent 3,730,182

AEROSEB–HC® ℞
(hydrocortisone)
Topical aerosol spray

Description: The topical corticosteroids constitute a class of primarily synthetic steroids used as anti-inflammatory and anti-pruritic agents.
Chemical Name: Pregn-4-ene-3, 20-dione, 11, 17, 21-trihydroxy-, (11β)-.
Contains:
hydrocortisone 0.5%
alcohol 68%
with: isopropyl myristate and propellant (butane).
Each 1 second of spray dispenses approximately 1 mg of hydrocortisone.
Clinical Pharmacology: Topical corticosteroids share anti-inflammatory, antipruritic and vasoconstrictive actions.
The mechanism of anti-inflammatory activity of the topical corticosteroids is unclear. Various laboratory methods, including vasoconstrictors assays, are used to compare and predict potencies and/or clinical efficacies of the topical corticosteroids. There is some evidence to suggest that a recognizable correlation exists between vasoconstrictor potency and therapeutic efficacy in man.
Pharmacokinetics: The extent of percutaneous absorption of topical corticosteroids is determined by many factors including the vehicle, the integrity of the epidermal barrier and the use of occlusive dressings.
Topical corticosteroids can be absorbed from normal intact skin. Inflammation and/or other disease processes in the skin increase percutaneous absorption. Occlusive dressings substantially increase the percutaneous absorption of topical corticosteroids. Thus, occlusive dressings may be a valuable therapeutic adjunct for treatment of resistant dermatoses (see DOSAGE AND ADMINISTRATION).
Once absorbed through the skin, topical corticosteroids are handled through pharmacokinetic pathways similar to systemically administered corticosteroids. Corticosteroids are bound to plasma proteins in varying degrees. Corticosteroids are metabolized primarily in the liver and are then excreted by the kidneys. Some of the topical corticosteroids and their metabolites are also excreted into the bile.
Indications and Usage: Topical corticosteroids are indicated for the relief of the inflammatory and pruritic manifestations of corticosteroid-responsive dermatoses. Aeroseb-HC is particularly useful in treating conditions of the scalp such as seborrheic dermatitis.
Contraindications: Topical corticosteroids are contraindicated in those patients with a history of hypersensitivity to any of the components of the preparation.
Precautions:
General: Systemic absorption of topical corticosteroids has produced reversible hypothalamic-pituitary-adrenal (HPA) axis suppression, manifestations of Cushing's syndrome, hyperglycemia and glucosuria in some patients.
Conditions which augment systemic absorption include the application of more potent steroids, use over large surface areas, prolonged use and the addition of occlusive dressings.
Therefore, patients receiving a large dose of a potent topical steroid applied to a large surface area or under an occlusive dressing should be evaluated periodically for evidence of HPA axis suppression by using the urinary free cortisol and ACTH stimulation tests. If HPA axis suppression is noted, an attempt should be made to withdraw the drug, to reduce the frequency of application, or to substitute a less potent steroid.
Recovery of HPA axis function is generally prompt and complete upon discontinuation of the drug. Infrequently, signs and symptoms of steroid withdrawal may occur, requiring supplemental systemic corticosteroids.
Children may absorb proportionally larger amounts of topical corticosteroids and thus be more susceptible to systemic toxicity (see PRECAUTIONS - Pediatric Use).
This medication contains alcohol. It may produce irritation or burning sensations in open lesions. If irritation develops, topical corticosteroids should be discontinued and appropriate therapy instituted.
In the presence of dermatological infections, the use of an appropriate antifungal or antibacterial agent should be instituted. If a favorable response does not occur promptly, the corticosteroid should be discontinued until the infection has been adequately controlled.
Information for the Patient: Patients using topical corticosteroids should receive the following information and instructions:
1. This medication is to be used as directed by the physician. It is for external use only. Avoid contact with the eyes. When used about the face, the eyes should be covered and inhalation of the spray should be avoided.
2. Patients should be advised not to use this medication for any disorder other than for which it was prescribed.
3. The treated skin area should not be bandaged or otherwise covered or wrapped as to be occlusive unless directed by the physician.
4. Patients should report any signs of local adverse reactions especially under occlusive dressing.
5. Parents of pediatric patients should be advised not to use tight-fitting diapers or plastic pants on a child being treated in the diaper area, as these garments may constitute occlusive dressings.

Laboratory Tests: The urinary free cortisol test and the ACTH stimulation test may be helpful in evaluating the HPA axis suppression.
Carcinogenesis, mutagenesis, impairment of fertility: Long-term animal studies have not been performed to evaluate the carcinogenic potential or the effect of topical corticosteroids on fertility.
Studies to determine mutagenicity with prednisolone and hydrocortisone have revealed negative results.
Pregnancy Category C: Corticosteroids are generally teratogenic in laboratory animals when administered systemically at relatively low dosage levels. The more potent corticosteroids have been shown to be teratogenic after dermal application in laboratory animals. There are no adequate and well-controlled studies in pregnant women on teratogenic effects from topically applied corticosteroids. Therefore, topical corticosteroids should be used during pregnancy only if the potential benefit justifies the potential risk to the fetus. Drugs of this class should not be used extensively on pregnant patients, in large amounts, or for prolonged periods of time.
Nursing Mothers: It is not known whether topical administration of corticosteroids could result in sufficient systemic absorption to produce detectable quantities in breast milk. Systemically administered corticosteroids are secreted into breast milk in quantities not likely to have a deleterious effect on the infant. Nevertheless, caution should be exercised when topical corticosteroids are administered to a nursing woman.
Pediatric Use: Pediatric patients may demonstrate greater susceptibility to topical corticosteroid-induced HPA axis suppression and Cushing's syndrome than mature patients because of a larger skin surface area to body weight ratio.
Hypothalamic-pituitary-adrenal (HPA) axis suppression, Cushing's syndrome and intracranial hypertension have been reported in children receiving topical corticosteroids. Manifestations of adrenal suppression in children include linear growth retardation, delayed weight gain, low plasma cortisol levels and absence of response to ACTH stimulation. Manifestations of intracranial hypertension include bulging fontanelles, headaches and bilateral papilledema.
Administration of topical corticosteroids to children should be limited to the least amount compatible with an effective therapeutic regimen. Chronic corticosteroid therapy may interfere with the growth and development of children.
Adverse Reactions: The following local adverse reactions are reported infrequently with topical corticosteroids, but may occur more frequently with the use of occlusive dressings. These reactions are listed in an approximate decreasing order of occurrence:

Burning	Perioral dermatitis
Itching	Allergic contact dermatitis
Irritation	Maceration of the skin
Dryness	Secondary infection
Folliculitis	Skin atrophy
Hypertrichosis	Striae
Acneiform eruptions	Miliaria
Hypopigmentation	

Overdosage: Topically applied corticosteroids can be absorbed in sufficient amounts to produce systemic effects (see PRECAUTIONS).
Dosage and Administration: Aeroseb-HC® should be applied to the affected area from two or three times daily depending on the severity of the condition.
Occlusive dressings may be used for management of psoriasis or recalcitrant conditions.
If an infection develops, the use of occlusive dressings should be discontinued and appropriate antimicrobial therapy instituted.
For use on the scalp: Apply to dry scalp after shampoo. Shake well before spraying.
1. Hold aerosol upright. Slide applicator tube under the hair so that it touches scalp. Spray while moving tube to all affected areas, keeping tube under hair and in contact with scalp throughout treatment. Spraying should take 1 to 2 seconds.
2. If some areas of the scalp are not covered adequately, they may be "spot" sprayed by

sliding applicator tube through hair to touch scalp—press and immediately release spray button.
3. It is unnecessary to massage medication into the scalp.
4. Be sure that the tip of the applicator tube stops at the hairline so that forehead and eyes are not sprayed.

For other dermatoses: Remove applicator tube. Shake well before spraying. Hold the can upright, approximately six inches from the area to be treated. Spray each four-inch square of affected area for one or two seconds, two or three times a day.
Note: For best results and to avoid wasting medication, it is important to follow the application instructions carefully (application instructions appear on the carton; however, it is preferable that the physician demonstrate the proper application method to the patient).
Caution: Flammable. Do not spray near flame or heated surfaces. If medication accidentally gets in the eyes, wash thoroughly with water and contact physician immediately. Keep out of the reach of children. Contents under pressure. Do not puncture, incinerate, or expose to temperatures above 120°F.
How Supplied: In a 58 gm aerosol with applicator tube.* On prescription only.
*U.S. Patent 3,730,182

EXSEL® ℞
(selenium sulfide 2.5%)
Lotion

Description: Exsel Lotion is an antiseborrheic dermatitis preparation for dermatological use.
Contains:
selenium sulfide 2.5%
with: edetate disodium; bentonite; sodium dodecylbenzene sulfonate; sodium C14-16 olefin sulfonate; glyceryl ricinoleate; dimethicone copolyol; titanium dioxide; citric acid monohydrate; sodium phosphate monobasic, monohydrate; perfume; and purified water.
Clinical Pharmacology: The mechanism of action of selenium sulfide in seborrheic dermatitis is unknown. Its antidandruff effectiveness is thought to result from its antimitotic activity and substantivity to the skin.
Indications and Usage: Selenium sulfide is indicated in the treatment of seborrheic dermatitis of the scalp, including dandruff.
Contraindications: This product should not be used by patients who are allergic to any of its components.
Warnings: Chemical conjunctivitis may result if this preparation comes in contact with the eyes.
Precautions:
General: This product should be used with caution when acute inflammation or exudation is present as an increase in absorption may occur.
Information for Patients: Avoid contact with eyes or eyelids. Do not take internally. Keep out of the reach of children.
Carcinogenesis, mutagenesis, impairment of fertility: Animal studies are in progress to evaluate the potential of these effects.
Pregnancy Category C: Animal reproduction studies have not been conducted with selenium sulfide. It is also not known whether selenium sulfide can cause fetal harm when administered to a pregnant woman or can affect reproduction capacity. Selenium sulfide should be given to a pregnant woman only if clearly needed.
Pediatric Use: Safety and effectiveness in children have not been established.
Adverse Reactions: Exact incidence figures are not available since no denominator of treated patients is available.
1. Hair loss has been reported with the use of selenium sulfide shampoos.
2. Discoloration of the hair may follow the use of selenium sulfide shampoo. This can be minimized by careful rinsing of the hair after treatment.
3. Oiliness of the hair and scalp may increase following the use of selenium sulfide shampoos.

Dosage and Administration:
1. Massage about 1 or 2 teaspoons of the medicated shampoo into the wet scalp. Avoid contact with the eyes.
2. Allow product to remain on the scalp for 2 to 3 minutes.
3. Rinse the scalp thoroughly.
4. Repeat application and rinse thoroughly.
5. After treatment, wash hands well.
6. Repeat treatments as directed by physician.

The preparation should not be applied more frequently than required to maintain control of symptoms.
Accidental Oral Ingestion: Selenium sulfide is highly toxic if ingested. Nausea and vomiting usually occur after oral ingestion. Treatment is to induce vomiting or if necessary perform gastric lavage, together with general supportive measures as required. Administer a purgative to hasten elimination.
How Supplied: In 4 oz plastic bottles. On prescription only. Protect from heat. For external use only. Keep out of reach of children.

FLUONID® ℞
(fluocinolone acetonide)
Ointment 0.025%
Cream 0.01%
Cream 0.025%
Topical Solution 0.01%

Description: The topical corticosteroids constitute a class of primarily synthetic steroids used as anti-inflammatory and anti-pruritic agents.
Chemical Name: Pregna-1, 4-diene-3, 20-dione, 6,9-difluoro-11, 21-dihydroxy-16, 17-[1-methylethylidene)bis (oxy)]-, ($6\alpha,11\beta,16\alpha$)-.
Fluonid® Cream contains:
fluocinolone acetonide 0.01%, 0.025%
with: methylparaben, propylparaben, stearic acid, propylene glycol, sorbitan monostearate, sorbitan monooleate, polyoxyethylene sorbitan monostearate, citric acid and purified water.
Fluonid® Ointment contains:
fluocinolone acetonide 0.025%
in white petrolatum.
Fluonid® Topical Solution contains:
fluocinolone acetonide 0.01%
with: propylene glycol and citric acid.
Clinical Pharmacology: Topical corticosteroids share anti-inflammatory, antipruritic and vasoconstrictive actions.
The mechanism of anti-inflammatory activity of the topical corticosteroids is unclear. Various laboratory methods, including vasoconstrictor assays, are used to compare and predict potencies and/or clinical efficacies of the topical corticosteroids. There is some evidence to suggest that a recognizable correlation exists between vasoconstrictor potency and therapeutic efficacy in man.
Pharmacokinetics: The extent of percutaneous absorption of topical corticosteroids is determined by many factors including the vehicle, the integrity of the epidermal barrier and the use of occlusive dressings.
Topical corticosteroids can be absorbed from normal intact skin. Inflammation and/or other disease processes in the skin increase percutaneous absorption. Occlusive dressings substantially increase the percutaneous absorption of topical corticosteroids. Thus, occlusive dressings may be a valuable therapeutic adjunct for treatment of resistant dermatoses. (see DOSAGE AND ADMINISTRATION).
Once absorbed through the skin, topical corticosteroids are handled through pharmacokinetic pathways similar to systemically administered corticosteroids. Corticosteroids are bound to plasma proteins in varying degrees. Corticosteroids are metabolized primarily in the liver and are then excreted by the kidneys. Some of the topical corticosteroids and their metabolites are also excreted into the bile.
Indications and Usage: Topical corticosteroids are indicated for the relief of the inflammatory and pruritic manifestations of corticosteroid-responsive dermatoses. Fluonid Cream 0.01% and 0.025% are useful in corticosteroid responsive dermatoses that require a mid-potency corticosteroid particularly when large areas are treated.
Fluonid Ointment 0.025% is useful in such conditions as atopic dermatitis where an emollient effect is desired.
Fluonid Solution 0.01% is useful in hairy sites such as the scalp, particularly in treating seborrheic dermatitis.
Contraindications: Topical corticosteroids are contraindicated in those patients with a history of hypersensitivity to any of the components of the preparation.
Precautions:
General: Systemic absorption of topical corticosteroids has produced reversible hypothalamic-pituitary-adrenal (HPA) axis suppression, manifestations of Cushing's syndrome, hyperglycemia and glucosuria in some patients.
Conditions which augment systemic absorption include the application of more potent steroids, use over large surface areas, prolonged use and the addition of occlusive dressings.
Therefore, patients receiving a large dose of a potent topical steroid applied to a large surface area or under an occlusive dressing should be evaluated periodically for evidence of HPA axis suppression by using the urinary free cortisol and ACTH stimulation tests. If HPA axis suppression is noted, an attempt should be made to withdraw the drug, to reduce the frequency of application, or to substitute a less potent steroid.
Recovery of HPA axis function is generally prompt and complete upon discontinuation of the drug. Infrequently, signs and symptoms of steroid withdrawal may occur, requiring supplemental systemic corticosteroids.
Children may absorb proportionally larger amounts of topical corticosteroids and thus be more susceptible to systemic toxicity (see PRECAUTIONS—Pediatric Use).
In the presence of dermatological infections, the use of an appropriate antifungal or antibacterial agent should be instituted. If a favorable response does not occur promptly, the corticosteroid should be discontinued until the infection has been adequately controlled.
Information for the Patient: Patients using topical corticosteroids should receive the following information and instructions:
1. This medication is to be used as directed by the physician. It is for external use only. Avoid contact with the eyes.
2. Patients should be advised not to use this medication for any disorder other than for which it was prescribed.
3. The treated skin area should not be bandaged or otherwise covered or wrapped as to be occlusive unless directed by the physician.
4. Patients should report any signs of local adverse reactions especially under occlusive dressing.
5. Parents of pediatric patients should be advised not to use tight-fitting diapers or plastic pants on a child being treated in the diaper area, as these garments may constitute occlusive dressings.

Laboratory Tests: The urinary free cortisol test and the ACTH stimulation test may be helpful in evaluating the HPA axis suppression.
Carcinogenesis, mutagenesis, impairment of fertility: Long-term animal studies have not been performed to evaluate the carcinogenic

Continued on next page

Herbert—Cont.

potential or the effect of topical corticosteroids on fertility.
Studies to determine mutagenicity with prednisolone and hydrocortisone have revealed negative results.
Pregnancy Category C: Corticosteroids are generally teratogenic in laboratory animals when administered systemically at relatively low dosage levels. The more potent corticosteroids have been shown to be teratogenic after dermal application in laboratory animals. There are no adequate and well-controlled studies in pregnant women on teratogenic effects from topically applied corticosteroids. Therefore, topical corticosteroids should be used during pregnancy only if the potential benefit justifies the potential risk to the fetus. Drugs of this class should not be used extensively on pregnant patients, in large amounts, or for prolonged periods of time.
Nursing Mothers: It is not known whether topical administration of corticosteroids could result in sufficient systemic absorption to produce detectable quantities in breast milk. Systemically administered corticosteroids are secreted into breast milk in quantities not likely to have a deleterious effect on the infant. Nevertheless, caution should be exercised when topical corticosteroids are administered to a nursing woman.
Pediatric Use: Pediatric patients may demonstrate greater susceptibility to topical corticosteroid-induced HPA axis suppression and Cushing's syndrome than mature patients because of a larger skin surface area to body weight ratio.
Hypothalamic-pituitary-adrenal (HPA) axis suppression, Cushing's syndrome and intracranial hypertension have been reported in children receiving topical corticosteroids. Manifestations of adrenal suppression in children include linear growth retardation, delayed weight gain, low plasma cortisol levels and absence of response to ACTH stimulation. Manifestations of intracranial hypertension include bulging fontanelles, headaches and bilateral papilledema.
Administration of topical corticosteroids to children should be limited to the least amount compatible with an effective therapeutic regimen. Chronic corticosteroid therapy may interfere with the growth and development of children.
Adverse Reactions: The following local adverse reactions are reported infrequently with topical corticosteroids, but may occur more frequently with the use of occlusive dressings. These reactions are listed in an approximate decreasing order of occurrence:

Burning	Perioral dermatitis
Itching	Allergic contact dermatitis
Irritation	Maceration of the skin
Dryness	Secondary infection
Folliculitis	Skin atrophy
Hypertrichosis	Striae
Acneiform eruptions	Miliaria
Hypopigmentation	

Overdosage: Topically applied corticosteroids can be absorbed in sufficient amounts to produce systemic effects (see PRECAUTIONS).
Dosage and Administration: Fluonid® (fluocinolone acetonide) should be applied to the affected area two to four times daily depending on the severity of the condition.
Fluonid® Cream 0.01% and 0.025% may be used over long periods of time in specific conditions when deemed necessary. Where an emollient effect is desired, as in atopic dermatitis, Fluonid® Ointment 0.025% may be preferred. When large areas are involved, Fluonid Cream 0.01% is recommended. The cream should be massaged gently and thoroughly until it disappears.
Fluonid® Topical Solution should be applied directly on the lesion, taking note that small quantities are adequate. It should be rubbed in thoroughly but gently at each application. In hairy sites, the hair should be parted to allow direct contact with the lesion.
In some cases treated with Fluonid Topical Solution, it has been observed that saprophytic or low-grade infections may clear spontaneously as the skin recovers its integrity under the influence of Fluonid Topical Solution alone. This may be partially attributed to the inherent antimicrobial activity of the solution base, propylene glycol.
Occlusive dressings may be used for the management of psoriasis or recalcitrant conditions. If an infection develops, the use of occlusive dressings should be discontinued and appropriate antimicrobial therapy instituted.
How Supplied: Fluonid (fluocinolone acetonide)

- Cream 0.01%—15 gm and 60 gm collapsible tubes and 425 gm jars.
- Cream 0.025%—15 gm and 60 gm collapsible tubes.
- Ointment 0.025%—15 gm and 60 gm collapsible tubes.
- Topical Solution 0.01%—20 ml and 60 ml plastic squeeze bottles.

These preparations are available on prescription only.
U.S. Patent 3,126,375
Manufactured by
Marion Laboratories, Inc.
Kansas City, Missouri 64137
for
Herbert Laboratories
Dermatology Division of
Allergan Pharmaceuticals, Inc.
Irvine, CA 92713, U.S.A.

FLUOROPLEX® ℞
(fluorouracil)
1% Topical Solution
and 1% Topical Cream

Description: Fluoroplex (fluorouracil) 1% Topical Cream is a stable, standardized cream formulation of fluorouracil in an emulsion base with the following formula:
fluorouracil..................1.0%
with: benzyl alcohol (0.5%), ethoxylated stearyl alcohol, mineral oil, isopropyl myristate, sodium hydroxide, purified water.
Fluoroplex (fluorouracil) 1% Topical Solution is a stable, standardized solution of fluorouracil in a clear propylene glycol base with the following formula:
fluorouracil..................1.0%
with: propylene glycol, sodium hydroxide, hydrochloric acid to adjust to pH 9, purified water.
Fluorouracil is a modified pyrimidine similar to uracil and thymine, with whose metabolism it competes. It is a white, crystalline substance with a melting point of 283±2° C., an empirical formula of $C_4H_3FN_2O_2$ and a molecular weight of 130.08. It has a characteristic ultraviolet absorption maximum at 266±1 millimicrons in 0.1N HCl.
Actions: There is evidence that fluorouracil (or its biological metabolites) blocks the methylation reaction of deoxyuridylic acid to thymidylic acid. In this fashion fluorouracil interferes with the synthesis of deoxyribonucleic acid (DNA) and to a lesser extent inhibits the formation of ribonucleic acid (RNA).
Indications: Fluoroplex (fluorouracil) 1% Topical Solution and Fluoroplex® (fluorouracil) 1% Topical Cream are indicated for the topical treatment of multiple actinic (solar) keratoses.
Contraindications: Should not be used in patients with known hypersensitivity to any of the components of the drug.
Warnings:

1. If an occlusive dressing is used there may be an increase in the incidence of inflammatory reactions to the adjacent normal skin.
2. The patient should avoid prolonged exposure to sunlight or other forms of ultraviolet irradiation during treatment with Fluoroplex as the intensity of the reaction may be increased.

USE IN PREGNANCY: Safety for use in pregnancy has not been established.
Precautions: The medication should be applied with care near the eyes, nose and mouth. Excessive reaction in these areas may occur due to irritation from accumulation of drug. To rule out the presence of a frank neoplasm, a biopsy should be made of those areas failing to respond to treatment or recurring after treatment.
Adverse Reactions: Pain, pruritus, burning, irritation, inflammation, dermatitis and telangiectasia have been reported. Occasionally, hyperpigmentation and scarring have also been reported.
Dosage and Administration: The patient should be instructed to apply sufficient medication to cover the entire face or other affected areas.
Apply medication twice daily with non-metallic applicator or fingertips and wash hands afterwards. A treatment period of 2-6 weeks is usually required.
Increasing frequency of application and a longer period of administration with Fluoroplex may be required on areas other than the head and neck.
When Fluoroplex is applied to keratotic skin, a response occurs with the following sequence: erythema, usually followed by scaling, tenderness, erosion, ulceration, necrosis and re-epithelialization. When the inflammatory reaction reaches the erosion, necrosis and ulceration stage, the use of the drug should be terminated. Responses may sometimes occur in areas which appear clinically normal. These may be sites of subclinical actinic (solar) keratoses which the medication is affecting.
How Supplied: Fluoroplex (fluorouracil) 1% Topical Solution is available in 30 ml plastic dropper bottles. On prescription only. Fluoroplex (fluorouracil) 1% Topical Cream is available in 30 gm tubes. On prescription only.
Avoid freezing.
Store at controlled room temperature (59°-86°F).

MAXIFLOR® ℞
(diflorasone diacetate)
Cream 0.05%

Description: Each gram of Maxiflor Cream (diflorasone diacetate) contains 0.5 mg diflorasone diacetate in a cream base.
Chemically, diflorasone diacetate is: 6α,9α-difluoro 11β,17,21 trihydroxy-16β-methylpregna-1,4-diene-3,20-dione 17,21 diacetate.
Maxiflor Cream contains diflorasone diacetate in an emulsified and hydrophilic cream base consisting of propylene glycol, stearic acid, polyoxyethylene 20 sorbitan monostearate, sorbitan monostearate and monooleate, sorbic acid, citric acid and water. The corticosteroid is formulated as a solution in the vehicle using 15 percent propylene glycol to optimize drug delivery.
Actions: Maxiflor Cream (diflorasone diacetate) is effective because of its anti-inflammatory, antipruritic and vasoconstrictor actions.
Indications: Maxiflor Cream (diflorasone diacetate) is intended for topical use as adjunctive therapy for the relief of inflammatory manifestations of acute and chronic corticosteroid-responsive dermatoses.
Contraindications: Topical steroids are contraindicated in vaccinia and varicella. Topical steroids are contraindicated in those pa-

tients with a history of hypersensitivity to any of the components of the preparations.
Precautions: If irritation develops, the cream should be discontinued and appropriate therapy instituted.
In the presence of an infection, the use of an appropriate antifungal or antibacterial agent should be instituted. If a favorable response does not occur promptly, the corticosteroid cream should be discontinued until the infection has been adequately controlled.
If extensive areas are treated, the possibility exists of increased systemic absorption and suitable precautions should be taken.
Although topical steroids have not been reported to have an adverse effect on human pregnancy, the safety of their use in pregnant females has not been absolutely established. Studies in rats show increased numbers of fetal abnormalities in groups treated with topical corticosteroids. Therefore, they should not be used extensively on pregnant patients, in large amounts or for prolonged periods of time.
Occlusive Dressing Technique: The use of occlusive dressings increases the percutaneous absorption of corticosteroids; their extensive use increases the possibility of systemic effects. For patients with extensive lesions it may be preferable to use a sequential approach, occluding one portion of the body at a time. The patient should be kept under close observation if treated with the occlusive technique over large areas and over a considerable period of time. Occasionally, a patient who had been on prolonged therapy, especially occlusive therapy, may develop symptoms of steroid withdrawal when the medication is stopped. Thermal homeostasis may be impaired if large areas of the body are covered. Use of the occlusive dressing should be discontinued if elevation of the body temperature occurs. Occasionally, a patient may develop a sensitivity reaction to a particular occlusive dressing material or adhesive and a substitute material may be necessary. If infection develops, discontinue the use of the occlusive dressing and institute appropriate antimicrobial therapy.
Maxiflor Cream (diflorasone diacetate) is not for ophthalmic use.
Adverse Reactions: The following adverse reactions have been reported with topical corticosteroids: burning, itching, irritation, striae, skin atrophy, secondary infection, dryness, folliculitis, hypertrichosis, acneiform eruptions and hypopigmentation. The following may occur more frequently with occlusive dressings: maceration of the skin, secondary infection, skin atrophy, striae and miliaria.
Dosage and Administration: A small amount of cream should be gently massaged into the affected area one to four times daily, as needed.
How Supplied: Maxiflor Cream 0.05% is available in collapsible tubes in the following sizes:
15 gram NDC 0023-0766-15
30 gram NDC 0023-0766-30
60 gram NDC 0023-0766-60
Caution: Federal law prohibits dispensing without prescription.
Manufactured by
The Upjohn Company
Kalamazoo, Michigan 49001
For
Herbert Laboratories
Dermatology Division of
Allergan Pharmaceuticals, Inc.
Irvine, California 92713, U.S.A.

MAXIFLOR®
(diflorasone diacetate)
Ointment 0.05%

Description: Each gram of Maxiflor Ointment (diflorasone diacetate) contains 0.5 mg diflorasone diacetate in an ointment base.
Chemically, diflorasone diacetate is: 6α,9α-difluoro 11β,17,21 trihydroxy-16β-methylpregna-1,4-diene-3,20-dione 17,21 diacetate.
Maxiflor Ointment contains 0.5 mg/gram of diflorasone diacetate in an emollient, occlusive base consisting of polyoxypropylene 15-stearyl ether, stearic acid, lanolin alcohol and white petrolatum.
Actions: Maxiflor Ointment (diflorasone diacetate) is effective because of its anti-inflammatory, antipruritic and vasoconstrictor actions.
Indications: Maxiflor Ointment (diflorasone diacetate) is intended for topical use as adjunctive therapy for the relief of inflammatory manifestations of corticosteroid-responsive dermatoses.
Contraindications: Topical steroids are contraindicated in vaccinia and varicella and in those patients with a history of hypersensitivity to any of the components of the preparations. Maxiflor Ointment (diflorasone diacetate) is not for ophthalmic use.
Precautions: If irritation develops, the ointment should be discontinued and appropriate therapy instituted.
In the presence of an infection, the use of an appropriate antifungal or antibacterial agent should be instituted. If a favorable response does not occur promptly, the corticosteroid ointment should be discontinued until the infection has been adequately controlled.
If extensive areas are treated, the possibility exists of increased systemic absorption and suitable precautions should be taken.
Although topical steroids have not been reported to have an adverse effect on pregnancy, the safety of their use in pregnant females has not been absolutely established. Studies in rats show increased numbers of fetal abnormalities in groups treated with topical corticosteroids. Therefore, they should not be used extensively on pregnant patients, in large amounts or for prolonged periods of time.
Adverse Reactions: The following adverse reactions have been reported with topical corticosteroids: burning, itching, irritation, striae, skin atrophy, secondary infection, dryness, folliculitis, hypertrichosis, acneiform eruptions and hypopigmentation. The following may occur more frequently with occlusive dressings: maceration of the skin, secondary infection, skin atrophy, striae and miliaria.
Dosage and Administration: Apply a thin film of Maxiflor Ointment (diflorasone diacetate) to the affected skin areas one to three times a day.
Occlusive Dressing Technique: The use of occlusive dressings increases the percutaneous absorption of corticosteroids; their extensive use increases the possibility of systemic effects. For patients with extensive lesions it may be preferable to use a sequential approach, occluding one portion of the body at a time. The patient should be kept under close observation if treated with occlusive technique over large areas and over a considerable period of time. Occasionally, a patient who had been on prolonged therapy, especially occlusive therapy, may develop symptoms of steroid withdrawal when the medication is stopped. Thermal homeostasis may be impaired if large areas of the body are covered. Use of occlusive dressing should be discontinued if elevation of the body temperature occurs. Occasionally, a patient may develop a sensitivity reaction to a particular occlusive dressing material or adhesive and a substitute material may be necessary. If infection develops, discontinue the use of the occlusive dressing and institute appropriate antimicrobial therapy.
How Supplied: Maxiflor Ointment 0.05% is available in collapsible tubes in the following sizes:
15 gram NDC 0023-0770-15
30 gram NDC 0023-0770-30
60 gram NDC 0023-0770-60
Caution: Federal law prohibits dispensing without prescription.
Manufactured by
The Upjohn Company
Kalamazoo, Michigan 49001
For
Herbert Laboratories
Dermatology Division of
Allergan Pharmaceuticals, Inc.
Irvine, California 92713, U.S.A.

Dow B. Hickam, Inc.
P.O. BOX 35413
HOUSTON, TX 77035

GRANULEX ℞

Composition: Each 0.82 cc. of medication delivered to the wound site contains Trypsin crystallized 0.1 mg., Balsam Peru 72.5 mg., Castor Oil 650.0 mg., and an emulsifier.
Action: Trypsin is intended for debridement of eschar and other necrotic tissue. It appears that in many instances removal of wound debris strengthens humoral defense mechanisms sufficiently to retard proliferation of local pathogens. Balsam Peru is an effective capillary bed stimulant used to increase circulation in the wound site area. Also, Balsam Peru has a mildly bactericidal action. Castor Oil is used to improve epithelialization by reducing premature epithelial desiccation and cornification. Also, it can act as a protective covering and aids in the reduction of pain.
Indications: For the treatment of decubitus ulcers, varicose ulcers, debridement of eschar, dehiscent wounds and sunburn.
Uses: Granulex is in aerosol form which can be important to healing. It must be remembered, healing starts with a thin sheath of epithelium no more than a cell or two thick. Any rough movement or trauma can quickly destroy the healing tissue. Aerosols have the advantage of eliminating all extraneous physical contact with the wound. Granulex is easy to apply and quickly reduces odor frequently accompanying a decubitus ulcer. The wound may be left open or a wet bandage may be applied. As a suggestion; keep in mind wounds heal poorly in the presence of hemoglobin or zinc deficiency.
Warning: Do not spray on fresh arterial clots. Avoid spraying in eyes. Flammable, do not expose to fire or open flame. Contents under pressure. Do not puncture or incinerate. Do not store at temperature above 120°F. Keep out of reach of children. Use only as directed. Intentional misuse by deliberately concentrating and inhaling the contents can be harmful or fatal.
Dosage: Apply a minimum of twice daily or as often as necessary. Shake well, press the aerosol valve and coat the wound rapidly but not excessively.
How Supplied:
2 oz. Aerosol NDC 0514-0001-01
4 oz. Aerosol NDC 0514-0001-02

Products are cross-indexed by generic and chemical names in the **YELLOW SECTION**

High Chemical Co.

Div. Day & Frick, Inc.
1760 N. HOWARD ST.
PHILADELPHIA, PA 19122

SARAPIN ℞

Composition: An aqueous distillate of Sarracenia purpurea, pitcher plant, prepared for parenteral administration.
Action and Uses: Local injection therapy for the relief of pain of neuro-muscular or neuralgic origin.
Administration and Dosage: Paravertebral nerve injection—2 to 10 cc. Local neuromuscular infiltration—5 to 10 cc.
Side Effects: None.
Precautions: Non-toxic.
Contraindications: Local inflammation.
How Supplied: One dozen 10 cc. ampuls and 50 cc. multi-dose vials.
Literature Available: Booklet "SARAPIN, Injection Technique in Pain Control."

Hill Dermaceuticals, Inc.

P.O. BOX 19283
ORLANDO, FL 32814

BURDEO®

Contains: Aluminum Acetate Basic, Boric Acid, and Hexachlorophene in a non-greasy gel base (NDC 28105-0098-08).

DERMA-SMOOTHE® OIL

Contains: Refined peanut oil-mineral oil blend and is a lipophilic, neutral, non-ionic skin cleanser (NDC 28105-0048-06).

DERMA-SMOOTHE/FS ℞

Contains: Fluocinolone Acetonide 0.01% in a blend of oils (NDC 28105 148-04).

DERMA-SONE® CREAM 1% ℞
Paraben Free

Contains: Hydrocortisone 1%, Pramoxine HCl 1% (NDC 28105-162-04).

FLORIDA FOAM® IMPROVED

Contains: Benzalkonium Chloride, Aluminum Acetate Basic, Boric Acid, Biodegradable Protein and Non-ionic Detergent in a Dermoat (Oat Powder) base (NDC 28105-069-08).

HILL CORTAC® LOTION ℞

Contains: Hydrocortisone 0.5%, Sulfur 5%, Zinc Oxide 20%, Isopropyl Alcohol 5% (NDC 28105-149-02).

HILL-SHADE LOTION

Contains: Para-aminobenzoic Acid 5%, Alcohol 65% (NDC 28105-0160-04).

R.S. LOTION NO. 2

Contains: Sulfur 8%, Resorcinol Monoacetate 4%, in a special clay-free, inert, drying, CLEAR ON APPLICATION, adhering jell base (NDC 28105-0054-02).

Products are

listed alphabetically

in the

PINK SECTION.

Hoechst-Roussel Pharmaceuticals Inc.

SOMERVILLE, NJ 08876

A/T/S™ ℞
(erythromycin)
2% Acne Topical Solution

Description: A/T/S™ (erythromycin) is an antibiotic produced from a strain of *Streptomyces erythraeus.* It is basic and readily forms salts with acids. Each mL of A/T/S (erythromycin) topical solution contains 20 mg of erythromycin base in a vehicle consisting of alcohol, propylene glycol, and citric acid. The alcohol content is 66%.
Actions: Although the mechanism by which A/T/S (erythromycin) acts in reducing inflammatory lesions of acne vulgaris is unknown, it is presumably due to its antibiotic action.
Indications: A/T/S (erythromycin) is indicated for the topical control of acne vulgaris.
Contraindications: A/T/S (erythromycin) is contraindicated in persons who have shown hypersensitivity to any of its ingredients.
Warning: The safe use of A/T/S (erythromycin) during pregnancy or lactation has not been established.
Precautions: A/T/S (erythromycin) is for external use only and should be kept away from the eyes, nose, mouth, and mucous membranes. Concomitant topical acne therapy should be used with caution because a cumulative irritant effect may occur, especially with the use of peeling, desquamating, or abrasive agents.
The use of antimicrobial agents may be associated with the overgrowth of antibiotic-resistant organisms; in such a case, antibiotic administration should be stopped and appropriate measures taken.
Adverse Reactions: Of a total of 90 patients exposed to the drug during clinical effectiveness studies, 17 experienced some type of adverse effect. These included dry skin, scaly skin, pruritus, irritation of the eye, and burning sensation.
Dosage and Administration: A/T/S (erythromycin) should be applied to the affected area twice a day after the skin is thoroughly washed with warm water and soap. Moisten the applicator or a pad with A/T/S (erythromycin), then rub over the entire facial area. Acne lesions on the neck, shoulder, chest, and back may also be treated in this manner.
How Supplied: Topical Solution—60 mL. Store at controlled room temperature. 15° to 30°C (59°–86°F).
Manufactured by Eli Lilly and Company, Indianapolis, Indiana 46206 for Hoechst-Roussel Pharmaceuticals Inc.
[*Shown in Product Identification Section*]

CLAFORAN® ℞
(cefotaxime sodium)
Sterile

Description: Sterile Claforan® (cefotaxime sodium) is a semisynthetic, broad spectrum cephalosporin antibiotic for parenteral administration. It is the sodium salt of 7-[2-(2-amino-4-thiazolyl) glyoxylamido]-3-(hydroxymethyl)-8-oxo-5-thia-1-azabicyclo [4.2.0] oct-2-ene-2-carboxylate 7^2-(Z)-(O-methyloxime), acetate (ester). Claforan contains approximately 50.5 mg (2.2 mEq) of sodium per gram of cefotaxime activity. Solutions of Claforan range from light yellow to amber depending on the concentration and the diluent used. The pH of freshly reconstituted solutions usually ranges from 4.5 to 6.5.
Clinical Pharmacology: Following IM administration of a single 500 mg or 1 g dose of Claforan to normal volunteers, mean peak serum concentrations of 11.7 and 20.5 μg/mL respectively are attained within 30 minutes and decline with an elimination half-life of approximately 1 hour. There is a dose-dependent increase in serum levels after the IV administration of 500 mg, 1 g and 2 g of Claforan (38.9, 101.7, and 214.4 μg/mL respectively) without alteration in the elimination half-life. There is no evidence of accumulation following repetitive IV infusion of 1 g doses every 6 hours for 14 days as there are no alterations of serum or renal clearance. About 60% of the administered dose was recovered from urine during the first 6 hours following the start of the infusion. Approximately 20–36% of an intravenously administered dose of ^{14}C-cefotaxime is excreted by the kidney as unchanged cefotaxime and 15–25% as the desacetyl derivative, the major metabolite. The desacetyl metabolite has been shown to contribute to the bactericidal activity. Two other urinary metabolites (UP1 and UP2) account for about 20–25%. They lack bactericidal activity.
A single 50 mg/kg dose of Claforan was administered as an intravenous infusion over a 10- to 15-minute period to 29 newborn infants grouped according to birth weight and age. The mean half-life of cefotaxime in infants with lower birth weights (≤ 1500 grams), regardless of age, was longer (4.6 hours) than the mean half-life (3.4 hours) in infants whose birth weight was greater than 1500 grams. Mean serum clearance was also smaller in the lower birth weight infants. Although the differences in mean half-life values are statistically significant for weight, they are not clinically important. Therefore, dosage should be based solely on age. (See **Dosage and Administration** section.)
Additionally, no disulfiram-like reactions were reported in a study conducted in 22 healthy volunteers administered Claforan and ethanol.

Microbiology
The bactericidal activity of cefotaxime sodium results from inhibition of cell wall synthesis. Cefotaxime sodium has *in vitro* activity against a wide range of gram-positive and gram-negative organisms. Claforan has a high degree of stability in the presence of beta-lactamases, both penicillinases and cephalosporinases, of gram-negative and gram-positive bacteria. Cefotaxime sodium has been shown to be a potent inhibitor of β-lactamases produced by certain gram-negative bacteria. Cefotaxime sodium is usually active against the following microorganisms both *in vitro* and in clinical infections (see **Indications and Usage**).
Aerobes, Gram-positive: *Staphylococcus aureus,* including penicillinase and non-penicillinase producing strains, *Staphylococcus epidermidis, Streptococcus pyogenes* (Group A beta-hemolytic streptococci), *Streptococcus agalactiae* (Group B streptococci), (NOTE: Most strains of enterococci, e.g., *S. faecalis* are resistant), *Streptococcus pneumoniae* (formerly *Diplococcus pneumoniae*).
Aerobes, Gram-negative: *Citrobacter* species, *Enterobacter* species, *Escherichia coli, Haemophilus influenzae* (including ampicillin-resistant *H. influenzae*), *Klebsiella* species (including *K. pneumoniae*), *Neisseria gonorrhoeae* (including penicillinase and non-penicillinase producing strains), *Neisseria meningitidis, Proteus mirabilis, Proteus morganii, Proteus rettgeri, Proteus vulgaris, Serratia* species.
NOTE: Many strains of the above organisms that are multiply resistant to other antibiotics, e.g., penicillins, cephalosporins, and aminoglycosides, are susceptible to cefotaxime sodium.
Cefotaxime sodium is active against some strains of *Pseudomonas aeruginosa.*
Anaerobes: *Bacteroides* species, including some strains of *B. fragilis, Clostridium* species (NOTE: Most strains of *C. difficile* are resistant), *Peptococcus* species, *Peptostreptococcus* species.
Cefotaxime sodium is highly stable *in vitro* to four of the five major classes of β-lactamases described by Richmond et al., including type IIIa (TEM) which is produced by many gram-

negative bacteria. The drug is also stable to β-lactamase (penicillinase) produced by staphylococci. In addition, cefotaxime sodium shows high affinity for penicillin-binding proteins in the cell wall, including PBP, Ib and III.

Cefotaxime sodium also demonstrates *in vitro* activity against the following microorganisms although clinical significance is unknown: *Salmonella* species (including *S. typhi*), *Providencia* species, and *Shigella* species.

Cefotaxime sodium and aminoglycosides have been shown to be synergistic *in vitro* against some strains of *Pseudomonas aeruginosa.*

Susceptibility Tests

Quantitative methods that require measurement of zone diameters give the most precise estimate of antibiotic susceptibility. One such procedure[1] has been recommended for use with discs to test susceptibility to cefotaxime sodium. Interpretation involves correlation of the diameters obtained in the disc test with minimum inhibitory concentration (MIC) values for cefotaxime sodium.

Reports from the laboratory giving results of the standardized single-disc susceptibility test using a 30-μg cefotaxime sodium disc should be interpreted according to the following criteria:

Susceptible organisms produce zones of 20 mm or greater, indicating that the tested organism is likely to respond to therapy.

Organisms that produce zones of 15 to 19 mm are expected to be susceptible if high dosage is used or if the infection is confined to tissues and fluids (e.g., urine) in which high antibiotic levels are attained.

Resistant organisms produce zones of 14 mm or less, indicating that other therapy should be selected.

Organisms should be tested with the cefotaxime sodium disc, since cefotaxime sodium has been shown by *in vitro* tests to be active against certain strains found resistant when other beta lactam discs are used. The cefotaxime sodium disc should not be used for testing susceptibility to other cephalosporins. Organisms having zones of less than 18 mm around the cephalothin disc are not necessarily of intermediate susceptibility or resistant to cefotaxime sodium.

A bacterial isolate may be considered susceptible if the MIC value for cefotaxime sodium is not more than 16 μg/mL. Organisms are considered resistant to cefotaxime sodium if the MIC is equal to or greater than 64 μg/mL. Organisms having an MIC value of less than 64 μg/mL but greater than 16μg/mL are expected to be susceptible if high dosage is used or if the infection is confined to tissues and fluids (e.g., urine) in which high antibiotic levels are attained.

Indications and Usage:

Treatment

Claforan is indicated for the treatment of patients with serious infections caused by susceptible strains of the designated microorganisms in the diseases listed below.

(1) **Lower respiratory tract infections,** including pneumonia, caused by *Streptococcus pneumoniae* (formerly *Diplococcus pneumoniae*), *Streptococcus pyogenes* (Group A streptococci) and other streptococci (excluding enterococci, e.g., *Streptococcus faecalis*), *Staphylococcus aureus* (penicillinase and non-penicillinase producing), *Escherichia coli, Klebsiella* species, *Haemophilus influenzae* (including ampicillin resistant strains), *Proteus mirabilis, Serratia marcescens,* and *Enterobacter* species.

(2) **Genitourinary infections.** Urinary tract infections caused by *Enterococcus* species, *Staphylococcus epidermidis, Staphylococcus aureus* (penicillinase and non-penicillinase producing), *Citrobacter* species, *Enterobacter* species, *Escherichia coli, Klebsiella* species, *Proteus mirabilis,* indole positive *Proteus (i.e., Proteus morganii, Proteus rettgeri,* and *Proteus vulgaris*), and *Serratia marcescens.* Also, uncomplicated gonorrhea of single or multiple sites caused by *Neisseria gonorrhoeae,* including penicillinase producing strains.

(3) **Gynecologic infections,** including pelvic inflammatory disease, endometritis and pelvic cellulitis caused by *Staphylococcus epidermidis, Streptococcus* species, *Enterococcus* species, *Escherichia coli, Proteus mirabilis, Bacteroides* species (including *B. fragilis*), *Clostridium* species, and anaerobic cocci (including *Peptostreptococcus* species and *Peptococcus* species).

(4) **Bacteremia/Septicemia** caused by *Escherichia coli, Klebsiella* species, and *Serratia marcescens.*

(5) **Skin and skin structure infections** caused by *Staphylococcus aureus* (penicillinase and non-penicillinase producing), *Staphylococcus epidermidis, Streptococcus pyogenes* (Group A streptococci) and other streptococci, *Enterococcus* species, *Escherichia coli, Enterobacter* species, *Klebsiella* species, *Proteus mirabilis,* and indole positive *Proteus* (i.e., *Proteus morganii, Proteus rettgeri,* and *Proteus vulgaris*), *Pseudomonas* species, *Serratia marcescens, Bacteroides* species, and anaerobic cocci (including *Peptostreptococcus* species and *Peptococcus* species).

(6) **Intra-abdominal infections** including peritonitis caused by *Escherichia coli, Klebsiella* species, *Bacteroides* species, and anaerobic cocci (including *Peptostreptococcus* species and *Peptococcus species*).

(7) **Bone and/or joint infections** caused by *Staphylococcus aureus* (penicillinase and non-penicillinase producing strains).

(8) **Central nervous system infections,** e.g. meningitis and ventriculitis, caused by *Neisseria meningitidis, Haemophilus influenzae, Streptococcus pneumoniae, Klebsiella pneumoniae,* and *Escherichia coli.*

Although many strains of enterococci (e.g., *S. faecalis*) and *Pseudomonas* species are resistant to cefotaxime sodium *in vitro,* Claforan has been used successfully in treating patients with infections caused by susceptible organisms.

Specimens for bacteriologic culture should be obtained prior to therapy in order to isolate and identify causative organisms and to determine their susceptibilities to Claforan. Therapy may be instituted before results of susceptibility studies are known; however, once these results become available, the antibiotic treatment should be adjusted accordingly.

In certain cases of confirmed or suspected gram-positive or gram-negative sepsis or in patients with other serious infections in which the causative organism has not been identified, Claforan may be used concomitantly with an aminoglycoside. The dosage recommended in the labeling of both antibiotics may be given and depends on the severity of the infection and the patient's condition. Renal function should be carefully monitored, especially if higher dosages of the aminoglycosides are to be administered or if therapy is prolonged, because of the potential nephrotoxicity and ototoxicity of aminoglycoside antibiotics. Some β-lactam antibiotics also have a certain degree of nephrotoxicity. Although, to date, this has not been noted when Claforan was given alone, it is possible that nephrotoxicity may be potentiated if Claforan is used concomitantly with an aminoglycoside.

Prevention

The administration of Claforan perioperatively (preoperatively, intraoperatively, and postoperatively) may reduce the incidence of certain infections in patients undergoing elective surgical procedures (e.g. abdominal or vaginal hysterectomy, gastrointestinal and genitourinary tract surgery) that may be classified as contaminated or potentially contaminated.

In patients undergoing cesarean section, intraoperative (after clamping the umbilical cord) and postoperative use of Claforan may also reduce the incidence of certain postoperative infections. See **Dosage and Administration** section.

Effective perioperative use for elective surgery depends on the time of administration. To achieve effective tissue levels, Claforan should be given ½ to 1½ hours before surgery and intraoperatively ½ to 2 hours after the first dose. Additional intraoperative doses may be administered. The final dose should be administered within 2 hours following surgery. See **Dosage and Administration** section. Continued use beyond 2 hours does not necessarily reduce the incidence of subsequent infections.

For patients undergoing gastrointestinal surgery, preoperative bowel preparation by mechanical cleansing as well as with a non-absorbable antibiotic (e.g., neomycin) is recommended.

If there are signs of infection, specimens for culture should be obtained for identification of the causative organism so that appropriate therapy may be instituted.

Contraindications: Claforan is contraindicated in patients who have shown hypersensitivity to cefotaxime sodium or the cephalosporin group of antibiotics.

Warnings: BEFORE THERAPY WITH CLAFORAN IS INSTITUTED, CAREFUL INQUIRY SHOULD BE MADE TO DETERMINE WHETHER THE PATIENT HAS HAD PREVIOUS HYPERSENSITIVITY REACTIONS TO CEFOTAXIME SODIUM, CEPHALOSPORINS, PENICILLINS, OR OTHER DRUGS. THIS PRODUCT SHOULD BE GIVEN WITH CAUTION TO PATIENTS WITH TYPE 1 HYPERSENSITIVITY REACTIONS TO PENICILLIN. ANTIBIOTICS SHOULD BE ADMINISTERED WITH CAUTION TO ANY PATIENT WHO HAS DEMONSTRATED SOME FORM OF ALLERGY, PARTICULARLY TO DRUGS. IF AN ALLERGIC REACTION TO CLAFORAN OCCURS, DISCONTINUE TREATMENT WITH THE DRUG. SERIOUS HYPERSENSITIVITY REACTIONS MAY REQUIRE EPINEPHRINE AND OTHER EMERGENCY MEASURES.

Pseudomembranous colitis has been reported with the use of cephalosporins (and other broad spectrum antibiotics); therefore, it is important to consider its diagnosis in patients who develop diarrhea in association with antibiotic use.

Treatment with broad spectrum antibiotics alters normal flora of the colon and may permit overgrowth of Clostridia. Studies indicate a toxin produced by *Clostridium difficile* is one primary cause of antibiotic-associated colitis. Cholestyramine and colestipol resins have been shown to bind the toxin *in vitro.*

Mild cases of colitis may respond to drug discontinuance alone.

Moderate to severe cases should be managed with fluid, electrolyte, and protein supplementation as indicated.

When the colitis is not relieved by drug discontinuance or when it is severe, oral vancomycin is the treatment of choice for antibiotic-associated pseudomembranous colitis produced by *C. difficile.* Other causes of colitis should also be considered.

Precautions: Claforan® (cefotaxime sodium) should be prescribed with caution in individuals with a history of gastrointestinal disease, particularly colitis.

Claforan has not been shown to be nephrotoxic; however, because high and prolonged serum antibiotic concentrations can occur from usual doses in patients with transient or persistent reduction of urinary output because of renal insufficiency, the total daily dosage should be reduced when Claforan is administered to such patients. Continued dosage should be determined by degree of renal impairment, severity

Continued on next page

Hoechst-Roussel—Cont.

of infection, and susceptibility of the causative organism.

Although there is no clinical evidence supporting the necessity of changing the dosage of cefotaxime sodium in patients with even profound renal dysfunction, it is suggested that, until further data are obtained, the dose of cefotaxime sodium be halved in patients with estimated creatinine clearances of less than 20 mL/min/1.73 m^2.

When only serum creatinine is available, the following formula[2] (based on sex, weight, and age of the patient) may be used to convert this value into creatinine clearance. The serum creatinine should represent a steady state of renal function.

Males $\frac{\text{Weight (kg)} \times (140 - \text{age})}{72 \times \text{serum creatinine}}$

Females 0.85 × above value

As with other antibiotics, prolonged use of Claforan may result in overgrowth of nonsusceptible organisms. Repeated evaluation of the patient's condition is essential. If superinfection occurs during therapy, appropriate measures should be taken.

Drug Interactions: Increased nephrotoxicity has been reported following concomitant administration of cephalosporins and aminoglycoside antibiotics.

Carcinogenesis, Mutagenesis: Long-term studies in animals have not been performed to evaluate carcinogenic potential. Mutagenic tests included a micronucleus and an Ames test. Both tests were negative for mutagenic effects.

Pregnancy (Category B): Reproduction studies have been performed in mice and rats at doses up to 30 times the usual human dose and have revealed no evidence of impaired fertility or harm to the fetus because of cefotaxime sodium. However, there are no well-controlled studies in pregnant women. Because animal reproductive studies are not always predictive of human response, this drug should be used during pregnancy only if clearly needed.

Nonteratogenic Effects: Use of the drug in women of child-bearing potential requires that the anticipated benefit be weighed against the possible risks.

In perinatal and postnatal studies with rats, the pups in the group given 1200 mg/kg of Claforan were significantly lighter in weight at birth and remained smaller than pups in the control group during the 21 days of nursing.

Nursing Mothers: Claforan is excreted in human milk in low concentrations. Caution should be exercised when Claforan is administered to a nursing woman.

Adverse Reactions: Claforan is generally well tolerated. The most common adverse reactions have been local reactions following IM or IV injection. Other adverse reactions have been encountered infrequently.

The most frequent adverse reactions (greater than 1%) are:

Local (4.7%) - Injection site inflammation with IV administration. Pain, induration, and tenderness after IM injection.

Hypersensitivity (1.8%) - Rash, pruritus, and fever.

Gastrointestinal (1.7%) - Colitis, diarrhea, nausea, and vomiting.

Symptoms of pseudomembranous colitis can appear during or after antibiotic treatment.

Nausea and vomiting have been reported rarely.

Less frequent adverse reactions (less than 1%) are:

Hemic and Lymphatic System - Granulocytopenia, transient leukopenia, eosinophilia, and neutropenia have been reported. Some individuals have developed positive direct

Strength	Amount of Diluent To Be Added (mL)	Approximate Withdrawable Volume (mL)	Approximate Average Concentration (mg/mL)
Intramuscular			
500 mg vial	2	2.2	230
1 g vial	3	3.4	300
2 g vial	5	6.0	330
Intravenous			
500 mg vial	10	10.2	50
1 g vial	10	10.4	95
2 g vial	10	11.0	180

Coombs Tests during treatment with the cephalosporin antibiotics.

Genitourinary System - Moniliasis, vaginitis.

Central Nervous System - Headache.

Liver - Transient elevations in SGOT, SGPT, serum LDH, and serum alkaline phosphatase levels have been reported.

Kidney - As with some other cephalosporins, transient elevations of BUN have been occasionally observed with Claforan.

Dosage and Administration:

Adults

The usual adult dosage for Claforan is 1 gram every six to eight hours. Dosage and route of administration should be determined by susceptibility of the causative organisms, severity of the infection, and the condition of the patient (see table for dosage guideline). Claforan may be administered IM or IV after reconstitution.

[See table below].

To prevent postoperative infection in contaminated or potentially contaminated surgery, recommended doses are as follows:

a. 1 gram IM or IV administered 30 to 90 minutes prior to start of surgery.

b. 1 gram IM or IV administered 30 to 120 minutes following the first dose. (For lengthy operative procedures, additional intraoperative doses may be given.)

c. 1 gram IM or IV administered within 2 hours following surgery.

Cesarean Section Patients

The first dose of 1 gram is administered intravenously as soon as the umbilical cord is clamped. The second and third doses should be given as 1 gram intravenously or intramuscularly at 6 and 12 hours after the first dose.

Neonates, Infants and Children

The following dosage schedule is recommended:

Neonates (birth to 1 month):

0–1 week of age	50 mg/kg IV q 12 h
1–4 weeks of age	50 mg/kg IV q 8 h

It is not necessary to differentiate between premature and normal-gestational age infants.

Infants and Children (1 month to 12 years): For body weights less than 50 kg, the recommended daily dose is 50 to 180 mg/kg IM or IV of body weight divided into four to six equal doses. The higher dosages should be used for more severe or serious infections, including meningitis. For body weights 50 kg or more, the usual adult dosage should be used; the maximum daily dosage should not exceed 12 grams.

Impaired Renal Function - see **Precautions** section.

NOTE: As with antibiotic therapy in general, administration of Claforan should be continued for a minimum of 48 to 72 hours after the patient defervesces or after evidence of bacterial eradication has been obtained; a minimum of 10 days of treatment is recommended for infections caused by Group A beta-hemolytic streptococci in order to guard against the risk of rheumatic fever or glomerulonephritis; frequent bacteriologic and clinical appraisal is necessary during therapy of chronic urinary tract infection and may be required for several months after therapy has been completed; persistent infections may require treatment of several weeks and doses smaller than those indicated above should not be used.

Preparation of Solution: Claforan for IM or IV administration should be reconstituted as follows:

[See table above].

Shake to dissolve; inspect for particulate matter and discoloration prior to use. Solutions of Claforan range from light yellow to amber, depending on concentration, diluent used, and length and condition of storage.

For intramuscular use: Reconstitute with Sterile Water for Injection or Bacteriostatic Water for Injection as described above.

For intravenous use: Reconstitute all strengths with at least 10 mL of Sterile Water for Injection. Infusion bottles may be reconstituted with 50 or 100 mL of 0.9% Sodium Chloride Injection or 5% Dextrose Injection. For other diluents see **Compatibility and Stability.**

NOTE: Solutions of Claforan must not be admixed with aminoglycoside solutions. If Claforan and aminoglycosides are to be administered to the same patient, they must be administered separately and not as mixed injection.

A SOLUTION OF 1 G CLAFORAN IN 14 ML OF STERILE WATER FOR INJECTION IS ISOTONIC.

IM Administration: As with all IM preparations, Claforan should be injected well within the body of a relatively large muscle such as the upper outer quadrant of the buttock (i.e., gluteus maximus); aspiration is necessary to avoid inadvertent injection into a blood vessel. Individual IM doses of 2 grams may be given if the dose is divided and is administered in different intramuscular sites.

IV Administration: The IV route is preferable for patients with bacteremia, bacterial septicemia, peritonitis, meningitis, or other severe or life-threatening infections, or for patients who may be poor risks because of lowered resis-

GUIDELINES FOR DOSAGE OF CLAFORAN

Type of Infection	Daily Dose (grams)	Frequency and Route
Gonorrhea	1	1 gram IM (single dose)
Uncomplicated infections such as pneumococcal pneumonia or acute urinary infection	2	1 gram every 12 hours IM or IV
Moderate to severe infections	3–6	1–2 grams every 6–8 hours IM or IV
Infections commonly needing antibiotics in higher dosage (e.g., septicemia)	6–8	2 grams every 6–8 hours IV
Life-threatening infections	up to 12	2 grams every 4 hours IV

The maximum daily dosage should not exceed 12 grams.

tance resulting from such debilitating conditions as malnutrition, trauma, surgery, diabetes, heart failure, or malignancy, particularly if shock is present or impending.

For intermittent IV administration, a solution containing 1 gram or 2 grams in 10 mL of Sterile Water for Injection can be injected over a period of three to five minutes. With an infusion system, it may also be given over a longer period of time through the tubing system by which the patient may be receiving other IV solutions. However, during infusion of the solution containing Claforan, it is advisable to discontinue temporarily the administration of other solutions at the same site.

For the administration of higher doses by continuous IV infusion, a solution of Claforan may be added to IV bottles containing the solutions discussed below.

Compatibility and Stability: Claforan reconstituted as described above (**Preparation of Solution**) maintains satisfactory potency for 24 hours at room temperature (25°C), for 10 days under refrigeration (below 5°C), and for at least 13 weeks in the frozen state.

After reconstitution Claforan may be stored in disposable glass or plastic syringes for 24 hours at room temperature, 5 days under refrigeration and 13 weeks frozen.

Reconstituted solutions may be further diluted to 50 to 1000 mL with the following solutions and maintain potency for 24 hours at room temperature and at least 5 days under refrigeration: 0.9% Sodium Chloride Injection; 5 or 10% Dextrose Injection; 5% Dextrose and 0.9% Sodium Chloride Injection; 5% Dextrose and 0.45% Sodium Chloride Injection; 5% Dextrose and 0.2% Sodium Chloride Injection; Lactated Ringers Solution; Sodium Lactate Injection (M/6); 10% Invert Sugar Injection, FREAMINE® II Injection.

Solutions of Claforan in 0.9% Sodium Chloride Injection and 5% Dextrose Injection in VIAFLEX® intravenous bags are stable for 24 hours at room temperature, 5 days under refrigeration, and 13 weeks frozen.

Frozen samples should not be heated but should be thawed at room temperature before use. After the periods mentioned above, any unused solutions or frozen materials should be discarded. DO NOT REFREEZE. NOTE: Claforan solutions exhibit maximum stability in the pH 5–7 range. Solutions of Claforan should not be prepared with diluents having a pH above 7.5, such as Sodium Bicarbonate Injection.

How Supplied: Sterile Claforan is a dry white to off-white powder supplied in vials and infusion bottles containing cefotaxime sodium as follows:

500 mg cefotaxime free acid equivalent in vials (NDC 0039 0017 01)

1 gram cefotaxime free acid equivalent in vials (NDC 0039 0018 01) and in infusion bottles (NDC 0039 0018 02)

2 gram cefotaxime free acid equivalent in vials (NDC 0039 0019 01) and in infusion bottles (NDC 0039 0019 02)

NOTE: Claforan in the dry state should be stored below 30°C. The dry material as well as solutions tend to darken depending on storage conditions and should be protected from elevated temperatures and excessive light.

References:

1) Bauer, A.W.; Kirby, W.M.M.; Sherris, J.C.; and Turck, M.: Antibiotic Susceptibility Testing by a Standardized Single Disk Method, Am. J. Clin. Pathol., 45:493, 1966; Standardized Disc Susceptibility Test, Federal Register, 39:19182-4, 1974. National Committee for Clinical Laboratory Standards, Approved Standard: ASM-2, Performance Standards for Antimicrobial Disc Susceptibility Tests, July, 1975.

2) Cockcroft, D.W. and Gault, M.H.: Prediction of Creatinine Clearance from Serum Creatinine. Nephron 16:31-41, 1976.

CLAFORAN® REG TM ROUSSEL-UCLAF

DOXIDAN®

Composition: Doxidan is a combination of 60 mg docusate calcium USP, 50 mg danthron USP and up to 1.5% alcohol (w/w). This combination has a highly effective stool softener and a mild peristaltic stimulant that acts mainly in the lower bowel.

Action and Uses: Doxidan is a safe, gentle laxative for the relief and management of constipation. Due to the effectiveness of the stool softening component, Doxidan produces soft, formed, easily evacuated stools, with the least possible disturbance of normal body physiology. Doxidan has proved clinically effective in the management of constipation in geriatric or inactive patients, obstetric patients, and following surgery, particularly anorectal procedures. It may be used as a safe and effective evacuant prior to x-ray examination of the colon in preparing patients for barium enema.

Dosages: Adults and children over 12—one or two capsules daily. Children 6 to 12—one capsule daily. Give at bedtime for two or three days or until bowel movements are normal. For children under 6 consult a physician.

Warning: Do not use when abdominal pain, nausea, or vomiting is present. Frequent or prolonged use of this preparation may result in dependence on laxatives. A harmless pink or orange discoloration may appear in urine. In some patients occasional cramping may occur. If pregnant or nursing, consult your physician or pharmacist before taking this or any medicine.

How Supplied: Packs of 10; bottles of 30, 100 (NSN 6505-00-074-3169) and 1000 (NSN 6505-00-890-1247) maroon, soft-gelatin capsules, and Unit Dose 100's (10×10 strips) (NSN 6505-00-118-1700).

[*Shown in Product Identification Section*]

FESTAL®

Composition: Each enteric-coated tablet contains the following: Lipase 6,000 NF units, Amylase 30,000 NF units and Protease 20,000 NF units.

Action and Uses: Festal provides a high degree of protected digestive activity in a formula of standardized enzymes. Enteric coating of the tablet protects potency from inactivation in the stomach so that high enzymatic potency is delivered to the site in the intestinal tract where digestion normally takes place.

Festal is indicated in any condition where normal digestion is impaired by insufficiency of natural digestive enzymes, or when additional digestive enzymes may be beneficial. These conditions often manifest complaints of discomfort due to excess intestinal gas, such as bloating, cramps and flatulence. The following are conditions or situations where Festal may be helpful: pancreatic insufficiency, enteritis, postgastrectomy syndrome, chronic pancreatitis, pancreatic necrosis, chronic hepatitis, gallbladder disease, surgical patients following cholecystectomy, subtotal gastrectomy, pancreatectomy and other surgery of the upper gastrointestinal tract, removal of gas prior to x-ray examination; and in the healthy individual who may experience temporary digestive deficiency due to over-indulgence in excessively fatty meals.

Dosage: *Adults*—one or two tablets with each meal, or as directed by a physician.

Contraindications: None.

How Supplied: Bottles of 100 and 500 white, enteric-coated tablets for oral use.

Literature Available: Yes.

[*Shown in Product Identification Section*]

FESTALAN® ℞

Description: A tablet consisting of digestive enzymes in an enteric-coated core with atropine methyl nitrate in the outer coating. In the outer layer: Atropine Methyl Nitrate 1 mg. In the enteric coated core: Lipase 6,000 NF units, Amylase 30,000 NF units and Protease 20,000 NF units.

The enzymes Lipase, Amylase and Protease in Festalan® are obtained from porcine pancreas. Although allergic reactions to the animal protein in this preparation occur only rarely, these enzymes should be used cautiously in patients with known sensitivity.

Clinical Pharmacology: Pharmacologic and biochemical effects of Lipase, Amylase and Protease are limited to their actions upon the contents of the gastrointestinal tract. None of these enzymes are known to exert systemic pharmacologic effects after oral administration.

Atropine, atropine methyl nitrate and related belladonna alkaloids block the parasympathomimetic (muscarinic) effects of acetylcholine. These drugs are variously known as anticholinergic, parasympatholytic or antispasmodic agents. They act distally on parasympathetic nerve endings to inhibit the action of acetylcholine on smooth muscle, exocrine glands and the heart. Atropine does not block transmission at the neuromuscular junction of skeletal muscle. Atropine is readily absorbed from the gastrointestinal tract and crosses the blood-brain barrier. Most is excreted in the urine within the first 12 hours.

It reduces both motility and secretory activity of the gastrointestinal system. Atropine does not cause CNS depression at usual oral clinical doses, but may decrease heart rate slightly without changing blood pressure. Most of the pharmacologic effects reported with atropine and its analogs are attributable to its cholinergic blockade of parasympathetic effectors.

Indications and Usage: Festalan® is indicated for the treatment of functional gastrointestinal disorders involving disturbed motor function, hypermotility and spasticity as in patients with irritable colon syndrome. Atropine methyl nitrate reduces gastrointestinal tone and spasm. The enzyme content is helpful in reducing symptoms of postprandial intestinal distress in conditions involving digestive enzyme insufficiency.

Contraindications: Festalan® should not be used in patients with glaucoma, reflux esophagitis (gastric retention), prostate hypertrophy, pyloric obstruction, obstruction of the bladder neck, congestive heart failure with tachycardia and achalasia (cardiospasm). Festalan® should not be given to patients sensitive to protein of porcine origin or to atropine.

Warnings: Serious adverse reactions to atropine usually occur at higher doses and are extensions of known pharmacologic effects such as signs of CNS stimulation followed by depression, orthostatic hypotension and respiratory arrest. Children are more susceptible to the toxic effects than adults.

Precautions:

General: Festalan® should be used with caution in patients with cardiac disease. Patients using Festalan® should be warned of signs of atropine intoxication, particularly with doses exceeding the usual recommended dose. These may include dry mouth, difficulty with speech and swallowing and marked thirst. Vision may be blurred and skin may feel hot, dry and flushed. Usage of the drug should be discontinued and a physician consulted if any of the above symptoms appear.

This product contains FD & C Yellow No. 5 (tartrazine) which may cause allergic-type reactions (including bronchial asthma) in certain susceptible individuals. Although the overall incidence of FD & C Yellow No. 5 (tartrazine) sensitivity in the general population is low, it is frequently seen in patients who also have aspirin hypersensitivity.

Drug Interactions: Antacids may interfere with absorption of atropine and should not be given with this drug.

Continued on next page

Hoechst-Roussel—Cont.

Pregnancy: Pregnancy Category C. Animal reproduction studies have not been conducted with Festalan®. It is also not known whether Festalan® can cause fetal harm when administered to a pregnant woman or can effect reproduction capacity. Festalan® should be given to a pregnant woman only if clearly needed.

Atropine has negligible effects on the human uterus and the fetus is not adversely affected nor is respiration of the newborn depressed.*

Nursing Mothers: Traces of atropine are found in human milk. Caution should be observed when Festalan® is administered to a nursing woman.

Pediatric Use: The safety and effectiveness of Festalan® in children have not been established. See WARNINGS section.

Adverse Reactions: Adverse reactions associated with Festalan® may be of two main types: those due to allergic manifestations to pork proteins and those due to pharmacologic properties of atropine methyl nitrate. Allergic reactions occur only rarely and patients with known sensitivity should not be treated with Festalan®.

The most frequent adverse reactions seen after atropine are primarily due to the anticholinergic effects on various organs and systems. Dryness of the mouth, anhidrosis, mydriasis, cycloplegia, tachycardia (sometimes preceded by slowing), constipation, dysuria, and acute urinary retention may occur at clinical doses. At higher doses, marked dryness of the mouth, thirst, cardiac acceleration, blurring of vision, and speech difficulties may be encountered. Larger doses produce more marked development of symptoms, including CNS stimulation.

Overdosage: Symptoms of overdosage with atropine may comprise signs of CNS stimulation followed by depression, orthostatic hypotension and respiratory arrest. Children are more susceptible to the toxic effects than adults. Overdosage with atropine should be treated by gastric lavage to limit absorption. Physostigmine is an antidote for atropine poisoning and 1 to 4 mg (0.5 to 1.0 mg in children) may be given by slow intravenous injection to reduce or abolish delirium and coma caused by large doses of atropine. Phenothiazines should not be used for treatment of overdosage.

Dosage and Administration: Usual adult dose is one or two tablets with each meal. Pediatric dosage has not been established.

How Supplied: Festalan® is available in bottles of 100 and 1,000 orange, enteric coated tablets. Store at controlled room temperature—59° to 86°F.

Reference: *Goodman and Gilman, *The Pharmacological Basis of Therapeutics,* 1975, 5th Edition, p. 521.

[*Shown in Product Identification Section*]

LASIX® ℞
(furosemide)
Oral Solution
Tablets/Injection
Diuretic

> **WARNING: Lasix (furosemide) is a potent diuretic which, if given in excessive amounts, can lead to a profound diuresis with water and electrolyte depletion. Therefore, careful medical supervision is required, and dose and dose schedule have to be adjusted to the individual patient's needs. (See under "DOSAGE AND ADMINISTRATION.")**

Description: Lasix (furosemide) is an anthranilic acid derivative. Chemically, it is 4-chloro-N-furfuryl-5-sulfamoylanthranilic acid.

Actions: Investigations into the mode of action of Lasix (furosemide) have utilized micropuncture studies in rats, stop flow experiments in dogs, and various clearance studies in both humans and experimental animals.

It has been demonstrated that Lasix (furosemide) inhibits primarily the reabsorption of sodium and chloride not only in the proximal and distal tubules but also in the loop of Henle. The high degree of efficacy is largely due to this unique site of action. The action on the distal tubule is independent of any inhibitory effect on carbonic anhydrase and aldosterone.

The onset of diuresis following oral administration is within 1 hour. The peak effect occurs within the first or second hour. The duration of diuretic effect is 6 to 8 hours.

The onset of diuresis following intravenous administration is within 5 minutes and somewhat later after intramuscular administration. The peak effect occurs within the first half hour. The duration of diuretic effect is approximately 2 hours.

Indications:

Edema—Oral Lasix (furosemide) is indicated for the treatment of edema associated with congestive heart failure, cirrhosis of the liver, and renal disease, including the nephrotic syndrome. Lasix (furosemide) is particularly useful when an agent with greater diuretic potential than that of those commonly employed is desired.

Lasix (furosemide) is indicated as adjunctive therapy in acute pulmonary edema. The intravenous administration of Lasix (furosemide) is indicated when a rapid onset of diuresis is desired, eg, in acute pulmonary edema.

If gastrointestinal absorption is impaired or oral medication is not practical for any reason, Lasix (furosemide) is indicated by the intravenous or intramuscular route. Parenteral use should be replaced with oral Lasix (furosemide) as soon as practical.

Hypertension—Oral Lasix (furosemide) may be used for the treatment of hypertension alone or in combination with other antihypertensive agents. Hypertensive patients who cannot be adequately controlled with thiazides will probably also not be adequately controlled with Lasix (furosemide) alone.

Contraindications: Lasix (furosemide) is contraindicated in anuria. It is contraindicated in patients with a history of hypersensitivity to this compound.

Warnings: Excessive diuresis may result in dehydration and reduction in blood volume with circulatory collapse and with the possibility of vascular thrombosis and embolism, particularly in elderly patients. Excessive loss of potassium in patients receiving digitalis glycosides may precipitate digitalis toxicity. Care should also be exercised in patients receiving potassium-depleting steroids.

Frequent serum electrolyte, CO_2, and BUN determinations should be performed during the first few months of therapy and periodically thereafter, and abnormalities corrected or the drug temporarily withdrawn.

In patients with hepatic cirrhosis and ascites, initiation of therapy with Lasix (furosemide) is best carried out in the hospital. In hepatic coma and in states of electrolyte depletion, therapy should not be instituted until the basic condition is improved. Sudden alterations of fluid and electrolyte balance in patients with cirrhosis may precipitate hepatic coma; therefore, strict observation is necessary during the period of diuresis. Supplemental potassium chloride and, if required, an aldosterone antagonist are helpful in preventing hypokalemia and metabolic alkalosis.

If increasing azotemia and oliguria occur during treatment of severe progressive renal disease, the drug should be discontinued.

As with many other drugs, patients should be observed regularly for the possible occurrence of blood dyscrasias, liver damage, or other idiosyncratic reactions.

Patients with known sulfonamide sensitivity may show allergic reactions to Lasix (furosemide).

Lasix (furosemide) may add to or potentiate the therapeutic effect of other antihypertensive drugs. Potentiation occurs with ganglionic or peripheral adrenergic blocking drugs.

The possibility exists of exacerbation or activation of systemic lupus erythematosus.

Lasix (furosemide) appears in breast milk. If use of the drug is deemed essential, the patient should stop nursing.

Parenterally administered Lasix (furosemide) may increase the ototoxic potential of aminoglycoside antibiotics. Especially in the presence of impaired renal function, the use of parenterally administered Lasix (furosemide) in patients to whom aminoglycoside antibiotics are also being given should be avoided, except in life-threatening situations.

When parenteral use of Lasix (furosemide) precedes its oral use, it should be kept in mind that cases of tinnitus and reversible hearing impairment have been reported. There have also been some reports of cases in which irreversible hearing impairment occurred. Usually, ototoxicity has been reported when Lasix (furosemide) was injected rapidly in patients with severe impairment of renal function at doses exceeding several times the usual recommended dose and in whom other drugs known to be ototoxic were given. If the physician elects to use high dose parenteral therapy in patients with severely impaired renal function, controlled intravenous infusion is advisable [for adults, an infusion rate not exceeding 4 mg Lasix (furosemide) per minute has been used].

Because of the amount of sorbitol present in the vehicle for Lasix (furosemide) Oral Solution, the possibility of diarrhea, especially in the pediatric population, exists when the formulation is given at higher doses.

Precautions: As with any effective diuretic, electrolyte depletion may occur during therapy with Lasix (furosemide), especially in patients receiving higher doses and a restricted salt intake. Periodic determinations of serum electrolytes to detect possible imbalance should be performed at appropriate intervals.

All patients receiving Lasix (furosemide) therapy should be observed for signs of fluid or electrolyte imbalance, namely, hyponatremia, hypochloremic alkalosis, and hypokalemia. Serum and urine electrolyte determinations are particularly important when the patient is vomiting excessively or receiving parenteral fluids. Medications such as digitalis may also influence serum electrolytes. Warning signs, irrespective of cause, are: dryness of mouth, thirst, weakness, lethargy, drowsiness, restlessness, muscle pains or cramps, muscular fatigue, hypotension, oliguria, tachycardia, arrhythmia, and gastrointestinal disturbances such as nausea and vomiting.

Hypokalemia may develop with Lasix (furosemide) as with any other potent diuretic, especially with brisk diuresis, when cirrhosis is present, or during concomitant use of corticosteroids or ACTH.

Interference with adequate oral electrolyte intake will also contribute to hypokalemia. Digitalis therapy may exaggerate metabolic effects of hypokalemia, especially with reference to myocardial activity.

Asymptomatic hyperuricemia can occur and gout may rarely be precipitated.

Periodic checks on urine and blood glucose should be made in diabetics and even those suspected of latent diabetes when receiving Lasix (furosemide). Increases in blood glucose and alterations in glucose tolerance tests with abnormalities of the fasting and 2-hour postprandial sugar have been observed and rare cases of precipitation of diabetes mellitus have been reported.

Lasix (furosemide) may lower serum calcium levels and rare cases of tetany have been reported. Accordingly, periodic serum calcium levels should be obtained.

Reversible elevations of BUN may be seen. These have been observed in association with dehydration, which should be avoided, particularly in patients with renal insufficiency.

Patients receiving high doses of salicylates, as in rheumatic disease, in conjunction with Lasix (furosemide) may experience salicylate toxicity at lower doses because of competitive renal excretory sites.

Lasix (furosemide) has a tendency to antagonize the skeletal muscle relaxing effect of tubocurarine and may potentiate the action of succinylcholine.

Lithium generally should not be given with diuretics because they reduce its renal clearance and add a high risk of lithium toxicity.

It has been reported in the literature that diuretics such as furosemide may enhance the nephrotoxicity of cephaloridine. Therefore, Lasix (furosemide) and cephaloridine should not be administered simultaneously.

Lasix (furosemide) may decrease arterial responsiveness to norepinephrine. This diminution is not sufficient to preclude effectiveness of the pressor agent for therapeutic use.

It has been reported in the literature that coadministration of indomethacin may reduce the natriuretic and antihypertensive effects of Lasix (furosemide) in some patients. This effect has been attributed to inhibition of prostaglandin synthesis by indomethacin. Indomethacin may also affect plasma renin levels and aldosterone excretion; this should be borne in mind when a renin profile is evaluated in hypertensive patients. Patients receiving both indomethacin and Lasix (furosemide) should be observed closely to determine if the desired diuretic and/or antihypertensive effect of Lasix (furosemide) is achieved.

Lasix (furosemide) Oral Solution contains FD & C Yellow No. 5 (tartrazine) which may cause allergic-type reactions (including bronchial asthma) in certain susceptible individuals. Although the overall incidence of FD & C Yellow No. 5 (tartrazine) sensitivity in the general population is low, it is frequently seen in patients who also have aspirin sensitivity.

Pregnancy

Pregnancy Category C. Furosemide has been shown to cause unexplained maternal deaths and abortions in rabbits at 2, 4 and 8 times the human dose. There are no adequate and well-controlled studies in pregnant women. Furosemide should be used during pregnancy only if the potential benefit justifies the potential risk to the fetus.

The effects of furosemide on embryonic and fetal development and on pregnant dams were studied in mice, rats and rabbits.

Furosemide caused unexplained maternal deaths and abortions in the rabbit when 50 mg/kg (4 times the maximal recommended human dose of 600 mg per day) was administered between days 12 and 17 of gestation. In a previous study the lowest dose of only 25 mg/kg (2 times the maximal recommended human dose of 600 mg per day) caused maternal deaths and abortions. In a third study, none of the pregnant rabbits survived a dose of 100 mg/kg. Data from the above studies indicate fetal lethality that can precede maternal deaths.

The results of the mouse study and one of the three rabbit studies also showed an increased incidence of hydronephrosis (distention of the renal pelvis and, in some cases, of the ureters) in fetuses derived from treated dams as compared to the incidence in fetuses from the control group.

Adverse Reactions

Gastrointestinal System Reactions

1. anorexia
2. oral and gastric irritation
3. nausea
4. vomiting
5. cramping
6. diarrhea
7. constipation
8. jaundice (intrahepatic cholestatic jaundice)
9. pancreatitis

Central Nervous System Reactions

1. dizziness
2. vertigo
3. paresthesias
4. headache
5. xanthopsia
6. blurred vision
7. tinnitus and hearing loss

Hematologic Reactions

1. anemia
2. leukopenia
3. agranulocytosis (rare)
4. thrombocytopenia
5. aplastic anemia (rare)

Dermatologic—Hypersensitivity Reactions

1. purpura
2. photosensitivity
3. rash
4. urticaria
5. necrotizing angiitis (vasculitis, cutaneous vasculitis)
6. exfoliative dermatitis
7. erythema multiforme
8. pruritus

Cardiovascular Reaction

Orthostatic hypotension may occur and be aggravated by alcohol, barbiturates, or narcotics.

Other

1. hyperglycemia
2. glycosuria
3. hyperuricemia
4. muscle spasm
5. weakness
6. restlessness
7. urinary bladder spasm
8. thrombophlebitis
9. transient pain at the injection site following intramuscular injection

Whenever adverse reactions are moderate or severe, Lasix (furosemide) dosage should be reduced or therapy withdrawn.

Dosage and Administration:

Oral Administration

Edema—Therapy should be individualized according to patient response. This therapy should be titrated to gain maximal therapeutic response as well as the minimal dose possible to maintain that therapeutic response.

ADULTS—The usual initial daily dose of oral Lasix (furosemide) is 20 to 80 mg given as a single dose. Ordinarily a prompt diuresis ensues. Depending on the patient's response, a second dose can be administered 6 to 8 hours later.

If the diuretic response to a single dose of 20 to 80 mg is not satisfactory, increase this dose by increments of 20 or 40 mg not sooner than 6 to 8 hours after the previous dose until the desired diuretic effect has been obtained. This individually determined single dose should then be given once or twice daily (eg, at 8:00 a.m. and 2:00 p.m.). The dose of Lasix (furosemide) may be carefully titrated up to 600 mg/day in those patients with severe clinical edematous states.

The mobilization of edema may be most efficiently and safely accomplished by utilizing an intermittent dosage schedule in which the diuretic is given for 2 to 4 consecutive days each week.

When doses exceeding 80 mg/day are given for prolonged periods, careful clinical and laboratory observations are particularly advisable.

INFANTS AND CHILDREN—The usual initial dose of oral Lasix (furosemide) in infants and children is 2 mg/kg body weight, given as a single dose. If the diuretic response is not satisfactory after the initial dose, dose may be increased by 1 or 2 mg/kg no sooner than 6 to 8 hours after the previous dose. Doses greater than 6 mg/kg body weight are not recommended.

For maintenance therapy in infants and children, the dose should be adjusted to the minimum effective level.

Hypertension—Therapy should be individualized according to the patient's response. This therapy should be titrated to gain maximal therapeutic response as well as the minimal dose possible to maintain that therapeutic response.

ADULTS—The usual initial daily dose of Lasix (furosemide) for antihypertensive therapy is 80 mg, usually divided into 40 mg twice a day. Dosage should then be adjusted according to response. If the patient does not respond, add other antihypertensive agents.

Careful observations for changes in blood pressure must be made when this compound is used with other antihypertensive drugs, especially during initial therapy. The dosage of other agents must be reduced by at least 50 percent as soon as Lasix (furosemide) is added to the regimen, to prevent excessive drop in blood pressure. As the blood pressure falls under the potentiating effect of Lasix (furosemide), a further reduction in dosage or even discontinuation of other antihypertensive drugs may be necessary.

Parenteral Administration

ADULTS—Parenteral therapy should be reserved for patients for whom oral medication is not practical or in emergency situations where prompt diuresis is desired. Parenteral therapy should be replaced by oral therapy as soon as this is practical for continued mobilization of edema.

Edema—The usual initial dose of Lasix (furosemide) is 20 to 40 mg given as a single dose, injected intramuscularly or intravenously. The intravenous injection should be given slowly (1 to 2 minutes). Ordinarily, a prompt diuresis ensues. Depending on the patient's response, a second dose can be administered 2 hours after the first dose or later.

If the diuretic response with a single dose of 20 to 40 mg is not satisfactory, increase this dose by increments of 20 mg not sooner than 2 hours after the previous dose until the desired diuretic effect has been obtained. This individually determined single dose should then be given once or twice daily.

If the physician elects to use high dose parenteral therapy it should be administered as a controlled infusion at a rate not exceeding 4 mg/min. Lasix (furosemide) Injection is a mildly buffered alkaline solution which should not be mixed with acidic solutions of pH below 5.5. To prepare infusion solutions, isotonic saline and lactated Ringer's injection and 5% dextrose injection have been used after pH has been adjusted when necessary.

Therapy should be individualized according to patient response. This therapy should be titrated to gain maximal therapeutic response as well as the minimal dose possible to maintain that therapeutic response. Close medical supervision is necessary.

Acute Pulmonary Edema—The usual initial dose of Lasix (furosemide) is 40 mg injected intravenously. The injection should be given slowly (1 to 2 minutes). If 40 mg Lasix (furosemide) does not produce a satisfactory response within 1 hour the dose may be increased to 80 mg given intravenously (over 1 to 2 minutes). If deemed necessary, additional therapy (eg, digitalis, oxygen) can be administered concomitantly.

INFANTS AND CHILDREN—Parenteral therapy should be reserved for patients for whom oral medication is not practical or in emergency situations where prompt diuresis is desired. Parenteral therapy should be replaced by oral therapy as soon as this is practical for continued mobilization of edema.

The usual initial dose of Lasix (furosemide) Injection (intravenously or intramuscularly) in infants and children is 1 mg/kg body weight and should be given slowly under close medical supervision. If the diuretic response after the initial dose is not satisfactory, dosage may be increased by 1 mg/kg not sooner than 2 hours after the previous dose, until the desired diuretic effect has been obtained. Doses greater than 6 mg/kg body weight are not recommended.

How Supplied: Lasix (furosemide) Tablets are supplied as white, round, monogrammed,

Continued on next page

Hoechst-Roussel—Cont.

scored tablets of 40 mg in amber bottles of 100 (NSN 6505-00-062-3336), 500 (NSN 6505-00-254-5546; 5546A), and 1,000 (NSN 6505-01-095-3600A); unit dose 100s (20 strips of 5) (NSN 6505-00-117-5982; 5982A); and Unit of Use trays of 12 × 100, 25 × 30 (NSN 6505-01-105-7485A) and 25 × 60 (NSN 6505-01-105-7484A); white, oval, monogrammed tablets of 20 mg in amber bottles of 100, 500 and 1000, and unit dose 100s (10 strips of 10); and white, round, monogrammed, facetted-edge tablets of 80 mg in amber bottles of 50 (NSN 6505-01-086-1994A) and 500, and unit dose 100s (20 strips of 5).

Note: **Dispense in well-closed, light-resistant containers. Exposure to light may cause slight discoloration. Discolored tablets should not be dispensed.**

Lasix (furosemide) Oral Solution is supplied as an orange-flavored liquid containing furosemide 10 mg/mL in bottles of 60 mL (accompanied by graduated dropper) and bottles of 120 mL (accompanied by graduated dispensing spoon).

Note: **Store in a cold place (refrigerator, 36–46°F). Dispense in light-resistant containers. Protect from freezing.**

Lasix (furosemide) Injection is supplied as a sterile solution in 2 mL amber ampuls, boxes of 5 (NSN 6505-00-435-0377) and 50 (NSN 6505-00-933-8704A); 4 mL amber ampuls, boxes of 5 and 25; 10 mL amber ampuls, boxes of 5 (NSN 6505-00-148-9814) and 25 (NSN 6505-00-516-0515A); 2 mL prefilled syringes, boxes of 5; 4 mL prefilled syringes, boxes of 5 (NSN 6505-01-083-7833); and 10 mL prefilled syringes, boxes of 5. Each mL contains 10 mg furosemide. Syringes supplied with 22 gauge × 1¼″ needle.

Note: **Store at controlled room temperature. (59°–86°F). Do not use if solution is discolored. Protect syringes from light. Do not remove syringes from individual package until time of use.**

[*Shown in Product Identification Section*]

STREPTASE® ℞
(streptokinase)

Description: Streptase® (streptokinase) is a sterile, purified preparation of a bacterial protein elaborated by group C β-hemolytic streptococci. It is supplied as a lyophilized white powder containing 25 mg cross-linked gelatin polypeptides, 25 mg sodium L-glutamate and 100 mg Normal Serum Albumin (Human) as stabilizers for intravenous and intracoronary administration.

Clinical Pharmacology: Streptase® (streptokinase) acts with plasminogen to produce an "activator complex" that converts plasminogen to the proteolytic enzyme plasmin. Plasmin degrades fibrin clots as well as fibrinogen and other plasma proteins (1). Intravenous infusion of streptokinase is followed by increased fibrinolytic activity. This hyperfibrinolytic effect disappears within a few hours after discontinuation, but a prolonged thrombin time, especially with prolonged administration, may persist for up to 24 hours due to a decrease in plasma levels of fibrinogen and an increase in the amount of circulating fibrin(ogen) degradation products (FDP). The thrombin time will usually decrease to less than two times normal control value within 4 hours.

Indications and Usage: STREPTASE® (STREPTOKINASE) IS INDICATED FOR THE LYSIS OF THROMBI IN SEVERAL CONDITIONS. THE ROUTE (METHOD) OF ADMINISTRATION, DURATION, AND DOSAGE VARY WITH EACH CONDITION (SEE DOSAGE AND ADMINISTRATION).

Pulmonary Embolism

With Streptase® (streptokinase) therapy, angiographic, lung scan and/or hemodynamic improvement is more rapid and complete than with heparin therapy (2-4).

Streptase® (streptokinase) is indicated in adults for:

- the lysis of acute pulmonary emboli, involving obstruction of blood flow to a lobe or multiple segments (5), or
- the lysis of pulmonary emboli accompanied by unstable hemodynamics, i.e., failure to maintain blood pressure without supportive measures.

The diagnosis should be confirmed by objective means, such as pulmonary angiography via an upper extremity vein, or noninvasive procedures such as lung scanning.

Deep Vein Thrombosis

Streptase® (streptokinase) is indicated in adults for lysis of acute, extensive thrombi of the deep veins, such as those involving the popliteal and more proximal vessels. Diagnosis should be confirmed by objective means, preferably ascending venography. Studies have demonstrated better salvage of valvular function and prevention of postphlebitic syndrome by streptokinase plus heparin than by heparin alone (6-8).

Arterial Thrombosis and Embolism

Streptase® (streptokinase) is indicated in adults for the lysis of acute arterial thrombi and for the lysis of arterial emboli (9-11). However, the use of Streptase® (streptokinase) in arterial emboli originating from the left side of the heart (e.g., in mitral stenosis accompanied by atrial fibrillation) should be avoided due to the danger of new embolic phenomena, including those to cerebral vessels.

Arteriovenous Cannulae Occlusion

Streptase® (streptokinase) is indicated for clearing of totally or partially occluded arteriovenous cannulae as an alternative to surgical revision when acceptable flow cannot otherwise be achieved (12).

Coronary Artery Thrombosis

Streptase® (streptokinase) has been reported to lyse acute thrombi obstructing coronary arteries, associated with evolving transmural myocardial infarction. Diagnosis of acute myocardial infarction has been confirmed, and the site of coronary thrombosis identified by selective coronary angiography (13,14). Other studies (15-21) have demonstrated that (a) a thrombus is present in approximately 90% of patients evaluated within four hours of onset of symptoms; (b) when compared to concurrent or historical controls, the majority of patients who received intracoronary streptokinase within 6 hours of onset of symptoms, showed a more immediate recanalization (within a few minutes vs hours/days) of the involved vessel.

IT HAS NOT BEEN ESTABLISHED THAT INTRACORONARY ADMINISTRATION OF STREPTOKINASE DURING EVOLVING TRANSMURAL MYOCARDIAL INFARCTION RESULTS IN SALVAGE OF MYOCARDIAL TISSUE, NOR THAT IT REDUCES MORTALITY. CONTROLLED STUDIES ADDRESSING THESE PARAMETERS ARE IN PROGRESS (22) AND UNTIL COMPLETED, THOSE PATIENTS WHO MIGHT BENEFIT FROM THIS THERAPY CANNOT BE DEFINED.

Contraindications: Because thrombolytic therapy increases the risk of bleeding, Streptase® (streptokinase) is contraindicated in the following situations:

- active internal bleeding
- recent (within 2 months) cerebrovascular accident, intracranial or intraspinal surgery (see **Warnings**)
- intracranial neoplasm

Warnings:

Bleeding

The aim of Streptase® (streptokinase) therapy is the production of sufficient amounts of plasmin for the lysis of intravascular deposits of fibrin; however, fibrin deposits which provide hemostasis, for example, at sites of needle punctures, are also lysed and bleeding from such sites may occur.

Intramuscular injections and nonessential handling of the patient must be avoided during treatment with Streptase® (streptokinase). Venipunctures should be performed carefully and as infrequently as possible.

Should an arterial puncture be necessary during intravenous therapy, upper extremity vessels are preferable. Pressure should be applied for at least 30 minutes, a pressure dressing applied and the puncture site checked frequently for evidence of bleeding.

When internal bleeding occurs, it may be more difficult to manage than that which occurs with conventional anticoagulant therapy.

In the following conditions the risks of therapy may be increased and should be weighed against the anticipated benefits.

- Recent (within 10 days) major surgery, obstetrical delivery, organ biopsy, previous puncture of noncompressible vessels
- Recent serious gastrointestinal bleeding (within 10 days)
- Recent trauma including cardiopulmonary resuscitation
- Severe, uncontrolled arterial hypertension
- High likelihood of left heart thrombus, e.g., mitral stenosis with atrial fibrillation
- Subacute bacterial endocarditis
- Hemostatic defects including those secondary to severe hepatic or renal disease
- Pregnancy
- Cerebrovascular disease
- Diabetic hemorrhagic retinopathy
- Prior severe allergic reaction to streptokinase
- Septic thrombophlebitis or occluded AV cannula at seriously infected site
- Any other condition in which bleeding constitutes a significant hazard or would be particularly difficult to manage because of its location.

Should serious spontaneous bleeding (not controllable by local pressure) occur, the infusion of Streptase® (streptokinase) should be terminated immediately and treatment instituted as described under **Adverse Reactions.**

Use of Anticoagulants

Concurrent use of anticoagulants with intravenous administration of Streptase® (streptokinase) is not recommended. However, concurrent use of heparin may be required during intracoronary administration of Streptase® (streptokinase). Clinical studies with concurrent use of heparin and lower Streptase® (streptokinase) dosages employed during intracoronary administration have demonstrated no tendency toward increased bleeding that would not be attributable to the procedure or Streptase® (streptokinase) alone. Nevertheless, careful monitoring for excessive bleeding is advised.

Arrhythmias

Rapid lysis of coronary thrombi has been reported occasionally to cause reperfusion atrial or ventricular dysrhythmias requiring immediate treatment. During studies, careful monitoring for arrhythmia was maintained during and immediately following intracoronary administration of Streptase® (streptokinase).

Precautions:

Use in Pregnancy and Children

Safety and effectiveness of Streptase® (streptokinase) therapy in children and during pregnancy has not been established. Therefore, treatment of such patients is not recommended.

Drug Interactions

The interaction of Streptase® (streptokinase) with other drugs has not been studied. Drugs that alter platelet function should not be used during therapy. Common examples are: aspirin, indomethacin, and phenylbutazone (6).

Patient Monitoring

Before commencing thrombolytic therapy, it is desirable to obtain a thrombin time (TT), activated partial thromboplastin time (APTT), prothrombin time (PT), hematocrit and platelet count to obtain hemostatic status of the patient.

Intracoronary Artery Infusion

During studies, laboratory monitoring of hemostatic parameters during intracoronary artery infusion showed minimal changes, if any. Heparin was continued during therapy or instituted following therapy and monitored accordingly.

Intravenous Infusion

If heparin has been given, it should be discontinued and the TT or APTT should be less than twice the normal control value before thrombolytic therapy is started.

During the infusion, decreases in the plasminogen and fibrinogen level and an increase in the level of FDP (the latter two serving to prolong the clotting times of coagulation tests) will generally confirm the existence of a lytic state. Therefore, therapy can be monitored by performing the TT or PT, approximately 4 hours after initiation of therapy.

Following the infusion, **before (re)instituting heparin**, the TT should be less than twice the normal control value.

Adverse Reactions: The following adverse reactions have been frequently associated with intravenous therapy but may also occur with intracoronary artery infusion:

Bleeding

Minor bleeding occurs often with thrombolytic therapy mainly at invaded or disturbed sites. When lytic therapy is continued while local measures are used to control minor bleeding, do **not** reduce the dose as this will increase lytic activity since more plasminogen will be available for conversion to plasmin. Severe internal bleeding involving gastrointestinal, genitourinary, retroperitoneal or intracerebral sites, may occur. Several fatalities due to cerebral and other serious internal hemorrhage have occurred during intravenous thrombolytic therapy.

Should uncontrollable bleeding occur, Streptase® (streptokinase) infusion should be discontinued and, if necessary, blood loss and reversal of the bleeding tendency can be effectively managed with whole blood (fresh blood preferable), packed red blood cells and cryoprecipitate or fresh frozen plasma. Although the use of aminocaproic acid (ACA, AMICAR®) in humans as an antidote for streptokinase has not been documented, it may be considered in an emergency situation.

Allergic Reactions

Reactions attributed to possible anaphylaxis have been observed rarely in patients treated with Streptase® (streptokinase) intravenously. These ranged in severity from minor breathing difficulty to bronchospasm, periorbital swelling or angioneurotic edema. Other milder allergic effects such as urticaria, itching, flushing, nausea, headache and musculoskeletal pain have also been observed.

Mild or moderate reactions may be managed with concomitant antihistamine and/or corticosteroid therapy. Severe allergic reactions require immediate discontinuation of Streptase® (streptokinase), with adrenergics, antihistamines, or corticosteroids administered intravenously as required.

Fever

Although Streptase® (streptokinase) is nonpyrogenic in standard animal tests, approximately one-third of patients treated with Streptase® (streptokinase) intravenously have shown increases in body temperature of ≥ 1.5°F. Symptomatic treatment is usually sufficient to alleviate discomfort. The use of acetaminophen rather than aspirin is recommended.

Dosage and Administration:

A. Lysis of Coronary Artery Thrombi (15-20)

During clinical studies, Streptase® (streptokinase) was administered selectively into the thrombosed coronary artery via coronary catheter placed by the Judkins or Sones Technique. When administered within 6 hours of onset of symptoms of acute transmural myocardial infarction, at a bolus dose averaging 20,000 IU and a maintenance dose averaging 2,000 IU/min for 60 minutes, greater than 75% of occlusions were opened in less than 1 hour.

B. Treatment of Deep Vein Thrombosis, Pulmonary or Arterial Embolism or Arterial Thrombosis (23,24)

Streptokinase treatment should be instituted as soon as possible after onset of thrombotic event, preferably no later than seven days after onset. Any delay in instituting lytic therapy to evaluate the effect of heparin therapy decreases the potential for optimal efficacy (25). Reconstituted streptokinase solution may alter drop size which will influence the accuracy of drop counting infusion devices, either manually or instrument controlled. Use of volumetric or syringe infusion pumps is recommended.

Loading Dose

Since human exposure to streptococci is common, antibodies to streptokinase (streptokinase resistance) are found normally. Thus, a loading dose of Streptase® (streptokinase) sufficient to neutralize the resistance is required. A dose of 250,000 IU Streptase® (streptokinase) infused into a peripheral vein over 30 minutes has been found appropriate in over 90% of patients.

Maintenance Dose*

A maintenance dose infusion of 100,000 IU/hr is given following the loading dose. Administer this maintenance dose for 24 hours for the treatment of pulmonary embolism (up to 72 hours if concurrent deep vein thrombosis is suspected), 24-72 hours for the treatment of arterial thrombosis and arterial embolism, and 72 hours for the treatment of deep vein thrombosis.

If the thrombin time or any other parameter of lysis after 4 hours of therapy is less than approximately 1½ times the normal control value, discontinue Streptase® (streptokinase) as excessive resistance to streptokinase is present.

*A variable dosage of Streptase® (streptokinase) and frequent laboratory monitoring were recommended in the past (26). However, since experience shows that these do not increase the efficacy or safety of Streptase® (streptokinase) therapy, they are no longer recommended.

Anticoagulation after Terminating Intravenous Streptokinase Treatment

At the end of Streptase® (streptokinase) therapy, treatment with heparin by continuous intravenous infusion is recommended to prevent recurrent thrombosis (3). Heparin treatment (without a loading dose) should not begin until the thrombin time has decreased to **less than twice** the normal control value (approximately 3 to 4 hours). (See manufacturer's prescribing information for proper use of heparin.) This should be followed by oral anticoagulation in the conventional manner.

C. Treatment of Arteriovenous Cannula Occlusion:

1. Before Treatment:
   Before using Streptase® (streptokinase), an attempt should be made to clear the cannula by careful syringe technique, using heparinized saline solution. If adequate flow is not reestablished, Streptase® (streptokinase) may be employed. Allow the effect of any pretreatment anticoagulants to diminish.
2. Streptase® (streptokinase) Administration:
   Instill 250,000 IU Streptase® (streptokinase) in 2 mL intravenous solution into each occluded limb of the cannula slowly. Clamp off cannula limb(s) for 2 hours. Observe the patient closely for possible adverse effects.
3. After Treatment:
   Aspirate contents of infused cannula limb(s), flush with saline, reconnect cannula.

Reconstitution and Dilution:

For Intracoronary Artery and Intravenous Administration

Slight flocculation (described as thin translucent fibers) of reconstituted Streptase® (streptokinase) occurred occasionally during clinical trials but did not interfere with safe use of the solution. Do not add any other medication to the container of Streptase® (streptokinase).

The following reconstitution and dilution procedure will minimize flocculation:

1. Slowly add 5 mL Sodium Chloride Injection, USP or Dextrose (5%) Injection, USP, directing it at the side of the vacuum packed vial rather than into the Streptase® (streptokinase).
2. Roll and tilt the vial gently to reconstitute. **Avoid shaking.** (Shaking may cause foaming and/or increase flocculation.)
3. Further dilute the entire reconstituted contents of the vial slowly and carefully to a total volume as recommended in Table 1. Avoid shaking and agitation on dilution. (If necessary, total volume may be increased to a maximum of 500 mL with the infusion pump rate in Table 1 increased accordingly. To facilitate setting the infusion pump rate, a total volume of 45 mL, or multiple thereof, is recommended.)
4. The solution may be filtered through a 0.22 μm or a 0.45 μm filter.
5. Solutions containing **large amounts** of flocculation should be discarded.
6. If not used soon after reconstitution, store Streptase® (streptokinase) at 2-4°C. Discard reconstituted drug if not administered within 24 hours.

[See table on next page].

For Use in Arteriovenous Cannulae

Slowly reconstitute the contents of 250,000 IU Streptase® (streptokinase) vacuum packed vial with 2 mL Sodium Chloride Injection, USP or Dextrose (5%) Injection, USP.

How Supplied: Streptase® (streptokinase) is supplied as a lyophilized white powder in 6.5 mL vials (in packages of 10) with color-coded labels corresponding to the amount of purified Streptase® (streptokinase) in each vial as follows:

green-250,000 IU blue-750,000 IU

Store unopened vials at controlled room temperature (15-30°C).

References:

1. McNicol, G.P.: The fibrinolytic system. Postgrad Med J 49 (Suppl): 10-2, 1973.
2. Brogden, R.N., Speight, T.M., Avery, G.S.: Streptokinase: A review of its clinical pharmacology, mechanism of action and therapeutic uses. Drugs 5:357-445, 1973.
3. Fratantoni, J.C., Ness, P., Simon, T.L.: Thrombolytic therapy: Current status. N Engl J Med 293:1073-8, 1975.
4. Urokinase Pulmonary Embolism Study Group: Urokinase-streptokinase embolism trial. JAMA 229:1606-13, 1974.
5. Sharma, G.V.R.K., Burleson, V.A. Sasahara, A.A.: Effect of thrombolytic therapy on pulmonary-capillary blood volume in patients with pulmonary embolism. N Engl J Med 303:842-5. 1980.
6. Common, H.H., Seaman, A.J., Rosch, J., et al: Deep vein thrombosis treated with streptokinase or heparin. Follow-up of a randomized study. Angiology 27:645-54, 1976.
7. Marder, V.J., Soulen, R.L., Atichartakarn, V., et al: Quantitative venographic assessment of deep vein thrombosis in the evaluation of streptokinase and heparin therapy. J Lab Clin Med 89:1018-29, 1977.

Continued on next page

Hoechst-Roussel—Cont.

8. Johansson, L., Nylander, G., Hedner, U., et al: Comparison of streptokinase with heparin: Late results in the treatment of deep venous thrombosis. Acta Med Scand 206:93-8, 1979.
9. Dotter, C.T., Rosch, J., Seaman, A.J., et al: Streptokinase treatment of thromboembolic disease. Radiology 102:283-90, 1972.
10. Persson, A.V., Thompson, J.E., Patman, R.D.: Acute arterial occlusions. Vasc Surg 11:359-63, 1977.
11. Reichle, F.A., Rao, N.A., Chang, K.H., et al: Thrombolysis of acute or subacute nonembolic arterial thrombosis. J Surg Res 22:202-208, 1977.
12. Data on File for Arteriovenous Cannulae Occlusion. Hoechst-Roussel Pharmaceuticals Inc.
13. Mathey, D.G., Kuck, K.H., Tilsner, V., et al: Nonsurgical coronary artery recanalization in acute transmural myocardial infarction. Circulation 63: 489-97, 1981.
14. Rentrop, P., Blanke H., Karsch, K.R., et al: Selective intracoronary thrombolysis in acute myocardial infarction and unstable angina pectoris. Circulation 63: 307-17, 1981.
15. Cowley, M.J., Hastillo, A., Vetrovec, G.W., et al: Effects of intracoronary streptokinase in acute myocardial infarction. Am Heart J 102:1149-1158, 1981.
16. Mathey, D.G., Rodewald, G., Rentrop, P., et al: Intracoronary streptokinase thrombolytic recanalization and subsequent surgical bypass of remaining atherosclerotic stenosis in acute myocardial infarction: Complimentary combined approach effecting reduced infarct size, preventing reinfarction, and improving left ventricular function. Am Heart J 102:1194-1201, 1981.
17. Merx, W., Doerr, R., Rentrop, P., et al: Evaluation of the effectiveness of intracoronary streptokinase infusion in acute myocardial infarction: Postprocedure management and hospital course in 204 patients. Am Heart J 102:1181-1187, 1981.
18. Reduto, L.A., Freund, G.C., Gaeta, J.M., et al: Coronary artery reperfusion in acute myocardial infarction: Beneficial effects of intracoronary streptokinase on left ventricular salvage and performance. Am Heart J 102:1168-1177, 1981.
19. Rentrop, K.P., Karsch, K.R., Blanke H., et al: Changes in left ventricular function after intracoronary streptokinase infusion in clinically evolving myocardial infarction. Am Heart J 102:1188-1193, 1981.
20. Rutsch, W., Schartl, M., Mathey, D., et al: Percutaneous transluminal coronary recanalization: Procedure, results and acute complications. Am Heart J 102:1178-1180, 1981.
21. De Wood, M.A.; Spores J; Notske R; et al: Prevalence of total coronary occlusion during the early hours of transmural myocardial infarction. New Eng J. Med 303:897-902, 1980.
22. Workshop on Limitations of Infarct Size with Thrombolytic Agents. NIH, Bethesda, Maryland, 1981.
23. Marder, V.J.: The use of thrombolytic agents: Choice of patient, drug administration, laboratory monitoring. Ann Intern Med 90:802-8, 1979.
24. Bell, W.R., Meek, A.G.: Guidelines for the use of thrombolytic agents. N Eng J Med 301:1266-70, 1979.
25. Sherry, S., Bell, W.R., Duckert, F.H., et al: Thrombolytic Therapy in Thrombosis: A National Institutes of Health Consensus Development Conference. Ann Intern Med 93:141-4, 1980.
26. Porter, J.M., Seaman, A.J., Common, H.H., et al: Comparison of heparin and streptokinase in the treatment of venous thrombosis. Am Surg 40:511-19, 1975.

TABLE I
Suggested Dilutions and Infusion Rates

Streptase® (streptokinase) Dosage/Infusion Rate	Streptase® (streptokinase) Vial Content Needed	Total Volume of Solution (mL)	Infusion Pump Rate
I. Intracoronary Artery Administration			
A. Bolus Injection 20,000 IU	1 vial, 250,000 IU*	125	Inject 10 mL
B. Maintenance Dose 2,000 IU/min			60 mL per hour
*sufficient for Bolus Injection and Maintenance Dose			
II. Intravenous Administration			
A. Loading Dose 250,000 IU/30 min	a) 1 vial, 250,000 IU	45	90 mL per hour for 30 min
	or		
	b) 1 vial, 750,000 IU	45	30 mL per hour for 30 min
B. Maintenance Dose 100,000 IU/hr	1 vial, 750,000 IU	45**	6 mL per hour

** If necessary, total volume may be increased, in increments of 45 mL, to a maximum of 500 mL with the infusion pump rate increased accordingly. The total volume of 45 mL or multiple thereof is recommended.

SURFAK®
(docusate calcium USP)

Composition: Surfak is the stool softening agent, docusate calcium USP. Each 240 mg capsule contains 240 mg docusate calcium USP and up to 3% alcohol (w/w). Each 50 mg capsule contains 50 mg docusate calcium USP and up to 1.3% alcohol (w/w).
Action and Uses: Surfak is useful in patients where prevention of hard stools is essential to treatment, or in those conditions where laxative therapy is undesirable or contraindicated. Surfak is indicated for patients who require only fecal softening without propulsive action to accomplish defecation, such as obstetric, geriatric, surgical, and cardiac patients, those with anorectal conditions and after proctologic surgery. Surfak provides homogenization and formation of soft, easily evacuated stools without disturbance of body physiology, discomfort of bowel distention, oily leakage or interference with vitamin absorption.
Dosages: Adults—one red 240 mg capsule daily for several days or until bowel movements are normal. Children and adults with minimal needs—one to three orange 50 mg capsules daily. For use in children under 6, consult a physician.
Adverse Reactions: Surfak is non-habit forming. It has no known side effects or disadvantages, except for the unusual occurrence of mild, transitory cramping pains. Overdosage does not lead to systemic toxicity.
Caution: If cramping pain occurs, discontinue the medication. If pregnant or nursing, consult your physician or pharmacist before taking this or any medicine.
Contraindications: None.
How Supplied: 240 mg red, soft gelatin capsules—bottles of 30 (NSN 6505-00-117-8607), 100 (NSN 6505-00-926-8844), 500 (NSN 6505-00-148-9815) and Unit Dose 100's (10 x 10 strips) (NSN 6505-00-118-1449), 50 mg orange, soft gelatin capsules—bottles of 30 and 100.
Literature Available: Yes.
[*Shown in Product Identification Section*]

TOPICORT® ℞
(desoximetasone)
EMOLLIENT CREAM 0.25%

TOPICORT® LP
(desoximetasone)
EMOLLIENT CREAM 0.05%

Description: Topicort® (desoximetasone) Emollient Cream 0.25% and Topicort® LP (desoximetasone) Emollient Cream 0.05% contain the active synthetic corticosteroid desoximetasone. The topical corticosteroids constitute a class of primarily synthetic steroids used as anti-inflammatory and anti-pruritic agents.
Each gram of Topicort® (desoximetasone) Emollient Cream 0.25% contains 2.5 mg of desoximetasone in an emollient cream consisting of isopropyl myristate, cetylstearyl alcohol, white petrolatum, mineral oil, lanolin alcohol and purified water.
Each gram of Topicort® LP (desoximetasone) Emollient Cream 0.05% contains 0.5 mg of desoximetasone in an emollient cream consisting of isopropyl myristate, cetylstearyl alcohol, white petrolatum, mineral oil, lanolin alcohol, edetate disodium, lactic acid and purified water.
The chemical name of desoximetasone is Pregna-1, 4-diene-3, 20-dione, 9-fluoro-11, 21-dihydroxy-16-methyl-, (11β,16α)-.
Desoximetasone has the empirical formula $C_{22}H_{29}FO_4$ and a molecular weight of 376.47. The CAS Registry Number is 382-67-2.
Clinical Pharmacology: Topical corticosteroids share anti-inflammatory, anti-pruritic and vasoconstrictive actions.
The mechanism of anti-inflammatory activity of the topical corticosteroids is unclear. Various laboratory methods, including vasoconstrictor assays, are used to compare and predict potencies and/or clinical efficacies of the topical corticosteroids. There is some evidence to suggest that a recognizable correlation exists between vasoconstrictor potency and therapeutic efficacy in man.

Pharmacokinetics
The extent of percutaneous absorption of topical corticosteroids is determined by many factors including the vehicle, the integrity of the epidermal barrier, and the use of occlusive dressings.
Topical corticosteroids can be absorbed from normal intact skin. Inflammation and/or other disease processes in the skin increase percutaneous absorption. Occlusive dressings substantially increase the percutaneous absorption of topical corticosteroids. Thus, occlusive dressings may be a valuable therapeutic adjunct for treatment of resistant dermatoses.
Once absorbed through the skin, topical corticosteroids are handled through pharmacokinetic pathways similar to systemically administered corticosteroids. Corticosteroids are bound to plasma proteins in varying degrees. Corticosteroids are metabolized primarily in the liver and are then excreted by the kidneys. Some of the topical corticosteroids and their metabolites are also excreted into the bile.
Pharmacokinetic studies in men with Topicort® (desoximetasone) Emollient Cream 0.25% with tagged desoximetasone showed a total of 5.2% ± 2.9% excretion in urine (4.1% ± 2.3%) and feces (1.1% ± 0.6%) and no detectable level (limit of sensitivity: 0.005 µg/mL) in the blood when it was applied topi-

cally on the back followed by occlusion for 24 hours. Seven days after application, no further radioactivity was detected in urine or feces. The half-life of the material was 15 ± 2 hours (for urine) and 17 ± 2 hours (for feces) between the third and fifth trial day. Studies with other similarly structured steroids have shown that predominant metabolite reaction occurs through conjugation to form the glucuronide and sulfate ester.

Indications and Usage: Topicort® (desoximetasone) Emollient Cream 0.25% and Topicort® LP (desoximetasone) Emollient Cream 0.05% are indicated for the relief of the inflammatory and pruritic manifestations of corticosteroid-responsive dermatoses.

Contraindications: Topical corticosteroids are contraindicated in those patients with a history of hypersensitivity to any of the components of the preparation.

Precautions:

General

Systemic absorption of topical corticosteroids has produced reversible hypothalamic-pituitary-adrenal (HPA) axis suppression, manifestations of Cushing's syndrome, hyperglycemia, and glucosuria in some patients.

Conditions which augment systemic absorption include the application of the more potent steroids, use over large surface areas, prolonged use, and the addition of occlusive dressings.

Therefore, patients receiving a large dose of a potent topical steroid applied to a large surface area or under an occlusive dressing should be evaluated periodically for evidence of HPA axis suppression by using the urinary free cortisol and ACTH stimulation tests. If HPA axis suppression is noted, an attempt should be made to withdraw the drug, to reduce the frequency of application, or to substitute a less potent steroid.

Recovery of HPA axis function is generally prompt and complete upon discontinuation of the drug. Infrequently, signs and symptoms of steroid withdrawal may occur, requiring supplemental systemic corticosteroids.

Children may absorb proportionally larger amounts of topical corticosteroids and thus be more susceptible to systemic toxicity (See **Precautions—Pediatric Use**)

If irritation develops, topical corticosteroids should be discontinued and appropriate therapy instituted.

In the presence of dermatological infections, the use of an appropriate antifungal or antibacterial agent should be instituted. If a favorable response does not occur promptly, the corticosteroid should be discontinued until the infection has been adequately controlled.

Information for the Patient

Patients using topical corticosteroids should receive the following information and instructions:

1. This medication is to be used as directed by the physician. It is for external use only. Avoid contact with the eyes.
2. Patients should be advised not to use this medication for any disorder other than for which it was prescribed.
3. The treated skin area should not be bandaged or otherwise covered or wrapped as to be occlusive unless directed by the physician.
4. Patients should report any signs of local adverse reactions especially under occlusive dressing.
5. Parents of pediatric patients should be advised not to use tight-fitting diapers or plastic pants on a child being treated in the diaper area, as these garments may constitute occlusive dressings.

Laboratory Tests

The following tests may be helpful in evaluating the HPA axis suppression:

Urinary free cortisol test
ACTH stimulation test

Carcinogenesis, Mutagenesis, and Impairment of Fertility

Long-term animal studies have not been performed to evaluate the carcinogenic potential or the effect on fertility of topical corticosteroids.

Studies to determine mutagenicity with prednisolone and hydrocortisone have revealed negative results.

Pregnancy Category C

Corticosteroids are generally teratogenic in laboratory animals when administered systemically at relatively low dosage levels. The more potent corticosteroids have been shown to be teratogenic after dermal application in laboratory animals.

Desoximetasone has been shown to be teratogenic and embryotoxic in mice, rats, and rabbits when given by subcutaneous or dermal routes of administration in doses 3 to 30 times the human dose of Topicort® (desoximetasone) Emollient Cream 0.25% or 15 to 150 times the human dose of Topicort® LP (desoximetasone) Emollient Cream 0.05%.

There are no adequate and well-controlled studies in pregnant women on teratogenic effects from topically applied corticosteroids. Therefore, Topicort® (desoximetasone) Emollient Cream 0.25% and Topicort® LP (desoximetasone) Emollient Cream 0.05% should be used during pregnancy only if the potential benefit justifies the potential risk to the fetus. Drugs of this class should not be used extensively on pregnant patients, in large amounts, or for prolonged periods of time.

Nursing Mothers

It is not known whether topical administration of corticosteroids could result in sufficient systemic absorption to produce detectable quantities in breast milk. Systemically administered corticosteroids are secreted into breast milk in quantities not likely to have a deleterious effect on the infant. Nevertheless, caution should be exercised when topical corticosteroids are administered to a nursing woman.

Pediatric Use

Pediatric patients may demonstrate greater susceptibility to topical corticosteroid-induced HPA axis suppression and Cushing's syndrome than mature patients because of a larger skin surface area to body weight ratio.

Hypothalamic-pituitary-adrenal (HPA) axis suppression, Cushing's syndrome, and intracranial hypertension have been reported in children receiving topical corticosteroids. Manifestations of adrenal suppression in children include linear growth retardation, delayed weight gain, low plasma cortisol levels, and absence of response to ACTH stimulation. Manifestations of intracranial hypertension include bulging fontanelles, headaches, and bilateral papilledema.

Administration of topical corticosteroids to children should be limited to the least amount compatible with an effective therapeutic regimen. Chronic corticosteroid therapy may interfere with the growth and development of children.

Adverse Reactions: The following local adverse reactions are reported infrequently with topical corticosteroids, but may occur more frequently with the use of occlusive dressings. These reactions are listed in an approximate decreasing order of occurrence:

Burning	Perioral dermatitis
Itching	Allergic contact dermatitis
Irritation	Maceration of the skin
Dryness	Secondary infection
Folliculitis	Skin Atrophy
Hypertrichosis	Striae
Acneiform eruptions	Miliaria
Hypopigmentation	

In controlled clinical studies the incidence of adverse reactions was low (0.8%) for Topicort® (desoximetasone) Emollient Cream 0.25% and included burning, folliculitis and folliculo-pustular lesions. The incidence of adverse reactions was also 0.8% for Topicort® LP (desoximetasone) Emollient Cream 0.05% and included pruritus, erythema, vesiculation and burning sensation.

Overdosage: Topically applied corticosteroids can be absorbed in sufficient amounts to produce systemic effects (See **Precautions**).

Dosage and Administration: Apply a thin film of Topicort® (desoximetasone) Emollient Cream 0.25% or Topicort® LP (desoximetasone) Emollient Cream 0.05% to the affected skin areas twice daily. Rub in gently.

How Supplied: Topicort® (desoximetasone) Emollient Cream 0.25% is supplied in 15 gram, 60 gram, and 4 ounce tubes.

Topicort® LP (desoximetasone) Emollient Cream 0.05% is supplied in 15 gram and 60 gram tubes.

Store at controlled room temperature (59°-86°F).

"CAUTION: FEDERAL LAW PROHIBITS DISPENSING WITHOUT A PRESCRIPTION."

Topicort® REG TM Roussel Uclaf

[*Shown in Product Identification Section*]

Holland-Rantos Company, Inc.

P.O. BOX 385
865 CENTENNIAL AVE.
PISCATAWAY, NJ 08854

See YOUNGS DRUG PRODUCTS CORPORATION

Hoyt Laboratories

Division of Colgate-Palmolive Co.
575 UNIVERSITY AVENUE
NORWOOD, MASSACHUSETTS 02062

LURIDE® Drops ℞
brand of Sodium Fluoride

Description: Each drop contains 0.125 (1/8) mg fluoride ion (F^-) from 0.275 mg sodium fluoride (NaF) for use as a dental caries preventive in children. Sugar-free. Saccharin-free.

Clinical Pharmacology: Sodium fluoride acts systemically (before tooth eruption) and topically (post-eruption) by increasing tooth resistance to acid dissolution, by promoting remineralization, and by inhibiting the cariogenic microbial process.

Indications and Usage: It has been established that ingestion of fluoridated drinking water (1 ppm F) during the period of tooth development results in a significant decrease in the incidence of dental caries.[1] LURIDE Drops was developed to provide systemic fluoride for use as a supplement in infants and children from birth to age 3 and older, living in areas where the drinking water fluoride level does not exceed 0.7 ppm.

Contraindications: Do not use in areas where the drinking water exceeds 0.7 ppm F.

Warnings: See "Contraindications" above. As in the case of all medications, keep out of reach of children.

Precautions: See "Overdosage" section below. Incompatibility of fluoride with dairy foods has been reported due to formation of calcium fluoride which is poorly absorbed.

Adverse Reactions: Allergic rash and other idiosyncrasies have been rarely reported.

Overdosage: Prolonged daily ingestion of excessive fluoride will result in varying degrees of dental fluorosis. (The total amount of sodium fluoride in a bottle of 30 ml LURIDE Drops (120 mg F) conforms with the recommen-

Continued on next page

Hoyt—Cont.

dations of the American Dental Association for the maximum to be dispensed at one time for safety purposes.)

Dosage[2] and Administration:

F-Content of Drinking Water	Daily Dosage Birth to Age 2	Age 2–3	Age 3–12
<0.3 ppm	2 drops	4 drops	8 drops
0.3–0.7 ppm	One-half above dosage.		
>0.7 ppm	Fluoride supplements contra-indicated.		

LURIDE Drops may be administered orally undiluted or mixed with fluids.

How Supplied: Squeeze-bottles of 30 ml. (peach flavor—NDC#0126-0004-31)

Caution: Federal (U.S.A.) law prohibits dispensing without prescription.

References:

1. *Accepted Dental Therapeutics*, Ed. 38, American Dental Association, Chicago, 1979, p.318.
2. Ibid., p.321; American Academy of Pediatrics, Pediatrics 63:150–152, 1979.

LURIDE® Lozi-Tabs® Tablets ℞

brand of Sodium Fluoride

Full-strength 1.0 mg F

Luride-SF (no artificial flavor or color) 1.0 mg F

Half-strength 0.5 mg F

Quarter-strength 0.25 mg F

Description: LURIDE® brand of sodium fluoride Lozi-Tabs® brand of lozenge/chewable tablets for use as a dental caries preventive in children. Sugar-free. Saccharin-free.

Each LURIDE 1.0 mg F tablet (full-strength) contains 1.0 mg fluoride (F) from 2.2 mg sodium fluoride (NaF).

Each LURIDE -SF 1.0 mg F tablet (SF for Special Formula: no artificial color or flavor) contains 1.0 mg F from 2.2 mg NaF.

Each LURIDE 0.5 mg F tablet (half-strength) contains 0.5 mg F from 1.1 mg NaF.

Each Luride 0.25 mg F tablet (quarter-strength) contains 0.25 mg F from 0.55 mg NaF.

Clinical Pharmacology: Sodium fluoride acts systemically (before tooth eruption) and topically (post-eruption) by increasing tooth resistance to acid dissolution, by promoting remineralization, and by inhibiting the cariogenic microbial process.

Indications and Usage: It is well established that ingestion of fluoridated drinking water (1 ppm F) during the period of tooth development results in a significant decrease in the incidence of dental caries.[1] LURIDE tablets were developed to provide fluoride for children living in areas where the water fluoride level is 0.7 ppm or less.

Contraindications: LURIDE and LURIDE-SF 1.0 mg F tablets are contraindicated when the F-content of drinking water is 0.3 ppm or more and should not be administered to children under age 3. LURIDE 0.5 mg F and .25 mg F tablets are contraindicated when the F-content of drinking water exceeds 0.7 ppm.

Warnings: Do not use LURIDE or LURIDE-SF 1.0 mg F tablets for children under age 3, nor in areas where the F-content of the drinking water is 0.3 ppm or more. Do not use LURIDE 0.5 mg F or LURIDE 0.25 mg F in areas where the F-content of the drinking water is more than 0.7 ppm. As in the case of all medications, keep out of reach of children.

Precautions: See "Overdosage" section below. Incompatibility of fluoride with dairy foods has been reported due to formation of calcium fluoride which is poorly absorbed.

Adverse Reactions: Allergic rash and other idiosyncrasies have been rarely reported.

Overdosage: Prolonged daily ingestion of excessive fluoride will result in varying degrees of dental fluorosis. (The total amount of sodium fluoride in a bottle of 120 LURIDE tablets (all strengths) conforms with the recommendations of the American Dental Association for the maximum to be dispensed at one time for safety purposes.)

Dosage[2] and Administration:

F-Content of Drinking Water	Daily Dosage (F ion) Birth to Age 2	Age 2–3	Age 3–12
<0.3 ppm	0.25 mg	0.5 mg	1.0 mg.
0.3–0.7 ppm	One-half above dosages.		
>0.7 ppm	Fluoride supplements contra-indicated.		

One tablet daily, to be dissolved in the mouth or chewed before swallowing, preferably at bedtime after brushing teeth.

How Supplied:

[See table below].

(1) cherry, orange, lemon, lime

(2) Special Formula: no artificial flavor or coloring

* FOR DISPENSING ONLY

Caution: Federal (U.S.A.) law prohibits dispensing without prescription.

References:

1. *Accepted Dental Therapeutics*, Ed. 38, American Dental Association, Chicago, 1979, p. 318.
2. Ibid., p. 321; American Academy of Pediatrics, Pediatrics 63:150–152, 1979

[*Shown in Product Identification Section*]

Strength (F ion)	Tablets per Bottle	Flavor	NDC Number 0126-
1.0mg F (full strength)	120	cherry	0006-21
		assorted(1)	0143-21
		SF(2)	0007-21
	1000*	cherry	0006-10
		assorted(1)	0143-10
	5000*	cherry	0006-51
0.5mg F (half-strength)	120	grape	0014-21
	1200*	grape	0014-81
0.25mg F (quarter-strength)	120	vanilla	0186-21

ORABASE® Plain
"THE ORAL BANDAGE" ™
Oral Protective Paste

Description: Unique preparation designed for the temporary relief and protection of minor irritations of the mouth and gums. It combines gelatin, pectin, and sodium carboxymethylcellulose in a plasticized hydrocarbon gel (a polyethylene and mineral oil gel base). Imitation vanilla flavor.

Action and Uses: Provides a protective soothing covering for minor mouth irritations, and because of its adhesive qualities (it adheres tenaciously to oral mucous membranes), helps protect involved area against further irritation from chewing, swallowing, and other normal mouth activity.

Nonirritating, nontoxic, and harmless if swallowed. It contains no antibiotic, analgesic, nor antiseptic, and is essentially odorless and tasteless.

Indications: Orabase is indicated for minor lesions of the oral mucosa such as abrasions caused by toothbrushing, chewing or facial injuries; irritation from orthodontic appliances; denture irritations; and sensitive post-infection ulcerated sites.

Administration and Dosage: Press small dabs into place until the involved area is coated with a thin film of the paste. Attempting to spread this preparation may result in a granular, gritty sensation, causing it to crumble. After application, however, a smooth slippery film develops.

Use as often as needed for relief-particularly after eating-or as directed by a dentist or a physician.

Precautions and Contraindications: Not intended for use in the presence of infections. If an infection is suspected, or if any mouth irritation does not heal within 7 days, a dentist or physician should be consulted. If irritation is due to dentures that do not fit properly, a dentist should be consulted.

How Supplied: Net Wt. 0.17 oz. (5 gram) tubes and Net Wt. ½ oz. (15 gram) tubes. Tube is filled by weight not by volume. Available for office use in 0.75 gram chair-side packets—boxes of 100.

Also Available: ORABASE® with Benzocaine, analgesic oral protective paste and ORABASE® HCA, oral paste (hydrocortisone acetate 0.5%).

ORABASE® with Benzocaine
"THE ORAL BANDAGE" ™
Analgesic Oral Protective Paste

Description: Unique preparation designed for the temporary relief of pain and protection of minor irritations of the mouth and gums. It combines benzocaine, gelatin, pectin, and sodium carboxymethylcellulose in a plasticized hydrocarbon gel (a polyethylene and mineral oil gel base). Imitation vanilla flavor.

Action and Uses: Provides temporary relief of pain and a unique, protective covering for minor oral irritations. Because it adheres tenaciously to the oral mucous membranes, it holds pain relief at the site of the lesion to promote healing and prevents further irritation from chewing and other normal mouth activity.

Indications: For minor lesions of the oral mucosa such as denture irritations; abrasions caused by toothbrushing, chewing or facial injuries; irritation from orthodontic appliances; and sensitive post-infection ulcerated sites.

Administration and Dosage: Press small dabs into place until the involved area is coated with a thin film of the paste. Attempting to spread this preparation may result in a granular, gritty sensation, causing it to crumble. After application, however, a smooth slippery film develops.

Use as often as needed for relief-particularly after eating-or as directed by a dentist or a physician.

Precautions and Contraindications: Do not use in the eyes. Not for use in children under six years of age unless under professional direction. Not intended for use in the presence of infections. If an infection is suspected, or if any mouth irritation does not heal within 7 days, a dentist or physician should be consulted. If

irritation is due to dentures that do not fit properly, a dentist should be consulted.
Keep this and all medications out of reach of children.
As with any drug, if you are pregnant or nursing a baby, seek professional advice before using this product.
How Supplied: Net Wt. 0.17 oz. (5 gram) tubes and Net Wt. ½ oz. (15 gram) tubes. Tube is filled by weight not by volume. Available for office use in 0.75 gram chair-side packets—boxes of 100.
Also Available: ORABASE® Plain, oral protective paste and ORABASE® HCA, oral paste (hydrocortisone acetate 0.5%).

ORABASE® HCA ℞
Oral Paste

Description: ORABASE HCA is an adrenocorticoid topical dental paste for application to the oral mucosa. Each gram contains hydrocortisone acetate 5mg (0.5%) in a paste vehicle containing pectin, gelatin, sodium carboxymethylcellulose dispersed in a plasticized hydrocarbon gel composed of 5% polyethylene in mineral oil, flavored with imitation vanilla. Hydrocortisone is also known as cortisol, 11β, 17α, 21-trihydroxy-Δ^4-pregnene-3, 20-dione.
Clinical Pharmacology: Hydrocortisone acetate is a natural corticosteroid and possesses properties of an anti-inflammatory, antipruritic, and antiallergic nature. The paste acts as an adhesive vehicle for applying the active medication to oral tissues. The protective action of the adhesive vehicle may serve to reduce the pain associated with oral irritation.
Indications and Usage: Indicated for adjunctive treatment and for temporary relief of symptoms associated with oral inflammatory lesions and ulcerative lesions resulting from trauma.
Contraindications: Fungal, viral, or bacterial infections of the oral mucosa. Hypersensitivity to any component. This preparation is not for ophthalmic use.
Warnings: Patients with tuberculosis, peptic ulcer, or diabetes mellitus should not be routinely treated with this steroid preparation.
If significant regeneration or repair of oral tissues does not occur within 7 days of treatment, additional investigation of the oral lesion is advised.
Keep Out of Reach of Children
Precautions: It should be borne in mind that the normal defensive responses of the oral tissues are depressed in patients receiving topical corticosteroid therapy. Virulent strains of oral microorganisms may multiply without producing the usual warning symptoms of oral infections.
Pregnancy Category C. Animal reproduction studies have not been conducted with ORABASE HCA. It is also not known whether ORABASE HCA can cause fetal harm when administered to a pregnant woman or can affect reproduction capacity. ORABASE HCA should be given to a pregnant woman only if clearly needed.
Nursing mothers: It is not known whether this drug is excreted in human milk. Because many drugs are excreted in human milk, caution should be exercised when ORABASE HCA is administered in a nursing woman.
Adverse Reactions: Prolonged administration may elicit the adverse reactions known to occur with systemic hydrocortisone preparations; for example, adrenal suppression, alteration of glucose metabolism, protein catabolism, peptic ulcer activations, and others. These are usually reversible and disappear when the drug is discontinued.
Dosage and Administration: Dab, do not rub, on the lesion until the paste adheres. (Rubbing this preparation on lesions may result in a granular, gritty sensation.) After application, a smooth, slippery film develops.
Usual adult dose: Topical, to the oral mucous membrane, 2 or 3 times a day following meals and at bedtime.
Usual pediatric dose: Dosage has not been established.
How Supplied: Net weight 5-Gm. tubes (NDC #0126-0101-45). Available for office use in 0.75-Gm. chair-side packets in boxes of 100 (NDC #0126-0101-01).
Caution: Federal (U.S.A.) law prohibits dispensing without prescription.

PEROXYL™
brand of Hydrogen Peroxide MOUTHRINSE

1.5% Hydrogen Peroxide in a pleasantly flavored aqueous solution containing 6% (v/v) alcohol.
Directions: PerOxyl comes ready to use. Swish one capful (two teaspoonfuls) around in the mouth over the affected area for at least one minute and then expel. Use up to 4 times daily (after meals and at bedtime) for a maximum of 7 days or as directed by a dentist or physician. Children under 12 years of age should be supervised in the use of this product. For children under 2 years of age, there is no recommended dosage except under the advice and supervision of a dentist or physician.
Indications: For temporary use in the cleansing of wounds caused by minor oral irritation or injury, such as that following minor dental procedures, or from dentures or orthodontic appliances.
For temporary use in the cleansing of gum irritation due to erupting teeth (teething).
Warnings: Not to be used for a period exceeding 7 days. Discontinue use and see your dentist or physician promptly if irritation persists, inflammation develops, or if fever and infection develop. Do not swallow. **Keep out of reach of children.**

PHOS–FLUR® Oral Rinse/Supplement ℞
brand of Acidulated Phosphate Fluoride

Description: Each teaspoonful (5 ml) contains 1.0 mg fluoride ion (F^-) from 2.2 mg sodium fluoride (NaF), in a 0.1 Molar phosphate solution at pH 4, for use as a dental caries preventive in children and to treat dental cervical hypersensitivity. Cherry, orange, lime–sugar and saccharin free. Cinnamon–contains saccharin but is sugar free.
Clinical Pharmacology: Sodium fluoride acts systemically (before tooth eruption) and topically (post-eruption) by increasing tooth resistance to acid dissolution, by promoting remineralization, and by inhibiting the cariogenic microbial process. Acidulation provides greater topical fluoride uptake by dental enamel than neutral solutions.[1] Phosphate protects enamel from demineralization by the acidulated formulation (common ion effect).[1] When topical fluoride is applied to hypersensitive exposed dentin, it results in the formation of insoluble materials within the dentinal tubules and this, in turn, is believed to block the transmission of offending stimuli.
Indications and Usage: It has been well established that ingestion of fluoridated drinking water (1 ppm F) during the period of tooth development results in a significant decrease in the incidence of dental caries.[2] PHOS-FLUR was developed to provide topical and systemic fluoride for use as a rinse/supplement (rinse-and-swallow) in children age 3 and older living in areas where the water fluoride level does not exceed 0.7 ppm. Where the drinking water contains more than 0.7 ppm F, PHOS-FLUR provides benefits as a topical fluoride dental rinse only (rinse-and-expectorate) for children age 6 and older.[3] Pioneering clinical studies on PHOS-FLUR were published by Frankl et al.[4] and Aasenden et al,[5] in 1972.
The use of sodium fluoride for desensitizing exposed root surfaces of teeth was first reported in the 1940's.[6–10] Since then, various sodium fluoride preparations have been used for this purpose,[11–17] including PHOS-FLUR Rinse.[18]
Contraindications: DO NOT SWALLOW in areas where the F-content of drinking water exceeds 0.7 ppm, nor in children under age 3.
Warnings: Do not use as a rinse in children under age 6. Do not use as a supplement in children under age 3, nor in areas where the drinking water exceeds 0.7 ppm F. As in the case of all medications, keep out of reach of children.
Precautions: See "Overdosage" section below. Incompatibility of systemic fluoride with dairy foods has been reported due to formation of calcium fluoride which is poorly absorbed.
Adverse Reactions: Allergic reactions and other idiosyncrasies have been rarely reported. Lime flavored PHOS-FLUR contains FD&C Yellow No. 5 (tartrazine), a color additive, which may cause allergic-type reactions (including bronchial asthma) in certain susceptible individuals. Although the overall incidence of FD&C Yellow No. 5 (tartrazine) sensitivity in the general population is low, it frequently seen in patients who also have aspirin hypersensitivity.
Overdosage: Prolonged daily ingestion of excessive fluoride will result in varying degrees of dental fluorosis. (The total amount of sodium fluoride in a bottle of 500ml PHOS-FLUR Rinse/Supplement conforms to the recommendations of the American Dental Association for the maximum to be dispensed at one time for safety purposes).
Dosage and Administration:
As A Daily Dental Rinse—Children age 6 and over, preferably at bedtime after thoroughly brushing the teeth, rinse one teaspoonful (5 ml) or two teaspoonfuls (10 ml) vigorously around and between teeth for one minute, then expectorate. DO NOT SWALLOW.
As A Daily Supplement—Children age 3 and over, in areas where the drinking water contains less than 0.3 ppm F, rinse one teaspoonful (5 ml) as above and swallow. When drinking water contains 0.3 to 0.7 ppm F, inclusive, reduce dosage to ½ teaspoonful.
For Hypersensitivity, after the usual brushing and flossing at bedtime, rinse nightly over the affected areas for one minute, then expectorate.
How Supplied:

Bottles of	Flavors	NDC# 0126
250 ml	cherry	0129-99
500 ml	cherry	0129-46
	cinnamon	0126-46
	lime	0017-46
	orange	0128-46
1 gallon (with pump dispenser)	cherry	0129-28
	lime	0017-28
	orange	0128-28
30 ml (patient starter)	cherry	0129-31
	cinnamon	0126-31
	lime	0017-31
	orange	0128-31

Caution: Federal (U.S.A.) law prohibits dispensing without prescription.
References:
[1]F. Brudevold et al. Arch. Oral Biol. 8:167–177, 1963. [2]Accepted Dental Therapeutics, American Dental Association, Chicago, 1979, p.318. [3]Ibid., p. 323. [4]S.N. Frankl, S. Fleisch, and R. P. Diodati. J.A.D.A. 85:882–886, 1972. [5]R. Aasenden, P.F. DePaola, and F. Brudevold. Arch. Oral Biol. 17:1705–1714, 1972. [6]E.H. Lukomsky. J. Dent. Res. 20:649, 1941. [7]W. H. Hoyt and B. G. Bibby. J.A.D.A. 30:1372–1376, 1943. [8]S. Sorin. N.Y.J. Dent. 13:399, 1943. [9]A. J.

Continued on next page

Hoyt—Cont.

Clement. Brit. Dent. J. 82:168, 1947. [10]Council on Dental Therapeutics, American Dental Association. J.A.D.A. 38:762–763, 1949. [11]M. M. Manning. Dent. Surv. 37:731–734, 1961. [12]F. G. Everett. Dent. Clin. North Am. 3:221–230, 1964. [13]K. S. Murthy et al. Oral Surg. 36:448–458, 1973. [14]B. Minkov et al. J. Periodontol. 46:246–249, 1975. [15]J. Ehrlich et al. J. Dent. Res. 54:897–900, 1975. [16]R. Squillaro et al. J. Dent. Res. 60 (Special Issue A):461, 1981. [17]L.L. Zeldow. ADA Daily Bulletin (A.D.A. Meeting, Anaheim, 1978) 27:2(Oct. 23) 1978.

POINT-TWO® Dental Rinse ℞
brand of Sodium Fluoride

Description: 0.2% sodium fluoride (NaF) in a mint-flavored, neutral aqueous solution containing 6% alcohol. For weekly use as a caries preventive in children and to treat dental cervical hypersensitivity.

Clinical Pharmacology: Topical application of sodium fluoride increases tooth resistance to acid dissolution, promotes remineralization, and inhibits the cariogenic microbial process.

When topical fluoride is applied to hypersensitive exposed dentin, it results in the formation of insoluble materials within the dentinal tubules and this, in turn, is believed to block the transmission of offending stimuli.

Indications and Usage: It has been established that weekly rinsing with a neutral 0.2% sodium fluoride solution protects against dental caries in children.[1] POINT-TWO Rinse was developed to provide a ready-to-use, flavored preparation for convenient administration and favorable compliance.

The use of sodium fluoride for desensitizing exposed root surfaces of teeth was first reported in the 1940's.[3–7] Since then, various sodium fluoride preparations have been used for this purpose.[8–14]

Contraindications: None. (May be used whether drinking water is fluoridated or not, since **topical** fluoride cannot produce fluorosis).

Warnings: **DO NOT SWALLOW.** Do not use in children under age 6, since younger children frequently cannot perform the rinse process without significant swallowing. As in the case of all medications, keep out of reach of children.

Precautions: Not for systemic use. (Each 5 ml contains 5 mg fluoride ion).

Adverse Reactions: In patients with mucositis, gingival tissues may be hypersensitive to flavor or alcohol present in formulation.

Overdosage: In the event a dose is accidentally swallowed, nausea and/or vomiting may result (treat with milk or antacids).

Dosage and Administration: **For caries,**[2] children age 6 to 12, one teaspoonful (5 ml); over age 12, 2 teaspoonfuls (10 ml). Once a week, preferably at bedtime after thoroughly brushing the teeth, rinse vigorously around and between the teeth for one minute, then expectorate. DO NOT SWALLOW. For maximum benefit, do not eat, drink, or rinse mouth for at least 30 minutes afterwards.

For Hypersensitivity, after the usual brushing and flossing at bedtime, rinse nightly over the affected areas for one minute, then expectorate.

How Supplied:
Bottles of 30ml (Patient starter) (Mint—NDC #0126-0178-31)
Bottles of 4 fl. oz. (120ml) (Mint—NDC #0126-0178-04)
Bottles of 8 fl. oz. with child-resistant closure. (Mint—NDC #0126-0178-99)
Gallon (with pump dispenser) (Mint—NDC #0126-0178-28)

Caution. Federal (U.S.A.) law prohibits dispensing without prescription.

References: [1]Accepted Dental Therapeutics, Ed. 38, American Dental Association, Chicago, 1979, p.324. [2]Ibid. [3]E. H. Lukomsky. J. Dent. Res. 20:649, 1941. [4]W. H. Hoyt and B. G. Bibby, J.A.D.A. 30:1372–1376, 1943. [5]S. Sorin. N.Y.J. Dent. 13:399, 1943. [6]A. J. Clement. Brit. Dent. J. 82:168, 1947. [7]Council on Dental Therapeutics, American Dental Association. J.A.D.A. 38:762–763, 1949. [8]M. M. Manning. Dent. Surv. 37:731–734, 1961. [9]F. G. Everett. Dent. Clin. North Am. 3:221–230, 1964. [10]K. S. Murthy et al: Oral Surg. 36:448–458, 1973. [11]B. Minkov et al: J. Periodontol. 46:246–249, 1975. [12]J. Ehrlich et al. J. Dent. Res. 54:897–900, 1975. [13]L. L. Zeldow. ADA Daily Bulletin (A.D.A. Meeting, Anaheim, 1978) 27:2(Oct. 23) 1978. [14]R. Squillaro et al. J. Dent. Res. 60 (Special Issue A): 461, 1981.

THERA-FLUR® Topical Gel-Drops ℞
THERA-FLUR®-N Topical Gel-Drops ℞
brands of Acidulated Phosphate Fluoride

Description: THERA-FLUR (acidulated) gel-drops contains 0.5% fluoride ion (F^-) from 1.1% sodium fluoride (NaF) in a lime-flavored aqueous solution containing 0.1 Molar phosphate at pH 4.5. THERA-FLUR-N (neutral) also contains 0.5% (F^-) from 1.1% NaF, but with no acid phosphate, nor artificial flavor or color, at neutral pH. For daily self-topical use as a dental caries preventive and to treat dental cervical hypersensitivity.

Clinical Pharmacology: High-potency, high-frequency topical applications of sodium fluoride to the teeth increase tooth resistance to acid dissolution. Acidulation of topical fluoride increases deposition and penetration of the fluoride ion into tooth enamel. Phosphate acts as a common ion to inhibit demineralization of enamel by acidulated fluoride. Release of enamel-deposited fluoride inhibits the cariogenic microbial process and stimulates remineralization.

Neutral fluoride provides less fluoride uptake by enamel, but diminished clinical efficacy has not been detected after high-potency, high-frequency treatment. When topical fluoride is applied to hypersensitive exposed dentin, it results in the formation of insoluble materials within the dentinal tubules and this, in turn, is believed to block the transmission of offending stimuli.

Indications and Usage: It is well established that 1.1% sodium fluoride is a safe and effective caries preventive when applied frequently with mouthpiece applicators.[1] Pioneering clinical studies with THERA-FLUR and THERA-FLUR-N Gel-Drops in schoolchildren were conducted by Englander et al.[2,3,4]

Both neutral and acidulated phosphate fluoride gels have been effective in controlling rampant dental decay which frequently follows xerostomia-producing radiotherapy of tumors in the head and neck region.[5,6] The use of topical sodium fluoride for desensitizing exposed root surfaces of teeth was first reported in the 1940's.[7–11] Since that time, various sodium fluoride preparations have been used for this purpose.[12–16] In 1979, there was a report on successful treatment with THERA-FLUR Gel-Drops.[18] This was later confirmed in a 1981 report on a double-blind study with 1.1% sodium fluoride.[17]

Contraindications: None (May be used in areas where drinking water is fluoridated or not, because **topical** fluoride cannot produce fluorosis).

Warnings: As with all medications, keep out of reach of children.

Precautions: Laboratory tests indicate that use of acidulated fluoride may cause dulling of porcelain and ceramic restorations. Therefore, THERA-FLUR-N (neutral) is recommended for this type of patient.

Adverse Reactions: In patients with mucositis, gingival tissues may be hypersensitive to the acidity of THERA-FLUR, but will tolerate THERA-FLUR-N (neutral).

Overdosage: Accidental ingestion of a usual treatment dose (2–4 mg F) is not harmful.

Dosage and Administration: Age 3 and older. For daily use with applicators supplied by the dentist.[2] Apply 4 to 8 drops as required to cover inner surface of each applicator. Spread gel-drops with tip of bottle. Place applicators over upper and lower teeth at the same time. Bite down lightly for 6 minutes. Remove applicators and rinse mouth. Clean applicators with cold water.

For use in hypersensitivity, after the usual brushing and flossing at bedtime, apply a few drops to a toothbrush and brush nightly onto the affected areas.

How Supplied: 24 ml and 60 ml plastic squeeze bottles.

	NDC# 0126
THERA-FLUR (lime flavor)	24ml 0048-54
	60ml 0048-02
THERA-FLUR-N (no artificial flavor or color)	24ml 0196-54
	60ml 0196-02

Caution: Federal (U.S.A.) law prohibits dispensing without prescription.

References:
[1]Accepted Dental Therapeutics, Ed.38, American Dental Association, Chicago, 1979, p.325, 327. [2]H. R. Englander, P. H. Keyes, and M. Gestwicki. J.A.D.A. 75:638–644, 1967. [3]H. R. Englander et al. J.A.D.A. 78:783–787, 1969. [4]H. R. Englander et al. J.A.D.A. 82:354–358, 1971. [5]E. Johansen and T. O. Olsen in "Continuing Evaluation of the Use of Fluorides" (AAAS Selected Symposium 11), Westview Press, Boulder, CO, 1979, p.66. [6]S. Dreizen et al. J. Dent. Res. 56:99–104, 1977. [7]E. H. Lukomsky. J. Dent. Res. 20:649, 1941. [8]W. H. Hoyt and B. G. Bibby. J.A.D.A. 30:1372–1376, 1943. [9]S. Sorin. N.Y.J. Dent. 13:399, 1943. [10]A. J. Clement. Brit. Dent. J. 82:168, 1947. [11]Council on Dental Therapeutics, American Dental Association. J.A.D.A. 38:762–763, 1949. [12]M. M. Manning. Dent. Surv. 37:731–734, 1961. [13]F. G. Everett. Dent. Clin. North Am. 3:221–230, 1964. [14]K. S. Murthy et al. Oral Surg. 36:448–458, 1973. [15]B. Minkov et al. J. Periodontol. 46–246–249, 1975. [16]J. Ehrlich et al. J. Dent. Res. 54:897–900, 1975. [17]R. Squillaro et al. J. Dent. Res. 60 (Special Issue A):461, 1981. [18]L. L. Zeldow. ADA Daily Bulletin (A.D.A. Meetiing, Anaheim, 1978) 27:2(Oct. 23) 1978.

Hyland Therapeutics Division

TRAVENOL LABORATORIES, INC.
444 W. GLENOAKS BLVD.
GLENDALE, CA 91202

AUTOPLEX™ ℞
Anti-Inhibitor Coagulant Complex

Supplied in single dose 30 ml vials (Factor VIII correctional activity is stated on label of each vial) with sterile diluent and needles for reconstitution and withdrawal.

BUMINATE® 5% ℞
Normal Serum Albumin (Human), U.S.P., 5% Solution

Supplied as a 5% solution in 250 ml and 500 ml bottles. For use with intravenous administration set.

BUMINATE® 25% ℞
Normal Serum Albumin (Human), U.S.P., 25% Solution

Supplied as a 25% solution in 20 ml, 50 ml, and 100 ml vials. For use with intravenous administration set.

HEMOFIL® ℞
Antihemophilic Factor (Human), Factor VIII, AHF, AHG
Method Four, Dried

Supplied in single dose 10 ml, 20 ml, and 30 ml vials (AHF activity is stated on label of each vial) with sterile diluent and needles for reconstitution and withdrawal.

HU–TET® ℞
Tetanus Immune Globulin (Human), U.S.P.

Supplied in 250 units single dose vial or prefilled disposable syringe.

IMMUNE SERUM GLOBULIN (HUMAN), U.S.P. ℞
GAMMA GLOBULIN

Supplied in 2 ml and 10 ml vials.

PROPLEX® ℞
Factor IX Complex (Human)
(Factors II, VII, IX, and X), Dried

Supplied in single dose 30 ml vials (Factor IX activity is stated on label of each vial) with sterile diluent and needles for reconstitution and withdrawal.

PROTENATE® 5% ℞
Plasma Protein Fraction (Human), U.S.P., 5% Solution

Supplied as a 5% solution in 250 ml and 500 ml bottles. For use with intravenous administration set.

Hynson, Westcott & Dunning

Division of Becton Dickinson and Co.
CHARLES & CHASE STS.
BALTIMORE, MD 21201

BAL IN OIL AMPULES ℞
(Dimercaprol Injection, USP)

Description: Dimercaprol (2,3-dimercapto-1-propanol) is a colorless or almost colorless liquid, having a disagreeable, mercaptan-like odor. Each 1 ml sterile BAL in Oil contains 100 mg Dimercaprol in 200 mg benzyl benzoate and 700 mg peanut oil. The slight sediment which may be noticed in some ampules develops during sterilization. It is not an indication that the solution is deteriorating.
Action: Dimercaprol promotes the excretion of arsenic, gold and mercury in cases of poisoning. It is also used in combination with Edetate Calcium Disodium Injection, USP to promote the excretion of lead.
Indications: BAL in Oil (Dimercaprol Injection, USP) is indicated in the treatment of arsenic, gold and mercury poisoning. It is indicated in acute lead poisoning when used concomitantly with Edetate Calcium Disodium Injection, USP.
Dimercaprol Injection, USP is effective for use in acute poisoning by mercury salts if therapy is begun within one or two hours following ingestion. It is not very effective for chronic mercury poisoning.
Dimercaprol Injection, USP is of questionable value in poisoning caused by other heavy metals such as antimony and bismuth. It should not be used in iron, cadmium, or selenium poisoning because the resulting dimercaprol-metal complexes are more toxic than the metal alone, especially to the kidneys.
Contraindications: BAL in Oil is contraindicated in most instances of hepatic insufficiency with the exception of postarsenical jaundice. The drug should be discontinued or used only with extreme caution if acute renal insufficiency develops during therapy.
Warnings: There may be local pain at the site of the injection. A reaction apparently peculiar to children is fever which may persist during therapy. It occurs in approximately 30% of children. A transient reduction of the percentage of polymorphonuclear leukocytes may also be observed.
Precautions: Because the dimercaprol-metal complex breaks down easily in an acid medium, production of an alkaline urine affords protection to the kidney during therapy. Medicinal iron should not be administered to patients under therapy with BAL. Data is not available regarding the use of dimercaprol during pregnancy and it should not be used unless judged by the physician to be necessary in the treatment of life threatening acute poisoning.
Adverse Reactions: One of the most consistent responses to Dimercaprol Injection, USP is a rise in blood pressure accompanied by tachycardia. This rise is roughly proportional to the dose administered. Doses larger than those recommended may cause other transitory signs and symptoms in approximate order of frequency as follows: (1) nausea and, in some instances, vomiting; (2) headache; (3) a burning sensation in the lips, mouth and throat; (4) a feeling of constriction, even pain, in the throat, chest, or hands; (5) conjunctivitis, lacrimation, blepharal spasm, rhinorrhea, and salivation; (6) tingling of the hands; (7) a burning sensation in the penis; (8) sweating of the forehead, hands and other areas; (9) abdominal pain; and (10) occasional appearance of painful sterile abscesses. Many of the above symptoms are accompanied by a feeling of anxiety, weakness, and unrest and often are relieved by administration of an antihistamine.
Dosage and Administration: By deep intramuscular injection only. For mild arsenic or gold poisoning, 2.5 mg/kg of body weight four times daily for two days, two times on the third day, and once daily thereafter for ten days; for severe arsenic or gold poisoning, 3 mg/kg every four hours for two days, four times on the third day, then twice daily thereafter for ten days. For mercury poisoning, 5 mg/kg initially, followed by 2.5 mg/kg one or two times daily for ten days. For acute lead encephalopathy 4 mg/kg body weight is given alone in the first dose and thereafter at four hour intervals in combination with Edetate Calcium Disodium Injection, USP administered at a separate site. For less severe poisoning the dose can be reduced to 3 mg/kg after the first dose. Treatment is maintained for two to seven days depending on clinical response. Successful treatment depends on beginning injections at the earliest possible moment and on the use of adequate amounts at frequent intervals. Other supportive measures should always be used in conjunction with BAL in Oil therapy.
How Supplied: 3 ml (100 mg/ml, ampules, box of 10, NDC 0011-8341-09).

LACTINEX® TABLETS AND GRANULES
(See PDR For Nonprescription Drugs)

Important Notice

Before prescribing or administering any product described in PHYSICIANS' DESK REFERENCE always consult the PDR Supplement for possible new or revised information.

Hyrex Pharmaceuticals

3494 DEMOCRAT RD.
MEMPHIS, TN 38118

GLUKOR INJECTION ℞

Composition: When mixed, each ml contains: Chorionic Gonadotropin 200 U.S.P. units, Mannitol, Benzyl Alcohol 0.9%, Water for injection with Sodium Phosphate Dibasic and Sodium Phosphate Monobasic.
Available: 10 ml and 25 ml vials with diluent.

HYREX-105 Ⓒ ℞

Composition: Phendimetrazine Tartrate 105 mg. In special slow release capsule.
Supplied: Bottles of 30 and 100 capsules.

HYTINIC CAPSULES AND ELIXIR
(polysaccharide-iron complex)

Composition: HYTINIC is a highly water-soluble complex of iron and a low molecular weight polysaccharide. Each HYTINIC Capsule contains 150 mg. elemental iron. Each 5 ml. (teaspoonful) HYTINIC Elixir contains 100 mg. elemental iron, alcohol 10% (sugar free).
Action and Uses: HYTINIC is an easily assimilated source of iron for treatment of uncomplicated iron deficiency anemia. Because HYTINIC is a polysaccharide bound iron complex, it is relatively nontoxic and there are relatively few, if any, of the gastrointestinal side effects associated with iron therapy, thus permitting full therapeutic dosage (150 to 300 mg. elemental iron daily) in a single dose if desirable. There is no staining of teeth and no metallic aftertaste.
Indications: For treatment of uncomplicated iron deficiency anemia.
Contraindications: In patients with hemochromatosis and hemosiderosis, and in those with a known hypersensitivity to any of the ingredients.
Administration and Dosage: ADULTS: One or two HYTINIC Capsules daily, or one or two teaspoonfuls HYTINIC Elixir daily. CHILDREN 6 to 12 years of age: One teaspoonful HYTINIC Elixir daily; Children 2 to 6 years of age: ½ teaspoonful HYTINIC Elixir daily. For younger children, consult physician.
How Supplied: HYTINIC Capsules: (Green and white) Bottles of 50 and 500 and Unit Dose 100's: HYTINIC Elixir: Bottles of 8 ounces.
Product Identification Mark: Hyrex.

HYTUSS TABLETS (100 mg)
HYTUSS-2X CAPSULES (200 mg)
Brand of quaifenesin U.S.P. (formerly called glyceryl guaiacolate)

Composition: Each sugar-free Hytuss Tablet contains guaifenesin 100 mg. Each sugar-free Hytuss-2X Capsule contains guaifenesin 200 mg.
Action and Uses: This preparation utilizes the effective expectorant action of guaifenesin U.S.P. (formerly called glyceryl guaicolate) which significantly stimulates the secretion of respiratory tract fluid. The increased flow of less viscid fluid favors expectoration and has a demulcent effect on the tracheobronchial mucosa. The primary usefulness of Hytuss Tablets is to promote the change from a dry, unproductive cough to a productive cough. Hytuss is therefore useful in treating coughs due to the common cold, bronchitis, laryngitis, tracheitis, pharyngitis, influenza and the measles. The expectorant action of Hytuss may also provide symptomatic relief in some chronic respiratory disorders when the patient experiences spasms of dry nonproductive coughing.
Precautions: Extremely large amounts may cause nausea and vomiting.

Continued on next page

Hyrex—Cont.

Dosage: HYTUSS TABLETS—*Adults*—1 or 2 tablets four times daily. *Children 6-12 years of age*—½ tablet three or four times daily.
Dosage: HYTUSS-2X CAPSULES—*Adults*—1 or 2 capsules four times daily.
How Supplied: 100 mg. Tablet — White, scored, sugar-free, bottles of 100 — 1,000 — 5,000. Also 200 mg. Capsule, red and white, sugar-free, bottles of 100 — 1,000.
Product Identification Mark: Tablet—Hy. Capsule—Hyrex.

TRAC TABS ℞
TRAC TABS 2X

Composition: TRAC TABS: Each tablet contains Atropine Sulfate 0.03 mg, Hyoscyamine (as the sulfate) 0.03 mg, Methenamine 40.8 mg, Methylene Blue 5.4 mg, Phenyl Salicylate 18.1 mg. Benzoic Acid 4.5 mg.
TRAC TABS 2X: Each blue tablet coded Hy-408 contains Atropine Sulfate 0.06 mg, Hyoscyamine Sulfate 0.03 mg, Methenamine 120 mg, Methylene Blue 6 mg, Phenyl Salicylate 30 mg, Benzoic Acid 7.5 mg.
Supplied: Bottles of 100 and 1,000. Trac 2X tablet coded Hy-408.

TWO-DYNE™ ℞

Composition: Butalbital 50 mg, Caffeine 40 mg, Acetaminophen 325 mg.
Supplied: Capsules—bottles of 100 and 1,000.

ICN Pharmaceuticals, Inc.
222 NORTH VINCENT AVENUE
COVINA, CA 91722

TESTRED® ℞
brand of Methyltestosterone

Description: Each capsule contains 10 mg of USP Methyltestosterone, a synthetic androgen occurring as white or creamy white crystals or powder.
It is soluble in various organic solvents but is practically insoluble in water.
Clinical Pharmacology: 17 α-Methyltestosterone, a 17 α-substituted alkyl derivative of testosterone, is unique in retaining androgenic potency when given by mouth, this efficacy being attributed to the fact that the molecule is sufficiently stable to escape extensive inactivation in the liver.
The androgenic activity of methyltestosterone is responsible for maintenance of secondary sexual characteristics as well as for development of accessory sexual organs in the male. Methyltestosterone also exerts stimulating effects upon the spermatogenic cells and stimulates the development of bone, muscle, skin, and hair growth, and emotional responses to produce the characteristic adult masculine traits.
Indications and Usage: Methyltestosterone is indicated for treatment of the following:
In the Male:
1. Eunuchoidism and eunuchism.
2. Male climacteric when symptoms are secondary to androgen deficiency.
3. Impotence resulting from androgen deficiency.
4. Postpubertal cryptorchidism with evidence of hypogonadism.

In the Female:
1. Prevention of postpartum breast pain and engorgement in the non-nursing mother. There is no satisfactory evidence that this drug prevents or suppresses lactation per se.
2. Palliation of androgen-responsive, advancing, inoperable breast cancer in women who are more than 1, but less than 5 years postmenopausal or who have been proven to have a hormone-dependent tumor as shown by previous beneficial response to castration.

Refer to Dosage and Administration section.
Contraindications: Male patients with known or suspected prostatic carcinoma; in elderly patients in whom overstimulation is to be avoided; cases of benign prostatic hypertrophy with obstructive symptoms; carcinoma of the male breast; history of hypersensitivity or toxic reactions to androgens; cardiac, hepatic or renal impairment; patients with nephrosis or the nephrotic phase of nephritis; hypercalcemia; prepubertal males.
Contraindicated in pregnancy and lactation because masculinization of the female fetus or breasted infant may occur.
Warnings: Female patients should be watched carefully for symptoms or signs of virilization, such as hoarseness or deepening of the voice, oily skin, acne, hirsutism, enlarged clitoris, stimulation of libido, and menstrual irregularities. At the dosage necessary to achieve an antitumor response, androgens will cause virilization of the female; occasionally a sensitive female may exhibit one or more of these signs on smaller doses. Some of these changes may be irreversible even after the drug is stopped.
Do not give to elderly asthenic males who may react adversely to overstimulation by androgens.
Hypercalcemia may occur in immobilized patients and in patients with breast cancer. In patients with cancer this may indicate progression of bone metastasis. If this occurs, the drug should be discontinued.
Discontinue the drug if cholestatic hepatitis with jaundice appears or liver tests become abnormal.
Precautions:
General: If symptomatic hypercalcemia occurs, discontinue androgen therapy and institute appropriate measures.
In treating males for symptoms of climacteric, avoid stimulation to the point of increasing the nervous, mental, and physical activities beyond the patient's cardiovascular capacity. If priapism or other signs of excessive sexual stimulation develop, discontinue therapy.
If abnormal vaginal bleeding develops, discontinue therapy until the etiology is determined.
In the male, prolonged administration or excessive dosage may cause inhibition of testicular function, resulting in oligospermia and decrease in ejaculatory volume.
A clinically significant PBI decrease may occur in patients receiving androgens.
Prolonged administration may result in sodium and fluid retention. This may present a problem in patients with compromised cardiac reserve or renal disease.
Care should be taken in the treatment of adolescent or preadolescent males so that premature epiphyseal closure or precocious sexual development may be avoided.
Serum cholesterol may increase or decrease during therapy. Because of their hypercholesterolemic effects, caution is required when administering these drugs to patients with a history of myocardial infarction or coronary artery disease. Serial determinations of serum cholesterol should be made and therapy adjusted accordingly. A cause and effect relationship between myocardial infarction and hypercholesterolemia has not been established.
Testosterone has been reported to precipitate attacks of acute intermittent porphyria (AIP); use with caution in patients with known AIP.
Drug Interactions: Anabolic steroids may increase sensitivity to anticoagulants. The 17-alkylated agents (methyltestosterone, etc.) are most likely to interact with anticoagulants. Dosage of the anticoagulant may have to be decreased in order to maintain the prothrombin time at the desired therapeutic level.
Anabolic steroids have been shown to alter glucose tolerance tests. Diabetics should be followed closely and the insulin or oral hypoglycemic dosage adjusted accordingly.
Concomitant use of androgens with adrenal steroids or ACTH may add to edema resulting from androgen use.
Pregnancy: Category X. See "Contraindications" section. Methyltestosterone can cause fetal harm when administered to a pregnant woman, i.e., masculinization of the female fetus may occur. Methyltestosterone is contraindicated in women who are or who may become pregnant. If this drug is used during pregnancy, or if the patient becomes pregnant while taking this drug, the patient should be apprised of the potential hazard to the fetus.
Nursing mothers: See "Contraindications" section. Methyltestosterone may cause serious adverse reactions in nursing infants.
Pediatric use: See "Contraindications" section. The adverse consequences of giving androgens to young children are not fully understood, but the possibility of causing serious disturbances of growth and of sexual and osseous development makes highly questionable the use of androgens for their anabolic effects in childhood.
Adverse Reactions: In males, the following postpubertal adverse reactions have occurred: inhibition of testicular function, testicular atrophy and oligospermia; impotence; chronic priapism; gynecomastia; epididymitis; bladder irritability. Prepubertal adverse reactions consist of phallic enlargement and increased frequency of erection.
In females, hirsutism, male-pattern baldness; deepening of the voice, and clitoral enlargement may occur. These changes are usually irreversible even after prompt discontinuance of therapy and are not prevented by concomitant use of estrogens. Menstrual irregularities may also develop.
In both sexes, the following have occurred: Increased or decreased libido; flushing of the skin, acne (especially in females and prepubertal males); habituation; excitation and sleeplessness; chills; leukopenia; bleeding in patients on concomitant anticoagulant therapy; premature closure of epiphyses in children. Hypercalcemia may occur, particularly in immobile patients and in patients with metastatic breast carcinoma. Oral preparations have been associated with nausea, vomiting, and diarrhea, as well as with symptoms resembling those of peptic ulcer. Jaundice may occur, but is usually reversible with prompt discontinuance of therapy. Occasionally hepatic necrosis and death may result from treatment with 17-alpha alkyl substituted anabolic steroids. There have been rare reports of hepatocellular neoplasms and peliosis hepatis associated with long-term androgenic-anabolic steroid therapy.
Alterations may occur in the following clinical laboratory tests: Metyrapone test; fasting blood surgar (FBS) and glucose tolerance test; thyroid function tests (decrease in protein bound iodine (PBI), thyroxine-binding capacity, radioactive iodine uptake, and an increase in T3 uptake by the red blood cells or resin; free thyroxine levels remain normal and the altered tests usually persist for 2 to 3 weeks after stopping anabolic therapy); electrolytes (retention of sodium, chloride, water, potassium, calcium, and inorganic phosphates); blood coagulation tests (increase in clotting factors II, V, VII, and X); miscellaneous laboratory tests (decreased creatinine and creatinine excretion lasting up to 2 weeks after discontinuing therapy and increased 17-ketosteroid excretion).
Dosage and Administration: Dosage must be strictly individualized. Daily requirements are best administered in divided doses. The following chart is suggested as an average daily dosage guide. Duration of therapy will depend upon the response of the condition being treated and the appearance of adverse reactions.

Indications In the Male:	Average Daily Dosage
Eunuchism and eunuchoidism	10 to 40 mg
Male climacteric and male impotence	10 to 40 mg
Cryptorchidism-postpubertal	30 mg
In the Female:	
Postpartum breast pain and engorgement (3 to 5 days).	80 mg
Breast cancer	200 mg

How Supplied: Red capsules branded on both sections ICN 0901 containing 10 mg of methyltestosterone in bottles of 100, 500, and 1000 capsules.
Caution: Federal (U.S.A.) law prohibits dispensing without prescription.

I.C.P. Pharmaceuticals

A Division of Wisconsin Medical Enterprises, Inc.
P.O. BOX 294
CUDAHY, WISCONSIN 53110

DECUBITEX™ OINTMENT ℞

Ingredients: Biebrich Scarlet Red, Sulfonated, Water Soluble 0.1% in an ointment base containing Peruvian Balsam, Zinc Oxide, Starch, Castor Oil, Petrolatum, Sodium Propionate, Methylparaben, Propylparaben, Propylene Glycol and Water.
Indications: As an aid in the management of decubitus ulcers.
Administration: Pour a small amount of 3% Hydrogen Peroxide or Sterile Normal Saline onto the affected area. Cleanse thoroughly and apply ointment. Cover with dry sterile gauze. Dressing should be changed twice daily.
Contraindications: Known hypersensitivity to any of the ingredients.
Adverse Reactions: Gastroenteritis and renal irritation have been reported following percutaneous absorption over a massive area.
Caution: Federal law prohibits dispensing without prescription.
How Supplied: Jars ½ oz. NDC-51244-501-04, 2 oz. NDC-51244-501-60, ½ oz. in 4 oz. pack of 8 × ½ oz. NDC-51244-501-14, 4 oz. BULK NDC-51244-501-12, ½ oz. in 16 oz. pack of 32 × ½ oz. NDC-51244-501-44, 16 oz. BULK NDC-51244-501-48.

DECUBITEX™ POWDER ℞

Ingredients: Micronized Biebrich Scarlet Red, Sulfonated, Water Soluble 0.1% in a powder base containing Biosorb™ brand of Starch, Zinc Oxide, Sodium Propionate, Methylparaben and Propylparaben.
Indication: As an aid in the management of decubitus ulcers, especially in early stages where abundant secretions are present.
Administration: Pour a small amount of 3% Hydrogen Peroxide or Sterile Normal Saline onto the affected area. Cleanse thoroughly and powder. Cover with dry sterile gauze. Dressing should be changed twice daily.
Contraindications: Known hypersensitivity to any of the ingredients.
Adverse Reactions: Gastroenteritis and renal irritation have been reported following percutaneous absorption over a massive area.
Dispensing Instructions: Dispense in original container.
Caution: Federal law prohibits dispensing without prescription.
How Supplied:
10 gram Bulk Shaker Jar NDC 51244-301-10
30 gram Bulk Shaker Jar NDC 51244-301-30
30 gram Unit-Dose Foil Packets in Dispenser Roll of
30 × 1 gram Packet NDC 51244-301-33
100 gram Unit-Dose Foil Packets in Dispenser Roll of
100 × 1 gram Packet NDC 51244-301-99

HISTORAL™ ℞

Ingredients: Each capsule contains in a sustained-release form: Chlorpheniramine Maleate 12 mg., Pseudoephedrine HCl 60 mg., Methscopolamine Nitrate 2.5 mg.
Each 5cc contains: Chlorpheniramine Maleate 2 mg., Pseudoephedrine HCl 30 mg., Methcopolamine Nitrate 0.5 mg., in a dye-free liquid.
Action: Antihistaminic-Decongestant; Chlorpheniramine Maleate is a potent antihistamine with an excellent therapeutic index and low incidence of side effects, particularly the sedation associated with many other antihistamines. Pseudoephedrine hydrochloride provides a rapid and sustained decongestant effect on swollen mucosa of the respiratory tract. It does this by vasoconstriction and opens obstructed airways through direct action on the smooth muscle of the bronchi. The vasoconstrictor action of pseudoephedrine is similar to that of ephedrine. In the usual oral dosage, it has minimal vasopressor effects. Methscopolamine Nitrate affords atropine-like action without the deep CNS stimulation associated with scopolamine (Goodman and Gilman: "Pharmacological Basic of Therapeutics") September, 1969.
The liquid is dye-free.
Indication: For relief of upper respiratory and bronchial congestion associated with; the common cold, hay fever and allergies, sinusitis, influenza, and vasomotor and allergic rhinitis.
Contraindications: Sensitivity to antihistamines or sympathomimetic agents. It should not be used in patients with severe hypertension or coronary artery disease. Capsules should not be given to children under 12 years of age.
Warnings: Use with caution in patients suffering from hypertension, cardiac disease, or hyperthyroidism. Patients susceptible to the soporific effects of chlorpheniramine should be warned against driving or operating machinery should drowsiness occur.
Precautions: Use with caution in the presence of hypertension, coronary artery disease, narrow-angle glaucoma, prostatic hypertrophy, hyperthyroidism and diabetes. Patients should be cautioned about possible additive effects with alcohol and other central nervous system depressants (hypnotics, sedatives, tranquilizers), and should be cautioned against hazardous occupations requiring complete mental alertness such as operating machinery or driving a motor vehicle. If a sensitivity reaction or idiosyncrasy should occur, withdraw the drug.
Adverse Reactions: Most patients will have no side effects at the usual dosage. However, certain patients may exhibit mild stimulation or mild sedation. Although rare, hypersensitivity to either the antihistamine or decongestant may occur.
The liquid is dye-free.
Dosage: Capsules—Adults and children over 12, one capsule every 12 hours. Liquid—Adults and children over 12, 1 or 2 teaspoonsful; children 6 to 12, 1 teaspoonful; children 3 to 6 years, ½ teaspoonful. May be repeated in 4 to 6 hours if required for relief.
How Supplied: Bottles of 100 NDC-51244-102-01 and 1000 NDC-51244-102-10. Liquid in 16 oz. NDC-51244-302-16 and gallon NDC-51244-302-28.

HISTORAL™ PEDIATRIC ORAL DROPS ℞

Ingredients: Each 1.0 ml. contains Pseudoephedrine hydrochloride 30 mg decongestant effect on swollen mucosa of the respiratory tract. It does this by vasoconstriction and opens obstructed airways through direct action on the smooth muscle of the bronchi. The vasoconstrictor action of pseudoephedrine is similar to that of ephedrine. In the usual oral dosage, it has minimal vasopressor effects.
Indications: HISTORAL™ PEDIATRIC ORAL DROPS is indicated when mucosal decongestion and bronchodilation are desired in the following upper and lower respiratory tract disorders of allergic, infection or nonspecific etiology.
allergic rhinitis, nasopharyngitis, common cold, bronchitis, sinusitis, otitis media, eustachian tube obstruction, laryngitis, tracheitis, croup
In patients with nasopharyngitis and a history of otitis media. HISTORAL™ PEDIATRIC ORAL DROPS may be used prophylactically to permit better drainage through the eustachian tube.
Contraindications: There is no known contraindications to the use of HISTORAL™ PEDIATRIC ORAL DROPS as adjunctive therapy to antibiotics in the treatment of respiratory infections when relief of mucosal congestion is desired.
Warnings: Do not exceed recommended doses because at higher doses nervousness, dizziness or sleeplessness may occur. Patients having heart disease, high blood pressure, diabetes, thyroid disease or patients taking antihypertensive or antidepressant drugs containing a monoamine oxidase inhibitor should not use this preparation or should be carefully monitored. If a sensitivity reaction or idiosyncrasy should occur, withdraw the drug.
Precautions: Although pseudoephedrine causes virtually no pressor effects in normotensive patients, use with caution in hypersensitives.
Adverse Reactions: While the majority of patients will experience no side effects from pseudoephedrine, those particularly sensitive to sympathomimetic amines may note mild central nervous system stimulation.
Dispensing: Dispense in original container.
Dosage and Administration. USUAL DOSAGE:
1—3 months, 0.25 ml. 4 times a day BY MOUTH ONLY.
4—6 months, 0.50 ml. 4 times a day BY MOUTH ONLY.
7—9 months, 0.75 ml. 4 times a day BY MOUTH ONLY
10—18 months, 1.00 ml. 4 times a day BY MOUTH ONLY
How Supplied: 30 ml. bottle with accompanying calibrated dropper in box, NDC-51244-502-01

Ives Laboratories Inc.

685 THIRD AVENUE
NEW YORK, NY 10017

CERUBIDINE® ℞
(daunorubicin hydrochloride)
For Injection

WARNINGS

1. Cerubidine must be given into a rapidly flowing intravenous infusion. It must *never* be given by the intramuscular or subcutaneous route. Severe local tissue necrosis will occur if there is extravasation during administration.
2. Myocardial toxicity manifested in its most severe form by potentially fatal congestive heart failure may be encountered when total cumulative dosage exceeds 550 mg/m^2. This may occur either during therapy or several months after termination of therapy. Treatment with digitalis, diuretics, sodium restriction and bed-rest is indicated.

Continued on next page

Ives—Cont.

3. Severe myelosuppression occurs when used in therapeutic doses.
4. It is recommended that Cerubidine be administered only by physicians who are experienced in leukemia chemotherapy and in facilities with laboratory and supportive resources adequate to monitor drug tolerance and protect and maintain a patient compromised by drug toxicity. The physician and institution must be capable of responding rapidly and completely to severe hemorrhagic conditions, and/or overwhelming infection.
5. Dosage should be reduced in patients with impaired hepatic or renal function.

Description: Cerubidine (daunorubicin hydrochloride) is the hydrochloride salt of an anthracycline cytotoxic antibiotic produced by a strain of *Streptomyces coeruleorubidus.* It is soluble in water when adequately agitated and produces a reddish solution. It has the following structural formula which may be described with the chemical name of 7-(3-amino-2, 3, 6-trideoxy—L—lyxohexosyloxy) 9-acetyl-7, 8, 9, 10-tetrahydro-6, 9, 11-trihydroxy-4-methoxy-5, 12-naphthacenequinone hydrochloride. Its empirical formula is $C_{27}H_{29}NO_{10} \cdot HCl$ with a molecular weight of 563.99. It is a hygroscopic crystalline powder. The pH of a 5 mg/ml aqueous solution is 4.5–6.5.

Action: Cerubidine inhibits the synthesis of nucleic acids; its effect on deoxyribonucleic acid is particularly rapid and marked. Cerubidine has antimitotic and cytotoxic activity although the precise mode of action is unknown. Cerubidine displays an immunosuppressive effect. It has been shown to inhibit the production of heterohemagglutinins in mice. *In vitro,* it inhibits blast cell transformation of canine lymphocytes at 0.01 mcg/ml.

Cerubidine possesses a potent antitumor effect against a wide spectrum of animal tumors either grafted or spontaneous.

Pharmacology: Following intravenous injection of Cerubidine, plasma levels of daunorubicin decline rapidly indicating rapid tissue uptake and concentration. Thereafter, plasma levels decline slowly with a half-life of 18.5 hours. By 1 hour after drug administration, the predominant plasma species is daunorubicinol, an active metabolite, which disappears with a half-life of 26.7 hours. Further metabolism via reduction cleavage of the glycosidic bond, 4–0 demethylation, and conjugation with both sulfate and glucuronide have been demonstrated. Simple glycosidic cleavage of daunorubicin or daunorubicinol is not a significant metabolic pathway in man. Twenty-five percent of an administered dose of Cerubidine is eliminated in an active form by urinary excretion, and an estimated 40% by biliary excretion.

There is no evidence that Cerubidine crosses the blood-brain barrier.

Indications: Cerubidine is indicated for remission induction in acute non-lymphocytic leukemia (myelogenous, monocytic, erythroid) in adults.

Once complete remission has been achieved, an appropriate maintenance program should be instituted.

In the treatment of acute non-lymphocytic leukemia, Cerubidine used as a single agent has produced complete remission rates of 40–50%, and in combination with cytarabine, has produced complete remission rates of 53–65%.

Warnings: Therapy with Cerubidine should not be started in patients with pre-existing drug-induced bone marrow suppression unless the benefit from such treatment warrants the risk.

Pre-existing heart disease and previous therapy with doxorubicin are co-factors of increased risk of Cerubidine-induced cardiac toxicity, and the benefit to risk ratio of Cerubidine therapy in such patients should be weighed before starting Cerubidine.

Bone Marrow—Cerubidine is a potent bone marrow suppressant. Suppression will occur in all patients given a therapeutic dose of this drug.

Cardiac Effects—Special attention must be given to the cardiac toxicity of Cerubidine. At total cumulative doses less than 550 mg/m^2, acute congestive heart failure is seldom encountered. However, rare instances of pericarditis-myocarditis, not dose-related, have been reported. At cumulative doses exceeding 550 mg/m^2, there is an increased incidence of drug-induced congestive heart failure. Based on prior clinical experience with doxorubicin, this limit appears lower, namely 400 mg/m^2, in patients who received radiation therapy that encompassed the heart. Furthermore, the total dose of Cerubidine administered should also take into account any previous or concomitant therapy with other potentially cardiotoxic agents or related compounds such as doxorubicin.

There is absolutely no reliable method for predicting the patients in whom acute congestive heart failure will develop as a result of the cardiac toxic effect of Cerubidine. However, certain changes in the electrocardiogram and a decrease in the systolic ejection fraction from pre-treatment baseline may help to recognize those patients at greatest risk to develop congestive heart failure. On the basis of the electrocardiogram, a decrease equal to or greater than 30% in limb lead QRS voltage has been associated with a significant risk of drug-induced cardiomyopathy. Therefore, an electrocardiogram and/or determination of systolic ejection fraction should be performed before each course of Cerubidine. In the event that one or the other of these predictive parameters should occur, the benefit of continued therapy must be weighed against the risk of producing cardiac damage.

Early clinical diagnosis of drug-induced congestive heart failure appears to be essential for successful treatment with digitalis, diuretics, sodium restriction, and bed rest.

Evaluation of Hepatic and Renal Function—Significant hepatic or renal impairment can enhance the toxicity of the recommended doses of Cerubidine; therefore, prior to administration, evaluation of hepatic function and renal function using conventional clinical laboratory tests is recommended (See Dosage and Administration).

Pregnancy—Cerubidine can cause fetal harm when administered to a pregnant woman because of its teratogenic potential. If this drug is used during pregnancy, or if the patient becomes pregnant while taking this drug, the patient should be apprised of the potential hazard to the fetus.

Extravasation At Injection Site—Extravasation of Cerubidine at the site of intravenous administration can cause severe local tissue necrosis.

Precautions: Therapy with Cerubidine requires close observation of the patient and extensive chemical and laboratory monitoring. Cerubidine may induce hyperuricemia secondary to rapid lysis of leukemic cells. Blood uric acid levels should be monitored and appropriate therapy initiated in the event that hyperuricemia develops.

Appropriate measures must be taken to control any systemic infection before beginning therapy with Cerubidine.

Cerubidine may transiently impart a red coloration to the urine after administration, and patients should be advised to expect this.

Carcinogenesis, mutagenesis, impairment of fertility: Cerubidine, when injected subcutaneously into mice, causes fibrosarcomas to develop at the injection site. When administered to mice orally or intraperitoneally, no carcinogenic effect was noted after 22 months of observation.

In male dogs at a daily dose of 0.25 mg/kg administered intravenously, testicular atrophy was noted at autopsy. Histologic examination revealed total aplasia of the spermatocyte series in the seminiferous tubules with complete aspermatogenesis.

PREGNANCY CATEGORY D. See Warnings Section.

Adverse Reactions: Dose-limiting toxicity includes myelosuppression and cardiotoxicity (see Warnings). Other reactions include:

Cutaneous—Reversible alopecia occurs in most patients.

Gastrointestinal—Acute nausea and vomiting occur but are usually mild. Antiemetic therapy may be of some help. Mucositis may occur three to seven days after administration. Diarrhea has occasionally been reported.

Local—If extravasation occurs during administration, tissue necrosis can result at the site.

Acute Reactions—Rarely fever, chills, and skin rash can occur.

Dosage and Administration:

Principles—In order to eradicate the leukemic cells and induce a complete remission, a profound suppression of the bone marrow is usually required. Evaluation of both the peripheral blood and bone marrow are mandatory in the formulation of appropriate treatment plans.

In the treatment of acute non-lymphocytic leukemia, Cerubidine is effective either alone or in combination with certain other antileukemic drugs. Combinations incorporating Cerubidine improve the complete remission frequency. Appropriate maintenance therapy should be instituted following the successful induction of a complete remission.

It is recommended that the dosage of Cerubidine be reduced in instances of hepatic or renal impairment. For example, using serum bilirubin and serum creatinine as indicators of liver and kidney function, the following dose modifications are recommended:

Serum Bilirubin	Serum Creatinine	Recommended Dose
1.2–3.0 mg %		¾ normal dose
> 3 mg %	> 3 mg %	½ normal dose

Representative dose schedules and combination for the approved indication of adult acute non-lymphocytic leukemia:

As a Single Agent[1] — Cerubidine 60 mg/m^2/day IV on days 1,2,3 every 3—4 weeks.

In Combination[2,3]—Cerubidine 45 mg/m^2/day IV on days 1,2,3 of the first course and on days 1,2 of subsequent courses **AND** cytosine arabinoside 100 mg/m^2/day IV infusion daily for 7 days for the first course and for 5 days for subsequent courses.

The attainment of a normal appearing bone marrow may require up to three courses of induction therapy. The evaluation of the bone marrow following recovery from the previous course of induction therapy determines whether a further course of induction treatment is required.

The contents of a vial should be reconstituted with 4 ml of sterile water for injection, U.S.P., and agitated gently until the material has completely dissolved. The withdrawable vial contents provide 20 mg of daunorubicin activity, with 5 mg of daunorubicin activity per ml. The desired dose is withdrawn into a syringe containing 10–15 ml of normal saline and then injected into the tubing or sidearm of a rapidly flowing i.v. infusion of 5 percent glucose or normal saline solution. Cerubidine should not be administered mixed with other drugs or heparin. The reconstituted solution is stable for 24 hours at room temperature and 48 hours under refrigeration. It should be protected from exposure to sunlight.

How Supplied: Cerubidine (daunorubicin hydrochloride) for injection is available in butyl rubber-stoppered vials, each containing 20 mg of base activity (21.4 mg as the hydrochloride salt) and 100 mg of mannitol as a sterile reddish lyophilized powder. When reconstituted with 4 ml of sterile water for injection, U.S.P., each ml contains 5 mg of daunorubicin activity. Each package contains 10 vials. Storage (+15° to +25°C).

References:

1. Wiernik, P. H., Schimpff, S. C., Schiffer, C. A., et al: Randomized Clinical Comparison of Daunorubicin (NSC-82151) Alone with a Combination of Daunorubicin, Cytosine Arabinoside (NSC-63878), 6-Thioguanine (NSC-752) and Pyrimethamine (NSC-3061) for the Treatment of Acute Non-lymphocytic Leukemia. Cancer Treat Rep. 60: 41–53, 1979.
2. Yates, J. W., Wallace, J. H., Ellison, R. R., Holland, J. F.: Cytosine Arabinoside (NSC-63878) and Daunorubicin (NSC-83142) Therapy in Acute Non-lymphocytic Leukemia. Cancer Chemo Rep. 57: 485–488, 1973.
3. Rai, K. R., Holland, J. F., Glidewell, O.: Improvement in Remission Induction Therapy of Acute Myelocytic Leukemia. Proc. Am. Assoc. Cancer Res., Am. Soc. Clin. Oncol. 16: 265, 1975.

Literature Available: Yes

[Cir. CI 3052-1 6/26/80]

CYCLOSPASMOL® ℞
(cyclandelate)
Capsules-Tablets

Composition: Each *blue* and *red* capsule contains 400 mg. of cyclandelate, and each *blue* capsule contains 200 mg. of cyclandelate. Each *orange* tablet contains 100 mg. cyclandelate.

Actions: CYCLOSPASMOL is an orally acting vasodilator. The activity of this drug, as measured by pharmacological tests against various types of smooth-muscle spasm produced by acetylcholine, histamine, and barium chloride, exceeds that of papaverine, particularly in regard to the neurotropic component produced by the acetylcholine. Cyclandelate is musculotropic, acting directly on vascular smooth muscle, and has no significant adrenergic stimulating or blocking actions.

The drug is not intended to substitute for other appropriate medical or surgical programs in the treatment of peripheral or cerebral vascular disease.

Indications

Based on a review of this drug by the National Academy of Sciences—National Research Council and/or other information, FDA has classified the indications as follows:

"Possibly" effective: CYCLOSPASMOL is indicated for adjunctive therapy in intermittent claudication; arteriosclerosis obliterans; thrombophlebitis (to control associated vasospasm and muscular ischemia); nocturnal leg cramps; Raynaud's phenomenon; and for selected cases of ischemic cerebral vascular disease.

Final classification of the less-than-effective indications requires further investigation.

Contraindications: CYCLOSPASMOL is contraindicated in cases of known hypersensitivity to the drug.

Warnings: 1. Cyclandelate should be used with extreme caution in patients with severe obliterative coronary artery or cerebral-vascular disease, since there is a possibility that these diseased areas may be compromised by vasodilatory effects of the drug elsewhere. 2. **Use In Pregnancy:** The safety of cyclandelate for use during pregnancy or lactation has not been established; therefore, it should not be used in pregnant women or in women of childbearing age unless, in the judgment of the physician, its use is deemed absolutely essential to the welfare of the patient. 3. Although no prolongation of bleeding time has been demonstrated in humans in therapeutic dosages, it has been demonstrated in animals at very large doses. Therefore, the hazard of a prolonged bleeding time should be carefully considered when administering cyclandelate to a patient with active bleeding or a bleeding tendency.

Precautions: Since CYCLOSPASMOL (cyclandelate) is a vasodilator, it should be used with caution in patients having glaucoma.

Adverse Reactions: Gastrointestinal distress (pyrosis, pain, and eructation) may occur with CYCLOSPASMOL. These symptoms occur infrequently and are usually mild. Relief can often be obtained by taking the medication with meals or by the concomitant use of antacids.

Mild flush, headache, feeling of weakness, or tachycardia may occur, especially during the first weeks of administration.

Dosage and Administration: It is often advantageous to initiate therapy at higher dosage; e.g.: 1200-1600 mg. per day, given in divided doses before meals and at bedtime. When a clinical response is noted, the dosage can be decreased in 200-mg. decrements until the maintenance dosage is reached. The usual maintenance dosage of CYCLOSPASMOL (cyclandelate) is between 400 and 800 mg. per day given in two to four divided doses.

Although objective signs of therapeutic benefit may be rapid and dramatic, more often, this improvement occurs gradually over weeks of therapy. It is strongly recommended that the patient be educated to the fact that prolonged use may be necessary. Short-term use of CYCLOSPASMOL is rarely beneficial, nor is it likely to be of any permanent value.

How Supplied: 400 mg. blue and red capsules in bottles of 100, and 500; and Clinipak®, Unit Dose Medication, 100 capsules (20 strips of 5). 200 mg. blue capsules in bottles of 100, 500, and 1000; and Clinipak®, Unit Dose Medication, 100 capsules (20 strips of 5); 100 mg. orange tablets in bottles of 100 and 500.

Literature Available: Yes.

[Cir. 3016-2 7/14/80]

[*Shown in Product Identification Section*]

ISORDIL® ℞
(isosorbide dinitrate)
(10 Dosage Forms)

Actions: The basic action of ISORDIL is that of all nitrates, the relaxation of smooth muscle. How this relates to its clinical usefulness in the treatment of angina pectoris (pain of coronary artery disease) is not clear, since the exact cause of this pain is also obscure.

The objective of therapy is a decrease in the frequency and severity of attacks of angina pectoris and a decrease in the need to use nitroglycerin. This is the only practical way to judge the effects of therapy, especially since there is a wide variation in symptomatic response to treatment. ISORDIL is widely accepted as a safe and useful therapeutic agent in the treatment of angina pectoris.

Indications

Based on a review of this drug by the National Academy of Sciences—National Research Council and/or other information, FDA has classified the indications as follows:

"Probably" effective: When taken by the sublingual or chewable route, ISORDIL SUBLINGUAL and CHEWABLE tablets are indicated for the treatment of acute anginal attacks and for prophylaxis in situations likely to provoke such attacks.

"Possibly" effective: When taken by the oral route, ISORDIL is indicated for the relief of angina pectoris (pain of coronary artery disease). It is not intended to abort the acute anginal episode, but is widely regarded as useful in the prophylactic treatment of angina pectoris.

Final classification of the less-than-effective indications requires further investigation.

Contraindication: Idiosyncrasy to this drug.

Warning: Data supporting the use of nitrites during the early days of the acute phase of myocardial infarction (the period during which clinical and laboratory findings are unstable) are insufficient to establish safety.

Precautions: 1. Tolerance to this drug, and cross-tolerance to other nitrites and nitrates may occur. 2. In patients with functional or organic gastrointestinal hypermotility or malabsorption syndrome, it is suggested that either the ISORDIL 5 mg., 10 mg., 20 mg., or 30 mg. Oral TITRADOSE® tablets, ISORDIL 2.5 mg., 5 mg., or 10 mg. SUBLINGUAL tablets, 10 mg. ISORDIL CHEWABLE tablets, or 40 mg. ISORDIL TEMBIDS® **capsules** be the preferred therapy. The reason for this is that a few patients have reported passing partially dissolved ISORDIL TEMBIDS **tablets** in their stools. This phenomenon is believed to be on the basis of physiologic variability and to reflect rapid gastrointestinal transit of the tablet.

Adverse Reactions: 1. Cutaneous vasodilation with flushing. 2. Headache is common and may be severe and persistent. 3. Transient episodes of dizziness and weakness, as well as other signs of cerebral ischemia associated with postural hypotension, may occasionally develop. 4. This drug can act as a physiological antagonist to norepinephrine, acetylcholine, histamine, and many other agents. 5. An occasional individual exhibits marked sensitivity to the hypotensive effects of nitrite, and severe responses (nausea, vomiting, weakness, restlessness, pallor, perspiration, and collapse) can occur even with the usual therapeutic dose. Alcohol may enhance this effect. 6. Drug rash and/or exfoliative dermatitis may occasionally occur.

Dosage and Administration: ISORDIL (isosorbide dinitrate) 2.5 mg., 5 mg., and 10 mg. SUBLINGUAL tablets. The basic dosage is one 5 mg. or 10 mg. tablet every 2 to 3 hours. The 2.5 mg. tablet facilitates adjustment of dosage in patients who may require it. All dosage forms are used sublingually for treatment of an angina pectoris attack (including angina decubitus) or prophylactically in situations likely to provoke such attacks.

ISORDIL 10 mg. CHEWABLE tablets. The smallest effective dose should be used. The initial dose should be no more than 5 mg (½ tablet) as an occasional severe hypotensive response may occur. The low dose may be effective in relieving the acute attack, but if no significant hypotension is seen, an increase in dose may permit more effective prevention of attacks. The chewable tablet is scored to permit dosage adjustment. For relief of the acute attack, the medication may be taken p.r.n. For prophylaxis, it may be taken every 2–3 hours.

ISORDIL 5 mg., 10 mg., 20 mg., or 30 mg. ORAL TITRADOSE tablets with E.Z. SPLIT® scoring are administered orally. The dosage range is 5 mg. to 30 mg. q.i.d., with the usual dosage being 10 mg. to 20 mg. q.i.d., before meals and at bedtime.

The uniquely designed and patented **TITRADOSE E.Z. SPLIT** Oral Tablet dosage forms permit clean-cut splitting of the tablet into equal halves to simplify more accurate

Continued on next page

Ives—Cont.

dosage titration. Thus, the physician may prescribe (or adjust) a dosage regimen to include half-tablet units for optimal relief. To break the tablet into two even halves, the patient has only to place the tablet on a hard, flat surface, scored side up, and then press the scored surface lightly with the index finger or thumb. Isordil Oral 5, 10, 20, and 30 mg. **TITRADOSE** Tablets replace the former, conventionally-scored tablets.

ISORDIL (10 mg.) with PHENOBARBITAL (15 mg.) tablets are indicated when anxiety or emotional disturbances are important factors in the clinical picture. The dosage regimen is one tablet four times daily, before meals and at bedtime. **(Warning: Phenobarbital may be habit-forming.)**

ISORDIL TEMBIDS *TABLETS* 40 mg. and ISORDIL TEMBIDS *CAPSULES* 40 mg.: These sustained-action medications are administered orally every 6 to 12 hours according to need. They are indicated for sustained prophylaxis against angina pectoris attacks including nocturnal angina. Although the latter condition is relatively infrequent, it is nonetheless angina, i.e., pain of coronary artery disease. The drug is gradually released over a 6-hour period to provide 8–10 hours of sustained effect. Although experiencing a reduction in the number of anginal attacks while under TEMBIDS therapy, patients may still have an attack under stressful conditions. In such cases, the therapy should be supplemented with Sublingual ISORDIL Tablets or nitroglycerin. ISORDIL TEMBIDS SHOULD NOT BE CHEWED.

How Supplied: ISORDIL SUBLINGUAL 2.5 mg.: Supplied in bottles of 100 and 500 yellow tablets. ISORDIL SUBLINGUAL 5 mg.: Supplied in bottles of 100, 250, and 500 pink tablets. ISORDIL SUBLINGUAL 10 mg.: Supplied in bottle of 100 white tablets. ISORDIL CHEWABLE 10 mg.: Supplied in bottles of 100 scored, yellow tablets. ISORDIL ORAL TITRADOSE 5 mg.: Supplied in bottles of 100, 500, and 1000 scored, pink tablets. ISORDIL ORAL TITRADOSE 10 mg.: Supplied in bottles of 100, 500, and 1000 scored, white tablets. ISORDIL ORAL TITRADOSE 20 mg.: Supplied in bottles of 100 and 500 scored, green tablets. ISORDIL ORAL TITRADOSE 30 mg.: Supplied in bottles of 100 scored, blue tablets. ISORDIL (10 mg.) WITH PHENOBARBITAL (15 mg.): Supplied in bottles of 100 and 500 scored, orange tablets. ISORDIL TEMBIDS Tablets 40 mg.: Supplied in bottles of 100, 500, and 1000 scored, green, sustained-action tablets. ISORDIL TEMBIDS Capsules, 40 mg.: Supplied in bottles of 100 and 500 sustained-action capsules (opaque blue cap and colorless, transparent body).

Clinipak® Unit Dose Medication, Boxes of 100 Tablets (20 strips of 5), is available as:

Isordil Sublingual Tablets, 2.5 mg
Isordil Sublingual Tablets, 5 mg
Isordil Sublingual Tablets, 10 mg.
Isordil Chewable Tablets, 10 mg
Isordil Oral Titradose, 5 mg
Isordil Oral Titradose, 10 mg
Isordil Oral Titradose, 20 mg

Clinical Studies: ISORDIL (isosorbide dinitrate) is widely regarded as an effective, long-acting coronary vasodilator for the management of angina pectoris associated with coronary insufficiency. It may significantly reduce the number, duration, and severity of angina attacks. Exercise tolerance may be increased in some patients with all forms of ISORDIL. The 5 mg. sublingual tablet, however, provides greater benefit both in regard to the number of patients who respond to it and the amount of exercise tolerated. Clinical improvement has been customarily measured subjectively by reduction in number of angina attacks and by the change in nitroglycerin requirements.

The 5 mg. ISORDIL SUBLINGUAL tablet has been evaluated clinically, and by employing exercise tolerance tests, it has been found that this dosage has an onset of action within the range of 2 to 5 minutes, which in some instances is not as rapid as nitroglycerin (but almost equal in magnitude). Duration of action, however, ranges from 1 to 2 hours, which compares with a duration of action of 20 to 30 minutes in the case of nitroglycerin.

Kinetocardiographic clinical studies indicate that the 10 mg. oral tablet and 40 mg. TEMBID tablet are effective for prolonged periods. Exercise tolerance tests have similarly shown that 40 mg. TEMBIDS capsules are effective for at least 6 hours.

In patients subjected to emotional or physical stress, the oral 5 mg., 10 mg., 20 mg., 30 mg., and 40 mg. ISORDIL medications are of limited effectiveness. In situations where the patient may be exposed to unusual stress, it is suggested that the 2.5 mg., 5 mg., or 10 mg. ISORDIL SUBLINGUAL tablet or 10 mg. chewable tablet be used supplementally as required.

Cinecoronary arteriographic studies have demonstrated that ISORDIL can produce a marked dilatation of the larger branches of the coronary arteries (larger than 200 microns). Dilatation of these coronary arteries and collateral coronary arteries persists for more than two hours after Sublingual ISORDIL, as demonstrated by cinecoronary arteriography. The correlation of this demonstrated dilation to increased coronary flow or improvement in clinical angina has not been established.

Literature Available: Yes.

TEMBIDS®—Trademark for sustained action capsules and tablets.

[Cir. 3020-4—Rev. 9/11/'81]

[*Shown in Product Identification Section*]

SURMONTIL® ℞
(trimipramine maleate)

Description: SURMONTIL® (trimipramine maleate) is 5 - (3 - dimethylamino-2-methylpropyl)-10,11-dihydro-5H-dibenz (b,f) azepine acid maleate (racemic form).

Trimipramine maleate is prepared as a racemic mixture which can be resolved into levorotatory and dextrorotatory isomers. Trimipramine maleate is an almost odorless, white or slightly cream-colored crystalline substance melting at 140–144° C. It is very slightly soluble in ether and water, is slightly soluble in ethyl alcohol and acetone, and freely soluble in chloroform and methanol at 20° C.

Clinical Pharmacology: SURMONTIL® is an antidepressant with an anxiety-reducing, sedative component to its action. The mode of action of SURMONTIL® on the central nervous system is not known. However, unlike amphetamine-type compounds it does not act primarily by stimulation of the central nervous system. It does not act by inhibition of the monoamine oxidase system.

Indications: SURMONTIL® is indicated for the relief of symptoms of depression. Endogenous depression is more likely to be alleviated than other depressive states. In studies with neurotic out-patients, the drug appeared to be equivalent to amitripytyline in the less depressed patients but somewhat less effective than amitriptyline in the more severely depressed patients. In hospitalized depressed patients, trimipramine and imipramine were equally effective in relieving depression.

Contraindications: SURMONTIL® is contraindicated in cases of known hypersensitivity to the drug. The possibility of cross-sensitivity to other dibenzazepine compounds should be kept in mind. SURMONTIL® should not be given in conjunction with drugs of the monoamine oxidase inhibitor class (e.g.: tranylcypromine, isocarboxazid or phenelzine sulfate). The concomitant use of monoamine oxidase inhibitors (MAOI) and tricyclic compounds similar to SURMONTIL® has caused severe hyperpyretic reactions, convulsive crises, and death in some patients. At least two weeks should elapse after cessation of therapy with MAOI before instituting therapy with SURMONTIL®. Initial dosage should be low and increased gradually with caution and careful observation of the patient. The drug is contraindicated during the acute recovery period after a myocardial infarction.

Warnings:

Use in Children—This drug is not recommended for use in children, since safety and effectiveness in the pediatric age group have not been established.

General Consideration for Use—Extreme caution should be used when this drug is given to patients with any evidence of cardiovascular disease because of the possibility of conduction defects, arrhythmias, myocardial infarction, strokes, and tachycardia.

Caution is advised in patients with increased intraocular pressure, history of urinary retention, or history of narrow-angle glaucoma because of the drug's anticholinergic properties; hyperthyroid patients or those on thyroid medication because of the possibility of cardiovascular toxicity; patients with a history of seizure disorder because this drug has been shown to lower the seizure threshold; patients receiving guanethidine or similar agents since SURMONTIL® may block the pharmacologic effects of these drugs.

Since the drug may impair the mental and/or physical abilities required for the performance of potentially hazardous tasks, such as operating an automobile or machinery, the patient should be cautioned accordingly.

Precautions: The possibility of suicide is inherent in any severely depressed patient, and persists until a significant remission occurs. When a patient with a serious suicidal potential is not hospitalized, the prescription should be for the smallest amount feasible.

In schizophrenic patients activation of the psychosis may occur and require reduction of dosage or the addition of a major tranquilizer to the therapeutic regime.

Manic or hypomanic episodes may occur in some patients, in particular those with cyclic-type disorders. In some cases therapy with SURMONTIL® must be discontinued until the episode is relieved, after which therapy may be reinstituted at lower dosages if still required.

Concurrent administration of SURMONTIL® and electroshock therapy may increase the hazards of therapy. Such treatment should be limited to those patients for whom it is essential. When possible, discontinue the drug for several days prior to elective surgery.

Patients should be warned that the concomitant use of alcoholic beverages may be associated with exaggerated effects.

It has been reported that tricyclic antidepressants can potentiate the effects of catecholamines. Similarly, atropine-like effects may be more pronounced in patients receiving anticholinergic therapy. Therefore, particular care should be exercised when it is necessary to administer tricyclic antidepressants with sympathomimetic amines, local decongestants, local anesthetics containing epinephrine, atropine or drugs with an anticholinergic effect. In resistant cases of depression in adults, a dose of 2.5 mg/kg/day may have to be exceeded. If a higher dose is needed, ECG monitoring should be maintained during the initiation of therapy and at appropriate intervals during stabilization of dose.

Usage in Pregnancy—Pregnancy Category C. SURMONTIL® has shown evidence of embryo-toxicity and/or increased incidence of major anomalies in rats or rabbits at doses 20 times the human dose. There are no adequate and well-controlled studies in pregnant women. SURMONTIL® should be used during

pregnancy only if the potential benefit justifies the potential risk to the fetus.
Semen studies in man (four schizophrenics and nine normal volunteers) revealed no significant changes in sperm morphology. It is recognized that drugs having a parasympathetic effect, including tricyclic antidepressants, may alter the ejaculatory response.
Chronic animal studies showed occasional evidence of degeneration of seminiferous tubules at the highest dose of 60 mg/kg/day.
SURMONTIL® should be used with caution in patients with impaired liver function.
Chronic animal studies showed occasional occurrence of hepatic congestion, fatty infiltration, or increased serum liver enzymes at the highest dose of 60 mg/kg/day.
Both elevation and lowering of blood sugar have been reported with tricyclic antidepressants.

Adverse Reactions:
Note: The pharmacological similarities among the tricyclic antidepressants require that each of the reactions be considered when SURMONTIL® is administered. Some of the adverse reactions included in this listing have not in fact been reported with SURMONTIL®.
Cardiovascular—Hypotension, hypertension, tachycardia, palpitation, myocardial infarction, arrhythmias, heart block, stroke.
Psychiatric—Confusional states (especially the elderly) with hallucinations, disorientation, delusions; anxiety, restlessness, agitation; insomnia and nightmares; hypomania; exacerbation of psychosis.
Neurological—Numbness, tingling, paresthesias of extremities; incoordination, ataxia, tremors; peripheral neuropathy; extrapyramidal symptoms; seizures, alterations in EEG patterns; tinnitus.
Anticholinergic—Dry mouth and, rarely, associated sublingual adenitis; blurred vision, disturbances of accommodation, mydriasis, constipation, paralytic ileus; urinary retention, delayed micturition, dilation of the urinary tract.
Allergic—Skin rash, petechiae, urticaria, itching, photo-sensitization, edema of face and tongue.
Hematologic—Bone-marrow depression including agranulocytosis, eosinophilia; purpura; thrombocytopenia. Leukocyte and differential counts should be performed in any patient who develops fever and sore throat during therapy; the drug should be discontinued if there is evidence of pathological neutrophil depression.
Gastrointestinal—Nausea and vomiting, anorexia, epigastric distress, diarrhea, peculiar taste, stomatitis, abdominal cramps, black tongue.
Endocrine—Gynecomastia in the male; breast enlargement and galactorrhea in the female; increased or decreased libido, impotence; testicular swelling; elevation or depression of blood-sugar levels.
Other—Jaundice (simulating obstructive); altered liver function; weight gain or loss; perspiration; flushing; urinary frequency; drowsiness, dizziness, weakness, and fatigue; headache; parotid swelling; alopecia.
Withdrawal Symptoms—Though not indicative of addiction, abrupt cessation of treatment after prolonged therapy may produce nausea, headache, and malaise.

Dosage and Administration: Dosage should be initiated at a low level and increased gradually, noting carefully the clinical response and any evidence of intolerance.
Lower dosages are recommended for elderly patients and adolescents. Lower dosages are also recommended for outpatients as compared to hospitalized patients who will be under close supervision. It is not possible to prescribe a single dosage schedule of SURMONTIL® that will be therapeutically effective in all patients. The physical psychodynamic factors contributing to depressive symptomatology are very complex; spontaneous remissions or exacerbations of depressive symptoms may occur with or without drug therapy. Consequently, the recommended dosage regimens are furnished as a guide which may be modified by factors such as the age of the patient, chronicity and severity of the disease, medical condition of the patient, and degree of psychotherapeutic support.
Most antidepressant drugs have a lag period of ten days to four weeks before a therapeutic response is noted. Increasing the dose will not shorten this period, but rather increase the incidence of adverse reactions.

Usual Adult Dose:
Outpatients and Office Patients—Initially, 75 mg/day in divided doses, increased to 150 mg/day. Dosages over 200 mg/day are not recommended. Maintenance therapy is in the range of 50–150 mg/day. For convenient therapy and to facilitate patient compliance, the total dosage requirement may be given at bedtime.
Hospitalized Patients—Initially, 100 mg/day in divided doses. This may be increased gradually in a few days to 200 mg/day depending upon individual response and tolerance. If improvement does not occur in 2–3 weeks, the dose may be increased to the maximum recommended dose of 250–300 mg/day.
Adolescent and Geriatric Patients—Initially, a dose of 50 mg/day daily is recommended, with gradual increments up to 100 mg/day depending upon patient response and tolerance.
Maintenance—Following remission, maintenance medication may be required for a longer period of time, at the lowest dose that will maintain remission. Maintenance therapy is preferably administered as a single dose at bedtime. To minimize relapse, maintenance therapy should be continued for about three months.

Overdosage:
Signs and Symptoms—The response of the patient to toxic overdosage of tricyclic antidepressants may vary in severity and is conditioned by factors such as age, amount ingested, amount absorbed, interval between ingestion and start of treatment. SURMONTIL® is not recommended for infants or young children. Should accidental ingestion occur in any amount, it should be regarded as serious and potentially fatal.
CNS abnormalities may include drowsiness, stupor, coma, ataxia, restlessness, agitation, hyperactive reflexes, muscle rigidity, athetoid and choreiform movements and convulsions. Cardiac abnormalities may include arrhythmia, tachycardia, ECG evidence of impaired conduction, and signs of congestive failure. Other symptoms may include respiratory depression, cyanosis, hypotension, shock, vomiting, hyperpyrexia, mydriasis, and diaphoresis.
Treatment is supportive and symptomatic, as no specific antidote is known. Depending upon need the following measures can be considered:

1. SURMONTIL® is not recommended for use in infants and children. Hospitalization with continuous cardiac monitoring for up to 4 days is recommended for children who have ingested SURMONTIL® in any amount. This is based on the reported greater sensitivity of children to acute overdosage with tricyclic antidepressants.
2. Blood and urine levels may not reflect the severity of the poisoning and are mostly of diagnostic value.
3. CNS involvement, respiratory depression, or cardiac arrhythmia can occur suddenly; hospitalization and close observation are necessary, even when the amount ingested is thought to be small or initial toxicity appears slight. Patients with any alteration of ECG should have continuous cardiac monitoring for at least 72 hours and be observed until well after the cardiac status has returned to normal; relapses may occur after apparent recovery.
4. The slow intravenous administration of physostigmine salicylate has been reported to reverse most of the cardiovascular and CNS effects of overdosage with tricyclic antidepressants. In adults, 1 to 3 mg has been reported to be effective. In children, start with 0.5 mg and repeat at 5-minute intervals to determine the minimum effective dose; do not exceed 2.0 mg. Avoid rapid injection, to reduce the possibility of physostigmine-induced convulsions. Because of the short duration of action of physostigmine, it may be necessary to repeat doses at 30- to 60-minute intervals as necessary.
5. In the alert patient, empty the stomach rapidly by induced emesis, followed by lavage. In the obtunded patient, secure the airway with a cuffed endotracheal tube before beginning lavage (do not induce emesis). Instillation of activated-charcoal slurry may help reduce absorption of trimipramine.
6. Minimize external stimulation to reduce the tendency to convulsions. If anticonvulsants are necessary, diazepam, short-acting barbiturates, paraldehyde, or methocarbamol may be useful. Do not use barbiturates if MAO inhibitors have been taken recently.
7. Maintain adequate respiratory exchange. Do not use respiratory stimulants.
8. Shock should be treated with supportive measures, such as intravenous fluids, oxygen, and corticosteroids. Digitalis may increase conduction abnormalities and further irritate an already sensitized myocardium. If congestive heart failure necessitates rapid digitalization, particular care must be exercised.
9. Hyperpyrexia should be controlled by whatever external means available, including ice packs and cooling sponge baths if necessary.
10. Hemodialysis, peritoneal dialysis, exchange transfusions, and forced diuresis have been generally reported as ineffective in tricyclic poisoning.

How Supplied: SURMONTIL® (trimipramine maleate) Capsules are available as:
25 mg: in bottles of 100 opaque blue and yellow capsules.
50 mg: in bottles of 100 opaque blue and orange capsules.
100 mg. in bottles of 100 opaque blue and white capsules marked "Ives" and "4158".
Note: 100 mg. capsules approved too late to appear in Product Identification Section for 1983.
[Cir. CI 3059-2 Revised 7/15/82]
[*Shown in Product Identification Section*]

SYNALGOS® Capsules ℞

Composition: Each maroon and gray capsule contains:

Promethazine hydrochloride	6.25 mg.
Aspirin	356.4 mg.
Caffeine	30.0 mg.

Actions: Promethazine is a phenothiazine with sedative actions. Synalgos also contains the non-narcotic antipyretic-analgesic, aspirin.

Indications
Based on a review of this drug by the National Academy of Sciences-National Research Council and/or other information, FDA has classified the indications as follows:
"Possibly" effective for the relief of mild to moderate pain in those situations where the physician wishes to add a mild sedative effect.

Continued on next page

Ives—Cont.

> Final classification of the less-than-effective indications requires further investigation.

Contraindications: Hypersensitivity to aspirin or promethazine.
Warnings: Salicylates should be used with extreme caution in the presence of peptic ulcer or coagulation abnormalities. Promethazine may impair the mental and/or physical abilities required for the performance of potentially hazardous tasks such as driving a car or operating machinery. The patient using Synalgos should be cautioned accordingly.
Use with CNS Depressants: Synalgos may have additive effects with other CNS depressants (hypnotics, sedatives, tranquilizers, antianxiety agents). Patients who have demonstrated a hypersensitivity reaction (e.g. blood dyscrasia, jaundice) with a phenothiazine should not be re-exposed to any phenothiazine, including Synalgos, unless in the judgment of the physician the potential benefits of treatment outweigh the possible hazards.
Usage in Pregnancy: Reproduction studies have not been performed in animals. There is no adequate information on whether this drug may affect fertility in human males or females or has teratogenic potential or other adverse effect on the fetus.
Usage in Children: Since there is no experience in children who have received this drug, safety and efficacy in children have not been established.
Precautions: Promethazine should be administered cautiously to patients with cardiovascular or liver disease.
Adverse Reactions: Drowsiness, dizziness, light-headedness, sedation, skin reactions, nausea, vomiting, constipation, and rarely hypotension.
Dosage and Administration: Dosage should be adjusted according to the severity of the pain and the response of the patient. Synalgos is given orally. The usual adult dose is two capsules every 4 hours as needed for pain.
Drug Interactions: The CNS depressant effects of Synalgos may be additive with that of other CNS depressants. See Warnings. Aspirin may enhance the effects of anti-coagulants and inhibit the uricosuric effects of uricosuric agents.
How Supplied: Synalgos capsules: Supplied in bottles of 100 and 500 capsules.
Literature Available: Yes.
[Cir. CI 3061-1—3/20/81]
[*Shown in Product Identification Section*]

SYNALGOS®-DC Capsules ℞

Composition: Each blue and gray capsule contains:
Drocode (dihydrocodeine) bitartrate...16.0 mg.
Warning: May be habit-forming
Promethazine hydrochloride...............6.25 mg.
Aspirin...356.4 mg.
Caffeine...30.0 mg.
Actions: Dihydrocodeine is a semisynthetic narcotic analgesic, related to codeine, with multiple actions qualitatively similar to those of codeine; the most prominent of these involve the central nervous system and organs with smooth muscle components. The principal actions of therapeutic value are analgesia and sedation.
Promethazine is a phenothiazine with sedative actions.
Synalgos-DC also contains the non-narcotic antipyretic-analgesic, aspirin.

> **Indications**
> Based on a review of this drug by the National Academy of Sciences-National Research Council and/or other information, FDA has classified the indications as follows:
> "Possibly" effective for the relief of moderate to moderately severe pain in those situations where the physician wishes to add a mild sedative effect.
> Final classification of the less-than-effective indications requires further investigation.

Contraindications: Hypersensitivity to dihydrocodeine, codeine, promethazine, or aspirin.
Warnings: Salicylates should be used with extreme caution in the presence of peptic ulcer or coagulation abnormalities.
Drug Dependence: Dihydrocodeine can produce drug dependence of the codeine type and therefore has the potential of being abused. Psychic dependence, physical dependence and tolerance may develop upon repeated administration of dihydrocodeine and it should be prescribed and administered with the same degree of caution appropriate to the use of other oral narcotic containing medications.
Like other narcotic-containing medications, dihydrocodeine is subject to the provisions of the Federal Controlled Substances Act.
Usage in Ambulatory Patients: Dihydrocodeine and promethazine may impair the mental and/or physical abilities required for the performance of potentially hazardous tasks such as driving a car or operating machinery. The patient using Synalgos-DC should be cautioned accordingly.
Interactions with other Central Nervous System Depressants: Patients receiving other narcotic analgesics, general anesthetics, other phenothiazines, tranquilizers, sedative-hypnotics or other CNS depressants (including alcohol) concomitantly with Synalgos-DC may exhibit an additive CNS depression. When such combined therapy is contemplated, the dose of one or both agents should be reduced. Patients who have demonstrated a hypersensitivity reaction (e.g. blood dyscrasia, jaundice) with a phenothiazine should not be re-exposed to any phenothiazine, including Synalgos-DC, unless in the judgment of the physician the potential benefits of the treatment outweigh the possible hazards.
Usage in Pregnancy: Reproduction studies have not been performed in animals. There is no adequate information on whether this drug may affect fertility in human males and females or has a teratogenic potential or other adverse effect on the fetus.
Usage in Children: Since there is no experience in children who have received this drug, safety and efficacy in children have not been established.
Precautions: Promethazine should be administered cautiously to patients with cardiovascular or liver disease. Synalgos-DC should be given with caution to certain patients such as the elderly or debilitated, and those with hypothyroidism, Addison's disease and prostatic hypertrophy and urethral stricture.
Adverse Reactions: The most frequently observed reactions include lightheadedness, dizziness, drowsiness, sedation, nausea, vomiting, constipation, pruritus, skin reactions, and rarely hypotension.
Dosage and Administration: Dosage should be adjusted according to the severity of the pain and the response of the patient. Synalgos-DC is given orally. The usual adult dose is two capsules every 4 hours as needed for pain.
Drug Interactions: The CNS depressant effects of Synalgos-DC may be additive with that of other CNS depressants.
See Warnings.
Aspirin may enhance the effects of anticoagulants and inhibit the uricosuric effects of uricosuric agents.
How Supplied: Synalgos-DC capsules: Supplied in bottles of 100 and 500 capsules (DEA Schedule III).
Literature Available: Yes
[Cir. CI 3062-1 3/20/81]
[*Shown in Product Identification Section*]

TRECATOR®-SC ℞
(ethionamide)
Sugar-Coated Tablets

Action: Bacteriostatic against *Mycobacterium tuberculosis.*
Indications: Failure after adequate treatment with primary drugs (i.e. isoniazid, streptomycin, aminosalicylic acid) in any form of active tuberculosis. Ethionamide should only be given with other effective antituberculous agents.
Contraindications:
Severe hypersensitivity.
Severe hepatic damage.
Warning:
USE IN PREGNANCY: Teratogenic effects have been demonstrated in animals (rabbits, rats) receiving doses in excess of those recommended in humans. Use of the drug should be avoided during pregnancy or in women of childbearing potential, unless the benefits outweigh its possible hazard.
USE IN CHILDREN: Optimum dosage for children has not been established. This, however, does not preclude use of the drug when its use is crucial to therapy.
Precautions: Pretreatment examinations should include *in vitro* susceptibility tests of recent cultures of *M. tuberculosis* from the patient as measured against ethionomide and the usual primary antituberculous drugs.
Determinations of serum transaminase (SGOT, SGPT) should be made prior to and every 2 to 4 weeks during therapy.
In patients with diabetes mellitus, management may be more difficult and hepatitis occurs more frequently.
Ethionamide may intensify the adverse effects of the other antituberculous drugs administered concomitantly. Convulsions have been reported and special care should be taken, particularly when ethionamide is administered with cycloserine.
Adverse Reactions: The most common side effect is gastrointestinal intolerance.
Other adverse effects similar to those seen with isoniazid have been reported: peripheral neuritis, optic neuritis, psychic disturbances (including mental depression), postural hypotension, skin rashes, thrombocytopenia, pellagra-like syndrome, jaundice and/or hepatitis, increased difficulty in management of diabetes mellitus, stomatitis, gynecomastia, and impotence.
Dosage and Administration: Ethionamide should be administered with at least one other effective antituberculous drug.
Average adult dose: 0.5 gram to 1.0 gram/day in divided doses.
Concomitant administration of pyridoxine is recommended.
How Supplied: Trecator®-SC (ethionamide) is supplied as 250 mg. *orange*, sugar-coated tablets in bottles of 100.
Bibliography available upon request
[Cir. 3038-3—Revised 8/5/81]

Products are cross-indexed

by product classifications

in the

BLUE SECTION

Jacobus Pharmaceutical Co., Inc.
**37 CLEVELAND LANE
PRINCETON, NJ 08540**

DAPSONE USP ℞
25 mg. & 100 mg.

Description: Dapsone-USP, 4-4′ diaminodiphenylsulfone (DDS), is a primary treatment for Dermatitis herpetiformis. It is an effective antibacterial drug which has proved satisfactory in the treatment of leprosy. It is issued on prescription in tablets of 25 mg. and 100 mg. for oral administration.

NH_2–⟨C₆H₄⟩–SO_2–⟨C₆H₄⟩–NH_2

Clinical Pharmacology:
Actions: The mechanism of action in Dermatitis herpetiformis has not been established. By the kinetic method in mice, Dapsone is bactericidal as well as bacteriostatic against M. leprae.
Absorption and Excretion: Dapsone, when given orally, is rapidly and almost completely absorbed. About 85 percent of the daily intake is recoverable from the urine mainly in the form of water-soluble metabolities. Excretion of the drug is slow and a constant blood level can be maintained with the usual dosage.
Blood Levels: Detected a few minutes after ingestion, the drug reaches peak concentration in 4–8 hours. Daily administration for at least eight days is necessary to achieve a plateau level. With doses of 200 mg. daily, this level averaged 2.3 μgm/ml with a range of 0.1–7.0 μgm.
In man there are large individual differences in the rate of Dapsone clearance from the body. The half-life in the plasma in different individuals varies from ten hours to fifty hours and averages twenty eight hours. Repeat tests in the same individual show the clearance rate to be constant. Dapsone acetylation rates have been used to measure the acetylation phenotype. Daily administration (50–100 mg.) in leprosy patients will provide blood levels in excess of the usual minimum inhibitory concentration even for patients with a short Dapsone half-life.
Rifampicin lowers Dapsone levels 7 to 10 fold by accelerating plasma clearance.
Indications and Usage: Dermatitis herpetiformis (DH)
All forms of leprosy except for cases of proven Dapsone resistance.
Contraindication: Hypersensitivity to Dapsone and/or its derivatives.
Warnings: The patient should be warned to respond to the presence of clinical signs such as sore throat, fever, pallor, purpura or jaundice. Deaths associated with the administration of Dapsone have been reported from agranulocytosis, aplastic anemia and other blood dyscrasias.
Complete blood counts should be done frequently in patients receiving Dapsone. The FDA Dermatology Advisory Committee recommended that, when feasible, counts be done weekly for the first month, monthly for six months and semi-annually thereafter. If a significant reduction in leucocytes, platelets or hemopoiesis is noted, Dapsone should be discontinued and the patient followed intensively. Severe anemia should be treated prior to initiation of therapy and hemoglobin monitored. Hemolysis and methemoglobin may be poorly tolerated by patients with severe cardio-pulmonary disease.
Dapsone has been found carcinogenic (sarcomagenic) for male rats and female mice causing mesenchymal tumors in the spleen and peritoneum, and thyroid carcinoma in female rats.
Cutaneous reactions, especially bullous, include exfoliative dermatitis and are probably one of the most serious, though rare, complications of sulfone therapy. They are directly due to drug sensitization. Such reactions include toxic erythema, erythema multiforme, toxic epidermal necrolysis, morbilliform and scarlatiniform reactions, urticaria and erythema nodosum. If new or toxic dermatologic reactions occur, sulfone therapy must be promptly discontinued and appropriate therapy instituted.
Leprosy reactional states, including cutaneous, are not hypersensitivity reactions to Dapsone and do not require discontinuation. See special section.
Precautions: Hemolysis and Heinz body formation may be exaggerated in individuals with glucose-6-phosphate dehydrogenase (G6PD) deficiency, or methemoglobin reductase deficiency, or hemoglobin M. This reaction is frequently dose-related. Dapsone should be given with caution to these patients or if the patient is exposed to other agents or conditions such as infection or diabetic ketosis capable of producing hemolysis. Drugs or chemicals which have produced significant hemolysis in G6PD or methemoglobin reductase deficient patients include Dapsone, sulfanilamide, nitrite, aniline, pheylhydrazine, naphthalene, niridazole, nitrofurantoin and 8-amino-antimalarials such as primaquine.
Toxic hepatitis and cholestatic jaundice have been reported early in therapy. Hyperbilirubinema may occur more often in G6PD deficient patients. When feasible, baseline and subsequent monitoring of liver function is recommended. If abnormal, Dapsone should be discontinued until the source of abnormality is established.
Pregnancy Category A: Extensive, but uncontrolled, experience and two published surveys on the use of Dapsone in pregnant women have not shown that Dapsone increases the risk of fetal abnormalities if administered during all trimesters of pregnancy. If this drug is used during pregnancy, the possibility of fetal harm appears remote. Because studies cannot rule out the possibility of harm, however, Dapsone should be used during pregnancy only if really needed. In general, for leprosy, USPHS at Carville recommends maintenance of Dapsone. Dapsone has been important for the management of some pregnant D.H. patients. Dapsone is generally not considered to have an effect on the later growth, development and functional maturation of the child. Because of the potential for tumorgenicity shown for Dapsone in animal studies, a decision should be made whether to discontinue nursing or discontinue the drug, taking into account the importance of the drug to the mother.
Adverse Reactions: In addition to the warnings listed above, the following syndromes and serious reactions have been reported in patients on Dapsone:
Dose-related hemolysis is the most common adverse effect and is seen in patients with or without G6PD deficiency. Almost all patients demonstrate the interrelated changes of a loss of a 1–2 gms. HB, an increase in the reticulocytes (2–12%), a shortened red cell life span and a rise in methemoglobin. G6PD deficient patients have greater responses.
Peripheral neuropathy is a definite but unusual complication of Dapsone therapy in nonleprosy patients. Motor loss is predominant. If muscle weakness appears, Dapsone should be withdrawn. Recovery on withdrawal is usually substantially complete. The mechanism of recovery is reportedly by axonal regeneration. In leprosy this complication has not been reported and may be difficult to distinguish from a leprosy reactional state.
In addition to the warnings and adverse effects reported above, additional adverse reactions include: nausea, vomiting, abdominal pains, vertigo, blurred vision, tinnitus, insomnia, fever, headache, psychosis, phototoxicity, hyperpigmented macules, tachycardia, albuminuria, the nephrotic syndrome, hypoalbuminemia without proteinuria, renal papillary necrosis, male infertility, drug-induced Lupus erythematosus and an infectious mononucleosis-like syndrome. In general, these adverse reactions have regressed off drug.
Dosage and Administration:
Dermatitis herpetiformis: The dosage should be individually titrated starting in adults with 50 mg. daily and correspondingly smaller doses in children. If full control is not achieved within the range of 50–300 mg. daily, higher doses may be tried. Dosage should be reduced to a minimum maintenance level as soon as possible. In responsive patients there is a prompt reduction in pruritus followed by clearance of skin lesions. There is no effect on the gastro-intestinal component of the disease.
Dapsone levels are influenced by acetylation rates. Patients with high acetylation rates or who are receiving treatment affecting acetylation may require an adjustment in dosage. Maintenance Dapsone dosage often can be reduced (approximately 50%) after six months on a gluten-free diet.
Leprosy: In order to reduce secondary Dapsone resistance the WHO Expert Committee on Leprosy has recommended that Dapsone should be commenced and maintained at full dosage without interruption. The recommended dosage is 6–10 mg/kg of body weight per week. This schedule amounts to 50–100 mg. daily in full-size adults with correspondingly smaller doses for children.
In bacteriologically negative tuberculoid and indeterminate type leprosy patients, an adult dosage of 50 mg. daily is usually sufficient. After all signs of clinical activity are controlled, therapy should be continued a minimum of 3 years for tuberculoid and indeterminate patients.
In lepromatous and border line lepromatous patients, Dapsone therapy in full dosage should be administered for many years, perhaps for life. The WHO Committee recommends administration for at least 10 years after a patient is bacteriologically negative. More than five years of continuous therapy is required to render most patients with lepromatous leprosy bacteriologically negative.
Secondary Dapsone resistance should be suspected whenever a lepromatous or border-line lepromatous patient receiving Dapsone treatment relapses clinically and bacteriologically, solid staining bacilli being found in the smears taken from the new active lesions. If such cases show no response to regular and supervised Dapsone therapy within three to six months, Dapsone resistance should be considered confirmed clinically. Determination of drug sensitivity using the mouse footpad method is recommended and, after prior arrangement, is available without charge from the USPHS at Carville, LA. Patients with proven Dapsone resistance should be treated with other drugs.
Leprosy Reactional States: Abrupt changes in clinical activity occur in leprosy with any effective treatment and are known as reactional states. The majority can be classified into two groups.
Erythema nodosum leprosum (ENL) (lepromatous lepra reaction) (Type 2 reaction) occurs mainly in lepromatous patients and small numbers of borderline patients. Approximately 50 percent of treated patients show this reaction in the first year. The principal clinical features are fever and tender erythematous skin nodules sometimes associated with malaise, neuritis, orchitis, albuminuria, joint swelling, iritis, epistaxis or depression. Skin lesions can become pustular and/or ulcerate. Histologically there is a vasculitis with an intense polymorphonuclear infiltrate. Elevated

Continued on next page

Jacobus—Cont.

circulating immune complexes are considered to be the mechanism of the reaction. If severe, patients should be hospitalized. In general, anti-leprosy treatment is continued.

Analgesics, steroids and other agents available from USPHS Carville, LA, are used to suppress the reaction.

The "Reversal" reaction (Type 1) may occur in borderline or tuberculoid leprosy patients often soon after chemotherapy is started. The mechanism is presumed to result from a reduction in the antigenic load: the patient is able to mount an enhanced delayed hypersentitivity response to residual infection leading to swelling ("Reversal") of existing skin and nerve lesions. If severe, or if neuritis is present, large doses of steroids should always be used. If severe, the patient should be hospitalized. In general, anti-leprosy treatment is continued and therapy to suppress the reaction is indicated such as analgesics, steroids, or surgical decompression of swollen nerve trunks. USPHS at Carville, LA should be contacted for advice in management.

Overdosage: Symptoms of nausea, vomiting, hyperexcitability can appear a few minutes up to 24 hours after ingestion of an overdose. Methemoglobin induced depression, convulsions and severe cyanosis require prompt treatment. In normal and methemoglobin reductase deficient patients, methylene blue 1–2 mg/kg of body weight given slowly intravenously is the treatment of choice. The effect is complete in 30 minutes, but may have to be repeated if methemoglobin reaccumulates. For non-emergencies, if treatment is needed, methylene blue may be given orally in doses of 3–5 mg/kg every 4–6 hours.

Methylene blue reduction depends on G6PD and should not be given to fully expressed G6PD-deficient patients.

Properties: Dapsone is a white odorless crystalline powder, practically insoluble in water and insoluble in fixed and vegetable oils. The drug is not self-sterilizing but it may be sterilized by dry heat at 150°C for one hour.

How Supplied: Rx: 25 mg. and 100 mg. white scored tablets in light resistant, child proof bottles of 100. (25 mg. — NDC 49938-102-01) and (100 mg. — NDC 49938-101-01).

Distributed by: Jacobus Pharmaceutical Co., Inc., 37 Cleveland Lane, Princeton, NJ 08540.
Manufactured by: Rowell Laboratories, Inc., Baudette, MN 56623 2 E March, 1980

Jamol Laboratories Inc.
13 ACKERMAN AVENUE
EMERSON, NEW JERSEY 07630

PONARIS
Nasal Mucosal Emollient

Composition: Essential oils of cajeput, eucalyptus, and peppermint in a specially prepared iodized cottonseed oil. (Total Iodine 0.6%) Assimilable hence NON-lipoid potential.

Indications and Uses: Nasal emollient, for relief of nasal congestion due to colds, nasal irritations, atrophic rhinitis, (dry inflamed nasal passages), nasal mucosal encrustations and allergy manifestations.

Also nasal intubations and sterile gauze impregnated for epistaxis packing.

Administration and Dosage: 3 to 4 drops in each nostril 3 to 4 times daily. May be used in a compressed air nebulizer or a DeVilbiss nebulizer No. 33 or 40.

Childrens Dosage: As directed by physician.

How Supplied: One ounce bottle with dropper.

ROMA-NOL

Active Ingredient: An iodine solution for external use having none of the toxic, escharotic, or precipitating nature of usual iodine preparations.

Indications: For all skin and some mucous membrane infections.

Actions: By the J-R process the iodine is highly subdivided thus making **Roma-nol** the highest form of a water soluble iodine. The color density is increased by its high solubility. Hospital studies have proven unusual penetration qualities.

Dosage and Administration: The first 2 or 3 applications of **Roma-nol** act more like cleansers, the iodine color slowly disappearing as it combines with the infected organic matter, pus, mucous, etc. With the additional applications 2 to 4 times more, the impurities being eliminated, the iodine stain will remain. The infected parts have received the full compatible treatment with **Roma-nol** ending the treatment.

How Supplied: Bottles of 30 cc. each.

Janssen Pharmaceutica Inc.
501 GEORGE STREET
NEW BRUNSWICK, NJ 08903

IMODIUM® Ⓒ
(loperamide HCl)
Capsules

Description: IMODIUM® (loperamide hydrochloride), 4-(*p*-chlorophenyl)-4-hydroxy-N, N-dimethyl-α, α-diphenyl-1-piperidinebutyramide monohydrochloride, is a synthetic antidiarrheal for oral use.

IMODIUM® is available in 2 mg capsules.

Important Information: IMODIUM® Capsules are classified as a Schedule V controlled substance by federal law (*see* Overdosage Section).

KEEP THIS AND ALL MEDICATIONS OUT OF THE REACH OF CHILDREN.

Clinical Pharmacology: *In vitro* and animal studies show that IMODIUM® acts by slowing intestinal motility and by effecting water and electrolyte movement through the bowel. It inhibits peristaltic activity by a direct effect on the circular and longitudinal muscles of the intestinal wall.

In man, IMODIUM® prolongs the transit time of the intestinal contents. It reduces the daily fecal volume, increases the viscosity and bulk density, and diminishes the loss of fluid and electrolytes. Tolerance to the antidiarrheal effect has not been observed. Studies in morphine-dependent monkeys demonstrated that loperamide hydrochloride at doses above those recommended for humans prevented signs of morphine withdrawal. However, in humans, the naloxone challenge pupil test, which when positive indicates opiate-like effects, performed after a single high dose, or after more than two years of therapeutic use of IMODIUM®, was negative.

Clinical studies have indicated that the apparent elimination half-life of loperamide in man is 10.8 hours with a range of 9.1–14.4 hours. Plasma levels of unchanged drug remain below 2 nanograms per ml after the intake of a 2 mg capsule of IMODIUM®. Plasma levels are highest approximately five hours after the administration of the capsule dosage form. Of the total excreted in urine and feces, most of the administered drug was excreted in feces.

In those patients in whom biochemical and hematological parameters were monitored during clinical trials, no trends toward abnormality during IMODIUM® therapy were noted. Similarly, urinalyses, EKG and clinical ophthalmological examinations did not show trends toward abnormality. There was no evidence in clinical trials of drug interaction with concurrent medications.

Indications: IMODIUM® is indicated for the control and symptomatic relief of acute nonspecific diarrhea and of chronic diarrhea associated with inflammatory bowel disease. IMODIUM® is also indicated for reducing the volume of discharge from ileostomies.

Contraindications: IMODIUM® is contraindicated in patients with known hypersensitivity to the drug and in those in whom constipation must be avoided.

Warnings: Antiperistaltic agents should not be used in acute diarrhea associated with organisms that penetrate the intestinal mucosa, e.g., enteroinvasive *E. coli, Salmonella, Shigella,* and in pseudomembranous colitis associated with broad-spectrum antibiotics.

Fluid and electrolyte depletion may occur in patients who have diarrhea. The use of IMODIUM® does not preclude the administration of appropriate fluid and electrolyte therapy. In some patients with acute ulcerative colitis, agents which inhibit intestinal motility or delay intestinal transit time have been reported to induce toxic megacolon. IMODIUM® therapy should be discontinued promptly if abdominal distention occurs or if other untoward symptoms develop in patients with acute ulcerative colitis.

Precautions: In acute diarrhea, if clinical improvement is not observed in 48 hours, the administration of IMODIUM® should be discontinued.

Abuse and Dependence: Physical dependence to IMODIUM® in humans has not been observed. However, studies in monkeys demonstrated that loperamide hydrochloride at high doses produced symptoms of physical dependence of the morphine type.

Carcinogenesis: In an 18-month rat study with doses up to 133 times the maximum human dose (on a mg/kg basis) there was no evidence of carcinogenesis.

Pregnancy: Safe use of IMODIUM® during pregnancy has not been established. Reproduction studies performed in rats and rabbits with dosage levels up to 30 times the human therapeutic dose did not demonstrate evidence of impaired fertility or harm to the offspring due to IMODIUM®. Higher doses impaired maternal and neonate survival, but no dose level up to 30 times the human dose demonstrated teratogenicity. Such experience cannot exclude the possibility of damage to the fetus. IMODIUM® should be used in pregnant women only when clearly needed.

Nursing Mothers: It is not known whether IMODIUM® is excreted in human milk. As a general rule, nursing should not be undertaken while a patient is on a drug since many drugs are excreted in human milk.

Pediatric Use: Safety and effectiveness in children have not been established. Therefore, use of IMODIUM® is not recommended in the pediatric age group (under the age of 12). In case of accidental ingestion of IMODIUM® by children, *see* Overdosage Section for suggested treatment.

Adverse Reactions: The adverse effects reported during clinical investigations of IMODIUM® are difficult to distinguish from symptoms associated with the diarrheal syndrome. Adverse experiences recorded during clinical studies with IMODIUM® were generally of a minor and self-limiting nature. They were more commonly observed during the treatment of chronic diarrhea.

The following patient complaints have been reported:

Abdominal pain, distention or discomfort
Constipation
Drowsiness or dizziness
Dry mouth

Nausea and vomiting
Tiredness
Hypersensitivity Reactions (including skin rash), however, have been reported with IMODIUM® use.

Overdosage: Animal pharmacological and toxicological data indicate that overdosage in man may result in constipation, CNS depression, and gastrointestinal irritation. Clinical trials have demonstrated that a slurry of activated charcoal administered promptly after ingestion of loperamide hydrochloride can reduce the amount of drug which is absorbed into the systemic circulation by as much as ninefold. If vomiting occurs spontaneously upon ingestion, a slurry of 100 gms of activated charcoal should be administered orally as soon as fluids can be retained.

If vomiting has not occurred, gastric lavage should be performed followed by administration of 100 gms of the activated charcoal slurry through the gastric tube. In the event of overdosage, patients should be monitored for signs of CNS depression for at least 24 hours. If CNS depression is observed, naloxone may be administered. If responsive to naloxone, vital signs must be monitored carefully for recurrence of symptoms of drug overdose for at least 24 hours after the last dose of naloxone.

In view of the prolonged action of loperamide and the short duration (one to three hours) of naloxone, the patient must be monitored closely and treated repeatedly with naloxone as indicated. Based on the fact that relatively little drug is excreted in urine, forced diuresis is not expected to be effective for IMODIUM® overdosage.

In clinical trials an adult who took three 20 mg doses within a 24-hour period was nauseated after the second dose and vomited after the third dose. In studies designed to examine the potential for side-effects, intentional ingestion of up to 60 mg of loperamide hydrochloride in a single dose to healthy subjects resulted in no significant adverse effects.

Dosage and Administration:

Acute diarrhea: The recommended initial dose of IMODIUM® is two capsules (4 mg) followed by one capsule (2 mg) after each unformed stool. Daily dosage should not exceed eight capsules (16 mg). Clinical improvement is usually observed within 48 hours.

Chronic diarrhea: The recommended initial dosage of IMODIUM® is two capsules (4 mg) followed by one capsule (2 mg) after each unformed stool until diarrhea is controlled, after which the dosage of IMODIUM® should be reduced to meet individual requirements. When the optimal daily dosage has thus been established, this amount should then be administered as a single dose or in divided doses. The average daily maintenance dosage in clinical trials was two to four capsules (4–8 mg). A dosage of eight capsules (16 mg) was rarely exceeded. If clinical improvement is not observed after treatment with eight capsules (16 mg) of IMODIUM® per day for at least 10 days, symptoms are unlikely to be controlled by further administration. IMODIUM® administration may be continued if diarrhea cannot be adequately controlled with diet or specific treatment.

How Supplied: IMODIUM® is available as 2 mg capsules of loperamide hydrochloride. The capsules have a light green body and a dark green cap, with "JANSSEN" imprinted on one segment and "IMODIUM®" on the other segment. IMODIUM® capsules are supplied in bottles of 100 and 500 and in blister packs of 10 × 10 capsules.
NDC 50458-400-01
10 × 10 capsules-blister)
NDC 50458-400-10
100 capsules)
NDC 50458-400-50
500 capsules)
August 1982

An original product of
JANSSEN PHARMACEUTICA, n.v.
B-2340 Beerse
Belgium
Manufactured by
ORTHO PHARMACEUTICAL CORP.
Raritan
New Jersey 08869
Distributed by:
JANSSEN PHARMACEUTICA INC.
New Brunswick
New Jersey 08903
USA
U.S. Patent 3,714,159
[*Shown in Product Identification Section*]

INAPSINE® (droperidol) Injection ℞

(Protect from light—store at room temperature)

FOR INTRAVENOUS OR INTRAMUSCULAR USE ONLY

Droperidol is a neuroleptic (tranquilizer) agent.

Description:

2 ml. and 5 ml. ampoules
Each ml. contains:
Droperidol .... 2.5 mg.
Lactic acid for pH adjustment to 3.4 ± 0.4.

10 ml. vials
Each ml. contains:
Droperidol .... 2.5 mg.
With 1.8 mg. methylparaben and 0.2 mg. propylparaben, and lactic acid for pH adjustment to 3.4 ± 0.4.

Actions: INAPSINE (droperidol) produces marked tranquilization and sedation. It also produces an antiemetic effect as evidenced by the antagonism of the emetic effect of apomorphine in dogs. It potentiates other CNS depressants. It also produces mild alpha-adrenergic blockade, peripheral vascular dilatation and reduction of the pressor effect of epinephrine. INAPSINE (droperidol) can produce hypotension and decreased peripheral vascular resistance. It may decrease pulmonary arterial pressure (particularly if it is abnormally high). It may reduce the incidence of epinephrine-induced arrhythmias but it does not prevent other cardiac arrhythmias. The onset of action is from three to ten minutes following intravenous or intramuscular administration. The full effect, however, may not be apparent for 30 minutes. The duration of the sedative and tranquilizing effects of INAPSINE (droperidol) generally is two to four hours. Alteration of consciousness may persist as long as 12 hours.

Indications: INAPSINE (droperidol) is indicated:

- to produce tranquilization and to reduce the incidence of nausea and vomiting in surgical and diagnostic procedures;
- for premedication, induction, and as an adjunct in the maintenance of general and regional anesthesia;
- in neuroleptanalgesia in which INAPSINE (droperidol) is given concurrently with a narcotic analgesic, such as *SUBLIMAZE®* (fentanyl) injection, to aid in producing tranquility and decreasing anxiety and pain.

Contraindications: INAPSINE (droperidol) is contraindicated in patients with known intolerance to the drug.

Warnings: FLUIDS AND OTHER COUNTERMEASURES TO MANAGE HYPOTENSION SHOULD BE READILY AVAILABLE.

As with other CNS depressant drugs, patients who have received INAPSINE (droperidol) should have appropriate surveillance.

If INAPSINE (droperidol) is administered with a narcotic analgesic such as *SUBLIMAZE* (fentanyl), the user should familiarize himself with the special properties of each drug, particularly the widely differing durations of action. In addition, when such a combination is used, *resuscitative equipment and a narcotic antagonist should be readily available to manage apnea.* See package insert for fentanyl before using.

Narcotic analgesics such as *SUBLIMAZE* (fentanyl) may cause muscle rigidity, particularly involving the muscles of respiration. This effect is related to the speed of injection. Its incidence can be reduced by the use of slow intravenous injection. Once this effect occurs, it is managed by the use of assisted or controlled respiration and, if necessary, by a neuromuscular blocking agent compatible with the patient's condition.

The respiratory depressant effect of narcotics persists longer than their measured analgesic effect. When used with INAPSINE (droperidol), the total dose of all narcotic analgesics administered should be considered by the practitioner before ordering narcotic analgesics during recovery from anesthesia. It is recommended that narcotics, when required, be used initially in reduced doses as low as 1/4 to 1/3 those usually recommended.

Usage in Children—The safety of INAPSINE (droperidol) in children younger than two years of age has not been established.

Usage in Pregnancy—The safe use of INAPSINE (droperidol) has not been established with respect to possible adverse effects upon fetal development. Therefore, it should be used in women of childbearing potential only when, in the judgment of the physician, the potential benefits outweigh the possible hazards. There are insufficient data regarding placental transfer and fetal effects; therefore, safety for the infant in obstetrics has not been established.

Precautions: *The initial dose of INAPSINE (droperidol) should be appropriately reduced in elderly, debilitated and other poor-risk patients. The effect of the initial dose should be considered in determining incremental doses.*

Certain forms of conduction anesthesia, such as spinal anesthesia and some peridural anesthetics, can cause peripheral vasodilatation and hypotension because of sympathetic blockade. Through other mechanisms (see Actions), INAPSINE (droperidol) can also alter circulation. Therefore, when INAPSINE (droperidol) is used to supplement these forms of anesthesia, the anesthetist should be familiar with the physiological alterations involved, and be prepared to manage them in the patients selected for this form of anesthesia.

If hypotension occurs, the possibility of hypovolemia should be considered and managed with appropriate parenteral fluid therapy. Repositioning the patient to improve venous return to the heart should also be considered when operative conditions permit. It should be noted that in spinal and peridural anesthesia, tilting the patient into a head down position may result in a higher level of anesthesia than is desirable, as well as impair venous return to the heart. Care should be exercised in moving and positioning of patients because of the possibility of orthostatic hypotension. If volume expansion with fluids plus other countermeasures do not correct the hypotension, then the administration of pressor agents other than epinephrine should be considered. Epinephrine may paradoxically decrease the blood pressure in patients treated with INAPSINE (droperidol) due to the alpha-adrenergic blocking action of droperidol.

Since INAPSINE (droperidol) may decrease pulmonary arterial pressure, this fact should be considered by those who conduct diagnostic or surgical procedures where interpretation of pulmonary arterial pressure measurements might determine final management of the patient.

Vital signs should be monitored routinely.

Other CNS depressant drugs (e.g. barbiturates, tranquilizers, narcotics, and general anesthetics) have additive or potentiating effects with INAPSINE (droperidol). When patients have received such drugs, the dose of INAPSINE (droperidol) required will be less than usual. Likewise,

Continued on next page

Janssen—Cont.

following the administration of INAPSINE (droperidol), the dose of other CNS depressant drugs should be reduced.

INAPSINE (droperidol) should be administered with caution to patients with liver and kidney dysfunction because of the importance of these organs in the metabolism and excretion of drugs.

When the EEG is used for postoperative monitoring, it may be found that the EEG pattern returns to normal slowly.

Since INAPSINE (droperidol) is frequently used with the narcotic analgesic *SUBLIMAZE* (fentanyl), it should be noted that fentanyl may produce bradycardia, which may be treated with atropine; however, fentanyl should be used with caution in patients with cardiac bradyarrhythmias.

Adverse Reactions: The most common adverse reactions reported to occur with INAPSINE (droperidol) are mild to moderate hypotension and occasionally tachycardia, but these effects usually subside without treatment. If hypotension occurs and is severe or persists, the possibility of hypovolemia should be considered and managed with appropriate parenteral fluid therapy. Postoperative drowsiness is also frequently reported.

Extrapyramidal symptoms (dystonia, akathisia, and oculogyric crisis) have been observed following administration of INAPSINE (droperidol). Restlessness, hyperactivity, and anxiety, which can be either the result of inadequate dosage of INAPSINE (droperidol) or a part of the symptom complex of akathisia, may occur. When extrapyramidal symptoms occur, they can usually be controlled with anti-parkinson agents.

Other adverse reactions that have been reported are dizziness, chills and/or shivering, laryngospasm, bronchospasm and postoperative hallucinatory episodes (sometimes associated with transient periods of mental depression).

When INAPSINE (droperidol) is used with a narcotic analgesic such as *SUBLIMAZE* (fentanyl), respiratory depression, apnea, and muscular rigidity can occur; if these remain untreated respiratory arrest could occur.

Elevated blood pressure, with or without preexisting hypertension has been reported following administration of INAPSINE (droperidol) combined with *SUBLIMAZE* (fentanyl) or other parenteral analgesics. This might be due to unexplained alterations in sympathetic activity following large doses; however, it is also frequently attributed to anesthetic or surgical stimulation during light anesthesia.

Dosage and Administration: *Dosage should be individualized.* Some of the factors to be considered in determining the dose are age, body weight, physical status, underlying pathological condition, use of other drugs, type of anesthesia to be used, and the surgical procedure involved.

Vital signs should be monitored routinely.

Usual Adult Dosage

I. *Premedication*—(to be appropriately modified in the elderly, debilitated, and those who have received other depressant drugs) 2.5 to 10 mg. (1 to 4 ml.) may be administered intramuscularly 30 to 60 minutes preoperatively.

II. *Adjunct to General Anesthesia*
Induction–2.5 mg. (1 ml.) per 20 to 25 pounds may be administered (usually intravenously) along with an analgesic and/or general anesthetic. Smaller doses may be adequate. The total amount of INAPSINE (droperidol) administered should be titrated to obtain the desired effect based on the individual patient's response.
Maintenance—1.25 to 2.5 mg. (0.5 to 1 ml.) usually intravenously (see warning regarding use with concomitant narcotic analgesic medication and the possibility of widely differing durations of action).
If *INNOVAR®* injection is administered in addition to INAPSINE (droperidol), the calculation of the recommended dose of INAPSINE (droperidol) should include the droperidol contained in the *INNOVAR* injection. See *INNOVAR* injection Package Insert for full prescribing information.

III. *Use Without A General Anesthetic In Diagnostic Procedures*—Administer the usual I.M. premedication 2.5 to 10 mg. (1 to 4 ml.) 30 to 60 minutes before the procedure. Additional 1.25 to 2.5 mg. (0.5 to 1 ml) amounts of INAPSINE (droperidol) may be administered, usually intravenously (see warning regarding use with concomitant narcotic analgesic medication and the possibility of widely differing durations of action).
Note: When INAPSINE (droperidol) is used in certain procedures, such as bronchoscopy, appropriate topical anesthesia is still necessary.

IV. *Adjunct to Regional Anesthesia*—2.5 to 5 mg. (1 to 2 ml.) may be administered intramuscularly or slowly intravenously when additional sedation is required.

Usual Children's Dosage

For children two to 12 years of age, a reduced dose as low as 1.0 to 1.5 mg. (0.4 to 0.6 ml.) per 20 to 25 pounds is recommended for premedication or for induction of anesthesia.

See Warnings and Precautions for use of INAPSINE (droperidol) with other CNS depressants, and in patients with altered response.

Overdosage:

Manifestations: The manifestations of INAPSINE (droperidol) overdosage are an extension of its pharmacologic actions.

Treatment: In the presence of hypoventilation or apnea, oxygen should be administered and respiration should be assisted or controlled as indicated. A patent airway must be maintained; an oropharyngeal airway or endotracheal tube might be indicated. The patient should be carefully observed for 24 hours; body warmth and adequate fluid intake should be maintained. If hypotension occurs and is severe or persists, the possibility of hypovolemia should be considered and managed with appropriate parenteral fluid therapy.

How Supplied: 2 ml. and 5 ml. ampoules—packages of 10; 10 ml. multiple-dose vials—packages of 10.

NDC 50458-010-02
NDC 50458-010-05
NDC 50458-010-10
U.S. Patent No. 3,161,645
Manufactured by McNEILAB, Inc. for
JANSSEN Pharmaceutica Inc.
New Brunswick, NJ 08903
March 1980/Rev. June 1980

INNOVAR® Injection ℂ ℞

FOR INTRAVENOUS OR INTRAMUSCULAR USE ONLY

(Protect from light–store at room temperature)

Description: Each ml. contains (in a 1:50 ratio):

Fentanyl ....0.05 mg.
as the citrate
Warning: May be habit forming
Droperidol ....2.5 mg.
Lactic acid for adjustment of pH to 3.5 ± 0.3

> The two components of INNOVAR injection, fentanyl and droperidol, have different pharmacologic actions. Before administering INNOVAR injection, the user should familiarize himself with the special properties of each drug, particularly the widely differing durations of action.

Actions: INNOVAR injection is a combination drug containing a narcotic analgesic, fentanyl, and a neuroleptic (major tranquilizer), droperidol. The combined effect, sometimes referred to as neuroleptanalgesia, is characterized by general quiescence, reduced motor activity, and profound analgesia; complete loss of consciousness usually does not occur from use of INNOVAR injection alone. The incidence of early postoperative pain and emesis may be reduced.

A. Fentanyl is a narcotic analgesic with actions qualitatively similar to those of morphine and meperidine. Fentanyl in a dose of 0.1 mg. (2.0 ml.) is approximately equivalent in analgesic activity to 10 mg. of morphine or 75 mg. of meperidine. The principal actions of therapeutic value are analgesia and sedation. Alterations in respiratory rate and alveolar ventilation, associated with narcotic analgesics, may last longer than the analgesic effect. As the dose of narcotic is increased, the decrease in pulmonary exchange becomes greater. Large doses may produce apnea. Fentanyl appears to have less emetic activity than other narcotic analgesics. Histamine assays, and skin wheal testing in man, as well as *in vivo* testing in dogs indicate that histamine release rarely occurs with fentanyl.
Fentanyl may cause muscle rigidity, particularly involving the muscles of respiration. It may also produce other signs and symptoms characteristic of narcotic analgesics including euphoria, miosis, bradycardia, and bronchoconstriction.
The onset of action of fentanyl is almost immediate when the drug is given intravenously; however, maximal analgesic and respiratory depressant effect may not be noted for several minutes. The usual duration of action of the analgesic effect is 30 to 60 minutes after a single I.V. dose of up to 0.1 mg. Following intramuscular administration, the onset of action is from seven to eight minutes, and the duration of action is from one to two hours.
As with longer-acting narcotic analgesics, the duration of the respiratory depressant effect of *SUBLIMAZE®* (fentanyl) may be longer than the analgesic effect. The following observations have been reported concerning altered respiratory response to CO_2 stimulation following administration of fentanyl to man:
1. DIMINISHED SENSITIVITY TO CO_2 STIMULATION MAY PERSIST LONGER THAN DEPRESSION OF RESPIRATORY RATE. Fentanyl frequently slows the respiratory rate but this effect is seldom noted for over 30 minutes regardless of the dose administered.
2. Duration and degree of respiratory depression is dose related.
3. The peak respiratory depressant effect of a single intravenous dose of fentanyl is noted 5 to 15 minutes following injection.
4. Altered sensitivity to CO_2 stimulation has been demonstrated for up to four hours following a single intravenous dose of 0.6 mg. (12 ml.) fentanyl to healthy volunteers.
See also WARNINGS and PRECAUTIONS concerning respiratory depression.

B. Droperidol produces marked tranquilization and sedation. It also produces an antiemetic effect as evidenced by the antagonism of apomorphine in dogs. It potentiates other CNS depressants. It also produces mild alpha-adrenergic blockade, peripheral vascular dilatation and reduction of the pressor effect of epinephrine. Droperidol can produce hypotension and decreased peripheral vascular resistance. It may decrease pulmonary arterial pressure (particularly if it is abnormally high). It may reduce the incidence of epinephrine-induced arrhythmias but it does not prevent other cardiac arrhythmias. The onset of action is from three to ten minutes following intravenous or intramuscular administration. The full effect, however, may not be apparent for 30 minutes. The duration of the sedative and tranquilizing effects generally is two to four hours. Alteration of consciousness may persist as long as 12 hours. This is in contrast to the much shorter duration of fentanyl.

Indications: INNOVAR injection is indicated to produce tranquilization and analgesia for surgical and diagnostic procedures. It may be used as an anesthetic premedication, for the induction of anesthesia, and as an adjunct in the maintenance of general and regional anesthesia. If the supplementation of analgesia is necessary, *SUBLIMAZE* (fentanyl) injection alone rather than the combination drug INNOVAR injection, should usually be used; see Dosage and Administration Section.

Contraindications: INNOVAR injection is contraindicated in patients with known intolerance to either component.

Warnings: AS WITH OTHER CNS DEPRESSANTS, PATIENTS WHO HAVE RECEIVED *INNOVAR* INJECTION SHOULD HAVE APPROPRIATE SURVEILLANCE. RESUSCITATIVE EQUIPMENT AND A NARCOTIC ANTAGONIST SHOULD BE READILY AVAILABLE TO MANAGE APNEA.

See also discussion of narcotic antagonists in PRECAUTIONS and OVERDOSAGE.

FLUIDS AND OTHER COUNTERMEASURES TO MANAGE HYPOTENSION SHOULD ALSO BE AVAILABLE.

The respiratory depressant effect of narcotics persists longer than the measured analgesic effect. When used with INNOVAR *injection, the total dose of all narcotic analgesics administered should be considered by the practitioner before ordering narcotic analgesics during recovery from anesthesia. It is recommended that narcotics, when required, be used in reduced doses initially, as low as ¼ to ⅓ those usually recommended.*

INNOVAR *injection may cause muscle rigidity, particularly involving the muscles of respiration. This effect is due to the fentanyl component and is related to the speed of injection. Its incidence can be reduced by the use of slow intravenous injection. Once the effect occurs, it is managed by the use of assisted or controlled respiration and, if necessary, by a neuromuscular blocking agent compatible with the patient's condition.*

Drug Dependence: *Fentanyl, the narcotic analgesic component, can produce drug dependence of the morphine type and therefore has the potential for being abused.*

Severe and unpredictable potentiation by MAO inhibitors has been reported with narcotic analgesics. Since the safety of fentanyl in this regard has not been established, the use of INNOVAR injection or *SUBLIMAZE* (fentanyl) in patients who have received MAO inhibitors within 14 days is not recommended.

Head injuries and Increased Intracranial Pressure: INNOVAR injection should be used with caution in patients who may be particularly susceptible to respiratory depression such as comatose patients who may have a head injury or brain tumor. In addition, INNOVAR injection may obscure the clinical course of patients with head injury.

Usage in Children: The safety of INNOVAR injection in children younger than two years of age has not been established.

Usage in Pregnancy: The safe use of INNOVAR injection has not been established with respect to possible adverse effects upon fetal development. Therefore, it should be used in women of childbearing potential only when, in the judgment of the physician, the potential benefits outweigh the possible hazards. There are insufficient data regarding placental transfer and fetal effects; therefore, safety for the infant in obstetrics has not been established.

Precautions: *The initial dose of* INNOVAR *injection should be appropriately reduced in elderly, debilitated and other poor-risk patients. The effect of the initial dose should be considered in determining incremental doses.*

Certain forms of conduction anesthesia, such as spinal anesthesia and some peridural anesthetics, can alter respiration by blocking intercostal nerves, and can cause peripheral vasodilation and hypotension because of sympathetic blockade. Through other mechanisms (see Actions), fentanyl and droperidol also depress respiration and blood pressure. Therefore, when INNOVAR injection is used to supplement these forms of anesthesia, the anesthetist must be familiar with the physiological alterations involved, and be prepared to manage them in the patients selected for this form of anesthesia.

If hypotension occurs, the possibility of hypovolemia should be considered and managed with appropriate parenteral fluid therapy. Repositioning the patient to improve venous return to the heart should be considered when operative conditions permit. It should be noted that in spinal and peridural anesthesia, tilting the patient into a head down position may result in a higher level of anesthesia than is desirable, as well as impair venous return to the heart. Care should be exercised in the moving and positioning of patients because of a possibility of orthostatic hypotension. If volume expansion with fluids plus these other countermeasures do not correct the hypotension, then the administration of pressor agents other than epinephrine should be considered. Epinephrine may paradoxically decrease the blood pressure in patients treated with INNOVAR injection due to the alpha-adrenergic blocking action of droperidol.

The droperidol component of INNOVAR injection may decrease pulmonary arterial pressure. This fact should be considered by those who conduct diagnostic or surgical procedures where interpretation of pulmonary arterial pressure measurements might determine final management of the patient.

Vital signs should be monitored routinely.

INNOVAR injection, and *SUBLIMAZE* (fentanyl), should be used with caution in patients with chronic obstructive pulmonary disease, patients with decreased respiratory reserve, and others with potentially compromised ventilation. In such patients narcotics may additionally decrease respiratory drive and increase airway resistance. During anesthesia this can be managed by assisted or controlled respiration. Postoperative respiratory depression caused by narcotic analgesics can be reversed by narcotic antagonists. Appropriate surveillance should be maintained because the duration of respiratory depression of doses of fentanyl (as *SUBLIMAZE* (fentanyl) or INNOVAR) employed during anesthesia may be longer than the duration of the narcotic antagonist action. Consult individual prescribing information (levallorphan, nalorphine and naloxone) before employing narcotic antagonists.

Should respiration be compromised by muscle rigidity, assisted or controlled respiration and possibly a neuromuscular blocking agent will be required. The occurrence of muscle rigidity is related to the speed of intravenous injection and the incidence can be reduced by slow intravenous injection.

Other CNS depressant drugs (e.g. barbiturates, tranquilizers, narcotics, and general anesthetics) have additive or potentiating effects with INNOVAR injection. When patients have received such drugs, the dose of INNOVAR injection required will be less than usual. Likewise, following the administration of INNOVAR injection, the dose of other CNS depressant drugs should be reduced.

INNOVAR injection should be administered with caution to patients with liver and kidney dysfunction because of the importance of these organs in the metabolism and excretion of drugs.

The fentanyl component may produce bradycardia, which may be treated with atropine; however, INNOVAR injection should be used with caution in patients with cardiac bradyarrhythmias.

When the EEG is used for postoperative monitoring, it may be found that the EEG pattern returns to normal slowly.

Adverse Reactions: The most common serious adverse reactions reported to occur with INNOVAR injection are respiratory depression, apnea, muscular rigidity, and hypotension; if these remain untreated, respiratory arrest, circulatory depression or cardiac arrest could occur.

Extrapyramidal symptoms (dystonia, akathisia, and oculogyric crisis) have been observed following administration of INNOVAR injection. Restlessness, hyperactivity and anxiety which can be either the result of inadequate tranquilization or part of the symptom complex of akathisia may occur. When extrapyramidal symptoms occur, they can usually be controlled with anti-Parkinson agents.

Elevated blood pressure, with and without preexisting hypertension, has been reported following administration of INNOVAR injection. This might be due to unexplained alterations of sympathetic activity following large doses; however, it is also frequently attributed to anesthetic or surgical stimulation during light anesthesia.

Other adverse reactions that have been reported are dizziness, chills and/or shivering, twitching, blurred vision, laryngospasm, bronchospasm, bradycardia, tachycardia, nausea and emesis, diaphoresis, emergence delirium, and postoperative hallucinatory episodes (sometimes associated with transient periods of mental depression).

Postoperative drowsiness is also frequently reported.

Dosage and Administration: *Dosage should be individualized.* Some of the factors to be considered in determining dose are age, body weight, physical status, underlying pathological condition, use of other drugs, the type of anesthesia to be used, and the surgical procedure involved.

Vital signs should be monitored routinely.

Most patients who have received INNOVAR injection do not require narcotic analgesics during the immediate postoperative period. It is recommended that narcotic analgesics, when required, be used initially in reduced doses, as low as ¼ to ⅓ those usually recommended.

Usual Adult Dosage:

I. *Premedication*—(to be appropriately modified in the elderly, debilitated, and those who have received other depressant drugs)—0.5 to 2.0 ml. may be administered *intramuscularly* 45 to 60 minutes prior to surgery with or without atropine.

II. *Adjunct to General Anesthesia—*
Induction—1 ml. per 20 to 25 pounds of body weight may be administered slowly intravenously. Smaller doses may be adequate.
The total amount of INNOVAR injection administered should be carefully titrated to obtain the desired effect based on the individual patient's response.
There are several methods of administration of INNOVAR injection for induction of anesthesia.
A. Intravenous injection—To allow for the variable needs of patients INNOVAR injection may be administered intravenously in fractional parts of the calculated dose. With the onset of somnolence, the general anesthetic may be administered.

Continued on next page

Janssen—Cont.

B. Intravenous drip—10 ml. of INNOVAR injection are added to 250 ml. of 5% dextrose in water and the drip given rapidly until the onset of somnolence. At that time, the drip may be either slowed or stopped and the general anesthetic administered.

Maintenance—INNOVAR injection is not indicated as the sole agent for the maintenance of surgical anesthesia. It is customarily used in combination with other measures such as nitrous oxide-oxygen, other inhalation anesthetics, and/or topical or regional anesthesia.

To prevent the possibility of excessive accumulation of the relatively long-acting droperidol component, *SULBIMAZE* (fentanyl) alone should be used in increments of 0.025 to 0.05 mg. (0.5 to 1.0 ml.) for the maintenance of analgesia in patients initially given INNOVAR injection as an adjunct to general anesthesia. (See *SUBLIMAZE* (fentanyl) package insert for additional prescribing information.) However, in prolonged operations, additional 0.5 to 1.0 ml. amounts of INNOVAR injection may be administered with caution intravenously if changes in the patient's condition indicate lightening of tranquilization and analgesia.

III. *Use Without a General Anesthetic in Diagnostic Procedures*—Administer the usual I.M. premedication (0.5 to 2.0 ml.) 45 to 60 minutes before the procedure. To prevent the possibility of excessive accumulation of the relatively long-acting droperidol component, *SUBLIMAZE* (fentanyl) alone should be used in increments of 0.025 to 0.05 mg. (0.5 to 1.0 ml.) for the maintenance of analgesia in patients initially given INNOVAR injection. (See *SUBLIMAZE* (fentanyl) package insert for additional information). However, in prolonged operations, additional 0.5 to 1.0 ml. amounts of INNOVAR injection may be administered with caution intravenously if changes in the patient's condition indicate lightening of tranquilization and analgesia.
Note: When INNOVAR injection is used in certain procedures such as bronchoscopy, appropriate topical anesthesia is still necessary.

IV. *Adjunct to Regional Anesthesia*—1 to 2 ml. may be administered intramuscularly or slowly intravenously when additional sedation and analgesia are required.

Usual Children's Dosage:

I. *Premedication*—0.25 ml. per 20 lbs. body weight administered *intramuscularly* 45 to 60 minutes prior to surgery with or without atropine.

II. *Adjunct to General Anesthesia*—The total combined dose for induction and maintenance averages 0.5 ml. per 20 lbs. body weight. Following induction with INNOVAR injection, *SUBLIMAZE* (fentanyl) alone in a dose of 1/4 to 1/3 that recommended in the adult dosage section should usually be used when indicated to avoid the possibility of excessive accumulation of droperidol. However, in prolonged operations, additional increments of INNOVAR injection may be administered with caution when changes in the patient's condition indicate lightening of tranquilization and analgesia.

See Warnings and Precautions for use of INNOVAR injection with other CNS depressants, and in patients with altered response.

Overdosage: *Manifestations:* The manifestations of INNOVAR injection overdosage are an extension of its pharmacologic actions.

Treatment: In the presence of hypoventilation or apnea, oxygen should be administered and respiration should be assisted or controlled as indicated. A patent airway must be maintained; an oropharyngeal airway or endotracheal tube might be indicated. If depressed respiration is associated with muscular rigidity, an intravenous neuromuscular blocking agent might be required to facilitate assisted or controlled respiration. The patient should be carefully observed for 24 hours; body warmth and adequate fluid intake should be maintained. If hypotension occurs and is severe or persists, the possibility of hypovolemia should be considered and managed with appropriate parenteral fluid therapy. A specific narcotic antagonist such as nalorphine, levallorphan or naloxone should be available for use as indicated to manage respiratory depression caused by the narcotic component fentanyl. This does not preclude the use of more immediate countermeasures. The duration of respiratory depression following overdose of fentanyl may be longer than the duration of narcotic antagonist action. Consult the package inserts of the individual narcotic antagonists for details about use.

How Supplied: INNOVAR® injection is supplied in 2 ml. and 5 ml. ampoules, in packages of 10.

NDC 50458-020-02
NDC 50458-020-05
U.S. Patent No. 3,141,823
Manufactured by McNEILAB, Inc. for
JANSSEN Pharmaceutica Inc.
New Brunswick, NJ 08903
March, 1980/Rev. June 1980

MONISTAT i.v.™ ℞

(miconazole for intravenous infusion)

Description: MONISTAT i.v., (miconazole), 1- {2-(2, 4-dichlorophenyl)-2- [(2, 4-dichlorophenyl) methoxyl] ethyl}-1H-imidazole, is a synthetic antifungal supplied as a sterile solution for intravenous infusion. Each ml of this solution contains 10 mg of miconazole with 0.115 ml PEG 40 castor oil, 1.0 mg lactic acid USP, 0.5 mg methylparaben USP, 0.05 mg propylparaben USP in water for injection. Miconazole i.v. is a clear colorless to slightly yellow solution having a pH of 3.7 to 5.7.

Clinical Pharmacology: MONISTAT i.v. is rapidly metabolized in the liver and about 14% to 22% of the administered dose is excreted in the urine, mainly as inactive metabolites. The pharmacokinetic profile fits a three-compartment open model with the following biologic half-life: 0.4, 2.1, and 24.1 hours for each phase respectively. The pharmacokinetic profile of MONISTAT i.v. is unaltered in patients with renal insufficiency, including those patients on hemodialysis. The in-vitro antifungal activity of MONISTAT i.v. is very broad. Clinical efficacy has been demonstrated in patients with the following species of fungi: *Coccidioides immitis, Candida albicans, Cryptococcus neoformans, Petriellidium boydii (Allescheria boydii),* and *Paracoccidioides brasiliensis.*

Recommended doses of MONISTAT i.v. produce serum concentrations of drug which exceed the in-vitro MIC values for the fungal species noted above. Doses above 9 mg/kg of MONISTAT i.v. produce peak blood levels above 1μg/ml in most cases. The drug penetrates into joints.

Indications: MONISTAT i.v. is indicated for the treatment of the following severe systemic fungal infections: coccidioidomycosis, candidiasis, cryptococcosis, petriellidiosis (allescheriosis), paracoccidioidomycosis, and for the treatment of chronic mucocutaneous candidiasis. However, in the treatment of fungal meningitis and urinary bladder infections an intravenous infusion alone is inadequate. It must be supplemented with intrathecal administration and bladder irrigation. Appropriate diagnostic procedures should be followed and MIC's should be determined.

MONISTAT i.v. should not be used to treat common trivial forms of fungal diseases.

Contraindications: MONISTAT i.v. is contraindicated in those patients who have shown hypersensitivity to it.

Warnings: Rapid injection of undiluted MONISTAT i.v. may produce transient tachycardia or arrhythmia.

Precautions: Before a treatment course of MONISTAT i.v. is started, the physician should make sure that the patient is not hypersensitive to the drug product. MONISTAT i.v. should be given by intravenous infusion. The treatment should be started under stringent conditions of hospitalization but subsequently may be given to suitable patients under ambulatory conditions with close clinical monitoring. It is recommended that an initial dose of 200 mg be given with the physician in attendance. It is also recommended that clinical laboratory monitoring including hemoglobin, hematocrit, electrolytes and lipids be performed.

It should be borne in mind that systemic fungal mycoses may be complications of chronic underlying conditions which in themselves may require appropriate measures.

Since Petriellidium boydii is difficult to histologically distinguish from species of aspergillus, it is strongly recommended that cultures be grown.

Pregnancy: Reproductive studies with MONISTAT i.v. in rats and rabbits revealed no evidence of impaired fertility or harm to the fetus. There are no data, however, on the use of the drug in pregnant women.

Children: Since the safety of miconazole i.v. in children under one year of age has not been extensively studied, its benefits in this age group must be weighed against the possible risks involved.

Adverse Reactions: Adverse reactions which have been observed with MONISTAT i.v. therapy include phlebitis, pruritus, rash, nausea, vomiting, febrile reactions, drowsiness, diarrhea, anorexia and flushes. In the U.S. studies, 29% of 209 patients studied had phlebitis, 21% pruritus, 18% nausea, 10% fever and chills, 9% rash, and 7% emesis. Transient decreases in hematocrit and serum sodium values have been observed following infusion of MONISTAT i.v. Thrombocytopenia has also been reported. No serious renal or hepatic toxicity has been reported. If pruritus and skin rashes are severe, discontinuation of treatment may be necessary. Nausea and vomiting can be mitigated with antihistaminic or antiemetic drugs given prior to MONISTAT i.v. infusion, or by reducing the dose, slowing the rate of infusion, or avoiding administration at mealtime.

Aggregation of erythrocytes or rouleau formation on blood smears has been reported. Hyperlipemia has occurred in patients and is reported to be due to the vehicle, Cremophor EL (PEG 40 castor oil).

Drug Interactions: Drugs containing cremophor type vehicles are known to cause electrophoretic abnormalities of the lipoprotein. These effects are reversible upon discontinuation of treatment but are usually not an indication that treatment should be discontinued.

Interaction with the coumarin drugs resulting in an enhancement of the anticoagulant effect has also been reported. In cases of simultaneous treatment with MONISTAT i.v. and coumarin drugs, the anticoagulant effect should be carefully titrated since reductions of the anticoagulant doses may be indicated.

Dosage and Administration:

DOSAGE

Adults. The doses may vary with the diagnosis and with the infective agent, from 200 to 1200 mg per infusion. The following daily doses, which may be divided over 3 infusions, are recommended:

[See table on next page].

Repeated courses may be necessitated by relapse or reinfection.

Children. A total daily dose of about 20 to 40 mg/kg is generally adequate. However, a dose of 15 mg/kg body weight per infusion should not be exceeded.

ADMINISTRATION

MONISTAT i.v. should be diluted by adding at least 200 ml of diluent. The diluent of choice is 0.9% sodium chloride or alternatively Dextrose 5% injectable solution. The intravenous infusion should be given over a period of 30 to 60 minutes.

Generally, treatment should be continued until all clinical and laboratory tests no longer indicate that active fungal infection is present. Inadequate periods of treatment may yield poor response and lead to early recurrence of clinical symptoms. The dosing intervals and sites and the duration of treatment vary from patient to patient and depend on the causative organism.

OTHER MODES OF ADMINISTRATION

Intrathecal: Administration of the undiluted injectable solution of MONISTAT i.v. by the various intrathecal routes (20 mg per dose) is indicated as an adjunct to intravenous treatment in fungal meningitis. Succeeding intrathecal injections may be alternated between lumbar and cisternal punctures every 3 to 7 days.

Bladder instillation: 200 mg of miconazole in a diluted solution is indicated in the treatment of mycoses of the urinary bladder.

Store at controlled room temperatures (15° to 30°C/59° to 86°F)

How Supplied: MONISTAT i.v. is supplied in 20 ml ampoules. (**NDC** 50458-200-20).

U.S. Patent No. 3,717,655; 3,839,574

March 1980/Rev. May 1981/Rev. Jan 1982

MONISTAT i.v. (miconazole) is an original product of Janssen Pharmaceutica, N.V., Belgium.

Manufactured by McNEILAB, Inc. for JANSSEN Pharmaceutica Inc.
New Brunswick, NJ 08903

[*Shown in Product Indentification Section*]

NIZORAL® Tablets ℞
(ketoconazole)

Description: NIZORAL (ketoconazole) is a synthetic broad-spectrum antifungal agent available in scored white tablets, each containing 200 mg ketoconazole. Ketoconazole is *cis*-1-acetyl-4-[4-[[2-(2,4-dichlorophenyl)-2-(1*H*-imidazol-1-ylmethyl)-1,3-dioxolan-4-yl]methoxy] phenyl]piperazine.

NIZORAL is a white to slightly beige, odorless powder, soluble in acids, with a molecular weight of 531.44.

Clinical Pharmacology: Mean peak plasma levels of approximately 3.5 μg/ml are reached within 1 to 2 hours, following oral administration of a single 200 mg dose taken with a meal. Subsequent plasma elimination is biphasic with a half-life of 2 hours during the first 10 hours and 8 hours thereafter. Following absorption from the gastrointestinal tract, NIZORAL is converted into several inactive metabolites. The major identified metabolic pathways are oxidation and degradation of the imidazole and piperazine rings, oxidative O-dealkylation and aromatic hydroxylation. About 13% of the dose is excreted in the urine, of which 2 to 4% is unchanged drug. The major route of excretion is through the bile into the intestinal tract. *In vitro*, the plasma protein binding is about 99%, mainly to the albumin fraction. Only a negligible proportion of NIZORAL reaches the cerebral spinal fluid. NIZORAL is a weak dibasic agent and thus requires acidity for dissolution and absorption.

NIZORAL is active against clinical infections with *Candida* spp., *Coccidioides immitis, Histoplasma capsulatum, Paracoccidioides brasiliensis*, and *Phialophora* spp. Development of resistance to NIZORAL has not yet been reported.

The following preclinical data are available; however, their clinical significance is unknown. NIZORAL is active *in vitro* against dermatophytes, dimorphic fungi, eumycetes,

Organism	Dosage Range*	Duration of Successful Therapy (weeks)
Candidiasis	600 to 1800 mg per day	1 to > 20
Cryptococcosis	1200 to 2400 mg per day	3 to > 12
Coccidioidomycosis	1800 to 3600 mg per day	3 to > 20
Petriellidiosis (Allescheriosis)	600 to 3000 mg per day	5 to > 20
Paracoccidioidomycosis	200 to 1200 mg per day	2 to > 16

*May be divided over 3 infusions.

yeasts, actinomycetes, phycomycetes and various other fungi. In animal models, activity has been demonstrated against *Candida* spp., dermatophytes *(Trichophyton* spp., *Microsporum* spp., *Epidermophyton floccosum), Blastomyces dermatitidis, Histoplasma capsulatum, Malassezia furfur, Coccidioides immitis*, and *Cryptococcus neoformans.*

Mode of Action: *In vitro* studies suggest that NIZORAL impairs the synthesis of ergosterol, which is a vital component of fungal cell membranes. Tests in animals suggest this mechanism is not important in mammalian cells.

Indications and Usage: NIZORAL is indicated for the treatment of the following fungal infections: candidiasis, chronic mucocutaneous candidiasis, oral thrush, candiduria, coccidioidomycosis, histoplasmosis, chromomycosis, and paracoccidioidomycosis. NIZORAL should not be used for fungal meningitis because it penetrates poorly into the cerebral-spinal fluid.

For the initial diagnosis, the infective organism should be identified; however, therapy may be initiated prior to obtaining laboratory results.

Contraindications: NIZORAL is contraindicated in patients who have shown hypersentivity to the drug.

Warnings: Several cases of possible idiosyncratic hepatocellular dysfunction have been reported during NIZORAL treatment. It is important to recognize that liver disorders may occur with NIZORAL therapy. The rare occurrences of liver disorders could be potentially fatal unless properly recognized and managed.

It is desirable to perform liver function tests, such as SGGT, alkaline phosphatase, SGPT, SGOT and bilirubin, before treatment and at periodic intervals during treatment (monthly or more frequent), particularly in patients who will be on prolonged therapy or who have a history of liver disease. Instances of minor elevations of liver enzyme levels in patients on NIZORAL have been shown to normalize during therapy, and may not necessitate discontinuation of treatment. However, if liver function tests are significantly elevated or other signs and symptoms are suggestive of hepatocellular dysfunction, ketoconazole should be discontinued.

In female rats treated three to six months with ketoconazole at dose levels of 80 mg/kg and higher, increased fragility of long bones, in some cases leading to fracture, was seen. The maximum "no effect" dose level in these studies was 20 mg/kg (2.5 times the maximum recommended human dose). The mechanism responsible for this phenomenon is obscure. Limited studies in dogs failed to demonstrate such an effect on the metacarpals and ribs.

Precautions:

General: In four subjects with drug-induced achlorhydria, a marked reduction in NIZORAL absorption was observed. NIZORAL requires acidity for dissolution. If concomitant antacids, anticholinergics, and H_2-blockers are needed, they should be given at least two hours after NIZORAL administration. In cases of achlorhydria, the patients should be instructed to dissolve each tablet in 4 ml aqueous solution of 0.2 N HCl. For ingesting the resulting mixture, they should use a glass or plastic straw so as to avoid contact with the teeth. This administration should be followed with a cup of tap water.

Drug Interactions: There is no evidence for clinically significant interaction with oral anticoagulant or oral hypoglycemic agents.

Carcinogeneis, Mutagenesis, Impairment of Fertility: The dominant lethal mutation test in male and female mice revealed that single oral doses of NIZORAL as high as 80 mg/kg produced no mutation in any stage of germ cell development. The Ames *Salmonella* microsomal activator assay was also negative.

Pregnancy: Teratogenic effect: *Pregnancy Category C.* NIZORAL has been shown to be teratogenic (syndactylia and oligodactylia) in the rat when given in the diet at 80 mg/kg/day, (10 times the maximum recommended human dose). However, these effects may be related to maternal toxicity, evidence of which also was seen at this and higher dose levels.

There are no adequate and well controlled studies in pregnant women. NIZORAL should be used during pregnancy only if the potential benefit justifies the potential risk to the fetus.

Nonteratogenic effects: NIZORAL has also been found to be embryotoxic in the rat when given in the diet at doses higher than 80 mg/kg during the first trimester of gestation.

In addition, dystocia (difficult labor) was noted in rats administered NIZORAL during the third trimester of gestation. This occurred when NIZORAL was administered at doses higher than 10 mg/kg (higher than 1.25 times the maximum human dose).

It is likely that both the malformations and the embryotoxicity resulting from the administration of NIZORAL during gestation are a reflection of the particular sensitivity of the female rat to this drug. For example, the oral LD_{50} of NIZORAL given by gavage to the female rate is 166 mg/kg, whereas in the male rat the oral LD_{50} is 287 mg/kg.

Nursing Mothers: Since NIZORAL is probably excreted in the milk, mothers who are under NIZORAL treatment should not breastfeed the child.

Pediatric Use: Safety in children under two years of age has been documented in a limited number of cases.

Adverse Reactions: NIZORAL is usually well tolerated. Most adverse reactions reported have been mild and transient and have only rarely required withdrawal of therapy.

The most frequent adverse reactions were nausea and/or vomiting, which occurred in approximately 3% of patients. Abdominal pain was reported in approximately 1.2% of patients, pruritis in approximately 1.5% of patients. The following have been reported in less than 1% of patients: headache, dizziness, somnolence, fever and chills, photophobia, and diarrhea, jaundice and gynecomastia. Transient increases in serum liver enzymes have been observed. In the majority of cases, these increases have normalized during therapy or shortly after drug has been discontinued. However, several cases of idiosyncratic hepatocellular dysfunction have been reported (see WARNINGS).

Overdosage: In the event of accidental overdosage, supportive measures, including gastric lavage with sodium bicarbonate should be employed.

Continued on next page

Janssen—Cont.

Dosage and Administration:
Adults: The recommended starting dose of NIZORAL is a single daily administration of 200 mg (one tablet). In very serious infections or if clinical responsiveness is insufficient within the expected time, the dose of NIZORAL may be increased to 400 mg (two tablets) once daily.
Children:
Children weighing 20 kg or less ......50 mg (1/4 tablet) once daily
Children weighing 20–40 kg ...100 mg (1/2 tablet) once daily
Children weighing over 40 kg ....200 mg (1 tablet) once daily
Generally, treatment should be continued until all clinical and laboratory tests indicate that active fungal infection has subsided. Inadequate periods of treatment may yield poor response and lead to early recurrence of clinical symptoms. Minimum treatment for candidiasis is one or two weeks. Patients with chronic mucocutaneous candidiasis usually require maintenance therapy. Minimum treatment for the other indicated systemic mycoses is six months.
How Supplied: NIZORAL is available as white, scored tablets containing 200 mg of ketoconazole debossed "JANSSEN" and on the reverse side debossed "K" and "200". They are supplied in bottles of 60 tablets and in blister packs of 10 × 10 tablets.
U.S. Patent 4,335,125
NDC 50458-220-06 (60 tablets)
NDC 50458-220-01 (10 × 10 tablets-blister)
May 1981/Rev. Nov. 1981/Rev. Feb. 1982
Manufactured by
Janssen Pharmaceutica n.v.
B-2340 Beerse, Belgium
For:
Janssen Pharmaceutica Inc.
New Brunswick, New Jersey 08903 USA

SUBLIMAZE® ℂ ℞
(fentanyl) as the citrate
INJECTION

Protect from light. Store at room temperature.

FOR INTRAVENOUS OR INTRAMUSCULAR USE ONLY

Description: Each ml. contains:
Fentanyl ......50 mcg. (0.05 mg.) as the citrate
Warning: May be habit forming.
Sodium hydroxide for adjustment of pH to 4.0–7.5.
[See table below].
Actions: SUBLIMAZE (fentanyl) is a narcotic analgesic. SUBLIMAZE (fentanyl) in a dose of 100 mcg. (0.1 mg.)(2.0 ml.) is approximately equivalent in analgesic activity to 10 mg. of morphine or 75 mg. of meperidine. The principal actions of therapeutic value are analgesia and sedation. Alterations in respiratory rate and alveolar ventilation, associated with narcotic analgesics, may last longer than the analgesic effect. As the dose of narcotic is increased, the decrease in pulmonary exchange becomes greater. Large doses may produce apnea. SUBLIMAZE (fentanyl) appears to have less emetic activity than other narcotic analgesics. Histamine assays and skin wheal testing in man, as well as in *in vivo* testing in dogs, indicate that clinically significant histamine release rarely occurs with SUBLIMAZE (fentanyl). Recent assays in man show no clinically significant histamine release in dosages up to 50 mcg./kg. (.05 mg./kg.)(1 ml./kg.). SUBLIMAZE (fentanyl) preserves cardiac stability, and obtunds stress-related hormonal changes at higher doses.
SUBLIMAZE (fentanyl) may cause muscle rigidity, particularly involving the muscles of respiration. It may also produce other signs and symptoms characteristic of narcotic analgesics including euphoria, miosis, bradycardia, and bronchoconstriction.
The onset of action of SUBLIMAZE (fentanyl) is almost immediate when the drug is given intravenously; however, the maximal analgesic and respiratory depressant effect may not be noted for several minutes. The usual duration of action of the analgesic effect is 30 to 60 minutes after a single I.V. dose of up to 100 mcg. (0.1 mg.)(2.0 ml.). Following intramuscular administration, the onset of action is from seven to eight minutes, and the duration of action is one to two hours. As with longer acting narcotic analgesics, the duration of the respiratory depressant effect of SUBLIMAZE (fentanyl) may be longer than the analgesic effect. The following observations have been reported concerning altered respiratory response to CO_2 stimulation following administration of fentanyl to man.
1. DIMINISHED SENSITIVITY TO CO_2 STIMULATION MAY PERSIST LONGER THAN DEPRESSION OF RESPIRATORY RATE. (Altered sensitivity to CO_2 stimulation has been demonstrated for up to four hours following a single intravenous dose of 600 mcg. (0.6 mg.)(12 ml.) fentanyl to healthy volunteers.) Fentanyl frequently slows the respiratory rate, duration and degree of respiratory depression being dose related.
2. The peak respiratory depressant effect of a single intravenous dose of fentanyl is noted 5 to 15 minutes following injection.
See also WARNINGS and PRECAUTIONS concerning respiratory depression.
Indications: SUBLIMAZE (fentanyl) is indicated:
—for analgesic action of short duration during the anesthetic periods, premedication, induction, and maintenance, and in the immediate postoperative period (recovery room) as the need arises.
—for use as a narcotic analgesic supplement in general or regional anesthesia.
—for administration with a neuroleptic such as *INAPSINE*® (droperidol) injection as an anesthetic premedication, for the induction of anesthesia and as an adjunct in the maintenance of general and regional anesthesia.
—for use as an anesthetic agent with oxygen in selected high risk patients, such as those undergoing open heart surgery or certain complicated neurological or orthopedic procedures.
Contraindications: SUBLIMAZE (fentanyl) is contraindicated in patients with known intolerance to the drug.
Warnings: AS WITH OTHER CNS DEPRESSANTS, PATIENTS WHO HAVE RECEIVED *SUBLIMAZE* (FENTANYL) SHOULD HAVE APPROPRIATE SURVEILLANCE.
RESUSCITATION EQUIPMENT AND A NARCOTIC ANTAGONIST SHOULD BE READILY AVAILABLE TO MANAGE APNEA.
See also discussion of narcotic antagonists in Precautions and Overdosage.
If SUBLIMAZE (fentanyl) is administered with a tranquilizer such as *INAPSINE* (droperidol), the user should familiarize himself with the special properties of each drug, particularly the widely differing duration of action. In addition, when such a combination is used, *fluids and other countermeasures to manage hypotension should be available.*
As with other potent narcotics, the respiratory depressant effect of SUBLIMAZE (fentanyl) may persist longer than the measured analgesic effect. The total dose of all narcotic analgesics administered should be considered by the practitioner before ordering narcotic analgesics during recovery from anesthesia. It is recommended that narcotics, when required, should be used in reduced doses initially, as low as 1/4 to 1/3 those usually recommended. SUBLIMAZE (fentanyl) may cause muscle rigidity, particularly involving the muscles of respiration. The effect is related to the speed of injection and its incidence can be reduced by the use of slow intravenous injection. Once the effect occurs, it is managed by the use of assisted or controlled respiration and, if necessary, by a neuromuscular blocking agent compatible with the patient's condition. Where moderate or high doses are used (above 10 mcg./kg.), there must be adequate facilities for postoperative observation, and ventilation if necessary, of patients who have received SUBLIMAZE (fentanyl). It is essential that these facilities be fully equipped to handle all degrees of respiratory depression.

DOSAGE RANGE CHART

TOTAL DOSAGE

Low dose—2 mcg./kg. (.002 mg./kg.)(.04 ml./kg.) SUBLIMAZE® injection. Fentanyl in small doses is most useful for minor, but painful, surgical procedures. In addition to the analgesia during surgery, fentanyl may also provide some pain relief in the immediate post-operative period.	**Moderate dose**—2-20 mcg./kg. (.002–.02 mg./kg.)(.04–0.4 ml./kg.) SUBLIMAZE® injection. Where surgery becomes more major, a larger dose is required. With this dose, in addition to adequate analgesia, one would expect to see some abolition of the stress response. However, respiratory depression will be such that artificial ventilation during anesthesia is necessary, and careful observation of ventilation post-operatively is essential.	**High dose**—20–50 mcg./kg. (.02–.05 mg./kg.)(0.4–1 ml./kg.) SUBLIMAZE® injection. During open heart surgery and certain more complicated neurosurgical and orthopedic procedures where surgery is more prolonged, and in the opinion of the anesthesiologist, the stress response to surgery would be detrimental to the well being of the patient, dosages of 20–50 mcg./kg. (.02–.05 mg.)(0.4–1 ml.) of SUBLIMAZE® injection with nitrous oxide oxygen have been shown to attenuate the	stress response as defined by increased levels of circulating growth hormone, catecholamine, ADH, and prolactin. When dosages in this range have been used during surgery, post-operative ventilation and observation are essential due to extended post-operative respiratory depression. The main objective of this technique would be to produce "stress free" anesthesia.

Drug Dependence—SUBLIMAZE (fentanyl) can produce drug dependence of the morphine type and, therefore, has the potential for being abused.

Severe and unpredictable potentiation by MAO inhibitors has been reported with narcotic analgesics. Since the safety of fentanyl in this regard has not been established, the use of SUBLIMAZE (fentanyl) in patients who have received MAO inhibitors within 14 days is not recommended.

Head Injuries and Increased Intracranial Pressure—SUBLIMAZE (fentanyl) should be used with caution in patients who may be particularly susceptible to respiratory depression, such as comatose patients who may have a head injury or brain tumor. In addition, SUBLIMAZE (fentanyl) may obscure the clinical course of patients with head injury.

Usage in Children—The safety of SUBLIMAZE (fentanyl) in children younger than two years of age has not been established.

Usage in Pregnancy—The safe use of SUBLIMAZE (fentanyl) has not been established with respect to possible adverse effects upon fetal development. Therefore, it should be used in women of childbearing potential only when, in the judgment of the physician, the potential benefits outweigh the possible hazards. There are insufficient data regarding placental transfer and fetal effects; therefore, safety for the infant in obstetrics has not been established.

Precautions: *The initial dose of SUBLIMAZE (fentanyl) should be appropriately reduced in elderly and debilitated patients. The effect of the initial dose should be considered in determining incremental doses. Nitrous oxide has been reported to produce cardiovascular depression when given with higher doses of fentanyl.*

Certain forms of conduction anesthesia, such as spinal anesthesia and some peridural anesthetics, can alter respiration by blocking intercostal nerves. Through other mechanisms (see Actions) SUBLIMAZE (fentanyl) can also alter respiration. Therefore, when SUBLIMAZE (fentanyl) is used to supplement these forms of anesthesia, the anesthetist should be familiar with the physiological alterations involved, and be prepared to manage them in the patients selected for these forms of anesthesia.

When used with a tranquilizer such as *INAPSINE* (droperidol), blood pressure may be altered and hypotension can occur.

Vital signs should be monitored routinely.

SUBLIMAZE (fentanyl) should be used with caution in patients with chronic obstructive pulmonary disease, patients with decreased respiratory reserve, and others with potentially compromised respiration. In such patients, narcotics may additionally decrease respiratory drive and increase airway resistance. During anesthesia, this can be managed by assisted or controlled respiration. Respiratory depression caused by narcotic analgesics can be reversed by narcotic antagonists. Appropriate surveillance should be maintained because the duration of respiratory depression of doses of fentanyl employed during anesthesia may be longer than the duration of the narcotic antagonist action. Consult individual prescribing information (levallorphan, nalorphine and naloxone) before employing narcotic antagonists.

When a tranquilizer such as *INAPSINE* (droperidol) is used with SUBLIMAZE (fentanyl) pulmonary arterial pressure may be decreased. This fact should be considered by those who conduct diagnostic and surgical procedures where interpretation of pulmonary arterial pressure measurements might determine final management of the patient. When high dose or anesthetic dosages of SUBLIMAZE (fentanyl) are employed, even relatively small dosages of diazepam may cause cardiovascular depression.

Other CNS depressant drugs (e.g. barbiturates, tranquilizers, narcotics, and general anesthetics) will have additive or potentiating effects with SUBLIMAZE (fentanyl). When patients have received such drugs, the dose of SUBLIMAZE (fentanyl) required will be less than usual. Likewise, following the administration of SUBLIMAZE (fentanyl), the dose of other CNS depressant drugs should be reduced.

SUBLIMAZE (fentanyl) should be administered with caution to patients with liver and kidney dysfunction because of the importance of these organs in the metabolism and excretion of drugs.

SUBLIMAZE (fentanyl) may produce bradycardia, which may be treated with atropine; however, SUBLIMAZE (fentanyl) should be used with caution in patients with cardiac bradyarrhythmias.

When SUBLIMAZE (fentanyl) is used with a tranquilizer such as *INAPSINE* (droperidol) hypotension can occur. If this occurs, the possibility of hypovolemia should also be considered and managed with appropriate parenteral fluid therapy. Repositioning the patient to improve venous return to the heart should be considered when operative conditions permit. Care should be exercised in moving and positioning of patients because of the possibility of orthostatic hypotension. If volume expansion with fluids plus other countermeasures do not correct hypotension, the administration of pressor agents other than epinephrine should be considered. Because of the alpha-adrenergic blocking action of *INAPSINE* (droperidol), epinephrine may pardoxically decrease the blood pressure in patients treated with *INAPSINE* (droperidol).

When *INAPSINE* (droperidol) is used with SUBLIMAZE (fentanyl) and the EEG is used for postoperative monitoring, it may be found that the EEG pattern returns to normal slowly.

Adverse Reactions: As with other narcotic analgesics, the most common serious adverse reactions reported to occur with SUBLIMAZE (fentanyl) are respiratory depression, apnea, muscular rigidity, and bradycardia; if these remain untreated, respiratory arrest, circulatory depression or cardiac arrest could occur. Other adverse reactions that have been reported are hypotension, dizziness, blurred vision, nausea, emesis, laryngospasm, and diaphoresis.

It has been reported that secondary rebound respiratory depression may occasionally occur postoperatively. Patients should be monitored for this possibility and appropriate countermeasures taken as necessary.

When a tranquilizer such as *INAPSINE* (droperidol) is used with SUBLIMAZE (fentanyl), the following adverse reactions can occur: chills and/or shivering, restlessness, and postoperative hallucinatory episodes (sometimes associated with transient periods of mental depression); extrapyramidal symptoms (dystonia, akathisia, and oculogyric crisis) have been observed up to 24 hours postoperatively. When they occur, extrapyramidal symptoms can usually be controlled with anti-parkinson agents. Postoperative drowsiness is also frequently reported following the use of *INAPSINE* (droperidol).

Elevated blood pressure, with and without preexisting hypertension, has been reported following administration of SUBLIMAZE (fentanyl) combined with *INAPSINE* (droperidol). This might be due to unexplained alterations in sympathetic activity following large doses; however, it is also frequently attributed to anesthetic and surgical stimulation during light anesthesia.

Dosage and Administration:

50 mcg. = .05 mg. = 1 ml.

Dosage should be individualized. Some of the factors to be considered in determining the dose are age, body weight, physical status, underlying pathological condition, use of other drugs, type of anesthesia to be used, and the surgical procedure involved.

Vital signs should be monitored routinely.

I. *Premedication*—Premedication (to be appropriately modified in the elderly, debilitated, and those who have received other depressant drugs)—50 to 100 mcg. (0.05 to 0.1 mg.)(1 to 2 ml.) may be administered *intramuscularly* 30 to 60 minutes prior to surgery.

II. *Adjunct to General Anesthesia*—See Dosage Range Chart.

III. *Adjunct to Regional Anesthesia*—50 to 100 mcg. (0.05 to 0.1 mg.)(1 to 2 ml.) may be administered intramuscularly or slowly intravenously, over one to two minutes, when additional analgesia is required.

IV. *Postoperatively (recovery room)*—50 to 100 mcg. (0.05 to 0.1 mg.)(1 to 2 ml.) may be administered intramuscularly for the control of pain, tachypnea and emergence delirium. The dose may be repeated in one to two hours as needed.

Usual Children's Dosage: For induction and maintenance in children 2 to 12 years of age, a reduced dose as low as 20 to 30 mcg. (0.02 to 0.03 mg.)(0.4 to 0.6 ml.) per 20 to 25 pounds is recommended.

As a General Anesthetic

When attenuation of the responses to surgical stress is especially important, doses of 50 to 100 mcg./kg. (.05 to 0.1 mg./kg.)(1 to 2 ml./kg.) may be administered with oxygen and a muscle relaxant. This technique has been reported to provide anesthesia without the use of additional anesthetic agents. In certain cases, doses

DOSAGE RANGE CHART

MAINTENANCE DOSE

Low dose—2 mcg./kg. (.002 mg./kg.)(.04 ml./kg.) SUBLIMAZE® injection.	**Moderate dose**—2–20 mcg./kg.) (.002–.02 mg./kg.)(.04–0.4 ml./kg.) SUBLIMAZE® injection.	**High dose**—20–50 mcg./kg. (.02–.05 mg./kg.)(0.4–1 ml./kg.) SUBLIMAZE® injection.
Additional dosages of SUBLIMAZE® injection are infrequently needed in these minor procedures.	25 to 100 mcg. (0.025 to 0.1 mg.)(0.5 to 2.0 ml.) may be administered intravenously or intramuscularly when movement and/or changes in vital signs indicate surgical stress or lightening of analgesia.	Maintenance dosage (ranging from 25 mcg. (.025 mg.)(0.5 ml.) to one half the initial loading dose) will be dictated by the changes in vital signs which indicate stress and lightening of analgesia. However, the additional dosage selected must be individualized especially if the anticipated remaining operative time is short.

Continued on next page

Janssen—Cont.

up to 150 mcg./kg. (.15 mg./kg.)(3 ml./kg.) may be necessary to produce this anesthetic effect. It has been used for open heart surgery and certain other major surgical procedures in patients for whom protection of the myocardium from excess oxygen demand is particularly indicated, and for certain complicated neurological and orthopedic procedures.
(See table on preceding page)
As noted above, it is essential that qualified personnel and adequate facilities be available for the management of respiratory depression. See Warnings and Precautions for use of SUBLIMAZE (fentanyl) with other CNS depressants, and in patients with altered response.

Overdosage:
Manifestations: The manifestations of SUBLIMAZE (fentanyl) overdosage are an extension of its pharmacologic actions.
Treatment: In the presence of hypoventilation or apnea, oxygen should be administered and respiration should be assisted or controlled as indicated. A patent airway must be maintained; an oropharyngeal airway or endotracheal tube might be indicated. If depressed respiration is associated with muscular rigidity, an intravenous neuromuscular blocking agent might be required to facilitate assisted or controlled respiration. The patient should be carefully observed for 24 hours; body warmth and adequate fluid intake should be maintained. If hypotension occurs and is severe or persists, the possibility of hypovolemia should be considered and managed with appropriate parenteral fluid therapy. A specific narcotic antagonist such as nalorphine, levallorphan, or naloxone should be available for use as indicated to manage respiratory depression. This does not preclude the use of more immediate countermeasures. The duration of respiratory depression following overdosage of fentanyl may be longer than the duration of narcotic antagonist action. Consult the package insert of the individual narcotic antagonists for details about use.

How Supplied:
2 ml. and 5 ml. ampoules—packages of 10.
NDC 50458-030-02 **NDC** 50458-030-05
10 ml. and 20 ml. ampoules—packages of 5.
NDC 50458-030-10 **NDC** 50458-030-20
(FOR INTRAVENOUS USE BY HOSPITAL PERSONNEL SPECIFICALLY TRAINED IN THE USE OF NARCOTIC ANALGESICS)
U.S. Patent No. 3,164,600
Manufactured by McNEILAB, Inc. for
JANSSEN Pharmaceutica Inc.
New Brunswick, NJ 08903
March 1980/Rev. June 1980/Rev. Jan. 1981
[*Shown in Product Identification Section*]

VERMOX® Chewable Tablets ℞
(mebendazole)

Description: VERMOX (mebendazole) is methyl 5-benzoylbenzimidazole-2-carbamate.
Actions: VERMOX exerts its anthelmintic effect by blocking glucose uptake by the susceptible helminths, thereby depleting the energy level until it becomes inadequate for survival.
In man, approximately 2% of administered mebendazole is excreted in urine as unchanged drug or a primary metabolite. Following administration of 100 mg of mebendazole twice daily for three consecutive days, plasma levels of mebendazole and its primary metabolite, the 2-amine, never exceeded 0.03 μg/ml and 0.09 μg/ml, respectively.
Indications: VERMOX is indicated for the treatment of *Trichuris trichiura* (whipworm), *Enterobius vermicularis* (pinworm), *Ascaris lumbricoides* (roundworm), *Ancylostoma duodenale* (common hookworm), *Necator americanus* (American hookworm) in single or mixed infections.
Efficacy varies as a function of such factors as pre-existing diarrhea and gastrointestinal transit time, degree of infection and helminth strains. Efficacy rates derived from various studies are shown in the table below:
[See table above].

	Efficacy Rates			
	Whipworm	Common Roundworm	Hookworm	Pinworm
cure rates				
mean	68%	98%	96%	95%
(range)	(61–75%)	(91–100%)	—	(90–100%)
egg reduction				
mean	93%	99.7%	99.9%	—
(range)	(70–99%)	(99.5–100%)	—	—

Contraindications: VERMOX is contraindicated in pregnant women (see: Pregnancy Precautions) and in persons who have shown hypersensitivity to the drug.
Precautions:
PREGNANCY:
VERMOX has shown embryotoxic and teratogenic activity in pregnant rats at single oral doses as low as 10 mg/kg. Since VERMOX may have a risk of producing fetal damage if administered during pregnancy, it is contraindicated in pregnant women.
PEDIATRIC USE:
The drug has not been extensively studied in children under two years; therefore, in the treatment of children under two years the relative benefit/risk should be considered.
Adverse Reactions: Transient symptoms of abdominal pain and diarrhea have occurred in cases of massive infection and expulsion of worms.
Dosage and Administration: The same dosage schedule applies to children and adults. The tablet may be chewed, swallowed or crushed and mixed with food. For the control of pinworm (enterobiasis), a single tablet is administered orally, one time. For the control of common roundworm (ascariasis), whipworm (trichuriasis), and hookworm infection, one tablet of VERMOX is administered, orally, morning and evening, on three consecutive days.
If the patient is not cured three weeks after treatment, a second course of treatment is advised. No special procedures, such as fasting or purging, are required.
How Supplied: VERMOX is available as chewable tablets, each containing 100 mg of mebendazole, and is supplied in boxes of twelve tablets. (**NDC** 50458-110-01)
U.S. Patent 3,657,267 December 1979
VERMOX (mebendazole) is an original product of Janssen Pharmaceutica, Belgium.
Tableted by Janssen Pharmaceutica, Beerse, Belgium for Janssen Pharmaceutica Inc. New Brunswick, NJ 08903 USA
[*Shown in Product Identification Section*]

IDENTIFICATION PROBLEM?

Consult PDR's

Product Identification Section

where you'll find over 900

products pictured actual size

and in full color.

Johnson & Johnson Products Inc.
PATIENT CARE DIVISION
501 GEORGE STREET
NEW BRUNSWICK, NJ 08903

DEBRISAN®
wound cleaning beads and paste.
Draws Exudate from Wet Ulcers and Wounds

Description: DEBRISAN® consists of spherical hydrophilic beads of dextranomer, 0.1–0.3mm in diameter; the paste is a mixture of the beads and polyethylene glycol. The beads are composed of a three dimensional network of macromolecular chains of cross-linked dextran which is large enough to allow substances with a molecular weight of less than 1000 to enter freely. Substances with a molecular weight of 1000–5000 enter the beads less freely, while those with a molecular weight greater than 5000 remain in the interspaces between the beads.
Characteristics: Because of its hydrophilic properties, each gram of DEBRISAN® beads absorbs approximately 4 ml. of fluid. The beads swell to approximately four times their original size. This swelling causes significant suction forces and capillary action in the spaces between the beads. This action is continuous as long as unsaturated beads or paste is in proximity to the ulcer or wound.
When DEBRISAN® beads or paste are applied to the surface of wet ulcers or wounds their suction forces immediately begin removing various exudates and particles that tend to impede tissue repair. For example, low molecular weight components of wound exudates are drawn up within the DEBRISAN® beads or paste, while higher molecular weight components, such as plasma proteins, and fibrinogen are found between the swollen beads. Removal of these latter components, particularly fibrin and fibrinogen, retards eschar formation. Additionally, there is *in vitro* evidence that the suction forces created by the beads remove bacteria and inflammatory exudates from the surface of the wound.
The use of DEBRISAN® beads or paste to remove exudates rapidly and continuously from the surface of the wound results in a concomitant reduction of inflammation and edema.
Indications: DEBRISAN® beads and paste are indicated for use in cleaning wet ulcers and wounds such as venous stasis ulcers, decubitus ulcers, and infected traumatic and surgical wounds. DEBRISAN® beads are also indicated for use in cleaning infected burns.
Precautions: To minimize the possibility of cross-contamination, contents of a DEBRISAN® bead container should be limited to use in one patient.
When treating cratered decubitus ulcers, do not pack the wounds tightly. Allow for expansion of the beads. Do not use DEBRISAN® beads or paste in deep fistulas, sinus tracts, or any body cavity where complete removal is not assured.
Once the DEBRISAN® is saturated it should be removed. This avoids encrustation of beads which makes removal more difficult. A DEBRISAN® must be removed before an

surgical procedure to close the wound (*ie* graft or flap).

Wounds may appear larger during the first few days of treatment due to the reduction of edema.

DEBRISAN® beads and paste are not effective in cleaning dry wounds.

Not all wounds require treatment with DEBRISAN® to complete healing. When the wound is no longer wet and a healthy granulation base has been established, the application of DEBRISAN® beads or paste should be discontinued.

Treatment of the underlying condition (venous or arterial flow, pressure, etc.) should be addressed, in addition to using DEBRISAN® beads or paste.

Adverse Reactions: Upon application and/or removal of DEBRISAN® beads, transitory pain, bleeding, blistering and erythema have been reported in isolated cases.

Directions for Use:

Applying DEBRISAN®

Debride and wash the area in the usual manner. **DEBRISAN® beads and paste are not enzymes and will not debride.** Leave the area moist since this facilitates the action of DEBRISAN®

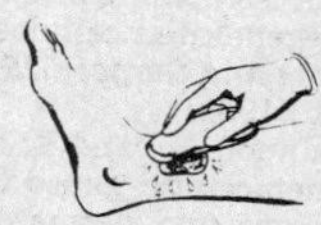

Apply DEBRISAN® beads or paste to at least ¼ inch (6mm) thickness. At least ¼ inch thickness is required to achieve desired suction effects.

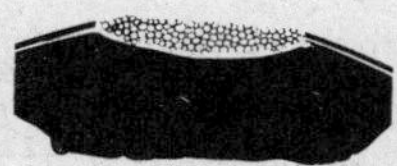

Apply a dressing. Close all four sides.

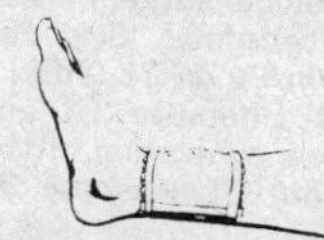

Removing DEBRISAN®

When DEBRISAN® beads or paste become saturated, a color change will be noted indicating that they should be removed. Removal should be as complete as possible and is best achieved by irrigation. Occasionally vigorous irrigation, soaking, or whirlpool may be required to remove patches of DEBRISAN® that adhere to the wound.

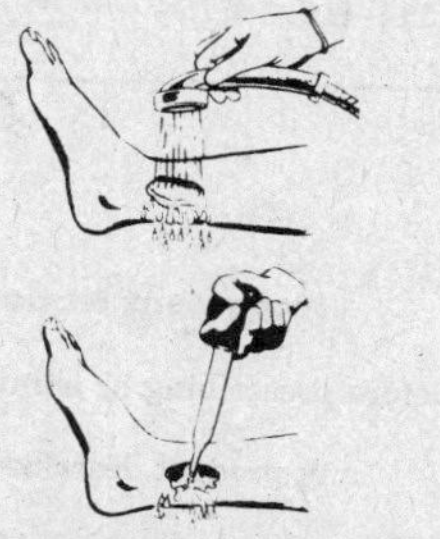

Reapply DEBRISAN® beads or paste every 12 hours, or more frequently if necessary. Reduce the number of applications as the exudate diminishes.

A paste mixture of DEBRISAN® beads may be prepared for application on irregular body surfaces or hard to reach areas. Two methods of application are possible:

1. Carefully pour a small amount of glycerin on a dry dressing large enough to cover the

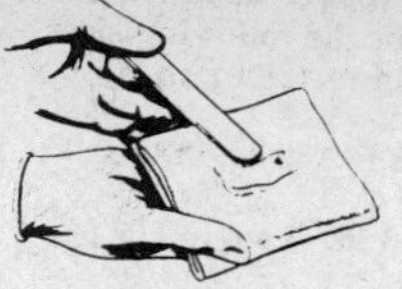

wound and add a sufficient amount of DEBRISAN® beads to make a layer at least ¼″ thick.
2. Or, DEBRISAN® beads (3 parts) may be mixed with glycerin (1 part) in a receptacle and applied directly to the wound with a spatula. Do not mix with any substance other than glycerin.

In either case, dress the wound in the usual manner. Mix a fresh paste for each application. Do not reuse.

When to Discontinue:

When the area is free of exudate and edema.

When a healthy granulation base is present.

The patient should consult the physician if the condition worsens or persists beyond the expected length of treatment (normally 14–21 days).

How Supplied: DEBRISAN® beads are supplied sterile, in containers of 25, 60, 120 grams each and 4 gram packets in boxes of 7 or 14. DEBRISAN® paste is also available in a pre-mixed sterile form, in 10 gram foil packets, six per box.

Store in a dry place below 85°F.

Avoid contact with eyes.

For external use only.

Spilling beads or paste onto the floor will result in a slippery surface.

MANUFACTURED IN SWEDEN FOR
JOHNSON & JOHNSON PRODUCTS INC.
NEW BRUNSWICK, NEW JERSEY 08903
©J&JPI82

SURGICEL® Absorbable Hemostat ℞
(oxidized regenerated cellulose)

For surgical use

(For dental application of this product, reference should be made to the package insert for dental use.)

Description: SURGICEL® Absorbable Hemostat is a sterile, absorbable knitted fabric prepared by the controlled oxidation of regenerated cellulose. The fabric is white with a pale yellow cast and has a faint, caramel-like aroma. It is strong and can be sutured or cut without fraying. It is stable and can be stored at controlled room temperature. A slight discoloration may occur with age, but this does not affect performance.

Actions: The mechanism of action whereby SURGICEL® Absorbable Hemostat accelerates clotting is not completely understood, but it appears to be a physical effect rather than any alteration of the normal physiologic clotting mechanism. After SURGICEL has been saturated with blood, it swells into a brownish or black gelatinous mass which aids in the formation of a clot, thereby serving as a hemostatic adjunct in the control of local hemorrhage. When used properly in minimal amounts, SURGICEL is absorbed from the sites of implantation with practically no tissue reaction. Absorption depends upon several factors including the amount used, degree of saturation with blood, and the tissue bed.

In addition to its local hemostatic properties, SURGICEL Absorbable Hemostat is bactericidal **in vitro** against a wide range of gram positive and gram negative organisms including aerobes and anaerobes. SURGICEL is bactericidal **in vitro** against strains of species including those of:

Staphylococcus aureus
Staphylococcus epidermidis
Micrococcus luteus
Streptococcus pyogenes Group A
Streptococcus pyogenes Group B
Bacillus subtilis
Proteus vulgaris
Corynebacterium serosis
Mycobacterium phlei
Clostridium tetani
Streptococcus salivarius
Branhamella catarrhalis
Escherichia coli
Klebsiella aerogenes
Lactobacillus sp.
Salmonella enteritidis
Shigella dysenteriae
Serratia marscescens
Clostridium perfringens
Bacteroides fragilis
Enterococcus
Enterbacter cloacae
Pseudomonas aeruginosa
Pseudomonas stutzeri
Proteus mirabilis

Studies conducted in animals show that SURGICEL in contrast to other hemostatic agents does not tend to enhance experimental infection.

Indications: SURGICEL® Absorbable Hemostat (oxidized regenerated cellulose) is used adjunctively in surgical procedures to assist in the control of capillary, venous, and small arterial hemorrhage when ligation or other conventional methods of control are impractical or ineffective.

Contraindications: Although packing or wadding sometimes is medically necessary, SURGICEL® Absorbable Hemostat should not be used in this manner unlss it is to be removed after hemostasis is achieved.

SURGICEL should not be used for implantation in bone defects, such as fractures, since there is a possibility of interference with callus formation and a theoretical chance of cyst formation.

When SURGICEL is used to help achieve hemostasis around the spinal cord in laminectomies, or around the optic nerve and chiasm, it must always be removed after hemostasis is achieved since it will swell and could exert unwanted pressure.

SURGICEL should not be used to control hemorrhage from large arteries.

SURGICEL should not be used on non-hemorrhagic serous oozing surfaces, since body fluids other than whole blood, such as serum, do not react with SURGICEL to produce satisfactory hemostatic effect.

Warnings: SURGICEL® Absorbable Hemostat is supplied sterile and should not be autoclaved because autoclaving causes physical breakdown of the product.

SURGICEL is not intended as a substitute for careful surgery and the proper use of sutures and ligatures.

Closing SURGICEL in a contaminated wound without drainage may lead to complications and should be avoided.

The hemostatic effect of SURGICEL is greater when it is applied dry; therefore it should not be moistened with water or saline.

SURGICEL should not be impregnated with anti-infective agents or with other materials such as buffering or hemostatic substances. Its hemostatic effect is not enhanced by the addition of thrombin, the activity of which is destroyed by the low pH of the product.

Although SURGICEL Absorbable Hemostat may be left in situ when necessary, it is advisable to remove it once hemostasis is achieved. It must always be removed from the site of application after use in laminectomy procedures and from foramina in bone when hemostasis is obtained. This is because SURGICEL, by swelling, may cause nerve damage by pressure in a bony confine. Paralysis has been reported

Continued on next page

Johnson & Johnson—Cont.

when used around the spinal cord, particularly in surgery for herniated intervertebral disc.
Although SURGICEL is bactericidal against a wide range of pathogenic microorganisms, it is not intended as a substitute for systemically administered therapeutic or prophylactic antimicrobial agents to control or prevent postoperative infections.

Precautions: Use only as much SURGICEL® Absorbable Hemostat as is necessary for hemostasis, holding it in place until bleeding stops. Remove any excess before surgical closure in order to facilitate absorption and minimize the possibility of foreign body reaction.

SURGICEL should be applied loosely against the bleeding surface Wadding or packing should be avoided, especially within rigid cavities where swelling may intefere with normal function or possibly cause necrosis.

In urological procedures, minimal amounts of SURGICEL should be used and care must be exercised to prevent plugging of the urethra, ureter, or a catheter by dislodged portions of the product.

Since absorption of SURGICEL could be prevented in chemically cauterized areas, its use should not be preceded by application of silver nitrate or any other escharotic chemicals.

If SURGICEL is used temporarily to line the cavity of large open wounds, it should be placed so as not to overlap the skin edges. It should also be removed from open wounds by forceps or by irrigation with sterile water or saline solution after bleeding has stopped.

Precautions should be taken in otorhinolaryngologic surgery to assure that none of the material is aspirated by the patient. (Examples: controlling hemorrhage after tonsillectomy and controlling epistaxis.)

Care should be taken not to apply SURGICEL too tightly when it is used as a wrap during vascular surgery (See "ADVERSE REACTIONS" section).

Adverse Reactions: "Encapsulation" of fluid and foreign body reactions have been reported.

There have been two reports of stenotic effect when SURGICEL® Absorbable Hemostat has been applied as a wrap during vascular surgery. Although it has not been established that the stenosis was directly related to the use of SURGICEL, it is important to be cautious and avoid applying the material tightly as a wrapping.

Possible prolongation of drainage in cholecystectomies and difficulty passing urine per urethra after prostatectomy have been reported.

There has been one report of a blocked ureter after kidney resection, in which postoperative catheterization was required.

Occasional reports of "burning" and "stinging" sensations and sneezing when SURGICEL has been used as packing in epistaxis, are believed due to the low pH of the product.

Burning has been reported when SURGICEL was applied after nasal polyp removal and after hemorrhoidectomy. Headache, burning, stinging, and sneezing in epistaxis and other rhinological procedures, and stinging when SURGICEL was applied on surface wounds (varicose ulcerations, dermabrasions, and donor sites) also have been reported.

Dosage and Administration: Sterile technique should be observed in removing SURGICEL® Absorbable Hemostat from its envelope. Minimal amounts of SURGICEL in appropriate size are laid on the bleeding site or held firmly against the tissues until hemostasis is obtained.

Opened, unused SURGICEL should be discarded, because it cannot be resterilized.

How Supplied: Sterile SURGICEL® Absorbable Hemostat (oxidized regenerated cellulose) is supplied as knitted fabric strips in envelopes in the following sizes.

2 in. × 14 in. (28 sq. in.) (5.1 × 35.6 cm. (180.6 sq. cm.))
4 in. × 8 in. (32 sq. in.) (10.2 × 20.3 cm. (206.5 sq. cm.))
2 in. × 3 in. (6 sq. in.) (5.1 × 7.6 cm. (38.7 sq. cm.))
½ in. × 2 in. (1 sq. in.) (1.3 × 5.1 cm. (6.5 sq. cm.))

Clinical Studies: SURGICEL® Absorbable Hemostat (oxidized regenerated cellulose) has been found useful in helping to control capillary or venous bleeding in a variety of surgical applications, including abdominal, thoracic, neurosurgical, and orthopedic, as well as in otorhinolaryngologic procedures. Examples include gallbladder surgery, partial hepatectomy, hemorrhoidectomy, resections or injuries of the pancreas, spleen, kidney, prostate, bowel, breast or thyroid, and in amputations. (1,3)

SURGICEL has been applied as a surface dressing on donor sites and superficial open wounds, controlling bleeding adequately, and causing no delay in healing or interference with epithelization (4,6). It also has been applied after dermabrasion, punch biopsy, excision biopsy, curettage, finger and toenail removal, and to traumatic wounds. In the foregoing applications, bleeding was controlled and the SURGICEL was absorbed from the sites where it was applied. (5)

In cardiovascular surgery, investigators have found SURGICEL useful in helping to control bleeding from implanted textile grafts, including those of the abdominal aorta. (2,7) Such grafts may leak or weep considerably, even when pre-clotted, but this seepage can be controlled by covering the graft with a layer or two of SURGICEL after the graft is in place and before releasing the proximal and distal clamps. When the flow has been reestablished and all the bleeding controlled, the fabric either can be removed or left in situ, since absorption of SURGICEL has been shown to occur without constriction of the graft or other untoward incident when proper wrapping technique is employed.

Otorhinolaryngologic experience with SURGICEL includes adjunctive use in controlling bleeding resulting from epistaxis, tonsillectomy, adenoidectomy, removal of nasal polyps, repair of deviated septum, tympanoplasty, stapes surgery, surgery for sinusitis, and removal of tumors. (8,9)

SURGICEL has been reported useful as a hemostatic adjunct in such gynecologic procedures as oophorectomy, hysterectomy, conization of the cervix, and repair of cystorectocele. (1,10)

Animal Pharmacology: The effects of SURGICEL® Absorbable Hemostat, absorbable gelatin sponge, and microfibrillar collagen hemostat were compared in a standardized infection model consisting of intra-abdominal and intrahepatic abscesses in mice. This infection mimics the common characteristics of human infection with nonspore-forming anaerobic bacteria, including a chronic and progressive course. SURGICEL did not increase the infectivity of normally subinfectious inocula of mixed anaerobic species in mice. With the other hemostatic agents, microfibrillar collagen hemostat and absorbable gelatin sponge, an enhancement of infectivity of anaerobic mixtures has been shown. SURGICEL Absorbable Hemostat, in contrast to these hemostatic agents, did not enhance or provide a site for bacterial growth.

It was also found that aerobic pathogens did not grow in the presence of SURGICEL Absorbable Hemostat. In these studies (11), SURGICEL® Absorbable Hemostat was placed in contaminated incisions of guinea pigs and markedly reduced bacterial growth of three different strains of common pathogens.

In a dog model (12), it was shown that bacterial contamination of implanted teflon patches in the aorta could be reduced by wrapping the area of the patch with SURGICEL prior to pathogen challenge. Also, in another study (13), SURGICEL® Absorbable Hemostat and an absorbable gelatin sponge were placed in two splenotomy sites in large mongrel dogs and the animals were then challenged intravenously and the number of organisms from the splenotomy sites were measured over a period of time. The number of organisms at the site of SURGICEL Absorbable Hemostat was significantly lower than that in the control, or the absorbable gelatin sponge site.

References:

1. Degenshein, G., Hurwitz, A., and S. Ribacoff: Experience with regenerated oxidized celluose. ***New York State Journal of Medicine 63***(18):2639–2643, 1963.
2. Hurwitt, E.: A new absorbable hemostatic packing. ***Bulletin de la Societe Internationale de Chirurgle XXI***(3):237–242, 1962.
3. Venn, R.: Reduction of postsurgical blood-replacement needs with SURGICEL hemostasis. ***Medical Times 93***(10):1113–1116, 1965.
4. Miller, J., Ginsberg, M., McElfatrick, G., and H. Johnson: Clinical experience with oxidized regenerated cellulose. ***Experimental Medicine and Surgery 19***(2–3):202–206, (June-Sept.) 1961.
5. Blau, S., Kanof, N., and L. Simonson: Absorbable hemostatic gauze SURGICEL in dermabrasions and dermatologic surgery. ***Acta Dermato-Venerelogica 40***:358–361, 1960.
6. Shea, P., Jr.: Management of the donor site: a new dressing technic ***Journal of the Medical Associaion of Georgia 51***(9):437–440, 1962.
7. Denck, H.: Use of resorbable oxycellulose in surgery. ***Chirurg 33***(11):486–488, 1962.
8. Tibbels, E., Jr.: Evaluation of a new method of epistaxis management ***Laryngoscope LXXIII***(3):306–314, 1963.
9. Huggins, S.: Control of hemorrhage in otorhinolaryngologic surgery with oxidized regenerated cellulose. ***Eye, Ear, Nose and Throat Monthly 48***(7): (July) 1969.
10. Crisp, W.E., Shalauta, H., and W.A. Bennett: Shallow conization of the cervix. ***Obstetrics and Gynecology 31***(6):755–758, 1968.
11. Dineen, P.: Antibacterial activity of oxidized regenerated cellulose. ***Surgery, Gynecology and Obstetrics 142***:481–486, 1976.
12. Dineen, P.: The effect of oxidized regenerated cellulose on experimental intravascular infection. ***Surgery 82***:576–579, 1977.
13. Dineen, P.: The effect of oxidized regenerated cellulose on experimental infected splenotomies. ***Journal of Surgical Research 23***:114–116, 1977.

Important Notice

Before prescribing or administering

any product described in

PHYSICIANS' DESK REFERENCE

always consult the PDR Supplement for

possible new or revised information.

Keighley Proctological Instruments, Inc.

359 FOREST AVENUE
DAYTON, OH 45405

K-HC™ RECTAL SUPPOSITORIES ℞
Hemorrhoidal Suppositories

Caution: Federal law prohibits dispensing without prescription.

Composition: Each suppository contains:

Hydrocortisone Acetate	10 mg.
Bismuth Subgallate	60 mg.
Benzocaine	60 mg.
Zinc Oxide	80 mg.
Balsam Peru	20 mg.
Resorcin	5 mg.
Lanolin	12 mg.
Cod Liver Oil	12 mg.

in Hydrogenated Vegetable Oil Base

Action and Uses: K-HC™ suppositories reduce and alleviate anorectal inflammation, swelling, itching, and discomfort while lubricating the anorectal canal to facilitate smoother fecal evacuation, and accelerating the normal healing process. Useful in the therapy of hemorrhoids, proctitis, post operative pain and edema, cryptitis, and pruritus ani. Also, a valuable adjunct during hemorrhoidal ligation.

ANESTHETIC — ANTI-INFLAMMATORY
ANTIPRURITIC — ANTIBACTERIAL

Administration and Dosage: Adults—start therapy with one K-HC™ suppository inserted into the rectum (after removal of foil) in the morning and one at bed time for three to six days or until inflammation subsides.

Precautions: Definitive diagnosis should be made by complete proctological examination to ascertain the patients exact disease entity when use of hydorcortisone is considered. Prolonged or excessive use might produce systemic corticosteroid effects. Skin sensitization may be caused by benzocaine. The use of K-HC™ suppositories would be contraindicated in patients with known allergies to any of the ingredients. If irritation of the anoderm occurs during therapy with these suppositories the therapy should be discontinued at once and appropriate therapy instituted. The use of topical steroids during pregnancy is exceedingly questionable and should not be used unnecessarily. Care should be taken when using the hydrocortisone acetate in children and infants.

Contraindications: Do not use in the presence of tubercular, fungal, and most viral lesions, especially herpes simplex, vaccinia and varicella.

How Supplied: K-HC™ suppositories—Boxes of twelve individually foil wrapped, cream colored suppositories (NDC 50393-250-12).

Kenwood Laboratories, Inc.

490-A MAIN STREET
NEW ROCHELLE, NY 10801

GLUTOFAC Tablets™

Composition: Each tablet contains: Saccharomyces Siccum (a selected Brewer's Yeast)—390 mg. (contains Glucose Tolerance Factor—Chromium Complex)

		% U.S. RDA
Vitamin C (Ascorbic Acid)	250 mg.	416
Thiamine Hydrochloride (Vitamin B1)	15 mg.	1000
Riboflavin (Vitamin B2)	10 mg.	588
Niacinamide	50 mg.	250
Vitamin B6 (Pyridoxine Hydrochloride)	50 mg.	2500
Calcium Pantothenate	20 mg.	200
Magnesium Sulfate*	70 mg.	17.5
Zinc Sulfate+	80 mg.	533

* AS 50 mg. Dried Magnesiium Sulfate
\+ AS 50 mg. Dried Zinc Sulfate

Indication: For patients with nutritional deficiencies resulting from diabetes mellitus, physiologic stress, alcoholism and for other acute and chronic depletional states.

Dosage: Adults: One (1) tablet three (3) times daily or as directed by a physician.

Supplied: Green (film coated) tablets in bottles of 90 and 500.

I.L.X.™ B_{12} Elixir Crystalline

Composition:
Each (15 cc) contain:

Elemental Iron (from Iron Ammonium Citrate, Brown)	102 mg
Liver Fraction 1	98 mg
Thiamine Hydrochloride (Vitamin B1)	5 mg
Riboflavin (Vitamin B2)	2 mg
Nicotinamide	10 mg
Vitamin B12 Crystalline (Cyanocobalamin)	10 mcg
Alcohol 8% by Volume	

Action and Uses: A readily assimilated elixir for oral therapy in the treatment of iron deficiency anemias.

Administration and Dosage: As a hematinic. One teaspoonful 3 times daily or as directed by physician.

How Supplied: 12 ounce bottles.

I.L.X.™ B_{12} Tablets

Each tablet contains:

Elemental Iron (from Ferrous Gluconate)	38 mg.
Vitamin C	60 mg.
Cyanocobalamin USP (Vit. B12 Cryst.)	10 mcg.
Liver (Desiccated) N.F.	2 gr.
Thiamine Hydrochloride	2 mg.
Riboflavin	2 mg.
Niacinamide	20 mg.

Indications: A readily assimilated oral hematinic for the treatment of nutritional and iron deficiency anemias such as those commonly seen in older patients, in convalescense from surgical procedures or medical diseases, and anemias of pregnancy.

Administration and Dosage: One tablet 3 times a day or as directed by physician.

How Supplied: I.L.X. B_{12}™ tablets are supplied in bottles of 100.

Key Pharmaceuticals, Inc.

18425 N.W. 2ND AVE.
MIAMI, FL 33169

IRCON®-FA ℞

Description: IRCON-FA contains 1.0 mg of folic acid, and 250 mg of ferrous fumarate equivalent to 82 mg of elemental iron.

Clinical Pharmacology: IRCON-FA is a prenatal supplemental hematinic agent specifically intended for prophylaxis against two common types of anemia developing as a result of pregnancy. The use of prophylactic iron and prophylactic folic acid during pregnancy is well accepted. Child-bearing (per pregnancy) has an iron "cost" of about 725 mg. It has been shown that 78 mg of elemental iron, taken orally each day during the last half of pregnancy, will protect against iron deficiency anemia; half this dose is insufficient to maintain iron stores. Two hundred fifty mg of ferrous fumarate contain approximately 82 mg of iron. Absorption characteristics of ferrous fumarate are identical to those of ferrous sulfate.

A deficiency of folic acid, typically during pregnancy, has long been known to cause a megaloblastic anemia, similar in some respects to Addisonian pernicious anemia. The vitamin is not storable in the body and the combination of fetal demand during pregnancy and misnourishment can lead to a deficiency, hence anemia. The average daily requirement of folic acid during pregnancy is unknown. It has been found that a dosage of 20 mcg/day is inadequate. In other instances doses of 1000 mcg/day orally have been found to produce a prompt hematological response in megaloblastic anemia of pregnancy.

Daily doses of folic acid greater than 1.0 mg/day have not been shown to be necessary, even in cases of overt folate deficiency anemia. The estimated minimum daily requirement for folic acid in late pregnancy when folate depletion is present is said to be greater than 200 mcg and possibly 400 mcg or more. IRCON-FA contains 1000 mcg. Folic acid is nontoxic and has commonly been given in several times this daily dose. Though folic acid dietary deficiency in the United States is rare, prophylaxis during pregnancy is considered to be justified in view of the possibly serious consequences of its depletion, both for the mother (megaloblastic anemia) and the fetus.

Finally, it has been observed that the rapid production of red blood cells following treatment with iron alone may deplete the body of folate if there is inadequate intake; combining the two substances avoids this complication.

Indications and Usage: For maintenance of maternal hematopoiesis during pregnancy, particularly when diet is abnormal or substandard.

Contraindications:

1) Pernicious anemia. Although rare in the population likely to receive IRCON-FA this megaloblastic anemia must be borne in mind. It is due to faulty or blocked absorption of vitamin B_{12}, or extrinsic factor, on either a genetic, immunologic or surgical basis. The particular danger of missing a diagnosis of pernicious anemia—in relation to folic acid therapy—is that folic acid can mask PA by causing a hematologic remission while allowing the neurological complications of the disease to proceed apace. Thus, before IRCON-FA is prescribed for megaloblastic anemia in pregnancy, appropriate diagnostic exclusion of Addisonian pernicious anemia should be carried out.

2) Anemias other than those due to iron deficiency.

Warning: Folic acid alone is improper therapy in the treatment of pernicious anemia and other megaloblastic anemias where vitamin B_{12} is deficient.

Precautions:

1) If, at the time of initial examination, definite anemia is found, a diagnosis of its cause should be made.

2) IRCON-FA is primarily intended to prevent the development of anemia due to a deficiency of either iron or folic acid by reason of the demands of pregnancy. It is not intended for the treatment of these disorders in fully developed form.

3) Blood examinations including hemoglobin and hematocrit should be done at the usual intervals to make certain that therapy is adequate.

4) Use with care in the presence of peptic ulcer, regional enteritis and ulcerative colitis.

5) Folic acid especially in doses above 1.0 mg. daily may obscure pernicious anemia, in that hematologic remission may occur while neurological manifestations remain progressive.

Adverse Reactions:

1) Ferrous fumarate gastric distress, abdominal cramps, diarrhea.

2) Folic acid allergic sensitization has been reported following both oral and parenteral administration of folic acid.

Administration and Dosage: The usual dose in the second and third trimester of pregnancy is one tablet daily, taken in the morning

Continued on next page

Key—Cont.

between breakfast and lunch with a glass of water or milk. If hyperemesis gravidarum is a problem, the dose may be taken in mid-afternoon.
How Supplied: IRCON-FA tablets are available in bottles of 100.
Caution: FEDERAL LAW PROHIBITS DISPENSING WITHOUT A PRESCRIPTION.

NICO-SPAN® ℞
(niacin)
Sustained Action Capsules

Description: NICO-SPAN, formulated as sustained action capsules, contains 400 mg of niacin in a specially prepared form to permit prolonged release.
Clinical Pharmacology: Niacin functions in the body as a component of two hydrogen transporting coenzymes: Coenzyme I [Nicotinamide Adenine Dinucleotide (NAD), sometimes called Diphosphopyridine Nucleotide (DPN)] and Coenzyme II [Nicotinamide Adenine Dinucleotide Phosphate (NADP), sometimes called Triphosphopyridine Nucleotide (TPN)]. Niacin in addition to its functions as a vitamin, exerts several distinctive pharmacologic effects which vary according to the dosage level employed.
Niacin in large doses, causes a reduction in serum lipids. The exact mechanism of this action is unknown.
Indications and Usage: As adjunctive therapy in addition to diet and other measures in the treatment of hypercholesterolemia and hyperbetalipoproteinemia. Because NICO-SPAN has prolonged release, it minimizes flushing, pruritus and gastrointestinal irritation and permits adequate dosage with maximum patient cooperation.

> **Notice:**
> It has not been established whether the drug-induced lowering of serum cholesterol or triglyceride levels has a beneficial effect, no effect, or a detrimental effect on the morbidity or mortality due to atherosclerosis including coronary heart disease. Investigations now in progress may yield an answer to this question.

Contraindications: Niacin is contraindicated in patients with hepatic dysfunction or in patients with active acute peptic ulcer.
Warnings: Use of this drug in pregnancy, during lactation, or in women of child-bearing age requires that the potential benefits of the drug should be weighed against its possible hazards to the mother and child. Although fetal abnormalities have not been reported with this drug, its use as an antilipidemic agent requires high dosages, and animal reproduction or teratology studies have not been done. There are insufficient studies done for usage in children.
Precautions: Patients with gall bladder disease, or those with a past history of jaundice, liver disease or peptic ulcer should be observed closely while taking the medication. Frequent monitoring of liver function tests and blood glucose should be performed during therapy to ascertain that the drug has no adverse effects on these organ systems. Diabetic or potential diabetic patients should be observed closely in the event of decreased tolerance. Adjustment of diet and/or hypoglycemic therapy may be necessary. Antihypertensive drugs of the adrenergic-blocking type may have an additive vasodilating effect and produce postural hypotension.
Elevated uric acid levels have occurred; therefore, use with caution in patients predisposed to gout.
Adverse Reactions: Severe flushing, decreased glucose tolerance, activation of peptic ulcer, abnormal liver function tests, jaundice, gastrointestinal disorders, dry skin, keratosis nigricans, pruritus, hyperuricemia, toxic amblyopia, hypotension, transient headache.
Dosage and Administration: The dose and frequency for the administration of NICO-SPAN should be adjusted to the response of the patient. Slow build-up of dosage in gradual increments is recommended to observe efficacy and/or adverse effects. One or two capsules three times a day is the usual dosage. The maximum dosage is 6 g per day.
Caution: FEDERAL LAW PROHIBITS DISPENSING WITHOUT PRESCRIPTION.
How Supplied: NICO-SPAN 400 mg sustained action capsules are available in bottles of 100, and 1000.
[*Shown in Product Identification Section*]

NITRO–DUR™
(nitroglycerin)
Transdermal Infusion System

Description: The Nitro-Dur Transdermal Infusion System contains nitroglycerin in a gel-like matrix composed of glycerin, water (purified), lactose, polyvinyl alcohol, povidone and sodium citrate to provide a continuous source of the active ingredient. Nitro-Dur is available in dosage sizes $10cm^2$, $15cm^2$ and $20cm^2$, containing 51 mg, 77 mg and 104 mg of nitroglycerin, respectively, thereby providing precise dosing levels of nitroglycerin. Nitro-Dur has a rated release *in vivo* of approximately $0.5mg/cm^2/24$ hours. Each unit is sealed in a polyester-foil-polyethylene laminate. The bandage portion consists of a medical grade non-woven, heat sealable, microporous tape.
Clinical Pharmacology: When the Nitro-Dur system is applied to the skin, nitroglycerin is absorbed continuously through the skin into the systemic circulation. This results in active drug reaching the target organs (heart, extremities) before deactivation by the liver. Nitroglycerin is a smooth muscle relaxant with vascular effects manifested predominantly by venous dilation and pooling. The major beneficial effect of nitroglycerin in angina pectoris is a reduction in myocardial oxygen consumption secondary to vascular smooth muscle relaxation with resultant reduction in cardiac preload and afterload. In recent years there has been an increasing recognition of a direct vasodilator effect of nitroglycerin on the coronary vessels.
In bioavailability studies[1], transdermal absorption of nitroglycerin from the gel-like matrix achieved steady state venous plasma levels comparable to that of sublingual nitroglycerin and maintained these levels for 24 hours. Therapeutic effect is achieved within 30 minutes after application of the unit, and persists about 30 minutes after removal of the unit.
Indications and Usage: Prevention and treatment of angina pectoris due to coronary artery disease.
Contraindications: Intolerance of organic nitrate drugs, marked anemia, increased intraocular pressure or increased intracranial pressure.
Warnings: The Nitro-Dur system should be used under careful clinical and/or hemodynamic monitoring in patients with acute myocardial infarction or congestive heart failure.
In terminating treatment of anginal patients, both the dosage and frequency of application must be gradually reduced over a period of 4 to 6 weeks in order to prevent sudden withdrawal reactions, which are characteristic of all vasodilators in the nitroglycerin class.
Usage in Pregnancy: Safe use in pregnancy has not been established relative to possible adverse effects on fetal development, but neither have adverse effects on fetal development been established. Therefore, use of nitroglycerin in pregnant women should be balanced against the risk of uncontrolled angina pectoris.
Precautions: Symptoms of hypotension, such as faintness, weakness or dizziness, particularly orthostatic hypotension, may be due to overdosage. If during the course of treatment these symptoms occur, the dosage should be reduced.
Nitro-Dur is not intended for use in the treatment of acute anginal attacks. For this purpose, occasional use of sublingual nitroglycerin may be necessary.
Adverse Reactions: Transient headache is the most common side effect, especially when higher doses of the drug are administered. Headaches should be treated with mild analgesics while continuing Nitro-Dur therapy. If headache persists, the Nitro-Dur dosage should be reduced.
Adverse reactions reported less frequently include hypotension, increased heart rate, faintness, flushing, dizziness, nausea, vomiting, and dermatitis. Except for dermatitis, these symptoms are attributed to the pharmacologic effects of nitroglycerin. However, they may be symptoms of overdosage. When they persist, the Nitro-Dur dosage should be reduced or use of the product discontinued.
Dosage and Administration: To apply the Nitro-Dur system, tear away the printed foil surface, then peel away the sectioned release liner as you would an adhesive bandage. Apply the Nitro-Dur system firmly to the skin surface. The initial starting dose is a $10cm^2$ system. To achieve optimum therapeutic effect in some patients, it may be necessary to titrate to a higher dosing strength. Dosage should be titrated while monitoring clinical response, i.e., blood pressure, episodes of angina and subsequent use of sublingual nitroglycerin. The Nitro-Dur system may remain in place for periods up to 24 hours as required to provide continuous prophylactic levels of nitroglycerin.
The Nitro-Dur system may be applied to any convenient skin area; a recommended site of application is the arm or chest. A suitable area may be shaved if necessary. Do not apply the Nitro-Dur system to the distal part of the extremities.
Storage Conditions: Store at controlled room temperature 15–30°C (59–86°F).
How Supplied: Nitro-Dur Transdermal Infusion System, $10cm^2$, $15cm^2$, and $20cm^2$, is available in unit dose packages of 28.
Caution: Federal law prohibits dispensing without a prescription.
Patient Instructions for Application: Patient Instructions are furnished with each unit dose package.

Revised 0882

[1]Data on file: Key Pharmaceuticals, Inc. Miami, Florida (USA) 33169
[*Shown in Product Identification Section*]

NITROGLYN® ℞
(nitroglycerin)
Sustained Action Tablets

Description: NITROGLYN, formulated as sustained action tablets, contains nitroglycerin (glyceryl trinitrate). NITROGLYN is available in two strengths: 1/25 gr (2.6 mg) and 1/10 gr (6.5 mg).
Clinical Pharmacology: The principal action of nitroglycerin is to relax all smooth muscle, most prominently on vascular smooth muscle. The action on small post-capillary vessels dominates the hemodynamic picture. The resulting increase in cardiac output is transient, and followed by a moderate decrease due to reduced venous return, associated with peripheral vasodilation. The mean arterial pressure may not be affected, or may be decreased. The speed and magnitude of response depend on the dose, the rate of release from the tablet, the rate of absorption, and individual susceptibility. Availability of nitroglycerin at 3 dosage

levels permits tailoring the required dose to the need of each patient with angina pectoris. The release of nitroglycerin from NITROGLYN is gradual but the rate of absorption from the gastrointestinal tract in patients with angina pectoris has not been estabished. Dilation of the coronary arteries has been established in some anginal patients following sublingual administration but not in others. More often patients with coronary artery disease show no change or decrease in coronary flow. Nitroglycerin can act as physiological antagonist to norepinephrine, acetylcholine and histamine. While the mechanism of action of nitroglycerin in the treatment of patients with angina pectoris is still to be established, its use has been well documented for more than a century and is considered the drug of choice.

Indications and Usage:
Based on a review of this drug by the National Academy of Sciences-National Research Council and/or other information FDA has classified the indications as follows: "Possibly" Effective.
Sustained action tablets of nitroglycerin are possibly effective for indications relating to the management, prophylaxis or treatment of anginal attacks. This possibly effective classification applies also to conventional or extended action oral forms of all other organic nitrate antianginal drugs alone or in combination.

Contraindications: Data supporting the use of organic nitrates during the course of acute myocardial infarction are not sufficient to establish safety. Caution should be used in administration to anginal patients with postural hypotension or with closed-angle glaucoma.
Precautions: Use the smallest dose which proves effective. Tablets must be swallowed whole. FOR ORAL, NOT SUBLINGUAL USE. Store in cool, dry place and keep container tightly capped. Cross tolerance may develop to other organic nitrates. Continued treatment is not recommended unless the patient is benefited.
Adverse Reactions: Some patients exhibit hypersensitivity to the hypotensive effects of nitroglycerin, as shown by nausea, vomiting, restlessness, pallor, perspiration and collapse, from the usual dose. Other patients may develop severe and persistent headaches, cutaneous flushing, dizziness and weakness; occasionally drug rash or exfoliative dermatitis; these responses may disappear with decrease in dosage. Adverse effects are enhanced by ingestion of alcohol, which appears to increase absorption from the gastrointestinal tract.
Dosage and Administration: Administer the smallest effective dose 2 or 3 times daily unless clinical response suggests a different regimen. Discontinue if not effective.
How Supplied: NITROGLYN 1/25 gr (2.6 mg) and 1/10 gr (6.5 mg) sustained action tablets are available in bottles of 100 and 1000.
Caution: FEDERAL LAW PROHIBITS DISPENSING WITHOUT PRESCRIPTION.
[*Shown in Product Identification Section*]

PAVAKEY-300® ℞
(papaverine hydrochloride, 300 mg.)
Sustained Action Capsules

PAVAKEY®
(papaverine hydrochloride, 150 mg.)
Sustained Action Capsules

Description: PAVAKEY, formulated as sustained action capsules, contains papaverine hydrochloride. PAVAKEY is available in two strengths: PAVAKEY contains 150 mg of papaverine hydrochloride and PAVAKEY-300 contains 300 mg of papaverine hydrochloride; both in a specially prepared form to permit sustained action for prolonged activity.
Clinical Pharmacology: The main actions of papaverine are exerted on cardiac and smooth muscle. Like quinidine, papaverine acts directly on the heart muscle to depress conduction and prolong the refractory period. Papaverine relaxes various smooth muscles. This relaxation may be prominent if spasm exists. The muscle cell is not paralyzed by papaverine, and still responds to drugs and other stimuli causing contraction. The antispasmodic effect is a direct one, and unrelated to muscle innervation. Papaverine is practically devoid of effects on the central nervous system. Papaverine relaxes the smooth musculature of the larger blood vessels, especially coronary, systemic, peripheral, and pulmonary arteries. Perhaps by its direct vasodilating action on cerebral blood vessels, papaverine increases cerebral blood flow and decreases cerebral vascular resistance in normal subjects; oxygen consumption is unaltered. These effects may explain the benefit reported from the drug in cerebral vascular encephalopathy.
The direct actions of papaverine on the heart to depress conduction and irritability and to prolong the refractory period of the myocardium provide the basis for its clinical trial in abrogating atrial and ventricular premature systoles and ominous ventricular arrhythmias. The coronary vasodilator action could be an additional factor of therapeutic value when such rhythms are secondary to insufficiency or occlusion of the coronary arteries. In patients with acute coronary thrombosis, the occurence of ventricular rhythms is serious and requires measures designed to decrease myocardial irritability. Papaverine may have advantages over quinidine, used for a similar purpose, in that it may be given in an emergency by the intravenous route, does not depress myocardial contraction or cause cinchonism, and produces coronary vasodilation.
Indications and Usage: For the relief of cerebral and peripheral ischemia associated with arterial spasm and myocardial ischemia complicated by arrhythmias.
Precautions: Use with caution in patients with glaucoma. Hepatic hypersensitivity has been reported with gastrointestinal symptoms, jaundice, eosinophilia and altered liver function tests. Discontinue medication if these occur.
Adverse Reactions: Although occurring rarely, the reported side effects of papaverine include nausea, abdominal distress, anorexia, constipation, malaise, drowsiness, vertigo, sweating, headache, diarrhea and skin rash.
Dosage and Administration:
PAVAKEY—One capsule every 12 hours. In difficult cases administration may be increased to one capsule every 8 hours, or two capsules every 12 hours.
PAVAKEY-300—One capsule every twelve hours for difficult cases.
How Supplied: PAVAKEY sustained action capsules are available in bottles of 100 and 1000.
PAVAKEY-300 sustained action capsules are available in bottles of 100.
Caution: FEDERAL LAW PROHIBITS DISPENSING WITHOUT PRESCRIPTION.

QUINORA® ℞
(quinidine sulfate tablets U.S.P.)

Description: QUINORA tablets contain quinidine sulfate with no color additives in the base. QUINORA is available in two strengths, 200 mg and 300 mg.
Clinical Pharmacology: Quinidine is generally regarded as a myocardial depressant drug, because it depresses excitability, conduction velocity, and contractility of the myocardium. Besides these direct effects quinidine exerts some indirect effects on the heart through an anticholinergic action. Large oral doses may reduce the arterial pressure due to peripheral vasodilation. Hypotension of a serious degree is more likely with the parenteral use of the drug.
Quinidine is essentially completely absorbed after oral administration; maximal effects occur within 1 to 3 hours and persist for 6 to 8 or more hours. Blood levels of quinidine can be measured; the average therapeutic range is between 3 and 6 mg per liter of plasma; toxic reactions are almost certain to appear at levels above 8 mg per liter.
Indications and Usage: Quinidine sulfate is indicated in the treatment of premature atrial and ventricular contractions, paroxysmal atrial tachycardia, paroxysmal A-V junctional rhythm, atrial flutter, paroxysmal atrial fibrillation, established atrial fibrillation when therapy is appropriate, and paroxysmal ventricular tachycardia when not associated with complete heartblock, and for maintenance therapy after electrical conversion of atrial fibrillation and/ or flutter.
Contraindications: Hypersensitivity or idiosyncrasy to the drug. History of thrombocytopenic purpura associated with previous quinidine administration. Digitalis intoxication manifested by A-V conduction disorders. Complete A-V block with an A-V nodal or idioventricular pacemaker. Ectopic impulses and rhythms due to escape mechanisms.
Warnings: In the treatment of atrial flutter, reversion to sinus rhythm may be preceded by a progressive reduction in the degree of A-V block to a 1:1 ratio resulting in extremely rapid ventricular rate. This possible hazard may be decreased by digitalization prior to giving quinidine. Evidence of quinidine cardiotoxicity (50% widening of QRS, frequent ventricular ectopic beats) mandates immediate discontinuation of the drug followed with close observation (ECG-monitoring) of the patient.
Usage in Pregnancy: The use of quinidine in pregnancy should be reserved only for those cases where the benefits outweigh the possible hazards to patient and fetus.
Precautions: Use quinidine with extreme caution in the presence of incomplete A-V block since complete block and asystole may result. Quinidine may cause unpredictable abnormalities of rhythm in digitalized hearts and it should be used with special caution in the presence of digitalis intoxication. **Note:** Quinidine effect is enhanced by potassium and reduced in the presence of hypokalemia.
The depressant actions of quinidine on cardiac contractility and arterial blood pressure limit its use in congestive heart failure and in hypotensive states unless these conditions are due to, or aggravated by, the arrhythmia. The potential disadvantage and benefits must be weighed. Continuous ECG-monitoring and determination of plasma quinidine levels are indicated when large doses, more than 2 g/day, are used.
Adverse Reactions:
Symptoms of cinchonism: (ringing in the ears, headache, nausea, disturbed vision) may appear (in sensitive patients) after a single dose of the drug.
Cardiovascular: widening of QRS-complex, cardiac asystole, ventricular ectopic beats, idioventricular rhythms including ventricular tachycardia and fibrillation, paradoxical tachycardia, arterial embolism.
Gastrointestinal: nausea, vomiting, abdominal pain, diarrhea.
Hematologic: acute hemalytic anemia, hypoprothrombinemia, thrombocytopenic purpura, agranulocytosis.
CNS: headache, fever, vertigo, apprehension, excitement, confusion, delirium and syncope, disturbed hearing (tinnitus, decreased auditory acuity), disturbed vision (mydriasis, blurred vision, disturbed color perception, photophobia, diplopia, night blindness, scotomata), optic neuritis.

Continued on next page

Key—Cont.

Dermatologic: cutaneous flushing with intense pruritus.
Hypersensitivity reactions: Angioedema, acute asthmatic episode, vascular collapse, respiratory arrest.

Dosage and Administration: A preliminary test dose of a single tablet of quinidine sulfate should be administered to determine whether the patient has an idiosyncrasy to it. Continuous ECG-monitoring is recommended in all cases, where quinidine is used in large doses.

Usual Adult Dose: Premature atrial and ventricular contractions: 200 to 300 mg three or four times daily.
Paroxysmal supraventricular tachycardias: 400 to 600 mg every 2 or 3 hours until the paroxysm is terminated.
Atrial flutter: Quinidine should be administered after digitalization for this indication. Dosage is to be individualized.
Conversion of atrial fibrillation: Various schedules of quinidine administration have been in clinical use. A widely used technique is the administration of 200 mg of quinidine orally every 2 or 3 hours for 5 to 8 doses, with subsequent daily increase of the individual dose until sinus rhythm is restored or toxic effects occur. The total daily dose should not exceed 3 to 4 g, given by any schedule. Prior to quinidine administration the ventricular rate and congestive failure (if present) should be brought under control by digitalis therapy.
Maintenance therapy: 200 to 300 mg three or four times daily.

Overdosage: Cardiotoxic effects of quinidine may be reversed in part by sodium lactate; the hypotension by vasoconstrictors and by catecholamines (since the vasodilation is partly due to α adrenergic blockade).

How Supplied: QUINORA 200 mg and 300 mg tablets are available in bottles of 100 and 1000.

Caution: FEDERAL LAW PROHIBITS DISPENSING WITHOUT A PRESCRIPTION.

THEO-DUR® ℞
theophylline (anhydrous)
Sustained Action Tablets

Description: THEO-DUR Sustained Action Tablets contain anhydrous theophylline, with no color additives. THEO-DUR is available in three strengths: 100 mg, 200 mg and 300 mg: each tablet is scored for flexibility of dose. Theophylline, a xanthine compound, is a white, odorless crystalline powder, having a bitter taste.

Clinical Pharmacology: The pharmacologic actions of theophylline are as a bronchodilator, pulmonary vasodilator and smooth muscle relaxant since the drug directly relaxes the smooth muscle of the bronchial airways and pulmonary blood vessels. Theophylline also possesses other actions typical of the xanthine derivatives: coronary vasodilator, diuretic, cardiac stimulant, cerebral stimulant and skeletal muscle stimulant. The actions of theophylline may be mediated through inhibition of phosphodiesterase and a resultant increase in intracellular cyclic AMP which could mediate smooth muscle relaxation.
No development of tolerance appears to occur with chronic use of theophylline.
The half-life is shortened with cigarette smoking and prolonged in alcoholism, reduced hepatic or renal function, congestive heart failure, and in patients receiving certain antibiotics (see DRUG INTERACTIONS). High fever for prolonged periods may decrease theophylline elimination. Children over six months of age have rapid clearances with average half-lives of approximately 3–5 hours. Newborn infants have extremely slow clearances and half-lives exeeding 24 hours. Older adults with chronic obstructive pulmonary disease, any patients with cor pulmonale or other causes of heart failure, and patients with liver pathology may have much lower clearances with half-lives that exceed 24 hours. The half-life of theophylline in smokers (1–2 packs per day) averages 4–5 hours; the half-life in non-smokers averages 7–9 hours.
In single dose studies, THEO-DUR, administered at 8 mg/kg body weight, produced mean peak theophylline blood levels of 7.5 $\pm$ 1.9 mcg/ml at 9.2 $\pm$ 1.9 hours following administration. In the multiple dose, steady-state, 3 and 5 day studies, THEO-DUR achieved remarkably constant intra-subject theophylline levels with an average peak-trough difference of only 4 mcg/ml. This is indicative of smooth and stable maintenance therapeutic theophylline levels throughout a q12h dosing interval.

Indications and Usage: Symptomatic relief and/or prevention of asthma and reversible bronchospasm associated with chronic bronchitis and emphysema.

Contraindications: THEO-DUR is contraindicated in individuals who have shown hypersensitivity to any of its components or xanthine derivatives.

Warnings: Excessive theophylline doses may be associated with toxicity; serum theophylline levels should be monitored to assure maximum benefit with minimum risk. Incidence of toxicity increases at serum levels greater than 20 mcg/ml. High blood levels of theophylline resulting from conventional doses are correlated with clinical manifestations of toxicity in: patients with lowered body plasma clearances; patients with liver dysfunction or chronic obstructive lung disease, and patients who are older than 55 years of age, particularly males. There are often no early signs of less serious theophylline toxicity such as nausea and restlessness, which may appear in up to 50% of patients prior to onset of convulsions. Ventricular arrhythmias or seizures may be the first signs of toxicity. Many patients who have higher theophylline serum levels exhibit a tachycardia. Theophylline products may worsen pre-existing arrhythmias.

Usage in Pregnancy: Safe use in pregnancy has not been established relative to possible adverse effects on fetal development, but neither have adverse effects on fetal development been established. This is, unfortunately, true for most antiasthmatic medications. Therefore, use of theophylline in pregnant women should be balanced against the risk of uncontrolled asthma.

Precautions: THEO-DUR TABLETS SHOULD NOT BE CHEWED OR CRUSHED. Theophyllines should not be administered concurrently with other xanthine medications. It should be used with caution in patients with severe cardiac disease, severe hypoxemia, hypertension, hyperthyroidism, acute myocardial injury, cor pulmonale, congestive heart failure, liver disease and in the elderly, particularly males, and in neonates. Great caution should be used in giving theophylline to patients in congestive heart failure since these patients show markedly prolonged theophylline blood level curves. Use theophylline cautiously in patients with history of peptic ulcer. Theophylline may occasionally act as a local irritant to G.I. tract although gastrointestinal symptoms are more commonly central and associated with high serum concentrations above 20 mcg/ml.

Adverse Reactions: The most consistent adverse reactions are usually due to overdose and are:
Gastrointestinal: Nausea, vomiting, epigastric pain, hematemesis, diarrhea.
Central Nervous System: Headaches, irritability, restlessness, insomnia, reflex hyperexcitability, muscle twitching, clonic and tonic generalized convulsions.
Cardiovascular: Palpitation, tachycardia, extrasystoles, flushing, hypotension, circulatory failure, life threatening ventricular arrhythmias.
Respiratory: Tachypnea.
Renal: Albuminuria, increased excretion of renal tubular cells and red blood cells; potentiation of diuresis.
Others: Hyperglycemia and inappropriate ADH syndrome.

Drug Interactions:

Drug	Effect
Theophylline with Furosemide	Increased Diuresis
Theophylline with Hexamethonium	Decreased Chronotropic Effect
Theophylline with Reserpine	Tachycardia
Theophylline with Cyclamycin (TAO), Erythromycin, or Lincomycin.	Increased Theophylline Blood Levels

Overdosage:
Management:
A. If potential oral overdose is established and seizure has not occurred;
 1) Induce vomiting.
 2) Administer a cathartic (this is particularly important if sustained release preparations have been taken).
 3) Administer activated charcoal.
B. If patient is having a seizure:
 1) Establish an airway.
 2) Administer O_2.
 3) Treat the seizure with intravenous diazepam, 0.1 to 0.3 mg/kg up to 10 mg.
 4) Monitor vital signs, maintain blood pressure and provide adequate hydration.
C. Post-Seizure Coma:
 1) Maintain airway and oxygenation.
 2) If a result of oral medication, follow above recommendations to prevent absorption of drug, but intubation and lavage will have to be performed instead of inducing emesis, and the cathartic and charcoal will need to be introduced via a large bore gastric lavage tube.
 3) Continue to provide full supportive care and adequate hydration while waiting for drug to be metabolized. In general, the drug is metabolized sufficiently rapidly so as to not warrant consideration of dialysis.

Dosage and Administration: Therapeutic serum levels associated with optimal likelihood for benefit and minimal risk of toxicity are considered to be between 10 and 20 mcg/ml. There is a great variation from patient to patient in dosage needed in order to achieve a therapeutic blood level due to variable rates of elimination. Because of this wide variation from patient to patient, and the relatively narrow therapeutic range, dosage must be individualized.
THE AVERAGE INITIAL CHILDREN'S (15 to 20 kg) DOSE IS ONE THEO-DUR 100 mg TABLET q12h.
THE AVERAGE INITIAL CHILDREN's (20 to 25 kg) DOSE IS ONE-HALF (150 mg) OF A THEO-DUR 300 mg TABLET q12h.
THE AVERAGE INITIAL ADULT AND CHILDREN'S (OVER 25 kg) DOSE IS ONE THEO-DUR 200 mg TABLET q12h.
If the desired response is not achieved with the above AVERAGE INITIAL DOSAGE recommendations, and there are no adverse reactions, the dose may be increased, after 3 days, to the following MAXIMUM DOSE WITHOUT MEASUREMENT OF SERUM CONCENTRATION.

MAXIMUM DOSE WITHOUT MEASUREMENT OF SERUM CONCENTRATION

	Dose Per Interval
Children (15–20 kg)	150 mg q12h
Children (20–25 kg)	200 mg q12h
Children (25–35 kg)	250 mg q12h
Adults and Children (over 35 kg)	300 mg q12h

If increased dose is not tolerated because of headaches or stomach upset (nausea, vomiting, diarrhea, etc.), decrease dose to AVERAGE INITIAL DOSE. If tolerated, the dose may be increased, after 3 days, to the following MINIMUM DOSE REQUIRING MEASUREMENT OF SERUM CONCENTRATION.

MINIMUM DOSE REQUIRING MEASUREMENT OF SERUM CONCENTRATION

	Dose Per Interval
Children (15–20 kg)	200 mg q12h
Children (20–30 kg)	250 mg q12h
Children (30–35 kg)	300 mg q12h
Children (35–40 kg)	350 mg q12h
Adults and Children (over 40 kg)	400 mg q12h

CHECK SERUM CONCENTRATION BETWEEN 3 AND 8 HOURS AFTER A DOSE WHEN NONE HAVE BEEN MISSED OR ADDED FOR AT LEAST 3 DAYS

If serum theophylline concentration is between 10 and 20 mcg/ml, maintain dose if tolerated. RECHECK SERUM THEOPHYLLINE CONCENTRATION AT 6 TO 12 MONTH INTERVALS.*

Take the following action if the serum theophylline concentration is too high.

20 to 25 mcg/ml—Decrease dose by 50 mg q12h

25 to 30 mcg/ml—Skip next dose and decrease subsequent doses by 25% to the nearest 50 mg q12h.

Over 30 mcg/ml—Skip next 2 doses and decrease subsequent doses by 50% to nearest 50 mg q12h. RECHECK SERUM THEOPHYLLINE CONCENTRATION.

Take the following action if the serum theophylline concentration is too low

7.5 to 10 mcg/ml—Increase dose by 25% to the nearest 50 mg.**

5 to 7.5 mcg/ml—Increase dose by 25% to the nearest 50 mg and RECHECK SERUM THEOPHYLLINE FOR GUIDANCE IN FURTHER DOSAGE ADJUSTMENT.

*Finer adjustments in dosage may be needed for some patients.

**Dividing the daily dosage into 3 doses administered at 8 hour intervals may be indicated if symptoms occur repeatedly at the end of a dosing interval.

DOSAGE ADJUSTMENT BASED ON SERUM THEOPHYLLINE CONCENTRATION MEASUREMENTS WHEN THESE INSTRUCTIONS HAVE NOT BEEN FOLLOWED, MAY RESULT IN RECOMMENDATIONS THAT PRESENT RISK OF TOXICITY TO THE PATIENT.

How Supplied: THEO-DUR 100 mg. 200 mg. and 300 mg Sustained Action Tablets are available in bottles of 100, 500, 1000, and 5000, and in unit dose packages of 100.

Storage Conditions: Keep tightly closed. Store at controlled room temperature 15–30°C (59–86°F).

Caution: Federal law prohibits dispensing without a prescription.

[Shown in Product Identification Section]

THEO-DUR® SPRINKLE ℞

(anhydrous theophylline)
Sustained Action Capsules

Description: THEO-DUR SPRINKLE Sustained Action Capsules contain anhydrous theophylline with no color additives. Theophylline, a xanthine compound, is a white, odorless crystalline powder, having a bitter taste. THEO-DUR SPRINKLE is available in four strengths: 50, 75, 125, and 200 mg. THEO-DUR SPRINKLE capsules contain theophylline which has been microencapsulated in a proprietary coating of polymers to mask the bitter taste associated with the drug, while providing a prolonged therapeutic effect. THEO-DUR SPRINKLE capsules may be swallowed whole. In addition, the microencapsulation technique makes THEO-DUR SPRINKLE ideal for children and other patients who are unable to swallow a tablet or capsule. The entire contents of a THEO-DUR SPRINKLE capsule should be sprinkled on a small amount of soft food immediately prior to ingestion. SUBDIVIDING THE CONTENTS OF A CAPSULE IS NOT RECOMMENDED. Each capsule is oversized to allow ease of opening.

Pharmacologic Actions: The pharmacologic actions of theophylline are as a bronchodilator; pulmonary vasodilator and smooth muscle relaxant since the drug directly relaxes the smooth muscle of the bronchial airways and pulmonary blood vessels. Theophylline also possesses other actions typical of the xanthine derivatives: coronary vasodilator, diuretic, cardiac stimulant, cerebral stimulant and skeletal muscle stimulant. The actions of theophylline may be mediated through inhibition of phosphodiesterase and a resultant increase in intracellular cyclic AMP which could mediate smooth muscle relaxation.

No development of tolerance appears to occur with chronic use of theophylline. The half-life is shortened with cigarette smoking and prolonged in alcoholism, reduced hepatic or renal function, congestive heart failure, and in patients receiving certain antibiotics (see DRUG INTERACTIONS). High fever for prolonged periods may decrease theophylline elimination. Children over six months of age have rapid clearances with average half-lives of approximately 3–5 hours. Newborn infants have extremely slow clearances and half-lives exceeding 24 hours. Older adults with chronic obstructive pulmonary disease, any patients with cor pulmonale or other causes of heart failure, and patients with liver pathology may have much lower clearances with half-lives that exceed 24 hours. The half-life of theophylline in smokers (1–2 packs per day) averages 4–5 hours; the half-life in non-smokers averages 7–9 hours.

Indications: Symptomatic relief and/or prevention of asthma and reversible bronchospasm associated with chronic bronchitis and emphysema.

Contraindications: THEO-DUR Sprinkle is contraindicated in individuals who have shown hypersensitivity to any of its components or xanthine derivatives.

Warnings: Excessive theophylline doses may be associated with toxicity; serum theophylline levels should be monitored to assure maximum benefit with minimum risk. Incidence of toxicity increases at serum levels greater than 20 mcg/ml. High blood levels of theophylline resulting from conventional doses are correlated with clinical manifestations of toxicity in patients with lowered body plasma clearances; patients with liver dysfunction or chronic obstructive lung disease, and patients who are older than 55 years of age, particularly males. There are often no early signs of less serious theophylline toxicity such as nausea and restlessness, which may appear in up to 50% of patients prior to onset of convulsions. Ventricular arrhythmias or seizures may be the first signs of toxicity. Many patients who have higher theophylline serum levels exhibit a tachycardia. Theophylline products may worsen preexisting arrhythmias.

Usage in Pregnancy: Safe use in pregnancy has not been established relative to possible adverse effects on fetal development but neither have adverse effects on fetal development been established. This is, unfortunately, true for most antiasthmatic medications. Therefore, use of theophylline in pregnant women should be balanced against the risk of uncontrolled asthma.

Precautions: THE CONTENTS OF A THEO-DUR SPRINKLE CAPSULE SHOULD NOT BE CHEWED OR CRUSHED.

Theophyllines should not be administered concurrently with other xanthine medications, it should be used with caution in patients with severe cardiac disease, severe hypoxemia, hypertension, hyperthyroidism, acute myocardial injury, cor pulmonale, congestive heart failure, liver disease and in the elderly, particularly males, and in neonates. Great caution should be used in giving theophylline to patients in congestive heart failure since these patients show markedly prolonged theophylline blood level curves. Use theophylline cautiously in patients with history of peptic ulcer. Theophylline may occasionally act as a local irritant to G.I. tract although gastrointestinal symptoms are more commonly central and associated with high serum concentrations above 20 mcg/ml.

Adverse Reactions: The most consistent adverse reactions are usually due to overdose and are:

Gastrointestinal: Nausea, vomiting, epigastric pain, hematernesis, diarrhea

Central Nervous System: Headaches, irritability, restlessness, insomnia, reflex hyperexcitability, muscle twitching, clonic and tonic generalized convulsions.

Cardiovascular: Palpitation, tachycardia, extrasystoles, flushing, hypotension, circulatory failure, life threatening ventricular arrhythmias.

Respiratory: Tachpnea

Renal: Albuminuria, increased excretion of renal tubular cells and red blood cells; potentiation of diuresis.

Other: Hyperglycemia and inappropriate ADH syndrome.

Drug Interactions:

Drug:	Effect:
Theophylline with Furosemide	Increased diuresis
Theophylline with Hexamethonium	Decreased Chronotropic Effect
Theophylline with Reserpine	Tachycardia
Theophylline with Cyclamycin (TAO) Erythromycin or Lincomycin	Increased Theophylline Blood Levels

Overdosage:

Management:

A. If potential oral overdose is established and seizure has not occurred:
1. Induce vomiting
2. Administer a cathartic (this is particularly important if sustained release preparations have been taken).
3. Administer activated charcoal.

B. If patient is having a seizure:
1. Establish an airway
2. Administer 0_2
3. Treat the seizure with intravenous diazepam, 0.1 to 0.3 mg/kg up to 10 mg.
4. Monitor vital signs, maintain blood pressure and provide adequate hydration.

C. Post-Seizure Coma:
1. Maintain airway and oxygenation.
2. If a result of oral medication, follow above recommendations to prevent absorption of drug but intubation and lavage will have to be performed instead of inducing ernesis, and the cathartic and charcoal will need to be introduced via a large bore gastric lavage tube.
3. Continue to provide full supportive care and adequate hydration while waiting for drug to be metabolized. In general, the

Continued on next page

Key—Cont.

drug is metabolized sufficiently rapidly so as to not warrant consideration of dialysis.

Dosage and Administration: Therapeutic serum levels associated with likelihood for optimum benefit and minimal risk of toxicity are considered to be between 10 and 20 mcg/ml. There is a great variation from patient to patient in dosage needed to achieve a therapeutic blood level due to variable rates of elimination. Because of this wide variation from patient to patient, and the relatively narrow therapeutic range, dosage must be individualized.

If the calculated dose falls between two available strengths of a capsule or combination of capsules, the lower strength should be utilized.

If the calculated dose is less than 50 mg, alternate means of theophylline therapy should be considered.

The initial dose should be determined on the basis of body weight and patient history. The following guidelines may be used to determine an average initial dose.

AVERAGE INITIAL DOSE REQUIREMENTS*

Daily Dose	Dose Per 12 Hours**
CHILDREN:	
16 mg/kg/day	8 mg/kg/12 hr
(Not to exceed 400 mg)	
ADULTS:	
9 mg/kg/day	4.5 mg/kg/12 hr

* Use ideal body weight for obese patients.

**Some patients may require dosing every 8 hours.

If the desired response is not achieved with the above AVERAGE INITIAL DOSAGE recommendations and there are no adverse reactions the dose may be safely increased by 2–3 mg/kg body weight per day at 3 day intervals until the following MAXIMUM DOSE WITHOUT MEASUREMENT OF SERUM CONCENTRATION or maximum of 900 mg in any 24 hour period, whichever is less, is attained:

MAXIMUM DOSE WITHOUT MEASUREMENT OF SERUM CONCENTRATION*

Daily Dose	Dose Per 12 Hr**
CHILDREN (6 mo–9 yrs):†	
24 mg/kg/day	12 mg/kg/12 hr
CHILDREN (9–12 yrs):	
20 mg/kg/day	10 mg/kg/12 hr
ADOLESCENTS (12–16 yrs):	
18 mg/kg/day	9 mg/kg/12 hr
ADULTS:	
13 mg/kg/day	6.5 mg/kg/12 hr

* Use ideal body weight for obese patients.

**Some patients may require dosing every 8 hours.

† Children under 1 year require lower doses and caution should be exercised in titration to a therapeutic level.

Nassif EG, et al, "Theophylline Disposition in Infancy", **J. Peds. 98**:158-161, 1981

If higher than those contained in the above MAXIMUM DAILY DOSE WITHOUT MEASUREMENT OF SERUM CONCENTRATION are necessary, it is recommended that serum theophylline levels be monitored. Check serum theophylline levels between 3 and 8 hours after a dose. It is important that the patient will have missed no doses during the previous 72 hours and that dosing intervals will have been reasonably typical with no added doses during that period of time.

DOSAGE ADJUSTMENT BASED ON SERUM THEOPHYLLINE MEASUREMENTS WHEN THESE INSTRUCTIONS HAVE NOT BEEN FOLLOWED MAY RESULT IN RECOMMENDATIONS THAT PRESENT RISK OF TOXICITY TO THE PATIENT.

How Supplied: THEO-DUR SPRINKLE 50 mg, 75 mg, 125 mg and 200 mg Sustained Action Capsules are available in bottles of 100.

Storage Conditions: Keep tightly closed. Store at controlled room temperture 15–30°C (59–86°F).

Caution: Federal law prohibits dispensing without a prescription.

Revised 0782

[*Shown in Product Identification Section*]

TYZINE® ℞
(tetrahydrozoline hydrochloride)
0.1% NASAL SOLUTION
and
0.05% PEDIATRIC NASAL DROPS

Clinical Pharmacology: Tyzine (tetrahydrozoline hydrochloride), a sympathomimetic amine, possesses vasoconstrictor and decongestant actions when applied to the nasal mucosa, resulting in constriction of the smaller arterioles of the nasal passages effecting a decongesting action. Tyzine administered systemically has a central depressant rather than stimulant effect.

Indications and Usage: For decongestion of nasal and nasopharyngeal mucosa.

Contraindications: Tyzine is contraindicated for patients who have shown previous hypersensitivity to its components. The 0.1% solution is contraindicated in children under six years of age. Tyzine is not to be used for infants under two years of age. Tyzine Pediatric Solution should be used for children between the ages of 2 and 6 years. (See "Dosage and Administration".) Tyzine should not be used by patients under treatment with MAO inhibitors.

Warnings: Clinical data in human beings are inadequate to establish conditions for safe use in pregnancy. Therefore, Tyzine Nasal Solution should not be used during pregnancy unless, in the judgement of the physician, the expected benefits outweigh the possible hazards.

Overdosage in children may produce profound sedation. This may be accompanied by profuse sweating. (See "Management Of Overdosage".)

Precautions: Avoid doses greater or more frequent than those recommended below. Excessive dosage in children may, on rare occasions, cause severe drowsiness. Profuse sweating may accompany this effect. Overdosage may also cause marked hypotension or even shock.

Use cautiously in patients with cardiovascular disease (e.g., coronary artery disease, hypertension), and metabolic-endocrine disease (e.g., hyperthyroidism, diabetes).

Adverse Reactions: The most frequent adverse reactions are burning, stinging, sneezing, dryness, headache, drowsiness, weakness, tremors, lightheadedness, insomnia, and palpitations. Prolonged or excessive use may cause rebound congestion.

If adverse reactions occur, discontinue use.

Overdosage: The administration or ingestion of overdoses of Tyzine may result in oversedation in young children. Very occasionally in adults with very excessive overdoses, a shock-like syndrome with hypotension and bradycardia may occur. In either case, the treatment of overdosage is usually that of watchful expectancy and general supportive measures. The patient should be kept warm, fluid balance should be maintained orally, if possible, and parenterally, if necessary. If the respiratory rate drops to 10 or below, the patient should be given oxygen, and respiration assisted. Blood pressure should be watched carefully to prevent a hypotensive crisis.

There is no known antidote for Tyzine (tetrahydrozoline hydrochloride). The use of stimulants is contraindicated. To date, we have had no reports of fatalities resulting from overdosages of Tyzine and while the symptoms resulting from Tyzine overdosage may be alarming, they are self-limiting and the patient recovers with no sequelae.

Dosage and Administration:

Adults and Children 6 years and over:

It is recommended that 2 to 4 drops of Tyzine 0.1% Nasal Solution be instilled in each nostril as needed, never more often than every three hours. Less frequent administration is usually sufficient since relief is maintained for four hours or longer in most cases, and often for as long as eight hours. Bedtime instillation usually assures sleep undisturbed by the need for remedication before morning, or by insomnia from central stimulation.

Children 2 to 6 years of age:

It is recommended that 2 to 3 drops of Tyzine 0.05% Pediatric Nasal Drops be instilled in each nostril as needed and never more often than every three hours. Relief usually lasts for several hours so that instillations are usually needed only every four to six hours.

Instillation of nose drops can be most conveniently accomplished with the patient in the lateral head-low position.

How Supplied:

Tyzine

Nasal Solution (0.1%)
—1 fl. oz. (30 cc.) and 1 pint bottles
—½ fl. oz. (15 cc.) plastic squeeze bottles
Pediatric Nasal Drops (0.05%)—½ fl. oz. (15 cc.) bottles

Caution: FEDERAL LAW PROHIBITS DISPENSING WITHOUT A PRESCRIPTION.

Knoll Pharmaceutical Company
WHIPPANY, NJ 07981

AKINETON® TABLETS AND AMPULES ℞
(biperiden hydrochloride and biperiden lactate)

Description: Each AKINETON® Tablet for oral administration contains 2 mg biperiden hydrochloride. Each 1 ml AKINETON Ampule for intramuscular or intravenous administration contains 5 mg biperiden lactate in an aqueous 1.4 percent sodium lactate solution. No added preservative. AKINETON is an anticholinergic agent. Biperiden is α-5-Norbornen-2-yl-α-phenyl-1-piperidine-propanol. It is a white, crystalline, odorless powder, slightly soluble in water and alcohol. It is stable in air at normal temperatures.

Clinical Pharmacology: AKINETON is a weak visceral anticholinergic agent which is somewhat more potent than atropine on a dosage basis in terms of its ability to block nicotine-induced extensor spasm and death in mice. The mechanism of action of centrally acting anticholinergic drugs such as AKINETON in parkinsonism is thought to relate to their partial blocking effect on the striatal cholinergic receptors which predominate in parkinsonism, in which the inhibitory control by the nigrostriatal dopaminergic pathways is gradually lost. Thus, the balance of excitation and inhibition returns toward normal. Another possibility is that anticholinergic drugs block the re-uptake of dopamine by nerve terminals in the striatum, making more of the transmitter available to the receptors.

The parenteral form of AKINETON is an effective and reliable agent for the treatment of acute episodes of extrapyramidal disturbances during treatment with reserpine and the phenothiazines. Akathisia, akinesia, dyskinetic tremors, rigor, oculogyric crisis, spasmodic torticollis, and profuse sweating are markedly reduced or eliminated. With parenteral AKINETON, these drug-induced disturbances are rapidly brought under control. Subsequently, this can usually be maintained with oral doses which may be given with tranquilizer therapy in psychotic and other conditions requiring an uninterrupted program with phenothiazines or reserpine. This regimen can be particularly useful when drug-induced extrapyramidal disturbances interfere with indicated convulsant therapy.

The pharmacokinetics of AKINETON in humans have not been established. Six hours after an oral dose of 250 mg/kg in rats, 87% of the drug had been absorbed. Cardiovascular and respiratory studies in the dog and cat using large doses of biperiden hydrochloride reveal that the drug has only minor actions on these systems. When given subcutaneously its drying effect on the salivary glands of rabbits and its mydriatic effect on the mouse pupil are relatively weak compared with those of atropine. Biperiden lactate (10 mg/ml) was not irritating to the tissue of rabbits when injected intramuscularly (1.0 ml) into the sacrospinalis muscles and intradermally (0.25 ml) and subcutaneously (0.5 ml) into the shaved abdominal skin.

Indications and Usage: For use as an adjunct in the therapy of all forms of parkinsonism (post-encephalitic, arteriosclerotic, idiopathic). Useful in the control of extrapyramidal disorders due to central nervous system drugs such as reserpine and phenothiazines.

Contraindications: Hypersensitivity to biperiden.

Warnings: Isolated instances of mental confusion, euphoria, agitation and disturbed behavior have been reported in susceptible patients. Also, the central anticholinergic syndrome can occur as an adverse reaction to properly prescribed anticholinergic medication, although it is more frequently due to overdosage. It may also result from concomitant administration of an anticholinergic agent and a drug that has secondary anticholinergic actions (see Drug Interactions and Overdosage sections). Caution should be observed in patients with manifest glaucoma, though no prohibitive rise in intraocular pressure has been noted following either oral or parenteral administration. Patients with prostatism or cardiac arrhythmia should be given this drug with caution.

Precautions

Drug Interactions: The central anticholinergic syndrome can occur when anticholinergic agents such as AKINETON are administered concomitantly with drugs that have secondary anticholinergic actions, e.g., certain narcotic analgesics such as meperidine, the phenothiazines and other antipsychotics, tricyclic antidepressants, certain antiarrhythmics such as the quinidine salts, and antihistamines. See Overdosage section for signs and symptoms of the central anticholinergic syndrome, and for treatment.

Pregnancy: Pregnancy Category C. Animal reproduction studies have not been conducted with AKINETON. It is also not known whether AKINETON can cause fetal harm when administered to a pregnant woman or can affect reproduction capacity. AKINETON should be given to a pregnant woman only if clearly needed.

Nursing Mothers: It is not known whether this drug is excreted in human milk. Because many drugs are excreted in human milk, caution should be exercised when AKINETON is administered to a nursing woman.

Pediatric Use: Safety and effectiveness in children have not been established.

Adverse Reactions: Dry mouth; blurred vision; drowsiness; euphoria or disorientation; urinary retention; postural hypotension; constipation; agitation; disturbed behavior. There have been no significant changes in blood pressure levels or pulse rate in patients who have been given the parenteral form of AKINETON although mild transient postural hypotension may occur. These side effects can be minimized or avoided by slow intravenous administration. No local tissue reactions have been reported following intramuscular injection. If gastric irritation occurs following oral administration, it can be avoided by administering the drug during or after meals.

The central anticholinergic syndrome can occur as an adverse reaction to properly prescribed anticholinergic medication. See Overdosage section for signs and symptoms of the central anticholinergic syndrome, and for treatment.

Overdosage

Signs and Symptoms: Overdosage with AKINETON produces typical central symptoms of atropine intoxication (the central anticholinergic syndrome). Correct diagnosis depends upon recognition of the peripheral signs of parasympathetic blockade including dilated and sluggish pupils; warm, dry skin; facial flushing; decreased secretions of the mouth, pharynx, nose, and bronchi; foul-smelling breath; elevated temperature, tachycardia, decreased bowel sounds, and urinary retention. Neuropsychiatric signs such as delirium, disorientation, anxiety, hallucinations, illusions, confusion, incoherence, agitation, hyperactivity, ataxia, loss of memory, paranoia, combativeness, and seizures may be present. The condition can progress to stupor, coma, and cardiac and respiratory arrest.

Treatment: If AKINETON was administered orally, gastric lavage or other measures to limit absorption should be instituted. A small dose of diazepam or a short acting barbiturate may be administered if CNS excitation is observed. Phenothiazines are contraindicated because the toxicity may be intensified due to their antimuscarinic action, causing coma. Respiratory support, artificial respiration or vasopressor agents may be necessary. Hyperpyrexia must be reversed, fluid volume replaced and acid-base balance maintained. Physostigmine salicylate may be administered to treat this syndrome. One mg (half this amount for the children or elderly) may be given intramuscularly or by slow intravenous infusion. If there is no response within 20 minutes, an additional 1 mg dose may be given; this may be repeated until a total of 4 mg has been administered or excessive cholinergic signs are seen. Frequent monitoring of clinical signs should be done. Since physostigmine is rapidly destroyed, additional injections may be required every one or two hours to maintain control. The relapse intervals tend to lengthen as the toxic anticholinergic agent is metabolized, so the patient should be carefully observed for 8 to 12 hours following the last relapse.

Toxicity in Animals: The acute subcutaneous toxicity (LD_{50}) of biperiden hydrochloride in mice was found to be 195 mg/kg and the intravenous toxicity (LD_{50}), 72 mg/kg. The acute oral toxicity (LD_{50}) in rats is 750 mg/kg. The intraperitoneal toxicity (LD_{50}) of biperiden lactate in rats was 270 mg/kg, and the intravenous toxicity (LD_{50}) in dogs was 222 mg/kg.

Dosage and Administration

Drug-Induced Extrapyramidal Symptoms:

Parenteral: The average adult dose is 2 mg intramuscularly or intravenously. May be repeated every half-hour until there is resolution of symptoms, but not more than four consecutive doses should be given in a 24-hour period.

Note: Parenteral drug products should be inspected visually for particulate matter and discoloration prior to administration, whenever solution and container permit.

Oral: One tablet one to three times daily.

Parkinson's Disease: Oral: One tablet three or four times daily.

How Supplied:

AKINETON Tablets, 2 mg each, white, embossed on one face with a triangle, bisected on the reverse and imprinted with the number "11".

Bottles of 100—NDC #0044-0120-02.

Bottles of 1000—NDC #0044-0120-04.

[*Shown in Product Identification Section*]

AKINETON Ampules, 1 ml each containing 5 mg biperiden lactate per ml.

Boxes of 10—NDC #0044-0110-01.

Storage: All dosage forms of AKINETON should be stored at 59°–86°F, 15°–30°C.

DILAUDID® Ⓒ ℞

(hydromorphone hydrochloride)

Description: DILAUDID (hydromorphone hydrochloride) (**WARNING:** May be habit forming), a hydrogenated ketone of morphine, is a narcotic analgesic. It is available in ampules (for parenteral administration) containing 1 mg, 2 mg, 3 mg and 4 mg hydromorphone hydrochloride per ml with 0.2% sodium citrate, 0.2% citric acid solution; in multiple dose vials (for parenteral administration) of 10 ml and 20 ml solutions, each ml containing 2 mg hydromorphone hydrochloride and 0.5 mg edetate disodium with 1.8 mg methylparaben and 0.2 mg propylparaben as preservatives and pH adjusted with sodium hydroxide or hydrochloric acid; in color coded tablets (for oral administration) containing 1 mg, 2 mg, 3 mg and 4 mg hydromorphone hydrochloride; in suppositories (for rectal administration) containing 3 mg hydromorphone hydrochloride in cocoa butter base with 1% colloidal silica as an inactive ingredient; and in powder for prescription compounding. DILAUDID ampules and multiple dose vials are sterile.

Clinical Pharmacology: DILAUDID is a narcotic analgesic; its principal therapeutic effect is relief of pain. The precise mechanism of action of DILAUDID and other opiates is not known, although it is believed to relate to the existence of opiate receptors in the central nervous system. There is no intrinsic limit to the analgesic effect of DILAUDID; like morphine, adequate doses will relieve even the most severe pain. Clinically, however, dosage limitations are imposed by the adverse effects, primarily respiratory depression, nausea, and vomiting, which can result from high doses.

DILAUDID has diverse additional actions. It may produce drowsiness, changes in mood and mental clouding, depress the respiratory center and the cough center, stimulate the vomiting center, produce pinpoint constriction of the pupil, enhance parasympathetic activitiy, elevate cerebrospinal fluid pressure, increase biliary pressure, produce transient hyperglycemia.

Generally, the analgesic action of parenterally administered DILAUDID is apparent within 15 minutes and usually remains in effect for more than five hours. The onset of action of oral DILAUDID is somewhat slower, with measurable analgesia occurring within 30 minutes. Radioimmunoassay techniques have recently been developed for the analysis of DILAUDID in human plasma. In humans the half-life of a DILAUDID 4 mg tablet is 2.6 hours. In a random crossover study in six subjects, 4mg of oral DILAUDID produced a mean concentration/time curve similar to that of 2mg DILAUDID I.V., after the first hour.

Indications and Usage: DILAUDID is indicated for the relief of moderate to severe pain such as that due to:

- Surgery
- Cancer
- Trauma (soft tissue & bone)
- Biliary Colic
- Myocardial Infarction
- Burns
- Renal Colic

Contraindications: As is morphine, DILAUDID is contraindicated in patients known to have a hypersensitivity to it; in the presence of an intracranial lesion associated with increased intracranial pressure; and whenever ventilatory function is depressed (chronic obstructive pulmonary disease, cor pulmonale, emphysema, kyphoscoliosis, status asthmaticus).

Continued on next page

Knoll—Cont.

Warnings

Respiratory Depression: DILAUDID produces dose-related respiratory depression by acting directly on brain stem respiratory centers. DILAUDID also affects centers that control respiratory rhythm, and may produce irregular and periodic breathing.

Head Injury and Increased Intracranial Pressure: The respiratory depressant effects of narcotics and their capacity to elevate cerebrospinal fluid pressure may be markedly exaggerated in the presence of head injury, other intracranial lesions or a pre-existing increase in intracranial pressure. Furthermore, narcotics produce effects which may obscure the clinical course of patients with head injuries.

Acute Abdominal Conditions: The administration of narcotics may obscure the diagnosis or clinical course of patients with acute abdominal conditions.

Precautions

Special Risk Patients: DILAUDID should be used with caution in elderly or debilitated patients and those with impaired renal or hepatic function, hypothyroidism, Addison's disease, prostatic hypertrophy or urethral stricture. As with any narcotic analgesic agent, the usual precautions should be observed and the possibility of respiratory depression should be kept in mind.

Cough Reflex: DILAUDID suppresses the cough reflex; as with all narcotics, caution should be exercised when DILAUDID is used postoperatively and in patients with pulmonary disease.

Usage in Ambulatory Patients: Narcotics may impair the mental and/or physical abilities required for the performance of potentially hazardous tasks such as driving a car or operating machinery; patients should be cautioned accordingly.

Drug Interactions: Patients receiving other narcotic analgesics, general anesthetics, phenothiazines, tranquilizers, sedative-hypnotics, tricyclic antidepressants or other CNS depressants (including alcohol) concomitantly with DILAUDID may exhibit an additive CNS depression. When such combined therapy is contemplated, the dose of one or both agents should be reduced.

Parenteral Administration: The parenteral form of DILAUDID may be given intravenously, but the injection should be given very slowly. Rapid intravenous injection of narcotic analgesics increases the possibility of side effects such as hypotension and respiratory depression.

Usage in Pregnancy: Pregnancy Category C. DILAUDID has been shown to be teratogenic in hamsters when given in doses 600 times the human dose. There are no adequate and well-controlled studies in pregnant women. DILAUDID should be used during pregnancy only if the potential benefit justifies the potential risk to the fetus.

Nonteratogenic effects: Babies born to mothers who have been taking opioids regularly prior to delivery will be physically dependent. The withdrawal signs include irritability and excessive crying, tremors, hyperactive reflexes, increased respiratory rate, increased stools, sneezing, yawning, vomiting, and fever. The intensity of the syndrome does not always correlate with the duration of maternal opioid use or dose. There is no consensus on the best method of managing withdrawal. Chlorpromazine 0.7 to 1.0 mg/kg q6h, phenobarbital 2 mg/kg q6h, and paregoric 2–4 drops/kg q4h, have been used to treat withdrawal symptoms in infants. The duration of therapy is 4 to 28 days, with the dosages decreased as tolerated.

Labor and Delivery: As with all narcotics, administration of DILAUDID to the mother shortly before delivery may result in some degree of respiratory depression in the newborn, especially if higher doses are used.

Nursing Mothers: It is not known whether this drug is excreted in human milk. Because many drugs are excreted in human milk and because of the potential for serious adverse reactions in nursing infants from DILAUDID, a decision should be made whether to discontinue nursing or to discontinue the drug, taking into account the importance of the drug to the mother.

Pediatric Use: Safety and effectiveness in children have not been established.

FD&C Yellow No. 5: DILAUDID 1 mg, 2 mg and 4 mg color coded tablets contain FD&C Yellow No. 5 (tartrazine) dye which may cause allergic-type reactions (including bronchial asthma) in certain susceptible individuals. Although the overall incidence of FD&C Yellow No. 5 (tartrazine) dye sensitivity in the general population is low, it is frequently seen in patients who also have aspirin hypersensitivity.

Adverse Reactions

Central Nervous System: Sedation, drowsiness, mental clouding, lethargy, impairment of mental and physical performance, anxiety, fear, dysphoria, dizziness, psychic dependence, mood changes.

Gastrointestinal System: Nausea and vomiting occur more frequently in ambulatory than in recumbent patients. The antiemetic phenothiazines are useful in suppressing these effects; however, some phenothiazine derivatives seem to be antianalgesic and to increase the amount of narcotic required to produce pain relief, while other phenothiazines reduce the amount of narcotic required to produce a given level of analgesia. Prolonged administration of DILAUDID may produce constipation.

Cardiovascular System: Circulatory depression, peripheral circulatory collapse and cardiac arrest have occurred after rapid intravenous injection. Orthostatic hypotension and fainting may occur if a patient stands up suddenly after receiving an injection of DILAUDID.

Genitourinary System: Ureteral spasm, spasm of vesical sphincters and urinary retention have been reported.

Respiratory Depression: DILAUDID produces dose-related respiratory depression by acting directly on brain stem respiratory centers. DILAUDID also affects centers that control respiratory rhythm, and may produce irregular and periodic breathing. If significant respiratory depression occurs, it may be antagonized by the use of naloxone hydrochloride, 0.005 mg/kg intravenously. Apply other supportive measures when indicated.

Drug Abuse and Dependence: DILAUDID is a Schedule Ⓒ narcotic. Psychic dependence, physical dependence, and tolerance may develop upon repeated administration of narcotics; therefore, DILAUDID should be prescribed and administered with caution. However, psychic dependence is unlikely to develop when DILAUDID is used for a short time for the treatment of pain. Physical dependence, the condition in which continued administration of the drug is required to prevent the appearance of a withdrawal syndrome, assumes clinically significant proportions only after several weeks of continued narcotic use, although some mild degree of physical dependence may develop after a few days of narcotic therapy. Tolerance, in which increasingly large doses are required in order to produce the same degree of analgesia, is manifested initially by a shortened duration of analgesic effect, and subsequently by decreases in the intensity of analgesia. The rate of development of tolerance varies among patients.

Overdosage

Signs and Symptoms: Serious overdosage with DILAUDID is characterized by respiratory depression (a decrease in respiratory rate and/or tidal volume, Cheyne-Stokes respiration, cyanosis), extreme somnolence progressing to stupor or coma, skeletal muscle flaccidity, cold and clammy skin, and sometimes bradycardia and hypotension. In severe overdosage, particularly by the intravenous route, apnea, circulatory collapse, cardiac arrest, and death may occur.

Treatment: Primary attention should be given to the reestablishment of adequate respiratory exchange through provision of a patent airway and institution of assisted or controlled ventilation. The narcotic antagonist naloxone hydrochloride is a specific antidote against respiratory depression which may result from overdosage or unusual sensitivity to narcotics, including DILAUDID. Therefore, naloxone hydrochloride, 0.005 mg/kg should be administered intravenously simultaneously with ventilatory assistance.

Since the duration of action of DILAUDID may exceed that of the antagonist, the patient should be kept under continued surveillance; repeated doses of the antagonist may be required to maintain adequate respiration. An antagonist should not be administered in the absence of clinically significant respiratory or cardiovascular depression. Oxygen, intravenous fluids, vasopressors, and other supportive measures should be employed as indicated.

In cases of overdosage with oral DILAUDID, gastric lavage or induced emesis may be useful in removing unabsorbed drug from conscious patients.

Dosage and Administration

Parenteral: The usual dose is 2 mg intramuscularly every 4 to 6 hours as necessary. The dose must be individually adjusted according to severity of pain, patient response and patient size. The subcutaneous route of administration may be utilized, if desired. Intravenous or subcutaneous administration is usually not painful. Should intravenous administration be necessary, the injection should be given very slowly (taking at least 2 to 3 minutes to administer). If the pain increases in severity, analgesia is not adequate or tolerance occurs, a gradual increase in dosage may be required. The first sign of beginning tolerance is usually a reduced duration of effect.

NOTE: Parenteral drug products should be inspected visually for particulate matter and discoloration prior to administration, whenever solution and container permit. A slight yellowish discoloration may develop in DILAUDID ampules and multiple dose vials. No loss of potency has been demonstrated.

Oral: The usual oral dose is 2 mg every 4 to 6 hours as necessary. The dose must be individually adjusted according to severity of pain, patient response and patient size. More severe pain may require 4 mg or more every 4 to 6 hours. If the pain increases in severity, analgesia is not adequate or tolerance occurs, a gradual increase in dosage may be required. If pain is exceedingly severe, or if prompt response is desired, parenteral DILAUDID should be used initially in adequate amounts to control the pain.

Rectal: DILAUDID suppositories (3 mg) may provide longer duration of relief which could obviate additional medication during the sleeping hours. The usual adult dose is 1 suppository inserted rectally every 6 to 8 hours or as directed by physician.

How Supplied

Ampules: 1 mg, 2 mg, 3 mg, and 4 mg hydromorphone hydrochloride per ml with 0.2% sodium citrate, 0.2% citric acid solution. No added preservative.

1 mg/ml ampules—Boxes of 10—
NDC# 0044-1011-01.

2 mg/ml ampules—Boxes of 10—
NDC# 0044-1012-01.
Boxes of 25—NDC# 0044-1012-09.

3 mg/ml ampules—Boxes of 10—
NDC# 0044-1013-01.

4 mg/ml ampules—Boxes of 10—
NDC# 0044-1014-01.

Multiple Dose Vials: 10 ml and 20 ml sterile solutions, each ml contains 2 mg hydromorphone hydrochloride and 0.5 mg edetate disodium with 1.8 mg methylparaben and 0.2 mg propylparaben as preservatives. pH adjusted with sodium hydroxide or hydrochloric acid.

2 mg/ml—10 ml multiple dose vials—
NDC# 0044-1062-01.

2 mg/ml—20 ml multiple dose vials—
NDC# 0044-1062-05.

Oral Color Coded Tablets: (NOT FOR INJECTION)

1 mg tablet (green)—Bottles of 100—
NDC# 0044-1021-02.

2 mg tablet (orange)—Bottles of 100—
NDC# 0044-1022-02.
Strip Pack of 100 (4 × 25)—
NDC# 0044-1022-45
Bottles of 500—NDC# 0044-1022-03.

3 mg tablet (pink)—Bottles of 100—
NDC# 0044-1023-02.

4 mg tablet (yellow)—Bottles of 100—
NDC# 0044-1024-02.
Strip Pack of 100 (4 × 25)—
NDC# 0044-1024-45
Bottles of 500—NDC# 0044-1024-03.

Rectal Suppositories: 3 mg hydromorphone hydrochloride in cocoa butter base with 1% colloidal silica as an inactive ingredient.
Boxes of 6—NDC# 0044-1053-01.

Powder: For prescription compounding.
15 grain vial—NDC# 0044-1040-01.

Storage: Parenteral and oral dosage forms of DILAUDID should be stored at 59°–86°F, 15°–30°C.

DILAUDID suppositories should be stored in a refrigerator.

DEA order form required.

A Schedule Ⓒ Narcotic.

[*Shown in Product Identification Section*]

DILAUDID® COUGH SYRUP Ⓒ ℞
(hydromorphone hydrochloride)

Description: Each 5 ml (1 teaspoonful) contains 1 mg DILAUDID (hydromorphone hydrochloride) (**WARNING:** May be habit forming) and 100 mg guaifenesin in a peach-flavored syrup containing 5% alcohol. DILAUDID is a hydrogenated ketone of morphine; it is a narcotic analgesic and antitussive.

Clinical Pharmacology: DILAUDID (hydromorphone hydrochloride) is a centrally acting narcotic antitussive which acts directly on the cough reflex center. DILAUDID is also an analgesic and has diverse additional actions. It may produce drowsiness, changes in mood and mental clouding, depress the respiratory center, stimulate the vomiting center, produce pinpoint constriction of the pupil, enhance parasympathetic activity, elevate cerebrospinal fluid pressure, increase biliary pressure, and produce transient hyperglycemia, depending on the amount administered and individual patient sensitivity.

Radioimmunoassay techniques have recently been developed for the analysis of DILAUDID in human plasma. However, little is known as yet about the bioavailability or pharmacokinetics of DILAUDID in humans, except that the half-life of a 4 mg DILAUDID tablet is 2.6 hours.

Guaifenesin (glyceryl guaiacolate) reduces the viscosity of secretions, thereby increasing the efficiency of the cough reflex and of ciliary action in removing accumulated secretions from the trachea and bronchi. Unlike many other expectorants, guaifenesin rarely causes gastric irritation.

Indications and Usage: DILAUDID Cough Syrup is indicated for the control of persistent, exhausting cough or dry, non-productive cough.

Contraindications: DILAUDID Cough Syrup is contraindicated in patients known to have a hypersensitivity to it; in the presence of an intracranial lesion associated with increased intracranial pressure; and whenever ventilatory function is depressed (chronic obstructive pulmonary disease, cor pulmonale, emphysema, kyphoscoliosis, status asthmaticus).

Warnings

Respiratory Depression: DILAUDID may produce dose-related respiratory depression by acting directly on brain stem respiratory centers in susceptible individuals or when used in excessive doses.

Head Injury and Increased Intracranial Pressure: The respiratory depressant effects of narcotics and their capacity to elevate cerebrospinal fluid pressure may be markedly exaggerated in the presence of head injury, other intracranial lesions or a preexisting increase in intracranial pressure. Furthermore, narcotics produce effects which may obscure the clinical course of patients with head injuries.

Acute Abdominal Conditions: The administration of narcotics may obscure the diagnosis or clinical course of patients with acute abdominal conditions.

Precautions

Special Risk Patients: As with any narcotic, DILAUDID Cough Syrup should be used with caution in elderly or debilitated patients and those with impaired renal or hepatic function, hypothyroidism, Addison's disease, prostatic hypertrophy or urethral stricture. The usual precautions should be observed and the possibility of respiratory depression should be kept in mind.

Cough Reflex: DILAUDID Cough Syrup suppresses the cough reflex; as with all narcotics, caution should be exercised when DILAUDID Cough Syrup is used postoperatively and in patients with pulmonary disease.

Usage in Ambulatory Patients: Narcotics may impair the mental and/or physical abilities required for the performance of potentially hazardous tasks such as driving a car or operating machinery; patients should be cautioned accordingly.

Drug Interactions: Patients receiving other narcotics, general anesthetics, phenothiazines, tranquilizers, sedative-hypnotics, tricyclic antidepressants or other CNS depressants (including alcohol) concomitantly with DILAUDID Cough Syrup may exhibit an additive CNS depression. When such combined therapy is contemplated, the dose of one or both agents should be reduced.

Usage in Pregnancy: Pregnancy Category C. DILAUDID has been shown to be teratogenic in hamsters when given in doses 600 times the human dose. There are no adequate and well-controlled studies in pregnant women. DILAUDID Cough Syrup should be used during pregnancy only if the potential benefit justifies the potential risk to the fetus.

Nonteratogenic effects: Babies born to mothers who have been taking opioids regularly prior to delivery will be physically dependent. The withdrawal signs include irritability and excessive crying, tremors, hyperactive reflexes, increased respiratory rate, increased stools, sneezing, yawning, vomiting, and fever. The intensity of the syndrome does not always correlate with the duration of maternal opioid use or dose. There is no consensus on the best method of managing withdrawal. Chlorpromazine 0.7 to 1.0 mg/kg q6h, phenobarbital 2 mg/kg q6h, and paregoric 2 to 4 drops/kg q4h, have been used to treat withdrawal symptoms in infants. The duration of therapy is 4 to 28 days, with the dosage decreased as tolerated.

Labor and Delivery: As with all narcotics, administration of DILAUDID Cough Syrup to the mother shortly before delivery may result in some degree of respiratory depression in the newborn, especially if higher doses are used.

Nursing Mothers: It is not known whether this drug is excreted in human milk. Because many drugs are excreted in human milk and because of the potential for serious adverse reactions in nursing infants from DILAUDID Cough Syrup, a decision should be made whether to discontinue nursing or to discontinue the drug, taking into account the importance of the drug to the mother.

Pediatric Use: Safety and effectiveness in children have not been established.

FD&C Yellow No. 5: DILAUDID Cough Syrup contains FD&C Yellow No. 5 (tartrazine) dye which may cause allergic-type reactions (including bronchial asthma) in certain susceptible individuals. Although the overall incidence of FD&C Yellow No. 5 (tartrazine) dye sensitivity in the general population is low, it is frequently seen in patients who also have aspirin hypersensitivity.

Adverse Reactions

Central Nervous System: Sedation, drowsiness, mental clouding, lethargy, impairment of mental and physical performance, anxiety, fear, dysphoria, dizziness, psychic dependence, mood changes.

Gastrointestinal System: Nausea and vomiting occur more frequently in ambulatory than in recumbent patients. Some of the antiemetic phenothiazines are useful in suppressing these effects. Prolonged administration of DILAUDID Cough Syrup may produce constipation.

Genitourinary System: Ureteral spasm, spasm of vesical sphincters and urinary retention have been reported.

Respiratory Depression: DILAUDID may produce dose-related respiratory depression by acting directly on brain stem respiratory centers in susceptible individuals or when used in excessive doses. DILAUDID also affects centers that control respiratory rhythm, and may produce irregular and periodic breathing. If significant respiratory depression occurs, it can be antagonized by the use of naloxone hydrochloride, 0.005 mg/kg intravenously. Apply other supportive measures when indicated.

Drug Abuse and Dependence: DILAUDID is a Schedule Ⓒ narcotic. Psychic dependence, physical dependence, and tolerance may develop upon repeated administration of narcotics; therefore, DILAUDID Cough Syrup should be prescribed and administered with caution.

Overdosage

Signs and Symptoms: Serious overdosage with DILAUDID Cough Syrup is characterized by respiratory depression (a decrease in respiratory rate and/or tidal volume, Cheyne-Stokes respiration, cyanosis), extreme somnolence progressing to stupor or coma, skeletal muscle flaccidity, cold and clammy skin, and sometimes bradycardia and hypotension. In severe overdosage, apnea, circulatory collapse, cardiac arrest and death may occur.

Treatment: Primary attention should be given to the reestablishment of adequate respiratory exchange through provision of a patent airway and the institution of assisted or controlled ventilation. The narcotic antagonist naloxone hydrochloride is a specific antidote against respiratory depression which may result from overdosage or unusual sensitivity to narcotics. Therefore, naloxone hydrochloride 0.005 mg/kg should be administered intravenously simultaneously with ventilatory assistance.

Since the duration of action of the narcotic may exceed that of the antagonist, the patient should be kept under continued surveillance and repeated doses of the antagonist should be administered as needed to maintain adequate respiratory function. An antagonist should not be administered in the absence of clinically significant respiratory or cardiovascular depression. Oxygen, intravenous fluids, vasopressors and other supportive measures should be employed as indicated. Gastric lavage or induced emesis may be useful in removing unabsorbed drug from conscious patients.

Continued on next page

Knoll—Cont.

Dosage and Administration: The usual adult dose of DILAUDID Cough Syrup is one teaspoonful (5 ml) every 3 to 4 hours.

How Supplied: Bottles of 1 pint (473 ml)—NDC #0044-1080-01.

Storage: Store at 59°–86°F, 15°–30°C.

A Schedule Ⓒ Narcotic.

DEA order form required.

ISOPTIN® ℞
(verapamil hydrochloride)
for Intravenous Injection

Description: ISOPTIN (verapamil hydrochloride) is a slow-channel inhibitor or calcium antagonist. Each 2 ml sterile ampule (for intravenous administration) contains 5 mg verapamil HCl and 17 mg sodium chloride in water for injection. Hydrochloric acid is used for pH adjustment. The pH of the solution is between 4.1 and 6.0. Protect contents from light.

The structural formula of verapamil HCl is given below:

CH_3O, CH_3O (3,4-dimethoxyphenyl)—$C(CN)(CH(CH_3)_2)(CH_2)_3N(CH_3)CH_2CH_2$—(3,4-dimethoxyphenyl, OCH_3, OCH_3) $\cdot HCl$

$C_{27}H_{38}N_2O_4 \cdot HCl$ M.W. = 491.08

Benzeneacetonitrile, α-[3-[[2-(3,4-dimethoxyphenyl) ethyl] methylamino] propyl] - 3,4-dimethoxy-α-(1-methylethyl) hydrochloride

Verapamil HCl is an almost white, crystalline powder, practically free of odor, with a bitter taste. It is soluble in water, chloroform and methanol. Verapamil HCl is not chemically related to other antiarrhythmic drugs.

Clinical Pharmacology

Mechanism of Action: ISOPTIN (verapamil HCl) inhibits the calcium ion (and possibly sodium ion) influx through slow channels into conductile and contractile myocardial cells and vascular smooth muscle cells. The antiarrhythmic effect of ISOPTIN appears to be due to its effect on the slow channel in cells of the cardiac conductile system.

Electrical activity through the SA and AV nodes depends, to a significant degree, upon calcium influx through the slow channel. By inhibiting this influx, ISOPTIN slows AV conduction and prolongs the effective refractory period within the AV node in a rate-related manner, reducing elevated ventricular rate in patients with supraventricular tachycardia due to atrial flutter and/or atrial fibrillation. By interrupting reentry at the AV node, ISOPTIN can restore normal sinus rhythm in patients with paroxysmal supraventricular tachycardias (PSVT), including Wolff-Parkinson-White syndrome. ISOPTIN has no effect on conduction across accessory bypass tracts. ISOPTIN does not alter the normal atrial action potential or intraventricular conduction time, but depresses amplitude, velocity of depolarization and conduction in depressed atrial fibers.

In the isolated rabbit heart, concentrations of ISOPTIN that markedly affect SA nodal fibers or fibers in the upper and middle regions of the AV node, have very little effect on fibers in the lower AV node (NH region) and no effect on atrial action potentials or His bundle fibers.

ISOPTIN does not induce bronchoconstriction or peripheral arterial spasm.

ISOPTIN has a local anesthetic action that is 1.6 times that of procaine on an equimolar basis. It is not known whether this action is important at the doses used in man.

ISOPTIN does not alter total serum calcium levels.

Hemodynamics: In animals and man, ISOPTIN (verapamil HCl) reduces afterload and myocardial contractility. In most patients, including those with organic cardiac disease, the negative inotropic action of ISOPTIN is countered by reduction of afterload and cardiac index is usually not reduced, but in patients with moderately severe to severe cardiac dysfunction (pulmonary wedge pressure above 20 mm Hg, ejection fraction less than 20%), acute worsening of heart failure may be seen. Peak therapeutic effects occur within 3 to 5 minutes after a bolus injection. The commonly used intravenous doses of 5–10 mg ISOPTIN produce transient, usually asymptomatic, reduction in normal systemic arterial pressure, systemic vascular resistance and contractility; left ventricular filling pressure is slightly increased.

Pharmacokinetics: Intravenously administered ISOPTIN (verapamil HCl) has been shown to be rapidly metabolized in both humans and animals. Following intravenous infusion in man, verapamil is eliminated bi-exponentially, with a rapid early distribution phase (half-life about 4 minutes) and a slower terminal elimination phase (half-life 2–5 hours). In healthy men, orally administered ISOPTIN undergoes extensive metabolism in the liver with 12 metabolites having been identified, most in only trace amounts. The major metabolites have been identified as various N- and O-dealkylated products of ISOPTIN. Approximately 70% of an administered dose is excreted in the urine and 16% or more in the feces within 5 days. About 3–4% is excreted as unchanged drug.

Indications and Usage: ISOPTIN (verapamil HCl) is indicated for the treatment of supraventricular tachyarrhythmias, including:

- Rapid conversion to sinus rhythm of paroxysmal supraventricular tachycardias, including those associated with accessory bypass tracts (Wolff-Parkinson-White [W-P-W] and Lown-Ganong-Levine [L-G-L] syndromes). When clinically advisable, appropriate vagal maneuvers (e.g. Valsalva maneuver) should be attempted prior to ISOPTIN administration.
- Temporary control of rapid ventricular rate in atrial flutter or atrial fibrillation.

In controlled studies in the United States, about 60% of patients with supraventricular tachycardia converted to normal sinus rhythm within 10 minutes after intravenous ISOPTIN. Uncontrolled studies reported in the world literature describe a conversion rate of about 80%. About 70% of patients with atrial flutter and/or fibrillation with a fast ventricular rate respond with a decrease in heart rate of at least 20%. Conversion of atrial flutter or fibrillation to sinus rhythm is uncommon (about 10%) after ISOPTIN and may reflect the spontaneous conversion rate, since the conversion rate after placebo was similar. The effect of a single injection lasts for 30–60 minutes when conversion to sinus rhythm does not occur.

Because a small fraction (< 1.0%) of patients treated with ISOPTIN respond with life-threatening adverse responses (rapid ventricular rate in atrial flutter/fibrillation, marked hypotension, or extreme bradycardia/asystole—see Warnings), the initial use of intravenous ISOPTIN should, if possible, be in a treatment setting with monitoring and resuscitation facilities, including D.C.-cardioversion capability. As familiarity with the patient's response is gained, an office setting would be acceptable.

Contraindications: Verapamil HCl is contraindicated in:

1. Severe hypotension or cardiogenic shock
2. Second- or third-degree AV block
3. Sick sinus syndrome (except in patients with a functioning artificial ventricular pacemaker)
4. Severe congestive heart failure (unless secondary to a supraventricular tachycardia amenable to verapamil therapy)
5. Patients receiving **intravenous** beta adrenergic blocking drugs (e.g., propranolol). **Intravenous** verapamil and **intravenous** beta adrenergic blocking drugs should not be administered in close proximity to each other (within a few hours), since both may have a depressant effect on myocardial contractility and AV conduction.

Warnings: ISOPTIN SHOULD BE GIVEN AS A SLOW INTRAVENOUS INJECTION OVER AT LEAST A TWO MINUTE PERIOD OF TIME. (See Dosage and Administration)

Hypotension: Intravenous verapamil often produces a decrease in blood pressure below baseline levels that is usually transient and asymptomatic but may result in dizziness. Systolic pressure less than 90 mm Hg and/or diastolic pressure less than 60 mm Hg was seen in 5–10% of patients in controlled U.S. trials in supraventricular tachycardia and in about 10% of the patients with atrial flutter/fibrillation. The incidence of symptomatic hypotension observed in studies conducted in the U.S. was approximately 1.5%. Three of the five symptomatic patients required pharmacologic treatment (levarterenol bitartrate I.V., metaraminol bitartrate I.V., or 10% calcium gluconate I.V.). All recovered without sequelae.

Rapid Ventricular Response in Atrial Flutter/Fibrillation: Patients with atrial flutter/fibrillation and an accessory AV pathway (e.g., Wolff-Parkinson-White or Lown-Ganong-Levine syndromes) may develop increased antegrade conduction across the aberrant pathway bypassing the AV node, producing a very rapid ventricular response after receiving verapamil (or digitalis). This has been reported in 1% of the patients treated in controlled double-blind trials in the United States. Treatment is usually D.C.-cardioversion. Cardioversion has been used safely and effectively after intravenous ISOPTIN. (See Adverse Reactions and Treatment of Adverse Reactions)

Extreme Bradycardia/Asystole: Verapamil slows conduction across the AV node and rarely may produce second- or third-degree AV block, bradycardia and, in extreme cases, asystole. This is more likely to occur in patients with a sick sinus syndrome (SA nodal disease), which is more common in older patients. Bradycardia associated with sick sinus syndrome was reported in 0.3% of the patients treated in controlled double-blind trials in the United States. The total incidence of bradycardia (ventricular rate less than 60 beats/min) was 1.2% in these studies. Asystole in patients other than those with sick sinus syndrome is usually of short duration (few seconds or less), with spontaneous return to AV nodal or normal sinus rhythm. If this does not occur promptly, appropriate treatment should be initiated immediately. (See Adverse Reactions and Treatment of Adverse Reactions)

Heart Failure: When heart failure is not severe or rate related, it should be controlled with optimum digitalization and diuretics, as appropriate, before ISOPTIN is used.

In patients with moderately severe to severe cardiac dysfunction (pulmonary wedge pressure above 20 mm Hg, ejection fraction less than 20%), acute worsening of heart failure may be seen.

Concomitant Antiarrhythmic Therapy:

Digitalis

Intravenous verapamil has been used concomitantly with digitalis preparations without the occurrence of serious adverse effects. However, since both drugs slow AV conduction, patients should be monitored for AV block or excessive bradycardia.

Quinidine—Procainamide

Intravenous verapamil has been administered to a small number of patients receiving oral quinidine and oral procainamide without the occurrence of serious adverse effects.

Beta Adrenergic Blocking Drugs

Intravenous verapamil has been administered to patients receiving **oral** beta blockers without the development of serious adverse effects. However, since both drugs may depress myocardial contractility or AV conduction, these possibilities should be considered. On rare occasions, the concomitant adminis-

Suggested Treatment of Acute Cardiovascular Adverse Reactions*

The frequency of these adverse reactions was quite low and experience with their treatment has been limited.

Adverse Reaction	Proven Effective Treatment	Treatment with Good Theoretical Rationale	Supportive Treatment
1. Symptomatic hypotension requiring treatment	Calcium chloride (I.V.) Levarterenol bitartrate (I.V.) Metaraminol bitartrate (I.V.) Isoproterenol HCl (I.V.) Dopamine (I.V.)	Dobutamine (I.V.)	Intravenous fluids Trendelenburg position
2. Bradycardia, AV block, Asystole	Isoproterenol HCl (I.V.) Calcium chloride (I.V.) Cardiac pacing Levarterenol bitartrate (I.V.) Atropine (I.V.)	———	Intravenous fluids (slow drip)
3. Rapid ventricular rate (due to antegrade conduction in flutter/fibrillation with W-P-W or L-G-L syndromes)	D.C. -cardioversion (high energy may be required) Procainamide (I.V.) Lidocaine (I.V.)	———	Intravenous fluids (slow drip)

* Actual treatment and dosage should depend on the severity of the clinical situation and the judgment and experience of the treating physician.

tration of **intravenous** beta blockers and **intravenous** verapamil has resulted in serious adverse reactions (see Contraindications), especially in patients with severe cardiomyopathy, congestive heart failure or recent myocardial infarction.

Disopyramide

Until data on possible interactions between verapamil and all forms of disopyramide phosphate are obtained, disopyramide should not be administered within 48 hours before or 24 hours after verapamil administration.

Heart Block: ISOPTIN prolongs AV conduction time. While high degree AV block has not been observed in controlled clinical trials in the U.S., a low percentage (less than 0.5%) has been reported in the world literature. Development of second- or third-degree AV block or unifascicular, bifascicular or trifascicular bundle branch block requires reduction in subsequent doses or discontinuation of verapamil and institution of appropriate therapy, if needed. (See Adverse Reactions and Concomitant Antiarrhythmic Therapy)

Hepatic and Renal Failure: Significant hepatic and renal failure should not increase the effects of a single intravenous dose of ISOPTIN but may prolong its duration. Repeated injections of intravenous ISOPTIN in such patients may lead to accumulation and an excessive pharmacologic effect of the drug. There is no experience to guide use of multiple doses in such patients and this generally should be avoided If repeated injections are essential, blood pressure and PR interval should be closely monitored and smaller repeat doses should be utilized. Data on the clearance of verapamil by dialysis are not yet available.

Premature Ventricular Contractions: During conversion to normal sinus rhythm, or marked reduction in ventricular rate, a few benign complexes of unusual appearance (sometimes resembling premature ventricular contractions) may be seen after treatment with verapamil. Similar complexes are seen during spontaneous conversion of supraventricular tachycardias, after D.C.-cardioversion and other pharmacologic therapy. These complexes appear to have no clinical significance.

Precautions

Drug interactions: (See Warnings: Concomitant Antiarrhythmic Therapy) Intravenous ISOPTIN (verapamil HCl) has been used concomitantly with other cardioactive drugs (especially digitalis and quinidine) without evidence of serious negative drug interactions, except, in rare instances, when patients with severe cardiomyopathy, congestive heart failure or recent myocardial infarction were given **intravenous** beta-adrenergic blocking agents or disopyramide. Drug interaction studies are ongoing. As verapamil is highly bound to plasma proteins, it should be administered with caution to patients receiving other highly protein bound drugs.

Pregnancy: Pregnancy Category B. Reproduction studies have been performed in rats and rabbits. At doses up to 2.5 and 1.5 times the human **oral** dose, respectively, no evidence of impaired fertility or harm to the fetus due to verapamil was revealed. There are, however, no adequate and well-controlled studies in pregnant women. Because animal reproduction studies are not always predictive of human response, this drug should be used during pregnancy only if clearly needed.

Labor and Delivery: There have been few controlled studies to determine whether the use of verapamil during labor or delivery has immediate or delayed adverse effects on the fetus, or whether it prolongs the duration of labor or increases the need for forceps delivery or other obstetric intervention. Such adverse experiences have not been reported in the literature, despite a long history of use of intravenous ISOPTIN in Europe in the treatment of cardiac side effects of beta-adrenergic agonist agents used to treat premature labor.

Nursing Mothers: It is not known whether this drug is excreted in human milk. Because many drugs are excreted in human milk and because of the potential for adverse reactions in nursing infants from verapamil, nursing should be discontinued while verapamil is administered.

Pediatrics: Controlled studies with verapamil have not been conducted in pediatric patients, but uncontrolled experience with intravenous administration in more than 250 patients, about half under 12 months of age and about 25% newborn, indicates that results of treatment are similar to those in adults. The most commonly used single doses in patients up to 12 months of age have ranged from 0.1 to 0.2 mg/kg of body weight, while in patients aged 1 to 15 years, the most commonly used single doses ranged from 0.1 to 0.3 mg/kg of body weight. Most of the patients received the lower dose of 0.1 mg/kg once, but in some cases, the dose was repeated once or twice every 10 to 30 minutes.

Adverse Reactions: The following reactions were reported with intravenous ISOPTIN use in controlled U.S. clinical trials involving 324 patients:

Cardiovascular: Symptomatic hypotension (1.5%); bradycardia (1.2%); severe tachycardia (1.0%). The worldwide experience in open clinical trials in more than 7,900 patients was similar.

Central Nervous System Effects: Dizziness (1.2%); headache (1.2%).

Gastrointestinal: Nausea (0.9%); abdominal discomfort (0.6%).

The following reactions were reported in single patients: emotional depression, rotary nystagmus, sleepiness, vertigo, muscle fatigue or diaphoresis.

[See table above].

Overdosage: Treatment of overdosage should be supportive. Beta-adrenergic stimulation or parenteral administration of calcium solutions (calcium chloride) may increase calcium ion flux across the slow channel. These pharmacologic interventions have been effectively used in treatment of deliberate overdosage with oral verapamil. Clinically significant hypotensive reactions or high degree AV block should be treated with vasopressor agents or cardiac pacing, respectively. Asystole should be handled by the usual measures including isoproterenol hydrochloride, other vasopressor agents or cardiopulmonary resuscitation. (See Treatment of Cardiovascular Adverse Reactions)

Dosage and Administration (For Intravenous Use Only) ISOPTIN SHOULD BE GIVEN AS A SLOW INTRAVENOUS INJECTION OVER AT LEAST A TWO MINUTE PERIOD OF TIME.

The recommended intravenous doses of ISOPTIN are as follows:

ADULT: Initial dose: 5-10 mg (0.075—0.15 mg/kg body weight) given as an intravenous bolus over 2 minutes.

Repeat dose: 10 mg (0.15 mg/kg body weight) 30 minutes after the first dose if the initial response is not adequate.

Older Patients: The dose should be administered over at least 3 minutes to minimize the risk of untoward drug effects.

PEDIATRIC: Initial dose

0—1 year: 0.1—0.2 mg/kg body weight (usual single dose range: 0.75—2 mg) should be administered as an intravenous bolus over 2 minutes **under continuous ECG monitoring.**

1—15 years: 0.1—0.3 mg/kg body weight (usual single dose range: 2—5 mg) should be

Continued on next page

Knoll—Cont.

administered as an intravenous bolus over 2 minutes. **Do not exceed 5 mg.**

Repeat dose

0—1 year: 0.1—0.2 mg/kg body weight (usual single dose range: 0.75—2 mg) 30 minutes after the first dose if the initial response is not adequate **(under continuous ECG monitoring).**

1—15 years: 0.1—0.3 mg/kg body weight (usual single dose range: 2—5 mg) 30 minutes after the first dose if the initial response is not adequate. **Do not exceed 10 mg as a single dose.**

Note: Parenteral drug products should be inspected visually for particulate matter and discoloration prior to administration, whenever solution and container permit.

How Supplied: Each ISOPTIN 2 ml sterile ampule contains 5 mg verapamil HCl and 17 mg sodium chloride. pH is adjusted with hydrochloric acid.

5 mg/2 ml ampule—Individual unit carton —NDC 0044-1815-01

Space saver pack of 5 ampules—
NDC 0044-1815-05

Storage: 15°–30°C, 59°–86°F. Protect from light.

[*Shown in Product Identification Section*]

ISOPTIN® ℞

(verapamil hydrochloride)
Oral Tablets

Description: ISOPTIN (verapamil hydrochloride) is a calcium ion influx inhibitor (slow channel blocker or calcium ion antagonist). ISOPTIN is available for oral administration in sugar-coated tablets containing 80 mg or 120 mg verapamil hydrochloride.

The structural formula of verapamil HCl is given below:

[Structural formula: CH_3O, CH_3O – phenyl – C(CN)($CH(CH_3)_2$)$(CH_2)_3$ – N(CH_3)CH_2CH_2 – phenyl(OCH_3)(OCH_3) · HCl]

$C_{27}H_{38}N_2O_4 \cdot HCl$ M.W. = 491.08
Benzeneacetonitrile,
α-[3-[[2-(3,4-dimethoxyphenyl) ethyl] methylamino]
propyl]-3,4-dimethoxy-α-(1-methylethyl) hydrochloride

Verapamil HCl is an almost white, crystalline powder, practically free of odor, with a bitter taste. It is soluble in water, chloroform and methanol. Verapamil HCl is not chemically related to other cardioactive drugs.

Clinical Pharmacology: ISOPTIN is a calcium ion influx inhibitor (slow channel blocker or calcium ion antagonist) which exerts its pharmacologic effects by modulating the influx of ionic calcium across the cell membrane of the arterial smooth muscle as well as in conductile and contractile myocardial cells.

Mechanism of Action: The precise mechanism of action of ISOPTIN as an antianginal agent remains to be fully determined but includes the following mechanisms:

1. **Relaxation and prevention of coronary artery spasm**
   ISOPTIN dilates the main coronary arteries and coronary arterioles, both in normal and ischemic regions, and is a potent inhibitor of coronary artery spasm, whether spontaneous or ergonovine-induced. This property increases myocardial oxygen delivery in patients with coronary artery spasm, and is responsible for the effectiveness of ISOPTIN in vasospastic (Prinzmetal's or variant) as well as unstable angina at rest. Whether this effect plays any role in classical effort angina is not clear, but studies of exercise tolerance have not shown an increase in the maximum exercise rate-pressure product, a widely accepted measure of oxygen utilization. This suggests that, in general, relief of spasm or dilation of coronary arteries is not an important factor in classical angina.
2. **Reduction of oxygen utilization**
   ISOPTIN regularly reduces arterial pressure at rest and at a given level of exercise by dilating peripheral arterioles and reducing the total peripheral resistance (afterload) against which the heart works. This unloading of the heart reduces myocardial energy consumption and oxygen requirements and probably accounts for the effectiveness of ISOPTIN in chronic stable effort angina.

Electrical activity through the SA and AV nodes depends, to a significant degree, upon calcium influx through the slow channel. By inhibiting this influx, ISOPTIN slows AV conduction and prolongs the effective refractory period within the AV node in a rate-related manner. It can interfere with sinus node impulse generation and induce sinus arrest in patients with sick sinus syndrome and also can induce atrioventricular block, although this has been seen rarely in clinical use.

ISOPTIN may shorten the antegrade effective refractory period of accessory bypass tracts. ISOPTIN does not alter the normal atrial action potential or intraventricular conduction time, but depresses amplitude, velocity of depolarization and conduction in depressed atrial fibers.

ISOPTIN has a local anesthetic action that is 1.6 times that of procaine on an equimolar basis. It is not known whether this action is important at the doses used in man.

ISOPTIN does not alter total serum calcium levels.

Pharmacokinetics and Metabolism: More than 90% of the orally administered dose of ISOPTIN is absorbed. Because of rapid biotransformation of verapamil during its first pass through the portal circulation, absolute bioavailability ranges from 20% to 35%. Peak plasma concentrations are reached between 1 and 2 hours after oral administration. Chronic oral administration of 120 mg of ISOPTIN every 6 hours resulted in plasma levels of verapamil ranging from 125 to 400 ng/ml with higher values reported occasionally. A close relationship exists between verapamil plasma concentration and prolongation of the PR interval. The mean elimination half-life in single dose studies ranged from 2.8 to 7.4 hours. In these same studies, after repetitive dosing, the half-life increased to a range from 4.5 to 12.0 hours (after less than 10 consecutive doses given 6 hours apart). Half-life may increase during titration due to saturation of hepatic enzyme systems as plasma verapamil levels rise. A linear correlation between the verapamil dose administered and verapamil plasma levels seems to exist.

In healthy men, orally administered ISOPTIN undergoes extensive metabolism in the liver. Twelve metabolites have been identified in plasma; all except norverapamil are present in trace amounts only. Norverapamil can reach steady-state plasma concentrations approximately equal to those of verapamil itself. The major metabolites of verapamil have been identified as various N- and O-dealkylated products of ISOPTIN. Approximately 70% of an administered dose is excreted as metabolites in the urine and 16% or more in the feces within 5 days. About 3% to 4% is excreted in the urine as unchanged drug. Approximately 90% is bound to plasma proteins. In patients with hepatic insufficiency, metabolism is delayed and elimination half-life prolonged up to 14 to 16 hours (see Precautions); the volume of distribution is increased and plasma clearance reduced to about 30% of normal. Verapamil clearance values suggest that patients with liver dysfunction may attain therapeutic verapamil plasma concentrations with one-third of the oral daily dose required for patients with normal liver function.

Hemodynamics and Myocardial Metabolism: In animals and man, ISOPTIN reduces afterload and myocardial contractility. In most patients, including those with organic cardiac disease, the negative inotropic action of ISOPTIN is countered by reduction of afterload and cardiac index is usually not reduced. In patients with severe left ventricular dysfunction however, (e.g., pulmonary wedge pressure above 20 mm Hg or ejection fraction lower than 30%), or in patients on beta-adrenergic blocking agents or other cardiodepressant drugs, deterioration of ventricular function may occur (see Drug Interactions).

Pulmonary Function: ISOPTIN does not induce bronchoconstriction and hence, does not impair ventilatory function.

Indications and Usage: ISOPTIN is indicated for the treatment of angina pectoris including:

1. Angina at rest including:
   - Vasospastic (Prinzmetal's variant) angina
   - Unstable (crescendo, pre-infarction) angina
2. Chronic stable angina (classic effort-associated angina)

Contraindications: Verapamil HCl is contraindicted in:

1. Severe left ventricular dysfunction (see Warnings)
2. Hypotension (less than 90 mm Hg systolic pressure) or cardiogenic shock
3. Sick sinus syndrome (except in patients with a functioning artificial ventricular pacemaker)
4. Second- or third-degree AV block

Warnings

Heart Failure: Verapamil has a negative inotropic effect which, in most patients, is compensated by its afterload reduction (decreased peripheral vascular resistance) properties without a net impairment of ventricular performance. In clinical experience with 1166 patients, 11 (0.9%) developed congestive heart failure or pulmonary edema. Congestive heart failure/pulmonary edema led to discontinuation or reduction in dosage of verapamil in 6 (0.5%) patients. Verapamil should be avoided in patients with severe left ventricular dysfunction (e.g., ejection fraction less than 30% or moderate to severe symptoms of cardiac failure) and in patients with any degree of ventricular dysfunction if they are receiving a beta blocker (see Drug Interactions). Patients with milder ventricular dysfunction should, if possible, be controlled with optimum doses of digitalis and/or diuretics before verapamil treatment (**Note interactions with digoxin under: Precautions).**

Hypotension: Occasionally, the pharmacologic action of verapamil may produce a decrease in blood pressure below normal levels which may result in dizziness or symptomatic hypotension. Hypotension is usually asymptomatic, orthostatic, mild and can be controlled by a decrease in the ISOPTIN dose. The incidence of hypotension observed in 1166 patients enrolled in clinical trials was 2.9%.

Elevated Liver Enzymes: Occasional elevations of transaminases and alkaline phosphatase have been reported. Two patients had marked elevation of transaminase with recurrent elevation upon rechallenge with verapamil. Although these patients were not biopsied, the potential for hepatocellular-type injury with verapamil appears to exist. Worldwide experience has not revealed similar cases and the incidence of this injury is not known. Patients receiving verapamil should have liver enzymes monitored periodically.

Atrial Flutter/Fibrillation with Accessory Bypass Tract: Patients with atrial flutter or fibrillation and an accessory AV pathway (e.g., Wolff-Parkinson-White or Lown-Ganong-Levine syndromes) may develop increased antegrade conduction across the aberrant pathway bypassing the AV node, producing a very rapid ventricular response after receiving verapamil (or digitalis). Treatment is usually D.C.-cardioversion. Cardioversion has been used safely and effectively after oral ISOPTIN.

Atrioventricular Block: The effect of verapamil on AV conduction and the SA node leads to first-degree AV block and transient bradycardia, sometimes accompanied by nodal escape rhythms, fairly commonly during the peaks of serum concentration. Higher degrees of AV block, however, were infrequently (0.8%) observed. Marked first-degree block or progressive development to second- or third-degree AV block requires a reduction in dosage or, in rare instances, discontinuation of verapamil HCl and institution of appropriate therapy depending upon the clinical situation.

Patients with Hypertrophic Cardiomyopathy (IHSS): In 120 patients with hypertrophic cardiomyopathy (most of them refractory or intolerant to propranolol) who received therapy with verapamil at doses up to 720 mg/day, a variety of serious adverse effects were seen. Three patients died in pulmonary edema; all had severe left ventricular outflow obstruction and a past history of left ventricular dysfunction. Eight other patients had pulmonary edema and/or severe hypotension; abnormally high (over 20 mm Hg) capillary wedge pressure and a marked left ventricular outflow obstruction were present in most of these patients. Concomitant administration of quinidine preceded the severe hypotension in 3 of the 8 patients (2 of whom developed pulmonary edema). Sinus bradycardia occurred in 11% of the patients, second-degree AV block in 4% and sinus arrest in 2%. It must be appreciated that this group of patients had a serious disease with a high mortality rate. Most adverse effects responded well to dose reduction and only rarely did verapamil have to be discontinued.

Precautions

General:

Use in Patients with Impaired Hepatic Function: Since verapamil is highly metabolized by the liver, it should be administered cautiously to patients with impaired hepatic function. Severe liver dysfunction prolongs the elimination half-life of verapamil to about 14 to 16 hours; hence, approximately 30% of the dose given to patients with normal liver function should be administered to these patients. Careful monitoring for abnormal prolongation of the PR interval or other signs of excessive pharmacologic effects (See Overdosage) should be carried out.

Use in Patients with Impaired Renal Function: About 70% of an administered dose of verapamil is excreted as metabolites in the urine. Until further data are available, verapamil should be administered cautiously to patients with impaired renal function. These patients should be carefully monitored for abnormal prolongation of the PR interval or other signs of overdosage (see Overdosage).

Drug Interactions:

Beta Blockers: Controlled studies in small numbers of patients suggest that the concomitant use of ISOPTIN and beta-blocking agents may be beneficial in patients with chronic stable angina but available information is not sufficient to predict with confidence the effects of concurrent treatment, especially in patients with left ventricular dysfunction or cardiac conduction abnormalities.

The combination can have adverse effects on cardiac function. In one study of 15 patients treated with high doses of propranolol (median dose: 480 mg/day, range 160 to 1280 mg/day) for severe angina, with preserved left ventricular function (ejection fraction greater than 35%), the hemodynamic effects of additional therapy with ISOPTIN (verapamil HCl) were assessed using invasive methods. The addition of verapamil to high dose beta blockers induced modest negative inotropic and chronotropic effects which were not severe enough to limit short-term (48 hours) combination therapy in this study. These modest cardiodepressant effects persist for greater than 6, but less than 30 hours after abrupt withdrawal of beta blockers and were closely related to plasma levels of propranolol. The primary verapamil/beta-blocker interaction in this study appeared to be hemodynamic rather than electrophysiologic.

In three other studies involving 51 patients, verapamil did not induce negative inotropic or chronotropic effects in patients with preserved left ventricular function receiving low or moderate doses of propranolol (less than or equal to 320 mg/day). Because of the still limited experience with combination therapy verapamil should be used alone, if possible. If combined therapy is used, close surveillance of vital signs and clinical status should be carried out and the need for concomitant treatment with propranolol reassessed periodically. Combined therapy should usually be avoided in patients with atrioventricular conduction abnormalities and those with depressed left ventricular function.

Digitalis: Chronic verapamil treatment increases serum digoxin levels by 50% to 70% during the first week of therapy and this can result in digitalis toxicity. Maintenance digitalization doses should be reduced when verapamil is administered and the patient should be carefully monitored to avoid over- or underdigitalization. Whenever overdigitalization is suspected, the daily dose of digoxin should be reduced or temporarily discontinued. Upon discontinuation of ISOPTIN (verapamil HCl), the patient should be monitored to avoid underdigitalization.

Antihypertensive Agents: Verapamil administered concomitantly with oral antihypertensive agents (e.g., vasodilators, diuretics) may have an additive effect on lowering blood pressure. Patients receiving these combinations should be appropriately monitored. In patients who have recently received drugs such as methyldopa, which attenuate alpha-adrenergic response, combined therapy of verapamil and propranolol should probably be avoided (severe hypotension may occur).

Disopyramide: Until data on possible interactions between verapamil and disopyramide phosphate are obtained, disopyramide should not be administered within 48 hours before or 24 hours after verapamil administration.

Quinidine: In a small number of patients with hypertrophic cardiomyopathy (IHSS), concomitant use of verapamil and quinidine resulted in significant hypotension. Until further data are obtained, combined therapy of verapamil and quinidine in patients with hypertrophic cardiomyopathy should probably be avoided.

Nitrates: Verapamil has been given concomitantly with short- and long-acting nitrates without any undesirable drug interactions. The pharmacologic profile of both drugs and the clinical experience suggest beneficial interactions.

Carcinogenesis, Mutagenesis, Impairment of Fertility: Adequate animal carcinogenicity studies have not been performed with verapamil. An 18 month toxicity study in rats, at a low multiple (6 fold) of the maximum recommended human dose, and not the maximum tolerated dose, did not suggest a tumorigenic potential. A two year carcinogenicity study will be carried out in rats.

Verapamil was not mutagenic in the Ames test in 5 test strains at 3 mg per plate, with or without metabolic activation.

Studies in female rats at daily dietary doses up to 5.5 times (55 mg/kg/day) the maximum recommended human dose did not show impaired fertility. Effects on male fertility have not been determined.

Pregnancy: Pregnancy Category C. Reproduction studies have been performed in rabbits and rats at oral doses up to 1.5 (15 mg/kg/day) and 6 (60 mg/kg/day) times the human oral daily dose, respectively, and have revealed no evidence of teratogenicity. In the rat, however, this multiple of the human dose was embryocidal and retarded fetal growth and development, probably because of adverse maternal effects reflected in reduced weight gains of the dams. This oral dose has also been shown to cause hypotension in rats. There are no adequate and well-controlled studies in pregnant women. Because animal reproduction studies are not always predictive of human response, this drug should be used during pregnancy only if clearly needed.

Labor and Delivery: It is not known whether the use of verapamil during labor or delivery has immediate or delayed adverse effects on the fetus, or whether it prolongs the duration of labor or increases the need for forceps delivery or other obstetric intervention. Such adverse experiences have not been reported in the literature, despite a long history of use of ISOPTIN in Europe in the treatment of cardiac side effects of beta-adrenergic agonist agents used to treat premature labor.

Nursing Mothers: It is not known whether this drug is excreted in human milk. Because many drugs are excreted in human milk and because of the potential for adverse reactions in nursing infants from verapamil, nursing should be discontinued while verapamil is administered. Studies in rats at 2.5 times the maximum recommended human dose revealed no evidence of an effect of verapamil on lactation or weaning.

Animal Pharmacology and/or Animal Toxicology: Chronic animal toxicology studies indicate that verapamil causes lenticular and/or suture line changes at 30 mg/kg/day or greater and frank cataracts at 62.5 mg/kg/day or greater in the beagle dog but not the rat. These effects are thought to be species-specific. Development of cataracts due to verapamil has not been reported in man.

Adverse Reactions: Serious adverse reactions are rare when ISOPTIN therapy is initiated with upward dose titration within the recommended single and total daily dose. The following reactions to orally administered ISOPTIN were reported from clinical experience in 1166 patients with angina or arrhythmia. Adverse reactions occurred at a similar rate in controlled clinical trials and uncontrolled clinical experience.

Cardiovascular: Hypotension (2.9%), peripheral edema (1.7%), AV block (third-degree)(0.8%), bradycardia (HR <50/min, 1.1%), congestive heart failure or pulmonary edema (0.9%).

Central Nervous System: Dizziness (3.6%), headache (1.8%), fatigue (1.1%).

Gastrointestinal: Constipation (6.3%), nausea (1.6%).

The following reactions, reported in less than 0.5%, occurred under circumstances where a causal relationship is uncertain and are therefore mentioned to alert the physician to a possible relationship: confusion, paresthesia, insomnia, somnolence, equilibrium disorder, blurred vision, syncope, muscle cramp, shakiness, claudication, hair loss, macules, spotty menstruation. In addition, more serious adverse events were observed, not readily distinguishable from the natural history of the disease in these patients. Of the 1166 patients evaluated 16 (1.4%) had myocardial infarctions. Nine of these 16 patients had myocardial infarctions while being treated for unstable angina, 4 of these were receiving placebo, the remaining 5 received verapamil.

The daily dose of verapamil was reduced in 6.3% and discontinued in 5.5% of the 1166 patients. In general, the highest incidence of adverse reactions was seen in the dose titration periods in all the studies.

Continued on next page

Knoll—Cont.

Treatment of Acute Cardiovascular Adverse Reactions: The frequency of cardiovascular adverse reactions which require therapy is rare; hence, experience with their treatment is limited. Whenever severe hypotension or complete AV block occur following oral administration of verapamil, the appropriate emergency measures should be applied immediately, e.g., intravenously administered isoproterenol HCl, levarterenol bitartrate, atropine (all in the usual doses), or calcium chloride (13.5 millequivalents or 1 ampule) in 50 cc of 5% dextrose in water. In patients with hypertrophic cardiomyopathy (IHSS), alpha-adrenergic agents (phenylephrine, metaraminol bitartrate or methoxamine) should be used to maintain blood pressure and isoproterenol and levarterenol should be avoided. If further support is necessary, inotropic agents (dopamine or dobutamine) may be administered. Actual treatment and dosage should depend on the severity of the clinical situation and the judgment and experience of the treating physician.

Overdosage: Treatment of overdosage should be supportive. Beta-adrenergic stimulation or parenteral administration of calcium solutions (calcium chloride) may increase calcium ion flux across the slow channel, and have been used effectively in treatment of deliberate overdosage with verapamil. Clinically significant hypotensive reactions or fixed high degree AV block should be treated with vasopressor agents or cardiac pacing, respectively. Asystole should be handled by the usual measures including cardiopulmonary resuscitation.

Dosage and Administration: The dose of verapamil must be individualized by titration. ISOPTIN is available in 80 mg and 120 mg tablets. The usual initial dose is 80 mg three or four times a day. Dosage may be increased at daily (e.g., patients with unstable angina) or weekly intervals until optimum clinical response is obtained. In general, maximum effects of any given dosage would be apparent during the first 24 to 48 hours of therapy, but note that between 24 to 48 hours the half-life of verapamil increases, hence maximum response may be delayed. The total daily dose ranges from 240 to 480 mg. The optimum daily dose for most patients ranges from 320 to 480 mg. The usefulness and safety of dosages exceeding 480 mg per day in angina pectoris have not been established.

How Supplied: ISOPTIN tablets are supplied as sugar-coated, round tablets containing either 80 mg or 120 mg of verapamil hydrochloride and imprinted with "Knoll" on one side and "ISOPTIN 80" or "ISOPTIN 120" on the other side.

80 mg (yellow)—
- Bottle of 100—NDC #0044-1822-02
- Bottle of 500—NDC #0044-1822-05
- Hospital Unit Dose (100 tablets—Strips of 10)—NDC #0044-1822-10

120 mg (white)—
- Bottle of 100—NDC #0044-1823-02
- Bottle of 500—NDC #0044-1823-05
- Hospital Unit Dose (100 tablets—Strips of 10)—NDC #0044-1823-10

Storage: 15° to 30°C, 59° to 86°F.

Manufactured for
Knoll Pharmaceutical Company
Whippany, New Jersey 07981
by Knoll AG., Ludwigshafen/Rhine,
West Germany

[*Shown in Product Identification Section*]

QUADRINAL™ Tablets and Suspension ℞

Description: Each QUADRINAL™ Tablet contains ephedrine hydrochloride 24 mg; phenobarbital 24 mg [**Warning:** May be habit forming]; theophylline calcium salicylate 130 mg (equivalent to 65 mg anhydrous theophylline); potassium iodide 320 mg. Each 5 ml (1 teaspoonful) of the fruit-flavored Suspension is equivalent to ½ tablet.

QUADRINAL contains two bronchodilators, theophylline and ephedrine. Phenobarbital serves as a mild sedative to help counteract central nervous system stimulation which may be caused by ephedrine. Wheezing and coughing are relieved by improved bronchodilation while the expectorant action of potassium iodide helps to remove secretions from the bronchial tree. Dyspnea is thus relieved or prevented and acute episodes of bronchospasm are often eliminated with consequent lessening of apprehension and distress.

Clinical Pharmacology: Theophylline directly relaxes the smooth muscle of the bronchial airways and pulmonary blood vessels, thus acting mainly as a bronchodilator, pulmonary vasodilator and smooth muscle relaxant. It also possesses other actions typical of the xanthine derivatives: coronary vasodilator, diuretic, and cardiac, cerebral, and skeletal muscle stimulant. The actions of theophylline may be mediated through inhibition of phosphodiesterase and a resultant increase in intracellular cyclic AMP which could mediate smooth muscle relaxation.

In vitro, theophylline has been shown to react synergistically with beta agonists (such as isoproterenol) that increase intracellular cyclic AMP through the stimulation of adenyl cyclase, but synergism has not been demonstrated in clinical studies and more data are needed to determine if theophylline and beta agonists have clinically important additive effects **in vivo**.

Apparently, tolerance does not develop with chronic use of theophylline.

The half-life is shortened with cigarette smoking. The half-life is prolonged in alcoholism, reduced hepatic or renal function, congestive heart failure, and in patients receiving cimetidine or antibiotics such as troleandomycin (TAO, Cyclamycin), erythromycin, lincomycin and clindamycin. High fever for prolonged periods may decrease theophylline elimination.

Theophylline Elimination Characteristics

	Theophylline Clearance Rates (mean ± S.D.)	Half-life Average (mean ± S.D.)
Children (over 6 months of age)	1.45 ± 0.58 ml/kg/min	3.7 ± 1.1 hrs.
Adult non-smokers with uncomplicated asthma	0.65 ± 0.19 ml/kg/min	8.7 ± 2.2 hrs.

Newborn infants have extremely slow clearances with half-lives exceeding 24 hours. These approach those seen for older children after about 3–6 months.

Older adults with chronic obstructive pulmonary disease, patients with cor pulmonale or other causes of heart failure, and patients with liver pathology may have much lower clearances with half-lives that may exceed 24 hours.

The half-life is prolonged in alcoholism, reduced hepatic or renal function, congestive heart failure, and in patients receiving cimetidine or antibiotics such as troleandomycin (TAO, Cyclamycin), erythromycin, lincomycin and clindamycin. High fever for prolonged periods may decrease theophylline elimination.

The half-life of theophylline in smokers (1 to 2 packs/day) averaged 4 to 5 hours in various studies, much shorter than the 7 to 9 hour half-life in nonsmokers. The increase in theophylline clearance caused by smoking is probably the result of induction of drug-metabolizing enzymes that do not readily normalize after cessation of smoking. It appears that between 3 months and 2 years may be necessary for normalization of the effect of smoking on theophylline pharmacokinetics.

Indications: For chronic respiratory disease in which tenacious mucus and bronchospasm are dominant symptoms, such as bronchial asthma, chronic bronchitis and pulmonary emphysema.

Contraindications: Use of QUADRINAL is contraindicated in patients with enlarged thyroid or goiter or with known sensitivity to theophylline, potassium iodide, ephedrine or sympathomimetics, or barbiturates.

The iodide in QUADRINAL can cause fetal harm when administered to a pregnant woman. Development of goiter has been reported in infants whose mothers received iodide-containing medications during pregnancy. A few neonatal deaths resulting from tracheal obstruction due to congenital goiters have been reported. Use of barbiturates during pregnancy may cause physical dependence with resulting withdrawal symptoms in the neonate; may cause birth defects; may be associated with neonatal hemorrhage due to reduction in levels of vitamin K-dependent clotting factors in the neonate; may cause respiratory depression in the neonate.

QUADRINAL is contraindicated in women who are or may become pregnant. If this drug is used during pregnancy, or if the patient becomes pregnant while taking this drug, the patient should be apprised of the potential hazard to the fetus.

Warnings: Excessive theophylline doses may be associated with toxicity; determination of serum theophylline levels is recommended to assure maximal benefit without excessive risk. Incidence of toxicity increases at serum levels greater than 20 mcg/ml. Because of the theophylline content of QUADRINAL, it is unlikely that toxic levels of theophylline would be reached unless a serious overdosage occurs.

Morphine, curare, and stilbamidine should be used with caution in patients with airflow obstruction since they stimulate histamine release and can induce asthmatic attacks. They may also suppress respiration leading to respiratory failure. Alternative drugs should be chosen whenever possible.

There is an excellent correlation between clinical manifestations of toxicity and high blood levels of theophylline resulting from conventional doses in patients with lowered body plasma clearances (due to transient cardiac decompensation), patients with liver dysfunction or chronic obstructive lung disease, and patients who are older than 55 years of age, particularly males. In about 50% of patients, nausea and restlessness precede more severe manifestations of toxicity. In other patients, ventricular arrhythmias or seizures may be the first signs of toxicity. These more serious side effects are more likely to occur after intravenous administration of theophylline. Many patients who have high theophylline serum levels exhibit a tachycardia, and theophylline may worsen pre-existing arrhythmias.

Precautions: Mean half-life in smokers is shorter than in nonsmokers; therefore, smokers may require larger doses of theophylline. QUADRINAL, like all theophylline products, should not be administered concurrently with other xanthine medications. Use with caution in patients with severe cardiac disease, severe hypoxemia, hypertension, hyperthyroidism, acute myocardial injury, cor pulmonale, congestive heart failure, liver disease, peptic ulcer and in the elderly (especially males) and in neonates. Great caution should be used especially in giving theophylline to patients in congestive heart failure; such patients have shown markedly prolonged theophylline blood level curves with theophylline persisting in serum for long periods following discontinuation of the drug.

Theophylline may occasionally act as a local irritant to the G.I. tract although gastrointestinal symptoms are more commonly central in origin and associated with serum concentrations over 20 mcg/ml.

Ephedrine-containing medications should be used with caution in patients with cardiovascular disease, diabetes mellitus, predisposition to

glaucoma, hypertension, hyperthyroidism, or prostatic hypertrophy.
Potassium iodide may aggravate acne in adolescents and adults.
Phenobarbital should be used with caution in patients with a history of drug abuse or dependence, impaired renal or hepatic function, hyperkinesis, uncontrolled pain, or history of porphyria.
Usage in Pregnancy: Pregnancy Category X. See "Contraindications" section.
Nursing Mothers: Because of the potential for serious adverse reactions in nursing infants from the potassium iodide, ephedrine and phenobarbital in QUADRINAL, a decision should be made whether to discontinue nursing or to discontinue the drug, taking into account the importance of the drug to the mother.
Pediatric Use: QUADRINAL is indicated for use in children on a short term basis. Chronic use should be reserved for patients in whom other expectorants have not been effective. If QUADRINAL is used chronically in children, the patient should be observed for signs of thyroid enlargement and worsening of acne.
Geriatric Patients: Geriatric patients may be more sensitive to the effects of ephedrine.
Adverse Reactions: The most frequent adverse reactions to theophylline are usually due to overdose (serum levels in excess of 20 mcg/ml) and are: nausea, vomiting, epigastric pain, hematemesis, diarrhea, headaches, irritability, restlessness, insomnia, reflex hyperexcitability, muscle twitching, clonic and tonic generalized convulsions, palpitations, tachycardia, extra systoles, flushing, hypotension, circulatory failure, ventricular arrhythmias, tachypnea, albuminuria, increased excretion of renal tubular cells and red blood cells, potentiation of diuresis, hyperglycemia and inappropriate ADH syndrome.
Thyroid adenoma, goiter and myxedema are possible side effects of potassium iodide.
Hypersensitivity to iodides may be manifested by angio-neurotic edema, cutaneous and mucosal hemorrhages, and symptoms resembling serum sickness, such as fever, arthralgia, lymph node enlargement and eosinophilia.
Chronic ingestion of iodides may result in chronic iodide poisoning, or iodism. Initial symptoms include an unpleasant brassy taste, burning in the mouth and throat, soreness of the teeth and gums, increased salivation, coryza, sneezing, irritation of the eyes with swelling of the eyelids, headache, cough, skin lesions, diarrhea, gastric irritation, anorexia, fever and depression. The symptoms of iodism disappear spontaneously within a few days after stopping the administration of iodide. Therefore, treatment consists of stopping QUADRINAL therapy and providing supportive measures as indicated by the symptoms. Abundant fluid and sodium chloride intake may hasten iodide elimination. In severe cases, the use of mannitol to establish an osmotic diuresis may be appropriate. Potassium iodide may produce hyperkalemia and, if ingested chronically, may lead to goiter.
Adverse reactions to ephedrine include nervousness, restlessness, trouble in sleeping, irregular heartbeat, difficult or painful urination, dizziness or light-headedness, headache, loss of appetite, nausea or vomiting, trembling, troubled breathing, unusual increase in sweating, unusual paleness, feeling of warmth, and weakness. Tolerance to ephedrine may develop with prolonged or excessive use.
Adverse reactions to phenobarbital include mental confusion or depression, shortness of breath or troubled breathing, skin rash, hives, swelling of eyelids, face or lips, wheezing or tightness in chest, sore throat and fever, unusual bleeding or bruising, unusual excitement, tiredness or weakness, unusually slow heartbeat, yellowing of eyes or skin.
Drug Interactions: Toxic synergism of theophylline with ephedrine has been documented and may occur with some other sympathomimetic bronchodilators.
[See table below].

Drug	Effect
Aminophylline with lithium carbonate	Increased excretion of lithium carbonate
Potassium iodide with lithium	Increased hypothyroid and goiterogenic effects
Aminophylline with propranolol	Antagonism of propranolol effect
Theophylline with furosemide	Increased diuresis
Theophylline with hexamethonium	Decreased hexamethonium-induced chronotropic effect
Theophylline with reserpine	Reserpine-induced tachycardia
Theophylline with chlordiazepoxide	Chlordiazepoxide-induced fatty acid mobilization
Theophylline with troleandomycin (TAO, Cyclamycin), erythromycin, lincomycin, clindamycin	Increased theophylline plasma levels
Theophylline with phenytoin	Decreased phenytoin levels
Theophylline with cimetidine	Increased theophylline blood levels
Ephedrine with digitalis glycosides or anesthetics	May cause cardiac arrhythmias
Ephedrine with ergonovine, methylergonovine or oxytocin	Hypertension
Ephedrine with guanethidine	Decreased hypotensive effect
Ephedrine with MAO inhibitors	Potentiation of pressor effect of ephedrine
Ephedrine with reserpine	Decreased pressor effect of ephedrine
Ephedrine with other sympathomimetics	Increased effects of either medication
Ephedrine with tricyclic antidepressants	May antagonize the pressor action of ephedrine
Phenobarbital with alcohol, general anesthetics, other CNS depressants, or MAO inhibitors	Increased effects of either medication
Phenobarbital with oral anticoagulants	Decreased anticoagulant effects
Phenobarbital with corticosteroids, digitalis, digitoxin, doxycycline, tricyclic antidepressants, griseofulvin or phenytoin	Decreased effects of these drugs

Overdosage:
A. If potential overdose is established and seizure has not occurred and patient is conscious:
1) Induce vomiting.
2) Administer a cathartic.
3) Administer activated charcoal.
B. If patient is having a seizure:
1) Establish an airway.
2) Administer oxygen.
3) Treat the seizure with intravenous diazepam, 0.1 to 0.3 mg/kg up to 10 mg.
4) Monitor vital signs, maintain blood pressure and provide adequate hydration.
C. Post-seizure coma:
1) Maintain airway and oxygenation.
2) Following above recommendations to prevent absorption of drug, but intubation and lavage will have to be performed instead of inducing emesis, and introduce the cathartic and charcoal via a large bore gastric lavage tube.
3) Continue to provide full supportive care and adequate hydration while waiting for drug to be metabolized. In general, the drug is metabolized sufficiently rapidly so as not to require dialysis.

Dosage and Administration: When rapidly absorbed products such as solutions and uncoated tablets with rapid dissolution are used, dosing to maintain "around the clock" blood levels generally requires administration every 6 hours in children; dosing intervals up to 8 hours may be satisfactory for adults because of their slower elimination rate.
Pulmonary function measurements before and after a period of treatment permit an objective assessment of response to QUADRINAL.
Usual dose:
Adults—One tablet or two teaspoonfuls (10 ml) of the Suspension 3 or 4 times daily; if needed, an additional one tablet or two teaspoonfuls upon retiring for nighttime relief. In severe attacks, the usual dose may be increased by one half.
Children 6 to 12 years—one half tablet, or one teaspoonful (5 ml) of the Suspension three times daily.
Children under 6 years—dose is proportionately less.
How Supplied: QUADRINAL Tablets—white, round, bi-convex tablets, engraved with a triangle on one side, bisected on the other side and imprinted with the number "14".
Bottles of 100—NDC #0044-4520-02.
Bottles of 1000—NDC #0044-4520-04.
QUADRINAL Suspension—Reddish-pink in color, fruit-like flavor.
Bottles of 1 pint (473 ml)—NDC #0044-4580-01.
Storage: Store at 59°–86°F, 15°–30°C.
[*Shown in Product Identification Section*]

SANTYL® Ointment ℞
(collagenase)

Description: SANTYL® OINTMENT is a sterile enzymatic debriding ointment which contains 250 collagenase units per gram of white petrolatum USP. The enzyme collagenase is derived from the fermentation by *Clostridium histolyticum.* It possesses the unique ability to digest native and denatured collagen in necrotic tissue.
Clinical Pharmacology: Since collagen accounts for 75% of the dry weight of skin tissue, the ability of collagenase to digest collagen in the physiological pH range and temperature makes it particularly effective in the removal of detritus.[1] Collagenase thus contributes towards the formation of granulation tissue and subsequent epithelization of dermal ulcers and severely burned areas.[2,3,4,5,6] Collagen in healthy tissue or in newly formed granulation tissue is not attacked.[2,3,4,5,6,7,8]

Continued on next page

Knoll—Cont.

Indications: Santyl Ointment is indicated for debriding chronic dermal ulcers[2,3,4,5,6,8,9,10,11,12,13,14,15,16,17,18] and severely burned areas.[3,4,5,7,16,19,20,21]

Contraindications: Santyl Ointment is contraindicated in patients who have shown local or systemic hypersensitivity to collagenase.

Precautions: The optimal pH range of collagenase is 6 to 8. Higher or lower pH conditions will decrease the enzyme's activity and appropriate precautions should be taken. The enzymatic activity is also adversely affected by detergents, hexachlorophene and heavy metal ions such as mercury and silver which are used in some antiseptics. When it is suspected such materials have been used, the site should be carefully cleansed by repeated washings with normal saline before Santyl Ointment is applied. Soaks containing metal ions or acidic solutions such as Burow's solution should be avoided because of the metal ion and low pH. Cleansing materials such as hydrogen peroxide, Dakin's solution, and sterile saline are compatible with Santyl Ointment.

Debilitated patients should be closely monitored for systemic bacterial infections because of the theoretical possibility that debriding enzymes may increase the risk of bacteremia.

A slight transient erythema has been noted occasionally in the surrounding tissue, particularly when Santyl Ointment was not confined to the lesion. Therefore, the ointment should be applied carefully within the area of the lesion.

Adverse Reactions: No allergic sensitivity or toxic reactions have been noted in the recorded clinical investigations. However, one case of systemic manifestations of hypersensitivity to collagenase in a patient treated for more than one year with a combination of collagenase and cortisone has been reported to us.

Overdosage: Action of the enzyme may be stopped, should this be desired, by the application of Burow's solution USP (pH 3.6–4.4) to the lesion.

Dosage and Administration: Santyl Ointment should be applied once daily (or more frequently if the dressing becomes soiled, as from incontinence) in the following manner:

(1) Prior to application the lesion should be cleansed of debris and digested material by gently rubbing with a gauze pad saturated with hydrogen peroxide or Dakin's solution followed by sterile normal saline.

(2) Whenever infection is present it is desirable to use an appropriate topical antibacterial agent. Neomycin-Bacitracin-Polymyxin B (Neosporin) powder has been found to be compatible with Santyl Ointment. The antibiotic should be applied to the lesion prior to the application of Santyl Ointment. Should the infection not respond, therapy with Santyl Ointment should be discontinued until remission of the infection.

(3) Santyl Ointment should be applied directly to deep lesions with a wooden tongue depressor or spatula. For shallow lesions, Santyl Ointment may be applied to a sterile gauze pad which is then applied to the wound and properly secured.

(4) Crosshatching thick eschar with a #10 blade allows collagenase more surface contact with necrotic debris. It is also desirable to remove, with forceps and scissors, as much loosened detritus as can be done readily.

(5) All excess ointment should be removed each time dressing is changed.

(6) Use of Santyl Ointment should be terminated when debridement of necrotic tissue is complete and granulation tissue is well established.

How Supplied: Santyl Ointment contains 250 units of collagenase enzyme per gram of white petrolatum USP. The potency assay of collagenase is based on the digestion of undenatured collagen (from bovine Achilles tendon) at pH 7.2 and 37°C for 24 hours. The number of peptide bonds cleaved are measured by reaction with ninhydrin. Amino groups released by a trypsin digestion control are subtracted. One net collagenase unit will solubilize ninhydrin reactive material equivalent to 4 micromoles of leucine.

References:

1— Mandl, I., Adv. Enzymol. 23:163, 1961.
2— Boxer, A.M., Gottesman, N., Bernstein, H., & Mandl, I., Geriatrics 24:75, 1969.
3— Mazurek, I., Med. Welt 22:150, 1971.
4— Zimmerman, W.E., in "Collagenase," I. Mandl, ed., Gordon & Breach, Science Publishers, New York, 1971, p. 131, p. 185.
5— Vetra, H., & Whittaker, D., Geriatrics 30:53, 1975.
6— Rao, D.B., Sane, P.G., & Georgiev, E.L., J. Am. Geriatrics Soc. 23:22, 1975.
7— Vrabec, R., Moserova, J., Kõnickova, Z., Behounkova, E., & Blaha, J., J. Hyg. Epidemiol. Microbiol. Immunol. 18:496, 1974.
8— Lippmann, H.I., Arch. Phys. Med. Rehabil. 54:588, 1973.
9— German, F.M., in "Collagenase," I., Mandl, ed. Gordon & Breach, Science Publishers, New York, 1971, p. 165.
10— Haimovici, H. & Strauch, B., in "Collagenase," I. Mandl, ed., Gordon & Breach, Science Publishers, New York, 1971, p. 177.
11— Lee, L.K., & Ambrus, J.L., Geriatrics 30:91, 1975.
12— Locke, R.K., & Heifitz, N.M., J. Am. Pod. Assoc. 65:242, 1975.
13— Varma, A.O., Bugatch, E., & German, F.M., Surg. Gynecol. Obstet. 136:281, 1973.
14— Barrett, D., Jr., & Klibanski, A., Am. J. Nurs. 73:849, 1973.
15— Bardfeld, L.A., J. Pod. Ed. 1:41, 1970.
16— Blum, G., Schweiz. Rundschau Med. Praxis 62:820, 1973. Abstr. in Dermatology Digest, Feb. 1974, p. 36.
17— Zaruba, F., Lettl, A., Brozkova, L., Skrdlantova, H., & Krs, V., J. Hyg. Epidemiol. Microbiol. Immunol. 18:499, 1974.
18— Altman, M.I., Goldstein, L., Horowitz, S., J. Am. Pod. Assoc. 68:11, 1978.
19— Rehn, V.J., Med. Klin. 58:799, 1963.
20— Krauss, H., Koslowski, L., & Zimmermann, W.E., Langenbecks Arch. Klin. Chir. 303:23, 1963.
21— Gruenagel, H.H., Med. Klin. 58:442, 1963.

[*Shown in Product Identification Section*]

VICODIN® TABLETS Ⓒ ℞

Description: Each VICODIN® tablet contains:

hydrocodone bitartrate .... 5 mg
(**WARNING**: may be habit forming.)
acetaminophen .... 500 mg

Hydrocodone bitartrate is an opioid analgesic and antitussive and occurs as fine, white crystals or as a crystalline powder. It is affected by light. The structural formula of hydrocodone bitartrate is:

Acetaminophen is a nonopiate, nonsalicylate analgesic and antipyretic which occurs as a white, odorless, crystalline powder possessing a slightly bitter taste. It may be represented by the following structural formula:

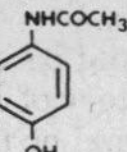

Clinical Pharmacology: Hydrocodone is a semisynthetic narcotic analgesic and antitussive with multiple actions qualitatively similar to those of codeine. Most of these involve the central nervous system and smooth muscle. The precise mechanism of action of hydrocodone and other opiates is not known, although it is believed to relate to the existence of opiate receptors in the central nervous system. In addition to analgesia, narcotics may produce drowsiness, changes in mood and mental clouding.

Radioimmunoassay techniques have recently been developed for the analysis of hydrocodone in human plasma. After a 10 mg oral dose of hydrocodone bitartrate, a mean peak serum drug level of 23.6 ng/ml and an elimination half-life of 3.8 hours were found.

The analgesic action of acetaminophen involves peripheral and central influences, but the specific mechanism is as yet undetermined. Antipyretic activity is mediated through hypothalamic heat regulating centers. Acetaminophen inhibits prostaglandin synthetase. Therapeutic doses of acetaminophen have negligible effects on the cardiovascular or respiratory systems; however, toxic doses may cause circulatory failure and rapid, shallow breathing.

Acetaminophen is rapidly and almost completely absorbed from the gastrointestinal tract, producing maximum serum concentrations within 30 minutes to one hour. The plasma half-life in adults and children ranges from 0.90 hours to 3.25 hours with an average of approximately 2 hours. The drug distributes uniformly in most body fluids and is approximately 25% protein bound. Acetaminophen is conjugated in the liver, with less than 3% of the dose excreted unchanged in 24 hours. The primary metabolic pathway is conjugation to sulfate and glucuronide by-products. A minor oxidative pathway forms cysteine and mercapturic acid. These compounds are subsequently excreted by the kidneys into the urine.

Indications and Usage: For the relief of moderate to moderately severe pain.

Contraindications: Hypersensitivity to acetaminophen or hydrocodone.

Warnings

Respiratory Depression: At high doses or in sensitive patients, hydrocodone may produce dose-related respiratory depression by acting directly on brain stem respiratory centers. Hydrocodone also affects centers that control respiratory rhythm, and may produce irregular and periodic breathing. If significant respiratory depression occurs, it may be antagonized by the use of naloxone hydrochloride, 0.005 mg/kg intravenously. Since the duration of action of hydrocodone may exceed that of the antagonist, the patient should be kept under continued surveillance and repeated doses of the antagonist should be administered as needed to maintain adequate respiration. Apply other supportive measures when indicated.

Head Injury and Increased Intracranial Pressure: The respiratory depressant effects of narcotics and their capacity to elevate cerebrospinal fluid pressure may be markedly exaggerated in the presence of head injury, other intracranial lesions or a preexisting increase in intracranial pressure. Furthermore, narcotics produce adverse reactions which may obscure the clinical course of patients with head injuries.

Acute Abdominal Conditions: The administration of narcotics may obscure the diagnosis or clinical course of patients with acute abdominal conditions.

Precautions

Special Risk Patients: As with any narcotic analgesic agent, VICODIN should be used with caution in elderly or debilitated patients and those with severe impairment of hepatic or renal function, hypothyroidism, Addison's disease, prostatic hypertrophy or urethral stricture. The usual precautions should be observed and the possibility of respiratory depression should be kept in mind.

Information for Patients: VICODIN, like all narcotics, may impair the mental and/or physical abilities required for the performance of potentially hazardous tasks such as driving a car or operating machinery; patients should be cautioned accordingly.

Cough Reflex: Hydrocodone suppresses the cough reflex; as with all narcotics, caution should be exercised when VICODIN is used postoperatively and in patients with pulmonary disease.

Drug Interactions: Patients receiving other narcotic analgesics, antipsychotics, antianxiety agents, or other CNS depressants (including alcohol) concomitantly with VICODIN may exhibit an additive CNS depression. When combined therapy is contemplated, the dose of one or both agents should be reduced.

The use of MAO inhibitors or tricyclic antidepressants with hydrocodone preparations may increase the effect of either the antidepressant or hydrocodone.

The concurrent use of anticholinergics with hydrocodone may produce paralytic ileus.

Usage in Pregnancy: Pregnancy Category C. Hydrocodone has been shown to be teratogenic in hamsters when given in doses 700 times the human dose. There are no adequate and well-controlled studies in pregnant women. VICODIN should be used during pregnancy only if the potential benefit justifies the potential risk to the fetus.

Nonteratogenic effects: Babies born to mothers who have been taking opioids regularly prior to delivery will be physically dependent. The withdrawal signs include irritability and excessive crying, tremors, hyperactive reflexes, increased respiratory rate, increased stools, sneezing, yawning, vomiting, and fever. The intensity of the syndrome does not always correlate with the duration of maternal opioid use or dose. There is no consensus on the best method of managing withdrawal. Chlorpromazine 0.7 to 1.0 mg/kg q6h, and paregoric 2 to 4 drops/kg q4h, have been used to treat withdrawal symptoms in infants. The duration of therapy is 4 to 28 days, with the dosage decreased as tolerated.

Labor and Delivery: As with all narcotics, administration of VIDODIN to the mother shortly before delivery may result in some degree of respiratory depression in the newborn, especially if higher doses are used.

Nursing Mothers: It is not known whether this drug is excreted in human milk. Because many drugs are excreted in human milk and because of the potential for serious adverse reactions in nursing infants from VICODIN, a decision should be made whether to discontinue nursing or to discontinue the drug, taking into account the importance of the drug to the mother.

Pediatric Use: Safety and effectiveness in children have not been established.

Adverse Reactions

Central Nervous System: Sedation, drowsiness, mental clouding, lethargy, impairment of mental and physical performance, anxiety, fear, dysphoria, dizziness, psychic dependence, mood changes.

Gastrointestinal System: Nausea and vomiting may occur; they are more frequent in ambulatory than in recumbent patients. The antiemetic phenothiazines are useful in suppressing these effects; however, some phenothiazine derivatives seem to be antianalgesic and to increase the amount of narcotic required to produce pain relief, while other phenothiazines reduce the amount of narcotic required to produce a given level of analgesia. Prolonged administration of VICODIN may produce constipation.

Genitourinary System: Ureteral spasm, spasm of vesical sphincters and urinary retention have been reported.

Respiratory Depression: VICODIN may produce dose-related respiratory depression by acting directly on brain stem respiratory centers. Hydrocodone also affects centers that control respiratory rhythm, and may produce irregular and periodic breathing. If significant respiratory depression occurs, it may be antagonized by the use of naloxone hydrochloride, 0.005 mg/kg intravenously. Since the duration of action of hydrocodone may exceed that of the antagonist, the patient should be kept under continued surveillance and repeated doses of the antagonist should be administered as needed to maintain adequate respiration. Apply other supportive measures when indicated.

Drug Abuse and Dependence: VICODIN is subject to the Federal Controlled Substance Act (Schedule Ⓒ).

Psychic dependence, physical dependence, and tolerance may develop upon repeated administration of narcotics; therefore, VICODIN should be prescribed and administered with caution. However, psychic dependence is unlikely to develop when VICODIN is used for a short time for the treatment of pain. Physical dependence, the condition in which continued administration of the drug is required to prevent the appearance of a withdrawal syndrome, assumes clinically significant proportions only after several weeks of continued narcotic use, although some mild degree of physical dependence may develop after a few days of narcotic therapy. Tolerance, in which increasingly large doses are required in order to produce the same degree of analgesia, is manifested initially by a shortened duration of analgesic effect, and subsequently by decreases in the intensity of analgesia. The rate of development of tolerance varies among patients.

Overdosage

Hydrocodone

Signs and Symptoms: Serious overdose with hydrocodone is characterized by respiratory depression (a decrease in respiratory rate and /or tidal volume, Cheyne-Stokes respiration, cyanosis), extreme somnolence progressing to stupor or coma, skeletal muscle flaccidity, cold and clammy skin, and sometimes bradycardia and hypotension. In severe overdosage, apnea, circulatory collapse, cardiac arrest and death may occur.

Treatment: Primary attention should be given to the reestablishment of adequate respiratory exchange through provision of a patent airway and the institution of assisted or controlled ventilation. The narcotic antagonist naloxone is a specific antidote against respiratory depression which may result from overdosage or unusual sensitivity to narcotics, including hydrocodone. Therefore, 0.005 mg/kg of naloxone should be administered, preferably by the intravenous route, and simultaneously with efforts at respiratory resuscitation. Since the duration of action of hydrocodone may exceed that of the antagonist, the patient should be kept under continued surveillance and repeated doses of the antagonist should be administered as needed to maintain adequate respiration.

An antagonist should not be administered in the absence of clinically significant respiratory or cardiovascular depression. Oxygen, intravenous fluids, vasopressors and other supportive measures should be employed as indicated.

Gastric emptying may be useful in removing unabsorbed drug.

Acetaminophen

Signs and Symptoms: Acetaminophen in massive overdosage may cause hepatic toxicity in some patients. In all cases of suspected overdose, immediately call your Regional Poison Center or the Rocky Mountain Poison Center's toll free number (800/525-6115) for assistance in diagnosis and for directions in the use of N-acetylcysteine as an antidote, a use currently restricted to investigational status.

In adults, hepatic toxicity has rarely been reported with acute overdoses of less than 10 grams and fatalities with less than 15 grams. Importantly, young children seem to be more resistant than adults to the hepatotoxic effect of an acetaminophen overdose. Despite this, the measures outlined below should be initiated in any adult or child suspected of having ingested an acetaminophen overdose.

Early symptoms following a potentially hepatotoxic overdose may include: nausea, vomiting, diaphoresis and general malaise. Clinical and laboratory evidence of hepatic toxicity may not be apparent until 48 to 72 hours post-ingestion.

Treatment: The stomach should be emptied promptly by lavage or by induction of emesis with syrup of ipecac. Patients' estimates of the quantity of a drug ingested are notoriously unreliable. Therefore, if an acetaminophen overdose is suspected, a serum acetaminophen assay should be obtained as early as possible, but no sooner than four hours following ingestion. Liver function studies should be obtained initially and repeated at 24-hour intervals.

The antidote, N-acetylcysteine, should be administered as early as possible, and within 16 hours of the overdose ingestion for optimal results. Following recovery, there are no residual, structural or functional hepatic abnormalities.

Dosage and Administration: Dosage should be adjusted according to the severity of the pain and the response of the patient. However, tolerance to hydrocodone can develop with continued use and the incidence of untoward effects is dose related.

The usual dose is one tablet every six hours as needed for pain. If necessary, this dose may be repeated at four hour intervals. In cases of more severe pain, two tablets every six hours (up to 8 tablets in 24 hours) may be required.

How Supplied: White, flat, capsule shaped, bisected tablets inscribed with a double K logo on one side and the number "24" on the other side.

Bottles of 100—NDC #0044-0727-02.

Hospital Unit Dose Package—100 tablets (4×25 tablets)—NDC #0044-0727-41.

Storage: VICODIN should be stored at 59°–86°F, 15°–30°C.

A Schedule Ⓒ Narcotic.

[*Shown in Product Identification Section*]

Kremers-Urban Company

BOX 2038
MILWAUKEE, WI 53201

CALCIFEROL™ ℞
(Ergocalciferol, Vitamin D_2)
50,000 USP Unit Tablets
500,000 USP Units/cc in Oil
8,000 USP Units/cc in Propylene Glycol

Description: CALCIFEROL™, also known as ergocalciferol or Vitamin D_2 is a Vitamin D analog. It occurs as white crystals and is insoluble in water and soluble in alcohol and in fatty oils. CALCIFEROL Tablets contain 1.25 mg (50,000 USP units) of Ergocalciferol (Vitamin D_2). CALCIFEROL In Oil Injection is a sterile solution of Vitamin D_2 in sesame oil for intramuscular use only. Each c.c. of CALCIFEROL In Oil contains 500,000 U.S.P. units of Ergocalciferol. CALCIFEROL Drops, oral solution, contains 8,000 units of Vitamin D_2 in Propylene Glycol.

Pharmacology: CALCIFEROL in its activated form (1,25-dihydroxy ergocalciferol)

Continued on next page

Kremers-Urban—Cont.

along with parathyroid hormone and calcitonin, regulates calcium metabolism. Vitamin D deficiency leads to rickets in children and osteomalacia in adults. The administration of Vitamin D completely reverses the symptoms of nutritional rickets or osteomalacia unless permanent deformities have already occurred. In humans, activated CALCIFEROL functions primarily to increase intestinal absorption of calcium and phosphorus. It is also required for normal mineralization of bone and stimulates resorption of bone matrix.
CALCIFEROL is readily absorbed from the gastrointestinal tract if fat absorption is normal. The presence of bile is necessary for absorption of Vitamin D and its analogs. In patients with hepatic, biliary, or GI disease, the absorption of Vitamin D may decrease. Once absorbed, ergocalciferol appears in chylomicrons of lymph and then associates primarily with a specific alphaglobulin and with albumin. The plasma half-life of ergocalciferol is approximately 24 hours. Ergocalciferol is stored in the liver, fat, and muscle for prolonged periods.
Indications and Uses: CALCIFEROL is indicated for use in the treatment of hypoparathyroidism and refractory rickets. CALCIFEROL is used to increase serum calcium concentration to prevent or treat rickets or osteomalacia. Patients with gastrointestinal, liver or biliary disease associated with malabsorption of Vitamin D require intramuscular administration of Vitamin D.
Contraindications: CALCIFEROL should not be given to patients with hypercalcemia or evidence of Vitamin D toxicity.
Warning: Overdosage of any form of Vitamin D is dangerous. Progressive hypercalcemia due to overdosage of Vitamin D and its metabolites may be so severe as to require emergency attention. Chronic hypercalcemia can lead to generalized vascular calcification, nephrocalcinosis and other soft tissue calcification. Radiographic evaluation of suspect anatomical regions may be useful in the early detection of this condition.
Precautions: Treatment of patients with coronary disease, impaired renal function, and arteriosclerosis, especially in the elderly, should be cautious.
Large doses of Vitamin D are potentially dangerous; therefore, early in treatment or during dosage adjustment, serum calcium should be determined twice weekly. Similarly, phosphate, magnesium, and alkaline phosphatase and 24 hour urinary calcium and phosphate should be determined periodically. A fall in serum alkaline phosphatase levels usually precedes the appearance of hypercalcemia and may be an indication of impending hypercalcemia. Should hypercalcemia develop, the drug should be discontinued immediately.
Adverse Reactions: Excessive Vitamin D intake can produce vitamin toxicity. The early and late signs and symptoms of Vitamin D intoxication associated with hypercalcemia may include weakness and headache, vomiting, muscle pain, bone pain, anorexia, weight loss, hypertension, and cardiac arrhythmias.
Overdosage: Use of CALCIFEROL in excessive quantities in patients can cause hypercalcemia, hypercalciuria and hyperphosphatemia. High intake of calcium and phosphate concomitant with CALCIFEROL can lead to similar abnormalities.
Treatment of Vitamin D intoxication consists of withdrawal of the drug and calcium supplements, administration of low-calcium diet, oral or parenteral fluids, and if needed, glucocorticoids or other drugs to decrease serum calcium levels. When serum calcium levels have returned to within normal limits, CALCIFEROL therapy may be reinstituted at a dose lower than prior therapy. Serum calcium levels should be determined at least twice weekly after all dosage changes and subsequent dosage titration. Persistent or markedly elevated serum calcium levels may be corrected by dialysis against a calcium free dialysate.
Dosage and Administration: The optimal daily dose of CALCIFEROL must be carefully determined for each patient. Patients with refractory rickets may need 50,000 to 500,000 units per day. After oral therapy with CALCIFEROL is instituted, normal serum calcium and phosphate levels may be observed within 2 weeks. Roentgenographic evidence of healing of bone may be seen within 4 weeks after administration of a fixed maintenance dose. During therapy with CALCIFEROL, the dosage must be individualized and carefully adjusted to avoid hypercalcemia. Determinations of serum calcium, phosphate, alkaline phosphatase, total protein, creatine and BUN should be made every two weeks or more frequently as needed. Until the condition stabilizes, monthly radiographic evaluation is helpful. In treatment of hypoparathyroidism, 50,000 to 400,000 units per day are recommended. In recommending CALCIFEROL, it is assumed that each patient is receiving an adequate daily intake of calcium. The recommended daily allowance for calcium in adults is 1 gram.
How Supplied: 50,000 unit tablets, bottles of 100 (NDC 0091-3150-01).
CALCIFEROL in Oil Injection is supplied in 1cc ampuls containing 500,000 units per cc in oil. Packaged in boxes of 5 (NDC 0091-1150-05).
CALCIFEROL Drops, oral solution, contains 8,000 units/ml in 60 ml bottle (NDC 0091-4150-60).
[*Shown in Product Identification Section*]

KUDROX® SUSPENSION (DOUBLE STRENGTH) ANTACID — OTC

Composition: A pleasantly flavored SUSPENSION containing a concentrated combination of aluminum hydroxide gel and magnesium hydroxide in d-sorbitol.
One teaspoonful of KUDROX Liquid contains not more than 0.65 mEq (15 mg.) of sodium.
Action and Uses: A palatable antacid to alleviate acid indigestion, heartburn and/or sour stomach, or whenever antacid therapy is the treatment indicated for symptomatic relief of hyperacidity associated with the diagnosis of peptic ulcer, gastritis, peptic esophagitis, gastric hyperacidity, and hiatal hernia. The ratio of aluminum hydroxide to magnesium hydroxide is such that undesirable bowel effects are minimal. Each 5cc dose of SUSPENSION will neutralize approximately 25 mEq of HCl. High concentration of the active ingredients produces prompt, long lasting neutralization without the acid rebound associated with calcium carbonate containing antacids.
Dosage: KUDROX SUSPENSION, half that ordinarily employed with other liquid antacids. Usual dose only 1 teaspoonful 30 minutes after meals and at bedtime. May be taken undiluted or mixed with water or milk. In peptic ulcer, 2 to 4 teaspoonfuls after meals and at bedtime.
Warning: Antacids containing magnesium hydroxide or magnesium salts should be administered cautiously in patients with renal insufficiency.
Drug Interaction Precaution: This product should not be taken if the patient is currently taking a prescription drug containing any form of tetracycline.
Supplied: KUDROX SUSPENSION, 12 oz. plastic bottles (NDC 0091-4475-42).

KUTRASE® CAPSULES — ℞

Description: KUTRASE® is a unique formulation containing 4 digestive enzymes, an antispasmodic-anticholinergic agent and a non-barbiturate sedative.
Each green and white capsule contains:

STANDARDIZED ENZYMES

Amylolytic	30 mg.
Proteolytic	6 mg.
Lipolytic	75 mg.
Cellulolytic	2 mg.
Phenyltoloxamine citrate	15 mg.
LEVSIN (Hyoscyamine Sulfate)	0.0625 mg.

Clinical Pharmacology: Diminution of secretions from exocrine glands is often a result of normal aging process. KUTRASE provides a balanced combination of natural proteolytic, amylolytic, cellulolytic and lipolytic enzymes to enhance digestion of proteins, starch and fat in the gastrointestinal tract. These enzymes do not exert any systemic pharmacologic effects. KUTRASE should be considered an enzyme supplement and not an enzyme replacement therapy. Enzymes in KUTRASE are basically derived from vegetable sources and possess a broad spectrum of pH activity. Enzymes are promptly released from the capsule and are bioavailable for digestion of food in the stomach and intestines. LEVSIN (Hyoscyamine Sulfate) provides a potent spasmolytic effect in reducing gastrointestinal hypermotility and intestinal spasm. A mild sedative effect is provided by Phenyltoloxamine Citrate.
Indications and Usage: KUTRASE is indicated for the relief of the symptoms of functional indigestion devoid of organic pathology commonly referred to as nervous indigestion and colloquially as "butterflies". The symptoms are bloating, gas, and fullness.
Contraindications: Glaucoma, obstructive uropathy, obstructive disease of the gastrointestinal tract (as in achalasia, pyloroduodenal stenosis); paralytic ileus, intestinal atony of the elderly or debilitated patients; unstable cardiovascular status in acute hemorrhage; severe ulcerative colitis; toxic megacolon, complicating ulcerative colitis; myasthenia gravis, or a hypersensitivity to any of the ingredients.
Warnings: In the presence of high environmental temperature, heat prostration can occur with drug use (fever and heat stroke due to decreased sweating). Diarrhea may be an early symptom of incomplete intestinal obstruction, especially in patients with ileostomy or colostomy. In this instance, treatment with this drug would be inappropriate. KUTRASE may produce drowsiness or blurred vision. In this event, the patient should be warned not to engage in activities requiring mental alertness such as operating a motor vehicle or other machinery or to perform hazardous work while taking this drug.
Precautions: Use with caution in patients with autonomic neuropathy, hyperthyroidism, coronary heart disease, congestive heart failure, cardiac arrhythmias, and hypertension. Investigate any tachycardia before giving any anticholinergic drugs since they may increase the heart rate. Use with caution in patients with hiatal hernia associated with reflux esophagitis.
Carcinogenesis, mutagenesis — Long-term studies in animals have not been performed to evaluate carcinogenic potential.
Pregnancy Category C—Animal reproduction studies have not been conducted with KUTRASE. It is not known whether KUTRASE can cause fetal harm when administered to a pregnant woman or can affect reproduction capacity. KUTRASE should be given to a pregnant woman only if clearly needed.
Adverse Reactions: Occasionally a slight looseness of the stools may be noticed. Other adverse reactions may include dryness of the mouth; urinary hesitancy and retention; blurred vision and tachycardia; palpitations; mydriasis; cycloplegia; increased ocular tension; headache; nervousness; drowsiness; weakness; suppression of lactation, and allergic reactions or drug idiosyncrasies, urticaria and other dermal manifestations and decreased sweating.

Drug Abuse and Dependence: The information on drug abuse and dependence is limited to uncontrolled data derived from marketing experience. Such experience has revealed no evidence of drug abuse and dependence associated with KUTRASE.
Overdosage: The signs and symptoms of overdose are headache, nausea, vomiting, blurred vision, dilated pupils, hot dry skin, dizziness, dryness of the mouth, difficulty in swallowing. Measures to be taken are immediate lavage of the stomach and injection of physostigmine 0.5 to 2 mg intravenously and repeated as necessary up to a total of 5 mg. Fever may be treated symptomatically. Excitement to a degree which demands attention may be managed with sodium thiopental 2% solution given slowly intravenously. In the event of paralysis of the respiratory muscles, artificial respiration should be instituted.
Administration and Dosage: The dosage of KUTRASE should be adjusted to the needs of the individual patient to assure symptomatic control with a minimum of adverse effects. The usual dose is one or two capsules at meal times, preferably taken during the course of the meal.
Supplied: KUTRASE capsules are green and white with a "Kremers-Urban 475" imprint.

Bottles of 100 capsules	NDC 0091-3475-01
Bottles of 500 capsules	NDC 0091-3475-05

Store at controlled room temperature, between 15°C and 30°C (59°F and 86°F).
Dispense in tight container.
[Shown in Product Identification Section]

KU-ZYME® CAPSULES ℞

Description: KU-ZYME® is a digestive aid containing 4 digestive enzymes which are highly purified, accurately standardized and potent.
Each yellow and white capsule contains:

STANDARDIZED ENZYMES	
Amylolytic	30 mg.
Proteolytic	6 mg.
Lipolytic	75 mg.
Cellulolytic	2 mg.

Clinical Pharmacology: Diminution of secretions from exocrine glands is often a result of normal aging process. KU-ZYME provides a balanced combination of natural proteolytic, amylolytic, cellulolytic and lipolytic enzymes to enhance digestion of proteins, starch and fat in the gastrointestinal tract. These enzymes do not exert any systemic pharmacologic effects. KU-ZYME should be considered an enzyme supplement and not an enzyme replacement therapy. Enzymes in KU-ZYME are basically derived from vegetable sources and possess a broad spectrum of pH activity. Enzymes are promptly released from the capsule and are bioavailable for digestion of food in the stomach and intestines.
Indications and Usage: For the relief of functional indigestion when due to enzyme deficiency or imbalance. KU-ZYME relieves symptoms due to faulty digestion including the sensation of fullness after meals, dyspepsia, flatulence, abdominal distention and intolerance to certain foods.
Contraindications: There are no known contraindications to the administration of digestive enzymes. These enzymes do not attack living tissues and do not present any danger to the patient with ulceration or inflammation in the digestive tract.
Warnings: Do not administer to patients who are allergic to pork products.
Precautions: Long-term studies in animals have not been performed to evaluate carcinogenic potential.
Pregnancy Category C—Animal reproduction studies have not been conducted with KU-ZYME. It is not known whether KU-ZYME can cause fetal harm when administered to a pregnant woman or can affect reproduction capacity. KU-ZYME should be given to a pregnant woman only if clearly needed.
Adverse Reactions: Virtually unknown. Occasionally a slight looseness of stools may be noticed. If so, dosage should be reduced.
Overdosage: No systemic toxicity occurs. Excessive dosage may, however produce a laxative effect.
Dosage and Administration: For most patients, one capsule of KU-ZYME taken during the course of a meal will relieve symptoms due to a digestive deficiency. In patients (especially children) who experience difficulty in swallowing the capsule, it may be opened and the contents sprinkled on the food. In a few cases, where enzyme deficiency is marked (e.g. following gastrectomy, pancreatitis) the dosage may be doubled.
Supplied: KU-ZYME capsules are yellow and white with a "Kremers-Urban 522" imprint.
Bottles of 100 capsules
(NDC 0091-3522-01)
Bottles of 500 capsules
(NDC 0091-3522-05)
Store at controlled room temperature, between 15°C and 30°C (59°F and 86°F).
Dispense in tight container.
[Shown in Product Identification Section]

KU-ZYME® HP ℞
(Pancrelipase Capsules USP)

Description: KU-ZYME HP (Pancrelipase USP) is a standardized concentrate of pancreatic enzymes. Each white capsule contains:

Lipase	8,000 USP units
Protease	30,000 USP units
Amylase	30,000 USP units

Clinical Pharmacology: Pancrelipase USP is a pancreatic enzyme concentrate, which hydrolyzes fats to glycerol and fatty acids, changes protein into proteoses and derived substances, and converts starch into dextrins and sugars. The administration of Pancrelipase reduces the fat and nitrogen content in the stool. Pancreatic enzymes are normally secreted in great excess. Generally, steatorrhea and malabsorption occur only after a 90 percent or greater reduction in secretion of lipase and proteolytic enzymes. It has been estimated that approximately 8,000 units of lipase per hour should be delivered into the duodenum postprandially. Even if all the enzymes taken orally reached the proximal intestine in active form, ingestion of 24,000 units of lipase (8,000 units per hour) for 3 postprandial hours would be required. If one could deliver sufficient pancreatic enzymes to the small intestine, malabsorption could be corrected. It is rarely possible to achieve complete relief of steatorrhea although major improvement in fat absorption can be achieved in most patients.
Indications: KU-ZYME HP is effective in patients with deficient exocrine pancreatic secretions. Thus, KU-ZYME HP may be used as enzyme replacement therapy in cystic fibrosis, chronic pancreatitis, post pancreatectomy, in ductal obstructions caused by cancer of the pancreas, pancreatic insufficiency and for steatorrhea of malabsorption syndrome and post gastrectomy (Billroth II and Total). May also be used as a presumptive test for pancreatic function, especially in pancreatic insufficiency due to chronic pancreatitis.
Contraindications: There are no known contraindications for the use of pancrelipase although sensitivity to pork protein may preclude its use.
Warnings: Pancreatic exocrine replacement therapy should not delay or supplant treatment of the primary disorder. Use with caution in patients known to be hypersensitive to pork or enzymes.
Precautions: Drug interactions—The serum iron response to oral iron may be decreased by concomitant administration of pancreatic extracts.
Carcinogenicity, Mutagenicity, and Impairment of Fertility—There have been no studies in animals to evaluate the carcinogenic, mutagenic or impairment of fertility potential of pancrelipase.
Adverse Reactions: High doses may cause nausea, abdominal cramps and/or diarrhea in certain patients.
Dosage and Administration: Dosage should be adjusted to individual patient needs. 1 to 3 capsules with meals and 1 capsule with any food between meals. In severe deficiencies, the dose may be increased to 8 capsules with meals or the frequency of administration may increase to hourly intervals if nausea, cramps and/or diarrhea do not occur.
Caution: Federal law prohibits dispensing without prescription.
Supplied: White capsules, bottles of 100.
NDC 0091-3525-01
[Shown in Product Identification Section]

LEVSIN® ℞
(Hyoscyamine Sulfate U.S.P.)

LEVSIN® Tablets
LEVSIN® Injection
LEVSIN® Elixir
LEVSIN® Drops (Oral Solution)
LEVSINEX™ TIMECAPS™

Description: LEVSIN® Tablets contain Hyoscyamine Sulfate 0.125 mg. They are white scored tablets with K-U logo and 531 imprint.
LEVSIN® Injection contains 0.5 mg/ml of hyoscyamine sulfate.
LEVSIN® Elixir contains Hyoscyamine Sulfate 0.125 mg/5cc (Teaspoonful). It is orange colored and flavored and contains alcohol 20%.
LEVSIN® Drops contain Hyoscyamine Sulfate 0.125 mg/cc. It is orange colored and flavored and contains alcohol 5%. Supplied in a dropper bottle.
LEVSINEX™ TIMECAPS™ contain Hyocyamine Sulfate 0.375 mg in a sustained release formulation designed for b.i.d. dosage. They are brown and clear capsules containing brown and white beadlets.
Clinical Pharmacology: LEVSIN is a chemically pure hyoscyamine sulfate, one of the principle anticholinergic/antispasmodic components of Belladonna alkaloids. LEVSIN inhibits specifically the actions of acetylcholine on structures innervated by postganglionic cholinergic nerves and on smooth muscles that respond to acetylcholine but lack cholinergic innervation. These peripheral cholinergic receptors are present in the autonomic effector cells of the smooth muscle, cardiac muscle, the sinoatrial node, the atrioventricular node and exocrine glands. It is completely devoid of any action in the autonomic ganglia. LEVSIN inhibits gastrointestinal propulsive motility and decreases gastric acid secretion. LEVSIN also controls excessive pharyngeal, tracheal, and bronchial secretions. LEVSIN is absorbed totally and completely by sublingual administration as well as oral administration. Once absorbed, LEVSIN disappears rapidly from the blood and is distributed throughout the entire body. The half-life of LEVSIN is 3½ hours and the majority of drug is excreted in the urine unchanged within the first 12 hours. Only traces of this drug are found in breast milk.
Indications and Usage: LEVSIN is effective as adjunctive therapy in the treatment of peptic ulcer. It can also be used to control gastric secretion, visceral spasm and hyper-motility in spastic colitis, cystitis, pylorospasm, and associated abdominal cramps. May be used in functional intestinal disorders to reduce symptoms such as those seen in mild dysenteries and diverticulitis. For use as adjunctive ther-

Continued on next page

Kremers-Urban—Cont.

apy in the treatment of irritable bowel syndrome (irritable colon, spastic colon, mucous colitis, acute enterocolitis and functional gastrointestinal disorders). Also as adjunctive therapy in the treatment of neurogenic bowel disturbances (including the splenic flexure syndrome and neurogenic colon). Also used in the treatment of infant colic (elixir and drops). LEVSIN is indicated along with morphine and other narcotics in symptomatic relief of biliary and renal colic; as a "drying agent" in the relief of symptoms of acute rhinitis; in the therapy of Parkinsonism to reduce rigidity and tremors and to control associated sialorrhea, and hyperhydrosis. May be used in the therapy of poisoning of anticholinesterase agents.

Contraindications: Glaucoma, obstructive uropathy (for example, bladder neck obstruction due to prostatic hypertrophy); obstructive disease of the gastrointestinal tract (as in achalasia, pyloroduodenal stenosis); paralytic ileus; intestinal atony of the elderly or debilitated patients; unstable cardiovascular status in acute hemorrhage; severe ulcerative colitis; toxic megacolon, complicating ulcerative colitis; myasthenia gravis.

Warnings: In the presence of high environmental temperature, heat prostration can occur with drug use (fever and heat stroke due to decreased sweating). Diarrhea may be an early symptom of incomplete intestinal obstruction, especially in patients with ileostomy or colostomy. In this instance, treatment with this drug would be inappropriate and possibly harmful. Like other anticholinergic agents, LEVSIN may produce drowsiness or blurred vision. In this event, the patient should be warned not to engage in activities requiring mental alertness such as operating a motor vehicle or other machinery or to perform hazardous work while taking this drug.

Precautions: Use with caution in patients with autonomic neuropathy, hyperthyroidism, coronary heart disease, congestive heart failure, cardiac arrhythmias, and hypertension. Investigate any tachycardia before giving any anticholinergic drugs since they may increase the heart rate. Use with caution in patients with hiatal hernia associated with reflux esophagitis.

Adverse Reactions: Adverse reactions may include dryness of the mouth; urinary hesitancy and retention; blurred vision and tachycardia; palpitations; mydriasis; cycloplegia; increased ocular tension; headache; nervousness; drowsiness; weakness; suppression of lactation, and allergic reactions or drug idiosyncrasies, urticaria and other dermal manifestations and decreased sweating.

Drug Abuse and Dependence: The information on drug abuse and dependence is limited to uncontrolled data derived from marketing experience. Such experience has revealed no evidence of drug abuse and dependence associated with LEVSIN.

Overdosage: The signs and symptoms of overdose are headache, nausea, vomiting, blurred vision, dilated pupils, hot/dry skin, dizziness, dryness of the mouth, difficulty in swallowing. Overdosage may be treated with immediate lavage of the stomach and injection of physostigmine 0.5 to 2 mg intravenously and repeated as necessary up to a total of 5 mg. Fever may be treated symptomatically (alcohol sponging, icepacks). Excitement to a degree which demands attention may be managed with sodium thiopental 2% solution given slowly intravenously or chloral hydrate (100–200 ml of a 2% solution) by rectal infusion. In the event of progression of the curare-like effect to paralysis of the respiratory muscles, artificial respiration should be instituted and maintained until effective respiratory action returns.

Dosage and Administration: The dosage of LEVSIN products should be adjusted to the needs of the individual patient to assure symptomatic control with a minimum of adverse effects.

LEVSIN Tablets: One or two tablets three to four times a day according to condition and severity of symptoms. May be taken orally or sublingually.

LEVSIN Elixir: Adults, one or two teaspoonfuls of elixir three to four times a day according to conditions and severity of symptoms.

Children (Elixir)

Body Weight	Starting Dosage
10 lb.	0.5 ml to 0.75 ml
20 lb.	1.25 ml (1/4 tsp) to 2.0 ml
30 lb.	2.5 ml (1/2 tsp)
50 lb.	3/4 tsp to 1 tsp
75–80 lb.	1 tsp to 1 1/2 tsp

Doses may be repeated every 4 hours as needed; dosage adjustment may be necessary.

LEVSIN Drops:

Infants

Body Weight	Starting Dosage (in drops)
5 lb.	3
7.5 lb.	4
10 lb.	6
15 lb.	7
20 lb.	9

Children 1–10 years: 1/2–1cc

Adults: 1–2cc

Doses may be repeated every 4 hours as needed; dosage adjustment may be necessary according to conditions and severity of symptoms.

LEVSIN Injection may be administered subcutaneously, intramuscularly, or intravenously without dilution. The usual recommended dose of LEVSIN in the treatment of gastrointestinal disorders is 0.5 or 1.0 ml (0.25 to 0.5 mg) administered at four hour intervals three to four times daily. Some patients may need only a single dose, others may require administration 2, 3, or 4 times a day. For hypotonic duodenography, LEVSIN Injection may be used five to ten minutes prior to the diagnostic procedure. The usual dose is 0.5 to 1.0 ml (0.25 mg to 0.5 mg).

IN ANESTHESIA:

As pre-anesthetic medication, the recommended dose of LEVSIN Injection is 5 mcg/kg of body weight, given thirty to sixty minutes prior to the anticipated time of induction of anesthesia, or at the time the pre-anesthetic narcotic or sedatives are administered. In intraoperative medication, LEVSIN Injectable may be used during surgery to counteract drug induced bradycardia. It should be administered intravenously in increments of 0.25 ml and repeated as needed. To achieve reversal of neuromuscular blockage, the recommended dose of LEVSIN Injectable is 0.2 mg for each 1 mg of neostigmine or the equivalent dose of physostigmine and pyridostigmine.

LEVSINEX TIMECAPS:

Adults

The usual dose is one TIMECAP every 12 hours. For patients requiring higher anticholinergic therapy, the dosage may be increased to two TIMECAPS every 12 hours or one TIMECAP every 8 hours.

Supplied:

LEVSIN Tablets (0.125 mg. hyoscyamine sulfate tablets, U.S.P.) white, scored tablets; bottles of 100 (NDC 0091-3531-01), bottles of 500 (NDC 0091-3531-05).

[Shown in Product Indentification Section]

LEVSIN with Phenobarbital Tablets (0.125 mg. hyoscyamine sulfate and 15 mg. Phenobarbital) pink, scored tablets; bottles of 100 (NDC 0091-3534-01), and 500 (NDC 0091-3534-05).

[Shown in Product Identification Section]

LEVSIN Elixir (0.125 mg. hyoscyamine sulfate per 5 cc.) orange colored and flavored; pints. (NDC 0091-4532-16).

LEVSIN with Phenobarbital Elixir (0.125 mg. hyoscyamine sulfate and 15 mg. Phenobarbital per 5 cc.) red, raspberry flavored; pints. (NDC 0091-4530-16).

LEVSIN DROPS (0.125 mg. hyoscyamine sulfate per cc.), orange colored and flavored, 15 cc. (NDC 0091-4538-15).

LEVSIN-PB DROPS (0.125 mg hyoscyamine sulfate and 15 mg. phenobarbital per cc.), red, cherry flavored, 15 cc. (NDC 0091-4536-15).

LEVSIN Injection (0.5 mg hyoscyamine sulfate per ml.) Single dose ampuls, boxes of 5. (NDC 0091-1536-05) and multiple dose 10 ml vial (NDC 0091-1536-10).

LEVSINEX TIMECAPS (0.375 mg. hyoscyamine sulfate) brown and white sustained release beadlets in brown and clear capsules; bottles of 100. (NDC 0091-3537-01).

[Shown in Product Identification Section]

LEVSINEX with Phenobarbital TIMECAPS (0.375 mg. hyoscyamine sulfate and 45 mg. Phenobarbital) pink and white sustained release beadlets in pink and clear capsules; bottles of 100. (NDC 0091-3539-01).

[Shown in Product Identification Section]

MILKINOL® OTC

Composition: MILKINOL is a unique formulation containing liquid petrolatum for lubrication, a special emulsifier to aid in penetration and softening of the fecal mass, and to make oil and water mix for complete dispersion.

Action and Uses: Pleasant, dependable MILKINOL provides safe, gentle lubrication for the constipation problem. No oily taste, no purgative griping, not habit forming, sugar free. MILKINOL is an agent of choice for the correction of simple constipation in older children and adults. At the discretion of the physician it may also be employed in the management of constipation in younger children, in pregnant patients and in elderly or bedridden persons.

Dosage: Adults 1 to 2 tablespoonfuls. Children over 6: 1 to 2 teaspoonfuls. Infants, young children, expectant mothers, aged or bedridden patients, use only as directed by physician.

Directions: Pour desired dosage of MILKINOL into a dry drinking glass. Add just a small amount (about 1/4 glass or less) of water, milk, fruit juice or soft drink. Stir and drink. Follow with additional liquid if desired.

Precautions: Prolonged usage, without intermission is not advised. Should be given at bedtime ONLY.

Supplied: 8 oz. glass bottles (NDC 0091-7580-08).

NITROL® Ointment ℞

Description: NITROL Ointment contains 2% nitroglycerin and lactose in a special absorptive lanolin and white petrolatum base formulated to provide a controlled-release of the active ingredient. Each inch, as squeezed from the tube, contains approximately 15 mg nitroglycerin.

Action: When the ointment is spread on the skin, the active ingredient (nitroglycerin) is continuously absorbed through the skin into the circulation, thus exerting prolonged vasodilator effect. Nitroglycerin ointment is effective in the control of angina pectoris, regardless of the site of application.

Nitroglycerin relaxes smooth muscles, principally in the smaller blood vessels and dilates the arterioles and capillaries, especially in the coronary circulation. Nitroglycerin ointment reduces the workload of the heart by virtue of its smooth muscle relaxation. This results predominantly in peripheral venous dilitation which reduces preload, but also to a lesser degree in peripheral arteriolar dilitation which reduces afterload. These hemodynamic effects have been advanced as explanations for the beneficial actions of nitroglycerin ointment in angina pectoris. Nitroglycerin exerts a favorable influence on myocardial oxygen consumption, resulting in increased myocardial efficiency and significant improvement in left ventricular function. Computerized digital plethysmographic studies have shown the duration of action of nitroglycerin ointment (2 inches applied to the chest) to be eight hours in comparison to placebo; the onset of action occurred within thirty minutes of administration. Controlled clinical studies have demonstrated that nitroglycerin ointment increased measured exercise tolerance in patients with angina pectoris up to three hours after application (the maximal time interval studied).

Indications: For the prevention and treatment of angina pectoris due to coronary artery disease.

Contraindications: In patients known to be intolerant of the organic nitrate drugs.

Warnings: In acute myocardial infarction or congestive heart failure, nitroglycerin ointment should be used under careful clinical and/or hemodynamic monitoring.

Precautions: Nitroglycerin ointment should not be used for treatment of acute anginal attacks. Symptoms of hypotension, particularly when suddenly arising from the recumbent position, are signs of overdosage. When they occur, the dosage should be reduced.

Adverse Reactions: Transient headaches are the most common side effect, especially at higher dosages. Headaches should be treated with mild analgesics, and nitroglycerin ointment continued. Only with untreatable headaches should the dosage be reduced. Although uncommon, hypotension, an increase in heart rate, faintness, flushing, dizziness, and nausea may occur. These are all attributable to the pharmacologic effects of nitroglycerin on the cardiovascular system, and are symptoms of overdosage. When they occur and persist, the dosage should be reduced. Occasionally, contact dermatitis has been reported with continuous use of topical nitroglycerin. Such incidences may be reduced by changing the site of application or by using topical corticosteroids.

Management of Overdosage: Severe hypotension may result from overdosage of nitroglycerin ointment. Should hypotension develop, quickly remove the ointment. Severe hypotension usually responds to the administration of Phenylephrine HCl or Levarterenol Bitartrate.

Dosage and Administration: When applying the ointment, use the specially designed dose determining applicator supplied with the package and squeeze the necessary amount of ointment from the tube onto the applicator. Then place the applicator with the ointment side down onto the desired area of skin, usually the chest (although other areas can be used). Spread the ointment over at least a 2 × 3 inch area in a thin uniform layer using the applicator. Cover the area with plastic wrap which can be held in place by adhesive tape. The applicator allows the patient to measure the necessary amount of ointment and to spread it without being absorbed through the fingers while applying it to the skin surface.

The usual therapeutic dose is 1 to 2 inches (50 mm) applied every eight hours, although some patients may require as much as 4 to 5 inches (100 to 125 mm) and/or application every four hours.

Start at ½ inch (12.5 mm) every eight hours and increase the dose by ½ inch (12.5 mm) with each successive application to achieve the desired clinical effects. The optimal dosage should be selected based upon the clinical responses, side effects, and the effects of therapy upon blood pressure. The greatest attainable decrease in resting blood pressure which is not associated with clinical symptoms of hypotension especially during orthostasis indicates the optimal dosage. To decrease adverse reactions, the dose and frequency of application should be tailored to the individual patient's needs.

Keep the tube tightly closed and store at room temperature 59° to 86°F (15° to 30°C).

How Supplied:

30 gram tube (NDC 0091-5617-31)
60 gram tube (NDC 0091-5617-02)
30 gram 6 Pack Unit (NDC 0091-5617-61)
60 gram 6 Pack Unit (NDC 0091-5617-62)
Unit Dose (1″ Equivalent) - Box of 10 (NDC 0091-5617-10)
Titratable Unit Dose 50 × 3 g Tubes (NDC 0091-5617-53)
[*Shown in Product Identification Section*]

PRE-PEN® ℞
(Benzylpenicilloyl-polylysine)
Skin Test Antigen

Description: PRE-PEN® is a sterile solution of benzylpenicilloyl-polylysine in a concentration of 6.0×10^{-5}M. (penicilloyl) in 0.01 M phosphate buffer and 0.15 M sodium chloride. The benzylpenicilloyl-polylysine in PRE-PEN® is a derivative of poly-l-lysine, where the epsilon amino groups are substituted with benzylpenicilloyl groups (50-70%) forming benzylpenicilloyl alpha amide. Each single dose ampule contains 0.25 ml of PRE-PEN®.

Action: PRE-PEN® (benzylpenicilloyl-polylysine) reacts specifically with benzylpenicilloyl skin sensitizing antibodies (reagins: IgE class) to initiate release of chemical mediators which produce an immediate wheal and flare reaction at a skin test site. All individuals exhibiting a positive skin test to PRE-PEN® possess reagins against the benzylpenicilloyl group which is a haptene. A haptene is a low molecular weight chemical which, when conjugated to a carrier, e.g., poly-l-lysine, has the properties under appropriate conditions of an antigen with the haptene's specificity.

It is to be noted that individuals who have previously received therapeutic penicillin may have positive skin test reactions to PRE-PEN® as well as to a number of other non-benzylpenicilloyl haptenes. The latter are designated as minor determinants, in that they are present in lesser amounts than the major determinant, benzylpenicilloyl. The minor determinants may nevertheless be associated with examples of significant clinical hypersensitivity. Virtually everyone who receives penicillin develops specific antibodies to the drug as measured by hemagglutination studies, but (a) positive skin tests to various penicillin and penicillin-derived reagents become positive in less than 10% of patients who have tolerated penicillin in the past and (b) allergic responses are infrequent (less than 1%).

Many individuals reacting positively to PRE-PEN® will not develop a systemic allergic reaction on subsequent exposure to therapeutic penicillin. Thus, the PRE-PEN® skin test facilitates assessing the local allergic skin reactivity of a patient to benzylpenicilloyl.

Indications: PRE-PEN® is useful as an adjunct in assessing the risk of administering penicillin (benzylpenicillin or penicillin G) when it is the preferred drug of choice in adult patients who have previously received penicillin and have a history of clinical penicillin hypersensitivity. In this situation, a negative skin test to PRE-PEN® is associated with an incidence of allergic reactions of less than 5% after the administration of therapeutic penicillin, whereas the incidence may be more than 20% in the presence of a positive skin test to PRE-PEN®.

These allergic reactions are predominantly dermatologic. Because of the extremely low incidence of anaphylactic reactions, there are insufficient data at present to document that a decreased incidence of anaphylactic reactions following the administration of penicillin will occur in patients with a negative skin test to PRE-PEN®. Similarly, when deciding the risk of proposed penicillin treatment, there are not enough data at present to permit relative weighting in individual cases of a history of clinical penicillin hypersensitivity as compared to positive skin tests to PRE-PEN® and/or minor penicillin determinants.

It should be borne in mind that no reagent, test, or combination of tests will completely assure that a reaction to penicillin therapy will not occur.

Contraindications: PRE-PEN® is contraindicated in those patients who have exhibited either a systemic or marked local reaction to its previous administration. Patients known to be extremely hypersensitive to penicillin should not be skin tested.

Warnings: There are insufficient data to assess the potential danger of sensitization to penicillin from repeated skin testing with PRE-PEN®.

Rarely, a systemic allergic reaction (see below) may follow a skin test with PRE-PEN®. This can be avoided by making the first application by scratch test and very carefully following the instructions below in administering the intradermal test, using the intradermal route only if the scratch test has been entirely negative. Skin testing with penicillin and/or other penicillin-derived reagents should not be performed simultaneously.

No controlled studies have been made of the safety of PRE-PEN® skin testing in pregnant women and therefore, the hazard of skin testing of such patients should be weighed against the hazards of penicillin therapy without skin testing.

Precautions: There are insufficient data derived from well-controlled studies to determine the value of the PRE-PEN® skin test as a means of assessing the risk of administering therapeutic penicillin (when penicillin is the preferred drug of choice) in the following situations:

(1) Adult patients who give no history of clinical penicillin hypersensitivity.
(2) Pediatric patients.

In addition, there are no data at present to assess the clinical value of PRE-PEN® where exposure to penicillin is suspected as a cause of a drug reaction and in patients who are undergoing routine allergy evaluation.

Furthermore, there are no data relating the clinical value of PRE-PEN® skin tests to the risk of administering semi-synthetic penicillins (phenoxymethyl penicillin, ampicillin, carbenicillin, dicloxacillin, methicillin, nafcillin, oxacillin, phenethicillin) and cephalosporin-derived antibiotics.

Recognition that the following clinical outcomes are possible makes it imperative for the physician to weigh risk to benefit in every instance where the decision to administer or not to administer penicillin is based in part on a PRE-PEN® skin test.

(1) An allergic reaction to therapeutic penicillin may occur in a patient with a negative skin test to PRE-PEN®.
(2) It is possible for a patient to have an anaphylactic reaction to therapeutic penicillin in the presence of a negative PRE-PEN® skin test and a negative history of clinical penicillin hypersensitivity.
(3) If penicillin is the absolute drug of choice in a life-threatening situation, successful desensitization with therapeutic penicillin may be possible irrespective of a positive skin test and/or a positive history of clinical penicillin hypersensitivity.

Adverse Reactions: Occasionally, patients may develop an intense local inflammatory response at the skin test site. Rarely, patients will develop a systemic allergic reaction, manifested by generalized erythema, pruritus, angioneurotic edema, urticaria, dyspnea, and/or hypotension. The usual methods of treating a skin test antigen induced reaction—the application of a venous occlusion tourniquet proximal to the skin test site and administration of epinephrine (and, at times, an injection of an

Continued on next page

Kremers-Urban—Cont.

antihistamine) — are recommended and will usually control the reaction. As a rule, systemic allergic reactions following skin test procedures are of short duration and controllable, but the patient should be kept under observation for several hours.

Skin Testing Dosage and Technique:
SCRATCH TESTING
Skin testing is usually performed on the inner volar aspect of the forearm. The skin test material should **always** be applied first by the scratch technique. After preparing the skin surface, a sterile 20 gauge needle should be used to make a 3–5 mm scratch of the epidermis. Very little pressure is required to break the epidermal continuity. If bleeding occurs, prepare a second site and scratch more lightly with the needle—sufficient to produce a non-bleeding scratched surface. Apply a small drop of PRE-PEN® solution to the scratch and rub gently with an applicator, toothpick, or the side of the needle. Observe for the appearance of a wheal, erythema, and the occurrence of itching at the test site during the succeeding 15 minutes at which time the solution over the scratch is wiped off. A positive reaction is unmistakable and consists of the development within 10 minutes of a pale wheal, usually with pseudopods, surrounding the scratch site and varying in diameter from 5 to 15 mm (or more). This wheal may be surrounded by a variable diameter of erythema, and accompanied by a variable degree of itching. The most sensitive individuals develop itching almost instantly, and the wheal and erythema are prompt in their appearance. As soon as a positive response as defined above is clearly evident, the solution over the scratch should be immediately wiped off. If the scratch test is either negative or equivocally positive (less than 5 mm wheal and little or no erythema, and no itching), an intradermal test may be performed.

THE INTRADERMAL TEST
Using a tuberculin syringe with a $^3/_8$" to $^5/_8$" long, 26 to 30 gauge, short bevel needle, withdraw the contents of the ampule. Prepare a sterile skin test area on the upper, outer arm, sufficiently below the deltoid muscle to permit proximal application of a tourniquet later, if necessary. Be sure to eject all air from the syringe through the needle, then insert the needle, bevel up immediately below the skin surface. Inject an amount of PRE-PEN® sufficient to raise the smallest possible perceptible bleb. This volume will be between 0.01 and 0.02 ml. Using a separate syringe and needle, inject a like amount of saline as a control at least 1½ inches removed from the test site. Most skin reactions will develop within 5–15 minutes and response to the skin test is read as follows:

(—) Negative response—no increase in size of original bleb and/or no greater reaction than the control site.
(±) Ambiguous response—wheal being only slightly larger than initial injection bleb, with or without accompanying erythematous flare and larger than the control site.
(+) Positive response—itching and marked increase in size of original bleb. Wheal may exceed 20 mm in diameter and exhibit pseudopods.

The control site should be completely reactionless. If it exhibits a wheal greater than 2–3 mm, repeat the test, and if the same reaction is observed, a physician experienced with allergy skin testing should be consulted.

How Supplied: PRE-PEN® is supplied in ampules containing 0.25 ml. and packaged in boxes of 5 (NDC 0091-1640-05).
PRE-PEN® is stable only when kept under refrigeration. It is, therefore, recommended that test materials subjected to ambient temperatures for over a day be discarded.

Further information on these and other Kremers-Urban products will be furnished upon request to our Professional Service Department.

LactAid Inc.
600 FIRE ROAD
P.O. BOX 111
PLEASANTVILLE, NJ 08232-0111

LACTAID®
(lactase enzyme)

Description: Each 5 drop dosage contains not less than 1000 NLU (Neutral Lactase Units) of Beta-D-galactosidase derived from Kluyveromyces lactis yeast. The enzyme is in a liquid carrier of glycerol (50%), water (30%), and inert yeast dry matter (20%) 4–5 drops hydrolyzes approximately 70% of the lactose in 1 quart of milk at refrigerator temperature, @ 42°F–6°C in 24 hours, or will do the same in 2 hours @ 85°F–30°C. Additional time and/or enzyme required for 100% lactose conversion. 1 U.S. quart of milk will contain approximately 50 gm lactose prior to lactose hydrolysis and will contain 15 gm or less, after. Hydrolysis converts the lactose into its simple sugar components, glucose and galactose.
Actions: Converts the disaccharide lactose into its monosugar components, glucose and galactose.
Indications: Lactase insufficiency in the patient, suspected from g.i. disturbances after consumption of milk or milk content products: e.g., bloat, distension, flatulence, diarrhea; or identified by a lactose tolerance test.
Precautions: Diabetics should be aware that the milk sugar will now be metabolically available and must be taken into account (25 gm glucose and 25 gm galactose per quart). No reports received of any diabetics' reactions. Galactosemics may not have milk in any form, lactase enzyme modified or not.
Usage: Added to milk. 4–10 drops per quart of milk depending on level of lactose conversion desired.
Toxicity: Animal studies @ 4% of enzyme by body weight (equivalent of 24,000-5 drop dosages in a 50-kilo human) showed no effects. LD_{50} not achievable. LactAid is not a drug but a food which modifies another food to make it more digestible.
Other Uses: Veterinary indications: treatment of milk for animals with gastric surgery; sick young animals; sick or healthy older animals.
How Supplied: Sold in 3 forms:
(1) Lactase enzyme in a stable liquid form, in sales units of 4, 12 or 30 one-quart dosages at 5 drops per dose. This form also available in bulk packs for institutions, e.g., 100/4-quart size, 100/30-quart size, etc.
(2) In some areas of the U.S.: Fresh hydrolyzed lowfat milk from dairies, ready to drink, sold in food markets. Lactose hydrolysis level: 70%. Brand name: LactAid.
(3) Sterile canned hydrolyzed lowfat milk, single strength, ready to drink, in cases of 12/1-quart and 24/8-oz. size, for institutions and sold individually in food markets and drug stores. Lactose hydrolysis level: 70%. Brand name: LactAid.

If desired, further conversion of the treated milks (2) and (3) can be done at home or institution with the LactAid liquid enzyme. Any person or institution unable to locate LactAid enzyme or canned milk locally can order direct from LactAid Inc. at retail or wholesale. Sample and full product information to doctors, nutritionists and institutions on request.
[*Shown in Product Identification Section*]

Lambda Pharmacal Corporation
Subsidiary of A. J. Bart, Inc.
PLAINVIEW, NY 11803

MIGRALAM™ CAPSULES ℞

Description: Each white MIGRALAM capsule contains: Isometheptene Mucate 65 mg., Caffeine 100 mg., Acetaminophen 325 mg.
Actions: Isometheptene Mucate, a sympathomimetic amine, acts by constricting dilated cranial and cerebral arterioles, thus reducing the stimuli that lead to vascular headaches. It is particularly desirable in patients predisposed to nausea and vomiting and where ergotamines are precluded. Its action is similar to ergotamine but possessed of a low order of toxicity. Caffeine, also a cranial vasoconstrictor, is added to further enhance the vasoconstrictor effect. Acetaminophen, an effective non-narcotic analgesic, reduces the perception of pain impulses originating from dilated cerebral vessels. It is unlikely to produce many of the side effects associated with aspirin.
Indications: For relief of vascular and tension headaches.

> Based on a review for this drug (isometheptene mucate), The National Academy of Sciences-National Research Council and/or other information, FDA has classified the other indications as "Possibly" effective in the treatment of migraine headache.
> Final classification of the less-than-effective indication requires further investigation.

Contraindications: MIGRALAN is contraindicated in Glaucoma and/or severe cases of renal disease, hypertension, organic heart disease, hepatic disease and in those patients who are on monoamine-oxidase (MAO) inhibitor therapy.
Precautions: Caution should be observed in hypertension, peripheral vascular disease and after recent cardiovascular attacks.
Adverse Reactions: Transient dizziness and skin rash may appear in hypersensitive patients. This can usually be eliminated by reducing the dose.
Dosage and Administration: **FOR RELIEF OF MIGRAINE HEADACHE.** The usual adult dosage is two capsules at once, followed by one capsule every hour until relieved, up to 5 capsules within a twelve hour period.
FOR RELIEF OF TENSION HEADACHE. The usual adult dose is one or two capsules every four hours up to 8 capsules a day.
How Supplied: Bottles of 100 capsules (NDC 49326-116-90) and 500 capsules (NDC 49326-116-75).

NEURO™ B-12 INJECTABLE ℞
(B-12, B-1)

Description: Each cc in NEURO B-12 contains: Cyanocobalamin (Vitamin B-12) 1000 mcg., Thiamine HCl. (Vitamin B-1) 100 mg., Benzyl Alcohol 1.5% and Disodium E.D.T.A. 0.5 mg. in a sterile aqueous solution.
How Supplied: NEURO B-12 Injectable is supplied in a 10 cc multidose vial (NDC 49326-114-10).

NEURO™ B-12 FORTE INJECTABLE ℞
(B-12, B-1, B-6)

Description: Each cc in NEURO B-12 FORTE contains: Cyanocobalamin 1000 mcg., Thiamine HCl 100 mg., Pyridoxine HCl 100 mg., Benzyl Alcohol 1.5% in a physiological salt solution q.s.
How Supplied: NEURO B-12 FORTE Injectable is supplied in 10 cc multidose vials (NDC 49326-115-10).

VITA-NUMONYL INJECTABLE ℞
(Expectorant and Antiseptic)

Description: Each ml. contains:
Vitamin A Palmitate ....2,500 I.U.
Vitamin D_2 (Ergocalciferol) ....250 I.U.
Eucaliptol ....75 mg.
Oil of Niaouli ....15 mg.
Oil of Arachida ....C.s.h. 1.0 ml.
Pharmacological Use and Action: The balsamics exert and expectorant and antiseptic action of the respiratory tracks. The prophylactic properties of Vitamins "A" and "D" are added to this action.
Dosage: Adults: 2 ml. intramuscular daily for 5 days or according to physician.
Children: 1 ml. intramuscular daily for 5 days.
How Supplied: In 1 ml. and 2 ml. ampoules, boxes of 25.

The Lannett Company, Inc.
9000 STATE ROAD
PHILADELPHIA, PA 19136

ACNEDERM™ LOTION
(See PDR For Nonprescription Drugs)

CODALAN™ ℞

Composition: Each tablet contains: Codeine Phosphate* gr. 1/8 in No. 1; gr. 1/4 in No. 2; gr. 1/2 in No. 3; Acetaminophen 2½ grs.; Salicylamide 3½ grs.; and caffeine ½ gr.
*Warning: May be habit-forming.
Action and Uses: Analgesic, antitussive. Indicated for the relief of pain of all degrees of severity up to that which requires morphine.
Administration and Dosage: One (No. 1, No. 2 or No. 3) as required to relieve pain.
How Supplied: No. 1 orange color, No. 2 white color, No. 3 green color; all strengths in bottles of 100 and 500. No. 2 and No. 3 also available in bottles of 1000.
Literature Available: Complete Data Card.

DISONATE™ Capsules and Liquid
(dioctyl sodium sulfosuccinate)

Composition: Dioctyl sodium sulfosuccinate, an effective stool-softener.
Action and Uses: Disonate keeps stools soft for easy passage. It is not a laxative and does not irritate the intestinal tract. Useful in treating constipation due to hard stools, in painful anorectal conditions, in cardiac and other patients who must avoid straining at stool.
Dosage: Adults and older children 60 to 240 mg. daily. Children 6 to 12 years of age 40 to 120 mg. daily. Higher doses are recommended for initial therapy and the effect on stools is usually apparent one to three days after the initial dose. Divided dosage may be used and dosage should be adjusted to individual response.
How Supplied: Capsules of 60 mg., 100 mg., and 240 mg. Bottles of 100, 500 and 1000 capsules. Solution, 10 mg/cc Pint Bottle. Syrup, 20 mg/5 cc Pint and Gallon Bottle.
Literature Available: Yes.

MAGNATRIL™ SUSPENSION AND TABLETS
(See PDR For Nonprescription Drugs)

Products are cross-indexed by

generic and chemical names

in the

YELLOW SECTION

LaSalle Laboratories, Inc.
Subsidiary of Mallard, Inc.
3021 WABASH AVENUE
DETROIT, MI 48216

AQUEX ℞
(benzthiazide)

Each tablet contains: 50 mg. Benzthiazide (3-benzylthiomethyl-6-chloro-7-sulfamyl -1,2,4-benzothiadiazine-1, 1-dioxide)
How Supplied: Bottles of 100 tablets.
Literature: Available on request.

DYTUSS ℞
Antihistaminic Expectorant

Description: Each 30 ml (fl. oz.) contains:
Diphenhydramine HCl .... 80 mg.
Ammonium Chloride ....778 mg.
Sodium Citrate ....324 mg.
Menthol ....6.4 mg.
Alcohol ....5% U.S.P.
How Supplied: Available in 16 fl. oz. (1 pint) bottles.
Literature: Available upon request.

FETRIN ℞
Hematinic with Vitamins B-12 & C

Description: Each sustained release capsule contains:
Ferrous Fumarate (equivalent to 66 mg. elemental Iron) ....200 mg.
Ascorbic Acid .... 60 mg.
Cyanocobalamin ....5 mcg.
With Intrinsic Factor
How Supplied: Bottles of 100 capsules.
Literature: Available on request.

ORABEX-TF ℞
Therapeutic B-Complex Vitamins with Vitamin C and Folic Acid.

Description: Each coated tablet contains:
Vitamin A (Acetate) ....6000 I.U.
Vitamin D (Ergocalciferol) .... 400 I.U.
Vitamin E (as 25 mg. d-Alpha Tocopherol Succinate) .... 30 I.U.
Folic Acid .... 1.0 mg.
Ascorbic Acid .... 60 mg.
Thiamine Mononitrate .... 1.1 mg.
Riboflavin .... 1.8 mg.
Pyridoxine Hydrochloride .... 2.5 mg.
Vitamin B-12 (Cyanocobalamin) .... 5 mcg.
Niacin (as Niacinamide) .... 15 mg.
Calcium (as Calcium Carbonate) ...... 125 mg.
Iron (as Ferrous Fumarate) .... 65 mg.
How Supplied: Bottle of 100 tablets.
Literature: Available on request.

PACAPS ℞

Description: Each capsule contains:
Butalbital ....50 mg.
(May be habit forming)
Caffeine ....40 mg.
Acetaminophen ....325 mg.
How Supplied: Available in bottles of 100 capsules.
Literature: Available on request.

PROTID ℞

Description: Each timed release tablet contains:
Acetaminophen ....300 mg.
Chlorpheniramine Maleate ....8 mg.
Phenylephrine HCl ....10 mg.
Phenylpropanolamine HCl ....20 mg.
How Supplied: Bottles of 100 tablets.
Literature: Available on request.

SUL-AZO

Each coated tablet represents:
Phenylazodiaminopyridine Hydrochloride ....50 mg.
Sulfamethizole ....250 mg.
How Supplied: Bottles of 100 tablets.
Literature: Available on request.

Laser, Inc.
2000 N. MAIN ST.
P.O. BOX 905
CROWN POINT, IN 46307

DALLERGY® Syrup, Tablets and Sustained-Release Capsules ℞

Composition: Each 5 ml. (teaspoonful) of purple, grape flavored syrup contains: chlorpheniramine maleate 2 mg., phenylephrine hydrochloride 10 mg., methscopolamine nitrate 0.625 mg. Each white scored tablet contains: chlorpheniramine maleate 4 mg., phenylephrine hydrochloride 10 mg., methscopolamine nitrate 1.25 mg. Each pink and white sustained-release capsule contains: chlorpheniramine maleate 8 mg., phenylephrine hydrochloride 20 mg., methscopolamine nitrate 2.5 mg.

DONATUSSIN DC SYRUP Ⓒ ℞

Composition: Each 5 ml. (teaspoonful) of red syrup contains: hydrocodone bitartrate 2.5 mg. (WARNING: May be habit forming), phenylephrine hydrochloride 7.5 mg., guaifenesin 50 mg.

DONATUSSIN DROPS ℞

Composition: Each ml. of orange syrup contains: chlorpheniramine maleate 1 mg., phenylephrine hydrochloride 2 mg., guaifenesin 20 mg.

KIE® SYRUP ℞

Composition: Each 5 ml. (teaspoonful) of green syrup contains: potassium iodide 150 mg., ephedrine hydrochloride 8 mg.

RESPAIRE-SR CAPSULES ℞

Composition: Each sustained - release RESPAIRE-SR Capsule (opaque orange and clear capsule with white and orange pellets) contains pseudoephedrine hydrochloride 120 mg. and guaifenesin 250 mg.

THEOSPAN® -SR CAPSULES 65 mg. ℞
(theophylline anhydrous USP)

THEOSPAN® -SR CAPSULES 130 mg. ℞
(theophylline anhydrous USP)

THEOSPAN® -SR CAPSULES 260 mg. ℞
(theophylline anhydrous USP)

Composition: Each sustained-release THEOSPAN-SR Capsule 65 mg. (dye-free, white and clear capsule with white pellets) contains theophylline anhydrous USP 65 mg. Each sustained-release THEOSPAN-SR Capsule 130 mg. (white and clear capsule with orange and white pellets) contains theophylline anhydrous USP 130 mg. Each sustained-release THEOSPAN-SR Capsule 260 mg. (dye-free, white and clear capsule with white pellets) contains theophylline anhydrous USP 260 mg.

THEOSTAT® 80 SYRUP ℞
(theophylline anhydrous USP)

THEOSTAT® TABLETS, 100 mg. ℞
(theophylline anhydrous USP)

THEOSTAT® TABLETS, 200 mg. ℞
(theophylline anhydrous USP)

Composition: Each 15 ml. (tablespoonful) of dye-free THEOSTAT Syrup contains theophylline anhydrous USP 80 mg., alcohol 1%. Each

Continued on next page

Laser—Cont.

white, dye-free, quad-scored THEOSTAT Tablet, 100 mg. contains theophylline anhydrous USP 100 mg. Each white, dye-free, quad-scored THEOSTAT Tablet, 200 mg. contains theophylline anhydrous USP 200 mg.

TRIMSTAT® TABLETS Ⓒ℞
(phendimetrazine tartrate)

Composition: Each tan tablet contains: phendimetrazine tartrate 35 mg.

Lederle Laboratories

A Division of American Cyanamid Co.
ONE CYANAMID PLAZA
WAYNE, NJ 07470

Lederle Parenterals, Inc.

CAROLINA, PUERTO RICO 00630

Lederle Piperacillin, Inc.

CAROLINA, PUERTO RICO 00630

LEDERMARK™ Product Identification Code

To provide quick and positive identification of Lederle products, we have imprinted an alphanumeric code on the tablet and capsule products. In order that you may quickly identify a product by its code, following is an alphanumeric list of LEDERMARK codes with their corresponding product names.

A1 ARISTOCORT® Tabs., 1 mg.
A2 ARISTOCORT® Tabs., 2 mg.
A3 ACHROMYCIN® V Caps., 250 mg.
A4 ARISTOCORT® Tabs., 4 mg.
A4 ARISTO-PAK® Tabs., 4 mg.
A5 ACHROMYCIN® V Caps., 500 mg.
A8 ARISTOCORT® Tabs., 8 mg.
A9 ARTANE® SEQUELS®, 5 mg.
A10 AMICAR® Tabs., 500 mg.
A11 ARTANE® Tabs., 2 mg.
A12 ARTANE® Tabs., 5 mg.
A15 ASENDIN® Tabs., 50 mg.
A16 ARISTOCORT® Tabs., 16 mg.
A17 ASENDIN® Tabs., 100 mg.
A18 ASENDIN® Tabs., 150 mg.
A20 Acetaminophen Caps., 500 mg.
A21 Acetaminophen Tabs., USP, 325 mg.
A23 Acetaminophen w/Codeine Tabs., 30 mg.
A24 Amitriptyline HCl Tabs., USP, 10 mg.
A25 Amitriptyline HCl Tabs., USP, 25 mg.
A26 Amitriptyline HCl Tabs., USP, 50 mg.
A27 Amitriptyline HCl Tabs., USP, 75 mg.
A28 Amitriptyline HCl Tabs., USP, 100 mg.
A31 Ampicillin Trihydrate Caps., USP, 250 mg.
A32 Ampicillin Trihydrate Caps., USP, 500 mg.
A36 Ascorbic Acid Tabs., USP, 250 mg.
A37 Ascorbic Acid Tabs., USP, 500 mg.
A38 Ascorbic Acid Tabs., USP, 1000 mg.
B6 Butalbital with APC Tabs.
C1 CENTRUM®, Advanced Formula
C2 CENTRUM,® JR.
C7 Chlorthalidone Tabs., USP, 25 mg.
C9 Chlordiazepoxide HCl Caps., USP, 5 mg.
C10 Chlordiazepoxide HCl Caps., USP, 10 mg.
C11 Chlordiazepoxide HCl Caps., USP, 25 mg.
C13 Chlorothiazide Tabs., USP, 250 mg.
C14 Chlorothiazide Tabs., USP, 500 mg.
C15 Chlorthalidone Tabs., USP, 50 mg.
C16 Chlorpheniramine Maleate Tabs., USP, 4 mg.
C17 Chlorpheniramine Maleate T.D. Caps., 8 mg.
C18 Chlorpheniramine Maleate T.D. Caps., 12 mg.
C19 Chlorzoxazone w/Acetaminophen Tabs., 250 mg./300 mg.
C22 Chlorpromazine HCl Tabs., USP, 25 mg.
C23 Chlorpromazine HCl Tabs., USP, 50 mg.
C24 Chlorpromazine HCl Tabs., USP, 100 mg.
C25 Chlorpromazine HCl Tabs., USP, 200 mg.
C30 Cloxacillin Sodium Caps., USP, 250 mg.
C31 Cloxacillin Sodium Caps., USP, 500 mg.
D1 DIAMOX® Tabs., 125 mg.
D2 DIAMOX® Tabs., 250 mg.
D3 DIAMOX® SEQUELS® 500 mg.
D9 DECLOMYCIN® Caps., 150 mg.
D11 DECLOMYCIN® Tabs., 150 mg.
D12 DECLOMYCIN® Tabs., 300 mg.
D22 Doxycycline Hyclate Caps., USP, 50 mg.
D23 Dicyclomine HCl Caps, USP, 10 mg.
D24 Dicyclomine HCl Tabs., USP, 20 mg.
D25 Doxycycline Hyclate Caps., USP, 100 mg.
D27 Ergoloid Mesylates Sublingual Tabs., 0.5 mg. (Dihydroergotoxine Methanesulfonate)
D28 Ergoloid Mesylates Sublingual Tabs., 1.0 mg. (Dihydroergotoxine Methanesulfonate)
D29 Dexbrompheniramine Maleate NF w/pseudoephedrine Sulfate Tabs., 6 mg./120 mg.
D31 Diphenoxylate HCl 2.5 mg. and Atropine Sulfate 0.025 mg. Tabs., USP
D32 Docusate Sodium (DSS), USP, Caps., 100 mg.
D33 Docusate Sodium (DSS), USP, Caps., 250 mg.
D34 Docusate Sodium (DSS), 100 mg., USP, w/Casanthranol 30 mg., Caps.
D35 DOLENE® AP-65 Tabs.
D36 DOLENE® Caps., USP, 65 mg.
D37 DOLENE® Compound-65 Caps.
D38 Diphenhydramine HCl Caps., USP, 25 mg.
D39 Diphenhydramine HCl Caps., USP, 50 mg.
D44 Dipyridamole Tabs., 25 mg.
E2 Erythromycin Stearate Tabs., USP, 250 mg.
E3 Ergoloid Mesylates Tabs., oral, 1.0 mg.
E5 Erythromycin Stearate Tabs., USP, 500 mg.
F1 FOLVITE® Tabs., 1 mg.
F2 FERRO-SEQUELS®
F4 FILIBON® Tabs.
F5 FILIBON® F.A. Tabs.
F6 FILIBON® FORTE Tabs.
F7 FILIBON® OT Tabs.
F8 FOLBESYN® Tabs.
F10 FOLVRON® Caps.
F11 Furosemide Tabs., USP, 20 mg.
F12 Furosemide Tabs., USP, 40 mg.
F20 Ferrous Sulfate Tabs., USP, 300 mg.
F21 Ferrous Gluconate Iron Supplment Tabs., USP, 300 mg.
G1 GEVRAL® Tabs.
G2 GEVRAL® T Tabs.
G4 GEVRITE® Tabs.
H1 HYDROMOX® Tabs., 50 mg.
H2 HYDROMOX® R Tabs.
H11 Hydralazine HCl Tabs., USP, 25 mg.
H12 Hydralazine HCl Tabs., USP, 50 mg.
H14 Hydrochlorothiazide Tabs., USP, 25 mg.
H15 Hydrochlorothiazide Tabs., USP, 50 mg.
H22 Reserpine 0.1 mg. Hydrochlorothiazide 15 mg. Hydralazine HCl 25 mg. (Formerly R-HCTZ-H™)
I11 Imipramine HCl Tabs., USP, 10 mg.
I12 Imipramine HCl Tabs., USP, 25 mg.
I13 Imipramine HCl Tabs., USP, 50 mg.
I15 Isosorbide Dinitrate Tabs., 5 mg.
I16 Isosorbide Dinitrate Tabs., 10 mg.
I17 Isosorbide Dinitrate Tab., USP, 2.5 mg. Sublingual
I18 Isosorbide Dinitrate Tabs., USP, 5 mg. Sublingual
I21 Isoxsuprine HCl Tabs., USP, 10 mg.
I22 Isoxsuprine HCl Tabs., USP, 20 mg.
L1 LOXITANE® Caps., 5 mg.
L2 LOXITANE® Caps., 10 mg.
L3 LOXITANE® Caps., 25 mg.
L4 LOXITANE® Caps., 50 mg.
L6 LEDERPLEX® Caps.
L7 LEDERPLEX® Tabs.
L9 LEDERCILLIN® VK Tabs., USP, 500 mg.
L10 LEDERCILLIN® VK Tabs., USP, 250 mg.
L11 Levothyroxine Sodium Tabs., USP, 0.1 mg.
L12 Levothyroxine Sodium Tabs., USP, 0.2 mg.
L13 Levothyroxine Sodium Tabs., USP, 0.3 mg.
L15 Brompheniramine maleate 12 mg., phenylephrine HCl 15 mg., and phenylpropanolamine 15 mg. SEQUELS® Sustained Release Tablets (Formerly LEDER-BP™ SEQUELS®)
M1 Methotrexate Tabs., 2.5 mg.
M2 MINOCIN® Caps, 50 mg.
M3 MINOCIN® Tabs., 50 mg.
M4 MINOCIN® Caps, 100 mg.
M5 MINOCIN® Tabs., 100 mg.
M6 MYAMBUTOL® Tabs., 100 mg.
M7 MYAMBUTOL® Tabs., 400 mg.
M10 MATERNA® 1· 60 Tabs.
M12 Meclizine HCl Tabs., USP, 12.5 mg.
M13 Meclizine HCl Tabs., USP, 25 mg.
M19 Methocarbamol Tabs., USP, 500 mg.
M20 Methocarbamol Tabs., USP, 750 mg.
N1 NEPTAZANE® Tabs., 50 mg.
N5 NILSTAT® Oral Tabs.
N6 NILSTAT® Vaginal Tabs.
N10 Neomycin Sulfate Tabs., USP, 500 mg.
N20 Nitroglycerin T.D. Caps., 2.5 mg.
N21 Nitroglycerin T.D. Caps., 6.5 mg.
N23 Nylidrin HCl Tabs., USP, 6 mg.
N24 Nylidrin HCl Tabs., USP, 12 mg.
P1 PATHIBAMATE® 200 Tabs.
P2 PATHIBAMATE® 400 Tabs.
P3 PATHILON® SEQUELS®, 75 mg.
P7 PERIHEMIN® Caps.
P8 PERITINIC® Tabs.
P9 PRONEMIA® Caps.
P11 Papaverine HCl Time Release Caps., 150 mg.
P13 Papaverine HCl Tabs., USP, 100 mg.
P17 Penicillin G Potassium Tabs., USP, 400,000 Units
P19 Pyridoxine HCl (Vitamin B-6) Tabs., USP, 100 mg.
P21 Phenobarbital Tabs., USP, 30 mg.
P24 Prednisone Tabs., USP, 5 mg.
P25 Probenecid Tabs., USP, 500 mg.
P26 Probenecid with Colchicine Tabs., 500 mg./0.5 mg.
P29 Procainamide HCl Caps., USP, 250 mg.
P30 Procainamide HCl Caps., USP, 375 mg.
P31 Procainamide HCl Caps., USP, 500 mg.
P32 Propantheline Bromide Tabs., USP, 15 mg.
P33 Propylthiouracil Tabs., USP, 50 mg.
P34 Pseudoephedrine HCl Tabs., USP, 60 mg.
P35 Pseudoephedrine HCl Tabs., USP, 30 mg.
P36 Pyrazinamide Tabs., 500 mg.
P37 Pyridoxine HCl (Vitamin B-6) Tabs., USP, 25 mg.
P38 Pyridoxine HCl (Vitamin B-6) Tabs., USP, 50 mg.

Q11	Quinidine Sulfate Tabs., USP, 200 mg.
Q15	Quinine Sulfate Caps., USP, 325 mg.
S1	STRESSTABS® 600, Advanced Formula
S2	STRESSTABS® 600 w/Iron, Advanced Formula
S3	STRESSTABS® 600 w/Zinc, Advanced Formula
S5	STRESSCAPS®
S12	Spironolactone with Hydrochlorothiazide Tabs., 25 mg/25 mg.
S13	Spironolactone Tabs., USP, 25 mg.
S14	Sulfasalazine Tabs., 0.5 Gram
S15	Sulfisoxazole Tabs., USP, 500 mg.
T1	TriHEMIC® 600 Tabs.
T11	Thiamine HCl (Vitamin B-1) Tabs., 50 mg.
T12	Thiamine HCl (Vitamin B-1) Tabs., 100 mg.
T14	Thyroid Tabs., USP, 60 mg.
T17	Tolbutamide Tabs., USP, 500 mg.
T21	Triple Sulfas (Trisulfapyrimidines USP) Tabs.
T23	Triprolidine HCl and Pseudoephedrine HCl Tabs., 2.5 mg./60 mg.
V3	VI-MAGNA® Caps.
V11	Vitamin A Caps., Natural USP, 25,000 I.U.
V14	Vitamin C Chewable Tabs., 250 mg.
V15	Vitamin C Chewable Tabs., 500 mg.
V19	Vitamin E Caps., Natural, USP, 400 I.U.
V21	Vitamin E Caps., USP., 200 I.U.
V22	Vitamin E Caps., USP., 400 I.U.
V23	Vitamin E Caps., USP, 600 I.U.
V24	Vitamin E Caps., USP, 1,000 I.U.

LEDERLE STANDARD PRODUCTS

PRODUCT IDENTITY CODE NO.	PRODUCT
—	Acetaminophen Elixir, USP, 120mg/5ml
A20	Acetaminophen Capsules, USP, 500mg
A21	Acetaminophen Tablets, USP, 325mg
A23	Acetaminophen w/Codeine Tablets, 30mg
A24	Amitriptyline HCl Tablets, USP, 10mg
A25	Amitriptyline HCl Tablets, USP, 25mg
A26	Amitriptyline HCl Tablets, USP, 50mg
A27	Amitriptyline HCl Tablets, USP, 75mg
A28	Amitriptyline HCl Tablets, USP, 100mg
A31	Ampicillin Trihydrate Capsules, 250mg
A32	Ampicillin Trihydrate Capsules, 500mg
—	Ampicillin Trihydrate for Oral Suspension, 125mg/5ml
—	Ampicillin Trihydrate for Oral Suspension, 250mg/5ml
A36	Ascorbic Acid Tablets, USP, 250mg
A37	Ascorbic Acid Tablets, USP, 500mg
A38	Ascorbic Acid Tablets, USP, 1,000mg
—	Brompheniramine Compound Elixir
L15	Brompheniramine Maleate, N.F., 12 mg, Phenylephrine HCl 15 mg, and Phenylpropanolamine HCl 15 mg SEQUELS® Sustained Release Tablets (Formerly LEDER-BP™ SEQUELS®)
—	Brompheniramine Maleate With Codeine, D.C., Expectorant
B 6	Butalbital w/APC Tablets
C 9	Chlordiazepoxide HCl Capsules, USP, 5mg
C10	Chlordiazepoxide HCl Capsules, USP, 10mg
C11	Chlordiazepoxide HCl Capsules, USP, 25mg
C13	Chlorothiazide Tablets, USP 250mg
C14	Chlorothiazide Tablets, USP 500mg
C16	Chlorpheniramine Maleate Tablets, USP, 4mg
C17	Chlorpheniramine Maleate T.D. Capsules, 8mg
C18	Chlorpheniramine Maleate T.D. Capsules, 12 mg
C22	Chlorpromazine HCl Tablets, 25mg
C23	Chlorpromazine HCl Tablets, 50mg
C24	Chlorpromazine HCl Tablets, 100 mg
C25	Chlorpromazine HCl Tablets, 200 mg
—	Chlorpromazine HCl Liquid Concentrate 100mg/ml
C 7	Chlorthalidone Tablets, 25mg
C15	Chlorthalidone Tablets, 50mg
C19	Chlorzoxazone w/Acetaminophen Tablets 250mg/300mg
C30	Cloxacillin Sodium Capsules, 250 mg
C31	Cloxacillin Sodium Capsules, 500 mg
D29	Dexbrompheniramine Maleate, USP, and Pseudoephedrine Sulfate SEQUELS® P.A., 6mg/120 mg
D23	Dicyclomine HCl Capsules, USP, 10mg
D24	Dicyclomine HCl Tablets, USP, 20mg
D38	Diphenhydramine HCl Capsules, USP, 25mg
D39	Diphenhydramine HCl Capsules, USP, 50mg
—	Diphenhydramine HCl Elixir, USP, 12.5mg/5ml
—	Diphenhydramine HCl Cough Syrup, 12.5 mg/5ml
D31	Diphenoxylate HCl 2.5mg + Atropine Sulfate 0.025mg Tablets, USP
D44	Dipyridamole Tablets, 25mg
D32	Docusate Sodium, USP, Capsules, 100mg
D33	Docusate Sodium, USP, Capsules, 250mg
D34	Docusate Sodium, 100mg, w/Casanthranol, 30mg, Capsules
—	Docusate Sodium Syrup, N.F., 20mg/5ml
—	Docusate Sodium Syrup, 60mg/15ml, w/Casanthranol, 30 mg /15 ml
D36	DOLENE®, Propoxyphene HCl, Plain, 65mg
D35	DOLENE®, Propoxyphene HCl, AP-65
D37	DOLENE®, Compound 65 Capsules
D22	Doxycycline Hyclate Capsules, 50 mg
D25	Doxycycline Hyclate Capsules, 100 mg
D27	Ergoloid Mesylates Tablets, Sublingual, 0.5mg
D28	Ergoloid Mesylates Tablets, Sublingual, 1.0mg
E 3	Ergoloid Mesylates Tablets, Oral 1mg
E 2	Erythromycin Stearate Tablets, USP, 250mg
E 5	Erythromycin Stearate Tablets, USP, 500mg
—	Erythromycin Ethylsuccinate Oral Suspension, 200mg/5ml
—	Erythromycin Ethylsuccinate Oral Suspension, 400mg/5ml
F21	Ferrous Gluconate Iron Supplement Tabs., N.F., 300mg
—	Ferrous Sulfate Elixir, 220mg/5ml
F20	Ferrous Sulfate Tablets, USP, 300mg
F11	Furosemide Tablets, USP, 20mg
F12	Furosemide Tablets, USP, 40mg
—	Guaifenesin Syrup, N.F., 100mg/5ml
—	Guaifenesin, 100mg, w/D-Methorphan Hydrobromide Syrup, 15 mg/5ml
H11	Hydralazine HCl Tablets, USP, 25 mg
H12	Hydralazine HCl Tablets, USP, 50 mg
H14	Hydrochlorothiazide Tablets, USP, 25mg
H15	Hydrochlorothiazide Tablets, USP, 50mg
I11	Imipramine HCl Tablets, USP, 10mg
I12	Imipramine HCl Tablets, USP, 25mg
I13	Imipramine HCl Tablets, USP, 50mg
I15	Isosorbide Dinitrate Tablets, oral, 5mg
I16	Isosorbide Dinitrate Tablets, oral, 10mg
I17	Isosorbide Dinitrate Tablets, Sublingual, 2.5mg
I18	Isorsorbide Dinitrate Tablets, Sublingual, 5.0mg
I21	Isoxsuprine HCl Tablets, USP, 10mg
I22	Isoxsuprine HCl Tablets, USP, 20mg
—	LEDERCILLIN® VK, for Oral Solution, 125mg/5ml
—	LEDERCILLIN® VK, for Oral Solution, 250mg/5ml
L10	LEDERCILLIN® VK, USP, Tablets, 250mg
L 9	LEDERCILLIN® VK, USP, Tablets, 500mg
L11	Levothyroxine Sodium Tabs., USP, 0.1mg
L12	Levothyroxine Sodium Tabs., USP, 0.2mg
L13	Levothyroxine Sodium Tabs., USP, 0.3mg
M12	Meclizine HCl Tablets, USP, 12.5mg
M13	Meclizine HCl Tablets, USP, 25mg
—	Methenamine Mandelate Suspension, 500mg/5ml
M19	Methocarbamol Tablets, N.F., 500mg
M20	Methocarbamol Tablets, N.F., 750mg
N10	Neomycin Sulfate Tablets, USP, 500mg
N20	Nitroglycerin T.D. Capsules, 2.5mg
N21	Nitroglycerin T.D. Capsules, 6.5mg
N23	Nylidrin HCl Tablets, N.F., 6mg
N24	Nylidrin HCl Tablets, N.F., 12mg
P11	Papaverine HCl T.R. Capsules, 150mg
P13	Papaverine HCl Capsules, 100mg
P17	Penicillin G Potassium Tablets, USP, 400,000 Units
P21	Phenobarbital Tablets, USP, 30mg (½ gr)
—	Potassium Chloride Liquid 10%
—	Potassium Chloride Liquid 20%
—	Potassium Gluconate Elixir, N.F., 4.68gm/15ml

Continued on next page

The information on each product appearing here is based on labelling effective in August, 1982 and is either the entire official brochure or an accurate condensation therefrom. Offical brochures are enclosed in product packages. Information concerning all Lederle products may be obtained from the Professional Services Department, Lederle Laboratories, Pearl River, New York, 10965.

Lederle—Cont.

P24	Prednisone Tablets, 5mg
P25	Probenecid Tablets, USP, 500mg
P26	Probenecid w/Colchicine Tablets, 500 mg/0.5 mg
P29	Procainamide HCl Capsules, USP, 250mg
P30	Procainamide HCl Capsules, USP, 375mg
P31	Procainamide HCl Capsules, USP, 500mg
—	Promethazine HCl Expectorant, Plain, 5mg/5ml
—	Promethazine HCl Expectorant w/Codeine, 10mg/5ml
—	Promethazine HCl Expectorant VC w/Codeine, 10mg/5ml
—	Promethazine HCl Expectorant VC, Plain
P32	Propantheline Bromide Tablets, USP, 15 mg
P33	Propylthiouracil Tablets, USP, 50 mg
—	Pseudoephedrine HCl N.F. Syrup, 30mg/5ml
P35	Pseudoephedrine HCl Tablets, 30mg
P34	Pseudoephedrine HCl Tablets, 60 mg
P36	Pyrazinamide Tablets, 500mg
P37	Pyridoxine HCl (Vitamin B-6) Tablets, USP, 25mg
P38	Pyridoxine HCl (Vitamin B-6) Tablets, USP, 50mg
P19	Pyridoxine HCl (Vitamin B-6) Tablets, USP, 100mg
Q11	Quinidine Sulfate Tablets, USP, 200mg
Q15	Quinine Sulfate Capsules, USP, 325mg
H22	Reserpine 0.1mg, Hydrochlorthiazide 15mg and Hydralazine HCl 25mg Combination Tablets
S12	Spironolactone/Hydrochlorothiazide Tablets, 25 mg/25mg
S13	Spironolactone Tablets, 25mg
S14	Sulfasalazine Tablets, 0.5gm
S15	Sulfisoxazole Tablets, USP, 500mg
T11	Thiamine HCl (Vitamin B-1) Tablets, 50mg
T12	Thiamine HCl (Vitamin B-1) Tablets, 100mg
T14	Thyroid Tablets, USP, 60mg
T17	Tolbutamide Tablets USP, 500mg
—	Triprolidine HCl with Pseudoephedrine HCl Syrup 1.25mg/30mg per 5ml
T23	Triprolidine HCl with Pseudoephedrine HCl Tablets 2.5mg/60mg
—	Trisulfapyrimidines (Triple Sulfas) USP, Suspension
T21	Trisulfapyrimidines (Triple Sulfas) USP, Tablets
V11	Vitamin A Capsules, Natural, USP, 25,000 I.U.
V14	Vitamin C Chewable Tablets, 250mg
V15	Vitamin C Chewable Tablets, 500mg
V19	Vitamin E Capsules, Natural, N.F., 400 I.U.
V21	Vitamin E Capsules, N.F., 200 I.U.
V22	Vitamin E Capsules, N.F., 400 I.U.
V23	Vitamin E Capsules, N.F., 600 I.U.
V24	Vitamin E Capsules, N.F., 1000 I.U.

ACHROMYCIN® V ℞
tetracycline HCl
Capsules and Oral Suspension
ACHROMYCIN Intramuscular
ACHROMYCIN Intravenous

Description: ACHROMYCIN *tetracycline HCl* is an antibiotic isolated from *Streptomyces aureofaciens.* Chemically it is the hydrochloride of 4-dimethylamino-1,4,4a,5,5a,6,11, 12a-octahydro-3, 6, 10, 12, 12a-pentahydroxy-6-methyl-1, 11-dioxo-2-naphthacenecarboxamide.

Actions: The tetracyclines are primarily bacteriostatic and are thought to exert their antimicrobial effect by the inhibition of protein synthesis. Tetracyclines are active against a wide range of gram-negative and gram-positive organisms.

The drugs in the tetracycline class have closely similar antimicrobial spectra, and cross-resistance among them is common. Microorganisms may be considered susceptible if the M.I.C. (minimum inhibitory concentration) is not more than 4.0 mcg./ml. and intermediate if the M.I.C. is 4.0 to 12.5 mcg./ml.

Susceptibility plate testing: A tetracycline disc may be used to determine microbial susceptibility to drugs in the tetracycline class. If the Kirby-Bauer method of disc susceptibility testing is used, a 30 mcg. tetracycline HCl disc should give a zone of at least 19 mm. when tested against a tetracycline-susceptible bacterial strain.

Tetracyclines are readily absorbed and are bound to plasma proteins in varying degree. They are concentrated by the liver in the bile and excreted in the urine and feces at high concentrations and in a biologically active form.

Indications: ACHROMYCIN *tetracycline HCl* is indicated in infections caused by the following micro-organisms:

Rickettsiae: (Rocky Mountain spotted fever, typhus fever and the typhus group, Q fever, rickettsialpox, tick fevers.)
Mycoplasma pneumoniae (PPLO, Eaton agent).
Agents of psittacosis and ornithosis.
Agents of lymphogranuloma venereum and granuloma inguinale.
The spirochetal agent of relapsing fever *(Borrelia recurrentis).*
The following gram-negative micro-organisms:
Haemophilus ducreyi (chancroid),
Pasteurella pestis and *Pasteurella tularensis,*
Bartonella bacilliformis,
Bacteroides species,
Vibrio comma and *Vibrio fetus.*
Brucella species (in conjunction with streptomycin).

Because many strains of the following groups of micro-organisms have been shown to be resistant to tetracyclines, culture and susceptibility testing are recommended.

Tetracycline is indicated for treatment of infections caused by the following gram-negative micro-organisms, when bacteriologic testing indicates appropriate susceptibility to the drug:

Escherichia coli,
Enterobacter aerogenes (formerly *Aerobacter aerogenes*),
Shigella species,
Mima species and *Herellea* species,
Haemophilus influenzae (respiratory infections),
Klebsiella species (respiratory and urinary infections).

Tetracycline is indicated for treatment of infections caused by the following gram-positive micro-organisms when bacteriologic testing indicates appropriate susceptibility to the drug:

Streptococcus species:

Up to 44 percent of strains of *Streptococcus pyogenes* and 74 percent of *Streptococcus faecalis* have been found to be resistant to tetracycline drugs. Therefore, tetracyclines should not be used for streptococcal disease unless the organism has been demonstrated to be sensitive.

For upper respiratory infections due to group A beta-hemolytic streptococci, penicillin is the usual drug of choice, including prophylaxis of rheumatic fever.

Diplococcus pneumoniae,
Staphylococcus aureus, skin and soft tissue infections. Tetracyclines are not the drug of choice in the treatment of any type of staphylococcal infection.

When penicillin is contraindicated, tetracyclines are alternative drugs in the treatment of infections due to:

Neisseria gonorrhoeae,
Neisseria meningitidis (IV only)
Treponema pallidum and *Treponema pertenue* (syphilis and yaws),
Listeria monocytogenes,
Clostridium species,
Bacillus anthracis,
Fusobacterium fusiforme (Vincent's infection),
Actinomyces species.

In acute intestinal amebiasis, the tetracyclines may be a useful adjunct to amebicides.

In severe acne, the tetracyclines may be useful adjunctive therapy. (This indication is for the Oral Use only. Not for IM or IV.)

Tetracyclines are indicated in the treatment of trachoma, although the infectious agent is not always eliminated, as judged by immunofluorescence.

Inclusion conjunctivitis may be treated with oral tetracyclines or with a combination of oral and topical agents.

Contraindications: This drug is contraindicated in persons who have shown hypersensitivity to any of the tetracyclines.

Warnings: In the presence of renal dysfunction, particularly in pregnancy, intravenous tetracycline therapy in daily doses exceeding 2 grams has been associated with deaths through liver failure.

When the need for intensive treatment outweighs its potential dangers (mostly during pregnancy or in individuals with known or suspected renal or liver impairment), it is advisable to perform renal and liver function tests before and during therapy. Also tetracycline serum concentrations should be followed.

If renal impairment exists, even usual oral or parenteral doses may lead to excessive systemic accumulation of the drug and possible liver toxicity. Under such conditions, lower than usual total doses are indicated, and if therapy is prolonged, serum level determinations of the drug may be advisable. This hazard is of particular importance in the parenteral administration of tetracyclines to pregnant or postpartum patients with pyelonephritis. When used under these circumstances, the blood level should not exceed 15 micrograms/ml. and liver function tests should be made at frequent intervals. Other potentially hepatotoxic drugs should not be prescribed concomitantly.

THE USE OF DRUGS OF THE TETRACYCLINE CLASS DURING TOOTH DEVELOPMENT (LAST HALF OF PREGNANCY, INFANCY, AND CHILDHOOD TO THE AGE OF 8 YEARS) MAY CAUSE PERMANENT DISCOLORATION OF THE TEETH (YELLOW-GRAY-BROWN). This adverse reaction is more common during long-term use of the drugs but has been observed following repeated short-term courses. Enamel hypoplasia has also been reported. TETRACYCLINES, THEREFORE, SHOULD NOT BE USED IN THIS AGE GROUP UNLESS OTHER DRUGS ARE NOT LIKELY TO BE EFFECTIVE OR ARE CONTRAINDICATED.

Photosensitivity manifested by an exaggerated sunburn reaction has been observed in some individuals taking tetracyclines. Patients apt to be exposed to direct sunlight or ultraviolet light should be advised that this reaction can occur with tetracycline drugs, and treatment should be discontinued at the first evidence of skin erythema.

The antianabolic action of the tetracyclines may cause an increase in BUN. While this is not a problem in those with normal renal function, in patients with significantly impaired function, higher serum levels of tetracycline may lead to azotemia, hyperphosphatemia, and acidosis.

Usage in pregnancy: (See above "Warnings" about use during tooth development.)

Results of animal studies indicate that tetracyclines cross the placenta, are found in fetal tissues and can have toxic effects on the developing fetus (often related to retardation of skeletal development). Evidence of embryotoxicity has also been noted in animals treated early in pregnancy.

Usage in newborns, infants, and children: (See above "Warnings" about use during tooth development.)

All tetracyclines form a stable calcium complex in any bone forming tissue. A decrease in the fibula growth rate has been observed in prematures given oral tetracycline in doses of 25 mg./kg. every 6 hours. This reaction was shown to be reversible when the drug was discontinued.

Tetracyclines are present in the milk of lactating women who are taking a drug in this class.

Precautions: As with other antibiotic preparations, use of this drug may result in overgrowth of nonsusceptible organisms, including fungi. If superinfection occurs, the antibiotic should be discontinued and appropriate therapy instituted.

In venereal diseases when coexistent syphilis is suspected, darkfield examination should be done before treatment is started and the blood serology repeated monthly for at least 4 months.

Because the tetracyclines have been shown to depress plasma prothrombin activity, patients who are on anticoagulant therapy may require downward adjustment of their anticoagulant dosage.

In long-term therapy, periodic laboratory evaluation of organ systems, including hematopoietic, renal and hepatic studies should be performed.

All infections due to Group A beta hemolytic streptococci should be treated for at least 10 days.

Since bacteriostatic drugs may interfere with the bactericidal action of penicillin, it is advisable to avoid giving tetracycline in conjunction with penicillin.

Adverse Reactions: Local irritation may be present after intramuscular injection. The injection should be deep, with care taken not to injure the sciatic nerve nor inject intravascularly.

Gastrointestinal: Anorexia, nausea, vomiting, diarrhea, glossitis, dysphagia, enterocolitis, and inflammatory lesions (with monilial overgrowth) in the anogenital region. These reactions have been caused by both the oral and parenteral administration of tetracyclines.

Skin: Maculopapular and erythematous rashes. Exfoliative dermatitis has been reported but is uncommon. Photosensitivity is discussed above. (See "Warnings".)

Renal toxicity: Rise in BUN has been reported and is apparently dose related. (See "Warnings".)

Hypersensitivity reactions: Urticaria, angioneurotic edema, anaphylaxis, anaphylactoid purpura, pericarditis and exacerbation of systemic lupus erythematosus.

Bulging fontanels have been reported in young infants following full therapeutic dosage. This sign disappeared rapidly when the drug was discontinued.

Blood: Hemolytic anemia, thrombocytopenia, neutropenia and eosinophilia have been reported.

When given over prolonged periods, tetracyclines have been reported to produce brown-black microscopic discoloration of thyroid glands. No abnormalities of thyroid function studies are known to occur.

ORAL FORMS:

Dosage and Administration: Therapy should be continued for at least 24-48 hours after symptoms and fever have subsided.

Concomitant therapy: Antacids containing aluminum, calcium, or magnesium impair absorption and should not be given to patients taking oral tetracycline.

Foods and some dairy products also interfere with absorption. Oral forms of tetracycline should be given 1 hour before or 2 hours after meals. Pediatric oral dosage forms should not be given with milk formulas and should be given at least 1 hour prior to feeding.

In patients with renal impairment: (See "Warnings".) Total dosage should be decreased by reduction of recommended individual doses and/or by extending time intervals between doses.

In the treatment of streptococcal infections, a therapeutic dose of tetracycline should be administered for at least 10 days.

Adults: Usual daily dose, 1-2 Grams divided in two or four equal doses, depending on the severity of the infection.

For children above eight years of age: Usual daily dose, 10-20 mg. (25-50 mg./kg.) per pound of body weight divided in two or four equal doses.

For treatment of brucellosis, 500 mg. tetracycline four times daily for 3 weeks should be accompanied by streptomycin, 1 gram intramuscularly twice daily the first week and once daily the second week.

For treatment of syphilis, a total of 30-40 grams in equally divided doses over a period of 10-15 days should be given. Close followup, including laboratory tests, is recommended.

Gonorrhea patients sensitive to penicillin may be treated with tetracycline, administered as an initial oral dose of 1.5 grams followed by 0.5 grams every 6 hours for 4 days to a total dosage of 9 grams.

INTRAMUSCULAR:

Preparation of Solution: Add 2 ml. of Sterile Water for Injection U.S.P. (or Sodium Chloride Injection U.S.P.) to the 100 mg. or 250 mg. vial. The resulting solution may be stored at room temperature and should not be used after 24 hours.

Dosage and Administration:

Intramuscular administration, Adults: The usual daily dose is 250 mg. administered once every 24 hours or 300 mg. given in divided doses at 8-to 12-hour intervals.

For children above eight years of age: 15-25 mg./kg. body weight up to a maximum of 250 mg. per single daily injection. Dosage may be divided and given at 8- to 12-hour intervals.

Gonorrhea patients sensitive to penicillin may be treated with tetracycline administered as an initial oral dose of 1.5 grams followed by 0.5 grams every 6 hours for 4 days, a total dosage of 9 grams. Intramuscular therapy should be reserved for situations in which oral therapy is not feasible.

In patients with renal impairment: (See "Warnings".)

Total dosage should be decreased by reduction of recommended individual doses and/or by extending time intervals between doses.

The intramuscular administration of ACHROMYCIN *sterile tetracycline hydrochloride* produces lower blood levels than oral administration in the recommended dosages. Patients placed on intramuscular tetracyclines should be changed to the oral dosage form as soon as possible. If rapid, high blood levels are needed, ACHROMYCIN should be administered intravenously.

Administration: ACHROMYCIN Intramuscular should be injected deeply into a large muscle mass such as the gluteal region. Inadvertent injection into the subcutaneous or fat layers may cause pain and induration, which can be relieved by applying an ice pack.

INTRAVENOUS:

Preparation of Solution: The vials should be initially reconstituted by adding 5 ml. of Sterile Water for Injection to the 250 mg. vial and 10 ml. of Sterile Water for Injection to the 500 mg. vial, and then further diluted prior to administration to at least 100 ml. (up to 1000 ml.) with any of the following diluents:

Ringer's Injection, U.S.P.
Sodium Chloride Injection, U.S.P.
Dextrose Injection, U.S.P. (5% Dextrose in Sterile Water for Injection, U.S.P.)
Dextrose and Sodium Chloride Injection, U.S.P. (5% in Sodium Chloride Injection U.S.P.)
Lactated Ringer's Injection, U.S.P.
Protein Hydrolysate Injection, Low Sodium, U.S.P. 5%, 5% with Dextrose 5%, 5% with Invert Sugar 10%

The initial reconstituted solutions are stable at room temperature for twelve hours without significant loss of potency. The final dilution for administration should be administered immediately.

Note: The use of solutions containing calcium should be avoided as these tend to form precipitates (especially in neutral to alkaline solution) and, therefore, should not be used unless necessary. However, Ringer's Injection, U.S.P. and Lactated Ringer's Injection, U.S.P. can be used with caution since the calcium ion content in these diluents does not normally precipitate tetracycline in an acid media.

Dosage and Administration:

Note: Rapid administration is to be avoided. Parenteral therapy is indicated only when oral therapy is not adequate or tolerated. Oral therapy should be instituted as soon as possible. If intravenous therapy is given over prolonged periods of time, thrombophlebitis may result.

Adults: The usual adult dose: 250 to 500 mg. every 12 hours and should not exceed 500 mg. every 6 hours. The drug may be dissolved and then diluted in 100-1,000 ml. of Dextrose 5 percent in water, Isotonic Sodium Chloride Solution or Ringer's solution, but not in other solutions containing calcium (a precipitate may form).

For children above eight years of age: The usual dose: 12 mg./kg./day, divided into 2 doses, but from 10 to 20 mg./kg./day may be given, depending on the severity of the infection.

Gonorrhea patients sensitive to penicillin may be treated with tetracycline administered as an initial oral dose of 1.5 grams followed by 0.5 grams every 6 hours for 4 days, a total dosage of 9 grams. Intravenous therapy should be reserved for situations in which oral therapy is not feasible.

In patients with renal impairment: (See "Warnings".)

Total dosage should be decreased by reduction of recommended individual doses and/or by extending time intervals between doses.

How Supplied:

CAPSULES:

500 mg. Tetracycline HCl (hard shell yellow and blue) printed Lederle 500-A5 bottles of 100 and 1000. Unit Dose 10-10's, Unit of Issue 50 x 20's.

250 mg. Tetracycline HCl (hard shell yellow and blue) printed Lederle A3 bottles of 100, 1000, Unit Dose 10 x 10's, Unit of Issue 50 x 20, 28 and 40.

The information on each product appearing here is based on labelling effective in August, 1982 and is either the entire official brochure or an accurate condensation therefrom. Offical brochures are enclosed in product packages. Information concerning all Lederle products may be obtained from the Professional Services Department, Lederle Laboratories, Pearl River, New York, 10965.

Continued on next page

Lederle—Cont.

ORAL SUSPENSION:
Tetracycline equivalent to 125 mg. Tetracycline HCl per teaspoonful (5 ml.). Preserved with Methylparaben 0.12% and Propylparaben 0.03%. Cherry-flavored in bottles of 2 fl. oz. and 16 fl. oz.

INTRAMUSCULAR:

Sterile Tetracycline HCl	100 mg./vial	250 mg./vial
Procaine HCl	40 mg./vial	40 mg./vial
Magnesium Chloride	46.84 mg./vial	46.84 mg./vial
Ascorbic Acid	250 mg./vial	275 mg./vial
	packages of 1 and 100 vials.	packages of 1 and 100 vials.

INTRAVENOUS:
Sterile Tetracycline HCl 250 mg. with 625 mg. ascorbic acid/vial.
Sterile Tetracycline HCl 500 mg. with 1250 mg. ascorbic acid/vial.

A.H.F.S. 8:12.24

ACHROMYCIN® V Capsules, 250 mg
Military Depot: NSN 6505-00-117-8544, 40's

[*Capsules shown in Product Identification Section*]

ACHROMYCIN®
tetracycline

is also supplied in a number of other dosage forms and combinations for special purposes (for details of indications, dosage, administration and precautions, see circular in package.)

ACHROMYCIN ℞
tetracycline HCl
Ophthalmic Ointment 1% (sterile)
1/8 oz. tube

ACHROMYCIN
tetracycline HCl
3% Ointment
(For topical use)—1/2 and 1 oz. tubes. ℞ not required.

ACHROMYCIN ℞
tetracycline HCl
Ophthalmic Suspension 1% (sterile)
4 ml. plastic dropper bottle.

AMICAR® ℞
aminocaproic acid
Intravenous, Syrup, and Tablets

Description: AMICAR *aminocaproic acid Lederle* is a monaminocarboxylic acid which acts as an effective inhibitor of fibrinolysis.

Actions: The beneficial fibrinolysis-inhibitory effects of AMICAR appear to be principally via inhibition of plasminogen activator substances and, to a lesser degree, through antiplasmin activity. The drug is absorbed rapidly following oral administration. Whether administered by the oral or intravenous route, a major portion of the compound is recovered unmetabolized in the urine. The renal clearance of AMICAR is high (about 75 percent of the creatinine clearance). Thus the drug is excreted rapidly. After prolonged administration, AMICAR distributes throughout both the extravascular and intravascular compartments of the body and readily penetrates human red blood and other tissue cells.

Indications: AMICAR has proved useful, in many instances, in the treatment of excessive bleeding which results from *systemic hyperfibrinolysis and urinary fibrinolysis.* In life-threatening situations, fresh whole blood transfusions, fibrinogen infusions, and other emergency measures may be required.

Systemic hyperfibrinolysis, a pathological condition, may frequently be associated with *surgical complications* following heart surgery (with or without cardiac bypass procedures) and portacaval shunt; *hematological disorders* such as aplastic anemia, *abruptio placentae, hepatic cirrhosis, neoplastic disease* such as carcinoma of the prostate, lung, stomach, and cervix.

Urinary fibrinolysis, usually a normal physiological phenomenon, may frequently be associated with life-threatening complications following severe trauma, anoxia, and shock. Symptomatic of such complications is *surgical hematuria* (following prostatectomy and nephrectomy) or *non-surgical hematuria* (accompanying polycystic or neoplastic diseases of the genitourinary system).

Contraindications: AMICAR should not be used when there is evidence of an active intravascular clotting process.

Warnings: Safe use of AMICAR has not been established with respect to adverse effects upon fetal development. Therefore, it should not be used in women of childbearing potential and particularly during early pregnancy, unless in the judgment of the physician the potential benefits outweigh the possible hazards.

Precautions: AMICAR *aminocaproic acid* has a very specific action in that it inhibits both plasminogen activator substances and, to a lesser degree, plasmin activity. The drug should NOT be administered without a definite diagnosis, and/or laboratory findings indicative of hyperfibrinolysis (hyperplasminemia).*

The use of AMICAR should be accompanied by tests designed to determine the amount of fibrinolysis present. There are presently available (a) general tests, such as those for the determination of the lysis of a clot of blood or plasma and (b) more specific tests for the study of various phases of fibrinolytic mechanisms. These latter tests include both semi-quantitative and quantitative technics for the determination of profibrinolysin, fibrinolysin, and antifibrinolysin.

Animal experiments indicate particular caution should be taken in administering AMICAR to patients with cardiac, hepatic or renal diseases.

Demonstrable animal pathology in some cases have shown endocardial hemorrhages and myocardial fat degeneration. The use of this drug should thus be restricted to patients in whom the benefit hoped for would outweigh the hazard. Physicians are cautioned in the use of this product because of animal data showing rat teratogenicity and kidney concretions.

Rapid intravenous administration of the drug should be avoided since this may induce hypotension, bradycardia and/or arrhythmia.

One case of *cardiac* and *hepatic lesions* observed in man has been reported. The patient received 2 grams of aminocaproic acid every 6 hours for a total dose of 26 grams. Death was due to continued cerebral vascular hemorrhage. Necrotic changes in the heart and liver were noted at autopsy.

If it is accepted that fibrinolysis is a normal process, potentially active at all times to ensure the fluidity of blood, then it must also be accepted that inhibition of fibrinolysis by aminocaproic acid *may* result in clotting or thrombosis. However, there is no definite evidence that administration of aminocaproic acid has been responsible for the few reported cases of *intravascular clotting* which followed this treatment. Rather, it appears that such intravascular clotting was most likely a result of the fibrinolytic disease being treated.

It has been postulated that *extravascular clots* formed *in vivo* with incorporated aminocaproic acid may not undergo spontaneous lysis as do normal clots.

Adverse Reactions: Occasionally nausea, cramps, diarrhea, hypotension, dizziness, tinnitus, malaise, conjunctival suffusion, nasal stuffiness, headache, and skin rash have been reported as results of the administration of aminocaproic acid. Only rarely has it been necessary to discontinue or reduce medication because of one or more of these effects.

Thrombophlebitis, a possibility with all intravenous therapy, should be guarded against by strict attention to the proper insertion of the needle and the fixing of its position.

Dosage and Administration: Initial Therapy—An initial priming dose of 5 grams of AMICAR administered either orally or intravenously followed by 1 to 1¼ gram doses at hourly intervals thereafter should achieve and sustain plasma levels of 0.130 mg./ml. of the drug. This is the concentration apparently necessary for the inhibition of systemic hyperfibrinolysis. Administration of more than 30 grams in any 24-hour period is not recommended.

Intravenous—AMICAR *aminocaproic acid* Intravenous is administered by infusion, utilizing the usual compatible intravenous vehicles (e.g. Sterile Water for Injection, physiologic saline, 5% dextrose or Ringer's solution). RAPID INJECTION OF AMICAR INTRAVENOUS UNDILUTED INTO A VEIN IS NOT RECOMMENDED.

For the treatment of *acute* bleeding syndromes due to elevated fibrinolytic activity, it is suggested that 16 to 20 ml. (4 to 5 grams) of AMICAR Intravenous be administered by infusion during the first hour of treatment, followed by a continuing infusion at the rate of 4 ml. (1.0 gram) per hour. This method of treatment would ordinarily be continued for about 8 hours or until the bleeding situation has been controlled.

Oral Therapy—If the patient is able to take medication by mouth, an identical dosage regimen may be followed by administering AMICAR Tablets or 25% Syrup as follows: For the treatment of *acute* bleeding syndromes due to elevated fibrinolytic activity, it is suggested that 10 tablets (5 grams) or 4 teaspoonfuls of syrup (5 grams) of AMICAR be administered during the first hour of treatment, followed by a continuing rate of 2 tablets (1 gram) or 1 teaspoonful of syrup (1¼ grams) per hour. This method of treatment would ordinarily be continued for about 8 hours or until the bleeding situation has been controlled.

How Supplied:
AMICAR *Lederle 25% Syrup*
Each ml of raspberry flavored syrup contains 250 mg of Aminocaproic Acid with 0.1% Sodium Benzoate and 0.2% Potassium Sorbate as preservative. 16 Fl. Oz. bottles.
AMICAR *Lederle Tablets*
Each tablet contains 500 mg of Aminocaproic Acid. Scored-white A10 Bottles of 100.

Also Available:
AMICAR *Lederle Intravenous*
Each 20 ml vial contains 5.0 Grams of Aminocaproic Acid (250 mg per ml) as an aqueous solution, with 0.9% benzyl alcohol as a preservative. The pH is adjusted to approx. 6.8 with Hydrochloric Acid. 20/ml vials.
A.H.F.S. 20:12.16

Intravenous
Military Depot NSN 6505-00-926-1442
V.A. Depot System NSN 6505-00-926-1442A

Manufactured for
LEDERLE LABORATORIES DIVISION
American Cyanamid Company
Pearl River, NY 10965
by
LEDERLE PARENTERALS INC.
Carolina, Puerto Rico 00630

*Stefanini, M. and Dameshek, W.: The Hemorrhagic Disorders, Ed. 2, New York, Grune and Stratton, pp. 510–514, 1962.

[*Shown in Product Identification Section*]

ARISTOCORT® ℞
triamcinolone
TABLETS
ARISTOCORT®
triamcinolone diacetate
SYRUP

Description: ARISTOCORT *triamcinolone* is a synthetic adrenocorticosteroid. The tablets contain Triamcinolone, 9α-fluoro-16α-hydroxyprednisolone, Syrup contains Triamcinolone Diacetate, 9α-fluoro-16α-hydroxyprednisolone diacetate. It is readily absorbed from the gastrointestinal tract.

Action: ARISTOCORT is primarily glucocorticoid in action and has potent anti-inflammatory, hormonal and metabolic effects common to cortisone-like drugs. It is essentially devoid of mineralocorticoid activity when administered in therapeutic doses, causing little or no sodium retention, with potassium excretion minimal or absent. The body's immune responses to diverse stimuli is also modified by its action.

Indications:

1. Endocrine Disorders:
Primary or secondary adrenocortical insufficiency (hydrocortisone or cortisone is the first choice; synthetic analogs may be used in conjunction with mineralocorticoids where applicable. In infancy mineralocorticoid supplementation is of particular importance).
Congenital adrenal hyperplasia.
Nonsuppurative thyroiditis.
Hypercalcemia associated with cancer.

2. Rheumatic Disorders:
As adjunctive therapy for short-term administration (to tide the patient over an acute episode or exacerbation) in:
Psoriatic arthritis.
Rheumatoid arthritis including juvenile rheumatoid arthritis (selected cases may require low-dose maintenance therapy).
Ankylosing spondylitis.
Acute and subacute bursitis.
Acute nonspecific tenosynovitis.
Acute gouty arthritis.
Post-traumatic osteoarthritis.
Synovitis of osteoarthritis.
Epicondylitis.

3. Collagen Diseases:
During an exacerbation or as maintenance therapy in selected cases of—
Systemic lupus erythematosus.
Acute rheumatic carditis.

4. Dermatologic Diseases:
Pemphigus.
Bullous dermatitis herpetiformis.
Severe erythema multiforme (Stevens-Johnson syndrome).
Exfoliative dermatitis.
Mycosis fungoides.
Severe psoriasis.
Severe seborrheic dermatitis.

5. Allergic States:
Control of severe or incapacitating allergic conditions intractable to adequate trials of conventional treatment:
Seasonal or perennial allergic rhinitis.
Bronchial asthma.
Contact dermatitis.
Atopic dermatitis.
Serum sickness.
Drug hypersensitivity reactions.

6. Ophthalmic Diseases:
Severe acute and chronic allergic and inflammatory processes involving the eye and its adnexa such as—
Allergic conjunctivitis.
Keratitis.
Allergic corneal marginal ulcers.
Herpes zoster ophthalmicus.
Iritis and iridocyclitis.
Chorioretinitis.
Anterior segment inflammation.
Diffuse posterior uveitis and choroiditis.
Optic neuritis.
Sympathetic ophthalmia.

7. Respiratory Diseases:
Symptomatic sarcoidosis.
Loeffler's syndrome not manageable by other means.
Berylliosis.
Fulminating or disseminated pulmonary tuberculosis when used concurrently with appropriate antituberculous chemotherapy.
Aspiration pneumonitis.

8. Hematologic Disorders:
Idiopathic thrombocytopenic purpura in adults.
Secondary thrombocytopenia in adults.
Acquired (autoimmune) hemolytic anemia.
Erythroblastopenia (RBC anemia).
Congenital (erythroid) hypoplastic anemia.

9. Neoplastic Diseases:
For palliative management of:
Leukemias and lymphomas in adults.
Acute leukemia of childhood.

10. Edematous States:
To induce a diuresis or remission of proteinuria in the nephrotic syndrome, without uremia, of the idiopathic type or that due to lupus erythematosus.

11. Gastrointestinal Diseases:
To tide the patient over a critical period of the disease in:
Ulcerative Colitis.
Regional enteritis.

12. Nervous System:
Acute exacerbations of multiple sclerosis.

13. Miscellaneous:
Tuberculous meningitis with subarachnoid block or impending block when used concurrently with appropriate antituberculous chemotherapy.
Trichinosis with neurologic or myocardial involvement.

Contraindications:
Systemic fungal infections.
Sensitivity to the drug or any of its components.

Warnings: In patients on corticosteroid therapy subjected to unusual stress, increased dosage of rapidly acting corticosteroids before, during, and after the stressful situation is indicated.

Corticosteroids may mask some signs of infection, and new infections may appear during their use. There may be decreased resistance and inability to localize infection when corticosteroids are used.

Prolonged use of corticosteroids may produce posterior subcapsular cataracts, glaucoma with possible damage to the optic nerves, and may enhance the establishment of secondary ocular infections due to fungi or viruses.

Usage in pregnancy: Since adequate human reproduction studies have not been done with corticosteroids, the use of these drugs in pregnancy, nursing mothers or women of childbearing potential requires that the possible benefits of the drug be weighed against the potential hazards to the mother and embryo or fetus. Infants born of mothers who have received substantial doses of corticosteroids during pregnancy should be carefully observed for signs of hypoadrenalism.

Average and large doses of hydrocortisone or cortisone can cause elevation of blood pressure, salt and water retention, and increased excretion of potassium. These effects are less likely to occur with ARISTOCORT *triamcinolone* except when used in large doses. Dietary salt restriction and potassium supplementation may be necessary. All corticosteroids increase calcium excretion.

While on Corticosteroid Therapy Patients Should Not Be Vaccinated Against Smallpox. Other Immunization Procedures Should Not Be Undertaken in Patients Who are on Corticosteroids, Especially on High Dose, Because of Possible Hazards of Neurological Complications and a Lack of Antibody Response.

The use of Triamcinolone in active tuberculosis should be restricted to those cases of fulminating or disseminated tuberculosis in which the corticosteroid is used for the management of the disease in conjunction with an appropriate antituberculous regimen.

If corticosteroids are indicated in patients with latent tuberculosis or tuberculin reactivity, close observation is necessary as reactivation of the disease may occur. During prolonged corticosteroid therapy, these patients should receive chemoprophylaxis.

Precautions: Drug-induced secondary adrenocortical insufficiency may be minimized by gradual reduction of dosage. This type of relative insufficiency may persist for months after discontinuation of therapy; therefore, in any situation of stress occurring during that period, hormone therapy should be reinstituted. Since mineralocorticoid secretion may be impaired, salt and/or a mineralocorticoid should be administered concurrently.

There is an enhanced effect of corticosteroids on patients with hypothyroidism and in those with cirrhosis.

Corticosteroids should be used cautiously in patients with ocular herpes simplex because of possible corneal perforation.

The lowest possible dose of corticosteroid should be used to control the condition under treatment, and when reduction in dosage is possible, the reduction should be gradual.

Psychic derangements may appear when corticosteroids are used, ranging from euphoria, insomnia, mood swings, personality changes, and severe depression, to frank psychotic manifestations. Also, existing emotional instability or psychotic tendencies may be aggravated by corticosteroids.

Aspirin should be used cautiously in conjunction with corticosteroids in hypoprothrombinemia.

Steroids should be used with caution in nonspecific ulcerative colitis if there is a probability of impending perforation, abscess or other pyogenic infection; diverticulitis; fresh intestinal anastomoses; active or latent peptic ulcer; renal insufficiency; hypertension; osteoporosis; and myasthenia gravis.

Growth and development of infants and children on prolonged corticosteroid therapy should be carefully observed.

Although controlled clinical trials have shown corticosteroids to be effective in speeding the resolution of acute exacerbations of multiple sclerosis they do not show that they affect the ultimate outcome or natural history of the disease. The studies do show relatively high doses of corticosteroids are necessary to demonstrate a significant effect. (See Dosage and Administration).

Since complications of treatment with glucocorticoid are dependent on the size of the dose and the duration of treatment a risk/benefit decision must be made in each individual case as to dose and duration of treatment and as to whether daily or intermittent therapy should be used.

Adverse Reactions:
Fluid and Electrolyte Disturbances.
Sodium retention.
Fluid retention.
Congestive heart failure in susceptible patients.
Potassium loss.
Hypokalemic alkalosis.
Hypertension.

Continued on next page

The information on each product appearing here is based on labelling effective in August, 1982 and is either the entire official brochure or an accurate condensation therefrom. Offical brochures are enclosed in product packages. Information concerning all Lederle products may be obtained from the Professional Services Department, Lederle Laboratories, Pearl River, New York, 10965.

Lederle—Cont.

Musculoskeletal.
Muscle weakness.
Steroid myopathy.
Loss of muscle mass.
Osteoporosis.
Vertebral compression fractures.
Aseptic necrosis of femoral and humeral heads.
Pathologic fracture of long bones.

Gastrointestinal.
Peptic ulcer with possible perforation and hemorrhage.
Pancreatitis.
Abdominal distention.
Ulcerative esophagitis.

Dermatologic.
Impaired wound healing.
Thin fragile skin.
Petechiae and ecchymoses.
Facial erythema.
Increased sweating.
May suppress reactions to skin tests.

Neurological.
Convulsions.
Increased intracranial pressure with papilledema (pseudotumor cerebri) usually after treatment.
Vertigo.
Headache.

Endocrine.
Menstrual irregularities.
Development of Cushingoid state.
Suppression of growth in children.
Secondary adrenocortical and pituitary unresponsiveness, particularly in times of stress, as in trauma, surgery or illness.
Decreased carbohydrate tolerance.
Manifestations of latent diabetes mellitus.
Increased requirements for insulin or oral hypoglycemic agents in diabetics.

Ophthalmic.
Posterior subcapsular cataracts.
Increased intraocular pressure.
Glaucoma.
Exophthalmos.

Metabolic.
Negative nitrogen balance due to protein catabolism.

Dosage and Administration:

General Principles:

1. The initial dosage of ARISTOCORT *triamcinolone* may vary from 4 mg. to 48 mg. per day depending on the specific disease entity being treated. In situations of less severity lower doses will generally suffice while in selected patients higher initial doses may be required. The initial dosage should be maintained or adjusted until a satisfactory response is noted. If after a reasonable period of time there is a lack of satisfactory clinical response, the drug should be discontinued and the patient transferred to other appropriate therapy. *IT SHOULD BE EMPHASIZED THAT DOSAGE REQUIREMENTS ARE VARIABLE AND MUST BE INDIVIDUALIZED ON THE BASIS OF THE DISEASE UNDER TREATMENT AND THE RESPONSE OF THE PATIENT.* After a favorable response is noted, the proper maintenance dosage should be determined by decreasing the initial drug dosage in small increments at appropriate time intervals until the lowest dosage which will maintain an adequate clinical response is reached. It should be kept in mind that constant monitoring is needed in regard to drug dosage. Included in the situations which may make dosage adjustments necessary are changes in clinical status secondary to remissions or exacerbations in the disease process, the patient's individual drug responsiveness, and the effect of patient exposure to stressful situations not directly related to the disease entity under treatment; in this latter situation it may be necessary to increase the dosage of ARISTOCORT for a period of time consistent with the patient's condition. If after long-term therapy the drug is to be stopped, it is recommended that it be withdrawn gradually rather than abruptly.

2. Dosage should be individualized according to the severity of the disease and the response of the patient. For infants and children, the recommended dosage should be governed by the same considerations rather than by strict adherence to the ratio indicated by age or body weight.

3. Hormone therapy is an adjunct to, and not a replacement for, conventional therapy.

4. The severity, prognosis and expected duration of the disease and the reaction of the patient to medication are primary factors in determining dosage.

5. If a period of spontaneous remission occurs in a chronic condition, treatment should be discontinued.

6. Blood pressure, body weight, routine laboratory studies, including 2-hour postprandial blood glucose and serum potassium, and a chest X-ray should be obtained at regular intervals during prolonged therapy. Upper GI X-rays are desirable in patients with known or suspected peptic ulcer disease.

7. Suppression of autogenous pituitary function, a common effect of exogenous corticosteroid administration, may be reduced, modified or minimized by revision of dose schedules. The time of maximum corticoid effect is from midnight to 8 a.m. and minimal during the intervening hours. Use of a single daily dose beginning at or after 8 a.m. will be effective in most conditions, will lower corticoid overload and will cause the least interference with the diurnal system of endogenous secretion and hypothalamopituitary-adrenal function; alternate-day dosage in some conditions and intermittent administration in certain severe disorders requiring long-term and/or high dose maintenance levels have proven both clinically effective and less likely to produce adverse reactions. The maximum daily morning dose not associated with lasting adrenocorticoid suppression is 8 mg.

8. *Alternate-Day Therapy.* After the conventional dose has been established, some patients may be maintained on alternate day therapy. It has been shown that the activity of the adrenal cortex varies throughout the day, being greatest from about midnight to 8:00 a.m. Exogenous corticoid suppresses this activity least when given at the time of maximum activity. A 48-hour interval appears to be necessary since shorter intervals are accompanied by adrenal suppression similar to that of conventional daily divided doses. Therefore, with the alternate day dose plan, a total 48-hour requirement is given every other day at 8:00 a.m. As with other regimens, the minimum effective dose level should be sought.

Specific Dosage Recommendations:

1. *Endocrine Disorders:* Wide variation in dosage requirements for the endocrine disorders such as *congenital adrenal hyperplasia, non-suppurative thyroiditis,* and *hypercalcemia associated* with *cancer* precludes specific recommendation except for *adrenocortical insufficiency* where the dose is usually 4-12 mg. daily in addition to mineralocorticoid therapy.

2. *Rheumatic Disorders: Rheumatoid arthritis; acute gouty arthritis; ankylosing spondylitis;* and *selected cases of psoriatic arthritis;* in *acute* and *subacute bursitis;* and in *acute nonspecific tenosynovitis.* The initial suppressive dose of ARISTOCORT in these conditions ranges from 8 mg. to 16 mg. per day, although the occasional patient may require higher doses. Patients may show an early or a delayed effect, characterized by a reduction in the inflammatory reaction and in joint swelling, together with alleviation of pain and stiffness, resulting in an increased range of motion of the affected joints or tissues. Maintenance doses are adjusted to keep symptoms at a level tolerable to the patient. Rapid reduction of the steroid or its abrupt discontinuance may result in recurrence or even exacerbation of signs and symptoms. Short-term administration is desirable as a rule. ARISTOCORT *triamcinolone* is ordinarily administered as a single morning dose daily or on alternate days, depending on the need of the patient. Occasional patients may secure more effective relief on divided daily doses, either 2 to 4 times daily.

3. *Collagen Diseases: Systemic Lupus Erythematosus:* The initial dose is usually 20 mg. to 32 mg. daily continued until the desired response is obtained, when reduced maintenance levels are sought. Patients with more severe symptoms may require higher initial doses, 48 mg. or more daily, and higher maintenance doses. Although some patients with systemic lupus erythematosus appear to have spontaneous remissions or to tolerate the disorder in its milder forms for prolonged periods of time, adjustment of dosage scheduling to reduce adverse suppression of the pituitary-adrenal axis may be useful.

Acute Rheumatic Carditis: In severely ill patients with carditis, pericardial effusion and/or congestive heart failure, corticosteroid therapy is effective in the control of the acute and severe inflammatory changes and may be lifesaving. Initial doses of ARISTOCORT may be from 20 mg. to 60 mg. daily, and clinical response is usually rapid and the drug can then be reduced. Maintenance therapy should be continued for at least 6 to 8 weeks and is seldom required beyond a period of 3 months. Corticosteroid therapy does not preclude conventional treatment, including antibiotics and salicylization.

4. *Dermatological Disorders: Pemphigus; bullous dermatitis herpetiformis, severe erythema multiforme* (Stevens-Johnson Syndrome); *exfoliative dermatitis;* and *mycosis fungoides.* The initial dose is 8 mg. to 16 mg. daily. In these conditions, as well as in certain allergic dermatoses, *alternate-day* administration has been found effective and apparently less likely to produce adverse side effects.

Severe psoriasis: ARISTOCORT may produce reduction or remission of the disabling skin manifestations following initial doses of 8 mg. to 16 mg. daily. The period of maintenance is dependent on the clinical response. Corticosteroid reduction or discontinuation of therapy should be attempted with caution since relapse may occur and may appear in a more aggravated form, the so-called "rebound phenomenon".

5. *Allergic States:* ARISTOCORT *triamcinolone* is administered in doses of 8 mg. to 12 mg. daily in acute seasonal or perennial *allergic rhinitis.* Intractable cases may require high initial and maintenance doses. In *bronchial asthma,* 8 mg. to 16 mg. daily are usually effective. The usual therapeutic measures for control of bronchial asthma should be carried out in addition to ARISTOCORT therapy. In both allergic rhinitis and bronchial asthma, therapy is directed at alleviation of acute distress and chronic long-term use of corticosteroids is neither desirable nor often essential. Some patients may be maintained on alternate day therapy. In such conditions as *contact dermatitis* and *atopic dermatitis,* topical therapy may be supplemented with short courses of ARISTOCORT by mouth in doses of 8 mg. to 16 mg. daily. In severely ill patients with *serum sickness,* epinephrine may be the drug of choice for immediate therapy, often supplemented by antihistamines. ARISTOCORT is frequently useful as adjunctive treatment in such cases, with the dosage determined by the severity of the disorder, the speed with which therapeutic response is desired and the response of the patient to initial therapy.

6. *Ophthalmological Disease: Allergic conjunctivitis; keratitis; allergic corneal marginal ulcers, iritis* and *iridocyclitis; chorioretinitis; anterior segment inflammation; diffuse poste-*

rior uveitis and *choroiditis; optic neuritis* and *sympathetic ophthalmia.* Initial doses range from 12 mg. to 40 mg. daily depending on the severity of the condition, the nature and degree of involvement of ocular structure, but response is usually rapid and therapy of short-term duration.

7. *Respiratory Diseases: Symptomatic sarcoidosis; Loeffler's Syndrome; berylliosis;* and in certain cases of *fulminating* or *disseminated pulmonary tuberculosis* when concurrently accompanied by appropriate antituberculous chemotherapy. Initial doses are usually in the range of 16 mg. to 48 mg. daily.

8. *Hematologic Disorders: Idiopathic* and *secondary thrombocytopenia* in *adults, acquired (autoimmune) hemolytic anemia; erythroblastopenia (RBC anemia); congenital (erythroid) hypoplastic anemia.* ARISTOCORT is used to produce a remission of symptoms and may, in some instances, produce an apparent regression of abnormal cellular blood elements to normal states, temporary or permanent. The recommended dose varies between 16 mg. and 60 mg. daily, with reduction after adequate clinical response.

9. *Neoplastic Diseases: Acute leukemia in childhood.* The usual dose of ARISTOCORT is 1 mg. per kilogram of body weight daily, although as much as 2 mg. per kilogram may be necessary. Initial response is usually seen within 6 to 21 days and therapy continued from 4 to 6 weeks.

Acute leukemia and *lymphoma in adults.* The usual dose of ARISTOCORT is 16 mg. to 40 mg. daily, although it may be necessary to give as much as 100 mg. daily in leukemia. ARISTOCORT therapy in these neoplasias is only palliative and not curative. Other therapeutic and supportive measures must be used when appropriate.

10. *Edematous States: Nephrotic Syndrome:* ARISTOCORT may be used to induce a diuresis or remission of proteinuria in the *nephrotic syndrome,* without uremia, of the idiopathic type or that due to *lupus erythematosus.* The average dose is 16 to 20 mg. (up to 48 mg.) daily until diuresis occurs. The diuresis may be massive and usually occurs by the 14th day, but occasionally may be delayed. After diuresis begins it is advisable to continue treatment until maximal or complete chemical and clinical remission occurs, at which time the dosage should be reduced gradually and then discontinued. In less severe cases maintenance dosages of as little as 4 mg. daily may be adequate. Alternatively and when maintenance therapy may be prolonged, ARISTOCORT may be administered on alternate-day dose schedules.

Equivalence Table

	Anti-inflammatory Relative Potency		Frequently Used Tablet Strength (mg)		Tablet × Potency Equivalent Value
Hydrocortisone	1	×	20	=	20
Prednisolone	4	×	5	=	20
ARISTOCORT® Triamcinolone	5	×	4	=	20
Dexamethasone	25	×	0.75	=	18.75

11. *Miscellaneous: Tuberculous meningitis:* ARISTOCORT may be useful when accompanied by appropriate antituberculous therapy when there is subarachnoid block or impending block. The average dosage is 32 to 48 mg. daily in either single or divided doses.

[See table above].

How Supplied:

1 mg. Tablets-Scored yellow; Engraved LL A1 bottles of 50.

2 mg. Tablets-Scored pink; Engraved LL A2 bottles of 100.

4 mg. Tablets-Scored white; Engraved LL A4 bottles of 30, 100, 500 and ARISTO-PAK® *triamcinolone* 16's Engraved LL 4 (for 6 days' therapy).

8 mg. Tablets-Scored yellow; Engraved LL A8 bottles of 50.

16 mg. Tablets-Scored white: Engraved LL A16 bottles of 30.

Syrup 2 mg./5 ml. triamcinolone diacetate; cherry flavored; bottles of 4 fl. oz. Preservatives: Methylparaben 0.08% and Propylparaben 0.02%.

A.H.F.S. 68:04

[*Tablets, and ARISTO-PAK 4 mg. Shown in Product Identification Section*]

ARISTOCORT® ℞
triamcinolone acetonide
Topical Products

[See table below].

ARISTOCORT *triamcinolone acetonide* Topicals contain the highly active steroid, Triamcinolone Acetonide, which is a derivative of triamcinolone.

Actions: Topical steroids are primarily effective because of their anti-inflammatory, antipruritic and vasoconstrictive actions.

Indications: For relief of the inflammatory manifestations of corticosteroid-responsive dermatoses.

Contraindications: Topical steroids are contraindicated in those patients with a history of hypersensitivity to any of the components of the preparation.

Precautions: If irritation develops, the product should be discontinued and appropriate therapy instituted.

In the presence of an infection the use of appropriate antifungal or antibacterial agents should be instituted. If a favorable response does not occur promptly, the corticosteroid should be discontinued until the infection has been adequately controlled.

If extensive areas are treated or if the occlusive technique is used there will be increased systemic absorption of the corticosteroid and suitable precautions should be taken, particularly in children and infants.

Although topical steroids have not been reported to have an adverse effect on human pregnancy, the safety of their use in pregnant women has not absolutely been established. In laboratory animals, increases in incidence of fetal abnormalities have been associated with exposure of gestating females to topical corticosteroids, in some cases at rather low dosage levels. Therefore, drugs of this class should not be used extensively on pregnant patients, in large amounts, or for prolonged periods of time.

The product is not for ophthalmic use.

Adverse Reactions: The following local adverse reactions have been reported with topical corticosteroids, especially under occlusive dressings.

1. Burning 2. Itching 3. Irritation 4. Dryness 5. Folliculitis 6. Hypertrichosis 7. Acneiform eruptions 8. Hypopigmentation 9. Perioral dermatitis 10. Allergic Contact Dermatitis 11. Maceration of the skin 12. Secondary infection 13. Skin atrophy 14. Striae 15. Miliaria

A.H.F.S. 84:06

[*Shown in Product Identification Section*]

ARISTOCORT® Triamcinolone Acetonide TOPICAL PRODUCTS

	Cream 0.025%	Cream 0.1%	Cream 0.5%	Ointment 0.1%	Ointment 0.5%
Each gram contains Triamcinolone Acetonide	0.25 mg.	1 mg.	5 mg.	1 mg.	5 mg.
Preservatives:					
Sorbic Acid	0.1%	0.1%	0.1%		
Potassium Sorbate	0.1%	0.1%	0.1%		
Inactive Ingredients:	In a water base: Mono and Diglycerides, Squalane NF, Polysorbate 80 NF, Cetyl Esters Wax NF, Polysorbate 60 NF, Stearyl Alcohol NF, Tenox II, and Sorbitol Solution USP			white petroleum	
Dosage and Administration	Apply to the affected areas 3 or 4 times daily. The cream should be rubbed in gently and thoroughly until it disappears.			Apply to the affected areas 3 or 4 times daily.	
How Supplied	15 and 60 gram tubes, 240 gram and 5.25 lb. jars	15 and 60 gram tubes 240 gram and 5.25 lb. jars	15 gram tubes and 240 gram jars	15 and 60 gram tubes, 240 gram and 5 lb. jars	15 gram tubes, 240 gram jars

Suspensions
ARISTOCORT® ℞
triamcinolone diacetate
Forte parenteral
Intralesional

NOT FOR INTRAVENOUS USE

FORTE PARENTERAL:

Description: A suspension of 40 mg./ml. of *triamcinolone diacetate* micronized in:

Polysorbate 80 NF 0.20%
Polyethylene Glycol 4000 NF 3%
Sodium Chloride 0.85%

Continued on next page

The information on each product appearing here is based on labelling effective in August, 1982 and is either the entire official brochure or an accurate condensation therefrom. Offical brochures are enclosed in product packages. Information concerning all Lederle products may be obtained from the Professional Services Department, Lederle Laboratories, Pearl River, New York, 10965.

Lederle—Cont.

Benzyl Alcohol....................0.90%
Water for Injection q.s. 100%
Hydrochloric Acid and Sodium Hydroxide to approx. pH 6

This preparation is a slightly soluble suspension suitable for parenteral administration through a 24-gauge needle (or larger), but NOT suitable for intravenous use. It may be administered by the intramuscular, intra-articular, or intrasynovial routes, depending upon the situation. The response to each glucocorticoid varies considerably with each type of disease indication and each corticosteroid prescribed. Irreversible clumping occurs when product is frozen.

Chemically Triamcinolone Diacetate NF is Pregna - 1, 4 - diene - 3, 20 - dione, 16, 21-bis-(acetyloxy) - 9 - fluoro-11, 17- dihydroxy-, (11β, 16α) - 9 - Fluoro-11β, 16α, 17,21-tetrahydroxy-pregna-1, 4-diene-3, 20-dione 16, 21-diacetate. Molecular weight is 478.51.

Action: ARISTOCORT is primarily glucocorticoid in action and has potent anti-inflammatory, hormonal and metabolic effects common to cortisone-like drugs. It is essentially devoid of mineralocorticoid activity when administered in therapeutic doses, causing little or no sodium retention, with potassium excretion minimal or absent. The body's immune responses to diverse stimuli is also modified by its action.

Indications: Where oral therapy is not feasible or temporarily desirable in the judgment of the physician, ARISTOCORT *triamcinolone diacetate* FORTE 40 mg./ml. is indicated for intramuscular use as follows:

1. Endocrine disorders.
   Primary or secondary adrenocortical insufficiency (hydrocortisone or cortisone is the drug of choice; synthetic analogs may be used in conjunction with mineralocorticoids where applicable; in infancy, mineralocorticoid supplementation is of particular importance).
   Preoperatively and in the event of serious trauma or illness, in patients with known adrenal insufficiency or when adrenocortical reserve is doubtful.
   Congenital adrenal hyperplasia.
   Nonsuppurative thyroiditis.
   Hypercalcemia associated with cancer.
2. Rheumatic disorders. As adjunctive therapy for short-term administration to tide the patient over an acute episode or exacerbation) in:
   Post-traumatic osteoarthritis.
   Synovitis of osteoarthritis.
   Rheumatoid arthritis including juvenile rheumatoid arthritis (selected cases may require low-dose maintenance therapy).
   Acute and subacute bursitis.
   Epicondylitis.
   Acute nonspecific tenosynovitis.
   Acute gouty arthritis.
   Psoriatic arthritis.
   Ankylosing spondylitis.
3. Collagen diseases. During an exacerbation or as maintenance therapy in selected cases of:
   Systemic lupus erythematosus.
   Acute rheumatic carditis.
4. Dermatologic diseases. Pemphigus.
   Severe erythema multiforme (Stevens-Johnson syndrome).
   Exfoliative dermatitis.
   Bullous dermatitis herpetiformis.
   Severe seborrheic dermatitis.
   Severe psoriasis.
   Mycosis fungoides.
5. Allergic states. Control of severe or incapacitating allergic conditions intractable to adequate trials of conventional treatment in:
   Bronchial asthma.
   Contact dermatitis.
   Seasonal or perennial allergic rhinitis.
   Drug hypersensitivity reactions.
   Urticarial transfusion reactions.
   Atopic dermatitis.
   Serum sickness.
   Acute noninfectious laryngeal edema (epinephrine is the drug of first choice).
6. Ophthalmic diseases. Severe acute and chronic allergic and inflammatory processes involving the eye, such as:
   Herpes zoster ophthalmicus.
   Iritis, iridocyclitis.
   Chorioretinitis.
   Sympathetic ophthalmia.
   Diffuse posterior uveitis and choroiditis.
   Optic neuritis.
   Keratitis.
   Allergic conjunctivitis.
   Allergic corneal marginal ulcers.
7. Gastrointestinal diseases. To tide the patient over a critical period of disease in:
   Ulcerative colitis - (Systemic therapy).
   Regional enteritis - (Systemic therapy).
8. Respiratory diseases.
   Symptomatic sarcoidosis.
   Berylliosis.
   Fulminating or disseminated pulmonary tuberculosis when used concurrently with appropriate antituberculous chemotherapy.
   Aspiration pneumonitis.
   Loeffler's syndrome not manageable by other means.
9. Hematologic disorders.
   Acquired (autoimmune) hemolytic anemia.
   Secondary thrombocytopenia in adults.
   Erythroblastopenia (RBC anemia).
   Congenital (erythroid) hypoplastic anemia.
10. Neoplastic diseases. For palliative management of:
   Leukemias and lymphomas in adults.
   Acute leukemia of childhood.
11. Edematous state. To induce diuresis or remission of proteinuria in the nephrotic syndrome, without uremia, of the idiopathic type or that due to lupus erythematosus.
12. Nervous System.
   Acute exacerbations of multiple sclerosis.
13. Miscellaneous. Tuberculosis meningitis with subarachnoid block or impending block when used concurrently with appropriate antituberculous chemotherapy.
   Trichinosis with neurologic or myocardial involvement.

ARISTOCORT *triamcinolone diacetate* FORTE 40 mg./ml. is indicated for intra-articular or soft tissue use as follows:
As adjunctive therapy for short-term administration (to tide the patient over an acute episode or exacerbation) in:
  Synovitis of osteoarthritis.
  Rheumatoid arthritis.
  Acute and subacute bursitis.
  Acute gouty arthritis.
  Epicondylitis.
  Acute nonspecific tenosynovitis.
  Post-traumatic osteoarthritis.

ARISTOCORT FORTE is indicated for intralesional use as follows:
  Keloids
  Localized hypertrophic, infiltrated, inflammatory lesions of: lichen planus, psoriatic plaques, granuloma annulare and lichen simplex chronicus (neurodermatitis).
  Discoid lupus erythematosus.
  Necrobiosis lipoidica diabeticorum.
  Alopecia areata.
  It may also be useful in cystic tumors of an aponeurosis or tendon (ganglia).

INTRALESIONAL:

Description: ARISTOCORT *triamcinolone diacetate,* 9α fluoro 16α hydroxy prednisolone diacetate possesses glucocorticoid properties while being essentially devoid of mineralocorticoid activity thus causing little or no sodium retention.

A suspension of 25 mg./ml. micronized in:
  Polysorbate 80 USP....................0.20%
  Polyethylene Glycol 4000 USP................3%
  Sodium Chloride....................0.85%
  Benzyl Alcohol....................0.90%
  Water for Injection q.s....................100%
  Hydrochloric Acid to approx. pH 6

Chemically triamcinolone diacetate NF is Pregna - 1, 4 - diene - 3, 20 - dione, 16, 21 - bis-(acetyloxy) - 9 - fluoro - 11, 17-dihydroxy-,(11β, 16α)- or 9-Fluoro-11β, 16α, 17, 21-tetrahydro-xypregna-1, 4-diene-3,20-dione 16,21-diacetate. Molecular weight is 478.51.

Actions: Naturally occurring glucocorticoids (hydrocortisone), which also have salt-retaining properties, are used as replacement therapy in adrenocortical deficiency states. Their synthetic analogs are primarily used for their potent anti-inflammatory effects in disorders of many organ systems.

Glucocorticoids cause profound and varied metabolic effects. In addition, they modify the body's immune responses to diverse stimuli.

Indications: ARISTOCORT INTRALESIONAL is indicated by the intralesional route for:
  Keloids
  Localized hypertrophic, infiltrated, inflammatory lesions of:
  lichen planus, psoriatic plaques, granuloma annulare and lichen simplex chronicus (neurodermatitis).
  Discoid lupus erythematosus.
  Necrobiosis lipoidica diabeticorum.
  Alopecia areata.

It may also be useful in cystic tumors of an aponeurosis or tendon (ganglia).

When used intra-articularly it is also indicated for:
Adjunctive therapy for short-term administration (to tide the patient over an acute episode or exacerbation) in:
  Synovitis of osteoarthritis.
  Rheumatoid arthritis.
  Acute and subacute bursitis.
  Acute gouty arthritis.
  Epicondylitis.
  Acute nonspecific tenosynovitis.
  Post-traumatic osteoarthritis.

FORTE AND INTRALESIONAL:

Contraindications: Systemic fungal infections.

Warnings: In patients on corticosteroid therapy subjected to any unusual stress, increased dosage of rapidly acting corticosteroids before, during, and after the stressful situation is indicated.

Corticosteroids may mask some signs of infection, and new infections may appear during their use. There may be decreased resistance and inability to localize infection when corticosteroids are used.

Prolonged use of corticosteroids may produce posterior subcapsular cataracts, glaucoma with possible damage to the optic nerves, and may enhance the establishment of secondary ocular infections due to fungi or viruses.

Usage in pregnancy

Since adequate human reproduction studies have not been done with corticosteroids, the use of these drugs in pregnancy, nursing mothers, or women of childbearing potential requires that the possible benefits of the drug be weighed against the potential hazards to the mother and embryo or fetus. Infants born of mothers who have received substantial doses of corticosteroids during pregnancy should be carefully observed for signs of hypoadrenalism.

Average and large doses of cortisone or hydrocortisone can cause elevation of blood pressure, salt and water retention, and increased excretion of potassium. These effects are less likely to occur with the synthetic derivatives except when used in large doses. Dietary salt restriction and potassium supplementation may be necessary. All corticosteroids increase calcium excretion.

While on Corticosteroid Therapy Patients Should Not Be Vaccinated Against Smallpox. Other Immunization Procedures Should Not Be Undertaken in Patients Who Are on Corticosteroids, Especially in High Doses, Because of Possible Hazards of Neurological Complications and Lack of Antibody Response.

The use of ARISTOCORT *triamcinolone diacetate* in active tuberculosis should be restricted to those cases of fulminating or disseminated tuberculosis in which the corticosteroid is used for the management of the disease in conjunction with appropriate antituberculous regimen.

If corticosteroids are indicated in patients with latent tuberculosis or tuberculin reactivity, close observation is necessary as reactivation of the disease may occur. During prolonged corticosteroid therapy, these patients should receive chemoprophylaxis.

Because rare instances of anaphylactoid reactions have occurred in patients receiving parenteral corticosteroid therapy, appropriate precautionary measures should be taken prior to administration, especially when the patient has a history of allergy to any drug.

Postinjection flare (following intra-articular) and Charcot-like arthropathy have been associated with parenteral corticosteroid therapy.

Intralesional or Sublesional injection of excessive dosage whether by single or multiple injection into any given area may cause cutaneous or subcutaneous atrophy.

Precautions: Drug-induced secondary adrenocortical insufficiency may be minimized by gradual reduction of dosage. This type of relative insufficiency may persist for months after discontinuation of therapy; therefore, in any situation of stress occurring during that period, hormone therapy should be reinstituted.

Since mineralocorticoid secretion may be impaired, salt and/or a mineralocorticoid should be administered concurrently.

There is an enhanced effect of corticosteroids in patients with hypothyroidism and in those with cirrhosis.

Corticosteroids should be used cautiously in patients with ocular herpes simplex for fear of corneal perforation.

The lowest possible dose of corticosteroid should be used to control the condition under treatment, and when reduction in dosage is possible, the reduction must be gradual.

Psychic derangements may appear when corticosteroids are used, ranging from euphoria, insomnia, mood swings, personality changes, and severe depression to frank psychotic manifestations. Also, existing emotional instability or psychotic tendencies may be aggravated by corticosteroids.

Aspirin should be used cautiously in conjunction with corticosteroids in hypoprothrombinemia.

Steroids should be used with caution in nonspecific ulcerative colitis, if there is a probability of impending perforation, abscess or other pyogenic infection, also in diverticulitis, fresh intestinal anastomoses, active or latent peptic ulcer, renal insufficiency, hypertension, osteoporosis, and myasthenia gravis.

Growth and development of infants and children on prolonged corticosteroid therapy should be carefully followed.

The following additional precautions apply for parenteral corticosteroids. Intra-articular injection of a corticosteroid may produce systemic as well as local effects.

Appropriate examination of any joint fluid present is necessary to exclude a septic process.

A marked increase in pain accompanied by local swelling, further restriction of joint motion, fever, and malaise are suggestive of septic arthritis. If this complication occurs and the diagnosis of sepsis is confirmed, appropriate antimicrobial therapy should be instituted.

Local injection of a steroid into a previously infected joint is to be avoided.

Corticosteroids should not be injected into unstable joints.

The slower rate of absorption by intramuscular administration should be recognized.

Routine laboratory studies, such as urinalysis, two-hour postprandial blood sugar, determination of blood pressure and body weight, and a chest x-ray should be made at regular intervals during prolonged therapy. Upper GI x-rays are desirable in patients with an ulcer history or significant dyspepsia.

Accidental injection into soft tissue during intra-articular administration decreases local effectiveness in the joint and, by increasing rate of absorption, may produce systemic effects.

Although controlled clinical trials have shown corticosteroids to be effective in speeding the resolution of acute exacerbations of multiple sclerosis they do not show that they affect the ultimate outcome or natural history of the disease. The studies do show that relatively high doses of corticosteroids are necessary to demonstrate a significant effect. (See Dosage and Administration).

Since complications of treatment with glucocorticoid are dependent on the size of the dose and the duration of treatment a risk/benefit decision must be made in each individual case as to dose and duration of treatment and as to whether daily or intermittent therapy should be used.

Adverse Reactions:

Fluid and electrolyte disturbances:
- Sodium retention.
- Fluid retention.
- Congestive heart failure in susceptible patients.
- Potassium loss.
- Hypokalemic alkalosis.
- Hypertension.

Musculoskeletal:
- Muscle weakness.
- Steroid myopathy.
- Loss of muscle mass.
- Osteoporosis.
- Vertebral compression fractures.
- Aseptic necrosis of femoral and humeral heads.
- Pathologic fracture of long bones.

Gastrointestinal:
- Peptic ulcer with possible subsequent perforation and hemorrhage.
- Pancreatitis.
- Abdominal distention.
- Ulcerative esophagitis.

Dermatologic:
- Impaired wound healing.
- Thin fragile skin.
- Petechiae and ecchymoses.
- Facial erythema.
- Increased sweating.
- May suppress reactions to skin tests.

Neurological:
- Increased intracranial pressure with papilledema (pseudotumor cerebri) usually after treatment.
- Convulsions.
- Vertigo.
- Headache.

Endocrine:
- Menstrual irregularities.
- Development of Cushingoid state.
- Suppression of growth in children.
- Secondary adrenocortical and pituitary unresponsiveness, particularly in times of stress, as in trauma, surgery, or illness.
- Decreased carbohydrate tolerance.
- Manifestations of latent diabetes mellitus.
- Increased requirements for insulin or oral hypoglycemic agents in diabetics.

Ophthalmic:
- Posterior subcapsular cataracts.
- Increased intraocular pressure.
- Glaucoma.
- Exophthalmos.

Metabolic:
- Negative nitrogen balance due to protein catabolism.

The following additional adverse reactions are related to parenteral and intralesional corticosteroid therapy:
- Rare instances of blindness associated with intralesional therapy around the orbit or intranasally.
- Hyperpigmentation or hypopigmentation.
- Subcutaneous and cutaneous atrophy.
- Sterile abscess.

Dosage and Administration:

General

The initial dosage of ARISTOCORT *triamcinolone diacetate* may vary from 3 to 48 mg. per day depending on the specific disease entity being treated. In situations of less severity, lower doses will generally suffice while in selected patients higher initial doses may be required. Usually the parenteral dosage ranges are one-third to one-half the oral dose given every 12 hours. However, in certain overwhelming, acute, life-threatening situations, administration in dosages exceeding the usual dosages may be justified and may be in multiples of the oral dosages.

The initial dosage should be maintained or adjusted until a satisfactory response is noted. If after a reasonable period of time there is a lack of satisfactory clinical response, ARISTOCORT *triamcinolone diacetate* should be discontinued and the patient transferred to other appropriate therapy. It Should Be Emphasized That Dosage Requirements Are Variable and Must Be Individualized on the Basis of the Disease Under Treatment and the Response of the Patient. After a favorable response is noted, the proper maintenance dosage should be determined by decreasing the initial drug dosage in small increments at appropriate time intervals until the lowest dosage which will maintain an adequate clinical response is reached. It should be kept in mind that constant monitoring is needed in regard to drug dosage. Included in the situations which may make dosage adjustments necessary are changes in clinical status secondary to remissions or exacerbations in the disease process, the patient's individual drug responsiveness, and the effect of patient exposure to stressful situations not directly related to the disease entity under treatment; in this latter situation, it may be necessary to increase the dosage of ARISTOCORT *triamcinolone diacetate* for a period of time consistent with the patient's condition. If after long-term therapy the drug is to be stopped, it is recommended that it be withdrawn gradually rather than abruptly.

For intra-articular, intralesional and soft tissue use, a lesser initial dosage range of Triamcinolone Diacetate may produce the desired effect when the drug is administered to provide a localized concentration. The site of the injection and the volume of the injection should be carefully considered when Triamcinolone Diacetate is administered for this purpose.

Specific

Forte:

ARISTOCORT FORTE Parenteral is a suspension of 40 mg./ml. of *triamcinolone diacetate.* The full-strength suspension may be employed. If preferred, the suspension may be diluted

Continued on next page

The information on each product appearing here is based on labelling effective in August, 1982 and is either the entire official brochure or an accurate condensation therefrom. Offical brochures are enclosed in product packages. Information concerning all Lederle products may be obtained from the Professional Services Department, Lederle Laboratories, Pearl River, New York, 10965.

Lederle—Cont.

with normal saline or water. The diluent may also be prepared by mixing equal parts of normal saline and 1% procaine hydrochloride or other similar local anesthetics. The use of diluents containing preservatives such as methylparaben, propylparaben, phenol, etc. must be avoided as these preparations tend to cause flocculation of the steroid. These dilutions retain full potency for at least one week. Topical ethyl chloride spray may be used locally prior to injection.

Intramuscular: Although ARISTOCORT FORTE Parenteral may be administered intramuscularly for initial therapy, most physicians prefer to adjust the dose orally until adequate control is attained. Intramuscular administration provides a sustained or depot action which can be used to supplement or replace initial oral therapy. With intramuscular therapy, greater supervision of the amount of steroid used is made possible in the patient who is inconsistent in following an oral dosage schedule. In maintenance therapy, the patient-to-patient response is not uniform and, therefore, the dose must be individualized for optimal control.

Although triamcinolone diacetate may possess greater anti-inflammatory potency than many glucocorticoids, this is only dose-related since side effects, such as osteoporosis, peptic ulcer, etc. related to glucocorticoid activity, have not been diminished.

The average dose is 40 mg. (1 ml.) administered intramuscularly once a week for conditions in which anti-inflammatory action is desired.

In general, a single parenteral dose 4 to 7 times the oral daily dose may be expected to control the patient from 4 to 7 days up to 3 to 4 weeks. Dosage should be adjusted to the point where adequate but not necessarily complete relief of symptoms is obtained.

Intra-Articular and Intrasynovial: The usual dose varies from 5 to 40 mg. The average for the knee, for example, is 25 mg. The duration of effect varies from one week to 2 months. However, acutely inflamed joints may require more frequent injections.

A lesser initial dosage range of Triamcinolone Diacetate may produce the desired effect when the drug is administered to provide a localized concentration. The site of the injection and the volume of the injection should be carefully considered when Triamcinolone Diacetate is administered for this purpose.

A specific dose depends largely on the size of the joint.

Strict surgical asepsis is mandatory. The physician should be familiar with anatomical relationships as described in standard text books. ARISTOCORT FORTE Parenteral may be used in any accessible joint except the intervertebrals. In general, intrasynovial therapy is suggested under the following circumstances:

1. When systemic steroid therapy is contraindicated because of side effects such as peptic ulcer.
2. When it is desirable to secure relief in one or two specific joints.
3. When good systemic maintenance fails to control flare-ups in a few joints and it is desirable to secure relief without increasing oral therapy.

Such treatment should not be considered to constitute a cure; although this method will ameliorate the joint symptoms, it does not preclude the need for the conventional measures usually employed.

It is suggested that infiltration of the soft tissue by local anesthetic precede intra-articular injection. A 24-gauge or larger needle on a dry syringe may be inserted into the joint and excess fluid aspirated. For the first few hours following injection, there may be local discomfort in the joint but this is usually followed rapidly by effective relief of pain and improvement in local function.

[See table below].

Intralesional

When ARISTOCORT INTRALESIONAL is administered by injection strict aseptic technique is mandatory. Full strength suspensions may be employed, or if preferred, the suspension may be diluted, either to a 1:1 or 1:10 concentration, thus obtaining a working concentration of 12.5 mg./ml. or approximately 2.5 mg./ml. respectively. Normal (isotonic) saline solution alone or equal parts of normal (isotonic saline solution and 1% procaine or other local anesthetics, may be used as diluents. These dilutions usually retain full potency for at least one week. Topical ethyl chloride spray may be used as a local anesthetic. The use of diluents containing preservatives such as methylparaben, propylparaben, phenol, etc. must be avoided as these preparations tend to cause flocculations of the steroid.

Intralesional or Sublesional: For small lesions, injection is usually well tolerated and a local anesthetic is not necessary. The location and type of lesion will determine the route of injection: intralesional, sublesional, intradermal, subdermal, intracutaneous, or subcutaneous. The size of the lesion will determine: the total amount of drug needed, the concentration used, and the number and pattern of injection sites utilized (e.g. from a total of 5 mg. ARISTOCORT INTRALESIONAL in a 2 ml. volume divided over several locations in small lesions, ranging up to 48 mg. total ARISTOCORT INTRALESIONAL for large psoriatic plaques). Avoid injecting too superficially. In general, no more than 12.5 mg. per injection site should be used. An average of 25 mg. is the usual limit for any one lesion. Large areas require multiple injections with smaller doses per injection.

For a majority of conditions, sublesional injection directly through the lesion into the deep dermal tissue is suggested. In cases where it is difficult to inject intradermally, the suspension may be introduced subcutaneously, as superficially as possible.

Two or three injections at one to two week intervals may suffice as an average course of treatment for many conditions. Within 5-7 days after initial injection involution of the lesion can usually be seen, with pronounced clearing towards normal tissue after 12-14 days. Multiple injections of small amounts of equal strength may be convenient in alopecia areata and in psoriasis where there are large or confluent lesions. This is best accomplished by a series of fan-like injections ½ to 1 inch apart.

Alopecia areata and totalis require an average dose of 25 mg. to 30 mg. in a concentration of 10 mg./ml. subcutaneously 1 to 2 times a week, to stimulate hair regrowth. Results may be expected in 3 to 6 weeks on this dosage, and hair growth may last 3-6 months after initial injection. No more than 0.5 ml. should be given in any one site, because excessive deposition may produce local skin atrophy. Continued periodic local injections may be necessary to maintain response and continued hair growth. Use of more dilute solutions diminish the incidence and degree of local atrophy in the injection site.

In keloids and similar dense scars, injections are usually made directly into the lesion.

Injections may be repeated as required, but probably a total of no more than 75 mg. of ARISTOCORT *triamcinolone* a week should be given to any one patient. The need for repeated injections is best determined by clinical response. Remissions may be expected to last from a few weeks up to eleven months.

Intra-articular or Intrasynovial: Strict surgical asepsis is mandatory. The physician should be familiar with anatomical relationships as described in standard text books. A recent paper details the anatomy and the technical approach in arthrocentesis.

It is usually recommended that infiltration by local anesthetic of the soft tissue precede intra-articular injection. A 22-gauge or larger needle on a dry syringe should be inserted into the joint and excess fluid if present should be aspirated. The specific dose depends primarily on the size of the joint. The usual dose varies from 5 mg. to 40 mg. with the average for the knee being 25 mg. Smaller joints as in the fingers require 2 mg. to 5 mg. The duration of effect varies from one week to two months. However, acutely inflamed joints may require more frequent injections. Accidental injection into soft tissue is usually not harmful but decreases the local effectiveness and, because the drug is more rapidly absorbed, may produce a systemic effect. Injection into subcutaneous lipoid tissue may produce "pseudo-atrophy" with a persistent depression of the overlying dermis, lasting several weeks or months.

Administration and dosage of ARISTOCORT INTRALESIONAL must be individualized according to the nature, severity and chronicity of the disease or disorder treated, and should be undertaken with a view of the patient's entire clinical condition. Corticosteroid therapy is considered an adjunct to and not usually a replacement for conventional therapy. Therapy with ARISTOCORT INTRALESIONAL, as with all steroids, is of the suppressive type, related to its anti-inflammatory effect. The dose should be regulated during therapy according to the degree of therapeutic response, and should be reduced gradually to maintenance levels, whereby the patient obtains adequate or acceptable control of symptoms. When such control occurs, consideration should be given to gradual decrease in dosage and eventual cessation of therapy. Remission of symptoms may be due to therapy or may be spontaneous and a therapeutic test of gradual withdrawal of steroid treatment is usually indicated.

How Supplied:

*__Intralesional:__ (25 mg./ml.); 5 ml. Vials.

*__Forte:__ (40 mg./ml.); 1 ml. and 5 ml. Vials.

A.H.F.S. 68:04

*Manufactured for
LEDERLE LABORATORIES DIVISION
American Cyanamid Company
Pearl River, NY 10965
by
LEDERLE PARENTERALS INC.
Carolina, Puerto Rico 00630

Equivalence Table

	Anti-inflammatory Relative Potency		Frequently Used Tablet Strength (mg)		Tablet × Potency Equivalent Value
Hydrocortisone	1	×	20	=	20
Prednisolone	4	×	5	=	20
ARISTOCORT® triamcinolone	5	×	4	=	20
Dexamethasone	25	×	0.75	=	18.75

ARISTOCORT® A ℞

Triamcinolone Acetonide
Topical Products

[See table on next page].

Actions: Topical steroids are primarily effective because of their anti-inflammatory, antipruritic and vasoconstrictive actions.

Indications: For relief of the inflammatory manifestations of corticosteroid-responsive dermatoses.

Contraindications: Topical steroids are contraindicated in those patients with a history of hypersensitivity to any of the components of the preparation.

Precautions: If irritation develops, the product should be discontinued and appropriate therapy instituted.

In the presence of an infection the use of an appropriate antifungal or antibacterial agent should be instituted. If a favorable response does not occur promptly, the corticosteroid should be discontinued until the infection has been adequately controlled.

If extensive areas are treated or if the occlusive technique is used there will be increased systemic absorption of the corticosteroid and suitable precautions should be taken, particularly in children and infants.

Although topical steroids have not been reported to have an adverse effect on human pregnancy, the safety of their use in pregnant women has not absolutely been established. In laboratory animals, increases in incidence of fetal abnormalities have been associated with exposure of gestating females to topical corticosteroids, in some cases at rather low dosage levels. Therefore, drugs of this class should not be used extensively on pregnant patients, in large amounts, or for prolonged periods of time.

The product is not for ophthalmic use.

Adverse Reactions: The following local adverse reactions have been reported with topical corticosteroids, especially under occlusive dressings.

1. Burning 2. Itching 3. Irritation 4. Dryness 5. Folliculitis 6. Hypertrichosis 7. Acneiform eruptions 8. Hypopigmentation 9. Perioral dermatitis 10. Allergic Contact Dermatitis 11. Maceration of the skin 12. Secondary infection 13. Skin atrophy 14. Striae 15. Miliaria

0.1% cream

Military Depots: NSN 6505-01-107-1731, 60 Gm. tube

VA Depots: NSN 6505-01-107-1731A, 60 Gm. tube

[*Shown in Product Identification Section*]

ARISTOCORT® A Triamcinotone Acetonide TOPICAL PRODUCTS

	Cream 0.025%	Cream 0.1%	Cream 0.5%	Ointment 0.1%	Ointment 0.5%
Each gram contains Triamcinolone Acetonide	0.25 mg	1 mg	5 mg	1 mg	5 mg
Base	AQUATAIN™ Hydrophilic Base Emulsifying wax NF, isopropyl palmitate, glycerin USP, sorbitol solution USP, lactic acid, 2% benzyl alcohol, purified water. AQUATAIN is non-staining, water-washable, paraben-free, spermaceti-free and has a light texture and consistency.			Emulsifying wax NF, white petrolatum, propylene glycol, Tenox II, lactic acid.	
Dosage and Administration	Apply to affected areas 3 or 4 times daily. The cream should be rubbed in gently and thoroughly until it disappears.			Apply to affected areas 3 or 4 times daily.	
How Supplied	15 and 60 gram tubes	15 and 60 gram tubes, 240 gram jar	15 gram tube, 240 gram jar	15 and 60 gram tubes	15 gram tube

ARISTOSPAN® ℞

Sterile Triamcinolone Hexacetonide Suspension, USP

For Intralesional Administration

5 mg./ml.—Parenteral

For Intra-articular Administration

20 mg./ml.—Parenteral

NOT FOR INTRAVENOUS USE

Description:

Intralesional:

A sterile suspension containing 5 mg./ml. of micronized triamcinolone hexacetonide in the following inactive ingredients:

Polysorbate 80 NF........................0.20% w/v
Sorbitol Solution USP ....50.00% v/v
Water for Injection qs ad ....100.00% V
Preservative:
Benzyl Alcohol..............................0.90% w/v

Intra-articular:

A sterile suspension containing 20 mg./ml. of micronized triamcinolone hexacetonide in the following inactive ingredients:

Polysorbate 80 NF........................0.40% w/v
Sorbitol Solution USP ....50.00% v/v
Water for Injection qs ad ....100.00% V
Preservative:
Benzyl Alcohol.............................. 0.90% w/v

The hexacetonide ester of the potent glucocorticoid triamcinolone is relatively insoluble (0.0002% at 25° C. in water). When injected intralesionally, sublesionally, or intra-articularly, it can be expected to be absorbed slowly from the injection site.

Chemically triamcinolone hexacetonide USP is 9-Fluoro-11β, 16α, 17,21-tetrahydroxypregna-1,4-diene-3,20-dione cyclic 16,17-acetal with acetone 21-(3,3-dimethylbutyrate). Molecular weight 532.65.

Actions: Naturally occurring glucocorticoids (hydrocortisone), which also have salt-retaining properties, are used as replacement therapy in adrenocortical deficiency states. Their synthetic analogs are primarily used for their potent anti-inflammatory effects in disorders of many organ systems.

Glucocorticoids cause profound and varied metabolic effects. In addition, they modify the body's immune responses to diverse stimuli.

Indications:

Intralesional or sublesional ARISTOSPAN *sterile triamcinolone hexacetonide suspension* is indicated for the following:

Keloids.
Localized hypertrophic, infiltrated, inflammatory lesions of: lichen planus, psoriatic plaques, granuloma annulare and lichen simplex chronicus (neurodermatitis).
Discoid lupus erythematosus.
Necrobiosis lipoidica diabeticorum.
Alopecia areata.

They may also be useful in cystic tumors of an aponeurosis or tendon (ganglia).

Intra-articular:

As adjunctive therapy for short-term administration (to tide the patient over an acute episode or exacerbation) in:

Synovitis of osteoarthritis
Acute and subacute bursitis
Epicondylitis
Posttraumatic osteoarthritis
Rheumatoid arthritis
Acute gouty arthritis
Acute nonspecific tenosynovitis

Contraindications: Systemic fungal infections.

Warnings: In patients on corticosteroid therapy subjected to any unusual stress, increased dosage of rapidly acting corticosteroids before, during, and after the stressful situation is indicated.

Corticosteroids may mask some signs of infection, and new infections may appear during their use. There may be decreased resistance and inability to localize infection when corticosteroids are used.

Prolonged use of corticosteroids may produce posterior subcapsular cataracts, glaucoma with possible damage to the optic nerves and may enhance the establishment of secondary ocular infections due to fungi or viruses.

Usage in pregnancy

Since adequate human reproduction studies have not been done with corticosteroids, the use of these drugs in pregnancy, nursing mothers, or women of childbearing potential requires that the possible benefits of the drug be weighed against the potential hazards to the mother and embryo or fetus.

Infants born of mothers who have received substantial doses of corticosteroids during pregnancy should be carefully observed for signs of hypoadrenalism.

Average and large doses of cortisone or hydrocortisone can cause elevation of blood pressure, salt and water retention, and increased excretion of potassium. These effects are less likely to occur with the synthetic derivatives except when used in large doses. Dietary salt restriction and potassium supplementation may be necessary. All corticosteroids increase calcium excretion.

While on Corticosteroid Therapy Patients Should Not Be Vaccinated Against Smallpox. Other Immunization Procedures Should Not Be Undertaken in Patients Who Are on Corticosteroids, Especially in High Doses, Because of Possible Hazards of Neurological Complications and Lack of Antibody Response.

The use of ARISTOSPAN *sterile triamcinolone hexacetonide suspension* in active tuberculosis should be restricted to those cases of fulminating or disseminated tuberculosis in which the corticosteroid is used for the management of the disease in conjunction with appropriate antituberculous regimen.

If corticosteroids are indicated in patients with latent tuberculosis or tuberculin reactivity, close observation is necessary as reactivation of the disease may occur. During prolonged corticosteroid therapy, these patients should receive chemoprophylaxis.

Because rare instances of anaphylactoid reactions have occurred in patients receiving parenteral corticosteroid therapy, appropriate precautionary measures should be taken prior to administration, especially when the patient has a history of allergy to any drug.

Continued on next page

The information on each product appearing here is based on labelling effective in August, 1982 and is either the entire official brochure or an accurate condensation therefrom. Offical brochures are enclosed in product packages. Information concerning all Lederle products may be obtained from the Professional Services Department, Lederle Laboratories, Pearl River, New York, 10965.

Lederle—Cont.

Intralesional or sublesional injection of excessive dosage whether by single or multiple injection into any given area may cause cutaneous or subcutaneous atrophy.
Post-injection flare (following intra-articular use) and charcot-like arthropathy have been associated with parenteral corticosteroid therapy.

Precautions: Drug-induced secondary adrenocortical insufficiency may be minimized by gradual reduction of dosage. This type of relative insufficiency may persist for months after discontinuation of therapy; therefore, in any situation of stress occurring during that period, hormone therapy should be reinstituted. Since mineralocorticoid secretion may be impaired, salt and/or a mineralocorticoid should be administered concurrently.
There is an enhanced effect of corticosteroids in patients with hypothyroidism and in those with cirrhosis.
Corticosteroids should be used cautiously in patients with ocular herpes simplex for fear of corneal perforation.
The lowest possible dose of corticosteroid should be used to control the condition under treatment, and when reduction in dosage is possible, the reduction must be gradual.
Psychic derangements may appear when corticosteroids are used, ranging from euphoria, insomnia, mood swings, personality changes, and severe depression to frank psychotic manifestations. Also, existing emotional instability or psychotic tendencies may be aggravated by corticosteroids.
Aspirin should be used cautiously in conjunction with corticosteroids in hypoprothrombinemia.
Steroids should be used with caution in nonspecific ulcerative colitis, if there is a probability of impending perforation, abscess or other pyogenic infection, also in diverticulitis, fresh intestinal anastomoses, active or latent peptic ulcer, renal insufficiency, hypertension, osteoporosis, and myasthenia gravis.
Growth and development of infants and children on prolonged corticosteroid therapy should be carefully followed.
The following additional precautions apply for parenteral corticosteroids.
Intra-articular injection of a corticosteroid may produce systemic as well as local effects.
Appropriate examination of any joint fluid present is necessary to exclude a septic process..
A marked increase in pain accompanied by local swelling, further restriction of joint motion, fever, and malaise are suggestive of septic arthritis. If this complication occurs and the diagnosis of sepsis is confirmed, appropriate antimicrobial therapy should be instituted.
Local injection of a steroid into a previously infected joint is to be avoided.
Corticosteroids should not be injected into unstable joints.
The slower rate of absorption by intramuscular administration should be recognized.
Routine laboratory studies, such as urinalysis, two-hour postprandial blood sugar, determination of blood pressure and body weight, and a chest X-ray should be made at regular intervals during prolonged therapy. Upper GI X-rays are desirable in patients with an ulcer history or significant dyspepsia.

Adverse Reactions:
Fluid and electrolyte disturbances:
- Sodium retention.
- Fluid retention.
- Congestive heart failure in susceptible patients.
- Potassium loss.
- Hypokalemic alkalosis.
- Hypertension.

Musculoskeletal:
- Muscle weakness.
- Steroid myopathy.
- Loss of muscle mass.
- Osteoporosis.
- Vertebral compression fractures.
- Aseptic necrosis of femoral and humeral heads.
- Pathologic fracture of long bones.

Gastrointestinal:
- Peptic ulcer with possible subsequent perforation and hemorrhage.
- Pancreatitis.
- Abdominal distention.
- Ulcerative esophagitis.

Dermatologic:
- Impaired wound healing.
- Thin fragile skin.
- Petechiae and ecchymoses.
- Facial erythema.
- Increased sweating.
- May suppress reactions to skin tests.

Neurological:
- Convulsions
- Increased intracranial pressure with papilledema (pseudotumor cerebri) usually after treatment.
- Vertigo.
- Headache.

Endocrine:
- Menstrual irregularities.
- Development of Cushingoid state.
- Suppression of growth in children.
- Secondary adrenocortical and pituitary unresponsiveness, particularly in times of stress, as in trauma, surgery, or illness.
- Decreased carbohydrate tolerance.
- Manifestations of latent diabetes mellitus.
- Increased requirements for insulin or oral hypoglycemic agents in diabetics.

Ophthalmic:
- Posterior subcapsular cataracts.
- Increased intraocular pressure.
- Glaucoma.
- Exophthalmos.

Metabolic:
- Negative nitrogen balance due to protein catabolism.

The following additional adverse reactions are related to parenteral and intralesional corticosteroid therapy:
- Rare instances of blindness associated with intralesional therapy around the face and head.
- Hyperpigmentation or hypopigmentation.
- Sterile abscess.
- Subcutaneous and cutaneous atrophy.

Dosage and Administration:
General
The initial dosage of ARISTOPAN *sterile triamcinolone hexacetonide suspension* may vary from 2 to 48 mg. per day depending on the specific disease entity being treated. In situations of less severity, lower doses will generally suffice while in selected patients higher initial doses may be required. Usually the parenteral dosage ranges are one-third to one-half the oral dose given every 12 hours. However, in certain overwhelming, acute, life-threatening situations, administration in dosages exceeding the usual dosages may be justified and may be in multiples of the oral dosages.
The initial dosage should be maintained or adjusted until a satisfactory response is noted. If after a reasonable period of time there is a lack of satisfactory clinical response, ARISTOSPAN should be discontinued and the patient transferred to other appropriate therapy.
It Should Be Emphasized That Dosage Requirements Are Variable and Must Be Individualized on the Basis of the Disease Under Treatment and the Response of the Patient. After a favorable response is noted, the proper maintenance dosage should be determined by decreasing the initial drug dosage in small increments at appropriate time intervals until the lowest dosage which will maintain an adequate clinical response is reached. It should be kept in mind that constant monitoring is needed in regard to drug dosage. Included in the situations which may make dosage adjustments necessary are changes in clinical status secondary to remissions or exacerbations in the disease process, the patient's individual drug responsiveness, and the effect of patient exposure to stressful situations not directly related to the disease entity under treatment; in this latter situation it may be necessary to increase the dosage of ARISTOSPAN for a period of time consistent with the patient's condition. If after long-term therapy the drug is to be stopped, it is recommended that it be withdrawn gradually rather than abruptly.
Directions for Use
Strict aseptic administration technique is mandatory. Topical ethyl chloride spray may be used locally before injection.
The syringe should be gently agitated to achieve uniform suspension before use. Since ARISTOSPAN suspension has been designed for ease of administration, a small bore needle (25 or 26 gauge) may be used.
Dilution—Intralesional 5 mg./ml.
ARISTOSPAN suspension may be diluted, if desired, with Dextrose and Sodium Chloride Injection USP, (5% and 10% Dextrose), Sodium Chloride Injection USP, or Sterile Water for Injection USP.
The optimum dilution, i.e., 1:1, 1:2, 1:4, should be determined by the nature of the lesion, its size, the depth of injection, the volume needed, and location of the lesion. In general, more superficial injections should be performed with greater dilution. Certain conditions, such as keloids, require a less dilute suspension such as 5 mg./ml., with variation in dose and dilution as dictated by the condition of the individual patient. Subsequent dosage, dilution, and frequency of injections are best judged by the clinical response.
The suspension may also be mixed with 1% or 2% Lidocaine Hydrochloride, using the formulations which do not contain parabens. Similar local anesthetics may also be used. Diluents containing methylparaben, propylparaben, phenol, etc., should be avoided since these compounds may cause flocculation of the steroid. These dilutions will retain full potency for one week, but care should be exercised to avoid contamination of the vial's contents and the dilutions should be discarded after 7 days.

Intralesional or Sublesional
Average Dose—up to 0.5 mg. per square inch of affected skin injected intralesionally or sublesionally. The frequency of subsequent injections is best determined by the clinical response. If desired, the vial may be diluted as indicated under DIRECTIONS FOR USE.
A lesser initial dosage range of ARISTOSPAN may produce the desired effect when the drug is administered to provide a localized concentration. The site of the injection and the volume of the injection should be carefully considered when ARISTOSPAN is administered for this purpose.
Dilution—Intra-articular 20 mg./ml.
ARISTOSPAN suspension may be mixed with 1% or 2% Lidocaine Hydrochloride, using the formulations which do not contain parabens. Similar local anesthetics may also be used. Diluents containing methylparaben, propylparaben, phenol, etc., should be avoided since these compounds may cause flocculation of the steroid. These dilutions will retain full potency for one week, but care should be exercised to avoid contamination.

Intra-articular
Average dose—2 to 20 mg. (0.1 ml. to 1.0 ml.)
The dose depends on the size of the joint to be injected, the degree of inflammation, and the amount of fluid present. In general, large joints (such as knee, hip, shoulder) require 10 to 20 mg. For small joints (such as interphalangeal, metacarpophalangeal), 2 to 6 mg, may be employed. When the amount of synovial fluid is increased, aspiration may be performed before administering ARISTOSPAN. Subsequent

dosage and frequency of injections can best be judged by clinical response.
The usual frequency of injection into a single joint is every three or four weeks, and injection more frequently than that is generally not advisable. To avoid possible joint destruction from repeated use of intra-articular corticosteroids, injection should be as infrequent as possible, consistent with adequate patient care. Attention should be paid to avoiding deposition of drug along the needle path which might produce atrophy.

How Supplied:
*Intralesional, 5 ml. (in a 12.5 ml. vial).
*Intra-articular, 1 ml. vial and 5 ml. vial.
A.H.F.S. 68:04

Military Depots: NSN-6505-00-148-6985, 5 ml vial

VA Depots: NSN-6505-00-148-6985A, 5 ml vial

*Manufactured for
LEDERLE LABORATORIES DIVISION
American Cyanamid Company
Pearl River, NY 10965
by
LEDERLE PARENTERALS INC.
Carolina, Puerto Rico 00630

ARTANE® ℞
trihexyphenidyl HCl
Tablets, Elixir, and SEQUELS®
Sustained Release Capsules

Description: ARTANE *trihexyphenidyl HCl* is a synthetic antispasmodic drug available in the following forms:
TABLETS: 2 mg—round, flat, scored, white tablets; engraved ARTANE above 2 on one side and LL above A11 below the score on the other side. 2 mg—round, flat, scored, white tablets; engraved ARTANE above 5 on one side and LL above A12 below the score on the other side.
ELIXIR: 2 mg/5ml in a clear, colorless, limemint flavored preparation with 0.08% methylparaben, 0.02% propylparaben, and 5% alcohol as preservatives.
SEQUELS: The 5 mg Sustained Release Capsules are soft shelled, oval shaped, clear blue, printed A9L.
Actions: ARTANE *trihexyphenidyl HCl Lederle* is the substituted piperidine salt, 3-(1-piperidyl)-1-phenyl-cyclohexyl-1-propanol hydrochloride, which exerts a direct inhibitory effect upon the parasympathetic nervous system. It also has a relaxing effect on smooth musculature; exerted both directly upon the muscle tissue itself and indirectly through an inhibitory effect upon the parasympathetic nervous system. Its therapeutic properties are similar to those of atropine, although undesirable side effects are ordinarily less frequent and severe than with the latter.
Indications:
This drug is indicated as an adjunct in the treatment of all forms of parkinsonism (postencephalitic, arteriosclerotic, and idiopathic). It is often useful as adjuvant therapy when treating these forms of parkinsonism with levodopa. Additionally, it is indicated for the control of extrapyramidal disorders caused by central nervous system drugs such as the dibenoxazepines, phenothiazines, thioxanthenes, and butyrophenones.
SEQUELS—For maintenance therapy after patients have been stabilized on trihexyphenidyl hydrochloride in conventional dosage forms (tablets or elixir).
Warning: Patients to be treated with ARTANE should have a gonioscope evaluation and close monitoring of intraocular pressures at regular periodic intervals.
Precautions: Although trihexyphenidyl HCl is *not* contraindicated for patients with cardiac, liver, or kidney disorders, or with hypertension, such patients should be maintained under close observation.
Since the use of trihexyphenidyl HCl may, in some cases, continue indefinitely and since it has atropine-like properties, patients should be subjected to constant and careful long-term observation to avoid allergic and other untoward reactions. Inasmuch as trihexyphenidyl HCl possesses some parasympatholytic activity, it should be used with caution in patients with glaucoma, obstructive disease of the gastrointestinal or genitourinary tracts, and in elderly males with possible prostatic hypertrophy. Geriatric patients, particularly over the age of 60, frequently develop increased sensitivity to the actions of drugs of this type, and hence, require strict dosage regulation. Incipient glaucoma may be precipitated by parasympatholytic drugs such as trihexyphenidyl HCl.
Adverse Reactions: Minor side effects, such as dryness of the mouth, blurring of vision, dizziness, mild nausea or nervousness, will be experienced by 30 to 50 per cent of all patients. These sensations, however, are much less troublesome with ARTANE *trihexyphenidyl HCl* than with belladonna alkaloids and are usually less disturbing than unalleviated parkinsonism. Such reactions tend to become less pronounced, and even to disappear, as treatment continues. Even before these reactions have remitted spontaneously, they may often be controlled by careful adjustment of dosage form, amount of drug, or interval between doses.
Isolated instances of suppurative parotitis secondary to excessive dryness of the mouth, skin rashes, dilatation of the colon, paralytic ileus, and certain psychiatric manifestations such as delusions and hallucinations, plus one doubtful case of paranoia all of which may occur with any of the atropine-like drugs, have been rarely reported with ARTANE.
Patients with arteriosclerosis or with a history of idiosyncrasy to other drugs may exhibit reactions of mental confusion, agitation, disturbed behavior, or nausea and vomiting. Such patients should be allowed to develop a tolerance through the initial administration of a small dose and gradual increase in dose until an effective level is reached. If a severe reaction should occur, administration of the drug should be discontinued for a few days and then resumed at a lower dosage. Psychiatric disturbances can result from indiscriminate use (leading to overdosage) to sustain continued euphoria.
Potential side effects associated with the use of any atropine-like drugs include constipation, drowsiness, urinary hesitancy or retention, tachycardia, dilation of the pupil, increased intraocular tension, weakness, vomiting, and headache.
The occurrence of angle-closure glaucoma due to long-term treatment with trihexyphenidyl hydrochloride has been reported.
Dosage and Administration: Dosage should be individualized. The initial dose should be low and then increased gradually, especially in patients over 60 years of age. Whether ARTANE *trihexyphenidyl HCl* may best be given before or after meals should be determined by the way the patient reacts. Postencephalitic patients, who are usually more prone to excessive salivation, may prefer to take it after meals and may, in addition, require small amounts of atropine which, under such circumstances, is sometimes an effective adjuvant. If ARTANE tends to dry the mouth excessively, it may be better to take it before meals, unless it causes nausea. If taken after meals, the thirst sometimes induced can be allayed by mint candies, chewing gum or water.
ARTANE Trihexyphenidyl HCl in Idiopathic Parkinsonism
As initial therapy for parkinsonism, 1 mg of ARTANE in tablet or elixir form may be administered the first day. The dose may then be increased by 2 mg increments at intervals of three tc five days, until a total of 6 to 10 mg is given daily. The total daily dose will depend upon what is found to be the optimal level. Many patients derive maximum benefit from this daily total of 6 to 10 mg, but some patients, chiefly those in the postencephalitic group, may require a total daily dose of 12 to 15 mg.
ARTANE Trihexyphenidyl HCl in Drug-Induced Parkinsonism
The size and frequency of dose of ARTANE needed to control extrapyramidal reactions to commonly employed tranquilizers, notably the phenothiazines, thioxanthenes, and butyrophenones, must be determined empirically. The total daily dosage usually ranges between 5 and 15 mg although, in some cases, these reactions have been satisfactorily controlled on as little as 1 mg daily. It may be advisable to commence therapy with a single 1 mg dose. If the extrapyramidal manifestations are not controlled in a few hours, the subsequent doses may be progressively increased until satisfactory control is achieved. Satisfactory control may sometimes be more rapidly achieved by temporarily reducing the dosage of the tranquilizer on instituting ARTANE trihexyphenidyl HCl therapy and then adjusting dosage of both drugs until the desired ataractic effect is retained without onset of extrapyramidal reactions.
It is sometimes possible to maintain the patient on a reduced ARTANE dosage after the reactions have remained under control for several days. Instances have been reported in which these reactions have remained in remission for long periods after ARTANE therapy was discontinued.
Concomitant Use of ARTANE Trihexyphenidyl HCl with Levodopa
When ARTANE is used concomitantly with levodopa, the usual dose of each may need to be reduced. Careful adjustment is necessary, depending on side effects and degree of symptom control. ARTANE dosage of 3 to 6 mg daily, in divided doses, is usually adequate.
Concomitant Use of ARTANE Trihexyphenidyl HCl with Other Parasympathetic Inhibitors
ARTANE *trihexyphenidyl HCl* may be substituted, in whole or in part, for other parasympathetic inhibitors. The usual technique is partial substitution initially, with progressive reduction in the other medication as the dose of trihexyphenidyl HCl is increased.
ARTANE TABLETS and ELIXIR—The total daily intake of ARTANE tablets or elixir is tolerated best if divided into 3 doses and taken at mealtimes. High doses (> 10 mg daily) may be divided into 4 parts, with 3 doses administered at mealtimes and the fourth at bedtime.
ARTANE SEQUELS—Because of the relatively high dosage in each controlled release capsule, this dosage form should not be used for initial therapy. After patients are stabilized on trihexyphenidyl HCl in conventional dosage forms (tablet or elixir), for convenience of administration they may be switched to the controlled release capsules on a milligram per milligram total daily dose basis, as a single dose after breakfast or in two divided doses 12 hours apart. Most patients will be adequately maintained on the controlled release form, but some may develop an exacerbation of parkinsonism and have to be returned to the conventional form.
How Supplied:
ARTANE® Trihexyphenidyl HCl is available as follows:

Continued on next page

The information on each product appearing here is based on labelling effective in August, 1982 and is either the entire official brochure or an accurate condensation therefrom. Offical brochures are enclosed in product packages. Information concerning all Lederle products may be obtained from the Professional Services Department, Lederle Laboratories, Pearl River, New York, 10965.

Lederle—Cont.

TABLETS: 2 mg—round, flat, scored, white tablets; engraved ARTANE above 2 on one side and LL above A11 below the score on the other side, are supplied as follows:
NDC 0005-4434-23—Bottles of 100
NDC 0005-4434-34—Bottles of 1000
NDC 0005-4434-60—Unit Dose 10 × 10's
5 mg—round, flat, scored, white tablets; engraved ARTANE above 5 on one side and LL above A12 below the score on the other side, are supplied as follows:
NDC 0005-4436-23—Bottles of 100
NDC 0005-4436-34—Bottles of 1000
NDC 0005-4436-60—Unit Dose 10 × 10's
Store at Controlled Room Temperature 15–30° C (59–86° F)
ELIXIR: 2 mg/5ml—NDC 0005-4440-65—Bottles of 16 Fl. Oz.
Store at Controlled Room Temperature 15–30° C (59–86°F) DO NOT FREEZE
SEQUELS SUSTAINED RELEASE CAPSULES: 5 mg—soft shell, oval shaped, clear blue, printed A9L, are supplied as follows:
NDC 0005-4438-32—Unit-of-Issue 60's with CRC
NDC 0005-4438-31—Bottles of 500
Store at Controlled Room Temperature 15–30° C (59–86° F)
VA depot NSN 6505-00-890-1378A—16 oz.

ASENDIN® ℞
amoxapine

Description: ASENDIN *amoxapine* is an antidepressant of the dibenzoxazepine class, chemically distinct from the dibenzazepines, dibenzocycloheptenes, and dibenzoxepines.
It is designated chemically as 2-chloro-11-(1-piperazinyl)dibenz-[b,f][1,4] oxazepine. The molecular weight is 313.8. The empirical formula is $C_{17}H_{16}ClN_3O$.
ASENDIN is supplied for oral administration as 25 mg, 50 mg, 100 mg, and 150 mg tablets.
Clinical Pharmacology: ASENDIN is an antidepressant with a mild sedative component to its action. The mechanism of its clinical action in man is not well understood. In animals, amoxapine reduced the uptake of norepinephrine and serotonin and blocked the response of dopamine receptors to dopamine. Amoxapine is not a monoamine oxidase inhibitor.
ASENDIN is absorbed rapidly and reaches peak blood levels approximately 90 minutes after ingestion. It is almost completely metabolized. The main route of excretion is the kidney. *In vitro* tests show that amoxopine binding to human serum is approximately 90%.
In man, amoxapine serum concentration declines with a half-life of 8 hours. However, the major metabolite, 8-hydroxyamoxapine, has a biologic half-life of 30 hours. Metabolites are excreted in the urine in conjugated form as glucuronides.
Clinical studies have demonstrated that ASENDIN has a more rapid onset of action than either amitriptyline or imipramine. The initial clinical effect may occur within four to seven days and occurs within two weeks in over 80% of responders.
Indications and Usage: ASENDIN is indicated for the relief of symptoms of depression in patients with neurotic or reactive depressive disorders as well as endogenous and psychotic depressions. It is indicated for depression accompanied by anxiety or agitation.
Contraindications: ASENDIN is contraindicated in patients who have shown prior hypersensitivity to dibenzoxazepine compounds. It should not be given concomitantly with monoamine oxidase inhibitors. Hyperpyretic crises, severe convulsions, and deaths have occurred in patients receiving tricyclic antidepressants and monoamine oxidase inhibitors simultaneously. When it is desired to replace a monoamine oxidase inhibitor with ASENDIN, a minimum of 14 days should be allowed to elapse after the former is discontinued. ASENDIN should then be initiated cautiously with gradual increase in dosage until optimum response is achieved. The drug is not recommended for use during the acute recovery phase following myocardial infarction.
Warnings: ASENDIN should be used with caution in patients with a history of urinary retention, angle-closure glaucoma or increased intraocular pressure. Patients with cardiovascular disorders should be watched closely. Tricyclic antidepressant drugs, particularly when given in high doses, can induce sinus tachycardia, changes in conduction time, and arrhythmias. Myocardial infarction and stroke have been reported with drugs of this class.
Extreme caution should be used in treating patients with a history of convulsive disorder or those with overt or latent seizure disorders.
Precautions:
General:
In prescribing the drug it should be borne in mind that the possibility of suicide is inherent in any severely depressed patient, and persists until a significant remission occurs; the drug should be dispensed in the smallest suitable amount. Manic depressive patients may experience a shift to the manic phase. Schizophrenic patients may develop increased symptoms of psychosis; patients with paranoid symptomatology may have an exaggeration of such symptoms. This may require reduction of dosage or the addition of a major tranquilizer to the therapeutic regimen. Antidepressant drugs can cause skin rashes and/or "drug fever" in susceptible individuals. These allergic reactions may, in rare cases, be severe. They are more likely to occur during the first few days of treatment, but may also occur later. ASENDIN should be discontinued if rash and /or fever develop. Amoxapine possesses a degree of dopamine-blocking activity which may cause extrapyramidal symptoms in <1% of patients. Rarely, symptoms indicative of tardive dyskinesia have been reported, possibly related to treatment with amoxapine.
Information for the patient:
Patients should be warned of the possibility of drowsiness that may impair performance of potentially hazardous tasks such as driving an automobile or operating machinery.
Drug interactions:
See "Contraindications" about concurrent usage of tricyclic antidepressants and monoamine oxidase inhibitors. Paralytic ileus may occur in patients taking tricyclic antidepressants in combination with anticholenergic drugs. ASENDIN may enhance the response to alcohol and the effects of barbiturates and other CNS depressants.
Therapeutic interactions:
Concurrent administration with electroshock therapy may increase the hazards associated with such therapy.
Carcinogenesis, impairment of fertility:
In a 21-month toxicity study at 3 dose levels in rats, pancreatic islet cell hyperplasia occured with slightly increased incidence at doses 5–10 times the human dose. Pancreatic adenocarcinoma was detected in low incidence in the mid-dose group only, and may possibly have resulted from endocrine-mediated organ hyperfunction. The significance of these findings to man is not known.
Treatment of male rats with 5–10 times the human dose resulted in a slight decrease in the number of fertile matings. Female rats receiving oral doses within the therapeutic range displayed a reversible increase in estrous cycle length.
Pregnancy. Pregnancy category C:
Studies performed in mice, rats and rabbits have demonstrated no evidence of teratogenic effect due to ASENDIN. Embryotoxicity was seen in rats and rabbits given oral doses approximating the human dose. Fetotoxic effects (intrauterine death, stillbirth, decreased birth weight) were seen in animal studies at oral doses 3–10 times the human dose. Decreased postnatal survival (between days 0–4) was demonstrated in the offspring of rats at 5–10 times the human dose. There are no adequate and well-controlled studies in pregnant women. ASENDIN should be used during pregnancy only if the potential benefit justifies the potential risk to the fetus.
Nursing mothers:
ASENDIN, like many other systemic drugs, is excreted in human milk. Because effects of the drug on infants are unknown, caution should be exercised when ASENDIN is administered to nursing women.
Pediatric use:
Safety and effectiveness in children below the age of 16 have not been established.
Adverse Reactions: Adverse reactions reported in controlled studies in the United States are categorized with respect to incidence below. Following this is a listing of reactions known to occur with other antidepressant drugs of this class but not reported to date with ASENDIN.
INCIDENCE GREATER THAN 1%
The most frequent types of adverse reactions occurring with ASENDIN in controlled clinical trials were sedative and anticholinergic: these included drowsiness (14%), dry mouth (14%), constipation (12%), and blurred vision (7%).
Less frequently reported reactions were:
CNS and Neuromuscular—anxiety, insomnia, restlessness, nervousness, palpitations, tremors, confusion, excitement, nightmares, ataxia, alterations in EEG patterns.
Allergic—edema.
Gastrointenstinal—Nausea.
Other—dizziness, headache, fatigue, weakness, excessive appetite, increased perspiration.
INCIDENCE LESS THAN 1%
Anticholinergic—disturbances of accommodation, mydriasis, delayed micturition, urinary retention, nasal stuffiness.
Cardiovascular—hypotension, hypertension, syncope, tachycardia.
Allergic—drug fever with skin rash, photosensitization, pruritus, rarely vasculitis.
CNS and Neuromuscular—tingling, paresthesias of the extremities, tinnitus, disorientation, seizures, hypomania, numbness, incoordination, disturbed concentration, extrapyramidal symptoms, including, rarely, tardive dyskinesia.
Hematologic—Leukopenia.
Gastrointestinal—epigastric distress, vomiting, flatulence, abdominal pain, peculiar taste, diarrhea.
Endocrine—increased or decreased libido, impotence, menstrual irregularity, breast enlargement and galactorrhea in the female.
Other—lacrimation, weight gain or loss, altered liver function.
DRUG RELATIONSHIP UNKNOWN
The following reactions have been reported very rarely, and occurred under controlled circumstances where a drug relationship was difficult to assess. These observations are listed to serve as alerting information to physicians.
Allergic—urticaria and petechiae.
Anticholinergic—paralytic ileus.
Cardiovascular—atrial arrhythmias (including atrial fibrillation), myocardial infarction, stroke, heart block.
CNS *and Neuromuscular*—hallucinations, nightmares.
Hematologic—thrombocytopenia, purpura.
Gastrointestinal—parotic swelling.
Endocrine—change in blood glucose levels.
Other—pancreatitis, hepatitis, jaundice, urinary frequency, testicular swelling, anorexia.
ADDITIONAL ADVERSE REACTIONS
The following reactions have been reported with other antidepressant drugs, but not with ASENDIN.

Anticholinergic—sublingual adenitis, dilation of the urinary tract.
CNS *and Neuromuscular*—delusions, syndrome of inappropriate ADH secretion.
Hematologic—agranulocytosis, eosinophilia.
Gastrointestinal—stomatitis, black tongue.
Endocrine—gynecomastia.
Other—alopecia.

Overdosage:
Signs and Symptoms
Initial toxic manifestations of ASENDIN overdosage typically are CNS effects: delirium, lethargy with diminished deep tendon reflexes, and/or seizures. Cardiovascular effects, when they occur, are usually limited to sinus tachycardia and transient minor EKG changes. Serious hypotension, hypertension, or cardiac arrhythmias are rare. Respiratory acidosis may develop following repeated seizures, and metabolic acidosis has been reported.
Important
Renal impairment may develop three to five days after substantial overdosage in patients who may appear otherwise recovered. Oliguria, hematuria, and renal failure have been reported. Tubular necrosis and rhabdomyolysis with myoglobinuria may also occur in such cases. Treatment is the same as that for non-drug-induced renal dysfunction. In a limited series of cases of renal failure following overdosage, 70% have recovered with appropriate treatment.
In general, treatment of overdosage must be symptomatic and supportive. If the patient is conscious, induced emesis followed by gastric lavage with appropriate precautions to prevent pulmonary aspiration should be accomplished as soon as possible. Following lavage, activated charcoal may be administered to reduce absorption. An adequate airway should be established in comatose patients and assisted ventilation instituted if necessary. Convulsions, should they occur, may respond to standard anticonvulsant therapy; however, barbiturates may potentiate any respiratory depression. Specific treatment should be guided by the predominent symptoms which may suggest use of a particular pharmacologic agent. For example, the slow intravenous administration of physostigmine salicylate has been reported to reverse most of the serious cardiovascular and CNS effects of overdosage with tricyclic antidepressants, such as cardiac arryhthmias and convulsions. (Avoid rapid injection to reduce the possibility of physostigmin induced convulsions.) Convulsions may also be treated with intravenous diazepam. Acidosis may be treated by cautious intravenous administration of sodium bicarbonate.
A patient who has ingested a toxic overdose of a tricyclic antidepressant may remain medically and psychiatrically unstable for several days due to sustained excessive drug levels. Unexpected cardiac deaths have occurred up to six days post overdose with other antidepressants. The QRS interval of the electocardiogram appears a reliable correlate of the severity of overdosage. If the QRS interval exceeds 100 milliseconds anytime during the first 24 hours after overdose, cardiac function should be continuously monitored for five or six days. (Prolongation of the QRS interval beyond 100 milliseconds has not been reported with ASENDIN overdosage, and there have been no deaths due to primary cardiac toxicity.)
The smallest estimated lethal overdose reported has been 2.6 grams. On the other hand, some patients have survived much larger overdoses. Age and physical condition of the patient, concomitant ingestion of other drugs, and especially the interval between drug ingestion and initiation of emergency treatment, are important determining factors in the probability of survival.

Dosage and Administration: Effective dosage of ASENDIN may vary from one patient to another. Usual effective dosage is 200 mg to 300 mg daily. Three weeks constitutes an adequate period of trial providing dosage has reached 300 mg daily (or a lower level of tolerance) for at least two weeks. If no response is seen at 300 mg, dosage may be increased, depending upon tolerance, up to 400 mg daily. Hospitalized patients who have been refractory to antidepressant therapy and who have no history of convulsive seizures may have dosage raised cautiously up to 600 mg daily in divided doses.
ASENDIN may be given in a single daily dose, not to exceed 300 mg, preferably at bedtime. If the total daily dosage exceeds 300 mg, it should be given in divided doses.
Initial Dosage for Adults—Usual starting dosage is 50 mg three times daily. Depending upon tolerance, dosage may be increased to 100 mg three times daily on the third day of treatment. (Initial dosage of 300 mg daily may be given, but notable sedation may occur in some patients during the first few days of therapy at this level.) Increases above 300 mg daily should be made only if 300 mg daily has been ineffective during a trial period of at least two weeks. When effective dosage is established, the drug may be given in a single dose (not to exceed 300 mg) at bedtime.
Elderly Patients—In general, lower dosages of the tricyclic antidepressants are recommended for these patients. Recommended starting dosage of ASENDIN is 25 mg three times daily. If no intolerance is observed, dosage may be increased after three days to 50 mg three times daily. Although 100–150 mg daily may be adequate for many elderly patients, some may require higher dosage. Careful increases up to 300 mg daily are indicated in such cases.
Once an effective dosage is established, ASENDIN may conveniently be given in a single bedtime dose, not to exceed 300 mg.
Maintenance—Recommended maintenance dosage of ASENDIN is the lowest dose that will maintain remission. If symptoms reappear, dosage should be increased to the earlier level until they are controlled.
For maintenance therapy at dosage of 300 mg or less, a single dose at bedtime is recommended.

How Supplied: ASENDIN *Amoxapine* Tablets are supplied as follows:
25 mg—white, heptagon-shaped tablets, engraved on one side with LL above 25 and with A13 on the other scored side.
(Product No. NDC 0005-5389-23)—bottles of 100
50 mg—orange, heptagon-shaped tablets, engraved on one side with LL above 50 and with A15 on the other scored side.
(Product No. NDC 0005-5390-23)—bottles of 100
(Product No. NDC 0005-5390-31)—bottles of 500
(Product No. NDC 0005-5390-60)—10 × 10 Unit Dose
100 mg—Blue, heptagon-shaped tablets, engraved on one side with LL above 100 and with A17 on the other scored side.
(Product No. NDC 0005-5391-23)—bottles of 100
(Product No. NDC 0005-5391-60)—10 × 10 Unit Dose
150 mg—Peach, heptagon-shaped tablets, engraved on one side with LL above 150 and with A18 on the other scored side.
(Product No. NDC 0005-5392-38)—bottles of 30
Store at Controlled Room Temperature 15–30°C (59–86°F)
VA Depot: NSN 6505-01-111-3195A 50 mg-100's
NSN 6505-01-111-3194A 100 mg-100's
[*Shown in Product Identification Section*]

AUREOMYCIN®
chlortetracycline HCl
OINTMENT

Description: Each gram contains:
Chlortetracycline HCl ....30 mg. (3%)
in a white petrolatum-anhydrous lanolin base. AUREOMYCIN *chlortetracycline HCl* is one of the most versatile of the broad spectrum antibiotics and is effective against many Gram-positive and Gram-negative organisms, as well as rickettsial, viral and virus-like infections.
Indications: AUREOMYCIN Ointment, for topical application only, is indicated for the treatment of superficial pyogenic infections of the skin. It is effective against both Gram-positive cocci (streptococci, staphylococci and pneumococci) and Gram-negative bacteria (coli-aerogenes group).
Precautions: The use of antibiotics may result in the overgrowth of nonsusceptible organisms. If new infections appear during therapy, appropriate measures should be taken.
If adverse reaction or idiosyncrasy occurs, discontinue medication.
Administration and Dosage: In the treatment of local skin infections, apply the ointment directly to the involved area, preferably on sterile gauze, one or more times daily as the condition warrants. In severe local infection, topical application should be supplemented by oral administration of an appropriate antibiotic.
How Supplied: ½ and 1 oz. tubes. Rx not required.

Advanced Formula
CENTRUM®
High Potency
Multivitamin-Multimineral Formula
(See PDR For Nonprescription Drugs)

Children's Chewable
CENTRUM®, Jr.
Vitamin/Mineral Formula + Iron
(See PDR For Nonprescription Drugs)

CHOLERA VACCINE ℞
(India Strains)

How Supplied: 1 ml. vial (1 immunization)
COMPLETE INFORMATION FURNISHED IN THE PACKAGE.

CYCLOCORT® ℞
amcinonide cream 0.1% with
AQUATAIN™ hydrophilic base

Description: 0.1% topical cream with AQUATAIN™ hydrophilic base:
Each gram of CYCLOCORT topical cream contains 1 mg (0.1%) of the active steroid, amcinonide in AQUATAIN, a specially formulated base composed of emulsifying wax NF, isopropyl palmitate, glycerin USP, sorbitol solution USP, lactic acid, 2% benzyl alcohol and purified water.
Action: Topical steroids are primarily effective because of their anti-inflammatory, antipruritic, and vasoconstrictive actions.
Indications: For relief of the inflammatory manifestations of corticosteroid responsive dermatoses.

Continued on next page

The information on each product appearing here is based on labelling effective in August, 1982 and is either the entire official brochure or an accurate condensation therefrom. Offical brochures are enclosed in product packages. Information concerning all Lederle products may be obtained from the Professional Services Department, Lederle Laboratories, Pearl River, New York, 10965.

Lederle—Cont.

Contraindications: Topical steroids are contraindicated in those patients with a history of hypersensitivity to any of the components of the preparation.
Precautions: If irritation develops, the product should be discontinued and appropriate therapy instituted.
In the presence of an infection the use of an appropriate antifungal or antibacterial agent should be instituted. If a favorable response does not occur promptly, the corticosteroid should be discontinued until the infection has been adequately controlled.
If extensive areas are treated or if an occlusive technique is used there will be increased systemic absorption of the corticosteroid and suitable precautions should be taken, particularly in children and infants.
Although topical steroids have not been reported to have an adverse effect on human pregnancy, the safety of their use in pregnant women has not absolutely been established. In laboratory animals, increases in incidence of fetal abnormalities have been associated with exposure of gestating females to topical corticosteroids, in some cases at rather low dosage levels. Therefore, drugs of this class should not be used extensively on pregnant patients, in large amounts, or for prolonged periods of time.
The product is not for ophthalmic use.
Adverse Reactions: The following local adverse reactions have been reported with topical corticosteroids, especially under occlusive dressings: burning, itching, irritation, dryness, folliculitis, hypertrichosis, acneiform eruptions, hypopigmentation, perioral dermatitis, allergic contact dermatitis, maceration of the skin, secondary infection, skin atrophy, striae and miliaria.
Dosage and Administration: Apply a light film to affected areas 2 or 3 times daily. The cream should be rubbed in gently and thoroughly until it disappears.
How Supplied: 0.1% Topical Cream Available in 15, 30 and 60 Gram tubes.
[*Shown in Product Identification Section*]
VA Depots: NSN 6505-01-093-7968A
60 gm Tubes

CYCLOCORT® ℞
amcinonide
Ointment 0.1%

Description: 0.1% topical ointment.
Each gram of CYCLOCORT Ointment contains 1 mg of the active steroid amcinonide in a specially formulated base composed of petrolatum, white USP; benzyl alcohol NF, emulsifying wax NF; and Tenox II (butylated hydroxyanisole, propyl gallate, citric acid, propylene glycol). Amcinonide is (11β,16 α)-21-(acetyloxy)-16,17-[cyclopentylidenebis(oxy)]-9-fluoro-11-hydroxypregna-1,4-diene-3,20-dione.
The topical corticosteroids constitute a class of primarily synthetic steroids used as anti-inflammatory and anti-pruritic agents.
Clinical Pharmacology: Topical corticosteroids share anti-inflammatory, anti-pruritic and vasoconstrictive actions.
The mechanism of anti-inflammatory activity of the topical corticosteroids is unclear. Various laboratory methods, including vasoconstrictor assays, are used to compare and predict potencies and/or clinical efficacies of the topical corticosteroids. There is some evidence to suggest that a recognizable correlation exists between vasoconstrictor potency and therapeutic efficacy in man.
Pharmacokinetics
The extent of percutaneous absorption of topical corticosteroids is determined by many factors including the vehicle, the integrity of the epidermal barrier, and the use of occlusive dressings.
Topical corticosteroids can be absorbed from normal intact skin. Inflammation and/or other disease processes in the skin increase percutaneous absorption. Occlusive dressings substantially increase the percutaneous absorption of topical corticosteroids. Thus, occlusive dressings may be valuable therapeutic adjunct for treatment of resistant dermatoses. (See *DOSAGE AND ADMINISTRATION*).
Once absorbed through the skin, topical corticosteroids are handled through pharmacokinetic pathways similar to systemically administered corticosteroids. Corticosteroids are bound to plasma proteins in varying degrees. Corticosteroids are metabolized primarily in the liver and are then excreted by the kidneys. Some of the topical corticosteroids and their metabolites are also excreted into the bile.
Indications and Usage: Topical corticosteroids are indicated for the relief of the inflammatory and pruritic manifestations of corticosteroid-responsive dermatoses.
Contraindications: Topical corticosteroids are contraindicated in those patients with a history of hypersensitivity to any of the components of the preparation.
Precautions:
General
Systemic absorption of topical corticosteroids has produced reversible hypothalamic-pituitary-adrenal (HPA) axis suppression, manifestations of Cushing's syndrome, hyperglycemia, and glucosuria in some patients.
Conditions which augment systemic absorption include the application of the more potent steroids, use over large surface areas, prolonged use, and the addition of occlusive dressings.
Therefore, patients receiving a large dose of a potent topical steroid applied to a large surface area or under an occlusive dressing should be evaluated periodically for evidence of HPA axis suppression by using the urinary free cortisol and ACTH stimulation tests. If HPA axis suppression is noted, an attempt should be made to withdraw the drug, to reduce the frequency of application, or to substitute a less potent steroid.
Recovery of HPA axis function is generally prompt and complete upon discontinuation of the drug. Infrequently, signs and symptoms of steroid withdrawal may occur, requiring supplemental systemic corticosteroids.
Children may absorb proportionally larger amounts of topical corticosteroids and thus be more susceptible to systemic toxicity. (See *PRECAUTIONS—Pediatric Use*).
If irritation develops, topical corticosteroids should be discontinued and appropriate therapy instituted.
In the presence of dermatological infections, the use of an appropriate antifungal or antibacterial agent should be instituted. If a favorable response does not occur promptly, the corticosteroid should be discontinued until the infection has been adequately controlled.
The product is not for ophthalmic use.
Information for the Patient
Patients using topical corticosteroids should receive the following information and instructions:
1. This medication is to be used as directed by the physician. It is for external use only. Avoid contact with the eyes.
2. Patients should be advised not to use this medication for any disorder other than for which it was prescribed.
3. The treated skin area should not be bandaged or otherwise covered or wrapped as to be occlusive unless directed by the physician.
4. Patients should report any signs of local adverse reactions especially under occlusive dressing.
5. Parents of pediatric patients should be advised not to use tight-fitting diapers or plastic pants on a child being treated in the diaper area, as these garments may constitute occlusive dressings.

Laboratory Tests
The following tests may be helpful in evaluating the HPA axis suppression:
Urinary free cortisol test
ACTH stimulation test
Carcinogenesis, Mutagenesis, and Impairment of Fertility
Long-term animal studies have not been performed to evaluate the carcinogenic potential or the effect on fertility of topical corticosteroids.
Studies to determine mutagenicity with prednisolone and hydrocortisone have revealed negative results.
Pregnancy Category C
Corticosteroids are generally teratogenic in laboratory animals when administered systemically at relatively low dosage levels. The more potent corticosteroids have been shown to be teratogenic after dermal application in laboratory animals. There are no adequate and well-controlled studies in pregnant women on teratogenic effects from topically applied corticosteroids. Therefore, topical corticosteroids should be used during pregnancy only if the potential benefit justifies the potential risk to the fetus. Drugs of this class should not be used extensively on pregnant patients, in large amounts, or for prolonged periods of time.
Nursing Mothers
It is not known whether topical administration of corticosteroids could result in sufficient systemic absorption to produce detectable quantities in breast milk. Systemically administered, corticosteroids are secreted into breast milk in quantities *not* likely to have a deleterious effect on the infant. Nevertheless, caution should be exercised when topical corticosteroids are administered to a nursing woman.
Pediatric Use
Pediatric patients may demonstrate greater susceptibility to topical corticosteroid-induced HPA axis suppression and Cushing's syndrome than mature patients because of a larger skin surface area to body weight ratio.
Hypothalamic-pituitary-adrenal (HPA) axis suppression, Cushing's syndrome, and intracranial hypertension have been reported in children receiving topical corticosteroids. Manifestations of adrenal suppression in children include linear growth retardation, delayed weight gain, low plasma cortisol levels, and absence of response to ACTH stimulation. Manifestations of intracranial hypertension include bulging fontanelles, headaches, and bilateral papilledema.
Administration of topical corticosteroids to children should be limited to the least amount compatible with an effective therapeutic regimen. Chronic corticosteroid therapy may interefere with the growth and development of children.
Adverse Reactions: The following local adverse reactions are reported infrequently with topical corticosteroids, but may occur more frequently with the use of occlusive dressings. These reactions are listed in an approximate decreasing order of occurrence: Burning, Itching, Irritation, Dryness, Folliculitis, Hypertrichosis, Acneiform eruptions, Hypopigmentation, Perioral dermatitis, Allergic contact dermatitis, Maceration of the skin, Secondary infection, Skin Atrophy, Striae and Miliaria.
Overdosage: Topically applied corticosteroids can be absorbed in sufficient amounts to produce systemic effects (See *PRECAUTIONS*).
Dosage and Administration: Topical corticosteroids are generally applied to the affected area as a thin film twice daily, depending on the severity of the condition.
Occlusive dressings may be used for the management of psoriasis or recalcitrant conditions.
If an infection develops, the use of occlusive dressings should be discontinued and appropriate antimicrobial therapy instituted.

How Supplied: CYCLOCORT® Amcinonide Topical Ointment 0.1% (1 mg/gm) is available as follows:

15 gram tubes—NDC 0005-9345-09
60 gram tubes—NDC 0005-9345-40
30 gram tubes—NDC 0005-9345-32

Store at Controlled Room Temperature 15–30°C (59–86°F)

LEDERLE LABORATORIES DIVISION
American Cyanamid Company, Pearl River, N.Y. 10965

DECLOMYCIN® ℞

demeclocycline hydrochloride
For oral use

Description: DECLOMYCIN *demeclocycline hydrochloride* is an antibiotic isolated from a mutant strain of *Streptomyces aureofaciens*. Chemically it is the hydrochloride of 7-chloro-4-dimethylamino-1, 4, 4a, 5, 5a, 6, 11, 12a-octahydro-3, 6, 10, 12, 12a-pentahydroxy-1, 11-dioxo-2-naphthacenecarboxamide.

Actions: The tetracyclines are primarily bacteriostatic and are thought to exert their antimicrobial effect by the inhibition of protein synthesis. Tetracyclines are active against a wide range of gram-negative and gram-positive organisms.

The drugs in the tetracycline class have closely similar antimicrobial spectra, and cross-resistance among them is common. Micro-organisms may be considered susceptible if the M.I.C. (minimum inhibitory concentration) is not more than 4.0 mcg./ml. and intermediate if the M.I.C. is 4.0 to 12.5 mcg./ml.

Susceptibility plate testing: A tetracycline disc may be used to determine microbial susceptibility to drugs in the tetracycline class. If the Kirby-Bauer method of disc susceptibility testing is used, a 30 mcg. tetracycline disc should give a zone of at least 19 mm. when tested against a tetracycline-susceptible bacterial strain.

Tetracyclines are readily absorbed and are bound to plasma proteins in varying degree. They are concentrated by the liver in the bile and excreted in the urine and feces at high concentrations and in a biologically active form.

Indications: DECLOMYCIN *demeclocycline hydrochloride* is indicated in infections caused by the following micro-organisms:

Rickettsiae: (Rocky Mountain spotted fever, typhus fever and the typhus group, Q fever, rickettsialpox, tick fevers.)
Mycoplasma pneumoniae (PPLO, Eaton agent).
Agents of psittacosis and ornithosis.
Agents of lymphogranuloma venereum and granuloma inguinale.
The spirochetal agent of relapsing fever *(Borrelia recurrentis)*.

The following gram-negative micro-organisms:
Haemophilus ducreyi (chancroid),
Pasteurella pestis and *Pasteurella tularensis*,
Bartonella bacilliformis,
Bacteroides species,
Vibrio comma and *Vibrio fetus*.
Brucella species (in conjunction with streptomycin).

Because many strains of the following groups of micro-organisms have been shown to be resistant to tetracyclines, culture and susceptibility testing are recommended.

Demeclocycline is indicated for treatment of infections caused by the following gram-negative micro-organisms, when bacteriologic testing indicates appropriate susceptibility to the drug:
Escherichia coli,
Enterobacter aerogenes (formerly *Aerobacter aerogenes*),
Shigella species,
Mima species and *Herellea* species,
Haemophilus influenzae (respiratory infections),
Klebsiella species (respiratory and urinary infections).

Demeclocycline is indicated for treatment of infections caused by the following gram-positive micro-organisms when bacteriologic testing indicates appropriate susceptibility to the drug:
Streptococcus species:
Up to 44 percent of strains of *Streptococcus pyogenes* and 74 percent of *Streptococcus faecalis* have been found to be resistant to tetracycline drugs. Therefore, tetracyclines should not be used for streptococcal disease unless the organism has been demonstrated to be sensitive.
For upper respiratory infections due to group A beta-hemolytic streptococci, penicillin is the usual drug of choice, including prophyaxis of rheumatic fever.
Diplococcus pneumoniae,
Staphylococcus aureus, skin and soft tissue infections. Tetracyclines are not the drugs of choice in the treatment of any type of staphylococcal infection.

When penicillin is contraindicated, tetracyclines are alternative drugs in the treatment of infections due to:
Neisseria gonorrhoeae,
Treponema pallidum and *Treponema pertenue* (syphilis and yaws),
Listeria monocytogenes,
Clostridium species,
Bacillus anthracis,
Fusobacterium fusiforme (Vincent's infection),
Actinomyces species.

In acute intestinal amebiasis, the tetracyclines may be a useful adjunct to amebicides.

DECLOMYCIN *demeclocycline hydrochloride* is indicated in the treatment of trachoma, although the infectious agent is not always eliminated, as judged by immunofluorescence.

Inclusion conjunctivitis may be treated with oral tetracyclines or with a combination of oral and topical agents.

Contraindications: This drug is contraindicated in persons who have shown hypersensitivity to any of the tetracyclines.

Warnings: THE USE OF DRUGS OF THE TETRACYCLINE CLASS DURING TOOTH DEVELOPMENT (LAST HALF OF PREGNANCY, INFANCY AND CHILDHOOD TO THE AGE OF 8 YEARS) MAY CAUSE PERMANENT DISCOLORATION OF THE TEETH (YELLOW-GRAY-BROWN).

This adverse reaction is more common during long-term use of the drugs but has been observed following repeated short-term courses. Enamel hypoplasia has also been reported. TETRACYCLINE DRUGS, THEREFORE, SHOULD NOT BE USED IN THIS AGE GROUP UNLESS OTHER DRUGS ARE NOT LIKELY TO BE EFFECTIVE OR ARE CONTRAINDICATED.

If renal impairment exists, even usual oral or parenteral doses may lead to excessive systemic accumulation of the drug and possible liver toxicity. Under such conditions, lower than usual total doses are indicated and, if therapy is prolonged, serum level determinations of the drug may be advisable.

Phototoxic reactions can occur in individuals taking demeclocycline, and are characterized by severe burns of exposed surfaces resulting from direct exposure of patients to sunlight during therapy with moderate or large doses of demeclocycline. Patients apt to be exposed to direct sunlight or ultraviolet light should be advised that this reaction can occur, and treatment should be discontinued at the first evidence of skin erythema.

The anti-anabolic action of the tetracyclines may cause an increase in BUN. While this is not a problem in those with normal renal function, in patients with significantly impaired function, higher serum levels of tetracycline may lead to azotemia, hyperphosphatemia, and acidosis.

Administration of demeclocycline has resulted in appearance of the diabetes insipidus syndrome (polyuria, polydipsia and weakness) in some patients on long term therapy. The syndrome has been shown to be nephrogenic, dose-dependent and reversible on discontinuance of therapy.

Usage in pregnancy (See above "Warnings" about use during tooth development.)

Results of animal studies indicate that tetracyclines cross the placenta, are found in fetal tissues and can have toxic effects on the developing fetus (often related to retardation of skeletal development). Evidence of embryotoxicity has also been noted in animals treated early in pregnancy.

Usage in newborns, infants, and children (See above "Warnings" about use during tooth development.)

All tetracyclines form a stable calcium complex in any bone forming tissue. A decrease in the fibula growth rate has been observed in prematures given oral tetracycline in doses of 25 mg./kg. every 6 hours. This reaction was shown to be reversible when the drug was discontinued.

Tetracyclines are present in the milk of lactating women who are taking a drug in this class.

Precautions: As with other antibiotic preparations, use of this drug may result in overgrowth of nonsusceptible organisms, including fungi. If superinfection occurs, the antibiotic should be discontinued and appropriate therapy should be instituted.

In venereal diseases when coexistent syphilis is suspected, darkfield examination should be done before treatment is started and the blood serology repeated monthly for at least 4 months..

Because the tetracyclines have been shown to depress plasma prothrombin activity, patients who are on anticoagulant therapy may require downward adjustment of their anticoagulant dosage.

In long-term therapy, periodic laboratory evaluation of organ systems, including hematopoietic, renal and hepatic studies should be performed.

All infections due to Group A beta-hemolytic streptococci should be treated for at least 10 days.

Since bacteriostatic drugs may interfere with the bactericidal action of penicillin, it is advisable to avoid giving demeclocycline in conjunction with penicillin.

Interpretation of Bacteriologic Studies: Following a course of therapy, persistence for several days in both urine and blood of bacteriosuppressive levels of demeclocycline may interfere with culture studies. These levels should not be considered therapeutic.

Adverse Reactions: Gastrointestinal: Anorexia, nausea, vomiting, diarrhea, glossitis, dysphagia, enterocolitis, and inflammatory lesions (with monilial overgrowth) in the anogenital region. These reactions have been caused by both the oral and parenteral administration of tetracyclines.

Skin: Maculopapular and erythematous rashes. Exfoliative dermatitis has been reported but is uncommon. Photosensitivity is discussed above. (See "Warnings".)

Renal toxicity: Rise in BUN has been reported and is apparently dose related. Nephrogenic diabetes insipidus. (See "Warnings".)

Hypersensitivity reactions: Urticaria, angioneurotic edema, anaphylaxis, anaphylactoid

Continued on next page

The information on each product appearing here is based on labelling effective in August, 1982 and is either the entire official brochure or an accurate condensation therefrom. Offical brochures are enclosed in product packages. Information concerning all Lederle products may be obtained from the Professional Services Department, Lederle Laboratories, Pearl River, New York, 10965.

Lederle—Cont.

purpura, pericarditis and exacerbation of systemic lupus erythematosus.
Bulging fontanels have been reported in young infants following full therapeutic dosage. This sign disappeared rapidly when the drug was discontinued.
Blood: Hemolytic anemia, thrombocytopenia, neutropenia and eosinophilia have been reported.
When given over prolonged periods, tetracyclines have been reported to produce brown-black microscopic discoloration of thyroid glands. No abnormalities of thyroid function studies are known to occur.
Dosage and Administration: Therapy should be continued for at least 24-48 hours after symptoms and fever have subsided.
Concomitant therapy: Antacids containing aluminum, calcium, or magnesium impair absorption and should not be given to patients taking oral tetracycline.
Foods and some dairy products also interfere with absorption. Oral forms of tetracycline should be given 1 hour before or 2 hours after meals. Pediatric oral dosage forms should not be given with milk formulas and should be given at least 1 hour prior to feeding.
In patients with renal impairment: (See "Warnings.") Total dosage should be decreased by reduction of recommended individual doses and/or by extending time intervals between doses.
In the treatment of streptococcal infections, a therapeutic dose of demeclocycline should be administered for at least 10 days.
Adults: Usual daily dose—Four divided doses of 150 mg. each or two divided doses of 300 mg. each.
For children above eight years of age: Usual daily dose, 3-6 mg. per pound body weight per day, depending upon the severity of the disease, divided into 2 or 4 doses.
Gonorrhea patients sensitive to penicillin may be treated with demeclocycline administered as an initial oral dose of 600 mg. followed by 300 mg. every 12 hours for 4 days to a total of 3 grams.
How Supplied:
Capsules: 150 mg. *demeclocycline hydrochloride* (soft shell two tone coral) printed Lederle D9 bottles of 16 and 100.
Tablets: 150 mg. *demeclocycline hydrochloride* (Film Coated Red) D11 bottles of 16 and 100.
300 mg. *demeclocycline hydrochloride* (Film Coated Red) engraved LL D12 bottles of 12, 48 and Unit Dose 10 x 10's.
A.H.F.S. 8:12.24
[*Shown in Product Identification Section*]

DIAMOX® ℞
acetazolamide
TABLETS, PARENTERAL AND SEQUELS®
Sustained Release Capsules

Description: Tablets: 125 mg of acetazolamide, round, flat-faced, beveled, white tablets engraved with DIAMOX and 125 on one side and scored in half on the other side. Engraved with LL on the right of the score and D1 on the left. 250 mg of acetazolamide, round, convex, white tablets engraved with DIAMOX and 250 on one side and scored in quarters on the other side. Engraved with LL in the upper right quadrant and D2 in the lower left quadrant.
Parenteral: *Each vial contains acetazolamide 500 mg (as sodium salt) and pH adjusted to aproximately 9.2 with sodium hydroxide and, if necessary, hydrochloric acid.
SEQUELS: DIAMOX *acetazolamide* SEQUELS Lederle are sustained-release capsules each containing 500 mg. of acetazolamide.
Actions: DIAMOX is a potent carbonic anhydrase inhibitor, effective in the control of fluid secretion (e.g. some types of glaucoma), in the treatment of certain convulsive disorders (e.g. epilepsy) and in the promotion of diuresis in instances of abnormal fluid retention (e.g. cardiac edema).
DIAMOX is not a mercurial diuretic. Rather it is a nonbacteriostatic sulfonamide possessing a chemical structure and pharmacological activity distinctly different from the bacteriostatic sulfonamides.
DIAMOX is an enzyme inhibitor which acts specifically on carbonic anhydrase, the enzyme which catalyzes the reversible reaction involving the hydration of carbon dioxide and the dehydration of carbonic acid. In the eye, this inhibitory action of acetazolamide decreases the secretion of aqueous humor and results in a drop in intraocular pressure, a reaction considered desirable in cases of glaucoma and even in certain non-glaucomatous conditions. Evidence seems to indicate that DIAMOX has utility as an adjuvant in the treatment of certain dysfunctions of the central nervous system (e.g. epilepsy). Inhibition of carbonic anhydrase in this area appears to retard abnormal, paroxysmal, excessive discharge from central nervous system neurons. The diuretic effect of DIAMOX *acetazolamide* is due to its action in the kidney on the reversible reaction involving hydration of carbon dioxide and dehydration of carbonic acid. The result is renal loss of HCO_3 ion, which carries out sodium, water, and potassium. Alkalinization of the urine and promotion of diuresis are thus effected.
SEQUELS: DIAMOX Acetazolamide SEQUELS Sustained Release Capsules provide prolonged action to inhibit aqueous humor secretion for 18 to 24 hours after each dose, whereas tablets act for only 8 to 12 hours. The prolonged/continuous effect of SEQUELS permits a reduction in dosage frequency.
Blood level concentrations of acetazolamide peak between 8 to 12 hours after administration of DIAMOX SEQUELS, compared to 2 to 4 hours with tablets.
Indications—Tablets and Parenteral: For adjunctive treatment of: edema due to congestive heart failure; drug-induced edema; centrencephalic epilepsies (petit mal, unlocalized seizures); chronic simple (open angle) glaucoma, secondary glaucoma, and preoperatively in acute angle closure glaucoma where delay of surgery is desired in order to lower intraocular pressure.
Indications—SEQUELS: For adjunctive treatment of: chronic simple (open angle) glaucoma, secondary glaucoma, and preoperatively in acute angle closure glaucoma where delay of surgery is desired in order to lower intraocular pressure.
Contraindications: Acetazolamide therapy is contraindicated in situations in which sodium and/or potassium blood serum levels are depressed, in cases of marked kidney and liver disease or dysfunction, suprarenal gland failure, and hyperchloremic acidosis.
Long-term administration of DIAMOX *acetazolamide* is contraindicated in patients with chronic noncongestive angle closure glaucoma since it may permit organic closure of the angle to occur while the worsening glaucoma is masked by lowered intraocular pressure.
Warning: Studies of acetazolamide in rats and mice have demonstrated teratogenic and embryocidal effects at doses in excess of ten times those recommended in human beings. There is no evidence of these effects in human beings, however acetazolamide should not be used in pregnancy, especially during the first trimester, unless the benefits to be expected outweigh these potential adverse effects.
Precautions: Increasing the dose does not increase the diuresis and may increase the incidence of drowsiness and/or paresthesia. Increasing the dose often results in a decrease in diuresis. Under certain circumstances, however, very large doses have been given in conjunction with other diuretics in order to secure diuresis in complete refractory failure.
Adverse reactions common to all sulfonamide derivatives may occur: fever, rash, crystalluria, renal calculus, bone marrow depression, thrombocytopenic purpura, hemolytic anemia, leukopenia, pancytopenia and agranulocytosis. Precaution is advised for early detection of such reactions and the drug should be discontinued and appropriate therapy instituted.
In patients with pulmonary obstruction or emphysema where alveolar ventilation may be impaired, DIAMOX acetazolamide which may precipitate or aggravate acidosis, should be used with caution.
Adverse Reactions: Adverse reactions during short-term therapy are minimal. Those effects which have been noted include: paresthesias, particularly a "tingling" feeling in the extremities; some loss of appetite; polyuria and occasional instances of drowsiness and confusion.
During long-term therapy, an acidotic state may occasionally supervene. This can usually be corrected by the administration of bicarbonate.
Transient myopia has been reported. This condition invariably subsides upon diminution or discontinuance of the medication.
Other occasional adverse reactions include: urticaria; melena; hematuria; glycosuria; hepatic insufficiency; flaccid paralysis; and convulsions.
Dosage and Administration:
Preparation and Storage of Parenteral Solution:
Each 500 mg. vial containing DIAMOX *sterile acetazolamide sodium* Parenteral should be reconstituted with at least 5 ml. of Sterile Water for Injection prior to use. Reconstituted solutions retain potency for one week if refrigerated. Since this product contains no preservative, use within 24 hours of reconstitution is strongly recommended. The direct intravenous route of administration is preferred. Intramuscular administration may be employed but is painful, due to the alkaline pH of the solution.
Glaucoma: DIAMOX *acetazolamide* should be used as an adjunct to the usual therapy. The dosage employed in the treatment of *chronic simple (open-angle) glaucoma* ranges from 250 mg. to 1 Gram of DIAMOX per 24 hours, usually in divided doses for amounts over 250 mg. It has usually been found that a dosage in excess of 1 Gram per 24 hours does not produce an increased effect. In all cases, the dosage should be adjusted with careful individual attention both to symptomatology and ocular tension. Continuous supervision by a physician is advisable.
In the treatment of secondary glaucoma and in the preoperative treatment of some cases of *acute congestive (closed-angle) glaucoma,* the preferred dosage is 250 mg. every 4 hours, although some cases have responded to 250 mg. twice daily on short-term therapy. In some acute cases, it may be more satisfactory to administer an initial dose of 500 mg. followed by 125 or 250 mg. every 4 hours depending on the individual case. Intravenous therapy may be used for rapid relief of ocular tension in acute cases. A complementary effect has been noted when DIAMOX has been used in conjunction with miotics or mydriatics as the case demanded.
Epilepsy: It is not clearly known whether the beneficial effects observed in epilepsy are due to direct inhibition of carbonic anhydrase in the central nervous system or whether they are due to the slight degree of acidosis produced by the divided dosage. The best results to date have been seen in petit mal in children. Good results, however, have been seen in patients, both children and adult, in other types of seizures such as grand mal, mixed seizure patterns, myoclonic jerk patterns, etc. The suggested total daily dose is 8 to 30 mg. per Kg. in divided doses. Although some patients respond to a low dose, the optimum range appears to be from 375 to 1000 mg. daily. However, some investigators feel that daily doses in

excess of 1 Gram do not produce any better results than a 1 Gram dose. When DIAMOX is given in combination with other anti-convulsants, it is suggested that the starting dose should be 250 mg. once daily in addition to the existing medications. This can be increased to levels as indicated above.

The change from other medication to DIAMOX should be gradual in accordance with usual practice in epilepsy therapy.

Congestive Heart Failure: For diuresis in congestive heart failure, the starting dose is usually 250 to 375 mg. once daily in the morning (5 mg./Kg.). If after an initial response, the patient fails to continue to lose edema fluid, do not increase the dose but allow for kidney recovery by skipping medication for a day. DIAMOX *acetazolamide* yields best diuretic results when given on alternate days, or for 2 days alternating with a day of rest.

Failures in therapy may be due to overdosage or too frequent dosage. The use of DIAMOX does not eliminate the need for other therapy such as digitalis, bed rest, and salt restriction.

Drug-Induced Edema: Recommended dosage is 250 mg. to 375 mg. of DIAMOX once a day for 1 or 2 days, alternating with a day of rest.

Note: The dosage recommendations for glaucoma and epilepsy differ considerably from those for congestive heart failure, since the first two conditions are not dependent upon carbonic anhydrase inhibition in the kidney which requires intermittent dosage if it is to recover from the inhibitory effect of the therapeutic agent.

SEQUELS: The recommended dose is 1 capsule (500 mg.) 2 times a day. Usually 1 capsule is administered in the morning and 1 capsule in the evening. It may be necessary to adjust the dose but it has usually been found that dosage in excess of 2 capsules (1 Gram) does not produce an increased effect. The dosage should be adjusted with careful individual attention both to symptomatology and intraocular tension. In all cases, continuous supervision by a physician is advisable.

In those unusual instances where adequate control is not obtained by the twice-a-day administration of DIAMOX *acetazolamide* SEQUELS, sustained release capsules, the desired control may be established by means of DIAMOX (Tablets or Parenteral). Use tablets or parenteral in accordance with the more frequent dosage schedules recommended for these items, such as 250 mg. every 4 hours, or an initial dose of 500 mg. followed by 250 mg. or 125 mg. every 4 hours; depending on the case in question.

How Supplied: **Tablets** 125 mg—Round, flat-faced, beveled, white tablets engraved with DIAMOX and 125 on one side and scored in half on the other side. Engraved with LL on the right of the score and D1 on the left.

Bottles of 100—Product Number NDC 0005-4398

Tablets 250 mg—Round, convex, white tablets engraved with DIAMOX and 250 on one side and scored in quarters on the other side. Engraved with LL in the upper right quadrant and D2 in the lower left quadrant.

Bottles of 100, 1,000 unit dose 10 × 10's and Unit-of-Use 50 × 100's—Product Number NDC 0005-4469

***Parenteral**—500 mg vials of cryodesiccated powder—Product Number NDC 0005-4466

SEQUELS® sustained release capsules (soft shell, orange) printed with "DIAMOX" over D3, 500 mg.—bottles of 30 NDC 0005-4465-13 and 100 NDC 0005-4465-23.

Store at controlled room temperature 15–30°C (59–86°F).

A.H.F.S. 40:28

SEQUELS, 500 mg
Military Depot: NSN 6505-00-880-4949, 100's
VA Depot: NSN 6505-00-880-4949A, 100's

*Manufactured for
LEDERLE LABORATORIES DIVISION
American Cyanamid Company
Pearl River, NY 10965
by
LEDERLE PARENTERALS INC.
Carolina, Puerto Rico 00630

[Tablets and SEQUELS, Shown in Product Identification Section]

DIPHTHERIA AND TETANUS TOXOIDS, COMBINED PUROGENATED® ℞

How Supplied: 5 ml. vials (5 immunizations). COMPLETE INFORMATION FURNISHED IN THE PACKAGE.

FERRO-SEQUELS®
sustained release iron Capsules

Composition: Each capsule contains 150 mg. of ferrous fumarate equivalent to approximately 50 mg. of elemental iron, so prepared that it is released over a 5 to 6 hour period, and 100 mg. of docusate sodium (DSS) to counteract constipating effect of iron.

Indications: For the treatment of iron deficiency anemias.

Dosage: 1 capsule, once or twice daily or as prescribed by the physician.

Precautions: If pregnant or nursing, consult your physician or pharmacist before taking this or any medicine. Keep this and all medications out of the reach of children. In case of accidental overdose, seek professional assistance or contact a Poison Control Center immediately.

How Supplied: Capsules (green) Printed Lederle FERRO-SEQUELS®—F2—bottles of 30, 100, and 1,000; unit-dose 10 x 10's.

Military and USPHS depots
NSN-6505-00-149-0103, 30's
NSN 6505-00-074-2981, 1,000's
NSN 6505-00-131-8870, individually sealed 100's

A.H.F.S. 20:04.04

[Shown in Product Identification Section]

FILIBON®
prenatal tablets

Each tablet contains:

	For Pregnant or Lactating Women Percentage of U.S. Recommended Daily Allowance (U.S. RDA)
Vitamin A (as Acetate)	5000 I.U. (63%)
Vitamin D_2	400 I.U. (100%)
Vitamin E (as *dl*-Alpha Tocopheryl Acetate)	30 I.U. (100%)
Vitamin C (Ascorbic Acid)	60 mg (100%)
Folic Acid (Folacin)	0.4 mg (50%)
Vitamin B_1 (as Thiamine Mononitrate)	1.5 mg (88%)
Vitamin B_2 (as Riboflavin)	1.7 mg (85%)
Niacinamide	20 mg (100%)
Vitamin B_6 (as Pyridoxine Hydrochloride)	2 mg (80%)
Vitamin B_{12} (as Cyanocobalamin)	6 mcg (75%)
Calcium (as Calcium Carbonate)	125 mg (10%)
Iodine (as Potassium Iodide)	150 mcg (100%)
Iron (as Ferrous Fumarate)	18 mg (100%)
Magnesium (as Magnesium Oxide)	100 mg (22%)

A phosphorus-free vitamin and mineral dietary supplement for use in prenatal care and lactation.

Recommended Intake: 1 daily, or as prescribed by the physician.

How Supplied: Capsule-shaped tablets (film-coated, pink) engraved LL-F4—bottles of 100.

[Shown in Product Identification Section]

FILIBON® F.A. ℞
prenatal tablets

Each tablet contains:

	Percentage of U.S. Recommended Daily Allowance (U.S. RDA)
Vitamin A (as Acetate)	8000 I.U. (100%)
Vitamin D_2	400 I.U. (100%)
Vitamin E (as *dl*-Alpha Tocopheryl Acetate)	30 I.U. (100%)
Vitamin C (as Ascorbic Acid)	60 mg (100%)
Folic Acid (as Folacin)	1 mg (125%)
Vitamin B_1 (as Thiamine Mononitrate)	1.7 mg (100%)
Vitamin B_2 (as Riboflavin)	2 mg (100%)
Niacinamide	20 mg (100%)
Vitamin B_6 (as Pyridoxine Hydrochloride)	4.0 mg (160%)
Vitamin B_{12} (as Cyanocobalamin)	8 mcg (100%)
Calcium (as Calcium Carbonate)	250 mg (19%)
Iodine (as Potassium Iodide)	150 mcg (100%)
Iron (as Ferrous Fumarate)	45 mg (250%)
Magnesium (as Magnesium Oxide)	100 mg (22%)

Precaution: Folic acid may obscure pernicious anemia in that the peripheral blood picture may revert to normal while neurological manifestations remain progressive.

How Supplied: Capsule-shaped tablets (film-coated, pink) engraved LL-F5—bottles of 100.

[Shown in Product Identification Section]

FILIBON® FORTE ℞
prenatal tablets

Each tablet contains:

	Percentage of U.S. Recommended Daily Allowance (U.S. RDA)
Vitamin A (as Acetate)	8000 I.U. (100%)
Vitamin D_2	400 I.U. (100%)
Vitamin E (as *dl*-Alpha Tocopheryl Acetate)	45 I.U. (150%)
Vitamin C (Ascorbic Acid)	90 mg (150%)
Folic Acid (Folacin)	1 mg (125%)
Vitamin B_1 (as Thiamine Mononitrate)	2 mg (118%)
Vitamin B_2 (as Riboflavin)	2.5 mg (125%)
Niacinamide	30 mg (150%)
Vitamin B_6 (as Pyridoxine Hydrochloride)	3 mg (120%)
Vitamin B_{12} (as Cyanocobalamin)	12 mcg (150%)
Calcium (as Calcium Carbonate)	300 mg (23%)
Iodine (as Potassium Iodide)	200 mg (133%)
Iron (as Ferrous Fumarate)	45 mg (250%)
Magnesium (as Magnesium Oxide)	100 mg (22%)

Recommended Intake: 1 tablet daily. This dosage provides 23% and 22% the Recommended Daily Allowance of calcium and magnesium respectively, therefore, supplementation of the diet by milk or other sources of calcium may be advisable.

Precaution: Folic Acid may obscure pernicious anemia in that the peripheral blood pic-

Continued on next page

The information on each product appearing here is based on labelling effective in August, 1982 and is either the entire official brochure or an accurate condensation therefrom. Offical brochures are enclosed in product packages. Information concerning all Lederle products may be obtained from the Professional Services Department, Lederle Laboratories, Pearl River, New York, 10965.

Lederle—Cont.

ture may revert to normal while neurological manifestations remain progressive.
How Supplied: Tablets—film coated (pink) scored LL-F6—bottles of 100.
[*Shown in Product Identification Section*]

FILIBON® OT ℞
prenatal tablets

Each tablet contains:

	Percentage of U.S. Recommended Daily Allowance (U.S. RDA)
Vitamin A (as Acetate)	8000 I.U. (100%)
Vitamin D_2	400 I.U. (100%)
Vitamin E (as *dl*-Alpha Tocopheryl Acetate)	30 I.U. (100%)
Vitamin C (as Ascorbic Acid)	60 mg (100%)
Folic Acid (as Folacin)	1 mg (125%)
Vitamin B_1 (as Thiamine Mononitrate)	1.7 mg (100%)
Vitamin B_2 (as Riboflavin)	2 mg (100%)
Niacinamide	20 mg (100%)
Vitamin B_6 (as Pyridoxine Hydrochloride)	2.5 mg (100%)
Vitamin B_{12} (as Cyanocobalamin)	8 mcg (100%)
Calcium (as Calcium Carbonate)	250 mg (19%)
Iodine (as Potassium Iodide)	150 mcg (100%)
Iron (as Ferrous Fumarate)	30 mg (166%)
Magnesium (as Magnesium Oxide)	100 mg (22%)
Docusate Sodium USP (DSS)	100 mg

Precaution: Folic acid may obscure pernicious anemia in that the peripheral blood picture may revert to normal while neurological manifestations remain progressive.
How Supplied: Tablets (film-coated blue) scored LL-F7—bottles of 100.
[*Shown in Product Identification Section*]

FOLVITE® ℞
folic acid
Tablets—Parenteral Solution

Composition: Each Tablet contains 1 mg. of folic acid.
Each ml. of Parenteral Solution contains: Sodium folate equivalent to 5 mg. of folic acid. Inactive ingredients: Sequestrene sodium, 0.2%; Water for Injection, q.s. 100%; Sodium hydroxide to approx. pH 9. Preservative: Benzyl alcohol 1.5%.
How Supplied: Tablets (Scored, orange) engraved LL F1—1 mg.—bottles of 100 and 1,000; Unit-dose 10 x 10's. ***Parenteral Solution,** 5 mg./ml.—10 ml. vials.
A.H.F.S. 88:08
*Manufactured for
LEDERLE LABORATORIES DIVISION
American Cyanamid Company
Pearl River, NY 10965
by
LEDERLE PARENTERALS INC.
Carolina, Puerto Rico 00630

FOLVRON® ℞
folic acid and iron
Capsules

Composition: Each Capsule contains:

Folic acid	0.33 mg.
Dried ferrous sulfate	182 mg.
(Elemental iron 57 mg.)	

How Supplied: Capsules (soft shell, red) F10—bottles of 100.

GEVRABON®
(vitamin-mineral supplement)

(See PDR for Nonprescription Drugs)

GEVRAL®
Multivitamin and Multimineral Supplement for Adults and Children 4 or More Years of Age
TABLETS

(See PDR for Nonprescription Drugs)

GEVRAL® T
High Potency
Multivitamin and Multimineral Supplement for Adults and Children 4 or More Years of Age
TABLETS

(See PDR for Nonprescription Drugs)

HYDROMOX® ℞
quinethazone
Tablets

Description: Chemistry: HYDROMOX is a quinazoline derivative, in which a cyclic carbamyl group replaces the cyclic sulfamyl group present in the thiazide derivatives.
Chemical name: 7 - Chloro - 2 - ethyl - 1, 2, 3, 4-tetrahydro-4-oxo-6-sulfamyl-quinazoline
Tablet Size: 50 mg. scored
Actions: HYDROMOX produces urinary excretion of sodium and chloride in approximately equivalent amounts (saluresis), while potassium is excreted to a much lesser degree. The saluretic effect of HYDROMOX is rapid and relatively prolonged, beginning within 2 hours after administration, reaching a peak at 6 hours, and lasting for 18 to 24 hours. While HYDROMOX is chemically different, it is pharmacologically genetic to the benzothiadiazine group of drugs.
The dominant action of quinethazone is to increase the renal excretion of sodium and chloride and an accompanying volume of water. This results from inhibition of the tubular mechanism of electrolyte reabsorption. The renal effect is virtually independent of alterations in acid-base balance.
Quinethazone, like other drugs in this class, inhibits the proximal reabsorption of sodium and chloride. The excretion of potassium results from increased potassium secretion by the distal tubule where potassium is exchanged for sodium.
Quinethazone may exert its antihypertensive effect by diuresis and sodium loss and/or on vascular function to reduce peripheral resistance.
Indications: HYDROMOX *quinethazone* Lederle, a nonmercurial oral diuretic agent is indicated as adjunctive therapy in edema associated with congestive heart failure, hepatic cirrhosis and corticosteroid and estrogen therapy.
HYDROMOX has also been found useful in edema due to various forms of renal dysfunction such as: nephrotic syndrome; acute glomerulonephritis; and chronic renal failure.
HYDROMOX is indicated in the management of hypertension either as the sole therapeutic agent or to enhance the effectiveness of other antihypertensive drugs in the more severe forms of hypertension.
Usage in Pregnancy: The routine use of diuretics in an otherwise healthy woman is inappropriate and exposes mother and fetus to unnecessary hazard. Diuretics do not prevent development of toxemia of pregnancy, and there is no satisfactory evidence that they are useful in the treatment of developed toxemia. Edema during pregnancy may arise from pathological causes or from the physiologic and mechanical consequences of pregnancy. Diuretics are indicated in pregnancy when edema is due to pathologic causes, just as they are in the absence of pregnancy (however, see Warnings, below). Dependent edema in pregnancy, resulting from restriction of venous return by the expanded uterus, is properly treated through elevation of the lower extremities and use of support hose; use of diuretics to lower intravascular volume in this case is illogical and unnecessary. There is hypervolemia during normal pregnancy which is harmful to neither the fetus nor the mother (in the absence of cardiovascular disease), but which is associated with edema, including generalized edema, in the majority of pregnant women. If this edema produces discomfort, increased recumbency will often provide relief. In rare instances, this edema may cause extreme discomfort which is not relieved by rest. In these cases, a short course of diuretics may provide relief and may be appropriate.
Contraindications:
A. Anuria
B. Hypersensitivity to this or other sulfonamide derived drugs.
Warnings: Diuretics should be used with caution in severe renal disease. In patients with renal disease, diuretics may precipitate azotemia. Cumulative effects of the drug may develop in patients with impaired renal function.
Diuretics should be used with caution in patients with impaired hepatic function or progressive liver disease, since minor alterations of fluid and electrolyte balance may precipitate hepatic coma.
Quinethazone may add to or potentiate the action of other antihypertensive drugs. Potentiation occurs with ganglionic or peripheral adrenergic blocking drugs.
Sensitivity reactions may occur in patients with a history of allergy or bronchial asthma. The possibility of exacerbation or activation of systemic lupus erythematosus has been reported.
Usage in Pregnancy: Quinethazone crosses the placental barrier and appears in cord blood. The use of quinethazone in pregnant women requires that the anticipated benefit be weighed against possible hazards to the fetus. These hazards include fetal or neonatal jaundice, thrombocytopenia, and possible other adverse reactions which have occurred in the adult.
Nursing Mothers: Quinethazone appears in breast milk. If use of the drug is deemed essential, the patient should stop nursing.
Precautions: (1) Quinethazone should be used with caution in patients with impaired hepatic function or progressive liver disease, since minor alterations of fluid and electrolyte balance may precipitate hepatic coma. (2) Whereas electrolyte abnormalities are often present in such conditions as heart failure and cirrhosis as a result of underlying disease process, they may also be aggravated or may be produced independently by any potent diuretic affecting electrolyte excretion. Caution is especially important during prolonged or intensive therapy and when salt intake is restricted or during concomitant use of steroids or ACTH. Hypokalemia attributable to HYDROMOX *quinethazone* therapy has been mild and infrequent, and other electrolyte abnormalities have been rare.
The possibility of potassium depletion and its toxic sequelae must be kept in mind, particularly in cirrhotics and patients receiving digitalis. As a preventive measure the use of foods rich in potassium, such as orange juice, or supplements of potassium chloride may be desirable. (3) In patients with impaired renal function, azotemia and/or excessive drug accumulation may develop. (4) As with other potent diuretics, when HYDROMOX is added to a regimen that includes ganglionic-blocking agents, the dosage of these latter preparations should be reduced to avoid a sudden drop in blood pressure. Reduction of dosage is also necessary when one or more of these antihypertensive agents is added to an established HYDROMOX regimen. (5) As with the thiazide diuretics, increases of serum uric acid may occur but precipitation of gout has been rare. (6) A decreased glucose tolerance as evidenced by hyperglycemia and glycosuria thus aggravat-

ing or provoking diabetes mellitus has occurred. (7) Quinethazone may decrease arterial responsiveness to norepinephrine and therefore should be withdrawn 48 hours before elective surgery. If emergency surgery is indicated, pre-anesthetic and anesthetic agents should be administered in reduced dosage. Quinethazone may also increase the responsiveness to tubocurarine. The antihypertensive effects of the drug may be enhanced in the post-sympathectomy patient. (8) Sensitivity reactions may be more likely to occur in patients with a history of allergy or bronchial asthma. (9) The possibility of exacerbation or activation of systemic lupus erythematosus has been suggested for sulfonamide derived drugs.

Adverse Reactions: The following adverse reactions have been reported with the diuretic drugs some of which may be expected to occur with quinethazone:

A. *Gastrointestinal System reactions:* 1. anorexia, 2. gastric irritation, 3. nausea, 4. vomiting, 5. cramping, 6. diarrhea, 7. constipation, 8. jaundice (intrahepatic cholestatic jaundice), 9. pancreatitis, 10. hyperglycemia, 11. glycosuria.

B. *Central Nervous System reactions:* 1. dizziness, 2. vertigo, 3. paresthesias, 4. headache, 5. xanthopsia.

C. *Hematologic Reactions:* 1. leukopenia, 2. thrombocytopenia, 3. agranulocytosis, 4. aplastic anemia.

D. *Dermatologic—hypersensitivity reactions:* 1. purpura, 2. photosensitivity, 3. rash, 4. urticaria, 5. necrotizing angiitis (vasculitis) (cutaneous vasculitis).

E. *Cardiovascular Reactions:* 1. orthostatic hypotension may occur and may be potentiated by alcohol, barbiturates or narcotics.

F. *Miscellaneous:* 1. muscle spasm, 2. weakness, 3. restlessness. Whenever adverse reactions are moderate or severe, thiazide dosage should be reduced or therapy withdrawn.

Dosage: Average Adult Dosage: One or two 50 mg. tablets, orally, once a day. Because of its relatively prolonged duration of activity, a single daily dose is generally sufficient. Occasionally, 1 tablet (50 mg.) is administered twice a day. Infrequently, a total daily dose of 3 to 4 tablets (150 to 200 mg.) may be necessary. The dosage employed depends upon the severity of the condition being treated and the responsiveness of the patient, and often must be adjusted at the beginning or during the course of therapy. When HYDROMOX *quinethazone* is used in combination with other antihypertensive agents, the dosage of each drug may often be reduced because of potentiation. (see under Precautions concerning the necessity for dosage adjustment when one or more of these drugs is added to an already established therapeutic regimen.)

How Supplied: 50 mg. tablets (scored) engraved LL H1—bottles of 100 and 500.

[*Shown in Product Identification Section*]

HYDROMOX® R ℞

quinethazone with reserpine
TABLETS

Warnings:

> This fixed combination drug is not indicated for initial therapy of hypertension. Hypertension requires therapy titrated to the individual patient. If the fixed combination represents the dosage so determined, its use may be more convenient in patient management. The treatment of hypertension is not static, but must be reevaluated as conditions in each patient warrant.

Description: HYDROMOX R tablets each contain 50 mg. quinethazone and 0.125 mg. reserpine. *HYDROMOX® quinethazone Lederle is a nonmercurial oral diuretic agent, effective in the treatment of edema and hypertension. It is chemically distinct from the benzothiadiazine series of compounds.* Reserpine, an antihypertensive agent, has been combined with quinethazone in a dosage form designed to be useful in the treatment of hypertension with or without edema.

Chemistry: HYDROMOX is a quinazoline derivative, in which a cyclic carbamyl group replaces the cyclic sulfamyl group present in the thiazide derivatives.

Quinethazone is 7-Chloro-2-ethyl-1, 2, 3, 4- tetrahydro-4-oxo-6-sulfamyl-quinazoline.

Reserpine is 3, 4, 5 trimethoxybenzyl methyl reserpate.

Actions: HYDROMOX produces urinary excretion of sodium and chloride in approximately equivalent amounts (saluresis), while potassium is excreted to a much lesser degree. The saluretic effect of HYDROMOX is rapid and relatively prolonged, beginning within 2 hours after administration, reaching a peak at 6 hours, and lasting for 18 to 24 hours. While HYDROMOX is chemically different, it is pharmacologically genetic to the benzothiadiazine group of drugs.

The dominant action of quinethazone is to increase the renal excretion of sodium and chloride and an accompanying volume of water. This results from inhibition of the tubular mechanism of electrolyte reabsorption. The renal effect is virtually independent of alterations in acid-base balance.

Quinethazone, like other drugs in this class, inhibits the proximal reabsorption of sodium and chloride. The excretion of potassium results from increased potassium secretion by the distal tubule where potassium is exchanged for sodium.

Quinethazone may exert its antihypertensive effect by diuresis and sodium loss and/or on vascular function to reduce peripheral resistance.

Reserpine is an antihypertensive agent which produces a mild type of sedation that is tranquilizing rather than hypnotic. The most prominent actions of reserpine are upon the cardiovascular and central nervous systems. In clinical hypertension, reserpine produces a gradual and moderate fall in both systolic and diastolic blood pressures after oral administration for several days to 2-3 weeks. Its effects persist about 3-4 weeks after medication is withdrawn. With an increase in dose, a prolongation of hypotensive effect, rather than an intensification of blood pressure fall, tends to occur. The doses employed in the therapy of hypertension are smaller than those used in psychiatric disorders.

The dosage form combining quinethazone with reserpine is designed to provide effective antihypertensive action upon patients who have failed to show satisfactory response to the use of quinethazone or reserpine alone. This combination of quinethazone and reserpine frequently permits use of a lower dosage of each agent and hence tends to produce the desired antihypertensive effect while eliminating, or at least minimizing, adverse reactions. Blood pressure reductions averaging about –30/–15 have been demonstrated within the first 2 weeks of treatment. Continuation of therapy beyond 2 weeks may be expected to produce further *small* drops in blood pressure. The enhanced reduction in blood pressure produced by quinethazone with reserpine appears to be an additive rather than a potentiating effect.

Indications: HYDROMOX R is indicated in the management of hypertension (see box warnings) either as the sole therapeutic agent or to enhance the effectiveness of other antihypertensive drugs in the more severe forms of hypertension.

Usage in Pregnancy

The routine use of diuretics in an otherwise healthy woman is inappropriate and exposes mother and fetus to unnecessary hazard. Diuretics do not prevent development of toxemia of pregnancy, and there is no satisfactory evidence that they are useful in the treatment of developed toxemia.

Edema during pregnancy may arise from pathological causes or from the physiologic and mechanical consequences of pregnancy. Diuretics are indicated in pregnancy when edema is due to pathologic causes, just as they are in the absence of pregnancy (however, see WARNINGS, below). Dependent edema in pregnancy, resulting from restriction of venous return by the expanded uterus, is properly treated through elevation of the lower extremities and use of support hose; use of diuretics to lower intravascular volume in this case is illogical and unnecessary. There is hypervolemia during normal pregnancy which is harmful to neither the fetus nor the mother (in the absence of cardiovascular disease), but which is associated with edema, including generalized edema, in the majority of pregnant women. If this edema produces discomfort, increased recumbency will often provide relief. In rare instances, this edema may cause extreme discomfort which is not relieved by rest. In these cases, a short course of diuretics may provide relief and may be appropriate.

Contraindications:

A. Anuria

B. Hypersensitivity to this or other sulfonamide derived drugs.

C. Progressively impaired renal function. Since reserpine may increase gastric secretion and motility, its use alone or in combination requires caution and is sometimes contraindicated in patients with a history of peptic or duodenal ulcer or other gastrointestinal disorders.

D. HYDROMOX R should not be administered to patients with severe hepatic dysfunction. The use of the drug should be avoided in patients with a history of mental depression or psychosis. HYDROMOX R should not be used by patients who are known to be hypersensitive to either agent.

Warnings: Diuretics should be used with caution in severe renal disease. In patients with renal disease, diuretics may precipitate azotemia. Cumulative effects of the drug may develop in patients with impaired renal function.

Diuretics should be used with caution in patients with impaired hepatic function or progressive liver disease, since minor alterations of fluid and electrolyte balance may precipitate hepatic coma.

HYDROMOX R may add to or potentiate the action of other antihypertensive drugs. Potentiation occurs with ganglionic or peripheral adrenergic blocking drugs.

Sensitivity reactions may occur in patients with a history of allergy or bronchial asthma. The possibility of exacerbation or activation of systemic lupus erythematosus has been reported with sulfonamide-derived drugs.

Usage in Pregnancy

HYDROMOX R crosses the placental barrier and appears in cord blood. The use of HYDROMOX R in pregnant women requires that the anticipated benefit be weighed against possible hazards to the fetus. These hazards include fetal or neonatal jaundice, thrombocyto-

Continued on next page

The information on each product appearing here is based on labelling effective in August, 1982 and is either the entire official brochure or an accurate condensation therefrom. Offical brochures are enclosed in product packages. Information concerning all Lederle products may be obtained from the Professional Services Department, Lederle Laboratories, Pearl River, New York, 10965.

Lederle—Cont.

penia, and possibly other adverse reactions which have occurred in the adult.

Nursing Mothers

HYDROMOX R appears in breast milk. If use of drug is essential, the patient should stop nursing.

Reserpine has been reported to cause central nervous system depression of the newborn infant when given to the mother in the immediate ante partum period.

HYDROMOX R should be discontinued promptly if any symptoms of mental depression occur with the use of the drug.

Precautions:

Quinethazone:

(1) Quinethazone should be used with caution in patients with impaired hepatic function or progressive liver disease, since minor alterations of fluid and electrolyte balance may precipitate hepatic coma.

(2) Whereas electrolyte abnormalities are often present in such conditions as heart failure and cirrhosis as a result of underlying disease process, they may also be aggravated or may be produced independently by any potent diuretic affecting electrolyte excretion. Caution is especially important during prolonged or intensive therapy and when salt intake is restricted or during concomitant use of steroids or ACTH. Hypokalemia attributable to HYDROMOX *quinethazone* therapy has been mild and infrequent, and other electrolyte abnormalities have been rare.

The possibility of potassium depletion and its toxic sequelae must be kept in mind, particularly in cirrhotics and patients receiving digitalis. As a preventive measure the use of foods rich in potassium, such as orange juice, or supplements of potassium chloride may be desirable.

(3) In patients with impaired renal function, azotemia and/or excessive drug accumulation may develop.

(4) As with other potent diuretics, when HYDROMOX is added to a regimen that includes ganglionic-blocking agents, the dosage of these latter preparations should be reduced to avoid a sudden drop in blood pressure. Reduction of dosage is also necessary when one or more of these antihypertensive agents is added to an established HYDROMOX regimen.

(5) As with the thiazide diuretics, increases of serum uric acid may occur but precipitation of gout has been rare.

(6) A decreased glucose tolerance as evidenced by hyperglycemia and glycosuria thus aggravating or provoking diabetes mellitus has occurred.

(7) Quinethazone may decrease arterial responsiveness to norepinephrine and therefore should be withdrawn 48 hours before elective surgery. If emergency surgery is indicated, pre-anesthetic and anesthetic agents should be administered in reduced dosage. Quinethazone may also increase the responsiveness to tubocurarine. The antihypertensive effects of the drug may be enhanced in the post-sympathectomy patient.

(8) Sensitivity reactions may be more likely to occur in patients with a history of allergy or bronchial asthma.

(9) The possibility of exacerbation or activation of systemic lupus erythematosus has been suggested for sulfonamide derived drugs.

Reserpine:

Reserpine may precipitate biliary colic in patients with gallstones, or bronchial asthma in susceptible patients. Reserpine preparations should be used with caution in patients with a history of peptic ulcer, ulcerative colitis and other gastrointestinal disorders. It may cause severe depression and suicidal risk and may produce pseudoparkinsonism (a paralysis agitans-like syndrome). Administration of reserpine should be discontinued 2 weeks or more before electroconvulsant therapy if possible to preclude severe, even fatal, reactions.

Reserpine may cause cardiotoxic effects, e.g. premature ventricular contractions and other arrhythmias, possible sensitization to digitalis (which might be further complicated by any hypokalemic effects of quinethazone), fluid retention, and congestive failure.

Adverse Reactions: The following adverse reactions have been reported with the diuretic drugs some of which may be expected to occur with quinethazone:

A. Gastrointestinal System reactions

1. anorexia 2. gastric irritation 3. nausea 4. vomiting 5. cramping 6. diarrhea 7. constipation 8. jaundice (intrahepatic cholestatic jaundice) 9. pancreatitis 10. hyperglycemia 11. glycosuria

B. Central Nervous System reactions

1. dizziness 2. vertigo 3. paresthesias 4. headache 5. xanthopsia

C. Hematologic reactions

1. leukopenia 2. thrombocytopenia 3. agranulocytosis 4. aplastic anemia

D. Dermatologic-hypersensitivity reactions

1. purpura 2. photosensitivity 3. rash 4. urticaria 5. necrotizing angiitis (vasculitis) (cutaneous vasculitis)

E. Cardiovascular reactions

1. orthostatic hypotension may occur and may be potentiated by alcohol, barbiturates or narcotics.

F. Miscellaneous

1. muscle spasm 2. weakness 3. restlessness

Reserpine:

With reserpine, nasal congestion, weight gain, and diarrhea are the most frequently noted side effects. The drug may reactivate old peptic ulcers because it increases hydrochloric acid secretion by the stomach. More serious reactions are excessive drowsiness, fatigue, weakness, insomnia, nightmares, excitement, irrational behavior, and incipient parkinsonism. Sodium retention edema may occur when reserpine is used.

Whenever adverse reactions are moderate or severe, thiazide dosage should be reduced or therapy withdrawn.

Dosage and Administration:

Dosage: As determined by individual titration (see box warning).

Usual Initial Adult Loading Dosage: If considered necessary, 3 to 4 HYDROMOX R Tablets (150 mg. quinethazone with 0.375 mg. reserpine to 200 mg. quinethazone with 0.5 mg. reserpine) may be administered orally, once a day, for not more than 2 weeks.

Average (or Maintenance) Adult Dosage: 1 to 2 HYDROMOX R Tablets (50 mg. quinethazone with 0.125 mg. reserpine to 100 mg. quinethazone with 0.25 mg. reserpine) administered orally, once a day.

Because of the relatively prolonged effect of HYDROMOX R, a single daily dose is usually sufficient. Occasionally 1 tablet is administered twice a day, but ordinarily medication is administered only in the morning to avoid the inconvenience of nocturia.

With the exception of the initial loading phase, a total dose of 3 to 4 tablets of HYDROMOX R Quinethazone with Reserpine is not recommended since the 0.375 mg. to 0.5 mg. of reserpine thus provided is more than is routinely necessary for a hypotensive effect and serves to increase the risk of adverse reactions. If more than 100 mg. of quinethazone per day is desired, it is recommended that HYDROMOX Quinethazone Tablets be used to supplement HYDROMOX R.

The dosage of HYDROMOX R to be employed depends upon the severity of the condition being treated and the responsiveness of the individual patient and often must be adjusted at the beginning of, or during the course of, therapy. Reduction of dosage is often possible after 2 weeks, when as little as 1 tablet a day may be sufficient for maintenance.

When HYDROMOX R Tablets are used in combination with other antihypertensive drugs, the dosage of each drug may often be reduced because of potentiation. (See under Precautions concerning the necessity for dosage adjustment when one or more of these drugs is added to an already established therapeutic regimen).

How Supplied: Yellow Tablets Scored-engraved LL H2 Bottles of 100 and 500.

[*Shown in Product Identification Section*]

INCREMIN® WITH IRON • SYRUP

(vitamins B_1, B_6, B_{12}-lysine-iron)
Dietary Supplement

(See PDR for Nonprescription Drugs)

LEDERPLEX®

Dietary Supplement of B-Complex Vitamins for Adults and Children 4 or More Years of Age
Capsules—Liquid—Tablets

(See PDR For Nonprescription Drugs)

LEUCOVORIN CALCIUM INJECTION ℞

Description: Each 1 ml ampul of Leucovorin Calcium *Lederle* contains Leucovorin 3 mg as the calcium salt which is the form preferred for intramuscular injection. Preservative: Benzyl Alcohol 0.9% w/v. The inactive ingredients are Sodium Chloride 0.56% w/v, Water for Injection q.s. 100% and sodium hydroxide or hydrochloric acid is used to adjust the pH to approximately 7.7.

Each 50 mg vial of Leucovorin Calcium cryodesiccated powder when reconstituted with 5 ml of sterile diluent contains Leucovorin 10 mg per ml as the calcium salt which is the form preferred for intramuscular injection.

Contains no preservative. Dilute only with Bacteriostatic Water for Injection USP which contains benzyl alcohol. The inactive ingredients are sodium chloride 40 mg/vial, and sodium hydroxide or hydrochloric acid qs to pH approximately 8.1. When reconstituted as directed, the resulting solution must be used within 7 days. If the product is reconstituted with Water for Injection USP, use immediately.

Actions: Leucovorin (folinic acid) is the formyl derivative and active form of folic acid. Leucovorin Calcium is useful clinically in circumventing the action of folate reductase. There is no evidence that intramuscular doses of greater than 1 mg have greater efficacy than those of 1 mg.

Indications: Indicated (a) to diminish the toxicity and counteract the effect of inadvertently administered overdosages of folic acid antagonists. (See Warnings). (b) In the treatment of the megaloblastic anemias due to sprue, nutritional deficiency, pregnancy, and infancy when oral therapy is not feasible.

Contraindications: Not to be administered for the treatment of pernicious anemia or other megaloblastic anemias where Vitamin B_{12} is deficient.

Warnings: Leucovorin is improper therapy for pernicious anemia and other megaloblastic anemias secondary to lack of vitamin B_{12}. A hematologic remission may occur while neurologic manifestations remain progressive.

In the treatment of overdosage of folic acid antagonists, leucovorin must be administered within 1 hour, if possible, and is usually ineffective if administered after a delay of 4 hours.

Precautions: In the presence of pernicious anemia a hematologic remission may occur

while neurologic manifestations remain progressive.
Adverse Reactions: Allergic sensitization has been reported following both oral and parenteral administration of folic acid.
Dosage: Megaloblastic anemia: No more than or up to 1 mg daily. There is no evidence that intramuscular doses greater than 1 mg daily have greater efficacy than those of 1 mg; additionally, loss of folate in the urine becomes roughly logarithmic as the amount administered exceeds 1 mg.
For the treatment of overdosage of folic acid antagonists: To be given in amounts equal to the weight of the antagonist given.
How Supplied:
6 — 1 ml ampuls.
50 mg vials of cryodesiccated powder.
Military Depot
NSN 6505-01-054-7008, 50 mg/vial
Manufactured for
LEDERLE LABORATORIES DIVISION
American Cyanamid Company
Pearl River, NY 10965
by
LEDERLE PARENTERALS INC.
Carolina, Puerto Rico 00630

LOXITANE® ℞
loxapine succinate
Capsules

LOXITANE® C
loxapine hydrochloride
Oral Concentrate

LOXITANE® IM
loxapine hydrochloride
For Intramuscular Use Only

Description: LOXITANE *loxapine,* a dibenzoxazepine compound, represents a new subclass of tricyclic antipsychotic agent, chemically distinct from the thioxanthenes, butyrophenones, and phenothiazines. Chemically, it is 2-chloro-11-(4-methyl-1-piperazinyl)dibenz[b,f]-[1,4]oxazepine. It is present in capsules as the succinate salt, and in the concentrate and parenteral primarily as the HCl.
CAPSULES—Each capsule contains loxapine succinate equivalent to 5, 10, 25 or 50 mg of loxapine base.
ORAL CONCENTRATE—Each ml contains loxapine hydrochloride equivalent to 25 mg of loxapine base.
INTRAMUSCULAR—(Sterile)—Not for Intravenous Use—Each ml contains loxapine hydrochloride equivalent to 50 mg of loxapine base. Inactive Ingredients: polysorbate 80 NF 5% w/v; propylene glycol 70% v/v; and water for injection qs ad 100% v. Hydrochloric acid or Sodium hydroxide qs pH approx. 5.8.
Actions: Pharmacologically, loxapine is a tranquilizer for which the exact mode of action has not been established. However, changes in the level of excitability of subcortical inhibitory areas have been observed in several animal species in association with such manifestations of tranquilization as calming effects and suppression of aggressive behavior.
In normal human volunteers, signs of sedation were seen within 20 to 30 minutes after administration, were most pronounced within 1½ to 3 hours, and lasted through 12 hours. Similar timing of primary pharmacologic effects was seen in animals.
Absorption of loxapine following oral or parenteral administration is virtually complete. The drug is removed rapidly from the plasma and distributed in tissues. Animal studies suggest an initial preferential distribution in lungs, brain, spleen, heart, and kidney. Loxapine is metabolized extensively and is excreted mainly in the first 24 hours. Metabolites are excreted in the urine in the form of conjugates and in the feces unconjugated.
Indications: LOXITANE is indicated for the management of the manifestations of psychotic disorders. The antipsychotic efficacy of LOXITANE was established in clinical studies which enrolled newly hospitalized and chronically hospitalized acutely ill schizophrenic patients as subjects.
Contraindications: LOXITANE is contraindicated in comatose or severe drug-induced depressed states (alcohol, barbiturates, narcotics, etc.)
LOXITANE is contraindicated in individuals with known hypersensitivity to the drug.
Warnings:
Usage in Pregnancy: Safe use during pregnancy or lactation has not been established; therefore, its use in pregnancy, in nursing mothers, or in women of childbearing potential requires that the benefits of treatment be weighed against the possible risks to mother and child. No embryotoxicity or teratogenicity was observed in studies in rats, rabbits or dogs, although with the exception of one rabbit study, the highest dosage was only two times the maximum recommended human dose and in some studies it was below this dose. Perinatal studies have shown renal papillary abnormalities in offspring of rats treated from mid-pregnancy with doses of 0.6 and 1.8 mg/kg, doses which approximate the usual human dose but which are considerably below the maximum recommended human dose.
Usage in Children: Studies have not been performed in children; therefore, this drug is not recommended for use in children below the age of 16.
LOXITANE, like other tranquilizers, may impair mental and/or physical abilities, especially during the first few days of therapy. Therefore, ambulatory patients should be warned about activities requiring alertness (eg, operating vehicles or machinery), and about concomitant use of alcohol and other CNS depressants.
LOXITANE has not been evaluated for the management of behavioral complications in patients with mental retardation, and therefore, it cannot be recommended.
Precautions: LOXITANE should be used with extreme caution in patients with a history of convulsive disorders since it lowers the convulsive threshold. Seizures have been reported in epileptic patients receiving LOXITANE at antipsychotic dose levels, and may occur even with maintenance of routine anticonvulsant drug therapy.
Loxapine has an antiemetic effect in animals. Since this effect may also occur in man, loxapine may mask signs of overdosage of toxic drugs and may obscure conditions such as intestinal obstruction and brain tumor.
LOXITANE should be used with caution in patients with cardiovascular disease. Increased pulse rates have been reported in the majority of patients receiving antipsychotic doses; transient hypotension has been reported. In the presence of severe hypotension requiring vasopressor therapy, the preferred drugs may be norepinephrine or angiotensin. Usual doses of epinephrine may be ineffective because of inhibition of its vasopressor effect by loxapine.
The possibility of ocular toxicity from loxapine cannot be excluded at this time. Therefore, careful observation should be made for pigmentary retinopathy and lenticular pigmentation since these have been observed in some patients receiving certain other antipsychotic drugs for prolonged periods.
Because of possible anticholinergic action, the drug should be used cautiously in patients with glaucoma or a tendency to urinary retention, particularly with concomitant administration of anticholinergic-type anti-parkinson medication.
Experience to date indicates the possibility of a slightly higher incidence of extrapyramidal effects following intramuscular administration than normally anticipated with oral formulations. The increase may be attributable to higher plasma levels following intramuscular injection.
Neuroleptic drugs elevate prolactin levels; the elevation persists during chronic administration. Tissue culture experiments indicate that approximately one-third of human breast cancers are prolactin dependent in vitro, a factor of potential importance if the prescription of these drugs is contemplated in a patient with a previously detected breast cancer. Although disturbances such as galactorrhea, amenorrhea, gynecomastia, and impotence have been reported, the clinical significance of elevated serum prolactin levels is unknown for most patients. An increase in mammary neoplasms has been found in rodents after chronic administration of neuroleptic drugs. Neither clinical studies nor epidemiologic studies conducted to date, however, have shown an association between chronic administration of these drugs and mammary tumorigenesis; the available evidence is considered too limited to be conclusive at this time.
Adverse Reactions:
CNS Effects: Manifestations of adverse effects on the central nervous system, other than extrapyramidal effects, have been seen infrequently. Drowsiness, usually mild, may occur at the beginning of therapy or when dosage is increased.
It usually subsides with continued LOXITANE therapy. The incidence of sedation has been less than that of certain aliphatic phenothiazines and slightly more the piperazine phenothiazines. Dizziness, faintness, staggering gait, muscle twitching, weakness, and confusional states have been reported.
Extrapyramidal Reactions—Neuromuscular (extra-pyramidal) reactions during the administration of LOXITANE have been reported frequently, often during the first few days of treatment. In most patients, these reactions involved parkinsonian-like symptoms such as tremor, rigidity, excessive salivation, and masked facies. Akathisia (motor restlessness) also has been reported relatively frequently. These symptoms are usually not severe and can be controlled by reduction of LOXITANE dosage or by administration of antiparkinson drugs in usual dosage. Dystonic and dyskinetic reactions have occurred less frequently, but may be more severe. Dystonias include spasms of muscles of the neck and face, tongue protrusion, and oculogyric movement. Dyskinetic reaction has been described in the form of choreoathetoid movements. These reactions sometimes require reduction or temporary withdrawal of LOXITANE dosage in addition to appropriate counteractive drugs.
Persistent Tardive Dyskinesia—As with all antipsychotic agents, tardive dyskinesia may appear in some patients on long-term therapy or may appear after drug therapy has been discontinued. The risk appears to be greater in elderly patients on high-dose therapy, especially females. The symptoms are persistent and in some patients appear to be irreversible. The syndrome is characterized by rhythmical involuntary movement of the tongue, face, mouth, or jaw (eg, protrusion of tongue, puffing of cheeks, puckering of mouth, chewing movements). Sometimes these may be accompanied by involuntary movements of extremities.

Continued on next page

The information on each product appearing here is based on labelling effective in August, 1982 and is either the entire official brochure or an accurate condensation therefrom. Offical brochures are enclosed in product packages. Information concerning all Lederle products may be obtained from the Professional Services Department, Lederle Laboratories, Pearl River, New York, 10965.

Lederle—Cont.

There is no known effective treatment for tardive dyskinesia; antiparkinson agents usually do not alleviate the symptoms of this syndrome. It is suggested that all antipyschotic agents be discontinued if these symptoms appear. Should it be necessary to reinstitute treatment, or increase the dosage of the agent, or switch to a different antipsychotic agent, the syndrome may be masked. It has been suggested that fine vermicular movements of the tongue may be an early sign of the syndrome, and if the medication is stopped at that time the syndrome may not develop.

Cardiovascular Effects: Tachycardia, hypotension, hypertension, lightheadedness, and syncope have been reported.

A few cases of ECG changes similar to those seen with phenothiazines have been reported. It is not known whether these were related to loxapine administration.

Skin: Dermatitis, edema (puffiness of face), pruritus, and seborrhea have been reported with loxapine. The possibility of photosensitivity and/or phototoxicity occurring has not been excluded; skin rashes of uncertain etiology have been observed in a few patients during hot summer months.

Anticholinergic Effects: Dry mouth, nasal congestion, constipation, and blurred vision have occurred; these are more likely to occur with concomitant use of antiparkinson agents.

Gastrointestinal: Nausea and vomiting have been reported in some patients. Hepatocellular injury (i.e. SGOT/SGPT elevation) has been reported in association with loxapine administration.

Other Adverse Reactions: Weight gain, weight loss, dyspnea, ptosis, hyperpyrexia, flushed facies, headache, paresthesia, and polydipsia have been reported in some patients.

Rarely, galactorrhea and menstrual irregularity of uncertain etiology have been reported.

Dosage and Administration: LOXITANE is administered, usually in divided doses, two or four times a day. Daily dosage (in terms of base equivalents) should be adjusted to the individual patient's needs as assessed by the severity of symptoms and previous history of response to antipsychotic drugs.

Oral Administration

Initial dosage of 10 mg twice daily is recommended, although in severely disturbed patients initial dosage up to a total of 50 mg daily may be desirable. Dosage should then be increased fairly rapidly over the first seven to ten days until there is effective control of psychotic symptoms. The usual therapeutic and maintenance range is 60 mg to 100 mg daily. However, as with other antipsychotic drugs, some patients respond to lower dosage and others require higher dosage for optimal benefit. Daily dosage higher than 250 mg is not recommended.

LOXITANE C Oral Concentrate should be mixed with orange or grapefruit juice shortly before administration. Use only the enclosed calibrated (10 mg, 15 mg, 20 mg, 25 mg) dropper for dosage.

Maintenance Therapy

For maintenance therapy, dosage should be reduced to the lowest level compatible with symptom control; many patients have been maintained satisfactorily at dosages in the range of 20 mg to 60 mg daily.

Intramuscular Administration

LOXITANE IM is utilized for prompt symptomatic control in the acutely agitated patient and in patients whose symptoms render oral medication temporarily impractical. During clinical trial there were no reports of significant local tissue reaction.

LOXITANE IM is administered by intramuscular (not intravenous) injection in doses of 12.5 mg (1/4 ml) to 50 mg (1 ml) at intervals of four to six hours or longer, both dose and interval depending on patient response. Many patients have responded satisfactorily to twice-daily dosage. As described above for oral administration, attention is directed to the necessity for dosage adjustment on an individual basis over the early days of loxapine administration.

Once the desired symptomatic control is achieved and the patient is able to take medication orally, loxapine should be administered in capsule or oral concentrate form. Usually this should occur within five days.

Overdosage: Signs and symptoms of overdosage will depend on the amount ingested and individual patient tolerance. As would be expected from the pharmacologic actions of the drug, the clinical findings may range from mild depression of the CNS and cardiovascular systems to profound hypotension, respiratory depression, and unconsciousness. The possibility of occurrence of extrapyramidal symptoms and/or convulsive seizures should be kept in mind.

The treatment of overdosage is essentially symptomatic and supportive. Early gastric lavage and extended dialysis might be expected to be beneficial. Centrally acting emetics may have little effect because of the antiemetic action of loxapine. In addition, emesis should be avoided because of the possibility of aspiration of vomitus. Avoid analeptics, such as pentylenetetrazol, which may cause convulsions. Severe hypotension might be expected to respond to the administration of levarterenol or phenylephrine. EPINEPHRINE SHOULD NOT BE USED SINCE ITS USE IN A PATIENT WITH PARTIAL ADRENERGIC BLOCKADE MAY FURTHER LOWER THE BLOOD PRESSURE. Severe extrapyramidal reactions should be treated with anticholinergic antiparkinson agents or diphenhydramine hydrochloride, and anticonvulsant therapy should be initiated as indicated. Additional measures include oxygen and intravenous fluids.

How Supplied: LOXITANE *loxapine succinate* capsules are supplied in the following base equivalent strengths:

5 mg–Hard Shell, opaque, dark green capsules printed with Lederle over L1 on one half and 5 mg on the other; Bottles of 100 and unit dose 10 × 10's—Product Number 5359

10 mg–Hard Shell, opaque, with yellow body and a dark green cap, printed with Lederle over L2 on one half and 10 mg on the other; Bottles of 100, 1000, and unit dose 10 × 10's—Product Number 5360

25 mg–Hard Shell, opaque, with a light green body and a dark green cap, printed with Lederle over L3 one one half and 25 mg on the other; Bottles of 100, 1000, and unit dose 10 × 10's—Product Number 5361

50 mg–Hard Shell, opaque with a blue body and a dark green cap, printed with Lederle over L4 on one half and 50 mg on the other; Bottles of 100, 1000, and unit dose 10 × 10's—Product Number 5362.

LOXITANE C *loxapine hydrochloride* Oral Concentrate (Product Number 5387) is supplied in bottles of 4 fl. oz. (120 ml) with calibrated dropper. Each ml contains the equivalent of 25 mg loxapine base as the HCl.

*LOXITANE IM *loxapine hydrochloride* for Intramuscular use only (Product Number 5385) is supplied in sterile 10-1 ml ampuls and 10 ml multi-dose vials. Each ml contains the equivalent of 50 mg loxapine base as the HCl.

Keep package closed to protect from light. Intensification of the straw color to a light amber will not alter potency or therapeutic efficacy; if noticeably discolored, ampul or vial should not be used.

A.H.F.S. 28:16.08

Oral Concentrate

VA Depot NSN 6505-01-026-0101A, 4 oz

*Manufactured for
LEDERLE LABORATORIES DIVISION
American Cyanamid Company
Pearl River, NY 10965
by
LEDERLE PARENTERALS INC.
Carolina, Puerto Rico 00630

[*Shown in Product Identification Section*]

MATERNA® 1•60 ℞
Prenatal Tablets
(Film Coated)

Each tablet contains:	For Pregnant or Lactating Women	% of U.S. RDA
Vitamin A Acetate	8,000 I.U.	(100%)
Vitamin D	400 I.U.	(100%)
Vitamin E (as *dl*-Alpha Tocopheryl Acetate)	30 I.U.	(100%)
Vitamin C (Ascorbic Acid)	100 mg.	(167%)
Folic Acid	1 mg.	(125%)
Thiamine (as Thiamine Mononitrate Vitamin B_1)	3 mg.	(224%)
Riboflavin (Vitamin B_2)	3.4 mg.	(170%)
Vitamin B_6 (as Pyridoxine Hydrochloride)	4 mg.	(160%)
Niacinamide	20 mg.	(100%)
Vitamin B_{12} (Cyanocobalamin)	12 mcg.	(150%)
Calcium (as Calcium Carbonate)	250 mg.	(19%)
Iodine (as Potassium Idodide)	0.3 mg.	(200%)
Elemental Iron (as Ferrous Fumarate)	60 mg.	(333%)
Magnesium (as Magnesium Oxide)	25 mg.	(6%)
Copper (as Cupric Oxide)	2 mg.	(100%)
Zinc (as Zinc Sulfate)	25 mg.	(167%)
Docusate Sodium USP (DSS)	50 mg.	

Caution: Federal law prohibits dispensing without prescription.

A phosphorus-free vitamin and mineral dietary supplement with surfactant, for use during pregnancy and lactation. Recommended intake: 1 daily or as prescribed by physician.

Precaution: Folic acid may obscure pernicious anemia in that the peripheral blood picture may revert to normal while neurological manifestations remain progressive. Keep this and all medications out of the reach of children.

Allergic sensitization has been reported following both oral and parenteral administration of Folic Acid.

How Supplied: Tablets (film-coated, pink) Embossed Materna on one side and scored M10 on the other — bottles of 100.

[*Shown in Product Indentification Section*]

METHOTREXATE ℞
Tablets and Parenteral

WARNING

METHOTREXATE MUST BE USED ONLY BY PHYSICIANS EXPERIENCED IN ANTIMETABOLITE CHEMOTHERAPY.

BECAUSE OF THE POSSIBILITY OF FATAL OR SEVERE TOXIC REACTIONS THE PATIENT SHOULD BE FULLY INFORMED BY THE PHYSICIAN OF THE RISKS INVOLVED AND SHOULD BE UNDER HIS CONSTANT SUPERVISION.

DEATHS HAVE BEEN REPORTED WITH THE USE OF METHOTREXATE IN THE TREATMENT OF PSORIASIS.

IN THE TREATMENT OF PSORIASIS METHOTREXATE SHOULD BE RESTRICTED TO SEVERE, RECALCITRANT, DISABLING, PSORIASIS WHICH IS NOT ADEQUATELY RESPONSIVE TO OTHER FORMS OF THERAPY, BUT ONLY WHEN THE DIAGNOSIS HAS BEEN ESTABLISHED, AS BY BIOPSY AND/OR AFTER DERMATOLOGIC CONSULTATION.

1. Methotrexate may produce marked depression of bone marrow, anemia, leukopenia, thrombocytopenia and bleeding.
2. Methotrexate may be hepatotoxic, particularly at high dosage or with prolonged therapy. Liver atrophy, necrosis, cirrhosis, fatty changes, and periportal fibrosis have been reported. Since changes may occur without previous signs of gastrointestinal or hematologic toxicity, it is imperative that hepatic function be determined prior to initiation of treatment and monitored regularly throughout therapy. Special caution is indicated in the presence of preexisting liver damage or impaired hepatic function. Concomitant use of other drugs with hepatotoxic potential (including alcohol) should be avoided.
3. Methotrexate has caused fetal death and/or congenital anomalies, therefore, it is not recommended in women of childbearing potential unless there is appropriate medical evidence that the benefits can be expected to outweigh the considered risks. Pregnant psoriatic patients should not receive Methotrexate.
4. Impaired renal function is usually a contraindication.
5. Diarrhea and ulcerative stomatitis are frequent toxic effects and require interruption of therapy; otherwise hemorrhagic enteritis and death from intestinal perforation may occur.

METHOTREXATE HAS BEEN ADMINISTERED IN VERY HIGH DOSAGE FOLLOWED BY LEUCOVORIN RESCUE IN EXPERIMENTAL TREATMENT OF CERTAIN NEOPLASTIC DISEASES. THIS PROCEDURE IS INVESTIGATIONAL AND HAZARDOUS.

Description: Methotrexate Lederle (formerly A-methopterin) is an antimetabolite used in the treatment of certain neoplastic diseases. Chemically methotrexate is N-[p [[(2, 4-diamino-6-pteridinyl) methyl]-methylamino]benzoyl]glutamic acid.

Methotrexate Tablets contain 2.5 mg of Methotrexate.

Methotrexate Sodium Parenteral, preserved, is available both in 2.5 mg/ml and 25 mg/ml strengths each available in 2 ml vials.

Each 2.5 mg/ml (5.0 mg) vial contains per 2 ml: Methotrexate Sodium equivalent to 5 mg Methotrexate, 0.90% w/v of benzyl alcohol as a preservative, and the following Inactive Ingredients. Sodium Chloride 0.630% w/v and Water for Injection qs ad 100% V. Sodium Hydroxide and if necessary, Hydrochloric Acid to adjust pH to approx. 8.5.

Each 25 mg/ml (50 mg) vial contains per 2 ml: Methotrexate Sodium equivalent to 50 mg Methotrexate, 0.90% w/v of benzyl alcohol as a preservative, and the following Inactive Ingredients: Sodium Chloride 0.260% w/v and Water for Injection qs ad 100% V. Sodium Hydroxide and, if necessary, Hydrochloric Acid to adjust pH to approx. 8.5.

If desired, the solution may be further diluted with a compatible medium such as Sodium Chloride Injection USP. Storage for 24 hours at a temperature of 21° to 25° C results in a product which is within 90% of label potency.

Methotrexate LPF* Sodium Parenteral, Isotonic, preservative free, single use only, is available in 2 ml (50 mg), 4 ml (100 mg), and 8 ml (200 mg) vials.

Each 25 mg/ml, 2 ml (50 mg) vial contains: Methotrexate Sodium equivalent to 50 mg Methotrexate, and the following Inactive Ingredients: Sodium Chloride 0.490% w/v and Water for Injection qs ad 100% V. Sodium Hydroxide and, if necessary, Hydrochloric Acid to adjust pH to approx. 8.5. Contains approximately 0.43 milliequivalents of sodium per vial and is an isotonic solution.

Each 25 mg/ml, 4 ml (100 mg) vial contains: Methotrexate Sodium equivalent to 100 mg Methotrexate, and the following Inactive Ingredients: Sodium Chloride 0.490% w/v and Water for Injection qs ad 100% V. Sodium Hydroxide and, if necessary, Hydrochloric Acid to adjust pH to approx. 8.5. Contains approximately 0.86 milliequivalents of sodium per vial and is an isotonic solution.

Each 25 mg/ml, 8 ml (200 mg) vial contains: Methotrexate Sodium equivalent to 200 mg Methotrexate, and the following Inactive Ingredients: Sodium Chloride 0.490% w/v and Water for Injection qs ad 100% V. Sodium Hydroxide and, if necessary, Hydrochloric Acid to adjust pH to approx. 8.5. Contains approximately 1.72 milliequivalents of sodium per vial and is an isotonic solution.

If desired, the solution may be further diluted immediately prior to use with an appropriate sterile, preservative free medium such as Sterile Water for Injection, USP.

Each Low Sodium 20 mg vial of sterile cryodesiccated powder, for single use only, contains: Methotrexate Sodium equivalent to 20 mg Methotrexate. Contains no preservative. With Sodium Hydroxide and, if necessary, Hydrochloric Acid to adjust pH to approximately 8.5. Contains approximately 0.14 milliequivalents of sodium per vial. Each Low Sodium 50 mg vial of sterile cryodesiccated powder, for single use only, contains: Methotrexate Sodium equivalent to 50 mg Methotrexate. Contains no preservative. With Sodium Hydroxide and, if necessary, Hydrochloric Acid to adjust pH to approximately 8.5. Contains approximately 0.33 milliequivalents of sodium per vial.

Each Low Sodium 100 mg vial of sterile cryodesiccated powder, for single use only, contains: Methotrexate Sodium equivalent to 100 mg Methotrexate. Contains no preservative. With Sodium Hydroxide and, if necessary, Hydrochloric Acid to adjust pH to approximately 8.5. Contains approximately 0.65 milliequivalents of sodium per vial.

Action: Methotrexate has as its principal mechanism of action the competitive inhibition of the enzyme folic acid reductase. Folic acid must be reduced to tetrahydrofolic acid by this enzyme in the process of DNA synthesis and cellular replication. Methotrexate inhibits the reduction of folic acid and interferes with tissue-cell reproduction.

Actively proliferating tissues such as malignant cells, bone marrow, fetal cells, dermal epithelium, buccal and intestinal mucosa and cells of the urinary bladder are in general more sensitive to this effect of Methotrexate. Cellular proliferation in malignant tissue is greater than in most normal tissue and thus Methotrexate may impair malignant growth without irreversible damage to normal tissues.

Orally administered Methotrexate is absorbed rapidly in most, but not all patients, and reaches peak serum levels in 1–2 hours. After parenteral injection, peak serum levels are seen in about one-half this period. Approximately one-half the absorbed Methotrexate is reversibly bound to serum protein, but exchanges with body fluids easily and diffuses into the body tissue cells.

Excretion of single daily doses occurs through the kidneys in amounts from 55% to 88% or higher within 24 hours. Repeated doses daily result in more sustained serum levels and some retention of Methotrexate over each 24 hour period which may result in accumulation of the drug within the tissues. The liver cells appear to retain certain amounts of the drug for prolonged periods even after a single therapeutic dose. Methotrexate is retained in the presence of impaired renal function and may increase rapidly in the serum and in the tissue cells under such conditions. Methotrexate does not penetrate the blood cerebrospinal fluid barrier in therapeutic amounts when given orally or parenterally. High concentrations of the drug when needed may be attained by direct intrathecal administration.

In psoriasis, the rate of production of epithelial cells in the skin is greatly increased over normal skin. This differential in reproductive rates is the basis for the use of Methotrexate to control the psoriatic process.

Indications:

Anti-neoplastic Chemotherapy

Methotrexate is indicated for the treatment of gestational choriocarcinoma, and in patients with chorioadenoma destruens and hydatidiform mole.

Methotrexate is indicated for the palliation of acute lymphocytic leukemia. It is also indicated in the treatment and prophylaxis of meningeal leukemia. Greatest effect has been observed in palliation of acute lymphoblastic (stem-cell) leukemias in children. In combination with other anticancer drugs or suitable agents Methotrexate may be used for induction of remission, but it is most commonly used, as described in the literature, in the maintenance of induced remissions.

Methotrexate may be used alone or in combination with other anticancer agents in the management of breast cancer, epidermoid cancers of the head and neck, and lung cancer, particularly squamous cell and small cell types.

Methotrexate is also effective in the treatment of the advanced stages (III and IV, Peters Staging System) of lymphosarcoma, particularly in those cases in children; and in advanced cases of mycosis fungoides.

Psoriasis Chemotherapy **[See box warnings at top of Insert]** Because of high risk attending its use, Methotrexate is only indicated in the symptomatic control of severe, recalcitrant, disabling psoriasis which is not adequately responsive to other forms of therapy, *but only when the diagnosis has been established, as by biopsy and/or after dermatologic consultation.*

Contraindications: Pregnant psoriatic patients should not receive Methotrexate. Psoriatic patients with severe renal or hepatic disorders should not receive Methotrexate.

Psoriatic patients with pre-existing blood dyscrasias, such as bone marrow hypoplasia, leukopenia, thrombocytopenia or anemia, should not receive Methotrexate.

Warnings: See Box Warnings

Precautions: Methotrexate has a high potential toxicity, usually dose-related. The physician should be familiar with the various characteristics of the drug and its established clinical usage. Patients undergoing therapy should be subject to appropriate supervision so that signs or symptoms of possible toxic effects or adverse reactions may be detected and evaluated with minimal delay. Pretreatment and periodic hematologic studies are essential to the use of Methotrexate in chemotherapy because of its common effect of hematopoietic suppression. This may occur abruptly and on apparent safe dosage, and any profound drop in blood-cell count indicates immediate stopping of the drug and appropriate therapy. In patients with malignant disease who have preexisting bone marrow aplasia, leukopenia, thrombocytopenia or anemia, the drug should be used with caution, if at all.

Continued on next page

The information on each product appearing here is based on labelling effective in August, 1982 and is either the entire official brochure or an accurate condensation therefrom. Offical brochures are enclosed in product packages. Information concerning all Lederle products may be obtained from the Professional Services Department, Lederle Laboratories, Pearl River, New York, 10965.

Lederle—Cont.

Methotrexate is excreted principally by the kidneys. Its use in the presence of impaired renal function may result in accumulation of toxic amounts or even additional renal damage. The patient's renal status should be determined prior to and during Methotrexate therapy and proper caution exercised should significant renal impairment be disclosed. Drug dosage should be reduced or discontinued until renal function is improved or restored.

In general, the following laboratory tests are recommended as part of essential clinical evaluation and appropriate monitoring of patients chosen for or receiving Methotrexate therapy: complete hemogram; hematocrit; urinalysis; renal function tests; and liver function tests. A chest x-ray is also recommended. The purpose is to determine any existing organ dysfunction or system impairment. The tests should be performed prior to therapy, at appropriate periods during therapy and after termination of therapy. It may be useful or important to perform liver biopsy or bone marrow aspiration studies where high dose or long-term therapy is being followed.

Methotrexate is bound in part to serum albumin after absorption and toxicity may be increased because of displacement by certain drugs such as salicylates, sulfonamides, diphenylhydantoin, phenylbutazone, and some antibacterials as tetracycline, chloramphenicol and para-amino-benzoic acid. These drugs, especially salicylates, phenylbutazone, and sulfonamides, whether antibacterial, hypoglycemic or diuretic, should not be given concurrently until the significance of these findings is established.

Vitamin preparations containing folic acid or its derviatives may alter responses to Methotrexate.

Methotrexate should be used with extreme caution in the presence of infection, peptic ulcer, ulcerative colitis, debility, and in extreme youth and old age.

If profound leukopenia occurs during therapy, bacterial infection may occur or become a threat. Cessation of the drug and appropriate antibiotic therapy is usually indicated. In severe bone marrow depression, blood or platelet transfusions may be necessary.

Since it is reported that Methotrexate may have an immunosuppressive action, this factor must be taken into consideration in evaluating the use of the drug where immune responses in a patient may be important or essential.

In all instances where the use of Methotrexate is considered for chemotherapy, the physician must evaluate the need and usefulness of the drug against the risks of toxic effects or adverse reaction. Most such adverse reactions are reversible if detected early. When such effects or reactions do occur, the drug should be reduced in dosage or discontinued and appropriate corrective measures should be taken, according to the clinical judgment of the physician. Reinstitution of Methotrexate therapy should be carried out with caution, with adequate consideration of further need for the drug and alertness as to possible recurrence of toxicity.

Adverse Reactions: The most common adverse reactions include ulcerative stomatitis, leukopenia, nausea and abdominal distress. Others reported are malaise, undue fatigue, chills and fever, dizziness and decreased resistance to infection. In general, the incidence and severity of side effects are considered to be dose-related. Adverse reactions as reported for the various systems are as follows:

Skin: erythematous rashes, pruritus, urticaria, photosensitivity, depigmentation, alopecia, ecchymosis, telangiectasia, acne, furunculosis. Lesions of psoriasis may be aggravated by concomitant exposure to ultraviolet radiation.

Blood: bone marrow depression, leukopenia, thrombocytopenia, anemia, hypogammaglobulinemia, hemorrhage from various sites, septicemia.

Alimentary System: gingivitis, pharyngitis, stomatitis, anorexia, vomiting, diarrhea, hematemesis, melena, gastrointestinal ulceration and bleeding, enteritis, hepatic toxicity resulting in acute liver atrophy, necrosis, fatty metamorphosis, periportal fibrosis, or hepatic cirrhosis.

Urogenital System: renal failure, azotemia, cystitis, hematuria; defective oogenesis or spermatogenesis, transient oligospermia, menstrual dysfunction; infertility, abortion, fetal defects, severe nephropathy.

Pulmonary System: Interstitial Pneumonitis. Deaths have been reported and chronic interstitial obstructive pulmonary disease has occasionally occurred.

Central Nervous System: Headaches, drowsiness, blurred vision. Aphasia, hemiparesis, paresis and convulsions have also occurred following administration of Methotrexate.

There have been reports of leucoencephalopathy following intravenous administration of Methotrexate to patients who have had craniospinal irradiation.

After the intrathecal use of Methotrexate, the central nervous system toxicity which may occur can be classified as follows: (1) chemical arachnoiditis manifested by such symptoms as headache, back pain, nuchal rigidity, and fever; (2) paresis, usually transient, manifested by paraplegia associated with involvement with one or more spinal nerve roots; (3) leucoencephalopathy manifested by confusion, irritability, somnolence, ataxia, dementia, and occasionally major convulsions.

Other reactions related to or attributed to the use of Methotrexate such as metabolic changes, precipitating diabetes; osteoporotic effects, abnormal tissue cell changes, and even sudden death have been reported.

Dosage and Administration:

Anti-neoplastic chemotherapy

Oral administration in tablet form is often preferred since absorption is rapid and effective serum levels are obtained. Methotrexate sodium parenteral may be given by intramuscular, intravenous, intraarterial or intrathecal route. Initial treatment is usually undertaken with the patient under hospital care.

*For conversion of mg/kg b.w. to mg/M^2 of body surface or the reverse, a ratio of 1:30 is given as a guideline. The conversion factor varies between 1:20 and 1:40 depending on age and body build.

Choriocarcinoma and similar trophoblastic diseases: Methotrexate is administered orally or intramuscularly in doses of 15 to 30 mg daily for a 5 day course. Such courses are usually repeated for 3 to 5 times as required, with rest periods of one or more weeks interposed between courses, until any manifesting toxic symptoms subside. The effectiveness of therapy is ordinarily evaluated by 24 hour quantitative analysis of urinary chorionic gonadotropin hormone (CGH), which should return to normal or less than 50 IU/24 hr. usually after the 3rd or 4th course and usually be followed by a complete resolution of measurable lesions in 4 to 6 weeks. One to two courses of Methotrexate after normalization of CGH is usually recommended. Before each course of the drug careful clinical assessment is essential. Cyclic combination therapy of Methotrexate with other antitumor drugs has been reported as being useful. Since hydatidiform mole may precede or be followed by choriocarcinoma, prophylactic chemotherapy with Methotrexate has been recommended. Chorioadenoma destruens is considered to be an invasive form of hydatidiform mole. Methotrexate is administered in these disease states in doses similar to those recommended for choriocarcinoma.

Leukemia: acute lymphatic (lymphoblastic) leukemia in children and young adolescents is the most responsive to present day chemotherapy. In young adults and older patients, clinical remission is more difficult to obtain and early relapse is more common. In chronic lymphatic leukemia, the prognosis for adequate response is less encouraging.

Methotrexate alone or in combination with steroids was used initially for induction of remission of lymphoblastic leukemias. More recently corticosteroid therapy in combination with other antileukemic drugs or in cyclic combinations with Methotrexate included appear to produce rapid and effective remissions. When used for induction, Methotrexate in doses of 3.3 mg/M^2 in combination with prednisone 60 mg/M^2, given daily, produced remission in 50% of patients treated, usually within a period of 4 to 6 weeks. Methotrexate alone or in combination with other agents appears to be the drug of choice for securing maintenance of drug-induced remissions. When remission is achieved and supportive care has produced general clinical improvement, maintenance therapy is initiated, as follows: Methotrexate is administered 2 times weekly either by mouth or intramuscularly in doses of 30 mg/M^2. It has also been given in doses of 2.5 mg/kg intravenously every 14 days. If and when relapse does occur, reinduction of remission can again usually be obtained by repeating the initial induction regimen. Various experts have recently introduced a variety of dosage schedules for both induction and maintenance of remission with various combinations of alkylating and antifolic agents. Multiple drug therapy with several agents, including Methotrexate given concomitantly is gaining increasing support in both the acute and chronic forms of leukemia. The physician should familiarize himself with the new advances in antileukemic therapy.

Acute granulocytic leukemia is rare in children but common in adults. This form of leukemia responds poorly to chemotherapy and remissions are short with relapses common, and resistance to therapy develops rapidly.

Meningeal leukemia: Patients with leukemia are subject to leukemic invasion of the central nervous system. This may manifest characteristic signs or symptoms or may remain silent and be diagnosed only by examination of the cerebrospinal fluid which contains leukemic cells in such cases. Therefore, the CSF should be examined in all leukemic patients. Since passage of Methotrexate from blood serum to the cerebrospinal fluid is minimal, for adequate therapy the drug is administered intrathecally. It is now common practice because of the noted increased frequency of meningeal leukemia to administer Methotrexate intrathecally as prophylaxis in all cases of lymphocytic leukemia.

By intrathecal injection, the sodium salt of Methotrexate is administered in solution in doses of 12 mg per square meter of body surface or in an empirical dose of 15 mg. The solution is made in a strength of 1 mg per ml with an appropriate, sterile, preservative-free medium such as Sodium Chloride Injection, USP.

For the treatment of meningeal leukemia, Methotrexate is given at intervals of 2 to 5 days. Methotrexate is administered until the cell count of the cerebrospinal fluid returns to normal. At this point one additional dose is advisable.

For prophylaxis against meningeal leukemia, the dosage is the same as for treatment except for the intervals of administration.

On this subject, it is advisable for the physician to consult the medical literature.

Large doses may cause convulsions. Untoward side effects may occur with any given intrathecal injection and are commonly neurological in character. Methotrexate given by intrathecal route appears significantly in the systemic circulation and may cause systemic Methotrexate toxicity. Therefore systemic antileukemic therapy with the drug should be appropriately adjusted, reduced or discontinued. Focal luekemic involvement of the central nervous system may not respond to intrathecal chemotherapy and is best treated with radiotherapy.

Lymphomas: in Burkitt's Tumor, Stages I-II, Methotrexate has produced prolonged remissions in some cases. Recommended dosage is 10 to 25 mg per day orally for 4 to 8 days. In stage III, Methotrexate is commonly given concomitantly with other antitumor agents. Treatment in all stages usually consists of several courses of the drug interposed with 7 to 10 day rest periods. Lymphosarcomas in Stage III may respond to combined drug therapy with Methotrexate given in doses of 0.625 mg to 2.5 mg/kg daily. Hodgkin's Disease responds poorly to Methotrexate and to most types of chemotherapy.

Mycosis fungoides: therapy with Methotrexate appears to produce clinical remissions in one half of the cases treated. Dosage is usually 2.5 to 10 mg daily by mouth for weeks or months. Dose levels of drug and adjustment of dose regimen by reduction or cessation of drug are guided by patient response and hematologic monitoring. Methotrexate has also been given intramuscularly in doses of 50 mg once weekly or 25 mg 2 times weekly.

Psoriasis Chemotherapy

The patient should be fully informed of the risks involved and should be under constant supervision of the physician.

Assessment of renal function, liver function, and blood elements should be made by history, physical examination, and laboratory tests (such as CBC, urinalysis, serum creatinine, liver function studies, and liver biopsy if indicated) before beginning Methotrexate, periodically during Methotrexate therapy, and before reinstituting Methotrexate therapy after a rest period. Appropriate steps should be taken to avoid conception during and for at least eight weeks following Methotrexate therapy.

There are three commonly used general types of dosage schedules:

1) weekly oral or parenteral intermittent large doses
2) divided dose intermittent oral schedule over a 36 hour period
3) daily oral with a rest period

All schedules should be continually tailored to the individual patient. Dose schedules cited below pertain to an average 70 Kg adult. An initial test dose one week prior to initiation of therapy is recommended to detect any idiosyncrasy. A suggested dose range is 5–10 mg parenterally.

Recommended starting dose schedules:

1. Weekly single oral, IM or IV dose schedule: 10–25 mg per week until adequate response is achieved. With this dosage schedule, 50 mg per week should ordinarily not be exceeded.
2. Divided oral dose schedule: 2.5 mg at 12 hour intervals for three doses or at 8 hour intervals for four doses each week. With this dosage schedule, 30 mg per week should not be exceeded.
3. Daily oral dose schedule: 2.5 mg daily for five days followed by at least a two day rest period. With this dosage schedule, 6.25 mg per day should not be exceeded.

SPECIAL NOTE: Available data suggest that schedule 3 may carry an increased risk of serious liver pathology.

Dosages in each schedule may be gradually adjusted to achieve optimal clinical response, but not to exceed the maximum stated for each schedule.

Once optimal clinical response has been achieved, each dosage schedule should be reduced to the lowest possible amount of drug and to the longest possible rest period. The use of Methotrexate may permit the return to conventional topical therapy, which should be encouraged.

Antidote for Overdosage: Leucovorin (citrovorum factor) is a potent agent for neutralizing the immediate toxic effects of Methotrexate on the hematopoietic system. Where large doses or overdoses are given, Calcium Leucovorin may be administered by intravenous infusion in doses up to 75 mg within 12 hours, followed by 12 mg intramuscularly every 6 hours for 4 doses. Where average doses of Methotrexate appear to have an adverse effect, 2 to 4 ml (6 to 12 mg) of Calcium Leucovorin may be given intramuscularly every 6 hours for 4 doses. In general, where overdosage is suspected, the dose of Leucovorin should be equal to or higher than the offending dose of Methotrexate and should best be administered within the first hour. Use of Calcium Leucovorin after an hour delay is much less effective.

CAUTION: Pharmacist: Because of its potential to cause severe toxicity, Methotrexate therapy requires close supervision of the patient by the physician. Pharmacists should dispense no more than a seven (7) day supply of the drug at one time. Refill of such prescriptions should be by direct order (written or oral) of the physician only.

Reconstitution of Low Sodium Cryodesiccated Powders

Dilute immediately prior to use.

For IV or IM administration, dilute with 2 to 10 ml of an appropriate sterile, preservative free medium such as 5% Dextrose Solution, USP or Sodium Chloride Injection, USP.

For intrathecal injection, see special instructions under **Dosage and Administration.**

How Supplied:

***Parenterals:**

Low Sodium Cryodesiccated Powders—Preservative Free, Single Use Only

20 mg Vial—Product No. NDC 0205-4654-90 (Dark Blue Cap)

50 mg Vial—Product No. NDC 0205-9337-92 (Violet Cap)

100 mg Vial—Product No. NDC 0205-9338-94 (Green Cap)

Store at Controlled Room Temperature 15–30° C (59–86°F)

Isotonic Liquids—Preservative Free, Single Use Only Methotrexate LPF Sodium

25 mg/ml—2 ml (50 mg) Vials—Product No. NDC 0205-5325-26 (Brown Cap)

25 mg/ml—4 ml (100 mg) Vials—Product No. NDC 0205-5326-18 (Light Blue Cap)

25 mg/ml—8 ml (200 mg) Vials—Product No. NDC 0205-5327-30 (Orange Cap)

Store at Controlled Room Temperature 15–30° C (50–86°F)

Isotonic Liquids—Preserved

25 mg per ml—2 ml Vials—Product NDC 0205-4554-26 (Red Cap)

Store at Controlled Room Temperature 15–30° C (59–86°F)

***Parenterals:**

Isotonic Liquid—Preserved

2.5 mg per ml—2 ml Vials—Product No. NDC 0005-4554-26 (White Cap)

Store at Controlled Room Temperature 15–30° C (50–86°F)

*Lederle Parenterals, Inc.
Carlina, Puerto Rico 00630

Oral:

Description

Methotrexate tablets contain 2.5 mg of Methotrexate and are round, convex, yellow tablets, engraved with LL on one side, scored in half on the other side, and engraved with M above the score, and 1 below. 2.5 mg Tablets—Bottles of 100—Product No. NDC 0005-4507-23

Store at Controlled Room Temperature 15–30° C (59–86°F)

Lederle Laboratories Division
American Cyanamid Company,
Pearl River, N.Y. 10965

Military Depots

NSN 6505-01-020-2367, 25 mg/ml—2 ml vial

[Tablets Shown in Product Identification Section]

MINOCIN® ℞

minocycline hydrochloride
Oral and Intravenous

Description: MINOCIN *minocycline hydrochloride* is a semi-synthetic derivative of tetracycline, 7-dimethylamino-6-deoxy-6-demethyltetracycline hydrochloride.

Intravenous: Each vial, dried by cryodesiccation, contains sterile Minocycline Hydrochloride equivalent to 100 mg. Minocycline. When reconstituted with 5 ml. of Sterile Water For Injection the pH ranges from 2.0 to 2.8.

Actions: Microbiology—The tetracyclines are primarily bacteriostatic and are thought to exert their antimicrobial effect by the inhibition of protein synthesis. Minocycline HCl is a tetracycline with antibacterial activity comparable to other tetracyclines with activity against a wide range of gram-negative and gram-positive organisms.

Tube dilution testing: Microorganisms may be considered susceptible (likely to respond to minocycline therapy) if the minimum inhibitory concentration (M.I.C.) is not more than 4.0 mcg./ml. Microorganisms may be considered intermediate (harboring partial resistance) if the M.I.C. is 4.0 to 12.5 mcg./ml. and resistant (not likely to respond to minocycline therapy) if the M.I.C. is greater than 12.5 mcg./ml.

Susceptibility plate testing: If the Kirby-Bauer method of susceptibility testing (using a 30 mcg. tetracycline disc) gives a zone of 18 mm. or greater, the bacterial strain is considered to be susceptible to any tetracycline. Minocycline shows moderate *in vitro* activity against certain strains of staphylococci which have been found resistant to other tetracyclines. For such strains, minocycline susceptibility powder may be used for additional susceptibility testing.

Human Pharmacology: Oral—Following a single dose of two 100 mg. of Minocycline HCl capsules administered to ten normal adult volunteers, serum levels ranged from 0.74 to 4.45 mcg./ml. in one hour (average 2.24), after 12 hours they ranged from 0.34 to 2.36 mcg./ml. (average 1.25). The serum half-life following a single 200 mg. dose in 12 essentially normal volunteers ranged from 11 to 17 hours, in 7 patients with hepatic dysfunction ranged from 11 to 16 hours, and in 5 patients with renal dysfunction from 18 to 69 hours. The urinary and fecal recovery of minocycline when administered to 12 normal volunteers is one-half to one-third that of other tetracyclines.

Human Pharmacology: Intravenous—Following a single dose of 200 mg. administered intravenously to 10 healthy male volunteers, serum levels ranged from 2.52 to 6.63 mcg./ml. (average 4.18), after 12 hours they ranged from 0.82 to 2.64 mcg./ml. (average 1.38). In a group of 5 healthy male volunteers, serum levels of 1.4-1.8 mcg./ml. were maintained at 12 and 24 hours with doses of 100 mg. every 12 hours for three days. When given 200 mg. once daily for three days the serum levels had fallen to approximately 1 mcg./ml. at 24 hours. The serum half-life following I.V. doses of 100 mg. every 12 hours or 200 mg. once daily did not differ significantly and ranged from 15 to 23 hours. The serum half-life following a single 200 mg. oral dose in 12 essentially normal volunteers ranged from 11 to 17 hours, in 7 patients with hepatic dysfunction ranged from 11 to 16

Continued on next page

The information on each product appearing here is based on labelling effective in August, 1982 and is either the entire official brochure or an accurate condensation therefrom. Offical brochures are enclosed in product packages. Information concerning all Lederle products may be obtained from the Professional Services Department, Lederle Laboratories, Pearl River, New York, 10965.

Lederle—Cont.

hours, and in 5 patients with renal dysfunction from 18 to 69 hours.

Intravenously administered Minocycline appears similar to oral doses in excretion. The urinary and fecal recovery of oral minocycline when administered to 12 normal volunteers is one-half to one-third that of other tetracyclines.

Indications: MINOCIN *minocycline HCl* is indicated in infections caused by the following microorganisms:

Rickettsiae: (Rocky Mountain spotted fever, typhus fever and the typhus group, Q fever, rickettsialpox, tick fevers.)

Mycoplasma pneumoniae (PPLO, Eaton agent).

Agents of psittacosis and ornithosis.

Agents of lymphogranuloma venereum and granuloma inguinale. The spirochetal agent of relapsing fever *(Borrelia recurrentis).*

The following gram-negative microorganisms:

Hemophilus ducreyi (chancroid),
Pasteurella pestis and *Pasteurella tularensis,*
Bartonella bacilliformis,
Bacteroides species,
Vibrio comma and *Vibrio fetus,*
Brucella species (in conjunction with streptomycin).

Because many strains of the following groups of microorganisms have been shown to be resistant to tetracyclines, culture and susceptibility testing are recommended.

MINOCIN *minocycline hydrochloride* is indicated for treatment of infections caused by the following gram-negative microorganisms, when bacteriologic testing indicates appropriate susceptibility to the drug:

Escherichia coli,
Enterobacter aerogenes (formerly *Aerobacter aerogenes*),
Shigella species,
Mima species and *Herellea* species,
Haemophilus influenzae (respiratory infections).
Klebsiella species (respiratory and urinary infections).

MINOCIN is indicated for treatment of infections caused by the following gram-positive microorganisms when bacteriologic testing indicates appropriate susceptibility to the drug:

Streptococcus species:

Up to 44 percent of strains of *Streptococcus pyogenes* and 74 percent of *Streptococcus faecalis* have been found to be resistant to tetracycline drugs. Therefore, tetracyclines should not be used for streptococcal disease unless the organism has been demonstrated to be sensitive.

For upper respiratory infections due to group A beta-hemolytic streptococci, penicillin is the usual drug of choice, including prophylaxis of rheumatic fever.

Diplococcus pneumoniae,

Staphylococcus aureus, skin and soft tissue infections. Tetracyclines are not the drug of choice in the treatment of any type of staphylococcal infection.

When penicillin is contraindicated, tetracyclines are alternative drugs in the treatment of infections due to:

Neisseria gonorrhoeae,
Neisseria meningitidis (I.V. only)
Treponema pallidum and *Treponema pertenue* (syphilis and yaws),
Listeria monocytogenes,
Clostridium species,
Bacillus anthracis,
Fusobacterium fusiforme (Vincent's infection),
Actinomyces species.

In acute intestinal amebiasis, the tetracyclines may be a useful adjunct to amebicides.

In severe acne, the tetracyclines may be useful adjunctive therapy. (Oral Only)

MINOCIN is indicated in the treatment of trachoma, although the infectious agent is not always eliminated as judged by immunofluorescence.

Inclusion conjunctivitis may be treated with oral tetracyclines or with a combination of oral and topical agents.

Minocycline is indicated in the treatment of asymptomatic carriers of *N. meningitidis* to eliminate meningococci from the nasopharynx.

In order to preserve the usefulness of MINOCIN *minocycline HCl* in the treatment of asymptomatic meningococcal carriers, diagnostic laboratory procedures, including serotyping and susceptibility testing, should be performed to establish the carrier state and the correct treatment. It is recommended that the drug be reserved for situations in which the risk of meningococcal meningitis is high.

Minocycline by oral administration is not indicated for the treatment of meningococcal infection.

Although no controlled clinical efficacy studies have been conducted, limited clinical data show that oral minocycline hydrochloride has been used successfully in the treatment of infections caused by Mycobacterium marinum.

Contraindications: This drug is contraindicated in persons who have shown hypersensitivity to any of the tetracyclines.

Warnings: In the presence of renal dysfunction, particularly in pregnancy, intravenous tetracycline therapy in daily doses exceeding 2 grams has been associated with deaths through liver failure.

When the need for intensive treatment outweighs its potential dangers (mostly during pregnancy or in individuals with known or suspected renal or liver impairment), it is advisable to perform renal and liver function tests before and during therapy. Also tetracycline serum concentrations should be followed.

If renal impairment exists, even usual oral or parenteral doses may lead to excessive systemic accumulation of the drug and possible liver toxicity. Under such conditions, lower than usual total doses are indicated, and if therapy is prolonged, serum level determinations of the drug may be advisable. This hazard is of particular importance in the parenteral administration of tetracyclines to pregnant or postpartum patients with pyelonephritis. When used under these circumstances, the blood level should not exceed 15 micrograms/ml. and liver function tests should be made at frequent intervals. Other potentially hepatotoxic drugs should not be prescribed concomitantly.

THE USE OF TETRACYCLINES DURING TOOTH DEVELOPMENT (LAST HALF OF PREGNANCY, INFANCY AND CHILDHOOD TO THE AGE OF 8 YEARS) MAY CAUSE PERMANENT DISCOLORATION OF THE TEETH (YELLOW-GRAY-BROWN). This adverse reaction is more common during long-term use of the drugs but has been observed following repeated short-term courses. Enamel hypoplasia has also been reported. TETRACYCLINES, THEREFORE, SHOULD NOT BE USED IN THIS AGE GROUP UNLESS OTHER DRUGS ARE NOT LIKELY TO BE EFFECTIVE OR ARE CONTRAINDICATED.

Photosensitivity manifested by an exaggerated sunburn reaction has been observed in some individuals taking tetracyclines. Patients apt to be exposed to direct sunlight or ultraviolet light should be advised that this reaction can occur with tetracycline drugs, and treatment should be discontinued at the first evidence of skin erythema. Studies to date indicate that photosensitivity is rarely reported with MINOCIN *minocycline HCl.*

The antianabolic action of the tetracyclines may cause an increase in BUN. While this is not a problem in those with normal renal function, in patients with significantly impaired function, higher serum levels of tetracyclines may lead to azotemia, hyperphosphatemia, and acidosis.

CNS side effects including lightheadedness, dizziness or vertigo have been reported. Patients who experience these symptoms should be cautioned about driving vehicles or using hazardous machinery while on minocycline therapy. These symptoms may disappear during therapy and always disappear rapidly when the drug is discontinued.

Usage in Pregnancy—(See above "Warnings" about use during tooth development.) Results of animal studies indicate that tetracyclines cross the placenta, are found in fetal tissues and can have toxic effects on the developing fetus (often related to retardation of skeletal development). Evidence of embryotoxicity has also been noted in animals treated early in pregnancy.

The safety of minocycline HCl for use during pregnancy has not been established.

Usage in newborns, infants, and children—(See above "Warnings" about use during tooth development.)

All tetracyclines form a stable calcium complex in any bone forming tissue. A decrease in the fibula growth rate has been observed in prematures given oral tetracycline in doses of 25 mg./kg. every 6 hours. This reaction was shown to be reversible when the drug was discontinued.

Tetracyclines are present in the milk of lactating women who are taking a drug in this class.

Precautions: As with other antibiotic preparations, use of this drug may result in overgrowth of nonsusceptible organisms, including fungi. If superinfection occurs, the antibiotic should be discontinued and appropriate therapy should be instituted.

In venereal diseases when coexistent syphilis is suspected, darkfield examination should be done before treatment is started and the blood serology repeated monthly for at least 4 months.

Because tetracyclines have been shown to depress plasma prothrombin activity, patients who are on anticoagulant therapy may require downward adjustment of their anticoagulant dosage.

In long-term therapy, periodic laboratory evaluation of organ systems, including hematopoietic, renal and hepatic studies, should be performed.

All infections due to Group A beta-hemolytic streptococci should be treated for at least 10 days.

Since bacteriostatic drugs may interfere with the bactericidal action of penicillin, it is advisable to avoid giving tetracycline in conjunction with penicillin.

Adverse Reactions: Gastrointestinal: Anorexia, nausea, vomiting, diarrhea, glossitis, dysphagia, enterocolitis, and inflammatory lesions (with monilial overgrowth) in the anogenital region.

These reactions have been caused by both the oral and parenteral administration of tetracyclines.

Skin: Maculopapular and erythematous rashes. Exfoliative dermatitis has been reported but is uncommon. Photosensitivity is discussed above. (See "Warnings".) Pigmentation of skin and mucous membranes has been reported.

Renal toxicity: Rise in BUN has been reported and is apparently dose related. (See "Warnings".)

Hypersensitivity reactions: Urticaria, angioneurotic edema, anaphylaxis, anaphylactoid purpura, pericarditis and exacerbation of systemic lupus erythematosus.

Bulging fontanels have been reported in young infants following full therapeutic dosage. This sign disappeared rapidly when the drug was discontinued.

Blood: Hemolytic anemia, thrombocytopenia, neutropenia and eosinophilia have been reported.

CNS: (See "Warnings".)

When given over prolonged periods, tetracyclines have been reported to produce brown-black microscopic discoloration of thyroid glands. No abnormalities of thyroid function studies are known to occur.

Dosage and Administration: Oral—Therapy should be continued for at least 24-48 hours after symptoms and fever have subsided.

Concomitant therapy: Antacids containing aluminum, calcium, or magnesium impair absorption and should not be given to patients taking oral tetracycline.

Studies to date have indicated that the absorption of MINOCIN is not notably influenced by foods and dairy products.

In patients with renal impairment: (See "Warnings".) Total dosage should be decreased by reduction of recommended individual doses and/or by extending time intervals between doses.

In the treatment of streptococcal infections, a therapeutic dose of tetracycline should be administered for at least 10 days.

Adults: The usual dosage of MINOCIN *minocycline HCl* is 200 mg. initially followed by 100 mg. every 12 hours. Alternatively, if more frequent doses are preferred, two or four 50 mg. capsules may be given initially followed by one 50 mg. capsule four times daily.

For children above eight years of age: The usual dosage of MINOCIN *minocycline HCl* is 4 mg./kg. initially followed by 2 mg./kg. every 12 hours.

For treatment of syphilis, the usual dosage of MINOCIN should be administered over a period of 10-15 days. Close follow-up, including laboratory tests, is recommended.

Gonorrhea patients sensitive to penicillin may be treated with MINOCIN, administered as 200 mg. initially followed by 100 mg. every twelve hours for a minimum of 4 days, with post-therapy cultures within 2-3 days.

In the treatment of meningococcal carrier state recommended dose is 100 mg. every 12 hours for five days. *Mycobacterium Marinum* Infections–Although optimal doses have not been established, 100 mg twice a day for 6–8 weeks have been used successfully in a limited number of cases.

Dosage and Administration: Intravenous

Note: Rapid administration is to be avoided. Parenteral therapy is indicated only when oral therapy is not adequate or tolerated. Oral therapy should be instituted as soon as possible. If intravenous therapy is given over prolonged periods of time thrombophlebitis may result.

Adults: Usual adult dose: 200 mg. followed by 100 mg. every 12 hours and should not exceed 400 mg. in 24 hours. The drug should be initially dissolved and then further diluted to 500-1,000 ml. with either Sodium Chloride Injection USP, Dextrose Injection USP, Dextrose and Sodium Chloride Injection USP, Ringer's Injection USP, or Lactated Ringer's Injection USP but not in other solutions containing calcium (a precipitate may form).

The reconstituted solutions are stable at room temperature for 24 hours without significant loss of potency. Any unused portion must be discarded after that period. The final dilution for administration should be administered immediately.

For children above eight years of age: Usual pediatric dose: 4 mg./kg. followed by a 2 mg./kg. every 12 hours. In patients with renal impairment: (See "Warnings".)

Total dosage should be decreased by reduction of recommended individual doses and/or by extending time intervals between doses.

How Supplied: CAPSULES: Minocycline Hydrochloride equivalent to 100 mg. Minocycline. Hardshell purple and orange. Printed with Lederle over M4 on one half and MINOCIN over 100 mg on the other.

NDC 0005-5301-18—bottles of 50
NDC 0005-5301-23—bottles of 100
NDC 0005-5301-60—Unit Dose of 10 × 10's

Minocycline Hydrochloride equivalent to 50 mg Minocycline. Hardshell orange with Lederle over M2 on one half and MINOCIN over 50 mg on the other.

NDC 0005-5300-23 bottles of 100
NDC 0005-5300-60 Unit Dose 10 × 10's

Store at Controlled Room Temperature 15–30°C (50–86°F)

ORAL SUSPENSION: Minocycline Hydrochloride equivalent to 50 mg. Minocycline per teaspoonful (5 ml.) Preserved with propylparaben 0.10% and butylparaben 0.06% with Alcohol USP 5% v/v. Custard-flavored in bottles of 2 fl. oz. NDC 0005-5313-56

Store at Controlled Room Temperature 15–30°C (59–86°F)

DO NOT FREEZE

TABLETS—minocycline hydrochloride equivalent to 100 mg minocycline. Round, convex, orange film-coated tablet engraved with M over bisect and 5 under bisect on one side of the tablet and LL on the other.

NDC 0005-9376-18—bottles of 50

Store at Controlled Room Temperature 15–30° C (59–86°F)

Minocycline hydrochloride equivalent to 50 mg minocycline. Round, convex, orange film-coated tablet engraved with M3 on one side and LL on the other.

NDC 0005-9375-23—bottles of 100

Store at Controlled Room Temperature 15–30° C (59–86°F)

***INTRAVENOUS**—100 mg. vials of sterile cryodesiccated powder. NDC 0005-5305-94

Animal Pharmacology and Toxicology: MINOCIN *minocycline HCl* has been found to produce high blood concentrations following oral dosage to various animal species and to be extensively distributed to all tissues examined in ^{14}C-labeled drug studies in dogs. MINOCIN has been found experimentally to produce discoloration of the thyroid glands. This finding has been observed in rats and dogs. Changes in thyroid function have also been found in these animal species. However, no change in thyroid function has been observed in humans.

[*Shown in Product Identification Section*]

Capsules, 50 mg.
Military Depot NSN 6505-01-015-4147, 100's
VA Depot NSN 6505-01-015-4147A, 100's
Capsules, 100 mg
Military Depot NSN 6505-00-003-5112, 50's
VA Depot NSN 6505-01-108-9040A, 100's
Intravenous, 100 mg.
Military Depot NSN 6505-00-149-0574

*Manufactured for
LEDERLE LABORATORIES DIVISION
American Cyanamid Company
Pearl River, NY 10965
by
LEDERLE PARENTERALS INC.
Carolina, Puerto Rico 00630

MYAMBUTOL® ℞

ethambutol hydrochloride
Tablets

Description: MYAMBUTOL *ethambutol hydrochloride Lederle* is an oral chemotherapeutic agent which is specifically effective against actively growing microorganisms of the genus *Mycobacterium,* including *M. tuberculosis.*

Action: MYAMBUTOL, following a single oral dose of 25 mg./Kg. of body weight, attains a peak of 2 to 5 micrograms/ml. in serum 2 to 4 hours after administration. When the drug is administered daily for longer periods of time at this dose, serum levels are similar. The serum level of MYAMBUTOL falls to undetectable levels by 24 hours after the last dose except in some patients with abnormal renal function. The intracellular concentrations of erythrocytes reach peak values approximately twice those of plasma and maintain this ratio throughout the 24 hours.

During the 24-hour period following oral administration of MYAMBUTOL, approximately 50 percent of the initial dose is excreted unchanged in the urine, while an additional 8 to 15 percent appears in the form of metabolites. The main path of metabolism appears to be an initial oxidation of the alcohol to an aldehydic intermediate, followed by conversion to a dicarboxylic acid. From 20 to 22 percent of the initial dose is excreted in the feces as unchanged drug. No drug accumulation has been observed with consecutive single daily doses of 25 mg./Kg. in patients with normal kidney function, although marked accumulation has been demonstrated in patients with renal insufficiency.

MYAMBUTOL diffuses into actively growing *mycobacterium* cells such as tubercle bacilli. MYAMBUTOL appears to inhibit the synthesis of one or more metabolites, thus causing impairment of cell metabolism, arrest of multiplication, and cell death. No cross resistance with other available antimycobacterial agents has been demonstrated.

MYAMBUTOL has been shown to be effective against strains of *Mycobacterium tuberculosis* but does not seem to be active against fungi, viruses, or other bacteria.

Mycobacterium tuberculosis strains previously unexposed to MYAMBUTOL have been uniformly sensitive to concentrations of 8 or less micrograms/ml., depending on the nature of the culture media. When MYAMBUTOL has been used alone for treatment of tuberculosis, tubercle bacilli from these patients have developed resistance to MYAMBUTOL by *in vitro* susceptibility tests; the development of resistance has been unpredictable and appears to occur in a step-like manner. No cross resistance between MYAMBUTOL and other antituberculous drugs has been reported. MYAMBUTOL has reduced the incidence of the emergence of mycobacterial resistance to isoniazid when both drugs have been used concurrently.

An agar diffusion microbiologic assay, based upon inhibition of *Mycobacterium smegmatis* (ATCC 607) may be used to determine concentrations of MYAMBUTOL in serum and urine. This technique has not been published, but further information can be obtained upon inquiry to Lederle Laboratories.

Animal Pharmacology: Toxicological studies in dogs on high prolonged doses produced evidence of myocardial damage and failure, and depigmentation of the tapetum lucidum of the eyes, the significance of which is not known. Degenerative changes in the central nervous system, apparently not dose-related, have also been noted in dogs receiving ethambutol hydrochloride over a prolonged period.

In the rhesus monkey, neurological signs appeared after treatment with high doses given daily over a period of several months. These were correlated with specific serum levels of ethambutol hydrochloride and with definite neuro-anatomical changes in the central nervous system. Focal interstitial carditis was also noted in monkeys which received ethambutol hydrochloride in high doses for a prolonged period.

When pregnant mice or rabbits were treated with high doses of ethambutol hydrochloride, fetal mortality was slightly but not significantly ($P > 0.05$) increased. Female rats treated

Continued on next page

The information on each product appearing here is based on labelling effective in August, 1982 and is either the entire official brochure or an accurate condensation therefrom. Offical brochures are enclosed in product packages. Information concerning all Lederle products may be obtained from the Professional Services Department, Lederle Laboratories, Pearl River, New York, 10965.

Lederle—Cont.

with ethambutol hydrochloride displayed slight but insignificant ($P > 0.05$) decreases in fertility and litter size.

In fetuses born of mice treated with high doses of ethambutol hydrochloride during pregnancy, a low incidence of cleft palate, exencephaly and abnormality of the vertebral column were observed. Minor abnormalities of the cervical vertebra were seen in the newborn of rats treated with high doses of ethambutol hydrochloride during pregnancy. Rabbits receiving high doses of ethambutol hydrochloride during pregnancy gave birth to two fetuses with monophthalmia, one with a shortened right forearm accompanied by bilateral wrist-joint contracture and one with hare lip and cleft palate.

Indications: MYAMBUTOL *ethambutol hydrochloride* is indicated for the treatment of pulmonary tuberculosis. It should not be used as the sole antituberculous drug, but should be used in conjunction with at least one other antituberculous drug. Selection of the companion drug should be based on clinical experience, considerations of comparative safety and appropriate *in vitro* susceptibility studies.

In patients who have not received previous antituberculous therapy, i.e. initial treatment, the most frequently used regimens have been the following:

MYAMBUTOL plus isoniazid

MYAMBUTOL plus isoniazid plus streptomycin.

In patients who have received previous antituberculous therapy, mycobacterial resistance to other drugs used in initial therapy is frequent. Consequently in such retreatment patients, MYAMBUTOL should be combined with at least one of the second line drugs not previously administered to the patient and to which bacterial susceptibility has been indicated by appropriate *in vitro* studies. Antituberculous drugs used with MYAMBUTOL have included cycloserine, ethionamide, pyrazinamide, viomycin and other drugs. Isoniazid, aminosalicylic acid, and streptomycin have also been used in multiple drug regimens. Alternating drug regimens have also been utilized.

Contraindications: MYAMBUTOL is contraindicated in patients who are known to be hypersensitive to this drug. It is also contraindicated in patients with known optic neuritis unless clinical judgment determines that it may be used.

Precautions: The effects of combinations of ethambutol hydrochloride with other antituberculous drugs on the fetus is not known. While administration of this drug to pregnant human patients has produced no detectable effect upon the fetus, the possible teratogenic potential in women capable of bearing children should be weighed carefully against the benefits of therapy. There are published reports of five women who received the drug during pregnancy without apparent adverse effect upon the fetus.

MYAMBUTOL is not recommended for use in children under thirteen years of age since safe conditions for use have not been established.

Patients with decreased renal function need the dosage reduced as determined by serum levels of MYAMBUTOL, since the main path of excretion of this drug is by the kidneys.

Because this drug may have adverse effects on vision, physical examination should include ophthalmoscopy, finger perimetry and testing of color discrimination. In patients with visual defects such as cataracts, recurrent inflammatory conditions of the eye, optic neuritis, and diabetic retinopathy, the evaluation of changes in visual acuity is more difficult, and care should be taken to be sure the variations in vision are not due to the underlying disease conditions. In such patients, consideration should be given to relationship between benefits expected and possible visual deterioration since evaluation of visual changes is difficult. (For recommended procedures, see next paragraphs under Adverse Reactions.)

As with any potent drug, periodic assessment of organ system functions, including renal, hepatic, and hematopoietic, should be made during long-term therapy.

Adverse Reactions: MYAMBUTOL may produce decreases in visual acuity which appear to be due to optic neuritis and to be related to dose and duration of treatment. The effects are generally reversible when administration of the drug is discontinued promptly.

In rare cases recovery may be delayed for up to one year or more and the effect may possibly be irreversible in these cases.

Patients should be advised to report promptly to their physician any change of visual acuity.

The change in visual acuity may be unilateral or bilateral and hence *each eye must be tested separately and both eyes tested together.* Testing of visual acuity should be performed before beginning MYAMBUTOL *ethambutol hydrochloride* therapy and periodically during drug administration, except that it should be done monthly when a patient is on a dosage of more than 15 mg. per Kilogram per day. Snellen eye charts are recommended for testing of visual acuity. Studies have shown that there are definite fluctuations of one or two lines of the Snellen chart in the visual acuity of many tuberculous patients *not* receiving MYAMBUTOL.

The table may be useful in interpreting possible changes in visual acuity attributable to MYAMBUTOL.

[See table below].

In general, changes in visual acuity less than those indicated under "Significant Number of Lines" and "Decreases-Number of Points", may be due to chance variation, limitations of the testing method or physiologic variability. Conversely, changes in visual acuity equaling or exceeding those under "Significant Number of Lines" and "Decreases-Number of Points" indicate need for retesting and careful evaluation of the patient's visual status. If careful evaluation confirms the magnitude of visual change and fails to reveal another cause, MYAMBUTOL should be discontinued and the patient reevaluated at frequent intervals. Progressive decreases in visual acuity during therapy must be considered to be due to MYAMBUTOL.

If corrective glasses are used prior to treatment, these must be worn during visual acuity testing. During 1 to 2 years of therapy, a refractive error may develop which must be corrected in order to obtain accurate test results. Testing the visual acuity through a pinhole eliminates refractive error. Patients developing visual abnormality during MYAMBUTOL treatment may show subjective visual symptoms before, or simultaneously with, the demonstration of decreases in visual acuity, and all patients receiving MYAMBUTOL should be questioned periodically about blurred vision and other subjective eye symptoms.

Recovery of visual acuity generally occurs over a period of weeks to months after the drug has been discontinued. Patients have then received MYAMBUTOL again without recurrence of loss of visual acuity.

Other adverse reactions reported include: anaphylactoid reactions, dermatitis, pruritus and joint pain; anorexia, nausea, vomiting, gastrointestinal upset, abdominal pain; fever, malaise, headache, and dizziness; mental confusion, disorientation and possible hallucinations. Numbness and tingling of the extremities due to peripheral neuritis have been reported infrequently.

Elevated serum uric acid levels occur and precipitation of acute gout has been reported. Transient impairment of liver function as indicated by abnormal liver function tests is not an unusual finding. Since MYAMBUTOL is recommended for therapy in conjunction with one or more other antituberculous drugs, these changes may be related to the concurrent therapy.

Dosage and Administration: MYAMBUTOL should not be used alone, in initial treatment or in retreatment. MYAMBUTOL should be administered on a once every 24-hour basis only. Absorption is not significantly altered by administration with food. Therapy, in general, should be continued until bacteriological conversion has become permanent and maximal clinical improvement has occurred.

MYAMBUTOL is not recommended for use in children under thirteen years of age since safe conditions for use have not been established.

Initial Treatment: In patients who have not received previous antituberculous therapy, administer MYAMBUTOL 15 mg. per Kilogram (7 mg. per pound) of body weight, as a single oral dose once every 24 hours. In the more recent studies, isoniazid has been administered concurrently in a single, daily, oral dose.

Retreatment: In patients who have received previous antituberculous therapy, administer MYAMBUTOL 25 mg. per Kilogram (11 mg. per pound) of body weight, as a single oral dose once every 24 hours. Concurrently administer at least one other antituberculous drug to which the organisms have been demonstrated to be susceptible by appropriate *in vitro* tests. Suitable drugs usually consist of those not previously used in the treatment of the patient. After 60 days of MYAMBUTOL (ethambutol hydrochloride) administration, decrease the dose to 15 mg. per Kilogram (7 mg. per pound) of body weight, and administer as a single oral dose once every 24 hours.

During the period when a patient is on a daily dose of 25 mg./kg., monthly eye examinations are advised.

See Table for easy selection of proper weight-dose tablet(s).

Weight-Dose Table

15 mg./Kg. (7 mg./lb.) Schedule

Weight Range Pounds	Kilograms	Daily Dose In mg.
Under 85 lbs.	Under 37 Kg	500
85–94.5	37–43	600
95–109.5	43–50	700
110–124.5	50–57	800
125–139.5	57–64	900
140–154.5	64–71	1000
155–169.5	71–79	1100
170–184.5	79–84	1200
185–199.5	84–90	1300
200–214.5	90–97	1400
215 and Over	Over 97	1500

25 mg./Kg. (11 mg./lb.) Schedule

Pounds	Kilograms	Daily Dose In mg.
Under 85 lbs.	Under 38 Kg.	900
85–92.5	38–42	1000
93–101.5	42–45.5	1100
102–109.5	45.5–50	1200
110–118.5	50–54	1300

VISUAL ACUITY TABLE

Initial Snellen Reading	Reading Indicating Significant Decrease	Significant Number of Lines	Decreases Number of Points
20/13	20/25	3	12
20/15	20/25	2	10
20/20	20/30	2	10
20/25	20/40	2	15
20/30	20/50	2	20
20/40	20/70	2	30
20/50	20/70	1	20

119–128.5	54–58	1400
129–136.5	58–62	1500
137–146.5	62–67	1600
147–155.5	67–71	1700
156–164.5	71–75	1800
165–173.5	75–79	1900
174–182.5	79–83	2000
183–191.5	83–87	2100
192–199.5	87–91	2200
200–209.5	91–95	2300
210–218.5	95–99	2400
219 and Over	Over 99	2500

How Supplied: Tablets 100 mg round, convex, white, coated tablets engraved M6 on one side and LL on the other, are supplied as follows:

NDC 0005-5015-23 - bottles of 100
NDC 0005-5015-34 bottles of 1000

400 mg - round, convex, white scored, film coated tablets engraved with LL on one side and M to the left and 7 to the right of the score on the other side, are supplied as follows:

NDC 0005-5084-62 Unit-of-Issue 100's with CRC
NDC 0005-5084-34 bottles of 1000
NDC 0005-5084-60 - Unit Dose 10 × 10's

Store at Controlled Room Temperature 15–30°C (59–86°F)
A.H.F.S. 8:16

Tablets, 100 mg.
Military Depot NSN 6505-00-403-7645, 100's
Tablets 400 mg.
Military Depot NSN 6505-00-812-2579, 100's
VA Depot NSN 6505-00-812-2543A, 1000's

NEOLOID®
emulsified castor oil

Composition: NEOLOID Emulsified Castor Oil USP 36.4% (w/w) with 0.1% (w/w) Sodium Benzoate and 0.2% (w/w) Potassium Sorbate added as preservatives, emulsifying and flavoring agents in water. NEOLOID is an emulsion with an exceptionally bland, pleasant taste.
Indications: For the treatment of isolated bouts of constipation.
Administration and Dosage:
Infants—½ to 1½ teaspoonfuls.
Children—Adjust between infant and adult dose.
Adult—Average dose, 2 to 4 tablespoonfuls.
Precautions: Not to be used when abdominal pain, nausea, vomiting, or other symptoms of appendicitis are present. Frequent or continued use of this preparation may result in dependence on laxatives. Do not use during pregnancy except on a physician's advice. Keep this and all drugs out of the reach of children.
Caution: If pregnant or nursing, consult your physician or pharmacist before taking this or any medicine. In case of accidental overdose, seek professional assistance or contact a Poison Control Center immediately.
How Supplied: Bottles of 4 fl. oz. (peppermint flavor).

NEPTAZANE® ℞
methazolamide

Description: NEPTAZANE *methazolamide* is a white crystalline powder, weakly acid, slightly soluble in water, and is a complex sulfonamide derivative. It is available as a 50 mg white convex scored tablet.
Action: NEPTAZANE is a potent inhibitor of the enzyme carbonic anhydrase. It is absorbed somewhat slowly from the gastrointestinal tract and disappears more slowly from the plasma than does acetazolamide, which may account for the delay in onset and duration of its activity. It is distributed throughout the body, and can be assayed in the blood plasma, the cerebrospinal fluid, the aqueous humor of the eye, the red blood cell, in the bile and the extra-cellular fluid. Urinary excretion accounts for only 15% of NEPTAZANE in man. It is not cumulative in its concentration. The drug is considered nonbactericidal. Although concentration in the cerebrospinal fluid is high, it is not considered an effective anticonvulsant.
Methazolamide does have a diuretic effect, resulting in increase in urinary volume, with excretion of sodium and potassium and chloride, but it is less active than acetazolamide. This effect is transient and of low degree and the drug is not used as a diuretic. Serum electrolyte changes in sodium, potassium and chloride are minimal and return to pretreatment levels after daily administration for three to four days. Inhibition of renal bicarbonate reabsorption produces an alkaline urine. Plasma bicarbonate decreases temporarily and a relative and transient metabolic acidosis may occur due to a disequilibrium in CO_2 transport in the red cell. This is quickly restored to balance by the initiation of compensatory mechanisms. Urinary citrate excretion is decreased by 40% on doses of 100 mgs every 8 hours with variations in urinary volume output. Uric acid output was decreased 36% in the first 24 hour period and varied thereafter. The oral administration of the drug by inhibition of carbonic anhydrase in the various tissues of the eye causes a decrease in the rate of aqueous humor formation. Various authors differ somewhat as to the time of onset of intraocular pressure fall, of the peak of activity and the duration of the effect on the pressure, of a 24 hour period of ingestion, but on the average, th onset of fall in intraocular pressure occurs within 2-4 hours, with peak of fall in 6-8 hours, the effect lasting from 10-18 hours.
Indications: For adjunctive treatment of: chronic simple (open angle) glaucoma, secondary glaucoma, and preoperatively in acute angle closure glaucoma where delay of surgery is desired in order to lower intraocular pressure.
Contraindications: Severe or absolute glaucoma and chronic noncongestive angle closure glaucoma. It is of doubtful use in glaucoma due to severe peripheral anterior synechiae or hemorrhagic glaucoma.
NEPTAZANE *methazolamide* is contraindicated in patients with adrenocortical insufficiency, hepatic insufficiency, renal insufficiency, or an electrolyte imbalance state such as hyperchloremic acidosis, and sodium and potassium depletion states.
Warning: Studies in rats have demonstrated teratogenic effects (skeletal anomalies) at high doses. There is no evidence of these effects in human beings and no fetal defects have been reported. However, methazolamide should not be used in women of childbearing potential or in pregnancy, especially in the first trimester, unless the benefits to be gained in the control of glaucoma outweigh potential adverse effects.
Precautions: Potassium excretion is increased initially, upon administration of methazolamide and in patients with cirrhosis or hepatic insufficiency could precipitate an hepatic coma. It should be used with caution in patients on steroid therapy because of the potentiality of hypokalemic state.
Adequate and balanced electrolyte intake is essential in all patients whose concomitant clinical condition may occasion electrolyte imbalance.
In patients with pulmonary obstruction or emphysema where alveolar ventilation may be impaired, methazolamide, which may precipitate or aggravate acidosis, should be used with caution.
Adverse reactions common to all sulfonamide derivatives may occur: fever, rash, crystalluria, renal calculus, bone marrow depression, thrombocytopenic purpura, hemolytic anemia, leukopenia, pancytopenia and agranulocytosis. Precaution is advised for early detection of such reactions and the drug should be discontinued and appropriate therapy instituted.
Adverse Reactions: Most adverse reactions to methazolamide have been relatively mild in character and disappear upon withdrawal of the drug or adjustment of dosage. They are as follows: anorexia, nausea, vomiting; malaise, fatigue or drowsiness, headache; vertigo, mental confusion, depression, and paresthesias of fingers, toes, hands or feet and occasionally at the mucocutaneous junction of the lips, mouth and anus.
Urinary citrate excretion is decreased during the administration of NEPTAZANE *methazolamide* as is uric acid output, but urinary calculi clearly due to the drug have not been reported. The effect on citrate excretion is less than that reported from the administration of acetazolamide.
Dosage and Administration: The effective therapeutic dose administered in tablet form varies from 50 mg to 100 mg 2-3 times daily. The drug may be used concomitantly with miotic and osmotic agents. It is not available for parenteral use.
How Supplied: Tablets, 50 mg (scored white) embossed LL on one side and N on the left of a bisect and 1 on the right on the other side.—Bottles of 100
[*Shown in Product Identification Section*]

NILSTAT® ℞
Nystatin Oral Suspension

Description: This antifungal agent is obtained from *Streptomyces noursei*. It is a polyene antibiotic of undetermined structural formula.
Nystatin is an antibiotic with antifungal activity produced by a strain of *Streptomycès noursei*. NILSTAT *nystatin* Oral Suspension, Lederle, is a cherry flavored, ready-to-use suspension containing 100,000 units of nystatin per ml.-with methylparaben (0.12%) and propylparaben (0.03%) as preservatives.
Actions: Nystatin probably acts by binding to sterols in the cell membrane of the fungus with a resultant change in membrane permeability allowing leakage of intracellular components. It is absorbed very sparingly following oral administration, with no detectable blood levels when given in the recommended doses.
Indications: For the treatment of infections of the oral cavity caused by *Candida* (Monilia) *albicans*.
Contraindications: Hypersensitivity to the drug.
Adverse Reactions:
Nausea and vomiting, Gastrointestinal distress, Diarrhea.
Dosage and Administration:
Infants: 2 ml. (200,000 units) four times daily (1 ml. in each side of mouth).
Children and adults: 4-6 ml. (400,000 to 600,000 units) four times daily (one-half of dose in each side of mouth).
Note: Limited clinical studies in prematures and low birth weight infants indicate that 1 ml. four times daily is effective.
Local treatment should be continued at least 48 hours after perioral symptoms have disappeared and cultures returned to normal.
It is recommended that the drug be retained in the mouth as long as possible before swallowing.
How Supplied: 16 fl. oz. bottles and 60 ml. bottles with dropper.

Continued on next page

The information on each product appearing here is based on labelling effective in August, 1982 and is either the entire official brochure or an accurate condensation therefrom. Offical brochures are enclosed in product packages. Information concerning all Lederle products may be obtained from the Professional Services Department, Lederle Laboratories, Pearl River, New York, 10965.

Lederle—Cont.

NILSTAT® ℞
Nystatin Vaginal Tablets U.S.P.

Description: NILSTAT *nystatin Vaginal Tablets,* USP are oblong shaped vaginal tablets, each containing 100,000 units Nystatin, USP.
Nystatin is a polyene antibiotic of undetermined structural formula that is obtained from *streptomyces noursei.*
Clinical Pharmacology: Nystatin is an antifungal antibiotic which is both fungistatic and fungicidal *in vitro* against a wide variety of yeasts and yeast-like fungi. It probably acts by binding to sterols in the cell membrane of the fungus with a resultant change in membrane permeability allowing leakage of intracellular components. It exhibits no appreciable activity against bacteria or trichomonads.
Indications and Usage: NILSTAT *nystatin Vaginal Tablets,* USP are effective for the local treatment of vulvovaginal candidiasis (moniliasis). The diagnosis should be confirmed, prior to therapy, by KOH smears and/or cultures. Other pathogens commonly associated with vulvovaginitis (Trichomonas and *Haemophilus vaginalis)* do not respond to nystatin and should be ruled out by appropriate laboratory methods.
Contraindications: This preparation is contraindicated in patients with a history of hypersensitivity to any of its components.
Precautions:
General
Discontinue treatment if sensitization or irritation is reported during use.
Laboratory Tests:
If there is a lack of response to NILSTAT *nystatin Vaginal Tablets,* USP, appropriate microbiological studies should be repeated to confirm the diagnosis and rule out other pathogens, before instituting another course of antimycotic therapy.
Usage in Pregnancy:
No adverse effects or complications have been attributed to nystatin in infants born to women treated with nystatin vaginal tablets.
Adverse Reactions: Nystatin is virtually nontoxic and nonsensitizing and is well tolerated by all age groups, even on prolonged administration. Rarely, irritation or sensitization may occur (see PRECAUTIONS).
Dosage and Administration: The usual dosage is one tablet (100,000 units nystatin) daily for two weeks. The tablets should be deposited high in the vagina by means of the applicator. "Instructions for the Patient" are enclosed in each package.
Even though symptomatic relief may occur within a few days, treatment should be continued for the full course.
It is important that therapy be continued during menstruation. Adjunctive measures such as therapeutic douches are unnecessary and sometimes inadvisable. Cleansing douches may be used by nonpregnant women, if desired, for esthetic purposes.
How Supplied: Oblong shaped—pale yellow—engraved LL and N6 in packages of 15 and 30 Vaginal Tablets with Applicator.

NILSTAT ℞
nystatin
Oral Tablets (film-coated) pink—engraved LL and N5

500,000 Units per tablet, bottles of 100; unit-dose 10 x 10's.

NILSTAT ℞
nystatin
Topical Cream, 100,000 Units per Gm.
Inactive ingredients in a vanishing cream water base: Emulsifying Wax NF, Isopropyl Myristate, Glycerin, Lactic Acid and Sodium Hydroxide. Preservative: Sorbic Acid 0.2%.
How Supplied: 15 gm tube, 240 gm jar.
Military Depot
NSN 6505-01-063-1141, 240 gm jar

NILSTAT ℞
nystatin
Topical Ointment, 100,000 Units per Gm.
Inactive Ingredients: Light Mineral Oil and Plastibase 50 W.
15 Gm. tubes.

ORIMUNE® POLIOVIRUS VACCINE, LIVE, ORAL, TRIVALENT ℞
0.5 ml Dose Contains Sorbitol
SABIN STRAINS TYPES 1, 2 and 3
FOR ORAL ADMINISTRATION—NOT FOR INJECTION

Description: *Manufacture and Composition:* ORIMUNE® TRIVALENT VACCINE is a mixture of three types of attenuated polioviruses which have been propagated in cercopithecus monkey kidney cell culture. The cells are grown in the presence of Eagle's Basal Medium consisting of Earle's Balanced Salt Solution containing amino acids, antibiotics and calf serum. After cell growth, the medium is removed and replaced with fresh medium containing the inoculating virus but no calf serum. The final vaccine is diluted with a modified cell culture maintenance medium containing sorbitol. Each dose (0.5 ml) contains less than 25 micrograms of each of the antibiotics, streptomycin and neomycin.
The potency is expressed in terms of the amount of virus contained in the recommended dose as tissue culture infective doses (TCID50). The human dose of vaccine containing all three virus types shall be constituted to have infectivity titers in the final container material of $10^{5.4}$ to $10^{6.4}$ for Type 1, $10^{4.5}$ to $10^{5.5}$ for Type 2 and $10^{5.2}$ to $10^{6.2}$ for Type 3.[1]
Color Change: This vaccine contains phenol red as a pH indicator. The usual color of the vaccine is pink, although some containers of vaccine, shipped or stored in dry ice, may exhibit a yellow coloration due to the very low temperature or possible absorption of carbon dioxide. The color of the vaccine prior to use (red-pink-yellow) has no effect on the virus or efficacy of the vaccine.
Indications and Usage: The purpose of administering any attenuated, live, virus vaccine is to stimulate the body mechanism to produce an active immunity by simulating the natural infection without producing untoward symptoms of the disease. To accomplish this with live poliovirus vaccine, it is necessary for the virus to multiply in the intestinal tract. A primary series of this vaccine is designed to produce an antibody response to poliovirus Types 1, 2 and 3. This response is comparable to the immunity induced by the natural disease. The antibodies thus formed help protect the individual against clinical poliomyelitis infection by any of the three types of poliovirus. When used in the prescribed manner for primary immunization, type specific neutralizing antibodies will be induced in 90% or more of susceptibles.
This vaccine is indicated for use in the prevention of poliomyelitis caused by Poliovirus Types 1, 2 and 3.
Infants starting at six to twelve weeks of age, *all unimmunized children* and *adolescents* through age 18 are the usual candidates for routine prophylaxis.
The Immunization Practices Advisory Committee of the Public Health Service states that trivalent oral poliovirus vaccine (TOPV) and inactivated poliovirus vaccine (IPV) are both effective in preventing poliomyelitis. TOPV is the vaccine of choice for primary immunization of children in the United States when the benefits and risks for the entire population are considered. TOPV is preferred because it induces intestinal immunity, is simple to administer, is well accepted by patients, results in immunization of some contacts of vaccinated persons, and has a record of having essentially eliminated disease associated with wild poliovirus in this country.[2] The choice of TOPV as the preferred poliovirus vaccine in the United States has also been made by the committee on Infectious Diseases of the American Academy of Pediatrics and a special expert committee of the Institute of Medicine, National Academy of Science.[3,4] TOPV is also recommended for control of epidemic poliomyelitis.[2,3]
Past history of clinical poliomyelitis or prior vaccination with IPV in otherwise healthy individuals does not preclude the administration of TOPV when otherwise indicated.
Serologic evidence indicates that measles and rubella vaccines or combinations (measles-mumps-rubella vaccine) given simultaneously with trivalent oral poliovirus vaccine can be expected to give adequate antibody response.[5]
Routine poliomyelitis immunization for adults residing in the continental United States is not necessary because of extreme unlikelihood of exposure. However, primary immunization with IPV is recommended whenever feasible for those unimmunized adults subject to *increased risk* of exposure, as by travel to or contact with epidemic or endemic areas and for those employed in hospitals, medical laboratories, clinics or sanitation facilities. If less than 4 weeks are available before protection is needed, a single dose of TOPV is recommended, with IPV given later if the person remains at increased risk. Immunization with IPV may be indicated for unimmunized parents and those in other special situations where, in the judgment of the attending physician, protection may be needed.[2] (See Contraindications and Adverse Reactions.)
Contraindications: *Under no circumstances should this vaccine be administered parenterally.*
Administration of the vaccine should be postponed or avoided in those experiencing any acute illness and in those with any advanced debilitated condition or persistent vomiting or diarrhea.
ORIMUNE *must not* be administered to patients with immune deficiency diseases such as combined immunodeficiency, hypogammaglobulinemia and agammaglobulinemia. It would also be prudent to withhold ORIMUNE from siblings of a child known to have an immunodeficiency syndrome. Further, ORIMUNE *must not* be administered to patients with altered immune states such as those occurring in thymic abnormalities, leukemia, lymphoma or generalized malignancy or by lowered reistance from therapy with corticosteroids, alkylating drugs, antimetabolites or radiation. When possible, all persons with altered immune status should avoid close household-type contact with recipients of the vaccine for at least 6-8 weeks. IPV is preferred for immunizing all persons in this setting.[2,3,4,6,7]
Precautions: Other viruses (including poliovirus and other enterovirus) may interfere with the desired response to this vaccine, since their presence in the intestinal tract may interfere with the replication of the attenuated strains of poliovirus in the vaccine.
It would seem prudent not to administer TOPV shortly after Immune Serum Globulin (ISG) unless such a procedure is unavoidable, for example, with unexpected travel to or contact with epidemic areas or endemic areas. If TOPV is given with or shortly after ISG, the dose probably should be repeated after three months, if immunization is still indicated.
The vaccine will not be effective in modifying or preventing cases of existing and/or incubating poliomyelitis.
Use in Pregnancy: Although there is no convincing evidence documenting adverse effects of either TOPV or IPV on the developing fetus or pregnant woman, it is prudent on theoretical grounds to avoid vaccinating pregnant

women. However, if immediate protection against poliomyelitis is needed, TOPV is recommended.[2] (See Contraindications and Adverse Reactions.)

Adverse Reactions: **Paralytic disease following the ingestion of live poliovirus vaccines has been, on rare occasion, reported in individuals receiving the vaccine, as well as in persons who were in close contact with vaccinees.[2,3,4,8,9] Most Reports of paralytic disease following ingestion of the vaccine or contact with a recent vaccinee are based on epidemiological analysis and temporal association between vaccination or contact and the onset of symptoms. Most authorities believe that a causal relationship exists.[2,8,12,13]**

The Center for Disease Control reports that during the years 1969 through 1978 approximately 242 million does of TOPV were distributed in the United States. In the same 10 years, 18 "vaccine-associated" and 47 "contact vaccine-associated" paralytic cases were reported. Eleven other "vaccine-associated" cases have been reported in persons (recipients or contacts) with immune deficiency conditions.[2]

The risk of vaccine-associated paralysis is extremely small for vaccinees, susceptible family members and other close personal contacts. However, the attending physician should convey or specifically direct personnel acting under his authority to convey the warnings to the vaccinee, parent, guardian or other responsible person of the possibility of vaccine-associated paralysis prior to administration of the vaccine. When the attenuated vaccine strains are to be introduced into a household with adults who have never been vaccinated, some physicians may choose to give these adults at least two doses of IPV a month apart, if not a full primary series, before the children receive ORIMUNE.[2] The benefit of being protected against polio is believed to greatly outweigh any risk from polio vaccine.[14]

Administration: ORIMUNE is to be administered *orally, under the supervision of a physician. Under no circumstances should this vaccine be administered parenterally.* For convenience, the vaccine is supplied in a disposable pipette containing a single dose of 0.5 ml. The vaccine can be administered directly or mixed with distilled water, tap water free of chlorine, simple syrup USP or milk. Alternatively, it may be adsorbed on any one of a number of foods such as bread, cake or cube sugar.

Community Programs

Poliovirus Vaccine Live, Oral, Trivalent has been recommended for epidemic control. Within an epidemic area. TOPV should be provided for all persons over 6 weeks of age who have not been completely immunized or whose immunization status is unknown, with the exceptions noted under immunodeficiency.[2,3]

Dosage:

Dose: Each single dose consists of 0.5 ml of POLIOVIRUS VACCINE, LIVE, ORAL, TRIVALENT ORIMUNE.

Initial Administration (Primary Series)

Infants: The primary series is three doses. The Immunization Practices Advisory Committee (Public Health Service) recommends that the three dose immunization series be started at 6 to 12 weeks of age, commonly with the first DTP inoculation. The second dose should be given not less than 6 and preferably 8 weeks later. The third dose is an integral part of the primary immunization and should be administered 8 to 12 months after the second dose.[2]

The American Academy of Pediatrics recommends that the vaccine be administered at 2 months, 4 months, and at approximately 18 months of age. An optional dose of TOPV may be given at 6 months in areas where poliomyelitis is endemic.[3]

Administration to the newborn (under 6 weeks) is not generally recommended because of the varying persistence of maternal antibodies. However, in certain tropical endemic areas, where poliomyelitis has been increasing in recent years, the physician may wish to administer TOPV to the infant at birth, and complete the basic course during the first six months of life.[3] If the physician chooses to immunize the infant at birth, it may be wise to wait until the child is three days old, and it may be prudent to recommend abstention from breast-feeding for two to three hours before and after oral vaccination to permit establishment of the vaccine viruses in the gut.[15]

Older Children and Adolescents (through age 18): Two doses, given not less than 6 and preferably 8 weeks apart and the third dose 6 to 12 months after the second dose.[2,3]

Adults: See Indications and Adverse Reactions. Where ORIMUNE is given to unimmunized adults, the dosage is as indicated for children and adolescents.

Booster Doses—School Entrance: On entering elementary school, all children who have completed the primary series should be given a single follow-up dose of trivalent oral poliovirus vaccine.[2,3] All other should complete the primary series.

The Public Health Service Advisory Committee does not recommend routine booster doses of vaccine on the basis of current information, beyond that given at the time of entering school.[2] Recent data indicates that over 95% of children studied five years after full immunization with oral poliovirus vaccine had protective antibodies to all three types of poliovirus.[16]

Increased risk: If an individual who has completed a primary series is subjected to a substantially increased risk by virtue of contact, travel or occupation, a single dose of TOPV has been suggested.[2]

Storage: To maintain potency it is necessary to store this vaccine at a temperature which will maintain ice continuously in a solid state. This vaccine may remain fluid at temperatures above −14°C(+7°F) because of its sorbitol content. If frozen, the vaccine must be completely thawed prior to use. An *unopened* container of vaccine that has been frozen and then is thawed may be carried through a maximum of 10 freeze-thaw cycles; provided the temperaure does not exceed 8°C (46°F) during the periods of thaw, and provided the total cumulative duration of thaw does not exceed 24 hours. If the 24-hour period is exceeded, the vaccine then must be used within 30 days, during which time it must be stored at a temperature between 2-8°C(36-46°F).

Disclaimer of Representations and Warranties: **This vaccine has been produced and tested in accordance with the regulations of the United States Food and Drug Administration for the production of Poliovirus Vaccine, Live, Oral, Trivalent. The Manufacturer makes no representation or warranty, expressed or implied, with respect to the merchantability or fitness for use of this vaccine other than that the vaccine has been produced in accordance with the standards for its production prescribed by the United States Food and Drug Administration and applicable thereto at the time of its release by the manufacturer. While the use of this preparation and other measures described herein are consistent with accepted standards of medical practice, their use as described cannot be expected necessarily to assure a specific result.**

How Supplied:

2084-08—10 (0.5 ml) DISPETTES® Disposable Pipettes

2084-12—50 (0.5 ml) DISPETTES®

Also Available:

2 Drop Dose: 2044-25

10 dose vial with dropper

U.S.P.H.S. Depot:

NSN 6505-00-762-1056 10 × 1 dose

Military Depot NSN 6505-00-782-2650 10 dose vial

References:

1. Code of Federal Regulations. 21 CFR: 630.17(c) page 86, revised April 1, 1979.
2. Morbidity and Mortality Weekly Report: Recommendations of the Public Health Service Immunization Practices Advisory Committee (ACIP). *Vol. 28, No. 43:*510–520 (Nov. 2) 1979.
3. Report of the Committee on the Control of Infectious Diseases: *Amer. Acad. of Ped.* 18th Edition: 73–77, 1977.
4. Nightingale, E.O.: Recommendations for a National Policy on Poliomyelitis Vaccination. *New Eng. J. Med.* 297: 249–253, 1977.
5. Morbidity and Mortality Weekly Report: Recommendation of ACIP Simultaneous Administration of Certain Live Virus Vaccines. *Vol. 21, No. 47:*403 (Nov. 25) 1972.
6. Feigin, R.D. et. al.: Vaccine-Related Paralytic Poliomyelitis in an Immunodeficient Child. *The Journal of Pediatrics 79(4)* 642–647, 1971.
7. Riker, J.B. et. al.: Vaccine-Associated Poliomyelitis in a Child With Thymic Abnormality. *Pediatrics 48(6)* 923-929, 1971.
8. Henderson, D.A. et al.: Paralytic Disease Associated with Oral Polio Vaccines. *JAMA 190(1):*41–48 (Oct. 5) 1964.
9. Morse, L.J. et. al.: Vaccine-Acquired Paralytic Poliomyelitis in an Unvaccinated Mother. *JAMA 197:*1034–1035 (Sept. 19) 1966.
10. Swanson, P.D. et. al.: Poliomyelitis Associated with Type 2 Virus. *JAMA 201(10)* 771–773 (Sept. 4) 1967.
11. Balduzzi, P. et al.: Paralytic Poliomyelitis in a Contact of a Vaccinated Child. *New Eng. J. Med. 276(14)* 796–797, 1967.
12. Center for Disease Control: Neurotropic Diseases Surveillance Annual Poliomyelitis Summary 1971 (March 1973).
13. Evidence on the Safety and Efficacy of Live Poliomyelitis Vaccines Currently in Use, with Special Reference to Type 3 Poliovirus, *Memoranda, Bull. W.H.O. 40:*925–945, 1969.
14. Center for Disease Control: Brochures on Benefits and Risks of Vaccines. May 7, 1976.
15. Welsh, J.K. et. al.: Anti-infective Properties of Breast Milk. *The Journal of Pediatrics 94(1) 1–9, 1979.*
16. Krugman, R.D. et. al: Antibody Persistance After Primary Immunization With Trivalent Oral Poliovirus Vaccine. *Pediatrics 60(1)* 80–82, 1977.

PATHIBAMATE®-200 ℞

tridihexethyl chloride-meprobamate

PATHIBAMATE®-400 ℞

tridihexethyl chloride-meprobamate
Tablets

Description: PATHILON® *tridihexethyl chloride* is a synthetic quaternary ammonium compound. Meprobamate is 2-methyl-2-propyltrimethylene dicarbamate.

Actions: *PATHIBAMATE tridihexethyl chloride-meprobamate* combines tridihexethyl chloride, an anticholinergic agent with meprobamate, a tranquilizing agent.

Tridihexethyl chloride

Tridihexethyl chloride possesses antimuscarinic actions. Gastrointestinal actions include

Continued on next page

The information on each product appearing here is based on labelling effective in August, 1982 and is either the entire official brochure or an accurate condensation therefrom. Offical brochures are enclosed in product packages. Information concerning all Lederle products may be obtained from the Professional Services Department, Lederle Laboratories, Pearl River, New York, 10965.

Lederle—Cont.

reduction in both gastric secretion and gastrointestinal motility.

Meprobamate

Meprobamate is a carbamate derivative which has been shown in animal studies to have effects at multiple sites in the central nervous system, including the thalamus and limbic system.

INDICATIONS

Based on a review of this drug by the National Academy of Sciences-National Research Council and/or other information, FDA has classified the indications as follows:

Possibly Effective: as adjunctive therapy in peptic ulcer and in the irritable bowel syndrome (irritable colon, spastic colon, mucous colitis, and functional gastrointestinal disorders), especially when accompanied by anxiety or tension. It should be used as an adjunct to other appropriate measures such as proper diet and antacids.

Contraindications:

Tridihexethyl chloride

Allergic or idiosyncratic reactions to tridihexethyl chloride or related compounds; glaucoma; obstructive uropathy (e.g., bladder neck obstruction due to prostatic hypertrophy); obstructive disease of the gastrointestinal tract (as in achalasia, paralytic ileus, pyloroduodenal stenosis, etc.); intestinal atony of the elderly or debilitated patient; unstable cardiovascular status in acute hemorrhage; severe ulcerative colitis; toxic megacolon complicating ulcerative colitis; myasthenia gravis.

Meprobamate

Acute intermittent porphyria as well as allergic or idiosyncratic reactions to meprobamate or related compounds such as carisoprodol, mebutamate, tybamate, or carbromal.

Warnings:

Tridihexethyl chloride

In the presence of a high environment temperature, heat prostration can occur with drug use (fever and heat stroke due to decreased sweating).

Diarrhea may be an early symptom of incomplete intestinal obstruction, especially in patients with ileostomy or colostomy. In this instance treatment with this drug would be inappropriate and possibly harmful.

This drug may produce drowsiness or blurred vision. In this event, the patient should be warned not to engage in activities requiring mental alertness such as operating a motor vehicle or other machinery or perform hazardous work while taking this drug.

Meprobamate

Drug Dependence—Physical dependence, psychological dependence, and abuse have occurred. When chronic intoxication from prolonged use occurs, it usually involves ingestion of greater than recommended doses and is manifested by ataxia, slurred speech, and vertigo. Therefore, careful supervision of dose and amounts prescribed is advised, as well as avoidance of prolonged administration, especially for alcoholics and other patients with a known propensity for taking excessive quantities of drugs. Sudden withdrawal of the drug after prolonged and excessive use may precipitate recurrence of pre-existing symptoms, such as anxiety, anorexia, or insomnia, or withdrawal reactions, such as vomiting, ataxia, tremors, muscle twitching, confusional states, hallucinosis, and, rarely, convulsive seizures. Such seizures are more likely to occur in persons with central nervous system damage or pre-existent or latent convulsive disorders. Onset of withdrawal symptoms occurs usually within 12 to 48 hours after discontinuation of meprobamate; symptoms usually cease within the next 12 to 48 hours.

When excessive dosage has continued for weeks or months, dosage should be reduced gradually over a period of one or two weeks rather than abruptly stopped. Alternatively, a short-acting barbiturate may be substituted, then gradually withdrawn.

Potentially Hazardous Tasks—Patients should be warned that this drug may impair the mental and/or physical abilities required for the performance of potentially hazardous tasks such as driving a motor vehicle or operating machinery.

Additive Effects—Since the effects of meprobamate and alcohol or meprobamate and other CNS depressants or psychotropic drugs may be additive, appropriate caution should be exercised with patients who take more than one of these agents simultaneously.

***Usage in Pregnancy and Lactation*—An increased risk of congenital malformations associated with the use of minor tranquilizers (meprobamate, chlordiazepoxide, and diazepam) during the first trimester of pregnancy has been suggested in several studies. Because use of these drugs is rarely a matter of urgency, their use during this period should also always be avoided. The possibility that a woman of childbearing potential may be pregnant at the time of institution of therapy should be considered. Patients should be advised that if they become pregnant during therapy or intend to become pregnant, they should communicate with their physicians about the desirability of discontinuing the drug.**

Meprobamate passes the placental barrier. It is present both in umbilical cord blood at or near maternal plasma levels and in breast milk of lactating mothers at concentrations two to four times that of maternal plasma. When use of meprobamate is contemplated in breast-feeding patients, the drug's higher concentrations in breast milk as compared to maternal plasma levels should be considered.

Precautions:

Tridihexethyl chloride

Use with caution in patients with:

- Autonomic neuropathy.
- Hepatic or renal disease.
- Early evidence of ileus as in peritonitis.
- Ulcerative colitis-large doses may suppress intestinal motility to the point of producing a paralytic ileus and the use of this drug may precipitate or aggravate the serious complication of toxic megacolon.
- Hyperthyroidism, coronary heart disease, congestive heart failure, cardiac arrhythmias, hypertension and non-obstructing prostatic hypertrophy.
- Hiatal hernia associated with reflux esophagitis since anticholinergic drugs may aggravate this condition.
- It should be noted that the use of anticholinergic drugs in the treatment of gastric ulcer may produce a delay in gastric emptying time and may complicate such therapy (antral stasis).
- Do not rely on the use of the drug in the presence of complication of biliary tract disease.
- Investigate any tachycardia before giving anticholinergic (atropine-like) drugs since they may increase the heart rate.
- With overdosage, a curare-like action may occur.

Meprobamate

The lowest effective dose should be administered, particularly to elderly and/or debilitated patients, in order to preclude oversedation.

The possibility of suicide attempts should be considered and the least amount of drug feasible should be dispensed at any one time.

Meprobamate is metabolized in the liver and excreted by the kidney; to avoid its excess accumulation, caution should be exercised in administration to patients with compromised liver or kidney function.

Meprobamate occasionally may precipitate seizures in epileptic patients.

Adverse Reactions: In evaluating adverse reactions to this combination, consider the possibility of adverse reactions that can occur with either component, as listed below:

Tridihexethyl chloride

Adverse reactions may be physiologic or toxic, depending upon the individual patient's response, and may include xerostomia; urinary hesitancy and retention; tachycardia; palpitations; blurred vision; mydriasis; cycloplegia; increased ocular tension; loss of taste; headaches; nervousness; drowsiness; weakness; dizziness; insomnia; nausea; vomiting; impotence; suppression of lactation; constipation; bloated feeling; severe allergic reaction or drug idiosyncrasies including anaphylaxis; urticaria and other dermal manifestations; decreased sweating; some degree of mental confusion and/or excitement especially in elderly persons.

Meprobamate

Central Nervous System—Drowsiness, ataxia, dizziness, slurred speech, headache, vertigo, weakness, paresthesias, impairment of visual accommodation, euphoria, overstimulation, paradoxical excitement, fast EEG activity.

Gastrointestinal—Nausea, vomiting, diarrhea.

Cardiovascular—Palpitations, tachycardia, various forms of arrhythmia, transient ECG changes, syncope; also, hypotensive crises (including one fatal case).

Allergic or Idiosyncratic—Allergic or idiosyncratic reactions are usually seen within the period of the first to fourth dose in patients having had no previous contact with the drug. Milder reactions are characterized by an itchy, urticarial, or erythematous maculopapular rash which may be generalized or confined to the groin. Other reactions have included leukopenia, acute nonthrombocytopenic purpura, petechiae, ecchymoses, eosinophilia, peripheral edema, adenopathy, fever, fixed drug eruption with cross reaction to carisoprodol, and cross sensitivity between meprobamate/-mebutamate and meprobamate/carbromal.

More severe hypersensitivity reactions, rarely reported, include hyperpyrexia, chills, angioneurotic edema, bronchospasm, oliguria, and anuria. Also, anaphylaxis, erythema multiforme, exfoliative dermatitis, stomatitis, proctitis, Stevens-Johnson syndrome, and bullous dermatitis, including one fatal case of the latter following administration of meprobamate in combination with prednisolone.

In case of allergic or idiosyncratic reactions to meprobamate, discontinue the drug and initiate appropriate symptomatic therapy, which may include epinephrine, antihistamines, and in severe cases, corticosteroids. In evaluating possible allergic reactions, also consider allergy to excipients (information on excipients is available to physicians on request).

Hematologic (See also *Allergic or Idiosyncratic.*) —Agranulocytosis and aplastic anemia have been reported, although no causal relationship has been established. These cases rarely were fatal. Rare cases of thrombocytopenic purpura have been reported.

Other—Exacerbation of porphyric symptoms.

Dosage and Administration: The usual adult dose of PATHIBAMATE *tridihexethyl chloride-meprobamate*-400 (meprobamate 400 mg. + tridihexethyl chloride 25 mg.) is one tablet three times a day at mealtimes, and two tablets at bedtime. If a greater anticholinergic effect is desired, the usual adult dose is two PATHIBAMATE *tridihexethyl chloride-meprobamate*-200 (meprobamate 200 mg. + tridihexethyl chloride 25 mg.) tablets three times a day at mealtimes, and two tablets at bedtime. Doses of meprobamate above 2400 mg. daily are not recommended.

Not for use in children under age 12.

Overdosage: Overdosage information on this combination is lacking. However, consider the possibility of signs and symptoms that can occur with either component, as listed below:

Tridihexethyl chloride

Acute overdosage of anticholinergic agents can produce dry mouth, difficulty in swallowing, marked thirst; blurred vision, photophobia; flushed, hot, dry skin; rash; hyperthermia; palpitations, tachycardia with weak pulse, elevated blood pressure; urinary urgency with difficulty in micturition; abdominal distention; restlessness, confusion, delirium and other signs suggestive of an acute organic psychosis. Treatment should include removal of remaining drug from stomach after administration of Universal Antidote, and supportive and symptomatic therapy as indicated. Universal Antidote is a mixture of 2 parts activated charcoal, 1 part magnesium oxide, and 1 part tannic acid, given as ½ ounce in a half glass of warm water.

Meprobamate

Suicidal attempts with meprobamate have resulted in drowsiness, lethargy, stupor, ataxia, coma, shock, vasomotor and respiratory collapse. Some suicidal attempts have been fatal.

The following data on meprobamate tablets have been reported in the literature and from other sources. These data are not expected to correlate with each case (considering factors such as individual susceptibility and length of time from ingestion to treatment), but represent the *usual ranges* reported.

Acute simple overdose (meprobamate alone): Death has been reported with ingestion of as little as 12 Grams meprobamate and survival with as much as 40 Grams.

Blood Levels:

0.5-2.0 mg.% represents the usual blood level range of meprobamate after therapeutic doses. The level may occasionally be as high as 3.0 mg.%.

3-10 mg.% usually corresponds to findings of mild to moderate symptoms of overdosage, such as stupor or light coma.

10-20 mg.% usually corresponds to deeper coma, requiring more intensive treatment. Some fatalities occur.

At levels greater than 20 mg.%, more fatalities than survivals can be expected.

Acute combined overdose (meprobamate with alcohol or other CNS depressants or psychotropic drugs): Since effects can be additive, a history of ingestion of a low dose of meprobamate plus any of these compounds (or of a relatively low blood or tissue level) cannot be used as a prognostic indicator.

In cases where excessive doses have been taken, sleep ensues rapidly; and blood pressure, pulse, and respiratory rates are reduced to basal levels. Any drug remaining in the stomach should be removed and symptomatic therapy given. Should respiration or blood pressure become compromised, respiratory assistance, central nervous system stimulants, and pressor agents should be administered cautiously as indicated. Meprobamate is metabolized in the liver and excreted by the kidney. Diuresis, osmotic (mannitol) diuresis, peritoneal dialysis, and hemodialysis have been used successfully. Careful monitoring of urinary output is necessary and caution should be taken to avoid overhydration. Relapse and death, after initial recovery, have been attributed to incomplete gastric emptying and delayed absorption. Meprobamate can be measured in biological fluids by two methods: colorimetric (Hoffman, A.J. and Ludwig, B.J.: *J Amer Pharm Assn 48:*740,1959) and gas chromatographic (Douglas, J.F. et al: *Anal Chem 39:*956, 1967).

How Supplied: PATHIBAMATE *tridihexethyl chloride-meprobamate* is available in two formulations:

PATHIBAMATE-400: Yellow embossed Lederle P2

Each tablet contains:
meprobamate .... 400 mg.
tridihexethyl chloride........................ 25 mg.

Bottles of 100 and 1000; drum of 5000.

PATHIBAMATE-200: Yellow, coated tablets. Printed LL above P1

Each tablet contains:
meprobamate .... 200 mg.
tridihexethyl chloride........................ 25 mg.

Bottles of 100 and 1000.

A.H.F.S. 12:08

[*Shown in Product Identification Section*]

PATHILON® ℞
tridihexethyl chloride
Products

Description: PATHILON *tridihexethyl chloride* is a synthetic anticholinergic quaternary ammonium compound.

Phenobarbital is 5-Ethyl-5-phenylbarbituric acid.

The following dosage forms are available:
Tablets 25 mg. Tridihexethyl Chloride
SEQUELS Sustained Release Capsules 75 mg. Tridihexethyl Chloride
Tablets 25 mg. Tridihexethyl Chloride with 15 mg. Phenobarbital

Actions: PATHILON relieves pain by reducing spasm of the gastrointestinal tract. Phenobarbital is a hypnotic acid sedative drug with anticonvulsive properties. WARNING: May be habit forming.

INDICATIONS

Based on a review of these products by the National Academy of Sciences-National Research Council and/or other information, FDA has classified the indications as follows:

Tablets—Effective as adjunctive therapy in the treatment of peptic ulcer. Probably effective as adjunctive therapy in the irritable bowel syndrome (irritable colon, spastic colon, mucous colitis, acute enterocolitis, and functional gastrointestinal disorders).

SEQUELS—Probably effective as adjunctive therapy in the treatment of peptic ulcer. May also be useful in the irritable bowel syndrome (see above) and in neurogenic bowel disturbances (including the splenic flexure syndrome and neurogenic colon).

TABLETS with phenobarbital—Possibly effective for the indications for SEQUELS (above).

To be effective the dosage must be titrated to the individual patient's needs.

Contraindications: Glaucoma; obstructive uropathy (for example, bladder neck obstruction due to prostatic hypertrophy); obstructive disease of the gastrointestinal tract (as in achalasia, paralytic ileus, pyloroduodenal stenosis, etc.); intestinal atony of the elderly or debilitated patient; unstable cardiovascular status in acute hemorrhage; severe ulcerative colitis; toxic megacolon complicating ulcerative colitis; myasthenia gravis.

Phenobarbital is contraindicated in acute intermittent porphyria. A sensitivity to phenobarbital contraindicates the use of PATHILON *tridihexethyl chloride* with Phenobarbital Tablets and in those patients in whom phenobarbital produces restlessness and/or excitement.

Warnings: USE IN PREGNANCY—The use of any drug in pregnancy, lactation, or in women of child-bearing potential, requires that the potential benefit of the drug be weighed against its possible hazards to the mother and child. As with all anticholinergic drugs, an inhibiting effect on lactation may occur.

In the presence of a high environmental temperature, heat prostration can occur with drug use (fever and heat stroke due to decreased sweating). Diarrhea may be an early symptom of incomplete intestinal obstruction, especially in patients with ileostomy or colostomy. In this instance treatment with this drug would be inappropriate and possibly harmful.

PATHILON *tridihexethyl chloride* may produce drowsiness or blurred vision. In this event, the patient should be warned not to engage in activities requiring mental alertness such as operating a motor vehicle or other machinery or perform hazardous work while taking this drug.

Phenobarbital in patients taking anticoagulants may decrease the effect of the anticoagulant and thus require larger doses of the anticoagulant for optimal effect. When the phenobarbital is discontinued, the dose of the anticoagulant may have to be decreased. Barbiturates may thus decrease the action of anticoagulant drugs.

Phenobarbital may be habit forming and should not be administered to individuals known to be addiction prone or to those with a history of physical and/or psychological dependence upon habit forming drugs.

Since barbiturates are metabolized in the liver, use with initial small doses and caution in patients with hepatic dysfunction.

Precautions: Use with caution in patients with:
Autonomic neuropathy.
Hepatic or renal disease.
Early evidence of ileus as in peritonitis.
Ulcerative colitis—large doses may suppress intestinal motility to the point of producing a paralytic ileus and the use of this drug may precipitate or aggravate the serious complication of toxic megacolon.
Hyperthyroidism, coronary heart disease, congestive heart failure, cardiac arrhythmias, hypertension and non-obstructing prostatic hypertrophy.
Hiatal hernia associated with reflux esophagitis since anticholinergic drugs may aggravate this condition.

It should be noted that the use of anticholinergic drugs in the treatment of gastric ulcer may produce a delay in gastric emptying time and may complicate such therapy (antral stasis).

Do not rely on the use of the drug in the presence of complication of biliary tract disease.

Investigate any tachycardia before giving anticholinergic (atropine-like) drugs since they may increase the heart rate.

With overdosage, a curare-like action may occur.

Adverse Reactions: Anticholinergics produce certain effects which may be physiologic or toxic depending upon the individual patient's response. The physician must delineate these. Adverse reactions may include xerostomia; urinary hesitancy and retention; blurred vision and tachycardia; palpitations; mydriasis; dilatation of the pupil; cycloplegia; increased ocular tension; loss of taste; headaches; nervousness; drowsiness; weakness; dizziness; insomnia; nausea; vomiting; impotence; suppression of lactation; constipation; bloated feeling; severe allergic reaction or drug idiosyncrasies including anaphylaxis; urticaria and other

Continued on next page

The information on each product appearing here is based on labelling effective in August, 1982 and is either the entire official brochure or an accurate condensation therefrom. Offical brochures are enclosed in product packages. Information concerning all Lederle products may be obtained from the Professional Services Department, Lederle Laboratories, Pearl River, New York, 10965.

Lederle—Cont.

dermal manifestation; some degree of mental confusion and/or excitement especially in elderly persons.
Decreased sweating is another adverse reaction that may occur. It should be noted that adrenergic innervation of the eccrine sweat glands on the palms and soles make complete control of sweating impossible. An end point of complete anhidrosis cannot occur because large doses of drug would be required, and this would produce severe side effects from parasympathetic paralysis.
Phenobarbital may produce excitement in some patients rather than a sedative effect. An occasional patient may experience musculoskeletal pain. Some patients may acquire a sensitivity to barbiturates and experience allergic phenomena and/or dermatologic response.
In patients habituated to barbiturates, abrupt withdrawal may produce delirium or convulsions.
Dosage and Administration: For effective therapeutic results, in particular with anticholinergic drugs, it is absolutely necessary to titrate dosage against the patient's individual needs and response.
Tablets:
The average oral adult dose is 25 to 50 mg. of PATHILON *tridihexethyl chloride* (with or without 15 to 30 mg. of Phenobarbital) 3 to 4 times per day. The usual bedtime dose has been 50 mg. A few patients are well controlled on as little as 10 mg. 3 times per day, while some require as much as 75 mg. 4 times per day. The suggested initial dose is 25 mg. 3 times per day before meals and 50 mg. at bedtime.
SEQUELS:
PATHILON *tridihexethyl chloride* is available in a sustained release form which allows less frequent dosage administration with comparable clinical effect obtained by the usual dosage form. SEQUELS Sustained Release Capsules are prepared by a unique process whereby the basic drug is coated with an inert waxy material in a controlled manner. It is possible, therefore, to obtain 24-hour drug effects, including the anticholinergic activity, during the entire normal sleeping period. The average dosage is one 75 mg. capsule every 12 hours; however, if more anticholinergic effect is desired, the SEQUELS may be given as frequently as 1 capsule every 6 hours depending on tolerance.
Overdosage:
Tridihexethyl chloride:
Acute overdosage of anticholinergic agents can produce dry mouth, difficulty swallowing, marked thirst; blurred vision, photophobia; flushed, hot, dry skin; rash; hyperthermia; palpitations, tachycardia with weak pulse, elevated blood pressure; urinary urgency with difficulty in micturition; abdominal distention; restlessness, confusion, delirium and other signs suggestive of an acute organic psychosis. Treatment should include removal of remaining drug from stomach after administration of Universal Antidote, and supportive and symptomatic therapy as indicated. Universal Antidote is a mixture of 2 parts activated charcoal, 1 part magnesium oxide, and 1 part tannic acid, given as ½ ounce in a half glass of warm water.
Phenobarbital:
Early symptoms are sleepiness, mental confusion, and unsteadiness. These are followed by coma (which may last as long as 7 days), slow, shallow respiration, flaccid muscles and absent deep reflexes. Death occurs most often from pulmonary involvement. Shock should be treated with appropriate measures. Absorption of ingested drug should be delayed by giving tap water, milk, or "Universal Antidote", and then removing by thorough gastric lavage or emesis followed by catharsis. The probability of removing a significant amount of drug is good if treatment is started within two hours after ingestion. In comatose patients, care must be taken to prevent aspiration during gastric lavage and emesis.
If necessary to maintain adequate airway, mucous secretions should be removed from the trachea by suction with a soft rubber catheter, or an oropharyngeal airway may be used. If laryngeal stridor or laryngeal edema occurs, a laryngeal airway or tracheotomy may be necessary. It is important to maintain adequate oxygen intake and carbon dioxide removal. If respiration is depressed, moistened 40 to 60% oxygen may be administered. Mechanical assistance to respiration may be needed.
Experimental data have indicated that alkalinization reduces the penetration of phenobarbital into cells. Large quantities of hypertonic $NaHCO_3$ intravenously, usually in concentrations of 14% have produced satisfactory results and the average duration of the coma has been substantially reduced. Hemodialysis has been successfully employed in severe barbiturate intoxication.
How Suppled: *SEQUELS* (75 mg., two-tone pink)—printed Lederle and P3 bottles of 30; *Tablets* (25 mg., coated pink)—printed LL and P4 bottles of 100 and 1,000; *Tablets,* 25 mg. with phenobarbital, 15 mg. (coated blue)—printed LL and P6 bottles of 100 and 1,000.
A.H.F.S. 12:08
[*Tablets Shown in Product Identification Section*]

PERIHEMIN® ℞
hematinic
Capsules

Description: PERIHEMIN *hematinic* Capsules for children over 12 and adults.
Each capsule contains: Vitamin B_{12} (as Cyanocobalamin U.S.P.) 5 mcg.; Intrinsic Factor Concentrate 25 mg.; Ferrous Fumarate 168 mg., (Elemental Iron 55 mg.); Folic Acid 0.33 mg.; Ascorbic Acid (C) 50 mg.
Actions: PERIHEMIN *Lederle* is a general hematinic for the oral treatment of the common anemias. They contain the common substances used in the prevention and treatment of anemic conditions produced or aggravated by insufficient food intake.
Indications: PERIHEMIN is primarily indicated in the hypochromic, microcytic anemias due to insufficient iron intake or absorption. It is also useful in the treatment of macrocytic hyperchromic anemias where an increased intake of oral B_{12} or folic acid is desirable.
Warnings: Folic Acid alone is improper therapy in the treatment of pernicious anemia and other megaloblastic anemias where vitamin B_{12} is deficient.
Precautions: Some patients affected with pernicious anemia may not respond to orally administered Vitamin B_{12} with intrinsic factor concentrate and there is no known way to predict which patients will respond or which patients may cease to respond. Periodic examinations and laboratory studies of pernicious anemia patients are essential and recommended.
Folic acid especially in doses above 1.0 mg. daily may obscure pernicious anemia, in that hematologic remission may occur while neurological manifestations remain progressive.
Overdosage or accidental overingestion of iron-containing compounds may lead to gastrointestinal hemorrhage in children. If symptoms of intolerance develop, the drug should be temporarily or permanently discontinued.
PERIHEMIN *hematinic* preparations should not be relied on to correct the serious folic acid deficiency characterizing sprue or the malabsorption syndromes. In these conditions therapeutic amounts of folic acid should be administered.
Adverse Reactions: Allergic sensitization has been reported following both oral and parenteral administration of Folic Acid.
Dosage: PERIHEMIN Capsules for children over 12 and adults.
1 capsule 3 times daily with or after meals.
How Supplied: Capsules—soft shell red printed P7—Bottles of 100.

PERITINIC®
hematinic with vitamins and fecal softener
Tablets

Each tablet contains:

Elemental Iron .... (as Ferrous Fumarate)	100 mg.	
Docusate Sodium U.S.P. (DSS) (to counteract the constipating effect of iron)	100 mg.	
Vitamin B_1 .... (as Thiamine Mononitrate)	7.5 mg.	(7½ MDR)
Vitamin B_2 .... (Riboflavin)	7.5 mg.	(6¼ MDR)
Vitamin B_6 .... (Pyridoxine Hydrochloride)	7.5 mg.	
Vitamin B_{12} .... (Cyanocobalamin)	50 mcg.	
Vitamine C .... (Ascorbic Acid)	200 mg.	(6⅔ MDR)
Niacinamide	30 mg.	(3 MDR)
Folic Acid	0.05 mg.	
Pantothenic Acid .... (as D-Pantothenyl Alcohol)	15 mg.	

MDR—Adult Minimum Daily Requirement
Action and Uses: In the prevention of nutritional anemias, certain vitamin deficiencies, and iron-deficiency anemias.
Administration and Dosage:
Adults: 1 or 2 tablets daily.
How Supplied: Tablets (maroon capsule-shaped, film coated) embossed LL and P8 bottles of 60.

PIPRACIL™ ℞
sterile piperacillin sodium
For Intravenous and Intramuscular Use

Description: PIPRACIL™ sterile piperacillin sodium is a semisynthetic broad spectrum penicillin for parenteral use derived from *d*(-) α-aminobenzylpenicillin. The chemical name of piperacillin sodium is sodium [2*S*-[2α, 5α, 6β(*S**)]]-6-[[[[(4-ethyl-2, 3-dioxo-1-piperazinyl) carbonyl] amino] phenylacetyl] amino]-3, 3-dimethyl-7- oxo - 4 -thia-1-azabicyclo[3.2.0] heptane-2-carboxylate.
PIPRACIL is a white to off-white hygroscopic cryodesiccated crystalline powder which is readily soluble in water and gives a colorless to pale-yellow solution. The pH of the aqueous solution is 5.5 to 7.5. One gram contains 1.85 mEq (45.5 mg) of sodium (Na+).
Clinical Pharmacology:
Intravenous Administration. In healthy adult volunteers, mean serum levels immediately after a 2 to 3 minute intravenous injection of 2, 4 or 6 grams were 305, 412, and 775 mcg/ml. Serum levels lack dose proportionality.
[See table on next page].
A 30 minute infusion of 6 grams every 6 hours gave, on the fourth day, a mean peak serum concentration of 420 mcg/ml.
Intramuscular Administration. PIPRACIL™ is rapidly absorbed after intramuscular injection. In healthy volunteers, the mean peak serum concentration occurs approximately 30 minutes after a single dose of 2 g and is about 36 mcg/ml. The oral administration of 1 g probenecid before injection produces an increase in piperacillin peak serum level of about 30%. The area under the curve (AUC) is increased by approximately 60%.
General. PIPRACIL is not absorbed when given orally. Peak serum concentrations are attained approximately 30 minutes after intramuscular injections and immediately after completion of intravenous injection or infusion. The serum half-life in healthy volunteers

PIPERACILLIN SERUM LEVELS IN ADULTS (mcg/ml) after a 2-3 minute IV INJECTION

DOSE	0	10 min	20 min	30 min	1 hr	1.5 hr	2 hr	3 hr	4 hr	6 hr	8 hr
2	**305** (159–615)	**202** (164–225)	**156** (52–165)	**67** (41–88)	**40** (25–57)	**24** (18–31)	**20** (14–24)	**8** (3–11)	**3** (2–4)	**2** (<0.6–3)	—
4	**412** (389–484)	**344** (315–379)	**295** (269–330)	**117** (98–138)	**93** (78–110)	**60** (50–67)	**36** (26–51)	**20** (17–24)	**8** (7–11)	**4** (3.7–4.1)	**0.9** (0.7–1)
6	**775** (695–849)	**609** (530–670)	**563** (492–630)	**325** (292–363)	**208** (180–239)	**138** (115–175)	**90** (71–113)	**38** (29–53)	**33** (25–44)	**8** (3–19)	**3.2** (<2–6)

PIPERACILLIN SERUM LEVELS IN ADULTS (mcg/ml) after a 30 minute IV INFUSION

DOSE	0	5 min	10 min	15 min	30 min	45 min	1 hr	1.5 hr	2 hr	4 hr	6 hr	7.5 hr
4	**244** (155–298)	**215** (169–247)	**186** (140–209)	**177** (142–213)	**141** (122–156)	**146** (110–265)	**105** (85–133)	**72** (53–105)	**53** (36–69)	**15** (6–24)	**4** (1–9)	**2** (0.5–3)
6	**353** (324–371)	**298** (242–339)	**298** (232–331)	**272** (219–314)	**229** (185–249)	**180** (144–209)	**149** (117–171)	**104** (89–113)	**73** (66–94)	**22** (12–39)	**16** (5–49)	—

ranges from 36 minutes to 1 hour and 12 minutes. The mean elimination half-life of PIPRACIL in healthy adult volunteers is 54 minutes following administration of 2 grams and 63 minutes following 6 grams. As with other penicillins, PIPRACIL is eliminated primarily by glomerular filtration and tubular secretion; it is excreted rapidly as unchanged drug in high concentrations in the urine. Approximately 60 to 80% of the administered dose is excreted in the urine in the first 24 hours. Piperacillin urine concentrations, determined by microbioassay, were as high as 14,100 mcg/ml following a 6 g intravenous dose and 8,500 mcg/ml following a 4 g intravenous dose. These urine drug concentrations remained well above 1,000 mcg/ml throughout the dosing interval. The elimination half-life is increased two-fold in mild to moderate renal impairment and five- to six-fold in severe impairment.

PIPRACIL™ binding to human serum proteins is 16%. The drug is widely distributed in human tissues and body fluids, including bone, prostate, and heart and reaches high concentrations in bile. After a 4 gram bolus, maximum biliary concentrations averaged 3205 mcg/ml. It penetrates into the cerebral spinal fluid in the presence of inflamed meninges. Because PIPRACIL is excreted by the biliary route, as well as by the renal route, it can be used safely in appropriate dosage (see DOSAGE AND ADMINISTRATION) in patients with severely restricted kidney function, and can be used effectively in treatment of hepatobiliary infections.

Microbiology:

PIPRACIL is an antibiotic which exerts its bactericidal activity by inhiting both septum and cell wall synthesis. It is active against a variety of gram-positive and gram-negative aerobic and anaerobic bacteria. *In vitro,* piperacillin is active against most strains of clinical isolates of the following micro-organisms:

Aerobic and facultatively anaerobic organisms

Gram-negative bacteria

Escherichia coli
Proteus mirabilis
Proteus vulgaris
Morganella morganii (formerly *Proteus morganii)*
Providencia rettgerii (formerly *Proteus rettgerii)*
Serratia species including *S. marcescens* and *S. liquefaciens*
Klebsiella pneumoniae
Klebsiella species
Enterobacter species including *E. aerogenes* and *E. cloacae*
Citrobacter species including *C. freundii* and *C. diversus*
Salmonella species*
Shigella species*
Pseudomonas aeruginosa
Pseudomonas species including *P. cepacia,* *P. maltophilia** and *P fluorescens*
Acinetobacter species (formerly *Mima-Herellea)*
Haemophilus influenzae (non-β-lactamase-producing strains)
Neisseria gonorrhoeae
*Neisseria meningitidis**
Moraxella species*
Yersinia species* (formerly *Pasteurella)*

Gram-positive bacteria

Group D streptococci including
Enterococci *(Streptococcus faecalis, S. faecium)*
Non-enterococci*
Beta-hemolytic streptococci including
Streptococcus Group A *(S. pyogenes)*
Streptococcus Group B *(S. agalactiae)*
Streptococcus pneumoniae
Streptococcus viridans
Staphylococcus aureus (non-penicillinase-producing)*
Staphylococcus epidermidis (non-penicillinase-producing)*

Anaerobic bacteria

Actinomyces species*
Bacteroides species including
B. fragilis group *(B. fragilis, B. vulgatus)*
Non-*B. fragilis (B. melaninogenicus)*
*B. asaccharolyticus**
Clostridium species including
C. perfringens and *C. difficile**
Eubacterium species
Fusobacterium species including
F. nucleatum and *F. necrophorum*
Peptococcus species
Peptostreptococcus species
Veillonella species

*Piperacillin has been shown to be active *in vitro* against these organisms; however, clinical efficacy has not yet been established.

In vitro, PIPRACIL™ sterile piperacillin sodium is inactivated by staphylococcal β-lactamases, and β-lactamases produced by gram-negative bacteria. However, it is active against β-lactamase-producing gonococci.

Many strains of gram-negative organisms resistant to certain antibiotics have been found to be susceptible to PIPRACIL.

PIPRACIL has excellent activity against gram-positive organisms, including enterococci *(S. faecalis).* It is active against obligate anaerobes such as *Bacteroides* and also against *Clostridium difficile* (which has been associated with pseudomembranous colitis).

Piperacillin is active against many gram-negative bacteria including *Enterobacteriaceae, Klebsiella, Serratia, Pseudomonas, E coli, Proteus,* and *Citrobacter,* and in addition it is active against anaerobes and enterococci. *In vitro* tests show PIPRACIL to act synergistically with aminoglycoside antibiotics against most isolates of *Pseudomonas aeruginosa.*

Susceptibility Testing:

The use of antibiotic disc susceptibility test methods which measure zone diameter gives an accurate estimation of susceptibility of organisms to PIPRACIL. The following standard procedure** has been recommended for use with discs for testing antimicrobials. Piperacillin 100 mcg discs should be used for the determination of the susceptibility of organisms to piperacillin.

**NCCLS Approved Standard; M2-A2 (Formerly ASM-2) Performance Standards for Antimicrobic Disk Susceptibility Tests, Second Edition, available from the National Committee of Clinical Laboratory Standards.

With this type of procedure, a report of "susceptible" from the laboratory indicates that the infecting organism is likely to respond to therapy. A report of "intermediate susceptibility" suggests that the organism would be susceptible if high dosage is used or if the infection is confined to tissue and fluids (e.g., urine) in which high antibiotic levels are obtained. A report of "resistant" indicates that the infecting organism is not likely to respond to therapy. With the piperacillin disc, a zone of 18 mm or greater indicates susceptibility, zone sizes of 14 mm or less indicate resistance, and zone sizes of 15 to 17 mm indicate intermediate susceptibility.

Haemophilus and *Neisseria* species which give zones of ≥ 29 mm are susceptible; resistant strains give zones of ≤ 28 mm. The above interpretive criteria are based on the use of the standardized procedure. Antibiotic susceptibility testing requires carefully prescribed procedures. Susceptibility tests are biased to a considerable degree when different methods are used.

The standardized procedure requires the use of control organisms. The 100 mcg piperacillin disc should give zone diameters between 24 and 30 mm for *E coli* ATCC No. 25922 and between 25 and 33 mm for *Pseudomonas aeruginosa* ATCC No. 27853.

Dilution methods such as those described in the International Collaborative Study† have been used to determine susceptibility of the following organisms to PIPRACIL.

†Acta Pathal Microbiol Scand (B) Suppl. 217 (1971).

The information on each product appearing here is based on labelling effective in August, 1982 and is either the entire official brochure or an accurate condensation therefrom. Offical brochures are enclosed in product packages. Information concerning all Lederle products may be obtained from the Professional Services Department, Lederle Laboratories, Pearl River, New York, 10965.

Continued on next page

Lederle—Cont.

Enterobacteriaceae, Pseudomonas species and *Acinetobacter* spp. are considered susceptible if the minimal inhibitory concentration (MIC) of piperacillin is no greater than 64 mcg/ml and are considered resistant if the MIC is greater than 128 mcg/ml.

Haemophilus and *Neisseria* species are considered susceptible if the MIC of PIPRACIL is less than or equal to 1 mcg/ml.

When anaerobic organisms are isolated from infection sites, it is recommended that other tests such as the modified Broth-Disk Method* be used to determine the antibiotic susceptibility of these slow-growing organisms.

*Wilkins TD, Thiel T: *Antimicrob Agents Chemother 3*:350–356, March 1973.

Indications and Usage: PIPRACIL is indicated for the treatment of serious infections caused by susceptible strains of the designated organisms in the conditions as listed below.

Intra-abdominal Infections including hepatobiliary and surgical infections caused by *Escherichia coli, Pseudomonas aeruginosa,* enterococci, *Clostridium* spp., anaerobic cocci, and *Bacteroides* spp., including *B. fragilis.*

Urinary Tract Infections caused by *E coli, Klebsiella* spp., *P. aeruginosa, Proteus* spp. including *P. mirabilis* and enterococci.

Gynecologic Infections including endometritis, pelvic inflammatory disease, pelvic cellutitis caused by *Bacteroides* spp. including *B. fragilis,* anaerobic cocci, Neisseria gonorrhoeae, and enterococci *(Streptococcus faecalis).*

Septicemia, including bacteremia caused by *E coli, Klebsiella* spp., *Enterobacter* spp., *Serratia* spp., *P. mirabilis, S. pneumoniae,* enterococci, *Pseudomonas aeruginosa, Bacteroides* spp., and anaerobic cocci.

Lower Respiratory Tract Infections caused by *Escherichia coli, Klebsiella* spp., *Enterobacter* spp., *Pseudomonas aeruginosa, Serratia* spp., *Haemophilus influenzae, Bacteroides* species, and anaerobic cocci. Although improvement has been noted in patients with cystic fibrosis, lasting bacterial eradication may not necessarily be achieved.

Skin and Skin Structure Infections caused by *E coli, Klebsiella* spp., *Serratia* spp., *Acinetobacter* spp., *Enterobacter* spp., *Pseudomonas aeruginosa,* indolepositive *Proteus* spp., *Proteus mirabilis, Bacteroides* spp., including *B. fragilis,* anaerobic cocci, and enterococci.

Bone and Joint Infections caused by P. aeruginosa, enterococci, *Bacteroides* spp., and anaerobic cocci.

Gonococcal Infections PIPRACIL has been effective in the treatment of uncomplicated gonococcal urethritis.

PIPRACIL™ sterile piperacillin sodium has also been shown to be clinically effective for the treatment of infections at various sites caused by *Streptococcus* species including Group A β-hemolytic *Streptococcus* and *Streptococcus pneumoniae;* however, infections caused by these organisms are ordinarily treated with more narrow spectrum penicillins. Because of its broad spectrum of bactericidal activity against gram-positive and gram-negative aerobic and anaerobic bacteria, PIPRACIL is particularly useful for the treatment of mixed infections and presumptive therapy prior to the identification of the causative organisms.

Also, PIPRACIL may be administered as single drug therapy in some situations where normally two antibiotics might be employed.

PIPRACIL has been successfully used with aminoglycosides, especially in patients with impaired host defenses. Both drugs should be used in full therapeutic doses.

Appropriate cultures should be made for susceptibility testing before initiating therapy and therapy adjusted, if appropriate, once the results are known.

Contraindications: A history of allergic reactions to any of the penicillins and/or cephalosporins.

Warnings: Serious and occasionally fatal hypersensitivity (anaphylactic) reactions have been reported in patients receiving therapy with penicillins. These reactions are more apt to occur in persons with a history of sensitivity to multiple allergens.

There have been reports of patients with a history of penicillin hypersensitivity who have experienced severe hypersensitivity reactions when treated with a cephalosporin. Before initiating therapy with PIPRACIL, careful inquiry should be made concerning previous hypersensitivity reactions to penicillins, cephalosporins, and other allergens. If an allergic reactions occurs during therapy with PIPRACIL, the antibiotic should be discontinued. The usual agents (antihistamines, pressor amines, and corticosteroids) should be readily available. SERIOUS ANAPHYLACTOID REACTIONS REQUIRE IMMEDIATE EMERGENCY TREATMENT WITH EPINEPHRINE. OXYGEN AND INTRAVENOUS CORTICOSTEROIDS AND AIRWAY MANAGEMENT INCLUDING INTUBATION SHOULD ALSO BE ADMINISTERED AS NECESSARY.

Precautions:

General. While PIPRACIL possesses the characteristic low toxicity of the penicillin group of antibiotics, periodic assessment of organ system functions, including renal, hepatic, and hematopoietic, during prolonged therapy is advisable.

Bleeding manifestations have occurred in some patients receiving beta-lactam antibiotics including piperacillin. These reactions have sometimes been associated with abnormalities of coagulation tests such as clotting time, platelet aggregation and prothrombin time and are more likely to occur in patients with renal failure.

If bleeding manifestations occur, the antibiotic should be discontinued and appropriate therapy instituted.

The possibility of the emergence of resistant organisms which might cause superinfections should be kept in mind, particularly during prolonged treatment. If this occurs, appropriate measures should be taken.

As with other penicillins, patients may experience neuromuscular excitability or convulsions if higher than recommended doses are given intravenously.

PIPRACIL™ is a monosodium compound containing 1.85 milliequivalents of Na+ per gram. This should be considered when treating patients requiring restricted salt intake. Periodic electrolyte determinations should be made in patients with low potassium reserves, and the possibility of hypokalemia should be kept in mind with patients who have potentially low potassium reserves and who are receiving cytotoxic therapy or diuretics. Antimicrobials used in high doses for short periods to treat gonorrhea may mask or delay the symptoms of incubating syphilis. Therefore, prior to treatment, patients with gonorrhea should also be evaluated for syphilis. Specimens for darkfield examination should be obtained from patients with any suspected primary lesion, and serologic tests should be performed. In all cases where concomitant syphilis is suspected, monthly serological tests should be made for a minimum of 4 months.

Drug Interactions. The mixing of PIPRACIL™ with an aminoglycoside *in vitro* can result in substantial inactivation of the aminoglycosides.

Pregnancy—Pregnancy Category B. Although reproduction studies in mice and rats performed at doses up to 4 times the human dose have shown no evidence of impaired fertility or harm to the fetus, safety of PIPRACIL use in pregnant women has not been determined by adequate and well-controlled studies. Because animal reproduction studies are not always predictive of human response, this drug should be used during pregnancy only if clearly needed. It has been found to cross the placenta in rats.

Nursing Mothers. Caution should be exercised when PIPRACIL is administered to nursing mothers. It is excreted in low concentrations in milk.

Pediatric Use. Dosages for children under the age of 12 have not been established. The safety of PIPRACIL™ in neonates is not known. In dog neonates dilated renal tubules and peritubular hyalinization occurred following administration of PIPRACIL.

Adverse Effects: PIPRACIL is generally well tolerated. The most common adverse reactions have been local in nature, following intravenous or intramuscular injection. The following adverse reactions may occur.

Local Reactions. In clinical trials thrombophlebitis was noted in 4% of patients. Pain, erythema, and/or induration at the injection site occurred in 2% of patients. Less frequent reactions including ecchymosis, deep vein thrombosis and hematomas have also occurred.

Gastrointestinal. Diarrhea and loose stools were noted in 2% of patients. Other less frequent reactions included vomiting, nausea, increases in liver enzymes (LDH, SGOT, SGPT), hyperbilirubinemia, cholestatic hepatitis, bloody diarrhea.

Hypersensitivity Reactions. Rash was noted in 1% of patients. Other less frequent findings included pruritus, vesicular eruptions, positive Coombs' test.

Renal. Elevations of creatinine or BUN.

Central Nervous System. Headache, dizziness, fatigue.

Hemic and Lymphatic. Reversible leukopenia, neutropenia, thrombocytopenia and/or eosinophilia have been reported. As with other β-lactam antibiotics, reversible leukopenia (neutropenia) is more apt to occur in patients receiving prolonged therapy at high dosages or in association with drugs known to cause this reaction.

Serum Electrolytes. Individuals with liver disease or individuals receiving cytotoxic therapy or diuretics were reported rarely to demonstrate a decrease in serum potassium concentrations with high doses of PIPRACIL.™

Skeletal. Rarely, prolonged muscle relaxation.

Other. Superinfection, including candidiasis. Hemorrhagic manifestations.

Dosage and Administration: PIPRACIL may be administered by the intramuscular route or intravenously. It can be administered in a 3 to 5 minute intravenous injection. The usual dosage of PIPRACIL for serious infections is 3 to 4 grams given every 4 to 6 hours as a 20 to 30 minute infusion. For serious infections, the intravenous route of administration should be used.

PIPRACIL should not be mixed with an aminoglycoside in a syringe or infusion bottle since this can result in inactivation of the aminoglycoside.

The maximum daily dose for adults is usually 24 g/day, although higher doses have been used.

Intramuscular injections should be limited to 2 g per injection site. This route of administration has been used primarily in the treatment of patients with uncomplicated gonorrhea and urinary tract infections.

[See table on next page].

For patients with renal failure and hepatic insufficiency, measurement of serum levels of PIPRACIL™ sterile piperacillin sodium will provide additional guidance for adjusting dosage.

Infants and Children. Dosages in infants and children under 12 years of age have not been established.

The averge duration of PIPRACIL treatment is from 7 to 10 days, except in the treatment of gynecologic infections, in which it is from 3 to 10 days; the duration should be guided by the patient's clinical and bacteriological progress. For most acute infections, treatment should be continued for at least 48 to 72 hours after the patient becomes asymptomatic. Antibiotic therapy for Group A beta-hemolytic streptococcal infections should be maintained for at least 10 days to reduce the risk of rheumatic fever or glomerulonephritis.

When PIPRACIL is given concurrently with aminoglycosides, both drugs should be used in ful therapeutic doses.

Intravenous Administration

Directions. Reconstitute each gram of PIPRACIL with at least 5 ml of a suitable diluent such as Bacteriostatic Water for Injection, Bacteriostatic Sodium Chloride Injection, or diluents listed below. Shake well until dissolved. It may be further diluted to the desired volume.

Intravenous Injection—Following reconstitution in order to help avoid vein irritation, the solution should be administered slowly over a 3- to 5-minute period.

Intermittent Intravenous Infusion—Reconstitute as described above, using a suitable intravenous solution listed below, dilute the total content of the vial or infusion bottle, and then further dilute to the desired volume (at least 50 ml). Administer by infusion over a period of about 30 minutes. During infusion it is desirable to discontinue the primary intravenous solution.

Stability of PIPRACIL™ Following Reconstitution. PIPRACIL is stable in both glass and plastic containers when reconstituted with recommended diluents and diluted with the indicated intravenous solutions and intravenous admixtures.

Extensive stability studies have demonstrated chemical stability (potency, pH, and clarity) through 24 hours at room temperature, up to one week refrigerated, and up to one month frozen. Appropriate consideration of aseptic technique and individual hospital policy, however, may recommend the more conservative label instructions to discard unused portions after storage for 24 hours at room temperature or for 48 hours when refrigerated.

Diluents for IV Reconstitution.

Sterile Water for Injection, USP
†Bacteriostatic Water for Injection, USP
Sodium Chloride Injection, USP
†Bacteriostatic Sodium Chloride Injection, USP
**Lidocaine HCl 0.5-1% (without epinephrine)
**For Intramuscular Use Only
†Either Parabens or Benzyl Alcohol

Intravenous Solutions.

Dextrose 5% in Water.
0.9% Sodium Chloride
Dextrose 5% and 0.9% Sodium Chloride
Lactated Ringer's Injection, USP
Dextran 6% in 0.9% Sodium Chloride

Intravenous Admixtures.

Normal Saline [+ KCl 40 mEq]
5% Dextrose/Water D_5W [+ KCl 40 mEq]
5% Dextrose/Normal Saline D_5NS [+ KCl 40 mEq]
Ringer's Injection, USP [+ KCl 40 mEq]
Lactated Ringer's Injection, USP [+ KCl 40 mEq]

Intramuscular Administration

When indicated by clinical and bacteriological findings, intramuscular administration of 6 to 8 grams daily of PIPRACIL,™ in divided doses, may be utilized for initiation of therapy. In addition, intramuscular administration of the drug may be considered for maintenance therapy after clinical and bacteriologic improvement has been obtained with intravenous piperacillin sodium treatment. Intramuscular administration should not exceed 2 grams per injection at any one site.

The preferred site is the upper outer quadrant of the buttock (i.e., gluteus maximus).

The deltoid area should be used only if well-developed, and then only with caution to avoid radial nerve injury. Intramuscular injections should not be made into the lower or mid-third of the upper arm.

Reconstitution for Intramuscular Use

Directions. Recommended diluents for 2 g, 3 g and 4 g standard vials are listed below.

Each gram of PIPRACIL™ should be reconstituted with a minimum of 2 ml using one of the following diluents:

1. Sterile Water for Injection, USP
2. Bacteriostatic Water for Injection, USP
3. Sodium Chloride Injection, USP
4. Bacteriostatic Sodium Chloride Injection, USP
5. Sterile Lidocaine HCl Injection, USP, 0.5–1.0% for Intramuscular Use Only (without epinephrine). Lidocaine HCl is contraindicated in patients with a known history of hypersensitivity to local anesthetics of the amide type.

DOSAGE RECOMMENDATIONS

Type of Infections	Usual Total Daily Dosage	Frequency of Administration
Serious infections such as septicemia nosocomial pneumonia, intra-abdominal infections, aerobic and anaerobic gynecologic infections, and skin and soft-tissue infections	12–18 g IV (200–300 mg/kg)	Every four to six hours
Complicated urinary tract infections	8–16 g IV (125–200 mg/kg)	Every six to eight hours
Uncomplicated urinary tract infections and most community-acquired pneumonia	6–8 g IM or IV (100–125 mg/kg)	Every six to twelve hours
Uncomplicated gonorrhea infections	2 g IM*	Single dose

*One gram of probenecid given orally ½ hour prior to injection.

Dosage in renal impairment

Creatinine Clearance ml/min	Urinary Tract Infection (uncomplicated)	Urinary Tract Infection (complicated)	Serious Systemic Infection
>40	No dosage adjustment necessary		
20–40	No dosage adjustment necessary	9 g/day (3 g every 8 hr)	12 g/day (4 g every 8 hr)
<20	6 g/day (3 g every 12 hr)	6 g/day (3 g every 12 hr)	8 g/day (4 g every 12 hr)
Patients on Hemodialysis*	*Hemodialysis removes 30–50% of piperacillin in 4 hours; 1 g additional dose should be administered following each dialysis period		6 g/day (2 g every 8 hr)

Dilution Table for IM Use

Volume of Diluent for the Following Vial Size 2g	3g	4g	Volume to be Withdrawn for a 1g Dose
4.0 ml	6.0 ml	7.8 ml	2.5 ml

To expedite reconstitution, the vial contents should be shaken immediately after adding the diluent.

How Supplied: PIPRACIL™ sterile cryodesiccated piperacillin sodium is available in vials containing sterile freeze-dried piperacillin sodium powder equivalent to two, three and four grams of piperacillin. One gram of piperacillin (as a monosodium salt) contains approximately 1.85 mEq (45.5 mg) of sodium.

Product Numbers:

2 gram/vial—NDC 0206-3879-14
2 gram/vial—10 per box—NDC 0206-3879-16
3 gram/vial—NDC 0206-3882-06
3 gram/vial—25 per box—NDC 0206-3882-21
4 gram/vial—NDC 0206-3880-18
4 gram/vial—25 per box—NDC 0206-3880-22
3 gram infusion bottle in box—NDC 0206-3882-68
3 gram infusion bottle—10 per box—NDC 0206-3882-65
4 gram infusion bottle in box—NDC 0206-3880-69
4 gram infusion bottle—10 per box—NDC 0206-3880-66

This product should be stored at controlled room temperature, 15–30°C (59–86°F).

LEDERLE PIPERACILLIN, INC.
Carolina, Puerto Rico 00630

Rev. 4/82

[*Shown in Product Identification Section*]

PNU-IMUNE® ℞
pneumococcal vaccine, polyvalent

Description: PNU-IMUNE is a vaccine consisting of a mixture of purified capsular polysaccharides from 14 pneumococcal types:
[See table on next page].

It is indicated for immunization against infections caused by the 14 most prevalent types of pneumococci responsible for 80 or more percent of serious pneumococcal disease in the United States and the rest of the world.[1–4]

Each of the pneumococcal polysaccharide types is produced separately by Lederle Laboratories to give a high degree of purity. After an individual pneumococcal type is grown, the polysaccharide is separated from the cell and

Continued on next page

The information on each product appearing here is based on labelling effective in August, 1982 and is either the entire official brochure or an accurate condensation therefrom. Offical brochures are enclosed in product packages. Information concerning all Lederle products may be obtained from the Professional Services Department, Lederle Laboratories, Pearl River, New York, 10965.

Lederle—Cont.

purified by a series of steps including ethanol fractionation. The resultant 14 purified polysaccharides are combined in amounts to give 50 micrograms of each type per dose (0.5 ml) in the final vaccine. Thimerosal at a concentration of 0.01% is added as a preservative.

Actions: Pneumococci are the etiologic agents for a significant number of the pneumonias occurring throughout the world. The emergence of strains of pneumococci with increased resistance to one or more of the common antibiotics[4] and recent isolations of pneumococci with multiple-antibiotic resistance[5] emphasize the importance of vaccine prophylaxis against pneumococcal disease.

Based on projections from limited observations[2] in the United States, it has been estimated that 400,000 to 500,000 cases of pneumococcal pneumonia may occur annually. The overall case fatality rate ranges from 5–10%.[2] Populations at high risk are the elderly,[6–7] individuals with immune deficiencies, asplenics and patients with splenic deficiencies including sickle cell anemia and other severe hemoglobinopathies, alcoholics and patients with the following diseases: chronic respiratory illness, the nephrotic syndrome, multiple myeloma, Hodgkin's disease and cirrhosis. Antibiotics have only been partially effective in reducing the mortality of pneumococcal pneumonia. As many as 60 percent of all deaths among patients with pneumococcal bacteremia treated with penicillin or tetracycline occur within five days of onset of the illness.[5] Thus, vaccination offers an effective means for further reducing the mortality and morbidity of this disease. The pneumococcus is also the chief infectious agent in meningitis[8] and otitis media. Other illnesses caused by pneumococci include sinus infection, arthritis and conjunctivitis. The annual incidence of pneumococcal meningitis is approximately 1.5 to 2.5 per 100,000 population. One-half of the cases occur in children in whom the fatality rate is about 40%.[1,7]

The polysaccharide capsules of pneumococci endow these organisms with resistance to the phagocytic action of polymorphonuclear leukocytes and monocytes. The opsonin activity of type-specific antibody facilitates their destruction in the body by complement-mediated activities. The protection induced by the vaccine is of long duration but its extent is not yet known. Elevated antibody levels have been shown to persist for at least 5 years after immunization with other pneumococcal vaccines.[1] Studies with pneumococcal polysaccharide vaccines prepared in the immediate post-World War II era demonstrated persistence of antibody for as long as 5 years.[9] Children under 2 years of age do not respond adequately to some of the important polysaccharide types. Recipients of polyvalent vaccines acquired less nasopharyngeal carriage of pneumococcal types included in the vaccine.[2,10]

Until further information on duration of immunity becomes available, revaccination should not be considered at less than 5-year intervals, since protective antibody levels are believed to persist for substantial periods in most vaccinated persons. Available data suggest that revaccination before 5 years may result in more frequent and severe local reactions at the site of injection, especially in persons who have retained high antibody levels. Long-term surveillance of antibody levels in immunized individuals is continuing.

In recent clinical studies with PNU-IMUNE, at least 90% of all adults showed a 4-fold or greater increase in geometric mean antibody titer for each vaccine capsular type.[12]

Patients over the age of 2 years with anatomical or functional asplenia and otherwise intact lymphoid function responded to PNU-IMUNE *pneumococcal vaccine, polyvalent* and other comparable pneumococcal vaccines with a serological conversion comparable to that observed in healthy individuals of the same age.[13]

Polyvalent pneumococcal vaccines, from other sources, were shown to be effective in preventing pneumococcal disease. Controlled field trials in South Africa involving 12,000 gold miners have shown polyvalent vaccine to be 78.5% effective in preventing type-specific pneumococcal pneumonia and 82.3% effective in preventing pneumococcal bacteremia with the types in the vaccine.[14] In a preliminary study of an octavalent polysaccharide vaccine in a group consisting of 77 patients with sickle cell disease and 19 asplenic persons, there were no pneumococcal infections in the immunized patients within two years of immunization. There were eight cases of pneumococcal infection in 106 unimmunized, age-matched patients with sickle cell disease. Antibody response of the asplenic patients was comparable to normal controls.[15]

In a study carried out by Austrian et al.[14] with pneumococcal vaccines prepared for the National Institutes of Allergy and Infectious Disease, the reduction in pneumonias caused by the capsular types in the vaccines was 79%. Reduction in type-specific pneumococcal bacteremia was 82%.

In a double-blind study of a 14-valent pneumococcal vaccine carried out in Papua New Guinea, pneumococcal infection was less in the vaccinated group by 84%. Mortality from pneumonia was less by 44%.[16]

Indications: PNU-IMMUNE is indicated for immunization against pneumococcal disease caused by those pneumococcal types included in the vaccine.

Use in Selected Individuals as Follows: persons over 2 years of age as follows: (1) who have anatomical asplenia or who have splenic dysfunction due to sickle cell disease or other causes; (2) persons with chronic illnesses in which there is an increased risk of pneumococcal disease, such as diabetes mellitus, functional impairment of cardiorespiratory, hepatic and renal systems; (3) persons 50 years of age or older.

Use in Communities. Persons over 2 years of age as follows: (1) closed groups such as those in residential schools, nursing homes and other institutions; (2) groups epidemiologically at risk in the community when there is a generalized outbreak in the general population due to a single pneumococcal type included in the vaccine; (3) patients at high risk of influenza complications, particularly pneumonia.[10]

Simultaneous administration of pneumococcal polysaccharide vaccine and whole-virus influenza vaccine has been found to give satisfactory antibody response without increasing the incidence of side effects. Although not yet studied, simultaneous administration of the pneumococcal vaccine and split-virus influenza vaccine may also be expected to yield satisfactory results.[11]

Contraindications:

Pregnancy. Safety, immunogenicity and efficacy of the vaccine in pregnancy has not been established, and vaccination is not recommended during pregnancy.

Children below 2 years of age. Children in this age group respond poorly to the current vaccine, and vaccination of children in this age group *should not be undertaken.*

Hypersensitivity. Known hypersensitivity to any component of the vaccine including hypersensitivity to thimerosal. Remedial measures for anaphylactoid reactions, including epinephrine injection (1:1000), must be available for immediate use.

Warnings: *PNU-IMUNE is not an effective agent for prophylaxis against pneumococcal disease caused by types not present in the vaccine.*

The vaccine may not be effective in patients undergoing treatment causing therapeutic suppression of the immune-response system.

Patients who have received extensive chemotherapy and/or splenectomy for the treatment of Hodgkin's Disease have been shown to have an impaired serum antibody response to pneumococcal vaccine.[17]

Precautions: The vaccine should be injected deeply subcutaneously or intramuscularly. Do not inject intravenously.

In the presence of any febrile respiratory illness or other active infection, the vaccine should not be used.

The parenteral administration of any biological product should be surrounded by every known precaution for the prevention and arrest of allergic and other untoward reactions.

When administering this vaccine, a separate heat-sterilized syringe and needle or a new disposable equivalent should be used for each patient to prevent transmission of hepatitis B (homologous serum hepatitis) or other infectious agents.

Patients who have had episodes of pneumococcal pneumonia or other pneumococcal infection in the preceding three years may have high levels of pre-existing pneumococcal antibodies which may result in increased reactions to PNU-IMUNE, mostly local but occasionally systemic. Caution should be exercised if such patients are considered for vaccination with PNU-IMUNE.

Until further information on duration of immunity becomes available, revaccination should not be considered at less than 5-year intervals, since protective antibody levels are believed to persist for substantial periods in most vaccinated persons. Available data suggest that revaccination before 5 years may result in more frequent and severe local reactions at the site of injection, especially in persons who have retained high antibody levels. Long-term surveillance of antibody levels in immunized individuals is continuing. (See DOSAGE AND ADMINISTRATION.)

Adverse Reactions: PNU-IMUNE *pneumococcal vaccine, polyvalent* is associated with a relatively low incidence of adverse reactions as compared with injectable vaccines presently in use. The adverse reactivity observed in clinical studies was not serious and of short duration. In a study of 32 individuals who received PNU-IMUNE, 23 (72%) experienced local reaction characterized by local soreness at the injection site within 3 days after vaccination.

Low grade fever (less than 100° F) occurs occasionally with PNU-IMUNE and is usually confined to the 24-hour period following vaccination.

Although rare, fever over 102° and marked local swelling has been reported with pneumococcal polysaccharide vaccine.

Reactions of greater severity or extent are unusual. Rarely, anaphylactoid reactions have been reported.

Dosage and Administration: Do not inject intravenously. The immunization schedule consists of a single 0.5 ml dose given subcutaneously or intramuscularly.

Until further information on duration of immunity becomes available, revaccination should not be considered at less than 5-year intervals, since protective antibody levels are believed to persist for substantial periods in most vaccinated persons. Available data suggest that revaccination before 5 years may result in more frequent and severe local reac-

Nomenclature	Pneumococcal Types													
Danish	1	2	3	4	6A	7F	8	9N	12F	14	18C	19F	23F	25
U.S.	1	2	3	4	6	51	8	9	12	14	56	19	23	25

tions at the site of injection, especially in persons who have retained high antibody levels. Long-term surveillance of antibody levels in immunized individuals is continuing. (See ACTIONS.)

Directions for Use of the LEDERJECT® Disposable Syringe

1. Twist the plunger rod clockwise to be sure that rod is secure to rubber plunger base.
2. Hold needle shield in place with index finger and thumb of one hand while with other thumb exert light pressure on plunger rod until the plunger base has been freed and demonstrates slight movement when pressure is applied.
3. Grasp the rubber needle shield at its base; twist and pull to remove.
4. Pull back plunger rod slowly and carefully to insure smooth plunger operation.
5. Expel the air bubble.

Storage and Use: Store syringes and unopened or opened vials at 2–8° C (35.6—46.4° F). The vaccine is used directly as supplied. No dilution or reconstitution is necessary. Thimerosal in 0.01% concentration is present in the vaccine as preservative. Discard unused vials beyond expiration date.

How Supplied: PNU-IMUNE *pneumococcal vaccine, polyvalent* is supplied as follows:
5 Dose Vial. For use with syringe only.
5 × One Dose Vials. For use with syringe only.
5 × One Dose LEDERJECT® Disposable Syringes

References:

1. Austrian, R. "Surveillance of Pneumococcal Infection for Field Trials of Polyvalent Vaccines." Annual Contract Prog. Report to the Nat. Inst. of Allerg. and Inf. Dis. (1975) Updated to Dec. 1977, personal communication.
2. Editors. Pneumococcal Polysaccharide Vaccine. Morb. Mort. Weekly Report 27 (1978) 25.
3. Lund, E. "Distribution of Pneumococcal Types at Different Times and Different Areas" in *Bayer Symposium III. Bacterial Infections.* "Changes in Their Causative Agents, Trends and Possible Basis." M. Finland, W. Marget and K. Bartman (eds.) Berlin, Springer — Verlag (1971) 49.
4. Mufson, M.A., Kruss, D.M., Wasil, R.E. and Metzger, W.I. "Capsular Types and Outcome of Bacteremic Pneumococcal Disease in the Antibiotic Era." Arch. Int. Med., 134 (1974) 505.
5. Editors. Multiple-Antibiotic Resistance of Pneumococci-South Africa. Morb. Mort. Weekly Report 26 (1977) 285.
6. Austrian, R., and Gold, J. "Pneumococcal Bacteremia with Especial Reference to Bacteremic Pneumococcal Pneumonia." Ann. Int. Med., 60 (1964) 759.
7. Valenti, W.M., Jenzer, M. and Bently, W. "Type-Specific Pneumococcal Respiratory Disease in the Elderly and Chronically Ill." Am. Rev. Resp. Dis., 117 (1978) 233.
8. Fraser, D.W., Geil, C.C., and Feldman, R.A. "Meningitis in Bernalillo County, New Mexico. A Comparison with Three Other American Populations." Am. J. Epidemiol., 100 (1974) 29.
9. Heidelberger, M., Dilapi, M.M., Seigel, M. and Walter, A.N. "Persistence of Antibodies in Human Subjects Injected with Pneumococcal Polysaccharides." J. Immunol., 65 (1950) 535.
10. Mufson, M.A. and Krause, H.E. "Role of Antibody in Prevention of Acquisition of Pneumococcal Carriage Among Vaccinees." Clin. Res., 24 (1976) 577A.
11. Recommendation of the Advisory Committee on Immunization Practices, Morb. Mort. Weekly Report 29 (1980) 76.
12. Data on File, Lederle Laboratories.
13. Sullivan, J.L., Ochs, H.D., Schiffman, G., Hammerschlag, M.R., Miser, J., Vichinsky, E., and Wedgwood, R.J. "Immune Response After Splenectomy." Lancet, (1978) 178.
14. Austrian, R., Douglas, R.M., Schiffman, G., Coetzee, A.M., Koornhof, H.J., Hayden-Smith, S. and Reid, R.D.W. "Prevention of Pneumococcal Pneumonia by Vaccination." Trans Ass. Am. Physicians, 89 (1976) 184.
15. Amman, A.J., Addiego, K., Wara, D.W., Lubin, B., Smith, W.B. and Mentzer, W.C. "Polyvalent Pneumococcal-Polysaccharide Immunization of Patients with Sickle-Cell Anemia and Patients with Splenectomy." New Eng. J. Med., 297 (1977) 897.
16. Riley, I.D., Andrews, M., Howard, R., Tarr, P.I., Pfeiffer, M., Challands, P. and Jennison, G. "Immunization with Polyvalent Pneumococcal Vaccine." Lancet, (1977) 1338.
17. Siber, G.R. Weitzman, S.A., Aisenberg, A.C., Weinstein, H.J., and Schiffman, G. "Impaired Antibody Response to Pneumococcal Vaccine After Treatment for Hodgkin's Disease." New Eng J. Med., 299 (1978) 442.

PRONEMIA® ℞
hematinic
Capsules

Composition: Each capsule contains: Vitamin B_{12} (as Cobalamin Concentrate) 15 mcg.; Intrinsic Factor Concentrate 75 mg.; Ferrous Fumarate 350 mg. (Elemental Iron 115 mg.); Ascorbic Acid (Vitamin C) 150 mg. and Folic Acid 1 mg.

Indications: Indicated for treatment and maintenance in common anemias, including iron-deficiency anemia, megaloblastic anemias of pregnancy, and those of nutritional origin. All of the other means that are recognized as suited to the treatment of these anemias should also be employed. If cases prove resistant to this form of therapy, further exploration of the etiology and additional therapeutic measures should be instituted.

Warnings: Folic Acid alone is improper therapy in the treatment of pernicious anemia and other megaloblastic anemias where vitamin B_{12} is deficient.

Precautions: Some patients affected with pernicious anemia may not respond to orally administered Vitamin B_{12} with intrinsic factor concentrate and there is no known way to predict which patients will respond or which patients may cease to respond. Periodic examinations and laboratory studies of pernicious anemia patients are essential and recommended. If any symptoms of intolerance occur, the drug should be temporarily or permanently discontinued.

Folic acid in doses above 0.1 mg. daily may obscure pernicious anemia, in that hematologic remission can occur while neurological manifestations remain progressive.

Adverse Reactions: Allergic sensitization has been reported following both oral and parenteral administration of Folic Acid.

Administration and Dosage: One capsule daily with or after meals to treat and maintain the average uncomplicated case of anemia.

How Supplied: Capsules (red)—P9 bottles of 100.

RHULICAINE™
Anesthetic-Antiseptic Medicated Spray

(See PDR For Nonprescription Drugs)

RHULICREAM®
RHULIGEL®
RHULISPRAY®
analgesic-anesthetic

(See PDR For Nonprescription Drugs)

STRESSCAPS®
stress formula B+C vitamins

(See PDR For Nonprescription Drugs)

STRESSTABS® 600, Advanced Formula
High Potency
Stress Formula Vitamins

(See PDR For Nonprescription Drugs)

STRESSTABS® 600 with IRON,
Advanced Formula
High Potency
Stress Formula Vitamins

(See PDR For Nonprescription Drugs)

STRESSTABS® 600 with ZINC,
Advanced Formula
High Potency
Stress Formula Vitamins

(See PDR For Nonprescription Drugs)

TETANUS AND DIPHTHERIA TOXOIDS, ADSORBED PUROGENATED® ℞

How Supplied: 5 ml. vial; 10 x 0.5 ml. LEDERJECT® Disposable Syringe.
COMPLETE INFORMATION FURNISHED IN THE PACKAGE.

TETANUS TOXOID, ADSORBED PUROGENATED® ℞

How Supplied: 5 ml. vial (5 immunizations); 10 x 0.5 ml. and 100 x 0.5 ml. LEDERJECT® Disposable Syringe.
COMPLETE INFORMATION FURNISHED IN THE PACKAGE.

TETANUS TOXOID PUROGENATED® ℞
(Tetanus Toxoid fluid)

How Supplied: 7.5 ml. vial (5 immunizations); 10 x 0.5 ml. and 100 x 0.5 ml. LEDERJECT® Disposable Syringe.
COMPLETE INFORMATION FURNISHED IN THE PACKAGE.

THIOTEPA ℞
parenteral
Sterile

THIOTEPA Lederle is a polyfunctional alkylating agent used in the chemotherapy of certain neoplastic diseases.

Description: Thiotepa is the ethylenimine-type compound N, N′, N″-Triethylenethiophosphoramide and is available in powder form in vials which contain a sterile mixture of 15 mg. Thiotepa, 80 mg. NaCl, and 50 mg. $NaHCO_3$. Thiotepa has also been known as TESPA and TSPA and is not the same as TEPA. Thiotepa is stable in alkaline medium and unstable in acid medium. When reconstituted with Sterile Water for Injection, the resulting solution has a pH of approximately 7.6.

Action: Thiotepa is a cytotoxic agent of the polyfunctional alkylating type (more than one reactive ethylenimine group) related chemically and pharmacologically to nitrogen mustard. Its radiomimetic action is believed to occur through the release of ethylenimine radicals which, like irradiation, disrupt the bonds of DNA. One of the principal bond disruptions is initiated by alkylation of guanine at the N-7 position, which severs the linkage between the purine base and the sugar and liberates alkyl-

Continued on next page

The information on each product appearing here is based on labelling effective in August, 1982 and is either the entire official brochure or an accurate condensation therefrom. Offical brochures are enclosed in product packages. Information concerning all Lederle products may be obtained from the Professional Services Department, Lederle Laboratories, Pearl River, New York, 10965.

Lederle—Cont.

ated guanines. On the basis of tissue concentration studies, it is reported that Thiotepa has no differential affinity for neoplasms. Most of the drug appears to be excreted unchanged in the urine.

Indications: Thiotepa has been tried with varying results in the palliation of a wide variety of neoplastic diseases. However, the most consistent results have been seen in the following tumors:

1. Adenocarcinoma of the breast.
2. Adenocarcinoma of the ovary.
3. For controlling intracavitary effusions secondary to diffuse or localized neoplastic disease of various serosal cavities.
4. For the treatment of superficial papillary carcinoma of the urinary bladder.

While now largely superseded by other treatments, Thiotepa has been effective against other lymphomas, such as lymphosarcoma and Hodgkin's disease.

Contraindications: Therapy is probably contraindicated in cases of existing hepatic, renal, or bone-marrow damage. However, if the need overweighs the risk in such patients, Thiotepa may be used in low dosage, and accompanied by hepatic, renal, and hemopoietic function tests.

Thiotepa is contraindicated in patients with a known hypersensitivity (allergy) to this preparation.

Warnings: The administration of Thiotepa to pregnant women is not recommended except in cases where the benefit to be gained outweighs the risk of teratogenicity involved.

Thiotepa is highly toxic to the hematopoietic system. A rapidly falling white blood cell or platelet count indicates the necessity for discontinuing or reducing the dosage of Thiotepa. Weekly blood and platelet counts are recommended during therapy and for at least three weeks after therapy has been discontinued.

Thiotepa is a polyfunctional alkylating agent, capable of cross-linking the DNA within a cell and changing its nature. The replication of the cell is, therefore, altered, and Thiotepa may be described as mutagenic. An *in vitro* study has shown that it causes chromosomal aberrations of the chromatid type and that the frequency of induced aberrations increases with the age of the subject.

Like all alkylating agents, Thiotepa is carcinogenic. Carcinogenicity is shown most clearly in mouse studies, but there is strong circumstantial evidence of carcinogenicity in man.

Precautions: The serious complication of excessive Thiotepa therapy, or sensitivity to the effects of Thiotepa, is bone-marrow depression. If proper precautions are not observed Thiotepa may cause leukopenia, thrombocytopenia, and anemia. Death from septicemia and hemorrhage has occurred as a direct result of hematopoietic depression by Thiotepa.

It is not advisable to combine simultaneously or sequentially cancer chemotherapeutic agents or a cancer chemotherapeutic agent and a therapeutic modality having the same mechanism of action. Therefore, Thiotepa combined with other alkylating agents such as nitrogen mustard or cyclophosphamide or Thiotepa combined with irradiation would serve to intensify toxicity rather than to enhance therapeutic response. If these agents must follow each other, it is important that recovery from the first agent, as indicated by white blood cell count, be complete before therapy with the second agent is instituted.

The most reliable guide to Thiotepa toxicity is the white blood cell count. If this falls to 3000 or less, the dose should be discontinued. Another good index of Thiotepa toxicity is the platelet count; if this falls to 150,000, therapy should be discontinued. Red blood cell count is a less accurate indicator of Thiotepa toxicity. Other drugs which are known to produce bone-marrow depression should be avoided.

There is no known antidote for overdosage with Thiotepa. Transfusions of whole blood or platelets or leukocytes have proved beneficial to the patient in combatting hematopoietic toxicity.

Adverse Reactions: Apart from its effect on the blood-forming elements, Thiotepa may cause other adverse reactions. These include pain at the site of injection, nausea, vomiting, anorexia, dizziness, headache, amenorrhea, and interference with spermatogenesis.

Febrile reaction and weeping from a subcutaneous lesion may occur as the result of breakdown of tumor tissue.

Allergic reactions are rare, but hives and skin rash have been noted occasionally. One case of alopecia has been reported. In addition, a patient who had received Thiotepa and other anticancer agents experienced prolonged apnea after succinylcholine administered prior to surgery. It was theorized that this was caused by decrease of pseudocholinesterase activity caused by the anticancer drugs.

Dosage: Parenteral routes of administration are most reliable since absorption of Thiotepa from the gastrointestinal tract is variable.

Since Thiotepa is nonvesicant, intravenous doses may be given directly and rapidly without need for slow drip or large volumes of diluent. Some physicians prefer to give Thiotepa directly into the tumor mass. This may be effected transrectally, transvaginally, or intracerebrally. The technique is discussed in the appropriate section which follows. For the control of malignant effusions, Thiotepa is instilled directly into the cavity involved.

Dosage must be carefully individualized. A slow response to Thiotepa may be deceptive and may occasion unwarranted frequency of administration with subsequent signs of toxicity. After maximum benefit is obtained by initial therapy, it is necessary to continue patient on maintenance therapy (1 to 4 week intervals). In order to continue optimal effect, maintenance doses should be no more frequent than weekly in order to preserve correlation between dose and blood counts.

Initial and Maintenance Doses: Initially the higher dose in the given range is commonly administered. The maintenance dose should be adjusted weekly on the basis of pretreatment control blood counts and subsequent blood counts.

Intravenous Administration: Thiotepa may be given by rapid intravenous administration in doses of 0.3–0.4 mg/kg. Doses should be given at 1–4 week intervals.

For conversion of mg/kg of body weight to mg/M^2 of body surface or the reverse, a ratio of 1:30 is given as a guideline. The conversion factor varies between 1:20 and 1:40 depending on age and body build.

Intratumor Administration: Thiotepa in initial doses of 0.6–0.8 mg/kg may be injected directly into a tumor by means of a 22-gauge needle. A small amount of local anesthetic is injected first; then the syringe is removed and the Thiotepa solution is injected through the same needle. The drug is diluted in sterile water, 10 mg per 1 ml. Maintenance doses at one to four week intervals range from 0.07 mg/kg to 0.8 mg/kg depending on the condition of the patient.

Intracavitary Administration: The dosage recommended is 0.6–0.8 mg/kg. Administration is usually effected through the same tubing which is used to remove the fluid from the cavity involved.

Intravesical Administration: Patients with papillary carcinoma of the bladder are dehydrated for 8 to 12 hours prior to treatment. Then 60 mg of Thiotepa in 30–60 ml of distilled water is instilled into the bladder by catheter. For maximum effect, the solution should be retained for 2 hours. If the patient finds it impossible to retain 60 ml for 2 hours, the dose may be given in a volume of 30 ml. If desired, the patient may be positioned every 15 minutes for maximum area contact. The usual course of treatment is once a week for 4 weeks. The course may be repeated if necessary, but second and third courses must be given with caution since bone-marrow depression may be increased. Deaths have occurred after intravesical administration, caused by bone-marrow depression from systemically absorbed drug.

Preparation of Solution: The powder should be reconstituted preferably in Sterile Water for Injection. The amount of diluent most often used is 1.5 ml. resulting in a drug concentration of 5 mg. in each 0.5 ml. of solution. Larger volumes are usually employed for intracavity use, intravenous drip, or perfusion therapy. The 1.5 ml. reconstituted preparation may be added to larger volumes of other diluents: Sodium Chloride Injection USP, Dextrose Injection USP, Dextrose and Sodium Chloride Injection USP, Ringer's Injection USP, or Lactated Ringer's Injection USP. Reconstituted solutions should be clear to slightly opaque but solutions that are grossly opaque or precipitated should not be used.

Since the original powder form contains 15 mg. Thiotepa, 80 mg. NaCl, 50 mg. $NaHCO_3$, the addition of Sterile Water for Injection produces an isotonic solution. The addition of other diluents may result in hypertonic solutions, which may cause mild to moderate discomfort on injection.

For local use into single or multiple sites, Thiotepa may be mixed with procaine HCl 2%, epinephrine HCl 1:1000, or both.

Whether in its original powder form or in reconstituted solution, Thiotepa must be stored in the refrigerator at 2°–8° C. (35–46° F.).

Reconstituted solutions may be kept for 5 days in a refrigerator without substantial loss of potency.

How Supplied: 15 mg. vials, sterile.

A.H.F.S. 10:00

TriHEMIC® 600 ℞
hematinic
Tablets

Description:
Each tablet contains:

Vitamin C (Ascorbic Acid) ....600 mg.
Vitamin B_{12} (Cyanocobalamin) ....25 mcg.
Intrinsic Factor Concentrate ....75 mg.
Folic Acid (Folacin)....................................1 mg.
Vitamin E (*dl*-Alpha
Tocopheryl Acetate) ....30 Int. Units
Elemental Iron (as 350 mg. of
Ferrous Fumarate) ....115 mg.
Docusate Sodium USP (DSS) ....50 mg.

Actions: TriHEMIC 600 *hematinic* is a preparation containing those ingredients essential to normal erythropoiesis, plus a stool softener to counteract the constipating effects of iron.

Indications: TriHEMIC 600 is a multiphasic preparation for use in the treatment of most megaloblastic, macrocytic and iron-deficiency anemias, in the anemias of pregnancy, in those anemias occurring in a variety of malabsorption syndromes, and those of nutritional origin. It is a useful adjuvant in patients in whom erythropoiesis is suppressed due to severe infections, malignancies or to the toxic effects of certain chemotherapeutic agents. A deficiency of Vitamin E may increase the fragility of red blood cells, with resultant enhanced hemolysis. Vitamin C is present to aid in the absorption of iron.

Warnings: Folic Acid alone is improper therapy in the treatment of pernicious anemia and other megaloblastic anemias where Vitamin $B_{12}$is deficient.

Precautions: Some patients affected with pernicious anemia may not respond to orally administered Vitamin B_{12} with intrinsic factor concentrate and there is no known way to predict which patients will respond or which patients may cease to respond. Periodic examinations and laboratory studies of pernicious anemia patients are essential and recommended. If any symptoms of intolerance occur, the drug should be temporarily or permanently discontinued.

Folic Acid in doses above 0.1 mg. daily may obscure pernicious anemia, in that hematologic remission can occur while neurological manifestations remain progressive.

Adverse Reactions: Gastrointestinal intolerance may develop and be manifest by nausea, vomiting, diarrhea or abdominal pain. Skin rashes of various types may occur. Such reactions can necessitate temporary or permanent changes in dosage or usage.

Allergic sensitization has been reported following both oral and parenteral administration of Folic Acid.

Dosage and Administration: One tablet daily. Adjustment of dosage is dependent on patient response and the physician's clinical judgment.

How Supplied: Film coated, red; engraved LL T1 bottles of 30 tablets, and 500 tablets.

[Shown in Product Identification Section]

TRI-IMMUNOL® ℞
diphtheria and tetanus toxoids and pertussis vaccine adsorbed

How Supplied: 7.5 ml. vials. (5 immunizations).

COMPLETE INFORMATION FURNISHED IN THE PACKAGE.

ZINCON®, Improved Richer, Thicker Formula Dandruff Shampoo

(See PDR For Nonprescription Drugs)

Leeming Division

Pfizer, Inc.
100 JEFFERSON ROAD
PARSIPPANY, NJ 07054

BEN-GAY® EXTERNAL ANALGESIC PRODUCTS

(See PDR For Nonprescription Drugs)

DESITIN® OINTMENT

(See PDR For Nonprescription Drugs)

UNISOM® NIGHTTIME SLEEP-AID OTC
(doxylamine succinate)

Description: Pale blue oval scored tablets containing 25 mg. of doxylamine succinate, 2-(α-(2-dimethylaminoethoxy)α-methylbenzyl) pyridine succinate.

Action and Uses: Doxylamine succinate is an antihistamine of the ethanolamine class, which characteristically shows a high incidence of sedation. In a comparative clinical study of over 20 antihistamines on more than 3000 subjects, doxylamine succinate 25 mg. was one of the three most sedating antihistamines, producing a significantly reduced latency to end of wakefulness and comparing favorably with established hypnotic drugs such as secobarbital and pentobarbital in sedation activity. It was chosen as the antihistamine, based on dosage, causing the earliest onset of sleep. In another clinical study, doxylamine succinate 25 mg. scored better than secobarbital 100 mg. as a nighttime hypnotic. Two additional, identical clinical studies involving a total of 121 subjects demonstrated that doxylamine succinate 25 mg. reduced the sleep latency period by a third, compared to placebo. Duration of sleep was 26.6% longer with doxylamine succinate, and the quality of sleep was rated higher with the drug than with placebo. An EEG study on 6 subjects confirmed the results of these studies.

Administration and Dosage: One tablet 30 minutes before retiring. Not for children under 12 years of age.

Side Effects: Occasional anticholinergic effects may be seen.

Precautions: Unisom® should be taken only at bedtime.

Contraindications: Asthma, glaucoma, enlargement of the prostate gland. This product should not be taken by pregnant women, or those who are nursing a baby.

Warnings: Should be taken with caution if alcohol is being consumed. Product should not be taken if patient is concurrently on any other drug, without prior consultation with physician. Should not be taken for longer than two weeks unless approved by physician.

How Supplied: Boxes of 8, 16, 32 or 48 tablets.

Legere Pharmaceuticals, Inc.

7326 E. EVANS ROAD
SCOTTSDALE, AZ 85260

Product Number	Product	
1038	ACE + Z Tablets	OTC
	Vitamin A	5000 I.U.
	Vitamin C	1000 mg.
	Vitamin E (Succinate)	50 I.U.
	Magnesium (oxide)	100 mg.
	Zinc Sulfate	100 mg.
1066	ACETACO Tablets	℞ Ⓒ
	Acetaminophen	325 mg.
	Codeine Phosphate	30 mg.
094	ADENOSINE 30 ml	℞
	Adenosine 5 Monophosphate	25 mg.
005	B COMPLEX 100 30 ml	℞
	Thiamine HCl	100 mg.
	Riboflavin	2 mg.
	Pyridoxine HCl	2 mg.
	Panthenol	2 mg.
	Niacinamide	100 mg.
1027	CAFAMINE T.D. 2X Capsules	OTC
	Caffeine	150 mg.
	Phenylpropanolamine	50 mg.
007	CEE-500 50 ml	℞
	Sodium Ascorbate	500 mg.
1073	CEE-1000 T.D. Tablets	OTC
	Ascorbic Acid	1000 mg.
055	CINALONE 40 5 ml	℞
	Triamcinolone Diacetate	40 mg.
101	CINONIDE 40 5 ml	℞
	Triamcinolone Acetonide	40 mg.
062	DEPO-PREDATE 80 5 ml	℞
	Methylprednisolone Acetate	80 mg.
010	DEXASONE 4 5 ml	℞
	Dexamethasone Phosphate	4 mg.
011	DEXASONE L.A.	℞
	Dexamethasone Acetate	8 mg.
1058	DEXOL T.D. Tablets	OTC
	Pantothenic Acid	1000 mg.
065	DEXTRARON-50 10 ml	℞
	Iron Dextran	50 mg.
1111	DI-ATRO Tablets	℞ Ⓒ
	Diphenoxylate HCl	2.5 mg.
	Atropine Sulfate	0.025 mg.
1130	DIEUTRIM Capsule	OTC
	Phenylpropanolamine HCl	75 mg.
	Benzocaine	9 mg.
	Carboxymethylcellulose	75 mg.
080	E.D.T.A. 20 ml	℞
	Edetate Disodium	150 mg.
015	E-CYPIONATE 10 ml	℞
	Estradiol Cypionate	5 mg.
109	KABOLIN 2 ml	℞
	Nandrolone Decanoate	50 mg.
091	MAG-5 30 ml	℞
	Magnesium Sulfate	500 mg.
017	MENAVAL 20 10 ml	℞
	Estradiol Valerate	20 mg.
106	MYOTROL 2 ml	℞
	Orphenadrine Citrate	30 mg.
049	NEUCALM 50 10 ml	℞
	Hydroxyzine HCl	50 mg
1133	P T 105 Capsules	℞
	Phendimetrazine 105 mg	Ⓒ
1022	PHENAZINE Tablets & Capsules	℞ Ⓒ
	Phendimetrazine	35 mg.
090	PREDATE-100 10 ml	℞
	Prednisolone Acetate	100 mg.
066	PREDATE-L.A.S.A. 10 ml	℞
	Prednisolone Acetate	80 mg.
	Predisolone Sodium Phosphate	20 mg.
1132	PROBAHIST Capsules	℞
	Pseudoephedrine	120 mg
	Chlorpheniramine	8 mg
092	PROBOCON	℞
	Atropine Sulfate	0.2 mg.
	Chlorpheniramine Maleate	5 mg.
073	RODEX 30 ml	℞
	Pyridoxine HCl	100 mg
1037	RODEX T.D. Capsules	OTC
	Pyridoxine	150 mg
1025	TERAMINE Capsules	℞ Ⓒ
	Phentermine HCl	30 mg.
050	TESTAVAL 90/4 10 ml	℞
	Testosterone Enanthate	90 mg.
	Estradiol Valerate	4 mg.
2001	VAGIMIDE CREAM 4 oz	℞
	Sulfanilamide	15%
	Allantoin	2.0%
	Aminacrine HCl	0.2%

Lemmon Company

SELLERSVILLE, PA 18960

ADIPEX-P® Tablets Ⓒ ℞
(phentermine hydrochloride)

Description: Each tablet contains: Phentermine Hydrochloride, 37.5 mg. (equivalent to 30 mg. of Phentermine base)

Phentermine hydrochloride is designated chemically as phenyl-tert-butylamine hydrochloride. It is a white crystalline powder, very soluble in water and alcohol.

Actions: Phentermine hydrochloride is a sympathomimetic amine with pharmacologic activity similar to the prototype drugs of this class used in obesity, the amphetamines. Actions include central nervous system stimulation and elevation of blood pressure. Tachyphylaxis and tolerance have been demonstrated with all drugs of this class in which these phenomena have been looked for.

Drugs of this class used in obesity are commonly known as "anorectics" or "anorexigenics". It has not been established, however, that the action of such drugs in treating obesity is primarily one of appetite suppression. Other central nervous system actions, or metabolic effects, may be involved, for example.

Adult obese subjects instructed in dietary management and treated with "anorectic" drugs, lose more weight on the average than those treated with placebo and diet, as determined in relatively short-term clinical trials.

Continued on next page

Lemmon—Cont.

The magnitude of increased weight loss of drug-treated patients over placebo-treated patients is only a fraction of a pound a week. The rate of weight loss is greatest in the first weeks of therapy for both drug and placebo subjects and tends to decrease in succeeding weeks. The possible origins of the increased weight loss due to the various drug effects are not established. The amount of weight loss associated with the use of an "anorectic" drug varies from trial to trial, and the increased weight loss appears to be related in part to variables other than the drug prescribed, such as the physician-investigator, the population treated, and the diet prescribed. Studies do not permit conclusions as to the relative importance of the drug and non-drug factors on weight loss.

The natural history of obesity is measured in years, whereas, the studies cited are restricted to a few weeks duration; thus, the total impact of drug-induced weight loss over that of diet alone must be considered clinically limited.

Indications: Phentermine hydrochloride is indicated in the management of exogenous obesity as a short term adjunct (a few weeks) in a regimen of weight reduction based on caloric restriction.

The limited usefulness of agents of this class (see ACTIONS) should be measured against possible risk factors inherent in their use such as those described below.

Contraindications: Advanced arteriosclerosis, symptomatic cardiovascular disease, moderate to severe hypertension, hyperthyroidism, known hypersensitivity or idiosyncrasy to the sympathomimetic amines, glaucoma.

Agitated states.

Patients with a history of drug abuse.

During or within 14 days following the administration of monoamine oxidase inhibitors (hypertensive crisis may result).

Warnings: Tolerance to the anorectic effect usually develops within a few weeks. When this occurs, the recommended dose should not be exceeded in an attempt to increase the effect; rather, the drug should be discontinued. Phentermine hydrochloride may impair the ability of the patient to engage in potentially hazardous activities such as operating machinery or driving a motor vehicle; the patient should therefore be cautioned accordingly.

Drug Dependence: Phentermine hydrochloride is related chemically and pharmacologically to the amphetamines. Amphetamines and related stimulant drugs have been extensively abused, and the possibility of abuse of phentermine hydrochloride should be kept in mind when evaluating the desirability of including a drug as part of a weight reduction program. Abuse of amphetamines and related drugs may be associated with intense psychological dependence and severe social dysfunction. There are reports of patients who have increased the dosage to many times that recommended. Abrupt cessation following prolonged high dosage administration results in extreme fatigue and mental depression; changes are also noted in the sleep EEG. Manifestations of chronic intoxication with anorectic drugs include severe dermatoses, marked insomnia, irritability, hyperactivity, and personality changes. The most severe manifestation of chronic intoxications is psychosis, often clinically indistinguishable from schizophrenia.

Usage in Pregnancy: No reproduction studies or teratology studies of phentermine hydrochloride, in animals or humans, have been published. Therefore, use of phentermine hydrochloride by women who are or may become pregnant, requires that the potential benefit be weighed against the possible hazard to mother and infant.

Usage In Children: Phentermine hydrochloride is not recommended for use in children under 12 years of age.

Precautions: Caution is to be exercised in prescribing phentermine hydrochloride for patients with even mild hypertension.

Insulin requirements in diabetes mellitus may be altered in association with the use of phentermine hydrochloride and the concomitant dietary regimen.

Phentermine hydrochloride may decrease the hypotensive effect of guanethidine.

The least amount feasible should be prescribed or dispensed at one time in order to minimize the possibility of overdosage.

Adverse Reactions:

Cardiovascular: Palpitation, tachycardia, elevation of blood pressure.

Central Nervous System: Overstimulation, restlessness, dizziness, insomnia, euphoria, dysphoria, tremor, headache; rarely psychotic episodes at recommended doses.

Gastrointestinal: Dryness of the mouth, unpleasant taste, diarrhea, constipation, other gastrointestinal disturbances.

Allergic: Urticaria.

Endocrine: Impotence, changes in libido.

Dosage and Administration: The usual adult dose is one tablet daily, administered before breakfast or 1-2 hours after breakfast. Dosage may be adjusted to the patient's need. For some patients ½ tablet daily may be adequate, while in some cases it may be desirable to give ½ tablet two times a day.

Phentermine hydrochloride is not recommended for use in children under 12 years of age.

Overdosage: Manifestations of acute overdosage with phentermine hydrochloride include restlessness, tremor, hyperreflexia, rapid respiration, confusion, assaultive behavior hallucinations, panic states.

Fatigue and depression usually follow the central stimulation.

Cardiovascular effects include arrhythmias, hypertension or hypotension and circulatory collapse. Gastrointestinal symptoms include nausea, vomiting, diarrhea, and abdominal cramps. In fatal poisoning, death is usually preceded by convulsions and coma.

Management of acute phentermine hydrochloride intoxication is largely symptomatic and includes lavage and sedation with a barbiturate. Experience with hemodialysis or peritoneal dialysis is inadequate to permit recommendation in this regard. Acidification of the urine increases phentermine hydrochloride excretion. Intravenous phentolamine (Regitine) has been suggested for possible acute, severe hypertension, if this complicates phentermine hydrochloride overdosage.

How Supplied: Tablets (white with blue specks, oblong, $^{13}/_{32}''$ length, scored, engraved Lemmon /9) in bottles of 100, 400, and 1000 (NDC 0093-0009).

[*Shown in Product Identification Section*]

METRYL™ ℞
(metronidazole)

> **WARNING**
> Metronidazole has been shown to be carcinogenic in mice and rats. (SEE WARNINGS). Unnecessary use of this drug should be avoided. Its use should be reserved for the conditions described in the INDICATIONS section below.

Description: Metronidazole is 1-(beta-hydroxyethyl)-2-methyl-nitroimidazole. Metronidazole is classified therapeutically as an antiprotozoal (Trichomonas). It occurs as pale yellow crystals that are slightly soluble in water and alcohol.

Clinical Pharmacology: The major route of elimination of Metronidazole and its metabolites is via the urine (60%–80% of the dose), with fecal excretion accounting for 6–15% of the dose. The metabolites that appear in the urine result primarily from side chain oxidation (1-beta-hydroxyethyl)-2-hydroxymethyl-5-nitroimidazole and 2-methyl-5-nitroimidazole-1-yl-acetic acid) and glucuronide conjugation, with unchanged Metronidazole accounting for approximately 20% of the total. Renal clearance of Metronidazole is approximately 10 ml/min/1.73m^2.

Metronidazole is the major component appearing in the plasma, with lesser quantities of the 2-hydroxymethyl metabolite also being present. Less than 20% of the circulating metronidazole is bound to plasma proteins. Both the parent compound and the metabolite possess *in vitro* bactericidal activity against most strains of anaerobic bacteria and *in vitro* trichomonacidal activity.

Metronidazole appears in cerebrospinal fluid, saliva, and breast milk in concentrations similar to those found in plasma. Bactericidal concentrations of metronidazole have also been detected in pus from hepatic abscesses.

Following oral administration, metronidazole is well absorbed, with peak plasma concentration occurring between one and two hours after administration. Plasma concentrations of metronidazole are proportional to the administered dose. Oral administration of 250 mg, 500 mg, or 2,000 mg, produced peak plasma concentrations of 6 mcg/ml, 12 mcg/ml, and 40 mcg/ml respectively. Studies reveal no significant bioavailability differences between males and females; however, because of weight differences, the resulting plasma levels in males are generally lower.

Decreased renal function does not alter the single dose pharmacokinetics of metronidazole. However, plasma clearance of metronidazole is decreased in patients with decreased liver function.

Microbiology: Trichomonas vaginalis, Entamoeba histolytica: Metronidazole possesses direct trichomonacidal and amebacidal activity against *T. vaginalis* and *E. histolytica.* The *in vitro* minimal inhibitory concentration (MIC) for most strains of these organisms is 1 mcg/ml or less.

Indications and Usage: *Symptomatic Trichomoniasis:* Metronidazole is indicated for the treatment of symptomatic trichomoniasis in females and males when the presence of trichomonad has been confirmed by appropriate laboratory procedures (wet smears and/or cultures).

Asymptomatic Trichomoniasis: Metronidazole is indicated in the treatment of asymptomatic females when the organism is associated with endocervicitis, cervicitis, or cervical erosion. Since there is evidence that presence of the trichomonad can interfere with accurate assessment of abnormal cytological smears, additional smears should be performed after eradication of the parasite.

Treatment of Asymptomatic Consorts: T. vaginalis infection is a venereal disease. Therefore, asymptomatic sexual partners of treated patients should be treated simultaneously if the organism has been found to be present in order to prevent infection of the partner. The decision as to whether to treat an asymptomatic male partner with a negative culture or one in whom no culture has been attempted is an individual one. In making this decision, it should be noted that there is evidence that there can be considerable difficulty in isolating the organism from the asymptomatic male carrier, negative smears and cultures cannot be relied upon in this regard. In any event, the consort should be treated with Metronidazole in cases of reinfection.

Amebiasis: Metronidazole is indicated in the treatment of acute intestinal amebiasis (amebic dysentery) and amebic liver abscess.

In amebic liver abscess, Metronidazole therapy does not obviate the need for aspiration or drainage of pus.

Contraindications: Metronidazole is contraindicated in patients with active organic disease of the central nervous system (SEE ADVERSE REACTIONS).

Metronidazole is contraindicated during the first trimester of pregnancy (SEE WARNINGS).

Metronidazole is also contraindicated in patients with a prior history of hypersensitivity to Metronidazole.

Warnings: *Convulsive Seizures and Peripheral Neuropathy:* Convulsive seizures and peripheral neuropathy, the latter characterized mainly by numbness or paresthesia of an extremity, have been reported in patients treated with Metronidazole. The appearance of abnormal neurologic signs demands the prompt discontinuation of Metronidazole therapy. Metronidazole should be administered with caution to patients with central nervous system diseases.

Tumorigenicity Studies in Rodents: Metronidazole has shown evidence of carcinogenic activity in a number of studies involving chronic, oral administration in mice and rats. Prominent among the effects in the mouse was the promotion of pulmonary tumorigenesis. This has been observed in all six reported studies in that species, including one study in which the animals were dosed on an intermittent schedule (administration during every fourth week only). At very high dose levels (approx. 500 mg/kg/day) there was a statistically significant increase in the incidence of malignant liver tumors in males. Also, the published results of one of the mouse studies indicate an increase in the incidence of malignant lymphomas as well as pulmonary neoplasms associated with lifetime feeding of the drug. All these effects are statistically significant.

Several long-term oral-dosing studies in the rats have been completed. There was a statistically significant increase in the incidence of various neoplasms, particularly in mammary and hepatic tumors, among female rats administered Metronidazole over those noted in the concurrent female control groups.

Two lifetime tumorigenicity studies in hamsters have been performed and reported to be negative.

Mutagenicity Studies: Although Metronidazole has shown mutagenic activity in a number of *in vitro* assay systems, studies in mammal (*in vivo*) have failed to demonstrate a potential for genetic damage.

Precautions: *General:* Patients with severe hepatic disease metabolize Metronidazole slowly, with resultant accumulation of Metronidazole and its metabolites in the plasma. Accordingly, for such patients, doses below those usually recommended should be administered cautiously.

Known or previously unrecognized candidiasis may present more prominent symptoms during therapy with Metronidazole and requires treatment with a candicidal agent.

Laboratory Tests: Metronidazole is a nitroimidazole and should be used with care in patients with evidence of, or history of blood dyscrasia. A mild leukopenia has been observed during its administration; however no persistent hematologic abnormalities attributable to Metronidazole have been observed in clinical studies. Total and differential leukocyte counts are recommended before and after therapy for trichomoniasis and amebiasis, especially if a second course of therapy is necessary.

Drug Interactions: Metronidazole has been reported to potentiate the anticoagulent effect of coumadin and warfarin resulting in a prolongation of prothrombin time. This possible drug interaction should be considered when Metronidazole is prescribed for patients on this type of anticoagulant therapy.

Alcoholic beverages should not be consumed during Metronidazole therapy because abdominal cramps, nausea, vomiting, headache, and flushing may occur.

Drug/Laboratory Test Interactions: Metronidazole may interfere with certain chemical analyses for serum glutamic oxalacetic transaminase, resulting in decreased values. Values of zero may be observed.

Carcinogenesis: (SEE WARNINGS)

Pregnancy: Teratogenic Effects—*Pregnancy Category B:* Metronidazole crosses the placental barrier and enters the fetal circulation rapidly. Reproduction studies have been performed in rabbits and rats at doses up to five times the human dose and have revealed no evidence of impaired fertility or harm to the fetus due to Metronidazole. There are, however, no adequate and well-controlled studies in pregnant women. Because animal reproduction studies are not always predictive of human response, and because Metronidazole is a carcinogen in rodents, this drug should be used during pregnancy only if clearly needed (SEE CONTRAINDICATIONS).

Use of Metronidazole for trichomoniasis in the second and third trimesters should be restricted to those in whom local palliative treatment has been inadequate to control symptoms.

Nursing Mothers: Because of the potential for tumorigenicity shown for Metronidazole in mouse and rat studies, a decision should be made whether to discontinue nursing or to discontinue the drug, taking into account the importance of the drug to the mother. Metronidazole is secreted in breast milk in concentrations similar to those found in plasma.

Pediatric Use: Safety and effectiveness in children have not been established except for the treatment of amebiasis.

Adverse Reactions: By far the most common adverse reactions have been referable to the gastrointestinal tract, particularly nausea, sometimes accompanied by headache, anorexia, and occasionally vomiting, diarrhea, epigastric distress and abdominal cramping; constipation has also been reported. A metallic, sharp, unpleasant taste is not unusual. Furry tongue; glossitis and stomatitis have occurred; these may be associated with a sudden overgrowth of *Candida* which may occur during effective therapy. Proliferation of *Candida* also may occur in the vagina.

A moderate leukopenia may be observed occasionally. If this occurs, the total leukocyte count may be expected to return to normal after the course of medication is completed.

If patients receiving Metronidazole drink alcoholic beverages, they may experience abdominal distress, nausea, vomiting, flushing, or headache. A modification of the taste of alcoholic beverages has also been reported.

Dizziness, vertigo, uncoordination, ataxia, convulsive seizures, and peripheral neuropathy have been reported. Numbness or paresthesia of an extremity and fleeting joint pains sometimes resembling "serum sickness" have been experienced, as have confusion, irritability, depression, weakness, insomnia, and a mild erythematous eruption.

Urticaria, flushing, nasal congestion, dryness of the mouth (or vagina or vulva), pruritus, dysuria, cystitis, and a sense of pelvic pressure have been reported. Very rarely dyspareunia, fever, polyuria, incontinence, decrease of libido, proctitis, and pyuria have occurred in patients receiving the drug.

Instances of darkened urine have been reported and this manifestation has been the subject of a special investigation. Although the pigment which is probably responsible for this phenomenon has not been positively identified, it is almost certainly a metabolite of Metronidazole. It seems certain that it is of no clinical significance and may be encountered only when Metronidazole is administered in higher-than-recommended doses.

Flattening of the T-wave may be seen in electrocardiographic tracings.

Overdosage: Single oral doses of Metronidazole, up to 15 g, have been reported in suicide attempts and accidental overdoses. Symptoms reported include nausea, vomiting, and ataxia. Oral Metronidazole has been studied as a radiation sensitizer in the treating of malignant tumors. Neurotoxic effects, including seizures and peripheral neuropathy, have been reported after 5 to 7 doses of 6 to 10.4 g every other day.

Treatment: There is no specific antidote for Metronidazole overdose: therefore, management of the patient should consist of symptomatic and supportive therapy.

Dosage and Administration: *Trichomoniasis:*

In the female: The recommended dosage is one 250 mg tablet orally 3 times daily for 7 days. One-day therapy with 2 g of Metronidazole administered either as a single dose or divided doses (1 g twice a day) is efficacious. Cure rates may be higher for the 7 day regimen.

Selection of the appropriate treatment mode should be individualized. One day therapy often maximizes compliance, while 7 day therapy decreases the possibility of reinfection by her sexual partner(s). Certain patients may tolerate one form of therapy over the other.

Pregnant patients should not be treated during the first trimester with either regimen. If treated during the second or third trimester, the one day course of therapy should not be used, as it results in higher serum levels which reach the fetal circulation. (SEE CONTRAINDICATIONS AND PRECAUTIONS).

When repeat courses of the drug are required, it is recommended that an interval of 4 to 6 weeks elapse between courses and that the presence of the trichomonad be reconfirmed by appropriate laboratory measures. Total and differential leukocyte counts should be made before and after retreatment. (SEE PRECAUTIONS-LABORATORY TESTS).

In the male: One 250 mg tablet 3 times daily for 7 days is recommended as a course of treatment, however, treatment may be individualized as for the female.

Amebiasis:

Adults: For acute intestinal amebiasis (acute amebic dysentery): 750 mg orally 3 times daily for 5 to 10 days.

For Amebic Liver Abscess: 500 mg or 750 mg orally 3 times daily for 5 to 10 days.

Children: 35 to 50 mg/kg of body weight/24 hours, divided into 3 doses, orally for 10 days.

How Supplied: Metryl Tablets 250 mg (white, round, $^{11}/_{32}''$, engraved "Metryl" and "93") in bottles of 100, 250, 500, and 1000. (NDC 0093-0551). Metryl Tablets 500 mg (white, oblong, $^{5}/_{8}''$ length, scored, engraved "Metryl 500" and "93/93") in bottles of 100 and 500. (NDC 0093-0500).

[*Shown in Product Identification Section*]

POTAGE™ ℞
(potassium chloride for oral solution)
20 mEq (1.5g KCl)

Description: POTAGE is an oral potassium ($K+$) and chloride (Cl^-) supplement offered as a powder for reconstitution in individual packets. Each packet contains Potassium Chloride 1.5 g (20 mEq) in a pleasant tasting Beef or Chicken flavored base. When reconstituted as directed, makes a delicious broth which is low in sodium.

Clinical Pharmacology: Potassium ion is the principal intracellular cation of most body tissues. Potassium ions participate in a number of essential physiological processes, including the maintenance of intracellular tonicity, the transmission of nerve impulses, the contraction of cardiac, skeletal, and smooth mus-

Continued on next page

Lemmon—Cont.

cle and the maintenance of normal renal function.

Potassium depletion may occur whenever the rate of potassium loss through renal excretion and/or loss from the gastrointestinal tract exceeds the rate of potassium intake. Such depletion usually develops slowly as a consequence of prolonged therapy with oral diuretics, primary or secondary hyperaldosteronism, diabetic ketoacidosis, severe diarrhea, or inadequate replacement of potassium in patients on prolonged parenteral nutrition. Potassium depletion due to these causes is usually accompanied by a concomitant deficiency of chloride and is manifested by hypokalemia and metabolic alkalosis. Potassium depletion may produce weakness, fatigue, disturbances of cardiac rhythm (primarily ectopic beats), prominent U-waves in the electrocardiogram, and in advanced cases flaccid paralysis and/or impaired ability to concentrate urine.

Potassium depletion associated with metabolic alkalosis is managed by correcting the fundamental causes of the deficiency whenever possible and administering supplemental potassium chloride, in the form of high potassium food or potassium chloride solution or tablets. In rare circumstances, (e.g. patients with renal tubular acidosis) potassium depletion may be associated with metabolic acidosis and hyperchloremia. In such patients potassium replacement should be accomplished with potassium salts other than the chloride, such as potassium bicarbonate, potassium citrate, potassium gluconate, or potassium acetate.

Indications and Usage:

1. For therapeutic use in patients with hypokalemia with or without metabolic alkalosis; in digitalis intoxication and in patients with hypokalemia familial periodic paralysis.
2. For prevention of potassium depletion when the dietary intake of potassium is inadequate in the following conditions: patients receiving digitalis and diuretics for congestive heart failure; hepatic cirrhosis with ascites; states of aldosterone excess with normal renal function; potassium-losing nephropathy, and certain diarrheal states.
3. The use of potassium salts in patients receiving diuretics for uncomplicated essential hypertension is often unnecessary when such patients have a normal dietary pattern. Serum potassium should be checked periodically, however, if hypokalemia occurs, dietary supplementation with potassium-containing foods may be adequate to control milder cases. In more severe cases supplementation with potassium salts may be indicated.

Contraindications: Potassium supplements are contraindicated in patients with hyperkalemia since a further increase in serum potassium concentration in such patients can produce cardiac arrest. Hyperkalemia may complicate any of the following conditions: chronic renal failure; systemic acidosis such as diabetic acidosis, acute dehydration, extensive tissue breakdown as in severe burns or adrenal insufficiency. Potassium supplements are contraindicated in patients receiving potassium-sparing diuretics (e.g., spironolactone, triamterene), since such use may produce severe hyperkalemia.

Potassium chloride supplements are contraindicated in hypokalemic patients with metabolic acidosis. These patients should be treated with an alkalinizing potassium salt such as potassium bicarbonate, potassium citrate, potassium gluconate, or potassium acetate.

Warnings: Hyperkalemia: In patients with impaired mechanisms for excreting potassium, the administration of potassium salts can produce hyperkalemia and cardiac arrest. This occurs most commonly in patients given potassium by the intravenous route but may also occur in patients given potassium orally. Potentially fatal hyperkalemia can develop rapidly and be asymptomatic.

Interaction with Potassium-Sparing Diuretics: Hypokalemia should not be treated by the concomitant administration of potassium salts and a potassium-sparing diuretic (e.g., spironolactone or triamterene), since the simultaneous administration of these agents can produce severe hyperkalemia.

Precautions: The diagnosis of potassium depletion is ordinarily made by demonstrating hypokalemia in a patient with a clinical history suggesting some cause for potassium depletion. In interpreting the serum potassium level, the physician should bear in mind that acute alkalosis per se can produce hypokalemia in the absence of a deficit in total body potassium, while acute acidosis per se can increase the serum potassium concentration into the normal range even in the presence of a reduced total body potassium. The treatment of potassium depletion, particularly in the presence of cardiac disease, renal disease, or acidosis, requires careful attention to acid-base balance and appropriate monitoring of serum electrolytes, the electrocardiogram, and the clinical status of the patient.

The use of potassium salts with chronic renal disease, or any other condition which impairs potassium excretion, requires particularly careful monitoring of the serum potassium concentration and appropriate dosage adjustment.

Carcinogenesis: No data are available on long-term potential for carcinogenicity in animals or humans.

Pregnancy Category C: Animal reproduction studies have not been conducted with POTAGE. It is also not known whether POTAGE can cause fetal harm when administered to a pregnant woman or can affect reproduction capacity. POTAGE should be given to a pregnant woman only if clearly needed.

Nursing Mothers: Although no studies have been done, it is presumed that potassium chloride is excreted in human milk. Caution should be excised when POTAGE is administered to a nursing woman.

Pediatric Use: Safety and effectiveness in children have not been established.

Adverse Reactions: One of the most severe side effects is hyperkalemia (see CONTRAINDICATIONS, WARNINGS, AND OVERDOSAGE).

The most common adverse reactions to oral potassium salts are nausea, vomiting, abdominal discomfort, and diarrhea. These symptoms are due to irritation of the gastrointestinal tract and are best managed by diluting the preparation further, taking the dose with meals, or reducing the dose.

Skin rash has been reported rarely.

Overdosage: The administration of oral potassium salts to persons with normal excretory mechanisms for potassium rarely causes serious hyperkalemia. However, if excretory mechanisms are impaired or if potassium is administered too rapidly intravenously, potentially fatal hyperkalemia can result (see CONTRAINDICATIONS AND WARNINGS). It is important to recognize that hyperkalemia is usually asymptomatic and may be manifested only by an increased serum potassium concentration and characteristic electrocardiographic changes (peaking of T-waves, loss of P-waves, depression of S-T segments, and prolongation of QT intervals). Late manifestations include muscle paralysis and cardiovascular collapse from cardiac arrest.

Treatment measures for hyperkalemia include the following: (1) elimination of foods and medication containing potassium and of potassium-sparing diuretics; (2) intravenous administration of 300 to 500 ml/hr of dextrose solution (10-25%), containing 10 units of insulin/20 Gm dextrose; (3) correction of acidosis, if present, with intravenous sodium bicarbonate; (4) use of exchange resins, hemodialysis, or peritoneal dialysis. In treating hyperkalemia, it should be recalled that in patients who have been stabilized on digitalis, too rapid a lowering of the serum potassium concentration can produce digitalis toxicity.

Dosage and Administration: The usual adult dosage is the contents of one packet of POTAGE dissolved in four fluid ounces (about ½ cup) or more of hot water 1 to 2 times daily, preferably with meals. Consume while warm; do not reheat. Do not prepare in advance. This preparation, like other potassium supplements, must be properly diluted to avoid the possibility of gastrointestinal irritation. This supplies 20 to 40 mEq of elemental potassium and chloride. The approximate minimum adult daily requirement for potassium is 40 mEq. Deviations from the recommended dosage may be indicated, since no average total daily dose can be defined but must be governed by close observation for clinical effects. Potassium intoxication may result from any therapeutic dosage (see OVERDOSAGE AND PRECAUTIONS).

How Supplied: POTAGE™ (Potassium Chloride for Oral Solution). Each 5 g packet in solution provides 20 mEq of potassium and chloride. NDC 0093-0243-56 Beef Flavor. Boxes of 30 Unit-Dose Packets. NDC 0093-0242-56 Chicken Flavor. Boxes of 30 Unit-Dose Packets.

[*Shown in Product Identification Section*]

RHUS TOX ANTIGEN™ ℞
(poison ivy extract)

Composition: Each ml. of sterile solution contains 40 mg. poison ivy extract in a 35 per cent aqueous-alcoholic menstruum, with 4 per cent benzyl alcohol to reduce pain of injection; pH adjusted with lactic acid.

Indications: For prophylaxis and treatment of rhus dermatitis.

Precautions: Attention is directed to reports that renal complications may follow extensive dermatitis of various types, and that with severe rhus dermatitis there may be an aggravation of symptoms following administration of poison ivy extract.

Dosage and Administration: Specific Treatment of Rhus Dermatitis—1 ml. intramuscularly every 12 to 24 hours until symptoms are controlled. A minimum of four injections is recommended even if symptoms are alleviated within a few hours; the tendency to future attacks will be lessened. Children usually tolerate the same dose as adults.

Prophylactic Treatment—Susceptible persons can usually be protected against attacks of rhus dermatitis for a season or longer by preseasonal injections of RHUS TOX ANTIGEN. Dose: 1 ml. intramuscularly every 4 to 7 days for four or more injections. In very sensitive individuals it may be advisable to start with a smaller dose—0.25 to 0.5 ml.—and increase the dose gradually to 1 ml., giving a total of 4 ml. or more.

Note: The patient usually complains of a burning sensation at site of the injection. This is due to the alcohol and disappears in a few seconds. In some individuals, localized soreness or a dull ache may be noted for 24 to 48 hours.

How Supplied: Boxes of four 1 ml. vials. Refrigeration not required. Full prescribing information is available on request (NDC 0093-0401).

VAGILIA® Cream/Suppositories ℞

Composition: Vagilia Cream contains:

Sulfisoxazole	10.0%
Aminacrine Hydrochloride	0.2%
Allantoin	2.0%

in a water-miscible base made from stearic acid, mineral oil, polysorbate 60, sorbitan mon-

ostearate, sorbitol, methylparaben, propylparaben, and purified water.
Each Vagilia Suppository contains:
Sulfisoxazole .... 600 mg
Aminacrine Hydrochloride .... 12 mg
Allantoin .... 120 mg
with lactose, in a base made from polyethylene glycol 400, polyethylene glycol 3350, glycerin and polysorbate 80; buffered with lactic acid to an acid pH. The inert covering of the suppositories consists of gelatin, glycerin, water, methylparaben, propylparaben, and coloring. It dissolves promptly in the vagina.

Actions: Vagilia is designed to provide in one preparation treatment for a variety of infections of the vaginal tract. It combines the bacteriostatic effect of sulfisoxazole with the antibacterial-antifungal action of aminacrine hydrochloride. Sulfisoxazole is believed to block certain metabolic processes essential for the growth of susceptible bacteria. Aminacrine hydrochloride is thought to act by interfering or competing with hydrogen ions in microbial enzyme systems.
Allantoin is included to help liquefy pus and accelerate healing. The active ingredients are combined in a specially compounded base which provides an environment hostile to the invading organisms and favors eventual restoration of acid-producing organisms normally present in the vagina.

Indications: For the treatment of *Hemophilus vaginalis* vaginitis.

> Based on a review of this drug by the National Academy of Sciences—National Research Council and/or other information, FDA has classified the indications as follows:
> "Probably" effective: For the relief of symptoms of vulvovaginitis where isolation of the specific organism responsible (usually *Trichomonas vaginalis* or *Candida albicans*) is not possible.
> NOTE: When the offending organism is known, treatment with a specific agent known to be active against that microorganism is preferred.
> "Possibly" effective: For the treatment of trichomoniasis, vulvovaginal candidiasis, and vaginitis due to susceptible bacteria.
> Final classification of the less-than-effective indications requires further investigation.

Contraindications: Vagilia should not be used in patients known to be sensitive to sulfonamides.

Precautions: As with all sulfonamides, the usual precautions apply. Patients should be observed for manifestations such as skin rash or other evidence of systemic toxicity, and if these develop, the medication should be discontinued.
Vaginal applicators should not be used after the seventh month of pregnancy.

Adverse Reactions: Although some absorption of sulfisoxazole may occur through the vaginal mucosa, systemic manifestations attributable to this drug are infrequent. Local sensitivity reactions such as increased discomfort or a burning sensation have occasionally been reported following the use of topical sulfonamides. Treatment should be discontinued if either local or systemic manifestations of sulfonamide toxicity or sensitivity occur.

Dosage and Administration: One applicatorful (approximately 6 Gm) or 1 suppository intravaginally once or twice daily. Improvements in symptoms occur within a few days, but treatment should be continued through one complete menstrual cycle unless a definite diagnosis is made and specific therapy initiated.
If there is no response within a few days or if symptoms recur, Vagilia should be discontinued and another attempt made by appropriate laboratory methods to isolate the organism responsible (*Trichomonas vaginalis* or *Candida albicans*) and institute specific therapy.
Douching with a suitable solution before insertion may be recommended for hygienic purposes. A pad may be used to protect underclothing if necessary.

How Supplied: Cream (yellow) in 90 Gm tubes with reusable applicator. Store at room temperature (NDC 0093-0015). Suppositories (orange) in boxes of 16 with inserter. Store at room temperature; avoid excessive heat (NDC 0093-0315).

[Shown in Product Identification Section]

Eli Lilly and Company
307 E. McCARTY ST.
INDIANAPOLIS, IN 46285

LEGEND

Aspirol®—*Inhalant in an Ampoule, Lilly*
Disket®—*Dispersible Tablet, Lilly*
Enseal®—*Enteric-Release Tablet, Lilly*
Faspak™—*Flexible Plastic Bag, Lilly*
Gelseal®—*Filled Elastic Capsule, Lilly*
Hyporet®—*Disposable Syringe, Lilly*
Identi-Code®—*Formula Identification Code, Lilly*
Identi-Dose®—*Unit Dose Medication, Lilly*
Pulvule®—*Filled Gelatin Capsule, Lilly*
Redi Vial®—*Dual Compartment Vial, Lilly*
℞Pak—*Prescription Package, Lilly*
Solvet®—*Soluble Tablet, Lilly*
Traypak™—*Multivial Carton, Lilly*

IDENTI-CODE® Index

Illustrations of examples of products bearing Identi-Code® appear in Product Identification Section.

Identi-Code® **Product Name**

A01-A36 (Enseals®)

A01 **Ammonium Chloride**
Composition (Each Enseal®): Ammonium Chloride, USP, 7½ grs (500 mg)
A02 **Ferrous Sulfate**
Composition (Each Enseal®): Ferrous Sulfate, USP, 5 grs (325 mg) (equiv. to 65 mg elemental iron), Red
A04 **Pancreatin**
Composition (Each Enseal®): Pancreatin, Triple Strength, equivalent to 1 g Pancreatin, USP
A05 **Potassium Chloride**
Composition (Each Enseal®): Potassium chloride, 300 mg (5 grs)
A06 **Potassium Iodide**
Composition (Each Enseal®): Potassium Iodide, USP, 300 mg (5 grs)
A09 **Sodium Chloride**
Composition (Each Enseal®): Sodium Chloride, USP, 15½ grs (1 g)
A10 **Sodium Salicylate**
Composition (Each Enseal®): Sodium Salicylate, USP, 5 grs (325 mg)
A11 **Sodium Salicylate**
Composition (Each Enseal®): Sodium Salicylate, USP, 10 grs (650 mg)
A12 **Ammonium Chloride**
Composition (Each Enseal®): Ammonium Chloride, USP, 15 grs (1 g)
A14 **Thyroid**
Composition (Each Enseal®): Thyroid, USP, 30 mg (½ gr)
A15 **Thyroid**
Composition (Each Enseal®): Thyroid, USP, 60 mg (1 gr)
A16 **Thyroid**
Composition (Each Enseal®): Thyroid, USP, 120 mg (2 grs)
A17 **Thyroid**
Composition (Each Enseal®): Thyroid, USP, 200 mg (3 grs)
A19 **Diethylstilbestrol**
Composition (Each Enseal®): Diethylstilbestrol, USP, 0.1 mg
A20 **Diethylstilbestrol**
Composition (Each Enseal®): Diethylstilbestrol, USP, 0.25 mg
A21 **Diethylstilbestrol**
Composition (Each Enseal®): Diethylstilbestrol, USP, 0.5 mg
A22 **Diethylstilbestrol**
Composition (Each Enseal®): Diethylstilbestrol, USP, 1 mg
A24 **Seconal® Sodium**
Composition (Each Enseal®): Secobarbital sodium, 100 mg (1½ grs)
A25 **A.S.A.®**
Composition (Each Enseal®): Aspirin, USP, 5 grs (325 mg)
A26 **Ox Bile Extract**
Composition (Each Enseal®): Ox bile extract, 5 grs (325 mg)
A27 **Amesec®**
Composition (Each Enseal®): Aminophylline, 130 mg; ephedrine hydrochloride, 25 mg; amobarbital, 25 mg
A30 **Aminosalicylic Acid**
Composition (Each Enseal®): Aminosalicylic Acid, USP, 500 mg (7½ grs)
A31 **Potassium Chloride**
Composition (Each Enseal®): Potassium chloride, 1 g (15 grs)
A32 **A.S.A.®**
Composition (Each Enseal®): Aspirin, USP, 10 grs (650 mg)
A33 **Diethylstilbestrol**
Composition (Each Enseal®): Diethylstilbestrol, USP, 5 mg
A36 **Ferrous Sulfate**
Composition (Each Enseal®): Ferrous Sulfate, USP, 5 grs (325 mg) (equiv. to 65 mg elemental iron), Green

C06-C71 (Coated Tablets)

C06 **Cascara**
Composition (Each Coated Tablet): Cascara, USP, 5 grs (325 mg)
C07 **Cascara Compound**
Composition (Each Coated Tablet): Ext. cascara, 16 mg; aloin, 16 mg.; podophyllum resin, 10 mg; ext. belladonna, 8 mg (total alkaloids, 0.1 mg); oleoresin ginger, 4 mg
C09 **Digiglusin®**
Composition (Each Coated Tablet): Digitalis glucosides, 1 USP digitalis unit
C11 **Rhinitis, Full Strength**
Composition (Each Coated Tablet): Camphor, 32.5 mg; quinine sulfate, 32.5 mg; ext. belladonna leaf, 5.8 mg (total alkaloids, 1/960 gr)
C13 **Ferrous Sulfate**
Composition (Each Coated Tablet): Ferrous Sulfate, USP, 5 grs (325 mg) (equiv. to 65 mg elemental iron)
C15 **Menadione**
Composition (Each Coated Tablet): Menadione, USP, 5 mg
C16 **Pagitane® Hydrochloride**
Composition (Each Coated Tablet): Cycrimine Hydrochloride, USP, 1.25 mg

Continued on next page

*Identi-Code® symbol.

Lilly—Cont.

C17 Pagitane® Hydrochloride
Composition (Each Coated Tablet): Cycrimine Hydrochloride, USP, 2.5 mg

C27 V-Cillin K®
Composition (Each Coated Tablet): Penicillin V Potassium, USP, 125 mg

C29 V-Cillin K®
Composition (Each Coated Tablet): Penicillin V Potassium, USP, 250 mg

C36 Quinine Sulfate
Composition (Each Coated Tablet): Quinine Sulfate, USP, 5 grs (325 mg)

C46 V-Cillin K®
Composition (Each Coated Tablet): Penicillin V Potassium, USP, 500 mg

C47 Hepicebrin®
Composition (Each Coated Tablet): Vitamin A acetate, 5000 IU (1.5 mg); vitamin D (as ergocalciferol), 400 IU (10 mcg); ascorbic acid (vitamin C), 75 mg; thiamine mononitrate (vitamin B_1), 2 mg; riboflavin (vitamin B_2), 3 mg; niacinamide, 20 mg; (USP)

C51 Darvocet-N® 50
Composition (Each Coated Tablet): Propoxyphene napsylate, 50 mg; acetaminophen, 325 mg (USP)

C53 Darvon-N®
Composition (Each Coated Tablet): Propoxyphene Napsylate, USP, 100 mg

C54 Darvon-N® with A.S.A.®
Composition (Each Coated Tablet): Propoxyphene napsylate, 100 mg; aspirin, 325 mg (USP)

C63 Darvocet-N® 100
Composition (Each Coated Tablet): Propoxyphene napsylate, 100 mg; acetaminophen, 650 mg (USP)

C71 Multicebrin®
Composition (Each Coated Tablet): Thiamine (vitamin B_1), 3 mg; riboflavin (vitamin B_2), 3 mg; pyridoxine (vitamin B_6), 1.2 mg; pantothenic acid, 5 mg; niacinamide, 25 mg; vitamin B_{12} (activity equivalent), 3 mcg; ascorbic acid (vitamin C), 75 mg; *dl*-alpha tocopheryl acetate (vitamin E), 6.6 IU (6.6 mg); vitamin A, 10,000 IU (3 mg); vitamin D, 400 IU (10 mcg)

F03-H72 (Pulvules®)

F03 Zentinic®
Composition (Each Pulvule®): Iron, elemental (as ferrous fumarate), 100 mg; folic acid, 0.05 mg; thiamine mononitrate (vitamin B_1), 7.5 mg; riboflavin (vitamin B_2), 7.5 mg; pyridoxine hydrochloride (vitamin B_6), 7.5 mg; vitamin B_{12} (activity equivalent), 50 mcg; pantothenic acid (as calcium pantothenate), 15 mg; niacinamide, 30 mg; ascorbic acid (vitamin C), 200 mg

F04 Seromycin®
Composition (Each Pulvule®): Cycloserine, USP, 250 mg

F10 Amytal® and Aspirin
Composition (Each Pulvule®): Amobarbital, 50 mg; aspirin, 325 mg

F11 A.S.A.®
Composition (Each Pulvule®): Aspirin, USP, 5 grs (325 mg), Clear

F12 A.S.A.®
Composition (Each Pulvule®): Aspirin, USP, 5 grs (325 mg), Pink

F13 A.S.A.® Compound
Composition (Each Pulvule®): Aspirin, 227 mg; phenacetin, 160 mg; caffeine, 32.5 mg; White Opaque

F14 Ephedrine and Amytal®
Composition (Each Pulvule®): Ephedrine sulfate, 25 mg; amobarbital, 50 mg

F15 Lextron®
Composition (Each Pulvule®): Liver-stomach concentrate (as intrinsic powder), 50 mg; iron, elemental (as iron and ammonium citrates green), 30 mg; vitamin B_{12} (activity equivalent), 2 mcg; thiamine hydrochloride (vitamin B_1), 1 mg; riboflavin (vitamin B_2), 0.25 mg; with other factors of vitamin B complex present in the liver-stomach concentrate

F16 Lextron® Ferrous
Composition (Each Pulvule®): Liver-stomach concentrate (as intrinsic powder), 50 mg; iron, elemental (as ferrous sulfate), 35 mg; vitamin B_{12} (activity equivalent), 2 mcg; thiamine hydrochloride (vitamin B_1), 1 mg; riboflavin (vitamin B_2), 0.25 mg; with other factors of vitamin B complex present in the liver-stomach concentrate

F19 Extralin®
Composition (Each Pulvule®): Liver-stomach concentrate (as intrinsic powder), 50 mg

F20 Ephedrine and Seconal® Sodium
Composition (Each Pulvule®): Ephedrine sulfate, 25 mg; secobarbital sodium, 50 mg

F21 Extralin® B
Composition (Each Pulvule®): Liver-stomach concentrate (as intrinsic powder), 67 mg; vitamin B_{12} (activity equivalent), 3 mcg; thiamine hydrochloride (vitamin B_1), 1 mg; riboflavin (vitamin B_2), 0.25 mg; with other factors of vitamin B complex present in the liver-stomach concentrate

F22 Lextron® F. G.
Composition (Each Pulvule®): Liver-stomach concentrate (as intrinsic powder), 50 mg; iron, elemental (as ferrous gluconate), 20 mg; vitamin B_{12} (activity equivalent), 2 mcg; thiamine hydrochloride (vitamin B_1), 1 mg; riboflavin (vitamin B_2), 0.25 mg; with other factors of vitamin B complex present in the liver-stomach concentrate

F23 Amytal® Sodium
Composition (Each Pulvule®): Amobarbital Sodium, USP, 65 mg (1 gr)

F24 Ephedrine Sulfate
Composition (Each Pulvule®): Ephedrine Sulfate, USP, 25 mg (3/8 gr)

F25 Ephedrine Sulfate
Composition (Each Pulvule®): Ephedrine Sulfate, USP, 50 mg (3/4 gr)

F26 Quinine Sulfate
Composition (Each Pulvule®): Quinine Sulfate, USP, 2 grs (130 mg)

F27 Quinine Sulfate
Composition (Each Pulvule®): Quinine Sulfate, USP, 3 grs (200 mg)

F29 Quinine Sulfate
Composition (Each Pulvule®): Quinine Sulfate, USP, 5 grs (325 mg)

F30 A.S.A.® Compound
Composition (Each Pulvule®): Aspirin, 227 mg; phenacetin, 160 mg; caffeine, 32.5 mg; Pink

F31 Acidulin®
Composition (Each Pulvule®): Glutamic acid hydrochloride, 340 mg

F32 Digitalis
Composition (Each Pulvule®): Digitalis, USP, 100 mg (1 1/2 grs)

F33 Amytal® Sodium
Composition (Each Pulvule®): Amobarbital Sodium, USP, 200 mg (3 grs)

F34 Carbarsone
Composition (Each Pulvule®): Carbarsone, USP, 250 mg (4 grs)

F36 Copavin®
Composition (Each Pulvule®): Codeine sulfate, 15 mg; papaverine hydrochloride, 15 mg

F39 Quinidine Sulfate
Composition (Each Pulvule®): Quinidine Sulfate, USP, 200 mg (3 grs)

F40 Seconal® Sodium
Composition (Each Pulvule®): Secobarbital Sodium, USP, 100 mg (1 1/2 grs)

F41 Bilron®
Composition (Each Pulvule®): Iron bile salts, 300 mg (5 grs)

F42 Seconal® Sodium
Composition (Each Pulvule®): Secobarbital Sodium, USP, 50 mg (3/4 gr)

F43 Vitamin B Complex (Betalin® Compound)
Composition (Each Pulvule®): Thiamine (vitamin B_1), 1 mg; riboflavin (vitamin B_2), 2 mg; pyridoxine (vitamin B_6), 0.4 mg; pantothenic acid, 3.333 mg; niacinamide, 10 mg; vitamin B_{12} (activity equivalent), 1 mcg

F44 Ferrous Gluconate
Composition (Each Pulvule®): Ferrous Gluconate, USP, 5 grs (325 mg)

F45 Epragen™
Composition (Each Pulvule®): Ephedrine hydrochloride, 22 mg; aspirin, 130 mg; phenacetin, 227 mg; amobarbital, 50 mg

F46 Aminophylline and Amytal®
Composition (Each Pulvule®): Aminophylline, 100 mg; amobarbital, 32 mg

F47 Amesec®
Composition (Each Pulvule®): Aminophylline, 130 mg; ephedrine hydrochloride, 25 mg; amobarbital, 25 mg

F50 A.S.A.® and Codeine Compound, No. 2
Composition (Each Pulvule®): Codeine phosphate, 15 mg; phenacetin, 150 mg; aspirin, 230 mg; caffeine, 30 mg

F51 A.S.A.® and Codeine Compound, No. 3
Composition (Each Pulvule®): Codeine phosphate, 30 mg; phenacetin, 150 mg; aspirin, 230 mg; caffeine, 30 mg

F52 Dibasic Calcium Phosphate with Vitamin D
Composition (Each Pulvule®): Dibasic calcium phosphate, anhydrous, equivalent to 500 mg of dibasic calcium phosphate dihydrate; vitamin D synthetic, 33 IU (0.825 mcg)

F53 Trisogel®
Composition (Each Pulvule®): Magnesium trisilicate, 4 1/2 grs; aluminum hydroxide gel, desiccated, 1 1/2 grs

F54 Dicumarol
Composition (Each Pulvule®): Dicumarol, USP, 50 mg

F56 Calcium Gluconate with Vitamin D
Composition (Each Pulvule®): Calcium gluconate, 325 mg; vitamin D synthetic, 0.825 mcg

F61 Bilron®
Composition (Each Pulvule®): Iron bile salts, 150 mg (2 1/2 grs)

F63 Dibasic Calcium Phosphate with Vitamin D and Iron
Composition (Each Pulvule®): Dibasic calcium phosphate, anhydrous, equivalent to 500 mg of dibasic calcium phosphate dihydrate; vitamin D, 33 IU (0.825 mcg); iron (as iron pyrophosphate), 10 mg

F64 **Tuinal®**
Composition (Each Pulvule®): Secobarbital sodium, 25 mg; amobarbital sodium, 25 mg (USP)

F65 **Tuinal®**
Composition (Each Pulvule®): Secobarbital sodium, 50 mg; amobarbital sodium, 50 mg (USP)

F66 **Tuinal®**
Composition (Each Pulvule®): Secobarbital sodium, 100 mg; amobarbital sodium, 100 mg (USP)

F67 **A.S.A.® and Codeine Compound, No. 4**
Composition (Each Pulvule®): Codeine phosphate, 60 mg; phenacetin, 150 mg; aspirin, 230 mg; caffeine, 30 mg

F71 **Dicumarol**
Composition (Each Pulvule®): Dicumarol, USP, 25 mg

F72 **Seconal® Sodium**
Composition (Each Pulvule®): Secobarbital Sodium, USP, 30 mg (½ gr)

F74 **Tycopan®**
Composition: Three Pulvules® contain thiamine mononitrate (vitamin B_1), 10 mg; riboflavin (vitamin B_2), 8 mg; pyridoxine hydrochloride (vitamin B_6), 10 mg; pantothenic acid (as calcium pantothenate), 60 mg; niacinamide, 60 mg; vitamin B_{12} (activity equivalent), 15 mcg; ascorbic acid (vitamin C), 200 mg; *dl*-alpha tocopheryl acetate (vitamin E), 22 IU (22 mg); biotin, 0.16 mg; folic acid, 0.45 mg; aminobenzoic acid, 33 mg; inositol, 160 mg; choline (as choline bitartrate), 160 mg; lipoic acid, 0.3 mg; vitamin A synthetic, 20,000 IU (6 mg); vitamin D synthetic, 1000 IU (25 mcg)

F92 **Extralin® F**
Composition (Each Pulvule®): Special Liver-Stomach Concentrate, Lilly (containing intrinsic factor), 390 mg; Cobalamin Concentrate, USP, equivalent to cobalamin, 15 mcg (the total vitamin B_{12} activity in the Special Liver-Stomach Concentrate, Lilly, and the Cobalamin Concentrate, USP, is 30 mcg); folic acid, 1 mg

F96 **Reticulex®**
Composition (Each Pulvule®): Liver-stomach concentrate (as intrinsic powder), 222 mg; vitamin B_{12} (activity equivalent), 10 mcg; iron, elemental (as ferrous sulfate), 75 mg; ascorbic acid (vitamin C), 50 mg; folic acid, 0.3 mg

---

G01 **Vitamin A (Alphalin®)**
Composition (Each Pulvule®): Vitamin A synthetic (palmitate), 10,000 IU (3 mg)

H02 **Darvon®**
Composition (Each Pulvule®): Propoxyphene Hydrochloride, USP, 32 mg

H03 **Darvon®**
Composition (Each Pulvule®): Propoxyphene Hydrochloride, USP, 65 mg

H04 **Darvon® with A.S.A.®**
Composition (Each Pulvule®): Propoxyphene hydrochloride, 65 mg; aspirin, 325 mg

H05 **Darvon® Compound**
Composition (Each Pulvule®): Propoxyphene hydrochloride, 32 mg; aspirin, 389 mg; caffeine, 32.4 mg

H06 **Darvon® Compound-65**
Composition (Each Pulvule®): Propoxyphene hydrochloride, 65 mg; aspirin, 389 mg; caffeine, 32.4 mg

H10 **En-Cebrin® F**
Composition (Each Pulvule®): Vitamin A synthetic, 4000 IU (1.2 mg); thiamine mononitrate (vitamin B_1), 3 mg; riboflavin (vitamin B_2), 2 mg; niacinamide, 10 mg; pyridoxine hydrochloride (vitamin B_6), 2 mg; folic acid, 1 mg; vitamin B_{12} (activity equivalent), 5 mcg; pantothenic acid (as calcium pantothenate), 5 mg; ascorbic acid (vitamin C), 50 mg; vitamin D synthetic, 400 IU (10 mcg); calcium (as the carbonate), 250 mg; iron (as ferrous fumarate), 30 mg; iodine (as potassium iodide), 0.15 mg; copper (as the sulfate), 1 mg; magnesium (as the hydroxide), 5 mg; manganese (as the glycerophosphate), 1 mg; zinc (as the chloride), 1.5 mg

H12 **En-Cebrin®**
Composition (Each Pulvule®): Vitamin A, 4000 IU (1.2 mg); thiamine mononitrate (vitamin B_1), 3 mg; riboflavin (vitamin B_2), 2 mg; niacinamide, 10 mg; pyridoxine (vitamin B_6), 1.7 mg; vitamin B_{12} (activity equivalent), 5 mcg; pantothenic acid, 5 mg; ascorbic acid (vitamin C), 50 mg; vitamin D, 400 IU (10 mcg); calcium (as the carbonate), 250 mg; iron (as ferrous fumarate), 30 mg; iodine (as potassium iodide), 0.15 mg; copper (as the sulfate), 1 mg; magnesium (as the hydroxide), 5 mg; manganese (as the glycerophosphate), 1 mg; zinc (as the chloride), 1.5 mg

H14 **Novrad®**
Composition (Each Pulvule®): Levopropoxyphene Napsylate, USP, 100 mg (equivalent to levopropoxyphene)

H17 **Aventyl® HCl**
Composition (Each Pulvule®): Nortriptyline Hydrochloride, USP, 10 mg (equiv. to base)

H19 **Aventyl® HCl**
Composition (Each Pulvule®): Nortriptyline Hydrochloride, USP, 25 mg (equiv. to base)

H66 **Kafocin®**
Composition (Each Pulvule®): Cephaloglycin, USP, 250 mg

H69 **Keflex®**
Composition (Each Pulvule®): Cephalexin, USP, 250 mg

H71 **Keflex®**
Composition (Each Pulvule®): Cephalexin, USP, 500 mg

H72 **Theracebrin®**
Composition (Each Pulvule®): Thiamine (as the mononitrate) (vitamin B_1), 15 mg; riboflavin (vitamin B_2), 10 mg; pyridoxine (as the hydrochloride) (vitamin B_6), 2.5 mg; pantothenic acid (as *d*-calcium pantothenate), 20 mg; niacinamide, 150 mg; vitamin B_{12} (activity equivalent), 10 mcg; ascorbic acid (vitamin C), 150 mg; *dl*-alpha tocopheryl acetate (vitamin E), 18.5 IU (18.5 mg); vitamin A synthetic, 25,000 IU (7.5 mg); vitamin D synthetic, 1500 IU (37.5 mcg)

3061 **Ceclor®**
Composition (Each Pulvule®): Cefaclor, USP, 250 mg

3062 **Ceclor®**
Composition (Each Pulvule®): Cefaclor, USP, 500 mg

3074 **Hista-Clopane®**
Composition (Each Pulvule®): Chlorpheniramine maleate, 4 mg; cyclopentamine hydrochloride, 12.5 mg

3075 **Histadyl® and A.S.A.®**
Composition (Each Pulvule®): Chlorpheniramine maleate, 4 mg; aspirin, 325 mg

---

J02-J99 (Compressed Tablets)

J02 **Atropine Sulfate**
Composition (Each Compressed Tablet): Atropine Sulfate, USP, 0.4 mg (1/150 gr)

J03 **Belladonna Extract**
Composition (Each Compressed Tablet): Belladonna Extract, USP, 15 mg (¼ gr) (total alkaloids, 0.187 mg)

J04 **Bismuth Subcarbonate**
Composition (Each Compressed Tablet): Bismuth subcarbonate, 5 grs (325 mg)

J05 **Citrated Caffeine**
Composition (Each Compressed Tablet): Citrated caffeine, 1 gr (65 mg)

J09 **Codeine Sulfate**
Composition (Each Compressed Tablet): Codeine Sulfate, USP, 15 mg (¼ gr)

J10 **Codeine Sulfate**
Composition (Each Compressed Tablet): Codeine Sulfate, USP, 30 mg (½ gr)

J11 **Codeine Sulfate**
Composition (Each Compressed Tablet): Codeine Sulfate, USP, 60 mg (1 gr)

J13 **Colchicine**
Composition (Each Compressed Tablet): Colchicine, USP, 0.6 mg (1/100 gr)

J20 **Quinidine Sulfate**
Composition (Each Compressed Tablet): Quinidine Sulfate, USP, 200 mg (3 grs)

J23 **Soda Mint**
Composition (Each Compressed Tablet): Sodium bicarbonate, 5 grs; oil peppermint

J24 **Sodium Bicarbonate**
Composition (Each Compressed Tablet): Sodium Bicarbonate, USP, 5 grs (325 mg)

J25 **Thyroid**
Composition (Each Compressed Tablet): Thyroid, USP, 60 mg (1 gr)

J26 **Thyroid**
Composition (Each Compressed Tablet): Thyroid, USP, 120 mg (2 grs)

J29 **Thyroid**
Composition (Each Compressed Tablet): Thyroid, USP, 30 mg (½ gr)

J30 **Thyroid**
Composition (Each Compressed Tablet): Thyroid, USP, 15 mg (¼ gr)

J31 **Phenobarbital**
Composition (Each Compressed Tablet): Phenobarbital, USP, 15 mg (¼ gr)

J32 **Phenobarbital**
Composition (Each Compressed Tablet): Phenobarbital, USP, 30 mg (½ gr)

J33 **Phenobarbital**
Composition (Each Compressed Tablet): Phenobarbital, USP, 100 mg (1½ grs)

J34 **Copavin®**
Composition (Each Compressed Tablet): Codeine sulfate, 15 mg; papaverine hydrochloride, 15 mg

Continued on next page

*Identi-Code® symbol.

Lilly—Cont.

J36 Ergotrate® Maleate
Composition (Each Compressed Tablet): Ergonovine Maleate, USP, 0.2 mg (1/300 gr)

J37 Phenobarbital
Composition (Each Compressed Tablet): Phenobarbital, USP, 60 mg (1 gr)

J41 Niacin
Composition (Each Compressed Tablet): Niacin, USP, 20 mg

J42 Niacin
Composition (Each Compressed Tablet): Niacin, USP, 100 mg

J43 Niacin
Composition (Each Compressed Tablet): Niacin, USP, 50 mg

J45 Pyridoxine Hydrochloride (Hexa-Betalin®)
Composition (Each Compressed Tablet): Pyridoxine Hydrochloride, USP, 25 mg

J46 Niacinamide
Composition (Each Compressed Tablet): Niacinamide, USP, 50 mg

J47 Riboflavin
Composition (Each Compressed Tablet): Riboflavin, USP, 5 mg

J49 Diethylstilbestrol
Composition (Each Compressed Tablet): Diethylstilbestrol, USP, 0.1 mg

J50 Diethylstilbestrol
Composition (Each Compressed Tablet): Diethylstilbestrol, USP, 0.25 mg

J51 Diethylstilbestrol
Composition (Each Compressed Tablet): Diethylstilbestrol, USP, 0.5 mg

J52 Diethylstilbestrol
Composition (Each Compressed Tablet): Diethylstilbestrol, USP, 1 mg

J53 Pantholin®
Composition (Each Compressed Tablet): Calcium Pantothenate, USP, 10 mg

J54 Diethylstilbestrol
Composition (Each Compressed Tablet): Diethylstilbestrol, USP, 5 mg

J55 Phenobarbital and Belladonna, No. 1
Composition (Each Compressed Tablet): Phenobarbital, 30 mg; ext. belladonna, 8 mg (total alkaloids, 0.1 mg)

J56 Pyridoxine Hydrochloride (Hexa-Betalin®)
Composition (Each Compressed Tablet): Pyridoxine Hydrochloride, USP, 10 mg

J57 Crystodigin®
Composition (Each Compressed Tablet): Digitoxin, USP, 0.2 mg

J59 Phenobarbital and Belladonna, No. 2
Composition (Each Compressed Tablet): Phenobarbital, 15 mg; ext. belladonna, 4 mg (total alkaloids, 0.05 mg)

J60 Crystodigin®
Composition (Each Compressed Tablet): Digitoxin, USP, 0.1 mg

J61 Papaverine Hydrochloride
Composition (Each Compressed Tablet): Papaverine Hydrochloride, USP, 30 mg (½ gr)

J62 Papaverine Hydrochloride
Composition (Each Compressed Tablet): Papaverine Hydrochloride, USP, 60 mg (1 gr)

J63 Riboflavin
Composition (Each Compressed Tablet): Riboflavin, USP, 10 mg

J64 Dolophine® Hydrochloride
Composition (Each Compressed Tablet): Methadone Hydrochloride, USP, 5 mg

J69 Propylthiouracil
Composition (Each Compressed Tablet): Propylthiouracil, USP, 50 mg

J70 Phenobarbital and Belladonna, No. 3
Composition (Each Compressed Tablet): Phenobarbital, 15 mg; ext. belladonna, 8 mg (total alkaloids, 0.1 mg)

J72 Dolophine® Hydrochloride
Composition (Each Compressed Tablet): Methadone Hydrochloride, USP, 10 mg

J73 Methyltestosterone
Composition (Each Compressed Tablet): Methyltestosterone, USP, 10 mg

J74 Methyltestosterone
Composition (Each Compressed Tablet): Methyltestosterone, USP, 25 mg

J75 Crystodigin®
Composition (Each Compressed Tablet): Digitoxin, USP, 0.05 mg

J76 Crystodigin®
Composition (Each Compressed Tablet): Digitoxin, USP, 0.15 mg

J94 Tapazole®
Composition (Each Compressed Tablet): Methimazole, USP, 5 mg

J95 Tapazole®
Composition (Each Compressed Tablet): Methimazole, USP, 10 mg

J96 Tylosterone®
Composition (Each Compressed Tablet): Diethylstilbestrol, 0.25 mg; methyltestosterone, 5 mg

J97 Paveril® Phosphate
Composition (Each Compressed Tablet): Dioxyline phosphate, 100 mg (1½ grs)

J99 Sandril®
Composition (Each Compressed Tablet): Reserpine, USP, 0.1 mg

S04-S17 (Suppositories)

S04 Metycaine® Hydrochloride and Zinc Oxide Compound
Composition (Each Suppository): Piperocaine hydrochloride, 125 mg; extract belladonna, 12.5 mg (total alkaloids, 0.15 mg); bismuth subcarbonate, 125 mg; zinc oxide, 250 mg

S05 Seconal® Sodium
Composition (Each Suppository): Secobarbital sodium, 120 mg

S07 Diethylstilbestrol
Composition (Each Suppository): Diethylstilbestrol, USP, 0.1 mg

S09 Diethylstilbestrol
Composition (Each Suppository): Diethylstilbestrol, USP, 0.5 mg

S11 Seconal® Sodium
Composition (Each Suppository): Secobarbital sodium, 200 mg

S13 Surfacaine®
Composition (Each Suppository): Cyclomethycaine Sulfate, USP, 10 mg

S14 Seconal® Sodium
Composition (Each Suppository): Secobarbital sodium, 60 mg

S15 A.S.A.®
Composition (Each Suppository): Aspirin, USP, 5 grs (325 mg)

S16 A.S.A.®
Composition (Each Suppository): Aspirin, USP, 10 grs (650 mg)

S17 Seconal® Sodium
Composition (Each Suppository): Secobarbital sodium, 30 mg

T01-U60 (Compressed Tablets)

T01 Zentron® Chewable
Composition (Each Compressed Tablet): Iron, elemental (as ferrous fumarate), 20 mg; thiamine mononitrate (vitamin B_1), 1 mg; riboflavin (vitamin B_2), 1 mg; pyridoxine hydrochloride (vitamin B_6), 1 mg; cyanocobalamin (vitamin B_{12} crystalline), 5 mcg; pantothenic acid (as panthenol), 1 mg; niacinamide, 5 mg; ascorbic acid (vitamin C), 100 mg

T02 Novacebrin® Chewable
Composition (Each Compressed Tablet): Vitamin A, 4000 IU (1.2 mg); vitamin D, 400 IU (10 mcg); ascorbic acid (vitamin C), 60 mg; thiamine mononitrate (vitamin B_1), 1.5 mg; riboflavin (vitamin B_2), 2 mg; pyridoxine (vitamin B_6), 0.8 mg; vitamin B_{12} (activity equivalent), 3 mcg; niacinamide, 12 mg; pantothenic acid, 2.5 mg

T03 Novacebrin® c̄ Fluoride Chewable
Composition (Each Compressed Tablet): Fluoride (as sodium fluoride), 1 mg; vitamin A, 4000 IU (1.2 mg); vitamin D, 400 IU (10 mcg); vitamin C (as sodium ascorbate and ascorbic acid), 60 mg; thiamine mononitrate (vitamin B_1), 1.5 mg; riboflavin (vitamin B_2), 2 mg; pyridoxine hydrochloride (vitamin B_6), 1 mg; cyanocobalamin (vitamin B_{12}), 3 mcg; niacinamide, 12 mg; pantothenic acid (as panthenol), 2.5 mg

T04 Antiseptic No. 3, R. St. J. Perry
Composition (Each Compressed Tablet): Mercury cyanide, 0.5 g; sodium borate, 0.97 g

T05 A.S.A.®
Composition (Each Compressed Tablet): Aspirin, USP, 5 grs (325 mg)

T06 A.S.A.®
Composition (Each Compressed Tablet): Aspirin, USP, 5 grs (325 mg), Pink

T07 A.S.A.® Compound
Composition (Each Compressed Tablet): Aspirin, 227 mg; phenacetin, 160 mg; caffeine, 32.5 mg

T13 Calcium Lactate
Composition (Each Compressed Tablet): Calcium Lactate, USP, 5 grs (325 mg)

T14 Calcium Lactate
Composition (Each Compressed Tablet): Calcium Lactate, USP, 10 grs (650 mg)

T17 Diamond® Antiseptics
Composition (Each Compressed Tablet): Mercury bichloride, 475 mg

T20 Methenamine
Composition (Each Compressed Tablet): Methenamine, USP, 7½ grs (500 mg)

T21 Methenamine and Sodium Biphosphate
Composition (Each Compressed Tablet): Methenamine, 325 mg; sodium biphosphate, 325 mg; (USP)

T23 Sodium Chloride
Composition (Each Compressed Tablet): Sodium Chloride, USP, 2.25 g

T24 Sodium Chloride
Composition (Each Compressed Tablet): Sodium Chloride, USP, 1 g

T26 Pancreatin
Composition (Each Compressed Tablet): Pancreatin, Single Strength, equivalent to 325 mg Pancreatin, USP

T29 Sodium Bicarbonate
Composition (Each Compressed Tablet): Sodium Bicarbonate, USP, 10 grs (650 mg)

T32 **Amytal®**
Composition (Each Compressed Tablet): Amobarbital, USP, 100 mg ($1\frac{1}{2}$ grs)

T35 **Calcium Carbonate**
Composition (Each Compressed Tablet): Calcium Carbonate, USP, Aromatic, 10 grs (650 mg)

T36 **Calcium Gluconate**
Composition (Each Compressed Tablet): Calcium Gluconate, USP, 1 g ($15\frac{1}{2}$ grs)

T37 **Amytal®**
Composition (Each Compressed Tablet): Amobarbital, USP, 50 mg ($\frac{3}{4}$ gr)

T39 **Calcium Gluconate**
Composition (Each Compressed Tablet): Calcium Gluconate, USP, $7\frac{1}{2}$ grs (500 mg)

T40 **Amytal®**
Composition (Each Compressed Tablet): Amobarbital, USP, 15 mg ($\frac{1}{4}$ gr)

T42 **A.S.A.® and Codeine Compound, No. 2**
Composition (Each Compressed Tablet): Codeine phosphate, 15 mg; aspirin, 230 mg; phenacetin, 150 mg; caffeine, 30 mg

T44 **Calcium Gluconate with Vitamin D**
Composition (Each Compressed Tablet): Calcium gluconate, 1 g; vitamin D synthetic, 1.65 mcg

T45 **Vitamin C (Cevalin®)**
Composition (Each Compressed Tablet): Ascorbic Acid, USP, 100 mg

T46 **Sulfapyridine**
Composition (Each Compressed Tablet): Sulfapyridine, USP, 0.5 g (7.72 grs)

T47 **Vitamin C (Cevalin®)**
Composition (Each Compressed Tablet): Ascorbic Acid, USP, 50 mg

T49 **A.S.A.® and Codeine Compound, No. 3**
Composition (Each Compressed Tablet): Codeine phosphate, 30 mg; aspirin, 230 mg; phenacetin, 150 mg; caffeine, 30 mg

T50 **A.S.A.® Compound**
Composition (Each Compressed Tablet): Aspirin, 227 mg; phenacetin, 160 mg; caffeine, 32.5 mg; Pink

T52 **Betalin® S**
Composition (Each Compressed Tablet): Thiamine Hydrochloride, USP, 10 mg

T53 **Niacinamide**
Composition (Each Compressed Tablet): Niacinamide, USP, 100 mg

T54 **Sulfadiazine**
Composition (Each Compressed Tablet): Sulfadiazine, USP, 0.5 g (7.72 grs)

T55 **Papaverine Hydrochloride**
Composition (Each Compressed Tablet): Papaverine Hydrochloride, USP, 100 mg ($1\frac{1}{2}$ grs)

T56 **Amytal®**
Composition (Each Compressed Tablet): Amobarbital, USP, 30 mg ($\frac{1}{2}$ gr)

T59 **Betalin® S**
Composition (Each Compressed Tablet): Thiamine Hydrochloride, USP, 25 mg

T60 **Cevalin®**
Composition (Each Compressed Tablet): Ascorbic Acid, USP, 250 mg

T61 **Dibasic Calcium Phosphate**
Composition (Each Compressed Tablet): Dibasic calcium phosphate, anhydrous, equivalent to $7\frac{1}{2}$ grs (500 mg) of dibasic calcium phosphate dihydrate (USP)

T62 **Betalin® S**
Composition (Each Compressed Tablet): Thiamine Hydrochloride, USP, 50 mg

T63 **Betalin® S**
Composition (Each Compressed Tablet): Thiamine Hydrochloride, USP, 100 mg

T67 **Vitamin C (Cevalin®)**
Composition (Each Compressed Tablet): Ascorbic Acid, USP, 500 mg

T72 **Pyridoxine Hydrochloride (Hexa-Betalin®)**
Composition (Each Compressed Tablet): Pyridoxine Hydrochloride, USP, 50 mg

T73 **Papaverine Hydrochloride**
Composition (Each Compressed Tablet): Papaverine Hydrochloride, USP, 200 mg (3 grs)

T75 **Neotrizine®**
Composition (Each Compressed Tablet): Sulfadiazine, 167 mg; sulfamerazine, 167 mg; sulfamethazine, 167 mg; (USP)

T91 **Paveril® Phosphate**
Composition (Each Compressed Tablet): Dioxyline phosphate, 200 mg (3 grs)

T93 **Isoniazid**
Composition (Each Compressed Tablet): Isoniazid, USP, 100 mg

T96 **Neomycin Sulfate**
Composition (Each Compressed Tablet): Neomycin Sulfate, USP, 500 mg (equiv. to 350 mg base)

T99 **Haldrone®**
Composition (Each Compressed Tablet): Paramethasone Acetate, USP, 1 mg

---

U01 **Haldrone®**
Composition (Each Compressed Tablet): Paramethasone Acetate, USP, 2 mg

U03 **Dymelor®**
Composition (Each Compressed Tablet): Acetohexamide, USP, 250 mg

U07 **Dymelor®**
Composition (Each Compressed Tablet): Acetohexamide, USP, 500 mg

U09 **Anhydron®**
Composition (Each Compressed Tablet): Cyclothiazide, USP, 2 mg

U23 **Isoniazid**
Composition (Each Compressed Tablet): Isoniazid, USP, 300 mg

U29 **Sandril®**
Composition (Each Compressed Tablet): Reserpine, USP, 0.25 mg

U53 **Methadone Hydrochloride**
Composition (Each Disket®): Methadone Hydrochloride, USP, 40 mg

U56 **Folic Acid**
Composition (Each Compressed Tablet): Folic Acid, USP, 1 mg

U60 **Keflex®**
Composition (Each Compressed Tablet): Cephalexin, USP, 1 g

W07-W68 (Miscellaneous)

W07 **V-Cillin K®, for Oral Solution**
Composition (When Mixed as Directed): Each 5 ml contain penicillin V potassium equivalent to penicillin V, 125 mg (USP).

W10 **V-Cillin® Drops**
Composition (When Mixed as Directed): Each 0.6 ml contains penicillin V, 125 mg; buffered with citric acid (USP).

W16 **V-Cillin K®, for Oral Solution**
Composition (When Mixed as Directed): Each 5 ml contain penicillin V potassium equivalent to penicillin V, 250 mg (USP).

W21 **For Oral Suspension, Keflex®**
Composition (When Mixed as Directed): Each 5 ml contain cephalexin, 125 mg (USP).

W22 **For Pediatric Drops, Keflex®**
Composition (When Mixed as Directed): Each ml contains cephalexin, 100 mg (USP).

W68 **For Oral Suspension, Keflex®**
Composition (When Mixed as Directed): Each 5 ml contain cephalexin, 250 mg (USP).

5057 **For Oral Suspension, Ceclor®**
Composition (When Mixed as Directed): Each 5 ml contain cefaclor, 125 mg (USP).

5058 **For Oral Suspension, Ceclor®**
Composition (When Mixed as Directed): Each 5 ml contain cefaclor, 250 mg (USP).

UNIT-DOSE PACKAGING

Dispenser Strip
Hyporets® (disposable syringes, Lilly)
Identi-Dose® (unit dose medication, Lilly)
Reverse-Numbered Package
Closed-circuit control of medication from pharmacy to nurse to patient and return. Simplifies counting and dispensing whether in single-unit or prescription-size quantities. Fits into any dispensing system for ready identification and legibility, better inventory control, protection from contamination, easier handling and recording under Medicare, prevention of drug loss through pilferage or spilling, better control of Federal Controlled Substances, and less chance of medication errors.
The following products are available through normal channels of supply:

Dispenser Strip
Pulvules®
No.
(C-II) 240 Seconal® Sodium, 100 mg
(C-II) 303 Tuinal®, 100 mg

Identi-Dose® (ID100)
Pulvules®
No.
(C-II) 222 Amytal® Sodium, 200 mg
(C-II) 240 Seconal® Sodium, 100 mg
(C-II) 243 Seconal® Sodium, 50 mg
(C-III) 286 A.S.A.® and Codeine Compound, No. 3
(C-II) 303 Tuinal®, 100 mg
(C-II) 304 Tuinal®, 200 mg
(C-IV) 364 Darvon®, 32 mg
(C-IV) 365 Darvon®, 65 mg
(C-IV) 366 Darvon® with A.S.A.®
(C-IV) 368 Darvon® Compound
(C-IV) 369 Darvon® Compound-65
387 Aventyl® HCl, 10 mg
389 Aventyl® HCl, 25 mg
3061 Ceclor®, 250 mg
3062 Ceclor®, 500 mg

Tablets
No.
55 Hepicebrin®
100 Multicebrin®
186 A.S.A.®, 5 grs
189 A.S.A.® Compound
(C-II) 558 Codeine Sulfate, USP, 30 mg
1125 Quinidine Sulfate, USP, 200 mg
(C-IV) 1544 Phenobarbital, USP, 15 mg
(C-IV) 1545 Phenobarbital, USP, 30 mg
(C-IV) 1546 Phenobarbital, USP, 100 mg
1572 Ergotrate® Maleate, 0.2 mg
(C-IV) 1574 Phenobarbital, USP, 60 mg
1671 Papaverine Hydrochloride, USP, 100 mg

Continued on next page

*Identi-Code® symbol.

Lilly—Cont.

1685 Diethylstilbestrol, USP, 5 mg
1703 Crystodigin®, 0.1 mg, Pink
1803 Neomycin Sulfate, USP, 500 mg
1831 V-Cillin K®, 250 mg
1832 V-Cillin K®, 500 mg
1842 Dymelor®, 250 mg
1843 Dymelor®, 500 mg, Yellow
C-IV 1883 Darvon-N®, 100 mg
C-IV 1884 Darvon-N® with A.S.A.®
C-IV 1890 Darvocet-N® 50
C-IV 1893 Darvocet-N® 100

Miscellaneous

M-126 V-Cillin K®, for Oral Solution, 125 mg
M-142 V-Cillin K®, for Oral Solution, 250 mg

Reverse-Numbered Package (RN500)

Pulvules®

No.

C-IV **365** Darvon®, 65 mg
C-IV **369** Darvon® Compound-65

Tablets

No.

C-IV **1893** Darvocet-N® 100

Single-Cut Identi-Dose® (ID500)

Pulvules®

No.

C-IV **365** Darvon®, 65 mg
C-IV **369** Darvon® Compound-65

Tablets

No.

C-IV **1883** Darvon-N®, 100 mg
C-IV **1884** Darvon-N® with A.S.A.®
C-IV **1890** Darvocet-N® 50
C-IV **1893** Darvocet-N® 100

C-II, C-III, C-IV Federal Controlled Substances.

ACIDULIN® OTC
(glutamic acid hydrochloride)

Description: Each Pulvule® contains 340 mg glutamic acid hydrochloride and is equivalent to about 10 minims of Diluted Hydrochloric Acid, USP, or to about 16.8 ml of 0.1 *N* hydrochloric acid.

Hydrochloric acid deficiency can be corrected easily and safely with Pulvules Acidulin. The Pulvule form, unlike solutions, is tasteless, cannot injure mucous membranes or teeth, and is safe and convenient for the patient to carry when traveling or dining out.

Indications: Acidulin is administered to counterbalance deficiency of hydrochloric acid in the gastric juice and to destroy or inhibit the growth of putrefactive microorganisms in ingested food. A deficiency of hydrochloric acid is often associated with pernicious anemia, gastric carcinoma, congenital achlorhydria, and allergy.

Contraindications: Should not be used if gastric hyperacidity or peptic ulcers are present.

Dosage: 1 to 3 Pulvules three times daily before meals, or as directed by the physician.

Overdosage: *Symptoms*—Massive overdosage may produce systemic acidosis. *Treatment*—Alkalies, such as sodium bicarbonate or sodium *r*-lactate solution, one molar (to be diluted).

How Supplied: *Pulvules No. 213, Acidulin ® (glutamic acid hydrochloride, Lilly), F31,** 340 mg (No. 1, Pink), in bottles of 100 (NDC 0002-0631-02) and 1000 (NDC 0002-0631-04).

[030180]

AEROLONE® SOLUTION ℞
(isoproterenol hydrochloride inhalation)
(Not USP)

Description: Aerolone® Solution (isoproterenol hydrochloride inhalation, Lilly) is a bronchodilator. Each 100 ml contain isoproterenol hydrochloride, 0.25 g, with propylene glycol, ascorbic acid, coloring, and purified water, q.s. Sodium hydroxide is added during manufacture to adjust the pH.

This product differs from the USP Inhalation in that it contains 80 percent propylene glycol by volume instead of purified water and it is not isotonic.

Actions: Isoproterenol is an adrenergic (sympathomimetic) agent and relieves bronchospasm by relaxing the smooth muscle of the bronchioles.

Indications: Aerolone® Solution (isoproterenol hydrochloride inhalation, Lilly) is indicated for the treatment of bronchospasm associated with acute and chronic bronchial asthma, pulmonary emphysema, bronchitis, and bronchiectasis.

Contraindications: Aerolone® Solution (isoproterenol hydrochloride inhalation, Lilly) is contraindicated in patients with (1) known hypersensitivity to isoproterenol or (2) cardiac arrhythmia associated with tachycardia.

Warnings: Occasional patients have been reported to develop severe paradoxical airway resistance with repeated excessive use of isoproterenol inhalation preparations. The cause of this refractory state is unknown. It is advisable that, in such instances, the use of this preparation be discontinued immediately and alternative therapy instituted, since in the reported cases the patients did not respond to other forms of therapy until the drug was withdrawn.

Deaths have been reported following excessive use of isoproterenol inhalation preparations, and the exact cause is unknown. Cardiac arrest was noted in several instances.

Usage in Pregnancy—Safe use during pregnancy has not been established relative to possible adverse effects on fetal development. Therefore, Aerolone Solution should not be used in pregnant women unless, in the judgment of the physician, the potential benefits outweigh the possible hazards.

Precautions: Aerolone® Solution (isoproterenol hydrochloride inhalation, Lilly) should be used with caution in patients having serious cardiac disease, hypertension, or hyperthyroidism.

Adverse Reactions: Rarely, insomnia, nervousness, vertigo, tachycardia, and palpitation may occur.

Dosage and Administration: For use by aerosol only. The technique is the same as that for administering epinephrine, 1:100. A nebulizer which produces a fine mist is necessary. The mist is inhaled through the mouth, and the breath is held in momentarily. Usually, 6 to 12 inhalations will bring adequate relief. Mild cases may require only one treatment per day; severe cases may need the treatment repeatedly at intervals of 15 minutes. If relief is not noticeable after three such treatments at 15-minute intervals, consult a physician. Ordinarily, the number of such treatments for repeated attacks should not exceed eight per 24 hours.

Physicians prescribing isoproterenol for use in inhalation therapy equipment should bear in mind the fact that different dosages of medication are delivered into the patient's airways depending on the proficiency of the therapist and the type of inhalator used.

Proficiency in the use of any of these devices can be gained only by firsthand experience. Furthermore, some equipment can deliver 100 percent of the medication deep into the airways, whereas other inhalators may deliver considerably less than the prescribed dose. The number of inhalations per treatment and the frequency of re-treatment should, therefore, be titrated to the patient's response.

Overdosage: *Symptoms*—Insomnia, nervousness, vertigo, tachycardia, and palpitation resulting from C.N.S. stimulation.

Treatment—No specific treatment; general management consists in controlling symptoms of C.N.S. stimulation by the use of sedatives, such as the barbiturates.

How Supplied: (℞) *Solution No. 50, Aerolone® Solution (isoproterenol hydrochloride inhalation, Lilly),* in 1-fl-oz bottles (NDC 0002-2605-67).

[082380]

AMYTAL® C-II
(amobarbital)

WARNING: MAY BE HABIT-FORMING

Description: Amytal® (amobarbital, Lilly) is a white, friable, granular powder that is odorless, has a bitter taste, and is hygroscopic. It is very soluble in water, soluble in alcohol, and practically insoluble in ether and chloroform. Amytal is 5-ethyl-5-isopentylbarbiturate and has the empirical formula $C_{11}H_{17}N_2O_3$. Amytal is available as tablets and elixir for oral administration. The scored tablets contain 15 mg, 30 mg, 50 mg, or 100 mg amobarbital, and the elixir, 880 mg per 100 ml.

Clinical Pharmacology: Amobarbital, a short-acting barbiturate, is a central-nervous-system depressant. It is a rapid-acting sedative and hypnotic, with a duration of effect ranging from eight to 11 hours. It is detoxified in the liver.

Indications and Usage: Amytal® (amobarbital, Lilly) is indicated in any conditions that require degrees of sedation ranging from minimum doses for the relief of anxiety and tension to hypnotic doses for preanesthetic medication.

Contraindications: Amytal® (amobarbital, Lilly) is contraindicated in patients who are hypersensitive to barbiturates. It is also contraindicated in patients with a history of manifest or latent porphyria, marked impairment of liver function, or respiratory disease in which dyspnea or obstruction is evident. It should not be administered to persons with known previous addiction to sedative/hypnotics, since ordinary doses may be ineffectual and may contribute to further addiction. Amytal should not be administered in the presence of acute or chronic pain, because paradoxical excitement may be induced or important symptoms may be masked.

Precautions: *General Precautions* — Barbiturates induce liver microsomal enzyme activity. This accelerates the biotransformation of various drugs and is probably part of the mechanism of the tolerance encountered with barbiturates. Amytal® (amobarbital, Lilly) should, therefore, be used with caution in patients with decreased liver function. This drug should also be administered cautiously to patients with a history of drug dependence or abuse (*see* Drug Abuse and Dependence). Amytal may decrease the potency of coumarin anticoagulants; therefore, patients receiving such concomitant therapy should have more frequent prothrombin determinations.

As with other sedatives and hypnotics, elderly or debilitated patients may react to barbiturates with marked excitement or depression.

The systemic effects of exogenous hydrocortisone and endogenous hydrocortisone (cortisol) may be diminished by Amytal. Thus, this product should be administered with caution to patients with borderline hypoadrenal function, regardless of whether it is of pituitary or of primary adrenal origin.

Information for Patients—Amytal may impair the mental and/or physical abilities required for the performance of potentially hazardous tasks, such as driving a car or operating machinery. The patient should be cautioned accordingly.

Drug Interactions—Amytal in combination with alcohol, tranquilizers, and other central-nervous-system depressants has additive depressant effects, and the patient should be so advised. Patients taking this drug should be warned not to exceed the dosage recommended by their physician. Toxic effects and fatalities have occurred following overdoses of Amytal alone and in combination with other central-nervous-system depressants. Caution should be exercised in prescribing unnecessarily large amounts of Amytal for patients who have a history of emotional disturbances or suicidal ideation or who have misused alcohol and other C.N.S. drugs (*see* Overdosage).

Usage in Pregnancy—Pregnancy Category B—Reproduction studies have been performed in animals and have revealed no evidence of impaired fertility or harm to the fetus due to Amytal. There are, however, no adequate and well-controlled studies in pregnant women. Because animal reproduction studies are not always predictive of human response, this drug should be used during pregnancy only if clearly needed.

Labor and Delivery—Depression has been noted in infants born following the use of Amytal during labor.

Nursing Mothers—Caution should be exercised when Amytal is administered to a nursing woman.

Usage in Children—Safety and effectiveness have not been established in children below the age of six years.

Adverse Reactions: Idiosyncrasy, in the form of excitement, hangover, or pain, may appear. Hypersensitivity reactions occur in some patients, especially in those with asthma, urticaria, or angioneurotic edema.

Drug Abuse and Dependence: *Controlled Substance*—Amytal® (amobarbital, Lilly) is a Schedule II drug.

Dependence—Prolonged, uninterrupted use of barbiturates (particularly the short-acting drugs), even in therapeutic doses, may result in psychic and physical dependence. Withdrawal symptoms due to physical dependence following chronic use of large doses of barbiturates may include delirium, convulsions, and death.

Overdosage: *Symptoms* — The manifestations of overdosage are early hypothermia followed by fever, sluggish or absent reflexes, respiratory depression, gradual appearance of circulatory collapse, pulmonary edema, and coma.

Treatment—General management should consist in symptomatic and supportive therapy, including gastric lavage, administration of intravenous fluids, and maintenance of blood pressure, body temperature, and adequate respiratory exchange. Dialysis will increase the rate of removal of barbiturates from the body fluids. Antibiotics may be required to control pulmonary complications.

Dosage and Administration: Because of the wide variation in individual response to the barbiturates, the dosage range is relatively great, and doses must be individualized for each patient. The adult dosage range for daytime sedation may be from 15 to 120 mg two to four times a day. However, the usual adult dosage for daytime sedation is 30 to 50 mg two or three times a day. Dosage may be adjusted to relieve tension and anxiety without significant loss of mental acuity. The usual adult hypnotic dose is 100 to 200 mg. On occasion, a larger dose may be necessary to produce the desired degree of hypnosis.

How Supplied: Ⓒ *Elixir No. 237, Amytal® (amobarbital, Lilly)*, 880 mg per 100 ml (Not USP), in 16-fl-oz bottles (NDC 0002-2441-05). Alcohol, 34 percent. This product differs from the USP elixir in that it contains a greater proportion of alcohol than the USP drug.

Ⓒ *Tablets Amytal® (Amobarbital Tablets, USP)* (scored): *No. 1575, T40,** 15 mg, Light-Green, in bottles of 100 (NDC 0002-2040-02) and 500 (NDC 0002-2040-03); *No. 1678, T56,** 30 mg, Yellow, in bottles of 100 (NDC 0002-2056-02) and 1000 (NDC 0002-2056-04); *No. 1550, T37,** 50 mg, Orange, in bottles of 100 (NDC 0002-2037-02) and 500 (NDC 0002-2037-03); *No. 1462, T32,** 100 mg, Pink, in bottles of 100 (NDC 0002-2032-02) and 500 (NDC 0002-2032-03).

[111279]

[*Shown in Product Identification Section*]

AMYTAL® SODIUM Ⓒ

(amobarbital sodium)
Sterile, USP
AMPOULES

WARNING: MAY BE HABIT-FORMING

Caution: These products are to be used by the physician or under his direction. The intravenous administration of Amytal Sodium carries with it the potential dangers inherent in the intravenous use of any potent hypnotic.

Description: Amytal Sodium is a white, friable, granular powder that is odorless, has a bitter taste, and is hygroscopic. It is very soluble in water, soluble in alcohol, and practically insoluble in ether and chloroform. Amytal Sodium is sodium-5-ethyl-5-isopentylbarbiturate and has the empirical formula $C_{11}H_{17}N_2NaO_3$. Vials Amytal® Sodium (Sterile Amobarbital Sodium, USP, Lilly) are for parenteral administration. The vials contain 250 mg or 0.5 g sterile amobarbital sodium.

Clinical Pharmacology: Amobarbital sodium, a short-acting barbiturate, is a central-nervous-system depressant. It is a rapid-acting sedative and hypnotic, with a duration of effect ranging from eight to 11 hours. It is detoxified in the liver.

Indications and Usage: Amytal® Sodium (amobarbital sodium, Lilly) may be used intravenously or intramuscularly for the control of convulsive seizures such as may be due to chorea, eclampsia, meningitis, tetanus, procaine or cocaine reactions, or poisoning from such drugs as strychnine or picrotoxin. It may be administered for the management of catatonic and negativistic reactions, manic reactions, and epileptiform seizures. It is also useful in narcoanalysis and narcotherapy and as a diagnostic aid in schizophrenia.

Contraindications: Amytal® Sodium (amobarbital sodium, Lilly) is contraindicated in patients who are hypersensitive to barbiturates. It is also contraindicated in patients with a history of manifest or latent porphyria, marked impairment of liver function, or respiratory disease in which dyspnea or obstruction is evident. It should not be administered to persons with known previous addiction to the sedative/hypnotic group, since ordinary doses may be ineffectual and may contribute to further addiction. Amytal Sodium should not be administered in the presence of acute or chronic pain, because paradoxical excitement may be induced or important symptoms may be masked.

Warnings: The rate of intravenous injection must not exceed 1 ml/minute.

Either too-rapid injection or relative overdosage may cause apnea or hypotension. Respiratory depression is more likely to occur if other central-nervous-system agents have been used concurrently.

The maximum single dose should not exceed 1 g in adult patients. The maximum intramuscular dose should not exceed 0.5 g. No greater volume than 5 ml, irrespective of drug concentration, should be injected intramuscularly at any one site.

Several minutes may be required for the drug to dissolve completely, but under no circumstances should a solution be injected if it has not become absolutely clear within five minutes' time. Also, a solution that forms a precipitate after clearing should not be used. Amytal Sodium hydrolyzes in solution or upon exposure to air. Not more than 30 minutes should elapse from the time the vial is opened until its contents are injected. Amytal Sodium supplied in capsules should not be used for injection purposes.

Precautions: *General Precautions*—Barbiturates induce liver microsomal enzyme activity. This accelerates the biotransformation of various drugs and is probably part of the mechanism of the tolerance encountered with barbiturates. Amytal Sodium should, therefore, be used with caution in patients with decreased liver function. This drug should also be administered cautiously to patients with a history of drug dependence or abuse (*see* Drug Abuse and Dependence). Amytal Sodium may decrease the potency of coumarin anticoagulants; therefore, patients receiving such concomitant therapy should have more frequent prothrombin determinations.

As with other sedatives and hypnotics, elderly or debilitated patients may react to barbiturates with marked excitement or depression.

The systemic effects of exogenous hydrocortisone and endogenous hydrocortisone (cortisol) may be diminished by Amytal® Sodium (amobarbital sodium, Lilly). Thus, this product should be administered with caution to patients with borderline hypoadrenal function, regardless of whether it is of pituitary or of primary adrenal origin.

Information for Patients—Amytal Sodium may impair the mental and/or physical abilities required for the performance of potentially hazardous tasks, such as driving a car or operating machinery. The patient should be cautioned accordingly.

Drug Interactions—Amytal Sodium in combination with alcohol, tranquilizers, and other central-nervous-system depressants has additive depressant effects, and the patient should be so advised. Patients taking this drug should be warned not to exceed the dosage recommended by their physician. Toxic effects and fatalities have occurred following overdoses of Amytal Sodium alone and in combination with other central-nervous-system depressants. Caution should be exercised in prescribing unnecessarily large amounts of Amytal Sodium for patients who have a history of emotional disturbances or suicidal ideation or who have misused alcohol and other CNS drugs (*see* Overdosage).

Usage in Pregnancy—Pregnancy Category B—Reproduction studies have been performed in animals and have revealed no evidence of impaired fertility or harm to the fetus due to Amytal Sodium. There are, however, no adequate and well-controlled studies in pregnant women. Because animal reproduction studies are not always predictive of human response, this drug should be used during pregnancy only if clearly needed.

Labor and Delivery—Depression has been noted in infants born following the use of Amytal Sodium during labor.

Nursing Mothers—Caution should be exercised when Amytal Sodium is administered to a nursing woman.

Usage in Children—Safety and effectiveness have not been established in children below the age of six years.

Adverse Reactions: In the general use of barbiturates by the intravenous route, respiratory depression is the most serious side effect. Idiosyncrasy, in the form of excitement, hangover, or pain, may appear. Hypersensitivity reactions occur in some patients, especially in those with asthma, urticaria, or angioneurotic edema. Laryngospasm may develop during normal induction or as a result of improper dosage. Rapid intravenous administration may also induce vasodilation and some fall in blood pressure.

Nausea and vomiting, postoperative atelectasis, and circulatory disturbances are uncommon. When they occur, they are usually due to overdosage or extraneous factors. Embolism has not been reported following intravenous use of Amytal® Sodium (amobarbital sodium, Lilly).

Drug Abuse and Dependence: *Controlled Substance*—Amytal® Sodium (amobarbital sodium, Lilly) is a Schedule II drug.

Continued on next page

***Identi-Code® symbol.**

Lilly—Cont.

Dependence—Prolonged, uninterrupted use of barbiturates (particularly the short-acting drugs), even in therapeutic doses, may result in psychic and physical dependence. Withdrawal symptoms due to physical dependence following chronic use of large doses of barbiturates may include delirium, convulsions, and death.
Overdosage: *Symptoms*—The manifestations of overdosage are early hypothermia followed by fever, sluggish or absent reflexes, respiratory depression, gradual appearance of circulatory collapse, pulmonary edema, and coma. *Treatment*—General management should consist in symptomatic and supportive therapy, including gastric lavage, administration of intravenous fluids, and maintenance of blood pressure, body temperature, and adequate respiratory exchange. Dialysis will increase the rate of removal of barbiturates from the body fluids. Antibiotics may be required to control pulmonary complications.
Dosage and Administration: Solutions of Amytal® Sodium (amobarbital sodium, Lilly) should be made up aseptically with Sterile Water for Injection. The accompanying table will aid in preparing solutions of various concentrations. Ordinarily, a 10 percent solution is used; the maximum single dose for an adult is 1 g. After Sterile Water for Injection is added, the ampoule should be rotated to facilitate solution of the powder. **Do not shake the vial.** [See table below].
Intramuscular Use—No more than 5 ml should be injected at any one site. Depositions should be made deeply in large muscles, such as the gluteus maximus. Superficial intramuscular or subcutaneous injections may be painful and may produce sterile abscesses or sloughs.
The average intramuscular dose ranges from 65 mg to 0.5 g. Twenty percent solutions may be used so that a small volume can contain a large dose.
Intravenous Use—The rate of intravenous injection should not exceed 1 ml/minute. When the 10 percent solution is used, faster rates of administration may precipitate serious respiratory depression. Because of their higher metabolic rate, children tolerate comparatively larger doses. The final dosage is determined to a great extent by the patient's reaction to the slow administration of the drug. Ordinarily, 65 mg to 0.5 g may be given to a child six to 12 years of age.
How Supplied: Ⓒ *Ampoules Amytal® Sodium (Sterile Amobarbital Sodium, USP)* (Dry Powder): *No. 386,* 250 mg, in Traypak™ (multivial carton, Lilly) of 10 (NDC 0002-7214-10) and 25 (NDC 0002-7214-25); *No. 387,* 0.5 g, in Traypak of 10 (NDC 0002-7215-10) and 25 (NDC 0002-7215-25).

[020982]

AMYTAL® SODIUM Ⓒ
(amobarbital sodium)
PULVULES®
Capsules, USP

WARNING: MAY BE HABIT-FORMING

Description: Amytal® Sodium (Amobarbital Sodium, USP, Lilly) is a white, friable, granular powder that is odorless, has a bitter taste, and is hygroscopic. It is very soluble in water, soluble in alcohol, and practically insoluble in ether and chloroform. Amytal Sodium is sodium-5-ethyl-5-isopentylbarbiturate and has the empirical formula $C_{11}H_{17}N_2NaO_3$.
Each Pulvule contains 65 or 200 mg of amobarbital sodium for oral administration.
Clinical Pharmacology: Amobarbital sodium, a short-acting barbiturate, is a central-nervous-system depressant. It is a rapid-acting sedative and hypnotic, with a duration of effect ranging from eight to 11 hours. It is detoxified in the liver.
Indications and Usage: Amytal® Sodium (amobarbital sodium, Lilly) is indicated for sedation and relief of anxiety (in minimum doses); for hypnotic effects; as preanesthetic medication; and to control convulsive disorders. The prolonged administration of Amytal Sodium is not recommended, since it has not been shown to be effective for a period of more than 14 days. If insomnia persists, drug-free intervals of one or more weeks should elapse before re-treatment is considered. Attempts should be made to find alternative nondrug therapy for chronic insomnia.
Contraindications: Amytal® Sodium (amobarbital sodium, Lilly) is contraindicated in patients who are hypersensitive to barbiturates. It is also contraindicated in patients with a history of manifest or latent porphyria, marked impairment of liver function, or respiratory disease in which dyspnea or obstruction is evident. It should not be administered to persons with known previous addiction to the sedative/hypnotic group, since ordinary doses may be ineffectual and may contribute to further addiction. Amytal Sodium should not be administered in the presence of acute or chronic pain, because paradoxical excitement may be induced or important symptoms may be masked.
Precautions: *General Precautions*—Barbiturates induce liver microsomal enzyme activity. This accelerates the biotransformation of various drugs and is probably part of the mechanism of the tolerance encountered with barbiturates. Amytal® Sodium (amobarbital sodium, Lilly) should, therefore, be used with caution in patients with decreased liver function. This drug should also be administered cautiously to patients with a history of drug dependence or abuse (*see* Drug Abuse and Dependence). Amytal Sodium may decrease the potency of coumarin anticoagulants; therefore, patients receiving such concomitant therapy should have more frequent prothrombin determinations.
As with other sedatives and hypnotics, elderly or debilitated patients may react to barbiturates with marked excitement or depression.
The systemic effects of exogenous hydrocortisone and endogenous hydrocortisone (cortisol) may be diminished by Amytal Sodium. Thus, this product should be administered with caution to patients with borderline hypoadrenal function, regardless of whether it is of pituitary or of primary adrenal origin.
Information for Patients—Amytal Sodium may impair the mental and/or physical abilities required for the performance of potentially hazardous tasks, such as driving a car or operating machinery. The patient should be cautioned accordingly.
Drug Interactions—Amytal Sodium in combination with alcohol, tranquilizers, and other central-nervous-system depressants has additive depressant effects, and the patient should be so advised. Patients taking this drug should be warned not to exceed the dosage recommended by their physician. Toxic effects and fatalities have occurred following overdoses of Amytal Sodium alone and in combination with other central-nervous-system depressants. Caution should be exercised in prescribing unnecessarily large amounts of Amytal Sodium for patients who have a history of emotional disturbances or suicidal ideation or who have misused alcohol and other C.N.S. drugs (*see* Overdosage).
Usage in Pregnancy—Pregnancy Category B—Reproduction studies have been performed in animals and have revealed no evidence of impaired fertility or harm to the fetus due to Amytal Sodium. There are, however, no adequate and well-controlled studies in pregnant women. Because animal reproduction studies are not always predictive of human response, this drug should be used during pregnancy only if clearly needed.
Labor and Delivery—Depression has been noted in infants born following the use of Amytal® Sodium (amobarbital sodium, Lilly) during labor.
Nursing Mothers—Caution should be exercised when Amytal Sodium is administered to a nursing woman.
Usage in Children—Safety and effectiveness in children have not been established.
Adverse Reactions: The following adverse reactions have been reported:
C.N.S. Depression—Residual sedation or "hangover," drowsiness, lethargy.
Respiratory/Circulatory—Respiratory depression, apnea, circulatory collapse.
Allergic—Hypersensitivity reactions, especially in individuals with asthma, urticaria, angioneurotic edema, or similar conditions; skin eruptions.
Other—Nausea and vomiting; headache.
Drug Abuse and Dependence: *Controlled Substance*—Amytal® Sodium (amobarbital sodium, Lilly) is a Schedule II drug.
Dependence—Prolonged, uninterrupted use of barbiturates (particularly the short-acting drugs), even in therapeutic doses, may result in psychic and physical dependence. Withdrawal symptoms due to physical dependence following chronic use of large doses of barbiturates may include delirium, convulsions, and death.
Overdosage: *Symptoms* — The manifestations of overdosage are early hypothermia followed by fever, sluggish or absent reflexes, respiratory depression, gradual appearance of circulatory collapse, pulmonary edema, and coma. *Treatment* — General management should consist in symptomatic and supportive therapy, including gastric lavage, administration of intravenous fluids, and maintenance of blood pressure, body temperature, and adequate respiratory exchange. Dialysis will increase the rate of removal of barbiturates from the body fluids. Antibiotics may be required to control pulmonary complications.
Administration and Dosage: Because of the wide variation in individual response to the barbiturates, the dosage range is relatively great.
For insomnia, 65 to 200 mg by mouth at bedtime. For preanesthetic sedation, 200 mg one or two hours before surgery. In labor, the initial dose is 200 to 400 mg, and additional quantities of 200 to 400 mg may be given at one to three-hour intervals for a total dose of not more than 1 g.
How Supplied: (Ⓒ) *Pulvules Amytal® Sodium (Amobarbital Sodium Capsules, USP): No. 111, F23,** 65 mg (No. 4, Blue), in bottles of 100 (NDC 0002-0623-02) and 500 (NDC 0002-0623-03); *No. 222, F33,** 200 mg (No. 2, Blue), in bot-

Quantity of Sterile Water for Injection Required to Dilute
the Contents of a Given Vial of Amytal Sodium to Obtain the Percentages Listed.
Solutions Derived Will Be in Weight/Volume.

AMYTAL® SODIUM (amobarbital sodium, Lilly)

Vial Number	Content in Weight	1 Percent	2.5 Percent	5 Percent	10 Percent	20 Percent
386	250 mg	25 ml	10 ml	5 ml	2.5 ml	1.25 ml
387	0.5 g	50 ml	20 ml	10 ml	5 ml	2.5 ml

tles of 100 (NDC 0002-0633-02) and 500 (NDC 0002-0633-03) and in 10 strips of 10 individually labeled blisters each containing 1 Pulvule (ID100) (NDC 0002-0633-33).

[101679]

[*Shown in Product Identification Section*]

ANHYDRON® ℞
(cyclothiazide)
Tablets, USP

Description: Anhydron® (cyclothiazide, Lilly) is 6-chloro-3,4-dihydro-3-(5-norbornen-2-yl) - 7 - sulfamoyl - 1,2,4 - benzothiadiazine-1,1-dioxide. Cyclothiazide is a white crystalline solid with a melting point of approximately 220°C. It is moderately soluble in hot ethyl alcohol and hot dilute alcohol, very soluble in cold ethyl acetate (an ethyl acetate solvate is formed), and relatively insoluble in ether, benzene, or chloroform.

Action: The action of Anhydron® (cyclothiazide, Lilly) results in interference with electrolyte reabsorption by the renal tubules. At maximum therapeutic dosage, all thiazides have approximately equal diuretic potency. The mechanism by which thiazides function in the control of hypertension is unknown.

Indications: Anhydron® (cyclothiazide, Lilly) is indicated as adjunctive therapy in edema associated with congestive heart failure, hepatic cirrhosis, and corticosteroid and estrogen therapy.

Anhydron has also been found useful in edema due to various forms of renal dysfunction, such as nephrotic syndrome, acute glomerulonephritis, and chronic renal failure.

Anhydron is indicated in the management of hypertension either as the sole therapeutic agent or to enhance the effectiveness of other antihypertensive drugs in the more severe forms of hypertension.

Usage in Pregnancy—The routine use of diuretics in an otherwise healthy woman is inappropriate and exposes mother and fetus to unnecessary hazard. Diuretics do not prevent development of toxemia of pregnancy, and there is no satisfactory evidence that they are useful in the treatment of developed toxemia.

Edema during pregnancy may arise from pathologic causes or from the physiologic and mechanical consequences of pregnancy. Thiazides are indicated in pregnancy when edema is due to pathologic causes, just as they are in the absence of pregnancy (however, see Warnings below). Dependent edema in pregnancy, resulting from restriction of venous return by the expanded uterus, is properly treated through elevation of the lower extremities and use of support hose; use of diuretics to lower intravascular volume in this case is illogical and unnecessary. There is hypervolemia during normal pregnancy which is harmful to neither the fetus nor the mother (in the absence of cardiovascular disease) but which is associated with edema, including generalized edema, in the majority of pregnant women. If this edema produces discomfort, increased recumbency will often provide relief. In rare instances, such edema may cause extreme discomfort that is not relieved by rest. In these cases, a short course of diuretics may provide relief and may be appropriate.

Contraindications: Anhydron® (cyclothiazide, Lilly) is contraindicated in anuria and in patients who are hypersensitive to cyclothiazide or other sulfonamide-derived drugs.

Warnings: Thiazides should be used with caution in severe renal disease. In patients with renal disease, thiazides may precipitate azotemia. Cumulative effects of the drug may develop in patients with impaired renal function. Thiazides should be used with caution in patients with impaired hepatic function or progressive liver disease, since minor alterations of fluid and electrolyte balance may precipitate hepatic coma.

Thiazides may add to or potentiate the action of other antihypertensive drugs. Potentiation occurs with ganglionic or peripheral adrenergic blocking drugs.

Sensitivity reactions may occur in patients with a history of allergy or bronchial asthma. The possibility of exacerbation or activation of systemic lupus erythematosus has been reported.

Usage in Pregnancy—Thiazides cross the placental barrier and appear in cord blood. The use of thiazides in pregnant women requires that the anticipated benefit be weighed against possible hazards to the fetus. These hazards include fetal or neonatal jaundice, thrombocytopenia, and possibly other adverse reactions which have occurred in the adult.

Nursing Mothers—Thiazides appear in breast milk. If use of the drug is deemed essential, the patient should stop nursing.

Precautions: Determination of serum electrolytes to detect possible imbalance should be performed at appropriate intervals.

All patients receiving thiazides should be observed for clinical signs of fluid or electrolyte imbalance, e.g., hyponatremia, hypochloremic alkalosis, and hypokalemia. Serum and urine electrolyte determinations are particularly important when the patient is vomiting excessively or receiving parenteral fluids. Medication such as digitalis may also influence serum electrolytes. Warning signs, irrespective of cause, are dryness of mouth, thirst, weakness, lethargy, drowsiness, restlessness, muscle pains or cramps, muscular fatigue, hypotension, oliguria, tachycardia, and gastrointestinal disturbances, such as nausea and vomiting.

Hypokalemia may develop with use of thiazides as with any other potent diuretic, especially with brisk diuresis, in the presence of severe cirrhosis, or during concomitant use of corticosteroids or ACTH. Interference with adequate oral electrolyte intake will also contribute to hypokalemia. Digitalis therapy may exaggerate metabolic effects of hypokalemia, especially in regard to myocardial activity.

Any chloride deficit is generally mild and usually does not require specific treatment except under extraordinary circumstances (as in liver or renal disease). Dilutional hyponatremia may occur in edematous patients in hot weather. Appropriate therapy is water restriction instead of administration of salt (except in rare instances when the hyponatremia is life threatening). In actual salt depletion, appropriate replacement is the therapy of choice.

Hyperuricemia may occur or frank gout may be precipitated in certain patients receiving thiazide therapy.

Insulin requirements in diabetic patients may be increased, decreased, or unchanged. Latent diabetes mellitus may become manifest during thiazide administration.

Thiazide drugs may increase the responsiveness to tubocurarine.

The antihypertensive effects of the drug may be enhanced in postsympathectomy patients.

Thiazides may decrease arterial responsiveness to norepinephrine. This diminution is not sufficient to preclude effectiveness of the pressor agent for therapeutic use.

If progressive renal impairment becomes evident, as indicated by a rising nonprotein nitrogen or blood urea nitrogen, therapy should be carefully reappraised, because it may be necessary to withhold or discontinue diuretic therapy.

Thiazides may decrease serum PBI levels without signs of thyroid disturbance.

Adverse Reactions: *Gastrointestinal* —Anorexia, gastric irritation, nausea, vomiting, cramping, diarrhea, constipation, jaundice (intrahepatic cholestatic jaundice), pancreatitis

Central Nervous System—Dizziness, vertigo, paresthesias, headache, xanthopsia

Hematologic—Leukopenia, agranulocytosis, thrombocytopenia, aplastic anemia

Dermatologic and Hypersensitivity—Purpura, photosensitivity, rash, urticaria, necrotizing angiitis (vasculitis or cutaneous vasculitis)

Cardiovascular—Orthostatic hypotension may occur and may be aggravated by alcohol, barbiturates, or narcotics.

Other—Hyperglycemia, glycosuria, hyperuricemia, muscle spasm, weakness, restlessness

Whenever adverse reactions are moderate or severe, thiazide dosage should be reduced or therapy withdrawn.

Dosage and Administration: Therapy should be individualized according to patient response. This therapy should be titrated to gain maximum therapeutic response as well as the minimum dose possible to maintain that therapeutic response.

For Diuretic Effect—The usual adult dosage of Anhydron® (cyclothiazide, Lilly) is ½ or 1 tablet (1 or 2 mg) once a day, preferably given early in the morning in order to obtain diuresis predominantly during the day and avoid disturbing the patient's rest at night. After the edema is eliminated, the dosage should be reduced according to the patient's need; body weight is usually a very helpful guide. For maintenance therapy, ½ or 1 tablet given on alternate days or two or three times a week frequently may be sufficient. Such an intermittent dosage schedule reduces the possibility of excessive depletion of body sodium and chloride or of potassium deficiency.

For Antihypertensive Effect—The dosage of Anhydron, like that of other thiazides, is often greater than that required for diuresis. The usual dosage of Anhydron is 1 tablet (2 mg) once a day; in some cases, it may be necessary to give 1 tablet two or three times a day.

Since Anhydron augments the action of other antihypertensive drugs, dosage of the latter should be reduced—perhaps to 50 percent of the usually recommended dosage—at the start of treatment and carefully readjusted upward or downward according to the patient's response and need.

How Supplied: (℞) *Tablets No. 1850, Anhydron® (Cyclothiazide Tablets, USP), U09,** 2 mg, Pink (capsule-shaped, scored), in bottles of 100 and 1000. [032480]

AVENTYL® HCL ℞
(nortriptyline hydrochloride)
USP

Description: Aventyl® HCl (nortriptyline hydrochloride, Lilly) is 5-(3-methylaminopropylidene)-10,11-dihydro-5H-dibenzo [a,d] cycloheptene hydrochloride. Its molecular weight is 299.8, and its empirical formula is $C_{19}H_{21}N \cdot HCl$.

Actions: The mechanism of mood elevation by tricyclic antidepressants is at present unknown. Aventyl® HCl (nortriptyline hydrochloride, Lilly) is not a monoamine oxidase inhibitor. It inhibits the activity of such diverse agents as histamine, 5-hydroxytryptamine, and acetylcholine. It increases the pressor effect of norepinephrine but blocks the pressor response of phenethylamine. Studies suggest that Aventyl HCl interferes with the transport, release, and storage of catecholamines. Operant conditioning techniques in rats and pigeons suggest that Aventyl HCl has a combination of stimulant and depressant properties.

Indications: Aventyl® HCl (nortriptyline hydrochloride, Lilly) is indicated for the relief of symptoms of depression. Endogenous depressions are more likely to be alleviated than are other depressive states.

Contraindications: The use of Aventyl® HCl (nortriptyline hydrochloride, Lilly) or other tricyclic antidepressants concurrently with a

Continued on next page

*Identi-Code® symbol.

Lilly—Cont.

monoamine oxidase (MAO) inhibitor is contraindicated. Hyperpyretic crises, severe convulsions, and fatalities have occurred when similar tricyclic antidepressants were used in such combinations. It is advisable to have discontinued the MAO inhibitor for at least two weeks before treatment with Aventyl HCl is started.
Patients hypersensitive to Aventyl HCl should not be given the drug.
Cross-sensitivity between Aventyl HCl and other dibenzazepines is a possibility.
Aventyl HCl is contraindicated during the acute recovery period after myocardial infarction.
Warnings: Patients with cardiovascular disease should be given Aventyl® HCl (nortriptyline hydrochloride, Lilly) only under close supervision because of the tendency of the drug to produce sinus tachycardia and to prolong the conduction time. Myocardial infarction, arrhythmia, and strokes have occurred. The antihypertensive action of guanethidine and similar agents may be blocked. Because of its anticholinergic activity, Aventyl HCl should be used with great caution in patients who have glaucoma or a history of urinary retention. Patients with a history of seizures should be followed closely when Aventyl HCl is administered, inasmuch as this drug is known to lower the convulsive threshold. Great care is required if Aventyl HCl is given to hyperthyroid patients or to those receiving thyroid medication, since cardiac arrhythmias may develop.
Aventyl HCl may impair the mental and/or physical abilities required for the performance of hazardous tasks, such as operating machinery or driving a car; therefore, the patient should be warned accordingly.
Excessive consumption of alcohol in combination with nortriptyline therapy may have a potentiating effect, which may lead to the danger of increased suicidal attempts or overdosage, especially in patients with histories of emotional disturbances or suicidal ideation.
Use in Pregnancy—Safe use of Aventyl HCl during pregnancy and lactation has not been established; therefore, when the drug is administered to pregnant patients, nursing mothers, or women of childbearing potential, the potential benefits must be weighed against the possible hazards. Animal reproduction studies have yielded inconclusive results.
Use in Children—This drug is not recommended for use in children, since safety and effectiveness in the pediatric age group have not been established.
Precautions: The use of Aventyl® HCl (nortriptyline hydrochloride, Lilly) in schizophrenic patients may result in an exacerbation of the psychosis or may activate latent schizophrenic symptoms. If the drug is given to overactive or agitated patients, increased anxiety and agitation may occur. In manic-depressive patients, Aventyl HCl may cause symptoms of the manic phase to emerge.
Administration of reserpine during therapy with a tricyclic antidepressant has been shown to produce a "stimulating" effect in some depressed patients.
Troublesome patient hostility may be aroused by the use of Aventyl HCl. Epileptiform seizures may accompany its administration, as is true of other drugs of its class.
Close supervision and careful adjustment of the dosage are required when Aventyl HCl is used with other anticholinergic drugs and sympathomimetic drugs.
The patient should be informed that the response to alcohol may be exaggerated.
When it is essential, the drug may be administered with electroconvulsive therapy, although the hazards may be increased. Discontinue the drug for several days, if possible, prior to elective surgery.
The possibility of a suicidal attempt by a depressed patient remains after the initiation of treatment; in this regard, it is important that the least possible quantity of drug be dispensed at any given time.
Both elevation and lowering of blood sugar levels have been reported.
Adverse Reactions: Note—Included in the following list are a few adverse reactions that have not been reported with this specific drug. However, the pharmacologic similarities among the tricyclic antidepressant drugs require that each of the reactions be considered when nortriptyline is administered.
Cardiovascular—Hypotension, hypertension, tachycardia, palpitation, myocardial infarction, arrhythmias, heart block, stroke.
Psychiatric—Confusional states (especially in the elderly) with hallucinations, disorientation, delusions; anxiety, restlessness, agitation; insomnia, panic, nightmares; hypomania; exacerbation of psychosis.
Neurologic—Numbness, tingling, paresthesias of extremities; incoordination, ataxia, tremors; peripheral neuropathy; extrapyramidal symptoms; seizures, alteration in EEG patterns; tinnitus.
Anticholinergic—Dry mouth and, rarely, associated sublingual adenitis; blurred vision, disturbance of accommodation, mydriasis; constipation, paralytic ileus; urinary retention, delayed micturition, dilation of the urinary tract.
Allergic—Skin rash, petechiae, urticaria, itching, photosensitization (avoid excessive exposure to sunlight); edema (general or of face and tongue), drug fever, cross-sensitivity with other tricyclic drugs.
Hematologic—Bone-marrow depression, including agranulocytosis; eosinophilia; purpura; thrombocytopenia.
Gastrointestinal—Nausea and vomiting, anorexia, epigastric distress, diarrhea; peculiar taste, stomatitis, abdominal cramps, black-tongue.
Endocrine—Gynecomastia in the male; breast enlargement and galactorrhea in the female; increased or decreased libido, impotence; testicular swelling; elevation or depression of blood sugar levels.
Other—Jaundice (simulating obstructive); altered liver function; weight gain or loss; perspiration; flushing; urinary frequency, nocturia; drowsiness, dizziness, weakness, fatigue; headache; parotid swelling; alopecia.
Withdrawal Symptoms—Though these are not indicative of addiction, abrupt cessation of treatment after prolonged therapy may produce nausea, headache, and malaise.
Dosage and Administration: Aventyl® HCl (nortriptyline hydrochloride, Lilly) is not recommended for children.
Aventyl HCl is administered orally in the form of Pulvules® or liquid. Lower than usual dosages are recommended for elderly patients and adolescents. Lower dosages are also recommended for outpatients than for hospitalized patients who will be under close supervision. The physician should initiate dosage at a low level and increase it gradually, noting carefully the clinical response and any evidence of intolerance. Following remission, maintenance medication may be required for a longer period of time at the lowest dose that will maintain remission.
If a patient develops minor side effects, the dosage should be reduced. The drug should be discontinued promptly if adverse effects of a serious nature or allergic manifestations occur.
Usual Adult Dose—25 mg three or four times daily; dosage should begin at a low level and be increased as required. Doses above 100 mg per day are not recommended.
Elderly and Adolescent Patients—30 to 50 mg per day, in divided doses.
Overdosage: Toxic overdosage may result in confusion, restlessness, agitation, vomiting, hyperpyrexia, muscle rigidity, hyperactive reflexes, tachycardia, ECG evidence of impaired conduction, shock, congestive heart failure, stupor, coma, and C.N.S. stimulation with convulsions followed by respiratory depression. Deaths have occurred following overdosage with drugs of this class.
No specific antidote is known. General supportive measures are indicated, with gastric lavage. Respiratory assistance is apparently the most effective measure when indicated. The use of C.N.S. depressants may worsen the prognosis.
The administration of barbiturates for control of convulsions alleviates an increase in the cardiac workload but should be undertaken with caution to avoid potentiation of respiratory depression.
Intramuscular paraldehyde or diazepam provides anticonvulsant activity with less respiratory depression than do the barbiturates; diazepam seems to be preferred.
The use of digitalis and/or physostigmine may be considered in case of serious cardiovascular abnormalities or cardiac failure.
The value of dialysis has not been established.
How Supplied: (℞) *Liquid No. 38, Aventyl® HCl (Nortriptyline Hydrochloride Oral Solution, USP)*, 10 mg (equivalent to base) per 5 ml, in 16-fl-oz bottles (NDC 0002-2468-05). Alcohol, 4 percent.
(℞) *Pulvules Aventyl® HCl (Nortriptyline Hydrochloride Capsules, USP): No. 387, H17** (No. 3, White Opaque Body, Yellow Opaque Cap), 10 mg (equivalent to base), and *No. 389, H19** (No. 1, White Opaque Body, Yellow Opaque Cap), 25 mg (equivalent to base), in bottles of 100 (NDC 0002-0817-02 and 0819-02) and 500 (NDC 0002-0817-03 and 0819-03) and in 10 strips of 10 individually labeled blisters each containing 1 Pulvule (ID100) (NDC 0002-0817-33 and 0819-33). [102882]

[*Shown in Product Identification Section*]

BILRON® OTC
(iron bile salts)

Description: Pulvules® Bilron contain those naturally occurring bile salts from the gallbladder bile of cattle which, when combined with iron, are insoluble in an acid medium. Bilron is inactive in the stomach because it is insoluble in an acid medium. When Bilron enters the alkaline medium of the small intestine, the iron moiety separates, and the bile salts become soluble and physiologically active like endogenously produced bile salts. Bile from cattle is used because the bile-salt content (chiefly salts of cholic, deoxycholic, lithocholic, and sterocholic acids conjugated with glycine and taurine) is similar to that of human bile.
Indications: Bilron is indicated as a physiologic laxative in the symptomatic treatment of uncomplicated constipation.
Contraindications: Bilron is nontoxic in therapeutic doses, and no absolute contraindications to its use have been recognized. However, on theoretical grounds, Bilron should be withheld from patients with complete biliary obstruction.
Precautions: In marked hepatic insufficiency (as in viral hepatitis, suppurative cholangitis, and advanced cirrhosis), therapy with Bilron should be avoided except in the presence of malnutrition with steatorrhea and vitamin K deficiency with hypoprothrombinemia.
Adverse Reactions: Excessive doses can cause loose stools and mild cramping, which are indications for a reduction in dosage.
Dosage and Administration: In adults, the usual dose is 150 to 450 mg, with or after meals, until constipation is relieved.
Overdosage: *Symptoms*—Loose stools and gastrointestinal cramping. *Treatment*—For general management, symptomatic therapy should be employed.

How Supplied: *Pulvules Bilron® (iron bile salts, Lilly): No. 298, F61,** 150 mg (2½ grs) (No. 2, Green), in bottles of 100 (NDC 0002-0661-02); *No. 241, F41,** 300 mg (5 grs) (No. 0, Green), in bottles of 100 (NDC 0002-0641-02) and 500 (NDC 0002-0641-03). [030180]

BREVITAL® SODIUM ©

(methohexital sodium)
For Injection, USP
For Intravenous Use

WARNING
This drug should be administered by persons qualified in the use of intravenous anesthetics and with the ready availability of appropriate resuscitative equipment for prevention and treatment of anesthetic emergencies.

Description: Brevital® Sodium (Methohexital Sodium for Injection, USP, Lilly) is sodium α-*dl*-1-methyl-5-allyl-5-(1-methyl-2-pentynyl) barbiturate. It differs chemically from the established barbiturate anesthetics in that it contains no sulfur.

Action: Methohexital sodium is a rapid, ultrashort-acting barbiturate anesthetic agent.

Indications: For induction of anesthesia, for supplementing other anesthetic agents, as intravenous anesthesia for short surgical procedures with minimum painful stimuli, or as an agent for inducing a hypnotic state.

Contraindications: Methohexital sodium is contraindicated when general anesthesia is contraindicated, in patients with latent or manifest porphyria, or in patients with a known hypersensitivity to barbiturates.

Warnings: May be habit-forming.

Repeated or continuous infusion may cause cumulative effects resulting in prolonged somnolence and respiratory and circulatory depression.

Usage in Pregnancy—Safe use of methohexital sodium has not been established with respect to possible adverse effects on human fetal development. Therefore, if methohexital sodium is to be given to women who are pregnant, the benefits to the mother should be weighed against possible risks to the fetus. When administered to pregnant rabbits and rats at four and seven times the human dose respectively, methohexital sodium produced no evidence of teratogenicity and no fetal abnormalities.

Precautions: Respiratory depression, apnea, or hypotension may occur owing to variations in tolerance from individual to individual or to the physical status of the patient. Caution should be exercised in debilitated patients or in those with impaired function of respiratory, circulatory, renal, hepatic, or endocrine systems.

Methohexital sodium should be used with extreme caution in patients in status asthmaticus.

Extravascular injection may cause pain, swelling, ulceration, and necrosis. Intra-arterial injection is dangerous and may produce gangrene of an extremity. The central-nervous-system (CNS) depressant effect of methohexital sodium may be additive with that of other CNS depressants, including alcohol.

Adverse Reactions: The following reactions have been reported:

- Circulatory depression
- Thrombophlebitis
- Pain at injection site
- Respiratory depression, including apnea
- Laryngospasm
- Bronchospasm
- Salivation
- Hiccups
- Skeletal-muscle hyperactivity (twitching to convulsive-like movements)
- Emergence delirium
- Headache
- Injury to nerves adjacent to injection site
- Nausea
- Emesis

Acute allergic reactions, such as erythema, pruritus, urticaria, rhinitis, dyspnea, hypotension, restlessness, anxiety, abdominal pain, and peripheral vascular collapse, have been reported with the use of Brevital® Sodium (methohexital sodium, Lilly).

Dosage and Administration: Preanesthetic medication is generally advisable. Brevital® Sodium (methohexital sodium, Lilly) may be used with any of the recognized preanesthetic medications, but the phenothiazines are less satisfactory than the combination of an opiate and a belladonna derivative.

Facilities for assisting respirations and administering oxygen are necessary adjuncts for intravenous anesthesia.

[See table above].

Preparation of Solutions of Brevital® Sodium (methohexital sodium)

Preparation of Solution—FOLLOW DILUTING INSTRUCTIONS EXACTLY.

Diluents—DO NOT USE DILUENTS CONTAINING BACTERIOSTATS.

Sterile Water for Injection is the preferred diluent.

Dextrose Injection (5%) or Sodium Chloride Injection (0.9%) may be used.

(Brevital Sodium is not compatible with Lactated Ringer's Injection.)

Dilution Instructions—For a 1% solution (10 mg/ml), contents of vials should be diluted as follows:

Vials No. 660 (500 mg)—add 50 ml of diluent
Vials No. 760 (500 mg)—add 50 ml of accompanying diluent
Vials No. 664 (2.5 g)—add 250 ml of diluent
Vials No. 662 (5 g)—add 500 ml of diluent

Vial No.	Amount of Diluent to Be Added to the Vial	For 1% Solution Dilute to
663 (2.5 g)	15 ml	250 ml
659 (5 g)	30 ml	500 ml

When the first dilution is made with Vials No. 663 or No. 659, the solution in the vial will be yellow. When further diluted to make a 1% solution, it must be *clear and colorless* or should not be used.

For continuous drip anesthesia, prepare a 0.2% solution by adding 500 mg of Brevital Sodium to 250 ml of diluent. For this dilution, we recommend as solvents either 5% glucose solution or isotonic (0.9%) sodium chloride solution instead of distilled water in order to avoid extreme hypotonicity.

Administration—A 1% solution is recommended for induction of anesthesia and for maintenance by intermittent injection. Dosage of all intravenous barbiturates must be individualized according to the patient's response. The usual range for Brevital® Sodium (methohexital sodium, Lilly) is 5 to 12 ml of a 1% solution (50 to 120 mg). This induction dose will provide anesthesia for five to seven minutes. The rate of injection is not fixed, but it is usually found to be about 1 ml of the 1% solution (10 mg) in five seconds. If intermittent injection of a 1% solution is used for maintenance, additional amounts of about 2 to 4 ml (20 to 40 mg) will be required every four to seven minutes.

Some anesthesiologists have preferred the continuous drip method of maintenance with a 0.2% solution. The rate of flow must be individualized for each patient. As a guide, 1 drop per second may be used.

Storage—Brevital Sodium is stable in Sterile Water for Injection at room temperature (25°C or below) for at least *six weeks*. Dextrose Injection (5%) or isotonic (0.9%) sodium chloride injection may be used as diluents, but these solutions are not stable for much more than *24 hours*. Solutions may be stored and used as long as they remain clear and colorless.

Compatibility Information: Solutions of Brevital® Sodium (methohexital sodium, Lilly) should not be mixed with acid solutions such as atropine sulfate, Metubine® Iodide (Metocurine Iodide Injection, USP, Lilly), and succinylcholine chloride. However, because of numerous requests from anesthesiologists for information regarding the chemical compatibility of these mixtures, the following is provided.

The soluble sodium salts of barbiturates are the forms used for intravenous administration. Solubility is maintained only at a relatively high (basic) pH. The accompanying chart contains information obtained from compatibility studies in which a 1% solution of Brevital Sodium was mixed with therapeutic amounts of agents whose solutions have a low (acid) pH.

Solutions of Brevital Sodium are incompatible with silicone and should not be allowed to come in contact with rubber stoppers or parts of disposable syringes that have been treated with silicone.

[See table left].

Compatibility of Brevital® Sodium (methohexital sodium) with Solutions Having a Low pH

Active Ingredient	Potency per ml	Volume Used	Physical Change: Immediate	15 min	30 min	1 hr
BREVITAL SODIUM	10 mg	10 ml	CONTROL			
Atropine sulfate	1/150 gr	1 ml	None	Haze		
Atropine sulfate	1/100 gr	1 ml	None	Ppt.	Ppt.	
Succinylcholine chloride	0.5 mg	4 ml	None	None	Haze	
Succinylcholine chloride	1 mg	4 ml	None	None	Haze	
Metocurine iodide	0.5 mg	4 ml	None	None	Ppt.	
Metocurine iodide	1 mg	4 ml	None	None	Ppt.	
Scopolamine hydrobromide	1/120 gr	1 ml	None	None	None	Haze
Tubocurarine chloride	3 mg	4 ml	None	Haze		

How Supplied: *Vials Brevital® Sodium (Methohexital Sodium for Injection, USP)* are supplied as follows:

Continued on next page

*Identi-Code® symbol.

Lilly—Cont.

(©) *No. 660,* 500 mg, 50-ml size, multiple dose, rubber-stoppered (Dry Powder), in singles (10 per carton) (NDC 0002-1446-01) and in packages of 25 (NDC 0002-1446-25).
Each vial contains—
Brevital® Sodium (methohexital sodium, Lilly) ....500 mg
Anhydrous Sodium Carbonate .... 30 mg
Contains no preservative.
(©) *No. 760,* 500 mg, 50-ml size, multiple dose, rubber-stoppered (Dry Powder), in singles (10 per carton) (NDC 0002-1465-01). Each package contains one 50-ml vial of Sterile Water for Injection.
Each vial contains—
Brevital® Sodium (methohexital sodium, Lilly) ....500 mg
Anhydrous Sodium Carbonate .... 30 mg
Contains no preservative.
(©) *No. 663,* 2.5 g, rubber-stoppered (Dry Powder), in singles (10 per carton) (NDC 0002-1448-01) and in packages of 25 (NDC 0002-1448-25).
Each vial contains—
Brevital® Sodium (methohexital sodium, Lilly) ....2.5 g
Anhydrous Sodium Carbonate ....150 mg
Contains no preservative.
(©) *No. 664,* 2.5 g, 250-ml size, multiple dose, rubber-stoppered (Dry Powder), in singles (NDC 0002-1449-01) and in packages of 25 (NDC 0002-1449-25).
Each vial contains—
Brevital® Sodium (methohexital sodium, Lilly) ....2.5 g
Anhydrous Sodium Carbonate ....150 mg
Contains no preservative.
(©) *No. 659,* 5 g, rubber-stoppered (Dry Powder), in singles (10 per carton) (NDC 0002-1445-01).
Each vial contains—
Brevital® Sodium (methohexital sodium, Lilly) ....5 g
Anhydrous Sodium Carbonate ....300 mg
Contains no preservative.
(©) *No. 662,* 5 g, 500-ml size, multiple dose, rubber-stoppered (Dry Powder), in singles (NDC 0002-1447-01) and in packages of 25 (NDC 0002-1447-25).
Each vial contains—
Brevital® Sodium (methohexital sodium, Lilly) ....5 g
Anhydrous Sodium Carbonate ....300 mg
Contains no preservative. [102582]

CAPASTAT® SULFATE ℞

(capreomycin sulfate)
Sterile, USP
Not for Pediatric Use

Warnings

The use of capreomycin in patients with renal insufficiency or preexisting auditory impairment must be undertaken with great caution, and the risk of additional eighth-nerve impairment or renal injury should be weighed against the benefits to be derived from therapy.

Refer to animal pharmacology section for additional information.

Since other parenteral antituberculosis agents (streptomycin, viomycin) also have similar and sometimes irreversible toxic effects, particularly on eighth-cranial-nerve and renal function, simultaneous administration of these agents with capreomycin is not recommended. Use with nonantituberculosis drugs (polymyxin, colistin sulfate, gentamicin, tobramycin, vancomycin, kanamycin, and neomycin) having ototoxic or nephrotoxic potential should be undertaken only with great caution.

Usage in Pregnancy—The safety of the use of capreomycin in *pregnancy* has not been determined.

Pediatric Usage—Safety of the use of capreomycin in infants and children has not been established.

Description: Capastat® Sulfate (capreomycin sulfate, Lilly) is a polypeptide antibiotic isolated from *Streptomyces capreolus.* It is a complex of four microbiologically active components which have been characterized in part; however, complete structural determination of all the components has not been established. Capreomycin is supplied as the disulfate salt and is soluble in water. In complete solution, it is almost colorless.

Actions: *Human Pharmacology*—Capastat® Sulfate (capreomycin sulfate, Lilly) is not absorbed in significant quantities from the gastrointestinal tract and must be administered parenterally. In two studies of ten patients each, peak serum concentrations following 1 g of capreomycin given intramuscularly were achieved one to two hours after administration, and average peak levels reached were 28 and 32 mcg/ml respectively (range, 20 to 47 mcg/ml). Low serum concentrations were present at 24 hours. However, 1 g of capreomycin daily for 30 days or more produced no significant accumulation in subjects with normal renal function. Two patients with marked reduction of renal function had high serum concentrations 24 hours after administration of the drug. When a 1-g dose of capreomycin was given intramuscularly to normal volunteers, 52 percent was excreted in the urine within 12 hours.

Paper chromatographic studies indicated that capreomycin is excreted essentially unaltered. Urine concentrations averaged 1.68 mg/ml (average urine volume, 228 ml) during the six hours following a 1-g dose.

Microbiology—Capreomycin is active against human strains of *Mycobacterium tuberculosis.* The susceptibility of strains of *M. tuberculosis* in vitro varies with the media and techniques employed. In general, the minimum inhibitory concentrations for *M. tuberculosis* are lowest in liquid media that are free of egg protein (7H10 or Dubos) and range from 1 to 5 mcg/ml when the indirect method is used. Comparable inhibitory concentrations are obtained when 7H10 agar is used for direct susceptibility testing. When indirect susceptibility tests are performed on standard tube slants with 7H10 media, susceptible strains are inhibited by 10 to 25 mcg/ml. Egg-containing media, such as Löwenstein-Jensen or ATS, require concentrations of 25 to 50 mcg/ml to inhibit susceptible strains.

Cross-Resistance—Frequent cross-resistance occurs between capreomycin and viomycin. Varying degrees of cross-resistance between capreomycin and kanamycin and neomycin have been reported. No cross-resistance has been observed between capreomycin and isoniazid, aminosalicylic acid, cycloserine, streptomycin, ethionamide, or ethambutol.

Indications: Capreomycin, which is to be used concomitantly with other appropriate antituberculosis agents, is indicated in pulmonary infections caused by capreomycin-susceptible strains of *M. tuberculosis* when the primary agents (isoniazid, aminosalicylic acid, and streptomycin) have been ineffective or cannot be used because of toxicity or the presence of resistant tubercle bacilli.

Susceptibility studies should be performed to determine the presence of a capreomycin-susceptible strain of *M. tuberculosis.*

Contraindication: Capreomycin is contraindicated in those patients who are hypersensitive to it.

Precautions: Audiometric measurements and assessment of vestibular function should be performed prior to initiation of therapy with capreomycin and at regular intervals during treatment.

Regular tests of renal function should be made throughout the period of treatment, and reduced dosage should be employed in patients with known or suspected renal impairment.

Renal injury, with tubular necrosis, elevation of the blood urea nitrogen (BUN) or nonprotein nitrogen (NPN), and abnormal urinary sediment, has been noted. Renal function studies should be made both before capreomycin therapy is started and on a weekly basis during treatment. Slight elevation of the BUN or NPN has been observed in a significant number of patients receiving prolonged therapy. The appearance of casts, red cells, and white cells in the urine has been noted in a high percentage of these cases. Elevation of the BUN above 30 mg/100 ml or any other evidence of decreasing renal function with or without a rise in BUN levels calls for careful evaluation of the patient, and the dosage should be reduced or the drug completely withdrawn. The clinical significance of abnormal urine sediment and slight elevation in the BUN (or total NPN) observed during long-term capreomycin therapy has not been established.

Since hypokalemia may occur during capreomycin therapy, serum potassium levels should be determined frequently.

The peripheral neuromuscular blocking action that has been attributed to other polypeptide antibiotics (colistin sulfate, polymyxin A sulfate, paromomycin, and viomycin) and aminoglycoside antibiotics (streptomycin, dihydrostreptomycin, neomycin, and kanamycin) has been studied with capreomycin. A partial neuromuscular block was demonstrated after large intravenous doses of capreomycin. This action was enhanced by ether anesthesia (as has been reported for neomycin) and was antagonized by neostigmine.

Caution should be exercised in the administration of antibiotics, including capreomycin, to any patient who has demonstrated some form of allergy, particularly to drugs.

Adverse Reactions: *Nephrotoxicity*—In 36 percent of 722 patients treated with capreomycin, elevation of the BUN above 20 mg/100 ml and of the NPN above 35 mg/100 ml has been observed. In many instances, there was also depression of PSP excretion and abnormal urine sediment. In 10 percent of this series, the BUN elevation exceeded 30 mg/100 ml or the NPN exceeded 50 mg/100 ml.

Toxic nephritis was reported in one patient with tuberculosis and portal cirrhosis who was treated with capreomycin (1 g) and aminosalicylic acid daily for one month. This patient developed renal insufficiency and oliguria and died. Autopsy showed subsiding acute tubular necrosis.

Ototoxicity—Subclinical auditory loss was noted in approximately 11 percent of patients undergoing treatment with capreomycin. This has been a 5 to 10-decibel loss in the 4000 to 8000-CPS range. Clinically apparent hearing loss occurred in 3 percent of 722 subjects. Some audiometric changes were reversible. Other cases with permanent loss were not progressive following withdrawal of capreomycin. Tinnitus and vertigo have occurred.

Liver—Serial tests of liver function have demonstrated a decrease in BSP excretion without change in SGOT or SGPT in the presence of preexisting liver disease. Abnormal results in liver function tests have occurred in many persons receiving capreomycin in combination with other antituberculosis agents which also are known to cause changes in hepatic function. The role of capreomycin in producing these abnormalities is not clear; however, periodic determinations of liver function are recommended.

Blood—Leukocytosis and leukopenia have been observed. The majority of patients treated have had eosinophilia exceeding 5 percent while receiving daily injections of capreo-

mycin. This has subsided with reduction of the capreomycin dosage to 2 or 3 g weekly.
Pain and induration at the injection sites have been observed. Excessive bleeding at the injection site has been reported. Sterile abscesses have been noted.
Hypersensitivity—Urticaria and maculopapular skin rashes associated in some cases with febrile reactions have been reported when capreomycin and other antituberculosis drugs were given concomitantly.
Dosage and Administration: Capastat® Sulfate (capreomycin sulfate, Lilly) should be dissolved in 2 ml of 0.9% Sodium Chloride Injection or Sterile Water for Injection. Two to three minutes should be allowed for complete solution. For administration of a 1-g dose, the entire contents of the vial should be given. For dosages less than 1 g, the accompanying dilution table may be used.
[See table above].

DILUTION TABLE FOR CAPASTAT® SULFATE (capreomycin sulfate)

Diluent Added to 1-g Vial	Volume of Capastat Sulfate Solution	Concentration* (Approx.)
2.15 ml	2.85 ml	350 mg/ml
2.63 ml	3.33 ml	300 mg/ml
3.3 ml	4 ml	250 mg/ml
4.3 ml	5 ml	200 mg/ml

*Stated in terms of mg of capreomycin activity.

The solution may acquire a pale straw color and darken with time, but this is not associated with loss of potency or the development of toxicity. After reconstitution, solutions of Capastat Sulfate may be stored for 48 hours at room temperature and up to 14 days under refrigeration.
Capastat Sulfate should be given by deep intramuscular injection into a large muscle mass, since superficial injections may be associated with increased pain and the development of sterile abscesses.
Capreomycin is always administered in combination with at least one other antituberculosis agent to which the patient's strain of tubercle bacilli is susceptible. The usual dose is 1 g daily (not to exceed 20 mg/kg/day) given intramuscularly for 60 to 120 days, followed by 1 g intramuscularly two or three times weekly. (*Note*—Therapy for tuberculosis should be maintained for 18 to 24 months. If facilities for administering injectable medication are not available, a change to appropriate oral therapy is indicated on the patient's release from the hospital.)
Animal Pharmacology: In addition to renal and eighth-cranial-nerve toxicity demonstrated in animal toxicology studies, two dogs have developed cataracts while on doses of 62 mg/kg and 100 mg/kg for prolonged periods.
In teratology studies, a low incidence of "wavy ribs" was noted in litters of female rats treated with daily doses of 50 mg/kg or more of capreomycin.
How Supplied: (℞) *Vials No. 718, Capastat® Sulfate (Sterile Capreomycin Sulfate, USP),* equivalent to 1 g capreomycin activity, 10-ml size, rubber-stoppered (Dry Powder), in singles (NDC 0002-1485-01) (10 per carton).

[102682]

CARBARSONE ℞

(Arsenic Derivative)
Capsules, USP

Description: Carbarsone, USP, is a pentavalent organic arsenical containing approximately 29 percent arsenic. It is a white, crystalline, odorless solid that is stable in air and has a slightly acid taste. It is practically insoluble in water but is soluble in carbonate or bicarbonate solutions.
Chemically, Carbarsone is *p*-ureido-benzenearsonic acid with the empirical formula $C_7H_9AsN_2O_4$.
Clinical Pharmacology: Carbarsone is directly amebicidal by virtue of its arsenic content; it probably combines with thiol (SH) groups in essential enzyme systems in the parasite. The action of the drug on motile forms is not as rapid as that of emetine, and it has no value in the treatment of extraintestinal amebiasis. Carbarsone eradicates cysts by destroying the trophozoites that are the source of the cysts. Carbarsone is absorbed readily after oral administration and is excreted rather slowly in the urine. Rest periods between courses are therefore imperative to prevent cumulative toxic effects. In experimental animals, parenterally administered carbarsone has been found to be excreted into the small intestine, mostly by way of the bile.
Indications and Usage: Carbarsone is indicated in the treatment of intestinal amebiasis and is effective against the trophozoite form of *Entamoeba histolytica* in the lumen and shallow ulcers of the colon.
Contraindications: Carbarsone should not be used (1) as the initial agent when amebic hepatitis of any degree may be present, (2) when there is any other liver or kidney disease, (3) in the presence of contracted visual or color fields, or (4) when the patient is hypersensitive or intolerant to organic or inorganic arsenic given systemically or applied topically.
Warnings: Fatalities from exfoliative dermatitis, liver necrosis, and hemorrhagic encephalitis are on record.
Precautions: *General Precautions*—Since Carbarsone is absorbed readily from the gastrointestinal tract and excreted rather slowly by way of the kidneys, accumulation of the drug may result. Therefore, the following precautions should be observed. If prolonged treatment is indicated or contemplated, it is mandatory that the recommended daily dose not be exceeded, that a course of treatment be no longer than ten days, and that a rest interval of at least ten days be allowed before another treatment period is started. If there is any evidence of intolerance or toxicity (i.e., increase in severity of gastrointestinal symptoms already present; development of nausea, vomiting, abdominal pain or cramps, or diarrhea when these symptoms have not previously been present; urinary symptoms; dermatitis or other skin lesions suggesting sensitivity to arsenic; any central or peripheral nervous-system changes; or any of the signs or symptoms listed below or under Adverse Reactions), the drug should be discontinued at once. Since Carbarsone accumulates in the tissues and is eliminated slowly, the patient should be instructed to report any unusual signs or symptoms for a period of time after treatment has been discontinued.
Epstein (*Arch. Dermat. & Syph., 36:* 964, 1937) found that individuals who are sensitive to trivalent arsenicals may also exhibit positive skin reactions when tested with pentavalent arsenicals. Four of six such patients showed positive patch tests with Carbarsone. This author also reported a fatality which occurred following a course of therapy with Carbarsone, but he stated that, when correctly administered, this drug is less toxic than other related arsenical preparations. Smithies (*J.A.M.A., 103:* 258, 1934) observed sore throat, splenic enlargement, and edema of ankles, knees, and wrists in patients receiving Carbarsone and reported single instances of icterus, dermatitis, and papillitis with retinal edema.
Information for Patients—Substances such as arsenic, lead, mercury, cadmium disulfide, phosphorus, and carbon monoxide may cause deafness, tinnitus, and vertigo. Following the administration of arsenicals, a brownish discoloration of the skin, thrombocytopenia, aplastic anemia, and agranulocytosis may develop. (*See* sections on Contraindications, Warnings, General Precautions, and Adverse Reactions.)
Carcinogenesis, Mutagenesis, Impairment of Fertility—No long-term studies in animals have been performed to evaluate carcinogenic potential. However, the literature indicates that the use of arsenic has been associated with skin cancer.
Pregnancy—Pregnancy Category C—Animal reproduction studies have not been conducted with Carbarsone. It is also not known whether Carbarsone can cause fetal harm when administered to a pregnant woman or can affect reproduction capacity. Carbarsone should be given to a pregnant woman only if clearly needed.
Nursing Mothers—It is not known whether this drug is excreted in human milk. Because many drugs are excreted in human milk and because of the potential for serious adverse reactions in nursing infants from Carbarsone or tumorigenicity due to arsenic, a decision should be made whether to discontinue nursing or to discontinue the drug, taking into account the importance of the drug to the mother.
Usage in Children—Carbarsone is one of the most innocuous of the organic arsenicals. However, skin rashes may occur, but they are usually mild. Nausea, vomiting, abdominal pain, and diarrhea may also occur.
Chronic amebic infections that resist an adequate course of Carbarsone therapy will frequently respond to it after a several-day course of penicillin, erythromycin, or sulfisoxazole to reduce the bacterial pathogens in the large intestine.
Adverse Reactions: The following adverse reactions have been noted: sore throat, edema, splenomegaly, icterus, pruritus, skin eruptions, gastrointestinal irritation, hepatitis, neuritis, and visual disturbances.
If it is warranted, untoward reactions to Carbarsone may be treated with the specific antiarsenical compound dimercaprol (BAL).
Drug Abuse and Dependence: It is not likely that this drug will be abused or that dependence will develop.
Overdosage: *Symptoms*—Nausea, vomiting, abdominal pain, diarrhea, shock, coma, convulsions, ulceration of mucous membranes and skin, and kidney damage.
Treatment—Specifically, dimercaprol, 3 to 4 mg/kg (or 0.3 to 0.4 ml/kg) every six hours for the first two days and then twice daily for a total of ten days. General management should be symptomatic and supportive and may include gastric lavage, administration of oxygen, intravenous fluids, and maintenance of body temperature. If there is reason for rapid removal of the drug, asenicals are hemodialyzable.
Dosage and Administration:
Adults—The usual course of treatment consists in oral administration of 250 mg (4 grs) of Carbarsone two or three times daily for ten days. Additional courses of treatment are given as indicated following a rest period of ten to 14 days.
Children—The individual and total dosage may be reduced in proportion to weight. The

Continued on next page

*Identi-Code® symbol.

Lilly—Cont.

average total dose, based on body weight, is about 75 mg/kg.

The following dosage scale will be effective: ages two to four years, a total dose of 2 g of Carbarsone over a period of ten days, a dose of 66 mg being given three times a day in half a glass of milk or in orange juice; ages five to eight years, a total dose of 3 g of Carbarsone over a ten-day period in three daily doses; nine to 12 years, a total dose of 4 g in three daily doses for ten days; and from puberty on to young adulthood, a total dose of 5 g.

For children, it will be necessary to divide the contents of a Pulvule® and to give the Carbarsone as suggested above or in a small volume of sodium bicarbonate solution (1 percent), in jelly, or in some other food. The taste is not objectionable. If a solution is made of the Pulvule, it is to be remembered that it will not be clear, but the Carbarsone will be in solution.

Should toxic manifestations appear, discontinue therapy at once.

How Supplied: (℞) Pulvules, 250 mg, pink (No. 227), in bottles of 20 (NDC 0002-0634-20-20).

[030481]

CECLOR® ℞
(cefaclor)

Description: Ceclor® (cefaclor, Lilly) is a semisynthetic cephalosporin antibiotic for oral administration. It is chemically designated as 3-chloro-7-D-(2-phenylglycinamido)-3-cephem-4-carboxylic acid. Ceclor is available in 250-mg and 500-mg Pulvules® and in a powder for oral suspension containing 125 or 250 mg/5 ml.

Clinical Pharmacology: Cefaclor is well absorbed after oral administration to fasting subjects. Total absorption is the same whether the drug is given with or without food; however, when it is taken with food, the peak concentration achieved is 50 to 75 percent of that observed when the drug is administered to fasting subjects and generally appears from three-fourths to one hour later. Following administration of 250-mg, 500-mg, and 1-g doses to fasting subjects, average peak serum levels of approximately 7, 13, and 23 mcg/ml respectively were obtained within 30 to 60 minutes. Approximately 60 to 85 percent of the drug is excreted unchanged in the urine within eight hours, the greater portion being excreted within the first two hours. During this eight-hour period, peak urine concentrations following the 250-mg, 500-mg, and 1-g doses were approximately 600, 900, and 1900 mcg/ml respectively. The serum half-life in normal subjects is 0.6 to 0.9 hour. In patients with reduced renal function, the serum half-life of cefaclor is slightly prolonged. In those with complete absence of renal function, the biologic half-life of the intact molecule is 2.3 to 2.8 hours. Excretion pathways in patients with markedly impaired renal function have not been determined. Hemodialysis shortens the half-life by 25 to 30 percent.

Microbiology—In vitro tests demonstrate that the bactericidal action of the cephalosporins results from inhibition of cell-wall synthesis. Cefaclor is usually active against the following organisms in vitro and in clinical infections:

- Staphylococci, including coagulase-positive, coagulase-negative, and penicillinase-producing strains
- *Streptococcus pyogenes* (group A beta-hemolytic streptococci)
- *S. pneumoniae* (formerly *Diplococcus pneumoniae*)
- *Escherichia coli*
- *Proteus mirabilis*
- *Klebsiella* species
- *Haemophilus influenzae,* including some beta-lactamase-producing ampicillin-resistant strains

Note: Pseudomonas species, *Acinetobacter calcoaceticus* (formerly *Mima* and *Herellea* species), and most strains of enterococci (*S. faecalis,* group D streptococci), *Enterobacter* species, indole-positive *Proteus,* and *Serratia* species are resistant to cefaclor. When tested by in vitro methods, staphylococci exhibit cross-resistance between cefaclor and methicillin-type antibiotics.

Disc Susceptibility Tests—Quantitative methods that require measurement of zone diameters give the most precise estimates of antibiotic susceptibility. One such procedure* has been recommended for use with discs for testing susceptibility to cephalothin. The currently accepted zone diameter interpretative criteria for the cephalothin disc are appropriate for determining bacterial susceptibility to cefaclor. With this procedure, a report from the laboratory of "resistant" indicates that the infecting organism is not likely to respond to therapy. A report of "intermediate susceptibility" suggests that the organism would be susceptible if the infection is confined to tissues and fluids (e.g., urine) in which high antibiotic levels can be obtained or if high dosage is used.

Indications and Usage: Ceclor® (cefaclor, Lilly) is indicated in the treatment of the following infections when caused by susceptible strains of the designated microorganisms:

- Otitis media caused by *S. pneumoniae (D. pneumoniae), H. influenzae,* staphylococci, and *S. pyogenes* (group A beta-hemolytic streptococci)
- Lower respiratory infections, including pneumonia caused by *S. pneumoniae (D. pneumoniae), H. influenzae,* and *S. pyogenes* (group A beta-hemolytic streptococci)
- Upper respiratory infections, including pharyngitis and tonsillitis caused by *S. pyogenes* (group A beta-hemolytic streptococci)

  Note: Penicillin is the usual drug of choice in the treatment and prevention of streptococcal infections, including the prophylaxis of rheumatic fever. Ceclor is generally effective in the eradication of streptococci from the nasopharynx; however, substantial data establishing the efficacy of Ceclor in the subsequent prevention of rheumatic fever are not available at present.
- Urinary tract infections, including pyelonephritis and cystitis caused by *E. coli, P. mirabilis, Klebsiella* species, and coagulase-negative staphylococci
- Skin and skin-structure infections caused by *Staphylococcus aureus* and *S. pyogenes* (group A beta-hemolytic streptococci)

Appropriate culture and susceptibility studies should be performed to determine susceptibility of the causative organism to Ceclor.

Contraindication: Ceclor® (cefaclor, Lilly) is contraindicated in patients with known allergy to the cephalosporin group of antibiotics.

Warnings: IN PENICILLIN-SENSITIVE PATIENTS, CEPHALOSPORIN ANTIBIOTICS SHOULD BE ADMINISTERED CAUTIOUSLY. THERE IS CLINICAL AND LABORATORY EVIDENCE OF PARTIAL CROSS-ALLERGENICITY OF THE PENICILLINS AND THE CEPHALOSPORINS, AND THERE ARE INSTANCES IN WHICH PATIENTS HAVE HAD REACTIONS, INCLUDING ANAPHYLAXIS, TO BOTH DRUG CLASSES.

Antibiotics, including Ceclor® (cefaclor, Lilly), should be administered cautiously to any patient who has demonstrated some form of allergy, particularly to drugs.

Pseudomembranous colitis has been reported with virtually all broad-spectrum antibiotics (including macrolides, semisynthetic penicillins, and cephalosporins); therefore, it is important to consider its diagnosis in patients who develop diarrhea in association with the use of antibiotics. Such colitis may range in severity from mild to life-threatening.

Treatment with broad-spectrum antibiotics alters the normal flora of the colon and may permit overgrowth of clostridia. Studies indicate that a toxin produced by *Clostridium difficile* is one primary cause of antibiotic-associated colitis.

Mild cases of pseudomembranous colitis usually respond to drug discontinuance alone. In moderate to severe cases, management should include sigmoidoscopy, appropriate bacteriologic studies, and fluid, electrolyte, and protein supplementation. When the colitis does not improve after the drug has been discontinued, or when it is severe, oral vancomycin is the drug of choice for antibiotic-associated pseudomembranous colitis produced by *C. difficile.* Other causes of colitis should be ruled out.

Precautions: *General Precautions*—If an allergic reaction to cefaclor occurs, the drug should be discontinued, and, if necessary, the patient should be treated with appropriate agents, e.g., pressor amines, antihistamines, or corticosteroids.

Prolonged use of Ceclor® (cefaclor, Lilly) may result in the overgrowth of nonsusceptible organisms. Careful observation of the patient is essential. If superinfection occurs during therapy, appropriate measures should be taken.

Positive direct Coombs' tests have been reported during treatment with the cephalosporin antibiotics. In hematologic studies or in transfusion cross-matching procedures when antiglobulin tests are performed on the minor side or in Coombs' testing of newborns whose mothers have received cephalosporin antibiotics before parturition, it should be recognized that a positive Coombs' test may be due to the drug.

Ceclor should be administered with caution in the presence of markedly impaired renal function. Under such conditions, careful clinical observation and laboratory studies should be made because safe dosage may be lower than that usually recommended.

As a result of administration of Ceclor, a false-positive reaction for glucose in the urine may occur. This has been observed with Benedict's and Fehling's solutions and also with Clinitest® tablets but not with Tes-Tape® (Glucose Enzymatic Test Strip, USP, Lilly).

Broad-spectrum antibiotics should be prescribed with caution in individuals with a history of gastrointestinal disease, particularly colitis.

Usage in Pregnancy—Pregnancy Category B—Reproduction studies have been performed in mice and rats at doses up to 12 times the human dose and in ferrets given three times the maximum human dose and have revealed no evidence of impaired fertility or harm to the fetus due to Ceclor. There are, however, no adequate and well-controlled studies in pregnant women. Because animal reproduction studies are not always predictive of human response, this drug should be used during pregnancy only if clearly needed.

Nursing Mothers—Small amounts of Ceclor have been detected in mother's milk following administration of single 500-mg doses. Average levels were 0.18, 0.20, 0.21, and 0.16 mcg/ml at two, three, four, and five hours respectively. Trace amounts were detected at one hour. The effect on nursing infants is not known. Caution should be exercised when Ceclor is administered to a nursing woman.

Usage in Children—Safety and effectiveness of this product for use in infants less than one month of age have not been established.

Adverse Reactions: Adverse effects considered related to therapy with Ceclor® (cefaclor, Lilly) are uncommon and are listed below:

Gastrointestinal symptoms occur in about 2.5 percent of patients and include diarrhea (1 in 70).

Symptoms of pseudomembranous colitis may appear either during or after antibiotic treatment. Nausea and vomiting have been reported rarely.

Hypersensitivity reactions have been reported in about 1.5 percent of patients and include morbilliform eruptions (1 in 100). Pruritus, urticaria, and positive Coombs' tests each occur in less than 1 in 200 patients. Cases of serum-sickness-like reactions (erythema multiforme or the above skin manifestations accompanied by arthritis/arthralgia and, frequently, fever) have been reported. These reactions are apparently due to hypersensitivity and have usually occurred during or following a second course of therapy with Ceclor. Such reactions have been reported more frequently in children than in adults. Signs and symptoms usually occur a few days after initiation of therapy and subside within a few days after cessation of therapy. No serious sequelae have been reported. Antihistamines and corticosteroids appear to enhance resolution of the syndrome.

Cases of anaphylaxis have been reported, half of which have occurred in patients with a history of penicillin allergy.

Other effects considered related to therapy include eosinophilia (1 in 50 patients) and genital pruritus or vaginitis (less than 1 in 100 patients).

Causal Relationship Uncertain—Transitory abnormalities in clinical laboratory test results have been reported. Although they were of uncertain etiology, they are listed below to serve as alerting information for the physician.

Hepatic—Slight elevations in SGOT, SGPT, or alkaline phosphatase values (1 in 40).

Hematopoietic—Transient fluctuations in leukocyte count, predominantly lymphocytosis occurring in infants and young children (1 in 40).

Renal—Slight elevations in BUN or serum creatinine (less than 1 in 500) or abnormal urinalysis (less than 1 in 200).

Dosage and Administration: Ceclor® (cefaclor, Lilly) is administered orally.

Adults—The usual adult dosage is 250 mg every eight hours. For more severe infections (such as pneumonia) or those caused by less susceptible organisms, doses may be doubled. Doses of 4 g/day have been administered safely to normal subjects for 28 days, but the total daily dosage should not exceed this amount.

Children—The usual recommended daily dosage for children is 20 mg/kg/day in divided doses every eight hours, as indicated:

Child's Weight	Ceclor Suspension 125 mg/5 ml	250 mg/5 ml
9 kg	½ tsp t.i.d.	
18 kg	1 tsp t.i.d.	½ tsp t.i.d.

In more serious infections, otitis media, and infections caused by less susceptible organisms, 40 mg/kg/day are recommended, with a maximum dosage of 1 g/day.

Ceclor may be administered in the presence of impaired renal function. Under such a condition, the dosage usually is unchanged (*see* Precautions).

In the treatment of beta-hemolytic streptococcal infections, a therapeutic dosage of Ceclor should be administered for at least ten days.

How Supplied: (℞) *Ceclor® (Cefaclor, USP), for Oral Suspension, M-5057,* 125 mg/5 ml (strawberry flavor) and *M-5058,* 250 mg/5 ml (grape flavor), in 75 (NDC 0002-5057-18 and NDC 0002-5058-18) and 150-ml-size (NDC 0002-5057-68 and NDC 0002-5058-68) packages.

Directions for mixing are included on the label. After mixing, store in a refrigerator. Shake well before using. Keep tightly closed. The mixture may be kept for 14 days without significant loss of potency. Discard unused portion after 14 days.

(℞) *Pulvules® Ceclor® (Cefaclor, USP): No. 3061,* 250 mg (White Opaque Body, Purple Opaque Cap), and *No. 3062,* 500 mg (Gray Opaque Body, Purple Opaque Cap), in bottles of 15 (NDC 0002-3061-15 and NDC 0002-3062-15) and 100 (NDC 0002-3061-02 and NDC 0002-3062-02) in 10 strips of 10 individually labeled blisters each containing one Pulvule (ID100) (NDC 0002-3061-33 and NDC 0002-3062-33).

[*Shown in Product Identification Section*]

*Bauer, A. W., Kirby, W. M. M., Sherris, J. C., and Turck, M.: Antibiotic Susceptibility Testing by a Standardized Single Disk Method, Am. J. Clin. Pathol, *45:*493, 1966; Standardized Disc Susceptibility Test, Federal Register, *39:*19182–19184, 1974.

[061782]

CEFACLOR, *see* Ceclor® (cefaclor, Lilly).

CEFAMANDOLE NAFATE, *see* Mandol® (cefamandole nafate, Lilly).

CEFAZOLIN SODIUM, *see* Kefzol® (cefazolin sodium, Lilly).

CEPHALOTHIN SODIUM, *see* Keflin® (cephalothin sodium, Lilly).

COLCHICINE ℞
Injection, USP

This product to be used by the physician or under his direction.

Description: A phenanthrene derivative, colchicine is the active alkaloidal principle derived from various species of *Colchicum;* it appears as pale-yellow amorphorus scales or powder that darkens on exposure to light.

The empirical formula is $C_{22}H_{25}NO_6$ (399.45). One g dissolves in 25 ml of water and in 220 ml of ether. Colchicine is freely soluble in alcohol and chloroform.

Colchicine, an acetyltrimethylcolchicinic acid, is hydrolyzed in the presence of dilute acids or alkalies, with cleavage of a methyl group as methanol and formation of *colchiceine,* which has very little therapeutic activity. On hydrolysis with strong acids, colchicine is converted to trimethylcolchicinic acid.

Ampoules Colchicine Injection, USP, provide an aqueous solution of colchicine for intravenous use. Each ampoule contains 1 mg of colchicine in 2 ml of solution. Sodium hydroxide may have been added during manufacture to adjust the *p*H.

Clinical Pharmacology: The mechanism of the relief afforded by colchicine in acute attacks of gouty arthritis is not completely known, but studies on the processes involved in precipitation of an acute attack have helped elucidate how this drug may exert its effects. The drug is not an analgesic, does not relieve other types of pain or inflammation, and is of no value in other types of arthritis. It is not a diuretic and does not influence the renal excretion of uric acid or its level in the blood or the magnitude of the "miscible pool" of uric acid. It also does not alter the solubility of urate in the plasma.

Colchicine is not a uricosuric agent. An acute attack of gout apparently occurs as a result of an inflammatory reaction to crystals of monosodium urate that are deposited in the joint tissue from hyperuric body fluids; the reaction is aggravated as more urate crystals accumulate. The initial inflammatory response involves local infiltration of granulocytes that phagocytize the urate crystals. Interference with these processes will prevent the development of an acute attack. Colchicine apparently exerts its effect by reducing the inflammatory response to the deposited crystals and also by diminishing phagocytosis. The deposition of uric acid is favored by an acid *p*H. In synovial tissues and in leukocytes associated with inflammatory processes, lactic acid production is high, and this favors a local decrease in *p*H that enhances uric acid deposition. Colchicine diminishes lactic acid production by leukocytes directly and by diminishing phagocytosis and thereby interrupts the cycle of urate crystal deposition and inflammatory response that sustains the acute attack. The oxidation of glucose in phagocytizing as well as in nonphagocytizing leukocytes in vitro is suppressed by colchicine; this suppression may explain the diminished lactic acid production. The precise biochemical step that is affected by colchicine is not yet known. That the antimitotic activity of colchicine is unrelated to its effectiveness in the treatment of acute gout is indicated by the fact that trimethylcolchicinic acid, an analog of colchicine, has no antimitotic activity except in extremely high doses.

Indications and Usage: Colchicine is indicated for the treatment of gout. It is effective in relieving the pain of acute attacks, especially if therapy is begun early in the attack and in adequate dosage. Many therapists use colchicine as interval therapy to prevent acute attacks of gout. It has no effect on nongouty arthritis or on uric acid metabolism.

The intravenous use of colchicine is advantageous when a rapid response is desired or when gastrointestinal side effects interfere with oral administration of the medication. Occasionally, intravenous colchicine is effective when the oral preparation is not. After the acute attack has subsided, the patient can usually be given colchicine tablets by mouth.

Contraindications: Colchicine is contraindicated in patients with gout who also have serious gastrointestinal, renal, or cardiac disorders.

Warnings: Colchicine can cause fetal harm when administered to a pregnant woman. If this drug is used during pregnancy, or if the patient becomes pregnant while taking it, the woman should be apprised of the potential hazard to the fetus.

Precautions: *General Precautions*—Colchicine should be administered with great caution to aged and debilitated patients, especially those with renal, gastrointestinal, or heart disease. Reduction in dosage is indicated if weakness, anorexia, nausea, vomiting, or diarrhea appears. Rarely, thrombophlebitis occurs at the site of injection.

Drug Interactions—Colchicine has been shown to induce reversible malabsorption of vitamin B_{12}, apparently by altering the function of ileal mucosa. The possibility that colchicine may increase response to central-nervous-system depressants and to sympathomimetic agents is suggested by the results of experiments on animals.

Usage in Pregnancy—Pregnancy Category D—See Warnings.

Nursing Mothers—It is not known whether this drug is excreted in human milk. Because many drugs are excreted in human milk, caution should be exercised when colchicine is administered to a nursing woman.

Usage in Children—Safety and effectiveness in children have not been established.

Adverse Reactions: These are usually gastrointestinal in nature and consist of abdominal pain, nausea, vomiting, and diarrhea. The diarrhea may be severe. The gastrointestinal symptoms may occur even though the drug is given intravenously; however, such symptoms are unusual unless the recommended dose is exceeded.

Prolonged administration may cause bone-marrow depression, with agranulocytosis, thrombocytopenia, and aplastic anemia. Peripheral neuritis and depilation have also been reported.

Overdosage: There is usually a latent period between overdosage and the onset of symptoms, regardless of the route of administration. The lethal dose of colchicine has been esti-

Continued on next page

•Identi-Code® symbol.

Lilly—Cont.

mated to be 65 mg. However, deaths have been reported with as little as 8 mg, although higher doses have been taken without fatal results. The first symptoms to appear are gastrointestinal—nausea, vomiting, abdominal pain, and diarrhea. The diarrhea may be severe and bloody owing to hemorrhagic gastroenteritis. To control the diarrhea and cramps, paregoric is usually administered. Burning sensations in the throat, stomach, and skin may also occur. Extensive vascular damage may result in shock. The kidney may show evidence of damage by hematuria and oliguria, since it is an excretory site. Severe dehydration and hypotension develop. Muscular weakness is marked, and an ascending paralysis of the central nervous system may develop. The patient usually remains conscious. However, delirium and convulsions may occur. Death usually is the result of respiratory depression.
Recent studies[1,2] appear to support the use of hemodialysis or peritoneal dialysis as part of the treatment of acute overdosage. Shock must be combated. Atropine and morphine may relieve the abdominal pain. Respiratory assistance may be needed to insure proper oxygenation and ventilation.
Dosage and Administration: Colchicine Injection is for intravenous use only. Severe local irritation occurs if it is administered subcutaneously or intramuscularly.
It is extremely important that the needle be properly positioned in the vein before colchicine is injected. If leakage into surrounding tissue or outside the vein along its course should occur during intravenous administration, considerable irritation may follow. There is no specific antidote for the prevention of this irritation. Local application of heat or cold as well as administration of analgesics, may afford relief.
The injection should take two to five minutes for completion. Colchicine Injection should not be diluted with 5% Dextrose in Water. If a decrease in concentration of colchicine in solution is required, 0.9% Sodium Chloride Injection, which does not contain a bacteriostatic agent, should be used. Solutions which thereafter become turbid should not be injected.
In the treatment of acute gouty arthritis, the average initial dose of Colchicine Injection is 2 mg (4 ml). This may be followed by 0.5 mg (1 ml) every six hours until a satisfactory response is achieved. In general, the total dosage for a 24-hour period should not exceed 4 mg (8 ml). Some clinicians recommend a single intravenous dose of 3 mg, whereas others recommend not more than 1 mg of colchicine intravenously for the initial dose, followed by 0.5 mg once or twice daily if needed.
If pain recurs, it may be necessary to administer a daily dose of 1 to 2 mg (2 to 4 ml) for several days. Many patients can be transferred to the oral colchicine in a similar dosage to that being given intravenously.
In the prophylactic or maintenance therapy of recurrent or chronic gouty arthritis, a dosage of 0.5 to 1 mg (1 to 2 ml) once or twice daily may be used. However, in these cases, oral administration of colchicine is preferable, usually in conjunction with a uricosuric agent.
How Supplied: (℞) *Ampoules No. 656, Colchicine Injection, USP,* 1 mg, 2 ml, in packages of 6 (NDC 0002-1443-16).

[090382]

1. Donigian, D. W., and Owellen, R. J.: Interaction of Vinblastine, Vincristine, and Colchicine with Serum Proteins, Biochem. Pharmacol., *22:*2113, 1973.
2. Wolen, R. L.: Unpublished data, Lilly Research Laboratories, 1975.

COLCHICINE ℞
Tablets, USP

Description and Clinical Pharmacology: *See under* Colchicine Injection, USP.
Indications and Usage: Colchicine is indicated for the treatment of gout. It is effective in relieving the pain of acute attacks, especially if therapy is begun early in the attack and in adequate dosage. Many therapists use colchicine as interval therapy to prevent acute attacks of gout. It has no effect on nongouty arthritis or on uric acid metabolism.
Contraindications, Warnings, and Precautions: *See under* Colchicine Injection, USP.
Adverse Reactions: In full dosage, colchicine produces nausea, vomiting, or diarrhea. However, it is generally necessary to reach such dose levels for an adequate therapeutic effect. Paregoric may be given either concurrently or when diarrhea develops.
Prolonged administration may cause bone-marrow depression, with agranulocytosis, thrombocytopenia, and aplastic anemia. Peripheral neuritis and depilation have also been reported.
Overdosage: *See under* Colchicine Injection, USP.
Recent studies[1,2] would appear to support the use of hemodialysis or peritoneal dialysis as part of the treatment of acute overdosage in addition to gastric lavage. Shock must be combated. Atropine and morphine may relieve the abdominal pain. Respiratory assistance may be needed to insure proper oxygenation and ventilation.
Dosage and Administration: Colchicine should be started at the first warning of an acute attack; a delay of a few hours impairs its effectiveness. The usual adult dose is 1 or 2 tablets initially, followed by 1 tablet every one to two hours until pain is relieved or nausea, vomiting, or diarrhea develops. Some physicians use 2 tablets every two hours. Since the number of doses required may range from six to 16, the total dose is variable. As interval treatment, 1 tablet may be taken one to four times a week for the mild or moderate case, once or twice daily for the severe case.
How Supplied: (℞) *Tablets No. 560, Colchicine Tablets, USP, J13,** 0.6 mg, in bottles of 100 (NDC 0002-1013-02) and 1000 (NDC 0002-1013-04).

[052681]

1. Donigian, D. W., and Owellen, R. J.: Interaction of Vinblastine, Vincristine, and Colchicine with Serum Proteins, Biochem. Pharmacol., *22:*2113, 1973.
2. Wolen, R. L.: Unpublished data, Lilly Research Laboratories, 1975.

CRYSTODIGIN® ℞
(digitoxin)
Injection, USP
AMPOULES

Description: The cardiac (or digitalis) glycosides are a closely related group of drugs having in common specific and powerful effects on the myocardium. Typically, the glycosides are composed of three portions—a steroid nucleus, a lactone ring, and a sugar (hence, "glycosides").
Crystodigin® (digitoxin, Lilly) is a crystalline cardiac glycoside obtained from *Digitalis purpurea.* Crystodigin® Injection (Digitoxin Injection, USP, Lilly) is a sterile solution of digitoxin in water for injection and 49 percent (v/v) alcohol. Each ampoule contains 0.2 mg of digitoxin in each ml.
Actions: Qualitatively, digitalis glycosides have the same therapeutic effect on the heart. They increase the force of myocardial contraction, increase the refractory period of the atrioventricular (AV) node, and, to a lesser degree, affect the sinoatrial (SA) node and conduction system via the parasympathetic and sympathetic nervous systems.
Following intravenous injection of Crystodigin® (digitoxin, Lilly), the action starts in 25 minutes to two hours, is maximal in four to 12 hours, regresses in two to three days, and disappears in two to three weeks.
Indications: Crystodigin® (digitoxin, Lilly) Injection is indicated in the following conditions when the patient cannot take medication by mouth.
Congestive Heart Failure (All Degrees)—The increased cardiac output results in diuresis and general amelioration of the disturbances characteristic of right and left heart failure. Digitalis, generally, is most effective in "low-output" failure and less effective in "high-output" (bronchopulmonary insufficiency, infection, hyperthyroidism) heart failure. The drug should be continued after heart failure is abolished unless some known precipitating factor is corrected.
Atrial Fibrillation—Digitalis is especially indicated when the ventricular rate is elevated. It rapidly reduces ventricular rates and thus the pulse deficit. Digitalis is continued in doses necessary to maintain the desired ventricular rate and other clinical effects.
Atrial Flutter—Digitalis usually slows the heart, and regular sinus rhythm may appear. Flutter may be converted to atrial fibrillation with a slow ventricular rate. Stopping digitalis treatment at this point may result in restoration of sinus rhythm, especially if the flutter was of the paroxysmal type. It is preferable, however, to continue digitalis if failure ensues or if atrial flutter is a frequent occurrence.
Paroxysmal Atrial Tachycardia—Digitalis may be used, especially if the tachycardia is resistant to lesser measures. Depending on the urgency, a more rapidly acting parenteral digitalis preparation may be preferable. If failure has ensued or paroxysms recur frequently, the digitalis effect should be maintained by oral administration.
The value of digitalis is not established in cardiogenic shock.
Contraindications: The presence of toxic effects (*see* Overdosage and Toxic Effects) induced by any digitalis preparation is an absolute contraindication to all of the glycosides. Allergy, though rare, does occur.
Ventricular tachycardia is a contraindication. However, if congestive failure supervenes after a protracted episode of tachycardia and the patient has not already received digitalis, the drug may be used.
Warnings: Many of the arrhythmias for which digitalis is advised are identical with those reflecting digitalis intoxication. When the possibility of digitalis intoxication cannot be excluded, cardiac glycosides should be withheld temporarily if the clinical situation permits.
The patient with congestive heart failure may complain of nausea and vomiting. Since these symptoms may also be associated with digitalis intoxication, a clinical determination of their cause must be attempted before further administration of the drug.
Cases of idiopathic hypertrophic subaortic stenosis must be managed with extreme care. Unless cardiac failure is severe, it is doubtful whether digitalis should be employed.
Children—During the first month of life, infants have a sharply defined tolerance to digitalis. Impaired renal function must also be considered. Premature and immature infants are particularly sensitive, and reduction of dosage may be necessary.
The presence of acute glomerulonephritis accompanied by congestive failure requires extreme care in digitalization. A relatively low total dose, administered in divided doses, and concomitant use of reserpine or other antihypertensive agents have been recommended. Constant ECG monitoring is essential. Digitalis should be discontinued as soon as possible.

Patients with rheumatic carditis, especially when severe, are unusually sensitive to digitalis and prone to disturbances of rhythm. If heart failure develops, digitalization may be tried with relatively low doses; these must be cautiously increased until a beneficial effect is obtained. If a therapeutic trial does not result in improvement, the drug should be discontinued.

Note: Digitalis glycosides are an important cause of accidental poisoning in children.

Precautions: Great caution should be exercised when Crystodigin® (digitoxin, Lilly) Injection is given to patients still under the influence of digitalis from previous medication; to patients with hypercalcemia; and in the presence of multiple ventricular extrasystoles, hypersensitivity of the carotid sinus, Adams-Stokes syndrome, or heart block.

Potassium depletion sensitizes the myocardium to digitalis. Toxicity is apt to develop even with usual dosage. Hypokalemia also tends to reduce the positive inotropic effect of digitalis. Potassium wastage may result from diuretic, corticosteroid, hemodialysis, and other therapy and is liable to accompany malnutrition, old age, and long-standing congestive heart failure.

Patients with acute myocardial infarction, severe pulmonary disease, or far-advanced heart failure are likely to be more sensitive to digitalis and may be more prone to disturbances of rhythm.

Calcium may produce serious arrhythmias in digitalized patients and should not be given to them intravenously.

In myxedema, digitalis requirements are reduced because the excretion rate is decreased and blood levels are significantly higher.

Patients with incomplete atrioventricular block, especially those subject to Stokes-Adams attacks, may develop advanced or complete heart block. Heart failure in these patients can usually be controlled by other measures and by increasing the heart rate.

Patients with chronic constrictive pericarditis are likely to respond unfavorably.

Renal insufficiency delays the excretion of digitalis, and dosage must be adjusted accordingly in patients with renal disease.

Note: This applies also to potassium administration, should it become necessary.

Electrical conversion of arrhythmias may require adjustment of digitalis dosage.

Children—Dosage must be carefully titrated. Electrocardiographic monitoring may be necessary to avoid intoxication. Premonitory signs of toxicity in the newborn are undue slowing of the sinus rate, sinoatrial arrest, and prolongation of the P-R interval.

Adverse Reaction: Gynecomastia can occur, but it is uncommon.

Overdosage and Toxic Effects: *Gastrointestinal*—Anorexia, nausea, vomiting, and diarrhea are the most common early symptoms of overdosage in the adult (but are rarely conspicuous in infants). Uncontrolled heart failure may also produce such symptoms.

Central Nervous System—Headache, weakness, apathy, and visual disturbances may be present. Mental depression may be an early symptom; mental confusion, disorientation, and delirium may be seen with more severe intoxication.

Cardiovascular—The most common arrhythmia is ventricular premature beats (except in infants and young children). Paroxysmal and nonparoxysmal nodal rhythms, atrioventricular (interference) dissociation, and paroxysmal atrial tachycardia with block are also common arrhythmias due to digitalis overdosage.

Excessive slowing of the pulse is a clinical sign of digitalis overdosage. Atrioventricular block of increasing degree may proceed to complete heart block. The electrocardiogram is fundamental in determining the presence and nature of these arrhythmias. Other electrocardiographic changes (as of the S-T segment) provide no measure of the degree of digitalization.

Children—Cardiac arrhythmias are the more reliable and frequent signs of toxicity, whereas vomiting, diarrhea, and neurologic and ophthalmologic disturbances are rare as initial signs.

Premature ventricular systoles are rarely seen; nodal and atrial systoles are more frequent. Atrial arrhythmias, atrial ectopic rhythms, and paroxysmal atrial tachycardia (particularly with atrioventricular block) are more common manifestations of toxicity in children. Ventricular arrhythmias are rare.

Treatment of Toxic Arrhythmias: *Adults*—Digitalis should be discontinued until all signs of toxicity are abolished. This may be all that is necessary if toxic manifestations are not severe and appear after the time for peak effect of the drug.

Potassium salts are commonly used, e.g., potassium chloride in divided doses totaling 4 to 6 g, provided renal function is adequate. When correction of the arrhythmia is urgently needed, potassium may be administered intravenously in a solution of 5% dextrose in water, for a total dosage of 40 to 100 mEq (40 mEq/500 ml) at the rate of 40 mEq per hour, unless injection is limited because of pain due to local irritation. Additional amounts may be given if the arrhythmia is uncontrolled and the potassium is well tolerated. Electrocardiographic monitoring is indicated to avoid potassium toxicity, e.g., peaking of T waves. However, potassium should not be used and may be dangerous when severe or complete heart block is due to digitalis (and is not related to tachycardia).

Chelating agents to bind calcium may also be used to counteract the arrhythmia caused by digitalis toxicity, hypokalemia, or elevated serum calcium. Four g (0.8% solution) of the disodium salt of EDTA (ethylenediaminetetraacetic acid) are dissolved in 500 ml of 5% dextrose in water (50 mg/ml) and administered over a period of two hours, unless the arrhythmia is controlled before the infusion is completed. A continuous electrocardiogram should be observed so that the infusion may be stopped promptly when the desired effect is achieved. Other counteracting agents are quinidine, procainamide, and beta-adrenergic blocking agents.

Children—Potassium preparations may be given orally in divided doses totaling 1 to 2 g daily. When correction of the arrhythmia is urgent, 5 to 10 mEq of potassium/hour may be given; this amount should be dissolved in 100 ml of 5% dextrose in water. Additional amounts of potassium may be administered if necessary and if well tolerated by the child.

A chelating agent may be tried if other measures fail. EDTA has been recommended in an intravenous dose of 15 mg/kg per hour in 5% dextrose in water, with the total not to exceed 60 mg/kg per day. A continuous electrocardiogram should be observed so that the infusion can be stopped promptly when the desired effect is achieved.

Dosage and Administration: Crystodigin® (digitoxin, Lilly) Injection should be given intravenously.

Adults—Intravenous administration of Crystodigin should be used only when the drug cannot be taken orally.

The average digitalizing dose by the intravenous route is 1.2 to 1.6 mg; this is approximately the same as that used when digitoxin is given orally.

In a patient who has not received digitalis or any digitalis-like preparation during the preceding three weeks, digitalization may be accomplished by the slow intravenous injection of an initial dose of 0.6 mg Crystodigin, followed by 0.4 mg four to six hours later and by 0.2 mg every four to six hours thereafter until the full therapeutic effect becomes apparent. This should occur in eight to 12 hours. Daily intravenous or oral administration of 0.05 to 0.3 mg of Crystodigin will be needed as a maintenance dose. It should be emphasized that the dose of Crystodigin must be proportionately reduced for partially digitalized patients.

The administration of the average digitalizing dose in a single injection is not recommended.

Patients who have extensive myocardial damage or conduction defects may require a much smaller quantity of digitoxin than those with less abnormal hearts.

Children—Digitalization must be individualized. Generally, premature and immature infants are particularly sensitive and require reduced dosage that must be determined by careful titration. Intravenous doses should be given slowly with continuous electrocardiographic monitoring to avoid toxic doses.

The digitalizing dose for newborn infants under two weeks, premature infants, and those having reduced renal function or myocarditis is 0.022 mg/kg (0.3 to 0.35 mg/m^2).

After the neonatal period, the dose is as follows:

Under one year of age—0.045 mg/kg
One to two years of age—0.04 mg/kg
Over two years of age—0.03 mg/kg (0.75 mg/m^2)

The total dose should be divided into three, four, or more portions, with six hours or more between doses.

For a maintenance dose, the patient should be given one-tenth of the digitalizing dose.

How Supplied: (℞) *Ampoules No. 426, Crystodigin® (Digitoxin Injection, USP),* 0.2 mg, 1 ml, in packages of 6 (NDC 0002-1678-16) and 100 (NDC 0002-1678-02). [011681]

CRYSTODIGIN® ℞
(digitoxin)
Tablets, USP

Description: Crystodigin® (digitoxin, Lilly) is a crystalline-pure single cardiac glycoside obtained from *Digitalis purpurea* and is identical in pharmacologic action with whole-leaf digitalis.

Digitoxin is the most slowly excreted of all digitalis compounds (excretion time is 14 to 21 days). It is most useful in patients with impaired renal function, since excretion and metabolism are independent of renal function.

Crystodigin is noted for its uniform potency, complete absorption, and lack of gastrointestinal irritation. It permits accurate dosage adjustments to produce maximum therapeutic effect smoothly and dependably.

Crystodigin, for oral administration, is available in tablets containing 0.05, 0.1, 0.15, or 0.2 mg crystalline digitoxin.

Digitoxin is a cardiotonic glycoside. The chemical name is card-20 (22) - enolide,3-[(*O*-2,6-dideoxy-*β*- D -*ribo*-hexopyranosyl-(1→4)-*O*-2,6-dideoxy-*β*- D -*ribo*-hexopyranosyl - (1→4)-2,6-dideoxy - *β* - D -*ribo* - hexopyranosyl) oxy]-14-hydroxy, (3*β*,5*β*)-. The empirical formula of digitoxin is $C_{41}H_{64}O_{13}$.

Clinical Pharmacology: The cellular basis for the inotropic effects of digitalis is probably enhancement of excitation-contraction coupling, that process by which chemical energy is converted into mechanical energy when triggered by membrane depolarization. Most evidence relates this process to the entry of calcium ions into the cell during depolarization of the membrane and/or to the release of calcium from intracellular binding sites on the sarcoplasmic reticulum. The free calcium ion mediates the interaction of actin and myosin, resulting in contraction.

The amount of glycoside absorbed depends largely on its polarity, which is a function of the net electronic charge on the molecule. The

Continued on next page

*Identi-Code® symbol.

Lilly—Cont.

more nonpolar or lipid soluble, the better is the absorption, because of the greater permeability of lipid membrane of the intestinal mucosa for lipid-soluble substances. The nonpolar, lipophilic digitoxin is completely absorbed; the oral dose, therefore, is the same as the intravenous dose. Other glycosides are not as well absorbed.
Nonpolar digitoxin is over 90 percent bound to tissue proteins. The firm binding of digitoxin to protein is responsible for its long half-life (seven to nine days).
Digitoxin differs from other commonly used glycosides not only in its firm binding to protein but also because it is metabolized in the liver, with the only active metabolite being digoxin, which represents only a small fraction of the total metabolites. All other metabolites are inert and are probably excreted as such in the urine. The portion of digitoxin that is not metabolized is excreted in the bile to the intestines and recycled to the liver until it is completely metabolized. The portion of digitoxin that is bound to protein is in equilibrium with free digitoxin in the serum. Thus, as more and more of the free digitoxin is metabolized after a single dose, there is proportionately less bound digitoxin.
Indications and Usage: Crystodigin® (digitoxin, Lilly) is indicated in the treatment of heart failure, atrial flutter, atrial fibrillation, and supraventricular tachycardia. Parenteral administration of Crystodigin is indicated for neonates and immature infants.
Contraindications: If the indications are carefully observed, there are few contraindications to digitalis therapy except toxic response to digitalis or idiosyncrasy, ventricular tachycardia, beriberi heart disease, and some instances of the hypersensitive carotid sinus syndrome.
Patients already taking digitalis preparations must not be given the rapid digitalizing dose of Crystodigin® (digitoxin, Lilly) or parenteral calcium.
Warnings: Many of the arrhythmias for which digitalis is advised are identical with those reflecting digitalis intoxication. When the possibility of digitalis intoxication cannot be excluded, cardiac glycosides should be withheld temporarily if the clinical situation permits.
The patient with congestive heart failure may complain of nausea and vomiting. Since these symptoms may also be associated with digitalis intoxication, a clinical determination of their cause must be attempted before further administration of the drug.
Cases of idiopathic hypertrophic subaortic stenosis must be managed with extreme care. Unless cardiac failure is severe, it is doubtful whether digitalis should be employed.
Children—During the first month of life, infants have a sharply defined tolerance to digitalis. Impaired renal function must also be considered. Premature and immature infants are particularly sensitive, and reduction in dosage may be necessary.
The presence of acute glomerulonephritis accompanied by congestive failure requires extreme care in digitalization. A relatively low total dose, administered in divided doses, and concomitant use of reserpine or other antihypertensive agents have been recommended. Constant ECG monitoring is essential. Digitalis should be discontinued as soon as possible.
Patients with rheumatic carditis, especially when severe, are unusually sensitive to digitalis and prone to disturbances of rhythm. If heart failure develops, digitalization may be tried with relatively low doses; these must be cautiously increased until a beneficial effect is obtained. If a therapeutic trial does not result in improvement, the drug should be discontinued.
NOTE: Digitalis glycosides are an important cause of accidental poisoning in children.
Precautions: *General Precautions*—When the risk of digitalis intoxication is great, the use of a short-acting, rapidly eliminated glycoside, such as digoxin, is advisable. Although intoxication cannot always be prevented by the selection of one glycoside over another, certain glycosides may be preferred in patients who have fixed disabilities (e.g., liver impairment, drug intolerance). However, digitoxin can be used in patients with impaired renal function. Newborn infants with heart disease, especially prematures, are particularly susceptible to digitalis intoxication, and frequent electrocardiographic monitoring is essential in these patients. Special care must likewise be exercised in elderly patients receiving digitalis because their body mass tends to be small and renal clearance is likely to be reduced. In addition, digitalis must be used cautiously in the presence of active heart disease, such as acute myocardial infarction or acute myocarditis. In patients with acute or unstable chronic atrial fibrillation, digitalis may not normalize the ventricular rate even when the serum concentration exceeds the usual therapeutic level. Although these patients may be less sensitive to the toxic effects of digitalis than are patients with normal sinus rhythm, dosage should not be increased to potentially toxic levels.
Hypokalemia predisposes to digitalis toxicity, and even a moderate decrease in the concentration of serum potassium can precipitate serious arrhythmias.
Impaired liver function may necessitate reduction in dosage of any digitalis preparation, including digitoxin.
Sensitive radioimmunoassay techniques have been developed for measuring serum levels of digitoxin, and these procedures can be instituted in almost any hospital. Serum levels must, however, be evaluated in conjunction with clinical history and the results of the electrocardiogram and other laboratory tests. A therapeutic serum level for one patient may be excessive or inadequate for another patient.
Drug Interactions—The synthesis of microsomal enzymes that metabolize digitoxin in the liver is subject to stimulation by a number of drugs, such as antihistamines, anticonvulsants, barbiturates, oral hypoglycemic agents, and others.
When digitoxin is the glycoside used for digitalis maintenance, drugs that are liver-microsomal enzyme inducers should not be used at the same time. Phenobarbital, phenylbutazone, and diphenylhydantoin will increase the rate of metabolism of digitoxin. In patients receiving 60 mg of phenobarbital three times a day for 12 weeks, the steady-state concentration of digitoxin in plasma fell approximately 50 percent when the drugs were administered concurrently and returned to previous levels when phenobarbital was discontinued.
When drugs that increase the rate of metabolism of digitoxin in the liver are discontinued, toxicity may occur.
Hypokalemia is most frequently encountered in patients receiving concomitant diuretic therapy, because the most widely used and most effective diuretics (i.e., thiazides and furosemide) increase the urinary loss of potassium. Prescribing a potassium-sparing agent (spironolactone or triamterene) together with the potassium-wasting diuretic is a reliable means for maintaining the serum potassium level. Alternatively, potassium chloride supplements may be prescribed.
Mineralocorticoids (e.g., prednisone), and, rarely, certain antibiotics (e.g., amphotericin B) may also cause increased excretion of potassium.
Usage in Pregnancy—Pregnancy Category C—Animal reproduction studies have not been conducted with Crystodigin. It is also not known whether this drug can cause fetal harm when administered to a pregnant woman or can affect reproduction capacity. Crystodigin should be given to a pregnant woman only if clearly needed.
Labor and Delivery—No information is available concerning the use of Crystodigin in labor and delivery.
Nursing Mothers—It is not known whether this drug is excreted in human milk. Because many drugs are excreted in human milk, caution should be exercised when Crystodigin is administered to a nursing woman.
Adverse Reactions Anorexia, nausea, and vomiting have been reported. These effects are central in origin, but following large oral doses, there is also a local emetic action. Abdominal discomfort or pain and diarrhea may also occur.
Overdosage: Overdosage causes side effects, such as mental depression, anorexia, nausea, vomiting, premature beats, complete heart block, AV dissociation, ventricular tachycardia, ventricular fibrillation, restlessness, yellow vision, mental confusion, disorientation, and delirium.
Alterations in cardiac rate and rhythm occurring in digitalis poisoning may simulate almost any known type of arrhythmia seen clinically. Extrasystoles are probably the most frequent effect. An electrocardiogram is necessary in the clinical management of the patient to aid in the differentiation of arrhythmia due to digitalis poisoning from that due to heart disease. Older patients and particularly those with disease of the coronary arteries and impaired myocardial blood supply are more susceptible to these untoward effects. Sinus arrhythmia may occur early as a minor toxic effect. Paroxysmal atrial and ventricular tachycardia call for immediate cessation of the drug. Atrial fibrillation can occur following large doses of digitalis. Ventricular fibrillation is the most common cause of death from digitalis poisoning.
Potassium ion is probably the best agent for prompt suppression of digitalis arrhythmias. It can be administered intravenously in the form of potassium chloride at a rate of 0.5 mEq/minute in sodium chloride (isotonic) or dextrose (5 percent) solution containing 50 to 100 mEq of potassium per liter. Administration of the potassium salt in normal saline is preferred. Constant electrocardiographic monitoring is essential during injection of the solution. Since the action of potassium ion lasts only minutes after infusion is discontinued, oral therapy with potassium chloride may be given for prolonged suppression of arrhythmias. Potassium is contraindicated in the presence of renal failure. Diphenylhydantoin may be used if potassium fails or is contraindicated. If both potassium and diphenylhydantoin fail, procainamide and quinidine can be used. Disodium edetate has been used for terminating digitalis-induced ventricular arrhythmias and abnormalities of atrioventricular conduction.
Dosage and Administration: *Adults: Slow Digitalization*—0.2 mg twice daily for a period of four days, followed by maintenance dosage. *Rapid Digitalization*—Preferably 0.6 mg initially, followed by 0.4 mg and then 0.2 mg at intervals of four to six hours. *Maintenance Dosage*—Ranges from 0.05 to 0.3 mg daily, the most common dose being 0.15 mg daily.
Children: Digitalization must be individualized. Generally, premature and immature infants are particularly sensitive and require reduced parenteral dosage of Crystodigin that must be determined by careful titration.
After the neonatal period, the dose is as follows:

Under one year of age—0.045 mg/kg
One to two years of age—0.04 mg/kg
Over two years of age—0.03 mg/kg (0.75 mg/m^2)

The total dose should be divided into three, four, or more portions, with six hours or more between doses.
For a maintenance dose, the patient should be given one-tenth of the digitalizing dose.

How Supplied: (℞) *Tablets Crystodigin® (Digitoxin Tablets, USP)* (scored): *No. 1736, J75,** 0.05 mg, Orange, in bottles of 100 (NDC 0002-1075-02) and 500 (NDC 0002-1075-03); *No. 1703, J60,**0.1 mg, Pink, in bottles of 100 (NDC 0002-1060-02), 500 (NDC 0002-1060-03), and 5000 (NDC 0002-1060-31) and in 10 strips of 10 individually labeled blisters each containing 1 tablet (ID100) (NDC 0002-1060-33); *No. 1737, J76,** 0.15 mg, Yellow, and *No. 1694, J57,** 0.2 mg, White, in bottles of 100 (NDC 0002-1076 and 1057-02) and 500 (NDC 0002-1076 and 1057-03).

[090281]

[*Shown in Product Identification Section*]

CYCLOMETHYCAINE SULFATE, *see* Surfacaine® (cyclomethycaine sulfate, Lilly)

CYCLOSERINE, *see* Seromycin® (cycloserine, Lilly).

CYCLOTHIAZIDE, *see* Anhydron® (cyclothiazide, Lilly).

DARVOCET-N® 50 and DARVOCET-N® 100 (propoxyphene napsylate and acetaminophen) USP

Ⓒ

DARVON-N® (propoxyphene napsylate) USP

DARVON-N® WITH A.S.A.® (propoxyphene napsylate and aspirin) USP

Description: Propoxyphene napsylate (Darvon-N®) is an odorless white crystalline solid with a bitter taste. It is very slightly soluble in water and soluble in methanol, ethanol, chloroform, and acetone. Chemically, it is α-(+)-4-(Dimethylamino)-3-methyl-1, 2-diphenyl-2-butanol Propionate (ester) 2-Naphthalenesulfonate (salt) Hydrate.

Propoxyphene napsylate differs from propoxyphene hydrochloride in that it allows more stable liquid dosage forms and tablet formulations. Because of differences in molecular weight, a dose of 100 mg of propoxyphene napsylate is required to supply an amount of propoxyphene equivalent to that present in 65 mg of propoxyphene hydrochloride.

Each tablet of Darvocet-N 50 contains 50 mg propoxyphene napsylate and 325 mg acetaminophen.

Each tablet of Darvocet-N 100 contains 100 mg propoxyphene napsylate and 650 mg acetaminophen.

Each 5 ml of Suspension Darvon-N contain 50 mg propoxyphene napsylate.

Each tablet of Darvon-N contains 100 mg propoxyphene napsylate.

Each tablet of Darvon-N with A.S.A. contains 100 mg propoxyphene napsylate and 325 mg aspirin.

Clinical Pharmacology: Propoxyphene is a centrally acting narcotic analgesic agent. Equimolar doses of propoxyphene hydrochloride or napsylate provide similar plasma concentrations. Following administration of 65, 130, or 195 mg of propoxyphene hydrochloride, the bioavailability of propoxyphene is equivalent to that of 100, 200, or 300 mg respectively of propoxyphene napsylate. Peak plasma concentrations of propoxyphene are reached in two to two and one-half hours. After a 100-mg oral dose of propoxyphene napsylate, peak plasma levels of 0.05 to 0.1 mcg/ml are achieved. As shown in Figure 1, the napsylate salt tends to be absorbed more slowly than the hydrochloride. At or near therapeutic doses, this difference is small when compared with that among subjects and among doses.

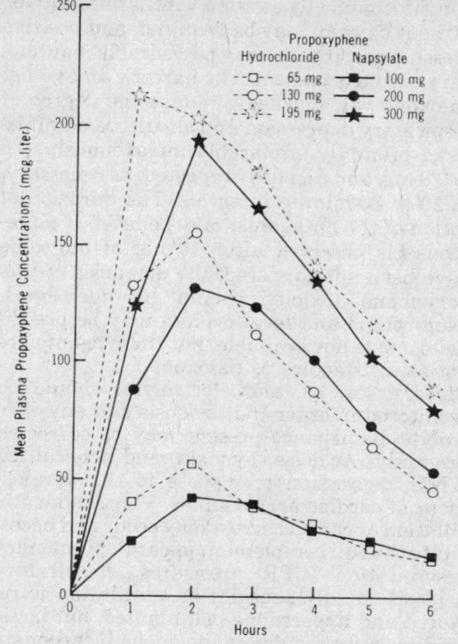

Figure 1. Mean plasma concentrations of propoxyphene in eight human subjects following oral administration of 65 and 130 mg of the hydrochloride salt and 100 and 200 mg of the napsylate salt and in seven given 195 mg of the hydrochloride and 300 mg of the napsylate salt

Because of this several hundredfold difference in solubility, the absorption rate of very large doses of the napsylate salt is significantly lower than that of equimolar doses of the hydrochloride.

Repeated doses of propoxyphene at six-hour intervals lead to increasing plasma concentrations, with a plateau after the ninth dose at 48 hours.

Propoxyphene is metabolized in the liver to yield norpropoxyphene. Propoxyphene has a half-life of six to 12 hours, whereas that of norpropoxyphene is 30 to 36 hours.

Norpropoxyphene has substantially less central - nervous - system - depressant effect than propoxyphene but a greater local anesthetic effect, which is similar to that of amitriptyline and antiarrhythmic agents, such as lidocaine and quinidine.

In animal studies in which propoxyphene and norpropoxyphene were continuously infused in large amounts, intracardiac conduction time (PR and QRS intervals) was prolonged. Any intracardiac conduction delay attributable to high concentrations of norpropoxyphene may be of relatively long duration.

Actions: Propoxyphene is a mild narcotic analgesic structurally related to methadone. The potency of propoxyphene napsylate is from two-thirds to equal that of codeine.

Darvocet-N 50 and Darvocet-N 100 provide the analgesic activity of propoxyphene napsylate and the antipyretic-analgesic activity of acetaminophen.

The combination of propoxyphene and acetaminophen produces greater analgesia than that produced by either propoxyphene or acetaminophen administered alone.

The combination of propoxyphene with aspirin produces greater analgesia than that produced by either drug administered alone.

Indications: Darvocet-N 50, Darvocet-N 100, and Darvon-N with A.S.A. are indicated for the relief of mild to moderate pain, either when pain is present alone or when it is accompanied by fever.

Darvon-N® (propoxyphene napsylate, Lilly) is indicated for the relief of mild to moderate pain.

Contraindications: Hypersensitivity to propoxyphene, acetaminophen, or aspirin.

WARNINGS

- **Do not prescribe propoxyphene for patients who are suicidal or addiction-prone.**
- **Prescribe propoxyphene with caution for patients taking tranquilizers or antidepressant drugs and patients who use alcohol in excess.**
- **Tell your patients not to exceed the recommended dose and to limit their intake of alcohol.**

Propoxyphene products in excessive doses, either alone or in combination with other C.N.S. depressants, including alcohol, are a major cause of drug-related deaths. Fatalities within the first hour of overdosage are not uncommon. In a survey of deaths due to overdosage conducted in 1975, in approximately 20 percent of the fatal cases, death occurred within the first hour (5 percent occurred within 15 minutes). Propoxyphene should not be taken in doses higher than those recommended by the physician. The judicious prescribing of propoxyphene is essential to the safe use of this drug. With patients who are depressed or suicidal, consideration should be given to the use of non-narcotic analgesics. Patients should be cautioned about the concomitant use of propoxyphene products and alcohol because of potentially serious C.N.S.-additive effects of these agents. Because of its added depressant effects, propoxyphene should be prescribed with caution for those patients whose medical condition requires the concomitant administration of sedatives, tranquilizers, muscle relaxants, antidepressants, or other C.N.S.-depressant drugs. Patients should be advised of the additive depressant effects of these combinations.

Many of the propoxyphene-related deaths have occurred in patients with previous histories of emotional disturbances or suicidal ideation or attempts as well as histories of misuse of tranquilizers, alcohol, and other C.N.S.-active drugs. Some deaths have occurred as a consequence of the accidental ingestion of excessive quantities of propoxyphene alone or in combination with other drugs. Patients taking propoxyphene should be warned not to exceed the dosage recommended by the physician.

Drug Dependence—Propoxyphene, when taken in higher-than-recommended doses over long periods of time, can produce drug dependence characterized by psychic dependence and, less frequently, physical dependence and tolerance. Propoxyphene will only partially suppress the withdrawal syndrome in individuals physically dependent on morphine or other narcotics. The abuse liability of propoxyphene is qualitatively similar to that of codeine although quantitatively less, and propoxyphene should be prescribed with the same degree of caution appropriate to the use of codeine.

Usage in Ambulatory Patients—Propoxyphene may impair the mental and/or physical abilities required for the performance of potentially hazardous tasks, such as driving a car or operating machinery. The patient should be cautioned accordingly.

Precautions: *General Precautions*— Salicylates should be used with extreme caution in the presence of peptic ulcer or coagulation abnormalities.

Continued on next page

*Identi-Code® symbol.

Lilly—Cont.

Drug Interactions—The C.N.S.-depressant effect of propoxyphene is additive with that of other C.N.S. depressants, including alcohol.
Salicylates may enhance the effect of anticoagulants and inhibit the uricosuric effect of uricosuric agents.
Usage in Pregnancy—Safe use in pregnancy has not been established relative to possible adverse effects on fetal development. Instances of withdrawal symptoms in the neonate have been reported following usage during pregnancy. Therefore, propoxyphene should not be used in pregnant women unless, in the judgment of the physician, the potential benefits outweigh the possible hazards.
Usage in Nursing Mothers—Low levels of propoxyphene have been detected in human milk. In postpartum studies involving nursing mothers who were given propoxyphene, no adverse effects were noted in infants receiving mother's milk.
Usage in Children—Propoxyphene is not recommended for use in children, because documented clinical experience has been insufficient to establish safety and a suitable dosage regimen in the pediatric age group.
A Patient Information Sheet is available for these products. See text following "How Supplied" section below.
Adverse Reactions: In a survey conducted in hospitalized patients, less than 1 percent of patients taking propoxyphene hydrochloride at recommended doses experienced side effects. The most frequently reported have been dizziness, sedation, nausea, and vomiting. Some of these adverse reactions may be alleviated if the patient lies down.
Other adverse reactions include constipation, abdominal pain, skin rashes, lightheadedness, headache, weakness, euphoria, dysphoria, and minor visual disturbances.
Cases of liver dysfunction have been reported.
Dosage and Administration: These products are given orally. The usual dose of Darvocet-N 50 or Darvocet-N 100 is 100 mg propoxyphene napsylate and 650 mg acetaminophen every four hours as needed for pain.
The usual dose of Darvon-N® (propoxyphene napsylate, Lilly) is 100 mg every four hours as needed for pain.
The usual dose of Darvon-N with A.S.A. is 100 mg propoxyphene napsylate and 325 mg aspirin every four hours as needed for pain.
The maximum recommended dose of propoxyphene napsylate is 600 mg per day.
Management of Overdosage: Initial consideration should be given to the management of the C.N.S. effects of propoxyphene overdosage. Resuscitative measures should be initiated promptly.
Symptoms of Propoxyphene Overdosage—The manifestations of acute overdosage with propoxyphene are those of narcotic overdosage. The patient is usually somnolent but may be stuporous or comatose and convulsing. Respiratory depression is characteristic. The ventilatory rate and/or tidal volume is decreased, which results in cyanosis and hypoxia. Pupils, initially pinpoint, may become dilated as hypoxia increases. Cheyne-Stokes respiration and apnea may occur. Blood pressure and heart rate are usually normal initially, but blood pressure falls and cardiac performance deteriorates, which ultimately results in pulmonary edema and circulatory collapse, unless the respiratory depression is corrected and adequate ventilation is restored promptly. Cardiac arrhythmias and conduction delay may be present. A combined respiratory-metabolic acidosis occurs owing to retained CO_2 (hypercapnea) and to lactic acid formed during anaerobic glycolysis. Acidosis may be severe if large amounts of salicylates have also been ingested. Death may occur.
Treatment of Propoxyphene Overdosage — Attention should be directed first to establishing a patent airway and to restoring ventilation. Mechanically assisted ventilation, with or without oxygen, may be required, and positive pressure respiration may be desirable if pulmonary edema is present. The narcotic antagonist naloxone will markedly reduce the degree of respiratory depression and should be administered promptly, preferably intravenously, 0.4 to 0.8 mg, and carefully repeated, as necessary, at 20 to 30-minute intervals. The duration of action of the antagonist may be brief. If no response is observed after 10 mg of naloxone have been administered, the diagnosis of propoxyphene toxicity should be questioned. (Nalorphine and levallorphan may be used if naloxone is not available, but these agents are not as satisfactory as naloxone.)
Blood gases, *p*H, and electrolytes should be monitored in order that acidosis and any electrolyte disturbance present may be corrected promptly. Acidosis, hypoxia, and generalized C.N.S. depression predispose to the development of cardiac arrhythmias. Ventricular fibrillation or cardiac arrest may occur and necessitate the full complement of cardiopulmonary resuscitation (CPR) measures. Respiratory acidosis rapidly subsides as ventilation is restored and hypercapnea eliminated, but lactic acidosis may require intravenous bicarbonate for prompt correction.
Electrocardiographic monitoring is essential. Prompt correction of hypoxia, acidosis, and electrolyte disturbance (when present) will help prevent these cardiac complications and will increase the effectiveness of agents administered to restore normal cardiac function.
In addition to the use of a narcotic antagonist, the patient may require careful titration with an anticonvulsant to control convulsions. Analeptic drugs (for example, caffeine or amphetamine) should not be used because of their tendency to precipitate convulsions.
General supportive measures, in addition to oxygen, include, when necessary, intravenous fluids, vasopressor-inotropic compounds, and, when infection is likely, anti-infective agents. Gastric lavage may be useful, and activated charcoal can adsorb a significant amount of ingested propoxyphene. Dialysis is of little value in poisoning due to propoxyphene. Efforts should be made to determine whether other agents, such as alcohol, barbiturates, tranquilizers, or other C.N.S. depressants, were also ingested, since these increase C.N.S. depression as well as cause specific toxic effects.
Symptoms of Acetaminophen Overdosage—Shortly after oral ingestion of an overdose of acetaminophen and for the next 24 hours, anorexia, nausea, vomiting, and abdominal pain have been noted. The patient may then present no symptoms, but evidence of liver dysfunction may be apparent during the next 24 to 48 hours, with elevated serum transaminase and lactic dehydrogenase levels, an increase in serum bilirubin concentrations, and a prolonged prothrombin time. Death from hepatic failure may result three to seven days after overdosage.
Treatment of Acetaminophen Overdosage—There is no specific antidote currently available for the treatment of acetaminophen intoxication. Subject to primary consideration of the C.N.S.-depressant effects of propoxyphene, gastric lavage should be instituted.
Symptoms of Salicylate Overdosage—Such symptoms include central nausea and vomiting, tinnitus and deafness, vertigo and headaches, mental dullness and confusion, diaphoresis, rapid pulse, and increased respiration and respiratory alkalosis.
Treatment of Salicylate Overdosage—When Darvon-N with A.S.A. has been ingested, the clinical picture may be complicated by salicylism.
The treatment of acute salicylate intoxication includes minimizing drug absorption, promoting elimination through the kidneys, and correcting metabolic derangements affecting body temperature, hydration, acid-base balance, and electrolyte balance. The technique to be employed for eliminating salicylate from the bloodstream depends on the degree of drug intoxication.
If the patient is seen within four hours of ingestion, the stomach should be emptied by inducing vomiting or by gastric lavage as soon as possible.
The nomogram of Done is a useful prognostic guide in which the expected severity of salicylate intoxication is based on serum salicylate levels and the time interval between ingestion and taking the blood sample.
Exchange transfusion is most feasible for a small infant. Intermittent peritoneal dialysis is useful for cases of moderate severity in adults. Intravenous fluids alkalinized by the addition of sodium bicarbonate or potassium citrate are helpful. Hemodialysis with the artificial kidney is the most effective means of removing salicylate and is indicated for the very severe cases of salicylate intoxication.
Animal Toxicology: The acute lethal doses of the hydrochloride and napsylate salts of propoxyphene were determined in four species. The results shown in Figure 2 indicate that, on a molar basis, the napsylate salt is less toxic than the hydrochloride. This may be due to the relative insolubility and retarded absorption of propoxyphene napsylate.
Figure 2. Acute oral toxicity of propoxyphene

	LD_{50} (mg/kg) ± SE / LD_{50} (mM/kg)	
Species	Propoxyphene Hydrochloride	Propoxyphene Napsylate
Mouse	282 ± 39 / 0.75	915 ± 163 / 1.62
Rat	230 ± 44 / 0.61	647 ± 95 / 1.14
Rabbit	ca. 82 / 0.22	>183 / >0.32
Dog	ca. 100 / 0.27	>183 / >0.32

Some indication of the relative insolubility and retarded absorption of propoxyphene napsylate was obtained by measuring plasma propoxyphene levels in two groups of four dogs following oral administration of equimolar doses of the two salts. As shown in Figure 3, the peak plasma concentration observed with propoxyphene hydrochloride was much higher than that obtained after administration of the napsylate salt.

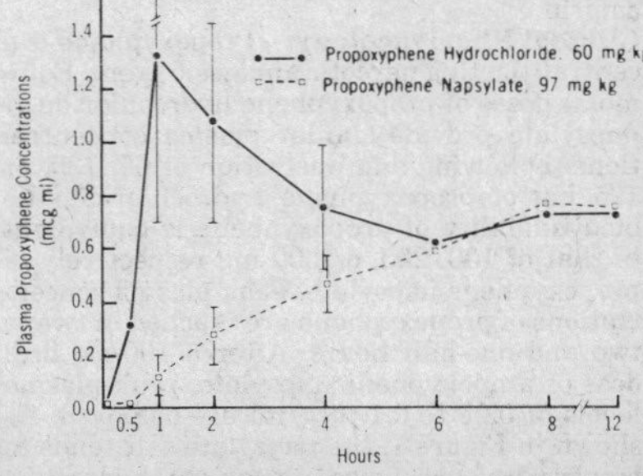

Figure 3. Plasma propoxyphene concentra-

tions in dogs following large doses of the hydrochloride and napsylate salts

Although none of the animals in this experiment died, three of the four dogs given propoxyphene hydrochloride exhibited convulsive seizures during the time interval corresponding to the peak plasma levels. The four animals receiving the napsylate salt were mildly ataxic but not acutely ill.

How Supplied: Ⓒ *Darvocet-N® 50 (Propoxyphene Napsylate and Acetaminophen, USP), Tablets No. 1890, C51,** Specially Coated, Dark-Orange, in bottles of 500 (NDC 0002-0351-03), in 10 strips of 10 individually labeled blisters each containing 1 tablet (ID100) (NDC 0002-0351-33), in 500 single-cut individually labeled blisters each containing 1 tablet (ID500) (NDC 0002-0351-43), and in ℞Paks (prescription packages, Lilly) in bottles of 100 (NDC 0002-0351-02) and in 20 packages of 50 (NDC 0002-0351-51). All ℞Paks have safety closures.
500's—6505-00-279-7469A.

Ⓒ *Darvocet-N® 100 (Propoxyphene Napsylate and Acetaminophen, USP), Tablets No. 1893, C63,** Specially Coated, Dark-Orange, in bottles of 500 (NDC 0002-0363-03), in 10 strips of 10 individually labeled blisters each containing 1 tablet (ID100) (NDC 0002-0363-33), in 500 single-cut individually labeled blisters each containing 1 tablet (ID500) (NDC 0002-0363-43), in 20 rolls, each consisting of 25 tablets in individual unit-dose packets, reverse-numbered (RN500) (NDC 0002-0363-46), and in ℞Paks in bottles of 100 (NDC 0002-0363-02), and in 25 packages of 30 (NDC 0002-0363-29). All ℞Paks have safety closures.
℞Pak 30—6505-00-111-8364; ID100—6505-00-111-8373; 500's—6505-00-111-8359 and 6505-00-111-8359A

Ⓒ *Darvon-N® (Propoxyphene Napsylate Oral Suspension, USP), Suspension No. M-135,* 50 mg per 5 ml, in 16-fl-oz (473-ml) bottles (NDC 0002-2371-05). *Avoid freezing.*

Ⓒ *Darvon-N® (Propoxyphene Napsylate Tablets, USP), Tablets No. 1883, C53,** 100 mg, Specially Coated, Buff, in bottles of 100 (℞Pak) (NDC 0002-0353-02) and 500 (NDC 0002-0353-03), in 10 strips of 10 individually labeled blisters each containing 1 tablet (ID100) (NDC 0002-0353-33), in 500 single-cut individually labeled blisters each containing 1 tablet (ID500) (NDC 0002-0353-43), and in ℞Paks in 25 packages of 30 (NDC 0002-0353-29) and 20 packages of 50 (NDC 0002-0353-51). All ℞Paks have safety closures.
ID100—6505-00-197-9201A; 500's—6505-00-111-8383 and 6505-00-111-8383A

Ⓒ *Darvon-N® with A.S.A.® (Propoxyphene Napsylate and Aspirin, USP), Tablets No. 1884, C54,** Specially Coated, Orange, in bottles of 100 (℞Pak) (NDC 0002-0354-02) and 500 (NDC 0002-0354-03), in 10 strips of 10 individually labeled blisters each containing 1 tablet (ID100) (NDC 0002-0354-33), in 500 single-cut individually labeled blisters each containing 1 tablet (ID500) (NDC 0002-0354-43), and in ℞Paks in 25 packages of 30 (NDC 0002-0354-29). All ℞Paks have safety closures.
500's—6505-00-212-6109A

---

*Identi-Code® symbol.

[*Shown in Product Identification Section*]

The following information, including illustrations of dosage forms and the maximum daily dosage of each, is available to patients receiving Darvon products.

Patient Information Sheet

YOUR PRESCRIPTION FOR A DARVON® (PROPOXYPHENE) PRODUCT Ⓒ

Summary: Products containing Darvon are used to relieve pain.

LIMIT YOUR INTAKE OF ALCOHOL WHILE TAKING THIS DRUG. Make sure your doctor knows that you are taking tranquilizers, sleep aids, antidepressants, antihistamines, or any other drugs that make you sleepy. Combining propoxyphene with alcohol or these drugs in excessive doses is dangerous. Use care while driving a car or using machines until you see how the drug affects you because propoxyphene can make you sleepy. Do not take more of the drug than your doctor prescribed. Dependence has occurred when patients have taken propoxyphene for a long period of time at doses greater than recommended.

The rest of this leaflet gives you more information about propoxyphene. Please read it and keep it for future use.

Uses of Darvon: Products containing Darvon are used for the relief of mild to moderate pain. Products which contain Darvon plus aspirin or acetaminophen are prescribed for the relief of pain or pain associated with fever.

Before Taking Darvon: Make sure your doctor knows if you have ever had an allergic reaction to propoxyphene, aspirin, or acetaminophen. Some forms of propoxyphene products contain aspirin to help relieve the pain. Your doctor should be advised if you have a history of ulcers or if you are taking an anticoagulant ("blood thinner"). The aspirin may irritate the stomach lining and may cause bleeding, particularly if an ulcer is present. Also, bleeding may occur if you are taking an anticoagulant. In a small group of people, aspirin may cause an asthma attack. If you are one of these people, be sure your drug does not contain aspirin.

The effect of propoxyphene in children under 12 has not been studied. Therefore, use of the drug in this age group is not recommended.

How to Take Darvon: Follow your doctor's directions exactly. Do not increase the amount you take without your doctor's approval. If you miss a dose of the drug, do not take twice as much the next time.

Pregnancy: Do not take propoxyphene during pregnancy unless your doctor knows you are pregnant and specifically recommends its use. Cases of temporary dependence in the newborn have occurred when the mother has taken propoxyphene consistently in the weeks before delivery. As a general principle, no drug should be taken during pregnancy unless it is clearly necessary.

General Cautions: Heavy use of alcohol with propoxyphene is hazardous and may lead to overdosage symptoms (see "Overdose" below). THEREFORE, LIMIT YOUR INTAKE OF ALCOHOL WHILE TAKING PROPOXYPHENE.

Combinations of excessive doses of propoxyphene, alcohol, and tranquilizers are dangerous. Make sure your doctor knows you are taking tranquilizers, sleep aids, antidepressant drugs, antihistamines, or any other drugs that make you sleepy. The use of these drugs with propoxyphene increases their sedative effects and may lead to overdosage symptoms, including death (see "Overdose" below).

Propoxyphene may cause drowsiness or impair your mental and/or physical abilities; therefore, use caution when driving a vehicle or operating dangerous machinery. DO NOT perform any hazardous task until you have seen your response to this drug.

Dependence: You can become dependent on propoxyphene if you take it in higher than recommended doses over a long period of time. Dependence is a feeling of need for the drug and a feeling that you cannot perform normally without it.

Overdose: An overdose of Darvon, alone or in combination with other drugs, including alcohol, may cause weakness, difficulty in breathing, confusion, anxiety, and more severe drowsiness and dizziness. Extreme overdosage may lead to unconsciousness and death.

If the propoxyphene product contains acetaminophen, the overdosage symptoms include nausea, vomiting, lack of appetite, and abdominal pain. Liver damage may occur.

When the propoxyphene product contains aspirin, symptoms of taking too much of the drug are headache, dizziness, ringing in the ears, difficulty in hearing, dim vision, confusion, drowsiness, sweating, thirst, rapid breathing, nausea, vomiting, and, occasionally, diarrhea. In any suspected overdosage situation, contact your doctor or nearest hospital emergency room. GET EMERGENCY HELP IMMEDIATELY.

KEEP THIS DRUG AND ALL DRUGS OUT OF THE REACH OF CHILDREN.

Possible Side Effects: When propoxyphene is taken as directed, side effects are infrequent. Among those reported are drowsiness, dizziness, nausea, and vomiting. If these effects occur, it may help if you lie down and rest.

Less frequently reported side effects are constipation, abdominal pain, skin rashes, lightheadedness, headache, weakness, minor visual disturbances, and feelings of elation or discomfort.

If side effects occur and concern you, contact your doctor.

Other Information: The safe and effective use of propoxyphene depends on your taking it exactly as directed. This drug has been prescribed specifically for you and your present condition. Do not give this drug to others who may have similar symptoms. Do not use it for any other reason.

If you would like more information about propoxyphene, ask your doctor or pharmacist. They have a more technical leaflet (professional labeling) you may read.

Keep this and all other drugs out of the reach of children.

Prescription Vial Sticker

Tell your doctor if you are taking tranquilizers, antidepressant drugs, or sleep aids. LIMIT alcohol use with Darvon-N® (propoxyphene napsylate) and Darvon® (propoxyphene hydrochloride) products.

[120481]

DARVON® Ⓒ
(propoxyphene hydrochloride) Capsules, USP

DARVON® COMPOUND and DARVON® COMPOUND–65
(propoxyphene hydrochloride, aspirin, and caffeine)

DARVON® WITH A.S.A®
(propoxyphene hydrochloride and aspirin)

Description: Darvon® (propoxyphene hydrochloride, Lilly) is an odorless white crystalline powder with a bitter taste. It is freely soluble in water. Chemically, it is alpha-(+)-4-(Dimethylamino) - 3 - methyl - 1, 2-diphenyl-2-butanol Propionate Hydrochloride.

Each Pulvule® Darvon contains 32 or 65 mg propoxyphene hydrochloride.

Pulvules No. 368 Darvon® Compound		Pulvules No. 369 Darvon® Compound-65
32 mg	Darvon® (propoxyphene hydrochloride, Lilly)	65 mg
389 mg	A.S.A.® (aspirin, Lilly)	389 mg
32.4 mg	Caffeine	32.4 mg

Each Pulvule Darvon with A.S.A. contains 65 mg propoxyphene hydrochloride and 325 mg aspirin.

Clinical Pharmacology: Propoxyphene is a centrally acting narcotic analgesic agent. Equimolar doses of propoxyphene hydrochloride or napsylate provide similar plasma concentrations. Following administration of 65, 130, or 195 mg of propoxyphene hydrochloride, the

Continued on next page

---

*Identi-Code® symbol.

Lilly—Cont.

bioavailability of propoxyphene is equivalent to that of 100, 200, or 300 mg respectively of propoxyphene napsylate. Peak plasma concentrations of propoxyphene are reached in two to two and one-half hours. After a 65-mg oral dose of propoxyphene hydrochloride, peak plasma levels of 0.05 to 0.1 mcg/ml are achieved.

Repeated doses of propoxyphene at six-hour intervals lead to increasing plasma concentrations, with a plateau after the ninth dose at 48 hours.

Propoxyphene is metabolized in the liver to yield norpropoxyphene. Propoxyphene has a half-life of six to 12 hours, whereas that of norpropoxyphene is 30 to 36 hours.

Norpropoxyphene has substantially less central-nervous-system-depressant effect than propoxyphene but a greater local anesthetic effect, which is similar to that of amitriptyline and antiarrhythmic agents, such as lidocaine and quinidine.

In animal studies in which propoxyphene and norpropoxyphene were continuously infused in large amounts, intracardiac conduction time (PR and QRS intervals) was prolonged. Any intracardiac conduction delay attributable to high concentrations of norpropoxyphene may be of relatively long duration.

Actions: Propoxyphene is a mild narcotic analgesic structurally related to methadone. The potency of propoxyphene hydrochloride is from two-thirds to equal that of codeine.

The combination of propoxyphene with a mixture of aspirin and caffeine produces greater analgesia than that produced by either propoxyphene or aspirin and caffeine administered alone.

Indications: Darvon® (propoxyphene hydrochloride, Lilly) is indicated for the relief of mild to moderate pain.

Darvon Compound, Darvon Compound-65, and Darvon with A.S.A. are indicated for the relief of mild to moderate pain, either when pain is present alone or when it is accompanied by fever.

Contraindication: Hypersensitivity to propoxyphene, aspirin, or caffeine.

WARNINGS

- **Do not prescribe propoxyphene for patients who are suicidal or addiction-prone.**
- **Prescribe propoxyphene with caution for patients taking tranquilizers or antidepressant drugs and patients who use alcohol in excess.**
- **Tell your patients not to exceed the recommended dose and to limit their intake of alcohol.**

Propoxyphene products in excessive doses, either alone or in combination with other CNS depressants, including alcohol, are a major cause of drug-related deaths. Fatalities within the first hour of overdosage are not uncommon. In a survey of deaths due to overdosage conducted in 1975, in approximately 20 percent of the fatal cases, death occurred within the first hour (5 percent occurred within 15 minutes). Propoxyphene should not be taken in doses higher than those recommended by the physician. The judicious prescribing of propoxyphene is essential to the safe use of this drug. With patients who are depressed or suicidal, consideration should be given to the use of non-narcotic analgesics. Patients should be cautioned about the concomitant use of propoxyphene products and alcohol because of potentially serious CNS-additive effects of these agents. Because of its added depressant effects, propoxyphene should be prescribed with caution for those patients whose medical condition requires the concomitant administration of sedatives, tranquilizers, muscle relaxants, antidepressants, or other CNS-depressant drugs. Patients should be advised of the additive depressant effects of these combinations.

Many of the propoxyphene-related deaths have occurred in patients with previous histories of emotional disturbances or suicidal ideation or attempts as well as histories of misuse of tranquilizers, alcohol, and other CNS-active drugs. Some deaths have occurred as a consequence of the accidental ingestion of excessive quantities of propoxyphene alone or in combination with other drugs. Patients taking propoxyphene should be warned not to exceed the dosage recommended by the physician.

Drug Dependence—Propoxyphene, when taken in higher-than-recommended doses over long periods of time, can produce drug dependence characterized by psychic dependence and, less frequently, physical dependence and tolerance. Propoxyphene will only partially suppress the withdrawal syndrome in individuals physically dependent on morphine or other narcotics. The abuse liability of propoxyphene is qualitatively similar to that of codeine although quantitatively less, and propoxyphene should be prescribed with the same degree of caution appropriate to the use of codeine.

Usage in Ambulatory Patients—Propoxyphene may impair the mental and/or physical abilities required for the performance of potentially hazardous tasks, such as driving a car or operating machinery. The patient should be cautioned accordingly.

Precautions: *General Precautions*—Salicylates should be used with extreme caution in the presence of peptic ulcer or coagulation abnormalities.

Drug Interactions—The CNS-depressant effect of propoxyphene is additive with that of other CNS depressants, including alcohol.

Salicylates may enhance the effect of anticoagulants and inhibit the uricosuric effect of uricosuric agents.

Usage in Pregnancy—Safe use in pregnancy has not been established relative to possible adverse effects on fetal development. Instances of withdrawal symptoms in the neonate have been reported following usage during pregnancy. Therefore, propoxyphene should not be used in pregnant women unless, in the judgment of the physician, the potential benefits outweigh the possible hazards.

Usage in Nursing Mothers—Low levels of propoxyphene have been detected in human milk. In postpartum studies involving nursing mothers who were given propoxyphene, no adverse effects were noted in infants receiving mother's milk.

Usage in Children—Propoxyphene is not recommended for use in children, because documented clinical experience has been insufficient to establish safety and a suitable dosage regimen in the pediatric age group.

A Patient Information Sheet is available for these products. See text following "How Supplied" section below.

Adverse Reactions: In a survey conducted in hospitalized patients, less than 1 percent of patients taking propoxyphene hydrochloride at recommended doses experienced side effects. The most frequently reported have been dizziness, sedation, nausea, and vomiting. Some of these adverse reactions may be alleviated if the patient lies down.

Other adverse reactions include constipation, abdominal pain, skin rashes, lightheadedness, headache, weakness, euphoria, dysphoria, and minor visual disturbances.

Cases of liver dysfunction have been reported.

Dosage and Administration: These products are given orally. The usual dosage of Darvon® (propoxyphene hydrochloride, Lilly) is 65 mg every four hours as needed for pain.

The usual dosage of Darvon Compound and Darvon Compound-65 is 32 or 65 mg propoxyphene hydrochloride, 389 mg aspirin, and 32.4 mg caffeine every four hours as needed for pain.

The usual dosage of Darvon with A.S.A. is 65 mg propoxyphene hydrochloride and 325 mg aspirin every four hours as needed for pain.

The maximum recommended dose of propoxyphene hydrochloride is 390 mg per day.

Management of Overdosage: Initial consideration should be given to the management of the CNS effects of propoxyphene overdosage. Resuscitative measures should be initiated promptly.

Symptoms of Propoxyphene Overdosage—The manifestations of acute overdosage with propoxyphene are those of narcotic overdosage. The patient is usually somnolent but may be stuporous or comatose and convulsing. Respiratory depression is characteristic. The ventilatory rate and/or tidal volume is decreased, which results in cyanosis and hypoxia. Pupils, initially pinpoint, may become dilated as hypoxia increases. Cheyne-Stokes respiration and apnea may occur. Blood pressure and heart rate are usually normal initially, but blood pressure falls and cardiac performance deteriorates, which ultimately results in pulmonary edema and circulatory collapse, unless the respiratory depression is corrected and adequate ventilation is restored promptly. Cardiac arrhythmias and conduction delay may be present. A combined respiratory-metabolic acidosis occurs owing to retained CO_2 (hypercapnea) and to lactic acid formed during anaerobic glycolysis. Acidosis may be severe if large amounts of salicylates have also been ingested. Death may occur.

Treatment of Propoxyphene Overdosage —Attention should be directed first to establishing a patent airway and to restoring ventilation. Mechanically assisted ventilation, with or without oxygen, may be required, and positive pressure respiration may be desirable if pulmonary edema is present. The narcotic antagonist naloxone will markedly reduce the degree of respiratory depression and should be administered promptly, preferably intravenously, 0.4 to 0.8 mg, and carefully repeated, as necessary, at 20 to 30-minute intervals. The duration of action of the antagonist may be brief. If no response is observed after 10 mg of naloxone have been administered, the diagnosis of propoxyphene toxicity should be questioned. (Nalorphine and levallorphan may be used if naloxone is not available, but these agents are not as satisfactory as naloxone.)

Blood gases, *p*H, and electrolytes should be monitored in order that acidosis and any electrolyte disturbance present may be corrected promptly. Acidosis, hypoxia, and generalized CNS depression predispose to the development of cardiac arrhythmias. Ventricular fibrillation or cardiac arrest may occur and necessitate the full complement of cardiopulmonary resuscitation (CPR) measures. Respiratory acidosis rapidly subsides as ventilation is restored and hypercapnea eliminated, but lactic acidosis may require intravenous bicarbonate for prompt correction.

Electrocardiographic monitoring is essential. Prompt correction of hypoxia, acidosis, and electrolyte disturbance (when present) will help prevent these cardiac complications and will increase the effectiveness of agents administered to restore normal cardiac function.

In addition to the use of a narcotic antagonist, the patient may require careful titration with an anticonvulsant to control convulsions. Analeptic drugs (for example, caffeine or amphetamine) should not be used because of their tendency to precipitate convulsions.

General supportive measures, in addition to oxygen, include, when necessary, intravenous fluids, vasopressor-inotropic compounds, and, when infection is likely, anti-infective agents. Gastric lavage may be useful, and activated charcoal can adsorb a significant amount of ingested propoxyphene. Dialysis is of little value in poisoning due to propoxyphene. Efforts should be made to determine whether other agents, such as alcohol, barbiturates, tranquilizers, or other CNS depressants, were also ingested, since these increase CNS depression as well as cause specific toxic effects.

Symptoms of Salicylate Overdosage—Such symptoms include central nausea and vomiting, tinnitus and deafness, vertigo and headaches, mental dullness and confusion, diaphoresis, rapid pulse, and increased respiration and respiratory alkalosis.

Treatment of Salicylate Overdosage—When Darvon Compound, Darvon Compound-65, or Darvon with A.S.A. has been ingested, the clinical picture may be complicated by salicylism. The treatment of acute salicylate intoxication includes minimizing drug absorption, promoting elimination through the kidneys, and correcting metabolic derangements affecting body temperature, hydration, acid-base balance, and electrolyte balance. The technique to be employed for eliminating salicylate from the bloodstream depends on the degree of drug intoxication.

If the patient is seen within four hours of ingestion, the stomach should be emptied by inducing vomiting or by gastric lavage as soon as possible.

The nomogram of Done is a useful prognostic guide in which the expected severity of salicylate intoxication is based on serum salicylate levels and the time interval between ingestion and taking the blood sample.

Exchange transfusion is most feasible for a small infant. Intermittent peritoneal dialysis is useful for cases of moderate severity in adults. Intravenous fluids alkalinized by the addition of sodium bicarbonate or potassium citrate are helpful. Hemodialysis with the artificial kidney is the most effective means of removing salicylate and is indicated for the very severe cases of salicylate intoxication.

How Supplied: Ⓒ *Pulvules Darvon® (Propoxyphene Hydrochloride Capsules, USP): No. 364, HO2,** 32 mg (No. 4, Light-Pink Opaque), in bottles of 100 (℞Pak) (NDC 0002-0802-02) and 500 (NDC 0002-0802-03) and in 10 strips of 10 individually labeled blisters each containing 1 Pulvule (ID100) (NDC 0002-0802-33); *No. 365, HO3,** 65 mg (No. 3, Light-Pink Opaque), in bottles of 100 (℞Pak) (NDC 0002-0803-02) and 500 (NDC 0002-0803-03), in 10 strips of 10 individually labeled blisters each containing 1 Pulvule (ID100) (NDC 0002-0803-33), in 500 single-cut individually labeled blisters each containing 1 Pulvule (ID500) (NDC 0002-0803-43), in 20 rolls, each consisting of 25 Pulvules in individual unit-dose packets, reverse-numbered (RN500) (NDC 0002-0803-46), and in ℞Paks (prescription packages, Lilly) in 25 packages of 30 (NDC 0002-0803-29) and 20 packages of 50 (NDC 0002-0803-51). All ℞Paks have safety closures.

Ⓒ *Darvon Compound, Pulvules No. 368, USP, HO5** (No. 0, Light-Pink Opaque Body, Light-Gray Opaque Cap), in bottles of 100 (℞Pak) (NDC 0002-3110-02) and 500 (NDC 0002-3110-03) and in 10 strips of 10 individually labeled blisters each containing 1 Pulvule (ID100) (NDC 0002-3110-33). All ℞Paks have safety closures.

Ⓒ *Darvon Compound-65, Pulvules No. 369, USP, HO6** (No. 0, Red Opaque Body, Light-Gray Opaque Cap), in bottles of 100 (℞Pak) (NDC 0002-3111-02) and 500 (NDC 0002-3111-03), in 10 strips of 10 individually labeled blisters each containing 1 Pulvule (ID100) (NDC 0002-3111-33), in 20 rolls, each consisting of 25 Pulvules in individual unit-dose packets, reverse-numbered (RN500) (NDC 0002-3111-46), and in ℞Paks in 20 packages of 50 (NDC 0002-3111-51). All ℞Paks have safety closures.

Ⓒ *Darvon with A.S.A., Pulvules No. 366, HO4** (No. 0, Red Opaque Body, Light-Pink Opaque Cap), in bottles of 100 (℞Pak) (NDC 0002-0804-02) and 500 (NDC 0002-0804-03) and in 10 strips of 10 individually labeled blisters each containing 1 Pulvule (ID100) (NDC 0002-0804-33). All ℞Paks have safety closures.

[*Shown in Product Identification Section*]

*Identi-Code® symbol.

The following information, including illustrations of dosage forms and the maximum daily dosage of each, is available to patients receiving Darvon products.

Patient Information Sheet

YOUR PRESCRIPTION FOR A DARVON® (PROPOXYPHENE) PRODUCT Ⓒ

Summary: Products containing Darvon are used to relieve pain.

LIMIT YOUR INTAKE OF ALCOHOL WHILE TAKING THIS DRUG. Make sure your doctor knows that you are taking tranquilizers, sleep aids, antidepressants, antihistamines, or any other drugs that make you sleepy. Combining propoxyphene with alcohol or these drugs in excessive doses is dangerous. Use care while driving a car or using machines until you see how the drug affects you because propoxyphene can make you sleepy. Do not take more of the drug than your doctor prescribed. Dependence has occurred when patients have taken propoxyphene for a long period of time at doses greater than recommended.

The rest of this leaflet gives you more information about propoxyphene. Please read it and keep it for future use.

Uses of Darvon: Products containing Darvon are used for the relief of mild to moderate pain. Products which contain Darvon plus aspirin or acetaminophen are prescribed for the relief of pain or pain associated with fever.

Before Taking Darvon: Make sure your doctor knows if you have ever had an allergic reaction to propoxyphene, aspirin, or acetaminophen. Some forms of propoxyphene products contain aspirin to help relieve the pain. Your doctor should be advised if you have a history of ulcers or if you are taking an anticoagulant ("blood thinner"). The aspirin may irritate the stomach lining and may cause bleeding, particularly if an ulcer is present. Also, bleeding may occur if you are taking an anticoagulant. In a small group of people, aspirin may cause an asthma attack. If you are one of these people, be sure your drug does not contain aspirin.

The effect of propoxyphene in children under 12 has not been studied. Therefore, use of the drug in this age group is not recommended.

How to Take Darvon: Follow your doctor's directions exactly. Do not increase the amount you take without your doctor's approval. If you miss a dose of the drug, do not take twice as much the next time.

Pregnancy: Do not take propoxyphene during pregnancy unless your doctor knows you are pregnant and specifically recommends its use. Cases of temporary dependence in the newborn have occurred when the mother has taken propoxyphene consistently in the weeks before delivery. As a general principle, no drug should be taken during pregnancy unless it is clearly necessary.

General Cautions: Heavy use of alcohol with propoxyphene is hazardous and may lead to overdosage symptoms (see "Overdose" below). THEREFORE, LIMIT YOUR INTAKE OF ALCOHOL WHILE TAKING PROPOXYPHENE.

Combinations of excessive doses of propoxyphene, alcohol, and tranquilizers are dangerous. Make sure your doctor knows you are taking tranquilizers, sleep aids, antidepressant drugs, antihistamines, or any other drugs that make you sleepy. The use of these drugs with propoxyphene increases their sedative effects and may lead to overdosage symptoms, including death (see "Overdose" below).

Propoxyphene may cause drowsiness or impair your mental and/or physical abilities: therefore, use caution when driving a vehicle or operating dangerous machinery. DO NOT perform any hazardous task until you have seen your response to this drug.

Dependence: You can become dependent on propoxyphene if you take it in higher than recommended doses over a long period of time. Dependence is a feeling of need for the drug and a feeling that you cannot perform normally without it.

Overdose: An overdose of Darvon, alone or in combination with other drugs, including alcohol, may cause weakness, difficulty in breathing, confusion, anxiety, and more severe drowsiness and dizziness. Extreme overdosage may lead to unconsciousness and death.

If the propoxyphene product contains acetaminophen, the overdosage symptoms include nausea, vomiting, lack of appetite, and abdominal pain. Liver damage may occur.

When the propoxyphene product contains aspirin, symptoms of taking too much of the drug are headache, dizziness, ringing in the ears, difficulty in hearing, dim vision, confusion, drowsiness, sweating, thirst, rapid breathing, nausea, vomiting, and, occasionally, diarrhea. In any suspected overdosage situation, contact your doctor or nearest hospital emergency room. GET EMERGENCY HELP IMMEDIATELY.

KEEP THIS DRUG AND ALL DRUGS OUT OF THE REACH OF CHILDREN.

Possible Side Effects: When propoxyphene is taken as directed, side effects are infrequent. Among those reported are drowsiness, dizziness, nausea, and vomiting. If these effects occur, it may help if you lie down and rest.

Less frequently reported side effects are constipation, abdominal pain, skin rashes, lightheadedness, headache, weakness, minor visual disturbances, and feelings of elation or discomfort.

If side effects occur and concern you, contact your doctor.

Other Information: The safe and effective use of propoxyphene depends on your taking it exactly as directed. This drug has been prescribed specifically for you and your present condition. Do not give this drug to others who may have similar symptoms. Do not use it for any other reason.

If you would like more information about propoxyphene, ask your doctor or pharmacist. They have a more technical leaflet (professional labeling) you may read.

Prescription Vial Sticker

Tell your doctor if you are taking tranquilizers, antidepressant drugs, or sleep aids. LIMIT alcohol use with Darvon-N® (propoxyphene napsylate) and Darvon® (propoxyphene hydrochloride) products.

[052782]

DIETHYLSTILBESTROL USP ℞

PROLONGED USE OF ESTROGENS HAS BEEN REPORTED TO INCREASE THE RISK OF ENDOMETRIAL CARCINOMA

Three independent case-control studies have reported an increased risk of endometrial cancer in postmenopausal women exposed to exogenous estrogens for prolonged periods. This risk was independent

Continued on next page

*Identi-Code® symbol.

Lilly—Cont.

of other known risk factors for endometrial cancer. These studies are further supported by the finding that, since 1969, the incidence rate of endometrial cancer has increased sharply in eight different areas of the United States which have population-based cancer reporting systems.
The three case-control studies reported that the risk of endometrial cancer in estrogen users was about 4.5 to 13.9 times greater than in nonusers. The risk appears to depend on both the duration of treatment and the dose of estrogen. In view of these findings, the lowest dose that will control symptoms should be utilized when estrogens are used for the treatment of menopausal symptoms, and medication should be discontinued as soon as possible. When prolonged treatment is medically indicated, a reassessment should be made on at least a semiannual basis to determine the need for continued therapy. Although the evidence must be considered preliminary, one study suggests that cyclic administration of low doses of estrogen may carry less risk than does continuous administration; it therefore appears prudent to utilize such a regimen.
Close clinical surveillance of all women taking estrogens is important. In all cases of undiagnosed persistent or recurring abnormal vaginal bleeding, adequate diagnostic measures should be undertaken to rule out malignancy.
At present, there is no evidence that "natural" estrogens are more or less hazardous than "synthetic" estrogens at equivalent estrogenic doses.
ESTROGENS SHOULD NOT BE USED DURING PREGNANCY
The use of female sex hormones, both estrogens and progestogens, during early pregnancy may affect the offspring. It has been reported that females exposed *in utero* to diethylstilbestrol, a nonsteroidal estrogen, may have an increased risk of developing later in life a rare form of vaginal or cervical cancer. This risk has been estimated to be 0.14 to 1.4 per 1000 exposures. Furthermore, from 30 to 90 percent of such exposed women have been found to have vaginal adenosis and epithelial changes of the vagina and cervix. Although these changes are histologically benign, it is not known whether they are precursors of malignancy. Even though similar data are not available with the use of other estrogens, it cannot be presumed that they would not induce similar changes.
Several reports suggest that there is an association between intrauterine exposure to female sex hormones and congenital anomalies, including congenital heart defects and limb-reduction defects. One case-control study estimated a 4.7-fold increased risk of limb-reduction defects in infants exposed *in utero* to sex hormones (oral contraceptives, hormone withdrawal tests for pregnancy, or attempted treatment for threatened abortion). Some of these exposures were very short and involved only a few days of treatment. The data suggest that the risk of limb-reduction defects in exposed fetuses is somewhat less than 1 per 1000.
In the past, female sex hormones have been used during pregnancy in an attempt to treat threatened or habitual abortion; however, their efficacy was never conclusively proved or disproved.
If diethylstilbestrol is administered during pregnancy, or if the patient becomes pregnant while taking this drug, she should be apprised of the potential risks to the fetus and of the advisability of pregnancy continuation.

THIS DRUG PRODUCT SHOULD NOT BE USED AS A POSTCOITAL CONTRACEPTIVE
Description: Diethylstilbestrol is a crystalline synthetic estrogenic substance capable of producing all the pharmacologic and therapeutic responses attributed to natural estrogens. Diethylstilbestrol may be administered orally (in the form of Enseals® [enteric-release tablets, Lilly] and tablets) or vaginally (in the form of suppositories). Chemically, diethylstilbestrol is α,α′-diethyl-4,4′-stilbenediol.
Indications: Diethylstilbestrol is indicated in the treatment of:
1. Moderate to severe *vasomotor* symptoms associated with the menopause (There is no evidence that estrogens are effective for nervous symptoms or depression which might occur during menopause, and they should not be used to treat these conditions.)
2. Atrophic vaginitis
3. Kraurosis vulvae
4. Female hypogonadism
5. Female castration
6. Primary ovarian failure
7. Breast cancer (for palliation only) in appropriately selected women and men with metastatic disease
8. Prostatic carcinoma—palliative therapy of advanced disease

DIETHYLSTILBESTROL SHOULD NOT BE USED FOR ANY PURPOSE DURING PREGNANCY. ITS USE MAY CAUSE SEVERE HARM TO THE FETUS (SEE BOXED WARNING).
Contraindications: Estrogens should not be used in women (or men) with any of the following conditions:
1. Known or suspected cancer of the breast, except in appropriately selected patients being treated for metastatic disease
2. Known or suspected estrogen-dependent neoplasia
3. Known or suspected pregnancy (see boxed warning)
4. Undiagnosed abnormal genital bleeding
5. Active thrombophlebitis or thromboembolic disorders
6. A past history of thrombophlebitis, thrombosis, or thromboembolic disorders associated with previous use of estrogen (except when used in treatment of breast or prostatic malignancy)

Warnings: 1. *Induction of Malignant Neoplasms*—In certain animal species, long-term continuous administration of natural and synthetic estrogens increases the frequency of carcinomas of the breast, cervix, vagina, kidney, and liver. There are now reports that prolonged use of estrogens increases the risk of carcinoma of the endometrium in humans (see boxed warning).
At the present time, there is no satisfactory evidence that administration of estrogens to postmenopausal women increases the risk of cancer of the breast. This possibility, however, has been raised by a recent long-term follow-up of one physician's practice. Because of the animal data, there is a need for caution in prescribing estrogens for women with a family history of breast cancer or for women who have breast nodules, fibrocystic disease, or abnormal mammograms.
2. *Gallbladder Disease*—A recent study reported a two-to-threefold increase in the risk of gallbladder disease occurring in women receiving postmenopausal estrogen therapy, similar to the twofold increased risk previously noted in women using oral contraceptives. In the case of oral contraceptives, this increased risk appeared after two years of use.
3. *Effects Similar to Those Caused by Estrogen-Progestogen Oral Contraceptives*—There are several serious adverse effects associated with the use of oral contraceptives; however, most of these adverse effects have not as yet been documented as consequences of postmenopausal estrogen therapy. This may reflect the comparatively low doses of estrogen used in postmenopausal women. It would be expected that these adverse effects are more likely to occur following administration of the larger doses of estrogen used for treating prostatic or breast cancer. It has, in fact, been shown that there is an increased risk of thrombosis with the administration of estrogens for prostatic cancer in men and for postpartum breast engorgement in women.
a. *Thromboembolic Disease*—It is now well established that women taking oral contraceptives run an increased risk of various thromboembolic and thrombotic vascular diseases, such as thrombophlebitis, pulmonary embolism, stroke, and myocardial infarction. Cases of retinal thrombosis, mesenteric thrombosis, and optic neuritis have been reported in users of oral contraceptives. There is evidence that the risk of several of these adverse reactions is related to the dose of the drug. An increased risk of postsurgical thromboembolic complications has also been reported in users of oral contraceptives. If feasible, estrogen therapy should be discontinued at least four weeks before any surgery that may be associated with an increased risk of thromboembolism or that may require periods of prolonged immobilization.
Although an increased rate of thromboembolic and thrombotic disease has not been noted in postmenopausal users of estrogen, this does not rule out the possiblity that such an increase may be present or that it exists in subgroups of women who have underlying risk factors or who are receiving relatively large doses of estrogens. Therefore, estrogens should not be used in persons with active thrombophlebitis or thromboembolic disorders, nor should they be used (except in treatment of malignancy) in persons with a history of such disorders associated with estrogen therapy. Estrogens should be administered cautiously to patients with cerebral vascular or coronary artery disease and only when such therapy is clearly needed.
In a large prospective clinical trial in men, large doses of estrogen (5 mg of conjugated estrogens per day), comparable to those used to treat cancer of the prostate and breast, have been shown to increase the risk of nonfatal myocardial infarction, pulmonary embolism, and thrombophlebitis. When such large doses of estrogen are used, any of the thromboembolic and thrombotic adverse effects associated with the use of oral contraceptives should be considered a clear risk.
b. *Hepatic Adenoma*—Benign hepatic adenomas appear to be associated with the use of oral contraceptives. Although these adenomas are benign and rare, they may rupture and may cause death by intra-abdominal hemorrhage. Such lesions have not yet been reported in association with the administration of other estrogen or progestogen preparations, but they should be considered when abdominal pain and tenderness, abdominal mass, or hypovolemic shock occurs in persons receiving estrogen therapy. Hepatocellular carcinoma has also been reported in women taking estrogen-containing oral contraceptives. The relationship of this malignancy to such drugs is not known at this time.
c. *Elevated Blood Pressure*—Increased blood pressure is not uncommon in women taking oral contraceptives. There is now one report that this may occur with use of estrogens in the menopause, and blood pressure should be monitored during estrogen therapy, especially if high doses are used.
d. *Glucose Tolerance*—A decrease in glucose tolerance has been observed in a significant percentage of patients on estrogen-con-

taining oral contraceptives. For this reason, diabetic patients should be carefully observed while receiving estrogen.

4. *Hypercalcemia*—Administration of estrogens may lead to severe hypercalcemia in patients with breast cancer and bone metastases. If this occurs, the drug should be stopped and appropriate measures taken to reduce the serum calcium level.

Precautions: A. General Precautions.

1. A complete medical and family history should be taken prior to initiation of any estrogen therapy. In the pretreatment and periodic physical examinations, special consideration should be given to blood pressure, breasts, abdomen, and pelvic organs, and a Papanicolaou smear should be performed. As a general rule, estrogen should not be prescribed for over a year without another physical examination.

2. Fluid retention—Because estrogens may cause some degree of fluid retention, conditions which might be influenced by this factor, such as epilepsy, migraine, and cardiac or renal dysfunction, require careful observation.

3. Certain patients may develop undesirable manifestations of excessive estrogenic stimulation, such as abnormal or excessive uterine bleeding, mastodynia, etc.

4. Oral contraceptives appear to be associated with an increased incidence of mental depression. Although it is not clear whether this is due to the estrogenic or progestogenic component of the contraceptive agent, patients with a history of depression should be carefully observed.

5. Preexisting uterine leiomyomata may increase in size with administration of estrogens.

6. The pathologist should be advised of estrogen therapy when relevant specimens are submitted.

7. Patients with a past history of jaundice during pregnancy run an increased risk of recurrence of jaundice while receiving estrogen-containing oral contraceptive therapy. If jaundice develops in any patient receiving estrogen, the medication should be discontinued while the cause is investigated.

8. Estrogens may be poorly metabolized in patients with impaired liver function, and they should therefore be administered with caution in such patients.

9. Because estrogens influence the metabolism of calcium and phosphorus, they should be used with caution in patients with metabolic bone diseases associated with hypercalcemia or in patients with renal insufficiency.

10. Because of the effects of estrogens on epiphyseal closure, they should be used judiciously in young patients in whom bone growth is not complete.

11. Certain endocrine and liver function tests may be affected by estrogen-containing oral contraceptives. The following similar changes may be expected with larger doses of estrogen:

a. Increased sulfobromophthalein retention

b. Increased prothrombin and factors VII, VIII, IX, and X; decreased antithrombin 3; increased norepinephrine-induced platelet aggregability

c. Increased thyroid-binding globulin (TBG) leading to increased circulating total thyroid hormone, as measured by PBI, T^4 by column, or T^4 by radioimmunoassay. Free T^3 resin uptake is decreased, reflecting the elevated TBG; free T^4 concentration is unaltered

d. Impaired glucose tolerance

e. Decreased pregnanediol excretion

f. Reduced response to metyrapone test

g. Reduced serum folate concentration

h. Increased serum triglyceride and phospholipid concentration

B. Information for the Patient. *See* text of Patient Package Insert.

C. Pregnancy Category X. *See* Contraindications and boxed warning.

D. Nursing Mothers. As a general principle, any drug should be administered to nursing mothers only when clearly necessary, since many drugs are excreted in human milk.

Adverse Reactions: (*See* Warnings regarding induction of neoplasia, adverse effects on the fetus, increased incidence of gallbladder disease, and adverse effects similar to those of oral contraceptives, including thromboembolism.) The following additional adverse reactions have been reported with estrogenic therapy, including oral contraceptives:

1. *Genitourinary System*
   Breakthrough bleeding, spotting, change in menstrual flow
   Dysmenorrhea
   Premenstrual-like syndrome
   Amenorrhea during and after treatment
   Increase in size of uterine fibromyomata
   Vaginal candidiasis
   Change in cervical eversion and in degree of cervical secretion
   Cystitis-like syndrome
2. *Breasts*
   Tenderness, enlargement, secretion
3. *Gastrointestinal*
   Nausea, vomiting
   Abdominal cramps, bloating
   Cholestatic jaundice
4. *Skin*
   Chloasma or melasma which may persist when drug is discontinued
   Erythema multiforme
   Erythema nodosum
   Hemorrhagic eruption
   Loss of scalp hair
   Hirsutism
5. *Eyes*
   Steepening of corneal curvature
   Intolerance to contact lenses
6. *C.N.S.*
   Headache, migraine, dizziness
   Mental depression
   Chorea
7. *Miscellaneous*
   Increase or decrease in weight
   Reduced carbohydrate tolerance
   Aggravation of porphyria
   Edema
   Changes in libido

Acute Overdosage: Numerous reports indicate that serious ill effects do not occur when large doses of estrogen containing oral contraceptives are ingested by young children. Overdosage of estrogen may cause nausea, and withdrawal bleeding may occur in females.

Dosage and Administration: 1. *Given Cyclically for Short-Term Use Only:*

For treatment of moderate to severe *vasomotor* symptoms, atrophic vaginitis, or kraurosis vulvae associated with the menopause.

The lowest dose that will control symptoms should be chosen, and medication should be discontinued as promptly as possible.

Administration should be cyclic (e.g., three weeks on and one week off).

Attempts to discontinue or taper medication should be made at three to six-month intervals.

The usual dosage range is 0.2 to 0.5 mg daily. Patients with atrophic vaginitis may require up to 2 mg daily, and cyclic administration may be necessary for several years. Patients with atrophic vaginitis may notice relief of symptoms sooner if up to 1 mg of the suppository form is administered daily for ten to 14 days concomitantly with oral diethylstilbestrol. Consideration should also be given to prescribing the suppository form as the only means of estrogenic therapy for patients with atrophic vaginitis or kraurosis vulvae, in which case the dosage may be increased to 5 to 7 mg weekly.

2. *Given Cyclically:*
   Female hypogonadism
   Female castration
   Primary ovarian failure
      0.2 to 0.5 mg daily
3. *Given Chronically:*
   Inoperable progressing prostatic cancer
      1 to 3 mg daily initially, increased in advanced cases; the dosage may later be reduced to an average of 1 mg daily.
   Inoperable progressing breast cancer in appropriately selected men and postmenopausal women (*see* Indications)
      15 mg daily

Patients with an intact uterus should be closely monitored for signs of endometrial cancer, and appropriate diagnostic measures should be taken to rule out malignancy in the event of persistent or recurring abnormal vaginal bleeding.

How Supplied: (℞) *Enseals—Diethylstilbestrol Tablets, USP (Enteric): No. 46, A19,** 0.1 mg, *No. 47, A20,** 0.25 mg, *No. 48, A21,** 0.5 mg, *No. 49, A22,** 1 mg, and *No. 85, A33,** 5 mg, in bottles of 100 and 1000.

(℞) *Diethylstilbestrol Suppositories, USP* (Vaginal): *No. 14, SO7,* *0.1 mg, and *No. 15, SO9,* *0.5 mg, in packages of 6. In addition to the diethylstilbestrol, the suppositories also contain glycerin, gelatin, polysorbate 20, and propylene glycol.

(℞) *Tablets—Diethylstilbestrol Tablets, USP: No. 1646, J49,** 0.1 mg, in bottles of 100 and 1000; *No. 1647, J50,** 0.25 mg, in bottles of 100; *No. 1648, J51,** 0.5 mg, and *No. 1649, J52,** 1 mg, in bottles of 100 and 1000; *No. 1685, J54,** 5 mg, in bottles of 100 and 1000 and in 10 strips of 10 individually labeled blisters each containing 1 tablet (ID100). [113081]

DOBUTREX® ℞
(dobutamine hydrochloride)
For Injection
USP

Description: Dobutrex® (dobutamine hydrochloride, Lilly) is (±)-4-[2-[[3-(*p*-hydroxyphenyl)-1-methylpropyl]amino]-ethyl] -pyrocatechol hydrochloride. It is a synthetic catecholamine.

The clinical formulation is supplied in a sterile lyophilized form for intravenous use only. Each vial contains 250 mg of dobutamine and 250 mg of mannitol. Hydrochloric acid is used to adjust the *p*H. The *p*H of the reconstituted solution is between 2.5 and 5.5.

Clinical Pharmacology: Dobutrex® (dobutamine hydrochloride, Lilly) is a direct-acting inotropic agent whose primary activity results from stimulation of the beta receptors of the heart while producing comparatively mild chronotropic, hypertensive, arrhythmogenic, and vasodilative effects. It does not cause the release of endogenous norepinephrine, as does dopamine. In animal studies, dobutamine produces less increase in heart rate and less decrease in peripheral vascular resistance for a given inotropic effect than does isoproterenol. In patients with depressed cardiac function, both dobutamine and isoproterenol increase the cardiac output to a similar degree. In the case of dobutamine, this increase is usually not accompanied by marked increases in heart rate (although tachycardia is occasionally observed), and the cardiac stroke volume is usually increased. In contrast, isoproterenol increases the cardiac index primarily by increasing the heart rate while stroke volume changes little or declines.

Facilitation of atrioventricular conduction has been observed in human electrophysiologic studies and in patients with atrial fibrillation.

Systemic vascular resistance is usually decreased with administration of dobutamine. Occasionally, minimum vasoconstriction has been observed.

Continued on next page

*Identi-Code® symbol.

Lilly—Cont.

Most clinical experience with dobutamine is short-term—up to several hours in duration. In the limited number of patients who were studied for 24, 48, and 72 hours, a persistent increase in cardiac output occurred in some, whereas the output of others returned toward base-line values.
The onset of action of Dobutrex is within one to two minutes; however, as much as ten minutes may be required to obtain the peak effect of a particular infusion rate.
The plasma half-life of dobutamine in humans is two minutes. The principal routes of metabolism are methylation of the catechol and conjugation. In human urine, the major excretion products are the conjugates of dobutamine and 3-O-methyl dobutamine. The 3-O-methyl derivative of dobutamine is inactive.
Alteration of synaptic concentrations of catecholamines with either reserpine or tricyclic antidepressants does not alter the actions of dobutamine in animals, which indicates that the actions of dobutamine are not dependent on presynaptic mechanisms.
Indications and Usage: Dobutrex® (dobutamine hydrochloride, Lilly) is indicated when parenteral therapy is necessary for inotropic support in the short-term treatment of adults with cardiac decompensation due to depressed contractility resulting either from organic heart disease or from cardiac surgical procedures.
In patients who have atrial fibrillation with rapid ventricular response, a digitalis preparation should be used prior to institution of therapy with Dobutrex.
Contraindication: Dobutrex® (dobutamine hydrochloride, Lilly) is contraindicated in patients with idiopathic hypertrophic subaortic stenosis.
Warnings: 1. *Increase in Heart Rate or Blood Pressure*—Dobutrex® (dobutamine hydrochloride, Lilly) may cause a marked increase in heart rate or blood pressure, especially systolic pressure. Approximately 10 percent of patients in clinical studies have had rate increases of 30 beats/minute or more, and about 7.5 percent have had a 50-mm Hg or greater increase in systolic pressure. Reduction of dosage usually reverses these effects promptly. Because dobutamine facilitates atrioventricular conduction, patients with atrial fibrillation are at risk of developing rapid ventricular response. Patients with preexisting hypertension appear to face an increased risk of developing an exaggerated pressor response.
2. *Ectopic Activity*—Dobutrex may precipitate or exacerbate ventricular ectopic activity, but it rarely has caused ventricular tachycardia.
Precautions: 1. During the administration of Dobutrex® (dobutamine hydrochloride, Lilly), as with any adrenergic agent, ECG and blood pressure should be continuously monitored. In addition, pulmonary wedge pressure and cardiac output should be monitored whenever possible to aid in the safe and effective infusion of Dobutrex.
2. Hypovolemia should be corrected with suitable volume expanders before treatment with Dobutrex is instituted.
3. Animal studies indicate that Dobutrex may be ineffective if the patient has recently received a beta-blocking drug. In such a case, the peripheral vascular resistance may increase.
4. No improvement may be observed in the presence of marked mechanical obstruction, such as severe valvular aortic stenosis.
Usage Following Acute Myocardial Infarction—Clinical experience with Dobutrex following myocardial infarction has been insufficient to establish the safety of the drug for this use. There is concern that any agent which increases contractile force and heart rate may increase the size of an infarction by intensifying ischemia, but it is not known whether dobutamine does so.
Usage in Pregnancy—Reproduction studies performed in rats and rabbits have revealed no evidence of impaired fertility, harm to the fetus, or teratogenic effects due to dobutamine. However, the drug has not been administered to pregnant women and should be used only when the expected benefits clearly outweigh the potential risks to the fetus.
Pediatric Use—The safety and effectiveness of Dobutrex for use in children have not been studied.
Drug Interactions—There was no evidence of drug interactions in clinical studies in which Dobutrex was administered concurrently with other drugs, including digitalis preparations, furosemide, spironolactone, lidocaine, glyceryl trinitrate, isosorbide dinitrate, morphine, atropine, heparin, protamine, potassium chloride, folic acid, and acetaminophen. Preliminary studies indicate that the concomitant use of dobutamine and nitroprusside results in a higher cardiac output and, usually, a lower pulmonary wedge pressure than when either drug is used alone.
Adverse Reactions: *Increased Heart Rate, Blood Pressure, and Ventricular Ectopic Activity*—A 10 to 20-mm increase in systolic blood pressure and an increase in heart rate of five to 15 beats/minute have been noted in most patients. (*See* Warnings regarding exaggerated chronotropic and pressor effects.) Approximately 5 percent of patients have had increased premature ventricular beats during infusions. These effects are dose related.
Miscellaneous Uncommon Effects—The following adverse effects have been reported in 1 to 3 percent of patients: nausea, headache, anginal pain, nonspecific chest pain, palpitations, and shortness of breath.
No abnormal laboratory values attributable to Dobutrex® (dobutamine hydrochloride, Lilly) have been observed.
Longer-Term Safety—Infusions of up to 72 hours have revealed no adverse effects other than those seen with shorter infusions.
Overdosage: In case of overdosage, as evidenced by excessive alteration of blood pressure or by tachycardia, reduce the rate of administration or temporarily discontinue Dobutrex® (dobutamine hydrochloride, Lilly) until the patient's condition stabilizes. Because the duration of action of Dobutrex is short, usually no additional remedial measures are necessary.
Dosage and Administration: *Reconstitution and Stability*—Dobutrex® (dobutamine hydrochloride, Lilly) is incompatible with alkaline solutions and should not be mixed with products such as 5% Sodium Bicarbonate Injection.
Dobutrex may be reconstituted with Sterile Water for Injection or 5% Dextrose Injection. To reconstitute, add 10 ml of diluent to Vial No. 7051, Dobutrex, 250 mg. If the material is not completely dissolved, add another 10 ml of diluent. The reconstituted solution may be stored under refrigeration for 48 hours or at room temperature for six hours.
Reconstituted Dobutrex must be further diluted to at least 50 ml prior to administration in 5% Dextrose Injection, 0.9% Sodium Chloride Injection, or Sodium Lactate Injection. Intravenous solutions should be used within 24 hours.
Solutions containing Dobutrex may exhibit a color that, if present, will increase with time. This color change is due to slight oxidation of the drug, but there is no significant loss of potency during the reconstituted time periods stated above.
Recommended Dosage—The rate of infusion needed to increase cardiac output usually ranges from 2.5 to 10 mcg/kg/min (see table). On rare occasions, infusion rates up to 40 mcg/kg/min have been required to obtain the desired effect.
[See table below].
The rate of administration and the duration of therapy should be adjusted according to the patient's response, as determined by heart rate, presence of ectopic activity, blood pressure, urine flow, and, whenever possible, measurement of central venous or pulmonary wedge pressure and cardiac output.
Concentrations up to 5000 mcg/ml have been administered to humans (250 mg/50 ml). The final volume administered should be determined by the fluid requirements of the patient.
How Supplied: (℞) *Vials No. 7051, Dobutrex® (Dobutamine Hydrochloride for Injection, USP), for Injection* (lyophilized), equivalent to 250 mg dobutamine, 20-ml size, rubber-stoppered, in singles (10 per carton) (NDC 0002-7051-01). [012282]

Dobutrex® (dobutamine hydrochloride)—Rates of Infusion for Concentrations of 250, 500, and 1000 mcg/ml

Drug Delivery Rate (mcg/kg/min)	Infusion Delivery Rate: 250 mcg/ml* (ml/kg/min)	500 mcg/ml† (ml/kg/min)	1000 mcg/ml‡ (ml/kg/min)
2.5	0.01	0.005	0.0025
5	0.02	0.01	0.005
7.5	0.03	0.015	0.0075
10	0.04	0.02	0.01
12.5	0.05	0.025	0.0125
15	0.06	0.03	0.015

*250 mg/liter of diluent
†500 mg/liter or 250 mg/500 ml of diluent
‡1000 mg/liter or 250 mg/250 ml of diluent

DOLOPHINE® HYDROCHLORIDE Ⓒ
(methadone hydrochloride)
Injection, USP

AMPOULES AND VIALS

CONDITIONS FOR DISTRIBUTION AND USE OF METHADONE PRODUCTS:
Code of Federal Regulations, Title 21, Sec. 291.505

METHADONE PRODUCTS, WHEN USED FOR THE TREATMENT OF NARCOTIC ADDICTION IN DETOXIFICATION OR MAINTENANCE PROGRAMS, SHALL BE DISPENSED ONLY BY APPROVED HOSPITAL PHARMACIES, APPROVED COMMUNITY PHARMACIES, AND MAINTENANCE PROGRAMS APPROVED BY THE FOOD AND DRUG ADMINISTRATION AND THE DESIGNATED STATE AUTHORITY.

APPROVED MAINTENANCE PROGRAMS SHALL DISPENSE AND USE METHADONE IN ORAL FORM ONLY AND ACCORDING TO THE TREATMENT REQUIREMENTS STIPULATED IN THE FEDERAL METHADONE REGULATIONS (21 CFR 291.505).
FAILURE TO ABIDE BY THE REQUIREMENTS IN THESE REGULATIONS MAY RESULT IN CRIMINAL PROSECUTION, SEIZURE OF THE DRUG SUPPLY, REVOCATION OF THE PROGRAM APPROVAL, AND INJUNCTION PRECLUDING OPERATION OF THE PROGRAM.
A METHADONE PRODUCT, WHEN USED AS AN ANALGESIC, MAY BE DISPENSED IN ANY LICENSED PHARMACY.

Description: Dolophine® Hydrochloride (Methadone Hydrochloride, USP, Lilly) (4,4-diphenyl-6-dimethylamino-heptanone-3 hydrochloride) is a white crystalline material which is water soluble.
Each ml contains methadone hydrochloride, 10 mg, and sodium chloride, 0.9 percent. Sodium hydroxide and/or hydrochloric acid may have been added during manufacture to adjust the *p*H. The 20-ml vials also contain chlorobutanol (chloroform derivative), 0.5 percent, as a preservative.
Actions: Methadone hydrochloride is a synthetic narcotic analgesic with multiple actions quantitatively similar to those of morphine, the most prominent of which involve the central nervous system and organs composed of smooth muscle. The principal actions of therapeutic value are analgesia and sedation and detoxification or temporary maintenance in narcotic addiction. The methadone abstinence syndrome, although qualitatively similar to that of morphine, differs in that the onset is slower, the course is more prolonged, and the symptoms are less severe.
A parenteral dose of 8 to 10 mg of methadone is approximately equivalent in analgesic effect to 10 mg of morphine. With single-dose administration, the onset and duration of analgesic action of the two drugs are similar.
When administered orally, methadone is approximately one-half as potent as when given parenterally. Oral administration results in a delay of the onset, a lowering of the peak, and an increase in the duration of analgesic effect.
Indications: (See Note below.)
For relief of severe pain.
For detoxification treatment of narcotic addiction.
For temporary maintenance treatment of narcotic addiction.

NOTE
If methadone is administered for treatment of heroin dependence for more than three weeks, the procedure passes from treatment of the acute withdrawal syndrome (detoxification) to maintenance therapy. Maintenance treatment is permitted to be undertaken only by approved methadone programs. This does not preclude the maintenance treatment of an addict who is hospitalized for medical conditions other than addiction and who requires temporary maintenance during the critical period of his stay or whose enrollment has been verified in a program which has approval for maintenance treatment with methadone.

Contraindication: Hypersensitivity to methadone.
Warnings: Methadone hydrochloride, a narcotic, is a Schedule II controlled substance under the Federal Controlled Substances Act. Appropriate security measures should be taken to safeguard stocks of methadone against diversion.
DRUG DEPENDENCE—METHADONE CAN PRODUCE DRUG DEPENDENCE OF THE MORPHINE TYPE AND, THEREFORE, HAS THE POTENTIAL FOR BEING ABUSED. PSYCHIC DEPENDENCE, PHYSICAL DEPENDENCE, AND TOLERANCE MAY DEVELOP UPON REPEATED ADMINISTRATION OF METHADONE, AND IT SHOULD BE PRESCRIBED AND ADMINISTERED WITH THE SAME DEGREE OF CAUTION APPROPRIATE TO THE USE OF MORPHINE.
Interaction with Other Central-Nervous-System Depressants—Methadone should be used with caution and in reduced dosage in patients who are concurrently receiving other narcotic analgesics, general anesthetics, phenothiazines, other tranquilizers, sedative-hypnotics, tricyclic antidepressants, and other CNS depressants (including alcohol). Respiratory depression, hypotension, and profound sedation or coma may result.
Anxiety—Since methadone, as used by tolerant subjects at a constant maintenance dosage, is not a tranquilizer, patients who are maintained on this drug will react to life problems and stresses with the same symptoms of anxiety as do other individuals. The physician should not confuse such symptoms with those of narcotic abstinence and should not attempt to treat anxiety by increasing the dosage of methadone. The action of methadone in maintenance treatment is limited to the control of narcotic symptoms and is ineffective for relief of general anxiety.
Head Injury and Increased Intracranial Pressure—The respiratory depressant effects of methadone and its capacity to elevate cerebrospinal-fluid pressure may be markedly exaggerated in the presence of increased intracranial pressure. Furthermore, narcotics produce side effects that may obscure the clinical course of patients with head injuries. In such patients, methadone must be used with caution and only if it is deemed essential.
Asthma and Other Respiratory Conditions—Methadone should be used with caution in patients having an acute asthmatic attack, in those with chronic obstructive pulmonary disease or cor pulmonale, and in individuals with a substantially decreased respiratory reserve, preexisting respiratory depression, hypoxia, or hypercapnia. In such patients, even usual therapeutic doses of narcotics may decrease respiratory drive while simultaneously increasing airway resistance to the point of apnea.
Hypotensive Effect—The administration of methadone may result in severe hypotension in an individual whose ability to maintain his blood pressure has already been compromised by a depleted blood volume or concurrent administration of such drugs as the phenothiazines or certain anesthetics.
Use in Ambulatory Patients—Methadone may impair the mental and/or physical abilities required for the performance of potentially hazardous tasks, such as driving a car or operating machinery. The patient should be cautioned accordingly.
Methadone, like other narcotics, may produce orthostatic hypotension in ambulatory patients.
Use in Pregnancy—Safe use in pregnancy has not been established in relation to possible adverse effects on fetal development. Therefore, methadone should not be used in pregnant women unless, in the judgment of the physician, the potential benefits outweigh the possible hazards.
Methadone is not recommended for obstetric analgesia because its long duration of action increases the probability of respiratory depression in the newborn.
Use in Children—Methadone is not recommended for use as an analgesic in children, since documented clinical experience has been insufficient to establish a suitable dosage regimen for the pediatric age group.
Precautions: Interaction with Pentazocine—**Patients who are addicted to heroin or who are on the methadone maintenance program may experience withdrawal symptoms when given pentazocine.**
Interaction with Rifampin—The concurrent administration of rifampin may possibly reduce the blood concentration of methadone to a degree sufficient to produce withdrawal symptoms. The mechanism by which rifampin may decrease blood concentrations of methadone is not fully understood, although enhanced microsomal drug-metabolized enzymes may influence drug disposition.
Acute Abdominal Conditions—The administration of methadone or other narcotics may obscure the diagnosis or clinical course in patients with acute abdominal conditions.
Interaction with Monoamine Oxidase (MAO) Inhibitors—Therapeutic doses of meperidine have precipitated severe reactions in patients concurrently receiving monoamine oxidase inhibitors or those who have received such agents within 14 days. Similar reactions thus far have not been reported with methadone; but if the use of methadone is necessary in such patients, a sensitivity test should be performed in which repeated small incremental doses are administered over the course of several hours while the patient's condition and vital signs are under careful observation.
Special-Risk Patients—Methadone should be given with caution and the initial dose should be reduced in certain patients, such as the elderly or debilitated and those with severe impairment of hepatic or renal function, hypothyroidism, Addison's disease, prostatic hypertrophy, or urethral stricture.
Adverse Reactions: THE MAJOR HAZARDS OF METHADONE, AS OF OTHER NARCOTIC ANALGESICS, ARE RESPIRATORY DEPRESSION AND, TO A LESSER DEGREE, CIRCULATORY DEPRESSION. RESPIRATORY ARREST, SHOCK, AND CARDIAC ARREST HAVE OCCURRED.
The most frequently observed adverse reactions include lightheadedness, dizziness, sedation, nausea, vomiting, and sweating. These effects seem to be more prominent in ambulatory patients and in those who are not suffering severe pain. In such individuals, lower doses are advisable. Some adverse reactions may be alleviated in the ambulatory patient if he lies down.
Other adverse reactions include the following:
Central Nervous System—Euphoria, dysphoria, weakness, headache, insomnia, agitation, disorientation, and visual disturbances.
Gastrointestinal—Dry mouth, anorexia, constipation, and biliary tract spasm.
Cardiovascular—Flushing of the face, bradycardia, palpitation, faintness, and syncope.
Genitourinary—Urinary retention or hesitancy, antidiuretic effect, and reduced libido and/or potency.
Allergic—Pruritus, urticaria, other skin rashes, edema, and, rarely, hemorrhagic urticaria.
In addition, pain at injection site; local tissue irritation and induration following subcutaneous injection, particularly when repeated.
Dosage and Administration: *For Relief of Pain*—Dosage should be adjusted according to the severity of the pain and the response of the patient. Occasionally it may be necessary to exceed the usual dosage recommended in cases of exceptionally severe pain or in those patients who have become tolerant to the analgesic effect of narcotics.

Continued on next page

*Identi-Code® symbol.

Lilly—Cont.

Although subcutaneous administration is suitable for occasional use, intramuscular injection is preferred when repeated doses are required.
The usual adult dosage is 2.5 to 10 mg intramuscularly or subcutaneously every three or four hours as necessary.
For Detoxification Treatment—THE DRUG SHALL BE ADMINISTERED DAILY UNDER CLOSE SUPERVISION AS FOLLOWS:
A detoxification treatment course shall not exceed 21 days and may not be repeated earlier than four weeks after completion of the preceding course.
The oral form of administration is preferred. However, if the patient is unable to ingest oral medication, he may be started on the parenteral form initially.
In detoxification, the patient may receive methadone when there are significant symptoms of withdrawal. The dosage schedules indicated below are recommended but could be varied in accordance with clinical judgment. Initially, a single dose of 15 to 20 mg of methadone will often be sufficient to suppress withdrawal symptoms. Additional methadone may be provided if withdrawal symptoms are not suppressed or if symptoms reappear. When patients are physically dependent on high doses, it may be necessary to exceed these levels. Forty mg/day in single or divided doses will usually constitute an adequate stabilizing dosage level. Stabilization can be continued for two to three days, and then the amount of methadone normally will be gradually decreased. The rate at which methadone is decreased will be determined separately for each patient. The dose of methadone can be decreased on a daily basis or at two-day intervals, but the amount of intake shall always be sufficient to keep withdrawal symptoms at a tolerable level. In hospitalized patients, a daily reduction of 20 percent of the total daily dose may be tolerated and may cause little discomfort. In ambulatory patients, a somewhat slower schedule may be needed. If methadone is administered for more than three weeks, the procedure is considered to have progressed from detoxification or treatment of the acute withdrawal syndrome to maintenance treatment, even though the goal and intent may be eventual total withdrawal.
Overdosage: *Symptoms*—Serious overdosage of methadone is characterized by respiratory depression (a decrease in respiratory rate and/or tidal volume, Cheyne-Stokes respiration, cyanosis), extreme somnolence progressing to stupor or coma, maximally constricted pupils, skeletal-muscle flaccidity, cold and clammy skin, and, sometimes, bradycardia and hypotension. In severe overdosage, particularly by the intravenous route, apnea, circulatory collapse, cardiac arrest, and death may occur.
Treatment—Primary attention should be given to the reestablishment of adequate respiratory exchange through provision of a patent airway and institution of assisted or controlled ventilation. If a nontolerant person, especially a child, takes a large dose of methadone, effective narcotic antagonists are available to counteract the potentially lethal respiratory depression. **The physician must remember, however, that methadone is a long-acting depressant (36 to 48 hours), whereas the antagonists act for much shorter periods (one to three hours).** The patient must, therefore, be monitored continuously for recurrence of respiratory depression and treated repeatedly with the narcotic antagonist as needed. If the diagnosis is correct and respiratory depression is due only to overdosage of methadone, the use of other respiratory stimulants is not indicated.
An antagonist should not be administered in the absence of clinically significant respiratory or cardiovascular depression. Intravenously administered narcotic antagonists (naloxone, nalorphine, and levallorphan) are the drugs of choice to reverse signs of intoxication. These agents should be given repeatedly until the patient's status remains satisfactory. The hazard that the narcotic antagonist will further depress respiration is less likely with the use of naloxone.
Oxygen, intravenous fluids, vasopressors, and other supportive measures should be employed as indicated.

NOTE: IN AN INDIVIDUAL PHYSICALLY DEPENDENT ON NARCOTICS, THE ADMINISTRATION OF THE USUAL DOSE OF A NARCOTIC ANTAGONIST WILL PRECIPITATE AN ACUTE WITHDRAWAL SYNDROME. THE SEVERITY OF THIS SYNDROME WILL DEPEND ON THE DEGREE OF PHYSICAL DEPENDENCE AND THE DOSE OF THE ANTAGONIST ADMINISTERED. THE USE OF A NARCOTIC ANTAGONIST IN SUCH A PERSON SHOULD BE AVOIDED IF POSSIBLE. IF IT MUST BE USED TO TREAT SERIOUS RESPIRATORY DEPRESSION IN THE PHYSICALLY DEPENDENT PATIENT, THE ANTAGONIST SHOULD BE ADMINISTERED WITH EXTREME CARE AND BY TITRATION WITH SMALLER THAN USUAL DOSES OF THE ANTAGONIST.

How Supplied: (Ⓒ) *Dolophine® Hydrochloride (Methadone Hydrochloride Injection, USP): Ampoules No. 456,* 10 mg, 1 ml, in packages of 12 (NDC 0002-1687-12) and 100 (NDC 0002-1687-02). *Vials No. 435,* 10 mg per ml, 20 ml, multiple dose, rubber-stoppered, in singles (10 per carton) (NDC 0002-1682-01) and in packages of 25 (NDC 0002-1682-25). [032382]

DOLOPHINE® HYDROCHLORIDE Ⓒ
(methadone hydrochloride)
Tablets, USP

CONDITIONS FOR DISTRIBUTION AND USE OF METHADONE PRODUCTS: *See under* Ampoules Dolophine Hydrochloride.
Description, Actions, Indications, and Contraindication: *See under* Ampoules Dolophine Hydrochloride.
Warnings:

Tablets Dolophine® Hydrochloride (methadone hydrochloride, Lilly) are for oral administration only and *must not* be used for injection. It is recommended that Tablets Dolophine Hydrochloride, if dispensed, be packaged in child-resistant containers and kept out of the reach of children to prevent accidental ingestion.

See also under Ampoules Dolophine Hydrochloride.
Precautions and Adverse Reactions: *See under* Ampoules Dolophine Hydrochloride.
Dosage and Administration: *For Relief of Pain*—Dosage should be adjusted according to the severity of the pain and the response of the patient. Occasionally it may be necessary to exceed the usual dosage recommended in cases of exceptionally severe pain or in those patients who have become tolerant to the analgesic effect of narcotics.
The usual adult dosage is 2.5 to 10 mg every three or four hours as necessary.
See also under Ampoules Dolophine Hydrochloride.
If the patient cannot ingest methadone orally, parenteral administration may be substituted.
Overdosage: *See under* Ampoules Dolophine Hydrochloride.
How Supplied: (Ⓒ) *Tablets Dolophine® Hydrochloride (Methadone Hydrochloride Tablets, USP): No. 1712, J64,** 5 mg, in bottles of 100 (NDC 0002-1064-02) and 1000 (NDC 0002-1064-04); *No. 1730, J72,**10 mg, in bottles of 100 (NDC 0002-1072-02).

[092981]

DROLBAN® ℞
(dromostanolone propionate)
Injection, USP

Description: Drolban® (dromostanolone propionate, Lilly) is a synthetic steroid, a variant of testosterone. It is 17β-hydroxy-2α-methyl-5α-androstan-3-one propionate and is also known as 2-α-methyl-dihydrotestosterone propionate.
Indications: Dromostanolone propionate is recommended for use in the palliative treatment of advanced or metastatic carcinoma of the breast in women who are inoperable and are one to five years postmenopausal at the time of diagnosis or who have been proved to have hormone-dependent cancer by previous beneficial response to castration.
Contraindications: Androgens are contraindicated in carcinoma of the male breast and in premenopausal women.
Precautions: In general, the usual precautions pertaining to testosterone propionate should apply to Drolban® (dromostanolone propionate, Lilly), although in the latter the androgenic effects appear to be significantly less marked.
Patients with edema may require diuretics before and during treatment with this steroid. In patients with bone metastases, the level of the serum calcium should be determined before and at intervals during the course of treatment with Drolban. Hypercalcemia may require other management, such as the use of corticosteroid therapy. Increase in libido appears to be unusual with this steroid; however, if it occurs, the use of sedation may be helpful. Objective evidence of tumor progression should be evaluated periodically by physical examination, x-rays of known or suspected metastases, and determinations of serum calcium and alkaline phosphatase levels. The latter determination may reflect improvement in osseous lesions if there is a slight to moderate rise after initiation of treatment, or it may be indicative of extensive hepatic metastases if the level is markedly elevated.
Drug-induced jaundice or masculinization of the fetus reported with the use of other anabolic agents has thus far not been seen with Drolban. There are no reports of the use of this agent in carcinoma of the breast during pregnancy or in carcinoma of the breast in males with or without associated carcinoma of the prostate.
Until further information is available, Drolban should be used with caution in the presence of any of the following: liver disease, cardiac decompensation, nephritis, nephrosis, pregnancy, and carcinoma of the prostate.
Adverse Reactions: Side effects are significantly less intense with Drolban® (dromostanolone propionate, Lilly) than with comparable doses of testosterone propionate. The most likely side effects are mild virilism, such as deepening of the voice, acne, facial hair growth, and enlargement of the clitoris. At times, marked virilism will occur after prolonged treatment. Edema occasionally occurs. Hypercalcemia was noted in a few cases but usually accompanied progression of the disease. Libido seldom seems to be affected. Goldenberg reported a single case of "severe CNS side effects, which cleared when the drug was stopped." Local reactions at the site of injection may occur rarely.
Dosage and Administration: It is recommended that 100 mg of Drolban® (dromostanolone propionate, Lilly) be administered by intramuscular injection three times weekly.

Treatment probably should be continued as long as satisfactory results are obtained. After treatment has begun, eight to 12 weeks should elapse before any conclusions are drawn as to the efficacy of this steroid. If a significant progression of the disease occurs during the first six to eight weeks of therapy, another form of treatment should be considered.

How Supplied: (℞) *Vials No. 691, Drolban® (Dromostanolone Propionate Injection, USP),* 50 mg per ml, 10 ml, rubber-stoppered, multiple dose, in singles (10 per carton) (NDC 0002-1453-01). Each ml provides 50 mg dromostanolone propionate and sesame oil, q.s., with 0.5 percent phenol as a preservative. *Do not refrigerate.* [060782]

DROMOSTANOLONE PROPIONATE, *see* Drolban® (dromostanolone propionate, Lilly).

DURACILLIN® A.S., *see* Penicillin G Procaine Suspension, Sterile.

DYMELOR® ℞
(acetohexamide)
Tablets, USP

Description: Dymelor® (acetohexamide, Lilly) is a sulfonylurea characterized by the presence of an acetyl group in the para position of the phenyl ring and the incorporation of a cyclohexyl group on the urea moiety. Chemically, it is N-(*p*-acetylphenylsulfonyl)-N′-cyclohexylurea.

Action: Dymelor® (acetohexamide, Lilly) is an oral antidiabetic agent which is effective in controlling the blood glucose in properly selected patients with maturity-onset diabetes.

The mode of action of Dymelor is stimulation of release of insulin from the beta cells of the pancreas. In addition, a number of extrapancreatic actions of this class of drug have been elucidated; the most important of these is a reduction in glucose output from the liver.

Indications: The principal clinical indication for Dymelor® (acetohexamide, Lilly) is diabetes mellitus of the stable type (without such complications as ketosis or acidosis), variously described as relatively mild adult, maturity-onset, or nonketotic type.

The use of Dymelor in insulin-dependent patients may reduce the insulin requirements.

Contraindications: Dymelor® (acetohexamide, Lilly) is contraindicated in patients with hyperglycemia and glycosuria which may be associated with primary renal disease. If reduction of the blood sugar becomes essential in these cases, insulin is indicated.

Warnings: *Use in Pregnancy*—Safe use in pregnancy *has not been* established at this time, from the standpoint of either the mother or the fetus. Therefore, the use of Dymelor® (acetohexamide, Lilly) is not recommended for the management of diabetes when complicated by pregnancy. The advisability of administering Dymelor to women of childbearing age should be considered with caution.

Dymelor is of no value in diabetes complicated by acidosis and coma. These conditions require insulin.

In times of stress to the patient, such as fever of any cause, trauma, infection, or surgical procedures, it may be necessary to return the patient to insulin therapy or to use insulin in addition to Dymelor.

Precautions: The principles of management of diabetes mellitus are necessary to insure optimum control with Dymelor® (acetohexamide, Lilly) and are the same as for patients requiring insulin.

In patients with impaired hepatic and/or renal function and in debilitated or malnourished individuals, careful observation of the patient and adjustment of dosage are mandatory to prevent the occurrence of hypoglycemia.

Thiazide-type diuretics may aggravate the diabetic state and alter the dosage of Dymelor required.

Preparations containing phenylbutazone interfere with the excretion of the active metabolite hydroxyhexamide; as a result, increased sulfonylurea levels depress the blood glucose. This may also be true of probenecid and the absorbed antimicrobial sulfas.

Nonsteroidal anti-inflammatory agents have an affinity for albumin and may displace other albumin-bound drugs from their binding sites; this may lead to drug interaction. Patients receiving both Dymelor and nonsteroidal anti-inflammatory agents should be observed for signs of toxicity to these drugs.

Sulfonylurea compounds, like antimicrobial sulfa drugs and barbiturates, may aggravate hepatic porphyria.

Patients receiving sulfonylureas may experience peculiar symptoms, referred to as the "disulfiram reaction," following the ingestion of alcohol.

Secondary failures and the spontaneous tendency of diabetes to fluctuate in severity may occur. Therefore, patients should be seen by their physicians at regular intervals and their diabetes evaluated in order to avoid hyperglycemic and hypoglycemic episodes.

Adverse Reactions: Hypoglycemia may occur in those patients who do not eat regularly or who exercise without caloric supplementation. It is most likely to appear during the period of transition from insulin to Dymelor® (acetohexamide, Lilly) and should be considered in patients who have hepatic or renal disease as well as those who are debilitated or malnourished. Other untoward reactions consist principally in gastrointestinal disturbances (nausea, epigastric fullness, heartburn) and headache, appear to be dose related, and may disappear when dosage is reduced.

Allergic skin manifestations (pruritus, erythema, urticaria, morbilliform or maculopapular eruptions) occur but are usually transient and may disappear with continued dosage. If the skin reactions persist, the drug should be stopped. Photosensitivity reactions may be noted. Jaundice of both the cholestatic and mixed hepatic types has been observed with Dymelor.

As with other sulfonylurea drugs, leukopenia, thrombocytopenia, pancytopenia, agranulocytosis, aplastic anemia, and hemolytic anemia may occur with Dymelor.

Dosage and Administration: Since diabetes may be of various degrees of severity, there can be no fixed dosage of either Dymelor® (acetohexamide, Lilly) or insulin. Daily oral dosage of Dymelor may range between 250 mg and 1.5 g. No loading dose is required. Patients who do not respond to 1.5 g daily usually will not respond to a higher dose. For this reason, doses in excess of 1.5 g daily are not recommended.

The majority of patients receiving 1 g or less per day can be controlled on a convenient once-daily dosage. Patients who need 1.5 g per day usually benefit from twice-daily dosage, given before the morning and evening meals.

Dymelor may be used in combination with insulin.

Various measures have been employed to establish patients on Dymelor, and the following procedures are suggested.

Patients Not Previously Receiving Insulin or Drug Therapy—In mild, stable diabetes (after dietary regulation), therapy may be initiated with 250 mg daily before breakfast; subsequent adjustment of the dosage may be made by increments of 250 to 500 mg every five to seven days as necessary. The 250-mg or the 500-mg tablet (scored and easily broken in half) may be used.

Because of reports of hyperresponsiveness of some elderly diabetics to Dymelor® (acetohexamide, Lilly), patients in this group should be started with a single dose of 250 mg before breakfast, and their blood and urine sugars should be checked during the first 24 hours of therapy. If control appears to be satisfactory, this dose may be continued on a daily basis or, if necessary, gradually increased. If, however, there appears to be a tendency toward hypoglycemia, this dose should be reduced or the drug should be discontinued.

Patients Receiving Other Oral Agents—When transfer is made from tolbutamide, the initial dose of Dymelor® (acetohexamide, Lilly) should be about half the tolbutamide dose (e.g., 250 mg of Dymelor in place of 500 mg of tolbutamide), up to a maximum of 1.5 g of Dymelor. When transfer is made from chlorpropamide, the initial dose of Dymelor should be about double the chlorpropamide dose (e.g., 500 mg of Dymelor in place of 250 mg of chlorpropamide). No transition period is required. Subsequent adjustment of dosage should be made according to clinical response. The maximum recommended dose of Dymelor is 1.5 g.

Clinical reports on the efficacy of once-daily dosage of Dymelor indicate that its effect on the blood sugar is better sustained than that of tolbutamide. However, patients requiring more than 1 g of Dymelor daily should be treated with divided doses.

Patients Receiving Insulin—In general, patients who were previously maintained on insulin in small dosage (e.g., up to 20 units per day) may be placed on Dymelor® (acetohexamide, Lilly) directly and their insulin administration abruptly discontinued. Patients requiring larger doses of insulin, such as 20 to 40 units or more per day, should have an initial reduction of insulin dosage by 25 to 30 percent daily or every other day and subsequent further reduction depending on the response to Dymelor. An initial dose of 250 mg of Dymelor can be used, with readjustment depending on response to therapy. Because of the potential hazards of hypoglycemia in the elderly, patients in this age group should be carefully observed during the transition from insulin to Dymelor.

During the period of insulin withdrawal, the patient should test his urine for sugar and acetone at least three times a day and report the results frequently to his physician so that appropriate adjustments of therapy may be made. In some cases, it may be advisable to consider hospitalization during the transition period from insulin to Dymelor.

It should be noted that, as with other sulfonylureas, primary and secondary failures may occur with Dymelor.

Overdosage: Hypoglycemia may appear in those patients who do not eat regularly or who exercise without caloric supplementation. This is treated in the usual manner, by supplying carbohydrate in various forms, dependent on the clinical status.

In patients with protracted hypoglycemia, treatment with 10 to 50 percent dextrose in water is advisable until the tendency toward hypoglycemia has subsided.

How Supplied: (℞) *Tablets Dymelor® (Acetohexamide Tablets, USP)* (capsule-shaped, scored): *No. 1842, U03,** 250 mg, White, and *No. 1843, U07,** 500 mg, Yellow, in bottles of 50 (NDC 0002-2103-50 and 2107-50), 200 (NDC 0002-2103-22 and 2107-22), and 500 (NDC 0002-2103-03 and 2107-03) and in 10 strips of 10 individually labeled blisters each containing 1 tablet (ID100) (NDC 0002-2103-33 and 2107-33). [081781]

[*Shown in Product Identification Section*]

Tablets No. 1843, 500 mg—50's—6505-00-765-0589; 500's—6505-00-765-2068A

EN-CEBRIN® OTC
(prenatal vitamin-minerals)

Description: En-Cebrin is a broad and potent vitamin-mineral formulation for use during pregnancy and lactation. Each Pulvule® contains phosphorus-free calcium in the form of calcium carbonate, plus liberal quantities of

*Identi-Code® symbol.

Continued on next page

Lilly—Cont.

important vitamins and minerals in well-balanced proportions.

Each Pulvule contains—
Vitamin A ....4000 IU (1.2 mg)
Thiamine Mononitrate
(Vitamin B_1) ....3 mg
Riboflavin (Vitamin B_2) ....2 mg
Niacinamide ....10 mg
Pyridoxine (Vitamin B_6) ....1.7 mg
Vitamin B_{12} (Activity Equivalent) ....5 mcg
Pantothenic Acid ....5 mg
Ascorbic Acid (Vitamin C) ....50 mg
Vitamin D ....400 IU (10 mcg)
Calcium (as the Carbonate) ....250 mg
Iron (as Ferrous Fumarate) ....30 mg
Iodine (as Potassium Iodide) ....0.15 mg
Copper (as the Sulfate) ....1 mg
Magnesium (as the Hydroxide) ....5 mg
Manganese (as the
Glycerophosphate) ....1 mg
Zinc (as the Chloride) ....1.5 mg

Indications: For use during pregnancy and lactation.

Adverse Reactions: Infrequently, nausea and vomiting have been reported after administration.

Dosage: 1 Pulvule a day, or as directed by the physician.

How Supplied: *Pulvules No. 382, En-Cebrin® (prenatal vitamin-minerals, Lilly), H12** (No. 0, Light-Pink Opaque Body, Light-Blue Opaque Cap), in bottles of 100 (NDC 0002-0812-02). [030180]

EN-CEBRIN® F ℞

(prenatal vitamins and minerals with folic acid)

Description: Each Pulvule® contains—

Vitamin A Synthetic	4000 IU	(1.2 mg)
Thiamine Mononitrate (Vitamin B_1)	3	mg
Riboflavin (Vitamin B_2)	2	mg
Niacinamide	10	mg
Pyridoxine Hydrochloride (Vitamin B_6)	2	mg
Folic Acid	1	mg
Vitamin B_{12} (Activity Equivalent)	5	mcg
Pantothenic Acid (as Calcium Pantothenate)	5	mg
Ascorbic Acid (Vitamin C)	50	mg
Vitamin D Synthetic	400 IU	(10 mcg)
Calcium (as the Carbonate)	250	mg
Iron (as Ferrous Fumarate)	30	mg
Iodine (as Potassium Iodide)	0.15	mg
Copper (as the Sulfate)	1	mg
Magnesium (as the Hydroxide)	5	mg
Manganese (as the Glycerophosphate)	1	mg
Zinc (as the Chloride)	1.5	mg

Each Pulvule supplies at least the minimum daily requirement of vitamins A and D, thiamine, riboflavin, niacinamide, ascorbic acid, iron, and iodine. In addition, the formula contains pyridoxine to help meet the increased need for this substance in pregnant women. Calcium (phosphorus-free) is also supplied, as well as other minerals for which the qualitative, but not quantitative, needs seem to be well established.

Clinical Pharmacology: The water-soluble vitamins are widely distributed in both plants and animals. They are absorbed in man by both diffusion and active transport mechanisms. These vitamins are structurally diverse (derivatives of sugar, pyridine, purines, pyrimidine, organic acid complexes, and nucleotide complex) and act as coenzymes, as oxidation-reduction agents, or possibly as mitochondrial agents. Metabolism is rapid, and the excess is excreted in the urine.

Thiamine is distributed in all tissues. The highest concentrations occur in liver, brain, kidney, and heart. When thiamine intake is greatly in excess of need, tissue stores increase two to three times. If intake is insufficient, tissues become depleted of their vitamin content. Absorption of thiamine following intramuscular administration is rapid and complete.

No overt pharmacodynamic actions accompany the oral or parenteral administration of riboflavin. It is readily absorbed from the gastrointestinal tract and parenteral sites of administration. Riboflavin is distributed in all tissues, but little is stored, and tissue concentrations are uniformly low. Highest concentrations are found in the kidney, liver, and heart. When riboflavin is ingested in amounts that approximate the minimum daily requirement, only about 9 percent appears in the urine. The metabolic fate of the remainder is unknown. As the intake of riboflavin is increased above minimum requirements, larger proportions are excreted unchanged in the urine.

Both nicotinic acid and nicotinamide (niacinamide) are readily absorbed from all portions of the intestinal tract and from parenteral sites of administration. The vitamin is distributed in all tissues. When therapeutic doses of nicotinic acid or its amide are administered, only small amounts of the unchanged vitamin appear in the urine. When extremely high doses of these vitamins are given, the unchanged vitamin represents the major urinary component.

Pantothenic acid exhibits no outstanding pharmacodynamic actions following its administration to experimental animals or man. The vitamin is essentially nontoxic. Pantothenic acid is readily absorbed from the gastrointestinal tract. It is present in all tissues; however, the highest concentrations are found in the liver, adrenal, heart, and kidney. Pantothenic acid apparently is not destroyed in the human body, since the intake and the excretion of the vitamin are approximately equal. About 70 percent of unchanged pantothenic acid is excreted in the urine and about 30 percent in the feces.

Pyridoxine elicits no outstanding pharmacodynamic actions after either oral or intravenous administration. It is readily absorbed from the gastrointestinal tract.

Ascorbic acid is readily absorbed, and, after tissue saturation occurs, the excess is excreted by the kidney.

Vitamin A is readily absorbed from the normal gastrointestinal tract. If the amount ingested is not much greater than the requirement, absorption is complete.

Vitamin D is usually given by mouth, and gastrointestinal absorption is adequate in most circumstances. Its metabolic fate is unknown. Vitamin D clearly augments gastrointestinal absorption of calcium, and data suggest that it increases the intestinal absorption of magnesium.

In general, the major portion of calcium absorption takes place in the gastrointestinal tract, and calcium is excreted in feces.

Iron is absorbed in the gastrointestinal tract and may be excreted in feces, sweat, nails, hair, and urine.

Iodine is absorbed in the gastrointestinal tract and may be excreted via sweat, feces, and milk; however, the kidney serves as the chief excretory organ for iodine.

Copper is absorbed from the gastrointestinal tract and excreted via feces and urine. Copper and iron metabolism are interrelated. Synthesis of heme may be diminished in copper deficiency.

Magnesium is absorbed from the gastrointestinal tract and is excreted in the urine.

Manganese is absorbed from the small intestine and is excreted in the bile; this constitutes the principal mechanism for regulating the amounts of manganese in the tissues.

Zinc is part of at least 18 enzymes and enzyme cofactors. It is involved in protein synthesis and nucleic acid synthesis. The mobilization of vitamin A from the liver into the plasma requires zinc. Zinc is distributed in bone, muscle, and blood and is excreted via the feces, urine, and skin.

Indications and Usage: En-Cebrin F is indicated whenever a wide-range vitamin-mineral preparation is needed during pregnancy.

En-Cebrin F contains 1 mg folic acid per Pulvule. Folic acid deficiency is the cause of most cases of megaloblastic anemia of pregnancy, a condition which may occur in 3 to 4 percent of patients in the temperate zone and in an even higher percentage of patients in the tropics. There is an increased requirement for folic acid during pregnancy, especially in the third trimester. In addition, recent studies suggest that absorption of this substance may be impaired in pregnancy.

A report based on bone-marrow biopsies of pregnant women indicates that megaloblastic erythropoiesis was found in about 4 percent of cases. It is significant that, clinically, many of the women had only a slight anemia.

Contraindications: En-Cebrin F should be administered cautiously, if at all, to individuals who are sensitive to thiamine.

Hemochromatosis and hemosiderosis are contraindications to therapy with preparations containing iron.

Precautions: *General Precautions*—Although administration of folic acid alone may produce a temporary hematologic remission in Addisonian pernicious anemia, neurologic progression may not be halted. Therefore, vitamin B_{12} in ample doses must be given to patients with this disease. However, true Addisonian pernicious anemia in pregnancy is extremely rare.

Drug Interactions—It has been reported that ascorbic acid shortens prothrombin time in animals receiving coumarin anticoagulants.

Usage in Pregnancy—Pregnancy Category A—Studies in pregnant women have not shown that En-Cebrin F increases the risk of fetal abnormalities when administered during pregnancy. If the drug is used during pregnancy, the possibility of fetal harm appears remote. Because studies cannot rule out the possibility of harm, however, En-Cebrin F should be used during pregnancy only if clearly needed.

Nursing Mothers—It is not known whether this drug is excreted in human milk. Because many drugs are excreted in human milk, caution should be exercised when En-Cebrin F is administered to a nursing woman.

Adverse Reactions: An occasional individual may develop a sensitivity or intolerance to thiamine.

Infrequently, nausea and vomiting have been reported after administration of En-Cebrin F.

Administration and Dosage: The usual dosage is 1 Pulvule daily.

How Supplied: (℞) *Pulvules No. 376, En-Cebrin® F (prenatal vitamins and minerals with folic acid, Lilly), H10** (No. 0, Light-Pink Opaque Body, Light-Blue Opaque Cap), in an ℞Pak (prescription package, Lilly) of 100 (NDC 0002-0723-02). ℞Paks have safety closures. [060380]

ERGOTRATE® MALEATE ℞

(ergonovine maleate)
Injection, USP
AMPOULES

Description: Ergonovine is the hydroxyisopropylamide of lysergic acid. It is somewhat soluble in water, and its salts are readily soluble. It is obtained from ergot and has been shown to possess all of the desirable oxytocic activity of ergot itself.

Each ampoule contains 0.2 mg of the active ingredient, ergonovine maleate, with ethyl lactate, 0.1 percent, lactic acid, 0.1 percent, and phenol, 0.25 percent, as a preservative.
The empirical formula of ergonovine maleate is $C_{19}H_{23}N_3O_2 \cdot C_4H_4O_4$. Chemically, it is 9,10-didehydro-*N* -[(*S*)-2-hydroxy-1-methylethyl] - 6-methylergoline-8β-carboxamide maleate (1:1) (salt).
Clinical Pharmacology: Injection Ergotrate® Maleate (Ergonovine Maleate Injection, USP, Lilly) produces a firm contraction of the uterus. Upon the initial tetanic contraction is superimposed a succession of minor relaxations and contractions. The extent of relaxation gradually increases over a period of about one and one-half hours, but vigorous rhythmic contractions continue for a period of three or more hours after injection. The prolonged initial contraction is the type necessary to control uterine hemorrhage.
Indications and Usage: Ergotrate® Maleate (ergonovine maleate, Lilly) is indicated for the prevention and treatment of postpartum and postabortal hemorrhage and of puerperal morbidity.
Contraindications: Ergotrate® Maleate (ergonovine maleate, Lilly) is contraindicated for the induction of labor and in cases of threatened spontaneous abortion. It should not be administered to those patients who have shown allergic or idiosyncratic reactions to it.
Warnings: All oxytocic agents are potentially dangerous. Mothers and infants have been injured, and some have died because of their injudicious use. Hyperstimulation of the uterus during labor may lead to uterine tetany with marked impairment of the uteroplacental blood flow, uterine rupture, cervical and perineal lacerations, amniotic fluid embolism, and trauma to the infant (e.g., hypoxia, intracranial hemorrhage). Because of these hazards which result from overdosage, oxytocic agents must be administered under conditions of meticulous observation.
Precautions: *General Precautions*—Because of the high uterine tone produced, Ergotrate® Maleate (ergonovine maleate, Lilly) is not recommended for routine use prior to the delivery of the placenta unless the operator is versed in the technique described by Davis and others and has adequate facilities and personnel at his disposal.
As is the case with all ergot preparations, prolonged use of Ergotrate Maleate is to be avoided. Discontinue Ergotrate Maleate if symptoms of ergotism appear.
Ergotrate Maleate should be used cautiously in patients with hypertension, heart disease, venoatrial shunts, mitral-valve stenosis, obliterative vascular disease, sepsis, or hepatic or renal impairment.
The character and amount of vaginal bleeding should be observed. Hypocalcemia may affect patient response to the drug. If the patient is not also taking digitalis, cautious administration of calcium gluconate IV may produce the desired oxytocic action.
Laboratory Tests—Blood pressure, pulse, and uterine response should be monitored. Sudden changes in vital signs or frequent periods of uterine relaxation should be noted.
Adverse Reactions: Nausea and vomiting may occur, but they are uncommon. Allergic phenomena, including shock, have been reported. Ergotism has also been reported. Elevation of blood pressure (sometimes extreme) may appear in a small percentage of patients, most frequently in association with regional anesthesia (caudal or spinal), previous administration of a vasoconstrictor, and the intravenous route of administration of the oxytocic. The mechanism of such hypertension is obscure, since it may occur in the absence of anesthesia, vasoconstrictors, and oxytocics. These elevations are no more frequent with Ergotrate® Maleate (ergonovine maleate, Lilly) than with other oxytocics. They usually subside promptly following intravenous administration of 15 mg of chlorpromazine.
Overdosage: *Symptoms*—The principal manifestations of serious overdosage are convulsions and gangrene. Symptoms of overdosage include the following: vomiting, diarrhea, dizziness, rise or fall in blood pressure, weak pulse, dyspnea, loss of consciousness, numbness and coldness of the extremities, tingling, pain in the chest, gangrene of the fingers and toes, and hypercoagulability.
Treatment—Treat convulsions. Control hypercoagulability by the administration of heparin, and maintain blood-clotting time at approximately three times the normal. Give a vasodilator such as tolazine as an antidote; the rate of administration may be controlled by monitoring pulse rate and blood pressure. For emergency measures, delay absorption of ingested Ergotrate® Maleate (ergonovine maleate, Lilly) by giving tap water, milk, or activated charcoal and then removing by gastric lavage or emesis followed by catharsis. Gangrene will require surgical amputation.
Dosage and Administration: Ergotrate® Maleate (ergonovine maleate, Lilly) is intended primarily for routine intramuscular injection in obstetric practice. By this route, it usually produces a firm contraction of the uterus within a few minutes.
Intravenous administration leads to a quicker response. However, because of the higher incidence of nausea and other side effects, it is recommended that the intravenous route be confined to emergencies such as excessive uterine bleeding.
The usual intramuscular (or emergency intravenous) dose of Ergotrate Maleate is 0.2 mg, one ampoule. Severe uterine bleeding may call for repeated doses, but injection will rarely be required more often than once in two to four hours.
In some calcium-deficient patients, the uterus may fail to respond to Ergotrate Maleate. In such instances, responsiveness can be immediately restored by the cautious intravenous injection of calcium salts. Calcium should not be given intravenously to patients under the influence of digitalis.
Tablets Ergotrate Maleate are available for oral administration.
Storage—Ampoules Ergotrate Maleate should be stored in a cold place (below 46°F). However, delivery-room stock may be kept at room temperature (although periods of more than 60 days at room temperature prior to use are not recommended).
How Supplied: (℞) *Ampoules No. 302, Ergotrate® Maleate (Ergonovine Maleate Injection, USP),* 0.2 mg, 1 ml, in packages of 6 (NDC 0002-1629-16) and 100 (NDC 0002-1629-02).
[032482]

ERGOTRATE® MALEATE ℞
(ergonovine maleate)
Tablets, USP

Description: Ergonovine is the hydroxyisopropylamide of lysergic acid. It is somewhat soluble in water, and its salts are readily soluble. It is obtained from ergot and has been shown to possess all of the desirable oxytocic activity of ergot itself.
The empirical formula of ergonovine maleate is $C_{19}H_{23}N_3O_2 \cdot C_4H_4O_4$.
Clinical Pharmacology: Within six to 15 minutes, Ergotrate® Maleate (ergonovine maleate, Lilly) produces a firm tetanic contraction of the postpartum uterus which, in the course of about 90 minutes, gradually changes to a series of clonic contractions that persist for another 90 minutes or more.
Indications and Usage: Ergotrate® Maleate (ergonovine maleate, Lilly) is indicated for the prevention and treatment of postpartum and postabortal hemorrhage due to uterine atony.
Contraindications, Warnings, Precautions, Adverse Reactions, and **Overdosage:** *See under* Ergotrate Maleate, Injection, USP.
Dosage and Administration: The immediate postpartum dose of Ergotrate® Maleate (ergonovine maleate, Lilly) is usually 0.2 mg. It is ordinarily administered parenterally. To minimize late postpartum bleeding, 1 or 2 tablets may be given orally two to four times daily (every six to 12 hours) until the danger of uterine atony has passed—usually 48 hours. Severe cramping is evidence of effectiveness but may justify reduction in dosage. Tablets Ergotrate Maleate may also be administered sublingually.
How Supplied: (℞) *Tablets No. 1572, Ergotrate® Maleate (Ergonovine Maleate Tablets, USP), J36,** 0.2 mg, in bottles of 100 (NDC 0002-1036-02) and 1000 (NDC 0002-1036-04) and in 10 strips of 10 individually labeled blisters each containing 1 tablet (ID100) (NDC 0002-1036-33).
[080282]

FOLIC ACID ℞
Tablets, USP

Description: Folic acid is a member of the vitamin B complex.
Action: Folic acid acts on megaloblastic bone marrow to produce a normoblastic marrow.
Indications: It is effective in the treatment of megaloblastic anemias due to a deficiency of folic acid (as may be seen in tropical or nontropical sprue) and in anemias of nutritional origin, pregnancy, infancy, or childhood.
Warning: Administration of folic acid alone is improper therapy for pernicious anemia and other megaloblastic anemias in which vitamin B_{12} is deficient.
Precaution: Folic acid in doses above 0.1 mg daily may obscure pernicious anemia in that hematologic remission can occur while neurologic manifestations remain progressive.
Adverse Reaction: Allergic sensitization has been reported following both oral and parenteral administration of folic acid.
Dosage and Administration: Folic acid is well absorbed and may be administered orally with satisfactory results except in severe instances of intestinal malabsorption.
The usual therapeutic dosage in adults and children (regardless of age) is up to 1 mg daily. Resistant cases may require larger doses.
When clinical symptoms have subsided and the blood picture has become normal, a daily maintenance level should be used, i.e., 0.1 mg for infants and up to 0.3 mg for children under four years of age, 0.4 mg for adults and children four or more years of age, and 0.8 mg for pregnant and lactating women, but never less than 0.1 mg/day. Patients should be kept under close supervision and adjustment of the maintenance level made if relapse appears imminent.
In the presence of alcoholism, hemolytic anemia, anticonvulsant therapy, or chronic infection, the maintenance level may need to be increased.
How Supplied: (℞) *Tablets No. 1897, Folic Acid, USP, U56,** 1 mg, in bottles of 100 (NDC 0002-2156-02).
[111880]

GLUCAGON FOR INJECTION ℞
USP

Description: Glucagon is produced in the pancreas (alpha cells of the islands of Langerhans). Purified and crystallized by scientists at the Lilly Research Laboratories, it is used in the treatment of hypoglycemic states and is effective in small doses.
Chemically unrelated to insulin, glucagon is a straight-chain polypeptide containing 29

Continued on next page

*Identi-Code® symbol.

Lilly—Cont.

amino acid residues and having a molecular weight of 3485.

Crystalline glucagon is a white powder containing less than 0.01 percent zinc. It is relatively insoluble in water but is soluble at a pH of less than 3 or more than 9.5. Glucagon is stable in lyophilized form at room temperatures. It will remain potent in solution for as long as three months if kept under refrigeration.

Actions: Glucagon causes an increase in blood glucose concentration and is used in the treatment of hypoglycemic states. It is effective in small doses, and no evidence of toxicity has been reported with its use. Glucagon acts only on liver glycogen, converting it to glucose.

Parenteral administration of glucagon produces relaxation of the smooth muscle of the stomach, duodenum, small bowel, and colon.

Indications: *For the treatment of hypoglycemia:* Glucagon is useful in counteracting severe hypoglycemic reactions in diabetic patients or during insulin shock therapy in psychiatric patients. Glucagon is helpful in hypoglycemia only if liver glycogen is available. It is of little or no help in states of starvation, adrenal insufficiency, or chronic hypoglycemia.

The patient with juvenile-type diabetes does not have as great a response in blood glucose levels as does the adult-type stable diabetic. Therefore, supplementary carbohydrate should be given as soon as possible to the juvenile patient especially.

For use as a diagnostic aid: Glucagon is indicated as a diagnostic aid in the radiologic examination of the stomach, duodenum, small bowel, and colon when a hypotonic state would be advantageous.

Glucagon is as effective for this examination as are the anticholinergic drugs, but it has fewer side effects. When glucagon is administered concomitantly with an anticholinergic agent, the response is not significantly greater than when either drug is used alone. However, the addition of the anticholinergic agent results in increased side effects.

Contraindication: Since glucagon is a protein, hypersensitivity is a possibility.

Warnings: Glucagon should be administered cautiously to patients with a history of insulinoma and/or pheochromocytoma. In patients with insulinoma, intravenous administration of glucagon will produce an initial increase in blood glucose but, because of its insulin-releasing effect, may subsequently cause hypoglycemia. Exogenous glucagon also stimulates the release of catecholamines, which can cause a marked increase in blood pressure in patients with pheochromocytoma.

Precautions: In the treatment of hypoglycemic shock with glucagon, liver glycogen must be available. Glucose by the intravenous route or by gavage should be considered in the hypoglycemic patient.

Adverse Reactions: Glucagon is relatively free of adverse reactions except for occasional nausea and vomiting, which may also occur with hypoglycemia.

Dosage and Administration: *For the treatment of hypoglycemia:* The diluent is provided for use only in the preparation of glucagon for *intermittent* parenteral injection and for no other use.

Directions for Use of Glucagon—1. Dissolve the lyophilized glucagon in the accompanying solvent.

2. Give 0.5 to 1 unit of glucagon by subcutaneous, intramuscular, or intravenous injection.

3. The patient will usually awaken in five to 20 minutes. If the response is delayed, there is no contraindication to the administration of one or two additional doses of glucagon; however, in view of the deleterious effects of cerebral hypoglycemia and depending on the duration and depth of coma, the use of parenteral glucose *must* be considered by the physician.

4. Intravenous glucose *must* be given if the patient fails to respond to glucagon.

5. When the patient responds, give supplemental carbohydrate to restore the liver glycogen and prevent secondary hypoglycemia.

General Management of Hypoglycemia—The following are helpful measures in the prevention of hypoglycemic reactions due to insulin:

1. Reasonable uniformity from day to day with regard to diet, insulin, and exercise.

2. Careful adjustment of the insulin program so that the type (or types) of insulin, dose, and time (or times) of administration are suited to the individual patient.

3. Frequent testing of the urine so that a change in insulin requirements can be foreseen.

4. Routine carrying of sugar, candy, or other readily absorbable carbohydrate by the patient so that it may be taken at the first warning of an oncoming reaction.

If the patient is unaware of the symptoms of hypoglycemia, he may lapse into insulin shock; therefore, the physician should instruct the patient in this regard when feasible.

It is important that the patient be aroused as quickly as possible, for prolonged hypoglycemic reactions may result in cortical damage. Glucagon or intravenous glucose will awaken the patient sufficiently so that oral carbohydrates may be taken.

Instructions to the Family—Instructions describing the method of using this preparation are included in the literature which accompanies the patient's package. It is advisable for the patient to become familiar with the technique of preparing glucagon for injection before an emergency arises.

CAUTION—Although glucagon may be used for the treatment of hypoglycemia by the patient during an emergency, the physician must still be notified when hypoglycemic reactions occur so that the dose of insulin may be adjusted more accurately.

Insulin Shock Therapy—Dissolve the lyophilized glucagon in the accompanying diluting solution.

After one hour of coma, inject 0.5 to 1 unit of glucagon by the subcutaneous, intramuscular, or intravenous route. Larger doses may be employed if desired.

The patient will usually awaken in ten to 25 minutes. If no response occurs within the desired interval, the dose may be repeated. Upon awakening, the patient should be fed orally as soon as possible and the usual dietary regimen followed.

In a very deep state of coma, such as Stage IV or Stage V of Himwich, intravenous glucose should be given in addition to glucagon for a more immediate response. Glucagon and glucose may be used together without decreasing the efficacy of glucose administration.

For use as a diagnostic aid: Dissolve the lyophilized glucagon in the accompanying diluting solution.

The doses in the accompanying chart may be administered for relaxation of the stomach, duodenum, and small bowel, depending on the time of onset of action and the duration of effect required for the examination. Since the stomach is less sensitive to the effect of glucagon, ½ unit I.V. or 2 units I.M. are recommended.

[See table below].

For examination of the colon, it is recommended that a 2-unit dose (2 mg) be administered intramuscularly approximately ten minutes prior to initiation of the procedure. Relaxation of the colon and reduction of discomfort to the patient will allow the radiologist to perform a more satisfactory examination.

How Supplied: (℞) *Vials Glucagon for Injection, USP: No. 666,* 1 unit (1 mg), rubber-stoppered (Dry Powder), with 49 mg of lactose, in single packages (10 per carton) (NDC 0002-1450-01). Vial No. 667, Diluting Solution for Glucagon for Injection, USP, 1 ml, included in this package, is not offered separately. It contains glycerin, 1.6 percent, with phenol, 0.2 percent, as a preservative. Sodium hydroxide and/or hydrochloric acid may have been added during manufacture to adjust the pH. *No. 668,* 10 units (10 mg), rubber-stoppered (Dry Powder), multiple dose, with 140 mg of lactose, in single packages (10 per carton) (NDC 0002-1451-01). Vial No. 669, Diluting Solution for Glucagon for Injection, USP, 10 ml, included in this package, is not offered separately. It contains glycerin, 1.6 percent, with phenol, 0.2 percent, as a preservative. Sodium hydroxide and/or hydrochloric acid may have been added during manufacture to adjust the pH. If properly refrigerated, Vials No. 668 may be used up to three months after reconstitution. [120981]

Dosage of Glucagon as a Diagnostic Aid

Dose	Route of Administration	Time of Onset of Action	Approximate Duration of Effect
¼–½ unit (0.25–0.5 mg)	I.V.	1 minute	9–17 minutes
1 unit (1 mg)	I.M.	8–10 minutes	12–27 minutes
2 units (2 mg)*	I.V.	1 minute	22–25 minutes
2 units (2 mg)*	I.M.	4–7 minutes	21–32 minutes

***Administration of 2-unit doses produces a higher incidence of nausea and vomiting than do lower doses.**

HALDRONE® ℞
(paramethasone acetate)
Tablets, USP

Description: Haldrone® (paramethasone acetate, Lilly) is 6α-fluoro-11β, 17,21-trihydroxy-16α-methylpregna-1,4 -diene-3,20-dione 21 acetate. It is a white crystalline compound with an elemental composition of $C_{24}H_{31}O_6F$. It is insoluble in water and soluble in chloroform, ether, and methanol.

Actions: Haldrone has anti-inflammatory activity, and within the usual dose range there is little effect on electrolyte metabolism. Haldrone compares favorably in its metabolic actions and side effects with other corticosteroids.

Naturally occurring glucocorticoids (hydrocortisone and cortisone), which have salt-retaining properties, are used as replacement therapy in adrenocortical deficiency states. Their synthetic analogs are used primarily for their potent anti-inflammatory effects in disorders of many organ systems.

Glucocorticoids cause profound and varied metabolic effects. In addition, they modify the body's immune responses to diverse stimuli.

Indications:

Endocrine Disorders

Primary or secondary adrenocortical insufficiency

(Hydrocortisone or cortisone is the first choice; synthetic analogs may be used in conjunction with mineralocorticoids when applicable; in infancy, mineralocorticoid supplementation is of particular importance.)

Congenital adrenal hyperplasia
Nonsuppurative thyroiditis
Hypercalcemia associated with cancer

Rheumatic Disorders

Psoriatic arthritis—Adjunctive therapy for short-term administration to tide the patient over an acute episode or exacerbation.
Rheumatoid arthritis, including juvenile rheumatoid arthritis—Selected cases may require low-dose maintenance therapy.
Ankylosing spondylitis
Bursitis—Use only in acute and subacute conditions. Not effective in chronic bursitis.
Acute nonspecific tenosynovitis
Acute gouty arthritis
Posttraumatic osteoarthritis
Synovitis of osteoarthritis
Epicondylitis

Collagen Diseases

During an exacerbation or as maintenance therapy in selected cases of the following:
Systemic lupus erythematosus
Acute rheumatic carditis

Dermatologic Diseases

Pemphigus
Bullous dermatitis herpetiformis
Severe erythema multiforme (Stevens-Johnson syndrome)
Exfoliative dermatitis
Mycosis fungoides
Severe psoriasis
Severe seborrheic dermatitis

Allergic States

Control of severe or incapacitating allergic conditions intractable to adequate trials of conventional treatment:
Seasonal or perennial allergic rhinitis
Bronchial asthma
Contact dermatitis
Atopic dermatitis
Serum sickness
Drug hypersensitivity reactions

Ophthalmic Diseases

Severe acute and chronic allergic and inflammatory processes involving the eye and its adnexa, such as:
Allergic conjunctivitis
Keratitis
Allergic corneal marginal ulcers
Herpes zoster ophthalmicus
Iritis and iridocyclitis
Chorioretinitis
Anterior segment inflammation
Diffuse posterior uveitis and choroiditis
Optic neuritis
Sympathetic ophthalmia

Respiratory Diseases

Symptomatic sarcoidosis
Loeffler's syndrome not manageable with other treatment
Pulmonary tuberculosis—Only in fulminating or disseminated disease in conjunction with appropriate and adequate antituberculosis chemotherapy
Berylliosis
Aspiration pneumonitis

Hematologic Disorders

Idiopathic thrombocytopenic purpura in adults
Secondary thrombocytopenia in adults
Acquired (autoimmune) hemolytic anemia
Erythroblastopenia (RBC anemia)
Congenital (erythroid) hypoplastic anemia

Neoplastic Diseases

For the palliative management of leukemias and lymphomas in adults and acute leukemia of childhood

Edematous States

To induce diuresis or a remission of proteinuria in nephrotic syndrome, without uremia, of the idiopathic type or that due to lupus erythematosus

Gastrointestinal Diseases

To tide the patient over a critical period of the disease in ulcerative colitis or regional enteritis

Nervous System Disease

Acute exacerbations of multiple sclerosis

Miscellaneous

Tuberculous meningitis with subarachnoid block or impending block when the patient is receiving appropriate and adequate antituberculosis chemotherapy
Trichinosis with neurologic or myocardial involvement

Contraindications: Therapy with Haldrone® (paramethasone acetate, Lilly) is contraindicated in the presence of systemic fungal infections.

Warnings: In patients on corticosteroid therapy subjected to unusual stress, increased dosage of rapidly acting corticosteroids is indicated before, during, and after the stressful situation.

Corticosteroids may mask some signs of infection, and new infections may appear during their use. There may be decreased resistance and inability to localize infection when corticosteroids are administered.

Prolonged use of corticosteroids may produce posterior subcapsular cataracts, may cause glaucoma with possible damage to the optic nerves, and may increase the possibility of secondary ocular infections due to fungi or viruses.

Usage in Pregnancy—Since adequate human reproduction studies have not been made with corticosteroids, the use of these drugs in pregnancy, nursing mothers, or women of childbearing potential requires that the possible benefits of the drug be weighed against the potential hazards to the mother and embryo or fetus. Infants born of mothers who have received substantial doses of corticosteroids during pregnancy should be carefully observed for signs of hypoadrenalism.

Average and large doses of hydrocortisone or cortisone can cause elevation of blood pressure, salt and water retention, and increased excretion of potassium. These effects are less likely to occur with the synthetic derivatives except when large doses are employed. Dietary salt restriction and potassium supplementation may be necessary. All corticosteroids increase calcium excretion.

PATIENTS ON CORTICOSTEROID THERAPY SHOULD NOT BE VACCINATED AGAINST SMALLPOX. OTHER IMMUNIZATION PROCEDURES SHOULD NOT BE UNDERTAKEN IN PATIENTS WHO ARE RECEIVING CORTICOSTEROIDS, ESPECIALLY WHEN HIGH DOSES ARE BEING GIVEN, BECAUSE OF POSSIBLE HAZARDS OF NEUROLOGIC COMPLICATIONS AND A LACK OF ANTIBODY RESPONSE.

The use of Haldrone® (paramethasone acetate, Lilly) in active tuberculosis should be restricted to cases of fulminating or disseminated disease in which the corticosteroid is used in conjunction with an appropriate antituberculosis regimen.

If corticosteroids are indicated in patients with latent tuberculosis or tuberculin reactivity, close observation is necessary, since reactivation of the disease may occur. During prolonged corticosteroid therapy, such individuals should receive chemoprophylaxis.

Precautions: Drug-induced secondary adrenocortical insufficiency may be minimized by gradual reduction of dosage. This type of relative insufficiency may persist for months after discontinuation of therapy; therefore, in any situation of stress occurring during that period, hormone therapy should be reinstituted. Since mineralocorticoid secretion may be impaired, salt and/or a mineralocorticoid should be administered concurrently.

Corticosteroids have an enhanced effect on patients with hypothyroidism and those with cirrhosis.

Corticosteroids should be used cautiously in patients with ocular herpes simplex because of possible corneal perforation.

The lowest possible dose of corticosteroid should be employed to control the condition under treatment; and when the dose is reduced, it should be done gradually.

Psychic derangements, ranging from euphoria, insomnia, mood swings, personality changes, and severe depression to frank psychotic manifestations, may appear when corticosteroids are given. Also, existing emotional instability or psychotic tendencies may be aggravated by corticosteroids.

Aspirin should be used cautiously in conjunction with corticosteroids in hypoprothrombinemia.

Steroids should be administered with caution in nonspecific ulcerative colitis if there is a probability of impending perforation, abscess, or other pyogenic infection; diverticulitis; fresh intestinal anastomoses; active or latent peptic ulcer; renal insufficiency; hypertension; osteoporosis; and myasthenia gravis.

Growth and development of infants and children on prolonged corticosteroid therapy should be carefully observed.

Although controlled clinical trials have shown that corticosteroids are effective in speeding the resolution of acute exacerbations of multiple sclerosis, they do not show that they affect the ultimate outcome or natural history of the disease. The studies do demonstrate that relatively high doses of corticosteroids are necessary to produce a significant effect. (*See* Dosage and Administration.)

Since complications of treatment with glucocorticoid are dependent on the size of the dose and the duration of treatment, a risk/benefit decision must be made in each individual case as to dose and duration of therapy and whether daily or intermittent therapy should be used.

Adverse Reactions:

Fluid and Electrolyte Disturbances

Sodium retention
Fluid retention
Congestive heart failure in susceptible patients
Potassium loss
Hypokalemic alkalosis
Hypertension

Musculoskeletal

Muscle weakness
Steroid myopathy
Loss of muscle mass
Osteoporosis
Vertebral compression fractures
Aseptic necrosis of femoral and humeral heads
Pathologic fracture of long bones

Gastrointestinal

Peptic ulcer with possible perforation and hemorrhage
Pancreatitis
Abdominal distention
Ulcerative esophagitis

Dermatologic

Impaired wound healing
Thin, fragile skin
Petechiae and ecchymoses
Facial erythema
Increased sweating
Suppression of reactions to skin tests

Neurologic

Convulsions
Increased intracranial pressure with papilledema (pseudotumor cerebri), usually after treatment
Vertigo
Headache

Endocrine

Menstrual irregularities
Development of Cushingoid state
Suppression of growth in children
Secondary adrenocortical and pituitary unresponsiveness, particularly in times of stress, as in trauma, surgery, or illness

Continued on next page

***Identi-Code® symbol.**

Lilly—Cont.

Decreased carbohydrate tolerance
Manifestations of latent diabetes mellitus
Increased requirements for insulin or oral hypoglycemic agents in diabetics

Ophthalmic
Posterior subcapsular cataracts
Increased intraocular pressure
Glaucoma
Exophthalmos

Metabolic
Negative nitrogen balance due to protein catabolism

Dosage and Administration: The initial dosage of Haldrone® (paramethasone acetate, Lilly) may vary from 2 to 24 mg per day, depending on the disease entity being treated. In situations of less severity, lower doses will generally suffice, although higher initial quantities may be required in selected patients. The initial regimen should be maintained or adjusted until a satisfactory response is noted. If a satisfactory response does not occur after a reasonable period of time, Haldrone should be discontinued and other appropriate therapy begun. DOSAGE REQUIREMENTS ARE VARIABLE AND MUST BE INDIVIDUALIZED ACCORDING TO THE DISEASE BEING TREATED AND THE RESPONSE OF THE PATIENT.

After a favorable response, the initial dosage should be decreased by small amounts at appropriate intervals until the lowest effective maintenance dosage is reached. Constant monitoring of dosage is needed. Adjustments may be necessary on the basis of clinical changes secondary to remission or exacerbation of the disease, the patient's individual response to the drug, or the effect of stress other than that of the disease under treatment; in the last situation, it may be necessary to increase the dosage for a period of time. If the drug is to be stopped after long-term therapy, it should be withdrawn gradually rather than abruptly.

In the treatment of acute exacerbations of multiple sclerosis, daily doses of 200 mg of prednisolone for one week followed by 80 mg of prednisolone or 4 to 8 mg of dexamethasone every other day for one month have been shown to be effective (2 mg of Haldrone are equivalent to 5 mg of prednisolone or to 0.75 mg of dexamethasone).

How Supplied: (℞) *Tablets Haldrone® (Paramethasone Acetate Tablets, USP)* (capsule-shaped, scored): *No. 1818, T99,** 1 mg, Yellow, in bottles of 100 (NDC 0002-2099-02); *No. 1819, U01,** 2 mg, Orange, in bottles of 30 (NDC 0002-2101-30) and 100 (NDC 0002-2101-02).

[061080]

HEPARIN SODIUM ℞
Injection, USP

WARNING—This is a potent drug, and serious consequences may result if used other than under constant medical supervision.

Description: Heparin Sodium Injection, USP, is a sterile solution of heparin sodium derived from porcine intestinal mucosa, standardized for use as an anticoagulant. Its potency is determined by biological assay with a USP reference standard based on units of heparin activity per milligram.

Each ml of Vial No. 405 contains 1000 USP heparin units (derived from porcine intestinal mucosa) and sodium chloride, 0.5%.

Each ml of Vial No. 520 contains 10,000 USP heparin units (derived from porcine intestinal mucosa) and sodium chloride, 0.1%.

Each ml of Vial No. 642 contains 20,000 USP heparin units (derived from porcine intestinal mucosa).

Each ml of Vial No. 622 contains 20,000 USP heparin units (derived from porcine intestinal mucosa).

During manufacture, 1% benzyl alcohol has been added as a preservative to each vial of heparin sodium. Sodium hydroxide and/or hydrochloric acid may have been added during manufacture to adjust the pH.

Actions: Heparin sodium inhibits reactions that lead to the clotting of blood and the formation of fibrin clots both in vitro and in vivo. Heparin acts at multiple sites in the normal coagulation system. Small amounts of heparin in combination with antithrombin III (heparin cofactor) can prevent the development of a hypercoagulable state by inactivating activated Factor X and inhibiting the conversion of prothrombin to thrombin. Once a hypercoagulable state exists, larger amounts of heparin in combination with antithrombin III can inhibit the coagulation process by inactivating thrombin and earlier clotting intermediates and thus prevent the conversion of fibrinogen to fibrin. Heparin also prevents the formation of a stable fibrin clot by inhibiting the activation of the fibrin stabilizing factor.

Bleeding time is usually unaffected by heparin. Clotting time is prolonged by full therapeutic doses of heparin; in most cases, it is not measurably affected by low doses of heparin.

Heparin does not have fibrinolytic activity; therefore, it will not lyse existing clots.

Indications: Heparin sodium is indicated for:

Anticoagulant therapy in prophylaxis and treatment of venous thrombosis and its extension

Low-dose regimen for prevention of postoperative deep venous thrombosis and pulmonary embolism in patients undergoing major abdominothoracic surgery who are at risk of developing thromboembolic disease (*see* Dosage and Administration)

Prophylaxis and treatment of pulmonary embolism

Atrial fibrillation with embolization

Diagnosis and treatment of acute and chronic consumption coagulopathies (disseminated intravascular coagulation)

Prevention of clotting in arterial and heart surgery

Prevention of cerebral thrombosis in evolving stroke

Heparin sodium is indicated as an adjunct both in treating coronary occlusion with acute myocardial infarction and in the prophylaxis and treatment of peripheral arterial embolism.

Heparin sodium may also be employed as an anticoagulant in blood transfusions, extracorporeal circulation, and dialysis procedures and in blood samples for laboratory purposes.

Contraindications: Heparin sodium is contraindicated in patients known to have a hypersensitivity to heparin.

It is also contraindicated when suitable blood coagulation tests—e.g., the whole-blood clotting time, partial thromboplastin time, etc.—cannot be performed at the required intervals. (There is usually no need to monitor the effect of low-dose heparin in patients with normal coagulation parameters.)

The drug is contraindicated during any uncontrollable active bleeding state (*see* Warnings).

Warnings:

> Heparin sodium should be used with extreme caution in disease states in which there is increased danger of hemorrhage.

When heparin sodium is administered in therapeutic amounts, its dosage should be regulated by frequent blood coagulation tests. If the coagulation test is unduly prolonged or if hemorrhage occurs, heparin sodium should be discontinued promptly (*see* Overdosage).

Some of the conditions in which increased danger of hemorrhage exists are as follows:

Cardiovascular—Subacute bacterial endocarditis; arterial sclerosis; increased capillary permeability; during and immediately following (a) spinal tap or spinal anesthesia or (b) major surgery, especially involving the brain, spinal cord, or eye.

Hematologic—Conditions associated with increased bleeding tendencies, such as hemophilia, some purpuras, and thrombocytopenia.

Gastrointestinal—Inaccessible ulcerative lesions and continuous tube drainage of the stomach or small intestine.

Heparin sodium may prolong the one-stage prothrombin time. Therefore, when heparin sodium is given with dicumarol or warfarin sodium, a period of at least five hours after the last intravenous dose or 24 hours after the last subcutaneous (intrafat, i.e., above the iliac crest or abdominal fat layer) dose should elapse before blood is drawn if a valid prothrombin time is to be obtained.

Drugs (such as acetylsalicylic acid, dextran, phenylbutazone, ibuprofen, indomethacin, dipyridamole, and hydroxychloroquine) that interfere with platelet-aggregation reactions (the main hemostatic defense of heparinized patients) may induce bleeding and should be used with caution in patients receiving heparin sodium.

Although there is experimental evidence that heparin sodium may antagonize the action of ACTH, insulin, or corticoids, this effect has not been clearly defined.

There is also evidence in experimental animals that heparin sodium may modify or inhibit allergic reactions. However, the application of these findings to human patients has not been fully defined.

It may be necessary to increase doses of heparin sodium in the febrile state.

Digitalis, tetracyclines, nicotine, or antihistamines may partially counteract the anticoagulant action of heparin sodium. An increased resistance to the drug is frequently encountered in thrombosis, thrombophlebitis, infections with thrombosing tendencies, myocardial infarction, cancer, and postsurgical patients.

Usage in Pregnancy—Heparin sodium injection should be used with caution during pregnancy, especially during the last trimester and in the immediate postpartum period.

There is no adequate information as to whether heparin may affect human fertility or have a teratogenic potential or other adverse effect on the fetus.

Heparin does not cross the placental barrier; it is not excreted in human milk.

Precautions: Because heparin sodium is derived from animal tissue, it should be used with caution in any patient with a history of allergy. Before a therapeutic dose is given to such a patient, a trial dose of 1000 units may be advisable.

Heparin sodium should be used with caution in the presence of hepatic or renal disease, in hypertension, during menstruation, or in patients with indwelling catheters.

A higher incidence of bleeding may be seen in women over 60 years of age.

Caution should be exercised when administering ACD-converted blood (i.e., blood collected in heparin sodium and later converted to ACD blood), since the anticoagulant activity of its heparin sodium content persists without loss for 22 days. ACD-converted blood may alter the coagulation system of the recipient, especially if it is given in multiple transfusions.

Adverse Reactions: Hemorrhage is the chief complication that may result from heparin sodium therapy. An overly prolonged clotting time or minor bleeding during therapy can usually be controlled by withdrawing the drug (*see* Overdosage).

The occurrence of significant gastrointestinal or urinary tract bleeding during anticoagulant therapy may indicate the presence of an underlying occult lesion.

Adrenal hemorrhage, with resultant acute adrenal insufficiency, has occurred during anticoagulant therapy. Therefore, such treatment should be discontinued in patients who develop signs and symptoms of acute adrenal hemorrhage and insufficiency. Plasma cortisol levels should be measured immediately, and vigorous therapy with intravenous corticosteroids should be instituted promptly. Initiation of therapy should not depend on laboratory confirmation of the diagnosis, since any delay in an acute situation may result in the patient's death.

Intramuscular injection of heparin sodium frequently causes local irritation, mild pain, or hematoma and, for these reasons, should be avoided. These effects are less often seen following deep subcutaneous (intrafat) injection. Histamine-like reactions have also been observed at the site of injection.

Hypersensitivity reactions have been reported, with chills, fever, and urticaria as the most usual manifestations. Asthma, rhinitis, lacrimation, and anaphylactoid reactions have also been reported. Vasospastic reactions may develop, independent of the origin of heparin, six to ten days after the initiation of therapy and may last for four to six hours. The affected limb is painful, ischemic, and cyanosed. An artery to this limb may have been recently catheterized. After repeated injections, the reaction may gradually increase to include generalized vasospasm, with cyanosis, tachypnea, feeling of oppression, and headache. Protamine sulfate treatment has no marked therapeutic effect. Itching and burning, especially on the plantar side of the feet, is possibly caused by a similar allergic vasospastic reaction. Chest pain, elevated blood pressure, arthralgias, and/or headache have also been reported in the absence of definite peripheral vasospasm. Anaphylactic shock has been reported rarely following the intravenous administration of heparin sodium. Acute reversible thrombocytopenia has been reported following the intravenous administration of heparin sodium. Osteoporosis and suppression of renal function following long-term administration of high doses, suppression of aldosterone synthesis, delayed transient alopecia, priapism, and rebound hyperlipemia on discontinuation of heparin sodium have also been reported.

Dosage and Administration: Heparin sodium is not effective by oral administration and should be given by intermittent intravenous injection, intravenous infusion, or deep subcutaneous (intrafat) injection. The intramuscular route of administration should be avoided because of the frequent occurrence of hematoma at the injection site.

The dosage of heparin sodium should be adjusted according to the patient's coagulation test results, which, during the first day of treatment, should be determined just prior to each injection. (There is usually no need to monitor the effect of low-dose heparin in patients with normal coagulation parameters.) Dosage is considered adequate when the whole-blood clotting time is elevated approximately two and one-half to three times the control value. When heparin sodium is given by continuous intravenous infusion, the coagulation time should be determined approximately every four hours in the early stages of treatment. When the drug is administered intermittently by intravenous or deep subcutaneous (intrafat) injection, coagulation tests should be performed before each injection during the early stages of treatment and daily thereafter.

When an oral anticoagulant of the coumadin or similar type is administered with heparin sodium, coagulation tests and prothrombin activity should be determined at the start of therapy. For an immediate anticoagulant effect, give heparin sodium in the usual therapeutic dosage. When the results of the initial prothrombin tests are known, administer the first dose of an oral anticoagulant in the usual initial amount. Thereafter, perform a coagulation test and determine the prothrombin activity at appropriate intervals. A period of at least five hours after the last intravenous dose or 24 hours after the last subcutaneous (intrafat) dose of heparin sodium should elapse before blood is drawn if a valid prothrombin time is to be obtained. When the oral anticoagulant shows its full effect and prothrombin activity is in the desired therapeutic range, heparin sodium may be discontinued and therapy continued with the oral anticoagulant.

Dosage Schedule Guidelines for Administration of Heparin Sodium

Method of Administration	Frequency	Recommended Dose*
Deep Subcutaneous (Intrafat) Injection	Initial dose	5000 units by I.V. injection, followed by 10,000–20,000 units of a concentrated solution, subcutaneously
	Every 8 hours	8000–10,000 units of a concentrated solution
	or	
	Every 12 hours	15,000–20,000 units of a concentrated solution
Intermittent Intravenous Injection	Initial dose	10,000 units, either undiluted or in 50–100 ml of isotonic Sodium Chloride Injection
	Every 4 to 6 hours	5000–10,000 units, either undiluted or in 50–100 ml of isotonic Sodium Chloride Injection
Intravenous Infusion	Initial dose	5000 units by I.V. injection
	Continuous	20,000–40,000 units/day in 1000 ml of isotonic Sodium Chloride Injection for infusion

*Based on 150-lb (68-kg) patient.

Therapeutic Anticoagulant Effect with Full-Dose Heparin—Although dosage must be adjusted for the individual patient according to the results of suitable laboratory tests, the dosage schedules in the accompanying chart may be used as guidelines.

1. *Deep Subcutaneous (Intrafat) Injection*—After an initial intravenous injection of 5000 units, inject 10,000 to 20,000 units of a concentrated heparin sodium solution subcutaneously, followed by 8000 to 10,000 units every eight hours or 15,000 to 20,000 units every 12 hours. A different site should be used for each injection to prevent the development of a massive hematoma.
2. *Intermittent Intravenous Injection*—Initially, 10,000 units; then, 5000 to 10,000 units every four to six hours. These amounts may be given undiluted or diluted with 50 to 100 ml of isotonic Sodium Chloride Injection.
3. *Continuous Intravenous Infusion*—After an initial intravenous injection of 5000 units, add 20,000 to 40,000 units of heparin sodium to 1000 ml of isotonic Sodium Chloride Injection for infusion. For most patients, the rate of flow should be adjusted to deliver approximately 20,000 to 40,000 units in 24 hours.

[See table above].

Surgery of the Heart and Blood Vessels—Patients undergoing total body perfusion for open-heart surgery should receive an initial dose of not less than 150 units of heparin sodium/kg of body weight. Frequently, a dose of 300 units/kg is used for procedures estimated to last less than 60 minutes or 400 units/kg for those estimated to last longer than 60 minutes.

Low-Dose Prophylaxis of Postoperative Thromboembolism—A number of well-controlled clinical trials have demonstrated that low-dose heparin prophylaxis, given just prior to and after surgery, will reduce the incidence of postoperative deep vein thrombosis in the legs (as measured by the I-125 fibrinogen technique and venography) and of clinical pulmonary embolism. The most widely used dosage has been 5000 units two hours before surgery and 5000 units every eight to 12 hours thereafter for seven days or until the patient is fully ambulatory, whichever is longer. The heparin is given by deep subcutaneous (intrafat) injection in the arm or abdomen with a fine (25 to 26-gauge) needle to minimize tissue trauma. A concentrated solution of heparin sodium is recommended. Such prophylaxis should be reserved for patients over the age of 40 who are undergoing major surgery. Patients with bleeding disorders and those having neurosurgery, spinal anesthesia, eye surgery, or potentially sanguineous operations should be excluded, as should patients receiving oral anticoagulants or platelet-active drugs (*see* Warnings). The value of such prophylaxis in hip surgery has not been established. The possibility of increased bleeding during surgery or postoperatively should be borne in mind. If such bleeding occurs, discontinuance of heparin and neutralization with protamine sulfate are advisable. If clinical evidence of thromboembolism develops despite low-dose prophylaxis, full therapeutic doses of anticoagulants should be given unless contraindicated. All patients should be screened prior to heparinization to rule out bleeding disorders, and monitoring with appropriate coagulation tests should be performed just prior to surgery. Coagulation test values should be normal or only slightly elevated. There is usually no need for daily monitoring of the effect of low-dose heparin in patients with normal coagulation parameters.

Extracorporeal Dialysis—Follow equipment manufacturers' operating directions carefully.

Blood Transfusion—Addition of 400 to 600 USP units/100 ml of whole blood. Usually, 7500 USP units of heparin sodium are added to 100 ml of Sterile Sodium Chloride Injection (or 75,000 USP units/1000 ml of Sterile Sodium Chloride Injection) and mixed; from this sterile solution, 6 to 8 ml are added/100 ml of whole blood. Leukocyte counts should be performed on heparinized blood within two hours after addition of the heparin. Heparinized blood should not be used for isoagglutinin, complement, or erythrocyte fragility tests or platelet counts.

Laboratory Samples—Addition of 70 to 150 units of heparin sodium per 10 to 20-ml sample of whole blood is usually employed to prevent coagulation of the sample. See comments under *Blood Transfusion.*

Continued on next page

*Identi-Code® symbol.

Lilly—Cont.

Overdosage: Protamine sulfate (1 percent solution) given by *slow infusion* will neutralize heparin sodium. *No more than 50 mg* should be administered, *very slowly,* in any ten-minute period. Each mg of protamine sulfate neutralizes approximately 100 USP heparin units (or injection of 1 to 1.5 mg neutralizes approximately 1 mg of heparin sodium). Heparins derived from various animal sources require different amounts of protamine sulfate for neutralization. This fact is of most importance during procedures of regional heparinization, including dialysis.
The amount of protamine required decreases as the time interval since the last heparin injection increases. Thirty minutes after a dose of heparin sodium, approximately 0.5 mg of protamine is sufficient to neutralize each 100 units of administered heparin. In some cases, blood or plasma transfusions may be necessary; these dilute but do not neutralize heparin sodium.
How Supplied: (℞) *Vials Heparin Sodium Injection, USP: No. 405,* 1000 USP units/ml, 10 ml (NDC 0002-7216-01); *No. 520,* 10,000 USP units/ml, 5 ml (NDC 0002-7217-01); *No. 622,* 20,000 USP units/ml, 1 ml (NDC 0002-7218-01); and *No. 642,* 20,000 USP units/ml, 2 ml, rubber-stoppered, in singles (10 per carton) (NDC 0002-7219-01).
[090782]

HEXA-BETALIN® ℞
(pyridoxine hydrochloride)
Injection, USP

Description: Injection Hexa-Betalin® (Pyridoxine Hydrochloride Injection, USP, Lilly) is a sterile solution of pyridoxine hydrochloride in Water for Injection with a *p*H between 2 and 3.8.
Each vial is preserved with chlorobutanol (chloroform derivative), 0.5 percent. Sodium hydroxide and/or hydrochloric acid may have been added during manufacture to adjust the *p*H.
Pyridoxine hydrochloride is a colorless or white crystal or a white crystalline powder. One g dissolves in 5 ml of water. It is stable in air and is slowly affected by sunlight.
Its chemical name is 2-methyl-3-hydroxy-4,5-bis(hydroxymethyl) pyridine hydrochloride.
Actions: Natural substances that have vitamin B_6 activity are pyridoxine in plants and pyridoxal or pyridoxamine in animals. All three are converted to pyridoxal phosphate by the enzyme pyridoxal kinase. The physiologically active forms of vitamin B_6 are pyridoxal phosphate (codecarboxylase) and pyridoxamine phosphate. Riboflavin is required for the conversion of pyridoxine phosphate to pyridoxal phosphate.
Vitamin B_6 acts as a coenzyme in the metabolism of protein, carbohydrate, and fat. In protein metabolism, it participates in the decarboxylation of amino acids, conversion of tryptophan to niacin or to serotonin (5-hydroxytryptamine), deamination, and transamination and transulfuration of amino acids. In carbohydrate metabolism, it is responsible for the breakdown of glycogen to glucose-1-phosphate.
The total adult body pool consists of 16 to 25 mg of pyridoxine. Its half-life appears to be 15 to 20 days. Vitamin B_6 is degraded to 4-pyridoxic acid in the liver. This metabolite is excreted in the urine.
The need for pyridoxine increases with the amount of protein in the diet. The tryptophan load test appears to uncover early vitamin B_6 deficiency by detecting xanthinuria. The average adult minimum daily requirement is about 1.25 mg. The "Recommended Dietary Allowance" of the National Academy of Sciences is estimated to be as much as 2 mg for adults and 2.5 mg for pregnant and lactating women. The requirements are more in persons having certain genetic defects or those being treated with isonicotinic acid hydrazide (INH) or oral contraceptives.
Indications: Pyridoxine hydrochloride injection is effective for the treatment of pyridoxine deficiency as seen in the following:
Inadequate dietary intake
Drug-induced deficiency, as from isoniazid (INH) or oral contraceptives
Inborn errors of metabolism, e.g., vitamin-B_6-dependent convulsions or vitamin-B_6-responsive anemia
The parenteral route is indicated when oral administration is not feasible, as in anorexia, nausea and vomiting, and preoperative and postoperative conditions. It is also indicated when gastrointestinal absorption is impaired.
Contraindication: A history of sensitivity to pyridoxine or to any of the ingredients in Hexa-Betalin® (pyridoxine hydrochloride, Lilly) is a contraindication.
Warning: This product should be protected from exposure to light.
Precautions: *General Precautions*—Single deficiency, as of pyridoxine alone, is rare. Multiple vitamin deficiency is to be expected in any inadequate diet. Patients treated with levodopa should avoid supplemental vitamins that contain more than 5 mg pyridoxine in the daily dose.
Women taking oral contraceptives may exhibit increased pyridoxine requirements.
Drug Interactions—Pyridoxine supplements should not be given to patients receiving levodopa, because the action of the latter drug is antagonized by pyridoxine. However, this vitamin may be used concurrently in patients receiving a preparation containing both carbidopa and levodopa.
Usage in Pregnancy—Pregnancy Category A—The requirement for pyridoxine appears to be increased during pregnancy. Pyridoxine is sometimes of value in the treatment of nausea and vomiting of pregnancy.
Nursing Mothers—The need for pyridoxine is increased during lactation.
It is not known whether this drug is excreted in human milk. Because many drugs are excreted in human milk, caution should be exercised, when Hexa-Betalin is administered to a nursing woman.
Usage in Children—Safety and effectiveness in children have not been established.
Adverse Reactions: Paresthesia, somnolence, and low serum folic acid levels have been reported.
Drug Abuse and Dependence: Symptoms of dependence have been noted in adults given only 200 mg daily, followed by withdrawal.
Overdosage: Pyridoxine given to animals in amounts of 3 to 4 g/kg of body weight produces convulsions and death. In man, a dose of 25 mg/kg of body weight is well tolerated.
Dosage and Administration: In cases of dietary deficiency, the dosage is 10 to 20 mg daily for three weeks. Follow-up treatment is recommended daily for several weeks with an oral therapeutic multivitamin preparation containing 2 to 5 mg pyridoxine. Poor dietary habits should be corrected, and an adequate, well-balanced diet should be prescribed.
The vitamin-B_6-dependency syndrome may require a therapeutic dosage of as much as 600 mg a day and a daily intake of 30 mg for life.
In deficiencies due to INH, the dosage is 100 mg daily for three weeks followed by a 30-mg maintenance dose daily.
In poisoning caused by ingestion of more than 10 g of INH, an equal amount of pyridoxine should be given—4 g intravenously followed by 1 g intramuscularly every 30 minutes.
How Supplied: (℞) *Vials (Multiple Dose) No. 479, Hexa-Betalin® (Pyridoxine Hydrochloride Injection, USP),* 100 mg/ml, 10 ml, rubber-stoppered, in singles (10 per carton) (NDC 0002-1694-01).
Also Available:
*Pyridoxine Hydrochloride Tablets, USP (Hexa-Betalin®): No. 1691, J56,** 10 mg (NDC 0002-1056-02), *No. 1632, J45,** 25 mg (NDC 0002-1045-02), and *No. 1728, T72,**50 mg (NDC 0002-2072-02), in bottles of 100. [120381]

ILETIN® (INSULIN, LILLY)— REGULAR AND MODIFIED INSULIN PRODUCTS

All of the insulins listed below are prepared from a mixture of insulin crystals extracted from beef and pork pancreas, except for Regular (Concentrated) Iletin® II *(purified pork insulin injection, Lilly), U-500, which is prepared from pork insulin only. Regular Iletin®* II *(purified insulin injection, Lilly), Lente® Iletin®* II *(purified insulin zinc suspension, Lilly), NPH Iletin®* II *(isophane purified insulin suspension, Lilly), and Protamine, Zinc & Iletin®* II *(protamine zinc purified insulin suspension, Lilly) made solely from beef or pork source are available on special order in U-100 strength only. When insulin is prepared from a single animal source, the species is indicated on the vial label and on the package.*

REGULAR ILETIN® I
(Beef-Pork)
(insulin injection)
USP

INFORMATION FOR THE PATIENT
WARNINGS:
ANY CHANGE OF INSULIN SHOULD BE MADE CAUTIOUSLY AND ONLY UNDER MEDICAL SUPERVISION. CHANGES IN REFINEMENT, PURITY, STRENGTH (U-40, U-100), BRAND (MANUFACTURER), TYPE (LENTE®, NPH, REGULAR, ETC.), AND SOURCE (BEEF, PORK, OR BEEF-PORK) MAY RESULT IN THE NEED FOR A CHANGE IN DOSAGE.
SOME PATIENTS TAKING THIS BEEF-PORK INSULIN WILL REQUIRE SUCH A CHANGE IN DOSAGE. IF AN ADJUSTMENT IS NEEDED, IT MAY OCCUR WITH THE FIRST DOSE OR OVER A PERIOD OF SEVERAL WEEKS.
Insulin and Diabetes: Your doctor has explained that you have diabetes. You have learned that the treatment of your diabetes requires injections of insulin.
Insulin is a hormone produced by the pancreas, a large gland that lies near the stomach. This hormone is necessary for the body's correct use of food, especially sugar. Diabetes occurs when the pancreas does not make enough insulin to meet the body's needs.
To control your diabetes, your doctor has prescribed injections of insulin to keep your blood sugar at a nearly normal level and to keep your urine as free of sugar as possible. Each case of diabetes is different. Your doctor has told you which insulin to use, how much, and when and how often to inject it. This schedule has been individualized for you. Proper control of your diabetes requires close and constant cooperation with your doctor.
In spite of diabetes, you can lead a fairly normal, healthy, and useful life if you eat a balanced diet daily, exercise regularly, and take your insulin injections exactly as prescribed by your doctor.
You have been instructed to test your urine and/or blood regularly for sugar. If your urine tests consistently show the presence of sugar or your blood tests consistently show above-normal sugar levels, your diabetes is not properly controlled and you must let your doctor know.
Use the Proper Type of Insulin: This insulin, manufactured by Eli Lilly and Company, has the trademark Iletin® I (insulin, Lilly) and is available in various types—Regular, NPH, Protamine Zinc, Lente, Semilente®, and Ultralente®.

These types of insulin differ mainly in the time they require to take effect and in the length of time their action lasts. Your doctor has prescribed the type of insulin that he/she believes is best for you. **Do not use any other type of insulin except on his/her advice and direction.**

Regular Beef-Pork Insulin: Regular Iletin I, consisting of zinc-insulin crystals dissolved in a clear fluid, is obtained from beef and pork pancreas. Regular beef-pork insulin is "unmodified" (that is, nothing has been added to change the speed or length of its action). It takes effect rapidly and has a relatively short duration of activity (six to eight hours) as compared with other insulins.

Regular beef-pork insulin should be clear and colorless. Do not use it if it is cloudy, unusually viscous, precipitated, or even slightly colored.

Storage: Insulin should be stored in a cold place, preferably in a refrigerator but not in the freezing compartment. Do not let it freeze or leave it in direct sunlight. If refrigeration is not possible, the bottle of insulin which you are currently using can be kept unrefrigerated as long as it is kept as cool as possible and away from heat and sunlight. Do not use a bottle of insulin after the expiration date stamped on the label.

Use the Correct Syringe: Doses of insulin are measured in **units.** The number of units in each cubic centimeter (cc) is clearly stated on the package. Two strengths are available for each type of insulin: U-40 (40 units per cc) and U-100 (100 units per cc). It is important that you understand the markings on your syringe, because the volume of insulin you inject depends on the strength, that is, the number of units per cc. For this reason, you should always use a syringe marked for the strength of insulin you are injecting. Failure to use the proper syringe can lead to a mistake in dosage, and you may receive too little or too much insulin. This can cause serious problems for you, ranging from a blood sugar that is too low or too high to coma (unconsciousness) or, rarely, death.

IMPORTANT: TO HELP AVOID CONTAMINATION AND POSSIBLE INFECTION, FOLLOW THESE INSTRUCTIONS EXACTLY.

Disposable Syringes: Disposable syringes and needles require no sterilization; they should be used only once and then discarded.

Sterilizing and Assembling Reusable Syringes: Your reusable syringe and needle must be sterilized before each injection—**follow the package directions supplied with your syringe.** Boiling, as described below, is the best method of sterilizing.

1. Put syringe, plunger, and needle in strainer, place in saucepan, and cover with water. Boil for five minutes.
2. Remove articles from water or alcohol. When they have cooled, insert plunger into barrel, and fasten needle to syringe with a slight twist.
3. Push plunger in and out several times until water is completely removed. (If the syringe, plunger, and needle cannot be boiled, as when you are traveling, they may be sterilized by immersion for at least five minutes in Isopropyl Alcohol, 91%. Do not use bathing, rubbing, or medicated alcohol for this sterilization. If the syringe is sterilized with alcohol, it must be absolutely dry before use.)

Preparing the Dose:

1. Wash your hands.
2. Flip off the colored protective cap on the bottle, but **do not** remove rubber stopper.
3. Wipe top of bottle with alcohol swab.
4. Draw air into the syringe by pulling back on the plunger. The amount of air should be equal to your insulin dose.
5. Remove the needle cover. Put the needle through rubber top of insulin bottle.
6. Push plunger in. The air injected into the bottle will allow insulin to be easily withdrawn into syringe.
7. Turn bottle and syringe upside down in one hand. Be sure tip of needle is in insulin. Your other hand will be free to move the plunger. Draw back on plunger slowly to draw the correct dose of insulin into syringe.
8. Check for air bubbles. The air is harmless, but too large an air bubble will reduce the insulin dose. To remove air bubbles, push insulin back into the bottle and measure your correct dose of insulin.
9. Double check your dose. Remove needle from bottle. Cover needle with guard or lay syringe down so that needle does not touch anything.

Injecting the Dose:

1. Clean the skin where the injection is to be made.
2. With one hand, stabilize the skin by spreading it or pinching up a large area of skin.
3. Pick up syringe with other hand, and hold it as you would a pencil. Insert needle straight into the skin (90° angle). Be sure to insert needle all the way.
4. To inject the insulin, push plunger all the way down, using less than five seconds to inject the dose.
5. Hold alcohol swab near the needle and pull needle straight out of skin. Press alcohol swab over injection site for several seconds.
6. Use disposable syringe only once to insure sterility of syringe and needle and accuracy of dose. Destroy syringes as directed.
7. To avoid tissue damage, always change the site for each injection.

Warnings—See Additional Warnings Above: Patients who have been directed by their physicians to mix two types of insulin should be aware that insulin hypodermic syringes of different manufacturers may vary in the amount of space between the bottom line and the needle.

Because of this, do not change:

1. The order of mixing that the physician has prescribed or
2. The model and brand of syringe or needle without first consulting your physician.

The mixing should be done immediately prior to injection. Failure to heed this warning could result in a dosage error.

Usage in Pregnancy: Pregnancy may make managing your diabetes more difficult. If you are pregnant or nursing a baby, consult your physician, pharmacist, or nurse-educator when using this product.

Insulin Reaction and Shock: Insulin reaction (too little sugar in the blood, also called "hypoglycemia") can be brought about by:

1. Taking too much insulin
2. Missing or delaying meals
3. Exercising or working too hard just before a meal
4. An infection or illness (especially with diarrhea or vomiting)
5. A change in the body's need for insulin

The first symptoms of insulin reaction usually come on suddenly and may include fatigue, nervousness or "shakiness," headache, rapid heartbeat, nausea, and a cold sweat. Eating sugar or a sugar-sweetened product will often correct the condition and prevent more serious symptoms. If the reaction becomes more severe, breathing will be shallow and the skin pale. Contact your doctor at once if you develop any of these symptoms.

Diabetic Acidosis and Coma: Diabetic acidosis may develop if your body has too little insulin. (This is the opposite of insulin reaction, which is the result of too much insulin in the blood.) Diabetic acidosis may be brought on if you omit your insulin or take less than the doctor has prescribed, eat significantly more than your diet calls for, or develop a fever or infection. With acidosis, urine tests show a large amount of sugar and acetone.

The first symptoms of diabetic acidosis usually come on gradually, over a period of hours or days, and include a drowsy feeling, flushed face, thirst, and loss of appetite. Heavy breathing and a rapid pulse are more severe symptoms. It is important that you notify your doctor immediately, because diabetic coma (unconsciousness) can follow.

Adverse Reactions: On rare occasions, the skin where insulin has been injected may become red, swollen, and itchy. If you have a local reaction, notify your doctor.

Insulin allergy occurs very rarely, but when it does, it may cause a serious reaction including a general skin rash over the body, shortness of breath, fast pulse, sweating, and a drop in blood pressure. If any of these symptoms develop, you should be seen immediately by your doctor.

Important Notes:

1. Never change from the insulin that has been prescribed for you to another insulin without instructions from your doctor. Changing the type, strength, species, or manufacturer of insulin can cause problems with your diabetes.
2. Your doctor will tell you what to do if you miss a dose of insulin or miss a meal because of illness. Always keep an extra supply of insulin, as well as spare syringe and needle, on hand. If you miss a meal, use a substitute of sugar, sugar-sweetened candy, fruit juice, or sugar-sweetened beverage according to your doctor's instructions.
3. If you become ill from any cause, especially with nausea and vomiting, your insulin requirement may change. Test your urine and/or blood and notify your doctor at once.
4. Consult your doctor if you notice anything unusual or have doubts about your condition or your use of insulin.
5. Always wear diabetic identification so that appropriate treatment can be given if complications occur away from home.
6. Understand how to manage your diabetes so that your life can be active and healthy.

How Supplied: *Regular Iletin ® I (Insulin Injection, USP) (Beef-Pork)* is supplied in rubber-stoppered vials as follows:

CP-240, U-40, forty units per cc, 10 cc (400 units).

CP-210, U-100, one hundred units per cc, 10 cc (1000 units).

The above products are supplied 10 per carton.

Refrigerate. Avoid freezing. [101482]

REGULAR (CONCENTRATED) ILETIN® II, U-500 ℞

(purified pork insulin injection)

WARNINGS: ANY CHANGE OF INSULIN SHOULD BE MADE CAUTIOUSLY AND ONLY UNDER MEDICAL SUPERVISION. CHANGES IN PURITY, STRENGTH (U-40, U-100), BRAND (MANUFACTURER), TYPE (LENTE®, NPH, REGULAR, ETC.), AND/OR SOURCE OF SPECIES (BEEF, PORK, OR BEEF-PORK) MAY RESULT IN THE NEED FOR A CHANGE IN DOSAGE. SEE BELOW. IT IS NOT POSSIBLE TO IDENTIFY WHICH PATIENTS WILL REQUIRE A REDUCTION IN DOSE TO AVOID HYPOGLYCEMIA WHEN USING THIS INSULIN. HOWEVER, IT IS KNOWN THAT A SMALL NUMBER OF PATIENTS MAY REQUIRE A SIGNIFICANT CHANGE.

ADJUSTMENT MAY BE NEEDED WITH THE FIRST DOSE OR OCCUR OVER A PERIOD OF SEVERAL WEEKS. BE AWARE OF THE POSSIBILITY OF SYMPTOMS OF EI-

Continued on next page

*Identi-Code® symbol.

Lilly—Cont.

THER HYPOGLYCEMIA OR HYPERGLYCEMIA. (SEE SECTIONS ENTITLED INSULIN REACTION AND SHOCK and DIABETIC ACIDOSIS AND COMA.)

This insulin is prepared from pork pancreas only. The dose of pork insulin for patients with insulin resistance due to antibodies to beef insulin may be only a fraction of that of beef insulin.

This insulin preparation contains 500 units of insulin in each milliliter. Extreme caution must be observed in the measurement of dosage because inadvertent overdose may result in irreversible insulin shock. Serious consequences may result if it is used other than under constant medical supervision.

Description: This Lilly pork insulin product differs from previous pork insulin preparations because it has undergone additional steps of chromatographic purification.

Regular (Concentrated) Iletin® II (purified pork insulin injection, Lilly), U-500, is an aqueous solution made from the antidiabetic principle of pork pancreas as stated on the label. Each milliliter contains 500 units of regular (unmodified) insulin and approximately 1.6 percent glycerin (w/v), with approximately 0.25 percent m-cresol (w/v) as a preservative. Sodium hydroxide and hydrochloric acid are added during manufacture to adjust the *p*H. All preparations of Iletin® II (purified pork insulin, Lilly) are made from zinc-insulin crystals.

Adequate insulin dosage permits the diabetic patient to utilize carbohydrates and fats in a comparatively satisfactory manner. Regardless of concentration, the action of insulin is basically the same: to enable carbohydrate metabolism to occur and thus to prevent the production of ketone bodies by the liver. Although, under usual circumstances, diabetes can be controlled with doses in the vicinity of 40 to 60 units or less, an occasional patient develops such resistance or becomes so unresponsive to the effect of insulin that daily doses of several hundred, or even several thousand, units are required. Fortunately, there seems to be no condition of absolute resistance; all resistant patients will apparently respond to some dose, if it is large enough.

Occasionally, a cause of the insulin resistance can be found (such as hemochromatosis, cirrhosis of the liver, some complicating disease of the endocrine glands other than the pancreas, allergy, or infection), but in other cases, no cause of the high insulin requirement can be determined.

Iletin II, U-500, is unmodified by any agent that might prolong its action; however, clinical experience has shown that it frequently has a time action similar to a repository insulin preparation and that a single dose may show activity over a 24-hour period. This effect has been credited to the high concentration of the preparation.

Indications: Iletin® II (purified pork insulin injection, Lilly), U-500, is especially useful for the treatment of diabetic patients with marked insulin resistance (daily requirements more than 200 units), since a large dose may be administered subcutaneously in a reasonable volume.

Precautions: Every patient exhibiting insulin resistance who requires Iletin® II (purified pork insulin injection, Lilly), U-500, for the control of diabetes should be held under close observation until dosage is established. The response will vary among patients. Some can be controlled with a single dose daily; others may require two or three injections per day.

Most patients will show a "tolerance" to insulin, so that minor variations in dosage can occur without the development of untoward symptoms of insulin shock.

Insulin resistance is frequently self-limited; after several weeks or months during which high dosage is required, responsiveness to the pharmacologic effect of insulin may be regained and dosage can be reduced.

Insulin should be kept in a cold place, preferably in a refrigerator. Do not inject insulin that is not water-clear. Discoloration, turbidity, or unusual viscosity indicates deterioration or contamination.

Use of a package of insulin should not be started after the expiration date stamped on it.

Adverse Reactions: As with other insulin preparations, hypoglycemic reactions may be associated with the administration of Iletin® II (purified pork insulin injection, Lilly), U-500. However, deep secondary hypoglycemic reactions may develop 18 to 24 hours after the original injection of Iletin II, U-500. Consequently, patients should be carefully observed, and prompt treatment of such reactions should be initiated with glucagon injections and/or with glucose by intravenous injection or gavage.

Administration and Dosage: Iletin® II (purified pork insulin injection, Lilly), U-500, can be administered by both the subcutaneous and the intramuscular routes. It is inadvisable to inject Iletin II, U-500, intravenously because of the possible development of allergic or anaphylactoid reactions.

It is recommended that a tuberculin type of syringe be utilized for the measurement of dosage. Variations in dosage are frequently possible in the insulin-resistant patient, since the individual is unresponsive to the pharmacologic effect of the insulin. Nevertheless, accuracy of measurement is to be encouraged because of the potential danger of the preparation.

How Supplied: (℞) *CP-2500, Regular (Concentrated) Iletin® II (purified pork insulin injection, Lilly), U-500,* five hundred units/cc, 20 cc, rubber-stoppered vials (10,000 units) (10 per carton) (NDC 0002-8500-01). *Refrigerate. Avoid freezing.*

[082382]

LENTE® ILETIN® I
(Beef-Pork)
(insulin zinc suspension)
USP

SEMILENTE® ILETIN® I
(Beef-Pork)
(prompt insulin zinc suspension)
USP

ULTRALENTE® ILETIN® I
(Beef-Pork)
(extended insulin zinc suspension)
USP

INFORMATION FOR THE PATIENT

WARNINGS, Insulin and Diabetes, and Use of Proper Type of Insulin: *See under* Regular Iletin® I.

Lente Beef-Pork Insulin: Lente beef-pork insulin is obtained from beef and pork pancreas. Insulin has been combined with zinc to form small crystals. Lente beef-pork insulin has an intermediate time of activity. Its action starts more slowly than does that of regular beef-pork insulin and lasts somewhat longer (slightly over 24 hours).

Lente beef-pork insulin should look uniformly cloudy or milky. If the insulin substance (the cloudy material) settles at the bottom of the vial, the vial must be carefully rotated before the injection so that the contents are uniformly mixed (see instructions under Preparing the Dose). Do not use a vial of insulin if you see lumps that float or stick to the sides. Also, the insulin should not be used if it is clear and remains clear after the vial is rotated.

Semilente Beef-Pork Insulin: Semilente beef-pork insulin comes from beef and pork pancreas. Insulin has been combined with zinc to form small crystals. Semilente beef-pork insulin has a short period of activity. Its action starts nearly as rapidly as that of regular insulin and lasts slightly longer (approximately 12 to 16 hours). This type of insulin will shorten the action time of Lente insulin (an intermediate-acting form) when they are mixed.

Semilente beef-pork insulin should look uniformly cloudy or milky. If the insulin substance (the cloudy material) settles at the bottom of the vial, the vial must be carefully rotated before the injection so that the contents are uniformly mixed (see instructions under Preparing the Dose). Do not use a vial of insulin if you see lumps that float or stick to the sides. Also, the insulin should not be used if it is clear and remains clear after the vial is rotated.

Ultralente Beef-Pork Insulin: Ultralente beef-pork insulin comes from beef and pork pancreas. Insulin has been combined with zinc to form small crystals. Ultralente beef-pork insulin takes effect very gradually and, in comparison with regular insulin, has a long period of activity (more than 36 hours). This type of insulin will lengthen the action time of Lente insulin (an intermediate-acting form) when they are mixed.

Ultralente beef-pork insulin should look uniformly cloudy or milky. If the insulin substance (the cloudy material) settles at the bottom of the vial, the vial must be carefully rotated before the injection so that the contents are uniformly mixed (see instructions under Preparing the Dose). Do not use a vial of insulin if you see lumps that float or stick to the sides. Also, the insulin should not be used if it is clear and remains clear after the vial is rotated.

Storage, Use the Correct Syringe, Disposable Syringes, and Sterilizing and Assembling Reusable Syringes: *See under* Regular Iletin® I.

Preparing the Dose:

1. Wash your hands.
2. Gently roll the insulin bottle several times to mix the insulin. Be sure it is completely mixed. Do not shake bottle. Flip off the colored protective cap on the bottle, but **do not** remove the rubber stopper. *See also under* Regular Iletin® I.

Injecting the Dose, Warnings, Usage in Pregnancy, Insulin Reaction and Shock, Diabetic Acidosis and Coma, Adverse Reactions, and **Important Notes:** *See under* Regular Iletin® I.

How Supplied: *Lente® Iletin® I (Insulin Zinc Suspension, USP)* is supplied in rubber-stoppered vials as follows:

CP-440, U-40, forty units per cc, 10 cc (400 units).

CP-410, U-100, one hundred units per cc, 10 cc (1000 units).

Semilente® Iletin® I (Prompt Insulin Zinc Suspension, USP) is supplied in rubber-stoppered vials as follows:

CP-540, U-40, forty units per cc, 10 cc (400 units).

CP-510, U-100, one hundred units per cc, 10 cc (1000 units).

Ultralente® Iletin® I (Extended Insulin Zinc Suspension, USP) is supplied in rubber-stoppered vials as follows:

CP-640, U-40, forty units per cc, 10 cc (400 units).

CP-610, U-100, one hundred units per cc, 10 cc (1000 units).

The above products are supplied 10 per carton. *Refrigerate. Avoid freezing.* [121180]

NPH ILETIN® I
(Beef-Pork)
(isophane insulin suspension)
USP

INFORMATION FOR THE PATIENT

WARNINGS, Insulin and Diabetes, and Use of Proper Type of Insulin: *See under* Regular Iletin® I.

NPH Beef-Pork Insulin: NPH beef-pork insulin is obtained from beef and pork pancreas. Insulin has been combined with protamine and zinc so that its action is similar to that of a mixture of Regular and Protamine Zinc insulins. The result is an intermediate-acting insulin with a slower speed of action than Regular insulin and a shorter time of activity than Protamine Zinc insulin. The effect of NPH beef-pork insulin lasts slightly more than 24 hours.

NPH beef-pork insulin should look uniformly cloudy or milky. If the insulin substance (the cloudy material) settles at the bottom of the vial, the vial must be carefully rotated before the injection so that the contents are uniformly mixed (see instructions under Preparing the Dose). Do not use a vial of insulin if you see lumps that float or stick to the sides. Also, the insulin should not be used if it is clear and remains clear after the vial is rotated.

Storage, Use the Correct Syringe, Disposable Syringes, and Sterilizing and Assembling Reusable Syringes: *See under* Regular Iletin® I.

Preparing the Dose: *See under* Lente® Iletin® I and Regular Iletin® I.

Injecting the Dose, Warnings, Usage in Pregnancy, Insulin Reaction and Shock, Diabetic Acidosis and Coma, Adverse Reactions, and Important Notes: *See under* Regular Iletin® I.

How Supplied: *NPH Iletin® I (Isophane Insulin Suspension, USP)* is supplied in rubber-stoppered vials as follows:

CP-340, U-40, forty units per cc, 10 cc (400 units).

CP-310, U-100, one hundred units per cc, 10 cc (1000 units).

The above products are supplied 10 per carton.

Refrigerate. Avoid freezing. [102282]

PROTAMINE, ZINC & ILETIN® I

(Beef-Pork)
(protamine zinc insulin suspension)
USP

INFORMATION FOR THE PATIENT

WARNINGS, Insulin and Diabetes, and Use of Proper Type of Insulin: *See under* Regular Iletin® I.

Protamine Zinc Beef-Pork Insulin: Protamine zinc beef-pork insulin is obtained from beef and pork pancreas. Protamine and zinc have been added to lengthen the time of action. Protamine zinc beef-pork insulin takes effect gradually and, in comparison with regular beef-pork insulin, has a long period of activity (well over 24 hours).

Protamine zinc beef-pork insulin should look uniformly cloudy or milky. If the insulin substance (the cloudy material) settles at the bottom of the vial, the vial must be carefully rotated before the injection so that the contents are uniformly mixed (see instructions under Preparing the Dose). Do not use a vial of insulin if you see lumps that float or stick to the sides. Also, the insulin should not be used if it is clear and remains clear after the vial is rotated.

Storage, Use the Correct Syringe, Disposable Syringes, and Sterilizing and Assembling Reusable Syringes: *See under* Regular Iletin® I.

Preparing the Dose: *See under* Lente® Iletin® I and Regular Iletin® I.

Injecting the Dose, Warnings, Usage in Pregnancy, Insulin Reaction and Shock, Diabetic Acidosis and Coma, Adverse Reactions, and **Important Notes:** *See under* Regular Iletin® I.

How Supplied: *Protamine, Zinc & Iletin® I (Protamine Zinc Insulin Suspension, USP)* is supplied in rubber-stoppered vials as follows:

CP-140, U-40, forty units per cc, 10 cc (400 units).

CP-110, U-100, one hundred units per cc, 10 cc (1000 units).

The above products are supplied 10 per carton.

Refrigerate. Avoid freezing. [102282]

IPECAC ℞

Syrup, USP

Description: Ipecac Syrup contains 7 g of ipecac/100 ml (32 grs/fl oz). Contains alcohol, 2 percent.

Ipecac syrup is an emetic for oral use.

Ipecac consists of the dried rhizome and roots of *Cephaelis ipecacuanha* (Brotero) A. Richard, known in commerce as Rio or Brazilian ipecac, or of *Cephaelis acuminata* Karsten, known in commerce as Cartagena, Nicaragua, or Panama ipecac (Fam. *Rubiaceae*). Ipecac yields not less than 2 percent of the ether-soluble alkaloids of ipecac.

Ipecac contains emetine (methylcephaeline) [$C_{29}H_{40}N_2O_4$], cephaeline, [$C_{28}H_{38}N_2O_4$], psychotrine [$C_{28}H_{36}N_2O_4$], emetamine [$C_{29}H_{36}N_2O_4$], ipecamine, also ipecacuanhic acid, pectin, starch, resin, sugar, etc. All of the alkaloids are interrelated and may be synthesized from one another. Brazilian roots yield as much as 2.5 percent of total alkaloids and Cartagena root, 2 percent.

Ipecac syrup is a clear amber hydroalcoholic syrup with a characteristic odor.

Clinical Pharmacology: Ipecac alkaloids act both locally on the gastric mucosa and centrally on the chemoreceptor trigger zone to induce vomiting. An adequate dose causes vomiting within 30 minutes in more than 90 percent of patients; the average time is usually less than 20 minutes. The emetic action is increased if 200 to 300 ml of water are taken immediately after administration of the syrup. In young and frightened children, giving water prior to the ipecac syrup may be more successful.

It should be recognized that an episode of vomiting does not necessarily completely empty the stomach.

Indications and Usage: Ipecac syrup is useful as an emetic (inducing vomiting) for emergency use in the treatment of drug overdosage and in certain cases of poisoning.

Contraindications: This drug should not be given to unconscious patients. It should not be used if strychnine, corrosives such as alkalies (lye) and strong acids, or petroleum distillates such as kerosene, gasoline, coal oil, fuel oil, paint thinner, or cleaning fluid have been ingested. (Some authorities consider emesis with ipecac syrup to be appropriate in certain instances of hydrocarbon ingestion.)

Warnings: IPECAC SYRUP SHOULD NOT BE CONFUSED WITH IPECAC FLUID EXTRACT, WHICH IS 14 TIMES STRONGER AND HAS CAUSED SOME DEATHS.

If ipecac syrup is not vomited, the alkaloid emetine may be absorbed; this has been associated with cardiotoxic effects in the long-term treatment of amebiasis.

Note to the Pharmacist:

The Food and Drug Administration has determined that, in the interest of public health, ipecac syrup should be available for sale without prescription provided it is packaged in a quantity of 1 fl oz (30 ml) and, in addition to other required labeling, contains the following:

1. A statement, conspicuously boxed and in red letters, to the effect: "For emergency use to cause vomiting in poisoning. Before using, call physician, the Poison Control Center, or hospital emergency room immediately for advice."

2. A warning to the effect: "Warning—Keep out of reach of children. Do not use in unconscious persons. Ordinarily, this drug should not be used if strychnine, corrosives such as alkalies (lye) and strong acids, or petroleum distillates such as kerosene, gasoline, coal oil, fuel oil, paint thinner, or cleaning fluid have been ingested."

3. Usual dosage: 1 tablespoonful (15 ml) in persons over one year of age.

Information for Patients—See Precautions.

Drug Interactions—Activated charcoal should not be given with ipecac syrup, because the charcoal adsorbs the ipecac and nullifies its emetic effect; however, it may be given after vomiting has occurred.

Usage in Pregnancy—Pregnancy Category C—Animal reproduction studies have not been conducted with ipecac syrup. It is not known whether the drug can cause harm when administered to a pregnant woman or can affect reproductive capacity. Minimal systemic absorption would be expected when ipecac syrup is used as directed (*See* Dosage and Administration). (The alkaloid emetine, obtained from ipecac, is used by injection for systemic treatment of disease, e.g., amebiasis. This use of emetine may be associated with significant toxicity and is not recommended in pregnancy.)

Nursing Mothers—It is not known whether the alkaloids of ipecac are excreted in human milk. Caution should be exercised if ipecac syrup is used for treatment of a nursing woman. (The alkaloid emetine, when used for treatment of systemic disease, is detoxicated and excreted from the body very slowly, over a period of several weeks.)

Adverse Reactions: When ipecac syrup does not cause emesis, absorption of the alkaloid emetine may occur. (In the treatment of amebiasis, emetine may cause heart conduction disturbances, atrial fibrillation, or fatal myocarditis.)

Overdosage: *See* **Warnings.**

Dosage and Administration: Children less than one year of age, 1 to 2 teaspoonfuls; children over one year of age and adults, 3 teaspoonfuls.

If vomiting does not occur within 20 minutes, a similar dose is repeated once. Then, if the patient does not vomit within 30 minutes, the dosage should be recovered (lavage).

How Supplied: (℞) *Syrup No. 37, Ipecac, USP,* in 16-fl-oz bottles (NDC 0002-2520-05).

[041382]

ISONIAZID ℞

Tablets, USP

WARNING

Severe and sometimes fatal hepatitis associated with isoniazid therapy has been reported and may occur or may develop even after many months of treatment. The risk of developing hepatitis is age related. Approximate case rates by age are 0 per 1000 for persons under 20 years of age, 3 per 1000 for persons in the 20 to 34-year age group, 12 per 1000 for persons in the 35 to 49-year age group, 23 per 1000 for persons in the 50 to 64-year age group, and 8 per 1000 for persons over 65 years of age. The risk of hepatitis is increased with daily consumption of alcohol. Precise data to provide a fatality rate for isoniazid-related hepatitis are not available; however, in a U.S. Public Health Service Surveillance Study of 13,838 persons taking isoniazid, there were eight deaths among 174 cases of hepatitis.

Therefore, patients given isoniazid should be carefully monitored and interviewed at monthly intervals. Serum transaminase concentration becomes elevated in about 10 to 20 percent of patients, usually during the first few months of therapy, but it can occur at any time. Usually, enzyme levels return to normal despite continuance of the drug, but in some cases progressive liver dysfunction occurs. Patients should be instructed to report immediately any of the prodromal symptoms of hepatitis, such as fatigue, weakness, malaise, anorexia, nausea, or vomiting. If these symptoms

Continued on next page

*Identi-Code® symbol.

Lilly—Cont.

appear or if signs suggestive of hepatic damage are detected, isoniazid should be discontinued promptly, since continued use of the drug in such cases has been reported to cause a more severe form of liver damage.
Patients with tuberculosis should be given appropriate treatment with alternative drugs. If isoniazid must be reinstituted, it should be done only after symptoms and laboratory abnormalities have cleared. The drug should be restarted in very small and gradually increasing doses and should be withdrawn immediately if there is any indication of recurrent liver involvement. Preventive treatment should be deferred in persons with acute hepatic diseases.

Description: Isoniazid, USP, the hydrazide of isonicotinic acid, is chemically isonicotinyl hydrazine, and the chemical formula is $C_6H_7N_3O$. It exists as colorless or white crystals or as a crystalline powder that is water soluble. It is slowly affected by exposure to air and light.

Actions: Isoniazid acts against actively growing tubercle bacilli.
After oral administraton, isoniazid produces peak blood levels within one or two hours; these decline to 50 percent or less within six hours. It diffuses readily into all body fluids (cerebrospinal, pleural, and ascitic), tissues, organs, and excreta (saliva, sputum, and feces). The drug also passes through the placental barrier and into milk in concentrations comparable to those in the plasma. From 50 to 70 percent of a dose of isoniazid is excreted in the urine within 24 hours.
Isoniazid is metabolized primarily by acetylation and dehydrazination. The rate of acetylation is genetically determined. Approximately 50 percent of blacks and Caucasians are "slow inactivators," and the rest are "rapid inactivators"; the majority of Eskimos and Orientals are "rapid inactivators."
The rate of acetylation does not significantly alter the effectiveness of isoniazid. However, slow acetylation may lead to higher blood levels of the drug and, thus, to an increase in toxic reactions.
Pyridoxine (vitamin B_6) deficiency is sometimes observed in adults taking high doses of isoniazid and is considered probably due to the drug's competition with pyridoxal phosphate for the enzyme apotryptophanase.

Indications: Isoniazid is recommended for all forms of tuberculosis in which organisms are susceptible.
Isoniazid is recommended as preventive therapy for the following individuals, in order of priority:

1. Household members and other close associates of persons with recently diagnosed tuberculous disease.
2. Positive tuberculin skin-test reactors for whom findings on the chest roentgenogram are consistent with nonprogressive tuberculous disease and in whom there are neither positive bacteriologic findings nor a history of adequate chemotherapy.
3. Newly infected persons.
4. Positive tuberculin skin-test reactors in the following special clinical situations:
   a. Prolonged therapy with adrenocorticosteroids
   b. Immunosuppressive therapy
   c. Some hematologic and reticuloendothelial diseases, such as leukemia or Hodgkin's disease
   d. Diabetes mellitus
   e. Silicosis
   f. After gastrectomy
5. Other positive tuberculin reactors who are less than 35 years of age.

The risk of hepatitis must be weighed against the risk of tuberculosis in positive tuberculin reactors over the age of 35. However, the use of isoniazid is recommended for those with the additional risk factors listed above (1–4) and, on an individual basis, in situations in which there is a likelihood of serious consequences to contacts who may become infected.

Contraindications: Isoniazid is contraindicated in patients with previous isoniazid-associated hepatic injury; severe adverse reactions to isoniazid, such as drug fever, chills, and arthritis; or acute liver disease of any etiology.

Warning: See the boxed warning.

Precautions: Use of isoniazid should be carefully monitored in the following:

1. Patients who are receiving phenytoin concurrently. Isoniazid may decrease the excretion of phenytoin or may enhance its effects. To avoid phenytoin intoxication, appropriate dosage adjustment of the anticonvulsant should be made.
2. Daily users of alcohol. Daily ingestion of alcohol may be associated with a higher incidence of isoniazid-related hepatitis.
3. Patients with active chronic liver disease or severe renal dysfunction.

Periodic ophthalmologic examinations during isoniazid therapy are recommended when visual symptoms occur.

Usage in Pregnancy and Lactation: It has been reported that isoniazid may exert an embryocidal effect in both rats and rabbits when administered orally during pregnancy, but no isoniazid-related congenital anomalies have been found in reproduction studies in mammalian species (mice, rats, and rabbits). Isoniazid should be prescribed during pregnancy only when therapeutically necessary. The benefit of preventive therapy should be weighed against a possible risk to the fetus. Preventive treatment generally should be started after delivery because the risk of tuberculosis for new mothers is increased during the postpartum period. Since isoniazid is known to cross the placental barrier and to pass into maternal breast milk, neonates and breast-fed infants of isoniazid-treated mothers should be carefully observed for any evidence of adverse effects.

Carcinogenesis: Isoniazid has been reported to induce pulmonary tumors in a number of strains of mice.

Adverse Reactions: The most frequent reactions are those affecting the nervous system and the liver.
Nervous System Reactions—Peripheral neuropathy is the most common toxic effect. It is dose related, occurs most often in the malnourished and in those predisposed to neuritis (e.g., alcoholics and diabetics), and is usually preceded by paresthesias of the feet and hands. The incidence is higher in "slow inactivators."
Other neurotoxic effects that are uncommon with conventional doses are convulsions, toxic encephalopathy, optic neuritis and atrophy, memory impairment, and toxic psychosis.
Gastrointestinal Reactions—Nausea, vomiting, and epigastric distress.
Hepatic Reactions—Elevated serum transaminase levels (SGOT, SGPT), bilirubinemia, bilirubinuria, jaundice, and occasionally severe and sometimes fatal hepatitis. The common prodromal symptoms are anorexia, nausea, vomiting, fatigue, malaise, and weakness. Mild hepatic dysfunction, evidenced by mild and transient elevation of serum transaminase levels, occurs in 10 to 20 percent of patients taking isoniazid. This abnormality usually appears in the first four to six months of treatment but can develop at any time during therapy. Enzyme levels return to normal in most instances, and there is no necessity to discontinue medication. Occasionally, progressive liver damage with accompanying symptoms may occur. In such cases, the drug should be discontinued immediately. The frequency of progressive liver damage increases with age. It is rare in individuals under 20 but is seen in as many as 2.3 percent of those over 50 years of age.
Hematologic Reactions—Agranulocytosis; hemolytic, sideroblastic, or aplastic anemia; thrombocytopenia; and eosinophilia.
Hypersensitivity Reactions—Fever, skin eruptions (morbilliform, maculopapular, purpuric, or exfoliative), lymphadenopathy, and vasculitis.
Metabolic and Endocrine Reactions—Pyridoxine deficiency, pellagra, hyperglycemia, metabolic acidosis, and gynecomastia.
Miscellaneous Reactions—Rheumatic syndrome and systemic lupus erythematosus-like syndrome.

Overdosage: *Signs and Symptoms*—Isoniazid overdosage produces signs and symptoms within 30 minutes to three hours after ingestion. Nausea, vomiting, dizziness, slurring of speech, blurring of vision, and visual hallucinations (including bright colors and strange designs) are among the early manifestations. With marked overdosage, respiratory distress and C.N.S. depression, progressing rapidly from stupor to profound coma, are to be expected along with severe, intractable seizures. Severe metabolic acidosis, acetonuria, and hyperglycemia are typical laboratory findings.
Treatment — Untreated or inadequately treated cases of gross isoniazid overdosage can terminate fatally, but good response has been reported in most patients brought under adequate therapy within the first few hours after drug ingestion.
Secure the airway and establish adequate respiratory exchange. Gastric lavage is advised within the first two to three hours, but it should not be attempted until convulsions are under control. To control convulsions, administer short-acting barbiturates intravenously, followed by pyridoxine intravenously (usually 1 mg per 1 mg of isoniazid ingested).
Obtain blood samples for immediate determination of gases, electrolytes, BUN, glucose, etc., and type and cross-match blood in preparation for possible hemodialysis.
Rapid control of metabolic acidosis is fundamental to management. Give sodium bicarbonate intravenously at once and repeat as needed, adjusting subsequent dosage on the basis of laboratory findings (i.e., serum sodium, pH, etc.).
Forced osmotic diuresis must be started early and should be continued for some hours after clinical improvement has been noted to hasten renal clearance of the drug and help prevent relapse; monitor fluid intake and output.
Hemodialysis is advised for severe cases; if this is not available, peritoneal dialysis can be used concomitantly with forced diuresis.
In conjunction with measures based on initial and repeated determination of blood gases and other laboratory tests as needed, utilize meticulous respiratory and other intensive care to protect against hypoxia, hypotension, aspiration pneumonitis, etc.
Note: For preventive therapy of tuberculous infection, it is recommended that physicians be familiar with the joint recommendations of the American Thoracic Society, American Lung Association, and the Center for Disease Control, as published in the *American Review of Respiratory Disease, 110:*306, 1974, or CDC's *Morbidity and Mortality Weekly Report, 24:*71, 1975.

Dosage and Administration: *For Treatment of Tuberculosis*—Isoniazid is used in conjunction with other effective antituberculosis agents. If the bacilli become resistant, therapy must be changed to agents to which the bacilli are susceptible.

Usual Oral Dosage

Adults: 5 mg per kg (up to 300 mg) daily in a single dose.

Infants and Children: 10 to 20 mg per kg (up to 300 to 500 mg) daily in a single dose, depending on the severity of the infection.

For Preventive Therapy

Adults: 300 mg daily in a single dose.

Infants and Children: 10 mg per kg (up to 300 mg) daily in a single dose.

Continuous administration of isoniazid for a sufficient period is an essential part of the regimen, because relapse rates are higher if chemotherapy is stopped prematurely. Resistant organisms may multiply in the treatment of tuberculosis, and their emergence during treatment may necessitate a change in the regimen.

Concomitant administration of pyridoxine (B_6) is recommended in the malnourished and in those predisposed to neuropathy (e.g., alcoholics and diabetics).

How Supplied: (℞) *Isoniazid Tablets, USP: No. 1795, T93,** 100 mg (scored), in bottles of 100 and 1000; *No. 1868, U23,** 300 mg, in bottles of 100.

[080480]

ISOPROTERENOL HYDROCHLORIDE INHALATION,

see Aerolone® Solution.

KEFLIN® ℞

(cephalothin sodium)
For Injection, USP
Neutral

Description: Keflin® (cephalothin sodium, Lilly), Neutral, is a semisynthetic cephalosporin antibiotic for parenteral use. It is the sodium salt of 7-(thiophene-2-acetamido) cephalosporanic acid. Sodium bicarbonate has been added to result in reconstituted solutions having a *p*H ranging between 6 and 8.5. The total sodium content is approximately 63 mg (2.8 mEq sodium ion) per g of Keflin.

Cephalothin was synthesized in the Lilly Research Laboratories by the reaction of thiophene-2-acetic acid with 7-aminocephalosporanic acid. The cephalosporanic acid nucleus is obtained from cephalosporin C, which is produced by the fungus *Cephalosporium.*

Cephalothin is supplied as the sodium salt of 7-(thiophene-2-acetamido) cephalosporanic acid.

Cephalothin is a cream-colored crystalline solid which is stable in the dry state and moderately soluble in distilled water (250 to 300 mg/ml).

Keflin, Neutral, contains 30 mg of sodium bicarbonate/g of cephalothin sodium. Free cephalothin acid does not form within this range, and the solubility and freezability are thereby enhanced.

The molecular weight of cephalothin sodium is 418.4.

Clinical Pharmacology: *Human Pharmacology*—Keflin® (cephalothin sodium, Lilly) is a broad-spectrum antibiotic for parenteral administration. After administration of a 500-mg dose intramuscularly to normal volunteers, the average peak serum antibiotic level was 10 mcg/ml at one-half hour; with a 1-g dose, the average was about 20 mcg/ml. Following a single 1-g intravenous dose of Keflin, blood levels have been about 30 mcg/ml at 15 minutes, have ranged from 3 to 12 mcg at one hour, and have declined to about 1 mcg at four hours. With continuous infusion, at the rate of 500 mg/hour, levels have been from 14 to 20 mcg/ml of serum. Dosages of 2 g given intravenously over a 30-minute period have produced serum concentrations of 80 to 100 mcg/ml one-half hour after the infusion; levels ranged from 10 to 40 mcg/ml at one hour and from 3 to 6 mcg/ml at two hours and were not assayable after five hours.

Sixty to 70 percent of an intramuscular dose is excreted by the kidneys in the first six hours; this results in high urine levels, e.g., 800 mcg/ml of urine after a 500-mg dose and 2500 mcg/ml following 1 g. Probenecid slows tubular excretion and almost doubles peak blood levels.

Spinal-fluid levels have ranged from 0.4 to 1.4 mcg/ml in a child and from 0.15 to 5 mcg/ml in adults with meningeal inflammatory states. The antibiotic passes readily into other body fluids, e.g., pleural, joint, and ascitic fluids. Studies of amniotic fluid and cord blood show prompt transfer of Keflin across the placenta. Following single 1-g intramuscular doses of cephalothin, peak maternal levels were reached between 31 and 45 minutes after injection; the peak levels in the infants occurred about 15 minutes later. All plasma levels in the infants were far below those of the mothers. Secondary aqueous-humor levels have averaged 0.5 mcg/ml 30 minutes after a single 1-g intravenous dose. The antibiotic has been detected in bile.

Microbiology—The in vitro bactericidal action of cephalothin results from inhibition of cell-wall synthesis.

Keflin is usually active against the following organisms in vitro:

- Beta-hemolytic and other streptococci (many strains of enterococci, e.g., *Streptococcus faecalis,* are relatively resistant)
- Staphylococci, including coagulase-positive, coagulase-negative, and penicillinase-producing strains
- *S. (Diplococcus) pneumoniae*
- *Haemophilus influenzae*
- *Escherichia coli* and other coliform bacteria
- *Klebsiella*
- *Proteus mirabilis*
- *Salmonella* sp.
- *Shigella* sp.

Pseudomonas organisms are resistant to Keflin, as are most indole-producing *Proteus* species and motile *Enterobacter* species.

Susceptibility Plate Tests—If the Bauer-Kirby-Sherris-Turck method of disc susceptibility testing is used (*Am. J. Clin. Pathol., 45:*493, 1966; *Federal Register, 39:*19182-19184, 1974), a disc containing 30 mcg cephalothin should give a zone of over 17 mm when tested against a cephalothin-susceptible bacterial strain and a zone of over 14 mm with an organism of intermediate susceptibility.

Indications and Usage: Keflin® (cephalothin sodium, Lilly) is indicated for the treatment of serious infections caused by susceptible strains of the designated microorganisms in the diseases listed below. Culture and susceptibility studies should be performed. Therapy may be instituted before results of susceptibility studies are obtained.

Respiratory tract infections caused by *S. pneumoniae,* staphylococci (penicillinase and non-penicillinase-producing), group A beta-hemolytic streptococci, *Klebsiella,* and *H. influenzae*

Skin and soft-tissue infections, including peritonitis, caused by staphylococci (penicillinase and non-penicillinase-producing), group A beta-hemolytic streptococci, *E. coli, P. mirabilis,* and *Klebsiella*

Genitourinary tract infections caused by *E. coli, P. mirabilis,* and *Klebsiella*

Septicemia, including endocarditis, caused by *S. pneumoniae,* staphylococci (penicillinase and non-penicillinase-producing), group A beta-hemolytic streptococci, *S. viridans, E. coli, P. mirabilis,* and *Klebsiella*

Gastrointestinal infections caused by *Salmonella* and *Shigella* species

Meningitis caused by *S. pneumoniae,* group A beta-hemolytic streptococci, and staphylococci (penicillinase and non-penicillinase-producing)

NOTE: Inasmuch as only low levels of Keflin are found in the cerebrospinal fluid, the drug is not reliable in the treatment of meningitis and cannot be recommended for that purpose. Keflin has, however, proved to be effective in a number of cases of meningitis and may be considered for unusual circumstances in which other, more reliably effective antibiotics cannot be used.

Bone and joint infections caused by staphylococci (penicillinase and non-penicillinase-producing)

The prophylactic administration of Keflin preoperatively, intraoperatively, and postoperatively may reduce the incidence of certain postoperative infections in patients undergoing surgical procedures (e.g., vaginal hysterectomy) that are classified as contaminated or potentially contaminated.

The perioperative use of Keflin also may be effective in surgical patients in whom infection at the operative site would present a serious risk, e.g., during open-heart surgery and prosthetic arthroplasty.

The prophylactic administration of Keflin should be discontinued within a 24-hour period after the surgical procedure. If there are signs of infection, specimens for culture should be obtained for the identification of the causative organism so that appropriate therapy may be instituted. (*See* Dosage and Administration.)

NOTE: If the susceptibility tests show that the causative organism is resistant to Keflin, other appropriate antibiotic therapy should be instituted.

Contraindication: Keflin® (cephalothin sodium, Lilly) is contraindicated in persons who have shown hypersensitivity to cephalosporin antibiotics.

Warnings: BEFORE CEPHALOTHIN THERAPY IS INSTITUTED, CAREFUL INQUIRY SHOULD BE MADE CONCERNING PREVIOUS HYPERSENSITIVITY REACTIONS TO CEPHALOSPORINS AND PENICILLIN. CEPHALOSPORIN C DERIVATIVES SHOULD BE GIVEN CAUTIOUSLY TO PENICILLIN-SENSITIVE PATIENTS.

SERIOUS ACUTE HYPERSENSITIVITY REACTIONS MAY REQUIRE EPINEPHRINE AND OTHER EMERGENCY MEASURES.

There is some clinical and laboratory evidence of partial cross-allergenicity of the penicillins and the cephalosporins. Patients have been reported to have had severe reactions (including anaphylaxis) to both drugs.

Any patient who has demonstrated some form of allergy, particularly to drugs, should receive antibiotics cautiously and then only when absolutely necessary. No exception should be made with regard to Keflin® (cephalothin sodium, Lilly).

Pseudomembranous colitis has been reported with virtually all broad-spectrum antibiotics (including macrolides, semisynthetic penicillins, and cephalosporins); therefore, it is important to consider its diagnosis in patients who develop diarrhea in association with the use of antibiotics. Such colitis may range in severity from mild to life-threatening.

Treatment with broad-spectrum antibiotics alters the normal flora of the colon and may permit overgrowth of clostridia. Studies indicate that a toxin produced by *Clostridium difficile* is one primary cause of antibiotic-associated colitis.

Mild cases of pseudomembranous colitis usually respond to drug discontinuance alone. In moderate to severe cases, management should include sigmoidoscopy, appropriate bacteriologic studies, and fluid, electrolyte, and protein supplementation. When the colitis does not improve after the drug has been discontinued, or when it is severe, oral vancomycin is the drug of choice for antibiotic-associated pseudomembranous colitis produced by *C. difficile.* Other causes of colitis should be ruled out.

Precautions: *General Precautions*—Patients should be followed carefully so that any side

Continued on next page

*Identi-Code® symbol.

Lilly—Cont.

effects or unusual manifestations of drug idiosyncrasy may be detected. If an allergic reaction to Keflin® (cephalothin sodium, Lilly) occurs, the drug should be discontinued and the patient treated with the usual agents (e.g., epinephrine or other pressor amines, antihistamines, or corticosteroids).

Although Keflin rarely produces alteration in kidney function, evaluation of renal status is recommended, especially in seriously ill patients receiving maximum doses. Patients with impaired renal function should be placed on the dosage schedule recommended under Administration and Dosage. Usual doses in such individuals may result in excessive serum concentrations.

When intravenous doses of cephalothin larger than 6 g daily are given by infusion for periods longer than three days, they may be associated with thrombophlebitis, and the veins may have to be alternated. The addition of 10 to 25 mg of hydrocortisone to intravenous solutions containing 4 to 6 g of cephalothin may reduce the incidence of thrombophlebitis. The use of small IV needles in the larger available veins may be preferred.

Prolonged use of Keflin may result in the overgrowth of nonsusceptible organisms. Constant observation of the patient is essential. If superinfection occurs during therapy, appropriate measures should be taken.

A false-positive reaction for glucose in the urine may occur with Benedict's or Fehling's solution or with Clinitest® tablets but not with Tes-Tape® (Glucose Enzymatic Test Strip, USP, Lilly).

An increased incidence of nephrotoxicity has been reported following concomitant administration of cephalosporins and aminoglycoside antibiotics.

Broad-spectrum antibiotics should be prescribed with caution in individuals with a history of gastrointestinal disease, particularly colitis.

Usage in Pregnancy—Pregnancy Category B—Reproduction studies have been performed in rabbits given doses of 200 mg/kg and have revealed no evidence of impaired fertility or harm to the fetus due to Keflin. There are, however, no adequate and well-controlled studies in pregnant women. Because animal reproduction studies are not always predictive of human response, this drug should be used during pregnancy only if clearly needed.

Nursing Mothers—Caution should be exercised when Keflin is administered to a nursing woman.

Adverse Reactions: *Hypersensitivity*—Maculopapular rash, urticaria, reactions resembling serum sickness, and anaphylaxis have been reported. Eosinophilia and drug fever have been observed to be associated with other allergic reactions. These reactions are most likely to occur in patients with a history of allergy, particularly to penicillin.

Blood—Neutropenia, thrombocytopenia, and hemolytic anemia have been reported. Some individuals, particularly those with azotemia, have developed positive direct Coombs' tests during cephalothin therapy.

Liver—Transient rise in SGOT and alkaline phosphatase has been noted.

Kidney—Rise in BUN and decreased creatinine clearance have been reported, particularly in patients with prior renal impairment. The role of Keflin® (cephalothin sodium, Lilly) in renal changes is difficult to assess, because other factors predisposing to prerenal azotemia or to acute renal failure usually have been present.

Local Reactions—Pain, induration, tenderness, and elevation of temperature have been reported following repeated intramuscular injections. Thrombophlebitis has occurred and is usually associated with daily doses of more than 6 g given by infusion for longer than three days.

Gastrointestinal—Symptoms of pseudomembranous colitis may appear either during or after antibiotic treatment. Nausea and vomiting have been reported rarely.

Dosage and Administration: *In adults*, the usual dosage range is 500 mg to 1 g of cephalothin every four to six hours. A dosage of 500 mg q. 6 h. is adequate in uncomplicated pneumonia, furunculosis with cellulitis, and most urinary tract infections. In severe infections, this may be increased by giving the injections q. 4 h. or, when the desired response is not obtained, by raising the dose to 1 g. In life-threatening infections, doses up to 2 g q. 4 h. may be required.

For perioperative prophylactic use to prevent postoperative infection in contaminated or potentially contaminated surgery in adults, the following doses are recommended:

(a) 1 to 2 g administered IV just prior to surgery (approximately one-half to one hour before the initial incision);

(b) 1 to 2 g during surgery (administration modified according to the duration of the operative procedure); and

(c) 1 to 2 g q. 6 h. postoperatively for 24 hours.

In children, 20 to 30 mg/kg may be given at the times designated above.

Since Keflin has a serum half-life of 30 to 50 minutes, it is important that (1) the preoperative dose be given just prior to the start of surgery so that adequate antibiotic levels are present in the serum and tissues at the time of initial surgical incision; and (2) Keflin be administered, if necessary, at appropriate intervals during surgery to provide sufficient levels of the antibiotic at the anticipated moments of greatest exposure to infective organisms.

When renal function is reduced, an intravenous loading dose of 1 to 2 g may be given. Continued dosage schedule should be determined by degree of renal impairment, severity of infection, and susceptibility of the causative organism. The maximum doses administered should be based on the following recommendations.

DOSAGE OF KEFLIN®
(CEPHALOTHIN SODIUM, LILLY)
WHEN RENAL FUNCTION IS IMPAIRED

STATUS OF RENAL FUNCTION	MAXIMUM ADULT DOSAGE (Maintenance)
Mild Impairment (C_{cr}=80–50 ml/min)	2 g q. 6 h.
Moderate Impairment (C_{cr}=50–25 ml/min)	1.5 g q. 6 h.
Severe Impairment (C_{cr}=25–10 ml/min)	1 g q. 6 h.
Marked Impairment (C_{cr}=10–2 ml/min)	0.5 g q. 6 h.
Essentially No Function (C_{cr}= $<$2 ml/min)	0.5 g q. 8 h.

In infants and children, the dosage should be proportionately less in accordance with age, weight, and severity of infection. Daily administration of 100 mg/kg (80 to 160 mg/kg or 40 to 80 mg/lb) in divided doses has been found effective for most infections susceptible to Keflin® (cephalothin sodium, Lilly).

Antibiotic therapy in beta-hemolytic streptococcal infections should continue for at least ten days. In staphylococcal infections, surgical procedures, such as incision and drainage, should be carried out in all cases when indicated.

Keflin may be given intravenously or by deep intramuscular injection into a large muscle mass, such as the gluteus or lateral aspect of the thigh, to minimize pain and induration.

Intramuscular—Each g of cephalothin should be diluted with 4 ml of Sterile Water for Injection. If the vial contents do not completely dissolve, an additional small amount of diluent (e.g., 0.2 to 0.4 ml) may be added and the contents warmed slightly.

Intravenous—The intravenous route may be preferable for patients with bacteremia, septicemia, or other severe or life-threatening infections who may be poor risks because of lowered resistance resulting from such debilitating conditions as malnutrition, trauma, surgery, diabetes, heart failure, or malignancy, particularly if shock is present or impending. For these infections in patients with normal renal function, the intravenous dosage is 4 to 12 g of cephalothin daily. In conditions such as septicemia, 6 to 8 g/day may be given intravenously for several days at the beginning of therapy; then, depending on the clinical response and laboratory findings, the dosage may gradually be reduced.

For patients who are to receive cephalothin intravenously, it is convenient to use the 1 or 2-g 100-ml-size vial (*see* Precautions).

For intermittent intravenous administration, a solution containing 1 g cephalothin in 10 ml of diluent may be slowly injected directly into the vein over a period of three to five minutes or may be given through the tubing when the patient is receiving parenteral solutions.

Intermittent intravenous infusion with a Y-type administration set can also be accomplished while bulk intravenous solutions are being infused. However, during infusion of the solution containing Keflin® (cephalothin sodium, Lilly), it is desirable to discontinue the other solution. When this technique is employed, careful attention should be paid to the volume of the solution containing Keflin so that the calculated dose will be infused.

For continuous intravenous infusion, 1 or 2 g of cephalothin, diluted and well mixed with at least 10 ml of Sterile Water for Injection, may be added to an IV bottle containing one of the following intravenous solutions: Acetated Ringer's Injection, 5% Dextrose Injection, 5% Dextrose in Lactated Ringer's Injection, Ionosol® B in D5-W, Isolyte® M with 5% Dextrose, Lactated Ringer's Injection, Normosol®-M in D5-W, Plasma-Lyte® Injection, Plasma-Lyte®-M Injection in 5% Dextrose, Ringer's Injection, or 0.9% Sodium Chloride Injection. The choice of solution and the volume to be employed are dictated by fluid and electrolyte management.

Intraperitoneal—In peritoneal dialysis procedures, cephalothin has been added to dialysis fluid in concentrations up to 6 mg/100 ml and instilled into the peritoneal space throughout an entire dialysis (16 to 30 hours). Careful assay procedures have shown that 44 percent of the administered drug was absorbed into the bloodstream. Serum levels of 10 mcg/ml were reported, with no evidence of accumulation and no untoward local or systemic reactions. The intraperitoneal administration of solutions containing 0.1 to 4 percent Keflin in saline has been used in treating patients with peritonitis or contaminated peritoneal cavities. (The total daily dosage of Keflin should take into account the amount given by the intraperitoneal route.)

Stability: While stored under *refrigeration*, the solution has a satisfactory potency for 96 hours after reconstitution. Solutions may precipitate; they can be redissolved by being warmed to room temperature with constant agitation. Kept at *room temperature*, solutions for intramuscular injection should be given within 12 hours after being mixed. Intravenous infusions should be started within 12 hours and completed within 24 hours. For prolonged infusions, replace with a freshly prepared solution at least every 24 hours.

The concentrated solution will darken, especially at room temperature. Slight discoloration of the solution is permissible.

Solutions of Keflin® (cephalothin sodium, Lilly) in Sterile Water for Injection, 5% Dextrose Injection, or 0.9% Sodium Chloride Injection that are frozen immediately after reconstitution in the original container are stable for as long as 12 weeks when stored at −20°C. **If the product is warmed, care should be taken to avoid heating it after the thawing is complete. Once thawed, the solution should not be refrozen.**

How Supplied: (℞) *Vials Keflin® (Cephalothin Sodium for Injection, USP), Neutral,* rubber-stoppered (Dry Powder): *No. 7001,* 1 g (equivalent to cephalothin), 10-ml size, in singles (NDC 0002-7001-01) (10 per carton) and Traypak™ (multivial carton, Lilly) of 25 (NDC 0002-7001-25); *No. 7000,* 1 g (equivalent to cephalothin), 100-ml size (NDC 0002-7000-10), *No. 7003,* 2 g (equivalent to cephalothin), 20-ml size (NDC 0002-7003-10), *No. 7002,* 2 g (equivalent to cephalothin), 100-ml size (NDC 0002-7002-10), and *No. 7004,* 4 g (equivalent to cephalothin), 50-ml size (NDC 0002-7004-10), in Traypak of 10; *No. 7020,* 20 g (equivalent to cephalothin), 200-ml size, in Traypak of 6 (NDC 0002-7020-16); *No. 7190,* 1 g (equivalent to cephalothin), in Faspak™ (flexible plastic bag, Lilly) of 96 (NDC 0002-7190-74); *No. 7191,* 2 g, in Faspak of 96 (NDC 0002-7191-74). [052682]

No. 7001, 1 g—1's—6505-00-000-0072

No. 7004, 4 g—Traypak of 10—6505-00-000-0074

KEFZOL® ℞

(cefazolin sodium)
Sterile, USP

Description: Kefzol® (cefazolin sodium, Lilly) is a semisynthetic cephalosporin for parenteral administration. It is the sodium salt of 3-[[(5-methyl-1,3,4-thiadiazol-2-yl) -thio] methyl]-7- [2- (1H-tetrazol-1-yl) acetamido] -3- cephem-4-carboxylic acid. The sodium content is 48.3 mg/g of cefazolin sodium. The molecular formula is $C_{14}H_{14}N_8O_4S_3$ (sodium salt). The molecular weight is 476.5.

The dry crystalline powder is stable for at least two years when stored at room temperature (25°C). After reconstitution, the solution should be stored in a refrigerator and used within 96 hours. If kept at room temperature, the solution should be used within 24 hours.

The *p*H of the reconstituted solution is between 4.5 and 6.

Clinical Pharmacology: *Microbiology*—In vitro tests demonstrate that the bactericidal action of cephalosporins results from inhibition of cell-wall synthesis. Kefzol® (cefazolin sodium, Lilly) is active against the following organisms in vitro:

- *Staphylococcus aureus* (penicillin-sensitive and penicillin-resistant)
- Group A beta-hemolytic streptococci and other strains of streptococci (many strains of enterococci are resistant)
- *Streptococcus (Diplococcus) pneumoniae*
- *Escherichia coli*
- *Proteus mirabilis*
- *Klebsiella* species
- *Enterobacter aerogenes*
- *Haemophilus influenzae*

Most strains of *E. cloacae* and indole-positive *Proteus* (*P. vulgaris, P. morganii, P. rettgeri*) are resistant. Methicillin-resistant staphylococci, *Serratia, Pseudomonas, Mima,* and *Herellea* species are almost uniformly resistant to cefazolin.

Human Pharmacology—Table 1 demonstrates the blood levels and duration of cefazolin following intramuscular administration.

TABLE 1. SERUM CONCENTRATIONS AFTER INTRAMUSCULAR ADMINISTRATION

Dose	Serum Concentrations (mcg/ml)					
	½ hr	1 hr	2 hr	4 hr	6 hr	8 hr
250 mg	15.5	17	13	5.1	2.5	
500 mg	36.2	36.8	37.9	15.5	6.3	3
1 g*	60.1	63.8	54.3	29.3	13.2	7.1

*Average of two studies

Clinical pharmacology studies in patients hospitalized with infections indicate that cefazolin produces mean peak serum levels approximately equivalent to those seen in normal volunteers.

In a study (using normal volunteers) of constant intravenous infusion with dosages of 3.5 mg/kg for one hour (approximately 250 mg) and 1.5 mg/kg the next two hours (approximately 100 mg), cefazolin produced a steady serum level at the third hour of approximately 28 mcg/ml. Table 2 shows the average serum concentrations after I.V. injection of a single 1-g dose; average half-life was 1.4 hours.

TABLE 2. SERUM CONCENTRATIONS AFTER 1-G INTRAVENOUS DOSE

Serum Concentrations (mcg/ml)					
5 min	15 min	30 min	1 hr	2 hr	4 hr
188.4	135.8	106.8	73.7	45.6	16.5

Controlled studies on adult normal volunteers receiving 1 g four times a day for ten days, monitoring CBC, SGOT, SGPT, bilirubin, alkaline phosphatase, BUN, creatinine, and urinalysis, indicated no clinically significant changes attributed to cefazolin.

Cefazolin is excreted unchanged in the urine primarily by glomerular filtration and, to a lesser degree, by tubular secretion. Following intramuscular injection of 500 mg, 56 to 89 percent of the administered dose is recovered within six hours and 80 to nearly 100 percent in 24 hours. Cefazolin achieves peak urine concentrations greater than 1000 mcg/ml and 4000 mcg/ml respectively following 500-mg and 1-g intramuscular doses.

When cefazolin is administered to patients with unobstructed biliary tracts, high concentrations well over serum levels occur in the gallbladder tissue and bile. In the presence of obstruction, however, concentration of the antibiotic is considerably lower in bile than in serum.

Cefazolin readily crosses an inflamed synovial membrane, and the concentration of the antibiotic achieved in the joint space is comparable to levels measured in the serum.

Cefazolin readily crosses the placental barrier into the cord blood and amniotic fluid. It is present in very low concentrations in the milk of nursing mothers.

Disc Susceptibility Tests—Quantitative methods that require measurement of zone diameters give the most precise estimates of antibiotic susceptibility. One such procedure *(Am. J. Clin. Pathol., 45:*493, 1966; *Federal Register, 39:*19182-19184, 1974) has been recommended for use with discs for testing susceptibility to cephalosporin-class antibiotics. Interpretations correlate diameters of the disc test with MIC values for Kefzol® (cefazolin sodium, Lilly). With this procedure, a report from the laboratory of "susceptible" indicates that the infecting organism is likely to respond to therapy. A report of "resistant" indicates that the infecting organism is not likely to respond to therapy. A report of "intermediate susceptibility" suggests that the organism would be susceptible if high dosage is used or if the infection is confined to tissues and fluids (e.g., urine) in which high antibiotic levels are attained.

Indications and Usage: Kefzol® (cefazolin sodium, Lilly) is indicated in the treatment of the following serious infections due to susceptible organisms:

Respiratory tract infections due to *S. pneumoniae, Klebsiella* species, *H. influenzae, S. aureus* (penicillin-sensitive and penicillin-resistant), and group A beta-hemolytic streptococci

Injectable penicillin G benzathine is considered to be the drug of choice in the treatment and prevention of streptococcal infections, including the prophylaxis of rheumatic fever. Kefzol is effective in the eradication of streptococci from the nasopharynx; however, data establishing the efficacy of Kefzol in the subsequent prevention of rheumatic fever are not available at present.

Genitourinary tract infections due to *E. coli, P. mirabilis, Klebsiella* species, and some strains of *Enterobacter* and enterococci

Skin and soft-tissue infections due to *S. aureus* (penicillin-sensitive and penicillin-resistant) and group A beta-hemolytic streptococci and other strains of streptococci

Biliary tract infections due to *E. coli,* various strains of streptococci, *P. mirabilis, Klebsiella* species, and *S. aureus*

Bone and joint infections due to *S. aureus*

Septicemia due to *S. pneumoniae, S. aureus* (penicillin-sensitive and penicillin-resistant), *P. mirabilis, E. coli,* and *Klebsiella* species

Endocarditis due to *S. aureus* (penicillin-sensitive and penicillin-resistant) and group A beta-hemolytic streptococci

Appropriate culture and susceptibility studies should be performed to determine susceptibility of the causative organism to Kefzol.

Perioperative Prophylaxis—The prophylactic administration of Kefzol preoperatively, intraoperatively, and postoperatively may reduce the incidence of certain postoperative infections in patients undergoing surgical procedures that are classified as contaminated or potentially contaminated (e.g., vaginal hysterectomy or cholecystectomy in high-risk patients such as those over 70 years of age, with acute cholecystitis, obstructive jaundice, or common-bile-duct stones).

The perioperative use of Kefzol also may be effective in surgical patients in whom infection at the operative site would present a serious risk (e.g., during open-heart surgery and prosthetic arthroplasty).

The prophylactic administration of Kefzol should usually be discontinued within a 24-hour period after the surgical procedure. In surgery in which the occurrence of infection may be particularly devastating (e.g., open-heart surgery and prosthetic arthroplasty), the prophylactic administration of Kefzol may be continued for three to five days following the completion of surgery. If there are signs of infection, specimens for culture should be obtained for the identification of the causative organism so that appropriate therapy may be instituted. (*See* Dosage and Administration.)

Contraindication: Kefzol® (cefazolin sodium, Lilly) is contraindicated in patients with known allergy to the cephalosporin group of antibiotics.

Warnings: BEFORE CEFAZOLIN THERAPY IS INSTITUTED, CAREFUL INQUIRY SHOULD BE MADE CONCERNING PREVIOUS HYPERSENSITIVITY REACTIONS TO CEPHALOSPORINS AND PENICILLIN. CEPHALOSPORIN C DERIVATIVES SHOULD BE GIVEN CAUTIOUSLY TO PENICILLIN-SENSITIVE PATIENTS.

Continued on next page

*Identi-Code® symbol.

Lilly—Cont.

SERIOUS ACUTE HYPERSENSITIVITY REACTIONS MAY REQUIRE EPINEPHRINE AND OTHER EMERGENCY MEASURES.
There is some clinical and laboratory evidence of partial cross-allergenicity of the penicillins and the cephalosporins. Patients have been reported to have had severe reactions (including anaphylaxis) to both drugs.
Antibiotics, including Kefzol® (cefazolin sodium, Lilly), should be administered cautiously to any patient who has demonstrated some form of allergy, particularly to drugs.
Pseudomembranous colitis has been reported with virtually all broad-spectrum antibiotics (including macrolides, semisynthetic penicillins, and cephalosporins); therefore, it is important to consider its diagnosis in patients who develop diarrhea in association with the use of antibiotics. Such colitis may range in severity from mild to life-threatening.
Treatment with broad-spectrum antibiotics alters the normal flora of the colon and may permit overgrowth of clostridia. Studies indicate that a toxin produced by *Clostridium difficile* is one primary cause of antibiotic-associated colitis.
Mild cases of pseudomembranous colitis usually respond to drug discontinuance alone. In moderate to severe cases, management should include sigmoidoscopy, appropriate bacteriologic studies, and fluid, electrolyte, and protein supplementation. When the colitis does not improve after the drug has been discontinued, or when it is severe, oral vancomycin is the drug of choice for antibiotic-associated pseudomembranous colitis produced by *C. difficile.* Other causes of colitis should be ruled out.
Usage in Infants—Safety for use in prematures and infants under one month of age has not been established.
Precautions: *General Precautions*—If an allergic reaction to Kefzol® (cefazolin sodium, Lilly) occurs, the drug should be discontinued and the patient treated with the usual agents (e.g., epinephrine or other pressor amines, antihistamines, or corticosteroids).
Prolonged use of Kefzol may result in the overgrowth of nonsusceptible organisms. Careful clinical observation of the patient is essential. If superinfection occurs during therapy, appropriate measures should be taken.
When Kefzol is administered to patients with low urinary output because of impaired renal function, lower daily dosage is required (see dosage instructions).
A false-positive reaction for glucose in the urine may occur with Benedict's or Fehling's solution or with Clinitest® tablets but not with Tes-Tape® (Glucose Enzymatic Test Strip, USP, Lilly).
An increased incidence of nephrotoxicity has been reported following concomitant administration of cephalosporins and aminoglycoside antibiotics.
Broad-spectrum antibiotics should be prescribed with caution in individuals with a history of gastrointestinal disease, particularly colitis.
Usage in Pregnancy—Pregnancy Category B—Reproduction studies have been performed in rats given doses of 500 mg or 1 g of cefazolin/kg and have revealed no evidence of impaired fertility or harm to the fetus due to Kefzol. There are, however, no adequate and well-controlled studies in pregnant women. Because animal reproduction studies are not always predictive of human response, this drug should be used during pregnancy only if clearly needed.
Nursing Mothers—The concentration of cefazolin in mothers' milk was very low. Levels of less than 0.9 mcg/ml were found only in isolated milk samples after intramuscular administration of 500 mg three times daily for two days.
Caution should be exercised when Kefzol is administered to a nursing woman.
Adverse Reactions: The following reactions have been reported:
Hypersensitivity—Drug fever, skin rash, vulvar pruritus, and eosinophilia have occurred.
Blood—Neutropenia, leukopenia, thrombocythemia, and positive direct and indirect Coombs' tests have occurred.
Hepatic and Renal—Transient rise in SGOT, SGPT, BUN, and alkaline phosphatase levels has been observed without clinical evidence of renal or hepatic impairment.
Gastrointestinal—Symptoms of pseudomembranous colitis may appear either during or after antibiotic treatment. Nausea and vomiting have been reported rarely. Anorexia, diarrhea, and oral candidiasis (oral thrush) have been reported.
Other—Pain on intramuscular injection, sometimes with induration, has occurred infrequently. Phlebitis at the site of injection has been noted. Other reactions have included genital and anal pruritus, genital moniliasis, and vaginitis.
Dosage and Administration: Kefzol® (cefazolin sodium, Lilly) may be administered intramuscularly or intravenously after reconstitution.
Intramuscular Administration—Reconstitute with 0.9% Sodium Chloride Injection, Sterile Water for Injection, or Bacteriostatic Water for Injection according to Table 3. Shake well until dissolved. Kefzol should be injected into a large muscle mass. Pain on injection is infrequent with Kefzol.
[See table below].

TABLE 3. DILUTION TABLE FOR KEFZOL® (CEFAZOLIN SODIUM)

Vial Size	Diluent to Be Added	Approximate Available Volume	Approximate Average Concentration
250 mg	2 ml	2 ml	125 mg/ml
500 mg	2 ml	2.2 ml	225 mg/ml
1 g	2.5 ml	3 ml	330 mg/ml

Intravenous Administration—Kefzol® (cefazolin sodium, Lilly) may be administered by intravenous injection or by continuous or intermittent infusion. Total daily dosages are the same as with intramuscular injection.
Intermittent intravenous infusion: Kefzol can be administered along with primary intravenous fluid management programs in a volume control set or in a separate, secondary I.V. bottle. Reconstituted 500 mg or 1 g of Kefzol may be diluted in 50 to 100 ml of one of the following intravenous solutions: 0.9% Sodium Chloride Injection, 5% or 10% Dextrose Injection, 5% Dextrose in Lactated Ringer's Injection, 5% Dextrose and 0.9% Sodium Chloride Injection (also may be used with 5% Dextrose and 0.45% or 0.2% Sodium Chloride Injection), Lactated Ringer's Injection, 5% or 10% Invert Sugar in Sterile Water for Injection, Ringer's Injection, Normosol®-M in D5-W, Ionosol® B with Dextrose 5%, or Plasma-Lyte® with 5% Dextrose.
Direct intravenous injection: Dilute the reconstituted 500 mg or 1 g of Kefzol in a minimum of 10 ml of Sterile Water for Injection. Inject solution slowly over three to five minutes. It may be administered directly into a vein or through the tubing for a patient receiving the above parenteral fluids.
Dosage—The usual adult dosages are given in Table 4.

TABLE 4. USUAL ADULT DOSAGE OF KEFZOL® (CEFAZOLIN SODIUM)

Type of Infection	Dose	Frequency
Pneumococcal pneumonia	500 mg	q. 12 h.
Mild infections caused by susceptible gram-positive cocci	250 to 500 mg	q. 8 h.
Acute uncomplicated urinary tract infections	1 g	q. 12 h.
Moderate to severe infections	500 mg to 1 g	q. 6 to 8 h.

Cefazolin has been administered in dosages of 6 to 12 g per day in life-threatening infections such as endocarditis and septicemia.
In adults with renal impairment, cefazolin is not readily excreted. After a loading dose of 500 mg, the following recommendations for *maintenance dosage* (Table 5) may be used as a guide.
[See Table 5 above].

TABLE 5. MAINTENANCE DOSAGE OF KEFZOL® (CEFAZOLIN SODIUM) IN ADULTS WITH REDUCED RENAL FUNCTION

Renal Function	BUN* (mg %)	Creatinine Clearance (ml/min)	Dosage: Mild to Moderate Infection	Dosage: Moderate to Severe Infection	Serum Half-Life (Hours)
Mild impairment	20–34	70–40	250 to 500 mg q. 12 h.	500 mg to 1.25 g q. 12 h.	3–5
Moderate impairment	35–49	40–20	125 to 250 mg q. 12 h.	250 to 600 mg q. 12 h.	6–12
Severe impairment	50–75	20–5	75 to 150 mg q. 24 h.	150 to 400 mg q. 24 h.	15–30
Essentially no function	> 75	< 5	37.5 to 75 mg q. 24 h.	75 to 200 mg q. 24 h.	30–40

*If used to estimate degree of renal impairment, BUN concentrations should reflect a steady state of renal azotemia.

Perioperative Prophylactic Use—To prevent postoperative infection in contaminated or potentially contaminated surgery, the recommended doses are as follows:

a. 1 g IV or IM administered one-half to one hour prior to the start of surgery.
b. For lengthy operative procedures (e.g., two hours or more), 0.5 to 1 g IV or IM during surgery (administration modified according to the duration of the operative procedure).
c. 0.5 to 1 g IV or IM every six to eight hours postoperatively.

It is important that (1) the preoperative dose be given just (one-half to one hour) prior to the start of surgery so that adequate antibiotic levels are present in the serum and tissues at the time of the initial surgical incision and (2) Kefzol be administered, if necessary, at appropriate intervals during surgery to provide sufficient levels of the antibiotic at the anticipated moments of greatest exposure to infective organisms.

In surgery in which the occurrence of infection may be particularly devastating (e.g., open-heart surgery and prosthetic arthroplasty), the prophylactic administration of Kefzol may be continued for three to five days following the completion of surgery.

In children, a total daily dosage of 25 to 50 mg/kg (approximately 10 to 20 mg/lb) of body weight, divided into three or four equal doses, is effective for most mild to moderately severe infections (Table 6). Total daily dosage may be increased to 100 mg/kg (45 mg/lb) of body weight for severe infections.

TABLE 6. PEDIATRIC DOSAGE GUIDE FOR KEFZOL® (CEFAZOLIN SODIUM)

Weight		**25 mg/kg/Day Divided into 3 Doses**		**25 mg/kg/Day Divided into 4 Doses**	
lb	kg	Approximate Single Dose (mg q. 8 h.)	Vol. (ml) Needed with Dilution of 125 mg/ml	Approximate Single Dose (mg q. 6 h.)	Vol. (ml) Needed with Dilution of 125 mg/ml
10	4.5	40 mg	0.35 ml	30 mg	0.25 ml
20	9	75 mg	0.6 ml	55 mg	0.45 ml
30	13.6	115 mg	0.9 ml	85 mg	0.7 ml
40	18.1	150 mg	1.2 ml	115 mg	0.9 ml
50	22.7	190 mg	1.5 ml	140 mg	1.1 ml

Weight		**50 mg/kg/Day Divided into 3 Doses**		**50 mg/kg/Day Divided into 4 Doses**	
lb	kg	Approximate Single Dose (mg q. 8 h.)	Vol. (ml) Needed with Dilution of 225 mg/ml	Approximate Single Dose (mg q. 6 h.)	Vol. (ml) Needed with Dilution of 225 mg/ml
10	4.5	75 mg	0.35 ml	55 mg	0.25 ml
20	9	150 mg	0.7 ml	110 mg	0.5 ml
30	13.6	225 mg	1 ml	170 mg	0.75 ml
40	18.1	300 mg	1.35 ml	225 mg	1 ml
50	22.7	375 mg	1.7 ml	285 mg	1.25 ml

In children with mild to moderate renal impairment (creatinine clearance of 70 to 40 ml/min), 60 percent of the normal daily dose given in divided doses every 12 hours should be sufficient. In patients with moderate impairment (creatinine clearance of 40 to 20 ml/min), 25 percent of the normal daily dose given in divided doses every 12 hours should be sufficient. In children with severe impairment (creatinine clearance of 20 to 5 ml/min), 10 percent of the normal daily dose given every 24 hours should be adequate. All dosage recommendations apply after an initial loading dose. Since safety for use in premature infants and in infants under one month of age has not been established, the use of Kefzol in these patients is not recommended.

Stability: Reconstituted Kefzol® (cefazolin sodium, Lilly) and dilutions of Kefzol in the recommended intravenous fluids are stable for 24 hours at room temperature and for 96 hours if stored under refrigeration (5°C).

Solutions of Kefzol in Sterile Water for Injection, 5% Dextrose Injection, or 0.9% Sodium Chloride Injection that are frozen immediately after reconstitution in the original container are stable for as long as 12 weeks when stored at −20°C. **If the product is warmed, care should be taken to avoid heating it after the thawing is complete. Once thawed, the solution should not be refrozen.**

How Supplied: (℞) *Vials Kefzol® (Sterile Cefazolin Sodium, USP),* rubber-stoppered (Dry Powder): *No. 766,* 250 mg (equivalent to cefazolin), 10-ml size (NDC 0002-1496-01), in singles (10 per carton); *No. 767,* 500 mg (equivalent to cefazolin), and *No. 768,* 1 g (equivalent to cefazolin), 10-ml size, in singles (NDC 0002-1497-01 and NDC 0002-1498-01) (10 per carton) and in Traypak™ (multivial carton, Lilly) of 25 (NDC 0002-1497-25 and NDC 0002-1498-25); *No. 7018,* 500 mg (equivalent to cefazolin) (NDC 0002-7018-10), and *No. 7011,* 1 g (equivalent to cefazolin) (NDC 0002-7011-10), 100-ml size, in Traypak of 10; *No. 7014,* 10 g (equivalent to cefazolin), 100-ml size, in Traypak of 6 (NDC 0002-7014-16).

(℞) *Redi Vial® (dual compartment vial, Lilly) Kefzol® (Sterile Cefazolin Sodium, USP): No. 7082,* 500 mg (equivalent to cefazolin), and *No. 7083,* 1 g (equivalent to cefazolin), in singles (NDC 0002-7082-01 and NDC 0002-7083-01) (10 per carton) and in Traypak of 10 (NDC 0002-7082-10 and NDC 0002-7083-10). [052782]

LENTE® ILETIN® I (insulin zinc suspension, Lilly), *see under* Iletin® (insulin, Lilly).

MANDOL® ℞
(cefamandole nafate)
For Injection
USP

Description: Mandol® (cefamandole nafate, Lilly) is a semisynthetic broad-spectrum cephalosporin antibiotic for parenteral administration. It is the sodium salt of 7-D-mandelamido-3-[[(1-methyl-1*H*-tetrazol-5-yl)-thio]-methyl]-3-cephem-4-carboxylic acid, formate (ester). Mandol also contains 63 mg sodium carbonate/g of cefamandole activity. The total sodium content is approximately 77 mg (3.3 mEq sodium ion)/g of cefamandole activity. After addition of diluent, cefamandole nafate rapidly hydrolyzes to cefamandole, and both compounds have microbiologic activity in vivo. Solutions of Mandol range from light-yellow to amber, depending on concentration and diluent used. The *p*H of freshly reconstituted solutions usually ranges from 6.0 to 8.5.

Clinical Pharmacology: After intramuscular administration of a 500-mg dose of cefamandole to normal volunteers, the mean peak serum concentration was 13 mcg/ml. After a 1-g dose, the mean peak concentration was 25 mcg/ml. These peaks occurred at 30 to 120 minutes. Following intravenous doses of 1, 2, and 3 g, serum concentrations were 139, 240, and 533 mcg/ml respectively at ten minutes. These concentrations declined to 0.8, 2.2, and 2.9 mcg/ml at four hours. Intravenous administration of 4-g doses every six hours produced no evidence of accumulation in the serum. The half-life after an intravenous dose is 32 minutes; after intramuscular administration, the half-life is 60 minutes.

Sixty-five to 85 percent of cefamandole is excreted by the kidneys over an eight-hour period, resulting in high urinary concentrations. Following intramuscular doses of 500 mg and 1 g, urinary concentrations averaged 254 and 1357 mcg/ml respectively. Intravenous doses of 1 and 2 g produced urinary levels averaging 750 and 1380 mcg/ml respectively. Probenecid slows tubular excretion and doubles the peak serum level and the duration of measurable serum concentrations.

The antibiotic reaches therapeutic levels in pleural and joint fluids and in bile and bone.

Microbiology—The bactericidal action of cefamandole results from inhibition of cell-wall synthesis. Cephalosporins have in vitro activity against a wide range of gram-positive and gram-negative organisms. Cefamandole is usually active against the following organisms in vitro and in clinical infections:

Gram-positive
- *Staphylococcus aureus,* including penicillinase and non-penicillinase-producing strains
- *S. epidermidis*
- Beta-hemolytic and other streptococci (Most strains of enterococci, e.g., *Streptococcus faecalis,* are resistant.)
- *S. pneumoniae* (formerly *Diplococcus pneumoniae*)

Gram-negative
- *Escherichia coli*
- *Klebsiella* species
- *Enterobacter* species (Initially susceptible organisms occasionally may become resistant during therapy.)
- *Haemophilus influenzae*
- *Proteus mirabilis*
- *P. rettgeri*
- *P. morganii*
- *P. vulgaris* (Some strains of *P. vulgaris* have been shown by in vitro tests to be resistant to cefamandole and other cephalosporins.)

Anaerobic organisms
- Gram-positive and gram-negative cocci (including *Peptococcus* and *Peptostreptococcus* species)
- Gram-positive bacilli (including *Clostridium* species)
- Gram-negative bacilli (including *Bacteroides* and *Fusobacterium* species). Most strains of *Bacteroides fragilis* are resistant.

Pseudomonas, Acinetobacter calcoaceticus (formerly *Mima* and *Herellea* species), and most *Serratia* strains are resistant to cephalosporins. Cefamandole is resistant to degradation by beta-lactamases from certain members of the *Enterobacteriaceae.*

Susceptibility Tests—Quantitative methods that require measurement of zone diameters give the most precise estimates of antibiotic susceptibility. One such procedure[1] has been recommended for use with discs to test susceptibility to cefamandole. Interpretation involves correlation of the diameters obtained in the disc test with minimum inhibitory concentration (MIC) values for cefamandole.

Reports from the laboratory giving results of the standardized single-disc susceptibility test[1] using a 30-mcg cefamandole disc should be interpreted according to the following criteria:

- Susceptible organisms produce zones of 18 mm or greater, indicating that the tested organism is likely to respond to therapy.
- Organisms of intermediate susceptibility produce zones of 15 to 17 mm, indicating that the tested organism would be susceptible if high dosage is used or if the infection is confined to tissues and fluids (e.g., urine), in which high antibiotic levels are attained.
- Resistant organisms produce zones of 14 mm or less, indicating that other therapy should be selected.

For gram-positive isolates, the test may be performed with either the cephalosporin-class disc

Continued on next page

*Identi-Code® symbol.

Lilly—Cont.

(30 mcg cephalothin) or the cefamandole disc (30 mcg cefamandole), and a zone of 18 mm is indicative of a cefamandole-susceptible organism.

Gram-negative organisms should be tested with the cefamandole disc (using the above criteria), since cefamandole has been shown by in vitro tests to have activity against certain strains of *Enterobacteriaceae* found resistant when tested with the cephalosporin-class disc. Gram-negative organisms having zones of less than 18 mm around the cephalothin disc are not necessarily of intermediate susceptibility or resistant to cefamandole.

The cefamandole disc should not be used for testing susceptibility to other cephalosporins.

A bacterial isolate may be considered susceptible if the MIC value for cefamandole[2] is not more than 16 mcg/ml. Organisms are considered resistant if the MIC is greater than 32 mcg/ml.

Indications and Usage: Mandol® (cefamandole nafate, Lilly) is indicated for the treatment of serious infections caused by susceptible strains of the designated microorganisms in the diseases listed below:

- Lower respiratory infections, including pneumonia caused by *S. pneumoniae (D. pneumoniae), H. influenzae, Klebsiella* species, *S. aureus* (penicillinase and non-penicillinase-producing), beta-hemolytic streptococci, and *P. mirabilis*
- Urinary tract infections caused by *E. coli, Proteus* species (both indole-negative and indole-positive), *Enterobacter* species, *Klebsiella* species, group D streptococci (*Note:* Most enterococci, e.g., *S. faecalis,* are resistant), and *S. epidermidis*
- Peritonitis caused by *E. coli* and *Enterobacter* species
- Septicemia caused by *E. coli, S. aureus* (penicillinase and non-penicillinase-producing), *S. pneumoniae, S. pyogenes* (group A beta-hemolytic streptococci), *H. influenzae,* and *Klebsiella* species
- Skin and skin-structure infections caused by *S. aureus* (penicillinase and non-penicillinase-producing), *S. pyogenes* (group A beta-hemolytic streptococci), *H. influenzae. E. coli, Enterobacter* species, and *P. mirabilis*
- Bone and joint infections caused by *S. aureus* (penicillinase and non-penicillinase-producing)

Clinical microbiologic studies in nongonococcal pelvic inflammatory disease in females, lower respiratory infections, and skin infections frequently reveal the growth of susceptible strains of both aerobic and anaerobic organisms. Mandol has been used successfully in these infections in which several organisms have been isolated. Most strains of *B. fragilis* are resistant in vitro; however, infections caused by susceptible strains have been treated successfully.

Specimens for bacteriologic cultures should be obtained in order to isolate and identify causative organisms and to determine their susceptibilities to cefamandole. Therapy may be instituted before results of susceptibility studies are known; however, once these results become available, the antibiotic treatment should be adjusted accordingly.

In certain cases of confirmed or suspected gram-positive or gram-negative sepsis or in patients with other serious infections in which the causative organism has not been identified, Mandol may be used concomitantly with an aminoglycoside (*see* Precautions). The recommended doses of both antibiotics may be given, depending on the severity of the infection and the patient's condition. The renal function of the patient should be carefully monitored, especially if higher dosages of the antibiotics are to be administered.

Antibiotic therapy of beta-hemolytic streptococcal infections should continue for at least ten days.

Preventive Therapy—The administration of Mandol preoperatively, intraoperatively, and postoperatively may reduce the incidence of certain postoperative infections in patients undergoing surgical procedures that are classified as contaminated or potentially contaminated (e.g., gastrointestinal surgery, cesarean section, vaginal hysterectomy, or cholecystectomy in high-risk patients such as those with acute cholecystitis, obstructive jaundice, or common-bile-duct stones).

In major surgery in which the risk of postoperative infection is low but serious (cardiovascular surgery, neurosurgery, or prosthetic arthroplasty), Mandol may be effective in preventing such infections.

The perioperative use of Mandol should be discontinued after 24 hours; however, in prosthetic arthroplasty, it is recommended that administration be continued for 72 hours. If signs of infection occur, specimens for culture should be obtained for identification of the causative organism so that appropriate antibiotic therapy may be instituted.

Contraindication: Mandol® (cefamandole nafate, Lilly) is contraindicated in patients with known allergy to the cephalosporin group of antibiotics.

Warnings: BEFORE THERAPY WITH MANDOL® (cefamandole nafate, Lilly) IS INSTITUTED, CAREFUL INQUIRY SHOULD BE MADE TO DETERMINE WHETHER THE PATIENT HAS HAD PREVIOUS HYPERSENSITIVITY REACTIONS TO CEPHALOSPORINS, PENICILLINS, OR OTHER DRUGS. THIS PRODUCT SHOULD BE GIVEN CAUTIOUSLY TO PENICILLIN-SENSITIVE PATIENTS. ANTIBIOTICS SHOULD BE ADMINISTERED WITH CAUTION TO ANY PATIENT WHO HAS DEMONSTRATED SOME FORM OF ALLERGY, PARTICULARLY TO DRUGS. SERIOUS ACUTE HYPERSENSITIVITY REACTIONS MAY REQUIRE EPINEPHRINE AND OTHER EMERGENCY MEASURES.

In newborn infants, accumulation of other cephalosporin-class antibiotics (with resulting prolongation of drug half-life) has been reported.

Pseudomembranous colitis has been reported with virtually all broad-spectrum antibiotics (including macrolides, semisynthetic penicillins, and cephalosporins); therefore, it is important to consider its diagnosis in patients who develop diarrhea in association with the use of antibiotics. Such colitis may range in severity from mild to life-threatening.

Treatment with broad-spectrum antibiotics alters the normal flora of the colon and may permit overgrowth of clostridia. Studies indicate that a toxin produced by *Clostridium difficile* is one primary cause of antibiotic-associated colitis.

Mild cases of pseudomembranous colitis usually respond to drug discontinuance alone. In moderate to severe cases, management should include sigmoidoscopy, appropriate bacteriologic studies, and fluid, electrolyte, and protein supplementation. When the colitis does not improve after the drug has been discontinued, or when it is severe, oral vancomycin is the drug of choice for antibiotic-associated pseudomembranous colitis produced by *C. difficile.* Other causes of colitis should be ruled out.

Precautions: *General Precautions*—Although Mandol® (cefamandole nafate, Lilly) rarely produces alteration in kidney function, evaluation of renal status is recommended, especially in seriously ill patients receiving maximum doses.

Prolonged use of Mandol may result in the overgrowth of nonsusceptible organisms. Careful observation of the patient is essential. If superinfection occurs during therapy, appropriate measures should be taken.

Nephrotoxicity has been reported following concomitant administration of aminoglycoside antibiotics and cephalosporins.

A false-positive reaction for glucose in the urine may occur with Benedict's or Fehling's solution or with Clinitest® tablets but not with Tes-Tape® (Glucose Enzymatic Test Strip, USP, Lilly). There may be a false-positive test for proteinuria with acid and denaturization-precipitation tests.

As with other broad-spectrum antibiotics, hypoprothrombinemia, with or without bleeding, has been reported rarely, but it has been promptly reversed by administration of vitamin K. Such episodes usually have occurred in elderly, debilitated, or otherwise compromised patients with deficient stores of vitamin K. Treatment of such individuals with antibiotics possessing significant gram-negative and/or anaerobic activity is thought to alter the number and/or type of intestinal bacterial flora, with consequent reduction in synthesis of vitamin K. Prophylactic administration of vitamin K may be indicated in such patients, especially when intestinal sterilization and surgical procedures are performed.

In a few patients receiving Mandol, nausea, vomiting, and vasomotor instability with hypotension and peripheral vasodilatation occurred following the ingestion of ethanol.

Cefamandole inhibits the enzyme acetaldehyde dehydrogenase in laboratory animals. This causes accumulation of acetaldehyde when ethanol is administered concomitantly.

Broad-spectrum antibiotics should be prescribed with caution in individuals with a history of gastrointestinal disease, particularly colitis.

Usage in Pregnancy—Pregnancy Category B—Reproduction studies have been performed in rats given doses of 500 or 1000 mg/kg/day and have revealed no evidence of impaired fertility or harm to the fetus due to Mandol. There are, however, no adequate and well-controlled studies in pregnant women. Because animal reproduction studies are not always predictive of human response, this drug should be used during pregnancy only if clearly needed.

Nursing Mothers—Caution should be exercised when Mandol is administered to a nursing woman.

Usage in Infancy—Mandol has been effectively used in this age group, but all laboratory parameters have not been extensively studied in infants between one and six months of age; safety of this product has not been established in prematures and infants under one month of age. Therefore, if Mandol is administered to infants, the physician should determine whether the potential benefits outweigh the possible risks involved.

Adverse Reactions: *Gastrointestinal*—Symptoms of pseudomembranous colitis may appear either during or after antibiotic treatment. Nausea and vomiting have been reported rarely.

Hypersensitivity—Maculopapular rash, urticaria, eosinophilia, and drug fever have been reported. These reactions are more likely to occur in patients with a history of allergy, particularly to penicillin.

Blood—Thrombocytopenia has been reported rarely. Neutropenia has been reported, especially in long courses of treatment. Some individuals have developed positive direct Coombs' tests during treatment with the cephalosporin antibiotics.

Liver—Transient rise in SGOT, SGPT, and alkaline phosphatase levels has been noted.

Kidney—Decreased creatinine clearance has been reported in patients with prior renal impairment. As with some other cephalosporins, transitory elevations of BUN have occasionally been observed with Mandol® (cefamandole nafate, Lilly); their frequency increases in patients over 50 years of age. In some of these cases, there was also a mild increase in serum creatinine.

Local Reactions—Pain on intramuscular injection is infrequent. Thrombophlebitis occurs rarely.

Dosage and Administration: *Dosage—Adults:* The usual dosage range for cefamandole is 500 mg to 1 g every four to eight hours. In infections of skin structures and in uncomplicated pneumonia, a dosage of 500 mg every six hours is adequate.

In uncomplicated urinary tract infections, a dosage of 500 mg every eight hours is sufficient. In more serious urinary tract infections, a dosage of 1 g every eight hours may be needed.

In severe infections, 1-g doses may be given at four to six-hour intervals.

In life-threatening infections or infections due to less susceptible organisms, doses up to 2 g every four hours (i.e., 12 g/day) may be needed.

Infants and Children: Administration of 50 to 100 mg/kg/day in equally divided doses every four to eight hours has been effective for most infections susceptible to Mandol® (cefamandole nafate, Lilly). This may be increased to a total daily dose of 150 mg/kg (not to exceed the maximum adult dose) for severe infections. (*See* Warnings and Precautions for this age group.)

Note: As with antibiotic therapy in general, administration of Mandol should be continued for a minimum of 48 to 72 hours after the patient becomes asymptomatic or after evidence of bacterial eradication has been obtained; a minimum of ten days of treatment is recommended in infections caused by group A beta-hemolytic streptococci in order to guard against the risk of rheumatic fever or glomerulonephritis; frequent bacteriologic and clinical appraisal is necessary during therapy of chronic urinary tract infection and may be required for several months after therapy has been completed; persistent infections may require treatment for several weeks; and doses smaller than those indicated above should not be used.

For perioperative use of Mandol, the following dosages are recommended:

Adults—1 or 2 g intravenously or intramuscularly one-half to one hour prior to the surgical incision followed by 1 or 2 g every six hours for 24 to 48 hours.

Children (three months of age and older)—50 to 100 mg/kg/day in equally divided doses by the routes and schedule designated above.

Note: In patients undergoing prosthetic arthroplasty, administration is recommended for as long as 72 hours.

In patients undergoing cesarean section, the initial dose may be administered just prior to surgery or immediately after the cord has been clamped.

Impaired Renal Function—When renal function is impaired, a reduced dosage must be employed and the serum levels closely monitored. After an initial dose of 1 to 2 g (depending on the severity of infection), a maintenance dosage schedule should be followed (see chart). Continued dosage should be determined by degree of renal impairment, severity of infection, and susceptibility of the causative organism.

[See table above].

When only serum creatinine is available, the following formula (based on sex, weight, and age of the patient) may be used to convert this value into creatinine clearance. The serum creatinine should represent a steady state of renal function.

$$\text{Males: } \frac{\text{Weight (kg)} \times (140 - \text{age})}{72 \times \text{serum creatinine}}$$

Females: $0.9 \times$ above value

Modes of Administration—Mandol® (cefamandole nafate, Lilly) may be given intravenously or by deep intramuscular injection into a large muscle mass (such as the gluteus or lateral part of the thigh) to minimize pain.

Intramuscular Administration—Each g of Mandol should be diluted with 3 ml of one of the following diluents: Sterile Water for Injection, Bacteriostatic Water for Injection, 0.9% Sodium Chloride Injection, or Bacteriostatic Sodium Chloride Injection. Shake well until dissolved.

Intravenous Administration—The intravenous route may be preferable for patients with bacterial septicemia, localized parenchymal abscesses (such as intra-abdominal abscess), peritonitis, or other severe or life-threatening infections when they may be poor risks because of lowered resistance. In those with normal renal function, the intravenous dosage for such infections is 3 to 12 g of Mandol daily. In conditions such as bacterial septicemia, 6 to 12 g/day may be given initially by the intravenous route for several days, and dosage may then be gradually reduced according to clinical response and laboratory findings.

If combination therapy with Mandol and an aminoglycoside is indicated, each of these antibiotics should be administered in different sites. *Do not mix an aminoglycoside with Mandol in the same intravenous fluid container.*

A SOLUTION OF 1 G MANDOL IN 22 ML OF STERILE WATER FOR INJECTION IS ISOTONIC.

The choice of saline, dextrose, or electrolyte solution and the volume to be employed are dictated by fluid and electrolyte management.

For direct intermittent intravenous administration, each g of cefamandole should be reconstituted with 10 ml of Sterile Water for Injection, 5% Dextrose Injection, or 0.9% Sodium Chloride Injection. Slowly inject the solution into the vein over a period of three to five minutes, or give it through the tubing of an administration set while the patient is also receiving one of the following intravenous fluids: 0.9% Sodium Chloride Injection; 5% Dextrose Injection; 10% Dextrose Injection; 5% Dextrose and 0.9% Sodium Chloride Injection; 5% Dextrose and 0.45% Sodium Chloride Injection; 5% Dextrose and 0.2% Sodium Chloride Injection; or Sodium Lactate Injection (M/6).

Intermittent intravenous infusion with a Y-type administration set or volume control set can also be accomplished while any of the above-mentioned intravenous fluids are being infused. However, during infusion of the solution containing Mandol® (cefamandole nafate, Lilly), it is desirable to discontinue the other solution. When this technique is employed, careful attention should be paid to the volume of the solution containing Mandol so that the calculated dose will be infused. When a Y-tube hookup is used, 100 ml of the appropriate diluent should be added to the 1 or 2-g piggyback (100-ml) vial. If Sterile Water for Injection is used as the diluent, reconstitute with approximately 20 ml/g to avoid a hypotonic solution.

For continuous intravenous infusion, each g of cefamandole should be diluted with 10 ml of Sterile Water for Injection. An appropriate quantity of the resulting solution may be added to an IV bottle containing one of the following fluids: 0.9% Sodium Chloride Injection; 5% Dextrose Injection; 10% Dextrose Injection; 5% Dextrose and 0.9% Sodium Chloride Injection; 5% Dextrose and 0.45% Sodium Chloride Injection; 5% Dextrose and 0.2% Sodium Chloride Injection; or Sodium Lactate Injection (M/6).

Stability: Reconstituted Mandol® (cefamandole nafate, Lilly) is stable for 24 hours at room temperature (25°C) and for 96 hours if stored under refrigeration (5°C). *During storage at room temperature, carbon dioxide develops inside the vial after reconstitution. This pressure may be dissipated prior to withdrawal of the vial contents, or it may be used to aid withdrawal if the vial is inverted over the syringe needle and the contents are allowed to flow into the syringe.*

Solutions of Mandol in Sterile Water for Injection, 5% Dextrose Injection, or 0.9% Sodium Chloride Injection that are frozen immediately after reconstitution in the original container are stable for six months when stored at −20°C. If the product is warmed (to a maximum of 37°C), care should be taken to avoid heating it after the thawing is complete. Once thawed, the solution should not be refrozen.

How Supplied: (℞) *Vials Mandol® (Cefamandole Nafate for Injection, USP),* rubber-stoppered (Dry Powder): *No. 7060,* 500 mg (equivalent to cefamandole activity) (NDC 0002-7060-25), and *No. 7061,* 1 g (equivalent to cefamandole activity) (NDC 0002-7061-25), 10-ml size, in Traypak™ (multivial carton, Lilly) of 25; *No. 7068,* 1 g (equivalent to cefamandole activity), 100-ml size (NDC 0002-7068-10), *No. 7064,* 2 g (equivalent to cefamandole activity), 20-ml size (NDC 0002-7064-10), and *No. 7069,* 2 g (equivalent to cefamandole activity), 100-ml

Continued on next page

*Identi-Code® symbol.

MANDOL® (CEFAMANDOLE NAFATE)—MAINTENANCE DOSAGE GUIDE FOR PATIENTS WITH RENAL IMPAIRMENT

Creatinine Clearance (ml/min/1.73 m²)	Renal Function	Life-Threatening Infections—Maximum Dosage	Less Severe Infections
>80	Normal	2 g q. 4 h.	1–2 g q. 6 h.
80–50	Mild Impairment	1.5 g q. 4 h. OR 2 g q. 6 h.	0.75–1.5 g q. 6 h.
50–25	Moderate Impairment	1.5 g q. 6 h. OR 2 g q. 8 h.	0.75–1.5 g q. 8 h.
25–10	Severe Impairment	1 g q. 6 h. OR 1.25 g q. 8 h.	0.5–1 g q. 8 h.
10–2	Marked Impairment	0.67 g q. 8 h. OR 1 g q. 12 h.	0.5–0.75 g q. 12 h.
<2	None	0.5 g q. 8 h. OR 0.75 g q. 12 h.	0.25–0.5 g q. 12 h.

Lilly—Cont.

size (NDC 0002-7069-10), in Traypak of 10. [061182]

1. Bauer, A. W., Kirby, W. M. M., Sherris, J. C., and Turck, M.: Antibiotic Susceptibility Testing by a Standardized Single Disk Method, Am. J. Clin. Pathol., *45*:493, 1966; Standardized Disc Susceptibility Test, Federal Register, *39*:19182-19184, 1974. National Committee for Clinical Laboratory Standards. Approved Standard: ASM-2, Performance Standards for Antimicrobial Disc Susceptibility Tests, July, 1975.
2. Determined by the ICS agar-dilution method (Ericsson, H. M., and Sherris, J. C.: Acta Pathol. Microbiol. Scand. [B], Supplement No. 217, 1971) or any other method that has been shown to give equivalent results.

METHADONE HYDROCHLORIDE Ⓒ
DISKETS® (dispersible tablets, Lilly)
Tablets, USP
(*See also* Dolophine® Hydrochloride)

CONDITIONS FOR DISTRIBUTION AND USE OF METHADONE PRODUCTS:

Code of Federal Regulations, Title 21, Sec. 291.505

METHADONE PRODUCTS, WHEN USED FOR THE TREATMENT OF NARCOTIC ADDICTION IN DETOXIFICATION OR MAINTENANCE PROGRAMS, SHALL BE DISPENSED ONLY BY APPROVED HOSPITAL PHARMACIES, APPROVED COMMUNITY PHARMACIES, AND MAINTENANCE PROGRAMS APPROVED BY THE FOOD AND DRUG ADMINISTRATION AND THE DESIGNATED STATE AUTHORITY.

APPROVED MAINTENANCE PROGRAMS SHALL DISPENSE AND USE METHADONE IN ORAL FORM ONLY AND ACCORDING TO THE TREATMENT REQUIREMENTS STIPULATED IN THE FEDERAL METHADONE REGULATIONS (21 CFR 291.505).

FAILURE TO ABIDE BY THE REQUIREMENTS IN THESE REGULATIONS MAY RESULT IN CRIMINAL PROSECUTION, SEIZURE OF THE DRUG SUPPLY, REVOCATION OF THE PROGRAM APPROVAL, AND INJUNCTION PRECLUDING OPERATION OF THE PROGRAM.

Description: Methadone Hydrochloride, USP (4, 4- diphenyl -6- dimethylamino - heptanone-3 hydrochloride), is a white crystalline material which is water soluble. However, the Disket preparation of methadone hydrochloride has been specially formulated with insoluble excipients to deter the use of this drug by injection.

Actions: Methadone hydrochloride is a synthetic narcotic analgesic with multiple actions quantitatively similar to those of morphine, the most prominent of which involve the central nervous system and organs composed of smooth muscle. The principal actions of therapeutic value are analgesia and sedation and detoxification or maintenance in narcotic addiction. The methadone abstinence syndrome, although qualitatively similar to that of morphine, differs in that the onset is slower, the course is more prolonged, and the symptoms are less severe.

When administered orally, methadone is approximately one-half as potent as when given parenterally. Oral administration results in a delay of the onset, a lowering of the peak, and an increase in the duration of analgesic effect.

Indications: 1. Detoxification treatment of narcotic addiction (heroin or other morphine-like drugs).

2. Maintenance treatment of narcotic addiction (heroin or other morphine-like drugs), in conjunction with appropriate social and medical services.

NOTE

If methadone is administered for treatment of heroin dependence for more than three weeks, the procedure passes from treatment of the acute withdrawal syndrome (detoxification) to maintenance therapy. Maintenance treatment is permitted to be undertaken only by approved methadone programs. This does not preclude the maintenance treatment of an addict who is hospitalized for medical conditions other than addiction and who requires temporary maintenance during the critical period of his stay or whose enrollment has been verified in a program which has approval for maintenance treatment with methadone.

Contraindication: Hypersensitivity to methadone.

Warnings:

Diskets Methadone Hydrochloride are for oral administration only. This preparation contains insoluble excipients and therefore *must not* be injected. It is recommended that Diskets Methadone Hydrochloride, if dispensed, be packaged in child-resistant containers to prevent accidental ingestion.

Methadone hydrochloride, a narcotic, is a Schedule II controlled substance under the Federal Controlled Substances Act. Appropriate security measures should be taken to safeguard stocks of methadone against diversion.

DRUG DEPENDENCE—**METHADONE CAN PRODUCE DRUG DEPENDENCE OF THE MORPHINE TYPE AND, THEREFORE, HAS THE POTENTIAL FOR BEING ABUSED. PSYCHIC DEPENDENCE, PHYSICAL DEPENDENCE, AND TOLERANCE MAY DEVELOP UPON REPEATED ADMINISTRATION OF METHADONE, AND IT SHOULD BE PRESCRIBED AND ADMINISTERED WITH THE SAME DEGREE OF CAUTION APPROPRIATE TO THE USE OF MORPHINE.**

Interaction with Other Central-Nervous-System Depressants—Methadone should be used with caution and in reduced dosage in patients who are concurrently receiving other narcotic analgesics, general anesthetics, phenothiazines, other tranquilizers, sedative-hypnotics, tricyclic antidepressants, and other C.N.S. depressants (including alcohol). Respiratory depression, hypotension, and profound sedation or coma may result.

Anxiety—Since methadone, as used by tolerant subjects at a constant maintenance dosage, is not a tranquilizer, patients who are maintained on this drug will react to life problems and stresses with the same symptoms of anxiety as do other individuals. The physician should not confuse such symptoms with those of narcotic abstinence and should not attempt to treat anxiety by increasing the dosage of methadone. The action of methadone in maintenance treatment is limited to the control of narcotic symptoms and is ineffective for relief of general anxiety.

Head Injury and Increased Intracranial Pressure —The respiratory depressant effects of methadone and its capacity to elevate cerebrospinal-fluid pressure may be markedly exaggerated in the presence of increased intracranial pressure. Furthermore, narcotics produce side effects that may obscure the clinical course of patients with head injuries. In such patients, methadone must be used with caution and only if it is deemed essential.

Asthma and Other Respiratory Conditions—Methadone should be used with caution in patients having an acute asthmatic attack, in those with chronic obstructive pulmonary disease or cor pulmonale, and in individuals with a substantially decreased respiratory reserve, preexisting respiratory depression, hypoxia, or hypercapnia. In such patients, even usual therapeutic doses of narcotics may decrease respiratory drive while simultaneously increasing airway resistance to the point of apnea.

Hypotensive Effect—The administration of methadone may result in severe hypotension in an individual whose ability to maintain his blood pressure has already been compromised by a depleted blood volume or concurrent administration of such drugs as the phenothiazines or certain anesthetics.

Use in Ambulatory Patients—Methadone may impair the mental and/or physical abilities required for the performance of potentially hazardous tasks, such as driving a car or operating machinery. The patient should be cautioned accordingly.

Methadone, like other narcotics, may produce orthostatic hypotension in ambulatory patients.

Use in Pregnancy—Safe use in pregnancy has not been established in relation to possible adverse effects on fetal development. Therefore, methadone should not be used in pregnant women unless, in the judgment of the physician, the potential benefits outweigh the possible hazards.

Precautions: ***Interaction with Pentazocine*—Patients who are addicted to heroin or who are on the methadone maintenance program may experience withdrawal symptoms when given pentazocine.**

Interaction with Rifampin—The concurrent administration of rifampin may possibly reduce the blood concentration of methadone to a degree sufficient to produce withdrawal symptoms. The mechanism by which rifampin may decrease blood concentrations of methadone is not fully understood, although enhanced microsomal drug-metabolized enzymes may influence drug disposition.

Acute Abdominal Conditions—The administration of methadone or other narcotics may obscure the diagnosis or clinical course in patients with acute abdominal conditions.

Interaction with Monoamine Oxidase (MAO) Inhibitors—Therapeutic doses of meperidine have precipitated severe reactions in patients concurrently receiving monoamine oxidase inhibitors or those who have received such agents within 14 days. Similar reactions thus far have not been reported with methadone; but if the use of methadone is necessary in such patients, a sensitivity test should be performed in which repeated small incremental doses are administered over the course of several hours while the patient's condition and vital signs are under careful observation.

Special-Risk Patients—Methadone should be given with caution and the initial dose should be reduced in certain patients, such as the elderly or debilitated and those with severe impairment of hepatic or renal function, hypothyroidism, Addison's disease, prostatic hypertrophy, or urethral stricture.

Adverse Reactions: *Heroin Withdrawal*—During the induction phase of methadone maintenance treatment, patients are being withdrawn from heroin and may therefore show typical withdrawal symptoms, which should be differentiated from methadone-induced side effects. They may exhibit some or all of the following symptoms associated with acute withdrawal from heroin or other opiates: lacrimation, rhinorrhea, sneezing, yawning, excessive perspiration, gooseflesh, fever, chilliness alternating with flushing, restlessness, irritability, "sleepy yen," weakness, anxiety, depression, dilated pupils, tremors, tachycardia, abdominal cramps, body aches, involuntary twitching and kicking movements, anorexia, nausea, vomiting, diarrhea, intestinal spasms, and weight loss.

Initial Administration—Initially, the dosage of methadone should be carefully titrated to the individual. Induction too rapid for the patient's sensitivity is more likely to produce the following effects.

THE MAJOR HAZARDS OF METHADONE, AS OF OTHER NARCOTIC ANALGESICS, ARE RESPIRATORY DEPRESSION AND, TO A LESSER DEGREE, CIRCULATORY DEPRESSION. RESPIRATORY ARREST, SHOCK, AND CARDIAC ARREST HAVE OCCURRED.

The most frequently observed adverse reactions include lightheadedness, dizziness, sedation, nausea, vomiting, and sweating. These effects seem to be more prominent in ambulatory patients and in those who are not suffering severe pain. In such individuals, lower doses are advisable. Some adverse reactions may be alleviated in the ambulatory patient if he lies down.

Other adverse reactions include the following:

Central Nervous System—Euphoria, dysphoria, weakness, headache, insomnia, agitation, disorientation, and visual disturbances.

Gastrointestinal—Dry mouth, anorexia, constipation, and biliary tract spasm.

Cardiovascular—Flushing of the face, bradycardia, palpitation, faintness, and syncope.

Genitourinary—Urinary retention or hesitancy, antidiuretic effect, and reduced libido and/or potency.

Allergic—Pruritus, urticaria, other skin rashes, edema, and, rarely, hemorrhagic urticaria.

Maintenance on a Stabilized Dose—During prolonged administration of methadone, as in a methadone maintenance treatment program, there is a gradual, yet progressive, disappearance of side effects over a period of several weeks. However, constipation and sweating often persist.

Dosage and Administration: *For Detoxification Treatment*—THE DRUG SHALL BE ADMINISTERED DAILY UNDER CLOSE SUPERVISION AS FOLLOWS:

A detoxification treatment course shall not exceed 21 days and may not be repeated earlier than four weeks after completion of the preceding course.

In detoxification, the patient may receive methadone when there are significant symptoms of withdrawal. The dosage schedules indicated below are recommended but could be varied in accordance with clinical judgment. Initially, a single oral dose of 15 to 20 mg of methadone will often be sufficient to suppress withdrawal symptoms. Additional methadone may be provided if withdrawal symptoms are not suppressed or if symptoms reappear. When patients are physically dependent on high doses, it may be necessary to exceed these levels. Forty mg per day in single or divided doses will usually constitute an adequate stabilizing dosage level. Stabilization can be continued for two to three days, and then the amount of methadone normally will be gradually decreased. The rate at which methadone is decreased will be determined separately for each patient. The dose of methadone can be decreased on a daily basis or at two-day intervals, but the amount of intake shall always be sufficient to keep withdrawal symptoms at a tolerable level. In hospitalized patients, a daily reduction of 20 percent of the total daily dose may be tolerated and may cause little discomfort. In ambulatory patients, a somewhat slower schedule may be needed. If methadone is administered for more than three weeks, the procedure is considered to have progressed from detoxification or treatment of the acute withdrawal syndrome to maintenance treatment, even though the goal and intent may be eventual total withdrawal.

For Maintenance Treatment—In maintenance treatment, the initial dosage of methadone should control the abstinence symptoms that follow withdrawal of narcotic drugs but should not be so great as to cause sedation, respiratory depression, or other effects of acute intoxication. It is important that the initial dosage be adjusted on an individual basis to the narcotic tolerance of the new patient. If such a patient has been a heavy user of heroin up to the day of admission, he may be given 20 mg four to eight hours later or 40 mg in a single oral dose. If he enters treatment with little or no narcotic tolerance (e.g., if he has recently been released from jail or other confinement), the initial dosage may be one-half these quantities. When there is any doubt, the smaller dose should be used initially. The patient should then be kept under observation, and, if symptoms of abstinence are distressing, additional 10-mg doses may be administered as needed. Subsequently, the dosage should be adjusted individually, as tolerated and required, up to a level of 120 mg daily. The patient will initially ingest the drug under observation daily, or at least six days a week, for the first three months. After demonstrating satisfactory adherence to the program regulations for at least three months, the patient may be permitted to reduce to three times weekly the occasions when he must ingest the drug under observation. He shall receive no more than a two-day take-home supply. With continuing adherence to the program's requirements for at least two years, he may then be permitted twice-weekly visits to the program for drug ingestion under observation, with a three-day take-home supply. A daily dose of 120 mg or more shall be justified in the medical record. Prior approval from state authority and the Food and Drug Administration is required for any dose above 120 mg administered at the clinic and for any dose above 100 mg to be taken at home. A regular review of dosage level should be made by the responsible physician, with careful consideration given to reduction of dosage as indicated on an individual basis. A new dosage level is only a test level until stability is achieved.

Special Considerations for a Pregnant Patient—Caution shall be taken in the maintenance treatment of pregnant patients. Dosage levels shall be kept as low as possible if continued methadone treatment is deemed necessary. It is the responsibility of the program sponsor to assure that each female patient be fully informed concerning the possible risks to a pregnant woman or her unborn child from the use of methadone.

Special Limitations—

Treatment of Patients under Age 18

1. The safety and effectiveness of methadone for use in the treatment of adolescents have not been proved by adequate clinical study. Special procedures are therefore necessary to assure that patients under age 16 will not be admitted to a program and that patients between 16 and 18 years of age will be admitted to maintenance treatment only under limited conditions.

2. Patients between 16 and 18 years of age who were enrolled and under treatment in approved programs on December 15, 1972, may continue in maintenance treatment. No new patients between 16 and 18 years of age may be admitted to a maintenance treatment program after March 15, 1973, unless a parent, legal guardian, or responsible adult designated by the state authority completes and signs Form FD 2635, "Consent for Methadone Treatment." Methadone treatment of new patients between the ages of 16 and 18 years will be permitted after December 15, 1972, only with a documented history of two or more unsuccessful attempts at detoxification and a documented history of dependence on heroin or other morphine-like drugs beginning two years or more prior to application for treatment. No patient under age 16 may be continued or started on methadone treatment after December 15, 1972, but these patients may be detoxified and retained in the program in a drug-free state for follow-up and aftercare.

3. Patients under age 18 who are not placed on maintenance treatment may be detoxified. Detoxification may not exceed three weeks. A repeat episode of detoxification may not be initiated until four weeks after the completion of the previous detoxification.

Overdosage: *Symptoms*—Serious overdosage of methadone is characterized by respiratory depression (a decrease in respiratory rate and/or tidal volume, Cheyne-Stokes respiration, cyanosis), extreme somnolence progressing to stupor or coma, maximally constricted pupils, skeletal-muscle flaccidity, cold and clammy skin, and, sometimes, bradycardia and hypotension. In severe overdosage, particularly by the intravenous route, apnea, circulatory collapse, cardiac arrest, and death may occur.

Treatment—Primary attention should be given to the reestablishment of adequate respiratory exchange through provision of a patent airway and institution of assisted or controlled ventilation. If a nontolerant person, especially a child, takes a large dose of methadone, effective narcotic antagonists are available to counteract the potentially lethal respiratory depression. **The physician must remember, however, that methadone is a long-acting depressant (36 to 48 hours), whereas the antagonists act for much shorter periods (one to three hours).** The patient must, therefore, be monitored continuously for recurrence of respiratory depression and treated repeatedly with the narcotic antagonist as needed. If the diagnosis is correct and respiratory depression is due only to overdosage of methadone, the use of respiratory stimulants is not indicated.

An antagonist should not be administered in the absence of clinically significant respiratory or cardiovascular depression. Intravenously administered narcotic antagonists (naloxone, nalorphine, and levallorphan) are the drugs of choice to reverse signs of intoxication. These agents should be given repeatedly until the patient's status remains satisfactory. The hazard that the narcotic antagonist will further depress respiration is less likely with the use of naloxone.

Oxygen, intravenous fluids, vasopressors, and other supportive measures should be employed as indicated.

NOTE: IN AN INDIVIDUAL PHYSICALLY DEPENDENT ON NARCOTICS, THE ADMINISTRATION OF THE USUAL DOSE OF A NARCOTIC ANTAGONIST WILL PRECIPITATE AN ACUTE WITHDRAWAL SYNDROME. THE SEVERITY OF THIS SYNDROME WILL DEPEND ON THE DEGREE OF PHYSICAL DEPENDENCE AND THE DOSE OF THE ANTAGONIST ADMINISTERED. THE USE OF A NARCOTIC ANTAGONIST IN SUCH A PERSON SHOULD BE AVOIDED IF POSSIBLE. IF IT MUST BE USED TO TREAT SERIOUS RESPIRATORY DEPRESSION IN THE PHYSICALLY DEPENDENT PATIENT, THE ANTAGONIST SHOULD BE ADMINISTERED WITH EXTREME CARE AND BY TITRATION WITH SMALLER THAN USUAL DOSES OF THE ANTAGONIST.

How Supplied: (Ⓒ) *Diskets No. 1, Methadone Hydrochloride Tablets, USP, U53,** 40 mg,

Continued on next page

*Identi-Code® symbol.

Lilly—Cont.

Peach-Colored (cross-scored), in bottles of 100 (NDC 0002-2153-02). [032681]

[*Shown in Product Identification Section*]

METUBINE® IODIDE ℞

(metocurine iodide)
Injection, USP

THIS DRUG SHOULD BE ADMINISTERED ONLY BY ADEQUATELY TRAINED INDIVIDUALS WHO ARE FAMILIAR WITH ITS ACTIONS, CHARACTERISTICS, AND HAZARDS.

Description: Metubine® Iodide (metocurine iodide, Lilly) is a nondepolarizing muscle relaxant and is presented as a sterile isotonic solution for intravenous injection.

Each ml contains 2 mg metocurine iodide and sodium chloride, 0.9 percent, with 0.5 percent phenol as a preservative. Sodium carbonate and/or hydrochloric acid may have been added during manufacture to adjust the pH in the range of 4 to 4.3.

The empirical formula is $C_{40}H_{48}I_2N_2O_6$, and the molecular weight is 906.64.

Clinical Pharmacology: Metubine® Iodide (metocurine iodide, Lilly) is a methyl analogue of tubocurarine which produces nondepolarizing (competitive) neuromuscular blockade at the myoneural junction. Recent animal studies suggest that Metubine Iodide does not produce the autonomic ganglionic blockade seen with other nondepolarizing muscle relaxants. Recent clinical findings suggest that Metubine Iodide reaches the neuromuscular junction more rapidly than does tubocurarine. After intravenous injection, there is rapid onset (one to four minutes) of muscle relaxation with maximum twitch inhibition (96 percent) in 1.5 to ten minutes. The maximum effect lasts 35 to 60 minutes. The time for recovery to 50 percent of control twitch response is in excess of three hours.

Following bolus injection of 0.05 mg/kg, the mean terminal half-life of Metubine Iodide was 3.6 hours (217 minutes). Approximately 50 percent of the dose was excreted as unchanged drug in the urine over 48 hours, and 2 percent was excreted unchanged in the bile. Approximately 35 percent is protein bound, mainly to the beta and gamma globulins.

The use of repeated doses may be accompanied by a cumulative effect. The duration of action and degree of muscle relaxation may be altered by dehydration, body temperature changes, hypocalcemia, excess magnesium, or acid-base imbalance. Concurrently administered general anesthetics, certain antibiotics, and neuromuscular disease may potentiate the neuromuscular blocking action of Metubine Iodide.

Histamine release with Metubine Iodide occurs less frequently than *d*-tubocurarine and is related to dosage and rapidity of administration. Effects on the cardiovascular system (e.g., changes in pulse rate, hypotension) are less than those reported with equipotent doses of *d*-tubocurarine and gallamine.

Because the main excretory pathway for Metubine Iodide is through the kidneys, severe renal disease or conditions associated with poor renal perfusion (shock states) may result in prolonged neuromuscular blockade.

Following intravenous injection in the mother, placental transfer of Metubine Iodide occurs rapidly, and, after six minutes, the fetal plasma concentration is approximately one-tenth the maternal level.

Indications and Usage: Metubine® Iodide (metocurine iodide, Lilly) is indicated as an adjunct to anesthesia to induce skeletal-muscle relaxation. It may be employed to reduce the intensity of muscle contractions in pharmacologically or electrically induced convulsions. It may also be employed to facilitate the management of patients undergoing mechanical ventilation.

Contraindications: Metubine® Iodide (metocurine iodide, Lilly) is contraindicated in those persons with known hypersensitivity to the drug or to its iodide content.

Warnings: METUBINE® IODIDE, (METOCURINE IODIDE, LILLY) SHOULD BE ADMINISTERED IN CAREFULLY ADJUSTED DOSES BY OR UNDER THE SUPERVISION OF EXPERIENCED CLINICIANS WHO ARE FAMILIAR WITH THE COMPLICATIONS WHICH MAY OCCUR WITH THE USE OF THIS DRUG. Metubine Iodide should not be administered unless facilities for intubation, artificial ventilation, oxygen therapy, and reversal agents are immediately available. The clinician must be prepared to assist or control respiration.

Metubine Iodide should be used with extreme caution in patients with myasthenia gravis. In such patients, a peripheral nerve stimulator may be valuable in assessing the effects of administration.

Precautions: *General Precautions*—Metubine® Iodide (metocurine iodide, Lilly) should be used with caution in patients with poor renal perfusion or severe renal disease (*see* Clinical Pharmacology).

Rapid administration of large doses of Metubine Iodide may produce changes in blood pressure or heart rate or signs of histamine release.

Metubine Iodide has no effect on consciousness, pain threshold, or cerebration; therefore, it should be used with adequate anesthesia.

Drug Interactions—Synergistic or antagonistic effects may result when depolarizing and nondepolarizing muscle relaxants are administered simultaneously or sequentially.

Parenteral administration of high doses of certain antibiotics may intensify or resemble the neuroblocking action of muscle relaxants. These include neomycin, streptomycin, bacitracin, kanamycin, gentamicin, dihydrostreptomycin, polymyxin B, colistin, sodium colistimethate, and tetracyclines. If muscle relaxants and antibiotics must be administered simultaneously, the patient should be observed closely for any unexpected prolongation of respiratory depression.

Certain general anesthetics have a synergistic action with neuromuscular blocking agents. Diethyl ether, halothane, and isoflurane potentiate the neuromuscular blocking action of other nondepolarizing agents and may be presumed to do so with Metubine Iodide.

Administration of quinidine shortly after recovery may produce recurrent paralysis.

The effect of diazepam on neuromuscular blockade by Metubine Iodide is not clear. Until more information is available, patients should be carefully monitored for unexpected drug response and prolongation of action.

The use of magnesium sulfate in preeclamptic patients potentiates the effects of both depolarizing and nondepolarizing muscle relaxants.

Usage in Pregnancy—Pregnancy Category C—Intrauterine growth retardation and limb deformities resembling clubfoot were produced by *d*-tubocurarine chloride and succinylcholine chloride when administered to the rat fetus between the sixteenth and nineteenth days of gestation or when injected in chick embryos from the fifth to the fifteenth day of incubation. When *d*-tubocurarine was injected intramuscularly into the interscapular region of the fetuses on the sixteenth to the nineteenth day of gestation, the incidence of growth retardation and limb deformity ranged from 21 to 23 percent and 7 to 8 percent respectively.

There are no adequate and well-controlled studies of Metubine Iodide in pregnant women. Metubine Iodide should be used during pregnancy only if the potential benefit justifies the risk to the fetus.

Labor and Delivery—It is not known whether the use of muscle relaxants during labor or delivery has immediate or delayed adverse effects on the fetus, prolongs the duration of labor, or increases the likelihood that forceps delivery, obstetric intervention, or resuscitation of the newborn will be necessary.

Nursing Mothers—It is not known whether Metubine Iodide is excreted in human milk. Because many drugs are excreted in human milk, caution should be excercised when Metubine Iodide is administered to a nursing woman.

Usage in Children—A clinical study has shown that Metubine Iodide is twice as potent as *d*-tubocurarine in children, but the rate of recovery is the same. There may be a slight increase in heart rate, but no change occurs in blood pressure or ECG. Doses calculated on the basis of body weight or body surface area may be applicable when the advantages of nondepolarizing neuromuscular blockade are desired.

Adverse Reactions: The most frequently noted adverse reaction is prolongation of the drug's pharmacologic action. Neuromuscular effects may range from skeletal-muscle weakness to a profound relaxation that produces respiratory insufficiency or apnea.

Possible adverse reactions include allergic or hypersensitivity reactions to the drug or its iodide content and histamine release when large doses are administered rapidly. Signs of histamine release include erythema, edema, flushing, tachycardia, arterial hypotension, bronchospasm, and circulatory collapse.

Prolonged apnea and respiratory depression have occurred following the use of muscle relaxants. Many physiologic factors, drug interactions, and individual sensitivities may contribute to the development of respiratory paralysis (*see* Clinical Pharmacology and Precautions).

Overdosage: An overdose of Metubine® Iodide (metocurine iodide, Lilly) may result in prolonged apnea, cardiovascular collapse, and sudden release of histamine.

Massive doses of metocurarine are not reversible by the antagonists edrophonium or neostigmine and atropine.

Overdosage may be avoided by the careful monitoring of response by means of a peripheral nerve stimulator.

The primary treatment for residual neuromuscular blockade with respiratory paralysis or inadequte ventilation is maintenance of the patient's airway and manual or mechanical ventilation.

Accompanying derangements of blood pressure, electrolyte imbalance, or circulating blood volume should be determined and corrected by appropriate fluid and electrolyte therapy.

Residual neuromuscular blockade following surgery may be reversed by the use of anticholinesterase inhibitors such as neostigmine or pyridostigmine bromide and atropine. Prescribing information should be consulted for the appropriate drug selection based on dosage and desired duration of action.

Dosage and Administration: Metubine® Iodide (metocurine iodide, Lilly) should be administered intravenously as a sustained injection over a period of 30 to 60 seconds. INTRAMUSCULAR ADMINISTRATION OF METUBINE IODIDE IS NOT RECOMMENDED. Care must be taken to avoid overdosage. The use of a peripheral nerve stimulator to monitor response will minimize the risk of overdosage. The type of anesthetic used and nature of the surgical procedure will influence the amount of Metubine Iodide required. Doses of 0.2 to 0.4 mg/kg have been found satisfactory for endotracheal intubation. Relaxation following the initial dose may be expected to be effective for periods of 25 to 90 minutes, with an average of approximately 60 minutes. Supplemental administration may be made as indicated to provide needed surgical relaxation. Supplemental doses average 0.5 to 1 mg. The use of strong anesthetics that potentiate the effect of neuromuscular blocking drugs such as halothane, diethyl ether, isoflurane, or enflurane reduces the requirement for Metubine Iodide. Incremental doses should be reduced by approximately one-third to one-half.

Recommended Doses for Use during Electroshock Therapy—Doses required for satisfactory relaxation range from 1.75 to 5.5 mg. When the patient is treated for the first time, the drug is administered slowly by the intravenous route as a sustained injection until a head-drop response ensues. After dosage has been established, subsequent injections are completed in 15 to 50 seconds. The average dose ranges from 2 to 3 mg.

Drug Incompatibilities—Metubine Iodide is unstable in alkaline solutions. When it is combined with barbiturate solutions, precipitation may occur. Solutions of barbiturates, meperidine, and morphine sulfate should not be administered from the same syringe.

How Supplied: (℞) *Vials (Multiple Dose) No. 586, Metubine® Iodide (Metocurine Iodide Injection, USP),* 2 mg per ml, 20 ml, rubber-stoppered, in singles (10 per carton) (NDC 0002-1421-01). Store at controlled room temperature, 59° to 86°F (15° to 30°C).

[021282]

MOXAM™ ℞

(moxalactam disodium)

Description: Moxam™ (moxalactam disodium, Lilly) is a semisynthetic broad-spectrum β-lactam antibiotic for parenteral administration. It is the disodium salt of (6R, 7R)-7-[[carboxy (4-hydroxyphenyl) acetyl] amino]-7-methoxy-3-[[(1-methyl-1*H*-tetrazol-5-yl)thio] methyl]-8-oxo-5-oxa-1-azabicyclo[4.2.0] oct-2-ene-2-carboxylic acid.

Moxam is a sterile dry powder which contains 150 mg mannitol/g of moxalactam activity. The total sodium content is approximately 88 mg (3.8 mEq sodium ion)/g of moxalactam activity. Sodium bicarbonate and/or sodium hydroxide may have been added during manufacture for neutralization. The *p*H of freshly reconstituted solutions usually ranges from 5.5 to 6.5.

Clinical Pharmacology: After rapid intravenous infusion (two minutes) of 500-mg and 1-g doses of moxalactam in normal adult volunteers, mean peak serum levels of 57 mcg/ml and 94 mcg/ml respectively were achieved. Average serum concentrations following intravenous doses of 0.25, 0.5, 1, 2, 3, and 4 g infused over a 20-minute period in adult volunteers are listed in Table 1. Intravenous administration of 4-g doses every eight hours for seven doses produced no evidence of accumulation in the serum. The half-life after an intravenous dose is approximately 1.9 hours (114 minutes).

TABLE 1. MOXALACTAM SERUM LEVELS IN ADULTS (MCG/ML)

IV Dose	20 Minutes*	4 Hours*	8 Hours*
0.25 g	24	4	1
0.5 g	48	7	2
1 g	101	13	3
2 g	204	31	8
3 g	262	40	9
4 g	443	61	13

* Time after beginning of infusion.

Following intramuscular administration of 250-mg, 500-mg, and 1-g doses of moxalactam to normal adult volunteers, the mean peak serum concentrations were 10, 16, and 27 mcg/ml respectively. These peaks occurred at 60 to 120 minutes. After intramuscular administration, the half-life is approximately 2.1 hours (126 minutes).

Sixty to 90 percent of an intramuscular or intravenous dose is excreted by the kidneys over a 24-hour period, which results in high urinary concentrations. No metabolite of moxalactam has been detected in the urine. Following intravenous doses of 250 mg, 500 mg, 1 g, and 2 g, urinary concentrations were highest during the first two hours and were 170, 446, 1820, and 4220 mcg/ml respectively. These levels decreased at ten to 12 hours to 14, 59, 96, and 156 mcg/ml respectively.

The mean renal clearance of moxalactam was approximately 78 ml/min, with a calculated mean total body clearance of 99.3 ml/min for a man weighing 70 kg.

In patients with reduced renal function, the serum half-life of moxalactam is significantly prolonged. Although serum concentrations in patients with normal renal function declined to 0 within 24 to 48 hours after a 1-g intravenous dose, serum concentrations in patients with severe renal impairment were approximately 25 and 10 percent of peak levels at 24 and 48 hours respectively.

Therapeutic levels of moxalactam are achieved in the following fluids: pleural fluid, interstitial fluid, aqueous humor, and the cerebrospinal fluid of patients with normal and inflamed meninges.

Microbiology—The bactericidal activity of moxalactam results from inhibition of cell-wall synthesis. Moxalactam has in vitro activity against a wide range of gram-negative and certain gram-positive organisms. Moxalactam has a high degree of stability in the presence of β-lactamases, both penicillinases and cephalosporinases produced by gram-negative and gram-positive bacteria. Because of its unique chemical structure, moxalactam is also a potent inhibitor of β-lactamases from certain gram-negative bacteria, e.g., *Enterobacter cloacae* and *Pseudomonas aeruginosa.* Moxalactam is usually active against the following microorganisms in vitro and in clinical infections (*see* Indications and Usage).

Aerobes, gram-negative: *Haemophilus influenzae,* including ampicillin-resistant strains; *Escherichia coli; Klebsiella* species, including *Klebsiella pneumoniae; Proteus mirabilis, P. vulgaris; Providencia rettgeri* (formerly *Proteus rettgeri*); *Morganella morganii* (formerly *Proteus morganii*); *Enterobacter* species; *P. aeruginosa* (some strains are resistant); *Serratia* species.

Note.: Many strains of the above organisms that are multiply resistant to other antibiotics, e.g., penicillins, cephalosporins, and aminoglycosides, are susceptible to moxalactam.

Aerobes, gram-positive: staphylococci, including penicillinase-producing strains (*Note:* Methicillin-resistant staphylococci as well as some strains of *Staphylococcus epidermidis* are resistant to moxalactam); *Streptococcus pyogenes* (group A β-hemolytic streptococci); *S. agalactiae* (group B streptococci); *S. pneumoniae* (formerly *Diplococcus pneumoniae*) (*Note:* Most strains of enterococci, e.g., *S. faecalis,* are resistant).

Anaerobes: *Bacteroides* species, including *Bacteroides fragilis; Fusobacterium* species; *Clostridium* species (*Note:* Most strains of *Clostridium difficile* are resistant); *Eubacterium* species; *Peptococcus* species; *Peptostreptococcus* species; *Veillonella* species.

Moxalactam also demonstrates in vitro activity against the following microorganisms, although its clinical significance is unknown: *Neisseria gonorrhoeae; N. meningitidis; Providencia* species; *Salmonella* species, including *Salmonella typhi; Shigella* species.

Moxalactam is highly resistant to hydrolysis by β-lactamases of Richmond Types I, II, III, IV, and V. These enzymes are frequently produced by strains of *Enterobacteriaceae, P. aeruginosa, Acinetobacter* species, *H. influenzae,* and *Neisseria* species. Furthermore, moxalactam is stable to some β-lactamases not classified as Richmond types, such as those produced by strains of *S. aureus* and *B. fragilis.*

Moxalactam and aminoglycosides have been shown to be synergistic in vitro against some strains of *Enterobacteriaceae* and *P. aeruginosa.*

Disc Susceptibility Tests—Quantitative methods that require measurement of zone diameters give the most precise estimate of antibiotic susceptibility. One such procedure[1] has been recommended for use with discs to test susceptibility to moxalactam.

Reports from the laboratory giving results of the standard single-disc susceptibility test with a 30-mcg moxalactam disc should be interpreted according to the following criteria:

Susceptible organisms produce zones of 20 mm or greater, indicating that the test organism is likely to respond to therapy.

Organisms that produce zones of 15 to 19 mm are expected to be susceptible if high dosage is used or if the infection is confined to tissues and fluids (e.g., urine) in which high antibiotic levels are attained.

Resistant organisms produce zones of 14 mm or less, indicating that other therapy should be selected.

Organisms should be tested with the moxalactam disc, since moxalactam has been shown by in vitro tests to be active against certain strains found resistant when other β-lactam discs are used.

In other susceptibility testing procedures, e.g., ICS agar dilution[2] or the equivalent, a bacterial isolate may be considered susceptible if the MIC value for moxalactam is not more than 16 mcg/ml. Organisms are considered resistant to moxalactam if the MIC is equal to or greater than 64 mcg/ml. Organisms having an MIC value of less than 64 mcg/ml but greater than 16 mcg/ml are expected to be susceptible if high dosage is used or if the infection is confined to tissues and fluids (e.g., urine) in which high antibiotic levels are attained.

Indications and Usage: Moxam™ (moxalactam disodium, Lilly) is indicated for the treatment of infections caused by susceptible strains of the designated microorganisms in the diseases listed below:

Lower respiratory infections, including pneumonia, caused by *S. pneumoniae, H. influenzae, Klebsiella* species, *Enterobacter* species, *S. aureus* (penicillin-sensitive and penicillin-resistant strains), *E. coli,* and *P. mirabilis.*

Urinary tract infections caused by *E. coli, Klebsiella* species, *Enterobacter* species, *Proteus* species (indole-positive and indole-negative), and *Serratia* species.

Intra-abdominal infections, such as peritonitis, endometritis, and pelvic cellulitis, caused by *E. coli; Peptostreptococcus* species; *Bacteroides* species, including *B. fragilis,* mixed aerobic and anaerobic organisms, such as *K. pneumoniae, S. agalactiae* (group B streptococci), *P. mirabilis, Enterobacter* species, *P. aeruginosa, Peptococcus* species, *Clostridium* species, *Fusobacterium* species, and *Eubacterium* species.

Bacterial septicemia caused by *S. aureus, E. coli, S. pneumoniae, Klebsiella* species, *Serratia* species, *Pseudomonas* species, and *B. fragilis.*

Central-nervous-system infections, e.g., meningitis and ventriculitis, caused by *E. coli* and *Klebsiella* species. Moxam has been used successfully in the treatment of a limited number of patients with meningitis and ventriculitis caused by other *Enterobacteriaceae* and *H. influenzae.*

Skin and skin-structure infections caused by *S. aureus* (penicillinase and non-penicillinase-producing); *S. pyogenes* (group A β-hemolytic streptococci); *E. coli; Serratia* species; mixed aerobic and anaerobic organisms, such as *Proteus* species, *Klebsiella* species, *Enterobacter* species, *Peptococcus* species, *Peptostreptococcus* species, *Bacteroides* species, and *Clostridium* species.

Continued on next page

*Identi-Code® symbol.

Lilly—Cont.

Bone and joint infections caused by *S. aureus* (penicillinase and non-penicillinase-producing), *P. aeruginosa,* and *Serratia* species.
Because of the serious nature of infections due to *P. aeruginosa* and because many strains of *Pseudomonas* species are moderately susceptible to moxalactam, higher dosage is recommended in serious systemic infections caused by this organism (*see* Dosage and Administration). Moxam has been used successfully in the treatment of some patients with serious lower respiratory tract infections caused by *P. aeruginosa* and *Serratia* species. In such cases, higher dosage is recommended, and other therapy should be instituted if the response is not prompt.
Moxam has been used successfully in surgical infections in cases where concomitant therapy with other antibiotics may be used.
Specimens for bacteriologic cultures should be obtained in order to isolate and identify causative organisms and to determine their susceptibilities to moxalactam. Therapy may be instituted before results of susceptibility studies are known; however, once these results become available, the antibiotic treatment should be adjusted accordingly.
In certain cases of confirmed or suspected gram-positive or gram-negative sepsis or in patients with other serious infections in which the causative organism has not been identified, Moxam may be used concomitantly with an aminoglycoside. The dosage recommended in the labeling of both antibiotics may be given and depends on the severity of the infection and the patient's condition. Renal function should be carefully monitored, especially if higher dosages of the aminoglycosides are to be administered or if therapy is prolonged, because of the potential nephrotoxicity and ototoxicity of aminoglycosidic antibiotics. Some β-lactam antibiotics also have a certain degree of nephrotoxicity. Although, to date, this has not been noted when Moxam was given alone, it is possible that nephrotoxicity may be potentiated if Moxam is used concomitantly with an aminoglycoside.

Contraindication: Moxam™ (moxalactam disodium, Lilly) is contraindicated in patients with known allergy to the drug.

Warnings: BEFORE THERAPY WITH MOXAM IS INSTITUTED, CAREFUL INQUIRY SHOULD BE MADE FOR A HISTORY OF HYPERSENSITIVITY REACTIONS TO MOXALACTAM DISODIUM, CEPHALOSPORINS, PENICILLINS, OR OTHER DRUGS. THIS PRODUCT SHOULD BE GIVEN WITH CAUTION TO PATIENTS WITH TYPE 1 HYPERSENSITIVITY REACTIONS TO PENICILLIN. ANTIBIOTICS SHOULD BE GIVEN WITH CAUTION TO ANY PATIENT WHO HAS HAD SOME FORM OF ALLERGY, PARTICULARLY TO DRUGS. IF AN ALLERGIC REACTION TO MOXALACTAM OCCURS, DISCONTINUE THE DRUG. SERIOUS HYPERSENSITIVITY REACTIONS MAY REQUIRE EPINEPHRINE AND OTHER EMERGENCY MEASURES.
Pseudomembranous colitis has been reported with virtually all broad-spectrum antibiotics (including macrolides, semisynthetic penicillins, and cephalosporins); therefore, it is important to consider its diagnosis in patients who develop diarrhea in association with the use of antibiotics. Such colitis may range in severity from mild to life-threatening.
Treatment with broad-spectrum antibiotics alters the normal flora of the colon and may permit overgrowth of clostridia. Studies indicate that a toxin produced by *Clostridium difficile* is one primary cause of antibiotic-associated colitis.
Mild cases of pseudomembranous colitis usually respond to drug discontinuance alone. In moderate to severe cases, management should include sigmoidoscopy, appropriate bacteriologic studies, and fluid, electrolyte, and protein supplementation. When the colitis does not improve after the drug has been discontinued, or when it is severe, oral vancomycin is the drug of choice for antibiotic-associated pseudomembranous colitis produced by *C. difficile.* Other causes of colitis should be ruled out.

Precautions: As with other broad-spectrum antibiotics, hypoprothrombinemia, occasionally resulting in significant hemorrhage, has been reported, but it has been promptly reversed by administration of vitamin K. Such episodes usually have occurred in elderly, debilitated, or otherwise compromised patients with deficient stores of vitamin K. Treatment of such individuals with antibiotics possessing significant activity against gram-negative organisms and/or anaerobes is thought to alter the number and/or type of intestinal bacterial flora, with consequent reduction in synthesis of vitamin K. In these patients with deficient stores of vitamin K, the prophylactic administration of 5 to 10 mg of vitamin K per week parenterally or orally may be indicated.
Inhibition of platelet function similar to the effect seen with penicillin G, carbenicillin, ticarcillin, and cephalothin has been observed in patients receiving high doses of moxalactam. Clinical bleeding which has occurred and which is associated with prolonged bleeding time and suppressed platelet function ceases on withdrawal of the antibiotic. Tests of platelet function return to normal 72 to 96 hours later.
A disulfiram-like reaction, i.e., nausea, vomiting, and vasomotor instability with hypotension and peripheral vasodilatation, has occurred following the ingestion of ethanol. The timing of the ingestion of alcohol is an important factor. When alcohol was ingested prior to the first dose of Moxam™ (moxalactam disodium, Lilly), this syndrome was not observed. It has been reported only when ethanol ingestion followed the administration of Moxam. This has been observed as late as 48 hours after the last dose of Moxam. Moxalactam inhibits the enzyme acetaldehyde dehydrogenase in laboratory animals. This causes accumulation of acetaldehyde when ethanol is administered concomitantly.
Prolonged use of Moxam may result in the overgrowth of nonsusceptible organisms (e.g., enterococci). Careful observation of the patient is essential. If superinfection occurs during therapy, appropriate measures should be taken.
Broad-spectrum antibiotics should be prescribed with caution in individuals with a history of gastrointestinal disease, particularly colitis.
Usage in Pregnancy—Pregnancy Category C—Reproduction studies have been performed in mice, rats, rabbits, and ferrets. Administration of Moxam at ten to 20 times the usual human dose has resulted in an increased incidence of birth defects or embryotoxicity in the ferret. Since the incidence of birth defects and embryotoxicity in control ferrets was high and variable, its significance in ferrets after the administration of Moxam is unknown. Studies in mice and rats at doses up to 20 times the usual human dose (eight times the maximum dose) have revealed no evidence of impaired fertility or teratogenicity. A decrease in offspring viability was noted in rats, perhaps due to drug-related growth depression and decrease in food consumption by the pregnant dams. There are no adequate and well-controlled studies in pregnant women. Moxam should be used during pregnancy only if the potential benefit justifies the potential risk to the fetus.
Nursing Mothers—It is not known whether this drug is excreted in human milk. Studies have shown that it is excreted in the milk of rats. Because many drugs are excreted in human milk, caution should be exercised when Moxam is administered to a nursing woman.

Adverse Reactions: In clinical studies, adverse effects considered related to moxalactam therapy or of uncertain etiology are listed below:
Hematopoietic abnormalities, half of which were of uncertain etiology, occurred in about 5 percent of patients and included eosinophilia (1 in 35), disturbances in vitamin K-dependent clotting function (decreased prothrombin), increased bleeding time, thrombocytopenia (1 in 276) (*see* Precautions), and reversible leukopenia (1 in 145). Reversible neutropenia has been reported in children who were three years of age or younger (1 in 23).
Local effects were reported in less than 4 percent of patients and included pain at the site of injection (1 in 70) and phlebitis (1 in 50).
Hypersensitivity reactions were reported in about 3 percent of patients and included morbilliform eruptions (1 in 60), fever (1 in 155), and positive Coombs' test (1 in 180). Two-thirds of the occurrences were considered related to therapy. Anaphylaxis occurred in one patient.
Gastrointestinal symptoms occurred in less than 3 percent of patients, the most frequent being diarrhea (1 in 60).
Symptoms of pseudomembranous colitis may appear either during or after antibiotic treatment. Nausea and vomiting have been reported rarely.
Hepatic enzyme elevations (SGOT, SGPT, alkaline phosphatase) occurred in about 1 in 25 patients. Ninety percent of the abnormalities were of uncertain etiology.
Causal Relationship Uncertain—Although of uncertain etiology, the following transient abnormalities in clinical laboratory renal function test results are listed to serve as alerting information for the physician:
Elevated BUN (1 in 150), pyuria and hematuria (1 of each in 250), and elevated serum creatinine (1 in 300).

Dosage and Administration: *Dosage: Adults*—The usual daily dose of Moxam™ (moxalactam disodium, Lilly) is 2 to 6 g administered in divided doses every eight hours for five to ten days or up to 14 days. Most mild to moderate infections can be expected to respond to a dosage of 500 mg to 2 g every 12 hours.
In mild skin and skin-structure infections and in uncomplicated pneumonia, a dosage of 500 mg every eight hours is recommended.
In mild, uncomplicated urinary tract infections, a dosage of 250 mg every 12 hours is adequate. In urinary tract infections that are more difficult to treat, a dosage of 500 mg every 12 hours may be needed. In serious urinary tract infections, the dosage frequency may be increased to every eight hours.
In life-threatening infections or infections due to less susceptible organisms (e.g., *P. aeruginosa*), doses up to 4 g every eight hours (i.e., 12 g/day) may be needed.
Neonates, Infants, and Children—The following dosage schedule is recommended:

PEDIATRIC DOSAGE SCHEDULE

Neonates	
0–1 week of age	50 mg/kg q. 12 h.
1–4 weeks of age	50 mg/kg q. 8 h.
Infants	50 mg/kg q. 6 h.
Children	50 mg/kg q. 6 h. or q. 8 h.

This may be increased to a total daily dose of 200 mg/kg (not to exceed the maximum adult dose) for serious infections.
In pediatric gram-negative meningitis, an initial loading dose of 100 mg/kg is recommended prior to the utilization of the above dosage schedule.
Impaired Renal Function—When renal function is impaired, a reduced dose must be employed and the serum levels closely monitored. After an intial dose of 1 to 2 g (depending on the severity of the infection), a maintenance dosage schedule should be followed. Continued dosage should be determined by the degree of renal impairment, the severity of infection, and the susceptibility of the causative organism.
When only serum creatinine is available, the following formula (based on sex, weight, and

age of the patient) may be used to convert this value into creatinine clearance. The serum creatinine should represent a steady state of renal function.

$$\text{Males: } \frac{\text{Weight (kg)} \times (140 - \text{age})}{72 \times \text{serum creatinine}}$$

Females: 0.9 × male value

[See table right].

The serum half-life of moxalactam during hemodialysis has ranged from two to five hours. Maintenance doses of Moxam should be repeated following regular hemodialysis.

Administration: Moxam™ (moxalactam disodium, Lilly) may be given intravenously or by deep intramuscular injection into a large muscle mass (such as the upper outer quadrant of the gluteus maximus or lateral part of the thigh).

Intramuscular Administration—Each g of Moxam should be diluted with 3 ml of one of the following diluents: Sterile Water for Injection, Bacteriostatic Water for Injection, 0.9% Sodium Chloride Injection, Bacteriostatic Sodium Chloride Injection, or 0.5% Lidocaine Injection. Shake well until dissolved.

Intravenous Administration—The intravenous route may be preferable for patients with bacterial septicemia, localized parenchymal abscesses (such as intra-abdominal abscess), peritonitis, meningitis, or other severe or life-threatening infections. In those with normal renal function, the intravenous dosage for such infections is 3 to 12 g of Moxam daily. In conditions such as septicemia, 6 to 12 g/day may be given initially by the intravenous route for several days, and the dosage may then be gradually reduced according to clinical response and laboratory findings.

For direct intermittent intravenous administration, add 10 ml of Sterile Water for Injection, 5% Dextrose Injection, or 0.9% Sodium Chloride Injection/g of moxalactam. Slowly inject directly into the vein over a period of three to five minutes or give through the tubing of an administration set while the patient is also receiving one of the following intravenous fluids: 0.9% Sodium Chloride Injection, 5% Dextrose Injection, 5% Dextrose and 0.9% Sodium Chloride Injection, 5% Dextrose and 0.45% Sodium Chloride Injection, 5% Dextrose and 0.2% Sodium Chloride Injection, 5% Dextrose and 0.15% Potassium Chloride Injection, 5% Osmitrol® in Water for Injection, Sodium Lactate Injection (M/6) Normosal®-M in D5-W, Ionosol® B in 5% Dextrose Injection, Plasma-Lyte®-M in 5% Dextrose Injection, Ringer's Injection, Acetated Ringer's Injection, or Lactated Ringer's in 5% Dextrose Injection.

Intravenous solutions containing alcohol should be avoided (*see* Precautions).

Intermittent intravenous infusion with a Y-type administration set or volume control set can also be accomplished while any of the above-mentioned intravenous fluids are being infused. However, during infusion of the solution containing Moxam, it is desirable to discontinue the other solution. When this technique is employed, careful attention should be paid to the volume of the solution containing moxalactam so that the calculated dose will be infused. When a Y-tube hookup is used, 100 ml of an appropriate diluent should be added to the 1 or 2-g piggyback (100-ml) vial. If Sterile Water for Injection is used as the diluent, reconstitute with approximately 20 ml/g to avoid a hypotonic solution.

For continuous intravenous infusion, each g of moxalactam should be diluted with 10 ml of Sterile Water for Injection. An appropriate quantity of the resulting solution may be added to an IV bottle containing one of the fluids listed above under Direct Intermittent Intravenous Administration.

Stability: Reconstituted Moxam is stable for 96 hours if stored under refrigeration (5°C) and for 24 hours at room temperature.

MOXAM™ (MOXALACTAM DISODIUM)—
MAINTENANCE DOSAGE GUIDE FOR PATIENTS WITH RENAL IMPAIRMENT

Creatinine Clearance (ml/min/1.73 m²)	Renal Function	Life-Threatening Infections—Maximum Dosage	Less Severe Infections
>80	Normal	4 g q. 8 h.	0.5–2 g q. 8–12 h.
50–80	Mild Impairment	3 g q. 8 h.	0.5–1 g q. 8 h.
25–50	Moderate Impairment	2 g q. 8 h. OR 3 g q. 12 h.	0.25–1 g q. 12 h.
2–25	Severe Impairment	1 g q. 8 h. OR 1.25 g q. 12 h.	0.25–0.5 g q. 8 h
<2	0	1 g q. 24 h.	0.25–0.5 g q. 12 h.

How Supplied: *Vials No. 7152,* Moxam™ (moxalactam disodium, Lilly) 1 g (equivalent to moxalactam activity), 10-ml size (NDC 0002-7152-10), and *Vials No. 7154,* 2 g (equivalent to moxalactam activity), 20-ml size (NDC 0002-7154-10), in Traypak™ (multivial carton, Lilly) of 10.

[081682]

1. Am. J. Clin. Pathol., *45:*493, 1966; Federal Register, *39:*19182–19184, 1974.
2. Ericsson, H. M., and Sherris, J. C.: Acta Pathol. Microbiol. Scand. [B], Supplement No. 217, 1971.

MULTICEBRIN® OTC
(pan-vitamins)

Description: Each tablet contains—

Thiamine (Vitamin B_1)	3 mg
Riboflavin (Vitamin B_2)	3 mg
Pyridoxine (Vitamin B_6)	1.2 mg
Pantothenic Acid	5 mg
Niacinamide	25 mg
Vitamin B_{12} (Activity Equivalent)	3 mcg
Ascorbic Acid (Vitamin C)	75 mg
dl-Alpha Tocopheryl Acetate (Vitamin E)	6.6 IU (6.6 mg)
Vitamin A	10,000 IU (3 mg)
Vitamin D	400 IU (10 mcg)

Indications: One tablet supplies the optimum requirements of six essential vitamins and significant amounts of other important factors for which optimum requirements have not been established. Tablets Multicebrin are indicated in the prophylaxis or treatment of multiple vitamin deficiencies, in patients on restricted diets, in pregnancy, in wasting diseases, and in any situation characterized by improper food intake, utilization, or absorption.

Dosage: 1 tablet a day, or as directed by the physician.

How Supplied: *Tablets No. 100, Multicebrin® (pan-vitamins, Lilly), C71,** Coated, Red, in bottles of 100 and 1000 and in 10 strips of 10 individually labeled blisters each containing 1 tablet (ID100). [030180]

NEOMYCIN SULFATE ℞
Tablets, USP

Description: Neomycin is an antibiotic obtained from the metabolic products of the actinomycete *Streptomyces fradiae.*

Actions: Neomycin is poorly absorbed from the normal gastrointestinal tract. The small absorbed fraction is rapidly excreted with normal kidney function. The unabsorbed portion of the drug (approximately 97 percent) is eliminated unchanged in the feces.

Growth of most intestinal bacteria is rapidly suppressed following oral administration of neomycin, and the suppression persists for 48 to 72 hours. Nonpathogenic yeasts and, occasionally, resistant strains of *Enterobacter aerogenes* replace the intestinal bacteria.

Indications: *Suppression of Intestinal Bacteria*—Neomycin may be indicated when suppression of the normal bacterial flora of the bowel is desirable for either short-term or long-term adjunctive therapy.

Hepatic Coma—Prolonged administration has been shown to be effective adjunctive therapy in hepatic coma because it reduces the ammonia-forming bacteria in the intestinal tract. The subsequent reduction in blood ammonia has resulted in neurologic improvement.

Diarrhea Due to Enteropathogenic Escherichia coli—Diarrhea caused by enteropathogenic *E. coli* may be effectively treated with neomycin sulfate. When this diarrhea occurs in epidemic form, all patients and carriers should be treated concurrently.

Contraindications: Neomycin sulfate tablets are contraindicated in the presence of intestinal obstruction and in individuals with a history of hypersensitivity to the drug.

Warnings: Patients treated with oral neomycin should be under close clinical observation because of the potential nephrotoxic and ototoxic effects. Patients with renal insufficiency may develop toxic blood levels of the drug unless doses are properly regulated. If renal insufficiency develops during treatment, the dosage should be reduced or the antibiotic discontinued. Urine and blood examinations and audiometric tests should be given prior to and during extended therapy in individuals with hepatic and/or renal disease to avoid nephrotoxicity and eighth-nerve damage from improper dosage.

Usage in Pregnancy—Safety of this product for use during pregnancy has not been established.

Precautions: Caution should be observed in the concurrent use of other ototoxic and/or nephrotoxic antimicrobial drugs while neomycin is being administered orally. These include streptomycin, kanamycin, polymyxin B, colistin, viomycin, gentamicin, cephaloridine, and tobramycin.

The concurrent use of potent diuretics, such as ethacrynic acid, furosemide, urea, and mannitol (particularly when given intravenously), should be avoided. They may cause cumulative adverse effects of the neomycin on the kidney and auditory nerve.

Prolonged oral use of neomycin may result in overgrowth of nonsusceptible organisms, particularly fungi. If this occurs, appropriate therapy should be instituted.

Adverse Reactions: The most common adverse reactions to neomycin given orally are nausea, vomiting, and diarrhea. The "malabsorption syndrome," characterized by increased fecal fat, decreased serum carotene, and fall in xylose absorption, has been reported

Continued on next page

*Identi-Code® symbol.

Lilly—Cont.

with prolonged therapy. Nephrotoxicity and ototoxicity have occurred following extended and high-dosage therapy in hepatic coma.
Administration and Dosage: *Adults*—For suppression of intestinal bacteria as an adjunct to mechanical cleansing of the large bowel in short-term therapy prior to bowel surgery, 40 mg/kg every 24 hours in six divided doses may be used. Duration of therapy should not exceed three days.
As adjunctive therapy in the treatment of hepatic coma, the recommended dosage schedule is 100 mg/kg in four divided doses the first 24 hours, followed by 50 mg/kg/day thereafter. The total daily dose should not exceed 3 g.
Infants and Children—Diarrhea due to enteropathogenic *E. coli* may be treated with 50 mg/kg given in four divided doses daily for two to three days.
How Supplied: (℞) *Tablets No. 1803, Neomycin Sulfate, USP, T96,** 500 mg (equivalent to 350 mg base), in bottles of 20 (NDC 0002-2096-20) and 100 (NDC 0002-2096-02) and in 10 strips of 10 individually labeled blisters each containing 1 tablet (ID100) (NDC 0002-2096-33).

[101580]

ONCOVIN® ℞
(vincristine sulfate)
For Injection, USP

Description: Oncovin® (vincristine sulfate, Lilly) is the salt of an alkaloid obtained from a common flowering herb, the periwinkle plant (*Vinca rosea* Linn.). Originally known as leurocristine, it has also been referred to as LCR and VCR. The empirical formula is $C_{46}H_{56}N_4O_{10} \cdot H_2SO_4$.
The vials contain either 1 mg Oncovin and 10 mg lactose or 5 mg Oncovin and 50 mg lactose. Each size is supplied in a combination package with an accompanying vial of diluting solution (Bacteriostatic Sodium Chloride Injection), 10 ml, containing 90 mg sodium chloride, with 0.9 percent benzyl alcohol as a preservative.
Action: The mode of action of Oncovin® (vincristine sulfate, Lilly) is unknown but is under investigation. Treatment of neoplastic cells in vitro with Oncovin demonstrated that it may cause an arrest of mitotic division at the stage of metaphase.
Central-nervous-system leukemia has been reported in patients undergoing otherwise successful therapy with Oncovin. This suggests that Oncovin does not penetrate well into the cerebrospinal fluid.
Indications: Oncovin® (vincristine sulfate, Lilly) is indicated in acute leukemia.
It has also been shown to be useful in combination with other oncolytic agents in Hodgkin's disease, lymphosarcoma, reticulum-cell sarcoma, rhabdomyosarcoma, neuroblastoma, and Wilms' tumor.
Contraindications: There are no contraindications to the use of Oncovin® (vincristine sulfate, Lilly), but careful attention should be given to those conditions listed under Warnings and Precautions.
Warnings: This preparation is for intravenous use only. The intrathecal administration of Oncovin is uniformly fatal.
Since reproduction studies have not been performed in animals, there is insufficient information as to whether this drug may affect fertility in men and women or have teratogenic or other adverse effects on the fetus. The physician should weigh the benefits in relation to the risks when using this and other chemotherapeutic agents in populations in which reproduction may be a factor.
Precautions: Acute uric acid nephropathy, which may occur after the administration of oncolytic agents, has also been reported with Oncovin® (vincristine sulfate, Lilly). In the presence of leukopenia or a complicating infection, administration of the next dose of Oncovin warrants careful consideration.
If central-nervous-system leukemia is diagnosed, additional agents may be required, since Oncovin does not appear to cross the blood-brain barrier in adequate amounts.
Particular attention should be given to dosage and neurologic side effects if Oncovin is administered to patients with preexisting neuromuscular disease and also when other drugs with neurotoxic potential are being used.
Adverse Reactions: In general, adverse reactions are reversible and are related to dosage. The most common adverse reaction is hair loss; the most troublesome are neuromuscular in origin.
When single weekly doses of the drug are employed, the adverse reactions of leukopenia, neuritic pain, constipation, and difficulty in walking are usually of short duration (i.e., less than seven days). When the dosage is reduced, these reactions may lessen or disappear. They seem to be increased when the calculated amount of drug is given in divided doses. Other adverse reactions, such as hair loss, sensory loss, paresthesia, slapping gait, loss of deep-tendon reflexes, and muscle wasting, may persist for at least as long as therapy is continued. In most instances, they have disappeared by about the sixth week after discontinuance of treatment, but in some patients the neuromuscular difficulties may persist for prolonged periods.
In addition to constipation (mentioned below), paralytic ileus may occur, particularly in young children. The ileus will reverse itself upon temporary discontinuance of Oncovin and with symptomatic care. It mimics the "surgical abdomen."
Frequently, there is a sequence in the development of neuromuscular side effects. Initially, only sensory impairment and paresthesias may be encountered. With continued treatment, neuritic pain may appear and, later, motor difficulties. No reports have yet been made of any agent that can reverse the neuromuscular manifestations accompanying therapy with Oncovin® (vincristine sulfate, Lilly).
Convulsions, frequently with hypertension, have been reported in a few patients receiving Oncovin.
Rare occurrences of the syndrome attributed to inappropriate antidiuretic hormone secretion have been observed in patients treated with Oncovin. The syndrome has been described in association with several disease states. There is high urinary sodium excretion in the presence of hyponatremia; renal or adrenal disease, hypotension, dehydration, azotemia, and clinical edema are absent. With fluid deprivation, improvement occurs in the hyponatremia and in the renal loss of sodium.
Constipation may take the form of upper-colon impaction, and, on physical examination, the rectum may be found to be empty. Colicky abdominal pain coupled with an empty rectum may mislead the physician. A flat film of the abdomen is useful in demonstrating this condition. All cases have responded to high enemas and laxatives. A routine prophylactic regimen against constipation is recommended for all patients receiving Onocovin.
Other adverse reactions that have been reported are abdominal cramps, ataxia, foot drop, weight loss, optic atrophy with blindness, transient cortical blindness, fever, cranial nerve manifestations, paresthesia and numbness of the digits, polyuria, dysuria, oral ulceration, headache, vomiting, diarrhea, and intestinal necrosis and/or perforation.
Oncovin does not appear to have any constant or significant effect upon the platelets or the red blood cells. Thrombocytopenia, if present when therapy with Oncovin is begun, may actually improve before the appearance of marrow remission.
Dosage and Administration: This preparation is for intravenous use only (*see Warnings*). Extreme care must be used in calculating and administering the dose of Oncovin® (vincristine sulfate, Lilly), since overdosage may have a very serious or fatal outcome.
The drug is administered intravenously *at weekly intervals.* The usual dose of Oncovin for children is 2 mg/m^2; for adults, 1.4 mg/m^2. Various dosage schedules have been used (see references in package insert).
Oncovin should be mixed with the diluting solution provided (Bacteriostatic Sodium Chloride Injection). The resulting solution of Oncovin may be stored in the refrigerator for 14 days without significant loss of potency.
Oncovin may also be diluted in sterile water or physiological saline to concentrations of 0.01 to 1 mg/ml.
The solution may be injected either directly into a vein or into the tubing of a running intravenous infusion. Injection of the Oncovin may be completed in about one minute.
Caution—It is extremely important that the needle be properly positioned in the vein before any vincristine is injected. If leakage into surrounding tissue should occur during intravenous administration of Oncovin, it may cause considerable irritation. The injection should be discontinued immediately, and any remaining portion of the dose should then be introduced into another vein. Local injection of hyaluronidase and the application of moderate heat to the area of leakage help disperse the drug and are thought to minimize discomfort and the possibility of cellulitis.
Overdosage: Side effects following the use of Oncovin® (vincristine sulfate, Lilly) are dose related. Therefore, following administration of an overdose, patients can be expected to experience side effects in an exaggerated fashion. Supportive care should include the following: (1) prevention of side effects resulting from the syndrome of inappropriate secretion of antidiuretic hormone (this would include restriction of fluid intake and perhaps the administration of a diuretic affecting the function of the loop of Henle and the distal tubule); (2) administration of anticonvulsant doses of phenobarbital; (3) use of enemas to prevent ileus (in some instances, decompression of the gastrointestinal tract may be necessary); (4) monitoring the cardiovascular system; and (5) determining daily blood counts for guidance in transfusion requirements.
Folinic acid has been observed to have a protective effect in normal mice which were administered lethal doses of Oncovin (Cancer Res., *23:*1390, 1963). Isolated case reports suggest that folinic acid may be helpful in treating humans who have received an overdose of Oncovin. A suggested schedule is to administer 15 mg of folinic acid intravenously every three hours for 24 hours and then every six hours for at least 48 hours. Theoretical tissue levels of Oncovin derived from pharmacokinetic data are predicted to remain significantly elevated for at least 72 hours. Treatment with folinic acid does not eliminate the need for the above-mentioned supportive measures.
How Supplied: (℞) *Vials (Multiple Dose) Oncovin® (Vincristine Sulfate for Injection, USP)* (Dry Powder): *No. 694,* 1 mg (NDC 0002-1455-01), and *No. 695,* 5 mg (NDC 0002-1456-01), rubber-stoppered, in singles (10 per carton). *Refrigerate.* [100782]
Vials No. 694, 1 mg—6505-00-904-0024
Vials No. 695, 5 mg—6505-00-903-9990

PAGITANE® HYDROCHLORIDE ℞
(cycrimine hydrochloride)
Tablets, USP

Description: Pagitane® Hydrochloride (cycrimine hydrochloride, Lilly) is α-cyclopentyl-α-phenyl-1-piperidinepropanol hydrochloride.
Actions: Pagitane® Hydrochloride (cycrimine hydrochloride, Lilly) has anticholinergic

activity. It has been suggested that this action may block the uptake of catecholamines into the corpus striatum.

Indications: Pagitane® Hydrochloride (cycrimine hydrochloride, Lilly) is useful as an adjunct in all three types of parkinsonism (postencephalitic, arteriosclerotic, or idiopathic).

Contraindication: Pagitane® Hydrochloride (cycrimine hydrochloride, Lilly) is contraindicated in individuals showing hypersensitivity to this drug.

Warning: Caution should be observed in treating patients with glaucoma, because the possible consequent dilation of the pupil might be harmful.

Usage in Pregnancy—Safety of this product for use during pregnancy has not been established.

Precautions: Use of Pagitane® Hydrochloride (cycrimine hydrochloride, Lilly) should be avoided in those conditions in which inhibition of the parasympathetic nervous system is undesirable.

Great care should be taken in the administration of Pagitane Hydrochloride to patients in the older age groups, particularly those with arteriosclerotic changes, because side effects are likely to be more severe. The drug should be used with caution in patients with tachycardia or any tendency toward urinary retention (such as may be produced by a benign enlargement of the prostate).

Adverse Reactions: Side effects appear to be related to the dosage and to individual sensitivity. Transient nausea associated with anorexia may occur about 30 to 60 minutes after the drug is taken. Some patients may also have blurring of vision and dryness of the mouth, occasionally in conjunction with soreness of the mouth and tongue. These minor side effects often disappear when the drug has been continued for one or two weeks. Epigastric distress can often be overcome if the medication is administered with meals or with a glass of milk. Sucking hard candy at intervals throughout the day usually relieves dryness of the mouth. Lightheadedness, weakness, tachycardia, elevated temperature, flushing, rash, and transitory confusional states have been reported. These side effects quickly disappeared when the drug was discontinued. The more significant side effects were observed in the older age groups, especially in those with arteriosclerotic changes.

Administration and Dosage: Pagitane® Hydrochloride (cycrimine hydrochloride, Lilly) is administered by mouth, preferably with meals. The dosage must be individualized; it is influenced by the type of the disease and by other factors, such as the patient's age. In general, patients with postencephalitic parkinsonism tolerate larger doses of the drug than do those suffering from the arteriosclerotic or idiopathic types of the disease. Elderly patients, particularly when their disease has an arteriosclerotic basis, do not tolerate large single doses. However, an adequate total daily dosage can often be reached in these patients by frequent administration of very small doses. The following are recommended starting doses.

Type of Parkinsonism

Postencephalitic................................5 mg t.i.d.
Idiopathic ....1.25 mg t.i.d.
Arteriosclerotic...............................1.25 mg t.i.d.

The maximum recommended dose is usually 20 mg daily; however, some postencephalitic patients may require more.

Overdosage: Symptoms of intoxication with Pagitane® Hydrochloride (cycrimine hydrochloride, Lilly) are similar to those of atropine overdosage. They include dryness of the mucous membranes, dilatation of pupils, hot, dry, and flushed skin, hyperpyrexia, tachycardia, nausea and vomiting, restlessness and confusion with coma, circulatory collapse, and respiratory depression. Treatment of overdosage is symptomatic. Gastric lavage should be performed with 4 percent tannic acid or other alkaloidal antidotes. To relieve the peripheral effects, 5 mg of pilocarpine may be given orally at repeated intervals. Artificial respiration and oxygen therapy may be needed for respiratory depression. Urinary retention may require catheterization. The hyperpyrexia is best treated with alcohol sponges. To counteract mydriasis, pilocarpine nitrate, 0.5 percent, may be used. Because of photophobia, the patient may be more comfortable in a darkened room.

How Supplied: (℞) *Tablets Pagitane® Hydrochloride (Cycrimine Hydrochloride Tablets, USP): No. 1783, C16,**1.25 mg (NDC 0002-0316-02), Sugar-Coated, Orange, and *No. 1784, C17,** 2.5 mg (NDC 0002-0317-02), Sugar-Coated, Brown, in bottles of 100. [061081]

PENICILLIN G PROCAINE SUSPENSION, STERILE, USP ℞

Duracillin® A.S.

Description: Duracillin® A.S. (Sterile Penicillin G Procaine Suspension, USP, Lilly) is a ready-to-use aqueous suspension of Duracillin® (Penicillin G Procaine, USP, Lilly), the original penicillin G procaine, which was developed in the Lilly laboratories to fill a need for a long-acting parenteral penicillin preparation. Penicillin G procaine is a stable crystalline salt which is only slightly soluble in water. When combined with certain dispersing agents and suspended in water, it is slowly absorbed (because of its low solubility in body fluids) from the injection site in the muscle.

Each ml contains 300,000 units crystalline penicillin G procaine; sodium citrate, 4%; lecithin, 1%; povidone, 0.1%; with methylparaben, 0.15%, propylparaben, 0.02%, benzyl alcohol, 1%, as preservatives; water for injection, q.s.

Actions and Pharmacology: Penicillin G is bactericidal against penicillin-susceptible microorganisms during the stage of active multiplication. It produces its effect by inhibiting biosynthesis of cell-wall mucopeptide. It is not active against the penicillinase-producing bacteria, which include many strains of staphylococci. Pencillin G exerts high in vitro activity against staphylococci (except penicillinase-producing strains), streptococci (groups A, C, G, H, L, and M), and pneumococci. Other organisms suspectible to penicillin G are *Neisseria gonorrhoeae, Corynebacterium diphtheriae, Bacillus anthracis, Clostridium, Actinomyces bovis, Streptobacillus moniliformis, Listeria monocytogenes,* and *Leptospira. Treponema pallidum* is extremely susceptible to the bactericidal action of penicillin G.

Disc Susceptibility Tests—Quantitative methods that require measurement of zone diameters give the most precise estimates of antibiotic susceptibility. One such procedure (*Am. J. Clin. Pathol., 45:*493, 1966; *Federal Register, 39:*19182–19184, 1974) has been recommended for use with discs for testing susceptibility to penicillin.

Penicillin G procaine is an equimolecular compound of procaine and penicillin G administered intramuscularly as a suspension. It dissolves slowly at the site of injection and gives a plateau type of blood level at about four hours, which falls slowly over a period of the next 15 to 20 hours.

Approximately 60 percent of penicillin G is bound to serum protein. The drug is distributed throughout the body tissues in widely varying amounts. Highest levels are found in the kidneys, and lesser amounts appear in the liver, skin, and intestines. Small concentrations are found in all other body tissues and the cerebrospinal fluid. With normal kidney function, the drug is excreted rapidly by tubular excretion. In neonates, young infants, and individuals with impaired kidney function, excretion is considerably delayed. Approximately 60 to 90 percent of a dose of parenteral penicillin G is excreted in the urine within 24 to 36 hours.

Indications: Penicillin G procaine is indicated in the treatment of moderately severe infections due to penicillin-G-susceptible microorganisms that are sensitive to the low and persistent serum levels common to this particular dosage form. Therapy should be guided by bacteriologic studies (including susceptibility tests) and by clinical response.

NOTE: When high, sustained serum levels are required, aqueous penicillin G should be used either intramuscularly or intravenously.

The following infections will usually respond to adequate dosages of intramuscular penicillin G procaine:

Streptococcal Infections (Group A) (without Bacteremia)—Moderately severe to severe infections of the upper respiratory tract, skin and soft-tissue infections, scarlet fever, and erysipelas.

NOTE: Streptococci in groups A, C, G, H, L, and M are very susceptible to penicillin G. Other groups, including group D (enterococcus), are resistant. Aqueous penicillin is recommended for streptococcal infections with bacteremia.

Pneumococcal Infections—Moderately severe infections of the respiratory tract.

NOTE: Severe pneumonia, empyema, bacteremia, pericarditis, meningitis, peritonitis, and arthritis of pneumococcal etiology are better treated with aqueous penicillin G during the acute stage.

Staphylococcal Infections Susceptible to Penicillin G—Moderately severe infections of the skin and soft tissues.

NOTE: Reports indicate an increasing number of strains of staphylococci resistant to penicillin G, which emphasizes the need for culture and susceptibility studies in treating suspected staphylococcal infections.

Indicated surgical procedures should be performed.

Fusospirochetosis (Vincent's Gingivitis and Pharyngitis)—Moderately severe infections of the oropharynx respond to therapy with penicillin G procaine.

NOTE: Necessary dental care should be accomplished in infections involving the gum tissue.

Syphilis (T. pallidum)—All stages

Acute and Chronic Gonorrhea (without Bacteremia) (N. gonorrhoeae)

Yaws, Bejel, Pinta

Diphtheria (C. diphtheriae)—Penicillin G procaine as an adjunct to antitoxin for prevention of the carrier stage.

Anthrax

Rat-Bite Fever (S. moniliformis and *Spirillum minus)*

Erysipeloid

Subacute Bacterial Endocarditis (Group A Streptococci)—Limited to extremely susceptible strains.

Although no controlled clinical efficacy studies have been conducted, aqueous crystalline penicillin G for injection and penicillin G procaine suspension have been suggested by the American Heart Association and the American Dental Association for use as part of a combined parenteral/oral regimen for prophylaxis against bacterial endocarditis in patients with congenital heart disease or rheumatic or other acquired valvular heart disease when they undergo dental procedures and surgical procedures of the upper respiratory tract.[1] Since alpha-hemolytic streptococci relatively resistant to penicillin may be found when patients are receiving continuous oral penicillin for secondary prevention of rheumatic fever, prophylactic agents other than penicillin may be

Continued on next page

*Identi-Code® symbol.

Lilly—Cont.

chosen for these patients and prescribed in addition to their continuous prophylactic regimen for rheumatic fever.

NOTE: When selecting antibiotics for the prevention of bacterial endocarditis, the physician or dentist should read the full joint statement of the American Heart Association and the American Dental Association.[1]

Contraindication: A previous hypersensitivity reaction to any penicillin is a contraindication.

Warnings: Serious and occasionally fatal hypersensitivity (anaphylactoid) reactions have been reported in patients receiving penicillin therapy. Although anaphylaxis is more frequent following parenteral therapy, it has occurred in patients given oral penicillins. These reactions are more likely in individuals with a history of sensitivity to multiple allergens.

There have been well-documented reports of individuals with a history of penicillin hypersensitivity who have experienced severe reactions when treated with a cephalosporin. Before therapy with a penicillin, careful inquiry should be made concerning previous hypersensitivity reactions to penicillins, cephalosporins, and other allergens. If an allergic reaction occurs, the drug should be discontinued and the patient treated with the usual agents (e.g., epinephrine or other pressor amines, antihistamines, or corticosteroids).

Immediate toxic reactions to procaine may occur in some individuals, particularly when a large single dose is administered in the treatment of gonorrhea (4,800,000 units). These reactions may be mainifested by mental disturbances, including anxiety, confusion, agitation, depression, weakness, seizures, hallucinations, combativeness, and expressed "fear of impending death." The reactions noted in carefully controlled studies occurred in approximately one of 500 patients treated for gonorrhea. Reactions are transient and last from 15 to 30 minutes.

Precautions: Penicillin should be used with caution in individuals having histories of significant allergies and/or asthma.

In intramuscular therapy, care should be taken to avoid accidental intravenous administration.

In suspected staphylococcal infections, proper laboratory studies, including susceptibility tests, should be performed.

A small percentage of patients are sensitive to procaine. If there is a history of sensitivity, make the usual test: Inject 0.1 ml of a 1 to 2 percent procaine solution intradermally. Development of an erythema, wheal, flare, or eruption indicates procaine sensitivity. Sensitivity should be treated by the usual methods, including barbiturates, and penicillin procaine preparations should not be used. Antihistamines appear beneficial in treatment of procaine reactions.

The use of antibiotics may result in overgrowth of nonsusceptible organisms. Constant observation of the patient is essential. If new infections due to bacteria or fungi appear during therapy, the drug should be discontinued and appropriate measures taken. Whenever allergic reactions occur, penicillin should be withdrawn unless, in the opinion of the physician, the condition being treated is life threatening and amendable only to penicillin therapy. In prolonged therapy with penicillin, and particularly with high dosage schedules, periodic evaluation of the renal and hematopoietic systems is recommended.

When gonococcal infections are treated in which primary or secondary syphilis may be suspected, proper diagnostic procedures, including darkfield examinations, should be performed. In all cases in which concomitant syphilis is suspected, monthly serologic tests should be made for at least four months.

Adverse Reactions: Penicillin is a substance of low toxicity but does have a significant index of sensitization. The following hypersensitivity reactions have been reported: skin rashes ranging from maculopapular eruptions to exfoliative dermatitis; urticaria; and reactions resembling serum sickness, including chills, fever, edema, arthralgia, and prostration. Severe and often fatal anaphylaxis has occurred (*see* Warnings). As with other treatments for syphilis, the Jarisch-Herxheimer reaction has been reported.

Manifestations of procaine toxicity have been reported (*see* Warnings). Procaine hypersensitivity reactions have not been reported with this drug.

Dosage and Administration: Penicillin G procaine (aqueous) is for intramuscular injection only.

Recommended dosage is as follows:

Pneumonia (Pneumococcus)—Moderately severe (uncomplicated): 600,000 to 1,000,000 units daily.

Streptococcal Infections (Group A)—Moderately severe to severe tonsillitis, erysipelas, scarlet fever, and upper respiratory tract, skin, and soft-tissue infections: 600,000 to 1,000,000 units daily for a minimum of ten days.

Staphylococcal Infections—Moderately severe to severe: 600,000 to 1,000,000 units daily.

For prophylaxis against bacterial endocarditis[1] in patients with congenital heart disease or rheumatic or other acquired valvular heart disease when undergoing dental procedures or surgical procedures of the upper respiratory tract, use a combined parenteral/oral regimen. One million units of aqueous crystalline penicillin G (30,000 units/kg in children) mixed with 600,000 units of procaine penicillin G (600,000 units for children) should be given intramuscularly one-half to one hour before the procedure. Oral penicillin V (phenoxymethyl penicillin), 500 mg for adults or 250 mg for children weighing less than 30 kg, should be given every six hours for eight doses. Doses for children should not exceed the recommendations for adults for a single dose or for a 24-hour period.

Syphilis—Primary, secondary, and latent with a negative spinal fluid in adults and children over 12 years of age: 600,000 units daily for eight days (total, 4,800,000 units.)

Late (tertiary and latent syphilis and neurosyphilis with positive spinal-fluid examination or no spinal fluid examination): 600,000 units daily for ten to 15 days (total, 6,000,000 to 9,000,000 units).

Congenital syphilis in a patient weighing less than 70 pounds: 10,000 units/kg/day for ten days.

Syphilis in pregnancy: Treatment should correspond to the stage of the disease.

Yaws, Bejel, and Pinta—Same treatment as for syphilis in corresponding stage of disease.

Gonorrheal Infections (Uncomplicated)—Men or women: 4,800,000 units intramuscularly, divided into at least two doses and injected at different sites during one visit, together with 1 g of oral probenecid, preferably given at least 30 minutes prior to the injection.

NOTE: Gonorrheal endocarditis should be treated intensively with aqueous penicillin G.

Diphtheria—Adjunctive therapy with antitoxin: 300,000 to 600,000 units daily.

Diphtheria Carrier State—300,000 units daily for ten days.

Anthrax (Cutaneous)—600,000 to 1,000,000 units/day.

Vincent's Infection (Fusospirochetosis)—600,000 to 1,000,000 units/day.

Erysipeloid—600,000 to 1,000,000 units/day.

Rat-Bite Fever (S. moniliformis and *S. minus)*—600,000 to 1,000,000 units/day.

Reference: 1. American Heart Association: Prevention of Bacterial Endocarditis, Circulation, *56:*139A, 1977.

How Supplied: (℞) *Vials (Multiple Dose) No. 554, Sterile Penicillin G Procaine Suspension, USP,* 300,000 units/ml, 10 ml, rubber-stoppered, in singles (10 per carton) (NDC 0002-7185-01) and in Traypak™ (multivial carton, Lilly) of 100 (NDC 0002-7185-02).

Refrigerate. Avoid freezing. [031682]

PENICILLIN V POTASSIUM PRODUCTS,

see V-Cillin K® (penicillin V potassium, Lilly).

POTASSIUM IODIDE ℞
USP

Description: Each Enseal® (enteric-release tablet, Lilly) Potassium Iodide, USP, contains 300 mg of the salt in a special coating designed to prevent disintegration in the stomach.

Potassium iodide occurs as hexahedral crystals, either transparent and colorless or somewhat opaque and white, or as a white, granular powder. It is stable in dry air but slightly hygroscopic in moist air. With prolonged storage, it may become yellowish because of oxidation. Potassium iodide is very soluble in water and even more soluble in boiling water, freely soluble in glycerin, and soluble in alcohol.

Clinical Pharmacology: Iodide is absorbed from the enteric tract as iodinated amino acids and distributed largely extracellularly. It is markedly accumulated by the thyroid gland, and its concentration is far greater in gastric and salivary solutions than in extracellular fluids. Most of plasma iodine is in the form of thyroid hormones. The kidney serves as the chief excretory organ for iodide.

Indications and Usage: Potassium iodide is used as an expectorant to liquefy the tenacious bronchial secretions often seen in chronic bronchitis, bronchiectasis, and asthma.

Contraindications: Known sensitivity to iodides is a contraindication to the use of potassium iodide. The drug should not be administered in the presence of acute bronchitis.

Warnings: There have been several reports, published and unpublished, concerning nonspecific small-bowel lesions (consisting of stenosis with or without ulceration) associated with the administration of enteric-coated thiazides with potassium salts. Such lesions may occur when enteric-coated potassium tablets are given alone, with non-enteric-coated thiazides, or with certain other oral diuretics.

These small-bowel lesions have caused obstruction, hemorrhage, and perforation. Surgery has frequently been required, and deaths have occurred.

Available information tends to implicate enteric-coated potassium salts, although lesions of this type also occur spontaneously. Therefore, coated potassium-containing formulations should be administered only when indicated and should be discontinued immediately if abdominal pain, distention, nausea, vomiting, or gastrointestinal bleeding occurs.

Coated potassium tablets should be used only when adequate dietary supplementation is not practical.

Potassium iodide can cause fetal harm when administered to a pregnant woman. Because of the possible development of fetal goiter, if this drug is used during pregnancy or if the patient becomes pregnant while taking it, the patient should be apprised of the potential hazard to the fetus.

Precautions: *General Precautions*—Occasionally, persons are markedly sensitive to iodides, and care should be used in administering the drug for the first time. Iodides should be given with great caution, if at all, in the presence of tuberculosis. *See* Warnings.

Laboratory Tests—Determinations in tests of thyroid function may be altered by the iodide in this product.

Drug Interactions—*See* Warnings.

Usage in Pregnancy—*Pregnancy Category D*—*See* Warnings.

Nursing Mothers—It is not known whether this drug is excreted in human milk. Because many drugs are excreted in human milk, caution should be exercised when potassium iodide is administered to a nursing woman.
Usage in Children—Safety and effectiveness in children have not been established.
Adverse Reactions: Thyroid adenoma, goiter, and myxedema are possible side effects.
Hypersensitivity to iodides may be manifested by angioneurotic edema, cutaneous and mucosal hemorrhages, and symptoms resembling serum sickness, such as fever, arthralgia, lymph node enlargement, and eosinophilia.
Iodism or chronic iodine poisoning may occur during prolonged treatment. The symptoms of iodism include a metallic taste, soreness of the mouth, increased salivation, coryza, sneezing, and swelling of the eyelids. There may be a severe headache, productive cough, pulmonary edema, and swelling and tenderness of the salivary glands. Acneform skin lesions are seen in the seborrheic areas. Severe and sometimes fatal skin eruptions may develop. Gastric disturbance and diarrhea are common. If iodism appears, the drug should be withdrawn and the patient given appropriate supportive therapy.
Overdosage: Acute toxicity from potassium iodide is relatively rare. An occasional individual, however, may show a marked sensitivity and the onset of acute poisoning can occur immediately or hours after administration. Angioedema, larygeal edema, and cutaneous hemorrhages may be manifested.
The symptoms of iodism disappear soon after administration of the drug is discontinued. Abundant fluid and salt intake aids in elimination of iodide.
Dosage and Administration: The usual adult daily dose of potassium iodide given to increase secretions is 1 or 2 Enseals three times a day. If symptoms of increased lacrimal and nasal secretions are noted, the dose should be decreased to 1 Enseal three times a day or less. The medication should be used no longer than is necessary to produce the desired effect. However, in chronic conditions, continuous administration may be required.
How Supplied: (℞) *Enseals No. 23, Potassium Iodide Tablets, USP (Enteric), A06,* * 300 mg, in bottles of 100 (NDC 0002-0106-02) and 1000 (NDC 0002-0106-04).

[071682]

POTASSIUM TRIPLEX, *see* Trikates Oral Solution, USP.

PROPYLTHIOURACIL ℞
Tablets, USP

Description: Propylthiouracil (6-propyl-2-thiouracil) is one of the thiocarbamide compounds. It is a white crystalline substance that has a bitter taste and is very slightly soluble in water.
Each tablet contains 50 mg propylthiouracil. Propylthiouracil is an antithyroid drug administered orally in the treatment of hyperthyroidism, either preoperatively or when thyroidectomy is contraindicated or not advisable. The molecular weight is 170.23, and the empirical formula is $C_7H_{10}N_2OS$.
Clinical Pharmacology: Propylthiouracil inhibits the synthesis of thyroid hormones and thus is effective in the treatment of hyperthyroidism. The drug does not inactivate existing thyroxine and triiodothyronine which is stored in the thyroid or is circulating in the blood, nor does it interfere with the effectiveness of thyroid hormones given by mouth or by injection. Propylthiouracil is readily absorbed from the gastrointestinal tract. It is metabolized rapidly and requires frequent administration. Approximately 35% of the drug is excreted in the urine, intact and in conjugated form, within 24 hours.
Indications and Usage: Propylthiouracil is indicated in the medical treatment of hyperthyroidism. Long-term therapy may lead to remission of the disease. Propylthiouracil may also be used to ameliorate hyperthyroidism in preparation for subtotal thyroidectomy or radioactive iodine therapy. Propylthiouracil is also used when thyroidectomy is contraindicated or not advisable.
Contraindications: Propylthiouracil is contraindicated in the presence of hypersensitivity to the drug and in nursing mothers, since the drug is excreted in milk.
Warnings: Propylthiouracil can cause fetal harm when administered to a pregnant woman. Because the drug readily crosses placental membranes and can induce goiter and even cretinism in the developing fetus, it is important that a sufficient, but not excessive, dose be given. In many pregnant women, the thyroid dysfunction diminishes as the pregnancy proceeds; consequently, a reduction of dosage may be possible. In some instances, propylthiouracil can be withdrawn two or three weeks before delivery.
If this drug is used during pregnancy, or if the patient becomes pregnant while taking this drug, the patient should be apprised of the potential hazard to the fetus.
Postpartum patients receiving propylthiouracil should not nurse their babies.
Agranulocytosis is potentially the most serious side effect of propylthiouracil therapy. Leukopenia and thrombocytopenia may also occur. Patients should be instructed to report any symptoms of agranulocytosis, such as fever or sore throat.
Precautions: *General Precautions*—Patients who receive propylthiouracil should be under close surveillance and should be impressed with the necessity of reporting immediately any evidence of illness, particularly sore throat, skin eruptions, fever, headache, or general malaise. In such cases, white-blood-cell and differential counts should be made to determine whether agranulocytosis has developed. Particular care should be exercised with patients who are receiving additional drugs known to cause agranulocytosis.
Laboratory Tests—Because propylthiouracil may cause hypoprothrombinemia and bleeding, prothrombin time should be monitored during therapy with the drug, especially before surgical procedures.
Drug Interactions—The activity of anticoagulants may be potentiated by anti-vitamin-K activity attributed to propylthiouracil.
Usage in Pregnancy—Pregnancy Category D—See Warnings.
Nursing Mothers—The drug appears in human milk and is contraindicated in nursing mothers. *See* Warnings.
Usage in Children—See Dosage and Administration.
Adverse Reactions: Adverse reactions probably occur in less than 1 percent of patients. Major adverse reactions (much less common than the minor adverse reactions) include inhibition of myelopoiesis (agranulocytosis, granulopenia, and thrombocytopenia), drug fever, a lupuslike syndrome, hepatitis, periarteritis, and hypoprothrombinemia and bleeding. Nephritis has been reported.
Minor adverse reactions include skin rash, urticaria, nausea, vomiting, epigastric distress, arthralgia, paresthesia, loss of taste, abnormal loss of hair, myalgia, headache, pruritus, drowsiness, neuritis, edema, vertigo, skin pigmentation, jaundice, sialadenopathy, and lymphadenopathy.
It should be noted that about 10 percent of patients with untreated hyperthyroidism have leukopenia (white-blood-cell count of less than 4000/mm^3), often with relative granulopenia.
Overdosage: Agranulocytosis is the most serious effect. Rarely, exfoliative dermatitis, hepatitis, neuropathies, or CNS stimulation or depression may occur.
Symptoms—Nausea, vomiting, epigastric distress, headache, fever, arthralgia, pruritus, edema, and pancytopenia. Prolonged therapy may result in hypothyroidism.
Treatment—For specific therapy, the drug should be discontinued in the presence of agranulocytosis, pancytopenia, hepatitis, fever, or exfoliative dermatitis.
For bone-marrow depression, use of an antibiotic and transfusions of fresh whole blood should be considered.
For hepatitis, rest and adequate diet may be indicated.
General management may consist in symptomatic and supportive therapy, including rest, analgesics, gastric lavage, intravenous fluids, and mild sedation.
Dosage and Administration: Propylthiouracil is administered orally. The total daily dosage is usually given in three equal doses at approximately eight-hour intervals.
Adult—The initial dosage is 300 mg daily. In patients with severe hyperthyroidism, very large goiters, or both, the beginning dosage usually should be 400 mg daily; an occasional patient will require 600 to 900 mg/day initially. The usual maintenance dosage is 100 to 150 mg daily.
Pediatric—For children six to ten years of age, the initial dosage is 50 to 150 mg daily. For children ten years and over, the initial dosage is 150 to 300 mg daily. The maintenance dosage is determined by the response of the patient.
How Supplied: (℞) *Tablets No. 1723, Propylthiouracil, USP, J69,* * 50 mg (scored), in bottles of 100 (NDC 0002-1069-02) and 1000 (NDC 0002-1069-04).

[040982]

PROTAMINE SULFATE ℞
Injection, USP

Description: Protamines are simple proteins of low molecular weight that are rich in arginine and strongly basic. They occur in the sperm of salmon and certain other species of fish.
Each 5-ml ampoule of Protamine Sulfate Injection, USP, contains protamine sulfate equivalent to 50 mg of activity, and each 25-ml vial contains protamine sulfate equivalent to 250 mg of activity. Both products also contain 0.9 percent sodium chloride. Sodium phosphate and/or sulfuric acid may have been added during manufacture to adjust the *p*H. Contains no preservative.
Actions: When administered alone, protamine has an anticoagulant effect. However, when it is given in the presence of heparin (which is strongly acidic), a stable salt is formed which results in the loss of anticoagulant activity of both drugs.
Indication: Protamine sulfate is indicated in the treatment of heparin overdosage.
Warnings: Hyperheparinemia or bleeding has been reported in experimental animals and in some patients 30 minutes to 18 hours after cardiac surgery (under cardiopulmonary bypass) in spite of complete neutralization of heparin by adequate doses of protamine sulfate at the end of the operation.
Therefore, it is important to keep the patient under close observation after cardiac surgery. Additional doses of protamine sulfate should be administered if indicated by coagulation studies, such as the heparin titration test with protamine and the determination of plasma thrombin time.
Too rapid administration of protamine sulfate can cause severe hypotensive and anaphylactoid-like reactions. Facilities to treat shock should be available. (*See* Dosage and Administration).

Continued on next page

*Identi-Code® symbol.

Lilly—Cont.

Usage in Pregnancy—Reproduction studies have not been performed in animals. There is no adequate information as to whether this drug may affect fertility in human males or females or have a teratogenic potential or other adverse effect on the fetus.

Precautions: Because of the anticoagulant effect of protamine, it is unwise to give more than 100 mg over a short period unless there is certain knowledge of a larger requirement.

Patients with a history of allergy to fish may develop hypersensitivity reactions to protamine, although to date no relationship has been established between allergic reactions to protamine and fish allergy. A number of individuals hypersensitive to fish have received protamine sulfate without developing allergic reactions.

Adverse Reactions: Intravenous injections of protamine may cause a sudden fall in blood pressure, bradycardia, dyspnea, or transitory flushing and a feeling of warmth. There have been reports of anaphylaxis that resulted in respiratory embarrassment (*see* Precautions).

Because fatal reactions often resembling anaphylaxis have been reported after administration of protamine sulfate, the drug should be given only when resuscitation techniques and treatment of anaphylactoid shock are readily available.

Dosage and Administration: Each mg of protamine sulfate neutralizes approximately 90 USP units of heparin activity derived from lung tissue or about 115 USP units of heparin activity derived from intestinal mucosa.

Protamine Sulfate Injection, USP, should be given by very slow intravenous injection in doses not to exceed 50 mg of protamine sulfate in any 10-minute period (*see* Warnings).

Protamine sulfate is intended for injection without further dilution; however, if further dilution is desired, D5W or normal saline may be used. Diluted solutions should not be stored since they contain no preservative.

Protamine sulfate should not be mixed with other drugs without knowledge of their compatibility, because protamine sulfate has been shown to be incompatible with certain antibiotics, including several of the cephalosporins and penicillins.

Because heparin disappears rapidly from the circulation, the dose of protamine sulfate required also decreases rapidly with the time elapsed following intravenous injection of heparin. For example, if the protamine sulfate is administered 30 minutes after the heparin, one-half the usual dose may be sufficient.

The dosage of protamine sulfate should be guided by blood coagulation studies (*see* Warnings).

How Supplied: (℞) *Protamine Sulfate Injection, USP: Ampoules No. 473,* 5 ml (equivalent to 50 mg of activity), in packages of 6 (NDC 0002-1691-16) and 25 (NDC 0002-1691-25); *Vials No. 735,* 25 ml (equivalent to 250 mg of activity), rubber-stoppered, in singles (10 per carton) (NDC 0002-1462-01). *Refrigerate. Avoid freezing.*

Both products should be stored in the refrigerator above freezing and below 50°F.

CAUTION—The total dose of protamine sulfate contained in Vials No. 735 (250 mg of activity in 25 ml) is five times greater than that in Ampoules No. 473 (50 mg of activity in 5 ml). The large-size vials (No. 735) are designed only for antiheparin treatment in certain cases in which large doses of heparin have been given during surgery and are to be neutralized by large doses of protamine sulfate after surgical procedures.

[020282]

Ampoules No. 473, 5 ml—6's—6505-00-299-9667

QUINIDINE GLUCONATE ℞
Injection, USP

Description: Quinidine gluconate, a white dextrorotatory salt, contains 62.3 percent anhydrous quinidine and 37.7 percent gluconic acid. Quinidine Gluconate Injection, USP, is suitable for parenteral use because of its high efficacy, local tolerance, and stability in solution.

Each vial contains 800 mg of the salt of the alkaloid in 10 ml of Sterile Water for Injection, with 0.005 percent edetate disodium and 0.25 percent phenol. This quantity of quinidine gluconate represents 500 mg of anhydrous quinidine.

Indications: Parenteral administration of quinidine is indicated in the treatment of the following conditions when oral therapy is not feasible or when rapid therapeutic effect is required:

- Premature atrial and ventricular contractions
- Paroxysmal atrial tachycardia
- Paroxysmal atrioventricular junctional rhythm
- Atrial flutter
- Paroxysmal atrial fibrillation
- Established atrial fibrillation when therapy is appropriate
- Paroxysmal ventricular tachycardia when not associated with complete heart block
- Maintenance therapy after electrical conversion of atrial fibrillation and/or flutter

Contraindications: Aberrant impulses and abnormal rhythms due to escape mechanisms should not be treated with quinidine.

The other absolute contraindication to the use of quinidine is the known presence of an idiosyncrasy or hypersensitivity to this alkaloid or to other derivatives of cinchona.

Warnings: In the treatment of atrial flutter, reversion to sinus rhythm may be preceded by a progressive reduction in the degree of atrioventricular block to a 1:1 ratio and a resulting extremely rapid ventricular rate.

The dangers of the parenteral use of quinidine are increased in the presence of atrioventricular heart block or in the absence of atrial activity. The administration of quinidine is more hazardous in patients with extensive myocardial damage than it is in persons with a normal heart who have a cardiac arrhythmia. Occasionally, a cardiac arrhythmia may have been produced by digitalis intoxication, and the use of quinidine in this situation is extremely dangerous because the cardiac glycoside may already have caused serious impairment of the intracardiac conduction system.

Adverse Reactions: As much as 500 mg of quinidine gluconate has been administered into the gluteal muscle without producing irritation.

It was reported that untoward subjective reactions, such as nausea, vomiting, cramps, an urge to defecate or urinate, cold sweat, and apprehensiveness, occurred in patients who received quinidine lactate by the intravenous route. Such symptoms were unrelated to the dosage and occurred when as little as 130 to 260 mg of this preparation was given. Signs of cinchonism, such as vertigo, tinnitus, headache, fever, and visual disturbances, can be produced by an overdose of quinidine, regardless of the route of administration.

The rate of injection into the vein is all-important. Too-rapid administration of as little as 200 mg of quinidine may cause a fall of 40 to 50 mm Hg in arterial pressure.

Large doses of the alkaloid may have a deleterious effect on the heart and result in heart block or standstill in diastole. Deaths have been reported during the intravenous administration of quinidine, but in every instance the patient was *in extremis* before this treatment was initiated. The undesirable effects are more likely to occur in the presence of a previously damaged myocardium than in the treatment of arrhythmia of a more normal heart.

Dosage and Administration: If the patient's condition is not critical, quinidine gluconate should be given intramuscularly. On the other hand, extreme palpitation, dyspnea, vomiting, and a shocklike state in patients with ventricular tachycardia are signs that the intravenous administration of quinidine may be required as a lifesaving measure.

The patient must be under close clinical observation. Frequent or continuous electrocardiograms are desirable, especially during intravenous injection, to detect any change in rate or rhythm.

Administration of the drug must be stopped when any one of the following occurs: (1) side effects of more than trivial nature, (2) restoration of sinus rhythm, (3) prolongation of QRS complex in excess of 25 percent beyond that observed prior to the injection, (4) disappearance of P waves, and (5) decrease in heart rate to 120 beats/minute.

In the treatment of cardiac arrhythmias with quinidine, therapy should be regulated in such a way that the drug is accumulated in the heart in sufficient quantities to abolish ectopic rhythm without disturbing the normal mechanism of the heartbeat. *The effective dose must be determined for each patient.*

If the patient has not received quinidine before and time permits, an initial dose of 200 mg of quinidine gluconate may be given intramuscularly as a test for idiosyncrasy. The test dose is given intramuscularly, regardless of whether subsequent administration is to be intramuscular or intravenous.

Intramuscular—In the treatment of acute tachycardia, the recommended initial dose is 600 mg. Subsequently, the injection of 400 mg of quinidine gluconate can be repeated as often as every two hours. The amount of each dose must be gauged by the effect of the preceding one.

Intravenous—It has been shown that in about 50 percent of patients who respond successfully to quinidine, the arrhythmia can be terminated by 330 mg or less of quinidine gluconate (or its equivalent in other salts). In some cases, the intravenous administration of as much as 500 to 750 mg may be required.

The quinidine gluconate solution must be injected *slowly.* It is advisable to dilute 10 ml of the preparation to 50 ml, using 5 percent glucose as the diluent. It has been suggested that the diluted quinidine gluconate be given at a rate of 1 ml/minute for maximum safety.

Clinical Reports: Intramuscular administration of quinidine gluconate was found by various investigators to be satisfactory in treating acute arrhythmias. Characteristic quinidine effect was observed as early as 15 minutes after injection, and conversion occurred within two hours. The maximum concentration of quinidine in the blood occurred after one hour, and the peak level was higher with a single dose of quinidine gluconate than with an equivalent intramuscular dose of quinidine sulfate in urea-antipyrine or in propylene glycol.

It has been repeatedly reported that the intravenous use of quinidine was successful in the treatment of urgent cases of tachycardias, particularly ventricular tachycardia. Normal rhythm was restored as quickly as four to six minutes after injection.

How Supplied: (℞) *Vials (Multiple Dose) No. 530, Quinidine Gluconate Injection, USP,* 80 mg/ml, 10 ml, rubber-stoppered, in singles (10 per carton) (NDC 0002-1407-01). [033082]

QUINIDINE SULFATE ℞
USP

Description: Quinidine sulfate occurs as minute needlelike white crystals (frequently cohering in masses) or fine white powder. It is odorless, has a very bitter taste, and darkens on exposure to light. It is slightly soluble in water, soluble in alcohol and in chloroform, and insoluble in ether. It contains not less than 99 percent and not more than 101 percent of total alkaloids, calculated as $(C_{20}H_{24}N_2O_2)_2 \cdot H_2SO_4$, on the anhydrous basis.

Clinical Pharmacology: Quinidine is generally regarded as a myocardial depressant drug, because it depresses excitability, conduction velocity, and contractility of the myocardium. Besides these direct effects, quinidine exerts some indirect activity on the heart through an anticholinergic action. Large oral doses may reduce the arterial pressure by means of peripheral vasodilation. Hypotension of a serious degree is more likely with the parenteral use of the drug.

Quinidine is rapidly absorbed from the gastrointestinal tract. The peak concentrations in plasma are attained in 60 to 90 minutes, and activity persists six to eight hours or more. Quinidine is metabolized in the liver and excreted by the kidney. Ten to 50 percent of quinidine is excreted in the urine as unchanged drug within 24 hours. Blood levels of quinidine can be measured; the average therapeutic range is between 3 and 6 mg/liter of plasma. Toxic reactions are almost certain to appear at levels above 8 mg/liter.

Indications and Usage: Quinidine sulfate is indicated in the treatment of:

- Premature atrial and ventricular contractions
- Paroxysmal atrial tachycardia
- Paroxysmal atrioventricular (AV) junctional rhythm
- Atrial flutter
- Paroxysmal atrial fibrillation
- Established atrial fibrillation when therapy is appropriate
- Paroxysmal ventricular tachycardia when not associated with complete heart block
- Maintenance therapy after electrical conversion of atrial fibrillation and/or flutter

Contraindications: Contraindications include hypersensitivity or idiosyncrasy to the drug, history of thrombocytopenic purpura associated with previous quinidine administration, digitalis intoxication manifested by AV conduction disorders, complete AV block with an AV nodal or idioventricular pacemaker, and ectopic impulses and rhythms due to escape mechanisms.

Warnings: In the treatment of atrial flutter, reversion to sinus rhythm may be preceded by a progressive reduction in the degree of AV block to a 1:1 ratio, which results in extremely rapid ventricular rate. This possible hazard may be decreased by digitalization prior to administration of quinidine.

Evidence of quinidine cardiotoxicity (50 percent widening of QRS complex, frequent ventricular ectopic beats) mandates immediate discontinuation of the drug and subsequent close observation (electrocardiographic monitoring) of the patient.

Precautions: *General Precautions*—Quinidine should be used with extreme caution when there is incomplete AV block, since complete block and asystole may result. The drug may cause unpredictable abnormalities of rhythm in digitalized hearts, and it should be used with special caution in the presence of digitalis intoxication.

Note—The effect of quinidine is enhanced by potassium and reduced if hypokalemia is present.

The depressant actions of quinidine on cardiac contractility and arterial blood pressure limit its use in congestive heart failure and in hypotensive states unless these conditions are due to or aggravated by the arrhythmia. The potential disadvantages and benefits must be weighed.

Laboratory Tests—Continuous electrocardiographic monitoring and determination of plasma quinidine levels are indicated when large doses (more than 2 g/day) are used.

Liver function should be monitored during the first four to eight weeks of therapy because of possible liver injury associated with the use of quinidine sulfate.

Usage in Pregnancy—Pregnancy Category C—Animal reproduction studies have not been conducted with quinidine sulfate. It is also not known whether quinidine sulfate can cause fetal harm when administered to a pregnant woman or can affect reproduction capacity. Quinidine sulfate should be given to a pregnant woman only if clearly needed.

Nursing Mothers—It is not known whether this drug is excreted in human milk. Because many drugs are excreted in human milk, caution should be exercised when quinidine sulfate is administered to a nursing woman.

Usage in Children—Safety and effectiveness in children have not been established.

Adverse Reactions: *Symptoms of Cinchonism* (ringing in the ears, headache, nausea, disturbed vision)—These may appear (in sensitive patients) after a single dose of the drug.

Cardiovascular—Widening of QRS complex, cardiac asystole, ventricular ectopic beats, idioventricular rhythms (including ventricular tachycardia and fibrillation), paradoxical tachycardia, arterial embolism.

Gastrointestinal—Nausea, vomiting, abdominal pain, diarrhea, hepatitis.

Hematologic—Acute hemolytic anemia, hypoprothrombinemia, thrombocytopenic purpura, agranulocytosis.

Central Nervous System—Headache, fever, vertigo, apprehension, excitement, confusion, delirium and syncope, disturbed hearing (tinnitus, decreased auditory acuity), disturbed vision (mydriasis, blurred vision, disturbed color perception, photophobia, diplopia, night blindness, scotomata), optic neuritis.

Dermatologic—Cutaneous flushing with intense pruritus.

Hypersensitivity Reactions—Angioedema, acute asthmatic episode, vascular collapse, respiratory arrest.

Overdosage: Cardiotoxic effects of quinidine may be reversed in part by molar sodium lactate; the hypotension, by vasoconstrictors and by catecholamines (since the vasodilatation is partly due to α adrenergic blockade).

Dosage and Administration: A preliminary test dose of a single tablet of quinidine sulfate should be administered to determine whether the patient has an idiosyncrasy to it. Continuous electrocardiographic monitoring is recommended in all cases in which quinidine is used in large doses.

Usual Adult Dose:

Premature Atrial and Ventricular Contractions—0.2 to 0.3 g three or four times daily.

Paroxysmal Supraventricular Tachycardias—0.4 to 0.6 g every two or three hours until the paroxysm is terminated.

Atrial Flutter—Quinidine should be administered after digitalization for this indication. Dosage is to be individualized.

Conversion of Atrial Fibrillation—Various schedules of quinidine administration have been in clinical use. A widely used technique is to give 0.2 g of quinidine orally every two or three hours for five to eight doses, with subsequent daily increase of the individual dose until sinus rhythm is restored or toxic effects occur. The total daily dose should not exceed 3 to 4 g in any regimen. Prior to quinidine administration, the ventricular rate and congestive failure (if present) should be brought under control by digitalis therapy.

Maintenance Therapy—0.2 to 0.3 g three or four times daily.

How Supplied: (℞) *Pulvules No. 239, Capsules, USP, F39,** 200 mg (No. 2, Pink), in bottles of 100 (NDC 0002-0639-02).

(℞) *Tablets No. 1125, USP, J20,** 200 mg (scored), in bottles of 100 (NDC 0002-1020-02) and 1000 (NDC 0002-1020-04) and in 10 strips of 10 individually labeled blisters each containing 1 tablet (ID100) (NDC 0002-1020-33).

[020282]

REGULAR ILETIN® I (insulin injection, Lilly), *see under* Iletin® (insulin, Lilly).

SECONAL® SODIUM ⓒ
(secobarbital sodium)
Capsules, USP

WARNING: MAY BE HABIT-FORMING

Description: Seconal® Sodium (Secobarbital Sodium, USP, Lilly) is a barbituric acid derivative and occurs as a white, odorless, bitter powder that is very soluble in water, soluble in alcohol, and practically insoluble in ether.

Each Pulvule contains 50 or 100 mg of secobarbital sodium.

Chemically, the drug is sodium 5-allyl-5-(1-methylbutyl)barbiturate, with the empirical formula $C_{12}H_{17}N_2NaO_3$.

Clinical Pharmacology: Seconal® Sodium (secobarbital sodium, Lilly), a short-acting barbiturate, is a central-nervous-system depressant. In ordinary doses, the drug acts as a sedative and hypnotic. Its onset of action is from 15 to 30 minutes, and the duration of action ranges from three to six hours. It is detoxified in the liver.

Indications and Usage: Seconal® Sodium (secobarbital sodium, Lilly) is indicated for intermittent use as a sedative or hypnotic. The prolonged administration of Seconal Sodium is not recommended, since it has not been shown to be effective for a period of more than 14 days. If insomnia persists, drug-free intervals of one or more weeks should elapse before retreatment is considered. Attempts should be made to find alternative nondrug therapy for chronic insomnia.

Contraindications: Seconal® Sodium (secobarbital sodium, Lilly) is contraindicated in patients who are hypersensitive to barbiturates. It is also contraindicated in patients with a history of manifest or latent porphyria, marked impairment of liver function, or respiratory disease in which dyspnea or obstruction is evident. It should not be administered to persons with known previous addiction to the sedative/hypnotic group, since ordinary doses may be ineffectual and may contribute to further addiction. Seconal Sodium should not be administered in the presence of acute or chronic pain, because paradoxical excitement may be induced or important symptoms may be masked.

Precautions: *General Precautions*—Barbiturates induce liver microsomal enzyme activity. This accelerates the biotransformation of various drugs and is probably part of the mechanism of the tolerance encountered with barbiturates. Seconal® Sodium (secobarbital sodium, Lilly) should, therefore, be used with caution in patients with decreased liver function. This drug should also be administered cautiously to patients with a history of drug dependence or abuse (*see* Drug Abuse and Dependence). Seconal may decrease the potency of coumarin anticoagulants; therefore, patients receiving such concomitant therapy should have more frequent prothrombin determinations.

As with other sedatives and hypnotics, elderly or debilitated patients may react to barbiturates with marked excitement or depression.

The systemic effects of exogenous hydrocortisone and endogenous hydrocortisone (cortisol) may be diminished by Seconal Sodium. Thus, this product should be administered with caution to patients with borderline hypoadrenal

Continued on next page

*Identi-Code® symbol.

Lilly—Cont.

function, regardless of whether it is of pituitary or of primary adrenal origin.
Information for Patients—Seconal Sodium may impair the mental and/or physical abilities required for the performance of potentially hazardous tasks, such as driving a car or operating machinery. The patient should be cautioned accordingly.
Drug Interactions—Seconal Sodium in combination with alcohol, tranquilizers, and other central-nervous-system depressants has additive depressant effects, and the patient should be so advised. Patients taking this drug should be warned not to exceed the dosage recommended by their physician. Toxic effects and fatalities have occurred following overdoses of Seconal Sodium alone and in combination with other central-nervous-system depressants. Caution should be exercised in prescribing unnecessarily large amounts of Seconal Sodium for patients who have a history of emotional disturbances or suicidal ideation or who have misused alcohol and other C.N.S. drugs (*see* Overdosage).
Usage in Pregnancy—Pregnancy Category B—Reproduction studies have been performed in animals and have revealed no evidence of impaired fertility or harm to the fetus due to Seconal Sodium. There are, however, no adequate and well-controlled studies in pregnant women. Because animal reproduction studies are not always predictive of human response, this drug should be used during pregnancy only if clearly needed.
Nursing Mothers—Caution should be exercised when Seconal Sodium is administered to a nursing woman.
Usage in Children—Safety and effectiveness in children have not been established.
Adverse Reactions: The following adverse reactions have been reported:
C.N.S. Depression—Residual sedation or "hangover," drowsiness, lethargy.
Respiratory/Circulatory—Respiratory depression, apnea, circulatory collapse.
Allergic—Hypersensitivity reactions, especially in individuals with asthma, urticaria, angioneurotic edema, or similar conditions; skin eruptions.
Other—Nausea and vomiting; headache.
Drug Abuse and Dependence: *Controlled Substance*—Seconal® Sodium (secobarbital sodium, Lilly) is a Schedule II drug.
Dependence—Prolonged, uninterrupted use of barbiturates (particularly the short-acting drugs), even in therapeutic doses, may result in psychic and physical dependence. Withdrawal symptoms due to physical dependence following chronic use of large doses of barbiturates may include delirium, convulsions, and death.
Overdosage: *Symptoms*—The manifestations of overdosage are early hypothermia followed by fever, sluggish or absent reflexes, respiratory depression, gradual appearance of circulatory collapse, pulmonary edema, and coma.
Treatment — General management should consist in symptomatic and supportive therapy, including gastric lavage, administration of intravenous fluids, and maintenance of blood pressure, body temperature, and adequate respiratory exchange. Dialysis will increase the rate of removal of barbiturates from the body fluids. Antibiotics may be required to control pulmonary complications.
Dosage and Administration: *Adults*—Insomnia, 100 mg at bedtime. Preoperatively, 200 to 300 mg one to two hours before surgery. *Children*—50 to 100 mg.
How Supplied: (Ⓒ) *Pulvules® Seconal® Sodium (Secobarbital Sodium Capsules, USP): No. 243, F42,* *50 mg (No. 4, Orange), in bottles of 100 (NDC 0002-0642-02) and 500 (NDC 0002-0642-03) and in 10 strips of 10 individually labeled blisters each containing 1 Pulvule (ID100) (NDC 0002-0642-33); *No. 240, F40,* *100 mg (No. 3, Orange), in bottles of 100 (NDC 0002-0640-02) and 500 (NDC 0002-0640-03), in 10 strips of 10 individually labeled blisters each containing 1 Pulvule (ID100) (NDC 0002-0640-33), and in strip packages of individually sealed Pulvules (DS1000) (NDC 0002-0640-35).
[101779]

[*Shown in Product Identification Section*]

SECONAL® SODIUM Ⓒ
(secobarbital sodium)
SUPPOSITORIES

WARNING: MAY BE HABIT-FORMING

Description: Seconal® Sodium (secobarbital sodium, Lilly) is a barbituric acid derivative and occurs as a white, odorless, bitter powder that is very soluble in water, soluble in alcohol, and practically insoluble in ether.
Suppositories Seconal Sodium contain white wax and cocoa butter.
Chemically, the drug is sodium 5-allyl-5-(1-methylbutyl)barbiturate, with the empirical formula $C_{12}H_{17}N_2NaO_3$.
Clinical Pharmacology: *See under* Seconal® Sodium, Capsules, USP.
Indications and Usage: Suppositories Seconal® Sodium (secobarbital sodium, Lilly) are indicated for intermittent use as a sedative or hypnotic whenever rectal administration of the drug is preferred. The prolonged administration of Seconal Sodium is not recommended, since it has not been shown to be effective for a period of more than 14 days. If insomnia persists, drug-free intervals of one or more weeks should elapse before re-treatment is considered. Attempts should be made to find alternative nondrug therapy for chronic insomnia.
Contraindications, Precautions, Adverse Reactions, Drug Abuse and Dependence, and Overdosage: *See under* Seconal Sodium, Capsules, USP.
Dosage and Administration: *Rectal*—Children up to six months of age, 15 to 60 mg; six months to three years, 60 mg; older children, 60 to 120 mg; adults, 120 to 200 mg. These suggested dosages should be considered approximate and should be adjusted according to the patient's general condition, degree of sedation or hypnosis desired, and clinical response.
How Supplied: (Ⓒ) *Suppositories Seconal® Sodium (secobarbital sodium, Lilly)* (Rectal): *No. 46, S17,* *30 mg (NDC 0002-1917-12), *No. 25, S14,** 60 mg (NDC 0002-1914-12), *No. 11, S05,** 120 mg (NDC 0002-1905-12), and *No. 17, S11,** 200 mg (NDC 0002-1911-12), in packages of 12. *Refrigerate.* [101679]

SECONAL® SODIUM (secobarbital sodium, Lilly) and
AMYTAL® SODIUM (amobarbital sodium, Lilly), *see* Tuinal® (secobarbital sodium and amobarbital sodium, Lilly).
SEMILENTE® ILETIN® I (prompt insulin zinc suspension, Lilly), *see under* Iletin® (insulin, Lilly).

SEROMYCIN® ℞
(cycloserine)
Capsules, USP

Description: Seromycin® (cycloserine, Lilly), D-4-amino-3-isoxazolidinone, is a broad-spectrum antibiotic which is produced by a strain of *Streptomyces orchidaceus* and has also been synthesized. A white powder that is soluble in water and stable in alkaline solution, it is rapidly destroyed at neutral or acid *p*H.
Actions: Cycloserine inhibits cell-wall synthesis in susceptible strains of gram-positive and gram-negative bacteria and in *Mycobacterium tuberculosis.*
Indications: Seromycin® (cycloserine, Lilly) is indicated in the treatment of active pulmonary and extrapulmonary tuberculosis (including renal disease) when the organisms are susceptible to this drug and after failure of adequate treatment with the primary medications (streptomycin, isoniazid, and ethambutol). Like all antituberculosis drugs, Seromycin should be administered in conjunction with other effective chemotherapy and not as the sole therapeutic agent.
Seromycin may be effective in the treatment of acute urinary tract infections caused by susceptible strains of gram-positive and gram-negative bacteria, especially *Enterobacter* and *Escherichia coli.* It is generally no more and is usually less effective than other antimicrobial agents in the treatment of urinary tract infections caused by bacteria other than mycobacteria. Use of Seromycin in these infections should be considered only when the more conventional therapy has failed and when the organism has been demonstrated to be sensitive to the drug.
Contraindications: Administration is contraindicated in patients with any of the following:
Hypersensitivity to cycloserine
Epilepsy
Depression, severe anxiety, or psychosis
Severe renal insufficiency
Excessive concurrent use of alcoholic beverages
Warnings: Administration of Seromycin® (cycloserine, Lilly) should be discontinued or the dosage reduced if the patient develops allergic dermatitis or symptoms of central-nervous-system toxicity, such as convulsions, psychosis, somnolence, depression, confusion, hyperreflexia, headache, tremor, vertigo, paresis, or dysarthria.
The toxicity of Seromycin is closely related to excessive blood levels (above 30 mcg/ml), which are determined by high dosage or inadequate renal clearance. The ratio of toxic dose to effective dose in tuberculosis is small.
The risk of convulsions is increased in chronic alcoholics.
Patients should be monitored by hematologic, renal excretion, blood level, and liver function studies.
Usage in Pregnancy—The safety of the use of Seromycin during pregnancy has not been established.
Usage in Children—Safety and dosage have not been established for pediatric use.
Precautions: Before treatment with Seromycin® (cycloserine, Lilly) is initiated, cultures should be taken and the organism's susceptibility to the drug should be established. In tuberculous infections, its sensitivity to the other antituberculosis agents in the regimen should also be demonstrated.
Blood levels should be determined at least weekly for patients having reduced renal function, for individuals receiving a daily dosage of more than 500 mg, and for those showing signs and symptoms suggestive of toxicity. The dosage should be adjusted to keep the blood level below 30 mcg/ml.
Anticonvulsant drugs or sedatives may be effective in controlling symptoms of central-nervous-system toxicity, such as convulsions, anxiety, and tremor. Patients receiving more than 500 mg of Seromycin daily should be closely observed for such symptoms. The value of pyridoxine in preventing C.N.S. toxicity from cycloserine has not been proved.
Administration of Seromycin and other antituberculosis drugs has been associated in a few instances with vitamin B_{12} and/or folic acid deficiency, megaloblastic anemia, and sideroblastic anemia. If evidence of anemia develops during treatment, appropriate studies and therapy should be instituted.
Adverse Reactions: Most adverse reactions occurring during therapy with Seromycin® (cycloserine, Lilly) involve the nervous system or are manifestations of drug hypersensitivity. The following side effects have been observed in patients receiving Seromycin:

Nervous system symptoms (which appear to be related to higher dosages of drug, i.e., more than 500 mg daily)
- Convulsions
- Drowsiness and somnolence
- Headache
- Tremor
- Dysarthria
- Vertigo
- Confusion and disorientation with loss of memory
- Psychoses, possibly with suicidal tendencies
  - Character changes
  - Hyperirritability
  - Aggression
- Paresis
- Hyperreflexia
- Paresthesias
- Major and minor (localized) clonic seizures
- Coma

Allergic (apparently not related to dosage)
- Skin rash

Miscellaneous
- Elevated serum transaminase, especially in patients with preexisting liver disease

Dosage and Administration: Seromycin® (cycloserine, Lilly) is effective orally and is currently administered only by this route. The usual dosage is 500 mg to 1 g daily in divided doses monitored by blood levels. The initial adult dosage most frequently given is 250 mg twice daily at 12-hour intervals for the first two weeks. The daily dosage of 1 g should not be exceeded.

Overdosage: *Symptoms*—C.N.S. depression with accompanying drowsiness, somnolence, dizziness, hyperreflexia, mental confusion, convulsions, and allergic dermatitis. *Treatment*—Pyridoxine (vitamin B_6), 300 mg or more daily, and anticonvulsants may be given to relieve convulsions. General management may include symptomatic and supportive therapy, such as gastric lavage, oxygen, artificial respiration, intravenous fluids, standard measures for management of circulatory shock, and maintenance of body temperature.

How Supplied: (℞) *Pulvules® No. 12, Seromycin® (Cycloserine Capsules, USP), F04,* *250 mg (No. 1, Light-Gray Opaque Body, Red Opaque Cap), in bottles of 40 (NDC 0002-0604-40).

[110680]

SILVER NITRATE ℞

Ophthalmic Solution, USP
One Percent (Buffered)
Wax Ampoules

This product is to be used by the physician or under his direction.

Description: Silver nitrate ophthalmic solution is a 1% solution of silver nitrate in a water medium. It contains not less than 0.95% and not more than 1.05% of $AgNO_3$. The solution may be buffered by the addition of sodium acetate.

Silver nitrate ophthalmic solution is an anti-infective (ophthalmic).

Clinical Pharmacology: Silver nitrate in weak solutions is used as a germicide and astringent to mucous membranes. The germicidal action is due to precipitation of bacterial proteins by liberated silver ions.

Indications and Usage: Silver nitrate ophthalmic solution is indicated for the prevention of gonorrheal ophthalmia neonatorum.

It has not been effective for prevention of neonatal chlamydial conjunctivitis.[1]

Contraindications: None known.

Warnings: A 1% solution is considered optimal; however, it must be used with caution, since cauterization of the cornea and blindness may result, especially with repeated applications.

When ingested, silver nitrate is highly toxic to the gastrointestinal tract and central nervous system. Swallowing can cause severe gastroenteritis that may end fatally. Sodium chloride may be used by gastric lavage to remove the chemical.

Silver nitrate is caustic and irritating to the skin and mucous membranes.

Precautions: *General Precautions*—Solutions of silver nitrate must be handled carefully, since they tend to stain skin and utensils. Silver nitrate stains may be removed from linen by applications of iodine tincture followed by sodium thiosulfate solution.

Adverse Reactions: A mild chemical conjunctivitis should result from a properly performed Credé prophylaxis using silver nitrate. With the 1% solution of silver nitrate, chemical conjunctivitis occurs in 20 percent or less of cases.

Overdosage: When a solution of 2% or higher silver nitrate concentration is used in the eye, conjunctivitis may be produced. The eye should be irrigated with an isotonic solution of sodium chloride after solutions of silver nitrate stronger than 1% are instilled.

Dosage and Administration: Immediately after the child is born, the eyelids should be cleaned with sterile absorbent cotton or gauze and sterile water. A separate pledget should be used for each eye, and the lids, without being opened, should be washed from the nose outward until quite free of all blood, mucus, or meconium.

Next, the lids should be separated, and two drops of 1% silver nitrate solution should be dropped into the eye. The lids should be separated and elevated away from the eyeball so that a lake of silver nitrate may lie for a half minute or longer between them, coming in contact with every portion of the conjunctival sac.

The American Academy of Pediatrics has endorsed a statement of the Committee on Ophthalmia Neonatorum of the National Society for the Prevention of Blindness which does not recommend irrigation of the eyes following instillation of the silver nitrate.

Method of Use: *See* the package literature for illustrations. Pierce the end of the ampoule with a needle, making sure that its entry into the interior of the ampoule is accomplished.

To express the contents of the ampoule, press between the thumb and first finger.

The ampoule should be kept at controlled room temperature, 59° to 86°F (15° to 30°C). Do not freeze. It should not be used when cold. Protect from light.

How Supplied: (℞) *Wax Ampoules No. 146, Silver Nitrate Ophthalmic Solution, USP, 1% (Buffered),* in packages of 100 (NDC 0002-1608-02). Sodium acetate and acetic acid are contained as buffers.

1. Schachter, J., *et al.:* Prospective Study of Chlamydial Infection in Neonates, Lancet, *2:*377-379, August 25, 1979.

[061482]

SURFACAINE® ℞

(cyclomethycaine sulfate)
Jelly, 0.75%, USP

Description: Surfacaine® (Cyclomethycaine Sulfate, USP, Lilly) is a topical anesthetic. It is a substituted piperidino-alkyl benzoate and is not a derivative of *p*-aminobenzoic acid.

Cyclomethycaine sulfate is 3-(2-methylpiperidino)-propyl *p*-(cyclohexyloxy) benzoate sulfate (1:1). The empirical formula is $C_{22}H_{33}NO_3 \cdot H_2SO_4$. The molecular weight is 457.58.

Each gram of Jelly Surfacaine contains 7.5 mg (0.75%) cyclomethycaine sulfate, sodium phosphate, hydroxypropylmethylcellulose 1500, polysorbate 80, propylene glycol, thimerosal, and purified water. The jelly base used in Surfacaine is water soluble. Jelly Surfacaine has a pH between 4.8 and 5.8.

Clinical Pharmacology: Surfacaine® (cyclomethycaine sulfate, Lilly) prevents the initiation and transmission of nerve impulses and thus effects local anesthetic action. Onset of anesthesia requires five to ten minutes. The vehicle provides lubrication for instrumentation.

No data are available on systemic absorption and toxicity of Jelly Surfacaine.

Indications and Usage: For use as a topical anesthetic and lubricant on nontraumatized, accessible mucous membranes prior to clinical examination and instrumentation.

Contraindications: Jelly Surfacaine® (cyclomethycaine sulfate, Lilly) is contraindicated in persons with an idiosyncrasy or allergy to any of the ingredients. Do not use in the eyes.

Precautions: *General Precautions*—Avoid application to extensive skin areas. If prolonged or indefinite use of Surfacaine® (cyclomethycaine sulfate, Lilly) is undertaken, observe periodically to detect possible development of allergic reaction. Increase in redness, itching, papules, or vesicles suggests possible allergy. Discontinue use if irritation or allergy develops.

Persons with a history of allergic asthma, rhinitis, or urticaria may have an increased risk of allergic reactions. One probable anaphylactoid reaction has occurred following the introduction of a cyclomethycaine sulfate suppository in a patient with a history of multiple allergies. No other case of systemic toxicity has been reported.

Urethral administration should be made only by the physician or persons under his direction. Extreme caution is imperative when any local anesthetic is injected into the traumatized urethra or under conditions in which trauma is likely to occur. Overdistention of the urethra by the jelly may produce trauma, with stinging and burning. These symptoms may recur following dissipation of the anesthetic effect if the injury to the mucosa is extensive.

Usage in Children—Safety and effectiveness in children have not been established.

Adverse Reactions: A transitory stinging and/or burning sensation is occasionally experienced before the onset of the anesthetic effect.

Contact dermatitis may occur in hypersensitive individuals. Unlike benzocaine and procaine, Surfacaine® (cyclomethycaine sulfate, Lilly) is not a *p*-aminobenzoic acid derivative, and allergic reactions are not common.

Dosage and Administration: To avoid contamination, employ only previously unused tubes.

For Surface Anesthesia of the Male Urethra—The outer orifice is washed and cleansed with a disinfectant. Before catheterization, instillation of small volumes (3.4 to 10 ml) of jelly is usually adequate.

If the 28-g tube is to be used, the plastic urethral tip is sterilized for five minutes in boiling water, cooled, and attached to the tube. The tip may be gas sterilized or cold sterilized, if preferred. The jelly is instilled slowly into the urethra until the patient has a feeling of tension or until half the tube is emptied. A penile clamp is then applied for several minutes at the corona, and subsequently the remaining contents of the tube are instilled.

Prior to sounding or cystoscopy, a penile clamp should be applied for five to ten minutes to obtain adequate anesthesia. Thirty ml of the jelly are usually required to fill and dilate the male urethra.

For Surface Anesthesia of the Female Urethra—The outer orifice is washed and cleansed with a disinfectant. Three to 7 ml of the jelly are instilled slowly into the urethra. If desired, jelly may also be deposited on a cotton swab and introduced into the urethra.

Continued on next page

*Identi-Code® symbol.

Lilly—Cont.

If the 28-g tube is to be used, the plastic urethral tip is sterilized for five minutes in boiling water, cooled, and attached to the tube. The tip may be gas sterilized or cold sterilized, if preferred.

In order to obtain adequate anesthesia, several minutes should be allowed before urologic procedures are performed.

Anus—Insert 10 ml into rectum five to ten minutes prior to anorectal, sigmoidoscopic, or prostatic examination. Apply a coating to gloved finger, anus, and instruments as needed for lubrication.

Vagina—Introduce 5 ml, using finger or vaginal applicator.

Nose and Throat—Apply to intubation apparatus, tracheal catheters, etc. Reflexes are reduced or abolished, and easier intubation may be achieved when the jelly is used in this manner. Jelly Surfacaine® (cyclomethycaine sulfate, Lilly) is not intended for use as the sole anesthetic agent prior to bronchoscopic examinations.

Maximum Dosage: No more than 30 ml should be given in any 12-hour period.

How Supplied: (℞) *Jelly No. 11, Surfacaine® (Cyclomethycaine Sulfate, USP), 0.75%*, in 28-g (26.9-ml) (NDC 0002-2458-67) and 142-g (136.5-ml) tubes (NDC 0002-2458-68). The 28-g package contains one nonsterile perforated urethral tip and one rectal pipe.

Store at controlled room temperature (59° to 86°F) (15° to 30°C). Keep tightly closed.

This product is not for use in the eyes.

[121581]

TAPAZOLE® ℞
(methimazole)
Tablets, USP

Description: Tapazole (1-methyl-2-mercaptoimidazole) is a white crystalline substance that is freely soluble in water. It differs chemically from the drugs of the thiouracil series primarily in that it has a five instead of a six-membered ring.

Actions: Tapazole® (methimazole, Lilly) inhibits the synthesis of thyroid hormones and thus is effective in the treatment of hyperthyroidism. The drug does not inactivate existing thyroxine and triiodothyronine which is stored in colloid or is circulating in the blood, nor does it interfere with the effectiveness of thyroid hormones given by mouth or by injection.

Indications: Tapazole® (methimazole, Lilly) is indicated in the medical treatment of hyperthyroidism. Long-term therapy may lead to remission of the disease. Tapazole may also be used to ameliorate hyperthyroidism in preparation for subtotal thyroidectomy or radioactive iodine therapy.

Contraindication: Tapazole® (methimazole, Lilly) is contraindicated in the presence of hypersensitivity to the drug.

Warnings: *Pregnancy*—Tapazole® (methimazole, Lilly), used judiciously, is an effective drug in hyperthyroidism complicated by pregnancy. Because the drug readily crosses placental membranes and can induce goiter and even cretinism in the developing fetus, it is important that a sufficient, but not excessive, dose be given. In many pregnant women, the thyroid dysfunction diminishes as the pregnancy proceeds; consequently, a reduction of dosage may be possible. In some instances, Tapazole can be withdrawn two or three weeks before delivery.

The administration of thyroid along with Tapazole to the pregnant hyperthyroid woman is also recommended in order to prevent hypothyroidism in the mother and her fetus. Administration should continue throughout the pregnancy and after delivery. Postpartum patients receiving Tapazole should not nurse their babies.

Precautions: Patients who receive Tapazole® (methimazole, Lilly) should be under close surveillance and should be impressed with the necessity of reporting immediately any evidence of illness, particularly sore throat, skin eruptions, fever, headache, or general malaise. In such cases, white-blood-cell and differential counts should be made to determine whether agranulocytosis has developed. Particular care should be exercised with patients who are receiving additional drugs known to cause agranulocytosis.

Adverse Reactions: Adverse reactions probably occur in less than 3 percent of patients.

Minor adverse reactions include skin rash, urticaria, nausea, vomiting, epigastric distress, arthralgia, paresthesia, loss of taste, abnormal loss of hair, myalgia, headache, pruritus, drowsiness, neuritis, edema, vertigo, skin pigmentation, jaundice, sialadenopathy, and lymphadenopathy.

Major adverse reactions (much less common than the minor adverse reactions) include inhibition of myelopoiesis (agranulocytosis, granulopenia, and thrombocytopenia), drug fever, a lupuslike syndrome, hepatitis (jaundice may persist for several weeks after discontinuation of the drug), periarteritis, and hypoprothrombinemia.

It should be noted that about 10 percent of patients with untreated hyperthyroidism have leukopenia (white-blood-cell count of less than 4000 per mm^3), often with relative granulopenia.

Dosage and Administration: Tapazole® (methimazole, Lilly) is administered orally. It is usually given in three equal doses at approximately eight-hour intervals.

Adult—The initial daily dosage is 15 mg for mild hyperthyroidism, 30 to 40 mg for moderately severe hyperthyroidism, and 60 mg for severe hyperthyroidism, divided into three doses at eight-hour intervals. The maintenance dosage is 5 to 15 mg daily.

Pediatric—Initially, the daily dosage is 0.4 mg/kg of body weight divided into three doses and given at eight-hour intervals. The maintenance dosage is approximately one-half of the initial dose.

Overdosage: Agranulocytosis is the most serious effect. Rarely, exfoliative dermatitis, hepatitis, neuropathies, or C.N.S. stimulation or depression may occur.

Symptoms—Nausea, vomiting, epigastric distress, headache, fever, arthralgia, pruritus, edema, and pancytopenia. Prolonged therapy may result in hypothyroidism.

Treatment—For specific therapy, the drug should be discontinued in the presence of agranulocytosis, pancytopenia, hepatitis, fever, or exfoliative dermatitis.

For bone-marrow depression, use of an antibiotic, transfusions of fresh whole blood, and a corticosteroid should be considered. For hepatitis, rest and adequate diet and, in severe cases, corticosteroid therapy may be indicated. General management may consist in symptomatic and supportive therapy, including rest, analgesics, gastric lavage, intravenous fluids, and mild sedation.

How Supplied: (℞) *Tablets Tapazole® (Methimazole Tablets, USP)* (scored): *No. 1765, J94,** 5 mg (NDC 0002-1094-02 and NDC 0002-1094-04), and *No. 1770, J95,** 10 mg (NDC 0002-1095-02 and NDC 0002-1095-04), in bottles of 100 and 1000.

[022680]

THERACEBRIN® ℞
(pan-vitamins)

Description: Each Pulvule® contains—

Thiamine (as the Mononitrate) (Vitamin B_1) .... 15 mg
Riboflavin (Vitamin B_2) .... 10 mg
Pyridoxine (as the Hydrochloride) (Vitamin B_6) .... 2.5 mg
Pantothenic Acid (as *d*-Calcium Pantothenate) .... 20 mg
Niacinamide .... 150 mg
Vitamin B_{12} (Activity Equivalent) .... 10 mcg
Ascorbic Acid (Vitamin C) .... 150 mg
dl-Alpha Tocopheryl Acetate (Vitamin E) .... 18.5 IU (18.5 mg)
Vitamin A Synthetic .... 25,000 IU (7.5 mg)
Vitamin D Synthetic .... 1500 IU (37.5 mcg)

Indications: For the treatment of multiple vitamin deficiencies, especially in gastrointestinal surgery, severe burns, or infectious hepatitis.

Precautions: Rarely, vitamins A and D in large doses (respectively, 50,000 IU and 25,000 IU or more daily for several months or longer) cause toxicity.

Dosage and Administration: *Prophylaxis*—1 Pulvule daily. *Treatment*—1 Pulvule twice daily.

How Supplied: (℞) *Pulvules No. 200, Theracebrin® (pan-vitamins, Lilly), H72** (No. 0, Black Body, Black Cap), in bottles of 30 and 100 (NDC 0002-0872-30 and NDC 0002-0872-02).

[100581]

TRIKATES ℞
Oral Solution, USP

Description: Trikates Oral Solution, USP, containing potassium acetate, potassium bicarbonate, and potassium citrate (each in 10 percent concentration), supplies approximately 15 mEq of potassium in each 5 ml.

Potassium acetate appears as colorless, monoclinic crystals or white crystalline powder. It is very soluble in water and freely soluble in alcohol. Potassium bicarbonate occurs as white granular powder. It is freely soluble in water but practically insoluble in alcohol. Potassium citrate occurs as transparent crystals or white granular powder. Freely soluble in water, it is almost insoluble in alcohol.

Contains in each 5 ml: Potassium, 15 mEq (approximately), provided by 0.5 g potassium acetate; 0.5 g potassium bicarbonate; and 0.5 g potassium citrate in a sugar-free vehicle containing glycerin, saccharin sodium, water, and aromatics.

Clinical Pharmacology: Potassium, the major intracellular cation, plays a significant part in the control of osmotic pressure and also serves as an essential activator in a number of enzymatic reactions. In addition, the potassium concentration of body fluids has an important influence on the excitability of both skeletal and cardiac muscle and on the structure and function of the kidneys. Disturbances in potassium equilibrium may, therefore, produce a wide range of clinical disorders.

The potassium concentration in extracellular fluid is normally 4 to 5 mEq/liter; that in intracellular fluid is approximately 150 mEq/liter. Since about 2 percent of body weight is extracellular fluid, it can readily be calculated that only a small fraction of the 2500 to 3000 mEq of potassium within the body is contained in the extracellular space. Changes in plasma potassium concentration often mirror those in cellular potassium content; thus, plasma concentration provides a useful clinical guide to disturbances in potassium balance. By producing large differences in the ratio of intracellular to extracellular potassium, relatively small absolute changes in extracellular concentration may have important effects on neuromuscular activity.

Despite wide variations in dietary intake of potassium (e.g., 40 to 120 mEq/day), plasma potassium concentration is normally stabilized within the narrow range of 4 to 5 mEq/liter by virtue of close renal regulation of potassium balance. Renal potassium excretion is accomplished largely, if not exclusively, by a process of potassium secretion in the distal portion of the nephron; essentially all filtered potassium is reabsorbed in the proximal tubule, and the potassium that appears in the urine is added to the filtrate by a distal process of sodium-cation exchange. Fecal excretion of potassium normally amounts to only a few milliequivalents/day and does not play a significant role in potassium homeostasis.

Indications and Usage: Trikates Oral Solution is indicated in the treatment of potassium deficiency which may occur in conjunction with (1) long-term diuretic therapy, (2) digitalis intoxication, (3) low dietary intake of potassium, (4) loss of potassium due to vomiting and diarrhea, (5) diabetic acidosis, (6) metabolic alkalosis, (7) corticosteroid therapy, and (8) familial periodic paralysis.

Symptoms and Signs of Potassium Deficiency—These include weakness, drowsiness, anorexia, nausea, chronic ileus with distention, edema, oliguria, shallow and infrequent respirations, dilatation of the heart, low blood pressure, ectopic rhythms, systolic murmurs, hypokalemia, and electrocardiographic changes showing prominent U wave, lengthening of the Q-U (Q-T) interval, depression of the S-T segment, and depression or inversion of the T wave.

Contraindications: Trikates Oral Solution is contraindicated in severe renal impairment with oliguria, anuria, or azotemia; untreated Addison's disease; adynamia episodica hereditaria; acute dehydration; heat cramps; and hyperkalemia from any cause. Potassium intensifies the symptoms of myotonia congenita.

Warnings: High plasma concentrations of potassium ion may cause death through cardiac depression, arrhythmias, or arrest.

Precautions: *General Precautions*—Trikates Oral Solution must be administered with caution, since the degree of potassium deficiency or the ideal daily dosage often is not accurately known. Excessive dosage may result in potassium intoxication. The drug should be used with caution in the presence of cardiac disease.

Laboratory Tests—Frequent checks of the clinical status of the patient, ECG, and/or plasma potassium levels should be made.

Usage in Pregnancy—Pregnancy Category C—Animal reproduction studies have not been conducted with Trikates Oral Solution. It is also not known whether Trikates Oral Solution can cause fetal harm when administered to a pregnant woman or can affect reproduction capacity. Trikates Oral Solution should be given to a pregnant woman only if clearly needed.

Nursing Mothers—It is not known whether this drug is excreted in human milk. Because many drugs are excreted in human milk and because of the potential for serious adverse reactions in nursing infants from Trikates Oral Solution, a decision should be made whether to discontinue nursing or to discontinue the drug, taking into account the importance of the drug to the mother.

Usage in Children—Safety and effectiveness in children have not been established.

Drug Interactions—Mineral acids liberate acetic acid, and, because of the feeble ionization of this acid, acetates act as buffers toward mineral acids, decreasing to some extent the hydrogen-ion concentration.

Aqueous solutions of potassium citrate are slightly alkaline and will react with acidic substances. Alkaloidal salts may be precipitated from their aqueous or hydroalcoholic solutions. Acidification or addition of alcohol will restore the solution. Calcium and strontium salts cause a precipitation of the corresponding citrates.

Potassium bicarbonate is decomposed by acids and salts having an acid reaction with the liberation of carbon dioxide. Acid-reacting vehicles are troublesome in this respect, as are some tinctures, fluid extracts, and solutions. Heating or agitating the aqueous solution partially converts it to the normal carbonate with evolution of carbon dioxide. Potassium bicarbonate intensifies the darkening that occurs in solutions of salicylates. Some alkaloids are precipitated from solutions of their salts.

In powder mixtures, atmospheric moisture or water of crystallization from another ingredient sometimes permits potassium bicarbonate to react with boric acid or a salt such as alum.

In liquid mixtures containing bismuth subnitrate, potassium bicarbonate reacts with the acid formed by hydrolysis of the bismuth salt.

Adverse Reactions: Trikates Oral Solution may cause gastric irritation if taken undiluted and on an empty stomach. Vomiting, diarrhea, nausea, and abdominal discomfort have been reported. The symptoms and signs of potassium intoxication include paresthesia of the extremities, flaccid paralysis, listlessness, mental confusion, weakness and heaviness of the legs, fall in blood pressure, cardiac arrhythmias, heart block, hyperkalemia, and electrocardiographic abnormalities (disappearance of the P wave, depression of the S-T segment, tall and peaked T waves, spreading and slurring of the QRS complex with development of a biphasic curve, and cardiac arrest).

Potassium intoxication may result from overdosage of Trikates Oral Solution or from therapeutic dosage in conditions stated under Contraindications. When detected, hyperkalemia must be treated immediately, because lethal levels can be reached in a few hours.

Overdosage: *Clinical Manifestations*—The clinical manifestations of potassium intoxication are related primarily to the heart and the neuromuscular system. Electrocardiographic abnormalities are the earliest and most frequent sign of disturbed membrane excitability and are characterized by the development of tall, "tent-shaped" T waves, by decreased amplitude of the P waves, and later by atrial asystole. Intraventricular block, with widening of the QRS complex, may lead to the development of a sine wave pattern and ultimately to ventricular standstill. Changes in the electrocardiogram usually appear when the serum potassium concentration reaches 7 to 8 mEq/liter, and cardiac standstill is likely to occur at a concentration of 9 to 10 mEq/liter. Weakness and flaccid paralysis, usually indistinguishable from that seen in hypokalemic paralysis, appear only in association with severe hyperkalemia, and death may occur from cardiac arrest before muscular weakness is evident. For this reason, the electrocardiogram is the single most important guide in appraising the threat posed by the hyperkalemia and in determining how aggressive a therapeutic approach is necessary.

Treatment—The treatment of severe potassium intoxication should be directed toward promoting rapid transfer of potassium into cells in order to lower serum potassium concentration and prevent cardiac arrest. Two approaches to this goal are likely to prove effective. Infusion of glucose and insulin induces the cellular deposition of glycogen and at the same time brings about a shift of potassium to the intracellular space; 1 liter of a 10 percent glucose solution with 50 units of insulin is generally employed for this purpose. A further redistribution of potassium can be achieved in the acidotic patient by the administration of sodium bicarbonate (150 to 300 mEq). In many cases, these measures will induce a striking reduction in plasma potassium concentration and prompt improvement in the electrocardiogram. In some instances, the administration of calcium (as 2 g of calcium lactate) is also useful because calcium, though it has no effect on the plasma potassium concentration, opposes the cardiotoxic effects of potassium. It should be noted, incidentally, that calcium cannot be given in the same solution with sodium bicarbonate because precipitation of the calcium ion will result.

Because the techniques described above do not remove potassium from the body and may be only temporarily effective, longer-term efforts should be directed toward promoting gastrointestinal losses of potassium. A cation-exchange resin in the sodium cycle, such as Kayexelate, will usually achieve this purpose if administered by mouth in a dose of 20 to 30 g every six hours. Each g of resin binds approximately 1 mEq of potassium, and within 24 hours a significant effect on plasma potassium concentration should be achieved. To enhance potassium loss and assure the rapid movement of the resin through the gastrointestinal tract, sorbitol, a nonreabsorbable polyhydric alcohol, should be given in quantities sufficient to induce a soft or semiliquid bowel movement every few hours. The usual dose for this purpose is 20 ml of a 70 percent solution three or four times a day. If the patient is unable to take medication by mouth, the resin can be administered by rectum as a retention enema of 100 g in several hundred ml of water.

Hemodialysis is an efficient alternative means of removing the excess potassium but usually will not be required if the program outlined above can be carried out effectively.

Dosage and Administration: Trikates Oral Solution is given orally after meals and is diluted with a glass of tomato juice, orange juice, or other readily available vehicle. The usual adult dosage is 5 ml (15 mEq) of potassium three or four times a day.

Since no average total daily dose can be defined, deviations from this recommendation may be indicated but must be governed by close observation for clinical effects. However, potassium intoxication may result from any therapeutic dosage. *See under* Precautions *and* Overdosage.

How Supplied: (℞) *Liquid No. 29, Trikates Oral Solution, USP,* in 16-fl-oz (NDC 0002-2463-05) and gallon bottles (NDC 0002-2463-06).

[040480]

TUBOCURARINE CHLORIDE ℞
Injection, USP

See also Metubine® Iodide (metocurine iodide, Lilly)

THIS DRUG SHOULD BE ADMINISTERED ONLY BY ADEQUATELY TRAINED INDIVIDUALS WHO ARE FAMILIAR WITH ITS ACTIONS, CHARACTERISTICS, AND HAZARDS.

Description: Tubocurarine Chloride Injection, USP, is a sterile isotonic solution for intravenous use. Each ml of the solution contains 3 mg (20 units) tubocurarine chloride, sodium bisulfite, 0.1 percent, and sodium chloride, 0.7 percent, with chlorobutanol (chloroform derivative), 0.5 percent, as a preservative. Sodium hydroxide and/or hydrochloric acid are sometimes added during manufacture to adjust the pH.

Actions: Tubocurarine chloride blocks nerve impulses to skeletal muscles at the myoneural junction. This is a nondepolarizing neuromuscular blockade. When it is administered intravenously (intramuscular injection is unpredictable), the onset of flaccid paralysis occurs within a few minutes.

Muscle paralysis may be expected for periods of 25 to 90 minutes. The use of repeated doses may be accompanied by a cumulative effect. Since tubocurarine chloride is excreted by the kidneys, severe renal disease or hypotension may result in a more prolonged action of this drug.

Concurrently administered general anesthetics, certain antibiotics, abnormal states (e.g., acidosis), electrolyte imbalance, and neuro-

Continued on next page

*Identi-Code® symbol.

Lilly—Cont.

muscular disease have been reported to cause a potentiation of this drug's activity.
Rapid intravenous injection may produce increased release of histamine with resultant decreased respiratory capacity due to bronchospasm and paralysis of the respiratory muscles. Hypotension may occur owing to ganglionic blockade, or it may be a complication of positive pressure respiration.
Tubocurarine chloride does not affect consciousness or cerebration, and it does not relieve pain. A patient in severe pain may not be able to communicate this to the anesthesiologist.
Indications: Tubocurarine chloride is indicated as an adjunct to anesthesia to induce skeletal-muscle relaxation. It may be employed to reduce the intensity of muscle contractions in pharmacologically or electrically induced convulsions. It may be used as a diagnostic agent for myasthenia gravis when the results of tests with neostigmine or edrophonium are inconclusive. It may also be employed to facilitate the management of patients undergoing mechanical ventilation.
Contraindications: Tubocurarine chloride is contraindicated in those persons who have shown an allergic reaction or hypersensitivity to the drug and in patients in whom histamine release is a definite hazard.
Warnings: TUBOCURARINE CHLORIDE IS A POTENT DRUG WHICH MAY CAUSE RESPIRATORY DEPRESSION. THEREFORE, IT SHOULD BE USED ONLY BY THOSE EXPERIENCED IN THE TECHNIQUE OF ARTIFICIAL RESPIRATION AND THE ADMINISTRATION OF OXYGEN UNDER POSITIVE PRESSURE. FACILITIES FOR THESE PROCEDURES SHOULD BE IMMEDIATELY AVAILABLE AT ALL TIMES.
Prolonged apnea with its attendant hazards due to hypoxia may result from overdosages of this preparation.
It should be employed with extreme caution in patients with known myasthenia gravis.
The administration of quinidine during postoperative recovery to patients who have received tubocurarine chloride may result in recurarization leading to respiratory paralysis.
Usage in Pregnancy—The safe use of tubocurarine chloride has not been established with respect to the possible adverse effects upon child development. Therefore, it should not be administered to women of childbearing potential and especially not during early pregnancy unless, in the judgment of the physician, the potential benefits outweigh the possible hazards.
Precautions: When sufficiently excessive dosage of curare has been administered, there is no antidote. It is again emphasized that dosage should be controlled so that emergency measures need not be instituted.
Tubocurarine chloride should be used with caution in patients with respiratory depression or with renal, hepatic, or pulmonary diseases. Hypotension can follow the administration of large doses.
Adverse Reactions: Adverse reactions consist primarily in extension of the drug's pharmacologic actions. Profound and prolonged muscle relaxation may occur, with consequent respiratory depression to the point of apnea.
Hypersensitivity to the drug may exist in rare instances.
Idiosyncrasy, interference with physical signs of anesthesia, circulatory depression, ganglionic blockade, and release of histamine are complications that can result from the use of this medication.
Drug Interaction: The intensity of blockade and duration of action of tubocurarine chloride are increased in patients receiving patent inhalational anesthetics such as halothane, diethyl ether, methoxyflurane, and enflurane. No increased intensity of blockade or duration of action is noted from the use of thiobarbiturates, narcotic analgesics, nitrous oxide, or droperidol.
Prior administration of succinylcholine chloride, such as that used for endotracheal intubation, may enhance the relaxant effect of tubocurarine chloride. If succinylcholine chloride is used before tubocurarine, the administration of tubocurarine should be delayed until the succinylcholine shows signs of wearing off.
Dosage and Administration:
Conversion Table for Calculating Dosage
20 units are contained in each ml
1 mg equals 7 units
1 unit is contained in 0.05 ml of this solution
Tubocurarine chloride is administered intravenously as a sustained injection over a period of 1 to 1½ minutes. As a precaution, the initial dose should be reduced to 20 units below the calculated amount. The speed of injection of the drug influences the amount administered. Although rapid injection may be dangerous, curarization can be accomplished with a smaller dose than that mentioned above if this is given more rapidly.
Tubocurarine chloride should be administered only by or under the supervision of experienced clinicians. The dosage must be individualized in each case after evaluation of the patient and consideration of factors that might alter the action of the drug in a particular case. If inhalational anesthetics known to enhance the action of curariform drugs are being used, the initial dose should be reduced and the response noted as a guide to incremental doses. If enhanced sensitivity is suspected, fractional dosage is advised initially to avoid overdosage. The following doses are for average patients without altered sensitivity.
Surgery—In the patient of average weight, 40 to 60 units of Tubocurarine Chloride Injection are administered intravenously at the time the skin incision is made, and 20 to 30 units in three to five minutes if required for further relaxation. For long operations, supplemental doses of 20 units may be given as required. As a general rule, dosage may be calculated on the basis of ½ unit/lb of body weight.
Electroshock Therapy—Tubocurarine chloride is administered just before electroshock therapy in the treatment of mental diseases. It reduces the severity of the convulsions and is useful as a means of preventing fractures. The patient should be observed closely until consciousness is regained in case respiratory failure should develop. A dose of ½ unit/lb of body weight is given intravenously and slowly as a sustained 1 to 1 ½-minute injection. Rapid administration is dangerous. The initial dose is 20 units less than this.
Diagnosis of Myasthenia Gravis—Tubocurarine chloride has been useful as a diagnostic agent in patients suspected of having myasthenia gravis. When small doses are given, a profound exaggeration of this syndrome occurs. The dosage is 1/15 to 1/5 of the average adult electroshock-therapy dose administered intravenously.
Every effort should be made to control dosage to the end that emergencies do not arise. It is important that physicians familiarize themselves with the dangers involved in using the drug and that preparations be made in advance for treating the patient if unwarranted side effects occur (*see* Contraindications *and* Adverse Reactions).
Tubocurarine chloride is adjusted to a *p*H sufficiently low to assure full stability for indefinite periods without the need for refrigeration; therefore, because of the high *p*H of barbiturate solutions, a precipitate will form when tubocurarine chloride is combined with such agents as Brevital® Sodium (Methohexital Sodium for Injection, USP, Lilly) and Thiopental Sodium. It is recommended that each component be given from a separate syringe to assure more uniform and predictable results with each of the drugs. A single needle and tube attached to a three-way stopcock apparatus can readily be adapted to this method if it is desirable to utilize as few of the patient's veins as possible.
Management of Adverse Reactions: If hypotension occurs, the etiology should be determined. When it is due to ganglionic blockade, hypotension may be treated with fluid and vasopressors which act at the adrenergic receptors as required. Apnea or prolonged curarization should be treated with controlled respiration. Edrophonium or neostigmine may antagonize the skeletal-muscle-relaxant action of tubocurarine chloride. Neostigmine injection should be accompanied or preceded by an injection of atropine sulfate or its equivalent. A nerve stimulator may be used to assess the nature and degree of the neuromuscular blockade. The optimum time to administer the antagonist is when the patient is being hyperventilated and the carbon-dioxide level of the blood is low. The effects of neostigmine given intravenously last from 30 to 90 minutes; the effects of edrophonium are usually dissipated within five minutes. The antagonists are merely adjuncts. Before they are used, the package inserts of these drugs should be consulted for prescribing information.
Pharmacology: Tubocurarine chloride blocks nervous impulses to skeletal muscles at the myoneural junction.
Renal excretion occurs fairly rapidly; therefore, the physiologic effect is of relatively short duration.
How Supplied: (Ɍ) *Vials (Multiple Dose) No. 449, Tubocurarine Chloride Injection, USP,* 3 mg/ml, 10 ml, rubber-stoppered, in singles (10/carton) (NDC 0002-1685-01). [011282]

TUINAL® Ⓒ
(secobarbital sodium and amobarbital sodium) Capsules, USP

WARNING: MAY BE HABIT-FORMING

Description: Tuinal is a combination of equal parts of Seconal® Sodium (secobarbital sodium, Lilly) and Amytal® Sodium (amobarbital sodium, Lilly), barbituric acid derivatives that occur as white, odorless, bitter powders. They are very soluble in water, soluble in alcohol, and practically insoluble in ether and in chloroform.
Each Pulvule No. 302 contains 25 mg Seconal Sodium and 25 mg Amytal Sodium.
Each Pulvule No. 303 contains 50 mg Seconal Sodium and 50 mg Amytal Sodium.
Each Pulvule No. 304 contains 100 mg Seconal Sodium and 100 mg Amytal Sodium.
Chemically, Seconal Sodium is sodium 5-allyl-5-(1-methylbutyl)barbiturate, with the empirical formula $C_{12}H_{17}N_2NaO_3$.
Amytal Sodium is sodium 5-ethyl-5-isopentylbarbiturate, with the empirical formula $C_{11}H_{17}N_2NaO_3$.
Clinical Pharmacology: Tuinal, a moderately long-acting barbiturate, is a central-nervous-system depressant. In ordinary doses, the drug acts as a hypnotic. Its onset of action occurs in 15 to 30 minutes, and the duration of action ranges from three to 11 hours. It is detoxified in the liver.
Indications and Usage: For use whenever prompt and moderately sustained hypnotic effect is required. Not suitable for continuous daytime sedation. The prolonged administration of Tuinal is not recommended, since it has not been shown to be effective for a period of more than 14 days. If insomnia persists, drug-free intervals of one or more weeks should elapse before re-treatment is considered.
Attempts should be made to find alternative nondrug therapy for chronic insomnia.

Contraindications: Tuinal is contraindicated in patients who are hypersensitive to barbiturates. It is also contraindicated in patients with a history of manifest or latent porphyria, marked impairment of liver function, or respiratory disease in which dyspnea or obstruction is evident. It should not be administered to persons with known previous addiction to the sedative/hypnotic group, since ordinary doses may be ineffectual and may contribute to further addiction. Tuinal should not be administered in the presence of acute or chronic pain, because paradoxical excitement may be induced or important symptoms may be masked.

Warnings: Prolonged, uninterrupted use of barbiturates (particularly the short-acting drugs), even in therapeutic doses, may result in psychic and physical dependence.

The central-nervous-system-depressant effect of secobarbital and amobarbital may be additive with that of other CNS depressants, including alcohol.

Precautions: *General Precautions*—Barbiturates induce liver microsomal enzyme activity. This accelerates the biotransformation of various drugs and is probably part of the mechanism of the tolerance encountered with barbiturates. Tuinal should, therefore, be used with caution in patients with decreased liver function. This drug should also be administered cautiously to patients with a history of drug dependence or abuse (*see* Drug Abuse and Dependence). Tuinal may decrease the potency of coumarin anticoagulants; therefore, patients receiving such concomitant therapy should have more frequent prothrombin determinations.

As with other sedatives and hypnotics, elderly or debilitated patients may react to barbiturates with marked excitement or depression.

The systemic effects of exogenous hydrocortisone and endogenous hydrocortisone (cortisol) may be diminished by Tuinal. Thus, this product should be administered with caution to patients with borderline hypoadrenal function, regardless of whether it is of pituitary or of primary adrenal origin.

Information for Patients—Tuinal may impair the mental and/or physical abilities required for the performance of potentially hazardous tasks, such as driving a car or operating machinery. The patient should be cautioned accordingly.

Drug Interactions—Tuinal in combination with alcohol, tranquilizers, and other central-nervous-system depressants has additive depressant effects, and the patient should be so advised. Patients taking this drug should be warned not to exceed the dosage recommended by their physician. Toxic effects and fatalities have occurred following overdoses of Tuinal alone and in combination with other central-nervous-system depressants. Caution should be exercised in prescribing unnecessarily large amounts of Tuinal for patients who have a history of emotional disturbances or suicidal ideation or who have misused alcohol and other CNS drugs (*see* Overdosage).

Usage in Pregnancy—Pregnancy Category B—Reproduction studies have been performed in animals and have revealed no evidence of impaired fertility or harm to the fetus due to Tuinal. There are, however, no adequate and well-controlled studies in pregnant women. Because animal reproduction studies are not always predictive of human response, this drug should be used during pregnancy only if clearly needed.

Labor and Delivery—Depression has been noted in infants born following the use of Tuinal during labor.

Nursing Mothers—Caution should be exercised when Tuinal is administered to a nursing woman.

Usage in Children—Safety and effectiveness in children have not been established.

Adverse Reactions: The following adverse reactions have been reported:

CNS Depression—Residual sedation or "hangover," drowsiness, and lethargy.

Respiratory/Circulatory—Respiratory depression, apnea, circulatory collapse.

Allergic—Hypersensitivity reactions, especially in individuals with asthma, urticaria, angioneurotic edema, or similar conditions; skin eruptions.

Other—Nausea and vomiting; headache.

Drug Abuse and Dependence: *Controlled Substance*—Tuinal is a Schedule II drug.

Dependence—Prolonged, uninterrupted use of barbiturates (particularly the short-acting drugs), even in therapeutic doses, may result in psychic and physical dependence. Withdrawal symptoms due to physical dependence following chronic use of large doses of barbiturates may include delirium, convulsions, and death (*see* Contraindications).

Overdosage: *Symptoms*—The manifestations of overdosage are early hypothermia followed by fever, sluggish or absent reflexes, respiratory depression, gradual appearance of circulatory collapse, pulmonary edema, and coma.

Treatment—General management should consist in symptomatic and supportive therapy, including gastric lavage, administration of intravenous fluids, and maintenance of blood pressure, body temperature, and adequate respiratory exchange. Dialysis will increase the rate of removal of barbiturates from the body fluids. Antibiotics may be required to control pulmonary complications.

Dosage and Administration: 50 to 200 mg at bedtime or one hour preoperatively.

How Supplied: (Ⓒ) *Pulvules® Tuinal® (Secobarbital Sodium and Amobarbital Sodium Capsules, USP), No. 302, F64,** 50 mg (No. 4, Blue Body, Orange Cap), in bottles of 100 (NDC 0002-0664-02); *No. 303, F65,** 100 mg (No. 3, Blue Body, Orange Cap), in bottles of 100 (NDC 0002-0665-02) and 1000 (NDC 0002-0665-04), in 10 strips of 10 individually labeled blisters each containing 1 Pulvule (ID100) (NDC 0002-0665-33), and in strip packages of individually sealed Pulvules (DS1000) (NDC 0002-0665-35); *No. 304, F66,** 200 mg (No. 2, Blue Body, Orange Cap), in bottles of 100 (NDC 0002-0666-02) and 1000 (NDC 0002-0666-04) and in 10 strips of 10 individually labeled blisters each containing 1 Pulvule (ID100) (NDC 0002-0666-33).

[042182]

[*Shown in Product Identification Section*]

ULTRALENTE® ILETIN® I

(extended insulin zinc suspension, Lilly), *see under* Iletin® (insulin, Lilly).

VANCOCIN® HCL ℞

(vancomycin hydrochloride)
Sterile, USP
IntraVenous

Description: Vancocin® HCl (vancomycin hydrochloride, Lilly), IntraVenous, is a glycopeptide antibiotic derived from *Streptomyces orientalis* which is bactericidal against many gram-positive bacteria. It should be administered intravenously, in dilute solution (*see* Dosage and Administration).

Actions: Vancocin® HCl (vancomycin hydrochloride, Lilly) is poorly absorbed by mouth, but an intravenous dose of 1 g produces serum levels averaging 25 mcg/ml at two hours. Its half-life in the circulation is about six hours. Many strains of streptococci, staphylococci, *Clostridium difficile,* and other gram-positive bacteria are susceptible in vitro to concentrations of 0.5 to 5 mcg/ml. Staphylococci are generally susceptible to less than 5 mcg of Vancocin HCl/ml, but a small proportion of *Staphylococcus aureus* strains require 10 or 20 mcg/ml for inhibition. If the Bauer-Kirby method of disc susceptibility testing is used, a 30-mcg disc of Vancocin HCl should produce a zone of more than 11 mm when tested against a vancomycin-susceptible bacterial strain.

Clinically effective concentrations of this antibiotic in the blood are usually achieved and maintained by its intravenous administration; moreover, inhibitory concentrations can be demonstrated in pleural, pericardial, ascitic, and synovial fluids and in urine. This antibiotic does not readily diffuse across normal meninges into the spinal fluid. However, when the meninges are inflamed as a result of infection, Vancocin HCl penetrates into the spinal fluid.

About 80 percent of injected Vancocin HCl is excreted by the kidneys. Concentrations are high in the urine. Impairment of renal function results in delayed excretion and in high blood levels associated with an increase in drug toxicity.

Indications: Vancocin® HCl (vancomycin hydrochloride, Lilly) is indicated in potentially life-threatening infections which cannot be treated with another effective, less toxic antimicrobial drug, including the penicillins and cephalosporins.

Vancocin HCl is useful in therapy of severe staphylococcal (including methicillin-resistant staphylococci) infections in patients who cannot receive or who have failed to respond to the penicillins and cephalosporins or who have infections with staphylococci that are resistant to other antibiotics, including methicillin. Vancocin HCl has been used successfully alone in the treatment of staphylococcal (including methicillin-resistant staphylococci) endocarditis. Its effectiveness has been documented in other infections due to staphylococci (including methicillin-resistant staphylococci), including osteomyelitis, pneumonia, septicemia, and soft-tissue infections. When staphylococcal infections are localized and purulent, antibiotics are used as adjuncts to appropriate surgical measures.

The parenteral form may be administered orally for treatment of staphylococcal enterocolitis and antiobiotic-associated pseudomembranous colitis produced by *C. difficile*. Parenteral antibiotic administration may be used concomitantly. Vancomycin is *not* effective by the oral route for other types of infection.

Contraindication: Vancocin® HCl (vancomycin hydrochloride, Lilly) is contraindicated in patients with known hypersensitivity to this antibiotic.

Warnings: Because of its ototoxicity and nephrotoxicity, Vancocin® HCl (vancomycin hydrochloride, Lilly) should be used with care in patients with renal insufficiency. The risk of toxicity is appreciably increased by high blood concentrations or prolonged therapy. If it is necessary to use Vancocin HCl in such patients, doses of less than 2 g/day usually will provide satisfactory blood levels.

Vancocin HCl should be avoided in patients with previous hearing loss. If it is used in such patients, the dose of Vancocin HCl should be regulated, if possible, by periodic determination of the drug level in the blood. Deafness may be preceded by tinnitus. The elderly are more susceptible to auditory damage. Experience with other antibiotics suggests that deafness may be progressive despite cessation of treatment.

Concurrent and sequential use of other neurotoxic and/or nephrotoxic antibiotics, particularly streptomycin, neomycin, kanamycin, gentamicin, cephaloridine, paromomycin, viomycin, polymyxin B, colistin, tobramycin, and amikacin, requires careful monitoring.

Continued on next page

***Identi-Code® symbol.**

Lilly—Cont.

Precautions: Patients with borderline renal function and individuals over the age of 60 should be given serial tests of auditory function and of vancomycin blood levels. (Vancomycin serum levels may be determined by use of the modified Rammelkamp serial twofold-dilution technique with streptococcus C203 as the indicator organism.) All patients receiving the drug should have periodic hematologic studies, urinalyses, and liver and renal function tests.
Vancocin® HCl (vancomycin hydrochloride, Lilly) is very irritating to tissue and causes necrosis when injected intramuscularly; it must be administered intravenously. Pain and thrombophlebitis occur in many patients receiving Vancocin HCl and are occasionally severe. The frequency and severity of thrombophlebitis can be minimized if the drug is administered in a volume of at least 200 ml of glucose or saline solution and if the sites of injection are rotated.
Adverse Reactions: Nausea, chills, fever, urticaria, and macular rashes have been associated with the administration of Vancocin® HCl (vancomycin hydrochloride, Lilly). It may also produce eosinophilia and anaphylactoid reactions.
The use of Vancocin HCl may result in overgrowth of nonsusceptible organisms. If new infections due to bacteria or fungi appear during therapy with this product, appropriate measures should be taken.
Dosage and Administration: *Adults*—The usual intravenous dose is 500 mg (in 0.9% Sodium Chloride Injection or 5% glucose in Sterile Water for Injection) every six hours or 1 g every 12 hours. The majority of patients with infections caused by organisms susceptible to the antibiotic show a therapeutic response by 48 to 72 hours. The total duration of therapy is determined by the type and severity of the infection and the clinical response of the patient. In staphylococcal endocarditis, therapy for three weeks or longer is recommended.
Children—The total daily dosage of Vancocin® HCl (vancomycin hydrochloride, Lilly), calculated on the basis of 20 mg/lb of body weight, can be divided and figured in with the child's 24-hour requirement of fluid.
PREPARATION OF SOLUTION:
At the time of use, add 10 ml of Sterile Water for Injection to the vial of dry, sterile Vancocin HCl powder.
FURTHER DILUTION IS REQUIRED. READ INSTRUCTIONS WHICH FOLLOW:

1. Intermittent Infusion (the preferred method of administration)
   The above solution (containing 500 mg Vancocin HCl) can be added to 100-200 ml of 0.9% Sodium Chloride Injection or 5% glucose in Sterile Water for Injection. This intravenous infusion may be given over a period of 20 to 30 minutes every six hours.
2. Continuous Infusion (should be used only when intermittent infusion is not feasible)
   Two to four vials of the above (1 to 2 g can be added to a sufficiently large volume of 0.9% Sodium Chloride Injection or 5% glucose in Sterile Water for Injection to permit the desired daily dose to be administered slowly by intravenous drip over a 24-hour period.

For Oral Administration—The contents of one vial (500 mg) may be diluted in 1 oz of water and given to the patient to drink, or the diluted material may be administered via nasogastric tube. The usual adult dosage for antibiotic-associated pseudomembranous colitis produced by *C. difficile* is 500 mg of vancomycin orally every six hours for a period of seven to ten days. For convenience of oral administration, Vancocin HCl is also available in a screw-cap container (No. M-206).
Stability of Prepared Solution: After reconstitution, the solution may be stored in a refrigerator for 96 hours without significant loss of potency.
How Supplied: (℞) *Vials No. 657, Vancocin® HCl (Sterile Vancomycin Hydrochloride, USP), IntraVenous,* equivalent to 500 mg vancomycin, 10-ml size, rubber-stoppered (Dry Powder), in singles (10 per carton) (NDC 0002-1444-01).
[010682]

VANCOCIN® HCl ℞
(vancomycin hydrochloride)
For Oral Solution, USP

> **This preparation is for oral use only. If parenteral vancomycin therapy is desired, use Vancocin® HCl (Sterile Vancomycin Hydrochloride, USP), IntraVenous, and consult package insert accompanying that preparation.**

Description: Vancocin® HCl (vancomycin hydrochloride, Lilly) is a glycopeptide antibiotic derived from *Streptomyces orientalis* which is bactericidal against many gram-positive bacteria.
Actions: Vancocin® HCl (vancomycin hydrochloride, Lilly) is poorly absorbed by mouth. Many strains of streptococci, staphylococci, *Clostridium difficile,* and other gram-positive bacteria are susceptible in vitro to concentrations of 0.5 to 5 mcg/ml. Staphylococci are generally susceptible to less than 5 mcg of Vancocin HCl per ml, but a small proportion of *Staphylococcus aureus* strains require 10 or 20 mcg/ml for inhibition. If the Bauer-Kirby method of disc susceptibility testing is used, a 30-mcg disc of Vancocin HCl should produce a zone of more than 11 mm when tested against a vancomycin-susceptible bacterial strain.
Indication: Vancocin® HCl (vancomycin hydrochloride, Lilly) may be administered orally for treatment of staphylococcal enterocolitis and antibiotic-associated pseudomembranous colitis produced by *C. difficile.* Parenteral antibiotic administration may be used concomitantly. Vancomycin is *not* effective by the oral route for other types of infection.
Contraindication: Vancocin® HCl (vancomycin hydrochloride, Lilly) is contraindicated in patients with known hypersensitivity to this antibiotic.
Warnings: Because of its ototoxicity and nephrotoxicity, Vancocin® HCl (vancomycin hydrochloride, Lilly) should be used with care in patients with renal insufficiency. During parenteral therapy, the risk of toxicity is appreciably increased by high blood concentrations or prolonged treatment. If it is necessary to use Vancocin HCl parenterally in such patients, doses of less than 2 g/day usually will provide satisfactory blood levels.
Vancocin HCl should also be avoided in patients with previous hearing loss. If it is used in such patients, the dose of Vancocin HCl should be regulated, if possible, by periodic determination of the drug level in the blood. Deafness may be preceded by tinnitus. The elderly are more susceptible to auditory damage. Experience with other antibiotics suggests that deafness may be progressive despite cessation of treatment.
Concurrent and sequential use of other neurotoxic and/or nephrotoxic antibiotics, particularly streptomycin, neomycin, kanamycin, gentamicin, cephaloridine, paromomycin, viomycin, polymyxin B, colistin, tobramycin, and amikacin, requires careful monitoring.
Precautions: Patients with borderline renal function and individuals over the age of 60 should be given serial tests of auditory function and of vancomycin blood levels. All patients receiving the drug should have periodic hematologic studies, urinalyses, and liver and renal function tests.
Adverse Reactions: Nausea, chills, fever, urticaria, and macular rashes have been associated with the administration of Vancocin HCl. It may also produce eosinophilia and anaphylactoid reactions.
The use of Vancocin® HCl (vancomycin hydrochloride, Lilly) may result in overgrowth of nonsusceptible organisms. If new infections due to bacteria or fungi appear during therapy with this product, appropriate measures should be taken.
Dosage and Administration: The contents of the container may be mixed with distilled or deionized water (115 ml) for oral administration. When mixed with 115 ml of water, each 6 ml provide approximately 500 mg of vancomycin. Mix thoroughly to dissolve. This mixture may be kept for one week in a refrigerator without significant loss of potency.
Adults—The usual dose is 500 mg every six hours or 1 g every 12 hours.
The usual adult dosage for antibiotic-associated pseudomembranous colitis produced by *C. difficile* is 500 mg to 2g of vancomycin orally/day in three or four divided doses administered for seven to ten days.
Children—The total daily dose is 20 mg/lb of body weight in divided doses.
How Supplied: (℞) *Vancocin® HCl (Vancomycin Hydrochloride for Oral Solution, USP), M-206,* 10 g (equivalent to vancomycin), in a screw-cap container (NDC 0002-2372-37).
[090982]

VANCOMYCIN HYDROCHLORIDE, *see* Vancocin® HC1 (vancomycin hydrochloride, Lilly).

V-CILLIN K® ℞
(penicillin V potassium)
USP

Description: V-Cillin K® (Penicillin V Potassium, USP, Lilly) is the potassium salt of V-Cillin® (Penicillin V, USP, Lilly). This chemically improved form combines acid stability with immediate solubility and rapid absorption.
Actions and Pharmacology: V-Cillin K® (penicillin V potassium, Lilly) is bactericidal against penicillin-sensitive microorganisms during the stage of active multiplication. It produces its effect by inhibiting biosynthesis of cell-wall mucopeptide. It is not active against the penicillinase-producing bacteria, which include many strains of staphylococci. The drug exerts high in vitro activity against staphylococci (except penicillinase-producing strains), streptococci (groups A, C, G, H, L, and M), and pneumococci. Other organisms sensitive in vitro to penicillin V are *Corynebacterium diphtheriae, Bacillus anthracis,* clostridia, *Actinomyces bovis, Streptobacillus moniliformis, Listeria monocytogenes, Leptospira,* and *Neisseria gonorrhoeae. Treponema pallidum* is extremely sensitive.
V-Cillin K has the distinct advantage over penicillin G in being resistant to inactivation by gastric acid. It may be given with meals; however, blood levels are slightly higher when the drug is given on an empty stomach. Average blood levels are two to five times higher than those following the same dose of oral penicillin G and also show much less individual variation.
Once absorbed, about 80 percent of V-Cillin K is bound to serum protein. Tissue levels are highest in the kidneys, and lesser amounts appear in the liver, skin, and intestines. Small concentrations are found in all other body tissues and the cerebrospinal fluid. The drug is excreted as rapidly as it is absorbed in individuals with normal kidney function; however, recovery of the drug from the urine indicates that only about 25 percent of the dose given is

absorbed. In neonates, young infants, and individuals with impaired kidney function, excretion is considerably delayed.

Indications: V-Cillin K® (penicillin V potassium, Lilly) is indicated in the treatment of mild to moderately severe infections due to microorganisms whose sensitivity to penicillin G is within the range of serum levels common to this particular dosage form. Therapy should be guided by bacteriologic studies (including susceptibility tests) and by clinical response.

NOTE: Severe pneumonia, empyema, bacteremia, pericarditis, meningitis, and arthritis should not be treated with penicillin V during the acute stage.

Indicated surgical procedures should be performed.

The following infections will usually respond to adequate dosage of penicillin V:

Streptococcal Infections (without Bacteremia)—Mild to moderate infections of the upper respiratory tract, scarlet fever, and mild erysipelas.

NOTE: Streptococci in groups A, C, G, H, L, and M are very sensitive to penicillin. Other groups, including group D (enterococcus), are resistant.

Pneumococcal Infections—Mild to moderately severe infections of the respiratory tract.

Staphylococcal Infections Sensitive to Penicillin G—Mild infections of the skin and soft tissues.

NOTE: Reports indicate an increasing number of strains of staphylococci resistant to penicillin G, which emphasizes the need for culture and susceptibility studies in treating suspected staphylococcal infections.

Fusospirochetosis (Vincent's Gingivitis and Pharyngitis)—Mild to moderately severe infections of the oropharynx usually respond to therapy with oral penicillin.

NOTE: Necessary dental care should be accomplished in infections involving the gum tissue.

Medical Conditions in Which Oral Penicillin Therapy Is Indicated as Prophylaxis—To prevent recurrence following rheumatic fever and/or chorea. Prophylaxis with oral penicillin on a continuing basis has proved effective in preventing recurrence of these conditions.

Although no controlled clinical efficacy studies have been conducted, penicillin V has been suggested by the American Heart Association and the American Dental Association for use as part of a parenteral/oral regimen and as an alternative oral regimen for prophylaxis against bacterial endocarditis in patients with congenital heart disease or rheumatic or other acquired valvular heart disease when they undergo dental procedures and surgical procedures of the respiratory tract.[1] Since alphahemolytic streptococci relatively resistant to penicillin may be found when patients are receiving continuous oral penicillin for secondary prevention of rheumatic fever, prophylactic agents other than penicillin may be chosen for these patients and prescribed in addition to their continuous prophylactic regimen for rheumatic fever. Oral penicillin should not be used as adjunctive prophylaxis for genitourinary instrumentation or surgery, lower intestinal tract surgery, sigmoidoscopy, and childbirth.

Note: When selecting antibiotics for the prevention of bacterial endocarditis, the physician or dentist should read the full joint statement of the American Heart Association and the American Dental Association.[1]

Contraindication: A previous hypersensitivity reaction to any penicillin is a contraindication.

Warnings: Serious and occasionally fatal hypersensitivity (anaphylactoid) reactions have been reported in patients receiving penicillin therapy. Although anaphylaxis is more frequent following parenteral therapy, it has occurred in patients given oral penicillins. These reactions are more likely in individuals with a history of sensitivity to multiple allergens.

There have been well-documented reports of individuals with a history of penicillin hypersensitivity who have experienced severe reactions when treated with a cephalosporin. Before therapy with a penicillin, careful inquiry should be made concerning previous hypersensitivity reactions to penicillins, cephalosporins, and other allergens. If an allergic reaction occurs, the drug should be discontinued and the patient treated with the usual agents (e.g., epinephrine or other pressor amines, antihistamines, or corticosteroids).

Precautions: Penicillin should be used with caution in individuals with histories of significant allergies and/or asthma.

The oral route of administration should not be relied on in patients with severe illness or with nausea, vomiting, gastric dilatation, cardiospasm, or intestinal hypermotility.

Occasional patients will not absorb therapeutic amounts of orally administered penicillin.

In streptococcal infections, therapy must be sufficient to eliminate the organism (a minimum of ten days); otherwise, the sequelae of streptococcal disease may occur. Cultures should be taken following completion of treatment to determine whether streptococci have been eradicated.

Prolonged use of antibiotics may promote the overgrowth of nonsusceptible organisms, including fungi. If superinfection occurs, appropriate measures should be taken.

Adverse Reactions: Although reactions have been reported much less frequently after oral than after parenteral penicillin therapy, it should be remembered that all degrees of hypersensitivity, including fatal anaphylaxis, have been observed with oral penicillin.

The most common reactions to oral penicillin are nausea, vomiting, epigastric distress, diarrhea, and black, hairy tongue. The hypersensitivity reactions noted are skin eruptions (ranging from maculopapular to exfoliative dermatitis); urticaria; reactions resembling serum sickness, including chills, fever, edema, arthralgia, and prostration; laryngeal edema; and anaphylaxis. Fever and eosinophilia may frequently be the only reactions observed. Hemolytic anemia, leukopenia, thrombocytopenia, neuropathy, and nephropathy are infrequent reactions and are usually associated with high doses of parenteral penicillin.

Dosage and Administration: The dosage of V-Cillin K® (penicillin V potassium, Lilly) should be determined according to the sensitivity of the causative microorganism and the severity of infection and should be adjusted to the clinical response of the patient.

The usual dosage recommendations for adults and children 12 years and over are as follows:

Streptococcal Infections—Mild to moderately severe infections of the upper respiratory tract, including scarlet fever and mild erysipelas: 200,000 to 500,000 units every six to eight hours for ten days.

Pneumococcal Infections—Mild to moderately severe infections of the respiratory tract, including otitis media: 400,000 to 500,000 units every six hours until the patient has been afebrile for at least two days.

Staphylococcal Infections—Mild infections of skin and soft tissue (culture and susceptibility tests should be performed): 400,000 to 500,000 units every six to eight hours.

Fusospirochetosis (Vincent's Infection) of the Oropharynx—Mild to moderately severe infections: 400,000 to 500,000 units every six to eight hours.

Prophylaxis in the Following Conditions—To prevent recurrence following rheumatic fever and/or chorea: 200,000 to 250,000 units twice daily on a continuing basis.

For prophylaxis against bacterial endocarditis[1] in patients with congenital heart disease or rheumatic or other acquired valvular heart disease when undergoing dental procedures or surgical procedures of the upper respiratory tract, one of two regimens may be selected:

(1) For the oral regimen, the usual adult dosage is 2 g of penicillin V (1 g for children under 30 kg) one-half to one hour before the procedure and then 500 mg (250 mg for children under 30 kg) every six hours for eight doses; or

(2) For the combined parenteral/oral regimen, the dosage schedule is 1,000,000 units of aqueous crystalline penicillin G (30,000 units/kg for children) intramuscularly mixed with 600,000 units procaine penicillin G (600,000 units for children) one-half to one hour before the procedure and then oral penicillin V, 500 mg for adults or 250 mg for children less than 30 kg, every six hours for eight doses. Doses for children should not exceed recommendations for adults for a single dose or for a 24-hour period.

NOTE: Therapy for children under 12 years of age is calculated on the basis of body weight. For infants and small children, the suggested daily dose is 25,000 to 90,000 units (15 to 50 mg)/kg in three to six divided doses.

How Supplied: (℞) *For Oral Solution, V-Cillin K® (Penicillin V Potassium for Oral Solution, USP): M-126, W07,** 125 mg (200,000 units) (equivalent to penicillin V) per 5 ml of solution, in 40 (NDC 0002-2307-77), 100 (NDC 0002-2307-48), 150 (NDC 0002-2307-68), and 200-ml-size (NDC 0002-2307-89) packages and in unit-dose bottles of 100 (ID100) (NDC 0002-2307-33); *M-142, W16,** 250 mg (400,000 units) (equivalent to penicillin V) per 5 ml of solution, in 100 (NDC 0002-2316-48), 150 (NDC 0002-2316-68), and 200-ml-size (NDC 0002-2316-89) packages and in unit-dose bottles of 100 (ID100) (NDC 0002-2316-33)

Each package consists of a bottle containing penicillin V potassium equivalent to penicillin V in a dry, pleasantly flavored mixture, buffered with sodium citrate and citric acid.

After being mixed, the solution should be stored in a refrigerator. It may be kept for 14 days without significant loss of potency. *Shake well before using. Keep tightly closed.*

(℞) *Tablets V-Cillin K® (Penicillin V Potassium Tablets, USP),* Specially Coated: *No. 1830, C27,** 125 mg (200,000 units) (equivalent to penicillin V), in bottles of 50 (NDC 0002-0327-50) and 100 (NDC 0002-0327-02); *No. 1831, C29,** 250 mg (400,000 units) (equivalent to penicillin V), in bottles of 24 (NDC 0002-0329-24), 100 (NDC 0002-0329-02), and 500 (NDC 0002-0329-03) and in 10 strips of 10 individually labeled blisters each containing 1 tablet (ID100) (NDC 0002-0329-33); and *No. 1832, C46,** 500 mg (800,000 units) (equivalent to penicillin V) in bottles of 24 (NDC 0002-0346-24), 100 (NDC 0002-0346-02), and 500 (NDC 0002-0346-03) and in 10 strips of 10 individually labeled blisters each containing 1 tablet (ID100) (NDC 0002-0346-33). [092782]

Reference: 1. American Heart Association: Prevention of Bacterial Endocarditis, Circulation, *56*:139A, 1977.

VELBAN® ℞

(vinblastine sulfate)
Sterile, USP

Description: Velban® (Vinblastine Sulfate, USP, Lilly) is the salt of an alkaloid extracted from *Vinca rosea* Linn., a common flowering herb known as the periwinkle (more properly known as *Catharanthus roseus* G. Don). Previously, the generic name was vincaleukoblastine, abbreviated VLB.

Chemical and physical evidence indicates that Velban has the empirical formula $C_{46}H_{58}O_9N_4 \cdot H_2SO_4$ and that it is a dimeric alkaloid containing both indole and dihydroindole moieties.

Continued on next page

*Identi-Code® symbol.

Lilly—Cont.

Vials of Velban contain 10 mg of vinblastine sulfate, in the form of a lyophilized plug, without excipients. When sodium chloride solution is added prior to injection, the *p*H of the resulting solution lies in the range of 3.5 to 5.

Actions: Velban® (vinblastine sulfate, Lilly) has been used for the palliative treatment of a variety of malignant neoplastic conditions. In susceptible clinical cases, Velban has produced temporary reduction in the size or temporary disappearance of some tumors. It has relieved pain and other symptoms and allowed some patients to regain appetite and weight.

Experimental data indicate that the action of Velban is different from that of other recognized antineoplastic agents. Tissue-culture studies suggest an interference with metabolic pathways of amino acids leading from glutamic acid to the citric acid cycle and to urea. In vivo experiments tend to confirm the in vitro results. A number of studies in vitro and in vivo have demonstrated that Velban produces a stathmokinetic effect and various atypical mitotic figures. The therapeutic responses, however, are not fully explained by the cytologic changes, since these changes are sometimes observed clinically and experimentally in the absence of any oncolytic effects.

Reversal of the antitumor effect of Velban by glutamic acid or tryptophan has been observed. In addition, glutamic acid and aspartic acid have protected mice from lethal doses of Velban. Aspartic acid was relatively ineffective in reversing the antitumor effect.

Other studies indicate that Velban has an effect on cell-energy production required for mitosis and interferes with nucleic acid synthesis.

Hematologic Effects—Clinically, leukopenia is an expected effect of Velban® (vinblastine sulfate, Lilly), and the level of the leukocyte count is an important guide to therapy with this drug. In general, the larger the dose employed, the more profound and longer lasting the leukopenia will be. The fact that the white-blood-cell count returns to normal levels after drug-induced leukopenia is an indication that the white-cell-producing mechanism is not permanently depressed. Usually, the white count has completely returned to normal after the virtual disappearance of white cells from the peripheral blood.

Following therapy with Velban, the nadir in white-blood-cell count may be expected to occur five to ten days after the last day of drug administration. Recovery of the white blood count is fairly rapid thereafter and is usually complete within another seven to 14 days. With the smaller doses employed for maintenance therapy, leukopenia may not be a problem.

Although the thrombocyte count ordinarily is not significantly lowered by therapy with Velban, patients whose bone marrow has been recently impaired by prior therapy with radiation or with other oncolytic drugs may show thrombocytopenia (less than 200,000 platelets/mm^3). When other chemotherapy or radiation has not been employed previously, thrombocyte reduction below the level of 200,000/mm^3 is rarely encountered, even when Velban may be causing significant leukopenia. Rapid recovery from thrombocytopenia within a few days is the rule.

The effect of Velban upon the red-cell count and hemoglobin is usually insignificant when other therapy does not complicate the picture. It should be remembered, however, that patients with malignant disease may exhibit anemia even in the absence of any therapy.

Indications: Vinblastine sulfate is indicated in the palliative treatment of the following:

I. *Frequently Responsive Malignancies*—
- Generalized Hodgkin's disease (Stages III and IV, Ann Arbor modification of Rye staging system)
- Lymphocytic lymphoma (nodular and diffuse, poorly and well differentiated)
- Histiocytic lymphoma
- Mycosis fungoides (advanced stages)
- Advanced carcinoma of the testis
- Kaposi's sarcoma
- Letterer-Siwe disease (histiocytosis X)

II. *Less Frequently Responsive Malignancies*—
- Choriocarcinoma resistant to other chemotherapeutic agents
- Carcinoma of the breast, unresponsive to appropriate endocrine surgery and hormonal therapy

Current principles of chemotherapy for many types of cancer include the concurrent administration of several antineoplastic agents. For enhanced therapeutic effect without additive toxicity, agents with different dose-limiting clinical toxicities and different mechanisms of action are generally selected. Therefore, although Velban® (vinblastine sulfate, Lilly) is effective as a single agent in the aforementioned indications, it is usually administered in combination with other antineoplastic drugs. Such combination therapy produces a greater percentage of response than does a single-agent regimen. These principles have been applied, for example, in the chemotherapy of Hodgkin's disease.

Hodgkin's Disease—Velban has been shown to be one of the most effective single agents for the treatment of Hodgkin's disease. Advanced Hodgkin's disease has also been successfully treated with several multiple-drug regimens that included Velban. Patients who had relapses after treatment with the MOPP program—mechlorethamine hydrochloride (nitrogen mustard), vincristine sulfate (Oncovin® [vincristine sulfate, Lilly]), prednisone, and procarbazine—have likewise responded to combination-drug therapy that included Velban. A protocol using cyclophosphamide in place of nitrogen mustard and Velban instead of Oncovin is an alternative therapy for previously untreated patients with advanced Hodgkin's disease.

Advanced testicular germinal-cell cancers (embryonal carcinoma, teratocarcinoma, and choriocarcinoma) are sensitive to Velban alone, but better clinical results are achieved when Velban is administered concomitantly with other antineoplastic agents. The effect of bleomycin is significantly enhanced if Velban is administered six to eight hours prior to the administration of bleomycin; this schedule permits more cells to be arrested during metaphase, the stage of the cell cycle in which bleomycin is active.

Contraindications: Velban® (vinblastine sulfate, Lilly) is contraindicated in patients who are leukopenic. It should not be used in the presence of bacterial infection. Such infections must be brought under control prior to the initiation of therapy with Velban.

Warnings: *Usage in Pregnancy*—Caution is necessary with the administration of all oncolytic drugs during pregnancy. Information on the use of Velban® (vinblastine sulfate, Lilly) during pregnancy is very limited. Although no abnormalities of the human fetus have been reported thus far, animal studies with Velban suggest that teratogenic effects may occur.

Aspermia has been reported in man. Animal studies show metaphase arrest and degenerative changes in germ cells.

Precautions: If leukopenia with less than 2000 white blood cells/mm^3 occurs following a dose of Velban® (vinblastine sulfate, Lilly), the patient should be watched carefully for evidence of infection until the white-blood-cell count has returned to a safe level.

When cachexia or ulcerated areas of the skin surface are present, there may be a more profound leukopenic response to the drug; therefore, its use should be avoided in older persons suffering from either of these conditions.

In patients with malignant-cell infiltration of the bone marrow, the leukocyte and platelet counts have sometimes fallen precipitously after moderate doses of Velban. Further use of the drug in such patients is inadvisable.

The use of small amounts of Velban daily for long periods is not advised, even though the resulting total weekly dosage may be similar to that recommended. Little or no added therapeutic effect has been demonstrated when such regimens have been used. *Strict adherence to the recommended dosage schedule is very important.* When amounts equal to several times the recommended weekly dosage were given in seven daily installments for long periods, convulsions, severe and permanent central-nervous-system damage, and even death occurred.

Care must be taken to avoid contamination of the eye with concentrations of Velban used clinically. If accidental contamination occurs, severe irritation (or, if the drug was delivered under pressure, even corneal ulceration) may result. The eye should be washed with water immediately and thoroughly.

Adverse Reactions: *Prior to the use of the drug, patients should be advised of the possibility of untoward symptoms.*

In general, the incidence of adverse reactions attending the use of Velban® (vinblastine sulfate, Lilly) appears to be related to the size of the dose employed. With the exception of epilation, leukopenia, and neurologic side effects, adverse reactions generally have not persisted for longer than 24 hours. Neurologic side effects are not common; but when they do occur, they often last for more than 24 hours. Leukopenia, the most common adverse reaction, is usually the dose-limiting factor.

The following are manifestations which have been reported as adverse reactions:

Gastrointestinal—Nausea, vomiting, constipation, vesiculation of the mouth, ileus, diarrhea, anorexia, abdominal pain, rectal bleeding, pharyngitis, hemorrhagic enterocolitis, bleeding from an old peptic ulcer

Neurologic—Numbness, paresthesias, peripheral neuritis, mental depression, loss of deep-tendon reflexes, headache, convulsions

Miscellaneous—Malaise, weakness, dizziness, pain in tumor site, vesiculation of the skin

Nausea and vomiting usually may be controlled with ease by antiemetic agents. When epilation develops, it frequently is not total; and, in some cases, hair regrows while maintenance therapy continues.

Extravasation during intravenous injection may lead to cellulitis and phlebitis. If the amount of extravasation is great, sloughing may occur.

Dosage and Administration: There are variations in the depth of the leukopenic response which follows therapy with Velban® (vinblastine sulfate, Lilly). For this reason, it is recommended that the drug be given no more frequently than *once every seven days.* It is wise to initiate therapy for adults by administering a single intravenous dose of 3.7 mg/m^2 of body surface area (bsa). Thereafter, white-blood-cell counts should be made to determine the patient's sensitivity to Velban.

A simplified and conservative incremental approach to dosage *at weekly intervals* may be outlined as follows:

	Adults	Children
First dose	3.7 mg/m^2 bsa	2.5 mg/m^2 bsa
Second dose	5.5 mg/m^2 bsa	3.75 mg/m^2 bsa
Third dose	7.4 mg/m^2 bsa	5.0 mg/m^2 bsa
Fourth dose	9.25 mg/m^2 bsa	6.25 mg/m^2 bsa
Fifth dose	11.1 mg/m^2 bsa	7.5 mg/m^2 bsa

The above-mentioned increases may be used until a maximum dose (not exceeding 18.5

mg/m^2 bsa for adults and 12.5 mg/m^2 bsa for children) is reached. The dose should not be increased after that dose which reduces the white-cell count to approximately 3000 $cells/mm^3$. In some adults, 3.7 mg/m^2 bsa may produce this leukopenia; other adults may require more than 11.1 mg/m^2 bsa; and, very rarely, as much as 18.5 mg/m^2 bsa may be necessary. For most adult patients, however, the weekly dosage will prove to be 5.5 to 7.4 mg/m^2 bsa.

When the dose of Velban which will produce the above degree of leukopenia has been established, a dose *one increment smaller* than this should be administered at weekly intervals for maintenance. Thus, the patient is receiving the maximum dose that does not cause leukopenia. *It should be emphasized that, even though seven days have elapsed, the next dose of Velban should not be given until the white-cell count has returned to at least 4000/mm³.* In some cases, oncolytic activity may be encountered before leukopenic effect. When this occurs, there is no need to increase the size of subsequent doses.

The duration of maintenance therapy varies according to the disease being treated and the combination of antineoplastic agents being used. There are differences of opinion regarding the duration of maintenance therapy with the same protocol for a particular disease; for example, various durations have been used with the MOPP program in treating Hodgkin's disease. Prolonged chemotherapy for maintaining remissions involves several risks, among which are life-threatening infectious diseases, sterility, and possibly the appearance of other cancers through suppression of immune surveillance. In some disorders, survival following complete remission may not be as prolonged as that achieved with shorter periods of maintenance therapy. On the other hand, failure to provide maintenance therapy in some patients may lead to unnecessary relapse; complete remissions in patients with testicular cancer, unless maintained for at least two years, often result in early relapse.

To prepare a solution containing 1 mg of Velban/ml, add 10 ml of Sodium Chloride Injection (preserved with phenol or benzyl alcohol) to the 10 mg of Velban in the sterile vial. Other solutions are not recommended. The drug dissolves instantly to give a clear solution. After a solution has been made in this way and a portion of it has been removed from a vial, the remainder of the vial's contents may be stored in a refrigerator for future use for 30 days without significant loss of potency.

The dose of Velban (calculated to provide the desired amount) may be injected either into the tubing of a running intravenous infusion or directly into a vein. The latter procedure is readily adaptable to outpatient therapy. In either case, the injection may be completed in about one minute. If care is taken to insure that the needle is securely within the vein and that no solution containing Velban is spilled extravascularly, cellulitis and/or phlebitis will not occur. To minimize further the possibility of extravascular spillage, it is suggested that the syringe and needle be rinsed with venous blood before withdrawal of the needle. The dose should not be diluted in large volumes of diluent (i.e., 100 to 250 ml) or given intravenously for prolonged periods (ranging from 30 to 60 minutes or more), since this frequently results in irritation of the vein and increases the chance of extravasation.

Because of the enhanced possibility of thrombosis, it is considered inadvisable to inject a solution of Velban into an extremity in which the circulation is impaired or potentially impaired by such conditions as compressing or invading neoplasm, phlebitis, or varicosity.

Caution—If leakage into surrounding tissue should occur during intravenous administration of Velban® (vinblastine sulfate, Lilly), it may cause considerable irritation. The injection should be discontinued immediately, and any remaining portion of the dose should then be introduced into another vein. Local injection of hyaluronidase and the application of moderate heat to the area of leakage help disperse the drug and are thought to minimize discomfort and the possibility of cellulitis.

How Supplied: (℞) *Vials No. 687, Velban® (Sterile Vinblastine Sulfate, USP),* 10 mg, 10-ml size, rubber-stoppered (Dry Powder), in singles (10 per carton) (NDC 0002-1452-01). *The vials should be stored in a refrigerator (2° to 8°C, or 36° to 46°F) to assure extended stability.*

[032682]

ZENTINIC® OTC
(multifactor hematinic with vitamins)

Description: Zentinic is a multifactor hematinic-vitamin formula.

Each Pulvule® contains—
Iron, Elemental
(as Ferrous Fumarate) ....100 mg
Folic Acid ....0.05 mg
Thiamine Mononitrate
(Vitamin B_1) ....7.5 mg
Riboflavin (Vitamin B_2) ....7.5 mg
Pyridoxine Hydrochloride
(Vitamin B_6) ....7.5 mg
Vitamin B_{12} (Activity Equivalent) ....50 mcg
Pantothenic Acid
(as Calcium Pantothenate) ....15 mg
Niacinamide ....30 mg
Ascorbic Acid (Vitamin C) ....200 mg

Indications: For the prevention of iron-deficiency anemia and certain nutritional anemias and vitamin deficiencies of the B complex.

Contraindications: Hemochromatosis and hemosiderosis are contraindications to iron therapy.

Precautions: Anemia is a manifestation that requires appropriate investigation to determine its cause. The ingredients in Zentinic are not sufficient nor are they intended for the treatment of pernicious anemia. The use of folic acid without adequate vitamin B_{12} therapy in patients with pernicious anemia may result in hematologic remission but neurologic progression. Adequate doses of vitamin B_{12} usually prevent, halt, or improve the neurologic changes.

Adverse Reactions: Iron in therapeutic doses may occasionally cause gastrointestinal disturbances, such as nausea, vomiting, diarrhea, or constipation.

Dosage: 1 or 2 Pulvules a day, or as directed by the physician.

Overdosage: *Symptoms*—Those of iron intoxication, which may include pallor and cyanosis, vomiting, hematemesis, diarrhea, melena, shock, drowsiness, and coma. *Treatment*—For specific therapy, exchange transfusion and chelating agents. For general management, gastric and rectal lavage with sodium bicarbonate solution or milk, administration of intravenous fluids and electrolytes, and use of oxygen.

How Supplied: *Pulvules No. 4, Zentinic® (multifactor hematinic with vitamins, Lilly), F03** (No. 0, Dark-Red), in bottles of 60 (NDC 0002-0719-60) and 500 (NDC 0002-0719-03).

[090182]

ZENTRON® OTC
and
ZENTRON® CHEWABLE
(iron, vitamin B complex, and vitamin C)

Description: Zentron is a liquid hematinic especially formulated for geriatric and pediatric patients. Zentron restores hemoglobin in patients with iron-deficiency anemia. It provides iron with B complex vitamins and vitamin C. A bright-yellow liquid with a wild-strawberry flavor, Zentron is readily accepted whether administered by spoon or mixed with formula, water, or fruit juice.

Each 5 ml (approximately one teaspoonful) of the liquid contain—
Iron, Elemental
(as Ferrous Sulfate) ....20 mg
Thiamine Hydrochloride
(Vitamin B_1) ....1 mg
Riboflavin (Vitamin B_2) ....1 mg
Pyridoxine Hydrochloride
(Vitamin B_6) ....1 mg
Cyanocobalamin (Vitamin B_{12}
Crystalline) ....5 mcg
Pantothenic Acid (as *d*-Panthenol) .... 1 mg
Niacinamide ....5 mg
Ascorbic Acid (Vitamin C) ....100 mg
Alcohol, 2 percent.

Zentron Chewable is a hematinic in chewable tablet form, especially formulated for pediatric patients. Zentron Chewable restores hemoglobin in patients with iron-deficiency anemia. It provides iron with B complex vitamins and vitamin C. A strawberry-flavored tablet, Zentron Chewable may be chewed, dissolved in the mouth, taken with liquid, or swallowed alone.

Each tablet contains—
Iron, Elemental
(as Ferrous Fumarate) ....20 mg
Thiamine Mononitrate
(Vitamin B_1) ....1 mg
Riboflavin (Vitamin B_2) ....1 mg
Pyridoxine Hydrochloride
(Vitamin B_6) ....1 mg
Cyanocobalamin (Vitamin B_{12}
Crystalline) ....5 mcg
Pantothenic Acid (as Panthenol) ....1 mg
Niacinamide ....5 mg
Ascorbic Acid (Vitamin C) ....100 mg

Indications: For the prevention and treatment of iron-deficiency anemia and the prevention of vitamin B complex and vitamin C deficiencies. Liquid Zentron is equally useful for pediatric and geriatric patients who may prefer liquid medication.

Contraindications: Hemochromatosis and hemosiderosis are contraindications to iron therapy.

Precaution: Like all medications, Zentron and Zentron Chewable should be kept out of the reach of children.

Adverse Reactions: Iron in therapeutic doses may occasionally cause gastrointestinal disturbances, such as nausea, vomiting, diarrhea, or constipation.

Dosage: *Zentron*—Infants and children, ½ to 1 teaspoonful one to three times daily, or as directed by the physician. Adults, 1 or 2 teaspoonfuls three times daily, or as directed by the physician.

Zentron Chewable—Children two years and older, 1 tablet one to three times a day, or as directed by the physician. Adults, 1 or 2 tablets three times a day, or as directed by the physician.

Overdosage: *See under* Zentinic®.

How Supplied: *Liquid No. 34, Zentron® (iron, vitamin B complex, and vitamin C, Lilly),* in 8-fl-oz bottles (NDC 0002-2466-88).

*Tablets No. 14, Zentron Chewable, T01,** Pink, in bottles of 50 (NDC 0002-2001-50).

[090182]

ZINC-INSULIN CRYSTALS, *see under* Iletin® (insulin, Lilly).

Products are cross-indexed by

generic and chemical names

in the

YELLOW SECTION

Macsil, Inc.
1326 FRANKFORD AVENUE
PHILADELPHIA, PA 19125

BALMEX® BABY POWDER
(See PDR For Nonprescription Drugs)

BALMEX® EMOLLIENT LOTION
(See PDR For Nonprescription Drugs)

BALMEX® OINTMENT
(See PDR For Nonprescription Drugs)

Mallard Incorporated
3021 WABASH AVE.
DETROIT, MI 48216

ALLERSONE OINTMENT ℞

Composition:
Representing:
Hydrocortisone 0.5%
Diperodon Hydrochloride 0.5%
Zinc Oxide 5.0%

Indications: Antiinflammatory, antipruritic and antiallergic, in the treatment of atopic dermatitis, dermatitis venenata or contact dermatitis, pruritus ani and vulvae, certain allergic skin diseases, eczemata, as infantile and chronic eczema of ear, neurodermatitides, intertrigo as chafing of opposing skin of thighs, axilla and below breasts. When used rectally, it helps to relieve discomfort due to uncomplicated hemmorrhoids as well as itching or pain associated with proctitis and pruritis ani.

Action: Hydrocortisone exhibits marked antiinflammatory activity and is of benefit in pruritic, allergic and atopic dermatitis. Diperodon Hydrochloride is a local anesthetic with little or negligible incidence of sensitivity. Zinc Oxide is well known for its mild astringent and protective actions.

Dosage and Administration: Distribute a small amount by gentle application over the affected area two or three times a day; frequency of application to be reduced with improvement.

Contraindications: Do not apply in the presence of herpes simplex of the eye or skin tuberculosis; in case there is a coexisting bacterial infection an antibacterial should be used concurrently.

Precautions: In rare instances local sensitivity reactions might occur. The safety of the use of topical steroid preparations during pregnancy has not been fully established. Therefore, they should not be used extensively on pregnant patients, in large amounts or for prolonged periods of time.

Advantages: Contains a local anesthetic which quickly ameliorates pain—while hydrocortisone reduces inflammation.

Caution: Federal law prohibits dispensing without prescription.

How Supplied: 0-90 Allersone, ointment in 15 gm. tubes and in pound jars.

Literature Available: Yes.

Products are cross-indexed
by product classifications
in the
BLUE SECTION

A. G. Marin Pharmaceuticals
POST OFFICE BOX 174
MIAMI, FL 33144

CODEGESIC Tablets Ⓒ
Analgesic

Description: Each tablet contains:
Codeine Phosphate .... 1 mg.
(Warning: May be habit forming)
Acetominophen .... 97.2 mg.
Aspirin .... 226.8 mg.
Salicylamide .... 32.4 mg.
Caffeine .... 32.4 mg.

How Supplied: Bottle of 24 tablets (NDC 12539-133-01).

COLIDROPS Pediatric Drops ℞
Antispasmodic-Sedative

Description: Each 1 ml. (30 drops) contains:
Phenobarbital .... 3.24 mg.
(Warning: May be habit forming)
Atropine Sulfate .... 0.00388 mg.
Hyoscyamine Sulfate .... 0.02074 mg.
Hyoscyne Hydrobromide .... 0.00130 mg.
Alcohol 23%

How Supplied: Bottle of 30 ml. with dropper (NDC 12539-115-01).

DRANOCHOL Tablets ℞
Hydrocholeretic and Antispasmodic

Description: Each tablet contains:
Dehydrocholic Acid .... 200 mg.
Homatropine Methylbromide .... 5 mg.

How Supplied: Bottle of 60 tablets (NDC 12539-101-01).

INTESTINEX Capsules OTC

Description: Each capsule contains: 50 million living Lactobacilli Acidophilus and Bulgaricus in a freeze-dried condition with goat milk.

How Supplied: Bottle of 24 capsules (NDC 12539–107–02).

MarEPA Capsules OTC

Description:
Marine Lipid Concentrate
Eicosapentaenoic Acid (EPA) .... 180 mg.
Docosahexaenoic Acid (DHA) .... 120 mg.
Total OMEGA—3 Fatty Acids ... 300 mg.

How Supplied: Bottle of 60 capsules (NDC 12539–300–01).

ORLENTA Capsules ℞
Decongestant plus Antihistamine

Description: Each timed action capsule contains:
Chlorpheniramine Maleate .... 8 mg.
d-Pseudoephedrine HCl .... 120 mg.

How Supplied: Bottle of 100 capsules (NDC 12539-108-01).

OTOCIDIN Otic Drops ℞

Description: Each ml. contains:
Neomycin Sulfate .... 5 mg.
Polymyxin B Sulfate .... 10,000 u.
Hydrocortisone (1%) .... 10 mg.

How Supplied: Bottle of 10 ml. of sterile solution (NDC 12539-140-01).

OTOMYCET-HC Otic Solution ℞

Description:
Hydrocortisone 1%
Acetic Acid-nonaqueous 2%

How Supplied: 10 ml. Measured-drop, safety tip plastic bottle (NDC 12539-01-125).

SIDEROL Syrup ℞

Description: A delicious, non-alcoholic Nutritional Supplement with chelated Iron, Vitamin B complex, Lipotropic factors, Folic Acid, essential Amino Acids, Trace Minerals.

How Supplied: Bottle of 8 fluid oz. (NDC 12539-013-01).

SOLU-PHYLLIN Liquid ℞

Description:
Theophylline anhydrous USP
150 mg/tablespoonful (15 ml.)
50 mg/teaspoonful (5 ml.)
10 mg/ml

How Supplied: Bottle of 8 fluid oz. (NDC 12539-017-03).

SUPPORT Liquid OTC

Description: Vitamin/Mineral Supplement with Zinc, Maganese, Magnesium, Vitamin B-12, B-Complex, and L-Lysine.

How Supplied: Bottle of 8 fluid oz. (NDC 12539–023–01).

SUPPORT-500 Capsules ℞

Description: Special Vitamin-Mineral formulation with therapeutic supplementation of Zinc, Vitamin A, B-complex 500 mg. of Vitamin C plus Vitamins D, E, Manganese and Magnesium.

How Supplied: Bottle of 60 capsules (NDC 12539-011-01).

TOLERASE Tablets ℞

Description: Each tablet contains:
Outer coating:
Pepsin .... 150 mg.
Enteric coated:
Pancreatic Enzyme .... 100 mg.
Ox bile extract .... 100 mg.
Cellulase .... 10 mg.

How Supplied: Bottle of 100 tablets (NDC 12539-103-01).

UTRETRON D/S Tablets ℞
Double strength Urinary antiseptic and antispasmodic

Description: Each tablet contains:
Atropine Sulfate .... 0.06 mg.
Hyoscyamine .... 0.03 mg.
Methenamine .... 120 mg.
Phenyl Salicylate .... 30 mg.
Benzoic Acid .... 7.5 mg.
Methylene Blue .... 6 mg.

How Supplied: Bottle of 100 tablets (NDC 12539-122-01).

VIGOREX Capsules ℞

Description: Each capsule contains:
Methyltestosterone .... 10 mg.
How Supplied: Bottle of 100 white and blue, hard-gelatine capsules (NDC 12539-106-01).

VIGOREX Injection ℞
Sterile Solution
For Intramuscular Use

Description:
Testosterone Cypionate ....200 mg./1 ml.

How Supplied: Vial of 1 ml. sterile solution (NDC 12539-127-01).

Products are
listed alphabetically
in the
PINK SECTION.

Marion Laboratories, Inc.

Pharmaceutical Products Division
MARION INDUSTRIAL PARK
10236 BUNKER RIDGE ROAD
KANSAS CITY, MO 64137

PRODUCT IDENTIFICATION NUMERICAL SUMMARY SOLID ORAL DOSAGE FORMS

Marion Laboratories, Inc.
Kansas City, MO 64137

To provide quick and positive identification of Marion Laboratories prescription drug products, we have imprinted an identifying number and the name MARION on the following tablets or capsules.

1350 TRITEN® Tablets, 2.5 mg (dimethindene maleate)
1375 DITROPAN® Tablets (oxybutynin chloride)
1525 DUOTRATE® Capsules, 30 mg (pentaerythritol tetranitrate)
1530 DUOTRATE® Capsules, 45 mg (pentaerythritol tetranitrate)
1550 NITRO-BID® Capsules, 2.5 mg (nitroglycerin)
1551 NITRO-BID® Capsules, 6.5 mg (nitroglycerin)
1553 NITRO-BID® Capsules, 9 mg (nitroglycerin)
1555 PAVABID® Capsules, 150 mg (papaverine hydrochloride)*
1712 CARAFATE® Tablets, 1 gm (sucralfate)

PAVABID® HP Capsulets, 300 mg (papaverine hydrochloride) is identified by the name MARION on one side and PAVABID HP on the reverse side.

* PAVABID Capsules, 150 mg (papaverine hydrochloride) also bears the brand name PAVABID.

Marion THYROID and THYROID STRONG Tablets bear the following identification numbers.

ML 626 THYROID STRONG Tablets (Coated), ½ grain
ML 627 THYROID STRONG Tablets (Coated), 1 grain
ML 628 THYROID STRONG Tablets (Coated), 2 grain
ML 629 THYROID STRONG Tablets (Coated), 3 grain
ML 674 THYROID STRONG Tablets (Plain), 1 grain
ML 675 THYROID STRONG Tablets (Plain), 2 grain
ML 686 THYROID STRONG Tablets (Plain), ½ grain
ML 775 THYROID Tablets, USP (Plain), 15 mg
ML 776 THYROID Tablets, USP (Plain), 30 mg
ML 777 THYROID Tablets, USP (Plain), 60 mg
ML 778 THYROID Tablets, USP (Plain), 125 mg

AMBENYL® EXPECTORANT ℭ ℞

Each 5 ml contains:

Codeine sulfate (Warning—May be habit-forming)	10 mg
Bromodiphenhydramine hydrochloride	3.75 mg
Diphenhydramine hydrochloride	8.75 mg
Ammonium chloride	80 mg
Potassium guaiacolsulfonate	80 mg
Menthol	0.5 mg
Alcohol, 5%	

Action: Ambenyl is a combination of two antihistaminic agents, along with well-recognized agents exhibiting expectorant and antitussive properties.

Diphenhydramine hydrochloride, in addition to being a potent antihistaminic agent, also possesses an antitussive action.

Indications: Ambenyl is indicated as an antitussive and expectorant for control of cough due to colds or allergy.
Based on a review of this drug by the National Academy of Sciences—National Research Council and/or other information, FDA has classified this indication as follows: There is a lack of substantial evidence that this fixed combination drug has the effect purported.
Final classification of the less-than-effective indication requires further investigation.

Contraindications: This preparation should not be used in premature or newborn infants.
Do not use in patients with:
Hypersensitivity to any of the components;
Asthmatic attack;
Narrow-angle glaucoma;
Prostatic hypertrophy;
Stenosing peptic ulcer;
Pyloroduodenal obstruction;
Bladder-neck obstruction.

Preparations containing bromodiphenhydramine hydrochloride and diphenhydramine hydrochloride should not be given to patients receiving monoamine oxidase inhibitors.

Warnings: Overdosage or accidental ingestion of large quantities of antihistamines may produce convulsions or death, especially in infants and children.

As in the case of other preparations containing central nervous system depressant drugs, patients receiving Ambenyl should be cautioned about probable additive effects with alcohol and other central nervous system depressants (hypnotics, sedatives, and tranquilizers).

Serious toxicity, including central nervous system and respiratory depression, and rarely death, have been reported in pediatric patients receiving overdosages of codeine, either alone or in combination with other CNS depressants.

Patients who become drowsy on antihistamine-containing preparations should be cautioned against engaging in activities requiring mental alertness, such as driving a car or operating heavy machinery or appliances, when taking Ambenyl.

Pregnancy Warning: Although there is no evidence that the use of Ambenyl is detrimental to the mother or fetus, the use of any drug in pregnancy or lactation should be carefully assessed.

Because of the anticholinergic effect of diphenhydramine hydrochloride, an inhibitory effect on lactation may occur.

Precautions: Bromodiphenhydramine and diphenhydramine have an atropine-like action which should be considered when prescribing Ambenyl. Use with caution in patients with a history of asthma.

Adverse Reactions: The following side effects may occur in patients taking Ambenyl: drowsiness; confusion; nervousness; restlessness; nausea; vomiting; diarrhea; blurring of vision; diplopia; difficulty in urination; constipation; nasal stuffiness; vertigo; palpitation; headache; insomnia; urticaria; drug rash; photosensitivity; hemolytic anemia; hypotension; epigastric distress; tightness of the chest and wheezing; thickening of bronchial secretions; dryness of mouth, nose, and throat; tingling, heaviness, weakness of hands.

Dosage and Administration: Adults—One or two teaspoonsful every four to six hours, not to exceed 12 teaspoonsful in 24 hours. Children (total intake of codeine sulfate should not exceed 1 mg/kg/24 hours)—Six to under 12 years of age—one-half to one teaspoonful every six hours; Two to under 6 years of age—one-quarter to one-half teaspoonful every six hours.

Not to be used in children under two years of age.

How Supplied: Ambenyl Expectorant is supplied in 4-fl-oz, 1-pt, and 1-gal bottles.

AMBENYL®-D OTC

Decongestant Cough Formula

Antitussive-Expectorant-Nasal Decongestant

Two teaspoonsful (10 ml) contain the following active ingredients:

Guaifenesin (glyceryl guaiacolate)	200 mg
Pseudoephedrine hydrochloride	60 mg
Dextromethorphan hydrobromide	30 mg

Also contains 9.5% alcohol.

Indications: AMBENYL®-D is for temporary relief of nasal congestion due to the common cold or associated with sinusitis, helps loosen phlegm, calms cough impulses without narcotics, and temporarily helps you cough less.

Directions for Use: Adult Dose (12 years and over)—Two teaspoonsful every six hours. Child Dose (6–12 years)—One teaspoonful every six hours. (2–6 years)—One-half teaspoonful every six hours.
No more than four doses per day.

Warnings: Do not give this product to children under two years except under the advice and supervision of a physician. Do not take this product for persistent or chronic cough such as occurs with smoking, asthma, or emphysema, or where cough is accompanied by excessive secretions except under the advice and supervision of a physician.

Do not exceed recommended dosage because at higher doses nervousness, dizziness, or sleeplessness may occur.

Caution: A persistent cough may be a sign of a serious condition. If cough persists for more than one week, tends to recur, or is accompanied by high fever, rash, or persistent headache, consult a physician.

If symptoms do not improve within seven days or are accompanied by high fever, consult a physician before continuing use. Do not take this product if you have high blood pressure, heart disease, diabetes, or thyroid disease, except under the advice and supervision of a physician.

If pregnant or nursing a baby, consult your physician or pharmacist before using this product.

Drug Interaction Precaution: Do not take this product if you are presently taking a prescription antihypertensive or antidepressant drug containing a monoamine oxidase inhibitor except under the advice and supervision of a physician.

Store at a controlled room temperature (59°–86°F).

Keep this and all drugs out of reach of children.

In case of accidental overdose, seek professional assistance or contact a poison control center immediately.

How Supplied: Ambenyl-D Decongestant Cough Formula is supplied in a 4-fl-oz bottle.

CARAFATE® Tablets ℞

(sucralfate) 1 gm

Description: CARAFATE® (sucralfate) is a complex of sulfated sucrose and aluminum hydroxide. The chemical name is beta-D-Fructofuranosyl-alpha-D-glucopyranoside octakis (hydrogen sulfate) aluminum hydroxide complex.

Tablets for oral administration contain 1 gm of sucralfate.

Therapeutic category: antiulcer

Clinical Pharmacology: Sucralfate is only minimally absorbed from the gastrointestinal tract. The small amounts of the sulfated disac-

Continued on next page

Marion—Cont.

charide that are absorbed are excreted primarily in the urine.

Although the mechanism of sucralfate's ability to accelerate healing of duodenal ulcers remains to be fully defined, it is known that it exerts its effect through a local, rather than systemic, action. The following observations also appear pertinent:

1. Studies in human subjects and with animal models of ulcer disease have shown that sucralfate forms an ulcer-adherent complex with proteinaceous exudate at the ulcer site.
2. *In vitro*, a sucralfate-albumin film provides a barrier to diffusion of hydrogen ions.
3. In human subjects, sucralfate given in doses recommended for ulcer therapy inhibits pepsin activity in gastric juice by 32%.
4. *In vitro*, sucralfate adsorbs bile salts.

These observations suggest that sucralfate's antiulcer activity is the result of formation of an ulcer-adherent complex that covers the ulcer site and protects it against further attack by acid, pepsin, and bile salts. Sucralfate has negligible acid-neutralizing capacity and its antiulcer effects cannot be attributed to neutralization of gastric acid.

Clinical Trials: Over 600 patients have participated in well-controlled clinical trials worldwide. Multicenter trials conducted in the United States, both of them placebo-controlled studies with endoscopic evaluation at 2 and 4 weeks, showed:

[See table below].

The sucralfate-placebo differences were statistically significant in both studies at 4 weeks but not at 2 weeks. The poorer result in the first study may have occurred because sucralfate was given two hours after meals and at bedtime rather than one hour before meals and at bedtime, the regimen used in international studies and in the second United States study. In addition, in the first study liquid antacid was utilized as needed, whereas in the second study antacid tablets were used.

Indications and Usage: CARAFATE (sucralfate) is indicated in the short-term (up to eight weeks) treatment of duodenal ulcer.

Antacids may be prescribed as needed for relief of pain.

Contraindications: There are no known contraindications to the use of sucralfate.

Precautions: Duodenal ulcer is a chronic recurrent disease. While short-term treatment with sucralfate can result in complete healing of the ulcer, a successful course of treatment with sucralfate should not be expected to alter the post-healing frequency or severity of duodenal ulceration.

Carcinogenesis, mutagenesis, impairment of fertility: Chronic oral toxicity studies of 24 months' duration were conducted in mice and rats at doses up to 1 gm/kg (12 times the human dose). There was no evidence of drug-related tumorigenicity. A reproduction study in rats at doses up to 38 times the human dose did not reveal any indication of fertility impairment. Mutagenicity studies were not conducted.

Pregnancy: Teratogenic effects. Pregnancy Category B. Teratogenicity studies have been performed in mice, rats, and rabbits at doses up to 50 times the human dose and have revealed no evidence of harm to the fetus due to sucralfate. There are, however, no adequate and well-controlled studies in pregnant women. Because animal reproduction studies are not always predictive of human response, this drug should be used during pregnancy only if clearly needed.

Nursing Mothers: It is not known whether this drug is excreted in human milk. Because many drugs are excreted in human milk, caution should be exercised when sucralfate is administered to a nursing woman.

Pediatric Use: Safety and effectiveness in children have not been established.

Adverse Reactions: Adverse reactions to sucralfate in clinical trials were minor and only rarely led to discontinuation of the drug. In studies involving over 2,500 patients treated with sucralfate, adverse effects were reported in 121 (4.7%).

Constipation was the most frequent complaint (2.2%). Other adverse effects, reported in no more than 1 of every 350 patients, were diarrhea, nausea, gastric discomfort, indigestion, dry mouth, rash, pruritus, back pain, dizziness, sleepiness, and vertigo.

Overdosage: There is no experience in humans with overdosage. Acute oral toxicity studies in animals, however, using doses up to 12 gm/kg body weight, could not find a lethal dose. Risks associated with overdosage should, therefore, be minimal.

Dosage and Administration: The recommended adult oral dosage for duodenal ulcer is 1 gm four times a day on an empty stomach (1 hour before each meal and at bedtime).

Antacids may be prescribed as needed for relief of pain but should not be taken within ½ hour before or after sucralfate.

While healing with sucralfate may occur during the first week or two, treatment should be continued for 4 to 8 weeks unless healing has been demonstrated by x-ray or endoscopic examination.

How Supplied: CARAFATE (sucralfate) 1-gm tablets are supplied in bottles of 100 (NDC 0088-1712-47) and in Unit Dose Identification Paks of 100 (NDC 0088-1712-49). Light pink, 1-gm tablets are embossed with Marion/1712.

Issued 10/82

[*Shown in Product Identification Section*]

CARDIZEM™ Tablets ℞
(diltiazem HCl)
30 mg and 60 mg

Description: CARDIZEM™ (diltiazem hydrochloride) is a calcium ion influx inhibitor (slow channel blocker or calcium antagonist). Chemically, diltiazem hydrochloride is 1, 5-Benzothiazepin-4(5H)one, 3-(acetyloxy)-5-[2-(dimethylamino)ethyl]-2, 3-dihydro-2-(4-methoxyphenyl)-,monohydrochloride,(+) -cis-.

Diltiazem hydrochloride is a white to off-white crystalline powder with a bitter taste. It is soluble in water, methanol, and chloroform. It has a molecular weight of 450.98. Each tablet of CARDIZEM contains either 30 mg or 60 mg diltiazem for oral administration.

Clinical Pharmacology: The therapeutic benefits achieved with CARDIZEM are believed to be related to its ability to inhibit the influx of calcium ions during membrane depolarization of cardiac and vascular smooth muscle.

Mechanism of Action. Although precise mechanisms of its antianginal actions are still being delineated, CARDIZEM is believed to act in the following ways:

1. Angina Due to Coronary Artery Spasm: CARDIZEM has been shown to be a potent dilator of coronary arteries both epicardial and subendocardial. Spontaneous and ergonovine-induced coronary artery spasm are inhibited by CARDIZEM.
2. Exertional Angina: CARDIZEM has been shown to produce increases in exercise tolerance probably due to its ability to reduce myocardial oxygen demand. This is accomplished via reductions in heart rate and systemic blood pressure at submaximal and maximal exercise work loads.

In animal models, diltiazem interferes with the slow inward (depolarizing) current in excitable tissue. It causes excitation-contraction uncoupling in various myocardial tissues without changes in the configuration of the action potential. Diltiazem produces relaxation of coronary vascular smooth muscle and dilation of both large and small coronary arteries at drug levels which cause little or no negative inotropic effect. The resultant increases in coronary blood flow (epicardial and subendocardial) occur in ischemic and nonischemic models and are accompanied by dose-dependent decreases in systemic blood pressure and decreases in peripheral resistance.

Hemodynamic and Electrophysiologic Effects. Like other calcium antagonists, diltiazem decreases sinoatrial and atrioventricular conduction in isolated tissues and has a negative inotropic effect in isolated preparations. In the intact animal, prolongation of the AH interval can be seen at higher doses.

In man, diltiazem prevents spontaneous and ergonovine-provoked coronary artery spasm. It causes a decrease in peripheral vascular resistance and a modest fall in blood pressure and, in exercise tolerance studies in patients with ischemic heart disease, reduces the heart rate/blood pressure product for any given work load. Studies to date, primarily in patients with good ventricular function, have not revealed evidence of a negative inotropic effect; cardiac output, ejection fraction, and left ventricular end diastolic pressure have not been affected. There are as yet few data on the interaction of diltiazem and beta-blockers. Resting heart rate is usually unchanged or slightly reduced by diltiazem.

Intravenous diltiazem in doses of 20 mg prolongs AH conduction time and AV node functional and effective refractory periods approximately 20%. In a study involving single oral doses of 300 mg of CARDIZEM in six normal volunteers, the average maximum PR prolongation was 14% with no instances of greater than first-degree AV block. Diltiazem-associated prolongation of the AH interval is not more pronounced in patients with first-degree heart block. In patients with sick sinus syndrome, diltiazem significantly prolongs sinus cycle length (up to 50% in some cases).

Chronic oral administration of CARDIZEM in doses of up to 240 mg/day has resulted in small increases in PR interval, but has not usually produced abnormal prolongation. There were, however, three instances of second-degree AV block and one instance of third-degree AV block in a group of 959 chronically treated patients.

Pharmacokinetics and Metabolism. Diltiazem is absorbed from the tablet formulation to about 80% of a reference capsule and is subject to an extensive first-pass effect, giving an absolute bioavailability (compared to intravenous dosing) of about 40%. CARDIZEM undergoes extensive hepatic metabolism in which 2% to 4% of the unchanged drug appears in the urine. In vitro binding studies show CARDIZEM is 70% to 80% bound to plasma proteins. Competitive ligand binding studies have also shown CARDIZEM binding is not altered by therapeutic concentrations of digoxin, hydrochlorothiazide, phenylbutazone, propranolol, salicylic acid, or warfarin. Single oral doses of 30 to 120 mg of CARDIZEM result

	Treatment Groups	Ulcer Healing/No. Patients	
		2 wk.	**4 wk. (Overall)**
Study 1	Sucralfate	37/105 (35.2%)	82/109 (75.2%)
	Placebo	26/106 (24.5%)	68/107 (63.6%)
		2 wk.	**4 wk. (Overall)**
Study 2	Sucralfate	8/24 (33%)	22/24 (92%)
	Placebo	4/31 (13%)	18/31 (58%)

in detectable plasma levels within 30 to 60 minutes and peak plasma levels 2 to 3 hours after drug administration. The plasma elimination half-life following single or multiple drug administration is approximately 3.5 hours. Desacetyl diltiazem is also present in the plasma at levels of 10% to 20% of the parent drug and is 25% to 50% as potent as a coronary vasodilator as diltiazem. Therapeutic blood levels of CARDIZEM appear to be in the range of 50 to 200 ng/ml. There is a departure from dose-linearity when single doses above 60 mg are given; a 120-mg dose gave blood levels three times that of the 60-mg dose. There is no information about the effect of renal or hepatic impairment on excretion or metabolism of diltiazem.

Indications and Usage:

1. **Angina Pectoris Due to Coronary Artery Spasm.** CARDIZEM is indicated in the treatment of angina pectoris due to coronary artery spasm. CARDIZEM has been shown effective in the treatment of spontaneous coronary artery spasm presenting as Prinzmetal's variant angina (resting angina with ST-segment elevation occurring during attacks).
2. **Chronic Stable Angina (Classic Effort-Associated Angina).** CARDIZEM is indicated in the management of chronic stable angina in patients who cannot tolerate therapy with beta-blockers and/or nitrates or who remain symptomatic despite adequate doses of these agents. CARDIZEM has been effective in short-term controlled trials in reducing angina frequency and increasing exercise tolerance, but confirmation of sustained effectiveness is incomplete.

There are no controlled studies of the effectiveness of the concomitant use of diltiazem and beta-blockers or of the safety of this combination in patients with impaired ventricular function or conduction abnormalities.

Contraindications: CARDIZEM is contraindicated in 1) patients with sick sinus syndrome except in the presence of a functioning ventricular pacemaker, 2) patients with second- or third-degree AV block, and 3) patients with hypotension (less than 90 mm Hg systolic).

Warnings:

1. **Cardiac Conduction.** CARDIZEM prolongs AV node refractory periods without significantly prolonging sinus node recovery time, except in patients with sick sinus syndrome. This effect may rarely result in abnormally slow heart rates (particularly in patients with sick sinus syndrome) or second- or third-degree AV block (4 of 959 patients for 0.42%). Concomitant use of diltiazem with beta-blockers or digitalis may result in additive effects on cardiac conduction. A patient with Prinzmetal's angina developed periods of asystole (2 to 5 seconds) after a single dose of 60 mg diltiazem.
2. **Congestive Heart Failure.** Although diltiazem has a negative inotropic effect in isolated animal tissue preparations, hemodynamic studies in humans with normal ventricular function have not shown a reduction in cardiac index nor consistent negative effects on contractility (dp/dt). Experience with the use of CARDIZEM alone or in combination with beta-blockers in patients with impaired ventricular function is very limited. Caution should be exercised when using the drug in such patients.
3. **Hypotension.** Decreases in blood pressure associated with CARDIZEM therapy may occasionally result in symptomatic hypotension.
4. **Acute Hepatic Injury.** There has been a single report in a patient receiving 120 mg of diltiazem t.i.d. of marked transaminase elevation (SGOT 4500, SGPT 2300) accompanied by hyperbilirubinemia (to 3 mg%), occurring after four days of treatment. The enzyme abnormalities resolved entirely, and enzymes were nearly normal a week after cessation of treatment. No rechallenge was carried out, but the patient had no evidence of viral hepatitis and received no other drugs but isosorbide dinitrate.

No other similar liver injury has been reported in clinical trials, but marketing experience in Europe has resulted in a rechallenge-confirmed instance of hepatocellular injury. However, it should be noted that there have been further episodes of raised transaminases in the absence of diltiazem in this patient, so that the relationship to diltiazem of the abnormalities is not completely clear. Other instances of transaminase elevation have been reported in Europe, but their relationship to drug is uncertain.

Precautions:

General. CARDIZEM is extensively metabolized by the liver and excreted by the kidneys and in bile. As with any new drug given over prolonged periods, laboratory parameters should be monitored at regular intervals. The drug should be used with caution in patients with impaired renal or hepatic function. In subacute and chronic dog and rat studies designed to produce toxicity, high doses of diltiazem were associated with hepatic damage. In special subacute hepatic studies, oral doses of 125 mg/kg and higher in rats were associated with histological changes in the liver which were reversible when the drug was discontinued. In dogs, doses of 20 mg/kg were also associated with hepatic changes; however, these changes were reversible with continued dosing.

Drug Interaction. Pharmacologic studies indicate that there may be additive effects in prolonging AV conduction when using beta-blockers or digitalis concomitantly with CARDIZEM. (See WARNINGS.)

Uncontrolled domestic studies suggest that concomitant use of CARDIZEM and beta-blockers or digitalis is usually well tolerated. Available data are not sufficient, however, to predict the effects of concomitant treatment, particularly in patients with left ventricular dysfunction or cardiac conduction abnormalities; the effect of diltiazem on serum digoxin levels has not been examined. The safety of the combination of CARDIZEM and beta-blockers or digitalis is currently being investigated in well-controlled studies.

Carcinogenesis, Mutagenesis, Impairment of Fertility. A 24-month study in rats and a 21-month study in mice showed no evidence of carcinogenicity. There was also no mutagenic response in in vitro bacterial tests. No intrinsic effect on fertility was observed in rats.

Pregnancy. Category C. Reproduction studies have been conducted in mice, rats, and rabbits. Administration of doses ranging from 5 to 10 times greater (on a mg/kg basis) than the daily recommended therapeutic dose has resulted in embryo and fetal lethality. These doses, in some studies, have been reported to cause skeletal abnormalities. In the perinatal/postnatal studies, there was some reduction in early individual pup weights and survival rates. There was an increased incidence of stillbirths at doses of 20 times the human dose or greater. There are no well-controlled studies in pregnant women; therefore, use CARDIZEM in pregnant women only if the potential benefit justifies the potential risk to the fetus.

Nursing Mothers. It is not known whether this drug is excreted in human milk. Because many drugs are excreted in human milk, exercise caution when CARDIZEM is administered to a nursing woman if the drug's benefits are thought to outweigh its potential risks in this situation.

Pediatric Use. Safety and effectiveness in children have not been established.

Adverse Reactions: Serious adverse reactions have been rare in studies carried out to date, but it should be recognized that patients with impaired ventricular function and cardiac conduction abnormalities have usually been excluded. Experience with an added beta-blocker is also extremely limited.

In domestic placebo-controlled trials, the incidence of adverse reactions reported during CARDIZEM therapy was not greater than that reported during placebo therapy.

In addition, the following have been reported infrequently and represent occurrences which can be at least reasonably associated with the pharmacology of calcium influx inhibition. In many cases, the relationship to CARDIZEM has not been established. The most common occurrences, as well as their frequency of presentation, are nausea (2.7%), swelling/edema (2.4%), arrhythmia (2.0%), headache (2.0%), rash (1.8%), and fatigue (1.1%). In addition, the following events were reported infrequently (< 1.0%). The order of presentation corresponds to the relative frequency of occurrence.

Cardiovascular: Flushing, congestive heart failure, bradycardia, hypotension, syncope, pounding heart.

Central Nervous System: Drowsiness, dizziness, lightheadedness, nervousness, depression, weakness, insomnia, confusion, hallucinations.

Gastrointestinal: Vomiting, diarrhea, gastric upset, constipation, indigestion, pyrosis.

Dermatologic: Pruritus, petechiae, urticaria.

Other: Photosensitivity, nocturia, thirst, paresthesias, polyuria, osteoarticular pain.

The following additional experiences have been noted:

A patient with Prinzmetal's angina experiencing episodes of vasospastic angina developed periods of transient asymptomatic asystole approximately five hours after receiving a single 60-mg dose of CARDIZEM.

Experience in 959 patients taking oral doses of CARDIZEM resulted in three cases (0.31%) of second-degree AV block and one case (0.10%) of third-degree AV block at doses of 240 to 360 mg daily.

In rare instances, mild to moderate transient elevations of alkaline phosphatase, SGOT, SGPT, LDH, and CPK have been noted during CARDIZEM therapy. A single incident of markedly elevated liver enzymes associated with symptoms was reported in a patient taking 360 mg per day for four days. Drug was discontinued and enzymes normalized within 1 week.

Overdosage or Exaggerated Response: Overdosage experiences with oral diltiazem have not been reported. Single oral doses of 300 mg of CARDIZEM have been well tolerated by healthy volunteers. In the event of overdosage or exaggerated response, appropriate supportive measures should be employed in addition to gastric lavage. The following measures may be considered:

Bradycardia: Administer atropine (0.60 to 1.0 mg). If there is no response to vagal blockade, administer isoproterenol cautiously.

High-Degree AV Block: Treat as for bradycardia above. Fixed high-degree AV block should be treated with cardiac pacing.

Cardiac Failure: Administer inotropic agents (isoproterenol, dopamine, or dobutamine) and diuretics.

Hypotension: Vasopressors (eg, dopamine or levarterenol bitartrate).

Actual treatment and dosage should depend on the severity of the clinical situation and the judgment and experience of the treating physician.

The oral LD_{50}'s in mice and rats range from 415 to 740 mg/kg and from 560 to 810 mg/kg, respectively. The intravenous LD_{50}'s in these species were 60 and 38 mg/kg, respectively. The oral LD_{50} in dogs is considered to be in excess of 50 mg/kg, while lethality was seen in monkeys at 360 mg/kg. The toxic dose in man is not known, but blood levels in excess of 800 ng/ml have not been associated with toxicity.

Continued on next page

Marion—Cont.

Dosage and Administration: Exertional Angina Pectoris Due to Atherosclerotic Coronary Artery Disease or Angina Pectoris at Rest Due to Coronary Artery Spasm. Dosage must be adjusted to each patient's needs. Starting with 30 mg four times daily, before meals and at bedtime, dosage should be increased gradually to 240 mg (given in divided doses three or four times daily) at one- to two-day intervals until optimum response is obtained. The effectiveness and safety of dosages exceeding 240 mg per day are currently being investigated. There are no available data concerning dosage requirements in patients with impaired renal or hepatic function. If the drug must be used in such patients, titration should be carried out with particular caution.

Concomitant Use With Other Antianginal Agents.

1. **Sublingual NTG** may be taken as required to abort acute anginal attacks during CARDIZEM therapy.
2. **Prophylactic Nitrate Therapy**—CARDIZEM may be safely coadministered with short- and long-acting nitrates, but there have been no controlled studies to evaluate the antianginal effectiveness of this combination.
3. **Beta-blockers.** (See WARNINGS and PRECAUTIONS.)

How Supplied: CARDIZEM 30-mg tablets are supplied in bottles of 100 (NDC 0088-1771-47). Each green tablet is engraved with MARION on one side and 1771 engraved on the other. CARDIZEM 60-mg scored tablets are supplied in bottles of 100 (NDC 0088-1772-47). Each yellow tablet is engraved with MARION on one side and 1772 on the other.

Issued 11/82

DEBROX® Drops OTC

Description: Carbamide peroxide 6.5% in specially prepared anhydrous glycerol.

Actions: DEBROX® penetrates, softens and facilitates removal of earwax, without causing the wax to swell.

Upon direct contact with earwax, carbamide peroxide releases oxygen to form a dense foam which helps to break up wax accumulations. These actions result in a chemomechanical cleansing, debriding effect. Any remaining wax may be removed by flushing with warm water, using a soft rubber bulb ear syringe. Avoid excessive pressure.

Indications: DEBROX provides a safe, nonirritating method of removing earwax. Aids in the prevention of ceruminosis. Used regularly, DEBROX Drops helps keep the ear canal free from blockage due to accumulated earwax.

Caution: Consult physician if redness, irritation, swelling or pain persists or increases.

Dosage and Administration: Use directly from bottle. Tilt head sideways and squeeze bottle gently so that 5-10 drops flow into ear. Tip of bottle should not enter ear canal. Keep drops in ear for several minutes while head remains tilted or by inserting cotton. Repeat twice daily for at least 3-4 days or as directed by physician. Any remaining wax may be removed by flushing with warm water, using a soft rubber bulb ear syringe.

AVOID CONTACT WITH EYES. Keep this and all drugs out of the reach of children. In case of accidental ingestion, seek professional assistance or contact a poison control center immediately. Protect from heat and direct sunlight.

How Supplied: DEBROX Drops in ½- or 1-fl-oz plastic squeeze bottles with applicator spouts.

DITROPAN® Tablets and Syrup ℞
(oxybutynin chloride)

Description: Each scored biconvex, engraved blue DITROPAN® Tablet contains 5 mg of oxybutynin chloride. Each 5 ml of DITROPAN® Syrup contains 5 mg of oxybutynin chloride. Chemically, oxybutynin chloride is the *dl*-(racemic) form of 4-diethylamino-2-butynyl phenylcyclohexylglycolate hydrochloride. The empirical formula of oxybutynin chloride is $C_{22}H_{32}Cl\ NO_3$. The structural formula appears below:

$$C_6H_5-C(C_6H_{11})(OH)-C(=O)-O-CH_2-C\equiv C-CH_2-N(C_2H_5)_2 \cdot HCl$$

Oxybutynin chloride is a white crystalline solid with a molecular weight of 393.9. It is readily soluble in water and acids, but relatively insoluble in alkalis.

Action: DITROPAN® (oxybutynin chloride) exerts direct antispasmodic effect on smooth muscle and inhibits the muscarinic action of acetylcholine on smooth muscle. DITROPAN exhibits only one-fifth of the anticholinergic activity of atropine on the rabbit detrusor muscle, but four to ten times the antispasmodic activity. No blocking effects occur at skeletal neuromuscular junctions or autonomic ganglia (antinicotinic effects).

In patients with uninhibited neurogenic and reflex neurogenic bladder, cystometric studies have demonstrated that DITROPAN increases vesical capacity, diminishes the frequency of uninhibited contractions of the detrusor muscle and delays the initial desire to void. These effects are more consistently improved in patients with uninhibited neurogenic bladder.

DITROPAN was well tolerated in patients administered the drug in controlled studies of 30 days' duration and in uncontrolled studies in which some of the patients received the drug for two years.

Indications: DITROPAN® (oxybutynin chloride) is indicated for the relief of symptoms associated with voiding in patients with uninhibited neurogenic and reflex neurogenic bladder.

Pretreatment examination should include cystometry and other appropriate diagnostic procedures.

Cystometry should be repeated at appropriate intervals to evaluate response to therapy. The appropriate antimicrobial therapy should be instituted in the presence of infection.

Contraindications: DITROPAN® (oxybutynin chloride) is contraindicated in patients with glaucoma. It is also contraindicated in partial or complete obstruction of the gastrointestinal tract, paralytic ileus, intestinal atony of the elderly or debilitated patient, megacolon, toxic megacolon complicating ulcerative colitis, severe colitis and myasthenia gravis. It is contraindicated in patients with obstructive uropathy and in patients with unstable cardiovascular status in acute hemorrhage.

Warnings: DITROPAN® (oxybutynin chloride), when administered in the presence of high environmental temperature, can cause heat prostration (fever and heat stroke due to decreased sweating).

Diarrhea may be an early symptom of incomplete intestinal obstruction, especially in patients with ileostomy or colostomy. In this instance treatment with DITROPAN would be inappropriate and possibly harmful.

DITROPAN may produce drowsiness or blurred vision. The patient should be cautioned regarding activities requiring mental alertness such as operating a motor vehicle or other machinery or performing hazardous work while taking this drug.

PREGNANCY: Reproduction studies in the hamster, rabbit, rat and mouse have shown no definite evidence of impaired fertility or harm to the animal fetus. The safety of DITROPAN administered to women who are or who may become pregnant has not been established. Therefore, DITROPAN should not be given to pregnant women unless, in the judgment of the physician, the probable clinical benefits outweight the possible hazards.

USAGE IN CHILDREN: The safety and efficacy of DITROPAN administration have been demonstrated for children five years of age and older (see "Dosage and Administration"). However, as there is insufficient clinical data for children under age five, DITROPAN is not recommended for this age group.

Precautions: DITROPAN® (oxybutynin chloride) should be used with caution in the elderly and in all patients with autonomic neuropathy, hepatic or renal disease. Administration of DITROPAN in large doses to patients with ulcerative colitis may suppress intestinal motility to the point of producing a paralytic ileus and precipitate or aggravate toxic megacolon, a serious complication of the disease.

The symptoms of hyperthyroidism, coronary heart disease, congestive heart failure, cardiac arrhythmias, tachycardia, hypertension and prostatic hypertrophy may be aggravated following administration of DITROPAN. DITROPAN should be administered with caution to patients with hiatal hernia associated with reflux esophagitis, since anticholinergic drugs may aggravate this condition.

Adverse Reactions: Following administration of DITROPAN® (oxybutynin chloride), the symptoms that can be associated with the use of other anticholinergic drugs may occur: dry mouth, decreased sweating, urinary hesitance and retention, blurred vision, tachycardia, palpitations, dilatation of the pupil, cycloplegia, increased ocular tension, drowsiness, weakness, dizziness, insomnia, nausea, vomiting, constipation, bloated feeling, impotence, suppression of lactation, severe allergic reactions or drug idiosyncrasies including urticaria and other dermal manifestations.

Dosage and Administration: Tablets—

Adults: The usual dose is one 5-mg tablet two to three times a day. The maximum recommended dose is one 5-mg tablet four times a day.

Children over 5 years of age: The usual dose is one 5-mg tablet two times a day. The maximum recommended dose is one 5-mg tablet three times a day.

Syrup—Adults: The usual dose is one teaspoon (5 mg/5 ml) syrup two to three times a day. The maximum recommended dose is one teaspoon (5 mg/5 ml) syrup four times a day.

Children over 5 years of age: The usual dose is one teaspoon (5 mg/5 ml) two times a day. The maximum recommended dose is one teaspoon (5 mg/5 ml) three times a day.

Overdosage: The symptoms of overdosage with DITROPAN® (oxybutynin chloride) progress from an intensification of the usual side effects of CNS disturbance (from restlessness and excitement to psychotic behavior), circulatory changes (flushing, fall in blood pressure, circulatory failure), respiratory failure, paralysis and coma.

Measures to be taken are (1) immediate lavage of the stomach and (2) injection of physostigmine 0.5 to 2 mg intravenously, and repeated as necessary up to a total of 5 mg. Fever may be treated symptomatically (alcohol sponging, ice packs). Excitement of a degree which demands attention may be managed with sodium thiopental 2% solution given slowly intravenously or chloral hydrate (100–200 ml of a 2% solution) by rectal infusion. In the event of progression of the curare-like effect to paralysis of the respiratory muscles, artificial respiration is required.

How Supplied: DITROPAN® (oxybutynin chloride) tablets are supplied in bottles of 100 tablets (NDC 0088-1375-47) and 1,000 tablets (NDC 0088-1375-58) and in Unit Dose Identifi-

cation Paks of 100 tablets (NDC 0088-1375-49). Blue scored tablets are engraved with Marion on one side and 1375 on the other side.
[*Shown in Product Identification Section*]
DITROPAN® Syrup is supplied in bottles of 16 fluid ounces (473 ml) (NDC 0088-1373-18).
Pharmacist: Dispense in tight, light-resistant container as defined in the USP.
Store at controlled room temperature (59°–86°F).
U.S. Patent 3,176,019
Issued 10/82

DUOTRATE® and DUOTRATE® 45 ℞
Plateau CAPS®
(pentaerythritol tetranitrate)

Each sustained-release capsule contains:
DUOTRATE® (pentaerythritol tetranitrate) .... 30 mg
White pellets in a black and clear capsule imprinted with MARION/1525.
DUOTRATE® 45 (pentaerythritol tetranitrate) .... 45 mg
White pellets in a black and light blue capsule imprinted with MARION/1530.
DUOTRATE® and DUOTRATE® 45 (pentaerythritol tetranitrate) are 2,2-Bishydroxymethyl-1,3-propanediol tetranitrate.
Action: The mechanism of action in the relief of angina pectoris is unknown at this time, although the basic pharmacologic action is to relax smooth muscle. The effect of pentaerythritol tetranitrate is usually measured by its ability to reduce the frequency, duration and severity of anginal attacks and reduce the need for sublingual nitroglycerin.

Indications:
Based on a review of this drug by the National Academy of Sciences-National Research Council and/or other information, FDA has classified the indications as follows:
Possibly effective: For the management, prophylaxis, or treatment of anginal attacks.
Final classification of the less-than-effective indications requires further investigation.

Contraindication: Idiosyncrasy to this drug.
Warnings: Data supporting the use of DUOTRATE® and DUOTRATE® 45 (pentaerythritol tetranitrate) during the early days of the acute phase of myocardial infarction (the period during which clinical and laboratory findings are unstable) are insufficient to establish safety.
Precautions: Intraocular pressure is increased; therefore, caution is required in administering to patients with glaucoma. Tolerance to this drug and cross-tolerance to other nitrites and nitrates may occur.
Adverse Reactions: Cutaneous vasodilation with flushing. Headache is common and may be severe and persistent. Transient episodes of dizziness and weakness, as well as other signs of cerebral ischemia associated with postural hypotension, may occasionally develop. This drug can act as a physiological antagonist to norepinephrine, acetylcholine, histamine, and many other agents. An occasional individual exhibits marked sensitivity to the hypotensive effects of nitrite and severe responses (nausea, vomiting, weakness, restlessness, pallor, perspiration and collapse) can occur, even with the usual therapeutic dose. Alcohol may enhance this effect. Drug rash and/or exfoliative dermatitis may occasionally occur.
Dosage and Administration: One capsule every 12 hours on an empty stomach. One capsule should be taken with an adequate amount of water before breakfast, and a second capsule approximately 12 hours later on an empty stomach. When medication is started, there is a delay from one to two hours before a significant change in pain level occurs. The selection of DUOTRATE® should be based on the patient's need for approximately 30 mg of pentaerythritol tetranitrate during a 12-hour period. The selection of DUOTRATE® 45 should be based on the patient's need for approximately 45 mg of pentaerythritol tetranitrate during a 12-hour period. Use the smallest dose that proves effective.
How Supplied: Each of the products described is available in bottles of 100 capsules. DUOTRATE® Capsules are imprinted with MARION/1525. DUOTRATE® 45 Capsules are imprinted with MARION/1530.
Caution: Federal law prohibits dispensing without a prescription.
Mfd. by:
KV Pharmaceutical Co.
St. Louis, MO 63144
Dist. by:
Marion Laboratories, Inc.
Kansas City, MO 64137
[*Shown in Product Identification Section*]

GAVISCON® Antacid Tablets OTC

Composition: Each chewable tablet contains the following active ingredients:
Aluminum hydroxide dried gel .... 80 mg
Magnesium trisilicate .... 20 mg
and the following inactive ingredients: sucrose, alginic acid, sodium bicarbonate, starch, calcium stearate, and flavoring.
Actions: Unique formulation produces soothing foam which floats on stomach contents. Foam containing antacid precedes stomach contents into the esophagus when reflux occurs to help protect the sensitive mucosa from further irritation. GAVISCON acts locally without neutralizing entire stomach contents to help maintain integrity of the digestive process. Endoscopic studies indicate that GAVISCON Antacid Tablets are equally as effective in the erect or supine patient.
Indications: For temporary relief of heartburn, sour stomach, and/or acid indigestion.
Directions: Chew two to four tablets four times a day or as directed by a physician. Tablets should be taken after meals and at bedtime or as needed. For best results follow by a half glass of water or other liquid. DO NOT SWALLOW WHOLE.
Warnings: Except under the advice and supervision of a physician: Do not take more than 16 tablets in a 24-hour period or 16 tablets daily for more than 2 weeks; do not use this product if you are on a sodium-restricted diet. Each GAVISCON Tablet contains approximately 0.8 mEq sodium.
Drug Interaction Precautions: Do not take this product if you are presently taking a prescription antibiotic drug containing any form of tetracycline.
STORE AT A CONTROLLED ROOM TEMPERATURE IN A DRY PLACE.
KEEP THIS AND ALL DRUGS OUT OF THE REACH OF CHILDREN. In case of accidental overdose, seek professional assistance or contact a poison control center immediately.
How Supplied: Available in bottle of 100 tablets and in foil-wrapped 2's in box of 30 tablets.
[*Shown in Product Identification Section*]

GAVISCON® Liquid Antacid OTC

Each tablespoonful (15 ml) contains the following active ingredients:
Aluminum hydroxide .... 95 mg
Magnesium carbonate .... 412 mg
and the following inactive ingredients: water, sorbitol solution, glycerin, sodium alginate, xanthan gum, edetate disodium, methylparaben, propylparaben, flavorings, and colors.
Indications: For the relief of heartburn, sour stomach, and/or acid indigestion and upset stomach associated with heartburn, sour stomach, and/or acid indigestion.
Directions: Shake well before using. Take one to two tablespoonful four times a day or as directed by a physician. GAVISCON Liquid should be taken after meals and at bedtime, followed by a half glass of water.
Warnings: Except under the advice and supervision of a physician: Do not take more than eight tablespoonsful in a 24-hour period or eight tablespoonsful daily for more than two weeks. May have laxative effect. Do not use this product if you have a kidney disease. Do not use this product if you are on a sodium-restricted diet. Each tablespoonful of GAVISCON Liquid contains approximately 1.7 mEq sodium.
Drug Interaction Precautions: Do not take this product if you are presently taking a prescription antibiotic drug containing any form of tetracycline.
KEEP TIGHTLY CLOSED. AVOID FREEZING. STORE AT A CONTROLLED ROOM TEMPERATURE.
KEEP THIS AND ALL DRUGS OUT OF THE REACH OF CHILDREN.
In case of accidental overdose, seek professional assistance or contact a poison control center immediately.
How Supplied: 12 fluid ounces (355 ml).
[*Shown in Product Identification Section*]

GAVISCON®-2 Antacid Tablets OTC

Each chewable tablet contains the following active ingredients:
Aluminum hydroxide dried gel .... 160 mg
Magnesium trisilicate .... 40 mg
and the following inactive ingredients: sucrose, alginic acid, sodium bicarbonate, starch, calcium stearate and flavoring.
Indications: For temporary relief of heartburn, sour stomach, and/or acid indigestion.
Directions: Chew one to two tablets four times a day or as directed by a physician. Tablets should be taken after meals and at bedtime or as needed. For best results follow by a half glass of water or other liquid. DO NOT SWALLOW WHOLE.
Warnings: Except under the advice and supervision of a physician: Do not take more than 8 tablets in a 24-hour period or 8 tablets daily for more than 2 weeks; do not use this product if you are on a sodium-restricted diet. Each GAVISCON-2 Tablet contains approximately 1.6 mEq sodium.
Drug Interaction Precautions: Do not take this product if you are presently taking a prescription antibiotic drug containing any form of tetracycline.
STORE AT A CONTROLLED ROOM TEMPERATURE IN A DRY PLACE.
KEEP THIS AND ALL DRUGS OUT OF THE REACH OF CHILDREN. In case of accidental overdose, seek professional assistance or contact a poison control center immediately.
How Supplied: Box of 48 foil-wrapped tablets.
[*Shown in Product Identification Section*]

GLY-OXIDE® Liquid OTC

Description: Carbamide peroxide 10% in specially prepared anhydrous glycerol. Artificial flavor added. Not NF.
Actions: GLY-OXIDE® is a safe, stabilized oxygenating agent. Specifically formulated for topical oral administration, it provides unique chemomechanical cleansing and debriding action which allows normal healing to occur.
Indications: Local treatment and hygienic prevention (as an aid to professional care) of minor oral inflammation such as canker sores, denture irritation and postdental procedure irritation. GLY-OXIDE Liquid provides effective aid to oral hygiene when normal cleansing measures are inadequate or impossible (eg, total-care geriatric patients). As an adjunct to

Continued on next page

Marion—Cont.

oral hygiene (orthodontics, dental appliances) after regular brushing.
Precautions: Severe or persistent oral inflammation or denture irritation may be serious. If these or unexpected effects occur, consult physician or dentist promptly.
Dosage and Administration: DO NOT DILUTE—use directly from the bottle. Apply 4 times daily after meals and at bedtime, or as directed by a dentist or physician. Place several drops on affected area; expectorate after 2-3 minutes, or place 10 drops onto tongue, mix with saliva, swish for several minutes, expectorate. Do not rinse. Foams on contact with saliva.
Avoid contact with eyes. Protect from heat and direct sunlight. Keep this and all drugs out of the reach of children. In case of accidental ingestion, seek professional assistance or contact a poison control center immediately.
How Supplied: GLY-OXIDE Liquid in ½-fl-oz and 2-fl-oz non-spill plastic squeeze bottles with applicator spouts.

NICO-400 ® OTC
(nicotinic acid)

A dietary supplement for 12-year-olds and older.
Each capsule contains:
Nicotinic acid (niacin) ....400 mg
equivalent to 20 times the Recommended Daily Allowance of niacin.
Directions: Take one capsule daily, as a dietary supplement for 12-year-olds and older.
Ingredients: Niacin, sugar, starch, povidone, pharmaceutical glaze, calcium stearate, talc.
Keep tightly closed.
Store between 59°–86°F.
Keep out of reach of children.
How Supplied: NICO-400 is available in bottles of 100 capsules. Capsules imprinted with MARION/1575.
Dist. by:
Marion Laboratories, Inc.
Kansas City, MO 64137
[*Shown in Product Identification Section*]

NITRO-BID® Plateau CAPS® ℞
(nitroglycerin) 2.5 mg, 6.5 mg, and 9 mg

Description: Each NITRO-BID® Controlled-Release Capsule contains:
2.5 mg nitroglycerin: Light purple and clear capsule with white beads; identification imprint MARION/1550.
6.5 mg nitroglycerin: Dark blue and yellow capsule with white beads; identification imprint MARION/1551.
9 mg nitroglycerin: Green and yellow capsule with white beads; identification imprint MARION/1553.
Action: The mechanism of action of nitroglycerin in the relief of angina pectoris is not as yet known. However, its main pharmacologic action is to relax smooth muscle, principally in the smaller blood vessels, thus dilating arterioles and capillaries, especially in the coronary circulation. In therapeutic doses, nitroglycerin is thought to increase the blood supply to the myocardium which may, in turn, relieve myocardial ischemia, the possible functional basis for the pain of angina pectoris. The sublingual administration of nitroglycerin is normally rapid and transient, but nitroglycerin in controlled-release NITRO-BID® 2.5, NITRO-BID® 6.5, and NITRO-BID® 9 produces a prolonged action.

Indications:
Based on a review of this drug and a related drug by the National Academy of Sciences—National Research Council and/or other information, FDA has classified the indications as follows:
"Possibly" effective:
For the management, prophylaxis or treatment of anginal attacks.
Final classification of the less-than-effective indications requires further investigation.

Contraindications: Acute or recent myocardial infarction, severe anemia, closed-angle glaucoma, postural hypotension, increased intracranial pressure, and idiosyncrasy to the drug.
Warnings: Capsules must be swallowed. FOR ORAL, NOT SUBLINGUAL, USE. NITRO-BID® 2.5, NITRO-BID® 6.5, and NITRO-BID® 9 Controlled-Release Capsules are not intended for immediate relief of anginal attacks.
Precautions: Intraocular pressure may be increased; therefore, caution is required in administering to patients with glaucoma. Tolerance to this drug and cross-tolerance to other organic nitrites and nitrates may occur. If blurring of vision, dryness of mouth, or lack of benefit occurs, the drug should be discontinued.
Adverse Reactions: Severe and persistent headaches, cutaneous flushing, dizziness, and weakness. Occasionally, drug rash or exfoliative dermatitis and nausea and vomiting may occur; these responses may disappear with a decrease in dosage. Adverse effects are enhanced by ingestion of alcohol, which appears to increase absorption from the gastrointestinal tract.
Dosage and Administration: Administer the smallest effective dose two or three times daily at 8- to 12-hour intervals, unless clinical response suggests a different regimen. Patient should be titrated to anginal relief or hemodynamic response. Hemodynamic response can be measured by drop in systolic blood pressure. Discontinue if not effective.
How Supplied: NITRO-BID® 2.5, 6.5, and 9 Controlled-Release Capsules are available in 60- and 100-count UNI-Rx® Paks.
Caution: Federal law prohibits dispensing without a prescription.
Storage: STORE AT A CONTROLLED ROOM TEMPERATURE. Dispense only in the original unopened container.
Issued 5/81
[*Shown in Product Identification Section*]

NITRO-BID™ IV ℞
(nitroglycerin)

NOT FOR DIRECT INTRAVENOUS INJECTION. NITRO-BID IV MUST BE DILUTED IN DEXTROSE (5%) INJECTION, USP OR SODIUM CHLORIDE (0.9%) INJECTION, USP BEFORE INTRAVENOUS ADMINISTRATION. THE ADMINISTRATION SET USED FOR INFUSION MAY AFFECT THE AMOUNT OF NITRO-BID IV DELIVERED TO THE PATIENT. (SEE WARNINGS AND DOSAGE AND ADMINISTRATION SECTIONS.)
CAUTION: SEVERAL PREPARATIONS OF NITROGLYCERIN FOR INJECTION ARE AVAILABLE. THEY DIFFER IN CONCENTRATION AND/OR VOLUME PER VIAL. WHEN SWITCHING FROM ONE PRODUCT TO ANOTHER, ATTENTION MUST BE PAID TO THE DILUTION AND DOSAGE AND ADMINISTRATION INSTRUCTIONS.
Description: NITRO-BID IV (nitroglycerin) is a clear, practically colorless additive solution for intravenous infusion after dilution. Each ml contains 5 mg nitroglycerin and 45 mg propylene glycol dissolved in 70% ethanol. The solution is sterile, nonpyrogenic, and nonexplosive. NITRO-BID IV, an organic nitrate, is a vasodilator. The chemical name for nitroglycerin is 1,2,3 propanetriol trinitrate.

Clinical Pharmacology: Relaxation of vascular smooth muscle is the principal pharmacologic action of NITRO-BID IV (nitroglycerin). Although venous effects predominate, nitroglycerin produces, in a dose-related manner, dilation of both arterial and venous beds. Dilation of the postcapillary vessels, including large veins, promotes peripheral pooling of blood and decreases venous return to the heart, reducing left ventricular end-diastolic pressure (preload). Arteriolar relaxation reduces systemic vascular resistance and arterial pressure (afterload). Myocardial oxygen consumption or demand (as measured by the pressure-rate product, tension-time index, and stroke-work index) is decreased by both the arterial and venous effects of nitroglycerin, and a more favorable supply-demand ratio can be achieved.
Therapeutic doses of intravenous nitroglycerin reduce systolic, diastolic, and mean arterial blood pressures. Effective coronary perfusion pressure is usually maintained, but can be compromised if blood pressure falls excessively or increased heart rate decreases diastolic filling time.
Elevated central venous and pulmonary capillary wedge pressures, pulmonary vascular resistance, and systemic vascular resistance are also reduced by nitroglycerin therapy. Heart rate is usually slightly increased, presumably a reflex response to the fall in blood pressure. Cardiac index may be increased, decreased, or unchanged. Patients with elevated left ventricular filling pressure and systemic vascular resistance values in conjunction with a depressed cardiac index are likely to experience an improvement in cardiac index. On the other hand, when filling pressures and cardiac index are normal, cardiac index may be slightly reduced by intravenous nitroglycerin.
Nitroglycerin is widely distributed in the body with an apparent volume of distribution of approximately 200 liters in adult male subjects, and is rapidly metabolized to dinitrates and mononitrates, with a short half-life, estimated at 1 to 4 minutes. This results in a low plasma concentration after intravenous infusion. At plasma concentrations of between 50 and 100 ng/ml, the binding of nitroglycerin to plasma proteins is approximately 60%, while that of 1,2 dinitroglycerin and 1,3 dinitroglycerin is 60% and 30%, respectively. The activity and half-life of the dinitroglycerins are not well characterized. The mononitrate is not active.
Indications and Usage: NITRO-BID IV (nitroglycerin) is indicated for:

1. **Control of blood pressure in perioperative hypertension,** ie, hypertension associated with surgical procedures, especially cardiovascular procedures, such as the hypertension seen during intratracheal intubation, anesthesia, skin incision, sternotomy, cardiac bypass, and in the immediate postsurgical period.
2. **Congestive heart failure associated with acute myocardial infarction.**
3. **Treatment of angina pectoris** in patients who have not responded to recommended doses of organic nitrates and/or a beta-blocker.
4. **Production of controlled hypotension during surgical procedures.**

Contraindications: NITRO-BID IV (nitroglycerin) should not be administered to individuals with:

1. A known hypersensitivity to nitroglycerin or a known idiosyncratic reaction to organic nitrates.
2. Hypotension or uncorrected hypovolemia, as the use of NITRO-BID IV in such states could produce severe hypotension or shock.
3. Increased intracranial pressure (eg, head trauma or cerebral hemorrhage).
4. Inadequate cerebral circulation, constrictive pericarditis, and pericardial tamponade.

Warnings:

1. Nitroglycerin readily migrates into many plastics. To avoid absorption of nitroglycerin into plastic parenteral solution containers, the dilution and storage of nitroglycerin for intravenous infusion should be made only in glass parenteral solution bottles.
2. Some filters also absorb nitroglycerin; they should be avoided.
3. Forty percent to 80% of the total amount of nitroglycerin in the final diluted solution for infusion is absorbed by the polyvinyl chloride (PVC) tubing of the intravenous administration sets currently in general use. The higher rates of absorption occur when flow rates are low, nitroglycerin concentrations are high, and tubing is long. Although the rate of loss is highest during the early phase of administration (when flow rates are lowest), the loss is neither constant nor self-limiting; consequently, no simple calculation or correction can be performed to convert the theoretical infusion rate (based on the concentration of the infusion solution) to the actual delivery rate. Because of this problem, Marion Laboratories recommends the use of the least absorptive infusion tubing available for infusions of NITRO-BID IV. DOSING INSTRUCTIONS MUST BE FOLLOWED WITH CARE. IT SHOULD BE NOTED THAT WHEN THESE INFUSION SETS ARE USED, THE CALCULATED DOSE WILL BE DELIVERED TO THE PATIENT DEPENDENT UPON THE LOSS OF NITROGLYCERIN DUE TO ABSORPTIVE TUBING. NOTE THAT THE DOSAGES COMMONLY USED IN PUBLISHED STUDIES UTILIZED GENERAL-USE PVC TUBING, AND RECOMMENDED DOSES BASED ON THIS EXPERIENCE ARE TOO HIGH IF NEW, LESS ABSORPTIVE INFUSION TUBING IS USED.

Precautions: NITRO-BID IV (nitroglycerin) should be used with caution in patients who have severe hepatic or renal disease.

Excessive hypotension, especially for prolonged periods of time, must be avoided because of possible deleterious effects on the brain, heart, liver, and kidney from poor perfusion and the attendant risk of ischemia, thrombosis, and altered function of these organs. Patients with normal or low pulmonary capillary wedge pressure are especially sensitive to the hypotensive effects of NITRO-BID IV. If pulmonary capillary wedge pressure is being monitored, it will be noted that a fall in wedge pressure precedes the onset of arterial hypotension, and the pulmonary capillary wedge pressure is thus a useful guide to safe titration of the drug.

Carcinogenesis, mutagenesis, impairment of fertility: No long-term studies in animals were performed to evaluate carcinogenic potential of NITRO-BID IV.

Pregnancy: Category C. Animal reproduction studies have not been conducted with NITRO-BID IV. It is also not known whether NITRO-BID IV can cause fetal harm when administered to a pregnant woman or can affect reproduction capacity. NITRO-BID IV should be given to a pregnant woman only if clearly needed.

Nursing Mothers: It is not known whether nitroglycerin is excreted in human milk. Because many drugs are excreted in human milk, caution should be exercised when NITRO-BID IV is administered to a nursing woman.

Pediatric Use: The safety and effectiveness of NITRO-BID IV in children have not been established.

Adverse Reactions: The most frequent adverse reaction in patients treated with nitroglycerin is headache, which occurs in approximately 2% of patients. Other adverse reactions occurring in less than 1% of patients are the following: tachycardia, nausea, vomiting, apprehension, restlessness, muscle twitching, retrosternal discomfort, palpitations, dizziness, and abdominal pain. Paradoxical bradycardia and increased angina pectoris may accompany nitroglycerin-induced hypotension. The following additional adverse reactions have been reported with the oral and/or topical use of nitroglycerin: cutaneous flushing, weakness, and, occasionally, drug rash or exfoliative dermatitis.

NITRO-BID IV Administration Table

Each 1 ml Amp = 5 mg nitroglycerin
Each 5 ml Amp = 25 mg nitroglycerin
Each 10 ml Amp = 50 mg nitroglycerin

Mixing Instructions	1 ml in 100 ml 5 ml in 500 ml 10 ml in 1000 ml	1 ml in 50 ml 5 ml in 250 ml 10 ml in 500 ml 20 ml in 1000 ml	2 ml in 50 ml 10 ml in 250 ml 20 ml in 500 ml 40 ml in 1000 ml	FLOW RATE milliliters/hour microdrops/minute
Concentration	50 mcg/ml	100 mcg/ml	200 mcg/ml	
Dosage	mcg/min	mcg/min	mcg/min	microdrops/min
	2.5	5	10	3
	5	10	20	6
	10	20	40	12
	20	40	80	24
	40	80	160	48
	60	120	240	72
	80	160	320	96

Overdosage: Accidental overdosage of nitroglycerin may result in severe hypotension and reflex tachycardia which can be treated by elevating the legs and decreasing or temporarily terminating the infusion until the patient's condition stabilizes. Since the duration of the hemodynamic effects following nitroglycerin administration is quite short, additional corrective measures are usually not required. However, if further therapy is indicated, administration of an intravenous alpha-adrenergic agonist (eg, methoxamine or phenylephrine) should be considered.

Dosage and Administration:

NOT FOR DIRECT INTRAVENOUS INJECTION.

NITRO-BID IV (NITROGLYCERIN) IS A CONCENTRATED, POTENT DRUG WHICH MUST BE DILUTED IN DEXTROSE (5%) INJECTION, USP, OR SODIUM CHLORIDE (0.9%) INJECTION, USP, PRIOR TO ITS INFUSION. NITRO-BID IV SHOULD NOT BE ADMIXED WITH OTHER DRUGS.

Dilution: It is important to consider the fluid requirements of the patient as well as the expected duration of infusion in selecting the appropriate dilution of NITRO-BID IV. [See table above].

Dosage: Dosage is affected by the type of infusion set used (see WARNINGS). Although the usual starting adult dose range reported in clinical studies was 25 mcg/min or more, those studies used PVC TUBING. **The use of nonabsorbing tubing will result in the need to use reduced doses.**

The dosage for NITRO-BID IV (nitroglycerin) infusion should initially be 5 mcg/min delivered through an infusion pump capable of exact and constant delivery of the drug. Subsequent titration must be adjusted to the clinical situation, with dose increments becoming more cautious as partial response is seen. Initial titration should be in 5 mcg/min increments, with increases every 3–5 minutes until some response is noted. If no response is seen at 20 mcg/min, increments of 10 and later 20 mcg/min can be used. Once a partial blood pressure response is observed, the dose increase should be reduced and the interval between increments should be lengthened. Patients with normal or low left ventricular filling pressure or pulmonary capillary wedge pressure (eg, angina patients without other complications) may be hypersensitive to the effects of NITRO-BID IV and may respond fully to doses as small as 5 mcg/min. These patients require especially careful titration and monitoring.

There is no fixed optimum dose of NITRO-BID IV. Due to variations in the responsiveness of individual patients to the drug, each patient must be titrated to the desired level of hemodynamic function. Therefore, continuous monitoring of physiologic parameters (eg, blood pressure, heart rate, and pulmonary capillary wedge pressure) MUST BE PERFORMED to achieve the correct dose. Adequate systemic blood pressure and coronary perfusion pressure must be maintained.

How Supplied: NITRO-BID IV is supplied in boxes of ten 1-ml ampules (NDC 0088-1800-07), each ampule containing 5 mg nitroglycerin (5 mg/ml); ten 5-ml ampules (NDC 0088-1800-08), each ampule containing 25 mg nitroglycerin (5 mg/ml); and five 10-ml ampules (NDC 0088-1800-13), each ampule containing 50 mg nitroglycerin (5 mg/ml).

Mfd. for
Marion Laboratories, Inc.
Mfd. by
Taylor Pharmacal Co.
Decatur, IL 62525

Issued 11/81

NITRO-BID® Ointment (nitroglycerin 2%) ℞

Description: NITRO-BID® Ointment contains 2% nitroglycerin and lactose in a special absorptive lanolin and white petrolatum base formulated to provide a controlled release of the active ingredient. Each inch, as squeezed from the tube, or the contents squeezed from the pouch, contains approximately 15 mg nitroglycerin.

Actions: When the ointment is spread on the skin, nitroglycerin is absorbed continuously into the systemic circulation. Nitroglycerin ointment reduces the work load of the heart by virtue of its smooth-muscle relaxation. This results predominantly in peripheral venous dilatation which reduces preload, but also to a lesser degree in peripheral arteriolar dilatation which reduces afterload. These hemodynamic effects have been advanced as explanations for the beneficial actions of nitroglycerin ointment in angina pectoris.

Computerized digital plethysmographic studies have shown the duration of action of nitroglycerin ointment (2 inches applied to the chest) to be eight hours in comparison to placebo; the onset of action occurred within thirty minutes of administration. Controlled clinical studies have demonstrated that nitroglycerin ointment increased measured exercise tolerance in patients with angina pectoris up to three hours after application (the maximal time interval studied).

Indications: For the prevention and treatment of angina pectoris due to coronary artery disease.

Contraindications: In patients known to be intolerant of the organic nitrate drugs.

Continued on next page

Marion—Cont.

Warnings: In acute myocardial infarction or congestive heart failure, nitroglycerin ointment should be used under careful clinical and/or hemodynamic monitoring.
Precautions: Nitroglycerin ointment should not be used for treatment of acute anginal attacks. Symptoms of hypotension, particularly when suddenly arising from the recumbent position, are signs of overdosage. When they occur, the dosage should be reduced.
Adverse Reactions: Transient headaches are the most common side effect, especially at higher dosages. Headaches should be treated with mild analgesics, and nitroglycerin ointment continued. Only with untreatable headaches should the dosage be reduced. Although uncommon, hypotension, an increase in heart rate, faintness, flushing, dizziness, and nausea may occur. These all are attributable to the pharmacologic effects of nitroglycerin on the cardiovascular system, but are symptoms of overdosage. When they occur and persist, the dosage should be reduced.
Occasionally, contact dermatitus has been reported with continuous use of topical nitroglycerin. Such incidence may be reduced by changing the site of application or by using topical corticosteroids.
Dosage and Administration: When applying the ointment, place the specially designed Dose Measuring Applicator supplied with the package printed side down and squeeze the necessary amount of ointment from the tube or pouch onto the applicator. Then place the applicator with the ointment side down onto the desired area of the skin, usually the chest (although other areas can be used). Spread the ointment over a 6x6-inch (150x150 mm) area in a thin, uniform layer using the applicator. Cover the area with plastic wrap which can be held in place by adhesive tape. The applicator allows the patient to measure the necessary amount of ointment and to spread it without its being absorbed through the fingers while applying it to the skin surface.
The usual therapeutic dose is 2 inches (50 mm) applied every eight hours, although some patients may require as much as 4 to 5 inches (100 to 125 mm) and/or application every four hours.
Tube: Start at 1/2 inch (12.5 mm) every eight hours and increase the dose by 1/2 inch (12.5 mm) with each successive application to achieve the desired clinical effects. The optimal dosage should be selected based upon the clinical response, side effects, and the effects of therapy upon blood pressure. The greatest attainable decrease in resting blood pressure which is not associated with clinical symptoms of hypotension, especially during orthostasis, indicates the optimal dosage. To decrease adverse reactions, the dose and frequency of application should be tailored to the individual patient's needs.
Keep the tube tightly closed and store at room temperature 59° to 86°F (15° to 30° C).
Foil Pouch: The 1-gram foil pouch is approximately equivalent to one inch as squeezed from a tube and is designed to be used in increments of one inch. Apply the ointment by squeezing the contents of the pouch onto a specially designed Dose Measuring Applicator supplied with the package printed side down.
Patient Instructions for Application: Information furnished with Dose Measuring Applicators.
How Supplied: NITRO-BID® Ointment is available in 20-gram and 60-gram UNI-Rx® Paks (six tubes per pack); in individual 20-gram, 60-gram, and 100-gram tubes; and in Unit Dose Identification Paks of 100 1-gram foil pouches.

Issued 5/82

[Shown in Product Identification Section]

OS-CAL® Tablets — OTC
Calcium with vitamin D

Each tablet contains: 625 mg of calcium carbonate from oyster shell which provides:
Elemental calcium .... 250 mg
Ergocalciferol (Vitamin D_2) 125 USP Units
Indications: OS-CAL® Tablets provide a source of calcium when it is desired to increase the dietary intake of this mineral. OS-CAL also contains Vitamin D_2 to aid in the absorption of calcium.
Directions: Take one tablet three times a day at mealtime. Three tablets daily provide:

	Quantity	%U.S.RDA* for Adults
Calcium	750 mg	75%
Vitamin D_2	375 units	94%

*Percent U.S. Recommended Daily Allowance
STORE AT ROOM TEMPERATURE.
Keep this and all drugs out of reach of children. In case of accidental overdose, seek professional assistance or contact a poison control center immediately.
How Supplied: Bottles of 100, 240, 500, and 1000 tablets.
[Shown in Product Identification Section]

OS-CAL® 500 Tablets — OTC
calcium supplement

Each tablet contains:
1,250 mg of calcium carbonate from oyster shell which provides:
Elemental calcium .... 500 mg
Indications: OS-CAL 500 Tablets provide a source of calcium where it is desired or recommended by a physician to increase the dietary intake of this mineral.
Directions: Take one tablet two or three times a day at mealtime or as directed. Two tablets daily provide:

	Quantity	%U.S.RDA†
Calcium	1,000 mg	100%*
		77%**

Three tablets daily provide:

	Quantity	%U.S.RDA†
Calcium	1,500 mg	150%*
		115%**

†Percent U.S. Recommended Daily Allowance.
*For adults and children 12 or more years of age.
**For pregnant and lactating women.
Keep this and all drugs out of reach of children. In case of accidental overdose, seek professional assistance or contact a poison control center immediately.
How Supplied: Bottles of 60 tablets.
[Shown in Product Identification Section]

OS-CAL FORTE® Tablets — OTC
multivitamin and mineral supplement

Each tablet contains:
Vitamin A (palmitate).......... 1668 USP Units
Ergocalciferol (Vitamin D_2).... 125 USP Units
Thiamine mononitrate (Vitamin B_1)... 1.7 mg
Riboflavin (Vitamin B_2)........................ 1.7 mg
Pyridoxine hydrochloride
(Vitamin B_6)........................ 2.0 mg
Cyanocobalamin (Vitamin B_{12}).......... 1.6 mcg
Ascorbic acid (Vitamin C)........................ 50 mg
dl-alpha-tocopherol acetate
(Vitamin E)........................ 0.8 IU
Niacinamide........................ 15 mg
Calcium (from oyster shell*) .... 250 mg
Iron (as ferrous fumarate)........................ 5 mg
Copper (as sulfate)........................ 0.3 mg
Iodine (as potassium iodide) .... 0.05 mg
Magnesium (as oxide)........................ 1.6 mg
Manganese (as sulfate) .... 0.3 mg
Zinc (as sulfate)........................ 0.5 mg
*Trace minerals from oyster shell: copper, iron, magnesium, manganese, silica and zinc.
Indication: Multivitamin and mineral supplement.
Dosage: One tablet three times daily or as directed by physician.
How Supplied: Bottles of 100 tablets.
Keep this and all drugs out of reach of children. In case of accidental overdose, seek professional assistance or contact a poison control center immediately.
Store at room temperature.
[Shown in Product Identification Section]

OS-CAL-GESIC® Tablets — OTC
antiarthritic

Each tablet contains:
Salicylamide .... 400 mg
Calcium (from oyster shell) .... 100 mg
Ergocalciferol (Vitamin D_2)..... 50 USP Units
Indication: For temporary relief of symptoms associated with arthritis.
Dosage: Initially–2 tablets hourly for 3 or 4 doses. Maintenance–1 or 2 tablets 4 times daily.
How Supplied: OS-CAL-GESIC® is available in bottles of 100 tablets.
Keep this and all drugs out of reach of children. In case of accidental overdose, seek professional assistance or contact a poison control center immediately.
Store at room temperature.
[Shown in Product Identification Section]

OS-CAL® Plus Tablets — OTC
multivitamin and multimineral supplement

Each tablet contains:
Calcium (from oyster shell*)............... 250 mg
Ergocalciferol (Vitamin D_2).... 125 USP Units
*Trace minerals from oyster shell: copper, iron, magnesium, manganese, silica and zinc.
Plus:
Vitamin A (palmitate).......... 1666 USP Units
Vitamin C (ascorbic acid)........................ 33 mg
Vitamin B_2 (riboflavin)........................ 0.66 mg
Vitamin B_1 (thiamine mononitrate).... 0.5 mg
Vitamin B_6 (pyridoxine HCl)............ 0.5 mg
Vitamin B_{12} (cyanocobalamin).......... 0.03 mcg
Niacinamide........................ 3.33 mg
Iron (as ferrous fumarate)................ 16.6 mg
Zinc (as the sulfate)........................ 0.75 mg
Manganese (as the sulfate)................ 0.75 mg
Copper (as the sulfate)........................ 0.036 mg
Iodine (as potassium iodide)............ 0.036 mg
Indications: As a multivitamin and multimineral supplement.
Dosage: One tablet three times a day before meals or as directed by a physician. For children under four years of age, consult a physician.
How Supplied: Bottles of 100 tablets.
Store at room temperature.
Keep this and all drugs out of reach of children. In case of accidental overdose, seek professional assistance or contact a poison control center immediately.
[Shown in Product Identification Section]

PAVABID® Capsules — ℞
(papaverine hydrochloride) 150 mg

Composition:
Each Pavabid capsule contains:
Papaverine hydrochloride .... 150 mg
in a specially prepared base to provide prolonged activity.
Actions and Uses: The main actions of papaverine are exerted on cardiac and smooth muscle. Like quinidine, papaverine acts directly on the heart muscle to depress conduction and prolong the refractory period. Papaverine relaxes various smooth muscles. This relaxation may be prominent if spasm exists. The muscle cell is not paralyzed by papaverine and still responds to drugs and other stimuli causing contraction. The antispasmodic effect is a direct one, and unrelated to muscle innervation. Papaverine is practically devoid of effects on the central nervous system.
Papaverine relaxes the smooth musculature of the larger blood vessels, especially coronary, systemic peripheral, and pulmonary arteries.

Perhaps by its direct vasodilating action on cerebral blood vessels, papaverine increases cerebral blood flow and decreases cerebral vascular resistance in normal subjects: oxygen consumption is unaltered. These effects may explain the benefit reported from the drug in cerebral vascular encephalopathy.
The direct actions of papaverine on the heart to depress conduction and irritability and to prolong the refractory period of the myocardium provide the basis for its clinical trial in abrogating atrial and ventricular premature systoles and ominous ventricular arrhythmias. The coronary vasodilator action could be an additional factor of therapeutic value when such rhythms are secondary to insufficiency or occlusion of the coronary arteries.
In patients with acute coronary thrombosis, the occurrence of ventricular rhythms is serious and requires measures designed to decrease myocardial irritability. Papaverine may have advantages over quinidine, used for a similar purpose, in that it may be given in an emergency by the intravenous route, does not depress myocardial contraction or cause cinchonism, and produces coronary vasodilation.
Indications: For the relief of cerebral and peripheral ischemia associated with arterial spasm and myocardial ischemia complicated by arrhythmias.
Precautions: Use with caution in patients with glaucoma. Hepatic hypersensitivity has been reported with gastrointestinal symptoms, jaundice, eosinophilia and altered liver function tests. Discontinue medication if these occur.
Adverse Reactions: Although occurring rarely, the reported side effects of papaverine include nausea, abdominal distress, anorexia, constipation, malaise, drowsiness, vertigo, sweating, headache, diarrhea and skin rash.
Dosage and Administration: One capsule every 12 hours. In difficult cases administration may be increased to one capsule every 8 hours, or two capsules every 12 hours.
How Supplied: Pavabid® Capsules are available in 60- and 100-count UNI-Rx® Paks, in bottles of 100, 250, 1000 and 5000 and in Unit Dose Identification Paks of 100 capsules. Capsules are imprinted with Marion/1555.
Caution: Federal law prohibits dispensing without prescription.
Keep out of reach of children.
Store at a controlled room temperature in a dry place.
[Shown in Product Identification Section]

PAVABID® HP Capsulets ℞
(papaverine hydrochloride) 300 mg

Composition: Each capsulet contains:
Papaverine hydrochloride .... 300 mg
Action and Uses: The main actions of papaverine are exerted on cardiac and smooth muscle. Like quinidine, papaverine acts directly on the heart muscle to depress conduction and prolong the refractory period. Papaverine relaxes various smooth muscles. This relaxation may be prominent if spasm exists. The muscle cell is not paralyzed by papaverine, and still responds to drugs and other stimuli causing contraction. The antispasmodic effect is a direct one, and unrelated to muscle innervation. Papaverine is practically devoid of effects on the central nervous system.
Papaverine relaxes the smooth musculature of the larger blood vessels, especially coronary, systemic peripheral, and pulmonary arteries. Perhaps by its direct vasodilating action on cerebral blood vessels, papaverine increases cerebral blood flow and decreases cerebral vascular resistance in normal subjects; oxygen consumption is unaltered. These effects may explain the benefit reported from the drug in cerebral vascular encephalopathy.
The direct actions of papaverine on the heart to depress conduction and irritability and to prolong the refractory period of the myocardium provide the basis for its clinical trial in abrogating atrial and ventricular premature systoles and ominous ventricular arrhythmias. The coronary vasodilator action could be an additional factor of therapeutic value when such rhythms are secondary to insufficiency or occlusion of the coronary arteries.
In patients with acute coronary thrombosis, the occurrence of ventricular rhythms is serious and requires measures designed to decrease myocardial irritability. Papaverine may have advantages over quinidine, used for a similar purpose, in that it may be given in an emergency by the intravenous route, does not depress myocardial contraction or cause cinchonism, and produces coronary vasodilation.
Indications: For the relief of cerebral and peripheral ischemia associated with arterial spasm and myocardial ischemia complicated by arrhythmias.
Precaution: Use with caution in patients with glaucoma. Hepatic hypersensitivity has been reported with gastrointestinal symptoms, jaundice, eosinophilia and altered liver function tests. Discontinue medication if these occur.
Adverse Reactions: Although occurring rarely, the reported side effects of papaverine include nausea, abdominal distress, anorexia, constipation, malaise, drowsiness, vertigo, sweating, headache, diarrhea and skin rash.
Dosage and Administration: Dosage should be started at 150 mg (one-half capsulet) two or three times daily and titrated upward to the desired level. The 300-mg capsulet breaks into two separate half-capsulets. To break: place capsulet on a hard surface with the embossed MARION M facing up, press down on the embossed M.
How Supplied: PAVABID® HP Capsulets are available in 60-count bottles. Each light orange capsulet is embossed with a raised M stamped MARION on one side and PAVABID HP on the other side.
Caution: Federal law prohibits dispensing without prescription.
Keep out of reach of children.
Store at a controlled room temperature in a dry place.
[Shown in Product Identification Section]

SILVADENE® Cream ℞
(1% silver sulfadiazine)

Description: SILVADENE Cream is a soft, white, water-miscible cream containing the antimicrobial agent, silver sulfadiazine in micronized form. Each gram of SILVADENE Cream contains 10 mg of micronized silver sulfadiazine. The cream vehicle consists of white petrolatum, stearyl alcohol, isopropyl myristate, sorbitan monooleate, polyoxyl 40 stearate, propylene glycol, and water, with methylparaben 0.3% as a preservative.
Actions: SILVADENE Cream (silver sulfadiazine) spreads easily and can be washed off readily with water.
Silver sulfadiazine, micronized, has broad antimicrobial activity. It is bactericidal for many gram-negative and gram-positive bacteria as well as being effective against yeast. Results from *in vitro* testing are listed below. Sufficient data have been obtained to demonstrate that silver sulfadiazine will inhibit bacteria that are resistant to other antimicrobial agents and that the compound is superior to sulfadiazine.

No. of Sensitive Strains/Total Strains Tested Concentration of silver sulfadiazine

Genus & Species	50 μg/ml	100 μg/ml
Pseudomonas aeruginosa	130/130	130/130
Pseudomonas maltophilia	7/7	7/7
Enterobacter species	48/50	50/50
Enterobacter cloacae	24/24	24/24
Klebsiella	53/54	54/54
Escherichia coli	63/63	63/63
Serratia	27/28	28/28
Proteus mirabilis	53/53	53/53
Proteus morganii	10/10	10/10
Proteus rettgeri	2/2	2/2
Proteus vulgaris	2/2	2/2
Providencia	1/1	1/1
Citrobacter	10/10	10/10
Herellea	8/9	9/9
Mima	2/2	2/2
Staphylococcus aureus	100/101	101/101
Staphylococcus epidermidis	51/51	51/51
β-hemolytic *Streptococcus*	4/4	4/4
Enterococcus (Group D *Streptococcus)*	52/53	53/53
Corynebacterium diphtheriae	2/2	2/2
Clostridium perfringens	0/2	2/2
Candida albicans	43/50	50/50

Studies utilizing radioactive micronized silver sulfadiazine, electron microscopy and elaborate biochemical techniques have revealed that the mechanism of action of silver sulfadiazine on bacteria differs from silver nitrate and sodium sulfadiazine. SILVADENE Cream (silver sulfadiazine) acts only on the cell membrane and cell wall to produce its bactericidal effect.
Silver sulfadiazine by its chemical nature is not a carbonic anhydrase inhibitor. **Acidosis in patients treated with SILVADENE Cream has not been reported.** Since it is not a carbonic anhydrase inhibitor, SILVADENE Cream may be particularly of value in treating pediatric burn patients.
Indications: SILVADENE Cream (silver sulfadiazine) is a topical antimicrobial drug indicated as an adjunct for the prevention and treatment of wound sepsis in patients with second- and third-degree burns.
Contraindications: Because sulfonamide therapy is known to increase the possibility of kernicterus, SILVADENE Cream should not be used at term pregnancy, on premature infants, or on newborn infants during the first month of life.
Warnings: SILVADENE Cream should be administered with great caution to patients with history of hypersensitivity to SILVADENE Cream. It is not known whether there is cross-sensitivity to other sulfonamides. If allergic reactions attributable to treatment with SILVADENE Cream occur, discontinuation of SILVADENE Cream must be considered. The use of SILVADENE Cream in some cases of glucose-6-phosphate dehydrogenase deficient individuals may be hazardous, as hemolysis may occur.
Use in Pregnancy: Safe use of SILVADENE Cream during pregnancy has not been established. Therefore, the preparation is not recommended for the treatment of women of childbearing potential, unless the burned area covers more than 20 percent of the total body surface area or the need for therapeutic benefit of SILVADENE Cream is, in the physician's judgment, greater than the possible risk to the fetus.
Fungal colonization in and below the eschar may occur concomitantly with reduction of bacterial growth in the burn wound. However, fungal dissemination is rare.

Continued on next page

Marion—Cont.

In the treatment of burn wounds involving extensive areas of the body, the serum sulfa concentration may approach adult therapeutic levels (8–12 mg%). Therefore, in these patients it would be advisable to monitor serum sulfa concentrations. Renal function should be carefully monitored and the urine should be checked for sulfa crystals.

Precautions: If hepatic and renal functions become impaired and elimination of drug decreases, accumulation may occur and discontinuation of SILVADENE Cream should be weighed against the therapeutic benefit being achieved.

In considering the use of topical proteolytic enzymes in conjunction with SILVADENE Cream, the possibility should be noted that silver may inactivate such enzymes.

Adverse Reactions: It is frequently difficult to distinguish between an adverse reaction due to SILVADENE Cream (silver sulfadiazine) and reactions that may occur due to the concomitant use of other therapeutic agents used in the treatment of a patient having a severe burn wound. In the aggregate of 2,297 patients treated with SILVADENE Cream, there were 59 drug-related reactions (2.5%). Of these there were 51 cases of burning, 5 of rash, 2 of itching, and 1 of interstitial nephritis. However, SILVADENE Cream therapy was discontinued in only 0.9% of the patient population. Since significant quantities of silver sulfadiazine are absorbed, it is possible that any of the adverse reactions attributable to sulfonamides may occur.

Dosage and Administration: Prompt institution of appropriate regimens for care of the burned patient is of prime importance and includes the control of shock and pain. The burn wounds are then cleansed and debrided and SILVADENE Cream (silver sulfadiazine) is applied with sterile, gloved hand. The burn areas should be covered with SILVADENE Cream at all times. The cream should be applied once to twice daily to a thickness of approximately 1/16 inch. Whenever necessary, the cream should be reapplied to any areas from which it has been removed by patient activity. Administration may be accomplished in minimal time because dressings are not required. However, if individual patient requirements make dressings necessary, they may be used.

When feasible, the patient should be bathed daily. This is an aid in debridement. A whirlpool bath is particularly helpful, but the patient may be bathed in bed or in a shower.

Reduction in bacterial growth after application of topical antibacterial agents has been reported to permit spontaneous healing of deep partial-thickness burns by preventing conversion of the partial thickness to full thickness by sepsis. However, reduction in bacterial colonization has caused delayed separation, in some cases necessitating escharotomy in order to prevent contracture.

Treatment with SILVADENE Cream should be continued until satisfactory healing has occurred or until the burn site is ready for grafting. **The drug should not be withdrawn from the therapeutic regimen while there remains the possibility of infection except if a significant adverse reaction occurs.**

How Supplied: SILVADENE Cream (silver sulfadiazine) is available in 50-mg, 400-gm, and 1000-gm jars; and 20-gm tubes.

U.S. Patent 3,761,590.

Issued 3/82

THROAT DISCS® OTC
Throat Lozenges

Description: Each lozenge contains capsicum, peppermint, anise, cubeb, glycyrrhiza extract (licorice), and linseed.

Indications: Effective for soothing, temporary relief of minor throat irritations from hoarseness and coughs due to colds.

Precautions: For severe or persistent cough or sore throat, or sore throat accompanied by high fever, headache, nausea, and vomiting, consult physician promptly. Not recommended for children under 3 years of age.

Dosage: Allow lozenge to dissolve slowly in mouth. One or two should give the desired relief. Do not use more than four lozenges per hour.

How Supplied: Box of 60 lozenges.

THYROID STRONG TABLETS ℞
THYROID TABLETS, USP ℞

Description: Thyroid Tablets are prepared from defatted, desiccated thyroid glands of edible animals. Thyroid, USP is standardized to contain 0.2% iodine. Thyroid Strong is standardized to contain 0.3% iodine. The standard of 0.3% iodine was adopted before the USP Standard was established and is 50% stronger than the USP specification. Each grain of Thyroid Strong is equivalent to 1½ grains of Thyroid USP. Thyroid is assayed both chemically and biologically to assure uniform potency. In this preparation the active thyroid hormones, thyroxine and liothyronine, are available in their natural state.

Action: The activity of thyroid is derived from its natural thyroid hormone content. Virtually every system of the body appears to be affected by the action of the thyroid hormones. The primary action of the thyroid hormones is the promotion of a generalized increase in the metabolic rate of the body tissues. The effect may be noted in increases in the following: oxygen consumption; respiratory rate; body temperature; cardiac output; heart rate; blood volume; rate of fat; protein and carbohydrate metabolism; enzyme system activity; and growth and maturation. The basic mechanism of action is not yet understood.

Following the administration of thyroid hormones, rapid and almost complete absorption takes place, but their effects develop slowly with initial effects being observed in 24 hours and full effect usually being achieved in 10 to 14 days.

The administration of small doses of thyroid to normal (euthyroid) individuals does not produce an increase in metabolic rate.

Indications: Thyroid is indicated for use in the treatment of thyroid deficiency states, especially cretinism and myxedema. In hypothyroidism, the administration of thyroid represents pure replacement therapy.

Thyroid is also indicated for administration as an adjunct to the use of thyroid-inhibiting agents when decreased release of thyrotrophic hormones is desired.

Contraindications: Thyroid preparations are contraindicated in the presence of uncorrected adrenal insufficiency and in acute myocardial infarction which is uncomplicated by hypothyroidism.

Warnings: Drugs with thyroid hormone activity, alone or together with other therapeutic agents, have been used for the treatment of obesity. In euthyroid patients, doses within the range of daily hormonal requirements are ineffective for weight reduction. Larger doses may produce serious or even life-threatening manifestations of toxicity, particularly when given in association with sympathomimetic amines such as those used for their anorectic effects.

The possibility of persons with coronary artery disease suffering an episode of coronary insufficiency following injections of epinephrine may be enhanced in persons on thyroid hormone.

Thyroid hormones may potentiate the effect of anticoagulant drugs and, consequently, special care is required in titrating the dosage for patients on such therapy.

Precautions: Patients with myxedema may be especially sensitive to the thyroid hormones. In such cases, treatment should be instituted with very small doses and the increments increasing dosage should be gradual.

Thyroid preparations should be administered with caution to persons with cardiovascular disease. If signs of aggravation of the cardiovascular disease develop, the dosage should be reduced.

The administration of thyroid preparations to persons with diabetes mellitus may affect insulin or hypoglycemic agent requirements and dosage of these agents should be adjusted as necessary.

Adverse Reactions: Excessive doses of thyroid produce signs and symptoms of thyrotoxicosis which include tachycardia, cardiac arrhythmias, palpitation, elevated pulse pressure, angina pectoris, tremors, nervousness, headache, insomnia, nausea, diarrhea, changes in appetite, excessive sweating, intolerance to heat and fever. Chronic overdosage causes emaciation.

Dosage and Administration: Each grain of Thyroid Strong is equivalent to 1½ grains of Thyroid, USP. The following listing indicates the equivalent USP Thyroid potency that corresponds to each strength of Thyroid Strong.

½ gr Thyroid Strong is equivalent to ¾ gr Thyroid, USP

1 gr Thyroid Strong is equivalent to 1½ gr Thyroid, USP

2 gr Thyroid Strong is equivalent to 3 gr Thyroid, USP

3 gr Thyroid Strong is equivalent to 4½ gr Thyroid, USP

The dose of thyroid must be established on an individual basis for each patient beginning with a small dose and increasing gradually until the desired effect is obtained. In order to standardize the expression of thyroid dosage, the dosages indicated are given in terms of USP thyroid. Where Thyroid Strong is desired for convenience or more precise dosing, conversion to potencies of that product may be made in accordance with the preceding listing of equivalents.

The usual maintenance dose in thyroid-deficient patients is ½ to 2 grains daily. In some individuals, titrated dosage may be well in excess of the usual dose because of variations in individual response.

In cretinism it is desired to have early diagnosis and treatment, with prompt establishment of a maintenance dosage level. This may be achieved by administering ¼ grain daily, to be increased in ¼-grain increments every two weeks to a maximum level of 1 grain for each 6 months of age, not to exceed 4 grains per day.

In adult myxedema, replacement therapy is usually initiated at the rate of ½ grain per day and then increased at monthly intervals to 1 to 1½ grains daily, as the individual response dictates.

The effects of thyroid therapy are highly cumulative, and no advantage occurs from dividing the daily dose, nor administering at a particular time.

How Supplied:

Thyroid Tablets, USP are supplied as:

Compressed Tablets (plain)

NDC 0088-0775-58	15 mg	1000's
NDC 0088-0776-58	30 mg	1000's
NDC 0088-0777-47	60 mg	100's
NDC 0088-0777-58	60 mg	1000's
NDC 0088-0778-58	125 mg	1000's

Thyroid Strong Tablets are supplied as:

Compressed Tablets (plain)

NDC 0088-0686-47	½ gr (32.5 mg)	100's

NDC 0088-0686-58	½ gr	(32.5 mg)	1000's
NDC 0088-0674-47	1 gr	(65 mg)	100's
NDC 0088-0674-58	1 gr	(65 mg)	1000's
NDC 0088-0675-47	2 gr	(0.13 gm)	100's
NDC 0088-0675-58	2 gr	(0.13 gm)	1000's
Compressed Tablets (sugar-coated)			
NDC 0088-0626-47	½ gr	(32.5 mg)	100's
NDC 0088-0626-58	½ gr	(32.5 mg)	1000's
NDC 0088-0627-47	1 gr	(65 mg)	100's
NDC 0088-0627-58	1 gr	(65 mg)	1000's
NDC 0088-0628-47	2 gr	(0.13 gm)	100's
NDC 0088-0629-47	3 gr	(0.2 gm)	100's

References:

1. DiPalma, J.R.: "Drill's Pharmacology in Medicine," 3rd Edition, New York, McGraw-Hill, 1965.
2. "New Drugs," AMA Council on Drugs, 1966 Edition.
3. Goodman, L.S. & Gilman, A: "The Pharmacological Basis of Therapeutics," 3rd Edition, New York, MacMillan, 1965.
4. Sellman, T.H.: "A Manual of Pharmacology and Its Applications to Therapeutics and Toxicology," 8th Edition, Philadelphia, Saunders, 1957.
5. Beckman, H.: "Pharmacology: The Nature, Action and Use of Drugs," 2nd Edition, Philadelphia, W.B. Saunders Co., 1961.
6. Goth, A.: "Medical Pharmacology, Principles and Concepts," 3rd Edition, St. Louis, The C.V. Mosby Co., 1966.
7. Duncan, G.G.: "Diseases of Metabolism. Detailed Methods of Diagnosis and Treatment," 5th Edition, Philadelphia, W.B. Saunders Co., 1964.

Mfd. for:
Pharmaceutical Division
Marion Laboratories, Inc.
Kansas City, Missouri 64137

by:
Western Research Laboratories, Inc.
Denver, Colorado 80223
[*Shown in Product Identification Section*]

TRITEN® Tablets ℞

(dimethindene maleate NF)
2.5 mg Tab-In™

Description: TRITEN is an antihistamine occurring as a white crystalline powder that is freely soluble in methanol, soluble in chloroform, and sparingly soluble in water. Chemically, it is 2-[1-[2-[2- (dimethylamino)ethyl]-inden-3-yl]- ethyl] pyridine maleate.

Actions: Antihistamines are competitive antagonists of histamine, which also produce central nervous system effects (both stimulant and depressant) and peripheral anticholinergic, atropine-like effects (eg, drying).

Indications:
Based on a review of this drug by the National Academy of Sciences—National Research Council and/or other information, FDA has classified the indications as follows:
"Probably" effective: Perennial and seasonal allergic rhinitis; vasomotor rhinitis; allergic conjunctivitis due to inhalant allergens and foods; mild, uncomplicated allergic skin manifestations of urticaria and angiodema; amelioration of allergic reactions to blood or plasma; dermographism; anaphylactic reactions as adjunctive therapy to epinephrine and other standard measures after the acute manifestations have been controlled.
Final classification of the less-than-effective indications requires further investigation.

Contraindications: TRITEN should not be used in premature infants, neonates, or nursing mothers; patients receiving MAO inhibitors; patients with narrow angle glaucoma, stenosing peptic ulcer, symptomatic prostatic hypertrophy, bladder neck obstruction, pyloroduodenal obstruction, lower respiratory tract symptoms (including asthma), or hypersensitivity to dimethindene or related compounds.

Warnings: Antihistamines often produce drowsiness and may reduce mental alertness in children and adults. Patients should be warned about engaging in activities requiring mental alertness (eg, driving a car, operating machinery or hazardous appliances). In elderly patients, approximately 60 years or older, antihistamines are more likely to cause dizziness, sedation, and hypotension.
Patients should be warned that the central nervous system effects of TRITEN may be additive with those of alcohol and other CNS depressants (eg, hypnotics, sedatives, tranquilizers, antianxiety agents).
Antihistamines may produce excitation, particularly in children.

Usage in Pregnancy: Although no Triten-related teratogenic potential or other adverse effects on the fetus have been observed in limited animal reproduction studies, the safe use of this drug in pregnancy or during lactation has not been established. Therefore, the drug should not be used during pregnancy or lactation unless, in the judgment of the physician, the expected benefits outweigh the potential hazards.

Usage in Children: In infants and children particularly, antihistamines in overdosage may produce hallucinations, convulsions and/or death.

Precautions: Triten, like other antihistamines, has atropine-like, anticholinergic activity and should be used with caution in patients with increased intraocular pressure, hyperthyroidism, cardiovascular disease, hypertension, or history of bronchial asthma.
This product contains FD&C Yellow No. 5 (tartrazine) which may cause allergic-type reactions (including bronchial asthma) in certain susceptible individuals. Although the overall incidence of FD&C Yellow No. 5 (tartrazine) sensitivity in the general population is low, it is frequently seen in patients who also have aspirin hypersensitivity.

Adverse Reactions: The most frequent reactions to antihistamines are sedation or drowsiness; sleepiness; dryness of the mouth, nose, and throat; thickening of bronchial secretions; dizziness; disturbed coordination; epigastric distress.
Other adverse reactions which may occur are: fatigue; chills; confusion; restlessness; excitation; hysteria; nervousness; irritability; insomnia; euphoria; anorexia; nausea; vomiting; diarrhea; constipation; hypotension; tightness in the chest; wheezing; blurred vision; diplopia; vertigo; tinnitus; convulsions; headache; palpitations; tachycardia; extrasystoles; nasal stuffiness; urinary frequency; difficult urination; urinary retention; leukopenia; hemolytic anemia; thrombocytopenia; agranulocytosis; aplastic anemia; allergic or hypersensitivity reactions, including drug rash, urticaria, anaphylactic shock, and photosensitivity. Although the following may have been reported to occur in association with some antihistamines, they have not been known to result from the use of Triten: excessive perspiration, tremor, paresthesias, acute labyrinthitis, neuritis and early menses.

Dosage and Administration:
Dosage should be individualized.
Adults and children over 6 years of age: one 2.5-mg Tab-In™ once or twice daily.

Overdosage: Signs and Symptoms— The greatest danger from acute overdosage with antihistamines is their central nervous system effects which produce depression and/or stimulation.
In children, stimulation predominates initially in a syndrome which may include excitement, hallucinations, ataxia, incoordination, athetosis, and convulsions followed by postictal depression. Dry mouth, fixed dilated pupils, flushing of the face, and fever are common and resemble the syndrome of atropine poisoning.
In adults, CNS depression (ie, drowsiness, coma) is more common. CNS stimulation is rare; fever and flushing are uncommon.
In both children and adults, there can be a terminal deepening of coma and cardiovascular collapse; death can occur, especially in infants and children.
Treatment— There is no specific therapy for acute overdosage with antihistamines. General symptomatic and supportive measures should be instituted promptly and maintained for as long as necessary.
In the conscious patient, vomiting should be induced even though it may have occurred spontaneously. If vomiting cannot be induced, gastric lavage is indicated. Adequate precautions must be taken to protect against aspiration, especially in infants and children. Charcoal slurry or other suitable agent should be instilled into the stomach after vomiting or lavage. Saline cathartics or milk of magnesia may be of additional benefit.
In the unconscious patient, the airway should be secured with a cuffed endotracheal tube before attempting to evacuate the gastric contents. Intensive supportive and nursing care is indicated, as for any comatose patient.
If breathing is significantly impaired, maintenance of an adequate airway and mechanical support of respiration is the safest and most effective means of providing for adequate oxygenation of tissues to prevent hypoxia (especially brain hypoxia during convulsions).
Hypotension is an early sign of impending cardiovascular collapse and should be treated vigorously. Although general supportive measures are important, specific treatment with intravenous infusion of a vasopressor (eg, levarterenol bitartrate) titrated to maintain adequate blood pressure may be necessary.
Do *not* use CNS stimulants.
Convulsions should be controlled by careful titration of a short-acting barbiturate, repeated as necessary.
Ice packs and cooling sponge baths can aid in reducing the fever commonly seen in children.

How Supplied: Tab-In™ 2.5 mg (yellow): bottles of 100.
Tab-In™ (Marion's brand of delayed-release tablet).

Mfd. for:
Marion Laboratories, Inc.
Kansas City, Mo. 64137
by:
Ciba-Geigy Corp.
Summit, N.J. 07901

Marlyn Pharmaceutical Co., Inc.

350 PAUMA PLACE
ESCONDIDO, CA 92025

HEP-FORTE®

Description: Hep Forte is a comprehensive formulation of protein, B factors and other nutritional factors which can be important in maintenance and support of normal hepatic function.

Composition: Each capsule contains:

Vitamin A (Palmitate)	1,200 I.U.
Vitamin E (d-Alpha Tocopherol)	10 I.U.
Vitamin C (Ascorbic Acid)	10 mg.
Folic Acid	0.06 mg.
VitaminB1(ThiamineMononitrate)	1 mg.
Vitamin B2 (Riboflavin)	1 mg.
Niacinamide	10 mg.
Vitamin B6 (Pyridoxine HCl)	0.5 mg.
Vitamin B12 (Cobalamin)	1 mcg.
Biotin	3.3 mg.
Pantothenic Acid	2 mg.

Continued on next page

Marlyn—Cont.

Choline Bitartrate	21 mg.
Zinc (Zinc Sulfate)	2 mg.
Desiccated Liver	194.4 mg.
Liver Concentrate	64.8 mg.
Liver Fraction Number 2	64.8 mg.
Yeast (Dried)	64.8 mg.
dl-Methionine	10 mg.
Inositol	10 mg.

Indications: Hep Forte is of value as supportive or adjunctive treatment in cases of: alcoholism, hepatic dysfunction due to hepatotoxic drugs and liver poisons, male and female infertility due to hormonal imbalance caused by hepatic dysfunction.
Contraindications: There are no known contraindications to Hep Forte.
Dosage: Three to six capsules daily.
How Supplied: Bottles of 100, 300 or 500 capsules.
Literature Available.

MARLYN FORMULA 50

Composition: Each capsule contains:

Amino Acids	0.5 Gm*
Vitamin B6 (pyridoxine HCl)	1.0 mg.

*Approximate analysis of the amino acids: indispensable amino acids (lysine, tryptophan, phenylalanine, methionine, threonine, leucine, isoleucine, valine), 35.30%; semi-dispensable amino acids (arginine, histidine, tyrosine, cystine, glycine), 19.18%; dispensable amino acids (glutamic acid, alanine, aspartic acid, serine, proline), 45.56%.
Amino acids: Protein "building blocks" important to growth and development of all protein containing tissue including nails, hair, and skin.
Dosage and Administration: The recommended daily dose is 6 capsules daily.
Supply: Bottles of 100, 250 and 1000 capsules.

Mason Pharmaceuticals, Inc.
POST OFFICE BOX 8330
NEWPORT BEACH, CA 92660

DAMASON-P® Ⓒ℞

Description: Each pink tablet of DAMASON-P® contains:

Hydrocodone Bitartrate	5 mg
(Warning: May be habit forming)	
Aspirin	224 mg
Caffeine	32 mg

Hydrocodone is a hydrogenated ketone of codeine available as bitartrate salt.
Actions: Hydrocodone bitartrate is a semisynthetic narcotic analgesic with multiple actions qualitatively similar to those of codeine. Most of these actions involve the central nervous system and organs composed of smooth muscle producing analgesia and sedation. DAMASON-P® also contains the non-narcotic anti-inflammatory, anti-pyretic analgesic, aspirin and caffeine.
Indications and Usage: For the relief of moderate to severe pain.
Contraindications: Hypersensitivity to aspirin or hydrocodone, intracranial lesion associated with increased intracranial pressure; status asthmaticus.
Warnings:
Respiratory Depression: As with all narcotics at high doses or in sensitive patients, DAMASON-P® may produce dose-related respiratory depression by acting directly on brain stem respiratory centers.
Head Injury and Increased Intracranial Pressure: The respiratory depressant effects of narcotics and their capacity to elevate cerebrospinal fluid pressure may be markedly exaggerated in the presence of head injury, other intracranial lesions or a pre-existing increase of intracranial pressure. Furthermore, narcotics produce effects which may obscure the clinical course of patients with head injuries.
Acute Abdominal Conditions: The administration of narcotics may obscure the diagnosis or clinical course of patients with acute abdominal conditions.
Use with CNS Depressants: DAMASON-P® may have additive effects with other CNS depressants (hypnotics, sedatives, tranquilizers, anti-anxiety agents).
Other: Salicylates should be used with extreme caution in the presence of peptic ulcer or coagulation abnormalities.
Precautions:
Special Risk Patients: As with any narcotic analgesic agent, DAMASON-P® should be used with caution in elderly or debilitated patients and those with severe impairment of hepatic or renal functions, hypothyroidism, Addison's disease, prostatic hypertrophy or urethral stricture. The usual precautions should be observed and the possibility of respiratory depression should be kept in mind.
Usage in Ambulatory Patients: Hydrocodone, like all narcotics, may impair the mental and /or physical abilities required for the performance of potentially hazardous tasks such as driving a car or operating machinery; patients should be cautioned accordingly.
Cough Reflex: Hydrocodone suppresses the cough reflex; as with all narcotics, caution should be exercised when DAMASON-P® is used postoperatively and in patients with pulmonary disease.
Drug Interactions: Patients receiving other narcotic analgesics, general anesthetics, phenothiazines, other tranquilizers, sedative-hypnotics or other CNS depressants (including alcohol) concomitantly with DAMASON-P® may exhibit an additive CNS depression. When such combined therapy is contemplated, the dose of one or both agents should be reduced. Aspirin may enhance the effects of anti-coagulants and inhibit the uricosuric effects of uricosuric agents.
Usage in Pregnancy: Hydrocodone has been shown to be teratogenic in hamsters when given in doses 700 times the human dose. There are no adequate and well-controlled studies in pregnant women. DAMASON-P® should be used during pregnancy only if the potential benefit justifies the potential risk to the fetus.
Nonteratogenic Effects: Babies born to mothers who have been taking opioids regularly prior to delivery will be physically dependent. The withdrawal signs include irritability and excessive crying, tremers, hyperactive reflexes, increased respiratory rate, increased stools, sneezing, yawning, vomiting, and fever. The intensity of the syndrome does not always correlate with the duration of maternal opioid use or dose. There is no consensus on the best method of managing withdrawal.
Labor and Delivery: As with all narcotics, administration of Hydrocodone Bitartrate to the mother shortly before delivery may result in some degree of respiratory depression in the newborn, especially if higher doses are used.
Nursing Mothers: It is not known whether this drug is excreted in human milk. Because many drugs are excreted in human milk and because of the potential for serious adverse reactions in nursing infants from DAMASON-P®, a decision should be made whether to discontinue nursing or to discontinue the drug, taking into account the importance of the drug in the mother. Hydrocodone is almost completely excreted within 72 hours.
Pediatric Use: Safety and efficacy in children have not been established.
Adverse Reactions:
Central Nervous System: As with all narcotics, sedation, drowsiness, mental clouding, lethargy, impairment of mental and physical performance, anxiety, fear, dysphoria, dizziness, psychic dependence, mood changes.
Gastrointestinal System: Nausea and vomiting occur infrequently, they are more frequent in ambulatory than in recumbent patients. Administration with meals may help reduce this problem. Prolonged administration of DAMASON-P® may produce constipation.
Genitourinary System: Ureteral spasm, spasm of vesical sphincters and urinary retention have been reported with codeine derivatives.
Respiratory Depression: As with all narcotics, DAMASON-P® produces dose-related respiratory depression by acting directly on brain stem respiratory centers. DAMASON-P® also affects centers that control respiratory rhythm, and may produce irregular and periodic breathing. If significant respiratory depression occurs, it may be antagonized by the use of naloxone hydrochloride, 0.55 mg/kg intravenously. Apply other supportive measures when indicated.
Drug Abuse and Dependence: Psychic dependence, physical dependence, and tolerance may develop upon repeated administration of narcotics; therefore, DAMASON-P® should be prescribed and administered with caution. However, psychjic dependence is unlikely to develop when used for a short time for the treatment of pain.
Physical dependence, the condition in which continued administration of the drug is required to prevent the appearance of a withdrawal syndrome, assumes clinically significant proportions only after several weeks of continued narcotic use, although some mild degree of physical dependence may develop after a few days of narcotic therapy. Tolerance, in which increasingly large doses are required in order to produce the same degree of analgesia, is manifested initially by a shortened duration of analgesic effect, and subsequently by decreases in the intensity of analgesia. The rate of development of tolerance varies among patients.
Overdosage:
Aspirin: *Signs and Symptoms:* Respiratory alkalosis is characteristic of the early phase of intoxication with aspirin while hyperventilation is occurring, and is quickly followed by metabolic acidosis in most people with severe intoxication. This occurs more readily in children. Hypoglycemia may occur in children who have taken large overdoses. Other laboratory findings associated with aspirin intoxication include ketonuria, hyponatremia, hypokalemia, and occasionally protein-uria. A slight rise in lactic dehydrogenase and hydroxybutyric dehydrogenase may occur.
Methemoglobin and sulfhemoglobin formation are seldom clinically significant in adults but may contribute to general toxicity. When prominent, they appear as a grayish cyanosis seen most clearly in the lips and nailbeds. Definitive diagnosis is made by spectroscopic analysis of a water-diluted (1:100) blood specimen, which shows an abnormal band at 630 m for methemoglobin and at 618 m for sulfhemoglobin.
Concentrations of aspirin in plasma above 30 mg/100 ml are associated with toxicity. The single lethal dose of aspirin in adults is probably about 25–30 g, but is not known with certainty.
Hydrocodone: *Signs and Symptoms:* Serious overdose with hydrocodone is characterized by respiratory depression (a decrease in respiratory rate and/or tidal volume, Cheyne-Stokes respiration, cyanosis), extreme somnolence progressing to stupor or coma, skeletal muscle flaccidity, cold and clammy skin, and sometimes bradycardia and hypotension. In severe overdosage, apnea, circulatory collapse, cardiac arrest and death may occur.
Treatment: Primary attention should be given to the reestablishment of adequate respiratory exchange through provision of a patent

airway and the institution of assisted or controlled ventilation. The narcotic antagonist naloxone is a specific antidote against respiratory depression which may result from overdosage or unusual sensitivity to narcotics, including hydrocodone. Therefore, an appropriate dose of naxolone (see package insert) should be administered, preferably by the intravenous route, and simultaneously with efforts at respiratory resuscitation. Since the duration of action of hydrocodone may exceed that of the antagonist, the patient should be kept under continued surveillance and repeated doses of the antagonist should be administered as needed to maintain adequate respiration.

Dosage and Administration:
The usual adult doses of DAMASON-P® is one or two tablets every four to six hours as needed for pain. Dosage should be adjusted according to the severity of pain and the response of the patient.

Caution: Federal Law prohibits dispensing without prescription.
DAMASON-P® has a schedule III classification which permits prescription refill up to six months or five times on physician's specification.

How Supplied: DAMASON-P® is supplied as 7/16 , round, pink mottled tablets with an "M" logo on one side and "D-P" on the other. Supplied in bottles of 100, NDC 12758-055-01, bottles of 500, NDC 12758-055-05.
Manufactured by:
Anabolic Inc.
Irvine, CA 92712
Manufactured expressly for:
Mason Pharmaceuticals, Inc.
Newport Beach, CA 92660
5815C–Revised June, 1982

Mastar Pharmaceutical Co., Inc.

P.O. Box 1122
BETHLEHEM, PA 18016

ADATUSS DC™ ℂ℞
Expectorant cough syrup

Actions: Hydrocodone bitartrate is an effective semisynthetic narcotic antitussive. Guaifenesin (glyceryl guaiacolate) is an expectorant which enhances the output of lower respiratory tract fluid.

Indications: Indicated in non-productive cough spasm. It is useful in the symptomatic relief of the upper respiratory tract due to allergic conditions, the common cold, and acute bronchitis.

Contraindications: Hypersensitivity to any of the ingredients.

Precautions: Continuous dosage over an extended period is generally contraindicated since Hydrocone may cause addiction. Since drowsiness may occur, patients should be cautioned about driving or operating machinery.

Adverse Reactions: ADATUSS DC™ Expectorant is generally well tolerated. Occasional drowsiness, dizziness, gastrointestinal upset, nausea or constipation may occur.

Dosage and Administration: Adults and children over 90 lbs., one to two teaspoonsful; children 50 to 90 lbs., 1/2 to one teaspoonful; children 25 to 50 lbs., 1/4 to 1/2 teaspoonful. May be given three or four times a day as needed.

How Supplied: As a black raspberry-flavored syrup containing sugar. Comes in pints NDC 50330-301-16 and in gallons NDC 50330-301-28.

MAXIGESIC® Capsules ℂ℞

Caution: Federal Law prohibits dispensing without prescription.

Description: Each gray and white capsule contains:

Codeine Phosphate*	30 mg (1/2 gr)
Acetaminophen	325 mg
Promethazine	6.25 mg

**Warning:* May be habit forming.

Codeine occurs as colorless or white crystals, effloresces slowly in dry air and is affected by light. Acetaminophen occurs as a white, odorless crystalline powder, possessing a slightly bitter taste. It is a non-salicylate. Promethazine is a phenothiazine with sedative actions.

Actions: Provide enhanced analgesia plus mild sedation. Codeine provides analgesic and antitussive actions. Acetaminophen is an effective analgesic and antipyretic. Promethazine is a phenothiazine derivative that has several different types of pharmacologic properties. In addition to its antihistaminic action, which is of marked potency and prolonged duration, it also provides antiemetic as well as sedative actions, so that it is useful in a variety of clinical situations such as:

Preoperative, postoperative, or obstetric sedation.
Prevention and control of nausea and vomiting associated with certain types of anesthesia and surgery.
Therapy adjunctive to meperidine or other analgesics for control of postoperative pain.
Sedation in both children and adults as well as relief of apprehension and production of light sleep from which the patient can be easily aroused.
Antiemetic effect in postoperative patients.

Indications
Based on a review of this drug by the National Academy of Sciences—National Research Council and/or other information, FDA has classified the indications as follows: "Possibly" effective for the relief of moderate to moderately severe pain in those situations where the physician wishes to add a mild sedative effect.
Final classification of the less-than-effective indications requires further investigation.

Contraindications: Hypersensitivity to acetaminophen, codeine or promethazine.

Warnings:
Drug Dependence: Codeine can produce drug dependence of the morphine type, and therefore has the potential for being abused. Psychic dependence, physical dependence and tolerance may develop upon repeated administration of this drug, and it should be prescribed and administered with the same degree of caution appropriate to the use of other oral narcotic-containing medications. Like other narcotic-containing medications, this drug is subject to the Federal Controlled Substances Act.
The sedative action of promethazine hydrochloride is additive to the sedative effects of central-nervous-system depressants; therefore, agents such as alcohol, barbiturates and narcotic analgesics should either be eliminated or given in reduced dosage in the presence of promethazine hydrochloride. When given concomitantly with promethazine hydrochloride the dose of barbiturates should be reduced by at least one-half and the dose of analgesic depressants, such as morphine or meperidine, should be reduced by one-quarter to one-half.
Usage in Ambulatory Patients: Acetaminophen, codeine and promethazine may impair the mental and/or physical abilities required for the performance of potentially hazardous tasks such as driving a car or operating machinery. The patients using this drug should be cautioned accordingly.
Interaction with other central nervous system depressants: Patients receiving other narcotic analgesics, general anesthetics, phenothiazines, other tranquilizers, sedative-hypnotics or other CNS depressants (including alcohol) concomitantly with this drug may exhibit an additive CNS depression. When such combined therapy is contemplated, the dose of one or both agents should be reduced. Patients who have demonstrated a hypersensitivity reaction (e.g. blood dyscrasia, jaundice) with a phenothiazine should not be re-exposed to any phenothiazine, including Maxigesic, unless in the judgment of the physician the potential benefits of the treatment outweigh the possible hazards.
Usage in Pregnancy: Safe use in pregnancy has not been established relative to possible adverse effects on fetal development. Therefore this drug should not be used in pregnant women unless, in the judgment of the physician, the potential benefits outweigh the possible hazards.
Pediatric Use: Safe dosage has not been established in children below the age of three: the capsules should not be administered to children under 12.

Precautions:
Head Injury and Increased Intracranial Pressure: The respiratory depressant effects of narcotics and their capacity to elevate cerebrospinal fluid pressure may be markedly exaggerated in the presence of head injury, other intracranial lesions or a pre-existing increase in intracranial pressure. Furthermore, narcotics produce adverse reactions which may obscure the clinical course of patients with head injuries.
Acute Abdominal Conditions: The administration of this product or other narcotics may obscure the diagnosis or clinical course of patients with acute abdominal conditions.
Special Risk Patients: This drug should be given with caution to certain patients such as the elderly or debilitated and those with severe impairment of hepatic or renal function, hypothyroidism, Addison's disease, prostatic hypertrophy or urethral stricture.
Promethazine Precautions: Ambulatory patients should be cautioned against driving automobiles or operating dangerous machinery until it is known that they do not become drowsy or dizzy from promethazine hydrochloride therapy.
Antiemetics may mask the symptoms of an unrecognized disease and thereby interfere with diagnosis.

Adverse Reactions:
Acetaminophen and Codeine
The most frequently observed adverse reactions include lightheadedness, dizziness, drowsiness, sedation, nausea and vomiting. These effects seem to be more prominent in ambulatory than in non-ambulatory patients and some of these adverse reactions may be alleviated if patient lies down. Other adverse reactions include euphoria, dysphoria, constipation and pruritus.
Promethazine
Patients may occasionally complain of autonomic reactions such as dryness of the mouth, blurring of vision and, rarely, dizziness.
Very rare cases have been reported where patients receiving promethazine have developed leukopenia. In one instance agranulocytosis has been reported. In nearly every instance reported, other toxic agents known to have caused these conditions have been associated with the administration of promethazine.
Cardiovascular by-effects from promethazine have been rare. Minor increases in blood pressure and occasional mild hypotension have been reported.
Photosensitivity, although extremely rare, has been reported. Occurrence of photosensitivity may be a contraindication to further treatment with promethazine or related drugs. In the presence of abraded or denuded rectal lesions the patient may experience initial local

Continued on next page

Mastar—Cont.

discomfort following administration of promethazine hydrochloride suppositories.
Attempted suicides with promethazine have resulted in deep sedation, coma, rarely convulsions and cardiorespiratory symptoms compatible with the depth of sedation present. A paradoxical reaction had been reported in children receiving single doses of 75 mg. to 125 mg. orally, characterized by hyperexcitability and nightmares.
Dosage and Administration: Dosage should be adjusted according to the severity of the pain and the response of the patient. It may occasionally be necessary to exceed the usual dosage recommended below in cases of more severe pain or in those patients who have become tolerant to the analgesic effect of narcotics. Maxigesic capsules are given orally. The usual adult dose is one to two capsules every 4 to 6 hours as required.
Drug Interactions: The CNS depressant effects of this drug may be additive with that of other CNS depressants. See WARNINGS.
Management of Overdosage:
Acetaminophen
Acetaminophen in massive overdosage may cause hepatic toxicity in some patients. In adults, hepatic toxicity has rarely been reported with less than 10 grams and fatalities with less than 15 grams, taken as single, massive overdoses. Importantly, for reasons not fully understood, young children seem to be more resistant than adults to the hepatotoxic effect of an acetaminophen overdose.
Early symptoms following a potentially hepatotoxic overdose may include: nausea, vomiting, diaphoresis and general malaise. Clinical and laboratory evidence of hepatic toxicity usually are not apparent until 48 to 72 hours postingestion. Following recovery there are no residual, structural or functional hepatic abnormalities.
Since patients' estimates of the quantity of a drug ingested are notoriously unreliable, if an acetaminophen overdose is suspected a serum acetaminophen assay should be obtained as early as possible, but no sooner than four hours following ingestion. Liver function studies should be obtained initially and repeated at 24 hour intervals.
Antidotal therapy with N-acetylcysteine appears effective in preventing and/or minimizing the toxic effect of acetaminophen. For optimal results, the antidote should be administered within 16 hours of ingestion of the overdose.
The Rocky Mountain Poison Center (303-629-1123) should be contacted for assistance in interpreting plasma levels and for directions on the administration of N-acetylcysteine as an antidote, a use currently restricted to investigational status.
Codeine
Signs and Symptoms: Serious overdose with codeine is characterized by respiratory depression (a decrease in respiratory rate and/or tidal volume, Cheyne-Stokes respiration, cyanosis), extreme somnolence progressing to stupor or coma, skeletal muscle flaccidity, cold and clammy skin, and sometimes bradycardia and hypotension. In severe overdosage, apnea, circulatory collapse, cardiac arrest and death may occur.
Treatment: Primary attention should be given to the reestablishment of adequate respiratory exchange through provision of a patent airway and the institution of assisted or controlled ventilation. The narcotic antagonist naloxone is a specific antidote against respiratory depression which may result from overdosage or unusual sensitivity to narcotics, including codeine. Therefore, an appropriate dose of naloxone (see package insert) should be administered, preferably by the intravenous route, and simultaneously with efforts at respiratory resuscitation. Since the duration of action of codeine may exceed that of the antagonist, the patient should be kept under continued surveillance and repeated doses of the antagonist should be administered as needed to maintain adequate respiration.
An antagonist should not be administered in the absence of clinically significant respiratory or cardiovascular depression. Oxygen, intravenous fluids, vasopressors and other supportive measures should be employed as indicated.
Gastric emptying may be useful in removing unabsorbed drugs."
Dispensing Instructions: Dispense in Tight, Light-Resistant container as per U.S.P.N.F. recommendations.
How Supplied: MAXIGESIC® capsules supplied in bottles of 100, NDC 50330-202-01 and in bottles of 1000, NDC 50330-202-10.
Distributed by:
Mastar Pharmaceutical Co., Inc.
P.O. Box 1122
Bethlehem, PA 18016

Mayrand, Inc.
P. O. BOX 8869
FOUR DUNDAS CIRCLE
GREENSBORO, NC 27419

ANAMINE T.D.* Caps ℞
ANAMINE Syrup
Sugar-Free/Alcohol-Free/Dye-Free

Description:
ANAMINE T.D. Caps
Each Capsule Contains:
Chlorpheniramine Maleate ....8 mg.
Pseudoephedrine Hydrochloride ....120 mg.
ANAMINE Syrup
Each 5 ml (teaspoonful) contains:
Chlorpheniramine Maleate ....2 mg.
Pseudoephedrine Hydrochloride ....30 mg.
*Mayrand brand of sustained release capsules.
How Supplied: ANAMINE T.D. Caps in bottles of 100. ANAMINE Syrup in bottles of 473 ml. (1 pint).

ANATUSS Tablets and Syrup ℞

Description:
Each ANATUSS Tablet contains:
Acetaminophen ....300 mg.
Guaifenesin ....50 mg.
Dextromethorphan Hydrobromide ....10 mg.
Phenylephrine HCl ....5 mg.
Phenylpropanolamine HCl ....25 mg.
Chlorpheniramine Maleate ....2 mg.
Each 5 ml. of ANATUSS Syrup contains:
Acetaminophen ....130 mg.
Guaifenesin ....25 mg.
Dextromethorphan Hydrobromide ....5 mg.
Phenylephrine HCl ....5 mg.
Phenylpropanolamine HCl ....12.5 mg.
Chlorpheniramine Maleate ....2 mg.
Alcohol 12%
How Supplied: Anatuss Tablets are available in bottles of 100 and 500 tablets. Anatuss Syrup is available in 4 fl. oz. (120 ml.) and pint (473 ml.) bottles.

ANATUSS Tablets and Syrup w/Codeine ℞

Anatuss Tablets w/Codeine Ⓒ
Description: Each tablet contains:
Acetaminophen ....300 mg.
Guaifenesin ....100 mg.
Phenylpropanolamine HCl ....25 mg.
Chlorpheniramine Maleate ....2 mg.
Codeine Phosphate ....10 mg.
(Warning: May Be Habit Forming.)
How Supplied: Bottles of 100.

Anatuss Syrup w/Codeine Ⓒ
Description: Each 5 ml (teaspoonful) contains:
Acetaminophen ....130 mg.
Guaifenesin ....25 mg.
Phenylpropanolamine HCl ....12.5 mg.
Chlorpheniramine Maleate ....2 mg.
Codeine Phosphate ....10 mg.
(Warning: May Be Habit Forming.)
Alcohol 12%
How Supplied: 4 oz. and pint bottles.

BUFF-A COMP TABLETS ℞
Buffered Analgesic-Relaxant
Phenacetin Free

Description: Each tablet contains:
Aspirin ....(10 gr.) 648 mg.
Caffeine .... 40 mg.
Butalbital .... 50 mg.
(Warning: May be habit forming.)
Buffered with calcium carbonate.
Indication and Usage: Buff-A Comp Tablets are indicated for the symptom complex of muscle contraction (tension headache). Buff-A Comp provides an effective analgesic/relaxant with caffeine to relieve tension headache. Aspirin helps alleviate pain while butalbital reduces the tension component of the muscle contraction headache syndrome.
Contraindications: Hypersensitivity to any of the components.
Warnings:
Use In Pregnancy: Adequate studies have not been performed to establish the safety of the drug during pregnancy. Therefore, Buff-A Comp should be used cautiously and only when absolutely necessary in pregnant women.
Drug Dependency: Prolonged use of barbiturates can produce drug dependence.
Precautions: Salicylates should be used with caution in the presence of peptic ulcer or coagulation abnormalities.
Adverse Reactions: Drowsiness, dizziness, lightheadedness, gastro-intestinal disturbances; ie. nausea, vomiting and flatulence may occur.
Dosage and Administration: The usual adult dose is one tablet 3 or 4 times daily.
How Supplied: Buff-A Comp Tablets are supplied in bottles of 100.

BUFF-A COMP #3 TABLETS Ⓒ

Description: Each tablet contains:
Aspirin ....(5 gr.) 325 mg.
Butalbital ....50 mg
(Warning: May be habit forming.)
Caffeine ....40 mg.
Codeine Phosphate ....30 mg.
(Warning: May be habit forming.)
How Supplied: Buff-A Comp #3 Tablets are supplied in bottles of 100.

ELDERCAPS ℞

Description: Each capsule contains:
Vitamin A Acetate ....4,000 I.U.
Vitamin D_2....................400 I.U.
Vitamin E ....25 I.U.
Ascorbic Acid ....200 mg.
Thiamine Mononitrate ....10 mg.
Riboflavin ....5 mg.
Pyridoxine HCl ....2 mg.
Niacinamide ....25 mg.
d-Calcium Pantothenate ....10 mg.
Zinc Sulfate ....110 mg.
Magnesium Sulfate ....70 mg.
Manganese Sulfate ....5 mg.
Folic Acid ....1 mg.
Indications: ELDERCAPS are indicated for the prophylaxis or treatment of vitamin and mineral deficiencies associated with restricted diets, improper food intake, and decreased absorption or utilization. ELDERCAPS are also indicated in patients with increased requirements for vitamins and minerals due to chronic disease, infection or the stress of surgery.
Warnings: Folic acid alone is improper therapy in the treatment of pernicious anemia and

other megaloblastic anemias where vitamin B_{12} is deficient.
Precautions: Folic acid, especially in doses above 1 mg. daily, may obscure pernicious anemia, that is, hematological remission may occur while neurologic manifestations remain progressive.
Dosage: One capsule daily or as directed by the physician.
How Supplied: Bottles of 100 capsules.

ELDERTONIC Elixir ℞
Description: Each 45 ml. contains:
Thiamine HCl ....1.5 mg.
Riboflavin ....1.7 mg.
Pyridoxine HCl ....2.0 mg.
Vitamin B-12 ....6.0 mcg.
(as Cobalamin Conc.)
Dexpanthenol ....10.0 mg.
Niacinamide ....20.0 mg.
Zinc (elemental) ....15 mg.
(as zinc sulfate)
Manganese ....2.0 mg.
(as manganese sulfate)
Magnesium ....2.0 mg.
(as magnesium sulfate)
Alcohol 13.5%
In special sherry wine base.
How Supplied: 8 oz, pints, gallons.

GLYTUSS Tablets
(Guaifenesin 200 mg.)
How Supplied: Bottles of 100 and 1,000.

NU-IRON 150 Caps
NU-IRON Elixir
(polysaccharide-iron complex)
Sugar Free
Description: NU-IRON is a highly water soluble complex of iron and a low molecular weight polysaccharide.
Each NU-IRON 150 Capsule contains:
Iron (elemental) ....150 mg.
(as polysaccharide Iron Complex)
Each 5 ml. of NU-IRON Elixir contains:
Iron (elemental) ....100 mg.
(as Polysaccharide Iron Complex)
Action and Uses: NU-IRON is a non-ionic, easily assimilated, relatively non-toxic form of iron. Full therapeutic doses may be achieved with virtually no gastrointestinal side effects. There is no metallic aftertaste and no staining of teeth.
Indications: For treatment of uncomplicated iron deficiency anemia.
Contraindications: Hemochromatosis, hemosiderosis or a known hypersensitivity to any of the ingredients.
Dosage: ADULTS; One or two NU-IRON 150 Caps daily, or one or two teaspoonfuls NU-IRON Elixir daily. CHILDREN; 6 to 12 years old; one teaspoonful NU-IRON Elixir daily; 2 to 6 years old: ½ teaspoonful daily; under 2 years: ¼ teaspoonful daily.
How Supplied: NU-IRON 150 Caps in bottles of 100. NU-IRON Elixir in 8 fl. oz. bottles.

NU-IRON-PLUS ELIXIR ℞
Composition: Each 5 ml (teaspoonful) contains:
Iron (Elemental) ....100 mg.
(as Polysaccharide Iron Complex)
Folic Acid ....1 mg.
Vitamin B_{12} ....25 mcg.
Alcohol 10%
How Supplied: Bottles of 8 fl. oz.

NU-IRON-V Tablets ℞
Description: Each film-coated tablet contains:
Iron (Elemental) ....60 mg.
(as Polysaccharide Iron Complex)
Folic Acid ....1 mg.
Ascorbic Acid ....50 mg.
(as sodium ascorbate)
Cyancobalamin ....3 mcg.
(Vitamin B-12)
Vitamin A ....4000 I.U.
Vitamin D-2 ....400 I.U.
Thiamine Mononitrate ....3 mg.
Riboflavin ....3 mg.
Pyridoxine HCl ....2 mg.
Niacinamide ....10 mg.
Calcium Carbonate ....312 mg.
Indications: For the prevention and/or treatment of dietary vitamin and iron deficiencies.
Dosage: Prophylactic—one tablet daily or as directed by a physician.
Contraindications: Sensitivity to any of the ingredients.
Precautions: The use of folic acid in patients having or who may develop pernicious anemia involves the hazard of treating the anemia characteristic of the disease while permitting progressive development of combined system disease of the spinal cord.
Parenteral Vitamin B_{12} is the drug of choice in pernicious anemia and should be used in patients receiving folic acid unless pernicious anemia has been ruled out.
How Supplied: Bottles of 100 tablets.

SEDAPAP-10 Tablets ℞
Description: Each white oblong tablet contains:
Acetaminophen .... 648 mg. (10 gr.)
Butalbital .... 50 mg.
(Warning: May be habit forming)
Indications and Usage: Sedapap-10 Tablets are indicated for the symptom complex of muscle contraction (tension headache). Sedapap-10 provides an effective analgesic/relaxant to relieve tension headache. Acetaminophen helps alleviate pain while butalbital reduces the tension component of the muscle contraction headache syndrome.
Contraindications: In patients with hepatic disease and in patients sensitive to either component.
Warnings:
Use in Pregnancy: Adequate studies have not been performed to establish the safety of the drug during pregnancy. Therefore, Sedapap-10 should be used cautiously and only when absolutely necessary in pregnant women.
Drug Dependency: Prolonged use of barbituates can produce drug dependence.
Adverse Reactions: Drowsiness, dizziness, lightheadedness, gastrointestinal disturbances; ie. nausea, vomiting and flatulence may occur.
Dosage and Administration: The usual adult dose is one tablet 3 or 4 times daily.
How Supplied: Sedapap-10 Tablets are supplied in bottles of 100.

SORBIDE ℞
(Isosorbide Dinitrate)
Available as:
SORBIDE T.D. * Capsules 40 mg.
*MAYRAND brand of sustained release Capsules.
How Supplied: Bottles of 100.

STERAPRED UNI-PAK ℞
(Prednisone 5 mg.)
Prednisone in convenient decremental dosage, for unit dispensing.
How Supplied: Box of 21 tablets.

TRIMCAPS Ⓒ ℞
(Phendimetrazine Tartrate 105 mg.)
Slow Release Capsule
How Supplied: Bottles of 30 and 100.

TRIMTABS Ⓒ ℞
(Phendimetrazine Tartrate 35 mg.)
How Supplied: Bottles of 100 and 500.

McGregor Pharmaceuticals
32580 GRAND RIVER AVENUE
FARMINGTON, MI 48024

ALL McGREGOR PRODUCTS ARE COMPLETELY DYE FREE.

Full prescribing information for all McGregor Pharmaceuticals products is available from your McGregor Pharmaceuticals representative.

Product Identification Codes
To provide quick and positive identification of McGregor Pharmaceuticals products, we have had imprinted the product identification number on our capsules. In order that you may quickly identify a product by its code number, we provide the following list of code numbers:

Product	Code Number
Rhinafed™ (Chlorpheniramine Maleate 8 mg, Pseudoephedrine HCl 120 mg, Methscopolamine Nitrate 2.5 mg) Sustained Release Capsules ℞	MCG 217
Rhinafed-EX™ (Chlorpheniramine Maleate 8 mg, Pseudoephedrine HCl 120 mg) Sustained Release Capsules ℞	MCG 216
Rhindecon™ (Phenylpropanolamine HCl, 75 mg) Sustained Release Capsules ℞	MCG 215
Rhindecon-G™ (Phenylpropanolamine HCl 50 mg, Guaifenesin 200 mg) Single Dose Capsule ℞	MCG 213
Rhinolar™ (Phenylpropanolamine HCl 75 mg, Chlorpheniramine Maleate 8 mg, Methscopolamine Nitrate 2.5 mg) Sustained Release Capsule ℞	MCG 219
Rhinolar-EX™ (Phenylpropanolamine HCl 75 mg, Chlorpheniramine Maleate 8 mg) Sustained Release Capsule ℞	MCG 210
Rhinolar-EX 12™ (Phenylpropanolamine HCl 75 mg, Chlorpheniramine Maleate 12 mg) Sustained Release Capsule ℞	MCG 211

McNeil Consumer Products Company
McNEILAB, INC.
FORT WASHINGTON, PA 19034

COTYLENOL® Cold Formula Tablets and Capsules OTC
Description: Each CoTYLENOL tablet or capsule contains acetaminophen 325 mg., chlorpheniramine maleate 2 mg., pseudoephedrine hydrochloride 30 mg. and dextromethorphan hydrobromide 15 mg.
Actions and Indications: CoTYLENOL Cold Formula Tablets and Capsules combine the non-salicylate analgesic-antipyretic acetaminophen with the decongestant pseudoephedrine hydrochloride, the cough suppressant dextromethorphan hydrobromide and the antihistamine chlorpheniramine maleate to help relieve nasal congestion and coughing, as well as fever, aches, pains and general discom-

Continued on next page

McNeil Consumer—Cont.

fort associated with colds and other upper respiratory infections.
While the acetaminophen component is equal to aspirin in analgesic and antipyretic effectiveness, it is unlikely to produce many of the side effects associated with aspirin and aspirin-containing products.
Usual Dosage: Adults: Two tablets or capsules every 6 hours, not to exceed 8 tablets or capsules per day. Children (6–12 years): One capsule or tablet every 6 hours, not to exceed 4 tablets or capsules per day.
Note: Since CoTYLENOL Cold Formula Tablets and Capsules are available without prescription, the following appears on the package label: "WARNING: Do not exceed the recommended dosage or administer to children under 6. Reduce dosage if nervousness, restlessness, or sleeplessness occurs. Persistent cough may indicate a serious condition. Persons with a high fever, rash, or persistent cough or headache or asthma, emphysema or with glaucoma, high blood pressure, heart disease, diabetes, thyroid disease, enlargement of the prostate gland, or who are presently taking a prescription drug for the treatment of high blood pressure or emotional disorders, do not take, except under the advice and supervision of a physician. This preparation may cause drowsiness. Do not drive or operate machinery while taking this medication. If symptoms do not improve within five days, consult a physician before continuing use. **Do not use if safety seal is broken. Keep this and all medication out of the reach of children. If pregnant or nursing, seek medical advice before taking this or any medicine. In case of accidental overdosage, contact a physician or poison control center immediately."**
Overdosage: Acetaminophen in massive overdosage may cause hepatic toxicity in some patients. In all cases of suspected overdose, immediately call your regional poison center or the Rocky Mountain Poison Center's toll-free number (800-525-6115) for assistance in diagnosis and for directions in the use of N-acetylcysteine as an antidote, a use currently restricted to investigational status.
In adults, hepatic toxicity has rarely been reported with acute overdoses of less than 10 grams and fatalities with less than 15 grams. Importantly, young children seem to be more resistant than adults to the hepatotoxic effect of an acetaminophen overdose. Despite this, the measures outlined below should be initiated in any adult or child suspected of having ingested an acetaminophen overdose.
Early symptoms following a potentially hepatotoxic overdose may include: nausea, vomiting, diaphoresis and general malaise. Clinical and laboratory evidence of hepatic toxicity may not be apparent until 48 to 72 hours post-ingestion.
The stomach should be emptied promptly by lavage or by induction of emesis with syrup of ipecac. Patients' estimates of the quantity of a drug ingested are notoriously unreliable. Therefore, if an acetaminophen overdose is suspected, a serum acetaminophen assay should be obtained as early as possible, but no sooner than four hours following ingestion. Liver function studies should be obtained initially and repeated at 24-hour intervals. The antidote, N-acetylcysteine, should be administered as early as possible, and within 16 hours of the overdose ingestion for optimal results. Following recovery, there are no residual, structural or functional hepatic abnormalities.
How Supplied: Tablets (colored yellow, imprinted "CoTYLENOL")—vials of 10, blister packs of 24, tamper-resistant bottles of 50 and 100. Capsules (colored dark green and light yellow, imprinted "CoTYLENOL")—blister packs of 20 and tamper-resistant bottles of 40.
[*Shown in Product Identification Section*]

COTYLENOL® LIQUID COLD FORMULA — OTC

Description: Each 30 ml (1 fl. oz.) contains acetaminophen 650 mg, chlorpheniramine maleate 4 mg, pseudoephedrine hydrochloride 60 mg, and dextromethorphan hydrobromide 30 mg (alcohol 7.5%).
Actions and Indications: CoTylenol Liquid Cold Formula combines the non-salicylate analgesic-antipyretic acetaminophen with the decongestant pseudoephedrine hydrochloride, the cough suppressant dextromethorphan hydrobromide and the antihistamine chlorpheniramine maleate to help relieve nasal congestion and coughing, as well as the fever, aches, pains and general discomfort associated with colds and other upper respiratory infections.
While the acetaminophen component is equal to aspirin in analgesic and antipyretic effectiveness, it is unlikely to produce many of the side effects associated with aspirin and aspirin-containing products.
Usual Dosage: Measuring cup is provided and marked for accurate dosing. Adults: 1 fluid ounce (2 tbsp.) every 6 hours as needed, not to exceed 4 doses in 24 hours. Children (6–12 yrs.): ½ the adult dose (1 tbsp.) as indicated on the measuring cup provided, not to exceed 4 doses in 24 hours.
Note: Since CoTylenol Liquid Cold Formula is available without a prescription, the following appears on the package label: "WARNING: Do not exceed the recommended dosage or administer to children under 6. Reduce dosage if nervousness, restlessness or sleeplessness occurs. Persistent cough may indicate a serious condition. Persons with a high fever, rash or persistent cough or headache or asthma, emphysema or with glaucoma, high blood pressure, heart disease, diabetes, thyroid disease, enlargement of the prostate gland, or who are presently taking a prescription drug for the treatment of high blood pressure or emotional disorders, do not take, except under the advice and supervision of a physician. This preparation may cause drowsiness. Do not drive or operate machinery while taking this medication. If symptoms do not improve within five days, consult a physician before continuing use. **Do not use if safety seals are broken. Keep this and all medication out of the reach of children. If pregnant or nursing, seek medical advice before taking this or any medicine. In case of accidental overdosage, contact a physician or poison control center immediately."**
Overdosage: Acetaminophen in massive overdosage may cause hepatic toxicity in some patients. In all cases of suspected overdose, immediately call your regional poison center or the Rocky Mountain Poison Center's toll-free number (800-525-6115) for assistance in diagnosis and for directions in the use of N-acetylcysteine as an antidote, a use currently restricted to investigational status.
In adults, hepatic toxicity has rarely been reported with acute overdoses of less than 10 grams and fatalities with less than 15 grams. Importantly, young children seem to be more resistant than adults to the hepatotoxic effect of an acetaminophen overdose. Despite this, the measures outlined below should be initiated in any adult or child suspected of having ingested an acetaminophen overdose.
Early symptoms following a potentially hepatotoxic overdose may include: nausea, vomiting, diaphoresis and general malaise. Clinical and laboratory evidence of hepatic toxicity may not be apparent until 48 to 72 hours post-ingestion.
The stomach should be emptied promptly by lavage or by induction of emesis with syrup of ipecac. Patients' estimates of the quantity of a drug ingested are notoriously unreliable. Therefore, if an acetaminophen overdose is suspected, a serum acetaminophen assay should be obtained as early as possible, but no sooner than four hours following ingestion. Liver function studies should be obtained initially and repeated at 24-hour intervals.
The antidote, N-acetylcysteine, should be administered as early as possible, and within 16 hours of the overdose ingestion for optimal results. Following recovery, there are no residual, structural or functional hepatic abnormalities.
How Supplied: Cherry/mint mentholated flavored (colored amber) bottles of 5 and 10 oz. with child-resistant safety cap, special dosage cup graded in ounces and tablespoons, and tamper-resistant packaging.

CHILDREN'S CoTYLENOL® — OTC
Chewable Cold Tablets and Liquid Cold Formula

Description: Each Children's CoTYLENOL Chewable Cold Tablet contains acetaminophen 80 mg, chlorpheniramine maleate 0.5 mg and phenylpropanolamine hydrochloride 3.125 mg. Children's CoTYLENOL Liquid Cold Formula is stable, cherry-flavored, red in color and contains 8.5% alcohol. Each teaspoon (5 ml) contains acetaminophen 160 mg, chlorpheniramine maleate 1 mg, and phenylpropanolamine hydrochloride 6.25 mg.
Actions and Indications: Children's CoTYLENOL Chewable Cold Tablets and Liquid Cold Formula combine the nonsalicylate analgesic-antipyretic acetaminophen with the decongestant phenylpropanolamine hydrochloride and the antihistamine chlorpheniramine maleate to help relieve nasal congestion, dry runny noses and prevent sneezing as well as to relieve the fever, aches, pains and general discomfort associated with colds and upper respiratory infections.
While the acetaminophen component is equal to aspirin in analgesic and antipyretic effectiveness, it is unlikely to produce the following side effects often associated with aspirin or aspirin-containing products: allergic reactions, even in aspirin-sensitive children or those with a history of allergy in general; "therapeutic toxicity" in feverish children, since electrolyte imbalance and acid-base changes are not likely to occur; gastric irritation even in children with an already upset stomach.
Dosage: Children's CoTYLENOL Chewable Cold Tablets: 2–3 years—2 tablets, 4–5 years—3 tablets; 6–8 years—4 tablets; 9–10 years—5 tablets; 11 years—6 tablets.
Children's CoTYLENOL Liquid Cold Formula: Measuring cup is provided and marked for accurate dosing. 2–3 years—1 teaspoonful; 4–5 years—1 ½ teaspoonfuls; 6–8 years—2 teaspoonfuls; 9–10 years—2 ½ teaspoonfuls; 11 years—3 teaspoonfuls.
Doses may be repeated every 4 hours as needed, not to exceed 4 doses in 24 hours.
Note: Since Children's CoTYLENOL Chewable Cold Tablets and Liquid Cold Formula are available without prescription, the following information appears on the package labels: "WARNING: Do not exceed the recommended dosage. Reduce dosage if nervousness, restlessness or sleeplessness occurs. Do not use if glaucoma, high blood pressure, heart disease, diabetes, or thyroid disease is present. This preparation may cause drowsiness, or in some instances, excitability. If presently taking a prescription drug for the treatment of high blood pressure or emotional disorders, or if you have asthma, do not use except under advice and supervision of a physician. Do not drive or operate machinery while taking this medication. If symptoms do not improve within seven days, or are accompanied by high fever or persistent cough, consult a physician before continuing use.
DO NOT USE IF SAFETY SEALS ARE BROKEN. KEEP THIS AND ALL MEDICINE OUT

OF THE REACH OF CHILDREN. IN CASE OF ACCIDENTAL OVERDOSAGE, CONTACT A PHYSICIAN OR POISON CONTROL CENTER IMMEDIATELY.

Overdosage: Acetaminophen in massive overdosage may cause hepatic toxicity in some patients. In all cases of suspected overdose, immediately call your regional poison center or the Rocky Mountain Poison Center's toll-free number (800-525-6115) for assistance in diagnosis and for directions in the use of N-acetylcysteine as an antidote, a use currently restricted to investigational status.

In adults, hepatic toxicity has rarely been reported with acute overdoses of less than 10 grams and fatalities with less than 15 grams. Importantly, young children seem to be more resistant than adults to the hepatotoxic effect of an acetaminophen overdose. Despite this, the measures outlined below should be initiated in any adult or child suspected of having ingested an acetaminophen overdose.

Early symptoms following a potentially hepatotoxic overdose may include: nausea, vomiting, diaphoresis and general malaise. Clinical and laboratory evidence of hepatic toxicity may not be apparent until 48 to 72 hours post-ingestion.

The stomach should be emptied promptly by lavage or by induction of emesis with syrup of ipecac. Patients' estimates of the quantity of a drug ingested are notoriously unreliable.

Therefore, if an acetaminophen overdose is suspected, a serum acetaminophen assay should be obtained as early as possible, but no sooner than four hours following ingestion. Liver function studies should be obtained initially and repeated at 24-hour intervals. The antidote, N-acetylcysteine, should be administered as early as possible, and within 16 hours of the overdose ingestion for optimal results. Following recovery, there are no residual, structural or functional hepatic abnormalities.

How Supplied: Chewable Tablets (colored orange, scored, imprinted "CoTYLENOL")—bottles of 24. Cold Formula—bottles (colored red) of 4 fl. oz.

[*Shown in Product Identification Section*]

SINE-AID® OTC
Sinus Headache Tablets

Description: Each SINE-AID Tablet contains acetaminophen 325 mg. and phenylpropanolamine hydrochloride 25 mg.

Actions: Acetaminophen is a clinically proven analgesic-antipyretic. Acetaminophen produces analgesia by elevation of the pain threshold and antipyresis through action on the hypothalamic heat-regulating center. Phenylpropanolamine hydrochloride is a sympathomimetic amine and provides vasoconstriction to the nasopharyngeal mucosa. Although similar in action to ephedrine, phenylpropanolamine HCl is less likely to cause CNS stimulation.

Indications: SINE-AID provides effective symptomatic relief from sinus headache pain and pressure caused by sinusitis. Since it contains no antihistamine, SINE-AID will not produce the drowsiness that may interfere with work, driving an automobile or operating dangerous machinery. SINE-AID is particularly well suited in patients with aspirin allergy, hemostatic disturbances (including anticoagulant therapy), and bleeding diatheses (e.g. hemophilia) and upper gastrointestinal disease (e.g. ulcer, gastritis, hiatus hernia).

Precautions and Adverse Reactions: Acetaminophen has rarely been found to produce any side effects. It is usually well tolerated by aspirin-sensitive patients. If a rare sensitivity reaction occurs, the drug should be stopped. In patients with high blood pressure, diabetes, or thyroid disease, phenylpropanolamine hydrochloride should be used with caution and only as directed by a physician. Do not use in patients receiving MAO inhibitors.

Usual Dosage: Adult dosage: Two tablets every four hours, no more than 6 tablets in any 24-hour period.

Note: Since SINE-AID tablets are available without a prescription, the following appears on the package labels: "CAUTION: Individuals with high blood pressure, heart disease, diabetes, thyroid disease, and children under 12 should use only as directed by a physician. Do not exceed recommended dosage unless directed by a physician. WARNING: If symptoms of sinusitis or colds persist after 3 days, consult a physician. **Keep this and all medications out of the reach of children. If pregnant or nursing, seek medical advice before taking this or any medicine. In case of accidental overdosage, contact a physician or poison control center immediately.**"

Overdosage: Acetaminophen in massive overdosage may cause hepatic toxicity in some patients. In all cases of suspected overdose, immediately call your regional poison center or the Rocky Mountain Poison Center's toll-free number (800-525-6115) for assistance in diagnosis and for directions in the use of N-acetylcysteine as an antidote, a use currently restricted to investigational status.

In adults, hepatic toxicity has rarely been reported with acute overdoses of less than 10 grams and fatalities with less than 15 grams. Importantly, young children seem to be more resistant than adults to the hepatotoxic effect of an acetaminophen overdose. Despite this, the measures outlined below should be initiated in any adult or child suspected of having ingested an acetaminophen overdose.

Early symptoms following a potentially hepatotoxic overdose may include: nausea, vomiting, diaphoresis and general malaise. Clinical and laboratory evidence of hepatic toxicity may not be apparent until 48 to 72 hours post-ingestion.

The stomach should be emptied promptly by lavage or by induction of emesis with syrup of ipecac. Patients' estimates of the quantity of a drug ingested are notoriously unreliable. Therefore, if an acetaminophen overdose is suspected, a serum acetaminophen assay should be obtained as early as possible, but no sooner than four hours following ingestion. Liver function studies should be obtained initially and repeated at 24-hour intervals.

The antidote, N-acetylcysteine, should be administered as early as possible, and within 16 hours of the overdose ingestion for optimal results. Following recovery, there are no residual, structural or functional hepatic abnormalities.

How Supplied: Tablets (colored white, imprinted "SINE-AID")—bottles of 24, 50 and 100.

CHILDREN'S TYLENOL® OTC
acetaminophen
Chewable Tablets, Elixir, Drops

Description: Each Children's TYLENOL Chewable Tablet contains 80 mg. acetaminophen in a fruit flavored tablet. Children's TYLENOL acetaminophen Elixir is stable, cherry flavored, red in color and contains 7% alcohol. Infants' TYLENOL Drops are stable, fruit flavored, orange in color and contain 7% alcohol. Children's TYLENOL Elixir: Each 5 ml. contains 160 mg. acetaminophen.

Infant's TYLENOL Drops: Each 0.8 ml. (one calibrated dropperful) contains 80 mg. acetaminophen.

Actions: TYLENOL acetaminophen is an antipyretic and analgesic clinically proven in pediatric use. TYLENOL acetaminophen produces antipyresis through action on the hypothalamic heat-regulating center and analgesia by elevation of the pain threshold.

Indications: Children's TYLENOL Chewable Tablets, Elixir and Drops are designed for treatment of infants and children with conditions requiring reduction of fever or relief of pain—such as mild upper respiratory infections (tonsillitis, common cold, "grippe"), headache, myalgia, post-immunization reactions, post-tonsillectomy discomfort and gastroenteritis. In conjunction with antibiotics or sulfonamides, TYLENOL acetaminophen is useful as an analgesic and antipyretic in many bacterial or viral infections, such as bronchitis, pharyngitis, tracheobronchitis, sinusitis, pneumonia, otitis media, and cervical adenitis.

Precautions and Adverse Reactions: If a rare sensitivity reaction occurs, the drug should be stopped. TYLENOL acetaminophen has rarely been found to produce any side effects. It is usually well tolerated by aspirin-sensitive patients.

Usual Dosage: Doses may be repeated 4 or 5 times daily, but not to exceed 5 doses in 24 hours. Children's TYLENOL Chewable Tablets: 1–2 years: one and one half tablets. 2–3 years: two tablets. 4–5 years: three tablets. 6–8 years: four tablets. 9–10 years: five tablets. 11–12 years: six tablets.

Children's TYLENOL Elixir: (special cup for measuring dosage is provided) 4–11 months: one-half teaspoon. 12–23 months: three-quarters teaspoon, 2–3 years: one teaspoon. 4–5 years: one and one-half teaspoons. 6–8 years: 2 teaspoons. 9–10 years: two and one-half teaspoons. 11–12 years: three teaspoons.

Infants' TYLENOL Drops: 0–3 months: 0.4 ml. 4–11 months: 0.8 ml. 12–23 months: 1.2 ml. 2–3 years: 1.6 ml. 4–5 years: 2.4 ml.

Note: Since Children's TYLENOL acetaminophen Chewable Tablets, Elixir and Drops are available without prescription as an analgesic, the following appears on the package labels: "WARNING: Consult your physician if fever persists for more than three days or if pain continues for more than five days. **Do not use if safety seals are broken. Keep this and all medication out of the reach of children. In cases of accidental overdosage, contact a physician or poison control center immediately.**"

Overdosage: Acetaminophen in massive overdosage may cause hepatic toxicity in some patients. In all cases of suspected overdose, immediately call your regional poison center or the Rocky Mountain Poison Center's toll-free number (800-525-6115) for assistance in diagnosis and for directions in the use of N-acetylcysteine as an antidote, a use currently restricted to investigational status.

The occurrence of acetaminophen overdose toxicity is uncommon in the pediatric age group. Even with large overdoses, children appear to be less vulnerable than adults to developing hepatotoxicity. This may be due to age-related differences that have been demonstrated in the metabolism of acetaminophen. Despite these differences, the measures outlined below should be immediately initiated in any child suspected of having ingested an overdose of acetaminophen.

Early symptoms following a potentially hepatotoxic overdose may include: nausea, vomiting, diaphoresis and general malaise. Clinical and laboratory evidence of hepatic toxicity may not be apparent until 48 to 72 hours post-ingestion. The stomach should be emptied promptly by lavage or by induction of emesis with syrup of ipecac. If an acute dose of 150 mg/kg body weight or greater was ingested, or if the dose cannot be accurately determined, a serum acetaminophen assay should be obtained as early as possible, but no sooner than four hours following ingestion. Liver function studies should be obtained initially and repeated at 24-hour intervals. The antidote, N-acetylcysteine, should be administered as early as possible, and within 16 hours of the overdose ingestion for optimal results. Following recovery, there are no residual, structural or functional hepatic abnormalities.

Continued on next page

McNeil Consumer—Cont.

How Supplied: Chewable Tablets (colored pink, scored, imprinted "TYLENOL")—Bottles of 30. Elixir (colored red)—bottles of 2 and 4 fl. oz. Drops (colored orange)—bottles of ½ oz. (15 ml.) with calibrated plastic dropper.
All packages listed above have child-resistant safety caps.
[Shown in Product Identification Section]

Regular Strength TYLENOL® acetaminophen Tablets and Capsules OTC

Description: Each Regular Strength TYLENOL Tablet or Capsule contains acetaminophen 325 mg.
Actions: TYLENOL acetaminophen is a clinically proven analgesic and antipyretic. TYLENOL acetaminophen produces analgesia by elevation of the pain threshold and antiypresis through action on the hypothalamic heat-regulating center.
Indications: TYLENOL acetaminophen provides effective analgesia in a wide variety of arthritic and rheumatic conditions involving musculoskeletal pain, as well as in other painful disorders such as headache, dysmenorrhea, myalgias and neuralgias. In addition, TYLENOL acetaminophen is indicated as an analgesic and antipyretic in diseases accompanied by discomfort and fever, such as the common cold and other viral infections. TYLENOL acetaminophen is particularly well suited as an analgesic-antipyretic in the presence of aspirin allergy, hemostatic disturbances (including anticoagulant therapy), and bleeding diatheses (e.g., hemophilia) and upper gastrointestinal disease (e.g., ulcer, gastritis, hiatus hernia).
Precautions and Adverse Reactions: If a rare sensitivity reaction occurs, the drug should be stopped. TYLENOL acetaminophen has rarely been found to produce any side effects. It is usually well tolerated by aspirin-sensitive patients.
Usual Dosage: Adults: One to two tablets or capsules every 4–6 hours. Not to exceed 12 tablets or capsules per day. Children (6 to 12): One-half to one tablet 3 or 4 times daily. (TYLENOL acetaminophen Chewable Tablets, Elixir and Drops are available for greater convenience in younger patients).
Note: Since TYLENOL acetaminophen tablets and capsules are available without prescription as an analgesic, the following appears on the package labels: "Caution: If pain persists for more than 10 days, or redness is present, or in arthritic or rheumatic conditions affecting children under 12 years, consult a physician immediately." "**WARNING: Do not use if safety seals are broken. Keep this and all medications out of the reach of children. If pregnant or nursing, seek medical advice before taking this or any medicine. In case of accidental overdosage, contact a physician or poison control center immediately.**"
Overdosage: Acetaminophen in massive overdosage may cause hepatic toxicity in some patients. In all cases of suspected overdose, immediately call your regional poison center or the Rocky Mountain Poison Center's toll-free number (800-525-6115) for assistance in diagnosis and for directions in the use of N-acetylcysteine as an antidote, a use currently restricted to investigational status.
In adults, hepatic toxicity has rarely been reported with acute overdoses of less than 10 grams and fatalities with less than 15 grams. Importantly, young children seem to be more resistant than adults to the hepatotoxic effect of an acetaminophen overdose. Despite this, the measures outlined below should be initiated in any adult or child suspected of having ingested an acetaminophen overdose.
Early symptoms following a potentially hepatotoxic overdose may include: nausea, vomiting, diaphoresis and general malaise. Clinical and laboratory evidence of hepatic toxicity may not be apparent until 48 to 72 hours post-ingestion.
The stomach should be emptied promptly by lavage or by induction of emesis with syrup of ipecac. Patients' estimates of the quantity of a drug ingested are notoriously unreliable. Therefore, if an acetaminophen overdose is suspected, a serum acetaminophen assay should be obtained as early as possible, but no sooner than four hours following ingestion. Liver function studies should be obtained initially and repeated at 24-hour intervals. The antidote, N-acetylcysteine, should be administered as early as possible, and within 16 hours of the overdose ingestion for optimal results. Following recovery, there are no residual, structural or functional hepatic abnormalities.
How Supplied: Tablets (colored white, scored, imprinted "TYLENOL")—tins and vials of 12, and tamper-resistant bottles of 24, 50, 100 and 200. Capsules (colored gray and white, imprinted "TYLENOL 325 mg.")—tamper-resistant bottles of 24, 50 and 100.
Also Available: For additional pain relief, Extra-Strength TYLENOL® Tablets and Capsules, 500 mg, and Extra-Strength TYLENOL® Adult Liquid Pain Reliever (colored green; 1 fl. oz. = 1000 mg.)
[Shown in Product Identification Section]

Extra-Strength TYLENOL® acetaminophen Tablets and Capsules OTC

Description: Each Extra-Strength TYLENOL Tablet or Capsule contains acetaminophen 500 mg.
Actions: TYLENOL acetaminophen is a clinically proven analgesic and antipyretic. Acetaminophen produces analgesia by elevation of the pain threshold and antipyresis through action on the hypothalamic heat-regulating center.
Indications: For relief of pain and fever. Extra-Strength TYLENOL acetaminophen Tablets and Capsules provide increased analgesic strength for minor conditions when the usual doses of mild analgesics are insufficient.
Precautions and Adverse Reactions: If a rare sensitivity reaction occurs, the drug should be stopped. TYLENOL acetaminophen has rarely been found to produce any side effects. It is usually well tolerated by aspirin-sensitive patients.
Usual Dosage: Adults: Two tablets or capsules 3 or 4 times daily. No more than a total of eight tablets or capsules in any 24-hour period.
Note: Since Extra-Strength TYLENOL acetaminophen Tablets or Capsules are available without a prescription, the following appears on the package labels: "Severe or recurrent pain or high or continued fever may be indicative of serious illness. Under these conditions, consult a physician. **WARNING: Do not use if safety seals are broken. Keep this and all medication out of the reach of children. If pregnant or nursing, seek medical advice before taking this or any medicine. In case of accidental overdosage, contact a physician or poison control center immediately.**"
Overdosage: Acetaminophen in massive overdosage may cause hepatic toxicity in some patients. In all cases of suspected overdose, immediately call your regional poison center or the Rocky Mountain Poison Center's toll-free number (800-525-6115) for assistance in diagnosis and for directions in the use of N-acetylcysteine as an antidote, a use currently restricted to investigational status.
In adults, hepatic toxicity has rarely been reported with acute overdoses of less than 10 grams and fatalities with less than 15 grams. Importantly, young children seem to be more resistant than adults to the hepatotoxic effect of an acetaminophen overdose. Despite this, the measures outlined below should be initiated in any adult or child suspected of having ingested an acetaminophen overdose.
Early symptoms following a potentially hepatotoxic overdose may include: nausea, vomiting, diaphoresis and general malaise. Clinical and laboratory evidence of hepatic toxicity may not be apparent until 48 to 72 hours post-ingestion.
The stomach should be emptied promptly by lavage or by induction of emesis with syrup of ipecac. Patients' estimates of the quantity of a drug ingested are notoriously unreliable. Therefore, if an acetaminophen overdose is suspected, a serum acetaminophen assay should be obtained as early as possible, but no sooner than four hours following ingestion. Liver function studies should be obtained initially and repeated at 24-hour intervals. The antidote, N-acetylcysteine, should be administered as early as possible, and within 16 hours of the overdose ingestion for optimal results. Following recovery, there are no residual, structural or functional hepatic abnormalities.
How Supplied: Tablets (colored white, imprinted "TYLENOL" and "500")—vials of 10 and tamper-resistant bottles of 30, 60, 100, and 200; Capsules (colored red and white, imprinted "TYLENOL 500 mg.")—vial of 8, tamper-resistant bottles of 24, 50, 100 and 165.
Also Available: For adults who prefer liquids or can't swallow solid medication, Extra-Strength TYLENOL® Adult Liquid Pain Reliever (colored green; 1 fl. oz. = 1000 mg.).
[Shown in Product Identification Section]

Extra-Strength TYLENOL® acetaminophen Adult Liquid Pain Reliever OTC

Description: Each 15 ml. (½ fl. oz. or one tablespoonful) contains 500 mg. acetaminophen (alcohol 8 ½%).
Actions: TYLENOL acetaminophen is a clinically proven analgesic and antipyretic. Acetaminophen produces analgesia by elevation of the pain threshold and antipyresis through action on the hypothalamic heat-regulating center.
Indications: TYLENOL acetaminophen provides fast, effective relief of pain and/or fever for adults who prefer liquids or can't swallow solid medication, e.g., the aged, patients with easily triggered gag reflexes, extremely sore throats, or those on liquid diets.
Precautions and Adverse Reactions: If a rare sensitivity reaction occurs, the drug should be stopped. TYLENOL acetaminophen has rarely been found to produce any side effects. It is usually well tolerated by aspirin-sensitive patients.
Usual Dosage: Extra-Strength TYLENOL Adult Liquid Pain Reliever is an adult preparation. Not for use in children under 12. Measuring cup is marked for accurate dosage.
Extra-Strength Dose—1 fl. oz. (30 ml or 2 tablespoonsful, 1000 mg) which is equivalent to two 500 mg Extra-Strength TYLENOL Tablets or Capsules. Take every 4–6 hours, no more than 4 doses in any 24–hour period.
Note: Since Extra-Strength TYLENOL Adult Liquid Pain Reliever is available without a prescription, the following appears on the package labels: "Severe or recurrent pain or high or continued fever may be indicative of serious illness. Under these conditions, consult a physician. **WARNING: Do not use if safety seals are broken. Keep this and all medication out of the reach of children. If pregnant or nursing, seek medical advice before taking this or any medicine. In case of accidental overdosage, contact a physician or poison control center immediately.**"
Overdosage: Acetaminophen in massive overdosage may cause hepatic toxicity in some patients. In all cases of suspected overdose, immediately call your regional poison center or the Rocky Mountain Poison Center's toll-free number (800-525-6115) for assistance in

diagnosis and for directions in the use of N-acetylcysteine as an antidote, a use currently restricted to investigational status.
In adults, hepatic toxicity has rarely been reported with acute overdoses of less than 10 grams and fatalitites with less than 15 grams. Importantly, young children seem to be more resistant than adults to the hepatotoxic effect of an acetaminophen overdose. Despite this, the measures outlined below should be initiated in any adult or child suspected of having ingested an acetaminophen overdose.
Early symptoms following a potentially hepatotoxic overdose may include: nausea, vomiting, diaphoresis and general malaise. Clinical and laboratory evidence of hepatic toxicity may not be apparent until 48 to 72 hours post-ingestion.
The stomach should be emptied promptly by lavage or by induction of emesis with syrup of ipecac. Patients' estimates of the quantity of a drug ingested are notoriously unreliable. Therefore, if an acetaminophen overdose is suspected, a serum acetaminophen assay should be obtained as early as possible, but no sooner than four hours following ingestion. Liver function studies should be obtained initially and repeated at 24-hour intervals.
The antidote, N-acetylcysteine, should be administered as early as possible, and within 16 hours of the overdose ingestion for optimal results. Following recovery, there are no residual, structural or functional hepatic abnormalities.
How Supplied: Mint-flavored liquid (colored green), 8 fl. oz. tamper-resistant bottle with child resistent safety cap and special dosage cup.

Maximum-Strength TYLENOL® Sinus Medication — OTC
Tablets and Capsules

Description: Each Maximum-Strength TYLENOL® Sinus Medication tablet or capsule contains acetaminophen 500 mg and pseudoephedrine hydrochloride 30 mg.
Actions: TYLENOL Sinus Medication contains a clinically proven decongestant and analgesic. Maximum allowable non-prescription levels of pseudoephedrine and acetaminophen provide temporary relief of sinus congestion and pain.
TYLENOL® Acetaminophen produces analgesia by elevation of the pain threshold. Pseudoephedrine hydrochloride is a sympathomimetic amine which promotes proper sinus cavity drainage by reducing nasopharyngeal mucosal congestion.
Indications: Maximum-Strength TYLENOL Sinus Medication provides safe and effective relief of sinusitis pain and congestion.
Adverse Reactions: While Maximum-Strength TYLENOL Sinus Medication's acetaminophen component is equal to aspirin in analgesic and antipyretic effectiveness, it is unlikely to produce many of the side effects associated with aspirin and aspirin-containing products. Since it contains no antihistamine, TYLENOL Sinus Medication will not produce the drowsiness that may interfere with work, driving an automobile or operating dangerous machinery. TYLENOL acetaminophen is usually well tolerated by aspirin-sensitive patients. If a rare sensitivity occurs, the drug should be stopped. TYLENOL acetaminophen has rarely been found to produce side effects. Although pseudoephedrine is virtually without pressor effect in normotensive patients, it should be used with caution in hypertensives.
Usual Dosage: Adult dosage: Two tablets or capsules every four to six hours. Do not exceed eight tablets or capsules in any 24 hour period.
Note: Since TYLENOL Sinus Medication tablets and capsules are available without a prescription, the following appears on the package labels: "WARNING: Do not exceed the recommended dosage or administer to children under 12. Reduce dosage if nervousness, dizziness or sleeplessness occurs. If you have high blood pressure, heart disease, diabetes, or thyroid disease, or are presently taking a prescription drug for the treatment of high blood pressure or emotional disorders, do not take except under the advice and supervision of a physician. If symptoms persist for 7 days or are accompanied by high fever, consult a physician." **Do not use if safety seals are broken. Keep this and all medication out of the reach of children. If pregnant or nursing, seek medical advice before taking this or any medicine. In case of accidental overdosage, contact a physician or poison control center immediately.**
Overdosage: Acetaminophen in massive overdosage may cause hepatic toxicity in some patients. In all cases of suspected overdose, immediately call your regional poison center or the Rocky Mountain Center's toll-free number (800-525-6115) for assistance in diagnosis and for directions in the use of N-acetylcysteine as an antidote, a use currently restricted to investigational status. In adults hepatic toxicity has rarely been reported with acute overdoses of less than 10 grams and fatalities with less than 15 grams. Importantly, young children seem to be more resistant than adults to the hepatotoxic effect of an acetaminophen overdose. Despite this, the measures outlined below should be initiated in any adult or child suspected of having ingested an acetaminophen overdose.
Early symptons following a potentially hepatotoxic overdose may include: nausea, vomiting, diaphoresis and general malaise. Clinical and laboratory evidence of hepatic toxicity may not be apparent until 48 to 72 hours postingestion.
The stomach should be emptied promptly by lavage or by induction of emesis with syrup of ipecac. Patients' estimates of the quanitity of a drug ingested are notoriously unreliable. Therefore, if an acetaminophen overdose is suspected, a serum acetaminophen assay should be obtained as early as possible, but no sooner than four hours following ingestion. Liver function studies should be obtained initially and repeated at 24-hour intervals. The antidote, N-acetylcysteine, should be administered as early as possible, and within 16 hours of the overdose ingestion for optimal results. Following recovery, there are no residual structural or functional hepatic abnormalities.
How Supplied: Tablets (colored light green, imprinted "Maximum-Strength TYLENOL Sinus")—tamper-resistant bottles of 24. Capsules (colored green and white, imprinted "Maximum-Strength TYLENOL Sinus")—tamper-resistant bottles of 20.
[Shown in Product Identification Section]

IDENTIFICATION PROBLEM?

Consult PDR's

Product Identification Section

where you'll find over 900

products pictured actual size

and in full color.

McNeil Pharmaceutical
McNEILAB, INC.
SPRING HOUSE, PA 19477

HALDOL® brand of haloperidol — ℞
tablets, concentrate, injection

1 mg (1000's):
Military NSN 6505-01-003-2415
VA NSN 6505-01-003-2415A
2 mg (1000's):
Military NSN 6505-00-876-7239
VA NSN 6505-00-876-7239A
5 mg (1000's):
Military NSN 6505-01-003-2416
VA NSN 6505-01-003-2416A
10 mg (1000's):
Military NSN 6505-01-003-2417
VA NSN 6505-01-003-2417A
Concentrate 120 ml:
Military NSN 6505-01-003-5341
VA NSN 6505-01-003-5341A
Injection 1 ml:
VA NSN 6505-00-268-8530A

Description: Haloperidol is the first of the butyrophenone series of major tranquilizers. The chemical designation is 4-[4-(p-chlorophenyl) -4-hydroxypiperidino] -4'-fluorobutyrophenone.
HALDOL haloperidol dosage forms include: tablets (½, 1*, 2, 5*, 10* mg and 20 mg); a concentrate with 2 mg per ml haloperidol (as the lactate); and a sterile parenteral form for intramuscular injection. The injection provides 5 mg haloperidol (as the lactate) with 1.8 mg methylparaben and 0.2 mg propylparaben per ml, and lactic acid for pH adjustment between 3.0–3.6.
* Contains FD&C Yellow No. 5 (see Precautions)
Actions: The precise mechanism of action has not been clearly established.
Indications: HALDOL haloperidol is indicated for use in the management of manifestations of psychotic disorders.
HALDOL is indicated for the control of tics and vocal utterances of Tourette's disorder in children and adults.
HALDOL is effective for the treatment of severe behavior problems in children of combative, explosive hyperexcitability (which cannot be accounted for by immediate provocation).
HALDOL is effective in the short-term treatment of hyperactive children who show excessive motor activity with accompanying conduct disorders consisting of some or all of the following symptoms: impulsivity, difficulty sustaining attention, aggressivity, mood lability, and poor frustration tolerance.
Contraindications: HALDOL haloperidol is contraindicated in severe toxic central nervous system depression or comatose states from any cause and in individuals who are hypersensitive to this drug or have Parkinson's disease.
Warnings: ***Usage in Pregnancy:*** Rodents given 2 to 20 times the usual maximum human dose of haloperidol by oral or parenteral routes showed an increase in incidence of resorption, reduced fertility, delayed delivery and pup mortality. No teratogenic effect has been reported in rats, rabbits or dogs at dosages within this range, but cleft palate has been observed in mice given 15 times the usual maximum human dose. Cleft palate in mice appears to be a non-specific response to stress or nutritional imbalance as well as to a variety of drugs, and there is no evidence to relate this phenomenon to predictable human risk for most of these agents.
There are no well controlled studies with HALDOL haloperidol in pregnant women. There are reports, however, of two cases of limb malformations observed following maternal use of HALDOL along with other drugs which have suspected teratogenic potential during the first

Continued on next page

McNeil Pharm.—Cont.

trimester of pregnancy. Causal relationships were not established in either case. Since such experience does not exclude the possibility of fetal damage due to HALDOL, this drug should be used during pregnancy or in women likely to become pregnant only if the benefit clearly justifies a potential risk to the fetus. Infants should not be nursed during drug treatment.

Combined Use of HALDOL and Lithium: An encephalopathic syndrome (characterized by weakness, lethargy, fever, tremulousness and confusion, extrapyramidal symptoms, leukocytosis, elevated serum enzymes, BUN, and FBS) followed by irreversible brain damage has occurred in a few patients treated with lithium plus HALDOL. A causal relationship between these events and the concomitant administration of lithium and HALDOL has not been established; however, patients receiving such combined therapy should be monitored closely for early evidence of neurological toxicity and treatment discontinued promptly if such signs appear.

General: A number of cases of bronchopneumonia, some fatal, have followed the use of major tranquilizers, including HALDOL. It has been postulated that lethargy and decreased sensation of thirst due to central inhibition may lead to dehydration, hemoconcentration and reduced pulmonary ventilation. Therefore, if the above signs and symptoms appear, especially in the elderly, the physician should institute remedial therapy promptly.

Although not reported with HALDOL, decreased serum cholesterol and/or cutaneous and ocular changes have been reported in patients receiving chemically-related drugs.

HALDOL may impair the mental and/or physical abilities required for the performance of hazardous tasks such as operating machinery or driving a motor vehicle. The ambulatory patient should be warned accordingly.

The use of alcohol with this drug should be avoided due to possible additive effects and hypotension.

Precautions: HALDOL haloperidol should be administered cautiously to patients:

—with severe cardiovascular disorders, because of the possibility of transient hypotension and/or precipitation of anginal pain. Should hypotension occur and a vasopressor be required, epinephrine should not be used since HALDOL may block its vasopressor activity and paradoxical further lowering of the blood pressure may occur.

—receiving anticonvulsant medication, because HALDOL may lower the convulsive threshold. Adequate anticonvulsant therapy should be maintained concomitantly.

—with known allergies, or with a history of allergic reactions to drugs.

—receiving anticoagulants, since an isolated instance of interference occurred with the effects of one anticoagulant (phenindione).

If concomitant antiparkinson medication is required, it may have to be continued after HALDOL is discontinued because of the difference in excretion rates. If both are discontinued simultaneously, extrapyramidal symptoms may occur. The physician should keep in mind the possible increase in intraocular pressure when anticholinergic drugs, including antiparkinson agents, are administered concomitantly with HALDOL.

When HALDOL is used to control mania in cyclic disorders, there may be a rapid mood swing to depression.

Severe neurotoxicity (ridigity, inability to walk or talk) may occur in patients with thyrotoxicosis who are also receiving antipsychotic medication, including HALDOL.

Neuroleptic drugs elevate prolactin levels; the elevation persists during chronic administration. Tissue culture experiments indicate that approximately one-third of human breast cancers are prolactin dependent *in vitro*, a factor of potential importance if the prescription of these drugs is contemplated in a patient with a previously detected breast cancer. Although disturbances such as galactorrhea, amenorrhea, gynecomastia, and impotence have been reported, the clinical significance of elevated serum prolactin levels is unknown for most patients. An increase in mammary neoplasms has been found in rodents after chronic administration of neuroleptic drugs. Neither clinical studies nor epidemiologic studies conducted to date, however, have shown an association between chronic administration of these drugs and mammary tumorigenesis: the available evidence is considered too limited to be conclusive at this time.

FD&C Yellow No. 5 (tartrazine) may cause allergic-type reactions (including bronchial asthma) in certain susceptible individuals. Although the overall incidence of FD&C Yellow No. 5 (tartrazine) sensitivity in the general population is low, it is frequently seen in patients who also have aspirin hypersensitivity.

Adverse Reactions: ***CNS Effects:*** *Extrapyramidal Reactions*—Neuromuscular (extrapyramidal) reactions during the administration of HALDOL haloperidol have been reported frequently, often during the first few days of treatment. In most patients, these reactions involved Parkinson-like symptoms which, when first observed, were usually mild to moderately severe and usually reversible. Other types of neuromuscular reactions (motor restlessness, dystonia, akathisia, hyperreflexia, opisthotonos, oculogyric crises) have been reported far less frequently, but were often more severe. Severe extrapyramidal reactions have been reported to occur at relatively low doses. Generally the occurrence and severity of most extrapyramidal symptoms are dose related since they occur at relatively high doses and have been shown to disappear or become less severe when the dose is reduced. Administration of antiparkinson drugs such as benztropine mesylate U.S.P. or trihexyphenidyl hydrochloride U.S.P. may be required for control of such reactions. It should be noted that persistent extrapyramidal reactions have been reported and that the drug may have to be discontinued in such cases.

Withdrawal Emergent Neurological Signs—Generally, patients receiving short term therapy experience no problems with abrupt discontinuation of antipsychotic drugs. However, some patients on maintenance treatment experience transient dyskinetic signs after abrupt withdrawal. In certain of these cases the dyskinetic movements are indistinguishable from the syndrome described below under "Persistent Tardive Dyskinesia" except for duration. It is not known whether gradual withdrawal of antipsychotic drugs will reduce the rate of occurrence of withdrawal emergent neurological signs but until further evidence becomes available, it seems reasonable to gradually withdraw use of HALDOL.

Persistent Tardive Dyskinesia—As with all antipsychotic agents HALDOL has been associated with persistent dyskinesias. Tardive dyskinesia may appear in some patients on long-term therapy or may occur after drug therapy has been discontinued. The risk appears to be greater in elderly patients on high-dose therapy, especially females. The symptoms are persistent and in some patients appear irreversible. The syndrome is characterized by rhythmical involuntary movements of tongue, face, mouth or jaw (e.g., protrusion of tongue, puffing of cheeks, puckering of mouth, chewing movements). Sometimes these may be accompanied by involuntary movements of extremities.

There is no known effective treatment for tardive dyskinesia; antiparkinson agents usually do not alleviate the symptoms of this syndrome. It is suggested that all antipsychotic agents be discontinued if these symptoms appear. Should it be necessary to reinstitute treatment, or increase the dosage of the agent, or switch to a different antipsychotic agent, this syndrome may be masked.

It has been reported that fine vermicular movement of the tongue may be an early sign of the syndrome and if the medication is stopped at that time the syndrome may not develop.

Other CNS Effects—Insomnia, restlessness, anxiety, euphoria, agitation, drowsiness, depression, lethargy, headache, confusion, vertigo, grand mal seizures, exacerbation of psychotic symptoms including hallucinations and catatonic-like behavorial states which may be responsive to drug withdrawal and/or treatment with anticholinergic drugs.

Body as a Whole: As with other neuroleptic drugs, hyperpyrexia, that is rarely associated with rhabdomyolysis and acute renal failure, has occurred.

Cardiovascular Effects: Tachycardia and hypotension.

Hematologic Effects: Reports have appeared citing the occurrence of mild and usually transient leukopenia and leukocytosis, minimal decreases in red blood cell counts, anemia, or a tendency toward lymphomonocytosis. Agranulocytosis has rarely been reported to have occurred with the use of HALDOL and then only in association with other medication.

Liver Effects: Impaired liver function and/or jaundice have been reported.

Dermatologic Reactions: Maculopapular and acneiform skin reactions and isolated cases of photosensitivity and loss of hair.

Endocrine Disorders: Lactation, breast engorgement, mastalgia, menstrual irregularities, gynecomastia, impotence, increased libido, hyperglycemia, hypoglycemia and hyponatremia.

Gastrointestinal Effects: Anorexia, constipation, diarrhea, hypersalivation, dyspepsia, nausea and vomiting.

Autonomic Reactions: Dry mouth, blurred vision, urinary retention and diaphoresis.

Respiratory Effects: Laryngospasm, bronchospasm and increased depth of respiration.

Other: Cases of sudden and unexpected death have been reported in association with the administration of HALDOL. The nature of the evidence makes it impossible to determine definitively what role, if any, HALDOL played in the outcome of the reported cases. The possibility that HALDOL caused death cannot, of course, be excluded, but it is to be kept in mind that sudden and unexpected death may occur in psychotic patients when they go untreated or when they are treated with other neuroleptic drugs.

Overdosage: ***Manifestations:*** In general, the symptoms of overdosage would be an exaggeration of known pharmacologic effects and adverse reactions, the most prominent of which would be: 1) severe extrapyramidal reactions, 2) hypotension, or 3) sedation. The patient would appear comatose with respiratory depression and hypotension which could be severe enough to produce a shock-like state. The extrapyramidal reaction would be manifest by muscular weakness or rigidity and a generalized or localized tremor as demonstrated by the akinetic or agitans types respectively. With accidental overdosage, hypertension rather than hypotension occurred in a two-year old child.

Treatment: Gastric lavage or induction of emesis should be carried out immediately followed by administration of activated charcoal. Since there is no specific antidote, treatment is primarily supportive. A patent airway must be established by use of an oropharyngeal airway or endotracheal tube or, in prolonged cases of coma, by tracheostomy. Respiratory depression may be counteracted by artificial respiration and mechanical respirators. Hypotension and circulatory collapse may be counteracted by use of intravenous fluids, plasma, or concentrated albumin, and vasopressor agents such as norepinephrine. Epinephrine should not be used. In case of severe extrapyramidal reactions, antiparkinson medication should be administered.

Dosage and Administration: There is considerable variation from patient to patient in the amount of medication required for treatment. As with all neuroleptic drugs, dosage should be individualized according to the needs and response of each patient. Dosage adjustments, either upward or downward, should be carried out as rapidly as practicable to achieve optimum therapeutic control.

To determine the initial dosage, consideration should be given to the patient's age, severity of illness, previous response to other neuroleptic drugs, and any concomitant medication or disease state. Children, debilitated or geriatric patients, as well as those with a history of adverse reactions to neuroleptic drugs may require less HALDOL haloperidol. The optimal response in such patients is usually obtained with more gradual dosage adjustments and at lower dosage levels, as recommended below.

Clinical experience suggests the following recommendations:

Oral Administration

Initial Dosage Range

Adults

Moderate Symptomatology	0.5 mg to 2.0 mg b.i.d. or t.i.d.
Severe Symptomatology	3.0 mg to 5.0 mg b.i.d. or t.i.d.
To achieve prompt control, higher doses may be required in some cases.	
Geriatric or Debilitated Patients	0.5 mg to 2.0 mg b.i.d. or t.i.d.
Chronic or Resistant Patients	3.0 mg to 5.0 mg b.i.d. or t.i.d.

Patients who remain severely disturbed or inadequately controlled may require dosage adjustment. Daily dosages up to 100 mg may be necessary in some cases to achieve an optimal response. Infrequently, HALDOL has been used in doses above 100 mg for severely resistant patients; however, the limited clinical usage has not demonstrated the safety of prolonged administration of such doses.

Children

The following recommendations apply to children between the ages of 3 and 12 years (weight range 15 to 40 kg). HALDOL is not intended for children under 3 years old. Therapy should begin at the lowest dose possible (0.5 mg per day). If required, the dose should be increased by an increment of 0.5 mg at 5 to 7 day intervals until the desired therapeutic effect is obtained. (See chart below).

The total dose may be divided, to be given b.i.d. or t.i.d.

Psychotic Disorders	0.05 mg/kg/day to 0.15 mg/kg/day
Non-Psychotic Behavior Disorders and Tourette's Disorder	0.05 mg/kg/day to 0.075 mg/kg/day

Severely disturbed psychotic children may require higher doses. In severely disturbed, non-psychotic children or in hyperactive children with accompanying conduct disorders, it should be noted that since these behaviors may be short-lived, short-term administration of HALDOL may suffice. There is no evidence establishing a maximum effective dosage. There is little evidence that behavior improvement is further enhanced in dosages beyond 6 mg per day.

Maintenance Dosage

Upon achieving a satisfactory therapeutic response, dosage should then be gradually reduced to the lowest effective maintenance level.

Intramuscular Administration

Adults

Parenteral medication, administered intramuscularly in doses of 2 to 5 mg, is utilized for prompt control of the acutely agitated patient with moderately severe to very severe symptoms. Depending on the response of the patient, subsequent doses may be given, administered as often as every hour, although 4 to 8 hour intervals may be satisfactory.

Controlled trials to establish the safety and effectiveness of intramuscular administration in children have not been conducted.

Switchover Procedure

The oral form should supplant the injectable as soon as practicable. In the absence of bioavailability studies establishing bioequivalence between these two dosage forms the following guidelines for dosage are suggested. For an initial approximation of the total daily dose required, the parenteral dose administered in the preceeding 24 hours may be used. Since this dose is only an initial estimate, it is recommended that careful monitoring of clinical signs and symptoms, including clinical efficacy, sedation, and adverse effects, be carried out periodically for the first several days following the initiation of switchover. In this way, dosage adjustments, either upward or downward, can be quickly accomplished. Depending on the patient's clinical status, the first oral dose should be given within 12–24 hours following the last parenteral dose.

(See table below)

HALDOL® brand of haloperidol Concentrate 2 mg per ml (as the lactate) Colorless, Odorless, and Tasteless Solution—**NDC** 0045-0250-15, bottles of 15 ml and **NDC** 0045-0250-04, bottles of 120 ml.

HALDOL® brand of haloperidol Injection 5 mg per ml (as the lactate)—**NDC** 0045-0255-01, units of 10 × 1 ml ampuls; **NDC** 0045-0255-49, 10 ml multiple-dose vial; **NDC** 0045-0255-31 units of 10 × 1 ml disposable Pre-filled Syringe.

Tablets and concentrate (120 ml) manufactured by McNeil Pharmaceutical Co., Dorado, Puerto Rico 00646.

[*Shown in Product Identification Section*]

How Supplied: HALDOL* brand of haloperidol Tablets Scored, Imprinted "McNEIL" and "HALDOL"

		Bottles containing 50	100	1000	Unit Dose Blister Pack 10 × 10
1/2mg white	NDC 0045-0240		x	x	x
1mg yellow	NDC 0045-0241		x	x	x
2mg pink	NDC 0045-0242		x	x	x
5mg green	NDC 0045-0245	x	x	x	x
10mg aqua	NDC 0045-0246	x	x	x	x
20mg salmon	NDC 0045-0248		x		x

PANCREASE® ℞
pancrelipase
ENTERIC COATED

Description: PANCREASE pancrelipase is a white, dye-free, orally administered capsule containing enteric coated microspheres of porcine pancreatic enzyme concentrate, predominately steapsin (pancreatic lipase), amylase and protease. Each capsule contains no less than:

Lipase	4,000 U.S.P. Units
Amylase	20,000 U.S.P. Units
Protease	25.000 U.S.P. Units

Clinical Pharmacology: PANCREASE pancrelipase resists gastric inactivation and delivers predictable, high levels of biologically active enzymes into the duodenum. The enzymes catalyze the hydrolysis of fats into glycerol and fatty acids, protein into proteoses and derived substances, and starch into dextrins and sugars. PANCREASE is effective in controlling steatorrhea and its consequences at low daily dosage levels.[1–9]

Indications and Usage: PANCREASE pancrelipase is indicated for patients with exocrine pancreatic enzyme deficiency as in:

- cystic fibrosis
- chronic pancreatitis
- post-pancreatectomy
- post-gastrointestinal bypass surgery (e.g. Billroth II gastroenterostomy)
- ductal obstruction from neoplasm (e.g. of the pancreas or common bile duct).

Contraindications: PANCREASE pancrelipase is contraindicated in patients known to be hypersensitive to pork protein.

Warnings: Should hypersensitivity occur, discontinue medication and treat symptomatically.

Precautions: TO PROTECT ENTERIC COATING, MICROSPHERES SHOULD NOT BE CRUSHED OR CHEWED.

Where swallowing of capsules is difficult, they may be opened and the microspheres shaken onto a small quantity of a soft food (e.g. aplesauce, gelatin, etc.), which does not require chewing, and swallowed immediately. Contact of the microspheres with foods having a pH greater than 5.5 can dissolve the protective enteric shell.

Pregnancy Category C. Diethylphthalate, an enteric coating component of PANCREASE pancrelipase has been shown with high intraperitoneal dosing to be tetratogenic in rats.[10] However, when this coating was administered orally to rats up to 100 times the human dose, no teratogenic or embryocidal effects were observed.[9] There were no adequate and well-controlled studies in pregnant women. PANCREASE should be used in pregnancy only if the potential benefit justifies the potential risk to the fetus.

Adverse Reactions: No adverse reactions have been reported with PANCREASE pancrelipase. However, it should be noted that extremely high doses of exogenous pancreatic enzymes have been associated with hyperuricosuria[11] and hyperuricemia.[12]

Dosage and Administration: Usual dosage: One or two capsules during each meal and one capsule with snacks. Occasionally a third capsule with meals may be required depending upon individual requirements for control of steatorrhea.

How Supplied: PANCREASE® pancrelipase capsules (white, dye-free, imprinted "McNeil" and "Pancrease") in bottles of:

100 ....NDC 0045-009

250 ....NDC 0045-00

Keep bottle tightly closed and store i place at controlled room tempera 86°F). Do not refrigerate after ope

Continue

McNeil Pharm.—Cont.

References:

1. Khaw, K.T., S. Adeniyi-Jones, D. Gordon, J. Palombo, R. Coryer, C. Schlaman, J. Watkins and R. Suskind, Comparative Effectiveness of Viokase, Cotazym and Pancrease in Children with Cystic Fibrosis, *Cystic Fibrosis Club Abstracts,* p. 57, April 26, 1977.
2. Valerio, D., E.H.A. Whyte, H.A. Schlamm and G.L. Blackburn: Enzyme Replacement Therapy in Pancreatic Insufficiency, *Journal of Parenteral and Enteral Nutrition,* 1:20A, 1977.
3. Khaw, K.T., S. Adeniyi-Jones, V. Pena-Cruz, D. Gordon, C. Bayerl, C. Batrus, J. Palombo, R. Suskind, The Effect of Caloric Supplementation Growth Parameters in Children with Cystic Fibrosis, *Cystic Fibrosis Club Abstracts,* p. 58, April 25, 1978.
4. Khaw, K.T., S. Adeniyi-Jones, D. Gordon, J. Palombo and R. M. Suskind, Efficacy of Panreatin Preparations on Fat and Nitrogen Absorptions in Cystic Fibrosis Patients, *Pediatric Research,* 12:444, 1978.
5. Suskind, R.S., Adeniyi-Jones, D. Gordon, C. Bayerl, J. Palombo, V. Pena-Cruz and K. Khaw, Nutritional Status, Nutrient Intake and Response to Enzyme Replacement in Children with Cystic Fibrosis, *Cystic Fibrosis Club Abstracts,* p. 95, April 25, 1978.
6. Holsclaw, D.S., J.C. Fahl and H.H. Keith, Enhancement of Enzyme Replacement Therapy in Cystic Fibrosis, *Cystic Fibrosis Club Abstracts,* p. 19, May 1, 1979.
7. Weber, A.M., B. de Gheldere, C.C. Ray, A Fontaine, O.L. Dufour, C.L. Morin and R. Lasalle, Effectiveness of Enteric Coated Pancrease in Cystic Fibrosis (CF) Children Under 4 Years Old, *Cystic Fibrosis Club Abstracts,* p. 18, May 1, 1979.
8. Salen, G. and A. Prakash, Evaluation of Enteric Coated Microspheres for Enzyme Replacement Therapy in Adults with Pancreatic Insufficiency, *Current Therapeutic Research,* 25:650–656, 1979.
9. Data on File, McNeil Pharmaceutical.
10. Singh, A.R., W.H. Laurence and J. Autian, Teratogenicity of Phthalate Esters in Rats, *Journal of Pharmaceutical Sciences,* 61:51–55, 1972.
11. Stapleton, F.D., et al: Hyperuricosuria Due to High Dose Pancreatic Extract Therapy in Cystic Fibrosis, *New England Journal of Medicine,* 295:246–248, 1976.
12. Davidson, G.P., F.M. Hassel, D. Crozier, M. Corey and G. Forstner, Iatrogenic Hyperuricemia in Children with Cystic Fibrosis, *Journal of Pediatrics,* 93:976–978, 1978.

Manufactured by:

McNEIL PHARMACEUTICAL
McNEILAB, INC.
SPRING HOUSE, PA 19477

PARAFLEX® (chlorzoxazone) tablets ℞

Description: Each tablet contains chlorzoxazone *250 mg. *5-chlorobenzoxazolinone

Actions: Chlorzoxazone is a centrally-acting agent for painful musculoskeletal conditions. Data available from animal experiments as well as human study indicate that chlorzoxazone acts primarily at the level of the spinal cord and subcortical areas of the brain where it inhibits multisynaptic reflex arcs involved in producing and maintaining skeletal muscle spasm of varied etiology. The clinical result is a reduction of the skeletal muscle spasm with relief of pain and increased mobility of the involved muscles. Blood levels of chlorzoxazone can be detected in man during the first hour fter administration and reach peak levels in third and fourth hours. Chlorzoxazone is dly metabolized and excreted in the urine, rily in a conjugated form as the glucuro- ess than one percent of a dose of chlorzoxazone is excreted unchanged in the urine in 24 hours.

Indications: PARAFLEX chlorzoxazone is indicated as an adjunct to rest, physical therapy, and other measures for the relief of discomfort associated with acute, painful musculoskeletal conditions. The mode of action of this drug has not been clearly identified, but may be related to its sedative properties. Chlorzoxazone does not directly relax tense skeletal muscles in man.

Contraindications: PARAFLEX chlorzoxazone is contraindicated in patients with known intolerance to the drug.

Warnings: The concomitant use of alcohol or other central nervous system depressants may have an additive effect.

Usage in Pregnancy: The safe use of PARAFLEX chlorzoxazone has not been established with respect to the possible adverse effects upon fetal development. Therefore, it should be used in women of childbearing potential only when, in the judgment of the physician, the potential benefits outweigh the possible risks.

Precautions: PARAFLEX chlorzoxazone should be used with caution in patients with known allergies or with a history of allergic reactions to drugs. If a sensitivity reaction occurs such as urticaria, redness, or itching of the skin, the drug should be stopped.

If any signs or symptoms suggestive of liver dysfunction are observed, the drug should be discontinued.

Adverse Reactions: After more than twenty-three years of extensive clinical use of PARAFLEX chlorzoxazone and other chlorzoxazone-containing products in an estimated thirty million patients, it is apparent that the drug is well tolerated and seldom produces undesirable side effects. Occasional patients may develop gastrointestinal disturbances. It is possible in rare instances that PARAFLEX chlorzoxazone may have been associated with gastrointestinal bleeding. Drowsiness, dizziness, lightheadedness, malaise, or overstimulation may be noted by an occasional patient. Rarely, allergic-type skin rashes, petechiae, or ecchymoses may develop during treatment. Angioneurotic edema or anaphylactic reactions are extremely rare. There is no evidence that the drug will cause renal damage. Rarely, a patient may note discoloration of the urine resulting from a phenolic metabolite of chlorzoxazone. This finding is of no known clinical significance.

Approximately twenty-seven patients have been reported in whom the administration of PARAFLEX chlorzoxazone or other chlorzoxazone-containing products was suspected as being the cause of liver damage. In one case, the jaundice was subsequently considered to be due to a carcinoma of the head of the pancreas rather than to the drug. In a second case, there was no jaundice but an elevated alkaline phosphatase and BSP retention. In this patient there was a malignancy with bony and liver metastases. The role of the drug was difficult to determine. A third and fourth case had cholelithiasis. Diagnosis in a fifth case was submassive hepatic necrosis possibly due to abusive use of the drug for approximately one year. The remaining cases had a clinical picture compatible with either a viral hepatitis or a drug-induced hepatitis. In all these latter cases the drug was stopped, and, with one exception, the patients recovered. It is not possible to state that the hepatitis in these patients was or was not drug-induced.

Dosage and Administration: ***Usual Adult Dosage:*** One tablet (250 mg) three or four times daily. Initial dosage for *painful musculoskeletal conditions* should be two tablets (500 mg) three or four times daily. If adequate response is not obtained with this dose, it may be increased to three tablets (750 mg) three or four times daily. As improvement occurs dosage can usually be reduced.

Usual Child's Dosage: One-half to two tablets (125 mg to 500 mg) three or four times daily given according to age and weight. The tablets may be crushed and mixed with food or a suitable vehicle for administration to children.

Overdosage:

Symptoms: Initially, gastrointestinal disturbances such as nausea, vomiting, or diarrhea together with drowsiness, dizziness, lightheadedness or headache may occur. Early in the course there may be malaise or sluggishness followed by marked loss of muscle tone, making voluntary movement impossible. The deep tendon reflexes may be decreased or absent. The sensorium remains intact, and there is no peripheral loss of sensation. Respiratory depression may occur with rapid, irregular respiration and intercostal and substernal retraction. The blood pressure is lowered, but shock has not been observed.

Treatment: Gastric lavage or induction of emesis should be carried out, followed by administration of activated charcoal. Thereafter, treatment is entirely supportive. If respirations are depressed, oxygen and artificial respiration should be employed and a patent airway assured by use of an oropharyngeal airway or endotracheal tube. Hypotension may be counteracted by use of dextran, plasma, concentrated albumin or a vasopressor agent such as norepinephrine. Cholinergic drugs or analeptic drugs are of no value and should not be used.

How Supplied: Tablets (colored orange, scored, imprinted "PARAFLEX" "McNEIL") —bottles of 100 **NDC** 0045-0317-60.

PARAFON FORTE® tablets ℞
500's:
Military NSN 6505-00-764-3313
VA NSN 6505-00-764-3313A

Description: Each tablet contains chlorzoxazone 250 mg and acetaminophen 300 mg.

Actions: PARAFON FORTE tablets provide symptomatic relief of pain, stiffness, and limitation of motion associated with most musculoskeletal disorders through (a) relaxation of muscle spasm by chlorzoxazone, an effective and well-tolerated centrally-acting agent; and (b) analgesia by acetaminophen, a nonsalicylate analgesic useful in skeletal muscle pain.

Data available from animal experiments, as well as human study, indicate that chlorzoxazone acts primarily at the level of the spinal cord and subcortical areas of the brain where it inhibits multisynaptic reflex arcs involved in producing and maintaining skeletal muscle spasm of varied etiology. Blood levels of chlorzoxazone can be detected in man during the first hour after administration and reach peak levels by the third to fourth hour. Chlorzoxazone is rapidly metabolized and is excreted in the urine, primarily in a conjugated form as the glucuronide. Less than one percent of a dose of chlorzoxazone is excreted unchanged in the urine in 24 hours.

Acetaminophen provides analgesic action to supplement that which results secondarily from muscle relaxation. Acetaminophen is rapidly absorbed after oral administration, with peak plasma levels occurring in one to two hours. After eight hours, only negligible amounts remain in the blood. Only 4 percent is excreted unchanged; 85 percent of the ingested dose is recovered in the urine in conjugated form as the glucuronide.

Indications: Based on a review of this drug by the National Academy of Sciences-National Research Council and/or other information, FDA has classified the indications as follows:

"Probably" effective as an adjunct to rest and physical therapy for the relief of discomfort associated with acute, painful musculoskeletal conditions. The mode of action of this drug has not been clearly identified, but may be related to its sedative properties. Chlorzoxazone does not directly relax tense skeletal muscles in man.

Contraindications: PARAFON FORTE tablets are contraindicated in patients sensitive to either component.

Warnings: The concomitant use of alcohol or other central nervous system depressants may have an additive effect.

Usage in Pregnancy: The safe use of PARAFON FORTE tablets has not been established with respect to the possible adverse effects upon fetal development. Therefore, it should be used in women of childbearing potential only when, in the judgment of the physician, the potential benefits outweigh the possible risks.

Precautions: PARAFON FORTE tablets should be used with caution in patients with known allergies or with a history of allergic reactions to drugs. If a sensitivity reaction occurs such as urticaria, redness, or itching of the skin, the drug should be stopped.

If any signs or symptoms suggestive of liver dysfunction are observed, the drug should be discontinued.

This product contains FD&C Yellow No. 5 (tartrazine) which may cause allergic-type reactions (including bronchial asthma) in certain susceptible individuals. Although the overall incidence of FD&C Yellow No. 5 (tartrazine) sensitivity in the general population is low, it is frequently seen in patients who also have aspirin hypersensitivity.

Adverse Reactions: After more than twenty-two years of extensive clinical use of PARAFLEX® (chlorzoxazone) tablets and other chlorzoxazone-containing products in an estimated twenty-seven million patients, it is apparent that the drug is well tolerated and seldom produces undesirable side effects. Occasional patients may develop gastrointestinal disturbances. It is possible in rare instances that chlorzoxazone may have been associated with gastrointestinal bleeding. Drowsiness, dizziness, lightheadedness, malaise, or overstimulation may be noted by an occasional patient. Rarely, allergic-type skin rashes, petechiae, or ecchymoses may develop during treatment. Angioneurotic edema or anaphylactic reactions are extremely rare. There is no evidence that the drug will cause renal damage. Rarely, a patient may note discoloration of the urine resulting from a phenolic metabolite of chlorzoxazone. This finding is of no known clinical significance.

Approximately twenty-seven patients have been reported in whom the administration of PARAFLEX chlorzoxazone or other chlorzoxazone-containing products was suspected as being the cause of liver damage. In one case, the jaundice was subsequently considered to be due to a carcinoma of the head of the pancreas rather than to the drug. In a second case, there was no jaundice but an elevated alkaline phosphatase and BSP retention. In this patient there was a malignancy with bony and liver metastases. The role of the drug was difficult to determine. A third and fourth case had cholelithiasis. Diagnosis in a fifth case was submassive hepatic necrosis possibly due to abusive use of the drug for approximately one year. The remaining cases had a clinical picture compatible with either a viral hepatitis or a drug-induced hepatitis. In all these latter cases the drug was stopped, and, with one exception, the patients recovered. It is not possible to state that the hepatitis in these patients was or was not drug induced.

Acetaminophen has rarely been found to produce any side effects.

Dosage and Administration *Usual Adult Dosage:* Two tablets 4 times daily.

Overdosage:

Acetaminophen

Acetaminophen in massive overdosage may cause hepatic toxicity in some patients. In adults, hepatic toxicity has rarely been reported with less than 10 grams and fatalities with less than 15 grams, taken as single, massive overdoses. Importantly, for reasons not fully understood, young children seem to be more resistant than adults to the hepatotoxic effect of acetaminophen overdose.

Early symptoms following a potentially hepatotoxic overdose may include: nausea, vomiting, diaphoresis and general malaise. Clinical and laboratory evidence of hepatic toxicity usually are not apparent until 48 to 72 hours post-ingestion. Following recovery there are no residual, structural or functional hepatic abnormalities.

Since patients' estimates of the quantity of a drug ingested are notoriously unreliable, if an acetaminophen overdose is suspected a serum acetaminophen assay should be obtained as early as possible, but no sooner than four hours following ingestion. Liver function studies should be obtained initially and repeated at 24 hour intervals.

Antidotal therapy with N-acetylcysteine appears effective in preventing and/or minimizing the toxic effects of acetaminophen. For optimal results, the antidote should be administered within 16 hours of ingestion of the overdose.

The Rocky Mountain Poison Center (800-525-6115) should be contacted for assistance in interpreting plasma levels and for directions on the administration of N-acetylcysteine as an antidote, a use currently restricted to investigational status.

Chlorzoxazone

Symptoms: Initially, gastrointestinal disturbances such as nausea, vomiting, or diarrhea together with drowsiness, dizziness, lightheadedness or headache may occur. Early in the course there may be malaise or sluggishness followed by marked loss of muscle tone, making voluntary movement impossible. The deep tendon reflexes may be decreased or absent. The sensorium remains intact, and there is no peripheral loss of sensation. Respiratory depression may occur with rapid, irregular respiration and intercostal and substernal retraction. The blood pressure is lowered, but shock has not been observed.

Treatment: Gastric lavage or induction of emesis should be carried out, followed by administration of activated charcoal. Thereafter, treatment is entirely supportive. If respirations are depressed, oxygen and artificial respiration should be employed and a patent airway assured by use of an oropharyngeal airway or endotracheal tube. Hypotension may be counteracted by use of dextran, plasma, concentrated albumin or a vasopressor agent such as norepinephrine. Cholinergic drugs or analeptic drugs are of no value and should not be used.

How Supplied: PARAFON FORTE® Tablets (colored green, imprinted "McNEIL" and "PARAFON FORTE")—bottles of 100 **NDC** 0045-0322-60 and 500 **NDC** 0045-0322-70; Unit dose of 200 **NDC** 0045-0322-58.

Tablets manufactured by McNeil Pharmaceutical Co., Dorado, PR 00646.

[*Shown in Product Identification Section*]

THEOPHYL® ℞

(anhydrous theophylline)

CHEWABLE TABLETS

for oral use

Description: Each double-scored white tablet contains not less than 94.0 percent and not more than 106.0 percent of 100 mg anhydrous theophylline USP. Theophylline ($C_7H_8N_4O_2$), a xanthine compound, is a white odorless crystalline powder having a bitter taste. The scoring of THEOPHYL® Chewable Tablets allows for titration in 25 mg (¼ tablet) increments.

Clinical Pharmacology: Theophylline directly relaxes the smooth muscle of the bronchial airways and pulmonary blood vessels, thus acting mainly as a bronchodilator, pulmonary vasodilator and smooth muscle relaxant. It also possesses other actions typical of the xanthine derivatives: coronary vasodilator, diuretic, and cardiac, cerebral, and skeletal muscle stimulant. The actions of theophylline may be mediated through inhibition of phosphodiesterase and a resultant increase in intracellular cyclic AMP which could mediate smooth muscle relaxation.

In vitro, theophylline has been shown to react synergistically with beta agonists (such as isoproterenol) that increase intracellular cyclic AMP through the stimulation of adenyl cyclase, but synergism has not been demonstrated in clinical studies and more data are needed to determine if theophylline and beta agonists have clinically important additive effects **in vivo.**

Apparently, tolerance does not develop with chronic use of theophylline.

The half-life is shortened with cigarette smoking. The half-life is prolonged in alcoholism, reduced hepatic or renal function, congestive heart failure, and in patients receiving cimetidine or certain antibiotics such as troleandomycin, (TAO, cyclamycin) erythromycin, lincomycin and clindamycin. High fever for prolonged periods may decrease theophylline elimination.

Theophylline Elimination Characteristics:

	Theophylline Clearance Rates (mean ± S.D.)	Half-Life Average (mean ± S.D.)
Children (over 6 months of age)	1.45 ± 0.58 ml/kg/min	3.7 ± 1.1 hours
Adult nonsmokers with uncomplicated asthma	0.65 ± 0.19 ml/kg/min	8.7 ± 2.2 hours

Newborn infants have extremely slow clearances with half-lives exceeding 24 hours. These approach those seen for older children after about 3–6 months.

Older adults with chronic obstructive pulmonary disease, patients with cor pulmonale or other causes of heart failure, and patients with liver pathology may have much lower clearances with half-lives that may exceed 24 hours. The half-life is prolonged in alcoholism, reduced hepatic or renal function, congestive heart failure, and in patients receiving cimetidine or certain antibiotics such as TAO (troleandomycin), erythromycin, and clindamycin. High fever for prolonged periods may decrease theophylline elimination.

The half-life of theophylline in smokers (1 to 2 packs/day) averaged 4 to 5 hours in various studies, much shorter than the 7 to 9 hour half-life in nonsmokers. The increase in theophylline clearance caused by smoking is probably the result of induction of drug-metabolizing enzymes that do not readily normalize after cessation of smoking. It appears that between 3 months and 2 years may be necessary for normalization of the effect of smoking on theophylline pharmacokinetics.

THEOPHYL® Chewable Tablets are a rapidly releasing form of theophylline. Bioavailability of these tablets has been shown to be 98% ± 5% when chewed and 101% ± 4% when swallowed whole.

Indications: For relief and/or prevention of symptoms of asthma and reversible bronchospasm associated with chronic bronchitis and emphysema.

Contraindications: Avoid using TH PHYL® Chewable Tablets in individua have shown hypersensitivity to any of ponents.

Continued

McNeil Pharm.—Cont.

Warnings: Status asthmaticus should be considered a medical emergency and is defined as the degree of bronchospasm which is not rapidly responsive to usual doses of conventional bronchodilators. Optimal therapy for such patients frequently requires both additional medication, parenterally administered, and close monitoring, preferably in an intensive care setting.

Although increasing the dose of theophylline may bring about relief, such treatment may be associated with toxicity. The likelihood of such toxicity developing increases significantly when the serum theophylline concentration exceeds 20 μg/ml. Therefore, determination of serum theophylline levels is recommended to assure maximal benefit without excessive risk.

Serum levels above 20 μg/ml are rarely found after appropriate administration of the recommended doses. However, in individuals in whom theophylline plasma clearance is reduced for any reason, even conventional doses may result in increased serum levels and potential toxicity. Reduced theophylline clearance has been documented in the following readily identifiable groups: 1) patients with impaired renal or liver function; 2) patients over 55 years of age, particularly males and those with chronic lung disease; 3) those with cardiac failure from any cause; 4) neonates; and 5) those patients taking certain drugs (macrolide antibiotics and cimetidine). Decreased clearance of theophylline may be associated with either influenza immunization or active infection with influenza.

Reduction of dosage and laboratory monitoring is especially appropriate in the above individuals.

Less serious signs of theophylline toxicity, i.e. nausea and restlessness, may appear in up to 50% of patients. Unfortunately however, serious side effects such as ventricular arrhythmias, convulsions or even death may appear as the first sign of toxicity without any previous warning. Stated differently: **serious toxicity is not reliably preceeded by less severe side effects.**

Many patients who require theophylline may exhibit tachycardia due to their underlying disease process so that the cause/effect relationship to elevated serum theophylline concentrations may not be appreciated.

Theophylline products may cause dysrhythmia and/or worsen pre-existing arrythmias and any significant change in rate and/or rhythm warrants monitoring and further investigation.

The occurrence of arrhythmias and sudden death (with histological evidence of necrosis of the myocardium) has been recorded in laboratory animals (minipigs, rodents and dogs) when theophylline and beta agonists were administered concomitantly, although not when either was administered alone. The significance of these findings when applied to human usage is currently unknown.

Usage in Pregnancy: Safe use in pregnancy has not been established relative to possible adverse effects on fetal development, but neither have adverse effects on fetal development been established. This is, unfortunately, true for most antiasthmatic medications. Therefore, use of theophylline in pregnant women should be balanced against the risk of uncontrolled asthma.

Precautions: Mean half-life in smokers is shorter than in nonsmokers; therefore, smokers may require larger doses of theophylline. THEOPHYL® Chewable Tablets, like all theo-hylline products, should not be administered ncurrently with other xanthine medications. with caution in patients with severe car- disease, severe hypoxemia, hypertension, thyroidism, acute myocardial injury, cor pulmonale, congestive heart failure, liver disease, peptic ulcer and in the elderly (especially males) and in neonates. Great caution should be used especially in giving theophylline to patients in congestive heart failure; such patients have shown markedly prolonged theophylline blood level curves with theophylline persisting in serum for long periods following discontinuation of the drug.

Theophylline may occasionally act as a local irritant to the GI tract although gastrointestinal symptoms are more commonly central in origin and associated with serum concentrations over 20 mcg/ml.

It has been reported that theophylline distributes readily into breast milk and may cause adverse effects in the infant. Caution must be used if prescribing xanthines to a mother who is nursing, taking into account the risk-benefit of this therapy.

Due to the marked variation in theophylline metabolism in infants under 6 months of age, this drug is not recommended for this age group.

Adverse Reactions: The most frequent adverse reactions to theophylline are usually due to overdose (serum levels in excess of 20 μg/ml) and are:

Gastrointestinal: nausea, vomiting, epigastric pain, hematemesis, diarrhea.

Central nervous system: headaches, irritability, restlessness, insomnia, reflex hyperexcitability, muscle twitching, clonic and tonic generalized convulsions.

Cardiovascular: palpitations, tachycardia, extra systoles, flushing, hypotension, circulatory failure, ventricular arrhythmias.

Respiratory: tachypnea.

Renal: albuminuria, increased excretion of renal tubular cells and red blood cells, potentiation of diuresis.

Others: hyperglycemia and inappropriate ADH syndrome.

Drug Interactions: Toxic synergism with ephedrine has been documented and may occur with some other sympathomimetic bronchodilators.

DRUG	EFFECT
Aminophylline with lithium carbonate	Increased excretion of lithium carbonate
Aminophylline with propranolol	Antagonism of propranolol effect
Theophylline with furosemide	Increased diuresis
Theophylline with hexamethonium	Decreased hexamethonium-induced chronotropic effect
Theophylline with reserpine	Reserpine-induced tachycardia
Theophylline with chlordiazepoxide	Chlordiazepoxide-induced fatty acid mobilization
Theophylline with cimetidine, troleandomycin, (TAO cyclamycin) erythromycin, lincomycin, clindamycin	Increased theophylline plasma levels
Theophylline with phenytoin	Decreased phenytoin levels

Management of Overdose:

A. If potential overdose is established and seizure has not occurred:
   1. Induce vomiting.
   2. Administer a cathartic.
   3. Administer activated charcoal.

B. If patient is having a seizure:
   1. Establish an airway.
   2. Administer O_2.
   3. Treat the seizure with intravenous diazepam, 0.1 to 0.3 mg/kg up to 10 mg.
   4. Monitor vital signs, maintain blood pressure and provide adequate hydration.

C. Post-seizure coma:
   1. Maintain airway and oxygenation.
   2. Follow above recommendations to prevent absorption of drug, but intubation and lavage will have to be performed instead of inducing emesis, and introduce the cathartic and charcoal via a large bore gastric lavage tube.
   3. Continue to provide full supportive care and adequate hydration while waiting for drug to be metabolized. In general, the drug is metabolized sufficiently rapidly so as not to require dialysis, however, if serum levels exceed 50 μg/ml, charcoal hemoperfusion may be indicated.

Dosage and Administration: Therapeutic serum levels associated with optimal likelihood for benefit and minimal risk of toxicity are considered to be between 10 μg/ml and 20 μg/ml. Levels above 20 μg/ml may produce toxic effects. There is great variation from patient to patient in dosage needed to achieve a therapeutic blood level because of variable rates of elimination. Therefore, dosage must be individualized and monitoring of theophylline serum levels is highly recommended. Serum theophylline measurement should be obtained at the time of peak absorption, which has been shown to be 2.0 ± 0.3 hours for THEOPHYL® Chewable Tablets when chewed and 2.2 ± 0.3 hours when swallowed whole. Samples for serum theophylline measurement should be taken after a patient has been on a given dose for at least 3 days and has missed no doses during the previous 48 hours. **Unless the above instructions with regard to serum theophylline measurement are followed, the results may be misleading and dosage adjustments based on these results may be incorrect, possibly increasing the risk of toxicity.**

As theophylline does not distribute into fatty tissue, dosage should be calculated on the basis of lean (ideal) body weight.

Giving theophylline with food may prevent the rare case of stomach irritation; though absorption may be slower, it is still complete.

When rapidly absorbed products such as solutions and uncoated tablets with rapid dissolution are used, dosing to maintain "around the clock" blood levels generally requires administration every 6 hours in children; dosing intervals up to 8 hours may be satisfactory for adults because of their slower elimination rate. Children, and adults requiring higher than average doses, may benefit from products with slower absorption, such as THEOPHYL SR Capsules, which may allow longer dosing intervals and/or less fluctuation in serum concentration over a dosing interval during chronic therapy.

Once a patient is stabilized on a particular dose of theophylline, his blood levels tend to remain constant with that dose.

Pulmonary function measurements before and after a period of treatment permit an objective assessment of response to THEOPHYL® Chewable Tablets.

> As a practical consideration, it is not always possible to obtain serum level determinations. Under such conditions, restriction of the daily dose (in otherwise healthy adults) to not greater than 16 mg/kg/day in divided doses will result in relatively few patients exceeding serum levels of 20 μg/ml and the resultant risk of toxicity.

I. Dosage of THEOPHYL® Chewable Tablets for Patients Exhibiting Acute Symptoms of Asthma Requiring Rapid Theophyllinization and Not Currently Receiving Theophylline Products.

[See table on next page].

II. Dosage for Patients Currently Receiving Theophylline Therapy.

Determine, where possible, the time, amount, route of administration and form of the patient's last dose. Ideally, the loading dose should be deferred if a serum theophylline determination can be rapidly obtained. If this is not possible, the clinician must exercise his judgment in selecting a dose based on the principle that each 0.5 μg/kg of theophylline administered as a loading dose will result in a 1 μg/ml increase in serum theophylline concentration. When there is sufficient respiratory distress to warrant a small risk, 2.5 mg/kg of theophylline is likely to increase the serum concentration by only about 5 μg/ml when administered as a loading dose. If the patient is not already experiencing theophylline toxicity, this is unlikely to result in dangerous adverse effects. Subsequent maintenance dosage recommendations are the same as those described above.

	Loading Dose	Maintenance Dose For Next 12 Hours	Maintenance Dose Beyond 12 Hours
1. Children 6 months to 9 years	6 mg/kg	4 mg/kg q4h	4 mg/kg q6h
2. Children age 9–16 and young adult smokers	6 mg/kg	3 mg/kg q4h	3 mg/kg q6h
3. Otherwise healthy nonsmoking adults	6 mg/kg	3 mg/kg q6h	3 mg/kg q8h
4. Older patients and patients with cor pulmonale	6 mg/kg	2 mg/kg q6h	2 mg/kg q8h
5. Patients with congestive heart failure, liver failure	6 mg/kg	2 mg/kg q8h	1–2 mg/kg q12h

III.Dosage for Chronic Asthma.

Theophyllinization is a treatment of first choice for the management of chronic asthma (to prevent symptoms and maintain patent airways). Slow clinical titration is generally preferred to assure acceptance and safety of the medication.

Initial Dose: 16 mg/kg/day or 450 mg/day (whichever is lower) in 3–4 divided doses at 6–8 hour intervals.

Increased Dose: The above dosage may be increased in approximately 25 percent increments at 2–3 day intervals so long as no intolerance is observed, until a maximum indicated below is reached.

Maximum Dose Without Measurement of Serum Concentration:

Not to exceed the following: **(WARNING: DO NOT ATTEMPT TO MAINTAIN ANY DOSE THAT IS NOT TOLERATED)**

Age Less than 9 years	–24 mg/kg/day
Age 9–12 years	–20 mg/kg/day
Age 12–16 years	–18 mg/kg/day
Age Greater than 16 years	–13 mg/kg/day or 900 mg/day
	(WHICHEVER IS LESS)

NOTE: Use ideal body weight for obese patients.

How Supplied: Each round white tablet (double bisected on one side, inscribed "Theophyl 100") contains 100 mg of anhydrous theophylline.

Bottles of 100—NDC 0045-0420-60.

Store at 59°–86°F (15°–30°C). Protect from moisture.

Dispense in a tight, light-resistant container as defined in the official compendium.

Manufactured by Knoll Pharmaceutical, Whippany, N.J. 07961 for:

McNEIL PHARMACEUTICAL
McNEILAB, INC.
SPRING HOUSE, PA 19477

THEOPHYL®-SR ℞

(anhydrous theophylline)
CAPSULES *
for oral use

Description: Each sustained release capsule contains not less than 94.0 percent and not more than 106.0 percent of 125 mg (yellow and clear capsules) or 250 mg (green and clear capsules) anhydrous theophylline in a coated bead timed-release formulation. Theophylline ($C_7H_8N_4O_2$), a xanthine compound, is a white odorless crystalline powder having a bitter taste.

Clinical Pharmacology: Theophylline directly relaxes the smooth muscle of the bronchial airways and pulmonary blood vessels, thus acting mainly as a bronchodilator, pulmonary vasodilator and smooth muscle relaxant. It also possesses other actions typical of the xanthine derivatives: coronary vasodilator, diuretic, and cardiac, cerebral, and skeletal muscle stimulant. The actions of theophylline may be mediated through inhibition of phosphodiesterase and a resultant increase in intracellular cyclic AMP which could mediate smooth muscle relaxation.

In vitro, theophylline has been shown to react synergistically with beta agonists (such as isoproterenol) that increase intracellular cyclic AMP through the stimulation of adenyl cyclase, but synergism has not been demonstrated in clinical studies and more data are needed to determine if theophylline and beta agonists have clinically important additive effects **in vivo.**

Apparently, tolerance does not develop with chronic use of theophylline.

The half-life is shortened with cigarette smoking. The half-life is prolonged in alcoholism, reduced hepatic or renal function, congestive heart failure, and in patients receiving cimetidine or antibiotics such as troleandomycin, (TAO, cyclamycin), erythromycin, lincomycin and clindamycin. High fever for prolonged periods may decrease theophylline elimination.

Theophylline Elimination Characteristics:

	Theophylline Clearance Rates (mean ± S.D.)	Half-Life Average (mean ± S.D.)
Children (over 6 months of age)	1.45 ± 0.58 ml/kg/min	3.7 ± 1.1 hours
Adult nonsmokers with uncomplicated asthma	0.65 ± 0.19 ml/kg/min	8.7 ± 2.2 hours

Newborn infants have extremely slow clearances with half-lives exceeding 24 hours. These approach those seen for older children after about 3–6 months.

Older adults with chronic obstructive pulmonary disease, patients with cor pulmonale or other causes of heart failure, and patients with liver pathology may have much lower clearances with half-lives that may exceed 24 hours.

The half-life is prolonged in alcoholism, reduced hepatic or renal function, congestive heart failure, and in patients receiving cimetidine or certain antibiotics such as TAO (troleandomycin), erythromycin, and clindamycin. High fever for prolonged periods may decrease theophylline elimination.

The half-life of theophylline in smokers (1 to 2 packs/day) averaged 4 to 5 hours in various studies, much shorter than the 7 to 9 hour half-life in nonsmokers. The increase in theophylline clearance caused by smoking is probably the result of induction of drug-metabolizing enzymes that do not readily normalize after cessation of smoking. It appears that between 3 months and 2 years may be necessary for normalization of the effect of smoking on theophylline pharmacokinetics.

Bioavailability of THEOPHYL SR Capsules is 99% ± 6%.

Indications: For relief and/or prevention of symptoms of asthma and reversible bronchospasm associated with chronic bronchitis and emphysema especially in patients requiring chronic therapy.

Contraindications: Avoid using THEOPHYL SR Capsules in individuals who have shown hypersensitivity to any of its components.

Warnings:

Status asthmaticus should be considered a medical emergency and is defined as the degree of bronchospasm which is not rapidly responsive to usual doses of conventional bronchodilators. Optimal therapy for such patients frequently requires both **additional medication,** parenterally administered, and **close monitoring,** preferably in an intensive care setting.

Although increasing the dose of theophylline may bring about relief, such treatment may be associated with toxicity. The likelihood of such toxicity developing increases significantly when the serum theophylline concentration exceeds 20 μg/ml. Therefore, determination of serum theophylline levels is recommended to assure maximal benefit without excessive risk.

Serum levels above 20 μg/ml are rarely found after appropriate administration of the recommended doses. However, in individuals in whom theophylline plasma clearance is reduced **for any reason,** even conventional doses may result in increased serum levels and potential toxicity. Reduced theophylline clearance has been documented in the following readily identifiable groups: 1) patients with impaired renal or liver function; 2) patients over 55 years of age, particularly males and those with chronic lung disease; 3) those with cardiac failure from any cause; 4) neonates; and 5) those patients taking certain drugs (macrolide antibiotics and cimetidine). Decreased clearance of theophylline may be associated with either influenza immunization or active infection with influenza.

Reduction of dosage and laboratory monitoring is especially appropoiate in the above individuals.

Less serious signs of theophylline toxicity, i.e. nausea and restlessness, may appear in up to 50% of patients. Unfortunately however, serious side effects such as ventricular arrhythmias, convulsions or even death may appear as the first sign of toxicity without any previous warning. Stated differently; **serious toxicity is not reliably preceded by less severe side effects.**

Many patients who require theophylline may exhibit tachycardia due to their underlying disease process so that the cause/effect relationship to elevated serum theophylline concentrations may not be appreciated.

Theophylline products may cause dysrhythmia and/or worsen pre-existing arrhythmias and any significant change in rate and/or rhythm warrants monitoring and further investigation.

The occurrence of arrhythmias and sudden death (with histological evidence of necrosis of the myocardium) has been recorded in laboratory animals (minipigs, rodents and dogs) when theophylline and beta agonists were administered concomitantly, although not when either was administered alone. The significance of these findings when applied to human usage is currently unknown.

Usage in Pregnancy: Safe use in pregnancy has not been established relative to possible adverse effects on fetal development, but neither have adverse effects on fetal development been established. This is, unfortunately, true for most antiasthmatic medications. Therefore, use of theophylline in pregnant women should be balanced against the risk of uncontrolled asthma.

Precautions: Mean half-life in smokers i shorter than in nonsmokers; therefore, sm ers may require larger doses of theophy THEOPHYL SR Capsules, like all th line products, should not be administ currently with other xanthine m

Continued o

McNeil Pharm.—Cont.

Use with caution in patients with severe cardiac disease, severe hypoxemia, hypertension, hyperthyroidism, acute myocardial injury, cor pulmonale, congestive heart failure, liver disease, peptic ulcer and in the elderly (especially males) and in neonates. Great caution should be used especially in giving theophylline to patients in congestive heart failure; such patients have shown markedly prolonged theophylline blood level curves with theophylline persisting in serum for long periods following discontinuation of the drug.

Theophylline may occasionally act as a local irritant to the GI tract although gastrointestinal symptoms are more commonly central in origin and associated with serum concentrations over 20 mcg/ml.

It has been reported that theophylline distributes readily into breast milk and may cause adverse effects in the infant. Caution must be used if prescribing xanthines to a mother who is nursing, taking into account the risk-benefit of this therapy.

Due to the marked variation in theophylline metabolism in infants under 6 months of age, this drug is not recommended for this age group.

Adverse Reactions: The most frequent adverse reactions to theophylline are usually due to overdose (serum levels in excess of 20 mcg/ml) and are:

Gastrointestinal: nausea, vomiting, epigastric pain, hematemesis, diarrhea.

Central nervous system: headaches, irritability, restlessness, insomnia, reflex hyperexcitability, muscle twitching, clonic and tonic generalized convulsions.

Cardiovascular: palpitations, tachycardia, extra systoles, flushing, hypotension, circulatory failure, ventricular arrhythmias.

Respiratory: tachypnea.

Renal: albuminuria, increased excretion of renal tubular cells and red blood cells, potentiation of diuresis.

Others: hyperglycemia and inappropriate ADH syndrome.

Drug Interactions: Toxic synergism with ephedrine has been documented and may occur with some other sympathomimetic bronchodilators.

DRUG	EFFECT
Aminophylline with lithium carbonate	Increased excretion of lithium carbonate
Aminophylline with propranolol	Antagonism of propranolol effect
Theophylline with furosemide	Increased diuresis
Theophylline with hexamethonium	Decreased hexamethonium-induced chronotropic effect
Theophylline with reserpine	Reserpine-induced tachycardia
Theophylline with chlordiazepoxide	Chlordiazepoxide-induced fatty acid mobilization
Theophylline with cimetidine, troleandomycin, (TAO, cyclamycin) erythromycin, lincomycin, clindamycin	Increased theophylline plasma levels
Theophylline with phenytoin	Decreased phenytoin levels

Management of Overdose:

A. If potential overdose is established and seizure has not occurred:
1. Induce vomiting.
2. Administer a cathartic.
3. Administer activated charcoal.

B. If patient is having a seizure:
1. Establish an airway.
2. Administer O_2.
3. Treat the seizure with intravenous diazepam, 0.1 to 0.3 mg/kg up to 10 mg.
4. Monitor vital signs, maintain blood pressure and provide adequate hydration.

C. Post-seizure coma:
1. Maintain airway and oxygenation.
2. Follow above recommendations to prevent absorption of drug, but intubation and lavage will have to be performed instead of inducing emesis, and introduce the cathartic and charcoal via a large bore gastric lavage tube.
3. Continue to provide full supportive care and adequate hydration while waiting for drug to be metabolized. In general, the drug is metabolized sufficiently rapidly so as not to require dialysis, however, if serum levels exceed 50 µg/ml, charcoal hemoperfusion may be indicated.

Dosage and Administration: Therapeutic serum levels associated with optimal likelihood for benefit and minimal risk of toxicity are considered to be between 10 mcg/ml and 20 mcg/ml. Levels above 20 mcg/ml may produce toxic effects. There is great variation from patient to patient in dosage needed to achieve a therapeutic blood level because of variable rates of elimination. Therefore, dosage must be individualized and monitoring of theophylline serum levels is highly recommended. Serum theophylline measurement should be obtained at the time of peak absorption. Average time to peak theophylline plasma concentrations in 14 patient volunteers after taking a dose of THEOPHYL® SR Capsules was 5.3 ± 0.5 hours (mean ± standard error). Samples for serum theophylline measurement should be taken after a patient has been on a given dose for at least 3 days and has missed no doses during the previous 48 hours. **Unless the above instructions with regard to serum theophylline measurement are followed, the results may be misleading and dosage adjustments based on these results may be incorrect, possibly increasing the risk of toxicity.**

As theophylline does not distribute into fatty tissue, dosage should be calculated on the basis of lean (ideal) body weight.

Giving theophylline with food may prevent the rare case of stomach irritation; though absorption may be slower, it is still complete.

When rapidly absorbed products such as solutions and uncoated tablets with rapid dissolution are used, dosing to maintain "around the clock" blood levels generally requires administration every 6 hours in children; dosing intervals up to 8 hours may be satisfactory for adults because of their slower elimination rate. Children, and adults requiring higher than average doses, may benefit from products with slower absorption, such as THEOPHYL SR Capsules, which may allow longer dosing intervals and/or less fluctuation in serum concentration over a dosing interval during chronic therapy.

Once a patient is stabilized on a particular dose of theophylline, his blood levels tend to remain constant with that dose.

Pulmonary function measurements before and after a period of treatment permit an objective assessment of response to THEOPHYL SR Capsules.

As a practical consideration, it is not always possible to obtain serum level determinations. Under such conditions, restriction of the daily dose (in otherwise healthy adults) to not greater than 16 mg/kg/day in divided doses will result in relatively few patients exceeding serum levels of 20 µg/ml and the resultant risk of toxicity.

I. Dosage of THEOPHYL® SR for Patients With Chronic Asthma **Not** Currently Receiving Theophylline Therapy

Patients not currently receiving theophylline therapy should be started on conventional rapidly absorbed theophylline products, such as THEOPHYL® Tablets—225 mg. Once the patient is stabilized on a particular dose of theophylline, therapy with THEOPHYL® SR Capsules should be initiated at the same total daily dose, with half the total daily dose administered every 12 hours. If satisfactory control of symptoms is not maintained for the full 12 hour period, or if unacceptable adverse effects occur, one third of the total daily dosage should be administered on an every 8 hour schedule.

If theophylline therapy is initiated with THEOPHYL® SR Capsules, the recommended starting dose is 250 mg twice daily. If this dosage is not effective after three days, the dosage may be increased to 375 mg every 12 hours or 250 mg every 8 hours.

II. Dosage of THEOPHYL® SR for Patients with Chronic Asthma Currently Receiving Theophylline Therapy.

Therapy with THEOPHYL® SR Capsules should be initiated at the patient's current total daily dosage, with half the total daily dose administered every 12 hours. If satisfactory control of symptoms is not maintained for the full 12 hours, or if unacceptable adverse effects occur, one third of the total daily dosage should be administered every 8 hours. If this dosage is not effective after three days, the dosage may be increased to 375 mg every 12 hours or 250 mg every 8 hours.

Maximum Dose Without Measurement of Serum Concentration:

Not to exceed the following: **(WARNING: DO NOT ATTEMPT TO MAINTAIN ANY DOSE THAT IS NOT TOLERATED)**

Age Less than 9 years	–24 mg/kg/day
Age 9–12 years	–20 mg/kg/day
Age 12–16 years	–18 mg/kg/day
Age Greater than 16 years	–13 mg/kg/day or 900 mg/day (WHICHEVER IS LESS)

Note: Use ideal body weight for obese patients.

How Supplied:

THEOPHYL®-SR capsules (yellow and clear, imprinted "Theophyl" and "125") contain 125 mg anhydrous theophylline-bottles of 100—NDC 0045-0422-60.

THEOPHYL®-SR capsules (green and clear, imprinted "Theophyl" and "250") contain 250 mg anhydrous theophylline—bottles of 100—NDC 0045-0423-60.

Store at 59°–86°F (15°–30°C). Protect from excessive moisture.

Dispense in a tight, light-resistant container as defined in the official compendium.

Manufactured by Cord Laboratories, Inc., Broomfield, CO 80020 for:

McNEIL PHARMACEUTICAL
McNEILAB, INC.
SPRING HOUSE, PA 19477

THEOPHYL®-225 ℞

(anhydrous theophylline)
TABLETS and ELIXIR
for oral use

Description: Each scored, white tablet contains not less than 94.0 percent and not more than 106.0 percent of 225 mg anhydrous theophylline USP.

Each 30 ml (two TABLESPOONfuls) of banana-mint flavored THEOPHYL® ELIXIR contains not less than 94.0 percent and not more than 106.0 percent of 225 mg anhydrous theophylline, USP, and 225 mg calcium salicylate as a solubilizing agent, with 5% alcohol.

Theophylline ($C_7H_8N_4O_2$), a xanthine compound, is a white odorless crystalline powder having a bitter taste.

Clinical Pharmacology: Theophylline directly relaxes the smooth muscle of the bronchial airways and pulmonary blood vessels, thus acting mainly as a bronchodilator, pulmonary vasodilator and smooth muscle relaxant. It also possesses other actions typical of the xanthine derivatives: coronary vasodilator, diuretic, and cardiac, cerebral, and skeletal muscle stimulant. The actions of theophylline may be mediated through inhibition of phosphodiesterase and a resultant increase in intracellular cyclic AMP which could mediate smooth muscle relaxation.

In vitro, theophylline has been shown to react synergistically with beta agonists (such as isoproterenol) that increase intracellular cyclic AMP through the stimulation of adenyl cyclase, but synergism has not been demonstrated in clinical studies and more data are needed to determine if theophylline and beta agonists have clinically important additive effects **in vivo.**

Apparently, tolerance does not develop with chronic use of theophylline. The half-life is shortened with cigarette smoking. The half-life is prolonged in alcoholism, reduced hepatic or renal function, congestive heart failure, and in patients receiving cimetidine or certain antibiotics such as troleandomycin, (TAO, cyclamycin) erythromycin, lincomycin and clindamycin. High fever for prolonged periods may decrease theophylline elimination.

Theophylline Elimination Characteristics:

	Theophylline Clearance Rates (mean ± S.D.)	Half-Life Average (mean ± S.D.)
Children (over 6 months of age)	1.45 ± 0.58 ml/kg/min	3.7 ± 1.1 hours
Adult nonsmokers with uncomplicated asthma	0.65 ± 0.19 ml/kg/min	8.7 ± 2.2 hours

Newborn infants have extremely slow clearances with half-lives exceeding 24 hours. These approach those seen for older children after about 3–6 months.

Older adults with chronic obstructive pulmonary disease, patients with cor pulmonale or other causes of heart failure, and patients with liver pathology may have much lower clearances with half-lives that may exceed 24 hours. The half-life is prolonged in alcoholism, reduced hepatic or renal function, congestive heart failure, and in patients receiving cimetidine or certain antibiotics such as (TAO) (troleandomycin), erythromycin, lincomycin, and clindamycin. High fever for prolonged periods may decrease theophylline elimination.

The half-life of theophylline in smokers (1 to 2 packs/day) averaged 4 to 5 hours in various studies, much shorter than the 7 to 9 hour half-life in nonsmokers. The increase in theophylline clearance caused by smoking is probably the result of induction of drug-metabolizing enzymes that do not readily normalize after cessation of smoking. It appears that between 3 months and 2 years may be necessary for normalization of the effect of smoking on theophylline pharmacokinetics.

THEOPHYL® Tablets and Elixir are rapidly releasing forms of theophylline. Bioavailability of the tablets has been shown to be 96% ± 3%. The availability of the elixir has been shown to be 99% ± 2%, with 85% of the drug absorbed within one hour.

Indications: For relief and/or prevention of symptoms of asthma and reversible bronchospasm associated with chronic bronchitis and emphysema.

Contraindications: Avoid using THEOPHYL® Tablets and Elixir in individuals who have shown hypersensitivity to any of its components.

Warnings: Status asthmaticus should be considered a medical emergency and is defined as the degree of bronchospasm which is not rapidly responsive to usual doses of conventional bronchodilators. Optimal therapy for such patients frequently requires both **additional medication,** parenterally administered, and **close monitoring,** preferably in an intensive care setting.

Although increasing the dose of theophylline may bring about relief, such treatment may be associated with toxicity. The likelihood of such toxicity developing increases significantly when the serum theophylline concentration exceeds 20 µg/ml. Therefore, determination of serum theophylline levels is recommended to assure maximal benefit without excessive risk. Serum levels above 20 µg/ml are rarely found after appropriate administration of the recommended doses. However, in individuals in whom theophylline plasma clearance is reduced **for any reason,** even conventional doses may result in increased serum levels and potential toxicity. Reduced theophylline clearance has been documented in the following readily identifiable groups: 1) patients with impaired renal or liver funtion; 2) patients over 55 years of age, particularly males and those with chronic lung disease; 3) those with cardiac failure from any cause; 4) neonates; and 5) those patients taking certain drugs (macrolide antibiotics and cimetidine). Decreased clearance of theophylline may be associated with either influenza immunization or active infection with influenza.

Reduction of dosage and laboratory monitoring is especially appropriate in the above individuals.

Less serious signs of theophylline toxicity, i.e. nausea and restlessness, may appear in up to 50% of patients. Unfortunately however, serious side effects such as ventricular arrhythmias, convulsions or even death may appear as the first sign of toxicity without any previous warning. Stated differently; **serious toxicity is not reliably preceded by less severe side effects.**

Many patients who require theophylline may exhibit tachycardia due to their underlying disease process so that the cause/effect relationship to elevated serum theophylline concentrations may not be appreciated.

Theophylline products may cause dysrhythmia and/or worsen pre-existing arrhthmias and any significant change in rate and/or rhythm warrants monitoring and further investigation.

The occurence of arrhythmias and sudden death (with histological evidence of necrosis of the myocardium) has been recorded in laboratory animals (minipigs, rodents and dogs) when theophylline and beta agonists were administered concomitantly, although not when either was administered alone. The significance of these findings when applied to human usage is currently unknown.

THEOPHYL Elixir contains 37.5 mg of calcium salicylate per cc as a solubilizing agent. Therefore, concomitant use of aspirin should either be avoided (by use of acetaminophen for analgesia and antipyresis) or should be confined to a dose that provides a total (aspirin and calcium salicylate) of no more than 15 mg/kg at intervals of 6 hours or longer.

Intolerance to aspirin is not intolerance to salicylates generally; aspirin-sensitive patients are not more likely to react to other salicylates such as calcium salicylate than to unrelated materials.

Usage in Pregnancy: Safe use in pregnancy has not been established relative to possible adverse effects on fetal development, but neither have adverse effects on fetal development been established. This is, unfortunately, true for most antiasthmatic medications. Therefore, use of theophylline in pregnant women should be balanced against the risk of uncontrolled asthma.

Precautions: Mean half-life in smokers is shorter than in nonsmokers; therefore, smokers may require larger doses of theophylline. THEOPHYL® Tablets and Elixir, like all theophylline products, should not be administered concurrently with other xanthine medications. Use with caution in patients with severe cardiac disease, severe hypoxemia, hypertension, hyperthyroidism, acute myocardial injury, cor pulmonale, congestive heart failure, liver disease, peptic ulcer and in the elderly (especially males) and in neonates. Great caution should be used especially in giving theophylline to patients in congestive heart failure; such patients have shown markedly prolonged theophylline blood level curves with theophylline persisting in serum for long periods following discontinuation of the drug.

Theophylline may occasionally act as a local irritant to the GI tract although gastrointestinal symptoms are more commonly central in origin and associated with serum concentrations over 20 µg/ml.

It has been reported that theophylline distributes readily into breast milk and may cause adverse effects in the infant. Caution must be used if prescribing xanthines to a mother who is nursing, taking into account the risk-benefit of this therapy.

Due to the marked variation in theophylline metabolism in infants under 6 months of age, this drug is not recommended for this age group.

Adverse Reactions: The most frequent adverse reactions to theophylline are usually due to overdose (serum levels in excess of 20 µg/ml and are:

Gastrointestinal: nausea, vomiting, epigastric pain, hematemesis, diarrhea.

Central nervous system: headaches, irritability, restlessness, insomnia, reflex hyperexcitability, muscle twitching, clonic and tonic generalized convulsions.

Cardiovascular: palpitations, tachycardia, extra systoles, flushing, hypotension, circulatory failure, ventricular arrhythmias.

Respiratory: tachypnea.

Renal: albuminuria, increased excretion of renal tubular cells and red blood cells, potentiation of diuresis.

Others: hyperglycemia and inappropriate ADH-syndrome.

Drug Interactions: Toxic synergism with ephedrine has been documented and may occur with some other sympathomimetic bronchodilators.

DRUG	EFFECT
Aminophylline with lithium carbonate	Increased excretion of lithium carbonate
Aminophylline with propranolol	Antagonism of propranolol effect
Theophylline with furosemide	Increased diuresis
Theophylline with hexamethonium	Decreased hexamethonium-induced chronotropic effect
Theophylline with reserpine	Reserpine-induced tachycardia
Theophylline with chlordiazepoxide	Chlordiazepoxide-induced fatty acid mobilization
Theophylline with cimetidine troleandomycin (TAO cyclamycin), erythromycin, lincomycin, clindamycin	Increased theophylline plasma levels
Theophylline with phenytoin	Decreased phenytoin levels

Management of Overdose:

A. If potential overdose is established and seizure has not occurred:
   1. Induce vomiting.
   2. Administer a cathartic.
   3. Administer activated charcoal.

B. If patient is having a seizure:
   1. Establish an airway.
   2. Administer O_2.
   3. Treat the seizure with intravenous diazepam, 0.1 to 0.3 mg/kg up to 10 mg.
   4. Monitor vital signs, maintain blood pressure and provide adequate hydration.

C. Post-seizure coma:
   1. Maintain airway and oxygenation.
   2. Follow above recommendations to prevent absorption of drug, but intubation and lavage will have to be performed instead of inducing emesis, and introduce the cathartic and charcoal via a large bore gastric lavage tube.
   3. Continue to provide full supportive care and adequate hydration while waiting f

Continued on next

McNeil Pharm.—Cont.

drug to be metabolized. In general, the drug is metabolized sufficiently rapidly so as not to require dialysis, however, if serum levels exceed 50μg/ml, charcoal hemoperfusion may be indicated.

Dosage and Administration: Therapeutic serum levels associated with optimal likelihood for benefit and minimal risk of toxicity are considered to be between 10 μg/ml and 20 μg/ml. Levels above 20 μg/ml may produce toxic effects. There is great variation from patient to patient in dosage needed to achieve a therapeutic blood level because of variable rates of elimination. Therefore, dosage must be individualized and monitoring of theophylline serum levels is highly recommended. Serum theophylline measurement should be obtained at the time of peak absorption. Average time to peak theophylline plasma concentrations in 14 patient volunteers after taking a dose of THEOPHYL Tablets was 2.0 ± 0.3 hours and 1.4 ± 0.3 hours for THEOPHYL Elixir (mean ± standard error). Samples for serum theophylline measurement should be taken after a patient has been on a given dose for at least 3 days and has missed no doses during the previous 48 hours. **Unless the above instructions with regard to serum theophylline measurement are followed, the results may be misleading and dosage adjustments based on these results may be incorrect, possibly increasing the risk of toxicity.**

As theophylline does not distribute into fatty tissue, dosage should be calculated on the basis of lean (ideal) body weight.

Giving theophylline with food may prevent the rare case of stomach irritation; though absorption may be slower, it is still complete.

When rapidly absorbed products such as solutions and uncoated tablets with rapid dissolution are used, dosing to maintain "around the clock" blood levels generally requires administration every 6 hours in children; dosing intervals up to 8 hours may be satisfactory for adults because of their slower elimination rate. Children, and adults requiring higher than average doses, may benefit from products with slower absorption, such as THEOPHYL SR Capsules, which may allow longer dosing intervals and/or less fluctuation in serum concentration over a dosing interval during chronic therapy.

Once a patient is stabilized on a particular dose of theophylline, his blood levels tend to remain constant with that dose.

Pulmonary function measurements before and after a period of treatment permit an objective assessment of response to THEOPHYL Tablets and Elixir.

As a practical consideration, it is not always possible to obtain serum level determinations. Under such conditions, restriction of the daily dose (in otherwise healthy adults) to not greater than 16 mg/kg/day in divided doses will result in relatively few patients exceeding serum levels of 20 μg/ml and the resultant risk of toxicity.

I. Dosage of THEOPHYL® Tablets and Elixir for Patients Exhibiting Acute Symptoms of Asthma Requiring Rapid Theophyllinization and Not Currently Receiving Theophylline Products.

[See table below].

II. Dosage for Patients Currently Receiving Theophylline Products.

Determine, where possible, the time, amount, route of administration and form of the patient's last dose. Ideally, the loading dose should be deferred if a serum theophylline determination can be rapidly obtained. If this is not possible, the clinician must exercise his judgment in selecting a dose based on the potential for benefit and risk. The loading dose of theophylline is based on the principle that each 0.5 mg/kg of theophylline administered as a loading dose will result in a 1 mcg/ml increase in serum theophylline concentration. When there is sufficient respiratory distress to warrant a small risk, 2.5 mg/kg of theophylline is likely to increase the serum concentration by only about 5 mcg/ml when administered as a loading dose. If the patient is not already experiencing theophylline toxicity, this is unlikely to result in dangerous adverse effects. Subsequent maintenance dosage recommendations are the same as those described above.

III. Dosage for Chronic Asthma.

Theophyllinization is a treatment of first choice for the management of chronic asthma (to prevent symptoms and maintain patent airways). Slow clinical titration is generally preferred to assure acceptance and safety of the medication.

Adult Dosage

Initial Dose: 16 mg/kg/day or 450 mg/day (whichever is lower) in 3–4 divided doses at 6–8 hour intervals.

Increased Dose: The above dosage may be increased in approximately 25 percent increments at 2–3 day intervals so long as no intolerance is observed, until a maximum indicated below is reached.

Pediatric Dosage

Approximate pediatric dosage may be determined by referring to the following table. (Note: this table utilizes TEASPOONSFUL (tsp) doses rather than TABLESPOONSFUL doses, since this involves a pediatric age group.) Children above age 9 require lower mg/kg doses than younger children.

Body Weight lbs.	kgs.	Approximate Pediatric Dose in TEASPOONSFUL (tsp) Initial 4 mg/kg	Maximum* 6 mg/kg
20	9	1 tsp	1½ tsp
30	14	1½ tsp	1 tsp
40	18	2 tsp	3 tsp
50	23	2½ tsp	3½ tsp
60	27	3 tsp	3½ tsp
70	32	3½ tsp	5 tsp
80	36	4 tsp	5½ tsp
90	41	4½ tsp	6½ tsp
100	45	5 tsp	7 tsp

administered every 6 hours

* Should not be exceeded unless Theophylline blood levels are obtained.

Maximum Dose Without Measurement of Serum Concentration:

Not to exceed the following: **(WARNING: DO NOT ATTEMPT TO MAINTAIN ANY DOSE THAT IS NOT TOLERATED)**

Age	
Age Less than 9 years	–24 mg/kg/day
Age 9–12 years	–20 mg/kg/day
Age 12–16 years	–18 mg/kg/day
Age Greater than 16 years	–13 mg/kg/day or 900 mg/day (WHICHEVER IS LESS)

NOTE: Use ideal body weight for obese patients.

How Supplied:

Each white triangle shaped tablet (bisected, inscribed with "Theophyl® 225") contains 225 mg of anhydrous theophylline. Bottles of 100—NDC 0045-0424-60

Each 30 ml (2 tablespoonsful) of the banana-mint flavored orange yellow elixir contains 225 mg of anhydrous theophylline. Available in pint bottles (473 ml)—NDC 0045-0421-16.

Store at 59°–86°F (15°–30°C).

Dispense in a tight, light-resistant container as defined in the official compendium.

Manufactured by Knoll Pharmaceutical, Whippany, N.J. 07981 for:

McNEIL PHARMACEUTICAL
McNEILAB, INC.
SPRING HOUSE, PA 19477

	Loading Dose	Maintenance Dose For Next 12 Hours	Maintenance Dose Beyond 12 Hours
1. Children 6 months to 9 years	6 mg/kg	4 mg/kg q4h	4 mg/kg q6h
2. Children age 9–16 and young adult smokers	6 mg/kg	3 mg/kg q4h	3 mg/kg q6h
3. Otherwise healthy nonsmoking adults	6 mg/kg	3 mg/kg q6h	3 mg/kg q8h
4. Older patients and patients with cor pulmonale	6 mg/kg	2 mg/kg q6h	2 mg/kg q8h
Patients with congestive heart failure, liver failure	6 mg/kg	2 mg/kg q8h	1–2 mg/kg q12h

TOLECTIN® DS (tolmetin sodium) capsules ℞

TOLECTIN® (tolmetin sodium) tablets

200 mg tablets—100's:

Military NSN 6505-01-038-7460

VA NSN 6505-01-038-7460A

400 mg capsules—100's:

VA NSN 6505-01-091-9624A

Description: TOLECTIN DS (tolmetin sodium) capsules for oral administration contain tolmetin sodium as the dihydrate in an amount equivalent to 400 mg of tolmetin. Each capsule contains 36 mg (1.568 mEq) of sodium.

TOLECTIN (tolmetin sodium) tablets for oral administration contain tolmetin sodium as the dihydrate in an amount equivalent to 200 mg of tolmetin (scored for 100 mg). Each tablet contains 18 mg (0.784 mEq) of sodium.

Tolmetin sodium is a non-steroidal anti-inflammatory agent.

Clinical Pharmacology: Studies in animals have shown TOLECTIN (tolmetin sodium) to possess anti-inflammatory, analgesic and antipyretic activity. In the rat, TOLECTIN prevents the development of experimentally induced polyarthritis and also decreases established inflammation.

The mode of action of TOLECTIN is not known. However, studies in laboratory animals and man have demonstrated that the anti-inflammatory action of TOLECTIN is *not* due to pituitary-adrenal stimulation. TOLECTIN inhibits prostaglandin synthetase *in vitro* and lowers the plasma level of prostaglandin E in man. This reduction in prostaglandin synthesis may be responsible for the anti-inflammatory action. TOLECTIN does not appear to alter the course of the underlying disease in man.

In patients with rheumatoid arthritis and in normal volunteers, TOLECTIN is rapidly and almost completely absorbed with peak plasma levels being reached within 30–60 minutes after an oral therapeutic dose. The drug is eliminated from the plasma with a mean half-life of one hour. Peak plasma levels of approximately 40 μg/ml are obtained with a 400 mg oral dose. Essentially all of the administered dose is recovered in the urine in 24 hours either as an inactive oxidative metabolite or as conjugates of TOLECTIN.

In two fecal blood loss studies of 4 to 6 days duration involving 15 subjects each, TOLECTIN did not induce an increase in blood loss over that observed during a 4-day drug-free control period. In the same studies, aspirin produced a greater blood loss than occurred during the drug-free control period, and a greater blood loss than occurred during the TOLECTIN treatment period. In one of the two studies, indomethacin produced a greater fecal blood loss than occurred during the drug-free control period; in the second study, indomethacin did not induce a significant increase in blood loss.

TOLECTIN does not interfere with the clinical assessment of the tuberculin skin test or the immediate-type hypersensitivity skin test. It appears that the drug does not interfere with the immune mechanism as measured by skin testing.

Indications and Usage: TOLECTIN (tolmetin sodium) is indicated for the relief of signs and symptoms of rheumatoid arthritis and osteoarthritis. TOLECTIN is indicated in the treatment of acute flares and the long-term management of the chronic disease. TOLECTIN is also indicated for treatment of juvenile rheumatoid arthritis.

The safety and effectiveness of TOLECTIN have not been established in those patients with rheumatoid arthritis who are designated by the American Rheumatism Association as Functional Class IV (incapacitated, largely or wholly bedridden or confined to a wheelchair; little or no self-care).

Improvement in patients treated with TOLECTIN for rheumatoid arthritis has been demonstrated by a reduction in joint swelling, a reduction in pain, a reduction in the number of inflamed joints, a reduction in the duration of morning stiffness, a decrease in disease activity as assessed by both the investigator and the patient, and improved functional capability as demonstrated by an increase in grip strength, a delay in the time to onset of fatigue and a decrease in the time to walk 50 feet.

Improvement in patients treated with TOLECTIN for osteoarthritis has been demonstrated by a reduction of pain at rest and pain on motion, a reduction of swelling, redness and tenderness, a reduction in the duration of morning stiffness and in the inflammation of Heberden's Nodes, a decrease in disease activity as assessed by both the investigator and patient, an increase in range of motion of affected joints, a decrease in the time to walk 50 feet and an improved functional capability as demonstrated by an increase in grip strength and performance of daily activities.

In clinical studies in patients with either rheumatoid arthritis or osteoarthritis, TOLECTIN has been shown to be comparable to aspirin and to indomethacin in controlling disease activity but the frequency of the milder gastrointestinal adverse effects and tinnitus was less than in aspirin-treated patients, and the incidence of central nervous system adverse effects was less than in indomethacin-treated patients. It is not known whether TOLECTIN causes less peptic ulceration than aspirin or indomethacin.

Clinical studies have shown that, when added to a regimen of gold salts or corticosteroids, TOLECTIN has produced additional therapeutic benefit, although this effect was somewhat less when patients were receiving gold salts than when they were receiving corticosteroids. The use of TOLECTIN in conjunction with salicylates is not recommended since there does not appear to be any greater benefit from the combination over that achieved with aspirin alone, and the potential for adverse reactions is increased.

In clinical studies in patients with juvenile rheumatoid arthritis, TOLECTIN has been shown to be comparable to aspirin in controlling disease activity, with a similar incidence of adverse reactions. In liver function tests, mean SGOT values, initially elevated in patients on previous aspirin therapy, remained elevated in the aspirin group and decreased in the TOLECTIN group. The safety and effectiveness of TOLECTIN have not been established in infants under 2 years of age.

Contraindications: TOLECTIN (tolmetin sodium) should not be used in patients who have previously exhibited intolerance to it. Because the potential exists for cross-sensitivity to aspirin and other non-steroidal anti-inflammatory drugs, TOLECTIN should not be given to patients in whom aspirin and other non-steroidal anti-inflammatory drugs induce symptoms of asthma, rhinitis or urticaria.

Warnings: TOLECTIN (tolmetin sodium) should be given under close supervision to patients with a history of upper gastrointestinal tract disease and only after consulting the "Adverse Reactions" section. Peptic ulceration and gastrointestinal bleeding, sometimes severe, have been reported in patients receiving TOLECTIN.

In patients with active peptic ulcer, attempts should be made to treat the arthritis with nonulcerogenic drugs, such as gold. If TOLECTIN must be given, the patient should be under close supervision for signs of ulcer perforation or severe gastrointestinal bleeding.

Precautions: ***General:*** Clinical studies of up to two years duration have shown no changes in the eyes attributable to TOLECTIN (tolmetin sodium) administration; however, because of microscopic changes in the lens in rats receiving TOLECTIN at doses about twice the maximum recommended dose in man and because of ocular changes observed clinically with other non-steroidal anti-inflammatory drugs, it is recommended that ophthalmologic examinations be carried out within a reasonable time after starting chronic therapy and at periodic intervals thereafter.

In a chronic study in rats, lesions of the renal papillae were observed at doses of TOLECTIN approximately twice the maximum recommended human dose. In a chronic study in mice, chronic nephritis and glomerular sclerosis occurred in animals receiving doses of one and a half times the human dose. In a chronic study in monkeys a single instance (one in eight) of renal papillary necrosis was observed at a dose more than three times the maximum recommended human dosage. There has been no evidence of renal toxicity to date in clinical studies; however, since TOLECTIN is eliminated primarily by the kidneys, patients with impaired renal function should be closely monitored, and they may require lower doses.

TOLECTIN prolongs bleeding time. Patients who may be adversely affected by prolongation of bleeding time should be carefully observed when TOLECTIN is administered.

In patients receiving concomitant TOLECTIN-steroid therapy, any reduction in steroid dosage should be gradual to avoid the possible complications of sudden steroid withdrawal.

TOLECTIN has been shown to cause some retention of water and sodium, and mild peripheral edema has been reported in about 7% of patients receiving TOLECTIN. Therefore, TOLECTIN should be used with caution in patients with compromised cardiac function.

The metabolites of tolmetin in urine have been found to give positive tests for proteinuria using tests which rely on acid precipitation as their endpoint (e.g. sulfosalicylic acid). No interference is seen in the tests for proteinuria using dye-impregnated commercially available reagent strips (e.g. Albustix®, Uristix®, etc.).

As with other nonsteroidal anti-inflammatory drugs, anaphylactoid reactions have been reported. Because of the possibility of cross-sensitivity due to structural relationships which exist among nonsteroidal anti-inflammatory drugs, anaphylactoid reactions may be more likely to occur in patients who have exhibited allergic reactions to these compounds, particularly zomepirac sodium. Patients who have had anaphylactoid reactions on TOLECTIN should be treated with conventional therapy, such as epinephrine, antihistamines, and/or steroids.

As with other nonsteroidal anti-inflammatory drugs, borderline elevations of one or more liver tests may occur in up to 15% of patients. These abnormalities may progress, may remain essentially unchanged, or may be transient with continued therapy. The SGPT (ALT) test is probably the most sensitive indicator of liver dysfunction. Meaningful (3 times the upper limit of normal) elevations of SGPT or SGOT (AST) occurred in controlled clinical trials in less than 1% of patients. A patient with symptoms and/or signs suggesting liver dysfunction, or in whom an abnormal liver test has occurred, should be evaluated for evidence of the development of more severe hepatic reaction while on therapy with TOLECTIN. Severe hepatic reactions, including jaundice and fatal hepatitis, have been reported with TOLECTIN as with other nonsteroidal anti-inflammatory drugs. Although such reactions are rare, if abnormal liver tests persist or worsen, if clinical signs and symptoms consistent with liver disease develop, or if systemic manifestations occur (e.g. eosinophilia, rash, etc.), TOLECTIN should be discontinued.

Usage in Pregnancy: Since TOLECTIN has not been studied in pregnant women, the use of TOLECTIN during pregnancy is not recommended. Reproduction studies in rats and rabbits at doses up to 1.7 times the maximum clinical dose revealed no evidence of impaired fertility or teratogenesis due to TOLECTIN. However, as with other non-steroidal anti-inflammatory drugs known to inhibit prostaglandin synthesis, an increased incidence of dystocia and delayed parturition occurs in rats. These effects were absent when TOLECTIN was discontinued 24 hours prior to expected delivery.

Nursing Mothers: It is not known whether TOLECTIN is secreted in human milk; however, it is secreted in the milk of lactating rats. As a general rule nursing should not be undertaken while a patient is on TOLECTIN since it may be excreted in human milk.

Drug Interactions: The *in vitro* binding of warfarin to human plasma proteins is unaffected by tolmetin, and tolmetin does not alter the prothrombin time of normal volunteers. However, in patients there have been rare reports that prothrombin time may increase and bleeding may occur.

In adult diabetic patients under treatment with either sulfonylureas or insulin there is no change in the clinical effects of either TOLECTIN or the hypoglycemic agents.

Adverse Reactions: The adverse reactions which have been observed in clinical trials encompass observations in about 4370 patients treated with TOLECTIN (tolmetin sodium), over 800 of whom have undergone at least one year of therapy. These adverse reactions, reported below by body system, are among those typical of nonsteroidal anti-inflammatory drugs and, as expected, gastrointestinal complaints were most frequent. In clinical trials with TOLECTIN, about 10% of patients dropped out because of adverse reactions, mostly gastrointestinal in nature.

Incidence Greater Than 1%

The following adverse reactions which occurred more frequently than 1 in 100 were reported in controlled clinical trials.

Gastrointestinal: Nausea (11%), dyspepsia,* gastrointestinal distress,* abdominal pain,* diarrhea,* flatulence,* vomiting,* constipation, gastritis, and peptic ulcer. Forty percent of the ulcer patients had a prior history of peptic ulcer disease and/or were receiving concomitant anti-inflammatory drugs including corticosteroids, which are known to produce peptic ulceration.

Body as a Whole: Headache,* asthenia,* chest pain

Cardiovascular: Elevated blood pressure,* edema*

Central Nervous System: Dizziness,* drows ness, depression

Metabolic/Nutritional: Weight gain,* w loss*

Continued on

McNeil Pharm.—Cont.

Dermatologic: Skin irritation
Special Senses: Tinnitus, visual disturbance
Hematologic: Small and transient decreases in hemoglobin and hematocrit not associated with gastrointestinal bleeding have occurred. These are similar to changes reported with other nonsteroidal anti-inflammatory drugs.
Urogenital: Elevated BUN, urinary tract infection

* Reactions occurring in 3% to 9% of patients treated with TOLECTIN. Reactions occurring in fewer than 3% of the patients are unmarked.

Incidence Less Than 1%
(Causal Relationship Probable)

The following adverse reactions were reported less frequently than 1 in 100 in controlled clinical trials or were reported since marketing. The probability exists that there is a causal relationship between TOLECTIN and these adverse reactions.
Gastrointestinal: Gastrointestinal bleeding with or without evidence of peptic ulcer, glossitis, stomatitis, hepatitis, liver function abnormalities
Body as a Whole: Anaphylactoid reactions, fever
Hematologic: Hemolytic anemia, thrombocytopenia, granulocytopenia, agranulocytosis
Cardiovascular: Congestive heart failure in patients with marginal cardiac function
Dermatologic: Urticaria, purpura, erythema multiforme
Urogenital: Hematuria, proteinuria, dysuria, acute renal failure

Incidence Less Than 1%
(Causal Relationship Unknown)

Other adverse reactions were reported less frequently than 1 in 100 in controlled clinical trials or were reported since marketing, but a causal relationship between TOLECTIN and the reaction could not be determined. These rarely reported reactions are being listed as alerting information for the physician since the possibility of a causal relationship cannot be excluded.
Body as Whole: Epistaxis

Management of Overdosage: In the event of overdosage, the stomach should be emptied by inducing vomiting or by gastric lavage followed by the administration of activated charcoal.

Dosage and Administration: In adults, the recommended starting dose is 400 mg three times daily (1200 mg daily), preferably including a dose on arising and a dose at bedtime. To achieve optimal therapeutic effect the dose should be adjusted according to the patient's response. For rheumatoid arthritis control is usually achieved at doses of 600–1800 mg daily in divided doses (t.i.d. or q.i.d.). For osteoarthritis control is usually achieved at doses of 600–1600 mg daily in divided doses (t.i.d. or q.i.d.). Doses larger than 2000 mg/day for rheumatoid arthritis and 1600 mg/day for osteoarthritis have not been studied and therefore are not recommended.

The recommended starting dose for children (two years and older) is 20 mg/kg/day in divided doses (t.i.d. or q.i.d.). When control has been achieved the usual dose ranges from 15 to 30 mg/kg/day. Doses higher than 30 mg/kg/day have not been studied and therefore are not recommended.

A therapeutic response to TOLECTIN (tolmetin sodium) can be expected in a few days to a week. Progressive improvement can be anticipated during succeeding weeks of therapy. If gastrointestinal symptoms occur, administer TOLECTIN with meals, milk or antacids, other than sodium bicarbonate.

How Supplied:
TOLECTIN® DS (tolmetin sodium) capsules 400 mg (colored orange opaque, with contrasting parallel bands imprinted "McNEIL" and "TOLECTIN DS"), **NDC** 0045-0414-60, bottles of 100.
TOLECTIN® (tolmetin sodium) tablets 200 mg (colored white, scored, imprinted "200", "McNeil" and "TOLECTIN"), bottles of 100 (**NDC** 0045-0412-60); bottles of 500 (**NDC** 0045-0412-70).

[*Shown in Product Identification Section*]

TYLENOL® with Codeine tablets ©, capsules © and elixir © ℞

Tablets:
No. 3 (100'S):
VA NSN 6505-00-400-2054
No. 3 (unit dose 20 × 25):
Military NSN 6505-01-086-2993
No. 3 (500's):
Military NSN 6505-00-147-8347
VA NSN 6505-01-074-8385

Description:
Tablets:
Each TYLENOL with codeine tablet contains:

No. 1 Codeine Phosphate*	7.5 mg (1/8 gr)
Acetaminophen	300 mg
No. 2 Codeine Phosphate*	15 mg (1/4 gr)
Acetaminophen	300 mg
No. 3 Codeine Phosphate*	30 mg (1/2 gr)
Acetaminophen	300 mg
No. 4 Codeine Phosphate*	60 mg (1 gr)
Acetaminophen	300 mg

Capsules:
Each TYLENOL with Codeine capsule contains:

No. 3 Codeine Phosphate*	30 mg (1/2 gr)
Acetaminophen	300 mg
No. 4 Codeine Phosphate*	60 mg (1 gr)
Acetaminophen	300 mg

Elixir:
Each 5 ml TYLENOL with Codeine elixir contains:

Codeine Phosphate*	12 mg
Acetaminophen	120 mg

Alcohol 7%

* *Warning*—May be habit forming.

Acetaminophen occurs as a white, odorless crystalline powder, possessing a slightly bitter taste. Codeine is an alkaloid obtained from opium or prepared from morphine by methylation. Codeine occurs as colorless or white crystals, effloresces slowly in dry air and is affected by light. Acetaminophen is a non-salicylate.

Actions: Acetaminophen is a non-narcotic analgesic and antipyretic; codeine is a narcotic with analgesic and antitussive actions. Codeine retains at least one-half of its analgesic activity when administered orally.

Indications: TYLENOL with Codeine tablets No. 1, No. 2, and No. 3 are indicated for the relief of mild to moderate pain. TYLENOL with Codeine No. 4 is indicated for the relief of moderate to severe pain. TYLENOL with Codeine elixir is indicated for the relief of mild to moderate pain.

Contraindications: Hypersensitivity to acetaminophen or codeine.

Warnings:
Drug Dependence: Codeine can produce drug dependence of the morphine type, and therefore has the potential for being abused. Psychic dependence, physical dependence and tolerance may develop upon repeated administration of this drug, and it should be prescribed and administered with the same degree of caution appropriate to the use of other oral narcotic-containing medications. Like other narcotic-containing medications, the drug is subject to the Federal Controlled Substances Act.
Usage in Ambulatory Patients: Codeine may impair the mental and/or physical abilities required for the performance of potentially hazardous tasks such as driving a car or operating machinery. The patient using this drug should be cautioned accordingly.
Interaction with other central nervous system depressants: Patients receiving other narcotic analgesics, general anesthetics, phenothiazines, other tranquilizers, sedative-hypnotics or other CNS depressants (including alcohol) concomitantly with this drug may exhibit an additive CNS depression. When such combined therapy is contemplated, the dose of one or both agents should be reduced.
Usage in Pregnancy: Safe use in pregnancy has not been established relative to possible adverse effects on fetal development. Therefore this drug should not be used in pregnant women unless, in the judgment of the physician, the potential benefits outweigh the possible hazards.
Pediatric use: Safe dosage of the elixir has not been established in children below the age of three; tablets or capsules should not be administered to children under 12.

Precautions:
Head injury and increased intracranial pressure: The respiratory depressant effects of narcotics and their capacity to elevate cerebrospinal fluid pressure may be markedly exaggerated in the presence of head injury, other intracranial lesions or a pre-existing increase in intracranial pressure. Furthermore, narcotics produce adverse reactions which may obscure the clinical course of patients with head injuries.
Acute abdominal conditions: The administration of this product or other narcotics may obscure the diagnosis or clinical course of patients with acute abdominal conditions.
Special risk patients: This drug should be given with caution to certain patients such as the elderly or debilitated, and those with severe impairment of hepatic or renal function, hypothyroidism, Addison's disease, and prostatic hypertrophy or urethral stricture.

Adverse Reactions: The most frequently observed adverse reactions include lightheadedness, dizziness, sedation, nausea and vomiting. These effects seem to be more prominent in ambulatory than in non-ambulatory patients, and some of these adverse reactions may be alleviated if the patient lies down.
Other adverse reactions include euphoria, dysphoria, constipation, skin rash, and pruritus.

Dosage and Administration: Dosage should be adjusted according to the severity of the pain and the response of the patient. It may occasionally be necessary to exceed the usual dosage recommended below in cases of more severe pain or in those patients who have become tolerant to the analgesic effect of narcotics. TYLENOL with Codeine tablets and capsules are given orally. The usual adult dose is: Tablets No. 1, No. 2, and No. 3 and Capsules No. 3: One or two tablets every four hours as required. Tablets and Capsules No. 4: One every four hours as required.
TYLENOL with Codeine elixir is given orally. The usual doses are: *Children (3 to 6 years):* 1 teaspoonful (5 ml) 3 or 4 times daily; *(7 to 12 years):* 2 teaspoonsful (10 ml) 3 or 4 times daily; *(under 3 years):* safe dosage has not been established. *Adults:* 1 tablespoonful (15 ml) every 4 hours as needed.

Drug Interactions: The CNS depressant effects of this drug may be additive with that of other CNS depressants. See WARNINGS.

Management of Overdosage:
Acetaminophen
Acetaminophen in massive overdosage may cause hepatic toxicity in some patients. In adults, hepatic toxicity has rarely been reported with less than 10 grams and fatalities with less than 15 grams, taken as single, massive overdoses. Importantly, for reasons not fully understood, young children seem to be more resistant than adults to the hepatotoxic effect of an acetaminophen overdose.
Early symptoms following a potentially hepatotoxic overdose may include: nausea, vomiting, diaphoresis and general malaise. Clinical and laboratory evidence of hepatic toxicity usually are not apparent until 48 to 72 hours post-ingestion. Following recovery there are no

residual, structural or functional hepatic abnormalities.

Since patients' estimates of the quantity of a drug ingested are notoriously unreliable, if an acetaminophen overdose is suspected a serum acetaminophen assay should be obtained as early as possible, but no sooner than four hours following ingestion. Liver function studies should be obtained initially and repeated at 24 hour intervals.

Antidotal therapy with N-acetylcysteine appears effective in preventing and/or minimizing the toxic effects of acetaminophen. For optimal results, the antidote should be administered within 16 hours of ingestion of the overdose.

The Rocky Mountain Poison Center (800-525-6115) should be contacted for assistance in interpreting plasma levels and for directions on the administration of N-acetylcysteine as an antidote, a use currently restricted to investigational status.

Codeine

Signs and Symptoms: Serious overdose with codeine is characterized by respiratory depression (a decrease in respiratory rate and/or tidal volume, Cheyne-Stokes respiration, cyanosis), extreme somnolence progressing to stupor or coma, skeletal muscle flaccidity, cold and clammy skin, and sometimes bradycardia and hypotension. In severe overdosage, apnea, circulatory collapse, cardiac arrest and death may occur.

Treatment: Primary attention should be given to the reestablishment of adequate respiratory exchange through provision of a patent airway and the institution of assisted or controlled ventilation. The narcotic antagonist naloxone is a specific antidote against respiratory depression which may result from overdosage or unusual sensitivity to narcotics, including codeine. Therefore, an appropriate dose of naloxone (see package insert) should be administered, preferably by the intravenous route, and simultaneously with efforts at respiratory resuscitation. Since the duration of action of codeine may exceed that of the antagonist, the patient should be kept under continued surveillance and repeated doses of the antagonist should be administered as needed to maintain adequate respiration.

An antagonist should not be administered in the absence of clinically significant respiratory or cardiovascular depression. Oxygen, intravenous fluids, vasopressors and other supportive measures should be employed as indicated.

Gastric emptying may be useful in removing unabsorbed drug.

How Supplied:

TYLENOL® with Codeine tablets (colored white, imprinted "McNEIL," "TYLENOL CODEINE," and either "1", "2", "3", "4"). No. 1 **NDC** 0045-0510—60, bottles of 100; No. 2 **NDC** 0045-0511, bottles of 100 & 500; No. 3 **NDC** 0045-0513, bottles of 100, 500 and 1000; and No. 4 **NDC** 0045-0515—bottles of 100 and 500. No. 2, No. 3, and No. 4 also available in a Unit Dose Dispensit (20 × 25).

TYLENOL® with Codeine capsules No. 3 (colored white with red bands, imprinted "McNEIL" and "TYLENOL 3 CODEINE")-**NDC** 0045-0521, bottles of 100 and unit dose of 100's; TYLENOL® with Codeine capsules No. 4 (colored red with white bands, imprinted "McNEIL" and "TYLENOL 4 CODEINE")-**NDC** 0045-0522, bottles of 100 and unit dose of 100's.

TYLENOL® with Codeine elixir (colored amber, cherry flavored) bottles of 1 pint; **NDC** 0045-0508-16.

TYLENOL with Codeine tablets and capsules are manufactured by McNeil Pharmaceutical Co., Dorado, PR 00646

[Shown in Product Identification Section]

TYLOX® capsules Ⓒ ℞
(oxycodone and acetaminophen)
100's
Military NSN 6505-01-053-8621
Unit Dose (100's) 6505-01-053-8622

Description: Each capsule contains:
Oxycodone Hydrocholoride .... 4.5 mg.
Warning—May be habit forming.
Oxycodone Terephthalate .... 0.38 mg
Warning—May be habit forming.
Acetaminophen .... 500 mg

Oxycodone, a semisynthetic narcotic, is a white, odorless crystalline powder which is derived from the opium alkaloid, thebaine. TYLOX capsules also contain the nonsalicylate analgesic-antipyretic acetaminophen. Acetaminophen occurs as a white, odorless crystalline powder possessing a slightly bitter taste.

Clinical Pharmacology: TYLOX capsules combine the analgesic effects of a potent centrally acting analgesic, oxycodone, with a peripherally acting analgesic, acetaminophen. This combination is well absorbed orally. Following oral administration of one TYLOX capsule, a peak oxycodone plasma level of 11.0 ng/ml is reached after 120 minutes. After 6 hours, 19% of this level remains in plasma. The plasma elimination half-life of oxycodone is 132 minutes. A peak plasma acetaminophen concentration of 5.8 μg/ml is reached 65 minutes following the administration of one TYLOX capsule. After 6 hours, 16% of this level of acetaminophen remains in plasma. The plasma elimination half-life of acetaminophen is 116 minutes.

TYLOX capsules have been shown in well-controlled clinical studies to significantly relieve pain as early as one-half hour after administration. This pain relief lasted for as long as six hours.

Acetaminophen is distributed throughout most tissues of the body. Acetaminophen is metabolized primarily in the liver. Little unchanged drug is excreted in the urine, but most metabolic products appear in the urine within 24 hours.

Indications and Usage: TYLOX capsules are indicated for the relief of moderate to moderately severe pain.

Contraindications: TYLOX capsules should not be administered to patients who have previously exhibited hypersensitivity to oxycodone or acetaminophen.

Warnings:

Drug dependence: Oxycodone can produce drug dependence of the morphine type and, therefore, has the potential for being abused. Psychic dependence, physical dependence, and tolerance may develop upon repeated administration of TYLOX capsules, and they should be prescribed and administered with the same degree of caution appropriate to the use of other oral narcotic-containing medications. Like other narcotic-containing medications, TYLOX capsules are subject to the Federal Controlled Substances Act.

Precautions:

General

Head Injury and Increased Intracranial Pressure: The respiratory depressant effects of narcotics and their capacity to elevate cerebrospinal fluid pressure may be markedly exaggerated in the presence of head injury, other intracranial lesions, or a pre-existing increase in intracranial pressure. Furthermore, narcotics produce adverse reactions which may obscure the clinical course of patients with head injuries.

Acute Abdominal Conditions: The administration of TYLOX capsules or other narcotics may obscure the diagnosis or clinical course in patients with acute abdominal conditions.

Special Risk Patients: TYLOX capsules should be given with caution to certain patients such as the elderly or debilitated, and those with severe impairment of hepatic or renal function, hypothyroidism, Addison's disease, and prostatic hypertrophy or urethral stricture.

Information for Patients

Oxycodone may impair the mental and/or physical abilities required for the performance of potentially hazardous tasks such as driving a car or operating machinery. The patient using TYLOX capsules should be cautioned accordingly.

Drug Interactions

Patients receiving other narcotic analgesics, antipsychotics, antianxiety agents, or other CNS depressants, including alcohol, concomitantly with TYLOX capsules, may exhibit additive CNS depression due to the oxycodone component. When such combined therapy is contemplated, the dose of one or both agents should be reduced.

The use of MAO inhibitors or tricyclic antidepressants with oxycodone preparations may increase the effect of either the antidepressant or oxycodone.

The concurrent use of anticholinergics with oxycodone may produce paralytic ileus.

Carcinogenesis, Mutagenesis, Impairment of Fertility

No long-term studies in animals have been performed with oxycodone to determine carcinogenic and mutagenic potential, or effects on fertility. Acetaminophen has been found to have no mutagenic potential using the Ames Salmonella-Microsomal Activation test, the Basc test on Drosophila germ cells, and the Micronucleus test on mouse bone marrow. In animals, acetaminophen has not been evaluated for carcinogenic potential or for effects on fertility.

Teratogenic Effects

Pregnancy Category C. Animal reproductive studies have not been conducted with TYLOX. It is also not known whether TYLOX can cause fetal harm when administered to a pregnant woman or can affect reproductive capacity. TYLOX should be given to a pregnant woman only if clearly needed.

Nursing Mothers

It is not known whether the components of this drug are excreted in human milk. Because many drugs are excreted in human milk, caution should be exercised when TYLOX is administered to a nursing woman.

Pediatric Use

TYLOX capsules should not be administered to children.

Adverse Reactions: The most frequently observed adverse reactions include lightheadedness, dizziness, sedation, nausea, and vomiting. These effects seem to be more prominent in ambulatory patients than in non-ambulatory patients, and some of these adverse reactions may be alleviated if the patient lies down. Other adverse reactions include euphoria, dysphoria, constipation, skin rash, and pruritus. At higher doses oxycodone has most of the disadvantages of morphine including respiratory depression.

Drug Abuse and Dependence: TYLOX capsules are a Schedule II controlled substance.

Oxycodone can produce drug dependence and has the potential for being abused. (see WARNINGS)

Overdosage:

Acetaminophen

Signs and Symptoms: Acetaminophen in massive overdosage may cause hepatic toxicity in some patients. In all cases of suspected overdose, immediately call your regional poison center or the Rocky Mountain Poison Center's toll-free number (800-525-6115) for assistance in diagnosis and for directions in the use of N-acetylcysteine as an antidote, a use currently restricted to investigational status.

Continued on next page

McNeil Pharm.—Cont.

In adults, hepatic toxicity has rarely been reported with acute overdoses of less than 10 grams and fatalities with less than 15 grams. Importantly, young children seem to be more resistant than adults to the hepatotoxic effect of an acetaminophen overdose. Despite this, the measures outlined below should be initiated in any adult or child suspected of having ingested an acetaminophen overdose.

Early symptoms following a potentially hepatotoxic overdose may include: nausea, vomiting, diaphoresis, and general malaise. Clinical and laboratory evidence of hepatic toxicity may not be apparent until 48 to 72 hours post-ingestion.

Treatment: The stomach should be emptied promptly by lavage or by induction of emesis with syrup of ipecac. Patients' estimates of the quantity of a drug ingested are notoriously unreliable. Therefore, if an acetaminophen overdose is suspected, a serum acetaminophen assay should be obtained as early as possible, but no sooner than four hours following ingestion. Liver function studies should be obtained initially and repeated at 24-hour intervals.

The antidote, N-acetylcysteine, should be administered as early as possible, and within 16 hours of the overdose ingestion for optimal results. Following recovery, there are no residual, structural, or functional hepatic abnormalities.

Oxycodone

Signs and symptoms: Serious overdosage with oxycodone is characterized by respiratory depression (a decrease in respiratory rate and/or tidal volume, Cheyne-Stokes respiration, cyanosis), extreme somnolence progressing to stupor or coma, skeletal muscle flaccidity, cold and clammy skin, and sometimes bradycardia and hypotension. In severe overdosage, apnea, circulatory collapse, cardiac arrest, and death may occur.

Treatment: Primary attention should be given to the reestablishment of adequate respiratory exchange through provision of a patent airway and the institution of assisted or controlled ventilation. The narcotic antagonist naloxone is a specific antidote against respiratory depression which may result from overdosage or unusual sensitivity to narcotics, including oxycodone. Therefore, an appropriate dose of naloxone should be administered (see package insert) preferably by the intravenous route and simultaneously with efforts at respiratory resuscitation. Since the duration of action of oxycodone may exceed that of the antagonist, the patient should be kept under continued surveillance, and repeated doses of the antagonist should be administered as needed to maintain adequate respiration.

An antagonist should not be administered in the absence of clinically significant respiratory or cardiovascular depression.

Oxygen, intravenous fluids, vasopressors, and other supportive measures should be employed as indicated.

Gastric emptying may be useful in removing unabsorbed drug.

Dosage and Administration: Dosage should be adjusted according to the severity of the pain and the response of the patient.

TYLOX capsules are given orally. The usual adult dose is one TYLOX capsule every 6 hours as needed for pain.

How Supplied: TYLOX® capsules (colored red, imprinted "TYLOX McNEIL") NDC 0045-0525—bottles of 100 and unit dose 25's.

Dispense in tight container as defined in the official compendium.

ZOMAX® ℞
(zomepirac sodium)
tablets

100 mg tablets–100's:
Military NSN 6505-01-106-7676
VA NSN 6505-01-106-7676A
100 mg tablets (unit dose)–100's:
VA NSN 6505-01-108-3281A

Description: ZOMAX (zomepirac sodium) is designated chemically as sodium 5-(4-chlorobenzoyl)-1, 4 - dimethyl -1*H*-pyrrole-2-acetate dihydrate. The pKa of zomepirac is 4.73, and zomepirac sodium is slightly soluble in water. Each ZOMAX 100 mg tablet contains zomepirac sodium salt dihydrate 120 mg equivalent to 100 mg of free acid (zomepirac). Each 100 mg tablet contains 8 mg (0.34 mEq) of sodium.

Clinical Pharmacology: ZOMAX (zomepirac sodium) is a nonsteroidal anti-inflammatory agent, which has been developed as an analgesic. It also possesses antipyretic properties. The mechanism of its activity is uncertain, but its pharmacological actions may be related to the observation that *in vitro* the drug is an inhibitor of prostaglandin synthesis. ZOMAX produces significant analgesia within ½ hour and maximum analgesia within 1 to 2 hours following oral administration. The duration of analgesia is generally 4 to 6 hours, but may be longer in some patients.

Zomepirac is rapidly and completely absorbed in man after oral administration of ZOMAX. The peak plasma concentration of zomepirac, approximately 4.5 mcg/ml after a single 100 mg dose, is achieved in approximately one hour, and the terminal plasma elimination half-life is approximately 4 hours. The primary route of excretion of the drug and its metabolites is the urine.

The pharmacokinetics of zomepirac changes with multiple dosing. Blood levels are approximately one third higher. The volume of distribution is approximately 75% greater, while clearance is decreased by about 25%. The net effect on half-life is to increase the half-life to 9.6 hours. The reasons for and clinical significance of these changes are not known.

The rate and extent of absorption of zomepirac are decreased by concomitant administration with food. However, the influence on efficacy and side effects, if any, is not known. Concomitant use of antacids does not affect the bioavailability of zomepirac.

Zomepirac sodium, like salicylates and other nonsteroidal anti-inflammatory agents, can cause fecal blood loss. In studies utilizing ^{51}Cr-tagged red blood cells, 300 mg of zomepirac sodium daily resulted in less fecal blood loss than 3900 mg of aspirin daily, and 600 mg of zomepirac sodium produced blood loss comparable to 4800 mg of aspirin. Zomepirac sodium prolongs bleeding time by decreasing platelet adhesiveness and platelet aggregation. These effects are normalized within 24 to 48 hours after the drug is discontinued. Zomepirac sodium does not affect platelet count or the humoral clotting mechanism.

Comparative and well-controlled short-term clinical studies have established the analgesic efficacy of ZOMAX relative to other analgesics. This information may serve as a guide for prescribing ZOMAX. Zomepirac sodium 50 mg is comparable in analgesic efficacy to aspirin 650 mg, and zomepirac sodium 100 mg is comparable to two APCs, each with 30 mg of codeine phosphate.

Indications and Usage: ZOMAX (zomepirac sodium) is indicated for the relief of mild to moderately severe pain.

Contraindications: ZOMAX (zomepirac sodium) should not be used in patients who have previously exhibited intolerance to it. Because of the possibility of cross-sensitivity, zomepirac sodium should not be given to patients in whom aspirin or other nonsteroidal anti-inflammatory drugs induce bronchospasm, rhinitis, or urticaria.

Warnings: ZOMAX (zomepirac sodium) should be given under close supervision to patients with a history of upper gastrointestinal tract disease and only after consulting the ADVERSE REACTIONS section. Peptic ulceration and gastrointestinal bleeding, sometimes severe, have been reported in patients receiving ZOMAX tablets.

In clinical studies in patients receiving long-term zomepirac sodium treatment for up to two years, peptic ulcers were reported at an incidence of almost one percent. Gastrointestinal bleeding without evidence of peptic ulceration has been reported at an incidence of about 3 per 1000.

Because of animal tumorigenicity findings (see PRECAUTIONS, Carcinogenesis section) and the possibility of adverse effects on the urinary tract from prolonged use in humans (see PRECAUTIONS), caution should be exercised in considering ZOMAX for chronic use.

Precautions: General: In a controlled multicenter clinical trial comparing zomepirac sodium and aspirin, patients were treated daily for more than 6 months. In these patients, the urinary tract signs and symptoms of dysuria, cystitis, urinary frequency, hematuria, pyuria, and urinary tract infection appeared at a greater incidence in the zomepirac sodium patients (6.8%) than in aspirin patients (1.4%). The probability that the difference observed in these two incidence rates is due to chance alone is 0.03. Although the cause of these signs and symptoms and their causal relationship to zomepirac sodium have not been adequately established, ZOMAX (zomepirac sodium) should be used with caution in patients treated for longer than 6 months (also see next paragraph for long-term renal effects in animals).

Long-term toxicological studies have been done in rodents and primates. Metabolic studies with zomepirac sodium suggest that monkeys provide the best animal model for man. In rats, dose-related renal papillary necrosis and papillary edema were observed. In mice, renal papillary necrosis was observed, usually associated with advanced amyloidosis. In two 12-month studies in monkeys, there were occurrences of multifocal chronic nephritis characterized by interstitial scarring in monkeys receiving 40 mg/kg/day of zomepirac sodium, and milder interstitial nephritis and edema after 20 mg/kg/day. Nephrotoxicity was not observed in monkeys given 10 mg/kg/day for 1 year.

As with other drugs which inhibit prostaglandin biosynthesis, elevations of BUN and serum creatinine have been reported in clinical studies with ZOMAX. Therefore, periodic kidney function tests are recommended for those patients undergoing long-term treatment with ZOMAX.

Since zomepirac is eliminated primarily by the kidneys, patients with significantly impaired renal function should be closely monitored and doses lowered to avoid drug accumulation.

Rarely, acute renal failure has been reported in patients receiving ZOMAX.

As with other nonsteroidal anti-inflammatory drugs, anaphylactoid reactions have been reported. Because of the possibility of cross-sensitivity due to structural relationships which exist among nonsteroidal anti-inflammatory drugs, anaphylactoid reactions may be more likely to occur in patients who have exhibited allergic reactions to these compounds, particularly tolmetin sodium. Patients presenting with an allergic reaction to ZOMAX should be evaluated as to the severity of the reaction and treated appropriately with conventional therapy. This may include the use of epinephrine, antihistamines, pressors, fluids, and/or steroids.

Mild peripheral edema has been reported in some patients receiving long-term ZOMAX therapy. Therefore, ZOMAX should be used with caution in patients with fluid retention, hypertension, and heart failure.

ZOMAX, like aspirin, inhibits platelet function and prolongs bleeding time; therefore, patients who have coagulation disorders should be carefully observed when ZOMAX tablets are administered.

Clinical studies of up to two years duration have shown no changes in the eyes attributable to ZOMAX administration; however, because of ocular changes observed in animals with other nonsteroidal anti-inflammatory drugs, it is recommended that ophthalmologic examinations be carried out if visual symptoms develop with zomepirac.

The antipyretic and anti-inflammatory activity of ZOMAX may reduce fever and inflammation, thus diminishing their utility as diagnostic signs in detecting complications of presumed non-infectious non-inflammatory painful conditions.

As with other nonsteroidal anti-inflammatory drugs, borderline elevations of one or more liver tests may occur in up to 15% of patients. These abnormalities may progress, may remain essentially unchanged, or may be transient with continued therapy. The SGPT (ALT) test is probably the most sensitive indicator of liver dysfunction. Meaningful (3 times the upper limit of normal) elevations of SGPT or SGOT (AST) occurred in controlled clinical trials in less than 1% of patients. A patient with symptoms and/or signs suggesting liver dysfunction, or in whom an abnormal liver test has occurred, should be evaluated for evidence of the development of more severe hepatic reaction while on therapy with ZOMAX. Severe hepatic reactions, including jaundice and hepatitis, have been reported with ZOMAX as with other nonsterodial anti-inflammatory drugs. Although such reactions are rare, if abnormal liver tests persist or worsen, if clinical signs and symptoms consistent with liver disease develop, or if systemic manifestations occur (e.g. eosinophilia, rash, etc.), ZOMAX should be discontinued.

Drug Interactions: The *in vitro* binding of warfarin to human plasma proteins is unaffected by zomepirac, and zomepirac does not alter the prothrombin time of normal volunteers. However, in patients there have been rare reports that prothrombin time may increase and bleeding may occur.

The *in vitro* binding of zomepirac to human plasma proteins is decreased by salicylate at salicylate concentrations as low as 5 mcg/ml, and the decrease is concentration dependent. *In vitro* studies indicated that at therapeutic concentrations of salicylates, the binding of zomepirac was reduced from approximately 98% to 96–93%. Since there have been no controlled clinical trials to demonstrate whether or not there is any beneficial effect or harmful interaction with the use of ZOMAX in conjunction with aspirin, the combination is not recommended.

Carcinogenesis, Mutagenesis, and Impairment of Fertility: In two 2-year studies in rats at doses up to 7.5 mg/kg/day (approximately the human dose in mg/kg), the incidence of adrenal tumors was increased. In two 18-month studies in mice at doses up to 10 mg/kg/day, zomepirac sodium did not show evidence of tumorigenicity.

No mutagenic potential of zomepirac sodium was found in the following standard laboratory tests: the Micronucleus Test for Mutagenicity in rats, the Liver Microsome Activated Bacterial Assay for Mutagenicity, and the Direct Chromosome Analysis Test in rats.

In classical studies in laboratory animals, zomepirac sodium did not show any teratogenic potential.

Reproductive studies revealed no impairment of fertility in animals, but zomepirac sodium did have an effect on parturition.

Pregnancy and Nursing Mothers: Because of the animal tumorigenicity findings (see PRECAUTIONS, Carcinogenesis section) ZOMAX is not recommended during pregnancy or for treatment of nursing mothers.

Pediatric Use: ZOMAX is not recommended for use in children because of animal tumorigenicity findings (see PRECAUTIONS, Carcinogenesis section) and the possibility of adverse effects on the urinary tract from prolonged use in humans (see PRECAUTIONS).

Adverse Reactions: The adverse reactions listed below by body system have been observed in clinical trials encompassing observations in about 3600 individuals who received ZOMAX (zomepirac sodium). The incidence of adverse reactions for patients receiving short-term therapy was in nearly all cases substantially lower than the long-term incidence.

Incidence Greater Than 1%

In approximately 1000 patients receiving therapy for one week or longer, the following adverse reactions occurred more frequently than 1 in 100.

Gastrointestinal: The most frequent adverse reaction occurring with ZOMAX administration was nausea which occurred in about 12% of the patients (6% in short-term therapy). Reported less frequently were gastrointestinal distress*, diarrhea*, abdominal pain*, dyspepsia*, constipation*, flatulence*, vomiting*, gastritis, and anorexia.

Central Nervous System: Dizziness*, insomnia*, drowsiness, paresthesia.

Cardiovascular/Respiratory: Edema*, elevated blood pressure*, cardiac irregularity, palpitations.

Dermatologic: Rash*, pruritus, skin irritation, sweating.

Body as a Whole: Asthenia*.

Urogenital: Urinary tract infection*, urinary frequency, elevated BUN, elevated creatinine, vaginitis.

Special Senses: Tinnitus, taste change.

Psychiatric: Nervousness, anxiety, depression.

*Reactions occurring in 3% to 9% of patients treated with ZOMAX. Reactions occurring in fewer than 3% of the patients are unmarked.

Incidence Less Than 1%
(Causal Relationship Probable)

The following adverse reactions occurred less frequently than 1 in 100. The probability exists that there is a causal relationship between ZOMAX and these adverse reactions.

Urogenital: Hematuria, acute renal failure, interstitial nephritis.

Dermatologic: Urticaria.

Gastrointestinal: Peptic ulcer, gastrointestinal bleeding, liver function abnormalities.

Body as a Whole: Periorbital edema, anaphylactoid reactions, Stevens-Johnson syndrome.

Incidence Less Than 1%
(Causal Relationship Unknown)

Other adverse reactions have been reported with a frequency of less than 1 in 100, but a causal relationship between ZOMAX and the reaction could not be determined. These rarely reported reactions are being listed as alerting information for the physician since the possibility of a causal relationship cannot be excluded.

Body as a Whole: Chills.

Drug Abuse and Dependence: ZOMAX (zomepirac sodium) is a non-narcotic, non-addicting analgesic drug. Classical animal studies which are reasonable predictors of addiction and dependency potential demonstrated that zomepirac sodium has no such potential. Patients receiving ZOMAX for six months or longer have not developed tolerance to the drug.

Overdosage: The absence of experience with acute overdosage precludes characterization of sequelae and assessment of antidotal efficacy at this time. It is reasonable to assume, however, that the standard practices of gastric evacuation, activated charcoal administration, and general supportive therapy would apply. Animal studies have indicated that bicarbonate alkalinization significantly enhances zomepirac elimination from the plasma and suggest that this measure would have benefit in a clinical overdosage situation.

Dosage and Administration: The recommended oral dose of ZOMAX (zomepirac sodium) tablets is 100 mg every 4 to 6 hours as required. In mild pain, 50 mg (one-half tablet) every 4 to 6 hours may be adequate.

In well controlled studies, single doses larger than 100 mg have not been more effective than 100 mg and are not recommended. Doses exceeding 600 mg per day have not been studied and are not recommended for even acute use. In treatment exceeding 3 months duration, doses greater than 400 mg per day have not been studied and are not recommended.

Patients who receive long-term treatment should be periodically monitored (see PRECAUTIONS). Since antacids do not interfere with the bioavailability of zomepirac, ZOMAX may be administered with antacids (other than sodium bicarbonate) if gastrointestinal symptoms occur.

ZOMAX is not recommended for use in children (see PRECAUTIONS, Pediatric Use).

How Supplied: ZOMAX® (zomepirac sodium) tablets are available as 100 mg hexagonal tablets (yellow, scored, imprinted "McNEIL" and "ZOMAX") NDC 0045-0938 bottles of 100 and unit dose of 100's.

[*Tablets Shown in Product Identification Section*]

Mead Johnson Nutritional Division

Mead Johnson & Company
2404 W. PENNSYLVANIA ST.
EVANSVILLE, INDIANA 47721

CASEC® powder
Calcium caseinate
Protein modifier

(See PDR For Nonprescription Drugs)

CE-VI-SOL®
Vitamin C supplement drops

(See PDR For Nonprescription Drugs)

CRITICARE™ HN
Ready to Use High Nitrogen Elemental Diet

(See PDR for Nonprescription Drugs)

ENFAMIL® concentrated liquid • powder
Infant formula

(See PDR For Nonprescription Drugs)

ENFAMIL® with Iron
concentrated liquid • powder
Infant formula

(See PDR For Nonprescription Drugs)

ENFAMIL NURSETTE®
Infant formula

(See PDR For Nonprescription Drugs)

ENFAMIL® ready-to-use
Infant formula

(See PDR For Nonprescription Drugs)

ENFAMIL® with Iron ready-to-use
Infant formula

(See PDR For Nonprescription Drugs)

Continued on next page

Mead Johnson—Cont.

FER-IN-SOL®
Iron supplement
- **drops**
- **syrup**
- **capsules**

Ferrous sulfate, Mead Johnson

(See PDR For Nonprescription Drugs)

ISOCAL®
Complete liquid diet

(See PDR For Nonprescription Drugs)

ISOCAL® HCN
High Calorie and Nitrogen Nutritionally Complete Liquid Tube Feeding Formula

(See PDR For Nonprescription Drugs)

LOFENALAC® powder
Low phenylalanine food

(See PDR For Nonprescription Drugs)

LONALAC® powder
Low sodium, high protein beverage mix

(See PDR For Nonprescription Drugs)

LYTREN®
Oral electrolyte solution

(See PDR For Nonprescription Drugs)

MCT® Oil
Medium chain triglycerides oil

(See PDR For Nonprescription Drugs)

MODUCAL® Dietary Carbohydrate

(See PDR For Nonprescription Drugs)

NUTRAMIGEN® powder
Protein hydrolysate formula

(See PDR For Nonprescription Drugs)

POLY-VI-FLOR® 1.0 mg ℞
Multivitamin and fluoride supplement chewable tablets

Description:
[See table below].

Ingredients: Vitamin A acetate, ergocalciferol, dl-alpha-tocopheryl acetate, ascorbic acid, sodium ascorbate, folic acid, thiamine mononitrate, riboflavin, niacinamide, pyridoxine hydrochloride, cyanocobalamin, and sodium fluoride.
Made with natural sweeteners.

Clinical Pharmacology: It is well established that fluoridation of the water supply (1 ppm fluoride) during the period of tooth development leads to a significant decrease in the incidence of dental caries.
Poly-Vi-Flor tablets provide sodium fluoride (1 mg fluoride), and ten essential vitamins in a chewable tablet. Because the tablets are chewable, they provide a *topical* as well as *systemic* source of fluoride.[1,2]
Hydroxyapatite is the principal crystal for all calcified tissue in the human body. The fluoride ion reacts with the *hydroxyapatite* in the tooth as it is formed to produce the more caries-resistant crystal, *fluorapatite*. The reaction may be expressed by the equation:[3]

$$Ca_{10}(PO_4)_6(OH)_2 + 2F^- \rightarrow Ca_{10}(PO_4)_6F_2 + 2OH^-$$

(Hydroxyapatite) (Fluorapatite)

Three stages of fluoride deposition in tooth enamel can be distinguished.[3]

1. Small amounts (reflecting the low levels of fluoride in tissue fluids) are incorporated into the enamel crystals while they are being formed.
2. After enamel has been laid down, fluoride deposition continues in the surface enamel. Diffusion of fluoride from the surface inward is apparently restricted.
3. After eruption, the surface enamel acquires fluoride from water, food, supplementary fluoride and smaller amounts from saliva.

Indications and Usage: Supplementation of the diet with ten essential vitamins.
Supplementation of the diet with the fluoride for caries prophylaxis.
The American Academy of Pediatrics recommends that children up to age 16, in areas where drinking water contains less than optimal levels of fluoride, receive daily fluoride supplementation.
Poly-Vi-Flor 1.0 mg chewable tablets provide fluoride in tablet form for children over 3 years in areas where the water fluoride level is less than 0.3 ppm.[8]
Poly-Vi-Flor chewable tablets supply significant amounts of vitamins A, D, E, C, thiamine, riboflavin, niacin, pyridoxine, cyanocobalamin and folic acid to supplement the diet, and to help assure that nutritional deficiencies of these vitamins will not develop. Thus, in a single easy-to-use preparation, children over three years of age obtain ten essential vitamins and the important mineral, fluoride.
A study of fluoride tablets given to 121 children revealed the efficacy of sodium fluoride in tablet form. The authors concluded that the caries reduction was comparable to that previously reported for children drinking fluoridated water.[5]
A comprehensive 5½ year series of studies of the effectiveness of Tri-Vi-Flor® and Poly-Vi-Flor® products in caries protection has been published.[1,2,6,7] Children in this continuing study lived in an area where the water supply contained only 0.05 ppm fluoride. The subjects were divided into two groups, one which used only non-fluoridated Vi-Sol® vitamin products and the other Tri-Vi-Flor and Poly-Vi-Flor vitamin-fluoride products.
The three-year interim report showed 63% fewer carious surfaces in primary teeth and 43% fewer carious surfaces in permanent teeth of the children taking Vi-Flor™ vitamin-fluoride products.[1]
After four years the studies continued to support the effectiveness of Tri-Vi-Flor and Poly-Vi-Flor, showing a reduction in carious surfaces of 68% in primary teeth and 46% in permanent teeth.[2]
Results at the end of 5½ years further confirmed the previous findings and indicated that significant reductions in dental caries are apparent with the continued use of Vi-Flor vitamin-fluoride products.[6]

Warnings: As in the case of all medications, keep out of the reach of children.

Precautions: The suggested dose *should not be exceeded*, since dental fluorosis may result from continued ingestion of large amounts of fluoride.
Before prescribing Vi-Flor products, the physician should:
1. determine the fluoride content of the drinking water.
2. make sure the child is not receiving significant amounts of fluoride from other medications.
3. periodically check to make sure that the child does not develop significant dental fluorosis.

The Council on Dental Therapeutics of the American Dental Association recommends that no more than 264 mg of sodium fluoride should be dispensed at one time.[4] Therefore, no more than 120 Poly-Vi-Flor 1.0 mg chewable tablets (2.2 mg sodium fluoride per tablet) should be dispensed at one time.

Adverse Reactions: Allergic rash and other idiosyncrasies have been rarely reported.

Dosage and Administration: One tablet daily or as prescribed by the physician.

How Supplied: Poly-Vi-Flor 1.0 mg (multivitamin and fluoride supplement) chewable tablets are available on prescription only in 100- and 1000-tablet bottles.
NDC 0087-0474-02 Bottles of 100
NDC 0087-0474-03 Bottles of 1000

Literature Available: Yes.

References:

1. Hennon, D.K..; Stookey, G.K., and Muhler, J.C.: The Clinical Anticariogenic Effectiveness of Supplementary Fluoride-Vitamin Preparations—Results at the End of Three Years, J. Dentistry for Children 33:3–12 (Jan.) 1966.
2. Hennon, D.K.; Stookey, G.K., and Muhler, J.C.: The Clinical Anticariogenic Effectiveness of Supplementary Fluoride-Vitamin Preparations—Results at the End of Four Years, J. Dentistry for Children 34:439–443 (Nov.) 1967.
3. Brudevold, F., and McCann, H.G.: Fluoride and Caries Control—Mechanism of Action, in Nizel, A.E.: The Science of Nutrition and Its Application in Clinical Dentistry, Philadelphia, W.B. Saunders Company, 1966, pp. 331–347.
4. Council on Dental Therapeutics, Am. Dental Assoc., Accepted Dental Therapeutics, 1977, 37th Edition, pp. 293.
5. Arnold, F.A., Jr.; McClure, F.J., and White, C.L.: Sodium Fluoride Tablets for Children, Dental Progress 1:12–16 (Oct.) 1960.
6. Hennon, D.K.; Stookey, G.K., and Muhler, J.C.: The Clinical Anticariogenic Effectiveness of Supplementary Fluoride-Vitamin Preparations—Results at the End of Five and a Half Years, Phar. and Ther. in Dent. 1:1, 1970.
7. Hennon, D.K.; Stookey, G.K., and Beiswanger, B.B.: Fluoride-vitamin supplements: Effects on Dental Caries and Fluorosis When Used in Areas With Suboptimum Fluoride in the Water Supply. J. Am. Dent. Assoc. 95:965, 1977.
8. American Academy of Pediatrics Committee on Nutrition: Fluoride Supplementation:

Each tablet supplies:		Percentage of U.S. Recommended Daily Allowance: Children Under 4	Adults & Children 4 or More
Vitamin A, IU	2500	100	50
Vitamin D, IU	400	100	100
Vitamin E, IU	15	150	50
Vitamin C (Ascorbic acid), mg	60	150	100
Folic acid (Folacin), mg	0.3	150	75
Thiamine (Vitamin B_1), mg	1.05	150	70
Riboflavin (Vitamin B_2), mg	1.2	150	70
Niacin, mg	13.5	150	68
Vitamin B_6, mg	1.05	150	53
Vitamin B_{12}, mcg	4.5	150	75
Fluoride, mg	1	*	*

* U.S. Recommended Daily Allowance has not been established.

Revised Dosage Schedule. Pediatrics 63:150, 1979.

POLY-VI-FLOR® 0.5 mg ℞
Multivitamin and fluoride supplement chewable tablets

Description:
[See table right].

Each tablet supplies:		Percentage of U.S. Recommended Daily Allowances — Children Under 4	Adults and Children 4 or More
Vitamin A, IU	2500	100	50
Vitamin D, IU	400	100	100
Vitamin E, IU	15	150	50
Vitamin C (Ascorbic acid), mg	60	150	100
Folic acid (Folacin), mg	0.3	150	75
Thiamine (Vitamin B_1), mg	1.05	150	70
Riboflavin (Vitamin B_2), mg	1.2	150	70
Niacin, mg	13.5	150	68
Vitamin B_6, mg	1.05	150	53
Vitamin B_{12}, mcg	4.5	150	75
Fluoride, mg	0.5	*	*

*U.S. Recommended Daily Allowance has not been established.

Ingredients: Vitamin A acetate, ergocalciferol, dl-alpha-tocopheryl acetate, ascorbic acid, sodium ascorbate, folic acid, thiamine mononitrate, riboflavin, niacinamide, pyridoxine hydrochloride, cyanocobalamin, and sodium fluoride.
Made with natural sweeteners.
Clinical Pharmacology: It is well established that fluoridation of the water supply (1 ppm fluoride) during the period of tooth development leads to a significant decrease in the incidence of dental caries.
Poly-Vi-Flor 0.5 mg tablets provide sodium fluoride (0.5 mg fluoride), and ten essential vitamins in a chewable tablet. Because the tablets are chewable, they provide a *topical* as well as *systemic* source of fluoride.[1,2]
Hydroxyapatite is the principal crystal for all calcified tissue in the human body. The fluoride ion reacts with the *hydroxyapatite* in the tooth as it is formed to produce the more caries-resistant crystal, *fluorapatite.* The reaction may be expressed by the equation:[3]

$$Ca_{10}(PO_4)_6(OH)_2 + 2F^- \rightarrow Ca_{10}(PO_4)_6F_2 + 2OH^-$$
(Hydroxyapatite) (Fluorapatite)

Three stages of fluoride deposition in tooth enamel can be distinguished:[3]

1. Small amounts (reflecting the low levels of fluoride in tissue fluids) are incorporated into the enamel crystals while they are being formed.
2. After enamel has been laid down, fluoride deposition continues in the surface enamel. Diffusion of fluoride from the surface inward is apparently restricted.
3. After eruption, the surface enamel acquires fluoride from water, food, supplementary fluoride and smaller amounts from saliva.

Indications and Usage: Supplementation of the diet with ten essential vitamins.
Supplementation of the diet with fluoride, for caries prophylaxis.
The American Academy of Pediatrics recommends that children up to age 16, in areas where drinking water contains less than optimal levels of fluoride, receive daily fluoride supplementation.
Poly-Vi-Flor 0.5 mg chewable tablets provide fluoride in tablet form for children 2-3 years of age where the drinking water has a fluoride content of 0.3 ppm or less, and for children 3 years of age and above where the drinking water has a fluoride level greater than 0.3 ppm and not more than 0.7 ppm.[4]
Poly-Vi-Flor 0.5 mg chewable tablets supply significant amounts of vitamins A, D, E, C, thiamine, riboflavin, niacin, pyridoxine, cyanocobalamin and folic acid to supplement the diet, and to help assure that nutritional deficiencies of these vitamins will not develop. Thus, in a single easy-to-use preparation, children obtain ten essential vitamins and fluoride.
Warnings: As in the case of all medications, keep out of the reach of children.
Precautions: The suggested dose *should not be exceeded,* since dental fluorosis may result from continued ingestion of large amounts of fluoride.
Before prescribing Vi-Flor products, the physician should:

1. determine the fluoride content of the drinking water,
2. make sure that the child is not taking fluoride-containing drugs, and
3. the physician should also periodically check to make sure that the child does not develop significant dental fluorosis.

Adverse Reactions: Allergic rash and other idiosyncrasies have been rarely reported.
Dosage and Administration: One tablet daily, or as prescribed by the physician.
How Supplied: Poly-Vi-Flor 0.5 mg (multivitamin and fluoride supplement) chewable tablets are available on prescription only in 100 tablet bottles.
NDC 0087-0468-41 Bottles of 100
Literature Available: Yes.
References:

1. Hennon, D.K.; Stookey, G.K., and Muhler, J.C.: The Clinical Anticariogenic Effectiveness of Supplementary Fluoride-Vitamin Preparations—Results at the End of Three Years, J. Dentistry for Children 33:3–12 (Jan.) 1966.
2. Hennon, D.K.; Stookey, G.K., and Muhler, J.C.: The Clinical Anticariogenic Effectiveness of Supplementary Fluoride-Vitamin Preparations—Results at the End of Four Years, J. Dentistry for Children 34:439–443 (Nov.) 1967.
3. Brudevold, F., and McCann, H.G.: Fluoride and Caries Control—Mechanism of Action, in Nizel, A.E.: The Science of Nutrition and Its Application in Clinical Dentistry, Philadelphia, W.B. Saunders Company, 1966, pp. 331–347.
4. American Academy of Pediatrics Committee on Nutrition: Fluoride Supplementation: Revised Dosage Schedule. Pediatrics 63:150, 1979.

POLY-VI-FLOR® 0.5 mg ℞
Multivitamin and fluoride supplement drops

Description:

Each 1.0 ml supplies:		Percentage of U.S. Recommended Daily Allowance — Infants	Children Under 4
Vitamin A, IU	1500	100	60
Vitamin D, IU	400	100	100
Vitamin E, IU	5	100	50
Vitamin C (Ascorbic acid), mg	35	100	88
Thiamine (Vitamin B_1), mg	0.5	100	71
Riboflavin (Vitamin B_2), mg	0.6	100	75
Niacin, mg	8	100	89
Vitamin B_6, mg	0.4	100	57
Vitamin B_{12}, mcg	2	100	67
Fluoride, mg	0.5	*	*

* U.S. Recommended Daily Allowance has not been established.
See INDICATIONS AND USAGE section below for use by infants and children under two years of age.
This product does not contain the essential vitamin folic acid.
Ingredients: Vitamin A palmitate, ergocalciferol, D-alpha-tocopheryl succinate, ascorbic acid, thiamine hydrochloride, riboflavin-5-phosphate sodium, niacinamide, pyridoxine hydrochloride, cyanocobalamin, and sodium fluoride.
Made with natural sweeteners.
Clinical Pharmacology: It is well established that fluoridation of the water supply (1 ppm fluoride) during the period of tooth development leads to a significant decrease in the incidence of dental caries.
Hydroxyapatite is the principal crystal for all calcified tissue in the human body. The fluoride ion reacts with the *hydroxyapatite* in the tooth as it is formed to produce the more caries-resistant crystal, *fluorapatite.* The reaction may be expressed by the equation:[1]

$$Ca_{10}(PO_4)_6(OH)_2 + 2F^- \rightarrow Ca_{10}(PO_4)_6F_2 + 2OH^-$$
(Hydroxyapatite) (Fluorapatite)

Three stages of fluoride deposition in tooth enamel can be distinguished.[1]

1. Small amounts (reflecting the low levels of fluoride in tissue fluids) are incorporated into the enamel crystals while they are being formed.
2. After enamel has been laid down, fluoride deposition continues in the surface enamel. Diffusion of fluoride from the surface inward is apparently restricted.
3. After eruption, the surface enamel acquires fluoride from water, food, supplementary fluoride and smaller amounts from saliva.

Indications and Usage: Supplementation of the diet with nine essential vitamins.
Supplementation of the diet with fluoride for caries prophylaxis.
The American Academy of Pediatrics recommends that children up to age 16, in areas where drinking water contains less than optimal levels of fluoride, receive daily fluoride supplementation.
Poly-Vi-Flor 0.5 mg (multivitamin and fluoride supplement) drops provide fluoride in drop form for children ages 2–3 years in areas where the drinking water contains less than 0.3 ppm fluoride; and for children over 3 years in areas where the drinking water contains 0.3 thru 0.7 ppm of fluoride.[6] Each 1.0 ml provides sodium fluoride (0.5 mg fluoride) plus nine essential vitamins.
The American Academy of Pediatrics[6] and the American Dental Association[7] currently recommend that infants and children under 2 years of age, in areas where drinking water contains less than 0.3 ppm of fluoride, and children 2-3, in areas where the drinking water contains 0.3 through 0.7 ppm of fluoride, receive 0.25 mg of supplemental fluoride daily which is provided in a full dose (1 ml) of Poly-Vi-Flor® 0.25 mg drops. A half dose (0.5 ml) of Poly-Vi-Flor 0.5 mg drops could also provide a daily fluoride intake of 0.25 mg; however, this dosage reduces vitamin supplementation by half.
Poly-Vi-Flor 0.5 mg drops supply significant amounts of vitamins A, D, E, C, thiamine, riboflavin, niacin, pyridoxine, and cyanocobalamin

Continued on next page

Mead Johnson—Cont.

to supplement the diet, and to help assure that nutritional deficiencies of these vitamins will not develop. Thus in a single easy-to-use preparation, children obtain nine essential vitamins and fluoride.

A comprehensive 5½ year series of studies of the effectiveness of Tri-Vi-Flor® and Poly-Vi-Flor® products in caries protection has been published.[2–5] Children in this continuing study lived in an area where the water supply contained only 0.05 ppm fluoride. The subjects were divided into two groups, one which used only nonfluoridated Vi-Sol® vitamin products and the other Tri-Vi-Flor and Poly-Vi-Flor vitamin-fluoride products.

The three-year interim report showed 63% fewer carious surfaces in primary teeth and 43% fewer carious surfaces in permanent teeth of the children taking Vi-Flor™ vitamin-fluoride products.[2]

After four years the studies continued to support the effectiveness of Tri-Vi-Flor and Poly-Vi-Flor, showing a reduction in carious surfaces of 68% in primary teeth and 46% in permanent teeth.[3]

Results at the end of 5½ years further confirmed the previous findings and indicated that significant reductions in dental caries are apparent with the continued use of Vi-Flor vitamin-fluoride products.[4]

Warnings: As in the case of all medications, keep out of the reach of children.

Precautions: The suggested dose should not be exceeded since dental fluorosis may result from continued ingestion of large amounts of fluoride.

When prescribing Vi-Flor products, the physician should:

1. determine the fluoride content of the drinking water.
2. make sure the child is not receiving significant amounts of fluoride from other medications.
3. periodically check to make sure that the child does not develop significant dental fluorosis.

Poly-Vi-Flor 0.5 mg drops should be dispensed in the original plastic container, since contact with glass leads to instability and precipitation. (The amount of sodium fluoride in both the 30- and 50-ml. sizes is well below the maximum to be dispensed at one time according to recommendations of the American Dental Association.)

Adverse Reactions: Allergic rash and other idiosyncrasies have been rarely reported.

Dosage and Administration: 1.0 ml daily for children 2 years of age or older, or as prescribed by the physician. May be dropped directly into mouth with 'Safti-Dropper', or mixed with cereal, fruit juice or other food.

How Supplied: Poly-Vi-Flor 0.5 mg (multivitamin and fluoride supplement) drops are available on prescription only in bottles of 30 and 50 ml.

NDC 0087-0472-01 Bottles of 1 fl. oz. (30 ml.)
NDC 0087-0472-02 Bottles of 1⅔ fl. oz. (50 ml.)
FSN 6505-080-0967 (50 ml.)

Literature Available: Yes.

References:

1. Brudevold, F., and McCann, H.G.: Fluoride and Caries Control—Mechanism of Action, in Nizel, A.E.: The Science of Nutrition and its Application in Clinical Dentistry, Philadelphia, W. B. Saunders Company, 1966, pp. 331–347.
2. Hennon, D.K.; Stookey, G.K., and Muhler, J.C.: The Clinical Anticariogenic Effectiveness of Supplementary Fluoride-Vitamin Preparations—Results at the End of Three Years, J. Dentistry for Children 33:3–12 (Jan.) 1966.
3. Hennon, D.K.; Stookey, G.K., and Muhler, J.C.: The Clinical Anticariogenic Effectiveness of Supplementary Fluoride-Vitamin Preparations—Results at the End of Four Years, J. Dentistry for Children 24:439–443 (Nov.) 1967.
4. Hennon, D.K.; Stookey, G.K., and Muhler, J.C.: The Clinical Anticariogenic Effectiveness of Supplementary Fluoride-Vitamin Preparations—Results at the End of Five and a Half Years, Phar. and Ther. In Dent. 1:1, 1970.
5. Hennon, D.K.; Stookey, G.K., and Beiswanger, B.B.: Fluoride vitamin supplements: Effects on dental caries and fluorosis when used in areas with suboptimum fluoride in the water supply. J.Am.Dent.Assoc.95:965, 1977.
6. American Academy of Pediatrics, Committee on Nutrition: Fluoride Supplementation: Revised Dosage Schedule, Pediatrics 63:150, 1979.
7. Accepted Dental Therapeutic, Ed. 38, Chicago, American Dental Association, 1979, p. 321.

POLY-VI-FLOR® 0.25 mg ℞
Multivitamin and fluoride supplement drops

Description:

Each 1.0 ml supplies:		Percentage of U.S. Recommended Daily Allowance Infants	Children Under 4
Vitamin A, IU	1500	100	60
Vitamin D, IU	400	100	100
Vitamin E, IU	5	100	50
Vitamin C (Ascorbic acid), mg	35	100	88
Thiamine (Vitamin B_1), mg	0.5	100	71
Riboflavin (Vitamin B_2), mg	0.6	100	75
Niacin, mg	8	100	89
Vitamin B_6, mg	0.4	100	57
Vitamin B_{12}, mcg	2	100	67
Fluoride, mg	0.25	*	*

*U.S. Recommended Daily Allowance has not been established.

This product does not contain the essential vitamin folic acid.

Ingredients: Vitamin A palmitate, ergocalciferol, D-alpha-tocopheryl succinate, ascorbic acid, thiamine hydrochloride, riboflavin-5-phosphate sodium, niacinamide, pyridoxine, hydrochloride, cyanocobalamin, and sodium fluoride.

Made with natural sweeteners.

Clinical Pharmacology: It is well established that fluoridation of the water supply (1 ppm fluoride) during the period of tooth development leads to a significant decrease in the incidence of dental caries.

Hydroxyapatite is the principal crystal for all calcified tissue in the human body. The fluoride ion reacts with the *hydroxyapatite* in the tooth as it is formed to produce the more caries-resistant crystal, *fluorapatite.* The reaction may be expressed by the equation:[1]

$$Ca_{10}(PO_4)_6(OH)_2 + 2F^- \rightarrow Ca_{10}(PO_4)_6F_2 + 2OH^-$$
(Hydroxyapatite) (Fluorapatite)

Three stages of fluoride deposition in tooth enamel can be distinguished.[1]

1. Small amounts (reflecting the low levels of fluoride in tissue fluids) are incorporated into the enamel crystals while they are being formed.
2. After enamel has been laid down, fluoride deposition continues in the surface enamel. Diffusion of fluoride from the surface inward is apparently restricted.
3. After eruption, the surface enamel acquires fluoride from water, food, supplementary fluoride and smaller amounts from saliva.

Indications and Usage: Supplementation of the diet with nine essential vitamins.

Supplementation of the diet with fluoride for caries prophylaxis.

The American Academy of Pediatrics recommends that children up to age 16, in areas where drinking water contains less than optimal levels of fluoride, receive daily fluoride supplementation.

POLY-VI-FLOR 0.25 mg (multivitamin and fluoride supplement) drops provide fluoride in drop form for infants and young children from birth to 2 years of age in areas where the drinking water contains less than 0.3 ppm of fluoride and for children ages 2–3 years in areas where the drinking water contains 0.3 thru 0.7 ppm of fluoride. Each 1.0 ml supplies sodium fluoride (0.25 mg fluoride) plus nine essential vitamins.[2]

POLY-VI-FLOR 0.25 mg drops supply significant amounts of vitamins A, D, E, C, thiamine, riboflavin, niacin, pyridoxine, and cyanocobalamin to supplement the diet, and to help assure that nutritional deficiencies of these vitamins will not develop. Thus, in a single easy-to-use preparation, infants obtain nine essential vitamins and fluoride.

Warnings: As in the case of all medications, keep out of the reach of children.

Precautions: The suggested dose should not be exceeded since dental fluorosis may result from continued ingestion of large amounts of fluoride.

When prescribing VI-FLOR products, the physician should:

1. determine the fluoride content of the drinking water.
2. make sure the child is not receiving significant amounts of fluoride from other medications.
3. periodically check to make sure that the child does not develop significant dental fluorosis.

POLY-VI-FLOR 0.25 mg. drops should be dispensed in the original plastic container, since contact with glass leads to instability and precipitation. (The amount of sodium fluoride in the 50-ml. size is well below the maximum to be dispensed at one time according to recommendations of the American Dental Association.)

Adverse Reactions: Allergic rash and other idiosyncrasies have been rarely reported.

Dosage and Administration: 1.0 ml daily or as prescribed by the physician. May be dropped directly into mouth with 'Safti-Dropper,' or mixed with cereal, fruit juice or other food.

How Supplied: POLY-VI-FLOR 0.25 mg (multivitamin and fluoride supplement) drops are available on prescription only in bottles of 50 ml.

NDC 0087-0451-41 Bottles of 50 ml.

Literature Available: Yes.

References:

1. Brudevold, F., and McCann, H. G.: Fluoride and caries control—mechanism of action, in Nizel, A. E.: The Science of Nutrition and Its Application in Clinical Dentistry, Philadelphia, WB Saunders Company, 1966, pp. 331–347.
2. American Academy of Pediatrics, Committee on Nutrition: Fluoride Supplementation: Revised Dosage Schedule, Pediatrics 63:150, 1979.

POLY-VI-FLOR® 1.0 mg with Iron ℞
Multivitamin, iron and fluoride supplement chewable tablets

Description:

[See table on top next page].

Ingredients: Vitamin A acetate, ergocalciferol, dl-alpha-tocopheryl acetate, ascorbic acid, sodium ascorbate, folic acid, thiamine mononitrate, riboflavin, niacinamide, pyridoxine hydrochloride, cyanocobalamin, ferrous fumarate, and sodium fluoride.

Made with natural sweeteners.

Clinical Pharmacology: It is well established that fluoridation of the water supply (1 ppm fluoride) during the period of tooth development leads to a significant decrease in the incidence of dental caries.

Poly-Vi-Flor tablets with iron provide sodium fluoride (1 mg fluoride), ferrous fumarate and ten essential vitamins in a chewable tablet. Because the tablets are chewable, they provide a *topical* as well as *systemic* source of fluoride.[1,2]

Hydroxyapatite is the principal crystal for all calcified tissue in the human body. The fluoride ion reacts with the *hydroxyapatite* in the tooth as it is formed to produce the more caries-resistant crystal, *fluorapatite.* The reaction may be expressed by the equation:[3]

$Ca_{10}(PO_4)_6(OH)_2 + 2F^- \rightarrow Ca_{10}(PO_4)_6F_2 + 2OH^-$
(Hydroxyapatite) (Fluorapatite)

Three stages of fluoride deposition in tooth enamel can be distinguished.[3]

1. Small amounts (reflecting the low levels of fluoride in tissue fluids) are incorporated into the enamel crystals while they are being formed.
2. After enamel has been laid down, fluoride deposition continues in the surface enamel. Diffusion of fluoride from the surface inward is apparently restricted.
3. After eruption, the surface enamel acquires fluoride from water, food, supplementary fluoride and smaller amounts from saliva.

Indications and Usage: Supplementation of the diet with ten essential vitamins and iron. Supplementation of the diet with fluoride, for caries prophylaxis.

The American Academy of Pediatrics recommends that children up to age 16, in areas where drinking water contains less than optimal levels of fluoride, receive daily fluoride supplementation.

Poly-Vi-Flor 1.0 mg chewable tablets with Iron were developed to provide fluoride in tablet form for children over 3 years in areas where the water fluoride level is less than 0.3 ppm.[6]

Poly-Vi-Flor 1.0 mg chewable tablets with Iron supply significant amounts of vitamins A, D, E, C, thiamine, riboflavin, niacin, pyridoxine, cyanocobalamin, folic acid, and ferrous fumarate to supplement the diet, and to help assure that deficiencies of these nutrients will not develop. Thus, in a single easy-to-use preparation, children over three years of age obtain ten essential vitamins, iron, and fluoride.

A comprehensive 5½ year series of studies of the effectiveness of Tri-Vi-Flor® and Poly-Vi-Flor® products in caries protection has been published.[1,2,4,5] Children in this continuing study lived in an area where the water supply contained only 0.05 ppm fluoride. The subjects were divided into two groups, one which used only non-fluoridated Vi-Sol® vitamin products and the other Tri-Vi-Flor and Poly-Vi-Flor vitamin-fluoride products.

The three-year interim report showed 63% fewer carious surfaces in primary teeth and 43% fewer carious surfaces in permanent teeth of the children taking Vi-Flor™ vitamin-fluoride products.[1]

Each tablet supplies:		Percentage of U.S. Recommended Daily Allowance: Children Under 4	Adults & Children 4 or More
Vitamin A, IU	2500	100	50
Vitamin D, IU	400	100	100
Vitamin E, IU	15	150	50
Vitamin C (Ascorbic acid), mg	60	150	100
Folic acid (Folacin), mg	0.3	150	75
Thiamine (Vitamin B_1), mg	1.05	150	70
Riboflavin (Vitamin B_2), mg	1.2	150	70
Niacin, mg	13.5	150	68
Vitamin B_6, mg	1.05	150	53
Vitamin B_{12}, mcg	4.5	150	75
Iron, mg	12	120	67
Fluoride, mg	1	*	*

*U.S. Recommended Daily Allowance has not been established.

After four years the studies continued to support the effectiveness of Tri-Vi-Flor and Poly-Vi-Flor, showing a reduction in carious surfaces of 68% in primary teeth and 46% in permanent teeth.[2]

Results at the end of 5½ years further confirmed the previous findings and indicated that significant reductions in dental caries are apparent with the continued use of Vi-Flor vitamin-fluoride products.[4]

Warnings: As in the case of all medications, keep out of the reach of children.

Precautions: The suggested dose *should not be exceeded,* since dental fluorosis may result from continued ingestion of large amounts of fluoride.

Before prescribing Vi-Flor products, the physician should:

1. determine the fluoride content of the drinking water.
2. make sure the child is not receiving significant amounts of fluoride from other medications.
3. periodically check to make sure that the child does not develop significant dental fluorosis.

The toxicity of ferrous fumarate is not established. However, to prevent possible serious harmful effects in the event of accidental overdosage, it is recommended that no more than 100 tablets be dispensed at one time.

Adverse Reactions: Allergic rash and other idiosyncrasies have been rarely reported.

Dosage and Administration: One tablet daily or as prescribed by the physician.

How Supplied: Poly-Vi-Flor 1.0 mg (multivitamin and fluoride supplement) chewable tablets with Iron are available by prescription only in 100- and 1000-tablet bottles.

NDC 0087-0476-03 Bottles of 100
NDC 0087-0476-04 Bottles of 1000

Literature Available: Yes.

References:

1. Hennon, D.K.; Stookey, G.K., and Muhler, J.C.: The Clinical Anticariogenic Effectiveness of Supplementary Fluoride-Vitamin Preparations—Results at the End of Three Years, J. Dentistry for Children 33:3–12 (Jan.) 1966.
2. Hennon, D.K.; Stookey, G.K., and Muhler, J.C.: The Clinical Anticariogenic Effectiveness of Supplementary Fluoride-Vitamin Preparations—Results at the End of Four Years, J. Dentistry for Children 34:439–443 (Nov.) 1967.
3. Brudevold, F., and McCann, H.G.: Fluoride and Caries Control—Mechanism of Action, in Nizel, A.E.: The Science of Nutrition and Its Application in Clinical Dentistry, Philadelphia, W.B. Saunders Company, 1966, pp. 331–347.
4. Hennon, D.K., Stookey, G.K., and Muhler, J.C.: The Clinical Anticariogenic Effectiveness of Supplementary Fluoride-Vitamin Preparations—Results at the End of Five and a Half Years, Phar. and Ther. in Dent. 1:1, 1970.
5. Hennon, D.K.; Stookey, G.K., and Beiswanger, B.B.: Fluoride-vitamin supplements: Effects on Dental Caries and Fluorosis When Used in Areas With Suboptimum Fluoride in the Water Supply, J. Am. Dent. Assoc. 95:965, 1977.
6. American Academy of Pediatrics Committee on Nutrition: Fluoride Supplementation: Revised Dosage Schedule. Pediatrics 63:150, 1979.

Each tablet supplies:		Percentage of U.S. Recommended Daily Allowance: Children Under 4	Adults & Children 4 or More
Vitamin A, IU	2500	100	50
Vitamin D, IU	400	100	100
Vitamin E, IU	15	150	50
Vitamin C (Ascorbic acid), mg	60	150	100
Folic acid (Folacin), mg	0.3	150	75
Thiamine (Vitamin B_1), mg	1.05	150	70
Riboflavin (Vitamin B_2), mg	1.2	150	70
Niacin, mg	13.5	150	68
Vitamin B_6, mg	1.05	150	53
Vitamin B_{12}, mcg	4.5	150	75
Iron, mg	12	120	67
Fluoride, mg	0.5	*	*

*U.S. Recommended Daily Allowance has not been established.

POLY-VI-FLOR® 0.5 mg with Iron ℞

Multivitamin, fluoride and iron supplement chewable tablets

Description:
[See table left].

Ingredients: Vitamin A acetate, ergocalciferol, dl-alpha-tocopheryl acetate, ascorbic acid, sodium ascorbate, folic acid, thiamine mononitrate, riboflavin, niacinamide, pyridoxine, hydrochloride, cyanocobalamin, ferrous fumarate and sodium fluoride.
Made with natural sweeteners.

Clinical Pharmacology: It is well established that fluoridation of the water supply (1 ppm fluoride) during the period of tooth development leads to a significant decrease in the incidence of dental caries.

Poly-Vi-Flor 0.5 mg chewable tablets with Iron provide sodium fluoride (0.5 mg fluoride), iron and ten essential vitamins in a chewable tablet. Because the tablets are chewable, they provide a *topical* as well as *systemic* source of fluoride.[1,2]

Hydroxyapatite is the principal crystal for all calcified tissue in the human body. The fluoride ion reacts with the *hydroxyapatite* in the

Continued on next page

Mead Johnson—Cont.

tooth as it is formed to produce the more caries-resistant crystal, *fluorapatite.* The reaction may be expressed by the equation:[3]

$Ca_{10}(PO_4)_6(OH)_2 + 2F \rightarrow CA_{10}(PO_4)_6F_2 + 2OH$
(Hydroxyapatite) (Fluorapatite)

Three stages of fluoride deposition in tooth enamel can be distinguished:[3]

1. Small amounts (reflecting the low levels of fluoride in tissue fluids) are incorporated into the enamel crystals while they are being formed.
2. After enamel has been laid down, fluoride deposition continues in the surface enamel. Diffusion of fluoride from the surface inward is apparently restricted.
3. After eruption, the surface enamel acquires fluoride from water, food, supplementary fluoride and smaller amounts from saliva.

Indications and Usage: Supplementation of the diet with ten essential vitamins and iron. Supplementation of the diet with fluoride, for caries prophylaxis, for children 2–3 years of age where the drinking water has a fluoride content of 0.3 ppm or less, and for children 3 years of age and above where the drinking water has a fluoride level greater than 0.3 ppm and not more than 0.7 ppm.[4]

The American Academy of Pediatrics recommends that children up to age 16, in areas where drinking water contains less than optimal levels of fluoride, receive daily fluoride supplementation.

Poly-Vi-Flor 0.5 mg chewable tablets with Iron supply significant amounts of vitamins A, D, E, C, thiamine, riboflavin, niacin, pyridoxine, cyanocobalamin, folic acid and iron to supplement the diet, and to help assure that deficiencies of these nutrients will not develop. Thus, in a single easy-to-use preparation, children obtain ten essential vitamins, iron and fluoride.

Children using Poly-Vi-Flor 0.5 mg chewable tablets with Iron regularly should receive semiannual dental examinations. The regular brushing of teeth and attention to good oral hygiene practices are also essential.

Warnings: As in the case of all medications, keep out of the reach of children.

Precautions: The suggested dose of Poly-Vi-Flor 0.5 mg chewable tablets with Iron *should not be exceeded,* since dental fluorosis may result from continued ingestion of large amounts of fluoride.

Before prescribing Poly-Vi-Flor 0.5 mg chewable tablets with Iron, the physician should:

1. determine the fluoride content of the drinking water.
2. make sure that the child is not taking fluoride-containing drugs, and
3. periodically check to make sure that the child does not develop significant dental fluorosis.

Adverse Reactions: Allergic rash and other idiosyncrasies have been rarely reported.

Dosage and Administration: One tablet daily, or as prescribed by the physician.

How Supplied: Poly-Vi-Flor 0.5 mg (multivitamin, fluoride and iron supplement) chewable tablets with Iron are available on prescription only in 100-tablet bottles.

References:

1. Hennon, D.K.; Stookey, G.K., and Muhler, J.C.: The Clinical Anticariogenic Effectiveness of Supplementary Fluoride-Vitamin Preparations—Results at the End of Three Years, J. Dentistry for Children 33:3–12 (Jan.) 1966.
2. Hennon, D.K.; Stookey, G.K., and Muhler, J.C.: The Clinical Anticariogenic Effectiveness of Supplementary Fluoride-Vitamin Preparations—Results at the End of Four Years, J. Dentistry for Children 34:439–443 (Nov.) 1967.
3. Brudevold, F., and McCann, H.G.: Fluoride and Caries Control—Mechanism of Action, in Nizel, A.E.: The Science of Nutrition and Its Application in Clinical Dentistry, Philadelphia, W.B. Saunders Company, 1966, pp. 331–347.
4. American Academy of Pediatrics Committee on Nutrition: Fluoride Supplementation: Revised Dosage Schedule. Pediatrics 63:150, 1979.

POLY-VI-FLOR® 0.5 mg with Iron ℞

Multivitamin, iron and fluoride supplement drops

Description:

Each 1.0 ml supplies		Percentage of U.S. Recommended Daily Allowance: Infants	Children Under 4
Vitamin A, IU	1500	100	60
Vitamin D, IU	400	100	100
Vitamin E, IU	5	100	50
Vitamin C (Ascorbic acid), mg	35	100	88
Thiamine (Vitamin B_1), mg	0.5	100	71
Riboflavin (Vitamin B_2), mg	0.6	100	75
Niacin, mg	8	100	89
Vitamin B_6, mg	0.4	100	57
Iron, mg	10	67	100
Fluoride, mg	0.5	*	*

*U.S. Recommended Daily Allowance has not been established.

See INDICATIONS AND USAGE section below for use by infants and children under two years of age.

This product does not contain the essential vitamins folic acid and B_{12}.

Ingredients: Vitamin A palmitate, ergocalciferol, D-alpha-tocopheryl succinate, ascorbic acid, thiamine hydrochloride, riboflavin-5-phosphate sodium, niacinamide, pyridoxine hydrochloride, ferrous sulfate and sodium fluoride. Made with natural sweeteners.

Clinical Pharmacology: It is well established that fluoridation of the water supply (1 ppm fluoride) during the period of tooth development leads to a significant decrease in the incidence of dental caries.

Hydroxyapatite is the principal crystal for all calcified tissue in the human body. The fluoride ion reacts with the *hydroxyapatite* in the tooth as it is formed to produce the more caries-resistant crystal, *fluorapatite.* The reaction may be expressed by the equation:[1]

$Ca_{10}(PO_4)_6(OH)_2 + 2F^- \rightarrow Ca_{10}(PO_4)_6F_2 + 2OH^-$
(Hydroxyapatite) (Fluorapatite)

Three stages of fluoride deposition in tooth enamel can be distinguished:[1]

1. Small amounts (reflecting the low levels of fluoride in tissue fluids) are incorporated into the enamel crystals while they are being formed.
2. After enamel has been laid down, fluoride deposition continues in the surface enamel. Diffusion of fluoride from the surface inward is apparently restricted.
3. After eruption, the surface enamel acquires fluoride from water, food, supplementary fluoride and smaller amounts from saliva.

Indications and Usage: Supplementation of the diet with eight essential vitamins and iron.

Supplementation of the diet with fluoride for caries prophylaxis.

The American Academy of Pediatrics recommends that children up to age 16, in areas where drinking water contains less than optimal levels of fluoride, receive daily fluoride supplementation.

Poly-Vi-Flor 0.5 mg (multivitamin, iron, and fluoride supplement) drops with Iron provide fluoride in drop form for children ages 2–3 years in areas where the drinking water contains less than 0.3 ppm fluoride; and for children over 3 years in areas where the drinking water contains 0.3 thru 0.7 ppm of fluoride.[6] Each 1.0 ml provides sodium fluoride (0.5 mg fluoride) plus eight essential vitamins and iron.

The American Academy of Pediatrics[6] and the American Dental Association[7] currently recommend that infants and children under 2 years of age, in areas where drinking water contains less than 0.3 ppm of fluoride, and children 2-3, in areas where the drinking water contains 0.3 through 0.7 ppm of fluoride, receive 0.25 mg of supplemental fluoride daily which is provided in a full dose (1 ml) of Poly-Vi-Flor® 0.25 mg drops with Iron. A half dose (0.5 ml) of Poly-Vi-Flor 0.5 mg drops with Iron could also provide a daily fluoride intake of 0.25 mg; however, this dosage reduces vitamin supplementation by half.

Poly-Vi-Flor 0.5 mg drops with Iron supply significant amounts of vitamins A, D, E, C, thiamine, riboflavin, niacin, pyridoxine, and ferrous sulfate to supplement the diet, and to help assure that deficiencies of these nutrients will not develop. Thus, in a single easy-to-use preparation, children obtain eight essential vitamins and iron, plus fluoride.

A comprehensive 5½ year series of studies of the effectiveness of Tri-Vi-Flor® and Poly-Vi-Flor® products in caries protection has been published.[2-5] Children in this continuing study lived in an area where the water supply contained only 0.05 ppm fluoride. The subjects were divided into two groups, one which used only nonfluoridated Vi-Sol® vitamin products and the other Tri-Vi-Flor and Poly-Vi-Flor vitamin-fluoride products.

The three-year interim report showed 63% fewer carious surfaces in primary teeth and 43% fewer carious surfaces in permanent teeth of the children taking Vi-Flor™ vitamin-fluoride products.[2]

After four years the studies continued to support the effectiveness of Tri-Vi-Flor and Poly-Vi-Flor, showing a reduction in carious surfaces of 68% in primary teeth and 46% in permanent teeth.[3]

Results at the end of 5½ years further confirmed the previous findings and indicated that significant reductions in dental caries are apparent with the continued use of Vi-Flor vitamin-fluoride products.[4]

Warnings: As in the case of all medications, keep out of the reach of children.

Precautions: The suggested dose should not be exceeded since dental fluorosis may result from continued ingestion of large amounts of fluoride.

When prescribing Vi-Flor products, the physician should:

1. determine the fluoride content of the drinking water.
2. make sure the child is not receiving significant amounts of fluoride from other medications.
3. periodically check to make sure that the child does not develop significant dental fluorosis.

Poly-Vi-Flor 0.5 mg drops with Iron should be dispensed in the original plastic container, since contact with glass leads to instability and precipitation. (The amount of sodium fluoride in the 50-ml. size is well below the maximum to be dispensed at one time according to recommendations of the American Dental Association.)

Adverse Reactions: Allergic rash and other idiosyncrasies have been reported rarely.

Dosage and Administration: 1.0 ml daily for children 2 years of age and older, or as prescribed by the physician. May be dropped directly into mouth with 'Safti-Dropper', or mixed with cereal, fruit juice or other food.

How Supplied: Poly-Vi-Flor 0.5 mg (multivitamin, fluoride and iron supplement) drops with Iron are available on prescription only in bottles of 50 ml.

NDC 0087-0469-41 Bottles of 1⅔ fl oz (50 ml)
Literature Available: Yes.

References:

1. Brudevold, F., and McCann, H.G.: Fluoride and Caries Control—Mechanism of Action, in Nizel, A.E.: The Science of Nutrition and its Application in Clinical Dentistry, Philadelphia, W.B. Saunders Company, 1966, pp. 331–347.
2. Hennon, D.K.; Stookey, G.K., and Muhler, J.C.: The Clinical Anticariogenic Effectiveness of Supplementary Fluoride-Vitamin Preparations—Results at the End of Three Years, J. Dentistry for Children 33:3–12 (Jan.) 1966.
3. Hennon, D.K.; Stookey, G.K., and Muhler, J.C.: The Clinical Anticariogenic Effectiveness of Supplementary Fluoride-Vitamin Preparations—Results at the End of Four Years, J. Dentistry for Children 34:439–443 (Nov.) 1967.
4. Hennon, D.K.; Stookey, G.K., and Muhler, J.C.: The Clinical Anticariogenic Effectiveness of Supplementary Fluoride-Vitamin Preparations—Results at the End of Five and a Half Years, Phar. and Ther. In Dent. 1:1, 1970.
5. Hennon, D.K.; Stookey, G.K., and Beiswanger, B.B.: Fluoride-vitamin supplements: Effects on Dental Caries and Fluorosis When Used in Areas With Suboptimum Fluoride in the Water Supply. J. Am. Dent. Assoc. 95:965, 1977.
6. American Academy of Pediatrics, Committee on Nutrition: Fluoride Supplementation: Revised Dosage Schedule, Pediatrics 63:150, 1979.
7. Accepted Dental Therapeutics, Ed. 38, Chicago, American Dental Association, 1979, p. 321.

POLY-VI-FLOR® 0.25 mg with Iron ℞

Multivitamin, fluoride and iron supplement drops

Each 1.0 ml supplies:		Percentage of U.S. Recommended Daily Allowance: Infants	Children Under 4
Vitamin A, IU	1500	100	60
Vitamin D, IU	400	100	100
Vitamin E, IU	5	100	50
Vitamin C (Ascorbic acid), mg	35	100	88
Thiamine (Vitamin B_1), mg	0.5	100	71
Riboflavin (Vitamin B_2), mg	0.6	100	75
Niacin, mg	8	100	89
Vitamin B_6, mg	0.4	100	57
Iron, mg	10	67	100
Fluoride, mg	0.25	*	*

*U.S. Recommended Daily Allowance has not been established.

Description:
[See table above].
This product does not contain the essential vitamins folic acid and B_{12}.
Ingredients: Vitamin A palmitate, ergocalciferol, D-alpha-tocopheryl succinate, ascorbic acid, thiamine hydrochloride, riboflavin-5-phosphate sodium, niacinamide, pyridoxine hydrochloride, ferrous sulfate, and sodium fluoride.
Made with natural sweeteners.
Clinical Pharmacology: It is well established that fluoridation of the water supply (1 ppm fluoride) during the period of tooth development leads to a significant decrease in the incidence of dental caries.
Hydroxyapatite is the principal crystal for all calcified tissue in the human body. The fluoride ion reacts with the *hydroxyapatite* in the tooth as it is formed to produce the more caries-resistant crystal, *fluorapatite.* The reaction may be expressed by the equation:[1]

$$Ca_{10}(PO_4)_6(OH)_2 + 2F \rightarrow Ca_{10}(PO_4)_6F_2 + 2\,OH$$
(Hydroxyapatite) (Fluorapatite)

Three stages of fluoride deposition in tooth enamel can be distinguished.[1]

1. Small amounts (reflecting the low levels of fluoride in tissue fluids) are incorporated into the enamel crystals while they are being formed.
2. After enamel has been laid down, fluoride deposition continues in the surface enamel. Diffusion of fluoride from the surface inward is apparently restricted.
3. After eruption, the surface enamel acquires fluoride from water, food, supplementary fluoride and small amounts from saliva.

Indications and Usage: Supplementation of the diet with eight essential vitamins and iron.
Supplementation of the diet with fluoride, for caries prophylaxis.
The American Academy of Pediatrics recommends that children up to age 16, in areas where drinking water contains less than optimal levels of fluoride, receive daily fluoride supplementation.
POLY-VI-FLOR 0.25 mg drops with Iron provide fluoride in drop form for infants and young children from birth to 2 years of age in areas where the drinking water contains less than 0.3 ppm of fluoride and for children ages 2-3 years in areas where the drinking water contains 0.3 thru 0.7 ppm of fluoride. Each 1.0 ml supplies sodium fluoride (0.25 mg fluoride) plus eight essential vitamins and iron.[2]
POLY-VI-FLOR 0.25 mg drops with Iron supply significant amounts of vitamins A, D, E, C, thiamine, riboflavin, niacin, pyridoxine, and iron to supplement the diet, and to help assure that deficiencies of these nutrients will not develop. Thus, in a single easy-to-use preparation, infants obtain eight essential vitamins and iron, plus fluoride.
Warnings: As in the case of all medications, keep out of the reach of children.
Precautions: The suggested dose should not be exceeded since dental fluorosis may result from continued ingestion of large amounts of fluoride.
When prescribing VI-FLOR products, the physician should:

1. determine the fluoride content of the drinking water.
2. make sure the child is not receiving significant amounts of fluoride from other medications.
3. periodically check to make sure that the child does not develop significant dental fluorosis.

POLY-VI-FLOR 0.25 mg drops with Iron should be dispensed in the original plastic container, since contact with glass leads to instability and precipitation. (The amount of sodium fluoride in the 50-ml size is well below the maximum to be dispensed at one time according to recommendations of the American Dental Association.)
Adverse Reactions: Allergic rash and other idiosyncrasies have been rarely reported.
Dosage and Administration: 1.0 ml daily or as prescribed by the physician. May be dropped directly into mouth with 'Safti-Dropper,' or mixed with cereal, fruit juice or other foods. **USE FULL DOSAGE.**
How Supplied: POLY-VI-FLOR 0.25 mg (multivitamin, fluoride and iron supplement) drops with Iron are available on prescription only in bottles of 50 ml.

REFERENCES:

1. Brudevold F and McCann HG: Fluoride and caries control—mechanism of action, in Nizel AE: The Science of Nutrition and Its Application in Clinical Dentistry, Philadelphia, WB Saunders Company, 1966, pp 331-347.
2. American Academy of Pediatrics, Committee on Nutrition: Fluoride Supplementation: Revised Dosage Schedule, Pediatrics 63:150, 1979.

POLY-VI-SOL®

Multivitamin supplement drops • chewable tablets

(See PDR For Nonprescription Drugs)

POLY-VI-SOL® with Iron

Multivitamin and Iron supplement chewable tablets

(See PDR For Nonprescription Drugs)

POLY-VI-SOL® with Iron

Multivitamin and Iron supplement drops

(See PDR For Nonprescription Drugs)

PORTAGEN®

Nutritionally complete dietary with Medium Chain Triglycerides and "Lactose-Free" (Less than 0.15% w/w Lactose)
U.S. Patent No. 3,450,819

(See PDR For Nonprescription Drugs)

PREGESTIMIL®

Protein hydrolysate formula with medium chain triglycerides and added amino acids

(See PDR For Nonprescription Drugs)

PROSOBEE® concentrated liquid • ready-to-use

Milk-free, sucrose-free formula with soy protein isolate

(See PDR For Nonprescription Drugs)

SUSTACAL®

• liquid (ready to use)
• powder (mix with milk)
• pudding (ready-to-eat)
Nutritionally complete food

(See PDR For Nonprescription Drugs)

SUSTACAL® HC

High Calorie Nutritionally Complete Food

(See PDR for Nonprescription Drugs)

SUSTAGEN® powder

Nutritional supplement

(See PDR For Nonprescription Drugs)

TEMPRA®

Acetaminophen

(See PDR For Nonprescription Drugs)

TRAUMACAL™

Nutritionally Complete Liquid for Traumatized Patients

(See PDR For Nonprescription Drugs)

TRIND® liquid

nasal decongestant • antihistamine

(See PDR For Nonprescription Drugs)

TRIND-DM® liquid

antitussive • nasal decongestant • antihistamine

(See PDR For Nonprescription Drugs)

Continued on next page

Mead Johnson—Cont.

TRI-VI-FLOR® 1.0 mg ℞
Vitamins A, D, C and fluoride chewable tablets

Description:
[See table below].

Each tablet supplies:		Percentage of U.S. Recommended Daily Allowance Children Under 4	Adults & Children 4 or More
Vitamin A, IU	2500	100	50
Vitamin D, IU	400	100	100
Vitamin C (Ascorbic acid), mg	60	150	100
Fluoride, mg	1.0	*	*

*U.S. Recommended Daily Allowance has not been established.

Ingredients: Vitamin A acetate, ergocalciferol, sodium ascorbate, ascorbic acid and sodium fluoride.
Made with natural sweeteners.
Clinical Pharmacology: It is well established that fluoridation of the water supply (1 ppm fluoride) during the period of tooth development leads to a significant decrease in the incidence of dental caries.
Tri-Vi-Flor tablets provide sodium fluoride (1 mg fluoride) and three basic vitamins in a chewable tablet. Because the tablets are chewable, they provide a *topical* as well as *systemic* source of fluoride.[1,2]
Hydroxyapatite is the principal crystal for all calcified tissue in the human body. The fluoride ion reacts with the *hydroxyapatite* in the tooth as it is formed to produce the more caries-resistant crystal, *fluorapatite*. The reaction may be expressed by the equation.[3]

$$Ca_{10}(PO_4)_6(OH)_2 + 2F^- \rightarrow Ca_{10}(PO_4)_6F_2 + 2OH^-$$

(Hydroxyapatite) *(Fluorapatite)*

Three stages of fluoride deposition in tooth enamel can be distinguished:[3]

1. Small amounts (reflecting the low levels of fluoride in tissue fluids) are incorporated into the enamel crystals while they are being formed.
2. After enamel has been laid down, fluoride deposition continues in the surface enamel. Diffusion of fluoride from the surface inward is apparently restricted.
3. After eruption, the surface enamel acquires fluoride from water, food, supplementary fluoride and smaller amounts from saliva.

Indications and Usage: Supplementation of the diet with vitamins A, D, and C.
Supplementation of the diet with fluoride for caries prophylaxis.
The American Academy of Pediatrics recommends that children up to age 16, in areas where drinking water contains less than optimal levels of fluoride, receive daily fluoride supplementation.
Tri-Vi-Flor 1.0 mg (vitamins A, D, C and fluoride) chewable tablets provide fluoride in tablet form for children 3 years of age and older where the drinking water contains less than 0.3 ppm of fluoride.[7]
Tri-Vi-Flor 1.0 mg chewable tablets supply vitamins A, D and C to help assure that nutritional deficiencies of these vitamins will not develop.
Tri-Vi-Flor 1.0 mg chewable tablets also provide the important mineral fluoride for caries prophylaxis. Thus in a single easy-to-use preparation, children over 3 years of age obtain three basic vitamins and the important mineral fluoride.
A study of fluoride tablets given to 121 children revealed the efficacy of sodium fluoride in tablet form. The authors concluded that the caries reduction was comparable to that previously reported for children drinking fluoridated water.[5]
A comprehensive 5½ year series of studies of the effectiveness of Tri-Vi-Flor® and Poly-Vi-Flor® products in caries protection has been published.[1,2,6] Children in this continuing study lived in an area where the water supply contained only 0.05 ppm fluoride. The subjects were divided into two groups, one which used only non-fluoridated Vi-Sol® vitamin products and the other Tri-Vi-Flor and Poly-Vi-Flor vitamin-fluoride products.
The three-year interim report showed 63% fewer carious surfaces in primary teeth and 43% fewer carious surfaces in permanent teeth of the children taking Vi-Flor™ vitamin-fluoride products.[1]
After four years the studies continued to support the effectiveness of Tri-Vi-Flor and Poly-Vi-Flor, showing a reduction in carious surfaces of 68% in primary teeth and 46% in permanent teeth.[2]
Results at the end of 5½ years further confirmed the previous findings and indicated that significant reductions in dental caries are apparent with the continued use of Vi-Flor vitamin-fluoride products.[6]
Warnings: As in the case of all medications, keep out of the reach of children.
Precautions: The suggested dose *should not be exceeded,* since dental fluorosis may result from continued ingestion of large amounts of fluoride.
When prescribing Vi-Flor products, the physician should:

1. determine the fluoride content of the drinking water.
2. make sure the child is not receiving significant amounts of fluoride from other medications.
3. periodically check to make sure that the child does not develop significant dental fluorosis.

The Council on Dental Therapeutics of the American Dental Association recommends that no more than 264 mg of sodium fluoride should be dispensed at one time.[4] Therefore, no more than 120 Tri-Vi-Flor 1.0 mg chewable tablets (2.2 mg sodium fluoride per tablet) should be dispensed at one time.
Adverse Reactions: Allergic rash and other idiosyncrasies have been rarely reported.
Dosage and Administration: One chewable tablet daily or as prescribed by the physician.
How Supplied: Tri-Vi-Flor 1.0 mg (vitamins A, D, C and fluoride) chewable tablets are available on prescription only in 100- and 1000-tablet bottles.
NDC 0087-0477-01 Bottles of 100
NDC 0087-0477-02 Bottles of 1000
Literature Available: Yes.
References:

1. Hennon DK, Stookey GK and Muhler JC: The Clinical Anticariogenic Effectiveness of Supplementary Fluoride-Vitamin Preparations—Results at the End of Three Years. J Dent for Children 33:3–12 (Jan) 1966.
2. Hennon DK, Stookey GK and Muhler JC: The Clinical Anticariogenic Effectiveness of Supplementary Fluoride-Vitamin Preparations—Results at the End of Four Years, J Dent for Children 34:439–443 (Nov) 1967.
3. Brudevold F and McCann HG: Fluoride and Caries Control—Mechanism of Action, In Nizel AE: The Science of Nutrition and Its Application in Clinical Dentistry, Philadelphia, WB Saunders Company, 1966, pp 331–347.
4. Council on Dental Therapeutics, Am Dental Assoc, Accepted Dental Therapeutics, 1977, 37th Edition, page 294.
5. Arnold FA, Jr, McClure FJ and White CL: Sodium Fluoride Tablets for Children, Dental Progress 1:12–16 (Oct) 1960.
6. Hennon DK, Stookey GK and Muhler JC: The Clinical Anticariogenic Effectiveness of Supplementary Fluoride-Vitamin Preparations—Results at the End of Five and a Half Years, Phar and Ther in Dent 1:1, 1970.
7. American Academy of Pediatrics, Committee on Nutrition: Fluoride supplementation: Revised Dosage Schedule. Pediatrics 63:150, 1979.

TRI-VI-FLOR® 0.5 mg ℞
Vitamins A, D, C and fluoride drops

Description:

Each 1.0 ml supplies:		Percentage of U.S. Recommended Daily Allowance Infants	Children Under 4
Vitamin A, IU	1500	100	60
Vitamin D, IU	400	100	100
Vitamin C (Ascorbic acid), mg	35	100	88
Fluoride, mg	0.5	*	*

*U.S. Recommended Daily Allowance has not been established.
See INDICATIONS AND USAGE section below for use by infants and children under two years of age.
Ingredients: Vitamin A palmitate, ergocalciferol, ascorbic acid and sodium fluoride. Made with natural sweeteners.
Clinical Pharmacology: It is well established that fluoridation of the water supply (1 ppm fluoride) during the period of tooth development leads to a significant decrease in the incidence of dental caries.
Hydroxyapatite is the principal crystal for all calcified tissue in the human body. The fluoride ion reacts with the *hydroxyapatite* in the tooth as it is formed to produce the more caries-resistant crystal, *fluorapatite*. The reaction may be expressed by the equation:[1]

$$Ca_{10}(PO_4)_6(OH)_2 + 2F^- \rightarrow Ca_{10}(PO_4)_6F_2 + 2OH^-$$

(Hydroxyapatite) (Fluorapatite)

Three stages of fluoride deposition in tooth enamel can be distinguished:[1]

1. Small amounts (reflecting the low levels of fluoride in tissue fluids) are incorporated into the enamel crystals while they are being formed.
2. After enamel has been laid down, fluoride deposition continues in the surface enamel. Diffusion of fluoride from the surface inward is apparently restricted.
3. After eruption, the surface enamel acquires fluoride from water, food, supplementary fluoride and smaller amounts from saliva.

Indications and Usage: Supplementation of the diet with vitamins A, D and C.
Tri-Vi-Flor 0.5 mg drops also provide fluoride for caries prophylaxis.
The American Academy of Pediatrics recommends that children up to age 16, in areas where drinking water contains less than optimal levels of fluoride, receive daily fluoride supplementation.
Tri-Vi-Flor 0.5 mg (vitamins A, D, C and fluoride) drops provide fluoride in drop form for children ages 2-3 years in areas where the drinking water contains less than 0.3 ppm fluoride; and for children over 3 years in areas where the drinking water contains 0.3 thru 0.7 ppm of fluoride. Each 1.0 ml provides sodium

fluoride (0.5 mg fluoride) plus three basic vitamins.

The American Academy of Pediatrics[6] and the American Dental Association[7] currently recommend that infants and children under 2 years of age, in areas where drinking water contains less than 0.3 ppm of fluoride, and children 2-3, in areas where the drinking water contains 0.3 through 0.7 ppm of fluoride, receive 0.25 mg of supplemental fluoride daily which is provided in a full dose (1 ml) of Tri-Vi-Flor® 0.25 mg drops. A half dose (0.5 ml) of Tri-Vi-Flor 0.5 mg drops could also provide a daily fluoride intake of 0.25 mg; however, this dosage reduces vitamin supplementation by half.

A comprehensive 5½ year series of studies of the effectiveness of Tri-Vi-Flor® and Poly-Vi-Flor® products in caries protection has been published.[2–5] Children in this continuing study lived in an area where the water supply contained only 0.05 ppm fluoride. The subjects were divided into two groups, one which used only nonfluoridated Vi-Sol® vitamin products and the other Tri-Vi-Flor and Poly-Vi-Flor vitamin-fluoride products.

The three-year interim report showed 63% fewer carious surfaces in primary teeth and 43% fewer carious surfaces in permanent teeth of the children taking Vi-Flor™ vitamin-fluoride products.[2]

After four years the studies continued to support the effectiveness of Tri-Vi-Flor and Poly-Vi-Flor, showing a reduction in carious surfaces of 68% in primary teeth and 46% in permanent teeth.[3]

Results at the end of 5½ years further confirmed the previous findings and indicated that significant reductions in dental caries are apparent with the continued use of Vi-Flor vitamin-fluoride products.[4]

Warnings: As in the case of all medications, keep out of the reach of children.

Precautions: The suggested dose should not be exceeded since dental fluorosis may result from continued ingestion of large amounts of fluoride.

When prescribing Vi-Flor products, the physician should:

1. determine the fluoride content of the drinking water.
2. make sure the child is not receiving significant amounts of fluoride from other medications.
3. periodically check to make sure that the child does not develop significant dental fluorosis.

Tri-Vi-Flor 0.5 mg drops should be dispensed in the original plastic container, since contact with glass leads to instability and precipitation. (The amount of sodium fluoride in both the 30- and 50-ml sizes is well below the maximum to be dispensed at one time acccording to recommendations of the American Dental Association.)

Adverse Reactions: Allergic rash and other idiosyncrasies have been rarely reported.

Dosage and Administration: 1.0 ml daily for children 2 years of age and older, or as prescribed by the physician. May be dropped directly into mouth with 'Safti-Dropper,' or mixed with cereal, fruit juice or other food.

How Supplied: Tri-Vi-Flor 0.5 mg (vitamins A,D,C, and fluoride) drops are available on prescription only in bottles of 30 and 50 ml.

NDC 0087-0473-01 Bottles of 1 fl oz (30 ml)

NDC 0087-0473-02 Bottles of 1⅔ fl oz (50 ml)

Literature Available: Yes.

References:

1. Brudevold, F., and McCann, H.G.: Fluoride and Caries Control—Mechanism of Action, in Nizel, A.E.: The Science of Nutrition and Its Application in Clinical Dentistry, Philadelphia, W.B. Saunders Company, 1966, pp. 331–347.

2. Hennon, D.K.; Stookey, G.K., and Muhler, J.C.: The Clinical Anticariogenic Effectiveness of Supplementary Fluoride-Vitamin Preparations—Results at the End of Three Years, J. Dentistry for Children 33:3–12 (Jan.) 1966.

3. Hennon, D.K.; Stookey, G.K., and Muhler, J.C.: The Clinical Anticariogenic Effectiveness of Supplementary Fluoride-Vitamin Preparations—Results at the End of Four Years, J. Dentistry for Children 34:439–443 (Nov.) 1967.

4. Hennon, D.K.; Stookey, G.K., and Muhler, J.C.: The Clinical Anticariogenic Effectiveness of Supplementary Fluoride-Vitamin Preparations—Results at the End of Five and a Half Years, Phar. and Ther. in Dent. 1:1, 1970.

5. Hennon, D.K.; Stookey, G.K., and Beiswanger, B.B.: Fluoride-vitamin supplements: Effects on dental caries and fluorosis when used in areas with suboptimum fluoride in the water supply. J Am Dent Assoc 95:965, 1977.

6. American Academy of Pediatrics, Committee on Nutrition: Fluoride Supplementation: Revised Dosage Schedule, Pediatrics 63:150, 1979.

7. Accepted Dental Therapeutics, Ed. 38, Chicago, American Dental Association, 1979, p. 321.

TRI-VI-FLOR® 0.25 mg ℞

Vitamins A, D, C and fluoride drops

Description:

		Percentage of U.S. Recommended Daily Allowance	
Each 1.0 ml supplies:		**Infants**	**Children Under 4**
Vitamin A, IU	1500	100	60
Vitamin D, IU	400	100	100
Vitamin C (Ascorbic acid), mg	35	100	88
Fluoride, mg	0.25	*	*

*U.S. Recommended Daily Allowance has not been established.

Ingredients: Vitamin A palmitate, ergocalciferol, ascorbic acid and sodium fluoride. Made with natural sweeteners.

Clinical Pharmacology: It is well established that fluoridation of the water supply (1 ppm fluoride) during the period of tooth development leads to a significant decrease in the incidence of dental caries.

Hydroxyapatite is the principal crystal for all calcified tissue in the human body. The fluoride ion reacts with the *hydroxyapatite* in the tooth as it is formed to produce the more caries-resistant crystal, *fluorapatite*. The reaction may be expressed by the equation:[1]

$Ca_{10}(PO_4)_6(OH)_2 + 2F^- \rightarrow Ca_{10}(PO_4)_6F_2 + 2OH^-$
(Hydroxyapatite) (Fluorapatite)

Three stages of fluoride deposition in tooth enamel can be distinguished:[1]

1. Small amounts (reflecting the low levels of fluoride in tissue fluids) are incorporated into the enamel crystals while they are being formed.
2. After enamel has been laid down, fluoride deposition continues in the surface enamel. Diffusion of fluoride from the surface inward is apparently restricted.
3. After eruption, the surface enamel acquires fluoride from water, food, supplementary fluoride and smaller amounts from saliva.

Indications and Usage: Supplementation of the diet with vitamins A, D and C.

Supplementation of the diet with fluoride for caries prophylaxis.

The American Academy of Pediatrics recommends that children up to age 16, in areas where drinking water contains less than optimal levels of fluoride, receive daily fluoride supplementation.

TRI-VI-FLOR 0.25 mg (vitamins A, D, C and fluoride) drops provide fluoride in drop form for infants and young children from birth to 2 years of age in areas where the drinking water contains less than 0.3 ppm of fluoride; and for children ages 2–3 years in areas where the drinking water contains 0.3 thru 0.7 ppm of fluoride. Each 1.0 ml supplies sodium fluoride (0.25 mg fluoride) plus three basic vitamins.[2]

Warnings: As in the case of all medications, keep out of the reach of children.

Precautions: The suggested dose should not be exceeded since dental fluorosis may result from continued ingestion of large amounts of fluoride.

When prescribing VI-FLOR products, the physician should:

1. determine the fluoride content of the drinking water.
2. make sure the child is not receiving significant amounts of fluoride from other medications.
3. periodically check to make sure that the child does not develop significant dental fluorosis.

TRI-VI-FLOR 0.25 mg drops should be dispensed in the original plastic container, since contact with glass leads to instability and precipitation. (The amount of sodium fluoride in the 50-ml size is well below the maximum to be dispensed at one time according to recommendations of the American Dental Association.)

Adverse Reactions: Allergic rash and other idiosyncrasies have been rarely reported.

Dosage and Administration: 1.0 ml daily, or as prescribed by the physician. May be dropped directly into mouth with 'Safti-Dropper', or mixed with cereal, fruit juice or other food.

How Supplied: TRI-VI-FLOR 0.25 mg (vitamins A, D, C and fluoride) drops are available on prescription only in bottles of 50 ml.

NDC 0087-0452-41 Bottles of 50 ml.

Literature Available: Yes.

References:

1. Brudevold F and McCann HG: Fluoride and caries control—mechanism of action, in Nizel AE: The Science of Nutrition and Its Application in Clinical Dentistry, Philadelphia, WB Saunders Company, 1966, pp 331–347.

2. American Academy of Pediatrics, Committee on Nutrition: Fluoride Supplementation: Revised Dosage Schedule, Pediatrics 63:150, 1979.

TRI-VI-FLOR® 0.25 mg with Iron ℞

Vitamins A, D, C, iron and fluoride drops

Description:

		Percentage of U.S. Recommended Daily Allowance	
Each 1.0 ml supplies:		**Infants**	**Children Under 4**
Vitamin A, IU	1500	100	60
Vitamin D, IU	400	100	100
Vitamin C (Ascorbic acid), mg	35	100	88
Iron, mg	10	67	100
Fluoride, mg	0.25	*	*

* U.S. Recommended Daily Allowance has not been established.

Ingredients: Vitamin A palmitate, ergocalciferol, ascorbic acid, ferrous sulfate and sodium fluoride. Made with natural sweeteners.

Clinical Pharmacology: It is well established that fluoridation of the water supply (1 ppm fluoride) during the period of tooth development leads to a significant decrease in the incidence of dental caries.

Hydroxyapatite is the principal crystal for all calcified tissue in the human body. The fluoride ion reacts with the hydroxyapatite in the tooth as it is formed to produce the more caries-resistant crystal, fluorapatite. The reaction may be expressed by the equation:[1]

$Ca_{10}(PO_4)_6(OH)_2 + 2F^- \rightarrow Ca_{10}(PO_4)_6F_2 + 2\,OH^-$
(Hydroxyapatite) (Fluorapatite)

Three stages of fluoride deposition in tooth enamel can be distinguished:[1]

1. Small amounts (reflecting the low levels of fluoride in tissue fluids) are incorporated

Continued on next page

Mead Johnson—Cont.

into the enamel crystals while they are being formed.

2. After enamel has been laid down, fluoride deposition continues in the surface enamel. Diffusion of fluoride from the surface inward is apparently restricted.
3. After eruption, the surface enamel acquires fluoride from water, food, supplementary fluoride and smaller amounts from saliva.

Indications and Usage: Supplementation of the diet with vitamins A, D, C and iron. Supplementation of the diet with fluoride for caries prophylaxis.

The American Academy of Pediatrics recommends that children up to age 16, in areas where drinking water contains less than optimal levels of fluoride, receive daily fluoride supplementation.

TRI-VI-FLOR 0.25 mg (vitamins A, D, C, iron and fluoride) drops with Iron provide fluoride in drop form for infants and young children from birth to 2 years of age in areas where the drinking water contains less than 0.3 ppm of fluoride; and for children ages 2-3 years in areas where the drinking water contains 0.3 thru 0.7 ppm of fluoride. Each 1.0 ml supplies sodium fluoride (0.25 mg fluoride) plus three basic vitamins and iron.[2]

Warnings: As in the case of all medications, keep out of the reach of children.

Precautions: The suggested dose should not be exceeded since dental fluorosis may result from continued ingestion of large amounts of fluoride.

When prescribing VI-FLOR products, the physician should:

1. determine the fluoride content of the drinking water.
2. make sure the child is not receiving significant amounts of fluoride from other medications.
3. periodically check to make sure that the child does not develop significant dental fluorosis.

TRI-VI-FLOR 0.25 mg drops with iron should be dispensed in the original plastic container, since contact with glass leads to instability and precipitation. (The amount of sodium fluoride in the 50-ml size is well below the maximum to be dispensed at one time according to recommendations of the American Dental Association.)

Adverse Reactions: Allergic rash and other idiosyncrasies have been rarely reported.

Dosage and Administration: 1.0 ml daily, or as prescribed by the physician. May be dropped directly into mouth with 'Safti-Dropper', or mixed with cereal, fruit juice or other food.

USE FULL DOSAGE.

How Supplied: TRI-VI-FLOR 0.25 mg (vitamins A, D, C, iron and fluoride) drops with Iron are available on prescription only in bottles of 50 ml.

References:

1. Brudevold F and McCann HG: Fluoride and caries control—mechanism of action, in Nizel AE: The Science of Nutrition and its Application in Clinical Dentistry, Philadelphia, WB Saunders Company, 1966, pp 332–347.

2. American Academy of Pediatrics, Committee on Nutrition: Fluoride Supplementation: Revised Dosage Schedule, Pediatrics 63:150, 1979.

TRI-VI-SOL®
Vitamin A, D and C Supplement
drops • chewable tablets

(See PDR For Nonprescription Drugs)

TRI-VI-SOL® with Iron
Vitamins A, D, C and Iron
Drops

(See PDR For Nonprescription Drugs)

Mead Johnson Pharmaceutical Division

Mead Johnson & Company
2404 W. PENNSYLVANIA ST.
EVANSVILLE, INDIANA 47721

COLACE®
Docusate sodium, Mead Johnson
capsules • syrup • liquid (drops)

Description: Colace (Docusate sodium) is a stool softener.

Actions and Uses: Colace, a surface-active agent, helps to keep stools soft for easy, natural passage. Not a laxative, thus not habit forming. Useful in constipation due to hard stools, in painful anorectal conditions, in cardiac and other conditions in which maximum ease of passage is desirable to avoid difficult or painful defecation, and when peristaltic stimulants are contraindicated. *Note:* When peristaltic stimulation is needed due to inadequate bowel motility, see Peri-Colace® (laxative and stool softener).

Contraindications: There are no known contraindications to Colace.

Side Effects: The incidence of side effects—none of a serious nature—is exceedingly small. Bitter taste, throat irritation, and nausea (primarily associated with the use of the syrup and liquid) are the main side effects reported. Rash has occurred.

Administration and Dosage: *Orally*—Suggested daily Dosage: *Adults and older children:* 50 to 200 mg. *Children 6 to 12:* 40 to 120 mg. *Children 3 to 6:* 20 to 60 mg. *Infants and children under 3:* 10 to 40 mg. The higher doses are recommended for initial therapy. Dosage should be adjusted to individual response. The effect on stools is usually apparent one to three days after the first dose. Give Colace liquid in half a glass of milk or fruit juice or in infant formula, to mask bitter taste. *In enemas*—Add 50 to 100 mg. Colace (5 to 10 ml. Colace liquid) to a retention or flushing enema.

How Supplied: Colace® capsules, 50 mg.

NDC 0087-0713-01 Bottles of 30
NDC 0087-0713-02 Bottles of 60
NDC 0087-0713-03 Bottles of 250
NDC 0087-0713-05 Bottles of 1000
NDC 0087-0713-07 Cartons of 100 single unit packs

Colace® capsules, 100 mg.

NDC 0087-0714-43 Cartons of 10 single unit packs
NDC 0087-0714-01 Bottles of 30
NDC 0087-0714-02 Bottles of 60
NDC 0087-0714-03 Bottles of 250
NDC 0087-0714-05 Bottles of 1000
NDC 0087-0714-07 Cartons of 100 single unit packs

Note: Colace capsules should be stored at controlled room temperature (15°–30°C. or 59°–86°F.)

Colace® liquid, 1% solution; 10 mg./ml. (with calibrated dropper)

NDC 0087-0717-04 Bottles of 16 fl. oz.
NDC 0087-0717-02 Bottles of 30 ml.
6505-00-045-7786 (Bottle of 30 ml) Defense

Colace® syrup, 20 mg./5-ml. teaspoon; contains not more than 1% alcohol

NDC 0087-0720-01 Bottles of 8 fl. oz.
NDC 0087-0720-02 Bottles of 16 fl. oz.

[*Shown in Product Identification Section*]

CYTOXAN® Oral tablets • injections ℞
(Cyclophosphamide)

Description: Cytoxan is a synthetic antineoplastic drug chemically related to the nitrogen mustards. It is a white crystalline powder which is soluble in water, physiological saline, or alcohol. **Store Cytoxan products at temperatures not to exceed 30° C. (86° F.), preferably below 25° C. (77° F.).**

Actions: Although it is classified generally as an alkylating agent, Cytoxan itself is not an alkylating agent or irritant. It interferes with the growth of susceptible neoplasms and, to some extent, certain normal tissues. Its mechanism of action is not known.

Cytoxan is absorbed from the gastrointestinal tract and parenteral sites. It is metabolized (the details of metabolism are not fully known) and the drug and its metabolites are distributed throughout the body, including the brain. Intravenously administered Cytoxan is reported to have a serum half-life of about four hours; however the drug and/or its metabolites may be detected in plasma up to seventy-two hours. Cytoxan and its metabolites are excreted by the kidneys, but the extent to which they are excreted by other routes is not known. Of three alkylating metabolites found in urine, only one (nor-nitrogen mustard) has been identified definitely.

Indications:

Cyclophosphamide, though effective alone in susceptible malignancies, is more frequently used concurrently or sequentially with other antineoplastic drugs. The following malignancies are often susceptible to cyclophosphamide treatment:

1. Malignant lymphomas (Stages III and IV of the Ann Arbor staging system); Hodgkin's disease; lymphocytic lymphoma (nodular or diffuse); mixed-cell type lymphoma; histiocytic lymphoma; Burkitt's lymphoma.
2. Multiple myeloma.
3. Leukemias: chronic lymphocytic leukemia; chronic granulocytic leukemia (it is ineffective in acute blastic crisis); acute myelogenous and monocytic leukemia; acute lymphoblastic (stem-cell) leukemia in children (cyclophosphamide given during remission is effective in prolonging its duration).
4. Mycosis fungoides (advanced disease).
5. Neuroblastoma (disseminated disease).
6. Adenocarcinoma of the ovary.
7. Retinoblastoma.
8. Carcinoma of the breast.

Warnings: Since Cytoxan has been reported to be more toxic in adrenalectomized dogs, adjustment of the doses of both replacement steroids and Cytoxan may be necessary for the adrenalectomized patient.

The rate of metabolism and the leukopenic activity of Cytoxan reportedly are increased by chronic administration of high doses of phenobarbital. The physician should be alert for possible combined drug actions, desirable or undesirable, involving Cytoxan even though Cytoxan has been used successfully concurrently with other drugs, including other cytotoxic drugs.

Cytoxan may interfere with normal wound healing.

Usage in Pregnancy. Cytoxan can be teratogenic or cause fetal resorption in experimental animals. It should not be used in pregnancy, particularly in early pregnancy, unless in the judgment of the physician the potential benefits outweigh the possible risks. Cytoxan is excreted in breast milk and breast-feeding should be terminated prior to institution of Cytoxan therapy.

Patients, male or female, capable of conception ordinarily should be advised of the mutagenic potential of Cytoxan. Adequate methods of contraception appear desirable for such patients receiving Cytoxan.

Precautions: Cytoxan should be given cautiously to patients with any of the following conditions.

1. Leukopenia
2. Thrombocytopenia
3. Tumor cell infiltration of bone marrow
4. Previous X-ray therapy
5. Previous therapy with other cytotoxic agents
6. Impaired hepatic function
7. Impaired renal function

Because Cytoxan may exert a suppressive action on immune mechanisms, the interruption or modification of dosage should be considered for patients who develop bacterial, fungal or viral infections. This is especially true for patients receiving concomitant steroid therapy and perhaps those with a recent history of steroid therapy, since infections in some of these patients have been fatal. Varicella-zoster infections appear to be particularly dangerous under these circumstances.

Cytoxan 25 mg and 50 mg tablets contain FD&C Yellow No. 5 (tartrazine) which may cause allergic-type reactions (including bronchial asthma) in certain susceptible individuals. Although the overall incidence of FD&C Yellow No. 5 (tartrazine) sensitivity in the general population is low, it is frequently seen in patients who also have aspirin hypersensitivity.

Adverse Reactions:

Secondary Neoplasia. Secondary malignancies have developed in some patients treated with cyclophosphamide alone or in association with other antineoplastic drugs and/or modalities. These malignancies most frequently have been urinary bladder, myeloproliferative, and lymphoproliferative malignancies. Secondary malignancies most frequently have developed in the cyclophosphamide-treated patients with primary myeloproliferative and lymphoproliferative malignancies and primary nonmalignant diseases in which immune processes are believed to be involved pathologically. In some cases, the secondary malignancy was detected up to several years after cyclophosphamide treatment was discontinued. The secondary urinary bladder malignancies generally have occurred in patients who previously developed hemorrhagic cystitis (see Genitourinary under Adverse Reactions). Although no cause-effect relationship has been established between cyclophosphamide and the development of malignancy in humans, the possibility of secondary malignancy, based on available data, should be considered in any benefit-to-risk assessment for the use of the drug.

Hematopoietic. Leukopenia is an expected effect and ordinarily is used as a guide to therapy. Thrombocytopenia or anemia may occur in a few patients. These effects are almost always reversible when therapy is interrupted.

Gastrointestinal. Anorexia, nausea, or vomiting are common and related to dose as well as individual susceptibility. There are isolated reports of hemorrhagic colitis, oral mucosal ulceration and jaundice occurring during therapy.

Genitourinary. Sterile hemorrhagic cystitis can result from the administration of Cytoxan. **This can be severe, even fatal, and is probably due to metabolites in the urine.** Nonhemorrhagic cystitis and/or fibrosis of the bladder also have been reported to result from Cytoxan administration. Atypical epithelial cells may be found in the urinary sediment. **Ample fluid intake and frequent voiding help to prevent the development of cystitis,** but when it occurs it is ordinarily necessary to interrupt Cytoxan therapy. Hematuria usually resolves spontaneously within a few days after Cytoxan therapy is discontinued, but may persist for several months. In severe cases replacement of blood loss may be required. The application of electrocautery to telangiectatic areas of the bladder and diversion of urine flow have been successful methods used in treatment of protracted cases. Cryosurgery has also been used. (See also Secondary Neoplasia under Adverse Reactions.) Nephrotoxicity, including hemorrhage and clot formation in the renal pelvis, have been reported.

Gonadal suppression, resulting in amenorrhea or azoospermia, has been reported in a number of patients treated with cyclophosphamide and appears to be related to dosage and duration of therapy. This side effect, possibly irreversible, should be anticipated in patients treated with Cytoxan. It is not known to what extent Cytoxan may affect prepuberal gonads. Fibrosis of the ovary following Cytoxan therapy has been reported also.

Integument. It is ordinarily advisable to inform patients in advance of possible alopecia, a frequent complication of Cytoxan therapy. Regrowth of hair can be expected although occasionally the new hair may be of a different color or texture. The skin and fingernails may become darker during therapy. Non-specific dermatitis has been reported to occur with Cytoxan.

Pulmonary. Interstitial pulmonary fibrosis has been reported in patients receiving high doses of Cytoxan over a prolonged period.

Dosage and Administration: Chemotherapy with Cytoxan, as with other drugs used in cancer chemotherapy, is potentially hazardous and fatal complications can occur. It is recommended that it be administered only by physicians aware of the associated risks. Therapy may be aimed at either induction or maintenance of remission.

Induction Therapy. The usual initial intravenous loading dose for patients with no hematologic deficiency is 40–50 mg/kg. This total initial intravenous loading dose usually is given in divided doses over a period of two to five days.

Patients with any previous treatment that may have compromised the functional capacity of the bone marrow, such as X ray or cytotoxic drugs, and patients with tumor infiltration of the bone marrow may require reduction of the initial loading dose by $\frac{1}{3}$ to $\frac{1}{2}$.

A marked leukopenia is usually associated with the above doses, but recovery usually begins after 7–10 days. The white blood cell count should be monitored closely during induction therapy.

If initial therapy is given orally, a dose of 1–5 mg/kg/day can be administered depending on tolerance by the patient.

Maintenance Therapy. It is frequently necessary to maintain chemotherapy in order to suppress or retard neoplastic growth. A variety of schedules has been used:

(1) 1–5 mg/kg p.o. daily
(2) 10–15 mg/kg i.v. every 7–10 days
(3) 3–5 mg/kg i.v. twice weekly

Unless the disease is unusually sensitive to Cytoxan, it is advisable to give the largest maintenance dose that can be reasonably tolerated by the patient. The total leukocyte count is a good objective guide for regulating the maintenance dose. Ordinarily a leukopenia of 3000–4000 cells/cu. mm. can be maintained without undue risk of serious infection or other complications.

Preparation and Handling of Solutions. Cytoxan for Injection should be prepared for parenteral use by adding **Sterile Water for Injection, U.S.P. or Bacteriostatic Water for Injection, U.S.P. (paraben preserved only)** to the vial and shaking to dissolve. Use 5 ml. for the 100-mg vial, 10 ml. for the 200-mg vial, 25 ml. for the 500-mg vial, 50 ml. for the 1.0-g. vial or 100 ml. for the 2.0-g. vial. Solutions of Cytoxan for Injection may be injected intravenously, intramuscularly, intraperitoneally or intrapleurally or they may be infused intravenously in Dextrose Injection, U.S.P. (5% dextrose) or Dextrose and Sodium Chloride Injection, U.S.P. (5% dextrose and 0.9% sodium chloride). These solutions should be used within 24 hours if stored at room temperature or within 6 days if stored under refrigeration. Cytoxan for Injection does not contain an antimicrobial agent and **care must be taken to insure the sterility of prepared solutions.**

Extemporaneous liquid preparations of Cytoxan for oral administration may be prepared by dissolving Cytoxan for Injection in Aromatic Elixir, U.S.P. Such preparations should be stored under refrigeration and used within 14 days.

Overdosage: No specific antidote for Cytoxan is known. Management of overdosage would include general supportive measures to sustain the patient through any period of toxicity that might occur.

How Supplied: Cytoxan for Injection contains 45 mg of sodium chloride per 100 mg of cyclophosphamide (anhydrous).

Cytoxan® (cyclophosphamide) for Injection. With sodium chloride.

NDC 0087-0500-41 100 mg vials, carton of 12, case of 1 carton
NDC 0087-0500-01 100 mg vials, carton of 12, case of 4 cartons
NDC 0087-0501-41 200 mg vials, carton of 12, case of 1 carton
NDC 0087-0501-01 200 mg vials, carton of 12, case of 4 cartons
NDC 0087-0502-41 500 mg vials, carton of 12, case of 1 carton
NDC 0087-0502-01 500 mg vials, carton of 12, case of 4 cartons
NDC 0087-0505-41 1.0 g vials, carton of 6
NDC 0087-0506-41 2.0 g vials, carton of 6
6505-00-767-3578 (200 mg, 20 ml vial) Defense
6505-01-037-9356 (500 mg, 30 ml vial) Defense
VA6505-00-767-3578A (200 mg, 20 ml vial)
VA6505-01-037-9356A (500 mg, 30 ml vial)

Cytoxan® (cyclophosphamide) tablets.

NDC 0087-0503-01 50 mg, bottles of 100
NDC 0087-0503-02 50 mg, bottles of 1000
NDC 0087-0503-03 50 mg, Unit Dose cartons of 100
NDC 0087-0504-01 25 mg, bottles of 100
6505-00-733-5246 (50 mg, 100's) Defense
VA6505-00-733-5246A (50 mg, 100's)

[*Shown in Product Identification Section*]

DEAPRIL-ST® ℞
(ergoloid mesylates)
SUBLINGUAL TABLETS

Description:
Each Deapril-ST **1.0 mg.** Sublingual Tablet contains dihydroergocornine 0.333 mg., dihydroergocristine 0.333 mg., and dihydroergocryptine 0.333 mg. (dihydro-alpha-ergocryptine and dihydro-beta-ergocryptine in the proportion of 2:1) as the methanesulfonates (mesylates), representing a total of 1.0 mg.

Actions: There is no specific evidence which clearly establishes the mechanism by which an ergoloid mesylates preparation such as Deapril-ST produces mental effects, nor is there conclusive evidence that it particularly affects cerebral arteriosclerosis or cerebrovascular insufficiency.

Indications: A proportion of individuals over sixty years of age who manifest signs and symptoms of an idiopathic decline in mental capacity (e.g., cognitive and interpersonal skills, mood, self-care, apparent motivation) can experience some symptomatic relief upon treatment with ergoloid mesylates preparations. The identity of the specific trait(s) or condition(s), if any, which would usefully predict a response to ergoloid mesylates therapy is not known. It appears, however, that those individuals who do respond come from groups of patients who may suffer from a disorder related in a poorly defined manner to the aging process or who have some underlying condition which compromises mental capacity (e.g., primary progressive dementia, Alzheimer's dementia, senile onset, or multi-infarct dementia).

Continued on next page

Mead Johnson Pharm.—Cont.

Before prescribing ergoloid mesylates therapy, the physician should exclude the possibility that the patient's signs and symptoms arise from a potentially reversible and treatable condition. Particular care should be taken to exclude delirium and dementiform illness secondary to systemic disease, primary neurological disease or primary disturbance of mood.
Ergoloid mesylates preparations are not indicated in the treatment of acute or chronic psychosis, regardless of etiology (see CONTRAINDICATIONS section).
The decision to use ergoloid mesylates therapy in the treatment of an individual with a symptomatic decline in mental capacity of unknown etiology should be continually reviewed since the presenting clinical picture may subsequently evolve sufficiently to allow a specific diagnosis and a specific alternative treatment. In addition, continued clinical evaluation is required to determine whether any initial benefit conferred by ergoloid mesylates therapy persists with time.
The efficacy of ergoloid mesylates therapy was evaluated using a special rating scale. The specific items on this scale on which modest but statistically significant changes were observed at the end of twelve weeks concerned mental alertness, confusion, recent memory, orientation, emotional lability, self-care, depression, anxiety/fears, cooperation, sociability, appetite, dizziness, fatigue, bothersome(ness), and an overall impression of clinical status.
Contraindications: Deapril-ST Sublingual Tablets are contraindicated in individuals who have previously shown hypersensitivity to the drug. Ergoloid mesylates preparations are also contraindicated in patients who have psychosis, acute or chronic, regardless of etiology.
Precautions: *Practitioners are advised that because the target symptoms are of unknown etiology careful diagnosis should be attempted before prescribing ergoloid mesylates sublingual tablets.*
This product contains FD&C Yellow No. 5 (tartrazine) which may cause allergic-type reactions (including bronchial asthma) in certain susceptible individuals. Although the overall incidence of FD&C Yellow No. 5 (tartrazine) sensitivity in the general population is low, it is frequently seen in patients who also have aspirin hypersensitivity.
Adverse Reactions: Deapril-ST Sublingual Tablets have not been found to produce serious side effects. Some sublingual irritation, transient nausea, and gastric disturbances have been reported. Ergoloid mesylates sublingual tablets do not possess the vasoconstrictor properties of the natural ergot alkaloids.
Dosage and Administration: One Deapril-ST 1.0 mg. Sublingual Tablet three times a day. Alleviation of symptoms is usually gradual and results may not be observed for 3–4 weeks.
How Supplied: Deapril-ST 1.0 mg, Sublingual Tablets
NDC 0087-0555-41 Bottles of 100
[*Shown in Product Identification Section*]

DESYREL® ℞
(trazodone HCl)

Description: DESYREL®, trazodone hydrochloride, is an antidepressant chemically unrelated to tricyclic, tetracyclic, or other known antidepressant agents. It is a triazolopyridine derivative designated as 2-[3-[4-(3-chlorophenyl) -1-piperazinyl]propyl]-1,2,4-thiazolo [4, 3-a]pyridin-3(2H)-one hydrochloride. DESYREL is a white odorless crystalline powder which is freely soluble in water. Its molecular weight is 408.3. The empirical formula is $C_{19}H_{22}ClN_5O \cdot HCl$ and the structural formula is represented as follows:

N — CH₂ — CH₂ — CH₂ — N N — •HCl Cl O

DESYREL is supplied for oral administration in 50 mg and 100 mg tablets.
Clinical Pharmacology: The mechanism of DESYREL's antidepressant action in man is not fully understood. In animals, DESYREL selectively inhibits serotonin uptake by brain synaptosomes and potentiates the behavioral changes induced by the serotonin precurser, 5-hydroxytryptophan. Cardiac conduction effects of DESYREL in the anesthetized dog are qualitatively dissimilar and quantitatively less pronounced than those seen with tricyclic antidepressants. DESYREL is not a monoamine oxidase inhibitor and, unlike amphetamine-type drugs, does not stimulate the central nervous system.
In man, DESYREL is well absorbed after oral administration without selective localization in any tissue. When DESYREL is taken shortly after ingestion of food, there may be a slight increase in the amount of drug absorbed, a decrease in maximum concentration and a lengthening in the time to maximum concentration. Peak plasma levels occur approximately one hour after dosing when DESYREL is taken on an empty stomach or two hours after dosing when taken with food. Elimination of DESYREL is biphasic, consisting of an initial phase (half-life 3–6 hours) followed by a slower phase (half-life 5–9 hours), and is unaffected by the presence or absence of food. Since the clearance of DESYREL from the body is sufficiently variable, in some subjects DESYREL may accumulate in the plasma.
For those patients who responded to DESYREL, one-third of the inpatients and one-half of the outpatients had a significant therapeutic response by the end of the first week of treatment. Three-fourths of all responders demonstrated a significant therapeutic effect by the end of the second week. One-fourth of responders required 2–4 weeks for a significant therapeutic response.
Indications and Usage: DESYREL is indicated for the treatment of depression. The efficacy of DESYREL has been demonstrated in both inpatient and outpatient settings and for depressed patients with and without prominent anxiety. The depressive illness of patients studied corresponds to the Major Depressive Episode criteria of the American Psychiatric Association's Diagnostic and Statistical Manual, III.[1]
Major Depressive Episode implies a prominent and relatively persistent (nearly every day for at least two weeks) depressed or dysphoric mood that usually interferes with daily functioning, and includes at least four of the following eight symptoms: change in appetite, change in sleep, psychomotor agitation or retardation, loss of interest in usual activities or decrease in sexual drive, increased fatigability, feelings of guilt or worthlessness, slowed thinking or impaired concentration, and suicidal ideation or attempts.
Contraindications: DESYREL is contraindicated in patients hypersensitive to DESYREL.
Warnings: Recent clinical studies in patients with preexisting cardiac disease indicate that DESYREL may be arrhythmogenic in some patients in that population. Arrhythmias identified include isolated PVCs, ventricular couplets, and in two patients short episodes (3-4 beats) of ventricular tachycardia. There have also been several post-marketing reports of arrhythmias in DESYREL-treated patients who had preexisting cardiac disease. Until the results of prospective studies are available, patients with preexisting cardiac disease should be closely monitored particularly for cardiac arrhythmias.
DESYREL is not recommended for use during the initial recovery phase of myocardial infarction.
Precautions:
General: The possibility of suicide in seriously depressed patients is inherent in the illness and may persist until significant remission occurs. Therefore, prescriptions should be written for the smallest number of tablets consistent with good patient management.
Little is known about the interaction between DESYREL and general anesthetics; therefore, prior to elective surgery, DESYREL should be discontinued for as long as clinically feasible.
Information for Patients: Antidepressants may impair the mental and/or physical abilities required for the performance of potentially hazardous tasks, such as operating an automobile or machinery; the patient should be cautioned accordingly.
DESYREL may enhance the response to alcohol, barbiturates, and other CNS depressants.
DESYREL should be given shortly after a meal or light snack. Within any individual patient, total drug absorption may be up to 20% higher when the drug is taken with food rather than on an empty stomach. The risk of dizziness/lightheadedness may increase under fasting conditions.
Laboratory Tests: Occasional low white blood cell and neutrophil counts have been noted in patients receiving DESYREL. These were not considered clinically significant and did not necessitate discontinuation of the drug; however, the drug should be discontinued in any patient whose white blood cell count or absolute neutrophil count falls below normal levels. White blood cells and differential counts are recommended for patients who develop fever and sore throat (or other signs of infection) during therapy.
Drug Interactions: Because DESYREL can cause hypotension concomitant administration of antihypertensive therapy with DESYREL may require a reduction in the dose of the antihypertensive drug.
Increased serum Dilantin levels have been reported to occur in patients receiving DESYREL and Dilantin concurrently.
It is not known whether interactions will occur between monoamine oxidase (MAO) inhibitors and DESYREL. Due to the absence of clinical experience, if MAO inhibitors are discontinued shortly before or are to be given concomitantly with DESYREL, therapy should be initiated cautiously with gradual increase in dosage until optimum response is achieved.
Therapeutic Interactions: Concurrent administration with electroshock therapy should be avoided because of the absence of experience in this area.
Carcinogenesis, Mutagenesis, Impairment of Fertility: No drug- or dose-related occurrence of carcinogenesis was evident in rats receiving DESYREL in daily oral doses up to 300 mg/kg for 18 months.
Pregnancy Category C: DESYREL has been shown to cause increased fetal resorption and other adverse effects on the fetus in two studies using the rat when given at dose levels approximately 30–50 times the proposed maximum human dose. There was also an increase in congenital anomalies in one of three rabbit studies at approximately 15–50 times the maximum human dose. There are no adequate and well-controlled studies in pregnant women. DESYREL should be used during pregnancy only if the potential benefit justifies the potential risk to the fetus.
Nursing Mothers: DESYREL and/or its metabolites have been found in the milk of lactating rats, suggesting that the drug may be secreted in human milk. Caution should be exercised when DESYREL is administered to a nursing woman.
Pediatric Use: Safety and effectiveness in children below the age of 18 have not been established.

Adverse Reactions: Because the frequency of adverse drug effects is affected by diverse factors (e.g., drug dose, method of detection, investigator judgment, disease under treatment, etc.) a single meaningful estimate of adverse event incidence is difficult to obtain. This problem is illustrated by the variation in adverse event incidence observed and reported from the inpatients and outpatients treated with DESYREL. It is impossible to determine precisely what accounts for the differences observed.

The table below is presented solely to indicate the relative frequency of adverse events reported in representative controlled clinical studies conducted to evaluate the safety and efficacy of DESYREL.

[See table right].

The figures cited cannot be used to predict precisely the incidence of untoward events in the course of usual medical practice where patient characteristics and other factors often differ from those which prevailed in the clinical trials. These incidence figures, also, cannot be compared with those obtained from other clinical studies involving related drug products and placebo as each group of drug trials is conducted under a different set of conditions.

Occasional sinus bradycardia has occurred in long-term studies.

In addition to the relatively common (i.e., greater than 1%) untoward events enumerated above, the following adverse events have been reported in association with the use of DESYREL: akathisia, allergic reaction, anemia, chest pain, delayed urine flow, early menses, flatulence, hallucinations/delusions, hematuria, hypersalivation, hypomania, impaired speech, impotence, increased appetite, increased libido, increased urinary frequency, missed periods, muscle twitches, numbness, and retrograde ejaculation.

Overdosage:

Animal Oral LD_{50}

The oral LD_{50} of the drug is 610 mg/kg in mice, 486 mg/kg in rats, and 560 mg/kg in rabbits.

Signs and Symptoms: Death by deliberate or accidental overdosage has not occurred with DESYREL. In one known suicide attempt, a patient was found unconscious ("passed out") and was hospitalized three hours after ingesting an apparently excessive amount (approximately 7.5 g, according to the patient) of DESYREL. At the time of hospitalization, the patient was arousable, and emesis was induced. Recovery was uneventful. In another known suicide attempt, a patient presented with symptoms of drowsiness and "numb in the head" and was hospitalized about 90 minutes after ingesting a moderate amount (approximately 1.25–1.50 g, according to the patient) of DESYREL. Emesis was induced. There was no disturbance of EKG, CBC, blood chemistry, or vital signs and recovery was uneventful. The amounts of DESYREL actually absorbed in these cases is unknown, since the dosage ingested was determined by patient report and emesis was induced in both cases. Therefore, these cases may not be generalizable to other instances of overdosage. Overdosage may cause an increase in incidence or severity of any of the reported adverse reactions.

Treatment: There is no specific antidote for DESYREL. Treatment should be symptomatic and supportive in the case of hypotension or excessive sedation. Any patient suspected of having taken an overdose should have the stomach emptied by gastric lavage. Forced diuresis may be useful in facilitating elimination of the drug.

Dosage and Administration: The dosage should be initiated at a low level and increased gradually, noting the clinical response and any evidence of intolerance. Occurrence of drowsiness may require the administration of a major portion of the daily dose at bedtime or a reduction of dosage. DESYREL should be taken shortly after a meal or light snack.

Treatment Emergent Symptom Incidence

	Inpts.		Outpts.	
	D	P	D	P
Number of Patients	142	95	157	158
% of Patients Reporting				
Allergic				
Skin Condition/Edema	2.8	1.1	7.0	1.3
Autonomic				
Blurred Vision	6.3	4.2	14.7	3.8
Constipation	7.0	4.2	7.6	5.7
Dry Mouth	14.8	8.4	33.8	20.3
Cardiovascular				
Hypertension	2.1	1.1	1.3	*
Hypotension	7.0	1.1	3.8	0.0
Shortness of Breath	*	1.1	1.3	0.0
Syncope	2.8	2.1	4.5	1.3
Tachycardia/Palpitations	0.0	0.0	7.0	7.0
CNS				
Anger/Hostility	3.5	6.3	1.3	2.5
Confusion	4.9	0.0	5.7	7.6
Decreased Concentration	2.8	2.1	1.3	0.0
Disorientation	2.1	0.0	*	0.0
Dizziness/Light-headedness	19.7	5.3	28.0	15.2
Drowsiness	23.9	6.3	40.8	19.6
Excitement	1.4	1.1	5.1	5.7
Fatigue	11.3	4.2	5.7	2.5
Headache	9.9	5.3	19.8	15.8
Insomnia	9.9	10.5	6.4	12.0
Impaired Memory	1.4	0.0	*	*
Nervousness	14.8	10.5	6.4	8.2
Gastrointestinal				
Abdominal/Gastric Disorder	3.5	4.2	5.7	4.4
Bad Taste in Mouth	1.4	0.0	0.0	0.0
Diarrhea	0.0	1.1	4.5	1.9
Nausea/Vomitjng	9.9	1.1	12.7	9.5
Musculoskeletal				
Musculoskeletal Aches/Pains	5.6	3.2	5.1	2.5
Neurological				
Incoordination	4.9	0.0	1.9	0.0
Paresthesia	1.4	0.0	0.0	*
Tremors	2.8	1.1	5.1	3.8
Sexual Function				
Decreased Libido	*	1.1	1.3	*
Other				
Decreased Appetite	3.5	5.3	0.0	*
Eyes Red/Tired/Itching	2.8	0.0	0.0	0.0
Head Full-Heavy	2.8	0.0	0.0	0.0
Malaise	2.8	0.0	0.0	0.0
Nasal/Sinus Congestion	2.8	0.0	5.7	3.2
Nightmares/Vivid Dreams	*	1.1	5.1	5.7
Sweating/Clamminess	1.4	1.1	*	*
Tinnitus	1.4	0.0	0.0	*
Weight Gain	1.4	0.0	4.5	1.9
Weight Loss	*	3.2	5.7	2.5

*Incidence less than 1%.

D = DESYREL   P = Placebo

Symptomatic relief may be seen during the first week, with optimal antidepressant effects typically evident within two weeks. Twenty-five percent of those who respond to DESYREL require more than two weeks (up to four weeks) of drug administration.

Usual Adult Dosage: An initial dose of 150 mg/day is suggested. The dose may be increased by 50 mg/day every three to four days. The maximum dose for outpatients usually should not exceed 400 mg/day in divided doses. Inpatients or more severely depressed subjects may be given up to but not in excess of 600 mg/day in divided doses.

Maintenance: Dosage during prolonged maintenance therapy should be kept at the lowest effective level. Once an adequate response has been achieved, dosage may be gradually reduced, with subsequent adjustment depending on therapeutic response.

How Supplied:

DESYREL® (trazodone hydrochloride)

Tablets, 50 mg—round, orange/scored, film-sealed (imprinted with MJ logo)

NDC 0087-0775-41 Bottles of 100
NDC 0087-0775-43 Bottles of 1000
NDC 0087-0775-42 Cartons of 100 Unit Doses

Tablets, 100 mg—round, white/scored, film-sealed (imprinted with MJ logo)

NDC 0087-0776-41 Bottles of 100
NDC 0087-0776-43 Bottles of 1000
NDC 0087-0776-42 Cartons of 100 Unit Doses

Store at room temperature. Protect from temperatures above 104° F (40° C).

Dispense in tight, light-resistant container (USP).

References:

1. Williams JBW, Ed: Diagnostic and Statistical Manual of Mental Disorders-III, American Psychiatric Association, May, 1980.

U.S. Pat. No. 3,381,009

[*Shown in Product Identification Section*]

Continued on next page

Mead Johnson Pharm.—Cont.

DURICEF® ℞
(Cefadroxil)

Description: DURICEF® (cefadroxil) is a semisynthetic cephalosporin antibiotic intended for oral administration. It is a white to yellowish-white crystalline powder. It is soluble in water and it is acid-stable. It is chemically designated as 7-[[D-2-amino-2-(4-hydroxyphenyl) acetyl]amino]-3-methyl-8-oxo -5-thia-1-azabicyclo [4.2.0] oct-2-ene-2-carboxylic acid monohydrate.

Clinical Pharmacology—DURICEF (cefadroxil) is rapidly absorbed after oral administration. Following single doses of 500 and 1000 mg., average peak serum concentrations were approximately 16 and 28 mcg./ml., respectively. Measurable levels were present 12 hours after administration. Over 90 percent of the drug is excreted unchanged in the urine within twenty-four hours. Peak urine concentrations are approximately 1800 mcg./ml. during the period following a single 500 mg. oral dose. Increases in dosage generally produce a proportionate increase in DURICEF urinary concentration. The urine antibiotic concentration, following a 1 gm. dose, was maintained well above the MIC of susceptible urinary pathogens for 20 to 22 hours.

Microbiology: *In vitro* tests demonstrate that the cephalosporins are bactericidal because of their inhibition of cell-wall synthesis. DURICEF is active against the following organisms *in vitro:*

Beta-hemolytic streptococci
Staphylococci, including coagulase-positive, coagulase-negative, and penicillinase-producing strains
Streptococcus (Diplococcus) pneumoniae
Escherichia coli.
Proteus mirabilis
Klebsiella species

Note:—Most strains of *Enterococci (Streptococcus faecalis* and *S. faecium)* are resistant to DURICEF. It is not active against most strains of *Enterobacter species, P. morganii,* and *P. vulgaris,* It has no activity against *Pseudomonas* sp. and *Acinetobacter calcoaceticus* (formerly *Mima* and *Herellea* sp.)

Disc Susceptibility Tests.—Quantitative methods that require measurement of zone diameters give the most precise estimates of antibiotic susceptibility. One recommended procedure (CFR Section 460.1) uses cephalosporin class disc for testing susceptibility; interpretations correlate zone diameters of this disc test with MIC values for DURICEF. With this procedure, a report from the laboratory of "resistant" indicates that the infecting organism is not likely to respond to therapy. A report of "intermediate susceptibility" suggests that the organism would be susceptible if the infection is confined to the urinary tract, as DURICEF produces high antibiotic levels in the urine.

Indications: DURICEF (cefadroxil) is indicated for the treatment of the following infections when caused by susceptible strains of the designated microorganisms:

Urinary tract infections caused by *E. coli, P. mirabilis,* and *Klebsiella* species
Skin and skin structure infections caused by staphylococci and/or streptococci
Pharyngitis and tonsillitis caused by Group A beta-hemolytic streptococci (Penicillin is the usual drug of choice in the treatment and prevention of streptococcal infections, including the prophylaxis of rheumatic fever. DURICEF is generally effective in the eradication of streptococci from the nasopharynx; however substantial data establishing the efficacy of DURICEF in the subsequent prevention of rheumatic fever are not available at present.)

Note: Culture and susceptibility tests should be initiated prior to and during therapy. Renal function studies should be performed when indicated.

Contraindications: DURICEF (cefadroxil) is contraindicated in patients with known allergy to the cephalosporin group of antibiotics.

WARNING: IN PENICILLIN-ALLERGIC PATIENTS, CEPHALOSPORIN ANTIBIOTICS SHOULD BE USED WITH GREAT CAUTION. THERE IS CLINICAL AND LABORATORY EVIDENCE OF PARTIAL CROSS-ALLERGENICITY OF THE PENICILLINS AND THE CEPHALOSPORINS, AND THERE ARE INSTANCES OF PATIENTS WHO HAVE HAD REACTIONS TO BOTH DRUGS (INCLUDING FATAL ANAPHYLAXIS AFTER PARENTERAL USE).

Any patient who has demonstrated a history of some form of allergy, particularly to drugs, should receive antibiotics cautiously and then only when absolutely necessary. No exception should be made with regard to DURICEF (cefadroxil).

Pseudomembranous colitis has been reported with the use of cephalosporins (and other broad spectrum antibiotics); therefore, it is important to consider its diagnosis in patients who develop diarrhea in association with antibiotic use.

Treatment with broad spectrum antibiotics alters normal flora of the colon and may permit overgrowth of clostridia. Studies indicate a toxin produced by *Clostridium difficile* is one primary cause of antibiotic-associated colitis. Cholestyramine and colestipol resins have been shown to bind the toxin *in vitro.*

Mild cases of colitis may respond to drug discontinuance alone.

Moderate to severe cases should be managed with fluid, electrolyte and protein supplementation as indicated.

When the colitis is not relieved by drug discontinuance or when it is severe, oral vancomycin is the treatment of choice for antibiotic-associated pseudomembranous colitis produced by *C. difficile.* Other causes of colitis should also be considered.

Precautions: Patients should be followed carefully so that any side-effects or unusual manifestations of drug idiosyncrasy may be detected. If a hypersensitivity reaction occurs, the drug should be discontinued and the patient treated with the usual agents (e.g., epinephrine or other pressor amines, antihistamines, or corticosteroids).

DURICEF (cefadroxil) should be used with caution in the presence of markedly impaired renal function (creatinine clearance rate of less than 50 ml/min/1.73 M^2). (See Dosage and Administration.) In patients with known or suspected renal impairment, careful clinical observation and appropriate laboratory studies should be made prior to and during therapy.

Prolonged use of DURICEF may result in the overgrowth of nonsusceptible organisms. Careful observation of the patient is essential. If superinfection occurs during therapy, appropriate measures should be taken.

Positive direct Coombs tests have been reported during treatment with the cephalosporin antibiotics. In hematologic studies or in transfusion cross-matching procedures when antiglobulin tests are performed on the minor side or in Coombs testing of newborns whose mothers have received cephalosporin antibiotics before parturition, it should be recognized that a positive Coombs test may be due to the drug.

DURICEF should be prescribed with caution in individuals with a history of gastrointestinal disease, particularly colitis.

Usage in Pregnancy: Pregnancy Category B: Reproduction studies have been performed in mice and rats at doses up to 11 times the human dose and have revealed no evidence of impaired fertility or harm to the fetus due to cefadroxil. There are, however, no adequate and well controlled studies in pregnant women. Because animal reproduction studies are not always predictive of human response, this drug should be used during pregnancy only if clearly needed.

Nursing Mothers: Caution should be exercised when cefadroxil is administered to a nursing mother.

Adverse Reactions: Gastrointestinal—Symptoms of pseudomembranous colitis can appear during antibiotic treatment. Nausea and vomiting have been reported rarely.

Hypersensitivity—Allergies (in the form of rash, urticaria, and angioedema) have been observed. These reactions usually subsided upon discontinuation of the drug.

Other reactions have included genital pruritus, genital moniliasis, vaginitis, and moderate transient neutropenia.

Dosage and Administration: DURICEF (cefadroxil) is acid stable and may be administered orally without regard to meals. Administration with food may be helpful in diminishing potential gastrointestinal complaints occasionally associated with oral cephalosporin therapy.

Adults—

Urinary Tract Infections

For uncomplicated lower urinary tract infections (i.e. cystitis) the usual dosage is one or two grams per day in single (q.d.) or divided doses (b.i.d.).

For all other urinary tract infections the usual dosage is two grams per day in divided doses (b.i.d.).

Skin and Skin Structure Infections

For skin and skin structure infections the usual dosage is one gram per day in single (q.d.) or divided doses (b.i.d.).

Pharyngitis and Tonsillitis

Treatment of Group A beta hemolytic streptococcal pharyngitis and tonsillitis—One gram per day in divided doses (b.i.d.) for ten days.

Children—

The recommended daily dosage for children is 30 mg/kg/day in divided doses every 12 hours as indicated:

[See table left].

In the treatment of beta-hemolytic streptococcal infections, a therapeutic dosage of Duricef should be administered for at least ten days.

In patients with renal impairment, the dosage of cefadroxil should be adjusted according to creatinine clearance rates to prevent drug accumulation. The following schedule is suggested. In adults, the initial dose is 1000 mg of DURICEF (cefadroxil) and the maintenance dose (based on the creatinine clearance rate [ml/min/1.73M^2]) is 500 mg at the time intervals listed below.

Duricef Suspension

Child's Weight lbs	kg	125 mg/5 ml	250 mg/5 ml	500 mg/5 ml
10	4.5	½ tsp b.i.d.		
20	9.1	1 tsp b.i.d.	½ tsp b.i.d.	
30	13.6	1½ tsp b.i.d.	¾ tsp b.i.d.	
40	18.2	2 tsp b.i.d.	1 tsp b.i.d.	½ tsp b.i.d.
50	22.7	2½ tsp b.i.d.	1¼ tsp b.i.d.	¾ tsp b.i.d.

Creatinine Clearances	Dosage Interval
0/10 ml/min	36 hours
10–25 ml/min	24 hours
25–50 ml/min	12 hours

Patients with creatinine clearance rates over 50 ml/min may be treated as if they were patients having normal renal function.

How Supplied:

DURICEF® (cefadroxil) for Oral Suspension
125 mg/5 ml 50 ml size (NDC 0087-0786-42)
100 ml size (NDC 0087-0786-41)
250 mg/5 ml 50 ml size (NDC 0087-0782-42)
100 ml size (NDC 0087-0782-41)
500 mg/5 ml 100 ml size (NDC 0087-0783-41)
All with orange-pineapple flavor. Directions for mixing are included on the label. Shake well before using. Keep container tightly closed. After mixing, store in refrigerator. Discard unused portion after 14 days.

DURICEF (cefadroxil) capsules, 500 mg, in bottles of 24 (NDC 0087-0784-41), 100 (NDC 0087-0784-42) and in 10 strips of 10 individually labeled blisters each containing 1 capsule (NDC 0087-0784-04).

DURICEF (cefodroxil) tablets, 1 gm, in bottles of 24 (NDC 0087-0785-41), 100 (NDC 0087-0785-42) and in 10 strips of 10 individually labeled blisters each containing 1 tablet (NDC 0087-0785-04).

U.S. Patent Re. 29,164

[*Shown in Product Identification Section*]

ESTRACE® ℞
(Estradiol)

WARNING

1. ESTROGENS HAVE BEEN REPORTED TO INCREASE THE RISK OF ENDOMETRIAL CARCINOMA.

Three independent case control studies have shown an increased risk of endometrial cancer in postmenopausal women exposed to exogenous estrogens for prolonged periods. This risk was independent of the other known risk factors for endometrial cancer. These studies are further supported by the finding that incidence rates of endometrial cancer have increased sharply since 1969 in eight different areas of the United States with population based cancer reporting systems, an increase which may be related to the rapidly expanding use of estrogens during the last decade.

The three case control studies reported that the risk of endometrial cancer in estrogen users was about 4.5 to 13.9 times greater than in nonusers. The risk appears to depend on both duration of treatment and on estrogen dose. In view of these findings, when estrogens are used for the treatment of menopausal symptoms, the lowest dose that will control symptoms should be utilized and medication should be discontinued as soon as possible. When prolonged treatment is medically indicated, the patient should be reassessed on at least a semiannual basis to determine the need for continued therapy. Although the evidence must be considered preliminary, one study suggests that cyclic administration of low doses of estrogen may carry less risk than continuous administration, it therefore appears prudent to utilize such a regimen.

Close clinical surveillance of all women taking estrogens is important. In all cases of undiagnosed persistent or recurring abnormal vaginal bleeding, adequate diagnostic measures should be undertaken to rule out malignancy.

There is no evidence at present that "natural" estrogens are more or less hazardous than "synthetic" estrogens at equiestrogenic doses.

2. ESTROGENS SHOULD NOT BE USED DURING PREGNANCY.

The use of female sex hormones, both estrogens and progestogens, during early pregnancy may seriously damage the offspring. It has been shown that females exposed *in utero* to diethylstilbestrol, a non-steroidal estrogen, have an increased risk of developing in later life a form of vaginal or cervical cancer that is ordinarily extremely rare. This risk has been estimated as not greater than 4 per 1000 exposures. Furthermore, a high percentage of such exposed women (from 30 to 90 percent) have been found to have vaginal adenosis, epithelial changes of the vagina and cervix. Although these changes are histologically benign, it is not known whether they are precursors of malignancy. Although similar data are not available with the use of other estrogens, it cannot be presumed they would not induce similar changes.

Several reports suggest an association between intrauterine exposure to female sex hormones and congenital anomalies, including congenital heart defects and limb reduction defects. One case control study estimated a 4.7-fold increased risk of limb reduction defects in infants exposed *in utero* to sex hormones (oral contraceptives, hormone withdrawal tests for pregnancy, or attempted treatment for threatened abortion). Some of these exposures were very short and involved only a few days of treatment. The data suggest that the risk of limb reduction defects in exposed fetuses is somewhat less than 1 per 1000.

In the past, female sex hormones have been used during pregnancy in an attempt to treat threatened or habitual abortion. There is considerable evidence that estrogens are ineffective for these indications, and there is no evidence from well controlled studies that progestogens are effective for these uses.

If Estrace® is used during pregnancy, or if the patient becomes pregnant while taking this drug, she should be apprised of the potential risks to the fetus and the advisability of pregnancy continuation.

Description: Estrace® oral tablets contain 1 or 2 mg. of micronized estradiol. Estradiol (17β-estradiol) is a white, crystalline solid, chemically described as estra-1,3,5(10)-triene-3,17β-diol. Estrace® oral tablets provide estrogen replacement therapy.

Clinical Pharmacology

17β-Estradiol is the most potent physiologic estrogen and, in fact, is the major estrogenic hormone secreted by the human. Estradiol in Estrace® has been micronized and demonstrated to be rapidly and effectively absorbed from the gastrointestinal tract.

Indications: Estrace® is indicated in the treatment of:

1. Moderate to severe *vasomotor* symptoms associated with the menopause. (There is no evidence that estrogens are effective for nervous symptoms or depression which might occur during menopause, and they should not be used to treat these conditions.)
2. Atrophic vaginitis.
3. Kraurosis vulvae.
4. Female hypogonadism.
5. Female castration.
6. Primary ovarian failure.
7. Breast cancer (for palliation only) in appropriately selected women and men with metastatic disease.
8. Prostatic carcinoma—palliative therapy of advanced disease.

ESTRACE® HAS NOT BEEN SHOWN TO BE EFFECTIVE FOR ANY PURPOSE DURING PREGNANCY AND ITS USE MAY CAUSE SEVERE HARM TO THE FETUS (SEE BOXED WARNING).

Contraindications: Estrogens should not be used in women (or men) with any of the following conditions:

1. Known or suspected cancer of the breast except in appropriately selected patients being treated for metastatic disease.
2. Known or suspected estrogen-dependent neoplasia.
3. Known or suspected pregnancy (See Boxed Warning).
4. Undiagnosed abnormal genital bleeding.
5. Active thrombophlebitis or thromboembolic disorders.
6. A past history of thrombophlebitis, thrombosis or thromboembolic disorders associated with previous estrogen use (except when used in treatment of breast or prostatic malignancy).

Warnings:

1. **Induction of malignant neoplasms.** Long term continuous administration of natural and synthetic estrogens in certain animal species increases the frequency of carcinomas of the breast, cervix, vagina, and liver. There is now evidence that estrogens increase the risk of carcinoma of the endometrium in humans. (See Boxed Warning).

At the present time there is no satisfactory evidence that estrogens given to postmenopausal women increase the risk of cancer of the breast, although a recent long-term followup of a single physician's practice has raised this possibility. Because of the animal data there is a need for caution in prescribing estrogens for women with a strong family history of breast cancer or who have breast nodules, fibrocystic disease, or abnormal mammograms.

2. **Gall bladder disease.** A recent study has reported a 2 to 3-fold increase in the risk of surgically confirmed gall bladder disease in women receiving postmenopausal estrogens, similar to the 2-fold increase previously noted in users of oral contraceptives. In the case of oral contraceptives, the increased risk appeared after two years of use.

3. **Effects similar to those caused by estrogen-progestogen oral contraceptives.** There are several serious adverse effects of oral contraceptives, most of which have not, up to now, been documented as consequences of postmenopausal estrogen therapy. This may reflect the comparatively low doses of estrogen used in postmenopausal women. It would be expected that the larger doses of estrogen used to treat prostatic or breast cancer or postpartum breast engorgement are more likely to result in these adverse effects, and, in fact, it has been shown that there is an increased risk of thrombosis in men receiving estrogens for prostatic cancer and women for postpartum breast engorgement.

a. **Thromboembolic disease.** It is now well established that users of oral contraceptives have an increased risk of various thromboembolic and thrombotic vascular diseases, such as thrombophlebitis, pulmonary embolism, stroke, and myocardial infarction. Cases of retinal thrombosis, mesenteric thrombosis, and optic neuritis have been reported in oral contraceptive users. There is evidence that the risk of several of these adverse reactions is related to the dose of the drug. An increased risk of post-surgery thromboembolic complications has also been reported in users of oral contraceptives. If feasible, estrogen should be discontinued at least 4 weeks before surgery of the type associated with an increased risk of thromboembolism, or during periods of prolonged immobilization.

While an increased rate of thromboembolic and thrombotic disease in postmenopausal users of estrogens has not been found, this does not rule out the possibility that such an increase may be present or that subgroups of women who have underlying risk factors or

Continued on next page

Mead Johnson Pharm.—Cont.

who are receiving relatively large doses of estrogens may have increased risk. Therefore estrogens should not be used in persons with active thrombophlebitis or thromboembolic disorders, and they should not be used (except in treatment of malignancy) in persons with a history of such disorders in association with estrogen use. They should be used with caution in patients with cerebral vascular or coronary artery disease and only for those in whom estrogens are clearly needed.

Large doses of estrogen (5 mg conjugated estrogens per day), comparable to those used to treat cancer of the prostate and breast, have been shown in a large prospective clinical trial in men to increase the risk of nonfatal myocardial infarction, pulmonary embolism and thrombophlebitis. When estrogen doses of this size are used, any of the thromboembolic and thrombotic adverse effects associated with oral contraceptive use should be considered a clear risk.

b. **Hepatic adenoma.** Hepatic adenomas appear to be associated with the use of oral contraceptives. Although rare, these may rupture and may cause death through intraabdominal hemorrhage. Such lesions have not yet been reported in association with other estrogen or progestogen preparations but should be considered in estrogen users having abdominal pain and tenderness, abdominal mass, or hypovolemic shock. Hepatocellular carcinoma has also been reported in women taking estrogen-containing oral contraceptives. The relationship of this malignancy to these drugs is not known at this time.

c. **Elevated blood pressure.** Increased blood pressure is not uncommon in women using oral contraceptives. There is now a report that this may occur with use of estrogens in the menopause and blood pressure should be monitored with estrogen use, especially if high doses are used.

d. **Glucose tolerance.** A worsening of glucose tolerance has been observed in a significant percentage of patients on estrogen-containing oral contraceptives. For this reason, diabetic patients should be carefully observed while receiving estrogen.

4. **Hypercalcemia.** Administration of estrogens may lead to severe hypercalcemia in patients with breast cancer and bone metastases. If this occurs, the drug should be stopped and appropriate measures taken to reduce the serum calcium level.

Precautions:

A. General Precautions.

1. A complete medical and family history should be taken prior to the initiation of any estrogen therapy. The pretreatment and periodic physical examinations should include special reference to blood pressure, breasts, abdomen, and pelvic organs, and should include a Papanicolaou smear. As a general rule, estrogen should not be prescribed for longer than one year without another physical examination being performed.
2. Fluid retention—Because estrogens may cause some degree of fluid retention, conditions which might be influenced by this factor such as epilepsy, migraine, and cardiac or renal dysfunction, require careful observation.
3. Certain patients may develop undesirable manifestations of excessive estrogenic stimulation, such as abnormal or excessive uterine bleeding, mastodynia, etc.
4. Oral contraceptives appear to be associated with an increased incidence of mental depression. Although it is not clear whether this is due to the estrogenic or progestogenic component of the contraceptive, patients with a history of depression should be carefully observed.
5. Preexisting uterine leiomyomata may increase in size during estrogen use.
6. The pathologist should be advised of estrogen therapy when relevant specimens are submitted.
7. Patients with a past history of jaundice during pregnancy have an increased risk of recurrence of jaundice while receiving estrogen-containing oral contraceptive therapy. If jaundice develops in any patient receiving estrogen, the medication should be discontinued while the cause is investigated.
8. Estrogens may be poorly metabolized in patients with impaired liver function and they should be administered with caution in such patients.
9. Because estrogens influence the metabolism of calcium and phosphorus, they should be used with caution in patients with metabolic bone diseases that are associated with hypercalcemia or in patients with renal insufficiency.
10. Because of the effects of estrogens on epiphyseal closure, they should be used judiciously in young patients in whom bone growth is not complete.
11. Certain endocrine and liver function tests may be affected by estrogen-containing oral contraceptives. The following similar changes may be expected with larger doses of estrogen:
    a. Increased sulfobromophthalein retention.
    b. Increased prothrombin and factors VII and VIII, IX, and X; decreased antithrombin 3; increased norepinephrine-induced platelet aggregability.
    c. Increased thyroid binding globulin (TBG) leading to increased circulating total thyroid hormone, as measured by PBI, T4 by column, or T4 by radioimmunoassay. Free T3 resin uptake is decreased, reflecting the elevated TBG; free T4 concentration is unaltered.
    d. Impaired glucose tolerance.
    e. Decreased pregnanediol excretion.
    f. Reduced response to metyrapone test.
    g. Reduced serum folate concentration.
    h. Increased serum triglyceride and phospholipid concentration.

B. Information for the Patient. See text of Patient Package Insert.

C. Pregnancy Category X. See Contraindications and Boxed Warning.

D. Nursing Mothers. As a general principle, the administration of any drug to nursing mothers should be done only when clearly necessary since many drugs are excreted in human milk.

Estrace 2 mg tablets contain FD&C Yellow No. 5 (tartrazine) which may cause allergic-type reactions (including bronchial asthma) in certain susceptible individuals. Although the overall incidence of FD&C Yellow No. 5 (tartrazine) sensitivity in the general population is low, it is frequently seen in patients who also have aspirin hypersensitivity.

Adverse Reactions: (See Warnings regarding induction of neoplasia, adverse effects on the fetus, increased incidence of gall bladder disease, and adverse effects similar to those of oral contraceptives, including thromboembolism.) The following additional adverse reactions have been reported with estrogenic therapy, including oral contraceptives:

1. **Genitourinary system.**
   Breakthrough bleeding, spotting, change in menstrual flow.
   Dysmenorrhea.
   Premenstrual-like syndrome.
   Amenorrhea during and after treatment.
   Increase in size of uterine fibromyomata.
   Vaginal candidiasis.
   Change in cervical eversion and in degree of cervical secretion.
   Cystitis-like syndrome.
2. **Breast.**
   Tenderness, enlargement, secretion.
3. **Gastrointestinal.**
   Nausea, vomiting.
   Abdominal cramps, bloating.
   Cholestatic jaundice.
4. **Skin.**
   Chloasma or melasma which may persist when drug is discontinued.
   Erythema multiforme.
   Erythema nodosum.
   Hemorrhagic eruption.
   Loss of scalp hair.
   Hirsutism.
5. **Eyes.**
   Steepening of corneal curvature.
   Intolerance to contact lenses.
6. **CNS.**
   Headache, migraine, dizziness.
   Mental depression.
   Chorea.
7. **Miscellaneous.**
   Increase or decrease in weight.
   Reduced carbohydrate tolerance.
   Aggravation of porphyria.
   Edema.
   Changes in libido.

Acute Overdosage: Numerous reports of ingestion of large doses of estrogen-containing oral contraceptives by young children indicate that serious ill effects do not occur. Overdosage of estrogen may cause nausea, and withdrawal bleeding may occur in females.

Dosage and Administration:

1. **Given cyclically for short term use only:**
   For treatment of moderate to severe **vasomotor** symptoms, atrophic vaginitis, or kraurosis vulvae associated with the menopause.
   The lowest dose that will control symptoms should be chosen and medication should be discontinued as promptly as possible.
   Administration should be cyclic (e.g., 3 weeks on and 1 week off).
   Attempts to discontinue or taper medication should be made at 3 to 6 month intervals.
   The usual initial dosage range is 1 or 2 mg. daily of micronized estradiol adjusted as necessary to control presenting symptoms. The minimal effective dose for maintenance therapy should be determined by titration.
2. **Given cyclically:**
   Female hypogonadism.
   Female castration.
   Primary ovarian failure.
   Treatment is usually initiated with a dose of 1 or 2 mg. daily of micronized estradiol, adjusted as necessary to control presenting symptoms; the minimal effective dose for maintenance therapy should be determined by titration.
3. Given chronically:
   Inoperable progressing prostatic cancer—Suggested dosage is 1 to 2 mg. three times daily. The effectiveness of therapy can be judged by phosphatase determinations as well as by symptomatic improvement of the patient.

Inoperable progessing breast cancer in appropriately selected men and postmenopausal women (see INDICATIONS)—Suggested dosage is 10 mg. three times daily for a period of at least three months.

Treated patients with an intact uterus should be monitored closely for signs of endometrial cancer and appropriate diagnostic measures should be taken to rule out malignancy in the event of persistent or recurring abnormal vaginal bleeding.

How Supplied:

Estrace 1 mg; lavender scored tablets
NDC 0087-0755-01 Bottles of 100
Estrace 2 mg; turquoise scored tablets
NDC 0087-0756-01 Bottles of 100

PATIENT LABELING

What You Should Know About Estrogens:

Estrogens are female hormones produced principally by the ovaries. The ovaries make several different kinds of estrogens. In addition, scientists have been able to make a variety of synthetic estrogens. As far as we know, all these estrogens have the same properties and therefore much the same usefulness, side effects, and risks. This leaflet is intended to help you understand what estrogens are used for, the risks involved in their use, and how to use them as safely as possible.

This leaflet includes important information about Estrace® (estradiol) and estrogens in general, but not all the information. If you want to know more you can ask your doctor or pharmacist to let you read the professional package insert.

Uses of Estrogen: Estrogens are prescribed by doctors for a number of purposes, including:

1. To provide estrogen during a period of adjustment when a woman's ovaries no longer produce it, in order to prevent certain uncomfortable symptoms of estrogen deficiency. (All women normally experience a decrease in the production of estrogens, generally between 45–55; this is called the menopause.)
2. To prevent symptoms of estrogen deficiency when a woman's ovaries have been removed surgically before the natural menopause.
3. To prevent pregnancy. (Some estrogens are given along with a progestogen, another female hormone; these combinations are called oral contraceptives or birth control pills. They will not be discussed in this leaflet.) However, Estrace is not intended for this use.
4. To treat certain cancers in women and men.
5. To prevent painful swelling of the breasts after pregnancy in women who choose not to nurse their babies.

THERE IS NO PROPER USE OF ESTROGENS IN A PREGNANT WOMAN.

Estrogens in The Menopause: In the natural course of their lives, all women eventually experience a decrease in estrogen production. This usually occurs between ages 45 and 55 but may occur earlier or later. Sometimes the ovaries may need to be removed before natural menopause by an operation, producing a "surgical menopause."

When the amount of estrogen in the blood begins to decrease, many women may develop typical symptoms: feelings of warmth in the face, neck, and chest or sudden intense episodes of heat and sweating throughout the body (called "hot flashes" or "hot flushes"). These symptoms are sometimes very uncomfortable. A few women eventually develop changes in the vagina (called "atrophic vaginitis") which cause discomfort, especially during and after intercourse.

Estrogens can be prescribed to treat these symptoms of the menopause. It is estimated that considerably more than half of all women undergoing the menopause have only mild symptoms or no symptoms at all and therefore do not need estrogens. Other women may need estrogens for a few months, while their bodies adjust to lower estrogen levels. Sometimes the need will be for periods longer than six months. In an attempt to avoid over-stimulation of the uterus (womb), estrogens are usually given cyclically during each month of use, that is three weeks of pills followed by one week without pills.

Sometimes women experience nervous symptoms or depression during menopause. There is no evidence that estrogens are effective for such symptoms and they should not be used to treat them, although other treatment may be needed.

You may have heard that taking estrogens for long periods (years) after the menopause will keep your skin soft and supple and keep you feeling young. There is no evidence that this is so, however, and such long-term treatment carries additional risks.

Estrogens To Prevent Swelling of The Breasts After Pregnancy: If you do not breast feed your baby after delivery, your breasts may fill up with milk and become painful and engorged. This usually begins about three to four days after delivery and may last for a few days to up to a week or more. Sometimes the discomfort is severe, but usually it is not and can be controlled by pain-relieving drugs such as aspirin and by binding the breasts up tightly. Estrogens can sometimes be used successfully to try to prevent the breasts from filling up. While this treatment is sometimes successful, in many cases the breasts fill up to some degree in spite of treatment. The dose of estrogens needed to prevent pain and swelling of the breasts is much larger than the dose needed to treat symptoms of the menopause and this may increase your chances of developing blood clots in the legs or lungs or other parts of the body (see below, 4. Abnormal Blood Clotting). Therefore, it is important that you discuss the benefits and the risks of estrogen use with your doctor, before using estrogen, if you have decided not to breast feed your baby.

The Dangers of Estrogens:

1. **Cancer of the uterus.** If estrogens are used in the postmenopausal period for more than a year, there is an increased risk of **cancer of the endometrium** (uterine lining). Women taking estrogens have roughly 5 to 15 times as great a chance of getting this cancer as women who take no estrogens. To put this another way, while a postmenopausal woman not taking estrogens has one chance in 1,000 each year of getting cancer of the uterus, a woman taking estrogens has 5 to 15 chances in 1,000 each year. For this reason **it is important to take estrogens only when you really need them.**

   The risk of this cancer is greater the longer estrogens are used and also seems to be greater when larger doses are taken. For this reason **it is important to take the lowest dose of estrogen that will control symptoms and to take it only as long as it is needed.** If estrogens are needed for longer periods of time, your doctor will want to reevaluate your need for estrogens at least every six months.

   Women using estrogens should report any irregular vaginal bleeding to their doctors; such bleeding may be of no importance, but it can be an early warning of cancer of the uterus. If you have undiagnosed vaginal bleeding, you should not use estrogens until a diagnosis is made and you are certain there is no cancer of the uterus. If you have had your uterus completely removed (total hysterectomy), there is no danger of developing cancer of the uterus.
2. **Other possible cancers.** Estrogens can cause development of other tumors in animals, such as tumors of the breast, cervix, vagina, or liver, when given for a long time. At present there is no satisfactory evidence that women using estrogens in the menopause have an increased risk of such tumors, but there is no way yet to be sure they do not; and one study raises the possibility that use of estrogens in the menopause may increase the risk of breast cancer many years later. This is a further reason to use estrogens only when clearly needed. While you are taking estrogens, it is important that you go to your doctor at least once a year for a physical examination. Also, if members of your family have had breast cancer or if you have breast nodules or abnormal mammograms (breast x-rays), your doctor may wish to carry out more frequent examinations.
3. **Gall bladder disease.** Women who use estrogens after menopause are two or three times more likely to develop gall bladder disease needing surgery than women who do not use estrogens. Birth control pills have a similar effect.
4. **Abnormal blood clotting.** Oral contraceptives increase the risk of blood clotting in various parts of the body. This can occur in different parts of the circulatory system causing thrombophlebitis (clot in the legs or pelvis), retinal thrombosis or optic neuritis (clots affecting vision, including blindness), mesenteric thrombosis (clots in the intestinal blood vessels), stroke (clot in the brain), heart attack (clot in a vessel of the heart) or a pulmonary embolism (clot which eventually lodges in the lungs). These can be fatal.

   At this time use of estrogens in the menopause is not known to cause increased blood clotting, this has not been fully studied and there could still prove to be such a risk. It is recommended that if you have had clotting in the legs or lungs or a heart attack or stroke while you were using estrogens or birth control pills, you should not use estrogens (unless they are being used to treat cancer of the breast or prostate). If you have had a stroke or heart attack or if you have angina pectoris, estrogens should be used with great caution and only if clearly needed (for example, if you have severe symptoms of the menopause).

   The larger doses of estrogen used to prevent swelling of the breasts after pregnancy have been reported to cause abnormal blood clotting **as indicated above.**

Special Warning About Pregnancy: You should not receive estrogen if you are pregnant.

If this should occur, there is a greater than usual chance that the developing child will be born with a birth defect, although the possibility remains fairly small. A female child may have an increased risk of developing cancer of the vagina or cervix later in life (in the teens or twenties). Every possible effort should be made to avoid exposure to estrogens during pregnancy. If exposure occurs, see your doctor.

Other Effects of Estrogens: In addition to the serious known risks of estrogens described above, estrogens have the following side effects and potential risks which, if occurring, should be discussed promptly with your doctor.

1. **Nausea and vomiting.** The most common side effect of estrogen therapy is nausea. Vomiting is less common.
2. **Effects on breasts.** Estrogens may cause breast tenderness or enlargement and may cause the breasts to secrete a liquid.
3. **Effects on the uterus.** Estrogens may cause benign fibroid tumors of the uterus to get larger. Some women will have menstrual bleeding when estrogens are stopped. But if the bleeding occurs on days you are still taking estrogens, you should report this to your doctor.
4. **Effects on liver.** Women taking oral contraceptives develop on rare occasions a tumor of the liver which can rupture, bleed into the abdomen, and cause death. So far, these tumors have not been reported in women using estrogens in the menopause, but you should report any swelling or unusual pain or tenderness in the abdomen to your doctor immediately.

   Women with a past history of jaundice (yellowing of the skin and white parts of the eyes) may get jaundice again during estrogen use. If this occurs, stop taking estrogens and see your doctor.
5. **Other effects.** Estrogens may cause excess fluid to be retained in the body. This may make some conditions worse, such as epilepsy, migraine, heart disease, or kidney disease. Mental depression or high blood pressure may occur. A spotty darkening of the skin, particularly of the face, is possible and may persist.

Summary: Estrogens have important uses, and they may have serious risks as well. You must decide, with your doctor, whether the risks are acceptable to you in view of the benefits of treatment. Except where your doctor has prescribed estrogens for use in special cases of cancer of the breast or prostate, you should not

Continued on next page

Mead Johnson Pharm.—Cont.

use estrogens if you have cancer of the breast or uterus, are pregnant, have undiagnosed abnormal vaginal bleeding, clotting in the legs or lungs or have had a stroke, heart attack or angina, or clotting in the legs or lungs in the past while you were taking estrogens.

You can use estrogens as safely as possible by understanding that your doctor will require regular physical examinations while you are taking them and will try to discontinue the drug as soon as possible and use the smallest dose possible. Be alert for signs of trouble including:

1. Abnormal bleeding from the vagina.
2. Pains in the calves or chest or sudden shortness of breath, or coughing blood (indicating possible clots in the legs, heart, or lungs).
3. Severe headache, dizziness, faintness, or changes in vision (indicating possible developing clots in the brain or eye).
4. Breast lumps (you should ask your doctor how to examine your own breasts).
5. Jaundice (yellowing of the skin).
6. Mental depression.

Based on his or her assessment of your medical needs, your doctor has prescribed this drug for you. Do not give the drug to anyone else.

List of references available upon request.

[*Shown in Product Identification Section*]

KLOTRIX® ℞

(Potassium Chloride)
Slow-Release Tablets 10 mEq

Description: KLOTRIX is a film-coated (not enteric-coated) tablet containing 750 mg potassium chloride (equivalent to 10 mEq) in a wax matrix. This formulation is intended to provide a controlled release of potassium from the matrix to minimize the likelihood of producing high localized concentrations of potassium within the gastrointestinal tract.

Actions: Potassium ion is the principal intracellular cation of most body tissues. Potassium ions participate in a number of essential physiological processes, including the maintenance of intracellular tonicity, the transmission of nerve impulses, the contraction of cardiac, skeletal, and smooth muscle and the maintenance of normal renal function.

Potassium depletion may occur whenever the rate of potassium loss through renal excretion and/or loss from the gastrointestinal tract exceeds the rate of potassium intake. Such depletion usually develops slowly as a consequence of prolonged therapy with oral diuretics, primary or secondary hyperaldosteronism, diabetic ketoacidosis, severe diarrhea, or inadequate replacement of potassium in patients on prolonged parenteral nutrition.

Potassium depletion due to these causes is usually accompanied by a concomitant deficiency of chloride and is manifested by hypokalemia and metabolic alkalosis. Potassium depletion may produce weakness, fatigue, disturbances of cardiac rhythm (primarily ectopic beats), prominent U-waves in the electrocardiogram, and in advanced cases flaccid paralysis and/or impaired ability to concentrate urine.

Potassium depletion associated with metabolic alkalosis is managed by correcting the fundamental causes of the deficiency whenever possible and administering supplemental potassium chloride, in the form of high potassium food or potassium chloride solution or tablets. In rare circumstances (e.g., patients with renal tubular acidosis) potassium depletion may be associated with metabolic acidosis and hyperchloremia. In such patients potassium replacement should be accomplished with potassium salts other than the chloride, such as potassium bicarbonate, potassium citrate, or potassium acetate.

Indications: BECAUSE OF REPORTS OF INTESTINAL AND GASTRIC ULCERATION AND BLEEDING WITH SLOW RELEASE POTASSIUM CHLORIDE PREPARATIONS, THESE DRUGS SHOULD BE RESERVED FOR THOSE PATIENTS WHO CANNOT TOLERATE OR REFUSE TO TAKE LIQUID OR EFFERVESCENT POTASSIUM PREPARATIONS OR FOR PATIENTS IN WHOM THERE IS A PROBLEM OF COMPLIANCE WITH THESE PREPARATIONS.

1. For therapeutic use in patients with hypokalemia with or without metabolic alkalosis; in digitalis intoxication and in patients with hypokalemic familial periodic paralysis.
2. For prevention of potassium depletion when the dietary intake of potassium is inadequate in the following conditions: Patients receiving digitalis and diuretics for congestive heart failure; hepatic cirrhosis with ascites; states of aldosterone excess with normal renal function; potassium-losing nephropathy, and certain diarrheal states.
3. The use of potassium salts in patients receiving diuretics for uncomplicated essential hypertension is often unnecessary when such patients have a normal dietary pattern. Serum potassium should be checked periodically, however, and, if hypokalemia occurs, dietary supplementation with potassium-containing foods may be adequate to control milder cases. In more severe cases supplementation with potassium salts may be indicated.

Contraindications: Potassium supplements are contraindicated in patients with hyperkalemia since a further increase in serum potassium concentration in such patients can produce cardiac arrest. Hyperkalemia may complicate any of the following conditions: chronic renal failure, systemic acidosis such as diabetic acidosis, acute dehydration, extensive tissue breakdown as in severe burns, adrenal insufficiency, or the administration of a potassium-sparing diuretic (e.g., spironolactone, triamterene).

Wax-matrix potassium chloride preparations have produced esophageal ulceration in certain cardiac patients with esophageal compression due to an enlarged left atrium.

All solid forms of potassium supplements are contraindicated in any patient in whom there is cause for arrest or delay in tablet passage through the gastrointestinal tract. In these instances, potassium supplementation should be with a liquid preparation.

Warnings:

Hyperkalemia

In patients with impaired mechanisms for excreting potassium, the administration of potassium salts can produce hyperkalemia and cardiac arrest. This occurs most commonly in patients given potassium by the intravenous route but may also occur in patients given potassium orally. Potentially fatal hyperkalemia can develop rapidly and be asymptomatic.

The use of potassium salts in patients with chronic renal disease, or any other condition which impairs potassium excretion, requires particularly careful monitoring of the serum potassium concentration and appropriate dosage adjustment.

Interaction with Potassium-Sparing Diuretics

Hypokalemia should not be treated by the concomitant administration of potassium salts and a potassium-sparing diuretic (e.g., spironolactone or triamterene), since the simultaneous administration of these agents can produce severe hyperkalemia.

Gastrointestinal lesions

Potassium chloride tablets have produced stenotic and/or ulcerative lesions of the small bowel and deaths. These lesions are caused by a high localized concentration of potassium ion in the region of a rapidly dissolving tablet, which injures the bowel wall and thereby produces obstruction, hemorrhage, or perforation. Klotrix is a wax-matrix tablet formulated to provide a controlled rate of release of potassium chloride and thus to minimize the possibility of a high local concentration of potassium ion near the bowel wall. While the reported frequency of small-bowel lesions is much less with wax-matrix tablets (less than one per 100,000 patient-years) than with enteric-coated potassium chloride tablets (40–50 per 100,000 patient-years) cases associated with wax-matrix tablets have been reported both in foreign countries and in the United States. In addition, perhaps because the wax-matrix preparations are not enteric-coated and release potassium in the stomach, there have been reports of upper gastrointestinal bleeding associated with these products. The total number of gastrointestinal lesions remains less than one per 100,000 patient-years. Klotrix should be discontinued immediately and the possibility of bowel obstruction or perforation considered if severe vomiting, abdominal pain, distention, or gastrointestinal bleeding occurs.

Metabolic acidosis

Hypokalemia in patients with metabolic acidosis should be treated with an alkalinizing potassium salt such as potassium bicarbonate, potassium citrate, or potassium acetate.

Precautions: The diagnosis of potassium depletion is ordinarily made by demonstrating hypokalemia in a patient with a clinical history suggesting some cause for potassium depletion. In interpreting the serum potassium level, the physician should bear in mind that acute alkalosis *per se* can produce hypokalemia in the absence of a deficit in total body potassium, while acute acidosis *per se* can increase the serum potassium concentration into the normal range even in the presence of a reduced total body potassium. The treatment of potassium depletion, particularly in the presence of cardiac disease, renal disease, or acidosis, requires careful attention to acid-base balance and appropriate monitoring of serum electrolytes, the electrocardiogram, and the clinical status of the patient.

Adverse Reactions: The most common adverse reactions to oral potassium salts are nausea, vomiting, abdominal discomfort, and diarrhea. These symptoms are due to irritation of the gastrointestinal tract and are best managed by diluting the preparation further, taking the dose with meals, or reducing the dose. One of the most severe adverse effects is hyperkalemia (see Contraindications, Warnings and Overdosage). There also have been reports of upper and lower gastrointestinal conditions including obstruction, bleeding, ulceration and perforation (see Contraindications and Warnings); other factors known to be associated with such conditions were present in many of these patients. Skin rash has been reported rarely.

Overdosage: The administration of oral potassium salts to persons with normal excretory mechanisms for potassium rarely causes serious hyperkalemia. However, if excretory mechanisms are impaired or if potassium is administered too rapidly intravenously, potentially fatal hyperkalemia can result (see Contraindications and Warnings). It is important to recognize that hyperkalemia is usually asymptomatic and may be manifested only by an increased serum potassium concentration and characteristic electrocardiographic changes (peaking of T-waves, loss of P-wave, depression of S-T segment, and prolongation of the QT interval). Late manifestations include muscle paralysis and cardiovascular collapse from cardiac arrest. Treatment measures for hyperkalemia include the following: (1) elimination of foods and medications containing potassium and of potassium-sparing diuretics: (2) intravenous administration of 300 to 500 ml/hr of 10% dextrose solution containing 10–20 units of insulin per 1,000 ml; (3) correction of acidosis, if present, with intravenous sodium bicarbonate; (4) use of exchange resins, hemodialysis, or peritoneal dialysis.

In treating hyperkalemia, it should be recalled that in patients who have been stabilized on digitalis, too rapid a lowering of the serum potassium concentration can produce digitalis toxicity.

Dosage and Administration: The usual dietary intake of potassium by the average adult is 40 to 80 mEq per day. Potassium depletion sufficient to cause hypokalemia usually requires the loss of 200 or more mEq of potassium from the total body store. Dosage must be adjusted to the individual needs of each patient but is typically in the range of 20 mEq per day for the prevention of hypokalemia to 40–100 mEq per day or more for the treatment of potassium depletion.

Note: Klotrix slow-release tablets must be swallowed whole and never crushed or chewed. Following release of the potassium chloride, the expended wax matrix, which is not absorbed, may be observed in the stool.

How Supplied: Tablets (light orange, film-coated) each containing 750 mg potassium chloride (equivalent to 10 mEq each of potassium and chloride).

NDC 0087-0770-41	Bottles of 100
NDC 0087-0770-42	Bottles of 1000
NDC 0087-0770-43	Unit Dose Cartons of 100
VA6505-01-099-0243A	(100's)
VA6505-01-103-0211B	(1000's)

U.S. Pat. No. 4,140,756

[*Shown in Product Identification Section*]

K–LYTE® ℞

Effervescent Tablets

Each tablet in solution supplies 25 mEq potassium as bicarbonate and citrate

K–LYTE®DS ℞

Effervescent Tablets

Each tablet in solution supplies 50 mEq potassium as bicarbonate and citrate

K–LYTE/CL® ℞

Effervescent Tablets and Powder

Each tablet in solution and each dose of powder in solution supply 25 mEq potassium and chloride

K–LYTE/CL® 50 ℞

Effervescent Tablets

Each tablet in solution provides 50 mEq potassium and chloride

Description:

[See table above].

	K-LYTE*	K-LYTE DS*	K-LYTE/CL*	K-LYTE/CL POWDER*†	K-LYTE/CL 50*
Potassium Chloride	—	—	1.5 gm	1.86 gm	2.24 gm
Potassium Bicarbonate	2.5 gm	2.5 gm	0.5 gm	—	2 gm
Potassium Citrate	—	2.7 gm	—	—	—
L-lysine Monohydrochloride	—	—	0.91 gm	—	3.65 gm
Citric Acid	2.1 gm	2.1 gm	0.55 gm	—	1 gm

* Also includes saccharin, natural and artificial flavor and color

† Also includes adipic acid

Clinical Pharmacology: Potassium ion is the principal intracellular cation of most body tissues and participates in a number of essential physiological processes. These include numerous enzymatic reactions in intermediary metabolism, the maintenance of intracellular tonicity, the transmission of nerve impulses, and the function of cardiac, skeletal, and smooth muscle. Disturbances in potassium metabolism may, therefore, elicit a broad range of clinical disorders. The normal serum potassium level is maintained principally by close renal regulation of potassium balance.

Potassium depletion may occur whenever potassium loss through renal excretion and/or loss from the gastrointestinal tract exceeds the potassium intake. Such depletion usually develops slowly as a consequence of prolonged therapy with oral diuretics, primary, or secondary, hyperaldosteronism, diabetic ketoacidosis, severe vomiting and diarrhea, or inadequate replacement of potassium in patients on prolonged parenteral nutrition. Potassium depletion may be accompanied by hypokalemia as well as hypochloremia and metabolic alkalosis.

Potassium deficiency may be manifested by generalized weakness, drowsiness, anorexia, and nausea; oliguria, edema, and chronic ileus with distention; shallow and infrequent respirations; low blood pressure, altered cardiac rhythms, and systolic murmurs; hypokalemia and such ECG changes as prominent U wave, lengthening of the Q-T interval, depression of the S-T segment, and depression or inversion of the T wave.

Indications and Usage: All K-LYTE® products are used for therapy or prophylaxis of potassium deficiency. They are useful when thiazide diuretics, corticosteroids, or vomiting and diarrhea cause excessive potassium loss; and when dietary potassium is low. These products may also be useful when potassium therapy is indicated in digitalis intoxication. K-LYTE/Cl and K-LYTE/Cl 50 are recommended in the management of hypokalemia accompanied by metabolic alkalosis and hypochloremia, e.g. as induced by vomiting.

Contraindications: Potassium supplements are contraindicated in patients with hyperkalemia since a further increase in serum potassium concentration in such patients can produce cardiac arrest. Hyperkalemia may complicate any of the following conditions; chronic renal impairment, metabolic acidosis such as diabetic acidosis, acute dehydration, extensive tissue breakdown as in severe burns or adrenal insufficiency. Hypokalemia should not be treated by the concomitant administration of potassium salts and a potassium-sparing diuretic (e.g.,spironolactone or triamterene), since the simultaneous administration of these agents can produce severe hyperkalemia.

Warnings: In patients with impaired mechanisms for excreting potassium, the administration of potassium salts can produce hyperkalemia and cardiac arrest. This occurs most commonly in patients given potassium by the intravenous route but may also occur in patients given potassium orally. Potentially fatal hyperkalemia can develop rapidly and may be asymptomatic. The use of potassium salts in patients with chronic renal disease, or any other condition which impairs potassium excretion, requires particularly careful monitoring of the serum potassium concentration and appropriate dosage adjustment.

Precautions: General precautions—The diagnosis of potassium depletion is ordinarily made by demonstrating hypokalemia in a patient with a clinical history suggesting some cause for potassium depletion. When interpreting the serum potassium level, the physician should bear in mind that acute alkalosis *per se* can produce hypokalemia in the absence of a deficit in total body potassium, while acute acidosis *per se* can increase the serum potassium concentration into the normal range even in the presence of a reduced total body potassium. Therefore, the treatment of potassium depletion requires careful attention to acid-base balance and appropriate monitoring of serum electrolytes, the ECG, and the clinical status of the patient.

Information for patients—To minimize the possibility of gastrointestinal irritation associated with the oral ingestion of concentrated potassium salt preparations, patients should be carefully directed to dissolve each dose completely in the stated amount of water.

Laboratory tests—Frequent clinical evaluation of the patient should include ECG and serum potassium determinations.

Drug interactions—The simultaneous administration of potassium supplements and a potassium-sparing diuretic can produce severe hyperkalemia (see Contraindications). Potassium supplements should be used cautiously in patients who are using salt substitutes because most of the latter contain substantial amounts of potassium. Such concomitant use could result in hyperkalemia.

Usage in Pregnancy—Pregnancy Category C —Animal reproduction studies have not been conducted with any of the K-LYTE products. It is also not known whether these products can cause fetal harm when administered to a pregnant woman or can affect reproduction capacity. They should be given to a pregnant woman only if clearly needed.

Nursing Mothers—Many drugs are excreted in human milk and because of the potential for serious adverse reactions in nursing infants from oral potassium supplements, a decision should be made whether to discontinue nursing or discontinue the drug, taking into account the importance of the drug to the mother.

Usage in Children—Safety and effectiveness in children have not been established.

Adverse Reactions: The most common adverse reactions to oral potassium supplements are nausea, vomiting, diarrhea and abdominal discomfort. These side effects occur more frequently when the medication is not taken with food or is not diluted properly or dissolved completely.

Hyperkalemia occurs only rarely in patients with normal renal function receiving potassium supplements orally. Signs and symptoms of hyperkalemia are cardiac arrhythmias, mental confusion, unexplained anxiety, numbness or tingling in hands, feet or lips, shortness of breath or difficult breathing, unusual tiredness or weakness and weakness or heaviness of legs (see Contraindications, Warnings and Overdosage).

Overdosage: The administration of oral potassium salts to persons with normal renal function rarely causes serious hyperkalemia. However, in patients with chronic renal disease, or any other condition which impairs potassium excretion or if potassium is administered too rapidly intravenously, potentially fatal hyperkalemia can result (see Contraindications and Warnings). The earliest clinical

Continued on next page

Mead Johnson Pharm.—Cont.

manifestations of this condition may be only increased serum potassium levels and characteristic ECG changes such as peaking of T-waves, loss of P-wave, depression of S-T segment and prolongation of the QT interval. These changes in the ECG usually appear when serum potassium concentration reaches 7 to 8 mEq per liter. Other clinical manifestations occurring at a concentration of 9 to 10 mEq per liter may include muscle paralysis and death from cardiac arrest.

The treatment of severe hyperkalemia should focus on reducing the serum potassium concentration by promoting the transfer of potassium from the extracellular to the intracellular space. The measures taken may include the following: a) intravenous administration of 1 liter of a 10 percent glucose solution containing 30-40 units of insulin; b) in the acidotic patient, intravenous administration of 150 mEq to 300 mEq of sodium bicarbonate. Other measures should incude the elimination of potassium-containing medications and potassium-sparing diuretics and frequently the oral administration of a cation exchange resin (such as sodium polystyrene sulfonate) to remove gastrointestinal potassium. To assure rapid movement of the resin through the gastrointestinal tract, a nonabsorbable polyhydric alcohol (e.g., sorbitol) should be given in quantities sufficient to induce a soft to semiliquid bowel movement every few hours.

Hemodialysis is an effective alternative means of removing excess potassium.

Dosage and Administration: Adults—One (1) K-LYTE/Cl 50 tablet (50 mEq potassium and chloride) or K-LYTE DS tablet (50 mEq potassium) completely dissolved in 6 to 8 ounces of cold or ice water; 1 to 2 times daily, depending on the requirements of the patient. One (1) K-LYTE/Cl tablet (25 mEq potassium and chloride) or one (1) K-LYTE tablet (25 mEq potassium) completely dissolved in 3 to 4 ounces of cold or ice water, 2 to 4 times daily, depending on the requirements of the patient. One dose (using measured scoop provided) (25 mEq potassium chloride) of K-LYTE/Cl powder completely dissolved in 6 ounces of cold or ice water, 2 to 4 times daily, depending on the requirements of the patient.

Note: It is suggested that all K-LYTE products be taken with meals and sipped slowly over a 5 to 10 minute period.

How Supplied:

K-LYTE® Effervescent Tablets, Each tablet in solution provides 25 mEq of potassium.

NDC 0087-0760-01 Lime-flavored, Boxes of 30

NDC 0087-0760-43 Lime-flavored, Boxes of 100

NDC 0087-0760-02 Lime-flavored, Boxes of 250

NDC 0087-0761-01 Orange-flavored, Boxes of 30

NDC 0087-0761-43 Orange-flavored, Boxes of 100

NDC 0087-0761-02 Orange-flavored, Boxes of 250

VA 6505-00-934-3477A (Box of 30) Lime
VA 6505-00-153-6904A (Box of 30) Orange
6505-00-934-3477 (Box of 30) Defense

K-LYTE® DS Effervescent Tablets. Each tablet provides 50 mEq potassium.

NDC 0087-0772-41 Lime-flavored, Boxes of 30

NDC 0087-0772-42 Lime-flavored, Boxes of 100

NDC 0087-0771-41 Orange-flavored, Boxes of 30

NDC 0087-0771-42 Orange-flavored, Boxes of 100

K-LYTE/CL® Effervecent Tablets. Each tablet in solution provides 25 mEq potassium and chloride.

NDC 0087-0766-41 Citrus-flavored, Boxes of 30

NDC 0087-0766-43 Citrus-flavored, Boxes of 100

NDC 0087-0766-42 Citrus-flavored, Boxes of 250

NDC 0087-0767-41 Fruit Punch-flavored, Boxes of 30

NDC 0087-0767-43 Fruit Punch-flavored, Boxes of 100

NDC 0087-0767-42 Fruit Punch-flavored, Boxes of 250

K-LYTE/CL® Powder. Each dose in solution provides 25 mEq potassium and chloride.

NDC 0087-0763-01 Fruit Punch-flavored, 225 g can (30 measured doses with scoop)

K-LYTE/CL® 50 mEq Effervescent Tablets. Each tablet in solution provides 50 mEq potassium and chloride.

NDC 0087-0757-41 Fruit Punch-flavored, Boxes of 30

NDC 0087-0757-42 Fruit Punch-flavored, Boxes of 100

NDC 0087-0758-41 Citrus-flavored, Boxes of 30

NDC 0087-0758-42 Citrus-flavored, Boxes of 100

[*Shown in Product Identification Section*]

MEGACE® tablets ℞
(megestrol acetate)
U.S. Patent No. 3,356,573

Description: Megestrol acetate is a white, crystalline solid chemically described as 17α-acetoxy-6-methylpregna-4, 6-diene-3, 20-dione. Its molecular weight is 384.5. The empirical formula is $C_{24}H_{32}O_4$.

Actions: While the precise mechanism by which Megace (megestrol acetate) produces its antineoplastic effects against endometrial carcinoma is unknown at the present time, an antiluteinizing effect mediated via the pituitary has been postulated. There is also evidence to suggest a local effect as a result of the marked changes brought about by the direct instillation of progestational agents into the endometrial cavity. Likewise, the antineoplastic action of Megace (megestrol acetate) on carcinoma of the breast is unclear.

Indications: Megace (megestrol acetate) is indicated for the palliative treatment of advanced carcinoma of the breast or endometrium (i.e., recurrent, inoperable, or metastatic disease). It should not be used in lieu of currently accepted procedures such as surgery, radiation, etc.

Contraindications: As a diagnostic test for pregnancy.

Warnings

THE USE OF PROGESTATIONAL AGENTS DURING THE FIRST FOUR MONTHS OF PREGNANCY IS NOT RECOMMENDED

Progestational agents have been used beginning with the first trimester of pregnancy in an attempt to prevent habitual abortion or treat threatened abortion. There is no adequate evidence that such use is effective and there is evidence of potential harm to the fetus when such drugs are given during the first four months of pregnancy.

Furthermore, in the vast majority of women, the cause of abortion is a defective ovum, which progestational agents could not be expected to influence. In addition, the use of progestational agents, with their uterine-relaxant properties, in patients with fertilized defective ova may cause a delay in spontaneous abortion. Therefore, the use of such drugs during the first four months of pregnancy is not recommended.

Several reports suggest an association between intrauterine exposure to female sex hormones and congenital anomalies, including congenital heart defects and limb reduction defects.[1–5] One study[4] estimated a 4.7-fold increased risk of limb reduction defects in infants exposed *in utero* to sex hormones (oral contraceptives, hormone withdrawal tests for pregnancy, or attempted treatment for threatened abortion).

Some of these exposures were very short and involved only a few days of treatment. The data suggest that the risk of limb reduction defects in exposed fetuses is somewhat less than 1 to 1,000.

If the patient is exposed to Megace during the first four months of pregnancy or if she becomes pregnant while taking this drug, she should be apprised of the potential risks to the fetus.

Administration for up to 7 years of megestrol acetate to female dogs is associated with an increased incidence of both benign and malignant tumors of the breast. Comparable studies in rats and ongoing studies in monkeys are not associated with an increased incidence of tumors. The relationship of the dog tumors to humans is unknown but should be considered in assessing the benefit-to-risk ratio when prescribing Megace and in surveillance of patients on therapy.

The use of Megace (megestrol acetate) in other types of neoplastic disease is not recommended.

Precautions: There are no specific precautions identified for the use of Megace (megestrol acetate) when used as recommended. Close, customary surveillance is indicated for any patient being treated for recurrent or metastatic cancer. Use with caution in patients with a history of thrombophlebitis.

This product contains FD&C Yellow No. 5 (tartrazine) which may cause allergic-type reactions (including bronchial asthma) in certain susceptible individuals. Although the overall incidence of FD&C Yellow No. 5 (tartrazine) sensitivity in the general population is low, it is frequently seen in patients who also have aspirin hypersensitivity.

Adverse Reactions: Untoward reactions that have been reported to occur in patients receiving Megace (megestrol acetate) include carpal tunnel syndrome, deep vein thrombophlebitis and alopecia. The relationship of these reactions to Megace therapy is not known at this time.

Overdosage: No serious side effects have resulted from studies involving Megace (megestrol acetate) administered in dosages as high as 800 mg/day.

Dosage and Administration:

Breast cancer: 160 mg/day (40 q.i.d.)
Endometrial carcinoma: 40—320 mg/day in divided doses.

At least two months of continuous treatment is considered an adequate period for determining the efficacy of Megace (megestrol acetate).

How Supplied: Megace® is available as light blue, scored tablets containing 20 mg or 40 mg megestrol acetate in bottles of 100 tablets each.

NDC 0087-0595-01, Bottles of 100 20 mg tablet
NDC 0087-0596-41, Bottles of 100 40 mg tablet
NDC 0087-0596-44, Bottles of 500 40 mg tablet
6505-01-070-1493 (Bottles of 100) (Defense)

References:

1. Gal I, Kirman B and Stern J: "Hormonal Pregnancy Tests and Congenital Malformation," Nature 216:83, 1967.
2. Levy EP, Cohen A and Fraser FC: "Hormone Treatment During Pregnancy and Congenital Heart Defects," Lancet 1:611, 1973.
3. Nora J and Nora A: "Birth Defects and Oral Contraceptives," Lancet 1:941, 1973.
4. Janerich DT, Piper JM and Glebatis DM: "Oral Contraceptives and Congenital Limb-Reduction Defects," N Eng J Med, 291:697, 1974.

5. Heinonen OP, Slone D, Monson RR, Hook EB and Shapiro S: "Cardiovascular Birth Defects and Antenatal Exposure to Female Sex Hormones," N Eng J Med, 296:67, 1977.

[*Shown in Product Identification Section*]

MUCOMYST® ℞

(Acetylcysteine)
U.S. Patent No. 3,091,569

Description: Mucomyst® is a solution of the sodium salt of acetylcysteine, and is used as a mucolytic agent. Acetylcysteine is the N-acetyl derivative of the naturally occurring amino acid, cysteine. The compound is a white crystalline powder with the molecular formula $C_5H_9NO_3S$, a molecular weight of 163.2, and chemical name of N-acetyl-L-cysteine.

Clinical Pharmacology: The viscosity of pulmonary mucous secretions depends on the concentrations of mucoprotein and to a lesser extent deoxyribonucleic acid (DNA). The latter increases with increasing purulence owing to the presence of cellular debris. The mucolytic action of acetylcysteine is related to the sulfhydryl group in the molecule. This group probably "opens" disulfide linkages in mucus thereby lowering the viscosity. The mucolytic activity of acetylcysteine is unaltered by the presence of DNA, and increases with increasing pH. Significant mucolysis occurs between pH 7 and 9.

Acetylcysteine undergoes rapid deacetylation *in vivo* to yield cysteine or oxidation to yield diacetylcystine.

Occasionally, patients exposed to the inhalation of an acetylcysteine aerosol respond with the development of increased airways obstruction of varying and unpredictable severity. Those patients who are reactors cannot be identified *a priori* from a random patient population. Even when patients are known to have reacted previously to the inhalation of an acetylcysteine aerosol, they may not react during a subsequent treatment. The converse is also true; patients who have had inhalation treatments of acetylcysteine without incident may still react to a subsequent inhalation with increased airways obstruction. Most patients with bronchospasm are quickly relieved by the use of a bronchodilator given by nebulization. If bronchospasm progresses, the medication should be discontinued immediately.

Indications and Usage: Mucomyst is indicated as adjuvant therapy for patients with abnormal, viscid, or inspissated mucous secretions in such conditions as:

- Chronic bronchopulmonary disease (chronic emphysema, emphysema with bronchitis, chronic asthmatic bronchitis, tuberculosis, bronchiectasis and primary amyloidosis of the lung)
- Acute bronchopulmonary disease (pneumonia, bronchitis, tracheobronchitis)
- Pulmonary complications of cystic fibrosis
- Tracheostomy care
- Pulmonary complications associated with surgery
- Use during anesthesia
- Post-traumatic chest conditions
- Atelectasis due to mucous obstruction
- Diagnostic bronchial studies (bronchograms, bronchospirometry, and bronchial wedge catheterization)

Contraindications: Mucomyst is contraindicated in those patients who are sensitive to it.

Warnings: After proper administration of Mucomyst, an increased volume of liquefied bronchial secretions may occur. When cough is inadequate, the airway must be maintained open by mechanical suction if necessary. When there is a mechanical block due to foreign body or local accumulation, the airway should be cleared by endotracheal aspiration, with or without bronchoscopy. Asthmatics under treatment with Mucomyst should be watched carefully. Most patients with bronchospasm are quickly relieved by the use of a bronchodilator given by nebulization. If bronchospasm progresses, the medication should be discontinued immediately.

Precautions: With the administration of Mucomyst, the patient may observe initially a slight disagreeable odor that is soon not noticeable. With a face mask there may be stickiness on the face after nebulization. This is easily removed by washing with water.

Under certain conditions, a color change may occur in Mucomyst in the opened bottle. The light purple color is the result of a chemical reaction which does not significantly affect safety or mucolytic effectiveness of Mucomyst. Continued nebulization of Mucomyst solution with a dry gas will result in an increased concentration of the drug in the nebulizer because of evaporation of the solvent. Extreme concentration may impede nebulization and efficient delivery of the drug. Dilution of the nebulizing solution with appropriate amounts of Sterile Water for Injection, USP, as concentration occurs, will obviate this problem.

Usage in Pregnancy: Pregnancy Category B. Reproduction studies have been performed in rats and rabbits at doses up to 17 times the human dose and have revealed no evidence of impaired fertility or harm to the fetus due to acetylcysteine. There are, however, no adequate and well-controlled studies in pregnant women. Because animal reproduction studies may not always be predictive of human responses, this drug should be used during pregnancy only if clearly needed.

Nursing Mothers

It is not known whether this drug is excreted in human milk. Because many drugs are excreted in human milk, caution should be exercised when Mucomyst is administered to a nursing woman.

Adverse Reactions: Adverse effects have included stomatitis, nausea, vomiting, fever, rhinorrhea, drowsiness, clamminess, chest tightness, and bronchoconstriction. Clinically overt acetylcysteine induced bronchospasm occurs infrequently and unpredictably even in patients with asthmatic bronchitis or bronchitis complicating bronchial asthma. Acquired sensitization to acetylcysteine has been reported rarely. Reports of sensitization in patients have not been confirmed by patch testing. Sensitization has been confirmed in several inhalation therapists who reported a history of dermal eruptions after frequent and extended exposure to acetylcysteine. Reports of irritation to the tracheal and bronchial tracts have been received and although hemoptysis has occurred in patients receiving acetylcysteine such findings are not uncommon in patients with bronchopulmonary disease and a causal relationship has not been established.

Dosage and Administration: Adults and Children: Mucomyst is available in plastic stoppered glass vials containing 4, 10, or 30 ml. The 20% solution may be diluted to a lesser concentration with either Sodium Chloride for Injection, USP, Sodium Chloride for Inhalation, USP, Sterile Water for Injection, USP, or Sterile Water for Inhalation, USP. The 10% solution may be used undiluted.

Nebulization—face mask, mouth piece, tracheostomy:

When nebulized into a face mask, mouth piece, or tracheostomy, 1 to 10 ml of the 20% solution or 2 to 20 ml of the 10% solution may be given every 2 to 6 hours; the recommended dose for most patients is 3 to 5 ml of the 20% solution or 6 to 10 ml of the 10% solution 3 to 4 times a day.

Nebulization—tent, Croupette:

In special circumstances it may be necessary to nebulize into a tent or Croupette, and this method of use must be individualized to take into account the available equipment and the patient's particular needs. This form of administration requires very large volumes of the solution, occasionally as much as 300 ml during a single treatment period. If a tent or Croupette must be used, the recommended dose is the volume of Mucomyst (using 10% or 20%) that will maintain a very heavy mist in the tent or Croupette for the desired period. Administration for intermittent or continuous prolonged periods, including overnight, may be desirable.

Direct Instillation:

When used by direct instillation, 1 to 2 ml of a 10 to 20% solution may be given as often as every hour.

When used for the routine nursing care of patients with tracheostomy, 1 to 2 ml of a 10 to 20% solution may be given every 1 to 4 hours by instillation into the tracheostomy.

Mucomyst may be introduced directly into a particular segment of the bronchopulmonary tree by inserting (under local anesthesia and direct vision) a small plastic catheter into the trachea. Two to 5 ml of the 20% solution may then be instilled by means of a syringe connected to the catheter.

Mucomyst may also be given through a percutaneous intratracheal catheter. One to 2 ml of the 20% or 2 to 4 ml of the 10% solution every 1 to 4 hours may then be given by a syringe attached to the catheter.

Diagnostic Bronchograms:

For diagnostic bronchial studies, 2 or 3 administrations of 1 to 2 ml of the 20% solution or 2 to 4 ml of the 10% solution should be given by nebulization or by instillation intratracheally, prior to the procedure.

Administration of Aerosol:

Materials:

Mucomyst may be administered using conventional nebulizers made of plastic or glass. Certain materials used in nebulization equipment react with acetylcysteine. The most reactive of these are certain metals (notably iron and copper) and rubber. Where materials may come into contact with Mucomyst solution, parts made of the following acceptable materials should be used: glass, plastic, aluminum, anodized aluminum, chromed metal, tantalum, sterling silver, or stainless steel. Silver may become tarnished after exposure, but this is not harmful to the drug action or the patient.

Nebulizing Gases:

Compressed tank gas (air) or an air compressor should be used to provide pressure for nebulizing the solution. Oxygen may also be used but should be used with the usual precautions in patients with severe respiratory disease and CO_2 retention.

Apparatus

Mucomyst is usually administered as a fine nebula and the nebulizer used should be capable of providing optimal quantities of a suitable range of particle sizes.

Commercially available nebulizers will produce nebulae of Mucomyst satisfactory for retention in the respiratory tract. Most of the nebulizers tested will supply a high proportion of the drug solution as particles of less than 10 micrometers in diameter. Mitchell[a] has shown that particles less than 10 micrometers should be retained in the respiratory tract satisfactorily.

---

[a]Amer. Rev. Resp. Dis. 82:627–639, 1960.

Units that nebulized this solution with satisfactory efficiency were the Maxi-Myst® Nebulizer (Mead Johnson Pharmaceutical Division, Evansville, Indiana), Hand-E-Vent intermittent positive pressure breathing device (Ohio Medical Products, 3030 Airco Drive, Madison, Wisconsin), and various other intermittent positive pressure breathing devices, No. 40 De Vilbiss (The De Vilbiss Co., Somerset, Pennsylvania), Bennett Twin-Jet Nebulizer (Puritan Bennett Corp. Oak at 13th St., Kansas City, Missouri).

Continued on next page

Mead Johnson Pharm.—Cont.

The nebulized solution may be inhaled directly from the nebulizer. Nebulizers may also be attached to plastic face masks or plastic mouthpieces. Suitable nebulizers may also be fitted for use with the various intermittent positive pressure breathing (IPPB) machines. The nebulizing equipment should be cleaned immediately after use because the residues may clog the smaller orifices or corrode metal parts.

Hand bulbs are not recommended for routine use for nebulizing Mucomyst because their output is generally too small. Also, some hand-operated nebulizers deliver particles that are larger than optimum for inhalation therapy.

Mucomyst should not be placed directly into the chamber of a heated (hot pot) nebulizer. A heated nebulizer may be part of the nebulization assembly to provide a warm saturated atmosphere if the Mucomyst aerosol is introduced by means of a separate unheated nebulizer. Usual precautions for administration of warm saturated nebulae should be observed.

The nebulized solution may be breathed directly from the nebulizer. Nebulizers may also be attached to plastic face masks, plastic face tents, plastic mouth pieces, conventional plastic oxygen tents, or head tents. Suitable nebulizers may also be fitted for use with the various intermittent positive pressure breathing (IPPB) machines.

The nebulizing equipment should be cleaned immediately after use, otherwise the residues may occlude the fine orifices or corrode metal parts.

Prolonged Nebulization:
When three-fourths of the initial volume of Mucomyst solution have been nebulized, a quantity of Sterile Water for Injection, USP (approximately equal to the volume of solution remaining) should be added to the nebulizer. This obviates any concentration of the agent in the residual solvent remaining after prolonged nebulization.

Storage of Opened Vials: Mucomyst does not contain an antimicrobial agent and care must be taken to minimize contamination of the sterile solution. If only a portion of the solution in a vial is used, store the remainder in a refrigerator and use within 96 hours.

Storage of Unopened Vials: Store unopened vials at controlled room temperature, 59° to 86°F (15° to 30°C).

How Supplied:

Mucomyst®20% acetylcysteine solution (200 mg Acetylcysteine per ml). Sterile, Not for injection

NDC 0087-0570-03	Cartons of three 10 ml vials, 1 plastic dropper
VA 6505-00-767-9111A	
6505-00-767-9111	Defense
NDC 0087-0570-09	Cartons of three 30 ml vials
VA 6505-00-782-2688A	
6505-00-782-2688	Defense
NDC 0087-0570-07	Cartons of twelve 4 ml vials

Mucomyst®-10, 10% acetylcysteine solution. (100 mg Acetylcysteine per ml). Sterile, Not for injection

NDC 0087-0572-01	Cartons of three 10 ml vials, 1 plastic dropper
NDC 0087-0572-02	Cartons of three 30 ml vials
NDC 0087-0572-03	Cartons of twelve 4 ml vials

MUCOMYST® WITH ISOPROTERENOL ℞
(10% acetylcysteine— 0.05% isoproterenol HCl solution)

Description: Mucomyst with Isoproterenol (10% acetylcysteine-0.05% isoproterenol·HCl) is a ready-to-use sterile aqueous solution of a mucolytic agent and a bronchodilator available as a convenience to physicians who wish to prescribe these agents concomitantly for use by nebulization into a face mask or mouthpiece.

Acetylcysteine, USP, is the N-acetyl derivative of the naturally occurring amino acid, L-cysteine. Acetylcysteine is a white crystalline powder, with the molecular formula $C_5H_9NO_3S$, a molecular weight of 163.2, and chemical name of N-acetyl-L-cysteine.

Isoproterenol hydrochloride, USP, is the nonproprietary name for the adrenergic bronchodilator 3,4-dihydroxy-α-[(isopropyl-amino) methyl]benzyl alcohol hydrochloride. It is a nearly white, odorless, crystalline powder with a slightly bitter taste. It has a molecular weight of 247.7 and a molecular formula of $C_{11}H_{17}NO_3 \cdot HCl$.

Clinical Pharmacology: The viscosity of pulmonary mucous secretions depends on the concentrations of mucoprotein and to a lesser extent deoxyribonucleic acid (DNA). The latter increases with increasing purulence owing to the presence of cellular debris. The mucolytic action of acetylcysteine is related to the sulfhydryl group in the molecule. This group probably "opens" disulfide linkages in mucus thereby lowering the viscosity. The mucolytic activity of acetylcysteine is unaltered by the presence of DNA, and increases with increasing pH. Significant mucolysis occurs between pH 7 and 9.

Acetylcysteine undergoes rapid deacetylation *in vivo* to yield cysteine or oxidation to yield diacetylcystine.

Occasionally, patients exposed to the inhalation of an acetylcysteine aerosol respond with the development of increased airways obstruction of varying and unpredictable severity. Those patients who are reactors cannot be identified *a priori* from a random patient population. Even when patients are known to have reacted previously to the inhalation of an acetylcysteine aerosol, they may not react during a subsequent treatment. The converse is also true; patients who have had inhalation treatments of acetylcysteine without incident may still react to a subsequent inhalation with increased airways obstruction. The presence of isoproterenol hydrochloride in the inhalation mixture generally reduces the severity of such reactions. However, it should be noted that (a) in some patients the isoproterenol may not reduce the acetylcysteine-induced airway obstruction and (b) in some patients the airway obstruction may return if the effect of the isoproterenol is dissipated prior to that of the acetylcysteine.

Indications and Usage: Mucomyst with Isoproterenol is indicated as adjuvant therapy for patients with viscid or inspissated mucous secretions who might react to an inhaled acetylcysteine aerosol with increased airways obstruction. Included among these patients are those with any of the following conditions who in the judgment of the physician may be placed at the risk of increased airways obstruction by inhalation therapy treatments using acetylcysteine:

- Chronic bronchopulmonary disease (chronic emphysema, emphysema with bronchitis, chronic asthmatic bronchitis, tuberculosis, bronchiectasis and primary amyloidosis of the lung)
- Acute bronchopulmonary disease (pneumonia, bronchitis, tracheobronchitis)
- Pulmonary complications of cystic fibrosis
- Pulmonary complications associated with surgery
- Post-traumatic chest conditions
- Atelectasis due to mucous obstruction

Mucomyst with Isoproterenol is not to be used as a routine bronchodilator since the isoproterenol component is only present to decrease possible increased airways obstruction caused by the acetylcysteine.

Contraindications: Mucomyst with Isoproterenol is contraindicated in those patients who are sensitive to it.

Use of isoproterenol in patients with a history of cardiac arrhythmias associated with tachycardia is generally contraindicated because the cardiac stimulant effect of the drug may aggravate such disorders.

Warnings: After proper administration of Mucomyst with Isoproterenol an increased volume of liquefied bronchial secretions may occur. When cough is inadequate, an airway must be maintained open by mechanical suction, if necessary. When there is a mechanical block due to foreign body or local accumulation, the airway should be cleared by endotracheal aspiration, with or without bronchoscopy.

Asthmatics under treatment with Mucomyst with Isoproterenol should be observed carefully. If bronchospasm does progress, the medication should be discontinued immediately.

Excessive or repetitive use of an adrenergic aerosol such as the isoproterenol in Mucomyst with Isoproterenol should be discouraged because it may lose its effectiveness.

Occasional patients have been reported to develop severe, paradoxical airway resistance following repeated, excessive use of isoproterenol inhalation preparations. The cause of this refractory state is unknown.

It is advisable that in such instances the use of this preparation be discontinued immediately and alternative therapy instituted, since in the reported cases the patients did not respond to other forms of therapy until the drug was withdrawn.

Deaths have been reported following excessive use of isoproterenol inhalation preparations and the exact cause is unknown. Cardiac arrest was noted in several instances.

Because insufficient experience exists with administration of Mucomyst with Isoproterenol by direct instillation or in tents or Croupettes, its use should be limited to nebulization and inhalation only using a face mask or mouthpiece delivery system.

Precautions: Continued nebulization of an acetylcysteine solution with a dry gas will result in an increased concentration of the drug in the nebulizer because of evaporation of the solvent. Extreme concentration may impede nebulization and efficient delivery of the drug. Dilution of the nebulizing solution with appropriate amounts of Sterile Water for Injection, USP, as concentration occurs, will obviate this problem.

With the administration of acetylcysteine, the patient may initially notice a slightly disagreeable odor. Any stickiness remaining on the face after nebulization using a face mask may be removed by washing with water.

Epinephrine should not be administered with isoproterenol because both drugs are direct cardiac stimulants, and their combined effects may induce serious arrhythmia. However, if desired, they may be alternated, provided an interval of at least four hours has elapsed between agents.

Isoproterenol should be used with caution in patients with hypertension, cardiovascular disorders including coronary insufficiency, diabetes, or hyperthyroidism, and in persons sensitive to sympathomimetic amines.

Patients should be screened by exposure to an isoproterenol aerosol prior to the administration of Mucomyst with Isoproterenol to detect those patients whose bronchospasm may paradoxically worsen with isoproterenol.

It has not been determined whether the administration of isoproterenol prior to acetylcysteine inhalation might be more advantageous to a given patient than the concomitant administration of the two medications.

Under certain conditions, a color change may occur in Mucomyst with Isoproterenol in the opened bottle. The light purple color is the result of a chemical reaction which does not significantly affect safety or effectiveness of the product.

Usage in Pregnancy: Reproduction studies have been performed in rats and rabbits. In pregnant rabbits exposure to nebulized Mucomyst with Isoproterenol for 35 minutes daily resulted in a decreased number of live pups per litter. In rats exposed to nebulized Mucomyst with Isoproterenol for the same period of time there was no evidence of impaired fertility or harm to the fetus.

There are no well controlled studies in pregnant women but clinical experience does not include any positive evidence of adverse effects on the fetus. Although there is no clearly defined risk, such experience cannot exclude the possibility of infrequent or subtle damage to the fetus. Mucomyst with Isoproterenol should be used in pregnant women only when clearly needed.

Nursing Mothers

It is not known whether these drugs are excreted in human milk. Because many drugs are excreted in human milk, caution should be exercised when Mucomyst with Isoproterenol is administered to a nursing woman.

Adverse Reactions: With acetylcysteine adverse effects have included stomatitis, nausea, vomiting, fever, rhinorrhea, drowsiness, clamminess, chest tightness, and bronchoconstriction. Clinically overt acetylcysteine-induced bronchospasm occurs infrequently and unpredictably even in patients with asthmatic bronchitis or bronchitis complicating bronchial asthma. Acquired sensitization to acetylcysteine has been reported rarely. Reports of sensitization in patients have not been confirmed by patch testing. Sensitization has been confirmed in several inhalation therapists who reported a history of dermal eruptions after frequent and extended exposure to acetylcysteine. Reports of irritation to the tracheal and bronchial tracts have been received and although hemoptysis has occurred in patients receiving acetylcysteine such findings are not uncommon in patients with bronchopulmonary disease and a causal relationship has not been established.

As with other sympathomimetic drugs, isoproterenol may produce some undesirable side effects such as nervousness, dizziness, palpitation, nausea, vomiting, headache, tremor, flushing, weakness, tachycardia, sweating, precordial distress, or anginal-type pain.

Adverse effects with Mucomyst with Isoproterenol have included drowsiness, jitteriness, lightheadness, and increased airways obstruction.

Dosage and Administration: Mucomyst with Isoproterenol is available in plastic stoppered glass vials containing 4 ml of solution. Should the solution require dilution, Sterile Water for Injection, USP or Sterile Water for Inhalation, USP may be used.

A critical determination in calculating the volume of Mucomyst with Isoproterenol to be given is the amount of isoproterenol contained in the volume of solution. The amount of isoproterenol present in 5 ml of this 10% acetylcysteine solution is equivalent to 0.5 ml of a 1:200 solution of isoproterenol.

Adult's Dosage: When nebulized into a face mask or mouthpiece, 3 to 5 ml of the solution may be given every 3 to 6 hours up to four times daily. Recommended dose, 4 ml four times a day.

CHILDREN DOSAGE—DUE TO THE ISOPROTERENOL COMPONENT, CAUTION SHOULD BE USED IN ADMINISTERING MUCOMYST WITH ISOPROTERENOL TO CHILDREN SIX YEARS AND YOUNGER.

While no formal studies have been undertaken to determine the optimal dosage in children of less than 15 years of age, retrospective studies have shown that combinations of acetylcysteine and isoproterenol are well tolerated by children. These studies and prior experience with the individual components of Mucomyst with Isoproterenol indicate the following dosages can serve as guides:

Children 2 to 6 years of age, 2 to 3 ml two times a day.

Children 7 to 14 years of age, 2 to 3 ml two or three times a day.

The duration of each treatment will vary with the type of nebulizing equipment and the capabilities and respiratory status of the patient but most often will be 15 to 30 minutes.

Because insufficient experience exists with administration of Mucomyst with Isoproterenol by direct instillation or in tents or Croupettes, its use should be limited to nebulization and inhalation only using a face mask or mouthpiece.

For direct instillation or for use in tents or Croupettes, Mucomyst® or Mucomyst®-10 should be used.

Administration of Aerosol:

Materials

Mucomyst with Isoproterenol may be administered using conventional nebulizers made of plastic or glass. Certain materials used in nebulization equipment react with acetylcysteine. The most reactive of these are certain metals (notably iron and copper) and most rubbers. Where materials may come into contact with acetylcysteine solution, parts made of the following acceptable materials should be used: glass, plastic, aluminum, anodized aluminum, chromed metal, tantalum, sterling silver, or stainless steel. Silver may become tarnished after exposure, but this is not deleterious to the drug action or the patient.

Nebulizing Gases

Compressed tank gas (air) or an air compressor should be used to provide pressure for nebulizing the solution. Oxygen may also be used but should be used with usual caution in patients with severe respiratory disease and CO_2 retention.

Apparatus

Mucomyst with Isoproterenol is usually administered as a fine nebula and the nebulizer used should be capable of providing optimal quantities of a suitable range of particle sizes. Commercially available nebulizers will produce nebulae of Mucomyst with Isoproterenol satisfactory for retention in the respiratory tract. Most of the nebulizers tested will supply a high proportion of the drug solution as particles of less than 10 micrometers in diameter. Mitchell[a] has shown that particles less than 10 micrometers should be retained in the respiratory tract satisfactorily.

[a] Amer. Rev. Resp. Dis. *82*:627–639 (1960)

Units that nebulized this solution with satisfactory efficiency were the Maxi-Myst® Nebulizer (Mead Johnson Pharmaceutical Division, Evansville, Indiana), Hand-E-Vent intermittent positive pressure breathing device (Ohio Medical Products, 3030 Airco Drive, Madison, Wisconsin), and various other intermittent positive pressure breathing devices, No. 40 De Vilbiss (The De Vilbiss Co., Somerset, Pennsylvania), Bennett Twin-Jet Nebulizer (Puritan Bennett Corp., Oak at 13th St., Kansas City, Missouri).

The nebulized solution may be inhaled directly from the nebulizer. Nebulizers may also be attached to plastic face masks or plastic mouthpieces. Suitable nebulizers may also be fitted for use with the various intermittent positive pressure breathing (IPPB) machines. The nebulizing equipment should be cleaned immediately after use because the residues may clog the smaller orifices or corrode metal parts.

Hand bulbs are not recommended for routine use for nebulizing Mucomyst with Isoproterenol because their output is generally too small. Also, some hand-operated nebulizers deliver particles that are larger than optimum for inhalation therapy.

Mucomyst with Isoproterenol should not be placed directly into the chamber of a heated (hot pot) nebulizer. A heated nebulizer may be part of the nebulization assembly to provide a warm saturated atmosphere if the aerosol is introduced by means of a separate unheated nebulizer. Usual precautions for administration of warm saturated nebulae should be observed.

Prolonged Nebulization

When three-fourths of the initial volume of Mucomyst with Isoproterenol solution have been nebulized, a quantity of Sterile Water for Injection USP (approximately equal to the volume of solution remaining) should be added to the nebulizer. This minimizes any concentration of the agent in the solvent remaining after prolonged nebulization.

Storage of Opened Vials: Mucomyst with Isoproterenol does not contain an antimicrobial agent and care must be taken to minimize contamination of the sterile solution. If only a portion of the solution in a vial is used, store the remainder in a refrigerator and use within 96 hours.

Storage of Unopened Vials: Store unopened vials at controlled room temperature, 59° to 86°F (15° to 30°C). Avoid exposure to temperatures above 104°F (40°C).

Compatibility: The physical and chemical compatibility of Mucomyst with Isoproterenol with other drugs commonly administered by nebulization, direct instillation or topical application has not been studied as it has for Mucomyst® (acetylcysteine). Nevertheless, all of the known incompatibilities of Mucomyst apply. These are listed in the following table.

EXPECTED IN VITRO INCOMPATIBILITIES OF MUCOMYST WITH ISOPROTERENOL

Product and/or Agent(s)	Manufacturer (Trademark)
Amphotericin B	Squibb (Fungizone® Intravenous)
Chlortetracycline HCl	Lederle (Aureomycin®)
Erythromycin lactobionate	Abbot (Erythrocin®)
Oxytetracycline HCl	Pfizer (Terramycin®)
Sodium Ampicillin	Bristol (Polycillin-N®)
Tetracycline HCl	Lederle (Achromycin®)
Iodized Oil USP	Fougera (Lipiodol®)
Chymotrypsin	Armour
Trypsin	Armour
Hydrogen peroxide	

How Supplied:

Mucomyst® with Isoproterenol: 10% acetylcysteine (100 mg acetylcysteine per ml) and 0.05% isoproterenol HCl solution. Sterile, not for injection.

NDC 0087-0573-47 Carton of twelve 4 ml vials

Mucomyst® 20% acetylcysteine solution (200 mg acetylcysteine per ml). Sterile, Not for injection

NDC 0087-0570-07 Cartons of twelve 4 ml vials

NDC 0087-0570-03 Cartons of three 10 ml vials
1 plastic dropper

NDC 0087-0570-09 Carton of three 30 ml vials

Mucomyst® -10, 10% acetylcysteine solution. (100 mg acetylcysteine per ml). Sterile, Not for injection

NDC 0087-0572-03 Cartons of twelve 4 ml vials

NDC 0087-0572-01 Cartons of three 10 ml vials
1 plastic dropper

NDC 0087-0572-02 Cartons of three 30 ml vials

Note To Pharmacist: Additional Warning to Patients

It is necessary for the protection of users that warning information to patients be included as

Continued on next page

Mead Johnson Pharm.—Cont.

part of the label and as part of any instructions to patients included in the package dispensed to the patient as follows.

Warning: Do not exceed the dose prescribed by your physician. If difficulty in breathing persists, contact your physician immediately.

NATALINS® tablets
Multivitamin and multimineral supplement

Composition: Each Natalins tablet supplies:

		% U.S. RDA Pregnant or Lactating Women
Vitamins		
Vitamin A, I.U.	8,000	100
Vitamin D, I.U.	400	100
Vitamin E, I.U.	30	100
Vitamin C (Ascorbic acid), mg.	90	150
Folic acid (Folacin), mg.	0.8	100
Thiamine (Vitamin B_1), mg.	1.7	100
Riboflavin (Vitamin B_2), mg.	2.0	100
Niacin, mg.	20	100
Vitamin B_6, mg.	4.0	160
Vitamin B_{12}, mcg.	8	100
Minerals		
Calcium, mg.	200	15
Iodine, mcg.	150	100
Iron, mg.	45	250
Magnesium, mg.	100	22

Ingredients: Calcium carbonate, magnesium hydroxide, polyvinylpyrrolidone USP, gum arabic, ion exchange resin, methyl cellulose, magnesium stearate, artificial color, ethyl cellulose, silicon dioxide, glycerin, titanium dioxide, artificial flavor, vitamin A acetate, ergocalciferol, dl-alpha-tocopheryl acetate, sodium ascorbate, folic acid, thiamine mononitrate, riboflavin, niacinamide, pyridoxine hydrochloride, cyanocobalamin, calcium iodate and ferrous fumarate.

Indications and Usage: Diet supplementation during pregnancy or lactation.

Dosage and Administration: One tablet a day or as indicated.

How Supplied:
Natalins® tablets
NDC 0087-0700-01 Bottles of 100
NDC 0087-0700-06 Bottles of 1000
[Shown in Product Identification Section]

NATALINS® RX ℞
Multivitamin and Multimineral Supplement Tablets with 1 mg. folic acid and 60 mg. Iron

Natalins Rx tablets provide twelve vitamins and six minerals to supplement the diet during pregnancy or lactation.

Composition: Each Natalins Rx tablet supplies:

		% U.S. RDA Pregnant Or Lactating Women
Vitamins		
Vitamin A, I.U.	8,000	100
Vitamin D, I.U.	400	100
Vitamin E, I.U.	30	100
Vitamin C (Ascorbic acid), mg.	90	150
Folic acid (Folacin), mg.	1.0	125
Thiamine (Vitamin B_1), mg.	2.55	150
Riboflavin (Vitamin B_2), mg.	3.0	150
Niacin, mg.	20	100
Vitamin B_6, mg.	10.0	400
Vitamin B_{12}, mcg.	8	100
Biotin, mg.	0.05	16
Pantothenic acid, mg.	15.0	150
Minerals		
Calcium, mg.	200	15
Iodine, mcg.	150	100
Iron, mg.	60	333
Magnesium, mg.	100	22
Copper, mg.	2.0	100
Zinc, mg.	15.0	100

Ingredients: Vitamin A acetate, ergocalciferol, dl-alpha-tocopheryl acetate, sodium ascorbate, folic acid, thiamine mononitrate, riboflavin, niacinamide, pyridoxine hydrochloride, cyanocobalamin, biotin, calcium pantothenate, calcium carbonate, calcium iodate, ferrous fumarate, magnesium hydroxide, cupric oxide and zinc oxide.

Indications and Usage: Natalins Rx tablets help assure an adequate intake of the vitamins and minerals listed above.
The folic acid helps prevent the development of megaloblastic anemia during pregnancy.

Contraindications: Supplemental vitamins and minerals should not be prescribed for patients with hemochromatosis or Wilson's disease.

Warning: Keep Natalins Rx tablets out of the reach of children.

Precautions:
General—pernicious anemia should be excluded before using this product since folic acid may mask the symptoms of pernicious anemia. The calcium content should be considered before prescribing for patients with kidney stones. Do not exceed the recommended dose.

Adverse Reactions: No adverse reactions or undesirable side effects have been attributed to the use of Natalins Rx tablets.

Dosage and Administration: One tablet daily, or as prescribed.

How Supplied:
Natalins® Rx Tablets: (Available on prescription.)
NDC 0087-0702-01 Bottles of 100
NDC 0087-0702-02 Bottles of 1000
[Shown in Product Identification Section]

OVCON®-50 ℞
21 tablets of norethindrone 1 mg and ethinyl estradiol 0.05 mg. Each green tablet in the 28 day regimen contains inert ingredients.

OVCON®-35 ℞
21 tablets of norethindrone 0.4 mg and ethinyl estradiol 0.035 mg. Each green tablet in the 28 day regimen contains inert ingredients.

Oral contraceptives

Description: 28-Day OVCON®-50 and OVCON®-35 tablets provide a continuous regimen for oral contraception derived from 21 tablets composed of norethindrone and ethinyl estradiol to be followed by 7 green tablets of inert ingredients.
21-Day OVCON®-50 and OVCON®-35 tablets provide a regimen for oral contraception derived from 21 tablets composed of norethindrone and ethinyl estradiol. The chemical name for norethindrone is 17-Hydroxy-19-nor-17α-pregn-4-en-20-yn-3-one and for ethinyl estradiol the chemical name is 19-Nor-17α-pregna-1,3,5 (10)-trien-20-yne-3, 17-diol.

Clinical Pharmacology: Combination oral contraceptives act primarily through the mechanism of gonadotropin suppression due to the estrogenic and progestational activity of the ingredients. Although the primary mechanism of action is inhibition of ovulation, alterations in the genital tract including changes in the cervical mucus (which increase the difficulty of sperm penetration) and the endometrium (which reduce the likelihood of implantation) may also contribute to contraceptive effectiveness.

Indications and Usage: OVCON is indicated for the prevention of pregnancy in women who elect to use oral contraceptives as a method of contraception.
Oral contraceptives are highly effective. The pregnancy rate in women using conventional combination oral contraceptives (containing 35 mcg or more of ethinyl estradiol or 50 mcg or more of mestranol) is generally reported as less than one pregnancy per 100 woman-years of use. Slightly higher rates (somewhat more than 1 pregnancy per 100 woman-years of use) are reported for some combination products containing 35 mcg or less of ethinyl estradiol, and rates on the order of 3 pregnancies per 100 woman-years are reported for the progestin-only oral contraceptives.
These rates are derived from separate studies conducted by different investigators in several population groups and cannot be compared precisely. Furthermore, pregnancy rates tend to be lower as clinical studies are continued, possibly due to selective retention in the longer studies of those patients who accept the treatment regimen and do not discontinue as a result of adverse reactions, pregnancy, or other reasons.
In clinical trials with OVCON-50, 1,126 patients completed 9,558 cycles and a total of 7 pregnancies were reported. This represents a pregnancy rate of 0.88 per 100 woman-years.
In clinical trials with OVCON-35, 2493 patients completed 35,881 cycles and a total of 33 pregnancies were reported. This represents a pregnancy rate of 1.10 per 100 woman-years.
The following table gives ranges of pregnancy rates reported in a standard textbook for other means of contraception. An individual patient may achieve higher or lower rates with any given method (except the IUD), depending upon the degree of adherence to the method.

Pregnancies per 100 Woman-Years: IUD, less than 1–6; Diaphragm with spermicidal product (creams or jellies), 2–20; Condom, 3–36; Aerosol foams, 2–29; Jellies and creams, 4–36; Rhythm (all types), less than 1–47: 1. Calendar method, 14–47; 2. Temperature method, 1–20; 3. Temperature method—intercourse only in post-ovulatory phase, less than 1–7; 4. Mucus method, 1–25; No contraception, 60–80.

Dose-Related Risk of Thromboembolism from Oral Contraceptives: Two studies have shown a positive association between the dose of estrogens in oral contraceptives and the risk of thromboembolism. For this reason, it is prudent and in keeping with good principles of therapeutics to minimize exposure to estrogen. The oral contraceptive product prescribed for any given patient should be that product which contains the least amount of estrogen that is compatible with an acceptable pregnancy rate and patient acceptance. It is recommended that new acceptors of oral contraceptives be started on preparations containing 50 mcg or less of estrogen.

Contraindications: Oral contraceptives should not be used in women with any of the following conditions:

1. Thrombophlebitis or thromboembolic disorders.
2. A past history of deep vein thrombophlebitis or thromboembolic disorders.
3. Cerebral vascular or coronary artery disease.
4. Known or suspected carcinoma of the breast.
5. Known or suspected estrogen dependent neoplasia.
6. Undiagnosed abnormal genital bleeding.
7. Known or suspected pregnancy (see warning No. 5).
8. Benign or malignant liver tumor which developed during the use of oral contraceptives or other estrogen containing products.

Warnings:

Cigarette smoking increases the risk of serious cardiovascular side effects from oral contraceptive use. This risk increases with age and with heavy smoking (15 or more cigarettes per day) and is quite marked in women over 35 years of age. Women who use oral contraceptives should be strongly advised not to smoke.

The use of oral contraceptives is associated with increased risk of several serious conditions including thromboembolism, stroke, myocardial infarction, hepatic adenoma, gall bladder disease, hypertension. Practitioners prescribing oral contraceptives should be familiar with the following information relating to these risks.

1. Thromboembolic Disorders and Other Vascular Problems An increased risk of thromboembolic and thrombotic disease associated with the use of oral contraceptives is well established. Three principal studies in Great Britain and three in the United States have demonstrated an increased risk of fatal and nonfatal venous thromboembolism and stroke, both hemorrhagic and thrombotic. These studies estimate that users of oral contraceptives are 4 to 11 times more likely than nonusers to develop these diseases without evident cause (Table 2).

Cerebrovascular Disorders: In a collaborative American study of cerebrovascular disorders in women with and without predisposing causes, it was estimated that the risk of hemorrhagic stroke was 2.0 times greater in users than nonusers and the risk of thrombotic stroke was 4 to 9.5 times greater in users than in nonusers (Table 2).

TABLE 2

SUMMARY OF RELATIVE RISK OF THROMBOEMBOLIC DISORDERS AND OTHER VASCULAR PROBLEMS IN ORAL CONTRACEPTIVE USERS COMPARED TO NONUSERS

	Relative risk, times greater
Idiopathic thromboembolic disease	4–11
Post surgery thromboembolic complications	4–6
Thrombotic stroke	4–9.5
Hemorrhagic stroke	2
Myocardial infarction	2–12

Myocardial Infarction: An increased risk of myocardial infarction associated with the use of oral contraceptives has been reported confirming a previously suspected association. These studies, conducted in the United Kingdom, found, as expected, that the greater the number of underlying risk factors for coronary artery disease (cigarette smoking, hypertension, hypercholesterolemia, obesity, diabetes, history of preeclamptic toxemia) the higher the risk of developing myocardial infarction, regardless of whether the patient was an oral contraceptive user or not. Oral contraceptives, however, were found to be a clear additional risk factor.

In terms of relative risk, it has been estimated that oral contraceptive users who do not smoke (smoking is considered a major predisposing condition to myocardial infarction) are about twice as likely to have a fatal myocardial infarction as nonusers who do not smoke. Oral contraceptive users who are also smokers have about a 5-fold increased risk of fatal infarction compared to users who do not smoke, but about a 10- to 12-fold increased risk compared to nonusers who do not smoke. Furthermore, the amount of smoking is also an important factor. In determining the importance of these relative risks, however, the baseline rates for various age groups, as shown in Table 3, must be given serious consideration. The importance of other predisposing conditions mentioned above in determining relative and absolute risks has not as yet been quantified; it is quite likely that the same synergistic action exists, but perhaps to a lesser extent.

Figure 1.
Estimated annual number of deaths associated with control of fertility and no control per 100,000 nonsterile women, by regimen of control and age of women.

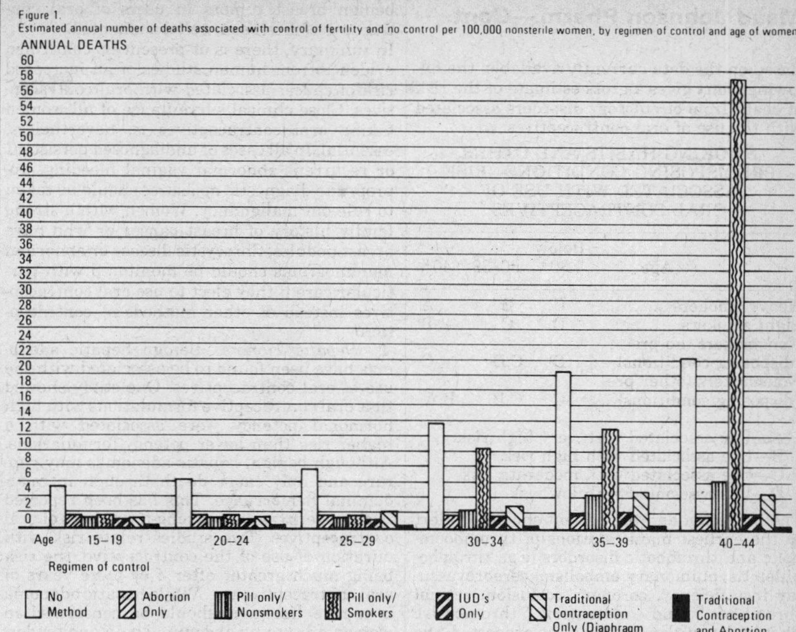

TABLE 3

ESTIMATED ANNUAL MORTALITY RATE PER 100,000 WOMEN FROM MYOCARDIAL INFARCTION BY USE OF ORAL CONTRACEPTIVES, SMOKING HABITS, AND AGE (IN YEARS)

	Myocardial infarction			
	Women aged 30–39		Women aged 40–44	
Smoking habits	Users	Non Users	Users	Non Users
All smokers	10.2	2.6	62.0	15.9
Heavy[1]	13.0	5.1	78.7	31.3
Light	4.7	.9	28.6	5.7
Nonsmokers	1.8	1.2	10.7	7.4
Smokers and nonsmokers	5.4	1.9	32.8	11.7

[1]Heavy smoker: 15 or more cigarettes per day. From Jain, A.K., Studies in Family Planning, 8:50, 1977.

Risk of Dose: In an analysis of data derived from several national adverse reaction reporting systems, British investigators concluded that the risk of thromboembolism including coronary thrombosis is directly related to the dose of estrogen used in oral contraceptives. Preparations containing 100 mcg or more of estrogen were associated with a higher risk of thromboembolism than those containing 50–80 mcg of estrogen. Their analysis did suggest, however, that the quantity of estrogen may not be the sole factor involved. This finding has been confirmed in the United States. Careful epidemiological studies to determine the degree of thromboembolic risk associated with progestogen-only oral contraceptives have not been performed. Cases of thromboembolic disease have been reported in women using these products, and they should not be presumed to be free of excess risk.

Estimate of Excess Mortality from Circulatory Diseases: A large prospective study carried out in the U.K. estimated the mortality rate per 100,000 women per year from diseases of the circulatory system for users and nonusers of oral contraceptives according to age, smoking habits, and duration of use. The overall excess death rate annually from circulatory diseases for oral contraceptive users was estimated to be 20 per 100,000 (ages 15–34—5/100,000; ages 35–44—33/100,000; ages 45–49—140/100,000), the risk being concentrated in older women, in those with a long duration of use, and in cigarette smokers. It was not possible, however, to examine the interrelationships of age, smoking and duration of use, nor to compare the effects of continuous versus intermittent use. Although the study showed a 10-fold increase in death due to circulatory diseases in users for 5 or more years, all of these deaths occurred in women 35 or older. Until larger numbers of women under 35 with continuous use for 5 or more years are available, it is not possible to assess the magnitude of the relative risk for this younger age group.

The available data from a variety of sources have been analyzed to estimate the risk of death associated with various methods of contraception. The estimates of risk of death for each method include the combined risk of the contraceptive method (e.g., thromboembolic and thrombotic disease in the case of oral contraceptives) plus the risk attributable to pregnancy or abortion in the event of method failure. This latter risk varies with the effectiveness of the contraceptive method. The findings of this analysis are shown in Figure 1 above. The study concluded that the mortality associated with all methods of birth control is low and below that associated with childbirth, with the exception of oral contraceptives in women over 40 who smoke. (The rates given for pill only/smokers for each age group are for smokers as a class. For "heavy" smokers [more than 15 cigarettes a day], the rates given would be about double; for "light" smokers [less than 15 cigarettes a day], about 50 percent.) The lowest mortality is associated with the condom or diaphragm backed up by early abortion.

The risk of thromboembolic and thrombotic disease associated with oral contraceptives increases with age after approximately age 30 and, for myocardial infarction, is further increased by hypertension, hypercholesterolemia, obesity, diabetes, or history of preeclamptic toxemia and especially by cigarette smoking.

Mead Johnson Pharm.—Cont.

Based on the data currently available, the following chart gives a gross estimate of the risk of death from circulatory disorders associated with the use of oral contraceptives:

SMOKING HABITS AND OTHER PREDISPOSING CONDITIONS—RISK ASSOCIATED WITH USE OF ORAL CONTRACEPTIVES

Age	Below 30	30–39	40+
Heavy smokers	C	B	A
Light smokers	D	C	B
Nonsmokers (no predisposing conditions) ..	D	C,D	C
Nonsmokers (other predisposing conditions) ..	C	C,B	B,A

A—Use associated with very high risk.
B—Use associated with high risk.
C—Use associated with moderate risk.
D—Use associated with low risk.

The physician and the patient should be alert to the earliest manifestations of thromboembolic and thrombotic disorders (e.g., thrombophlebitis, pulmonary embolism, cerebrovascular insufficiency, coronary occlusion, retinal thrombosis, and mesenteric thrombosis). Should any of these occur or be suspected, the drug should be discontinued immediately.
A four- to six-fold increased risk of post surgery thromboembolic complications has been reported in oral contraceptive users. If feasible, oral contraceptives should be discontinued at least 4 weeks before surgery of a type associated with an increased risk of thromboembolism or prolonged immobilization.
2. *Ocular Lesions.* There have been reports of neuro-ocular lesions such as optic neuritis or retinal thrombosis associated with the use of oral contraceptives. Discontinue oral contraceptive medication if there is unexplained, sudden or gradual, partial or complete loss of vision; onset of proptosis or diplopia; papilledema; or retinal vascular lesions and institute appropriate diagnostic and therapeutic measures.
3. *Carcinoma.* Long-term continuous administration of either natural or synthetic estrogen in certain animal species increases the frequency of carcinoma of the breast, cervix, vagina, and liver. Certain synthetic progestogens, none currently contained in oral contraceptives, have been noted to increase the incidence of mammary nodules, benign and malignant, in dogs.
In humans, three case control studies have reported an increased risk of endometrial carcinoma associated with the prolonged use of exogenous estrogen in post menopausal women. One publication reported on the first 21 cases submitted by physicians to a registry of cases of adenocarcinoma of the endometrium in women under 40 on oral contraceptives. Of the cases found in women without predisposing risk factors for adenocarcinoma of the endometrium (e.g., irregular bleeding at the time oral contraceptives were first given, polycystic ovaries), nearly all occurred in women who had used a sequential oral contraceptive. These products are no longer marketed. No evidence has been reported suggesting an increased risk of endometrial cancer in users of conventional combination or progestogen-only oral contraceptives.
Several studies have found no increase in breast cancer in women taking oral contraceptives or estrogens. One study however, while also noting no overall increased risk of breast cancer in women treated with oral contraceptives, found an excess risk in the subgroups of oral contraceptive users with documented benign breast disease. A reduced occurrence of benign breast tumors in users of oral contraceptives has been well-documented.
In summary, there is at present no confirmed evidence from human studies of an increased risk of cancer associated with oral contraceptives. Close clinical surveillance of all women taking oral contraceptives is, nevertheless, essential. In all cases of undiagnosed persistent or recurrent abnormal vaginal bleeding, appropriate diagnostic measures should be taken to rule out malignancy. Women with a strong family history of breast cancer or who have breast nodules, fibrocystic disease or abnormal mammograms should be monitored with particular care if they elect to use oral contraceptives instead of other methods of contraception.
4. *Hepatic Tumors.* Benign hepatic adenomas have been found to be associated with the use of oral contraceptives. One study showed that oral contraceptive formulations with high hormonal potency were associated with a higher risk than lower potency formulations. Although benign, hepatic adenomas may rupture and may cause death through intra-abdominal hemorrhage. This has been reported in short-term as well as long-term users of oral contraceptives. Two studies relate risk with duration of use of the contraceptive, the risk being much greater after 4 or more years of oral contraceptive use. While hepatic adenoma is a rare lesion, it should be considered in women presenting abdominal pain and tenderness, abdominal mass or shock.
A few cases of hepatocellular carcinoma have been reported in women taking oral contraceptives. The relationship of these drugs to this type of malignancy is not known at this time.
5. *Use in or Immediately Preceding Pregnancy, Birth Defects in Offspring, and Malignancy in Female Offspring.*
The use of female sex hormones—both estrogenic and progestational agents—during early pregnancy may seriously damage the offspring. It has been shown that females exposed **in utero** to diethylstilbestrol, a nonsteroidal estrogen, have an increased risk of developing in later life a form of vaginal or cervical cancer that is ordinarily extremely rare. This risk has been estimated to be of the order of 1 in 1,000 exposures or less. Although there is no evidence at the present time that oral contraceptives further enhance the risk of developing this type of malignancy, such patients should be monitored with particular care if they elect to use oral contraceptives instead of other methods of contraception.
Furthermore, a high percentage of such exposed women (from 30 to 90%) have been found to have epithelial changes of the vagina and cervix. Although these changes are histologically benign, it is not known whether this condition is a precursor of vaginal malignancy. Male children so exposed may develop abnormalities of the urogenital tract. Although similar data are not available with the use of other estrogens, it cannot be presumed that they would not induce similar changes.
An increased risk of congenital anomalies, including heart defects and limb defects, has been reported with the use of sex hormones, including oral contraceptives, in pregnancy. One case control study has estimated a 4.7-fold increase in risk of limb-reduction defects in infants exposed **in utero** to sex hormones (oral contraceptives, hormonal withdrawal tests for pregnancy or attempted treatment for threatened abortion). Some of these exposures were very short and involved only a few days of treatment. The data suggest that the risk of limb-reduction defects in exposed fetuses is somewhat less than one in 1,000 live births.
In the past, female sex hormones have been used during pregnancy in an attempt to treat threatened or habitual abortion. There is considerable evidence that estrogens are ineffective for these indications, and there is no evidence from well controlled studies that progestogens are effective for these uses.
There is some evidence that triploidy and possibly other types of polyploidy are increased among abortuses from women who become pregnant soon after ceasing oral contraceptives. Embryos with these anomalies are virtually always aborted spontaneously. Whether there is an overall increase in spontaneous abortion of pregnancies conceived soon after stopping oral contraceptives is unknown.
It is recommended that for any patient who has missed two consecutive periods, pregnancy should be ruled out before continuing the contraceptive regimen. If the patient has not adhered to the prescribed schedule, the possibility of pregnancy should be considered at the time of the first missed period (or after 45 days from the last menstrual period if the progestogen-only oral contraceptives are used), and further use of oral contraceptives should be withheld until pregnancy has been ruled out. If pregnancy is confirmed, the patient should be apprised of the potential risks to the fetus and the advisability of continuation of the pregnancy should be discussed in the light of these risks.
It is also recommended that women who discontinue oral contraceptives with the intent of becoming pregnant use an alternate form of contraception for a period of time before attempting to conceive. Many clinicians recommend 3 months although no precise information is available on which to base this recommendation.
The administration of progestogen-only or progestogen-estrogen combinations to induce withdrawal bleeding should not be used as a test of pregnancy.
6. *Gallbladder Disease.*
Studies report an increased risk of surgically confirmed gallbladder disease in users of oral contraceptives and estrogens. In one study, an increased risk appeared after 2 years of use and doubled after 4 or 5 years of use. In one of the other studies, an increased risk was apparent between 6 and 12 months of use.
7. *Carbohydrate and Lipid Metabolic Effects.*
A decrease in glucose tolerance has been observed in a significant percentage of patients on oral contraceptives. For this reason, prediabetic and diabetic patients should be carefully observed while receiving oral contraceptives.
An increase in triglycerides and total phospholipids has been observed in patients receiving oral contraceptives. The clinical significance of this finding remains to be defined.
8. *Elevated Blood Pressure.*
An increase in blood pressure has been reported in patients receiving oral contraceptives. In some women, hypertension may occur within a few months of beginning oral contraceptive use. In the first year of use, the prevalence of women with hypertension is low in users and may be no higher than that of a comparable group of nonusers. The prevalence in users increases, however, with longer exposure, and in the fifth year of use is two and a half to three times the reported prevalence in the first year. Age is also strongly correlated with the development of hypertension in oral contraceptive users. Women who previously have had hypertension during pregnancy may be more likely to develop elevation of blood pressure when given oral contraceptives. Hypertension that develops as a result of taking oral contraceptives usually returns to normal after discontinuing the drug.
9. *Headache.*
The onset or exacerbation of migraine or development of headache of a new pattern which is recurrent, persistent, or severe, requires discontinuation of oral contraceptives and evaluation of the cause.
10. *Bleeding Irregularities.*
Breakthrough bleeding, spotting, and amenorrhea are frequent reasons for patients discontinuing oral contraceptives. In breakthrough

bleeding, as in all cases of irregular bleeding from the vagina, nonfunctional causes should be borne in mind. In undiagnosed persistent or recurrent abnormal bleeding from the vagina, adequate diagnostic measures are indicated to rule out pregnancy or malignancy. If pathology has been excluded, time or a change to another formulation may solve the problem. Changing to an oral contraceptive with a higher estrogen content, while potentially useful in minimizing menstrual irregularity, should be done only if necessary since this may increase the risk of thromboembolic disease. Women with a past history of oligomenorrhea or secondary amenorrhea or young women without regular cycles may have a tendency to remain anovulatory or to become amenorrheic after discontinuation of oral contraceptives. Women with these preexisting problems should be advised of this possibility and encouraged to use other contraceptive methods. Post-use anovulation, possibly prolonged, may also occur in women without previous irregularities.

11. Ectopic Pregnancy.
Ectopic as well as intrauterine pregnancy may occur in contraceptive failures. However, in progestogen-only oral contraceptive failures, the ratio of ectopic to intrauterine pregnancies is higher than in women who are not receiving oral contraceptives, since the drugs are more effective in preventing intrauterine than ectopic pregnancies.

12. Breast Feeding.
Oral contraceptives given in the postpartum period may interfere with lactation. There may be a decrease in the quantity and quality of the breast milk. Furthermore, a small fraction of the hormonal agents in oral contraceptives has been identified in the milk of mothers receiving these drugs. The effects, if any, on the breast-fed child have not been determined. If feasible, the use of oral contraceptives should be deferred until the infant has been weaned.

Precautions:
General

1. A complete medical and family history should be taken prior to the initiation of oral contraceptives. The pretreatment and periodic physical examinations should include special reference to blood pressure, breasts, abdomen and pelvic organs, including Papanicolaou smear and relevant laboratory tests. As a general rule, oral contraceptives should not be prescribed for longer than 1 year without another physical examination being performed.
2. Under the influence of estrogen-progestogen preparations, preexisting uterine leiomyomata may increase in size.
3. Patients with a history of psychic depression should be carefully observed and the drug discontinued if depression recurs to a serious degree. Patients becoming significantly depressed while taking oral contraceptives should stop the medication and use an alternate method of contraception in an attempt to determine whether the symptom is drug related.
4. Oral contraceptives may cause some degree of fluid retention. They should be prescribed with caution, and only with careful monitoring, in patients with conditions which might be aggravated by fluid retention, such as convulsive disorders, migraine syndrome, asthma, or cardiac or renal insufficiency.
5. Patients with a past history of jaundice during pregnancy have an increased risk of recurrence of jaundice while receiving oral contraceptive therapy. If jaundice develops in any patient receiving such drugs, the medication should be discontinued.
6. Steroid hormones may be poorly metabolized in patients with impaired liver function and should be administered with caution in such patients.
7. Oral contraceptive users may have disturbances in normal tryptophan metabolism which may result from a relative pyridoxine deficiency. The clinical significance of this is yet to be determined.
8. Serum folate levels may be depressed by oral contraceptive therapy. Since the pregnant woman is predisposed to the development of folate deficiency and the incidence of folate deficiency increases with increasing gestation, it is possible that if a woman becomes pregnant shortly after stopping oral contraceptives, she may have a greater chance of developing folate deficiency, and complications attributed to this deficiency.
9. The pathologist should be advised of oral contraceptive therapy when relevant specimens are submitted.
10. Certain endocrine and liver function tests and blood components may be affected by estrogen-containing oral contraceptives:
    a. Increased sulfobromophthalein-retention.
    b. Increased prothrombin and factors VII, VIII, IX, and X; decreased antithrombin 3; increased norepinephrine-induced platelet aggregability.
    c. Increased thyroid binding globulin (TBG) leading to increased circulating total thyroid hormone, as measured by protein-bound iodine (PBI), T4 by column, or T4 by radioimmunoassay. Free T3 resin uptake is decreased, reflecting the elevated TBG, free T4 concentration is unaltered.
    d. Decreased pregnanediol excretion.
    e. Reduced response to metyrapone test.
11. The active yellow tablets and the inert green tablets in OVCON-50 (21 and 28 day regimens) and the inert green tablets in the 28 day regimen of OVCON-35 contain FD&C Yellow No. 5 (tartrazine) which may cause allergic-type reactions (including bronchial asthma) in certain susceptible individuals. Although the overall incidence of FD&C Yellow No. 5 (tartrazine) sensitivity in the general population is low, it is frequently seen in patients who also have aspirin hypersensitivity.

Information for the Patient: See Patient Labeling Printed below

Drug Interactions: Reduced efficacy and increased incidence of breakthrough bleeding have been associated with concomitant use of rifampin. A similar association has been suggested with barbiturates, phenylbutazone, phenytoin sodium, ampicillin, and tetracycline.

Carcinogenesis: See Warning section for information on the carcinogenic potential of oral contraceptives.

Pregnancy: Pregnancy category X. See Contraindications and Warnings.

Nursing Mothers: See Warnings.

Adverse Reactions: An increased risk of the following serious adverse reactions has been associated with the use of oral contraceptives (see Warnings):

Thrombophlebitis.
Pulmonary embolism.
Coronary thrombosis.
Cerebral thrombosis.
Cerebral hemorrhage.
Hypertension.
Gallbladder disease.
Benign hepatomas.
Congenital anomalies.

There is evidence of an association between the following conditions and the use of oral contraceptives, although additional confirmatory studies are needed:

Mesenteric thrombosis.
Neuro-ocular lesions, e.g., retinal thrombosis and optic neuritis.

The following adverse reactions have been reported in patients receiving oral contraceptives and are believed to be drug related:

Nausea and/or vomiting, usually the most common adverse reactions, occur in approximately 10% or less of patients during the first cycle. Other reactions, as a general rule, are seen much less frequently or only occasionally.

Gastrointestinal symptoms (such as abdominal cramps and bloating).
Breakthrough bleeding.
Spotting.
Change in menstrual flow.
Dysmenorrhea.
Amenorrhea during and after treatment.
Temporary infertility after discontinuance of treatment.
Edema.
Chloasma or melasma which may persist.
Breast changes: tenderness, enlargement, and secretion.
Change in weight (increase or decrease).
Change in cervical erosion and cervical secretion.
Possible diminution in lactation when given immediately postpartum.
Cholestatic jaundice.
Migraine.
Increase in size of uterine leiomyomata.
Rash (allergic).
Mental depression.
Reduced tolerance to carbohydrates.
Vaginal candidiasis.
Change in corneal curvature (steepening).
Intolerance to contact lenses.

The following adverse reactions have been reported in users of oral contraceptives, and the association has been neither confirmed nor refuted:

Premenstrual-like syndrome.
Cataracts.
Changes in libido.
Chorea.
Changes in appetite.
Cystitis-like syndrome.
Headache.
Nervousness.
Dizziness.
Hirsutism.
Loss of scalp hair.
Erythema multiforme.
Erythema nodosum.
Hemorrhagic Eruption.
Vaginitis.
Porphyria.

Acute Overdose: Serious ill effects have not been reported following acute ingestion of large doses of oral contraceptives by young children. Overdosage may cause nausea, and withdrawal bleeding may occur in females.

Dosage and Administration: To achieve maximum contraceptive effectiveness, OVCON-50 or OVCON-35 must be taken exactly as directed and at intervals not exceeding 24 hours.

28-DAY REGIMEN

The patient takes one tablet daily from a convenient package as follows: (yellow or peach tablet containing active ingredients, green tablet containing inert ingredients)

For the first cycle of use only, the first yellow or peach tablet is taken on day 5 of the menstrual cycle, counting the first day of bleeding as day 1. One tablet is taken daily in the same sequence as in the package—first the yellow or peach, then the green tablets. After the last green tablet is taken, the first yellow or peach tablet from a new package is taken **the following day.** Withdrawal bleeding will usually begin while the patient is taking the green tablets and may continue during the first few tablets from the next package.

21-DAY REGIMEN

The patient takes one tablet daily from a convenient package as follows: (yellow or peach)

For the first cycle of use only, the first yellow or peach tablet is taken on day 5 of the menstrual cycle, counting the first day of bleeding as day 1. Continue taking one tablet daily from the 5th through the 25th day of the menstrual cycle. If the first tablet is taken later than the fifth day of the first menstrual

Continued on next page

Mead Johnson Pharm.—Cont.

cycle an additional form of contraception should be used for at least one week. Withdrawal bleeding will normally begin within 2–3 days after taking the last tablet. The first tablet of the next package should be taken on the eighth day after the last tablet even if menstrual bleeding has not ceased. The dosage regimen then continues with one tablet daily for 21 days followed by 7 days of no medication, thus a cycle of three-weeks-on and one-week-off.

Patients should be cautioned to follow the dosage schedule strictly.

Evening administration is suggested. If the regimen is interrupted, an additional contraceptive method is recommended for the rest of the cycle. Should spotting or breakthrough bleeding occur, it is recommended that the patient continue medication. If bleeding is persistent or recurrent, the patient should consult her physician.

Use of oral contraceptives in the event of a missed menstrual period:

1. If the patient has not adhered to the prescribed dosage regimen, the possibility of pregnancy should be considered after the first missed period and oral contraceptives should be withheld until pregnancy has been ruled out.
2. If the patient has adhered to the prescribed regimen and misses two consecutive periods, pregnancy should be ruled out before continuing the contraceptive regimen.

How Supplied:

OVCON®-50 is available in 21 and 28 day regimens. Each package contains 21 yellow tablets of 1.0 mg. norethindrone and 0.05 mg. ethinyl estradiol. Each green tablet in the 28 day regimen contains inert ingredients.

NDC 0087-0584-40 Package of 21 tablets
NDC 0087-0584-42 Carton of 6 packages
NDC 0087-0579-40 Package of 28 tablets
NDC 0087-0579-41 Carton of 6 packages

OVCON®-35 is available in 21 and 28 day regimens. Each package contains 21 peach tablets of 0.4 mg. norethindrone and 0.035 mg. ethinyl estradiol. Each green tablet in the 28 day regimen contains inert ingredients.

NDC 0087-0583-40 Package of 21 tablets
NDC 0087-0583-42 Carton of 6 packages
6505-01-084-2667 (6 x 21) (Defense)
NDC 0087-0578-40 Package of 28 tablets
NDC 0087-0578-41 Carton of 6 packages

The Patient Labeling for oral contraceptive drug products is set forth below:

BRIEF SUMMARY
PATIENT PACKAGE INSERT

Warning:

Cigarette smoking increases the risk of serious adverse effects on the heart and blood vessels from oral contraceptive use. This risk increases with age and with heavy smoking (15 or more cigarettes per day) and is quite marked in women over 35 years of age. Women who use oral contraceptives should not smoke.

Oral contraceptives taken as directed are about 99% effective in preventing pregnancy. (The mini-pill, however, is somewhat less effective.) Forgetting to take your pills increases the chance of pregnancy. Various drugs, such as antibiotics, may also decrease the effectiveness of oral contraceptives.

Women who have or have had clotting disorders, cancer of the breast or sex organs, unexplained vaginal bleeding, a stroke, heart attack, angina pectoris, or who suspect they may be pregnant should not use oral contraceptives.

Most side effects of the pill are not serious. The most common side effects are nausea, vomiting, bleeding between menstrual periods, weight gain, and breast tenderness. However, proper use of oral contraceptives requires that they be taken under your doctor's continuous supervision, because they can be associated with serious side effects which may be fatal. Fortunately, these occur very infrequently. The serious side effects are:

1. Blood clots in the legs, lungs, brain, heart or other organs and hemorrhage into the brain due to bursting of a blood vessel.
2. Liver tumors, which may rupture and cause severe bleeding.
3. Birth defects if the pill is taken while you are pregnant.
4. High blood pressure.
5. Gallbladder disease.

The symptoms associated with these serious side effects are discussed in the detailed leaflet given you with your supply of pills. Notify your doctor if you notice any unusual physical disturbance while taking the pill.

The estrogen in oral contraceptives has been found to cause breast cancer and other cancers in certain animals. These findings suggest that oral contraceptives may also cause cancer in humans. However, studies to date in women taking currently marketed oral contraceptives have not confirmed that oral contraceptives cause cancer in humans.

The detailed leaflet describes more completely the benefits and risks of oral contraceptives. It also provides information on other forms of contraception. Read it carefully. If you have any questions, consult your doctor.

Caution: Oral contraceptives are of no value in the prevention or treatment of venereal disease.

Detailed Patient Labeling

What You Should Know About Oral Contraceptives: Oral contraceptives ("the pill") are the most effective way (except for sterilization) to prevent pregnancy. They are also convenient and, for most women, free of serious or unpleasant side effects. Oral contraceptives must always be taken under the continuous supervision of a physician.

It is important that any woman who considers using an oral contraceptive understand the risks involved. Although the oral contraceptives have important advantages over other methods of contraception, they have certain risks that no other method has. Only you can decide whether the advantages are worth these risks. This leaflet will tell you about the most important risks. It will explain how you can help your doctor prescribe the pill as safely as possible by telling him about yourself and being alert for the earliest signs of trouble. And it will tell you how to use the pill properly, so that it will be as effective as possible. There is more detailed information available in the leaflet prepared for doctors. Your pharmacist can show you a copy; you may need your doctor's help in understanding parts of it.

Who Should Not Use Oral Contraceptives:

A. If you have any of the following conditions you should not use the pill:

1. Clots in the legs or lungs.
2. Angina pectoris.
3. Known or suspected cancer of the breast or sex organs.
4. Unusual vaginal bleeding that has not yet been diagnosed.
5. Known or suspected pregnancy.

B. If you have had any of the following conditions you should not use the pill:

1. Heart attack or stroke.
2. Clots in the legs or lungs.

Warning:

C. Cigarette smoking increases the risk of serious adverse effects on the heart and blood vessels from oral contraceptive use. This risk increases with age and with heavy smoking (15 or more cigarettes per day) and is quite marked in women over 35 years of age. Women who use oral contraceptives should not smoke.

D. If you have scanty or irregular periods or are a young woman without a regular cycle, you should use another method of contraception because, if you use the pill, you may have difficulty becoming pregnant or may fail to have menstrual periods after discontinuing the pill.

Deciding to Use Oral Contraceptives: If you do not have any of the conditions listed above and are thinking about using oral contraceptives, to help you decide, you need information about the advantages and risks of oral contraceptives and of other contraceptive methods as well. This leaflet describes the advantages and risks of oral contraceptives. Except for sterilization, the IUD and abortion, which have their own exclusive risks, the only serious risks of other methods of contraception are those due to pregnancy should the method fail. Your doctor can answer questions you may have with respect to other methods of contraception. He can also answer any questions you may have after reading this leaflet on oral contraceptives.

1. What Oral Contraceptives Are and How They Work. Oral Contraceptives are of two types. The most common, often simply called "the pill" is a combination of an estrogen and a progestogen, the two kinds of female hormones. The amount of estrogen and progestogen can vary, but the amount of estrogen is most important because both the effectiveness and some of the dangers of oral contraceptives are related to the amount of estrogen. This kind of oral contraceptive works principally by preventing release of an egg from the ovary. When the amount of estrogen is 50 micrograms or more of mestranol or 35 micrograms or more of ethinyl estradiol and the pill is taken as directed, oral contraceptives are more than 99% effective (i.e., there would be less than one pregnancy if 100 women used the pill for 1 year). Pills that contain 20 to 35 micrograms of estrogen vary slightly in effectiveness, ranging from 98% to more than 99% effective.

The second type of oral contraceptive, often called the "mini-pill", contains only a progestogen. It works in part by preventing release of an egg from the ovary but also by keeping sperm from reaching the egg and by making the uterus (womb) less receptive to any fertilized egg that reaches it. The mini-pill is less effective than the combination oral contraceptive, about 97% effective. In addition, the progestogen-only pill has a tendency to cause irregular bleeding which may be quite inconvenient, or cessation of bleeding entirely. The progestogen-only pill is used despite its lower effectiveness in the hope that it will prove not to have some of the serious side effects of the estrogen-containing pill (see below) but it is not yet certain that the mini-pill does in fact have fewer serious side effects. The discussion below, while based mainly on information about the combination pills, should be considered to apply as well to the mini-pill.

2. Other Nonsurgical Ways to Prevent Pregnancy. As this leaflet will explain, oral contraceptives have several serious risks. Other methods of contraception have lesser risks or none at all. They are also less effective than oral contraceptives, but, used properly, may be effective enough for many women. The following table gives reported pregnancy rates (the number of women out of 100 who would become pregnant in 1 year) for these methods:

Pregnancies per 100 Women per year:
Intrauterine device (IUD), less than 1–6;
Diaphragm with spermicidal products (creams or jellies), 2–20;

Condom (rubber), 3–36;
Aerosol foams, 2–29;
Jellies and creams, 4–36;
Periodic abstinence (rhythm) all types, less than 1–47:

1. Calendar method, 14–47;
2. Temperature method, 1–20;
3. Temperature method—intercourse only in post-ovulatory phase, less than 1–7;
4. Mucus method, 1–25;

No contraception, 60–80.

The figures (except for the IUD) vary widely because people differ in how well they use each method. Very faithful users of the various methods obtain very good results, except for users of the calendar method of periodic abstinence (rhythm). Except for the IUD, effective use of these methods requires somewhat more effort than simply taking a single pill every morning, but it is an effort that many couples undertake successfully. Your doctor can tell you a great deal more about these methods of contraception.

3. The Dangers of Oral Contraceptives.

a. Circulatory disorders (abnormal blood clotting and stroke due to hemorrhage). Blood clots (in various blood vessels of the body) are the most common of the serious side effects of oral contraceptives. A clot can result in a stroke (if the clot is in the brain), a heart attack (if the clot is in a blood vessel of the heart), or a pulmonary embolus (a clot which forms in the legs or pelvis, then breaks off and travels to the lungs). Any of these can be fatal. Clots also occur rarely in the blood vessels of the eye, resulting in blindness or impairment of vision in that eye. There is evidence that the risk of clotting increases with higher estrogen doses. It is therefore important to keep the dose of estrogen as low as possible, so long as the oral contraceptive used has an acceptable pregnancy rate and doesn't cause unacceptable changes in the menstrual pattern. Furthermore, cigarette smoking by oral contraceptive users increases the risk of serious adverse effects on the heart and blood vessels. This risk increases with age and with heavy smoking (15 or more cigarettes per day) and begins to become quite marked in women over 35 years of age. For this reason women who use oral contraceptives should not smoke.

The risk of abnormal clotting increases with age in both users and nonusers of oral contraceptives, but the increased risk from the contraceptive appears to be present at all ages. For oral contraceptive users in general, it has been estimated that in women between the ages of 15 and 34 the risk of death due to a circulatory disorder is about 1 in 12,000 per year, whereas for nonusers the rate is about 1 in 50,000 per year. In the age group 35 to 44, the risk is estimated to be about 1 in 2,500 per year for oral contraceptive users and about 1 in 10,000 per year for nonusers.

Even without the pill the risk of having a heart attack increases with age and is also increased by such heart attack risk factors as high blood pressure, high cholesterol, obesity, diabetes, and cigarette smoking. Without any risk factors present, the use of oral contraceptives alone may double the risk of heart attack. However, the combination of cigarette smoking, especially heavy smoking, and oral contraceptive use greatly increases the risk of heart attack. Oral contraceptive users who smoke are about 5 times more likely to have a heart attack than users who do not smoke and about 10 times more likely to have a heart attack than nonusers who do not smoke. It has been estimated that users between the ages of 30 and 39 who smoke have about a 1 in 10,000 chance each year of having a fatal heart attack compared to about a 1 in 50,000 chance in users who do not smoke, and about a 1 in 100,000 chance in nonusers who do not smoke. In the age group 40 to 44, the risk is about 1 in 1,700 per year for users who smoke compared to about 1 in 10,000 for users who do not smoke and to about 1 in 14,000 per year for nonusers who do not smoke. Heavy smoking (about 15 cigarettes or more a day) further increases the risk. If you do not smoke and have none of the other heart attack risk factors described above, you will have a smaller risk than listed. If you have several heart attack risk factors, the risk may be considerably greater than listed.

In addition to blood-clotting disorders, it has been estimated that women taking oral contraceptives are twice as likely as nonusers to have a stroke due to rupture of a blood vessel in the brain.

b. Formation of tumors. Studies have found that when certain animals are given the female sex hormone estrogen, which is an ingredient of oral contraceptives, continuously for long periods, cancers may develop in the breast, cervix, vagina, and liver.

These findings suggest that oral contraceptives may cause cancer in humans. However, studies to date in women taking currently marketed oral contraceptives have not confirmed that oral contraceptives cause cancer in humans. Several studies have found no increase in breast cancer in users, although one study suggested oral contraceptives might cause an increase in breast cancer in women who already have benign breast disease (e.g., cysts).

Women with a strong family history of breast cancer or who have breast nodules, fibrocystic disease, or abnormal mammograms or who were exposed to DES (diethylstilbestrol), an estrogen, during their mother's pregnancy must be followed very closely by their doctors if they choose to use oral contraceptives instead of another method of contraception. Many studies have shown that women taking oral contraceptives have less risk of getting benign breast disease than those who have not used oral contraceptives. Recently, strong evidence has emerged that estrogens (one component of oral contraceptives), when given for periods of more than one year to women after the menopause, increase the risk of cancer of the uterus (womb). There is also some evidence that a kind of oral contraceptive which is no longer marketed, the sequential oral contraceptive, may increase the risk of cancer of the uterus. There remains no evidence, however, that the oral contraceptives now available increase the risk of this cancer.

Oral contraceptives do cause, although rarely, a benign (non-malignant) tumor of the liver. These tumors do not spread, but they may rupture and cause internal bleeding, which may be fatal. A few cases of cancer of the liver have been reported in women using oral contraceptives, but it is not yet known whether the drug caused them.

c. Dangers to a developing child if oral contraceptives are used in or immediately preceding pregnancy. Oral contraceptives should not be taken by pregnant women because they may damage the developing child. An increased risk of birth defects, including heart defects and limb defects, has been associated with the use of sex hormones, including oral contraceptives, in pregnancy. In addition, the developing female child whose mother has received DES (diethylstilbestrol), an estrogen, during pregnancy has a risk of getting cancer of the vagina or cervix in her teens or young adulthood. This risk is estimated to be about 1 in 1,000 exposures or less. Abnormalities of the urinary and sex organs have been reported in male offspring so exposed. It is possible that other estrogens, such as the estrogens in oral contraceptives, could have the same effect in the child if the mother takes them during pregnancy.

If you stop taking oral contraceptives to become pregnant, your doctor may recommend that you use another method of contraception for a short while. The reason for this is that there is evidence from studies in women who have had "miscarriages" soon after stopping the pill that the lost fetuses are more likely to be abnormal. Whether there is an overall increase in "miscarriage" in women who become pregnant soon after stopping the pill as compared with women who do not use the pill is not known, but it is possible that there may be. If, however, you do become pregnant soon after stopping oral contraceptives, and do not have a miscarriage, there is no evidence that the baby has an increased risk of being abnormal.

d. Gallbladder disease. Women who use oral contraceptives have a greater risk than nonusers of having gallbladder disease requiring surgery. The increased risk may first appear within 1 year of use and may double after 4 or 5 years of use.

e. Other side effects of oral contraceptives. Some women using oral contraceptives experience unpleasant side effects that are not dangerous and are not likely to damage their health. Some of these may be temporary. Your breasts may feel tender, nausea and vomiting may occur, you may gain or lose weight and your ankles may swell. A spotty darkening of the skin, particularly of the face, is possible and may persist. You may notice unexpected vaginal bleeding or changes in your menstrual period. Irregular bleeding is frequently seen when using the mini-pill or combination oral contraceptives containing less than 50 micrograms of estrogen.

More serious side effects include worsening of migraine, asthma, epilepsy, and kidney or heart disease because of a tendency for water to be retained in the body when oral contraceptives are used. Other side effects are growth of preexisting fibroid tumors of the uterus; mental depression; and liver problems with jaundice (yellowing of the skin). Your doctor may find that levels of sugar and fatty substances in your blood are elevated; the long-term effects of these changes are not known. Some women develop high blood pressure while taking oral contraceptives, which ordinarily returns to the original levels when the oral contraceptive is stopped.

Other reactions, although not proved to be caused by oral contraceptives, are occasionally reported. These include more frequent urination and some discomfort when urinating, nervousness, dizziness, some loss of scalp hair, an increase in body hair, an increase or decrease in sex drive, appetite changes, cataracts, and a need for a change in contact lens prescription or inability to use contact lenses.

After you stop using oral contraceptives there may be a delay before you are able to become pregnant or before you resume having menstrual periods. This is especially true of women who had irregular menstrual cycles prior to the use of oral contraceptives. As discussed previously, your doctor may recommend that you wait a short while after stopping the pill before you try to become pregnant. During this time, use another form of contraception. You should consult your physician before resuming use of oral contraceptives after childbirth, especially if you plan to nurse your baby. Drugs in oral contraceptives are known to appear in the milk, and the long-range effects on infants is not known at this time. Furthermore, oral contraceptives may cause a decrease in your milk supply as well as in the quality of the milk.

4. Comparison of the Risks of Oral Contraceptives and Other Contraceptive Methods. The many studies on the risks and effectiveness of oral contraceptives and other methods of contraception have been analyzed to estimate the risk of death associated with various methods of contraception. This risk has two parts: (a) the risk of the method itself (e.g., the risk that oral contraceptives will cause death due to abnormal clotting), and (b) the risk of death due to pregnancy or abortion in the event the method fails. The results of this analysis are

Continued on next page

Mead Johnson Pharm.—Cont.

shown in the bar graph below. The height of the bars is the number of deaths per 100,000 women each year. There are six sets of bars, each set referring to specific age groups of women. Within each set of bars there is a single bar for each of the different contraceptive methods. For oral contraceptives, there are two bars—one for smokers and the other for nonsmokers. The analysis is based on present knowledge and new information could, of course, alter it. The analysis shows that the risk of death from all methods of birth control is low and below that associated with child birth, except for oral contraceptives in women over 40 who smoke. It shows that the lowest risk of death is associated with the condom or diaphragm (traditional contraception) backed up by early abortion in case of failure of the condom or diaphragm to prevent pregnancy. Also, at any age the risk of death (due to unexpected pregnancy) from the use of traditional contraception, even without a backup of abortion, is generally the same as or less than that from use of oral contraceptives. (See Figure 1)

How to Use Oral Contraceptives as Safely and Effectively as Possible, Once You Have Decided to Use Them:

NOTE:
Reduced effectiveness and an increased incidence of breakthrough bleeding have been associated with the use of oral contraceptives with antibiotics such as rifampicin, ampicillin, and tetracycline or with certain other drugs, such as barbiturates, phenylbutazone or phenytoin sodium. You should use an additional means of contraception during any cycle in which any of these drugs are taken.

1. What to Tell your Doctor.
You can make use of the pill as safe as possible by telling your doctor if you have any of the following:

a. Conditions that mean you should not use oral contraceptives:
Clots in the legs or lungs.
Clots in the legs or lungs in the past.
A stroke, heart attack, or angina pectoris.
Known or suspected cancer of the breast or sex organs.
Unusual vaginal bleeding that has not yet been diagnosed.
Known or suspected pregnancy.

b. Conditions that your doctor will want to watch closely or which might cause him to suggest another method of contraception:
A family history of breast cancer.
Breast nodules, fibrocystic disease of the breast, or an abnormal mammogram.
Diabetes.
High blood pressure.
High cholesterol.
Cigarette smoking.
Migraine headaches.
Heart or kidney disease.
Epilepsy.
Mental depression.
Fibroid tumors of the uterus.
Gallbladder disease.

c. Once you are using oral contraceptives, you should be alert for signs of a serious adverse effect and call your doctor if they occur:
Sharp pain in the chest, coughing blood, or sudden shortness of breath (indicating possible clots in the lungs).
Pain in the calf (possible clot in the leg).
Crushing chest pain or heaviness (indicating possible heart attack).
Sudden severe headache or vomiting, dizziness or fainting, disturbance of vision or speech or weakness or numbness in an arm or leg (indicating a possible stroke).
Sudden partial or complete loss of vision (indicating a possible clot in the eye).
Breast lumps (you should ask your doctor to show you how to examine your own breasts).
Severe pain in the abdomen (indicating a possible ruptured tumor of the liver).
Severe depression.
Yellowing of the skin (jaundice).

2. How to Take the Pill So That It Is Most Effective.

Dosage and Administration: To achieve maximum contraceptive effectiveness, OVCON-50 or OVCON-35 must be taken exactly as directed and at intervals not exceeding 24 hours.

28-DAY REGIMEN
The patient takes one tablet daily from a convenient package as follows: (yellow or peach tablet containing active ingredients, green tablet containing inert ingredients)

For the first cycle of use only, the first yellow or peach tablet is taken on day 5 of the menstrual cycle, counting the first day of bleeding as day 1. One tablet is taken daily in the same sequence as in the package—first the yellow or peach, and then the green tablets. After the last green tablet is taken, the first yellow or peach tablet from a new package is taken **the following day.** Withdrawal bleeding will usually begin while the patient is taking the green tablets and may continue during the first few tablets from the next package.

21-DAY REGIMEN
The patient takes one tablet daily from a convenient package as follows: (yellow or peach)

For the first cycle of use only, the first yellow or peach tablet is taken on day 5 of the menstrual cycle, counting the first day of bleeding as day 1. Continue taking one tablet daily from the 5th through the 25th day of the menstrual cycle. If the first tablet is taken later than the fifth day of the first menstrual cycle an additional form of contraception should be used for at least one week. Withdrawal bleeding will normally begin within 2-3 days after taking the last tablet. The first tablet of the next package should be taken on the eighth day after the last tablet even if menstrual bleeding has not ceased. The dosage regimen then continues with one tablet daily for 21 days followed by 7 days of no medication, thus a cycle of three-weeks-on and one-week-off.

Patients should be cautioned to follow the dosage schedule strictly.

Evening administration is suggested. If the regimen is interrupted, an additional contraceptive method is recommended for the rest of the cycle. Should spotting or breakthrough bleeding occur, it is recommended that the patient continue medication. If bleeding is persistent or recurrent, the patient should consult her physician.

Use of oral contraceptives in the event of a missed menstrual period:

1. If the patient has not adhered to the prescribed dosage regimen, the possibility of pregnancy should be considered after the first missed period and oral contraceptives should be withheld until pregnancy has been ruled out.

2. If the patient has adhered to the prescribed regimen and misses two consecutive periods, pregnancy should be ruled out before continuing the contraceptive regimen.

At times there may be no menstrual period after a cycle of pills. Therefore, if you miss one menstrual period but have taken the pills **exactly as you were supposed to,** continue as usual into the next cycle. If you have not taken the pills correctly and miss a menstrual period, you may be pregnant and should stop taking oral contraceptives until your doctor determines whether or not you are pregnant. Until you can get to your doctor, use another form of contraception. If two consecutive menstrual periods are missed, you should stop taking pills until it is determined whether you are pregnant. If you do become pregnant while using oral contraceptives, you should discuss the risks to the developing child with your doctor.

3. Periodic Examination.
Your doctor will take a complete medical and family history before prescribing oral contraceptives. At that time and about once a year thereafter, he will generally examine your blood pressure, breasts, abdomen, and pelvic organs (including a Papanicolaou smear, i.e., test for cancer).

Summary: Oral contraceptives are the most effective method, except sterilization, for preventing pregnancy. Other methods, when used conscientiously, are also very effective and have fewer risks. The serious risks of oral contraceptives are uncommon and the "pill" is a

Figure 1
Estimated annual number of deaths associated with control of fertility and no control per 100,000 nonsterile women, by regimen of control and age of women

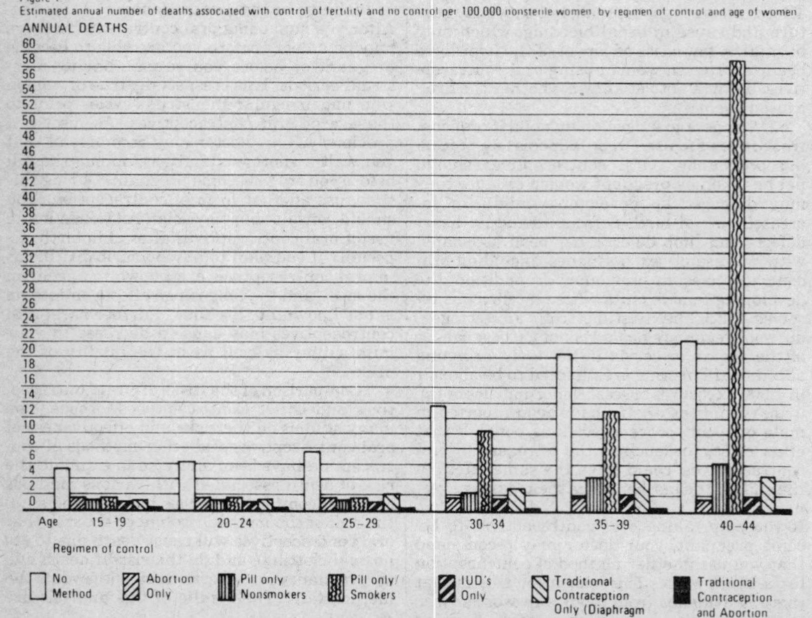

very convenient method of preventing pregnancy.
If you have certain conditions or have had these conditions in the past, you should not use oral contraceptives because the risk is too great. These conditions are listed in the leaflet. If you do not have these conditions, and decide to use the "pill," please read the leaflet carefully so that you can use the "pill" most safely and effectively.
Based on his or her assessment of your medical needs, your doctor has prescribed this drug for you. Do not give the drug to anyone else.
July, 1980
[*Shown in Product Identification Section*]

PERI–COLACE® capsules • syrup
Casanthranol and docusate sodium

Description: Peri-Colace is a combination of the mild stimulant laxative Peristim (casanthranol, Mead Johnson) and the stool-softener Colace (docusate sodium, Mead Johnson). Each capsule contains 30 mg of Peristim and 100 mg of Colace; the syrup contains 30 mg of Peristim and 60 mg of Colace per 15-ml tablespoon (10 mg of Peristim and 20 mg of Colace per 5-ml teaspoon) and 10% alcohol.
Action and Uses: Peri-Colace provides gentle peristaltic stimulation and helps to keep stools soft for easier passage. Bowel movement is induced gently—usually overnight or in 8 to 12 hours. Nausea, griping, abnormally loose stools, and constipation rebound are minimized. Useful in management of chronic or temporary constipation.
Note: To prevent hard stools when laxative stimulation is not needed or undesirable, see Colace (stool softener).
Side Effects: The incidence of side effects—none of a serious nature—is exceedingly small. Nausea, abdominal cramping or discomfort, diarrhea, and rash are the main side effects reported.
Administration and Dosage: *Adults*—1 or 2 capsules, or 1 or 2 tablespoons syrup at bedtime, or as indicated. In severe cases, dosage may be increased to 2 capsules or 2 tablespoons twice daily, or 3 capsules at bedtime. *Children*—1 to 3 teaspoons of syrup at bedtime, or as indicated.
Warning: Do not use when abdominal pain, nausea, or vomiting are present. Frequent or prolonged use of this preparation may result in dependence on laxatives.
Overdosage: In addition to symptomatic treatment, gastric lavage, if timely, is recommended in cases of large overdosage.
How Supplied: Peri-Colace® Capsules
NDC 0087-0715-43 Cartons of 10 single unit packs
NDC 0087-0715-01 Bottles of 30
NDC 0087-0715-02 Bottles of 60
NDC 0087-0715-03 Bottles of 250
NDC 0087-0715-05 Bottles of 1000
NDC 0087-0715-07 Cartons of 100 single unit packs
Note: Peri-Colace capsules should be stored at controlled room temperatures (15°–30° C or 59°–86° F).
Peri-Colace® Syrup
NDC 0087-0721-01 Bottles of 8 fl. oz.
NDC 0087-0721-02 Bottles of 16 fl. oz.
[*Shown in Product Identification Section*]

QUESTRAN® ℞
(Cholestyramine resin)

Description: Questran (cholestyramine resin), the chloride salt of a basic anion exchange resin, a cholesterol lowering agent, is intended for oral administration. Cholestyramine resin is quite hydrophilic, but insoluble in water. The cholestyramine resin in Questran is not absorbed from the digestive tract. Nine grams of Questran contain 4 grams of anhydrous cholestyramine resin.
Clinical Pharmacology: Cholesterol is probably the sole precursor of bile acids. During normal digestion, bile acids are secreted into the intestines. A major portion of the bile acids is absorbed from the intestinal tract and returned to the liver via the enterohepatic circulation. Only very small amounts of bile acids are found in normal serum.
Questran resin adsorbs and combines with the bile acids in the intestine to form an insoluble complex which is excreted in the feces. This results in a partial removal of bile acids from the enterohepatic circulation by preventing their absorption.
The increased fecal loss of bile acids due to Questran administration leads to an increased oxidation of cholesterol to bile acids, a decrease in beta lipoprotein or low density lipoprotein plasma levels and a decrease in serum cholesterol levels. Although in man Questran (cholestyramine resin) produces an increase in hepatic synthesis of cholesterol, plasma cholesterol levels fall.
In patients with partial biliary obstruction, the reduction of serum bile acid levels by Questran reduces excess bile acids deposited in the dermal tissue with resultant decrease in pruritus.
Indications: Since no drug is innocuous, strict attention should be paid to the indications and contraindications, particularly when selecting drugs for chronic long term use.

1) *Questran is indicated as adjunctive therapy to diet for the reduction of elevated serum cholesterol in patients with primary hypercholesterolemia (elevated low density lipoproteins). Questran may be useful to lower elevated cholesterol that occurs in patients with combined hypercholesterolemia and hypertriglyceridemia, but it is not indicated where hypertriglyceridemia is the abnormality of most concern.*

It has not been established whether the drug-induced lowering of serum cholesterol or triglyceride levels has a beneficial effect, no effect, or a detrimental effect on the morbidity or mortality due to atherosclerosis including coronary heart disease. Current investigations now in progress may yield an answer to this question.

2) For the relief of pruritus associated with partial biliary obstruction. Questran has been shown to have a variable effect on serum cholesterol in these patients. Patients with primary biliary cirrhosis may exhibit an elevated cholesterol as part of their desease.

Contraindications: Questran is contraindicated in patients with complete biliary obstruction where bile is not secreted into the intestine and in those individuals who have shown hypersensitivity to any of its components.
Warnings: In studies conducted in rats in which cholestyramine resin was used as a tool to investigate the role of various intestinal factors, such as fat, bile salts and microbial flora, in the development of intestinal tumors induced by potent carcinogens, the incidence of such tumors was observed to be greater in cholestyramine resin treated rats than in control rats.
The relevance of this laboratory observation from studies in rats to the clinical use of Questran is not known, especially in view of the absence of any suggestion of increased tumor incidence associated with the long-term use of the drug in man.
Precautions:
General
Before instituting therapy with Questran (cholestyramine resin) an attempt should be made to control serum cholesterol by appropriate dietary regimen, weight reduction, and the treatment of any underlying disorder which might be the cause of the hypercholesterolemia. Serum cholesterol levels should be determined frequently during the first few months of therapy and periodically thereafter. A favorable trend in cholesterol reduction should occur during the first month of Questran therapy. The therapy should be continued to sustain cholesterol reduction. Serum triglyceride levels should be measured periodically to detect whether significant changes have occurred.
Because cholestyramine binds bile acids, Questran may interfere with normal fat digestion and absorption and thus may prevent absorption of fat soluble vitamins such as A, D and K. When Questran is given for long periods of time, concomitant supplementation with a water-miscible (or parenteral) form of vitamins A and D should be considered. Chronic use of Questran may be associated with increased bleeding tendency due to hypoprothrombinemia associated with Vitamin K deficiency. This will usually respond promptly to parenteral Vitamin K_1 and recurrences can be prevented by oral administration of Vitamin K_1. Reduction of serum or red cell folate has been reported over long term administration of Questran. Supplementation with folic acid should be considered in these cases.
There is a possibility that prolonged use of Questran, since it is a chloride form of anion exchange resin, may produce hyperchloremic acidosis. This would especially be true in younger and smaller patients where the relative dosage may be higher.
Questran may produce or worsen pre-existing constipation. Dosage should be reduced or discontinued in such cases. Fecal impaction and aggravated hemorrhoids may occur. Every effort should be made to avert severe constipation and its inherent problems in those patients with clinically symptomatic coronary artery disease.
This product contains FD&C Yellow No. 5 (tartrazine) which may cause allergic-type reactions (including bronchial asthma) in certain susceptible individuals. Although the overall incidence of FD&C Yellow No. 5 (tartrazine) sensitivity in the general population is low, it is frequently seen in patients who also have aspirin hypersensitivity.
Drug Interactions
Questran may delay or reduce the absorption of concomitant oral medication such as phenylbutazone, warfarin, chlorothiazide (acidic), as well as tetracycline, penicillin G, phenobarbital, thyroid and thyroxine preparations, and digitalis. The discontinuance of the Questran (cholestyramine resin) could pose a hazard to health if a potentially toxic drug such as digitalis has been titrated to a maintenance level while the patient was taking Questran.
SINCE QUESTRAN MAY BIND OTHER DRUGS GIVEN CONCURRENTLY, PATIENTS SHOULD TAKE OTHER DRUGS AT LEAST ONE HOUR BEFORE OR 4–6 HOURS AFTER QUESTRAN TO AVOID IMPEDING THEIR ABSORPTION OR AT AS GREAT AN INTERVAL AS POSSIBLE.
Carcinogenesis, Mutagenesis and Impairment of fertility
See Warnings section.
Usage in Pregnancy
Since Questran is not absorbed systemically, it is not expected to cause fetal harm when administered during pregnancy in recommended dosages. There are, however, no adequate and well controlled studies in pregnant women and, the known interference with absorption of fat soluble vitamins may be detrimental even in the presence of supplementation.
Nursing Mothers
Caution should be exercised when Questran is administered to a nursing mother.
Pediatric Use
As experience in infants and children is limited, a practical dosage schedule has not been established.

Continued on next page

Mead Johnson Pharm.—Cont.

In calculating pediatric dosages, 44.4 mg of anhydrous cholestyramine resin are contained in 100 mg of Questran.
The effects of long term drug administration, as well as its effect in maintaining lowered cholesterol levels in pediatric patients, are unknown.
Adverse Reactions: The most common adverse reaction is constipation. Predisposing factors for most of these complaints when used as a cholesterol lowering agent are high dose and increased age (more than 60 years old). Most instances of constipation are mild, transient, and controlled with conventional therapy. Some patients require a temporary decrease in dosage or discontinuation of therapy.
Less Frequent Adverse Reactions: Abdominal discomfort, flatulence, nausea, vomiting, diarrhea, heartburn, anorexia, indigestive feeling and steatorrhea, bleeding tendencies due to hypoprothrombinemia (Vitamin K deficiency) as well as Vitamin A (one case of night blindness reported) and D deficiencies, hyperchloremic acidosis in children, and osteoporosis. Rash and irritation of the skin, tongue and perianal area. One ten month old baby with biliary atresia had an impaction presumed to be due to Questran (cholestyramine resin) after three days administration of 9 grams daily. She developed acute intestinal sepsis and died. Occasional calcified material has been observed in the biliary tree, including calcification of the gall bladder, in patients to whom cholestyramine resin has been given. However, this may be a manifestation of the liver disease and not drug related.
One patient experienced biliary colic on each of three occasions on which he took Questran. One patient diagnosed as acute abdominal symptom complex was found to have a "pasty mass" in the transverse colon on x-ray.
Other events (not necessarily drug-related) reported in patients taking Questran include: GI-rectal bleeding, black stools, hemorrhoidal bleeding, bleeding from known duodenal ulcer, dysphagia, hiccups, ulcer attack, sour taste, pancreatitis, rectal pain, diverticulitis.
Hematologic—Decreased prothrombin time, ecchymosis, anemia.
Hypersensitivity—Urticaria, asthma, wheezing, shortness of breath.
Musculoskeletal—Backache, muscle and joint pains, arthritis.
Neurologic—Headache, anxiety, vertigo, dizziness, fatigue, tinnitus, syncope, drowsiness, femoral nerve pain, paresthesia.
Eye—Uveitis.
Renal—Hematuria, dysuria, burnt odor to urine, diuresis.
Miscellaneous—Weight loss, weight gain, increased libido, swollen glands, edema, dental bleeding.
Overdosage: Overdosage of Questran has not been reported. Should overdosage occur, however, the chief potential harm would be obstruction of the gastrointestinal tract. The location of such potential obstruction, the degree of obstruction, and the presence or absence of normal gut motility would determine treatment.
Dosage and Administration: The recommended adult dose is one packet or one scoopful (9 grams of Questran contain 4 grams of anhydrous cholestyramine resin) three or four times daily. Dosage may be adjusted as required to meet the patient's needs.
Questran should not be taken in its dry form. Always mix Questran powder with water or other fluids before ingesting. See Preparation Instructions.
Preparation: The color of Questran (cholestyramine resin) may vary somewhat from batch to batch, but this variation does not affect the performance of the product. Mix contents of one packet or one level scoopful of Questran with 2 to 6 fluid ounces of the preferred beverage (water, milk, fruit juice or other noncarbonated beverage).
Questran may also be mixed with highly fluid soups or pulpy fruits with a high moisture content, such as applesauce or crushed pineapple.
How Supplied: Questran is available in cartons of fifty 9-gram packets and in cans containing 378 grams. Each nine grams of Questran contain 4 grams of anhydrous cholestyramine resin.
NDC0087-0580-01 Cartons of 50 packets
NDC0087-0580-05 Cans, 378 gm
6505-00-105-0372 (Cartons of 50 packets)
Defense
VA6505-00-105-0372A (Cartons of 50 packets)

QUIBRON® ℞
(Theophylline-Guaifenesin)

Description: Each Quibron® soft gelatin capsule or tablespoon (15 ml) of liquid contains 150 mg of theophylline (anhydrous) and 90 mg of guaifenesin, as an oral bronchodilator-expectorant.
Quibron Liquid contains no alcohol and is dye-free.

QUIBRON®-300 ℞
(Theophylline-Guaifenesin)

Description: Each Quibron®-300 soft gelatin capsule contains 300 mg of theophylline (anhydrous) and 180 mg of guaifenesin, as an oral bronchodilator-expectorant.
Theophylline, a xanthine compound, is a white, odorless crystalline powder, having a bitter taste.
Guaifenesin, a guaiacol compound, is a white to slightly yellow crystalline powder with a bitter, aromatic taste.
Clinical Pharmacology:
Theophylline
Mode of Action
Theophylline acts as a bronchodilator by direct relaxation of bronchial smooth muscle. Theophylline is a competitive inhibitor of cyclic nucleotide phosphodiesterase resulting in increased intracellular levels of cAMP which mediates smooth muscle relaxation. Like some other xanthines, theophylline acts as a coronary vasodilator, cardiac stimulant, skeletal muscle stimulant, central nervous system stimulant and diuretic.
Pharmacokinetics
As theophylline is released from the formulation it is, under usual conditions, absorbed completely and fairly rapidly. Excretion, principally as inactive metabolites, occurs primarily via the kidney. The half-life of theophylline varies among individuals with a wide range having been documented. Theophylline half-life is shortened in cigarette smokers. Half-life is prolonged in alcoholism, reduced hepatic or renal function, congestive heart failure and in patients receiving antibiotics such as troleandomycin or erythromycin. High fever for prolonged periods may decrease theophylline elimination. The theophylline half-life is generally shorter in children.
Representative Theophylline Serum Half-lives

	Half-life (hours)	
	Mean	Range
Adults		
non-smokers	8.7	6.1–12.8
smokers	5.5	4.0– 7.7
congestive heart failure	22.9	3.1–82.0
Children (6–16 yrs)	3.7	1.4– 7.9

Therapeutic serum theophylline levels are usually 10–20 μg/ml.
Binding to plasma proteins is not extensive and theophylline is not preferentially taken up by any particular organ.
Theophylline-containing products may increase the plasma levels of free fatty acids and the urinary levels of epinephrine and norepinephrine.
Apparently no development of tolerance occurs with chronic use of theophylline.
Clinical Pharmacology:
Guaifenesin
Mode of Action
Guaifenesin increases respiratory tract secretions, possibly by stimulating the goblet cells.
Pharmacokinetics
Guaifenesin appears to be well absorbed, but its pharmacokinetics has not been well studied.
Indications and Usage:
Quibron and Quibron-300 are indicated for the symptomatic treatment of bronchospasm associated with such conditions as bronchial asthma, chronic bronchitis and pulmonary emphysema.
Contraindications:
Quibron products are contraindicated in individuals who have shown hypersensitivity to any of their components or xanthine derivatives.
Warnings:
Excessive theophylline doses may be associated with toxicity; thus serum theophylline levels should be monitored to assure maximal benefit without excessive risk.
Serum levels of theophylline above the accepted therapeutic range (10–20 μg/ml) are associated with an increased incidence of toxicity. Such levels may be reached with customary doses in individuals who metabolize the drug slowly, especially patients (1) with lowered body plasma clearance (2) with liver dysfunction or chronic obstructive pulmonary disease or (3) older than 55 years of age, particularly males.
Serious toxicity, such as seizure or ventricular arrhythmias, is not necessarily preceded by less serious side-effects such as nausea, irritability or restlessness.
Many patients who have higher (greater than 20 μg/ml) theophylline serum levels exhibit tachycardia. Theophylline products may exacerbate pre-existing arrhythmias.
Precautions:
General
Use with caution in patients with severe cardiac disease, hypertension, acute myocardial injury, congestive heart failure, cor pulmonale, severe hypoxemia, hyperthyroidism, hepatic impairment, history of peptic ulcer, alcoholism and in the elderly. Concurrent administration with certain antibiotics (see DRUG INTERACTIONS section) may result in increased serum theophylline levels.
A decrease in serum half-life is seen in smokers (see Clinical Pharmacology/Pharmacokinetics).
Particular caution should be used in administering theophylline to patients in congestive heart failure. Reduced theophylline clearance in these patients may cause theophylline blood levels to persist long after discontinuing the drug.
Theophylline should not be administered concurrently with other xanthine medications.
Usage in Pregnancy
Teratogenic effects: Pregnancy Category C. Animal reproduction studies have not been conducted with Quibron products. It is also not known whether Quibron products can cause fetal harm when administered to a pregnant woman or can affect reproduction capacity. Quibron products should be given to a pregnant woman only if clearly indicated.
Nonteratogenic effects: It is not known whether use of this drug during labor or delivery has immediate or delayed adverse effects on the fetus, or whether it prolongs the duration of labor or increases the possibility of forceps delivery or other obstetrical intervention.
Nursing Mothers
Theophylline has been reported to be excreted in human milk and to have caused irritability in a nursing infant. Because of the potential for serious adverse reactions, a decision should be made whether to discontinue nursing or to dis-

continue Quibron or Quibron–300, taking into account the importance of this drug to the mother.

Drug Interactions

Drug	Effect
Theophylline with lithium carbonate	Increased renal excretion of lithium
Theophylline with propranolol	Mutual antagonism of therapeutic effects
Theophylline with cimetidine	Increased serum theophylline levels
Theophylline with clindamycin	Increased serum theophylline levels
Theophylline with lincomycin	Increased serum theophylline levels
Theophylline with troleandomycin or erythromycin	Increased serum theophylline levels

Drug/Laboratory Test Interactions

Theophylline may interfere with the assay of uric acid, especially the phosphotungstate method. Thus, serum uric acid levels may be overestimated. Metabolites of guaifenesin may contribute to increased 5–hydroxyindoleacetic acid readings when determined with nitrosonaphthol reagent.

Adverse Reactions: The frequency of adverse reactions is related to serum theophylline levels and is usually not a problem at levels below 20 μg/ml. The most consistent adverse reactions are usually due to overdosage and, while all have not been reported with Quibron or Quibron-300, the following reactions may be considered when theophylline is administered. Central nervous system: clonic and tonic generalized convulsions, muscle twitching, reflex hyperexcitability, headaches, insomnia, restlessness, and irritability. Cardiovascular: circulatory failure, ventricular arrhythmias, hypotension, extrasystoles, tachycardia, palpitation, and flushing. Gastrointestinal: hematemesis, vomiting, diarrhea, epigastric pain, and nausea. Renal: increased excretion of renal tubular cells and red blood cells, albuminuria, and diuresis. Respiratory: tachypnea. Others: hyperglycemia and inappropriate ADH syndrome.

Overdosage:

Symptoms

Nervousness, agitation, headache, insomnia, vomiting, tachycardia, extrasystoles, hyperreflexia, fasciculations and clonic and tonic convulsions. Children may be particularly prone to restlessness and hyperactivity that can proceed to convulsions.

Management

If potential oral overdose is established and seizure has **not** occurred.

1. Induce vomiting.
2. Administer a cathartic (this is particularly important if sustained release preparations have been taken).
3. Administer activated charcoal.
4. Monitor vital signs, maintain blood pressure and provide adequate hydration.

If patient is having seizure

1. Establish an airway.
2. Administer O_2.
3. Treat the seizure with intravenous diazepam 0.1 to 0.3 mg/kg up to 10 mg.
4. Monitor vital signs, maintain blood pressure and provide adequate hydration.

Post-Seizure Coma

1. Maintain airway and oxygenation.
2. If a result of oral medication, follow above recommendations to prevent absorption of drug, but intubation and lavage will have to be performed instead of inducing emesis and the cathartic and charcoal will need to be introduced via a large bore gastric lavage tube.
3. Continue to provide full supportive care and adequate hydration while waiting for drug to be metabolized. In general, the drug is metabolized rapidly enough so as to not warrant consideration of dialysis.

General

The oral LD_{50} of theophylline in mice is 350 mg/kg. The oral LD_{50} of guaifenesin in mice is 1725 mg/kg. In humans, adverse reactions often occur when serum theophylline levels exceed 20 μg/ml. Information on physiological variables which influence excretion of theophylline can be found under the heading "Clinical Pharmacology."

Dosage and Administration:

General

Therapeutic serum levels associated with optimal likelihood for benefit and minimal risk of toxicity are considered to be between 10 and 20 μg/ml, although levels of 5-10 μg/ml are reported to be effective for some patients. Levels above 20 μg/ml may produce toxic effects. There is great variation from patient to patient and dosage must be individualized because there is a relatively narrow range between therapeutic and toxic levels of theophylline. Monitoring of serum theophylline levels is highly recommended. Since theophylline does not distribute into fatty tissue, dosage should be calculated on the basis of ideal body weight. Giving theophylline with food may prevent the rare case of stomach irritation and, although absorption may be slower, it is still complete.

Quibron

Treatment should be *initiated* at a dose of 16 mg/kg/day or 400 mg/day, whichever is smaller. The usual adjusted dosages are—Adults: 1–2 capsules or 1–2 tablespoons (15 ml) liquid every 6–8 hours. Children 9 to 12: 4–5 mg theophylline/kg body weight every 6–8 hours. Children under 9: 4–6 mg theophylline/kg body weight every 6–8 hours.

Approximate mg/kg dosage by TEASPOON (5 ml) of Quibron Liquid may be determined from the following table:

BODY WEIGHT		AVERAGE DOSAGE IN TEASPOONS (5 ml) TO PROVIDE THE FOLLOWING MG OF THEOPHYLLINE/KG BODY WEIGHT/DOSE		
Lbs	Kgs	4 mg/kg	5 mg/kg	6 mg/kg
20	9	3/4	1	1
30	14	1	1½	1¾
40	18	1½	2	2¼
50	23	1¾	2¼	2¾
60	27	2	2¾	3¼
70	32	2½	3	3¾
80	36	3	3½	4¼
90	41	3¼	4	5
100	46	3½	4½	5½

If the desired response is not achieved with the recommended initial dose, and there are no adverse reactions, the dose may be cautiously adjusted upward in increments of no more than 25 percent at 2–3 day intervals until the following MAXIMUM DOSE WITHOUT MEASUREMENT OF SERUM CONCENTRATION or a maximum of 900 mg in any 24 hour period (whichever is less) is attained:

MAXIMUM DAILY DOSE WITHOUT MEASUREMENT OF SERUM CONCENTRATION

	mg per kg Body Weight*
Children (under 9)	24
Children (9–12)	20
Adolescents (12–16)	18
Adults	13

*Use ideal body weight for obese patients

Do not attempt to maintain any dose that is not tolerated. If doses higher than those contained in the above MAXIMUM DOSE WITHOUT MEASUREMENT OF SERUM CONCENTRATION are necessary, it is recommended that serum theophylline levels be monitored. For therapeutic levels, draw blood sample just before next dose is due; for toxic levels, draw blood sample when last dose peaks (~2 hours after dosing). It is important that the patient has missed no doses during the previous 72 hours and that dosing intervals have been reasonably typical with no added doses during that period of time. DOSAGE ADJUSTMENT BASED ON SERUM THEOPHYLLINE MEASUREMENTS WHEN THESE INSTRUCTIONS HAVE **NOT** BEEN FOLLOWED, MAY RESULT IN RECOMMENDATIONS THAT PRESENT RISK OF TOXICITY TO THE PATIENT.

Quibron-300 Capsules

Quibron-300 is appropriate therapy when higher theophylline dosages are required. The usual recommended dosages for Quibron-300 are **Adults:** 1 capsule every 6–8 hours for patients whose dosage has been adjusted upward to achieve therapeutic serum levels.

How Supplied:

Quibron® Capsules (yellow) in bottles of 100 (NDC 0087-0516-01); and 1000 (NDC 0087-0516-02, 6505-00-764-3366 Defense); Unit Dose 100's (NDC 0087-0516-03).

Quibron® Liquid in 1 pint (NDC 0087-0510-03) and 1 gallon (NDC 0087-0510-01).

Quibron®-300 Capsules (yellow and white) in bottles of 100 (NDC 0087-0515-41).

Store at controlled room temperature of 15–30°C (59–86°F).

[*Shown in Product Identification Section*]

QUIBRON PLUS® ℞

(Theophylline, Guaifenesin, Ephedrine and Butabarbital)

Description: Each Quibron Plus capsule or tablespoon (15 ml) of elixir contains theophylline (anhydrous) 150 mg, guaifenesin 100 mg, ephedrine HCl 25 mg, and butabarbital 20 mg (Warning: may be habit-forming) as an oral bronchodilator-expectorant. Elixir contains alcohol 15%.

Clinical Pharmacology:

Theophylline:

Mode of Action

Theophylline acts as a bronchodilator by direct relaxation of bronchial smooth muscle. Theophylline is a competitive inhibitor of cyclic nucleotide phosphodiesterase resulting in increased intracellular levels of cAMP which mediates smooth muscle relaxation. Like some other xanthines, theophylline acts as a coronary vasodilator, cardiac stimulant, skeletal muscle stimulant, central nervous system stimulant and diuretic.

Pharmacokinetics

Theophylline is, under usual conditions, absorbed completely and fairly rapidly. Excretion, principally as inactive metabolites, occurs primarily via the kidney. The half-life of theophylline varies among individuals with a wide range having been documented. Theophylline half-life is shortened in cigarette smokers. Half-life is prolonged in alcoholism, reduced hepatic or renal function, congestive heart failure and patients receiving antibiotics such as troleandomycin or erythromycin. High fever for prolonged periods may decrease theophylline elimination. The theophylline half-life is generally shorter in children.

Representative Theophylline Serum Half-Lives

	Half-life (hours) Mean	Range
Adults		
non-smokers	8.7	6.1 – 12.8
smokers	5.5	4.0 – 7.7
congestive heart failure	22.9	3.1 – 82.0
Children (6–16 yrs.)	3.7	1.4 – 7.9

Therapeutic serum theophylline levels are usually 10–20 μg/ml when theophylline is administered as the sole bronchodilator agent. Binding to plasma proteins is not extensive and theophylline is not preferentially taken up by any particular organ.

Theophylline-containing products may increase the plasma levels of free fatty acids and

Continued on next page

Mead Johnson Pharm.—Cont.

the urinary levels of epinephrine and norepinephrine. Apparently no development of tolerance occurs with chronic use of theophylline.

Guaifenesin:

Mode of Action

Guaifenesin increases respiratory tract secretions, possibly by stimulating the goblet cells.

Pharmacokinetics

Guaifenesin appears to be well absorbed, but its pharmacokinetics has not been well studied.

Ephedrine:

Mode of Action

Ephedrine acts as a bronchodilator by stimulating β-adrenergic receptors with a resulting increase in intracellular cAMP which mediates smooth muscle relaxation. Ephedrine stimulates both α- and β-adrenergic receptors and acts as a cardiac and CNS stimulant and a vasoconstrictor.

Pharmacokinetics

Ephedrine appears to be well-absorbed and has a reasonably long duration of action, but its pharmacokinetics has not been well-studied.

Butabarbital:

Mode of Action

Butabarbital reversibly depresses the activity of all excitable tissues probably by interfering with the chemical transmission across neuronal and neuroeffector junctions.

Pharmacokinetics

Barbiturates in general appear to be well-absorbed. The rate-limiting step in absorption is usually the dissolution and dispersal of the drug in the gastrointestinal contents. Food may decrease the rate of absorption, but not the amount absorbed. Otherwise, the specific pharmacokinetics of butabarbital has not been well studied.

Indications and Usage:

Indications

Based on a review of a similar drug by the National Academy of Sciences-National Research Council and/or other information, FDA has classified the indications as follows:

"Possibly" effective: bronchial asthma; bronchitis, bronchiectasis, and emphysema in which bronchospasm is present, or for the relief of bronchospasm. Final classification of the less-than-effective indications requires further investigation.

Contraindications: Quibron Plus is contraindicated in individuals who have shown hypersensitivity to any of its components or xanthine derivatives. Because of its ephedrine content Quibron Plus should not be administered within 14 days following administration of monoamine oxidase (MAO) inhibitors.

Warnings: Serum levels of theophylline above the accepted therapeutic range (10–20 μg/ml) are associated with an increased incidence of toxicity. Such levels may be reached with customary doses in individuals who metabolize the drug slowly, especially patients (1) with lowered body plasma clearance, (2) with liver dysfunction or chronic obstructive pulmonary disease, or (3) older than 55 years of age, particularly males.

Serious toxicity, such as a seizure or ventricular arrhythmia, is not necessarily preceded by less serious side effects such as nausea, irritability, or restlessness. Many patients who have higher (greater than 20 μg/ml) theophylline serum levels exhibit tachycardia. Theophylline products may exacerbate pre-existing arrhythmias.

Use cautiously in patients with degenerative heart disease (anginal pain may be induced in patients with angina pectoris) and in hyperthyroid or hypertensive individuals who are particularly susceptible to the pressor response to ephedrine. Butabarbital may be habit-forming.

Precautions:

General

Use with caution in patients with severe cardiac disease (including angina pectoris, cardiac arrhythmias and coronary insufficiency), hypertension, acute myocardial injury, congestive heart failure, cor pulmonale, severe hypoxemia, hyperthyroidism, hepatic impairment, history of peptic ulcer, alcoholism, drug-dependence or abuse, pain, porphyria, hyperkinesis, diabetes mellitus, prostatic hypertrophy, angle-closure glaucoma (or predisposition to it) and in the elderly.

Concurrent administration of barbiturates with several drugs (see DRUG INTERACTIONS) is known to decrease the effect of the principal drug because they induce the formation of drug-metabolizing, hepatic microsomal enzymes.

Concurrent administration with certain antibiotics (see DRUG INTERACTIONS section) may result in increased serum theophylline levels.

The incidence of side effects has been reported to be increased in patients receiving both theophylline and ephedrine.

A decrease in serum half-life is seen in smokers (see Clinical Pharmacology/Pharmacokinetics).

Particular caution should be used in administering theophylline to patients in congestive heart failure. Reduced theophylline clearance in these patients may cause theophylline blood levels to persist long after discontinuing the drug. Theophylline should not be administered concurrently with other xanthine medications.

Drug Interactions

Drug	Effect
Theophylline with lithium carbonate	Increased renal excretion of lithium
Theophylline with propranolol	Mutual antagonism of therapeutic effects
Theophylline with cimetidine	Increased serum theophylline levels
Theophylline with clindamycin	Increased serum theophylline levels
Theophylline with lincomycin	Increased serum theophylline levels
Theophylline with troleandomycin or erythromycin	Increased serum theophylline levels
Ephedrine with general anesthetics or digitalis glycosides	Cardiac arrhythmias
Ephedrine with ergonovine or methylergonovine or oxytocin	Severe hypertension
Ephedrine with guanethidine	Decreased hypotensive effect
Ephedrine with monoamine oxidase inhibitors	Potentiated pressor effect with hypertensive crisis
Ephedrine with other sympathomimetics	Increased sympathetic stimulation and potential for side effects
Butabarbital with alcohol, general anesthetics, CNS depressants, or monoamine oxidase inhibitors	Increased therapeutic effects
Butabarbital with oral anticoagulants, corticosteroid, digitalis, digitoxin or doxycycline or tricyclic antidepressants	Decreased therapeutic effects due to increased metabolism resulting from induction of hepatic microsomal enzymes
Butabarbital with griseofulvin	Decreased therapeutic effects due to impaired absorption

Drug/Laboratory Test Interactions

Theophylline may interfere with the assay of uric acid, especially the phosphotungstate method. Thus, serum uric acid levels may be overestimated. Metabolites of guaifenesin may contribute to increased 5-hydroxy-indoleacetic acid readings when determined with nitrosonaphthol reagent.

Carcinogenesis, Mutagenesis, Impairment of Fertility

Long-term animal studies have not been conducted to evaluate the carcinogenic potential of Quibron Plus.

Use in Pregnancy

Teratogenic effects: Pregnancy Category C. Animal reproduction studies have not been conducted with Quibron Plus. It is also not known whether Quibron Plus can cause fetal harm when administered to a pregnant woman or can affect reproduction capacity. Quibron Plus should be given to a pregnant woman only if clearly indicated.

Nonteratogenic Effects: Barbiturates such as butabarbital cross the placental barrier and may cause respiratory depression in the neonate or neonatal hemorrhage due to a reduced level of vitamin-K-dependent clotting factors. Chronic use may cause physical dependence in the neonate with resulting withdrawal symptoms.

Since barbiturates are known to cross the placenta, chronic use of one of this class of drugs during pregnancy may cause physical dependence with resulting withdrawal symptoms in the neonate. Use during late pregnancy or labor may cause respiratory depression in the neonate (especially the premature neonate) because of immature hepatic function.

Nursing Mothers: Theophylline, ephedrine, and barbiturates such as butabarbital have been reported to be excreted in human milk. Because of the potential for serious adverse reactions in nursing infants from Quibron Plus, a decision should be made whether to discontinue nursing or to discontinue the drug, taking into account the importance of the drug to the mother.

Adverse Reactions: The frequency of adverse reactions due to theophylline is related to serum levels and is usually not a problem at levels below 20 μg/ml. The most consistent adverse reactions are usually due to overdosage and, while all have not been reported with Quibron Plus, the following reactions may be considered when theophylline is administered.

Central nervous system: clonic and tonic generalized convulsions, muscle twitching, reflex hyperexcitability, headaches, insomnia, restlessness, and irritability. Cardiovascular: circulatory failure, ventricular arrhythmias, hypotension, extrasystoles, tachycardia, palpitation, and flushing. Gastrointestinal: hermatemesis, vomiting, diarrhea, epigastric pain, and nausea. Renal: increased excretion of renal tubular cells and red blood cells, albuminuria, and diuresis. Respiratory: tachypnea. Others: hyperglycemia and inappropriate ADH syndrome.

The following reactions may be considered when ephedrine is administered. Central nervous system: dizziness or lightheadedness, headache, nervousness, restlessness, trembling, trouble in sleeping, weakness. Cardiovascular: palpitation, chest pain, tachycardia, peripheral vasoconstriction, flushing. Gastrointestinal: epigastric pain, nausea, vomiting. Renal: difficulty of micturition. Respiratory: troubled breathing. Others: unusual increase in sweating.

The following reactions may be considered when butabarbital is administered: Central nervous system: mental confusion or depression, unusual excitement, clumsiness, unsteadiness, dizziness or lightheadedness, drowsiness, headache, joint or muscle pain, slurred speech, possible withdrawal symptoms including convulsions or seizures, feeling faint, hallucinations, increased dreaming, nightmares, trembling, trouble in sleeping, unusual restlessness, unusual weakness. Cardiovascular: unusually slow heart beat. Gastrointestinal: diarrhea, nausea, vomiting. Respiratory: shortness of breath, wheezing or tightness in chest. Other: Skin rash or hives or swelling of eyelids, face or lips, sore throat and fever, unusual bleeding or bruising, yellowing of eyes or skin, joint or muscle pain.

Overdosage:

Symptoms

Overdosage due to theophylline and ephedrine: nervousness, agitation, headache, insomnia, vomiting, tachycardia, extrasystoles, hyperreflexia, fasciculations and clonic and tonic convulsions.

Overdosage due to butabarbital: coma, early hypothermia, late fever, sluggish or absent reflexes, respiratory depression, gradual appearance of circulatory collapse and pulmonary edema.

Management

If potential overdosage is established and the patient is conscious:

1. Induce vomiting
2. Administer a cathartic
3. Administer activated charcoal
4. Monitor vital signs, maintain blood pressure and provide adequate hydration.

If the patient is having a seizure:

1. Establish an airway.
2. Administer O_2.
3. Treat seizure with intravenous diazepam 0.1 to 0.3 mk/kg up to 10 mg.
4. Monitor vital signs, maintain blood pressure and provide adequate hydration.

If the patient is in a coma:

1. Maintain airway and oxygenation.
2. Aspirate stomach contents, taking care to avoid pulmonary aspiration. Administer a cathartic and charcoal via a large bore gastric lavage tube.
3. Monitor vital signs and provide full supportive care and adequate hydration.
4. If renal function is normal, forced diuresis may aid in the elimination of the barbiturate.

General

The oral LD_{50} of theophylline in mice is 350 mg/kg. In humans, adverse reactions often occur when serum theophylline levels exceed 20 μg/ml. The oral LD_{50} of ephedrine in mice is 283 mg/kg. The oral LD_{50} of butabarbital in mice is 204 mg/kg, and the oral LD_{50} of guaifenesin in mice is 1725 mg/kg.

Dosage and Administration

Dosage should be adjusted on an individual basis. Administration with food may prevent the rare case of stomach irritation and absorption, although it may be slower, should still be complete.

Dosage:

Adults: 1–2 capsules or 1–2 tablespoons (15–30 ml) elixir 2–3 times daily.

Children 8–12: 1 capsule or 1 tablespoon (15 ml) elixir 2–3 times daily.

Children under 8: Up to ½ teaspoon (2–5 ml) elixir per 10 lb body weight 2–3 times daily.

How Supplied:

QUIBRON PLUS Capsules (green) in bottles of 100 (NDC-0087-0518-01).

QUIBRON PLUS Elixir in 1 pint bottles (NDC-0087-0511-01).

Store at controlled room temperature of 15–30°C (59–86°F).

[Shown in Product Identification Section]

QUIBRON®-T ℞

(Theophylline Anhydrous)

DIVIDOSE™ TABLETS

IMMEDIATE RELEASE BRONCHODILATOR

Description: Quibron®-T tablets provide 300 mg of anhydrous theophylline as an oral bronchodilator in an immediate release formulation combined with the convenience of the unique Dividose™ tablet design. With functional trisects and bisects, Quibron-T tablets can be conveniently and accurately divided into 100, 150, and 200 mg segments to provide a variety of dosing increments, as required.

QUIBRON-T tablets

One-third tablet	= 100 mg
One-half tablet	= 150 mg
Two-thirds tablet	= 200 mg
One tablet	= 300 mg

QUIBRON®-T/SR ℞

(Theophylline Anhydrous)

DIVIDOSE™ TABLETS

SUSTAINED RELEASE BRONCHODILATOR

Description: Quibron®-T/SR tablets provide 300 mg of anhydrous theophylline as an oral bronchodilator in a sustained release formulation combined with the convenience of the unique Dividose™ tablet design. With functional trisects and bisects, Quibron-T/SR tablets can be conveniently and accurately divided into 100, 150, and 200 mg segments to provide a variety of dosing increments, as required.

QUIBRON-T/SR tablets

One-third tablet	= 100 mg
One-half tablet	= 150 mg
Two-thirds tablet	= 200 mg
One tablet	= 300 mg

Theophylline is a white odorless crystalline powder which has a bitter taste. It is chemically related to caffeine.

Clinical Pharmacology:

Mode of Action

Theophylline acts as a bronchodilator by direct relaxation of bronchial smooth muscle. Theophylline is a competitive inhibitor of cyclic nucleotide phosphodiesterase resulting in increased intracellular levels of cAMP which mediates smooth muscle relaxation. Like some other xanthines, theophylline acts as a coronary vasodilator, cardiac stimulant, skeletal muscle stimulant, central nervous system stimulant and diuretic.

Pharmacokinetics

Theophylline is, under usual conditions, absorbed completely and fairly rapidly. Excretion, principally as inactive metabolites, occurs primarily via the kidney. The half-life of theophylline varies among individuals with a wide range having been documented. Theophylline half-life is shorter in cigarette smokers. Half-life is prolonged in alcoholism, reduced hepatic or renal function, congestive heart failure and in patients receiving antibiotics such as troleandomycin or erythromycin. High fever for prolonged periods may decrease theophylline elimination. The theophylline half-life is generally shorter in children.

Representative Theophylline Serum Half-Lives

	Half-life (hours) Mean	Range
Adults		
non-smokers	8.7	6.1–12.8
smokers	5.5	4.0–7.7
congestive heart failure	22.9	3.1–82.0
Children (6–16 yrs)	3.7	1.4–7.9

Therapeutic serum theophylline levels are usually 10–20 μg/ml.

Binding to plasma proteins is not extensive and theophylline is not preferentially taken up by any particular organ.

Theophylline-containing products may increase the plasma levels of free fatty acids and the urinary levels of epinephrine and norepinephrine.

Apparently no development of tolerance occurs with chronic use of theophylline.

Indications and Usage: Quibron-T tablets and Quibron-T/SR tablets are indicated for the symptomatic treatment of bronchospasm associated with such conditions as bronchial asthma, chronic bronchitis and pulmonary emphysema.

Contraindications: Quibron-T tablets and Quibron-T/SR tablets are contraindicated in individuals who have shown hypersensitivity to any of its components or xanthine derivatives.

Warnings: Excessive theophylline doses may be associated with toxicity; thus serum theophylline levels should be monitored to assure maximal benefit without excessive risk. Serum levels of theophylline above the accepted therapeutic range (10–20 μg/ml) are associated with an increased incidence of toxicity. Such levels may be reached with customary doses in individuals who metabolize the drug slowly, especially patients (1) with lowered body plasma clearance, (2) with liver dysfunction or chronic obstructive pulmonary disease, or (3) older than 55 years of age, particularly males.

Serious toxicity, such as seizure or ventricular arrhythmias, is not necessarily preceded by less serious side effects such as nausea, irritability or restlessness. Many patients who have higher (greater than 20 μg/ml) theophylline serum levels exhibit tachycardia. Theophylline products may exacerbate preexisting arrhythmias.

Precautions:

General

Quibron-T/SR tablets should not be chewed or crushed.

Use with caution in patients with severe cardiac disease, hypertension, acute myocardial injury, congestive heart failure, cor pulmonale, severe hypoxemia, hyperthyroidism, hepatic impairment, history of peptic ulcer, alcoholism and in the elderly. Concurrent administration with certain antibiotics (see DRUG INTERACTIONS section) may result in increased serum theophylline levels.

A decrease in serum half-life is seen in smokers (see Clinical Pharmacology/Pharmacokinetics).

Particular caution should be used in administering theophylline to patients in congestive heart failure. Reduced theophylline clearance in these patients may cause theophylline blood levels to persist long after discontinuing the drug.

Theophylline should not be administered concurrently with other xanthine medications.

Patients should be instructed carefully on how to divide Quibron-T tablets and Quibron-T/SR tablets along the appropriate tablet score.

Sustained release theophylline is not useful in status asthmaticus.

Usage in Pregnancy

Teratogenic effects: Pregnancy Category C. Animal reproduction studies have not been conducted with Quibron-T tablets and Quibron-T/SR tablets. It is also not known whether Quibron-T tablets and Quibron-T/SR tablets can cause fetal harm when administered to a pregnant woman or can affect reproduction capacity. Quibron-T tablets and Quibron-T/SR tablets should be given to a pregnant woman only if clearly indicated.

Nonteratogenic effects: it is not known whether use of this drug during labor or delivery has immediate or delayed adverse effects on the fetus, or whether it prolongs the duration of labor or increases the possibility of forceps delivery or other obstetrical intervention.

Nursing Mothers

Theophylline has been reported to be excreted in human milk and to have caused irritability in a nursing infant. Because of the potential for serious adverse reactions, a decision should be made whether to discontinue nursing or to discontinue Quibron-T tablets and Quibron-T/SR tablets, taking into account the importance of these drugs to the mother.

Drug Interactions

Drug	Effect
Theophylline with lithium carbonate	Increased renal excretion of lithium
Theophylline with propranolol	Mutual antagonism of therapeutic effects
Theophylline with cimetidine	Increased serum theophylline levels

Continued on next page

Mead Johnson Pharm.—Cont.

Theophylline with clindamycin	Increased serum theophylline levels
Theophylline with lincomycin	Increased serum theophylline levels
Theophylline with troleandomycin or erythromycin	Increased serum theophylline levels

Drug/Laboratory Test Interactions

Theophylline may interfere with the assay of uric acid, especially the phosphotungstate method. Thus, serum uric acid levels may be overestimated.

Adverse Reactions: The frequency of adverse reactions is related to serum theophylline levels and is usually not a problem at levels below 20 μg/ml. The most consistent adverse reactions are usually due to overdosage and, while not all have been reported with Quibron-T tablets and/or with Quibron-T/SR tablets, the following reactions may be considered when theophylline is administered. Central nervous system: clonic and tonic generalized convulsions, muscle twitching, reflex hyperexcitability, headaches, insomnia, restlessness, and irritability. Cardiovascular: circulatory failure, ventricular arrhythmias, hypotension, extrasystoles, tachycardia, palpitation, and flushing. Gastrointestinal: hematemesis, vomiting, diarrhea, epigastric pain, and nausea. Renal: increased excretion of renal tubular cells and red blood cells, albuminuria, and diuresis. Respiratory: tachypnea. Others: hyperglycemia and inappropriate ADH syndrome.

Overdosage:

Symptoms

Nervousness, agitation, headache, insomnia, nausea, vomiting, tachycardia, extrasystoles, hyperreflexia, fasciculations and clonic and tonic convulsions. Children may be particularly prone to restlessness and hyperactivity that can proceed to convulsions.

Management

If potential oral overdose is established and seizure has **not** occurred.

1. Induce vomiting.
2. Administer a cathartic (this is particularly important if a sustained release preparation has been taken).
3. Administer activated charcoal.
4. Monitor vital signs, maintain blood pressure and provide adequate hydration.

If patient is having a seizure.

1. Establish an airway.
2. Administer O_2.
3. Treat the seizure with intravenous diazepam 0.1 to 0.3 mg/kg up to total dose of 10 mg.
4. Monitor vital signs, maintain blood pressure and provide adequate hydration.

Post-seizure Coma.

1. Maintain airway and oxygenation.
2. If the reaction occurred after oral medication, follow above recommendations to prevent absorption of drug, but intubation and lavage will have to be performed instead of inducing emesis and the cathartic and charcoal will need to be introduced via a large bore gastric lavage tube.
3. Continue to provide full supportive care and adequate hydration while waiting for drug to be metabolized. In general, the drug is metabolized rapidly enough so as to not warrant consideration of dialysis.

General

The oral LD_{50} of theophylline in mice is 350 mg/kg. In humans, adverse reactions often occur when serum theophylline levels exceed 20 μg/ml. Information on physiological variables which influence excretion of theophylline can be found under the heading "Clinical Pharmacology."

Dosage and Administration:

General

Therapeutic serum levels associated with optimal likelihood for benefit and minimal risk of toxicity are considered to be between 10 μg/ml and 20 μg/ml, although levels of 5–10 μg/ml have been reported to be effective for some patients. Levels above 20 μg/ml may produce toxic effects. Because of the variable rates of theophylline elimination among patients the dose necessary to achieve the desired serum level of 10–20 μg theophylline per ml varies from patient to patient. Thus, dosage must be individualized (see CLINICAL PHARMACOLOGY and WARNINGS sections) because there is a relatively narrow range between therapeutic and toxic levels of theophylline. Monitoring of serum theophylline levels is highly recommended.

Since theophylline does not distribute into fatty tissue, dosage should be calculated on the basis of ideal body weight. Giving theophylline with food may prevent the rare case of stomach irritation and, although absorption may be slower, it is still complete.

Quibron-T Tablets

To maintain the desired serum level of theophylline generally requires dosing every six hours to obtain the optimal clinical benefit in children and some adult patients (e.g., heavy smokers) because of their rapid clearance of the drug. However, dosing intervals of eight hours may be satisfactory for most adults because of their slower elimination rate.

[See table below].

Note: Due to their slower rate of absorption, sustained-release theophylline products are *not* designed for use in conditions requiring rapid theophyllinization.

II. Patients currently receiving a theophylline product:

Determine, where possible, the time, amount, route of administration and form of the patient's last dose.

The loading dose for theophylline should be based on the principle that each 1 mg/kg of theophylline administered as a loading dose will result in a 2 mcg/ml increase in serum theophylline concentration. Ideally, then, the loading dose should be deferred if a serum theophylline concentration can be rapidly obtained. If this is not possible, the clinician should exercise his/her judgment in selecting a dose based on the potential for benefit and risk. When there is sufficient respiratory distress to warrant a small risk, 2.5 mg/kg of theophylline is likely to increase the serum concentration when administered as a loading dose in rapidly absorbed form by only about 5 mcg/ml. If the patient is not already experiencing theophylline toxicity, this is unlikely to result in dangerous adverse effects.

Subsequent to the modified decision regarding a loading dose in this group of patients, the subsequent maintenance dosage recommendations are the same as those described above.

Comments: To achieve optimal therapeutic theophylline dosage, it is recommended to monitor serum theophylline concentrations. However, it is not always possible or practical to obtain a serum theophylline level.

Patients should be closely monitored for signs of toxicity. The present data suggest that the above dosage recommendations will achieve therapeutic serum concentrations with minimal risk of toxicity for most patients. However, some risk of toxic serum concentrations is still present. Adverse reactions to theophylline often occur when serum theophylline levels exceed 20 mcg/ml.

CHRONIC ASTHMA

Theophyllinization is a treatment of first choice for the management of chronic asthma (to prevent symptoms and maintain patent airways). Slow clinical titration is generally preferred to assure acceptance and safety of the medication. Initial Dose: 16 mg/kg/day or 400 mg/day (whichever is less) in 3 or 4 divided doses at 6 to 8 hour intervals.

If the desired response is not achieved with the recommended initial dose, and there are no adverse reactions, the dose may be cautiously adjusted upward in increments of no more than 25 percent at 2–3 day intervals until the following MAXIMUM DOSE WITHOUT MEASUREMENT OF SERUM CONCENTRATION or, in the case of adults, a maximum of 900 mg in any 24 hour period (whichever is less) is attained:

MAXIMUM DAILY DOSE WITHOUT MEASUREMENT OF SERUM CONCENTRATION

	mg per kg Body Weight* per day
Children (under 9)	24
Children (9–12)	20
Adolescents (12–16)	18
Adults	13

*Use ideal body weight for obese patients.

Do not attempt to maintain any dose that is not tolerated. If doses higher than those contained in the above MAXIMUM DOSE WITHOUT MEASUREMENT OF SERUM CONCENTRATION are necessary, it is recommended that serum theophylline levels be monitored. For therapeutic levels, draw blood sample when last dose peaks (≃ 2 hours after dosing). It is important that the patient has missed no doses during the previous 72 hours and that dosing intervals have been reasonably typical with no doses added during that period of time. DOSE

DOSAGE FOR PATIENT POPULATION

ACUTE ASTHMA REQUIRING RAPID THEOPHYLLINIZATION

I. Patients not currently receiving a theophylline product:

Group	Oral Loading Dose (Theophylline)	Maintenance Dose for Next 12 Hours (Theophylline)	Maintenance Dose Beyond 12 Hours (Theophylline)
1. Children 6 months to 9 years	6 mg/kg	4 mg/kg q4h	4 mg/kg q6h
2. Children age 9–16 and young adult	6 mg/kg	3 mg/kg q4h	3 mg/kg q6h
3. Otherwise healthy non-smoking adults	6 mg/kg	3 mg/kg q6h	3 mg/kg q8h
4. Older patients and patients with cor pulmonale	6 mg/kg	2 mg/kg q6h	2 mg/kg q8h
5. Patients with congestive heart failure, liver failure	6 mg/kg	2 mg/kg q8h	1–2 mg/kg q12h

ADJUSTMENT BASED ON SERUM THEOPHYLLINE MEASUREMENTS MADE WHEN THESE INSTRUCTIONS HAVE NOT BEEN FOLLOWED MAY RESULT IN RECOMMENDATIONS THAT PRESENT RISK OF TOXICITY TO THE PATIENT.

Quibron-T/SR Tablets

The average initial dose for children (under 9 years of age) is one third (100 mg) of a Quibron-T/SR Tablet q 12 h.

The average initial dose for children (ages 9–12) is one half (150 mg) of a Quibron-T/SR Tablet q 12 h.

The average initial dose for adolescents (ages 12–16) is two thirds (200 mg) of a Quibron-T/SR Tablet q 12 h.

The average initial dose for adults is two thirds (200 mg) Quibron-T/SR Tablet q 12 h.

If the desired response is not achieved with the recommended initial dose, and there are no adverse reactions, the dose may be cautiously adjusted upward in increments of no more than 25 percent at 2–3 day intervals until the following MAXIMUM DOSE WITHOUT MEASUREMENT OF SERUM CONCENTRATION or, in the case of adults, a maximum of 900 mg in any 24 hour period (whichever is less) is attained:

MAXIMUM DOSE WITHOUT MEASUREMENT OF SERUM CONCENTRATION

	mg per kg Body Weight* per day**
Children (under 9)	24
Children (9–12)	20
Adolescents (12–16)	18
Adults	13

* Use ideal body weight for obese patients.
** Some patients who clear theophylline more rapidly (e.g., children and heavy smokers) may require dosing at intervals more frequent than 12 hours.

Do not attempt to maintain any dose that is not tolerated. If doses higher than those contained in the above MAXIMUM DOSE WTHOUT MEASUREMENT OF SERUM CONCENTRATION are necessary, it is recommended that serum theophylline levels be monitored. For therapeutic levels, draw blood sample when last dose peaks (4–5 hours after dosing). It is important that the patient has missed no doses during the previous 72 hours and that dosing intervals have been reasonably typical with no doses added during that period of time. DOSE ADJUSTMENT BASED ON SERUM THEOPHYLLINE MEASUREMENTS MADE WHEN THESE INSTRUCTIONS HAVE NOT BEEN FOLLOWED MAY RESULT IN RECOMMENDATIONS THAT PESENT RISK OF TOXICITY TO THE PATIENT.

How Supplied:

QUIBRON®-T tablets (ivory, in the Dividose™ tablet design) containing 300 mg anhydrous theophylline.

NDC 0087-0512-41 Bottles of 100

QUIBRON®-T/SR tablets (white, in the Dividose™ tablet design) containing 300 mg anhydrous theophylline.

NDC 0087-0519-41 Bottles of 100

Store below 86°F (30°C).

[*Shown in Product Identification Section*]

VASODILAN® ℞
(Isoxsuprine HCl) tablets • injection

Indications

Based on a review of this drug by the National Academy of Sciences—National Research Council and/or other information, the FDA has classified the indications as follows:

Possibly Effective:
1. For the relief of symptoms associated with cerebral vascular insufficiency.
2. In peripheral vascular disease of arteriosclerosis obliterans, thromboangiitis obliterans (Buerger's Disease) and Raynaud's disease.

Final classification of the less-than-effective indications requires further investigation.

Composition:

Vasodilan tablets, isoxsuprine HCl, 10 mg. and 20 mg.

Vasodilan injection, each ml. contains 5 mg. isoxsuprine hydrochloride and 2.5% Glycerin U.S.P., in Water for Injection U.S.P. pH adjusted with hydrochloric acid or sodium hydroxide.

Dosage and Administration:

Oral: 10 to 20 mg., three or four times daily.

Intramuscular: 5 to 10 mg. (1 to 2 ml.) two or three times daily. Intramuscular administration may be used initially in severe or acute conditions.

Contraindications and Cautions:

Oral

There are no known contraindications to oral use when administered in recommended doses. Should not be given immediately postpartum or in the presence of arterial bleeding.

Parenteral

Parenteral administration is not recommended in the presence of hypotension or tachycardia.

Intravenous administration should not be given because of increased likelihood of side effects.

Should not be given immediately postpartum or in the presence of arterial bleeding.

Adverse Reactions: On rare occasions oral administration of the drug has been associated in time with the occurrence of hypotension, tachycardia, chest pain, nausea, vomiting, dizziness, abdominal distress, and severe rash. If rash appears the drug should be discontinued. Although available evidence suggests a temporal association of these reactions with isoxsuprine, a causal relationship can be neither confirmed nor refuted.

Single doses of 10 mg intramuscularly may result in transient hypotension and tachycardia. These symptoms are more pronounced in higher doses. For these reasons single intramuscular doses exceeding 10 mg are not recommended. Repeated administration of 5 to 10 mg intramuscularly at suitable intervals may be employed.

β-Adrenergic receptor stimulants such as isoxsuprine hydrochloride have been used to inhibit preterm labor. Maternal and fetal tachycardia may occur under such use. Hypocalcemia, hypoglycemia, hypotension and ileus have been reported to occur in infants whose mothers received isoxsuprine. Pulmonary edema has been reported in mothers treated with β-stimulants. Vasodilan is neither approved nor recommended for use in the treatment of premature labor.

How Supplied: Tablets, 10 mg.
NDC 0087-0543-01 Bottles of 100
NDC 0087-0543-02 Bottles of 1000
NDC 0087-0543-07 Bottles of 5000
NDC 0087-0543-05 Unit Dose

Tablets, 20 mg.
NDC 0087-0544-01 Bottles of 100
NDC 0087-0544-02 Bottles of 500
NDC 0087-0544-06 Bottles of 1000
NDC 0087-0544-47 Bottles of 5000
NDC 0087-0544-03 Unit Dose

Injection, 10 mg. per 2 ml. ampul
NDC 0087-0540-01 Boxes of six 2 ml. ampuls

[*Shown in Product Identification Section*]

Medical Products Panamericana, Inc.
P.O. BOX 771
CORAL GABLES, FL 33134

VG CAPSULES™ ℞

Composition: Each capsule contains: Vitamin C (Ascorbic Acid) 500 mg.; Vitamin B1 (Thiamine) 15 mg.; Vitamin B2 (Riboflavin) 15 mg.; Niacinamide 100 mg.; Vitamin B6 (Pyridoxine) 5 mg.; Vitamin B12 5 mcg.; Calcium Pantothenate 20 mg.; Folic Acid 0.5 mg.; Vitamin E (d-alpha tocopheryl acetate) 30 I.U.; 1-lysine Hydrochloride (need in human nutrition established, but no U.S. RDA established) 25 mg.; Manganese Sulfate 4 mg.; Magnesium Sulfate 35 mg. (equivalent to 25 mg. dried $MgSO_4$); Zinc Sulfate 80 mg. (equivalent to 25 mg. dried $ZnSO_4$).

Indications: Indicated in the treatment of patients with deficiencies of, or increased requirements for Vitamin C and/or B-Complex Vitamins including Folic Acid, Zinc, Magnesium and/or Manganese.

Administration and Dosage: One Capsule Daily or as directed by a physician.

Precautions: Folic Acid may obscure pernicious anemia; the peripheral blood picture may revert to normal while neurological manifestations remain progressive.

Caution: Federal Law prohibits dispensing without prescription.

Supplied: NDC 0576-0506-30 Bottle of 30 Capsules.

Medicone Company
225 VARICK ST.
NEW YORK, NY 10014

DERMA MEDICONE® Ointment
(See PDR For Nonprescription Drugs)

DERMA MEDICONE®-HC Ointment ℞

Composition: Each gram contains:

Hydrocortisone acetate	10.0 mg.
Benzocaine	19.8 mg.
8-Hydroxyquinoline sulfate	10.4 mg.
Ephedrine hydrochloride	1.1 mg.
Menthol	4.8 mg.
Ichthammol	9.9 mg.
Zinc oxide	135.8 mg.
Petrolatum, Lanolin, perfume	q.s.

Action and Uses: Offers the advantage of quick, lasting comfort during treatment of severely inflamed dermatoses by affording prompt temporary local anesthetic action, inhibiting pain, burning, itching and controlling the scratch reflex. The hydrocortisone acetate reduces inflammation and swelling, aiding the normal healing process. The non-drying base will not disintegrate or liquefy at body temperature and is not washed off by exudate, perspiration or urine. Effectively suppresses inflammation, pain, swelling, burning and itching in contact dermatitis, eczematoid dermatitis, atopic dermatitis, neurodermatitis, seborrheic dermatitis, allergic dermatitis, rhus dermatitis, pruritus ani and pruritus vulvae.

Administration and Dosage: Apply to affected area 2 to 4 times daily. When adequate improvement is noted, reduce frequency of application or continue maintenance control with regular Derma Medicone ointment.

Precautions: Observe the usual adrenocorticosteroid precautions. Exercise care if the patient is on other corticosteroid therapy or if infection is present or if rash or irritation develops. Do not use in the eyes.

Continued on next page

Medicone—Cont.

Contraindications: Do not use in the presence of tuberculosis of the skin.
How Supplied: 7 gram and 20 gram tubes.

DioMEDICONE® Tablets

(See PDR For Nonprescription Drugs)

MEDICONE® DRESSING Cream

(See PDR For Nonprescription Drugs)

MEDICONET®
(medicated rectal wipes)

(See PDR For Nonprescription Drugs)

RECTAL MEDICONE® SUPPOSITORIES

(See PDR For Nonprescription Drugs)

RECTAL MEDICONE®-HC SUPPOSITORIES ℞

Composition: Each suppository contains:
Hydrocortisone acetate ....10 mg.
Benzocaine ....2 gr.
8-Hydroxyquinoline sulfate ....1/4 gr.
Zinc oxide ....3 gr.
Menthol ....1/7 gr.
Balsam Peru ....1 gr.
Cocoa butter—vegetable & petroleum oil base, Certified color added........q.s.
Action and Uses: The hydrocortisone acetate reduces and controls severe anorectal inflammation and swelling, effecting better management of the basic condition. Provides prompt, temporary relief from pain, burning and itching. Soothes, lubricates and protects; makes bowel evacuation more comfortable while accelerating the normal healing process. Useful as initial therapy in hemorrhoids, acute and chronic proctitis, post-operative edema, cryptitis, pruritus ani and inflamed post-operative scar tissue.

ANESTHETIC—ANTI-INFLAMMATORY
ANTIPRURITIC—ANTIBACTERIAL

Administration and Dosage: Start therapy with one Rectal Medicone-HC Suppository twice daily for a recommended period of three to six days. Continue maintenance control against recurring symptoms with regular Rectal Medicone Suppositories and/or Unguent as required.
Precautions: A thorough proctologic diagnosis should be made when use of hydrocortisone is considered. Care should be exercised if the patient is on other corticosteroid therapy or if infection is present or if rash or irritation develops.
Contraindications: Do not use in the presence of tuberculosis of the rectum.
How Supplied: Boxes of 12 individually foil-wrapped pink suppositories.

[Shown in Product Identification Section]

RECTAL MEDICONE® UNGUENT

(See PDR For Nonprescription Drugs)

Products are cross-indexed by generic and chemical names in the the **YELLOW SECTION**

Merck Sharp & Dohme
DIVISION OF MERCK & CO., INC.
WEST POINT, PA 19486

Product Identification Codes

To provide quick and positive identification of Merck Sharp & Dohme products, we have imprinted a code number on tablet and capsule products. In order that you may identify a product by its code number, we have compiled below a numerical list of code numbers with their corresponding product names. We are also listing the code numbers by alphabetical listing of products as a cross reference.
The code number as it appears on tablets and capsules bears the letters MSD plus the numerical code. Decadron® (Dexamethasone, MSD) tablets 0.25 mg is identified MSD 20.

Numerical Listing

MSD Code No.	Product	Product No.
20	Decadron® (Dexamethasone, MSD) Tablets 0.25 mg.	7592
21	Cogentin® (Benztropine Mesylate, MSD) Tablets 0.5 mg.	3297
23	Elavil® (Amitriptyline HCl, MSD) Tablets 10 mg.	3287
25	Indocin® (Indomethacin, MSD) Capsules 25 mg.	3316
26	Vivactil® (Protriptyline HCl, MSD) Tablets 5 mg.	3313
41	Decadron® (Dexamethasone, MSD) Tablets 0.5 mg.	7598
42	HydroDIURIL® (Hydrochlorothiazide, MSD) Tablets 25 mg.	3263
43	Mephyton® (Phytonadione, MSD) Tablets 5 mg.	7776
45	Elavil® (Amitriptyline HCl, MSD) Tablets 25 mg.	3288
47	Vivactil® (Protriptyline HCl, MSD) Tablets 10 mg.	3314
49	Daranide® (Dichlorphenamide, MSD) Tablets 50 mg.	3256
50	Indocin® (Indomethacin, MSD) Capsules 50 mg.	3317
52	Inversine® (Mecamylamine HCl, MSD) Tablets 2.5 mg.	3219
53	Hydropres® 25 (Reserpine-Hydrochlorothiazide, MSD) Tablets	3265
60	Cogentin® (Benztropine Mesylate, MSD) Tablets 2 mg.	3172
62	Periactin® (Cyproheptadine HCl, MSD) Tablets 4 mg.	3276
63	Decadron® (Dexamethasone, MSD) Tablets 0.75 mg.	7601
65	Edecrin® (Ethacrynic Acid, MSD) Tablets 25 mg.	3321
67	Timolide® 10/25 (Timolol Maleate-Hydrochlorothiazide, MSD) Tablets	3373
90	Edecrin® (Ethacrynic Acid, MSD) Tablets 50 mg.	3322
92	Midamor® (Amiloride HCl, MSD) Tablets 5 mg.	3381
95	Decadron® (Dexamethasone, MSD) Tablets 1.5 mg.	7638
97	Decadron® (Dexamethasone, MSD) Tablets 4 mg.	7645
102	Elavil® (Amitriptyline HCl, MSD) Tablets 50 mg.	3320
105	HydroDIURIL® (Hydrochlorothiazide, MSD) Tablets 50 mg.	3264
120	Inversine® (Mecamylamine HCl, MSD) Tablets 10 mg.	3220
127	Hydropres® 50 (Reserpine-Hydrochlorothiazide, MSD) Tablets	3266
135	Aldomet® (Methyldopa, MSD) Tablets 125 mg.	3341
136	Blocadren® (Timolol Maleate, MSD) Tablets 10 mg.	3344
214	Diuril® (Chlorothiazide, MSD) Tablets 250 mg.	3244
219	Cortone® (Cortisone Acetate, MSD) Tablets 25 mg.	7063
230	Diupres 250® Tablets	3261
401	Aldomet® (Methyldopa, MSD) Tablets 250 mg.	3290
403	Urecholine® (Bethanechol Chloride, MSD) Tablets 5 mg.	7785
405	Diupres 500® Tablets	3262
410	HydroDIURIL® (Hydrochlorothiazide, MSD) Tablets 100 mg.	3340
412	Urecholine® (Bethanechol Chloride, MSD) Tablets 10 mg.	7787
423	Aldoril® 15, Tablets	3294
430	Elavil® (Amitriptyline HCl, MSD) Tablets 75 mg.	3348
432	Diuril® (Chlorothiazide, MSD) Tablets 500 mg.	3245
435	Elavil® (Amitriptyline HCl, MSD) Tablets 100 mg.	3349
437	Blocadren® (Timolol Maleate, MSD) Tablets 20 mg.	3371
456	Aldoril® 25, Tablets	3295
457	Urecholine® (Bethanechol Chloride, MSD) Tablets 25 mg.	7788
460	Urecholine® (Bethanechol Chloride, MSD) Tablets 50 mg.	7790
501	Benemid® (Probenecid, MSD) Tablets 0.5 g.	3337
516	Aldomet® (Methyldopa, MSD) Tablets 500 mg.	3292
517	Triavil® 4-50 Tablets	3364
602	Cuprimine® (Penicillamine, MSD) Capsules 250 mg.	3299
605	Propadrine® (Phenylpropanolamine HCl, MSD) Capsules 25 mg.	2197
612	Aldoclor® 150, Tablets	3318
613	Propadrine® (Phenylpropanolamine HCl, MSD) Capsules 50 mg.	2198
614	ColBENEMID® Tablets	3283
619	Hydrocortone® (Hydrocortisone, MSD) Tablets 10 mg.	7604
625	Hydrocortone® (Hydrocortisone, MSD) Tablets 20 mg.	7602
634	Aldoclor® 250, Tablets	3319
635	Cogentin® (Benztropine Mesylate, MSD) Tablets 1 mg.	3334
647	Sinemet® 10/100 (Carbidopa-Levodopa, MSD) Tablets	3346
650	Sinemet® 25/100 (Carbidopa-Levodopa, MSD) Tablets	3365
654	Sinemet® 25/250 (Carbidopa-Levodopa, MSD) Tablets	3347
672	Cuprimine® (Penicillamine, MSD) Capsules 125 mg.	3350
673	Elavil® (Amitriptyline HCl, MSD) Tablets 150 mg.	3351
675	Dolobid® (Diflunisal, MSD) Tablets 250 mg.	3390
690	Demser® (Metyrosine, MSD) Capsules 250 mg.	3355
693	Indocin® SR (Indomethacin, MSD) Capsules 75 mg.	3370
694	Aldoril® D30 Tablets	3362
697	Dolobid® (Diflunisal, MSD) Tablets 500 mg.	3392
907	Mintezol® (Thiabendazole, MSD) Chewable Tablets 500 mg.	3332
914	Triavil® 2-10 Tablets	3328
917	Moduretic® (Amiloride HCl-Hydrochlorothiazide, MSD) Tablets	3385
921	Triavil® 2-25 Tablets	3311
931	Flexeril® (Cyclobenzaprine HCl, MSD) Tablets 10 mg.	3358
934	Triavil® 4-10 Tablets	3310
935	Aldoril® D50 Tablets	3363
941	Clinoril® (Sulindac, MSD) Tablets 150 mg.	3360
942	Clinoril® (Sulindac, MSD) Tablets 200 mg.	3353
946	Triavil® 4-25 Tablets	3312

Alphabetical Listing

MSD Code No.	Product	Product No.
612	Aldoclor® 150, Tablets	3318

634	Aldoclor® 250, Tablets	3319
135	Aldomet® (Methyldopa, MSD) Tablets 125 mg.	3341
401	Aldomet® (Methyldopa, MSD) Tablets 250 mg.	3290
516	Aldomet® (Methyldopa, MSD) Tablets 500 mg.	3292
423	Aldoril® 15, Tablets	3294
456	Aldoril® 25, Tablets	3295
694	Aldoril® D30 Tablets	3362
935	Aldoril® D50 Tablets	3363
501	Benemid® (Probenecid, MSD) Tablets 0.5 g.	3337
136	Blocadren® (Timolol Maleate, MSD) Tablets 10 mg.	3344
437	Blocadren® (Timolol Maleate, MSD) Tablets 20 mg.	3371
941	Clinoril® (Sulindac, MSD) Tablets 150 mg.	3360
942	Clinoril® (Sulindac, MSD) Tablets 200 mg.	3353
21	Cogentin® (Benztropine Mesylate, MSD) Tablets 0.5 mg.	3297
635	Cogentin® (Benztropine Mesylate, MSD) Tablets 1 mg.	3334
60	Cogentin® (Benztropine Mesylate, MSD) Tablets 2 mg.	3172
614	ColBENEMID® Tablets	3283
219	Cortone® (Cortisone Acetate, MSD) Tablets 25 mg.	7063
672	Cuprimine® (Penicillamine, MSD) Capsules 125 mg.	3350
602	Cuprimine® (Penicillamine, MSD) Capsules 250 mg.	3299
49	Daranide® (Dichlorphenamide, MSD) Tablets 50 mg.	3256
20	Decadron® (Dexamethasone, MSD) Tablets 0.25 mg.	7592
41	Decadron® (Dexamethasone, MSD) Tablets 0.5 mg.	7598
63	Decadron® (Dexamethasone, MSD) Tablets 0.75 mg.	7601
95	Decadron® (Dexamethasone, MSD) Tablets 1.5 mg.	7638
97	Decadron® (Dexamethasone, MSD) Tablets 4 mg.	7645
690	Demser® (Metyrosine, MSD) Capsules 250 mg.	3355
230	Diupres 250® Tablets	3261
405	Diupres 500® Tablets	3262
214	Diuril® (Chlorothiazide, MSD) Tablets 250 mg.	3244
432	Diuril® (Chlorothiazide, MSD) Tablets 500 mg.	3245
675	Dolobid® (Diflunisal, MSD) Tablets 250 mg.	3390
697	Dolobid® (Diflunisal, MSD) Tablets 500 mg.	3392
65	Edecrin® (Ethacrynic Acid, MSD) Tablets 25 mg.	3321
90	Edecrin® (Ethacrynic Acid, MSD) Tablets 50 mg.	3322
23	Elavil® (Amitriptyline HCl, MSD) Tablets 10 mg.	3287
45	Elavil® (Amitriptyline HCl, MSD) Tablets 25 mg.	3288
102	Elavil® (Amitriptyline HCl, MSD) Tablets 50 mg.	3320
430	Elavil® (Amitriptyline HCl, MSD) Tablets 75 mg.	3348
435	Elavil® (Amitriptyline HCl, MSD) Tablets 100 mg.	3349
673	Elavil® (Amitriptyline HCl, MSD) Tablets 150 mg.	3351
931	Flexeril® (Cyclobenzaprine HCl, MSD) Tablets 10 mg.	3358
619	Hydrocortone® (Hydrocortisone, MSD) Tablets 10 mg.	7604
625	Hydrocortone® (Hydrocortisone, MSD) Tablets 20 mg.	7602
42	HydroDIURIL® (Hydrochlorothiazide, MSD) Tablets 25 mg.	3263
105	HydroDIURIL® (Hydrochlorothiazide, MSD) Tablets 50 mg.	3264
410	HydroDIURIL® (Hydrochlorothiazide, MSD) Tablets 100 mg.	3340
53	Hydropres® 25 (Reserpine-Hydrochlorothiazide, MSD) Tablets	3265
127	Hydropres® 50 (Reserpine-Hydrochlorothiazide, MSD) Tablets	3266
25	Indocin® (Indomethacin, MSD) Capsules 25 mg.	3316
50	Indocin® (Indomethacin, MSD) Capsules 50 mg.	3317
693	Indocin® SR (Indomethacin, MSD) Capsules 75 mg.	3370
52	Inversine® (Mecamylamine HCl, MSD) Tablets 2.5 mg.	3219
120	Inversine® (Mecamylamine HCl, MSD) Tablets 10 mg.	3220
43	Mephyton® (Phytonadione, MSD) Tablets 5 mg.	7776
92	Midamor® (Amiloride HCl, MSD) Tablets 5 mg.	3381
907	Mintezol® (Thiabendazole, MSD) Chewable Tablets 500 mg.	3332
917	Moduretic® (Amiloride HCl-Hydrochlorothiazide, MSD) Tablets	3385
62	Periactin® (Cyproheptadine HCl, MSD) Tablets 4 mg.	3276
605	Propadrine® (Phenylpropanolamine HCl, MSD) Capsules 25 mg.	2197
613	Propadrine® (Phenylpropanolamine HCl, MSD) Capsules 50 mg.	2198
647	Sinemet® 10/100 (Carbidopa-Levodopa, MSD) Tablets	3346
650	Sinemet® 25/100 (Carbidopa-Levodopa, MSD) Tablets	3365
654	Sinemet® 25/250 (Carbidopa-Levodopa, MSD) Tablets	3347
67	Timolide® 10/25 (Timolol Maleate-Hydrochlorothiazide, MSD) Tablets	3373
914	Triavil® 2-10 Tablets	3328
921	Triavil® 2-25 Tablets	3311
934	Triavil® 4-10 Tablets	3310
946	Triavil® 4-25 Tablets	3312
517	Triavil® 4-50 Tablets	3364
403	Urecholine® (Bethanechol Chloride, MSD) Tablets 5 mg.	7785
412	Urecholine® (Bethanechol Chloride, MSD) Tablets 10 mg.	7787
457	Urecholine® (Bethanechol Chloride, MSD) Tablets 25 mg.	7788
460	Urecholine® (Bethanechol Chloride, MSD) Tablets 50 mg.	7790
26	Vivactil® (Protriptyline HCl, MSD) Tablets 5 mg.	3313
47	Vivactil® (Protriptyline HCl, MSD) Tablets 10 mg.	3314

ALDOCLOR® Tablets ℞
Antihypertensive

> **WARNING**
>
> This fixed combination drug is not indicated for initial therapy of hypertension. Hypertension requires therapy titrated to the individual patient. If the fixed combination represents the dosage so determined, its use may be more convenient in patient management. The treatment of hypertension is not static, but must be reevaluated as conditions in each patient warrant.

Description
ALDOCLOR® is a combination of methyldopa and chlorothiazide. The chemical name for methyldopa is levo-3-(3,4-dihydroxyphenyl)-2-methylalanine. Chlorothiazide is 6-chloro-*2H*-1, 2, 4-benzothiadiazine-7-sulfonamide 1, 1-dioxide.

Actions
ALDOMET® (Methyldopa, MSD)

Methyldopa, a unique antihypertensive, is an aromatic-amino-acid decarboxylase inhibitor in animals and in man. Although the mechanism of action has yet to be conclusively demonstrated, the antihypertensive effect of methyldopa probably is due to its metabolism to alpha-methylnorepinephrine, which then lowers arterial pressure by stimulation of central inhibitory alpha-adrenergic receptors, false neurotransmission, and/or reduction of plasma renin activity. Methyldopa has been shown to cause a net reduction in the tissue concentration of serotonin, dopamine, norepinephrine, and epinephrine.

Only methyldopa, the *L*-isomer of alpha-methyldopa, has the ability to inhibit dopa decarboxylase and to deplete animal tissues of norepinephrine. In man, the antihypertensive activity appears to be due solely to the *L*-isomer. About twice the dose of the racemate (*DL*-alpha-methyldopa) is required for equal antihypertensive effect.

Methyldopa has no direct effect on cardiac function and usually does not reduce glomerular filtration rate, renal blood flow, or filtration fraction. Cardiac output usually is maintained without cardiac acceleration. In some patients the heart rate is slowed.

Normal or elevated plasma renin activity may decrease in the course of methyldopa therapy.

Methyldopa reduces both supine and standing blood pressure. It usually produces highly effective lowering of the supine pressure with infrequent symptomatic postural hypotension. Exercise hypotension and diurnal blood pressure variations rarely occur.

DIURIL® (Chlorothiazide, MSD)

Chlorothiazide is a diuretic and antihypertensive. It affects the renal tubular mechanism of electrolyte reabsorption. At maximal therapeutic dosage all thiazides are approximately equal in their diuretic efficacy.

Chlorothiazide increases excretion of sodium and chloride in approximately equivalent amounts. Natriuresis may be accompanied by some loss of potassium and bicarbonate.

The mechanism of the antihypertensive effect of thiazides is unknown. Chlorothiazide does not affect normal blood pressure.

Chlorothiazide is eliminated rapidly by the kidney.

ALDOCLOR

The concomitant use of methyldopa and chlorothiazide, as provided in ALDOCLOR, frequently produces a more pronounced antihypertensive response than when either compound is the sole therapeutic agent. Particularly in those cases of hypertensive vascular disease where sodium and water retention is a problem, the coadministration of these two drugs in the form of ALDOCLOR will help control the fluid imbalance.

In severe essential hypertension and in malignant hypertension, ALDOCLOR may achieve effective lowering of blood pressure with fewer side effects than occur with other compounds used for this purpose.

ALDOCLOR reduces both supine and standing blood pressure; more effective lowering of the supine pressure with less frequent symptomatic postural hypotension can be obtained with ALDOCLOR than with most other antihypertensive agents. In patients treated with ALDOCLOR, exercise hypotension and diurnal blood pressure variations rarely occur.

Indication
Hypertension (see box warning).

Continued on next page

Information on the Merck Sharp & Dohme products listed on these pages is the full prescribing information from package circulars in use October 31, 1982.

Merck Sharp & Dohme—Cont.

Contraindications

Active hepatic disease, such as acute hepatitis and active cirrhosis.
If previous methyldopa therapy has been associated with liver disorders (see WARNINGS).
Anuria.
Hypersensitivity to methyldopa, or to chlorothiazide or other sulfonamide-derived drugs.

Warnings

Methyldopa
It is important to recognize that a positive Coombs test, hemolytic anemia, and liver disorders may occur with methyldopa therapy. The rare occurrences of hemolytic anemia or liver disorders could lead to potentially fatal complications unless properly recognized and managed. Read this section carefully to understand these reactions.
With prolonged methyldopa therapy, 10 to 20 percent of patients develop a positive direct Coombs test which usually occurs between 6 and 12 months of methyldopa therapy. Lowest incidence is at daily dosage of 1 g or less. This on rare occasions may be associated with hemolytic anemia, which could lead to potentially fatal complications. One cannot predict which patients with a positive direct Coombs test may develop hemolytic anemia.
Prior existence or development of a positive direct Coombs test is not in itself a contraindication to use of methyldopa. If a positive Coombs test develops during methyldopa therapy, the physician should determine whether hemolytic anemia exists and whether the positive Coombs test may be a problem. For example, in addition to a positive direct Coombs test there is less often a positive indirect Coombs test which may interfere with cross matching of blood.
At the start of methyldopa therapy, it is desirable to do a blood count (hematocrit, hemoglobin, or red cell count) for a baseline or to establish whether there is anemia. Periodic blood counts should be done during therapy to detect hemolytic anemia. It may be useful to do a direct Coombs test before therapy and at 6 and 12 months after the start of therapy.
If Coombs-positive hemolytic anemia occurs, the cause may be methyldopa and the drug should be discontinued. Usually the anemia remits promptly. If not, corticosteroids may be given and other causes of anemia should be considered. If the hemolytic anemia is related to methyldopa, the drug should not be reinstituted.
When methyldopa causes Coombs positivity alone or with hemolytic anemia, the red cell is usually coated with gamma globulin of the IgG (gamma G) class only. The positive Coombs test may not revert to normal until weeks to months after methyldopa is stopped.
Should the need for transfusion arise in a patient receiving methyldopa, both a direct and an indirect Coombs test should be performed on his blood. In the absence of hemolytic anemia, usually only the direct Coombs test will be positive. A positive direct Coombs test alone will not interfere with typing or cross matching. If the indirect Coombs test is also positive, problems may arise in the major cross match and the assistance of a hematologist or transfusion expert will be needed.
Occasionally, fever has occurred within the first three weeks of methyldopa therapy, associated in some cases with eosinophilia or abnormalities in one or more liver function tests, such as serum alkaline phosphatase, serum transaminases (SGOT, SGPT), bilirubin, cephalin cholesterol flocculation, prothrombin time, and bromsulphalein retention. Jaundice, with or without fever, may occur with onset usually within the first two to three months of therapy. In some patients the findings are consistent with those of cholestasis.
Rarely fatal hepatic necrosis has been reported after use of methyldopa. These hepatic changes may represent hypersensitivity reactions. Periodic determination of hepatic function should be done particularly during the first 6 to 12 weeks of therapy or whenever an unexplained fever occurs. If fever, abnormalities in liver function tests, or jaundice appear, stop therapy with methyldopa. If caused by methyldopa, the temperature and abnormalities in liver function characteristically have reverted to normal when the drug was discontinued. Methyldopa should not be reinstituted in such patients.
Rarely, a reversible reduction of the white blood cell count with a primary effect on the granulocytes has been seen. The granulocyte count returned promptly to normal on discontinuance of the drug. Rare cases of granulocytopenia have been reported. In each instance, upon stopping the drug, the white cell count returned to normal. Reversible thrombocytopenia has occurred rarely.
When methyldopa is used with other antihypertensive drugs, potentiation of antihypertensive effect may occur. Patients should be followed carefully to detect side reactions or unusual manifestations of drug idiosyncrasy.
Chlorothiazide
Use with caution in severe renal disease. In patients with renal disease, thiazides may precipitate azotemia. Cumulative effects of the drug may develop in patients with impaired renal function.
Thiazides should be used with caution in patients with impaired hepatic function or progressive liver disease, since minor alterations of fluid and electrolyte balance may precipitate hepatic coma.
Thiazides may add to or potentiate the action of other antihypertensive drugs.
Sensitivity reactions may occur in patients with or without a history of allergy or bronchial asthma.
The possibility of exacerbation or activation of systemic lupus erythematosus has been reported.
Lithium generally should not be given with diuretics because they reduce its renal clearance and add a high risk of lithium toxicity. Read circulars for lithium preparations before use of such concomitant therapy.

Pregnancy and Nursing

Use of any drug in women who are or may become pregnant requires that anticipated benefits be weighed against possible risks.
Methyldopa crosses the placental barrier and appears in cord blood. No unusual adverse reactions have been reported in association with the use of methyldopa during pregnancy. Though no obvious teratogenic effects have been reported, the possibility of fetal injury cannot be excluded.
Thiazides also cross the placental barrier and appear in cord blood. Hazards include fetal or neonatal jaundice, thrombocytopenia, and possibly other adverse reactions which have occurred in the adult.
Methyldopa and thiazides appear in breast milk. Patients taking ALDOCLOR should not nurse.

Precautions

Methyldopa
Methyldopa should be used with caution in patients with a history of previous liver disease or dysfunction (see WARNINGS).
Methyldopa may interfere with measurement of: urinary uric acid by the phosphotungstate method, serum creatinine by the alkaline picrate method, and SGOT by colorimetric methods. Interference with spectrophotometric methods for SGOT analysis has not been reported.
Since methyldopa causes fluorescence in urine samples at the same wave lengths as catecholamines, falsely high levels of urinary catecholamines may be reported. This will interfere with the diagnosis of pheochromocytoma. It is important to recognize this phenomenon before a patient with a possible pheochromocytoma is subjected to surgery. Methyldopa does not interfere with measurement of VMA (vanillylmandelic acid), a test for pheochromocytoma, by those methods which convert VMA to vanillin. Methyldopa is not recommended for the treatment of patients with pheochromocytoma. Rarely, when urine is exposed to air after voiding, it may darken because of breakdown of methyldopa or its metabolites.
Rarely, involuntary choreoathetotic movements have been observed during therapy with methyldopa in patients with severe bilateral cerebrovascular disease. Should these movements occur, stop therapy.
Patients may require reduced doses of anesthetics when on methyldopa. If hypotension does occur during anesthesia, it usually can be controlled by vasopressors. The adrenergic receptors remain sensitive during treatment with methyldopa.
Hypertension has recurred occasionally after dialysis in patients given methyldopa because the drug is removed by this procedure.
Chlorothiazide
Periodic determination of serum electrolytes to detect possible electrolyte imbalance should be performed at appropriate intervals.
All patients receiving diuretic therapy should be observed for evidence of fluid or electrolyte imbalance: namely, hyponatremia, hypochloremic alkalosis, and hypokalemia. Serum and urine electrolyte determinations are particularly important when the patient is vomiting excessively or receiving parenteral fluids. Warning signs or symptoms of fluid and electrolyte imbalance include dryness of mouth, thirst, weakness, lethargy, drowsiness, restlessness, muscle pains or cramps, muscular fatigue, hypotension, oliguria, tachycardia, and gastrointestinal disturbances such as nausea and vomiting.
Hypokalemia may develop, especially with brisk diuresis, when severe cirrhosis is present, during concomitant use of corticosteroids or ACTH, or after prolonged therapy.
Interference with adequate oral electrolyte intake will also contribute to hypokalemia. Hypokalemia can sensitize or exaggerate the response of the heart to the toxic effects of digitalis (e.g., increased ventricular irritability). Hypokalemia may be avoided or treated by use of potassium supplements such as foods with a high potassium content.
Although any chloride deficit is generally mild and usually does not require specific treatment except under extraordinary circumstances (as in liver disease or renal disease), chloride replacement may be required in the treatment of metabolic alkalosis.
Dilutional hyponatremia may occur in edematous patients in hot weather; appropriate therapy is water restriction, rather than administration of salt, except in rare instances when the hyponatremia is life threatening. In actual salt depletion, appropriate replacement is the therapy of choice.
Hyperuricemia may occur or acute gout may be precipitated in certain patients receiving thiazides.
Insulin requirements in diabetic patients may be increased, decreased, or unchanged. Latent diabetes mellitus may become manifest during thiazide therapy.
Thiazides may increase the responsiveness to tubocurarine.
The antihypertensive effects of the drug may be enhanced in the postsympathectomy patient. Thiazides may decrease arterial responsiveness to norepinephrine. This diminution is

not sufficient to preclude effectiveness of the pressor agent for therapeutic use.
If progressive renal impairment becomes evident, consider withholding or discontinuing diuretic therapy.
Thiazides may decrease serum PBI levels without signs of thyroid disturbance.
Thiazides may decrease urinary calcium excretion. Thiazides may cause intermittent and slight elevation of serum calcium in the absence of known disorders of calcium metabolism. Marked hypercalcemia may be evidence of hidden hyperparathyroidism. Thiazides should be discontinued before carrying out tests for parathyroid function.

Adverse Reactions

Methyldopa
Sedation, usually transient, may occur during the initial period of therapy or whenever the dose is increased. Headache, asthenia, or weakness may be noted as early and transient symptoms. However, significant adverse effects due to methyldopa have been infrequent and this agent usually is well tolerated.
Central nervous system: Sedation, headache, asthenia or weakness, dizziness, lightheadedness, symptoms of cerebrovascular insufficiency, paresthesias, parkinsonism, Bell's palsy, decreased mental acuity, involuntary choreoathetotic movements. Psychic disturbances including nightmares and reversible mild psychoses or depression.
Cardiovascular: Bradycardia, prolonged carotid sinus hypersensitivity, aggravation of angina pectoris. Orthostatic hypotension (decrease daily dosage). Edema (and weight gain) usually relieved by use of a diuretic. (Discontinue methyldopa if edema progresses or signs of heart failure appear.)
Gastrointestinal: Nausea, vomiting, distention, constipation, flatus, diarrhea, colitis, mild dryness of mouth, sore or "black" tongue, pancreatitis, sialadenitis.
Hepatic: Abnormal liver function tests, jaundice, liver disorders.
Hematologic: Positive Coombs test, hemolytic anemia. Bone marrow depression, leukopenia, granulocytopenia, thrombocytopenia. Positive tests for antinuclear antibody, LE cells, and rheumatoid factor.
Allergic: Drug-related fever, lupus-like syndrome, myocarditis.
Dermatologic: Rash as in eczema or lichenoid eruption; toxic epidermal necrolysis.
Other: Nasal stuffiness, rise in BUN, breast enlargement, gynecomastia, lactation, hyperprolactinemia, amenorrhea, impotence, decreased libido, mild arthralgia, myalgia.
Chlorothiazide
Gastrointestinal system: Anorexia, gastric irritation, nausea, vomiting, cramping, diarrhea, constipation, jaundice (intrahepatic cholestatic jaundice), pancreatitis, sialadenitis.
Central nervous system: Dizziness, vertigo, paresthesias, headache, xanthopsia.
Hematologic: Leukopenia, agranulocytosis, thrombocytopenia, aplastic anemia, hemolytic anemia.
Cardiovascular: Orthostatic hypotension (may be aggravated by alcohol, barbiturates, or narcotics).
Hypersensitivity: Purpura, photosensitivity, rash, urticaria, necrotizing angiitis (vasculitis) (cutaneous vasculitis), fever, respiratory distress including pneumonitis and pulmonary edema, anaphylactic reactions.
Other: Hyperglycemia, glycosuria, hyperuricemia, muscle spasm, weakness, restlessness, transient blurred vision.
Whenever adverse reactions are moderate or severe, thiazide dosage should be reduced or therapy withdrawn.

Dosage and Administration

Dosage: As determined by individual titration (see box warning).
The usual starting dosage is 1 tablet of ALDOCLOR 150 or 1 tablet of ALDOCLOR 250 two or three times a day in the first 48 hours. The daily dosage then may be increased or decreased, preferably at intervals of not less than two days, until an adequate response is achieved. To minimize the sedation associated with methyldopa, start dosage increases in the evening. By adjustment of dosage, morning hypotension may be prevented without sacrificing control of afternoon blood pressure.
When ALDOCLOR is given to patients on other antihypertensives, the dose of these agents may need to be adjusted to effect a smooth transition. When ALDOCLOR is given with antihypertensives other than thiazides, the initial dosage of methyldopa should be limited to 500 mg daily in divided doses.
Although occasional patients have responded to higher doses, the maximum recommended daily dosage is 3.0 g of methyldopa and 1.0 to 2.0 g of chlorothiazide. Once an effective dosage range is attained, a smooth blood pressure response occurs in most patients in 12 to 24 hours. If ALDOCLOR alone does not adequately control blood pressure, additional methyldopa may be given separately to obtain the maximum blood pressure response.
Since both components of ALDOCLOR have a relatively short duration of action, withdrawal is followed by return of hypertension usually within 48 hours. This is not complicated by an overshoot of blood pressure.
Occasionally tolerance may occur, usually between the second and third month of therapy. Increasing the dosage of either methyldopa or chlorothiazide separately or together frequently will restore effective control of blood pressure.
Methyldopa is largely excreted by the kidney and patients with impaired renal function may respond to smaller doses of ALDOCLOR. Syncope in older patients may be related to an increased sensitivity and advanced arteriosclerotic vascular disease. This may be avoided by lower doses.

How Supplied

No. 3318—Tablets ALDOCLOR 150 are beige, oval, film coated tablets coded MSD 612. Each tablet contains 250 mg of methyldopa and 150 mg of chlorothiazide. They are supplied as follows:
NDC 0006-0612-68 bottles of 100.
[*Shown in Product Identification Section*]
No. 3319—Tablets ALDOCLOR 250 are green, oval, film coated tablets coded MSD 634. Each tablet contains 250 mg of methyldopa and 250 mg of chlorothiazide. They are supplied as follows:
NDC 0006-0634-68 bottles of 100.
[*Shown in Product Identification Section*]
A.H.F.S. Category: 24:08
DC 6078621 Issued February 1982

ALDOMET® Tablets (methyldopa, MSD), U.S.P. ℞

ALDOMET® Oral Suspension (methyldopa, MSD) ℞

Description

Methyldopa is the *L*-isomer of alpha-methyldopa. Its chemical name is levo-3-(3,4 - dihydroxyphenyl) -2-methylalanine.
ALDOMET is supplied as 125 mg, 250 mg, and 500 mg tablets, and as an oral suspension containing 250 mg of methyldopa per 5 ml and alcohol 1 percent, with benzoic acid, 0.1 percent, added as preservative.

Actions

ALDOMET® (Methyldopa, MSD), a unique antihypertensive, is an aromatic-amino-acid decarboxylase inhibitor in animals and in man. Although the mechanism of action has yet to be conclusively demonstrated, the antihypertensive effect of methyldopa probably is due to its metabolism to alpha-methylnorepinephrine, which then lowers arterial pressure by stimulation of central inhibitory alpha-adrenergic receptors, false neurotransmission, and/or reduction of plasma renin activity. Methyldopa has been shown to cause a net reduction in the tissue concentration of serotonin, dopamine, norepinephrine, and epinephrine.
Only methyldopa, the *L*-isomer of alpha-methyldopa, has the ability to inhibit dopa decarboxylase and to deplete animal tissues of norepinephrine. In man the antihypertensive activity appears to be due solely to the *L*-isomer. About twice the dose of the racemate (*DL*-alpha-methyldopa) is required for equal antihypertensive effect.
Methyldopa has no direct effect on cardiac function and usually does not reduce glomerular filtration rate, renal blood flow, or filtration fraction. Cardiac output usually is maintained without cardiac acceleration. In some patients the heart rate is slowed.
Normal or elevated plasma renin activity may decrease in the course of methyldopa therapy.
ALDOMET reduces both supine and standing blood pressure. Methyldopa usually produces highly effective lowering of the supine pressure with infrequent symptomatic postural hypotension. Exercise hypotension and diurnal blood pressure variations rarely occur.

Indication

Hypertension.

Contraindications

Active hepatic disease, such as acute hepatitis and active cirrhosis.
If previous methyldopa therapy has been associated with liver disorders (see WARNINGS).
Hypersensitivity.

Warnings

It is important to recognize that a positive Coombs test, hemolytic anemia, and liver disorders may occur with methyldopa therapy. The rare occurrences of hemolytic anemia or liver disorders could lead to potentially fatal complications unless properly recognized and managed. Read this section carefully to understand these reactions.
With prolonged methyldopa therapy, 10 to 20 percent of patients develop a positive direct Coombs test which usually occurs between 6 and 12 months of methyldopa therapy. Lowest incidence is at daily dosage of 1 g or less. This on rare occasions may be associated with hemolytic anemia, which could lead to potentially fatal complications. One cannot predict which patients with a positive direct Coombs test may develop hemolytic anemia.
Prior existence or development of a positive direct Coombs test is not in itself a contraindication to use of methyldopa. If a positive Coombs test develops during methyldopa therapy, the physician should determine whether hemolytic anemia exists and whether the positive Coombs test may be a problem. For example, in addition to a positive direct Coombs test there is less often a positive indirect Coombs test which may interfere with cross matching of blood.
At the start of methyldopa therapy, it is desirable to do a blood count (hematocrit, hemoglo-

Continued on next page

Information on the Merck Sharp & Dohme products listed on these pages is the full prescribing information from package circulars in use October 31, 1982.

Merck Sharp & Dohme—Cont.

bin, or red cell count) for a baseline or to establish whether there is anemia. Periodic blood counts should be done during therapy to detect hemolytic anemia. It may be useful to do a direct Coombs test before therapy and at 6 and 12 months after the start of therapy.
If Coombs-positive hemolytic anemia occurs, the cause may be methyldopa and the drug should be discontinued. Usually the anemia remits promptly. If not, corticosteroids may be given and other causes of anemia should be considered. If the hemolytic anemia is related to methyldopa, the drug should not be reinstituted.
When methyldopa causes Coombs positivity alone or with hemolytic anemia, the red cell is usually coated with gamma globulin of the IgG (gamma G) class only. The positive Coombs test may not revert to normal until weeks to months after methyldopa is stopped.
Should the need for transfusion arise in a patient receiving methyldopa, both a direct and an indirect Coombs test should be performed on his blood. In the absence of hemolytic anemia, usually only the direct Coombs test will be positive. A positive direct Coombs test alone will not interfere with typing or cross matching. If the indirect Coombs test is also positive, problems may arise in the major cross match and the assistance of a hematologist or transfusion expert will be needed.
Occasionally, fever has occurred within the first 3 weeks of methyldopa therapy, associated in some cases with eosinophilia or abnormalities in one or more liver function tests, such as serum alkaline phosphatase, serum transaminases (SGOT, SGPT), bilirubin, cephalin cholesterol flocculation, prothrombin time, and bromsulphalein retention. Jaundice, with or without fever, may occur with onset usually within the first 2 to 3 months of therapy. In some patients the findings are consistent with those of cholestasis.
Rarely fatal hepatic necrosis has been reported after use of methyldopa. These hepatic changes may represent hypersensitivity reactions. Periodic determinations of hepatic function should be done particularly during the first 6 to 12 weeks of therapy or whenever an unexplained fever occurs. If fever, abnormalities in liver function tests, or jaundice appear, stop therapy with methyldopa. If caused by methyldopa, the temperature and abnormalities in liver function characteristically have reverted to normal when the drug was discontinued. Methyldopa should not be reinstituted in such patients.
Rarely, a reversible reduction of the white blood cell count with a primary effect on the granulocytes has been seen. The granulocyte count returned promptly to normal on discontinuance of the drug. Rare cases of granulocytopenia have been reported. In each instance, upon stopping the drug, the white cell count returned to normal. Reversible thrombocytopenia has occurred rarely.
When methyldopa is used with other antihypertensive drugs, potentiation of antihypertensive effect may occur. Patients should be followed carefully to detect side reactions or unusual manifestations of drug idiosyncrasy.
Pregnancy and Nursing
Use of any drug in women who are or may become pregnant or intend to nurse requires that anticipated benefits be weighed against possible risks.
Methyldopa crosses the placental barrier, appears in cord blood, and appears in breast milk. No unusual adverse reactions have been reported in association with the use of methyldopa during pregnancy. Though no obvious teratogenic effects have been reported, the possibility of fetal injury cannot be excluded. Also, the possibility of injury to a nursing infant cannot be excluded.

Precautions

Methyldopa should be used with caution in patients with a history of previous liver disease or dysfunction (see WARNINGS).
Methyldopa may interfere with measurement of: urinary uric acid by the phosphotungstate method, serum creatinine by the alkaline picrate method, and SGOT by colorimetric methods. Interference with spectrophotometric methods for SGOT analysis has not been reported.
Since methyldopa causes fluorescence in urine samples at the same wave lengths as catecholamines, falsely high levels of urinary catecholamines may be reported. This will interfere with the diagnosis of pheochromocytoma. It is important to recognize this phenomenon before a patient with a possible pheochromocytoma is subjected to surgery. Methyldopa does not interfere with measurement of VMA (vanillylmandelic acid), a test for pheochromocytoma, by those methods which convert VMA to vanillin. Methyldopa is not recommended for the treatment of patients with pheochromocytoma. Rarely, when urine is exposed to air after voiding, it may darken because of breakdown of methyldopa or its metabolites.
Rarely involuntary choreoathetotic movements have been observed during therapy with methyldopa in patients with severe bilateral cerebrovascular disease. Should these movements occur, stop therapy.
Patients may require reduced doses of anesthetics when on methyldopa. If hypotension does occur during anesthesia, it usually can be controlled by vasopressors. The adrenergic receptors remain sensitive during treatment with methyldopa.
Hypertension has recurred occasionally after dialysis in patients given methyldopa because the drug is removed by this procedure.

Adverse Reactions

Sedation, usually transient, may occur during the initial period of therapy or whenever the dose is increased. Headache, asthenia, or weakness may be noted as early and transient symptoms. However, significant adverse effects due to ALDOMET have been infrequent and this agent usually is well tolerated.
Central nervous system: Sedation, headache, asthenia or weakness, dizziness, lightheadedness, symptoms of cerebrovascular insufficiency, paresthesias, parkinsonism, Bell's palsy, decreased mental acuity, involuntary choreoathetotic movements. Psychic disturbances including nightmares and reversible mild psychoses or depression.
Cardiovascular: Bradycardia, prolonged carotid sinus hypersensitivity, aggravation of angina pectoris. Orthostatic hypotension (decrease daily dosage). Edema (and weight gain) usually relieved by use of a diuretic. (Discontinue methyldopa if edema progresses or signs of heart failure appear).
Gastrointestinal: Nausea, vomiting, distention, constipation, flatus, diarrhea, colitis, mild dryness of mouth, sore or "black" tongue, pancreatitis, sialadenitis.
Hepatic: Abnormal liver function tests, jaundice, liver disorders.
Hematologic: Positive Coombs test, hemolytic anemia. Bone marrow depression, leukopenia, granulocytopenia, thrombocytopenia. Positive tests for antinuclear antibody, LE cells, and rheumatoid factor.
Allergic: Drug-related fever, lupus-like syndrome, myocarditis.
Dermatologic: Rash as in eczema or lichenoid eruption; toxic epidermal necrolysis.
Other: Nasal stuffiness, rise in BUN, breast enlargement, gynecomastia, lactation, hyperprolactinemia, amenorrhea, impotence, decreased libido, mild arthralgia, myalgia.

Dosage and Administration

ADULTS
Initiation of Therapy
The usual starting dosage of ALDOMET is 250 mg two or three times a day in the first 48 hours. The daily dosage then may be increased or decreased, preferably at intervals of not less than two days, until an adequate response is achieved. To minimize the sedation, start dosage increases in the evening. By adjustment of dosage, morning hypotension may be prevented without sacrificing control of afternoon blood pressure.
When methyldopa is given to patients on other antihypertensives, the dose of these agents may need to be adjusted to effect a smooth transition. When ALDOMET is given with antihypertensives other than thiazides, the initial dosage of ALDOMET should be limited to 500 mg daily in divided doses; when ALDOMET is added to a thiazide, the dosage of thiazide need not be changed.
Maintenance Therapy
The usual daily dosage of ALDOMET is 500 mg to 2.0 g in two to four doses. Although occasional patients have responded to higher doses, the maximum recommended daily dosage is 3.0 g. Once an effective dosage range is attained, a smooth blood pressure response occurs in most patients in 12 to 24 hours. Since methyldopa has a relatively short duration of action, withdrawal is followed by return of hypertension usually within 48 hours. This is not complicated by an overshoot of blood pressure.
Occasionally tolerance may occur, usually between the second and third month of therapy. Adding a diuretic or increasing the dosage of methyldopa frequently will restore effective control of blood pressure. A thiazide may be added at any time during methyldopa therapy and is recommended if therapy has not been started with a thiazide or if effective control of blood pressure cannot be maintained on 2.0 g of methyldopa daily.
Methyldopa is largely excreted by the kidney and patients with impaired renal function may respond to smaller doses. Syncope in older patients may be related to an increased sensitivity and advanced arteriosclerotic vascular disease. This may be avoided by lower doses.
CHILDREN
Initial dosage is based on 10 mg/kg of body weight daily in two to four doses. The daily dosage then is increased or decreased until an adequate response is achieved. The maximum dosage is 65 mg/kg or 3.0 g daily, whichever is less.

How Supplied

No. 3341—Tablets ALDOMET, 125 mg, are yellow, film coated, round tablets, coded MSD 135. They are supplied as follows:
NDC 0006-0135-68 bottles of 100
[*Shown in Product Identification Section*]
No. 3290—Tablets ALDOMET, 250 mg, are yellow, film coated, round tablets, coded MSD 401. They are supplied as follows:
NDC 0006-0401-68 bottles of 100
(6505-00-890-1856, 250 mg 100's)
NDC 0006-0401-28 single unit packages of 100
(6505-00-149-0090, 250 mg individually sealed 100's)
NDC 0006-0401-78 unit of use bottles of 100
NDC 0006-0401-82 bottles of 1000.
(6505-00-931-6646, 250 mg 1000's)
[*Shown in Product Identification Section*]
No. 3292—Tablets ALDOMET, 500 mg, are yellow, film coated, round tablets, coded MSD 516. They are supplied as follows:
NDC 0006-0516-54 unit of use bottles of 60
NDC 0006-0516-68 bottles of 100
NDC 0006-0516-28 single unit packages of 100

NDC 0006-0516-78 unit of use bottles of 100
NDC 0006-0516-74 bottles of 500.
[*Shown in Product Identification Section*]
No. 3382—Oral Suspension ALDOMET, 250 mg per 5 ml, is an off-white, creamy suspension with a citric orange-pineapple flavor, and is supplied as follows:
NDC 0006-3382-74 bottles of 473 ml.
A.H.F.S. Category: 24:08
DC 6649716 Issued February 1982

ALDOMET® Ester HCl Injection ℞
(methyldopate hydrochloride, MSD), U.S.P.

Description

Injection ALDOMET® ester hydrochloride (Methyldopate Hydrochloride, MSD) is an antihypertensive agent for intravenous use, each 5 ml of which contains:

Methyldopate hydrochloride	250.0 mg
Citric acid anhydrous	25.0 mg
Sodium bisulfite	16.0 mg
Disodium edetate	2.5 mg
Monothioglycerol	10.0 mg
Sodium hydroxide to adjust pH	
Water for Injection, q.s. to	5.0 ml

Methylparaben 0.15% and propylparaben 0.02% added as preservatives.

Methyldopate hydrochloride [levo-3-(3,4-dihydroxyphenyl)-2-methylalanine, ethyl ester hydrochloride] is the ethyl ester of methyldopa, supplied as the hydrochloride salt. Methyldopate hydrochloride is more soluble and stable in solution than methyldopa and is the preferred form for intravenous use.

Actions

ALDOMET® (Methyldopa, MSD), a unique antihypertensive, is an aromatic-amino-acid decarboxylase inhibitor in animals and in man. Although the mechanism of action has yet to be conclusively demonstrated, the antihypertensive effect of methyldopa probably is due to its metabolism to alpha-methylnorepinephrine, which then lowers arterial pressure by stimulation of central inhibitory alpha-adrenergic receptors, false neurotransmission, and/or reduction of plasma renin activity. Methyldopa has been shown to cause a net reduction in the tissue concentration of serotonin, dopamine, norepinephrine, and epinephrine.

Only methyldopa, the *L*-isomer of alpha-methyldopa, has the ability to inhibit dopa decarboxylase and to deplete animal tissues of norepinephrine. In man the antihypertensive activity appears to be due solely to the *L*-isomer. About twice the dose of the racemate (*DL*-alpha-methyldopa) is required for equal antihypertensive effect.

Methyldopa has no direct effect on cardiac function and usually does not reduce glomerular filtration rate, renal blood flow, or filtration fraction. Cardiac output usually is maintained without cardiac acceleration. In some patients the heart rate is slowed.

Normal or elevated plasma renin activity may decrease in the course of methyldopa therapy.

Methyldopa reduces both supine and standing blood pressure. It usually produces highly effective lowering of the supine pressure with infrequent symptomatic postural hypotension. Exercise hypotension and diurnal blood pressure variations rarely occur.

Methyldopate hydrochloride is the ethyl ester of methyldopa hydrochloride and possesses the same pharmacologic attributes.

Indication

Hypertension, when parenteral medication is indicated.

The treatment of hypertensive crises may be initiated with injection ALDOMET ester hydrochloride.

Contraindications

Active hepatic disease, such as acute hepatitis and active cirrhosis.

If previous methyldopa therapy has been associated with liver disorders (see WARNINGS).

Hypersensitivity to any component of this product.

Warnings

It is important to recognize that a positive Coombs test, hemolytic anemia, and liver disorders may occur with methyldopa therapy. The rare occurrences of hemolytic anemia or liver disorders could lead to potentially fatal complications unless properly recognized and managed. Read this section carefully to understand these reactions.

With prolonged methyldopa therapy, 10 to 20 percent of patients develop a positive direct Coombs test which usually occurs between 6 and 12 months of methyldopa therapy. Lowest incidence is at daily dosage of 1 g or less. This on rare occasions may be associated with hemolytic anemia, which could lead to potentially fatal complications. One cannot predict which patients with a positive direct Coombs test may develop hemolytic anemia.

Prior existence or development of a positive direct Coombs test is not in itself a contraindication to use of methyldopa. If a positive Coombs test develops during methyldopa therapy, the physician should determine whether hemolytic anemia exists and whether the positive Coombs test may be a problem. For example, in addition to a positive direct Coombs test there is less often a positive indirect Coombs test which may interfere with cross matching of blood.

At the start of methyldopa therapy, it is desirable to do a blood count (hematocrit, hemoglobin, or red cell count) for a baseline or to establish whether there is anemia. Periodic blood counts should be done during therapy to detect hemolytic anemia. It may be useful to do a direct Coombs test before therapy and at 6 and 12 months after the start of therapy.

If Coombs-positive hemolytic anemia occurs, the cause may be methyldopa and the drug should be discontinued. Usually the anemia remits promptly. If not, corticosteroids may be given and other causes of anemia should be considered. If the hemolytic anemia is related to methyldopa, the drug should not be reinstituted.

When methyldopa causes Coombs positivity alone or with hemolytic anemia, the red cell is usually coated with gamma globulin of the lgG (gamma G) class only. The positive Coombs test may not revert to normal until weeks to months after methyldopa is stopped.

Should the need for transfusion arise in a patient receiving methyldopa, both a direct and an indirect Coombs test should be performed on his blood. In the absence of hemolytic anemia, usually only the direct Coombs test will be positive. A positive direct Coombs test alone will not interfere with typing or cross matching. If the indirect Coombs test is also positive, problems may arise in the major cross match and the assistance of a hematologist or transfusion expert will be needed.

Occasionally, fever has occurred within the first three weeks of methyldopa therapy, associated in some cases with eosinophilia or abnormalities in one or more liver function tests, such as serum alkaline phosphatase, serum transaminases (SGOT, SGPT), bilirubin, cephalin cholesterol flocculation, prothrombin time, and bromsulphalein retention. Jaundice, with or without fever, may occur with onset usually within the first two to three months of therapy. In some patients the findings are consistent with those of cholestasis.

Rarely fatal hepatic necrosis has been reported after use of methyldopa. These hepatic changes may represent hypersensitivity reactions. Periodic determination of hepatic function should be done particularly during the first 6 to 12 weeks of therapy or whenever an unexplained fever occurs. If fever, abnormalities in liver function tests, or jaundice appear, stop therapy with methyldopa. If caused by methyldopa, the temperature and abnormalities in liver function characteristically have reverted to normal when the drug was discontinued. Methyldopa should not be reinstituted in such patients.

Rarely, a reversible reduction of the white blood cell count with a primary effect on the granulocytes has been seen. The granulocyte count returned promptly to normal on discontinuance of the drug. Rare cases of granulocytopenia have been reported. In each instance, upon stopping the drug, the white cell count returned to normal. Reversible thrombocytopenia has occurred rarely.

When methyldopa is used with other antihypertensive drugs, potentiation of antihypertensive effect may occur. Patients should be followed carefully to detect side reactions or unusual manifestations of drug idiosyncrasy.

Pregnancy and Nursing

Use of any drug in women who are or may become pregnant or intend to nurse requires that anticipated benefits be weighed against possible risks.

Methyldopa crosses the placental barrier, appears in cord blood, and appears in breast milk. No unusual adverse reactions have been reported in association with the use of methyldopa during pregnancy. Though no obvious teratogenic effects have been reported, the possibility of fetal injury cannot be excluded. Also, the possibility of injury to a nursing infant cannot be excluded.

Precautions

Methyldopa should be used with caution in patients with a history of previous liver disease or dysfunction (see WARNINGS).

Methyldopa may interfere with measurement of: urinary uric acid by the phosphotungstate method, serum creatinine by the alkaline picrate method, and SGOT by colorimetric methods. Interference with spectrophotometric methods for SGOT analysis has not been reported.

A paradoxical pressor response has been reported with intravenous administration of ALDOMET ester hydrochloride.

Since methyldopa causes fluorescence in urine samples at the same wave lengths as catecholamines, falsely high levels of urinary catecholamines may be reported. This will interfere with the diagnosis of pheochromocytoma. It is important to recognize this phenomenon before a patient with a possible pheochromocytoma is subjected to surgery. Methyldopa does not interfere with measurement of VMA (vanillylmandelic acid), a test for pheochromocytoma, by those methods which convert VMA to vanillin. Methyldopa is not recommended for the treatment of patients with pheochromocytoma. Rarely, when urine is exposed to air after voiding, it may darken because of breakdown of methyldopa or its metabolites.

Rarely involuntary choreoathetotic movements have been observed during therapy with methyldopa in patients with severe bilateral cerebrovascular disease. Should these movements occur, stop therapy.

Patients may require reduced doses of anesthetics when on methyldopa. If hypotension does occur during anesthesia, it usually can be

Continued on next page

Information on the Merck Sharp & Dohme products listed on these pages is the full prescribing information from package circulars in use October 31, 1982.

Merck Sharp & Dohme—Cont.

controlled by vasopressors. The adrenergic receptors remain sensitive during treatment with methyldopa.
Hypertension has recurred occasionally after dialysis in patients given methyldopa because the drug is removed by this procedure.

Adverse Reactions

Sedation, usually transient, may occur during the initial period of therapy or whenever the dose is increased. Headache, asthenia, or weakness may be noted as early and transient symptoms. However, significant adverse effects due to methyldopa have been infrequent and this agent usually is well tolerated.
Central nervous system: Sedation, headache, asthenia or weakness, dizziness, lightheadedness, symptoms of cerebrovascular insufficiency, paresthesias, parkinsonism, Bell's palsy, decreased mental acuity, involuntary choreoathetotic movements. Psychic disturbances including nightmares and reversible mild psychoses or depression.
Cardiovascular: Bradycardia, prolonged carotid sinus hypersensitivity, aggravation of angina pectoris. Paradoxical pressor response with intravenous use. Orthostatic hypotension (decrease daily dosage). Edema (and weight gain) usually relieved by use of a diuretic. (Discontinue methyldopa if edema progresses or signs of heart failure appear.)
Gastrointestinal: Nausea, vomiting, distention, constipation, flatus, diarrhea, colitis, mild dryness of mouth, sore or "black" tongue, pancreatitis, sialadenitis.
Hepatic: Abnormal liver function tests, jaundice, liver disorders.
Hematologic: Positive Coombs test, hemolytic anemia. Bone marrow depression, leukopenia, granulocytopenia, thrombocytopenia. Positive tests for antinuclear antibody, LE cells, and rheumatoid factor.
Allergic: Drug-related fever, lupus-like syndrome, myocarditis.
Dermatologic: Rash as in eczema or lichenoid eruption; toxic epidermal necrolysis.
Other: Nasal stuffiness, rise in BUN, breast enlargement, gynecomastia, lactation, hyperprolactinemia, amenorrhea, impotence, decreased libido, mild arthralgia, myalgia.

Dosage and Administration

Injection ALDOMET ester hydrochloride, when given intravenously in effective doses, causes a decline in blood pressure that may begin in four to six hours and last 10 to 16 hours after injection.
Add the desired dose of injection ALDOMET ester hydrochloride to 100 ml of 5 percent Dextrose Injection U.S.P. Alternatively the desired dose may be given in 5% dextrose in water in a concentration of 100 mg/10 ml. Give this intravenous infusion slowly over a period of 30 to 60 minutes.

ADULTS

The usual adult dosage intravenously is 250 to 500 mg at six hour intervals as required. The maximum recommended intravenous dose is 1.0 g every six hours.
When control has been obtained, oral therapy with tablets ALDOMET (Methyldopa, MSD) may be substituted for intravenous therapy, starting with the same dosage schedule used for the parenteral route. The effectiveness and anticipated responses are described in the circular for tablets ALDOMET (Methyldopa, MSD).
Since methyldopa has a relatively short duration of action, withdrawal is followed by return of hypertension usually within 48 hours. This is not complicated by an overshoot of blood pressure.
Occasionally tolerance may occur, usually between the second and third month of therapy. Adding a diuretic or increasing the dosage of methyldopa frequently will restore effective control of blood pressure. A thiazide may be added at any time during methyldopa therapy and is recommended if therapy has not been started with a thiazide or if effective control of blood pressure cannot be maintained on 2.0 g of methyldopa daily.
Methyldopa is largely excreted by the kidney and patients with impaired renal function may respond to smaller doses. Syncope in older patients may be related to an increased sensitivity and advanced arteriosclerotic vascular disease. This may be avoided by lower doses.

CHILDREN

The recommended daily dosage is 20 to 40 mg/kg of body weight in divided doses every six hours. The maximum dosage is 65 mg/kg or 3.0 g daily, whichever is less. When the blood pressure is under control, continue with oral therapy using tablets ALDOMET (Methyldopa, MSD) in the same dosage as for the parenteral route.

How Supplied

No. 3293—Injection ALDOMET ester hydrochloride, 250 mg per 5 ml, is a clear, colorless solution and is supplied as follows:
NDC 0006-3293-05 in 5 ml vials.

A.H.F.S. Category: 24:08
DC 6112024 Issued February 1982

ALDORIL® Tablets ℞
Antihypertensive

WARNING

This fixed combination drug is not indicated for initial therapy of hypertension. Hypertension requires therapy titrated to the individual patient. If the fixed combination represents the dosage so determined, its use may be more convenient in patient management. The treatment of hypertension is not static, but must be reevaluated as conditions in each patient warrant.

Description

ALDORIL® is a combination of methyldopa and hydrochlorothiazide. The chemical name for methyldopa is levo - 3 - (3,4-dihydroxyphenyl)-2-methylalanine. Hydrochlorothiazide is 6-chloro-3, 4-dihydro-*2H*-1, 2, 4-benzothiadiazine-7-sulfonamide 1,1-dioxide.

Actions

ALDOMET® (Methyldopa, MSD)
Methyldopa, a unique antihypertensive, is an aromatic-amino-acid decarboxylase inhibitor in animals and in man. Although the mechanism of action has yet to be conclusively demonstrated, the antihypertensive effect of methyldopa probably is due to its metabolism to alpha-methylnorepinephrine, which then lowers arterial pressure by stimulation of central inhibitory alpha-adrenergic receptors, false neurotransmission, and/or reduction of plasma renin activity. Methyldopa has been shown to cause a net reduction in the tissue concentration of serotonin, dopamine, norepinephrine, and epinephrine.
Only methyldopa, the *L*-isomer of alpha-methyldopa, has the ability to inhibit dopa decarboxylase and to deplete animal tissues of norepinephrine. In man, the antihypertensive activity appears to be due solely to the *L*-isomer. About twice the dose of the racemate (*DL*-alpha-methyldopa) is required for equal antihypertensive effect.
Methyldopa has no direct effect on cardiac function and usually does not reduce glomerular filtration rate, renal blood flow, or filtration fraction. Cardiac output usually is maintained without cardiac acceleration. In some patients the heart rate is slowed.
Normal or elevated plasma renin activity may decrease in the course of methyldopa therapy.
Methyldopa reduces both supine and standing blood pressure. It usually produces highly effective lowering of the supine pressure with infrequent symptomatic postural hypotension. Exercise hypotension and diurnal blood pressure variations rarely occur.
HydroDIURIL®
(Hydrochlorothiazide, MSD)
Hydrochlorothiazide is a diuretic and antihypertensive. It affects the renal tubular mechanism of electrolyte reabsorption. At maximal therapeutic dosage all thiazides are approximately equal in their diuretic efficacy.
Hydrochlorothiazide increases excretion of sodium and chloride in approximately equivalent amounts. Natriuresis may be accompanied by some loss of potassium and bicarbonate.
The mechanism of the antihypertensive effect of thiazides is unknown. Hydrochlorothiazide does not affect normal blood pressure.
Hydrochlorothiazide is eliminated rapidly by the kidney.
ALDORIL
The concomitant use of methyldopa and hydrochlorothiazide, as provided in ALDORIL, frequently produces a more pronounced antihypertensive response than when either compound is the sole therapeutic agent. Particularly in those cases of hypertensive vascular disease where sodium and water retention is a problem, the coadministration of these two drugs in the form of ALDORIL will help control the fluid imbalance.
In severe essential hypertension and in malignant hypertension ALDORIL may achieve effective lowering of blood pressure with fewer side effects than occur with other compounds used for this purpose.
ALDORIL reduces both supine and standing blood pressure; more effective lowering of the supine pressure with less frequent symptomatic postural hypotension can be obtained with ALDORIL than with most other antihypertensive agents. In patients treated with ALDORIL, exercise hypotension and diurnal blood pressure variations rarely occur.

Indication

Hypertension (see box warning).

Contraindications

Active hepatic disease, such as acute hepatitis and active cirrhosis.
If previous methyldopa therapy has been associated with liver disorders (see WARNINGS).
Anuria.
Hypersensitivity to methyldopa, or to hydrochlorothiazide or other sulfonamide-derived drugs.

Warnings

Methyldopa
It is important to recognize that a positive Coombs test, hemolytic anemia, and liver disorders may occur with methyldopa therapy. The rare occurrences of hemolytic anemia or liver disorders could lead to potentially fatal complications unless properly recognized and managed. Read this section carefully to understand these reactions.
With prolonged methyldopa therapy, 10 to 20 percent of patients develop a positive direct Coombs test which usually occurs between 6 and 12 months of methyldopa therapy. Lowest incidence is at daily dosage of 1 g or less. This on rare occasions may be associated with hemolytic anemia, which could lead to potentially fatal complications. One cannot predict

which patients with a positive direct Coombs test may develop hemolytic anemia.
Prior existence or development of a positive direct Coombs test is not in itself a contraindication to use of methyldopa. If a positive Coombs test develops during methyldopa therapy, the physician should determine whether hemolytic anemia exists and whether the positive Coombs test may be a problem. For example, in addition to a positive direct Coombs test there is less often a positive indirect Coombs test which may interfere with cross matching of blood.
At the start of methyldopa therapy, it is desirable to do a blood count (hematocrit, hemoglobin, or red cell count) for a baseline or to establish whether there is anemia. Periodic blood counts should be done during therapy to detect hemolytic anemia. It may be useful to do a direct Coombs test before therapy and at 6 and 12 months after the start of therapy.
If Coombs-positive hemolytic anemia occurs, the cause may be methyldopa and the drug should be discontinued. Usually the anemia remits promptly. If not, corticosteroids may be given and other causes of anemia should be considered. If the hemolytic anemia is related to methyldopa, the drug should not be reinstituted.
When methyldopa causes Coombs positivity alone or with hemolytic anemia, the red cell is usually coated with gamma globulin of the IgG (gamma G) class only. The positive Coombs test may not revert to normal until weeks to months after methyldopa is stopped.
Should the need for transfusion arise in a patient receiving methyldopa, both a direct and an indirect Coombs test should be performed on his blood. In the absence of hemolytic anemia, usually only the direct Coombs test will be positive. A positive direct Coombs test alone will not interfere with typing or cross matching. If the indirect Coombs test is also positive, problems may arise in the major cross match and the assistance of a hematologist or transfusion expert will be needed.
Occasionally, fever has occurred within the first three weeks of methyldopa therapy, associated in some cases with eosinophilia or abnormalities in one or more liver function tests, such as serum alkaline phosphatase, serum transaminases (SGOT, SGPT), bilirubin, cephalin cholesterol flocculation, prothrombin time, and bromsulphalein retention. Jaundice, with or without fever, may occur with onset usually within the first two to three months of therapy. In some patients the findings are consistent with those of cholestasis.
Rarely fatal hepatic necrosis has been reported after use of methyldopa. These hepatic changes may represent hypersensitivity reactions. Periodic determination of hepatic function should be done particularly during the first 6 to 12 weeks of therapy or whenever an unexplained fever occurs. If fever, abnormalities in liver function tests, or jaundice appear, stop therapy with methyldopa. If caused by methyldopa, the temperature and abnormalities in liver function characteristically have reverted to normal when the drug was discontinued. Methyldopa should not be reinstituted in such patients.
Rarely, a reversible reduction of the white blood cell count with a primary effect on the granulocytes has been seen. The granulocyte count returned promptly to normal on discontinuance of the drug. Rare cases of granulocytopenia have been reported. In each instance, upon stopping the drug, the white cell count returned to normal. Reversible thrombocytopenia has occurred rarely.
When methyldopa is used with other antihypertensive drugs, potentiation of antihypertensive effect may occur. Patients should be followed carefully to detect side reactions or unusual manifestations of drug idiosyncrasy.

Hydrochlorothiazide
Use with caution in severe renal disease. In patients with renal disease, thiazides may precipitate azotemia. Cumulative effects of the drug may develop in patients with impaired renal function.
Thiazides should be used with caution in patients with impaired hepatic function or progressive liver disease, since minor alterations of fluid and electrolyte balance may precipitate hepatic coma.
Thiazides may add to or potentiate the action of other antihypertensive drugs.
Sensitivity reactions may occur in patients with or without a history of allergy or bronchial asthma.
The possibility of exacerbation or activation of systemic lupus erythematosus has been reported.
Lithium generally should not be given with diuretics because they reduce its renal clearance and add a high risk of lithium toxicity. Read circulars for lithium preparations before use of such concomitant therapy.

Pregnancy and Nursing

Use of any drug in women who are or may become pregnant requires that anticipated benefits be weighed against possible risks.
Methyldopa crosses the placental barrier and appears in cord blood. No unusual adverse reactions have been reported in association with the use of methyldopa during pregnancy. Though no obvious teratogenic effects have been reported, the possibility of fetal injury cannot be excluded.
Thiazides also cross the placental barrier and appear in cord blood. Hazards include fetal or neonatal jaundice, thrombocytopenia, and possibly other adverse reactions which have occurred in the adult.
Methyldopa and thiazides appear in breast milk. Patients taking ALDORIL should not nurse.

Precautions

Methyldopa
Methyldopa should be used with caution in patients with a history of previous liver disease or dysfunction (see WARNINGS).
Methyldopa may interfere with measurement of: urinary uric acid by the phosphotungstate method, serum creatinine by the alkaline picrate method, and SGOT by colorimetric methods. Interference with spectrophotometric methods for SGOT analysis has not been reported.
Since methyldopa causes fluorescence in urine samples at the same wave lengths as catecholamines, falsely high levels of urinary catecholamines may be reported. This will interfere with the diagnosis of pheochromocytoma. It is important to recognize this phenomenon before a patient with a possible pheochromocytoma is subjected to surgery. Methyldopa does not interfere with measurement of VMA (vanillylmandelic acid), a test for pheochromocytoma, by those methods which convert VMA to vanillin. Methyldopa is not recommended for the treatment of patients with pheochromocytoma. Rarely, when urine is exposed to air after voiding, it may darken because of breakdown of methyldopa or its metabolites.
Rarely, involuntary choreoathetotic movements have been observed during therapy with methyldopa in patients with severe bilateral cerebrovascular disease. Should these movements occur, stop therapy.
Patients may require reduced doses of anesthetics when on methyldopa. If hypotension does occur during anesthesia, it usually can be controlled by vasopressors. The adrenergic receptors remain sensitive during treatment with methyldopa.
Hypertension has recurred occasionally after dialysis in patients given methyldopa because the drug is removed by this procedure.

Hydrochlorothiazide
Periodic determination of serum electrolytes to detect possible electrolyte imbalance should be performed at appropriate intervals.
All patients receiving diuretic therapy should be observed for evidence of fluid or electrolyte imbalance: namely, hyponatremia, hypochloremic alkalosis, and hypokalemia. Serum and urine electrolyte determinations are particularly important when the patient is vomiting excessively or receiving parenteral fluids. Warning signs or symptoms of fluid and electrolyte imbalance include dryness of mouth, thirst, weakness, lethargy, drowsiness, restlessness, muscle pains or cramps, muscular fatigue, hypotension, oliguria, tachycardia, and gastrointestinal disturbances such as nausea and vomiting.
Hypokalemia may develop, especially with brisk diuresis, when severe cirrhosis is present, during concomitant use of corticosteroids or ACTH, or after prolonged therapy.
Interference with adequate oral electrolyte intake will also contribute to hypokalemia. Hypokalemia can sensitize or exaggerate the response of the heart to the toxic effects of digitalis (e.g., increased ventricular irritability). Hypokalemia may be avoided or treated by use of potassium supplements such as foods with a high potassium content.
Although any chloride deficit is generally mild and usually does not require specific treatment except under extraordinary circumstances (as in liver disease or renal disease), chloride replacement may be required in the treatment of metabolic alkalosis.
Dilutional hyponatremia may occur in edematous patients in hot weather; appropriate therapy is water restriction, rather than administration of salt, except in rare instances when the hyponatremia is life threatening. In actual salt depletion, appropriate replacement is the therapy of choice.
Hyperuricemia may occur or acute gout may be precipitated in certain patients receiving thiazides.
Insulin requirements in diabetic patients may be increased, decreased, or unchanged. Latent diabetes mellitus may become manifest during thiazide therapy.
Thiazides may increase the responsiveness to tubocurarine.
The antihypertensive effects of the drug may be enhanced in the postsympathectomy patient. Thiazides may decrease arterial responsiveness to norepinephrine. This diminution is not sufficient to preclude effectiveness of the pressor agent for therapeutic use.
If progressive renal impairment becomes evident, consider withholding or discontinuing diuretic therapy.
Thiazides may decrease serum PBI levels without signs of thyroid disturbance.
Thiazides may decrease urinary calcium excretion. Thiazides may cause intermittent and slight elevation of serum calcium in the absence of known disorders of calcium metabolism. Marked hypercalcemia may be evidence of hidden hyperparathyroidism. Thiazides should be discontinued before carrying out tests for parathyroid function.

Continued on next page

Information on the Merck Sharp & Dohme products listed on these pages is the full prescribing information from package circulars in use October 31, 1982.

Merck Sharp & Dohme—Cont.

Adverse Reactions

Methyldopa
Sedation, usually transient, may occur during the initial period of therapy or whenever the dose is increased. Headache, asthenia, or weakness may be noted as early and transient symptoms. However, significant adverse effects due to methyldopa have been infrequent and this agent usually is well tolerated.
Central nervous system: Sedation, headache, asthenia or weakness, dizziness, lightheadedness, symptoms of cerebrovascular insufficiency, paresthesias, parkinsonism, Bell's palsy, decreased mental acuity, involuntary choreoathetotic movements. Psychic disturbances including nightmares and reversible mild psychoses or depression.
Cardiovascular: Bradycardia, prolonged carotid sinus hypersensitivity, aggravation of angina pectoris. Orthostatic hypotension (decrease daily dosage). Edema (and weight gain) usually relieved by use of a diuretic. (Discontinue methyldopa if edema progresses or signs of heart failure appear.)
Gastrointestinal: Nausea, vomiting, distention, constipation, flatus, diarrhea, colitis, mild dryness of mouth, sore or "black" tongue, pancreatitis, sialadenitis.
Hepatic: Abnormal liver function tests, jaundice, liver disorders.
Hematologic: Positive Coombs test, hemolytic anemia. Bone marrow depression, leukopenia, granulocytopenia, thrombocytopenia. Positive tests for antinuclear antibody, LE cells, and rheumatoid factor.
Allergic: Drug-related fever, lupus-like syndrome, myocarditis.
Dermatologic: Rash as in eczema or lichenoid eruption; toxic epidermal necrolysis.
Other: Nasal stuffiness, rise in BUN, breast enlargement, gynecomastia, lactation, hyperprolactinemia, amenorrhea, impotence, decreased libido, mild arthralgia, myalgia.
Hydrochlorothiazide
Gastrointestinal system: Anorexia, gastric irritation, nausea, vomiting, cramping, diarrhea, constipation, jaundice (intrahepatic cholestatic jaundice), pancreatitis, sialadenitis.
Central nervous system: Dizziness, vertigo, paresthesias, headache, xanthopsia.
Hematologic: Leukopenia, agranulocytosis, thrombocytopenia, aplastic anemia, hemolytic anemia.
Cardiovascular: Orthostatic hypotension (may be aggravated by alcohol, barbiturates, or narcotics).
Hypersensitivity: Purpura, photosensitivity, rash, urticaria, necrotizing angiitis (vasculitis) (cutaneous vasculitis), fever, respiratory distress including pneumonitis and pulmonary edema, anaphylactic reactions.
Other: Hyperglycemia, glycosuria, hyperuricemia, muscle spasm, weakness, restlessness, transient blurred vision.
Whenever adverse reactions are moderate or severe, thiazide dosage should be reduced or therapy withdrawn.

Dosage and Administration

Dosage: As determined by individual titration (see box warning).
The usual dosage is 1 tablet of ALDORIL 15, ALDORIL 25, ALDORIL D30, or ALDORIL D50 two or three times a day in the first 48 hours. The daily dosage then may be increased or decreased, preferably at intervals of not less than two days, until an adequate response is achieved. To minimize the sedation associated with methyldopa, start dosage increases in the evening. By adjustment of dosage, morning hypotension may be prevented without sacrificing control of afternoon blood pressure.
When ALDORIL is given to patients on other antihypertensives, the dose of these agents may need to be adjusted to effect a smooth transition. When ALDORIL is given with antihypertensives other than thiazides, the initial dosage of methyldopa should be limited to 500 mg daily in divided doses.
Although occasional patients have responded to higher doses, the maximum recommended daily dosage is 3.0 g of methyldopa and 100 to 200 mg of hydrochlorothiazide. Once an effective dosage range is attained, a smooth blood pressure response occurs in most patients in 12 to 24 hours. If ALDORIL alone does not adequately control blood pressure, additional methyldopa may be given separately to obtain the maximum blood pressure response.
Since both components of ALDORIL have a relatively short duration of action, withdrawal is followed by return of hypertension usually within 48 hours. This is not complicated by an overshoot of blood pressure.
Occasionally tolerance may occur, usually between the second and third month of therapy. Increasing the dosage of either methyldopa or hydrochlorothiazide separately or together frequently will restore effective control of blood pressure.
Methyldopa is largely excreted by the kidney and patients with impaired renal function may respond to smaller doses of ALDORIL. Syncope in older patients may be related to an increased sensitivity and advanced arteriosclerotic vascular disease. This may be avoided by lower doses.

How Supplied

No. 3294—Tablets ALDORIL 15 are salmon, round, film coated tablets, coded MSD 423. Each tablet contains 250 mg of methyldopa and 15 mg of hydrochlorothiazide. They are supplied as follows:
NDC 0006-0423-68 bottles of 100
NDC 0006-0423-28 single unit package of 100
NDC 0006-0423-82 bottles of 1000
[*Shown in Product Identification Section*]
No. 3295—Tablets ALDORIL 25 are white, round, film coated tablets, coded MSD 456. Each tablet contains 250 mg of methyldopa and 25 mg of hydrochlorothiazide. They are supplied as follows:
NDC 0006-0456-68 bottles of 100
NDC 0006-0456-28 single unit package of 100
NDC 0006-0456-82 bottles of 1000.
[*Shown in Product Identification Section*]
No. 3362—Tablets ALDORIL D30 are salmon, oval, film coated tablets, coded MSD 694. Each tablet contains 500 mg of methyldopa and 30 mg of hydrochlorothiazide. They are supplied as follows:
NDC 0006-0694-68 bottles of 100.
NDC 0006-0694-28 single unit package of 100.
[*Shown in Product Identification Section*]
No. 3363—Tablets ALDORIL D50 are white, oval, film coated tablets, coded MSD 935. Each tablet contains 500 mg of methyldopa and 50 mg of hydrochlorothiazide. They are supplied as follows:
NDC 0006-0935-68 bottles of 100.
NDC 0006-0935-28 single unit package of 100.
[*Shown in Product Identification Section*]
A.H.F.S. Category: 24:08
DC 6086030 Issued February 1982

ANTIVENIN ℞
(latrodectus mactans), MSD
Black Widow Spider Antivenin
Equine Origin

Indications

Antivenin (Latrodectus mactans), MSD is used to treat patients with symptoms due to bites by the black widow spider (Latrodectus mactans). Early use of the Antivenin is emphasized for prompt relief.
Local muscular cramps begin from 15 minutes to several hours after the bite which usually produces a sharp pain similar to that caused by puncture with a needle. The exact sequence of symptoms depends somewhat on the location of the bite. The venom acts on the myoneural junctions or on the nerve endings, causing an ascending motor paralysis or destruction of the peripheral nerve endings. The groups of muscles most frequently affected at first are those of the thigh, shoulder, and back. After a varying length of time, the pain becomes more severe, spreading to the abdomen, and weakness and tremor usually develop. The abdominal muscles assume a boardlike rigidity, but tenderness is slight. Respiration is thoracic. The patient is restless and anxious. Feeble pulse, cold, clammy skin, labored breathing and speech, light stupor, and delirium may occur. Convulsions also may occur, particularly in small children. The temperature may be normal or slightly elevated. Urinary retention, shock, cyanosis, nausea and vomiting, insomnia, and cold sweats also have been reported. The syndrome following the bite of the black widow spider may be confused easily with any medical or surgical condition with acute abdominal symptoms.
The symptoms of black widow spider bite increase in severity for several hours, perhaps a day, and then very slowly become less severe, gradually passing off in the course of two or three days except in fatal cases. Residual symptoms such as general weakness, tingling, nervousness, and transient muscle spasm may persist for weeks or months after recovery from the acute stage.
If possible, the patient should be hospitalized. Other additional measures giving greatest relief are prolonged warm baths and intravenous injection of 10 ml of 10 percent solution of calcium gluconate repeated as necessary to control muscle pain. Morphine also may be required to control pain. Barbiturates may be used for extreme restlessness. However, as the venom is a neurotoxin, it can cause respiratory paralysis. This must be borne in mind when considering use of morphine or a barbiturate. Adrenocorticosteroids have been used with varying degrees of success. Supportive therapy is indicated by the condition of the patient. Local treatment of the site of the bite is of no value. Nothing is gained by applying a tourniquet or by attempting to remove venom from the site of the bite by incision and suction.
In otherwise healthy individuals between the ages of 16 and 60, the use of Antivenin may be deferred and treatment with muscle relaxants may be considered.

Precautions

Prior to treatment with any product prepared from horse serum, a careful review of the patient's history should be taken emphasizing prior exposure to horse serum or any allergies. Serious sickness and even death could result from the use of horse serum in a sensitive patient. A skin or conjunctival test should be performed prior to administration of Antivenin.
Skin test: Inject into (not under) the skin not more than 0.02 ml of the test material (1:10 dilution of normal horse serum in physiologic saline). Evaluate result in 10 minutes. A positive reaction is an urticarial wheal surrounded by a zone of erythema. A control test using Sodium Chloride Injection facilitates interpretation of the results.
Conjunctival test: For adults instill into the conjunctival sac one drop of a 1:10 dilution of horse serum and for children one drop of 1:100 dilution. Itching of the eye and reddening of the conjunctiva indicate a positive reaction, usually within 10 minutes.
Patients should be observed for serum sickness for an average of 8 to 12 days following administration of Antivenin.
Desensitization should be attempted only when the administration of Antivenin is considered necessary to save life. Epinephrine must be available in case of untoward reaction.

Desensitization: If the history is positive or the results of the sensitivity tests are mildly or questionably positive, Antivenin should be administered as follows to reduce the risk of an immediate severe allergic reaction:

1. In separate sterile vials or syringes prepare 1:10 or 1:100 dilutions of Antivenin in Sodium Chloride for Injection.
2. Allow at least 15 but preferably 30 minutes between injections and only proceed with the next dose if no reactions occurred following the previous dose.
3. Using a tuberculin syringe, inject subcutaneously 0.1, 0.2 and 0.5 ml of the 1:100 dilution at 15 or 30 minute intervals; repeat with the 1:10 dilution, and finally the undiluted Antivenin.
4. If there is a reaction after any of the injections, place a tourniquet proximal to the sites of injection and administer epinephrine, 1:1000 (0.3 to 1.0 ml subcutaneously, 0.05 to 0.1 ml intravenously), proximal to the tourniquet or into another extremity. Wait at least 30 minutes before giving another injection of Antivenin, the amount of which should be the same as the last one not evoking a reaction.
5. If no reaction has occurred after 0.5 ml of undiluted Antivenin has been given, it is probably safe to continue the dose at 15 minute intervals until the entire dose has been injected.

Method of Preparation

Antivenin (Latrodectus mactans), MSD is prepared from the blood serum of horses immunized against the venom of the black widow spider.

Each vial contains not less than 6000 Antivenin units. One unit of Antivenin will neutralize one average mouse lethal dose of black widow spider venom when the Antivenin and the venom are injected simultaneously in mice under suitable conditions.

Using a sterile syringe, remove from the accompanying vial 2.5 ml of Sterile Diluent for Antivenin and inject into the vial of Antivenin. With the needle still in the rubber stopper, shake the vial to dissolve the contents completely.

Dosage and Administration

The dose for adults and children is the entire contents of a restored vial (2.5 ml) of Antivenin. It may be given intramuscularly, preferably in the region of the anterolateral thigh so that a tourniquet may be applied in the event of a systemic reaction. Symptoms usually subside in 1 to 3 hours. Although one dose of Antivenin usually is adequate, a second dose may be necessary in some cases.

Antivenin also may be given intravenously in 10 to 50 ml of saline solution over a 15 minute period. It is the preferred route in severe cases, or when the patient is under 12, or in shock. One restored vial usually is enough.

How Supplied

No. 4084—Antivenin (Latrodectus mactans), MSD equine origin is supplied in a vial containing not less than 6000 Antivenin units. Thimerosal (mercury derivative) 1:10,000 is added as preservative, **NDC 0006-4084-00.** A 2.5 ml vial of Sterile Diluent for Antivenin is included. Also supplied is a 1 ml vial of normal horse serum (1:10 dilution) for sensitivity testing. Thimerosal (mercury derivative) 1:10,000 is added as preservative.

A.H.F.S. Category: 80:04

DC 6145211 Issued April 1975

AQUAMEPHYTON® Injection (phytonadione, MSD), U.S.P. ℞
Aqueous Colloidal Solution of Vitamin K_1

WARNING—INTRAVENOUS USE

Severe reactions, including fatalities, have occurred during and immediately after INTRAVENOUS injection of AquaMEPHYTON® (Phytonadione, MSD), even when precautions have been taken to dilute the AquaMEPHYTON and to avoid rapid infusion. Typically these severe reactions have resembled hypersensitivity or anaphylaxis, including shock and cardiac and/or respiratory arrest. Some patients have exhibited these severe reactions on receiving AquaMEPHYTON for the first time. Therefore the INTRAVENOUS route should be restricted to those situations where other routes are not feasible and the serious risk involved is considered justified.

Description

AquaMEPHYTON injection is a yellow, sterile, aqueous colloidal solution of vitamin K_1, available for injection by the intravenous, intramuscular, and subcutaneous routes. Each milliliter contains:

Phytonadione	2 mg or 10 mg
Inactive ingredients:	
Polyoxyethylated fatty acid derivative	70 mg
Dextrose	37.5 mg
Water for Injection, q.s.	1 ml
Added as preservative:	
Benzyl alcohol	0.9%

Actions

AquaMEPHYTON aqueous colloidal solution of vitamin K_1 for parenteral injection, possesses the same type and degree of activity as does naturally-occurring vitamin K, which is necessary for the production via the liver of active prothrombin (factor II), proconvertin (factor VII), plasma thromboplastin component (factor IX), and Stuart factor (factor X). The prothrombin test is sensitive to the levels of three of these four factors—II, VII, and X. The mechanism by which vitamin K promotes formation of these clotting factors in the liver is not known.

The action of the aqueous colloidal solution, when administered intravenously, is generally detectable within an hour or two and hemorrhage is usually controlled within 3 to 6 hours. A normal prothrombin level may often be obtained in 12 to 14 hours.

In the prophylaxis and treatment of hemorrhagic disease of the newborn, phytonadione has demonstrated a greater margin of safety than that of the water-soluble vitamin K analogues.

Indications

AquaMEPHYTON is indicated in the following coagulation disorders which are due to faulty formation of factors II, VII, IX and X when caused by vitamin K deficiency or interference with vitamin K activity.

AquaMEPHYTON injection is indicated in:
—anticoagulant-induced prothombin deficiency;
—prophylaxis and therapy of hemorrhagic disease of the newborn;
—hypoprothrombinemia due to antibacterial therapy;
—hypoprothrombinemia secondary to factors limiting absorption or synthesis of vitamin K, e.g., obstructive jaundice, biliary fistula, sprue, ulcerative colitis, celiac disease, intestinal resection, cystic fibrosis of the pancreas, and regional enteritis;
—other drug-induced hypoprothrombinemia where it is definitely shown that the result is due to interference with vitamin K metabolism, e.g., salicylates.

Contraindication

Hypersensitivity to any component of this medication.

Warnings

Benzyl alcohol as a preservative in Bacteriostatic Sodium Chloride Injection has been associated with toxicity in newborns. Data are unavailable on the toxicity of other preservatives in this age group. There is no evidence to suggest that the small amount of benzyl alcohol contained in AquaMEPHYTON, when used as recommended, is associated with toxicity.

An immediate coagulant effect should not be expected after administration of phytonadione. It takes a minimum of 1 to 2 hours for measurable improvement in the prothrombin time. Whole blood or component therapy may also be necessary if bleeding is severe.

Phytonadione will not counteract the anticoagulant action of heparin.

When vitamin K_1 is used to correct excessive anticoagulant-induced hypoprothrombinemia, anticoagulant therapy still being indicated, the patient is again faced with the clotting hazards existing prior to starting the anticoagulant therapy. Phytonadione is not a clotting agent, but overzealous therapy with vitamin K_1 may restore conditions which originally permitted thromboembolic phenomena. Dosage should be kept as low as possible, and prothrombin time should be checked regularly as clinical conditions indicate.

Repeated large doses of vitamin K are not warranted in liver disease if the response to initial use of the vitamin is unsatisfactory. Failure to respond to vitamin K may indicate that the condition being treated is inherently unresponsive to vitamin K.

Reproduction studies have not been performed in animals. There is no adequate information of whether this drug may affect fertility in human males or females or have a teratogenic potential or other adverse effect on the fetus.

Precautions

Protect from light at all times.

Temporary resistance to prothrombin-depressing anticoagulants may result, especially when larger doses of phytonadione are used. If relatively large doses have been employed, it may be necessary when reinstituting anticoagulant therapy to use somewhat larger doses of the prothrombin-depressing anticoagulant, or to use one which acts on a different principle, such as heparin sodium.

Adverse Reactions

Deaths have occurred after intravenous administration. (See Box Warning at beginning of circular).

Transient "flushing sensations" and "peculiar" sensations of taste have been observed, as well as rare instances of dizziness, rapid and weak pulse, profuse sweating, brief hypotension, dyspnea, and cyanosis.

Pain, swelling, and tenderness at the injection site may occur. The possibility of allergic sensitivity, including an anaphylactoid reaction, should be kept in mind.

Continued on next page

Information on the Merck Sharp & Dohme products listed on these pages is the full prescribing information from package circulars in use October 31, 1982.

Merck Sharp & Dohme—Cont.

Rarely, after repeated injections, reactions resembling erythema perstans have been reported.
Hyperbilirubinemia has been observed in the newborn following administration of phytonadione. This has occurred rarely and primarily with doses above those recommended.

Dosage and Administration

Whenever possible, AquaMEPHYTON should be given by the subcutaneous or intramuscular route. When intravenous administration is considered unavoidable, the drug should be injected very slowly, not exceeding 1 mg per minute.
The human minimum daily requirements for vitamin K have not been established officially but they have been estimated to be 1 to 5 mcg/kg of body weight for infants and 0.03 mcg/kg for adults. Usually, the dietary abundance of vitamin K will satisfy these requirements, except during the first five to eight days of the neonatal period.

Anticoagulant-Induced Prothrombin Deficiency

To correct excessively prolonged prothrombin time caused by oral anticoagulant therapy—2.5 to 10 mg or up to 25 mg initially is recommended. In rare instances 50 mg may be required. Frequency and amount of subsequent doses should be determined by prothrombin time response or clinical condition. If in 6 to 8 hours after parenteral administration the prothrombin time has not been shortened satisfactorily, the dose should be repeated.
In the event of shock or excessive blood loss, the use of whole blood or component therapy is indicated.
Smaller doses are recommended for patients being treated with the shorter-acting anticoagulants, and for those in need of continued anticoagulant therapy. The smallest effective dose should be sought to obviate the possibility of temporary refractoriness to further anticoagulant therapy, and to avoid lowering the prothrombin time too far below that indicating an effective level of anticoagulant activity.
Larger doses are recommended for patients on the longer-acting anticoagulants, for those with severe bleeding, and for those not needing further anticoagulant therapy. Although more than 25 mg may be necessary and a dose may need to be repeated, these courses of action are indicated *only rarely.*

Prophylaxis and Treatment of Hemorrhagic Disease of the Newborn

Prophylaxis

The Committee on Nutrition of the American Academy of Pediatrics recommends that vitamin K_1 be given to the newborn. A single intramuscular dose of AquaMEPHYTON 0.5 to 1.0 mg is recommended. Although less desirable, AquaMEPHYTON 1 to 5 mg may be given to the mother 12 to 24 hours before delivery.

Treatment

AquaMEPHYTON 1.0 mg should be given either subcutaneously or intramuscularly. Higher doses may be necessary if the mother has been receiving oral anticoagulants.
Empiric administration of vitamin K_1 should not replace proper laboratory evaluation of the coagulation mechanism. A prompt response (shortening of the prothrombin time in 2 to 4 hours) following administration of vitamin K_1 is usually diagnostic of hemorrhagic disease of the newborn, and failure to respond indicates another diagnosis or coagulation disorder.
Whole blood or component therapy may be indicated if bleeding is excessive. This therapy, however, does not correct the underlying disorder and AquaMEPHYTON should be given concurrently.

Hypoprothrombinemia Due to Other Causes

A dosage of 2.5 to 25 mg or more (rarely up to 50 mg) is recommended, the amount and route of administration depending upon the severity of the condition and response obtained.
If possible, discontinuation or reduction of the dosage of drugs interfering with coagulation mechanisms (such as salicylates, antibiotics) is suggested as an alternative to administering concurrent AquaMEPHYTON. The severity of the coagulation disorder should determine whether the immediate administration of AquaMEPHYTON is required in addition to discontinuation or reduction of interfering drugs.

Directions for Dilution

AquaMEPHYTON may be diluted with 0.9% Sodium Chloride Injection, 5% Dextrose Injection, or 5% Dextrose and Sodium Chloride Injection. Benzyl alcohol as a preservative has been associated with toxicity in newborns. *Therefore, all of the above diluents should be preservative-free* (See WARNINGS). *Other diluents should not be used.* When dilutions are indicated, administration should be started immediately after mixture with the diluent, and unused portions of the dilution should be discarded, as well as unused contents of the ampul.

How Supplied

Injection AquaMEPHYTON is a yellow, sterile, aqueous colloidal solution and is supplied in the following concentrations:
No. 7780—10 mg of vitamin K_1 per ml
NDC 0006-7780-64 boxes of 6–1 ml ampuls (6505-00-854-2499 10 mg 1.0 ml 6's)
NDC 0006-7780-66 boxes of 25–1 ml ampuls.
No. 7782—10 mg of vitamin K_1 per ml
NDC 0006-7782-30 in 2.5 ml multiple dose vials
NDC 0006-7782-03 in 5 ml multiple dose vials.
No. 7784—1 mg of vitamin K_1 per 0.5 ml
NDC 0006-7784-33 boxes of 25–0.5 ml ampuls (6505-00-180-6372 1 mg 0.5 ml 25's).

A.H.F.S. Category: 88:24
DC 6136713 Issued June 1982

ARAMINE® Injection (metaraminol bitartrate, MSD), U.S.P. ℞

Description

Injection ARAMINE® (Metaraminol Bitartrate, MSD) is a sterile solution, each ml of which contains:

Metaraminol bitartrate equivalent to metaraminol .... 10.0 mg
Inactive ingredients:
Sodium chloride .... 4.4 mg
Water for Injection q.s. ad .... 1.0 ml
Methylparaben 0.15%, propylparaben 0.02%, and sodium bisulfite 0.2% added as preservatives.

Metaraminol bitartrate is the generic name for levo-1-(m-hydroxyphenyl)-2-amino-1-propanol hydrogen D-tartrate. Metaraminol bitartrate is a white, crystalline powder, freely soluble in water, slightly soluble in alcohol, and practically insoluble in chloroform and in ether.

Actions

ARAMINE is a potent sympathomimetic amine that increases both systolic and diastolic blood pressure.
The pressor effect of ARAMINE begins in 1 to 2 minutes after intravenous infusion, in about 10 minutes after intramuscular injection, and in 5 to 20 minutes after subcutaneous injection. The effect lasts from about 20 minutes to one hour. ARAMINE has a positive inotropic effect on the heart and a peripheral vasoconstrictor action.
Renal, coronary, and cerebral blood flow are a function of perfusion pressure and regional resistance. In most instances of cardiogenic shock, the beneficial effect of sympathomimetic amines is attributable to their positive inotropic effect. In patients with insufficient or failing vasoconstriction, there is additional advantage to the peripheral action of ARAMINE, but in most patients with shock, vasoconstriction is adequate and any further increase is unnecessary. Therefore, blood flow to vital organs may decrease with ARAMINE if regional resistance increases excessively.
The pressor effect of ARAMINE is decreased but not reversed by alpha-adrenergic blocking agents. Primary or secondary fall in blood pressure and tachyphylactic response to repeated use are uncommon.

INDICATIONS

Based on a review of this drug by the National Academy of Sciences-National Research Council and/or other information, FDA has classified the indications as follows:
Effective: ARAMINE is indicated for prevention and treatment of the acute hypotensive state occurring with spinal anesthesia. Adjunctive treatment of hypotension due to hemorrhage; reactions to medications; surgical complications; and shock associated with brain damage due to trauma or tumor.
"Probably" effective: It may also be useful as an adjunct in the treatment of hypotension due to cardiogenic shock or septicemia.
Final classification of the less-than-effective indications requires further investigation.

Contraindications

Use of ARAMINE with cyclopropane or halothane anesthesia should be avoided, unless clinical circumstances demand such use.
Hypersensitivity to any component of this product.

Precautions

Caution should be used to avoid excessive blood pressure response. Rapidly induced hypertensive responses have been reported to cause acute pulmonary edema, arrhythmias, and cardiac arrest. ARAMINE should be used with caution in digitalized patients, since the combination of digitalis and sympathomimetic amines is capable of causing ectopic arrhythmic activity.
Patients with cirrhosis should be treated with caution, with adequate restoration of electrolytes if diuresis ensues. Fatal ventricular arrhythmia has been reported in one patient with Laennec's cirrhosis while receiving metaraminol bitartrate. In several instances, ventricular extrasystoles that appeared during infusion of this vasopressor subsided promptly when the rate of infusion was reduced.
With the prolonged action of ARAMINE, a cumulative effect is possible, and with an excessive vasopressor response there may be a prolonged elevation of blood pressure even with discontinuation of therapy. Monoamine oxidase inhibitors have been reported to potentiate the action of sympathomimetic amines.
When vasopressor amines are used for long periods, the resulting vasoconstriction may prevent adequate expansion of circulating volume and may cause perpetuation of the shock state. There is evidence that plasma volume may be reduced in all types of shock, and that the measurement of central venous pressure is useful in assessing the adequacy of the circulating blood volume. Therefore, blood or plasma volume expanders should be employed when the principal reason for hypotension or shock is decreased circulating volume.

Because of its vasoconstrictor effect ARAMINE should be given with caution in heart or thyroid disease, hypertension, or diabetes. Sympathomimetic amines may provoke a relapse in patients with a history of malaria.

Adverse Reactions

Sympathomimetic amines, including ARAMINE, may cause sinus or ventricular tachycardia, or other arrhythmias, especially in patients with myocardial infarction. See also PRECAUTIONS.
Also, in patients with a history of malaria, these compounds may provoke a relapse.
Abscess formation, tissue necrosis, or sloughing rarely may follow the use of ARAMINE. In choosing the site of injection, it is important to avoid those areas recognized as *not* suitable for use of any pressor agent and to discontinue the infusion immediately if infiltration or thrombosis occurs. Although the physician may be forced by the urgent nature of the patient's condition to choose injection sites that are not recognized as suitable, he should, when possible, use the preferred areas of injection. The larger veins of the antecubital fossa or the thigh are preferred to veins in the dorsum of the hand or ankle veins, particularly in patients with peripheral vascular disease, diabetes mellitus, Buerger's disease, or conditions with coexistent hypercoagulability.

Dosage and Administration

ARAMINE may be given intramuscularly, subcutaneously, or intravenously, the route depending on the nature and severity of the indication.
Allow at least 10 minutes to elapse before increasing the dose because the maximum effect is not immediately apparent. When the vasopressor is discontinued, observe the patient carefully as the effect of the drug tapers off, so that therapy can be reinitiated promptly if the blood pressure falls too rapidly. The response to vasopressors may be poor in patients with coexistent shock and acidosis. Established methods of shock management, such as blood or fluid replacement when indicated, and other measures directed to the specific cause of the shock state also should be used.
Intramuscular or Subcutaneous Injection (for prevention of hypotension—see INDICATIONS):
The recommended dose is 2 to 10 mg (0.2 to 1 ml). As with other agents given subcutaneously, only the preferred sites of injection, as set forth in standard texts, should be used.
Intravenous Infusion (for adjunctive treatment of hypotension—see INDICATIONS):
The recommended dose is 15 to 100 mg (1.5 to 10 ml) in 500 ml of Sodium Chloride Injection or 5% Dextrose Injection, adjusting the rate of infusion to maintain the blood pressure at the desired level. Higher concentrations of ARAMINE, 150 to 500 mg per 500 ml of infusion fluid, have been used.
If the patient needs more saline or dextrose solution at a rate of flow that would provide an excessive dose of the vasopressor, the recommended volume of infusion fluid (500 ml) should be increased accordingly. ARAMINE may also be added to *less* than 500 ml of infusion fluid if a smaller volume is desired.
Compatibility Information
In addition to Sodium Chloride Injection* and Dextrose Injection 5%*, the following infusion solutions were found physically and chemically compatible with injection ARAMINE when 5 ml of injection ARAMINE, 10 mg/ml (metaraminol equivalent), was added to 500 ml of infusion solution: Ringer's Injection*, Lactated Ringer's Injection*, Dextran 6% in Saline†, Normosol®-R pH 7.4†, and Normosol®-M in D5-W†.
When injection ARAMINE is mixed with an infusion solution, sterile precautions should be observed. Since infusion solutions generally do not contain preservatives, mixtures should be used within 24 hours.
Direct Intravenous Injection: In severe shock, where time is of great importance, this agent should be given by direct intravenous injection. The suggested dose is 0.5 to 5 mg (0.05 to 0.5 ml), followed by an infusion of 15 to 100 mg (1.5 to 10 ml) in 500 ml of infusion fluid as described previously.
If necessary, vials may be sterilized by autoclaving or by immersion in a sterilizing solution.

How Supplied

No. 3222X—Injection ARAMINE 1%, containing metaraminol bitartrate equivalent to 10 mg of metaraminol per ml, is a clear, colorless solution and is supplied as follows:
NDC 0006-3222-10 in 10 ml vials (6505-00-753-9601 10 ml vial)
NDC 0006-3222-17 in 12 × 1 ml vials.

*U.S.P.
†Product of Abbott Laboratories
A.H.F.S. Category: 12:12
DC 6019019 Issued December 1977

ATTENUVAX® ℞

(measles virus vaccine, live, attenuated, MSD), U.S.P.
(More Attenuated Enders' Line)
Prepared in Cell Cultures of Chick Embryo

Description

ATTENUVAX® (Measles Virus Vaccine, Live, Attenuated, MSD) is a live virus vaccine for immunization against measles (rubeola).
ATTENUVAX is a lyophilized preparation of a more attenuated line of measles virus derived from Enders' attenuated Edmonston strain. The further modification of the virus in ATTENUVAX was achieved in the Merck Institute for Therapeutic Research by multiple passage of Edmonston virus in cell cultures of chick embryo at low temperature.
When reconstituted as directed, the dose for injection contains not less than the equivalent of 1,000 $TCID_{50}$ (tissue culture infectious doses) of measles virus vaccine expressed in terms of the assigned titer of the FDA Reference Measles Virus. Each dose also contains approximately 25 mcg of neomycin.

Actions

ATTENUVAX produces a modified measles infection in susceptible persons. Fever and rash may appear. Extensive clinical trials have demonstrated that ATTENUVAX is highly immunogenic and generally well tolerated. A single injection of the vaccine has been shown to induce measles hemagglutination-inhibiting (HI) antibodies in 97 percent or more of susceptible persons. Vaccine-induced antibody levels have been shown to persist for at least eight years without substantial decline. If the present pattern continues, it will provide a basis for the expectation that immunity following the vaccine will be permanent. However, continued surveillance will be required to demonstrate this point.

Indications

ATTENUVAX is recommended for active immunization of children 15 months of age or older against measles (rubeola). A booster is not needed. Infants who are less than 15 months of age may fail to respond to the vaccine due to presence in the circulation of residual measles antibody of maternal origin; the younger the infant, the lower the likelihood of seroconversion. In geographically isolated or other relatively inaccessible populations for whom immunization programs are logistically difficult, and in population groups in which natural measles infection may occur in a significant proportion of infants before 15 months of age, it may be desirable to give the vaccine to infants at an earlier age. The advantage of early protection must be weighed against the chance for failure of response; infants vaccinated under these conditions should be revaccinated after reaching 15 months of age.
Children for whom ATTENUVAX is strongly recommended include those living in schools, orphanages, and similar institutions. It is also recommended for children with inactive tuberculosis or active tuberculosis under treatment, as well as for those with chronic diseases such as cystic fibrosis, heart disease, asthma, and other chronic pulmonary diseases, to minimize the risk of serious complications of natural measles.
ATTENUVAX given immediately after exposure to natural measles may provide some protection. If, however, the vaccine is given a few days before exposure, substantial protection may be provided.
Ordinarily, adults need not be immunized, since most are immune to measles. However, vaccination may be advisable for high school and college persons in epidemic situations and for adults in isolated communities where measles is not endemic.
Revaccination: Children vaccinated before 12 months of age—particularly if vaccine was administered with immune serum globulin or measles immune globulin, a standardized globulin preparation—should be revaccinated with live measles vaccine at about 15 months of age for optimal protection.
Based on available evidence, there is no reason to routinely revaccinate children originally vaccinated when 12 months of age or older. The decision to revaccinate should be based on evaluation of each individual case.
Despite the risk of local reaction (see ADVERSE REACTIONS), children who have previously been given inactivated vaccine alone or followed by live vaccine within 3 months should be revaccinated with live vaccine to avoid the severe atypical form of natural measles that may occur.
Use with Other Live Virus Vaccines
There are no data available concerning simultaneous use of ATTENUVAX with monovalent or trivalent poliovirus vaccine, live, oral, or with killed poliovirus vaccines. However, serologic evidence shows that when M-M-R® (Measles, Mumps and Rubella Virus Vaccine, Live, MSD), containing the HPV-77 rubella strain, is given simultaneously with trivalent poliovirus vaccine, live, oral, antibody responses can be expected to be comparable to those which follow administration of the vaccines at different times. From this it follows that when ATTENUVAX is given simultaneously with either monovalent or trivalent poliovirus vaccine, live, oral, MERUVAX® II (Rubella Virus Vaccine, Live, MSD) and/or MUMPSVAX® (Mumps Virus Vaccine, Live, MSD), antibody responses can be expected to be comparable to those which follow administration of the vaccines at different times.

Contraindications

ATTENUVAX is contraindicated in the following conditions:
Hypersensitivity to neomycin (each dose of reconstituted vaccine contains approximately 25 mcg of neomycin).
Any febrile respiratory illness, or other active febrile infection.

Continued on next page

Information on the Merck Sharp & Dohme products listed on these pages is the full prescribing information from package circulars in use October 31, 1982.

Merck Sharp & Dohme—Cont.

Active untreated tuberculosis.
Patients receiving therapy with ACTH, corticosteroids, irradiation, alkylating agents or antimetabolites.
This contraindication does not apply to patients who are receiving corticosteroids as replacement therapy, e.g., for Addison's disease.
Individuals with blood dyscrasias, leukemia, lymphomas of any type, or other malignant neoplasms affecting the bone marrow or lymphatic systems.
Primary immuno-deficiency states, including cellular immune deficiencies, hypogammaglobulinemic and dysgammaglobulinemic states.

Hypersensitivity to Eggs, Chicken, or Chicken Feathers

This vaccine is essentially devoid of potentially allergenic substances derived from host tissues (chick embryo).* However, because the attenuated virus in this vaccine is propagated in cell cultures of chick embryo, there is a potential risk of hypersensitivity reactions in patients allergic to eggs, chicken, or chicken feathers. Widespread use of the vaccine for more than a decade has resulted in only rare, isolated reports of minor allergic reactions attributed to allergens of this kind, possibly related to the vaccine. Significantly, when children with known allergies to eggs, chicken, and chicken feathers were given a similarly prepared vaccine in a clinical study, none experienced reactions other than those reactions previously observed in nonallergic children.

Pregnancy

The effects of ATTENUVAX on fetal development are unknown at this time. Therefore, live attenuated measles virus vaccine should not be given to persons known to be pregnant; furthermore, pregnancy should be avoided for three months following vaccination.
Reports have indicated that contracting of natural measles during pregnancy enhances fetal risk. Increased rates of spontaneous abortion, stillbirth, congenital defects and prematurity have been observed subsequent to natural measles during pregnancy. There are no adequate studies of the attenuated (vaccine) strain of measles virus in pregnancy. However, it would be prudent to assume that the vaccine strain of virus is also capable of inducing adverse fetal effects for up to three months following vaccination.
Vaccine administration to post-pubertal females entails a potential for inadvertent immunization during pregnancy. Theoretical risks involved should be weighed against the risks that measles poses to the unimmunized adolescent or adult. Advisory committees reviewing this matter have recommended vaccination of post-pubertal females who are presumed to be susceptible to measles and not known to be pregnant. If a measles exposure occurs during pregnancy, one should consider the possibility of providing temporary passive immunity through the administration of immune serum globulin (human).

Precautions

For subcutaneous administration; *do not give intravenously.*
Epinephrine should be available for immediate use should an anaphylactoid reaction occur.
ATTENUVAX may be given simultaneously with monovalent or trivalent poliovirus vaccine, live, oral, with MERUVAX$_{II}$ (Rubella Virus Vaccine, Live, MSD) and/or MUMPSVAX (Mumps Virus Vaccine, Live, MSD). ATTENUVAX should not be given less than one month before or after administration of other live virus vaccines.
Due caution should be employed in administration of measles vaccine to children with a history of febrile convulsions, or cerebral injury, or of any other condition in which stress due to fever should be avoided. The physician should be alert to the temperature elevation which may occur following vaccination.
The occurrence of thrombocytopenia and purpura associated with live virus measles vaccines has been extremely rare.
Vaccination should be deferred for at least 3 months following blood or plasma transfusions, or administration of human immune serum globulin.
It has been reported that attenuated measles virus vaccine, live, may result in a temporary depression of tuberculin skin sensitivity. Therefore, if a tuberculin test is to be done, it should be administered either before or simultaneously with ATTENUVAX.
Children under treatment for tuberculosis have not experienced exacerbation of the disease when immunized with live measles virus vaccine; no studies have been reported to date of the effect of measles virus vaccines on untreated tuberculous children.

*Morbidity and Mortality Weekly Report *25* (44): 350, Nov. 12, 1976.

Adverse Reactions

Because of the slightly acidic pH (6.2-6.6) of the vaccine, patients may complain of burning and/or stinging of short duration at the injection site.
Occasional
Moderate fever [101-102.9°F (38.3-39.4°C)] may occur during the month after vaccination. Generally, fever, rash, or both appear between the 5th and the 12th days. Rash, when it occurs, is usually minimal, but rarely may be generalized.
Less Common
High fever [over 103°F (39.4°C)].
Rare
Reactions at injection site. Allergic reactions such as wheal and flare at the injection site or urticaria have been reported.
Children developing fever may, on rare occasions, exhibit febrile convulsions.
Experience from more than 80 million doses of all live measles vaccines given in the U.S. through 1975 indicates that significant central nervous system reactions such as encephalitis and encephalopathy, occurring within 30 days after vaccination, have been temporally associated with measles vaccine approximately once for every million doses. In no case has it been shown that reactions were actually caused by vaccine. The Center for Disease Control has pointed out that "a certain number of cases of encephalitis may be expected to occur in a large childhood population in a defined period of time even when no vaccines are administered." However, the data suggest the possibility that some of these cases may have been caused by measles vaccines. The risk of such serious neurological disorders following live measles virus vaccine administration remains far less than that for encephalitis and encephalopathy with natural measles (one per thousand reported cases).
There have been isolated reports of ocular palsies and Guillain-Barre syndrome occurring after immunization with vaccines containing live attenuated measles virus. The ocular palsies have occurred approximately 3–24 days following vaccination. No definite causal relationship has been established between either of these events and vaccination.
There have been reports of subacute sclerosing panencephalitis (SSPE) in children who did not have a history of natural measles but did receive measles vaccine. Some of these cases may have resulted from unrecognized measles in the first year of life or possibly from the measles vaccination. Based on estimated nationwide measles vaccine distribution, the association of SSPE cases to measles vaccination is about one case per million vaccine doses distributed. This is far less than the association with natural measles, 5–10 cases of SSPE per million cases of measles. The results of a retrospective case-controlled study conducted by the Center for Disease Control suggest that the overall effect of measles vaccine has been to protect against SSPE by preventing measles with its inherent higher risk of SSPE.
Local reactions characterized by marked swelling, redness and vesiculation at the injection site of attenuated live virus measles vaccines have occurred in children who have previously received killed measles vaccine.

Dosage and Administration

After suitable cleansing of the immunization site, inject the total volume of reconstituted vaccine subcutaneously, preferably into the outer aspect of the upper arm. Do not inject intravenously.
The dosage of vaccine is the same for all patients. Inject the entire contents of the syringe (about 0.5 ml). *Do not give immune serum globulin (ISG) concurrently with* ATTENUVAX.
CAUTION: A new unused sterile disposable syringe with a 25 gauge ⅝" needle should be used for each injection of the vaccine because certain preservatives, antiseptics, and detergents will inactivate the live measles virus vaccine.

Shipment, Storage and Reconstitution

During shipment, to insure that there is no loss of potency, the vaccine must be maintained at a temperature of 10°C (50°F) or less.
Prior to reconstitution, store the vaccine in a refrigerator at 2–8° C (35.6–46.4° F). *Protect from light.*
The reconstituted vaccine should be protected from light, since such exposure may inactivate the virus.
To reconstitute, inject all the diluent in the syringe into the vial of lyophilized vaccine. Agitate to ensure thorough mixing. Draw the entire volume of reconstituted vaccine into the syringe. Each dose of ATTENUVAX contains not less than 1,000 $TCID_{50}$ (tissue culture infectious doses) of measles virus vaccine expressed in terms of the assigned titer of the FDA Reference Measles Virus.
Use only the diluent supplied and reconstitute ATTENUVAX just before using. Protect the vaccine from light at all times. If not used immediately, return the reconstituted vaccine to a dark place at 2–8° C (35.6–46.4° F). Discard if not used within eight hours.
Color: The color of the vaccine when reconstituted is yellow. It is acceptable for use only if clear.

How Supplied

No. 4588X—ATTENUVAX is supplied as a single-dose vial of lyophilized vaccine, **NDC** 0006-4588-00, and a diluent-containing disposable syringe with affixed 25 gauge, ⅝" needle.
No. 4589X/4590—ATTENUVAX is supplied as follows: (1) a box of 10 single-dose vials of lyophilized vaccine, **NDC** 0006-4589-00; and (2) a box of 10 diluent-containing disposable syringes with affixed 25 gauge, ⅝" needles. To conserve refrigerator space, the syringes may be stored separately at room temperature.

(6505-01-038-0794 Ten Pack)
A.H.F.S. Category: 80:12
DC 7075502 Issued September 1980

BENEMID® Tablets ℞
(probenecid, MSD), U.S.P.

Description

Probenecid is the generic name for 4-[(dipropylamino)sulfonyl] benzoic acid (molecular weight 285.36).
Probenecid is a white or nearly white, fine, crystalline powder. Probenecid is soluble in dilute alkali, in alcohol, in chloroform, and in acetone; it is practically insoluble in water and in dilute acids.

Actions

BENEMID® (Probenecid, MSD) is a uricosuric and renal tubular blocking agent. It inhibits the tubular reabsorption of urate, thus increasing the urinary excretion of uric acid and decreasing serum urate levels. Effective uricosuria reduces the miscible urate pool, retards urate deposition, and promotes resorption of urate deposits.
BENEMID inhibits the tubular secretion of penicillin and usually increases penicillin plasma levels by any route the antibiotic is given. A 2-fold to 4-fold elevation has been demonstrated for various penicillins.
BENEMID also has been reported to inhibit the renal transport of many other compounds including aminohippuric acid (PAH), aminosalicylic acid (PAS), indomethacin, sodium iodomethamate and related iodinated organic acids, 17-ketosteroids, pantothenic acid, phenolsulfonphthalein (PSP), sulfonamides, and sulfonylureas. See also DRUG INTERACTIONS.
BENEMID decreases both hepatic and renal excretion of sulfobromophthalein (BSP). The tubular reabsorption of phosphorus is inhibited in hypoparathyroid but not in euparathyroid individuals.
BENEMID does not influence plasma concentrations of salicylates, nor the excretion of streptomycin, chloramphenicol, chlortetracycline, oxytetracycline, or neomycin.

Indications

For treatment of the hyperuricemia associated with gout and gouty arthritis.
As an adjuvant to therapy with penicillin or with ampicillin, methicillin, oxacillin, cloxacillin, or nafcillin, for elevation and prolongation of plasma levels by whatever route the antibiotic is given.

Contraindications

Hypersensitivity to this product.
Children under 2 years of age.
Not recommended in persons with known blood dyscrasias or uric acid kidney stones.
Therapy with BENEMID should not be started until an acute gouty attack has subsided.

Warnings

Exacerbation of gout following therapy with BENEMID may occur; in such cases colchicine or other appropriate therapy is advisable.
BENEMID increases plasma concentrations of methotrexate in both animals and humans. In animal studies, increased methotrexate toxicity has been reported. If BENEMID is given with methotrexate, the dosage of methotrexate should be reduced and serum levels may need to be monitored.
In patients on BENEMID the use of salicylates in either small or large doses is contraindicated because it antagonizes the uricosuric action of BENEMID. The biphasic action of salicylates in the renal tubules accounts for the so-called "paradoxical effect" of uricosuric agents. In patients on BENEMID who require a mild analgesic agent the use of acetaminophen rather than small doses of salicylates would be preferred.
The appearance of hypersensitivity reactions requires cessation of therapy with BENEMID.
Use in Pregnancy: BENEMID crosses the placental barrier and appears in cord blood. The use of any drug in women of childbearing potential requires that the anticipated benefit be weighed against possible hazards.

Precautions

Hematuria, renal colic, costovertebral pain, and formation of uric acid stones associated with the use of BENEMID in gouty patients may be prevented by alkalization of the urine and a liberal fluid intake (*see* DOSAGE AND ADMINISTRATION). In these cases when alkali is administered, the acid-base balance of the patient should be watched.
Use with caution in patients with a history of peptic ulcer.
BENEMID has been used in patients with some renal impairment but dosage requirements may be increased. BENEMID may not be effective in chronic renal insufficiency particularly when the glomerular filtration rate is 30 ml/minute or less. Because of its mechanism of action, BENEMID is not recommended in conjunction with a penicillin in the presence of *known* renal impairment.
A reducing substance may appear in the urine of patients receiving BENEMID. This disappears with discontinuance of therapy. Suspected glycosuria should be confirmed by using a test specific for glucose.

Adverse Reactions

Headache, gastrointestinal symptoms (e.g., anorexia, nausea, vomiting), urinary frequency, hypersensitivity reactions (including anaphylaxis, dermatitis, pruritus, and fever), sore gums, flushing, dizziness, and anemia have occurred.
In gouty patients exacerbation of gout, and uric acid stones with or without hematuria, renal colic, or costovertebral pain, have been observed. Nephrotic syndrome, hepatic necrosis, and aplastic anemia occur rarely. Hemolytic anemia which in some instances could be related to genetic deficiency of glucose-6-phosphate dehydrogenase in red blood cells has been reported.

Drug Interactions

The use of salicylates antagonizes the uricosuric action of BENEMID (*see* WARNINGS). The uricosuric action of BENEMID is also antagonized by pyrazinamide.
BENEMID produces an insignificant increase in free sulfonamide plasma concentrations but a significant increase in total sulfonamide plasma levels. Since BENEMID decreases the renal excretion of conjugated sulfonamides, plasma concentrations of the latter should be determined from time to time when a sulfonamide and BENEMID are coadministered for prolonged periods. BENEMID may prolong or enhance the action of oral sulfonylureas and thereby increase the risk of hypoglycemia.
When BENEMID is given to patients receiving indomethacin, the plasma levels of indomethacin are likely to be increased. Therefore, a lower dosage of indomethacin may be required to produce a therapeutic effect, and increases in the dosage of indomethacin should be made cautiously and in small increments. BENEMID may increase plasma levels of rifampin. The clinical significance of this is not known.
In animals and in humans, BENEMID has been reported to increase plasma concentrations of methotrexate (*see* WARNINGS).
Falsely high readings for theophylline have been reported in an *in vitro* study, using the Schack and Waxler technic, when therapeutic concentrations of theophylline and BENEMID were added to human plasma.

Dosage and Administration

Gout
Therapy with BENEMID should not be *started* until an acute gouty attack has subsided. However, if an acute attack is precipitated *during* therapy, BENEMID may be continued without changing the dosage, and full therapeutic dosage of colchicine or other appropriate therapy should be given to control the acute attack.
The recommended adult dosage is 0.25 g (½ tablet of BENEMID) twice a day for one week, followed by 0.5 g (1 tablet) twice a day thereafter.
Some degree of renal impairment may be present in patients with gout. A daily dosage of 1 g may be adequate. However, if necessary, the daily dosage may be increased by 0.5 g increments every 4 weeks within tolerance (and usually not above 2 g per day) if symptoms of gouty arthritis are not controlled or the 24 hour uric acid excretion is not above 700 mg.
As noted, BENEMID may not be effective in chronic renal insufficiency particularly when the glomerular filtration rate is 30 ml/minute or less.
Gastric intolerance may be indicative of overdosage, and may be corrected by decreasing the dosage.
As uric acid tends to crystallize out of an acid urine, a liberal fluid intake is recommended, as well as sufficient sodium bicarbonate (3 to 7.5 g daily) or potassium citrate (7.5 g daily) to maintain an alkaline urine (*see* PRECAUTIONS).
Alkalization of the urine is recommended until the serum urate level returns to normal limits and tophaceous deposits disappear, i.e., during the period when urinary excretion of uric acid is at a high level. Thereafter, alkalization of the urine and the usual restriction of purine-producing foods may be somewhat relaxed.
BENEMID should be continued at the dosage that will maintain normal serum urate levels. When acute attacks have been absent for 6 months or more and serum urate levels remain within normal limits, the daily dosage may be decreased by 0.5 g every 6 months. The maintenance dosage should not be reduced to the point where serum urate levels tend to rise.
BENEMID *and Penicillin Therapy (General)*
Adults:
The recommended dosage is 2 g (4 tablets of BENEMID) daily in divided doses. This dosage should be reduced in older patients in whom renal impairment may be present.
Children 2-14 years of age:
Initial dose: 25 mg/kg body weight (*or* 0.7 g/square meter body surface).
Maintenance dose: 40 mg/kg body weight (*or* 1.2 g/square meter body surface) per day, divided into 4 doses.
For children weighing more than 50 kg (110 lb) the adult dosage is recommended.
BENEMID is contraindicated in children under 2 years of age.
The PSP excretion test may be used to determine the effectiveness of BENEMID in retarding penicillin excretion and maintaining therapeutic levels. The renal clearance of PSP is reduced to about one-fifth the normal rate when dosage of BENEMID is adequate.
Penicillin Therapy (Gonorrhea)
[See table on next page].

Continued on next page

Information on the Merck Sharp & Dohme products listed on these pages is the full prescribing information from package circulars in use October 31, 1982.

Merck Sharp & Dohme—Cont.

How Supplied

No. 3337—Tablets BENEMID, 0.5 g, are yellow, capsule shaped, scored, film coated tablets, coded MSD 501. They are supplied as follows:

NDC 0006-0501-68 bottles of 100 (6505-00-104-9735 100's)

NDC 0006-0501-28 single unit packages of 100.

NDC 0006-0501-82 bottles of 1000. (6505-00-181-8387 1000's)

[*Shown in Product Identification Section*]

A.H.F.S. Category: 40:40

DC 6103915 Issued September 1978

BIAVAX® II ℞

(rubella and mumps virus vaccine, live, MSD), U.S.P.

Description

BIAVAX® II (Rubella and Mumps Virus Vaccine, Live, MSD) is a live virus vaccine for immunization against rubella (German measles) and mumps.

BIAVAX II is a lyophilized preparation of MERUVAX®II (Rubella Virus Vaccine, Live, MSD), the Wistar RA 27/3 strain of live attenuated rubella virus grown in human diploid cell (WI-38) culture; and MUMPSVAX® (Mumps Virus Vaccine, Live, MSD), the Jeryl Lynn (B level) mumps strain grown in cell cultures of chick embryo. The two viruses are mixed before being lyophilized. The product contains no preservative.

When reconstituted as directed, the dose for injection is 0.5 ml and contains not less than 1,000 $TCID_{50}$ (tissue culture infectious doses) of Rubella Virus Vaccine, Live, and 5,000 $TCID_{50}$ of Mumps Virus Vaccine, Live, expressed in terms of the assigned titer of the FDA Reference Rubella and Mumps Viruses. Each dose contains approximately 25 mcg of neomycin.

Actions

Clinical studies of 73 double seronegative children 12 months to 2 years of age demonstrated that BIAVAX II is highly immunogenic and generally well tolerated. In these studies, a single injection of the vaccine induced rubella hemagglutination inhibition (HI) antibodies in 100 percent, and mumps neutralizing antibodies in 97 percent of the susceptible children.

The RA 27/3 rubella strain in BIAVAX II elicits higher immediate post-vaccination HI, complement-fixing and neutralizing antibody levels than other strains of rubella vaccine and has been shown to induce a broader profile of circulating antibodies including anti-theta and anti-iota precipitating antibodies. The RA 27/3 rubella strain immunologically simulates natural infection more closely than other rubella vaccine viruses. The increased levels and broader profile of antibodies produced by RA 27/3 strain rubella virus vaccine appear to correlate with greater resistance to subclinical reinfection with the wild virus, and provide greater confidence for lasting immunity.

Data relating to persistence of vaccine-induced antibodies are not available for BIAVAX II at this time; however, it is expected that the antibodies against rubella and mumps will be just as durable following administration of BIAVAX II as after the single vaccines given separately. Antibody levels after immuniza-

BENEMID® (Probenecid, MSD) Penicillin Therapy (Gonorrhea)*

	Recommended Regimens**	Remarks
Uncomplicated gonoococcal infection in men and women (urethral, cervical, rectal)	4.8 million units of aqueous procaine penicillin G† I.M., in at least 2 doses injected at different sites at one visit + 1 g of BENEMID (Probenecid, MSD) orally just before injections *or* 3.5 g of ampicillin† orally + 1 g of BENEMID orally given simultaneously.	Follow-up: Obtain urethral and other appropriate cultures from men, and cervical, anal, and other appropriate cultures from women, 7 to 14 days after completion of treatment. Treatment of sexual partners: Persons with known recent exposure to gonorrhea should receive same treatment as those known to have gonorrhea. Examination and treatment of male sex partners of persons with gonorrhea are essential because of high prevalence of nonsymptomatic urethral gonococcal infection in such men.
Pharyngeal gonococcal infection in men and women	4.8 million units of aqueous procaine penicillin G† I.M., in at least 2 doses injected at different sites at one visit + 1 g of BENEMID orally just before injections	Pharyngeal gonococcal infections may be more difficult to treat than anogenital gonorrhea. Posttreatment cultures are essential.
Uncomplicated gonorrhea in pregnant patients	4.8 million units of aqueous procaine penicillin G† I.M., in at least 2 doses injected at different sites at one visit *or* 3.5 g of ampicillin† orally + 1 g of BENEMID orally given simultaneously	
Acute gonococcal salpingitis	*Outpatients:* Aqueous procaine penicillin G† or ampicillin† with BENEMID as for gonorrhea in pregnancy, followed by 500 mg of ampicillin 4 times a day for 10 days *Hospitalized patients:* See details in CDC recommendations	Follow-up of patients with acute salpingitis is essential. All patients should receive repeat pelvic examinations and cultures for *Neisseria gonorrhoeae* after treatment. Examination and appropriate treatment of male sex partners are essential because of high prevalence of nonsymptomatic urethral gonorrhea in such men.
Disseminated gonococcal infection (arthritis-dermatitis syndrome)	10 million units of aqueous crystalline penicillin G† I.V. a day for 3 days or till significant clinical improvement occurs. May be followed with 500 mg of ampicillin† 4 times a day orally to complete 7 days of treatment *or* 3.5 g of ampicillin† orally with 1 g of BENEMID, followed by 500 mg of ampicillin† 4 times a day for at least 7 days	
Gonococcal infection in children	For postpubertal children and/or those weighing over 45 kg (100 lb) use the dosage regimens given above for adults Uncomplicated vulvovaginitis and urethritis: aqueous procaine penicillin G† 75,000—100,000 units/kg I.M., with BENEMID 23 mg/kg orally	See CDC recommendations for detailed information about prevention and treatment of neonatal gonococcal infection and gonococcal ophthalmia.

Note: Before treating gonococcal infections in patients with suspected primary or secondary syphilis, perform proper diagnostic procedures including darkfield examinations. If concomitant syphilis is suspected, perform monthly serological tests for at least 4 months.

* Recommended by Venereal Disease Control Advisory Committee, Center for Disease Control, U.S. Department of Health, Education, and Welfare, Public Health Service (Morbidity and Mortality Weekly Report, Vol. *23:* 341, 342, 347, 348, Oct. 11, 1974).

** See CDC recommendations for definition of regimens of choice. alternative regimens, treatment of hypersensitive patients, and other aspects of therapy.

† See package circulars of manufacturers for detailed information about contraindications, warnings, precautions, and adverse reactions.

tion with RA 27/3 strain rubella virus vaccine have persisted for at least six years without substantial decline, and for ten years after MUMPSVAX (Mumps Virus Vaccine, Live, MSD).

Indications

BIAVAX II is indicated for simultaneous immunization against rubella and mumps in children 12 months of age or older, and adults.
The vaccine is not recommended for infants younger than 12 months because they may retain maternal rubella and mumps neutralizing antibodies which may interfere with the immune response.
Previously unimmunized children of susceptible pregnant women should receive live attenuated rubella vaccine, because an immunized child will be less likely to acquire natural rubella and introduce the virus into the household.
Non-Pregnant Adolescent and Adult Females
Immunization of susceptible non-pregnant adolescent and adult females of child-bearing age with live attenuated rubella virus vaccine is indicated if certain precautions are observed (see below). Vaccinating susceptible postpubertal females confers individual protection against subsequently acquiring rubella infection during pregnancy, which in turn prevents infection of the fetus and consequent congenital rubella injury.
Pregnant females *must not* be given live attenuated rubella virus vaccine. It is not known to what extent infection of the fetus with attenuated virus might occur following vaccination, or whether damage to the fetus could result. Subjects should be considered for vaccination only if they agree that they will not become pregnant within three months following vaccination, and if they are informed of the reason for this precaution.* If a pregnant woman is inadvertently vaccinated or if she becomes pregnant within three months of vaccination, she should be counseled on the possible risks to the fetus.
It is recommended that rubella susceptibility be determined by serologic testing prior to immunization.** If immune, as evidenced by a specific rubella antibody titer of 1:8 or greater (hemagglutination inhibition test), vaccination is unnecessary. Congenital malformations do occur in up to seven percent of all live births. Their chance appearance after vaccination could lead to misinterpretation of the cause, particularly if the prior rubella-immune status of vaccinees is unknown.
Postpubertal females should be informed of the frequent occurrence of self-limited arthralgia and possible arthritis beginning 2 to 4 weeks after vaccination (See ADVERSE REACTIONS).
It has been found convenient in many instances to vaccinate rubella-susceptible women in the immediate postpartum period.
Revaccination: Based on available evidence, there is no reason to routinely revaccinate children originally vaccinated when 12 months of age or older; however, children vaccinated when younger than 12 months of age should be revaccinated. The decision to revaccinate should be based on evaluation of each individual case.
Use with Other Live Virus Vaccines
There are no data available concerning simultaneous use of BIAVAX II with monovalent or trivalent poliovirus vaccine, live, oral, or with killed poliovirus vaccines. However, serologic evidence shows that when M-M-R® (Measles, Mumps and Rubella Virus Vaccine, Live, MSD), containing the HPV-77 rubella strain, is given simultaneously with trivalent poliovirus vaccine, live, oral, antibody responses can be expected to be comparable to those which follow administration of the vaccines at different times. From this it follows that when BIAVAX II is given simultaneously with either monovalent or trivalent poliovirus vaccine, live, oral and/or ATTENUVAX® (Measles Virus Vaccine, Live, Attenuated, MSD), antibody responses can be expected to be comparable to those which follow administration of the vaccines at different times.

* NOTE: The Immunization Practices Advisory Committee (ACIP) has recommended "In view of the importance of protecting this age group against rubella, asking females if they are pregnant, excluding those who say they are, and explaining the theoretical risks to the others are reasonable precautions in a rubella immunization program."

**NOTE: The Immunization Practices Advisory Committee (ACIP) has stated "When practical, and when reliable laboratory services are available, potential vaccinees of childbearing age can have serologic tests to determine susceptibility to rubella. . . . However, routinely performing serologic tests for all females of childbearing age to determine susceptibility so that vaccine is given only to proven susceptibles is expensive and has been ineffective in some areas. Accordingly, the ACIP believes that rubella vaccination of a woman who is not known to be pregnant and has no history of vaccination is justifiable without serologic testing."

Contraindications

Do not give BIAVAX II to pregnant females; the possible effects of the vaccine on fetal development are unknown at this time. If vaccination of post-pubertal females is undertaken, pregnancy must be avoided for three months following vaccination.
Hypersensitivity to neomycin (each dose of reconstituted vaccine contains approximately 25 mcg of neomycin).
Any febrile respiratory illness or other active febrile infection.
Patients receiving therapy with ACTH, corticosteroids, irradiation, alkylating agents or antimetabolites. This contraindication does not apply to patients who are receiving corticosteroids as replacement therapy, e.g., for Addison's disease.
Individuals with blood dyscrasias, leukemia, lymphomas of any type, or other malignant neoplasms affecting the bone marrow or lymphatic systems.
Primary immuno-deficiency states, including cellular immune deficiencies, hypogammaglobulinemic and dysgammaglobulinemic states.

Hypersensitivity to Eggs, Chicken, or Chicken Feathers

This vaccine is essentially devoid of potentially allergenic substances derived from host tissues (chick embryos).* However, because the attenuated mumps virus in this vaccine is propagated in cell cultures of chick embryo, there is a potential risk of hypersensitivity reactions in patients allergic to eggs, chicken, or chicken feathers. Widespread use of the vaccine for more than a decade has resulted in only rare, isolated reports of minor allergic reactions attributed to allergens of this kind, possibly related to the vaccine. Significantly when children with known allergies to eggs, chicken, and chicken feathers were given a similarly prepared vaccine in a clinical study, none experienced reactions other than those reactions previously observed in nonallergic children.

Precautions

Administer BIAVAX II subcutaneously; *do not give intravenously.*
Epinephrine should be available for immediate use in case an anaphylactoid reaction occurs.
BIAVAX II may be given simultaneously with monovalent or trivalent poliovirus vaccine, live, oral and/or with ATTENUVAX (Measles Virus Vaccine, Live, Attenuated, MSD). BIAVAX II should not be given less than one month before or after administration of other live virus vaccines.
Vaccination should be deferred for at least 3 months following blood or plasma transfusions, or administration of human immune serum globulin.
Excretion of small amounts of the live attenuated rubella virus from the nose and throat has occurred in the majority of susceptible individuals 7–28 days after vaccination. There is no confirmed evidence to indicate that such virus is transmitted to susceptible persons who are in contact with the vaccinated individuals. Consequently, transmission, while accepted as a theoretical possibility, is not regarded as a significant risk.**
There are no reports of transmission of live attenuated mumps virus from vaccinees to susceptible contacts.
It has been reported that live attenuated rubella and mumps virus vaccines given individually may result in a temporary depression of tuberculin skin sensitivity. Therefore, if a tuberculin test is to be done, it should be administered either before or simultaneously with BIAVAX II.
As for any vaccine, vaccination with BIAVAX II may not result in seroconversion in 100% of susceptible subjects given the vaccine.

* Morbidity and Mortality Weekly Report *25*(44): 350, Nov. 12, 1976.

Adverse Reactions

Because of the slightly acidic pH (6.2–6.6) of the vaccine, patients may complain of burning and/or stinging of short duration at the injection site.
The adverse clinical reactions associated with the use of BIAVAX II are those expected to follow administration of the monovalent vaccines given separately. These may include malaise, sore throat, headache, fever, and rash; mild local reactions such as erythema, induration, tenderness and regional lymphadenopathy; parotitis; orchitis; thrombocytopenia and purpura; allergic reactions such as wheal and flare at the injection site or urticaria; and arthritis, arthralgia and polyneuritis.
Moderate fever [101–102.9°F (38.3–39.4°C)] occurs occasionally, and high fever [above 103°F (39.4°C)] occurs less commonly. On rare occasions, children developing fever may exhibit febrile convulsions. Rash occurs infrequently and is usually minimal, but rarely may be generalized.
Clinical experience with live attenuated rubella and mumps virus vaccines given individually indicates that encephalitis and other nervous system reactions have occurred very rarely. These might occur also with BIAVAX II.
Transient arthritis, arthralgia and polyneuritis are features of natural rubella and vary in frequency and severity with age and sex, being greatest in adult females and least in prepubertal children. This type of involvement has also been reported following administration of MERUVAX II (Rubella Virus Vaccine, Live, MSD). In children, joint reactions are rare and

** Recommendation of the Immunization Practices Advisory Committee (ACIP), Morbidity and Mortality Weekly Report *30*(4): 37–42, 47, Feb. 6, 1981.

Continued on next page

Information on the Merck Sharp & Dohme products listed on these pages is the full prescribing information from package circulars in use October 31, 1982.

Merck Sharp & Dohme—Cont.

of brief duration if they do occur. In women, incidence rates for arthritis and arthralgia are generally higher than those seen in children (children: 0–3%; women: 12–20%), and the reactions tend to be more marked and of longer duration. Rarely, symptoms may persist for a matter of months. In adolescent girls, the reactions appear to be intermediate in incidence between those seen in children and in adult women. Even in older women (35–45 years), these reactions are generally well tolerated and rarely interfere with normal activities.

Dosage and Administration

After suitably cleansing the immunization site, inject the total volume of reconstituted vaccine subcutaneously, preferably into the outer aspect of the upper arm. Do not inject BIAVAX II intravenously. *Do not give immune serum globulin (ISG) concurrently with* BIAVAX II.

Shipment, Storage, and Reconstitution

During shipment, to insure that there is no loss of potency, the vaccine must be maintained at a temperature of 10°C (50°F) or less.
Before reconstitution, store BIAVAX II at 2–8°C (35.6–46.4°F). *Protect from light.*
To reconstitute, use only the diluent supplied, since it is free of preservatives or other antiviral substances which might inactivate the vaccine. Inject all the diluent in the syringe into the vial of lyophilized vaccine, and agitate to mix thoroughly. Withdraw the entire contents into the syringe and inject the total volume of restored vaccine subcutaneously.
It is important to use a separate sterile syringe and needle for each individual patient to prevent transmission of hepatitis B and other infectious agents from one person to another.
The color of the vaccine when reconstituted is yellow.
It is recommended that the vaccine be used as soon as possible after reconstitution. Protect the vaccine from light at all times. Store reconstituted vaccine in a dark place at 2–8°C (35.6–46.4°F) and discard if not used within eight hours.

How Supplied

No. 4668—BIAVAX II is supplied as a single-dose vial of lyophilized vaccine with a disposable syringe containing diluent, and fitted with a 25 gauge, ⅝″ needle, **NDC** 0006-4668-00.
No. 4669/4590—BIAVAX II is supplied as follows: (1) a box of ten single-dose vials of lyophilized vaccine, **NDC** 0006-4669-00; and (2) a box of ten diluent-containing disposable syringes with affixed 25 gauge, ⅝″ needles. To conserve refrigerator space, the syringes may be stored separately at room temperature.

A.H.F.S. Category: 80:12
DC 7032303 Issued April 1981

BLOCADREN® Tablets (timolol maleate, MSD) ℞

Description

BLOCADREN® (Timolol Maleate, MSD) is a non-selective beta-adrenergic receptor blocking agent. The chemical name for timolol maleate is (S)-1-[(1,1-dimethylethyl)amino]-3-[[4-(4-morpholinyl)-1, 2, 5-thiadiazol-3-yl]oxy]-2-propanol, (Z)-butenedioate (1:1) salt. It possesses an asymmetric carbon atom in its structure and is provided as the levo isomer.
Timolol maleate has a molecular weight of 432.49. It is a water-soluble, white, crystalline solid. It is supplied as 10 mg and 20 mg tablets for oral administration.

Clinical Pharmacology

BLOCADREN is a $beta_1$ and $beta_2$ (non-selective) adrenergic receptor blocking agent that does not have significant intrinsic sympathomimetic, direct myocardial depressant, or local anesthetic activity.
Pharmacodynamics
Clinical pharmacology studies have confirmed the beta-adrenergic blocking activity as shown by (1) changes in resting heart rate and response of heart rate to changes in posture; (2) inhibition of isoproterenol-induced tachycardia; (3) alteration of the response to the Valsalva maneuver and amyl nitrite administration; and (4) reduction of heart rate and blood pressure changes on exercise.
BLOCADREN decreases the positive chronotropic, positive inotropic, bronchodilator, and vasodilator responses caused by beta-adrenergic receptor agonists. The magnitude of this decreased response is proportional to the existing sympathetic tone and the concentration of BLOCADREN at receptor sites.
In normal volunteers, the reduction in heart rate response to a standard exercise was dose dependent over the test range of 0.5 to 20 mg, with a peak reduction at 2 hours of approximately 30% at higher doses.
Beta-adrenergic receptor blockade reduces cardiac output in both healthy subjects and patients with heart disease. In patients with severe impairment of myocardial function beta-adrenergic receptor blockade may inhibit the stimulatory effect of the sympathetic nervous system necessary to maintain adequate cardiac function.
Beta-adrenergic receptor blockade in the bronchi and bronchioles results in increased airway resistance from unopposed parasympathetic activity. Such an effect in patients with asthma or other bronchospastic conditions is potentially dangerous.
Clinical studies indicate that BLOCADREN at a dosage of 20–60 mg/day reduces blood pressure without causing postural hypotension in most patients with essential hypertension. Administration of BLOCADREN to patients with hypertension results initially in a decrease in cardiac output, little immediate change in blood pressure, and an increase in calculated peripheral resistance. With continued administration of BLOCADREN blood pressure decreases within a few days, cardiac output usually remains reduced, and peripheral resistance falls toward pretreatment levels. Plasma volume may decrease or remain unchanged during therapy with BLOCADREN. In the majority of patients with hypertension BLOCADREN also decreases plasma renin activity. Dosage adjustment to achieve optimal antihypertensive effect may require a few weeks. When therapy with BLOCADREN is discontinued, the blood pressure tends to return to pretreatment levels gradually. In most patients the antihypertensive activity of BLOCADREN is maintained with long-term therapy and is well tolerated.
The mechanism of the antihypertensive effects of beta-adrenergic receptor blocking agents is not established at this time. Possible mechanisms of action include reduction in cardiac output, reduction in plasma renin activity, and a central nervous system sympatholytic action.
A Norwegian multi-center, double-blind study compared the effects of timolol maleate with placebo in 1,884 patients who had survived the acute phase of a myocardial infarction. Patients with systolic blood pressure below 100 mm Hg, sick sinus syndrome and contraindications to beta blockers, including uncontrolled heart failure, second or third degree AV block and bradycardia (< 50 beats per minute), were excluded from the multi-center trial. Therapy with BLOCADREN, begun 7 to 28 days following infarction, was shown to reduce overall mortality; this was primarily attributable to a reduction in cardiovascular mortality. The protective effect of BLOCADREN was consistent regardless of age, sex or site of infarction. The effect was clearest in patients with a first infarction who were considered at a high risk of dying, defined as those with one or more of the following characteristics during the acute phase: transient left ventricular failure, cardiomegaly, newly appearing atrial fibrillation or flutter, systolic hypotension, or SGOT (ASAT) levels greater than four times the upper limit of normal. Therapy with BLOCADREN also reduced the incidence of non-fatal reinfarction. The mechanism of the protective effect of BLOCADREN is unknown.
Pharmacokinetics and Metabolism
BLOCADREN is rapidly and nearly completely absorbed (about 90%) following oral ingestion. Detectable plasma levels of timolol occur within one-half hour and peak plasma levels occur in about one to two hours. The drug half-life in plasma is approximately 4 hours and this is essentially unchanged in patients with moderate renal insufficiency. Timolol is partially metabolized by the liver and timolol and its metabolites are excreted by the kidney. Timolol is not extensively bound to plasma proteins; i.e., < 10% by equilibrium dialysis and approximately 60% by ultrafiltration. An *in vitro* hemodialysis study, using ^{14}C timolol added to human plasma or whole blood, showed that timolol was readily dialyzed from these fluids; however, a study of patients with renal failure showed that timolol did not dialyze readily. Plasma levels following oral administration are about half those following intravenous administration indicating approximately 50% first pass metabolism. The level of beta sympathetic activity varies widely among individuals, and no simple correlation exists between the dose or plasma level of timolol maleate and its therapeutic activity. Therefore, objective clinical measurements such as reduction of heart rate and/or blood pressure should be used as guides in determining the optimal dosage for each patient.

Indications and Usage

Hypertension
BLOCADREN is indicated for the treatment of hypertension. It may be used alone or in combination with other antihypertensive agents, especially thiazide-type diuretics.
Myocardial Infarction
BLOCADREN is indicated in patients who have survived the acute phase of a myocardial infarction, and are clinically stable, to reduce cardiovascular mortality and the risk of reinfarction. It is recommended that treatment should be initiated within 1 to 4 weeks after infarction. Data are not available as to whether benefit would ensue if initiated later.

Contraindications

BLOCADREN is contraindicated in patients with: bronchospasm, including bronchial asthma, or severe chronic obstructive pulmonary disease; sinus bradycardia; second and third degree atrioventricular block; overt cardiac failure (see WARNINGS); cardiogenic shock; hypersensitivity to this product.

Warnings

Cardiac Failure
Sympathetic stimulation may be essential for support of the circulation in individuals with diminished myocardial contractility, and its inhibition by beta-adrenergic receptor blockade may precipitate more severe failure. Although beta-blockers should be avoided in overt congestive heart failure, they can be used, if necessary, with caution in patients with a history of failure who are well-compensated, usually with digitalis and diuretics. Both digitalis and timolol maleate slow AV conduction. If cardiac failure persists, therapy with BLOCADREN should be withdrawn.

In Patients Without a History of Cardiac Failure continued depression of the myocardium with beta-blocking agents over a period of time can, in some cases, lead to cardiac failure. At the first sign or symptom of cardiac failure, patients receiving BLOCADREN should be digitalized and/or be given a diuretic, and the response observed closely. If cardiac failure continues, despite adequate digitalization and diuretic therapy, BLOCADREN should be withdrawn.

Exacerbation of Ischemic Heart Disease Following Abrupt Withdrawal—Hypersensitivity to catecholamines has been observed in patients withdrawn from beta blocker therapy; exacerbation of angina and, in some cases, myocardial infarction have occurred after *abrupt* discontinuation of such therapy. When discontinuing chronically administered timolol maleate, particularly in patients with ischemic heart disease, the dosage should be gradually reduced over a period of one to two weeks and the patient should be carefully monitored. If angina markedly worsens or acute coronary insufficiency develops, timolol maleate administration should be reinstituted promptly, at least temporarily, and other measures appropriate for the management of unstable angina should be taken. Patients should be warned against interruption or discontinuation of therapy without the physician's advice. Because coronary artery disease is common and may be unrecognized, it may be prudent not to discontinue timolol maleate therapy abruptly even in patients treated only for hypertension.

Major Surgery
The necessity or desirability of withdrawal of beta-blocking therapy prior to major surgery is controversial. Beta-adrenergic receptor blockade impairs the ability of the heart to respond to beta-adrenergically mediated reflex stimuli. This may augment the risk of general anesthesia in surgical procedures. Some patients receiving beta-adrenergic receptor blocking agents have been subject to protracted severe hypotension during anesthesia. Difficulty in restarting and maintaining the heartbeat has also been reported. For these reasons, in patients undergoing elective surgery, some authorities recommend gradual withdrawal of beta-adrenergic receptor blocking agents.
If necessary during surgery, the effects of beta-adrenergic blocking agents may be reversed by sufficient doses of such agonists as isoproterenol, dopamine, dobutamine or levarterenol (see OVERDOSAGE).
Diabetes Mellitus
BLOCADREN should be administered with caution in patients subject to spontaneous hypoglycemia or to diabetic patients (especially those with labile diabetes) who are receiving insulin or oral hypoglycemic agents. Beta-adrenergic receptor blocking agents may mask the signs and symptoms of acute hypoglycemia.
Thyrotoxicosis
Beta-adrenergic blockade may mask certain clinical signs (e.g., tachycardia) of hyperthyroidism. Patients suspected of developing thyrotoxicosis should be managed carefully to avoid abrupt withdrawal of beta blockade which might precipitate a thyroid storm.

Precautions

General
Impaired Hepatic or Renal Function: Since BLOCADREN is partially metabolized in the liver and excreted mainly by the kidneys, dosage reductions may be necessary when hepatic and/or renal insufficiency is present.
Dosing in the Presence of Marked Renal Failure: Although the pharmacokinetics of BLOCADREN are not greatly altered by renal impairment, marked hypotensive responses have been seen in patients with marked renal impairment undergoing dialysis after 20 mg doses. Dosing in such patients should therefore be especially cautious.
Drug Interactions
Close observation of the patient is recommended when BLOCADREN is administered to patients receiving catecholamine-depleting drugs such as reserpine, because of possible additive effects and the production of hypotension and/or marked bradycardia, which may produce vertigo, syncope, or postural hypotension.
Carcinogenesis, Mutagenesis, Impairment of Fertility
In a two-year study of timolol maleate in rats, there was a statistically significant ($P \leq 0.05$) increase in the incidence of adrenal pheochromocytomas in male rats administered 300 times the maximum recommended human dose (1 mg/kg/day). Similar differences were not observed in rats administered doses equivalent to 25 or 100 times the maximum recommended human dose. In a lifetime study in mice, there were statistically significant ($P \leq 0.05$) increases in the incidence of benign and malignant pulmonary tumors and benign uterine polyps in female mice at 500 mg/kg/day, but not at 5 or 50 mg/kg/day. There was also a significant increase in mammary adenocarcinomas at the 500 mg/kg/day dose. This was associated with elevations in serum prolactin which occurred in female mice administered timolol at 500 mg/kg, but not at doses of 5 or 50 mg/kg/day. An increased incidence of mammary adenocarcinomas in rodents has been associated with administration of several other therapeutic agents which elevate serum prolactin, but no correlation between serum prolactin levels and mammary tumors has been established in man. Furthermore, in adult human female subjects who received oral dosages of up to 60 mg of timolol maleate, the maximum recommended human oral dosage, there were no clinically meaningful changes in serum prolactin.
There was a statistically significant increase ($P \leq 0.05$) in the overall incidence of neoplasms in female mice at the 500 mg/kg/day dosage level.
Timolol maleate was devoid of mutagenic potential when evaluated *in vivo* (mouse) in the micronucleus test and cytogenetic assay (doses up to 800 mg/kg) and *in vitro* in a neoplastic cell transformation assay (up to 100 μg/ml). In Ames tests the highest concentrations of timolol employed, 5000 or 10,000 μg/plate, were associated with statistically significant elevations ($P \leq 0.05$) of revertants observed with tester strain TA100 (in seven replicate assays), but not in the remaining three strains. In the assays with tester strain TA100, no consistent dose response relationship was observed, nor did the ratio of test to control revertants reach 2. A ratio of 2 is usually considered the criterion for a positive Ames test.
Reproduction and fertility studies in rats showed no adverse effect on male or female fertility at doses up to 150 times the maximum recommended human dose.
Pregnancy
Pregnancy Category C. Teratogenic studies with timolol in mice and rabbits at doses up to 50 mg/kg/day (50 times the maximum recommended human dose) showed no evidence of fetal malformations. Although delayed fetal ossification was observed at this dose in rats, there were no adverse effects on postnatal development of offspring. Doses of 1000 mg/kg/day (1,000 times the maximum recommended human dose) were maternotoxic in mice and resulted in an increased number of fetal resorptions. Increased fetal resorptions were also seen in rabbits at doses of 100 times the maximum recommended human dose, in this case without apparent maternotoxicity. There are no adequate and well-controlled studies in pregnant women. BLOCADREN should be used during pregnancy only if the potential benefit justifies the potential risk to the fetus.
Nursing Mothers
Because of the potential for serious adverse reactions from timolol in nursing infants, a decision should be made whether to discontinue nursing or to discontinue the drug, taking into account the importance of the drug to the mother.
Pediatric Use
Safety and effectiveness in children have not been established.

Adverse Reactions

BLOCADREN is usually well tolerated in properly selected patients. Most adverse effects have been mild and transient.
In a multicenter (12-week) clinical trial comparing timolol maleate and placebo, the following adverse reactions were reported spontaneously and considered to be causally related to timolol maleate:

	Timolol Maleate (n = 176) %	Placebo (n = 168) %
BODY AS A WHOLE		
fatigue/tiredness	3.4	0.6
headache	1.7	1.8
chest pain	0.6	0
asthenia	0.6	0
CARDIOVASCULAR		
bradycardia	9.1	0
arrhythmia	1.1	0.6
syncope	0.6	0
edema	0.6	1.2
DIGESTIVE		
dyspepsia	0.6	0.6
nausea	0.6	0
INTEGUMENTARY		
pruritus	1.1	0
NERVOUS SYSTEM		
dizziness	2.3	1.2
vertigo	0.6	0
paresthesia	0.6	0
PSYCHIATRIC		
decreased libido	0.6	0
RESPIRATORY		
dyspnea	1.7	0.6
bronchial spasm	0.6	0
rales	0.6	0
SPECIAL SENSES		
eye irritation	1.1	0.6
tinnitus	0.6	0

These data are representative of the incidence of adverse effects that may be observed in a properly selected hypertensive patient population, e.g., a group excluding patients with bronchospastic disease, congestive heart failure or other contraindications to beta blocker therapy. These adverse reactions can also occur in patients with coronary artery disease.
In a different population, the coronary artery disease population, studied in the Norwegian multi-center trial (see CLINICAL PHARMACOLOGY), the frequency of the principal adverse reactions and the frequency with which these resulted in discontinuation of therapy in the timolol and placebo groups were:
[See table on next page].
These adverse reactions can also occur in patients treated for hypertension.

Continued on next page

Information on the Merck Sharp & Dohme products listed on these pages is the full prescribing information from package circulars in use October 31, 1982.

Merck Sharp & Dohme—Cont.

The following additional adverse effects have been reported in clinical experience with the drug: *Body as a Whole:* extremity pain, decreased exercise tolerance, weight loss; *Cardiovascular:* cardiac failure, cerebral vascular accident, worsening of angina pectoris, worsening of arterial insufficiency, Raynaud's phenomenon, palpitations, vasodilatation; *Digestive:* gastrointestinal pain, hepatomegaly, vomiting, diarrhea, dyspepsia; *Endocrine:* hyperglycemia, hypoglycemia; *Integumentary:* rash, skin irritation, increased pigmentation, sweating; *Musculoskeletal:* arthralgia; *Nervous System:* local weakness; *Psychiatric:* depression, nightmares, somnolence, insomnia, nervousness, diminished concentration; *Respiratory:* cough; *Special Senses:* visual disturbances, dry eyes; *Urogenital:* impotence, urination difficulties.

Potential Adverse Effects: In addition, a variety of adverse effects not observed in clinical trials with BLOCADREN, but reported with other beta-adrenergic blocking agents, should be considered potential adverse effects of BLOCADREN: *Nervous System:* Reversible mental depression progressing to catatonia; hallucinations; an acute reversible syndrome characterized by disorientation for time and place, short-term memory loss, emotional lability, slightly clouded sensorium, and decreased performance on neuropsychometrics; *Cardiovascular:* Intensification of AV block (see CONTRAINDICATIONS); *Gastrointestinal:* Mesenteric arterial thrombosis, ischemic colitis; *Hematologic:* Agranulocytosis, nonthrombocytopenic purpura, thrombocytopenic purpura; *Allergic:* Erythematous rash, fever combined with aching and sore throat, laryngospasm and respiratory distress; *Miscellaneous:* Reversible alopecia, Peyronie's disease.

There have been reports of a syndrome comprising psoriasiform skin rash, conjunctivitis sicca, otitis, and sclerosing serositis attributed to the beta-adrenergic receptor blocking agent, practolol. This syndrome has not been reported with BLOCADREN.

Clinical Laboratory Test Findings: Clinically important changes in standard laboratory parameters were rarely associated with the administration of BLOCADREN. Slight increases in blood urea nitrogen, serum potassium, and serum uric acid, and slight decreases in hemoglobin and hematocrit occurred, but were not progressive or associated with clinical manifestations.

Overdosage

No data are available in regard to overdosage in humans.

The oral LD_{50} of the drug is 1190 and 900 mg/kg in female mice and female rats, respectively.

An *in vitro* hemodialysis study, using ^{14}C timolol added to human plasma or whole blood, showed that timolol was readily dialyzed from these fluids; however, a study of patients with renal failure showed that timolol did not dialyze readily.

The most common signs and symptoms to be expected with overdosage with a beta-adrenergic receptor blocking agent are symptomatic bradycardia, hypotension, bronchospasm, and acute cardiac failure. Therapy with BLOCADREN should be discontinued and the patient observed closely. The following additional therapeutic measures should be considered:

(1) *Gastric lavage*

(2) *Symptomatic bradycardia:* Use atropine sulfate intravenously in a dosage of 0.25 mg to 2 mg to induce vagal blockade. If bradycardia persists, intravenous isoproterenol hydrochloride should be administered cautiously. In refractory cases the use of a transvenous cardiac pacemaker may be considered.

(3) *Hypotension:* Use sympathomimetic pressor drug therapy, such as dopamine, dobutamine or levarterenol. In refractory cases the use of glucagon hydrochloride has been reported to be useful.

(4) *Bronchospasm:* Use isoproterenol hydrochloride. Additional therapy with aminophylline may be considered.

(5) *Acute cardiac failure:* Conventional therapy with digitalis, diuretics, and oxygen should be instituted immediately. In refractory cases the use of intravenous aminophylline is suggested. This may be followed if necessary by glucagon hydrochloride which has been reported to be useful.

(6) *Heart block (second or third degree):* Use isoproterenol hydrochloride or a transvenous cardiac pacemaker.

Dosage and Administration

Hypertension

The usual initial dosage of BLOCADREN is 10 mg twice a day, whether used alone or added to diuretic therapy. The usual total maintenance dosage is 20–40 mg per day. Depending on blood pressure and pulse rate, increases in dosage to a maximum of 60 mg per day divided into two doses may be necessary. There should be an interval of at least seven days between increases in dosages.

BLOCADREN may be used with a thiazide diuretic or with other antihypertensive agents. Patients should be observed carefully during initiation of such concomitant therapy.

Myocardial Infarction

The recommended dosage for long-term prophylactic use in patients who have survived the acute phase of a myocardial infarction is 10 mg given twice daily.

How Supplied

No. 3344—Tablets BLOCADREN, 10 mg, are light blue, round, scored, compressed tablets, with code MSD 136 on one side and BLOCADREN on the other. They are supplied as follows:

NDC 0006-0136-68 bottles of 100

NDC 0006-0136-28 single unit packages of 100.

[*Shown in Product Identification Section*]

No. 3371—Tablets BLOCADREN, 20 mg, are light blue, capsule shaped, scored, compressed tablets, with code MSD 437 on one side and BLOCADREN on the other. They are supplied as follows:

NDC 0006-0437-68 bottles of 100.

[*Shown in Product Identification Section*]

A.H.F.S. Category: 24:04, 24:08

DC 7117611 Issued January 1982

COPYRIGHT © MERCK & CO., INC., 1979
All rights reserved

CLINORIL® Tablets (sulindac, MSD), U.S.P. ℞

Description

Sulindac is a non-steroidal, anti-inflammatory indene derivative designated chemically as (Z)-5-fluoro-2-methyl - 1 - [[*p*- (methylsulfinyl) phenyl]methylene]-1*H*-indene-3-acetic acid. It is not a salicylate, pyrazolone or propionic acid derivative. Its empirical formula is $C_{20}H_{17}FO_3S$, with a molecular weight of 356.42. Sulindac, a yellow crystalline compound, is a weak organic acid practically insoluble in water below pH 4.5, but very soluble as the sodium salt or in buffers of pH 6 or higher. Following absorption, sulindac undergoes two major biotransformations—reversible reduction to the sulfide metabolite, and irreversible oxidation to the sulfone metabolite. Available evidence indicates that the biological activity resides with the sulfide metabolite.

Clinical Pharmacology

CLINORIL® (Sulindac, MSD) is a non-steroidal anti-inflammatory drug, also possessing analgesic and antipyretic activities. Its mode of action, like that of other non-steroidal, anti-inflammatory agents, is not known; however, its therapeutic action is not due to pituitary-adrenal stimulation. Inhibition of prostaglandin synthesis by the sulfide metabolite may be involved in the anti-inflammatory action of CLINORIL.

Sulindac is approximately 90% absorbed in man after oral administration. The peak plasma concentrations of the biologically active sulfide metabolite are achieved in about two hours when sulindac is administered in the fasting state, and in about three to four hours when sulindac is administered with food. The mean half-life of sulindac is 7.8 hours while the mean half-life of the sulfide metabolite is 16.4 hours. Sustained plasma levels of the sulfide metabolite are consistent with a prolonged anti-inflammatory action which is the rationale for a twice per day dosage schedule.

Sulindac and its sulfone metabolite undergo extensive enterohepatic circulation relative to the sulfide metabolite in animals. Similar enterohepatic circulation together with the reversible metabolism are probably major contributors to sustained plasma levels of the active drug in man.

The primary route of excretion in man is via the urine as both sulindac and its sulfone metabolite (free and glucuronide conjugates). Approximately 50% of the administered dose is excreted in the urine, with the conjugated sulfone metabolite accounting for the major portion. Less than 1% of the administered dose of sulindac appears in the urine as the sulfide metabolite. Approximately 25% is found in the feces, primarily as the sulfone and sulfide metabolites.

The bioavailability of sulindac, as assessed by urinary excretion, was not changed by concom-

	Adverse Reaction†		Withdrawal‡	
	Timolol (n = 945) %	Placebo (n = 939) %	Timolol (n = 945) %	Placebo (n = 939) %
Asthenia or Fatigue	5	1	<1	<1
Heart Rate <40 beats/minute	5	<1	4	<1
Cardiac Failure-Nonfatal	8	7	3	2
Hypotension	3	2	3	1
Pulmonary Edema-Nonfatal	2	<1	<1	<1
Claudication	3	3	1	<1
AV Block 2nd or 3rd degree	<1	<1	<1	<1
Sinoatrial Block	<1	<1	<1	<1
Cold Hands and Feet	8	<1	<1	0
Nausea or Digestive Disorders	8	6	1	<1
Dizziness	6	4	1	0
Bronchial Obstruction	2	<1	1	<1

† When an adverse reaction recurred in a patient, it is listed only once.

‡ Only principal reason for withdrawal in each patient is listed.

itant administration of an antacid containing magnesium and aluminum hydroxides (MAALOX®, William H. Rorer, Inc.).
In healthy men, the average fecal blood loss, measured over a two-week period during administration of 400 mg per day of CLINORIL, was similar to that for placebo, and was statistically significantly less than that resulting from 4800 mg per day of aspirin.
In controlled clinical studies CLINORIL was evaluated in the following five conditions:
1. *Osteoarthritis*
In patients with osteoarthritis of the hip and knee, the anti-inflammatory and analgesic activity of CLINORIL was demonstrated by clinical measurements that included: assessments by both patient and investigator of overall response; decrease in disease activity as assessed by both patient and investigator; improvement in ARA Functional Class; relief of night pain; improvement in overall evaluation of pain, including pain on weight bearing and pain on active and passive motion; improvement in joint mobility, range of motion, and functional activities; decreased swelling and tenderness; and decreased duration of stiffness following prolonged inactivity.
In clinical studies in which dosages were adjusted according to patient needs, CLINORIL 200 to 400 mg daily was shown to be comparable in effectiveness to aspirin 2400 to 4800 mg daily. CLINORIL was generally well tolerated, and patients on it had a lower overall incidence of total adverse effects, of milder gastrointestinal reactions, and of tinnitus than did patients on aspirin. (See ADVERSE REACTIONS.)
2. *Rheumatoid Arthritis*
In patients with rheumatoid arthritis, the anti-inflammatory and analgesic activity of CLINORIL was demonstrated by clinical measurements that included: assessments by both patient and investigator of overall response; decrease in disease activity as assessed by both patient and investigator; reduction in overall joint pain; reduction in duration and severity of morning stiffness; reduction in day and night pain; decrease in time required to walk 50 feet; decrease in general pain as measured on a visual analog scale; improvement in the Ritchie articular index; decrease in proximal interphalangeal joint size; improvement in ARA Functional Class; increase in grip strength; reduction in painful joint count and score; reduction in swollen joint count and score; and increased flexion and extension of the wrist.
In clinical studies in which dosages were adjusted according to patient needs, CLINORIL 300 to 400 mg daily was shown to be comparable in effectiveness to aspirin 3600 to 4800 mg daily. CLINORIL was generally well tolerated, and patients on it had a lower overall incidence of total adverse effects, of milder gastrointestinal reactions, and of tinnitus than did patients on aspirin. (See ADVERSE REACTIONS.)
In patients with rheumatoid arthritis, CLINORIL may be used in combination with gold salts at usual dosage levels. In clinical studies, CLINORIL added to the regimen of gold salts usually resulted in additional symptomatic relief but did not alter the course of the underlying disease.
3. *Ankylosing spondylitis*
In patients with ankylosing spondylitis, the anti-inflammatory and analgesic activity of CLINORIL was demonstrated by clinical measurements that included: assessments by both patient and investigator of overall response; decrease in disease activity as assessed by both patient and investigator; improvement in ARA Functional Class; improvement in patient and investigator evaluation of spinal pain, tenderness and/or spasm; reduction in the duration of morning stiffness; increase in the time to onset of fatigue; relief of night pain; increase in chest expansion; and increase in spinal mobility evaluated by fingers-to-floor distance, occiput to wall distance, the Schober Test, and the Wright Modification of the Schober Test. In a clinical study in which dosages were adjusted according to patient need, CLINORIL 200 to 400 mg daily was as effective as indomethacin 75 to 150 mg daily. In a second study, CLINORIL 300 to 400 mg daily was comparable in effectiveness to phenylbutazone 400 to 600 mg daily. CLINORIL was better tolerated than phenylbutazone. (See ADVERSE REACTIONS.)
4. *Acute painful shoulder (Acute subacromial bursitis/supraspinatus tendinitis)*
In patients with acute painful shoulder (acute subacromial bursitis/supraspinatus tendinitis), the anti-inflammatory and analgesic activity of CLINORIL was demonstrated by clinical measurements that included: assessments by both patient and investigator of overall response; relief of night pain, spontaneous pain, and pain on active motion; decrease in local tenderness; and improvement in range of motion measured by abduction, and internal and external rotation. In clinical studies in acute painful shoulder, CLINORIL 300 to 400 mg daily and oxyphenbutazone 400 to 600 mg daily were shown to be equally effective and well tolerated.
5. *Acute gouty arthritis*
In patients with acute gouty arthritis, the anti-inflammatory and analgesic activity of CLINORIL was demonstrated by clinical measurements that included: assessments by both the patient and investigator of overall response; relief of weight-bearing pain; relief of pain at rest and on active and passive motion; decrease in tenderness; reduction in warmth and swelling; increase in range of motion; and improvement in ability to function. In clinical studies, CLINORIL at 400 mg daily and phenylbutazone at 600 mg daily were shown to be equally effective. In these short-term studies in which reduction of dosage was permitted according to response, both drugs were equally well tolerated.

Indications and Usage

CLINORIL is indicated for acute or long-term use in the relief of signs and symptoms of the following:
1. Osteoarthritis
2. Rheumatoid arthritis*
3. Ankylosing spondylitis
4. Acute painful shoulder (Acute subacromial bursitis/supraspinatus tendinitis)
5. Acute gouty arthritis

Contraindications

CLINORIL should not be used in:
Patients who are hypersensitive to this product.
Patients in whom acute asthmatic attacks, urticaria, or rhinitis are precipitated by aspirin or other non-steroidal anti-inflammatory agents.

Warnings

Peptic ulceration and gastrointestinal bleeding have been reported in patients receiving CLINORIL. In patients with active gastrointestinal bleeding or an active peptic ulcer, an appropriate ulcer regimen should be instituted, and the physician must weigh the benefits of therapy with CLINORIL against possible hazards, and carefully monitor the patient's progress. When CLINORIL is given to patients with a history of upper gastrointestinal tract disease, it should be given under close supervision and only after consulting the ADVERSE REACTIONS section.
Rarely, fever and other evidence of hypersensitivity (see ADVERSE REACTIONS) including abnormalities in one or more liver function tests have occurred during therapy with CLINORIL. Fatalities have occurred in these patients. Hepatitis, jaundice, or both, with or without fever, may occur usually within the first one to three months of therapy. Determinations of liver function should be considered whenever a patient on therapy with CLINORIL develops unexplained fever, rash or other dermatologic reactions or constitutional symptoms. If unexplained fever or other evidence of hypersensitivity occurs, therapy with CLINORIL should be discontinued. The elevated temperature and abnormalities in liver function caused by CLINORIL characteristically have reverted to normal after discontinuation of therapy. Administration of CLINORIL should not be reinstituted in such patients.
In addition to hypersensitivity reactions involving the liver, in some patients the findings are consistent with those of cholestatic hepatitis. As with other non-steroidal anti-inflammatory drugs, borderline elevations of one or more liver tests without any other signs and symptoms may occur in up to 15% of patients. These abnormalities may progress, may remain essentially unchanged, or may be transient with continued therapy. The SGPT (ALT) test is probably the most sensitive indicator of liver dysfunction. Meaningful (3 times the upper limit of normal) elevations of SGPT or SGOT (AST) occurred in controlled clinical trials in less than 1% of patients. A patient with symptoms and/or signs suggesting liver dysfunction, or in whom an abnormal liver test has occurred, should be evaluated for evidence of the development of more severe hepatic reaction while on therapy with CLINORIL. Although such reactions as described above are rare, if abnormal liver tests persist or worsen, if clinical signs and symptoms consistent with liver disease develop, or if systemic manifestations occur (e.g. eosinophilia, rash, etc.), CLINORIL should be discontinued.

Precautions

General
Although CLINORIL has less effect on platelet function and bleeding time than aspirin, it is an inhibitor of platelet function; therefore, patients who may be adversely affected should be carefully observed when CLINORIL is administered.
Because of reports of adverse eye findings with non-steroidal anti-inflammatory agents, it is recommended that patients who develop eye complaints during treatment with CLINORIL have ophthalmologic studies.
Since CLINORIL is eliminated primarily by the kidneys, patients with significantly impaired renal function should be closely monitored and a reduction of daily dosage may be anticipated to avoid excessive drug accumulation.
In chronic studies in mice, rats and monkeys at high dosages, there were occasional occurrences of mild renal toxicity as evidenced by papillary edema or mild interstitial nephritis in some animals. Papillary necrosis occurred infrequently in mice and rats.
Edema has been observed in some patients taking CLINORIL. Therefore, as with other non-steroidal anti-inflammatory drugs, CLINORIL should be used with caution in patients with compromised cardiac function, hypertension,

Continued on next page

* The safety and effectiveness of CLINORIL have not been established in rheumatoid arthritis patients who are designated in the American Rheumatism Association classification as Functional Class IV (incapacitated, largely or wholly bedridden, or confined to wheelchair; little or no self-care).

Information on the Merck Sharp & Dohme products listed on these pages is the full prescribing information from package circulars in use October 31, 1982.

Merck Sharp & Dohme—Cont.

or other conditions predisposing to fluid retention.

CLINORIL may allow a reduction in dosage or the elimination of chronic corticosteroid therapy in some patients with rheumatoid arthritis. However, it is generally necessary to reduce corticosteroids gradually over several months in order to avoid an exacerbation of disease or signs and symptoms of adrenal insufficiency. Abrupt withdrawal of chronic corticosteroid treatment is generally not recommended even when patients have had a serious complication of chronic corticosteroid therapy.

Use in Pregnancy

CLINORIL is not recommended for use in pregnant women, since safety for use has not been established. In reproduction studies in the rat, a decrease in average fetal weight and an increase in numbers of dead pups were observed on the first day of the postpartum period at dosage levels of 20 and 40 mg/kg/day (2½ and 5 times the usual maximum daily dose in humans), although there was no adverse effect on the survival and growth during the remainder of the postpartum period. CLINORIL prolongs the duration of gestation in rats, as do other compounds of this class which also may cause dystocia and delayed parturition in pregnant animals. Visceral and skeletal malformations observed in low incidence among rabbits in some teratology studies did not occur at the same dosage levels in repeat studies, nor at a higher dosage level in the same species.

Nursing Mothers

Nursing should not be undertaken while a patient is on CLINORIL. It is not known whether sulindac is secreted in human milk; however, it is secreted in the milk of lactating rats.

Use in Children

Pediatric indications and dosage have not been established, but studies in juvenile rheumatoid arthritis are in progress.

Drug Interactions

Although sulindac and its sulfide metabolite are highly bound to protein, studies, in which CLINORIL was given at a dose of 400 mg daily, have shown no clinically significant interaction with oral anticoagulants or oral hypoglycemic agents. However, patients should be monitored carefully until it is certain that no change in their anticoagulant or hypoglycemic dosage is required. Special attention should be paid to patients taking higher doses than those recommended and to patients with renal impairment or other metabolic defects that might increase sulindac blood levels.

The concomitant administration of aspirin with sulindac significantly depressed the plasma levels of the active sulfide metabolite. A double-blind study compared the safety and efficacy of CLINORIL 300 or 400 mg daily given alone or with aspirin 2.4 g/day for the treatment of osteoarthritis. The addition of aspirin did not alter the types of clinical or laboratory adverse experiences for CLINORIL; however, the combination showed an increase in the incidence of gastrointestinal adverse experiences. Since the addition of aspirin did not have a favorable effect on the therapeutic response to CLINORIL, the combination is not recommended.

Probenecid given concomitantly with sulindac had only a slight effect on plasma sulfide levels, while plasma levels of sulindac and sulfone were increased. Sulindac was shown to produce a modest reduction in the uricosuric action of probenecid, which probably is not significant under most circumstances.

Neither propoxyphene hydrochloride nor acetaminophen had any effect on the plasma levels of sulindac or its sulfide metabolite.

Adverse Reactions

The following adverse reactions were reported in clinical trials or have been reported since the drug was marketed. The probability exists of a causal relationship between CLINORIL and these adverse reactions. The adverse reactions which have been observed in clinical trials encompass observations in 1,865 patients, including 232 observed for at least 48 weeks.

Incidence Greater Than 1%

Gastrointestinal

The most frequent types of adverse reactions occurring with CLINORIL are gastrointestinal; these include gastrointestinal pain (10%), dyspepsia*, nausea* with or without vomiting, diarrhea*, constipation*, flatulence, anorexia and gastrointestinal cramps.

Dermatologic

Rash*, pruritus.

Central Nervous System

Dizziness*, headache*, nervousness.

Special Senses

Tinnitus.

Miscellaneous

Edema (see PRECAUTIONS).

Incidence Less Than 1 in 100

Gastrointestinal

Gastritis or gastroenteritis. Peptic ulcer and gastrointestinal bleeding have been reported. GI perforation has been reported rarely.

Liver function abnormalities; jaundice, sometimes with fever; cholestasis; hepatitis.

Pancreatitis.

Dermatologic

Stomatitis, sore or dry mucous membranes, alopecia.

Erythema multiforme, toxic epidermal necrolysis, and Stevens-Johnson syndrome have been reported rarely.

Cardiovascular

Congestive heart failure in patients with marginal cardiac function; palpitation.

Hematologic

Thrombocytopenia; ecchymosis; purpura; leukopenia; bone marrow depression, including aplastic anemia; increased prothrombin time in patients on oral anticoagulants (see PRECAUTIONS).

Genitourinary

Urine discoloration.

Psychiatric

Depression; psychic disturbances including acute psychosis.

Nervous System

Vertigo; insomnia.

Special Senses

Blurred vision.

Hypersensitivity Reactions

Anaphylaxis and angioneurotic edema.

In a few patients, a potentially fatal apparent hypersensitivity syndrome has been reported. This has consisted of some or all of the following findings: fever, chills, skin rash or other dermatologic reactions (see above), changes in liver function, jaundice, pneumonitis, leukopenia, eosinophilia, anemia, adenitis, and renal impairment.

Causal Relationship Unknown

Other reactions have been reported in clinical trials or since the drug was marketed, but occurred under circumstances where a causal relationship could not be established. However, in these rarely reported events, that possibility cannot be excluded. Therefore, these observations are listed to serve as alerting information to physicians.

Cardiovascular

Hypertension.

Hematologic

Hemolytic anemia.

Nervous System

Paresthesias, neuritis.

Special Senses

Transient visual disturbances; decreased hearing.

Respiratory

Epistaxis.

Genitourinary

Vaginal bleeding, hematuria.

Renal impairment; interstitial nephritis; nephrotic syndrome.

* Incidence between 3% and 9%. Those reactions occurring in 1 to 3% of patients are not marked with an asterisk.

Management of Overdosage

In the event of overdosage, the stomach should be emptied by inducing vomiting or by gastric lavage, and the patient carefully observed and given symptomatic and supportive treatment. Animal studies show that absorption is decreased by the prompt administration of activated charcoal and excretion is enhanced by alkalinization of the urine.

Dosage and Administration

CLINORIL should be administered orally twice a day with food. In clinical studies to date, the usual maximum dosage was 400 mg per day. Although a few patients have received higher dosages, until further clinical experience is obtained, dosages above 400 mg per day are not recommended.

In osteoarthritis, rheumatoid arthritis, and ankylosing spondylitis, the recommended starting dosage is 150 mg twice a day. The dosage may be lowered or raised depending on the response.

A prompt response (within one week) can be expected in about one-half of patients with osteoarthritis, ankylosing spondylitis, and rheumatoid arthritis. Others may require longer to respond.

In acute painful shoulder (acute subacromial bursitis/supraspinatus tendinitis) and acute gouty arthritis, the recommended dosage is 200 mg twice a day. After a satisfactory response has been achieved, the dosage may be reduced according to the response. In acute painful shoulder, therapy for 7–14 days is usually adequate. In acute gouty arthritis, therapy for 7 days is usually adequate.

How Supplied

CLINORIL is available for oral administration as 150 mg yellow tablets, and as 200 mg scored yellow tablets.

No. 3360—Tablets CLINORIL 150 mg are yellow, hexagon-shaped, compressed tablets, coded MSD 941. They are supplied as follows:

NDC 0006-0941-54 unit of use bottles of 60
NDC 0006-0941-68 in bottles of 100
NDC 0006-0941-78 unit of use bottles of 100
NDC 0006-0941-28 single unit packages of 100.

[*Shown in Product Identification Section*]

No. 3353—Tablets CLINORIL 200 mg are yellow, hexagon-shaped, scored, compressed tablets, coded MSD 942. They are supplied as follows:

NDC 0006-0942-54 unit of use bottles of 60
NDC 0006-0942-68 in bottles of 100
NDC 0006-0942-78 unit of use bottles of 100
NDC 0006-0942-28 single unit packages of 100.

[*Shown in Product Identification Section*]

A.H.F.S. Category: 28:08

DC 7020016 Issued July 1982

COPYRIGHT© MERCK & CO., INC., 1977
All rights reserved

COGENTIN® Tablets ℞
(benztropine mesylate, MSD), U.S.P.
COGENTIN® Injection ℞
(benztropine mesylate, MSD), U.S.P.

Description

Benztropine mesylate is a synthetic compound resulting from the combination of the active portions of atropine and diphenhydramine.

It is a crystalline white powder, very soluble in water.

COGENTIN® (Benztropine Mesylate, MSD) is supplied as tablets in three strengths (0.5 mg, 1 mg, and 2 mg per tablet), and as an injection for intravenous and intramuscular use.

Each milliliter of the injection contains:

Benztropine mesylate	1.0 mg
Sodium chloride	9.0 mg
Water for injection q.s.	1.0 ml

Actions

COGENTIN possesses both anticholinergic and antihistaminic effects, although only the former have been established as therapeutically significant in the management of parkinsonism.

In the isolated guinea pig ileum, the anticholinergic activity of this drug is about equal to that of atropine; however, when administered orally to unanesthetized cats, it is only about half as active as atropine.

In laboratory animals, its antihistaminic activity and duration of action approach those of pyrilamine maleate.

Indications

For use as an adjunct in the therapy of all forms of parkinsonism.

Useful also in the control of extrapyramidal disorders (except tardive dyskinesia—see PRECAUTIONS) due to neuroleptic drugs (e.g., phenothiazines).

Contraindications

Hypersensitivity to COGENTIN tablets or to any component of COGENTIN injection.

Because of its atropine-like side effects, this drug is contraindicated in children under three years of age, and should be used with caution in older children.

Warnings

Safe use in pregnancy has not been established.

COGENTIN may impair mental and/or physical abilities required for performance of hazardous tasks, such as operating machinery or driving a motor vehicle.

When COGENTIN is given concomitantly with phenothiazines or other drugs with anticholinergic activity, patients should be advised to report gastrointestinal complaints promptly. Paralytic ileus, sometimes fatal, has occurred in patients taking anticholinergic-type antiparkinsonism drugs, including COGENTIN, in combination with phenothiazines and/or tricyclic antidepressants.

Since COGENTIN contains structural features of atropine, it may produce anhidrosis. For this reason, it should be administered with caution during hot weather, especially when given concomitantly with other atropine-like drugs to the chronically ill, the alcoholic, those who have central nervous system disease, and those who do manual labor in a hot environment. Anhidrosis may occur more readily when some disturbance of sweating already exists. If there is evidence of anhidrosis, the possibility of hyperthermia should be considered. Dosage should be decreased at the discretion of the physician so that the ability to maintain body heat equilibrium by perspiration is not impaired. Severe anhidrosis and fatal hyperthermia have occurred.

Precautions

Since COGENTIN has cumulative action, continued supervision is advisable. Patients with a tendency to tachycardia and patients with prostatic hypertrophy should be observed closely during treatment.

Dysuria may occur, but rarely becomes a problem.

In large doses, the drug may cause complaints of weakness and inability to move particular muscle groups. For example, if the neck has been rigid and suddenly relaxes, it may feel weak, causing some concern. In this event, dosage adjustment is required.

Mental confusion and excitement may occur with large doses, or in susceptible patients. Visual hallucinations have been reported occasionally. Furthermore, in the treatment of extrapyramidal disorders due to neuroleptic drugs (e.g., phenothiazines), in patients with mental disorders, occasionally there may be intensification of mental symptoms. In such cases, at times, increased doses of antiparkinsonian drugs can precipitate a toxic psychosis. These patients should be kept under careful observation, especially at the beginning of treatment or if dosage is increased.

Tardive dyskinesia may appear in some patients on long-term therapy with phenothiazines and related agents, or may occur after therapy with these drugs has been discontinued. Antiparkinsonism agents do not alleviate the symptoms of tardive dyskinesia, and in some instances may aggravate them. COGENTIN is not recommended for use in patients with tardive dyskinesia.

The physician should be aware of the possible occurrence of glaucoma. Although the drug does not appear to have any adverse effect on simple glaucoma, it probably should not be used in angle-closure glaucoma.

Adverse Reactions

Adverse reactions may be anticholinergic or antihistaminic in nature.

Dry mouth, blurred vision, nausea, and nervousness may develop. Adjustment of dosage or time of administration sometimes helps to control these reactions. If dry mouth is so severe that there is difficulty in swallowing or speaking, or loss of appetite and weight, reduce dosage, or discontinue the drug temporarily.

Vomiting occurs infrequently. Nausea unaccompanied by vomiting usually can be disregarded. Slight reduction in dosage may control the nausea and still give sufficient relief of symptoms. Vomiting may be controlled by temporary discontinuation, followed by resumption at a lower dosage.

Other adverse reactions include constipation, numbness of the fingers, listlessness and depression.

Occasionally, an allergic reaction, e.g., skin rash, develops. Sometimes this can be controlled by reducing dosage, but occasionally medication has to be discontinued.

Dosage and Administration

COGENTIN tablets should be used when patients are able to take oral medication.

The injection is especially useful for psychotic patients with acute dystonic reactions or other reactions that make oral medication difficult or impossible. It is recommended also when a more rapid response is desired than can be obtained with the tablets.

Since there is no significant difference in onset of effect after intravenous or intramuscular injection, usually there is no need to use the intravenous route. The drug is quickly effective after either route, with improvement sometimes noticeable a few minutes after injection. In emergency situations, when the condition of the patient is alarming, 1 to 2 ml of the injection normally will provide quick relief. If the parkinsonian effect begins to return, the dose can be repeated.

Because of cumulative action, therapy should be initiated with a low dose which is increased gradually at five or six-day intervals to the smallest amount necessary for optimal relief. Increases should be made in increments of 0.5 mg, to a maximum of 6 mg, or until optimal results are obtained without excessive adverse reactions.

Postencephalitic and Idiopathic Parkinsonism—

The usual daily dose is 1 to 2 mg, with a range of 0.5 to 6 mg orally or parenterally.

As with any agent used in parkinsonism, dosage must be individualized according to age and weight, and the type of parkinsonism being treated. Generally, older patients and thin patients cannot tolerate large doses. Most patients with postencephalitic parkinsonism need fairly large doses and tolerate them well. Patients with a poor mental outlook are usually poor candidates for therapy.

In idiopathic parkinsonism, therapy may be initiated with a single daily dose of 0.5 to 1 mg at bedtime. In some patients, this will be adequate; in others 4 to 6 mg a day may be required.

In postencephalitic parkinsonism, therapy may be initiated in most patients with 2 mg a day in one or more doses. In highly sensitive patients, therapy may be initiated with 0.5 mg at bedtime, and increased as necessary.

Some patients experience greatest relief by taking the entire dose at bedtime; others react more favorably to divided doses, two to four times a day. Frequently, one dose a day is sufficient, and divided doses may be unnecessary or undesirable.

The long duration of action of this drug makes it particularly suitable for bedtime medication when its effects may last throughout the night, enabling patients to turn in bed during the night more easily, and to rise in the morning.

When COGENTIN is started, do not terminate therapy with other antiparkinsonian agents abruptly. If the other agents are to be reduced or discontinued, it must be done gradually. Many patients obtain greatest relief with combination therapy.

COGENTIN may be used concomitantly with SINEMET® (a combination of carbidopa and levodopa), or with levodopa, in which case periodic dosage adjustment may be required in order to maintain optimum response.

Drug-Induced Extrapyramidal Disorders—In treating extrapyramidal disorders due to neuroleptic drugs (e.g., phenothiazines), the recommended dosage is 1 to 4 mg once or twice a day orally or parenterally. Dosage must be individualized according to the need of the patient. Some patients require more than recommended; others do not need as much.

In acute dystonic reactions, 1 to 2 ml of the injection usually relieves the condition quickly. After that, the tablets, 1 to 2 mg twice a day, usually prevent recurrence.

When extrapyramidal disorders develop soon after initiation of treatment with neuroleptic drugs (e.g., phenothiazines), they are likely to be transient. One to 2 mg of COGENTIN tablets two or three times a day usually provides relief within one or two days. After one or two weeks, the drug should be withdrawn to determine the continued need for it. If such disorders recur, COGENTIN can be reinstituted.

Certain drug-induced extrapyramidal disorders that develop slowly may not respond to COGENTIN.

Overdosage

Manifestations—May be any of those seen in atropine poisoning or antihistamine overdosage: CNS depression, preceded or followed by stimulation; confusion; nervousness; listlessness; intensification of mental symptoms or toxic psychosis in patients with mental illness

Continued on next page

Information on the Merck Sharp & Dohme products listed on these pages is the full prescribing information from package circulars in use October 31, 1982.

Merck Sharp & Dohme—Cont.

being treated with neuroleptic drugs (e.g., phenothiazines); hallucinations (especially visual); dizziness; muscle weakness; ataxia; dry mouth; mydriasis; blurred vision; palpitations; nausea; vomiting; dysuria; numbness of fingers; dysphagia; allergic reactions, e.g., skin rash; headache; hot, dry, flushed skin; delirium; coma; shock; convulsions; respiratory arrest; anhidrosis; hyperthermia; glaucoma; constipation.
Treatment—Physostigmine salicylate, 1 to 2 mg, sc or iv, reportedly will reverse symptoms of anticholinergic intoxication (Duvoisin, R.C.; Katz, R.: J. Amer. Med. Ass. *206*:1963-1965, Nov. 25, 1968). A second injection may be given after 2 hours if required. Otherwise treatment is symptomatic and supportive. Induce emesis or perform gastric lavage (contraindicated in precomatose, convulsive, or psychotic states). Maintain respiration. A short-acting barbiturate may be used for CNS excitement, but with caution to avoid subsequent depression; supportive care for depression (avoid convulsant stimulants such as picrotoxin, pentylenetetrazol, or bemegride); artificial respiration for severe respiratory depression; a local miotic for mydriasis and cycloplegia; ice bags or other cold applications and alcohol sponges for hyperpyrexia, a vasopressor and fluids for circulatory collapse. Darken room for photophobia.

How Supplied

No. 3297—Tablets COGENTIN, 0.5 mg, are white, round, scored, compressed tablets, coded MSD 21. They are supplied as follows:
NDC 0006-0021-68 in bottles of 100.
[*Shown in Product Identification Section*]
No. 3334—Tablets COGENTIN, 1 mg, are white, oval shaped, scored, compressed tablets, coded MSD 635. They are supplied as follows:
NDC 0006-0635-68 in bottles of 100.
NDC 0006-0635-28 single unit packages of 100.
[*Shown in Product Identification Section*]
No. 3172—Tablets COGENTIN, 2 mg, are white, round, scored, compressed tablets, coded MSD 60. They are supplied as follows:
NDC 0006-0060-68 in bottles of 100.
(6505-00-680-1907 2 mg 100's)
NDC 0006-0060-28 single unit packages of 100.
NDC 0006-0060-82 in bottles of 1000.
[*Shown in Product Identification Section*]
No. 3275—Injection COGENTIN, 1 mg per ml, is a clear, colorless solution and is supplied as follows:
NDC 0006-3275-16 in boxes of 6×2 ml ampuls.
A.H.F.S. Category: 12:08
DC 6460713 Issued September 1978

ColBENEMID® Tablets ℞
Uricosuric

Description

ColBENEMID® contains BENEMID® (Probenecid, MSD) and colchicine.
Probenecid is the generic name for 4-[(dipropylamino) sulfonyl] benzoic acid (molecular weight 285.36).
Probenecid is a white or nearly white, fine, crystalline powder. It is soluble in dilute alkali, in alcohol, in chloroform, and in acetone; it is practically insoluble in water and in dilute acids.
Colchicine is an alkaloid obtained from various species of Colchicum. The chemical name for colchicine is (*S*)-*N*-(5,6,7,9-tetrahydro-1,2,3,10-tetramethoxy-9-oxobenzo [*a*] heptalen-7-yl) acetamide (molecular weight 399.43).
Colchicine consists of pale yellow scales or powder; it darkens on exposure to light. Colchicine is soluble in water, freely soluble in alcohol and in chloroform, and slightly soluble in ether.

Actions

Probenecid is a uricosuric and renal tubular blocking agent. It inhibits the tubular reabsorption of urate, thus increasing the urinary excretion of uric acid and decreasing serum urate levels. Effective uricosuria reduces the miscible urate pool, retards urate deposition, and promotes resorption of urate deposits.
Probenecid inhibits the tubular secretion of penicillin and usually increases penicillin plasma levels by any route the antibiotic is given. A 2-fold to 4-fold elevation has been demonstrated for various penicillins.
Probenecid also has been reported to inhibit the renal transport of many other compounds including aminohippuric acid (PAH), aminosalicylic acid (PAS), indomethacin, sodium iodomethamate and related iodinated organic acids, 17-ketosteroids, pantothenic acid, phenolsulfonphthalein (PSP), sulfonamides, and sulfonylureas. See also DRUG INTERACTIONS.
Probenecid decreases both hepatic and renal excretion of sulfobromophthalein (BSP). The tubular reabsorption of phosphorus is inhibited in hypoparathyroid but not in euparathyroid individuals.
Probenecid does not influence plasma concentrations of salicylates, nor the excretion of streptomycin, chloramphenicol, chlortetracycline, oxytetracycline, or neomycin.
The mode of action of colchicine in gout is unknown. It is not an analgesic, though it relieves pain in acute attacks of gout. It is not a uricosuric agent and will not prevent progression of gout to chronic gouty arthritis. It does have a prophylactic, suppressive effect that helps to reduce the incidence of acute attacks and to relieve the residual pain and mild discomfort that patients with gout occasionally feel.
In man and certain other animals, colchicine can produce a temporary leukopenia that is followed by leukocytosis.
Colchicine has other pharmacologic actions in animals: It alters neuromuscular function, intensifies gastrointestinal activity by neurogenic stimulation, increases sensitivity to central depressants, heightens response to sympathomimetic compounds, depresses the respiratory center, constricts blood vessels, causes hypertension by central vasomotor stimulation, and lowers body temperature.

Indications

For the treatment of chronic gouty arthritis when complicated by frequent, recurrent acute attacks of gout.

Contraindications

Hypersensitivity to this product or to probenecid or colchicine.
Children under 2 years of age.
Not recommended in persons with known blood dyscrasias or uric acid kidney stones.
Therapy with ColBENEMID should not be started until an acute gouty attack has subsided.
Pregnancy: Probenecid crosses the placental barrier and appears in cord blood. Colchicine can arrest cell division in animals and plants. In certain species of animal under certain conditions, colchicine has produced teratogenic effects. The possibility of such effects in humans also has been reported. Because of the colchicine component, ColBENEMID is contraindicated in pregnant patients. The use of any drug in women of childbearing potential requires that the anticipated benefit be weighed against possible hazards.

Warnings

Exacerbation of gout following therapy with ColBENEMID may occur; in such cases additional colchicine or other appropriate therapy is advisable.
Probenecid increases plasma concentrations of methotrexate in both animals and humans. In animal studies, increased methotrexate toxicity has been reported. If ColBENEMID is given with methotrexate, the dosage of methotrexate should be reduced and serum levels may need to be monitored.
In patients on ColBENEMID the use of salicylates in either small or large doses is contraindicated because it antagonizes the uricosuric action of probenecid. The biphasic action of salicylates in the renal tubules accounts for the so-called "paradoxical effect" of uricosuric agents. In patients on ColBENEMID who require a mild analgesic agent the use of acetaminophen rather than small doses of salicylates would be preferred.
The appearance of hypersensitivity reactions requires cessation of therapy with ColBENEMID.
Colchicine has been reported to adversely affect spermatogenesis in animals. Reversible azoospermia has been reported in one patient.

Precautions

Hematuria, renal colic, costovertebral pain, and formation of uric acid stones associated with the use of ColBENEMID in gouty patients may be prevented by alkalization of the urine and a liberal fluid intake (*see* DOSAGE AND ADMINISTRATION). In these cases when alkali is administered, the acid-base balance of the patient should be watched.
Use with caution in patients with a history of peptic ulcer.
ColBENEMID has been used in patients with some renal impairment but dosage requirements may be increased. ColBENEMID may not be effective in chronic renal insufficiency particularly when the glomerular filtration rate is 30 ml/minute or less.
A reducing substance may appear in the urine of patients receiving probenecid. This disappears with discontinuance of therapy. Suspected glycosuria should be confirmed by using a test specific for glucose.
Adequate animal studies have not been conducted to determine the carcinogenicity potential of probenecid or this drug combination. Since colchicine is an established mutagen, its ability to act as a carcinogen must be suspected and administration of ColBENEMID should involve a weighing of the benefit-vs-risk when long-term administration is contemplated.

Adverse Reactions

Headache, gastrointestinal symptoms (e.g., anorexia, nausea, vomiting), urinary frequency, hypersensitivity reactions (including anaphylaxis, dermatitis, pruritus, and fever), sore gums, flushing, dizziness, and anemia have occurred following the use of probenecid. In gouty patients exacerbation of gout, and uric acid stones with or without hematuria, renal colic, or costovertebral pain, have been observed. Nephrotic syndrome, hepatic necrosis, and aplastic anemia occur rarely. Hemolytic anemia which in some instances could be related to genetic deficiency of glucose-6-phosphate dehydrogenase in red blood cells has been reported.
Side effects due to colchicine appear to be a function of dosage. The most prominent symptoms are referable to the gastrointestinal tract (e.g., nausea, vomiting, abdominal pain, diarrhea) and may be particularly troublesome in the presence of peptic ulcer or spastic colon. At toxic doses colchicine may cause severe diarrhea, generalized vascular damage, and renal damage with hematuria and oliguria. Muscular weakness, which disappears with discontinuance of therapy, urticaria, dermatitis, and purpura have also been reported. Hypersensitivity to colchicine is a very rare occurrence, but should be borne in mind. The appearance of any of the aforementioned symptoms may require reduction of dosage or discontinuance of the drug.

When given for prolonged periods, colchicine may cause agranulocytosis, aplastic anemia, and peripheral neuritis. Loss of hair attributable to colchicine therapy has been reported. The possibility of increased colchicine toxicity in the presence of hepatic dysfunction should be considered.

Drug Interactions

The use of salicylates antagonizes the uricosuric action of probenecid (*see* WARNINGS). The uricosuric action of probenecid is also antagonized by pyrazinamide.
Probenecid produces an insignificant increase in free sulfonamide plasma concentrations but a significant increase in total sulfonamide plasma levels. Since probenecid decreases the renal excretion of conjugated sulfonamides, plasma concentrations of the latter should be determined from time to time when a sulfonamide and ColBENEMID are coadministered for prolonged periods. Probenecid may prolong or enhance the action of oral sulfonylureas and thereby increase the risk of hypoglycemia.
When probenecid is given to patients receiving indomethacin, the plasma levels of indomethacin are likely to be increased. Therefore, a lower dosage of indomethacin may be required to produce a therapeutic effect, and increases in the dosage of indomethacin should be made cautiously and in small increments. Probenecid may increase plasma levels of rifampin. The clinical significance of this is not known.
In animals and in humans, probenecid has been reported to increase plasma concentrations of methotrexate (*see* WARNINGS).
Falsely high readings for theophylline have been reported in an *in vitro* study, using the Schack and Waxler technic, when therapeutic concentrations of theophylline and probenecid were added to human plasma.

Dosage and Administration

Therapy with ColBENEMID should not be *started* until an acute gouty attack has subsided. However, if an acute attack is precipitated *during* therapy, ColBENEMID may be continued without changing the dosage, and additional colchicine or other appropriate therapy should be given to control the acute attack.
The recommended adult dosage is 1 tablet of ColBENEMID daily for one week, followed by 1 tablet twice a day thereafter.
Some degree of renal impairment may be present in patients with gout. A daily dosage of 2 tablets may be adequate. However, if necessary, the daily dosage may be increased by 1 tablet every four weeks within tolerance (and usually not above 4 tablets per day) if symptoms of gouty arthritis are not controlled or the 24 hour uric acid excretion is not above 700 mg.
As noted, probenecid may not be effective in chronic renal insufficiency particularly when the glomerular filtration rate is 30 ml/minute or less.
Gastric intolerance may be indicative of overdosage, and may be corrected by decreasing the dosage.
As uric acid tends to crystallize out of an acid urine, a liberal fluid intake is recommended, as well as sufficient sodium bicarbonate (3 to 7.5 g daily) or potassium citrate (7.5 g daily) to maintain an alkaline urine (*see* PRECAUTIONS).
Alkalization of the urine is recommended until the serum urate level returns to normal limits and tophaceous deposits disappear, i.e., during the period when urinary excretion of uric acid is at a high level. Thereafter, alkalization of the urine and the usual restriction of purine-producing foods may be somewhat relaxed.
ColBENEMID (or probenecid) should be continued at the dosage that will maintain normal serum urate levels. When acute attacks have been absent for six months or more and serum urate levels remain within normal limits, the daily dosage of ColBENEMID may be decreased by 1 tablet every six months. The maintenance dosage should not be reduced to the point where serum urate levels tend to rise.

How Supplied

No. 3283—Tablets ColBENEMID are white to off-white, capsule-shaped, scored tablets, coded MSD 614. Each tablet contains 0.5 g of probenecid and 0.5 mg of colchicine. They are supplied as follows:
NDC 0006-0614-68 bottles of 100.
[*Shown in Product Identification Section*]
A.H.F.S. Category: 40:40
DC 6213020 Issued December 1979

COSMEGEN® Injection (dactinomycin, MSD), U.S.P. ℞

WARNING

Dactinomycin is extremely corrosive to soft tissue. If extravasation occurs during intravenous use, severe damage to soft tissues will occur. In at least one instance, this has led to contracture of the arms.

DOSAGE

The dosage of COSMEGEN® (Dactinomycin, MSD) is calculated in micrograms (mcg). The usual adult dosage is 500 micrograms (0.5 mg) daily intravenously for a maximum of five days. The dosage for adults or children should not exceed 15 mcg/kg or 400–600 mcg/square meter of body surface daily intravenously for five days. Calculation of the dosage for obese or edematous patients should be on the basis of surface area in an effort to relate dosage to lean body mass.

Description

Dactinomycin is one of the actinomycins, a group of antibiotics produced by various species of *Streptomyces.* Dactinomycin is the principal component of the mixture of actinomycins produced by *Streptomyces parvullus.* Unlike other species of *Streptomyces,* this organism yields an essentially pure substance that contains only traces of similar compounds differing in the amino acid content of the peptide side chains.

Actions

Generally, the actinomycins exert an inhibitory effect on gram-positive and gram-negative bacteria and on some fungi. However, the toxic properties of the actinomycins (including dactinomycin) in relation to antibacterial activity are such as to preclude their use as antibiotics in the treatment of infectious diseases.
Because the actinomycins are cytotoxic, they have an antineoplastic effect which has been demonstrated in experimental animals with various types of tumor implant. This cytotoxic action is the basis for their use in the palliative treatment of certain types of cancer.
Dactinomycin is minimally metabolized. Its plasma clearance half-life is 36 hours. It tends to concentrate in nucleated cells and does not cross the blood brain barrier.

Indications

Wilms's Tumor
The neoplasm responding most frequently to COSMEGEN is Wilms's tumor. With low doses of both dactinomycin and radiotherapy, temporary objective improvement may be as good as and may last longer than with higher doses of each given alone. In the National Wilms's Tumor study, combination therapy with dactinomycin and vincristine together with surgery and radiotherapy, was shown to have significantly improved the prognosis of patients in groups II and III. Dactinomycin and vincristine were given for a total of seven cycles, so that maintenance therapy continued for approximately 15 months.
Postoperative radiotherapy in group I patients and optimal combination chemotherapy for those in group IV are unsettled issues. About 70 percent of lung metastases have disappeared with an appropriate combination of radiation, dactinomycin and vincristine.
Rhabdomyosarcoma
Temporary regression of the tumor and beneficial subjective results have occurred with dactinomycin in rhabdomyosarcoma which, like most soft tissue sarcomas, is comparatively radio-resistant.
Several groups have reported successful use of cyclophosphamide, vincristine, dactinomycin and doxorubicin hydrochloride in various combinations. Effective combinations have included vincristine and dactinomycin; vincristine, dactinomycin and cyclophosphamide (VAC therapy) and all four drugs in sequence. At present, the most effective treatment for children with inoperable or metastatic rhabdomyosarcoma has been VAC chemotherapy. Two thirds of these children were doing well without evidence of disease at a median time of three years after diagnosis.
Carcinoma of Testis and Uterus
The sequential use of dactinomycin and methotrexate, along with meticulous monitoring of human chorionic gonadotropin levels until normal, has resulted in survival in the majority of women with metastatic choriocarcinoma. Sequential therapy is used if there is:

1. Stability in gonadotropin titers following two successive courses of an agent.
2. Rising gonadotropin titers during treatment.
3. Severe toxicity preventing adequate therapy.

In patients with nonmetastatic choriocarcinoma, dactinomycin or methotrexate or both, have been used successfully, with or without surgery.
Dactinomycin has been beneficial as a single agent in the treatment of metastatic nonseminomatour testicular carcinoma when used in cycles of 500 mcg/day for five consecutive days, every 6–8 weeks for periods of four months or longer.
Other Neoplasms
Dactinomycin has been given intravenously or by regional perfusion, either alone or with other antineoplastic compounds or x-ray therapy, in the palliative treatment of Ewing's sarcoma and sarcoma botryoides. For nonmetastatic Ewing's sarcoma, promising results were obtained when dactinomycin (45 mcg/m^2) and cyclophosphamide (1200 mg/m^2) were given sequentially and with radiotherapy, over an 18 month period. Those with metastatic disease remain the subject of continued investigation with a more aggressive chemotherapeutic regimen employed initially.
Temporary objective improvement and relief of pain and discomfort have followed the use of dactinomycin usually in conjunction with radiotherapy for sarcoma botryoides. This palliative effect ranges from transitory inhibition of tumor growth to a considerable but temporary regression in tumor size.

Continued on next page

Information on the Merck Sharp & Dohme products listed on these pages is the full prescribing information from package circulars in use October 31, 1982.

Merck Sharp & Dohme—Cont.

COSMEGEN (Dactinomycin, MSD) and Radiation Therapy
Much evidence suggests that dactinomycin potentiates the effects of x-ray therapy. The converse also appears likely; i.e., dactinomycin may be more effective when radiation therapy also is given.
With combined dactinomycin-radiation therapy, the normal skin, as well as the buccal and pharyngeal mucosa, show early erythema. A smaller than usual x-ray dose when given with dactinomycin causes erythema and vesiculation, which progress more rapidly through the stages of tanning and desquamation. Healing may occur in four to six weeks rather than two to three months. Erythema from previous x-ray therapy may be reactivated by dactinomycin alone, even when irradiation occurred many months earlier, and especially when the interval between the two forms of therapy is brief. This potentiation of radiation effect represents a special problem when the irradiation treatment area includes the mucous membrane. When irradiation is directed toward the nasopharynx, the combination may produce severe oropharyngeal mucositis. *Severe reactions may ensue if high doses of both dactinomycin and radiation therapy are used or if the patient is particularly sensitive to such combined therapy.*
Because of this potentiating effect, dactinomycin may be tried in radio-sensitive tumors not responding to doses of x-ray therapy that can be tolerated. Objective improvement in tumor size and activity may be observed when lower, better tolerated doses of both types of therapy are employed.
COSMEGEN (Dactinomycin, MSD) and Perfusion Technic
Dactinomycin alone or with other antineoplastic agents has also been given by the isolation-perfusion technic, either as palliative treatment or as an adjunct to resection of a tumor. Some tumors considered resistant to chemotherapy and radiation therapy may respond when the drug is given by the perfusion technic. Neoplasms in which dactinomycin has been tried by this technic include various types of sarcoma, carcinoma, and adenocarcinoma. In some instances tumors regressed, pain was relieved for variable periods, and surgery made possible. On other occasions, however, the outcome has been less favorable. Nevertheless, in selected cases, the drug by perfusion may provide more effective palliation than when given systemically.
Dactinomycin by the isolation-perfusion technic offers certain advantages, provided leakage of the drug through the general circulation into other areas of the body is minimal. By this technic the drug is in continuous contact with the tumor for the duration of treatment. The dose may be increased well over that used by the systemic route, usually without adding to the danger of toxic effects. If the agent is confined to an isolated part, it should not interfere with the patient's defense mechanism. Systemic absorption of toxic products from neoplastic tissue can be minimized by removing the perfusate when the procedure is finished.

Contraindications

If dactinomycin is given at or about the time of infection with chicken pox or herpes zoster, a severe generalized disease, which may result in death, may occur.

Warning

COSMEGEN should be administered only under the supervision of a physician who is experienced in the use of cancer chemotherapeutic agents.

Precautions

As with all antineoplastic agents, dactinomycin is a toxic drug and very careful and frequent observation of the patient for adverse reactions is necessary. These reactions may involve any tissue of the body. The possibility of an anaphylactoid reaction should be borne in mind.
The greater frequency of toxic effects of dactinomycin peculiar to infants suggest that this drug should be given to infants only over the age of 6 to 12 months.
A variety of abnormalities of renal, hepatic, and bone marrow function have been reported in patients with neoplastic disease and receiving dactinomycin. It is advisable to make frequent checks of renal, hepatic, and bone marrow function.
Increased incidence of gastrointestinal toxicity and marrow suppression has been reported when dactinomycin was given with x-ray therapy.
Particular caution is necessary when administering dactinomycin in the first two months after irradiation for the treatment of right-sided Wilms's tumor, since hepatomegaly and elevated SGOT levels have been noted.
Nausea and vomiting due to dactinomycin make it necessary to give this drug intermittently. It is extremely important to observe the patient daily for toxic side effects when multiple chemotherapy is employed, since a full course of therapy occasionally is not tolerated. If stomatitis, diarrhea, or severe hemopoietic depression appear during therapy, these drugs should be discontinued until the patient has recovered.
Recent reports indicate an increased incidence of second primary tumors following treatment with radiation and anti-neoplastic agents, such as dactinomycin. Multi-modal therapy creates the need for careful, long-term observation of cancer survivors.
Use in pregnancy: When administration of this drug during pregnancy is considered necessary, the danger for the fetus should be taken into consideration. The need for this precaution is based on published data showing teratogenic effects of dactinomycin in animals.
Nursing Mothers
Although breast milk studies have not been performed in animals or humans, breast feeding should be stopped before beginning treatment with COSMEGEN.

Adverse Reactions

Toxic effects (excepting nausea and vomiting) usually do not become apparent until two to four days after a course of therapy is stopped, and may not be maximal before one to two weeks have elapsed. Deaths have been reported. However, adverse reactions are usually reversible on discontinuance of therapy. They include the following:
Miscellaneous (malaise, fatigue, lethargy, fever, myalgia, proctitis, hypocalcemia).
Oral (cheilitis, dysphagia, esophagitis, ulcerative stomatitis, pharyngitis).
Gastrointestinal (anorexia, nausea, vomiting, abdominal pain, diarrhea, gastrointestinal ulceration). Nausea and vomiting, which occur early during the first few hours after administration, may be alleviated by giving antiemetics.
Hematologic (anemia, even to the point of aplastic anemia, agranulocytosis, leukopenia, thrombopenia, pancytopenia, reticulopenia). Platelet and white cell counts should be done *daily* to detect severe hemopoietic depression. If either count markedly decreases, the drug should be withheld to allow marrow recovery. This often takes up to three weeks.
Dermatologic (alopecia, skin eruptions, acne, flare-up of erythema or increased pigmentation of previously irradiated skin).
Soft tissues. Dactinomycin is extremely corrosive. If extravasation occurs during intravenous use, severe damage to soft tissues will occur. In at least one instance, this has led to contracture of the arms.

Dosage and Administration

Toxic reactions due to dactinomycin are frequent and may be severe (see ADVERSE REACTIONS), thus limiting in many instances the amount that may be given. However, the severity of toxicity varies markedly and is only partly dependent on the dose employed. The drug must be given in short courses.
Intravenous Use
The dosage of dactinomycin varies depending on the tolerance of the patient, the size and location of the neoplasm, and the use of other forms of therapy. It may be necessary to decrease the usual dosages suggested below when other chemotherapy or x-ray therapy is used concomitantly or has been used previously.
The dosage for adults or children should not exceed 15 mcg/kg or 400–600 mcg/square meter of body surface daily intravenously for five days. Calculation of the dosage for obese or edematous patients should be on the basis of surface area in an effort to relate dosage to lean body mass.
Adults: The usual adult dosage is 500 mcg (0.5 mg) daily intravenously for a maximum of five days.
Children: In children 15 mcg (0.015 mg) per kilogram of body weight is given intravenously daily for five days. An alternative schedule is a total dosage of 2500 mcg (2.5 mg) per square meter of body surface given intravenously over a one week period.
In both adults and children, a second course may be given after at least three weeks have elapsed, provided all signs of toxicity have disappeared.
Reconstitute COSMEGEN by adding 1.1 ml of **Sterile Water for Injection (without preservative)** using aseptic precautions. The resulting solution of dactinomycin will contain approximately 500 mcg or 0.5 mg per ml.
Once reconstituted, the solution of dactinomycin can be added to infusion solutions of Dextrose Injection 5 percent or Sodium Chloride Injection either directly or to the tubing of a running intravenous infusion.
Although reconstituted COSMEGEN is chemically stable, the product does not contain a preservative and accidental microbial contamination might result. Any unused portion should be discarded. Use of water containing preservatives (benzyl alcohol or parabens) to reconstitute COSMEGEN for injection, results in the formation of a precipitate.
Partial removal of dactinomycin from intravenous solutions by cellulose ester membrane filters used in some intravenous in-line filters has been reported.
Since dactinomycin is extremely corrosive to soft tissue, precautions for materials of this nature should be observed.
If the drug is given directly into the vein without the use of an infusion, the "two-needle technic" should be used. Reconstitute and withdraw the calculated dose from the vial with one sterile needle. Use another sterile needle for direct injection into the vein.
Discard any unused portion of the dactinomycin solution.
Isolation-Perfusion Technic
The dosage schedules and the technic itself vary from one investigator to another; the published literature, therefore, should be consulted for details. In general, the following doses are suggested:

50 mcg (0.05 mg) per kilogram of body weight for lower extremity or pelvis.

35 mcg (0.035 mg) per kilogram of body weight for upper extremity.

It may be advisable to use lower doses in obese patients, or when previous chemotherapy or radiation therapy has been employed.
Complications of the perfusion technic are related mainly to the amount of drug that escapes into the systemic circulation and may consist of hemopoietic depression, absorption of toxic products from massive destruction of neoplastic tissue, increased susceptibility to infection, impaired wound healing, and superficial ulceration of the gastric mucosa. Other side effects may include edema of the extremity involved, damage to soft tissues of the perfused area, and (potentially) venous thrombosis.

How Supplied

No. 3298—Injection COSMEGEN is a lyophilized powder and is supplied as follows: **NDC** 0006-3298-22 in vials containing 0.5 mg (500 micrograms) of dactinomycin with 20.0 mg of mannitol. In the dry form the compound is an amorphous yellow powder. The solution is clear and gold-colored.

A.H.F.S. Category: 10:00
DC 6059219 Issued September 1979

CUPRIMINE® Capsules (penicillamine, MSD), U.S.P. ℞

> Physicians planning to use penicillamine should thoroughly familiarize themselves with its toxicity, special dosage considerations, and therapeutic benefits. Penicillamine should never be used casually. Each patient should remain constantly under the close supervision of the physician. Patients should be warned to report promptly any symptoms suggesting toxicity.

Description

Penicillamine is 3-mercapto-D-valine. It is a white or practically white, crystalline powder, freely soluble in water, slightly soluble in alcohol, and insoluble in ether, acetone, benzene, and carbon tetrachloride. Although its configuration is D, it is levorotatory as usually measured:

$[\alpha]^{25°}_{D} = -63° \pm 5°$ (C = 1, 1N NaOH).

The empirical formula is $C_5H_{11}NO_2S$, giving it a molecular weight of 149.21.
It reacts readily with formaldehyde or acetone to form a thiazolidine-carboxylic acid.

Clinical Pharmacology

Penicillamine is a chelating agent recommended for the removal of excess copper in patients with Wilson's disease. From *in vitro* studies which indicate that one atom of copper combines with two molecules of penicillamine, it would appear that one gram of penicillamine should be followed by the excretion of about 200 milligrams of copper; however, the actual amount excreted is about one percent of this.
Penicillamine also reduces excess cystine excretion in cystinuria. This is done, at least in part, by disulfide interchange between penicillamine and cystine, resulting in formation of penicillamine-cysteine disulfide, a substance that is much more soluble than cystine and is excreted readily.
Penicillamine interferes with the formation of cross-links between tropocollagen molecules and cleaves them when newly formed.
The mechanism of action of penicillamine in rheumatoid arthritis is unknown although it appears to suppress disease activity. Unlike cytotoxic immunosuppressants, penicillamine markedly lowers IgM rheumatoid factor but produces no significant depression in absolute levels of serum immunoglobulins. Also unlike cytotoxic immunosuppressants which act on both, penicillamine *in vitro* depresses T-cell activity but not B-cell activity.
In vitro, penicillamine dissociates macroglobulins (rheumatoid factor) although the relationship of the activity to its effect in rheumatoid arthritis is not known.
In rheumatoid arthritis, the onset of therapeutic response to CUPRIMINE® (Penicillamine, MSD) may not be seen for two or three months. In those patients who respond, however, the first evidence of suppression of symptoms such as pain, tenderness, and swelling is generally apparent within three months. The optimum duration of therapy has not been determined. If remissions occur, they may last from months to years, but usually require continued treatment (see DOSAGE AND ADMINISTRATION).
In patients with rheumatoid arthritis, it is important that CUPRIMINE be given on an empty stomach, at least one hour before meals and at least one hour apart from any other drug, food, or milk. This permits maximum absorption and reduces the likelihood of inactivation by metal binding.
Methodology for determining the bioavailability of penicillamine is not available; however, penicillamine is known to be a very soluble substance.

Indications

CUPRIMINE is indicated in the treatment of Wilson's disease, cystinuria, and in patients with severe, active rheumatoid arthritis who have failed to respond to an adequate trial of conventional therapy. Available evidence suggests that CUPRIMINE is not of value in ankylosing spondylitis.
Wilson's Disease—Wilson's disease (hepatolenticular degeneration) results from the interaction of an inherited defect and an abnormality in copper metabolism. The metabolic defect, which is the consequence of the autosomal inheritance of one abnormal gene from each parent, manifests itself in a greater positive copper balance than normal. As a result, copper is deposited in several organs and appears eventually to produce pathologic effects most prominently seen in the brain, where degeneration is widespread; in the liver, where fatty infiltration, inflammation, and hepatocellular damage progress to postnecrotic cirrhosis; in the kidney, where tubular and glomerular dysfunction results; and in the eye, where characteristic corneal copper deposits are known as Kayser-Fleischer rings.
Two types of patients require treatment for Wilson's disease: (1) the symptomatic, and (2) the asymptomatic in whom it can be assumed the disease will develop in the future if the patient is not treated.
Diagnosis, suspected on the basis of family or individual history, physical examination, or a low serum concentration of ceruloplasmin*, is confirmed by the demonstration of Kayser-Fleischer rings or, particularly in the asymptomatic patient, by the quantitative demonstration in a liver biopsy specimen of a concentration of copper in excess of 250 mcg/g dry weight.
Treatment has two objectives:
(1) to minimize dietary intake and absorption of copper.
(2) to promote excretion of copper deposited in tissues.

*For quantitative test for serum ceruloplasmin see: Morell, A.G.; Windsor, J.; Sternlieb, I.; Scheinberg, I.H.: Measurement of the concentration of ceruloplasmin in serum by determination of its oxidase activity, in "Laboratory Diagnosis of Liver Disease", F.W. Sunderman; F.W. Sunderman, Jr. (eds.), St. Louis, Warren H. Green, Inc., 1968, pp. 193-195.

The first objective is attained by a daily diet that contains no more than one or two milligrams of copper. Such a diet should exclude, most importantly, chocolate, nuts, shellfish, mushrooms, liver, molasses, broccoli, and cereals enriched with copper, and be composed to as great an extent as possible of foods with a low copper content. Distilled or demineralized water should be used if the patient's drinking water contains more than 0.1 mg of copper per liter.
For the second objective, a copper chelating agent is used. Penicillamine is the only one of these agents that is orally effective.
In symptomatic patients this treatment usually produces marked neurologic improvement, fading of Kayser-Fleischer rings, and gradual amelioration of hepatic dysfunction and psychic disturbances.
Clinical experience to date suggests that life is prolonged with the above regimen.
Noticeable improvement may not occur for one to three months. Occasionally, neurologic symptoms become worse during initiation of therapy with CUPRIMINE. Despite this, the drug should not be discontinued permanently, although temporary interruption may result in clinical improvement of the neurological symptoms but it carries an increased risk of developing a sensitivity reaction upon resumption of therapy (see WARNINGS).
Treatment of asymptomatic patients has been carried out for over ten years. Symptoms and signs of the disease appear to be prevented indefinitely if daily treatment with CUPRIMINE can be continued.
Cystinuria—Cystinuria is characterized by excessive urinary excretion of the dibasic amino acids, arginine, lysine, ornithine, and cystine, and the mixed disulfide of cysteine and homocysteine. The metabolic defect that leads to cystinuria is inherited as an autosomal, recessive trait. Metabolism of the affected amino acids is influenced by at least two abnormal factors: (1) defective gastrointestinal absorption and (2) renal tubular dysfunction.
Arginine, lysine, ornithine, and cysteine are soluble substances, readily excreted. There is no apparent pathology connected with their excretion in excessive quantities.
Cystine, however, is so slightly soluble at the usual range of urinary pH that it is not excreted readily, and so crystallizes and forms stones in the urinary tract. Stone formation is the only known pathology in cystinuria.
Normal daily output of cystine is 40 to 80 mg. In cystinuria, output is greatly increased and may exceed 1 g/day. At 500 to 600 mg/day, stone formation is almost certain. When it is more than 300 mg/day, treatment is indicated.
Conventional treatment is directed at keeping urinary cystine diluted enough to prevent stone formation, keeping the urine alkaline enough to dissolve as much cystine as possible, and minimizing cystine production by a diet low in methionine (the major dietary precursor of cystine). Patients must drink enough fluid to keep urine specific gravity below 1.010, take enough alkali to keep urinary pH at 7.5 to 8, and maintain a diet low in methionine. This diet is not recommended in growing children and probably is contraindicated in pregnancy because of its low protein content (see PRECAUTIONS).
When these measures are inadequate to control recurrent stone formation, CUPRIMINE may be used as additional therapy. When patients refuse to adhere to conventional treatment, CUPRIMINE may be a useful substitute.

Continued on next page

Information on the Merck Sharp & Dohme products listed on these pages is the full prescribing information from package circulars in use October 31, 1982.

Merck Sharp & Dohme—Cont.

It is capable of keeping cystine excretion to near normal values, thereby hindering stone formation and the serious consequences of pyelonephritis and impaired renal function that develop in some patients.
Bartter and colleagues depict the process by which penicillamine interacts with cystine to form penicillamine-cysteine mixed disulfide as:

CSSC + PS′ ⇌ CS′ + CSSP
PSSP + CS′ ⇌ PS′ + CSSP
CSSC + PSSP ⇌ 2CSSP
CSSC = cystine
CS′ = deprotonated cysteine
PSSP = penicillamine
PS′ = deprotonated penicillamine sulfhydryl
CSSP = penicillamine-cysteine mixed disulfide

In this process, it is assumed that the deprotonated form of penicillamine, PS′, is the active factor in bringing about the disulfide interchange.
Rheumatoid Arthritis—Because CUPRIMINE can cause severe adverse reactions, its use in rheumatoid arthritis should be restricted to patients who have severe, active disease and who have failed to respond to an adequate trial of conventional therapy. Even then, benefit-to-risk ratio should be carefully considered. Other measures, such as rest, physiotherapy, salicylates, and corticosteroids should be used, when indicated, in conjunction with CUPRIMINE (see PRECAUTIONS).

Contraindications

Penicillamine should not be administered to patients with rheumatoid arthritis who are pregnant (see PRECAUTIONS).
Patients with a history of penicillamine-related aplastic anemia or agranulocytosis should not be restarted on penicillamine (see WARNINGS and ADVERSE REACTIONS).
Because of its potential for causing renal damage, penicillamine should not be administered to rheumatoid arthritis patients with a history or other evidence of renal insufficiency.

Warnings

The use of penicillamine has been associated with fatalities due to certain diseases such as aplastic anemia, agranulocytosis, thrombocytopenia, Goodpasture's syndrome, and myasthenia gravis.
Because of the potential for serious hematological and renal adverse reactions to occur at any time, routine urinalysis, white and differential blood cell count, hemoglobin determination, and direct platelet count must be done every two weeks for at least the first six months of penicillamine therapy and monthly thereafter. Patients should be instructed to report promptly the development of signs and symptoms of granulocytopenia and/or thrombocytopenia such as fever, sore throat, chills, bruising or bleeding. The above laboratory studies should then be promptly repeated.
Leukopenia and thrombocytopenia have been reported to occur in up to five percent of patients during penicillamine therapy. Leukopenia is of the granulocytic series and may or may not be associated with an increase in eosinophils. A confirmed reduction in WBC below 3500 mandates discontinuance of penicillamine therapy. Thrombocytopenia may be on an idiosyncratic basis, with decreased or absent megakaryocytes in the marrow, when it is part of an aplastic anemia. In other cases the thrombocytopenia is presumably on an immune basis since the number of megakaryocytes in the marrow has been reported to be normal or sometimes increased. The development of a platelet count below 100,000, even in the absence of clinical bleeding, requires at least temporary cessation of penicillamine therapy. A progressive fall in either platelet count or WBC in three successive determinations, even though values are still within the normal range, likewise requires at least temporary cessation.
Proteinuria and/or hematuria may develop during therapy and may be warning signs of membranous glomerulopathy which can progress to a nephrotic syndrome. Close observation of these patients is essential. In some patients the proteinuria disappears with continued therapy; in others, penicillamine must be discontinued. When a patient develops proteinuria or hematuria the physician must ascertain whether it is a sign of drug-induced glomerulopathy or is unrelated to penicillamine.
Rheumatoid arthritis patients who develop moderate degrees of proteinuria may be continued cautiously on penicillamine therapy, provided that quantitative 24-hour urinary protein determinations are obtained at intervals of one to two weeks. Penicillamine dosage should not be increased under these circumstances. Proteinuria which exceeds 1 g/24 hours, or proteinuria which is progressively increasing, requires either discontinuance of the drug or a reduction in the dosage. In some patients, proteinuria has been reported to clear following reduction in dosage.
In rheumatoid arthritis patients, penicillamine should be discontinued if unexplained gross hematuria or persistent microscopic hematuria develops.
In patients with Wilson's disease or cystinuria the risks of continued penicillamine therapy in patients manifesting potentially serious urinary abnormalities must be weighed against the expected therapeutic benefits.
When penicillaminne is used in cystinuria, an annual x-ray for renal stones is advised. Cystine stones form rapidly, sometimes in six months.
Up to one year or more may be required for any urinary abnormalities to disappear after penicillamine has been discontinued.
Because of rare reports of intrahepatic cholestasis and toxic hepatitis, liver function tests are recommended every six months for the duration of therapy.
Goodpasture's syndrome has occurred rarely. The development of abnormal urinary findings associated with hemoptysis and pulmonary infiltrates on x-ray requires immediate cessation of penicillamine.
Obliterative bronchiolitis has been reported rarely. The patient should be cautioned to report immediately pulmonary symptoms such as exertional dyspnea, unexplained cough or wheezing. Pulmonary function studies should be considered at that time.
Myasthenic syndrome sometimes progressing to myasthenia gravis has been reported. In the majority of cases, symptoms of myasthenia have receded after withdrawal of penicillamine.
Pemphigoid-type reactions characterized by bullous lesions clinically indistinguishable from pemphigus have occurred and have required discontinuation of penicillamine and treatment with corticosteroids.
Once instituted for Wilson's disease or cystinuria, treatment with penicillamine should, as a rule, be continued on a daily basis. Interruptions for even a few days have been followed by sensitivity reactions after reinstitution of therapy.

Precautions

Some patients may experience drug fever, a marked febrile response to penicillamine, usually in the second to third week following initiation of therapy. Drug fever may sometimes be accompanied by a macular cutaneous eruption.
In the case of drug fever in patients with Wilson's disease or cystinuria, because no alternative treatment is available, penicillamine should be temporarily discontinued until the reaction subsides. Then penicillamine should be reinstituted with a small dose that is gradually increased until the desired dosage is attained. Systemic steroid therapy may be necessary, and is usually helpful, in such patients in whom toxic reactions develop a second or third time.
In the case of drug fever in rheumatoid arthritis patients, because other treatments are available, penicillamine should be discontinued and another therapeutic alternative tried since experience indicates that the febrile reaction will recur in a very high percetage of patients upon readministration of penicillamine.
The skin and mucous membranes should be observed for allergic reactions. Early and late rashes have occurred. Early rash occurs during the first few months of treatment and is more common. It is usually a generalized pruritic, erythematous, maculopapular or morbilliform rash and resembles the allergic rash seen with other drugs. Early rash usually disappears within days after stopping penicillamine and seldom recurs when the drug is restarted at a lower dosage. Pruritus and early rash may often be controlled by the concomitant administration of antihistamines. Less commonly, a late rash may be seen, usually after six months or more of treatment, and requires discontinuation of penicillamine. It is usually on the trunk, is accompanied by intense pruritus, and is usually unresponsive to topical corticosteroid therapy. Late rash may take weeks to disappear after penicillamine is stopped and usually recurs if the drug is restarted.
The appearance of a drug eruption accompanied by fever, arthralgia, lymphadenopathy or other allergic manifestations usually requires discontinuation of penicillamine.
Certain patients will develop a positive antinuclear antibody (ANA) test and some of these may show a lupus erythematosus-like syndrome similar to drug-induced lupus associated with other drugs. The lupus erythematosus-like syndrome is not associated with hypocomplementemia and may be present without nephropathy. The development of a positive ANA test does not mandate discontinuance of the drug; however, the physician should be alerted to the possibility that a lupus erythematosus-like syndrome may develop in the future.
Some patients may develop oral ulcerations which in some cases have the appearance of aphthous stomatitis. The stomatitis usually recurs on rechallenge but often clears on a lower dosage. Although rare, cheilosis, glossitis and gingivostomatitis have also been reported. These oral lesions are frequently dose-related and may preclude further increase in penicillamine dosage or require discontinuation of the drug.
Hypogeusia (a blunting or diminution in taste perception) has occurred in some patients. This may last two to three months or more and may develop into a total loss of taste; however, it is usually self-limited despite continued penicillamine treatment. Such taste impairment is rare in patients with Wilson's disease.
Penicillamine should not be used in patients who are receiving concurrently gold therapy, antimalarial or cytotoxic drugs, oxyphenbutazone or phenylbutazone because these drugs are also associated with similar serious hematologic and renal adverse reactions. Patients who have had gold salt therapy discontinued due to a major toxic reaction may be at greater risk of serious adverse reactions with penicillamine but not necessarily of the same type.
Patients who are allergic to penicillin may theoretically have cross-sensitivity to penicillamine. The possibility of reactions from contamination of penicillamine by trace amounts of penicillin has been eliminated now that peni-

cillamine is being produced synthetically rather than as a degradation product of penicillin.

Because of their dietary restrictions, patients with Wilson's disease and cystinuria should be given 25 mg/day of pyridoxine during therapy, since penicillamine increases the requirement for this vitamin. Patients also may receive benefit from a multivitamin preparation, although there is no evidence that deficiency of any vitamin other than pyridoxine is associated with penicillamine. In Wilson's disease, multivitamin preparations must be copper-free.

Rheumatoid arthritis patients whose nutrition is impaired should also be given a daily supplement of pyridoxine. Mineral supplements should not be given, since they may block the response to penicillamine.

Iron deficiency may develop, especially in children and in menstruating women. In Wilson's disease, this may be a result of adding the effects of the low copper diet, which is probably also low in iron, and the penicillamine to the effects of blood loss or growth. In cystinuria, a low methionine diet may contribute to iron deficiency, since it is necessarily low in protein. If necessary, iron may be given in short courses, but a period of two hours should elapse between administration of penicillamine and iron, since orally administered iron has been shown to reduce the effects of penicillamine.

Penicillamine causes an increase in the amount of soluble collagen. In the rat this results in inhibition of normal healing and also a decrease in tensile strength of intact skin. In man this may be the cause of increased skin friability at sites especially subject to pressure or trauma, such as shoulders, elbows, knees, toes, and buttocks. Extravasations of blood may occur and may appear as purpuric areas, with external bleeding if the skin is broken, or as vesicles containing dark blood. Neither type is progressive. There is no apparent association with bleeding elsewhere in the body and no associated coagulation defect has been found. Therapy with penicillamine may be continued in the presence of these lesions. They may not recur if dosage is reduced. Other reported effects probably due to the action of penicillamine on collagen are excessive wrinkling of the skin and development of small, white papules at venipuncture and surgical sites.

The effects of penicillamine on collagen and elastin make it advisable to consider a reduction in dosage to 250 mg/day, when surgery is contemplated. Reinstitution of full therapy should be delayed until wound healing is complete.

Carcinogenesis—Long-term animal carcinogenicity studies have not been done with penicillamine. There is a report that five of ten autoimmune disease-prone NZB hybrid mice developed lymphocytic leukemia after 6 months' intraperitoneal treatment with a dose of 400 mg/kg penicillamine 5 days per week.

Use in Pregnancy—Penicillamine has been shown to be teratogenic in rats when given in doses several times higher than the highest dose recommended for human use. Skeletal defects, cleft palates and fetal toxicity (resorptions) have been reported.

Wilson's Disease—There are no controlled studies in pregnant women with Wilson's disease, but experience does not include any positive evidence of adverse effects on the fetus. Reported experience* shows that continued treatment with penicillamine throughout pregnancy protects the mother against relapse of the Wilson's disease, and that discontinuation of penicillamine has deleterious effects on the mother. It indicates that the drug does not increase the risks of fetal abnormalities, but it does not exclude the possibility of infrequent or subtle damage to the fetus.

*Scheinberg, I.H., Sternlieb, I.: N. Engl. J. Med. *293*: 1300-1302, Dec. 18, 1975.

If penicillamine is administered during pregnancy to patients with Wilson's disease, it is recommended that the daily dosage be limited to 1 g. If cesarean section is planned, the daily dosage should be limited to 250 mg during the last six weeks of pregnancy and postoperatively until wound healing is complete.

Cystinuria—If possible, penicillamine should not be give during pregnancy to women with cystinuria. There is a report of a woman with cystinuria treated with 2 g/day of penicillamine during pregnancy who gave birth to a child with a generalized connective tissue defect that may have been caused by penicillamine. If stones continue to form in these patients, the benefits of therapy to the mother must be evaluated against the risk to the fetus.

Rheumatoid Arthritis—Penicillamine should not be administered to rheumatoid arthritis patients who are pregnant (see CONTRAINDICATIONS) and should be discontinued promptly in patients in whom pregnancy is suspected or diagnosed. Penicillamine should be used in women of childbearing potential only when the expected benefits outweigh possible hazards. Women of childbearing potential should be informed of the possible hazards of penicillamine to the developing fetus and should be advised to report promptly any missed menstrual periods or other indications of possible pregnancy.

There is a report that a woman with rheumatoid arthritis treated with less than one gram a day of penicillamine during pregnancy gave birth (cesarean delivery) to an infant with growth retardation, flattened face with broad nasal bridge, low set ears, short neck with loose skin folds, and unusually lax body skin.

Usage in Children—The efficacy of CUPRIMINE in juvenile rheumatoid arthritis has not been established.

Adverse Reactions

Penicillamine is a drug with a high incidence of untoward reactions, some of which are potentially fatal. Therefore, it is mandatory that patients receiving penicillamine therapy remain under close medical supervision throughout the period of drug administration (see WARNINGS and PRECAUTIONS).

Reported incidences (%) for the most commonly occurring adverse reactions in rheumatoid arthritis patients are noted, based on 17 representative clinical trials reported in the literature (1270 patients).

Allergic—Generalized pruritus, early and late rashes (5%), pemphigoid-type reactions, and drug eruptions which may be accompanied by fever, arthralgia, or lymphadenopathy have occurred (see WARNINGS and PRECAUTIONS). Some patients may show a lupus erythematosus-like syndrome similar to drug-induced lupus produced by other pharmacological agents (see PRECAUTIONS).

Urticaria and exfoliative dermatitis have occurred.

Thyroiditis has been reported but is extremely rare.

Some patients may develop a migratory polyarthralgia, often with objective synovitis (see DOSAGE AND ADMINISTRATION).

Gastrointestinal—Anorexia, epigastric pain, nausea, vomiting, or occasional diarrhea may occur (17%).

Isolated cases of reactivated peptic ulcer have occurred, as have hepatic dysfunction and pancreatitis. Intrahepatic cholestasis and toxic hepatitis have been reported rarely. There have been a few reports of increased serum alkaline phosphatase, lactic dehydrogenase, and positive cephalin flocculation and thymol turbidity tests.

Some patients may report a blunting, diminution, or total loss of taste perception (12%), or may develop oral ulcerations. Although rare, cheilosis, glossitis, and gingivostomatitis have been reported (see PRECAUTIONS).

Gastrointestinal side effects are usually reversible following cessation of therapy.

Hematological—Penicillamine can cause bone marrow depression (see WARNINGS). Leukopenia (2%) and thrombocytopenia (4%) have occurred. Fatalities have been reported as a result of thrombocytopenia, agranulocytosis, and aplastic anemia.

Thrombotic thrombocytopenic purpura, hemolytic anemia, red cell aplasia, monocytosis, leukocytosis, eosinophilia, and thrombocytosis have also been reported.

Renal—Patients on penicillamine therapy may develop proteinuria (6%) and/or hematuria which, in some, may progress to the development of the nephrotic syndrome as a result of an immune complex membranous glomerulopathy (see WARNINGS).

Central Nervous System—Tinnitus has been reported. Reversible optic neuritis has been reported following administration of penicillamine.

Other—Adverse reactions that have been reported rarely include thrombophlebitis; hyperpyrexia (see PRECAUTIONS); falling hair or alopecia; lichen planus; myasthenia gravis (see WARNINGS); polymyositis; dermatomyositis; mammary hyperplasia; elastosis perforans serpiginosa; toxic epidermal necrolysis; anetoderma (cutaneous macular atrophy); and Goodpasture's syndrome, a severe and ultimately fatal glomerulonephritis associated with intra-alveolar hemorrhage (see WARNINGS). Fatal renal vasculitis has also been reported. Allergic alveolitis, obliterative bronchiolitis, interstitial pneumonitis and pulmonary fibrosis have been reported in patients with severe rheumatoid arthritis, some of whom were receiving penicillamine. Bronchial asthma also has been reported.

Increased skin friability, excessive wrinkling of skin, and development of small white papules at venipuncture and surgical sites have been reported (see PRECAUTIONS).

The chelating action of the drug may cause increased excretion of other heavy metals such as zinc, mercury and lead.

Dosage and Administration

Wilson's Disease—CUPRIMINE capsules should be given on an empty stomach, four times a day; one-half to one hour before meals and at bedtime—at least two hours after the evening meal.

Optimal dosage can be determined only by measurement of urinary copper excretion. The urine must be collected in copper-free glassware, and should be quantitatively analyzed for copper before and soon after initiation of therapy with CUPRIMINE. Continued therapy should be monitored by doing a 24-hour urinary copper analysis every three months or so for the duration of therapy. Since a low copper diet should keep copper absorption down to less than one milligram a day, the patient probably will be in negative copper balance if 0.5 to one milligram of copper is present in a 24-hour collection of urine.

To achieve this, the suggested initial dosage of CUPRIMINE in the treatment of Wilson's disease is 1 g/day for children or adults. This may be increased, as indicated by the urinary copper analyses, but it is seldom necessary to exceed a dosage of 2 g/day.

In patients who cannot tolerate as much as 1 g/day initially, initiating dosage with 250 mg/day, and increasing gradually to the requi-

Continued on next page

Information on the Merck Sharp & Dohme products listed on these pages is the full prescribing information from package circulars in use October 31, 1982.

Merck Sharp & Dohme—Cont.

site amount, gives closer control of the effects of the drug and may help to reduce the incidence of adverse reactions.

Cystinuria—It is recommended that CUPRIMINE be used along with conventional therapy. By reducing urinary cystine, it decreases crystalluria and stone formation. In some instances, it has been reported to decrease the size of, and even to dissolve, stones already formed.

The usual dosage of CUPRIMINE in the treatment of cystinuria is 2 g/day for adults, with a range of 1 to 4 g/day. For children, dosage can be based on 30 mg/kg/day. The total daily amount should be divided into four doses. If four equal doses are not feasible, give the larger portion at bedtime. If adverse reactions necessitate a reduction in dosage, it is important to retain the bedtime dose.

Initiating dosage with 250 mg/day, and increasing gradually to the requisite amount, gives closer control of the effects of the drug and may help to reduce the incidence of adverse reactions.

In addition to taking CUPRIMINE, patients should drink copiously. It is especially important to drink about a pint of fluid at bedtime and another pint once during the night when urine is more concentrated and more acid than during the day. The greater the fluid intake, the lower the required dosage of CUPRIMINE.

Dosage must be individualized to an amount that limits cystine excretion to 100–200 mg/day in those with no history of stones, and below 100 mg/day in those who have had stone formation and/or pain. Thus, in determining dosage, the inherent tubular defect, the patient's size, age, and rate of growth, and his diet and water intake all must be taken into consideration.

The standard nitroprusside cyanide test has been reported useful as a qualitative measure of the effective dose *: Add 2 ml of freshly prepared 5 percent sodium cyanide to 5 ml of a 24-hour aliquot of protein-free urine and let stand ten minutes. Add 5 drops of freshly prepared 5 percent sodium nitroprusside and mix. Cystine will turn the mixture magenta. If the result is negative, it can be assumed that cystine excretion is less than 100 mg/g creatinine.

Although penicillamine is rarely excreted unchanged, it also will turn the mixture magenta. If there is any question as to which substance is causing the reaction, a ferric chloride test can be done to eliminate doubt: Add 3 percent ferric chloride dropwise to the urine. Penicillamine will turn the urine an immediate and quickly fading blue. Cystine will not produce any change in appearance.

Rheumatoid Arthritis—The principal rule of treatment with CUPRIMINE in rheumatoid arthritis is patience. The onset of therapeutic response is typically delayed. Two or three months may be required before the first evidence of a clinical response is noted (see CLINICAL PHARMACOLOGY).

When treatment with CUPRIMINE has been interrupted because of adverse reactions or other reasons, the drug should be reintroduced cautiously by starting with a lower dosage and increasing slowly.

Initial Therapy—The currently recommended dosage regimen in rheumatoid arthritis begins with a single daily dose of 125 mg or 250 mg which is thereafter increased at one to three month intervals, by 125 mg or 250 mg/day, as patient response and tolerance indicate. If a satisfactory remission of symptoms is achieved, the dose associated with the remission should be continued (see *Maintenance Therapy*). If there is no improvement and there are no signs of potentially serious toxicity after two to three months of treatment with doses of 500–750 mg/day, increases of 250 mg/day at two to three month intervals may be continued until a satisfactory remission occurs (see *Maintenance Therapy*) or signs of toxicity develop (see WARNINGS and PRECAUTIONS). If there is no discernible improvement after three to four months of treatment with 1000 to 1500 mg of penicillamine/day, it may be assumed the patient will not respond and CUPRIMINE should be discontinued.

It is important that CUPRIMINE be given on an empty stomach at least one hour before meals and at least one hour apart from any other drug, food or milk (see CLINICAL PHARMACOLOGY).

Maintenance Therapy—The maintenance dosage of CUPRIMINE must be individualized, and may require adjustment during the course of treatment. Many patients respond satisfactorily to a dosage within the 500–750 mg/day range. Some need less.

Changes in maintenance dosage levels may not be reflected clinically or in the erythrocyte sedimentation rate for two to three months after each dosage adjustment.

Some patients will subsequently require an increase in the maintenance dosage to achieve maximal disease suppression. In those patients who do respond, but who evidence incomplete suppression of their disease after the first six to nine months of treatment, the daily dosage of CUPRIMINE may be increased by 125 mg or 250 mg/day at three-month intervals. It is unusual in current practice to employ a dosage in excess of 1 g/day, but up to 1.5 g/day has sometimes been required.

Management of Exacerbations—During the course of treatment some patients may experience an exacerbation of disease activity following an initial good response. These may be self-limited and can subside within twelve weeks. They are usually controlled by the addition of nonsteroidal anti-inflammatory drugs, and only if the patient has demonstrated a true "escape" phenomenon (as evidenced by failure of the flare to subside within this time period) should an increase in the maintenance dose ordinarily be considered.

In the rheumatoid patient, migratory polyarthralgia due to penicillamine is extremely difficult to differentiate from an exacerbation of the rheumatoid arthritis. Discontinuance or a substantial reduction in dosage of CUPRIMINE for up to several weeks will usually determine which of these processes is responsible for the arthralgia.

Duration of Therapy—The optimum duration of therapy with CUPRIMINE in rheumatoid arthritis has not been determined. If the patient has been in remission for six months or more, a gradual, stepwise dosage reduction in decrements of 125 mg or 250 mg/day at approximately three month intervals may be attempted.

Concomitant Drug Therapy—CUPRIMINE should not be used in patients who are receiving gold therapy, antimalarial or cytotoxic drugs, oxyphenbutazone, or phenylbutazone (see PRECAUTIONS). Other measures, such as salicylates, other nonsteroidal anti-inflammatory drugs, or systemic corticosteroids, may be continued when penicillamine is initiated. After improvement commences, analgesic and anti-inflammatory drugs may be slowly discontinued as symptoms permit. Steroid withdrawal must be done gradually, and many months of treatment with CUPRIMINE may be required before steroids can be completely eliminated.

Dosage Frequency—Based on clinical experience dosages up to 500 mg/day can be given as a single daily dose. Dosages in excess of 500 mg/day should be administered in divided doses.

*Lotz, M., Potts, J.T. and Bartter, F.C.: Brit. Med. J. *2*:521, Aug. 28, 1965 (in Medical Memoranda).

How Supplied

No. 3299—Capsules CUPRIMINE, 250 mg, are ivory-colored capsules containing a white or nearly white powder, and are coded MSD 602. They are supplied as follows:
NDC 0006-0602-68 in bottles of 100.
[*Shown in Product Identification Section*]

No. 3350—Capsules CUPRIMINE, 125 mg, are opaque yellow and gray capsules containing a white or nearly white powder, and are coded MSD 672. They are supplied as follows:
NDC 0006-0672-68 in bottles of 100.
[*Shown in Product Identification Section*]

A.H.F.S. Category: 64:00
DC 6177828 Issued May 1981

DECADRON® Elixir (dexamethasone, MSD), U.S.P. ℞

Description

Glucocorticoids are adrenocortical steroids, both naturally occurring and synthetic, which are readily absorbed from the gastrointestinal tract.

Dexamethasone, a synthetic adrenocortical steroid, is a white to practically white, odorless, crystalline powder. It is stable in air. It is practically insoluble in water. The molecular weight is 392.47. It is designated chemically as 9-fluoro-11β, 17, 21-trihydroxy-16α-methylpregna-1,4-diene-3,20-dione. The empirical formula is $C_{22}H_{29}FO_5$.

DECADRON® (Dexamethasone, MSD) elixir contains 0.5 mg of dexamethasone in each 5 ml. Benzoic acid, 0.1%, is added as a preservative. It also contains alcohol 5%.

Actions

Naturally occurring glucocorticoids (hydrocortisone and cortisone), which also have salt-retaining properties, are used as replacement therapy in adrenocortical deficiency states. Their synthetic analogs, including dexamethasone, are primarily used for their potent anti-inflammatory effects in disorders of many organ systems.

Glucocorticoids cause profound and varied metabolic effects. In addition, they modify the body's immune responses to diverse stimuli.

At equipotent anti-inflammatory doses, dexamethasone almost completely lacks the sodium-retaining property of hydrocortisone and closely related derivatives of hydrocortisone.

Indications

1. *Endocrine Disorders*

Primary or secondary adrenocortical insufficiency (hydrocortisone or cortisone is the first choice; synthetic analogs may be used in conjunction with mineralocorticoids where applicable; in infancy mineralocorticoid supplementation is of particular importance)
- Congenital adrenal hyperplasia
- Nonsuppurative thyroiditis
- Hypercalcemia associated with cancer

2. *Rheumatic Disorders*

As adjunctive therapy for short-term administration (to tide the patient over an acute episode or exacerbation) in:
- Psoriatic arthritis
- Rheumatoid arthritis, including juvenile rheumatoid arthritis (selected cases may require low-dose maintenance therapy)
- Ankylosing spondylitis
- Acute and subacute bursitis
- Acute nonspecific tenosynovitis
- Acute gouty arthritis
- Post-traumatic osteoarthritis
- Synovitis of osteoarthritis
- Epicondylitis

3. *Collagen Diseases*

During an exacerbation or as maintenance therapy in selected cases of—

Systemic lupus erythematosus
Acute rheumatic carditis

4. *Dermatologic Diseases*
Pemphigus
Bullous dermatitis herpetiformis
Severe erythema multiforme (Stevens-Johnson syndrome)
Exfoliative dermatitis
Mycosis fungoides
Severe psoriasis
Severe seborrheic dermatitis

5. *Allergic States*
Control of severe or incapacitating allergic conditions intractable to adequate trials of conventional treatment:
Seasonal or perennial allergic rhinitis
Bronchial asthma
Contact dermatitis
Atopic dermatitis
Serum sickness
Drug hypersensitivity reactions

6. *Ophthalmic Diseases*
Severe acute and chronic allergic and inflammatory processes involving the eye and its adnexa, such as—
Allergic conjunctivitis
Keratitis
Allergic corneal marginal ulcers
Herpes zoster ophthalmicus
Iritis and iridocyclitis
Chorioretinitis
Anterior segment inflammation
Diffuse posterior uveitis and choroiditis
Optic neuritis
Sympathetic ophthalmia

7. *Respiratory Diseases*
Symptomatic sarcoidosis
Loeffler's syndrome not manageable by other means
Berylliosis
Fulminating or disseminated pulmonary tuberculosis when used concurrently with appropriate antituberculous chemotherapy
Aspiration pneumonitis

8. *Hematologic Disorders*
Idiopathic thrombocytopenic purpura in adults
Secondary thrombocytopenia in adults
Acquired (autoimmune) hemolytic anemia
Erythroblastopenia (RBC anemia)
Congenital (erythroid) hypoplastic anemia

9. *Neoplastic Diseases*
For palliative management of:
Leukemias and lymphomas in adults
Acute leukemia of childhood

10. *Edematous States*
To induce a diuresis or remission of proteinuria in the nephrotic syndrome, without uremia, of the idiopathic type or that due to lupus erythematosus

11. *Gastrointestinal Diseases*
To tide the patient over a critical period of the disease in:
Ulcerative colitis
Regional enteritis

12. *Miscellaneous*
Tuberculous meningitis with subarachnoid block or impending block when used concurrently with appropriate antituberculous chemotherapy
Trichinosis with neurologic or myocardial involvement

13. *Diagnostic testing of adrenocortical hyperfunction.*

Contraindications

Systemic fungal infections
Hypersensitivity to this product

Warnings

In patients on corticosteroid therapy subjected to unusual stress, increased dosage of rapidly acting corticosteroids before, during, and after the stressful situation is indicated.

Drug-induced secondary adrenocortical insufficiency may result from too rapid withdrawal of corticosteroids and may be minimized by gradual reduction of dosage. This type of relative insufficiency may persist for months after discontinuation of therapy; therefore, in any situation of stress occurring during that period, hormone therapy should be reinstituted. If the patient is receiving steroids already, dosage may have to be increased. Since mineralocorticoid secretion may be impaired, salt and/or a mineralocorticoid should be administered concurrently.

Corticosteroids may mask some signs of infection, and new infections may appear during their use. There may be decreased resistance and inability to localize infection when corticosteroids are used. Moreover, corticosteroids may affect the nitroblue-tetrazolium test for bacterial infection and produce false negative results.

Corticosteroids may activate latent amebiasis. Therefore, it is recommended that latent or active amebiasis be ruled out before initiating corticosteroid therapy in any patient who has spent time in the tropics or any patient with unexplained diarrhea.

Prolonged use of corticosteroids may produce posterior subcapsular cataracts, glaucoma with possible damage to the optic nerves, and may enhance the establishment of secondary ocular infections due to fungi or viruses.

Usage in pregnancy: Since adequate human reproduction studies have not been done with corticosteroids, use of these drugs in pregnancy or in women of childbearing potential requires that the anticipated benefits be weighed against the possible hazards to the mother and embryo or fetus. Infants born of mothers who have received substantial doses of corticosteroids during pregnancy should be carefully observed for signs of hypoadrenalism.

Corticosteroids appear in breast milk and could suppress growth, interfere with endogenous corticosteroid production, or cause other unwanted effects. Mothers taking pharmacologic doses of corticosteroids should be advised not to nurse.

Average and large doses of hydrocortisone or cortisone can cause elevation of blood pressure, salt and water retention, and increased excretion of potassium. These effects are less likely to occur with the synthetic derivatives except when used in large doses. Dietary salt restriction and potassium supplementation may be necessary. All corticosteroids increase calcium excretion.

Administration of live virus vaccines, including smallpox, is contraindicated in individuals receiving immunosuppressive doses of corticosteroids. If inactivated viral or bacterial vaccines are administered to individuals receiving immunosuppressive doses of corticosteroids, the expected serum antibody response may not be obtained. However, immunization procedures may be undertaken in patients who are receiving corticosteroids as replacement therapy, e.g., for Addison's disease.

The use of DECADRON elixir in active tuberculosis should be restricted to those cases of fulminating or disseminated tuberculosis in which the corticosteroid is used for the management of the disease in conjunction with an appropriate antituberculous regimen.

If corticosteroids are indicated in patients with latent tuberculosis or tuberculin reactivity, close observation is necessary as reactivation of the disease may occur. During prolonged corticosteroid therapy, these patients should receive chemoprophylaxis.

Precautions

Following prolonged therapy, withdrawal of corticosteroids may result in symptoms of the corticosteroid withdrawal syndrome including fever, myalgia, arthralgia, and malaise. This may occur in patients even without evidence of adrenal insufficiency.

There is an enhanced effect of corticosteroids in patients with hypothyroidism and in those with cirrhosis.

Corticosteroids should be used cautiously in patients with ocular herpes simplex because of possible corneal perforation.

The lowest possible dose of corticosteroid should be used to control the condition under treatment, and when reduction in dosage is possible, the reduction should be gradual.

Psychic derangements may appear when corticosteroids are used, ranging from euphoria, insomnia, mood swings, personality changes, and severe depression, to frank psychotic manifestations. Also, existing emotional instability or psychotic tendencies may be aggravated by corticosteroids.

Aspirin should be used cautiously in conjunction with corticosteroids in hypoprothrombinemia.

Steroids should be used with caution in nonspecific ulcerative colitis, if there is a probability of impending perforation, abscess, or other pyogenic infection; diverticulitis; fresh intestinal anastomoses; active or latent peptic ulcer; renal insufficiency; hypertension; osteoporosis; and myasthenia gravis. Signs of peritoneal irritation following gastrointestinal perforation in patients receiving large doses of corticosteroids may be minimal or absent. Fat embolism has been reported as a possible complication of hypercortisonism.

When large doses are given, some authorities advise that corticosteroids be taken with meals and antacids taken between meals to help to prevent peptic ulcer.

Growth and development of infants and children on prolonged corticosteroid therapy should be carefully observed.

Steroids may increase or decrease motility and number of spermatozoa in some patients.

Phenytoin, phenobarbital, ephedrine, and rifampin may enhance the metabolic clearance of corticosteroids, resulting in decreased blood levels and lessened physiologic activity, thus requiring adjustment in corticosteroid dosage. These interactions may interfere with dexamethasone suppression tests which should be interpreted with caution during administration of these drugs.

The prothrombin time should be checked frequently in patients who are receiving corticosteroids and coumarin anticoagulants at the same time because of reports that corticosteroids have altered the response to these anticoagulants. Studies have shown that the usual effect produced by adding corticosteroids is inhibition of response to coumarins, although there have been some conflicting reports of potentiation not substantiated by studies.

When corticosteroids are administered concomitantly with potassium-depleting diuretics, patients should be observed closely for development of hypokalemia.

Adverse Reactions

Fluid and Electrolyte Disturbances
Sodium retention
Fluid retention
Congestive heart failure in susceptible patients
Potassium loss
Hypokalemic alkalosis
Hypertension

Musculoskeletal
Muscle weakness
Steroid myopathy

Continued on next page

Information on the Merck Sharp & Dohme products listed on these pages is the full prescribing information from package circulars in use October 31, 1982.

Merck Sharp & Dohme—Cont.

Loss of muscle mass
Osteoporosis
Vertebral compression fractures
Aseptic necrosis of femoral and humeral heads
Pathologic fracture of long bones
Tendon rupture

Gastrointestinal
Peptic ulcer with possible perforation and hemorrhage
Perforation of the small and large bowel, particularly in patients with inflammatory bowel disease
Pancreatitis
Abdominal distention
Ulcerative esophagitis

Dermatologic
Impaired wound healing
Thin fragile skin
Petechiae and ecchymoses
Erythema
Increased sweating
May suppress reactions to skin tests
Other cutaneous reactions, such as allergic dermatitis, urticaria, angioneurotic edema

Neurologic
Convulsions
Increased intracranial pressure with papilledema (pseudotumor cerebri) usually after treatment
Vertigo
Headache

Endocrine
Menstrual irregularities
Development of cushingoid state
Suppression of growth in children
Secondary adrenocortical and pituitary unresponsiveness, particularly in times of stress, as in trauma, surgery, or illness
Decreased carbohydrate tolerance
Manifestations of latent diabetes mellitus
Increased requirements for insulin or oral hypoglycemic agents in diabetics

Ophthalmic
Posterior subcapsular cataracts
Increased intraocular pressure
Glaucoma
Exophthalmos

Metabolic
Negative nitrogen balance due to protein catabolism

Other
Hypersensitivity
Thromboembolism
Weight gain
Increased appetite
Nausea
Malaise

Dosage and Administration

For oral administration

DOSAGE REQUIREMENTS ARE VARIABLE AND MUST BE INDIVIDUALIZED ON THE BASIS OF THE DISEASE AND THE RESPONSE OF THE PATIENT.

The initial dosage varies from 0.75 to 9 mg a day depending on the disease being treated. In less severe diseases doses lower than 0.75 mg may suffice, while in severe diseases doses higher than 9 mg may be required. The initial dosage should be maintained or adjusted until the patient's response is satisfactory. If satisfactory clinical response does not occur after a reasonable period of time, discontinue DECADRON elixir and transfer the patient to other therapy.

After a favorable initial response, the proper maintenance dosage should be determined by decreasing the initial dosage in small amounts to the lowest dosage that maintains an adequate clinical response.

Patients should be observed closely for signs that might require dosage adjustment, including changes in clinical status resulting from remissions or exacerbations of the disease, individual drug responsiveness, and the effect of stress (e.g., surgery, infection, trauma). During stress it may be necessary to increase dosage temporarily.

If the drug is to be stopped after more than a few days of treatment, it usually should be withdrawn gradually.

The following milligram equivalents facilitate changing to DECADRON from other glucocorticoids:

DECADRON	Methylprednisolone and Triamcinolone	Prednisolone and Prednisone	Hydrocortisone	Cortisone
0.75 mg =	4 mg =	5 mg =	20 mg =	25 mg

Dexamethasone suppression tests

1. Tests for Cushing's syndrome
   Give 1.0 mg of DECADRON orally at 11:00 p.m. Blood is drawn for plasma cortisol determination at 8:00 a.m. the following morning.
   For greater accuracy, give 0.5 mg of DECADRON orally every 6 hours for 48 hours. Twenty-four hour urine collections are made for determination of 17-hydroxycorticosteroid excretion.
2. Test to distinguish Cushing's syndrome due to pituitary ACTH excess from Cushing's syndrome due to other causes
   Give 2.0 mg of DECADRON orally every 6 hours for 48 hours. Twenty-four hour urine collections are made for determination of 17-hydroxycorticosteroid excretion.

How Supplied

No. 7622—Elixir DECADRON, 0.5 mg dexamethasone per 5 ml, is a clear, red liquid and is supplied as follows:

NDC 0006-7622-55 bottles of 100 ml with calibrated dropper assembly.

NDC 0006-7622-66 bottles of 237 ml without dropper assembly.

A.H.F.S. Category: 68:04
DC 6030723 Issued August 1981

DECADRON® Tablets (dexamethasone, MSD), U.S.P. ℞

Description

Glucocorticoids are adrenocortical steroids, both naturally occurring and synthetic, which are readily absorbed from the gastrointestinal tract.

Dexamethasone, a synthetic adrenocortical steroid, is a practically white, odorless, crystalline powder. It is stable in air. It is practically insoluble in water. The molecular weight is 392.47. It is designated chemically as 9-fluoro-11β,17,21-trihydroxy-16α-methylpregna-1, 4-diene-3,20-dione. The empirical formula is $C_{22}H_{29}FO_5$.

DECADRON® (Dexamethasone, MSD) tablets are supplied in five potencies, 0.25 mg, 0.5 mg, 0.75 mg, 1.5 mg, and 4 mg.

Actions

Naturally occurring glucocorticoids (hydrocortisone and cortisone), which also have salt-retaining properties, are used as replacement therapy in adrenocortical deficiency states. Their synthetic analogs including dexamethasone are primarily used for their potent anti-inflammatory effects in disorders of many organ systems.

Glucocorticoids cause profound and varied metabolic effects. In addition, they modify the body's immune responses to diverse stimuli.

At equipotent anti-inflammatory doses, dexamethasone almost completely lacks the sodium retaining property of hydrocortisone and closely related derivatives of hydrocortisone.

Indications

1. *Endocrine Disorders*
   Primary or secondary adrenocortical insufficiency (hydrocortisone or cortisone is the first choice; synthetic analogs may be used in conjunction with mineralocorticoids where applicable; in infancy mineralocorticoid supplementation is of particular importance).
   Congenital adrenal hyperplasia
   Nonsuppurative thyroiditis
   Hypercalcemia associated with cancer
2. *Rheumatic Disorders*
   As adjunctive therapy for short-term administration (to tide the patient over an acute episode or exacerbation) in:
   Psoriatic arthritis
   Rheumatoid arthritis, including juvenile rheumatoid arthritis (selected cases may require low-dose maintenance therapy)
   Ankylosing spondylitis
   Acute and subacute bursitis
   Acute nonspecific tenosynovitis
   Acute gouty arthritis
   Post-traumatic osteoarthritis
   Synovitis of osteoarthritis
   Epicondylitis
3. *Collagen Diseases*
   During an exacerbation or as maintenance therapy in selected cases of—
   Systemic lupus erythematosus
   Acute rheumatic carditis
4. *Dermatologic Diseases*
   Pemphigus
   Bullous dermatitis herpetiformis
   Severe erythema multiforme (Stevens-Johnson syndrome)
   Exfoliative dermatitis
   Mycosis fungoides
   Severe psoriasis
   Severe seborrheic dermatitis
5. *Allergic States*
   Control of severe or incapacitating allergic conditions intractable to adequate trials of conventional treatment:
   Seasonal or perennial allergic rhinitis
   Bronchial asthma
   Contact dermatitis
   Atopic dermatitis
   Serum sickness
   Drug hypersensitivity reactions
6. *Ophthalmic Diseases*
   Severe acute and chronic allergic and inflammatory processes involving the eye and its adnexa, such as—
   Allergic conjunctivitis
   Keratitis
   Allergic corneal marginal ulcers
   Herpes zoster ophthalmicus
   Iritis and iridocyclitis
   Chorioretinitis
   Anterior segment inflammation
   Diffuse posterior uveitis and choroiditis
   Optic neuritis
   Sympathetic ophthalmia
7. *Respiratory Diseases*
   Symptomatic sarcoidosis
   Loeffler's syndrome not manageable by other means
   Berylliosis
   Fulminating or disseminated pulmonary tuberculosis when used concurrently with appropriate antituberculous chemotherapy
   Aspiration pneumonitis
8. *Hematologic Disorders*
   Idiopathic thrombocytopenic purpura in adults

Secondary thrombocytopenia in adults
Acquired (autoimmune) hemolytic anemia
Erythroblastopenia (RBC anemia)
Congenital (erythroid) hypoplastic anemia

9. *Neoplastic Diseases*
For palliative management of:
Leukemias and lymphomas in adults
Acute leukemia of childhood

10. *Edematous States*
To induce a diuresis or remission of proteinuria in the nephrotic syndrome, without uremia, of the idiopathic type or that due to lupus erythematosus

11. *Gastrointestinal Diseases*
To tide the patient over a critical period of the disease in:
Ulcerative colitis
Regional enteritis

12. *Cerebral Edema* associated with primary or metastatic brain tumor, craniotomy, or head injury. Use in cerebral edema is not a substitute for careful neurosurgical evaluation and definitive management such as neurosurgery or other specific therapy.

13. *Miscellaneous*
Tuberculous meningitis with subarachnoid block or impending block when used concurrently with appropriate antituberculous chemotherapy
Trichinosis with neurologic or myocardial involvement

14. *Diagnostic testing of adrenocortical hyperfunction.*

Contraindications

Systemic fungal infections
Hypersensitivity to this drug

Warnings

In patients on corticosteroid therapy subjected to unusual stress, increased dosage of rapidly acting corticosteroids before, during, and after the stressful situation is indicated.

Drug-induced secondary adrenocortical insufficiency may result from too rapid withdrawal of corticosteroids and may be minimized by gradual reduction of dosage. This type of relative insufficiency may persist for months after discontinuation of therapy; therefore, in any situation of stress occurring during that period, hormone therapy should be reinstituted. If the patient is receiving steroids already, dosage may have to be increased. Since mineralocorticoid secretion may be impaired, salt and/or a mineralocorticoid should be administered concurrently.

Corticosteroids may mask some signs of infection, and new infections may appear during their use. There may be decreased resistance and inability to localize infection when corticosteroids are used. Moreover, corticosteroids may affect the nitroblue-tetrazolium test for bacterial infection and produce false negative results.

Corticosteroids may activate latent amebiasis. Therefore, it is recommended that latent or active amebiasis be ruled out before initiating corticosteroid therapy in any patient who has spent time in the tropics or any patient with unexplained diarrhea.

Prolonged use of corticosteroids may produce posterior subcapsular cataracts and glaucoma with possible damage to the optic nerves, and may enhance the establishment of secondary ocular infections due to fungi or viruses.

Usage in pregnancy: Since adequate human reproduction studies have not been done with corticosteroids, use of these drugs in pregnancy or in women of childbearing potential requires that the anticipated benefits be weighed against the possible hazards to the mother and embryo or fetus. Infants born of mothers who have received substantial doses of corticosteroids during pregnancy should be carefully observed for signs of hypoadrenalism.

Corticosteroids appear in breast milk and could suppress growth, interfere with endogenous corticosteroid production, or cause other unwanted effects. Mothers taking pharmacologic doses of corticosteroids should be advised not to nurse.

Average and large doses of hydrocortisone or cortisone can cause elevation of blood pressure, salt and water retention, and increased excretion of potassium. These effects are less likely to occur with the synthetic derivatives except when used in large doses. Dietary salt restriction and potassium supplementation may be necessary. All corticosteroids increase calcium excretion.

Administration of live virus vaccines, including smallpox, is contraindicated in individuals receiving immunosuppressive doses of corticosteroids. If inactivated viral or bacterial vaccines are administered to individuals receiving immunosuppressive doses of corticosteroids, the expected serum antibody response may not be obtained. However, immunization procedures may be undertaken in patients who are receiving corticosteroids as replacement therapy, e.g., for Addison's disease.

The use of DECADRON tablets in active tuberculosis should be restricted to those cases of fulminating or disseminated tuberculosis in which the corticosteroid is used for the management of the disease in conjunction with an appropriate antituberculous regimen.

If corticosteroids are indicated in patients with latent tuberculosis or tuberculin reactivity, close observation is necessary as reactivation of the disease may occur. During prolonged corticosteroid therapy, these patients should receive chemoprophylaxis.

Precautions

Following prolonged therapy, withdrawal of corticosteroids may result in symptoms of the corticosteroid withdrawal syndrome including fever, myalgia, arthralgia, and malaise. This may occur in patients even without evidence of adrenal insufficiency.

There is an enhanced effect of corticosteroids in patients with hypothyroidism and in those with cirrhosis.

Corticosteroids should be used cautiously in patients with ocular herpes simplex because of possible corneal perforation.

The lowest possible dose of corticosteroid should be used to control the condition under treatment, and when reduction in dosage is possible, the reduction should be gradual.

Psychic derangements may appear when corticosteroids are used, ranging from euphoria, insomnia, mood swings, personality changes, and severe depression, to frank psychotic manifestations. Also, existing emotional instability or psychotic tendencies may be aggravated by corticosteroids.

Aspirin should be used cautiously in conjunction with corticosteroids in hypoprothrombinemia.

Steroids should be used with caution in nonspecific ulcerative colitis, if there is a probability of impending perforation, abscess, or other pyogenic infection, diverticulitis, fresh intestinal anastomoses, active or latent peptic ulcer, renal insufficiency, hypertension, osteoporosis, and myasthenia gravis. Signs of peritoneal irritation following gastrointestinal perforation in patients receiving large doses of corticosteroids may be minimal or absent. Fat embolism has been reported as a possible complication of hypercortisonism.

When large doses are given, some authorities advise that corticosteroids be taken with meals and antacids taken between meals to help to prevent peptic ulcer.

Growth and development of infants and children on prolonged corticosteroid therapy should be carefully observed.

Steroids may increase or decrease motility and number of spermatozoa in some patients.

Phenytoin, phenobarbital, ephedrine, and rifampin may enhance the metabolic clearance of corticosteroids, resulting in decreased blood levels and lessened physiologic activity, thus requiring adjustment in corticosteroid dosage. These interactions may interfere with dexamethasone suppression tests which should be interpreted with caution during administration of these drugs.

The prothrombin time should be checked frequently in patients who are receiving corticosteroids and coumarin anticoagulants at the same time because of reports that corticosteroids have altered the response to these anticoagulants. Studies have shown that the usual effect produced by adding corticosteroids is inhibition of response to coumarins, although there have been some conflicting reports of potentiation not substantiated by studies.

When corticosteroids are administered concomitantly with potassium-depleting diuretics, patients should be observed closely for development of hypokalemia.

Adverse Reactions

Fluid and Electrolyte Disturbances
Sodium retention
Fluid retention
Congestive heart failure in susceptible patients
Potassium loss
Hypokalemic alkalosis
Hypertension

Musculoskeletal
Muscle weakness
Steroid myopathy
Loss of muscle mass
Osteoporosis
Vertebral compression fractures
Aseptic necrosis of femoral and humeral heads
Pathologic fracture of long bones
Tendon rupture

Gastrointestinal
Peptic ulcer with possible perforation and hemorrhage
Perforation of the small and large bowel, particularly in patients with inflammatory bowel disease
Pancreatitis
Abdominal distention
Ulcerative esophagitis

Dermatologic
Impaired wound healing
Thin fragile skin
Petechiae and ecchymoses
Erythema
Increased sweating
May suppress reactions to skin tests
Other cutaneous reactions, such as allergic dermatitis, urticaria, angioneurotic edema

Neurologic
Convulsions
Increased intracranial pressure with papilledema (pseudotumor cerebri) usually after treatment
Vertigo
Headache

Endocrine
Menstrual irregularities
Development of cushingoid state
Suppression of growth in children
Secondary adrenocortical and pituitary unresponsiveness, particularly in times of stress, as in trauma, surgery, or illness
Decreased carbohydrate tolerance
Manifestations of latent diabetes mellitus
Increased requirements for insulin or oral hypoglycemic agents in diabetics

Continued on next page

Information on the Merck Sharp & Dohme products listed on these pages is the full prescribing information from package circulars in use October 31, 1982.

Merck Sharp & Dohme—Cont.

Ophthalmic
Posterior subcapsular cataracts
Increased intraocular pressure
Glaucoma
Exophthalmos
Metabolic
Negative nitrogen balance due to protein catabolism
Other
Hypersensitivity
Thromboembolism
Weight gain
Increased appetite
Nausea
Malaise

Dosage and Administration

For oral administration
DOSAGE REQUIREMENTS ARE VARIABLE AND MUST BE INDIVIDUALIZED ON THE BASIS OF THE DISEASE AND THE RESPONSE OF THE PATIENT.
The initial dosage varies from 0.75 to 9 mg a day depending on the disease being treated. In less severe diseases doses lower than 0.75 mg may suffice, while in severe diseases doses higher than 9 mg may be required. The initial dosage should be maintained or adjusted until the patient's response is satisfactory. If satisfactory clinical response does not occur after a reasonable period of time, discontinue DECADRON tablets and transfer the patient to other therapy.
After a favorable initial response, the proper maintenance dosage should be determined by decreasing the initial dosage in small amounts to the lowest dosage that maintains an adequate clinical response.
Patients should be observed closely for signs that might require dosage adjustment, including changes in clinical status resulting from remissions or exacerbations of the disease, individual drug responsiveness, and the effect of stress (e.g., surgery, infection, trauma). During stress it may be necessary to increase dosage temporarily.
If the drug is to be stopped after more than a few days of treatment, it usually should be withdrawn gradually.
The following milligram equivalents facilitate changing to DECADRON from other glucocorticoids:

DECADRON	Methylprednisolone and Triamcinolone	Prednisolone and Prednisone	Hydrocortisone	Cortisone
0.75 mg =	4 mg =	5 mg =	20 mg =	25 mg

In *acute, self-limited allergic disorders or acute exacerbations of chronic allergic disorders,* the following dosage schedule combining parenteral and oral therapy is suggested:
DECADRON® phosphate (Dexamethasone Sodium Phosphate, MSD) injection, 4 mg per ml:
First Day
1 or 2 ml, intramuscularly
DECADRON tablets, 0.75 mg:
Second Day
4 tablets in two divided doses
Third Day
4 tablets in two divided doses
Fourth Day
2 tablets in two divided doses
Fifth Day
1 tablet
Sixth Day
1 tablet
Seventh Day
No treatment
Eighth Day
Follow-up visit
This schedule is designed to ensure adequate therapy during acute episodes, while minimizing the risk of overdosage in chronic cases.
In *cerebral edema,* DECADRON phosphate (Dexamethasone Sodium Phosphate, MSD) injection is generally administered initially in a dosage of 10 mg intravenously followed by 4 mg every six hours intramuscularly until the symptoms of cerebral edema subside. Response is usually noted within 12 to 24 hours and dosage may be reduced after two to four days and gradually discontinued over a period of five to seven days. For palliative management of patients with recurrent or inoperable brain tumors, maintenance therapy with either DECADRON phosphate (Dexamethasone Sodium Phosphate, MSD) injection or DECADRON tablets in a dosage of two mg two or three times daily may be effective.
Dexamethasone suppression tests

1. Tests for Cushing's syndrome
Give 1.0 mg of DECADRON orally at 11:00 p.m. Blood is drawn for plasma cortisol determination at 8:00 a.m. the following morning.
For greater accuracy, give 0.5 mg of DECADRON orally every 6 hours for 48 hours. Twenty-four hour urine collections are made for determination of 17-hydroxycorticosteroid excretion.
2. Test to distinguish Cushing's syndrome due to pituitary ACTH excess from Cushing's syndrome due to other causes
Give 2.0 mg of DECADRON orally every 6 hours for 48 hours. Twenty-four hour urine collections are made for determination of 17-hydroxycorticosteroid excretion.

How Supplied

Tablets DECADRON are compressed, pentagonal-shaped tablets, colored to distinguish potency. They are scored on one side and are available as follows:
No. 7645—4 mg, white in color and coded MSD 97.
NDC 0006-0097-50 bottles of 50.
NDC 0006-0097-28 single unit packages of 100.
[*Shown in Product Identification Section*]
No. 7638—1.5 mg, pink in color and coded MSD 95.
NDC 0006-0095-50 bottles of 50.
NDC 0006-0095-28 single unit packages of 100.
[*Shown in Product Identification Section*]
No. 7601—0.75 mg, bluish-green in color and coded MSD 63.
NDC 0006-0063-12 5-12 PAK® (package of 12).
NDC 0006-0063-68 bottles of 100.
NDC 0006-0063-28 single unit packages of 100.
NDC 0006-0063-82 bottles of 1000.
[*Shown in Product Identification Section*]
No. 7598—0.5 mg, yellow in color and coded MSD 41.
NDC 0006-0041-68 bottles of 100.
(6505-00-687-8482 0.5 mg 100's).
NDC 0006-0041-28 single unit packages of 100.
NDC 0006-0041-82 bottles of 1000.
[*Shown in Product Identification Section*]
No. 7592—0.25 mg, orange in color and coded MSD 20.
NDC 0006-0020-68 bottles of 100.
[*Shown in Product Identification Section*]
A.H.F.S. Category: 68:04
DC 6025239 Issued August 1981

DECADRON® Phosphate Injection (dexamethasone sodium phosphate, MSD), U.S.P. ℞

Description

Dexamethasone sodium phosphate, a synthetic adrenocortical steroid, is a white or slightly yellow, crystalline powder. It is freely soluble in water and is exceedingly hygroscopic. The molecular weight is 516.14. It is designated chemically as 9-fluoro-11β, 17-dihydroxy-16α-methyl-21-(phosphonooxy)pregna-1, 4-diene-3, 20-dione disodium salt. The empirical formula is $C_{22}H_{28}FNa_2O_8P$.
DECADRON® phosphate (Dexamethasone Sodium Phosphate, MSD) injection is a sterile solution (pH 7.0 to 8.5) of dexamethasone sodium phosphate, and is supplied in two concentrations: 4 mg/ml and 24 mg/ml. The 24 mg/ml concentration offers the advantage of less volume in indications where high doses of corticosteroids by the intravenous route are needed.
Each milliliter of DECADRON phosphate injection, 4 mg/ml, contains dexamethasone sodium phosphate equivalent to 4 mg dexamethasone phosphate or 3.33 mg dexamethasone. Inactive ingredients per ml: 8 mg creatinine, 10 mg sodium citrate, sodium hydroxide to adjust pH, and Water for Injection q.s., with 1 mg sodium bisulfite, 1.5 mg methylparaben, and 0.2 mg propylparaben added as preservatives.
Each milliliter of DECADRON phosphate injection, 24 mg/ml, contains dexamethasone sodium phosphate equivalent to 24 mg dexamethasone phosphate or 20 mg dexamethasone. Inactive ingredients per ml: 8 mg creatinine, 10 mg sodium citrate, 0.5 mg disodium edetate, sodium hydroxide to adjust pH, and Water for Injection q.s., with 1 mg sodium bisulfite, 1.5 mg methylparaben, and 0.2 mg propylparaben added as preservatives.

Actions

DECADRON phosphate injection has a rapid onset but short duration of action when compared with less soluble preparations. Because of this, it is suitable for the treatment of acute disorders responsive to adrenocortical steroid therapy.
Naturally occurring glucocorticoids (hydrocortisone and cortisone), which also have salt-retaining properties, are used as replacement therapy in adrenocortical deficiency states. Their synthetic analogs, including dexamethasone, are primarily used for their potent anti-inflammatory effects in disorders of many organ systems.
Glucocorticoids cause profound and varied metabolic effects. In addition, they modify the body's immune responses to diverse stimuli.
At equipotent anti-inflammatory doses, dexamethasone almost completely lacks the sodium-retaining property of hydrocortisone and closely related derivatives of hydrocortisone.

Indications

A. By intravenous or intramuscular injection when oral therapy is not feasible:
1. *Endocrine disorders*
Primary or secondary adrenocortical insufficiency (hydrocortisone or cortisone is the drug of choice; synthetic analogs may be used in conjunction with mineralocorticoids where applicable; in infancy, mineralocorticoid supplementation is of particular importance)
Acute adrenocortical insufficiency (hydrocortisone or cortisone is the drug of choice; mineralocorticoid supplementation may be necessary, particularly when synthetic analogs are used)
Preoperatively, and in the event of serious trauma or illness, in patients with known

adrenal insufficiency or when adrenocortical reserve is doubtful
Shock unresponsive to conventional therapy if adrenocortical insufficiency exists or is suspected
Congenital adrenal hyperplasia
Nonsuppurative thyroiditis
Hypercalcemia associated with cancer

2. *Rheumatic disorders*

As adjunctive therapy for short-term administration (to tide the patient over an acute episode or exacerbation) in:
Post-traumatic osteoarthritis
Synovitis of osteoarthritis
Rheumatoid arthritis, including juvenile rheumatoid arthritis (selected cases may require low-dose maintenance therapy)
Acute and subacute bursitis
Epicondylitis
Acute nonspecific tenosynovitis
Acute gouty arthritis
Psoriatic arthritis
Ankylosing spondylitis

3. *Collagen diseases*

During an exacerbation or as maintenance therapy in selected cases of:
Systemic lupus erythematosus
Acute rheumatic carditis

4. *Dermatologic diseases*

Pemphigus
Severe erythema multiforme (Stevens-Johnson syndrome)
Exfoliative dermatitis
Bullous dermatitis herpetiformis
Severe seborrheic dermatitis
Severe psoriasis
Mycosis fungoides

5. *Allergic states*

Control of severe or incapacitating allergic conditions intractable to adequate trials of conventional treatment in:
Bronchial asthma
Contact dermatitis
Atopic dermatitis
Serum sickness
Seasonal or perennial allergic rhinitis
Drug hypersensitivity reactions
Urticarial transfusion reactions
Acute noninfectious laryngeal edema (epinephrine is the drug of first choice)

6. *Ophthalmic diseases*

Severe acute and chronic allergic and inflammatory processes involving the eye, such as:
Herpes zoster ophthalmicus
Iritis, iridocyclitis
Chorioretinitis
Diffuse posterior uveitis and choroiditis
Optic neuritis
Sympathetic ophthalmia
Anterior segment inflammation
Allergic conjunctivitis
Keratitis
Allergic corneal marginal ulcers

7. *Gastrointestinal diseases*

To tide the patient over a critical period of the disease in:
Ulcerative colitis (Systemic therapy)
Regional enteritis (Systemic therapy)

8. *Respiratory diseases*

Symptomatic sarcoidosis
Berylliosis
Fulminating or disseminated pulmonary tuberculosis when used concurrently with appropriate antituberculous chemotherapy
Loeffler's syndrome not manageable by other means
Aspiration pneumonitis

9. *Hematologic disorders*

Acquired (autoimmune) hemolytic anemia
Idiopathic thrombocytopenic purpura in adults (I.V. only; I.M. administration is contraindicated)
Secondary thrombocytopenia in adults
Erythroblastopenia (RBC anemia)
Congenital (erythroid) hypoplastic anemia

10. *Neoplastic diseases*

For palliative management of:
Leukemias and lymphomas in adults
Acute leukemia of childhood

11. *Edematous states*

To induce diuresis or remission of proteinuria in the nephrotic syndrome, without uremia, of the idiopathic type, or that due to lupus erythematosus

12. *Miscellaneous*

Tuberculous meningitis with subarachnoid block or impending block when used concurrently with appropriate antituberculous chemotherapy
Trichinosis with neurologic or myocardial involvement

13. *Diagnostic testing of adrenocortical hyperfunction*

14. *Cerebral Edema* associated with primary or metastatic brain tumor, craniotomy, or head injury. Use in cerebral edema is not a substitute for careful neurosurgical evaluation and definitive management such as neurosurgery or other specific therapy.

B. By intra-articular or soft tissue injection:
As adjunctive therapy for short-term administration (to tide the patient over an acute episode or exacerbation) in:
Synovitis of osteoarthritis
Rheumatoid arthritis
Acute and subacute bursitis
Acute gouty arthritis
Epicondylitis
Acute nonspecific tenosynovitis
Post-traumatic osteoarthritis

C. By intralesional injection:
Keloids
Localized hypertrophic, infiltrated, inflammatory lesions of: lichen planus, psoriatic plaques, granuloma annulare, and lichen simplex chronicus (neurodermatitis)
Discoid lupus erythematosus
Necrobiosis lipoidica diabeticorum
Alopecia areata
May also be useful in cystic tumors of an aponeurosis or tendon (ganglia)

Contraindications

Systemic fungal infections (See WARNINGS re amphotericin B)
Hypersensitivity to any component of this product

Warnings

Corticosteroids may exacerbate systemic fungal infections and therefore should not be used in the presence of such infections unless they are needed to control drug reactions due to amphotericin B. Moreover, there have been cases reported in which concomitant use of amphotericin B and hydrocortisone was followed by cardiac enlargement and congestive failure.

In patients on corticosteroid therapy subjected to any unusual stress, increased dosage of rapidly acting corticosteroids before, during, and after the stressful situation is indicated.

Drug-induced secondary adrenocortical insufficiency may result from too rapid withdrawal of corticosteroids and may be minimized by gradual reduction of dosage. This type of relative insufficiency may persist for months after discontinuation of therapy; therefore, in any situation of stress occurring during that period, hormone therapy should be reinstituted. If the patient is receiving steroids already, dosage may have to be increased. Since mineralocorticoid secretion may be impaired, salt and/or a mineralocorticoid should be administered concurrently.

Corticosteroids may mask some signs of infection, and new infections may appear during their use. There may be decreased resistance and inability to localize infection when corticosteroids are used. Moreover, corticosteroids may affect the nitroblue-tetrazolium test for bacterial infection and produce false negative results.

Corticosteroids may activate latent amebiasis. Therefore, it is recommended that latent or active amebiasis be ruled out before initiating corticosteroid therapy in any patient who has spent time in the tropics or any patient with unexplained diarrhea.

Prolonged use of corticosteroids may produce posterior subcapsular cataracts, glaucoma with possible damage to the optic nerves, and may enhance the establishment of secondary ocular infections due to fungi or viruses.

Usage in pregnancy. Since adequate human reproduction studies have not been done with corticosteroids, use of these drugs in pregnancy or in women of childbearing potential requires that the anticipated benefits be weighed against the possible hazards to the mother and embryo or fetus. Infants born of mothers who have received substantial doses of corticosteroids during pregnancy should be carefully observed for signs of hypoadrenalism.

Corticosteroids appear in breast milk and could suppress growth, interfere with endogenous corticosteroid production, or cause other unwanted effects. Mothers taking pharmacologic doses of corticosteroids should be advised not to nurse.

Average and large doses of cortisone or hydrocortisone can cause elevation of blood pressure, salt and water retention, and increased excretion of potassium. These effects are less likely to occur with the synthetic derivatives except when used in large doses. Dietary salt restriction and potassium supplementation may be necessary. All corticosteroids increase calcium excretion.

Administration of live virus vaccines, including smallpox, is contraindicated in individuals receiving immunosuppressive doses of corticosteroids. If inactivated viral or bacterial vaccines are administered to individuals receiving immunosuppressive doses of corticosteroids, the expected serum antibody response may not be obtained. However, immunization procedures may be undertaken in patients who are receiving corticosteroids as replacement therapy, e.g., for Addison's disease.

The use of DECADRON phosphate injection in active tuberculosis should be restricted to those cases of fulminating or disseminated tuberculosis in which the corticosteroid is used for the management of the disease in conjunction with an appropriate antituberculous regimen.

If corticosteroids are indicated in patients with latent tuberculosis or tuberculin reactivity, close observation is necessary as reactivation of the disease may occur. During prolonged corticosteroid therapy, these patients should receive chemoprophylaxis.

Because rare instances of anaphylactoid reactions have occurred in patients receiving parenteral corticosteroid therapy, appropriate precautionary measures should be taken prior to administration, especially when the patient has a history of allergy to any drug.

Precautions

This product, like many other steroid formulations, is sensitive to heat. Therefore, it should not be autoclaved when it is desirable to sterilize the exterior of the vial.

Following prolonged therapy, withdrawal of corticosteroids may result in symptoms of the corticosteroid withdrawal syndrome including fever, myalgia, arthralgia, and malaise. This may occur in patients even without evidence of adrenal insufficiency.

Continued on next page

Information on the Merck Sharp & Dohme products listed on these pages is the full prescribing information from package circulars in use October 31, 1982.

Merck Sharp & Dohme—Cont.

There is an enhanced effect of corticosteroids in patients with hypothyroidism and in those with cirrhosis.
Corticosteroids should be used cautiously in patients with ocular herpes simplex for fear of corneal perforation.
The lowest possible dose of corticosteroid should be used to control the condition under treatment, and when reduction in dosage is possible, the reduction must be gradual.
Psychic derangements may appear when corticosteroids are used, ranging from euphoria, insomnia, mood swings, personality changes, and severe depression to frank psychotic manifestations. Also, existing emotional instability or psychotic tendencies may be aggravated by corticosteroids.
Aspirin should be used cautiously in conjunction with corticosteroids in hypoprothrombinemia.
Steroids should be used with caution in nonspecific ulcerative colitis, if there is a probability of impending perforation, abscess, or other pyogenic infection, also in diverticulitis, fresh intestinal anastomoses, active or latent peptic ulcer, renal insufficiency, hypertension, osteoporosis, and myasthenia gravis. Signs of peritoneal irritation following gastrointestinal perforation in patients receiving large doses of corticosteroids may be minimal or absent. Fat embolism has been reported as a possible complication of hypercortisonism.
When large doses are given, some authorities advise that antacids be administered between meals to help to prevent peptic ulcer.
Growth and development of infants and children on prolonged corticosteroid therapy should be carefully followed.
Steroids may increase or decrease motility and number of spermatozoa in some patients.
Phenytoin, phenobarbital, ephedrine, and rifampin may enhance the metabolic clearance of corticosteroids, resulting in decreased blood levels and lessened physiologic activity, thus requiring adjustment in corticosteroid dosage. These interactions may interfere with dexamethasone suppression tests which should be interpreted with caution during administration of these drugs.
The prothrombin time should be checked frequently in patients who are receiving corticosteroids and coumarin anticoagulants at the same time because of reports that corticosteroids have altered the response to these anticoagulants. Studies have shown that the usual effect produced by adding corticosteroids is inhibition of response to coumarins, although there have been some conflicting reports of potentiation not substantiated by studies.
When corticosteroids are administered concomitantly with potassium-depleting diuretics, patients should be observed closely for development of hypokalemia.
Intra-articular injection of a corticosteroid may produce systemic as well as local effects. Appropriate examination of any joint fluid present is necessary to exclude a septic process. A marked increase in pain accompanied by local swelling, further restriction of joint motion, fever, and malaise is suggestive of septic arthritis. If this complication occurs and the diagnosis of sepsis is confirmed, appropriate antimicrobial therapy should be instituted.
Injection of a steroid into an infected site is to be avoided.
Corticosteroids should not be injected into unstable joints.
Patients should be impressed strongly with the importance of not overusing joints in which symptomatic benefit has been obtained as long as the inflammatory process remains active.
Frequent intra-articular injection may result in damage to joint tissues.
The slower rate of absorption by intramuscular administration should be recognized.

Adverse Reactions

Fluid and electrolyte disturbances
Sodium retention
Fluid retention
Congestive heart failure in susceptible patients
Potassium loss
Hypokalemic alkalosis
Hypertension
Musculoskeletal
Muscle weakness
Steroid myopathy
Loss of muscle mass
Osteoporosis
Vertebral compression fractures
Aseptic necrosis of femoral and humeral heads
Pathologic fracture of long bones
Tendon rupture
Gastrointestinal
Peptic ulcer with possible subsequent perforation and hemorrhage
Perforation of the small and large bowel, particularly in patients with inflammatory bowel disease
Pancreatitis
Abdominal distention
Ulcerative esophagitis
Dermatologic
Impaired wound healing
Thin fragile skin
Petechiae and ecchymoses
Erythema
Increased sweating
May suppress reactions to skin tests
Burning or tingling, especially in the perineal area (after I.V. injection)
Other cutaneous reactions, such as allergic dermatitis, urticaria, angioneurotic edema
Neurologic
Convulsions
Increased intracranial pressure with papilledema (pseudotumor cerebri) usually after treatment
Vertigo
Headache
Endocrine
Menstrual irregularities
Development of cushingoid state
Suppression of growth in children
Secondary adrenocortical and pituitary unresponsiveness, particularly in times of stress, as in trauma, surgery, or illness
Decreased carbohydrate tolerance
Manifestations of latent diabetes mellitus
Increased requirements for insulin or oral hypoglycemic agents in diabetics
Ophthalmic
Posterior subcapsular cataracts
Increased intraocular pressure
Glaucoma
Exophthalmos
Metabolic
Negative nitrogen balance due to protein catabolism
Other
Anaphylactoid or hypersensitivity reactions
Thromboembolism
Weight gain
Increased appetite
Nausea
Malaise

The following *additional* adverse reactions are related to parenteral corticosteroid therapy:
Rare instances of blindness associated with intralesional therapy around the face and head
Hyperpigmentation or hypopigmentation
Subcutaneous and cutaneous atrophy
Sterile abscess
Postinjection flare (following intra-articular use)
Charcot-like arthropathy

Dosage and Administration

DECADRON phosphate injection, 4 mg/ml—*For intravenous, intramuscular, intra-articular, intralesional, and soft tissue injection.*
DECADRON phosphate injection, 24 mg/ml—*For intravenous injection only.*
DECADRON phosphate injection can be given directly from the vial or the disposable syringe, or it can be added to Sodium Chloride Injection or Dextrose Injection and administered by intravenous drip.
When it is mixed with an infusion solution, sterile precautions should be observed. Since infusion solutions generally do not contain preservatives, mixtures should be used within 24 hours.
DOSAGE REQUIREMENTS ARE VARIABLE AND MUST BE INDIVIDUALIZED ON THE BASIS OF THE DISEASE AND THE RESPONSE OF THE PATIENT.

Intravenous and Intramuscular Injection
The initial dosage of DECADRON phosphate injection varies from 0.5 to 9 mg a day depending on the disease being treated. In less severe diseases doses lower than 0.5 mg may suffice, while in severe diseases doses higher than 9 mg may be required.
The initial dosage should be maintained or adjusted until the patient's response is satisfactory. If a satisfactory clinical response does not occur after a reasonable period of time, discontinue DECADRON phosphate injection and transfer the patient to other therapy.
After a favorable initial response, the proper maintenance dosage should be determined by decreasing the initial dosage in small amounts to the lowest dosage that maintains an adequate clinical response.
Patients should be observed closely for signs that might require dosage adjustment, including changes in clinical status resulting from remissions or exacerbations of the disease, individual drug responsiveness, and the effect of stress (e.g., surgery, infection, trauma). During stress it may be necessary to increase dosage temporarily.
If the drug is to be stopped after more than a few days of treatment, it usually should be withdrawn gradually.
When the intravenous route of administration is used, dosage usually should be the same as the oral dosage. In certain overwhelming, acute, life-threatening situations, however, administration in dosages exceeding the usual dosages may be justified and may be in multiples of the oral dosages. The slower rate of absorption by intramuscular administration should be recognized.

Shock
There is a tendency in current medical practice to use high (pharmacologic) doses of corticosteroids for the treatment of unresponsive shock. The following dosages of DECADRON phosphate injection have been suggested by various authors:

*Author**	*Dosage*
Cavanagh[1]	3 mg/kg of body weight per 24 hours by constant intravenous infusion after an initial intravenous injection of 20 mg
Dietzman[2]	2 to 6 mg/kg of body weight as a single intravenous injection
Frank[3]	40 mg initially followed by repeat intravenous injection every 4 to 6 hours while shock persists
Oaks[4]	40 mg initially followed by repeat intravenous injection every 2 to 6 hours while shock persists
Schumer[5]	1 mg/kg of body weight as a single intravenous injection

Administration of high dose corticosteroid therapy should be continued only until the patient's condition has stabilized and usually not longer than 48 to 72 hours.
Although adverse reactions associated with high dose, short term corticosteroid therapy are uncommon, peptic ulceration may occur.

*1. Cavanagh, D.; Singh, K. B.: Endotoxin shock in pregnancy and abortion, in "Corticosteroids in the Treatment of Shock", Schumer, W.; Nyhus, L. M., Editors, Urbana, University of Illinois Press, 1970, pp. 86-96.
2. Dietzman, R. H.; Ersek, R. A.; Bloch, J. M.; Lillehei, R. C.: High-output, low-resistance gram-negative septic shock in man, Angiology *20:*691-700, Dec. 1969.
3. Frank, E.: Clinical observations in shock and management (In: Shields, T. F., ed.: Symposium on current concepts and management of shock), J. Maine Med. Ass. *59:*195-200, Oct. 1968.
4. Oaks, W. W.; Cohen, H. E.: Endotoxin shock in the geriatric patient, Geriat. *22:*120-130, Mar. 1967.
5. Schumer, W.; Nyhus, L. M.: Corticosteroid effect on biochemical parameters of human oligemic shock, Arch. Surg. *100:*405-408, Apr. 1970.

Cerebral Edema
DECADRON phosphate injection is generally administered initially in a dosage of 10 mg intravenously followed by 4 mg every six hours intramuscularly until the symptoms of cerebral edema subside. Response is usually noted within 12 to 24 hours and dosage may be reduced after two to four days and gradually discontinued over a period of five to seven days. For palliative management of patients with recurrent or inoperable brain tumors, maintenance therapy with two mg two or three times a day may be effective.
Acute Allergic Disorders
In acute, self-limited allergic disorders or acute exacerbations of chronic allergic disorders, the following dosage schedule combining parenteral and oral therapy is suggested:
DECADRON phosphate injection, 4 mg/ml: *first day,* 1 or 2 ml (4 or 8 mg), intramuscularly.
DECADRON® (Dexamethasone, MSD) tablets, 0.75 mg: *second and third days,* 4 tablets in two divided doses each day; *fourth day,* 2 tablets in two divided doses; *fifth and sixth days,* 1 tablet each day; *seventh day,* no treatment; *eighth day,* follow-up visit.
This schedule is designed to ensure adequate therapy during acute episodes, while minimizing the risk of overdosage in chronic cases.

Intra-articular, Intralesional, and Soft Tissue Injection
Intra-articular, intralesional, and soft tissue injections are generally employed when the affected joints or areas are limited to one or two sites. Dosage and frequency of injection varies depending on the condition and the site of injection. The usual dose is from 0.2 to 6 mg. The frequency usually ranges from once every three to five days to once every two to three weeks. Frequent intra-articular injection may result in damage to joint tissues.
Some of the usual single doses are:

Site of Injection	Amount of Dexamethasone Phosphate (mg)
Large Joints (e.g., Knee)	2 to 4
Small Joints (e.g., Interphalangeal, Temporomandibular)	0.8 to 1
Bursae	2 to 3
Tendon Sheaths	0.4 to 1
Soft Tissue Infiltration	2 to 6
Ganglia	1 to 2

DECADRON phosphate injection is particularly recommended for use in conjunction with one of the less soluble, longer-acting steroids for intra-articular and soft tissue injection.

How Supplied

No. 7628X—Injection DECADRON phosphate, 4 mg per ml, is a clear, colorless solution, and is available in 1 ml and 2.5 ml disposable syringes and in 1 ml, 5 ml, and 25 ml vials as follows:
NDC 0006-7628-01, 1 ml single dose disposable syringe
(6505-00-935-4117, 1 ml syringe)
NDC 0006-7628-66, boxes of 25 × 1 ml vials
NDC 0006-7628-30, 2.5 ml single dose disposable syringe
NDC 0006-7628-03, 5 ml vial
(6505-00-963-5355, 5 ml vial)
NDC 0006-7628-25, 25 ml vial
FOR INTRAVENOUS USE ONLY:
No. 7646—Injection DECADRON phosphate, 24 mg per ml, is a clear, colorless to light yellow solution and is available in 5 ml and 10 ml vials as follows:
NDC 0006-7646-03, 5 ml vial
NDC 0006-7646-10, 10 ml vial.
A.H.F.S. Category: 68:04
DC 6597119 Issued November 1981

DECADRON® Phosphate ℞
(dexamethasone sodium phosphate, MSD), U.S.P.
0.05% Dexamethasone Phosphate Equivalent
Sterile Ophthalmic Ointment

Description

Sterile Ophthalmic Ointment DECADRON® Phosphate (Dexamethasone Sodium Phosphate, MSD) is a topical steroid ointment containing dexamethasone sodium phosphate equivalent to 0.5 mg (0.05%) dexamethasone phosphate in each gram. Inactive ingredients: white petrolatum and mineral oil.
Dexamethasone sodium phosphate is an inorganic ester of dexamethasone.

Action

Inhibition of inflammatory response to inciting agents of mechanical, chemical or immunological nature. No generally accepted explanation of this steroid property has been advanced.

Indications

For the treatment of the following conditions: Steroid responsive inflammatory conditions of the palpebral and bulbar conjunctiva, cornea, and anterior segment of the globe, such as allergic conjunctivitis, acne rosacea, superficial punctate keratitis, herpes zoster keratitis, iritis, cyclitis, selected infective conjunctivitis when the inherent hazard of steroid use is accepted to obtain an advisable diminution in edema and inflammation; corneal injury from chemical or thermal burns, or penetration of foreign bodies.

Contraindications

Acute superficial herpes simplex keratitis.
Fungal diseases of ocular structures.
Acute infectious stages of vaccinia, varicella and most other viral diseases of the cornea and conjunctiva.
Tuberculosis of the eye.
Hypersensitivity to a component of this medication.

Warnings

Employment of steroid medication in the treatment of stromal herpes simplex requires great caution; frequent slit-lamp microscopy is mandatory.
Prolonged use may result in elevated intraocular pressure and/or glaucoma, damage to the optic nerve, defects in visual acuity and fields of vision, posterior subcapsular cataract formation, or may result in secondary ocular infections.
Viral, bacterial, and fungal infections of the cornea may be exacerbated by the application of steroids.
Acute purulent untreated infection of the eye may be masked or activity enhanced by the presence of steroid medication.
In those diseases causing thinning of the cornea or sclera, perforation has been known to occur with the use of topical steroids.
Usage in Pregnancy
Safety of intensive or protracted use of topical steroids during pregnancy has not been substantiated.

Precautions

As fungal infections of the cornea are particularly prone to develop coincidentally with long-term local steroid applications, fungus invasion must be considered in any persistent corneal ulceration where a steroid has been used or is in use.
Intraocular pressure should be checked frequently.

Adverse Reactions

Glaucoma with optic nerve damage, visual acuity and field defects, posterior subcapsular cataract formation, secondary ocular infection from pathogens including herpes simplex, perforation of the globe.
Rarely, filtering blebs have been reported when topical steroids have been used following cataract surgery.
Rarely, stinging or burning may occur.

Dosage and Administration

The duration of treatment will vary with the type of lesion and may extend from a few days to several weeks, according to therapeutic response. Relapses, more common in chronic active lesions than in self-limited conditions, usually respond to retreatment.
Apply a thin coating of ointment three or four times a day. When a favorable response is observed, reduce the number of daily applications to two, and later to one a day as a maintenance dose if this is sufficient to control symptoms.
Ophthalmic ointment DECADRON phosphate is particularly convenient when an eye pad is used. It may also be the preparation of choice for patients in whom therapeutic benefit depends on prolonged contact of the active ingredients with ocular tissues.

How Supplied

No. 7615—0.05% Sterile Ophthalmic Ointment DECADRON phosphate is a clear unctuous ointment and is supplied as follows:
NDC 0006-7615-04 in 3.5 g tubes.
A.H.F.S. Category: 52:08
DC 6033125 Issued May 1981

Continued on next page

Information on the Merck Sharp & Dohme products listed on these pages is the full prescribing information from package circulars in use October 31, 1982.

Merck Sharp & Dohme—Cont.

DECADRON® Phosphate ℞
(dexamethasone sodium phosphate, MSD), U.S.P.
0.1% Dexamethasone Phosphate Equivalent
Sterile Ophthalmic Solution

Description

Ophthalmic Solution DECADRON® Phosphate (Dexamethasone Sodium Phosphate, MSD) in the 2.5 ml and 5 ml glass bottles with dropper assembly is a topical steroid solution containing dexamethasone sodium phosphate equivalent to 1 mg (0.1%) dexamethasone phosphate in each milliliter of buffered solution. Inactive ingredients: creatinine, sodium citrate, sodium borate, polysorbate 80, sodium hydroxide to adjust pH, and water for injection. Sodium bisulfite 0.32%, phenylethanol 0.25%, and benzalkonium chloride 0.02% added as preservatives.
Each milliliter of buffered ophthalmic solution DECADRON phosphate in the OCUMETER® ophthalmic dispenser contains: dexamethasone sodium phosphate equivalent to 1 mg (0.1%) dexamethasone phosphate. Inactive ingredients: creatinine, sodium citrate, sodium borate, polysorbate 80, disodium edetate, hydrochloric acid to adjust pH, and water for injection. Sodium bisulfite 0.1%, phenylethanol 0.25% and benzalkonium chloride 0.02% added as preservatives.
Dexamethasone sodium phosphate is a water soluble, inorganic ester of dexamethasone. It is approximately three thousand times more soluble in water at 25°C than hydrocortisone.

Action

Inhibition of inflammatory response to inciting agents of mechanical, chemical or immunological nature. No generally accepted explanation of this steroid property has been advanced.

Indications

For the treatment of the following conditions:
Ophthalmic:
Steroid responsive inflammatory conditions of the palpebral and bulbar conjunctiva, cornea, and anterior segment of the globe, such as allergic conjunctivitis, acne rosacea, superficial punctate keratitis, herpes zoster keratitis, iritis, cyclitis, selected infective conjunctivitis when the inherent hazard of steroid use is accepted to obtain an advisable diminution in edema and inflammation; corneal injury from chemical or thermal burns, or penetration of foreign bodies.
Otic:
Steroid responsive inflammatory conditions of the external auditory meatus, such as allergic otitis externa, selected purulent and nonpurulent infective otitis externa when the hazard of steroid use is accepted to obtain an advisable diminution in edema and inflammation.

Contraindications

Acute superficial herpes simplex keratitis.
Fungal diseases of ocular or auricular structures.
Acute infectious stages of vaccinia, varicella and most other viral diseases of the cornea and conjunctiva.
Tuberculosis of the eye.
Hypersensitivity to a component of this medication.
Perforation of a drum membrane.

Warnings

Employment of steroid medication in the treatment of stromal herpes simplex requires great caution; frequent slit-lamp microscopy is mandatory.
Prolonged use may result in elevated intraocular pressure and/or glaucoma, damage to the optic nerve, defects in visual acuity and fields of vision, posterior subcapsular cataract formation, or may result in secondary ocular infections.
Viral, bacterial, and fungal infections of the cornea may be exacerbated by the application of steroids.
Acute purulent untreated infection of the eye or ear may be masked or activity enhanced by the presence of steroid medication.
In those diseases causing thinning of the cornea or sclera, perforation has been known to occur with the use of topical steroids.
Usage in Pregnancy
Safety of intensive or protracted use of topical steroids during pregnancy has not been substantiated.

Precautions

As fungal infections of the cornea are particularly prone to develop coincidentally with long-term local steroid applications, fungus invasion must be considered in any persistent corneal ulceration where a steroid has been used or is in use.
Intraocular pressure should be checked frequently.

Adverse Reactions

Glaucoma with optic nerve damage, visual acuity and field defects, posterior subcapsular cataract formation, secondary ocular infection from pathogens including herpes simplex, perforation of the globe.
Rarely, filtering blebs have been reported when topical steroids have been used following cataract surgery.
Rarely, stinging or burning may occur.

Dosage and Administration

The duration of treatment will vary with the type of lesion and may extend from a few days to several weeks, according to therapeutic response. Relapses, more common in chronic active lesions than in self-limited conditions, usually respond to retreatment.
Eye—Instill one or two drops of solution into the conjunctival sac every hour during the day and every two hours during the night as initial therapy. When a favorable response is observed, reduce dosage to one drop every four hours. Later, further reduction in dosage to one drop three or four times daily may suffice to control symptoms.
Ear—Clean the aural canal thoroughly and sponge dry. Instill the solution directly into the aural canal. A suggested initial dosage is three or four drops two or three times a day. When a favorable response is obtained, reduce dosage gradually and eventually discontinue.
If preferred, the aural canal may be packed with a gauze wick saturated with solution. Keep the wick moist with the preparation and remove from the ear after 12 to 24 hours. Treatment may be repeated as often as necessary at the discretion of the physician.

How Supplied

Sterile ophthalmic solution DECADRON phosphate is a clear, colorless to pale yellow solution.
No. 7610—Ophthalmic solution DECADRON phosphate is supplied as follows:
NDC 0006-7610-30 in 2.5 ml glass bottles with dropper assembly.
NDC 0006-7610-03 in 5 ml glass bottles with dropper assembly.
No. 7643—Ophthalmic solution DECADRON phosphate is supplied as follows:
NDC 0006-7643-03 in 5 ml white, opaque, plastic OCUMETER ophthalmic dispenser with a controlled drop tip.
(6505-00-007-4536 0.1% 5 ml)
A.H.F.S. Category: 52:08
DC 6460011 Issued May 1981

DECADRON® Phosphate ℞
RESPIHALER®
(dexamethasone sodium phosphate, MSD), U.S.P.

Description

RESPIHALER® DECADRON® Phosphate (Dexamethasone Sodium Phosphate, MSD) is an aerosol for oral inhalation which contains dexamethasone sodium phosphate, an inorganic ester of dexamethasone, a synthetic adrenocortical steroid with basic glucocorticoid actions and effects.
Each RESPIHALER DECADRON Phosphate contains an amount sufficient to deliver at least 170 sprays. The metering valve of the aerosol-mechanism of the RESPIHALER dispenses dexamethasone sodium phosphate equivalent to approximately 0.1 mg of dexamethasone phosphate or approximately 0.084 mg of dexamethasone with each activation. On a regimen of 12 inhalations daily, it has been determined that the patient absorbs approximately 0.4-0.6 mg of dexamethasone. The inactive ingredients are fluorochlorohydrocarbons included as propellants. Alcohol 2%.
Dexamethasone sodium phosphate, a synthetic adrenocortical steroid, is a white or slightly yellow, crystalline powder. It is freely soluble in water and is exceedingly hygroscopic. It is prepared by a special process to produce particles in the range of 0.5 to 4 microns in size. The molecular weight is 516.41. It is designated chemically as 9-fluoro-11β, 17-dihydroxy-16α-methyl-21-(phosphono-oxy)pregna-1, 4-diene-3, 20-dione disodium salt. The empirical formula is $C_{22}H_{28}FNa_2O_8P$.

Actions

Because of the high water solubility of dexamethasone sodium phosphate, the aerosolized particles dissolve readily in the secretions of the bronchial and bronchiolar mucous membrane.

Indications

RESPIHALER DECADRON Phosphate is indicated for the treatment of bronchial asthma and related corticosteroid responsive bronchospastic states intractable to adequate trial of conventional therapy.

Contraindications

Systemic fungal infections.
Hypersensitivity to any component of this medication.
Persistently positive cultures of the sputum for *Candida albicans.*

Warnings

Rare instances of laryngeal and pharyngeal fungal infections have been observed in patients using RESPIHALER DECADRON Phosphate. These have usually responded promptly to discontinuation of therapy and institution of antifungal treatment.
In patients on therapy with RESPIHALER DECADRON Phosphate subjected to unusual stress, increased dosage of rapidly acting corticosteroids before, during, and after the stressful situation is indicated.
Drug-induced secondary adrenocortical insufficiency may result from too rapid withdrawal of corticosteroids and may be minimized by gradual reduction of dosage. This type of relative insufficiency may persist for months after discontinuation of therapy; therefore, in any

situation of stress occurring during that period, hormone therapy should be reinstituted. If the patient is receiving steroids already, dosage may have to be increased. Since mineralocorticoid secretion may be impaired, salt and /or a mineralocorticoid should be administered concurrently.

Dexamethasone may mask some signs of infection, and new infections may appear during its use. There may be decreased resistance and inability to localize infection when corticosteroids are used. Moreover, dexamethasone may affect the nitroblue-tetrazolium test for bacterial infection and produce false negative results.

Corticosteroids may activate latent amebiasis. Therefore, it is recommended that latent or active amebiasis be ruled out before initiating corticosteroid therapy in any patient who has spent time in the tropics or any patient with unexplained diarrhea.

Prolonged use of RESPIHALER DECADRON Phosphate may produce posterior subcapsular cataracts, glaucoma with possible damage to the optic nerves, and may enhance the establishment of secondary ocular infections due to fungi or viruses.

Usage in pregnancy: Since adequate human reproduction studies have not been done with RESPIHALER DECADRON Phosphate, use of this drug in pregnancy or in women of childbearing potential requires that the anticipated benefits be weighed against the possible hazards to the mother and embryo or fetus. Infants born of mothers who have received substantial doses of dexamethasone during pregnancy, should be carefully observed for signs of hypoadrenalism.

Dexamethasone appears in breast milk and could suppress growth, interfere with endogenous corticosteroid production, or cause other unwanted effects. Mothers taking pharmacologic doses of dexamethasone should be advised not to nurse.

Average and large doses of hydrocortisone or cortisone can cause elevation of blood pressure, salt and water retention, and increased excretion of potassium. These effects are less likely to occur with the synthetic derivatives and with RESPIHALER DECADRON Phosphate, except when used in large doses. Dietary salt restriction and potassium supplementation may be necessary. All corticosteroids increase calcium excretion.

Administration of live virus vaccines, including smallpox, is contraindicated in individuals receiving immunosuppressive doses of corticosteroids. If inactivated viral or bacterial vaccines are administered to individuals receiving immunosuppressive doses of corticosteroids, the expected serum antibody response may not be obtained.

If RESPIHALER DECADRON Phosphate is indicated in patients with latent tuberculosis or tuberculin reactivity, close observation is necessary as reactivation of the disease may occur. During prolonged therapy with RESPIHALER DECADRON Phosphate, these patients should receive chemoprophylaxis.

Precautions

RESPIHALER DECADRON Phosphate is *not* indicated for relief of the occasional mild and isolated attack of asthma which is readily responsive to the immediate, though short-lived, action of epinephrine, isoproterenol, aminophylline, etc. Nor should it be employed for the treatment of severe status asthmaticus where intensive measures are required. RESPIHALER DECADRON should be considered only for the following classes of patients: patients not on corticosteroid therapy who have not responded adequately to other treatment; patients already on systemic corticosteroid therapy—in an attempt to reduce or eliminate systemic administration.

Although systemic absorption is low when RESPIHALER DECADRON Phosphate is used in the recommended dosage, adrenal suppression may occur. In addition, other systemic effects of steroid administration must be considered as a possibility.

Following prolonged therapy, withdrawal of corticosteroids may result in symptoms of the corticosteroid withdrawal syndrome including fever, myalgia, arthralgia, and malaise. This may occur in patients even without evidence of adrenal insufficiency.

There is an enhanced effect of dexamethasone in patients with hypothyroidism and in those with cirrhosis.

RESPIHALER DECADRON Phosphate should be used cautiously in patients with ocular herpes simplex for fear of corneal perforation.

The lowest possible dose of RESPIHALER DECADRON Phosphate should be used to control the condition under treatment, and when reduction in dosage is possible, the reduction must be gradual.

Psychic derangements may appear when dexamethasone is used, ranging from euphoria, insomnia, mood swings, personality changes, and severe depression, to frank psychotic manifestations. Also, existing emotional instability or psychotic tendencies may be aggravated.

Aspirin should be used cautiously in conjunction with RESPIHALER DECADRON Phosphate in hypoprothrombinemia.

RESPIHALER DECADRON Phosphate should be used with caution in nonspecific ulcerative colitis, if there is a probability of impending perforation, abscess or other pyogenic infection; also in diverticulitis; fresh intestinal anastomoses; active or latent peptic ulcer; renal insufficiency; hypertension; osteoporosis; and myasthenia gravis. Signs of peritoneal irritation following gastrointestinal perforation in patients receiving large doses of corticosteroids may be minimal or absent. Fat embolism has been reported as a possible complication of hypercortisonism.

Growth and development of infants and children on prolonged therapy with RESPIHALER DECADRON Phosphate should be carefully followed.

Dexamethasone may increase or decrease motility and number of spermatozoa in some patients.

Phenytoin, phenobarbital, ephedrine and rifampin may enhance the metabolic clearance of dexamethasone, resulting in decreased blood levels and lessened physiologic activity, thus requiring adjustment in dexamethasone dosage.

The prothrombin time should be checked frequently in patients who are receiving RESPIHALER DECADRON Phosphate and coumarin anticoagulants at the same time because of reports that corticosteroids have altered the response to these anticoagulants. Studies have shown that the usual effect produced by adding corticosteroids is inhibition of response to coumarins, although there have been some conflicting reports of potentiation, not substantiated by studies.

When RESPIHALER DECADRON Phosphate is used concomitantly with potassium-depleting diuretics, patients should be observed closely for development of hypokalemia.

Since the contents of RESPIHALER DECADRON Phosphate are under pressure, the container should not be broken, stored in extreme heat, or incinerated. It should be stored at a temperature below 120°F.

Adverse Reactions

Side effects which may occur in patients treated with RESPIHALER DECADRON Phosphate include throat irritation, hoarseness, coughing, and laryngeal and pharyngeal fungal infections.

Patients should be observed for the hormonal effects described below:

Fluid and Electrolyte Disturbances
Sodium retention
Fluid retention
Congestive heart failure in susceptible patients
Potassium loss
Hypokalemic alkalosis
Hypertension

Musculoskeletal
Muscle weakness
Steroid myopathy
Loss of muscle mass
Osteoporosis
Vertebral compression fractures
Aseptic necrosis of femoral and humeral heads
Pathologic fracture of long bones
Tendon rupture

Gastrointestinal
Peptic ulcer with possible subsequent perforation and hemorrhage
Perforation of the small and large bowel, particularly in patients with inflammatory bowel disease
Pancreatitis
Abdominal distention
Ulcerative esophagitis

Dermatologic
Impaired wound healing
Thin fragile skin
Petechiae and ecchymoses
Erythema
Increased sweating
May suppress reactions to skin tests
Other cutaneous reactions, such as allergic dermatitis, urticaria, angioneurotic edema

Neurologic
Convulsions
Increased intracranial pressure with papilledema (pseudotumor cerebri) usually after treatment
Vertigo
Headache

Endocrine
Menstrual irregularities
Development of cushingoid state
Suppression of growth in children
Secondary adrenocortical and pituitary unresponsiveness, particularly in times of stress, as in trauma, surgery, or illness
Decreased carbohydrate tolerance
Manifestations of latent diabetes mellitus
Increased requirements for insulin or oral hypoglycemic agents in diabetics

Ophthalmic
Posterior subcapsular cataracts
Increased intraocular pressure
Glaucoma
Exophthalmos

Metabolic
Negative nitrogen balance due to protein catabolism

Other
Hypersensitivity
Thromboembolism
Weight gain
Increased appetite
Nausea
Malaise

Dosage and Administration

Recommended *initial dosage:*
Adults —3 inhalations 3 or 4 times per day.
Children —2 inhalations 3 or 4 times per day.

Continued on next page

Information on the Merck Sharp & Dohme products listed on these pages is the full prescribing information from package circulars in use October 31, 1982.

Merck Sharp & Dohme—Cont.

Maximum dosage:
Adults —3 inhalations *per dose;* 12 inhalations *per day.*
Children —2 inhalations *per dose;* 8 inhalations *per day.*
When a favorable response is attained, the dose may be gradually reduced. In patients on systemic corticosteroids, it is recommended that systemic therapy be reduced or eliminated before reduction of RESPIHALER dosage is begun. Gradual reduction of systemic corticosteroid therapy must be emphasized to avoid withdrawal symptoms.

How Supplied

No. 7626X—RESPIHALER DECADRON Phosphate, aerosol for oral inhalation, is supplied as follows: **NDC** 0006-7626-13 in a pressurized container, and includes a plastic adapter.
No. 7640—Refill Unit RESPIHALER DECADRON Phosphate is supplied as follows: **NDC** 0006-7640-13 in a pressurized container.
A.H.F.S. Category: 84:06
DC 6055714 Issued August 1981

DECADRON® Phosphate TURBINAIRE® ℞
(dexamethasone sodium phosphate, MSD), U.S.P.

Description

TURBINAIRE® DECADRON® Phosphate (Dexamethasone Sodium Phosphate, MSD) is an aerosol for intranasal application. The inactive ingredients are fluorochlorohydrocarbons as propellants and alcohol 2%. One cartridge delivers an amount sufficient to ensure delivery of 170 metered sprays, each containing dexamethasone sodium phosphate equivalent to approximately 0.1 mg dexamethasone phosphate or to approximately 0.084 mg dexamethasone. Twelve sprays deliver a theoretical maximum of 1.0 mg dexamethasone.
Dexamethasone sodium phosphate, a synthetic adrenocortical steroid, is a white or slightly yellow, crystalline powder. It is freely soluble in water and is exceedingly hygroscopic. The molecular weight is 516.41. It is designated chemically as 9-fluoro-11β, 17-dihydroxy-16α-methyl-21-(phosphonooxy) pregna-1, 4-diene-3, 20-dione disodium salt. The empirical formula is $C_{22}H_{28}FNa_2O_8P$.

Action

Inhibition of inflammatory response to inciting agents of mechanical, chemical or immunological nature.

Indications

Allergic or inflammatory nasal conditions, and nasal polyps (excluding polyps originating within the sinuses).

Contraindications

Systemic fungal infections.
Hypersensitivity to components.
Tuberculous, viral and fungal nasal conditions, ocular herpes simplex.

Warnings

In patients on therapy with TURBINAIRE DECADRON Phosphate subjected to unusual stress, increased dosage of rapidly acting corticosteroids before, during, and after the stressful situation is indicated.
Drug-induced secondary adrenocortical insufficiency may result from too rapid withdrawal of corticosteroids and may be minimized by gradual reduction of dosage. This type of relative insufficiency may persist for months after discontinuation of therapy; therefore, in any situation of stress occurring during that period, hormone therapy should be reinstituted. If the patient is receiving steroids already, dosage may have to be increased. Since mineralocorticoid secretion may be impaired, salt and/or a mineralocorticoid should be administered concurrently.
Dexamethasone may mask some signs of infection, and new infections may appear during its use. There may be decreased resistance and inability to localize infection when corticosteroids are used. Therefore, patients with bacterial infections should also be given appropriate antibiotic therapy if TURBINAIRE DECADRON Phosphate is used. Moreover, dexamethasone may affect the nitroblue-tetrazolium test for bacterial infection and produce false negative results.
Corticosteroids may activate latent amebiasis. Therefore, it is recommended that latent or active amebiasis be ruled out before initiating corticosteroid therapy in any patient who has spent time in the tropics or any patient with unexplained diarrhea.
Prolonged use of TURBINAIRE DECADRON Phosphate may produce posterior subcapsular cataracts, glaucoma with possible damage to the optic nerves, and may enhance the establishment of secondary ocular infections due to fungi or viruses.
Usage in pregnancy: Since adequate human reproduction studies have not been done with TURBINAIRE DECADRON Phosphate, use of this drug in pregnancy or in women of childbearing potential requires that the anticipated benefits be weighed against the possible hazards to the mother and embryo or fetus. Infants born of mothers who have received substantial doses of dexamethasone during pregnancy, should be carefully observed for signs of hypoadrenalism.
Dexamethasone appears in breast milk and could suppress growth, interfere with endogenous corticosteroid production, or cause other unwanted effects. Mothers taking pharmacologic doses of dexamethasone should be advised not to nurse.
Average and large doses of hydrocortisone or cortisone can cause elevation of blood pressure, salt and water retention, and increased excretion of potassium. These effects are less likely to occur with the synthetic derivatives and with TURBINAIRE DECADRON Phosphate, except when used in large doses. Dietary salt restriction and potassium supplementation may be necessary. All corticosteroids increase calcium excretion.
Administration of live virus vaccines, including smallpox, is contraindicated in individuals receiving immunosuppressive doses of corticosteroids. If inactivated viral or bacterial vaccines are administered to individuals receiving immunosuppressive doses of corticosteroids, the expected serum antibody response may not be obtained.
If TURBINAIRE DECADRON Phosphate is indicated in patients with latent tuberculosis or tuberculin reactivity, close observation is necessary as reactivation of the disease may occur. During prolonged therapy with TURBINAIRE DECADRON Phosphate, these patients should receive chemoprophylaxis.

Precautions

During local corticosteroid therapy, the possibility of pharyngeal candidiasis should be kept in mind.
Although systemic absorption is low when TURBINAIRE DECADRON Phosphate is used in the recommended dosage, adrenal suppression may occur. In addition, other systemic effects of steroid administration must be considered as a possibility.
Following prolonged therapy, withdrawal of corticosteroids may result in symptoms of the corticosteroid withdrawal syndrome including fever, myalgia, arthralgia, and malaise. This may occur in patients even without evidence of adrenal insufficiency. Replacement of systemic steroid with TURBINAIRE DECADRON Phosphate should be gradual and carefully monitored by the physician.
There is an enhanced effect of dexamethasone in patients with hypothyroidism and in those with cirrhosis.
TURBINAIRE DECADRON Phosphate should be used cautiously in patients with ocular herpes simplex for fear of corneal perforation.
The lowest possible dose of TURBINAIRE DECADRON Phosphate should be used to control the condition under treatment, and when reduction in dosage is possible, the reduction must be gradual. If beneficial effect is not evident within 7 days after initiation of therapy, the patient should be re-evaluated.
Psychic derangements may appear when dexamethasone is used, ranging from euphoria, insomnia, mood swings, personality changes, and severe depression, to frank psychotic manifestations. Also, existing emotional instability or psychotic tendencies may be aggravated.
Aspirin should be used cautiously in conjunction with TURBINAIRE DECADRON Phosphate in hypoprothrombinemia.
TURBINAIRE DECADRON Phosphate should be used with caution in patients with nonspecific ulcerative colitis, if there is a probability of impending perforation, abscess or other pyogenic infection; also in diverticulitis; fresh intestinal anastomoses; active or latent peptic ulcer; renal insufficiency; hypertension; osteoporosis; and myasthenia gravis. Signs of peritoneal irritation following gastrointestinal perforation in patients receiving large doses of corticosteroids may be minimal or absent. Fat embolism has been reported as a possible complication of hypercortisonism.
Because clinical studies have not been done, the use of this product in children under the age of 6 years is not recommended. Growth and development of children 6 years of age or older on prolonged therapy with TURBINAIRE DECADRON Phosphate should be carefully followed.
Dexamethasone may increase or decrease motility and number of spermatozoa in some patients.
Phenytoin, phenobarbital, ephedrine and rifampin may enhance the metabolic clearance of dexamethasone, resulting in decreased blood levels and lessened physiologic activity, thus requiring adjustment in dexamethasone dosage.
The prothrombin time should be checked frequently in patients who are receiving TURBINAIRE DECADRON Phosphate and coumarin anticoagulants at the same time because of reports that corticosteroids have altered the response to these anticoagulants. Studies have shown that the usual effect produced by adding corticosteroids is inhibition of response to coumarins, although there have been some conflicting reports of potentiation, not substantiated by studies.
When TURBINAIRE DECADRON Phosphate is used concomitantly with potassium-depleting diuretics, patients should be observed closely for development of hypokalemia.
Since the contents of TURBINAIRE DECADRON Phosphate are under pressure, the container should not be broken, stored in extreme heat, or incinerated. It should be stored at a temperature below 120°F.

Adverse Reactions

Nasal irritation and dryness are the most common adverse reactions. The following have been reported: headache, lightheadedness, urticaria, nausea, epistaxis, rebound congestion, bronchial asthma, perforation of the nasal septum, and anosmia. Signs of adrenal hy-

percorticism may occur in some patients, especially with overdosage.
Systemic effects from therapy with TURBINAIRE DECADRON Phosphate are less likely to occur than with oral or parenteral corticosteroid therapy because of a lower total dose administered. Nevertheless, patients should be observed for the hormonal effects described below because of absorption of dexamethasone from the nasal mucosa.

Fluid and Electrolyte Disturbances
Sodium retention
Fluid retention
Congestive heart failure in susceptible patients
Potassium loss
Hypokalemic alkalosis
Hypertension

Musculoskeletal
Muscle weakness
Steroid myopathy
Loss of muscle mass
Osteoporosis
Vertebral compression fractures
Aseptic necrosis of femoral and humeral heads
Pathologic fracture of long bones
Tendon rupture

Gastrointestinal
Peptic ulcer with possible subsequent perforation and hemorrhage
Perforation of the small and large bowel, particularly in patients with inflammatory bowel disease
Pancreatitis
Abdominal distention
Ulcerative esophagitis

Dematologic
Impaired wound healing
Thin fragile skin
Petechiae and ecchymoses
Erythema
Increased sweating
May suppress reactions to skin tests
Other cutaneous reactions, such as allergic dermatitis, urticaria, angioneurotic edema.

Neurologic
Convulsions
Increased intracranial pressure with papilledema (pseudotumor cerebri) usually after treatment
Vertigo
Headache

Endocrine
Menstrual irregularities
Development of cushingoid state
Suppression of growth in children
Secondary adrenocortical and pituitary unresponsiveness, particularly in times of stress, as in trauma, surgery, or illness
Decreased carbohydrate tolerance
Manifestations of latent diabetes mellitus
Increased requirements for insulin or oral hypoglycemic agents in diabetics

Ophthalmic
Posterior subcapsular cataracts
Increased intraocular pressure
Glaucoma
Exophthalmos

Metabolic
Negative nitrogen balance due to protein catabolism

Other
Hypersensitivity
Thromboembolism
Weight gain
Increased appetite
Nausea
Malaise

Dosage and Administration

DO NOT EXCEED THE RECOMMENDED DOSAGE.
The usual initial dosage of TURBINAIRE DECADRON Phosphate is:
Adults—2 sprays in each nostril 2 or 3 times a day.
Children (6 to 12 years of age)—1 or 2 sprays in each nostril 2 times a day depending on age.
See accompanying instructions on the proper use of TURBINAIRE.
When improvement occurs the dosage should be gradually reduced. Some patients will be symptom-free on one spray in each nostril 2 times a day. The maximum daily dosage for adults is 12 sprays, and for children, 8 sprays. Therapy should be discontinued as soon as feasible. It may be reinstituted if recurrence of symptoms occurs.

How Supplied

No. 7634—TURBINAIRE DECADRON Phosphate, aerosol for intranasal application, is supplied as follows: **NDC** 0006-7634-13 in a pressurized container and includes a plastic adapter.
(6505-00-885-6302, 12.6 Grams, 170 Metered Doses)
No. 7642—Refill unit for TURBINAIRE DECADRON Phosphate aerosol for intranasal application is supplied as follows: **NDC** 0006-7642-13 in a pressurized container.
A.H.F.S. Category: 52:08
DC 6006419 Issued August 1981

DECADRON-LA® Suspension ℞
(dexamethasone acetate, MSD), U.S.P.

NOT FOR INTRAVENOUS USE

Description

Dexamethasone acetate, a synthetic adrenocortical steroid, is a white to practically white, odorless powder. It is a practically insoluble ester of dexamethasone.
Dexamethasone acetate is present in DECADRON-LA® (Dexamethasone Acetate, MSD) suspension as the monohydrate, with the empirical formula, $C_{24}H_{31}FO_6 \cdot H_2O$, and molecular weight, 452.52. Dexamethasone acetate is designated chemically as 21-(acetyloxy)-9-fluoro-11β, 17-dihydroxy-16α-methylpregna-1,4-diene-3,20-dione.
DECADRON-LA suspension is a sterile white suspension (pH 5.0 to 7.5) that settles on standing, but is easily resuspended by mild shaking. Each milliliter contains dexamethasone acetate equivalent to 8 mg dexamethasone. Inactive ingredients per ml: 6.67 mg sodium chloride; 5 mg creatinine; 0.5 mg disodium edetate; 5 mg sodium carboxymethylcellulose; 0.75 mg polysorbate 80; sodium hydroxide to adjust pH; and Water for Injection, q.s. 1 ml, with 9 mg benzyl alcohol, and 1 mg sodium bisulfite added as preservatives.

Actions

DECADRON-LA suspension is a long-acting, repository adrenocorticosteroid preparation with a prompt onset of action. It is suitable for intramuscular or local injection, but not when an immediate effect of short duration is desired.
Naturally occurring glucocorticoids (hydrocortisone and cortisone), which also have salt-retaining properties, are used as replacement therapy in adrenocortical deficiency states. Their synthetic analogs, including dexamethasone, are primarily used for their potent anti-inflammatory effects in disorders of many organ systems.
Glucocorticoids cause profound and varied metabolic effects. In addition, they modify the body's immune responses to diverse stimuli.
At equipotent anti-inflammatory doses, dexamethasone almost completely lacks the sodium-retaining property of hydrocortisone.

Indications

A. By intramuscular injection when oral therapy is not feasible:

1. *Endocrine disorders*
Congenital adrenal hyperplasia
Nonsuppurative thyroiditis
Hypercalcemia associated with cancer

2. *Rheumatic disorders*
As adjunctive therapy for short-term administration (to tide the patient over an acute episode or exacerbation) in:
Post-traumatic osteoarthritis
Synovitis of osteoarthritis
Rheumatoid arthritis, including juvenile rheumatoid arthritis (selected cases may require low-dose maintenance therapy)
Acute and subacute bursitis
Epicondylitis
Acute nonspecific tenosynovitis
Acute gouty arthritis
Psoriatic arthritis
Ankylosing spondylitis

3. *Collagen diseases*
During an exacerbation or as maintenance therapy in selected cases of:
Systemic lupus erythematosus
Acute rheumatic carditis

4. *Dermatologic diseases*
Pemphigus
Severe erythema multiforme (Stevens-Johnson syndrome)
Exfoliative dermatitis
Bullous dermatitis herpetiformis
Severe seborrheic dermatitis
Severe psoriasis
Mycosis fungoides

5. *Allergic states*
Control of severe or incapacitating allergic conditions intractable to adequate trials of conventional treatment in:
Bronchial asthma
Contact dermatitis
Atopic dermatitis
Serum sickness
Seasonal or perennial allergic rhinitis
Drug hypersensitivity reactions
Urticarial transfusion reactions

6. *Ophthalmic diseases*
Severe acute and chronic allergic and inflammatory processes involving the eye, such as:
Herpes zoster ophthalmicus
Iritis, Iridocyclitis
Chorioretinitis
Diffuse posterior uveitis and choroiditis
Optic neuritis
Sympathetic ophthalmia
Anterior segment inflammation
Allergic conjunctivitis
Keratitis
Allergic corneal marginal ulcers

7. *Gastrointestinal diseases*
To tide the patient over a critical period of the disease in:
Ulcerative colitis (Systemic therapy)
Regional enteritis (Systemic therapy)

8. *Respiratory diseases*
Symptomatic sarcoidosis
Berylliosis
Loeffler's syndrome not manageable by other means
Aspiration pneumonitis

9. *Hematologic disorders*
Acquired (autoimmune) hemolytic anemia
Secondary thrombocytopenia in adults
Erythroblastopenia (RBC anemia)
Congenital (erythroid) hypoplastic anemia

10. *Neoplastic diseases*
For palliative management of:
Leukemias and lymphomas in adults

Continued on next page

Information on the Merck Sharp & Dohme products listed on these pages is the full prescribing information from package circulars in use October 31, 1982.

Merck Sharp & Dohme—Cont.

Acute leukemia of childhood
11. *Edematous states*
To induce diuresis or remission of proteinuria in the nephrotic syndrome, without uremia, of the idiopathic type, or that due to lupus erythematosus
12. *Miscellaneous*
Trichinosis with neurologic or myocardial involvement
B. By intra-articular or soft tissue injection as adjunctive therapy for short-term administration (to tide the patient over an acute episode or exacerbation) in:
Synovitis of osteoarthritis
Rheumatoid arthritis
Acute and subacute bursitis
Acute gouty arthritis
Epicondylitis
Acute nonspecific tenosynovitis
Post-traumatic osteoarthritis
C. By intralesional injection in:
Keloids
Localized hypertrophic, infiltrated, inflammatory lesions of: lichen planus, psoriatic plaques, granuloma annulare, and lichen simplex chronicus (neurodermatitis)
Discoid lupus erythematosus
Necrobiosis lipoidica diabeticorum
Alopecia areata
May also be useful in cystic tumors of an aponeurosis or tendon (ganglia)

Contraindications

Systemic fungal infections
Hypersensitivity to any component of this product

Warnings

DO NOT INJECT INTRAVENOUSLY.
In patients on corticosteroid therapy subjected to any unusual stress, increased dosage of rapidly acting corticosteroids before, during, and after the stressful situation is indicated.
Drug-induced secondary adrenocortical insufficiency may result from too rapid withdrawal of corticosteroids and may be minimized by gradual reduction of dosage. This type of relative insufficiency may persist for months after discontinuation of therapy; therefore, in any situation of stress occurring during that period, hormone therapy should be reinstituted. If the patient is receiving steroids already, dosage may have to be increased. Since mineralocorticoid secretion may be impaired, salt and/or a mineralocorticoid should be administered concurrently.
Corticosteroids may mask some signs of infection, and new infections may appear during their use. There may be decreased resistance and inability to localize infection when corticosteroids are used. Moreover, corticosteroids may affect the nitroblue-tetrazolium test for bacterial infection and produce false negative results.
Corticosteroids may activate latent amebiasis. Therefore, it is recommended that latent or active amebiasis be ruled out before initiating corticosteroid therapy in any patient who has spent time in the tropics or any patient with unexplained diarrhea.
Prolonged use of corticosteroids may produce posterior subcapsular cataracts, glaucoma with possible damage to the optic nerves, and may enhance the establishment of secondary ocular infections due to fungi or viruses.
Usage in pregnancy. Since adequate human reproduction studies have not been done with corticosteroids, use of these drugs in pregnancy or in women of childbearing potential requires that the anticipated benefits be weighed against the possible hazards to the mother and embryo or fetus. Infants born of mothers who have received substantial doses of corticosteroids during pregnancy should be carefully observed for signs of hypoadrenalism.
Corticosteroids appear in breast milk and could suppress growth, interfere with endogenous corticosteroid production, or cause other unwanted effects. Mothers taking pharmacologic doses of corticosteroids should be advised not to nurse.
Average and large doses of cortisone or hydrocortisone can cause elevation of blood pressure, salt and water retention, and increased excretion of potassium. These effects are less likely to occur with the synthetic derivatives except when used in large doses. Dietary salt restriction and potassium supplementation may be necessary. All corticosteroids increase calcium excretion.
Administration of live virus vaccines, including smallpox, is contraindicated in individuals receiving immunosuppressive doses of corticosteroids. If inactivated viral or bacterial vaccines are administered to individuals receiving immunosuppressive doses of corticosteroids, the expected serum antibody response may not be obtained.
If corticosteroids are indicated in patients with latent tuberculosis or tuberculin reactivity, close observation is necessary as reactivation of the disease may occur. During prolonged corticosteroid therapy, these patients should receive chemoprophylaxis.
Because rare instances of anaphylactoid reactions have occurred in patients receiving parenteral corticosteroid therapy, appropriate precautionary measures should be taken prior to administration, especially when the patient has a history of allergy to any drug.
Repository adrenocorticosteroid preparations may cause atrophy at the site of injection. To minimize the likelihood and/or severity of atrophy, do not inject subcutaneously, avoid injection into the deltoid muscle, and avoid repeated intramuscular injections into the same site if possible.
Dosage in children under 12 has not been established.

Precautions

DECADRON-LA suspension is not recommended as initial therapy in acute, life-threatening situations.
This product, like many other steroid formulations, is sensitive to heat. Therefore, it should not be autoclaved when it is desirable to sterilize the exterior of the vial.
Following prolonged therapy, withdrawal of corticosteroids may result in symptoms of the corticosteroid withdrawal syndrome including fever, myalgia, arthralgia, and malaise. This may occur in patients even without evidence of adrenal insufficiency.
There is an enhanced effect of corticosteroids in patients with hypothyroidism and in those with cirrhosis.
Corticosteroids should be used cautiously in patients with ocular herpes simplex for fear of corneal perforation.
Psychic derangements may appear when corticosteroids are used, ranging from euphoria, insomnia, mood swings, personality changes, and severe depression to frank psychotic manifestations. Also, existing emotional instability or psychotic tendencies may be aggravated by corticosteroids.
Aspirin should be used cautiously in conjunction with corticosteroids in hypoprothrombinemia.
Steroids should be used with caution in nonspecific ulcerative colitis, if there is a probability of impending perforation, abscess, or other pyogenic infection, also in diverticulitis, fresh intestinal anastomoses, active or latent peptic ulcer, renal insufficiency, hypertension, osteoporosis, and myasthenia gravis. Signs of peritoneal irritation following gastrointestinal perforation in patients receiving large doses of corticosteroids may be minimal or absent. Fat embolism has been reported as a possible complication of hypercortisonism.
When large doses are given, some authorities advise that antacids be administered between meals to help to prevent peptic ulcer.
Growth and development of infants and children on prolonged corticosteroid therapy should be carefully followed.
Steroids may increase or decrease motility and number of spermatozoa in some patients.
Phenytoin, phenobarbital, ephedrine, and rifampin may enhance the metabolic clearance of corticosteroids, resulting in decreased blood levels and lessened physiologic activity, thus requiring adjustment in corticosteroid dosage.
The prothrombin time should be checked frequently in patients who are receiving corticosteroids and coumarin anticoagulants at the same time because of reports that corticosteroids have altered the response to these anticoagulants. Studies have shown that the usual effect produced by adding corticosteroids is inhibition of response to coumarins, although there have been some conflicting reports of potentiation not substantiated by studies.
When corticosteroids are administered concomitantly with potassium-depleting diuretics, patients should be observed closely for development of hypokalemia.
Intra-articular injection of a corticosteroid may produce systemic as well as local effects.
Appropriate examination of any joint fluid present is necessary to exclude a septic process.
A marked increase in pain accompanied by local swelling, further restriction of joint motion, fever, and malaise is suggestive of septic arthritis. If this complication occurs and the diagnosis of sepsis is confirmed, appropriate antimicrobial therapy should be instituted.
Injection of a steroid into an infected site is to be avoided.
Corticosteroids should not be injected into unstable joints.
Patients should be impressed strongly with the importance of not overusing joints in which symptomatic benefit has been obtained as long as the inflammatory process remains active.
Frequent intra-articular injection may result in damage to joint tissues.

Adverse Reactions

Fluid and electrolyte disturbances
Sodium retention
Fluid retention
Congestive heart failure in susceptible patients
Potassium loss
Hypokalemic alkalosis
Hypertension
Musculoskeletal
Muscle weakness
Steroid myopathy
Loss of muscle mass
Osteoporosis
Vertebral compression fractures
Aseptic necrosis of femoral and humeral heads
Pathologic fracture of long bones
Tendon rupture
Gastrointestinal
Peptic ulcer with possible subsequent perforation and hemorrhage
Perforation of the small and large bowel, particularly in patients with inflammatory bowel disease
Pancreatitis
Abdominal distention
Ulcerative esophagitis
Dermatologic
Impaired wound healing
Thin fragile skin
Petechiae and ecchymoses
Erythema
Increased sweating
May suppress reactions to skin tests
Other cutaneous reactions, such as allergic dermatitis, urticaria, angioneurotic edema

Neurologic
Convulsions
Increased intracranial pressure with papilledema (pseudotumor cerebri) usually after treatment
Vertigo
Headache
Endocrine
Menstrual irregularities
Development of cushingoid state
Suppression of growth in children
Secondary adrenocortical and pituitary unresponsiveness, particularly in times of stress, as in trauma, surgery, or illness
Decreased carbohydrate tolerance
Manifestations of latent diabetes mellitus
Increased requirements for insulin or oral hypoglycemic agents in diabetics
Ophthalmic
Posterior subcapsular cataracts
Increased intraocular pressure
Glaucoma
Exophthalmos
Metabolic
Negative nitrogen balance due to protein catabolism
Other
Anaphylactoid or hypersensitivity reactions
Thromboembolism
Weight gain
Increased appetite
Nausea
Malaise

The following *additional* adverse reactions are related to parenteral corticosteroid therapy:
Rare instances of blindness associated with intralesional therapy around the face and head
Hyperpigmentation or hypopigmentation
Subcutaneous and cutaneous atrophy
Sterile abscess
Postinjection flare (following intra-articular use)
Charcot-like arthropathy
Scarring
Induration
Inflammation
Paresthesia
Delayed pain or soreness
Muscle twitching, ataxia, hiccups, and nystagmus have been reported in low incidence after injection of DECADRON-LA suspension.

Dosage and Administration

For intramuscular, intralesional, intra-articular, and soft tissue injection.
Dosage Requirements Are Variable and Must Be Individualized on the Basis of the Disease and the Response of the Patient.
Dosage in children under 12 has not been established.
Intramuscular Injection
Dosage ranges from 1 to 2 ml, equivalent to 8 to 16 mg of dexamethasone. If further treatment is needed, dosage may be repeated at intervals of 1 to 3 weeks.
Intralesional Injection
The usual dose is 0.1 to 0.2 ml, equivalent to 0.8 to 1.6 mg of dexamethasone, per injection site.
Intra-articular and Soft Tissue Injection
The dose varies, depending on the location and the severity of inflammation. The usual dose is 0.5 to 2 ml, equivalent to 4 to 16 mg of dexamethasone. If further treatment is needed, dosage may be repeated at intervals of 1 to 3 weeks. Frequent intra-articular injection may result in damage to joint tissues.

How Supplied

No. 7644—Suspension DECADRON-LA, 8 mg dexamethasone equivalent per ml, is a sterile white suspension, and is supplied as follows:
NDC 0006-7644-01 in 1 ml vials
NDC 0006-7644-03 in 5 ml vials.

A.H.F.S. Category: 68:04
DC 6626711 Issued August 1981

DECASPRAY® Topical Aerosol (dexamethasone, MSD), U.S.P. ℞

Description

Topical Aerosol DECASPRAY® (Dexamethasone, MSD) is a topical steroid preparation, each 25 g of which contains 10 mg of dexamethasone. The inactive ingredients are isopropyl myristate, and isobutane. Each second of spray dispenses approximately 0.075 mg of dexamethasone.

Actions

Topical steroids are primarily effective because of their anti-inflammatory, antipruritic and vasoconstrictive actions.

Indications

DECASPRAY Topical Aerosol is indicated for relief of the inflammatory manifestations of corticosteroid-responsive dermatoses.

Contraindications

Topical steroids are contraindicated in those patients with a history of hypersensitivity to any of the components of the preparation.
Topical steroids are contraindicated in vaccinia and varicella; herpes simplex; in fungal infections; when tuberculosis of the skin is present; and in the ear if the drum is perforated.

Warnings

Avoid spraying in eyes or nose. Contents under pressure. Do not puncture or burn. Keep out of reach of children. Use only as directed. Intentional misuse by deliberately concentrating and inhaling the contents can be harmful or fatal.

Precautions

If irritation develops, the product should be discontinued and appropriate therapy instituted.
In the presence of an infection, the use of an appropriate antifungal or antibacterial agent should be instituted. If a favorable response does not occur promptly, the corticosteroid should be discontinued until the infection has been adequately controlled.
If extensive areas are treated or if the occlusive technique is used, there will be increased systemic absorption of the corticosteroid and suitable precautions should be taken, particularly in children and infants.
Although topical steroids have not been reported to have an adverse effect on human pregnancy, the safety of their uses in pregnant women has not absolutely been established. In laboratory animals, increases in incidence of fetal abnormalities have been associated with exposure of gestating females to topical corticosteroids, in some cases at rather low dosage levels. Therefore, drugs of this class should not be used extensively on pregnant patients, in large amounts, or for prolonged periods of time.
The product is not for ophthalmic use.
A few individuals may be sensitive to one or more of the components of this product. If any reaction indicating sensitivity is observed, discontinue use.
Generally, occlusive dressings should not be used on weeping or exudative lesions.
If the occlusive dressing technique is employed, caution should be exercised with regard to the use of plastic films which are often flammable and may pose a suffocation hazard for children.
If occlusive dressing therapy is used, inspect lesions between dressings for development of infection. If infection develops, the technique should be discontinued and appropriate antimicrobial therapy instituted.
When large areas of the body are covered with an occlusive dressing, thermal homeostasis may be impaired. If elevation of body temperature occurs, use of the occlusive dressing should be discontinued.
CAUTION: Flammable. Do not use around open flame or while smoking.

Adverse Reactions

The following local adverse reactions have been reported with topical corticosteroids: burning, itching, irritation, dryness, folliculitis, hypertrichosis, acneiform eruptions, hypopigmentation, perioral dermatitis, allergic contact dermatitis, maceration of the skin, secondary infection, skin atrophy, striae, and miliaria.
Contact sensitivity to a particular dressing or adhesive may occur occasionally.

Dosage and Administration

Patients should be instructed in the correct way to use DECASPRAY. The preparation is readily applied, even on hairy areas. It does not have to be rubbed into the skin.
Optimal effects will be obtained with DECASPRAY when these directions are followed:

1. Keep the affected area clean to reduce the possibility of infection.
2. Shake the container *gently* once or twice each time before using. Hold it about six inches from the area to be treated. Effective medication may be obtained with the container held either upright or inverted, since it is fitted with a special valve that dispenses approximately the same dosage in either position.
3. Spray each four inch square of affected area for one or two seconds three or four times a day, depending on the nature of the condition and the response to therapy.
4. When a favorable response is obtained, reduce dosage gradually and eventually discontinue.

How Supplied

No. 7623X—DECASPRAY is supplied as follows:
NDC 0006-7623-25 in a 25 g pressurized container.

A.H.F.S. Category: 84:06
DC 6005317 Issued January 1980

DEMSER® Capsules (metyrosine, MSD) ℞

Description

DEMSER® (Metyrosine, MSD) is (—)-α-methyl-*L*-tyrosine.
Metyrosine [(—)-α-methyl-*L*-tyrosine](α-MPT) is a white, crystalline compound of molecular weight 195. It is very slightly soluble in water, acetone, and methanol, and insoluble in chloroform and benzene. It is soluble in acidic aqueous solutions. It is also soluble in alkaline aqueous solutions, but is subject to oxidative degradation under these conditions.
Each capsule of DEMSER contains 250 mg metyrosine.

Clinical Pharmacology

DEMSER inhibits tyrosine hydroxylase, which catalyzes the first transformation in catecholamine biosynthesis, i.e., the conversion of tyrosine to dihydroxyphenylalanine (DOPA). Because the first step is also the rate-limiting

Continued on next page

Information on the Merck Sharp & Dohme products listed on these pages is the full prescribing information from package circulars in use October 31, 1982.

Merck Sharp & Dohme—Cont.

step, blockade of tyrosine hydroxylase activity results in decreased endogenous levels of catecholamines, usually measured as decreased urinary excretion of catecholamines and their metabolites.

In patients with pheochromocytoma, who produce excessive amounts of norepinephrine and epinephrine, administration of one to four grams of DEMSER per day has reduced catecholamine biosynthesis from about 35 to 80 percent as measured by the total excretion of catecholamines and their metabolites (metanephrine and vanillylmandelic acid). The maximum biochemical effect usually occurs within two to three days, and the urinary concentration of catecholamines and their metabolites usually returns to pretreatment levels within three to four days after DEMSER is discontinued. In some patients the total excretion of catecholamines and catecholamine metabolites may be lowered to normal or near normal levels (less than 10 mg/24 hours). In most patients the duration of treatment has been two to eight weeks, but several patients have received DEMSER for periods of one to 10 years.

Most patients with pheochromocytoma treated with DEMSER experience decreased frequency and severity of hypertensive attacks with their associated headache, nausea, sweating, and tachycardia. In patients who respond, blood pressure decreases progressively during the first two days of therapy with DEMSER; after withdrawal, blood pressure usually increases gradually to pretreatment values within two to three days.

Metyrosine is well absorbed from the gastrointestinal tract in animals and in man. In the dog, about 70 percent of an oral dose was recovered unchanged in the urine within 24 hours after administration. In man, from 53 to 88 percent (mean 69 percent) was recovered in the urine as unchanged drug following maintenance oral dosages of 600 to 4000 mg/24 hours. A very small percentage of administered drug was recovered as catechol metabolites, consisting of alpha-methyldopa, alpha-methyldopamine, and alpha-methylnorepinephrine. Although it is estimated that the sum of all catechol metabolites of metyrosine accounts for less than 0.5 percent of the administered dose, this is sufficient to interfere with accurate determination of urinary catecholamines in normal individuals. The catechol metabolites probably are not present in sufficient amounts to contribute to the biochemical effects of metyrosine.

For further information refer to: Sjoerdsma, A.; Engelman, K.; Waldman, T. A.; Cooperman, L. H.; Hammond, W. G.: Pheochromocytoma: Current concepts of diagnosis and treatment, Ann. Intern. Med. *65:* 1302–1326, Dec. 1966.

Indications

DEMSER is indicated in the treatment of patients with pheochromocytoma for:

1. preoperative preparation of patients for surgery
2. management of patients when surgery is contraindicated
3. chronic treatment of patients with malignant pheochromocytoma.

DEMSER is not recommended for the control of essential hypertension.

Contraindications

DEMSER is contraindicated in persons known to be hypersensitive to this compound.

Warnings

1. *Maintain fluid volume during and after surgery*

When DEMSER is used preoperatively, alone or especially in combination with alpha-adrenergic blocking drugs, adequate intravascular volume must be maintained intraoperatively (especially after tumor removal) and postoperatively to avoid hypotension and decreased perfusion of vital organs resulting from vasodilatation and expanded volume capacity. Following tumor removal, large volumes of plasma may be needed to maintain blood pressure and central venous pressure within the normal range.

In addition, life-threatening arrhythmias may occur during anesthesia and surgery, and may require treatment with a beta blocker or lidocaine. During surgery, patients should have continuous monitoring of blood pressure and electrocardiogram.

2. *Intraoperative Effects*

While the preoperative use of DEMSER in patients with pheochromocytoma is thought to decrease intraoperative problems with blood pressure control, DEMSER does not eliminate the danger of hypertensive crises or arrhythmias during manipulation of the tumor, and the alpha-adrenergic blocking drug, phentolamine, may be needed.

Precautions

1. ***Metyrosine Crystalluria***

Crystalluria and urolithiasis have been found in dogs treated with DEMSER (Metyrosine, MSD) at doses similar to those used in humans, and crystalluria has also been observed in a few patients. To minimize the risk of crystalluria, patients should be urged to maintain water intake sufficient to achieve a daily urine volume of 2000 ml or more, particularly when doses greater than 2 g per day are given. Routine examination of the urine should be carried out. Metyrosine will crystallize as needles or rods. If metyrosine crystalluria occurs, fluid intake should be increased further. If crystalluria persists, the dosage should be reduced or the drug discontinued.

2. *Interaction with phenothiazines or butyrophenones*

Caution should be observed in administering DEMSER to patients receiving phenothiazines or haloperidol because the extrapyramidal effects of these drugs can be expected to be potentiated by inhibition of catecholamine synthesis; this has been documented to date only for haloperidol.

3. *Relatively little data regarding long-term use*

Although no evidence of adverse effects on hepatic, hematologic, or other functions, except for a few instances of increased SGOT levels, has been noted during clinical trials of DEMSER, the total human experience with the drug is quite limited (approximately 300 patients as of 1979) and few patients have been studied long-term. Chronic animal studies have not been carried out. Therefore, suitable laboratory tests should be carried out periodically in patients requiring prolonged use of DEMSER and caution should be observed in patients with impaired hepatic or renal function.

4. *Interference with urinary catecholamine measurements*

Spurious increases in urinary catecholamines may be observed in patients receiving DEMSER due to the presence of metabolites of the drug.

5. *Usage in Pregnancy*

Complete reproduction studies have not been performed in animals to determine whether DEMSER affects fertility in males or females, has teratogenic potential, or has other adverse effects on the fetus. There are no well-controlled studies of DEMSER in pregnant women. The use of DEMSER in pregnant women should be avoided, if possible, but may be appropriate when anticipated benefits outweigh the potential risks.

6. *Nursing Mothers*

It is not known whether DEMSER is excreted in human milk. If use of this drug is necessary, nursing should be discontinued.

Adverse Reactions

Central Nervous System

1. *Sedation*

The most common adverse reaction to DEMSER is moderate to severe sedation, which has been observed in almost all patients. It occurs at both low and high dosages. Sedative effects begin within the first 24 hours of therapy, are maximal after two to three days, and tend to wane during the next few days. Sedation usually is not obvious after one week unless the dosage is increased, but at dosages greater than 2000 mg/day some degree of sedation or fatigue may persist.

When receiving DEMSER, patients should be warned about engaging in activities requiring mental alertness and motor coordination, such as driving a motor vehicle or operating machinery. DEMSER may have additive effects with alcohol and other CNS depressants, e.g., hypnotics, sedatives, tranquilizers, antianxiety agents.

In most patients who experience sedation, temporary changes in sleep pattern occur following withdrawal of the drug. Changes consist of insomnia that may last for two or three days and feelings of increased alertness and ambition. Even patients who do not experience sedation while on DEMSER may report symptoms of psychic stimulation when the drug is discontinued.

2. *Extrapyramidal Signs*

Extrapyramidal signs such as drooling, speech difficulty, and tremor have been reported in approximately 10 percent of patients. These occasionally have been accompanied by trismus and frank parkinsonism.

3. *Anxiety and Psychic Disturbances*

Anxiety and psychic disturbances such as depression, hallucinations, disorientation, and confusion may occur. These effects seem to be dose-dependent and may disappear with reduction of dosage.

Diarrhea

Diarrhea occurs in about 10 percent of patients and may be severe. Antidiarrheal agents may be required if continuation of DEMSER is necessary.

Miscellaneous

Infrequently, slight swelling of the breast, galactorrhea, nasal stuffiness, decreased salivation, dry mouth, headache, nausea, vomiting, abdominal pain, and impotence or failure of ejaculation may occur. Crystalluria (see PRECAUTIONS) and transient dysuria and hematuria have been observed in a few patients. Eosinophilia, increased SGOT levels, peripheral edema, and hypersensitivity reactions such as urticaria and pharyngeal edema have been reported rarely.

Dosage and Administration

The recommended initial dosage of DEMSER for adults and children 12 years of age and older is 250 mg orally four times daily. This may be increased by 250 mg to 500 mg every day to a maximum of 4.0 g/day in divided doses. When used for preoperative preparation, the optimally effective dosage of DEMSER should be given for at least five to seven days.

Optimally effective dosages of DEMSER usually are between 2.0 and 3.0 g/day, and the dose should be titrated by monitoring clinical symptoms and catecholamine excretion. In patients who are hypertensive, dosage should be titrated to achieve normalization of blood pressure and control of clinical symptoms. In patients who are usually normotensive, dosage should be titrated to the amount that will re-

duce urinary metanephrines and/or vanillylmandelic acid by 50 percent or more.
If patients are not adequately controlled by the use of DEMSER, an alpha-adrenergic blocking agent (phenoxybenzamine) should be added.
Use of DEMSER in children under 12 years of age has been limited and a dosage schedule for this age group cannot be given.

How Supplied

No. 3355—Capsules DEMSER, 250 mg, are opaque, two-toned blue capsules coded MSD 690 on one side and DEMSER on the other. They are supplied as follows:
NDC 0006-0690-68 bottles of 100.

[*Shown in Product Identification Section*]

A.H.F.S. Category: 92:00

DC 7111501 Issued May 1979

COPYRIGHT© MERCK & CO., INC., 1979
All rights reserved

DIUPRES® Tablets ℞
Antihypertensive

> **WARNING**
>
> This fixed combination drug is not indicated for initial therapy of hypertension. Hypertension requires therapy titrated to the individual patient. If the fixed combination represents the dosage so determined, its use may be more convenient in patient management. The treatment of hypertension is not static, but must be re-evaluated as conditions in each patient warrant.

Description

DIUPRES® combines two antihypertensive agents: DIURIL® (Chlorothiazide, MSD) and reserpine. The chemical name for chlorothiazide is 6-chloro-2*H*-1,2,4-benzothiadiazine-7-sulfonamide 1,1-dioxide. Reserpine (11,17α-dimethoxy-18β-[(3,4,5-trimethoxybenzoyl)oxy]-3β,20α-yohimban-16β-carboxylic acid methyl ester) is a crystalline alkaloid derived from Rauwolfia serpentina.

Actions

Chlorothiazide
Chlorothiazide is a diuretic and antihypertensive. It affects the renal tubular mechanism of electrolyte reabsorption. At maximal therapeutic dosage all thiazides are approximately equal in their diuretic efficacy.
Chlorothiazide increases excretion of sodium and chloride in approximately equivalent amounts. Natriuresis may be accompanied by some loss of potassium and bicarbonate.
The mechanism of the antihypertensive effect of thiazides is unknown. Chlorothiazide does not affect normal blood pressure.
Chlorothiazide is eliminated rapidly by the kidney.
Reserpine
Reserpine has antihypertensive, bradycardic, and tranquilizing properties. It lowers arterial blood pressure by depletion of catecholamines.
Reserpine is beneficial in relieving anxiety, tension, and headache in the hypertensive patient. It acts at the hypothalamic level of the central nervous system to promote relaxation without hypnosis or analgesia. The sleep pattern shown by the electroencephalogram following barbiturates does not occur with this drug. In laboratory animals spontaneous activity and response to external stimuli are decreased, but confusion or difficulty of movement is not evident.
The bradycardic action of reserpine promotes relaxation and may eliminate sinus tachycardia. It is most pronounced in subjects with sinus tachycardia and usually is not prominent in persons with a normal pulse rate.
Miosis, relaxation of the nictitating membrane, ptosis, hypothermia, and increased gastrointestinal activity are noted in animals given reserpine, sometimes in subclinical doses. None of these effects, except increased gastrointestinal activity, has been found to be clinically significant in man with therapeutic doses.

Indication

Hypertension (see box warning)

Contraindications

Chlorothiazide is contraindicated in anuria.
DIUPRES is contraindicated in hypersensitivity to chlorothiazide or other sulfonamide-derived drugs or to reserpine.
Electroshock therapy should not be given to patients while on reserpine, as severe and even fatal reactions have been reported with minimal convulsive electroshock dosage. After discontinuing reserpine, allow at least seven days before starting electroshock therapy.
Active peptic ulcer, ulcerative colitis, and active mental depression, especially suicidal tendencies, are contraindications to reserpine therapy.

Warnings

Chlorothiazide
Use with caution in severe renal disease. In patients with renal disease, thiazides may precipitate azotemia. Cumulative effects of the drug may develop in patients with impaired renal function.
Thiazides should be used with caution in patients with impaired hepatic function or progressive liver disease, since minor alterations of fluid and electrolyte balance may precipitate hepatic coma.
Thiazides may add to or potentiate the action of other antihypertensive drugs.
Sensitivity reactions may occur in patients with or without a history of allergy or bronchial asthma.
The possibility of exacerbation or activation of systemic lupus erythematosus has been reported.
Lithium generally should not be given with diuretics because they reduce its renal clearance and add a high risk of lithium toxicity. Read circulars for lithium preparations before use of such concomitant therapy.
Reserpine
The occurrence of mental depression due to reserpine in doses of 0.25 mg daily or less is unusual. In any event, DIUPRES should be discontinued at the first sign of depression.
Use in Pregnancy
Reserpine has been demonstrated to cross the placental barrier in guinea pigs with depression of adrenal catecholamine stores in the newborn. There is some evidence that side effects such as nasal congestion, lethargy, depressed Moro reflex, and bradycardia may appear in infants born of reserpine-treated mothers.
Thiazides cross the placental barrier and appear in cord blood. The use of thiazides in pregnancy requires that the anticipated benefit be weighed against possible hazards to the fetus. These hazards include fetal or neonatal jaundice, thrombocytopenia, and possibly other adverse reactions which have occurred in the adult.
Nursing Mothers
Thiazides and reserpine appear in breast milk. If use of the drug is deemed essential, the patient should stop nursing.

Precautions

Chlorothiazide
Periodic determination of serum electrolytes to detect possible electrolyte imbalance should be performed at appropriate intervals.
All patients receiving diuretic therapy should be observed for evidence of fluid or electrolyte imbalance: namely, hyponatremia, hypochloremic alkalosis, and hypokalemia. Serum and urine electrolyte determinations are particularly important when the patient is vomiting excessively or receiving parenteral fluids. Warning signs or symptoms of fluid and electrolyte imbalance include dryness of mouth, thirst, weakness, lethargy, drowsiness, restlessness, muscle pains or cramps, muscular fatigue, hypotension, oliguria, tachycardia, and gastrointestinal disturbances such as nausea and vomiting.
Hypokalemia may develop, especially with brisk diuresis, when severe cirrhosis is present, during concomitant use of corticosteroids or ACTH, or after prolonged therapy.
Interference with adequate oral electrolyte intake will contribute to hypokalemia. Hypokalemia can sensitize or exaggerate the response of the heart to the toxic effects of digitalis (e.g., increased ventricular irritability). Hypokalemia may be avoided or treated by use of potassium supplements such as foods with a high potassium content.
Although any chloride deficit is generally mild and usually does not require specific treatment except under extraordinary circumstances (as in liver disease or renal disease), chloride replacement may be required in the treatment of metabolic alkalosis.
Dilutional hyponatremia may occur in edematous patients in hot weather. Appropriate therapy is water restriction, rather than administration of salt, except in rare instances when the hyponatremia is life threatening. In actual salt depletion, appropriate replacement is the therapy of choice.
Hyperuricemia may occur or acute gout may be precipitated in certain patients receiving thiazides.
Insulin requirements in diabetic patients may be increased, decreased, or unchanged. Latent diabetes mellitus may become manifest during thiazide therapy.
Thiazides may increase the responsiveness to tubocurarine.
The antihypertensive effect of the drug may be enhanced in the postsympathectomy patient.
Thiazides may decrease arterial responsiveness to norepinephrine. This diminution is not sufficient to preclude effectiveness of the pressor agent for therapeutic use.
If progressive renal impairment becomes evident, consider withholding or discontinuing diuretic therapy.
Thiazides may decrease serum PBI levels without signs of thyroid disturbance.
Thiazides may decrease urinary calcium excretion. Thiazides may cause intermittent and slight elevation of serum calcium in the absence of known disorders of calcium metabolism. Marked hypercalcemia may be evidence of hidden hyperparathyroidism. Thiazides should be discontinued before carrying out tests for parathyroid function.
Reserpine
Since reserpine may increase gastric secretion and motility, it should be used cautiously in patients with a history of peptic ulcer, ulcerative colitis, or other gastrointestinal disorder. This compound may precipitate biliary colic in patients with gallstones, or bronchial asthma in susceptible persons.

Continued on next page

Information on the Merck Sharp & Dohme products listed on these pages is the full prescribing information from package circulars in use October 31, 1982.

Merck Sharp & Dohme—Cont.

Reserpine may case hypotension including orthostatic hypotension.
In hypertensive patients on reserpine therapy significant hypotension and bradycardia may develop during surgical anesthesia. The anesthesiologist should be aware that reserpine has been taken, since it may be necessary to give vagal blocking agents parenterally to prevent or reverse hypotension and/or bradycardia.
Anxiety or depression, as well as psychosis, may develop during reserpine therapy. If depression is present when therapy is begun, it may be aggravated. Mental depression is unusual with reserpine doses of 0.25 mg daily or less. In any case, DIUPRES should be discontinued at the first sign of depression. Extreme caution should be used in treating patients with a history of mental depression, and the possibility of suicide should be kept in mind.
As with most antihypertensive therapy, caution should be exercised when treating hypertensive patients with renal insufficiency, since they adjust poorly to lowered blood pressure levels. Use reserpine cautiously with digitalis and quinidine; cardiac arrhythmias have occurred with reserpine preparations.
When two or more antihypertensives are given, the individual dosages may have to be reduced to prevent excessive drop in blood pressure. In hypertensive patients with coronary artery disease, it is important to avoid a precipitous drop in blood pressure.

Adverse Reactions

Chlorothiazide
Gastrointestinal: Anorexia, gastric irritation, nausea, vomiting, cramping, diarrhea, constipation, jaundice (intrahepatic cholestatic jaundice), pancreatitis, sialadenitis.
Central nervous system: Dizziness, vertigo, paresthesias, headache, xanthopsia.
Hematologic: Leukopenia, agranulocytosis, thrombocytopenia, aplastic anemia, hemolytic anemia.
Cardiovascular: Orthostatic hypotension (may be aggravated by alcohol, barbiturates, or narcotics).
Allergic: Purpura, photosensitivity, rash, urticaria, necrotizing angiitis (vasculitis) (cutaneous vasculitis), fever, respiratory distress including pneumonitis and pulmonary edema, anaphylactic reactions.
Other: Hyperglycemia, glycosuria, hyperuricemia, muscle spasm, weakness, restlessness, transient blurred vision.
Whenever adverse reactions are moderate or severe, thiazide dosage should be reduced or therapy withdrawn.
Reserpine
Central nervous system: Excessive sedation, mental depression, nightmares, headache, dizziness, syncope, nervousness, paradoxical anxiety, central nervous system sensitization (dull sensorium, deafness, glaucoma, uveitis, optic atrophy), parkinsonism (usually reversible with decreased dosage or discontinuance of therapy).
Respiratory: Nasal congestion, dyspnea, epistaxis.
Cardiovascular: Bradycardia, angina pectoris, arrhythmia, premature ventricular contractions, and other direct cardiac effects (e.g., fluid retention, congestive failure).
Gastrointestinal: Hypersecretion and increased motility, nausea, vomiting, anorexia, diarrhea, dryness of mouth, increased salivation.
Hematologic: Excessive bleeding following prostatic surgery, thrombocytopenic purpura.
Allergic: Flushing of skin, pruritus, rash.
Other: Conjunctival injection, enhanced susceptibility to colds, muscular aches, weight gain, blurred vision, dysuria, nonpuerperal lactation, impotence, decreased libido.

Dosage and Administration

The initial dosage of DIUPRES should conform to the dosages of the individual components established during titration (see box warning). The usual adult dosage of DIUPRES 250 is 1 or 2 tablets once or twice a day; that of DIUPRES 500 is 1 tablet once or twice a day. Dosage may require adjustment according to the blood pressure response of the patient.
Careful observations for changes in blood pressure must be made when DIUPRES is used with other antihypertensive drugs.

How Supplied

No. 3261—Tablets DIUPRES 250 are pink, round, scored, compressed tablets, coded MSD 230. Each tablet contains 250 mg of chlorothiazide and 0.125 mg of reserpine. They are supplied as follows:
NDC 0006-0230-68 in bottles of 100
NDC 0006-0230-82 in bottles of 1000.
[*Shown in Product Identification Section*]
No. 3262—Tablets DIUPRES 500 are pink, round, scored, compressed tablets, coded MSD 405. Each tablet contains 500 mg of chlorothiazide and 0.125 mg of reserpine. They are supplied as follows:
NDC 0006-0405-68 in bottles of 100
NDC 0006-0405-82 in bottles of 1000.
[*Shown in Product Identification Section*]
A.H.F.S. Category: 24:08
DC 6053128 Issued May 1980

DIURIL® Intravenous Sodium (chlorothiazide sodium, MSD), U.S.P. ℞

Description

DIURIL® (Chlorothiazide, MSD) is 6-chloro-2*H*-1,2,4-benzothiadiazine-7-sulfonamide 1,1-dioxide.
It is a white, or practically white, crystalline compound very slightly soluble in water, but readily soluble in dilute aqueous sodium hydroxide. It is soluble in urine to the extent of about 150 mg per 100 ml at pH 7.
Intravenous Sodium DIURIL® (Chlorothiazide Sodium, MSD) is supplied in a vial containing:
Chlorothiazide sodium equivalent to chlorothiazide.................................0.5 g
Inactive ingredients:
Mannitol...0.25 g
Sodium hydroxide to adjust pH, with 0.4 mg thimerosal added as preservative.

Actions

DIURIL is a diuretic and antihypertensive.
DIURIL affects the renal tubular mechanism of electrolyte reabsorption. At maximal therapeutic dosage all thiazides are approximately equal in their diuretic efficacy.
DIURIL increases excretion of sodium and chloride in approximately equivalent amounts. Natriuresis may be accompanied by some loss of potassium and bicarbonate.
After oral use diuresis begins within 2 hours, peaks in about 4 hours and lasts about 6 to 12 hours. Following intravenous use of Sodium DIURIL, onset of the diuretic action occurs in 15 minutes and the maximal action in 30 minutes. DIURIL is eliminated rapidly by the kidney.
The mechanism of the antihypertensive effect of thiazides is unknown. DIURIL does not affect normal blood pressure.

Indications

Intravenous Sodium DIURIL is indicated as adjunctive therapy in edema associated with congestive heart failure, hepatic cirrhosis, and corticosteroid and estrogen therapy.
Intravenous Sodium DIURIL has also been found useful in edema due to various forms of renal dysfunction such as nephrotic syndrome, acute glomerulonephritis, and chronic renal failure.
Use in Pregnancy. Routine use of diuretics during normal pregnancy is inappropriate and exposes mother and fetus to unnecessary hazard. Diuretics do not prevent development of toxemia of pregnancy and there is no satisfactory evidence that they are useful in the treatment of toxemia.
Edema during pregnancy may arise from pathologic causes or from the physiologic and mechanical consequences of pregnancy. Thiazides are indicated in pregnancy when edema is due to pathologic causes, just as they are in the absence of pregnancy (however, see WARNINGS). Dependent edema in pregnancy, resulting from restriction of venous return by the gravid uterus, is properly treated through elevation of the lower extremities and use of support stockings. Use of diuretics to lower intravascular volume in this instance is illogical and unnecessary. During normal pregnancy there is hypervolemia which is not harmful to the fetus or the mother in the absence of cardiovascular disease. However, it may be associated with edema, rarely generalized edema. If such edema causes discomfort, increased recumbency will often provide relief. Rarely this edema may cause extreme discomfort which is not relieved by rest. In these instances, a short course of diuretic therapy may provide relief and be appropriate.

Contraindications

Anuria.
Hypersensitivity to any component of this product or to other sulfonamide-derived drugs.

Warnings

Intravenous use in infants and children has been limited and is not generally recommended.
Use with caution in severe renal disease. In patients with renal disease, thiazides may precipitate azotemia. Cumulative effects of the drug may develop in patients with impaired renal function.
Thiazides should be used with caution in patients with impaired hepatic function or progressive liver disease, since minor alterations of fluid and electrolyte balance may precipitate hepatic coma.
Thiazides may add to or potentiate the action of other antihypertensive drugs.
Sensitivity reactions may occur in patients with or without a history of allergy or bronchial asthma.
The possibility of exacerbation or activation of systemic lupus erythematosus has been reported.
Lithium generally should not be given with diuretics because they reduce its renal clearance and add a high risk of lithium toxicity. Read circulars for lithium preparations before use of such concomitant therapy.
Use in Pregnancy. Thiazides cross the placental barrier and appear in cord blood. The use of thiazides in pregnancy requires that the anticipated benefit be weighed against possible hazards to the fetus. These hazards include fetal or neonatal jaundice, thrombocytopenia, and possibly other adverse reactions which have occurred in the adult.
Nursing Mothers. Thiazides appear in breast milk. If use of the drug is deemed essential, the patient should stop nursing.

Precautions

Periodic determination of serum electrolytes to detect possible electrolyte imbalance should be performed at appropriate intervals.
All patients receiving diuretic therapy should be observed for evidence of fluid or electrolyte imbalance: namely, hyponatremia, hypochloremic alkalosis, and hypokalemia. Serum and urine electrolyte determinations are particu-

larly important when the patient is vomiting excessively or receiving parenteral fluids. Warning signs or symptoms of fluid and electrolyte imbalance include dryness of mouth, thirst, weakness, lethargy, drowsiness, restlessness, muscle pains or cramps, muscular fatigue, hypotension, oliguria, tachycardia, and gastrointestinal disturbances such as nausea and vomiting.

Hypokalemia may develop especially with brisk diuresis, when severe cirrhosis is present, during concomitant use of corticosteroids or ACTH, or after prolonged therapy.

Interference with adequate oral electrolyte intake will also contribute to hypokalemia. Hypokalemia can sensitize or exaggerate the response of the heart to the toxic effects of digitalis (e.g., increased ventricular irritability). Hypokalemia may be avoided or treated by use of potassium supplements such as foods with a high potassium content.

Although any chloride deficit is generally mild and usually does not require specific treatment except under extraordinary circumstances (as in liver disease or renal disease), chloride replacement may be required in the treatment of metabolic alkalosis.

Dilutional hyponatremia may occur in edematous patients in hot weather; appropriate therapy is water restriction, rather than administration of salt, except in rare instances when the hyponatremia is life threatening. In actual salt depletion, appropriate replacement is the therapy of choice.

Hyperuricemia may occur or acute gout may be precipitated in certain patients receiving thiazides.

Insulin requirements in diabetic patients may be increased, decreased, or unchanged. Latent diabetes mellitus may become manifest during thiazide therapy.

Thiazides may increase the responsiveness to tubocurarine.

The antihypertensive effects of the drug may be enhanced in the postsympathectomy patient. Thiazides may decrease arterial responsiveness to norepinephrine. This diminution is not sufficient to preclude effectiveness of the pressor agent for therapeutic use.

If progressive renal impairment becomes evident, consider withholding or discontinuing diuretic therapy.

Thiazides may decrease serum PBI levels without signs of thyroid disturbance.

Thiazides may decrease urinary calcium excretion. Thiazides may cause intermittent and slight elevation of serum calcium in the absence of known disorders of calcium metabolism. Marked hypercalcemia may be evidence of hidden hyperparathyroidism. Thiazides should be discontinued before carrying out tests for parathyroid function.

Adverse Reactions

A. *Gastrointestinal System*
  1. anorexia
  2. gastric irritation
  3. nausea
  4. vomiting
  5. cramping
  6. diarrhea
  7. constipation
  8. jaundice (intrahepatic cholestatic jaundice)
  9. pancreatitis
  10. sialadenitis

B. *Central Nervous System*
  1. dizziness
  2. vertigo
  3. paresthesias
  4. headache
  5. xanthopsia

C. *Hematologic*
  1. leukopenia
  2. agranulocytosis
  3. thrombocytopenia
  4. aplastic anemia
  5. hemolytic anemia

D. *Cardiovascular*
  Orthostatic hypotension (may be aggravated by alcohol, barbiturates, or narcotics)

E. *Hypersensitivity*
  1. purpura
  2. photosensitivity
  3. rash
  4. urticaria
  5. necrotizing angiitis (vasculitis) (cutaneous vasculitis)
  6. fever
  7. respiratory distress including pneumonitis and pulmonary edema
  8. anaphylactic reactions

F. *Other*
  1. hyperglycemia
  2. glycosuria
  3. hyperuricemia
  4. muscle spasm
  5. weakness
  6. restlessness
  7. transient blurred vision
  8. hematuria (one case following intravenous use)

Whenever adverse reactions are moderate or severe, thiazide dosage should be reduced or therapy withdrawn.

Dosage and Administration

Intravenous Sodium DIURIL should be reserved for patients unable to take oral medication or for emergency situations.

Therapy should be individualized according to patient response. Use the smallest dosage necessary to achieve the required response.

Intravenous use in infants and children has been limited and is not generally recommended.

When medication can be taken orally, therapy with DIURIL tablets or oral suspension may be substituted for intravenous therapy, using the same dosage schedule as for the parenteral route.

Add 18 ml of Sterile Water for Injection to the vial to form an isotonic solution for intravenous injection. Never add less than 18 ml. Unused solution may be stored at room temperature for 24 hours, after which it must be discarded. The solution is compatible with dextrose or sodium chloride solutions for intravenous infusion. Avoid simultaneous administration of solutions of chlorothiazide with whole blood or its derivatives.

Extravasation must be rigidly avoided. Do not give subcutaneously or intramuscularly.

The usual adult dosage is 0.5 to 1.0 g once or twice a day. Many patients with edema respond to intermittent therapy, i.e., administration on alternate days or on three to five days each week. With an intermittent schedule, excessive response and the resulting undesirable electrolyte imbalance are less likely to occur.

How Supplied

No. 3250—Intravenous Sodium DIURIL is a dry, white powder usually in plug form, supplied in vials containing chlorothiazide sodium equivalent to 0.5 g of chlorothiazide. **NDC** 0006-3250-32.

A.H.F.S. Category: 40:28
DC 6435018 Issued May 1980

DIURIL® Tablets (chlorothiazide, MSD), U.S.P. ℞
DIURIL® Oral Suspension (chlorothiazide, MSD), U.S.P. ℞

Description

DIURIL® (Chlorothiazide, MSD) is 6-choro-2*H*-1,2,4-benzothiadiazine-7-sulfonamide 1,1-dioxide.

It is a white, or practically white, crystalline compound very slightly soluble in water, but readily soluble in dilute aqueous sodium hydroxide. It is soluble in urine to the extent of about 150 mg per 100 ml at pH 7.

DIURIL is supplied as 250 mg and 500 mg tablets, and as an oral suspension containing 250 mg per 5 ml, alcohol 0.5 percent, with methylparaben 0.12 percent, propylparaben 0.02 percent, and benzoic acid 0.1 percent added as preservatives.

Actions

DIURIL is a diuretic and antihypertensive.

DIURIL affects the renal tubular mechanism of electrolyte reabsorption. At maximal therapeutic dosage all thiazides are approximately equal in their diuretic efficacy.

DIURIL increases excretion of sodium and chloride in approximately equivalent amounts. Natriuresis may be accompanied by some loss of potassium and bicarbonate.

After oral use diuresis begins within 2 hours, peaks in about 4 hours and lasts about 6 to 12 hours. DIURIL is eliminated rapidly by the kidney.

The mechanism of the antihypertensive effect of thiazides is unknown. DIURIL does not affect normal blood pressure.

Indications

DIURIL is indicated as adjunctive therapy in edema associated with congestive heart failure, hepatic cirrhosis, and corticosteroid and estrogen therapy.

DIURIL has also been found useful in edema due to various forms of renal dysfunction such as nephrotic syndrome, acute glomerulonephritis, and chronic renal failure.

DIURIL is indicated in the management of hypertension either as the sole therapeutic agent or to enhance the effectiveness of other antihypertensive drugs in the more severe forms of hypertension.

Use in Pregnancy. Routine use of diuretics during normal pregnancy is inappropriate and exposes mother and fetus to unnecessary hazard. Diuretics do not prevent development of toxemia of pregnancy and there is no satisfactory evidence that they are useful in the treatment of toxemia.

Edema during pregnancy may arise from pathologic causes or from the physiologic and mechanical consequences of pregnancy. Thiazides are indicated in pregnancy when edema is due to pathologic causes, just as they are in the absence of pregnancy (however, see WARNINGS, below). Dependent edema in pregnancy, resulting from restriction of venous return by the gravid uterus, is properly treated through elevation of the lower extremities and use of support stockings. Use of diuretics to lower intravascular volume in this instance is illogical and unnecessary. During normal pregnancy there is hypervolemia which is not harmful to the fetus or the mother in the absence of cardiovascular disease. However, it may be associated with edema, rarely generalized edema. If such edema causes discomfort, increased recumbency will often provide relief. Rarely this edema may cause extreme discomfort which is not relieved by rest. In these instances, a short course of diuretic therapy may provide relief and be appropriate.

Contraindications

Anuria.

Hypersensitivity to this product or to other sulfonamide-derived drugs.

Information on the Merck Sharp & Dohme products listed on these pages is the full prescribing information from package circulars in use October 31, 1982.

Continued on next page

Merck Sharp & Dohme—Cont.

Warnings

Use with caution in severe renal disease. In patients with renal disease, thiazides may precipitate azotemia. Cumulative effects of the drug may develop in patients with impaired renal function.

Thiazides should be used with caution in patients with impaired hepatic function or progressive liver disease, since minor alterations of fluid and electrolyte balance may precipitate hepatic coma.

Thiazides may add to or potentiate the action of other antihypertensive drugs.
Sensitivity reactions may occur in patients with or without a history of allergy or bronchial asthma.
The possibility of exacerbation or activation of systemic lupus erythematosus has been reported.

Lithium generally should not be given with diuretics because they reduce its renal clearance and add a high risk of lithium toxicity. Read circulars for lithium preparations before use of such concomitant therapy.

Use in Pregnancy. Thiazides cross the placental barrier and appear in cord blood. The use of thiazides in pregnancy requires that the anticipated benefit be weighed against possible hazards to the fetus. These hazards include fetal or neonatal jaundice, thrombocytopenia, and possibly other adverse reactions which have occurred in the adult.

Nursing Mothers. Thiazides appear in breast milk. If use of the drug is deemed essential, the patient should stop nursing.

Precautions

Periodic determination of serum electrolytes to detect possible electrolyte imbalance should be performed at appropriate intervals.
All patients receiving diuretic therapy should be observed for evidence of fluid or electrolyte imbalance: namely, hyponatremia, hypochloremic alkalosis, and hypokalemia. Serum and urine electrolyte determinations are particularly important when the patient is vomiting excessively or receiving parenteral fluids. Warning signs or symptoms of fluid and electrolyte imbalance include dryness of mouth, thirst, weakness, lethargy, drowsiness, restlessness, muscle pains or cramps, muscular fatigue, hypotension, oliguria, tachycardia, and gastrointestinal disturbances such as nausea and vomiting.
Hypokalemia may develop, especially with brisk diuresis, when severe cirrhosis is present, during concomitant use of corticosteroids or ACTH, or after prolonged therapy.
Interference with adequate oral electrolyte intake will also contribute to hypokalemia. Hypokalemia can sensitize or exaggerate the response of the heart to the toxic effects of digitalis (e.g., increased ventricular irritability). Hypokalemia may be avoided or treated by use of potassium supplements such as foods with a high potassium content.
Although any chloride deficit is generally mild and usually does not require specific treatment except under extraordinary circumstances (as in liver disease or renal disease), chloride replacement may be required in the treatment of metabolic alkalosis.
Dilutional hyponatremia may occur in edematous patients in hot weather; appropriate therapy is water restriction, rather than administration of salt, except in rare instances when the hyponatremia is life threatening. In actual salt depletion, appropriate replacement is the therapy of choice.
Hyperuricemia may occur or acute gout may be precipitated in certain patients receiving thiazides.
Insulin requirements in diabetic patients may be increased, decreased, or unchanged. Latent diabetes mellitus may become manifest during thiazide therapy.
Thiazides may increase the responsiveness to tubocurarine.
The antihypertensive effects of the drug may be enhanced in the postsympathectomy patient. Thiazides may decrease arterial responsiveness to norepinephrine. This diminution is not sufficient to preclude effectiveness of the pressor agent for therapeutic use.
If progressive renal impairment becomes evident, consider withholding or discontinuing diuretic therapy.
Thiazides may decrease serum PBI levels without signs of thyroid disturbance.
Thiazides may decrease urinary calcium excretion. Thiazides may cause intermittent and slight elevation of serum calcium in the absence of known disorders of calcium metabolism. Marked hypercalcemia may be evidence of hidden hyperparathyroidism. Thiazides should be discontinued before carrying out tests for parathyroid function.

Adverse Reactions

A. *Gastrointestinal System*
1. anorexia
2. gastric irritation
3. nausea
4. vomiting
5. cramping
6. diarrhea
7. constipation
8. jaundice (intrahepatic cholestatic jaundice)
9. pancreatitis
10. sialadenitis

B. *Central Nervous System*
1. dizziness
2. vertigo
3. paresthesias
4. headache
5. xanthopsia

C. *Hematologic*
1. leukopenia
2. agranulocytosis
3. thrombocytopenia
4. aplastic anemia
5. hemolytic anemia

D. *Cardiovascular*
Orthostatic hypotension (may be aggravated by alcohol, barbiturates, or narcotics)

E. *Hypersensitivity*
1. purpura
2. photosensitivity
3. rash
4. urticaria
5. necrotizing angiitis (vasculitis) (cutaneous vasculitis)
6. fever
7. respiratory distress including pneumonitis and pulmonary edema
8. anaphylactic reactions

F. *Other*
1. hyperglycemia
2. glycosuria
3. hyperuricemia
4. muscle spasm
5. weakness
6. restlessness
7. transient blurred vision

Whenever adverse reactions are moderate or severe, thiazide dosage should be reduced or therapy withdrawn.

Dosage and Administration

Therapy should be individualized according to patient response. Use the smallest dosage necessary to achieve the required response.

Adults
For Diuresis
The usual adult dosage is 0.5 to 1.0 g once or twice a day. Many patients with edema respond to intermittent therapy, i.e., administration on alternate days or on three to five days each week. With an intermittent schedule, excessive response and the resulting undesirable electrolyte imbalance are less likely to occur.
For Control of Hypertension
The usual adult starting dosage is 0.5 or 1.0 g a day as a single or divided dose. Dosage is increased or decreased according to blood pressure response. Rarely some patients may require up to 2.0 g a day in divided doses.
When thiazides are used with other antihypertensives, the dose of the latter may need to be reduced to prevent excessive decrease in blood pressure.
Infants and Children
The usual oral pediatric dosage is based on 10 mg of DIURIL per pound of body weight per day in two doses. Infants under 6 months of age may require up to 15 mg per pound per day in two doses.
On this basis, infants up to 2 years of age may be given 125 to 375 mg daily in two doses (2.5 to 7.5 ml, or ½ to 1½ teaspoonfuls of the oral suspension daily). Children from 2 to 12 years of age may be given 375 mg to 1.0 g daily in two doses (7.5 to 20 ml, or 1½ to 4 teaspoonfuls of oral suspension daily). Dosage in both age groups should be based on body weight.

How Supplied

No. 3244—Tablets DIURIL, 250 mg, are white, round, scored, compressed tablets, coded MSD 214. They are supplied as follows:
NDC 0006-0214-68 bottles of 100
NDC 0006-0214-28 single unit packages of 100
NDC 0006-0214-82 bottles of 1000
[*Shown in Product Identification Section*]
No. 3245—Tablets DIURIL, 500 mg, are white, round, scored, compressed tablets, coded MSD 432. They are supplied as follows:
NDC 0006-0432-68 bottles of 100
NDC 0006-0432-28 single unit packages of 100
NDC 0006-0432-82 bottles of 1000
NDC 0006-0432-86 bottles of 5000
[*Shown in Product Identification Section*]
No. 3239—Oral Suspension DIURIL, 250 mg per 5 ml, is a yellow, creamy suspension, and is supplied as follows:
NDC 0006-3239-66 bottles of 237 ml.
A.H.F.S. Category: 40:28
DC 6020741 Issued May 1980

DOLOBID® Tablets ℞
(diflunisal, MSD)

Description

Diflunisal is 2′, 4′-difluoro-4-hydroxy-3-biphenylcarboxylic acid. Its empirical formula is $C_{13}H_8F_2O_3$.
Diflunisal has a molecular weight of 250.20. It is a stable, white, crystalline compound with a melting point of 211–213°C. It is practically insoluble in water at neutral or acidic pH. Because it is an organic acid, it dissolves readily in dilute alkali to give a moderately stable solution at room temperature. It is soluble in most organic solvents including ethanol, methanol, and acetone.
DOLOBID® (Diflunisal, MSD) is available in 250 and 500 mg tablets for oral administration.

Clinical Pharmacology

Action
DOLOBID is a non-steroidal drug with analgesic, anti-inflammatory and antipyretic properties. It is a peripherally-acting non-narcotic analgesic drug. Habituation, tolerance and addiction have not been reported.
Diflunisal is a difluorophenyl derivative of salicylic acid. Chemically, diflunisal differs

from aspirin (acetylsalicylic acid) in two respects. The first of these two is the presence of a difluorophenyl substituent at carbon 1. The second difference is the removal of the 0-acetyl group from the carbon 4 position. Diflunisal is not metabolized to salicylic acid, and the fluorine atoms are not displaced from the difluorophenyl ring structure.
The precise mechanism of the analgesic and anti-inflammatory actions of diflunisal is not known. Diflunisal is a prostaglandin synthetase inhibitor. In animals, prostaglandins sensitize afferent nerves and potentiate the action of bradykinin in inducing pain. Since prostaglandins are known to be among the mediators of pain and inflammation, the mode of action of diflunisal may be due to a decrease of prostaglandins in peripheral tissues.

Pharmacokinetics and Metabolism

DOLOBID is rapidly and completely absorbed following oral administration with peak plasma concentrations occurring between 2 to 3 hours. The drug is excreted in the urine as two soluble glucuronide conjugates accounting for about 90% of the administered dose. Little or no diflunisal is excreted in the feces. Diflunisal appears in human milk in concentrations of 2–7% of those in plasma. More than 99% of diflunisal in plasma is bound to proteins.
As is the case with salicylic acid, concentration-dependent pharmacokinetics prevail when DOLOBID is administered; a doubling of dosage produces a greater than doubling of drug accumulation. The effect becomes more apparent with repetitive doses. Following single doses, peak plasma concentrations of 41 ± 11 μg/ml (mean $\pm$ S.D.) were observed following 250 mg doses, 87 ± 17 μg/ml were observed following 500 mg and 124 ± 11 μg/ml following single 1,000 mg doses. However, following administration of 250 mg b.i.d., a mean peak level of 56 ± 14 μg/ml was observed on day 8, while the mean peak level after 500 mg b.i.d. for 11 days was 190 ± 33 μg/ml. In contrast to salicylic acid which has a plasma half-life of 2½ hours, the plasma half-life of diflunisal is 3 to 4 times longer (8 to 12 hours), because of a difluorophenyl substituent at carbon 1. Because of its long half-life and nonlinear pharmacokinetics, several days are required for diflunisal plasma levels to reach steady state following multiple doses. For this reason, an initial loading dose is necessary to shorten the time to reach steady state levels, and 2 to 3 days of observation are necessary for evaluating changes in treatment regimens if a loading dose is not used.
Studies in baboons to determine passage across the blood brain barrier have shown that only small quantities of diflunisal, under normal or acidotic conditions are transported into the cerebrospinal fluid (CSF). The ratio of blood/CSF concentrations after intravenous doses of 50 mg/kg or oral doses of 100 mg/kg of diflunisal was 100:1. In contrast, oral doses of 500 mg/kg of aspirin resulted in a blood/CSF ratio of 5:1.

Mild to Moderate Pain

DOLOBID is a peripherally-acting analgesic agent with a long duration of action. DOLOBID produces significant analgesia within 1 hour and maximum analgesia within 2 to 3 hours. Consistent with its long half-life, clinical effects of DOLOBID mirror its pharmacokinetic behavior, which is the basis for recommending a loading dose when instituting therapy. Patients treated with DOLOBID, on the first dose, tend to have a slower onset of pain relief when compared with drugs achieving comparable peak effects. However, DOLOBID produces longer-lasting responses than the comparative agents.
Comparative single dose clinical studies have established the analgesic efficacy of DOLOBID at various dose levels relative to other analgesics. Analgesic effect measurements were derived from hourly evaluations by patients during eight and twelve-hour postdosing observation periods. The following information may serve as a guide for prescribing DOLOBID.
DOLOBID 500 mg was comparable in analgesic efficacy to aspirin 650 mg, acetaminophen 600 mg or 650 mg, and acetaminophen 650 mg with propoxyphene napsylate 100 mg. Patients treated with DOLOBID had longer lasting responses than the patients treated with the comparative analgesics.
DOLOBID 1000 mg was comparable in analgesic efficacy to acetaminophen 600 mg with codeine 60 mg. Patients treated with DOLOBID had longer lasting responses than the patients who received acetaminophen with codeine.
A loading dose of 1000 mg provides faster onset of pain relief, shorter time to peak analgesic effect, and greater peak analgesic effect than an initial 500 mg dose.
In contrast to the comparative analgesics, a significantly greater proportion of patients treated with DOLOBID did not remedicate and continued to have a good analgesic effect eight to twelve hours after dosing. Seventy-five percent (75%) of patients treated with DOLOBID continued to have a good analgesic response at four hours. When patients having a good analgesic response at four hours were followed, 78% of these patients continued to have a good analgesic response at eight hours and 64% at twelve hours.

Osteoarthritis

The effectiveness of DOLOBID for the treatment of osteoarthritis was studied in patients with osteoarthritis of the hip and/or knee. The activity of DOLOBID was demonstrated by clinical improvement in the signs and symptoms of disease activity.
In a double-blind multicenter study of 12 weeks' duration in which dosages were adjusted according to patient response, DOLOBID, 500 or 750 mg daily, was shown to be comparable in effectiveness to aspirin, 2,000 or 3,000 mg daily. Patients treated with DOLOBID had a lower overall incidence of digestive system adverse experiences, and of dizziness, edema, and tinnitus. In open-label extensions of this study to 24 or 48 weeks, DOLOBID continued to show similar effectiveness and generally was well tolerated.

Antipyretic Activity

DOLOBID is not recommended for use as an antipyretic agent. In single 250 mg, 500 mg, or 750 mg doses, DOLOBID produced measurable but not clinically useful decreases in temperature in patients with fever; however, the possibility that it may mask fever in some patients, particularly with chronic or high doses, should be considered.

Uricosuric Effect

In normal volunteers, an increase in the renal clearance of uric acid and a decrease in serum uric acid was observed when DOLOBID was administered at 500 mg or 750 mg daily in divided doses. Patients on long-term therapy taking DOLOBID at 500 mg to 1000 mg daily in divided doses showed a prompt and consistent reduction across studies in mean serum uric acid levels, which were lowered as much as 1.4 mg%. It is not known whether DOLOBID interferes with the activity of other uricosuric agents.

Effect on Platelet Function

As an inhibitor of prostaglandin synthetase, DOLOBID has a dose-related effect on platelet function and bleeding time. In normal volunteers, 250 mg b.i.d. for 8 days had no effect on platelet function, and 500 mg b.i.d., the usual recommended dose, had a slight effect. At 1000 mg b.i.d., which exceeds the maximum recommended dosage, however, DOLOBID inhibited platelet function. In contrast to aspirin, these effects of DOLOBID were reversible, because of the absence of the chemically labile and biologically reactive 0-acetyl group at the carbon 4 position. Bleeding time was not altered by a dose of 250 mg b.i.d., and was only slightly increased at 500 mg b.i.d. At 1000 mg b.i.d., a greater increase occurred, but was not statistically significantly different from the change in the placebo group.

Effect on Fecal Blood Loss

When DOLOBID was given to normal volunteers at the usual recommended dose of 500 mg twice daily, fecal blood loss was not significantly different from placebo. Aspirin at 1000 mg four times daily produced the expected increase in fecal blood loss. DOLOBID at 1000 mg twice daily (NOTE: exceeds the recommended dosage) caused a statistically significant increase in fecal blood loss, but this increase was only one-half as large as that associated with aspirin 1300 mg twice daily.

Effect on Blood Glucose

DOLOBID did not affect fasting blood sugar in diabetic patients who were receiving tolbutamide or placebo.

Indications and Usage

DOLOBID is indicated for acute or long-term use for symptomatic treatment of the following:

1. Mild to moderate pain
2. Osteoarthritis

Contraindications

Patients who are hypersensitive to this product.
Patients in whom acute asthmatic attacks, urticaria, or rhinitis are precipitated by aspirin or other nonsteroidal anti-inflammatory drugs.

Warnings

Peptic ulceration and gastrointestinal bleeding have been reported in patients receiving DOLOBID. In patients with active gastrointestinal bleeding or an active peptic ulcer, the physician must weigh the benefits of therapy with DOLOBID against possible hazards, institute an appropriate ulcer regimen, and carefully monitor the patient's progress. When DOLOBID is given to patients with a history of upper gastrointestinal tract disease, it should be given only after consulting the ADVERSE REACTIONS section and under close supervision.

Precautions

General

Although DOLOBID has less effect on platelet function and bleeding time than aspirin, at higher doses it is an inhibitor of platelet function; therefore, patients who may be adversely affected should be carefully observed when DOLOBID is administered (see CLINICAL PHARMACOLOGY).
Because of reports of adverse eye findings with agents of this class, it is recommended that patients who develop eye complaints during treatment with DOLOBID have ophthalmologic studies.
Since DOLOBID is eliminated primarily by the kidneys, patients with significantly impaired renal function should be closely monitored; a lower daily dosage should be anticipated to avoid excessive drug accumulation.
In studies in rats and dogs at high dosages, there was an occasional occurrence of mild renal toxicity as evidenced by papillary edema in some animals. Papillary necrosis occurred in mice in long-term studies.
Peripheral edema has been observed in some patients taking DOLOBID. Therefore, as with other drugs in this class, DOLOBID should be used with caution in patients with compro-

Continued on next page

Information on the Merck Sharp & Dohme products listed on these pages is the full prescribing information from package circulars in use October 31, 1982.

Merck Sharp & Dohme—Cont.

mised cardiac function, hypertension, or other conditions predisposing to fluid retention.

Laboratory Tests

As with other non-steroidal anti-inflammatory drugs, borderline elevations of one or more liver tests may occur in up to 15% of patients. These abnormalities may progress, may remain essentially unchanged, or may be transient with continued therapy. The SGPT (ALT) test is probably the most sensitive indicator of liver dysfunction. Meaningful (3 times the upper limit of normal) elevations of SGPT or SGOT (AST) occurred in controlled clinical trials in less than 1% of patients. A patient with symptoms and/or signs suggesting liver dysfunction, or in whom an abnormal liver test has occurred, should be evaluated for evidence of the development of more severe hepatic reaction while on therapy with DOLOBID. Severe hepatic reactions, including jaundice and cases of fatal hepatitis, have been reported with other non-steroidal anti-inflammatory drugs. Although such reactions are rare, if abnormal liver tests persist or worsen, if clinical signs and symptoms consistent with liver disease develop, or if systemic manifestations occur (e.g. eosinophilia, rash, etc.), DOLOBID should be discontinued.

Drug Interactions

DOLOBID prolongs the prothrombin time in patients who are on oral anticoagulants. DOLOBID has not been shown to interact with tolbutamide. DOLOBID interacts with hydrochlorothiazide, furosemide, acetaminophen, aspirin, indomethacin, sulindac and naproxen (see below).

Oral Anticoagulants: In some normal volunteers, the concomitant administration of DOLOBID and warfarin, acenocoumarol, or phenprocoumon resulted in prolongation of prothrombin time. This may occur because diflunisal competitively displaces coumarins from protein binding sites. Accordingly, when DOLOBID is administered with oral anticoagulants, the prothrombin time should be closely monitored during and for several days after concomitant drug administration. Adjustment of dosage of oral anticoagulants may be required.

Tolbutamide: In diabetic patients receiving DOLOBID and tolbutamide, no significant effects were seen on tolbutamide plasma levels or fasting blood glucose.

Hydrochlorothiazide: In normal volunteers, concomitant administration of DOLOBID and hydrochlorothiazide resulted in significantly increased plasma levels of hydrochlorothiazide. DOLOBID decreased the hyperuricemic effect of hydrochlorothiazide.

Furosemide: In normal volunteers, the concomitant administration of DOLOBID and furosemide had no effect on the diuretic activity of furosemide. DOLOBID decreased the hyperuricemic effect of furosemide.

Antacids: Concomitant administration of antacids may reduce plasma levels of DOLOBID. This effect is small with occasional doses of antacids, but may be clinically significant when antacids are used on a continuous schedule.

Acetaminophen: Concomitant administration of DOLOBID and acetaminophen to normal volunteers resulted in significantly increased plasma levels of acetaminophen. Acetaminophen had no effect on plasma levels of DOLOBID.

Drug Interactions: Non-steroidal Anti-inflammatory Drugs

The administration of diflunisal to normal volunteers receiving indomethacin decreased the renal clearance and significantly increased the plasma levels of indomethacin. Further, the combined use of indomethacin and DOLOBID has been associated with fatal gastrointestinal hemorrhage. Therefore, indomethacin and DOLOBID should not be used concomitantly.

Since no further clinical data are available about the safety and effectiveness of DOLOBID when used in combination with other non-steroidal anti-inflammatory drugs, no recommendation for their concomitant use can be made. The following information was obtained from studies in normal volunteers.

Aspirin: In normal volunteers, a small decrease in diflunisal levels was observed when multiple doses of DOLOBID and aspirin were administered concomitantly.

Sulindac: The concomitant administration of DOLOBID and sulindac in normal volunteers resulted in substantial but not statistically significant lowering of the plasma levels of the active sulindac sulfide metabolite.

Naproxen: The concomitant administration of DOLOBID and naproxen in normal volunteers had no effect on the plasma levels of naproxen, but significantly decreased the urinary excretion of naproxen and its glucuronide metabolite. Naproxen had no effect on plasma levels of DOLOBID.

Carcinogenesis, Mutagenesis, Impairment of Fertility

In a two-year study in the mouse, there was an apparent but not statistically significant increase in the incidence of pulmonary adenoma and hepatocellular adenoma. Since findings were inconclusive, the study is being repeated. Diflunisal did not affect the type or incidence of neoplasia in a 105-week study in the rat.

Diflunisal passes the placental barrier to a minor degree in the rat. Diflunisal had no mutagenic activity after oral administration in the dominant lethal assay, in the Ames microbial mutagen test or in the V-79 Chinese hamster lung cell assay.

No evidence of impaired fertility was found in reproduction studies in rats at doses up to 50 mg/kg/day.

Pregnancy

Pregnancy Category C. A dose of 60 mg/kg/day of diflunisal (equivalent to two times the maximum human dose) was maternotoxic, embryotoxic, and teratogenic in rabbits. In three of six studies in rabbits, evidence of teratogenicity was observed at doses ranging from 40 to 50 mg/kg/day. Teratology studies in mice, at doses up to 50 mg/kg/day, and in rats at doses up to 100 mg/kg/day, revealed no harm to the fetus due to diflunisal. Aspirin and other salicylates have been shown to be teratogenic in a wide variety of species, including the rat and rabbit, at doses ranging from 50 to 400 mg/kg/day (approximately one to eight times the human dose). There are no adequate and well controlled studies with diflunisal in pregnant women. DOLOBID should be used during the first two trimesters of pregnancy only if the potential benefit justifies the potential risk to the fetus. Because of the known effect of drugs of this class on the human fetal cardiovascular system (closure of ductus arteriosus), use during the third trimester of pregnancy is not recommended.

In rats at a dose of one and one-half times the maximum human dose, there was an increase in the average length of gestation. Similar increases in the length of gestation have been observed with aspirin, indomethacin, and phenylbutazone, and may be related to inhibition of prostaglandin synthetase. Drugs of this class may cause dystocia and delayed parturition in pregnant animals.

Nursing Mothers

Diflunisal is excreted in human milk in concentrations of 2–7% of those in plasma. Because of the potential for serious adverse reactions in nursing infants from DOLOBID, a decision should be made whether to discontinue nursing or to discontinue the drug, taking into account the importance of the drug to the mother.

Pediatric Use

The adverse effects observed following diflunisal administration to neonatal animals appear to be species, age, and dose-dependent. At dose levels approximately 3 times the usual human therapeutic dose, both aspirin (200 to 400 mg/kg/day) and diflunisal (80 mg/kg/day) resulted in death, leukocytosis, weight loss, and bilateral cataracts in neonatal (4 to 5-day-old) beagle puppies after 2 to 10 doses. Administration of an 80 mg/kg/day dose of diflunisal to 25-day-old puppies resulted in lower mortality, and did not produce cataracts. In newborn rats, a 400 mg/kg/day dose of aspirin resulted in increased mortality and some cataracts, whereas the effects of diflunisal administration at doses up to 140 mg/kg/day were limited to a decrease in average body weight gain.

Safety and effectiveness in infants and children have not been established, and use of the drug in children below the age of 12 years is not recommended.

Adverse Reactions

The adverse reactions observed in controlled clinical trials encompass observations in 2,427 patients.

Listed below are the adverse reactions reported in the 1,314 of these patients who received long-term treatment. Five hundred thirteen patients were treated for at least 24 weeks, 255 patients were treated for at least 48 weeks, and 46 patients were treated for 96 weeks. In general, the adverse reactions listed below were 2 to 14 times less frequent in the 1,113 patients who received short-term treatment for mild to moderate pain.

Incidence Greater Than 1%

Gastrointestinal

The most frequent types of adverse reactions occurring with DOLOBID are gastrointestinal: these include nausea*, vomiting, dyspepsia*, gastrointestinal pain*, diarrhea*, constipation, and flatulence.

Psychiatric

Somnolence, insomnia.

Central Nervous System

Dizziness.

Special Senses

Tinnitus.

Dermatologic

Rash*.

Miscellaneous

Headache*, fatigue/tiredness.

Incidence Less Than 1 in 100

The following adverse reactions, occurring less frequently than 1 in 100, were reported in clinical trials. The probability exists of a causal relationship between DOLOBID and these adverse reactions.

Dermatologic

Pruritus, sweating, dry mucous membranes, stomatitis.

Gastrointestinal

Peptic ulcer, gastrointestinal bleeding, anorexia, eructation.

Psychiatric

Nervousness.

Central Nervous System

Vertigo.

Miscellaneous

Asthenia, edema.

Causal Relationship Unknown

Other reactions have been reported in clinical trials or since the drug was marketed abroad, but occurred under circumstances where a causal relationship could not be established. However, in these rarely reported events, that possibility cannot be excluded. Therefore, these observations are listed to serve as alerting information to physicians.

*Incidence between 3% and 9%. Those reactions occurring in 1% to 3% are not marked with an asterisk.

Dermatologic
Erythema multiforme and Stevens-Johnson Syndrome.
Respiratory
Dyspnea.
Cardiovascular
Palpitation, syncope.
Special Senses
Transient visual disturbances.
Nervous System
Paresthesias.
Musculoskeletal
Muscle cramps.
Psychiatric
Depression.
Genitourinary
Dysuria.
Miscellaneous
Chest pain, fever, malaise, hypersensitivity (including interstitial nephritis with renal failure), anaphylactic reaction with bronchospasm.

Potential Adverse Effects

In addition, a variety of adverse effects not observed with DOLOBID in clinical trials or in marketing experience abroad, but reported with other non-steroidal analgesic/anti-inflammatory agents, should be considered potential adverse effects of DOLOBID.

Overdosage

Cases of overdosage have occurred and deaths have been reported. Most patients recovered without evidence of permanent sequelae. The most common signs and symptoms observed with overdosage were drowsiness, disorientation or stupor. A dose that is usually fatal has not yet been identified.
The oral LD_{50} of the drug is 439 and 826 mg/kg in female mice and female rats, respectively.
In the event of overdosage, the stomach should be emptied by inducing vomiting or by gastric lavage, and the patient carefully observed and given symptomatic and supportive treatment. Because of the high degree of protein binding, hemodialysis may not be effective.

Dosage and Administration

Concentration-dependent pharmacokinetics prevail when DOLOBID is administered; a doubling of dosage produces a greater than doubling of drug accumulation. The effect becomes more apparent with repetitive doses.
For mild to moderate pain, an initial dose of 1000 mg followed by 500 mg every 12 hours is recommended for most patients. Following the initial dose, some patients may require 500 mg every 8 hours.
A lower dosage may be appropriate depending on such factors as pain severity, patient response, weight, or advanced age; for example, 500 mg initially, followed by 250 mg every 8–12 hours.
For osteoarthritis, the suggested dosage range is 500 mg to 1000 mg daily in two divided doses. The dosage of DOLOBID may be increased or decreased according to patient response.
Maintenance doses higher than 1500 mg a day are not recommended.
DOLOBID may be administered with water, milk or meals. Tablets should be swallowed whole, not crushed or chewed.

How Supplied

Tablets DOLOBID are capsule-shaped, film-coated tablets supplied as follows:
No. 3390—250 mg peach colored, coded MSD 675
NDC 0006-0675-28 single unit package of 100
NDC 0006-0675-61 unit of use bottles of 60.
No. 3392—500 mg orange colored, coded MSD 697
NDC 0006-0697-28 single unit package of 100
NDC 0006-0697-61 unit of use bottles of 60.
A.H.F.S. Category: 28:08
DC 7170706 Issued July 1982

COPYRIGHT ©MERCK & CO., INC., 1980
All rights reserved

EDECRIN® Tablets ℞
(ethacrynic acid, MSD), U.S.P.
Intravenous
SODIUM EDECRIN® ℞
(ethacrynate sodium, MSD), U.S.P.

Warning

EDECRIN® (Ethacrynic Acid, MSD) is a potent diuretic which, if given in excessive amounts, may lead to profound diuresis with water and electrolyte depletion. Therefore, careful medical supervision is required, and dose and dose schedule must be adjusted to the individual patient's needs (see DOSAGE AND ADMINISTRATION).

Description

Ethacrynic acid is an unsaturated ketone derivative of an aryloxyacetic acid. Its chemical name is [2,3-dichloro-4-(2-methylenebutyryl) phenoxy]acetic acid. It is a white, or practically white, crystalline powder, only very slightly soluble in water, but is soluble in most organic solvents such as alcohols, chloroform, and benzene. The sodium salt of ethacrynic acid is soluble in water at 25°C to the extent of about 7 percent. Solutions of the sodium salt are relatively stable at about pH 7 at room temperature for short periods, but as the pH or temperature increases the solutions are less stable.

Actions

EDECRIN acts on the ascending limb of the loop of Henle and on the proximal and distal tubules. Urinary output is usually dose dependent and related to the magnitude of fluid accumulation. Water and electrolyte excretion may be increased several times over that observed with thiazide diuretics, since EDECRIN inhibits reabsorption of a much greater proportion of filtered sodium than most other diuretic agents. Therefore, EDECRIN is effective in many patients who have significant degrees of renal insufficiency (see ADDITIONAL WARNINGS concerning deafness). EDECRIN has little or no effect on glomerular filtration or on renal blood flow, except following pronounced reductions in plasma volume when associated with rapid diuresis.
The electrolyte excretion pattern of ethacrynic acid varies from that of the thiazides and mercurial diuretics. Initial sodium and chloride excretion is usually substantial and chloride loss exceeds that of sodium. With prolonged administration, chloride excretion declines, and potassium and hydrogen ion excretion may increase. EDECRIN is effective whether or not there is clinical acidosis or alkalosis.
Although EDECRIN, in carefully controlled studies in animals and experimental subjects, produces a more favorable sodium/potassium excretion ratio than the thiazides, in patients with increased diuresis excessive amounts of potassium may be excreted.
Onset of action is rapid, usually within 30 minutes after an oral dose of EDECRIN or within 5 minutes after an intravenous injection of SODIUM EDECRIN® (Ethacrynate Sodium, MSD). Duration of action following oral administration is 6 to 8 hours, with peak activity occurring in about 2 hours.
The sulfhydryl binding propensity of ethacrynic acid differs somewhat from that of the organomercurials; its mode of action is not by carbonic anhydrase inhibition.

Indications

EDECRIN is especially useful in patients who require an agent with greater diuretic potential than those commonly employed.

1. Treatment of the edema associated with congestive heart failure, cirrhosis of the liver, and renal disease, including the nephrotic syndrome.
2. Short term management of ascites due to malignancy, idiopathic edema, and lymphedema.
3. Short term management of hospitalized pediatric patients with congenital heart disease or the nephrotic syndrome. Information in infants is insufficient to recommend therapy with EDECRIN.
4. Intravenous administration of SODIUM EDECRIN is indicated when a rapid onset of diuresis is desired, e.g., in acute pulmonary edema, or when gastrointestinal absorption is impaired or oral medication is not practicable.

Contraindications

All diuretics, including ethacrynic acid, are contraindicated in anuria. If increasing electrolyte imbalance, azotemia, and/or oliguria occur during treatment of severe, progressive renal disease, the diuretic should be discontinued.
In a few patients this diuretic has produced severe, watery diarrhea. If this occurs, it should be discontinued and not readministered.
Until further experience in infants is accumulated, therapy with oral and parenteral EDECRIN is contraindicated.
See also *Use in Pregnancy* under ADDITIONAL WARNINGS.
Hypersensitivity to any component of this product.

Additional Warnings

Frequent serum electrolyte, CO_2 and BUN determinations should be performed early in therapy and periodically thereafter during active diuresis. Any electrolyte abnormalities should be corrected or the drug temporarily withdrawn.
Initiation of diuretic therapy with EDECRIN in the cirrhotic patient with ascites is best carried out in the hospital. When maintenance therapy has been established, the individual can be satisfactorily followed as an outpatient. EDECRIN should be given with caution to patients with advanced cirrhosis of the liver, particularly those with a history of previous episodes of electrolyte imbalance or hepatic encephalopathy. Like other diuretics it may precipitate hepatic coma and death.
Too vigorous a diuresis, as evidenced by rapid and excessive weight loss, may induce an acute hypotensive episode. In elderly cardiac patients, rapid contraction of plasma volume and the resultant hemoconcentration should be avoided to prevent the development of thromboembolic episodes, such as cerebral vascular thromboses and pulmonary emboli which may be fatal. Excessive loss of potassium in patients receiving digitalis glycosides may precipitate digitalis toxicity. Care should also be exercised in patients receiving potassium-depleting steroids.
The effects of EDECRIN on electrolytes are related to its renal pharmacologic activity and are dose dependent. The possibility of profound electrolyte and water loss may be avoided by weighing the patient throughout the treatment period, by careful adjustment of dosage, by initiating treatment with small doses, and by using the drug on an intermittent schedule when possible. When excessive diuresis occurs,

Continued on next page

Information on the Merck Sharp & Dohme products listed on these pages is the full prescribing information from package circulars in use October 31, 1982.

Merck Sharp & Dohme—Cont.

the drug should be withdrawn until homeostasis is restored. When excessive electrolyte loss occurs, the dosage should be reduced or the drug temporarily withdrawn.
A number of possibly drug-related deaths have occurred in critically ill patients refractory to other diuretics. These generally have fallen into two categories: (1) patients with severe myocardial disease who have been receiving digitalis and presumably developed acute hypokalemia with fatal arrhythmia; (2) patients with severely decompensated hepatic cirrhosis with ascites, with or without accompanying encephalopathy, who were in electrolyte imbalance and died because of intensification of the electrolyte defect.
Deafness, tinnitus, and vertigo with a sense of fullness in the ears have occurred, most frequently in patients with severe impairment of renal function. These symptoms have been associated most often with intravenous administration and with doses in excess of those recommended. The deafness has usually been reversible and of short duration (one to 24 hours). However, in some patients the hearing loss has been permanent. A number of these patients were also receiving drugs known to be ototoxic.
Furthermore, EDECRIN may increase the ototoxic potential of other drugs such as aminoglycoside antibiotics. Their concurrent use should be avoided.
Lithium generally should not be given with diuretics because they reduce its renal clearance and add a high risk of lithium toxicity. Read circulars for lithium preparations before use of such concomitant therapy.
Nonspecific small bowel lesions consisting of stenosis with or without ulceration may occur in association with administration of enteric coated potassium tablets alone or in conjunction with diuretic therapy. Surgery was frequently required and deaths have occurred. Therefore, enteric coated potassium tablets should not be used when supplementary potassium administration is needed.

Use in Pregnancy
EDECRIN is not recommended for use in pregnant patients. Use of the drug in women of the childbearing age requires that its potential benefits be weighed against the possible hazards to the fetus. The safety and efficacy of the drug in toxemia of pregnancy have not been established. EDECRIN is contraindicated in nursing mothers. If use of the drug is deemed essential, the patient should stop nursing.

Precautions

Weakness, muscle cramps, paresthesias, thirst, anorexia, and signs of hyponatremia, hypokalemia, and/or hypochloremic alkalosis may occur following vigorous or excessive diuresis and these may be accentuated by rigid salt restriction. Rarely tetany has been reported following vigorous diuresis. *During therapy with ethacrynic acid, liberalization of salt intake and supplementary potassium chloride are often necessary.*
When a metabolic alkalosis may be anticipated, e.g., in cirrhosis with ascites, the use of potassium chloride with or without an aldosterone antagonist before and continuously during therapy with EDECRIN may mitigate or prevent the hypokalemia.
The safety and efficacy of ethacrynic acid in hypertension have not been established. However, the dosage of coadministered antihypertensive agents may require adjustment.
Orthostatic hypotension may occur in patients receiving other antihypertensive agents when given ethacrynic acid.
EDECRIN has little or no effect on glomerular filtration or on renal blood flow, except following pronounced reductions in plasma volume when associated with rapid diuresis. A transient increase in serum urea nitrogen may occur. Usually, this is readily reversible when the drug is discontinued.
As with other diuretics used in the treatment of renal edema, hypoproteinemia may reduce responsiveness to ethacrynic acid and the use of salt-poor albumin should be considered.
A number of drugs, including ethacrynic acid, have been shown to displace warfarin from plasma protein; a reduction in the usual anticoagulant dosage may be required in patients receiving both drugs.
EDECRIN may increase the risk of gastric hemorrhage associated with corticosteroid treatment.

Adverse Reactions

Gastrointestinal
Anorexia, malaise, abdominal discomfort or pain, dysphagia, nausea, vomiting, and diarrhea have occurred. These are more frequent with large doses or after one to three months of continuous therapy. A few patients have had sudden onset of watery, profuse diarrhea. Discontinue EDECRIN if diarrhea is severe and do not readminister it. Gastrointestinal bleeding has occurred in some patients.
Rarely, acute pancreatitis has been reported in patients receiving diuretics, including EDECRIN.
Renal
Reversible hyperuricemia and acute gout have been reported. Acute symptomatic hypoglycemia with convulsions occurred in two uremic patients who received doses above those recommended.
Carbohydrate Metabolism
Hyperglycemia has been reported in a few patients, most of whom had decompensated cirrhosis. However, patients who developed hyperglycemia on thiazide therapy have not done so when given EDECRIN.
Hemopoietic System
Agranulocytosis or severe neutropenia has been reported in a few critically ill patients also receiving agents known to produce this effect. Thrombocytopenia has been reported rarely. Rare instances of Henoch-Schönlein purpura have been reported in patients with rheumatic heart disease receiving many drugs, including EDECRIN.
Hepatic
Rarely, jaundice and abnormal liver function tests have been reported in seriously ill patients on multiple drug therapy that included EDECRIN.
Miscellaneous
Deafness, tinnitus, and vertigo, with a sense of fullness in the ears, have occurred (see ADDITIONAL WARNINGS). Infrequently, skin rash, headache, fever, chills, hematuria, blurred vision, fatigue, apprehension, and confusion have occurred.
SODIUM EDECRIN occasionally has caused local irritation and pain after intravenous use.

Dosage and Administration

Dosage must be regulated carefully to prevent a more rapid or substantial loss of fluid or electrolyte than is indicated or necessary. The magnitude of diuresis and natriuresis is largely dependent on the degree of fluid accumulation present in the patient. Similarly, the extent of potassium excretion is determined in large measure by the presence and magnitude of aldosteronism.
Oral Use
EDECRIN is available for oral use as 25 mg and 50 mg tablets.
Dosage: To Initiate Diuresis
The smallest dose required to produce gradual weight loss (about 1 to 2 pounds per day) is recommended. Onset of diuresis usually occurs at 50 to 100 mg for adults. After diuresis has been achieved, the minimally effective dose (usually from 50 to 200 mg daily) may be given on a continuous or intermittent dosage schedule. Dosage adjustments are usually in 25 to 50 mg increments to avoid derangement of water and electrolyte excretion.
The patient should be weighed under standard conditions before and during the institution of diuretic therapy with this compound. Small alterations in dose should effectively prevent a massive diuretic response. The following schedule may be helpful in determining the smallest effective dose.

Day 1— 50 mg (single dose) after a meal
Day 2— 50 mg twice daily after meals, if necessary
Day 3— 100 mg in the morning and 50 to 100 mg following the afternoon or evening meal, depending upon response to the morning dose

A few patients may require initial and maintenance doses as high as 200 mg twice daily. These higher doses, which should be achieved gradually, are most often required in patients with severe, refractory edema.
In children, the initial dose should be 25 mg. Careful stepwise increments in dosage of 25 mg should be made to achieve effective maintenance. A dosage for *infants* has not been established.

Maintenance Therapy
It is usually possible to reduce the dosage and frequency of administration once dry weight has been achieved.
EDECRIN (Ethacrynic Acid, MSD) may be given intermittently after an effective diuresis is obtained with the regimen outlined above. Dosage may be on an alternate daily schedule or more prolonged periods of diuretic therapy may be interspersed with rest periods. Such an intermittent dosage schedule allows time for correction of any electrolyte imbalance and may provide a more efficient diuretic response.
The chloruretic effect of this agent may give rise to retention of bicarbonate and a metabolic alkalosis. This may be corrected by giving chloride (ammonium chloride or arginine chloride). Ammonium chloride should not be given to cirrhotic patients.
EDECRIN has additive effects when used with other diuretics. For example, a patient who is on maintenance dosage of an oral diuretic may require additional intermittent diuretic therapy, such as an organomercurial, for the maintenance of basal weight. The intermittent use of EDECRIN orally may eliminate the need for injections of organomercurials. Small doses of EDECRIN may be added to existing diuretic regimens to maintain basal weight. This drug may potentiate the action of carbonic anhydrase inhibitors, with augmentation of natriuresis and kaliuresis. Therefore, when adding EDECRIN the initial dose and changes of dose should be in 25 mg increments, to avoid electrolyte depletion. Rarely, patients who failed to respond to ethacrynic acid have responded to older established agents.
While many patients do not require supplemental potassium, the use of potassium chloride or aldosterone antagonists, or both, during treatment with EDECRIN is advisable, especially in cirrhotic or nephrotic patients and in patients receiving digitalis.
Salt liberalization usually prevents the development of hyponatremia and hypochloremia. During treatment with EDECRIN, salt may be liberalized to a greater extent than with other diuretics. Cirrhotic patients, however, usually require at least moderate salt restriction concomitant with diuretic therapy.

Intravenous Use
INTRAVENOUS SODIUM EDECRIN is for intravenous use when oral intake is impractical or in urgent conditions, such as acute pulmonary edema.

Each vial contains:
Ethacrynate sodium equivalent
to ethacrynate acid .... 50 mg
Inactive ingredients:
Mannitol ....62.5 mg
with 0.1 mg thimerosal added as preservative

The usual intravenous dose for the average sized adult is 50 mg, or 0.5 to 1.0 mg per kg of body weight. Usually only one dose has been necessary; occasionally a second dose at a new injection site, to avoid possible thrombophlebitis, may be required. A single intravenous dose not exceeding 100 mg has been used in critical situations. Insufficient pediatric experience precludes recommendation for this age group.
To reconstitute the dry material, add 50 ml of 5 percent Dextrose Injection, or Sodium Chloride Injection to the vial. Occasionally, some 5 percent Dextrose Injection solutions may have a low pH (below 5). The resulting solution with such a diluent may be hazy or opalescent. Intravenous use of such a solution is not recommended.
The solution may be given slowly through the tubing of a running infusion or by direct intravenous injection over a period of several minutes. Do not mix this solution with whole blood or its derivatives. Discard unused reconstituted solution after 24 hours.
SODIUM EDECRIN should not be given subcutaneously or intramuscularly because of local pain and irritation.

How Supplied

No. 3321—Tablets EDECRIN, 25 mg, are white, capsule shaped, scored tablets, coded MSD 65. They are supplied as follows:
NDC 0006-0065-68 in bottles of 100
[*Shown in Product Identification Section*]
No. 3322—Tablets EDECRIN, 50 mg, are green, capsule shaped, scored tablets, coded MSD 90. They are supplied as follows:
NDC 0006-0090-68 in bottles of 100
(6505-00-834-0473 50 mg 100's)
[*Shown in Product Identification Section*]
No. 3330—INTRAVENOUS SODIUM EDECRIN is a dry white material either in a plug form or as a powder. It is supplied in vials containing ethacrynate sodium equivalent to 50 mg of ethacrynic acid, **NDC** 0006-3330-50.
(6505-00-875-7941 50 mg 50 ml vial)
A.H.F.S. Category: 40:28
DC 6073020 Issued September 1980

ELAVIL® Tablets (amitriptyline HCl, MSD), U.S.P. ℞
ELAVIL® Injection (amitriptyline HCl, MSD), U.S.P. ℞

Description

Amitriptyline HCl, a dibenzocycloheptadiene derivative, is a white or practically white, crystalline compound that is freely soluble in water.
It is designated chemically as 10,11-dihydro-*N,N*-dimethyl-5*H*-dibenzo [*a,d*] cycloheptene-Δ^5,γ-propylamine hydrochloride. The molecular weight is 313.87. The empirical formula is $C_{20}H_{23}N{\bullet}HCl$.
ELAVIL® (Amitriptyline HCl, MSD) is supplied as 10 mg, 25 mg, 50 mg, 75 mg, 100 mg, and 150 mg tablets and as a sterile solution for intramuscular use. Each milliliter of the sterile solution contains:
Amitriptyline hydrochloride....................10 mg
Dextrose ....44 mg
Water for Injection, q.s. ....1 ml
Added as preservatives:
Methylparaben ....1.5 mg
Propylparaben ....0.2 mg

Actions

ELAVIL is an antidepressant with sedative effects. Its mechanism of action in man is not known. It is not a monoamine oxidase inhibitor and it does not act primarily by stimulation of the central nervous system.
Amitriptyline inhibits the membrane pump mechanism responsible for uptake of norepinephrine and serotonin in adrenergic and serotonergic neurons. Pharmacologically this action may potentiate or prolong neuronal activity since reuptake of these biogenic amines is important physiologically in terminating transmitting activity. This interference with the reuptake of norepinephrine and/or serotonin is believed by some to underlie the antidepressant activity of amitriptyline.

Indications

For the relief of symptoms of depression. Endogenous depression is more likely to be alleviated than are other depressive states.

Contraindications

ELAVIL is contraindicated in patients who have shown prior hypersensitivity to it.
It should not be given concomitantly with monoamine oxidase inhibitors. Hyperpyretic crises, severe convulsions, and deaths have occurred in patients receiving tricyclic antidepressant and monoamine oxidase inhibiting drugs simultaneously. When it is desired to replace a monoamine oxidase inhibitor with ELAVIL, a minimum of 14 days should be allowed to elapse after the former is discontinued. ELAVIL should then be initiated cautiously with gradual increase in dosage until optimum response is achieved.
This drug is not recommended for use during the acute recovery phase following myocardial infarction.

Warnings

ELAVIL may block the antihypertensive action of guanethidine or similarly acting compounds.
It should be used with caution in patients with a history of seizures and, because of its atropine-like action, in patients with a history of urinary retention, angle-closure glaucoma or increased intraocular pressure. In patients with angle-closure glaucoma, even average doses may precipitate an attack.
Patients with cardiovascular disorders should be watched closely. Tricyclic antidepressant drugs, including ELAVIL, particularly when given in high doses, have been reported to produce arrhythmias, sinus tachycardia, and prolongation of the conduction time. Myocardial infarction and stroke have been reported with drugs of this class.
Close supervision is required when ELAVIL is given to hyperthyroid patients or those receiving thyroid medication.
This drug may impair mental and/or physical abilities required for performance of hazardous tasks, such as operating machinery or driving a motor vehicle.
ELAVIL may enhance the response to alcohol and the effects of barbiturates and other CNS depressants. In patients who may use alcohol excessively, it should be borne in mind that the potentiation may increase the danger inherent in any suicide attempt or overdosage.
Usage in Pregnancy—Safe use of ELAVIL during pregnancy and lactation has not been established; therefore, in administering the drug to pregnant patients, nursing mothers, or women who may become pregnant, the possible benefits must be weighed against the possible hazards to mother and child.
Animal reproduction studies have been inconclusive and clinical experience has been limited.
Usage in Children—In view of the lack of experience with the use of this drug in children, it is not recommended at the present time for patients under 12 years of age.

Precautions

Schizophrenic patients may develop increased symptoms of psychosis; patients with paranoid symptomatology may have an exaggeration of such symptoms. Depressed patients, particularly those with known manic-depressive illness, may experience a shift to mania or hypomania. In these circumstances the dose of amitriptyline may be reduced or a major tranquilizer such as perphenazine may be administered concurrently.
When ELAVIL is given with anticholinergic agents or sympathomimetic drugs, including epinephrine combined with local anesthetics, close supervision and careful adjustment of dosages are required.
Paralytic ileus may occur in patients taking tricyclic antidepressants in combination with anticholinergic-type drugs.
Caution is advised if patients receive large doses of ethchlorvynol concurrently. Transient delirium has been reported in patients who were treated with one gram of ethchlorvynol and 75-150 mg of ELAVIL.
The possibility of suicide in depressed patients remains until significant remission occurs. Potentially suicidal patients should not have access to large quantities of this drug. Prescriptions should be written for the smallest amount feasible.
Concurrent administration of ELAVIL and electroshock therapy may increase the hazards associated with such therapy. Such treatment should be limited to patients for whom it is essential.
When possible, the drug should be discontinued several days before elective surgery.
Both elevation and lowering of blood sugar levels have been reported.
ELAVIL should be used with caution in patients with impaired liver function.

Adverse Reactions

Note: Included in the listing which follows are a few adverse reactions which have not been reported with this specific drug. However, pharmacological similarities among the tricyclic antidepressant drugs require that each of the reactions be considered when amitriptyline is administered.
Cardiovascular: Hypotension, particularly orthostatic hypotension; hypertension; tachycardia; palpitation; myocardial infarction; arrhythmias; heart block; stroke.
CNS and Neuromuscular: Confusional states; disturbed concentration; disorientation; delusions; hallucinations; excitement; anxiety; restlessness; insomnia; nightmares; numbness, tingling, and paresthesias of the extremities; peripheral neuropathy; incoordination; ataxia; tremors; seizures; alteration in EEG patterns; extrapyramidal symptoms; tinnitus; syndrome of inappropriate ADH (antidiuretic hormone) secretion.
Anticholinergic: Dry mouth, blurred vision, disturbance of accommodation, increased intraocular pressure, constipation, paralytic ileus, urinary retention, dilatation of urinary tract.
Allergic: Skin rash, urticaria, photosensitization, edema of face and tongue.
Hematologic: Bone marrow depression including agranulocytosis, leukopenia, eosinophilia, purpura, thrombocytopenia.
Gastrointestinal: Nausea, epigastric distress, vomiting, anorexia, stomatitis, peculiar taste, diarrhea, parotid swelling, black tongue. Rarely hepatitis (including altered liver function and jaundice).
Endocrine: Testicular swelling and gynecomastia in the male, breast enlargement and

Continued on next page

Information on the Merck Sharp & Dohme products listed on these pages is the full prescribing information from package circulars in use October 31, 1982.

Merck Sharp & Dohme—Cont.

galactorrhea in the female, increased or decreased libido, elevation and lowering of blood sugar levels.
Other: Dizziness, weakness, fatigue, headache, weight gain or loss, edema, increased perspiration, urinary frequency, mydriasis, drowsiness, alopecia.
Withdrawal Symptoms: Abrupt cessation of treatment after prolonged administration may produce nausea, headache, and malaise. These are not indicative of addiction. Rare instances have been reported of mania or hypomania occurring within 2–7 days following cessation of chronic therapy with tricyclic antidepressants.

Dosage and Administration

Oral Dosage
Dosage should be initiated at a low level and increased gradually, noting carefully the clinical response and any evidence of intolerance.
Initial Dosage for Adults—For outpatients 75 mg of amitriptyline HCl a day in divided doses usually is satisfactory. If necessary, this may be increased to a total of 150 mg per day. Increases are made preferably in the late afternoon and/or bedtime doses. A sedative effect may be apparent before the antidepressant effect is noted, but an adequate therapeutic effect may take as long as 30 days to develop. An alternate method of initiating therapy in outpatients is to begin with 50 to 100 mg amitriptyline HCl at bedtime. This may be increased by 25 or 50 mg as necessary in the bedtime dose to a total of 150 mg per day.
Hospitalized patients may require 100 mg a day initially. This can be increased gradually to 200 mg a day if necessary. A small number of hospitalized patients may need as much as 300 mg a day.
Adolescent and Elderly Patients—In general, lower dosages are recommended for these patients. Ten mg 3 times a day with 20 mg at bedtime may be satisfactory in adolescent and elderly patients who do not tolerate higher dosages.
Maintenance—The usual maintenance dosage of amitriptyline HCl is 50 to 100 mg per day. In some patients 40 mg per day is sufficient. For maintenance therapy the total daily dosage may be given in a single dose preferably at bedtime. When satisfactory improvement has been reached, dosage should be reduced to the lowest amount that will maintain relief of symptoms. It is appropriate to continue maintenance therapy 3 months or longer to lessen the possibility of relapse.
Intramuscular Dosage
Initially, 20 to 30 mg (2 to 3 ml) four times a day.
When ELAVIL injection is administered intramuscularly, the effects may appear more rapidly than with oral administration.
When ELAVIL injection is used for initial therapy in patients unable or unwilling to take ELAVIL tablets, the tablets should replace the injection as soon as possible.
Usage in Children
In view of the lack of experience with the use of this drug in children, it is not recommended at the present time for patients under 12 years of age.
Plasma Levels
Because of the wide variation in the absorption and distribution of tricyclic antidepressants in body fluids, it is difficult to directly correlate plasma levels and therapeutic effect. However, determination of plasma levels may be useful in identifying patients who appear to have toxic effects and may have excessively high levels, or those in whom lack of absorption or noncompliance is suspected. Adjustments in dosage should be made according to the patient's clinical response and not on the basis of plasma levels.*

Overdosage

Manifestations—High doses may cause temporary confusion, disturbed concentration, or transient visual hallucinations. Overdosage may cause drowsiness; hypothermia; tachycardia and other arrhythmic abnormalities, such as bundle branch block; ECG evidence of impaired conduction; congestive heart failure; dilated pupils; disorders of ocular motility; convulsions; severe hypotension; stupor; and coma. Other symptoms may be agitation, hyperactive reflexes, muscle rigidity, vomiting, hyperpyrexia, or any of those listed under ADVERSE REACTIONS.
All patients suspected of having taken an overdosage should be admitted to a hospital as soon as possible. *Treatment* is symptomatic and supportive. Empty the stomach as quickly as possible by emesis followed by gastric lavage upon arrival at the hospital. Following gastric lavage, activated charcoal may be administered. Twenty to 30 g of activated charcoal may be given every four to six hours during the first 24 to 48 hours after ingestion. An ECG should be taken and close monitoring of cardiac function instituted if there is any sign of abnormality. Maintain an open airway and adequate fluid intake; regulate body temperature.
The intravenous administration of 1–3 mg of physostigmine salicylate is reported to reverse the symptoms of tricyclic antidepressant poisoning. Because physostigmine is rapidly metabolized, the dosage of physostigmine should be repeated as required particularly if life threatening signs such as arrhythmias, convulsions, and deep coma recur or persist after the initial dosage of physostigmine. Because physostigmine itself may be toxic, it is not recommended for routine use.
Standard measures should be used to manage circulatory shock and metabolic acidosis. Cardiac arrhythmias may be treated with neostigmine, pyridostigmine, or propranolol. Should cardiac failure occur, the use of digitalis should be considered. Close monitoring of cardiac function for not less than five days is advisable. Anticonvulsants may be given to control convulsions. Amitriptyline increases the CNS depressant action but not the anticonvulsant action of barbiturates; therefore, an inhalation anesthetic, diazepam, or paraldehyde is recommended for control of convulsions.
Dialysis is of no value because of low plasma concentrations of the drug.
Since overdosage is often deliberate, patients may attempt suicide by other means during the recovery phase.
Deaths by deliberate or accidental overdosage have occurred with this class of drugs.

How Supplied

No. 3287—Tablets ELAVIL, 10 mg, are blue, round, film coated tablets, coded MSD 23. They are supplied as follows:
NDC 0006-0023-68 bottles of 100
(6505-00-079-7453, 10 mg 100's)
NDC 0006-0023-28 single unit packages of 100
NDC 0006-0023-82 bottles of 1000
NDC 0006-0023-86 bottles of 5000.
[*Shown in Product Identification Section*]
No. 3288—Tablets ELAVIL, 25 mg, are yellow, round, film coated tablets, coded MSD 45. They are supplied as follows:
NDC 0006-0045-68 bottles of 100
(6505-00-082-2659, 25 mg 100's)
NDC 0006-0045-28 single unit packages of 100
(6505-00-118-2509, 25 mg individually sealed 100's)
NDC 0006-0045-82 bottles of 1000
(6505-00-724-6358, 25 mg 1000's)
NDC 0006-0045-86 bottles of 5000.
[*Shown in Product Identification Section*]
No. 3320—Tablets ELAVIL, 50 mg, are beige, round, film coated tablets, coded MSD 102. They are supplied as follows:
NDC 0006-0102-68 bottles of 100
NDC 0006-0102-28 single unit packages of 100
NDC 0006-0102-82 bottles of 1000.
[*Shown in Product Identification Section*]
No. 3348—Tablets ELAVIL, 75 mg, are orange, round, film coated tablets, coded MSD 430. They are supplied as follows:
NDC 0006-0430-68 bottles of 100
NDC 0006-0430-28 single unit packages of 100.
[*Shown in Product Identification Section*]
No. 3349—Tablets ELAVIL, 100 mg, are mauve, round, film coated tablets, coded MSD 435. They are supplied as follows:
NDC 0006-0435-68 bottles of 100
NDC 0006-0435-28 single unit packages of 100.
[*Shown in Product Identification Section*]
No. 3351—Tablets ELAVIL, 150 mg, are blue, capsule shaped, film coated tablets, coded MSD 673. They are supplied as follows:
NDC 0006-0673-30 bottles of 30
NDC 0006-0673-68 bottles of 100
NDC 0006-0673-28 single unit packages of 100.
[*Shown in Product Identification Section*]
No. 3286—Injection ELAVIL, 10 mg/ml, is a clear, colorless solution, and is supplied as follows:
NDC 0006-3286-10 in 10 ml vials.

Metabolism

Studies in man following oral administration of ^{14}C-labeled drug indicated that amitriptyline is rapidly absorbed and metabolized. Radioactivity of the plasma was practically negligible, although significant amounts of radioactivity appeared in the urine by 4 to 6 hours and one-half to one-third of the drug was excreted within 24 hours.
Amitriptyline is metabolized by N-demethylation and bridge hydroxylation in man, rabbit, and rat. Virtually the entire dose is excreted as glucuronide or sulfate conjugate of metabolites, with little unchanged drug appearing in the urine. Other metabolic pathways may be involved.

A.H.F.S. Category: 28:16:04
DC 6613122 Issued October 1981

*Hollister, L. E., J. Amer. Med. Ass. *241:* 2530–2533, June 8, 1979.

ELSPAR® ℞
(asparaginase, MSD)

Warning

IT IS RECOMMENDED THAT ASPARAGINASE BE ADMINISTERED TO PATIENTS ONLY IN A HOSPITAL SETTING UNDER THE SUPERVISION OF A PHYSICIAN WHO IS QUALIFIED BY TRAINING AND EXPERIENCE TO ADMINISTER CANCER CHEMOTHERAPEUTIC AGENTS, BECAUSE OF THE POSSIBILITY OF SEVERE REACTIONS, INCLUDING ANAPHYLAXIS AND SUDDEN DEATH. THE PHYSICIAN MUST BE PREPARED TO TREAT ANAPHYLAXIS AT EACH ADMINISTRATION OF THE DRUG.
IN THE TREATMENT OF EACH PATIENT THE PHYSICIAN MUST WEIGH CAREFULLY THE POSSIBILITY OF ACHIEVING THERAPEUTIC BENEFIT VERSUS THE RISK OF TOXICITY. THE FOLLOWING DATA SHOULD BE THOROUGHLY REVIEWED BEFORE ADMINISTERING THE COMPOUND.

Description

ELSPAR® (Asparaginase, MSD) contains the enzyme L-asparagine amidohydrolase, type EC-2, derived from *Escherichia coli.* It is a white crystalline powder that is freely soluble in water and practically insoluble in methanol, acetone and chloroform. Its activity is expressed in terms of International Units (I.U.) according to the recommendation of the International Union of Biochemistry. The specific activity of ELSPAR is at least 225 I.U. per milligram of protein and each vial contains 10,000 I.U. of asparaginase and 80 mg of mannitol, an inactive ingredient, as a sterile, white lyophilized plug or powder for intravenous or intramuscular injection after reconstitution.

Clinical Pharmacology

Action
In a significant number of patients with acute leukemia, particularly lymphocytic, the malignant cells are dependent on an exogenous source of asparagine for survival. Normal cells, however, are able to synthesize asparagine and thus are affected less by the rapid depletion produced by treatment with the enzyme asparaginase. This is a unique approach to therapy based on a metabolic defect in asparagine synthesis of some malignant cells. ELSPAR, derived from *Escherichia coli*, is effective in inducing remissions in some patients with acute lymphocytic leukemia.

Asparagine Dependence Test
An asparagine dependence test has been utilized during the investigational studies. In this test leukemic cells obtained from some marrow cultures could be shown to require asparagine *in vitro*, suggesting sensitivity to asparaginase therapy *in vivo*. However, present data indicate that the correlation between asparagine dependence in such tests and the final response to therapy is sufficiently poor that the test is not recommended as a basis for selection of patients for treatment.

Pharmacokinetics and Metabolism
In a study in patients with metastatic cancer and leukemia, initial plasma levels of L-asparaginase following intravenous administration were correlated to dose. Daily administration resulted in a cumulative increase in plasma levels. Plasma half-life varied from 8 to 30 hours; it did not appear to be influenced by dosage, either single or repetitive, and could not be correlated with age, sex, surface area, renal or hepatic function, diagnosis or extent of disease. Apparent volume of distribution was approximately 70–80% of estimated plasma volume. There was some slow movement of asparaginase from vascular to extravascular, extracellular space. L-asparaginase was detected in the lymph. Cerebrospinal fluid levels were less than 1% of concurrent plasma levels. Only trace amounts appeared in the urine.
In a study in which patients with leukemia and metastatic cancer received intramuscular L-asparaginase, peak plasma levels of asparaginase were reached 14 to 24 hours after dosing. Plasma half-life was 39 to 49 hours. No asparaginase was detected in the urine.

Indications and Usage

ELSPAR is indicated in the therapy of patients with acute lymphocytic leukemia. This agent is useful primarily in combination with other chemotherapeutic agents in the induction of remissions of the disease in children. ELSPAR should not be used as the sole induction agent unless combination therapy is deemed inappropriate. ELSPAR is not recommended for maintenance therapy.

Contraindications

ELSPAR is contraindicated in patients with pancreatitis or a history of pancreatitis. Acute hemorrhagic pancreatitis, in some instances fatal, has been reported following asparaginase administration. Asparaginase is also contraindicated in patients who have had previous anaphylactic reactions to it.

Warnings

Allergic reactions to asparaginase are frequent and may occur during the primary course of therapy. They are not completely predictable on the basis of the intradermal skin test. Anaphylaxis and death have occurred even in a hospital setting with experienced observers. Once a patient has received ELSPAR as part of a treatment regimen, retreatment with this agent at a later time is associated with increased risk of hypersensitivity reactions. In patients found by skin testing to be hypersensitive to asparaginase, and in any patient who has received a previous course of therapy with asparaginase, therapy with this agent should be instituted or reinstituted only after successful desensitization, and then only if in the judgement of the physician the possible benefit is greater than the increased risk. Desensitization itself may be hazardous. (See DOSAGE AND ADMINISTRATION, *Intradermal Skin Test.*)
In view of the unpredictability of the adverse reactions to asparaginase, it is recommended that this product be used in a hospital setting.
Asparaginase has an adverse effect on liver function in the majority of patients. Therapy with asparaginase may increase pre-existing liver impairment caused by prior therapy or the underlying disease. Because of this there is a possibility that asparaginase may increase the toxicity of other medications.
The administration of ELSPAR *intravenously concurrently with or immediately before* a course of vincristine and prednisone may be associated with increased toxicity. (See DOSAGE AND ADMINISTRATION, *Recommended Induction Regimens.*)

Precautions

General
Asparaginase has been reported to have immunosuppressive activity in animal experiments. Accordingly, the possibility that use of the drug in man may predispose to infection should be considered.
Asparaginase toxicity is reported to be greater in adults than in children.

Laboratory Tests
The fall in circulating lymphoblasts often is quite marked; normal or below normal leukocyte counts are noted frequently within the first several days after initiating therapy. This may be accompanied by a marked rise in serum uric acid. The possible development of uric acid nephropathy should be borne in mind. Appropriate preventive measures should be taken, e.g., allopurinol, increased fluid intake, alkalization of urine. As a guide to the effects of therapy, the patient's peripheral blood count and bone marrow should be monitored frequently.
Frequent serum amylase determinations should be obtained to detect early evidence of pancreatitis. If pancreatitis occurs, therapy should be stopped and not reinstituted.
Blood sugar should be monitored during therapy with ELSPAR because hyperglycemia may occur.

Drug Interactions
Tissue culture and animal studies indicate that ELSPAR can diminish or abolish the effect of methotrexate on malignant cells. This effect on methotrexate activity persists as long as plasma asparagine levels are suppressed. These results would seem to dictate against the clinical use of methotrexate with ELSPAR, or during the period following ELSPAR therapy when plasma asparagine levels are below normal.

Drug/Laboratory Test Interactions
L-asparaginase has been reported to interfere with the interpretation of thyroid function tests by producing a rapid and marked reduction in serum concentrations of thyroxine-binding globulin within two days after the first dose. Serum concentrations of thyroxine-binding globulin returned to pretreatment values within four weeks of the last dose of L-asparaginase.

Animal Toxicology
A one-month intravenous toxicity study of ELSPAR in dogs at doses of 250, 1000, and 2000 I.U./kg/day revealed reduced serum total protein and albumin with loss of body weight at the highest dose level and anorexia, emesis, and diarrhea at all dosage levels. A similar study in monkeys at doses of 100, 300, and 1000 I.U./kg/day also revealed reduction of serum total protein and albumin and body weight loss at all dosage levels. Bromsulfalein retention and fatty changes in the liver were noted in monkeys that were given 300 and 1000 I.U./kg/day. The rabbit was unusually sensitive to ELSPAR since a single intravenous dose of 1000 I.U./kg caused hypocalcemia associated with necrosis of the parathyroid cells, convulsions, and death in about one third of the animals. Some rabbits that died showed small thymic and lymph node hemorrhages and necrosis of the germinal centers in the lymph nodes and spleen. The intravenous administration of calcium gluconate alleviated or prevented the adverse effects.
Changes in the pancreatic islets (not pancreatitis) ranging from edema to necrosis were observed in the rabbits in the acute intravenous toxicity studies (doses of 12,500 to 50,000 I.U./kg) but not in rabbits that received 1000 I.U./kg. The anatomical changes and the hypocalcemia found in the rabbits were not observed in the subacute intravenous studies in the dogs and monkeys.

Carcinogenesis, Mutagenesis, Impairment of Fertility
The intraperitoneal injection of 2500 I.U./kg/day for 4 days in newborn Swiss mice resulted in a small increase in pulmonary adenomas; lymphatic leukemia was not increased.
L-asparaginase at concentrations of 152-909 I.U./plate was not mutagenic in the Ames microbial mutagen test with or without metabolic activation.
There are no adequate studies on the effects of asparaginase on fertility.

Pregnancy
Pregnancy Category C. In mice and rats ELSPAR has been shown to retard the weight gain of mothers and fetuses when given in doses of more than 1000 I.U./kg (the recommended human dose). Resorptions, gross abnormalities and skeletal abnormalities were observed. The intravenous administration of 50 or 100 I.U./kg (one-twentieth or one-tenth of the human dose) to pregnant rabbits on Day 8 and 9 of gestation resulted in dose dependent embryotoxicity and gross abnormalities. There are no adequate and well-controlled studies in pregnant women. ELSPAR should be used during pregnancy only if the potential benefit justifies the potential risk to the fetus.

Nursing Mothers
It is not known whether this drug is secreted in human milk. Because many drugs are secreted in human milk and because of the potential for serious adverse reactions in nursing infants from ELSPAR, a decision should be made whether to discontinue nursing or to discontinue the drug, taking into account the importance of the drug to the mother.

Adverse Reactions

Allergic reactions, including skin rashes, urticaria, arthralgia, respiratory distress, and acute anaphylaxis have been reported. (See

Continued on next page

Information on the Merck Sharp & Dohme products listed on these pages is the full prescribing information from package circulars in use October 31, 1982.

Merck Sharp & Dohme—Cont.

WARNINGS.) Acute reactions have occurred in the absence of a positive skin test and during continued maintenance of therapeutic serum levels of ELSPAR.

In children with advanced leukemia, a lower incidence of anaphylaxis has been reported with intramuscular administration, although there was a higher incidence of milder hypersensitivity reactions than with intravenous administration.

Fatal hyperthermia has been reported.

Pancreatitis, sometimes fulminant, has occurred during or following therapy with ELSPAR.

Hyperglycemia with glucosuria and polyuria has been reported in low incidence. Serum and urine acetone usually have been absent or negligible in these patients; this syndrome thus resembles hyperosmolar, nonketotic, hyperglycemia induced by a variety of other agents. This complication usually responds to discontinuance of ELSPAR, judicious use of intravenous fluid, and insulin, but may be fatal on occasion.

In addition to hypofibrinogenemia, depression of various other clotting factors has been reported. Most marked has been a decrease in plasma levels of factors V and VIII with a variable decrease in factors VII and IX. A decrease in circulating platelets has occurred in low incidence which, together with the increased levels of fibrin degradation products in the serum, may indicate development of a consumption coagulopathy. Bleeding has been a problem in only a minority of patients with demonstrable coagulopathy. However, fatal bleeding associated with low fibrinogen levels has been reported. Increased fibrinolytic activity, apparently compensatory in nature, also has occurred.

Some patients have shown central nervous system effects consisting of depression, somnolence, fatigue, coma, confusion, agitation, and hallucinations varying from mild to severe. Rarely, a Parkinson-like syndrome has occurred, with tremor and a progressive increase in muscular tone. These side effects usually have reversed spontaneously after treatment was stopped. Therapy with ELSPAR is associated with an increase in blood ammonia during the conversion of asparagine to asparatic acid by the enzyme. No clear correlation exists between the degree of elevation of blood ammonia levels and the appearance of CNS changes.

Chills, fever, nausea, vomiting, anorexia, abdominal cramps, weight loss, headache, and irritability may occur and usually are mild.

Azotemia, usually pre-renal, occurs frequently. Acute renal shut down and fatal renal insufficiency have been reported during treatment. Proteinuria has occurred infrequently.

A variety of liver function abnormalities have been reported, including elevations of SGOT, SGPT, alkaline phosphatase, bilirubin (direct and indirect), and depression of serum albumin, cholesterol (total and esters), and plasma fibrinogen. Increases and decreases of total lipids have occurred. Marked hypoalbuminemia associated with peripheral edema has been reported. However, these abnormalities usually are reversible on discontinuance of therapy and some reversal may occur during the course of therapy. Fatty changes in the liver have been documented by biopsy. Malabsorption syndrome has been reported.

Rarely, transient bone marrow depression has been observed, as evidenced by a delay in return of hemoglobin or hematocrit levels to normal in patients undergoing hematologic remission of leukemia. Marked leukopenia has been reported.

Overdosage

The acute intravenous LD_{50} of ELSPAR for mice was about 500,000 I.U./kg and for rabbits about 22,000 I.U./kg.

Dosage and Administration

As a component of selected multiple agent induction regimens, ELSPAR may be administered by either the intravenous or the intramuscular route. When administered intravenously this enzyme should be given over a period of not less than thirty minutes through the side arm of an already running infusion of Sodium Chloride Injection or Dextrose Injection 5% (D_5W). ELSPAR has little tendency to cause phlebitis when given intravenously. Anaphylactic reactions require the immediate use of epinephrine, oxygen, and intravenous steroids.

When administering ELSPAR intramuscularly, the volume at a single injection site should be limited to 2 ml. If a volume greater than 2 ml is to be administered two injection sites should be used.

Unfavorable interactions of ELSPAR with some antitumor agents have been demonstrated. It is recommended therefore, that ELSPAR be used in combination regimens only by physicians familiar with the benefits and risks of a given regimen. During the period of its inhibition of protein synthesis and cell replication ELSPAR may interfere with the action of drugs such as methotrexate which require cell replication for their lethal effect. ELSPAR may interfere with the enzymatic detoxification of other drugs, particularly in the liver.

Recommended Induction Regimens:

When using chemotherapeutic agents in combination for the induction of remissions in patients with acute lymphocytic leukemia, regimens are sought which provide maximum chance of success while avoiding excessive cumulative toxicity or negative drug interactions.

One of the following combination regimens incorporating ELSPAR is recommended for acute lymphocytic leukemia in children:

In the regimens below, Day 1 is considered to be the first day of therapy.

Regimen I

Prednisone 40 mg/square meter of body surface area per day orally in three divided doses for 15 days, followed by tapering of the dosage as follows:

20 mg/square meter for 2 days, 10 mg/square meter for 2 days, 5 mg/square meter for 2 days, 2.5 mg/square meter for 2 days and then discontinue.

Vincristine sulfate 2 mg/square meter of body surface area intravenously once weekly on Days 1, 8, and 15 of the treatment period. The maximum single dose should not exceed 2.0 mg.

Asparaginase 1,000 I.U./kg/day intravenously for ten successive days beginning on Day 22 of the treatment period.

Regimen II

Prednisone 40 mg/square meter of body surface area per day orally in three divided doses for 28 days (the total daily dose should be to the nearest 2.5 mg), following which the dosage of prednisone should be discontinued gradually over a 14 day period.

Vincristine sulfate 1.5 mg/square meter of body surface area intravenously weekly for four doses, on Days 1, 8, 15, and 22 of the treatment period. The maximum single dose should not exceed 2.0 mg.

Asparaginase 6,000 I.U./square meter of body surface area intramuscularly on Days 4, 7, 10, 13, 16, 19, 22, 25, and 28 of the treatment period. When a remission is obtained with either of the above regimens, appropriate maintenance therapy must be instituted. ELSPAR should not be used as part of a maintenance regimen. The above regimens do not preclude a need for special therapy directed toward the prevention of central nervous system leukemia.

It should be noted that ELSPAR has been used in combination regimens other than those recommended above. It is important to keep in mind that ELSPAR administered intravenously concurrently with or immediately before a course of vincristine and prednisone may be associated with increased toxicity. Physicians using a given regimen should be thoroughly familiar with its benefits and risks. Clinical data are insufficient for a recommendation concerning the use of combination regimens in adults. Asparaginase toxicity is reported to be greater in adults than in children.

Use of ELSPAR as the sole induction agent should be undertaken only in an unusual situation when a combined regimen is inappropriate because of toxicity or other specific patient-related factors, or in cases refractory to other therapy. When ELSPAR is to be used as the sole induction agent for children or adults the recommended dosage regimen is 200 I.U./kg/day intravenously for 28 days. When complete remissions were obtained with this regimen, they were of short duration, 1 to 3 months. ELSPAR has been used as the sole induction agent in other regimens. Physicians using a given regimen should be thoroughly familiar with its benefits and risks.

Patients undergoing induction therapy must be carefully monitored and the therapeutic regimen adjusted according to response and toxicity.

Such adjustments should always involve decreasing dosages of one or more agents or discontinuation depending on the degree of toxicity. Patients who have received a course of ELSPAR, if retreated, have an increased risk of hypersensitivity reactions. Therefore, retreatment should be undertaken only when the benefit of such therapy is weighed against the increased risk.

Intradermal Skin Test:

Because of the occurrence of allergic reactions, an intradermal skin test should be performed prior to the initial administration of ELSPAR and when ELSPAR is given after an interval of a week or more has elapsed between doses. The skin test solution may be prepared as follows: Reconstitute the contents of a 10,000 I.U. vial with 5.0 ml of diluent. From this solution (2,000 I.U./ml) withdraw 0.1 ml and inject it into another vial containing 9.9 ml of diluent, yielding a skin test solution of approximately 20.0 I.U./ml. Use 0.1 ml of this solution (about 2.0 I.U.) for the intradermal skin test. The skin test site should be observed for at least one hour for the appearance of a wheal or erythema either of which indicates a positive reaction. An allergic reaction even to the skin test dose in certain sensitized individuals may rarely occur. A negative skin test reaction does not preclude the possibility of the development of an allergic reaction.

Desensitization:

Desensitization should be performed before administering the first dose of ELSPAR on initiation of therapy in positive reactors, and on retreatment of any patient in whom such therapy is deemed necessary after carefully weighing the increased risk of hypersensitivity reactions. Rapid desensitization of the patient may be attempted with progressively increasing amounts of intravenously administered ELSPAR provided adequate precautions are taken to treat an acute allergic reaction should it occur. One reported schedule begins with a total of 1 I.U. given intravenously and doubles the dose every 10 minutes, provided no reaction has occurred, until the accumulated total amount given equals the planned doses for that day.

For convenience the following table is included to calculate the number of doses necessary to reach the patient's total dose for that day:

Injection Number	ELSPAR Dose in I.U.	Accumulated Total Dose
1	1	1
2	2	3
3	4	7
4	8	15
5	16	31
6	32	63
7	64	127
8	128	255
9	256	511
10	512	1023
11	1024	2047
12	2048	4095
13	4096	8191
14	8192	16383
15	16384	32767
16	32768	65535
17	65536	131071
18	131072	262143

For example: A patient weighing 20 kg who is to receive 200 I.U./kg (total dose 4000 I.U.) would receive injections 1 through 12 during desensitization.

Directions for Reconstitution

Parenteral drug products should be inspected visually for particulate matter and discoloration prior to administration whenever solution and container permit. When reconstituted, ELSPAR should be a clear, colorless solution. If the solution becomes cloudy, discard.

For Intravenous Use

Reconstitute with Sterile Water for Injection or with Sodium Chloride Injection. The volume recommended for reconstitution is 5 ml for the 10,000 unit vials. Ordinary shaking during reconstitution does not inactivate the enzyme. This solution may be used for direct intravenous administration within an eight hour period following restoration. For administration by infusion, solutions should be diluted with the isotonic solutions, Sodium Chloride Injection or Dextrose Injection 5%. These solutions should be infused within eight hours and only if clear.

Occasionally, a very small number of gelatinous fiber-like particles may develop on standing. Filtration through a 5.0 micron filter during administration will remove the particles with no resultant loss in potency. Some loss of potency has been observed with the use of a 0.2 micron filter.

For Intramuscular Use

When ELSPAR is administered intramuscularly according to the schedule cited in the induction regimen, reconstitution is carried out by adding 2 ml Sodium Chloride Injection to the 10,000 unit vial. The resulting solution should be used within eight hours and only if clear.

How Supplied

No. 4612 — ELSPAR is a white lyophilized plug or powder supplied as follows:

NDC 0006-4612-00 in a sterile 10 ml vial containing 10,000 I.U. of asparaginase and 80 mg mannitol, an inactive ingredient.

Store below 8°C (46°F). ELSPAR does not contain a preservative. Unused, reconstituted solution should be stored at 2 to 8°C (36 to 46°F) and discarded after eight hours, or sooner if it becomes cloudy.

A.H.F.S. Category: 44:00

DC 6680206 Issued March 1982

Copyright © MERCK & CO., INC., 1977. All rights reserved.

FLEXERIL® Tablets ℞

(cyclobenzaprine HCl, MSD), U.S.P.

Description

Cyclobenzaprine hydrochloride is a white, crystalline tricyclic amine salt with the empirical formula $C_{20}H_{21}N \cdot HCl$ and a molecular weight of 311.9. It has a melting point of 217°C, and a pK_a of 8.47 at 25°C. It is freely soluble in water and alcohol, sparingly soluble in isopropanol, and insoluble in hydrocarbon solvents. If aqueous solutions are made alkaline, the free base separates. Cyclobenzaprine HCl is designated chemically as 3-(5*H*-dibenzo[*a,d*]cyclohepten-5-ylidene)-*N, N*-dimethyl-1-propanamine hydrochloride.

FLEXERIL® (Cyclobenzaprine HCl, MSD) is supplied as 10 mg tablets for oral administration.

Clinical Pharmacology

Cyclobenzaprine HCl relieves skeletal muscle spasm of local origin without interfering with muscle function. It is ineffective in muscle spasm due to central nervous system disease.

Cyclobenzaprine reduced or abolished skeletal muscle hyperactivity in several animal models. Animal studies indicate that cyclobenzaprine does not act at the neuromuscular junction or directly on skeletal muscle. Such studies show that cyclobenzaprine acts primarily within the central nervous system at brain stem as opposed to spinal cord levels, although its action on the latter may contribute to its overall skeletal muscle relaxant activity. Evidence suggests that the net effect of cyclobenzaprine is a reduction of tonic somatic motor activity, influencing both gamma (γ) and alpha (α) motor systems.

Pharmacological studies in animals showed a similarity between the effects of cyclobenzaprine and the structurally related tricyclic antidepressants, including reserpine antagonism, norepinephrine potentiation, potent peripheral and central anticholinergic effects, and sedation. Cyclobenzaprine caused slight to moderate increase in heart rate in animals.

Cyclobenzaprine is well absorbed after oral administration, but there is a large intersubject variation in plasma levels. Cyclobenzaprine is eliminated quite slowly with a half-life as long as one to three days. It is highly bound to plasma proteins, is extensively metabolized primarily to glucuronide-like conjugates, and is excreted primarily via the kidneys.

No significant effect on plasma levels or bioavailability of FLEXERIL or aspirin was noted when single or multiple doses of the two drugs were administered concomitantly. Concomitant administration of FLEXERIL and aspirin is usually well tolerated and no unexpected or serious clinical or laboratory adverse effects have been observed. No studies have been performed to indicate whether FLEXERIL enhances the clinical effect of aspirin or other analgesics, or whether analgesics enhance the clinical effect of FLEXERIL in acute musculoskeletal conditions.

Clinical Studies

Controlled clinical studies show that FLEXERIL significantly improves the signs and symptoms of skeletal muscle spasm as compared with placebo. The clinical responses include improvement in muscle spasm as determined by palpation, reduction in local pain and tenderness, increased range of motion, and less restriction in activities of daily living. When daily observations were made, clinical improvement was observed as early as the first day of therapy.

Eight double-blind controlled clinical studies were performed in 642 patients comparing FLEXERIL, diazepam*, and placebo. Muscle spasm, local pain and tenderness, limitation of motion, and restriction in activities of daily living were evaluated. In three of these studies there was a significantly greater improvement with FLEXERIL than with diazepam, while in the other studies the improvement following both treatments was comparable.

Although the frequency and severity of adverse reactions observed in patients treated with FLEXERIL were comparable to those observed in patients treated with diazepam, dry mouth was observed more frequently in patients treated with FLEXERIL and dizziness more frequently in those treated with diazepam. The incidence of drowsiness, the most frequent adverse reaction, was similar with both drugs.

Analysis of the data from controlled studies shows that FLEXERIL produces clinical improvement whether or not sedation occurs.

Surveillance Program

A post-marketing surveillance program was carried out in 7607 patients with acute musculoskeletal disorders, and included 297 patients treated for 30 days or longer. The overall effectiveness of FLEXERIL was similar to that observed in the double-blind controlled studies; the overall incidence of adverse effects was less (see ADVERSE REACTIONS).

Indications and Usage

FLEXERIL is indicated as an adjunct to rest and physical therapy for relief of muscle spasm associated with acute, painful musculoskeletal conditions.

Improvement is manifested by relief of muscle spasm and its associated signs and symptoms, namely, pain, tenderness, limitation of motion, and restriction in activities of daily living.

FLEXERIL (Cyclobenzaprine HCl, MSD) should be used only for short periods (up to two or three weeks) because adequate evidence of effectiveness for more prolonged use is not available and because muscle spasm associated with acute, painful musculoskeletal conditions is generally of short duration and specific therapy for longer periods is seldom warranted.

FLEXERIL has not been found effective in the treatment of spasticity associated with cerebral or spinal cord disease, or in children with cerebral palsy.

Contraindications

Hypersensitivity to the drug.

Concomitant use of monoamine oxidase inhibitors or within 14 days after their discontinuation.

Acute recovery phase of myocardial infarction, and patients with arrhythmias, heart block or conduction disturbances, or congestive heart failure.

Hyperthyroidism.

Warnings

Cyclobenzaprine is closely related to the tricyclic antidepressants, e.g., amitriptyline and imipramine. In short term studies for indications other than muscle spasm associated with acute musculoskeletal conditions, and usually at doses somewhat greater than those recommended for skeletal muscle spasm, some of the more serious central nervous system reactions noted with the tricyclic antidepressants have occurred (see WARNINGS, below, and ADVERSE REACTIONS).

FLEXERIL may interact with monoamine oxidase (MAO) inhibitors. Hyperpyretic crisis, severe convulsions, and deaths have occurred

Continued on next page

*VALIUM® (diazepam, Roche)

Information on the Merck Sharp & Dohme products listed on these pages is the full prescribing information from package circulars in use October 31, 1982.

Merck Sharp & Dohme—Cont.

in patients receiving tricyclic antidepressants and MAO inhibitor drugs.
Tricyclic antidepressants have been reported to produce arrhythmias, sinus tachycardia, prolongation of the conduction time leading to myocardial infarction and stroke.
FLEXERIL may enhance the effects of alcohol, barbiturates, and other CNS depressants.

Precautions

General
Because of its atropine-like action, FLEXERIL should be used with caution in patients with a history of urinary retention, angle-closure glaucoma, increased intraocular pressure, and in patients taking anticholinergic medication.
Information for Patients
FLEXERIL may impair mental and/or physical abilities required for performance of hazardous tasks, such as operating machinery or driving a motor vehicle.
Drug Interactions
FLEXERIL may enhance the effects of alcohol, barbiturates, and other CNS depressants.
Tricyclic antidepressants may block the antihypertensive action of guanethidine and similarly acting compounds.
Carcinogenesis, Mutagenesis, Impairment of Fertility
In rats treated with FLEXERIL for up to 67 weeks at doses of approximately 5 to 40 times the maximum recommended human dose, pale, sometimes enlarged, livers were noted and there was a dose-related hepatocyte vacuolation with lipidosis. In the higher dose groups this microscopic change was seen after 26 weeks and even earlier in rats which died prior to 26 weeks; at lower doses, the change was not seen until after 26 weeks.
Cyclobenzaprine did not affect the onset, incidence or distribution of neoplasia in an 81-week study in the mouse or in a 105-week study in the rat.
At oral doses of up to 10 times the human dose, cyclobenzaprine did not adversely affect the reproductive performance or fertility of male or female rats. Cyclobenzaprine did not demonstrate mutagenic activity in the male mouse at dose levels of up to 20 times the human dose.
Pregnancy
Pregnancy Category B: Reproduction studies have been performed in rats, mice and rabbits at doses up to 20 times the human dose, and have revealed no evidence of impaired fertility or harm to the fetus due to FLEXERIL. There are, however, no adequate and well-controlled studies in pregnant women. Because animal reproduction studies are not always predictive of human response, this drug should be used during pregnancy only if clearly needed.
Nursing Mothers
It is not known whether this drug is excreted in human milk. Because cyclobenzaprine is closely related to the tricyclic antidepressants, some of which are known to be excreted in human milk, caution should be exercised when FLEXERIL is administered to a nursing woman.
Pediatric Use
Safety and effectiveness of FLEXERIL in children below the age of 15 have not been established.

Adverse Reactions

The following list of adverse reactions is based on the experience in 473 patients treated with FLEXERIL in controlled clinical studies, 7607 patients in the post-marketing surveillance program, and reports received since the drug was marketed. The overall incidence of adverse reactions among patients in the surveillance program was less than the incidence in the controlled clinical studies.
The adverse reactions reported most frequently with FLEXERIL were drowsiness, dry mouth and dizziness. The incidence of these common adverse reactions was lower in the surveillance program than in the controlled clinical studies:

	Clinical Studies	*Surveillance Program*
drowsiness	39%	16%
dry mouth	27%	7%
dizziness	11%	3%

Among the less frequent adverse reactions, there was no appreciable difference in incidence in controlled clinical studies or in the surveillance program. Adverse reactions which were reported in 1% to 3% of the patients were: fatigue/tiredness, asthenia, nausea, constipation, dyspepsia, unpleasant taste, blurred vision, headache, nervousness, and confusion.

Incidence Less Than 1 in 100

The following adverse reactions have been reported at an incidence of less than 1 in 100:
Cardiovascular: Tachycardia; syncope; arrhythmia; vasodilatation; palpitation; hypotension.
Nervous System: Ataxia; vertigo; dysarthria; paresthesia; tremors; hypertonia.
Psychiatric: Disorientation; insomnia; depressed mood; abnormal sensations; anxiety; agitation; abnormal thinking and dreaming; hallucinations; excitement.
Gastrointestinal: Vomiting; anorexia; diarrhea; gastrointestinal pain; gastritis; thirst; flatulence.
Genitourinary: Urinary frequency and/or retention.
Integumentary: Sweating.
Musculoskeletal: Muscle twitching; local weakness.
Special Senses: Ageusia; tinnitus.
Hypersensitivity: Allergic reactions including skin rash, urticaria, and edema of face and tongue.
Miscellaneous: Malaise.

Causal Relationship Unknown

Other reactions have been reported rarely under circumstances where a causal relationship could not be established. These rarely reported events are listed to serve as alerting information to physicians: hypertension; chest pain; abnormal gait; convulsions; decreased or increased libido; paralytic ileus; hepatitis; jaundice; abnormal liver function; tongue discoloration; edema; weight gain or loss; pruritus; alopecia; myalgia; impaired urination; impotence; and dyspnea.
Pharmacologic similarities among the tricyclic drugs require that certain other adverse reactions be considered when FLEXERIL is administered, even though they have not been reported to occur with this drug: myocardial infarction; heart block; stroke; delusions; peripheral neuropathy; alteration in EEG patterns; extrapyramidal symptoms; inappropriate ADH syndrome; dilatation of urinary tract; photosensitization; bone marrow depression; leukopenia; eosinophilia; purpura; thrombocytopenia; stomatitis; parotid swelling; testicular swelling; gynecomastia; breast enlargement; galactorrhea; and elevation and lowering of blood sugar levels.

Drug Abuse and Dependence

Pharmacologic similarities among the tricyclic drugs require that certain withdrawal symptoms be considered when FLEXERIL is administered, even though they have not been reported to occur with this drug. Abrupt cessation of treatment after prolonged administration may produce nausea, headache, and malaise. These are not indicative of addiction.

Overdosage

Manifestations: High doses may cause temporary confusion, disturbed concentration, transient visual hallucinations, agitation, hyperactive reflexes, muscle rigidity, vomiting, or hyperpyrexia, in addition to anything listed under ADVERSE REACTIONS. Based on the known pharmacologic actions of the drug, overdosage may cause drowsiness, hypothermia, tachycardia and other cardiac rhythm abnormalities such as bundle branch block, ECG evidence of impaired conduction, and congestive heart failure. Other manifestations may be dilated pupils, convulsions, severe hypotension, stupor, and coma.
The acute oral LD_{50} of FLEXERIL is approximately 338 and 425 mg/kg in mice and rats, respectively.
Treatment: Treatment is symptomatic and supportive. Empty the stomach as quickly as possible by emesis, followed by gastric lavage. After gastric lavage, activated charcoal may be administered. Twenty to 30 g of activated charcoal may be given every four to six hours during the first 24 to 48 hours after ingestion. An ECG should be taken and close monitoring of cardiac function must be instituted if there is any evidence of dysrhythmia. Maintenance of an open airway, adequate fluid intake, and regulation of body temperature are necessary. The intravenous administration of 1-3 mg of physostigmine salicylate is reported to reverse symptoms of poisoning by atropine and other drugs with anticholinergic activity. Physostigmine may be helpful in the treatment of cyclobenzaprine overdose. Because physostigmine is rapidly metabolized, the dosage of physostigmine should be repeated as required, particularly if life-threatening signs such as arrhythmias, convulsions, and deep coma recur or persist after the initial dosage of physostigmine. Because physostigmine itself may be toxic, it is not recommended for routine use.
Standard medical measures should be used to manage circulatory shock and metabolic acidosis. Cardiac arrhythmias may be treated with neostigmine, pyridostigmine, or propranolol. When signs of cardiac failure occur, the use of a short-acting digitalis preparation should be considered. Close monitoring of cardiac function for not less than five days is advisable.
Anticonvulsants may be given to control seizures.
Dialysis is probably of no value because of low plasma concentrations of the drug.
Since overdosage is often deliberate, patients may attempt suicide by other means during the recovery phase. Deaths by deliberate or accidental overdosage have occurred with this class of drugs.

Dosage and Administration

The usual dosage of FLEXERIL is 10 mg three times a day, with a range of 20 to 40 mg a day in divided doses. Dosage should not exceed 60 mg a day. Use of FLEXERIL for periods longer than two or three weeks is not recommended. (See INDICATIONS AND USAGE).

How Supplied

No. 3358—Tablets FLEXERIL, 10 mg, are butterscotch yellow, D-shaped, film coated tablets, coded MSD 931. They are supplied as follows:
NDC 0006-0931-68 in bottles of 100.
NDC 0006-0931-28 single unit packages of 100.
NDC 0006-0931-30 BACK-PACK® unit-of-use package of 30.

[*Shown in Product Identification Section*]

A.H.F.S. Category: 12:20

DC 6919206 Issued December 1981

Copyright © MERCK & CO., Inc., 1977
All Rights Reserved

HEP-B-GAMMAGEE® ℞

(hepatitis B immune globulin [human], MSD), U.S.P.

Description

HEP-B-GAMMAGEE® [Hepatitis B Immune

Globulin (Human), MSD] is a sterile solution of human immunoglobulin (10–18% protein) prepared by Cohn cold ethanol fractionation of pooled plasma drawn from individuals with high titers of antibody to the hepatitis B surface antigen (anti-HBs). HEP-B-GAMMAGEE is prepared from human plasma that was nonreactive when tested for hepatitis B surface antigen (HBsAg). The product is dissolved in 0.3 molar glycine and contains thimerosal (mercury derivative) 1:10,000 added as a preservative. The solution has a pH of 6.8 $\pm$ 0.4 adjusted with hydrochloric acid or sodium hydroxide. Each vial of HEP-B-GAMMAGEE contains anti-HBs equivalent to or exceeding the potency of anti-HBs in a U.S. reference Hepatitis B Immune Globulin (Bureau of Biologics, FDA).

Clinical Pharmacology

Hepatitis B Immune Globulin (Human) provides passive immunization for individuals exposed to the hepatitis B virus (HBV) as evidenced by a reduction in the attack rate of hepatitis B following its use. The administration of the usual recommended dose of HEP-B-GAMAGEE generally results in a detectable level of circulating antibody to hepatitis B surface antigen (anti-HBs) which persists for approximately 2 months or longer. The possibility of hepatitis B transmission is remote, as it is with other immune globulins prepared by the cold ethanol process.

Indications and Usage

HEP-B-GAMMAGEE is indicated for post-exposure prophylaxis following either parenteral exposure, direct mucous membrane contact, or oral ingestion involving HBsAg-positive materials such as blood, plasma or serum. Such exposures might occur by accidental "needlestick", accidental splash, or a pipetting accident. HEP-B-GAMMAGEE is also indicated for post-exposure prophylaxis in infants born to hepatitis B-positive (HBsAg-positive) mothers. Use of Hepatitis B Immune Globulin (Human) has been and continues to be evaluated in other situations which include nonparenteral exposure to hepatitis B, in dialysis patients and among hospital staffs. In addition, it has been tested as a prophylactic measure for susceptible individuals in close association with HBsAg-positive persons. These studies are still in progress and there are insufficient data at present on effectiveness, dosage and schedule for any of these uses to be included as definite indications.

Contraindications

None known.

Warnings

Persons with isolated immunoglobulin A deficiency have the potential for developing antibodies to immunoglobulin A and could have anaphylactic reactions to subsequent administration of blood products that contain immunoglobulin A. Therefore, as with any immune globulin preparation, Hepatitis B Immune Globulin (Human) should be given to such persons only if the expected benefits outweigh the potential risks.
In patients who have severe thrombocytopenia or any coagulation disorder that would contraindicate intramuscular injections, Hepatitis B Immune Globulin (Human) should be given only if the expected benefits outweigh the potential risks.

Precautions

General

HEP-B-GAMMAGEE should be given with caution to patients with a history of prior systemic allergic reactions following the administration of human immune globulin preparations. Hypersensitivity reactions to injections of immune serum globulin occur rarely. The incidence of these reactions may be increased in patients receiving large intramuscular doses or in patients receiving repeated injections of immune serum globulin.
HEP-B-GAMMAGEE *must not be administered intravenously* because of the potential for serious reactions. Injections should be made intramuscularly. Care should be taken to draw back on the plunger of the syringe before injection in order to be certain that the needle is not in a blood vessel.
Epinephrine should be available for treatment of acute allergic symptoms.

Drug Interactions

Antibodies present in immune globulin preparations may interfere with the immune response to live virus vaccines such as measles, mumps, and rubella. Therefore, vaccination with live virus vaccines should be deferred until approximately three months after administration of Hepatitis B Immune Globulin. It may be necessary to revaccinate persons who received Hepatitis B Immune Globulin shortly after live virus vaccination.

Pregnancy

Pregnancy Category C. Animal reproduction studies have not been conducted with HEP-B-GAMMAGEE. Clinical experience with other immunoglobulin preparations administered during pregnancy suggests that there are no known adverse effects on the fetus from immune globulins per se. However, it is not known whether HEP-B-GAMMAGEE can cause fetal harm when administered to a pregnant woman or can affect reproduction capacity. HEP-B-GAMMAGEE should be given to a pregnant woman only if clearly needed.

Nursing Mothers

It is not known whether this drug is excreted in human milk. Because many drugs are excreted in human milk, caution should be exercised when HEP-B-GAMMAGEE is administered to a nursing woman.

Adverse Reactions

Local pain and tenderness at the injection site, urticaria and angioedema may occur. Anaphylactic reactions, although rare, have been reported following the injection of human immune globulin preparations. Anaphylaxis is more likely to occur if Hepatitis B Immune Globulin (Human) is given intravenously; therefore, Hepatitis B Immune Globulin (Human) must be administered *only* intramuscularly. In highly allergic individuals, repeated injections may lead to anaphylactic shock.

Overdosage

Although no data are available, clinical experience with other immunoglobulin preparations suggests that the only manifestations would be pain and tenderness at the injection site.

Dosage and Administration

Parenteral drug products should be inspected visually for particulate matter and discoloration prior to administration, whenever solution and container permit. HEP-B-GAMMAGEE is a clear, very slightly amber, moderately viscous liquid.
HEP-B-GAMMAGEE is administered *intramuscularly. It must not be injected intravenously.*
It is important to use a separate sterile syringe and needle for each individual patient to prevent transmission of hepatitis B and other infectious agents from one person to another.

Adults

The recommended dose is 0.06 ml per kilogram of body weight; the usual adult dose is 3 to 5 ml administered intramuscularly, preferably in the gluteal or deltoid region. The appropriate dose should be administered as soon after exposure as possible (preferably within 7 days) and repeated 28–30 days after exposure.

Newborns

The immunization regimen for infants born to hepatitis B-positive (HBsAg-positive) mothers consists of three doses. A dose of 0.5 ml should be administered intramuscularly in the anterolateral thigh as soon after birth as possible and repeated at 3 months and 6 months of age. Administration of the first dose later than 24 hours after birth results in a progressive loss of efficacy.

How Supplied

No. 4692—HEP-B-GAMMAGEE is supplied as follows:
NDC 0006-4692-00 in 5 ml vials.
Store at 2–8° C (35.6–46.4° F). Do not freeze. Do not use after expiration date.
A.H.F.S. Category: 80:04
DC 7062004 Issued February 1982
COPYRIGHT© MERCK & CO., Inc., 1978.
All Rights Reserved.

HEPTAVAX-B® ℞
(hepatitis B vaccine, MSD)

Description

HEPTAVAX-B® (Hepatitis B Vaccine, MSD) is a non-infectious formalin-inactivated subunit viral vaccine derived from surface antigen (HBsAg or Australia antigen) of hepatitis B virus (Dane particles). The antigen is harvested and purified from the plasma of human carriers of hepatitis B virus according to methods developed by Merck, Sharp and Dohme Research Laboratories. HEPTAVAX-B is a sterile suspension for intramuscular injection. Each 1.0 ml dose of vaccine contains 20 mcg of hepatitis B surface antigen formulated in an alum adjuvant, and thimerosal (mercury derivative) 1:20,000 added as a preservative. The vaccine is prepared without regard to subtype. HEPTAVAX-B is indicated for immunization of persons at risk of infection from hepatitis B virus including all known subtypes.

Clinical Pharmacology

Hepatitis B virus is one of at least three hepatitis viruses that cause a systemic infection, with a major pathology in the liver. The others are hepatitis A virus, and non-A, non-B hepatitis viruses.
Hepatitis B virus is an important cause of viral hepatitis. There is no specific treatment for this disease. The incubation period for type B hepatitis is relatively long; six weeks to six months may elapse between exposure and the onset of clinical symptoms. The prognosis following infection with hepatitis B virus is variable and dependent on at least three factors: (1) Age—Infants and younger children usually experience milder initial disease than older persons; (2) Dose of Virus—The higher the dose, the more likely acute icteric hepatitis B will result; and, (3) Severity of Associated Underlying Disease—Underlying malignancy or pre-existing hepatic disease predisposes to increased mortality and morbidity.

Continued on next page

Information on the Merck Sharp & Dohme products listed on these pages is the full prescribing information from package circulars in use October 31, 1982.

Merck Sharp & Dohme—Cont.

Persistence of viral infection (the chronic hepatitis B virus carrier state) occurs in 5–10% of persons following acute hepatitis B, and occurs more frequently after initial anicteric hepatitis B than after initial icteric disease. Consequently, carriers of HBsAg frequently give no history of recognized acute hepatitis. It has been estimated that more than 170 million people in the world today are persistently infected with hepatitis B virus. The Centers for Disease Control (CDC) estimates that there are approximately 0.7 to 1.0 million chronic carriers of hepatitis B virus in the USA and that this pool of carriers grows by 2%–3% (8,000 to 16,000 individuals) annually. Chronic carriers represent the largest human reservoir of hepatitis B virus.

The serious complications and sequelae of HBV infection include massive hepatic necrosis, cirrhosis of the liver, chronic active hepatitis, and hepatocellular carcinoma. Chronic carriers of HBsAg appear to be at increased risk of developing hepatocellular carcinoma, which accounts for 80 to 90 percent of primary liver carcinomas. Although a number of etiologic factors are associated with development of hepatocellular carcinoma, the single most important etiologic factor appears to be active infection with the hepatitis B virus.

There is also evidence that several diseases other than hepatitis have been associated with hepatitis B virus infection through an immunologic mechanism involving antigen-antibody complexes. Such diseases include a syndrome with rash, urticaria, and arthralgia resembling serum sickness; polyarteritis nodosa; membranous glomerulonephritis; and infantile papular acrodermatitis.

Although the vehicles for transmission of the virus are predominantly blood and blood products, viral antigen has also been found in tears, saliva, breast milk, urine, semen and vaginal secretions. Hepatitis B virus is quite stable and capable of surviving for days on environmental surfaces. Infection may occur when hepatitis B virus, transmitted by infected body fluids, is implanted via mucous surfaces or percutaneously introduced through accidental or deliberate breaks in the skin.

Transmission of hepatitis B virus infection is often associated with close interpersonal contact with an infected individual and with crowded living conditions. In such circumstances, transmission by inoculation via routes other then overt parenteral ones may be quite common.

Hepatitis B is endemic throughout the world and is a serious medical problem in population groups at increased risk. (Refer to INDICATIONS AND USAGE)

Numerous epidemiological studies have shown that persons who develop anti-HBs following active infection with the hepatitis B virus are protected against the disease on re-exposure to the virus. Clinical studies have established that HEPTAVAX-B characteristically induces neutralizing antibody (anti-HBs) in most individuals 3 months of age and older. Responsiveness is age-dependent, with children showing a more vigorous response than adults. Immunocompromised and immunosuppressed persons respond less well than do healthy individuals.

The protective efficacy of HEPTAVAX-B has been demonstrated in human populations. In one study involving individuals with a high risk of contracting hepatitis B virus infection, HEPTAVAX-B was shown to reduce the incidence of infection by 92%. The vaccine protected against acute hepatitis B, asymptomatic infection, and chronic antigenemia. There was evidence of immunity (neutralizing antibody) in 87% of vaccinated subjects after administration of two doses of the 3-dose vaccine regimen. However, the third dose was necessary to attain both a higher percentage of responses to the vaccine (96%) and a long-term protective effect (i.e., vaccine-induced antibody persisting during the entire 24-month follow-up period). In a second study of similar design, administration of three doses of vaccine induced immunity (neutralizing antibody) in 85% of recipients. In both studies, the vaccine was virtually 100% effective in preventing hepatitis B in those who developed anti-HBs.

Although the duration of protective effect of HEPTAVAX-B is unknown at present, available data suggest that immunity will last for about 5 years in patients who have received all 3 doses, after which time a single booster dose of vaccine might be necessary to maintain immunity.

Further study is required to determine the effectiveness of HEPTAVAX-B in preventing hepatitis B when the vaccine regimen is begun after an exposure to the hepatitis B virus has already occurred (i.e., use for post-exposure prophylaxis). Until those studies are complete, Hepatitis B Immune Globulin remains the treatment of choice for post-exposure prophylaxis. However, it has been demonstrated that doses up to 3 ml of Hepatitis B Immune Globulin, when administered simultaneously with HEPTAVAX-B at separate body sites, do not interfere with the induction of neutralizing antibodies against hepatitis B virus.

Indications and Usage

HEPTAVAX-B is indicated for immunization against infection caused by all known subtypes of hepatitis B virus.

HEPTAVAX-B will not prevent hepatitis caused by other agents, such as hepatitis A virus, non-A, non-B hepatitis viruses, or other viruses known to infect the liver.

Vaccination is recommended in persons 3 months of age or older, especially those who are at increased risk of infection with hepatitis B virus, for example:

A. *Health Care Personnel*
  Dentists and oral surgeons.
  Physicians and surgeons.
  Nurses.
  Paramedical personnel and custodial staff who may be exposed to the virus via blood or other patient specimens.
  Dental hygienists and dental nurses.
  Laboratory personnel handling blood, blood products and other patient specimens.
  Dental, medical and nursing students.

B. *Selected Patients and Patient Contacts*
  Patients and staff in hemodialysis units and hematology/oncology units.
  Patients requiring frequent and/or large volume blood transfusions or clotting factor concentrates (e.g., persons with hemophilia, thalassemia).
  Clients (residents) and staff of institutions for the mentally handicapped.
  Classroom contacts of deinstitutionalized mentally handicapped persons who have persistent hepatitis B antigenemia and who show aggressive behavior.
  Household and other intimate contacts of persons with persistent hepatitis B antigenemia.

C. *Populations with high incidence of the disease,* such as:
  Alaskan Eskimos.
  Indochinese refugees.
  Haitian refugees.

D. *Military Personnel identified as being at increased risk*

E. *Morticians and Embalmers*

F. *Blood bank and plasma fractionation workers*

G. *Persons at Increased Risk of the Disease Due to Their Sexual Practices,* such as:
  Persons who repeatedly contract sexually transmitted diseases.
  Homosexually active males.
  Female prostitutes.

H. *Prisoners*

I. *Users of illicit injectable drugs*

Revaccination

See CLINICAL PHARMACOLOGY

Contraindications

Hypersensitivity to any component of the vaccine.

Warnings

Persons with immuno-deficiency or those receiving immunosuppressive therapy may require larger vaccine doses to develop adequate circulating antibody levels. Refer to DOSAGE AND ADMINISTRATION for use in such individuals.

Because of the long incubation period for hepatitis B, it is possible for unrecognized infection to be present at the time HEPTAVAX-B is given. HEPTAVAX-B may not prevent hepatitis B in such patients.

Precautions

General

As with any parenteral vaccine, epinephrine should be available for immediate use should an anaphylactoid reaction occur.

Any serious active infection is reason for delaying use of HEPTAVAX-B, except when, in the opinion of the physician, withholding the vaccine entails a greater risk.

Caution and appropriate care should be exercised in administering HEPTAVAX-B to individuals with severely compromised cardiopulmonary status or to others in whom a febrile or systemic reaction could pose a significant risk.

Pregnancy

Pregnancy Category C. Animal reproduction studies have not been conducted with HEPTAVAX-B. It is also not known whether HEPTAVAX-B can cause fetal harm when administered to a pregnant woman or can affect reproductive capacity. HEPTAVAX-B is not recommended for use in pregnant women.

Nursing Mothers

It is not known whether this drug is secreted in human milk. Because many drugs are secreted in human milk, caution should be exercised when HEPTAVAX-B is administered to a nursing woman.

Pediatric Use

Safety and effectiveness in children below the age of 3 months have not been established. Use of this vaccine in children below the age of 3 months is not recommended at present.

Adverse Reactions

HEPTAVAX-B is generally well tolerated. No serious adverse reactions attributable to vaccination have been reported during the course of clinical trials involving administration of HEPTAVAX-B to over 6,000 individuals. As with any vaccine, there is the possibility that broad use of the vaccine could reveal rare adverse reactions not observed in clinical trials. In two double-blind placebo-controlled studies among 2,485 persons, the overall rates of adverse reactions reported by vaccine recipients (24.3% and 21.5%) did not differ significantly from those of placebo recipients (21.4% and 18.7%). Approximately half of all reported reactions were injection site soreness, which occurred somewhat more frequently among vaccine recipients.

Other less common local reactions have included erythema, swelling, warmth, or induration. These signs and symptoms of local inflammation are generally well tolerated and usually subside within 2 days of vaccination.

Low-grade fever (less than 101°F) occurs occasionally and is usually confined to the 48-hour period following vaccination. Although uncommon, fever over 102°F has been reported.

Systemic complaints including malaise, fatigue, headache, nausea, dizziness, myalgia, and arthralgia are infrequent and have been limited to the first few days following vaccination. Rash has been reported rarely.

Dosage and Administration

FOR INTRAMUSCULAR USE ONLY
Do not inject intravenously, subcutaneously or intradermally.
Shake well before withdrawal and use. Thorough agitation at the time of administration is necessary to maintain suspension of the vaccine.
Parenteral drug products should be inspected visually for particulate matter and discoloration prior to administration. After thorough agitation, HEPTAVAX-B is a slightly opaque, white suspension.
The immunization regimen consists of 3 doses of vaccine given *intramuscularly:*

1st dose: at elected date
2nd dose: 1 month later
3rd dose: 6 months after the first dose

The volume of vaccine to be given on each occasion is as follows:
[See table above].

Group	Initial	1 month	6 months
Younger Children (3 months to 10 years of age)	0.5 ml	0.5 ml	0.5 ml
Adults and Older Children	1.0 ml	1.0 ml	1.0 ml
Dialysis Patients and Immunocompromised Patients	2.0 ml*	2.0 ml*	2.0 ml*

*Two 1.0 ml doses given at different sites.

Revaccination (booster)—See CLINICAL PHARMACOLOGY.
Store unopened and opened vials at 2–8°C (35.6–46.4°F).
Do not freeze since freezing destroys potency. The vaccine is used as supplied; no dilution or reconstitution is necessary.
It is important to use a separate sterile syringe and needle for each individual patient to prevent transmission of hepatitis and other infectious agents from one person to another.
3.0 ml Vial
For Syringe Use Only: Withdraw the recommended dose from the vial using a sterile needle and syringe free of preservatives, antiseptics, and detergents.

How Supplied

No. 4720—HEPTAVAX-B is supplied as follows:
NDC 0006-4720-00 in a 3 ml vial.
A.H.F.S. Category: 80:12
DC 7207000 Issued May 1982
COPYRIGHT © MERCK & CO., INC., 1981
All rights reserved

HYDELTRA-T.B.A.® Suspension (prednisolone tebutate, MSD), U.S.P. ℞

For intra-articular, intralesional, and soft tissue injection only.

Description

Prednisolone tebutate, a synthetic adrenocortical steroid, is a white to slightly yellow powder sparingly soluble in alcohol, freely soluble in chloroform, and very slightly soluble in water. The molecular weight is 476.61 (monohydrate). It is designated chemically as 11β,17-dihydroxy - 21 - [(3,3-dimethyl-1-oxobutyl)oxy] pregna-1,4-diene-3,20-dione. The empirical formula is $C_{27}H_{38}O_6$.
HYDELTRA-T.B.A.® (Prednisolone Tebutate, MSD) suspension is a white to slightly yellow suspension (pH 6.0 to 8.0) that settles upon standing. Each ml contains prednisolone tebutate, 20 mg. Inactive ingredients per ml: sodium citrate, 1 mg; polysorbate 80, 1 mg; sorbitol solution, 0.5 ml (equal to 450 mg d-sorbitol); Water for Injection, q.s., 1 ml. Benzyl alcohol, 9 mg, added as preservative.

Actions

HYDELTRA-T.B.A. has a slow onset but long duration of action when compared with more soluble preparations. Because of its slight solubility, it is suitable for intraarticular, intralesional, and soft tissue injection where its anti-inflammatory effects are confined mainly to the area in which it has been injected, although it is capable of producing systemic hormonal effects.
Naturally occurring glucocorticoids (hydrocortisone and cortisone), which also have salt-retaining properties, are used as replacement therapy in adrenocortical deficiency states. Their synthetic analogs, including prednisolone, are primarily used for their potent anti-inflammatory effects in disorders of many organ systems.
Glucocorticoids cause profound and varied metabolic effects. In addition, they modify the body's immune responses to diverse stimuli.

Indications

A. By intra-articular or soft tissue injection:
As adjunctive therapy for short-term administration (to tide the patient over an acute episode or exacerbation) in:

Synovitis of osteoarthritis
Rheumatoid arthritis
Acute and subacute bursitis
Acute gouty arthritis
Epicondylitis
Acute nonspecific tenosynovitis
Post-traumatic osteoarthritis

B. By intralesional injection:
May be useful in cystic tumors of an aponeurosis or tendon (ganglia).

Contraindications

Systemic fungal infections
Hypersensitivity to any component of this product

Warnings

In patients on corticosteroid therapy subjected to any unusual stress, increased dosage of rapidly acting corticosteroids before, during, and after the stressful situation is indicated.
Drug-induced secondary adrenocortical insufficiency may result from too rapid withdrawal of corticosteroids and may be minimized by gradual reduction of dosage. This type of relative insufficiency may persist for months after discontinuation of therapy; therefore, in any situation of stress occurring during that period, hormone therapy should be reinstituted. If the patient is receiving steroids already, dosage may have to be increased. Since mineralocorticoid secretion may be impaired, salt and/or a mineralocorticoid should be administered concurrently.
Corticosteroids may mask some signs of infection, and new infections may appear during their use. There may be decreased resistance and inability to localize infection when corticosteroids are used. Moreover, corticosteroids may affect the nitroblue-tetrazolium test for bacterial infection and produce false negative results.
Corticosteroids may activate latent amebiasis. Therefore, it is recommended that latent or active amebiasis be ruled out before initiating corticosteroid therapy in any patient who has spent time in the tropics or any patient with unexplained diarrhea.
Prolonged use of corticosteroids may produce posterior subcapsular cataracts, glaucoma with possible damage to the optic nerves, and may enhance the establishment of secondary ocular infections due to fungi or viruses.
Usage in pregnancy. Since adequate human reproduction studies have not been done with corticosteroids, use of these drugs in pregnancy or in women of childbearing potential requires that the anticipated benefits be weighed against the possible hazards to the mother and embryo or fetus. Infants born of mothers who have received substantial doses of corticosteroids during pregnancy should be carefully observed for signs of hypoadrenalism.
Corticosteroids appear in breast milk and could suppress growth, interfere with endogenous corticosteroid production, or cause other unwanted effects. Mothers taking pharmacologic doses of corticosteroids should be advised not to nurse.
Average and large doses of cortisone or hydrocortisone can cause elevation of blood pressure, salt and water retention, and increased excretion of potassium. These effects are less likely to occur with the synthetic derivatives except when used in large doses. Dietary salt restriction and potassium supplementation may be necessary. All corticosteroids increase calcium excretion.
Administration of live virus vaccines, including smallpox, is contraindicated in individuals receiving immunosuppressive doses of corticosteroids. If inactivated viral or bacterial vaccines are administered to individuals receiving immunosuppressive doses of corticosteroids, the expected serum antibody response may not be obtained.
If corticosteroids are indicated in patients with latent tuberculosis or tuberculin reactivity, close observation is necessary as reactivation of the disease may occur. During prolonged corticosteroid therapy, these patients should receive chemoprophylaxis.
Because rare instances of anaphylactoid reactions have occurred in patients receiving parenteral corticosteroid therapy, appropriate precautionary measures should be taken prior to administration, especially when the patient has a history of allergy to any drug.

Precautions

This product, like many other steroid formulations, is sensitive to heat. Therefore, it should not be autoclaved when it is desirable to sterilize the exterior of the vial.
Following prolonged therapy, withdrawal of corticosteroids may result in symptoms of the corticosteroid withdrawal syndrome including fever, myalgia, arthralgia, and malaise. This

Continued on next page

Information on the Merck Sharp & Dohme products listed on these pages is the full prescribing information from package circulars in use October 31, 1982.

Merck Sharp & Dohme—Cont.

may occur in patients even without evidence of adrenal insufficiency.

There is an enhanced effect of corticosteroids in patients with hypothyroidism and in those with cirrhosis.

Corticosteroids should be used cautiously in patients with ocular herpes simplex for fear of corneal perforation.

Psychic derangements may appear when corticosteroids are used, ranging from euphoria, insomnia, mood swings, personality changes, and severe depression to frank psychotic manifestations. Also, existing emotional instability or psychotic tendencies may be aggravated by corticosteroids.

Aspirin should be used cautiously in conjunction with corticosteroids in hypoprothrombinemia.

Steroids should be used with caution in nonspecific ulcerative colitis, if there is a probability of impending perforation, abscess, or other pyogenic infection, also in diverticulitis, fresh intestinal anastomoses, active or latent peptic ulcer, renal insufficiency, hypertension, osteoporosis, and myasthenia gravis. Signs of peritoneal irritation following gastrointestinal perforation in patients receiving large doses of corticosteroids may be minimal or absent. Fat embolism has been reported as a possible complication of hypercortisonism.

When large doses are given, some authorities advise that antacids be administered between meals to help to prevent peptic ulcer.

Growth and development of infants and children on prolonged corticosteroid therapy should be carefully followed.

Steroids may increase or decrease motility and number of spermatozoa in some patients.

Phenytoin, phenobarbital, ephedrine, and rifampin may enhance the metabolic clearance of corticosteroids, resulting in decreased blood levels and lessened physiologic activity, thus requiring adjustment in corticosteroid dosage.

The prothrombin time should be checked frequently in patients who are receiving corticosteroids and coumarin anticoagulants at the same time because of reports that corticosteroids have altered the response to these anticoagulants. Studies have shown that the usual effect produced by adding corticosteroids is inhibition of response to coumarins, although there have been some conflicting reports of potentiation not substantiated by studies.

When corticosteroids are administered concomitantly with potassium-depleting diuretics, patients should be observed closely for development of hypokalemia.

Intra-articular injection of a corticosteroid may produce systemic as well as local effects.

Appropriate examination of any joint fluid present is necessary to exclude a septic process.

A marked increase in pain accompanied by local swelling, further restriction of joint motion, fever, and malaise is suggestive of septic arthritis. If this complication occurs and the diagnosis of sepsis is confirmed, appropriate antimicrobial therapy should be instituted.

Injection of a steroid into an infected site is to be avoided.

Corticosteroids should not be injected into unstable joints.

Patients should be impressed strongly with the importance of not overusing joints in which symptomatic benefit has been obtained as long as the inflammatory process remains active.

Frequent intra-articular injection may result in damage to joint tissues.

Adverse Reactions

Fluid and electrolyte disturbances
- Sodium retention
- Fluid retention
- Congestive heart failure in susceptible patients
- Potassium loss
- Hypokalemic alkalosis
- Hypertension

Musculoskeletal
- Muscle weakness
- Steroid myopathy
- Loss of muscle mass
- Osteoporosis
- Vertebral compression fractures
- Aseptic necrosis of femoral and humeral heads
- Pathlogic fracture of long bones
- Tendon rupture

Gastrointestinal
- Peptic ulcer with possible subsequent perforation and hemorrhage
- Perforation of the small and large bowel, particularly in patients with inflammatory bowel disease
- Pancreatitis
- Abdominal distention
- Ulcerative esophagitis

Dematologic
- Impaired wound healing
- Thin fragile skin
- Petechiae and ecchymoses
- Erythema
- Increased sweating
- May suppress reactions to skin tests
- Other cutaneous reactions, such as allergic dermatitis, urticaria, angioneurotic edema

Neurologic
- Convulsions
- Increased intracranial pressure with papilledema (pseudotumor cerebri) usually after treatment
- Vertigo
- Headache

Endocrine
- Menstrual irregularities
- Development of cushingoid state
- Suppression of growth in children
- Secondary adrenocortical and pituitary unresponsiveness, particularly in times of stress, as in trauma, surgery, or illness
- Decreased carbohydrate tolerance
- Manifestations of latent diabetes mellitus
- Increased requirements for insulin or oral hypoglycemic agents in diabetics

Ophthalmic
- Posterior subcapsular cataracts
- Increased intraocular pressure
- Glaucoma
- Exophthalmos

Metabolic
- Negative nitrogen balance due to protein catabolism

Other
- Anaphylactoid or hypersensitivity reactions
- Thromboembolism
- Weight gain
- Increased appetite
- Nausea
- Malaise

Foreign body granulomatous reactions involving the synovium have been reported with repeated injections of HYDELTRA-T.B.A.

Localized pain and swelling, sometimes distal to the site of injection and persisting for several days, have been reported.

The following *additional* adverse reactions are related to injection of corticosteroids:
- Rare instances of blindness associated with intralesional therapy around the face and head
- Hyperpigmentation or hypopigmentation
- Subcutaneous and cutaneous atrophy
- Sterile abscess
- Postinjection flare (following intra-articular use)
- Charcot-like arthropathy

Dosage and Administration

For intra-articular, intralesional, and soft tissue injection only.

DOSAGE AND FREQUENCY OF INJECTION ARE VARIABLE AND MUST BE INDIVIDUALIZED ON THE BASIS OF THE DISEASE AND THE RESPONSE OF THE PATIENT.

The initial dose varies from 4 to 40 mg depending on the disease being treated and the size of the area to be injected. Frequency of injection depends on symptomatic response, and usually is once every two or three weeks. Severe conditions may require injection once a week. Frequent intra-articular injection may result in damage to joint tissues. If satisfactory clinical response does not occur after a reasonable period of time, discontinue HYDELTRA-T.B.A. suspension and transfer the patient to other therapy.

Patients should be observed closely for signs that might require dosage adjustment, including changes in clinical status resulting from remissions or exacerbations of the disease, and individual drug responsiveness.

For rapid onset of action, a soluble adrenocortical hormone preparation, such as DECADRON® phosphate (Dexamethasone Sodium Phosphate, MSD) injection or HYDELTRASOL® (Prednisolone Sodium Phosphate, MSD) injection, may be given with HYDELTRA-T.B.A.

If desired, a local anesthetic may be used, and may be injected before HYDELTRA-T.B.A., or mixed in a syringe with HYDELTRA-T.B.A. and given simultaneously.

If used prior to intra-articular injection of the steroid, inject most of the anesthetic into the soft tissues of the surrounding area and instill a small amount into the joint.

If given together, mixing should be done in the injection syringe by drawing the steroid in *first,* then the anesthetic. In this way, the anesthetic will not be introduced inadvertently into the vial of steroid. *The mixture must be used immediately and any unused portion discarded.*

Some of the usual single doses are:

Large Joints (e.g., Knee)	20 mg (1 ml), occasionally 30 mg (1.5 ml). Doses over 40 mg (2 ml) not recommended.
Small Joints (e.g., Interphalangeal, Temporomandibular)	8 to 10 mg (0.4 to 0.5 ml).
Bursae	20 to 30 mg (1 to 1.5 ml).
Tendon Sheaths	4 to 10 mg (0.2 to 0.5 ml).
Ganglia	10 to 20 mg (0.5 to 1 ml).

How Supplied

No. 7572—Suspenson HYDELTRA-T.B.A., 20 mg per ml, is a white, milky suspension, and is supplied as follows:

NDC 0006-7572-01 in 1 ml vials (6505-00-225-7499 1 ml vial)

NDC 0006-7572-03 in 5 ml vials (6505-00-890-1353 5 ml vial).

A.H.F.S. Category: 68:04

DC 6138621 Issued August 1981

HYDELTRASOL® Sterile Ophthalmic Solution (prednisolone sodium phosphate, MSD), U.S.P. ℞

Description

Ophthalmic Solution HYDELTRASOL® (Prednisolone Sodium Phosphate, MSD) is a topical steroid solution containing prednisolone sodium phosphate equivalent to 5 mg

(0.5%) of prednisolone phosphate in each milliliter of buffered solution. Inactive ingredients: creatinine, sodium citrate, polysorbate 80, disodium edetate, potassium phosphate, hydrochloric acid to adjust pH, and water for injection. Benzalkonium chloride 0.02% and phenylethanol 0.25% added as preservatives. Prednisolone sodium phosphate is an inorganic ester of prednisolone. It is approximately two thousand times more soluble in water at 25° C than hydrocortisone.

Action

Inhibition of inflammatory response to inciting agents of mechanical, chemical or immunological nature. No generally accepted explanation of this steroid property has been advanced.

Indications

For the treatment of the following conditions:
Ophthalmic:
Steroid responsive inflammatory conditions of the palpebral and bulbar conjunctiva, cornea, and anterior segment of the globe, such as allergic conjunctivitis, acne rosacea, superficial punctate keratitis, herpes zoster keratitis, iritis, cyclitis, selected infective conjunctivitis when the inherent hazard of steroid use is accepted to obtain an advisible diminution in edema and inflammation; corneal injury from chemical or thermal burns, or penetration of foreign bodies.
Otic:
Steroid responsive inflammatory conditions of the external auditory meatus, such as allergic otitis externa, selected purulent and nonpurulent infective otitis externa when the hazard of steroid use is accepted to obtain an advisable diminution in edema and inflammation.

Contraindications

Acute superficial herpes simplex keratitis.
Fungal diseases of ocular or auricular structures.
Acute infectious stages of vaccinia, varicella and most other viral diseases of the cornea and conjunctiva.
Tuberculosis of the eye.
Hypersensitivity to a component of this medication.
Perforation of a drum membrane.

Warnings

Employment of steroid medication in the treatment of stromal herpes simplex requires great caution; frequent slit-lamp microscopy is mandatory.
Prolonged use may result in elevated intraocular pressure and/or glaucoma, damage to the optic nerve, defects in visual acuity and fields of vision, posterior subcapsular cataract formation, or may result in secondary ocular infections.
Viral, bacterial, and fungal infections of the cornea may be exacerbated by the application of steroids.
Acute purulent untreated infection of the eye or ear may be masked or activity enhanced by the presence of steroid medication.
In those diseases causing thinning of the cornea or sclera, perforation has been known to occur with the use of topical steroids.
Usage in Pregnancy
Safety of intensive or protracted use of topical steroids during pregnancy has not been substantiated.

Precautions

As fungal infections of the cornea are particularly prone to develop coincidentally with long-term local steroid applications, fungus invasion must be considered in any persistent corneal ulceration where a steroid has been used or is in use.
Intraocular pressure should be checked frequently.

Adverse Reactions

Glaucoma with optic nerve damage, visual acuity and field defects, posterior subcapsular cataract formation, secondary ocular infection from pathogens including herpes simplex, perforation of the globe.
Rarely, filtering blebs have been reported when topical steroids have been used following cataract surgery.
Rarely, stinging or burning may occur.

Dosage and Administration

The duration of treatment will vary with the type of lesion and may extend from a few days to several weeks, according to therapeutic response. Relapses, more common in chronic active lesions than in self-limited conditions, usually respond to retreatment.
Eye—Instill one or two drops of solution into the conjunctival sac every hour during the day and every two hours during the night as initial therapy. When a favorable response is observed, reduce dosage to one drop every four hours. Later, further reduction in dosage to one drop three or four times daily may suffice to control symptoms.
Ear—Clean the aural canal thoroughly and sponge dry. Instill the solution directly into the aural canal by means of a dropper. A suggested initial dosage is three or four drops two or three times a day. When a favorable response is obtained, reduce dosage gradually and eventually discontinue.
If preferred, the aural canal may be packed with a gauze wick saturated with solution. Keep the wick moist with the preparation and remove from the ear after 12 to 24 hours. Treatment may be repeated as often as necessary at the discretion of the physician.

How Supplied

No. 7574X — 0.5% Ophthalmic Solution HYDELTRASOL is a clear, colorless to pale-yellow, sterile solution and is supplied as follows:
NDC 0006-7574-03 in 5 ml bottles with dropper assembly.
(6505-00-616-9517 5 ml bottle)

A.H.F.S. Category: 52:08
DC 6026117 Issued May 1981

HYDROCORTONE® Acetate ℞
Sterile Ophthalmic Ointment
(hydrocortisone acetate, MSD), U.S.P.
HYDROCORTONE® Acetate ℞
Sterile Ophthalmic Suspension
(hydrocortisone acetate, MSD), U.S.P.

Description

Sterile Ophthalmic Ointment HYDROCORTONE® Acetate (Hydrocortisone Acetate, MSD) 1.5% is a topical steroid preparation containing 15 mg of hydrocortisone acetate in a white petrolatum and mineral oil base in each gram.
Sterile Ophthalmic Suspension HYDROCORTONE® Acetate 2.5% contains 25 mg of hydrocortisone acetate in each milliliter. Inactive ingredients: sodium citrate, dibasic sodium phosphate, monobasic sodium phosphate, sodium chloride, polyethylene glycol 4000, polysorbate 80, and water for injection. Benzyl alcohol 0.5%, and benzalkonium chloride, 0.02%, are added as preservatives.

Action

Inhibition of inflammatory response to inciting agents of mechanical, chemical or immunological nature. No generally accepted explanation of this steroid property has been advanced.

Indications

For the treatment of the following conditions:
Ophthalmic:
Steroid responsive inflammatory conditions of the palpebral and bulbar conjunctiva, cornea, and anterior segment of the globe, such as allergic conjunctivitis, acne rosacea, superficial punctate keratitis, herpes zoster keratitis, iritis, cyclitis, selected infective conjunctivitis when the inherent hazard of steroid use is accepted to obtain an advisable diminution in edema and inflammation; corneal injury from chemical or thermal burns, or penetration of foreign bodies.
Otic:
Steroid responsive inflammatory conditions of the external auditory meatus, such as allergic otitis externa, selected purulent and nonpurulent infective otitis externa when the hazard of steroid use is accepted to obtain an advisable diminution in edema and inflammation.

Contraindications

Acute superficial herpes simplex keratitis.
Fungal diseases of ocular or auricular structures.
Acute infectious stages of vaccinia, varicella and most other viral diseases of the cornea and conjunctiva.
Tuberculosis of the eye.
Hypersensitivity to a component of this medication.
Perforation of a drum membrane.

Warnings

Employment of steroid medication in the treatment of stromal herpes simplex requires great caution; frequent slit-lamp microscopy is mandatory.
Prolonged use may result in elevated intraocular pressure and/or glaucoma, damage to the optic nerve, defects in visual acuity and fields of vision, posterior subcapsular cataract formation, or may result in secondary ocular infections.
Viral, bacterial, and fungal infections of the cornea may be exacerbated by the application of steroids.
Acute purulent untreated infection of the eye or ear may be masked or activity enhanced by the presence of steroid medication.
In those diseases causing thinning of the cornea or sclera, perforation has been known to occur with the use of topical steroids.
Usage in Pregnancy
Safety of intensive or protracted use of topical steroids during pregnancy has not been substantiated.

Precautions

As fungal infections of the cornea are particularly prone to develop coincidentally with long-term local steroid applications, fungus invasion must be considered in any persistent corneal ulceration where a steroid has been used or is in use.
Intraocular pressure should be checked frequently.

Adverse Reactions

Glaucoma with optic nerve damage, visual acuity and field defects, posterior subcapsular cataract formation, secondary ocular infection from pathogens including herpes simplex, perforation of the globe.

Continued on next page

Information on the Merck Sharp & Dohme products listed on these pages is the full prescribing information from package circulars in use October 31, 1982.

Merck Sharp & Dohme—Cont.

Rarely, filtering blebs have been reported when topical steroids have been used following cataract surgery.
Rarely, stinging or burning may occur.

Dosage and Administration

The duration of treatment will vary with the type of lesion and may extend from a few days to several weeks, according to therapeutic response. Relapses, more common in chronic active lesions than in self-limited conditions, usually respond to retreatment.
Ophthalmic Suspension HYDROCORTONE Acetate (Hydrocortisone Acetate, MSD)
Eye—Instill one or two drops into the conjunctival sac every hour during the day and every two hours during the night as initial therapy. When a favorable response is observed, reduce dosage to one drop every four hours. Later, further reduction in dosage to one drop three or four times daily may suffice to control symptoms.
Ear—Clean the aural canal thoroughly and sponge dry. Instill ophthalmic suspension HYDROCORTONE acetate directly into the aural canal by use of the dropper. A suggested initial dosage is three or four drops two or three times a day. When a favorable response is obtained, reduce dosage gradually and eventually discontinue.
If preferred, the aural canal may be packed with a gauze wick saturated with ophthalmic suspension HYDROCORTONE acetate. Keep the wick moist with the preparation and remove from the ear after 12 to 24 hours. Treatment may be repeated as often as necessary at the discretion of the physician.
Ophthalmic Ointment HYDROCORTONE Acetate (Hydrocortisone Acetate, MSD)
Eye—Apply a thin coating to the affected area three or four times a day. When a favorable response is observed, reduce the number of daily applications to two, and later to one a day as a maintenance dose if this proves sufficient to control symptoms.
Ophthalmic ointment HYDROCORTONE acetate is particularly convenient when an eye pad is used. It may also be the preparation of choice for patients in whom therapeutic benefit depends on prolonged contact of the active ingredients with ocular tissues.
Ear—Clean the aural canal thoroughly and sponge dry. With a cotton-tipped applicator, apply a thin coating of ophthalmic ointment HYDROCORTONE acetate to the affected canal area two or three times a day. When a favorable response is obtained, reduce the number of daily applications to one or two, and eventually discontinue.

Storage

Ophthalmic suspension HYDROCORTONE acetate should be protected from freezing to avoid the possibility of the formation of aggregates or larger crystals which may render the product unsuitable for use. It is supplied as a sterile preparation. Care should be exercised to avoid contamination.

How Supplied

No. 7504—1.5% Sterile Ophthalmic Ointment HYDROCORTONE Acetate, is a clear, unctuous ointment, supplied as follows:
NDC 0006-7504-04 in 3.5 g tubes, each gram containing 15 mg hydrocortisone acetate in a white petrolatum and mineral oil base.
No. 7506—2.5% Sterile Ophthalmic Suspension HYDROCORTONE Acetate, is a sterile, white suspension supplied as follows:
NDC 0006-7506-03 in 5 ml dropper bottles, each milliliter containing 25 mg hydrocortisone acetate.

A.H.F.S. Category: 52:08
DC 6007521 Issued May 1981

HydroDIURIL® Tablets ℞
(hydrochlorothiazide, MSD), U.S.P.

Description

HydroDIURIL® (Hydrochlorothiazide, MSD) is the 3,4-dihydro derivative of chlorothiazide. Its chemical name is 6-chloro-3,4-dihydro-2*H*-1,2,4-benzothiadiazine- 7-sulfonamide 1,1-dioxide.

It is a white, or practically white, crystalline compound slightly soluble in water, but freely soluble in sodium hydroxide solution.

Actions

HydroDIURIL is a diuretic and antihypertensive.

HydroDIURIL affects the renal tubular mechanism of electrolyte reabsorption. At maximal therapeutic dosage all thiazides are approximately equal in their diuretic efficacy.

HydroDIURIL increases excretion of sodium and chloride in approximately equivalent amounts. Natriuresis may be accompanied by some loss of potassium and bicarbonate.
After oral use diuresis begins within 2 hours, peaks in about 4 hours and lasts about 6 to 12 hours. HydroDIURIL is eliminated rapidly by the kidney.

The mechanism of the antihypertensive effect of thiazides is unknown. HydroDIURIL does not affect normal blood pressure.

Indications

HydroDIURIL is indicated as adjunctive therapy in edema associated with congestive heart failure, hepatic cirrhosis, and corticosteroid and estrogen therapy.

HydroDIURIL has also been found useful in edema due to various forms of renal dysfunction such as nephrotic syndrome, acute glomerulonephritis, and chronic renal failure.

HydroDIURIL is indicated in the management of hypertension either as the sole therapeutic agent or to enhance the effectiveness of other antihypertensive drugs in the more severe forms of hypertension.

Use in Pregnancy. Routine use of diuretics during normal pregnancy is inappropriate and exposes mother and fetus to unnecessary hazard. Diuretics do not prevent development of toxemia of pregnancy and there is no satisfactory evidence that they are useful in the treatment of toxemia.

Edema during pregnancy may arise from pathologic causes or from the physiologic and mechanical consequences of pregnancy. Thiazides are indicated in pregnancy when edema is due to pathologic causes, just as they are in the absence of pregnancy (however, see WARNINGS). Dependent edema in pregnancy, resulting from restriction of venous return by the gravid uterus, is properly treated through elevation of the lower extremities and use of support stockings. Use of diuretics to lower intravascular volume in this instance is illogical and unnecessary. During normal pregnancy there is hypervolemia which is not harmful to the fetus or the mother in the absence of cardiovascular disease. However, it may be associated with edema, rarely generalized edema. If such edema causes discomfort, increased recumbency will often provide relief. Rarely this edema may cause extreme discomfort which is not relieved by rest. In these instances, a short course of diuretic therapy may provide relief and be appropriate.

Contraindications

Anuria.
Hypersensitivity to this product or to other sulfonamide-derived drugs.

Warnings

Use with caution in severe renal disease. In patients with renal disease, thiazides may precipitate azotemia. Cumulative effects of the drug may develop in patients with impaired renal function.
Thiazides should be used with caution in patients with impaired hepatic function or progressive liver disease, since minor alterations of fluid and electrolyte balance may precipitate hepatic coma.
Thiazides may add to or potentiate the action of other antihypertensive drugs.
Sensitivity reactions may occur in patients with or without a history of allergy or bronchial asthma.
The possibility of exacerbation or activation of systemic lupus erythematosus has been reported.
Lithium generally should not be given with diuretics because they reduce its renal clearance and add a high risk of lithium toxicity. Read circulars for lithium preparations before use of such concomitant therapy.
Use in Pregnancy. Thiazides cross the placental barrier and appear in cord blood. The use of thiazides in pregnancy requires that the anticipated benefit be weighed against possible hazards to the fetus. These hazards include fetal or neonatal jaundice, thrombocytopenia, and possibly other adverse reactions which have occurred in the adult.
Nursing Mothers. Thiazides appear in breast milk. If use of the drug is deemed essential, the patient should stop nursing.

Precautions

Periodic determination of serum electrolytes to detect possible electrolyte imbalance should be performed at appropriate intervals.
All patients receiving diuretic therapy should be observed for evidence of fluid or electrolyte imbalance: namely, hyponatremia, hypochloremic alkalosis, and hypokalemia. Serum and urine electrolyte determinations are particularly important when the patient is vomiting excessively or receiving parenteral fluids. Warning signs or symptoms of fluid and electrolyte imbalance include dryness of mouth, thirst, weakness, lethargy, drowsiness, restlessness, muscle pains or cramps, muscular fatigue, hypotension, oliguria, tachycardia, and gastrointestinal disturbances such as nausea and vomiting.
Hypokalemia may develop, especially with brisk diuresis, when severe cirrhosis is present, during concomitant use of corticosteroids or ACTH, or after prolonged therapy.
Interference with adequate oral electrolyte intake will also contribute to hypokalemia. Hypokalemia can sensitize or exaggerate the response of the heart to the toxic effects of digitalis (e.g., increased ventricular irritability). Hypokalemia may be avoided or treated by use of potassium supplements such as foods with a high potassium content.
Although any chloride deficit is generally mild and usually does not require specific treatment except under extraordinary circumstances (as in liver disease or renal disease), chloride replacement may be required in the treatment of metabolic alkalosis.
Dilutional hyponatremia may occur in edematous patients in hot weather; appropriate therapy is water restriction, rather than administration of salt, except in rare instances when the hyponatremia is life threatening. In actual salt depletion, appropriate replacement is the therapy of choice.
Hyperuricemia may occur or acute gout may be precipitated in certain patients receiving thiazides.
Insulin requirements in diabetic patients may be increased, decreased, or unchanged. Latent

diabetes mellitus may become manifest during thiazide therapy.

Thiazides may increase the responsiveness to tubocurarine.

The antihypertensive effects of the drug may be enhanced in the postsympathectomy patient. Thiazides may decrease arterial responsiveness to norepinephrine. This diminution is not sufficient to preclude effectiveness of the pressor agent for therapeutic use.

If progressive renal impairment becomes evident, consider withholding or discontinuing diuretic therapy.

Thiazides may decrease serum PBI levels without signs of thyroid disturbance.

Thiazides may decrease urinary calcium excretion. Thiazides may cause intermittent and slight elevation of serum calcium in the absence of known disorders of calcium metabolism. Marked hypercalcemia may be evidence of hidden hyperparathyroidism. Thiazides should be discontinued before carrying out tests for parathyroid function.

Adverse Reactions

A. *Gastrointestinal System*
1. anorexia
2. gastric irritation
3. nausea
4. vomiting
5. cramping
6. diarrhea
7. constipation
8. jaundice (intrahepatic cholestatic jaundice)
9. pancreatitis
10. sialadenitis

B. *Central Nervous System*
1. dizziness
2. vertigo
3. paresthesias
4. headache
5. xanthopsia

C. *Hematologic*
1. leukopenia
2. agranulocytosis
3. thrombocytopenia
4. aplastic anemia
5. hemolytic anemia

D. *Cardiovascular*
Orthostatic hypotension (may be aggravated by alcohol, barbiturates, or narcotics)

E. *Hypersensitivity*
1. purpura
2. photosensitivity
3. rash
4. urticaria
5. necrotizing angiitis (vasculitis) (cutaneous vasculitis)
6. fever
7. respiratory distress including pneumonitis and pulmonary edema
8. anaphylactic reactions

F. *Other*
1. hyperglycemia
2. glycosuria
3. hyperuricemia
4. muscle spasm
5. weakness
6. restlessness
7. transient blurred vision

Whenever adverse reactions are moderate or severe, thiazide dosage should be reduced or therapy withdrawn.

Dosage and Administration

Therapy should be individualized according to patient response. Use the smallest dosage necessary to achieve the required response.

Adults
For Diuresis
The usual adult dosage is 50 to 100 mg once or twice a day. Many patients with edema respond to intermittent therapy, i.e., administration on alternate days or on three to five days each week. With an intermittent schedule, excessive response and the resulting undesirable electrolyte imbalance are less likely to occur.

For Control of Hypertension
The usual adult starting dosage is 50 or 100 mg a day as a single or divided dose. Dosage is increased or decreased according to blood pressure response. Rarely some patients may require up to 200 mg a day in divided doses.

When thiazides are used with other antihypertensives, the dose of the latter may need to be reduced to prevent excessive decrease in blood pressure.

Infants and Children
The usual pediatric dosage is based on 1.0 mg of HydroDIURIL per pound of body weight per day in two doses. Infants under 6 months of age may require up to 1.5 mg per pound per day in two doses.

On this basis, infants up to 2 years of age may be given 12.5 to 37.5 mg daily in two doses. Children from 2 to 12 years of age may be given 37.5 to 100 mg daily in two doses. Dosage in both age groups should be based on body weight.

How Supplied

No. 3263—Tablets HydroDIURIL, 25 mg, are peach-colored, round, scored, compressed tablets, coded MSD 42. They are supplied as follows:

NDC 0006-0042-68 bottles of 100
NDC 0006-0042-28 single unit packages of 100
NDC 0006-0042-82 bottles of 1000

[*Shown in Product Identification Section*]

No. 3264—Tablets HydroDIURIL, 50 mg, are peach-colored, round, scored, compressed tablets, coded MSD 105. They are supplied as follows:

NDC 0006-0105-68 bottles of 100
NDC 0006-0105-28 single unit packages of 100
NDC 0006-0105-82 bottles of 1000
NDC 0006-0105-86 bottles of 5000

[*Shown in Product Identification Section*]

No. 3340—Tablets HydroDIURIL, 100 mg, are peach-colored, round, scored, compressed tablets, coded MSD 410. They are supplied as follows:

NDC 0006-0410-68 bottles of 100.

[*Shown in Product Identification Section*]

A.H.F.S. Category: 40:28
DC 6028532 Issued May 1980

HYDROPRES® Tablets ℞
(reserpine-hydrochlorothiazide, MSD), U.S.P.

WARNING

This fixed combination drug is not indicated for initial therapy of hypertension. Hypertension requires therapy titrated to the individual patient. If the fixed combination represents the dosage so determined, its use may be more convenient in patient management. The treatment of hypertension is not static, but must be reevaluated as conditions in each patient warrant.

Description

HYDROPRES® (Reserpine-Hydrochlorothiazide, MSD) combines two antihypertensive agents: HydroDIURIL® (Hydrochlorothiazide, MSD) and reserpine. The chemical name for hydrochlorothiazide is 6-chloro-3, 4-dihydro- 2*H*-1, 2, 4 - benzothiadiazine - 7 - sulfonamide 1,1-dioxide. Reserpine (11,17α-dimethoxy-18β-[(3, 4, 5-trimethoxybenzoyl) oxy]-3β, 20α-yohimban-16β-carboxylic acid methyl ester) is a crystalline alkaloid derived from Rauwolfia serpentina.

Actions

Hydrochlorothiazide
Hydrochlorothiazide is a diuretic and antihypertensive. It affects the renal tubular mechanism of electrolyte reabsorption. At maximal therapeutic dosage all thiazides are approximately equal in their diuretic efficacy.

Hydrochlorothiazide increases excretion of sodium and chloride in approximately equivalent amounts. Natriuresis may be accompanied by some loss of potassium and bicarbonate.

The mechanism of the antihypertensive effect of thiazides is unknown. Hydrochlorothiazide does not affect normal blood pressure.

Hydrochlorothiazide is eliminated rapidly by the kidney.

Reserpine
Reserpine has antihypertensive, bradycardic, and tranquilizing properties. It lowers arterial blood pressure by depletion of catecholamines. Reserpine is beneficial in relieving anxiety, tension, and headache in the hypertensive patient. It acts at the hypothalamic level of the central nervous system to promote relaxation without hypnosis or analgesia. The sleep pattern shown by the electroencephalogram following barbiturates does not occur with this drug. In laboratory animals spontaneous activity and response to external stimuli are decreased, but confusion or difficulty of movement is not evident.

The bradycardic action of reserpine promotes relaxation and may eliminate sinus tachycardia. It is most pronounced in subjects with sinus tachycardia and usually is not prominent in persons with a normal pulse rate.

Miosis, relaxation of the nictitating membrane, ptosis, hypothermia, and increased gastrointestinal activity are noted in animals given reserpine, sometimes in subclinical doses. None of these effects, except increased gastrointestinal activity, has been found to be clinically significant in man with therapeutic doses.

Indication

Hypertension (see box warning).

Contraindications

Hydrochlorothiazide is contraindicated in anuria.

HYDROPRES is contraindicated in hypersensitivity to hydrochlorothiazide or other sulfonamide-derived drugs or to reserpine.

Electroshock therapy should not be given to patients while on reserpine, as severe and even fatal reactions have been reported with minimal convulsive electroshock dosage. After discontinuing reserpine, allow at least seven days before starting electroshock therapy.

Active peptic ulcer, ulcerative colitis, and active mental depression, especially suicidal tendencies, are contraindications to reserpine therapy.

Warnings

Hydrochlorothiazide
Use with caution in severe renal disease. In patients with renal disease, thiazides may precipitate azotemia. Cumulative effects of the drug may develop in patients with impaired renal function.

Continued on next page

Information on the Merck Sharp & Dohme products listed on these pages is the full prescribing information from package circulars in use October 31, 1982.

Merck Sharp & Dohme—Cont.

Thiazides should be used with caution in patients with impaired hepatic function or progressive liver disease, since minor alterations of fluid and electrolyte balance may precipitate hepatic coma.
Thiazides may add to or potentiate the action of other antihypertensive drugs.
Sensitivity reactions may occur in patients with or without a history of allergy or bronchial asthma.
The possibility of exacerbation or activation of systemic lupus erythematosus has been reported.
Lithium generally should not be given with diuretics because they reduce its renal clearance and add a high risk of lithium toxicity. Read circulars for lithium preparations before use of such concomitant therapy.
Reserpine
The occurrence of mental depression due to reserpine in doses of 0.25 mg daily or less is unusual. In any event, HYDROPRES should be discontinued at the first sign of depression.
Use in Pregnancy
Reserpine has been demonstrated to cross the placental barrier in guinea pigs with depression of adrenal catecholamine stores in the newborn. There is some evidence that side effects such as nasal congestion, lethargy, depressed Moro reflex, and bradycardia may appear in infants born of reserpine-treated mothers.
Thiazides cross the placental barrier and appear in cord blood. The use of thiazides in pregnancy requires that the anticipated benefit be weighed against possible hazards to the fetus. These hazards include fetal or neonatal jaundice, thrombocytopenia, and possibly other adverse reactions which have occurred in the adult.
Nursing Mothers
Thiazides and reserpine appear in breast milk. If use of the drug is deemed essential, the patient should stop nursing.

Precautions

Hydrochlorothiazide
Periodic determination of serum electrolytes to detect possible electrolyte imbalance should be performed at appropriate intervals.
All patients receiving diuretic therapy should be observed for evidence of fluid or electrolyte imbalance: namely, hyponatremia, hypochloremic alkalosis, and hypokalemia. Serum and urine electrolyte determinations are particularly important when the patient is vomiting excessively or receiving parenteral fluids. Warning signs or symptoms of fluid and electrolyte imbalance include dryness of mouth, thirst, weakness, lethargy, drowsiness, restlessness, muscle pains or cramps, muscular fatigue, hypotension, oliguria, tachycardia, and gastrointestinal disturbances such as nausea and vomiting.
Hypokalemia may develop, especially with brisk diuresis, when severe cirrhosis is present, during concomitant use of corticosteroids or ACTH, or after prolonged therapy.
Interference with adequate oral electrolyte intake will contribute to hypokalemia. Hypokalemia can sensitize or exaggerate the response of the heart to the toxic effects of digitalis (e.g., increased ventricular irritability). Hypokalemia may be avoided or treated by use of potassium supplements such as foods with a high potassium content.
Although any chloride deficit is generally mild and usually does not require specific treatment except under extraordinary circumstances (as in liver disease or renal disease), chloride replacement may be required in the treatment of metabolic alkalosis.
Dilutional hyponatremia may occur in edematous patients in hot weather. Appropriate therapy is water restriction, rather than administration of salt, except in rare instances when the hyponatremia is life threatening. In actual salt depletion, appropriate replacement is the therapy of choice.
Hyperuricemia may occur or acute gout may be precipitated in certain patients receiving thiazides.
Insulin requirements in diabetic patients may be increased, decreased, or unchanged. Latent diabetes mellitus may become manifest during thiazide therapy.
Thiazides may increase the responsiveness to tubocurarine.
The antihypertensive effect of the drug may be enhanced in the postsympathectomy patient.
Thiazides may decrease arterial responsiveness to norepinephrine. This diminution is not sufficient to preclude effectiveness of the pressor agent for therapeutic use.
If progressive renal impairment becomes evident, consider withholding or discontinuing diuretic therapy.
Thiazides may decrease serum PBI levels without signs of thyroid disturbance.
Thiazides may decrease urinary calcium excretion. Thiazides may cause intermittent and slight elevation of serum calcium in the absence of known disorders of calcium metabolism. Marked hypercalcemia may be evidence of hidden hyperparathyroidism. Thiazides should be discontinued before carrying out tests for parathyroid function.
Reserpine
Since reserpine may increase gastric secretion and motility, it should be used cautiously in patients with a history of peptic ulcer, ulcerative colitis, or other gastrointestinal disorder. This compound may precipitate biliary colic in patients with gallstones, or bronchial asthma in susceptible persons.
Reserpine may cause hypotension including orthostatic hypotension.
In hypertensive patients on reserpine therapy significant hypotension and bradycardia may develop during surgical anesthesia. The anesthesiologist should be aware that reserpine has been taken, since it may be necessary to give vagal blocking agents parenterally to prevent or reverse hypotension and/or bradycardia.
Anxiety or depression, as well as psychosis, may develop during reserpine therapy. If depression is present when therapy is begun, it may be aggravated. Mental depression is unusual with reserpine doses of 0.25 mg daily or less. In any case, HYDROPRES should be discontinued at the first sign of depression. Extreme caution should be used in treating patients with a history of mental depression, and the possibility of suicide should be kept in mind.
As with most antihypertensive therapy, caution should be exercised when treating hypertensive patients with renal insufficiency, since they adjust poorly to lowered blood pressure levels. Use reserpine cautiously with digitalis and quinidine; cardiac arrhythmias have occurred with reserpine preparations.
When two or more antihypertensives are given, the individual dosages may have to be reduced to prevent excessive drop in blood pressure. In hypertensive patients with coronary artery disease, it is important to avoid a precipitous drop in blood pressure.

Adverse Reactions

Hydrochlorothiazide
Gastrointestinal: Anorexia, gastric irritation, nausea, vomiting, cramping, diarrhea, constipation, jaundice (intrahepatic cholestatic jaundice), pancreatitis, sialadenitis.
Central nervous system: Dizziness, vertigo, paresthesias, headache, xanthopsia.
Hematologic: Leukopenia, agranulocytosis, thrombocytopenia, aplastic anemia, hemolytic anemia.
Cardiovascular: Orthostatic hypotension (may be aggravated by alcohol, barbiturates, or narcotics).
Allergic: Purpura, photosensitivity, rash, urticaria, necrotizing angiitis (vasculitis) (cutaneous vasculitis), fever, respiratory distress including pneumonitis and pulmonary edema, anaphylactic reactions.
Other: Hyperglycemia, glycosuria, hyperuricemia, muscle spasm, weakness, restlessness, transient blurred vision.
Whenever adverse reactions are moderate or severe, the thiazide dosage should be reduced or therapy withdrawn.
Reserpine
Central nervous system: Excessive sedation, mental depression, nightmares, headache, dizziness, syncope, nervousness, paradoxical anxiety, central nervous system sensitization (dull sensorium, deafness, glaucoma, uveitis, optic atrophy), parkinsonism (usually reversible with decreased dosage or discontinuance of therapy).
Respiratory: Nasal congestion, dyspnea, epistaxis.
Cardiovascular: Bradycardia, angina pectoris, arrhythmia, premature ventricular contractions, and other direct cardiac effects (e.g., fluid retention, congestive failure).
Gastrointestinal: Hypersecretion and increased motility, nausea, vomiting, anorexia, diarrhea, dryness of mouth, increased salivation.
Hematologic: Excessive bleeding following prostatic surgery, thrombocytopenic purpura.
Allergic: Flushing of skin, pruritus, rash.
Other: Conjunctival injection, enhanced susceptibility to colds, muscular aches, weight gain, blurred vision, dysuria, nonpuerperal lactation, impotence, decreased libido.

Dosage and Administration

The initial dosage of HYDROPRES should conform to the dosages of the individual components established during titration (see box warning).
The usual adult dosage of HYDROPRES 25 is 1 or 2 tablets once or twice a day; that of HYDROPRES 50 is 1 tablet once or twice a day. Dosage may require adjustment according to the blood pressure response of the patient. Careful observations for changes in blood pressure must be made when HYDROPRES is used with other antihypertensive drugs.

How Supplied

No. 3265—Tablets HYDROPRES 25 are green, round, scored, compressed tablets, coded MSD 53. Each tablet contains 25 mg of hydrochlorothiazide and 0.125 mg of reserpine. They are supplied as follows:
NDC 0006-0053-68 in bottles of 100.
NDC 0006-0053-82 in bottles of 1000.
[*Shown in Product Identification Section*]
No. 3266—Tablets HYDROPRES 50 are green, round, scored, compressed tablets, coded MSD 127. Each tablet contains 50 mg of hydrochlorothiazide and 0.125 mg of reserpine. They are supplied as follows:
NDC 0006-0127-68 in bottles of 100.
NDC 0006-0127-82 in bottles of 1000.
[*Shown in Product Identification Section*]
A.H.F.S. Category: 24:08
DC 6053228 Issued May 1980

INDOCIN® Capsules ℞
(indomethacin, MSD), U.S.P.

INDOCIN® SR Capsules ℞
(indomethacin, MSD)

Description

INDOCIN® (Indomethacin, MSD) cannot be considered a simple analgesic and should not be used in conditions other than those recommended under INDICATIONS.

INDOCIN is supplied in two dosage forms: Capsules INDOCIN for oral administration containing either 25 mg or 50 mg of indomethacin, and Capsules INDOCIN SR for sustained release oral administration containing 75 mg of indomethacin. Indomethacin is a non-steroidal anti-inflammatory indole derivative designated chemically as 1-(4-chlorobenzoyl)-5-methoxy-2-methyl-1 *H*-indole-3-acetic acid.

Clinical Pharmacology

INDOCIN is a non-steroidal drug with anti-inflammatory, antipyretic and analgesic properties. Its mode of action, like that of other anti-inflammatory drugs, is not known. However, its therapeutic action is not due to pituitary-adrenal stimulation.

INDOCIN is a potent inhibitor of prostaglandin synthesis *in vitro*. Concentrations are reached during therapy which have been demonstrated to have an effect *in vivo* as well. Prostaglandins sensitize afferent nerves and potentiate the action of bradykinin in inducing pain in animal models. Moreover, prostaglandins are known to be among the mediators of inflammation. Since indomethacin is an inhibitor of prostaglandin synthesis, its mode of action may be due to a decrease of prostaglandins in peripheral tissues.

INDOCIN has been shown to be an effective anti-inflammatory agent, appropriate for long-term use in rheumatoid arthritis, ankylosing spondylitis, and osteoarthritis.

INDOCIN affords relief of symptoms; it does not alter the progressive course of the underlying disease.

INDOCIN suppresses inflammation in rheumatoid arthritis as demonstrated by relief of pain, and reduction of fever, swelling and tenderness. Improvement in patients treated with INDOCIN for rheumatoid arthritis has been demonstrated by a reduction in joint swelling, average number of joints involved, and morning stiffness; by increased mobility as demonstrated by a decrease in walking time; and by improved functional capability as demonstrated by an increase in grip strength.

Capsules INDOCIN have been found effective in relieving the pain, reducing the fever, swelling, redness, and tenderness of acute gouty arthritis. Capsules INDOCIN rather than Capsules INDOCIN SR are recommended for treatment of acute gouty arthritis—see INDICATIONS.

Following single oral doses of Capsules INDOCIN 25 mg or 50 mg, indomethacin is readily absorbed, attaining peak plasma concentrations of about 1 and 2 mcg/ml, respectively, at about 2 hours. Orally administered Capsules INDOCIN are virtually 100% bioavailable, with 90% of the dose absorbed within 4 hours. Capsules INDOCIN SR 75 mg are designed to release 25 mg of the drug initially and the remaining 50 mg over an extended time period. When measured over a 24-hour period, the cumulative amount and time-course of indomethacin absorption from a single Capsule INDOCIN SR are comparable to those of 3 doses of 25 mg Capsules INDOCIN given at 4-6 hour intervals. Absorption into the systemic circulation continues over an extended period with 90% of the dose absorbed by 12 hours.

Plasma concentrations of indomethacin fluctuate less and are more sustained following administration of Capsules INDOCIN SR than following administration of 25 mg Capsules INDOCIN given at 4-6 hour intervals. In multiple-dose comparisons, the mean steady-state plasma level of indomethacin attained with daily administration of Capsules INDOCIN SR 75 mg was indistinguishable from that following Capsules INDOCIN 25 mg given at 0, 6 and 12 hours daily.

Controlled clinical studies of safety and efficacy have shown that one Capsule INDOCIN SR was clinically comparable to one 25 mg Capsule INDOCIN t.i.d.; and one Capsule INDOCIN SR taken in the morning and one in the evening were clinically indistinguishable from one 50 mg Capsule INDOCIN t.i.d.

Indomethacin is eliminated via renal excretion, metabolism, and biliary excretion. Indomethacin undergoes appreciable enterohepatic circulation. The mean half-life of indomethacin is estimated to be about 4.5 hours. With a typical therapeutic regimen of 25 or 50 mg t.i.d., the steady-state plasma concentrations of indomethacin are an average 1.4 times those following the first dose.

Indomethacin exists in the plasma as the parent drug and its desmethyl, desbenzoyl, and desmethyl-desbenzoyl metabolites, all in the unconjugated form. About 60 percent of an oral dosage is recovered in urine as drug and metabolites (26 percent as indomethacin and its glucuronide), and 33 percent is recovered in feces (1.5 percent as indomethacin).

About 90% of indomethacin is bound to protein in plasma over the expected range of therapeutic plasma concentrations.

Indications

Because of its potential to cause adverse reactions, particularly at high dose levels, the use of INDOCIN in rheumatoid arthritis and osteoarthritis in adults should be carefully considered for active disease unresponsive to adequate trial with salicylates and other measures of established value, such as appropriate rest. In accord with this important concept indomethacin has been found effective in active stages of the following:

1. Moderate to severe rheumatoid arthritis including acute flares of chronic disease.
2. Moderate to severe ankylosing spondylitis.
3. Moderate to severe osteoarthritis.
4. Acute painful shoulder (bursitis and/or tendinitis).
5. Acute gouty arthritis.

Capsules INDOCIN SR are recommended for all of the indications for Capsules INDOCIN except acute gouty arthritis.

INDOCIN may enable the reduction of steroid dosage in patients receiving steroids for the more severe forms of rheumatoid arthritis. In such instances the steroid dosage should be reduced slowly and the patients followed very closely for any possible adverse effects.

The use of INDOCIN in conjunction with aspirin or other salicylates is not recommended. Controlled clinical studies have shown that the combined use of INDOCIN and aspirin does not produce any greater therapeutic effect than the use of INDOCIN alone. Furthermore, in one of these clinical studies, the incidence of gastrointestinal side effects was significantly increased with combined therapy. (See DRUG INTERACTIONS)

Contraindications

INDOCIN is contraindicated in patients who are allergic to INDOCIN or who have nasal polyps associated with angioedema or a bronchospastic reaction to aspirin or other non-steroidal anti-inflammatory drugs.

Warnings

General:

Because of the variability of the potential of INDOCIN to cause adverse reactions in the individual patient, the following are strongly recommended:

1. The lowest possible effective dose for the individual patient should be prescribed. Increased dosage tends to increase adverse effects, particularly in doses over 150-200 mg/day, without corresponding increase in clinical benefits.
2. Careful instructions to, and observations of, the individual patient are essential to the prevention of serious adverse reactions. As advancing years appear to increase the possibility of adverse reactions, INDOCIN should be used with greater care in the aged.
3. Safe conditions for use in children have not been established; therefore, INDOCIN should not be prescribed for children 14 years of age and under except under circumstances where lack of efficacy or toxicity associated with other drugs warrants the risk. Such patients should be monitored closely.

Gastrointestinal Effects:

Single or multiple ulcerations, including perforation and hemorrhage of the esophagus, stomach, duodenum or small intestine, have been reported to occur with INDOCIN. Fatalities have been reported in some instances. Rarely, intestinal ulceration has been associated with stenosis and obstruction.

Gastrointestinal bleeding without obvious ulcer formation and perforation of pre-existing sigmoid lesions (diverticulum, carcinoma, etc.) have occurred. Increased abdominal pain in ulcerative colitis patients or the development of ulcerative colitis and regional ileitis have been reported to occur rarely.

Because of the occurrence, and at times severity, of gastrointestinal reactions to INDOCIN, the prescribing physician must be continuously alert for any sign or symptom signaling a possible gastrointestinal reaction. The risks of continuing therapy with INDOCIN in the face of such symptoms must be weighed against the possible benefits to the individual patient.

INDOCIN should not be given to patients with active gastrointestinal lesions or with a history of recurrent gastrointestinal lesions except under circumstances which warrant the very high risk and where patients can be monitored very closely.

The gastrointestinal effects may be reduced by giving INDOCIN immediately after meals, with food, or with antacids.

Ocular Effects:

Corneal deposits and retinal disturbances, including those of the macula, have been observed in some patients who had received prolonged therapy with INDOCIN. The prescribing physician should be alert to the possible association between the changes noted and INDOCIN. It is advisable to discontinue therapy if such changes are observed. Blurred vision may be a significant symptom and warrants a thorough ophthalmological examination. Since these changes may be asymptomatic, ophthalmologic examination at periodic intervals is desirable in patients where therapy is prolonged.

Central Nervous System Effects:

INDOCIN may aggravate depression or other psychiatric disturbances, epilepsy, and parkinsonism, and should be used with considerable caution in patients with these conditions. If severe CNS adverse reactions develop, INDOCIN should be discontinued.

INDOCIN may cause drowsiness; therefore, patients should be cautioned about engaging in activities requiring mental alertness and motor coordination, such as driving a car. INDOCIN may also cause headache. Headache which persists despite dosage reduction requires cessation of therapy with INDOCIN.

Use in Pregnancy and the Neonatal Period

The safe use of INDOCIN in pregnant women has not been established. Administration of INDOCIN is not recommended during pregnancy.

Teratogenic studies were conducted in mice and rats at dosages of 0.5, 1.0, 2.0, and 4.0 mg/kg/day. Except for retarded fetal ossification at 4 mg/kg/day considered secondary to

Continued on next page

Information on the Merck Sharp & Dohme products listed on these pages is the full prescribing information from package circulars in use October 31, 1982.

Merck Sharp & Dohme—Cont.

the decreased average fetal weights, no increase in fetal malformations was observed as compared with control groups. Other studies in mice reported in the literature using higher doses (5 to 15 mg/kg/day) have described maternal toxicity and death, increased fetal resorptions, and fetal malformations. Comparable studies in rodents using high doses of aspirin have shown similar maternal and fetal effects.

As with other non-steroidal anti-inflammatory agents which inhibit prostaglandin synthesis, indomethacin has been found to delay parturition in rats.

In rats and mice, 4.0 mg/kg/day given during the last three days of gestation caused a decrease in maternal weight gain and some maternal and fetal deaths. An increased incidence of neuronal necrosis in the diencephalon in the live-born fetuses was observed. At 2.0 mg/kg/day, no increase in neuronal necrosis was observed as compared to the control groups. Administration of 0.5 or 4.0 mg/kg/day during the first three days of life did not cause an increase in neuronal necrosis at either dose level.

Use in Nursing Mothers

INDOCIN is excreted in the milk of lactating mothers. INDOCIN is not recommended for use in nursing mothers.

Precautions

INDOCIN may mask the usual signs and symptoms of infection. Therefore, the physician must be continually on the alert for this and should use the drug with extra care in the presence of existing controlled infection.

INDOCIN, like other non-steroidal anti-inflammatory agents, can inhibit platelet aggregation. This effect is of shorter duration than that seen with aspirin and usually disappears within 24 hours after discontinuation of INDOCIN. INDOCIN has been shown to prolong bleeding time (but within the normal range) in normal subjects. Because this effect may be exaggerated in patients with underlying hemostatic defects, INDOCIN should be used with caution in persons with coagulation defects.

INDOCIN and other prostaglandin inhibitors should be used with caution in patients with impairment of renal function. There have been reports of worsening of renal impairment in such patients, some of whom developed hyperkalemia. Similarly, in patients with sodium retention associated with hepatic disease or congestive heart failure, there are reports of the precipitation of acute renal failure. Most of the renal abnormalities reported have been reversible.

As with other non-steroidal anti-inflammatory drugs, borderline elevations of one or more liver tests may occur in up to 15% of patients. These abnormalities may progress, may remain essentially unchanged, or may be transient with continued therapy. The SGPT (ALT) test is probably the most sensitive indicator of liver dysfunction. Meaningful (3 times the upper limit of normal) elevations of SGPT or SGOT (AST) occurred in controlled clinical trials in less than 1% of patients. A patient with symptoms and/or signs suggesting liver dysfunction, or in whom an abnormal liver test has occurred, should be evaluated for evidence of the development of more severe hepatic reaction while on therapy with INDOCIN. Severe hepatic reactions, including jaundice and cases of fatal hepatitis, have been reported with INDOCIN as with other non-steroidal anti-inflammatory drugs. Although such reactions are rare, if abnormal liver tests persist or worsen, if clinical signs and symptoms consistent with liver disease develop, or if systemic manifestations occur (e.g. eosinophilia, rash, etc.), INDOCIN should be discontinued.

Incidence greater than 1%	*Incidence less than 1%*	
GASTROINTESTINAL		
nausea* with or without vomiting dyspepsia* (including indigestion, heartburn and epigastric pain) diarrhea abdominal distress or pain constipation	anorexia bloating (includes distention) flatulence peptic ulcer gastro-enteritis rectal bleeding proctitis perforation and hemorrhage of the esophagus, stomach, duodenum or small intestines intestinal ulceration associated with stenosis and obstruction	gastrointestinal bleeding without obvious ulcer formation and perforation of pre-existing sigmoid lesions (diverticulum, carcinoma, etc.) development of ulcerative colitis and regional ileitis ulcerative stomatitis toxic hepatitis and jaundice (some fatal cases have been reported)
CENTRAL NERVOUS SYSTEM		
headache** dizziness* vertigo somnolence depression and fatigue (including malaise and listlessness)	anxiety (includes nervousness) muscle weakness involuntary muscle movements insomnia muzziness psychic disturbances including psychotic episodes mental confusion drowsiness	light-headedness syncope paresthesia aggravation of epilepsy and parkinsonism depersonalization coma peripheral neuropathy convulsions
SPECIAL SENSES		
tinnitus	ocular-corneal deposits and retinal disturbances, including those of the macula, have been reported in some patients on prolonged therapy with INDOCIN.	blurred vision hearing disturbances, deafness
CARDIOVASCULAR		
none	hypertension tachycardia chest pain	arrhythmia; palpitations BUN elevation
METABOLIC		
none	edema weight gain flushing or sweating	hyperglycemia glycosuria hyperkalemia
INTEGUMENTARY		
none	pruritus rash; urticaria petechiae or ecchymosis	exfoliative dermatitis erythema nodosum loss of hair
HEMATOLOGIC		
none	leukopenia bone marrow depression anemia secondary to obvious or occult gastrointestinal bleeding	aplastic anemia hemolytic anemia agranulocytosis thrombocytopenic purpura
HYPERSENSITIVITY		
none	acute respiratory distress rapid fall in blood pressure resembling a shock-like state angioedema	dyspnea asthma purpura angiitis
GENITOURINARY		
none	hematuria vaginal bleeding	
MISCELLANEOUS		
none	epistaxis	

* Reactions occurring in 3% to 9% of patients treated with INDOCIN. (Those reactions occurring in less than 3% of the patients are unmarked.)

** Reactions occurring in over 10% of patients treated with INDOCIN.

Drug Interactions

In normal volunteers receiving indomethacin, the administration of diflunisal decreased the renal clearance and significantly increased the plasma levels of indomethacin. Further, combined use of INDOCIN and diflunisal has been associated with fatal gastrointestinal hemorrhage. Therefore, diflunisal and INDOCIN should not be used concomitantly.

In a study in normal volunteers, it was found that chronic concurrent administration of 3.6 g of aspirin per day decreases indomethacin blood levels approximately 20%.

Clinical studies have shown that INDOCIN does not influence the hypoprothrombinemia produced by anticoagulants. However, when any additional drug, including INDOCIN, is added to the treatment of patients on anticoagulant therapy, the patient should be observed for alterations of the prothrombin time.

When INDOCIN is given to patients receiving probenecid, the plasma levels of indomethacin are likely to be increased. Therefore, a lower total daily dosage of INDOCIN may produce a satisfactory therapeutic effect. When increases in the dose of INDOCIN are made, they should be made carefully and in small increments.

Capsules INDOCIN 50 mg t.i.d. produced a clinically relevant elevation of plasma lithium and reduction in renal lithium clearance in psychiatric patients and normal subjects with steady state plasma lithium concentrations. This effect has been attributed to inhibition of prostaglandin synthesis. As a consequence, when INDOCIN and lithium are given concomitantly, the patient should be carefully observed for signs of lithium toxicity. (Read circulars for lithium preparations before use of such concomitant therapy.) In addition, the frequency of monitoring serum lithium concentration should be increased at the outset of such combination drug treatment.

Clinical studies have shown that the administration of INDOCIN can reduce the natriuretic and anti-hypertensive effect of furosemide and thiazides in some patients. This response has been attributed to inhibition of renal prostaglandin synthesis by non-steroidal anti-inflammatory drugs. Therefore, when INDOCIN is added to the treatment of a patient receiving furosemide or thiazides, or furosemide or thiazides are added to the treatment of a patient receiving INDOCIN, the patient should be observed closely to determine if the desired effect of furosemide or thiazides is obtained.

There is a report of a clinical pharmacology study in which triamterene was added to a maintenance schedule of INDOCIN for four healthy volunteers. Two of the subjects developed azotemia and reduced creatinine clearance after several days of combined drug administration. This effect was reversible and may be mediated by prostaglandin inhibition. Nonetheless, INDOCIN and triamterene should not be used together.

Blunting of the antihypertensive effect of beta-adrenoceptor blocking agents by non-steroidal anti-inflammatory drugs including INDOCIN has been reported. Therefore, when using these blocking agents to treat hypertension, patients should be observed carefully in order to confirm that the desired therapeutic effect has been obtained.

INDOCIN blocks the furosemide-induced increase in plasma renin activity. This fact should be kept in mind when evaluating plasma renin activity in hypertensive patients.

Adverse Reactions

The adverse reactions listed in the following table have been arranged into two groups: (1) incidence greater than 1%; and (2) incidence less than 1%. The incidence for group (1) was obtained from 33 double-blind controlled clinical trials reported in the literature (1,092 patients). The incidence for group (2) was based on reports in clinical trials, in the literature, and on voluntary reports since marketing. The probability of a causal relationship exists between INDOCIN and these adverse reactions, some of which have been reported only rarely.

In controlled clinical trials, the incidence of adverse reactions to Capsules INDOCIN SR and equal 24-hour doses of Capsules INDOCIN were similar. (See table on preceding page)

Causal relationship unknown: Other reactions have been reported but occurred under circumstances where a causal relationship could not be established. However, in these rarely reported events, the possibility cannot be excluded. Therefore, these observations are being listed to serve as alerting information to physicians:

Hematologic: Although there have been several reports of leukemia, the supporting information is weak.

Integumentary: Stevens-Johnson syndrome, erythema multiforme.

Genitourinary: Urinary frequency.

Miscellaneous: Breast changes including enlargement and tenderness.

Dosage and Administration

INDOCIN is available as 25 and 50 mg Capsules INDOCIN and 75 mg Capsules INDOCIN SR for oral use. Capsules INDOCIN SR once a day can be used as an alternate dosage form for Capsules INDOCIN 25 mg t.i.d. In addition, one Capsule INDOCIN SR b.i.d. can be substituted for Capsules INDOCIN 50 mg t.i.d. Capsules INDOCIN SR may be substituted for all the indications for Capsules INDOCIN except acute gouty arthritis.

Adverse reactions appear to correlate with the size of the dose of INDOCIN in most patients but not all. Therefore, every effort should be made to determine the smallest effective dosage for the individual patient.

Always give INDOCIN with food, immediately after meals, or with antacids to reduce gastric irritation.

INDOCIN should not ordinarily be prescribed for children 14 years of age and under because safe conditions for use have not been established. (See WARNINGS.)

Dosage Recommendations for Active Stages of the Following:

1. Moderate to severe rheumatoid arthritis including acute flares of chronic disease; moderate to severe ankylosing spondylitis; and moderate to severe osteoarthritis.
   Suggested Dosage:
   Capsules INDOCIN 25 mg b.i.d. or t.i.d. If this is well tolerated, increase the daily dosage by 25 or by 50 mg, if required by continuing symptoms, at weekly intervals until a satisfactory response is obtained or until a total daily dose of 150-200 mg is reached. DOSES ABOVE THIS AMOUNT GENERALLY DO NOT INCREASE THE EFFECTIVENESS OF THE DRUG.

In patients who have persistent night pain and/or morning stiffness, the giving of a large portion, up to a maximum of 100 mg, of the total daily dose at bedtime may be helpful in affording relief. The total daily dose should not exceed 200 mg. In acute flares of chronic rheumatoid arthritis, it may be necessary to increase the dosage by 25 mg or, if required, by 50 mg daily.

The usual starting dose for Capsules INDOCIN SR is one capsule daily, given either in the morning or at bedtime. Provided the patient tolerates the drug in this dosage, but symptoms persist, the dosage can be increased to one Capsule INDOCIN SR b.i.d.

If minor adverse effects develop as the dosage is increased, reduce the dosage rapidly to a tolerated dose and OBSERVE THE PATIENT CLOSELY.

If severe adverse reactions occur, STOP THE DRUG. After the acute phase of the disease is under control, an attempt to reduce the daily dose should be made repeatedly until the patient is receiving the smallest effective dose or the drug is discontinued.

Careful instructions to, and observations of, the individual patient are essential to the prevention of serious, irreversible, including fatal, adverse reactions.

As advancing years appear to increase the possibility of adverse reactions, INDOCIN should be used with greater care in the aged.

2. Acute painful shoulder (bursitis and/or tendinitis).
   Initial Dose:
   75-150 mg daily in 3 or 4 divided doses.
   The drug should be discontinued after the signs and symptoms of inflammation have been controlled for several days. The usual course of therapy is 7-14 days.
3. Acute gouty arthritis.
   Suggested Dosage:
   Capsules INDOCIN 50 mg t.i.d. until pain is tolerable. The dose should then be rapidly reduced to complete cessation of the drug. Definite relief of pain has been reported within 2 to 4 hours. Tenderness and heat usually subside in 24 to 36 hours, and swelling gradually disappears in 3 to 5 days.

How Supplied

No. 3316–Capsules INDOCIN, 25 mg are opaque blue and white capsules, coded MSD 25. They are supplied as follows:

NDC 0006-0025-68 bottles of 100
(6505-00-926-2154, 25 mg 100's)
NDC 0006-0025-78 unit of use bottles of 100
NDC 0006-0025-28 single unit packages of 100
(6505-00-118-2776, 25 mg individually sealed 100's)
NDC 0006-0025-82 bottles of 1000
(6505-00-931-0680, 25 mg 1000's).

[*Shown in Product Identification Section*]

No. 3317–Capsules INDOCIN, 50 mg are opaque blue and white capsules, coded MSD 50. They are supplied as follows:

NDC 0006-0050-54 unit of use bottles of 60
NDC 0006-0050-68 bottles of 100
NDC 0006-0050-78 unit of use bottles of 100
NDC 0006-0050-28 single unit packages of 100.

[*Shown in Product Identification Section*]

No. 3370–Capsules INDOCIN SR, 75 mg each, are capsules with an opaque blue cap and clear body containing a mixture of blue and white pellets, coded MSD 693. They are supplied as follows:

NDC 0006-0693-31 unit of use bottles of 30
NDC 0006-0693-61 unit of use bottles of 60.

[*Shown in Product Identification Section*]

A.H.F.S. Category: 28:08

DC 6473230 Issued August 1982

COPYRIGHT© MERCK & CO., INC., 1977
All rights reserved

LACRISERT® Sterile Ophthalmic Insert ℞
(hydroxypropyl cellulose ophthalmic insert, MSD)

Description

LACRISERT® (Hydroxypropyl Cellulose Ophthalmic Insert, MSD) is a rod-shaped, water soluble, ophthalmic preparation made of hydroxypropyl cellulose, 5 mg. LACRISERT contains no preservatives or other ingredients. It is about 1.27 mm in diameter by about 3.5 mm long.

LACRISERT is supplied in packages of 60 units, together with illustrated instructions and a special applicator for removing LACRISERT from the unit dose blister and inserting

Information on the Merck Sharp & Dohme products listed on these pages is the full prescribing information from package circulars in use October 31, 1982.

Continued on next page

Merck Sharp & Dohme—Cont.

it into the eye. A spare applicator is included in each package.

Actions

LACRISERT acts to stabilize and thicken the precorneal tear film and prolong the tear film breakup time which is usually accelerated in patients with dry eye states. LACRISERT also acts to lubricate and protect the eye. LACRISERT usually reduces the signs and symptoms resulting from moderate to severe dry eye syndromes.

Indications

LACRISERT is indicated in patients with moderate to severe dry eye syndromes, including keratoconjunctivitis sicca. LACRISERT is indicated especially in patients who remain symptomatic after an adequate trial of therapy with artificial tear solutions.
LACRISERT is also indicated for patients with:

Exposure keratitis
Decreased corneal sensitivity
Recurrent corneal erosions

LACRISERT usually reduces the signs and symptoms resulting from moderate to severe dry eye syndromes, such as conjunctival hyperemia, corneal and conjunctival staining with rose bengal, exudation, itching, burning, foreign body sensation, smarting, photophobia, dryness and blurred or cloudy vision. Progressive visual deterioration which occurs in some patients may be retarded, halted, or sometimes reversed.
In a multicenter crossover study the 5 mg LACRISERT administered once a day during the waking hours was compared to artificial tears used four or more times daily. There was a significant prolongation of tear film breakup time and a significant decrease in foreign body sensation associated with dry eye syndrome in patients during treatment with inserts as compared to artificial tears. Improvement, as measured by amelioration of symptoms, by slit lamp examination and by rose bengal staining of the cornea and conjunctiva, was greater in most patients with moderate to severe symptoms during treatment with LACRISERT. Patient comfort was usually better with LACRISERT than with artificial tears solution, and most patients preferred LACRISERT.
In most patients treated with LACRISERT for over one year, improvement was observed as evidenced by amelioration of symptoms generally associated with keratoconjunctivitis sicca such as burning, tearing, foreign body sensation, itching, photophobia and blurred or cloudy vision.
During studies in healthy volunteers, a thickened precorneal tear film was usually observed through the slit lamp while LACRISERT was present in the conjunctival sac.

Contraindications

LACRISERT is contraindicated in patients who are hypersensitive to hydroxypropyl cellulose.

Warnings

Instructions for inserting and removing LACRISERT should be carefully followed.

Precautions

Because this product may produce transient blurring of vision, patients should be instructed to exercise caution when operating hazardous machinery or driving a motor vehicle.

Adverse Reactions

The following adverse reactions have been reported in patients treated with LACRISERT, but were in most instances mild and transient:

Transient blurring of vision (See PRECAUTIONS)
Ocular discomfort or irritation
Matting or stickiness of eyelashes
Photophobia
Hypersensitivity
Edema of the eyelids
Hyperemia

Dosage and Administration

One LACRISERT ophthalmic insert in each eye once daily is usually sufficient to relieve the symptoms associated with moderate to severe dry eye syndromes. Individual patients may require more flexibility in the use of LACRISERT; some patients may require twice daily use for optimal results.
Clinical experience with LACRISERT indicates that in some patients several weeks may be required before satisfactory improvement of symptoms is achieved.
LACRISERT is inserted into the inferior cul-de-sac of the eye beneath the base of the tarsus. Illustrated instructions are included in each package. While in the licensed practitioner's office, the patient should read the instructions, then practice insertion and removal of LACRISERT until proficiency is achieved.
NOTE: Occasionally LACRISERT is inadvertently expelled from the eye, especially in patients with shallow conjunctival fornices. The patient should be cautioned against rubbing the eye(s) containing LACRISERT, especially upon awakening, so as not to dislodge or expel the insert. If required, another LACRISERT ophthalmic insert may be inserted. If experience indicates that transient blurred vision develops in an individual patient, the patient may want to remove LACRISERT a few hours after insertion to avoid this. Another LACRISERT ophthalmic insert may be inserted if needed.
If LACRISERT causes worsening of symptoms, the patient should be instructed to inspect the conjunctival sac to make certain LACRISERT is in the proper location, deep in the inferior cul-de-sac of the eye beneath the base of the tarsus. If these symptoms persist, LACRISERT should be removed and the patient should contact the practitioner.

How Supplied

No. 3380—LACRISERT, a rod-shaped, water-soluble, ophthalmic preparation made of hydroxypropyl cellulose, 5 mg, is supplied as follows:
NDC 0006-3380-60 in packages containing 60 unit doses, two reusable applicators and a storage container.
Store below 30°C (86°F).
DC 7189404 Issued November 1981
Copyright © MERCK & CO., Inc., 1979
All rights reserved

M-M-R®$_{II}$ ℞

(measles, mumps and rubella virus vaccine, live, MSD), U.S.P.

Description

M-M-R®$_{II}$ (Measles, Mumps and Rubella Virus Vaccine, Live, MSD) is a live virus vaccine for immunization against measles (rubeola), mumps and rubella (German measles).
M-M-R$_{II}$ is a lyophilized preparation of (1) ATTENUVAX® (Measles Virus Vaccine, Live, Attenuated, MSD), a more attenuated line of measles virus, derived from Enders' attenuated Edmonston strain and grown in cell cultures of chick embryo; (2) MUMPSVAX® (Mumps Virus Vaccine, Live, MSD), the Jeryl Lynn (B level) mumps strain grown in cell cultures of chick embryo; and (3) MERUVAX®$_{II}$ (Rubella Virus Vaccine, Live, MSD), the Wistar RA 27/3 strain of live attenuated rubella virus grown in human diploid cell (WI-38) culture. The three viruses are mixed before being lyophilized. The product contains no preservative.
When reconstituted as directed, the dose for injection is 0.5 ml and contains not less than 1,000 $TCID_{50}$ (tissue culture infectious doses) of Measles Virus Vaccine, Live, Attenuated; 5,000 $TCID_{50}$ of Mumps Virus Vaccine, Live; and 1,000 $TCID_{50}$ of Rubella Virus Vaccine, Live, expressed in terms of the assigned titer of the FDA Reference Measles, Mumps and Rubella Viruses. Each dose contains approximately 25 mcg of neomycin.

Actions

Clinical studies of 279 triple seronegative children, 11 months to 7 years of age, demonstrated that M-M-R$_{II}$ is highly immunogenic and generally well tolerated. In these studies, a single injection of the vaccine induced measles hemagglutination-inhibition (HI) antibodies in 95 percent, mumps neutralizing antibodies in 96 percent, and rubella HI antibodies in 99 percent of susceptible persons.
The RA 27/3 rubella strain in M-M-R$_{II}$ elicits higher immediate postvaccination HI, complement-fixing and neutralizing antibody levels than other strains of rubella vaccine and has been shown to induce a broader profile of circulating antibodies including anti-theta and anti-iota precipitating antibodies. The RA 27/3 rubella strain immunologically simulates natural infection more closely than other rubella vaccine viruses. The increased levels and broader profile of antibodies produced by RA 27/3 strain rubella virus vaccine appear to correlate with greater resistance to subclinical reinfection with the wild virus, and provide greater confidence for lasting immunity.
Data relating to persistence of vaccine-induced antibodies are not available for M-M-R$_{II}$ at this time; however, it is expected that the antibodies against measles, mumps and rubella will be just as durable following administration of M-M-R$_{II}$ as after the single vaccines given separately. Antibody levels after immunization with ATTENUVAX (Measles Virus Vaccine, Live, Attenuated, MSD) have persisted for at least eight years without substantial decline; for ten years after MUMPSVAX (Mumps Virus Vaccine, Live, MSD); and for at least six years after administration of RA 27/3 strain rubella virus vaccine.

Indications

M-M-R$_{II}$ is indicated for simultaneous immunization against measles, mumps, and rubella in children 15 months of age or older, and adults. Infants who are less than 15 months of age may fail to respond to one or all three components of the vaccine due to presence in the circulation of residual measles and/or mumps and/or rubella antibody of maternal origin; the younger the infant, the lower the likelihood of seroconversion. In geographically isolated or other relatively inaccessible populations for whom immunization programs are logistically difficult, and in population groups in which natural measles infection may occur in a significant proportion of infants before 15 months of age, it may be desirable to give the vaccine to infants at an earlier age. The advantage of early protection must be weighed against the chance for failure of response; infants vaccinated under these conditions should be revaccinated after reaching 15 months of age.
Previously unimmunized children of susceptible pregnant women should receive live attenuated rubella vaccine, because an immunized child will be less likely to acquire natural rubella and introduce the virus into the household.

Non-Pregnant Adolescent and Adult Females
Immunization of susceptible non-pregnant adolescent and adult females of child-bearing age with live attenuated rubella virus vaccine is indicated if certain precautions are observed (see below). Vaccinating susceptible postpubertal females confers individual protection against subsequently acquiring rubella infection during pregnancy, which in turn prevents infection of the fetus and consequent congenital rubella injury.
Pregnant females *must not* be given live attenuated rubella virus vaccine. It is not known to what extent infection of the fetus with attenuated virus might occur following vaccination, or whether damage to the fetus could result. Subjects should be considered for vaccination only if they agree that they will not become pregnant within three months following vaccination, and if they are are informed of the reason for this precaution.* If a pregnant woman is inadvertently vaccinated or if she becomes pregnant within three months of vaccination, she should be counseled on the possible risks to the fetus.
It is recommended that rubella susceptibility be determined by serologic testing prior to immunization.** If immune, as evidenced by a specific rubella antibody titer of 1:8 or greater (hemagglutination inhibition test), vaccination is unnecessary. Congenital malformations do occur in up to seven percent of all live births. Their chance appearance after vaccination could lead to misinterpretation of the cause, particularly if the prior rubella-immune status of vaccinees is unknown.
Postpubertal females should be informed of the frequent occurrence of self-limited arthralgia and possible arthritis beginning 2 to 4 weeks after vaccination (See ADVERSE REACTIONS).
It has been found convenient in many instances to vaccinate rubella-susceptible women in the immediate post-partum period.

Revaccination: Based on available evidence, there is no reason to routinely revaccinate children originally vaccinated when 12 months of age or older; however, children vaccinated when younger than 12 months of age should be revaccinated. The decision to revaccinate should be based on evaluation of each individual case.

Use with Other Live Virus Vaccines
There are no data available concerning simultaneous use of M-M-R_{II}, containing the RA 27/3 rubella strain, with monovalent or trivalent poliovirus vaccine, live, oral, or with killed poliovirus vaccines. However, serologic evidence shows that when M-M-R, containing the HPV-77 rubella strain, is given simultaneously with trivalent poliovirus vaccine, live, oral, antibody responses can be expected to be comparable to those which follow administration of the vaccines at different times.

* NOTE: The Immunization Practices Advisory Committee (ACIP) has recommended "In view of the importance of protecting this age group against rubella, asking females if they are pregnant, excluding those who say they are, and explaining the theoretical risks to the others are reasonable precautions in a rubella immunization program."

** NOTE: The Immunization Practices Advisory Committee (ACIP) has stated "When practical, and when reliable laboratory services are available, potential vaccinees of childbearing age can have serologic tests to determine susceptibility to rubella. . . . However, routinely performing serologic tests for all females of childbearing age to determine susceptibility so that vaccine is given only to proven susceptibles is expensive and has been ineffective in some areas. Accordingly, the ACIP believes that rubella vaccination of a woman who is not known to be pregnant and has no history of vaccination is justifiable without serologic testing."

Contraindications

Do not give M-M-R_{II} to pregnant females; the possible effects of the vaccine on fetal development are unknown at this time. If vaccination of post-pubertal females is undertaken, pregnancy must be avoided for three months following vaccination.
Hypersensitivity to neomycin (each dose of reconstituted vaccine contains approximately 25 mcg of neomycin).
Any febrile respiratory illness or other active febrile infection.
Active untreated tuberculosis.
Patients receiving therapy with ACTH, corticosteroids, irradiation, alkylating agents or antimetabolites. This contraindication does not apply to patients who are receiving corticosteroids as replacement therapy, e.g., for Addison's disease.
Individuals with blood dyscrasias, leukemia, lymphomas of any type, or other malignant neoplasms affecting the bone marrow or lymphatic systems.
Primary immuno-deficiency states, including cellular immune deficiencies, hypogammaglobulinemic and dysgammaglobulinemic states.

Hypersensitivity to Eggs, Chicken, or Chicken Feathers

This vaccine is essentially devoid of potentially allergenic substances derived from host tissues (chick embryos).* However, because the attenuated measles and mumps viruses in this vaccine are propagated in cell cultures of chick embryo, there is a potential risk of hypersensitivity reactions in patients allergic to eggs, chicken or chicken feathers. Widespread use of the vaccine for more than a decade has resulted in only rare, isolated reports of minor allergic reactions attributed to allergens of this kind, possibly related to the vaccine. Significantly, when children with known allergies to eggs, chicken and chicken feathers were given a similarly prepared vaccine in a clinical study, none experienced reactions other than those reactions previously observed in non-allergic children.

Precautions

Administer M-M-R_{II} subcutaneously; *do not give intravenously.*
Epinephrine should be available for immediate use in case an anaphylactoid reaction occurs.
M-M-R_{II} may be given simultaneously with monovalent or trivalent poliovirus vaccine, live, oral. M-M-R_{II} should not be given less than one month before or after administration of other live virus vaccines.
Due caution should be employed in administration of M-M-R_{II} to children with a history of febrile convulsions, cerebral injury or any other condition in which stress due to fever should be avoided. The physician should be alert to the temperature elevation which may occur 5 to 12 days following vaccination.
Vaccination should be deferred for at least 3 months following blood or plasma transfusions, or administration of human immune serum globulin.
Excretion of small amounts of the live attenuated rubella virus from the nose or throat has occurred in the majority of susceptible individuals 7–28 days after vaccination. There is no confirmed evidence to indicate that such virus is transmitted to susceptible persons who are in contact with the vaccinated individuals. Consequently, transmission, while accepted as a theoretical possibility, is not regarded as a significant risk.**
There are no reports of transmission of live attenuated measles or mumps viruses from vaccinees to susceptible contacts.
It has been reported that live attenuated measles, mumps and rubella virus vaccines given individually may result in a temporary depression of tuberculin skin sensitivity. Therefore, if a tuberculin test is to be done, it should be administered either before or simultaneously with M-M-R_{II}.
As for any vaccine, vaccination with M-M-R_{II} may not result in seroconversion in 100% of susceptible subjects given the vaccine.

Adverse Reactions

Because of the slightly acidic pH (6.2–6.6) of the vaccine, patients may complain of burning and/or stinging of short duration at the injection site.
The adverse clinical reactions associated with the use of M-M-R_{II} are those expected to follow administration of the monovalent vaccines given separately. These may include malaise, sore throat, headache, fever, and rash; mild local reactions such as erythema, induration, tenderness and regional lymphadenopathy; parotitis; orchitis; thrombocytopenia and purpura; allergic reactions such as wheal and flare at the injection site or urticaria; and arthritis, arthralgia and polyneuritis.
Moderate fever [101–102.9°F (38.3–39.4°C)] occurs occasionally, and high fever [above 103°F (39.4°C)] occurs less commonly. On rare occasions, children developing fever may exhibit febrile convulsions. Rash occurs infrequently and is usually minimal, but rarely may be generalized.
Clinical experience with live attenuated measles, mumps and rubella virus vaccines given individually indicates that encephalitis and other nervous system reactions have occurred very rarely. These might occur also with M-M-R_{II}.
Experience from more than 80 million doses of all live measles vaccines given in the U.S. through 1975 indicates that significant central nervous system reactions such as encephalitis and encephalopathy, occurring within 30 days after vaccination, have been temporally associated with measles vaccine approximately once for every million doses. In no case has it been shown that reactions were actually caused by vaccine. The Center for Disease Control has pointed out that "a certain number of cases of encephalitis may be expected to occur in a large childhood population in a defined period of time even when no vaccines are administered". However, the data suggest the possibility that some of these cases may have been caused by measles vaccines. The risk of such serious neurological disorders following live measles virus vaccine administration remains far less than that for encephalitis and encephalopathy with natural measles (one per thousand reported cases).
There have been isolated reports of ocular palsies and Guillain-Barre syndrome occurring after immunization with vaccines containing live attenuated measles virus. The ocular palsies have occurred approximately 3–24 days following vaccination. No definite causal rela-

* Morbidity and Mortality Weekly Report *25*(44): 350, Nov. 12, 1976.

** Recommendation of the Immunization Practices Advisory Committee (ACIP), Morbidity and Mortality Weekly Report 30(4): 37–42, 47, Feb. 6, 1981.

Information on the Merck Sharp & Dohme products listed on these pages is the full prescribing information from package circulars in use October 31, 1982.

Continued on next page

Merck Sharp & Dohme—Cont.

tionship has been established between either of these events and vaccination.

There have been reports of subacute sclerosing panencephalitis (SSPE) in children who did not have a history of natural measles but did receive measles vaccine. Some of these cases may have resulted from unrecognized measles in the first year of life or possibly from the measles vaccination. Based on estimated nationwide measles vaccine distribution, the association of SSPE cases to measles vaccination is about one case per million vaccine doses distributed. This is far less than the association with natural measles, 5–10 cases of SSPE per million cases of measles. The results of a retrospective case-controlled study conducted by the Center for Disease Control suggest that the overall effect of measles vaccine has been to protect against SSPE by preventing measles with its inherent higher risk of SSPE.

Local reactions characterized by marked swelling, redness and vesiculation at the injection site of attenuated live measles virus vaccines have occurred in children who received killed measles vaccine previously. M-M-R_{II} was not given under this condition in clinical trials.

Transient arthritis, arthralgia and polyneuritis are features of natural rubella and vary in frequency and severity with age and sex, being greatest in adult females and least in prepubertal children. This type of involvement has also been reported following administration of $MERUVAX_{II}$ (Rubella Virus Vaccine, Live, MSD). In children, joint reactions are rare and of brief duration if they do occur. In women, incidence rates for arthritis and arthralgia are generally higher than those seen in children (children: 0–3%; women: 12–20%), and the reactions tend to be more marked and of longer duration. Rarely, symptoms may persist for a matter of months. In adolescent girls, the reactions appear to be intermediate in incidence between those seen in children and in adult women. Even in older women (35–45 years), these reactions are generally well tolerated and rarely interfere with normal activities.

Dosage and Administration

After suitably cleansing the immunization site, inject the total volume of reconstituted vaccine subcutaneously, preferably into the outer aspect of the upper arm. Do not inject M-M-R_{II} intravenously. *Do not give immune serum globulin (ISG) concurrently with* M-M-R_{II}.

Shipment, Storage, and Reconstitution

During shipment, to insure that there is no loss of potency, the vaccine must be maintained at a temperature of 10°C (50°F) or less.

Before reconstitution, store M-M-R_{II} at 2–8°C (35.6–46.4°F). *Protect from light.*

To reconstitute, use only the diluent supplied, since it is free of preservatives or other antiviral substances which might inactivate the vaccine. Inject all the diluent in the syringe into the vial of lyophilized vaccine, and agitate to mix thoroughly. Withdraw the entire contents into the syringe and inject the total volume of restored vaccine subcutaneously.

It is important to use a separate sterile syringe and needle for each individual patient to prevent transmission of hepatitis B and other infectious agents from one person to another.

The color of the vaccine when reconstituted is yellow.

It is recommended that the vaccine be used as soon as possible after reconstitution. Protect vaccine from light at all times. Store reconstituted vaccine in a dark place at 2–8°C (35.6–46.4°F) and discard if not used within 8 hours.

How Supplied

No. 4680—M-M-R_{II} is supplied as a single-dose vial of lyophilized vaccine with a disposable syringe containing diluent, and fitted with a 25 gauge, ⅝" needle, **NDC** 0006-4680-00.

No. 4681/4590—M-M-R_{II} is supplied as follows: (1) a box of ten single-dose vials of lyophilized vaccine, **NDC** 0006-4681-00; and (2) a box of ten diluent-containing disposable syringes with affixed 25 gauge, ⅝" needles. To conserve refrigerator space, the syringes may be stored separately at room temperature.

A.H.F.S. Category: 80:12

DC 7034402 Issued April 1981

Copyright © MERCK & CO., INC., 1978
All rights reserved.

M–R–VAX®$_{II}$ ℞

(measles and rubella virus vaccine, live, MSD), U.S.P.

Description

M-R-VAX®$_{II}$ (Measles and Rubella Virus Vaccine, Live, MSD) is a live virus vaccine for immunization against measles (rubeola) and rubella (German measles).

M-R-VAX_{II} is a lyophilized preparation of (1) ATTENUVAX® (Measles Virus Vaccine, Live, Attenuated, MSD), a more attenuated line of measles virus, derived from Enders' attenuated Edmonston strain and grown in cell cultures of chick embryo; and (2) MERUVAX®$_{II}$ (Rubella Virus Vaccine, Live, MSD), the Wistar RA 27/3 strain of live attenuated rubella virus grown in human diploid cell (WI-38) culture. The two viruses are mixed before being lyophilized. The product contains no preservative.

When reconstituted as directed, the dose for injection is 0.5 ml and contains not less than 1,000 $TCID_{50}$ (tissue culture infectious doses) of Measles Virus Vaccine, Live, Attenuated; and 1,000 $TCID_{50}$ of Rubella Virus Vaccine, Live, expressed in terms of the assigned titer of the FDA Reference Measles and Rubella Viruses. Each dose contains approximately 25 mcg of neomycin.

Actions

Clinical studies of 237 double seronegative children, 10 months to 10 years of age, demonstrated that M-R-VAX_{II} is highly immunogenic and generally well tolerated. In these studies, a single injection of the vaccine induced measles hemagglutination-inhibition (HI) antibodies in 95 percent and rubella HI antibodies in 99 percent of susceptible persons.

The RA 27/3 rubella strain in M-R-VAX_{II} elicits higher immediate post-vaccination HI, complement-fixing and neutralizing antibody levels than other strains of rubella vaccine and has been shown to induce a broader profile of circulating antibodies including anti-theta and anti-iota precipitating antibodies. The RA 27/3 rubella strain immunologically simulates natural infection more closely than other rubella vaccine viruses. The increased levels and broader profile of antibodies produced by RA 27/3 strain rubella virus vaccine appear to correlate with greater resistance to subclinical reinfection with the wild virus, and provide greater confidence for lasting immunity.

Data relating to persistence of vaccine-induced antibodies are not available for M-R-VAX_{II} at this time; however, it is expected that the antibodies against measles and rubella will be just as durable following administration of M-R-VAX_{II} as after the single vaccines given separately. Antibody levels after immunization with ATTENUVAX (Measles Virus Vaccine, Live, Attenuated, MSD) have persisted for at least eight years without substantial decline; and for at least six years after administration of RA 27/3 strain rubella virus vaccine.

Indications

M-R-VAX_{II} is indicated for simultaneous immunization against measles and rubella in children 15 months of age or older, and adults.

Infants who are less than 15 months of age may fail to respond to one or both components of the vaccine due to presence in the circulation of residual measles and/or rubella antibody of maternal origin; the younger the infant, the lower the likelihood of seroconversion. In geographically isolated or other relatively inaccessible populations for whom immunization programs are logistically difficult, and in population groups in which natural measles infection may occur in a significant proportion of infants before 15 months of age, it may be desirable to give the vaccine to infants at an earlier age. The advantage of early protection must be weighed against the chance for failure of response; infants vaccinated under these conditions should be revaccinated after reaching 15 months of age.

Previously unimmunized children of susceptible pregnant women should receive live attenuated rubella vaccine, because an immunized child will be less likely to acquire natural rubella and introduce the virus into the household.

Non-Pregnant Adolescent and Adult Females

Immunization of susceptible non-pregnant adolescent and adult females of childbearing age with live attenuated rubella virus vaccine is indicated if certain precautions are observed (see below). Vaccinating susceptible postpubertal females confers individual protection against subsequently acquiring rubella infection during pregnancy, which in turn prevents infection of the fetus and consequent congenital rubella injury.

Pregnant females *must not* be given live attenuated rubella virus vaccine. It is not known to what extent infection of the fetus with attenuated virus might occur following vaccination, or whether damage to the fetus could result. Subjects should be considered for vaccination only if they agree that they will not become pregnant within three months following vaccination, and if they are informed of the reason for this precaution.* If a pregnant woman is inadvertently vaccinated or if she becomes pregnant within three months of vaccination, she should be counseled on the possible risks to the fetus.

It is recommended that rubella susceptibility be determined by serologic testing prior to immunization.** If immune, as evidenced by a specific rubella antibody titer of 1:8 or greater (hemagglutination inhibition test), vaccination is unnecessary. Congenital malformations do occur in up to seven percent of all live births. Their chance appearance after vaccination could lead to misinterpretation of the cause, particularly if the prior rubella-immune status of vaccinees is unknown.

* NOTE: The Immunization Practices Advisory Committee (ACIP) has recommended "In view of the importance of protecting this age group against rubella, asking females if they are pregnant, excluding those who say they are, and explaining the theoretical risks to the others are reasonable precautions in a rubella immunization program."

** NOTE: The Immunization Practices Advisory Committee (ACIP) has stated "When practical, and when reliable laboratory services are available, potential vaccinees of childbearing age can have serologic tests to determine susceptibility to rubella. . . . However, routinely performing serologic tests for all females of childbearing age to determine susceptibility so that vaccine is given only to proven susceptibles is expensive and has been ineffective in some areas. Accordingly, the ACIP believes that rubella vaccination of a woman who is not known to be pregnant and has no history of vaccination is justifiable without serologic testing."

Postpubertal females should be informed of the frequent occurrence of self-limited arthralgia and possible arthritis beginning 2 to 4 weeks after vaccination (See ADVERSE REACTIONS).

It has been found convenient in many instances to vaccinate rubella-susceptible women in the immediate postpartum period.

Revaccination: Based on available evidence, there is no reason to routinely revaccinate children originally vaccinated when 12 months of age or older; however, children vaccinated when younger than 12 months of age should be revaccinated. The decision to revaccinate should be based on evaluation of each individual case.

Use with Other Live Virus Vaccines

There are no data available concerning simultaneous use of M-R-VAX$_{II}$ with monovalent or trivalent poliovirus vaccine, live, oral, or with killed poliovirus vaccines. However, serologic evidence shows that when M-M-R® (Measles, Mumps and Rubella Virus Vaccine, Live, MSD) containing the HPV-77 rubella strain, is given simultaneously with trivalent poliovirus vaccine, live, oral, antibody responses can be expected to be comparable to those which follow administration of the vaccines at different times. From this it follows that when M-R-VAX$_{II}$ is given simultaneously with either monovalent or trivalent poliovirus vaccine, live, oral and/or MUMPSVAX® (Mumps Virus Vaccine, Live, MSD), antibody responses can be expected to be comparable to those which follow administration of the vaccines at different times.

Contraindications

Do not give M-R-VAX$_{II}$ to pregnant females; the possible effects of the vaccine on fetal development are unknown at this time. If vaccination of post-pubertal females is undertaken, pregnancy must be avoided for three months following vaccination.

Hypersensitivity to neomycin (each dose of reconstituted vaccine contains approximately 25 mcg of neomycin).

Any febrile respiratory illness or other active febrile infection.

Active untreated tuberculosis.

Patients receiving therapy with ACTH, corticosteroids, irradiation, alkylating agents or antimetabolites. This contraindication does not apply to patients who are receiving corticosteroids as replacement therapy, e.g., for Addison's disease.

Individuals with blood dyscrasias, leukemia, lymphomas of any type, or other malignant neoplasms affecting the bone marrow or lymphatic systems.

Primary immuno-deficiency states, including cellular immune deficiencies, hypogammaglobulinemic and dysgammaglobulinemic states.

Hypersensitivity to Eggs, Chicken, or Chicken Feathers

This vaccine is essentially devoid of potentially allergenic substances derived from host tissues (chick embryos).* However, because the attenuated measles virus in this vaccine is propagated in cell cultures of chick embryo, there is a potential risk of hypersensitivity reactions in patients allergic to eggs, chicken, or chicken feathers. Widespread use of the vaccine for more than a decade has resulted in only rare, isolated reports of minor allergic reactions attributed to allergens of this kind, possibly related to the vaccine. Significantly, when children with known allergies to eggs, chicken, and chicken feathers were given a similarly prepared vaccine in a clinical study, none experienced reactions other than those reactions previously observed in non-allergic children.

Precautions

Administer M-R-VAX$_{II}$ subcutaneously; *do not give intravenously.*

Epinephrine should be available for immediate use in case an anaphylactoid reaction occurs.

M-R-VAX$_{II}$ may be given simultaneously with monovalent or trivalent poliovirus vaccine, live, oral and/or with MUMPSVAX (Mumps Virus Vaccine, Live, MSD). M-R-VAX$_{II}$ should not be given less than one month before or after administration of other live virus vaccines.

Due caution should be employed in administration of M-R-VAX$_{II}$ to children with a history of febrile convulsions, cerebral injury or any other condition in which stress due to fever should be avoided. The physician should be alert to the temperature elevation which may occur 5 to 12 days following vaccination.

Vaccination should be deferred for at least 3 months following blood or plasma transfusions, or administration of human immune serum globulin.

Excretion of small amounts of the live attenuated rubella virus from the nose or throat has occurred in the majority of susceptible individuals 7–28 days after vaccination. There is no confirmed evidence to indicate that such virus is transmitted to susceptible persons who are in contact with the vaccinated individuals. Consequently, transmisson, while accepted as a theoretical possibility, is not regarded as a significant risk.**

There are no reports of transmission of live attenuated measles virus from vaccinees to susceptible contacts.

It has been reported that live attenuated measles and rubella virus vaccines given individually may result in a temporary depression of tuberculin skin sensitivity. Therefore, if a tuberculin test is to be done, it should be administered either before or simultaneously with M-R-VAX$_{II}$.

As for any vaccine, vaccination with M-R-VAX$_{II}$ may not result in seroconversion in 100% of susceptible subjects given the vaccine.

Adverse Reactions

Because of the slightly acidic pH (6.2–6.6) of the vaccine, patients may complain of burning and/or stinging of short duration at the injection site.

The adverse clinical reactions associated with the use of M-R-VAX$_{II}$ are those expected to follow administration of the monovalent vaccines given separately. These may include malaise, sore throat, headache, fever and rash; mild local reactions such as erythema, induration, tenderness and regional lymphadenopathy; thrombocytopenia and purpura; allergic reactions such as wheal and flare at the injection site or urticaria; and arthritis, arthralgia and polyneuritis.

Moderate fever [101–102.9°F (38.3–39.4°C)] occurs occasionally, and high fever [above 103°F (39.4°C)] occurs less commonly. On rare occasions, children developing fever may exhibit febrile convulsions. Rash occurs infrequently and is usually minimal, but rarely may be generalized.

Clinical experience with live attenuated measles and rubella virus vaccines given individually indicates that encephalitis and other nervous system reactions have occurred very rarely. These might occur also with M-R-VAX$_{II}$.

Experience from more than 80 million doses of all live measles vaccines given in the U.S. through 1975 indicates that significant central nervous system reactions such as encephalitis and encephalopathy, occurring within 30 days after vaccination, have been temporally associated with measles vaccine approximately once for every million doses. In no case has it been shown that reactions were actually caused by vaccine. The Center for Disease Control has pointed out that "a certain number of cases of encephalitis may be expected to occur in a large childhood population in a defined period of time even when no vaccines are administered". However, the data suggest the possibility that some of these cases may have been caused by measles vaccines. The risk of such serious neurological disorders following live measles virus vaccine administration remains far less than that for encephalitis and encephalopathy with natural measles (one per thousand reported cases).

There have been isolated reports of ocular palsies and Guillain-Barre syndrome occurring after immunization with vaccines containing live attenuated measles virus. The ocular palsies have occurred approximately 3–24 days following vaccination. No definite causal relationship has been established between either of these events and vaccination.

There have been reports of subacute sclerosing panencephalitis (SSPE) in children who did not have a history of natural measles but did receive measles vaccine. Some of these cases may have resulted from unrecognized measles in the first year of life or possibly from the measles vaccination. Based on estimated nationwide measles vaccine distribution, the association of SSPE cases to measles vaccination is about one case per million vaccine doses distributed. This is far less than the association with natural measles, 5–10 cases of SSPE per million cases of measles. The results of a retrospective case-controlled study conducted by the Center for Disease Control suggest that the overall effect of measles vaccine has been to protect against SSPE by preventing measles with its inherent higher risk of SSPE.

Local reactions characterized by marked swelling, redness and vesiculation at the injection site of attenuated live measles virus vaccines have occurred in children who received killed measles vaccine previously. M-R-VAX$_{II}$ was not given under this condition in clinical trials.

Transient arthritis, arthralgia and polyneuritis are features of natural rubella and vary in frequency and severity with age and sex, being greatest in adult females and least in prepubertal children. This type of involvement has also been reported following administration of MERUVAX$_{II}$ (Rubella Virus Vaccine, Live, MSD). In children, joint reactions are rare and of brief duration if they do occur. In women, incidence rates for arthritis and arthralgia are generally higher than those seen in children (children: 0–3%; women: 12–20%), and the reactions tend to be more marked and of longer duration. Rarely, symptoms may persist for a matter of months. In adolescent girls, the reactions appear to be intermediate in incidence between those seen in children and in adult women. Even in older women (35–45 years), these reactions are generally well tolerated and rarely interfere with normal activities.

Dosage and Administration

After suitably cleansing the immunization site, inject the total volume of reconstituted vaccine subcutaneously, preferably into the outer aspect of the upper arm. Do not inject M-R-VAX$_{II}$ intravenously. *Do not give immune*

Continued on next page

Information on the Merck Sharp & Dohme products listed on these pages is the full prescribing information from package circulars in use October 31, 1982.

* Morbidity and Mortality Weekly Report *25*(44): 350, Nov. 12, 1976.

** Recommendation of the Immunization Practices Advisory Committee (ACIP), Morbidity and Mortality Weekly Report 30(4): 37–42, 47, Feb. 6, 1981.

Merck Sharp & Dohme—Cont.

serum globulin (ISG) concurrently with M-R-VAX$_{II}$.

Shipment, Storage, and Reconstitution

During shipment, to insure that there is no loss of potency, the vaccine must be maintained at a temperature of 10°C (50°F) or less.
Before reconstitution, store M-R-VAX$_{II}$ at 2–8°C (35.6–46.4°F). *Protect from light.*
To reconstitute, use only the diluent supplied, since it is free of preservatives or other antiviral substances which might inactivate the vaccine. Inject all the diluent in the syringe into the vial of lyophilized vaccine, and agitate to mix thoroughly. Withdraw the entire contents into the syringe and inject the total volume of restored vaccine subcutaneously.
It is important to use a separate sterile syringe and needle for each individual patient to prevent transmission of hepatitis B and other infectious agents from one person to another.
The usual color of the vaccine when reconstituted is yellow.
It is recommended that the vaccine be used as soon as possible after reconstitution. Protect vaccine from light at all times. Store reconstituted vaccine in a dark place at 2–8°C (35.6–46.4°F) and discard if not used within 8 hours.

How Supplied

No. 4676—M-R-VAX$_{II}$ is supplied as a single-dose vial of lyophilized vaccine with a disposable syringe containing diluent, and fitted with a 25 gauge, 5/8″ needle, **NDC** 0006-4676-00.
No. 4677/4590—M-R-VAX$_{II}$ is supplied as follows: (1) a box of ten single-dose vials of lyophilized vaccine, **NDC** 0006-4677-00; and (2) a box of ten diluent-containing disposable syringes with affixed 25 gauge, 5/8″ needles. To conserve refrigerator space, the syringes may be stored separately at room temperature.

A.H.F.S. Category: 80:12
DC 7032903 Issued April 1981
Copyright © MERCK & CO., INC., 1978
All rights reserved

MEFOXIN® ℞
(cefoxitin sodium, MSD), U.S.P.

Description

MEFOXIN® (Sterile Cefoxitin Sodium, MSD) is a semi-synthetic, broad-spectrum cepha antibiotic for parenteral administration. It is derived from cephamycin C, which is produced by *Streptomyces lactamdurans*. It is the sodium salt of 3-(hydroxymethyl)-7α-methoxy-8-oxo-7-[2- (2-thienyl) acetamido]-5-thia-1-azabicyclo [4.2.0] oct-2-ene-2-carboxylate carbamate (ester). MEFOXIN contains approximately 53.8 mg (2.3 milliequivalents) of sodium per gram of cefoxitin activity. Solutions of MEFOXIN range from clear to light amber in color. The pH of freshly constituted solutions usually ranges from 4.2 to 7.0.

Actions

Clinical Pharmacology
After intramuscular administration of a 1 gram dose of MEFOXIN to normal volunteers, the mean peak serum concentration was 24 mcg/ml. The peak occurred at 20 to 30 minutes. Following an intravenous dose of 1 gram, serum concentrations were 110 mcg/ml at 5 minutes, declining to less than 1 mcg/ml at 4 hours. The half-life after an intravenous dose is 41 to 59 minutes; after intramuscular administration, the half-life is 64.8 minutes. Approximately 85 percent of cefoxitin is excreted unchanged by the kidneys over a 6-hour period, resulting in high urinary concentrations. Following an intramuscular dose of 1 gram, urinary concentrations greater than 3000 mcg/ml were observed. Probenecid slows tubular excretion and produces higher serum levels and increases the duration of measurable serum concentrations.
Cefoxitin passes into pleural and joint fluids and is detectable in antibacterial concentrations in bile.
Clinical experience has demonstrated that MEFOXIN can be administered to patients who are also receiving carbenicillin, kanamycin, gentamicin, tobramycin, or amikacin (see PRECAUTIONS and ADMINISTRATION).
Microbiology
The bactericidal action of cefoxitin results from inhibition of cell wall synthesis. Cefoxitin has *in vitro* activity against a wide range of gram-positive and gram-negative organisms. The methoxy group in the 7α position provides MEFOXIN with a high degree of stability in the presence of beta-lactamases, both penicillinases and cephalosporinases, of gram-negative bacteria. Cefoxitin is usually active against the following organisms *in vitro* and in clinical infections:
Gram-positive
Staphylococcus aureus, including penicillinase and non-penicillinase producing strains.
Staphylococcus epidermidis
Beta-hemolytic and other streptococci (most strains of enterococci, e.g., *Streptococcus faecalis,* are resistant)
Streptococcus pneumoniae (formerly *Diplococcus pneumoniae)*
Gram-negative
Escherichia coli
Klebsiella species (including *K. pneumoniae)*
Hemophilus influenzae
Neisseria gonorrhoeae, including penicillinase and non-penicillinase producing strains
Proteus mirabilis
Proteus rettgeri
Proteus morganii
Proteus vulgaris
Providencia species
Anaerobic organisms
Peptococcus species
Peptostreptococcus species
Clostridium species
Bacteroides species, including the *B. fragilis* group (includes *B. fragilis, B. distasonis, B. ovatus, B. thetaiotaomicron, B. vulgatus)*
MEFOXIN is inactive *in vitro* against most strains of *Pseudomonas aeruginosa* and enterococci and many strains of *Enterobacter cloacae.* Methicillin-resistant staphylococci are almost uniformly resistant to MEFOXIN.
Susceptibility Tests
For fast-growing aerobic organisms, quantitative methods that require measurements of zone diameters give the most precise estimates of antibiotic susceptibility. One such procedure* has been recommended for use with discs to test susceptibility to cefoxitin. Interpretation involves correlation of the diameters obtained in the disc test with minimal inhibitory concentration (MIC) values for cefoxitin.
Reports from the laboratory giving results of the standardized single disc susceptibility test* using a 30 mcg cefoxitin disc should be interpreted according to the following criteria:
Organisms producing zones of 18 mm or greater are considered susceptible, indicating that the tested organism is likely to respond to therapy.

*Bauer, A. W.; Kirby, W. M. M.; Sherris, J. C.; Turck, M.: Antibiotic susceptibility testing by a standardized single disc method, Amer. J. Clin. Path. *45*: 493–496, Apr. 1966. Standardized disc susceptibility test, Federal Register *37*: 20527–20529, 1972. National Committee for Clinical Laboratory Standards: Approved Standard: ASM-2, Performance Standards for Antimicrobial Disc Susceptibility Tests, July 1975.

Organisms of intermediate susceptibility produce zones of 15 to 17 mm, indicating that the tested organism would be susceptible if high dosage is used or if the infection is confined to tissues and fluids (e.g., urine) in which high antibiotic levels are attained.
Resistant organisms produce zones of 14 mm or less, indicating that other therapy should be selected.
The cefoxitin disc should be used for testing cefoxitin susceptibility.
Cefoxitin has been shown by *in vitro* tests to have activity against certain strains of *Enterobacteriaceae* found resistant when tested with the cephalosporin class disc. For this reason, the cefoxitin disc should not be used for testing susceptibility to cephalosporins, and cephalosporin discs should not be used for testing susceptibility to cefoxitin.
Dilution methods, preferably the agar plate dilution procedure, are most accurate for susceptibility testing of obligate anaerobes.
A bacterial isolate may be considered susceptible if the MIC value for cefoxitin† is not more than 16 mcg/ml. Organisms are considered resistant if the MIC is greater than 32 mcg/ml.

Indications and Usage

Treatment
MEFOXIN is indicated for the treatment of serious infections caused by susceptible strains of the designated microorganisms in the diseases listed below.
(1) Lower respiratory tract infections, including pneumonia and lung abscess, caused by *Streptococcus pneumoniae* (formerly *Diplococcus pneumoniae),* other streptococci (excluding enterococci, e.g., *Streptococcus faecalis), Staphylococcus aureus* (penicillinase and non-penicillinase producing), *Escherichia coli, Klebsiella* species, *Hemophilus influenzae,* and *Bacteroides* species.
(2) Genitourinary infections. Urinary tract infections caused by *Escherichia coli, Klebsiella* species, *Proteus mirabilis,* indole-positive Proteus (i.e., *Proteus morganii, rettgeri,* and *vulgaris*), and *Providencia* species. Uncomplicated gonorrhea due to *Neisseria gonorrhoeae* (penicillinase and non-penicillinase producing).
(3) Intra-abdominal infections, including peritonitis and intra-abdominal abscess, caused by *Escherichia coli, Klebsiella* species, *Bacteroides* species including the *Bacteroides fragilis* group**, and *Clostridium* species.
(4) Gynecological infections, including endometritis, pelvic cellulitis, and pelvic inflammatory disease caused by *Escherichia coli, Neisseria gonorrhoeae* (penicillinase and non-penicillinase producing), *Bacteroides* species including the *Bacteroides fragilis* group**, *Clostridium* species, *Peptococcus* species, *Peptostreptococcus* species, and Group B streptococci.
(5) Septicemia caused by *Streptococcus pneumoniae* (formerly *Diplococcus pneumoniae), Staphylococcus aureus* (penicillinase and non-penicillinase producing), *Escherichia coli, Klebsiella* species, and *Bacteroides* species including the *Bacteroides fragilis* group.**
(6) Bone and joint infections caused by *Staphylococcus aureus* (penicillinase and non-penicillinase producing).
(7) Skin and skin structure infections caused by *Staphylococcus aureus* (penicillinase and non-penicillinase producing), *Staphylococcus epidermidis,* streptococci (excluding entero-

†Determined by the ICS agar dilution method (Ericsson and Sherris, Acta Path. Microbiol. Scand. (B) Suppl. No. 217, 1971) or any other method that has been shown to give equivalent results.

** *B. fragilis, B. distasonis, B. ovatus, B. thetaiotaomicron, B. vulgatus.*

cocci, e.g., *Streptococcus faecalis*), *Escherichia coli*, *Proteus mirabilis*, *Klebsiella* species, *Bacteroides* species including the *Bacteroides fragilis* group**, *Clostridium* species, *Peptococcus* species, and *Peptostreptococcus* species.

Appropriate culture and susceptibility studies should be performed to determine the susceptibility of the causative organisms to MEFOXIN. Therapy may be started while awaiting the results of these studies.

In randomized comparative studies, MEFOXIN and cephalothin were comparably safe and effective in the management of infections caused by gram-positive cocci and gram-negative rods susceptible to the cephalosporins. MEFOXIN has a high degree of stability in the presence of bacterial beta-lactamases, both penicillinases and cephalosporinases.

Many infections caused by aerobic and anaerobic gram-negative bacteria resistant to some cephalosporins respond to MEFOXIN. Similarly, many infections caused by aerobic and anaerobic bacteria resistant to some penicillin antibiotics (ampicillin, carbenicillin, penicillin G) respond to treatment with MEFOXIN. Many infections caused by mixtures of susceptible aerobic and anaerobic bacteria respond to treatment with MEFOXIN.

Prevention

When compared to placebo in randomized controlled studies in patients undergoing gastrointestinal surgery, vaginal hysterectomy and cesarean section, the prophylactic use of MEFOXIN resulted in a significant reduction in the number of postoperative infections.

The prophylactic administration of MEFOXIN perioperatively (preoperatively, intraoperatively, and postoperatively) may reduce the incidence of certain postoperative infections in patients undergoing surgical procedures (e.g., vaginal hysterectomy, gastrointestinal surgery and transurethral prostatectomy) that are classified as contaminated or potentially contaminated.

The perioperative use of MEFOXIN may be effective in surgical patients in whom infection at the operative site would present a serious risk, e.g., prosthetic arthroplasty.

In patients undergoing cesarean section, intraoperative (after clamping the umbilical cord) and postoperative use of MEFOXIN may reduce the incidence of certain postoperative infections.

Effective prophylactic use depends on the time of administration. MEFOXIN usually should be given one-half to one hour before the operation, which is sufficient time to achieve effective levels in the wound during the procedure. Prophylactic administration should usually be stopped within 24 hours since continuing administration of any antibiotic increases the possibility of adverse reactions but, in the majority of surgical procedures, does not reduce the incidence of subsequent infection. However, in patients undergoing prosthetic arthroplasty, it is recommended that MEFOXIN be continued for 72 hours after the surgical procedure.

If there are signs of infection, specimens for culture should be obtained for identification of the causative organism so that appropriate therapy may be instituted.

Contraindications

MEFOXIN is contraindicated in patients who have shown hypersensitivity to cefoxitin and the cephalosporin group of antibiotics.

Warnings

BEFORE THERAPY WITH MEFOXIN IS INSTITUTED, CAREFUL INQUIRY SHOULD BE MADE TO DETERMINE WHETHER THE PATIENT HAS HAD PREVIOUS HYPERSENSITIVITY REACTIONS TO CEFOXITIN, CEPHALOSPORINS, PENICILLINS, OR OTHER DRUGS. THIS PRODUCT SHOULD BE GIVEN WITH CAUTION TO PENICILLIN-SENSITIVE PATIENTS. ANTIBIOTICS SHOULD BE ADMINISTERED WITH CAUTION TO ANY PATIENT WHO HAS DEMONSTRATED SOME FORM OF ALLERGY, PARTICULARLY TO DRUGS. IF AN ALLERGIC REACTION TO MEFOXIN OCCURS, DISCONTINUE THE DRUG. SERIOUS HYPERSENSITIVITY REACTIONS MAY REQUIRE EPINEPHRINE AND OTHER EMERGENCY MEASURES.

Pseudomembranous colitis has been reported with virtually all antibiotics (including cephalosporins); therefore, it is important to consider its diagnosis in patients who develop diarrhea in association with antibiotic use. This colitis may range from mild to life threatening in severity.

Treatment with broad-spectrum antibiotics alters normal flora of the colon and may permit overgrowth of clostridia. Studies indicate a toxin produced by *Clostridium difficile* is one primary cause of antibiotic-associated colitis. Mild cases of pseudomembranous colitis may respond to drug discontinuance alone. In more severe cases, management may include sigmoidoscopy, appropriate bacteriological studies, fluid, electrolyte and protein supplementation, and the use of a drug such as oral vancomycin as indicated. Isolation of the patient may be advisable. Other causes of colitis should also be considered.

Precautions

The total daily dose should be reduced when MEFOXIN is administered to patients with transient or persistent reduction of urinary output due to renal insufficiency (see DOSAGE), because high and prolonged serum antibiotic concentrations can occur in such individuals from usual doses.

Antibiotics (including cephalosporins) should be prescribed with caution in individuals with a history of gastrointestinal disease, particularly colitis.

As with other antibiotics, prolonged use of MEFOXIN may result in overgrowth of nonsusceptible organisms. Repeated evaluation of the patient's condition is essential. If superinfection occurs during therapy, appropriate measures should be taken.

Increased nephrotoxicity has been reported following concomitant administration of cephalosporins and aminoglycoside antibiotics.

Interference with Laboratory Tests

As with cephalothin, high concentrations of cefoxitin (>100 micrograms/ml) may interfere with measurement of serum and urine creatinine levels by the Jaffé reaction, and produce false increases of modest degree in the levels of creatinine reported. Serum samples from patients treated with cefoxitin should not be analyzed for creatinine if withdrawn within 2 hours of drug administration.

A false-positive reaction for glucose in the urine may occur. This has been observed with CLINITEST* reagent tablets.

Pregnancy

Reproduction and teratologic studies have been performed in mice and rats and have revealed no evidence of impaired fertility or harm to the fetus due to MEFOXIN. There are no well controlled studies with MEFOXIN in pregnant women. Use of the drug in women of childbearing potential requires that the anticipated benefit be weighed against the possible risks.

Nursing Mothers

MEFOXIN is excreted in human milk in low concentrations.

Infants and Children

Safety and efficacy in infants from birth to three months of age have not yet been established. In children three months of age and older, higher doses of MEFOXIN have been associated with an increased incidence of eosinophilia and elevated SGOT.

*Registered trademark of Ames Company, Division of Miles Laboratories, Inc.

Adverse Reactions

MEFOXIN is generally well tolerated. The most common adverse reactions have been local reactions following intravenous or intramuscular injection. Other adverse reactions have been encountered infrequently.

Local Reactions

Thrombophlebitis has occurred with intravenous administration. Pain, induration, and tenderness after intramuscular injections have been reported.

Allergic Reactions

Rash, pruritus, eosinophilia, fever, and other allergic reactions have been noted.

Gastrointestinal

Symptoms of pseudomembranous colitis can appear during or after antibiotic treatment. Nausea, vomiting, and diarrhea have been reported rarely.

Blood

Transient eosinophilia, leukopenia, neutropenia, hemolytic anemia, and thrombocytopenia have been reported. A positive direct Coombs test may develop in some individuals, especially those with azotemia.

Liver Function

Transient elevations in SGOT, SGPT, serum LDH, and serum alkaline phosphatase have been reported.

Renal Function

Elevations in serum creatinine and/or blood urea nitrogen levels have been observed. As with the cephalosporins, acute renal failure has been reported rarely. The role of MEFOXIN in changes in renal function tests is difficult to assess, since factors predisposing to prerenal azotemia or to impaired renal function usually have been present.

Dosage

TREATMENT

Adults

The usual adult dosage range is 1 gram to 2 grams every six to eight hours. Dosage and route of administration should be determined by susceptibility of the causative organisms, severity of infection, and the condition of the patient (see Table 1 for dosage guidelines).

[See table on next page].

MEFOXIN may be used in patients with reduced renal function with the following dosage adjustments:

In adults with renal insufficiency, an initial loading dose of 1 gram to 2 grams may be given. After a loading dose, the recommendations for *maintenance dosage* (Table 2) may be used as a guide.

[See table on next page].

When only the serum creatinine level is available, the following formula (based on sex, weight, and age of the patient) may be used to convert this value into creatinine clearance. The serum creatinine should represent a steady state of renal function.

$$\text{Males: } \frac{\text{Weight (kg)} \times (140 - \text{age})}{72 \times \text{serum creatinine (mg/100 ml)}}$$

Females: 0.85 × above value

In patients undergoing hemodialysis, the loading dose of 1 to 2 grams should be given after each hemodialysis, and the maintenance dose should be given as indicated in Table 2.

Continued on next page

Information on the Merck Sharp & Dohme products listed on these pages is the full prescribing information from package circulars in use October 31, 1982.

Merck Sharp & Dohme—Cont.

Antibiotic therapy for group A beta-hemolytic streptococcal infections should be maintained for at least 10 days to guard against the risk of rheumatic fever or glomerulonephritis. In staphylococcal and other infections involving a collection of pus, surgical drainage should be carried out where indicated.

The recommended dosage of MEFOXIN **for uncomplicated gonorrhea** is 2 grams intramuscularly, with 1 gram of BENEMID® (Probenecid, MSD) given by mouth at the same time or up to ½ hour before MEFOXIN.

Infants and Children

The recommended dosage in children three months of age and older is 80 to 160 mg/kg of body weight per day divided into four to six equal doses. The higher dosages should be used for more severe or serious infections. The total daily dosage should not exceed 12 grams.

At this time no recommendation is made for children from birth to three months of age (See PRECAUTIONS).

In children with renal insufficiency the dosage and frequency of dosage should be modified consistent with the recommendations for adults (see Table 2).

PREVENTION

For prophylactic use, the following doses are recommended:

Adults:

1) 2 grams administered intravenously or intramuscularly just prior to surgery (approximately one-half to one hour before the initial incision).
2) 2 grams every 6 hours after the first dose for no more than 24 hours (continued for 72 hours after prosthetic arthroplasty).

Children (3 months and older):

30 to 40 mg/kg doses may be given at the time designated above.

Cesarean section patients:

The first dose of 2.0 grams is administered intravenously as soon as the umbilical cord is clamped. The second and third doses should be given as 2.0 grams intravenously or intramuscularly 4 hours and 8 hours after the first dose. Subsequent doses may be given every 6 hours for no more than 24 hours.

Transurethral prostatectomy patients:

One gram administered just prior to surgery; 1 gram every 8 hours for up to five days.

Table 1—Guidelines for Dosage of MEFOXIN

Type of Infection	Daily Dosage	Frequency and Route
Uncomplicated forms* of infections such as pneumonia, urinary tract infection, cutaneous infection	3–4 grams	1 gram every 6–8 hours IV or IM
Moderately severe or severe infections	6–8 grams	1 gram every 4 hours *or* 2 grams every 6–8 hours IV
Infections commonly needing antibiotics in higher dosage (e.g., gas gangrene)	12 grams	2 grams every 4 hours *or* 3 grams every 6 hours IV

*Including patients in whom bacteremia is absent or unlikely

Preparation of Solution

Table 3 is provided for convenience in constituting MEFOXIN for both intravenous and intramuscular administration.

[See table on next page].

For intravenous use, 1 gram should be constituted with at least 10 ml of Sterile Water for Injection, and 2 grams, with 10 or 20 ml. One or 2 grams of MEFOXIN may be constituted with 50 or 100 ml of 0.9 percent Sodium Chloride Injection, 5 percent or 10 percent Dextrose Injection, or any of the solutions listed under the *Intravenous* portion of the COMPATIBILITY AND STABILITY section.

For intramuscular use, each gram of MEFOXIN may be constituted with 2 ml of Sterile Water for Injection *or*

For intramuscular use ONLY: each gram of MEFOXIN may be constituted with 2 ml of 0.5 percent lidocaine hydrochloride solution* (without epinephrine) to minimize the discomfort of intramuscular injection.

Administration

MEFOXIN may be administered intravenously or intramuscularly after constitution.

Intravenous Administration

The intravenous route is preferable for patients with bacteremia, bacterial septicemia, or other severe or life-threatening infections, or for patients who may be poor risks because of lowered resistance resulting from such debilitating conditions as malnutrition, trauma, surgery, diabetes, heart failure, or malignancy, particularly if shock is present or impending.

For intermittent intravenous administration, a solution containing 1 gram or 2 grams in 10 ml of Sterile Water for Injection can be injected over a period of three to five minutes. Using an infusion system, it may also be given over a longer period of time through the tubing system by which the patient may be receiving other intravenous solutions. However, during infusion of the solution containing MEFOXIN, it is advisable to temporarily discontinue administration of any other solutions at the same site.

For the administration of higher doses by continuous intravenous infusion, a solution of MEFOXIN may be added to an intravenous bottle containing 5 percent Dextrose Injection, 0.9 percent Sodium Chloride Injection, 5 percent Dextrose and 0.9 percent Sodium Chloride Injection, or 5 percent Dextrose Injection with 0.02 percent sodium bicarbonate solution. BUTTERFLY** or scalp vein-type needles are preferred for this type of infusion.

Solutions of MEFOXIN, like those of most beta-lactam antibiotics, should not be added to aminoglycoside solutions (e.g., gentamicin sulfate, tobramycin sulfate, amikacin sulfate) because of potential interaction. However, MEFOXIN and aminoglycosides may be administered separately to the same patient.

Intramuscular Administration

As with all intramuscular preparations, MEFOXIN should be injected well within the body of a relatively large muscle such as the upper outer quadrant of the buttock (i.e., gluteus maximus); aspiration is necessary to avoid inadvertent injection into a blood vessel.

*See package circular of manufacturer for detailed information concerning contraindications, warnings, precautions, and adverse reactions.

** Registered trademark of Abbott Laboratories.

Compatibility and Stability

Intravenous

MEFOXIN, as constituted to 1 gram/10 ml with Sterile Water for Injection, Bacteriostatic Water for Injection, 0.9 percent Sodium Chloride Injection, or 5 percent Dextrose Injection, maintains satisfactory potency for 24 hours at room temperature, for one week under refrigeration (below 5°C), and for at least 30 weeks in the frozen state.

These primary solutions may be further diluted in 50 to 1000 ml of the following solutions and maintain potency for 24 hours at room temperature and at least 48 hours under refrigeration:

- Sterile Water for Injection‡
- 0.9 percent Sodium Chloride Injection
- 5 percent or 10 percent Dextrose Injection‡
- 5 percent Dextrose and 0.9 percent Sodium Chloride Injection
- 5 percent Dextrose Injection with 0.02 percent sodium bicarbonate solution
- 5 percent Dextrose Injection with 0.2 percent or 0.45 percent saline solution
- Ringer's Injection
- Lactated Ringer's Injection‡
- 5 percent dextrose in Lactated Ringer's Injection‡
- 5 percent or 10 percent invert sugar in water
- 10 percent invert sugar in saline solution
- 5 percent Sodium Bicarbonate Injection
- Neut (sodium bicarbonate)*‡
- M/6 sodium lactate solution
- AMINOSOL* 5 percent Solution
- NORMOSOL-M in D5-W*‡
- IONOSOL B w/Dextrose 5 percent*‡
- POLYONIC M 56 in 5 percent Dextrose**
- Mannitol 5% and 2.5%
- Mannitol 10%‡
- ISOLYTE E***
- ISOLYTE E*** with 5% dextrose

Limited studies with solutions of MEFOXIN in 0.9 percent Sodium Chloride Injection, Lactated Ringer's Injection, and 5 percent Dextrose Injection in VIAFLEX† intravenous bags show stability for 24 hours at room temperature, 48 hours under refrigeration, 26 weeks in the frozen state, and 24 hours at room temperature thereafter. Also, solutions of MEFOXIN in 0.9 percent Sodium Chloride Injection show similar stability in plastic tubing, drip chambers, and volume control devices of common intravenous infusion sets.

* Registered trademark of Abbott Laboratories.

** Registered trademark of Cutter Laboratories, Inc.

*** Registered trademark of Baxter Laboratories.

† Registered trademark of Travenol Laboratories, Inc.

‡ In these solutions, MEFOXIN has been found to be stable for period of one week under refrigeration.

Table 2—Maintenance Dosage of MEFOXIN in Adults with Reduced Renal Function

Renal Function	Creatinine Clearance (ml/min)	Dose (grams)	Frequency
Mild impairment	50–30	1–2	every 8–12 hours
Moderate impairment	29–10	1–2	every 12–24 hours
Severe impairment	9–5	0.5–1	every 12–24 hours
Essentially no function	<5	0.5–1	every 24–48 hours

After constitution with Sterile Water for Injection and subsequent storage in disposable plastic syringes, MEFOXIN is stable for 24 hours at room temperature and 48 hours under refrigeration.
After the periods mentioned above, any unused solutions or frozen material should be discarded. Do not refreeze.

Intramuscular
MEFOXIN, as constituted with Sterile Water for Injection, Bacteriostatic Water for Injection, or 0.5 percent or 1 percent lidocaine hydrochloride solution (without epinephrine), maintains satisfactory potency for 24 hours at room temperature, for one week under refrigeration (below 5°C), and for at least 30 weeks in the frozen state.
After the periods mentioned above, any unused solutions or frozen material should be discarded. Do not refreeze.
MEFOXIN has also been found compatible when admixed in intravenous infusions with the following:
Heparin 0.1 units/ml at room temperature—8 hours
Heparin 100 units/ml at room temperature—24 hours
M.V.I.†† concentrate at room temperature 24 hours; under refrigeration 48 hours
BEROCCA††† C-500 at room temperature 24 hours; under refrigeration 48 hours
Insulin in Normal Saline at room temperature 24 hours; under refrigeration 48 hours
Insulin in 10% invert sugar at room temperature 24 hours; under refrigeration 48 hours

Note: MEFOXIN in the dry state should be stored below 30°C. Avoid exposure to temperatures above 50°C. The dry material as well as solutions tend to darken, depending on storage conditions; product potency, however, is not adversely affected.

How Supplied

Sterile MEFOXIN is a dry white to off-white powder supplied in vials and infusion bottles containing cefoxitin sodium as follows:
No. 3356—1 gram cefoxitin equivalent
NDC 0006-3356-02 in vials
NDC 0006-3356-45 in trays of 25 vials.
No. 3368—1 gram cefoxitin equivalent
NDC 0006-3368-02 in infusion bottles.
NDC 0006-3368-71 in trays of 10 infusion bottles.
No. 3357—2 gram cefoxitin equivalent
NDC 0006-3357-03 in vials
NDC 0006-3357-53 in trays of 25 vials.
No. 3369—2 gram cefoxitin equivalent
NDC 0006-3369-03 in infusion bottles.
NDC 0006-3369-73 in trays of 10 infusion bottles.

A.H.F.S. Category: 8:12.28
DC 7057114 Issued February 1982
COPYRIGHT© MERCK & CO., INC., 1977
All rights reserved

Table 3—Preparation of Solution

Strength	Amount of Diluent to be Added (ml)*	Approximate Withdrawable Volume (ml)	Approximate Average Concentration (mg/ml)
1 gram Vial	2 (Intramuscular)	2.5	400
2 gram Vial	4 (Intramuscular)	5	400
1 gram Vial	10 (IV)	10.5	95
2 gram Vial	10 or 20 (IV)	11.1 or 21.0	180 or 95
1 gram Infusion Bottle	50 to 100 (IV)	50 to 100	20 to 10
2 gram Infusion Bottle	50 to 100 (IV)	50 to 100	40 to 20

*Shake to dissolve and let stand until clear.

MERUVAX® II ℞

(rubella virus vaccine, live, MSD), U.S.P.
(Wistar RA 27/3 Strain
Prepared in WI-38 Human Diploid Cells)

Description

MERUVAX® II (Rubella Virus Vaccine, Live, MSD) is a live virus vaccine for immunization against rubella (German measles).
MERUVAX II is a lyophilized preparation of the Wistar Institute RA 27/3 strain of live attenuated rubella virus. The virus was adapted to and propagated in human diploid cell (WI-38) culture.

When reconstituted as directed, the dose for injection is 0.5 ml and contains not less than the equivalent of 1,000 $TCID_{50}$ (tissue culture infective doses) of rubella virus vaccine expressed in terms of the assigned titer of the FDA Reference Rubella Virus. Each dose also contains approximately 25 mcg of neomycin.

Actions

Extensive clinical trials of rubella virus vaccines, prepared using RA 27/3 strain rubella virus, have been carried out in more than 28,000 human subjects (approximately 11,000 with MERUVAX II) in the U.S.A. and more than 20 additional countries. Following subcutaneous inoculation, the vaccines have been shown to induce rubella hemagglutination-inhibiting (HI) antibodies in over 97% of susceptible subjects. The RA 27/3 rubella strain elicits higher immediate post-vaccination HI, complement-fixing and neutralizing antibody levels than other strains of rubella vaccine and has been shown to induce a broader profile of circulating antibodies including anti-theta and anti-iota precipitating antibodies. The RA 27/3 rubella strain immunologically simulates natural infection more closely than other rubella vaccine viruses. The increased levels and broader profile of antibodies produced by RA 27/3 strain rubella virus vaccine appear to correlate with greater resistance to subclinical reinfection with the wild virus, and provide greater confidence for lasting immunity.
Vaccine induced antibody levels have been shown to persist for at least six years without substantial decline. If the present pattern continues, it will provide a basis for the expectation that immunity following the vaccine will be permanent. However, continued surveillance will be required to demonstrate this point.

Indications†

1. *Children Between 12 Months of Age and Puberty*
MERUVAX II is indicated for immunization against rubella in boys and girls from 12 months of age to puberty. No booster is needed. It is not recommended for infants younger than 12 months because persons of that age may retain maternal rubella neutralizing antibodies that may interfere with the immune response. Children in kindergarten and the first grades of elementary school deserve priority for vaccination because often they are epidemiologically the major source of virus dissemination in the community. A history of rubella illness is usually not reliable enough to exclude children from immunization.
Previously unimmunized children of susceptible pregnant women should receive live attenuated rubella vaccine, because an immunized child will be less likely to acquire natural rubella and introduce the virus into the household.
2. *Adolescent and Adult Males*
Vaccination of adolescent or adult males may be a useful procedure in preventing or controlling outbreaks of rubella in circumscribed population groups (e.g., military bases and schools).
3. *Non-Pregnant Adolescent and Adult Females*
Immunization of susceptible non-pregnant adolescent and adult females of childbearing age with live attenuated rubella virus vaccine is indicated if certain precautions are observed (see below). Vaccinating susceptible postpubertal females confers individual protection against subsequently acquiring rubella infection during pregnancy, which in turn prevents infection of the fetus and consequent congenital rubella injury.
Pregnant females *must not* be given live attenuated rubella virus vaccine. It is not known to what extent infection of the fetus with attenuated virus might occur following vaccination, or whether damage to the fetus could result. Subjects should be considered for vaccination only if they agree that they will not become pregnant within three months following vaccination, and if they are informed of the reason for this precaution.* If a pregnant woman is inadvertently vaccinated or if she becomes pregnant within three months of vaccination, she should be counseled on the possible risks to the fetus.
It is recommended that rubella susceptibility be determined by serologic testing prior to immunization.** If immune, as evidenced by a specific rubella antibody titer of 1:8 or greater

†† Registered trademark of USV Pharmaceutical Corp.
††† Registered trademark of Roche Laboratories.

† Based in part on the recommendation for rubella vaccine use of the Immunization Practices Advisory Committee (ACIP), Morbidity and Mortality Weekly Report 30(4): 37–42, 47, Feb. 6, 1981.

* NOTE: The Immunization Practices Advisory Committee (ACIP) has recommended "In view of the importance of protecting this age group against rubella, asking females if they are pregnant, excluding those who say they are, and explaining the theoretical risks to the others are reasonable precautions in a rubella immunization program."

** NOTE: The Immunization Practices Advisory Committee (ACIP) has stated "When practical, and when reliable laboratory services are available, potential vaccinees of childbearing age can have serologic tests to determine susceptibility to rubella. . . . However, routinely performing serologic tests for all females of childbearing age to determine susceptibility so that vaccine is given only to proven susceptibles is expensive and has been ineffective in some areas. Accordingly, the ACIP believes that rubella vaccination of a woman who is not known to be pregnant and has no history of vaccination is justifiable without serologic testing."

Continued on next page

Information on the Merck Sharp & Dohme products listed on these pages is the full prescribing information from package circulars in use October 31, 1982.

Merck Sharp & Dohme—Cont.

(hemagglutination inhibition test), vaccination is unnecessary. Congenital malformations do occur in up to seven percent of all live births. Their chance appearance after vaccination could lead to misinterpretation of the cause, particularly if the prior rubella-immune status of vaccinees is unknown.
Postpubertal females should be informed of the frequent occurrence of self-limited arthralgia and possible arthritis beginning 2 to 4 weeks after vaccination (See ADVERSE REACTIONS).
It has been found convenient in many instances to vaccinate rubella-susceptible women in the immediate postpartum period.

Revaccination
Based on available evidence, there is no reason to revaccinate children who were vaccinated originally when 12 months of age or older; however, children vaccinated when younger than 12 months of age should be revaccinated.

Use with Other Live Virus Vaccines
There are no data available concerning simultaneous use of MERUVAX II with monovalent or trivalent poliovirus vaccine, live, oral, or with killed poliovirus vaccines. However, serologic evidence shows that when M-M-R® (Measles, Mumps and Rubella Virus Vaccine, Live, MSD), containing the HPV-77 rubella strain, is given simultaneously with trivalent poliovirus vaccine, live, oral, antibody responses can be expected to be comparable to those which follow administration of the vaccines at different times. From this it follows that when MERUVAX II is given simultaneously with either monovalent or trivalent poliovirus vaccine, live, oral, ATTENUVAX® (Measles Virus Vaccine, Live, Attenuated, MSD) and/or MUMPSVAX® (Mumps Virus Vaccine, Live, MSD), antibody responses can be expected to be comparable to those which follow administration of the vaccines at different times.

Contraindications

Do not give MERUVAX II to pregnant females; the possible effects of the vaccine on fetal development are unknown at this time. When vaccination of post-pubertal females is undertaken, pregnancy must be avoided for three months following vaccination.
Hypersensitivity to neomycin (each dose of reconstituted vaccine contains approximately 25 mcg of neomycin).
Any febrile respiratory illness, or other active febrile infection.
Patients receiving therapy with ACTH, corticosteroids, irradiation, alkylating agents or antimetabolites. This contraindication does not apply to patients who are receiving corticosteroids as replacement therapy, e.g., for Addison's disease.
Individuals with blood dyscrasias, leukemia, lymphomas of any type, or other malignant neoplasms affecting the bone marrow or lymphatic systems.
Primary immuno-deficiency states, including cellular immune deficiencies, hypogammaglobulinemic and dysgammaglobulinemic states.

Precautions

The vaccine is to be given subcutaneously; *do not give intravenously.*
Epinephrine should be available for immediate use should an anaphylactoid reaction occur.
MERUVAX II may be given simultaneously with monovalent or trivalent poliovirus vaccine, live, oral, with ATTENUVAX (Measles Virus Vaccine, Live, Attenuated, MSD) and/or MUMPSVAX (Mumps Virus Vaccine, Live, MSD). MERUVAX II should not be given less than one month before or after administration of other live virus vaccines.
Excretion of small amounts of the live attenuated rubella virus from the nose or throat has occurred in the majority of susceptible individuals 7–28 days after vaccination. There is no confirmed evidence to indicate that such virus is transmitted to susceptible persons who are in contact with the vaccinated individuals. Consequently, transmission, while accepted as a theoretical possibility, is not regarded as a significant risk.*
There is no evidence that live rubella virus vaccine given after exposure to natural rubella virus will prevent illness. There is, however, no contraindication to vaccinating children already exposed to natural rubella.
Vaccination should be deferred for at least three months following blood or plasma transfusions, or administration of human immune serum globulin. However, susceptible postpartum patients who received blood products may receive MERUVAX II prior to discharge provided that a repeat HI titer is drawn 6–8 weeks after vaccination to insure seroconversion. Similarly, although studies with other live rubella virus vaccines suggest that MERUVAX II may be given in the immediate postpartum period to those non-immune women who have received anti-Rho (D) globulin (human) without interfering with vaccine effectiveness, a follow-up post-vaccination HI titer should also be determined.
It has been reported that attenuated rubella virus vaccine, live, may result in a temporary depression of tuberculin skin sensitivity. Therefore, if a tuberculin test is to be done, it should be administered either before or simultaneously with MERUVAX II.
As for any vaccine, vaccination with MERUVAX II may not result in seroconversion in 100% of susceptible subjects given the vaccine.

Adverse Reactions

Because of the slightly acidic pH (6.2–6.6) of the vaccine, patients may complain of burning and/or stinging of short duration at the injection site.
Adverse reactions are uncommon, but symptoms of the same kind as those seen following natural rubella may occur after vaccination. These include regional lymphadenopathy, urticaria, wheal and flare at the injection site, rash, malaise, sore throat, fever, headache, polyneuritis, and occasionally temporary arthralgia that is infrequently associated with signs of inflammation. Local pain, induration, and erythema may occur at the site of injection.
Moderate fever [101–102.9°F (38.3–39.4°C)] occurs occasionally, and high fever [above 103°F (39.4°C)] occurs less commonly.
Reactions are usually mild and transient.
In children, joint reactions are rare and of brief duration if they do occur. In women, incidence rates for arthritis and arthralgia are generally higher than those seen in children (children: 0–3%; women: 12–20%) and the reactions tend to be more marked and of longer duration. Rarely, symptoms may persist for a matter of months. In adolescent girls, the reactions appear to be intermediate in incidence between those seen in children and in adult women. Even in older women (35–45 years), these reactions are generally well tolerated and rarely interfere with normal activities.
Clinical experience with live virus rubella vaccines thus far indicates that encephalitis and other nervous system reactions have occurred very rarely in subjects who were given the vaccines, but a cause and effect relationship has not been established.

* Recommendation of the Immunization Practices Advisory Committee (ACIP), Morbidity and Mortality Weekly Report 30(4): 37–42, 47, Feb. 6, 1981.

In view of the decreases in platelet counts that have been reported, thrombocytopenic purpura is a theoretical hazard.

Dosage and Administration

Inject the total volume of reconstituted vaccine subcutaneously, preferably into the outer aspect of the upper arm, after suitable cleansing of the immunization site. MERUVAX II should not be injected intravenously, or administered intranasally. *Do not give immune serum globulin (ISG) concurrently with* MERUVAX II.

Shipment, Storage and Reconstitution

To insure that there is no loss of potency during shipment, the vaccine must be maintained at a temperature of 10°C (50°F) or less.
Before reconstitution, store MERUVAX II at 2–8°C (35.6–46.4°F). *Protect from light.*
To reconstitute, inject all of the diluent in the syringe into the vial of lyophilized vaccine, and agitate to ensure thorough mixing. Withdraw the entire contents into the syringe and inject the total volume of restored vaccine subcutaneously.
It is important to use a separate sterile syringe and needle for each individual patient to prevent transmission of hepatitis B and other infectious agents from one person to another.
Each dose of reconstituted vaccine contains not less than 1000 $TCID_{50}$ (tissue culture infectious doses) of rubella virus vaccine expressed in terms of the assigned titer of the FDA Reference Rubella Virus.
The color of the vaccine when reconstituted is yellow.
Use only the diluent supplied to reconstitute the vaccine. It is recommended that the vaccine be used as soon as possible after reconstitution. Protect vaccine from light, at all times. Store reconstituted vaccine in a dark place at 2–8°C (35.6–46.4°F) and discard if not used within 8 hours.

How Supplied

No. 4672 MERUVAX II is supplied as a single-dose vial of lyophilized vaccine, **NDC** 0006-4672-00, with a disposable syringe containing diluent and fitted with a 25 gauge, 5/8″ needle.
No. 4673/4590 MERUVAX II is supplied as follows: (1) a box of 10 single-dose vials of lyophilized vaccine, **NDC** 0006-4673-00, and (2) a box of 10 diluent-containing disposable syringes with affixed 25 gauge, 5/8″ needles. To conserve refrigerator space, the syringes may be stored separately at room temperature.

A.H.F.S. Category: 80:12
DC 7030804 Issued April 1981

MIDAMOR® Tablets ℞
(amiloride HCl, MSD)

Description

Amiloride HCl, an antikaliuretic-diuretic agent, is a pyrazinecarbonyl-guanidine that is unrelated chemically to other known antikaliuretic or diuretic agents. It is the salt of a moderately strong base (pKa 8.7). Its chemical name is 3,5-diamino-6-chloro-*N*-(diaminomethylene)pyrazinecarboxamide monohydrochloride. Its empirical formula is $C_6H_8ClN_7O \cdot HCl$. MIDAMOR® (Amiloride HCl, MSD) is available for oral use as tablets containing 5 mg of amiloride HCl.

Clinical Pharmacology

MIDAMOR is a potassium-conserving (antikaliuretic) drug that possesses weak (compared with thiazide diuretics) natriuretic, diuretic, and antihypertensive activity. These effects have been partially additive to the effects of thiazide diuretics in some clinical studies. MIDAMOR has potassium-conserving activity in patients receiving kaliuretic-diuretic agents.

MIDAMOR is not an aldosterone antagonist and its effects are seen even in the absence of aldosterone.

MIDAMOR usually begins to act within 2 hours after an oral dose. Its effect on electrolyte excretion reaches a peak between 6 and 10 hours and lasts about 24 hours. Peak plasma levels are obtained in 3 to 4 hours and the plasma half-life varies from 6 to 9 hours. Effects on electrolytes increase with single doses of amiloride HCl up to approximately 15 mg. Amiloride HCl is not metabolized by the liver but is excreted unchanged by the kidneys. About 50 percent of a 20 mg dose of MIDAMOR is excreted in the urine and 40 percent in the stool within 72 hours. MIDAMOR has little effect on glomerular filtration rate or renal blood flow. Because amiloride HCl is not metabolized by the liver, drug accumulation is not anticipated in patients with hepatic dysfunction, but accumulation can occur if the hepatorenal syndrome develops.

Indications and Usage

MIDAMOR is indicated as adjunctive treatment with thiazide diuretics or other kaliuretic-diuretic agents in congestive heart failure or hypertension to:

a. help restore normal serum potassium levels in patients who develop hypokalemia on the kaliuretic diuretic
b. prevent development of hypokalemia in patients who would be exposed to particular risk if hypokalemia were to develop, e.g., digitalized patients or patients with significant cardiac arrhythmias.

The use of potassium-conserving agents is often unnecessary in patients receiving diuretics for uncomplicated essential hypertension when such patients have a normal diet. MIDAMOR has little additive diuretic or antihypertensive effect when added to a thiazide diuretic.

MIDAMOR should rarely be used alone. It has weak (compared with thiazides) diuretic and antihypertensive effects. Used as single agents, potassium sparing diuretics, including MIDAMOR, result in an increased risk of hyperkalemia (approximately 10% with amiloride). MIDAMOR should be used alone only when persistent hypokalemia has been documented and only with careful titration of the dose and close monitoring of serum electrolytes.

Contraindications

Hyperkalemia

MIDAMOR should not be used in the presence of elevated serum potassium levels (greater than 5.5 mEq per liter).

Antikaliuretic Therapy or Potassium Supplementation

MIDAMOR should not be given to patients receiving other potassium-conserving agents, such as spironolactone or triamterene. Potassium supplementation in the form of medication or a potassium-rich diet should not be used with MIDAMOR except in severe and/or refractory cases of hypokalemia. Such concomitant therapy can be associated with rapid increases in serum potassium levels. If potassium supplementation is used, careful monitoring of the serum potassium level is necessary.

Impaired Renal Function

Anuria, acute or chronic renal insufficiency, and evidence of diabetic nephropathy are contraindications to the use of MIDAMOR. Patients with evidence of renal functional impairment (blood urea nitrogen [BUN] levels over 30 mg per 100 ml or serum creatinine levels over 1.5 mg per 100 ml) or diabetes mellitus should not receive the drug without careful, frequent and continuing monitoring of serum electrolytes, creatinine, and BUN levels. Potassium retention associated with the use of an antikaliuretic agent is accentuated in the presence of renal impairment and may result in the rapid development of hyperkalemia.

Hypersensitivity

MIDAMOR is contraindicated in patients who are hypersensitive to this product.

Warnings

Hyperkalemia

Like other potassium-conserving agents, amiloride may cause hyperkalemia (serum potassium levels greater than 5.5 mEq per liter) which, if uncorrected, is potentially fatal. Hyperkalemia occurs commonly (about 10%) when amiloride is used without a kaliuretic diuretic. This incidence is greater in patients with renal impairment, diabetes mellitus (with or without recognized renal insufficiency), and in the elderly. When MIDAMOR is used concomitantly with a thiazide diuretic in patients without these complications, the risk of hyperkalemia is reduced to about 1–2%. It is thus essential to monitor serum potassium levels carefully in any patient receiving amiloride, particularly when it is first introduced, at the time of diuretic dosage adjustments, and during any illness that could affect renal function.

Warning signs or symptoms of hyperkalemia include paresthesias, muscular weakness, fatigue, flaccid paralysis of the extremities, bradycardia, shock, and ECG abnormalities. Monitoring of the serum potassium level is essential because mild hyperkalemia is not usually associated with an abnormal ECG.

When abnormal, the ECG in hyperkalemia is characterized primarily by tall, peaked T waves or elevations from previous tracings. There may also be lowering of the R wave and increased depth of the S wave, widening and even disappearance of the P wave, progressive widening of the QRS complex, prolongation of the PR interval, and ST depression.

Treatment of hyperkalemia: If hyperkalemia occurs in patients taking MIDAMOR, the drug should be discontinued immediately. If the serum potassium level exceeds 6.5 mEq per liter, active measures should be taken to reduce it. Such measures include the intravenous administration of sodium bicarbonate solution or oral or parenteral glucose with a rapid-acting insulin preparation. If needed, a cation exchange resin such as sodium polystyrene sulfonate may be given orally or by enema. Patients with persistent hyperkalemia may require dialysis.

Diabetes Mellitus

In diabetic patients, hyperkalemia has been reported with the use of all potassium-conserving diuretics, including MIDAMOR, even in patients without evidence of diabetic nephropathy. Therefore, MIDAMOR should be avoided, if possible, in diabetic patients and, if it is used, serum electrolytes and renal function must be monitored frequently.

MIDAMOR should be discontinued at least 3 days before glucose tolerance testing.

Metabolic or Respiratory Acidosis

Antikaliuretic therapy should be instituted only with caution in severely ill patients in whom respiratory or metabolic acidosis may occur, such as patients with cardiopulmonary disease or poorly controlled diabetes. If MIDAMOR is given to these patients, frequent monitoring of acid-base balance is necessary. Shifts in acid-base balance alter the ratio of extracellular/intracellular potassium, and the development of acidosis may be associated with rapid increases in serum potassium levels.

Precautions

General

Electrolyte Imbalance and BUN Increases

Hyponatremia and hypochloremia may occur when MIDAMOR is used with other diuretics and increases in BUN levels have been reported. These increases usually have accompanied vigorous fluid elimination, especially when diuretic therapy was used in seriously ill patients, such as those who had hepatic cirrhosis with ascites and metabolic alkalosis, or those with resistant edema. Therefore, when MIDAMOR is given with other diuretics to such patients, careful monitoring of serum electrolytes and BUN levels is important. In patients with pre-existing severe liver disease, hepatic encephalopathy, manifested by tremors, confusion, and coma, and increased jaundice, have been reported in association with diuretics, including amiloride HCl.

Drug Interactions

Lithium generally should not be given with diuretics because they reduce its renal clearance and add a high risk of lithium toxicity. Read circulars for lithium preparations before use of such concomitant therapy.

Carcinogenicity, Mutagenicity

There was no evidence of a tumorigenic effect when amiloride HCl was administered for 92 weeks to mice at doses up to 10 mg/kg/day (25 times the maximum daily human dose). Amiloride HCl has also been administered for 104 weeks to male and female rats at doses up to 6 and 8 mg/kg/day (15 and 20 times the maximum daily dose for humans, respectively) and showed no evidence of carcinogenicity.

Amiloride HCl was devoid of mutagenic activity in various strains of *Salmonella typhimurium* with or without a mammalian liver microsomal activation system (Ames test).

Pregnancy

Pregnancy Category B

Teratologic studies with amiloride HCl in rabbits and mice given 20 and 25 times the maximum human dose, respectively, revealed no evidence of harm to the fetus, although studies showed that the drug crossed the placenta in modest amounts. Reproduction studies in rats at 20 times the expected maximum daily dose for humans showed no evidence of impaired fertility. At approximately 5 or more times the expected maximum daily dose for humans, some toxicity was seen in adult rats and rabbits and a decrease in rat pup growth and survival occurred.

There are, however, no adequate and well-controlled studies in pregnant women. Because animal reproduction studies are not always predictive of human response, this drug should be used during pregnancy only if clearly needed.

Nursing Mothers

Studies in rats have shown that amiloride is excreted in milk in concentrations higher than that found in blood, but it is not known whether MIDAMOR is excreted in human milk. Because many drugs are excreted in human milk and because of the potential for serious adverse reactions in nursing infants from MIDAMOR, a decision should be made whether to discontinue nursing or to discontinue the drug, taking into account the importance of the drug to the mother.

Pediatric Use

Safety and effectiveness in children have not been established.

Adverse Reactions

MIDAMOR is usually well tolerated and, except for hyperkalemia (serum potassium levels greater than 5.5 mEq per liter—see WARNINGS), significant adverse effects have been reported infrequently. Minor adverse reactions were reported relatively frequently

Continued on next page

Information on the Merck Sharp & Dohme products listed on these pages is the full prescribing information from package circulars in use October 31, 1982.

Merck Sharp & Dohme—Cont.

(about 20%) but the relationship of many of the reports to amiloride HCl is uncertain and the overall frequency was similar in hydrochlorothiazide treated groups. Nausea/anorexia, abdominal pain, flatulence, and mild skin rash have been reported and probably are related to amiloride. Other adverse experiences that have been reported with amiloride are generally those known to be associated with diuresis, or with the underlying disease being treated. The clinical adverse reactions listed in the following table have been arranged into two groups: 1) incidence greater than 1%; and 2) incidence equal to or less than 1%. The incidence was determined from clinical studies conducted in the United States (837 patients treated with MIDAMOR).

Incidence > 1%	*Incidence ≤ 1%*
Body as a Whole	
Headache*	Back pain
Weakness	Chest pain
Fatigability	Neck/shoulder ache
	Pain, extremities
Cardiovascular	
None	Angina pectoris
	Orthostatic hypotension
	Arrhythmia
	Palpitation
Digestive	
Nausea/anorexia*	Jaundice
Diarrhea*	GI bleeding
Vomiting*	Abdominal fullness
Abdominal pain	GI disturbance
Gas pain	Thirst
Appetite changes	Heartburn
Constipation	Flatulence
	Dyspepsia
Metabolic	
Elevated serum potassium levels (> 5.5 mEq per liter)†	None
Integumentary	
None	Skin rash
	Itching
	Dryness of mouth
	Pruritus
	Alopecia
Musculoskeletal	
Muscle cramps	Joint pain
	Leg ache
Nervous	
Dizziness	Paresthesia
Encephalopathy	Tremors
	Vertigo
Psychiatric	
None	Nervousness
	Mental confusion
	Insomnia
	Decreased libido
	Depression
	Somnolence
Respiratory	
Cough	Shortness of breath
Dyspnea	
Special Senses	
None	Visual disturbances
	Nasal congestion
	Tinnitus
	Increased intraocular pressure
Urogenital	
Impotence	Polyuria
	Dysuria
	Urinary frequency
	Bladder spasms

* Reactions occurring in 3% to 8% of patients treated with MIDAMOR. (Those reactions occurring in less than 3% of the patients are unmarked.)

† See WARNINGS.

Causal Relationship Unknown
Other reactions have been reported but occurred under circumstances where a causal relationship could not be established. However, in these rarely reported events, that possibility cannot be excluded. Therefore, these observations are listed to serve as alerting information to physicians.

- Activation of probable pre-existing peptic ulcer
- Aplastic anemia
- Neutropenia
- Abnormalities of liver function tests

Overdosage

No data are available in regard to overdosage in humans.
The oral LD_{50} of amiloride hydrochloride (calculated as the base) is 56 mg/kg in mice and 36 to 85 mg/kg in rats, depending on the strain. It is not known whether the drug is dialyzable. The most likely signs and symptoms to be expected with overdosage are dehydration and electrolyte imbalance. These can be treated by established procedures. Therapy with MIDAMOR should be discontinued and the patient observed closely. There is no specific antidote. Emesis should be induced or gastric lavage performed. Treatment is symptomatic and supportive. If hyperkalemia occurs, active measures should be taken to reduce the serum potassium levels.

Dosage and Administration

MIDAMOR should be administered with food. MIDAMOR, one 5 mg tablet daily, should be added to the usual antihypertensive or diuretic dosage of a kaliuretic diuretic. The dosage may be increased to 10 mg per day, if necessary. More than two 5 mg tablets of MIDAMOR daily usually are not needed, and there is little controlled experience with such doses. If persistent hypokalemia is documented with 10 mg, the dose can be increased to 15 mg, then 20 mg, with careful monitoring of electrolytes.
In treating patients with congestive heart failure after an initial diuresis has been achieved, potassium loss may also decrease and the need for MIDAMOR should be reevaluated. Dosage adjustment may be necessary. Maintenance therapy may be on an intermittent basis.
If it is necessary to use MIDAMOR alone (see INDICATIONS), the starting dosage should be one 5 mg tablet daily. This dosage may be increased to 10 mg per day, if necessary. More than two 5 mg tablets usually are not needed, and there is little controlled experience with such doses. If persistent hypokalemia is documented with 10 mg, the dose can be increased to 15 mg, then 20 mg, with careful monitoring of electrolytes.

How Supplied

No. 3381—Tablets MIDAMOR, 5 mg, are yellow, diamond-shaped, compressed tablets, coded MSD 92. They are supplied as follows:
NDC 0006-0092-68 bottles of 100.

[*Shown in Product Identification Section*]

A.H.F.S. Category: 40:28
DC 7130004 Issued September 1981

COPYRIGHT© MERCK & CO., INC., 1978
All rights reserved

MINTEZOL® Chewable Tablets (thiabendazole, MSD) ℞
MINTEZOL® Suspension (thiabendazole, MSD), U.S.P. ℞

Description

MINTEZOL® (Thiabendazole, MSD) is provided as 500 mg chewable tablets, and as a suspension, containing 500 mg thiabendazole per 5 ml. The suspension also contains sorbic acid 0.1% added as a preservative. Thiabendazole, an anthelmintic, is a white to off-white odorless powder, practically insoluble in water. It is designated chemically as 2-(4-thiazolyl)-1*H*-benzimidazole. The empirical formula is $C_{10}H_7N_3S$.

Action

Thiabendazole is vermicidal against *Enterobius vermicularis* (pinworm), *Ascaris lumbricoides* ("common roundworm"), *Strongyloides stercoralis* (threadworm), *Necator americanus*, and *Ancylostoma duodenale* (hookworm), *Trichuris trichiura* (whipworm), and *Ancylostoma braziliense* (dog and cat hookworm).
Its effect on larvae of *Trichinella spiralis* that have migrated to muscle is questionable.
Thiabendazole also suppresses egg and/or larval production and may inhibit the subsequent development of those eggs or larvae which are passed in the feces. The anthelmintic activity against *Trichuris trichiura* (whipworm) is least predictable.
In man, an oral dose of thiabendazole is rapidly absorbed and peak plasma concentration is reached within 1 to 2 hours after the dose. It is metabolized almost completely to the 5-hydroxy form which appears in the urine as glucuronide or sulfate conjugates. In 48 hours, about 5% of the administered dose is recovered from the feces and about 90% from the urine. Most is excreted in the first 24 hours.

Indications

Thiabendazole is indicated in the treatment of enterobiasis, strongyloidiasis, ascariasis, uncinariasis (*Necator americanus* and *Ancylostoma duodenale* infections), trichuriasis, and cutaneous larva migrans (creeping eruption).
Therapeutic effect of this drug in trichuriasis, however, is limited. Thiabendazole is also indicated for alleviating symptoms of trichinosis during the invasive phase of the disease.

Contraindication

History of hypersensitivity to this product.

Warnings

If hypersensitivity reactions occur, the drug should be discontinued immediately and not be resumed. Erythema multiforme has been associated with thiabendazole therapy; in severe cases (Stevens-Johnson syndrome), fatalities have occurred.
Because CNS side effects may occur quite frequently, activities requiring mental alertness should be avoided.
Usage in Pregnancy
Safety for use of this drug in pregnancy and lactation has not been established.

Precautions

Ideally, supportive therapy is indicated for anemic, dehydrated or malnourished patients prior to initiation of the anthelmintic therapy. In the presence of hepatic or renal dysfunction, patients should be carefully monitored.

Adverse Reactions

The most frequently encountered side effects are anorexia, nausea, vomiting and dizziness. Less frequently, diarrhea, epigastric distress, pruritus, weariness, drowsiness, giddiness, and headache have occurred.
Side effects which have occurred rarely are:
tinnitus, hyperirritability, numbness, abnormal sensation in eyes, blurring of vision, xanthopsia; hypotension, collapse; enuresis; transient rise in cephalin flocculation and SGOT; jaundice, cholestasis and parenchymal liver damage; hyperglycemia; transient leukopenia; perianal rash; malodor of the urine, crystalluria, hematuria; appearance of live Ascaris in the mouth and nose.
Hypersensitivity reactions include: fever, facial flush, chills, conjunctival injection, angio-

edema, anaphylaxis, skin rashes, erythema multiforme (including Stevens-Johnson syndrome), and lymphadenopathy.

Dosage and Administration

The recommended maximum daily dose of MINTEZOL *is 3 grams.*
MINTEZOL should be given after meals if possible. Dietary restriction, complementary medications and cleansing enemas are not needed. The usual dosage schedule for all conditions is two doses per day. The size of the dose is determined by the patient's weight.

(1) Patients weighing less than 150 lbs —10 mg (0.1 ml)/lb, or 25 mg (0.25 ml)/kg.
(2) Patients weighing 150 lbs and over —1.5 g (15 ml).

A weight-dose chart based on these recommendations follows:
[See table above right].
The regimen for each indication follows:
[See table below].

How Supplied

No. 3331 — MINTEZOL Suspension, 500 mg per 5 ml, is white to off-white and is supplied as follows:
NDC 0006-3331-60 in bottles of 120 ml (6505-00-935-5835 0.5 g/5 ml 120 ml).
No. 3332 — MINTEZOL Chewable Tablets, 500 mg, are white to off-white, orange-flavored, round, scored, compressed tablets, coded MSD 907. They are supplied as follows:
NDC 0006-0907-36 in boxes of 36 strip packaged, individually foil-wrapped tablets.
[*Shown in Product Identification Section*]
A.H.F.S. Category: 8:08
DC 6857704 Issued January 1978

Weight	Each Dose g		Each Dose ml
25 lb	0.25	(½ tablet)	2.5 (½ teaspoon)
50 lb	0.5	(1 tablet)	5.0 (1 teaspoon)
75 lb	0.75	(1 ½ tablets)	7.5 (1 ½ teaspoons)
100 lb	1.0	(2 tablets)	10.0 (2 teaspoons)
125 lb	1.25	(2 ½ tablets)	12.5 (2 ½ teaspoons)
150 lb & over	1.5	(3 tablets)	15.0 (3 teaspoons)

Therapeutic Regimens

Indication	*Regimen*	*Comments*
I. *Intestinal Parasitosis* ENTEROBIASIS (Pinworm Infection)	2 doses per day for 1 day. Repeat in 7 days.	If this is not practical, give 2 doses per day for 2 successive days. This regimen is designed to reduce the risk of reinfection.
*STRONGYLOIDIASIS *ASCARIASIS ("Common Roundworm" Infection) *UNCINARIASIS (Hookworm Infection—both Necator americanus and Ancylostoma Duodenale) *TRICHURIASIS (Whipworm Infection)	2 doses per day for 2 successive days.	A single dose of 20 mg/lb or 50 mg/kg may be employed as an alternative schedule, but a higher incidence of side effects should be expected.
II. CUTANEOUS LARVA MIGRANS (Creeping Eruption)	2 doses per day for 2 successive days.	If active lesions are still present 2 days after completion of therapy, a second course is recommended.
III.* TRICHINOSIS	2 doses per day for 2–4 successive days according to the response of the patient.	The optimal dosage for the treatment of trichinosis has not been established.

*Clinical experience with thiabendazole for treatment of each of these conditions in children weighing less than 30 lbs has been limited.

MODURETIC® Tablets ℞
(amiloride HCl-hydrochlorothiazide, MSD)

Description

MODURETIC® (Amiloride HCl-Hydrochlorothiazide, MSD) combines the potassium-conserving action of amiloride HCl with the natriuretic action of hydrochlorothiazide. Each tablet contains 5 mg of amiloride HCl and 50 mg of hydrochlorothiazide.
Amiloride HCl is 3,5-diamino-6-chloro-*N*-(diaminomethylene)pyrazine-carboxamide monohydrochloride. Its empirical formula is $C_6H_8ClN_7O \cdot HCl$.
Hydrochlorothiazide is 6-chloro-3,4-dihydro-2*H*-1,2,4-benzothiadiazine-7-sulfonamide 1, 1-dioxide. Its empirical formula is $C_7H_8Cl N_3O_4S_2$.
MODURETIC is available for oral use as tablets containing 5 mg of amiloride HCl and 50 mg of hydrochlorothiazide.

Clinical Pharmacology

MODURETIC provides diuretic and antihypertensive activity (principally due to the hydrochlorothiazide component), while acting through the amiloride component to prevent the excessive potassium loss that may occur in patients receiving a thiazide diuretic. The onset of the diuretic action of MODURETIC is within 1 to 2 hours and this action appears to be sustained for approximately 24 hours.

Amiloride HCl
Amiloride HCl is a potassium-conserving (antikaliuretic) drug that possesses weak (compared with thiazide diuretics) natriuretic, diuretic, and antihypertensive activity. These effects have been partially additive to the effects of thiazide diuretics in some clinical studies. Amiloride HCl has potassium-conserving activity in patients receiving kaliuretic-diuretic agents.
Amiloride HCl is not an aldosterone antagonist and its effects are seen even in the absence of aldosterone.
Amiloride HCl usually begins to act within 2 hours after an oral dose. Its effect on electrolyte excretion reaches a peak between 6 and 10 hours and lasts about 24 hours. Peak plasma levels are obtained in 3 to 4 hours and the plasma half-life varies from 6 to 9 hours. Effects on electrolytes increase with single doses of amiloride HCl up to approximately 15 mg.
Amiloride HCl is not metabolized by the liver but is excreted unchanged by the kidneys. About 50 percent of a 20 mg dose of amiloride HCl is excreted in the urine and 40 percent in the stool within 72 hours. Amiloride HCl has little effect on glomerular filtration rate or renal blood flow. Because amiloride HCl is not metabolized by the liver, drug accumulation is not anticipated in patients with hepatic dysfunction, but accumulation can occur if the hepatorenal syndrome develops.

Hydrochlorothiazide
Hydrochlorothiazide is a diuretic and antihypertensive agent. It affects the renal tubular mechanism of electrolyte reabsorption.
Hydrochlorothiazide increases excretion of sodium and chloride in approximately equivalent amounts. Natriuresis may be accompanied by some loss of potassium and bicarbonate.
The onset of the diuretic action of hydrochlorothiazide occurs in 2 hours and the peak action in about 4 hours. Diuretic activity lasts about 6 to 12 hours. Hydrochlorothiazide is eliminated rapidly by the kidney.
The mechanism of the antihypertensive effect of thiazides may be related to the excretion and redistribution of body sodium. Hydrochlorothiazide usually does not cause clinically important changes in normal blood pressure.

Indications and Usage

MODURETIC is indicated in those patients with hypertension or with congestive heart failure who develop hypokalemia when thiazides or other kaliuretic diuretics are used alone, or in whom maintenance of normal serum potassium levels is considered to be clinically important, e.g., digitalized patients, or patients with significant cardiac arrhythmias.
The use of potassium conserving agents is often unnecessary in patients receiving diuretics for uncomplicated essential hypertension when such patients have a normal diet.
MODURETIC may be used alone or as an adjunct to other antihypertensive drugs, such as

Continued on next page

Information on the Merck Sharp & Dohme products listed on these pages is the full prescribing information from package circulars in use October 31, 1982.

Merck Sharp & Dohme—Cont.

methyldopa or beta blockers. Since MODURETIC enhances the action of these agents, dosage adjustments may be necessary to avoid an excessive fall in blood pressure and other unwanted side effects.

This fixed combination drug is not indicated for initial therapy of edema or hypertension. If the fixed combination represents the dose titrated to an individual patient's needs, it may be more convenient than the separate components.

Contraindications

Hyperkalemia
MODURETIC should not be used in the presence of elevated serum potassium levels (greater than 5.5 mEq per liter).

Antikaliuretic Therapy or Potassium Supplementation
MODURETIC should not be given to patients receiving other potassium-conserving agents, such as spironolactone or triamterene. Potassium supplementation in the form of medication or a potassium-rich diet should not be used with MODURETIC except in severe and/or refractory cases of hypokalemia. Such concomitant therapy can be associated with rapid increases in serum potassium levels. If potassium supplementation is used, careful monitoring of the serum potassium level is necessary.

Impaired Renal Function
Anuria, acute or chronic renal insufficiency, and evidence of diabetic nephropathy are contraindications to the use of MODURETIC. Patients with evidence of renal functional impairment (blood urea nitrogen [BUN] levels over 30 mg per 100 ml or serum creatinine levels over 1.5 mg per 100 ml) or diabetes mellitus should not receive the drug without careful, frequent and continuing monitoring of serum electrolytes, creatinine, and BUN levels. Potassium retention associated with the use of an antikaliuretic agent is accentuated in the presence of renal impairment and may result in the rapid development of hyperkalemia.

Hypersensitivity
MODURETIC is contraindicated in patients who are hypersensitive to this product, or to other sulfonamide-derived drugs.

Warnings

Hyperkalemia

> Like other potassium-conserving diuretic combinations, MODURETIC may cause hyperkalemia (serum potassium levels greater than 5.5 mEq per liter). In patients without renal impairment or diabetes mellitus, the risk of hyperkalemia with MODURETIC is about 1-2%. This risk is higher in patients with renal impairment or diabetes mellitus (even without recognized diabetic nephropathy). Since hyperkalemia, if uncorrected, is potentially fatal, it is essential to monitor serum potassium levels carefully in any patient receiving MODURETIC, particularly when it is first introduced, at the time of dosage adjustments, and during any illness that could affect renal function.

Warning signs or symptoms of hyperkalemia include paresthesias, muscular weakness, fatigue, flaccid paralysis of the extremities, bradycardia, shock, and ECG abnormalities. Monitoring of the serum potassium level is essential because mild hyperkalemia is not usually associated with an abnormal ECG.
When abnormal, the ECG in hyperkalemia is characterized primarily by tall, peaked T waves or elevations from previous tracings. There may also be lowering of the R wave and increased depth of the S wave, widening and even disappearance of the P wave, progressive widening of the QRS complex, prolongation of the PR interval, and ST depression.

Treatment of hyperkalemia: If hyperkalemia occurs in patients taking MODURETIC, the drug should be discontinued immediately. If the serum potassium level exceeds 6.5 mEq per liter, active measures should be taken to reduce it. Such measures include the intravenous administration of sodium bicarbonate solution or oral or parenteral glucose with a rapid-acting insulin preparation. If needed, a cation exchange resin such as sodium polystyrene sulfonate may be given orally or by enema. Patients with persistent hyperkalemia may require dialysis.

Diabetes Mellitus
In diabetic patients, hyperkalemia has been reported with the use of all potassium-conserving diuretics, including amiloride HCl, even in patients without evidence of diabetic nephropathy. Therefore, MODURETIC should be avoided, if possible, in diabetic patients and, if it is used, serum electrolytes and renal function must be monitored frequently.
MODURETIC should be discontinued at least 3 days before glucose tolerance testing.

Metabolic or Respiratory Acidosis
Antikaliuretic therapy should be instituted only with caution in severely ill patients in whom respiratory or metabolic acidosis may occur, such as patients with cardiopulmonary disease or poorly controlled diabetes. If MODURETIC is given to these patients, frequent monitoring of acid-base balance is necessary. Shifts in acid-base balance alter the ratio of extracellular/intracellular potassium, and the development of acidosis may be associated with rapid increases in serum potassium levels.

Precautions

General

Electrolyte Imbalance and BUN Increases
Determination of serum electrolytes to detect possible electrolyte imbalance should be performed at appropriate intervals.
Patients should be observed for clinical signs of fluid or electrolyte imbalance: i.e., hyponatremia, hypochloremic alkalosis, and hypokalemia. Serum and urine electrolyte determinations are particularly important when the patient is vomiting excessively or receiving parenteral fluids. Warning signs or symptoms of fluid and electrolyte imbalance include dryness of mouth, thirst, weakness, lethargy, drowsiness, restlessness, muscle pains or cramps, muscular fatigue, hypotension, oliguria, tachycardia, and gastrointestinal disturbances such as nausea and vomiting.
Hyponatremia and hypochloremia may occur during the use of thiazides and other diuretics. Any chloride deficit during thiazide therapy is generally mild and may be lessened by the amiloride HCl component of MODURETIC. Hypochloremia usually does not require specific treatment except under extraordinary circumstances (as in liver disease or renal disease). Dilutional hyponatremia may occur in edematous patients in hot weather; appropriate therapy is water restriction, rather than administration of salt, except in rare instances when the hyponatremia is life threatening. In actual salt depletion, appropriate replacement is the therapy of choice.
Hypokalemia may develop during thiazide therapy, especially with brisk diuresis, when severe cirrhosis is present, during concomitant use of corticosteroids or ACTH, or after prolonged therapy. However, this usually is prevented by the amiloride HCl component of MODURETIC.
Interference with adequate oral electrolyte intake will also contribute to hypokalemia. Hypokalemia can sensitize or exaggerate the response of the heart to the toxic effects of digitalis (e.g., increased ventricular irritability).
Increases in BUN levels have been reported with amiloride HCl and with hydrochlorothiazide. These increases usually have accompanied vigorous fluid elimination, especially when diuretic therapy was used in seriously ill patients, such as those who had hepatic cirrhosis with ascites and metabolic alkalosis, or those with resistant edema. Therefore, when MODURETIC is given to such patients, careful monitoring of serum electrolyte and BUN levels is important. In patients with pre-existing severe liver disease, hepatic encephalopathy, manifested by tremors, confusion, and coma, and increased jaundice, have been reported in association with diuretic therapy including amiloride HCl and hydrochlorothiazide.
In patients with renal disease, diuretics may precipitate azotemia. Cumulative effects of the components of MODURETIC may develop in patients with impaired renal function. If renal impairment becomes evident, MODURETIC should be discontinued (see CONTRAINDICATIONS and WARNINGS).

Drug Interactions
Thiazides may add to or potentiate the action of other antihypertensive drugs.
Thiazides may increase the responsiveness to tubocurarine.
Lithium generally should not be given with diuretics because they reduce its renal clearance and add a high risk of lithium toxicity. Read circulars for lithium preparations before use of such concomitant therapy.

Metabolic and Endocrine Effects
Thiazides may decrease serum PBI levels without signs of thyroid disturbance.
In diabetic patients, insulin requirements may be increased, decreased, or unchanged due to the hydrochlorothiazide component. Diabetes mellitus that has been latent may become manifest during administration of thiazide diuretics.
Because calcium excretion is decreased by thiazides, MODURETIC should be discontinued before carrying out tests for parathyroid function. Pathologic changes in the parathyroid glands, with hypercalcemia and hypophosphatemia have been observed in a few patients on prolonged thiazide therapy; however, the common complications of hyperparathyroidism such as renal lithiasis, bone resorption, and peptic ulceration have not been seen.
Hyperuricemia may occur or acute gout may be precipitated in certain patients receiving thiazide therapy.

Other Precautions
In patients receiving thiazides, sensitivity reactions may occur with or without a history of allergy or bronchial asthma. The possibility of exacerbation or activation of systemic lupus erythematosus has been reported with the use of thiazides.

Carcinogenicity, Mutagenicity
There was no evidence of a tumorigenic effect when amiloride HCl was administered for 92 weeks to mice at doses up to 10 mg/kg/day (25 times the maximum daily human dose). Amiloride HCl has also been administered for 104 weeks to male and female rats at doses up to 6 and 8 mg/kg/day (15 and 20 times the maximum daily dose for humans, respectively) and showed no evidence of carcinogenicity.
Amiloride HCl was devoid of mutagenic activity in various strains of *Salmonella typhimurium* with or without a mammalian liver microsomal activation system (Ames test).

Pregnancy

Pregnancy Category B
Teratologic studies have been performed with combinations of amiloride HCl and hydrochlorothiazide in rabbits and mice at doses up to 25 times the expected maximum daily dose for humans and have revealed no evidence of harm to the fetus. No evidence of impaired fertility in rats was apparent at dosage levels up to 25 times the expected maximum human daily dose. A perinatal and postnatal study in rats showed a reduction in maternal body weight gain during and after gestation at a daily dose of 25 times the expected maximum

daily dose for humans. The body weights of alive pups at birth and at weaning were also reduced at this dose level. There are no adequate and well controlled studies in pregnant women. Because animal reproduction studies are not always predictive of human responses, use of this drug in pregnant women or in women of childbearing potential requires that the anticipated benefits be weighed against possible hazards.

Amiloride HCl

Teratologic studies with amiloride HCl in rabbits and mice given 20 and 25 times the maximum human dose, respectively, revealed no evidence of harm to the fetus, although studies showed that the drug crossed the placenta in modest amounts. Reproduction studies in rats at 20 times the expected maximum daily dose for humans showed no evidence of impaired fertility. At approximately 5 or more times the expected maximum daily dose for humans, some toxicity was seen in adult rats and rabbits and a decrease in rat pup growth and survival occurred. There are, however, no adequate and well-controlled studies in pregnant women. Because animal reproduction studies are not always predictive of human response, this drug should be used during pregnancy only if clearly needed.

Hydrochlorothiazide

Thiazides cross the placental barrier and appear in cord blood. The use of thiazides in pregnancy requires that the anticipated benefit be weighed against possible hazards to the fetus. These hazards include fetal or neonatal jaundice, thrombocytopenia, and possibly other adverse reactions which have occurred in the adult.

Nursing Mothers

Studies in rats have shown that amiloride is excreted in milk in concentrations higher than that found in blood, but it is not known whether amiloride HCl is excreted in human milk. However, thiazides appear in breast milk. Because of the potential for serious adverse reactions in nursing infants, if the use of MODURETIC is deemed essential, the patient should stop nursing.

Pediatric Use

Safety and effectiveness in children have not been established.

Adverse Reactions

MODURETIC is usually well tolerated and significant clinical adverse effects have been reported infrequently. The risk of hyperkalemia (serum potassium levels greater than 5.5 mEq per liter) with MODURETIC is about 1–2% in patients without renal impairment or diabetes mellitus (see WARNINGS). Minor adverse reactions to amiloride HCl have been reported relatively frequently (about 20%) but the relationship of many of the reports to amiloride HCl is uncertain and the overall frequency was similar in hydrochlorothiazide treated groups. Nausea/anorexia, abdominal pain, flatulence, and mild skin rash have been reported and probably are related to amiloride. Other adverse experiences that have been reported with MODURETIC are generally those known to be associated with diuresis, thiazide therapy, or with the underlying disease being treated. Clinical trials have not demonstrated that combining amiloride and hydrochlorothiazide increases the risk of adverse reactions over those seen with the individual components. The clinical adverse reactions listed in the following table have been arranged into two groups: 1) incidence greater than 1%; and 2) incidence equal to or less than 1%. The incidence was obtained from clinical studies conducted in the United States (607 patients treated with MODURETIC).

Incidence > 1%	*Incidence ≤ 1%*
Body as a Whole	
Headache*	Malaise
Weakness*	Chest pain
Fatigue/tiredness	Back pain
Cardiovascular	
Arrhythmia	Tachycardia
	Digitalis toxicity
	Orthostatic hypotension
	Angina pectoris
Digestive	
Nausea/anorexia*	Constipation
Diarrhea	GI bleeding
Gastrointestinal pain	GI disturbance
Abdominal pain	Appetite changes
	Abdominal fullness
	Hiccups
	Thirst
	Vomiting
	Anorexia
	Flatulence
Metabolic	
Elevated serum potassium levels (> 5.5 mEq per liter)†	Gout
	Dehydration
Integumentary	
Rash*	Flushing
Pruritus	
Musculoskeletal	
Leg ache	Muscle cramps/spasm
	Joint pain
Nervous	
Dizziness*	Paresthesia/numbness
	Stupor
	Vertigo
Psychiatric	
None	Insomnia
	Nervousness
	Depression
	Sleepiness
	Mental confusion
Respiratory	
Dyspnea	None
Special Senses	
None	Bad taste
	Visual disturbance
	Nasal congestion
Urogenital	
None	Impotence
	Nocturia
	Dysuria
	Incontinence

Other adverse reactions that have been reported with the individual components are listed below:

Amiloride

Digestive
- Abnormal liver function
- Activation of probable pre-existing peptic ulcer

Metabolic
- Elevated serum potassium levels (> 5.5 mEq per liter)

Integumentary
- Dry mouth

Hematologic
- Aplastic anemia
- Neutropenia

Hydrochlorothiazide

Body as a Whole
- Anaphylactic reactions
- Fever

Cardiovascular
- Necrotizing angiitis (vasculitis, cutaneous vasculitis)

Digestive
- Cramping
- Gastric irritation
- Jaundice (intrahepatic cholestatic jaundice)
- Pancreatitis

Endocrine/Metabolic
- Glycosuria
- Hyperglycemia
- Hyperuricemia

Integumentary
- Photosensitivity
- Sialadenitis
- Urticaria

Psychiatric
- Restlessness

Respiratory
- Respiratory distress including pneumonitis

Special Senses
- Transient blurred vision
- Xanthopsia

Hematologic
- Agranulocytosis
- Aplastic anemia
- Hemolytic anemia
- Leukopenia
- Purpura
- Thrombocytopenia

* Reactions occurring in 3% to 8% of patients treated with MODURETIC. (Those reactions occurring in less than 3% of the patients are unmarked.)

† See WARNINGS.

Overdosage

No data are available in regard to overdosage in humans. The oral LD_{50} of the combination drug is 189 and 422 mg/kg for female mice and female rats, respectively.

It is not known whether the drug is dialyzable. No specific information is available on the treatment of overdosage with MODURETIC, and no specific antidote is available. Treatment is symptomatic and supportive. Therapy with MODURETIC should be discontinued and the patient observed closely. Suggested measures include induction of emesis and/or gastric lavage.

Amiloride HCl

No data are available in regard to overdosage in humans.

The oral LD_{50} of amiloride hydrochloride (calculated as the base) is 56 mg/kg in mice and 36 to 85 mg/kg in rats, depending on the strain. The most common signs and symptoms to be expected with overdosage are dehydration and electrolyte imbalance. If hyperkalemia occurs, active measures should be taken to reduce the serum potassium levels.

Hydrochlorothiazide

The oral LD_{50} of hydrochlorothiazide is greater than 10.0 g/kg in both mice and rats.

The most common signs and symptoms observed are those caused by electrolyte depletion (hypokalemia, hypochloremia, hyponatremia) and dehydration resulting from excessive diuresis. If digitalis has also been administered, hypokalemia may accentuate cardiac arrhythmias.

Dosage and Administration

MODURETIC should be administered with food.

The usual starting dosage is 1 tablet a day. The dosage may be increased to 2 tablets a day, if necessary. More than 2 tablets of MODURETIC daily usually are not needed and there is no controlled experience with such doses. The daily dose is usually given as a single dose but may be given in divided doses. Once an initial diuresis has been achieved, dosage adjustment may be necessary. Maintenance therapy may be on an intermittent basis.

Information on the Merck Sharp & Dohme products listed on these pages is the full prescribing information from package circulars in use October 31, 1982.

Continued on next page

Merck Sharp & Dohme—Cont.

How Supplied

No. 3385—Tablets MODURETIC are peach-colored, diamond-shaped, compressed tablets, coded MSD 917. Each tablet contains 5 mg of amiloride HCl and 50 mg of hydrochlorothiazide. They are supplied as follows:
NDC 0006-0917-68 in bottles of 100
NDC 0006-0917-28 single unit packages of 100.
[*Shown in Product Identification Section*]
A.H.F.S. Category: 40:28
DC 7130504 Issued October 1981
COPYRIGHT © MERCK & CO., INC., 1978
All rights reserved

MUMPSVAX® ℞
(mumps virus vaccine, live, MSD), U.S.P.
Jeryl Lynn Strain

Usually, mumps is a mild disease. However, it may occasionally be severe and produce serious complications. For example, meningoencephalitis has been estimated to occur in about 10 percent of patients, and unilateral orchitis in about 20 to 30 percent of postpubertal males. Post-infectious encephalitis, oophoritis, pancreatitis, muscular weakness, myelitis, myocarditis, facial neuritis, arthritis, hepatitis, and deafness may also occur. The relationship of endocardial fibroelastosis in infants, and mumps in the mother during pregnancy, has not been conclusively established.
Studies in susceptible children and adults have assessed the safety and efficacy of MUMPSVAX® (Mumps Virus Vaccine, Live, MSD). A single dose induced an effective antibody response in approximately 97 percent of susceptible children and approximately 93 percent of susceptible adults. There were few reports of soreness at the site of injection during clinical studies. There was no significant difference in the incidence of fever in clinical trials when children vaccinated with mumps vaccine were compared with unvaccinated subjects studied concurrently. In studies which included more than 200 susceptible male adults inoculated with mumps vaccine, no significant clinical side effects were reported. (See ADVERSE REACTIONS.)
No reports have been received of transmission of mumps from vaccinees to susceptible contacts.
Adequate antibody levels, with continuing protection of vaccinated children exposed to mumps, have persisted for ten years without substantial decline. The pattern of antibody closely resembles that observed for natural mumps although the antibody level is significantly lower than that following the natural infection. If this pattern continues it will provide a basis for expectation that immunity following the vaccine will be permanent. However, continued surveillance will be required to demonstrate this point.

Preparation

This vaccine is prepared from the Jeryl Lynn (B level) strain, named after the patient from whom the virus was initially recovered.
MUMPSVAX is grown in cell cultures of chick embryos, free of Avian leukosis, according to the general procedures used to prepare Enders' measles virus vaccine, live, attenuated. The vaccine is tested for safety and efficacy.

Indications

MUMPSVAX induces protective antibodies in essentially all non-immune recipients, provides protection against natural mumps in most cases, and has not been shown to cause significant systemic or local reactions. Evidence indicates that the mumps virus infection initiated by the vaccine is not contagious.
The vaccine is indicated for immunization against mumps in children 12 months of age or older, and adults. It is not recommended for infants younger than 12 months because they may retain maternal mumps neutralizing antibodies which may interfere with the immune response.
Evidence indicates that the vaccine will not offer protection when given after exposure to natural mumps. It has been reported that immune serum globulin (human) in a dosage of .01 to .02 ml/lb did not prevent the antibody response to the live vaccine when the two were administered simultaneously in opposite arms. However, protection afforded with this regimen has not been established.
Revaccination: Based on available evidence, there is no reason to routinely revaccinate children originally vaccinated when 12 months of age or older.
Use with Other Live Virus Vaccines
There are no data available concerning simultaneous use of MUMPSVAX with monovalent or trivalent poliovirus vaccine, live, oral, or with killed poliovirus vaccines. However, serologic evidence shows that when M-M-R® (Measles, Mumps and Rubella Virus Vaccine, Live, MSD), containing the HPV-77 rubella strain, is given simultaneously with trivalent oral poliovirus vaccine, live, oral, antibody responses can be expected to be comparable to those which follow administration of the vaccines at different times. From this it follows that when MUMPSVAX is given simultaneously with either monovalent or trivalent poliovirus vaccine, live, oral, ATTENUVAX® (Measles Virus Vaccine, Live, Attenuated, MSD) and/or MERUVAX®$_{II}$ (Rubella Virus Vaccine, Live, MSD), antibody responses can be expected to be comparable to those which follow administration of the vaccines at different times.

Contraindications

Hypersensitivity to neomycin (each dose of reconstituted vaccine contains approximately 25 micrograms of neomycin).
Individuals with blood dyscrasias, leukemia, lymphomas of any type, or other malignant neoplasms affecting the bone marrow or lymphatic systems.
Patients receiving therapy with ACTH, corticosteroids, irradiation, alkylating agents or antimetabolites.
This contraindication does not apply to patients who are receiving corticosteroids as replacement therapy, e.g., for Addison's disease.
Primary immuno-deficiency states, including cellular immune deficiencies, hypogammaglobulinemic and dysgammaglobulinemic states.
Any active infection is reason for delaying mumps vaccination.

Hypersensitivity to Eggs, Chicken, or Chicken Feathers

This vaccine is essentially devoid of potentially allergenic substances derived from host tissues (chick embryo)*. However, because the attenuated virus in this vaccine is propagated in cell cultures of chick embryo, there is a potential risk of hypersensitivity reactions in patients allergic to eggs, chicken, or chicken feathers. Widespread use of the vaccine for more than a decade has resulted in only rare, isolated reports of minor allergic reactions attributed to allergens of this kind, possibly related to the vaccine. Significantly, when children with known allergies to eggs, chicken, and chicken feathers were given a similarly prepared vaccine in a clinical study, none experienced reactions other than those reactions previously observed in non-allergic children.

*Morbidity and Mortality Weekly Report *25*(44): 350, Nov. 12, 1976.

Pregnancy

Do not give MUMPSVAX to pregnant females; the possible effects of the vaccine on fetal development are unknown at this time. When vaccination of post-pubertal females is undertaken, pregnancy at the time of vaccination must be ruled out and in addition, the possibility of pregnancy occurring in the three months following vaccination must be eliminated by medically acceptable methods.

Precautions

For subcutaneous use; *do not give intravenously.*
MUMPSVAX may be given simultaneously with monovalent or trivalent poliovirus vaccine, live, oral, with ATTENUVAX (Measles Virus Vaccine, Live, Attenuated, MSD) and/or MERUVAX$_{II}$ (Rubella Virus Vaccine, Live, MSD). MUMPSVAX should not be given less than one month before or after administration of other live virus vaccines.
Vaccination should be deferred for at least 3 months following blood or plasma transfusions, or administration of human immune serum globulin.
It has been reported that mumps virus vaccine, live, may result in a temporary depression of tuberculin skin sensitivity. Therefore, if a tuberculin test is to be done, it should be administered either before or simultaneously with MUMPSVAX.
Epinephrine should be available for immediate use if needed.

Adverse Reactions

Because of the slightly acidic pH (6.2–6.6) of the vaccine, patients may complain of burning and/or stinging of short duration at the injection site.
Mild fever occurs occasionally. Fever above 103°F (39.4°C) is uncommon.
Parotitis has been reported to occur in very low incidence, and orchitis rarely, in persons who were vaccinated. In most instances investigated, prior exposure to natural mumps was established. In other instances, whether or not this was due to vaccine or to prior natural mumps exposure or to other causes has not been established.
Reports of purpura and allergic reactions such as wheal and flare at the injection site or urticaria have been extremely rare.
Very rarely encephalitis and other nervous system reactions have occurred in vaccinees. A cause-effect relationship has not been established.

Shipment, Storage, and Reconstitution

During shipment, to insure that there is no loss of potency, the vaccine must be maintained at a temperature of 10°C (50°F) or less.
Prior to reconstitution, store the vaccine in a refrigerator at 2–8°C (35.6–46.4°F). *Protect from light.*
To reconstitute the vaccine, inject all the diluent in the syringe into the vial of lyophilized vaccine, and agitate to ensure thorough mixing. Draw back entire contents into the syringe and inject total volume of restored vaccine subcutaneously. Each dose of reconstituted vaccine contains not less than 5,000 $TCID_{50}$ (tissue culture infectious doses) of mumps virus vaccine expressed in terms of the assigned titer of the FDA Reference Mumps Virus.
Use only the diluent supplied and reconstitute the vaccine just before using. It is recommended that the vaccine be used as soon as possible after reconstitution. Protect the vaccine from light at all times. Store the reconstituted vaccine in a dark place at 2–8°C (35.6–46.4°F) and discard if not used within 8 hours.

Color: The color of the vaccine when reconstituted is yellow.

Dosage and Administration

After suitably cleansing the immunization site, inject total volume of reconstituted vaccine subcutaneously, preferably into the outer aspect of the upper arm. Do not inject intravenously.
The dosage of vaccine is the same for all patients. *Do not give immune serum globulin (ISG) concurrently with* MUMPSVAX.

How Supplied

No. 4582X—MUMPSVAX—a single-dose vial of lyophilized vaccine packed with a disposable syringe containing diluent, **NDC** 0006-4582-00. (6505-00-142-9203 Single dose).
No. 4584X/4590—MUMPSVAX—a box of 10 single dose vials of lyophilized vaccine, **NDC** 0006-4584-00; and a box of 10 diluent-containing disposable syringes with affixed 25 gauge, 5/8" needles supplied in an accompanying separate package. To conserve refrigerator space, the syringes may be stored at room temperature.

A.H.F.S. Category: 80:12
DC 7075402 Issued February 1981

MUSTARGEN®, Trituration of (mechlorethamine HCl for injection, MSD), U.S.P. ℞

Description

MUSTARGEN® (Mechlorethamine HCl, MSD) a nitrogen mustard also known as HN2 hydrochloride, is a nitrogen analog of sulfur mustard. It is a white, crystalline, hygroscopic powder that is very soluble in water and also soluble in alcohol.
Mechlorethamine hydrochloride is designated chemically as 2-chloro- *N*-(2-chloroethyl)- *N*-methylethanamine hydrochloride. The molecular weight is 192.52 and the melting point is 109–110°C. The empirical formula is $C_5H_{11}Cl_2N \cdot HCl$, and the structural formula is: $CH_3N(CH_2CH_2Cl)_2 \cdot HCl$.
Trituration of MUSTARGEN is a white crystalline powder. Each vial of MUSTARGEN contains 10 mg of mechlorethamine hydrochloride triturated with sodium chloride.

Actions

Mechlorethamine, a biologic alkylating agent, has a cytotoxic action which inhibits rapidly proliferating cells.

Indications

Before using MUSTARGEN *see Contraindications, Warnings, Precautions, Adverse Reactions, and Dosage and Administration.*
MUSTARGEN, administered intravenously, is indicated for the palliative treatment of Hodgkin's disease (Stages III and IV), lymphosarcoma, chronic myelocytic or chronic lymphocytic leukemia, polycythemia vera, mycosis fungoides, and bronchogenic carcinoma.
MUSTARGEN, administered intrapleurally, intraperitoneally, or intrapericardially, is indicated for the palliative treatment of metastatic carcinoma resulting in effusion.

Contraindications

Because of the toxicity of MUSTARGEN, and the unpleasant side effects following its use, the potential risk and discomfort from the use of this drug in patients with inoperable neoplasms or in the terminal stage of the disease must be balanced against the limited gain obtainable. These gains will vary with the nature and the status of the disease under treatment. The routine use of MUSTARGEN in all cases of widely disseminated neoplasms is to be discouraged.
The use of MUSTARGEN in patients with leukopenia, thrombocytopenia, and anemia, due to invasion of the bone marrow by tumor carries a greater risk. In such patients a good response to treatment with disappearance of the tumor from the bone marrow may be associated with improvement of bone marrow function. However, in the absence of a good response or in patients who have been previously treated with chemotherapeutic agents, hematopoiesis may be further compromised, and leukopenia, thrombocytopenia and anemia may become more severe and lead to the demise of the patient.
Tumors of bone and nervous tissue have responded poorly to therapy. Its use is contraindicated in the presence of known infectious diseases. Results are unpredictable in disseminated and malignant tumors of different types.

Warnings

Extravasation of the drug into subcutaneous tissues results in a painful inflammation. The area usually becomes indurated and sloughing may occur. If leakage of drug is obvious, prompt infiltration of the area with sterile isotonic sodium thiosulfate (1/6 molar) and application of an ice compress for 6 to 12 hours may minimize the local reaction. For a 1/6 molar solution of sodium thiosulfate, use 4.14 g of sodium thiosulfate per 100 ml of Sterile Water for Injection or 2.64 g of anhydrous sodium thiosulfate per 100 ml, or dilute 4 ml of Sodium Thiosulfate Injection U.S.P. (10%) with 6 ml of Sterile Water for Injection U.S.P.

Before using MUSTARGEN, *an accurate histologic diagnosis of the disease, a knowledge of its natural course, and an adequate clinical history are important. The hematologic status of the patient must first be determined. It is essential to understand the hazards and therapeutic effects to be expected. Careful clinical judgment must be exercised in selecting patients. If the indication for its use is not clear, the drug should not be used.*
As nitrogen mustard therapy may contribute to extensive and rapid development of amyloidosis, it should be used only if foci of acute and chronic suppurative inflammation are absent.
Usage in Pregnancy
There is evidence that the nitrogen mustards have induced fetal abnormalities particularly when used early in pregnancy. The possible benefits of administration of MUSTARGEN in women of childbearing potential must be weighed against the considered risks; patients should be apprised of the risks involved. In pregnant patients requiring treatment for a life-threatening progressive tumor, use of MUSTARGEN should be avoided at least until the third trimester.
Nursing Mothers
Although breast milk studies have not been performed in animals or humans, breast feeding should be stopped before beginning treatment with MUSTARGEN.

Precautions

This drug is highly toxic and both powder and solution must be handled and administered with care. Since MUSTARGEN is a powerful vesicant, it is intended primarily for intravenous use, and in most instances is given by this route. Inhalation of dust or vapors and contact with skin or mucous membranes, especially that of the eyes, must be avoided. Should accidental eye contact occur, copious irrigation with normal saline or a balanced salt ophthalmic irrigating solution should be instituted immediately, followed by prompt ophthalmologic consultation. Should accidental skin contact occur, the affected part must be irrigated immediately with copious amounts of water, for at least 15 minutes, followed by 2 percent sodium thiosulfate solution. (See also box warning.)
Do not use if the solution is discolored or if droplets of water are visible within the vial. Prepare fresh solution for injection and dispose of the unused portion after neutralization. (See DOSAGE AND ADMINISTRATION.)
Precautions must be observed with the use of MUSTARGEN and x-ray therapy or other chemotherapy in alternating courses. Hematopoietic function is characteristically depressed by either form of therapy, and neither MUSTARGEN following x-ray therapy nor x-ray therapy subsequent to the drug should be given until bone marrow function has recovered. In particular, irradiation of such areas as sternum, ribs, and vertebrae shortly after a course of nitrogen mustard may lead to hematologic complications.
Therapy with alkylating agents such as MUSTARGEN may be associated with an increased incidence of a second malignant tumor, especially when such therapy is combined with other antineoplastic agents or radiation therapy.
Hyperuricemia may develop during therapy with MUSTARGEN. The problem of urate precipitation should be anticipated, particularly in the treatment of the lymphomas, and adequate methods for control of hyperuricemia should be instituted and careful attention directed toward adequate fluid intake before treatment.
Since drug toxicity, especially sensitivity to bone marrow failure, seems to be more common in chronic lymphatic leukemia than in other conditions, the drug should be given in this condition with great caution, if at all.

Adverse Reactions

Clinical use of MUSTARGEN *usually is accompanied by toxic manifestations.*
Local Toxicity
Thrombosis and thrombophlebitis may result from direct contact of the drug with the intima of the injected vein. Avoid high concentration and prolonged contact with the drug, especially in cases of elevated pressure in the antebrachial vein (e.g., in mediastinal tumor compression from severe vena cava syndrome).
Systemic Toxicity
Nausea, vomiting and depression of formed elements in the circulating blood are dose-limiting side effects and usually occur with the use of full doses of MUSTARGEN. Jaundice, alopecia, vertigo, tinnitus and diminished hearing may occur infrequently. Rarely, hemolytic anemia associated with such diseases as the lymphomas and chronic lymphocytic leukemia may be precipitated by treatment with alkylating agents including MUSTARGEN. Also, various chromosomal abnormalities have been reported in association with nitrogen mustard therapy.
MUSTARGEN is given preferably at night in case sedation for side effects is required. Nausea and vomiting usually occur 1 to 3 hours after use of the drug. Emesis may disappear in the first 8 hours, but nausea may persist for 24 hours. Nausea and vomiting may be so severe as to precipitate vascular accidents in patients with a hemorrhagic tendency. Premedication with antiemetics, in addition to sedatives, may

Continued on next page

Information on the Merck Sharp & Dohme products listed on these pages is the full prescribing information from package circulars in use October 31, 1982.

Merck Sharp & Dohme—Cont.

help control severe nausea and vomiting. Anorexia, weakness and diarrhea may also occur. The usual course of MUSTARGEN (total dose of 0.4 mg/kg either given as a single intravenous dose or divided into two or four daily doses of 0.2 or 0.1 mg/kg respectively) generally produces a lymphocytopenia within 24 hours after the first injection; significant granulocytopenia occurs within 6 to 8 days and lasts for 10 days to 3 weeks. Agranulocytosis appears to be relatively infrequent and recovery from leukopenia in most cases is complete within two weeks of the maximum reduction. Thrombocytopenia is variable but the time course of the appearance and recovery from reduced platelet counts generally parallels the sequence of granulocyte levels. In some cases severe thrombocytopenia may lead to bleeding from the gums and gastrointestinal tract, petechiae, and small subcutaneous hemorrhages; these symptoms appear to be transient and in most cases disappear with return to a normal platelet count. However, a severe and even uncontrollable depression of the hematopoietic system occasionally may follow the usual dose of MUSTARGEN, particularly in patients with widespread disease and debility and in patients previously treated with other antineoplastic agents or x-ray. Persistent pancytopenia has been reported. In rare instances, hemorrhagic complications may be due to hyperheparinemia. Erythrocyte and hemoglobin levels may decline during the first 2 weeks after therapy but rarely significantly. Depression of the hematopoietic system may be found up to 50 days or more after starting therapy.

MUSTARGEN has been reported to have immunosuppressive activity. Therefore, it should be borne in mind that use of the drug may predispose the patient to bacterial, viral or fungal infection. This is more likely to occur when concomitant steroid therapy is employed.

Occasionally, a maculopapular skin eruption occurs, but this may be idiosyncratic and does not necessarily recur with subsequent courses of the drug. In one patient erythema multiforme has been observed. Herpes zoster, a common complicating infection in patients with lymphomas, may first appear after therapy is instituted and on occasion may be precipitated by treatment. Further treatment should be discontinued during the acute phase of this illness to avoid progression to generalized herpes zoster.

Since the gonads are susceptible to MUSTARGEN, treatment may be followed by delayed catamenia, oligomenorrhea, or temporary or permanent amenorrhea. Impaired spermatogenesis, azoospermia, and total germinal aplasia have been reported in male patients treated with alkylating agents, especially in combination with other drugs. In some instances spermatogenesis may return in patients in remission, but this may occur only several years after intensive chemotherapy has been discontinued. Patients should be warned of the potential risk to their reproductive capacity.

With total doses exceeding 0.4 mg/kg of body weight for a single course, severe leukopenia, anemia, thrombocytopenia and a hemorrhagic diathesis with subsequent delayed bleeding may develop. Death may follow. The only treatment in instances of excessive dosage appears to be repeated blood product transfusions, antibiotic treatment of complicating infections and general supportive measures. *Extreme caution must be used in exceeding the average recommended dose.*

Dosage and Administration

Intravenous Administration

The dosage of MUSTARGEN varies with the clinical situation, the therapeutic response and the magnitude of hematologic depression. A total dose of 0.4 mg/kg of body weight for each course usually is given either as a single dose or in divided doses of 0.1 to 0.2 mg/kg per day. Dosage should be based on ideal dry body weight. The presence of edema or ascites must be considered so that dosage will be based on actual weight unaugmented by these conditions.

Within a few minutes after intravenous injection, MUSTARGEN undergoes chemical transformation, combines with reactive compounds, and is no longer present in its active form in the blood stream. Subsequent courses should not be given until the patient has recovered hematologically from the previous course; this is best determined by repeated studies of the peripheral blood elements awaiting their return to normal levels. It is often possible to give repeated courses of MUSTARGEN as early as three weeks after treatment.

The margin of safety in therapy with MUSTARGEN *is narrow and considerable care must be exercised in the matter of dosage.* Repeated examinations of blood are *mandatory* as a guide to subsequent therapy.

Preparation of Solution and Intravenous Administration

Each vial of MUSTARGEN contains 10 mg of mechlorethamine hydrochloride triturated with sodium chloride q.s. 100 mg. In neutral or alkaline aqueous solution it undergoes rapid chemical transformation and is highly unstable. Although solutions prepared according to instructions are acidic and do not decompose as rapidly, they should be prepared immediately before each injection since they will decompose on standing.

Using a sterile 10 ml syringe, inject 10 ml of Sterile Water for Injection or 10 ml Sodium Chloride Injection into a vial of MUSTARGEN. With the needle still in the rubber stopper, shake the vial several times to dissolve the drug completely. The resultant solution contains 1 mg of mechlorethamine hydrochloride per ml.

Withdraw into the syringe the calculated volume of solution required for a single injection. *Dispose of any remaining solution after neutralization* (see below). Although the drug may be injected directly into any suitable vein, it is injected preferably into the rubber or plastic tubing of a flowing intravenous infusion set. This reduces the possibility of severe local reactions due to extravasation or high concentration of the drug. Injecting the drug into the tubing rather than adding it to the entire volume of the infusion fluid minimizes a chemical reaction between the drug and the solution. The rate of injection apparently is not critical provided it is completed within a few minutes.

Intracavitary Administration

Nitrogen mustard has been used by intracavitary administration with varying success in certain malignant conditions for the control of pleural, peritoneal, and pericardial effusions caused by malignant cells.

The technic and the dose used by any of these routes varies. Therefore, if MUSTARGEN is given by the intracavitary route, the published articles concerning such use should be consulted. *Because of the inherent risks involved, the physician should be experienced in the appropriate injection technics, and be thoroughly aware of the indications, dosages, hazards, and precautions as set forth in the published literature. When using* MUSTARGEN *by the intracavitary route, the general precautions concerning this agent should be borne in mind.*

As a general guide, reference is made especially to the technics of Weisberger et al. Intracavitary use is indicated in the presence of pleural, peritoneal, or pericardial effusion due to metastatic tumors. Local therapy with nitrogen mustard is used only when malignant cells are demonstrated in the effusion. Intracavitary injection is not recommended when the accumulated fluid is chylous in nature, since results are likely to be poor.

Paracentesis is first performed with most of the fluid being removed from the pleural or peritoneal cavity. The intracavitary use of MUSTARGEN may exert at least some of its effect through production of a chemical poudrage. Therefore, the removal of excess fluid allows the drug to more easily contact the peritoneal and pleural linings. For intrapleural or intrapericardial injection nitrogen mustard is introduced directly through the thoracentesis needle. For intraperitoneal injection it is given through a rubber catheter inserted into the trocar used for paracentesis or through a No. 18 gauge needle inserted at another site. This drug should be injected slowly, with frequent aspiration to ensure that a free flow of fluid is present. If fluid cannot be aspirated, pain and necrosis due to injection of solution outside the cavity may occur. Free flow of fluid also is necessary to prevent injection into a loculated pocket and to ensure adequate dissemination of nitrogen mustard.

The usual dose of nitrogen mustard for intracavitary injection is 0.4 mg/kg of body weight, though 0.2 mg/kg (or 10 to 20 mg) has been used by the intrapericardial route. The solution is prepared, as previously described for intravenous injection, by adding 10 ml of Sterile Water for Injection or 10 ml of Sodium Chloride Injection to the vial containing 10 mg of mechlorethamine hydrochloride. (Amounts of diluent of 50 to 100 ml of normal saline have also been used.) The position of the patient should be changed every 5 to 10 minutes for an hour after injection to obtain more uniform distribution of the drug throughout the serous cavity. The remaining fluid may be removed from the pleural or peritoneal cavity by paracentesis 24 to 36 hours later. The patient should be followed carefully by clinical and x-ray examination to detect reaccumulation of fluid.

Pain occurs rarely with intrapleural use; it is common with intraperitoneal injection and is often associated with nausea, vomiting, and diarrhea of 2 to 3 days duration. Transient cardiac irregularities may occur with intrapericardial injection. Death, possibly accelerated by nitrogen mustard, has been reported following the use of this agent by the intracavitary route. Although absorption of MUSTARGEN when given by the intracavitary route is probably not complete because of its rapid deactivation by body fluids, the systemic effect is unpredictable. The acute side effects such as nausea and vomiting are usually mild. Bone marrow depression is generally milder than when the drug is given intravenously. Care should be taken to avoid use by the intracavitary route when other agents which may suppress bone marrow function are being used systemically.

Neutralization of Equipment and Unused Solution

To clean rubber gloves, tubing, glassware, etc., after giving MUSTARGEN, soak them in an aqueous solution containing equal volumes of sodium thiosulfate (5%) and sodium bicarbonate (5%) for 45 minutes. Excess reagents and reaction products are washed away easily with water. Any unused injection solution should be neutralized by mixing with an equal volume of sodium thiosulfate/sodium bicarbonate solution. Allow the mixture to stand for 45 minutes. Vials that have contained MUSTARGEN should be treated in the same way with thiosulfate/bicarbonate solution before disposal.

How Supplied

No. 7753—Trituration of MUSTARGEN is a white crystalline powder, each vial containing 10 mg mechlorethamine hydrochloride with sodium chloride q.s. 100 mg, and is supplied as follows:

NDC 0006-7753-31 in treatment sets of 4 vials.

A.H.F.S. Category: 10:00

DC 6382423 Issued June 1979

MYOCHRYSINE® Injection ℞
(gold sodium thiomalate, MSD), U.S.P.

Physicians planning to use MYOCHRYSINE® (Gold Sodium Thiomalate, MSD) should thoroughly familiarize themselves with its toxicity and its benefits. The possibility of toxic reactions should always be explained to the patient before starting therapy. Patients should be warned to report promptly any symptoms suggesting toxicity. Before each injection of MYOCHRYSINE, *the physician should review the results of laboratory work, and see the patient to determine the presence or absence of adverse reactions since some of these can be severe or even fatal.*

Description

MYOCHRYSINE is a sterile aqueous solution of gold sodium thiomalate. It contains 0.5 percent benzyl alcohol added as a preservative. The pH of the product is 5.8–6.5.
Gold sodium thiomalate is a mixture of the mono- and di-sodium salts of gold thiomalic acid.
The molecular weight for $C_4H_3AuNa_2O_4S$ (the disodium salt) is 390.07 and for $C_4H_4AuNaO_4S$ (the monosodium salt) is 368.09.
MYOCHRYSINE is supplied as a solution for intramuscular injection containing 10 mg, 25 mg, 50 mg or 100 mg of gold sodium thiomalate per ml.

Clinical Pharmacology

The mode of action of gold sodium thiomalate is unknown. The predominant action appears to be a suppressive effect on the synovitis of active rheumatoid disease.

Indications and Usage

MYOCHRYSINE is indicated in the treatment of selected cases of active rheumatoid arthritis—both adult and juvenile type. The greatest benefit occurs in the early active stage. In late stages of the illness when cartilage and bone damage have occurred, gold can only check the progression of rheumatoid arthritis and prevent further structural damage to joints. It cannot repair damage caused by previously active disease.
MYOCHRYSINE should be used only as *one part* of a complete program of therapy; alone it is not a complete treatment.

Contraindications

Severe toxicity resulting from previous exposure to gold or other heavy metals.
Severe debilitation.
Systemic lupus erythematosus.

Warnings

Before treatment is started, the patient's hemoglobin, erythrocyte, white blood cell, differential and platelet counts should be determined, and urinalysis should be done to serve as basic reference. Urine should be analyzed for protein and sediment changes prior to each injection. Complete blood counts including platelet estimation should be made before every second injection throughout treatment. The occurrence of purpura or ecchymoses at any time always requires a platelet count.
Danger signals of possible gold toxicity include: rapid reduction of hemoglobin, leukopenia below 4000 WBC/cu ml, eosinophilia above 5 percent, platelet decrease below 100,000/cu ml, albuminuria, hematuria, pruritus, skin eruption, stomatitis, or persistent diarrhea. No additional injections of MYOCHRYSINE should be given unless further studies show these abnormalities to be caused by conditions other than gold toxicity.

Precautions

General
Gold salts should not be used concomitantly with penicillamine.
The safety of coadministration with cytotoxic drugs has not been established.
Caution is indicated in the use of MYOCHRYSINE in patients with the following:
1. a history of blood dyscrasias such as granulocytopenia or anemia caused by drug sensitivity,
2. allergy or hypersensitivity to medications,
3. skin rash,
4. previous kidney or liver disease,
5. marked hypertension,
6. compromised cerebral or cardiovascular circulation.

Diabetes mellitus or congestive heart failure should be under control before gold therapy is instituted.
Carcinogenicity
Renal adenomas have been reported in long-term toxicity studies of rats receiving MYOCHRYSINE at high dose levels (2 mg/kg weekly for 45 weeks, followed by 6 mg/kg daily for 47 weeks), approximately 2 to 42 times the usual human dose. These adenomas are histologically similar to those produced in rats by chronic administration of experimental gold compounds and other heavy metals, such as lead. No reports have been received of renal adenomas in man in association with the use of MYOCHRYSINE.
Pregnancy
Pregnancy Category C.
MYOCHRYSINE has been shown to be teratogenic during the organogenetic period in rats and rabbits when given in doses, respectively, of 140 and 175 times the usual human dose. Hydrocephaly and microphthalmia were the malformations observed in rats when MYOCHRYSINE was administered subcutaneously at a dose of 25 mg/kg/day from day 6 through day 15 of gestation. In rabbits, limb malformations and gastroschisis were the malformations observed when MYOCHRYSINE was administered subcutaneously at doses of 20–45 mg/kg/day from day 6 through day 18 of gestation.
There are no adequate and well-controlled studies in pregnant women. MYOCHRYSINE should be used during pregnancy only if the potential benefit to the mother justifies the potential risk to the fetus.
Nursing Mothers
The presence of gold has been demonstrated in the milk of lactating mothers. In addition, gold has been found in the serum and red blood cells of a nursing infant. In view of the above findings and because of the potential for serious adverse reactions in nursing infants from MYOCHRYSINE, a decision should be made whether to discontinue nursing or to discontinue the drug, taking into account the importance of the drug to the mother. The slow excretion and persistence of gold in the mother, even after therapy is discontinued, must also be kept in mind.

Adverse Reactions

A variety of adverse reactions may develop during the initial phase (weekly injections) of therapy or during maintenance treatment. Adverse reactions are observed most frequently when the cumulative dose of MYOCHRYSINE administered is between 400 and 800 mg. Very uncommonly, complications occur days to months after cessation of treatment.
Cutaneous reactions: Dermatitis is the most common reaction. *Any eruption, especially if pruritic, that develops during treatment with* MYOCHRYSINE *should be considered a reaction to gold until proven otherwise.* Pruritus often exists before dermatitis becomes apparent, and therefore should be considered a warning signal of impending cutaneous reaction. The most serious form of cutaneous reaction is generalized exfoliative dermatitis which may lead to alopecia and shedding of nails. Gold dermatitis may be aggravated by exposure to sunlight or an actinic rash may develop.
Mucous membrane reactions: Stomatitis is the second most common adverse reaction. Shallow ulcers on the buccal membranes, on the borders of the tongue, and on the palate or in the pharynx may occur as the only adverse reaction, or along with dermatitis. Sometimes diffuse glossitis or gingivitis develops. A metallic taste may precede these oral mucous membrane reactions and should be considered a warning signal.
Conjunctivitis is a rare reaction.
Renal reactions: Gold may be toxic to the kidney and produce a nephrotic syndrome or glomerulitis with hematuria. These renal reactions are usually relatively mild and subside completely if recognized early and treatment is discontinued. They may become severe and chronic if treatment is continued after onset of the reaction. Therefore, it is important to perform a *urinalysis before every injection,* and to discontinue treatment promptly if proteinuria or hematuria develops.
Hematologic reactions: Blood dyscrasia due to gold toxicity is rare, but because of the potential serious consequences it must be constantly watched for and recognized early by frequent blood examinations done throughout treatment. Granulocytopenia; thrombocytopenia, with or without purpura; hypoplastic and aplastic anemia have all been reported. These hematologic disorders may occur separately or in combinations.
Nitritoid and allergic reactions: Reactions of the "nitritoid type" which may resemble anaphylactoid effects have been reported. Flushing, fainting, dizziness and sweating are most frequently reported. Other symptoms that may occur include: nausea, vomiting, malaise and weakness.
More severe, but less common effects include: anaphylactic shock, syncope, bradycardia, thickening of the tongue, difficulty in swallowing and breathing, and angioneurotic edema. These effects may occur almost immediately after injection or as late as 10 minutes following injection. They may occur at any time during the course of therapy and if observed, treatment with MYOCHRYSINE should be discontinued.
Miscellaneous reactions: Gastrointestinal reactions have been reported, including nausea, vomiting, anorexia, abdominal cramps and diarrhea. Ulcerative enterocolitis, which can be severe or even fatal, has been reported rarely.
There have been rare reports of reactions involving the eye such as iritis, corneal ulcers, and gold deposits in ocular tissues.
Hepatitis with jaundice, peripheral neuritis, gold bronchitis, pulmonary injury manifested by interstitial pneumonitis and fibrosis, partial or complete hair loss and fever have also been reported.
Sometimes arthralgia occurs for a day or two after an injection of MYOCHRYSINE; this reaction usually subsides after the first few injections.

Management of Adverse Reactions

Continued on next page

Information on the Merck Sharp & Dohme products listed on these pages is the full prescribing information from package circulars in use October 31, 1982.

Merck Sharp & Dohme—Cont.

Treatment with MYOCHRYSINE should be discontinued immediately when toxic reactions occur. Minor complications such as localized dermatitis, mild stomatitis, or slight proteinuria generally require no other therapy and resolve spontaneously with suspension of MYOCHRYSINE. Moderately severe skin and mucous membrane reactions often benefit from topical corticosteroids, oral antihistaminics, and soothing or anesthetic lotions.
If stomatitis or dermatitis becomes severe or more generalized, systemic corticosteroids (generally, prednisone 10 to 40 mg daily in divided doses) may provide symptomatic relief.
For serious renal, hematologic, pulmonary, and enterocolitic complications, high doses of systemic corticosteroids (prednisone 40 to 100 mg daily in divided doses) are recommended. The optimum duration of corticosteroid treatment varies with the response of the individual patient. Therapy may be required for many months when adverse effects are unusually severe or progressive.
In patients whose complications do not improve with high-dose corticosteroid treatment, or who develop significant steroid-related adverse reactions, a chelating agent may be given to enhance gold excretion. Dimercaprol (BAL) has been used successfully, but patients must be monitored carefully as numerous untoward reactions may attend its use. Corticosteroids and a chelating agent may be used concomitantly.
MYOCHRYSINE *should not be reinstituted after severe or idiosyncratic reactions.*
MYOCHRYSINE may be readministered following resolution of mild reactions, using a reduced dosage schedule. If an initial test dose of 5 mg MYOCHRYSINE is well-tolerated, progressively larger doses (5 to 10 mg increments) may be given at weekly to monthly intervals until a dose of 25 to 50 mg is reached.

Dosage and Administration

MYOCHRYSINE should be administered only by intramuscular injection, preferably intragluteally. It should be given with the patient lying down. He should remain recumbent for approximately 10 minutes after the injection.
Therapeutic effects from MYOCHRYSINE occur slowly. Early improvement, often limited to a reduction in morning stiffness, may begin after six to eight weeks of treatment, but beneficial effects may not be observed until after months of therapy.
Parenteral drug products should be inspected visually for particulate matter and discoloration prior to administration. Do not use if material has darkened. Color should not exceed pale yellow.
For the adult of average size the following dosage schedule is suggested:

Weekly Injections
1st injection ....10 mg
2nd injection ....25 mg
3rd and subsequent injections .....25 to 50 mg

until there is toxicity or major clinical improvement, or, in the absence of either of these, the cumulative dose of MYOCHRYSINE reaches one gram.
MYOCHRYSINE is continued until the cumulative dose reaches one gram unless toxicity or major clinical improvement occurs. If significant clinical improvement occurs before a cumulative dose of one gram has been administered, the dose may be decreased or the interval between injections increased as with maintenance therapy. Maintenance doses of 25 to 50 mg every other week for two to 20 weeks are recommended. If the clinical course remains stable, injections of 25 to 50 mg may be given every third and subsequently every fourth week indefinitely. Some patients may require maintenance treatment at intervals of one to three weeks. Should the arthritis exacerbate during maintenance therapy, weekly injections may be resumed temporarily until disease activity is suppressed.
Should a patient fail to improve during initial therapy (cumulative dose of one gram), several options are available:

1—the patient may be considered to be unresponsive and MYOCHRYSINE is discontinued
2—the same dose (25 to 50 mg) of MYOCHRYSINE may be continued for approximately ten additional weeks
3—the dose of MYOCHRYSINE may be increased by increments of 10 mg every one to four weeks, not to exceed 100 mg in a single injection.

If significant clinical improvement occurs using option 2 or 3, the maintenance schedule described above should be initiated. If there is no significant improvement or if toxicity occurs, therapy with MYOCHRYSINE should be stopped. The higher the individual dose of MYOCHRYSINE, the greater the risk of gold toxicity. Selection of one of these options for chrysotherapy should be based upon a number of factors, including the physician's experience with gold salt therapy, the course of the patient's condition, the choice of alternative treatments, and the availability of the patient for the close supervision required.
Juvenile Rheumatoid Arthritis
The pediatric dose of MYOCHRYSINE is proportional to the adult dose on a weight basis. After the initial test dose of 10 mg, the recommended dose for children is one mg per kilogram body weight, not to exceed 50 mg for a single injection. Otherwise, the guidelines given above for administration to adults also apply to children.
Concomitant Drug Therapy—Gold salts should not be used concomitantly with penicillamine.
The safety of coadministration with cytotoxic drugs has not been established. Other measures, such as salicylates, other non-steroidal anti-inflammatory drugs, or systemic corticosteroids, may be continued when MYOCHRYSINE is initiated. After improvement commences, analgesic and anti-inflammatory drugs may be discontinued slowly as symptoms permit.

How Supplied

Injection MYOCHRYSINE is a clear colorless to light yellow solution, depending on potency, which must be protected from light. It is supplied as follows:
No. 7763—10 mg of gold sodium thiomalate per ml as
NDC 0006-7763-64 in boxes of 6 x 1 ml ampuls.
No. 7764—25 mg of gold sodium thiomalate per ml as
NDC 0006-7764-64 in boxes of 6 x 1 ml ampuls.
No. 7762—50 mg of gold sodium thiomalate per ml as
NDC 0006-7762-64 in boxes of 6 x 1 ml ampuls.
NDC 0006-7762-10 in 10 ml vials.
No. 7761—100 mg of gold sodium thiomalate per ml as
NDC 0006-7761-64 in boxes of 6 x 1 ml ampuls.

A.H.F.S. Category: 60:00
DC 6015520 Revised December 1980

NEODECADRON® Sterile Ophthalmic Ointment ℞
Neomycin sulfate-dexamethasone sodium phosphate ointment

Description

Sterile ophthalmic ointment NEODECADRON® is a topical corticosteroid-antibiotic ointment for use in certain disorders of the anterior segment of the eye.
Ophthalmic ointment NEODECADRON contains in each gram: dexamethasone sodium phosphate equivalent to 0.5 mg (0.05%) dexamethasone phosphate and neomycin sulfate equivalent to 3.5 mg neomycin base. Inactive ingredients: white petrolatum and mineral oil.
Dexamethasone sodium phosphate is an inorganic ester of dexamethasone. Its empirical formula is $C_{22}H_{28}FNa_2O_8P$.
Neomycin sulfate is the sulfate salt of neomycin, an antibacterial substance produced by the growth of *Streptomyces fradiae* Waksman (Fam. Streptomycetaceae).

Clinical Pharmacology

Dexamethasone sodium phosphate, a corticosteroid, suppresses the inflammatory response to a variety of agents, and it probably delays or slows healing. Since corticosteroids may inhibit the body's defense mechanism against infection, a concomitant antimicrobial drug may be used when this inhibition is considered to be clinically significant in a particular case.
Neomycin sulfate, the anti-infective component in the combination, is included to provide action against specific organisms susceptible to it. Neomycin sulfate is considered active mainly against gram-negative organisms, except *Bacteroides* spp. and *Pseudomonas aeruginosa*, which are resistant. Gram-positive organisms except for *Staphylococcus aureus* are usually resistant.
When a decision to administer both a corticosteroid and an antimicrobial is made, the administration of such drugs in combination has the advantage of greater patient compliance and convenience, with the added assurance that the appropriate dosage of both drugs is administered, plus assured compatibility of ingredient when both types of drug are in the same formulation and, particularly, that the correct volume of drug is delivered and retained.
The relative potency of corticosteroids depends on the molecular structure, concentration, and release from the vehicle.

Indications and Usage

For steroid-responsive inflammatory ocular conditions for which a corticosteroid is indicated and where bacterial infection or a risk of bacterial ocular infection exists.
Ocular steroids are indicated in inflammatory conditions of the palpebral and bulbar conjunctiva, cornea, and anterior segment of the globe where the inherent risk of steroid use in certain infective conjunctivitides is accepted to obtain a diminution in edema and inflammation. They are also indicated in chronic anterior uveitis and corneal injury from chemical, radiation, or thermal burns, or penetration of foreign bodies.
The use of a combination drug with an anti-infective component is indicated where the risk of infection is high or where there is an expectation that potentially dangerous numbers of bacteria will be present in the eye.
The particular anti-infective drug in this product is active against the following common bacterial eye pathogens:

Staphylococcus aureus
Escherichia coli
Haemophilus influenzae
Klebsiella/Enterobacter species
Neisseria species

The product does not provide adequate coverage against:

Pseudomonas aeruginosa
Serratia marcescens
Streptococci, including *Streptococcus pneumoniae*

Contraindications

Epithelial herpes simplex keratitis (dendritic keratitis), acute infectious stages of vaccinia, varicella, and many other viral diseases of the

cornea and conjunctiva. Mycobacterial infection of the eye. Fungal diseases of ocular structures. Hypersensitivity to a component of the medication (hypersensitivity to the antibiotic component occurs at a higher rate than for other components).
The use of these combinations is always contraindicated after uncomplicated removal of a corneal foreign body.

Warnings

Prolonged use may result in glaucoma, with damage to the optic nerve, defects in visual acuity and fields of vision, and posterior subcapsular cataract formation. Prolonged use may suppress the host response and thus increase the hazard of secondary ocular infections. In those diseases causing thinning of the cornea or sclera, perforations have been known to occur with the use of topical corticosteroids. In acute purulent conditions of the eye, corticosteroids may mask infection or enhance existing infection. If these products are used for 10 days or longer, intraocular pressure should be routinely monitored even though it may be difficult in children and uncooperative patients.
Employment of corticosteroid medication in the treatment of herpes simplex requires great caution: periodic slit-lamp microscopy is recommended.
Any substance (e.g. neomycin sulfate) may occasionally cause cutaneous sensitization. If any reaction indicating such sensitivity is observed, discontinue use.

Precautions

The initial prescriptions and renewal of the medication order beyond 8 grams should be made by a physician only after examination of the patient with the aid of magnification, such as slit lamp biomicroscopy and, where appropriate, fluorescein staining.
The possibility of persistent fungal infections of the cornea should be considered after prolonged corticosteroid dosing.
Usage in Pregnancy
Safety of intensive or protracted use of topical corticosteroids during pregnancy has not been substantiated.

Adverse Reactions

Adverse reactions have occurred with corticosteroid/anti-infective combination drugs which can be attributed to the corticosteroid component, the anti-infective component, or the combination. Exact incidence figures are not available since no denominator of treated patients is available.
Reactions occurring most often from the presence of the anti-infective ingredient are allergic sensitizations. The reactions due to the corticosteroid component in decreasing order of frequency are: elevation of intraocular pressure (IOP) with possible development of glaucoma, and infrequent optic nerve damage; posterior subcapsular cataract formation; and delayed wound healing.
Secondary Infection: The development of secondary infection has occurred after use of combinations containing corticosteroids and antimicrobials. Fungal infections of the cornea are particularly prone to develop coincidentally with long-term applications of corticosteroid. The possibility of fungal invasion must be considered in any persistent corneal ulceration where corticosteroid treatment has been used. Secondary bacterial ocular infection following suppression of host responses also occurs.

Dosage and Administration

The duration of treatment will vary with the type of lesion and may extend from a few days to several weeks, according to therapeutic response. Relapses, more common in chronic active lesions than in self-limited conditions, usually respond to retreatment.
Apply a thin coating of ophthalmic ointment NEODECADRON three or four times a day. When a favorable response is observed, reduce the number of daily applications to two, and later to one a day as maintenance dose if this is sufficient to control symptoms.
Not more than 8 grams should be prescribed initially and the prescription should not be refilled without further evaluation as outlined in PRECAUTIONS above.
Ophthalmic ointment NEODECADRON is particularly convenient when an eye pad is used. It may also be the preparation of choice for patients in whom therapeutic benefit depends on prolonged contact of the active ingredients with ocular tissues.

How Supplied

No. 7617—Sterile Ophthalmic Ointment NEODECADRON is a clear, unctuous ointment, and is supplied as follows:
NDC 0006-7617-04 in 3.5 g tubes
(6505-00-823-7956 0.05% 3.5 g)
A.H.F.S. Category: 52:08
DC 6167721 Issued June 1982

NEODECADRON® Sterile ℞
Ophthalmic Solution
Neomycin sulfate-dexamethasone sodium phosphate ophthalmic solution

Description

Ophthalmic solution NEODECADRON® is a topical corticosteroid-antibiotic solution for use in certain disorders of the anterior segment of the eye.
Each milliliter of buffered ophthalmic solution NEODECADRON contains: dexamethasone sodium phosphate equivalent to 1 mg (0.1%) dexamethasone phosphate, and neomycin sulfate equivalent to 3.5 mg neomycin base. Inactive ingredients: creatinine, sodium citrate, sodium borate, polysorbate 80, sodium hydroxide to adjust pH to 6.6–7.8, and water for injection. Benzalkonium chloride 0.02% and sodium bisulfite 0.32% added as preservatives.
Each milliliter of buffered ophthalmic solution NEODECADRON in the OCUMETER® ophthalmic dispenser contains: dexamethasone sodium phosphate equivalent to 1 mg (0.1%) dexamethasone phosphate, and neomycin sulfate equivalent to 3.5 mg neomycin base. Inactive ingredients: creatinine, sodium citrate, sodium borate, polysorbate 80, disodium edetate, hydrochloric acid to adjust pH to 6.6–7.8, and water for injection. Benzalkonium chloride 0.02% and sodium bisulfite 0.1% added as preservatives.
Dexamethasone sodium phosphate is a water soluble, inorganic ester of dexamethasone. Its empirical formula is $C_{22}H_{28}FNa_2O_8P$. It is approximately three thousand times more soluble in water at 25°C than hydrocortisone.
Neomycin sulfate is the sulfate salt of neomycin, an antibacterial substance produced by the growth of *Streptomyces fradiae* Waksman (Fam. Streptomycetaceae).

Clinical Pharmacology

Dexamethasone sodium phosphate, a corticosteroid, suppresses the inflammatory response to a variety of agents, and it probably delays or slows healing. Since corticosteroids may inhibit the body's defense mechanism against infection, a concomitant antimicrobial drug may be used when this inhibition is considered to be clinically significant in a particular case.
Neomycin sulfate, the anti-infective component in the combination, is included to provide action against specific organisms susceptible to it. Neomycin sulfate is considered active mainly against gram-negative organisms, except *Bacteroides* spp. and *Pseudomonas aeruginosa,* which are resistant. Gram-positive organisms except for *Staphylococcus aureus* are usually resistant.
When a decision to administer both a corticosteroid and an antimicrobial is made, the administration of such drugs in combination has the advantage of greater patient compliance and convenience, with the added assurance that the appropriate dosage of both drugs is administered, plus assured compatibility of ingredients when both types of drug are in the same formulation and, particularly, that the correct volume of drug is delivered and retained.
The relative potency of corticosteroids depends on the molecular structure, concentration, and release from the vehicle.

Indications and Usage

For steroid-responsive inflammatory ocular conditions for which a corticosteroid is indicated and where bacterial infection or a risk of bacterial ocular infection exists.
Ocular steroids are indicated in inflammatory conditions of the palpebral and bulbar conjunctiva, cornea, and anterior segment of the globe where the inherent risk of steroid use in certain infective conjunctivitides is accepted to obtain a diminution in edema and inflammation. They are also indicated in chronic anterior uveitis and corneal injury from chemical, radiation, or thermal burns, or penetration of foreign bodies.
The use of a combination drug with an anti-infective component is indicated where the risk of infection is high or where there is an expectation that potentially dangerous numbers of bacteria will be present in the eye.
The particular anti-infective drug in this product is active against the following common bacterial eye pathogens:
Staphylococcus aureus
Escherichia coli
Haemophilus influenzae
Klebsiella/Enterobacter species
Neisseria species
The product does not provide adequate coverage against:
Pseudomonas aeruginosa
Serratia marcescens
Streptococci, including *Streptococcus pneumoniae*

Contraindications

Epithelial herpes simplex keratitis (dendritic keratitis), acute infectious stages of vaccinia, varicella, and many other viral diseases of the cornea and conjunctiva. Mycobacterial infection of the eye. Fungal diseases of ocular structures. Hypersensitivity to a component of the medication (hypersensitivity to the antibiotic component occurs at a higher rate than for other components).
The use of these combinations is always contraindicated after uncomplicated removal of a corneal foreign body.

Warnings

Prolonged use may result in glaucoma, with damage to the optic nerve, defects in visual acuity and fields of vision, and posterior subcapsular cataract formation. Prolonged use may suppress the host response and thus increase the hazard of secondary ocular infections. In those diseases causing thinning of the cornea or sclera, perforations have been known to occur with the use of topical corticosteroids. In acute purulent conditions of the eye, corticosteroids may mask infection or en-

Continued on next page

Information on the Merck Sharp & Dohme products listed on these pages is the full prescribing information from package circulars in use October 31, 1982.

Merck Sharp & Dohme—Cont.

hance existing infection. If these products are used for 10 days or longer, intraocular pressure should be routinely monitored even though it may be difficult in children and uncooperative patients.
Employment of corticosteroid medication in the treatment of herpes simplex requires great caution: periodic slit-lamp microscopy is recommended.
Any substance (e.g. neomycin sulfate) may occasionally cause cutaneous sensitization. If any reaction indicating such sensitivity is observed, discontinue use.

Precautions

The initial prescription and renewal of the medication order beyond 20 milliliters should be made by a physician only after examination of the patient with the aid of magnification, such as slit lamp biomicroscopy and, where appropriate, fluorescein staining.
The possibility of persistent fungal infections of the cornea should be considered after prolonged corticosteroid dosing.
Usage in Pregnancy
Safety of intensive or protracted use of topical corticosteroids during pregnancy has not been substantiated.

Adverse Reactions

Adverse reactions have occurred with corticosteroid/anti-infective combination drugs which can be attributed to the corticosteroid component, the anti-infective component, or the combination. Exact incidence figures are not available since no denominator of treated patients is available.
Reactions occurring most often from the presence of the anti-infective ingredient are allergic sensitizations. The reactions due to the corticosteroid component in decreasing order of frequency are: elevation of intraocular pressure (IOP) with possible development of glaucoma, and infrequent optic nerve damage; posterior subcapsular cataract formation; and delayed wound healing.
Secondary Infection: The development of secondary infection has occurred after use of combinations containing corticosteroids and antimicrobials. Fungal infections of the cornea are particularly prone to develop coincidentally with long-term applications of corticosteroid. The possibility of fungal invasion must be considered in any persistent corneal ulceration where corticosteroid treatment has been used. Secondary bacterial ocular infection following suppression of host responses also occurs.

Dosage and Administration

The duration of treatment will vary with the type of lesion and may extend from a few days to several weeks, according to therapeutic response. Relapses, more common in chronic active lesions than in self-limited conditions, usually respond to retreatment.
Instill one or two drops of ophthalmic solution NEODECADRON into the conjunctival sac every hour during the day and every two hours during the night as initial therapy. When a favorable response is observed, reduce dosage to one drop every four hours. Later, further reduction in dosage to one drop three or four times daily may suffice to control symptoms.
Not more than 20 milliliters should be prescribed initially and the prescription should not be refilled without further evaluation as outlined in PRECAUTIONS above.

How Supplied

Sterile ophthalmic solution NEODECADRON is a clear, colorless to pale yellow solution.
No. 7612—Ophthalmic solution NEODECADRON is supplied as follows:
NDC 0006-7612-30 in 2.5 ml bottles with dropper assembly.
NDC 0006-7612-03 in 5 ml bottles with dropper assembly.
No. 7639—Ophthalmic solution NEODECADRON is supplied as follows:
NDC 0006-7639-03 in 5 ml white opaque, plastic OCUMETER ophthalmic dispenser with a controlled drop tip.
(6505-01-039-4325 0.1% 5 ml).

A.H.F.S. Category: 52:08
DC 6361412 Issued June 1982

NEO-HYDELTRASOL® Sterile Ophthalmic Solution ℞
Neomycin sulfate-prednisolone sodium phosphate ophthalmic solution

Description

Ophthalmic solution NEO-HYDELTRASOL® is a topical corticosteroid-antibiotic solution for use in certain disorders of the anterior segment of the eye.
Ophthalmic solution NEO-HYDELTRASOL contains in each milliliter of a nonirritating buffered solution: prednisolone sodium phosphate equivalent to 5 mg (0.5%) prednisolone phosphate and neomycin sulfate equivalent to 3.5 mg neomycin base. Inactive ingredients: creatinine, sodium citrate, polysorbate 80, disodium edetate, potassium phosphate, hydrochloric acid to adjust pH to 6.0 - 6.5, and water for injection. Benzalkonium chloride 0.02% added as preservative.
Prednisolone sodium phosphate is an inorganic ester of prednisolone. Its empirical formula is $C_{21}H_{27}Na_2O_8P$. It is approximately two thousand times more soluble in water at 25°C than hydrocortisone.
Neomycin sulfate is the sulfate salt of neomycin, an antibacterial substance produced by the growth of *Streptomyces fradiae* Waksman (Fam. Streptomycetaceae).

Clinical Pharmacology

Prednisolone sodium phosphate, a corticosteroid, suppresses the inflammatory response to a variety of agents, and it probably delays or slows healing. Since corticosteroids may inhibit the body's defense mechanism against infection, a concomitant antimicrobial drug may be used when this inhibition is considered to be clinically significant in a particular case.
Neomycin sulfate, the anti-infective component in the combination, is included to provide action against specific organisms susceptible to it. Neomycin sulfate is considered active mainly against gram-negative organisms, except *Bacteroides* spp. and *Pseudomonas aeruginosa*, which are resistant. Gram-positive organisms except for *Staphylococcus aureus* are usually resistant.
When a decision to administer both a corticosteroid and an antimicrobial is made, the administration of such drugs in combination has the advantage of greater patient compliance and convenience, with the added assurance that the appropriate dosage of both drugs is administered, plus assured compatibility of ingredients when both types of drug are in the same formulation and, particularly, that the correct volume of drug is delivered and retained.
The relative potency of corticosteroids depends on the molecular structure, concentration, and release from the vehicle.

Indications and Usage

For steroid-responsive inflammatory ocular conditions for which a corticosteroid is indicated and where bacterial infection or a risk of bacterial ocular infection exists.
Ocular steroids are indicated in inflammatory conditions of the palpebral and bulbar conjunctiva, cornea, and anterior segment of the globe where the inherent risk of steroid use in certain infective conjunctivitides is accepted to obtain a diminution in edema and inflammation. They are also indicated in chronic anterior uveitis and corneal injury from chemical, radiation, or thermal burns, or penetration of foreign bodies.
The use of a combination drug with an anti-infective component is indicated where the risk of infection is high or where there is an expectation that potentially dangerous numbers of bacteria will be present in the eye.
The particular anti-infective drug in this product is active against the following common bacterial eye pathogens:

Staphylococcus aureus
Escherichia coli
Haemophilus influenzae
Klebsiella/Enterobacter species
Neisseria species

The product does not provide adequate coverage against:

Pseudomonas aeruginosa
Serratia marcescens
Streptococci, including *Streptococcus pneumoniae*

Contraindications

Epithelial herpes simplex keratitis (dendritic keratitis), acute infectious stages of vaccinia, varicella, and many other viral diseases of the cornea and conjunctiva. Mycobacterial infection of the eye. Fungal diseases of ocular structures. Hypersensitivity to a component of the medication (hypersensitivity to the antibiotic component occurs at a higher rate than for other components).
The use of these combinations is always contraindicated after uncomplicated removal of a corneal foreign body.

Warnings

Prolonged use may result in glaucoma, with damage to the optic nerve, defects in visual acuity and fields of vision, and posterior subcapsular cataract formation. Prolonged use may suppress the host response and thus increase the hazard of secondary ocular infections. In those diseases causing thinning of the cornea or sclera, perforations have been known to occur with the use of topical corticosteroids. In acute purulent conditions of the eye, corticosteroids may mask infection or enhance existing infection. If these products are used for 10 days or longer, intraocular pressure should be routinely monitored even though it may be difficult in children and uncooperative patients.
Employment of corticosteroid medication in the treatment of herpes simplex requires great caution: periodic slit-lamp microscopy is recommended.
Any substance (e.g. neomycin sulfate) may occasionally cause cutaneous sensitization. If any reaction indicating such sensitivity is observed, discontinue use.

Precautions

The initial prescription and renewal of the medication order beyond 20 milliliters should be made by a physician only after examination of the patient with the aid of magnification, such as slit lamp biomicroscopy and, where appropriate, fluorescein staining.
The possibility of persistent fungal infections of the cornea should be considered after prolonged corticosteroid dosing.
Usage in Pregnancy
Safety of intensive or protracted use of topical corticosteroids during pregnancy has not been substantiated.

Adverse Reactions

Adverse reactions have occurred with corticosteroid/anti-infective combination drugs which can be attributed to the corticosteroid component, the anti-infective component, or the combination. Exact incidence figures are not available since no denominator of treated patients is available.

Reactions occurring most often from the presence of the anti-infective ingredient are allergic sensitizations. The reactions due to the corticosteroid component in decreasing order of frequency are: elevation of intraocular pressure (IOP) with possible development of glaucoma, and infrequent optic nerve damage; posterior subcapsular cataract formation; and delayed wound healing.

Secondary Infection: The development of secondary infection has occurred after use of combinations containing corticosteroids and antimicrobials. Fungal infections of the cornea are particularly prone to develop coincidentally with long-term applications of corticosteroid. The possibility of fungal invasion must be considered in any persistent corneal ulceration where corticosteroid treatment has been used. Secondary bacterial ocular infection following suppression of host responses also occurs.

Dosage and Administration

The duration of treatment will vary with the type of lesion and may extend from a few days to several weeks, according to therapeutic response. Relapses, more common in chronic active lesions than in self-limited conditions, usually respond to retreatment.

Instill one or two drops of ophthalmic solution NEO-HYDELTRASOL into the conjunctival sac every hour during the day and every two hours during the night as initial therapy. When a favorable response is observed, reduce dosage to one drop every four hours. Later, further reduction in dosage to one drop three or four times daily may suffice to control symptoms.

Not more than 20 milliliters should be prescribed initially and the prescription should not be refilled without further evaluation as outlined in PRECAUTIONS above.

How Supplied

No. 7580Z—Ophthalmic Solution NEO-HYDELTRASOL is a clear, colorless to pale yellow, sterile liquid and is supplied as follows:

NDC 0006-7580-30 in 2.5 ml bottles with dropper assembly.

NDC 0006-7580-03 in 5 ml bottles with dropper assembly.

A.H.F.S. Category: 52:08

DC 6163019 Issued June 1982

PERIACTIN® Tablets ℞
(cyproheptadine HCl, MSD), U.S.P.
PERIACTIN® Syrup ℞
(cyproheptadine HCl, MSD), U.S.P.

Description

Cyproheptadine hydrochloride is a white to slightly yellowish, crystalline solid. It is the sesquihydrate of 4-(5*H*-dibenzo[*a,d*]cyclohepten - 5 - ylidene)-1-methylpiperidine hydrochloride. The empirical formula of the anhydrous salt is $C_{21}H_{21}N \cdot HCl$.

Actions

PERIACTIN® (Cyproheptadine HCl, MSD) is a serotonin and histamine antagonist with anticholinergic and sedative effects. Antiserotonin and antihistamine drugs appear to compete with serotonin and histamine, respectively, for receptor sites.

Indications

Perennial and seasonal allergic rhinitis
Vasomotor rhinitis
Allergic conjunctivitis due to inhalant allergens and foods
Mild, uncomplicated allergic skin manifestations of urticaria and angioedema
Amelioration of allergic reactions to blood or plasma
Cold urticaria
Dermatographism
As therapy for anaphylactic reactions *adjunctive* to epinephrine and other standard measures after the acute manifestations have been controlled

Contraindications

Newborn or Premature Infants
This drug should *not* be used in newborn or premature infants.

Nursing Mothers
Because of the higher risk of antihistamines for infants generally and for newborns and prematures in particular, antihistamine therapy is contraindicated in nursing mothers.

Lower Respiratory Disease
Antihistamines should not be used to treat lower respiratory tract symptoms including asthma.

Other Conditions
Hypersensitivity to cyproheptadine and other drugs of similar chemical structure:

- Monoamine oxidase inhibitor therapy (see DRUG INTERACTIONS)
- Angle-closure glaucoma
- Stenosing peptic ulcer
- Symptomatic prostatic hypertrophy
- Bladder neck obstruction
- Pyloroduodenal obstruction
- Elderly, debilitated patients

Warnings

Children
Overdosage of antihistamines, particularly in infants and children, may produce hallucinations, central nervous system depression, convulsions, and death.

Antihistamines may diminish mental alertness; conversely, particularly, in the young child, they may occasionally produce excitation.

Pregnancy
The use of any drug in pregnancy or in women of childbearing potential requires that the anticipated benefit be weighed against possible hazards to the embryo or fetus.

CNS Depressants
Antihistamines may have additive effects with alcohol and other CNS depressants, e.g., hypnotics, sedatives, tranquilizers, antianxiety agents.

Activities Requiring Mental Alertness
Patients should be warned about engaging in activities requiring mental alertness and motor coordination, such as driving a car or operating machinery.

Antihistamines are more likely to cause dizziness, sedation, and hypotension in elderly patients.

Precautions

Cyproheptadine has an atropine-like action and, therefore, should be used with caution in patients with:

- History of bronchial asthma
- Increased intraocular pressure
- Hyperthyroidism
- Cardiovascular disease
- Hypertension

Drug Interactions

MAO Inhibitors prolong and intensify the anticholinergic effects of antihistamines.

Adverse Reactions

The most frequent adverse reactions to antihistamines are:

Sedation and sleepiness (often transient); dryness of mouth, nose, and throat; thickening of bronchial secretions, dizziness, epigastric distress, disturbed coordination.

Other adverse reactions which may occur with antihistamines:

Fatigue, confusion, restlessness, excitation, nervousness, tremor, irritability, paresthesias, acute labyrinthitis, hysteria, neuritis, convulsions, excessive perspiration, chills, hallucinations, insomnia, euphoria, anorexia, nausea, vomiting, diarrhea, constipation, faintness, hypotension, extrasystoles, tightness of chest and wheezing, urticaria, allergic manifestations of rash and edema, anaphylactic shock, blurred vision, diplopia, vertigo, tinnitus, headache, palpitation, tachycardia, nasal stuffiness, urinary frequency, difficult urination, urinary retention, early menses, photosensitivity, hemolytic anemia, leukopenia, agranulocytosis, thrombocytopenia.

Management of Overdosage

Antihistamine overdosage reactions may vary from central nervous system depression to stimulation especially in children. Also, atropine-like signs and symptoms (dry mouth; fixed, dilated pupils; flushing, etc.) as well as gastrointestinal symptoms may occur.

If vomiting has not occurred spontaneously the patient should be induced to vomit. This is best done by having him drink a glass of water after which he should be made to gag. Precautions against aspiration must be taken especially in infants and children.

If patient is unable to vomit, gastric lavage is indicated. Isotonic or ½ isotonic saline is the lavage of choice.

Saline cathartics, as milk of magnesia, by osmosis draw water into the bowel and, therefore, are valuable for their action in rapid dilution of bowel content.

Stimulants should *not* be used.

Vasopressors may be used to treat hypotension.

Dosage and Administration

DOSAGE SHOULD BE INDIVIDUALIZED ACCORDING TO THE NEEDS AND THE RESPONSE OF THE PATIENT.

Each PERIACTIN tablet contains 4 mg of cyproheptadine hydrochloride. Each 5 ml of PERIACTIN syrup contains 2 mg of cyproheptadine hydrochloride.

Although intended primarily for administration to children, the syrup is also useful for administration to adults who cannot swallow tablets.

Children
The total daily dosage for children may be calculated on the basis of body weight or body area using approximately 0.25 mg/kg/day (0.11 mg/lb/day) or 8 mg per square meter of body surface (8 mg/M²). In small children for whom the calculation of dosage based upon body size is most important, it may be necessary to use PERIACTIN syrup to permit accurate dosage.

Age 2 to 6 years
The usual dose is 2 mg (½ tablet or 1 teaspoon) two or three times a day, adjusted as necessary to the size and response of the patient. The dose is not to exceed 12 mg a day.

Age 7 to 14 years
The usual dose is 4 mg (1 tablet or 2 teaspoons) two or three times a day, adjusted as necessary to the size and response of the patient. The dose is not to exceed 16 mg a day.

Continued on next page

Information on the Merck Sharp & Dohme products listed on these pages is the full prescribing information from package circulars in use October 31, 1982.

Merck Sharp & Dohme—Cont.

Adults
The total daily dose for adults should not exceed 0.5 mg/kg/day (0.23 mg/lb/day).
The therapeutic range is 4 to 20 mg a day, with the majority of patients requiring 12 to 16 mg a day. An occasional patient may require as much as 32 mg a day for adequate relief. It is suggested that dosage be initiated with 4 mg (1 tablet or 2 teaspoons) three times a day and adjusted according to the size and response of the patient.

How Supplied

No. 3276—Tablets PERIACTIN, containing 4 mg of cyproheptadine hydrochloride each, are white, round, scored compressed tablets, coded MSD 62. They are supplied as follows:
NDC 0006-0062-68 bottles of 100.
(6505-00-890-1884 4 mg 100's)
[*Shown in Product Identification Section*]
No. 3289X—Syrup PERIACTIN, 2 mg per 5 ml is a clear, yellow, syrupy liquid. Contains alcohol 5%, with sorbic acid 0.1% added as preservative and is supplied as follows:
NDC 0006-3289-74 bottles of 473 ml.
A.H.F.S. Category: 4:00
DC 6589611 Issued August 1978

PNEUMOVAX® ℞
(pneumococcal vaccine, polyvalent, MSD)

Description

PNEUMOVAX® (Pneumococcal Vaccine, Polyvalent, MSD), is a sterile, liquid vaccine for intramuscular or subcutaneous injection. It consists of a mixture of highly purified capsular polysaccharides from the 14 most prevalent or invasive pneumococcal types accounting for at least 80% of pneumococcal disease isolates as determined by on-going surveillance.
PNEUMOVAX is manufactured according to methods developed by the MERCK SHARP & DOHME Research Laboratories. Each 0.5 ml dose of vaccine contains 50 μg of each polysaccharide type dissolved in isotonic saline solution containing 0.25% phenol as preservative.

14 Pneumococcal Capsular Types Included in PNEUMOVAX

Nomenclature	Pneumococcal Types						
U.S.	1	2	3	4	6	8	9
	12	14	19	23	25	51	56
Danish	1	2	3	4	6A	8	9N
	12F	14	19F	23F	25	7F	18C

Clinical Pharmacology

Pneumococcal infection is a leading cause of death throughout the world and a major cause of pneumonia, meningitis, and otitis media. The emergence of strains of pneumococci with increased resistance to one or more of the common antibiotics and recent isolations of pneumococci with multiple antibiotic resistance emphasize the importance of vaccine prophylaxis against pneumococcal disease. Based on projection from limited observations in the United States, it has been estimated that 400,000 to 500,000 cases of pneumococcal pneumonia may occur annually. The overall case fatality rate ranges from 5–10%. Populations at high risk are the elderly; individuals with immune deficiencies; patients with diabetes mellitus; patients with asplenia or splenic deficiencies, including sickle cell anemia and other severe hemoglobinopathies; alcoholics; and patients with the following diseases: Hodgkin's disease, multiple myeloma and nephrotic syndrome. About 25% of all persons with pneumococcal pneumonia develop bacteremia. Death occurs in about 28% of these bacteremic patients over 50 years of age. Of all patients with pneumococcal bacteremia who died despite treatment with penicillin or tetracycline, as many as 60% died within five days of onset of the illness.
The annual incidence of pneumococcal meningitis is approximately 1.5 to 2.5 per 100,000 population. One-half of the cases occur in children, in whom the fatality rate is about 40%. Within the first two years of life, about 15 to 20% of all children develop otitis media caused by pneumococci, and 50% of all children develop such illness within the first 10 years of life (see under INDICATIONS AND USAGE). Other illnesses caused by pneumococci include acute exacerbations of chronic bronchitis, sinusitis, arthritis and conjunctivitis.
Invasive pneumococcal disease causes high morbidity and mortality in spite of effective antimicrobial control by antibiotics. These effects of pneumococcal disease appear due to irreversible physiologic damage caused by the bacteria during the first 5 days following onset of illness, and irrespective of antimicrobial therapy. Vaccination offers an effective means of further reducing the mortality and morbidity of this disease.
At present, there are 83 known pneumococcal capsular types. However, the preponderance of pneumococcal diseases is caused by only some capsular types. For example, a 10-year (1952–1962) surveillance at a New York medical center showed that 56% of all deaths due to pneumococcal pneumonia were caused by 6 capsular types and that approximately 78% of all pneumococcal pneumonias were caused by 12 capsular types. Such unequal distribution of pneumococcal capsular types causing disease has been shown throughout the world. It is on the basis of this information that the pneumococcal vaccine is composed of 14 capsular types.
It has been established that the purified pneumococcal capsular polysaccharides induce antibody production and that such antibody is effective in preventing pneumococcal disease. Studies in humans have demonstrated the immunogenicity (antibody-stimulating capability) of each of the 14 capsular types when tested in polyvalent vaccines. Adults of all ages and children 2 years of age or older responded immunologically to the vaccines. Protective capsular type-specific antibody levels develop by the third week following vaccination.
The protective efficacy of pneumococcal vaccines containing 6 and 12 capsular polysaccharides was investigated in controlled studies of gold miners in South Africa, in whom there is a high attack rate for pneumococcal pneumonia. Capsular type-specific attack rates for pneumococcal pneumonia were observed for the period from 2 weeks through about 1 year after vaccination. The rates for pneumonia caused by the same capsular types represented in the vaccines are given in the table. Protective efficacy was 76% and 92%, respectively, in the two studies for the capsular types represented. [See table below].
In similar studies carried out by Dr. R. Austrian and associates using similar pneumococcal vaccines prepared for the National Institute of Allergy and Infectious Diseases, the reduction in pneumonias caused by the capsular types contained in the vaccines was 79%. Reduction in type-specific pneumococcal bacteremia was 82%. A preliminary report suggests that in patients with sickle cell anemia and/or anatomical or functional asplenia, the vaccine was highly effective in persons over two years of age in preventing severe pneumococcal disease and bacteremia.
The duration of protective effect of PNEUMOVAX is presently unknown, but it has been shown in previous studies with other pneumococcal vaccines that antibody induced by the vaccine may persist for as long as 5 years. Type-specific antibody levels induced by PNEUMOVAX have been observed to decline over a 42-month period of observation, but remain significantly above prevaccination levels in almost all recipients who manifest an initial response.

Number of Capsular Types in Pneumococcal Vaccine	Rate/1000 for Pneumonia Caused by Homologous Capsular Types		Protective Efficacy
	Vaccinated Group	Control Group	
6	9.2	38.3	76%
12	1.8	22.0	92%

Indications and Usage

PNEUMOVAX is indicated for immunization against pneumococcal disease caused by those pneumococcal types included in the vaccine. Effectiveness of the vaccine in the prevention of pneumococcal pneumonia and pneumococcal bacteremia has been demonstrated in controlled trials.
PNEUMOVAX *will not immunize against capsular types of pneumococcus other than those contained in the vaccine.*
Use in selected individuals over 2 years of age as follows: (1) patients who have anatomical asplenia or who have splenic dysfunction due to sickle cell disease or other causes; (2) persons with chronic illnesses in which there is an increased risk of pneumococcal disease, such as diabetes mellitus, functional impairment of cardiorespiratory, hepatic and renal systems; (3) persons 50 years of age or older.
Use in communities. Persons over 2 years of age as follows: (1) closed groups such as those in residential schools, nursing homes and other institutions; (2) groups epidemiologically at risk in the community when there is a generalized outbreak in the population due to a single pneumococcal type included in the vaccine; (3) patients at high risk of influenza complications, particularly pneumonia.
PNEUMOVAX may not be effective in preventing infection resulting from basilar skull fracture or from external communication with cerebrospinal fluid. Studies are under way to determine the effectiveness of the vaccine for preventing pneumococcal otitis media in infants.
Simultaneous administration of PNEUMOVAX and FLUAX® (Influenza Virus Vaccine, MSD), a killed whole virus vaccine, has been studied. When given simultaneously in separate extremities, antibody response and adverse effects were comparable to those which followed administration of the vaccines at different times. Before administering, see full prescribing information for FLUAX (Influenza Virus Vaccine, MSD). Studies have not been done to determine the effects of concomitant administration of PNEUMOVAX and other types of influenza virus vaccines. **NOTE**: Revaccination with PNEUMOVAX should not be carried out at intervals of less than 5 years (see PRECAUTIONS).
Revaccination
(See DOSAGE AND ADMINISTRATION.)

Contraindications

Hypersensitivity to any component of the vaccine. Epinephrine injection (1:1000) must be

immediately available should an acute anaphylactoid reaction occur due to any component of the vaccine.
Patients with Hodgkin's disease who have received extensive chemotherapy and/or nodal irradiation have been shown to have an impaired antibody response to a 12-valent pneumococcal vaccine. Because, in some intensively treated patients, administration of that vaccine depressed pre-existing levels of antibody to some pneumococcal types, PNEUMOVAX is not recommended at this time for patients who have received these forms of therapy for Hodgkin's disease.

Warnings

If the vaccine is used in persons receiving immunosuppressive therapy, the expected serum antibody response may not be obtained.
Intradermal administration may cause severe local reactions.

Precautions

General
Caution and appropriate care should be exercised in administering PNEUMOVAX to individuals with severely compromised cardiac and/or pulmonary function in whom a systemic reaction would pose a significant risk.
Any febrile respiratory illness or other active infection is reason for delaying use of PNEUMOVAX, except when, in the opinion of the physician, withholding the agent entails even greater risk.
In patients who require penicillin (or other antibiotic) prophylaxis against pneumococcal infection, such prophylaxis should not be discontinued after vaccination with PNEUMOVAX.
Revaccination should not be considered at less than 5-year intervals. Available data suggest that revaccination before 5 years may result in more frequent and severe local reactions at the site of injection. (See DOSAGE AND ADMINISTRATION.)
Pregnancy
Pregnancy Category C: Animal reproduction studies have not been conducted with PNEUMOVAX. It is also not known whether PNEUMOVAX can cause fetal harm when administered to a pregnant woman or can affect reproduction capacity. PNEUMOVAX is not recommended for use in pregnant women.
Nursing Mothers
It is not known whether this drug is excreted in human milk. Because many drugs are excreted in human milk, caution should be exercised when PNEUMOVAX is administered to a nursing woman.
Pediatric Use
Children less than 2 years of age do not respond satisfactorily to the capsular types of PNEUMOVAX that are most often the cause of pneumococcal disease in this age group. Safety and effectiveness in children below the age of 2 years have not been established. Accordingly, PNEUMOVAX is not recommended in this age group.

Adverse Reactions

Local erythema and soreness at the injection site, usually of less than 48 hours duration, occurs commonly; local induration occurs less commonly. In a study of PNEUMOVAX (containing 14 capsular types) in 26 adults, 24 (92%) showed local reaction characterized principally by local soreness and/or induration at the injection site within 2 days after vaccination.
Low grade fever (less than 100.9°F) occurs occasionally and is usually confined to the 24-hour period following vaccination. Although rare, fever over 102°F has been reported.
Reactions of greater severity, duration, or extent are unusual. Rarely, anaphylactoid reactions have been reported.

Dosage and Administration

Do not inject intravenously. Intradermal administration should be avoided.
Parenteral drug products should be inspected visually for particulate matter and discoloration prior to administration, whenever solution and container permit. PNEUMOVAX is a clear, colorless liquid.
Administer a single 0.5 ml dose of PNEUMOVAX subcutaneously or intramuscularly (preferably in the deltoid muscle or lateral midthigh), with appropriate precautions to avoid intravascular administration.
Single-Dose Prefilled Syringe
Inject contents of syringe to effect a single dose.
Single-Dose and 5-Dose Vials
For Syringe Use Only: Withdraw 0.5 ml from the vial using a sterile needle and syringe free of preservatives, antiseptics, and detergents.
It is important to use a separate sterile syringe and needle for each individual patient to prevent transmission of hepatitis B and other infectious agents from one person to another.
Because of the decline in antibody levels, revaccination may be considered. Available data suggest that revaccination should not be carried out at less than 5-year intervals so as to minimize the frequency and severity of local reactions, especially in persons who have retained high antibody levels. Long-term surveillance of antibody levels in immunized individuals is continuing.
Store single-dose prefilled syringes and unopened and opened vials at 2–8°C (35.6–46.4°F).
The vaccine is used directly as supplied. No dilution or reconstitution is necessary. Phenol 0.25% added as preservative. All vaccine must be discarded after the expiration date.

How Supplied

No. 4666—PNEUMOVAX contains one 5-dose vial of liquid vaccine, **NDC** 0006-4666-00. For use with syringe only.
No. 4689—PNEUMOVAX is supplied as follows: **NDC** 0006-4689-00. A box of 5 individual cartons, each containing a single-dose vial of vaccine.
No. 4670—PNEUMOVAX contains five single-dose 0.5 ml prefilled syringes, **NDC** 0006-4670-38.

A.H.F.S. Category: 80:12
DC 7014805 Issued November 1980
COPYRIGHT © MERCK & CO., INC., 1977
All rights reserved

SINEMET® Tablets ℞
(carbidopa-levodopa, MSD), U.S.P.

Description

When SINEMET® (Carbidopa-Levodopa, MSD) is to be given to patients who are being treated with levodopa, levodopa must be discontinued at least eight hours before therapy with SINEMET is started. In order to reduce adverse reactions, it is necessary to individualize therapy. See the WARNINGS and DOSAGE AND ADMINISTRATION sections before initiating therapy.
Carbidopa, an inhibitor of aromatic amino acid decarboxylation, is a white, crystalline compound, slightly soluble in water, with a molecular weight of 244.3. It is designated chemically as (—)-L-α-hydrazino-α-methyl-β-(3,4-dihydroxybenzene) propanoic acid monohydrate.
Tablet content is expressed in terms of anhydrous carbidopa which has a molecular weight of 226.3.
Levodopa, an aromatic amino acid, is a white, crystalline compound, slightly soluble in water, with a molecular weight of 197.2. It is designated chemically as (—)-L-α-amino-β-(3,4-dihydroxybenzene) propanoic acid.
SINEMET is supplied as tablets in three strengths:
SINEMET 10/100, containing 10 mg of carbidopa and 100 mg of levodopa
SINEMET 25/100, containing 25 mg of carbidopa and 100 mg of levodopa
SINEMET 25/250, containing 25 mg of carbidopa and 250 mg of levodopa

Actions

Current evidence indicates that symptoms of Parkinson's disease are related to depletion of dopamine in the corpus striatum. Administration of dopamine is ineffective in the treatment of Parkinson's disease apparently because it does not cross the blood-brain barrier. However, levodopa, the metabolic precursor of dopamine, does cross the blood-brain barrier, and presumably is converted to dopamine in the basal ganglia. This is thought to be the mechanism whereby levodopa relieves symptoms of Parkinson's disease.
When levodopa is administered orally it is rapidly converted to dopamine in extracerebral tissues so that only a small portion of a given dose is transported unchanged to the central nervous system. For this reason, large doses of levodopa are required for adequate therapeutic effect and these may often be attended by nausea and other adverse reactions, some of which are attributable to dopamine formed in extracerebral tissues.
Carbidopa inhibits decarboxylation of peripheral levodopa. It does not cross the blood-brain barrier and does not affect the metabolism of levodopa within the central nervous system.
Since its decarboxylase inhibiting activity is limited to extracerebral tissues, administration of carbidopa with levodopa makes more levodopa available for transport to the brain.
In dogs, reduced formation of dopamine in extracerebral tissues, such as the heart, provides protection against the development of dopamine-induced cardiac arrhythmias. Clinical studies tend to support the hypothesis of a similar protective effect in humans although controlled data are too limited at the present time to draw firm conclusions.
Carbidopa reduces the amount of levodopa required by about 75 percent and, when administered with levodopa, increases both plasma levels and the plasma half-life of levodopa, and decreases plasma and urinary dopamine and homovanillic acid.
In clinical pharmacologic studies, simultaneous administration of carbidopa and levodopa produced greater urinary excretion of levodopa in proportion to the excretion of dopamine than administration of the two drugs at separate times.
Pyridoxine hydrochloride (vitamin B_6), in oral doses of 10 mg to 25 mg, may reverse the effects of levodopa by increasing the rate of aromatic amino acid decarboxylation. Carbidopa inhibits this action of pyridoxine.

Indications

SINEMET, a combination of carbidopa and levodopa, is indicated in the treatment of the symptoms of idiopathic Parkinson's disease (paralysis agitans), postencephalitic parkinsonism, and symptomatic parkinsonism which may follow injury to the nervous system by carbon monoxide intoxication and manganese intoxication. SINEMET is indicated in these conditions to permit the administration of lower doses of levodopa with reduced nausea and vomiting, with more rapid dosage titration, with a somewhat smoother response, and with supplemental pyridoxine (vitamin B_6).
The incidence of levodopa-induced nausea and vomiting is less with SINEMET than with

Continued on next page

Information on the Merck Sharp & Dohme products listed on these pages is the full prescribing information from package circulars in use October 31, 1982.

Merck Sharp & Dohme—Cont.

levodopa. In many patients this reduction in nausea and vomiting will permit more rapid dosage titration.
In some patients a somewhat smoother antiparkinsonian effect results from therapy with SINEMET than with levodopa. However, patients with markedly irregular ("on-off") responses to levodopa have not been shown to benefit from SINEMET.
Since carbidopa prevents the reversal of levodopa effects caused by pyridoxine, SINEMET can be given to patients receiving supplemental pyridoxine (vitamin B_6).
Although the administration of carbidopa permits control of parkinsonism and Parkinson's disease with much lower doses of levodopa, there is no conclusive evidence at present that this is beneficial other than in reducing nausea and vomiting, permitting more rapid titration, and providing a somewhat smoother response to levodopa. *Carbidopa does not decrease adverse reactions due to central effects of levodopa. By permitting more levodopa to reach the brain, particularly when nausea and vomiting is not a dose-limiting factor, certain adverse CNS effects, e.g., dyskinesias, may occur at lower dosages and sooner during therapy with* SINEMET *than with levodopa.*
Certain patients who responded poorly to levodopa have improved when SINEMET was substituted. This is most likely due to decreased peripheral decarboxylation of levodopa which results from administration of carbidopa rather than to a primary effect of carbidopa on the nervous system. Carbidopa has not been shown to enhance the intrinsic efficacy of levodopa in parkinsonian syndromes.
In considering whether to give SINEMET to patients already on levodopa who have nausea and/or vomiting, the practitioner should be aware that, while many patients may be expected to improve, some do not. Since one cannot predict which patients are likely to improve, this can only be determined by a trial of therapy. It should be further noted that in controlled trials comparing SINEMET with levodopa, about half of the patients with nausea and/or vomiting on levodopa improved spontaneously despite being retained on the same dose of levodopa during the controlled portion of the trial.

Contraindications

Monoamine oxidase inhibitors and SINEMET should not be given concomitantly. These inhibitors must be discontinued at least two weeks prior to initiating therapy with SINEMET.
SINEMET is contraindicated in patients with known hypersensitivity to this drug, and in narrow angle glaucoma.
Because levodopa may activate a malignant melanoma, it should not be used in patients with suspicious, undiagnosed skin lesions or a history of melanoma.

Warnings

When patients are receiving levodopa, it must be discontinued at least eight hours before SINEMET is started. SINEMET should be substituted at a dosage that will provide approximately 25 percent of the previous levodopa dosage (see DOSAGE AND ADMINISTRATION). Patients who are taking SINEMET should be instructed not to take additional levodopa unless it is prescribed by the physician.
As with levodopa, SINEMET may cause involuntary movements and mental disturbances. These reactions are thought to be due to increased brain dopamine following administration of levodopa. All patients should be observed carefully for the development of depression with concomitant suicidal tendencies. Patients with past or current psychoses should be treated with caution. *Because carbidopa permits more levodopa to reach the brain and, thus, more dopamine to be formed, dyskinesias may occur at lower dosages and sooner with* SINEMET *than with levodopa.* The occurrence of dyskinesias may require dosage reduction.
SINEMET should be administered cautiously to patients with severe cardiovascular or pulmonary disease, bronchial asthma, renal, hepatic or endocrine disease.
Care should be exercised in administering SINEMET, as with levodopa, to patients with a history of myocardial infarction who have residual atrial, nodal, or ventricular arrhythmias. In such patients, cardiac function should be monitored with particular care during the period of initial dosage adjustment, in a facility with provisions for intensive cardiac care.
As with levodopa there is a possibility of upper gastrointestinal hemorrhage in patients with a history of peptic ulcer.
Usage in Pregnancy and Lactation: Although the effects of SINEMET on human pregnancy and lactation are unknown, both levodopa and combinations of carbidopa and levodopa have caused visceral and skeletal malformations in rabbits. Use of SINEMET in women of childbearing potential requires that the anticipated benefits of the drug be weighed against possible hazards to mother and child. SINEMET should not be given to nursing mothers.
Usage in Children: The safety of SINEMET in patients under 18 years of age has not been established.

Precautions

As with levodopa, periodic evaluations of hepatic, hematopoietic, cardiovascular, and renal function are recommended during extended therapy.
Patients with chronic wide angle glaucoma may be treated cautiously with SINEMET provided the intraocular pressure is well controlled and the patient is monitored carefully for changes in intraocular pressure during therapy.
Symptomatic postural hypotension can occur. For this reason, SINEMET should be given cautiously to patients on antihypertensive drugs. When SINEMET is started, dosage adjustment of the antihypertensive drug may be required. (For patients receiving pargyline, see the contraindication on monoamine oxidase inhibitors.)
Since phenothiazines and butyrophenones may reduce the therapeutic effects of levodopa, they should be administered with caution if concomitant administration with SINEMET is necessary. Also, the beneficial effects of levodopa in Parkinson's disease have been reported to be reversed by phenytoin and papaverine. Patients taking these drugs with SINEMET should be carefully observed for loss of antiparkinsonian effect.

Adverse Reactions

The most common serious adverse reactions occurring with SINEMET are choreiform, dystonic, and other involuntary movements. Other serious adverse reactions are mental changes including paranoid ideation and psychotic episodes, depression with or without development of suicidal tendencies, and dementia. Convulsions also have occurred; however, a causal relationship with SINEMET has not been established.
A common but less serious effect is nausea.
Less frequent adverse reactions are cardiac irregularities and/or palpitations, orthostatic hypotensive episodes, bradykinetic episodes (the "on-off" phenomenon), anorexia, vomiting, and dizziness.
Rarely, gastrointestinal bleeding, development of duodenal ulcer, hypertension, phlebitis, hemolytic anemia, leukopenia, and agranulocytosis have occurred.
Other adverse reactions that have been reported with levodopa include dry mouth, dysphagia, sialorrhea, abdominal pain and distress, ataxia, increased hand tremor, headache, numbness, weakness and faintness, bruxism, confusion, insomnia and nightmares, hallucinations and delusions, agitation and anxiety, malaise, fatigue, euphoria, muscle twitching, and blepharospasm (which may be taken as an early sign of excess dosage; consideration of dosage reduction may be made at this time), trismus, burning sensation of tongue, bitter taste, diarrhea, constipation, flatulence, flushing, skin rash, increased sweating, bizarre breathing patterns, urinary retention, urinary incontinence, diplopia, blurred vision, dilated pupils, hot flashes, weight gain or loss, dark sweat and/or urine, oculogyric crises, sense of stimulation, hiccups, edema, loss of hair, hoarseness, priapism, and activation of latent Horner's syndrome.
Abnormalities in laboratory tests may include elevations of blood urea nitrogen, SGOT, SGPT, lactic dehydrogenase, bilirubin, alkaline phosphatase, protein-bound iodine and positive Coombs test. More commonly, levels of blood urea nitrogen, creatinine, and uric acid are lower during administration of SINEMET than with levodopa.

Dosage and Administration

The optimum daily dosage of SINEMET must be determined by careful titration in each patient. SINEMET tablets are available in a 1:4 ratio of carbidopa to levodopa (SINEMET 25/100) as well as a 1:10 ratio (SINEMET 25/250 and SINEMET 10/100). Tablets of the two ratios may be given separately or combined as needed to provide the optimum dosage.
Studies show that peripheral dopa decarboxylase is saturated by carbidopa at approximately 70 to 100 mg a day. Patients receiving less than this amount of carbidopa are more likely to experience nausea and vomiting.
Usual Initial Dosage
Dosage is best initiated with one tablet of SINEMET 25/100 three times a day. This dosage schedule provides 75 mg of carbidopa per day. Dosage may be increased by one tablet every day or every other day, as necessary, until a dosage of six tablets of SINEMET 25/100 a day is reached. If SINEMET 10/100 is used, dosage may be initiated with one tablet three or four times a day and increased by one tablet every day or every other day until a total of eight tablets (2 tablets q.i.d.) is reached.
How to Transfer Patients from Levodopa
Levodopa must be discontinued at least eight hours before starting SINEMET (Carbidopa-Levodopa, MSD). A daily dosage of SINEMET should be chosen that will provide approximately 25 percent of the previous levodopa dosage. Patients who are taking less than 1500 mg of levodopa a day should be started on one tablet of SINEMET 25/100 three or four times a day. The suggested starting dosage for most patients taking more than 1500 mg of levodopa is one tablet of SINEMET 25/250 three or four times a day.
Maintenance
Therapy should be individualized and adjusted according to the desired therapeutic response. When a greater proportion of carbidopa is required, one tablet of SINEMET 25/100 may be substituted for each tablet of SINEMET 10/100. When more levodopa is required, SINEMET 25/250 should be substituted at a dosage of one tablet three or four times a day. If necessary, the dosage may be increased by one-half or one tablet every day or every other day to a maximum of eight tablets a day. Experience with total daily dosages of carbidopa greater than 200 mg is limited.
Because both therapeutic and adverse responses occur more rapidly with SINEMET than with levodopa alone, patients should be monitored closely during the dose adjustment

period. Specifically, involuntary movements will occur more rapidly with SINEMET than with levodopa. The occurrence of involuntary movements may require dosage reduction. Blepharospasm may be a useful early sign of excess dosage in some patients.
Current evidence indicates that other standard drugs for Parkinson's disease (except levodopa) may be continued while SINEMET is being administered, although their dosage may have to be adjusted.
If general anesthesia is required, SINEMET may be continued as long as the patient is permitted to take fluids and medication by mouth. If therapy is interrupted temporarily, the usual daily dosage may be administered as soon as the patient is able to take oral medication.

Overdosage

Management of acute overdosage with SINEMET is basically the same as management of acute overdosage with levodopa; however, pyridoxine is not effective in reversing the actions of SINEMET.
General supportive measures should be employed, along with immediate gastric lavage. Intravenous fluids should be administered judiciously and an adequate airway maintained. Electrocardiographic monitoring should be instituted and the patient carefully observed for the development of arrhythmias; if required, appropriate antiarrhythmic therapy should be given. The possibility that the patient may have taken other drugs as well as SINEMET should be taken into consideration. To date, no experience has been reported with dialysis; hence, its value in overdosage is not known.

How Supplied

No. 3346—Tablets SINEMET 10/100 are dark dapple-blue, oval, scored, uncoated tablets, coded MSD 647. They are supplied as follows:
NDC 0006-0647-68 bottles of 100
(6505-01-020-8280 100's)
NDC 0006-0647-28 single unit packages of 100.
NDC 0006-0647-78 unit of use bottles of 100.
[*Shown in Product Identification Section*]
No. 3365—Tablets SINEMET 25/100 are yellow, oval, scored tablets, coded MSD 650. They are supplied as follows:
NDC 0006-0650-68 bottles of 100
NDC 0006-0650-28 single unit packages of 100.
NDC 0006-0650-78 unit of use bottles of 100.
[*Shown in Product Identification Section*]
No. 3347—Tablets SINEMET 25/250 are light dapple-blue, oval, scored, uncoated tablets, coded MSD 654. They are supplied as follows:
NDC 0006-0654-68 bottles of 100
(6505-01-020-8279 100's)
NDC 0006-0654-28 single unit packages of 100.
NDC 0006-0654-78 unit of use bottles of 100.
[*Shown in Product Identification Section*]
A.H.F.S. Category: 92:00
DC6834810 Issued March 1982

TIMOLIDE® Tablets ℞
(timolol maleate-hydrochlorothiazide, MSD)

Description

TIMOLIDE® (Timolol Maleate-Hydrochlorothiazide, MSD) is for the treatment of hypertension. It combines the antihypertensive activity of two agents: a non-selective beta-adrenergic receptor blocking agent (timolol maleate) and a diuretic (hydrochlorothiazide). Each tablet of TIMOLIDE contains 10 mg of timolol maleate and 25 mg of hydrochlorothiazide.
Timolol maleate is (S)-1-[(1, 1-dimethylethyl) amino]-3-[[4-(4-morpholinyl)-1,2,5-thiadiazol-3-yl]oxy]-2-propanol, (Z)-butenedioate (1:1) salt.
Hydrochlorothiazide is 6-chloro-3,4-dihydro-2*H*-1,2,4-benzothiadiazine-7-sulfonamide 1, 1-dioxide.
TIMOLIDE is supplied as tablets containing 10 mg of timolol maleate and 25 mg of hydrochlorothiazide for oral administration.

Clinical Pharmacology

TIMOLIDE
Timolol maleate and hydrochlorothiazide have been used singly and concomitantly for the treatment of hypertension. The antihypertensive effects of these agents are additive. The two components of TIMOLIDE have similar dosage schedules, and studies have shown that there is no interference with bioavailability when these agents are given together in the single combination tablet. Therefore, this combination provides a convenient formulation for the concomitant administration of these two entities.
In controlled clinical trials with TIMOLIDE in selected patients with mild to moderate essential hypertension, about 90 percent had a good to excellent response. In patients with more severe hypertension, TIMOLIDE may be administered with other antihypertensives such as ALDOMET® (Methyldopa, MSD) or a vasodilator.
Although the mechanisms of action of timolol maleate and hydrochlorothiazide in the treatment of hypertension have not been established, they are thought to be different; for example, hydrochlorothiazide increases plasma renin activity while timolol maleate reduces plasma renin activity.
Timolol Maleate
Timolol maleate is a $beta_1$ and $beta_2$ (non-selective) adrenergic receptor blocking agent that does not have significant intrinsic sympathomimetic, direct myocardial depressant, or local anesthetic activity.
Pharmacodynamics
Clinical pharmacology studies have confirmed the beta-adrenergic blocking activity as shown by (1) changes in resting heart rate and response of heart rate to changes in posture; (2) inhibition of isoproterenol-induced tachycardia; (3) alteration of the response to the Valsalva maneuver and amyl nitrite administration; and (4) reduction of heart rate and blood pressure changes on exercise.
Timolol maleate decreases the positive chronotropic, positive inotropic, bronchodilator, and vasodilator responses caused by beta-adrenergic receptor agonists. The magnitude of this decreased response is proportional to the existing sympathetic tone and the concentration of timolol maleate at receptor sites.
In normal volunteers, the reduction in heart rate response to a standard exercise was dose dependent over the test range of 0.5 to 20 mg, with a peak reduction at 2 hours of approximately 30% at higher doses.
Beta-adrenergic receptor blockade reduces cardiac output in both healthy subjects and patients with heart disease. In patients with severe impairment of myocardial function beta-adrenergic receptor blockade may inhibit the stimulatory effect of the sympathetic nervous system necessary to maintain adequate cardiac function.
Beta-adrenergic receptor blockade in the bronchi and bronchioles results in increased airway resistance from unopposed parasympathetic activity. Such an effect in patients with asthma or other bronchospastic conditions is potentially dangerous.
Clinical studies indicate that timolol maleate at a dosage of 20–60 mg/day reduces blood pressure without causing postural hypotension in most patients with essential hypertension. Administration of timolol maleate to patients with hypertension results initially in a decrease in cardiac output, little immediate change in blood pressure, and an increase in calculated peripheral resistance. With continued administration of timolol maleate blood pressure decreases within a few days, cardiac output usually remains reduced, and peripheral resistance falls toward pretreatment levels. Plasma volume may decrease or remain unchanged during therapy with timolol maleate. In the majority of patients with hypertension timolol maleate also decreases plasma renin activity. Dosage adjustment to achieve optimal antihypertensive effect may require a few weeks. When therapy with timolol maleate is discontinued, the blood pressure tends to return to pretreatment levels gradually. In most patients the antihypertensive activity of timolol maleate is maintained with long-term therapy and is well tolerated.
The mechanism of the antihypertensive effects of beta-adrenergic receptor blocking agents is not established at this time. Possible mechanisms of action include reduction in cardiac output, reduction in plasma renin activity, and a central nervous system sympatholytic action.
Pharmacokinetics and Metabolism
Timolol maleate is rapidly and nearly completely absorbed (about 90%) following oral ingestion. Detectable plasma levels of timolol occur within one-half hour and peak plasma levels occur in about one to two hours. The drug half-life in plasma is approximately 4 hours and this is essentially unchanged in patients with moderate renal insufficiency. Timolol is partially metabolized by the liver and timolol and its metabolites are excreted by the kidney. Timolol is not extensively bound to plasma proteins; i.e., <10% by equilibrium dialysis and approximately 60% by ultrafiltration. An *in vitro* hemodialysis study, using ^{14}C timolol added to human plasma or whole blood, showed that timolol was readily dialyzed from these fluids; however, a study of patients with renal failure showed that timolol did not dialyze readily. Plasma levels following oral administration are about half those following intravenous administration indicating approximately 50% first pass metabolism. The level of beta sympathetic activity varies widely among individuals, and no simple correlation exists between the dose or plasma level of timolol maleate and its therapeutic activity. Therefore, objective clinical measurements such as reduction of heart rate and/or blood pressure should be used as guides in determining the optimal dosage for each patient.
Hydrochlorothiazide
Hydrochlorothiazide is a diuretic and antihypertensive agent. It affects the renal tubular mechanism of electrolyte reabsorption. Hydrochlorothiazide increases excretion of sodium and chloride in approximately equivalent amounts. Natriuresis may be accompanied by some loss of potassium and bicarbonate. The mechanism of the antihypertensive effect of thiazides may be related to the excretion and redistribution of body sodium. Hydrochlorothiazide usually does not cause clinically important changes in normal blood pressure.

Indications and Usage

TIMOLIDE is indicated for the treatment of hypertension.
This fixed combination drug is not indicated for initial therapy of hypertension. If the fixed combination represents the dose titrated to an individual patient's needs, it may be more convenient than the separate components.

Contraindications

TIMOLIDE is contraindicated in patients with: bronchospasm, including bronchial asthma, or severe chronic obstructive pulmonary disease; sinus bradycardia; second and third degree

Continued on next page

Information on the Merck Sharp & Dohme products listed on these pages is the full prescribing information from package circulars in use October 31, 1982.

Merck Sharp & Dohme—Cont.

atrioventricular block; overt cardiac failure (see WARNINGS); cardiogenic shock; anuria; hypersensitivity to this product or to sulfonamide-derived drugs.

Warnings

Cardiac Failure
Sympathetic stimulation may be essential for support of the circulation in individuals with diminished myocardial contractility, and its inhibition by beta-adrenergic receptor blockade may precipitate more severe failure. Although beta-blockers should be avoided in overt congestive heart failure, they can be used, if necessary, with caution in patients with a history of failure who are well-compensated, usually with digitalis and diuretics. Both digitalis and timolol maleate slow AV conduction. If cardiac failure persists, therapy with TIMOLIDE should be withdrawn.
In Patients Without a History of Cardiac Failure continued depression of the myocardium with beta-blocking agents over a period of time can, in some cases, lead to cardiac failure. At the first sign or symptom of cardiac failure, patients receiving TIMOLIDE should be digitalized and/or be given additional diuretic therapy. Observe the patient closely. If cardiac failure continues, despite adequate digitalization and diuretic therapy, TIMOLIDE should be withdrawn.
Renal and Hepatic Disease and Electrolyte Disturbances
Since timolol maleate is partially metabolized in the liver and excreted mainly by the kidneys, dosage reductions may be necessary when hepatic and/or renal insufficiency is present.
Although the pharmacokinetics of timolol maleate are not greatly altered by renal impairment, marked hypotensive responses have been seen in patients with marked renal impairment undergoing dialysis after 20 mg doses. Dosing in such patients should therefore be especially cautious.
In patients with renal disease, thiazides may precipitate azotemia, and cumulative effects may develop in the presence of impaired renal function. If progressive renal impairment becomes evident, TIMOLIDE should be discontinued.
In patients with impaired hepatic function or progressive liver disease, even minor alterations in fluid and electrolyte balance may precipitate hepatic coma. Hepatic encephalopathy, manifested by tremors, confusion, and coma, has been reported in association with diuretic therapy including hydrochlorothiazide.

Exacerbation of Ischemic Heart Disease Following Abrupt Withdrawal—Hypersensitivity to catecholamines has been observed in patients withdrawn from beta blocker therapy; exacerbation of angina and, in some cases, myocardial infarction have occurred after *abrupt* discontinuation of such therapy. When discontinuing chronically administered timolol maleate, particularly in patients with ischemic heart disease, the dosage should be gradually reduced over a period of one to two weeks and the patient should be carefully monitored. If angina markedly worsens or acute coronary insufficiency develops, timolol maleate administration should be reinstituted promptly, at least temporarily, and other measures appropriate for the management of unstable angina should be taken. Patients should be warned against interruption or discontinuation of therapy without the physician's advice. Because coronary artery disease is common and may be unrecognized, it may be prudent not to discontinue timolol maleate therapy abruptly even in patients treated only for hypertension.

Major Surgery
The necessity or desirability of withdrawal of beta-blocking therapy prior to major surgery is controversial. Beta-adrenergic receptor blockade impairs the ability of the heart to respond to beta-adrenergically mediated reflex stimuli. This may augment the risk of general anesthesia in surgical procedures. Some patients receiving beta-adrenergic receptor blocking agents have been subject to protracted severe hypotension during anesthesia. Difficulty in restarting and maintaining the heartbeat has also been reported. For these reasons, in patients undergoing elective surgery, some authorities recommend gradual withdrawal of beta-adrenergic receptor blocking agents.
If necessary during surgery, the effects of beta-adrenergic blocking agents may be reversed by sufficient doses of such agonists as isoproterenol, dopamine, dobutamine or levarterenol (see OVERDOSAGE).
Metabolic and Endocrine Effects
Beta-adrenergic blockade may mask certain clinical signs (e.g., tachycardia) of hyperthyroidism. Patients suspected of developing thyrotoxicosis should be managed carefully to avoid abrupt withdrawal of beta blockade which might precipitate a thyroid storm. Thiazides may decrease serum PBI levels without signs of thyroid disturbance.
Beta-adrenergic receptor blocking agents may mask the signs and symptoms of acute hypoglycemia. Therefore, TIMOLIDE should be administered with caution to patients subject to spontaneous hypoglycemia, or to diabetic patients (especially those with labile diabetes) who are receiving insulin or oral hypoglycemic agents. Insulin requirements in diabetic patients may be increased, decreased, or unchanged by thiazides. Diabetes mellitus which has been latent may become manifest during administration of thiazide diuretics.
Because calcium excretion is decreased by thiazides, TIMOLIDE should be discontinued before carrying out tests for parathyroid function. Pathologic changes in the parathyroid glands, with hypercalcemia and hypophosphatemia, have been observed in a few patients on prolonged thiazide therapy; however, the common complications of hyperparathyroidism such as renal lithiasis, bone resorption, and peptic ulceration have not been seen.
Hyperuricemia may occur or acute gout may be precipitated in certain patients receiving thiazide therapy.

Precautions

General
Electrolyte and Fluid Balance Status: Periodic determination of serum electrolytes to detect possible electrolyte imbalance should be performed at appropriate intervals.
Patients should be observed for clinical signs of fluid or electrolyte imbalance, i.e., hyponatremia, hypochloremic alkalosis, and hypokalemia. Serum and urine electrolyte determinations are particularly important when the patient is vomiting excessively or receiving parenteral fluids. Warning signs or symptoms of fluid and electrolyte imbalance include dryness of the mouth, thirst, weakness, lethargy, drowsiness, restlessness, muscle pains or cramps, muscular fatigue, hypotension, oliguria, tachycardia, and gastrointestinal disturbances such as nausea and vomiting.
Hypokalemia may develop, especially with brisk diuresis, when severe cirrhosis is present, or during concomitant use of corticosteroids or ACTH.
Interference with adequate oral electrolyte intake will also contribute to hypokalemia. Hypokalemia can sensitize or exaggerate the response of the heart to the toxic effects of digitalis (e.g., increased ventricular irritability). Hypokalemia may be avoided or treated by use of potassium supplements or foods with a high potassium content.
Any chloride deficit during thiazide therapy is generally mild and usually does not require specific treatment except under extraordinary circumstances (as in liver disease or renal disease). Dilutional hyponatremia may occur in edematous patients in hot weather; appropriate therapy is water restriction rather than administration of salt except in rare instances when the hyponatremia is life threatening. In actual salt depletion, appropriate replacement is the therapy of choice.
Drug Interactions
TIMOLIDE may potentiate the action of other antihypertensive agents used concomitantly. Close observation of the patient is recommended when TIMOLIDE is administered to patients receiving catecholamine-depleting drugs such as reserpine, because of possible additive effects and the production of hypotension and/or marked bradycardia, which may produce vertigo, syncope, or postural hypotension.
Thiazides may decrease arterial responsiveness to norepinephrine. This diminution is not sufficient to preclude the therapeutic effectiveness of norepinephrine. Thiazides may increase the responsiveness to tubocurarine.
Lithium generally should not be given with diuretics because they reduce its renal clearance and add a high risk of lithium toxicity. Read circulars for lithium preparations before use of such preparations with TIMOLIDE.
Other Precautions
In patients receiving thiazides, sensitivity reactions may occur with or without a history of allergy or bronchial asthma. The possible exacerbation or activation of systemic lupus erythematosus has been reported. The antihypertensive effects of thiazides may be enhanced in the post-sympathectomy patient.
Carcinogenesis, Mutagenesis, Impairment of Fertility
In two-year study of timolol maleate in rats, there was a statistically significant ($P \leq 0.05$) increase in the incidence of adrenal pheochromocytomas in male rats administered 300 times the maximum recommended human dose (1 mg/kg/day). Similar differences were not observed in rats administered doses equivalent to 25 or 100 times the maximum recommended human dose. In a lifetime study in mice, there were statistically significant ($P \leq 0.05$) increases in the incidence of benign and malignant pulmonary tumors and benign uterine polyps in female mice at 500 mg/kg/day, but not at 5 or 50 mg/kg/day. There was also a significant increase in mammary adenocarcinomas at the 500 mg/kg/day dose. This was associated with elevations in serum prolactin which occurred in female mice administered timolol at 500 mg/kg, but not at doses of 5 or 50 mg/kg/day. An increased incidence of mammary adenocarcinomas in rodents has been associated with administration of several other therapeutic agents which elevate serum prolactin, but no correlation between serum prolactin levels and mammary tumors has been established in man. Furthermore, in adult human female subjects who received oral dosages of up to 60 mg of timolol maleate, the maximum recommended human oral dosage, there were no clinically meaningful changes in serum prolactin.
There was a statistically significant increase ($P \leq 0.05$) in the overall incidence of neoplasms in female mice at the 500 mg/kg/day dosage level.
Timolol maleate was devoid of mutagenic potential when evaluated *in vivo* (mouse) in the micronucleus test and cytogenetic assay (doses up to 800 mg/kg) and *in vitro* in a neoplastic cell transformation assay (up to 100 μg/ml). In Ames tests the highest concentrations of timo-

lol employed, 5000 or 10,000 μg/plate, were associated with statistically significant elevations ($P \leq 0.05$) of revertants observed with tester strain TA100 (in seven replicate assays), but not in the remaining three strains. In the assays with tester strain TA100, no consistent dose response relationship was observed, nor did the ratio of test to control revertants reach 2. A ratio of 2 is usually considered the criterion for a positive Ames test.

Reproduction and fertility studies in rats showed no adverse effect on male or female fertility at doses up to 150 times the maximum recommended human dose.

Pregnancy

Pregnancy Category C. Combinations of timolol maleate and hydrochlorothiazide were studied for teratogenic potential in the mouse and rabbit. The timolol maleate/hydrochlorothiazide combinations were administered orally to pregnant mice and pregnant rabbits at dosage levels of 1/2.5, 4/10, or 8/10 mg/kg/day. No teratogenic, embryotoxic, fetotoxic, or maternotoxic effects attributable to treatment were observed in either species.

Timolol Maleate

Teratogenic studies with timolol maleate in mice and rabbits at doses up to 50 mg/kg/day (50 times the maximum recommended human dose) showed no evidence of fetal malformations. Although delayed fetal ossification was observed at this dose in rats, there were no adverse effects on postnatal development of offspring. Doses of 1000 mg/kg/day (1,000 times the maximum recommended human dose) were maternotoxic in mice and resulted in an increased number of fetal resorptions. Increased fetal resorptions were also seen in rabbits at doses of 100 times the maximum recommended human dose, in this case without apparent maternotoxicity. There are no adequate and well-controlled studies in pregnant women. TIMOLIDE should be used during pregnancy only if the potential benefit justifies the potential risk to the fetus.

Hydrochlorothiazide

TIMOLIDE contains hydrochlorothiazide. Thiazides cross the placental barrier and appear in cord blood. The use of thiazides in pregnancy requires that the anticipated benefit be weighed against possible hazards to the fetus. These hazards include fetal or neonatal jaundice, thrombocytopenia, and possibly other adverse reactions which have occurred in the adult.

Nursing Mothers

Because of the potential for serious adverse reactions from timolol and hydrochlorothiazide in nursing infants, a decision should be made whether to discontinue nursing or to discontinue the drug, taking into account the importance of the drug to the mother.

Pediatric Use

Safety and effectiveness in children have not been established.

Adverse Reactions

TIMOLIDE is usually well tolerated in properly selected patients. Most adverse effects have been mild and transient.

The adverse reactions listed in the following table were spontaneously reported and have been arranged into two groups: (1) incidence greater than 1%; and (2) incidence less than 1%. The incidence was obtained from clinical studies conducted in the United States (257 patients treated with TIMOLIDE).

Incidence Greater Than 1%	*Incidence Less Than 1%*
BODY AS A WHOLE	
fatigue/tiredness (1.9%)	chest pain
asthenia (1.9%)	headache
CARDIOVASCULAR	
hypotension (1.6%)	arrhythmia
bradycardia (1.2%)	syncope
	cardiac failure
DIGESTIVE SYSTEM	
none	diarrhea
	dyspepsia
	nausea
	gastrointestinal pain
	constipation
INTEGUMENTARY	
none	rash
	increased pigmentation
	dry mucous membranes
MUSCULOSKELETAL	
none	myalgia
NERVOUS SYSTEM	
dizziness (1.2%)	none
PSYCHIATRIC	
none	insomnia
	decreased libido
	nervousness
	confusion
	trouble concentrating
	somnolence
RESPIRATORY	
bronchial spasm (1.6%)	rales
dyspnea (1.2%)	
UROGENITAL	
none	renal colic

The following additional adverse effects have been reported in clinical experience with the drug: cerebral ischemia, cerebral vascular accident, gout, muscle cramps, oculogyric crisis, worsening of chronic obstructive pulmonary disease, earache, and impotence.

Other adverse reactions that have been reported with the individual components are listed below:

Timolol Maleate—Body as a Whole: extremity pain, decreased exercise tolerance, weight loss; *Cardiovascular:* cerebral vascular accident, worsening of angina pectoris, sinoatrial block, AV block, worsening of arterial insufficiency, Raynaud's phenomenon, claudication, palpitations, vasodilatation, cold hands and feet, edema; *Digestive:* hepatomegaly, vomiting; *Endocrine:* hyperglycemia, hypoglycemia; *Integumentary:* skin irritation, pruritus, sweating; *Musculoskeletal:* arthralgia; *Nervous System:* local weakness, vertigo, paresthesia; *Psychiatric:* depression, nightmares; *Respiratory:* cough; *Special Senses:* visual disturbances, eye irritation, dry eyes, tinnitus; *Urogenital:* urination difficulties.

Hydrochlorothiazide—Gastrointestinal: anorexia, gastric irritation, vomiting, cramping, jaundice (intrahepatic cholestatic jaundice), pancreatitis, sialadenitis; *Central nervous system:* vertigo, paresthesias, xanthopsia; *Hematologic:* Leukopenia, agranulocytosis, thrombocytopenia, aplastic anemia, hemolytic anemia; *Cardiovascular:* orthostatic hypotension (may be aggravated by alcohol, barbiturates, or narcotics); *Hypersensitivity:* purpura, photosensitivity, urticaria, necrotizing angiitis (vasculitis, cutaneous vasculitis), fever, respiratory distress including pneumonitis and pulmonary edema, anaphylactic reactions; *Miscellaneous:* hyperglycemia, glycosuria, hyperuricemia, muscle spasm, weakness, restlessness, transient blurred vision.

Potential Adverse Effects: In addition, a variety of adverse effects not observed in clinical trials with timolol maleate, but reported with other beta-adrenergic blocking agents, should be considered potential adverse effects of timolol maleate: *Nervous System:* Reversible mental depression progressing to catatonia; hallucinations; an acute reversible syndrome characterized by disorientation for time and place, short-term memory loss, emotional lability, slightly clouded sensorium, and decreased performance on neuropsychometrics; *Cardiovascular:* Intensification of AV block (see CONTRAINDICATIONS); *Gastrointestinal:* Mesenteric arterial thrombosis, ischemic colitis; *Hematologic:* Agranulocytosis, nonthrombocytopenic purpura, thrombocytopenic purpura; *Allergic:* Erythematous rash, fever combined with aching and sore throat, laryngospasm and respiratory distress; *Miscellaneous:* Reversible alopecia, Peyronie's disease.

There have been reports of a syndrome comprising psoriasiform skin rash, conjunctivitis sicca, otitis, and sclerosing serositis attributed to the beta-adrenergic receptor blocking agent, practolol. This syndrome has not been reported with TIMOLIDE or BLOCADREN® (Timolol Maleate, MSD).

Clinical Laboratory Test Findings: Clinically important changes in standard laboratory parameters were rarely associated with the administration of TIMOLIDE. The changes in laboratory parameters were not progressive and usually were not associated with clinical manifestations. The most common changes were increases in serum triglycerides and uric acid and decreases in serum potassium and chloride.

Overdosage

No data are available in regard to overdosage in humans. Pretreatment of mice with hydrochlorothiazide (5 mg/kg) did not alter the LD_{50} of timolol (1320 mg/kg compared to 1300 mg/kg without pretreatment).

No specific information is available on the treatment of overdosage with TIMOLIDE, and no specific antidote is available. Treatment is symptomatic and supportive. Therapy with TIMOLIDE should be discontinued and the patient observed closely. Suggested measures include induction of emesis and/or gastric lavage, and correction of dehydration, electrolyte imbalance, and hypotension by established procedures.

Timolol Maleate

No data are available in regard to overdosage in humans.

The oral LD_{50} of the drug is 1190 and 900 mg/kg in female mice and female rats, respectively.

An *in vitro* hemodialysis study, using ^{14}C timolol added to human plasma or whole blood, showed that timolol was readily dialyzed from these fluids; however, a study of patients with renal failure showed that timolol did not dialyze readily.

The most common signs and symptoms to be expected with overdosage with a beta-adrenergic receptor blocking agent are symptomatic bradycardia, hypotension, bronchospasm, and acute cardiac failure. If overdosage occurs the following therapeutic measures should be considered:

(1) *Gastric lavage.*

(2) *Symptomatic bradycardia:* Use atropine sulfate intravenously in a dosage of 0.25 mg to 2 mg to induce vagal blockade. If bradycardia persists, intravenous isoproterenol hydrochloride should be administered cautiously. In refractory cases the use of a transvenous cardiac pacemaker may be considered.

(3) *Hypotension:* Use sympathomimetic pressor drug therapy, such as dopamine, dobutamine or levarterenol. In refractory cases the use of glucagon hydrochloride has been reported to be useful.

(4) *Bronchospasm:* Use isoproterenol hydrochloride. Additional therapy with aminophylline may be considered.

(5) *Acute cardiac failure:* Conventional therapy with digitalis, diuretics, and oxygen should be instituted immediately. In refractory cases the use of intravenous aminophylline is sug-

Continued on next page

Information on the Merck Sharp & Dohme products listed on these pages is the full prescribing information from package circulars in use October 31, 1982.

Merck Sharp & Dohme—Cont.

gested. This may be followed, if necessary, by glucagon hydrochloride which has been reported to be useful.

(6) *Heart block (second or third degree):* Use isoproterenol hydrochloride or a transvenous cardiac pacemaker.

Hydrochlorothiazide

The most common signs and symptoms observed with hydrochlorothiazide overdosage are those caused by electrolyte depletion (hypokalemia, hypochloremia, hyponatremia) and dehydration resulting from excessive diuresis. If digitalis has also been administered, hypokalemia may accentuate cardiac arrhythmias.

Dosage and Administration

The recommended starting and maintenance dosage is 1 tablet twice a day. If the antihypertensive response is not satisfactory, another antihypertensive agent may be added.

How Supplied

No. 3373—Tablets TIMOLIDE 10/25 are light blue, flat, hexagonal-shaped, compressed tablets, with MSD 67 code on one side and TIMOLIDE on the other. Each tablet contains 10 mg of timolol maleate and 25 mg of hydrochlorothiazide. They are supplied as follows:

NDC 0006-0067-68 bottles of 100

NDC 0006-0067-28 single unit packages of 100.

[*Shown in Product Identification Section*]

A.H.F.S. Category: 24:08

DC 7119514 Issued January 1982

COPYRIGHT © MERCK & CO., INC., 1979
All rights reserved

TIMOPTIC® Sterile Ophthalmic Solution (timolol maleate, MSD), U.S.P. ℞

Description

TIMOPTIC® (Timolol Maleate, MSD) Ophthalmic Solution is a non-selective beta-adrenergic receptor blocking agent. Its chemical name is (S)-1-[(1,1-dimethylethyl)amino]-3-[[4-(4-morpholinyl)-1,2,5-thiadiazol-3-yl]oxy]-2-propanol, (Z)-butenedioate (1:1) salt. Timolol maleate possesses an asymmetric carbon atom in its structure and is provided as the levo isomer. The nominal optical rotation of timolol maleate is

$[\alpha]^{25°}_{405\ nm}$ in 0.1 N HCl (C = 5%) = −12.2°.

Its empirical formula is $C_{13}H_{24}N_4O_3S \cdot C_4H_4O_4$.

TIMOPTIC Ophthalmic Solution is supplied as a sterile, isotonic, buffered, aqueous solution of timolol maleate in two dosage strengths: Each ml of TIMOPTIC 0.25% contains 2.5 mg of timolol (3.4 mg of timolol maleate). Each ml of TIMOPTIC 0.5% contains 5.0 mg of timolol (6.8 mg of timolol maleate). Inactive ingredients: monobasic and dibasic sodium phosphate, sodium hydroxide to adjust pH, and water for injection. Benzalkonium chloride 0.01% is added as preservative.

Timolol maleate has a molecular weight of 432.49. It is a white, odorless, crystalline powder which is soluble in water, methanol, and alcohol. TIMOPTIC is stable at room temperature.

Clinical Pharmacology

Timolol maleate is a $beta_1$ and $beta_2$ (non-selective) adrenergic receptor blocking agent that does not have significant intrinsic sympathomimetic, direct myocardial depressant, or local anesthetic (membrane-stabilizing) activity.

TIMOPTIC Ophthalmic Solution, when applied topically in the eye, has the action of reducing elevated as well as normal intraocular pressure, whether or not accompanied by glaucoma. Elevated intraocular pressure is a major risk factor in the pathogenesis of glaucomatous visual field loss. The higher the level of intraocular pressure, the greater the likelihood of glaucomatous visual field loss and optic nerve damage.

The onset of reduction in intraocular pressure following administration of TIMOPTIC can usually be detected within one-half hour after a single dose. The maximum effect usually occurs in one to two hours and significant lowering of intraocular pressure can be maintained for periods as long as 24 hours with a single dose. Repeated observations over a period of one year indicate that the intraocular pressure-lowering effect of TIMOPTIC is well maintained.

The precise mechanism of the ocular hypotensive action of TIMOPTIC is not clearly established at this time. Tonography and fluorophotometry studies in man suggest that its predominant action may be related to reduced aqueous formation. However, in some studies a slight increase in outflow facility was also observed. Unlike miotics, TIMOPTIC reduces intraocular pressure with little or no effect on accommodation or pupil size. Thus, changes in visual acuity due to increased accommodation are uncommon, and dim or blurred vision and night blindness produced by miotics are not evident. In addition, in patients with cataracts the inability to see around lenticular opacities when the pupil is constricted is avoided.

In controlled multiclinic studies in patients with untreated intraocular pressures of 22 mmHg or greater, TIMOPTIC 0.25 percent or 0.5 percent administered twice a day produced a greater reduction in intraocular pressure than 1, 2, 3, or 4 percent pilocarpine solution administered four times a day or 0.5, 1, or 2 percent epinephrine hydrochloride solution administered twice a day.

In the multiclinic studies comparing TIMOPTIC with pilocarpine, 61 percent of patients treated with TIMOPTIC had intraocular pressure reduced to less than 22 mmHg compared to 32 percent of patients treated with pilocarpine. For patients completing these studies, the mean reduction in pressure at the end of the study from pretreatment was 30.7 percent for patients treated with TIMOPTIC and 21.7 percent for patients treated with pilocarpine.

In the multiclinic studies comparing TIMOPTIC with epinephrine, 69 percent of patients treated with TIMOPTIC had intraocular pressure reduced to less than 22 mmHg compared to 42 percent of patients treated with epinephrine. For patients completing these studies, the mean reduction in pressure at the end of the study from pretreatment was 33.2 percent for patients treated with TIMOPTIC and 28.1 percent for patients treated with epinephrine.

In these studies, TIMOPTIC was generally well tolerated and produced fewer and less severe side effects than either pilocarpine or epinephrine.

TIMOPTIC has also been used in patients with glaucoma wearing conventional (PMMA) hard contact lenses, and has generally been well tolerated. TIMOPTIC has not been studied in patients wearing lenses made with materials other than PMMA.

Indications and Usage

TIMOPTIC Ophthalmic Solution has been shown to be effective in lowering intraocular pressure and may be used in:

Patients with chronic open-angle glaucoma

Patients with aphakic glaucoma

Some patients with secondary glaucoma

Other patients with elevated intraocular pressure who are at sufficient risk to require lowering of the ocular pressure.

Clinical trials have also shown that in patients who respond inadequately to multiple antiglaucoma drug therapy the addition of TIMOPTIC may produce a further reduction of intraocular pressure.

Contraindications

Bronchospasm, including bronchial asthma, or severe chronic obstructive pulmonary disease

Uncontrolled cardiac failure

Hypersensitivity to any component of this product

Warnings

As with other topically applied ophthalmic drugs, this drug may be absorbed systemically.

Precautions

General

TIMOPTIC Ophthalmic Solution should be used with caution in patients with known contraindications to systemic use of beta-adrenergic receptor blocking agents. These include sinus bradycardia and greater than first degree block and cardiogenic shock. Cardiac failure should be adequately controlled before beginning therapy with TIMOPTIC. In patients with a history of severe cardiac disease, signs of cardiac failure should be watched for and pulse rates should be checked.

TIMOPTIC Ophthalmic Solution should also be used with caution in patients with diabetes, especially labile diabetes.

Patients who are receiving a beta-adrenergic blocking agent orally and TIMOPTIC should be observed for a potential additive effect either on the intraocular pressure or on the known systemic effects of beta blockade.

In patients with angle-closure glaucoma, the immediate objective of treatment is to reopen the angle. This requires constricting the pupil with a miotic. TIMOPTIC has little or no effect on the pupil. When TIMOPTIC is used to reduce elevated intraocular pressure in angle-closure glaucoma, it should be used with a miotic and not alone.

As with the use of other antiglaucoma drugs, diminished responsiveness to TIMOPTIC after prolonged therapy has been reported in some patients. However, in one long-term study in which 96 patients have been followed for at least 3 years, no significant difference in mean intraocular pressure has been observed after initial stabilization.

Drug Interactions

Although TIMOPTIC used alone has little or no effect on pupil size, mydriasis resulting from concomitant therapy with TIMOPTIC and epinephrine has been reported occasionally.

Close observation of the patient is recommended when a beta blocker is administered to patients receiving catecholamine-depleting drugs such as reserpine, because of possible additive effects and the production of hypotension and/or marked bradycardia, which may produce vertigo, syncope, or postural hypotension.

Animal Studies

No adverse ocular effects were observed in rabbits and dogs administered TIMOPTIC topically in studies lasting one and two years respectively.

Carcinogenesis, Mutagenesis, Impairment of Fertility

In a two-year oral study of timolol maleate in rats, there was a statistically significant ($P \leq 0.05$) increase in the incidence of adrenal pheochromocytomas in male rats administered 300 times the maximum recommended human oral dose* (1 mg/kg/day). Similar differences were not observed in rats administered oral doses equivalent to 25 or 100 times the maxi-

*The maximum recommended single oral dose is 30 mg of timolol. One drop of TIMOPTIC 0.5% contains about 1/150 of this dose which is about 0.2 mg.

mum recommended human oral dose. In a lifetime oral study in mice, there were statistically significant ($P \leq 0.05$) increases in the incidence of benign and malignant pulmonary tumors and benign uterine polyps in female mice at 500 mg/kg/day, but not at 5 or 50 mg/kg/day. There was also a significant increase in mammary adenocarcinomas at the 500 mg/kg/day dose. This was associated with elevations in serum prolactin which occurred in female mice administered timolol at 500 mg/kg, but not at doses of 5 or 50 mg/kg/day. An increased incidence of mammary adenocarcinomas in rodents has been associated with administration of several other therapeutic agents which elevate serum prolactin, but no correlation between serum prolactin levels and mammary tumors has been established in man. Furthermore, in adult human female subjects who received oral dosages of up to 60 mg of timolol maleate, the maximum recommended human oral dosage, there were no clinically meaningful changes in serum prolactin.

There was a statistically significant increase ($P \leq 0.05$) in the overall incidence of neoplasms in female mice at the 500 mg/kg/day dosage level.

Timolol maleate was devoid of mutagenic potential when evaluated *in vivo* (mouse) in the micronucleus test and cytogenetic assay (doses up to 800 mg/kg) and *in vitro* in a neoplastic cell transformation assay (up to 100 μg/ml). In Ames tests the highest concentrations of timolol employed, 5000 or 10,000 μg/plate, were associated with statistically significant elevations ($P \leq 0.05$) of revertants observed with tester strain TA100 (in seven replicate assays), but not in the remaining three strains. In the assays with tester strain TA100, no consistent dose response relationship was observed, nor did the ratio of test to control revertants reach 2. A ratio of 2 is usually considered the criterion for a positive Ames test.

Reproduction and fertility studies in rats showed no adverse effect on male or female fertility at doses up to 150 times the maximum recommended human oral dose.

Pregnancy

Pregnancy Category C. Teratogenic studies with timolol in mice and rabbits at doses up to 50 mg/kg/day (50 times the maximum recommended human oral dose) showed no evidence of fetal malformations. Although delayed fetal ossification was observed at this dose in rats, there were no adverse effects on postnatal development of offspring. Doses of 1000 mg/kg/day (1,000 times the maximum recommended human oral dose) were maternotoxic in mice and resulted in an increased number of fetal resorptions. Increased fetal resorptions were also seen in rabbits at doses of 100 times the maximum recommended human oral dose, in this case without apparent maternotoxicity. There are no adequate and well-controlled studies in pregnant women. TIMOPTIC should be used during pregnancy only if the potential benefit justifies the potential risk to the fetus.

Nursing Mothers

Because of the potential for serious adverse reactions from timolol in nursing infants, a decision should be made whether to discontinue nursing or to discontinue the drug, taking into acccount the importance of the drug to the mother.

Pediatric Use

Safety and effectiveness in children have not been established by adequate and well-controlled studies.

Adverse Reactions

TIMOPTIC Ophthalmic Solution is usually well tolerated. The following adverse reactions have been reported either in clinical trials of up to 3 years duration prior to release in 1978 or since the drug has been marketed:

Signs and symptoms of ocular irritation, including conjunctivitis, blepharitis, keratitis, and blepharoptosis, have been reported occasionally.

Hypersensitivity reactions, including localized and generalized rash, and urticaria have been reported rarely.

Visual disturbances including refractive changes (due to withdrawal of miotic therapy in some cases), have been infrequently associated with therapy with TIMOPTIC. Rarely, aphakic cystoid macular edema has been reported, but a causal relationship to therapy with TIMOPTIC has not been established.

Aggravation or precipitation of certain cardiovascular, pulmonary and other disorders, presumably related to effects of systemic beta blockade has been reported (see CONTRAINDICATIONS and PRECAUTIONS). These include bradyarrhythmia, hypotension, syncope, and bronchospasm (predominantly in patients with pre-existing bronchospastic disease). Respiratory failure; congestive heart failure; and in insulin-dependent diabetics, masked symptoms of hypoglycemia; have been reported rarely. In clinical trials, slight reduction of the resting heart rate in some patients (mean reduction 2.9 beats/minute, standard deviation 10.2) has been observed.

The following adverse effects have been reported rarely, and a causal relationship to therapy with TIMOPTIC has not been established: headache, dry mouth, anorexia, dyspepsia, nausea, dizziness, decreased corneal sensitivity, CNS effects (e.g., fatigue, confusion, depression, somnolence and anxiety), palpitation, and hypertension.

Dosage and Administration

TIMOPTIC Ophthalmic Solution is available in concentrations of 0.25 and 0.5 percent. The usual starting dose is one drop of 0.25 percent TIMOPTIC in the affected eye(s) twice a day. If the clinical response is not adequate, the dosage may be changed to one drop of 0.5 percent solution in the affected eye(s) twice a day.

Since in some patients the pressure-lowering response to TIMOPTIC may require a few weeks to stabilize, evaluation should include a determination of intraocular pressure after approximately 4 weeks of treatment with TIMOPTIC.

If the intraocular pressure is maintained at satisfactory levels, the dosage schedule may be changed to one drop once a day in the affected eye(s). Because of diurnal variations in intraocular pressure, satisfactory response to the once-a-day dose is best determined by measuring the intraocular pressure at different times during the day.

Dosages above one drop of 0.5 percent TIMOPTIC twice a day generally have not been shown to produce further reduction in intraocular pressure. If the patient's intraocular pressure is still not at a satisfactory level on this regimen, concomitant therapy with pilocarpine and other miotics, and/or epinephrine, and/or systemically administered carbonic anhydrase inhibitors, such as acetazolamide, can be instituted.

When a patient is transferred from a single antiglaucoma agent, continue the agent already being used and add one drop of 0.25 percent TIMOPTIC in the affected eye(s) twice a day. On the following day, discontinue the previously used antiglaucoma agent completely and continue with TIMOPTIC. If a higher dosage of TIMOPTIC is required, substitute one drop of 0.5 percent solution in the affected eye(s) twice a day.

When a patient is transferred from several concomitantly administered antiglaucoma agents, individualization is required. Adjustments should involve one agent at a time and usually should be made at intervals of not less than one week. A recommended approach is to continue the agents being used and to add one drop of 0.25 percent TIMOPTIC in the affected eye(s) twice a day. On the following day, discontinue one of the other antiglaucoma agents. The remaining antiglaucoma agents may be decreased or discontinued according to the patient's response to treatment. If a higher dosage of TIMOPTIC is required, substitute one drop of 0.5 percent solution in the affected eye(s) twice a day. The physician may be able to discontinue some or all of the other antiglaucoma agents.

How Supplied

Sterile Ophthalmic Solution TIMOPTIC is a clear, colorless to light yellow solution.

No. 3366—TIMOPTIC Ophthalmic Solution, 0.25% timolol equivalent, is supplied in a white, opaque, plastic OCUMETER® ophthalmic dispenser with a controlled drop tip as follows:

NDC 0006-3366-03, 5 ml
NDC 0006-3366-10, 10 ml
NDC 0006-3366-12, 15 ml.

No. 3367—TIMOPTIC Ophthalmic Solution, 0.5% timolol equivalent, is supplied in a white, opaque, plastic OCUMETER ophthalmic dispenser with a controlled drop tip as follows:

NDC 0006-3367-03, 5 ml
NDC 0006-3367-10, 10 ml
NDC 0006-3367-12, 15 ml.

A.H.F.S. Category: 52:36

DC 7046016 Issued February 1982

COPYRIGHT © MERCK & CO., INC., 1978
All rights reserved

TRIAVIL® Tablets ℞

Tranquilizer-antidepressant

Description

TRIAVIL®, a broad-spectrum psychotherapeutic agent for the management of outpatients and hospitalized patients with psychoses or neuroses characterized by mixtures of anxiety or agitation with symptoms of depression, is a combination of perphenazine and ELAVIL® (Amitriptyline HCl, MSD). Since such mixed syndromes can occur in patients with various degrees of intensity of mental illness, TRIAVIL tablets are provided in multiple combinations to afford dosage flexibility for optimum management.

Actions

Perphenazine—In common with all members of the piperazine group of phenothiazine derivatives, perphenazine has greater behavioral potency than phenothiazine derivatives of other groups without a corresponding increase in autonomic, hematologic, or hepatic side effects.

Extrapyramidal effects, however, may occur more frequently. These effects are interpreted as neuropharmacologic. They usually regress after discontinuation of the drug.

Perphenazine is a potent tranquilizer and also a potent antiemetic. Orally, its milligram potency is about five or six times that of chlorpromazine with respect to behavorial effects. It is capable of alleviating symptoms of anxiety, tension, psychomotor excitement, and other manifestations of emotional stress without apparent dulling of mental acuity.

ELAVIL (Amitriptyline HCl, MSD) is an antidepressant with sedative effects. Its mechanism of action in man is not known. It is not a monoamine oxidase inhibitor and it does not act primarily by stimulation of the central nervous system.

Continued on next page

Information on the Merck Sharp & Dohme products listed on these pages is the full prescribing information from package circulars in use October 31, 1982.

Merck Sharp & Dohme—Cont.

Indications

TRIAVIL is recommended for treatment of (1) patients with *moderate to severe anxiety and/or agitation and depressed mood,* (2) patients with *depression in whom anxiety and/or agitation are severe,* and (3) patients with *depression and anxiety in association with chronic physical disease.* In many of these patients, anxiety masks the depressive state so that, although therapy with a tranquilizer appears to be indicated, the administration of a tranquilizer alone will not be adequate.
Schizophrenic patients who have associated depressive symptoms should be considered for therapy with TRIAVIL.
Many patients presenting symptoms such as agitation, anxiety, insomnia, psychomotor retardation, functional somatic complaints, a feeling of tiredness, loss of interest, and anorexia have responded well to therapy with TRIAVIL.

Contraindications

TRIAVIL is contraindicated in depression of the central nervous system from drugs (barbiturates, alcohol, narcotics, analgesics, antihistamines); in the presence of evidence of bone marrow depression; and in patients known to be hypersensitive to phenothiazines or amitriptyline.
It should not be given concomitantly with monoamine oxidase inhibitors. Hyperpyretic crises, severe convulsions, and deaths have occurred in patients receiving tricyclic antidepressants and monoamine oxidase inhibitors simultaneously. When it is desired to replace a monoamine oxidase inhibitor with TRIAVIL, a minimum of 14 days should be allowed to elapse after the former is discontinued. TRIAVIL should then be initiated cautiously with gradual increase in dosage until optimum response is achieved.
Amitriptyline HCl is not recommended for use during the acute recovery phase following myocardial infarction.

Warnings

TRIAVIL should not be given concomitantly with guanethidine or similarly acting compounds, since amitriptyline, like other tricyclic antidepressants, may block the antihypertensive effect of these compounds.
Because of the atropine-like activity of amitriptyline, TRIAVIL should be used with caution in patients with a history of urinary retention, or with angle-closure glaucoma or increased intraocular pressure. In patients with angle-closure glaucoma, even average doses may precipitate an attack.
It should be used with caution also in patients with convulsive disorders. Dosage of anticonvulsive agents may have to be increased.
Patients with cardiovascular disorders should be watched closely. Tricyclic antidepressants, including amitriptyline HCl, particularly when given in high doses, have been reported to produce arrhythmias, sinus tachycardia, and prolongation of the conduction time. Myocardial infarction and stroke have been reported with drugs of this class.
Close supervision is required when amitriptyline HCl is given to hyperthyroid patients or those receiving thyroid medication.
This drug may impair mental and/or physical abilities required for performance of hazardous tasks, such as operating machinery or driving a motor vehicle.
TRIAVIL may enhance the response to alcohol and the effects of barbiturates and other CNS depressants. In patients who may use alcohol excessively, it should be borne in mind that the potentiation may increase the danger inherent in any suicide attempt or overdosage.
Usage in Pregnancy—TRIAVIL is not recommended for use in pregnant patients at this time. Reproduction studies in rats have shown no fetal abnormalities; however, clinical experience and follow-up in pregnancy have been limited, and the possibility of adverse effects on fetal development must be considered.
Usage in Children—Since dosage for children has not been established, TRIAVIL is not recommended for use in children.

Precautions

The possibility of suicide in depressed patients remains during treatment and until significant remission occurs. Such patients should not have access to large quantities of this drug.

Perphenazine
As with all phenothiazine compounds, perphenazine should not be used indiscriminately. Caution should be observed in giving it to patients who have previously exhibited severe adverse reactions to other phenothiazines.
Some of the untoward actions of perphenazine tend to appear more frequently when high doses are used. However, as with other phenothiazine compounds, patients receiving perphenazine in any dosage should be kept under close supervision.
The antiemetic effect of perphenazine may obscure signs of toxicity due to overdosage of other drugs, or render more difficult the diagnosis of disorders such as brain tumors or intestinal obstruction.
A significant, not otherwise explained, rise in body temperature may suggest individual intolerance to perphenazine, in which case TRIAVIL should be discontinued.
If hypotension develops, epinephrine should not be employed, as its action is blocked and partially reversed by perphenazine.
Phenothiazines may potentiate the action of central nervous system depressants (opiates, analgesics, antihistamines, barbiturates, alcohol) and atropine. In concurrent therapy with any of these, TRIAVIL should be given in reduced dosage. Phenothiazines also may potentiate the action of heat and phosphorous insecticides.
Neuroleptic drugs elevate prolactin levels; the elevation persists during chronic administration. Tissue culture experiments indicate that approximately one-third of human breast cancers are prolactin dependent in vitro, a factor of potential importance if the prescription of these drugs is contemplated in a patient with a previously detected breast cancer. Although disturbances such as galactorrhea, amenorrhea, gynecomastia, and impotence have been reported, the clinical significance of elevated serum prolactin levels is unknown for most patients. An increase in mammary neoplasms has been found in rodents after chronic administration of neuroleptic drugs. Neither clinical studies nor epidemiologic studies conducted to date, however, have shown an association between chronic administration of these drugs and mammary tumorigenesis; the available evidence is considered too limited to be conclusive at this time.

ELAVIL (Amitriptyline HCl, MSD)
Depressed patients, particularly those with known manic depressive illness, may experience a shift to mania or hypomania. Patients with paranoid symptomatology may have an exaggeration of such symptoms. The tranquilizing effect of TRIAVIL seems to reduce the likelihood of these effects.
When ELAVIL (Amitriptyline HCl, MSD) is given with anticholinergic agents or sympathomimetic drugs, including epinephrine combined with local anesthetics, close supervision and careful adjustment of dosages are required.
Paralytic ileus may occur in patients taking tricyclic antidepressants in combination with anticholinergic-type drugs.
Caution is advised if patients receive large doses of ethchlorvynol concurrently. Transient delirium has been reported in patients who were treated with 1 g of ethchlorvynol and 75-150 mg of ELAVIL (Amitriptyline HCl, MSD).
Concurrent administration of amitriptyline HCl and electroshock therapy may increase the hazards associated with such therapy. Such treatment should be limited to patients for whom it is essential.
Discontinue the drug several days before elective surgery if possible.
Both elevation and lowering of blood sugar levels have been reported.
ELAVIL (Amitriptyline HCl, MSD) should be used with caution in patients with impaired liver function.

Adverse Reactions

To date, clinical evaluation of TRIAVIL has not revealed any adverse reactions peculiar to the combination. The adverse reactions that occurred were limited to those that have been reported previously for perphenazine and amitriptyline.

Perphenazine
Extrapyramidal symptoms (opisthotonus, oculogyric crisis, hyper-reflexia, dystonia, akathisia, acute dyskinesia, ataxia, parkinsonism) have been reported. Their incidence and severity usually increase with an increase in dosage, but there is considerable individual variation in the tendency to develop such symptoms. Extrapyramidal symptoms can usually be controlled by the concomitant use of effective antiparkinsonian drugs, such as benztropine mesylate, and/or by reduction in dosage. In some instances, they may persist after discontinuation of the drug.
Tardive dyskinesia may appear in some patients on long-term therapy or may occur after drug therapy with phenothiazines and related agents has been discontinued. The risk appears to be greater in elderly patients on high-dose therapy, especially females. The symptoms are persistent and in some patients appear to be irreversible. The syndrome is characterized by rhythmical involuntary movements of the tongue, face, mouth or jaw (e.g., protrusion of tongue, puffing of cheeks, puckering of mouth, chewing movements). Involuntary movements of the extremities sometimes occur. There is no known treatment for tardive dyskinesia; antiparkinsonism agents usually do not alleviate the symptoms. It is advised that all antipsychotic agents be discontinued if the above symptoms appear. If treatment is reinstituted, or dosage of the particular drug increased, or another drug substituted, the syndrome may be masked. It has been suggested that fine vermicular movements of the tongue may be an early sign of the syndrome, and that the full-blown syndrome may not develop if medication is stopped when lingual vermiculation appears.
Skin disorders have occurred with phenothiazine compounds (photosensitivity, itching, erythema, urticaria, eczema, up to exfoliative dermatitis); as well as other allergic reactions (asthma, laryngeal edema, angioneurotic edema, anaphylactoid reactions); peripheral edema; reversed epinephrine effect; hyperglycemia; endocrine disturbances (lactation, galactorrhea, gynecomastia, disturbances in the menstrual cycle); altered cerebrospinal fluid proteins; paradoxical excitement; hypertension, hypotension, tachycardia, and EKG abnormalities (quinidine-like effect). Reactivation of psychotic processes and the production of catatonic-like states have been described.
Autonomic reactions, such as dry mouth or salivation, headache, anorexia, nausea, vomiting, constipation, obstipation, urinary fre-

quency or incontinence, blurred vision, nasal congestion, and a change in the pulse rate occasionally may occur.

Other adverse reactions reported with various phenothiazine compounds, but not with perphenazine, include grand mal convulsions, cerebral edema, polyphagia, photophobia, skin pigmentation, and failure of ejaculation.

The phenothiazine compounds have produced blood dyscrasias (pancytopenia, thrombocytopenic purpura, leukopenia, agranulocytosis, eosinophilia); and liver damage (jaundice, biliary stasis).

Pigmentary retinopathy has been reported to occur after administration of some phenothiazines with a piperidylethyl side chain, but not with perphenazine which has a piperazine side chain.

Pigmentation of the cornea and lens has been reported to occur after long-term administration of some phenothiazines. Although it has not been reported in patients receiving TRIAVIL, the possibility that it might occur should be considered.

Hypnotic effects appear to be minimal, particularly in patients who are permitted to remain active.

A few patients have reported lassitude, muscle weakness, and mild insomnia.

False positive pregnancy tests, including immunologic, have been reported with phenothiazines.

ELAVIL (Amitriptyline HCl, MSD)

Note: Included in the listing which follows are a few adverse reactions which have not been reported with this specific drug. However, pharmacological similarities among the tricyclic antidepressant drugs require that each of the reactions be considered when amitriptyline is administered.

Cardiovascular: Hypotension, particularly orthostatic hypotension; hypertension; tachycardia; palpitation; myocardial infarction; arrhythmias; heart block; stroke.

CNS and Neuromuscular: Confusional states; disturbed concentration; disorientation; delusions; hallucinations; excitement; anxiety; restlessness; insomnia; nightmares; numbness, tingling, and paresthesias of the extremities; peripheral neuropathy; incoordination; ataxia; tremors; seizures; alteration in EEG patterns; extrapyramidal symptoms; tinnitus; syndrome of inappropriate ADH (antidiuretic hormone) secretion.

Anticholinergic: Dry mouth, blurred vision, disturbance of accommodation, increased intraocular pressure, constipation, paralytic ileus, urinary retention, dilatation of urinary tract.

Allergic: Skin rash, urticaria, photosensitization, edema of face and tongue.

Hematologic: Bone marrow depression including agranulocytosis, leukopenia, eosinophilia, purpura, thrombocytopenia.

Gastrointestinal: Nausea, epigastric distress, vomiting, anorexia, stomatitis, peculiar taste, diarrhea, parotid swelling, black tongue. Rarely hepatitis (including altered liver function and jaundice).

Endocrine: Testicular swelling and gynecomastia in the male, breast enlargement and galactorrhea in the female, increased or decreased libido, elevation and lowering of blood sugar levels.

Other: Dizziness, weakness, fatigue, headache, weight gain or loss, edema, increased perspiration, urinary frequency, mydriasis, drowsiness, alopecia.

Withdrawal Symptoms: Abrupt cessation of treatment after prolonged administration may produce nausea, headache, and malaise. These are not indicative of addiction. Rare instances have been reported of mania or hypomania occurring within 2–7 days following cessation of chronic therapy with tricyclic antidepressants.

Dosage and Administration

TRIAVIL tablets are provided as:

TRIAVIL 2-25, containing 2 mg of perphenazine and 25 mg of amitriptyline HCl.

TRIAVIL 4-25, containing 4 mg of perphenazine and 25 mg of amitriptyline HCl.

TRIAVIL 4-50, containing 4 mg of perphenazine and 50 mg of amitriptyline HCl.

TRIAVIL 2-10, containing 2 mg of perphenazine and 10 mg of amitriptyline HCl.

TRIAVIL 4-10, containing 4 mg of perphenazine and 10 mg of amitriptyline HCl.

Since dosage for children has not been established, TRIAVIL is not recommended for use in children.

The total daily dose of TRIAVIL should not exceed four tablets of the 4-50 or eight tablets of any other dosage strength.

Initial Dosage

In psychoneurotic patients when anxiety and depression are of such a degree as to warrant combined therapy, one tablet of TRIAVIL 2-25 or TRIAVIL 4-25 three or four times a day or one tablet of TRIAVIL 4-50 twice a day is recommended.

In more severely ill patients with schizophrenia, TRIAVIL 4-25 is recommended in an initial dose of two tablets three times a day. If necessary, a fourth dose may be given at bedtime.

In elderly patients and adolescents, and some other patients in whom anxiety tends to predominate, TRIAVIL 4-10 may be administered three or four times a day initially, then adjusted as required for subsequent adequate therapy.

Maintenance Dosage

Depending on the condition being treated, therapeutic response may take from a few days to a few weeks or even longer. After a satisfactory response is noted, dosage should be reduced to the smallest amount necessary to obtain relief from the symptoms for which TRIAVIL is being administered. A useful maintenance dosage is one tablet of TRIAVIL 2-25 or 4-25 two to four times a day or one tablet of TRIAVIL 4-50 twice a day. TRIAVIL 2-10 and 4-10 can be used to increase flexibility in adjusting maintenance dosage to the lowest amount consistent with relief of symptoms. In some patients, maintenance dosage is required for many months.

Overdosage

Manifestations—High doses may cause temporary confusion, disturbed concentration, or transient visual hallucinations. Overdosage may cause drowsiness; hypothermia; tachycardia and other arrhythmic abnormalities, such as bundle branch block; ECG evidence of impaired conduction; congestive heart failure; dilated pupils; disorders of ocular motility; convulsions; severe hypotension; stupor; and coma. Other symptoms may be agitation, hyperactive reflexes, muscle rigidity, vomiting, hyperpyrexia, or any of the adverse reactions listed for perphenazine or amitriptyline.

Levarterenol (norepinephrine) may be used to treat hypotension, but not epinephrine.

All patients suspected of having taken an overdosage should be admitted to a hospital as soon as possible. *Treatment* is symptomatic and supportive. Empty the stomach as quickly as possible by emesis followed by gastric lavage upon arrival at the hospital. Saline emetics should not be used as the antiemetic effect of perphenazine may cause retention of the saline load and subsequent hypernatremia. Following gastric lavage, activated charcoal may be administered. Twenty to 30 g of activated charcoal may be given every four to six hours during the first 24 to 48 hours after ingestion. An ECG should be taken and close monitoring of cardiac function instituted if there is any sign of abnormality. Maintain an open airway and adequate fluid intake; regulate body temperature.

The intravenous administration of 1–3 mg of physostigmine salicylate is reported to reverse the symptoms of tricyclic antidepressant poisoning. Because physostigmine is rapidly metabolized, the dosage of physostigmine should be repeated as required particularly if life threatening signs such as arrhythmias, convulsions, and deep coma recur or persist after the initial dosage of physostigmine. On this basis, in severe overdosage with perphenazine-amitriptyline combinations, symptomatic treatment of central anticholinergic effects with physostigmine salicylate should be considered. Because physostigmine itself may be toxic, it is not recommended for routine use.

Standard measures should be used to manage circulatory shock and metabolic acidosis. Cardiac arrhythmias may be treated with neostigmine, pyridostigmine, or propranolol. Should cardiac failure occur, the use of digitalis should be considered. Close monitoring of cardiac function for not less than five days is advisable.

Anticonvulsants may be given to control convulsions. Amitriptyline and perphenazine increase the CNS depressant action but not the anticonvulsant action of barbiturates; therefore, an inhalation anesthetic, diazepam, or paraldehyde is recommended for control of convulsions. The management of acute symptoms of parkinsonism resulting from perphenazine intoxication may be treated with appropriate doses of COGENTIN® (Benztropine Mesylate, MSD) or diphenhydramine hydrochloride.*

Dialysis is of no value because of low plasma concentrations of the drug.

Since overdosage is often deliberate, patients may attempt suicide by other means during the recovery phase.

Deaths by deliberate or accidental overdosage have occurred with this class of drugs.

How Supplied

No. 3328—Tablets TRIAVIL 2–10 are blue, triangular, film coated tablets, coded MSD 914. They are supplied as follows:

NDC 0006-0914-68 bottles of 100

NDC 0006-0914-28 single unit package of 100

NDC 0006-0914-74 bottles of 500.

[*Shown in Product Identification Section*]

No. 3311—Tablets TRIAVIL 2–25 are orange, triangular, film coated tablets, coded MSD 921. They are supplied as follows:

NDC 0006-0921-68 bottles of 100

NDC 0006-0921-28 single unit package of 100

NDC 0006-0921-74 bottles of 500

(6505-00-931-4303 500's)

[*Shown in Product Identification Section*]

No. 3310—Tablets TRIAVIL 4–10 are salmon, triangular, film coated tablets, coded MSD 934. They are supplied as follows:

NDC 0006-0934-68 bottles of 100

NDC 0006-0934-28 single unit package of 100

NDC 0006-0934-74 bottles of 500.

[*Shown in Product Identification Section*]

No. 3312—Tablets TRIAVIL 4–25 are yellow, triangular, film coated tablets, coded MSD 946. They are supplied as follows:

NDC 0006-0946-68 bottles of 100

(6505-01-012-7558 100's)

NDC 0006-0946-28 single unit package of 100

*BENADRYL® (Diphenhydramine Hydrochloride), Parke, Davis & Co.

Continued on next page

Information on the Merck Sharp & Dohme products listed on these pages is the full prescribing information from package circulars in use October 31, 1982.

Merck Sharp & Dohme—Cont.

NDC 0006-0946-74 bottles of 500.
[*Shown in Product Identification Section*]
No. 3364—Tablets TRIAVIL 4-50 are orange, diamond shaped, film coated tablets, coded MSD 517. They are supplied as follows:
NDC 0006-0517-60 bottles of 60
NDC 0006-0517-68 bottles of 100
NDC 0006-0517-28 single unit package of 100
[*Shown in Product Identification Section*]
A.H.F.S. Categories: 28:16:04, 28:16:08
DC 6613219 Issued October 1981

TURBINAIRE®—see under DECADRON® Phosphate, TURBINAIRE® (dexamethasone sodium phosphate, MSD)

URECHOLINE® Tablets ℞
(bethanechol chloride, MSD), U.S.P.
URECHOLINE® Injection ℞
(bethanechol chloride, MSD), U.S.P.

Description

Bethanechol chloride is an ester of a choline-like compound.
It is designated chemically as 2-[(amino-carbonyl) oxy] -*N, N, N*-trimethyl-1-propan-aminium chloride.
It is a white, hygroscopic crystalline compound having a slight amine-like odor and is freely soluble in water.
URECHOLINE® (Bethanechol Chloride, MSD) is available as 5 mg, 10 mg, 25 mg, and 50 mg tablets for oral use, and as a sterile solution for subcutaneous use only.
The sterile solution is essentially neutral. Each milliliter contains bethanechol chloride, 5 mg, and Water for Injection, q.s., 1 ml. It may be autoclaved at 120° C for 20 minutes without discoloration or loss of potency.

Actions

Bethanechol chloride acts principally by producing the effects of stimulation of the parasympathetic nervous system. It increases the tone of the detrusor urinae muscle, usually producing a contraction sufficiently strong to initiate micturition and empty the bladder. It stimulates gastric motility, increases gastric tone, and often restores impaired rhythmic peristalsis.
Stimulation of the parasympathetic nervous system releases acetylcholine at the nerve endings. When spontaneous stimulation is reduced and therapeutic intervention is required, acetylcholine can be given, but it is rapidly hydrolyzed by cholinesterase, and its effects are transient. Bethanechol chloride is not destroyed by cholinesterase and its effects are more prolonged than those of acetylcholine.
It has predominant muscarinic action and only feeble nicotinic action. Doses that stimulate micturition and defecation and increase peristalsis do not ordinarily stimulate ganglia or voluntary muscles. Therapeutic test doses in normal human subjects have little effect on heart rate, blood pressure, or peripheral circulation.
A clinical study* was conducted on the relative effectiveness of oral and subcutaneous doses of bethanechol chloride on the stretch response of bladder muscle in patients with urinary retention. Results showed that 5 mg of the drug given subcutaneously stimulated a response that was more rapid in onset and of larger magnitude than an oral dose of 50 mg, 100 mg, or 200 mg. All the oral doses, however, had a longer duration of effect than the subcutaneous dose. Although the 50 mg oral dose caused little change in intravesical pressure in this study, this dose has been found in other studies to be clinically effective in the rehabilitation of patients with decompensated bladders.

*Diokno, A. C.; Lapides, J., Urol. *10:* 23–24, July 1977.

Indications

For the treatment of acute postoperative and postpartum nonobstructive (functional) urinary retention and for neurogenic atony of the urinary bladder with retention.

Contraindications

Hypersensitivity to URECHOLINE tablets or to any component of URECHOLINE injection, hyperthyroidism, pregnancy, peptic ulcer, latent or active bronchial asthma, pronounced bradycardia or hypotension, vasomotor instability, coronary artery disease, epilepsy, and parkinsonism.
URECHOLINE should not be employed when the strength or integrity of the gastrointestinal or bladder wall is in question, or in the presence of mechanical obstruction; when increased muscular activity of the gastrointestinal tract or urinary bladder might prove harmful, as following recent urinary bladder surgery, gastrointestinal resection and anastomosis, or when there is possible gastrointestinal obstruction; in bladder neck obstruction, spastic gastrointestinal disturbances, acute inflammatory lesions of the gastrointestinal tract, or peritonitis; or in marked vagotonia.

Warning

The sterile solution is for subcutaneous use only. It should never be given intramuscularly or intravenously. Violent symptoms of cholinergic over-stimulation, such as circulatory collapse, fall in blood pressure, abdominal cramps, bloody diarrhea, shock, or sudden cardiac arrest are likely to occur if the drug is given by either of these routes. Although rare, these same symptoms have occurred after subcutaneous injection, and may occur in cases of hypersensitivity or overdosage.

Precautions

Special care is required if this drug is given to patients receiving ganglion blocking compounds because a critical fall in blood pressure may occur. Usually, severe abdominal symptoms appear before there is such a fall in the blood pressure.
In urinary retention, if the sphincter fails to relax as URECHOLINE contracts the bladder, urine may be forced up the ureter into the kidney pelvis. If there is bacteriuria, this may cause reflux infection.

Adverse Reactions

Abdominal discomfort, salivation, flushing of the skin ("hot feeling"), sweating.
Large doses more commonly result in effects of parasympathetic stimulation, such as malaise, headache, sensation of heat about the face, flushing, colicky pain, diarrhea, nausea and belching, abdominal cramps, borborygmi, asthmatic attacks, and fall in blood pressure.
Atropine is a specific antidote. The recommended dose for adults is 0.6 mg (1/100 grain). The recommended dosage in infants and children up to 12 years of age is 0.01 mg/kg repeated every two hours as needed until the desired effect is obtained, or adverse effects of atropine preclude further usage. The maximum single dose should not exceed 0.4 mg. Subcutaneous injection of atropine is preferred except in emergencies when the intravenous route may be employed.
When URECHOLINE is administered subcutaneously, a syringe containing a dose of atropine sulfate should always be available to treat symptoms of toxicity.

Dosage and Administration

Dosage and route of administration must be individualized, depending on the type and severity of the condition to be treated.
Preferably give the drug when the stomach is empty. If taken soon after eating, nausea and vomiting may occur.
Oral—The usual adult dosage is 10 to 50 mg three or four times a day. The minimum effective dose is determined by giving 5 or 10 mg initially and repeating the same amount at hourly intervals until satisfactory response occurs or until a maximum of 50 mg has been given. The effects of the drug sometimes appear within 30 minutes and usually within 60 to 90 minutes. They persist for about an hour.
Subcutaneous—The usual dose is 1 ml (5 mg), although some patients respond satisfactorily to as little as 0.5 ml (2.5 mg). The minimum effective dose is determined by injecting 0.5 ml (2.5 mg) initially and repeating the same amount at 15 to 30 minute intervals to a maximum of four doses until satisfactory response is obtained, unless disturbing reactions appear. The minimum effective dose may be repeated thereafter three or four times a day as required.
Rarely, single doses up to 2 ml (10 mg) may be required. Such large doses may cause severe reactions and should be used only after adequate trial of single doses of 0.5 to 1 ml (2.5 to 5 mg) has established that smaller doses are not sufficient.
URECHOLINE is usually effective in 5 to 15 minutes after subcutaneous injection.
If necessary, the effects of the drug can be abolished promptly by atropine (see ADVERSE REACTIONS).

How Supplied

Tablets URECHOLINE are round, compressed tablets, scored on one side. They are supplied as follows:
No. 7785—5 mg, white in color, coded MSD 403.
NDC 0006-0403-68 in bottles of 100.
NDC 0006-0403-28 single unit packages of 100.
[*Shown in Product Identification Section*]
No. 7787—10 mg, pink in color, coded MSD 412.
NDC 0006-0412-68 in bottles of 100.
(6505-00-616-7856 10 mg 100's)
NDC 0006-0412-28 single unit packages of 100.
[*Shown in Product Identification Section*]
No. 7788—25 mg, yellow in color, coded MSD 457.
NDC 0006-0457-68 in bottles of 100.
NDC 0006-0457-28 single unit packages of 100.
[*Shown in Product Identification Section*]
No. 7790 — 50 mg, yellow in color, coded MSD 460.
NDC 0006-0460-68 in bottles of 100.
NDC 0006-0460-28 in single unit packages of 100.
[*Shown in Product Identification Section*]
No. 7786—Injection URECHOLINE, 5 mg per ml, is a clear, colorless solution, and is supplied as follows:
NDC 0006-7786-29 in box of 6 × 1 ml vials.
A.H.F.S. Category: 12:04
DC 6208426 Issued May 1980

VIVACTIL® Tablets ℞
(protriptyline HCl, MSD), U.S.P.

Description

Protriptyline HCl, a dibenzocycloheptene derivative, is a white to yellowish powder freely soluble in water.
It is designated chemically as N-methyl-5H-dibenzo[a,d]cycloheptene-5-propylamine hydrochloride.
The molecular weight is 299.8. The empirical formula is $C_{19}H_{21}N \bullet HCl$.
VIVACTIL® (Protriptyline HCl, MSD) is supplied as 5 mg and 10 mg film coated tablets.

Actions

VIVACTIL is an antidepressant agent. The mechanism of its antidepressant action in man is not known. It is not a monoamine oxidase inhibitor, and it does not act primarily by stimulation of the central nervous system.
VIVACTIL has been found in some studies to have a more rapid onset of action than imipramine or amitriptyline. The initial clinical effect may occur within one week. Sedative and tranquilizing properties are lacking. The rate of excretion is slow.

Indications

VIVACTIL is indicated for the treatment of symptoms of mental depression in patients who are under close medical supervision. Its activating properties make it particularly suitable for withdrawn and anergic patients.

Contraindications

VIVACTIL is contraindicated in patients who have shown prior hypersensitivity to it.
It should not be given concomitantly with a monoamine oxidase inhibiting compound. Hyperpyretic crises, severe convulsions, and deaths have occurred in patients receiving tricyclic antidepressant and monoamine oxidase inhibiting drugs simultaneously. When it is desired to substitute VIVACTIL for a monoamine oxidase inhibitor, a minimum of 14 days should be allowed to elapse after the latter is discontinued. VIVACTIL should then be initiated cautiously with gradual increase in dosage until optimum response is achieved.
This drug should not be used during the acute recovery phase following myocardial infarction.

Warnings

VIVACTIL may block the antihypertensive effect of guanethidine or similarly acting compounds.
It may impair mental and/or physical abilities required for the performance of hazardous tasks, such as operating machinery or driving a motor vehicle.
VIVACTIL should be used with caution in patients with a history of seizures, and, because of its autonomic activity, in patients with a tendency to urinary retention, or increased intraocular tension.
Tachycardia and postural hypotension may occur more frequently with VIVACTIL than with other antidepressant drugs. VIVACTIL should be used with caution in elderly patients and patients with cardiovascular disorders; such patients should be observed closely because of the tendency of the drug to produce tachycardia, hypotension, arrhythmias, and prolongation of the conduction time. Myocardial infarction and stroke have occurred with drugs of this class.
On rare occasions, hyperthyroid patients or those receiving thyroid medication may develop arrhythmias when this drug is given.
In patients who may use alcohol excessively, it should be borne in mind that the potentiation may increase the danger inherent in any suicide attempt or overdosage.

Usage in Children

This drug is not recommended for use in children because safety and effectiveness in the pediatric age group have not been established.

Usage in Pregnancy

Safe use in pregnancy and lactation has not been established; therefore, use in pregnant women, nursing mothers or women who may become pregnant requires that possible benefits be weighed against possible hazards to mother and child.
In mice, rats, and rabbits, doses about ten times greater than the recommended human doses had no apparent adverse effects on reproduction.

Precautions

When protriptyline HCl is used to treat the depressive component of schizophrenia, psychotic symptoms may be aggravated. Likewise, in manic-depressive psychosis, depressed patients may experience a shift toward the manic phase if they are treated with an antidepressant drug. Paranoid delusions, with or without associated hostility, may be exaggerated. In any of these circumstances, it may be advisable to reduce the dose of VIVACTIL or to use a major tranquilizing drug concurrently.
Symptoms, such as anxiety or agitation, may be aggravated in overactive or agitated patients.
When VIVACTIL is given with anticholinergic agents or sympathomimetic drugs, including epinephrine combined with local anesthetics, close supervision and careful adjustment of dosages are required.
It may enhance the response to alcohol and the effects of barbiturates and other CNS depressants.
The possibility of suicide in depressed patients remains during treatment and until significant remission occurs. This type of patient should not have access to large quantities of the drug.
Concurrent administration of VIVACTIL and electroshock therapy may increase the hazards of therapy. Such treatment should be limited to patients for whom it is essential.
Discontinue the drug several days before elective surgery, if possible.
Both elevation and lowering of blood sugar levels have been reported.

Adverse Reactions

Note: Included in the listing which follows are a few adverse reactions which have not been reported with this specific drug. However, the pharmacological similarities among the tricyclic antidepressant drugs require that each of the reactions be considered when protriptyline is administered. VIVACTIL is more likely to aggravate agitation and anxiety and produce cardiovascular reactions such as tachycardia and hypotension.
Cardiovascular: hypotension, particularly orthostatic hypotension; hypertension; tachycardia; palpitation; myocardial infarction; arrhythmias; heart block; stroke.
Psychiatric: confusional states (especially in the elderly) with hallucinations, disorientation, delusions, anxiety, restlessness, agitation; insomnia, panic, and nightmares; hypomania; exacerbation of psychosis.
Neurological: numbness, tingling, and paresthesias of extremities; incoordination, ataxia, tremors, peripheral neuropathy; extrapyramidal symptoms; seizures; alteration in EEG patterns, tinnitus.
Anticholinergic: dry mouth and rarely associated sublingual adenitis; blurred vision, disturbance of accommodation, increased intraocular pressure, mydriasis; constipation, paralytic ileus; urinary retention, delayed micturition, dilatation of the urinary tract.
Allergic: skin rash, petechiae, urticaria, itching, photosensitization (avoid excessive exposure to sunlight), edema (general, or of face and tongue), drug fever.
Hematologic: bone marrow depression; agranulocytosis; leukopenia; eosinophilia; purpura; thrombocytopenia.
Gastrointestinal: nausea and vomiting, anorexia, epigastric distress, diarrhea, peculiar taste, stomatitis, abdominal cramps, black tongue.
Endocrine: gynecomastia in the male; breast enlargement and galactorrhea in the female; increased or decreased libido, impotence; testicular swelling; elevation or depression of blood sugar levels.
Other: jaundice (simulating obstructive); altered liver function; weight gain or loss; perspiration; flushing; urinary frequency, nocturia; drowsiness, dizziness, weakness and fatigue; headache; parotid swelling; alopecia.
Withdrawal Symptoms: Though not indicative of addiction, abrupt cessation of treatment after prolonged therapy may produce nausea, headache, and malaise.

Dosage and Administration

Dosage should be initiated at a low level and increased gradually, noting carefully the clinical response and any evidence of intolerance.
Usual Adult Dosage—Fifteen to 40 mg a day divided into 3 or 4 doses. If necessary, dosage may be increased to 60 mg a day. Dosages above this amount are not recommended. Increases should be made in the morning dose.
Adolescent and Elderly Patients—In general, lower dosages are recommended for these patients. Five mg 3 times a day may be given initially, and increased gradually if necessary. In elderly patients, the cardiovascular system must be monitored closely if the daily dose exceeds 20 mg.
When satisfactory improvement has been reached, dosage should be reduced to the smallest amount that will maintain relief of symptoms.
Minor adverse reactions require reduction in dosage. Major adverse reactions or evidence of hypersensitivity require prompt discontinuation of the drug.
Usage in Children—This drug is not recommended for use in children because safety and effectiveness in the pediatric age group have not been established.

Overdosage

Manifestations—High doses may cause temporary confusion, disturbed concentration, or transient visual hallucinations. Overdosage may cause drowsiness; hypothermia; tachycardia and other arrhythmic abnormalities, for example, bundle branch block; ECG evidence of impaired conduction; congestive heart failure; dilated pupils; convulsions; severe hypotension; stupor; and coma. Other symptoms may be agitation, hyperactive reflexes, muscle rigidity, vomiting, hyperpyrexia, or any of those listed under ADVERSE REACTIONS.
Experience in the management of overdosage with protriptyline is limited. The following recommendations are based on the management of overdosage with other tricyclic antidepressants.
All patients suspected of having taken an overdosage should be admitted to a hospital as soon as possible. *Treatment* is symptomatic and supportive. Empty the stomach as quickly as possible by emesis followed by gastric lavage upon arrival at the hospital. Following gastric lavage, activated charcoal may be administered. Twenty to 30 g of activated charcoal may be given every four to six hours during the first 24 to 48 hours after ingestion. An ECG should be taken and close monitoring of cardiac function instituted if there is any sign of abnormality. Maintain an open airway and adequate fluid intake; regulate body temperature.
The intravenous administration of 1-3 mg of physostigmine salicylate is reported to reverse the symptoms of other tricyclic antidepressant poisoning in humans. Because physostigmine

Continued on next page

Information on the Merck Sharp & Dohme products listed on these pages is the full prescribing information from package circulars in use October 31, 1982.

Merck Sharp & Dohme—Cont.

is rapidly metabolized, the dosage of physostigmine should be repeated as required particularly if life threatening signs such as arrhythmias, convulsions, and deep coma recur or persist after the initial dosage of physostigmine. Because physostigmine itself may be toxic, it is not recommended for routine use.
Standard measures should be used to manage circulatory shock and metabolic acidosis. Cardiac arrhythmias may be treated with neostigmine, pyridostigmine, or propranolol. Should cardiac failure occur, the use of digitalis should be considered. Close monitoring of cardiac function for not less than five days is advisable.
Anticonvulsants may be given to control convulsions.
Dialysis is of no value because of low plasma concentrations of the drug.
Since overdosage is often deliberate, patients may attempt suicide by other means during the recovery phase.
Deaths by deliberate or accidental overdosage have occurred with this class of drugs.

How Supplied

No. 3313—Tablets VIVACTIL, 5 mg, are orange, oval, film coated tablets, coded MSD 26. They are supplied as follows:
NDC 0006-0026-68 bottles of 100
NDC 0006-0026-82 bottles of 1000.
[*Shown in Product Identification Section*]
No. 3314—Tablets VIVACTIL, 10 mg, are yellow, oval, film coated tablets, coded MSD 47. They are supplied as follows:
NDC 0006-0047-68 bottles of 100
NDC 0006-0047-28 single unit packages of 100
NDC 0006-0047-82 bottles of 1000.
[*Shown in Product Identification Section*]

Metabolism

Metabolic studies indicate that protriptyline is well absorbed from the gastrointestinal tract and is rapidly sequestered in tissues. Relatively low plasma levels are found after administration, and only a small amount of unchanged drug is excreted in the urine of dogs and rabbits. Preliminary studies indicate that demethylation of the secondary amine moiety occurs to a significant extent, and that metabolic transformation probably takes place in the liver. It penetrates the brain rapidly in mice and rats, and moreover that which is present in the brain is almost all unchanged drug.
Studies on the disposition of radioactive protriptyline in human test subjects showed significant plasma levels within 2 hours, peaking at 8 to 12 hours, then declining gradually.
Urinary excretion studies in the same subjects showed significant amounts of radioactivity in 2 hours. The rate of excretion was slow. Cumulative urinary excretion during 16 days accounted for approximately 50% of the drug. The fecal route of excretion did not seem to be important.

A.H.F.S. Category: 28:16:04
DC 6380614 Issued October 1981

Information on the Merck Sharp & Dohme products listed on these pages is the full prescribing information from package circulars in use October 31, 1982.

Products are cross-indexed by generic and chemical names in the **YELLOW SECTION**

Mericon Industries, Inc.
POST OFFICE BOX 5759
PEORIA, IL 61601

ORAZINC CAPSULES OTC
(zinc sulfate USP)
(See PDR For Nonprescription Drugs)

ZINC TABLETS OTC
(zinc sulfate USP)
(See PDR For Nonprescription Drugs)

Merieux Institute, Inc.
1200 N.W. 78TH AVENUE
SUITE 109
MIAMI, FL 33126

IMOGAM™ RABIES ℞
(Rabies Immune Globulin-Human)
NDC 50361-180200 2ml (300IU) pediatric vial
NDC 50361-181000 10ml (1500IU) adult vial

IMOVAX™ RABIES
(Rabies Vaccine Human Diploid Cell)
NDC 50361-250100 1ml IM pre-exposure/post-exposure dose vial

MONO-VACC® ℞
TUBERCULIN, MONO-VACC®TEST
(old tuberculin)
Multiple Puncture Device
NDC 50361-772425 25 test per box

Merrell Dow Pharmaceuticals Inc.

Subsidiary of The Dow Chemical Company
CINCINNATI, OH 45215

AVC™ Cream/Suppositories ℞
AVAILABLE ONLY ON PRESCRIPTION
Description:
AVC Cream
Each tube contains:
Sulfanilamide 15.0%
Aminacrine hydrochloride 0.2%
Allantoin 2.0%
with lactose, in a water-miscible base made from propylene glycol, stearic acid, diglycol stearate, and trolamine; buffered with lactic acid to an acid pH.
AVC Suppositories
Each suppository contains:
Sulfanilamide ....1.05 g
Aminacrine hydrochloride ....0.014 g
Allantoin ....0.14 g
with lactose, in a base made from polyethylene glycol 400, polysorbate 80, polyethylene glycol 4000, and glycerin; buffered with lactic acid to an acid pH. AVC Suppositories have an inert covering, which dissolves promptly in the vagina. The covering is composed of gelatin, glycerin, water, methylparaben, and propylparaben. Contains color additives including FD&C Yellow No. 5 (tartrazine).
Actions: AVC is a vaginal preparation combining aminacrine hydrochloride and sulfanilamide. Sulfanilamide is believed to block certain metabolic processes essential for the growth of susceptible bacteria. Aminacrine hydrochloride, a highly ionized acridine derivative, is thought to act by interfering or competing with certain hydrogen ions in microbial enzyme systems.
These ingredients are combined in a specially compounded base buffered to the pH of the normal vagina to encourage the presence of the normally occurring Döderlein's bacilli of the vagina.

Indications
Based on a review of AVC by the National Academy of Sciences—National Research Council and/or other information, FDA has classified the indications as follows:
"Probably" effective: For the relief of symptoms of vulvovaginitis where isolation of the specific organism responsible (usually *Trichomonas vaginalis, Candida albicans,* or *Hemophilus vaginalis*) is not possible.
NOTE: When the offending organism is known, treatment with a specific agent known to be active against that microorganism is preferred.
"Possibly" effective: For the treatment of trichomoniasis, vulvovaginal candidiasis, and vaginitis due to *Hemophilus vaginalis* or other susceptible bacteria.
Final classification of the less-than-effective indications requires further investigation.

Contraindications: AVC should not be used in patients known to be sensitive to the sulfonamides.
Precautions: As with all sulfonamides, the usual precautions apply. Patients should be observed for manifestations such as skin rash or other evidence of systemic toxicity, and if these develop, the medication should be discontinued.
AVC Suppositories contain FD&C Yellow No. 5 (tartrazine), which may cause allergic-type reactions (including bronchial asthma) in certain susceptible individuals. Although the overall incidence of FD&C Yellow No. 5 (tartrazine) sensitivity in the general population is low, it is frequently seen in patients who also have aspirin hypersensitivity.
Adverse Reactions: Although some absorption of sulfanilamide may occur through the vaginal mucosa, systemic manifestations attributable to this drug are infrequent. Local sensitivity reactions such as increased discomfort or a burning sensation have occasionally been reported following the use of topical sulfonamides. Treatment should be discontinued if either local or systemic manifestations of sulfonamide toxicity or sensitivity occur.
Dosage and Administration: 1 applicatorful (about 6 g) or 1 suppository intravaginally once or twice daily. Improvements in symptoms should occur within a few days, but treatment should be continued through one complete menstrual cycle unless a definite diagnosis is made and specific therapy initiated.
If there is no response within a few days or if symptoms recur, AVC should be discontinued and another attempt made by appropriate laboratory methods to isolate the organism responsible (*Trichomonas vaginalis, Candida albicans, Hemophilus vaginalis*) and institute specific therapy.
Douching with a suitable solution before insertion may be recommended for hygienic purposes. A pad may be used to prevent staining of clothing.
How Supplied:
AVC Cream
0068-0110-13: 4 oz. tube with applicator
AVC Suppositories
0068-0111-16: Box of 16 suppositories with inserter
Product Information as of August, 1979
Suppositories are
Manufactured by
R. P. Scherer, North America
Clearwater, Florida 33518 for
MERRELL DOW PHARMACEUTICALS INC.
Subsidiary of The Dow Chemical Company
Cincinnati, Ohio 45215, U.S.A.

ACCURBRON™ ℞
(theophylline)

Description: Each ml of ACCURBRON (theophylline) elixir for oral use contains anhydrous theophylline 10 mg (50 mg per 5 ml teaspoonful) and alcohol 7.5% in a pleasant-tasting vehicle. Theophylline is a bronchodilator. Chemically theophylline is 1,3-dimethylxanthine.

Clinical Pharmacology: Theophylline is rapidly absorbed when given as an elixir. It acts by inhibiting the enzyme phosphodiesterase which degrades cyclic AMP. Its plasma half-life ($T^1/_2$) varies widely because of differences in the rate of metabolism. The approximate average half-life of theophylline is 4 hours with a range for children of 2 to 10 hours, and up to 16 hours for adults. Steady state levels are reached in approximately three days. Theophylline relaxes the smooth muscle of the respiratory tract and relieves bronchospasm. Its bronchodilator effect is minimal in the absence of bronchospasm.

Other actions of theophylline include dilation of pulmonary, coronary and renal arteries, increased cardiac output and CNS stimulation. Usual doses increase blood pressure only slightly. Theophylline also has a mild diuretic action.

Indications and Usage: For the relief of bronchial asthma and reversible bronchospasm associated with obstructive pulmonary diseases such as chronic bronchitis and emphysema. Epinephrine is the drug of choice in severe acute asthma attacks.

Theophylline relieves the shortness of breath, wheezing and dyspnea associated with asthma and improves pulmonary function (increases flow rates and vital capacity). In doses sufficient to produce therapeutic serum concentrations (10–20 μg/ml), theophylline may also prevent the symptoms of chronic asthma and suppress exercise-induced asthma. It is especially useful for long-term treatment of bronchospasm because tolerance to the bronchodilator effect of theophylline rarely occurs.

Corticosteroids may be given in conjunction with theophylline, if needed.

Contraindications: Patients with peptic ulcers, active gastritis, and hypersensitivity or idiosyncrasy to theophylline and other methylxanthines.

Warnings: Should not be given concomitantly with other xanthine-containing drugs because of the potential for serious toxicity from elevated xanthine serum levels. Patients who exhibit idiosyncratic reactions to other xanthines (coffee, tea, colas, cocoas, chocolates, etc.) may also have similar reactions to theophylline and ACCURBRON should be used with caution for these patients.

Precautions: *General:* Use with caution in patients with cardiovascular disease, young children and the elderly, and patients with liver, kidney and heart disease.

Laboratory Tests: Serum theophylline levels may be helpful in following the patient's response to therapy with ACCURBRON.

Drug Interactions: Theophylline increases the excretion of lithium carbonate and may enhance the sensitivity and toxicity of digitalis derivatives and sympathomimetic amines. Doses higher than usual may increase the effect of oral anticoagulants. Concomitant use with erythromycin, clindamycin, lincomycin and troleandomycin may increase theophylline serum levels.

Drug/Laboratory Test Interactions: Colorimetric methods for serum uric acid are affected by theophylline. Spectrophotometric methods for theophylline in serum are affected by furosemide, sulfathiazole, phenylbutazone, probenecid and theobromine.

Pregnancy Category C: Animal reproduction studies have not been conducted with ACCURBRON. It is also not known whether ACCURBRON can cause fetal harm when administered to a pregnant women or can affect reproduction capacity. ACCURBRON may be given to a pregnant woman only if clearly needed.

Nursing Mothers: Theophylline is excreted in the milk. Use during lactation and in women of childbearing potential requires that benefits be weighed against possible hazards to fetus or child.

Adverse Reactions: *Gastrointestinal:* loss of appetite, nausea, vomiting, gastric irritation.

CNS: irritability, especially in children, insomnia, headache, dizziness and convulsions. These side effects are usually associated with high theophylline serum levels (exceeding 20 μg/ml).

Cardiovascular: palpitations, sinus tachycardia and increased pulse rate, usually mild and transient.

Other side-effects may include increased irritation with dehydration, muscle twitching and increased SGOT levels.

Overdosage: Theophylline has a narrow therapeutic index and toxicity is likely to occur when serum levels exceed 20 μg/ml. Usual signs of overdosage are anorexia, nausea, vomiting, irritability, headache. Gross overdosage, especially in children, may lead to seizures and death without preceding symptoms of toxicity. Treatment is symptomatic (prompt induction of emesis and gastric lavage, supportive therapy, hemodialysis, etc.).

Dosage and Administration: Dosage must be individualized. Accepted therapeutic serum levels of theophylline are 10–20 μg/ml. Its metabolism may vary greatly with age, among individuals and in patients with liver, kidney and heart disease. Metabolism may be stable within the same individual. Careful monitoring for manifestations of toxicity and periodic determinations of theophylline serum levels are necessary, especially for prolonged therapy and with high doses.

Children: The following table may be used with the graduated measuring spoon for ACCURBRON:

[See table above].

Adults: Recommended starting dose is 100 to 200 mg (10 to 20 ml) every 6 hours. The adequacy of the dose should be determined by clinical response and periodic monitoring of theophylline serum levels.

May be given after meals with water to minimize possible G.I. irritation.

Caution: Federal law prohibits dispensing without prescription.

How Supplied: As a dye-free liquid in pint bottles (NDC 0068-5002-16) with a graduated measuring spoon for ACCURBRON.

ACCURBRON™ (theophylline) - PEDIATRIC DOSAGE CALCULATION TABLE

Starting dosage: (All ages for first 3 days) — 4 mg/kg body wt every 6 hours not to exceed 100 mg (10 ml Accurbron)

Age	Body Weight		Dose/6 hours				
	lbs	kgs	3 mg/kg	4 mg/kg	5 mg/kg	6 mg/kg	7 mg/kg
Under 9 years*	10	4.5	1 ml	2 ml	2 ml	3 ml	3 ml
average dose	20	9	3 ml	4 ml	5 ml	5 ml	6 ml
4–6 mg/kg/6 hrs.	30	14	4 ml	6 ml	7 ml	8 ml	10 ml
	40	18	5 ml	7 ml	9 ml	11 ml	13 ml
	50	23	7 ml	9 ml	12 ml	14 ml	16 ml
	60	27	8 ml	11 ml	14 ml	16 ml	19 ml
	70	32	10 ml	13 ml	16 ml	19 ml	22 ml
9—12 years*	80	36	11 ml	14 ml	18 ml	22 ml	25 ml
average dose	90	41	12 ml	16 ml	20 ml	25 ml	29 ml
4–5 mg/kg/6 hrs.	100	45	14 ml	18 ml	22 ml	27 ml	32 ml

ACCURBRON contains 10 mg theophylline (anhydrous) per ml.

*Do not exceed this dosage without careful clinical monitoring or checking theophylline serum level because of the increased risk of side effects when serum levels exceed 20 μg/ml.

BENDECTIN® ℞

AVAILABLE ONLY ON PRESCRIPTION

Description:
Each specially coated tablet contains:
Decapryn® (doxylamine succinate)—antihistamine .... 10 mg
Pyridoxine hydrochloride .... 10 mg

Actions: Bendectin provides the action of 2 unrelated compounds. Doxylamine succinate, an antihistamine, provides anti-nauseant and anti-emetic activity; the pyridoxine hydrochloride provides vitamin B_6 supplementation to help avoid pyridoxine deficiency that may occur during pregnancy. Also, studies indicate B_6 has an anti-nauseant activity. The anti-emetic action of Bendectin is delayed by a special coating that permits the nighttime dose to be effective in the morning hours when the patient needs it most.

Indication: Bendectin is indicated only for nausea and vomiting of pregnancy which are unresponsive to conservative measures such as eating soda crackers or drinking hot and cold liquids, which interfere with normal eating habits or daily activities, and are sufficiently distressing to require drug intervention. (See Precautions –Pregnancy.)

Precautions:
Because of potential drowsiness, Bendectin should be prescribed with caution for patients who must drive automobiles or operate machinery.

Pregnancy:

Animal Studies:
Teratology studies with Bendectin or its two components (doxylamine succinate and pyridoxine hydrochloride) have been reported in various animal species, including: Sprague-Dawley and Wistar rats, New Zealand and Dutch-belted rabbits, NMRI mice, rhesus (*M. mulatta*) and cynomolgus (*M. fascicularis*) monkeys. The majority of studies did not demonstrate a teratogenic effect of Bendectin or its components. However, two of the most recent studies, although preliminary and unconfirmed, raise the possibility that Bendectin or doxylamine succinate may have a teratogenic potential in some species, as indicated below. Studies of Bendectin in Sprague-Dawley rats and New Zealand rabbits at doses up to 90 times the maximum human dose (MHD) gave no indication of drug-induced fetal abnormalities.

A small study in pregnant cynomolgus monkeys treated throughout organogenesis with Bendectin (10–20 times the MHD) indicated

Continued on next page

Information on Merrell Dow products is based on labeling in effect in October, 1982.

Merrell Dow—Cont.

defects in the interventricular septum of the heart in 4 of 7 fetuses that were delivered on day 100 of gestation (total gestation time approximately 160 days). Two fetuses from aborted pregnancies on day 46 and 56 appeared to be developing normally. Three additional fetuses allowed to go to term were normal.

In other experiments, pregnant rhesus and cynomolgus monkeys treated with Bendectin for shorter periods of time delivered normal fetuses.

Studies of doxylamine succinate at doses up to 60 times the MHD in Wistar rats and NMRI mice, and up to 125 times the MHD in Sprague-Dawley rats and Dutch-belted rabbits gave no indication of observable congenital abnormalities. At doses of 125 to 375 times the MHD in Wistar rats, wavy ribs (7–10%) and diaphragmatic hernias (2–6%) were noted. An overall increase in fetal wastage which varied from zero to 3-fold was reported for a majority of rodent species given doses of 125 times the MHD or more.

Human Studies:

Bendectin has been the subject of many epidemiologic studies (case control and cohort) designed to detect possible teratogenicity. A review of the results of these studies leads to the conclusion that the existing data do not demonstrate an association between Bendectin use and birth defects. In a few of these studies an association of Bendectin use with a specific congenital defect was suggested. However, in each such study, the associated defect was different. Because these results emerged after multiple analyses of the same data (i.e. looking at many drugs or many possible defects) and for other reasons, these findings were viewed as hypotheses and not as definitive findings. Some of these defects were specifically looked for in other epidemiologic studies and an association with Bendectin use was not confirmed. Studies are ongoing to help clarify the matter. The design of the cohort studies was generally adequate to have detected a small increase (less than a doubling*) in the overall malformation rate, if it existed, but was not sufficient to rule out a doubling of a specific malformation type, for example, 1 per 1000 to 2 per 1000. For the above reasons, Bendectin should be used only when clearly needed for the treatment of nausea and vomiting of pregnancy not responsive to conservative (non-drug) measures.

When a decision has been made to use drug therapy in the treatment of nausea and vomiting of pregnancy, the physician should be aware that Bendectin has been the subject of a considerably larger number of epidemiologic studies searching for a risk of birth defects than have other antinauseants (a bibliography on Bendectin is available to prescribers on request).

* Doubling is the level of sensitivity many epidemiologists regard as feasible to detect in the design of studies of this type.

A patient product information leaflet is available from pharmacists who carry this product and from the company upon request.

Adverse Reactions: The adverse reactions that may occur are those of the individual ingredients. Doxylamine succinate may cause drowsiness, vertigo, nervousness, epigastric pain, headache, palpitation, diarrhea, disorientation, or irritability.

Pyridoxine hydrochloride is a vitamin that is generally recognized as having no adverse effects.

Dosage and Administration: 2 Bendectin tablets at bedtime. In severe cases or when nausea occurs during the day: 1 additional Bendectin tablet in the morning and another in midafternoon.

How Supplied:

NDC 0068-0155-30: White tablets imprinted MERRELL 155 in cartons of 90 tablets as 3 dispensing cartons of 30 tablets each

Product Information as of July, 1982

[*Shown in Product Identification Section*]

BENTYL® ℞

(dicyclomine hydrochloride USP)
Capsules, Tablets, Syrup, Injection

AVAILABLE ONLY ON PRESCRIPTION

Description:

1. Bentyl 10 mg capsules
   10 mg dicyclomine hydrochloride USP in each blue capsule.
2. Bentyl 20 mg tablets
   20 mg dicyclomine hydrochloride USP in each blue tablet.
3. Bentyl syrup
   10 mg dicyclomine hydrochloride USP in each 5 ml (1 teaspoonful) pink syrup.
4. Bentyl Injection
   Ampul—2 ml—Each ml contains 10 mg dicyclomine hydrochloride USP, in water for injection, made isotonic with sodium chloride.
   Vial—10 ml—Each ml contains 10 mg dicyclomine hydrochloride USP, in water for injection, made isotonic with sodium chloride. 0.5% chlorobutanol hydrous (chloral derivative) added as a preservative.
   Prefilled Syringe—2 ml—Each ml contains 10 mg dicyclomine hydrochloride USP, in water for injection, made isotonic with sodium chloride.

Actions: Bentyl relieves smooth muscle spasm of the gastrointestinal tract.

Indications

Based on a review of this drug by the National Academy of Sciences—National Research Council and/or other information, FDA has classified the following indications as "probably" effective:

For the treatment of functional bowel/irritable bowel syndrome (irritable colon, spastic colon, mucous colitis) and acute enterocolitis.

THESE FUNCTIONAL DISORDERS ARE OFTEN RELIEVED BY VARYING COMBINATIONS OF SEDATIVE, REASSURANCE, PHYSICIAN INTEREST, AMELIORATION OF ENVIRONMENTAL FACTORS.

For use in the treatment of infant colic (syrup).

Final classification of the less-than-effective indications requires further investigation.

Contraindications: Obstructive uropathy (for example, bladder neck obstruction due to prostatic hypertrophy); obstructive disease of the gastrointestinal tract (as in achalasia, pyloroduodenal stenosis); paralytic ileus, intestinal atony of the elderly or debilitated patient; unstable cardiovascular status in acute hemorrhage; severe ulcerative colitis; toxic megacolon complicating ulcerative colitis; myasthenia gravis.

Warnings: In the presence of a high environmental temperature, heat prostration can occur with drug use (fever and heat stroke due to decreased sweating).

Diarrhea may be an early symptom of incomplete intestinal obstruction, especially in patients with ileostomy or colostomy. In this instance treatment with this drug would be inappropriate and possibly harmful.

Bentyl may produce drowsiness or blurred vision. In this event, the patient should be warned not to engage in activities requiring mental alertness such as operating a motor vehicle or other machinery or perform hazardous work while taking this drug.

There are rare reports of infants, 6 weeks of age and under, administered dicyclomine hydrochloride syrup, who have evidenced respiratory symptoms (breathing difficulty, shortness of breath, breathlessness, respiratory collapse, apnea), as well as seizures, syncope, asphyxia, pulse rate fluctuations, muscular hypotonia, and coma. The above symptoms have occurred within minutes of ingestion and lasted 20 to 30 minutes. The timing and nature of the reactions suggest that they were a consequence of local irritation and/or aspiration rather than a direct pharmacologic effect. No known deaths or permanent adverse effects have been reported. Bentyl syrup should be used with caution in this age group.

Precautions: Although studies have failed to demonstrate adverse effects of dicyclomine hydrochloride in glaucoma or in patients with prostatic hypertrophy, it should be prescribed with caution in patients known to have or suspected of having glaucoma or prostatic hypertrophy.

Use with caution in patients with:

- Autonomic neuropathy.
- Hepatic or renal disease.
- Ulcerative colitis. Large doses may suppress intestinal motility to the point of producing a paralytic ileus and the use of this drug may precipitate or aggravate the serious complication of toxic megacolon.
- Hyperthyroidism, coronary heart disease, congestive heart failure, cardiac arrhythmias, and hypertension.
- Hiatal hernia associated with reflux esophagitis since anticholinergic drugs may aggravate this condition.

Do not rely on the use of the drug in the presence of complication of biliary tract disease.

Investigate any tachycardia before giving anticholinergic (atropine-like) drugs since they may increase the heart rate.

With overdosage, a curare-like action may occur.

Adverse Reactions: Anticholinergics/antispasmodics produce certain effects which may be physiologic or toxic depending upon the individual patient's response. The physician must delineate these.

Adverse reactions may include xerostomia; urinary hesitancy and retention; blurred vision and tachycardia; palpitations; mydriasis; cycloplegia; increased ocular tension; loss of taste; headache; nervousness; drowsiness; weakness; dizziness; insomnia; nausea; vomiting; impotence; suppression of lactation; constipation; bloated feeling; severe allergic reaction or drug idiosyncrasies including anaphylaxis; urticaria and other dermal manifestations; some degree of mental confusion and/or excitement, especially in elderly persons; and decreased sweating.

With the injectable form there may be a temporary sensation of lightheadedness and occasionally local irritation.

Dosage and Administration: Dosage must be adjusted to individual patient's needs.

Usual Dosage

Bentyl 10 mg capsule and syrup:

Adults: 1 or 2 capsules or teaspoonfuls syrup three or four times daily.

Children: 1 capsule or teaspoonful syrup three or four times daily.

Infants: ½ teaspoonful syrup three or four times daily. (Dilute with equal volume of water.)

Bentyl 20 mg:

Adults: 1 tablet three or four times daily.

Bentyl Injection:

Adults: 2 ml (20 mg) every four to six hours intramuscularly only.

NOT FOR INTRAVENOUS USE.

Management of Overdose: The signs and symptoms of overdose are headache, nausea, vomiting, blurred vision, dilated pupils, hot, dry skin, dizziness, dryness of the mouth, difficulty in swallowing, CNS stimulation. Treatment should consist of gastric lavage, emetics, and activated charcoal. Barbiturates may be used either orally or intramuscularly for sedation but they should not be used if Bentyl with Phenobarbital has been ingested. If indicated, parenteral cholinergic agents such as Urecholine® (bethanecol chloride USP) should be used.

How Supplied:

10 mg Capsules imprinted MERRELL 120/BENTYL®

Bottles of 100, 500, and 1000 and unit dose dispenser of 100

[*Shown in Product Identification Section*]

Syrup

16-ounce bottles

20 mg Tablets debossed MERRELL 123

Bottles of 100, 500, and 1000 and unit dose dispenser of 100

[*Shown in Product Identification Section*]

Injection

10 ml multiple dose vials

Boxes of five 2 ml ampuls

Cartons of five 2 ml prefilled syringes

Product Information as of July, 1980

Injectable dosage forms manufactured by
CONNAUGHT LABORATORIES, INC.
Swiftwater, Pennsylvania 18370 or
TAYLOR PHARMACAL COMPANY
Decatur, Illinois 62525 for
MERRELL DOW PHARMACEUTICALS INC.
Subsidiary of The Dow Chemical Company
Cincinnati, Ohio 45215, U.S.A.

BRICANYL® ℞
(terbutaline sulfate)
Injection

Name of Drug: Bricanyl® (terbutaline sulfate) Subcutaneous Injection

Description: Terbutaline sulfate, a synthetic sympathomimetic amine, may be chemically described as α-[(tert-butylamine) methyl]-3,5-dihydroxybenzyl alcohol sulfate. The structural formula is as follows:

$$\left[(HO)_2C_6H_3\text{-}CH(OH)CH_2NHC(CH_3)_3 \right]_2 \cdot H_2SO_4$$

Terbutaline sulfate is a water soluble, colorless, crystalline solid. Solutions are sensitive to excessive heat and light. Ampules should therefore be stored at controlled room temperature with protection from light by storage in their original carton until dispensed. Solutions should not be used if discolored.

Each milliliter of sterile isotonic solution contains 1.0 mg of terbutaline sulfate (equivalent to 0.82 mg of the free base), 8.9 mg of sodium chloride, and hydrochloric acid to adjust the pH to 3.0–5.0.

Actions: Bricanyl, brand of terbutaline sulfate, is a β-adrenergic receptor agonist which has been shown by *in vitro* and *in vivo* pharmacological studies in animals to exert a preferential effect on β_2 adrenergic receptors such as those located in bronchial smooth muscle. Controlled clinical studies in patients who were administered the drug orally have revealed proportionally greater changes in pulmonary function parameters than in heart rate or blood pressure. While this suggests a relative preference for the β_2 receptor in man, the usual cardiovascular effects commonly associated with sympathomimetic agents were also observed with terbutaline sulfate.

Bricanyl (terbutaline sulfate) Subcutaneous Injection has been shown in controlled clinical studies to relieve acute bronchospasm in acute and chronic obstructive pulmonary disease, resulting in a clinically significant increase in pulmonary flow rates, e.g., an increase of 15% or greater in FEV_1. Following administration of 0.25 mg by subcutaneous injection, a measurable change in flow rate is usually observed within five minutes, and a clinically significant increase in FEV_1 occurs by 15 minutes following the injection. The maximum effect usually occurs within 30–60 minutes and clinically significant bronchodilator activity has been observed to persist for 90 minutes to four hours. The duration of clinically significant improvement is comparable to that found with equimilligram doses of epinephrine.

Indications: Bricanyl (terbutaline sulfate) Subcutaneous Injection is indicated as a bronchodilator for bronchial asthma and for reversible bronchospasm which may occur in association with bronchitis and emphysema.

Contraindications: Bricanyl (terbutaline sulfate) Subcutaneous Injection is contraindicated when there is known hypersensitivity to sympathomimetic amines.

Warnings:

Usage in Pregnancy: Animal reproductive studies have been negative with respect to adverse effects on fetal development. The safe use of terbutaline sulfate has not, however, been established in human pregnancy. As with any medication, the use of the drug in pregnancy, lactation, or women of childbearing potential requires that the expected therapeutic benefit of the drug be weighed against its possible hazards to the mother or child.

Usage in Pediatrics: Bricanyl (terbutaline sulfate) Subcutaneous Injection is not presently recommended for children below the age of twelve years due to insufficient clinical data in this pediatric group.

Usage in Labor and Delivery: Serious adverse reactions have been reported following administration of terbutaline sulfate to women in labor. These reports have included transient hypokalemia, pulmonary edema and hypoglycemia in the mother and hypoglycemia in the neonatal children of women treated with terbutaline parenterally.

Precautions: Bricanyl (terbutaline sulfate) Subcutaneous Injection should be used with caution in patients with diabetes, hypertension, hyperthyroidism, and history of seizures. As with other sympathomimetic bronchodilator agents, Bricanyl (terbutaline sulfate) Subcutaneous Injection should be administered cautiously to cardiac patients, especially those with associated arrhythmias.

The concomitant use of Bricanyl (terbutaline sulfate) Subcutaneous Injection with other sympathomimetic agents is not recommended, since their combined effect on the cardiovascular system may be deleterious to the patient.

Preparation of Other Dosage Forms: Use of the subcutaneous injection for preparation of other dosage forms, i.e., IV infusion, is inappropriate. Sterility and accurate dosing cannot be assured if the ampules are not used in accordance with *Dosage and Administration.*

Adverse Reactions: Commonly observed side effects include increases in heart rate, nervousness, tremor, palpitations and dizziness. These occur more frequently at doses in excess of 0.25 mg. Other reported reactions include headache, nausea, vomiting, anxiety, and muscle cramps. These reactions are transient in nature and usually do not require treatment. In general, all side effects are characteristic of those commonly seen with sympathomimetic amines such as epinephrine.

Dosage and Administration: The usual subcutaneous dose of Bricanyl, brand of terbutaline sulfate, is 0.25 mg injected into the lateral deltoid area. If significant clinical improvement does not occur by 15–30 minutes, a second dose of 0.25 mg may be administered. A total dose of 0.5 mg should not be exceeded within a four hour period. If a patient fails to respond to a second 0.25 mg dose within 15–30 minutes, other therapeutic measures should be considered.

Overdosage: Overdosage experience is limited. Excessive β-adrenergic receptor stimulation may augment the signs or symptoms listed under Adverse Reactions and they may be accompanied by other adrenergic effects. In the case of terbutaline overdosage, the patient should be treated symptomatically for the sympathomimetic overdosage with careful consideration to the appropriateness of any chosen therapy and possible effect on the patient's underlying disease state.

How Supplied: Bricanyl (terbutaline sulfate) Subcutaneous Injection is supplied in packages of ten 2 ml size ampules each containing one ml of solution [1.0 mg of Bricanyl (terbutaline sulfate)]. Thus, 0.25 ml of solution will provide the usual clinical dose of 0.25 mg. Ampules are expiration dated.

Product Information as of June, 1982

Manufactured by
Astra Pharmaceutical Products, Inc.
Worcester, Mass. 01606, U.S.A. for
MERRELL DOW PHARMACEUTICALS INC.
Subsidiary of The Dow Chemical Company
Cincinnati, Ohio 45215, U.S.A.
U.S. Patent No. 3,937,838

BRICANYL® ℞
(terbutaline sulfate)
Tablets

Name of Drug: Bricanyl® (terbutaline sulfate) tablets

Description: Terbutaline sulfate, a synthetic sympathomimetic amine, may be chemically described as α-[(tert-butylamino) methyl]-3,5-dihydroxybenzyl alcohol sulfate. The structural formula is as follows:

$$\left[(HO)_2C_6H_3\text{-}CH(OH)CH_2NHC(CH_3)_3 \right]_2 \cdot H_2SO_4$$

Terbutaline sulfate is a water soluble, colorless, crystalline solid. Tablets containing Bricanyl (terbutaline sulfate) should be stored at controlled room temperature.

Tablets containing 2.5 mg (equivalent to 2.05 mg of free base) and 5 mg (equivalent to 4.1 mg of free base) of terbutaline sulfate are white in color, and carry an inscription which represents the last 3 digits of the NDC product code (i.e., 725 for 2.5 mg tablets, and 750 for 5 mg tablets).

Actions: Bricanyl brand of terbutaline sulfate is a β-adrenergic receptor agonist which has been shown by *in vitro* and *in vivo* pharmacological studies in animals to exert a preferential effect on adrenergic receptors such as those located in bronchial smooth muscle. Controlled clinical studies in patients who were administered the drug orally have revealed proportionally greater changes in pulmonary function parameters than in heart rate or blood pressure. While this suggests a relative preference for the β_2 receptor in man, the usual cardiovascular effects commonly associated with sympathomimetic agents were also observed with terbutaline sulfate.

Bricanyl (terbutaline sulfate) tablets have been shown in controlled clinical studies to relieve bronchospasm in chronic obstructive pulmonary disease. This action is manifested by a clinically significant increase in pulmonary function as demonstrated by an increase of 15% or more in FEV_1 and FEF_{25-75}%. Following administration of Bricanyl tablets, a measurable change in pulmonary function occurs at 60–120 minutes. The maximum effect usually occurs within 120–180 minutes. There is a clinically significant decrease in airway and pulmonary resistance which persists for at least 4 hours or longer. Significant bronchodilator action, as measured by various pulmonary function determinations (airway resistance, MMEFR, PEFR) has been demonstrated in studies for periods up to 8 hours.

Clinical studies were conducted in which the effectiveness of Bricanyl brand of terbutaline

Continued on next page

Merrell Dow—Cont.

sulfate was evaluated in comparison with ephedrine over periods up to 3 months. Both drugs continued to produce significant improvement in pulmonary function throughout this period of treatment.

Indications: Bricanyl, brand of terbutaline sulfate, is indicated as a bronchodilator for bronchial asthma and for reversible bronchospasm which may occur in association with bronchitis and emphysema.

Contraindications: Bricanyl (terbutaline sulfate) tablets are contraindicated when there is known hypersensitivity to sympathomimetic amines.

Warnings:

Usage in Pregnancy: Animal reproductive studies have been negative with respect to adverse effects on fetal development. The safe use of terbutaline sulfate has not, however, been established in human pregnancy. As with any medication, the use of the drug in pregnancy, lactation, or women of childbearing potential requires that the expected therapeutic benefit of the drug be weighed against its possible hazards to the mother or child.

Usage in Pediatrics: Bricanyl (terbutaline sulfate) tablets are not presently recommended for children below the age of twelve years due to insufficient clinical data in this pediatric group.

Precautions: Bricanyl (terbutaline sulfate) tablets should be used with caution in patients with diabetes, hypertension, hyperthyroidism, and a history of seizures.

As with other sympathomimetic bronchodilator agents, Bricanyl (terbutaline sulfate) tablets should be administered cautiously to cardiac patients, especially those with associated arrhythmias.

The concomitant use of terbutaline sulfate with other sympathomimetic agents is not recommended, since their combined effect on the cardiovascular system may be deleterious to the patient. However, this does not preclude the use of an aerosol bronchodilator of the adrenergic stimulant type for the relief of an acute bronchospasm in patients receiving chronic oral terbutaline sulfate therapy.

Adverse Reactions: Commonly observed side effects include nervousness and tremor. The frequency of these side effects appears to diminish with continued therapy. Other reported reactions include headache, increased heart rate, palpitations, drowsiness, nausea, vomiting, sweating, and muscle cramps. These reactions are generally transient in nature and usually do not require treatment. In general, all the side effects observed are characteristic of those commonly seen with sympathomimetic amines.

Dosage and Administration: The usual oral dose of Bricanyl (terbutaline sulfate) tablets for adults is 5 mg administered at approximately six-hour intervals three times daily, during the hours the patient is usually awake. If side effects are particularly disturbing, the dose may be reduced to 2.5 mg three times daily and still provide a clinically significant improvement in pulmonary function. A dose of 2.5 mg three times daily also is recommended for children in the 12–15 year group. Bricanyl is not recommended at present for use in children below the age of twelve years. In adults, a total dose of 15 mg should not be exceeded in a 24-hour period.

Overdosage: Overdosage experience is limited. Excessive β-adrenergic receptor stimulation may augment the signs or symptoms listed under Adverse Reactions and they may be accompanied by other adrenergic effects. Treat the alert patient who has taken excessive oral medication by emptying the stomach by means of induced emesis, followed by gastric lavage. In the unconscious patient, secure the airway with a cuffed endotracheal tube before beginning lavage (do not induce emesis). Instillation of activated charcoal slurry may help reduce absorption of terbutaline sulfate. Maintain adequate respiratory exchange. Provide cardiac and respiratory support as needed. Continue observation until symptom-free.

How Supplied: Both 2.5 mg and 5 mg Bricanyl® (terbutaline sulfate) tablets are supplied in bottles of 100 and 1,000 and in hospital (unit dose) packs of 100 individually packaged tablets.

Product Information as of June, 1982

Manufactured by
Astra Pharmaceutical Products, Inc.
Worcester, Mass. 01606, U.S.A. for
MERRELL DOW PHARMACEUTICALS INC.
Subsidiary of The Dow Chemical Company
Cincinnati, Ohio 45215, U.S.A.
U.S. Patent No. 3,937,838

CANTIL® ℞
(mepenzolate bromide USP)
Tablets

Caution: Federal law prohibits dispensing without prescription.

Description: Cantil (mepenzolate bromide USP) chemically is 3-[(hydroxydiphenylacetyl) oxy]-1,1-dimethylpiperidinium bromide.

Mepenzolate bromide occurs as a white or light cream-colored powder, which is freely soluble in methanol, slightly soluble in water and chloroform, and practically insoluble in ether.

Each yellow tablet contains 25 mg mepenzolate bromide USP.

Clinical Pharmacology: Cantil diminishes gastric acid and pepsin secretion. Cantil also suppresses spontaneous contractions of the colon. Pharmacologically, it is a post-ganglionic parasympathetic inhibitor.

Radiotracer studies in which Cantil-^{14}C was used in animals and humans indicate that absorption following oral administration, as with other quaternary ammonium compounds, is low. Between 3 and 22% of an orally administered dose is excreted in the urine over a 5-day period, with the majority of the radioactivity appearing on Day 1. The remainder appears in the next 5 days in the feces and presumably has not been absorbed.

Indication: Cantil is indicated for use as adjunctive therapy in the treatment of peptic ulcer. Cantil has not been shown to be effective in contributing to the healing of peptic ulcer, decreasing the rate of recurrence or preventing complications.

Contraindications: Glaucoma, obstructive uropathy (for example, bladder neck obstruction due to prostatic hypertrophy), obstructive disease of the gastrointestinal tract (for example, pyloroduodenal stenosis, achalasia), paralytic ileus, intestinal atony of the elderly or debilitated patient, unstable cardiovascular status in acute hemorrhage, severe ulcerative colitis, toxic megacolon complicating ulcerative colitis, myasthenia gravis, allergic or idiosyncratic reactions to Cantil or related compounds.

Warnings: In the presence of high environmental temperature, heat prostration (fever and heat stroke due to decreased sweating) can occur with use of Cantil.

Cantil may produce drowsiness or blurred vision. The patient should be cautioned regarding activities requiring mental alertness such as operating a motor vehicle or other machinery or performing hazardous work while taking this drug.

With overdosage, a curare-like action may occur, i.e., neuromuscular blockade leading to muscular weakness and possible paralysis.

It should be noted that the use of anticholinergic drugs in the treatment of gastric ulcer may produce a delay in gastric emptying time and may complicate such therapy (antral stasis).

Pregnancy

Reproduction studies in rats and rabbits have shown no evidence of impaired fertility or harm to the animal fetus. Information on possible adverse effects in the pregnant female is limited to uncontrolled data derived from marketing experience. Such experience has revealed no reports of the effect of Cantil on human pregnancies. No controlled studies to establish the safety of the drug in pregnancy have been performed.

Pediatric Use

Since there is no adequate experience in children who have received this drug, safety and efficacy in children have not been established. Newborn animal studies have been undertaken that show that younger animals are more sensitive to the toxic effects of mepenzolate bromide than are older animals.

Precautions: Use Cantil with caution in the elderly and in all patients with:

- Autonomic neuropathy
- Hepatic or renal disease
- Ulcerative colitis. Large doses may suppress intestinal motility to the point of producing a paralytic ileus and for this reason precipitate or aggravate "toxic megacolon," a serious complication of the disease.

Hyperthyroidism, coronary heart disease, congestive heart failure, "cardiac tachyarrhythmias," tachycardia, hypertension, and prostatic hypertrophy.

Hiatal hernia associated with reflux esophagitis, since anticholinergic drugs may aggravate this condition.

This product contains FD&C Yellow No. 5 (tartrazine), which may cause allergic-type reactions (including bronchial asthma) in certain susceptible individuals. Although the overall incidence of FD&C Yellow No. 5 (tartrazine) sensitivity in the general population is low, it is frequently seen in patients who also have aspirin hypersensitivity.

Nursing Mothers

It is not known whether this drug is secreted in human milk. As a general rule, nursing should not be undertaken while a patient is on a drug since many drugs are excreted in human milk.

Adverse Reactions: Xerostomia, decreased sweating, urinary hesitancy and retention, blurred vision, tachycardia, palpitations, dilatation of the pupil, cycloplegia, increased ocular tension, loss of taste, headaches, nervousness, mental confusion, drowsiness, weakness, dizziness, insomnia, nausea, vomiting, constipation, bloated feeling, impotence, suppression of lactation, severe allergic reaction or drug idiosyncrasies including anaphylaxis, urticaria and other dermal manifestations.

Overdosage: The symptoms of overdosage with Cantil progress from an intensification of the usual adverse effects to CNS disturbances (from restlessness and excitement to psychotic behavior), circulatory changes (flushing, fall in blood pressure, circulatory failure), respiratory failure, paralysis, and coma.

Measures to be taken are (1) immediate lavage of the stomach and (2) injection of physostigmine 0.5 to 2 mg intravenously, repeated as necessary up to a total of 5 mg. Fever may be treated symptomatically (alcohol sponging, ice packs). Excitement of a degree that demands attention may be managed with sodium thiopental 2% solution given slowly intravenously or chloral hydrate (100–200 ml of a 2% solution) by rectal infusion. In the event of progression of the curare-like effect to paralysis of the respiratory muscles, artificial respiration should be instituted and maintained until effective respiratory action returns.

Dosage and Administration: Usual Adult Dose: 1 or 2 tablets three times a day preferably with meals and 1 or 2 tablets at bedtime. Begin with the lower dosage when possible and adjust subsequently according to the patient's response.

Since there is no adequate experience in children who have received this drug, safety and efficacy in children have not been established.
Drug Interactions: Concomitant administration of anticholinergic drugs and any other drugs which would increase the anticholinergic effects of Cantil is to be avoided.
How Supplied: Tablets (25 mg) debossed MERRELL 037: bottles of 100 and 1000

Product Information as of July, 1979
[*Shown in Product Identification Section*]

CĒPACOL® Mouthwash/Gargle

(See PDR For Nonprescription Drugs)

CĒPACOL® Throat Lozenges

(See PDR For Nonprescription Drugs)

CĒPACOL® Anesthetic Lozenges (Troches)

(See PDR For Nonprescription Drugs)

CĒPASTAT®
sore throat spray and lozenges

(See PDR For Nonprescription Drugs)

Cherry Flavor
CĒPASTAT®
sore throat lozenges

(See PDR For Nonprescription Drugs)

CEPHULAC® (lactulose) Syrup ℞
FOR ORAL OR RECTAL ADMINISTRATION

AVAILABLE ONLY ON PRESCRIPTION

Description: Lactulose is 4-O-β-D-galactopyranosyl-D-fructofuranose. The structural formula is:

The molecular formula is $C_{12}H_{22}O_{11}$ and the molecular weight is 342.30. Each 15 ml of Cephulac contains: 10 g lactulose (and less than 2.2 g galactose, less than 1.2 g lactose, and 1.2 g or less of other sugars), water, flavoring, and coloring. Sodium hydroxide used to adjust pH.
Clinical Pharmacology: Lactulose causes a decrease in blood ammonia concentration and reduces the degree of portal-systemic encephalopathy. These actions are considered to be results of the following:

Bacterial degradation of lactulose in the colon acidifies the colonic contents.
This acidification of colonic contents results in the retention of ammonia in the colon as the ammonium ion. Since the colonic contents are then more acid than the blood, ammonia can be expected to migrate from the blood into the colon to form the ammonium ion.
The acid colonic contents convert NH_3 to the ammonium ion $[NH_4]+$, trapping it and preventing its absorption.
The laxative action of the metabolites of lactulose then expels the trapped ammonium ion from the colon.

Experimental data indicate that lactulose is poorly absorbed. Lactulose given orally to man and experimental animals resulted in only small amounts reaching the blood. Urinary excretion has been determined to be 3% or less and is essentially complete within 24 hours.
When incubated with extracts of human small intestinal mucosa, lactulose was not hydrolyzed during a 24-hour period and did not inhibit the activity of these extracts on lactose.
Lactulose reaches the colon essentially unchanged. There it is metabolized by bacteria with the formation of low molecular weight acids that acidify the colonic contents.
Indications: For the prevention and treatment of portal-systemic encephalopathy, including the stages of hepatic pre-coma and coma.
Controlled studies have shown that lactulose syrup therapy reduces the blood ammonia levels by 25–50%; this is generally paralleled by an improvement in the patients' mental state and by an improvement in EEG patterns. The clinical response has been observed in about 75% of patients, which is at least as satisfactory as that resulting from neomycin therapy.
An increase in patients' protein tolerance is also frequently observed with lactulose therapy. In the treatment of chronic portal-systemic encephalopathy, Cephulac has been given for over 2 years in controlled studies.
Contraindications: Since Cephulac contains galactose (less than 2.2 g/15 ml), it is contraindicated in patients who require a low galactose diet.
Warnings:
A theoretical hazard may exist for patients being treated with lactulose syrup who may be required to undergo electrocautery procedures during proctoscopy or colonoscopy. Accumulation of H_2 gas in significant concentration in the presence of an electrical spark may result in an explosive reaction. Although this complication has not been reported with lactulose, patients on lactulose therapy undergoing such procedures should have a thorough bowel cleansing with a non-fermentable solution. Insufflation of CO_2 as an additional safeguard may be pursued but is considered to be a redundant measure.
Use in Pregnancy
Studies in laboratory animals have not revealed a teratogenic potential of lactulose. The safety of lactulose syrup during pegnancy and its effect on the mother or the fetus have not been evaluated in humans. The physician and patient should understand that the possibility that lactulose syrup might cause damage to the human fetus cannot be excluded. Lactulose syrup should not be given during pregnancy unless, in the opinion of the physician, the possible benefits outweigh the possible risks.
Precautions: Lactulose syrup contains galactose (less than 2.2 g/15 ml) and lactose (less than 1.2 g/15 ml) and it should be used with caution in diabetics.
There have been conflicting reports about the concomitant use of neomycin and lactulose syrup. Theoretically, the elimination of certain colonic bacteria by neomycin and possibly other anti-infective agents may intefere with the desired degradation of lactulose and thus prevent the acidification of colonic contents. Thus the status of the lactulose-treated patient should be closely monitored in the event of concomitant oral anti-infective therapy.
Other laxatives should not be used especially during the initial phase of therapy for portal-systemic encephalopathy because the loose stools resulting from their use may falsely suggest that adequate Cephulac dosage has been achieved.
In the overall management of portal-systemic encephalopathy it should be recognized that there is serious underlying liver disease with complications such as electrolyte disturbance (e.g., hypokalemia) for which other specific therapy may be required.

Adverse Reactions: Cephulac may produce gaseous distention with flatulence or belching and abdominal discomfort such as cramping in about 20% of patients. Excessive dosage can lead to diarrhea. Nausea and vomiting have been reported infrequently.
Overdosage: There have been no reports of accidental overdosage. In the event of overdosage it is expected that diarrhea and abdominal cramps would be the major symptoms.
Dosage and Administration:
Oral
Adult: The usual adult, oral dosage is 2 to 3 tablespoonfuls (30 to 45 ml, containing 20 g to 30 g of lactulose) three or four times daily. The dosage may be adjusted every day or two to produce 2 or 3 soft stools daily.
Hourly doses of 30 to 45 ml of Cephulac may be used to induce the rapid laxation indicated in the initial phase of the therapy of portal-systemic encephalopathy. When the laxative effect has been achieved, the dose of Cephulac may then be reduced to the recommended daily dose. Improvement in the patient's condition may occur within 24 hours but may not begin before 48 hours or even later.
Continuous long-term therapy is indicated to lessen the severity and prevent the recurrence of portal-systemic encephalopathy. The dose of Cephulac for this purpose is the same as the recommended daily dose.
Pediatric: Very little information on the use of lactulose in young children and adolescents has been recorded. As with adults, the subjective goal in proper treatment is to produce 2 or 3 soft stools daily. On the basis of information available, the recommended initial daily oral dose in infants is 2.5 to 10 ml in divided doses. For older children and adolescents the total daily dose is 40 to 90 ml. If the initial dose causes diarrhea, the dose should be reduced immediately. If diarrhea persists, lactulose should be discontinued.
Rectal
When the adult patient is in the impending coma or coma stage of portal-systemic encephalopathy and the danger of aspiration exists, or when the necessary endoscopic or intubation procedures physically interfere with the administration of the recommended oral doses, Cephulac may be given as a retention enema via a rectal balloon catheter. Cleansing enemas containing soap suds or other alkaline agents should not be used.
Three hundred ml of Cephulac should be mixed with 700 ml of water or physiologic saline and retained for 30 to 60 minutes. Cephulac enema may be repeated every 4 to 6 hours. If the enema is inadvertently evacuated too promptly, it may be repeated immediately.
The goal of treatment is reversal of the coma stage in order that the patient may be able to take oral medication. Reversal of coma may take place within 2 hours of the first enema in some patients. Cephulac given orally in the recommended doses should be started before Cephulac by enema is stopped entirely.
How Supplied:
1 pint (473 ml containing 315 g of lactulose)
2 quarts (1.89 liters containing 1260 g or 1.26 kg of lactulose)
15 ml (containing 10 g of lactulose) unit dose containers
30 ml (containing 20 g of lactulose) unit dose containers

Product Information as of April, 1981

Store at room temperature, below 86°F (30°C). Do not freeze.
Under recommended storage conditions, a normal darkening of color may occur. Such darkening is characteristic of sugar solutions and

Continued on next page

Information on Merrell Dow products is based on labeling in effect in October, 1982.

Merrell Dow—Cont.

does not affect therapeutic action. Prolonged exposure to temperatures above 86°F (30°C) or to direct light may cause extreme darkening and turbidity which may be pharmaceutically objectionable. If this condition develops do not use.
Prolonged exposure to freezing temperatures may cause change to a semisolid, too viscous to pour. Viscosity will return to normal upon warming to room temperature.
[*Shown in Product Identification Section*]

CHRONULAC® ℞
(lactulose)
Syrup

Caution: Federal law prohibits dispensing without a prescription.

Description: Chronulac is 4-O-β-D-galactopyranosyl-D-fructofuranose.
The molecular formula is $C_{12}H_{22}O_{11}$ and the molecular weight is 342.30. Each 15 ml of Chronulac contains: 10 g lactulose (and less than 2.2 g galactose, less than 1.2 g lactose, and 1.2 g or less of other sugars).
Clinical Pharmacology: Chronulac is poorly absorbed from the gastrointestinal tract and no enzyme capable of hydrolysis of this disaccharide is present in human gastrointestinal tissue. As a result, oral doses of Chronulac reach the colon virtually unchanged. In the colon, Chronulac is broken down primarily to lactic acid, and also to small amounts of formic and acetic acids, by the action of colonic bacteria, which results in an increase in osmotic pressure and slight acidification of the colonic contents. This in turn causes an increase in stool water content and softens the stool.
Since Chronulac does not exert its effect until it reaches the colon, and since transit time through the colon may be slow, 24 to 48 hours may be required to produce a normal bowel movement.
Chronulac given orally to man and experimental animals resulted in only small amounts reaching the blood. Urinary excretion has been determined to be 3% or less and is essentially complete within 24 hours.
Indication: For the treatment of constipation. In patients with a history of chronic constipation, lactulose syrup (Chronulac) therapy increases the number of bowel movements per day and the number of days on which bowel movements occur.
Contraindications: Since Chronulac contains galactose (less than 2.2 g/15 ml), it is contraindicated in patients who require a low galactose diet.
Warnings:
A theoretical hazard may exist for patients being treated with lactulose syrup who may be required to undergo electrocautery procedures during proctoscopy or colonoscopy. Accumulation of H_2 gas in significant concentration in the presence of an electrical spark may result in an explosive reaction. Although this complication has not been reported with lactulose, patients on lactulose therapy undergoing such procedures should have a thorough bowel cleansing with a non-fermentable solution. Insufflation of CO_2 as an additional safeguard may be pursued but is considered to be a redundant measure.
Use in Pregnancy
Studies in laboratory animals (mice, rats, rabbits) have not revealed a teratogenic potential of Chronulac. The safety of Chronulac syrup during pregnancy and its effect on the mother or the fetus have not been evaluated in humans.
The physician and patient should understand that the possibility that Chronulac might cause damage to the human fetus cannot be excluded. Chronulac should not be given during pregnancy unless, in the opinion of the physician, the possible benefits outweigh the possible risks.
Use in Nursing Mothers
There are no data on secretion of Chronulac in human milk or effect on the nursing infant.
Use in Children
There is insufficient experience to recommend a dose of Chronulac that is safe and effective for treatment of constipation in children.
Precautions: Elderly, debilitated patients who receive Chronulac for more than six months should have serum electrolytes (potassium, chloride, carbon dioxide) measured periodically. Also, since Chronulac contains galactose (less than 2.2 g/15 ml) and lactose (less than 1.2 g/15 ml), it should be used with caution in diabetics.
Adverse Reactions: Initial dosing may produce flatulence and intestinal cramps, which are usually transient. Excessive dosage can lead to diarrhea. Nausea has been reported.
Overdosage: There have been no reports of accidental overdosage. In the event of overdosage it is expected that diarrhea and abdominal cramps would be the major symptoms. Medication should be terminated.
Dosage and Administration: The usual dose is 1 to 2 tablespoonfuls (15 to 30 ml, containing 10 g to 20 g of lactulose) daily. The dose may be increased to 60 ml daily if necessary. Twenty-four to 48 hours may be required to produce a normal bowel movement.
Note: Some patients have found that Chronulac may be more acceptable when mixed with fruit juice, water, or milk.
How Supplied:
8 fl. oz. bottles (237 ml)
15 ml unit dose cups (containing 10 g of lactulose) in trays of 10 cups
30 ml unit dose cups (containing 20 g of lactulose) in trays of 10 cups
1 quart bottles (946 ml)
Product Information as of April, 1981
Store at room temperature, below 86°F (30°C). Do not freeze.
Under recommended storage conditions, a normal darkening of color may occur. Such darkening is characteristic of sugar solutions and does not affect therapeutic action. Prolonged exposure to temperatures above 86°F (30°C) or to direct light may cause extreme darkening and turbidity which may be pharmaceutically objectionable. If this condition develops do not use.
Prolonged exposure to freezing temperatures may cause change to a semisolid, too viscous to pour. Viscosity will return to normal upon warming to room temperature.
[*Shown in Product Identification Section*]

CLOMID® ℞
(clomiphene citrate)

For prescribing information, write to:
Manager, Professional Services
MERRELL DOW PHARMACEUTICALS INC.
Subsidiary of The Dow Chemical Company
Cincinnati, Ohio 45215, U.S.A.

DV® (dienestrol USP) ℞
Cream/Suppositories

AVAILABLE ONLY ON PRESCRIPTION

Warnings:

1. ESTROGENS HAVE BEEN REPORTED TO INCREASE THE RISK RATIO FOR ENDOMETRIAL CARCINOMA.
Three independent case control studies have reported an increased risk ratio of endometrial cancer in postmenopausal women exposed to exogenous estrogens for prolonged periods.[1–3] This reported risk was independent of the other risk factors studied. Additionally, the incidence rates of endometrial cancer have increased since 1969 in 8 different areas of the United States with population-based cancer reporting systems, an increase that may [or may not] be related to the expanded use of estrogens during the last decade.[4]
The 3 case control studies reported that the estimated risk ratio for endometrial cancer in estrogen users was about 4.5 to 13.9 times greater than in nonusers. The risk appeared to depend on both duration of treatment[1] and on estrogen dose.[3] In view of these reports, when estrogens are used for the treatment of menopausal symptoms, the lowest dose that will control symptoms should be utilized and medication should be discontinued as soon as possible. When prolonged treatment is medically indicated, the patient should be reassessed on at least a semiannual basis to determine the need for continued therapy. Although the evidence must be considered preliminary, one study suggests that cyclic administration of low doses of estrogen may carry less risk than continuous administration;[3] it therefore appears prudent to utilize such a regimen.
Close clinical surveillance of all women taking estrogens is important. In all cases of undiagnosed persistent or recurring abnormal vaginal bleeding, adequate diagnostic measures should be undertaken to rule out malignancy.
There is no evidence at present that "natural" estrogens are more or less hazardous than "synthetic" estrogens at equiestrogenic doses.
2. ESTROGENS SHOULD NOT BE USED DURING PREGNANCY.
The use of exogenous estrogens and progestagens during early pregnancy has been reported to damage the offspring. An association has been reported between *in utero* exposure of the female fetus to diethylstilbestrol, a non-steroidal estrogen, and an increased risk of the post-pubertal development of an ordinarily rare form of vaginal or cervical cancer.[5,6] This risk for diethylstilbestrol was recently estimated to be in the range of 0.14 to 1.4 per 1000 exposures,[7] consistent with a previous risk estimate of not greater than 4 per 1000 exposures.[8] Furthermore, a high percentage of such females exposed *in utero* (30 to over 90%) has been reported to have vaginal adenosis, epithelial changes of the vagina and cervix.[9–12] Although these changes are histologically benign, it is not known whether they are precursors of adenocarcinoma. Although similar data are not available with the use of other estrogens, it cannot be presumed they would not induce similar changes.
Several reports suggest a possible association between fetal exposure to exogenous estrogens and progestagens and congenital anomalies, including congenital heart defects and limb reduction defects.[13–16] One case control study[16] estimated a 4.7 fold increased risk of limb reduction defects in infants exposed *in utero* to exogenous steroids (oral contraceptives, hormone withdrawal tests for pregnancy, or attempted treatment for threatened abortion). Some of these exposures were very short and involved only a few days of treatment. The data suggest that the risk of limb reduction defects in exposed fetuses is somewhat less than 1 per 1000.
This product is not for use in therapy of threatened or habitual abortion.
If DV (dienestrol USP) Cream or Suppositories are used during pregnancy, or if the patient becomes pregnant while using this drug, she should be apprised of the poten-

tial risks to the fetus, and the advisability of pregnancy continuation.

Description: DV (dienestrol USP) is a synthetic estrogen in cream and suppository form suitable for vaginal administration.

DV Cream (dienestrol cream USP)—Each tube contains:

Dienestrol USP ....0.01% with lactose, in a water-miscible base made from propylene glycol, stearic acid, diglycol stearate, trolamine, benzoic acid, butylated hydroxytoluene and disodium edetate; buffered with lactic acid to an acid pH.

DV Suppositories—Each suppository contains:

Dienestrol USP ....0.70 mg with lactose, in a base made from polyethylene glycol 400, polysorbate 80, polyethylene glycol 4000, glycerin, and butylated hydroxytoluene; buffered with lactic acid to an acid pH. DV Suppositories have an inert covering, which dissolves promptly in the vagina. The covering is composed of gelatin, glycerin, water, methylparaben, and propylparaben. Contains color additives including FD&C Yellow No. 5 (tartrazine).

Chemistry

Generic name: Dienestrol USP

Chemical name: Phenol,4,4′-(1,2-diethylidene-1,2-ethanediyl)bis,(*E,E*)-. 4,4 -(Diethylideneethylene)diphenol.

Dienestrol occurs as colorless, white, or practically white needlelike crystals or as a white or practically white crystalline powder. It is odorless. It is practically insoluble in water, is slightly soluble in chloroform and fatty oils, and is soluble in alcohol, acetone, ether, and propylene glycol.

Indications: For the treatment of atrophic vaginitis and kraurosis vulvae.

DV (dienestrol USP) CREAM AND SUPPOSITORIES HAVE NOT BEEN SHOWN TO BE EFFECTIVE FOR ANY PURPOSE DURING PREGNANCY AND THE USE MAY HAVE POTENTIAL RISKS TO THE FETUS. (SEE BOXED WARNING.)

Contraindications: DV (dienestrol USP) should not be used in patients with any of the following conditions:

1. Known or suspected cancer of the breast except in appropriately selected patients being treated for metastatic disease.
2. Known or suspected estrogen-dependent neoplasia.
3. Known or suspected pregnancy. (See Boxed Warning.)
4. Undiagnosed abnormal genital bleeding.
5. Active thrombophlebitis or thromboembolic disorders.
6. A past history of thrombophlebitis, thrombosis, or thromboembolic disorders.
7. Hypersensitivity to the ingredients of the cream or suppositories.

Warnings:

1. *Induction of malignant neoplasms.* Long-term continuous administration of natural and synthetic estrogens in certain animal species increases the frequency of carcinomas of the breast, cervix, vagina, and liver. There are now reports that estrogens increase the risk of carcinoma of the endometrium in humans. (See Boxed Warning.)

At the present time there is no satisfactory evidence that estrogens given to postmenopausal women increase the risk of cancer of the breast,[17] although a recent long-term followup of a single physician's practice has raised this possibility.[18] Because of the animal data, there is a need for caution in prescribing estrogens for women with a strong family history of breast cancer or who have breast nodules, fibrocystic disease, or abnormal mammograms.

2. *Gallbladder disease.* A recent study has reported a two to threefold increase in the risk of surgically confirmed gallbladder disease in women receiving postmenopausal estrogens,[17] similar to the twofold increase previously noted in users of oral contraceptives.[19] In the case of oral contraceptives the increased risk appeared after a period of use.[19]

3. *Effects similar to those caused by estrogen-progestagen oral contraceptives.* There are several adverse effects reported in association with oral contraceptives, most of which have not been documented as consequences of postmenopausal estrogen therapy, although it has been reported that there is an increased risk of thrombosis in men receiving high doses of estrogens for prostatic cancer and in women receiving estrogens for postpartum breast engorgement.[20–23] The possibility that the adverse effects reported in association with oral contraceptives may be associated with larger doses of estrogen cannot be excluded.

a. *Thromboembolic disease.* Studies have now shown that users of oral contraceptives have an increased risk of various thromboembolic, thrombotic, and vascular diseases, such as thrombophlebitis, pulmonary embolism, stroke, and myocardial infarction.[24–31] Cases of retinal thrombosis, mesenteric thrombosis, and optic neuritis have been reported in oral contraceptive users. There is evidence that the risk of several of these adverse reactions is related to the dose of the drug.[32,33] An increased risk of post-surgery thromboembolic complications has also been reported in users of oral contraceptives.[34,35] If feasible, estrogen should be discontinued at least 4 weeks before surgery of the type associated with an increased risk of thromboembolism, or during periods of prolonged immobilization.

While an increased rate of thromboembolic and thrombotic disease in postmenopausal users of estrogens has not been found,[17,36] this does not rule out the possibility that such an increase may be present, or that subgroups of women who have underlying risk factors, or who are receiving relatively large doses of estrogens may have an increased risk. Therefore, estrogens should not be used in persons with active thrombophlebitis or thromboembolic disorders, and they should not be used (except in treatment of malignancy) in persons with a history of such disorders. They should be used with caution in patients with cerebral vascular or coronary artery disease and only for those in whom estrogens are needed.

Doses of estrogen (5 mg. conjugated estrogens per day), comparable to those used to treat cancer of the prostate and breast, have been reported in a large prospective clinical trial in men[37] to increase the risk of nonfatal myocardial infarction, pulmonary embolism, and thrombophlebitis. When estrogen doses of this size are used, any of the thromboembolic and thrombotic adverse effects associated with oral contraceptive use should be considered as a risk.

b. *Hepatic adenoma.* Benign hepatic adenomas have been reported to be associated with the use of oral contraceptives.[38–40] Although benign and rare, these may rupture and may cause death through intra-abdominal hemorrhage. Such lesions have not yet been reported in association with other estrogen or progestagen preparations but should be considered in estrogen users having abdominal pain and tenderness, abdominal mass, or hypovolemic shock. Hepatocellular carcinoma has also been reported in women taking estrogen-containing oral contraceptives.[39] The relationship of this malignancy to these drugs is not known at this time.

c. *Elevated blood pressure.* Increased blood pressure is not uncommon in women using oral contraceptives and there is now a report that this may occur with use of estrogens in the menopause[41] and blood pressure should be monitored with estrogen use, especially if high doses are used.

d. *Glucose tolerance.* A worsening of glucose tolerance has been observed in a significant percentage of patients on estrogen-containing oral contraceptives. For this reason diabetic patients should be carefully observed while receiving estrogen.

4. *Hypercalcemia.* Administration of estrogens may lead to hypercalcemia in patients with breast cancer and bone metastases. If this occurs, the drug should be stopped and appropriate measures taken to reduce the serum calcium level.

Precautions:

A. General Precautions

1. A complete medical and family history should be taken prior to the initiation of any estrogen therapy. The pretreatment and periodic physical examinations should include special reference to blood pressure, breasts, abdomen, and pelvic organs, and should include a Papanicolaou smear. As a general rule, estrogen should not be prescribed for longer than 1 year without another physical examination being performed.
2. For conditions due to infection with known organisms, specific treatment should be given for the organism responsible.
3. Fluid retention—Because estrogens may cause some degree of fluid retention, conditions that might be influenced by this factor such as epilepsy, migraine, and cardiac or renal dysfunction require careful observation.
4. Certain patients may develop undesirable manifestations of excessive estrogenic stimulation, such as abnormal or excessive uterine bleeding, mastodynia, etc. In order to avoid this, the dosage should be reduced or the estrogens should be administered intermittently in the menopausal or hypogonadal patient.
5. The age of the patient constitutes no absolute limiting factor, although treatment with estrogens may mask the onset of the climacteric.
6. Oral contraceptives have been reported to be associated with an increased incidence of mental depression. Although it is not clear whether this is possibly due to the estrogenic or progestagenic component of the contraceptive, patients with a history of depression should be carefully observed.
7. Patients having pre-existing uterine leiomyomata should be observed for increased growth of myomata during estrogen therapy.
8. The pathologist should be advised of estrogen therapy when relevant specimens are submitted.
9. Patients with a past history of jaundice during pregnancy have an increased risk of recurrence of jaundice while receiving estrogen-containing oral contraceptive therapy. If jaundice develops in any patient receiving estrogen, the medication should be discontinued while the cause is investigated.
10. Estrogens may be poorly metabolized in patients with impaired liver function and they should be administered with caution in such patients.
11. Because estrogens influence the metabolism of calcium and phosphorus, they should be used with caution in patients with metabolic bone diseases that are associated with hypercalcemia or in patients with renal insufficiency.
12. Because of the effects of estrogens on epiphyseal closure, they should be used judiciously in young patients in whom bone growth is not complete.
13. Judicious assessment of the following changes in certain endocrine and liver function tests is necessary for patients receiving large doses of estrogen:

a. Increased sulfobromophthalein retention.
b. Increased prothrombin and factors VII, VIII, IX, and X; decreased antithrombin 3;

Continued on next page

Information on Merrell Dow products is based on labeling in effect in October, 1982.

Merrell Dow—Cont.

increased norepinephrine-induced platelet aggregability.

c. Increased thyroid binding globulin (TBG) leading to increased circulating total thyroid hormone, as measured by PBI, T4 by column, or T4 by radioimmunoassay. Free T3 resin uptake is decreased, reflecting the elevated TBG; free T4 concentration is unaltered.

d. Impaired glucose tolerance.

e. Decreased pregnanediol excretion.

f. Reduced response to metyrapone test.

g. Reduced serum folate concentration.

h. Increased serum triglyceride, phospholipid, or cholesterol.

14. DV Suppositories contain FD&C Yellow No. 5 (tartrazine), which may cause allergic-type reactions (including bronchial asthma) in certain susceptible individuals. Although the overall incidence of FD&C Yellow No. 5 (tartrazine) sensitivity in the general population is low, it is frequently seen in patients who also have aspirin hypersensitivity.

B. Information For The Patient

A patient package insert accompanies this drug product. This insert is available from pharmacists who carry this product and from the company upon request.

C. Pregnancy Category X

See Contraindications and Boxed Warning.

D. Nursing Mothers

As a general principle, the administration of any drug to nursing mothers should be done only when clearly necessary since many drugs are excreted in human milk.

Adverse Reactions: (See Warnings regarding reports of induction of neoplasia, adverse effects on the fetus, increased incidence of gallbladder disease, and adverse effects similar to those of oral contraceptives, including thromboembolism.)

Since there is a possibility of dienestrol absorption through the vaginal mucosa, uterine bleeding might be provoked by excessive administration of dienestrol in menopausal women. Cytologic study or D & C may be required to differentiate this uterine bleeding from carcinoma. Tenderness of the breasts and vaginal discharge due to mucus hypersecretion may result from excessive estrogenic stimulation; endometrial withdrawal bleeding may occur if use of dienestrol is suddenly discontinued. Such reactions indicate overdosage.

Menstrual irregularity may be made worse by dienestrol if a sufficient amount is absorbed. Dienestrol may cause serious bleeding in a woman sterilized because of endometriosis and in whom remaining foci of endometrium could be activated.

The following additional adverse reactions have been reported with estrogenic therapy including oral contraceptives:

1. *Genitourinary system*

Breakthrough bleeding, spotting, change in menstrual flow and cycle.
Dysmenorrhea.
Premenstrual-like syndrome.
Amenorrhea during and after treatment.
Increase in size of uterine fibromyomata.
Vaginal candidiasis.
Change in cervical eversion and in degree of cervical secretion.
Cystitis-like syndrome.

2. *Breasts*

Tenderness, enlargement, secretion.

3. *Gastrointestinal*

Nausea, vomiting.
Abdominal cramps, bloating.
Cholestatic jaundice.

4. *Skin*

Chloasma or melasma which may persist when drug is discontinued.
Erythema multiforme.
Erythema nodosum.
Hemorrhagic eruption.
Loss of scalp hair.
Hirsutism.
Urticaria.

5. *Eyes*

Steepening of corneal curvature.
Intolerance to contact lenses.

6. *CNS*

Headache, migraine, dizziness.
Mental depression.
Chorea.

7. *Miscellaneous*

Increase or decrease in weight.
Reduced carbohydrate tolerance.
Aggravation of porphyria.
Edema.
Changes in libido and/or potency.

Acute Overdosage: Numerous reports of ingestion of large doses of estrogen-containing oral contraceptives by young children indicate that serious ill effects usually do not occur. Overdosage of estrogen may cause nausea, and withdrawal bleeding may occur in females.

Dosage and Administration: 1 or 2 applicatorfuls of cream or 1 or 2 suppositories intravaginally per day for 1 or 2 weeks, then reduced to either one-half initial dosage or 1 applicatorful (about 6 g) or 1 suppository every other day for a similar period.

Maintenance Dose

1 applicatorful of cream or 1 suppository one to three times a week may be used after restoration of the vaginal mucosa has been effected.

How Supplied:

DV Cream

NDC 0068-0293-13: 3 oz. tube with applicator

DV Suppositories

NDC 0068-0294-16: box of 16 with inserter

References:

1. Ziel, H.K. and Finkel, W.D.: Increased risk of endometrial carcinoma among users of conjugated estrogens. New Eng. J. Med. 293:1167-1170, 1975.
2. Smith, D.C., Prentice, R., Thompson, D.J., and Hermann, W.L.: Association of exogenous estrogen and endometrial carcinoma. New Eng. J. Med. 293:1164-1167, 1975.
3. Mack, T.M., Pike, M.C., Henderson, B.E., Pfeffer, R.I., Gerkins, V.R., Arthur, M., and Brown, S.E.: Estrogens and endometrial cancer in a retirement community. New Eng. J. Med. 294:1262-1267, 1976.
4. Weiss, N.S., Szekely, D.R., and Austin, D.F.: Increasing incidence of endometrial cancer in the United States. New Eng. J. Med. 294:1259-1262, 1976.
5. Herbst, A.L., Ulfelder, H., and Poskanzer, D.C.: Adenocarcinoma of the vagina. New Eng. J. Med. 284:878-881, 1971.
6. Greenwald, P., Barlow, J.J., Nasca, P.C., and Burnett, W.S.: Vaginal cancer after maternal treatment with synthetic estrogens. New Eng. J. Med. 285:390-392, 1971.
7. Herbst, A.L., Cole, P., Colton, T., Robboy, S.J., and Scully, R.E.: Age-incidence and risk of diethylstilbestrol-related clear cell adenocarcinoma of the vagina and cervix. Amer. J. Obstet. Gynec. 128:43-50, 1977.
8. Lanier, A.P., Noller, K.L., Decker, D.G., Elveback, L.R., and Kurland, L.T.: Cancer and stilbestrol. A follow-up of 1719 persons exposed to estrogens in utero and born 1943-1959. Mayo Clin. Proc. 48:793-799, 1973.
9. Herbst, A.L., Kurman, R.J., and Scully, R.E.: Vaginal and cervical abnormalities after exposure to stilbestrol in utero. Obstet. Gynec. 40:287-298, 1972.
10. Herbst, A.L., Poskanzer, D.C., Robboy, S.J., Friedlander, L., and Scully, R.E.: Prenatal exposure to stilbestrol. A prospective comparison of exposed female offspring with unexposed controls. New Eng. J. Med. 292:334-339, 1975.
11. Stafl, A., Mattingly, R.F., Foley, D.V., and Fetherston, W.C.: Clinical diagnosis of vaginal adenosis. Obstet. Gynec. 43:118-128, 1974.
12. Sherman, A.I., Goldrath, M., Berlin, A., Vakhariya, V., Banooni, F., Michaels, W., Goodman, P., and Brown, S.: Cervical-vaginal adenosis after *in utero* exposure to synthetic estrogens. Obstet. Gynec. 44:531-545, 1974.
13. Gal, I., Kirman, B., and Stern, J.: Hormone pregnancy tests and congenital malformation. Nature 216:83, 1967.
14. Levy, E.P., Cohen, A., and Fraser, F.C.: Hormone treatment during pregnancy and congenital heart defects. Lancet 1:611, 1973.
15. Nora, J.J. and Nora, A.H.: Birth defects and oral contraceptives. Lancet 1:941-942, 1973.
16. Janerich, D.T., Piper, J.M., and Glebatis, D.M.: Oral contraceptives and congenital limb-reduction defects. New Eng. J. Med. 291:697-700, 1974.
17. Boston Collaborative Drug Surveillance Program: Surgically confirmed gall bladder disease, venous thromboembolism, and breast tumors in relation to post menopausal estrogen therapy. New Eng. J. Med. 290:15-19, 1974.
18. Hoover, R., Gray, L.A., Sr., Cole, P., and MacMahon, B.: Menopausal estrogens and breast cancer. New Eng. J. Med. 295:401-405, 1976.
19. Boston Collaborative Drug Surveillance Program: Oral contraceptives and venous thromboembolic disease, surgically confirmed gall-bladder disease, and breast tumors. Lancet 1:1399-1404, 1973.
20. Daniel, D.G., Campbell, H., and Turnbull, A.C.: Puerperal thromboembolism and suppression of lactation. Lancet 2:287-289, 1967.
21. Bailar, J.C., III: Thromboembolism and oestrogen therapy. Lancet 2:560, 1967.
22. The Veterans Administration Cooperative Urological Research Group: Carcinoma of the prostate: Treatment comparisons. J. Urol. 98:516-522, 1967.
23. Blackard, C.E., Doe, R.P., Mellinger, G.T., and Byar, D.P.: Incidence of cardiovascular disease and death in patients receiving diethylstilbestrol for carcinoma of the prostate. Cancer 26:249-256, 1970.
24. Royal College of General Practitioners: Oral contraception and thromboembolic disease. J. Roy. Coll. Gen. Pract. 13:267-269, 1967.
25. Inman, W.H.W. and Vessey, M.P.: Investigation of deaths from pulmonary, coronary, and cerebral thrombosis and embolism in women of child-bearing age. Brit. Med. J. 2:193-199, 1968.
26. Vessey, M.P. and Doll, R.: Investigation of relation between use of oral contraceptives and thromboembolic disease. A further report. Brit. Med. J. 2:651-657, 1969.
27. Sartwell, P.E., Masi, A.T., Arthes, F.G., Greene, G.R., and Smith, H.E.: Thromboembolism and oral contraceptives: An epidemiological case-control study. Amer. J. Epidem. 90:365-380, 1969.
28. Collaborative Group for the Study of Stroke in Young Women: Oral contraception and increased risk of cerebral ischemia or thrombosis. New Eng. J. Med. 288:871-878, 1973.
29. Collaborative Group for the Study of Stroke in Young Women: Oral contraceptives and stroke in young women: Associated risk factors. J.A.M.A. 231:718-722, 1975.
30. Mann, J.I. and Inman, W.H.W.: Oral contraceptives and death from myocardial infarction. Brit. Med. J. 2:245-248, 1975.
31. Mann, J.I., Vessey, M.P., Thorogood, M., and Doll, R.: Myocardial infarction in young women with special reference in oral contraceptive practice. Brit. Med. J. 2:241-245, 1975.
32. Inman, W.H.W., Vessey, M.P., Westerholm, B., and Engelund, A.: Thromboembolic disease and the steroidal content of oral contraceptives. A report to the Committee on Safety of Drugs. Brit. Med. J. 2:203-209, 1970.
33. Stolley, P.D., Tonascia, J.A., Tockman, M.S., Sartwell, P.E., Rutledge, A.H., and Jacobs, M.P.: Thrombosis with low-estrogen oral

contraceptives. Amer. J. Epidem. 102:197-208, 1975.
34. Vessey, M.P., Doll, R., Fairbairn, A.S., and Glober, G.: Post-operative thromboembolism and the use of the oral contraceptives. Brit. Med. J. 3:123-126, 1970.
35. Greene, G.R. and Sartwell, P.E.: Oral contraceptive use in patients with thromboembolism following surgery, trauma, or infection. Amer. J. Public Health 62:680-685, 1972.
36. Rosenberg, L., Armstrong, B., Phil, D., and Jick, H.: Myocardial infarction and estrogen therapy in post-menopausal women. New Eng. J. Med. 294:1256-1259, 1976.
37. Coronary Drug Project Research Group: The coronary drug project: Initial findings leading to modifications of its research protocol. J.A.M.A. 214:1303-1313, 1970.
38. Baum, J., Holtz, F., Bookstein, J.J., and Klein, E.W.: Possible association between benign hepatomas and oral contraceptives. Lancet 2:926-928, 1973.
39. Mays, E.T., Christopherson, W.M., Mahr, M.M., and Williams, H.C.: Hepatic changes in young women ingesting contraceptive steroids. Hepatic hemorrhage and primary hepatic tumors. J.A.M.A. 235:730-732, 1976.
40. Edmondson, H., Henderson, A.B., and Benton, B.: Liver-cell adenomas associated with the use of oral contraceptives. New Eng. J. Med. 294:470-472, 1976.
41. Pfeffer, R.I. and Van Den Noort, S.: Estrogen use and stroke risk in postmenopausal women. Amer. J. Epidem. 103:445-456, 1976.

Product Information as of August, 1979

DV Suppositories are manufactured by
R. P. Scherer, North America
Clearwater, Florida 33518 for
MERRELL DOW PHARMACEUTICALS INC.
Subsidiary of The Dow Chemical Company
Cincinnati, Ohio 45215, U.S.A.

HIPREX® ℞
(methenamine hippurate)

AVAILABLE ONLY ON PRESCRIPTION

Description: Hiprex (methenamine hippurate) is the hippuric acid salt of methenamine (hexamethylenetetramine).

Actions: Microbiology: Hiprex (methenamine hippurate) has antibacterial activity because the methenamine component is hydrolyzed to formaldehyde in acid urine. Hippuric acid, the other component, has some antibacterial activity and also acts to keep the urine acid. The drug is generally active against *E. coli,* enterococci and staphylococci. *Enterobacter aerogenes* is generally resistant. The urine must be kept sufficiently acid for urea-splitting organisms such as *Proteus* and *Pseudomonas* to be inhibited.

Human Pharmacology: Within ½ hour after ingestion of a single 1-gram dose of Hiprex, antibacterial activity is demonstrable in the urine. Urine has continuous antibacterial activity when Hiprex is administered at the recommended dosage schedule of 1 gram twice daily. Over 90% of methenamine moiety is excreted in the urine within 24 hours after administration of a single 1-gram dose. Similarly, the hippurate moiety is rapidly absorbed and excreted, and it reaches the urine by both tubular secretion and glomerular filtration. This action may be important in older patients or in those with some degree of renal impairment.

Indications: Hiprex is indicated for prophylactic or suppressive treatment of frequently recurring urinary tract infections when long-term therapy is considered necessary. This drug should only be used after eradication of the infection by other appropriate antimicrobial agents.

Contraindications: Hiprex (methenamine hippurate) is contraindicated in patients with renal insufficiency, severe hepatic insufficiency, or severe dehydration. Methenamine preparations should not be given to patients taking sulfonamides because some sulfonamides may form an insoluble precipitate with formaldehyde in the urine.

Warnings: Large doses of methenamine (8 grams daily for 3 to 4 weeks) have caused bladder irritation, painful and frequent micturition, albuminuria, and gross hematuria.

Precautions:

1. Care should be taken to maintain an acid pH of the urine, especially when treating infections due to urea-splitting organisms such as *Proteus* and strains of *Pseudomonas.*
2. In a few instances in one study, the serum transaminase levels were slightly elevated during treatment but returned to normal while the patients were still taking Hiprex. Because of this report, it is recommended that liver function studies be performed periodically on patients taking the drug, especially those with liver dysfunction.
3. *Use in pregnancy:* In early pregnancy the safe use of Hiprex is not established. In the last trimester, safety is suggested, but not definitely proved. No adverse effects on the fetus were seen in studies in pregnant rats and rabbits.

Hiprex taken during pregnancy can interfere with laboratory tests of urine estriol (resulting in unmeasurably low values) when acid hydrolysis is used in the laboratory procedure. This interference is due to the presence in the urine of methenamine and/or formaldehyde. Enzymatic hydrolysis, in place of acid hydrolysis, will circumvent this problem.

4. This product contains FD&C Yellow No. 5 (tartrazine), which may cause allergic-type reactions (including bronchial asthma) in certain susceptible individuals. Although the overall incidence of FD&C Yellow No. 5 (tartrazine) sensitivity in the general population is low, it is frequently seen in patients who also have aspirin hypersensitivity.

Adverse Reactions: Minor adverse reactions have been reported in less than 3.5% of patients treated. These reactions have included nausea, upset stomach, dysuria, and rash.

Dosage and Administration:

1 tablet (1.0 g) twice daily (morning and night) for adults and children over 12 years of age.
½ to 1 tablet (0.5 to 1.0 g) twice daily (morning and night) for children 6 to 12 years of age.
Since the antibacterial activity of Hiprex is greater in acid urine, restriction of alkalinizing foods and medications is desirable. If necessary, as indicated by urinary pH and clinical response, supplemental acidification of the urine should be instituted. The efficacy of therapy should be monitored by repeated urine cultures.

How Supplied: 1-gram scored, capsule-shaped yellow tablets debossed MERRELL 277 in bottles of 100 and 500

Product Information as of August, 1979
[Shown in Product Identification Section]

IMFERON® ℞
(iron dextran injection USP)

AVAILABLE ONLY ON PRESCRIPTION

Warning:

THE PARENTERAL USE OF COMPLEXES OF IRON AND CARBOHYDRATES HAS RESULTED IN FATAL ANAPHYLACTIC-TYPE REACTIONS. DEATHS ASSOCIATED WITH SUCH ADMINISTRATION HAVE BEEN REPORTED. THEREFORE, IMFERON SHOULD BE USED ONLY IN THOSE PATIENTS IN WHOM THE INDICATIONS HAVE BEEN CLEARLY ESTABLISHED AND LABORATORY INVESTIGATIONS CONFIRM AN IRON DEFICIENT STATE NOT AMENABLE TO ORAL IRON THERAPY.

Description: Imferon is a dark brown, slightly viscous liquid complex of ferric hydroxide and dextran in a 0.9% sodium chloride solution for injection. It contains the equivalent of 50 mg elemental iron (as an iron dextran complex) per ml. Multiple dose vial also contains 0.5% phenol.

Action: The iron dextran complex is dissociated by the reticuloendothelial system, and the ferric iron is transported by transferrin and incorporated into hemoglobin.

Indications: Intravenous or intramuscular injections of iron dextran USP are advisable solely for use in those patients in whom an iron deficiency state is present, its cause has been determined, and, if possible, corrected, and in whom oral administration of iron is unsatisfactory or impossible.

Contraindications: Hypersensitivity to the product. All anemias other than iron deficiency anemia.

WARNINGS: Two ml of undiluted iron dextran is the maximum recommended daily dose for intravenous use. (See DOSAGE AND ADMINISTRATION.) Large intravenous doses, such as those used in Total Dose Infusions, may be associated with an increased incidence of adverse effects, particularly, delayed reactions typified by arthralgia, myalgia, and fever.

This preparation should be used with extreme care in patients with serious impairment of liver function.

A risk of carcinogenesis may attend the intramuscular injection of iron-carbohydrate complexes. Such complexes have been found under experimental conditions to produce sarcomas when large doses are injected in rats, mice, and rabbits, and, possibly in hamsters. The number of tumors produced was relatively small. Such tumors have not been produced in guinea pigs. The long latent period between the injection of a potential carcinogen and the appearance of a tumor makes it impossible to measure the risk in man accurately. There have, however, been several reports in the literature describing tumors at the injection site in humans who had previously received intramuscular injections of iron-carbohydrate complexes.

Use in Pregnancy

Animal studies have shown that administration of iron dextran injection USP during pregnancy caused an increase in the number of stillbirths and fetal anomalies, and a decrease in neonatal survival. Thus, iron dextran injection USP should not be used in pregnancy, or in women of childbearing potential unless, in the judgment of the physician, the potential benefits outweigh the possible hazards.

Precautions: Unwarranted therapy with parenteral iron will cause excess storage of iron with the consequent possibility of exogenous hemosiderosis. Such iron overload is particularly apt to occur in patients with hemoglobinopathies and other refractory anemias that might be erroneously diagnosed as iron deficiency anemias.

Imferon should be used with caution in individuals with histories of significant allergies and/or asthma.

Epinephrine should be immediately available in the event of acute hypersensitivity reactions. (Usual adult dose: 0.5 ml of a 1:1000 solution, by subcutaneous or intramuscular injection.)

Patients with both iron deficiency anemia and rheumatoid arthritis may have an acute exacerbation of joint pain and swelling following the intravenous administration of Imferon.

Continued on next page

Information on Merrell Dow products is based on labeling in effect in October, 1982.

Merrell Dow—Cont.

Reports in the literature from countries outside the United States (in particular, New Zealand) have suggested that the use of intramuscular iron dextran in neonates has been associated with an increased incidence of gram-negative sepsis, primarily due to *E. coli.* This effect from the use of Imferon in the United States has not been reported.

Drug/Laboratory Test Interactions
Interactions described below have been reported with intravenous doses of Imferon larger than the maximum dose (2 ml) in the currently approved labeling. (See Warnings.)

A. Serum iron: Caution should be used in interpreting results of serum iron values when blood samples are obtained within 1 or 2 weeks following administration of large doses of Imferon.
B. Serum discoloration: An intravenous injection of 5 ml of Imferon has been reported to impart a brownish color to serum from a blood sample drawn 4 hours after Imferon administration.

Interference with Laboratory Tests
Bone scans involving Tc-99 m diphosphonate have been reported to show dense, crescentic areas of activity following the contour of the iliac crest, visualized 1 to 6 days after intramuscular injections of Imferon.

Adverse Reactions: Anaphylactic reactions including fatal anaphylaxis; other hypersensitivity reactions including dyspnea, urticaria, other rashes and itching, arthralgia, myalgia, febrile episodes, and sweating; variable degree of soreness and inflammation at or near injection site, including sterile abscesses (IM injection); brown skin discoloration at injection site IM injection); lymphadenopathy; local phlebitis at injection site (IV injection); peripheral vascular flushing with overly rapid IV administration; hypotensive reaction; convulsions; possible arthritic reactivation in patients with quiescent rheumatoid arthritis; leucocytosis, frequently with fever; headache, transitory paresthesias, nausea, vomiting, and shivering.

Dosage and Administration:
Oral iron should be discontinued prior to administration of Imferon.

Dosage
Serum ferritin assays have been shown to correlate satisfactorily with iron stores. It is recommended that periodic serum ferritin testing be done in patients who are administered Imferon over prolonged periods.

Iron Deficiency Anemia
Periodic hematologic determinations should be used as a guide in therapy. It should be recognized that iron storage may lag behind the appearance of normal blood morphology. Although there are significant variations in body build and weight distribution among males and females, the accompanying table and formula represent a simple and convenient means for estimating the total iron required. This total iron requirement reflects the amount of iron needed to restore hemoglobin to normal or near normal levels plus an additional 50% allowance to provide adequate replenishment of iron stores in most individuals with moderately or severely reduced levels of hemoglobin. Factors contributing to the formula are shown below.*
[See table below].

Total Amount of Imferon Required (to the nearest ml) for Restoration of Hemoglobin and Replacement of Depleted Iron Stores, Based on Observed Hemoglobin and Body Weight

Patient Weight		Milliliter Requirement Based on Observed Hemoglobin of			
lb	kg	4.0 (g /dl)	6.0 (g /dl)	8.0 (g /dl)	10.0 (g /dl)
10	4.5	3 ml	3 ml	2 ml	2 ml
20	9.1	7	6	4	3
30	13.6	10	8	7	5
40	18.1	18	14	11	8
50	22.7	22	18	14	10
60	27.2	26	21	17	12
70	31.8	31	25	19	14
80	36.3	35	28	22	16
90	40.8	39	32	25	18
100	45.4	44	35	28	20
110	49.9	48	39	30	21
120	54.4	53	42	33	23
130	59.0	57	46	36	25
140	63.5	61	50	39	27
150	68.1	66	53	41	29
160	72.6	70	57	44	31
170	77.1	74	60	47	33
180	81.7	79	64	50	35

The total amount of iron (in mg) required to restore hemoglobin to normal levels and to replenish iron stores may be approximated from the formula:

$$0.3 \times \text{Body Weight in Pounds} \times \left(100 - \frac{\text{hemoglobin in g /dl} \times 100}{14.8}\right)$$

(To calculate dose in ml of Imferon, divide this result by 50.)

Based on the above factors, individuals with normal hemoglobin levels will have approximately 20 mg of blood iron per pound of body weight.

The formula should not be used for patients weighing 30 pounds or less. (Adjustments have been made in the table values to account for the lower normal hemoglobins for those weighing 30 pounds or less.)

Note: The table and accompanying formula are applicable for dosage determinations only in patients with *iron deficiency anemia;* they are not to be used for dosage determinations in patients requiring *iron replacement for blood loss.*
[See table above].

Iron Replacement for Blood Loss
Some individuals sustain blood losses on an intermittent or repetitive basis. Such blood losses may occur periodically in patients with hemorrhagic diatheses (familial telangiectasia; hemophilia; gastrointestinal bleeding) and on a repetitive basis from procedures such as renal hemodialysis.

Iron therapy in these patients should be directed toward replacement of the equivalent amount of iron represented in the blood loss. The table and formula described under iron deficiency anemia are *not* applicable for simple iron replacement values.

Quantitative estimates of the individual's periodic blood loss and hematocrit during the bleeding episode provide a convenient method for the calculation of the required iron dose.

The formula shown below is based on the approximation that 1 ml of normocytic, normochromic red cells contains 1 mg of elemental iron:

Replacement iron (in mg) = Blood loss (in ml) × hematocrit

Example: Blood loss of 500 ml with 20% hematocrit

Replacement Iron = 500 × 0.20 = 100 mg

$$\text{Imferon dose} = \frac{100 \text{ mg}}{50} = 2 \text{ ml}$$

Administration
The total amount of Imferon required for the treatment of *iron deficiency anemia* or *iron replacement for blood loss* is determined from the table or appropriate formula. (See Dosage.)

Intravenous Injection
Test dose: Prior to receiving their first Imferon therapeutic dose, all patients should be given an intravenous test dose of 0.5 ml. Although anaphylactic reactions known to occur following Imferon administration are usually evident within a few minutes, or sooner, it is recommended that a period of an hour or longer elapse before the remainder of the initial therapeutic dose is given.

Individual doses of 2 ml or less may be given on a daily basis until the calculated total amount required has been reached.

Imferon is given undiluted and *slowly* (1 ml or less per minute).

Intramuscular Injection
Test dose: Prior to receiving their first Imferon therapeutic dose, all patients should be given an intramuscular test dose of 0.5 ml administered in the same recommended test site and by the same technique as described in the last paragraph of this section. Although anaphylactic reactions known to occur following Imferon administration are usually evident within a few minutes or sooner, it is recommended that a period of an hour or longer elapse before the remainder of the initial therapeutic dose is given.

If no adverse reactions are observed, Imferon can be given according to the following schedule until the calculated total amount required

*

$$\frac{\text{mg blood iron}}{\text{lb body weight}} = \frac{\text{ml blood}}{\text{lb body weight}} \times \frac{\text{g hemoglobin}}{\text{ml blood}} \times \frac{\text{mg iron}}{\text{g hemoglobin}}$$

a) Blood volume .... 8.5% body weight
b) Normal hemoglobin (males and females)
   over 30 pounds .... 14.8 g /dl
   (30 pounds or less .... 12.0 g /dl)
c) Iron content of hemoglobin 0.34%
d) Hemoglobin deficit
e) Weight

has been reached. Each day's dose should ordinarily not exceed 0.5 ml (25 mg of iron) for infants under 10 lb; 1.0 ml (50 mg of iron) for children under 20 lb; 2.0 ml (100 mg of iron) for patients under 110 lb; and 5 ml (250 mg of iron) for others.

Imferon should be injected only into the muscle mass of the upper outer quadrant of the buttock—never into the arm or other exposed areas—and should be injected deeply, with a 2-inch or 3-inch 19 or 20 gauge needle. If the patient is standing, he should be bearing his weight on the leg opposite the injection site, or if in bed, he should be in the lateral position with injection site uppermost. To avoid injection or leakage into the subcutaneous tissue, a Z-track technique (displacement of the skin laterally prior to injection) is recommended.

How Supplied:

For intramuscular or intravenous use

2 ml ampuls
NDC 0068-0050-09: boxes of 10
5 ml ampuls
NDC 0068-0050-55: boxes of 5

For intramuscular use ONLY

10 ml multiple dose vial containing 0.5% phenol as a preservative
NDC 0068-0052-22: boxes of 2

Imferon is distributed under license from Fisons Pharmaceuticals, Ltd.

Product Information as of September, 1981

Manufactured by
Fisons Limited
Pharmaceutical Division
Loughborough, England for
MERRELL DOW PHARMACEUTICALS INC.
Subsidiary of The Dow Chemical Company
Cincinnati, Ohio 45215, U.S.A.

LORELCO® ℞
(probucol)

Description: LORELCO is an agent for the reduction of elevated serum cholesterol. The chemical name is 4,4′-(isopropylidenedithio) bis (2,6-di-t-butylphenol). Its chemical structure does not resemble that of any other available cholesterol-lowering agent. It is lipophilic.

Clinical Pharmacology: LORELCO lowers serum cholesterol and has relatively little effect on serum triglycerides. Patients responding to probucol exhibit a decrease in low density lipoprotein cholesterol. Cholesterol is reduced not only in the low density lipoprotein fraction, but also in some high density lipoprotein fractions with proportionately greater effect on the high density portion in some patients. Epidemiological studies have shown that both low HDL-cholesterol and high LDL-cholesterol are independent risk factors for coronary heart disease. The risk of lowering HDL-cholesterol while lowering LDL-cholesterol remains unknown. There is little or no effect reported on very low density lipoprotein. Studies on the mode of action of LORELCO indicate that it increases the fractional rate of catabolism of low density lipoproteins. This effect may be linked to the observed increased excretion of fecal bile acids, a final metabolic pathway for the elimination of cholesterol from the body. LORELCO also exhibits inhibition of early stages of cholesterol synthesis and slight inhibition of absorption of dietary cholesterol. There is no increase in the cyclic precursors of cholesterol, namely, desmosterol and 7-dehydro-cholesterol. On this basis, it is concluded that LORELCO does not affect the later stages of cholesterol biosynthesis.

Absorption of LORELCO from the gastrointestinal tract is limited and variable. When it is administered with food, peak blood levels are higher and less variable. With continuous administration in a dosage of 500 mg b.i.d., the blood levels of an individual gradually increase over the first three to four months and thereafter remain fairly constant. In 116 patients treated with LORELCO for periods of 3 months to one year, the mean blood level was 23.6 ± 17.2 mcg/ml (± S.D.) ranging to 78.3 mcg/ml. Levels observed after seven years of treatment in 40 patients yielded an average value of 21.5 ± 16.5 mcg/ml (± S.D.) ranging to 62.0 mcg/ml.

At the end of 12 months of treatment in eight patients blood levels averaged 19.0 mcg/ml. Six weeks after cessation of therapy, the average had fallen by 60 percent. After six months the average had fallen by 80 percent.

Indications and Usage: Serious animal toxicity has been encountered with probucol. See WARNINGS and ANIMAL PHARMACOLOGY AND TOXICOLOGY sections. Probucol is not an innocuous drug and strict attention should be paid to the INDICATIONS and WARNINGS.

Drug therapy should not be used for the routine treatment of elevated blood lipids for the prevention of coronary heart disease. Dietary therapy specific for the type of hyperlipidemia is the initial treatment of choice. Excess body weight may be an important factor and should be addressed prior to any drug therapy. Physical exercise can be an important ancillary measure. Contributory diseases such as hypothyroidism or diabetes mellitus should be looked for and adequately treated. The use of drugs should be considered only when reasonable attempts have been made to obtain satisfactory results with non-drug methods. If the decision ultimately is to use drugs, the patient should be instructed that this does not reduce the importance of adhering to diet.

The selection of patients for cholesterol-lowering drug therapy should take into account other important coronary risk factors such as smoking, hypertension, and diabetes mellitus. Consideration should be given to the efficacy, safety, and compliance factors for each of the cholesterol-lowering drugs prior to selecting the one most appropriate for an individual patient.

LORELCO may be indicated for the reduction of elevated serum cholesterol in patients with primary hypercholesterolemia (elevated low density lipoproteins) who have not responded adequately to diet, weight reduction, and control of diabetes mellitus. LORELCO may be useful to lower elevated cholesterol that occurs in patients with combined hypercholesterolemia and hypertriglyceridemia but it is not indicated where hypertriglyceridemia is the abnormality of most concern.

It is not always possible to predict from the lipoprotein type or other factors which patients will exhibit favorable results. Lipid levels should be periodically assessed. Small or transient changes in high density lipoprotein cholesterol may be due to inaccuracies in the method of determination. Substantial changes are sometimes seen with diet. If satisfactory lipid alteration is not achieved, the drug should be discontinued.

The effect of drug-induced reduction of serum cholesterol or triglyceride levels or alteration of HDL-cholesterol levels on morbidity or mortality due to coronary heart disease has not been established. Several years may be required before ongoing long-term investigations will resolve this question.

Contraindications: (See also PRECAUTIONS.) LORELCO is contraindicated in patients who are known to have a hypersensitivity to it.

Warnings: SERIOUS ANIMAL TOXICITY HAS BEEN ENCOUNTERED WITH PROBUCOL IN RHESUS MONKEYS FED AN ATHEROGENIC DIET AND IN BEAGLE DOGS (SEE ANIMAL PHARMACOLOGY AND TOXICOLOGY SECTION OF THIS INSERT). Although QT prolongation can occur in patients on probucol, the arrhythmias observed in monkeys fed large doses of probucol added to an atherogenic diet have not been reported in man; nevertheless, the following precautions are deemed prudent:

1. At the start of treatment with LORELCO and throughout the treatment period, patients should be advised to adhere to a low cholesterol, low fat diet.
2. As part of an overall evaluation, a baseline, 6 month, and 1 year repeat ECG tracing should be considered. If marked prolongation of the QT interval (after correction for rate) occurs, the possible benefits and risks should be carefully considered before making the decision to continue the probucol administration.

LORELCO should not be used in patients with evidence of recent or progressive myocardial damage or findings suggestive of ventricular arrhythmias.

No instances of increase in ectopy attributed to LORELCO have been reported. However, patients with unexplained syncope while on LORELCO should have ECG surveillance.

Precautions: Because LORELCO is intended for long-term administration, adequate baseline studies should be performed to determine that the patient has elevated serum cholesterol levels. Serum lipid levels should be determined before treatment and repeated during the first few months of treatment and periodically thereafter. A favorable trend in cholesterol reduction should be evident during the first three to four months of administration of LORELCO. In evaluating response, the effect of probucol on LDL-cholesterol and HDL-cholesterol should be considered. (See CLINICAL PHARMACOLOGY). If satisfactory lipid alteration is not achieved, the drug should be discontinued.

Neither oral hypoglycemic agents nor oral anticoagulants alter the effect of LORELCO on serum cholesterol. The dosage of these agents is not usually modified when given with LORELCO.

Use in Pregnancy: Reproduction studies have been performed in rats and rabbits and have revealed no evidence of impaired fertility or harm to the fetus due to LORELCO. Because there are no adequate studies in pregnant women, use of this drug in pregnancy is not recommended. Furthermore, if a patient wishes to become pregnant, it is recommended that the drug be withdrawn, and birth control procedures be used for at least six months because of persistence of the drug in the body for prolonged periods. (See CLINICAL PHARMACOLOGY.)

Use in Nursing Mothers: It is not known whether this drug is secreted in human milk, but it is likely to be since such excretion has been shown in animals. It is recommended that nursing not be undertaken while a patient is on LORELCO.

Use in Children: Safety and effectiveness in children have not been established.

Adverse Reactions: LORELCO may produce a prolongation of the QT interval on ECG in some patients. (See WARNINGS.)

Other adverse reactions associated with LORELCO are generally mild to moderate and of short duration.

The most commonly affected system is the gastrointestinal tract. Diarrhea or loose stools occurs in about one in ten patients. Other adverse gastrointestinal reactions in descending

Continued on next page

Information on Merrell Dow products is based on labeling in effect in October, 1982.

Merrell Dow—Cont.

order of frequency are flatulence, abdominal pain, nausea and vomiting. These reactions are usually transient and seldom require the drug to be discontinued. During the clinical studies LORELCO was discontinued in about 2% of the patients because of adverse gastrointestinal reactions.
An idiosyncratic reaction observed with initiation of therapy and characterized by dizziness, palpitations, syncope, nausea, vomiting, and chest pain has been reported.
Other events have been reported in patients treated with LORELCO. The relationship between these events and probucol is not well established. The most frequent were headaches, dizziness, paresthesias and eosinophilia observed in about one of each fifty subjects. Consistently low hemoglobin and/or hematocrit values were observed in about one of each one hundred patients. Less frequent were rash, pruritus, impotency, insomnia, conjunctivitis, tearing, blurred vision, tinnitus, diminished sense of taste and smell, enlargement of a multinodular goiter, anorexia, heartburn, indigestion, gastrointestinal bleeding, ecchymosis and petechiae, thrombocytopenia, nocturia, peripheral neuritis, hyperhidrosis, fetid sweat and angioneurotic edema. These were observed in the range of one to six per thousand subjects.
Elevations of the serum transaminases (glutamic-oxalacetic and glutamic-pyruvic), bilirubin, alkaline phosphatase, creatine phosphokinase, uric acid, blood urea nitrogen and blood glucose above the normal range were observed on one or more occasions in various patients treated with LORELCO. Most often these were transient and/or could have been related to the patient's clinical state or other modes of therapy. Although the basis for the relationship between probucol and these abnormalities is not firm, the possibility that some of these are drug-related cannot be excluded. In the controlled trials the incidence of abnormal laboratory values was no higher in the patients treated with probucol than in the patients who received placebo.
Dosage and Administration: For adult use only. The recommended and maximal dose is 500 mg (2 tablets of 250 mg each) twice daily with the morning and evening meals.
CAUTION: Federal law prohibits dispensing without prescription.
How Supplied: Each film-coated tablet contains 250 mg probucol and is imprinted with the DOW diamond trademark over the code number 51.
Bottles of 120 tablets, a 30-day supply for one patient (NDC 0068-0051-52)
Keep well closed. Store in a dry place, avoid excessive heat, and dispense in light-resistant containers.
Animal Pharmacology and Toxicology: In rhesus monkeys administration of probucol in diets containing unusually high amounts of cholesterol and saturated fat resulted in the death of 4 of 8 animals after several weeks. Premonitory syncope was frequently observed and was associated with a pronounced prolongation of the QT intervals (30–50% longer than that observed in untreated monkeys). Serum levels of probucol greater than 20 mcg/ml were generally associated with some prolongation in the QT interval in the cholesterol-fed monkey. A 75 msec or greater increase in QT interval from control values was usually seen at 40 mcg/ml and above. Blood levels in humans receiving probucol average approximately 20 mcg/ml and not uncommonly reach levels of 40 mcg/ml and higher. Rhesus monkeys fed normal (low fat) chow and receiving probucol three to thirty times the human dose equivalent achieved blood levels only one-third those of many human subjects. No adverse effects were detected in these monkeys over an eight-year period of continuous drug administration.
In another study in rhesus monkeys, an atherogenic diet was fed for two years and daily treatment with probucol, separated in time from the atherogenic meal, was carried out during the second year. Serum probucol levels ranged 20–50 mcg/ml in five of ten monkeys and less in the remaining animals. Marked prolongation of the QT_c interval in the electrocardiogram or syncopal behavior was never observed over the entire one-year treatment period. Regression of gross aortic lesions comparable to that observed in a parallel group of monkeys receiving cholestyramine was seen in animals receiving probucol. It should be emphasized that both HDL-cholesterol and LDL-cholesterol were markedly reduced in this regression study. During the performance of a two-year chronic study involving 32 probucol-treated dogs (beagles) there were 12 fatalities. Subsequent experiments have indicated that probucol sensitizes the canine myocardium to epinephrine resulting in ventricular fibrillation in many dogs. Among the animal species in which probucol has been studied, the dog is peculiar with respect to the phenomenon of sudden death due to the sensitization of the myocardium to epinephrine. In contrast to findings in the dog, injections of epinephrine to probucol-treated monkeys did not induce ventricular fibrillation.
In other studies, monkeys were given probucol either before and after, or only after myocardial infarction induced by coronary artery ligation. In these studies there was no difference between probucol- and placebo-treated groups with respect to either survival or detailed blind quantitation of myocardial changes (gross and histopathologic).
Probucol has shown no identifiable toxicity in mice and rats. In these animals the LD_{50} (oral) is in excess of five grams per kilogram of body weight. In chronic studies of two years duration in rats, no toxicity or carcinogenicity was observed.
From studies in rats, dogs and monkeys it is known that probucol accumulates slowly in adipose tissue. Approximately 90% of probucol administered orally is unabsorbed. For that which is absorbed, the biliary tract is the major pathway for clearance from the body and very little is excreted by way of the kidneys.
Myocardial injury was produced in various groups of rats by one of the following procedures: aortic coarctation, coronary ligation, or cobalt or isoproterenol injection. After probucol administration no deleterious effects related to treatment occurred as measured by survival and microscopic examination of myocardial damage.
Probucol was administered to minipigs beginning 10 days before ligation of a coronary artery and continued for 60 days post surgery. Challenge wth epinephrine at the end of 60 days failed to induce ventricular fibrillation in any of the coronary-ligated, probucol-treated minipigs.

Product Information as of June, 1982
[*Shown in Product Identification Section*]

METAHYDRIN® ℞
(trichlormethiazide USP)

AVAILABLE ONLY ON PRESCRIPTION

Description: Metahydrin is an oral diuretic and antihypertensive of the thiazide class. Differing from other thiazides by the inclusion of a dichloromethyl radical at the 3 position on the benzothiadiazine structure.
Action: The mechanism of action results in an interference with the renal tubular mechanism of electrolyte reabsorption. At maximal therapeutic dosage all thiazides are approximately equal in their diuretic potency. The mechanism whereby thiazides function in the control of hypertension is unknown.
Indications: Metahydrin is indicated as adjunctive therapy in edema associated with congestive heart failure, hepatic cirrhosis, and corticosteroid and estrogen therapy.
Metahydrin has also been found useful in edema due to various forms of renal dysfunction as:
Nephrotic syndrome;
Acute glomerulonephritis; and
Chronic renal failure.
Metahydrin is indicated in the management of hypertension either as the sole therapeutic agent or to enhance the effectiveness of other antihypertensive drugs in the more severe forms of hypertension.
Usage in Pregnancy. The routine use of diuretics in an otherwise healthy woman is inappropriate and exposes mother and fetus to unnecessary hazard. Diuretics do not prevent development of toxemia of pregnancy, and there is no satisfactory evidence that they are useful in the treatment of developed toxemia.
Edema during pregnancy may arise from pathologic causes or from the physiologic and mechanical consequences of pregnancy. Thiazides are indicated in pregnancy when edema is due to pathologic causes, just as they are in the absence of pregnancy. (However, see Warnings, below.) Dependent edema in pregnancy, resulting from restriction of venous return by the expanded uterus, is properly treated through elevation of the lower extremities and use of support hose; use of diuretics to lower intravascular volume in this case is illogical and unnecessary. There is hypervolemia during normal pregnancy, which is harmful to neither the fetus nor the mother (in the absence of cardiovascular disease), but which is associated with edema, including generalized edema, in the majority of pregnant women. If this edema produces discomfort, increased recumbency will often provide relief. In rare instances, this edema may cause extreme discomfort which is not relieved by rest. In these cases, a short course of diuretics may provide relief and may be appropriate.
Contraindications:
Anuria.
Hypersensitivity to this or other sulfonamide-derived drugs.
Warnings: Thiazides should be used with caution in severe renal disease. In patients with renal disease, thiazides may precipitate azotemia. Cumulative effects of the drug may develop in patients with impaired renal function.
Thiazides should be used with caution in patients with impaired hepatic function or progressive liver disease, since minor alterations of fluid and electrolyte balance may precipitate hepatic coma.
Thiazides may add to or potentiate the action of other antihypertensive drugs. Potentiation occurs with ganglionic or peripheral adrenergic blocking drugs.
Sensitivity reactions may occur in patients with a history of allergy or bronchial asthma.
The possibility of exacerbation or activation of systemic lupus erythematosus has been reported.
Usage in Pregnancy. Thiazides cross the placental barrier and appear in cord blood. The use of thiazides in pregnant women requires that the anticipated benefit be weighed against possible hazards to the fetus. These hazards include fetal or neonatal jaundice, thrombocytopenia, and possibly other adverse reactions which have occurred in the adult.
Nursing Mothers. Thiazides appear in the breast milk. If use of the drug is deemed essential, the patient should stop nursing.
Precautions: Periodic determination of serum electrolytes to detect possible electrolyte imbalance should be performed at appropriate intervals.
All patients receiving thiazide therapy should be observed for clinical signs of fluid or electrolyte imbalance; namely, hyponatremia, hypo-

chloremic alkalosis, and hypokalemia. Serum and urine electrolyte determinations are particularly important when the patient is vomiting excessively or receiving parenteral fluids. Medication such as digitalis may also influence serum electrolytes. Warning signs, irrespective of cause, are: dryness of mouth, thirst, weakness, lethargy, drowsiness, restlessness, muscle pains or cramps, muscular fatigue, hypotension, oliguria, tachycardia, and gastrointestinal disturbances such as nausea and vomiting.

Hypokalemia may develop with thiazides as with any other potent diuretic, especially with brisk diuresis, when severe cirrhosis is present, or during concomitant use of corticosteroids or ACTH.

Interference with adequate oral electrolyte intake will also contribute to hypokalemia. Digitalis therapy may exaggerate metabolic effects of hypokalemia especially with reference to myocardial activity.

Any chloride deficit is generally mild and usually does not require specific treatment except under extraordinary circumstances (as in liver disease or renal disease). Dilutional hyponatremia may occur in edematous patients in hot weather; appropriate therapy is water restriction, rather than administration of salt except in rare instances when the hyponatremia is life threatening. In actual salt depletion, appropriate replacement is the therapy of choice.

Hyperuricemia may occur or frank gout may be precipitated in certain patients receiving thiazide therapy.

Insulin requirements in diabetic patients may be increased, decreased, or unchanged. Latent diabetes mellitus may become manifest during thiazide administration.

Thiazide drugs may increase the responsiveness to tubocurarine.

The antihypertensive effects of the drug may be enhanced in the postsympathectomy patient.

Thiazides may decrease arterial responsiveness to norepinephrine. This diminution is not sufficient to preclude effectiveness of the pressor agent for therapeutic use.

If progressive renal impairment becomes evident, as indicated by a rising nonprotein nitrogen or blood urea nitrogen, a careful reappraisal of therapy is necessary with consideration given to withholding or discontinuing diuretic therapy.

Thiazides may decrease serum PBI levels without signs of thyroid disturbance.

This product contains FD&C Yellow No. 5 (tartrazine), which may cause allergic-type reactions (including bronchial asthma) in certain susceptible individuals. Although the overall incidence of FD&C Yellow No. 5 (tartrazine) sensitivity in the general population is low, it is frequently seen in patients who also have aspirin hypersensitivity.

Adverse Reactions:

1. Gastrointestinal System Reactions: anorexia, gastric irritation, nausea, diarrhea, constipation, jaundice (intrahepatic cholestatic jaundice), vomiting, cramping, pancreatitis.
2. Central Nervous System Reactions: dizziness, vertigo, parasthesias, headache, xanthopsia.
3. Hematologic Reactions: leukopenia, agranulocytosis, thrombocytopenia, aplastic anemia.
4. Dermatologic-Hypersensitivity Reactions: purpura, photosensitivity, rash, urticaria, necrotizing angiitis (vasculitis) (cutaneous vasculitis).
5. Cardiovascular Reaction: orthostatic hypotension may occur and may be aggravated by alcohol, barbiturates, or narcotics.
6. Other: hyperglycemia, glycosuria, hyperuricemia, muscle spasm, weakness, restlessness.

Whenever adverse reactions are moderate or severe, Metahydrin dosage should be reduced or therapy withdrawn.

Dosage and Administration: Therapy should be individualized according to patient response. This therapy should be titrated to gain maximal therapeutic response as well as the minimal dose possible to maintain that therapeutic response.

The usual daily doses of Metahydrin for antihypertensive and diuretic effect are as follows:

The usual dose is one 2 mg or 4 mg tablet once daily.

In initiating therapy, these doses may be given twice daily.

How Supplied:

2 mg pink tablets debossed MERRELL 62: bottles of 100 and 1000

4 mg aqua blue tablets debossed MERRELL 63: bottles of 100 and 1000

Product Information as of August, 1979

[*Shown in Product Identification Section*]

METATENSIN® ℞

(trichlormethiazide USP and reserpine)

AVAILABLE ONLY ON PRESCRIPTION

Warning

This fixed combination drug is not indicated for initial therapy of hypertension. Hypertension requires therapy titrated to the individual patient. If the fixed combination represents the dosage so determined, its use may be more convenient in patient management. The treatment of hypertension is not static, but must be re-evaluated as conditions in each patient warrant.

Description: Each tablet contains Metahydrin® (trichlormethiazide USP) 2 mg or 4 mg and reserpine 0.1 mg.

Metahydrin (trichlormethiazide USP) is an orally effective diuretic and antihypertensive of the thiazide class. Differing from other thiazides by the inclusion of a dichloromethyl radical at the 3 position on the benzothiadiazine structure.

Reserpine is a pure crystalline alkaloid derived from the root of Rauwolfia serpentina.

Action:

Trichlormethiazide

The mechanism of action results in an interference with the renal tubular mechanism of electrolyte reabsorption. At maximal therapeutic dosage all thiazides are approximately equal in their diuretic potency. The mechanism whereby thiazides function in the control of hypertension is unknown.

Reserpine

Reserpine probably produces its antihypertensive effects through depletion of tissue stores of epinephrine and norepinephrine from peripheral sites. By contrast, its sedative and tranquilizing properties are thought to be related to depletion of 5-hydroxytryptamine from the brain.

Reserpine is characterized by slow onset of action and sustained effect. Both its cardiovascular and central nervous system effects may persist following withdrawal of the drug.

Indications: Hypertension (See box Warning.)

Usage in Pregnancy. The routine use of diuretics in an otherwise healthy woman is inappropriate and exposes mother and fetus to unnecessary hazard. Diuretics do not prevent development of toxemia of pregnancy, and there is no satisfactory evidence that they are useful in the treatment of developed toxemia. Edema during pregnancy may arise from pathologic causes or from the physiologic and mechanical consequences of pregnancy. Thiazides are indicated in pregnancy when edema is due to pathologic causes, just as they are in the absence of pregnancy. (However, see Warnings, below.) Dependent edema in pregnancy, resulting from restriction of venous return by the expanded uterus, is properly treated through elevation of the lower extremities and use of support hose; use of diuretics to lower intravascular volume in this case is illogical and unnecessary. There is hypervolemia during normal pregnancy, which is harmful to neither the fetus nor the mother (in the absence of cardiovascular disease), but which is associated with edema, including generalized edema, in the majority of pregnant women. If this edema produces discomfort, increased recumbency will often provide relief. In rare instances, this edema may cause extreme discomfort which is not relieved by rest. In these cases, a short course of diuretics may provide relief and may be appropriate.

Contraindications:

Trichlormethiazide

Trichlormethiazide is contraindicated in patients with anuria and in patients known to be hypersensitive to this or other sulfonamide derived drugs.

Reserpine

Hypersensitivity, mental depression especially with suicidal tendencies, active peptic ulcer and ulcerative colitis.

Warnings:

Trichlormethiazide

Use with caution in severe renal disease. In patients with renal disease, thiazides may precipitate azotemia. Cumulative effects of the drug may develop in patients with impaired renal function.

Thiazides should be used with caution in patients with impaired hepatic function or progressive liver disease, since minor alterations of fluid and electrolyte balance may precipitate hepatic coma.

Thiazides may add to or potentiate the action of other antihypertensive drugs. Potentiation occurs with ganglionic or peripheral adrenergic blocking drugs. Sensitivity reactions may occur in patients with a history of allergy or bronchial asthma. Exacerbation or activation of systemic lupus erythematosis has been reported.

Reserpine

As suicide is always a possible result of mental depression, discontinue treatment if mood depression develops.

Reserpine may induce peptic ulceration; discontinue use if peptic ulcer develops.

Electroshock therapy should not be given to patients taking reserpine, since severe and even fatal reactions have been reported. The drug should be discontinued for two weeks before giving electroshock therapy.

MAO inhibitors should be avoided or used with extreme caution.

Usage in Pregnancy. Trichlormethiazide: Thiazides cross the placental barrier and appear in cord blood. The use of thiazides in pregnant women requires that the anticipated benefit be weighed against possible hazards to the fetus. These hazards include fetal or neonatal jaundice, thrombocytopenia, and possibly other adverse reactions which have occurred in the adult.

Reserpine: The safety of reserpine for use during pregnancy or lactation has not been established; therefore, the drug should be used in pregnant patients or in women of childbearing potential only when, in the judgement of the physician, it is essential to the welfare of the patient.

Increased respiratory secretions, nasal congestion, cyanosis, and anorexia may occur in infants born to reserpine-treated mothers, since reserpine crosses the placental barrier and appears in maternal breast milk.

Nursing Mothers. Thiazides and reserpine appear in breast milk. If use of Metatensin is deemed essential, the patient should stop nursing.

Continued on next page

Information on Merrell Dow products is based on labeling in effect in October, 1982.

Merrell Dow—Cont.

Precautions: The #2 tablet contains FD&C Yellow No. 5 (tartrazine), which may cause allergic-type reactions (including bronchial asthma) in certain susceptible individuals. Although the overall incidence of FD&C Yellow No. 5 (tartrazine) sensitivity in the general population is low, it is frequently seen in patients who also have aspirin hypersensitivity.
Trichlormethiazide
Periodic determinations of serum electrolytes to detect possible electrolyte imbalance should be performed at appropriate intervals.
All patients receiving thiazide therapy should be observed for clinical signs of fluid or electrolyte imbalance; namely, hyponatremia, hypochloremic alkalosis, and hypokalemia. Serum and urine electrolyte determinations are particularly important when the patient is vomiting excessively or receiving parenteral fluids. Medication such as digitalis may also influence serum electrolytes. Warning signs, irrespective of cause, are: dryness of mouth, thirst, weakness, lethargy, drowsiness, restlessness, muscle pains or cramps, muscular fatigue, hypotension, oliguria, tachycardia, and gastrointestinal disturbances such as nausea and vomiting.
Hypokalemia may develop with thiazides as with any other potent diuretic, especially with brisk diuresis, when severe cirrhosis is present, or during concomitant use of corticosteroids or ACTH.
Interference with adequate oral electrolyte intake will also contribute to hypokalemia. Digitalis therapy may exaggerate metabolic effects of hypokalemia especially with reference to myocardial activity.
Any chloride deficit is generally mild and usually does not require specific treatment except under extraordinary circumstances (as in liver disease or renal disease). Dilutional hyponatremia may occur in edematous patients in hot weather; appropriate therapy is water restriction, rather than administration of salt except in rare instances when the hyponatremia is life threatening. In actual salt depletion, appropriate replacement is the therapy of choice.
Hyperuricemia may occur or frank gout may be precipitated in certain patients receiving thiazide therapy.
Insulin requirements in diabetic patients may be increased, decreased, or unchanged. Latent diabetes mellitus may become manifest during thiazide administration.
Thiazide drugs may increase the responsiveness to tubocurarine.
The antihypertensive effects of the drug may be enhanced in the postsympathectomy patient.
Thiazides may decrease arterial responsiveness to norepinephrine. This diminution is not sufficient to preclude effectiveness of the pressor agent for therapeutic use.
If progressive renal impairment becomes evident, as indicated by a rising non-protein nitrogen or blood urea nitrogen, a careful reappraisal of therapy is necessary with consideration given to withholding or discontinuing diuretic therapy.
Thiazides may decrease serum PBI levels without signs of thyroid disturbance.
Reserpine
Caution should be used in treating hypertensive patients with renal insufficiency.
Cardiac arrhythmias have occurred in patients receiving digitalis and quinidine with reserpine.
Reserpine potentiates many anesthetic agents; hypotension and bradycardia have been noted during anesthesia. In addition, a relative sensitivity to norepinephrine or other pressor agents may exist due to the previous action of reserpine; thus usual amounts of the pressor agent may be excessive.
Use with caution in patients with a previous history of depression, peptic ulcer or other gastrointestinal disorders and in hypertensive patients with functionally severe coronary artery disease.

Adverse Reactions:
Trichlormethiazide
1. Gastrointestinal System Reactions: anorexia, gastric irritation, nausea, diarrhea, constipation, jaundice (intrahepatic cholestatic jaundice), vomiting, cramping, pancreatitis.
2. Central Nervous System Reactions: dizziness, vertigo, paresthesias, headache, xanthopsia.
3. Hematologic Reactions: leukopenia, agranulocytosis, thrombocytopenia, aplastic anemia.
4. Dermatologic-Hypersensitivity Reactions: purpura, photosensitivity, rash, urticaria, necrotizing angiitis (vasculitis) (cutaneous vasculitis).
5. Cardiovascular Reaction: orthostatic hypotension may occur and may be aggravated by alcohol, barbiturates, or narcotics.
6. Other: hyperglycemia, glycosuria, hyperuricemia, muscle spasm, weakness, restlessness.
Reserpine
Gastric hypersecretion; vomiting; nervousness; paradoxical anxiety, CNS sensitization manifested by deafness, glaucoma, uveitis, and optic atrophy; purpura; nasal stuffiness; loose stools; reversible parkinsonism; muscular fatigue and weakness; and nightmares. Mental depression particularly when doses of reserpine of over 1.0 mg. daily are used has been reported. Other side effects of reserpine reported include anorexia, nausea, dizziness, headaches, impotence, flushing of the skin, dryness of the mouth, biliary colic, blurring of vision, muscular aches and pruritus. Hypotension, including the orthostatic variety, may occur in some patients. Angina pectoris, arrhythmias and congestive heart failure have also been reported but are uncommon.
After the onset of therapy with reserpine, a turbulent phase of short duration may occur.
Very rare additional adverse effects that have been observed in association with reserpine therapy include epistaxis, skin eruptions and edema due to sodium retention. Bradycardia may occur as an exaggerated response related to the pharmacodynamic effect of reserpine.
Dosage: As determined by individual titration. (See box Warning.)
In the stabilized hypertensive patient, administration may be continued on a once-daily basis administered in the morning. The maximum single effective dose of Metatensin is 8 mg. (in some patients 4 mg.). Doses in excess of 8 mg. normally will not produce any increase in sodium and water excretion and in refractory patients may increase excretion of potassium.
How Supplied:
Metatensin #2
(trichlormethiazide 2.0 mg and reserpine 0.1 mg)
Bottles of 100 and 1000 yellow tablets debossed MERRELL 64
Metatensin #4
(trichlormethiazide 4.0 mg and reserpine 0.1 mg)
Bottles of 100 and 1000 lavender tablets debossed MERRELL 65
Product Information as of August, 1979
[*Shown in Product Identification Section*]

NEO-POLYCIN®
neomycin sulfate, polymyxin B sulfate and bacitracin zinc ointment
Topical Antibiotic

Description: Each gram of Neo-Polycin topical antibiotic ointment contains: neomycin sulfate equivalent to 3.5 mg neomycin; polymyxin B sulfate, 5000 units; bacitracin zinc, 400 units in a unique Fuzene® ointment base. Inert ingredients are polyethylene glycol dilaurate, polyethylene glycol distearate, light liquid petrolatum, white petrolatum and synthetic glyceride wax.
Actions: All three antibiotics in Neo-Polycin meet most criteria for ideal topical agents. They are rarely used systemically and there is apparently minimal risk of systemic toxicity from their topical use because they are not absorbed to an appreciable extent from denuded skin or mucous membranes. They are essentially non-irritating to the tissues. They are active in the presence of blood or pus, and they diffuse readily into tissue exudates.
Neomycin acts against most of the bacteria that cause topical infection and is especially active against species of *Proteus* and *Staphylococcus.* Bacitracin is primarily effective against gram-positive bacteria, and is especially effective against hemolytic streptococci. Polymyxin is primarily effective against gram-negative bacteria, particularly *Pseudomonas aeruginosa.* This combination of antibiotics makes Neo-Polycin effective against practically all pyogenic bacteria that cause topical infections. Because the Fuzene base is miscible with both tissue exudate and the oils and waxes of the skin, Neo-Polycin can be used in weeping exudative lesions.
Indications: Neo-Polycin may be used in the treatment of bacterial infections of the skin and mucous membrane caused by susceptible bacteria. These include such pyogenic conditions as impetigo, folliculitis, paronychia, and sycosis barbae. It is also effective in controlling secondary bacterial infections in skin carcinoma, burns, eczemas, contact dermatitis, fungal infections, acne, psoriasis, varicose ulcers and neurodermatitis. Its broad antibacterial spectrum and special base make Neo-Polycin especially useful for treating chronic lesions, where mixed infections with relatively resistant bacteria may be present and difficult to identify for definitive therapy.
Neo-Polycin is also indicated as a non-irritating, non-staining dressing for the prevention of bacterial infection of traumatic lesions and surgical incisions.
Contraindications: Hypersensitivity to product ingredients. Not for use in the eyes. Do not use in external ear canal if the eardrum is perforated.
Warning: Because of the potential hazard of nephrotoxicity and ototoxicity due to neomycin, care should be exercised when using Neo-Polycin in treating extensive burns, trophic ulceration and other extensive conditions where absorption of neomycin is possible. Not more than one application a day is recommended where widespread body surfaces are affected, especially if the patient has impaired renal function or is receiving other aminoglycoside antibiotics concurrently.
Precautions: As with any antibacterial preparation, prolonged use may result in overgrowth of nonsusceptible organisms, including fungi. If this occurs, treatment should be discontinued and appropriate therapy instituted.
Adverse Reactions: Sensitivity, especially to the neomycin ingredient, may develop after continuous, chronic therapy. If itching, burning or inflammation follows application, usage should be discontinued. Articles in the current medical literature indicate an increase in the prevalence of persons sensitive to neomycin.
Administration: Spread Neo-Polycin thinly, with or without a dressing. Reapplication 2 or 3 times daily may be desirable. Avoid using excessive amounts of ointment since it is unnecessary and tends to result in the deposition of undesirable residue.
How Supplied: In ½ ounce tubes (NDC 0068-2010-93), ounce tubes (NDC 0068-2010-01).

NORPRAMIN® ℞
(desipramine hydrochloride tablets USP)

AVAILABLE ONLY ON PRESCRIPTION

Description: Norpramin (desipramine hydrochloride USP) is an antidepressant drug of the tricyclic type, and is chemically: 5*H*-Dibenz[*b,f*]azepine-5-propanamine, 10, 11-dihydro-N-methyl-, monohydrochloride.

Clinical Pharmacology:

Mechanism of Action

Available evidence suggests that many depressions have a biochemical basis in the form of a relative deficiency of neurotransmitters such as norepinephrine and serotonin. Norepinephrine deficiency may be associated with relatively low urinary 3-methoxy-4-hydroxyphenyl glycol (MHPG) levels, while serotonin deficiencies may be associated with low spinal fluid levels of 5-hydroxyindolacetic acid.

While the precise mechanism of action of the tricyclic antidepressants is unknown, a leading theory suggests that they restore normal levels of neurotransmitters by blocking the re-uptake of these substances from the synapse in the central nervous system. Evidence indicates that the secondary amine tricyclic antidepressants, including Norpramin, may have greater activity in blocking the re-uptake of norepinephrine. Tertiary amine tricyclic antidepressants, such as amitriptyline, may have greater effect on serotonin re-uptake.

Norpramin (desipramine hydrochloride) is not a monoamine oxidase (MAO) inhibitor and does not act primarily as a central nervous system stimulant. It has been found in some studies to have a more rapid onset of action than imipramine. Earliest therapeutic effects may occasionally be seen in 2 to 5 days, but full treatment benefit usually requires 2 to 3 weeks to obtain.

Metabolism

Tricyclic antidepressants, such as desipramine hydrochloride, are rapidly absorbed from the gastrointestinal tract. Tricyclic antidepressants or their metabolites are to some extent excreted through the gastric mucosa and reabsorbed from the gastrointestinal tract. Desipramine is metabolized in the liver and approximately 70% is excreted in the urine.

The rate of metabolism of tricyclic antidepressants varies widely from individual to individual, chiefly on a genetically determined basis. Up to a thirty-sixfold difference in plasma level may be noted among individuals taking the same oral dose of desipramine. In general, the elderly metabolize tricyclic antidepressants more slowly than do younger adults.

Certain drugs, particularly the psychostimulants and the phenothiazines, increase plasma levels of concomitantly administered tricyclic antidepressants through competition for the same metabolic enzyme systems. Other substances, particularly barbiturates and alcohol, induce liver enzyme activity and thereby reduce tricyclic antidepressant plasma levels. Similar effects have been reported with tobacco smoke.

Research on the relationship of plasma level to therapeutic response with the tricyclic antidepressants has produced conflicting results. While some studies report no correlation, many studies cite therapeutic levels for most tricyclics in the range of 50 to 300 nanograms per milliliter. The therapeutic range is different for each tricyclic antidepressant. For desipramine, an optimal range of therapeutic plasma levels has not been established.

Indications: Norpramin (desipramine hydrochloride) is indicated for relief of symptoms in various depressive syndromes, especially endogenous depression.

Contraindications: Desipramine hydrochloride should not be given in conjunction with, or within 2 weeks of, treatment with an MAO inhibitor drug; hyperpyretic crises, severe convulsions, and death have occurred in patients taking MAO inhibitors and tricyclic antidepressants. When Norpramin (desipramine hydrochloride) is substituted for an MAO inhibitor, at least 2 weeks should elapse between treatments. Norpramin should then be started cautiously and should be increased gradually. The drug is contraindicated in the acute recovery period following myocardial infarction. It should not be used in those who have shown prior hypersensitivity to the drug. Cross sensitivity between this and other dibenzazepines is a possibility.

Warnings:

1. Extreme caution should be used when this drug is given in the following situations:
   a. In patients with cardiovascular disease, because of the possibility of conduction defects, arrhythmias, tachycardias, strokes, and acute myocardial infarction.
   b. In patients with a history of urinary retention or glaucoma, because of the anticholinergic properties of the drug.
   c. In patients with thyroid disease or those taking thyroid medication, because of the possibility of cardiovascular toxicity, including arrhythmias.
   d. In patients with a history of seizure disorder, because this drug has been shown to lower the seizure threshold.
2. This drug is capable of blocking the antihypertensive effect of guanethidine and similarly acting compounds.
3. USE IN PREGNANCY
Safe use of desipramine hydrochloride during pregnancy and lactation has not been established; therefore, if it is to be given to pregnant patients, nursing mothers, or women of childbearing potential, the possible benefits must be weighed against the possible hazards to mother and child. Animal reproductive studies have been inconclusive.
4. USE IN CHILDREN
Norpramin (desipramine hydrochloride) is not recommended for use in children since safety and effectiveness in the pediatric age group have not been established.
5. The patient should be cautioned that this drug may impair the mental and/or physical abilities required for the performance of potentially hazardous tasks such as driving a car or operating machinery.
6. In patients who may use alcohol excessively, it should be borne in mind that the potentiation may increase the danger inherent in any suicide attempt or overdosage.

Precautions:

1. It is important that this drug be dispensed in the least possible quantities to depressed outpatients, since suicide has been accomplished with this class of drug. Ordinary prudence requires that children not have access to this drug or to potent drugs of any kind; if possible this drug should be dispensed in containers with child-resistant safety closures. Storage of this drug in the home must be supervised responsibly.
2. If serious adverse effects occur, dosage should be reduced or treatment should be altered.
3. Norpramin (desipramine hydrochloride) therapy in patients with manic-depressive illness may induce a hypomanic state after the depressive phase terminates.
4. The drug may cause exacerbation of psychosis in schizophrenic patients.
5. Close supervision and careful adjustment of dosage are required when this drug is given concomitantly with anticholinergic or sympathomimetic drugs.
6. Patients should be warned that while taking this drug their reponse to alcoholic beverages may be exaggerated.
7. Clinical experience in the concurrent administration of ECT and antidepressant drugs is limited. Thus, if such treatment is essential, the possibility of increased risk relative to benefits should be considered.
8. If Norpramin (desipramine hydrochloride) is to be combined with other psychotropic agents such as tranquilizers or sedative/hypnotics, careful consideration should be given to the pharmacology of the agents employed since the sedative effects of Norpramin and benzodiazepines (e.g., chlordiazepoxide or diazepam) are additive. Both the sedative and anticholinergic effects of the major tranquilizers are also additive to those of Norpramin.
9. This drug should be discontined as soon as possible prior to elective surgery because of the possible cardiovascular effects. Hypertensive episodes have been observed during surgery in patients taking desipramine hydrochloride.
10. Both elevation and lowering of blood sugar levels have been reported.
11. Leukocyte and differential counts should be performed in any patient who develops fever and sore throat during therapy; the drug should be discontinued if there is evidence of pathologic neutrophil depression.
12. Norpramin 25, 50, 75, and 100 mg tablets contain FD&C Yellow No. 5 (tartrazine), which may cause allergic-type reactions (including bronchial asthma) in certain susceptible individuals. Although the overall incidence of FD&C Yellow No. 5 (tartrazine) sensitivity in the general population is low, it is frequently seen in patients who also have aspirin hypersensitivity.

Adverse Reactions:

Note: Included in the following listing are a few adverse reactions that have not been reported with this specific drug. However, the pharmacologic similarities among the tricyclic antidepressant drugs require that each of the reactions be considered when Norpramin (desipramine hydrochloride) is given.

Cardiovascular: hypotension, hypertension, tachycardia, palpitation, arrhythmias, heart block, myocardial infarction, stroke.

Psychiatric: confusional states (especially in the elderly) with hallucinations, disorientation, delusions; anxiety, restlessness, agitation; insomnia and nightmares; hypomania; exacerbation of psychosis.

Neurologic: numbness, tingling, paresthesias of extremities; incoordination, ataxia, tremors; peripheral neuropathy; extrapyramidal symptoms; seizures; alteration in EEG patterns; tinnitus.

Anticholinergic: dry mouth, and rarely associated sublingual adenitis; blurred vision, disturbance of accommodation, mydriasis, increased intraocular pressure; constipation, paralytic ileus; urinary retention, delayed micturition, dilatation of urinary tract.

Allergic: skin rash, petechiae, urticaria, itching, photosensitization (avoid excessive exposure to sunlight), edema (of face and tongue or general), drug fever, cross sensitivity with other tricyclic drugs.

Hematologic: Bone marrow depressions including agranulocytosis, eosinophilia, purpura, thrombocytopenia.

Gastrointestinal: anorexia, nausea and vomiting, epigastric distress, peculiar taste, abdominal cramps, diarrhea, stomatitis, black tongue.

Endocrine: gynecomastia in the male, breast enlargement and galactorrhea in the female; increased or decreased libido, impotence, testicular swelling; elevation or depression of blood sugar levels.

Other: jaundice (simulating obstructive), altered liver function; weight gain or loss; perspiration, flushing; urinary frequency, nocturia; parotid swelling; drowsiness, dizziness, weakness and fatigue, headache; alopecia.

Withdrawal Symptoms: Though not indicative of addiction, abrupt cessation of treatment

Continued on next page

Information on Merrell Dow products is based on labeling in effect in October, 1982.

Merrell Dow—Cont.

after prolonged therapy may produce nausea, headache, and malaise.

Dosage and Administration: Not recommended for use in children.

Lower dosages are recommended for elderly patients and adolescents. Lower dosages are also recommended for outpatients compared to hospitalized patients, who are closely supervised. Dosage should be initiated at a low level and increased according to clinical response and any evidence of intolerance. Following remission, maintenance medication may be required for a period of time and should be at the lowest dose that will maintain remission.

Usual Adult Dose:

The usual adult dose is 100 to 200 mg per day. In more severely ill patients, dosage may be further increased gradually to 300 mg/day if necessary. Dosages above 300 mg/day are not recommended.

Dosage should be initiated at a lower level and increased according to tolerance and clinical response.

Treatment of patients requiring as much as 300 mg should generally be initiated in hospitals, where regular visits by the physician, skilled nursing care, and frequent electrocardiograms (ECG's) are available.

The best available evidence of impending toxicity from very high doses of Norpramin is prolongation of the QRS or QT intervals on the ECG. Prolongation of the PR interval is also significant, but less closely correlated with plasma levels. Clinical symptoms of intolerance, especially drowsiness, dizziness, and postural hypotension, should also alert the physician to the need for reduction in dosage. Plasma desipramine measurement would constitute the optimal guide to dosage monitoring.

Initial therapy may be administered in divided doses or a single daily dose.

Maintenance therapy may be given on a once-daily schedule for patient convenience and compliance.

Adolescent and Geriatric Dose:

The usual adolescent and geriatric dose is 25 to 100 mg daily.

Dosage should be initiated at a lower level and increased according to tolerance and clinical response to a usual maximum of 100 mg daily. In more severely ill patients, dosage may be further increased to 150 mg/day. Doses above 150 mg/day are not recommended in these age groups.

Initial therapy may be administered in divided doses or a single daily dose.

Maintenance therapy may be given on a once-daily schedule for patient convenience and compliance.

Overdosage: There is no specific antidote for desipramine, nor are there specific phenomena of diagnostic value characterizing poisoning by the drug.

Within an hour of ingestion the patient may become agitated or stuporous and then comatose. Hypotension, shock, and renal shutdown may ensue. Grand mal seizures, both early and late after ingestion, have been reported. Hyperactive reflexes, hyperpyrexia, muscle rigidity, vomiting, and ECG evidence of impaired conduction may occur. Serious disturbances of cardiac rate, rhythm, and output can occur.

The precepts of early evacuation of the ingested material and subsequent support of respiration (airway and movement), circulation, and renal output apply.

The principles of management of coma and shock by means of the mechanical respirator, cardiac pacemaker, monitoring of central venous pressure, and regulation of fluid and acid-base balance are well known in most medical centers and are not further discussed here.

Because CNS involvement, respiratory depression, and cardiac arrhythmia can occur suddenly, hospitalization and close observation are generally advisable, even when the amount ingested is thought to be small or the initial degree of intoxication appears slight or moderate. Most patients with ECG abnormalities should have continuous cardiac monitoring for at least 72 hours and be closely observed until well after cardiac status has returned to normal; relapses may occur after apparent recovery.

The slow intravenous administration of physostigmine salicylate has been reported to reverse most of the anticholinergic cardiovascular and CNS effects of overdose with tricyclic antidepressants. In adults, 1 to 3 mg has been reported to be effective. In children, the dose should be started with 0.5 mg and repeated at 5-minute intervals to determine the minimum effective dose; no more than 2 mg. should be given. Because of the short duration of action of physostigmine, the effective dose should be repeated at 30-minute to 60-minute intervals, as necessary. Rapid injection should be avoided to reduce the possibility of physostigmine-induced convulsions.

Other possible therapeutic considerations include:

(a) Dialysis: Desipramine is found in low concentration in the serum, even after a massive oral dose. *In vitro* experiments in which blood bank blood was used indicate that it is very poorly dialyzed. Because of indications that the drug is secreted in gastric juice, constant gastric lavage has been suggested.

(b) Pharmacologic treatment of shock: Since desipramine potentiates the action of such vasopressor agents as levarterenol and metaraminol, they should be used only with caution.

(c) Pharmacologic control of seizures: Intravenous barbiturates are the treatment of choice for the control of grand mal seizures. One may, alternately, consider the parenteral use of diphenylhydantoin, which has less central depressant effect but also has an effect on heart rhythm that has not yet been fully defined.

(d) Pharmacologic control of cardiac function: Severe disturbances of cardiac rate, rhythm, and output are probably the initiating events in shock. Intravascular volume must be maintained by i.v. fluids. Digitalization should be carried out early in view of the fact that a positive inotropic effect can be achieved without increase in cardiac work. Many of the cardiodynamic effects of digitalis are the exact opposite of those of massive doses of desipramine (animal studies).

How Supplied:

10 mg blue coated tablets imprinted 68-7

25 mg yellow coated tablets imprinted MERRELL 11

Bottles of 100 and 1000 and unit dose dispenser of 100

50 mg green coated tablets imprinted MERRELL 15

Bottles of 100 and 1000 and unit dose dispenser of 100

75 mg orange coated tablets imprinted MERRELL 19

Bottles of 100

100 mg peach coated tablets imprinted MERRELL 20

Bottles of 100

150 mg white coated tablets imprinted MERRELL 21

Bottles of 50

U.S. Patent Numbers 3,454,554
3,454,698

Product Information as of May, 1980
(10 mg tablet added July, 1982)

[*Shown in Product Identification Section*]

NOVAFED® Capsules ℞

pseudoephedrine hydrochloride

Controlled-Release Decongestant

Description: Each Novafed capsule contains 120 mg of pseudoephedrine hydrochloride in specially formulated pellets designed to provide continuous therapeutic effect for 12 hours. About one-half of the active ingredient is released soon after administration and the rest slowly over the remaining time period.

Actions: Pseudoephedrine (a sympathomimetic) is an orally effective nasal decongestant with peripheral effects similar to epinephrine and central effects similar to, but less intense than, amphetamines. It has the potential for excitatory side effects. At the recommended oral dosage, it has little or no pressor effect in normotensive adults. Patients have not been reported to experience the rebound congestion sometimes experienced with frequent, repeated use of topical decongestants.

Indications: Relief of nasal congestion or eustachian tube congestion. May be given concomitantly with analgesics, antihistamines, expectorants and antibiotics.

Contraindications: Patients with severe hypertension, severe coronary artery disease, and patients on MAO inhibitor therapy. Also contraindicated in patients with hypersensitivity or idiosyncrasy to sympathomimetic amines which may be manifested by insomnia, dizziness, weakness, tremor or arrhythmias.

Children under 12: Should not be used by children under 12 years.

Nursing Mothers: Contraindicated because of the higher than usual risk for infants from sympathomimetic amines.

Warnings: Use judiciously and sparingly in patients with hypertension, diabetes mellitus, ischemic heart disease, increased intraocular pressure, hyperthyroidism or prostatic hypertrophy. See, however, Contraindications. Sympathomimetics may produce central nervous stimulation with convulsions or cardiovascular collapse with accompanying hypotension.

Do not exceed recommended dosage.

Use in Pregnancy: Safety in pregnancy has not been established.

Use in Elderly: The elderly (60 years and older) are more likely to have adverse reactions to sympathomimetics. Overdosage of sympathomimetics in this age group may cause hallucinations, convulsions, CNS depression, and death. Safe use of a short-acting sympathomimetic should be demonstrated in the individual elderly patient before considering the use of a sustained-action formulation.

Precautions: Patients with diabetes, hypertension, cardiovascular disease and hyper-reactivity to ephedrine.

Adverse Reactions: Hyper-reactive individuals may display ephedrine-like reactions such as tachycardia, palpitations, headache, dizziness or nausea. Sympathomimetics have been associated with certain untoward reactions including fear, anxiety, tenseness, restlessness, tremor, weakness, pallor, respiratory difficulty, dysuria, insomnia, hallucinations, convulsions, CNS depression, arrhythmias, and cardiovascular collapse with hypotension.

Drug Interactions: MAO inhibitors and beta adrenergic blockers increase the effects of pseudoephedrine. Sympathomimetics may reduce the antihypertensive effects of methyldopa, mecamylamine, reserpine and veratrum alkaloids.

Dosage and Administration: One capsule every 12 hours. Do not give to children under 12 years of age.

Caution: Federal law prohibits dispensing without prescription.

How Supplied: Brown and orange colored hard gelatin capsules, monogrammed with the Dow diamond followed by the number 104. Bottle of 100 capsules (NDC 0068-0104-61).

Manufactured by KV Pharmaceutical Company, St. Louis, MO 63144
[*Shown in Product Identification Section*]

NOVAFED® Liquid
pseudoephedrine hydrochloride
Decongestant

Description: Each 5 ml teaspoonful of NOVAFED liquid contains 30 mg of pseudoephedrine hydrochloride, the salt of a pharmacologically active stereoisomer of ephedrine (1-phenyl-2-methylamino propanol). The formulation also contains 7.5% alcohol.
Actions: Pseudoephedrine hydrochloride is an orally effective nasal decongestant. Pseudoephedrine is a sympathomimetic amine with peripheral effects similar to epinephrine and central effects similar to, but less intense than, amphetamines. Therefore, it has the potential for excitatory side effects. At the recommended oral dosage, pseudoephedrine has little or no pressor effect in normotensive adults. Patients taking pseudoephedrine orally have not been reported to experience the rebound congestion sometimes experienced with frequent, repeated use of topical decongestants. Pseudoephedrine is not known to produce drowsiness.
Indications: NOVAFED liquid is indicated for the relief of nasal congestion associated, for example, with the common cold, acute upper respiratory infections, sinusitis, and hay fever or upper respiratory allergies. Decongestants have been used for many years to relieve eustachian tube congestion associated with acute eustachian salpingitis, aerotitis media, acute otitis media and serous otitis media. NOVAFED liquid may be given concurrently, when indicated, with analgesics, antihistamines, expectorants and antibiotics.
Contraindications: Patients with severe hypertension, severe coronary artery disease and patients on MAO inhibitor therapy. Also contraindicated in patients with hypersensitivity or idiosyncrasy to sympathomimetic amines which may be manifested by insomnia, dizziness, weakness, tremor or arrythmias.
Nursing Mothers: Contraindicated because of the higher than usual risk for infants from sympathomimetic amines.
Warnings: Use judiciously and sparingly in patients with hypertension, diabetes mellitus, ischemic heart disease, increased intraocular pressure, hyperthyroidism, or prostatic hypertrophy. See, however, Contraindications. Sympathomimetics may produce central nervous stimulation with convulsions or cardiovascular collapse with accompanying hypotension.
Do not exceed recommended dosage.
Use in Pregnancy: Safety has not been established.
Use in Elderly: The elderly (60 years and older) are more likely to have adverse reactions to sympathomimetics. Overdosage of sympathomimetics in this age group may cause hallucinations, convulsions, CNS depression, and death.
Precautions: Patients with diabetes, hypertension, cardiovascular disease and hyper-reactivity to ephedrine.
Adverse Reactions: Hyper-reactive individuals may display ephedrine-like reactions such as tachycardia, palpitations, headache, dizziness, or nausea. Sympathomimetics have been associated with certain untoward reactions including fear, anxiety, tenseness, restlessness, tremor, weakness, pallor, respiratory difficulty, dysuria, insomnia, hallucinations, convulsions, CNS depression, arrhythmias, and cardiovascular collapse with hypotension.
Drug Interactions: MAO inhibitors and beta adrenergic blockers increase the effects of pseudoephedrine. Sympathomimetics may reduce the anti-hypertensive effects of methyldopa, mecamylamine, reserpine and veratrum alkaloids.
Dosage and Administration: Adults, and children over 12 years of age, 2 teaspoonfuls; children 6 to 12 years, 1 teaspoonful, and children under 6 years, ½ teaspoonful, every 4 hours, not to exceed 4 doses in a 24-hour period. However, this dosage may be modified at the discretion of the physician.
Note: NOVAFED liquid does not require a prescription. The package label has dosage instructions as follows: Adults, and children over 12 years of age, 2 teaspoonfuls, every four hours. Children 6 to 12 years, 1 teaspoonful, every four hours. Children 2 to 5 years, ½ teaspoonful, every four hours. Do not exceed four doses in a 24-hour period. For children younger than 2 years, consult a physician.
How Supplied: As a lime green liquid in 4 fluid ounce bottles (NDC 0068-1011-04).

NOVAFED® A CAPSULES ℞
Controlled-Release
Decongestant plus Antihistamine

Description: Each NOVAFED A capsule for oral use contains 120 mg pseudoephedrine hydrochloride, and 8 mg of chlorpheniramine maleate. The specially formulated pellets in each capsule are designed to provide continuous therapeutic effect for about 12 hours. Nearly one-half of the active ingredients is released soon after administration and the remainder is released slowly over the remaining time period.
Pseudoephedrine hydrochloride is a nasal decongestant. Chemically it is α-[1-(methylamino)ethyl]-benzenemethanol hydrochloride. Chlorpheniramine maleate is an antihistamine. Chemically it is α-(4-chlorophenyl)-N,N-dimethyl-2-pyridinepropanamine.
Clinical Pharmacology: Pseudoephedrine is an orally active sympathomimetic amine and exerts a decongestant action on the nasal mucosa. Pseudoephedrine produces peripheral effects similar to those of ephedrine and central effects similar to, but less intense than amphetamines. It has the potential for excitatory side effects. At the recommended oral dosages it has little or no pressor effect in normotensive adults. The serum half-life (T-½) of pseudoephedrine is approximately 4 to 6 hours. T-½ is decreased with increased excretion of drug at urine pH lower than 6 and may be increased with decreased excretion at urine pH higher than 8.
Chlorpheniramine is an antihistaminic that possesses anticholinergic and sedative effects. It is considered one of the most effective and least toxic of the histamine antagonists. Chlorpheniramine is an H_1 receptor antagonist. It antagonizes many of the pharmacologic actions of histamine. It prevents released histamine from dilating capillaries and causing edema of the respiratory mucosa. Chlorpheniramine has a duration of action of 4 to 6 hours in clinical studies. Its half-life in serum, however, is 12 to 16 hours.
Indications and Usage: Relief of nasal congestion and eustachian tube congestion associated with the common cold, sinusitis and acute upper respiratory infections. It is also indicated for symptomatic relief of perennial and seasonal allergic rhinitis, vasomotor rhinitis, allergic conjunctivitis due to inhalant allergens and foods and mild, uncomplicated allergic skin manifestations of urticaria and angioedema. Decongestants in combination with antihistamines have been used for many years to relieve eustachian tube congestion associated with acute eustachian salpingitis, aerotitis media, acute otitis media and serous otitis media. May be given concomitantly with analgesics and antibiotics.
Contraindications: Patients with severe hypertension, severe coronary artery disease, and in patients on MAO inhibitor therapy. Antihistamines are contraindicated in patients with narrow-angle glaucoma, urinary retention, peptic ulcer, during an asthmatic attack, and in patients receiving MAO inhibitors.
Hypersensitivity: Contraindicated in patients with hypersensitivity or idiosyncrasy to sympathomimetic amines or phenanthrene derivatives.
Nursing Mothers: Contraindicated because of the higher than usual risk for infants from sympathomimetic amines.
Warnings: Sympathomimetic amines should be used judiciously and sparingly in patients with hypertension, diabetes mellitus, ischemic heart disease, increased intraocular pressure, hyperthyroidism or prostatic hypertrophy (see CONTRAINDICATIONS). Sympathomimetics may produce CNS stimulation with convulsions or cardiovascular collapse with accompanying hypotension.
Chlorpheniramine maleate has an atropine-like action and should be used with caution in patients with increased intraocular pressure, cardiovascular disease, hypertension or in patients with a history of bronchial asthma (see CONTRAINDICATIONS). Do not exceed recommended dose.
Use in Elderly: The elderly (60 years and older) are more likely to have adverse reactions to sympathomimetics. Overdosage of sympathomimetics in this age group may cause hallucinations, convulsions, CNS depression and death.
Precautions: *General:* Should be used with caution in patients with diabetes, hypertension, cardiovascular disease and hyperreactivity to ephedrine. The antihistaminic may cause drowsiness and ambulatory patients who operate machinery or motor vehicles should be cautioned accordingly.
Information for Patients: Antihistamines may impair mental and physical abilities required for the performance of potentially hazardous tasks, such as driving a vehicle or operating machinery, and mental alertness in children.
Drug Interactions: MAO inhibitors and beta adrenergic blockers increase the effect of sympathomimetics. Sympathomimetics may reduce the antihypertensive effects of methyldopa, mecamylamine, reserpine and veratrum alkaloids. Concomitant use of antihistamines with alcohol, tricyclic antidepressants, barbiturates and other CNS depressants may have an additive effect.
Pregnancy Category C: Animal reproduction studies have not been conducted with NOVAFED A capsules. It is also not known whether NOVAFED A capsules can cause fetal harm when administered to a pregnant woman or can affect reproduction capacity. NOVAFED A capsules may be given to a pregnant woman only if clearly needed.
Nursing Mothers: Pseudoephedrine is contraindicated in nursing mothers because of the higher than usual risk for infants from sympathomimetic amines.
Adverse Reactions: Hyperreactive individuals may display ephedrine-like reactions such as tachycardia, palpitations, headache, dizziness, or nausea. Patients sensitive to antihistamines may experience mild sedation. Sympathomimetic drugs have been associated with certain untoward reactions including fear, anxiety, tenseness, restlessness, tremor, weakness, pallor, respiratory difficulty, dysuria, insomnia, hallucinations, convulsions, CNS depression, arrhythmias, and cardiovascular collapse with hypotension.
Possible side effects of antihistamines are drowsiness, restlessness, dizziness, weakness, dry mouth, anorexia, nausea, headache, nervousness, blurring of vision , heartburn, dysuria and very rarely dermatitis. Patient idiosyncrasy to adrenergic agents may be mani-

Continued on next page

Information on Merrell Dow products is based on labeling in effect in October, 1982.

Merrell Dow—Cont.

fested by insomnia, dizziness, weakness, tremor, or arrhythmias.

Overdosage: Acute overdosage with NOVAFED A capsules may produce clinical signs of CNS stimulation and variable cardiovascular effects. Pressor amines should be used with great caution in the presence of pseudoephedrine. Patients with signs of stimulation should be treated conservatively.

Dosage and Administration: One capsule every 12 hours. Do not give to children under 12 years of age.

Caution: Federal law prohibits dispensing without prescription.

How Supplied: NOVAFED A is supplied in red and orange colored hard gelatin capsules monogrammed with the Dow diamond followed by the number 106, in bottles of 100 capsules (NDC 0068-0106-61).

Manufactured by KV Pharmaceutical Company, St. Louis, MO 63144

[*Shown in Product Identification Section*]

NOVAFED® A

Decongestant Plus Antihistamine Liquid

Description: Each 5 ml teaspoonful of NOVAFED A liquid contains: pseudoephedrine hydrochloride, 30 mg and chlorpheniramine maleate, 2 mg. Pseudoephedrine hydrochloride is the salt of a pharmacologically active stereoisomer of ephedrine (1-phenyl-2-methylamino propanol). Chlorpheniramine is an antihistamine drug of the alkylamine type. Other ingredients include alcohol 5%.

Actions: Combines the actions of an orally effective nasal decongestant, pseudoephedrine, and an antihistamine, chlorpheniramine. The antihistamine also possesses anticholinergic and sedative effects.

Indications: NOVAFED A liquid is indicated for the relief of nasal congestion associated, for example, with the common cold, acute upper respiratory infections, sinusitis, and hay fever or upper respiratory allergies. Decongestants in combination with antihistamines have been used for many years to relieve eustachian tube congestion associated with acute eustachian salpingitis, aerotitis media, acute otitis media and serous otitis media. NOVAFED A liquid may be given concurrently, when indicated, with analgesics and antibiotics.

Contraindications: Patients with severe hypertension, severe coronary artery disease; patients on MAO inhibitor therapy; patients with narrow-angle glaucoma, urinary retention, peptic ulcer and during an asthmatic attack. Also contraindicated in patients with hypersensitivity or idiosyncrasy to sympathomimetic amines or antihistamines which may be manifested by insomnia, dizziness, weakness, tremor or arrhythmias, dry mouth, drowsiness and vomiting.

Nursing Mothers: Contraindicated because of the higher than usual risk for infants from sympathomimetic amines.

Warnings: Sympathomimetic amines should be used judiciously and sparingly in patients with hypertension, diabetes mellitus, ischemic heart disease, increased intraocular pressure, hyperthyroidism or prostatic hypertrophy. See, however, Contraindications. Sympathomimetics may produce central nervous system stimulation with convulsions or cardiovascular collapse with accompanying hypotension.

Antihistamines may impair mental and physical abilities required for the performance of potentially hazardous tasks, such as driving a vehicle or operating machinery, and may impair mental alertness in children. Chlorpheniramine has an atropine-like action and should be used with caution in patients with increased intraocular pressure, cardiovascular disease, hypertension or in patients with a history of bronchial asthma. See, however, Contraindications.

Do not exceed recommended dosage.

Use in Pregnancy: Safety of pseudoephedrine has not been established.

Use in Elderly: The elderly (60 years and older) are more likely to have adverse reactions to sympathomimetics. Overdosage of sympathomimetics in this age group may cause hallucinations, convulsions, CNS depression, and death.

Precautions: Patients with diabetes, hypertension, cardiovascular disease and hyper-reactivity to ephedrine. The antihistamine may cause drowsiness and ambulatory patients who operate machinery or motor vehicles should be cautioned accordingly.

Adverse Reactions: Hyper-reactive individuals may display ephedrine-like reactions such as tachycardia, palpitations, headache, dizziness or nausea. Patients sensitive to antihistamines may experience mild sedation.

Sympathomimetics have been associated with certain untoward reactions including fear, anxiety, tenseness, restlessness, tremor, weakness, pallor, respiratory difficulty, dysuria, insomnia, hallucinations, convulsions, CNS depression, arrhythmias, and cardiovascular collapse with hypotension.

Possible side effects of antihistamines are drowsiness, dry mouth, anorexia, nausea, vomiting, headache and nervousness, blurring of vision, polyuria, heartburn, dysuria and very rarely, dermatitis.

Drug Interactions: MAO inhibitors and beta adrenergic blockers increase the effects of sympathomimetics. Sympathomimetics may reduce the antihypertensive effects of methyldopa, mecamylamine, reserpine and veratrum alkaloids. Concomitant use of antihistamines with alcohol, tricyclic antidepressants, barbiturates and other CNS depressants may have an additive effect.

Dosage: Adults, and children over 12 years of age, 2 teaspoonfuls; children 6 to 12 years, 1 teaspoonful, and children under 6 years, ½ teaspoonful, every four hours, not to exceed 4 doses in a 24-hour period. However, this dosage may be modified at the discretion of the physician.

Note: NOVAFED A liquid does not require a prescription. The package label has dosage instructions as follows: adults, and children over 12 years of age, 2 teaspoonfuls every 4 hours. Children 6 to 12 years, 1 teaspoonful, every 4 hours. For children under 6 years of age, consult a physician. Do not exceed 4 doses in a 24-hour period.

How Supplied: As a green liquid in 4 fluid ounce bottles (NDC 0068-1010-04).

NOVAHISTINE® COUGH FORMULA

(See PDR For Nonprescription Drugs)

NOVAHISTINE® COUGH & COLD FORMULA

(See PDR For Nonprescription Drugs)

NOVAHISTINE® DH Ⓒ

Antitussive-Decongestant-Antihistamine

Description: Each 5 ml teaspoonful contains codeine phosphate, 10 mg (Warning: May be habit forming), phenylpropanolamine hydrochloride, 18.75 mg chlorpheniramine maleate, 2 mg, and alcohol, 5%.

Actions: Antitussive, decongestant and antihistaminic actions.

Codeine, at the recommended dose, causes suppression of the cough reflex by a direct effect on the cough center in the medulla of the brain. Codeine has antitussive, mild analgesic and sedative effects.

Phenylpropanolamine is a sympathomimetic amine similar in action to ephedrine but with less central nervous system stimulation.

Chlorpheniramine possesses antihistaminic, mild anticholinergic and sedative effects. It antagonizes many of the pharmacologic actions of histamine. It prevents released histamine from dilating capillaries and causing edema of the respiratory mucosa.

Indications: For the temporary relief of cough associated with minor throat and bronchial irritation or nasal congestion due to the common cold, sinusitis, and hay fever (allergic rhintis).

A minimum dosage of codeine is provided for the symptomatic relief of nonproductive cough. Phenylpropanolamine is one of the most commonly used oral nasal decongestants. Decongestants have been used to relieve eustachian tube congestion associated with acute eustachian salpingitis, aerotitis, otitis and serous otitis media. Chlorpheniramine maleate provides temporary relief from runny nose, sneezing, itching of nose or throat and itchy and watery eyes as may occur in hay fever (allergic rhinitis).

May be used as supportive therapy for acute otitis media and relief of mild otalgia.

May be given concomitantly, when indicated, with analgesics and antibiotics.

Contraindications: Patients with severe hypertension, severe coronary artery disease, narrow-angle glaucoma, urinary retention, peptic ulcer, during an asthmatic attack, and in patients on MAO inhibitor therapy and nursing mothers. Also contraindicated in patients with hypersensitivity or idiosyncrasy to its ingredients.

Warnings: Codeine should be prescribed and administered with the same degree of caution as all oral medications containing a narcotic analgesic. Codeine appears in the milk of nursing mothers.

If sympathomimetic amines are used in patients with hypertension, diabetes mellitus, ischemic heart disease, hyperthyroidism, increased intraocular pressure or prostatic hypertrophy, judicious caution should be exercised. See, however, Contraindications.

The elderly (60 years and older) are more likely to have adverse reactions to sympathomimetics. Safety for use during pregnancy has not been established.

Antihistamines may cause excitablity, especially in children.

Precautions: If cough persists for more than one week, tends to recur or is accompanied by fever, rash or headache, discontinue treatment. Other medications containing a narcotic analgesic, phenothiazines, tranquilizers, sedatives, hypnotics and other CNS depressants, including alcohol, may have an additive CNS depressant effect when used concomitantly. The dose should be reduced when such combined therapy is contemplated.

Caution should be exercised if used in patients with high blood pressure, heart disease, asthma, emphysema, diabetes or thyroid disease.

The antihistamine may cause drowsiness, and ambulatory patients who operate machinery or motor vehicles should be cautioned accordingly.

Adverse Reactions: Nausea, vomiting, constipation, dizziness, sedation, palpitations or pruritus may occur. More frequent or higher than recommended dosage may cause respiratory depression, especially in patients with respiratory disease associated with carbon dioxide retention.

Drugs containing sympathomimetic amines have been associated with certain untoward reactions including fear, anxiety, tenseness, restlessness, tremor, weakness, pallor, respiratory difficulty, dysuria, insomnia, hallucinations, convulsions, CNS depression, arrhythmias and cardiovascular collapse with hypotension.

Phenylpropanolamine is considered safe when taken at recommended dosage and is relatively free of unpleasant side effects. However, there

have been isolated reports of individuals experiencing an acute hypertensive episode after taking therapeutic doses of phenylpropanolamine-containing preparations.
Patients sensitive to antihistamine drugs may experience mild sedation. Other side effects from antihistamines may include dry mouth, dizziness, weakness, anorexia, nausea, vomiting, headache, nervousness, polyuria, heartburn, diplopia, dysuria, and, very rarely, dermatitits.
Drug Interactions: Codeine may potentiate the effects of other narcotics, general anesthetics, tranquilizers, sedatives and hypnotics, tricyclic antidepressants, MAO inhibitors, alcohol and other CNS depressants.
Beta adrenergic blockers and MAO inhibitors potentiate the sympathomimetic effects of phenylpropanolamine. Sympathomimetics may reduce the antihypertensive effects of methyldopa, mecamylamine, reserpine and veratrum alkaloids.
Antihistamines have been shown to enhance one or more of the effects of alcohol, tricyclic antidepressants, barbiturates and other CNS depressants.
Dosage: Adults, 2 teaspoonfuls. Children 50–90 lbs., ½ to 1 teaspoonful; 25–50 lbs., ¼ to ½ teaspoonful. May be given to children under 2 at the discretion of the physician at a dosage of 3 drops/kg. body weight every 4 hours. *Do not exceed 4 doses in a 24-hour period.*
Product label dosage is as follows: Adults, 2 teaspoonfuls; children 6 to 12 years, 1 teaspoonful. May be given every 4 hours, but *do not exceed 4 doses in 24 hours.* For children under 6 years, consult a physician.
How Supplied: In 4 fluid ounce bottles (NDC 0068-1027-04), and pints (NDC 0068-1027-16).
[*Shown in Product Identification Section*]

NOVAHISTINE® DMX
Antitussive-Decongestant
Liquid

(See PDR For Nonprescription Drugs)

NOVHASTINE® ELIXIR
NOVAHISTINE® COLD TABLETS
Decongestant—Antihistaminic

(See PDR For Nonprescription Drugs)

NOVAHISTINE® EXPECTORANT ©
Antitussive-Decongestant-Expectorant

Description: Each 5 ml teaspoonful contains codeine phosphate, 10 mg (Warning: may be habit forming), phenylpropanolamine hydrochloride, 18.75 mg, guaifenesin (glyceryl guaiacolate), 100 mg, and alcohol 7.5%.
Actions: Expectorant, antitussive and decongestant actions. Codeine, at the recommended dose, causes suppression of the cough reflex by a direct effect on the cough center in the medulla of the brain. Codeine has antitussive and mild analgesic and sedative effects.
Phenylpropanolamine is a sympathomimetic amine similar in action to ephedrine but with less central nervous system stimulation.
Guaifenesin helps drainage of bronchial tubes by thinning the mucus, and facilitates expectoration by loosening phlegm and bronchial secretions.
Indications: For loosening tenacious pulmonary secretions associated with cough and respiratory congestion.
A minimum dosage of codeine is provided for the symptomatic relief of nonproductive cough. Phenylpropanolamine is one of the most commonly used oral nasal decongestants. Decongestants have been used to relieve eustachian tube congestion associated with acute eustachian salpingitis, aerotitis, otitis and serous otitis media. Guaifenesin helps loosen phlegm (sputum) and bronchial secretions.
May be used as supportive therapy for acute otitis media and relief of mild otalgia.
May be given concomitantly, when indicated, with analgesics and antibiotics.
Contraindications: Patients with severe hypertension, severe coronary artery disease, in patients on MAO inhibitor therapy and in nursing mothers. Also contraindicated in patients with hypersensitivity or idiosyncrasy to its ingredients.
Warnings: Codeine should be prescribed and administered with the same degree of caution as all oral medications containing a narcotic analgesic. Codeine appears in the milk of nursing mothers.
If sympathomimetic amines are used in patients with hypertension, diabetes mellitus, ischemic heart disease, hyperthyroidism, increased intraocular pressure and prostatic hypertrophy, judicious caution should be exercised. See, however, Contraindications.
The elderly (60 years and older) are more likely to have adverse reactions to sympathomimetics. Safety for use during pregnancy has not been established.
Precautions: If cough persists for more than one week, tends to recur or is accompanied by fever, rash or headache, discontinue treatment.
Other medications containing a narcotic analgesic, phenothiazines, tranquilizers, sedatives, hypnotics, and other CNS depressants, including alcohol, may have an additive CNS depressant effect when used concomitantly. The dose should be reduced when such combined therapy is contemplated.
Caution should be exercised if used in patients with high blood pressure, heart disease, asthma, emphysema, diabetes or thyroid disease.
Adverse Reactions: Nausea, vomiting, constipation, dizziness, sedation, palpitations, or pruritus may occur. More frequent or higher than recommended dosage may cause respiratory depression, especially in patients with respiratory disease associated with carbon dioxide retention.
Drugs containing sympathomimetic amines have been associated with certain untoward reactions including fear, anxiety, tenseness, restlessness, tremor, weakness, pallor, respiratory difficulty, dysuria, insomnia, hallucinations, convulsions, CNS depression, arrhythmias and cardiovascular collapse with hypotension.
Phenylpropanolamine is considered safe when taken at recommended dosage and is relatively free of unpleasant side effects. However, there have been isolated reports of individuals experiencing an acute hypertensive episode after taking therapeutic doses of phenylpropanolamine-containing preparations.
Note: Guaifenesin interferes with the colorimetric determination of 5-hydroxyindoleacetic acid (5-HIAA) and vanilmandelic acid (VMA).
Drug Interactions: Codeine may potentiate the effects of other narcotics, general anesthetics, tranquilizers, sedatives and hypnotics, tricyclic antidepressants, MAO inhibitors, alcohol and other CNS depressants.
Beta adrenergic blockers and MAO inhibitors potentiate the sympathomimetic effects of phenylpropanolamine. Sympathomimetics may reduce the antihypertensive effects of methyldopa, mecamylamine, reserpine and veratrum alkaloids.
Dosage: Adults, 2 teaspoonfuls; children 50–90 lbs., ½ to 1 teaspoonful; 25–50 lbs., ¼ to ½ teaspoonful. May be given to children under 2 at the discretion of the physician at a dosage of 3 drops/kg. body weight every 4 hours. **Do not exceed 4 doses in a 24-hour period.**
Product label dosage is as follows: Adults, 2 teaspoonfuls; children 6 to 12 years, 1 teaspoonful; children 2 to 5 years, ½ teaspoonful. May be given every 4 hours but **do not exceed 4 doses in 24 hours.** For children under 2 years, consult a physician.
How Supplied: As a liquid in 4 fluid ounce bottles (NDC 0068-1028-04) and pints (NDC 0068-1028-16).
[*Shown in Product Identification Section*]

NOVAHISTINE®
SINUS TABLETS
Analgesic-Decongestant-Antihistamine

(See PDR For Nonprescription Drugs)

ORENZYME® ℞
(Oral enteric coated enzyme tablet)
ORENZYME® BITABS™
(Double strength oral enteric coated enzyme tablet)

AVAILABLE ONLY ON PRESCRIPTION

Description:
Orenzyme
Each red, enteric coated tablet of Orenzyme contains:

trypsin	50,000 USP Units
chymotrypsin	4,000 USP Units

equivalent in tryptic activity to 20 mg of USP trypsin.
Orenzyme Bitabs
Each yellow, enteric coated tablet of Orenzyme Bitabs contains:

trypsin	100,000 USP Units
chymotrypsin	8,000 USP Units

equivalent in tryptic activity to 40 mg of USP trypsin.
The tablets have a special enteric coating designed to permit intact passage through the stomach, followed by disintegration in the intestinal tract.
Action: The mode of action of Orenzyme has not been established.

Indications:
Based on a review of this drug by the National Academy of Sciences—National Research Council and/or other information, FDA has classified the indications as follows:
"Possibly" effective: Relief of symptomatology related to episiotomy.
Lack of substantial evidence of effectiveness: Adjunctive therapy for the resolution of inflammation and edema resulting from serious accidental trauma or surgical trauma.
Final classification of the less-than-effective indications requires further investigation.

Contraindications: Orenzyme should not be given to patients with a known sensitivity to trypsin or chymotrypsin.
Precautions: Orenzyme should be used with caution in patients with abnormality of the blood clotting mechanism such as hemophilia or with severe hepatic or renal disease. Safe use in pregnancy has not been established.
This product contains FD&C Yellow No. 5 (tartrazine), which may cause allergic-type reactions (including bronchial asthma) in certain susceptible individuals. Although the overall incidence of FD&C Yellow No. 5 (tartrazine) sensitivity in the general population is low, it is frequently seen in patients who also have aspirin hypersensitivity.
Adverse Reactions: Adverse reactions with Orenzyme have been reported infrequently. Reports include allergic manifestations (rash, urticaria, itching), gastrointestinal upset, and increased speed of dissolution of animal-origin surgical sutures. There have been isolated reports of anaphylactic shock, albuminuria, and hematuria. Increased tendency to bleed has

Continued on next page

Information on Merrell Dow products is based on labeling in effect in October, 1982.

Merrell Dow—Cont.

also been reported, but in controlled studies it has been seen with equal incidence in placebo-treated groups. (See Precautions.)

It is recommended that if side effects occur, medication be discontinued.

Dosage and Administration:

Orenzyme: 1 or 2 tablets q.i.d.

Orenzyme Bitabs: 1 tablet q.i.d.

How Supplied:

Orenzyme Tablets imprinted MERRELL 441
NDC 0068-0441-13: bottles of 48
NDC 0068-0441-16: bottles of 500

Orenzyme Bitabs imprinted MERRELL 442
NDC 0068-0442-15: bottles of 100

Product Information as of August, 1979

QUIDE® ℞
piperacetazine

Description: Quide (piperacetazine) is a piperidine derivative of phenothiazine having the following chemical designation: 10-{3-[4-(2-Hydroxyethyl)-piperidino] propyl}phenothiazin-2-yl methyl ketone.

Actions: The exact mode of action of the phenothiazines is unclear, but drugs of this class produce changes at all levels of the central nervous system, as well as on multiple organ systems.

Indications: Quide is indicated for use in the management of the manifestations of psychotic disorders.

Quide has not been shown effective in the management of behavioral complications in patients with mental retardation.

Contraindications: Quide is contraindicated in patients who are comatose or markedly depressed from any cause and in the presence of preexisting thrombocytopenia and other blood dyscrasias, bone marrow depression and in patients with significant liver disease. Quide is contraindicated in women who are or may become pregnant since animal reproductive studies adequate to establish safety during pregnancy have not been carried out. Quide is contraindicated in patients who have shown hypersensitivity to the drug. Cross sensitivity between phenothiazine derivatives may occur.

Warnings: Like other phenothiazines, Quide may impair the mental and/or physical abilities required for the performance of potentially hazardous tasks such as driving a car or operating machinery, especially during the first few days of therapy. Therefore, patients should be cautioned accordingly. Concomitant use with alcohol should be avoided due to the potential additive effect. Patients with known suicidal tendencies should not be given Quide except under strict medical supervision.

Use in Children: The use of Quide (piperacetazine) in children under 12 years of age is not recommended because safe conditions for its use have not been established.

Precautions: Use with caution in persons who:

1. are receiving barbiturates or narcotics, because of additive effects on central nervous system depression. The dosage of the narcotic or barbiturate should be reduced when given concomitantly with Quide.
2. are receiving atropine or related drugs, because of additive anticholinergic effects.
3. have a history of epilepsy, because this drug may lower the convulsive threshold. Adequate anticonvulsant therapy must be maintained concomitantly.
4. are exposed to extreme heat or phosphorus insecticides.
5. have cardiovascular disease.
6. have respiratory impairment due to acute pulmonary infections or chronic respiratory disorders such as severe asthma or emphysema.

Keep in mind that the antiemetic effect may mask the toxicity of other drugs or obscure the diagnosis of such conditions as intestinal obstruction or brain tumor.

Any sign of blood dyscrasias requires immediate discontinuance of the drug and the institution of appropriate therapy.

The possibility of liver damage, pigmentary retinopathy, lenticular or corneal deposits, and development of irreversible dyskinesias should be kept in mind when patients are on prolonged therapy.

Neuroleptic drugs elevate prolactin levels; the elevation persists during chronic administration. Tissue culture experiments indicate that approximately one-third of human breast cancers are prolactin dependent in vitro, a factor of potential importance if the prescription of these drugs is contemplated in a patient with a previously detected breast cancer. Although disturbances such as galactorrhea, amenorrhea, gynecomastia, and impotence have been reported, the clinical significance of elevated serum prolactin levels is unknown for most patients. An increase in mammary neoplasms has been found in rodents after chronic administration of neuroleptic drugs. Neither clinical studies nor epidemiologic studies conducted to date, however, have shown an association between chronic administration of these drugs and mammary tumorigenesis; the available evidence is considered too limited to be conclusive at this time.

Abrupt Withdrawal: In general, phenothiazines do not produce psychic dependence, but gastritis, nausea and vomiting, dizziness and tremulousness have been reported following abrupt cessation of high-dose therapy. Reports suggest that these symptoms can be reduced if concomitant antiparkinson agents are continued for several weeks after the phenothiazine is withdrawn.

Both QUIDE 10 mg and QUIDE 25 mg tablets contain FD&C Yellow No. 5 (tartrazine) which may cause allergic-type reactions (including bronchial asthma) in certain susceptible individuals. Although the overall incidence of FD&C Yellow No. 5 (tartrazine) sensitivity in the general population is low, it is frequently seen in patients who also have aspirin hypersensitivity.

Adverse Reactions: Not all of the following adverse reactions have been reported with Quide (piperacetazine) but pharmacological similarities among various phenothiazine derivatives require that each be considered.

Note: Sudden Death has occasionally been reported in patients who have received phenothiazines. In some cases death was apparently due to cardiac arrest, in others the cause appeared to be asphyxia due to failure of the cough reflex. In some patients the cause could not be determined, nor could it be established that death was due to the phenothiazine.

Drowsiness: May occur particularly during the first or second week, after which it generally disappears. If troublesome, lower the dosage.

Jaundice: Incidence is low. When it occurs (usually between the second and fourth weeks of therapy) it is generally regarded as a sensitivity reaction. The clinical picture resembles infectious hepatitis with laboratory features of obstructive jaundice It is usually reversible although chronic jaundice has been reported with phenothiazine therapy.

Hematological Disorders: Agranulocytosis, eosinophilia, leukopenia, hemolytic anemia, thrombocytopenic purpura, aplastic anemia and pancytopenia.

Agranulocytosis: Most cases have occurred between the fourth and tenth weeks of therapy. Patients should be watched closely during that period for the sudden appearance of sore throat or other signs of infection. If white blood count and differential show significant cellular depression, discontinue the drug and start appropriate therapy. A slightly lowered white count, however, is not in itself an indication to discontinue the drug.

Cardiovascular: Postural hypotension, tachycardia (especially following rapid increase in dosage), bradycardia, cardiac arrest, faintness and dizziness. Occasionally the hypotensive effect may produce a shock-like condition. In the event a vasoconstrictor is required, levarterenol and phenylephrine are the most suitable. Other pressor agents, including epinephrine, should not be used because a paradoxical further lowering of the blood pressure may ensue. EKG changes, nonspecific, usually reversible, have been observed in some patients receiving phenothiazine tranquilizers. Their relationship to myocardial damage has not been confirmed.

CNS Effects: Neuromuscular (extrapyramidal) Reactions: These are usually dose related and take three forms: (1) pseudoparkinsonism; (2) akathisia; and (3) dystonias (dystonias include spasms of the neck muscles, extensor rigidity of back muscles, carpopedal spasm, eyes rolled back, convulsions, trismus and swallowing difficulties). These resemble serious neurological disorders but usually subside within 48 hours. Management of the extrapyramidal symptoms, depending upon the type and severity, includes sedation, injectable diphenhydramine, and the use of antiparkinsonism agents. Hyperreflexia has been reported in the newborn when a phenothiazine was used during pregnancy.

Persistent Tardive Dyskinesia: As with all antipsychotic agents, tardive dyskinesia may appear in some patients on long-term therapy or may appear after drug therapy has been discontinued. The risk appears to be greater in elderly patients on high-dose therapy, especially females. The symptoms are persistent and in some patients appear to be irreversible. The syndrome is characterized by rhythmical involuntary movements of the tongue, face, mouth or jaw (e.g., protrusion of tongue, puffing of cheeks, puckering of the mouth, chewing movements). Sometimes these may be accompanied by involuntary movements of extremities.

There is no known effective treatment for tardive dyskinesia; anti-parkinsonism agents usually do not alleviate the symptoms of this syndrome. It is suggested that all antipsychotic agents be discontinued if these symptoms appear. Should it be necessary to reinstitute treatment, or increase the dosage of the agent, or switch to a different antipsychotic agent, the syndrome may be masked.

It has been reported that fine vermicular movements of the tongue may be an early sign of the syndrome and if the medication is stopped at that time the syndrome may not develop.

Other CNS Effects: Cerebral edema. Abnormality of cerebral spinal fluid proteins. Convulsive seizures, particularly in patients with EEG abnormalities or a history of such disorders. Hyperpyrexia.

Adverse Behavioral Effects: Paradoxical exacerbation of psychotic symptoms.

Allergic Reactions: Urticaria, itching, erythema, photosensitivity (avoid undue exposure to the sun), eczema. Severe reactions include: exfoliative dermatitis (rare); contact dermatitis in nursing personnel administering the drug; asthma; laryngeal edema; angioneurotic edema; and anaphylactoid reactions.

Endocrine Disorders: Lactation and moderate breast engorgement in females and gynecomastia in males on large doses; changes in libido; false-positive pregnancy tests; amenorrhea; hyperglycemia, hypoglycemia, glycosuria.

Autonomic Reactions: Dry mouth, nasal congestion, constipation, adynamic ileus, myosis, mydriasis, urinary retention.

Special Considerations in Long-term Therapy: After prolonged administration of phenothiazines, pigmentation of the skin has occurred chiefly in the exposed areas, especially in females on large doses. Ocular changes consisting of deposition of fine particulate matter in the cornea and lens, progressing in more severe cases to star-shaped lenticular opacities; epithelial keratopathies; pigmentary retinopathy.

Other Adverse Reactions: Increases in appetite and weight; peripheral edema; systemic lupus erythematosus-like syndrome.

Dosage and Administration: Dosage should be individualized, not only initially but during the course of therapy, and the minimal effective dose should always be employed.

A starting dosage of 10 mg two to four times daily is recommended for adults. The dose may be increased up to 160 mg daily within a three to five day period. Should side effects occur, dosage should be reduced or discontinued as indicated. For maintenance therapy, up to 160 mg daily in divided doses may be given.

Overdosage with Phenothiazines:

Manifestations: One of three clinical pictures may be seen.

1. Extreme somnolence; patient can usually be roused with prodding, but if permitted, will fall asleep. General condition is usually satisfactory. The skin, though pale, is warm and dry. Slight blood pressure, respiratory and pulse changes may occur but are not problems.
2. Mild to moderate drop in blood pressure (patient may be conscious or unconscious). Skin is markedly gray, but warm and dry. Nail beds are pink. Respiration is slow and regular. Pulse is strong but rate slightly increased.
3. Severe hypotension, possibly accompanied by weakness, cyanosis, perspiration, rapid, thready pulse and respiratory depression.

TREATMENT: Is essentially symptomatic and supportive. Early gastric lavage and intestinal purges may help. Centrally acting emetics may not help because of the possible antiemetic effect of Quide. Give hot tea or coffee. Severe hypotension usually responds to measures described under hypotensive effects (see ADVERSE REACTIONS: Cardiovascular). Additional measures include pressure bandages to lower limbs, oxygen and I.V. fluids.

Avoid stimulants that may cause convulsions (e.g., picrotoxin and pentylenetetrazol).

Limited experience with dialysis indicates that it is not helpful.

Caution: Federal law prohibits dispensing without prescription.

How Supplied:

Quide (piperacetazine) Tablets-10 mg (orange)-bottles of 100 (NDC 0068-0054-61). Quide (piperacetazine) Tablets-25 mg (yellow)-bottles of 100 (NDC 0068-0053-61).

Note: Dispense only in light-resistant containers; the coatings on the tablets contain light-sensitive colors.

QUINAMM™ ℞

(quinine sulfate tablets)

Description:

Quinamm

(quinine sulfate tablets)

Caution: Federal law prohibits dispensing without prescription.

Each white, beveled, compressed tablet for oral administration contains 260 mg quinine sulfate.

Neuromuscular Agent

Quinine sulfate has the following structural formula: (See above)

Quinine sulfate occurs as a white, crystalline powder, which darkens on exposure to light. It is odorless and has a persistent, very bitter taste. It is slightly soluble in water, alcohol, chloroform, and ether.

Clinical Pharmacology: Quinine, a cinchona alkaloid, acts on skeletal muscle by three mechanisms: it increases the refractory period by direct action on the muscle fiber, it decreases the excitability of the motor end-plate, an action similar to that of curare, and it affects the distribution of calcium within the muscle fiber.

Quinine is readily absorbed when given orally. Absorption occurs mainly from the upper part of the small intestine, and is almost complete even in patients with marked diarrhea.

The cinchona alkaloids in large measure are metabolically degraded in the body, especially in the liver; less than 5% of an administered dose is excreted unaltered in the urine. It is reported that there is no accumulation of the drugs in the body upon continued administration. The metabolic degradation products are excreted in the urine, where many of them have been identified as hydroxy derivatives, but small amounts also appear in the feces, gastric juice, bile, and saliva. Renal excretion of quinine is twice as rapid when the urine is acidic as when it is alkaline, due to the greater tubular reabsorption of the alkaloidal base that occurs in an alkaline media. Excretion is also limited by the binding of a large fraction of cinchona alkaloids to plasma proteins.

Peak plasma concentrations of cinchona alkaloids occur within 1 to 3 hours after a single oral dose. The half-life is 4 to 5 hours. After chronic administration of total daily doses of 1 g. of drug, the average plasma quinine concentration is approximately 7 μg/ml. After termination of quinine therapy, the plasma level falls rapidly and only a negligible concentration is detectable after 24 hours.

A large fraction (approximately 70%) of the plasma quinine is bound to proteins. This explains in part why the concentration of the alkaloid in cerebrospinal fluid is only 2 to 5% of that in the plasma. However, it can traverse the placental membrane and readily reach fetal tissues.

Tinnitus and impairment of hearing rarely should occur at plasma quinine concentrations of less than 10 μg/ml. While this level would not be anticipated from use of 1 or 2 tablets of Quinamm daily, an occasional patient may have some evidence of cinchonism on this dosage, such as tinnitus. (See WARNINGS section.)

Indications and Usage: For the prevention and treatment of nocturnal recumbency leg muscle cramps.

Contraindications: Quinamm may cause fetal harm when administered to a pregnant woman. Congenital malformations in the human have been reported with the use of quinine, primarily with large doses (up to 30 g) for attempted abortion. In about half of these reports the malformation was deafness related to auditory nerve hypoplasia. Among the other abnormalities reported were limb anomalies, visceral defects, and visual changes. In animal tests, teratogenic effects were found in rabbits and guinea pigs and were absent in mice, rats, dogs, and monkeys. Quinamm is contraindicated in women who are or may become pregnant. If this drug is used during pregnancy, or if the patient becomes pregnant while taking this drug, the patient should be apprised of the potential hazard to the fetus.

Because of the quinine content, Quinamm is contraindicated in patients with known quinine hypersensitivity and in patients with glucose-6-phosphate dehydrogenase (G-6-PD) deficiency.

Since thrombocytopenic purpura may follow the administration of quinine in highly sensitive patients, a history of this occurrence associated with previous quinine ingestion contraindicates its further use. Recovery usually occurs following withdrawal of the medication and appropriate therapy.

This drug should not be used in patients with tinnitus or optic neuritis or in patients with a history of blackwater fever.

Warnings: Repeated doses or overdosage of quinine in some individuals may precipitate a cluster of symptoms referred to as cinchonism. Such symptoms, in the mildest form, include ringing in the ears, headache, nausea, and slightly disturbed vision; however, when medication is continued or after large single doses, symptoms also involve the gastrointestinal tract, the nervous and cardiovascular systems, and the skin.

Hemolysis (with the potential for hemolytic anemia) has been associated with a G-6-PD deficiency in patients taking quinine. Quinamm should be stopped immediately if evidence of hemolysis appears.

If symptoms occur, drug should be discontinued and supportive measures instituted. In case of overdosage, see OVERDOSAGE section of pescribing information.

Precautions:

General

Quinamm should be discontinued if there is any evidence of hypersensitivity. (See CONTRAINDICATIONS.) Cutaneous flushing, pruritus, skin rashes, fever, gastric distress, dyspnea, ringing in the ears, and visual impairment are the usual expressions of hypersensitivity, particularly if only small doses of quinine have been taken. Extreme flushing of the skin accompanied by intense, generalized pruritus is the most common form. Hemoglobinuria and asthma from quinine are rare types of idiosyncrasy.

In patients with atrial fibrillation, the administration of quinine requires the same precautions as those for quinidine. (See Drug Interactions.)

Drug Interactions

Increased plasma levels of digoxin and digitoxin have been demonstrated in individuals after concomitant quinidine administration. Because of possible similar effects from use of quinine, it is recommended that plasma levels for digoxin and digitoxin be determined for those individuals taking these drugs and Quinamm concomitantly.

Concurrent use of aluminum-containing antacids may delay or decrease absorption of quinine.

Cinchona alkaloids, including quinine, have the potential to depress the hepatic enzyme system that synthesizes the vitamin K-dependent factors. The resulting hypoprothrombinemic effect may enhance the action of warfarin and other oral anticoagulants.

The effects of neuromuscular blocking agents (particularly pancuronium, succinylcholine, and tubocurarine) may be potentiated with quinine, and result in respiratory difficulties.

Urinary alkalizers (such as acetazolamide and sodium bicarbonate) may increase quinine blood levels with potential for toxicity.

Drug/Laboratory Interactions

Quinine may produce an elevated value for urinary 17-ketogenic steroids when the Zimmerman method is used.

Carcinogenesis, Mutagenesis, Impairment of Fertility

Continued on next page

Information on Merrell Dow products is based on labeling in effect in October, 1982.

Merrell Dow—Cont.

A study of quinine sulfate administered in drinking water (0.1%) to rats for periods up to 20 months showed no evidence of neoplastic changes.

Mutation studies of quinine (dihydrochloride) in male and female mice gave negative results by the micronucleus test. Intraperitoneal injections (0.5 mM./kg.) were given twice, 24 hours apart. Direct *Salmonella typhimurium* tests were negative; when mammalian liver hemogenate was added, positive results were found.

No information relating to the effect of quinine upon fertility in animal or in man has been found.

Pregnancy

Category X. See CONTRAINDICATIONS.

Nonteratogenic Effects

Because quinine crosses the placenta in humans, the potential for fetal effects is present. Stillbirths in mothers taking quinine have been reported in which no obvious cause for the fetal deaths was shown. Quinine in toxic amounts has been associated with abortion. Whether this action is always due to direct effect on the uterus is questionable.

Nursing Mothers

Caution should be exercised when Quinamm is given to nursing women because quinine is excreted in breast milk (in small amounts).

Adverse Reactions: The following adverse reactions have been reported with Quinamm in therapeutic or excessive dosage. (Individual or multiple symptoms may represent cinchonism or hypersensitivity.)

Hematologic: acute hemolysis, thrombocytopenic purpura, agranulocytosis, hypoprothrombinemia

CNS: visual disturbances, including blurred vision with scotomata, photophobia, diplopia, diminished visual fields, and disturbed color vision; tinnitus, deafness, and vertigo; headache, nausea, vomiting, fever, apprehension, restlessness, confusion, and syncope

Dermatologic/allergic: cutaneous rashes (urticarial, the most frequent type of allergic reaction, papular, or scarlatinal), pruritus, flushing of the skin, sweating, occasional edema of the face

Respiratory: asthmatic symptoms

Cardiovascular: anginal symptoms

Gastrointestinal: nausea and vomiting (may be CNS-related), epigastric pain

Drug Abuse and Dependence: Tolerance, abuse, or dependence with Quinamm has not been reported.

Overdosage: The more common signs and symptoms of overdosage are tinnitus, dizziness, skin rash, and gastrointestinal disturbance (intestinal cramping). With higher doses, cardiovascular and CNS effects may occur, including headache, fever, vomiting, apprehension, confusion, and convulsions. Other effects are listed in the ADVERSE REACTIONS section.

A fatal oral dose of quinine in adults has been reported as 8 grams. In a report of overdosage with a tablet containing quinine sulfate 260 mg and aminophylline 195 mg, a 43-year-old male ingested perhaps as many as 100 tablets but gastric lavage was performed within 5 to 6 hours. The clinical picture was described as normal but a massive elevation of the serum CPK was noted. Cardiac arrhythmias did not occur and the patient denied any symptoms of cinchonism. The CPK value was stated to have returned to normal in 4 days. Tinnitus and impaired hearing may occur at plasma quinine concentrations over 10 μg/ml. This level would not be normally attained with the use of 1 or 2 Quinamm tablets daily, but in a hypersensitive patient, as little as 0.3 g of quinine may produce tinnitus.

Treatment

Treatment for overdosage should include initially efforts to remove any residual Quinamm from the stomach by gastric lavage or by emesis induced with syrup of ipecac. The blood pressure should be supported and measures used to maintain renal function. Artificial respiration may be needed. Sedatives, oxygen, and other supportive measures should be used as necessary.

Fluid and electrolyte balance with intravenous fluids should be maintained. Acidification of the urine will promote renal excretion of quinine. In the presence of hemoglobinuria, however, acidification of the urine may augment renal blockade. Quinine should be readily dialyzable by hemodialysis and/or hemoperfusion procedures.

Evidence of angioedema or asthma may require the use of epinephrine, corticosteroids, and antihistamines. In the acute phase of toxic amaurosis caused by quinine, vasodilators administered intravenously may have a salutory effect. Stellate block has also been used effectively for quinine-associated blindness. Residual visual impairment occasionally yields to vasodilators.

Dosage and Administration:

1 tablet upon retiring. If needed, 2 tablets may be taken nightly—1 following the evening meal and 1 upon retiring.

After several consecutive nights in which recumbency leg cramps do not occur, Quinamm may be discontinued in order to determine whether continued therapy is needed.

How Supplied:

NDC 0068-0547-15: bottles of 100 white tablets debossed MERRELL 547

NDC 0068-0547-16: bottles of 500 white tablets debossed MERRELL 547

Product Information as of October, 1980

MERRELL DOW PHARMACEUTICALS INC.
Subsidiary of The Dow Chemical Company
Cincinnati, Ohio 45215, U.S.A.

[*Shown in Product Identification Section*]

RESOLVE™ COLD SORE & FEVER BLISTER RELIEF

(See PDR For Nonprescription Drugs)

RIFADIN® ℞
rifampin

Description: Rifadin (rifampin) is a semisynthetic antibiotic derivative of rifamycin B. Specifically, Rifadin is the hydrazone, 3-(4-methylpiperazinyliminomethyl) rifamycin SV.

Actions: Rifadin inhibits DNA-dependent RNA polymerase activity in susceptible cells. Specifically, it interacts with bacterial RNA polymerase, but does not inhibit the mammalian enzyme. This is the mechanism of action by which rifampin exerts its therapeutic effect. Cross resistance to Rifadin has only been shown with other rifamycins.

Peak blood levels in normal adults vary widely from individual to individual. Peak levels occur between 2 and 4 hours following the oral administration of a 600 mg dose. The average peak value is 7 mcg/ml; however, the peak level may vary from 4 to 32 mcg/ml.

In normal subjects the $T^{1/2}$ (biological half-life) of Rifadin in blood is approximately three hours. Elimination occurs mainly through the bile and, to a much lesser extent, the urine.

Indications: Pulmonary tuberculosis. In the initial treatment and in retreatment of patients with pulmonary tuberculosis Rifadin must be used in conjunction with at least one other antituberculosis drug. Frequently used regimens have been the following:

isoniazid and Rifadin
ethambutol and Rifadin
isoniazid, ethambutol and Rifadin

Neisseria meningitidis carriers: Rifadin is indicated for the treatment of asymptomatic carriers of *N. meningitidis* to eliminate meningococci from the nasopharynx.

Rifadin is not indicated for the treatment of meningococcal infection.

To avoid the indiscriminate use of Rifadin, diagnostic laboratory procedures, including serotyping and susceptibility testing, should be performed to establish the carrier state and the correct treatment. In order to preserve the usefulness of Rifadin in the treatment of asymptomatic meningococcal carriers, it is recommended that the drug be reserved for situations in which the risk of meningococcal meningitis is high.

Both in the treatment of tuberculosis and in the treatment of meningococcal carriers, small numbers of resistant cells, present within large populations of susceptible cells, can rapidly become the predominating type. Since rapid emergence of resistance can occur, culture and susceptibility tests should be performed in the event of persistent positive cultures.

Contraindications: A history of previous hypersensitivity reaction to any of the rifamycins.

Warnings: Rifampin has been shown to produce liver dysfunction. There have been fatalities associated with jaundice in patients with liver disease or receiving rifampin concomitantly with other hepatoxic agents. Since an increased risk may exist for individuals with liver disease, benefits must be weighed carefully against the risk of further liver damage. Periodic liver function monitoring is mandatory.

The possibility of rapid emergence of resistant meningococci restricts the use of Rifadin to short-term treatment of the asymptomatic carrier state. Rifadin is not to be used for the treatment of meningococcal disease.

Several studies of tumorigenicity potential have been done in rodents. In one strain of mice known to be particularly susceptible to the spontaneous development of hepatomas, rifampin given at a level 2–10 times the maximum dosage used clinically, resulted in a significant increase in the occurrence of hepatomas in female mice of this strain after one year of administration. There was no evidence of tumorigenicity in the males of this strain, in males or females of another mouse strain or in rats.

Usage in Pregnancy: Although rifampin has been reported to cross the placental barrier and appear in cord blood, the effect of Rifadin, alone or in combination with other antituberculosis drugs, on the human fetus is not known. An increase in congenital malformations, primarily spina bifida and cleft palate, has been reported in the offspring of rodents given oral doses of 150–250 mg/kg/day of rifampin during pregnancy.

The possible teratogenic potential in women capable of bearing children should be carefully weighed against the benefits of therapy.

Precautions: Rifadin is not recommended for intermittent therapy; the patient should be cautioned against intentional or accidental interruption of the daily dosage regimen since rare renal hypersensitivity reactions have been reported when therapy was resumed in such cases.

Rifampin has been observed to increase the requirement for anticoagulant drugs of the coumarin type. The cause of this phenomenon is unknown. In patients receiving anticoagulants and rifampin concurrently, it is recommended that the prothrombin time be performed daily or as frequently as necessary to establish and maintain the required dose of anticoagulant.

Urine, feces, saliva, sputum, sweat and tears may be colored red-orange by rifampin and its metabolites. Soft contact lenses may be permanently stained. Individuals to be treated should be made aware of these possibilities.

It has been reported that the reliability of oral contraceptives may be affected in some patients being treated for tuberculosis with rifampin in combination with at least one other antituberculosis drug. In such cases, alternative contraceptive measures may need to be considered.

It has also been reported that rifampin given in combination with other antituberculosis drugs may decrease the pharmacologic activity of methadone, oral hypoglycemics, digitoxin, quinidine, disopyramide, dapsone and corticosteroids. In these cases, dosage adjustment of the interacting drugs is recommended.

Therapeutic levels of rifampin have been shown to inhibit standard microbiological assays for serum folate and vitamin B_{12}. Alternative methods must be considered when determining folate and vitamin B_{12} concentrations in the presence of rifampin.

Since rifampin has been reported to cross the placental barrier and appear in cord blood, neonates of rifampin-treated mothers should be carefully observed for any evidence of adverse effects.

Adverse Reactions: Gastrointestinal disturbances such as heartburn, epigastric distress, anorexia, nausea, vomiting, gas, cramps, and diarrhea have been noted in some patients. Headache, drowsiness, fatigue, menstrual disturbances, ataxia, dizziness, inability to concentrate, mental confusion, visual disturbances, muscular weakness, fever, pains in the extremities and generalized numbness have also been noted.

Hypersensitivity reactions have been reported. Encountered occasionally have been pruritus, urticaria, rash, pemphigoid reaction, eosinophilia, sore mouth, sore tongue and exudative conjunctivitis. Rarely, hepatitis or a shock-like syndrome with hepatic involvement and abnormal liver function tests have been reported. Transient abnormalities in liver function tests (e.g., elevations in serum bilirubin, BSP, alkaline phosphatase, serum transaminases) have also been observed.

Thrombocytopenia, transient leukopenia, hemolytic anemia and decreased hemoglobin have been observed. Thrombocytopenia has occurred when Rifadin and ethambutol were administered concomitantly according to an intermittent dose schedule twice weekly, and in high doses.

Elevations in BUN and serum uric acid have occurred. Rarely, hemolysis, hemoglobinuria, hematuria, renal insufficiency or acute renal failure have been reported and are generally considered to be hypersensitivity reactions. These have usually occurred during intermittent therapy or when treatment was resumed following intentional or accidental interruption of a daily dosage regimen and were reversible when rifampin was discontinued and appropriate therapy instituted.

Although rifampin has been reported to have an immunosuppressive effect in some animal experiments, available human data indicate that this has no clinical significance.

Dosage and Administration: It is recommended that Rifadin be administered once daily, either one hour before, or two hours after a meal.

Data are not available for determination of dosage for children under 5.

Pulmonary tuberculosis:

Adults: 600 mg (two 300 mg or four 150 mg capsules) in a single daily administration.
Children: 10–20 mg/kg not to exceed 600 mg/day.

In the treatment of pulmonary tuberculosis, Rifadin must be used in conjunction with at least one other antituberculous agent. In general, therapy should be continued until bacterial conversion and maximal improvement have occurred.

Meningococcal carriers:

It is recommended that Rifadin be administered once daily for four consecutive days in the following doses:

Adults: 600 mg (two 300 mg or four 150 mg capsules) in a single daily administration.
Children: 10–20 mg/kg not to exceed 600 mg/day.

Preparation of Extemporaneous Oral suspension:

For pediatric and adult patients in whom capsule swallowing is difficult or when lower doses are needed a RIFADIN suspension can be prepared.

RIFADIN 1% (10 mg/ml) suspension can be compounded as follows:

1. Empty contents of four (4) RIFADIN 300 mg or eight (8) RIFADIN 150 mg capsules into a four (4) ounce amber glass prescription bottle.
2. Add 20 ml simple syrup (Syrup NF) and shake vigorously.
3. Add 100 ml simple syrup to fill bottle and shake vigorously.

This compounding procedure results in a 1% suspension containing 10 mg rifampin per ml. Stability studies indicate that the suspension is stable for six (6) weeks when stored in a refrigerator (2–8°C).

This extemporaneously prepared suspension must be shaken well prior to administration and then stored in the refrigerator.

Susceptibility testing: Pulmonary tuberculosis. Rifampin susceptibility powders are available for both direct and indirect methods of determining the susceptibility of strains of mycobacteria. The MIC's of susceptible clinical isolates when determined in 7H10 or other non-egg-containing media have ranged from 0.1 to 2 mcg/ml.

Meningococcal carriers: Susceptibility discs containing 5 mcg of rifampin are available for susceptibility testing of *N. meningitidis.* Quantitative methods that require measurement of zone diameters give the most precise estimates of antibiotic susceptibility. One such procedure* has been recommended for use with discs for testing susceptibility to rifampin. Interpretations correlate zone diameters from the disc test with MIC (minimal inhibitory concentration) values for rifampin. A range of MIC's from 0.1 to 1 mcg/ml has been found *in vitro* for susceptible strains of *N. meningitidis.* With this procedure, a report from the laboratory of "resistant" indicates that the organism is not likely to be eradicated from the nasopharynx of asymptomatic carriers.

Overdosage:

Signs and Symptoms:

Nausea, vomiting, and increasing lethargy will probably occur within a short time after ingestion; actual unconsciousness may occur with severe hepatic involvement. Brownish-red or orange discoloration of the skin, urine, sweat, saliva, tears, and feces is proportional to amount ingested.

Liver enlargement, possibly with tenderness, can develop within a few hours after severe overdosage and jaundice may develop rapidly. Hepatic involvement may be more marked in patients with prior impairment of hepatic function. Other physical findings remain essentially normal.

Direct and total bilirubin levels may increase rapidly with severe overdosage; hepatic enzyme levels may be affected, especially with prior impairment of hepatic function. A direct effect upon the hematopoietic system, electrolyte levels, or acid-base balance is unlikely.

Treatment:

Since nausea and vomiting are likely to be present, gastric lavage is probably preferable to induction of emesis. Activated charcoal slurry instilled into the stomach following evacuation of gastric contents can help absorb any remaining drug in the G.I. tract. Antiemetic medication may be required to control severe nausea/vomiting.

Active diuresis (with measured intake and output) will help promote excretion of the drug. Bile drainage may be indicated in presence of serious impairment of hepatic function lasting more than 24–48 hours; under these circumstances, extracorporeal hemodialysis may be required.

In patients with previously adequate hepatic function, reversal of liver enlargement and impaired hepatic excretory function probably will be noted within 72 hours, with rapid return toward normal thereafter.

Caution: Federal law prohibits dispensing without prescription.

How Supplied:

150 mg maroon and scarlet capsules imprinted with the Dow diamond trademark over the code number 510.

Bottles of 30 (NDC 0068-0510-30)

300 mg maroon and scarlet capsules imprinted with the Dow diamond trademark and the code number 508.

Bottles of 30 (NDC 0068-0508-30)
Bottles of 60 (NDC 0068-0508-60)
Bottles of 100 (NDC 0068-0508-61)

**Bauer, A.W., Kirby, W.M., Sherris, J.C., and Turck, M. Antibiotic susceptibility testing by a standardized single disk method. Am. J. Clin. Path. 45:493-496, 1966.*

Revised: October, 1981

Rifadin 150 mg capsules are manufactured by
DOW PHARMACEUTICALS
Dow Chemical of Canada, Limited
Richmond Hill, Ontario, L4C 5H2
Canada for
MERRELL DOW PHARMACEUTICALS INC.
Subsidiary of The Dow Chemical Company
Cincinnati, Ohio 45215, U.S.A.

[*Shown in Product Identification Section*]

RIFAMATE® ℞
rifampin-isoniazid
Capsules

WARNING

Severe and sometimes fatal hepatitis associated with isoniazid therapy may occur and may develop even after many months of treatment. The risk of developing hepatitis is age related. Approximate case rates by age are: 0 per 1,000 for persons under 20 years of age, 3 per 1,000 for persons in the 20–34 year age group, 12 per 1,000 for persons in the 35–49 year age group, 23 per 1,000 for persons in the 50–64 year age group, and 8 per 1,000 for persons over 65 years of age. The risk of hepatitis is increased with daily consumption of alcohol. Precise data to provide a fatality rate for isoniazid-related hepatitis are not available; however, in a U.S. Public Health Service Surveillance Study of 13,838 persons taking isoniazid, there were 8 deaths among 174 cases of hepatitis.

Therefore, patients given isoniazid should be carefully monitored and interviewed at monthly intervals. Serum transaminase concentration becomes elevated in about 10–20 percent of patients, usually during the first few months of therapy, but it can occur at any time. Usually enzyme levels return to normal despite continuance of drug, but in some cases progressive liver dysfunction occurs. Patients should be instructed to report immediately any of the prodromal symptoms of hepatitis, such as fatigue, weakness, malaise, anorexia, nausea, or vomiting. If these symptoms appear or if signs suggestive of hepatic damage are detected, isoniazid should be discontinued promptly, since continued use of the drug in these cases has been re-

Continued on next page

Information on Merrell Dow products is based on labeling in effect in October, 1982.

Merrell Dow—Cont.

ported to cause a more severe form of liver damage.
Patients with tuberculosis should be given appropriate treatment with alternative drugs. If isoniazid must be reinstituted, it should be reinstituted only after symptoms and laboratory abnormalities have cleared. The drug should be restarted in very small and gradually increasing doses and should be withdrawn immediately if there is any indication of recurrent liver involvement.
Treatment should be deferred in persons with acute hepatic diseases.

Description: Rifamate is a combination capsule contaning 300 mg rifampin and 150 mg isoniazid.
Rifampin is a semisynthetic antibiotic derivative of rifamycin B. Specifically, rifampin is the hydrazone, 3-(4-methylpiperazinyliminomethyl) rifamycin SV.
Isoniazid is the hydrazide of isonicotinic acid. It exists as colorless or white crystals or as a white, crystalline powder that is water soluble, ordorless, and slowly affected by exposure to air and light.

Actions:

Rifampin

Rifampin inhibits DNA-dependent RNA polymerase activity in susceptible cells. Specifically, it interacts with bacterial RNA polymerase but does not inhibit the mammalian enzyme. This is the mechanism of action by which rifampin exerts its therapeutic effect. Rifampin cross resistance has only been shown with other rifamycins.
In a study of 14 normal human adult males, peak blood levels of rifampin occured 1 ½ to 3 hours following oral administration of two Rifamate capsules. The peaks ranged from 6.9 to 14 mcg/ml with an average of 10 mcg/ml.
In normal subjects the $T^{1/2}$ (biological half-life) of rifampin in blood is approximately 3 hours. Elimination occurs mainly through the bile and, to a much lesser extent the urine.

Isoniazid

Isoniazid acts against actively growing tubercle bacilli.
After oral administration isoniazid produces peak blood levels within 1 to 2 hours which decline to 50% or less within 6 hours. It diffuses readily into all body fluids (cerebrospinal, pleural, and ascitic fluids), tissues, organs and excreta (saliva, sputum, and feces). The drug also passes through the placental barrier and into milk in concentrations comparable to those in the plasma. From 50 to 70% of a dose of isoniazid is excreted in the urine in 24 hours.
Isoniazid is metabolized primarily by acetylation and dehydrazination. The rate of acetylation is genetically determined. Approximately 50% of Blacks and Caucasians are "slow inactivators"; the majority of Eskimos and Orientals are "rapid inactivators."
The rate of acetylation does not significantly alter the effectiveness of isoniazid. However, slow acetylation may lead to higher blood levels of the drug, and thus an increase in toxic reactions.
Pyridoxine deficiency (B_6) is sometimes observed in adults with high doses of isoniazid and is considered probably due to its competition with pyridoxal phosphate for the enzyme apotryptophanase.

Indications: For pulmonary tuberculosis in which organisms are susceptible, and when the patient has been titrated on the individual components and it has therefore been established that this fixed dosage is therapeutically effective.
This fixed-dosage combination drug is not recommended for initial therapy of tuberculosis or for preventive therapy.
In the treatment of tuberculosis, small numbers of resistant cells, present within large populations of susceptible cells, can rapidly become the predominating type. Since rapid emergence of resistance can occur, culture and susceptibility tests should be performed in the event of persistent positive cultures.
This drug is *not* indicated for the treatment of meningococcal infections or asymptomatic carriers of *N. meningitidis* to eliminate meningococci from the nasopharynx.

Contraindications: Previous isoniazid-associated hepatic injury; severe adverse reactions to isoniazid, such as drug fever, chills, and arthritis; acute liver disease of any etiology.
A history of previous hypersensitivity reaction to any of the rifamycins or to isoniazid, including drug-induced hepatitis.

Warnings: Rifamate (rifampin-isoniazid) is a combination of two drugs, each of which has been associated with liver dysfunction. Liver function tests should be performed prior to therapy with Rifamate and periodically during treatment.

Rifampin

Rifampin has been shown to produce liver dysfunction. There have been fatalities associated with jaundice in patients with liver disease or receiving rifampin concomitantly with other hepatoxic agents. Since an increased risk may exist for individuals with liver disease, benefits must be weighed carefully against the risk of further liver damage.
Several studies of tumorigenicity potential have been done in rodents. In one strain of mice known to be particularly susceptible to the spontaneous development of hepatomas, rifampin given at a level 2–10 times the maximum dosage used clinically, resulted in a significant increase in the occurrence of hepatomas in female mice of this strain after one year of administration. There was no evidence of tumorigenicity in the males of this strain, in males or females of another mouse strain, or in rats.

Isoniazid

See the boxed warning.

Precautions:

Rifampin

Rifampin is not recommended for intermittent therapy; the patient should be cautioned against intentional or accidental interruption of the daily dosage regimen since rare renal hypersensitivity reactions have been reported when therapy was resumed in such cases.
Rifampin has been observed to increase the requirements for anticoagulant drugs of the coumarin type. The cause of the phenomenon is unknown. In patients receiving anticoagulants and rifampin concurrently, it is recommended that the prothrombin time be performed daily or as frequently as necessary to establish and maintain the required dose of anticoagulant.
Urine, feces, saliva, sputum, sweat and tears may be colored red-orange by rifamin and its metabolites. Soft contact lenses may be permanently stained. Individuals to be treated should be made aware of these possibilities.
It has been reported that the reliability of oral contraceptives may be affected in some patients being treated for tuberculosis with rifampin in combination with at least one other antituberculosis drug. In such cases, alternative contraceptive measures may need to be considered.
It has also been reported that rifampin given in combination with other antituberculosis drugs may affect the blood concentration of methadone, oral hypoglycemics, digitalis derivatives, dapsone and corticosteroids. In these cases, dosage adjustment of the interacting drugs is recommended.
Therapeutic levels of rifampin have been shown to inhibit standard assays for serum folate and vitamin B_{12}. Alternative methods must be considered when determining folate and vitamin B_{12} concentrations in the presence of rifampin.
Since rifampin has been reported to cross the placental barrier and appear in cord blood and in maternal milk, neonates and newborns of rifampin-treated mothers should be carefully observed for any evidence of untoward effects.

Isoniazid

All drugs should be stopped and an evaluation of the patient should be made at the first sign of a hypersensitivity reaction.
Use of isoniazid should be carefully monitored in the following:

1. Patients who are receiving phenytoin (diphenylhydantoin) concurrently. Isoniazid may decrease the excretion of phenytoin or may enhance its effects. To avoid phenytoin intoxication, appropriate adjustment of the anticonvulsant dose should be made.
2. Daily users of alcohol. Daily ingestion of alcohol may be associated with a higher incidence of isoniazid hepatitis.
3. Patients with current chronic liver disease or severe renal dysfunction.

Periodic ophthalmoscopic examination during isoniazid therapy is recommended when visual symptoms occur.

Usage in Pregnancy and Lactation

Rifampin

Although rifampin has been reported to cross the placental barrier and appear in cord blood, the effect of rifampin, alone or in combination with other antituberculosis drugs, on the human fetus is not known. An increase in congenital malformations, primarily spina bifida and cleft palate, has been reported in the offspring of rodents given oral doses of 150–250 mg/kg/day of rifampin during pregnancy.
The possible teratogenic potential in women capable of bearing children should be carefully weighed against the benefits of therapy.

Isoniazid

It has been reported that in both rats and rabbits, isoniazid may exert an embryocidal effect when administered orally during pregnancy, although no isoniazid-related congenital anomalies have been found in reproduction studies in mammalian species (mice, rats, and rabbits). Isoniazid should be prescribed during pregnancy only when therapeutically necessary. The benefit of preventive therapy should be weighed against a possible risk to the fetus. Preventive treatment generally should be started after delivery because of the increased risk of tuberculosis for new mothers.
Since isoniazid is known to cross the placental barrier and to pass into maternal breast milk, neonates and breast-fed infants of isoniazid treated mothers should be carefully observed for any evidence of adverse effects.

Carcinogenesis:

Isoniazid has been reported to induce pulmonary tumors in a number of strains of mice.

Adverse Reactions:

Rifampin

Nervous system reactions: headache, drowsiness, fatigue, ataxia, dizziness, inability to concentrate, mental confusion, visual disturbances, muscular weakness, pain in extremities and generalized numbness.
Gastrointestinal disturbances: in some patients heartburn, epigastric distress, anorexia, nausea, vomiting, gas, cramps, and diarrhea.
Hepatic reactions: transient abnormalities in liver function tests (e.g. elevations in serum bilirubin, BSP, alkaline phosphatase, serum transaminases) have been observed. Rarely, hepatitis or a shocklike syndrome with hepatic involvement and abnormal liver function tests.
Hematologic reactions: thrombocytopenia, transient leukopenia, hemolytic anemia, eosinophilia and decreased hemoglobin have been observed. Thrombocytopenia has occurred when rifampin and ethambutol were administered concomitantly according to an intermittent dose schedule twice weekly and in high doses.

Allergic and immunological reactions: occasionally pruritus, urticaria, rash, pemphigus, acneiform lesions, eosinophilia, sore mouth, sore tongue and exudative conjunctivitis. Rarely, hemolysis, hemoglobinuria, hematuria, renal insufficiency or acute renal failure have been reported which are generally considered to be hypersensitivity reactions. These have usually occurred during intermittent therapy or when treatment was resumed following intentional or accidental interruption of a daily dosage regimen and were reversible when rifampin was discontinued and appropriate therapy instituted.

Although rifampin has been reported to have an immunosuppressive effect in some animal experiments, available human data indicate that this has no clinical significance.

Metabolic reactions: elevations in BUN and serum uric acid have occurred.

Miscellaneous reactions: fever and menstrual distrubances have been noted.

Isoniazid

The most frequent reactions are those affecting the nervous system and the liver.

Nervous system reactions: Peripheral neuropathy is the most common toxic effect. It is dose-related, occurs most often in the malnourished and in those predisposed to neuritis (e.g., alcoholics and diabetics), and is usually preceded by paresthesias of the feet and hands. The incidence is higher in "slow inactivators".

Other neurotoxic effects, which are uncommon with conventional doses, are convulsions, toxic encephalopathy, optic neuritis and atrophy, memory impairment, and toxic psychosis.

Gastrointestinal reactions: Nausea, vomiting, and epigastric distress.

Hepatic reactions: Elevated serum transaminases (SGOT; SGPT), bilirubinemia, bilirubinuria, jaundice, and occasionally severe and sometimes fatal hepatitis. The common prodromal symptoms are anorexia, nausea, vomiting, fatigue, malaise, and weakness. Mild and transient elevation of serum transaminase levels occurs in 10 to 20 percent of persons taking isoniazid. The abnormality usually occurs in the first 4 to 6 months of treatment but can occur at any time during therapy. In most instances, enzyme levels return to normal with no necessity to discontinue medication. In occasional instances, progressive liver damage occurs, with accompanying symptoms. In these cases, the drug should be discontinued immediately. The frequency of progressive liver damage increases with age. It is rare in persons under 20, but occurs in up to 2.3 percent of those over 50 years of age.

Hematologic reactions: agranulocytosis, hemolytic sideroblastic or aplastic anemia, thrombocytopenia and eosinophilia.

Hypersensitivity reactions: fever, skin eruptions (morbilliform, maculopapular, purpuric, or exfoliative), lymphadenopathy and vasculitis.

Metabolic and endocrine reactions: pyridoxine deficiency, pellagra, hyperglycemia, metabolic acidosis, and gynecomastia.

Miscellaneous reactions: rheumatic syndrome and systemic lupus erythematosus-like syndrome.

Overdosage:

Rifampin

Signs and Symptoms

Nausea, vomiting, and increasing lethargy will probably occur within a short time after ingestion; actual unconsciousness may occur with severe hepatic involvement. Brownish-red or orange discoloration of the skin, urine, sweat, saliva, tears, and feces is proportional to amount ingested.

Liver enlargement, possibly with tenderness, can develop within a few hours after severe overdosage and jaundice may develop rapidly. Hepatic involvement may be more marked in patients with prior impairment of hepatic function. Other physical findings remain essentially normal.

Direct and total bilirubin levels may increase rapidly with severe overdosage; hepatic enzyme levels may be affected, especially with prior impairment of hepatic function. A direct effect upon hemopoietic system, electrolyte levels or acid-base balance is unlikely.

Isoniazid

Signs and Symptoms

Isoniazid overdosage produces signs and symptoms within 30 minutes to 3 hours. Nausea, vomiting, dizziness, slurring of speech, blurring of vision, visual hallucinations (including bright colors and strange designs), are among the early manifestations. With marked overdosage, respiratory distress and CNS depression, progessing rapidly from stupor to profound coma, are to be expected, along with severe, intractable seizures. Severe metabolic acidosis, acetonuria, and hyperglycemia are typical laboratory findings.

Rifamate (rifampin-isoniazid)

Treatment

The airway should be secured and adequate respiratory exchange established. Only then should gastric emptying (lavage-aspiration) be attempted; this may be difficult because of seizures. Since nausea and vomiting are likely to be present, gastric lavage is probably preferable to induction of emesis.

Activated charcoal slurry instilled into the stomach following evacuation of gastric contents can help absorb any remaining drug in the GI tract. Antiemetic medication may be required to control severe nausea and vomiting.

Blood samples should be obtained for immediate determination of gases, electrolytes, BUN, glucose, etc. Blood should be typed and cross-matched in preparation for possible hemodialysis.

Rapid control of metabolic acidosis is fundamental to management. Intravenous sodium bicarbonate should be given at once and repeated as needed, adjusting subsequent dosage on the basis of laboratory findings (i.e. serum sodium, pH, etc.). At the same time, anticonvulsants should be given intravenously (i.e. barbiturates, diphenylhydantoin, diazepam) as required, and large doses of intravenous pyridoxine.

Forced osmotic diuresis must be started early and should be continued for some hours after clinical improvement to hasten renal clearance of drug and help prevent relapse. Fluid intake and output should be monitored.

Bile drainage may be indicated in presence of serious impairment of hepatic function lasting more than 24–48 hours. Under these circumstances, and for severe cases extra-corporeal hemodialysis may be required; if this is not available, peritoneal dialysis can be used along with forced diuresis.

Along with measures based on initial and repeated determination of blood gases and other laboratory tests as needed, meticulous respiratory and other intensive care should be utilized to protect against hypoxia, hypotension, aspiration, pneumonitis, etc.

In patients with previously adequate hepatic function, reversal of liver enlargement and impaired hepatic excretory function probably will be noted within 72 hours, with rapid return toward normal thereafter.

Untreated or inadequately treated cases of gross isoniazid overdosage can terminate fatally, but good response has been reported in most patients brought under adequate treatment within the first few hours after drug ingestion.

Dosage and Administration: In general, therapy should be continued until bacterial conversion and maximal improvement have occured.

Adults: Two Rifamate (rifampin-isoniazid) capsules (600 mg rifampin, 300 mg isoniazid) once daily, administered one hour before or two hours after a meal.

Concomitant administration of pyridoxine (B_6) is recommended in the malnourished, in those predisposed to neuropathy (e.g. diabetics) and in adolescents.

Susceptibility Testing

Rifampin

Rifampin susceptibility powders are available for both direct and indirect methods of determining the susceptibility of strains of mycobacteria. The MIC's of susceptible clinical isolates when determined in 7H10 or other non-egg-containing media have ranged from 0.1 to 2 mcg/ml.

Quantitative methods that require measurement of zone diameters give the most precise estimates of antibiotic susceptibility. One such procedure has been recommended for use with discs for testing susceptibility to rifampin, Interpretations correlate zone diameters from the disc test with MIC (minimal inhibitory concentration) values for rifampin.

Caution: Federal law prohibits dispensing without prescription.

How Supplied: Capsules (opaque red), containing 300 mg rifampin and 150 mg isoniazid; bottles of 60 (NDC 0068-0509-60).

[*Shown in Product Identification Section*]

SINGLET® ℞

Long-Acting Tablets

Decongestant-Antihistamine-Analgesic

Description: Each SINGLET long-acting tablet for oral use contains phenylephrine hydrochloride 40 mg, chlorpheniramine maleate 8 mg, and acetaminophen 500 mg.

Phenylephrine hydrochloride is a nasal decongestant. Chemically it is: (R)-3-Hydroxy-α-[(methylamino)methyl] benzenemethanol hydrochloride.

Chlorpheniramine maleate is an anthihistamine. Chemically it is: α-(4-Chlorophenyl)-N,N-dimethyl-2-pyridinepropanamine.

Acetaminophen is an analgesic-antipyretic. Chemically it is: (N-acetyl-p-aminophenol).

Clinical Pharmacology: Phenylephrine is a nasal decongestant. Its effects are similar to epinephrine, but it is less potent on a weight basis, and has a longer duration of action. Phenylephrine produces peripheral effects similar to epinephrine, but has little or no central nervous system stimulation. After oral administration, nasal decongestion may occur within 15 to 20 minutes and persist for 2 to 4 hours.

Chlorpheniramine is an antihistaminic drug that possesses anticholinergic and sedative effects. It is considered one of the most effective and least toxic of the histamine antagonists. Chlorpheniramine is an H_1receptor antagonist. It antagonizes many of the pharmacologic actions of histamine. It prevents released histamine from dilating capillaries and causing edema of the respiratory mucosa. Chlorpheniramine has a duration of action of 4 to 6 hours. Its half-life in serum, however, is 12 to 16 hours.

Acetaminophen is an analgesic and antipyretic. Its actions are similar to salicylates, but it has a weak anti-inflammatory effect. Acetaminophen has a half-life of 1 to 3 hours.

Indications and Usage: For the relief of multiple symptoms of nasal and eustachian tube congestion, sneezing, runny nose, watery eyes, myalgia, headache and fever associated with colds and other viral infections, sinusitis, influenza, and seasonal and perennial nasal allergies.

May be given concomitantly, when indicated, with antibiotics.

Contraindications: Patients with severe hypertension, severe coronary artery disease,

Continued on next page

Merrell Dow—Cont.

on MAO inhibitor therapy, narrow angle glaucoma, urinary retention, peptic ulcer, during an asthmatic attack, and seriously impaired liver and kidney function. Contraindicated in children under 12 years.
Hypersensitivity: Contraindicated in patients with hypersensitivity or idiosyncrasy to sympathomimetic amines, phenanthrene derivatives, or to any other formula ingredients.
Nursing Mothers: Contraindicated because of the higher than usual risk for infants from sympathomimetic amines.
Warning: If sympathomimetic amines are used in patients with hypertension, diabetes mellitus, ischemic heart disease, hyperthyroidism, increased intraocular pressure, and prostatic hypertrophy, judicious caution should be exercised (see **Contraindications**).
Use in Elderly: The elderly (60 years and older) are more likely to have adverse reactions to sympathomimetics. Overdosage of sympathomimetics in this age group may cause hallucinations, convulsions, CNS depression, and death.
Precautions: *General:* Caution should be exercised if used in patients with diabetes, hypertension, cardiovascular disease, hyperreactivity to ephedrine or decreased respiratory drive (see **Contraindications**).
Information for Patient: Antihistamines may impair mental and physical abilities required for the performance of potentially hazardous tasks, such as driving a vehicle or operating machinery, and mental alertness in children. Do not exceed the prescribed dosage.
Drug Interactions: MAO inhibitors and beta adrenergic blockers increase the effect of sympathomimetics and the anticholinergic (drying) effects of antihistamines. Sympathomimetics may reduce the antihypertensive effects of methyldopa, mecamylamine, reserpine and veratrum alkaloids. Concomitant use of antihistamines with alcohol, tricyclic antidepressants, barbiturates and other CNS depressants may have an additive effect.
Pregnancy Category C: Animal reproduction studies have not been conducted with SINGLET. It is also not known whether SINGLET can cause fetal harm when administered to a pregnant woman or can affect reproduction capacity. SINGLET may be given to a pregnant woman only if clearly needed.
Nursing Mothers: Because of the potential for serious adverse reactions in nursing infants from sympathomimetic amines, phenylephrine is contraindicated in nursing mothers.
Adverse Reactions: Individuals hyperreactive to phenylephrine may display ephedrine-like reactions such as tachycardia, palpitation, headache, dizziness, or nausea. Sympathomimetic drugs have been associated with certain untoward reactions including fear, anxiety, tenseness, restlessness, tremor, weakness, pallor, respiratory difficulty, dysuria, insomnia, hallucinations, convulsions, CNS depression, arrhythmias, and cardiovascular collapse with hypotension. Possible side effects of antihistamines are drowsiness, restlessness, dizziness, weakness, dry mouth, anorexia, nausea, headache, nervousness, blurring of vision, heartburn, dysuria and very rarely dermatitis.
Patient idiosyncrasy to adrenergic agents may be manifested by insomnia, dizziness, weakness, tremor or arrhythmias.
Overdosage: Pressor amines should be used with great caution in the presence of phenylephrine. Patients with signs of stimulation should be treated conservatively. Acetaminophen in massive overdosage has caused liver damage and fatal hepatic necrosis.
Recent studies have indicated that n-acetylcysteine may prevent hepatic damage if given within 24 hours of acetaminophen ingestion. Since n-acetylcysteine has not yet been approved for use as an antidote, except as an investigational drug, consult the Rocky Mountain Poison Center (toll-free number (800) 526-6115).[1]
Dosage and Administration: Adults: one table three times daily. In severe cases, a fourth dose may be indicated. The interval between doses should not be less than six hours. (NOTE: This product is specifically formulated to provide therapeutic effect for up to eight hours. Do not break or crush the tablets.)
Caution: Federal law prohibits dispensing without prescription.
How Supplied: The long-acting, pink, capsule-shaped tablet is monogrammed with the Dow diamond and 103 for positive identification. In bottles of 100 tablets (NDC 0068-0103-61).

---

[1] Peterson R G and Rumack BH: Toxicity of acetaminophen overdose. *JACEP* 7:5, 202, 1978.
Glynn JP and Kendall SE: *Lancet,* 1147-48, May 17, 1975.

[*Show in Product Identification Section*]

SUSADRIN™ ℞
(nitroglycerin)
Transmucosal Tablets

Caution: Federal law prohibits dispensing without prescription.
Description: Nitroglycerin (glyceryl trinitrate) $C_3H_5N_3O_9$: mol wt 227.09

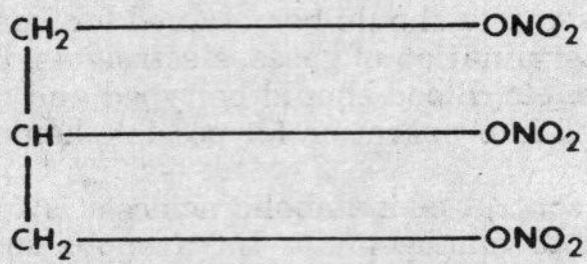

Susadrin tablets contain nitroglycerin in a patented* inert polymer base which releases nitroglycerin for absorption by the oral mucosa over a sustained period of time. When administered under the upper lip or buccally (in the buccal pouch), Susadrin tablets adhere comfortably to the mucosa. Patients may eat, drink, and talk while tablet is present.
*Synchron System (U.S. Patents 3,870,790, 4,226,849 and patents pending) provides an inert polymer vehicle which permits a metered release that is independent of the pH and avoids a "dumping action".
Clinical Pharmacology: The significant pharmacological action of nitroglycerin is relaxation of vascular smooth muscle. It has a greater relative effect on systemic veins than arteries, and on collateral and larger than smaller coronary arterioles. The favorable effects of nitroglycerin in angina are the result of (1) decreased preload, (2) decreased myocardial oxygen consumption, and (3) redistribution of blood flow to increase oxygen in the endocardium and ischemic areas.
Like sublingual nitroglycerin, transmucosal nitroglycerin passes directly into the blood stream through oral mucosa. It avoids the substantial and rapid deactivation by the liver that occurs with oral nitroglycerin products following gastrointestinal absorption. Computerized digital plethysmographic studies have shown that Susadrin tablets have demonstrated activity at 3 minutes, the earliest period measured, and duration of action up to 6 hours. Controlled clinical studies have demonstrated that Susadrin increased measured exercise tolerance in patients with angina pectoris up to 5 hours after administration, which was the longest period measured.

Indications
Based on a review of this drug by the National Academy of Sciences-National Research Council and/or other information, FDA has classified the indication as follows:

"Possibly" effective: For the prophylaxis, treatment, and management of patients with angina pectoris.

Final classification of the less-than-effective indication requires further investigation.

Contraindications: Acute or recent myocardial infarction, severe anemia, postural hypotension, and known idiosyncrasy to the drug.
Warning: Susadrin tablets should be placed under the upper lip or in a buccal pouch and permitted to dissolve, and should not be chewed or swallowed.
Precautions: The smallest dose needed for effective relief of angina pectoris should be used. As with other nitrates, orthostatic hypotension may occur, particularly during the initial dose titration process if stepwise titration is not observed. Intracranial pressure may be increased; therefore, caution is required in administering to patients with increased intracranial pressure. Tolerance to this drug and cross-tolerance to other organic nitrates may occur. If blurring of vision, dryness of mouth, or lack of benefit occurs, the drug should be discontinued.
Only limited data are available on the use of Susadrin during sleep; therefore, the benefits of Susadrin should be weighed against the possible risk of aspiration during sleep if the drug is used.
Adverse Reactions: Susadrin appears to have the adverse reactions characteristic of the nitrates and which relate to their vasodilating actions. Transient headache may be severe and persistent and may require lowering the dose or discontinuing medication. Vertigo, weakness, palpitation, nausea and vomiting and other signs of postural hypotension including syncope may develop. Nitroglycerin can act as a physiological antagonist to norepinephrine, acetylcholine, and histamine. Alcohol may accentuate cerebral ischemia symptoms.
Dosage and Administration: Susadrin (nitroglycerin) is available as 1 mg, 2 mg, and 3 mg transmucosal tablets. Patients, new to Susadrin, should receive a brief discussion of tablet placement in order to assure maximum effectiveness and comfort. Most patients will find it convenient and comfortable to place a tablet between the lip and gum above their upper incisors, while some will prefer the buccal areas between cheek and gum. Sites may be alternated from dose to dose. The tablet should be allowed to dissolve undisturbed. After a few doses, patients will develop favorite alternate sites and will readily adapt to the presence of the medication. The physical presence of the tablet, as it dissolves, provides reassurance of nitrate coverage.
THE USUAL DOSE IS ONE TABLET TID. (UPON ARISING, AFTER LUNCH, AND AFTER THE EVENING MEAL.)
Patients should be started at 1 mg tid. Dosage should be titrated upward, if necessary. Dosage may be adjusted as follows:

If angina occurs while the tablet is in place, increase the dose to the next tablet strength.
If angina occurs between tablet administration when no tablet is in place, increase the frequency of dosage to qid.

Tablet dissolution may be expected to vary from 3 to 5 hours in most patients. If continuous nitration is desirable, the next tablet should be taken within 1 hour after the previous one dissolves, unless clinical response suggests a different regimen.
Acute Prophylaxis Use: To cover periods of peak activity, place one tablet in as directed above, but not more than 1 tablet every 2 hours.
How Supplied: Susadrin Transmucosal Tablets are supplied in three strengths in bottles containing 100 tablets.

NDC 0068-0491-61: 1 mg: white, with "MERRELL" on one side, "1" on the other
NDC 0068-0503-61: 2 mg: white, with "MERRELL" on one side, "2" on the other
NDC 0068-0515-61: 3 mg: white, with "MERRELL" on one side, "3" on the other

Storage: Store at controlled temperatures below 86° F (30° C). Dispense only in original container.

Product Information as of March, 1982

Manufactured by
Forest Laboratories, Inc.
Inwood, New York 11696, U.S.A. for
MERRELL DOW PHARMACEUTICALS INC.
Subsidiary of The Dow Chemical Company
Cincinnati, Ohio 45215, U.S.A.

[*Shown in Product Identification Section*]

TACE® ℞
(CHLOROTRIANISENE USP)
12 mg and 25 mg
Capsules

AVAILABLE ONLY ON PRESCRIPTION

Warnings:

1. ESTROGENS HAVE BEEN REPORTED TO INCREASE THE RISK RATIO FOR ENDOMETRIAL CARCINOMA.
Three independent case control studies have reported an increased risk ratio of endometrial cancer in postmenopausal women exposed to exogenous estrogens for polonged periods.[1–3] This reported risk was independent of the other risk factors studied. Additionally, the incidence rates of endometrial cancer have increased since 1969 in 8 different areas of the United States with population-based cancer reporting systems, an increase that may [or may not] be related to the expanded use of estrogens during the last decade.[4]
The 3 case control studies reported that the estimated risk ratio for endomentrial cancer in estrogen users was about 4.5 to 13.9 times greater than in nonusers. The risk appeared to depend on both duration of treatment[1] and on estrogen dose.[3] In view of these reports, when estrogens are used for the treatment of menopausal symptoms, the lowest dose that will control symptoms should be utilized and medication should be discontinued as soon as possible. When prolonged treatment is medically indicated, the patient should be reassessed on at least a semiannual basis to determine the need for continued therapy. Although the evidence must be considered preliminary, one study suggests that cyclic administration of low doses of estrogen may carry less risk than continuous administration;[3] it therefore appears prudent to utilize such a regimen.
Close clinical surveillance of all women taking estrogens is important. In all cases of undiagnosed persistent or recurring abnormal vaginal bleeding, adequate diagnostic measures should be undertaken to rule out malignancy.
There is no evidence at present that "natural" estrogens are more or less hazardous than "synthetic" estrogens at equiestrogenic doses.
2. ESTROGENS SHOULD NOT BE USED DURING PREGNANCY.
The use of exogenous estrogens and progestagens during early pregnancy has been reported to damage the offspring. An association has been reported between *in utero* exposure of the female fetus to diethylstilbestrol, a nonsteroidal estrogen, and an increased risk of the post-pubertal development of an ordinarily rare form of vaginal or cervical cancer.[5,6] This risk for diethylstilbestrol was recently estimated to be in the range of 0.14 to 1.4 per 1000 exposures,[7] consistent with a previous risk estimate of not greater than 4 per 1000 exposures.[8] Furthermore, a high percentage of such females exposed *in utero* (30 to over 90%) has been reported to have vaginal adenosis, epithelial changes of the vagina and cervix.[9–12] Although these changes are histologically benign, it is not known whether they are precursors of adenocarcinoma. Although similar data are not available with the use of other estrogens, it cannot be presumed they would not induce similar changes.
Several reports suggest a possible association between fetal exposure to exogenous estrogens and progestagens and congenital anomalies, including congenital heart defects and limb reduction defects.[13–16] One case control study[16] estimated a 4.7 fold increased risk of limb reduction defects in infants exposed *in utero* to exogenous steroids (oral contraceptives, hormone withdrawal tests for pregnancy, or attempted treatment for threatened abortion). Some of these exposures were very short and involved only a few days of treatment. The data suggest that the risk of limb reduction defects in exposed fetuses is somewhat less than 1 per 1000.
This product is not for use in therapy of threatened or habitual abortion.
If TACE (CHLOROTRIANISENE USP) is used during pregnancy, or if the patient becomes pregnant while taking this drug, she should be apprised of the potential risks to the fetus, and the advisability of pregnancy continuation.

Description: TACE (CHLOROTRIANISENE USP) is a long-acting, synthetic estrogen in capsule form suitable for oral administration. Each green, soft gelatin capsule contains 12 mg of chlorotrianisene in corn oil. Each two-tone green, hard gelatin capsule contains 25 mg of chlorotrianisene in tristearin.

Chemistry
Generic name: Chlorotrianisene USP
Chemical name: Benzene, 1, 1′, 1″-(1-chloro-1-ethenyl-2-ylidene) tris [4-methoxy]-. Chlorotris (*p*-methoxyphenyl) ethylene.
Chlorotrianisene occurs as small, white crystals or as a crystalline powder. It is odorless. It is slightly soluble in alcohol and very slightly soluble in water.

Indications:
1. Postpartum breast engorgement—Although estrogens have been widely used for the prevention of postpartum breast engorgement, controlled studies have demonstrated that the incidence of significant painful engorgement in patients not receiving such hormonal therapy is low and usually responsive to appropriate analgesic or other supportive therapy. Consequently, the benefit to be derived from estrogen therapy for this indication must be carefully weighed against the potential risk of puerperal thromboembolism associated with the use of estrogens.[17]
2. Prostatic carcinoma—palliative therapy of advanced disease.
3. Moderate to severe *vasomotor* symptoms associated with the menopause. (There is no well-documented evidence that estrogens are effective for nervous symptoms or depression which might occur during menopause and they should not be used to treat these conditions.)
4. Atrophic vaginitis.
5. Kraurosis vulvae.
6. Female hypogonadism.

TACE (CHLOROTRIANISENE USP) HAS NOT BEEN SHOWN TO BE EFFECTIVE FOR ANY PURPOSE DURING PREGNANCY, AND ITS USE MAY HAVE POTENTIAL RISKS TO THE FETUS. (SEE BOXED WARNING.)

Contraindications: TACE (CHLOROTRIANISENE USP) should not be used in women or men with any of the following conditions:
1. Known or suspected cancer of the breast except in appropriately selected patients being treated for metastatic disease.
2. Known or suspected estrogen-dependent neoplasia.
3. Known or suspected pregnancy (See Boxed Warning.)
4. Undiagnosed abnormal genital bleeding.
5. Active thrombophlebitis or thromboembolic disorders.
6. A past history of thrombophlebitis, thrombosis, or thromboembolic disorders (except when used in treatment of prostatic malignancy).

Warnings:
1. *Induction of malignant neoplasms.* Long-term continuous administration of natural and synthetic estrogens in certain animal species increases the frequency of carcinomas of the breast, cervix, vagina, and liver. There are now reports that estrogens increase the risk of carcinoma of the endometrium in humans. (See Boxed Warning.)
At the present time there is no satisfactory evidence that estrogens given to postmenopausal women increase the risk of cancer of the breast,[18] although a recent long-term followup of a single physician's practice has raised this possibility.[19] Because of the animal data, there is a need for caution in prescribing estrogens for women with a strong family history of breast cancer or who have breast nodules, fibrocystic disease, or abnormal mammograms.
2. *Gallbladder disease.* A recent study has reported a two to threefold increase in the risk of surgically confirmed gallbladder disease in women receiving postmenopausal estrogens,[18] similar to the twofold increase previously noted in users of oral contraceptives.[20] In the case of oral contraceptives the increased risk appeared after a period of use.[20]
3. *Effects similar to those caused by estrogen-progestagen oral contraceptives.* There are several adverse effects reported in association with oral contraceptives, most of which have not been documented as consequences of postmenopausal estrogen therapy, although it has been reported that there is an increased risk of thrombosis in men receiving high doses of estrogens for prostatic cancer and in women receiving estrogens for postpartum breast engorgement.[17,21–23] The possibility that the adverse effects reported in association with oral contraceptives may be associated with larger doses of estrogen cannot be excluded.
a. *Thromboembolic disease.* Studies have now shown that users of oral contraceptives have an increased risk of various thromboembolic, thrombotic, and vascular diseases, such as thrombophlebitis, pulmonary embolism, stroke, and myocardial infarction.[24–31] Cases of retinal thrombosis, mesenteric thrombosis, and optic neuritis have been reported in oral contraceptive users. There is evidence that the risk of several of these adverse reactions is related to the dose of the drug.[32,33] An increased risk of post-surgery thromboembolic complications has also been reported in users of oral contraceptives.[34,35] If feasible, estrogen should be discontinued at least 4 weeks before surgery of the type associated with an increased risk of thromboembolism, or during periods of prolonged immobilization.
While an increased rate of thromboembolic and thrombotic disease in postmenopausal users of estrogens has not been found,[18,36] this does not rule out the possibility that such an increase may be present, or that subgroups of

Continued on next page

Information on Merrell Dow products is based on labeling in effect in October, 1982.

Merrell Dow—Cont.

women who have underlying risk factors, or who are receiving relatively large doses of estrogens may have an increased risk. Therefore, estrogens should not be used in persons with active thrombophlebitis or thromboembolic disorders, and they should not be used (except in treatment of malignancy) in persons with a history of such disorders. They should be used with caution in patients with cerebral vascular or coronary artery disease and only for those in whom estrogens are needed.

Doses of estrogen (5 mg conjugated estrogens per day), comparable to those used to treat cancer of the prostate and breast, have been reported in a large prospective clinical trial in men[37] to increase the risk of nonfatal myocardial infarction, pulmonary embolism, and thrombophlebitis. When estrogen doses of this size are used, any of the thromboembolic and thrombotic adverse effects associated with oral contraceptive use should be considered as a risk.

b. *Hepatic adenoma.* Benign hepatic adenomas have been reported to be associated with the use of oral contraceptives.[38–40] Although benign and rare, these may rupture and may cause death through intra-abdominal hemorrhage. Such lesions have not yet been reported in association with other estrogen or progestagen preparations but should be considered in estrogen users having abdominal pain and tenderness, abdominal mass, or hypovolemic shock. Hepatocellular carcinoma has also been reported in women taking estrogen-containing oral contraceptives.[39] The relationship of this malignancy to these drugs is not known at this time.

c. *Elevated blood pressure.* Increased blood pressure is not uncommon in women using oral contraceptives and there is now a report that this may occur with use of estrogens in the menopause[41] and blood pressure should be monitored with estrogen use, especially if high doses are used.

d. *Glucose tolerance.* A worsening of glucose tolerance has been observed in a significant percentage of patients on estrogen-containing oral contraceptives. For this reason diabetic patients should be carefully observed while receiving estrogen.

4. *Hypercalcemia.* Administration of estrogens may lead to hypercalcemia in patients with breast cancer and bone metastases. If this occurs, the drug should be stopped and appropriate measures taken to reduce the serum calcium level.

Precautions:

A. General Precautions

1. A complete medical and family history should be taken prior to the initiation of any estrogen therapy. The pretreatment and periodic physical examinations should include special reference to blood pressure, breasts, abdomen, and pelvic organs, and should include a Papanicolaou smear. As a general rule, estrogen should not be prescribed for longer than 1 year without another physical examination being performed.
2. Fluid retention—Because estrogens may cause some degree of fluid retention, conditions that might be influenced by this factor such as epilepsy, migraine, and cardiac or renal dysfunction require careful observation.
3. Certain patients may develop undesirable manifestations of excessive estrogenic stimulation, such as abnormal or excessive uterine bleeding, mastodynia, etc.
4. Oral contraceptives have been reported to be associated with an increased incidence of mental depression. Although it is not clear whether this is possibly due to the estrogenic or progestagenic component of the contraceptive, patients with a history of depression should be carefully observed.
5. Patients having pre-existing uterine leiomyomata should be observed for increased growth of myomata during estrogen therapy.
6. The pathologist should be advised of estrogen therapy when relevant specimens are submitted.
7. Patients with a past history of jaundice during pregnancy have an increased risk of recurrence of jaundice while receiving estrogen-containing oral contraceptive therapy. If jaundice develops in any patient receiving estrogen, the medication should be discontinued while the cause is investigated.
8. Estrogens may be poorly metabolized in patients with impaired liver function and they should be administered with caution in such patients.
9. Because estrogens influence the metabolism of calcium and phosphorus, they should be used with caution in patients with metabolic bone diseases that are associated with hypercalcemia or in patients with renal insufficiency.
10. Because of the effects of estrogens on epiphyseal closure, they should be used judiciously in young patients in whom bone growth is not complete.
11. Judicious assessment of the following changes in certain endocrine and liver function tests is necessary for patients receiving large doses of estrogen:

a. Increased sulfobromophthalein retention.

b. Increased prothrombin and factors VII, VIII, IX, and X; decreased antithrombin 3; increased norepinephrine-induced platelet aggregability.

c. Increased thyroid binding globulin (TBG) leading to increased circulating total thyroid hormone, as measured by PBI, T4 by column, or T4 by radioimmunoassay. Free T3 resin uptake is decreased, reflecting the elevated TBG; free T4 concentration is unaltered.

d. Impaired glucose tolerance.

e. Decreased pregnanediol excretion.

f. Reduced response to metyrapone test.

g. Reduced serum folate concentration.

h. Increased serum triglyceride, phospholipid, or cholesterol.

12. This product contains FD&C Yellow No. 5 (tartrazine), which may cause allergic-type reactions (including bronchial asthma) in certain susceptible individuals. Although the overall incidence of FD&C Yellow No. 5 (tartrazine) sensitivity in the general population is low, it is frequently seen in patients who also have aspirin hypersensitivity.

B. Information For The Patient

A patient package insert accompanies this drug product. This insert is available from pharmacists who carry this product and from the company upon request.

C. Pregnancy Category X

See Contraindications and Boxed Warning.

D. Nursing Mothers

As a general principle, the administration of any drug to nursing mothers should be done only when clearly necessary since many drugs are excreted in human milk.

Adverse Reactions: (See Warnings regarding reports of induction of neoplasia, adverse effects on the fetus, increased incidence of gallbladder disease, and adverse effects similar to those of oral contraceptives, including thromboembolism.) The following additional adverse reactions have been reported with estrogenic therapy including oral contraceptives:

1. *Genitourinary system*

Breakthrough bleeding, spotting, change in menstrual flow and cycle.
Dysmenorrhea.
Premenstrual-like syndrome.
Amenorrhea during and after treatment.
Increase in size of uterine fibromyomata.
Vaginal candidiasis.
Change in cervical eversion and in degree of cervical secretion.
Cystitis-like syndrome.

2. *Breasts*

Tenderness, enlargement, secretion.

3. *Gastrointestinal*

Nausea, vomiting.
Abdominal cramps, bloating.
Cholestatic jaundice.

4. *Skin*

Chloasma or melasma, which may persist when drug is discontinued.
Erythema multiforme.
Erythema nodosum.
Hemorrhagic eruption.
Loss of scalp hair.
Hirsutism.
Urticaria.

5. *Eyes*

Steepening of corneal curvature.
Intolerance to contact lenses.

6. *CNS*

Headache, migraine, dizziness.
Mental depression.
Chorea.

7. *Miscellaneous*

Increase or decrease in weight.
Reduced carbohydrate tolerance.
Aggravation of porphyria.
Edema.
Changes in libido and/or potency.

Acute Overdosage: Numerous reports of ingestion of large doses of estrogen-containing oral contraceptives by young children indicate that serious ill effects usually do not occur. Overdosage of estrogen may cause nausea, and withdrawal bleeding may occur in females.

Dosage and Administration:

Given for a few days

Prevention of postpartum breast engorgement.

The usual dosage is one 12 mg capsule four times daily for 7 days, or two 25 mg capsules every six hours for 6 doses. For immediate postpartum use, the first dose should be given within 8 hours after delivery.

Given chronically

Inoperable progressing prostatic cancer.

The usual dosage is 12 to 25 mg daily (one or two 12 mg capsules or one 25 mg capsule).

Given cyclically for short-term use only

For treatment of moderate to severe *vasomotor* symptoms, atrophic vaginitis, or kraurosis vulvae associated with the menopause.

The lowest dose that will control symptoms should be chosen and medication should be discontinued as promptly as possible.

Administration should be cyclic (*e.g.,* 3 weeks on and 1 week off).

Attempts to discontinue or taper medication should be made at 3-month to 6-month intervals.

The usual dosage range for vasomotor symptoms associated with the menopause is 12 to 25 mg daily (one or two 12 mg capsules or one 25 mg capsule) for 30 days; one or more courses may be prescribed.

The usual dosage range for atrophic vaginitis or kraurosis vulvae is 12 to 25 mg daily (one or two 12 mg capsules or one 25 mg capsule) for 30 to 60 days.

Given cyclically

For female hypogonadism.

The usual dosage is 12 to 25 mg daily (one or two 12 mg capsules or one 25 mg capsule) for 21 days. This course may, if desired, be followed immediately by the intramuscular injection of 100 mg of progesterone; alternatively, an oral progestogen such as medroxyprogesterone may be given during the last 5 days of TACE (CHLOROTRIANISENE USP) therapy. The next course may begin on the 5th day of the induced uterine bleeding.

Treated patients with an intact uterus should be monitored closely for signs of endometrial cancer, and appropriate diagnostic measures should be taken to rule out malignancy in the event of persistent or recurrent abnormal vaginal bleeding.

How Supplied:
TACE 12 mg (CHLOROTRIANISENE CAPSULES USP) green capsules imprinted MERRELL 690
NDC 0068-0690-61: bottles of 100
NDC 0068-0690-65: bottles of 500
TACE 25 mg (CHLOROTRIANISENE CAPSULES USP) two-tone green capsules imprinted MERRELL 691
NDC 0068-0691-60: bottles of 60

References:

1. Ziel, H.K. and Finkel, W.D.: Increased risk of endometrial carcinoma among users of conjugated estrogens. New Eng. J. Med. 293:1167–1170, 1975.
2. Smith, D.C., Prentice, R., Thompson, D.J., and Hermann, W.L.: Association of exogenous estrogen and endometrial carcinoma. New Eng. J. Med. 293:1164–1167, 1975.
3. Mack, T.M., Pike, M.C., Henderson, B.E., Pfeffer, R. I., Gerkins, V.R., Arthur, M., and Brown, S.E.: Estrogens and endometrial cancer in a retirement community. New Eng. J. Med. 294:1262–1267, 1976.
4. Weiss, N.S., Szekely, D.R., and Austin, D.F.: Increasing incidence of endometrial cancer in the United States. New Eng. J. Med. 294:1259–1262, 1976.
5. Herbst, A.L., Ulfelder, H., and Poskanzer, D.C.: Adenocarcinoma of the vagina. New Eng. J. Med. 284:878–881, 1971.
6. Greenwald, P., Barlow, J.J., Nasca, P.C., and Burnett, W.S.: Vaginal cancer after maternal treatment with synthetic estrogens. New Eng. J. Med. 285: 390–392, 1971.
7. Herbst, A.L., Cole, P., Colton, T., Robboy, S.J., and Scully, R.E.: Age-incidence and risk of diethylstilbestrol-related clear cell adenocarcinoma of the vagina and cervix. Amer. J. Obstet. Gynec. 128:43–50, 1977.
8. Lanier, A.P., Noller, K.L., Decker, D.G., Elveback, L.R., and Kurland, L.T.: Cancer and Stilbestrol. A follow-up of 1719 persons exposed to estrogens in utero and born 1943–1959. Mayo Clin. Proc. 48:793–799, 1973.
9. Herbst, A.L., Kurman, R.J., and Scully, R.E.: Vaginal and cervical abnormalities after exposure to stilbestrol in utero. Obstet. Gynec. 40:287-298, 1972.
10. Herbst, A.L., Poskanzer, D.C., Robboy, S.J., Friedlander, L. and Scully, R.E.: Prenatal exposure to stilbestrol. A prospective comparison of exposed female offspring with unexposed controls. New Eng. J. Med. 292:334–339, 1975.
11. Stafl, A., Mattingly, R.F., Foley, D.V., and Fetherston, W.C.: Clinical diagnosis of vaginal adenosis. Obstet. Gynec. 43:118–128, 1974.
12. Sherman, A.I., Goldrath, M., Berlin A., Vakhariya, V., Banooni, F., Michaels, W., Goodman, P., and Brown, S.: Cervical-vaginal adenosis after *in utero* exposure to synthetic estrogens. Obstet. Gynec. 44:531–545, 1974.
13. Gal, I., Kirman, B., Stern, J.: Hormone pregnancy tests and congenital malformation. Nature 216:83, 1967.
14. Levy, E.P., Cohen, A., and Fraser, F.C.: Hormone treatment during pregnancy and congenital heart defects. Lancet 1:611, 1973.
15. Nora, J.J. and Nora, A.H.: Birth defects and oral contraceptives. Lancet 1:941–942, 1973.
16. Janerich, D.T., Piper, J.M., and Glebatis, D.M.: Oral contraceptives and congenital limb-reduction defects. New Eng. J. Med. 291:697–700, 1974.
17. Daniel, D.G., Campbell, H., and Turnbull, A.C.: Puerperal thromboembolism and suppression of lactation. Lancet 2:287–289, 1967.
18. Boston Collaborative Drug Surveillance Program: Surgically confirmed gall bladder disease, venous thromboembolism, and breast tumors in relation to post menopausal estrogen therapy. New Eng. J. Med. 290:15–19, 1974.
19. Hoover, R., Gray, L.A., Sr., Cole, P., and MacMahon, B.: Menopausal estrogens and breast cancer. New Eng. J. Med. 295:401–405, 1976.
20. Boston Collaborative Drug Surveillance Program: Oral contraceptives and venous thromboembolic disease, surgically confirmed gall-bladder disease, and breast tumors. Lancet 1:1399–1404, 1973.
21. Bailar, J.C., III: thromboembolism and oestrogen therapy. Lancet 2:560, 1967.
22. The Veterans Administration Cooperative Urological Research Group: Carcinoma of the prostate: Treatment comparisons. J. Urol. 98:516–522, 1967.
23. Blackard, C.E., Doe, R.P., Mellinger, G.T., and Byar, D.P.: Incidence of cardiovascular disease and death in patients receiving diethylstilbestrol for carcinoma of the prostate. Cancer 26:249–256, 1970.
24. Royal College of General Practitioners: Oral contraception and thromboembolic disease. J. Roy. Coll. Gen. Pract. 13:267–269, 1967.
25. Inman, W.H.W. and Vessey, M.P.: Investigation of deaths from pulmonary, coronary, and cerebral thrombosis and embolism in women of child-bearing age. Brit. Med. J. 2:193–199, 1968.
26. Vessey, M.P. and Doll, R.: Investigation of relation between use of oral contraceptives and thromboembolic disease. A further report. Brit. Med. J. 2:651–657, 1969.
27. Sartwell, P.E., Masi, A.T., Arthes, F.G., Greene, G.R. and Smith, H.E.: Thromboembolism and oral contraceptives: An epidemiological case-control study. Amer. J. Epidem. 90:365-380, 1969.
28. Collaborative Group for the Study of Stroke in Young Women: Oral contraception and increased risk of cerebral ischemia or thrombosis. New Eng. J. Med. 288:871–878, 1973.
29. Collaborative Group for the Study of Stroke in Young Women: Oral contraceptives and stroke in young women: Associated risk factors. J.A.M.A. 231:718–722, 1975.
30. Mann, J.I. and Inman, W.H.W.: Oral contraceptives and death from myocardial infarction. Brit. Med. J. 2:245–248, 1975.
31. Mann, J.I., Vessey, M.P., Thorogood, M., and Doll, R.: Myocardial infarction in young women with special reference in oral contraceptive practice. Brit. Med. J. 2:241–245, 1975.
32. Inman, W.H.W., Vessey, M.P., Westerholm, B., and Engelund, A.: Thromboembolic disease and the steroidal content of oral contraceptives. A report to the Committee on Safety of Drugs. Brit. Med. J. 2:203–209, 1970.
33. Stolley, P.D., Tonascia, J.A., Tockman, M.S., Sartwell, P.E., Rutledge, A.H., and Jacobs, M.P.: Thrombosis with low-estrogen oral contraceptives. Amer. J. Epidem. 102:197–208, 1975.
34. Vessey, M.P., Doll, R., Fairbairn, A.S., and Glober, G.: Post-operative thromboembolism and the use of the oral contraceptives. Brit. Med. J. 3:123–126, 1970.
35. Greene, G.R. and Sartwell, P.E.: Oral contraceptive use in patients with thromboembolism following surgery, trauma, or infection. Amer. J. Public Health 62:680–685, 1972.
36. Rosenberg, L., Armstrong, B., Phil. D., and Jick H.: Myocardial infarction and estrogen therapy in post-menopausal women. New Eng. J. Med. 294:1256–1259, 1976.
37. Coronary Drug Project Research Group: The coronary drug project: initial findings leading to modifications of its research protocol. J.A.M.A. 214:1303–1313, 1970.
38. Baum, J., Holtz, F., Bookstein, J.J., and Klein, E.W.: Possible association between benign hepatomas and oral contraceptives. Lancet 2:926–928, 1973.
39. Mays, E.T., Christopherson, W.M., Mahr, M.M., and Williams, H.C.: Hepatic changes in young women ingesting contraceptive steroids. Hepatic hemorrhage and primary hepatic tumors. J.A.M.A. 235:730–732, 1976.
40. Edmondson, H., Henderson, A.B., and Benton, B.: Liver-cell adenomas associated with the use of oral contraceptives. New Eng. J. Med. 294:470–472, 1976.
41. Pfeffer, R.I. and Van Den Noort, S.: Estrogen use and stroke risk in postmenopausal women. Amer. J. Epidem. 103:445–456, 1976.

Product Information as of August, 1979

TACE 12 mg Capsules
Encapsulated by
R. P. Scherer, North America
Clearwater, Florida 33518 for
MERRELL DOW PHARMACEUTICALS INC.
Subsidiary of The Dow Chemical Company
Cincinnati, Ohio 45215, U.S.A.

[*Shown in Product Identification Section*]

TACE® (CHLOROTRIANISENE USP) 72 mg Capsules ℞

AVAILABLE ONLY ON PRESCRIPTION

Warnings

1. ESTROGENS HAVE BEEN REPORTED TO INCREASE THE RISK RATIO FOR ENDOMETRIAL CARCINOMA.
Three independent case control studies have reported an increased risk ratio of endometrial cancer in postmenopausal women exposed to exogenous estrogens for prolonged periods.[1-3] This reported risk was independent of the other risk factors studied. Additionally, the incidence rates of endometrial cancer have increased since 1969 in 8 different areas of the United States with population-based cancer reporting systems, an increase that may [or may not] be related to the expanded use of estrogens during the last decade.[4]
The 3 case control studies reported that the estimated risk ratio for endometrial cancer in estrogen users was about 4.5 to 13.9 times greater than in nonusers. The risk appeared to depend on both duration of treatment[1] and on estrogen dose.[3] In view of these reports, when estrogens are used for the treatment of menopausal symptoms, the lowest dose that will control symptoms should be utilized and medication should be discontinued as soon as possible. When prolonged treatment is medically indicated, the patient should be reassessed on at least a semiannual basis to determine the need for continued therapy. Although the evidence must be considered preliminary, one study suggests that cyclic administration of low doses of estrogen may carry less risk than continuous administration;[3] it therefore appears prudent to utilize such a regimen.
Close clinical surveillance of all women taking estrogens is important. In all cases of undiagnosed persistent or recurring abnormal vaginal bleeding, adequate diagnostic measures should be undertaken to rule out malignancy.
There is no evidence at present that "natural" estrogens are more or less hazardous than "synthetic" estrogens at equiestrogenic doses.
2. ESTROGENS SHOULD NOT BE USED DURING PREGNANCY.
The use of exogenous estrogens and progestagens during early pregnancy has been reported to damage the offspring. An association has been reported between *in utero* exposure of the female fetus to diethylstilbestrol, a non-steroidal estrogen, and an increased risk of the postpubertal development of an ordinarily rare form of vaginal or cervical cancer.[5,6] This risk for

Continued on next page

Information on Merrell Dow products is based on labeling in effect in October, 1982.

Merrell Dow—Cont.

diethylstilbestrol was recently estimated to be in the range of 0.14 to 1.4 per 1000 exposures,[7] consistent with a previous risk estimate of not greater than 4 per 1000 exposures.[8] Furthermore, a high percentage of such females exposed *in utero* (30 to over 90%) has been reported to have vaginal adenosis, epithelial changes of the vagina and cervix.[9-12] Although these changes are histologically benign, it is not known whether they are precursors of adenocarcinoma. Although similar data are not available with the use of other estrogens, it cannot be presumed they would not induce similar changes.

Several reports suggest a possible association between fetal exposure to exogenous estrogens and progestagens and congenital anomalies, including congenital heart defects and limb reduction defects.[13-16] One case control study[16] estimated a 4.7 fold increased risk of limb reduction defects in infants exposed *in utero* to exogenous steriods (oral contraceptives, hormone withdrawal tests for pregnancy, or attempted treatment for threatened abortion). Some of these exposures were very short and involved only a few days of treatment. The data suggest that the risk of limb reduction defects in exposed fetuses is somewhat less than 1 per 1000.

This product is not for use in therapy of threatened or habitual abortion.

If TACE (CHLOROTRIANISENE USP) is used during pregnancy, or if the patient becomes pregnant while taking this drug, she should be apprised of the potential risks to the fetus, and the advisability of pregnancy continuation.

Description:
TACE (CHLOROTRIANISENE USP) is a long-acting, synthetic estrogen in capsule form suitable for oral administration.

Each two-tone green and yellow soft gelatin capsule contains 72 mg of TACE (CHLOROTRIANISENE) in Dispex®, an emulsifiable vehicle containing corn oil, sorbitan trioleate, polysorbate 80, and benzyl benzoate.

Chemistry

Generic name: Chlorotrianisene USP

Chemical name: Benzene, 1, 1′, 1″-(1-chloro-1-ethenyl-2-ylidene) tris [4-methoxy]-. Chlorotris (*p*-methoxyphenyl) ethylene.

Chlorotrianisene occurs as small, white crystals or as a crystalline powder. It is odorless. It is slightly soluble in alcohol and very slightly soluble in water.

Indications: Postpartum breast engorgement—Although estrogens have been widely used for the prevention of postpartum breast engorgement, controlled studies have demonstrated that the incidence of significant painful engorgement in patients not receiving such hormonal therapy is low and usually responsive to appropriate analgesic or other supportive therapy. Consequently, the benefit to be derived from estrogen therapy for this indication must be carefully weighed against the potential risk of puerperal thromboembolism associated with the use of estrogens.[17]

TACE (CHLOROTRIANISENE USP) HAS NOT BEEN SHOWN TO BE EFFECTIVE FOR ANY PURPOSE DURING PREGNANCY, AND ITS USE MAY HAVE POTENTIAL RISKS TO THE FETUS. (SEE BOXED WARNING.)

Contraindications: TACE (CHLOROTRIANISENE USP) should not be used in women or men with any of the following conditions:

1. Known or suspected cancer of the breast except in appropriately selected patients being treated for metastatic disease.
2. Known or suspected estrogen-dependent neoplasia.
3. Known or suspected pregnancy. (See Boxed Warning.)
4. Undiagnosed abnormal genital bleeding.
5. Active thrombophlebitis or thromboembolic disorders.
6. A past history of thrombophlebitis, thrombosis, or thromboembolic disorders (except when used in treatment of prostatic malignancy).

Warnings:

1. *Induction of malignant neoplasms.* Long-term continuous administration of natural and synthetic estrogens in certain animal species increases the frequency of carcinomas of the breast, cervix, vagina, and liver. There are now reports that estrogens increase the risk of carcinoma of the endometrium in humans. (See Boxed Warning.)

At the present time there is no satisfactory evidence that estrogens given to postmenopausal women increase the risk of cancer of the breast,[18] although a recent long-term followup of a single physician's practice has raised this possibility.[19] Because of the animal data, there is a need for caution in prescribing estrogens for women with a strong family history of breast cancer or who have breast nodules, fibrocystic disease, or abnormal mammograms.

2. *Gallbladder disease.* A recent study has reported a two to threefold increase in the risk of surgically confirmed gallbladder disease in women receiving postmenopausal estrogens,[18] similar to the twofold increase previously noted in users of oral contraceptives.[20] In the case of oral contraceptives the increased risk appeared after a period of use.[20]

3. *Effects similar to those caused by estrogen-progestagen oral contraceptives.* There are several adverse effects reported in association with oral contraceptives, most of which have not been documented as consequences of postmenopausal estrogen therapy, although it has been reported that there is an increased risk of thrombosis in men receiving high doses of estrogens for prostatic cancer and in women receiving estrogens for postpartum breast engorgement.[17,21-23] The possibility that the adverse effects reported in association with oral contraceptives may be associated with larger doses of estrogen cannot be excluded.

a. *Thromboembolic disease.* Studies have now shown that users of oral contraceptives have an increased risk of various thromboembolic, thrombotic, and vascular diseases, such as thrombophlebitis, pulmonary embolism, stroke, and myocardial infarction.[24-31] Cases of retinal thrombosis, mesenteric thrombosis, and optic neuritis have been reported in oral contraceptive users. There is evidence that the risk of several of these adverse reactions is related to the dose of the drug.[32, 33] An increased risk of post-surgery thromboembolic complications has also been reported in users of oral contraceptives.[34,35] If feasible, estrogen should be discontinued at least 4 weeks before surgery of the type associated with an increased risk of thromboembolism, or during periods of prolonged immobilization.

While an increased rate of thromboembolic and thrombotic disease in postmenopausal users of estrogens has not been found,[18, 36] this does not rule out the possibility that such an increase may be present, or that subgroups of women who have underlying risk factors, or who are receiving relatively large doses of estrogens may have an increased risk. Therefore, estrogens should not be used in persons with active thrombophlebitis or thromboembolic disorders, and they should not be used (except in treatment of malignancy) in persons with a history of such disorders. They should be used with caution in patients with cerebral vascular or coronary artery disease and only for those in whom estrogens are needed.

Doses of estrogen (5 mg conjungated estrogens per day), comparable to those used to treat cancer of the prostate and breast, have been reported in a large prospective clinical trial in men[37] to increase the risk of nonfatal myocardial infarction, pulmonary embolism, and thrombophlebitis. When estrogen doses of this size are used, any of the thromboembolic and thrombotic adverse effects associated with oral contraceptive use should be considered as a risk.

b. *Hepatic adenoma.* Benign hepatic adenomas have been reported to be associated with the use of oral contraceptives.[38-40] Although benign and rare, these may rupture and may cause death through intra-abdominal hemorrhage. Such lesions have not yet been reported in association with other estrogen or progestagen preparations but should be considered in estrogen users having abdominal pain and tenderness, abdominal mass, or hypovolemic shock. Hepatocellular carcinoma has also been reported in women taking estrogen-containing oral contraceptives.[39] The relationship of this malignancy to these drugs is not known at this time.

c. *Elevated blood pressure.* Increased blood pressure is not uncommon in women using oral contraceptives and there is now a report that this may occur with use of estrogens in the menopause[41] and blood pressure should be monitored with estrogen use, especially if high doses are used.

d. *Glucose tolerance.* A worsening of glucose tolerance has been observed in a significant percentage of patients on estrogen-containing oral contraceptives. For this reason diabetic patients should be carefully observed while receiving estrogen.

4. *Hypercalcemia.* Administration of estrogens may lead to hypercalcemia in patients with breast cancer and bone metastases. If this occurs, the drug should be stopped and appropriate measures taken to reduce the serum calcium level.

Precautions:

A. General Precautions

1. A complete medical and family history should be taken prior to the initiation of any estrogen therapy. The pretreatment and periodic physical examinations should include special reference to blood pressure, breasts, abdomen, and pelvic organs, and should include a Papanicolaou smear. As a general rule, estrogen should not be prescribed for longer than 1 year without another physical examination being performed.
2. Fluid retention—Because estrogens may cause some degree of fluid retention, conditions that might be influenced by this factor such as epilepsy, migraine, and cardiac or renal dysfunction require careful observation.
3. Certain patients may develop undersirable manifestations of excessive estrogenic stimulation, such as abnormal or excessive uterine bleeding, mastodynia, etc.
4. Oral contraceptives have been reported to be associated with an increased incidence of mental depression. Although it is not clear whether this is possibly due to the estrogenic or progestagenic component of the contraceptive, patients with a history of depression should be carefully observed.
5. Patients having pre-existing uterine leiomyomata should be observed for increased growth of myomata during estrogen therapy.
6. The pathologist should be advised of estrogen therapy when relevant specimens are submitted.
7. Patients with a past history of jaundice during pregnancy have an increased risk of recurrence of jaundice while receiving estrogen-containing oral contraceptive therapy. If jaundice develops in any patient receiving estrogen, the medication should be discontinued while the cause is investigated.
8. Estrogens may be poorly metabolized in patients with impaired liver function and they should be administered with caution in such patients.

9. Because estrogens influence the metabolism of calcium and phosphorus, they should be used with caution in patients with metabolic bone diseases that are associated with hypercalcemia or in patients with renal insufficiency.
10. Because of the effects of estrogens on epiphyseal closure, they should be used judiciously in young patients in whom bone growth is not complete.
11. Judicious assessment of the following changes in certain endocrine and liver function tests is necessary for patients receiving large doses of estrogen:
a. Increased sulfobromophthalein retention.
b. Increased prothrombin and factors VII, VIII, IX and X; decreased antithrombin 3; increased norepinephrine-induced platelet aggregability.
c. Increased thyroid binding globulin (TBG) leading to increased circulating total thyroid hormone, as measured by PBI, T4 by column, or T4 by radioimmunoassay. Free T3 resin uptake is decreased, reflecting the elevated TBG; free T4 concentration is unaltered.
d. Impaired glucose tolerance.
e. Decreased pregnanediol excretion.
f. Reduced response to metyrapone test.
g. Reduced serum folate concentration.
h. Increased serum triglyceride, phospholipid, or cholesterol.
12. This product contains FD&C Yellow No. 5 (tartrazine), which may cause allergic-type reactions (including bronchial asthma) in certain susceptible individuals. Although the overall incidence of FD&C Yellow No. 5 (tartrazine) sensitivity in the general population is low, it is frequently seen in patients who also have aspirin hypersensitivity.
B. Information For The Patient
A patient package insert accompanies this drug product. This insert is available from pharmacists who carry this product and from the company upon request.
C. Pregnancy Category X
See Contraindications and Boxed Warning.
D. Nursing Mothers
As a general principle, the administration of any drug to nursing mothers should be done only when clearly necessary since many drugs are excreted in human milk.

Adverse Reactions: (See Warnings regarding reports of induction of neoplasia, adverse effects on the fetus, increased incidence of gallbladder disease, and adverse effects similar to those of oral contraceptives, including thromboembolism.) The following additional adverse reactions have been reported with estrogenic therapy including oral contraceptives:
1. *Genitourinary system*
Breakthrough bleeding, spotting, change in menstrual flow and cycle.
Dysmenorrhea.
Premenstrual-like syndrome.
Amenorrhea during and after treatment.
Increase in size of uterine fibromyomata.
Vaginal candidiasis.
Change in cervical eversion and in degree of cervical secretion.
Cystitis-like syndrome.
2. *Breasts*
Tenderness, enlargement, secretion.
3. *Gastrointestinal*
Nausea, vomiting.
Abdominal cramps, bloating.
Cholestatic jaundice.
4. *Skin*
Chloasma or melasma, which may persist when drug is discontinued.
Erythema multiforme.
Erythema nodosum.
Hemorrhagic eruption.
Loss of scalp hair.
Hirsutism.
Urticaria.
5. *Eyes*
Steepening of corneal curvature.
Intolerance to contact lenses.
6. *CNS*
Headache, migraine, dizziness.
Mental depression.
Chorea.
7. *Miscellaneous*
Increase or decrease in weight.
Reduced carbohydrate tolerance.
Aggravation of porphyria.
Edema.
Changes in libido and/or potency.

Acute Overdosage: Numerous reports of ingestion of large doses of estrogen-containing oral contraceptives by young children indicate that serious ill effects usually do not occur. Overdosage of estrogen may cause nausea, and withdrawal bleeding may occur in females.

Dosage and Administration:
Given for a few days
Prevention of postpartum breast engorgement.
The usual dosage is 1 TACE 72 mg capsule twice daily for 2 days. The first dose should be given as soon as possible after delivery but within 8 hours.

How Supplied:
TACE 72 mg (CHLOROTRIANISENE CAPSULES USP) green and yellow capsules imprinted MERRELL 692
NDC 0068-0692-48: packages of 48 capsules.

References:
1. Ziel, H. K. and Finkel, W. D.: Increased risk of endometrial carcinoma among users of conjugated estrogens. New Eng. J. Med. 293: 1167–1170, 1975.
2. Smith, D.C., Prentice, R., Thompson, D.J., and Hermann, W.L.: Association of exogenous estrogen and endometrial carcinoma. New Eng. J. Med. 293:1164–1167, 1975.
3. Mack, T.M., Pike, M.C., Henderson, B.E., Pfeffer, R.I., Gerkins, V.R., Arthur, M., and Brown, S.E.: Estrogens and endometrial cancer in a retirement community. New Eng. J. Med. 294:1262–1267, 1976.
4. Weiss, N.S., Szekely, D.R., and Austin, D.F.: Increasing incidence of endometrial cancer in the United States. New Eng. J. Med. 294:1259–1262, 1976.
5. Herbst, A.L., Ulfelder, H., and Poskanzer, D.C.: Adenocarcinoma of the vagina. New Eng. J. Med. 284:878–881, 1971.
6. Greenwald, P., Barlow, J.J., Nasca, P.C., and Burnett, W.S.: Vaginal cancer after maternal treatment with synthetic estrogens. New Eng. J. Med. 285:390–392, 1971.
7. Herbst, A.L., Cole, P., Colton, T., Robboy, S.J., and Scully, R.E.: Age-incidence and risk of diethylstilbestrol-related clear cell adenocarcinoma of the vagina and cervix. Amer. J. Obstet. Gynec. 128:43–50, 1977.
8. Lanier, A.P., Noller, K.L., Decker, D.G., Elveback, L.R., and Kurland, L.T.: Cancer and stilbestrol. A follow-up of 1719 persons exposed to estrogens in utero and born 1943-1959. Mayo Clin. Proc. 48:793–799, 1973.
9. Herbst, A.L., Kurman, R.J., and Scully, R.E.: Vaginal and cervical abnormalities after exposure to stilbestrol in utero. Obstet. Gynec. 40:287–298, 1972.
10. Herbst, A.L., Poskanzer, D.C., Robboy, S.J., Friedlander, L., and Scully, R.E.: Prenatal exposure to stilbestrol. A prospective comparison of exposed female offspring with unexposed controls. New Eng. J. Med. 292:334–339, 1975.
11. Stafl, A., Mattingly, R.F., Foley, D.V., and Fetherston, W.C.: Clincial diagnosis of vaginal adenosis. Obstet. Gynec. 43:118–128, 1974.
12. Sherman, A.I., Goldrath, M., Berlin, A., Vakhariya, V., Banooni, F., Michaels, W., Goodman, P., and Brown, S.: Cervical-vaginal adenosis after *in utero* exposure to synthetic estrogens. Obstet. Gynec. 44:531–545, 1974.
13. Gal, I., Kirman, B., and Stern. J.: Hormone pregnancy tests and congenital malformation, Nature 216:83, 1967.
14. Levy, E.P., Cohen, A., and Fraser, F.C.: Hormone treatment during pregnancy and congenital heart defects. Lancet 1:611, 1973.
15. Nora, J.J. and Nora, A.H.: Birth defects and oral contraceptives. Lancet 1:941–942, 1973.
16. Janerich, D.T., Piper, J.M., and Glebatis, D.M.: Oral contraceptives and congenital limb-reduction defects. New Eng. J. Med. 291:697–700, 1974.
17. Daniel, D.G., Campbell, H., and Turnbull, A.C.: Puerperal thromboembolism and suppression of lactation. Lancet 2:287–289, 1967.
18. Boston Collaborative Drug Surveillance Program: Surgically confirmed gall bladder disease, venous thromboembolism, and breast tumors in relation to post menopausal estrogen therapy. New Eng. J. Med. 290:15–19, 1974.
19. Hoover, R., Gray, L.A., Sr., Cole, P., and MacMahon, B.: Menopausal estrogens and breast cancer. New Eng. J. Med. 295:401–405, 1976.
20. Boston Collaborative Drug Surveillance Program: Oral contraceptives and venous thromboembolic disease, surgically confirmed gall-bladder disease, and breast tumors. Lancet 1:1399–1404, 1973.
21. Bailar, J.C., III: Thromboembolism and oestrogen therapy. Lancet 2:560, 1967.
22. The Veterans Adminstration Cooperative Urological Research Group: Carcinoma of the prostate: Treatment comparisons. J. Urol. 98:516–522, 1967.
23. Blackard, C.E., Doe, R.P., Mellinger, G.T., and Byar, D.P.: Incidence of cardiovascular disease and death in patients receiving diethylstilbestrol for carcinoma of the prostate. Cancer 26:249–256, 1970.
24. Royal College of General Practitioners: Oral contraception and thromboembolic disease. J. Roy. Coll. Gen. Pract. 13:267–269, 1967.
25. Inman, W.H.W. and Vessey, M.P.: Investigation of deaths from pulmonary, coronary, and cerebral thrombosis and embolism in women of child-bearing age. Brit. Med. J. 2:193–199, 1968.
26. Vessey, M.P. and Doll, R.: Investigation of relation between use of oral contraceptives and thromboembolic disease. A further report. Brit. Med. J. 2:651–657, 1969.
27. Sartwell, P.E., Masi, A.T., Arthes, F.G., Greene, G.R., and Smith, H.E.: Thromboembolism and oral contraceptives: An epidemiological case-control study. Amer. J. Epidem. 90:365–380, 1969.
28. Collaborative Group for the Study of Stroke in Young Women: Oral contraception and increased risk of cerebral ischemia or thrombosis. New Eng. J. Med. 288:871–878, 1973.
29. Collaborative Group for the Study of Stroke in Young Women: Oral contraceptives and stroke in young women: Associated risk factors. J.A.M.A. 231:718–722, 1975.
30. Mann, J.I. and Inman, W.H.W.: Oral contraceptives and death from myocardial infarction. Brit. Med. J. 2:245–248, 1975.
31. Mann, J.I., Vessey, M.P., Thorogood, M., and Doll, R.: Myocardial infarction in young women with special reference in oral contraceptive practice. Brit. Med. J. 2:241–245, 1975.
32. Inman, W.H.W., Vessey, M.P., Westerholm, B., and Engelund, A.: Thromboembolic disease and the steroidal content of oral contraceptives. A report to the Committee on Safety of Drugs. Brit. Med. J. 2:203–209, 1970.
33. Stolley, P.D., Tonascia, J.A., Tockman, M.S., Sartwell, P.E., Rutledge, A.H., and Jacobs, M.P.: Thrombosis with low-estrogen oral contraceptives. Amer. J. Epidem. 102:197–208, 1975.
34. Vessey, M.P., Doll, R., Fairbairn, A.S., and Glober, G.: Post-operative thromboembolism and the use of the oral contraceptives. Brit. Med. J. 3:123-126, 1970.

Continued on next page

Information on Merrell Dow products is based on labeling in effect in October, 1982.

Merrell Dow—Cont.

35. Greene, G.R. and Sartwell, P.E.: Oral contraceptive use in patients with thromboembolism following surgery, trauma, or infection. Amer. J. Public Health 62:680–685, 1972.
36. Rosenberg, L., Armstrong, B., Phil, D., and Jick, H.: Myocardial infarction and estrogen therapy in post-menopausal women. New Eng. J. Med. 294:1256–1259, 1976.
37. Coronary Drug Project Research Group: The coronary drug project: Initial findings leading to modifications of its research protocol. J.A.M.A. 214:1303–1313, 1970.
38. Baum, J., Holtz, F., Bookstein, J.J., and Klein, E.W.: Possible association between benign hepatomas and oral contraceptives. Lancet 2:926–928, 1973.
39. Mays, E.T., Christopherson, W.M., Mahr, M.M., and Williams, H.C.: Hepatic changes in young women ingesting contraceptive steroids. Hepatic hemorrhage and primary hepatic tumors. J.A.M.A. 235:730–732, 1976.
40. Edmondson, H., Henderson, A.B., and Benton, B.: Liver-cell adenomas associated with the use of oral contraceptives. New Eng. J. Med. 294:470–472, 1976.
41. Pfeffer, R.I. and Van Den Noort, S.: Estrogen use and stroke risk in postmenopausal women. Amer. J. Epidem. 103:445–456, 1976.

Product Information as of August, 1979

Encapsulated by
R. P. Scherer, North America
Clearwater, Florida 33518 for
MERRELL DOW PHARMACEUTICALS INC.
Subsidiary of The Dow Chemical Company
Cincinnati, Ohio 45215, U.S.A.

[*Shown in Product Indentification Section*]

TENUATE® ℭ ℞
(diethylpropion hydrochloride USP)
TENUATE DOSPAN®
(diethylpropion hydrochloride USP)
controlled-release tablets

AVAILABLE ONLY ON PRESCRIPTION

Description: Diethylpropion hydrochloride, a sympathomimetic agent, is 1-phenyl-2-diethylamino-1-propanone hydrochloride.

In Tenuate Dospan tablets, diethylpropion hydrochloride is dispersed in a hydrophilic matrix. On exposure to water the diethylpropion hydrochloride is released at a relatively uniform rate as a result of slow hydration of the matrix. The result is controlled release of the anorexic agent.

Actions: Tenuate is a sympathomimetic amine with some pharmacologic activity similar to that of the prototype drugs of this class used in obesity, the amphetamines. Actions include some central nervous system stimulation and elevation of blood pressure. Tolerance has been demonstrated with all drugs of this class in which these phenomena have been looked for.

Drugs of this class used in obesity are commonly known as "anorectics" or "anorexigenics." It has not been established, however, that the action of such drugs in treating obesity is primarily one of appetite suppression. Other central nervous system actions, or metabolic effects may be involved, for example.

Adult obese subjects instructed in dietary management and treated with "anorectic" drugs lose more weight on the average than those treated with placebo and diet, as determined in relatively short-term clinical trials. The magnitude of increased weight loss of drug-treated patients over placebo-treated patients is some fraction of a pound a week. However, some patients lose more weight than this and some lose less. The rate of weight loss is greatest in the first weeks of therapy for both drug and placebo subjects and tends to decrease in succeeding weeks. The possible origins of the increased weight loss due to the various drug effects are not established. The amount of weight loss associated with the use of an "anorectic" drug varies from trial to trial, and the increased weight loss appears to be related in part to variables other than the drug prescribed, such as the physician-investigator, the population treated, and the diet prescribed. Studies do not permit conclusions as to the relative importance of the drug and non-drug factors on weight loss.

The natural history of obesity is measured in years, whereas most studies cited are restricted to a few weeks duration; thus, the total impact of drug-induced weight loss over that of diet alone must be considered clinically limited.

The controlled-release characteristics of Tenuate Dospan have been demonstrated by studies in humans in which plasma levels of diethylpropion-related material were measured by phosphorescence analysis. Plasma levels obtained with the 75 mg Dospan formulation administered once daily indicated a more gradual release than the standard formulation. The formulation has not been shown superior in effectiveness to the same dosage of the standard, noncontrolled-release formulation.

Indication: Tenuate and Tenuate Dospan are indicated in the management of exogenous obesity as a short-term adjunct (a few weeks) in a regimen of weight reduction based on caloric restriction. The limited usefulness of agents of this class (see ACTIONS) should be measured against possible risk factors inherent in their use such as those described below.

Contraindications: Advanced arteriosclerosis, hyperthyroidism, known hypersensitivity, or idiosyncrasy to the sympathomimetic amines, glaucoma.

Agitated states.

Patients with a history of drug abuse.

During or within 14 days following the administration of monoamine oxidase inhibitors, (hypertensive crises may result).

Warnings: If tolerance develops, the recommended dose should not be exceeded in an attempt to increase the effect; rather, the drug should be discontinued. Tenuate may impair the ability of the patient to engage in potentially hazardous activities such as operating machinery or driving a motor vehicle; the patient should therefore be cautioned accordingly.

When central nervous system active agents are used, consideration must always be given to the possibility of adverse interactions with alcohol.

Drug Dependence

Tenuate has some chemical and pharmacologic similarities to the amphetamines and other related stimulant drugs that have been extensively abused. There have been reports of subjects becoming psychologically dependent on diethylpropion. The possibility of abuse should be kept in mind when evaluating the desirability of including a drug as part of a weight reduction program. Abuse of amphetamines and related drugs may be associated with varying degrees of psychologic dependence and social dysfunction which, in the case of certain drugs, may be severe. There are reports of patients who have increased the dosage to many times that recommended. Abrupt cessation following prolonged high dosage administration results in extreme fatigue and mental depression; changes are also noted on the sleep EEG. Manifestations of chronic intoxication with anorectic drugs include severe dermatoses, marked insomnia, irritability, hyperactivity, and personality changes. The most severe manifestation of chronic intoxications is psychosis, often clinically indistinguishable from schizophrenia.

Use in Pregnancy

Although rat and human reproductive studies have not indicated adverse effects, the use of Tenuate by women who are pregnant or may become pregnant requires that the potential benefits be weighed against the potential risks.

Use in Children

Tenuate is not recommended for use in children under 12 years of age.

Precautions: Caution is to be exercised in prescribing Tenuate for patients with hypertension or with symptomatic cardiovascular disease, including arrhythmias. Tenuate should not be administered to patients with severe hypertension.

Insulin requirements in diabetes mellitus may be altered in association with the use of Tenuate and the concomitant dietary regimen.

Tenuate may decrease the hypotensive effect of guanethidine.

The least amount feasible should be prescribed or dispensed at one time in order to minimize the possibiltiy of overdosage.

Reports suggest that Tenuate may increase convulsions in some epileptics. Therefore, epileptics receiving Tenuate should be carefully monitored. Titration of dose or discontinuance of Tenuate may be necessary.

Adverse Reactions:

Cardiovascular: Palpitation, tachycardia, elevation of blood pressure, precordial pain, arrhythmia. One published report described T-wave changes in the ECG of a healthy young male after ingestion of diethylpropion hydrochloride.

Central Nervous System: Overstimulation, nervousness, restlessness, dizziness, jitteriness, insomnia, anxiety, euphoria, depression, dysphoria, tremor, dyskinesia, mydriasis, drowsiness, malaise, headache; rarely psychotic episodes at recommended doses. In a few epileptics an increase in convulsive episodes has been reported.

Gastrointestinal: Dryness of the mouth, unpleasant taste, nausea, vomiting, abdominal discomfort, diarrhea, constipation, other gastrointestinal disturbances.

Allergic: Urticaria, rash, ecchymosis, erythema.

Endocrine: Impotence, changes in libido, gynecomastia, menstrual upset.

Hematopoietic System: Bone marrow depression, agranulocytosis, leukopenia.

Miscellaneous: A variety of miscellaneous adverse reactions has been reported by physicians. These include complaints such as dyspnea, hair loss, muscle pain, dysuria, increased sweating, and polyuria.

Dosage and Administration:

Tenuate (diethylpropion hydrochloride):

One 25 mg tablet three times daily, one hour before meals, and in midevening if desired to overcome night hunger.

Tenuate Dospan (diethylpropion hydrochloride) controlled-release:

One 75 mg tablet daily, swallowed whole, in midmorning.

Tenuate is not recommended for use in children under 12 years of age.

Overdosage: Manifestations of acute overdosage include restlessness, tremor, hyperreflexia, rapid respiration, confusion, assaultiveness, hallucinations, panic states.

Fatigue and depression usually follow the central stimulation.

Cardiovascular effects include arrhythmias, hypertension or hypotension and circulatory collapse. Gastrointestinal symptoms include nausea, vomiting, diarrhea, and abdominal cramps. Overdose of pharmacologically similar compounds has resulted in fatal poisoning, usually terminating in convulsions and coma. Management of acute Tenuate intoxication is largely symptomatic and includes lavage and sedation with a barbiturate. Experience with hemodialysis or peritoneal dialysis is inadequate to permit recommendation in this regard. Intravenous phentolamine (Regitine®) has been suggested on pharmacologic grounds for possible acute, severe hypertension, if this complicates Tenuate overdosage.

How Supplied: White 25 mg Tenuate tablets debossed MERRELL 697: bottles of 100 and 1000

White capsule-shaped 75 mg Tenuate Dospan tablets debossed MERRELL 698: bottles of 100 and 250

Product Information as of June, 1980

MERRELL DOW PHARMACEUTICALS INC.
Subsidiary of The Dow Chemcial Company
Cincinnati, Ohio 45215, U.S.A.

[*Shown in Product Identification Section*]

TRICLOS® ℞
(triclofos sodium)

Description: Triclos is a phosphate ester of trichlorethanol with hypnotic properties. Triclofos sodium is the sodium salt of trichlorethyl phosphate.

Actions: Triclos is rapidly dephosphorylated, principally in the gut, yielding high blood levels of trichlorethanol which is the same pharmacologically active metabolite obtained from chloral hydrate by enzymatic reduction. Triclos produces a peak serum level of trichlorethanol in about one hour and has a half-life of approximately eleven hours.

Triclos has minimal effects on the various stages of normal sleep, including REM sleep. The exact clinical significance of changes in REM sleep have not been established.

In animal studies Triclos increased the content of slow wave, high voltage spontaneous corticol EEG activity concomitant with behavioral sleep. The arousal threshold on electrical stimulation of the midbrain reticular formation was increased. Whether the latter effect is responsible for the hypnotic action of Triclos is not known.

Indications: Triclos is a hypnotic agent useful in the treatment of insomnia characterized by difficulty in falling asleep, frequent nocturnal awakenings and/or early morning awakening. Triclos has not been shown effective for more than 14 days except in persons over age 65 where it was effective for up to 42 days in one inpatient study.

Also, Triclos can be used as a pre-medication for obtaining sleep records in electroencephalography.

Contraindications: Triclos is contraindicated in patients with marked renal or hepatic impairment and in patients known to be sensitive or allergic to chloral hydrate or triclofos sodium.

Triclos is also contraindicated in women at labor and in the neonate because trichloroacetic acid, the principal metabolite in man of Triclos, frees bilirubin from albumin. Thus, by displacing protein-bound bilirubin, kernicterus could occur in the neonate.

Warnings:

Drug Dependency: Triclos may be habit forming. The relationship of Triclos to chloral hydrate suggests that the addiction liability would be similar. Therefore, caution should be exercised in administering Triclos to patients known to be addiction prone and repeated prescriptions are only advisable under careful medical supervision.

Drug Interactions: Response to concomitantly administered oral anticoagulants may be modified by Triclos in some patients; the anticoagulant effect may be either increased or decreased. Therefore, careful monitoring of prothrombin time with adjustment of anticoagulant dosage is advised throughout Triclos administration and following withdrawal of this drug.

Usage in Pregnancy: Triclos has been administered to three species of animals at various stages of pregnancy at levels as high as 700 mg/kg/day. No dose related effects were observed in these reproductive studies. The relevance to the human is not known. Since there is no experience in pregnant women who have received the drug, safety in pregnancy has not been established.

Nursing Mothers: There are no data on secretion of the drug in human milk or effect on the nursing infant.

Usage in Children: Except for single dose administration of Triclos Liquid for sleep induction in electroencephalography, the drug is not currently recommended for use in persons under 12 years of age.

Precautions: Triclos, like chloral hydrate, may increase the CNS depressant effects of other drugs such as alcohol, barbiturates, and tranquilizers. Therefore, patients taking Triclos should be cautioned accordingly.

Since Triclos may reduce alertness, it should be used cautiously in patients operating vehicles or machinery.

Triclos should be used with caution in patients with cardiac arrhythmias and with severe cardiac disease.

Most insomnias will be of brief duration and therefore long term chronic administration of Triclos is neither advised nor recommended. In cases where prolonged therapy with Triclos is necessary for treatment of insomnia, it is recommended that periodic blood counts be done. Studies of the efficacy of Triclos for periods exceeding six weeks have not been carried out.

Adverse Reactions: The following undesirable reactions have been reported in patients taking Triclos: headache, hangover, drowsiness, gastrointestinal upset, "gas," flatulence, nausea and vomiting, staggering gait, ataxia, "bad taste," ketonuria, relative eosinophilia, urticaria, light-headedness, vertigo, nightmares, malaise, and reduction in total white blood cell count. Excitement and delirium, since they have been observed with chloral hydrate, are possible.

Dosage and Administration: The usual hypnotic dosage of Triclos is 1500 mg (two 750 mg tablets or 15 ml of liquid) taken 15 to 30 minutes before bedtime.

The usual dose for sleep induction in electroencephalography in children under 12 years of age is 0.1 ml of Triclos Liquid per pound of body weight.

Overdosage: Accidental overdosage should be treated with gastric lavage or induce vomiting to empty the stomach. Supportive measures may be used.

How Supplied: TRICLOS (triclofos sodium), 750 mg film coated tablets debossed MERRELL 85, orange, capsule shaped.

NDC 0068-0085-01: bottles of 100 tablets.
NDC 0068-0085-05: bottles of 500 tablets.
TRICLOS (triclofos sodium) Liquid, 1.5 g/15 ml (100 mg/ml).
NDC 0068-0086-08: bottles containing 8 fl. oz.

Revised July, 1978

[*Shown in Product Identification Section*]

TUSSEND® Ⓔ ℞
Antitussive-Decongestant Liquid and Tablets

Description: Each 5 ml teaspoonful or tablet of TUSSEND for oral use contains hydrocodone bitartrate, 5 mg (Warning: may be habit forming) and pseudoephedrine hydrochloride 60 mg. The liquid also contains alcohol 5%.

Hydrocodone bitartrate is an antitussive. Chemically it is 4,5α-epoxy-3-methoxy-17-methylmorphinan-6-one tartrate (1:1) hydrate (2:5).

Pseudoephedrine hydrochloride is a nasal decongestant. Chemically it is α-[1-(methylamino) ethyl] - benzenemethanol hydrochloride.

Clinical Pharmacology: Hydrocodone is a narcotic-analgesic chemically and pharmacologically related to codeine. Hydrocodone suppresses the cough reflex by depressing the medullary cough center. The duration of antitussive action of hydrocodone in man after oral administration is 4 to 8 hours. Hydrocodone is approximately three times more potent than codeine on a weight basis.

Pseudoephedrine is an orally active sympathomimetic amine and exerts a decongestant action on the nasal mucosa. Pseudoephedrine produces peripheral effects similar to those of ephedrine and central effects similar to, but less intense than amphetamines. It has the potential for excitatory side effects. At the recommended oral dosages it has little or no pressor effect in normotensive adults. The serum half-life ($T^{1/2}$) of pseudoephedrine is approximately 4 to 6 hours. $T^{1/2}$ is decreased with increased excretion of drug at a urine pH lower than 6 and may be increased with decreased excretion at urine pH higher than 8.

Indications and Usage: For exhausting cough spasms accompanying upper respiratory tract congestion associated with the common cold, influenza, bronchitis and sinusitis.

Contraindications: Patients with severe hypertension, severe coronary artery disease, and in patients on MAO inhibitor therapy.

Hypersensitivity: Contraindicated in patients with hypersensitivity or idiosyncrasy to sympathomimetic amines, phenanthrene derivatives, or to any other formula ingredients.

Nursing Mothers: Contraindicated because of the higher than usual risk for infants from sympathomimetic amines.

Warnings: Hydrocodone should be prescribed and administered with the same degree of caution as all oral medications containing a narcotic-analgesic. Extreme caution should be exercised in the use of hydrocodone in patients with severe respiratory impairment or patients with impaired respiratory drive.

If sympathomimetic amines are used in patients with hypertension, diabetes mellitus, ischemic heart disease, hyperthyroidism, increased intraocular pressure or prostatic hypertrophy, judicious caution should be exercised (see CONTRAINDICATIONS).

Use in elderly: The elderly (60 years and older) are more likely to have adverse reactions to sympathomimetics. Overdosage of sympathomimetics in this age group may cause hallucinations, convulsions, CNS depression and death.

Precautions: *General:* Caution should be exercised if used in patients with diabetes, hypertension, cardiovascular disease, hyperreactivity to ephedrine, or decreased respiratory drive (see CONTRAINDICATIONS).

Information for Patients: Hydrocodone may produce drowsiness. Persons who perform hazardous tasks requiring mental alertness or physical coordination should be cautioned accordingly. Concomitant use of hydrocodone with tranquilizers, alcohol or other depressants may produce additive depressant effects. Do not exceed the prescribed dosage.

Drug Interactions: Hydrocodone may potentiate the effects of other narcotics, general anesthetics, tranquilizers, sedatives and hypnotics, tricyclic antidepressants, MAO inhibitors, alcohol, and other CNS depressants. Beta adrenergic blockers and MAO inhibitors potentiate the sympathomimetic effects of pseudoephedrine. Sympathomimetics may reduce the antihypertensive effects of methyldopa, mecamylamine, reserpine and veratrum alkaloids.

Pregnancy Category C: Animal reproduction studies have not been conducted with pseudoephedrine or hydrocodone. It is also not known whether pseudoephedrine or hydrocodone can cause fetal harm when administered to a pregnant woman or can affect reproduction capacity. Pseudoephedrine or hydrocodone may be given to a pregnant woman only if clearly needed.

Continued on next page

Information on Merrell Dow products is based on labeling in effect in October, 1982.

Merrell Dow—Cont.

Nursing Mothers: Because of the potential for serious adverse reactions in nursing infants from sympathomimetic amines, pseudoephedrine is contraindicated in nursing mothers.
Adverse Reactions: Gastrointestinal upset, nausea, drowsiness and constipation. A slight elevation in serum transaminase levels has been noted.
Individuals hyperreactive to pseudoephedrine may display ephedrine-like reactions such as tachycardia, palpitations, headache, dizziness or nausea. Sympathomimetic drugs have been associated with certain untoward reactions including fear, anxiety, tenseness, restlessness, tremor, weakness, pallor, respiratory difficulty, dysuria, insomnia, hallucinations, convulsions, CNS depression, arrhythmias, and cardiovascular collapse with hypotension.
Patient idiosyncrasy to adrenergic agents may be manifested by insomina, dizziness, weakness, tremor or arrhythmias.
Drug Abuse and Dependence:
Controlled Substance: Hydrocodone in TUSSEND mixture is controlled by the Drug Enforcement Administration. TUSSEND is a Schedule III controlled substance.
Abuse: Human experience indicates that abuse of TUSSEND is uncommon. However, hydrocodone is a narcotic drug related to codeine with roughly three times the abuse potential of codeine on a weight basis.
Dependence: Hydrocodone can produce drug dependence of the morphine type. Psychic dependence, physical dependence and tolerance may develop if dosage recommendations are greatly exceeded over a prolonged period of time.
Overdosage: Acute overdosage with TUSSEND may produce variable clinical signs as hydrocodone produces CNS depression and cardiovascular depression while pseudoephedrine produces CNS stimulation and variable cardiovascular effects. Hydrocodone is likely to be responsible for most of the severe reactions from overdosage. Pressor amines should be used with great caution when taking pseudoephedrine. Patients with signs of stimulation should be treated conservatively and depressant medications should be avoided if possible because of potential drug interaction with hydrocodone.
Dosage and Administration: Adults and children over 90 lbs, 1 tablet or one teaspoonful; children 50 to 90 lbs, ½ teaspoonful; children 25 to 50 lbs, ¼ teaspoonful. May be given four times a day as needed. May be taken with meals.
Caution: Federal law prohibits dispensing without prescription.
How Supplied: Tussend liquid is supplied in pints (NDC 0068-1018-16). Tussend tablets are supplied in bottles of 100 (NDC 0068-0042-61).
[*Shown in Product Identification Section*]

TUSSEND® EXPECTORANT ℞ Ⓒ
Antitussive-Decongestant
Liquid

Description: Each 5 ml teaspoonful of TUSSEND Expectorant liquid for oral use contains hydrocodone bitartrate, 5 mg (Warning: May be habit forming), pseudoephedrine hydrochloride 60 mg, guaifenesin (glyceryl guaiacolate) 200 mg, and alcohol 12.5%.
Hydrocodone bitartrate is an antitussive. Chemically it is 4,5α-epoxy-3-methoxy-17-methylmorphinan-6-one tartrate (1:1) hydrate (2:5).
Pseudoephedrine hydrochloride is a nasal decongestant. Chemically it is α-[1-(methylamino) ethyl]-benzenemethanol hydrochloride.
Guaifenesin is an expectorant. Chemically it is 3-(*O*-methoxyphenoxy)-1,2 propanediol.
Clinical Pharmacology: Hydrocodone is a narcotic-analgesic chemically and pharmacologically related to codeine. Hydrocodone suppresses the cough reflex by depressing the medullary cough center. The duration of antitussive action of hydrocodone in man after oral administration is 4 to 8 hours. Hydrocodone is approximately three times more potent than codeine on a weight basis.
Pseudoephedrine is an orally active sympathomimetic amine and exerts a decongestant action on the nasal mucosa. Pseudoephedrine produces peripheral effects similar to those of ephedrine and central effects similar to, but less intense than amphetamines. It has the potential for excitatory side effects. At the recommended oral dosages it has little or no pressor effect in normotensive adults. The serum half-life (T-½) of pseudoephedrine is approximately 4 to 6 hours. T-½ is decreased with increased excretion of drug at a urine pH lower than 6 and may be increased with decreased excretion at urine pH higher than 8.
Guaifenesin is used as an expectorant. On the basis of studies in animals, guaifenesin is thought to increase mucus flow in the lung by stimulation of gastric mucosal reflexes. Objective human data are lacking.
Indications and Usage: For exhausting, nonproductive cough accompanying respiratory tract congestion associated with the common cold, influenza, sinusitis and bronchitis.
Contraindications: Patients with severe hypertension, severe coronary artery disease, and in patients on MAO inhibitor therapy.
Hypersensitivity: Contraindicated in patients with hypersensitivity or idiosyncrasy to sympathomimetic amines, phenanthrene derivatives, or to any other formula ingredients.
Nursing Mothers: Contraindicated because of the higher than usual risk for infants for sympathomimetic amines.
Warnings: Hydrocodone should be prescribed and administered with the same degree of caution as all oral medications containing a narcotic analgesic. Extreme caution should be exercised in the use of hydrocodone in patients with severe respiratory impairment or patients with impaired respiratory drive.
If sympathomimetic amines are used in patients with hypertension, diabetes mellitus, ischemic heart disease, hyperthyroidism, increased intraocular pressure or prostatic hypertrophy, judicious caution should be exercised (see CONTRAINDICATIONS).
Use in Elderly: The elderly (60 years and older) are more likely to have adverse reactions to sympathomimetics. Overdosage of sympathomimetics in this age group may cause hallucinations, convulsions, CNS depression and death.
Precautions: *General:* Caution should be exercised if used in patients with diabetes, hypertension, cardiovascular diseases, hyperreactivity to ephedrine, or decreased respiratory drive (see CONTRAINDICATIONS).
Information for Patients: Hydrocodone may produce drowsiness. Persons who perform hazardous tasks requiring mental alertness or physical coordination should be cautioned accordingly. Concomitant use of hydrocodone with tranquilizers, alcohol or other depressants may produce additive depressant effects. Do not exceed the prescribed dosage.
Drug Interactions: Hydrocodone may potentiate the effects of other narcotics, general anesthetics, tranquilizers, sedatives and hypnotics, tricyclic antidepressants, MAO inhibitors, alcohol, and other CNS depressants. Beta adrenergic blockers and MAO inhibitors potentiate the sympathomimetic effects of pseudoephedrine. Sympathomimetics may reduce the antihypertensive effects of methyldopa, mecamylamine, reserpine and veratrum alkaloids.
Laboratory Test Interactions: Guaifenesin interferes with the colorimetric determination of 5-hydroxyindoleacetic acid (5-HIAA) and vanilmandelic acid (VMA).
Pregnancy Category C: Animal reproduction studies have not been conducted with pseudoephedrine, guaifenesin, or hydrocodone. It is also not known whether pseudoephedrine, guaifenesin or hydrocodone can cause fetal harm when administered to a pregnant woman or can affect reproduction capacity. Pseudoephedrine or hydrocodone may be given to a pregnant woman only if clearly needed.
Nursing Mothers: Because of the potential for serious adverse reactions in nursing infants from sympathomimetic amines, pseudoephedrine is contraindicated in nursing mothers.
Adverse Reactions: Gastrointestinal upset, nausea, drowsiness and constipation. A slight elevation in serum transaminase levels has been noted.
Individuals hyperreactive to pseudoephedrine may display ephedrine-like reactions such as tachycardia, palpitations, headache, dizziness or nausea. Sympathomimetic drugs have been associated with certain untoward reactions including fear, anxiety, tenseness, restlessness, tremor, weakness, pallor, respiratory difficulty, dysuria, insomnia, hallucinations, convulsions, CNS depression, arrhythmias, and cardiovascular collapse with hypotension.
Patient idiosyncrasy to adrenergic agents may be manifested by insomnia, dizziness, weakness, tremor or arrhythmias.
Drug Abuse and Dependence:
Controlled Substance: Hydrocodone in TUSSEND Expectorant mixture is controlled by the Drug Enforcement Administration. TUSSEND Expectorant is a Schedule III controlled substance.
Abuse: Human experience indicates that abuse of TUSSEND Expectorant is uncommon. However, hydrocodone is a narcotic drug related to codeine with roughly three times the abuse potential of codeine on a weight basis.
Dependence: Hydrocodone can produce drug dependence of the morphine type. Psychic dependence, physical dependence and tolerance may develop if dosage recommendations are greatly exceeded over a prolonged period of time.
Overdosage: Acute overdosage with TUSSEND Expectorant may produce variable clinical signs as hydrocodone produces CNS depression and cardiovascular depression while pseudoephedrine produces CNS stimulation and variable cardiovascular effects. Hydrocodone is likely to be responsible for most of the severe reactions from overdosage. Pressor amines should be used with great caution when taking pseudoephedrine. Patients with signs of stimulation should be treated conservatively and depressant medications should be avoided if possible because of potential drug interaction with hydrocodone.
Dosage and Administration: Adults and children over 90 lbs, 1 teaspoonful; children 50 to 90 lbs, ½ teaspoonful; children 25 to 50 lbs, ¼ teaspoonful. May be given four times a day as needed. May be taken with meals.
Caution: Federal law prohibits dispensing without prescription.
How Supplied: TUSSEND Expectorant is supplied in pints (NDC 0068-1016-16).
[*Shown in Products Identification Section*]

VANOBID® ℞
(candicidin USP)
Vaginal Ointment/Tablets

Description: Vanobid Vaginal Ointment and Vanobid Vaginal Tablets contain candicidin, a conjugated heptaene antibiotic complex, produced by a soil actinomycete similar to *Streptomyces griseus.* Vanobid Vaginal Ointment is a dispersion of candicidin in USP petrolatum. It contains 0.6 mg candicidin activity per 1 gram of ointment. Each Vanobid Vaginal Tablet contains 3 mg candicidin activity dispersed in starch, lactose, and magnesium stearate.

Action: Vanobid Vaginal Ointment and Vanobid Vaginal Tablets have anti-*Candida* activity.
Indications: For the treatment of vaginitis due to *Candida albicans* and other *Candida* species. Vanobid Vaginal Tablets are particularly suited for gravid patients.
Contraindications: Contraindicated for patients known to be sensitive to any of the components of Vanobid Vaginal Ointment and Vanobid Vaginal Tablets. During pregnancy, the use of an applicator may be contraindicated. The tablet inserter should be used only on advice of physician. Manual tablet insertion may be preferred.
Precautions: During treatment it is recommended that the patient refrain from sexual intercourse or the husband wear a condom to avoid re-infection.
A contraceptive diaphragm may deteriorate during prolonged contact with petrolatum-based products. The patient using a diaphragm should be advised to substitute another form of contraception during treatment with Vanobid Vaginal Ointment.
Adverse Reactions: Clinical reports of sensitization or temporary irritation with candicidin ointment or tablets have been extremely rare.
Dosage and Administration: 1 vaginal applicatorful of Vanobid Vaginal Ointment or 1 Vanobid Vaginal Tablet inserted high in the vagina twice daily, in the morning and at bedtime, for 14 days. Treatment may be repeated if symptoms persist or reappear.
How Supplied: A 14-day course of therapy of Vanobid Vaginal Ointment is supplied in a package containing two 75-gram tubes, two vaginal applicators, and patient instructions.
A 14-day course of therapy of Vanobid Tablets is supplied in packages of 28 individually foil-wrapped tablets debossed MERRELL 425 with vaginal inserter and patient instructions.
A pad may be used to protect clothing.
Store under refrigeration to ensure full potency.
Product Information as of November, 1974
[Shown in Product Identification Section]

Information on Merrell Dow products is based on labeling in effect in October, 1982.

Meyer Laboratories, Inc.
1900 WEST COMMERCIAL BLVD.
FT. LAUDERDALE, FL 33309

(See product listings under Glaxo Inc.)

Miles Laboratories, Inc.
P. O. BOX 340
ELKHART, IN 46515

ALKA-SELTZER® Effervescent Pain Reliever & Antacid
(See PDR For Nonprescription Drugs)

ALKA-SELTZER® Effervescent Antacid
(See PDR For Nonprescription Drugs)

ALKA-2® Chewable Antacid Tablets
(See PDR For Nonprescription Drugs)

ALKA-SELTZER PLUS® Cold Medicine
(See PDR For Nonprescription Drugs)

BACTINE® Antiseptic·Anesthetic First Aid Spray
(See PDR for Nonprescription Drugs)

BACTINE® Hydrocortisone (0.5%) Skin Care Cream
(See PDR for non-prescription drugs)

BUGS BUNNY® Children's Chewable Vitamins
(Multivitamin Supplement)
BUGS BUNNY® Children's Chewable Vitamins Plus Iron
(Multivitamin Supplement with Iron)
FLINTSTONES® Children's Chewable Vitamins Plus Iron
(Multivitamin Supplement with Iron)
FLINTSTONES® Children's Chewable Vitamins
(Multivitamin Supplement)
(See PDR For Nonprescription Drugs)

BUGS BUNNY® With Extra C
Multivitamin Supplement
(See PDR For Nonprescription Drugs)

FLINTSTONES® With Extra C
Multivitamin Supplement
(See PDR For Nonprescription Drugs)

MILES® NERVINE
NIGHTTIME SLEEP-AID
(See PDR For Nonprescription Drugs)

ONE-A-DAY® Vitamins
(Multivitamin Supplement)
ONE-A-DAY® Vitamins Plus Iron
(Multivitamin Supplement with Iron)
(See PDR For Nonprescription Drugs)

ONE-A-DAY® Vitamins Plus Minerals
(Multivitamin/Multimineral Supplement for adults and teens)
(See PDR For Nonprescription Drugs)

ONE-A-DAY® CORE C 500™ Vitamins
(Multivitamin Supplement for adults and children 12 or more years of age.)
ONE-A-DAY® Plus Extra C
High Potency 500 mg Vitamin C Plus 9 Essential Vitamins
(See PDR For Nonprescription Drugs)

ONE-A-DAY® STRESSGARD™ Vitamins
(B Complex Plus C Stress Formula)
High Potency
Multivitamin/Multimineral Supplement For Adults
(See PDR For Nonprescription Drugs)

Important Notice

Before prescribing or administering any product described in PHYSICIANS' DESK REFERENCE always consult the PDR Supplement for possible new or revised information.

Miles Pharmaceuticals
Division of Miles Laboratories, Inc.
400 MORGAN LANE
WEST HAVEN, CT 06516

PRODUCT IDENTIFICATION CODES

To provide an accurate identification of Miles Pharmaceuticals products, each solid dosage form is coded with the name Miles and a 3 digit product identification number.

PRODUCT	PRODUCT IDENTIFICATION CODE NUMBER
ORAL DOSAGE FORMS	
Decholin® Tablets 250 mg (dehydrocholic acid)	121
Lithane® Tablets 300 mg (lithium carbonate)	951
Niclocide® Chewable Tablets 500 mg (niclosamide)	721
Stilphostrol® Tablets 50 mg (diethylstilbestrol diphosphate)	132
NON-ORAL DOSAGE FORMS	
Domeboro® Tablets (aluminum sulfate, calcium acetate)	411
Mycelex®-G Vaginal Tablets (clotrimazole)	093

ACNE-DOME®
Creme and Lotion (acid pH)
(colloidal sulfur, resorcinol)

Composition: Colloidal sulfur and resorcinol in a compatible vehicle adjusted to the pH range for normal skin.
Action and Uses: Medicates acne blemishes. As an aid in drying and peeling acne blemishes.
Caution: If excessive drying or skin irritation develops or increases, discontinue use and consult physician. For external use only. Not for ophthalmic use. Store below 86°F. (30°C.), avoid freezing.
Administration and Dosage: Wash affected parts thoroughly, then dry. Apply sparingly twice daily, preferably in the morning and at bedtime. Follow advice of physician as to diet or other treatment. Shake lotion well.
How Supplied:

Creme	*Lotion*
1 oz. tube	2 fl. oz.

ACNE-DOME® Medicated Cleanser (acid pH)
(colloidal sulfur, salicylic acid)

Composition: Contains effective anti-acne medications: Colloidal sulfur—to dry excess skin oils. Salicylic acid—to peel away dead skin tissue.
Indications: Medicated skin cleanser as an aid in the treatment of acne.
Caution: WARNING: If excessive drying or skin irritation develops or increases, discontinue use and consult physician. For external use only. Keep away from children. Store below 86°F. (30°C.), avoid freezing. Keep away from eyes.
Administration and Dosage: Use twice daily, preferably in the morning and at bedtime. Wet the skin. Apply the cleanser to moist sponge. Work into lather. Massage for five minutes. Rinse.
How Supplied: In the exclusive 4 oz. DISPENSAJAR® with its "Personal Washcloth"—an applicator sponge so fingers never touch the cleanser.

Continued on next page

Miles Pharm.—Cont.

ALLPYRAL® allergenic extracts, alum-precipitated, for Subcutaneous Injection Pollens, Molds, Epithelia, House Dust and Other Inhalants, and Stinging Insects. ℞

Composition: Allpyral allergenic extracts are pyridine/aqueous alkaline solution extracted alum-precipitated antigens in saline suspension.

Indications: Allpyral allergenic extracts, alum-precipitated (pollens, molds, epithelia, house dust or other inhalants, and stinging insects) are indicated for hyposensitization of patients who have been shown by clinical history and/or skin testing to be allergic (hypersensitive) to one or more of these allergens and who have manifested signs and/or symptoms related to exposure to the allergen(s). These manifestations may be referable to the respiratory trace, for example rhinitis, asthma or airway obstruction or they may be ophthalmic such as non-infectious conjunctivitis, pruritus or edema of the eyelids.

Caution: Observe the usual precautions in preparing and administering allergenic extracts. Inject subcutaneously. Avoid depositing material intracutaneously or intravenously. Allpyral extracts may be combined with one another in any proportion. However, in mixing extracts, the total PNU injected shall not be more than the recommended dose (in PNU) of that component with the lowest maximum recommended PNU. This assures that the total aluminum injected shall not exceed 0.85mg. It is desirable to keep ALLPYRAL Mixed Stinging Insects separate from other ALLPYRAL antigens. Admixture with aqueous extracts is not recommended. Never attempt to switch a patient from treatment with Allpyral suspensions to aqueous solutions of allergens. If conversion to an aqueous preparation is necessary, start as though patient were coming for first treatment. Allpyral injections should not be administered more frequently than once a week in the early phases of treatment. Beyond the 1000 PNU dosage level, the interval should be increased to 2 weeks or more. The top dose should not be administered more frequently than every 4 weeks nor less frequently than every 8 weeks. Do not use phosphate-buffered saline or bicarbonate saline (Coca's solution) as a diluent.

Reactions: Should a local reaction occur, characterized by moderate edema, erythema and pain at the site of injection, the same or lower dose should be given at the next visit and no increase attempted. If the local reaction is marked, antihistamine drugs may be given. Reduce the dose at the next visit to a previous dose which did not elicit a reaction.

In the event that a delayed constitutional or systemic reaction characterized by urticaria, sneezing, itching, edema of the extremities, respiratory wheezing or asthma, or dyspnea occurs, this will generally appear slowly and gradually, and may last for 2 to 4 days due to continued slow release of the antigen. Injection of 0.3 ml to 0.5 ml of 1:1,000 epinephrine hydrochloride near the site of injection may be given. For children under 12 years of age, the dose of epinephrine 1:1000 is 0.1 ml to 0.3 ml. However, such reactions are rarely critical and are usually readily controlled with antihistamines and steroids. The patient should be supplied with medication and information to prevent undue apprehension and the dose of antigen at the next visit should be reduced.

Acute anaphylactic reactions characterized by difficulty in breathing, cyanosis and shock following Allpyral® therapy are extremely rare but if they do occur, emergency treatment measures must be adopted. Apply a tourniquet above the site of injection and administer 0.3 ml to 0.5 ml of 1:1,000 epinephrine hydrochloride intramuscularly at two sites: (a) at the site of injection and (b) in the opposite arm for systemic effect. In severe anaphylactic reactions, epinephrine may be given intravenously, using a 1:10,000 aqueous solution at a rate not exceeding 0.5 ml per minute and a total no greater than 0.25 mgm. If necessary, this may be repeated in 15 to 20 minutes. Intravenous antihistamine or adrenal corticosteroids should also be considered in severe cases. Oxygen therapy and artificial respiration may be necessary for respiratory failure. If bronchospasm is an important feature of the reaction, intravenous aminophylline may be required and the presence of laryngeal edema or laryngospasm may necessitate tracheotomy. For persistent hypotension an intravenous drip infusion of 5 percent dextrose in water with a vasopressor agent should be administered at a rate sufficient to maintain the blood pressure at reasonably normal levels.

If continuation of Allpyral® therapy is considered necessary in such patients, the dose at the next visit should be greatly reduced and extreme caution exercised.

As with all types of allergenic extracts, Allpyral grass antigens appear to be slightly more reactive than other categories of Allpyral allergens and should be administered on a more conservative basis.

Store at 5°C (± 3°C).

Administration and Dosage: Before administering, see package insert for complete product information.

Literature Available: Upon request.

AZLIN® ℞
Sterile azlocillin sodium for intravenous use.

Description: AZLIN® (sterile azlocillin sodium) is a semisynthetic broad spectrum penicillin antibiotic for parenteral administration. It is the monosodium salt of 6-D-2 (2-OXO-imidazolidine-1-carboxamido) -2- phenylacetamido -penicillanic acid.

Structural Formula:

Empirical Formula: $C_{20}H_{22}N_5O_6S$ Na

AZLIN® has a molecular weight of 483.5 and contains 49.8 mg (2.17 mEq) of sodium per one gram of azlocillin activity. The dosage form is supplied as a sterile white to pale yellow powder, which is freely soluble in water. When reconstituted, aqueous solutions of AZLIN® are clear and range from colorless to pale yellow with a pH of 6.0 to 8.0.

Clinical Pharmacology: Intravenous Administration. In healthy adult volunteers, means serum levels of azlocillin 30 minutes after a 5–10 minute intravenous injection of 1g, 2g, or 5g are 35, 106 and 256 mcg/ml, respectively. Serum levels, as noted below, lack dose proportionality:

[See table below].

After an intravenous infusion (30 min) of 2g or 3 g azlocillin, mean serum levels 5 minutes after dosing are 130 mcg/ml (73–189) and 180 mcg/ml (133–235), respectively.

[See table on next page].

Following intravenous infusion (30 min) of a 3g dose of azlocillin every 6 hours for 5 days, mean peak serum concentrations were higher than 150 mcg/ml; trough levels were between 4–12 mcg/ml. From the first to the last day of dosing, the serum half-life increased from 61 minutes to approximately 77 minutes.

General: As with other penicillins, azlocillin is excreted primarily by the kidney through glomerular filtration and tubular secretion. The rate of elimination is dose dependent and also related to the status of renal function. In patients with normal renal function, 50 to 70% of the administered dose is recovered from the urine within 24 hours after dosing. Two hours after an intravenous injection of 2g, concentrations of active drug in urine generally exceed 4000 mcg/ml. By 4–8 hours after injection, concentrations are still above 500 mcg/ml. The serum elimination half-life of azlocillin is dose dependent and ranges from approximately 55 minutes after an intravenous dose of 2g to about 70 minutes after intravenous dose of 5g. Probenecid interferes with the renal tubular secretion of azlocillin, thereby increasing serum concentrations and prolonging serum half-life of the antibiotic.

In patients with reduced renal function, the serum half-life of azlocillin is prolonged, depending on degree of renal impairment. Dosage adjustments are usually not necessary except in patients with moderate to severe renal impairment. (See Dosage and Administration). As with other penicillins, azlocillin is metabolized only slightly; less than 10% of the administered dose is found in the urine in the form of the penicilloate or penilloate. The drug is readily removed from the serum by hemodialysis.

Following an intravenous dose of 2g azlocillin, peak concentrations of active drug in bile generally exceed 1000 mcg/ml. The bile levels are approximately 15 times higher than the corresponding serum levels. Biliary excretion is reduced in patients with common bile duct obstruction.

Following parenteral administration, the apparent volume of distribution is approximately 20% of body weight. The drug is present in active form in the serum, urine, bile, bronchial and wound secretions, bone and other tissues. As with other penicillins, penetration into the cerebrospinal fluid (CSF) is generally poor, however, higher CSF concentrations are obtained in the presence of meningeal inflammation.

The serum level of uric acid has been noted to be depressed in some patients receiving azlocillin; this effect appears to be transient.

Protein binding studies indicate that the degree of azlocillin binding is low (25–45%) and

AZLOCILLIN SERUM LEVELS IN ADULTS (mcg/ml) 5–10 MIN IV INJECTION

DOSE	5 min	15 min	30 min	1 hr	2 hr	3 hr	4 hr	6 hr	8 hr
1g			**35** (29–41)	**22** (18–26)	**9.4** (7.2–14)	**4.3** (2.6–6.8)	**2.2** (1.2–4.0)		
2g	**239** (142–363)	**139** (85–188)	**106** (83–134)	**47** (30–60)	**19** (16–26)	**12** (8.7–13)	**7.4** (5.7–11)	**2.1** (1.8–2.9)	**0.5** (0–0.7)
5g	**527** (470–604)	**353** (258–440)	**256** (184–287)	**174** (116–231)	**85** (43–121)	**55** (26–91) 91	**33** (15–58)	**7.7** (1.6–19)	**4.1** (1.4–7.8)

AZLOCILLIN SERUM LEVELS IN ADULTS (mcg/ml) 30 MIN IV INFUSION

DOSE	0	5 min	15 min	30 min	45 min	1 hr	1.5 hr	2 hr	3 hr	4 hr	6 hr	8 hr
2g	**165** (55–278)	**130** (73–189)	**104** (62–175)	**85** (42–121)	**62** (23–85)	**49** (27–82)	**36** (19–57)	**26** (13–48)	**13** (5–25)	**6** (2–11)	**2** (1–4)	**1** (1–4)
3g	**214** (155–273)	**180** (133–235)	**139** (119–186)	**104** (61–159)	**82** (58–121)	**68** (38–94)	**58** (35–74)	**39** (17–53)	**24** (9–36)	**10** (3–14)	**3** (1–5)	**1** (1–4)

depends upon testing methods and concentrations of drug studied.

Microbiology

Azlocillin is a bactericidal antibiotic which acts by interfering with synthesis of cell wall components. It is active against *Pseudomonas aeruginosa* and other species of Pseudomonas, many of which are resistant to other broad spectrum antibiotics. Azlocillin is also active *in vitro* against many strains of the following organisms, however, clinical efficacy for infections other than those included in the indication section has not been documented:

Gram-negative bacteria

Escherichia coli
Proteus Mirabilis
Proteus vulgaris
Morganella morganii (formerly *P. morganii*)
Providencia rettgeri (formerly *P. rettgeri*)
Providencia stuartii
Enterobacter species
Shigella species
Haemophilus influenzae
Haemophilus parainfluenzae
Neisseria species
Citrobacter species

Some strains of *Klebsiella, Serratia, Salmonella,* and *Acinetobacter* are also susceptible.

Gram-positive bacteria

Staphylococcus aureus (non-penicillinase producing strains)
Beta-hemolytic streptococci (Groups A and B)
Streptococcus pneumoniae (formerly *Diplococcus pneumoniae*)
Streptococcus faecalis (enterococcus)
Listeria monocytogenes

Anaerobic Organisms

Peptococcus species
Peptostreptococcus species
Clostridium species
Bacteroides species (including *B. fragilis* group)
Fusobacterium species
Veillonella species
Eubacterium species

Azlocillin is inactive against penicillinase-producing strains of *Staphylococcus aureus* and is susceptible to inactivation by beta-lactamases produced by the Enterobacteriaceae.

In vitro studies have shown that azlocillin combined with an aminoglycoside (e.g., gentamicin, tobramycin, amikacin, sisomicin) acts synergistically against many strains of *Pseudomonas aeruginosa.*

Azlocillin is slightly more active when tested at alkaline pH and, as with other penicillins, has reduced activity when tested *in vitro* with increasing inoculum. The minimal bactericidal concentration (MBC) may exceed the minimal inhibitory concentration (MIC) by four-fold or more depending on medium used. Resistance to azlocillin *in vitro* develops slowly (multiple step mutation). Some strains of *Pseudomonas aeruginosa* have developed resistance fairly rapidly.

Susceptibility Tests

Quantitative methods that require measurement of zone diameters give good estimates of bacterial susceptibility. One such procedure* has been recommended for use with discs to test susceptibility to antimicrobials. When the causative organism is tested by the Kirby-Bauer disc diffusion method, a 75 mcg azlocillin disc should give a zone of 18 mm or greater to indicate susceptibility. Zone sizes of 14 mm or less indicate resistance. Zone sizes of 15 to 17 mm indicate intermediate susceptibility. With this procedure, a report from the laboratory of "Susceptible" indicates that the infecting organism is likely to respond to therapy. A report of "Resistant" indicates that the infecting organism is not likely to respond to therapy; other therapy should be selected. A report of "Intermediate Susceptibility" suggests that the organism may be susceptible if the infection is confined to tissues and fluids (e.g., urine), in which high antibiotic levels are attained. The azlocillin disc should be used for testing susceptibility to azlocillin. Standardized procedure requires use of control organisms. The 75 mcg azlocillin disc should give zone diameters between 24 and 30 mm for *P. aeruginosa* ATCC 27853. For *E. coli* ATCC 25922 the zone diameters should be between 21 and 24 mm.

* Bauer, A.W., Kirby, W.M., Sherris, J.C., and Turck, M.: Antibiotic Testing by a Standardized Single Disc Method, Am. J. Clin. Pathol., 45:493, 1966; Standardized Disc Susceptibility Test, FEDERAL REGISTER, 39: 19182–19184, 1974.

In certain conditions, it may be desirable to do additional susceptibility testing by broth or agar dilution techniques. Dilution methods, preferably the agar plate dilution procedure, are most accurate for susceptibility testing of obligate anaerobes. *Pseudomonas* species and the *Enterobacteriaceae* are considered susceptible if the MIC of azlocillin is no greater than 64 mcg/ml and are considered resistant if the MIC is greater than 128 mcg/ml. The MIC values of azlocillin for the control strains are the following:

P. aeruginosa ATCC 27853, 4–8 mcg/ml and
E. coli ATCC 25922, 8–16 mcg/ml.

Azlocillin standard is available for broth or agar dilution studies.

Indications and Usage: AZLIN® is indicated primarily for the treatment of serious infections caused by susceptible strains of *Pseudomonas aeruginosa* in the conditions listed below:

LOWER RESPIRATORY TRACT INFECTIONS including pneumonia and lung abscess.

URINARY TRACT INFECTIONS both complicated and uncomplicated of the lower and upper urinary tract.

SKIN AND SKIN STRUCTURE INFECTIONS including ulcers, abscesses, burns and severe external otitis.

BONE AND JOINT INFECTIONS including osteomyelitis.

BACTERIAL SEPTICEMIA

Azlocillin has also been shown to be effective for the treatment of Lower Respiratory Tract Infections caused by *Escherichia coli* and *Haemophilus influenzae;* Urinary Tract Infections and Skin Structure Infections caused by *Escherichia coli, Proteus mirabilis* or *Streptococcus faecalis;* and Septicemia caused by *Escherichia coli.*

Appropriate culture and susceptibility tests should be performed before treatment in order to isolate and identify organisms causing infections and to determine their susceptibility to azlocillin. Therapy with AZLIN® may be initiated before results of these tests are known; once results become available, appropriate therapy should be continued.

In certain severe infections, when the causative organisms are unknown and *Pseudomonas aeruginosa* is suspected, AZLIN® may be administered in conjunction with an aminoglycoside or a cephalosporin antibiotic as initial therapy. As soon as results of culture and susceptibility tests become available, antimicrobial therapy should be adjusted as indicated. Culture and susceptibility testing, performed periodically during therapy, will provide information on the therapeutic effect of the antimicrobial and will monitor for the possible emergence of bacterial resistance.

AZLIN® has been used effectively in combination with an aminoglycoside antibiotic for the treatment of life-threatening infections caused by *Pseudomonas aeruginosa* including acute pulmonary exacerbation in patients with cystic fibrosis. For the treatment of febrile episodes in immunosuppressed patients with granulocytopenia, AZLIN® should be combined with an aminoglycoside or a cephalosporin antibiotic.

Contraindications: AZLIN® is contraindicated in patients with a history of hypersensitivity reactions to any of the penicillins.

Warnings: Serious and occasionally fatal hypersensitivity (anaphylactic) reactions have occurred in patients receiving a penicillin. These reactions are more apt to occur in individuals with a history of sensitivity to multiple allergens. There have been reports of individuals with a history of penicillin hypersensitivity reactions who have experienced severe hypersensitivity reactions when treated with a cephalosporin. Before therapy with azlocillin is instituted, careful inquiry should be made to determine whether the patient has had previous hypersensitivity reactions to penicillins, cephalosporins or other drugs. Antibiotics should be used with caution in any patient who has demonstrated some form of allergy, particularly to drugs.

If an allergic reaction occurs during therapy with azlocillin, the drug should be discontinued. SERIOUS ANAPHYLACTOID REACTIONS REQUIRE IMMEDIATE EMERGENCY TREATMENT WITH EPINEPHRINE. OXYGEN, INTRAVENOUS STEROIDS, AND AIRWAY MANAGEMENT, INCLUDING INTUBATION, SHOULD ALSO BE PROVIDED AS INDICATED.

Precautions: Although AZLIN® shares with other penicillins the low potential for toxicity, as with any potent drug, periodic assessment of organ system functions, including renal, hepatic and hematopoietic, is advisable during prolonged therapy.

Bleeding manifestations have occurred in some patients receiving beta-lactam antibiotics. These reactions have been associated with abnormalities of coagulation tests, such as clotting time, platelet aggregation and prothrombin time and are more likely to occur in patients with renal impairment. Although AZLIN® has rarely been associated with any bleeding abnormalities, the possibility of this occurring should be kept in mind, particularly in patients with severe renal impairment receiving maximum doses of the drug.

AZLIN® has only rarely been reported to cause hypokalemia; however, the possibility of this occurring should also be kept in mind, particularly when treating patients with fluid and electrolyte imbalance. Periodic monitoring of serum potassium may be advisable in patients receiving prolonged therapy.

AZLIN® is a monosodium salt containing only 49.8 mg (2.17 mEq) of sodium per gram of azlocillin. This should be considered when treating patients requiring restricted salt intake.

Continued on next page

Miles Pharm.—Cont.

As with any penicillin, an allergic reaction, including anaphylaxis, may occur during AZLIN® administration, particularly in a hypersensitive individual.

The rapid intravenous administration of AZLIN® has been associated with transient chest discomfort. Therefore, the drug should not be infused over a period of less than five minutes.

As with other antibiotics, prolonged use of AZLIN® may result in overgrowth of nonsusceptible organisms. If this occurs, appropriate measures should be taken.

Interactions with Drugs and Laboratory Tests
As with other penicillins, the mixing of azlocillin with an aminoglycoside in solutions for parenteral administration can result in substantial inactivation of the aminoglycoside.

Probenecid interferes with the renal tubular secretion of azlocillin, thereby increasing serum concentrations and prolonging serum half-life of the antibiotic.

The serum level of uric acid has been noted to be depressed in some patients receiving azlocillin; this effect appears to be transient.

High urine concentrations of azlocillin may produce false positive protein reactions (pseudoproteinuria) with the following methods: sulfosalicylic acid and boiling test, acetic acid test, biuret reaction, and nitric acid test. The bromphenol blue (Multi-stix®) reagent strip test has been reported to be reliable.

Pregnancy Category B
Reproduction studies have been performed in rats and mice at doses up to 2 times the human dose, and have revealed no evidence of impaired fertility or harm to the fetus, due to AZLIN®. There are however no adequate and well controlled studies in pregnant women. Because animal reproductive studies are not always predictive of human response, this drug should be used during pregnancy only if clearly needed. Azlocillin crosses the placenta and is found in cord blood and amniotic fluid.

Nursing Mothers
Azlocillin is detected in low concentrations in the milk of nursing mothers, therefore caution should be exercised when AZLIN® is administered to a nursing woman.

Drug Abuse and Dependence
Neither AZLIN® abuse nor AZLIN® dependence has been reported.

Adverse Reactions: As with other penicillins, the following adverse reactions may occur:

Hypersensitivity reactions: skin rash, pruritus, urticaria, arthralgia, myalgia, drug fever, chills, chest discomfort, and anaphylactic reactions.

Central nervous system: headache, giddiness, neuromuscular hyperirritability or convulsive seizures.

Gastro-intestinal disturbances: disturbances of taste and smell, stomatitis, flatulence, nausea, vomiting and diarrhea, epigastric pain.

Hemic and Lymphatic Systems: thrombocytopenia, leukopenia, neutropenia, eosinophilia and reduction of hemoglobin or hematocrit. Prolongation of prothrombin time and bleeding time.

AZLIN® DOSAGE GUIDE FOR PATIENTS WITH IMPAIRED RENAL FUNCTION

Creatinine Clearance ml/min	Urinary Tract Infection (Uncomplicated)	Urinary Tract Infection (Complicated)	Serious Systemic Infection
>30	Usual Recommended Dosage		
10–30	1.5 g every 12 hours	1.5g every 8 hours	2g every 8 hours
<10	1.5 g every 12 hours	2g every 12 hours	3g every 12 hours

Abnormalities of hepatic and renal function tests: elevation of serum aspartate aminotransferase (SGOT), serum alanine aminotransferase (SGPT), serum alkaline phosphatase, serum LDH, serum bilirubin. Elevation of serum creatinine and/or BUN, hypernatremia. Reduction in serum potassium and uric acid.

Local reactions: pain and thrombophlebitis with intravenous administration.

Overdosage: As with other penicillins, AZLIN® in overdosage has the potential to cause neuromuscular hyperirritability or convulsive seizures. Hemodialysis, if necessary, will aid in removal of the drug from the blood.

Dosage and Administration: AZLIN® (sterile azlocillin sodium) may be administered by slow intravenous injection (5 min or longer) or by intravenous infusion (30 min).

The recommended adult dosage for serious infections is 200–300 mg/kg per day given in 4 to 6 divided doses. The usual dose is 3g given every 4 hours (18g/day). For life-threatening infections, up to 350 mg/kg per day may be administered, but the total daily dosage should ordinarily not exceed 24g.

[See table below].

For patients with life-threatening infections, 4g may be administered every 4 hours (24g/day).

Dosage for any individual patient must take into consideration the site and severity of infection, the susceptibility of the organisms causing infection, and the status of the patient's host defense mechanisms.

The duration of therapy depends upon the severity of infection. Generally, AZLIN® should be continued for at least 2 days after the signs and symptoms of infection have disappeared. The usual duration is 10 to 14 days; however, in difficult and complicated infections, more prolonged therapy may be required (e.g., osteomyelitis).

In certain deep-seated infections, involving abscess formation, appropriate surgical drainage should be performed in conjunction with antimicrobial therapy.

Patients with Impaired Renal Function
The rate of elimination of azlocillin is dose dependent and related to the degree of renal function impairment. After an intravenous dose of 5g, the serum half-life is approximately 1 hour in patients with creatinine clearances above 80 ml/min, 2.0 hr in those with clearances of 30–79 ml/min, 4.0 hr in those with clearances of 10–29 ml/min and approximately 5.9 hr in patients with clearances of less than 10 ml/min. Dosage adjustments of AZLIN® are not required in patients with mild impairment of renal function. For patients with a creatinine clearance of ≤ 30 ml/min (serum creatinine of approximately 3.0 mg% or greater), the following dosage guide may be used.

[See table above].

For patients undergoing hemodialysis for renal failure, 3g may be administered after each dialysis and then every 12 hours

For patients with renal failure, particularly those with concomitant hepatic insufficiency, measurement of serum levels of azlocillin will provide additional guidance for adjusting dosage.

Intravenous Administration
AZLIN® may be administered intravenously by intermittent infusion or by direct slow intravenous injection.

Infusion. Each gram of azlocillin should be reconstituted by vigorous shaking with at least 10 ml of Sterile Water for Injection, 5% Dextrose Injection or 0.9% Sodium Chloride Injection. The dissolved drug should be further diluted to desired volume (50-100 ml) with an appropriate intravenous solution. (See Compatibility and Stability section). The solution of reconstituted drug may then be administered over a period of 30 minutes by direct infusion or through a Y-type intravenous infusion set which may already be in place. If this method or the "piggyback" method of administration is used, it is advisable to discontinue temporarily the administration of any other solutions during the infusion of AZLIN®.

Injection. The reconstituted solution of AZLIN® may also be injected directly into a vein or into intravenous tubing; when administered in this way, the injection should be given slowly over a period of 5 minutes or longer. To minimize venous irritation, the concentration of drug should not exceed 10%.

When AZLIN® is given in combination with another antimicrobial, such as an aminoglycoside, each drug should be given separately in accordance with the recommended dosage and routes of administration for each drug.

After reconstitution and prior to administration, AZLIN® as with other parenteral drugs, should be inspected visually for particulate matter and discoloration.

Pediatric Use
Only limited data are available on the safety and effectiveness of AZLIN® in the treatment of infants with documented serious infection. Until further experience is gained, the drug should not be used in the newborn period.

In children with acute pulmonary exacerbation of cystic fibrosis, azlocillin may be administered at a dose of 75 mg/kg every 4 hours (450 mg/kg/day). The total daily dosage should not exceed 24g. The drug may be infused intravenously over a period of about 30 minutes.

Compatibility and Stability: AZLIN® at concentrations of 10 mg/ml and 50 mg/ml is stable (loss of potency less than 10%) when stored at room temperature in the following intravenous solutions for the time periods stated. When stored under refrigeration (below

AZLIN® DOSAGE GUIDE (ADULTS)

Condition	Daily Dosage Range	Usual Daily Dosage	Frequency and Route of Administration
Urinary tract infection (uncomplicated)	100–125 mg/kg	8g	2g every 6 hours IV
Urinary tract infection (complicated)	150–200 mg/kg	12g	3g every 6 hours IV
Lower respiratory tract infection			
Skin & skin structure infection			3g every 4 hours or 4g every 6 hours
Bone & joint infection Septicemia	225–300 mg/kg	16–18g	IV

8°C), AZLIN® at concentrations up to 100 mg/ml is stable for the time periods stated:

INTRAVENOUS SOLUTION	STABILITY
Sterile Water for Injection, U.S.P.	24 hours
0.9% Sodium Chloride Injection, U.S.P.	24 hours
5% Dextrose Injection, U.S.P.	24 hours
5% Dextrose in 0.225% Sodium Chloride Injection, U.S.P.	24 hours
Lactated Ringer's Injection, U.S.P.	24 hours
5% Dextrose in 0.45% Sodium Chloride Injection, U.S.P.	24 hours

Unused portion must be discarded after the time period stated

How Supplied: AZLIN® (sterile azlocillin sodium) is a white to pale yellow powder supplied in vials and infusion bottles. Each vial contains azlocillin sodium equivalent to 2g, 3g or 4g azlocillin. Each infusion bottle contains azlocillin sodium equivalent to 2g, 3g or 4g azlocillin.

AZLIN® vials and infusion bottles should be stored at or below 30°C (86°F). The powder as well as the reconstituted solution of drug may darken slightly, depending upon storage conditions, but potency is not affected.

Issued: June, 1982 PD 100565 18958

CANDEX® Lotion ℞
(nystatin)

Description: Candex® (nystatin) Lotion contains nystatin U.S.P. 100,000 units/ml in a base consisting of carboxy vinyl polymer, sodium lauryl sulfate, hexadecyl alcohol, cetyl alcohol, Dowicil® 200, sodium hydroxide, citric acid, sodium citrate, and purified water.

Actions: Nystatin is effective against Candida species (Monilia).

Indications: Candex® (nystatin) Lotion is indicated for the treatment of cutaneous or mucocutaneous mycotic infections caused by Candida species (Monilia). A lotion is preferred on oozing intertriginous areas.

Contraindications: Lesions caused by pathogens not susceptible to nystatin and hypersensitivity to any of the components.

Precautions: If irritation or sensitivity occurs and/or infection persists, discontinue use. If new infections appear, appropriate therapy should be instituted.

Caution: Federal (U.S.A.) law prohibits dispensing without prescription.

For external use only. Not for ophthalmic use. Store below 86° F. (30° C.), avoid freezing. Shake well.

Dosage and Administration: Apply two or three times daily. Continue use for one week after clinical cure.

How Supplied: Candex® (nystatin) Lotion in 30 ml plastic bottles.

CORT-DOME® ℞
1%, ½%, ¼% and ⅛%
(hydrocortisone)
creme **acid pH**

Description: Cort-Dome® Creme contains microdispersed hydrocortisone (the active ingredient) in a compatible vehicle buffered to the acid pH range of normal skin. Each gram of Cort-Dome® Creme contains 10.0mg/g (1%), 5.0mg/g (½%), 2.5mg/g (¼%) or 1.25 mg/g (⅛%) of hydrocortisone. Cort-Dome® Creme is applied topically. Hydrocortisone is a corticosteroid. Chemically, hydrocortisone is Pregn-4-ene-3, 20-dione,11,17,21-trihydroxy-,(11β)-. with the following structural formula:

[structural formula: CH2OH, C=O, HO, CH3, CH3, OH, O]

The vehicle for Cort-Dome® Creme 1%, ½%, and ¼% contains glycerin, calcium acetate, cetyl-stearyl alcohol-sodium lauryl sulfate, aluminum sulfate, purified water, synthetic beeswax (B-wax), white petrolatum, dextrin, and light mineral oil, preserved with methylparaben. The emollient vehicle for Cort-Dome® Creme ⅛% is composed of isopropyl myristate, cholesterol, white petrolatum, synthetic beeswax (B-wax), stearic acid, polyoxyethylene sorbitan monostearate, sorbitan monostearate, aluminum sulfate, propylene glycol, calcium acetate, dextrin, perfume, and purified water, preserved with methyl and propyl parabens.

EMPIRICAL FORMULA	MOLECULAR WEIGHT	CAS REGISTRY NUMBER
$C_{21}H_{30}O_5$	362.47	50-23-7

Clinical Pharmacology: Topical corticosteroids share anti-inflammatory, anti-pruritic and vasoconstrictive actions.

The mechanism of anti-inflammatory activity of the topical corticosteroids is unclear. Various laboratory methods, including vasoconstrictor assays, are used to compare and predict potencies and/or clinical efficacies of the topical corticosteroids. There is some evidence to suggest that a recognizable correlation exists between vasoconstrictor potency and therapeutic efficacy in man.

Pharmacokinetics

The extent of percutaneous absorption of topical corticosteroids is determined by many factors including the vehicle, the integrity of the epidermal barrier, and the use of occlusive dressings.

Topical corticosteroids can be absorbed from normal intact skin. Inflammation and/or other disease processes in the skin increase percutaneous absorption. Occlusive dressings substantially increase the percutaneous absorption of topical corticosteroids. Thus, occlusive dressings may be a valuable therapeutic adjunct for treatment of resistant dermatoses. (See DOSAGE AND ADMINISTRATION).

Once absorbed through the skin, topical corticosteroids are handled through pharmacokinetic pathways similar to systemically administered corticosteroids. Corticosteroids are bound to plasma proteins in varying degrees. Corticosteroids are metabolized primarily in the liver and are then excreted by the kidneys. Some of the topical corticosteroids and their metabolites are also excreted into the bile.

Indications and Usage: Topical corticosteroids are indicated for the relief of the inflammatory and pruritic manifestations of corticosteroid-responsive dermatoses.

Contraindications: Topical corticosteroids are contraindicated in those patients with a history of hypersensitivity to any of the components of the preparation.

Precautions:

General

Systemic absorption of topical corticosteroids has produced reversible hypothalamic-pituitary-adrenal (HPA) axis suppression, manifestations of Cushing's syndrome, hyperglycemia, and glucosuria in some patients.

Conditions which augment systemic absorption include the application of the more potent steroids, use over large surface areas, prolonged use, and the addition of occlusive dressings.

Therefore, patients receiving a large dose of a potent topical steroid applied to a large surface area or under an occlusive dressing should be evaluated periodically for evidence of HPA axis suppression by using the urinary free cortisol and ACTH stimulation tests. If HPA axis suppression is noted, an attempt should be made to withdraw the drug, to reduce the frequency of application, or to substitute a less potent steroid.

Recovery of HPA axis function is generally prompt and complete upon discontinuation of the drug. Infrequently, signs and symptoms of steroid withdrawal may occur, requiring supplemental systemic corticosteroids.

Children may absorb proportionally larger amounts of topical corticosteroids and thus be more susceptible to systemic toxicity. (See PRECAUTIONS—Pediatric Use).

If irritation develops, topical corticosteroids should be discontinued and appropriate therapy instituted.

In the presence of dermatological infections, the use of an appropriate antifungal or antibacterial agent should be instituted. If a favorable response does not occur promptly, the corticosteroid should be discontinued until the infection has been adequately controlled.

Information for the Patient

Patients using topical corticosteroids should receive the following information and instructions:

1. This medication is to be used as directed by the physician. It is for external use only. Avoid contact with the eyes.
2. Patients should be advised not to use this medication for any disorder other than for which it was prescribed.
3. The treated skin area should not be bandaged or otherwise covered or wrapped as to be occlusive unless directed by the physician.
4. Patients should report any signs of local adverse reactions especially under occlusive dressing.
5. Parents of pediatric patients should be advised not to use tight-fitting diapers or plastic pants on a child being treated in the diaper area, as these garments may constitute occlusive dressings.

Laboratory Tests

The following tests may be helpful in evaluating the HPA axis suppression:

Urinary free cortisol test

ACTH stimulation test

Carcinogenisis, Mutagenisis, and Impairment of Fertility

Long-term animal studies have not been performed to evaluate the carcinogenic potential or the effect on fertility of topical corticosteroids.

Studies to determine mutagenicity with prednisolone and hydrocortisone have revealed negative results.

Pregnancy Category C

Corticosteroids are generally teratogenic in laboratory animals when administered systemically at relatively low-dosage levels. The more potent corticosteroids have been shown to be teratogenic after dermal application in laboratory animals. There are no adequate and well-controlled studies in pregnant women on teratogenic effects from topically applied corticosteroids. Therefore, topical corticosteroids should be used during pregnancy only if the potential benefit justifies the potential risk to the fetus. Drugs of this class should not be used extensively on pregnant patients, in large amounts, or for prolonged periods of time.

Nursing Mothers

It is not known whether topical administration of corticosteroids could result in sufficient systemic absorption to produce detectable quantities in breast milk. Systemically administered corticosteroids are secreted into breast milk in quantities *not* likely to have a deleterious effect on the infant. Nevertheless, caution should be exercised when topical corticosteroids are administered to a nursing woman.

Pediatric Use

Pediatric patients may demonstrate greater susceptibility to topical corticosteroid-induced HPA axis suppression and Cushing's syndrome than mature patients because of a larger skin surface area to body weight ratio.

Hypothalamic-pituitary-adrenal (HPA) axis suppression, Cushing's syndrome, and intracranial hypertension have been reported in children receiving topical corticosteroids. Manifestations of adrenal suppression in children include linear growth retardation,

Continued on next page

Miles Pharm.—Cont.

delayed weight gain, low plasma cortisol levels, and absence of response to ACTH stimulation. Manifestations of intracranial hypertension include bulging fontanelles, headaches, and bilateral papilledema.

Administration of topical corticosteroids to children should be limited to the least amount compatible with an effective therapeutic regimen. Chronic corticosteroid therapy may interfere with the growth and development of children.

Adverse Reactions: The following local adverse reactions are reported infrequently with topical corticosteroids, but may occur more frequently with the use of occlusive dressings. These reactions are listed in an approximate decreasing order of occurrence:

Burning
Itching
Irritation
Dryness
Folliculitis
Hypertrichosis
Acneiform eruptions
Hypopigmentation
Perioral dermatitis
Allergic contact dermatitis
Maceration of the skin
Secondary infection
Skin atrophy
Striae
Miliaria

Overdosage: Topically applied corticosteroids can be absorbed in sufficient amounts to produce systemic effects. (See PRECAUTIONS).

Dosage and Administration: Topical corticosteroids are generally applied to the affected area as a thin film from two to four times daily depending on the severity of the condition.

Occlusive dressings may be used for the management of psoriasis or recalcitrant conditions.

If an infection develops, the use of occlusive dressings should be discontinued and appropriate antimicrobial therapy instituted.

How Supplied: Cort-Dome® (hydrocortisone) Creme ⅛%-1 oz. tube and 4 oz. dispensajar. Cort-Dome® Creme ¼%-1 oz. tube and 4 oz. dispensajar. Cort-Dome® Creme ½%-½ oz. tube, 1 oz tube and 4 oz. Cort-Dome® Creme 1%-½ oz. tube, 1 oz. tube.

Cort-Dome® Creme is a white semi-solid.

Store below 86°F (30°C), avoid freezing.

Caution: Federal (USA) law prohibits dispensing without a prescription.

July, 1982 PD100569 18876

CORT-DOME® ℞
1%, ½%, ¼% and ⅛%
(hydrocortisone)
lotion **acid pH**

Description: Cort-Dome® Lotion contains microdispersed hydrocortisone (the active ingredient) in a compatible vehicle buffered to the acid pH range of normal skin. Each ml of Cort-Dome® Lotion contains 10.0mg/ml (1%). 5.0mg/ml(½%), 2.5mg/ml (¼%) or 1.25mg/ml (⅛%) of hydrocortisone. Cort-Dome® Lotion is applied topically. Hydrocortisone is a corticosteroid. Chemically, hydrocortisone is Pregn-4-ene-3,20-dione,11,17,21-trihydroxy-(11β)-. with the following structural formula:

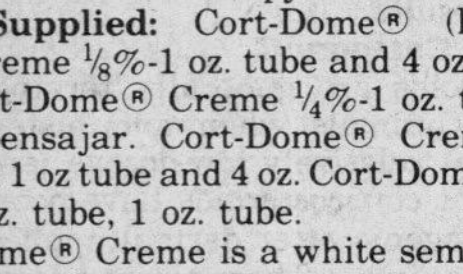

The vehicle for Cort-Dome® Lotion 1%, ½%, ¼% and ⅛% is composed of glyceryl monostearyl, cetyl-stearyl alcohol-sodium lauryl sulfate, butyl stearate, aluminum sulfate, calcium acetate, dextrin, isopropyl myristate, polyoxyethylene sorbitan monolaurate, glycerin, and purified water preserved with methyl and propyl parabens.

EMPIRICAL FORMULA	MOLECULAR WEIGHT	CAS REGISTRY NUMBER
$C_{21}H_{30}O_5$	362.47	50-23-7

Clinical Pharmacology: Topical corticosteroids share anti-inflammatory, anti-pruritic and vasoconstrictive actions.

The mechanism of anti-inflammatory activity of the topical corticosteroids is unclear. Various laboratory methods, including vasoconstrictor assays, are used to compare and predict potencies and/or clinical efficacies of the topical corticosteroids. There is some evidence to suggest that a recognizable correlation exists between vasoconstrictor potency and therapeutic efficacy in man.

Pharmacokinetics

The extent of percutaneous absorption of topical corticosteroids is determined by many factors including the vehicle, the integrity of the epidermal barrier, and the use of occlusive dressings.

Topical corticosteroids can be absorbed from normal intact skin. Inflammation and/or other disease processes in the skin increase percutaneous absorption. Occlusive dressings substantially increase the percutaneous absorption of topical corticosteroids. Thus, occlusive dressings may be a valuable therapeutic adjunct for treatment of resistant dermatoses. (See DOSAGE AND ADMINISTRATION).

Once absorbed through the skin, topical corticosteroids are handled through pharmacokinetic pathways similar to systemically administered corticosteroids. Corticosteroids are bound to plasma proteins in varying degrees. Corticosteroids are metabolized primarily in the liver and are then excreted by the kidneys. Some of the topical corticosteroids and their metabolites are also excreted into the bile.

Indications and Usage: Topical corticosteroids are indicated for the relief of the inflammatory and pruritic manifestations of corticosteroid-responsive dermatoses.

Contraindications: Topical corticosteroids are contraindicated in those patients with a history of hypersensitivity to any of the components of the preparation.

Precautions:

General

Systemic absorption of topical corticosteroids has produced reversible hypothalamic-pituitary-adrenal (HPA) axis suppression, manifestations of Cushing's syndrome, hyperglycemia, and glucosuria in some patients.

Conditions which augment systemic absorption include the application of the more potent steroids, use over large surface areas, prolonged use, and the addition of occlusive dressings.

Therefore, patients receiving a large dose of a potent topical steroid applied to a large surface area or under an occlusive dressing should be evaluated periodically for evidence of HPA axis suppression by using the urinary free cortisol and ACTH stimulation tests. If HPA axis suppression is noted, an attempt should be made to withdraw the drug, to reduce the frequency of application, or to substitute a less potent steroid.

Recovery of HPA axis function is generally prompt and complete upon discontinuation of the drug. Infrequently, signs and symptoms of steroid withdrawal may occur, requiring supplemental systemic corticosteroids.

Children may absorb proportionally larger amounts of topical corticosteroids and thus be more susceptible to systemic toxicity. (See PRECAUTIONS—Pediatric Use).

If irritation develops, topical corticosteroids should be discontinued and appropriate therapy instituted.

In the presence of dermatological infections, the use of an appropriate antifungal or antibacterial agent should be instituted. If a favorable response does not occur promptly, the corticosteroid should be discontinued until the infection has been adequately controlled.

Information for the Patient

Patients using topical corticosteroids should receive the following information and instructions:

1. This medication is to be used as directed by the physician. It is for external use only. Avoid contact with the eyes.
2. Patients should be advised not to use this medication for any disorder other than for which it was prescribed.
3. The treated skin area should not be bandaged or otherwise covered or wrapped as to be occlusive unless directed by the physician.
4. Patients should report any signs of local adverse reactions especially under occlusive dressing.
5. Parents of pediatric patients should be advised not to use tightfitting diapers or plastic pants on a child being treated in the diaper area, as these garments may constitute occlusive dressings.

Laboratory Tests

The following tests may be helpful in evaluating the HPA axis suppression:

Urinary free cortisol test
ACTH stimulation test

Carcinogenisis, Mutagenisis, and Impairment of Fertility

Long-term animal studies have not been performed to evaluate the carcinogenic potential or the effect on fertility of topical corticosteroids.

Studies to determine mutagenicity with prednisolone and hydrocortisone have revealed negative results.

Pregnancy Category C

Corticosteroids are generally teratogenic in laboratory animals when administered systemically at relatively low dosage levels. The more potent corticosteroids have been shown to be teratogenic after dermal application in laboratory animals. There are no adequate and well-controlled studies in pregnant women on teratogenic effects from topically applied corticosteroids. Therefore, topical corticosteroids should be used during pregnancy only if the potential benefit justifies the potential risk to the fetus. Drugs of this class should not be used extensively on pregnant patients, in large amounts, or for prolonged periods of time.

Nursing Mothers

It is not known whether topical administration of corticosteroids could result in sufficient systemic absorption to produce detectable quantities in breast milk. Systemically administered corticosteroids are secreted into breast milk in quantities *not* likely to have a deleterious effect on the infant. Nevertheless, caution should be exercised when topical corticosteroids are administered to a nursing woman.

Pediatric Use

Pediatric patients may demonstrate greater susceptibility to topical corticosteroid-induced HPA axis suppression and Cushing's syndrome than mature patients because of a larger skin surface area to body weight ratio.

Hypothalamic-pituitary-adrenal (HPA) axis suppression, Cushing's syndrome, and intracranial hypertension have been reported in children receiving topical corticosteroids. Manifestations of adrenal suppression in children include linear growth retardation, delayed weight gain, low plasma cortisol levels, and absence of response to ACTH stimulation. Manifestations of intracranial hypertension include bulging fontaneiles, headaches, and bilateral papilledema.

Administration of topical corticosteroids to children should be limited to the least amount compatible with an effective therapeutic regimen. Chronic corticosteroid therapy may interfere with the growth and development of children.

Adverse Reactions: The following local adverse reactions are reported infrequently with topical corticosteroids, but may occur more frequently with the use of occlusive dressings. These reactions are listed in an approximate decreasing order of occurrence:
Burning
Itching
Irritation
Dryness
Folliculitis
Hypertrichosis
Acneiform eruptions
Hypopigmentation
Perioral dermatitis
Allergic contact dermatitis
Maceration of the skin
Secondary infection
Skin atrophy
Striae
Miliaria
Overdosage: Topically applied corticosteroids can be absorbed in sufficient amounts to produce systemic effects. (See PRECAUTIONS).
Dosage and Administration: Topical corticosteroids are generally applied to the affected area as a thin film from two to four times daily depending on the severity of the condition.
Occlusive dressings may be used for the management of psoriasis or recalcitrant conditions. In an infection develops, the use of occlusive dressings should be discontinued and appropriate antimicrobial therapy instituted.
How Supplied: Cort-Dome® (hydrocortisone) Lotion 1/8%-6 fl. oz. bottle, Cort-Dome® Lotion 1/4%-4 fl. oz. bottles. Cort-Dome® Lotion 1/2%-4 fl. oz. bottles. Cort-Dome® Lotion 1%-1/2 oz. and 1 fl. oz. bottles.
Cort-Dome® Lotion is a white semi-fluid liquid.
Store below 86°F (30°C), avoid freezing.
Caution: Federal (USA) law prohibits dispensing without a prescription.
July, 1982 PD100570 18872

CORT-DOME® Suppositories ℞
(hydrocortisone acetate)

Composition: Regular: 15 mg. hydrocortisone acetate. High Potency: 25 mg. hydrocortisone acetate. Both are incorporated in a monoglyceride base.
Indications: For use in inflamed hemorrhoids, postirradiation (factitial) proctitis; as an adjunct in the treatment of chronic ulcerative colitis; cryptitis; other inflammatory conditions of anorectum; and pruritus ani.
Contraindications: Cort-Dome Suppositories are contraindicated in those patients with a history of hypersensitivity to any of the components.
Precautions: Do not use unless adequate proctologic examination is made.
If irritation develops, the product should be discontinued and appropriate therapy instituted. In the presence of an infection the use of an appropriate antifungal or antibacterial agent should be instituted. If a favorable response does not occur promptly, the corticosteroid should be discontinued until the infection has been adequately controlled.
Although topical steroids have not been reported to have an adverse effect on human pregnancy, the safety of their use in pregnant women has not absolutely been established. In laboratory animals, increases in incidence of fetal abnormalities have been associated with exposure of gestating females to topical corticosteroids, in some cases at rather low dosage levels. Therefore, drugs of this class should not be used extensively on pregnant patients in large amounts, or for prolonged periods of time.
Adverse Reactions: The following local adverse reactions have been reported with corticosteroids suppositories:

1. Burning
2. Itching
3. Irritation
4. Dryness
5. Folliculitis
6. Hypopigmentation
7. Allergic Contact Dermatitis
8. Secondary Infection

Caution: Federal (U.S.A.) law prohibits dispensing without prescription. Store below 86°F (30°C), avoid freezing.
Dosage and Administration: One suppository inserted in the rectum twice daily, morning and night for two weeks, in nonspecific proctitis. In more severe cases, one suppository three times daily; or, two suppositories twice daily. In factitial proctitis, recommended duration of therapy is six to eight weeks or less, according to response of individual case.
How Supplied: Boxes of 12.

DECHOLIN® Tablets
(dehydrocholic acid)

Composition: Dehydrocholic acid 250 mg. contained in each tablet.
Indications: For the temporary relief of constipation.
Average Adult Dose: One or two tablets, three times daily or as directed by physician.
Warning: Do not use when abdominal pain, nausea or vomiting are present. Frequent use of this preparation may result in dependence on laxatives.
Store at controlled room temperature (59°–86°F.).
KEEP THIS AND ALL MEDICATIONS OUT OF THE REACH OF CHILDREN.
How Supplied: White tablets coded with number 121-Miles in bottles of 100 and 500.
[*Shown in Product Identification Section*]

DOMEBORO® Powder Packets, Effervescent Tablets (acid pH)
Astringent Wet Dressing

One packet or tablet dissolved in a pint of water makes a modified Burow's Solution approximately equivalent to a 1:40 dilution, two packets or tablets a 1:20 dilution, and four packets or tablets a 1:10 dilution.
Buffered to an acid pH.
Contains: Aluminum sulfate and calcium acetate.
Indications: A soothing wet dressing for relief of inflammatory conditions of the skin such as insect bites, poison ivy, swellings and bruises or athlete's foot.
Directions: Dissolve one or two packets or tablets in a pint (large glass) of water and stir. When the powder disperses, shake resulting mixture. Do not strain or filter. Bandage the site of application loosely. Pour mixture on bandage every 15 to 30 minutes to keep dressing moist. Continue for 4 to 8 hours unless otherwise directed by physician. Do not use plastic or other impervious material to prevent evaporation without consulting your physician.
Caution: Keep away from eyes. For external use only. Store below 86°F. (30°C.), avoid freezing. Material in diluted form may be stored for 7 days at room temperature.
How Supplied:
Powder Packets: Boxes of 12 and 100. Each packet contains 2.2 gm. Individually foil-wrapped *Tablets:* Boxes of 12, 100 and 1000. White tablets coded with number 411-Miles.
[*Shown in Product Identification Section*]

DOME-PASTE® Bandage
3″ and 4″ Bandages
(Medicated Bandage for Leg or Arm, Improved Unna's boot)

Composition: Each medicated bandage is impregnated with zinc oxide, calamine and gelatin. No heating or painting necessary.
Indications: For those conditions of the extremities (e.g. varicose veins and associated ulcers, stasis edema, thrombophlebitis, lymphangitis).
Caution: If skin sensitivity or irritation develops discontinue use and consult a physician.
Administration and Dosage: Detailed instructions for application are supplied on each carton.
How Supplied: 3″ and 4″ cotton bandage by 360″ (10 yd.). Each carton contains one medicated bandage in polyethylene bag.

DOMOL® Bath and Shower Oil
(diisopropyl sebacate, isopropyl myristate)

Composition: Contains sebacate*, a special skin moisturizing agent, refined mineral oil and skin softener.
*Diisopropyl sebacate.
Action and Uses: Effective, pleasant way to lubricate skin and relieve itchy discomfort. It lubricates skin and restores the protective action of skin oils washed away by soaps and detergents. DOMOL helps maintain skin's normal condition by retarding evaporation of skin's moisture.
Directions for Use:
Bath—Add 1 or 2 capfuls to bathtub or water. Soak for 10-20 minutes.
Shower—Pour 1 capful on wet sponge or washcloth. Rub gently over body, rinse under shower.
Infant's Bath—Add 1 capful to basin or bathinette of water.
Sponge Bath—Add 1 or 2 capfuls to about a pint of water. Sponge body gently with washcloth or cellulose sponge. After bathing the skin should be patted dry rather than rubbed.
How Supplied: 8 fl. oz. unbreakable plastic bottle.

DTIC–Dome® ℞
(dacarbazine)
Sterile

Warning: It is recommended that DTIC-Dome (dacarbazine) be administered under the supervision of a qualified physician experienced in the use of cancer chemotherapeutic agents.
1. Hemopoietic depression is the most common toxicity with DTIC-Dome (See Warnings).
2. Hepatic necrosis has been reported (See Warnings).
3. Studies have demonstrated this agent to have a carcinogenic and teratogenic effect when used in animals.
4. In treatment of each patient, the physician must weigh carefully the possibility of achieving therapeutic benefit against the risk of toxicity.

Description: DTIC-Dome Sterile (dacarbazine) is a colorless to an ivory colored solid which is light sensitive. Each vial contains 100mg of dacarbazine, or 200mg of dacarbazine (the active ingredient), anhydrous citric acid and mannitol. DTIC-Dome is reconstituted and administered intravenously (pH 3-4) DTIC-Dome is an anticancer agent. Chemically, DTIC-Dome is 5-(3, 3-dimethyl-l-triazeno)-imidazole-4-carboxamide (DTIC).
Clinical Pharmacology: After intravenous administration of DTIC-Dome, the volume of distribution exceeds total body water content suggesting localization in some body tissue, probably the liver. Its disappearance from the plasma is biphasic with initial half-life of 19 minutes and a terminal half-life of 5 hours. In a patient with renal and hepatic dysfunctions, the half-lives were lengthened to 55 minutes and 7.2 hours. The average cumulative excre-

Continued on next page

Miles Pharm.—Cont.

tion of unchanged DTIC in the urine is 40% of the injected dose in 6 hours. DTIC is subject to renal tubular secretion rather than glomerular filtration. At therapeutic concentrations DTIC is not appreciably bound to human plasma protein.
In man, DTIC is extensively degraded. Besides unchanged DTIC, 5-aminoimidazole -4 carboxamide (AIC) is a major metabolite of DTIC excreted in the urine. AIC is not derived endogenously but from the injected DTIC, because the administration of radioactive DTIC labeled with ^{14}C in the imidazole portion of the molecule (DTIC-2-^{14}C) gives rise to AIC-2-^{14}C.
Although the exact mechanism of action of DTIC-Dome is not known, three hypotheses have been offered:
1. inhibition of DNA synthesis by acting as a purine analog
2. action as an alkylating agent
3. interaction with SH groups

Indications and Usage: DTIC-Dome is indicated in the treatment of metastatic malignant melanoma. In addition, DTIC-Dome is also indicated for Hodgkin's disease as a second-line therapy when used in combination with other effective agents.
Contraindications: DTIC-Dome is contraindicated in patients who have demonstrated a hypersensitivity to it in the past.
Warnings: Hemopoietic depression is the most common toxicity with DTIC-Dome and involves primarily the leukocytes and platelets, although, anemia may sometimes occur. Leukopenia and thrombocytopenia may be severe enough to cause death. The possible bone marrow depression requires careful monitoring of white blood cells, red blood cells, and platelet levels. Hemopoietic toxicity may warrant temporary suspension or cessation of therapy with DTIC-Dome.
Hepatic toxicity accompanied by hepatic vein thrombosis and hepatocellular necrosis resulting in death, has been reported. The incidence of such reactions has been low; approximately 0.01% of patients treated. This toxicity has been observed mostly when DTIC-Dome has been administered concomitantly with other anti-neoplastic drugs; however, it has also been reported in some patients treated with DTIC-Dome alone.
Anaphylaxis can occur following the administration of DTIC-Dome.
Precautions: Hospitalization is not always necessary but adequate laboratory study capability must be available. Extravasation of the drug subcutaneously during intravenous administration may result in tissue damage and severe pain. Local pain, burning sensation, and irritation at the site of injection may be relieved by locally applied hot packs.
Carcinogenicity of DTIC was studied in rats and mice. Proliferative endocardial lesions, including fibrosarcomas and sarcomas were induced by DTIC in rats. In mice, administration of DTIC resulted in the induction of angiosarcomas of the spleen.
Pregnancy Category C—DTIC-Dome has been shown to be teratogenic in rats when given in doses 20 times the human daily dose on day 12 of gestation. DTIC when administered in 10 times the human daily dose to male rats (twice weekly for 9 weeks) did not affect the male libido, although female rats mated to male rats had higher incidence of resorptions than controls. In rabbits, DTIC daily dose 7 times the human daily dose given on Days 6–15 of gestation resulted in fetal skeletal anomalies. There are no adequate and well controlled studies in pregnant women. DTIC-Dome should be used during pregnancy only if the potential benefit justifies the potential risk to the fetus.
It is not known whether this drug is excreted in human milk. Because many drugs are excreted in human milk and because of the potential for tumorigenicity shown for DTIC-Dome in animal studies, a decision should be made whether to discontinue nursing or to discontinue the drug, taking into account the importance of the drug to the mother.
Adverse Reactions: Symptoms of anorexia, nausea, and vomiting are the most frequently noted of all toxic reactions. Over 90% of patients are affected with the initial few doses. The vomiting lasts 1–12 hours and is incompletely and unpredictably palliated with phenobarbital and/or prochlorperazine. Rarely, intractable nausea and vomiting have necessitated discontinuance of therapy with DTIC-Dome. Rarely, DTIC-Dome has caused diarrhea. Some helpful suggestions include restricting the patient's oral intake of food for 4–6 hours prior to treatment. The rapid toleration of these symptoms suggests that a central nervous system mechanism may be involved, and usually these symptoms subside after the first 1 or 2 days.
There are a number of minor toxicities that are infrequently noted. Patients have experienced an influenza-like syndrome of fever to 39°C, myalgias and malaise. These symptoms occur usually after large single doses, may last for several days, and they may occur with successive treatments.
Alopecia has been noted as has facial flushing and facial paresthesia. There have been few reports of significant liver or renal function test abnormalities in man. However, these abnormalities have been observed more frequently in animal studies.
Erythematous and urticarial rashes have been observed infrequently after administration of DTIC-Dome. Rarely, photosensitivity reactions may occur.

Overdosage: Give supportive treatment and monitor blood cell counts.
Dosage and Administration: MALIGNANT MELANOMA—The recommended dosage is 2 to 4.5mg/kg/day for 10 days. Treatment may be repeated at 4 week intervals.
An alternate recommended dosage is 250mg/square meter body surface/day I.V. for 5 days. Treatment may be repeated every 3 weeks.
HODGKIN'S DISEASE: The recommended dosage of DTIC-Dome in the treatment of Hodgkin's Disease is 150mg/square meter body surface/day for 5 days, in combination with other effective drugs. Treatment may be repeated every 4 weeks. An alternative recommended dosage is 375mg/square meter body surface on day 1, in combination with other effective drugs, to be repeated every 15 days.
DTIC-Dome (dacarbazine) 100mg/vial and 200mg/vial are reconstituted with 9.9 ml and 19.7 ml, respectively, of Sterile Water for Injection, U.S.P. The resulting solution contains 10mg/ml of dacarbazine having a pH of 3.0 to 4.0. The calculated dose of the resulting solution is drawn into a syringe and administered *only* intravenously.
The reconstituted solution may be further diluted with 5% dextrose injection, U.S.P. or sodium chloride injection, U.S.P. and administered as an intravenous infusion.
After reconstitution and prior to use, the solution in the vial may be stored at 4°C for up to 72 hours or at normal room conditions (temperature and light) for up to 8 hours. If the reconstituted solution is further diluted in 5% dextrose, injection, U.S.P. or sodium chloride injection, U.S.P., the resulting solution may be stored at 4°C for up to 24 hours or at normal room conditions for up to 8 hours.
How Supplied: 10 ml vials containing 100mg or 20 ml vials containing 200 mg of DTIC-Dome as sterile dacarbazine in boxes of 12.
Manufactured by:
Ben Venue Laboratories
Bedford, Ohio 44146
Distributed by:
Miles Pharmaceuticals
Division of Miles Laboratories, Inc.
West Haven, Connecticut 06516 USA
PD100546 October 1981 18265

EXZIT® Medicated Cleanser
(acid pH)
(colloidal sulfur, salicylic acid)

Contains: Effective anti-acne medications: colloidal sulfur—to dry excess skin oils; salicylic acid—to peel away dead skin tissue.
Indication: Medicated skin cleanser as an aid in the treatment of acne.
Directions: Use twice daily, preferably in the morning and at bedtime. Wet the skin. Apply the cleanser to moist sponge. Work into lather. Massage for five minutes. Rinse.
Warnings: If excessive drying or skin irritation develops or increases, discontinue use and consult physician. For external use only. Avoid contact with eyes. Keep out of reach of children. Store below 86°F. (30°C.), avoid freezing.
How Supplied: Net weight 4 oz (114 g) in the exclusive **Dome Dispensajar**® with its "personal washcloth"—an applicator sponge so fingers never touch the cleanser. The DISPENSAJAR contains over 4 oz by weight to deliver a full 4 oz through the DISPENSAJAR disc.

EXZIT® Medicated Creme and Lotion
(acid pH)
(colloidal sulfur, resorcinal)

Contains: Colloidal sulfur and resorcinol in a compatible vehicle adjusted to the pH range for normal skin.
Indications: Creme—as an aid in drying and peeling acne blemishes. Lotion—as a colorless aid in drying and peeling blemishes in acne and related skin conditions.
Directions: Wash affected parts thoroughly, then dry. Apply creme or lotion sparingly twice daily, preferably in the morning and at bedtime. Follow advice of physician as to diet or other treatment.
Caution: If excessive drying or skin irritation develops or increases, discontinue use and consult physician. For external use only. Avoid contact with eyes. Keep out of reach of children. Store below 86°F. (30°C.), avoid freezing.
How Supplied: Creme—1 oz tube (28.4 g); Lotion—2 fl oz (60 cc).

LITHANE® ℞
(lithium carbonate)
TABLETS
For Control of Manic Episodes in Manic-Depressive Psychosis

Warning

Lithium toxicity is closely related to serum lithium levels, and can occur at doses close to therapeutic levels. Facilities for prompt and accurate serum lithium determinations should be available before initiating therapy.

Description: Lithium carbonate is a white, light, alkaline powder with molecular formula Li_2CO_3 and molecular weight 73.89. Lithium is an element of the alkali-metal group with atomic number 3, atomic weight 6.94, and an emission line at 671 nm on the flame photometer.
Actions: Preclinical studies have shown that lithium alters sodium transport in nerve and muscle cells and effects a shift toward intraneuronal metabolism of catecholamines, but the specific biochemical mechanism of lithium action in mania is unknown.
Indications: Lithium carbonate is indicated in the treatment of manic episodes of manic-depressive illness. Maintenance therapy prevents or diminishes the intensity of subsequent episodes in those manic-depressive patients with a history of mania.

Typical symptoms of mania include pressure of speech, motor hyperactivity, reduced need for sleep, flight of ideas, grandiosity, elation, poor judgment, aggressiveness, and possibly hostility. When given to a patient experiencing a manic episode, lithium may produce a normalization of symptomatology within 1 to 3 weeks.

Warnings: Lithium should generally not be given to patients with significant renal or cardiovascular disease, severe debilitation or dehydration, or sodium depletion, and to patients receiving diuretics, since the risk of lithium toxicity is very high in such patients. If the psychiatric indication is life-threatening, and if such a patient fails to respond to other measures, lithium treatment may be undertaken with extreme caution, including daily serum lithium determinations and adjustment to the usually low doses ordinarily tolerated by these individuals. In such instances, hospitalization is a necessity.

Lithium therapy has been reported in some cases to be associated with morphologic changes in the kidneys. The relationship between such changes and renal function has not been established.

An encephalopathic syndrome (characterized by weakness, lethargy, fever, tremulousness and confusion, extrapyramidal symptoms, leukocytosis, elevated serum enzymes, BUN and FBS) followed by irreversible brain damage has occurred in a few patients treated with lithium plus haloperidol. A causal relationship between these events and the concomitant administration of lithium and haloperidol has not been established; however, patients receiving such combined therapy should be monitored closely for early evidence of neurologic toxicity and treatment discontinued promptly if such signs appear. The possibility of similar adverse interactions with other antipsychotic medication exists.

Lithium toxicity is closely related to serum lithium levels, and can occur at doses close to therapeutic levels (see DOSAGE AND ADMINISTRATION).

Outpatients and their families should be warned that the patient must discontinue lithium carbonate therapy and contact his physician if such clinical signs of lithium toxicity as diarrhea, vomiting, tremor, mild ataxia, drowsiness, or muscular weakness occur.

Lithium carbonate may impair mental and/or physical abilities. Caution patients about activities requiring alertness (e.g., operating vehicles or machinery).

Lithium may prolong the effects of neuromuscular blocking agents. Therefore, neuromuscular blocking agents should be given with caution to patients receiving lithium.

Usage in Pregnancy: Adverse effects on nidation in rats, embryo viability in mice, and metabolism *in vitro* of rat testis and human spermatozoa have been attributed to lithium, as have teratogenicity in submammalian species and cleft palates in mice. Studies in rats, rabbits, and monkeys have shown no evidence of lithium-induced teratology.

There are lithium birth registries in the United States and elsewhere; however there is at the present time insufficient data to determine the effects of lithium carbonate on human fetuses. Therefore, at this point, lithium should not be used in pregnancy, especially the first trimester, unless in the opinion of the physician, the potential benefits outweigh the possible hazards.

Usage in Nursing Mothers: Lithium is excreted in human milk. Nursing should not be undertaken during lithium therapy except in rare and unusual circumstances where, in the view of the physician, the potential benefits to the mother outweigh possible hazards to the child.

Usage in Children: Since information regarding the safety and effectiveness of lithium carbonate in children under 12 years of age is not available, its use in such patients is not recommended at this time.

Precautions: The ability to tolerate lithium is greater during the acute manic phase and decreases when manic symptoms subside (see DOSAGE AND ADMINISTRATION).

The distribution space of lithium approximates that of total body water. Lithium is primarily excreted in urine with insignificant excretion in feces. Renal excretion of lithium is proportional to its plasma concentration. The half-life of elimination of lithium is approximately 24 hours. Lithium decreases sodium reabsorption by the renal tubules which could lead to sodium depletion. Therefore, it is essential for the patient to maintain a normal diet, including salt, and an adequate fluid intake (2500–3000 ml) at least during the initial stabilization period. Decreased tolerance to lithium has been reported to ensue from protracted sweating or diarrhea and, if such occur, supplemental fluid and salt should be administered.

In addition to sweating and diarrhea, concomitant infection with elevated temperatures may also necessitate a temporary reduction or cessation of medication.

Previously existing underlying thyroid disorders do not necessarily constitute a contraindication to lithium treatment; where hypothyroidism exists, careful monitoring of thyroid function during lithium stabilization and maintenance allows for correction of changing thyroid parameters, if any; where hypothroidism occurs during lithium stabilization and maintenance, supplemental thyroid treatment may be used.

This product contains FD&C Yellow No. 5 (tartrazine) which may cause allergic-type reactions (including bronchial asthma) in certain susceptible individuals. Although the over-all incidence of FD&C Yellow No. 5 (tartrazine) sensitivity in the general population is low, it is frequently seen in patients who also have aspirin hypersensitivity.

Adverse Reactions: Adverse reactions are seldom encountered at serum lithium levels below 1.5 mEq./l., except in the occasional patient sensitive to lithium. Mild to moderate toxic reactions may occur at levels from 1.5–2.5 mEq./l., and moderate to severe reactions may be seen at levels from 2.0–2.5 mEq./l., depending upon individual response to the drug.

Fine hand tremor, polyuria, and mild thirst may occur during initial therapy for the acute manic phase, and may persist throughout treatment. Transient and mild nausea and general discomfort may also appear during the first few days of lithium administration.

These side effects are an inconvenience rather than a disabling condition, and usually subside with continued treatment or a temporary reduction or cessation of dosage. If persistent, a cessation of dosage is indicated.

Diarrhea, vomiting, drowsiness, muscular weakness, and lack of coordination may be early signs of lithium intoxication, and can occur at lithium levels below 2.0 mEq./l. At higher levels, giddiness, ataxia, blurred vision, tinnitus, and a large output of dilute urine may be seen. Serum lithium levels above 3.0 mEq./l. may produce a complex clinical picture involving multiple organs and organ systems. Serum lithium levels should not be permitted to exceed 2.0 mEq./l, during the acute treatment phase.

The following reactions have been reported and appear to be related to serum lithium levels, including levels within the therapeutic range:

Neuromuscular: tremor, muscle hyperirritability (fasciculations, twitching, clonic movements of whole limbs), ataxia, choreo-athetotic movements, hyperactive deep tendon reflexes.

Central Nervous System: blackout spells, epileptiform seizures, slurred speech, dizziness, vertigo, incontinence of urine or feces, somnolence, psychomotor retardation, restlessness, confusion stupor, coma.

Cardiovascular: cardiac arrhythmia, hypotension, peripheral circulatory collapse.

Gastrointestinal: anorexia, nausea, vomiting, diarrhea.

Genitourinary: albuminuria, oliguria, polyuria, glycosuria.

Dermatologic: drying and thinning of hair, anesthesia of skin, chronic folliculitis, xerosis cutis, alopecia, and exacerbation of psoriasis.

Autonomic Nervous System: blurred vision, dry mouth.

Thyroid Abnormalities: Euthyroid goiter and/or hypothyroidism (including myxedema) accompanied by lower T_3 and T_4. I^{131} iodine uptake may be elevated. (See Precautions.) Paradoxically, rare cases of hyperthroidism have been reported.

EEG. Changes: diffuse slowing, widening of frequency spectrum, potentiation and disorganization of background rhythm.

EKG. Changes: reversible flattening, isoelectricity or inversion of T-waves.

Miscellaneous: fatigue, lethargy, tendency to sleep, dehydration, weight loss, transient scotomata.

Miscellaneous reactions unrelated to dosage are: transient electroencephalographic and electrocardiographic changes, leucocytosis, headache, diffuse non-toxic goiter with or without hypothyroidism, transient hyperglycemia, generalized pruritus with or without rash, cutaneous ulcers, albuminuria, worsening of organic brain syndromes, excessive weight gain, edematous swelling of ankles or wrists, and thirst or polyuria, sometimes resembling diabetes insipidus, and metallic taste. A single report has been received of the development of painful discoloration of fingers and toes and coldness of the extremities within one day of the starting of treatment of lithium. The mechanism through which these symptoms (resembling Raynaud's Syndrome) developed is not known. Recovery followed discontinuance.

Dosage and Administration:

Acute Mania: Optimal patient response to lithium carbonate usually can be established and maintained with 600 mg t.i.d. Such doses will normally produce an effective serum lithium level ranging between 1.0 and 1.5 mEq./l. Dosage must be individualized according to serum levels and clinical response. Regular monitoring of the patient's clinical state and of serum lithium levels is necessary. Serum levels should be determined twice per week during the acute phase, and until the serum level and clinical condition of the patient have been stabilized.

Long term Control: The desirable lithium levels are 0.6 to 1.2 mEq./l. Dosage will vary from one individual to another, but usually 300 mg t.i.d. or q.i.d. will maintain this level. Serum lithium levels in uncomplicated cases receiving maintenance therapy during remission should be monitored at least every two months.

Patients abnormally sensitive to lithium may exhibit toxic signs at serum levels of 1.0 to 1.5 mEq./l. Elderly patients often respond to reduced dosage, and may exhibit signs of toxicity at serum levels ordinarily tolerated by other patients.

N.B.: Blood samples for serum lithium determinations should be drawn immediately prior to the next dose when lithium concentrations are relatively stable (i.e., 8–12 hours after the previous dose). Total reliance must not be placed on serum levels alone. Accurate patient evaluation requires both clinical and laboratory analysis.

Overdosage: The toxic levels for lithium are close to the therapeutic levels. It is therefore important that patients and their families be cautioned to watch for early toxic symptoms and to discontinue the drug and inform the physician should they occur. Toxic symptoms

Continued on next page

MEZLOCILLIN SERUM LEVELS IN ADULTS (mcg/ml) 2–5 MIN IV INJECTION

DOSE	0	15 min	30 min	45 min	1 hr	2 hr	3 hr	4 hr	6 hr
4g	—	**254** (155–400)	**163** (99–260)	**122** (78–215)	**93** (67–133)	**47** (22–96)	**20** (8–45)	**9.1** (6–13)	**8.4** (5–17)

Miles Pharm.—Cont.

are listed in detail under ADVERSE REACTIONS.

Treatment: No specific antidote for lithium poisoning is known. Early symptoms of lithium toxicity can usually be treated by reduction or cessation of dosage of the drug and resumption of the treatment at a lower dose after 24 to 48 hours. In severe cases of lithium poisoning, the first and foremost goal of treatment consists of elimination of this ion from the organism.

Treatment is essentially the same as that used in barbiturate poisoning: 1) lavage, 2) correction of fluid and electrolyte imbalance, and 3) regulation of kidney functioning. Urea, mannitol, and aminophylline all produce significant increases in lithium excretion. Hemodialysis is an effective and rapid means of removing the ion from the severely toxic patient. Infection prophylaxis, regular chest X-rays, and preservation of adequate respiration are essential.

How Supplied: Lithane (lithium carbonate) is available as scored tablets, coded with the word "Miles" and number 951, containing 300 mg of lithium carbonate in bottles of 100 and 1000.

PD101501 Revised July 1982

©1980, Miles Laboratories, Inc.

[*Shown in Product Identification Section*]

MEZLIN® ℞

(sterile mezlocillin sodium)
for intravenous or intramuscular use.

Description: MEZLIN® (sterile mezlocillin sodium) is a semisynthetic broad spectrum penicillin antibiotic for parenteral administration. It is the monohydrate sodium salt of 6-{D-2 [3-(methyl-sulfonyl)-2-OXO-imidazolidine-1-carboxamido]-2-phenyl-acetamido} penicillanic acid.

Structural Formula:

Empirical Formula: $C_{21}H_{24}N_5O_8S_2Na \cdot H_2O$

MEZLIN® has a molecular weight of 579.6 and contains 42.6 mg (1.85 mEq) of sodium per one gram of mezlocillin activity. The dosage form is supplied as a sterile white to pale yellow crystalline powder, which is freely soluble in water. When reconstituted, solutions of MEZLIN® are clear and range from colorless to pale yellow with a pH of 4.5 to 8.0.

Clinical Pharmacology: Intravenous Administration. In healthy adult volunteers, mean serum levels of mezlocillin 5 minutes after a 5-minute intravenous injection of 1g, 2g, or 5g are 100, 253 or 411 mcg/ml, respectively. Serum levels, as noted below, lack dose proportionality.

[See table below].

Fifteen minutes after a 4g intravenous injection (2–5 min), the concentration in serum is 254 mcg/ml; 1 hour and 4 hours later levels are 93 mcg/ml and 9.1 mcg/ml, respectively:

[See table above].

After an intravenous infusion (15 min) of 3g, mean levels 15 minutes after dosing are 269 mcg/ml (170–280).

A 30-minute intravenous infusion of 3g produces mean peak concentrations of 263 mcg/ml; 1 hour and 4 hours later the concentrations are 57 mcg/ml and 4.4 mcg/ml, respectively:

[See table on next page].

Following intravenous infusion (2 hr) of a 3g dose of mezlocillin every 4 hours for 7 days, mean peak serum concentrations are higher than 100 mcg/ml, and levels above 50 mcg/ml are maintained throughout dosing.

Intramuscular Administration. MEZLIN® is rapidly absorbed after intramuscular injection. In healthy volunteers, the mean peak serum concentration occurs approximately 45 minutes after a single dose of 1g and is about 15 mcg/ml. The oral administration of 1g probenecid before injection produces an increase in mezlocillin serum levels of about 50%. After repetitive intramuscular doses of 1g mezlocillin every 6 hours, peak levels in the serum generally range between 35 and 45 mcg/ml. The relationship between the pharmacokinetics of intramuscular and intravenous dosing has not yet been clearly established.

General. As with other penicillins, mezlocillin is excreted primarily by glomerular filtration and tubular secretion. The rate of elimination is dose dependent and related to the degree of renal functional impairment. In patients with normal renal function, approximately 55% of the administered dose is recovered from the urine within the first 6 hours after dosing. Two hours after an intravenous injection of 2g, concentrations of active drug in urine generally exceed 4000 mcg/ml. By 4–6 hours after injection, concentrations usually decline to a range of about 50 to 200 mcg/ml. The serum elimination half-life of mezlocillin after intravenous dosing is approximately 55 minutes.

In patients with reduced renal function, the half-life is only slightly prolonged. Dosage adjustments are usually not necessary except in patients with severe renal impairment. (See Dosage and Administration). As with other penicillins, mezlocillin is metabolized only slightly; less than 10% of the drug excreted in the urine is in the form of the penicilloate or penilloate. The drug is readily removed from the serum by hemodialysis and, to a lesser extent, by peritoneal dialysis.

Up to 26% of a dose of mezlocillin is recovered from the bile of patients with normal liver function. Following intravenous doses of 2 to 5g, concentrations of active drug in bile generally range from 500 to 2500 mcg/ml. The biliary excretion of mezlocillin is reduced in patients with common bile duct obstruction.

Mezlocillin is not appreciably absorbed when given orally. Following parenteral administration, the apparent volume of distribution is approximately equal to the extracellular fluid volume. The drug is present in active form in the serum, urine, bile, peritoneal fluid, pleural fluid, bronchial and wound secretions, bone and other tissues. As with other penicillins, penetration into the cerebrospinal fluid (CSF) is generally poor, however higher CSF concentrations are obtained in the presence of meningeal inflammation.

Protein binding studies indicate that the degree of mezlocillin binding is low (16–42%) and depends upon testing methods and concentrations of drug studied.

Microbiology

Mezlocillin is a bactericidal antibiotic which acts by interfering with synthesis of cell wall components. It is active against a variety of gram-negative and gram-positive bacteria, including aerobic and anaerobic strains. Mezlocillin is usually active *in vitro* against most strains of the following organisms:

Gram-negative bacteria

Escherichia coli	*Klebsiella* species (including *K. pneumoniae*)
Proteus mirabilis	*Enterobacter* species
Proteus vulgaris	*Shigella* species*
Morganella morganii (formerly *P. morganii*)	*Pseudomonas aeruginosa* (*and other species*)
Providencia rettgeri (formerly *Proteus rettgeri*)	*Haemophilus influenzae*
Providencia stuartii	*Haemophilus parainfluenzae*
Citrobacter species*	*Neisseria* species

Many strains of *Serratia, Salmonella**, and *Acinetobacter** are also susceptible.

Gram-positive bacteria

Staphylococcus aureus (non-penicillinase producing strains)
Beta-hemolytic *streptococci* (Groups A and B)
Streptococcus pneumoniae (formerly *Diplococcus pneumoniae*)
Streptococcus faecalis (enterococcus)

Anaerobic Organisms

Peptococcus species	*Fusobacterium* species*
Peptostreptococcus species	*Veillonella* species*
Clostridium species*	*Eubacterium* species*

Bacteroides species (including *B. fragilis* group)

*Mezlocillin has been shown to be active *in vitro* against these organisms, however clinical efficacy has not yet been established.

Noteworthy is mezlocillin's broadened spectrum of *in vitro* activity against important pathogenic aerobic gram-negative bacteria, including strains of *Pseudomonas, Klebsiella, Enterobacter, Serratia, Proteus, Escherichia* and *Haemophilus*, as well as *Bacteroides* and other anaerobes; and its excellent inhibitory effect against gram-positive organisms including *Streptococcus faecalis* (enterococcus). It is inactive against penicillinase-producing strains of *Staphylococcus aureus*.

In vitro studies have shown that mezlocillin combined with an aminoglycoside (e.g., gentamicin, tobramycin, amikacin, sisomicin) acts

MEZLOCILLIN SERUM LEVELS IN ADULTS (mcg/ml) 5 MIN IV INJECTION

DOSE	0	5 min	10 min	20 min	30 min	1 hr	2 hr	3 hr	4 hr	6 hr	8 hr
1g	**149** (132–185)	**100** (64–143)	**66** (47–87)	**50** (31–87)	**40** (22–83)	**18** (8–31)	**5.3** (3.3–7.7)	**2.5** (1.7–3.7)	**1.7** (0.7–2.8)	**0.5** (0–1.2)	**0.1** (0–0.2)
2g	**314** (207–362)	**253** (161–364)	**161** (113–214)	**117** (76–174)	**82** (55–112)	**56** (23–88)	**20** (7.5–32)	**11** (3.8–16)	**4.4** (1.6–8.7)	**1.5** (0.5–2.6)	**0.6** (0.1–1.4)
5g	**547** (268–854)	**411** (199–597)	**357** (246–456)	**250** (203–353)	**226** (190–333)	**131** (104–193)	**76** (59–104)	**31** (20–40)	**13** (6.4–17)	**4.6** (2.1–9.4)	**1.9** (1.1–3.6)

MEZLOCILLIN SERUM LEVELS IN ADULTS (mcg/ml) 30 MIN IV INFUSION

DOSE	0	5 min	15 min	30 min	45 min	1 hr	2 hr	3 hr	4 hr	6 hr	8 hr
3g	**263** (87–489)	**170** (63–371)	**141** (75–301)	**109** (56–288)	**79** (41–135)	**57** (28–100)	**26** (14–55)	**12** (5.8–26)	**4.4** (2.2–6.5)	**1.6** (1.0–3.4)	<1

synergistically against strains of *Streptococcus faecalis* and *Pseudomonas aeruginosa*. In some instances, this combination also acts synergistically *in vitro* against other gram-negative bacteria such as *Serratia, Klebsiella* and *Acinetobacter* species.

Mezlocillin is slightly more active when tested at alkaline pH and, as with other penicillins, has reduced activity when tested *in vitro* with increasing inoculum. The minimum bactericidal concentration (MBC) generally exceeds the minimum inhibitory concentration (MIC) by a factor of 2 or 3. Resistance to mezlocillin *in vitro* develops slowly (multiple step mutation). Some strains of *Pseudomonas aeruginosa* have developed resistance fairly rapidly. Mezlocillin is not stable in the presence of penicillinase and strains of *Staphylococcus aureus* resistant to penicillin are also resistant to mezlocillin.

Susceptibility Tests

Quantitative methods that require measurement of zone diameters give good estimates of bacterial susceptibility. One such procedure* has been recommended for use with discs to test susceptibility to antimicrobials. When the causative organism is tested by the Kirby-Bauer method of disc susceptibility, a 75 mcg mezlocillin disc should give a zone of 18 mm or greater to indicate susceptibility. Zone sizes of 14 mm or less indicate resistance. Zone sizes of 15 to 17 mm indicate intermediate susceptibility. Susceptible strains of *Haemophilus* and *Neisseria* species give zones of ≥29 mm resistant strains ≤28 mm. With this procedure, a report from the laboratory of "Susceptible" indicates that the infecting organism is likely to respond to therapy. A report of "Resistant" indicates that the infecting organism is not likely to respond to therapy; other therapy should be selected. A report of "Intermediate Susceptibility" suggests that the organism may be susceptible if the infection is confined to tissues and fluids (e.g., urine), in which high antibiotic levels are attained. The mezlocillin disc should be used for testing susceptibility to mezlocillin. In certain conditions, it may be desriable to do additional susceptibility testing by broth or agar dilution techniques. Dilution methods, preferably the agar plate dilution procedure, are most accurate for susceptibility testing of obligate anaerobes. *Enterobacteriaceae Pseudomonas* species and *Acinetobacter* species are considered susceptible if the MIC of mezlocillin is no greater than 64 mcg/ml and are considered resistant if the MIC is greater than 128 mcg/ml. *Haemophilus* species and *Neisseria* species considered susceptible if the MIC of mezlocillin is less than or equal to 1 mcg/ml. Mezlocillin standard is available for broth or agar dilution studies.

*Bauer, A.W., Kirby, W.M., Sherris, J.C. and Turck, M.: Antibiotic Testing by a Standardized Single Disc Method, Am. J. Clin. Pathol., 45:493, 1966. Standardized Disc Susceptibility Test, FEDERAL REGISTER 39: 19182-19184, 1974.

Indications and Usage: MEZLIN® is indicated for the treatment of serious infections caused by susceptible strains of the designated microorganisms in the conditions listed below:

LOWER RESPIRATORY TRACT INFECTIONS including pneumonia and lung abscess caused by *Haemophilus influenzae, Klebsiella* species including *K. pneumoniae, Proteus mirabilis, Pseudomonas* species including *P. aeruginosa, E. Coli,* and *Baceroides* species including *B. fragilis.*

INTRA-ABDOMINAL INFECTIONS including acute cholecystitis, cholangitis, peritonitis, hepatic abscess and intra-abdominal abscess caused by susceptible *E. coli, Proteus mirabilis, Klebsiella* species, *Pseudomonas* species, *S. faecalis (enterococcus), Bacteroides* species, *Peptococcus* species, and *Peptostreptococcus* species.

URINARY TRACT INFECTIONS caused by susceptible *E. coli, Proteus mirabilis,* the indole positive *Proteus* species, *Morganella morganii; Klebsiella* species, *Enterobacter* species, *Serratia* species, *Pseudomonas* species *S. faecalis* (enterococcus).

Uncomplicated gonorrhea due to susceptible *Neisseria gonorrhoeae.*

GYNECOLOGICAL INFECTIONS including endometritis, pelvic cellulitis, and pelvic inflammatory disease associated with susceptible *Neisseria gonorrhoeae, Peptococcus* species, *Peptostreptococcus* species, *Bacteroides* species, *E. coli, Proteus mirabilis, Klebsiella* species, and *Enterobacter* species.

SKIN AND SKIN STRUCTURE INFECTIONS caused by susceptible *S. faecalis* (enterococcus), *E. coli, Proteus mirabilis,* the indole positive *Proteus* species, *Proteus vulgaris,* and *Providencia rettgeri; Klebsiella* species, *Enterobacter* species, *Pseudomonas* species, *Peptococcus* species, and *Bacteroides* species.

SEPTICEMIA including bacteremia caused by susceptible *E. coli, Klebsiella* species, *Enterobacter* species, *Pseudomonas* species, *Bacteroides* species, and *Peptoccoccus* species.

Mezlocillin has also been shown to be effective for the treatment of infections caused by *Streptococcus* species including Group A Beta-hemolytic *Streptococcus* and *Streptococcus pneumoniae* (formerly *Diplococcus pneumoniae*) however, infections caused by these organisms are ordinarily treated with more narrow spectrum penicillins.

Appropriate culture and susceptibility tests should be performed before treatment in order to isolate and identify organisms causing infection and to determine their susceptibility to mezlocillin Therapy with MEZLIN® may be initiated before results of these tests are known, once results become available, appropriate therapy should be continued.

Mezlocillin's broad spectrum of activity makes it particularly useful for treating mixed infections caused by susceptible strains of both gram-negative and gram-positive aerobic or anaerobic bacteria. It is not effective, however, against infections caused by penicillinase-producing *Staphylococcus-aureus.*

In certain severe infections, when the causative organisms are unknown, MEZLIN® may be administered in conjunction with an aminoglycoside or a cephalosporin antibiotic as initial therapy. As soon as results of culture and susceptibility tests become available, antimicrobial therapy should be adjusted if indicated. Culture and sensitivity testing, performed periodically during therapy, will provide information on the therapeutic effect of the antimicrobal and will monitor for the possible emergence of bacterial resistance.

MEZLIN® has been used effectively in combination with an aminoglycoside antibiotic for the treatment of life-threatening infections caused by *Pseudomonas aeruginosa.* For the treatment of febrile episodes in immunosuppressed patients with granulocytopenia. MEZLIN® should be combined with an aminoglycoside or a cephalosporin antibiotic.

Contraindications: MEZLIN® is contraindicated in patients with a history of hypersensitivity reactions to any of the penicillins.

Warnings: Serious and occasionally fatal hypersensitivity (anaphylactic) reactions have occurred in patients receiving a penicillin. These reactions are more apt to occur in individuals with a history of sensitivity to multiple allergens. There have been reports of individuals with a history of penicillin hypersensitivity reactions who have experienced severe hypersensitivity reactions when treated with a cephalosporin. Before therapy with mezlocillin is instituted, careful inquiry should be made to determine whether the patient has had previous hypersensitivity reactions to penicillins, cephalosporins or other drugs. Antibiotics should be used with caution in any patient who has demonstrated some form of allergy, particularly to drugs.

If an allergic reaction occurs during therapy with mezlocillin, the drug should be discontinued. SERIOUS ANAPHYLACTOID REACTIONS REQUIRE IMMEDIATE EMERGENCY TREATMENT WITH EPINEPHRINE, OXYGEN, INTRAVENOUS STERIODS, AND AIRWAY MANAGEMENT, INCLUDING INTUBATION, SHOULD ALSO BE PROVIDED AS INDICATED.

Precautions: Although MEZLIN™ shares with other pencillins the low potential for toxicity as with any potent drug, periodic assessment of organ system functions, including renal hepatic and hematopoietic, is advisable during prolonged therapy.

Bleeding manifestations have occurred in some patients receiving beta-lactam antibiotics. These reactions have been associated with abnormalities of coagulation tests such as clotting time, platelet aggregation and prothrombin time and are more likely to occur in patients with renal impairment. Although MEZLIN® has rarely been associated with any bleeding abnormalities, the possibility of this occurring should be kept in mind, particularly in patients with severe renal impairment receiving maximum doses of the drug.

MEZLIN® has only rarely been reported to cause hypokalemia, however, the possibility of this occurring should also be kept in mind particularly when treating patients with fluid and electrolyte imbalance. Periodic monitoring of serum potassium may be advisable in patients receiving prolonged therapy.

MEZLIN® is a monosodium salt containing only 42.6 mg (1.85 mEq) of sodium per gram of mezlocillin. This should be considered when treating patients requiring restricted salt intake.

As with any penicillin, an allergic reaction, including anaphylaxis, may occur during MEZLIN® administration, particularly in a hypersensitive individual.

As with other antibiotics prolonged use of MEZLIN® may result in overgrowth of nonsusceptible organisms. If this occurs, appropriate measures should be taken.

Antimicrobials used in high doses for short periods to treat gonorrhea may mask or delay the symptoms of incubating syphilis. Therefore, prior to treatment, patients with gonorrhea should also be evaluated for syphillis. Specimens for dark field examination should be obtained from any suspected primary lesion and serologic tests should be performed. Patients treated with MEZLIN® should undergo follow-up serologic tests three months after therapy.

Interactions with Drugs and Laboratory Tests

As with other penicillins, the mixing of mezlocillins with a aminoglycoside in solutions

Continued on next page

Miles Pharm.—Cont.

for parenteral administration can result in substantial inactivation of the aminoglycoside. Probenecid interferes with the renal tubular secretion of mezlocillin, therby increasing serum concentrations and prolonging serum half-life of the antibiotic.

High urine concentrations of mezlocillin may produce false positive protein reactions (pseudoproteinuria) with the following methods sulfosalicyclic acid and boiling test, acetic acid test, biuret reaction, and nitric acid test. The bromphenol blue (Multi-stix®) reagent strip test has been reported to be reliable.

Pregnancy Category B

Reproduction studies have been performed in rats and mice at doses up to 2 times the human dose, and have revealed no evidence of impaired fertility or harm to the fetus, due to MEZLIN®. There are however no adequate and well controlled studies in pregnant women. Because animal reproductive studies are not always predictive of human response, this drug should be used during pregnancy only if clearly needed. Mezlocillin crosses the placenta and is found in low concentrations in cord blood and amniotic fluid.

Nursing Mothers

Mezlocillin is detected in low concentrations in the milk of nursing mothers, therefore caution should be exercised when MEZLIN® is administered to a nursing woman.

Adverse Reactions: As with other penicillins, the following adverse reactions may occur.

Hypersensitivity reactions: skin rash, pruritus, urticaria, drug fever, and anaphylactic reactions.

Gastro-intestinal distrubances: abnormal taste sensation, nausea, vomiting and diarrhea.

Hemic and Lymphatic Systems: thrombocytopenia, leukopenia, neutropenia, eosinophilia and reduction of hemoglobin or hematocrit.

Abnormalities of hepatic and renal function tests: elevation of serum aspartate aminotransferase (SGOT), serum alanine aminotransferase (SGPT), serum alkaline phosphatase, serum bilirubin. Elevation of serum creatinine and/or BUN. Reduction in serum potassium.

Central nervous system: convulsive seizures or neuromuscular hyperirritability

Local reactions: thrombophlebitis with intravenous administration, pain with intramsucular injection.

Overdosage: As with other penicillins, MEZLIN® in overdosage has the potential to cause neuromusular hyperirritability or convulsive seizures. Hemodialysis, if necessary, will aid in removal of the drug from the blood.

Dosage and Administration: MEZLIN® (sterile mezlocillin sodium) may be administered intravenously or intramuscularly. For serious infections, the intravenous route of administration should be used. Intramuscular doses should not exceed 2g per injection.

The recommended adult dosage for serious infections is 200-300 mg/kg per day given in 4 to 6 divided doses. The usual dose is 3g given every 4 hours (18g/day) or 4g given every 6 hours (16g/day). For life-threatening infections, up to 350 mg/kg per day may be administered, but the total daily dosage should ordinarily not exceed 24g.

[See table below].

For patients with life-threatening infections, 4g may be administered every 4 hours (24g/day).

Dosage for any individual patient must take into consideration the site and severity of infection, the susceptibility of the organisms causing infection, and the status of the patient's host defense mechanism.

The duration of therapy depends upon the severity of infection. Generally, MEZLIN® should be continued for at least 2 days after the signs and symptoms of infection have disappeared. The usual duration is 7 to 10 days; however, in difficult and complicated infections, more prolonged therapy may be required. Antibiotic therapy for Group A beta-hemolytic streptococcal infections should be maintained for at least 10 days to reduce the risk of rheumatic fever or glomerulonephritis.

In certain deep-seated infections, involving abscess formation, appropriate surgical drainage should be performed in conjunction with antimicrobial therapy.

For acute, uncomplicated gonococcal urethritis, the usual dose is 1–2g given once intravenously or by intramuscular injection. Probenecid 1g may be given orally at the time of dosing or up to ½-hour before. (For full prescribing information, refer to probenecid package insert).

Patients with Impaired Renal Function

The rate of elimination of mezlocillin is dose dependent and related to the degree of renal function impairment. After an intravenous dose of 3g. the serum half-life is approximately 1 hour in patients with creatinine clearances above 60 ml/min, 1.3 hr in those with clearances of 30–59 ml/min, 1.6 hr in those with clearances of 10–29 ml/min and approximately 3.6 hr in patients with clearances of less than 10 ml/min. Dosage adjustments of MEZLIN® are not required in patients with mild impairment of renal function. For patients with a creatinine clearance of ≤30 ml/min (serum creatinine of approximately 3.0 mg% or greater), the following dosage guide may be used.

[See table above].

For life-threatening infections, 3g may be given every 6 hours to patients with creatinine clearances between 10–30 ml/min and 2g every 6 hours to those with clearances less than 10 ml/min.

For patients with serious systemic infection undergoing hemodialysis for renal failure, 3-4g may be administered after each dialysis and then every 12 hours. Patients undergoing peritoneal dialysis may receive 3g every 12 hours.

For patients with renal failure and hepatic insufficiency, measurement of serum levels of mezlocillin will provide additional guidance for adjusting dosage.

MEZLIN® DOSAGE GUIDE FOR PATIENTS WITH IMPAIRED RENAL FUNCTION

Creatinine Clearance ml/min	Urinary Tract Infection (Uncomplicated)	Urinary Tract Infection (Complicated)	Serious Systemic Infection
>30	Usual Recommended Dosage		
10–30	1.5g every 8 hours	1.5g every 6 hours	3g every 8 hours
<10	1.5g every 8 hours	1.5g every 8 hours	2g every 8 hours

MEZLIN® DOSAGE GUIDE (ADULTS)

Condition	Daily Dosage Range	Usual Daily Dosage	Frequency and Route of Administration
Urinary tract infection (uncomplicated)	100–125 mg/kg	6-8g	1.5–2g every 6 hours IV or IM
Urinary tract infection (complicated)	150–200 mg/kg	12g	3g every 6 hours IV
Lower respiratory tract infection Intra-abdominal infection Gynecological infection Skin & skin structure infection Septicemia	225–300 mg/kg	16–18g	4g every 6 hours or 3g every 4 hours IV

Intravenous Administration

MEZLIN® may be administered intravenously by intermittent infusion or by direct intravenous injection.

Infusion. Each gram of mezlocillin should be reconstituted by vigorous shaking with at least 10 ml of Sterile Water for injection, 5% Dextrose Injection or 0.9% Sodium Chloride Injection. The dissolved drug should be further diluted to desired volume (50-100 ml) with an appropriate intravenous solution (See Compatibility and Stability section). The solution of reconstituted drug may then be administered over a period of 30 minutes by direct infusion or through a Y-type intravenous infusion set which may already be in place. If this method or the "piggyback" method of administration is used, it is advisable to discontinue temporarily the administration of any other solutions during the infusion of MEZLIN®.

Injection. The reconstituted solution of MEZLIN® may also be injected directly into a vein or into intravenous tubing, when administered this way, the injection should be given slowly over a period of 3–5 minutes. To minimize venous irritation, the concentration of drug should not exceed 10%.

When MEZLIN®is given in combination with another antimicrobial, such as an aminoglycoside, each drug should be given separately in accordance with the recommended dosage and routes of administration for each drug.

Intramuscular Administration

Each gram of mezlocillin may be reconstituted by vigorous shaking with 3-4 ml of sterile water for injection or with 3-4 ml of 0.5 or 1.0% lidocaine hydrochloride solution (without epinephrine). (For Full prescribing information, refer to lidocaine package insert). Intramuscular doses of MEZLIN® should not exceed 2g per injection.

As with all intramuscular preparations, MEZLIN® should be injected well within the body of a relatively large muscle, such as the upper outer quadrant of the buttock (i.e., gluteus maximus), aspiration will help avoid unintentional injection into a blood vesel. Slow injection (12-15 sec) will minimize the discomfort associated with intramuscular administration.

Infants and Children

Only limited data are available on the safety and effectiveness of MEZLIN® in the treatment of infants and children with documented

serious infection. In the event a child has an infection for which MEZLIN® may be judged particularly appropriate, the following dosage guide may be used:
[See table right].
For infants beyond one month of age and children up to the age of 12 years, 50 mg/kg may be administered every 4 hours (300 mg/kg/day). The drug may be infused intravenously over 30-minutes or be given by intramuscular injection.
Compatibility and Stability: MEZLIN® at concentrations of 10 mg/ml and 100 mg/ml is stable (loss of potency less than 10%) in the following intravenous solutions for the time periods stated.
(See table below)
MEZLIN® at concentrations up to 250 mg/ml is stable for 24 hours at room temperature in the following diluents
Sterile Water for Injection, USP
0.9% Sodium Chloride Injection, USP
0.5% and 1.0% Lidocaine Hydrochloride solution (without epinephrine)
MEZLIN® is stable for up to 28 days when frozen at - 12 C at concentrations up to 100 mg/ml in the following diluents.
Sterile Water for Injection, USP
0.9% Sodium Chloride Injection, USP or 5% Dextrose Injection, USP
How Supplied: MEZLIN® (sterile mezolin sodium) is a white to pale yellow crystalline powder supplied in vials and infusion bottles. Each vial contains mezlocillin sodium equivalent to 1g, 2g, 3g or 4g mezlocillin. Each infusion bottle contains mezlocillin sodium equivalent to 2g, 3g or 4g mezlocillin.
MEZLIN® vials and infusion bottles should be stored at or below 30°C (86°F). The powder as well as the reconstituted solution of drug may darken-slightly, depending upon storage conditions, but potency is not affected.
Manufactured by Pfizer, Inc. New York, NY 10017 for Miles Pharmaceuticals, Division of Miles Laboratories, Inc., West Haven, Connecticut 06516 USA

MEZLIN® DOSAGE GUIDE (NEWBORNS)

BODY WEIGHT (gm)	AGE ≤7 DAYS	AGE >DAYS
≤2000	75 mg/kg every 12 hours (150 mg/kg/day)	75 mg/kg every 8 hours (225 mg/kg/day)
>2000	75 mg/kg every 12 hours (150 mg/kg/day)	75 mg/kg every 6 hours (300 mg/kg/day)

MITHRACIN® ℞
(plicamycin)
FOR INTRAVENOUS USE

Warning: IT IS RECOMMENDED THAT MITHRACIN (plicamycin) BE ADMINISTERED ONLY TO HOSPITALIZED PATIENTS BY OR UNDER THE SUPERVISION OF A QUALIFIED PHYSICIAN WHO IS EXPERIENCED IN THE USE OF CANCER CHEMOTHERAPEUTIC AGENTS, BECAUSE OF THE POSSIBILITY OF SEVERE REACTIONS. FACILITIES FOR THE DETERMINATION OF NECESSARY LABORATORY STUDIES MUST BE AVAILABLE.
SEVERE THROMBOCYTOPENIA, A HEMORRHAGIC TENDENCY AND EVEN DEATH MAY RESULT FROM THE USE OF MITHRACIN. ALTHOUGH SEVERE TOXICITY IS MORE APT TO OCCUR IN PATIENTS WHO HAVE FAR-ADVANCED DISEASE OR ARE OTHERWISE CONSIDERED POOR RISKS FOR THERAPY, SERIOUS TOXICITY MAY ALSO OCCASIONALLY OCCUR EVEN IN PATIENTS WHO ARE IN RELATIVELY GOOD CONDITION.
IN THE TREATMENT OF EACH PATIENT, THE PHYSICIAN MUST WEIGH CAREFULLY THE POSSIBILITY OF ACHIEVING THERAPEUTIC BENEFIT VERSUS THE RISK OF TOXICITY WHICH MAY OCCUR WITH MITHRACIN THERAPY, THE FOLLOWING DATA CONCERNING THE USE OF MITHRACIN IN THE TREATMENT OF TESTICULAR TUMORS, HYPERCALCEMIC AND/OR HYPERCALCIURIC CONDITIONS ASSOCIATED WITH VARIOUS ADVANCED MALIGNANCIES, SHOULD BE THOROUGHLY REVIEWED BEFORE ADMINISTERING THIS COMPOUND.
Description: Mithracin is a yellow crystalline compound which is produced by a microorganism, *Streptomyces plicatus.* It has an empirical formula of $C_{52}H_{75}O_{24}$.
Actions: Although the exact mechanism by which Mithracin causes tumor inhibition is not yet known, studies have indicated that this compound forms a complex with deoxyribonucleic acid (DNA) and inhibits cellular ribonucleic acid (RNA) and enzymic RNA synthesis. The binding of Mithracin to DNA in the presence of Mg^{11} (or other divalent cations) is responsible for the inhibition of DNA-dependent or DNA-directed RNA synthesis. This action presumably accounts for the biological properties of Mithracin.
Mithracin shows potent cytotoxicity against malignant cells of human origin (Hela cells) growing in tissue culture. Mithracin is lethal to Hela cells in 48 hours at concentrations as low as 0.5 micrograms per milliliter of tissue culture medium. Mithracin has shown significant anti-tumor activity against experimental leukemia in mice when administered intraperitoneally.
Indications: Mithracin is a potent antineoplastic agent which has been shown to be useful in the treatment of carefully selected hospitalized patients with malignant tumors of the testis in whom successful treatment by surgery and/or radiation is impossible. Also, on the basis of limited clinical experience to date, it may be considered in the treatment of certain symptomatic patients with hypercalcemia and hypercalciuria associated with a variety of advanced neoplasms.
The use of Mithracin in other types of neoplastic disease is not recommended at the present time.
Contraindications: Mithracin (plicamycin) is contraindicated in patients with thrombocytopenia, thrombocytopathy, coagulation disorder or an increased susceptibility to bleeding due to other causes. Mithracin should not be administered to any patient with impairment of bone marrow function.
Mithracin should not be used in the treatment of patients who are not hospitalized and who cannot be observed carefully and frequently during and after therapy, or whenever appropriate laboratory facilities are unavailable.
Precautions: Mithracin should be administered only to patients who are hospitalized and who can be observed carefully and frequently during and after therapy.
Severe thrombocytopenia, a hemorrhagic tendency and even death may result from the use of Mithracin. Although severe toxicity is more apt to occur in patients who have far-advanced disease or are otherwise considered poor risks for therapy, serious toxicity may also occasionally occur even in patients who are in relatively good condition.
Electrolyte imbalance, especially hypocalcemia, hypokalemia, and hypophosphatemia, should be corrected with appropriate electrolyte therapy prior to treatment with Mithracin.
Mithracin should be used with extreme caution in patients with significant impairment of renal or hepatic function.
In the treatment of each patient, the physician must weigh carefully the possiblity of achieving therapeutic benefit versus the risk of toxicity which may occur with Mithracin therapy.
The following laboratory studies should be obtained frequently during therapy and for several days following the last dose: platelet count, prothrombin time, bleeding time. The occurrence of thrombocytopenia or a significant prolongation of prothrombin time or bleeding time is an indication for the termination of therapy.
Adverse Reactions: THE MOST IMPORTANT FORM OF TOXICITY ASSOCIATED WITH THE USE OF MITHRACIN CONSISTS OF A BLEEDING SYNDROME WHICH USUALLY BEGINS WITH AN EPISODE OF EPISTAXIS. This bleeding tendency may only consist of a single or several episodes of epistaxis and progress no further. However, in some cases, this hemorrhagic syndrome can start with an episode of hematemesis which may progress to more wide-spread hemorrhage in the gastrointestinal tract or to a more generalized bleeding tendency. This hemorrhagic diathesis is most likely due to abnormalities in multiple clotting factors.
A detailed analysis of the clinical data in 1,160 patients treated with Mithracin indicates that the hemorrhagic syndrome is dose related. With doses of 30 mcg/kg/day or less for 10 or fewer doses, the incidence of bleeding episodes has been 5.4% with an associated drug-related mortality rate of 1.6%. With doses greater than 30 mcg/kg/day and/or for more than 10 doses, a significantly larger number of bleeding episodes occurred (11.9%) and the associ-

STABILITY

INTRAVENOUS SOLUTION	Controlled Room Temperature	Refrigeration
Sterile Water for Injection, USP	48 hours	7 days
0.9% Sodium Chloride Injection, USP	48 hours	7 days
5% Dextrose Injection, USP	48 hours	7 days
5% Dextrose in 0.225% Sodium Chloride Injection, USP	72 hours	7 days
Lactated Ringer's Injection, USP	72 hours	7 days
5% Dextrose in Electrolyte #75 Injection	72 hours	7 days
5% Dextrose in 0.45% Sodium Chloride Injection, USP*	48 hours	48 hours
Ringers Injection	24 hours	24 hours
10% Dextrose Injection	24 hours	24 hours
5% Fructose Injection	24 hours	24 hours

If precipitation should occur under refrigeration, the product should be warmed to 37°C for 20 minutes in a water bath and shaken well.
*This solution is stable from 10 mg/ml to 50 mg/ml under refrigeration.

Continued on next page

Miles Pharm.—Cont.

ated drug-related mortality rate was also significantly higher (5.7%).

The most common side effects reported with the use of Mithracin consist of gastrointestinal symptoms: anorexia, nausea, vomiting, diarrhea, and stomatitis. Other less frequently reported side effects include fever, drowsiness, weakness, lethargy, malaise, headache, depression, phlebitis, facial flushing, and skin rash.

The following laboratory abnormalities have been reported during therapy with Mithracin (plicamycin) and in most instances were reversible following cessation of treatment:

Hematologic Abnormalities: Depression of platelet count, white count, hemoglobin and prothrombin content; elevation of clotting time and bleeding time; abnormal clot retraction.

Thrombocytopenia may be rapid in onset and may occur at any time during therapy or within several days following the last dose. With the occurrence of severe thrombocytopenia, the infusion of platelet concentrates of platelet-rich plasma may be helpful in elevating the platelet count.

The occurrence of leukopenia with the use of Mithracin is relatively uncommon, occurring only in approximately 6% of patients.

It has been uncommon for abnormalities in clotting time or clot retraction to be demonstrated prior to the onset of an overt bleeding episode noted in some patients treated with Mithracin. Nevertheless, the performance of these tests periodically is recommended because in a few instances, an abnormality in one of these studies may have served as a warning to terminate therapy because of impeding serious toxicity.

Abnormal Liver Function Tests: Increased levels of serum glutamic oxalacetic transaminase, serum glutamic pyruvic transaminase, lactic dehydrogenase, alkaline phosphatase, serum bilirubin, ornithine carbamyl transferase, isocitric dehydrogenase, and increased retention of bromsulphalein.

Abnormal Renal Function Tests: Increased blood urea nitrogen and serum creatinine; proteinuria.

Abnormalities in Electrolyte Concentrations: Depression of serum calcium, phosphorus, and potassium.

Dosage: The daily dose of Mithracin is based on the patient's body weight. If a patient has abnormal fluid retention such as edema, hydrothorax or ascites, the patient's ideal weight rather than actual body weight should be used to calculate the dose.

Treatment of Testicular Tumors: In the treatment of patients with testicular tumors the recommended daily dose of Mithracin (plicamycin) is 25 to 30 micrograms per kilogram of body weight. Therapy should be continued for a period of 8 to 10 days unless significant side effects or toxicity occur during therapy. A course of therapy consisting of more than 10 daily doses is not recommended. Individual daily doses should not exceed 30 micrograms per kilogram of body weight.

In those patients with responsive tumors, some degree of tumor regression is usually evident within 3 or 4 weeks following the initial course of therapy. If tumor masses remain unchanged following an initial course of therapy, additional courses of therapy at monthly intervals are warranted.

When a significant tumor regression is obtained, it is suggested that additional courses of therapy be given at monthly intervals until a complete regression of tumor masses is achieved or until definite tumor progression or new tumor masses occur in spite of continued courses of therapy.

Treatment of Hypercalcemia and Hypercalciuria: Reversal of hypercalcemia and hypercalciuria can usually be achieved with Mithracin at doses considerably lower than those recommended for use in the treatment of testicular tumors.

In hypercalcemia and hypercalciuria associated with advanced malignancy the recommended course of treatment with Mithracin is 25 micrograms per kilogram of body weight per day for 3 or 4 days.

If the desired degree of reversal of hypercalcemia or hypercalciuria is not achieved with the initial course of therapy, additional courses of therapy may then be administered at intervals of one week or more to achieve the desired result or to maintain serum calcium and urinary calcium excretion at normal levels. It may be possible to maintain normal calcium balance with single, weekly doses or with a schedule of 2 or 3 doses per week.

NOTE: BECAUSE OF THE DRUG'S TOXICITY AND THE LIMITED CLINICAL EXPERIENCE TO DATE IN THESE INDICATIONS, THE FOLLOWING RECOMMENDATIONS SHOULD BE KEPT IN MIND BY THE PHYSICIAN.

1. **CONSIDER CASES OF HYPERCALCEMIA AND HYPERCALCIURIA NOT RESPONSIVE TO CONVENTIONAL TREATMENT.**
2. **APPLY SAME CONTRAINDICATIONS AND PRECAUTIONARY MEASURES AS IN ANTITUMOR TREATMENT.**
3. **RENAL FUNCTION SHOULD BE CAREFULLY MONITORED BEFORE, DURING, AND AFTER TREATMENT.**
4. **BENEFITS OF USE DURING PREGNANCY OR IN WOMEN OF CHILDBEARING AGE SHOULD BE WEIGHED AGAINST POTENTIAL TOXICITY TO EMBRYO OR FETUS.**

Administration: By IV administration only. The appropriate daily dose of Mithracin should be diluted in one liter of 5% Dextrose Injection, USP or Sodium Chloride Injection, USP and administered by slow intravenous infusion over a period of 4 to 6 hours. Rapid direct intravenous injection of Mithracin should be avoided as it may be associated with a higher incidence and greater severity of gastrointestinal side effects. Extravasation of solutions of Mithracin may cause local irritation and cellulitis at injection sites. Should thrombophlebitis or perivascular cellulitis occur, the infusion should be terminated and reinstituted at another site. The application of moderate heat to the site of extravasation may help to disperse the compound and minimize discomfort and local tissue irritation. The use of antiemetic compounds prior to and during treatment with Mithracin may be helpful in relieving nausea and vomiting.

How Supplied: Mithracin is available in vials as a freeze-dried preparation for intravenous administration. Each vial contains 2500 mcg of Mithracin with 100 mg of mannitol and sufficient disodium phosphate to adjust to pH 7. These vials should be stored at refrigerator temperatures between 2°C. to 8°C. (36°F. to 46°F.).

To reconstitute, add aseptically 4.9 ml of Sterile Water for Injection to the contents of the vial and shake to dissolve. Each ml of the resulting solution will then contain 500 mcg of Mithracin. AFTER REMOVAL OF THE APPROPRIATE DOSE, THE REMAINING UNUSED SOLUTION MUST BE DISCARDED, FRESH SOLUTIONS MUST BE PREPARED IN THE ABOVE MANNER EACH DAY OF THERAPY.

Pharmacology and Toxicology: In mice the average intravenous LD_{50} of Mithracin is 2,000 mcg/kg of body weight. When administered orally, it is not toxic to mice even at doses 100 times greater than the intravenous LD_{50}. In rats the average intravenous LD_{50} of Mithracin is 1,700 mcg/kg of body weight. It is not toxic to rats when administered orally at doses 17 times greater than the intravenous LD_{50}. In dogs and monkeys Mithracin is essentially non-toxic when administered intravenously for 24 days at daily doses as high as 50 and 24 mcg/kg of body weight, respectively. However, at higher doses of 100 mcg/kg/day intravenously it is lethal to dogs and monkeys. Signs of toxicity in dogs and monkeys included anorexia, vomiting, listlessness, melena, anemia, lymphopenia, elevated alkaline phosphatase, serum glutamic oxalacetic transaminase, serum glutamic pyruvic transaminase values, hypochloremia, and azotemia. Dogs also showed marked thrombocytopenia, hyponatremia, hypokalemia, hypocalcemia, and decreased prothrombin consumption. Necropsy findings consisted of necrosis of lymphoid tissue and multiple generalized hemorrhages. Mithracin (plicamycin) was only mildly irritating when injected intramuscularly in rabbits and subcutaneously in guinea pigs. Histologic evidence of inhibition of spermatogenesis was observed in a substantial number of male rats receiving doses of 0.6 mg/kg/day and above. This preclinical finding of selective drug effect constituted the scientific rationale for clinical trials in testicular tumors.

Clinical Reports:

Treatment of Patients with Inoperable Testicular Tumors: In a combined series of 305 patients with inoperable testicular tumors treated with Mithracin, 33 patients (10.8%) showed a complete disappearance of tumor masses and an additional 80 patients (26.2%) responded with significant partial regression of tumor masses. The longest duration of a continuing complete response is now over 8½ years. The therapeutic responses in this series of patients have been summarized by type of testicular tumor in the accompanying table. [See table left].

Mithracin may be useful in the treatment of patients with testicular tumors which are resistant to other chemotherapeutic agents. Prior radiation therapy or prior chemotherapy did not alter the response rate with Mithracin.

RESULTS IN 305 TESTICULAR TUMOR CASES BY TUMOR TYPE

TYPE OF TESTICULAR TUMOR	TOTAL	COMPLETE RESPONSE	PARTIAL RESPONSE	NO RESPONSE
EMBRYONAL CELL	173	26	42	105
TERATOMA	5	0	1	4
TERATOCARCINOMA	23	0	5	18
SEMINOMA	18	0	7	11
CHORIOCARCINOMA	13	1	6	6
MIXED TUMOR	73	6	19	48
TOTALS	305	33	80	192

This suggests that there is no significant cross resistance between Mithracin (plicamycin) and other chemotherapeutic agents.
Treatment of Patients with Hypercalcemia and Hypercalciuria: A limited number of patients with hypercalcemia (range: 12.0–25.8 mg%) and patients with hypercalciuria (range 215–492 mg/day) associated with malignant disease were treated with Mithracin. Hypercalcemia and hypercalciuria were promptly reversed in all patients. In some patients, the primary malignancy was of non-testicular origin.
Manufactured for
Miles Pharmaceuticals
Division of Miles Laboratories, Inc.
West Haven, Connecticut 06516 USA
by Pfizer Laboratories, New York, N.Y. 10017

MYCELEX® 1% ℞
(clotrimazole) cream
For dermatologic use only

Description: Mycelex is clotrimazole [1-(o-Chloro-α, α -diphenylbenzyl) imidazole], a synthetic anti-fungal agent having the chemical formula, $C_{22}H_{17}ClN_2$.
Each gram of Mycelex contains 10 mg clotrimazole in a vanishing cream base of sorbitan monostearate, polysorbate 60, cetyl esters wax, cetostearyl alcohol, 2-octyldodecanol, purified water and, as preservative, benzyl alcohol (1%).
Actions: Clotrimazole is a broad-spectrum, antifungal agent that inhibits the growth of pathogenic dermatophytes, yeasts, and *Malassezia furfur*. Clotrimazole exhibits fungicidal activity in vitro against isolates of *Trichophyton rubrum, Trichophyton mentagrophytes, Epidermophyton floccosum, Microsporum canis,* and *Candida albicans*.
No single-step or multiple-step resistance to clotrimazole has developed during successive passages of *Candida albicans* and *trichophyton mentagrophytes.*
Indications: Mycelex Cream is indicated for the topical treatment of the following dermal infections: tinea pedis, tinea cruris, and tinea corporis due to *Trichophyton rubrum, Trichophyton mentagrophytes, Epidermophyton folccosum,* and *Microsporum canis;* candidiasis due to *Candida albicans;* and tinea versicolor due to *Malassezia furfur.*
Contraindications: Mycelex Cream is contraindicated in individuals who have shown hypersensitivity to any of its components.
Warnings: Mycelex Cream is not for ophthalmic use.
Precautions: In the first trimester of pregnancy, Mycelex Cream should be used only when considered essential to the welfare of the patient.
If irritation or sensitivity develops with the use of Mycelex, treatment should be discontinued and appropriate therapy instituted.
Adverse Reactions: The following adverse reactions have been reported in connection with the use of this product: erythema, stinging, blistering, peeling, edema, pruritus, urticaria, and general irritation of the skin.
Dosage and Administration: Gently massage sufficient Mycelex Cream into the affected and surrounding skin areas twice a day, in the morning and evening.
Clinical improvement, with relief of pruritus, usually occurs within the first week of treatment. If a patient shows no clinical improvement after four weeks of treatment with Mycelex the diagnosis should be reviewed.
How Supplied: Mycelex Cream 1% is supplied in 15, 30 and 2 x 45 gram tubes.
DPSC Stocked:
15 gram—NSN 6505-01-023-5011
30 gram—NSN 6505-01-05-1405
VA Stocked: 15 gram—SN 6505-01-023-5011
30 gram—SN 6505-01-015-1405
Store between 35° and 86° F.
U.S. Patents No. 3,660,577 and 3,705,172.
April, 1981 PD 100504
Copyright © 1980, Miles Pharmaceuticals, Division Miles Laboratories, Inc.

MYCELEX® 1% ℞
(clotrimazole) Solution

For dermatologic use only

Description: Mycelex is clotrimazole [1-(o-Chloro-α, α-diphenylbenzyl) imidazole], a synthetic antifungal agent having the chemical formula $C_{22}H_{17}ClN_2$.
Each ml. of Mycelex Solution contains 10 mg. clotrimazole in a nonaqueous vehicle of polyethylene glycol 400.
Actions: Clotrimazole is a broad-spectrum, antifungal agent that inhibits the growth of pathogenic dermatophytes, yeasts and *Malassezia furfur.* Clotrimazole exhibits fungicidal activity *in vitro* against isolates of *Trichophyton rubrum, Trichophyton mentagrophytes, Epidermophyton floccosum, Microsporum canis,* and *Candida albicans.*
No single-step or multiple-step resistance to clotrimazole has developed during successive passages of *Candida albicans* and *Trichophyton mentagrophytes.*
Indications: Mycelex Solution is indicated for the topical treatment of the following dermal infections: tinea pedis, tinea cruris, and tinea corporis due to *Trichophyton rubum, Trichophyton mentagrophytes, Epidermophyton floccosum,* and *Microsporum canis;* candidiasis due to *Candida albicans;* and tinea versicolor due to *Malassezia furfur.*
Contraindications: Mycelex Solution is contraindicated in individuals who have shown hypersensitivity to any of its components.
Warnings: Mycelex Solution is not for ophthalmic use.
Precautions: In the first trimester of pregnancy, Mycelex Solution should be used only when considered essential to the welfare of the patient.
If irritation or sensitivity develops with the use of Mycelex, treatment should be discontinued and appropriate therapy instituted.
Adverse Reactions: The following adverse reactions have been reported in connection with the use of this product: erythema, stinging, blistering, peeling, edema, pruritus, urticaria, and general irritation of the skin.
Dosage and Administration: Gently massage sufficient Mycelex Solution into the affected and surrounding skin areas twice a day, in the morning and evening.
Clinical improvement, with relief of pruritus, usually occurs within the first week of treatment. If a patient shows no clinical improvement after four weeks of treatment with Mycelex the diagnosis should be reviewed.
How Supplied: Mycelex Solution 1% is supplied in 10 ml. and 30 ml. plastic bottles.
DPSC Stocked: 10 ml—NSN 6505-01-015-1406
VA Stocked: 10 ml—SN 6505-01-015-1406
30 ml—SN 6505-01-016-5675
Store between 35° and 86°F.
U.S. Patents No. 3,660,577 and 3,705,172.
PD100510 November, 1980 17370
Copyright© 1980, Miles Pharmaceuticals, Division of Miles Laboratories, Inc.

MYCELEX®-G 1% ℞
(clotrimazole) Vaginal Cream

Description: Mycelex-G is clotrimazole [1-(o-Chloro-α,α -diphenylbenzyl) imidazole], a synthetic antifungal agent having the chemical formula, $C_{22}H_{17}ClN_2$, and following chemical structure:

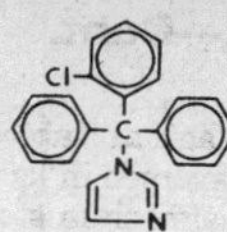

Each applicatorful of Mycelex-G Vaginal Cream contains approximately 50 mg. clotrimazole dispersed in sorbitan monostearate, polysorbate 60, cetyl esters wax, cetostearyl alcohol, 2-octyldodecanol, purified water, and as a preservative, benzyl alcohol (1%).
Actions: Clotrimazole is a broad spectrum antifungal agent that inhibits the growth of pathogenic yeasts. Clotrimazole exhibits fungicidal activity *in vitro* against *Candida albicans* and other species of the genus *Candida.*
No single-step or multiple-step resistance to clotrimazole has developed during successive passages of *Candida albicans.*
Indications: Mycelex-G Vaginal Cream is indicated for the local treatment of patients with vulvovaginal candidiasis (moniliasis). As Mycelex-G Vaginal Cream has been shown to be effective only for candidal vulvovaginitis, the diagnosis should be confirmed by KOH smears and/or cultures. Other pathogens commonly associated with vulvovaginitis (*Trichomonas* and *Hemophilus vaginalis*) should be ruled out by appropriate laboratory methods.
Studies have shown that women taking oral contraceptives had a cure rate similar to those not taking oral contraceptives.
Contraindications: Mycelex-G Vaginal Cream is contraindicated in women who have shown hypersensitivity to any of the components of the preparation.
Precautions: **Laboratory Tests:** If there is a lack of response to Mycelex-G Vaginal Cream, appropriate microbiological studies should be repeated to confirm the diagnosis and rule out other pathogens before instituting another course of antimycotic therapy.
Usage in Pregnancy: While Mycelex-G Vaginal Cream has not been studied in the first trimester of pregnancy, use in the second and third trimesters has not been associated with ill effects.
Application of ^{14}C labeled clotrimazole has shown negligible absorption (peak serum level of 0.01 mcg/ml 24 hours after insertion of vaginal cream containing 50 mg. of active drug) from both normal and inflamed human vaginal mucosa.
Adverse Reactions: Three (0.5%) of the 653 patients treated with Mycelex-G Vaginal Cream reported complaints during therapy that were possibly drug related. Vaginal burning occurred in one patient; erythema, irritation and burning in another; intercurrent cystitis was reported in the third.
Dosage and Administration: Mycelex-G Vaginal Cream has been found to be effective when used from seven to fourteen days; studies have shown that patients treated for fourteen days had a significantly higher cure rate. The recommended dose is one applicatorful a day for seven to fourteen consecutive days; using the applicator supplied, insert one applicatorful of cream (approximately 5 grams) intravaginally preferably at bedtime.
How Supplied: Mycelex-G Vaginal Cream 1% is supplied in 45 and 90 gram tubes with a measured-dose applicator; for seven-day and for fourteen-day treatments.
Store between 35° and 86° F (2° and 30° C).
February, 1981 PD100526
Copyright © 1980, Miles Pharmaceuticals, Division of Miles Laboratories, Inc.

MYCELEX®–G 100 mg ℞
(clotrimazole) Vaginal Tablets

Description: Mycelex-G is clotrimazole [1-(o-Chloro-α, α-diphenylbenzyl) imidazole], a synthetic antifungal agent having the chemical formula, $C_{22}H_{17}ClN_2$.

Continued on next page

Miles Pharm.—Cont.

Each Mycelex-G Vaginal Tablet contains 100 mg clotrimazole dispersed in lactose, povidone, corn starch and magnesium stearate.

Actions: Clotrimazole is a broad-spectrum antifungal agent that inhibits the growth of pathogenic yeasts. Clotrimazole exhibits fungicidal activity *in vitro* against *Candida albicans* and other species of the genus *Candida*.

No single-step or multiple-step resistance to clotrimazole has developed during successive passages of *Candida albicans*.

Indications: Mycelex-G Vaginal Tablets are indicated for the local treatment of vulvovaginal candidiasis. The diagnosis should be confirmed by KOH smears and/or cultures. Other pathogens commonly associated with vulvovaginits *(Trichomonas* and *Hemophilus vaginalis)* should be ruled out by appropriate laboratory methods.

Contraindications: Mycelex-G Vaginal Tablets are contraindicated in women who have shown hypersensitivity to any components of the preparation.

Precautions: **Laboratory Tests:** If there is a lack of response to Mycelex-G Vaginal Tablets, appropriate microbiological studies should be repeated to confirm the diagnosis and rule out other pathogens before instituting another course of antimycotic therapy.

Application of ^{14}C-labeled clotrimazole has shown negligible absorption (peak of 0.03 mcg/ml of serum 24 hours after insertion of a 100 mg tablet) from both normal and inflammed human vaginal mucosa.

Usage in Pregnancy: While Mycelex-G Vaginal Tablets have not been studied in the first trimester of pregnancy, use in the second and third trimesters has not been associated with ill effects. Follow-up reports now available on 71 neonates of 117 pregnant patients reveal no adverse effects or complications attributable to Mycelex-G therapy.

Adverse Reactions: Eighteen (1.6%) of the 1116 patients treated with Mycelex-G in double-blind studies reported complaints during therapy that were possibly drug-related. Mild burning occured in six patients while other complaints, such as skin rash, itching, vulval irritation, lower abdominal cramps and bloating, slight cramping, slight urinary frequency, and burning or irritation in the sexual partner, occurred rarely.

Dosage and Administration: The recommended dose is one tablet a day for seven consecutive days. Recent studies indicate that an alternative regimen of two tablets a day for three consecutive days is similarly effective in non-pregnant patients; however, in pregnant patients the three-day treatment course did not prove to be effective and is therefore not recommended. They should receive the seven-day treatment. Using the applicator supplied, insert one or two tablets intravaginally preferably at bedtime.

In the event of treatment failure, other pathogens commonly responsible for vaginitis should be ruled out before instituting another course of antimycotic therapy. There are no studies to show whether a second course of clotrimazole would be effective in patients who fail to respond to the initial course.

How Supplied: Mycelex-G Vaginal Tablets 100 mg, white, tear-drop-shaped, uncoated tablets coded with number 093-Miles, supplied in a strip of seven tablets with plastic applicator and patient leaflet of instructions.

DPSC Stocked: NSN 6505-01-090-6795

Do not store above 35°C [95°F].

U.S. Patent No. 3,660,577 and 3,705,172

PD100513 November, 1980 17372

[*Shown in Product Identification Section*]

NICLOCIDE™ ℞
(niclosamide)
Chewable Tablets

Description: NICLOCIDE (niclosamide) is an anthelmintic provided in chewable tablet form at a strength of 500 mg per tablet. Niclosamide is 2′, 5-Dichloro-4′-nitrosalicylanilide. The empirical formula is $C_{13}H_8Cl_2N_2O_4$ with the following structural formula.

OH Cl CONH NO₂ Cl

Clinical Pharmacology: NICLOCIDE inhibits oxidative phosphorylation in the mitochondria of cestodes. Both *in vitro* and *in vivo*, the scolex and proximal segments are killed on contact with the drug. The scolex of the tapeworm, loosened from the gut wall, may be digested in the intestine, and thus may not be identified in the feces even after extensive purging.

The use of NICLOCIDE has not been associated with the development of anemia, leukopenia or thrombocytopenia nor have there been any effects on normal renal and hepatic functions.

Indications and Usage: NICLOCIDE (niclosamide) is indicated for the treatment of tapeworm infections by *Taenia saginata* (beef tapeworm), *Diphyllobothrium latum* (fish tapeworm) and *Hymenolepis nana* (dwarf tapeworm).

Contraindications: NICLOCIDE™ Tablets are contraindicated in individuals who have shown hypersensitivity to any of its components.

Precautions: NICLOCIDE affects the cestodes of the intestine only. It is without effect in cysticercosis.

Drug Interactions: No data are available regarding interaction of niclosamide with other drugs.

Carcinogenesis, mutagenesis, impairment of fertility:

Carcinogenicity Potential: Although carcinogenicity studies on niclosamide *per se* have not been done, long-term feeding studies on its ethanolamine salt in rats and mice did not show carcinogenicity. Mutagenicity tests have not been performed.

Pregnancy: Pregnancy Category B: Reproduction studies in rabbits and rats at doses of 25 times the human therapeutic dose and in mice at 12 times the human therapeutic dose, have revealed no evidence of impaired fertility or harm to the fetus due to niclosamide. There are, however, no adequate and well-controlled studies in pregnant women. Because animal studies are not always predictive of human response, the drug should be used during pregnancy only if clearly needed.

Nursing Mothers: No studies are available.

Pediatric Use: In children under 2 years of age, the safety of the drug has not been established.

Adverse Reactions: The incidence of side effects has been reported as follows: nausea/-vomiting 4.1%, abdominal discomfort including loss of appetite 3.4%, diarrhea 1.6%, drowsiness, dizziness, and or headache 1.4%, and skin rash including pruritus ani 0.3%. Other side effects listed in decreasing order of frequency were: oral irritation, fever, rectal bleeding, weakness, bad taste in mouth, sweating, palpitations, constipation, alopecia, edema of an arm, backache and irritability. There was also one instance of a transient rise in SGOT in an i.v. narcotic addict. Two cases of urticaria reported may be related to the breakdown products of the tapeworm. All side effects were mild or moderate and transitory and did not necessitate discontinuation of the treatment.

Overdosage: Insufficient data are available. In the event of overdose a fast-acting laxative and enema should be given. Vomiting should not be induced.

Dosage and Administration:

1. *Taenia saginata* and *Diphyllobothrium latum*
   a. Adults: 4 tablets (2.0 g) chewed thoroughly in a single dose.
   b. Children weighing more than 34 kg (75 lbs): 3 tablets (1.5 g) chewed thoroughly in a single dose.
   c. Children weighing between 11 and 34 kg (25 to 75 lbs): 2 tablets (1.0 g) chewed throughly in a single dose.
2. *Hymenolepis nana*
   a. Adults: 4 tablets (2.0 g) chewed thoroughly as a single daily dose for 7 days.
   b. Children weighing more than 34 kg (75 lbs): 3 tablets (1.5g) chewed thoroughly on the first day, then 2 tablets (1.0 g) daily for next 6 days.
   c. Children weighing between 11 and 34 kg (25 to 75 lbs): 2 tablets (1.0 g) to be chewed thoroughly on the first day, then one tablet (0.5 g) daily for next 6 days.

   T. saginata and *D. latum* infections are usually due to a single adult worm and require an intermediate host in their life cycle. With *Hymenolepis nana* multiple infections are the rule. No intermediate host is required; both larval and adult stages of the worm may be found in the human intestine where the complete life cycle occurs. Since the drug is more effective against the mature than the larval stage, therapy must be extended over several days to cover all stages of maturation.

   Patients with *H. nana* must be instructed to observe strict personal and environmental hygiene to avoid autoinfection with this parasite.
3. NICLOCIDE™ must be thoroughly chewed and then swallowed with a little water. No special dietary restrictions are necessary before or after treatment. The best time to take the drug is after a light meal (e.g., breakfast). A mild laxative may be desirable in constipated patients to achieve a normal bowel movement.

   Young children should have the tablets crushed to a fine powder and mixed with a small amount of water to form a paste.

   NICLOCIDE has a vanilla taste which is not unpleasant to most persons.

   NICLOCIDE is suitable for administration on an ambulatory or outpatient basis.
4. Follow-up:

   As the vermicidal action of NICLOCIDE renders the tapeworm, especially the scolex and proximal segments, vulnerable to destruction during their passage through the gut, it is not always possible to identify the scolex in stools. The sooner the tapeworm is passed and examined after treatment, the better the chance of identification of the scolex. Segments and/or ova of beef or fish tapeworm may be present in the stool for up to 3 days after therapy. Persistent *T. saginata* or *D. latum* segments and/or ova on the seventh day post therapy indicate failure. A second identical course of treatment may be given at that time.

   No patient should be considered cured unless the stool has been negative for a minimum of three months.

How Supplied: NICLOCIDE is available as round, light yellow chewable tablets, scored on one side, embossed with the word Miles and number 721, each containing 500 mg of niclosamide, and is supplied in boxes of 4 tablets.

Storage Conditions: Store below 86°F (30°C), avoid freezing.

Manufactured: by
Bayvet Division Cutter Laboratories, Inc.
Shawnee, Kansas 66201

Distributed by:
Miles Pharmaceuticals
Division of Miles Laboratories, Inc.
West Haven, Connecticut 06516

April, 1982

NYSTAFORM® Ointment ℞
(nystatin-iodochlorhydroxyquin ointment)

Description: NYSTAFORM Ointment contains nystatin U.S.P. 100,000 units/Gm and iodochlorhydroxyquin 1% in a water-dispersible, white petrolatum base containing octylphenoxyethanol and paraffin wax.
Actions: Nystatin acts against Candida species (Monilia). Iodochlorhydroxyquin has antibacterial action against bacteria sensitive to this chemotherapeutic agent.
Indications: NYSTAFORM Ointment is indicated for the treatment of cutaneous or mucocutaneous mycotic infections caused by Candida species (Monilia) complicated by iodochlorhydroxyquin-sensitive bacteria.
Contraindications: Lesions caused by pathogens not susceptible to nystatin and iodochlorhydroxyquin and hypersensitivity to any of the components.
Precautions: If irritation or sensitivity occurs and/or infection persists, discontinue use. If new infections appear, appropriate therapy should be instituted. Trace amounts of iodochlorhydroxyquin present in the diaper or urine can yield a false positive test for phenylketonuria (PKU). Percutaneous absorption of iodochlorhydroxyquin may interfere with thyroid function tests. Therapy should be discontinued for one month before these tests are conducted.
Caution: Federal (U.S.A.) law prohibits dispensing without prescription. For external use only. Not for ophthalmic use. Store below 30°C (86°F), avoid freezing. May stain clothing and hair.
Dosage and Administration: Apply two or three times daily. Continue use for one week after clinical cure.
How Supplied: NYSTAFORM Ointment ½ oz. tube

Otic DOMEBORO® Solution (acid pH) ℞
(acetic acid 2%)

Composition: Acetic acid 2% in aluminum acetate (modified Burow's) solution.
Indications: For the treatment of superficial infections of the external auditory canal caused by organisms susceptible to the action of the antimicrobial.
Precautions: If undue irritation or sensitivity develops, discontinue treatment.
Caution: Federal (U.S.A.) law prohibits dispensing without prescription.
For external use only. Not for ophthalmic use. Store below 86°F (30°C), avoid freezing.
Administration and Dosage: 4 to 6 drops every 2 to 3 hours.
How Supplied: Packaged under sterile conditions in 2 fl. oz. (60 cc.) plastic squeeze bottle with otic tip.

OTIC NEO-CORT-DOME® ℞
Suspension 1% Sterile
(neomycin sulfate-hydrocortisone-acetic acid suspension)
ACID pH

Description: OTIC NEO-CORT-DOME Suspension contains neomycin sulfate (equivalent to 0.35% neomycin base), microdispersed hydrocortisone 1% and acetic acid 2% with emulsifiers, lubricants and preservatives in a compatible vehicle composed of glyceryl monostearate, stearic acid, propylene glycol, potassium sorbate, methyl and propyl parabens, sodium acetate, and purified water, buffered to the pH range for the normal ear.
Actions: Neomycin sulfate is active against a wide variety of gram-positive and gram-negative pathogens. Hydrocortisone has anti-inflammatory, anti-pruritic and anti-allergic properties.
Indications: For the treatment of superficial bacterial infections of the external auditory canal caused by organisms susceptible to the action of the antibacterials, and for the treatment of infections of mastoidectomy and fenestration cavities by organisms susceptible to the action of the antibacterials.
Contraindications: Tuberculous or fungal lesions of the skin or ear, acute herpes simplex, vaccinia or varicella and hypersensitivity to any of the components of the preparation. Perforated tympanic membranes are frequently considered a contra-indication to the use of external ear canal medication.
Precautions: Use with care in cases of chronic otitis media because of the possibility of ototoxicity. If sensitivity occurs and/or infection persists, discontinue use. If new infections appear, appropriate therapy should be instituted. Articles in the current medical literature indicate an increase in the prevalence of persons sensitive to neomycin.
Caution: Federal (U.S.A.) law prohibits dispensing without prescription. For external use only. Not for ophthalmic use.
Usual Dosage: Patient should lie on his side with affected ear uppermost. Gently cleanse and dry the infected ear. Instill 3 to 4 drops into the ear; maintain this position for five minutes. Repeat procedure 3 to 4 times daily. To obtain a uniform dispersion of the suspension, the bottle should be shaken before withdrawing each dose. If preferred, a gauze or cotton wick saturated with Otic Neo-Cort-Dome may be inserted in the ear canal and allowed to remain in situ. It should be kept moist by further addition of the suspension, when required.
Supplied: OTIC NEO-CORT-DOME Suspension 10 cc bottle with dropper.

STILPHOSTROL® ℞
(diethylstilbestrol diphosphate)

Actions: Although the mode of action is not known, diethylstilbestrol diphosphate acts in a similar fashion as estrogens and synthetic estrogens in the treatment of prostatic carcinoma.
Important Notes: An increased risk of thromboembolic disease associated with the use of estrogens has now been conclusively established. Retrospective studies have shown a statistically significant association between thrombophlebitis, pulmonary embolism, and cerebral thrombosis and embolism and the use of these drugs. There have been three principal studies in Great Britain[1-3] and one in the United States[4] leading to this conclusion. As a result of these studies, it has been estimated that users of estrogens are 4 to 7 times more likely than nonusers to develop thromboembolic disease without evident cause. The American study also indicated that the increased risk did not persist after discontinuance nor was it enhanced by long-continued administration.
In a more recent analysis of data derived from several national adverse reaction reporting system(s), British investigators concluded that the risk of thromboembolism, including coronary thrombosis, is directly related to the dose of estrogen. Their analysis did suggest, however, that the quantity of estrogen may not be the sole factor involved. Nevertheless, in view of this study, as well as others that have demonstrated a positive relationship between estrogens and thromboembolism, it would seem prudent and in keeping with basic therapeutic principles, to utilize, whenever feasible, the smallest effective dose of estrogen in treating patients.
Risks associated with certain other known adverse reactions, such as elevated blood pressure, liver dysfunction, and reduced tolerance to carbohydrate, have not as yet been quantitated.
Long-term administration of both natural and synthetic estrogens in subprimate animal species in multiples of the human dose increases the frequency for some animal carcinomas. These data cannot be transposed directly to man. The possible carcinogenicity due to the estrogens can neither be confirmed nor refuted at this time. Close clinical surveillance of all persons taking estrogens must be continued.
Indications: STILPHOSTROL (diethylstilbestrol diphosphate) is indicated for the treatment of inoperable progressing prostatic cancer (for palliation only when castration is not feasible or when castration failures or delayed escape following a response to castration have occurred).
Contraindications: 1. Patients with markedly impaired liver function.
2. Patients with thrombophlebitis, thromboembolic disorders, cerebral apoplexy or with a past history of these conditions.
Warning: 1. The physician should be alert to the earliest manifestations of thrombotic disorders (thrombophlebitis, cerebrovascular disorders, pulmonary embolism and retinal thrombosis). If these occur or are suspected, the drugs should be discontinued immediately.
2. Discontinue medication pending examination if there is sudden onset of proptosis, diplopia or migraine. If examination reveals papilledema or retinal vascular lesions, medication should be withdrawn.
Precautions: 1. Because of estrogen-induced salt and water retention, these drugs should be used with caution in patients with epilepsy, migraine, asthma, cardiac or renal disease.
2. Patients with a history of psychic depression should be carefully observed and the drug discontinued if the depression recurs to a serious degree.
3. Because of a possible decrease in glucose tolerance, diabetic patients should be followed closely.
4. Because estrogens influence the metabolism of calcium and phosphorus, they should be used with caution in patients with certain metabolic bone diseases that are associated with hypercalcemia or in patients with renal insufficiency.
5. The pathologist should be advised of estrogen therapy when relevant specimens are submitted.
6. Certain endocrine and liver function tests may be affected by treatment with estrogens. If such tests are abnormal in a patient taking these drugs it is recommended that they be repeated after the drug has been withdrawn for two months.
Adverse Reactions: A statistically significant association has been demonstrated between use of estrogen-containing drugs and the following serious reactions: thrombophlebitis, pulmonary embolism and cerebral thrombosis. Although available evidence is suggestive of an association, such a relationship has been neither confirmed nor refuted for the following serious reactions: coronary thrombosis and neuro-ocular lesions (e.g., retinal thrombosis and optic neuritis). The following adverse reactions are known to occur in patients receiving estrogens: nausea, vomiting, anorexia, gastrointestinal symptoms (such as abdominal cramps or bloating), edema, breast tenderness and enlargement, change in body weight (increase or decrease), headache, allergic rash, loss of libido and gynecomastia in the male, sterile abscess (injectable forms only), pain at the site of injection (injectable forms only), post-injection flare (injectable forms only), aggravation of migraine headaches, hepatic

Continued on next page

Miles Pharm.—Cont.

cutaneous porphyria becoming manifest, cholestatic jaundice, rise in blood pressure in susceptible individuals, mental depression, cystitis-like syndrome, loss of scalp hair, erythema nodosum, hemorrhagic eruption, changes in libido, changes in appetite, nervousness, dizziness, fatigue, backache, erythema multiforme, itching, irritability, malaise.

Dosage and Administration: TABLETS 50 mg: Start with one tablet t.i.d. and increase this dose level to four or more tablets t.i.d. depending on the tolerance of the patient. Alternatively, if relief is not obtained with high oral dosages, STILPHOSTROL (diethylstilbestrol diphosphate) may be administered intravenously. STILPHOSTROL (diethylstilbestrol diphosphate) solution must be diluted before intravenous infusion.

AMPULS 0.25 g: It is recommended that 0.5 g (2 ampuls) dissolved in 300 ml of saline or 5% dextrose be given intravenously the first day, and that each day thereafter 1 g (4 ampuls) be similarly administered in 300 ml of saline or dextrose. The infusion should be administered slowly (20–30 drops per minute) during the first 10–15 minutes and then the rate of flow adjusted so that the entire amount is given in a period of one hour. This procedure should be followed for five days or more depending on the response of the patient. Following the first intensive course of therapy, 0.25–0.5 g (1 or 2 ampuls) may be administered in a similar manner once or twice weekly or maintenance obtained with STILPHOSTROL (diethylstilbestrol diphosphate) Tablets.

How Supplied: STILPHOSTROL Tablets—Bottles of 50 tablets. Each mottled gray/white tablet contains diethylstilbestrol diphosphate 50 mg and is coded with number 132-Miles. Store at controlled room temperature (59°–86°F).

STILPHOSTROL Ampuls—Boxes of 20 ampuls. Each 5 ml ampul contains diethylstilbestrol diphosphate 0.25 g as a solution of its sodium salts. Store at controlled room temperature (59°–86°F).

Ampules manufactured by Taylor Pharmacal Co., Decatur, Illinois 62525

Distributed by Miles Pharmaceuticals, West Haven, Conn. 06516

References: 1. Royal College of General Practitioners: Oral contraception and thromboembolic disease. *J Coll Gen Pract* 13:267-279, 1967. 2. Inman WHW, Vessey MP: Investigation of deaths from pulmonary, coronary and cerebral thrombosis and embolism in women in childbearing age. *Brit Med J* 2:193-199, 1968. 3. Vessey MP, Doll R: Investigation of relation between use of oral contraceptives and thromboembolic disease. A further report. *Brit Med J* 2:651-657, 1969. 4. Sartwell PE, et al: Thromboembolism and oral contraceptives: An epidemiological case-control study. *Am J Epidemiol* 90:365-380, 1969. 5. Inman, WHW, et al: Thromboembolic disease and the steroidal content of oral contraceptives. *Brit Med J* 2:203-209, 1970. 6. Herbst AL, Ulfelder H, Poskanzer DR: Adenocarcinoma of the vagina. *N Engl J Med* 284:878-881, 1971.

[*Shown in Product Identification Section*]

TRIDESILON® 0.05% ℞
(desonide)
creme

Description: Tridesilon® Creme contains microdispersed desonide (the active ingredient) in a compatible vehicle buffered to the pH range of normal skin. Each gram of Tridesilon® Creme contains 0.5 milligrams of desonide. Tridesilon® Creme is applied topically. Tridesilon® (desonide) is a non-fluorinated corticosteroid. Chemically, desonide is Pregna-1,4-diene-3,20-dione,11,21-dihydroxy-16,17-[(1-methylethylidene)bis(oxy)]-,(11β,16α)- with the following structural formula:

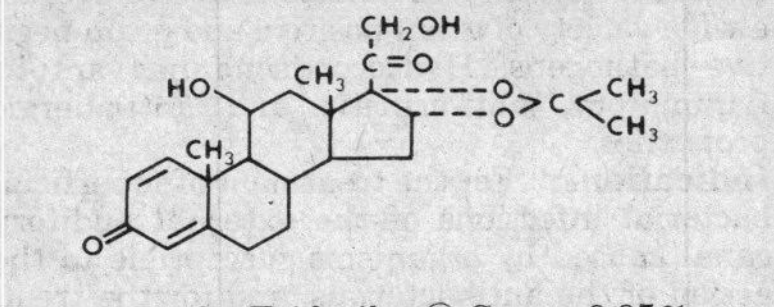

The vehicle for Tridesilon® Creme 0.05% contains glycerin, sodium lauryl sulfate, aluminum sulfate, calcium acetate, dextrin, purified water, cetyl stearyl alcohol, synthetic beeswax, (B-wax), white petrolatum, and light mineral oil. Preserved with methylparaben.

EMPIRICAL FORMULA	MOLECULAR WEIGHT	CAS REGISTRY NUMBER
$C_{24}H_{32}O_6$	416.51	638-94-8

Clinical Pharmacology: Topical corticosteroids share anti-inflammatory, anti-pruritic and vasoconstrictive actions.

The mechanism of anti-inflammatory activity of the topical corticosteroids is unclear. Various laboratory methods, including vasoconstrictor assays, are used to compare and predict potencies and/or clinical efficacies of the topical corticosteroids. There is some evidence to suggest that a recognizable correlation exists between vasoconstrictor potency and therapeutic efficacy in man.

Pharmacokinetics

The extent of percutaneous absorption of topical corticosteroids is determined by many factors including the vehicle, the integrity of the epidermal barrier, and the use of occlusive dressings.

Topical corticosteroids can be absorbed from normal intact skin. Inflammation and/or other disease processes in the skin increase percutaneous absorption. Occlusive dressings substantially increase the percutaneous absorption of topical corticosteroids. Thus, occlusive dressings may be a valuable therapeutic adjunct for treatment of resistant dermatoses. (See DOSAGE AND ADMINISTRATION).

Once absorbed through the skin, topical corticosteroids are handled through pharmacokinetic pathways similar to systemically administered corticosteroids. Corticosteroids are bound to plasma proteins in varying degrees. Corticosteroids are metabolized primarily in the liver and are then excreted by the kidneys. Some of the topical corticosteroids and their metabolites are also excreted into the bile.

Indications and Usage: Topical corticosteroids are indicated for the relief of the inflammatory and pruritic manifestations of corticosteroid-responsive dermatoses.

Contraindications: Topical corticosteroids are contraindicated in those patients with a history of hypersensitivity to any of the components of the preparation.

Precautions:

General

Systemic absorption of topical corticosteroids has produced reversible hypothalmic-pituitary-adrenal (HPA) axis suppression, manifestations of Cushing's syndrome, hyperglycemia, and glucose in some patients.

Conditions which augment systemic absorption include the application of the more potent steroids, use over large surface areas, prolonged use, and the addition of occlusive dressings.

Therefore, patients, receiving a large dose of a potent topical steroid applied to a large surface area or under an occlusive dressing should be evaluated periodically for evidence of HPA axis suppression by using the urinary free cortisol and ACTH stimulation tests. If HPA axis suppression is noted, an attempt should be made to withdraw the drug, to reduce the frequency of application, or to substitute a less potent steroid.

Recovery of HPA axis function is generally prompt and complete upon discontinuation of the drug. Infrequently, signs and symptoms of steroid withdrawal may occur, requiring supplemental systemic corticosteroids.

Children may absorb proportionally larger amounts of topical corticosteroids and thus be more susceptible to systemic toxicity. (See PRECAUTIONS—Pediatric Use).

If irritation develops, topical corticosteroids should be discontinued and appropriate therapy instituted.

In the presence of dermatological infections, the use of an appropriate antifungal or antibacterial agent should be instituted. If a favorable response does not occur promptly, the corticosteroid should be discontinued until the infection has been adequately controlled.

Information for the Patient

Patients using topical corticosteroids should receive the following information and instructions:

1. This medication is to be used as directed by the physician. It is for external use only. Avoid contact with eyes.
2. Patients should be advised not to use this medication for any disorder other than for which it was prescribed.
3. The treated skin area should not be bandaged or otherwise covered or wrapped as to be occlusive unless directed by the physician.
4. Patients should report any signs of local adverse reactions especially under occlusive dressing.
5. Parents of pediatric patients should be advised not to use tightfitting diapers or plastic pants on a child being treated in the diaper area, as these garments may constitute occlusive dressings.

Laboratory Tests

The following tests may be helpful in evaluating the HPA axis suppression:
Urinary free cortisol test
ACTH stimulation test

Carcinogenisis, Mutagenisis, and Impairment of Fertility

Long-term animal studies have not been performed to evaluate the carcinogenic potential or the effect on fertility of topical corticosteroids.

Studies to determine mutagenicity with prednisolone and hydrocortisone have revealed negative results.

Pregnancy Category C

Corticosteroids are generally teratogenic in laboratory animals when administered systemically at relatively low dosage levels. The more potent corticosteroids have been shown to be teratogenic after dermal application in laboratory animals. There are no adequate and well-controlled studies in pregnant women on teratogenic effects from topically applied corticosteroids. Therefore, topical corticosteroids should be used during pregnancy only if the potential benefit justifies the potential risk to the fetus. Drugs of this class should not be used extensively on pregnant patients, in large amounts, or for prolonged periods of time.

Nursing Mothers

It is not known whether topical administration of corticosteroids could result in sufficient systemic absorption to produce detectable quantities in breast milk. Systemically administered corticosteroids are secreted into breast milk in quantities *not* likely to have a deleterious effect on the infant. Nevertheless, caution should be exercised when topical corticosteroids are administered to a nursing woman.

Pediatric Use

Pediatric patients demonstrate greater susceptibility to topical corticosteroid-induced HPA axis suppression and Cushing's syndrome than mature patients because of a larger skin surface area to body weight ratio.

Hypothalamic-pituitary-adrenal (HPA) axis suppression. Cushing's syndrome, and intracranial hypertension have been reported in children receiving topical corticosteroids. Manifestations of adrenal supression in children include linear growth retardation, delayed weight gain, low plasma cortisol levels, and absence of response to ACTH stimulation. Manifestations of intracranial hypertension include bulging fontanelles, headaches, and bilateral papilledema.

Administration of topical corticosteroids to children should be limited to the least amount compatible with an effective therapeutic regimen. Chronic corticosteroid therapy may interfere with the growth and development of children.

Adverse Reactions: The following local adverse reactions are reported infrequently with topical corticosteroids, but may occur more frequently with the use of occlusive dressings. These reactions are listed in an approximate decreasing order of occurrence:

Burning
Itching
Irritation
Dryness
Folliculitis
Hypertrichosis
Acneiform eruptions
Hypopigmentation
Perioral dermatitis
Allergic contact dermatitis
Maceration of the skin
Secondary infection
Skin atrophy
Striae
Miliaria

Overdosage: Topically applied corticosteroids can be absorbed in sufficient amounts to produce systemic effects. (See PRECAUTIONS).

Dosage and Administration: Topical Corticosteroids are generally applied to the affected area as a thin film from two to four times daily depending on the severity of the condition.

Occlusive dressings may be used for management of psoriasis or recalcitrant conditions.

If an infection develops, the use of occlusive dressings should be discontinued and appropriate antimicrobial therapy instituted.

How Supplied: Tridesilon® (desonide) Creme 0.05% is supplied in 15 and 60 gram tubes and in 5 pound jars. It is a white semisolid.

DPSC Stocked:

15 gram—NSN 6505-00-148-6969
60 gram—NSN 6505-001-148-6968
5 pound—NSN 6505-01-004-9217

VA Stocked: 60 gram—SN 6505-01-027-6866A

Store below 86°F (30°C), avoid freezing.

Caution: Federal (USA) law prohibits dispensing without a prescription.

July, 1982 PD100573 18873

TRIDESILON® 0.05% ℞
(desonide)
ointment

Description: Tridesilon® Ointment contains microdispersed desonide (the active ingredient) in a compatible vehicle buffered to the pH range of normal skin. Each gram of Tridesilon® Ointment contains 0.5 miligrams of desonide. Tridesilon® Ointment is applied topically.

Tridesilon® (desonide) is a non-fluorinated corticosteroid. Chemically, desonide is Pregna-1,4-diene-3,20-dione,11,21-dihydroxy-16,17-[(1-methylethylidene)bis(oxy)]-,11β,16α)- with the following structural formula:

The vehicle for Tridesilon® Ointment is white petrolatum.

EMPIRICAL FORMULA	MOLECULAR WEIGHT	CAS REGISTRY NUMBER
$C_{24}H_{32}O_6$	416.51	638-94-8

Clinical Pharmacology: Topical corticosteroids share anti-inflammatory, anti-puritic and vasoconstrictive actions.

The mechanism of anti-inflammatory activity of the topical corticosteroids is unclear. Various laboratory methods, including vasoconstrictor assays, are used to compare and predict potencies and/or clinical efficacies of the topical corticosteroids. There is some evidence to suggest that a recognizable correlation exists between vasoconstrictor potency and therapeutic efficacy in man.

Pharmacokinetics

The extent of percutaneous absorption of topical corticosteroids is determined by many factors including the vehicle, the integrity of the epidermal barrier, and the use of occlusive dressings.

Topical corticosteroids can be absorbed from normal intact skin. Inflammation and/or other disease processes in the skin increase percutaneous absorption. Occlusive dressings substantially increase the percutaneous absorption of topical corticosteroids. Thus, occlusive dressings may be a valuable therapeutic adjunct for treatment of resistant dermatoses. (See DOSAGE AND ADMINISTRATION).

Once absorbed through the skin, topical corticosteroids are handled through pharmacokinetic pathways similar to systemically administered corticosteroids. Corticosteroids are bound to plasma proteins in varying degrees. Corticosteroids are metabolized primarily in the liver and are then excreted by the kidneys. Some of the topical corticosteroids and their metabolites are also excreted into the bile.

Indications and Usage: Topical corticosteroids are indicated for the relief of the inflammatory and pruritic manifestations of corticosteroid-responsive dermatoses.

Contraindications: Topical corticosteroids are contraindicated in those patients with a history of hypersensitivity to any of the components of the preparation.

Precautions:

General

Systemic absorption of topical corticosteroids has produced reversible hypothalamic-pituitary-adrenal (HPA) axis suppression, manifestations of Cushing's syndrome, hyperglycemia, and glucosuria in some patients.

Conditions which augment systemic absorption include the application of the more potent steroids, use over large surface areas, prolonged use, and the addition of occlusive dressings.

Therefore, patients receiving a large dose of a potent topical steroid applied to a large surface area or under an occlusive dressing should be evaluated periodically for evidence of HPA axis suppression by using the urinary free cortisol and ACTH stimulation tests. If HPA axis suppression is noted, an attempt should be made to withdraw the drug, to reduce the frequency of application, or to substitute a less potent steroid.

Recovery of HPA axis functions is generally prompt and complete upon discontinuation of the drug. Infrequently, signs and symptoms of steroid withdrawal may occur, requiring supplemental systemic corticosteroids.

Children may absorb proportionally larger amounts of topical corticosteroids and thus be more susceptible to systemic toxicity. (See PRECAUTIONS—Pediatric Use).

If irritation develops, topical corticosteroids should be discontinued and appropriate therapy instituted.

In the presence of dermatological infections, the use of an appropriate antifungal or antibacterial agent should be instituted. If a favorable response does not occur promptly, the corticosteroid should be discontinued until the infection has been adequately controlled.

Information for the Patient

Patients using topical corticosteroids should receive the following information and instructions:

1. This medication is to be used as directed by the physician. It is for external use only. Avoid contact with the eyes.
2. Patients should be advised not to use this medication for any disorder other than for which it was prescribed.
3. The treated skin area should not be bandaged or otherwise covered or wrapped as to be occlusive unless directed by the physician.
4. Patients should report any signs of local adverse reactions especially under occlusive dressing.
5. Parents of pediatric patients should be advised not to use tight-fitting diapers or plastic pants on a child being treated in the diaper area, as these garments may constitute occlusive dressings.

Laboratory Tests

The following tests may be helpful in evaluating the HPA axis suppression.

Urinary free cortisol test
ACTH stimulation test

Carcinogenisis, Mutagenisis, and Impairment of Fertility

Long-term animal studies have not been performed to evaluate the carcinogenic potential or the effect on fertility of topical corticosteroids.

Studies to determine mutagenicity with prednisolone and hydrocortisone have revealed negative results.

Pregnancy Category C

Corticosteroids are generally teratogenic in laboratory animals when administered systemically at relatively low dosage levels. The more potent corticosteroids have been shown to be teratogenic after dermal application in laboratory animals. There are no adequate and well-controlled studies in pregnant women on teratogenic effects from topically applied corticosteroids. Therefore, topical corticosteroids should be used during pregnancy only if the potential benefit justifies the potential risk to the fetus. Drugs of this class should not be used extensively on pregnant patients, in large amounts, or for prolonged periods of time.

Nursing Mothers

It is not known whether topical administration of corticosteroids could result in sufficient systemic absorption to produce detectable quantities in breast milk. Systemically administered corticosteroids are secreted into breast milk in quantities *not* likely to have a deleterious effect on the infant. Nevertheless, caution should be exercised when topical corticosteroids are administered to a nursing woman.

Pediatric Use

Pediatric patients may demonstrate greater susceptibility to topical corticosteroid-induced HPA axis and Cushing's syndrome than mature patients because of a larger skin surface area to body weight ratio.

Hypothalmic-pituitary-adrenal (HPA) axis suppression, Cushing's syndrome, and intracranial hypertension have been reported in children receiving topical corticosteroids. Manifestations of adrenal suppression in children include linear growth retardation, delayed weight gain, low plasma cortisol levels, and absence of response to ACTH stimulation. Manifestations of intracranial hypertension include bulging fontanelles, headaches, and bilateral papilledema.

Administration of topical costicosteroids to children should be limited to the least amount compatible with an effective therapeutic regimen. Chronic corticosteroid therapy may interfere with the growth and development of children.

Adverse Reactions. The following local adverse reactions are reported infrequently with

Continued on next page

Miles Pharm.—Cont.

topical corticosteroids, but may occur more frequently with the use of occlusive dressings. These reactions are listed in an approximate decreasing order of occurrence:
Burning
Itching
Irritation
Dryness
Folliculitis
Hypertrichosis
Acneiform eruptions
Hypopigmentation
Perioral dermatitis
Allergic contact dermatitis
Maceration of the skin
Secondary infection
Skin atrophy
Striae
Miliaria
Overdosage: Topically applied corticosteroids can be absorbed in sufficient amounts to produce systemic effects. (See PRECAUTIONS).
Dosage and Administration: Topical corticosteroids are generally applied to the affected area as a thin film from two to four times daily depending on the severity of the condition.
Occlusive dressings may be used for the management of psoriasis or recalcitrant conditions. In an infection develops, the use of occlusive dressings should be discontinued and appropriate antimicrobial therapy instituted.
How Supplied: Tridesilon® (desonide) Ointment 0.05% is supplied in 15 and 60 gram tubes. It is white or faintly yellowish, transparent semi-solid.
DPSC Stocked:
15 gram—NSN 6505-00-148-6969
60 gram—NSN 6505-00-148-6968
VA Stocked: 60 gram—SN 6505-01-027-6866A
Store below 86°F (30°C), avoid freezing.
Caution: Federal (USA) law prohibits dispensing without a prescription.
July, 1982 PD100574 18871

Otic TRIDESILON® ℞
Solution 0.05%
(desonide 0.05%—acetic acid 2%)

Description: Otic Tridesilon® Solution contains desonide 0.05% a non-fluorinated corticosteroid (16α- hydroxyprednisolone-16, 17-acetonide) and acetic acid 2% in a compatible vehicle composed of purified water, propylene glycol, sodium acetate, and citric acid.
Actions: Desonide is effective because of its anti-inflammatory, antipruritic and vasoconstrictive actions. Acetic acid has antibacterial and antifungal properties.
Indications: Otic Tridesilon Solution is indicated for the treatment of superficial infections of the external auditory canal caused by organisms susceptible to the action of the antimicrobial and accompanied by inflammation.
Contraindications: Otic Tridesilon Solution (desonide 0.05%—acetic acid 2%) is contraindicated in those patients who have shown hypersensitivity to any of the components of the preparation. Perforated tympanic membranes are frequently considered a contraindication to the use of external ear canal medication.
Precautions: If irritation develops, the product should be discontinued and appropriate therapy instituted.
If infection persists or new infection appears, appropriate therapy should be instituted.
If infection persists or new new infection appears, appropriate therapy should be instituted. If a favorable response does not occur promptly, the corticosteroid should be discontinued until the infection has been adequately controled.
Although topical steroids have not been reported to have an adverse effect on human pregnancy, the safety of their use in pregnant women has not absolutely been established. In laboratory animals, increases in incidence of fetal abnormalities have been associated with exposure of gestating females to topical corticosteroids, in some cases at rather low dosage levels. Therefore, drugs of this class should not be used extensively on pregnant patients, in large amounts, or for prolonged periods of time.
The product is not for ophthalmic use.
Adverse Reactions: The following local adverse reactions have been reported with otic topical corticosteroids:
1. Burning
2. Itching
3. Irritation
4. Dryness
5. Folliculitis
6. Hypertrichosis
7. Hypopigmentation
8. Allergic Contact Dermatitis
9. Maceration of the skin
10. Secondary Infection
11. Skin Atrophy

Administration and Dosage: All cerumінous material and debris should be carefully removed to permit Otic Tridesilon® Solution (desonide 0.05%—acetic acid 2%) to contact the infected surfaces. Instill 3 to 4 drops into the ear 3 to 4 times daily. If preferred, a gauze or cotton wick saturated with the solution may be inserted in the ear canal and allowed to remain in situ. It should be kept moist by further addition of the solution, as required.
Caution: Federal (U.S.A.) law prohibits dispensing without a prescription. For external use only. Store below 86°F (30°C), avoid freezing.
Supplied: Otic Tridesilon Solution (desonide 0.05%—acetic acid 2%) is supplied in 10 cc bottles with dropper.

Milex Products, Inc.
5915 NORTHWEST HIGHWAY
CHICAGO, IL 60631

AMINO-CERV™ ℞
pH 5.5 Cervical Creme

Active Ingredients: Urea 8.34%, Sodium Propionate 0.50%, Methionine 0.83%, Cystine 0.35%, Inositol 0.83%, Benzalkonium Chloride 0.000004%. Buffered to pH of 5.5 in a water-miscible creme base.
Description: An AMINO-ACID and UREA creme specifically formulated for cervical treatment: Cervicitis (mild), postpartum cervicitis, postpartum cervical tears, post cauterization, post cryosurgery and post conization.
Advantages: METHIONINE and CYSTINE are amino-acids necessary for wound healing and forming of epithelial tissue. INOSITOL acts as an essential growth factor and promotes epithelialization.
UREA aids in debridement, dissolves the coagulum and promotes epithelialization. Its solvent action on fibroblasts prevents the formation of excessive tissue—thus preventing stenosis when used as directed.
BENZALKONIUM CHLORIDE serves to lower surface tension and thus aids in spreading the medication. Along with SODIUM PROPIONATE it also exerts a bacteriostatic effect.
AMINO-CERV is geared to the higher pH of the healthy cervix in contrast with pH 4 vaginal preparations. With its pH factor of 5.5 Amino-Cerv promotes faster healing of the cervix, yet will not adversely affect a healthy vagina.
Directions: When immediate postpartum bleeding has subsided (usually from 24 to 48 hours after delivery), one Milex-Jector full of AMINO-CERV creme should be applied nightly for four weeks. In mild CERVICITIS (not requiring cautery or cryosurgery) one applicatorful of AMINO-CERV should be injected in the vagina nightly upon retiring for 2 weeks.
A small amount of AMINO-CERV should be applied immediately after HOT CAUTERIZATION, HOT CONIZATION and CRYOSURGERY. One applicatorful should be injected nightly upon retiring for 2 to 4 weeks (the duration of treatment depends on extent of cauterization or hot conization or cryosurgery). During the weekly office visit for (2 to 4 visits) the physician should again apply a small amount of AMINO-CERV with a probe or applicator. The canal is to be completely probed on the last visit.
After COLD CONING, one applicatorful should be injected upon retiring about 24 hours after surgery and nightly thereafter for four weeks. During the four weekly office visits following cold coning, a small amount of AMINO-CERV should be applied with a probe or applicator into the canal by the physician. The canal is to be completely probed on the last visit.
Reasons For Variation of Directions:
(1) After hot conization, cauterization and cryosurgery immediate use of AMINO-CERV is indicated to aid in dissolving dead or burned tissue.
(2) After cold coning, there is no dead tissue to slough off. Therefore, a wait of 24 hours or longer is desirable for normal healing to take place and for some fibroblasts to be laid down before applying the AMINO-CERV (which has a solvent action on both the fibroblasts and the absorbable sutures). When NONABSORBABLE sutures are used, AMINO-CERV can be used immediately.
Contraindications: Deleterious side effects have not been a problem at the doses recommended. The usual precautions against allergic reactions should be observed.
Storage: Store at room temperature.
Packaging: 2¾ oz. tube with Milex-Jector (2 weeks supply, 14 applications).
Available only on hospital direct orders: 5½ oz. tube with MILEX-JECTOR (4 weeks supply, 28 applications).

PRO-CEPTION

Description: PRO-CEPTION is a precoital douche to help promote conception. It provides in a convenient form supplementary nutrient immediately available to the sperm for metabolism and movement. Also effective for removal of a thick tenacious mucous plug of the cervix.
Directions: The screw cap is used as a measuring device and filled level with the powder which is then dissolved in eight ounces of lukewarm water. The woman is told to douche while in a recumbent position and to retain the solution (10 to 15 minutes). Following coitus the patient should remain recumbent for two hours or more. May be used as a companion with Milex Oligospermia Cups. Frequently used in connection with PRO-CEPTION Basal Thermometers.
Contraindications: None.
Packaging: Available in 12 douche container.

Products are

listed alphabetically

in the

PINK SECTION.

Mission Pharmacal Company
1325 E. DURANGO ST.
SAN ANTONIO, TX 78210

CALCET®
Calcium Supplement
NDC-0178-0251-01

Composition: Each tablet contains:

	% US RDA*	
Calcium Lactate		240 mg.
Calcium Gluconate		240 mg.
Calcium Carbonate		240 mg.
(Calcium	15	152.8 mg.)
Vitamin D2	25	100. Units

* Percent of U.S. Recommended Daily Allowance for adults and children 4 or more years of age.

Indications: CALCET® tablets are indicated as a daily supplement to provide a dietary source of calcium. CALCET® tablets are of particular value in people who have milk allergies, in people who have low calcium leg cramps or calcium deficiencies due to low dietary calcium.

Dosage: TWO CALCET® TABLETS AT BEDTIME as a general or prenatal supplement. In calcium deficiency states or in nocturnal leg cramping, dosage should be increased to TWO CALCET® TABLETS AT BEDTIME plus one tablet mid-morning and one tablet mid-afternoon.

How Supplied: CALCET® tablets are supplied as yellow, oval shaped, coated tablets in bottles of 100 tablets.

Literature Available: Yes.

COMPETE®
Multivitamins with Iron and Zinc
NDC-0178-0221-01

Description: COMPETE® is a multivitamin with iron and zinc formulated to provide an especially well tolerated group of nutritional components for the active, stressful lifestyle of the 1980's. COMPETE® provides 150% of the U.S.R.D.A. of all components except vitamins A and D, which have been maintained at a 100% level, and vitamin B_6 which is provided in a level of 1250% U.S.R.D.A. for the particular needs of today's active woman using birth control tablets.

Composition: Each tablet contains:

	Quantity/ Tablet	%USRDA
Vitamin A	5000 I.U.	100%
Vitamin D	400 I.U.	100%
Vitamin E	45 I.U.	150%
Vitamin C	90 mg	150%
Folic Acid	0.4 mg	150%
Thiamine Mononitrate	2.25 mg	150%
Riboflavin	2.6 mg	150%
Niacinamide	30 mg	150%
Pyridoxine HCl	25.0 mg	1250%
Vitamin B_{12}	9 mcg	150%
Iron (As Ferrous Gluconate 233 mg)	27 mg	150%
Zinc (As Zinc Sulfate)	22.5 mg	150%

Dosage: One tablet at bedtime as directed by your physician.

Warning: KEEP THIS AND ALL MEDICATIONS OUT OF THE REACH OF CHILDREN. In case of accidental overdose, seek professional assistance or contact a poison control center immediately.

Precaution: Folic Acid, especially in doses above 0.1 mg. daily, may obscure pernicious anemia in that hematologic remission may occur while neurological manifestations remain progressive.

How Supplied: COMPETE® is supplied as orange, football-shaped, sugar coated tablets in bottles of 100.

DILAX®-250
Docusate Sodium U.S.P. 250 mg.
NDC 0178-0242-01

Indications: DILAX® is a stool softener which works by softening and homogenizing bowel contents. DILAX® is safe because it has no systemic drug action and is not habit forming. DILAX® does not cause irritation of the bowel and is recommended by physicians for the prevention of constipation in heart conditions, anorectal conditions, in obstetrical patients and following surgical procedures. DILAX® is also helpful in ulcerative colitis, diverticulitis and in bedridden or hospitalized patients who must avoid constipation. DILAX® provides formation of soft easily evacuated stools without discomfort, oily leakage or interference with vitamin absorption.

Contraindications: DILAX® does not cause known side effects and overdosage does not cause toxic effect.

Dosage and Administration: Take one DILAX®-250 capsule at bedtime with a full glass of water. Dosage may be adjusted upward if necessary to achieve the desired result. In some individuals several days dosage may be necessary to provide proper softening actions.

EQUILET®
Antacid Compound
NDC-0178-0010-01

Composition: Each tablet contains:
Calcium Carbonate .... 500 mg.

Action and Uses: High capacity gastric antacid.

Administration and Dosage: One or two EQUILET® tablets as needed preferably between meals and at bedtime. EQUILET® tablets may be chewed or swallowed with water with equal effect according to the convenience or desire of the individual. Do not take more than 16 tablets in a 24-hour period except as may be directed by your physician.

How Supplied: EQUILET® is supplied as light yellow scored tablets in packages of 100 tablets.

Literature Available: Yes.

FERRALET®
Ferrous Gluconate
NDC-0178-0082-01

Composition: Each tablet contains:

		% US RDA*
Ferrous Gluconate	320 mg	
(Iron	37.0 mg.)	206.0

*Percent of U.S. recommended daily allowance for adults and children 4 or more years of age.

Description: The FERRALET® tablet contains only one active ingredient, iron, as ferrous gluconate. FERRALET® is particularly well tolerated in most patients because ferrous gluconate is non-astringent, non-irritating, and will not precipitate protein from aqueous media. FERRALET® provides a more efficient source of ferrous ion because of the low ionization constant of ferrous gluconate, coupled with high solubility and stability over the entire pH range of the gastrointestinal tract. FERRALET® provides utilizable iron throughout the entire length of the intestinal absorption bed. With FERRALET®, heavy iron loading is not necessary due to the superior efficiency of the iron component. The result of moderate ferrous ion dosage is usually improved patient acceptance and excellent dosage continuity. FERRALET® is manufactured in a unique, easy to swallow shape, to further enhance patient acceptance of the product. FERRALET® has a tailored disintegration rate to minimize gastric intoleration with a rapid dissolution rate to assure rapid availability for absorption.

Indications: Anemias amenable to iron therapy.

Dosage: One to three tablets a day depending upon the severity of the anemia and the particular toleration of the patient.

How Supplied: FERRALET® is packaged in bottles of 100 tablets.

Literature Available: Yes.

FOSFREE®
Calcium—Vitamins—Iron
NDC-0178-0031-01

Composition: Each tablet contains:

	One Tablet	% US RDA
Calcium Lactate	250.0 mg.	
Calcium Gluconate	250.0 mg.	
Calcium Carbonate	300.0 mg.	
(Calcium	175.7 mg.)	17
Ferrous Gluconate	125.0 mg.	
(Iron	14.5 mg.)	80
Vitamin D_2	150.0 USP U.	optional
Vitamin A Acetate	1500.0 USP U.	30
Ascorbic Acid (C)	50.0 mg.	83
Pyridoxine HCl (B_6)	3.0 mg.	150
Thiamine Mononitrate (B_1)	5.0 mg.	333
Riboflavin (B_2)	2.0 mg.	117
Niacinamide (B_3)	10.0 mg.	50
d-Calcium Pantothenate (B_5)	1.0 mg.	10
Vitamin B_{12} (Crystalline on resin)	2.0 mcg.	33

Action and Uses: FOSFREE® tablets are primarily indicated as a prenatal, postpartum or geriatric supplement particularly when soluble calcium salt supplementation is desired. FOSFREE® is a specific for hypocalcemic tetany (nocturnal leg cramping).

Administration and Dosage: One or two FOSFREE® tablets at bedtime as a general or prenatal supplement. In calcium deficiency states or in nocturnal leg cramping, dosage should be increased to two FOSFREE® tablets at bedtime plus one tablet mid-morning and one tablet mid-afternoon.

How Supplied: FOSFREE® is supplied as yellow capsule shaped coated tablets in bottles of 100 tablets.

Literature Available: Yes.

HOMAPIN® ℞
Homatropine Methylbromide

Description: Each tablet contains the following amounts of Homatropine Methylbromide, a synthetic quaternary ammonium derivative of belladona alkaloids:

Homapin- 5: Homatropine Methylbromide 5 mg

Homapin-10: Homatropine Methylbromide 10 mg

Actions: This drug diminishes gastric acid secretion and relieves smooth muscle spasm of the gastrointestinal tract.

Indications: Based on a review of this drug by the National Academy of Sciences—National Research Council and/or other information, FDA has classified the indications as "possibly" effective:
For use as adjunctive therapy in the treatment of peptic ulcer.
IT SHOULD BE NOTED AT THIS POINT IN TIME THAT THERE IS A LACK OF CONCURRENCE AS TO THE VALUE OF ANTICHOLINERGICS/ANTISPASMODICS IN THE TREATMENT OF GASTRIC ULCER. IT HAS NOT BEEN SHOWN CONCLUSIVELY WHETHER ANTICHOLINERGIC / ANTISPASMODIC DRUGS AID IN THE HEALING OF A PEPTIC ULCER, DECREASE THE RATE OF RECURRENCES, OR PREVENT COMPLICATION.

Continued on next page

Mission—Cont.

May also be useful in the irritable bowel syndrome (irritable colon, spastic colon, mucous colitis), and acute enterocolitis. Final classification of the less-than effective indications requires further investigation.

Contraindications: Glaucoma, obstructive uropathy (for example, bladder neck obstruction due to prostatic hypertrophy); obstructive disease of the gastrointestinal tract (as in achalasia, pyloroduodenal stenosis, etc.); paralytic ileus, intestinal atony of the elderly or debilitated patient; unstable cardiovascular status in acute hemorrhage; severe ulcerative colitis especially if complicated by toxic megacolon; myasthenia gravis; hiatal hernia associated with reflex esophagitis.

Warnings: Homatropine Methylbromide should be used in pregnancy, lactation, in women of childbearing age only when in the judgement of the physician, the expected benefits outweigh the potential hazards to the mother and child.

In the presence of a high environmental temperature, heat prostration can occur with drug use (fever and heatstroke due to decreased sweating).

Diarrhea may be an early symptom of incomplete intestinal obstruction, especially in patients with ileostomy or colostomy. In this instance treatment with this drug would be inappropriate and possibly harmful.

Homatropine Methylbromide may produce drowsiness or blurred vision. In this event, the patient should be warned not to engage in activities requiring mental alertness such as operating a motor vehicle or other machinery, or perform hazardous work while taking this drug.

Precautions: Use with caution in patients with:

Autonomic neuropathy.

Hepatic or renal disease.

Hyperthyroidism, coronary heart disease, congestive heart failure, cardiac arrhythmias, and hypertension.

It should be noted that the use of anticholinergic/antispasmodic drugs in the treatment of gastric ulcer may produce a delay in gastric emptying time and may complicate such therapy (antral stasis).

Do not rely on the use of the drug in the presence of complication of biliary tract disease.

Investigate any tachycardia before giving anticholinergic (atropine-like) drugs since they may increase the heart rate.

Adverse Reactions: Adverse reactions may include xerostomia; urinary hesitancy and retention; blurred vision and tachycardia; palpitation; mydriasis; cycloplegia; increased ocular tension, loss of taste, headache; nervousness; drowsiness; weakness; dizziness; insomnia; nausea; vomiting; impotency; suppression of lactation; constipation; bloated feeling; severe allergic reaction or drug idiosyncrasies including anaphylaxis; urticaria and other dermal manifestations; and decreased sweating. Elderly patients may react with symptoms of excitement, agitation, drowsiness, and other untoward manifestations to even small doses of the drug.

Dosage and Administration:

Usual Adult Dosage: One tablet half-hour before meals and at bedtime. Dosage should be adjusted to individual patient's needs.

Overdosage: A curare-like action may occur.

Management of Overdosage: Gastric lavage, emetics, universal antidote. Barbiturates for sedation, orally or intramuscularly. Parenteral cholinergic agents such as bethanechol chloride.

How Supplied: HOMAPIN® is supplied in bottles of 100 tablets in the following strengths:

PRODUCT	DOSAGE	COLOR
HOMAPIN® 5	5 mg. tablet NDC 0178-0041-01	White
HOMAPIN® 10	10 mg. tablet NDC 0178-0141-01	Blue

IROMIN-G®

Hematinic Supplement
NDC-0178-0081-01

Composition: Each tablet contains:

	% US RDA	
Ferrous Gluconate		333.3 mg.
(Iron	214	38.6 mg.)
Ascorbic Acid (C)	166	100.0 mg.
Thiamine Mononitrate (B_1)	333	5.0 mg.
Pyridoxine HCl (B_6)	1250	25.0 mg.
Riboflavin (B_2)	117	2.0 mg.
Niacinamide	50	10.0 mg.
Folic Acid	200	0.8 mg.
d-Calcium Pantothenate	10	1.0 mg.
Vitamin B_{12} (Crystalline on resin)	33	2.0 mcg.
Vitamin A Acetate	80	4000.0 USP U.
Vitamin D_2	Optional	400.0 USP U.
Calcium Carbonate		70.0 mg.
Calcium Gluconate		100.0 mg.
Calcium Lactate		100.0 mg.
(Calcium	5	50.0 mg.)

Action and Uses: Secondary anemias, and as a supplement for the prenatal, teenage and geriatric diet.

Administration and Dosage: One to three tablets daily after meals or as directed by a physician.

Precaution: Folic Acid, especially in doses above 0.1 mg. daily, may obscure pernicious anemia in that hematologic remission may occur while neurological manifestations remain progressive.

Side Effects: IROMIN-G® is virtually free of side effects when given in the recommended dosage. The rare constipation, diarrhea, or gastric upset can usually be controlled by dosage adjustment.

How Supplied: IROMIN-G® is supplied as red football shaped coated tablets in bottles of 100 tablets.

Literature Available: Yes.

MISSION PRENATAL SERIES

MISSION PRENATAL®

Vitamins—Iron—Calcium—.4 mg. Folic Acid
NDC 0178-132-01

MISSION PRENATAL® F.A.

Vitamins—Iron—Calcium—.8 mg. Folic Acid and Zinc
NDC 0178-0153-01

MISSION PRENATAL® H.P. ℞

Vitamins—Iron—Calcium—1.0 mg. Folic Acid
NDC 0178-0161-01

Composition: Each tablet contains:

	%U.S.R.D.A.	
Ferrous Gluconate		333.3 mg.
(Iron	214	38.6 mg.)
Ascorbic Acid (C)	167	100.0 mg.
Thiamine Mononitrate (B_1)	270	5.0 mg.
*† Pyridoxine HCl (B_6)	99	3.0 mg.
Riboflavin (B_2)	100	2.0 mg.
Niacinamide	50	10.0 mg.
d-Calcium Pantothenate	9	1.0 mg.
Vitamin B_{12} (Crystalline on Resin)	25	2.0 mcg.
*† Folic Acid	50	0.4 mg.
Vitamin A Acetate	50	4000.0 USPU
Vitamin D_2	100	400.0 USPU
Calcium Carbonate		70.0 mg.
Calcium Gluconate		100.0 mg.
Calcium Lactate		100.0 mg.
(Calcium	4	50.0 mg.)
Zinc (as Zinc Sulfate)		15.0 mg.

*Pyridoxine HCL—Mission® Prenatal F.A. =10mg., 329%U.S.R.D.A.

*Folic Acid—Mission® Prenatal F.A. =.8mg., 100%U.S.R.D.A.

†Pyridoxine HCL—Mission®Prenatal H.P. =25 mg., 1250%U.S.R.D.A.

†Folic Acid—Mission® Prenatal H.P. =1.0 mg., 125%U.S.R.D.A.

Zinc—only in Mission® Prenatal F.A.

Indications: ALL MISSION® PRENATALS are prenatal and postpartum supplements.

Dosage: Take one tablet at bedtime or as directed by your physician. Keep this and all medications out of the reach of children.

Caution: MISSION® PRENATAL H.P. prohibits dispensing without a prescription.

Precaution: Folic Acid, especially in doses above 0.1 mg. daily, may obscure pernicious anemia in that hematologic remission may occur while neurological manifestations remain progressive.

How Supplied: MISSION® PRENATAL is supplied as pink, football-shaped, sugar-coated tablets in bottles of 100.

MISSION® PRENATAL F.A. is supplied as blue, football-shaped, sugar coated tablets in bottles of 100.

MISSION® PRENATAL H.P. is supplied as green, football-shaped, sugar-coated tablets in bottles of 100.

MISSION® PRE-SURGICAL

A dietary supplement for pre-surgical and post-surgical patients. NDC 0178-0168-01

Composition: Each tablet contains:

		%USRDA*
Ascorbic Acid (C)	500.0 mg	833
Thiamine Mononitrate (B_1)	2.5 mg	150
Riboflavin(B_2)	2.6 mg	150
Niacinamide (B_3)	30.0 mg	150
Calcium Pantothenate (B_5)	16.3 mg	150
Pyridoxine Hydrochloride (B_6)	3.6 mg	150
Vitamin B_{12}	9.0 mcg	150
Vitamin A Acetate	5000 USPU	100
Vitamin D_2	400 USPU	100
Vitamin E Succinate	45 IU	150
Iron (as Ferrous Gluconate)	27.0 mg	150
Zinc (as Zinc Sulfate)	22.5 mg	150

*USRDA: U.S. Recommended Daily Allowance for adults and children 4 or more years of age.

Action and Uses: A dietary supplement specifically designed to provide the vitamin and mineral nutritional assistance needed by the pre- and post-surgical patient for optimal recovery from the stress of surgery.

Administration and Dosage: One tablet at bedtime or as directed by physician.

Warning: KEEP THIS AND ALL MEDICATIONS OUT OF THE REACH OF CHILDREN.

In case of accidental overdose, seek professional assistance or contact a poison control center immediately.

How Supplied: MISSION® PRE-SURGICAL is supplied as a light green, bolus-shaped, sugar coated tablet in bottles of 100.

Literature available: Yes.

PRULET®
White Phenolphthalein tablets N.F.
NDC 0178-0090-01

Composition: Each tablet contains:
White phenolphthalein N.F. .... 60 mg.
Action and Uses: PRULET® is a mild and gentle, effective laxative for patients with atonic or hypotonic bowel syndrome.
PRULET® is a chewable tablet in lemon—lime flavor.
Administration and Dosage: Take one to three tablets administered at bedtime; then adjust to need.
Contraindications: Not to be taken in the presence of nausea, vomiting, abdominal pains, or other symptoms of appendicitis.
Precautions: Phenolphthalein is known to produce skin eruptions in sensitized individuals. If a skin rash or eruption appears, do not take this or any other preparation containing phenolphthalein. PRULET® may cause pink to red urine coloration in patients with an alkaline urine.
How Supplied: PRULET® is supplied in green scored tablets in film strip packages of 12 and 40 tablets.
Literature Available: Yes.

PRULET® LIQUITAB®
White phenolphthalein tablets N.F.
NDC 0178-0120-50

Composition: Each tablet contains:
White phenolphthalein N.F. .... 30 mg.
Action and Uses: The PRULET® LIQUITAB® is a delicious fruit flavored, chewable laxative for adults and children (see PRULET®).
Administration and Dosage: Children: Chew or allow to dissolve in mouth 1 to 2 tablets at bedtime. Adults: Chew or allow to dissolve in mouth 1 to 3 tablets at bedtime. Adjust dosage to optimum level on following evening.
Contraindications: (See PRULET®)
Precautions: (See PRULET®)
How Supplied: PRULET® LIQUITABS® are supplied in packages of 100 tablets.
Literature Available: Yes.

SUPAC®
Analgesic Compound
NDC-0178-0100-01

Composition: Each tablet contains:
Acetaminophen..160 mg.
Aspirin ....230 mg.
Caffeine .... 33 mg.
Calcium Gluconate..................................... 60 mg.
Action and Uses: For temporary relief of pain accompanying simple head colds, temporary relief of pain accompanying menstruation, sinus and tension headache, minor traumatic pain, tooth extractions, arthritic and rheumatic pain syndromes.
Administration and Dosage: Adults—One or two tablets. This dose may be repeated in 4 hours. Do not exceed 4 tablets at a single dose or 16 tablets in a 24 hour period. Children—6 to 12 years of age, ½ of the maximum adult dose or dosage; 3 to 6 years of age, ⅓ of the maximum adult dose or dosage.
Precautions: If pain persists for more than 10 days, or redness is present, or in conditions affecting children under 12 years of age, physicians should be alert to other possible complications.
How Supplied: SUPAC® is supplied as white scored tablets in bottles of 100 and 1000 tablets.
Literature Available: Yes.

THERABID®
Therapeutic Multivitamin
NDC 0178-0171-01

Composition: Each Tablet Contains:

		% US RDA
Ascorbic Acid (Vitamin C)	500 mg.	833
Thiamine Mononitrate (Vitamin B_1)	15 mg.	1000
Riboflavin (Vitamin B_2)	10 mg.	588
Niacinamide (Vitamin B_3)	100 mg.	500
Calcium Pantothenate (Vitamin B_5)	20 mg.	200
Pyridoxine Hydrochloride (Vitamin B_6)	10 mg.	500
Vitamin B_{12}	5 mcg.	83
Vitamin A Acetate	5,000 U.	100
Vitamin D_2	200 U.	optional
Vitamin E (as a-tocopheryl acetate)	30 IU	100

Action and Uses: THERABID® is a therapeutic multivitamin preparation.
Administration and Dosage: One to two tablets per day or at the discretion of the physician.
Precautions: Do not exceed a dosage of four tablets per day.
How Supplied: THERABID® is supplied as green capsule shaped sugar coated tablets in bottles of 100 tablets.
Literature Available: Yes.

THERA–GESIC®
Analgesic Creme Balm
Methyl Salicylate and Menthol

Description: THERA-GESIC® contains Methyl Salicylate and Menthol in a rapidly absorbed greaseless base.
Actions: Topical analgesic, counter irritant.
Indications: For the temporary relief of pain associated with musculo-skeletal soreness and discomfort; additionally, as a topical adjunct in arthritis, rheumatism, and bursitis.
Contraindications: Do not use in patients with Aspirin or Salicylate idiosyncrasy.
Warnings: Use only as directed. Keep away from children to avoid accidental poisoning. Keep away from eyes, mucous membranes, broken or irritated skin. If skin irritation develops, or if pain lasts 10 days or more, or if redness is present, discontinue use and consult a physician. DO NOT SWALLOW. If swallowed, induce vomiting, call a physician.
Precautions: Do not use excessive amounts of THERA-GESIC® or occlude a fresh application of THERA-GESIC®. Do not heat pack THERA-GESIC® covered skin. For use by adults only.
Adverse Reactions: Adverse reactions related to the Salicylate and Menthol components are possible. These include excessive irritation, tinnitus, nausea or vomiting if excessive or extreme dosage is employed.
Dosage and Administration: Gently massage THERA-GESIC® in thin applications into the sore or painful area as well as into the area immediately surrounding the painful area. The number of thin applications applied controls the intensity of the action of THERA-GESIC®. One application provides a mild effect, two provide a strong effect and three applications provide a very strong effect. Once THERA-GESIC® has penetrated the skin, the area may be washed, leaving the area dry, clean and free from the typical wintergreen odor without decreasing the effectiveness of the product. If you intend to bandage or wrap the area, the area should be washed first to avoid excessive irritation.
How Supplied:
NDC-0178-0320-05 Tubes–5 oz.

Products are cross-indexed by generic and chemical names in the

YELLOW SECTION

Muro Pharmaceutical, Inc.
890 EAST STREET
TEWKSBURY, MA 01876

BROMFED™ CAPSULES ℞

A green and clear capsule containing white beads.
Each capsule contains:
Brompheniramine maleate .... 12 mg.
Pseudoephedrine hydrochloride .... 120 mg.
in a specially prepared base to provide prolonged action.

BROMFED™ PD CAPSULES ℞

A blue—green and clear capsule containing white beads.
Each capsule contains:
Brompheniramine maleate .... 6 mg.
Pseudoephedrine hydrochloride .... 60 mg.
in a specially prepared base to provide prolonged action.

BROMFED™ TABLETS ℞

A white scored tablet.
Each tablet contains:
Brompheniramine maleate .... 4 mg.
Pseudoephedrine hydrochloride .... 60 mg.
BROMFED contains ingredients of the following therapeutic classes: antihistamine and decongestant.
Clinical Pharmacology: Brompheniramine maleate is an alkylamine type antihistamine. This group of antihistamines are among the most active histamine antagonists and are generally effective in relatively low doses. The drugs are not so prone to produce drowsiness and are among the most suitable agents for day time use; but again, a significant proportion of patients do experience this effect. Pseudoephedrine hydrochloride is a sympathomimetic which acts predominently on alpha receptors and has little action on beta receptors. It therefore functions as an oral nasal decongestant with minimal CNS stimulation.
Indications: For the temporary relief of symptoms of the common cold, allergic rhinitis (hay fever) and sinusitis.
Contraindications: Hypersensitivity to any of the ingredients. Also contraindicated in patients with severe hypertension, severe coronary artery disease, patients on MAO inhibitor therapy, patients with narrow-angle glaucoma, urinary retention, peptic ulcer and during an asthmatic attack.
Warnings: Considerable caution should be exercised in patients with hypertension, diabetes mellitus, ischemic heart disease, hyperthyroidism, increased intraocular pressure and prostatic hypertrophy. The elderly (60 years or older) are more likely to exhibit adverse reactions.
Antihistamines may cause excitability, especially in children. At dosages higher than the recommended dose, nervousness, dizziness or sleeplessness may occur.
Precautions: General: Caution should be exercised in patients with high blood pressure, heart disease, diabetes or thyroid disease. The antihistamine in this product may exhibit additive effects with other CNS depressants, including alcohol.
Information for Patients: Antihistamine may cause drowsiness and ambulatory patients who operate machinery or motor vehicles should be cautioned accordingly.
Drug Interactions: MAO inhibitors and beta adrenergic blockers increase the effects of sympathomimetics. Sympathomimetics may reduce the antihypertensive effects of methyldopa, mecamylamine, reserpine and veratrum alkaloids. Concomitant use of antihistamines with alcohol and other CNS depressants may have an additive effect.

Continued on next page

Muro—Cont.

Pregnancy: The safety of use of this product in pregnancy has not been established.
Adverse Reactions: Adverse reactions include drowsiness, lassitude, nausea, giddiness, dryness of mouth, blurred vision, cardiac palpitations, flushing, increased irritability or excitement (especially in children).
Dosage and Administration:
BROMFED™ CAPSULES Adults and children over 12 years of age —1 capsule orally every 12 hours.
BROMFED™ PD CAPSULES Children 6 to 12 years of age —1 capsule orally every 12 hours. Adults —2 capsules every 12 hours.
BROMFED™ TABLETS Adults and children 12 and over: One tablet every 4 hours not to exceed 6 doses in 24 hours. Children 6 to 12 years: One-half tablet every 4 hours not to exceed 6 doses in 24 hours. Do not give to children under 6 years except under the advice and supervision of a physician.
How Supplied: Bottle of 100
Dispense in tight containers as defined in USP. Store between 59°–85°F.

LIQUID PRED Syrup ℞

Each teaspoonful contains:
Prednisone 5mg/5ml
How Supplied:
NDC-0451-1201-04–4 fl. oz. (120 ml)
NDC-0451-1202-08–8 fl. oz. (240 ml)

MURO TEARS™
Artificial Tears

(See PDR For Nonprescription Drugs)

SALINEX Nasal Mist
(Buffered isotonic sodium chloride solution)

(See PDR for Nonprescription Drugs)

Neutrogena Corporation
5755 W. 96TH STREET
P.O. BOX 45036
LOS ANGELES, CA 90045

NEUTROGENA®
Acne Cleansing Formula Soap

Composition: A mild, transparent, triethanolamine base soap containing no free alkali. Contains triethanolamine stearate, triethanolamine, sodium tallowate, glycerin, water, sodium cocoate, sodium castorate, TEA lauryl sulfate, triethanolamine oleate, acetylated lanolin alcohol, cocamide DEA, alcohol, fragrance, and tocopherol.
Actions and Uses: For use as a cleansing and drying adjunct to acne treatment. Neutrogena Acne-Cleansing Soap is based on the original Neutrogena Soap formulation with the addition of a lipid solvent, acetylated lanolin alcohol, and a surfactant, TEA lauryl sulfate. Aids in the cleansing and degreasing of the skin, and helps remove fatty or oily secretions. Extremely water soluble, Neutrogena Acne-Cleansing Soap is also non-medicated and will not interfere with other acne treatment, systemic or topical.
Administration and Dosage: For a mild drying effect, use once a day; for moderate drying, use twice a day; for more intensive drying, use three times a day; or use as physician directs.
How Supplied: 3.5 oz. Bar.

NEUTROGENA® Acne-Drying Gel

Composition: A clear gel base containing witch hazel, isopropyl alcohol, propylene glycol, carbomer 940, triethanolamine, EDTA, methylparaben, propylparaben, benzophenone-2, FD&C Yellow #5, FD&C Red #40, FD&C Blue #1. Contains 46% isopropyl alcohol, 7.5% alcohol (derived from witch hazel).
Actions and Uses: For use as a drying adjunct to acne treatment for the acne patient with sensitive skin. Helps degrease and reduce oily secretions on the skin, combining antisepsis and astringency. Neutrogena Acne-Drying Gel contains no perfume, is non-medicated and has a fresh, natural witch hazel scent. Can be applied under makeup.
Caution: Avoid contact with eyes and mouth. Should irritation occur, discontinue use.
Administration and Dosage: First wash with Neutrogena Acne-Cleansing Soap then apply Neutrogena Acne-Drying Gel. For mild to moderate drying effect, use once or twice a day; for more intensive drying, use three times a day; or use as physician directs.
How Supplied: ¾ oz. plastic tube.

NEUTROGENA®
Dry Skin Formula Soap

Composition: A mild, transparent, triethanolamine base soap containing no free alkali. Contains triethanolamine stearate, triethanolamine, sodium tallowate, glycerin, water, sodium cocoate, sodium castorate, triethanolamine oleate, laneth-10-acetate, nonoxynol-14 and PEG-4 octoate, cocamide DEA, fragrance (deleted for unscented formula) and tocopherol.
Action and Uses: Neutrogena Dry Skin Soap is specifically formulated to gently cleanse dry skin. Formulation is based on the original Neutrogena Soap formula with two added superfatting agents, nonoxynol-14 and PEG-4 octoate, plus laneth-10-acetate, and fatty acid esters to help retain moisture.
Administration and Dosage: Use daily in place of other soaps or as physician directs.
How Supplied: 3.5 and 5.5 oz. bars in Scented formula; 3.5 oz. bars in Unscented formula.

NEUTROGENA® MELANEX™ ℞
(3% hydroquinone topical solution)

Composition: Neutrogena Melanex™ is a 3% hydroquinone topical solution for the treatment of hyperpigmentation. Melanex™ in the Vehicle/N® delivery system contains 30 mg hydroquinone per ml in a vehicle of 47.3% alcohol, purified water, laureth-4, isopropyl alcohol 4%, propylene glycol and ascorbic acid, and is provided with the Appliderm™ Filter/Applicator Unit for ease of application.
Pharmacological class: Depigmenting agent.
Clinical Pharmacology: It has been suggested that the primary action of hydroquinone is directed at tyrosinase. The selective inhibition of the enzyme affects melanogenesis in the melanocytes resulting in cessation of melanin formation and subsequent reduction in pigmentation. Additional studies indicate that hydroquinone acts on the essential subcellular metabolic processes of melanocytes with resultant cytolysis, i.e. nonenzyme-medicated depigmentation.
Indications and Usage: Melanex™ is indicated in the temporary bleaching of hyperpigmented skin conditions such as chloasma, melasma, freckles, senile lentigines, and other forms of melanin hyperpigmentation.
If treatment is indicated, apply to affected areas twice daily, in the morning and before bedtime. During the day, an effective broad spectrum sunscreen should be used and unnecessary solar exposure avoided.
Contraindications: Melanex™ is contraindicated in persons who have shown hypersensitivity to hydroquinone or any of the other ingredients. The safety of topical treatment with hydroquinone during pregnancy has not been established.
Warning: Sun exposure should be minimized by using a sunscreen agent, or protective clothing to cover bleached skin in order to prevent repigmentation from occurring.
Precautions: For external use only. Hydroquinone preparations may produce skin irritation in susceptible individuals and have a slight potential to produce an allergic response. Therefore, the physician should use appropriate cautions. If rash or irritation develops, discontinue use. Do not use on children under 12.
If no improvement is seen after two months of treatment, use of product should be discontinued. Avoid contact with eyes. In case of accidental contact, patient should rinse eyes thoroughly with water and contact physician. A bitter taste and anesthetic effect may occur if applied to lips. Keep out of reach of children. Use of Melanex™ in paranasal and infraorbital areas increases the chance of irritation (see Adverse Reactions).
Adverse Reactions: The following have been reported: dryness and fissuring of paranasal and infraorbital areas, erythema and stinging. Hydroquinone has been known to produce irritation and sensitization in susceptible individuals.
Drug Abuse and Dependence: No drug abuse or dependence results from the use of Melanex™.
Overdosage: Not applicable.
How Supplied: 1.0 fl. oz. (30 ml) bottle with Appliderm™ Filter/Applicator Unit.
Note: Slight darkening of the Melanex™ solution is normal and will not affect potency. See expiration date on bottle.
Please contact Neutrogena Dermatologics for further information or questions: Toll free 800-421-6857 (in California 213-776-5223).
NDC# 10812-9300-1

NEUTROGENA®
Norwegian Formula Hand Cream

Composition: Neutrogena® Hand Cream is a highly concentrated, heavy duty protective cream containing water, glycerin, cetearyl alcohol, sodium cetearyl sulfate, fragrance (deleted for unscented formula), stearic acid, methylparaben, propylparaben, sodium sulfate, and dilauryl thiodipropionate.
Action and Uses: For use in dermatoses caused by over-exposure to water and weather and for extremely dry, chapped hands and skin. Effective as a barrier cream to protect hands and skin. Useful in the treatment of hand eczemas, as adjunct to topical steroids.
Administration and Dosage: Highly concentrated, use sparingly. Apply small quantity and rub in gently or as physician directs.
How Supplied: 2 oz. plastic tube. Scented or Unscented.

NEUTROGENA®
Original Formula Soap

Composition: A mild, transparent, triethanolamine base soap containing no free alkali. Contains triethanolamine stearate, triethanolamine, sodium tallowate, glycerin, water, sodium cocoate, sodium castorate, triethanolamine oleate, cocamide DEA, tochoperol and fragrance (deleted from unscented formula).
Action and Uses: Neutrogena Soap is formulated to gently cleanse sensitive skin. It is well tolerated in the cleansing care of post-dermatosis cutaneous irritation and inflammation, especially when washing with soap is contraindicated. Neutrogena Soap contains no free alkali and affects the pH of the skin no more than rinsing with plain water. It is extremely water soluble, resulting in reduced possibility of irritation due to soap residue on the skin. The heavy molecular structure of Neutrogena Soap minimizes epidermal penetration and therefore skin irritation.

Administration and Dosage: Use daily or as physician directs.
How Supplied: 3.5 and 5.5 oz. Bars. Scented or Unscented.

NEUTROGENA® Rainbath® Shower and Bath Gel

Composition: Rainbath is a gentle, soapless cleanser containing water, sodium laureth sulfate, oleyl betaine, lauramide DEA, fragrance (deleted from unscented formula), polysorbate 20, propylene glycol, sodium chloride, citric acid, methylparaben, propylparaben, FD&C Red No. 40, FD&C Yellow No. 5, FD&C Blue No. 1
Action and Uses: A lipid-free foaming gel cleanser for use in bath or shower. Indicated as a cleansing adjunct in atopic dermatitis and other conditions where soap is contraindicated. Produces a rich lather and cleanses with uncommon mildness. Satisfies patients that they are getting the cleansing quality of soap without soap, leaving skin smooth to touch.
Caution: Avoid contact with eyes.
Administration and Dosage: For shower, apply directly to wet skin or wash cloth and lather. Rinse and pat dry. May be used for foaming bath; pour one tablespoon into running water. Or use as physician directs.
How Supplied: 4 oz. plastic tube, 8 oz. and 32 oz. shatterproof plastic bottle in Scented formula. 8 oz. shatterproof plastic bottle in Unscented formula.

NEUTROGENA® Sesame Seed Body Oil

Composition: A light, non-greasy, easily applied oil with excellent patient acceptance. Contains isopropyl myristate, sesame oil, PEG-40 sorbitan peroleate, methylparaben, propylparaben, BHA, and fragrance (deleted from unscented formula).
Action and Uses: Effective as an adjunct in the management and maintenance therapy of xerotic dermatosis, pruritus, geriatric skin problems, and lichenification of the skin due to inflammation from chronic scratching or irritation. Neutrogena Body Oil helps skin retain its normal lipid/aqueous balance by retarding evaporation of moisture. Acts as an effective, easy-to-use adjunct in the nursing care of bedridden and/or elderly patients. Neutrogena Body Oil may be applied directly to damp skin and rinsing is not necessary.
Administration and Dosage: Apply directly to the skin immediately after bath, shower or sponge-bath, while the skin is still damp. Rub in gently. For use in the bath, pour two or three capfuls in the tub as it fills. Neutrogena Body Oil is easily dispersible in water. Will not leave the tub oily and slippery.
How Supplied: 8 oz. shatterproof plastic bottle in Scented and Unscented formula.

NEUTROGENA® Shampoo

Composition: A mild shampoo, especially formulated for everyday use.
Neutrogena® Shampoo contains Water, Ammonium lauryl sulfate, Cocamide DEA, Cocomidopropyl Betaine, Glycerine, Fragrance, Imidazolidinyl Urea, Methylparaben, Citric Acid, Propylparaben.
Actions and Uses: Neutrogena® Shampoo is a mild, gentle, nonmedicated shampoo recommended for thorough, gentle cleansing of even the most sensitive scalp and hair. Rinses quickly and easily, and will not strip hair of natural moisture or oils. Safe for color treated hair. Especially suited for both men and women with normal-to-oily hair and scalp.
Administration and Dosage: Use daily or as physician directs.
How Supplied: 3 oz. and 5.5 oz. plastic tubes.

NEUTROGENA T/Derm Therapeutic Tar Body Oil

Composition: T/Derm is a therapeutic body oil formulation containing 5% Neutar (solubilized coal tar extract in a light oil base, consisting of 2-ethylhexyloxystearate, PEG 40 Sorbitan Peroleate, Benzoic Acid, USP, and is applied with the Appliderm Filter/Applicator unit for easy, no-mess application.
Action and Uses: Neutrogena T/Derm is an effective aid in the topical treatment of psoriasis, eczema and atopic dermatitis and can be used effectively either by itself or in conjunction with ultraviolet (UV) light therapy performed under the direction of a physician.
Dosage and Administration (or use as physician directs): Use once per day before bed. Apply by tilting bottle and gently rubbing the applicator over the direction of hair growth. Allow to dry and absorb 15–20 minutes. Any excess may then be removed by blotting gently with tissue.
When T/Derm is used with UV light, follow the above procedure except apply at bedtime and again 30 minutes to one hour prior to UV light treatment.
NOTE: You should consult your physician prior to using T/Derm with ultraviolet light or in any other prescribed regimen.
Precautions: For external use only. Do not apply to acutely inflamed or broken skin. If irritation develops, discontinue use and consult physician. Treated areas should be protected from sunlight for 24 hours after application, especially if T/Derm has been applied to the face. Avoid contact with eyes. Slight staining of clothes may occur. Standard laundry procedures will usually remove stains. Keep this and all medication out of the reach of children.
How Supplied: 4 fl. oz. plastic bottle with applicator.
NDC#10812-9501-4

NEUTROGENA® T/Gel® Therapeutic Shampoo

Composition: T/Gel® is a potent therapeutic tar shampoo containing Neutar™ Solubilized Coal Tar Extract 2%, in a bland shampoo base consisting of: purified water, USP; sodium laureth sulfate; cocamide DEA; cocamidopropyl betaine; fragrance; imadazolidinyl urea; methylparaben; propylparaben tetrasodium EDTA; and citric acid.
Action and Uses: Neutrogena T/Gel Shampoo provides coal tar efficacy in a cosmetically elegant formulation that greatly enhances patient acceptance.
T/Gel is effective as an aid in the treatment of psoriasis, seborrheic dermatitis, dandruff and eczema. Regular use will help control itching, flaking and scaling while leaving hair lustrous and manageable. The unique, amber T/Gel formulation produces a rich lather with a pleasant fragrance and is gentle enough for everyday use.
Administration and Dosage: Wet hair thoroughly. Apply liberal amount of T/Gel and massage into scalp. Leave lather on scalp for several minutes. Rinse. Repeat application. Or Use as Physician Directs.
Precautions: For external use only. Do not apply to acutely inflamed or broken skin. If irritation develops discontinue use and consult physician. In rare instances temporary discoloration of blond, bleached or tinted hair may occur. Store away from direct sunlight. Avoid contact with eyes. Keep this and all medication out of the reach of children.
How Supplied: 4.4 oz. plastic bottle
NDC #10812-9200-4

NEUTROGENA® Vehicle/N®

Composition: Neutrogena® Vehicle/N® with Appliderm™ Filter/Applicator Unit is a topical vehicle system for extemporaneous compounding. Neutrogena® Vehicle/N® contains ethyl alcohol 47.5%, purified water, laureth-4, isopropyl alcohol 4%, and propylene glycol, a formulation which solubilizes selected dermatologic drugs and provides mild astringent and drying actions.
Action and Uses: Neutrogena® Vehicle/N® provides topical compounding convenience, economy and cosmetic elegance in an easy-to-use delivery system that greatly enhances patient acceptance.
Fifteen commonly used drugs have been found to be compatible with and soluble in Vehicle/N® in concentrations normally used in dermatology. These drugs have been shown to be stable in Vehicle/N® for a minimum of three months without refrigeration.
Call Neutrogena Dermatologics for compounding information or questions. 800-421-6857 toll free (in Calif. 213-776-5223).
Dosage and Administration: As physician directs. The Appliderm™ Filter/Applicator Unit removes any insoluble excipients from the compounded preparation and provides a convenient spill-proof container and topical application device which assures even, efficient coverage. The solution is applied directly to the skin by tilting the bottle and rubbing the Appliderm™ Applicator over the affected area.
Note: Laboratory and clinical evaluations necessary to determine the safety and efficacy of the preparations resulting from the addition of the drugs described to Neutrogena® Vehicle/N® have not been conducted. Neutrogena Corporation makes no claims regarding the safety or efficacy of extemporaneously prepared products utilizing Vehicle/N®.
Precautions: Do not use near fire or flame due to alcohol content. Neutrogena® Vehicle/N® contains substantial alcohol and is not suitable for use in acute dermatoses. Stinging may be noted if used on irritated or abraded skin. Avoid contact with eyes or eyelids. If the product accidentally comes in contact with eyes, rinse thoroughly with water, and consult physician. For external use only. Keep out of the reach of children.
Availability: 50 ml in plastic bottle with Appliderm™ Applicator.
NDC # 10812-9100-1
Patent Pending

NEUTROGENA® Vehicle/N® MILD

Composition: Neutrogena® Vehicle/N® MILD with Appliderm™ Filter/Applicator Unit is a gentle topical compounding formulation for patients with sensitive skin. Neutrogena® Vehicle/N® MILD contains alcohol 41.5%, purified water, isopropyl alcohol 6% and laureth-4.
Actions and Uses: Neutrogena® Vehicle/N® MILD is especially suited for patients who are susceptible to drying and irritation. Vehicle/N® MILD provides topical compounding convenience, economy, versatility and cosmetic elegance in an easy-to-use delivery system that greatly enhances patient acceptance.
Cumulative irritancy testing and clinical trials demonstrate a significant reduction in drying and irritancy with Vehicle/N® MILD.
Many commonly used dermatologic drugs have been found to be compatible with and soluble in Vehicle/N® MILD for a minimum of three months without refrigeration.
Call Neutrogena Dermatologics for compounding information or questions: Toll free 800-421-6857 (in California 213-776-5223).
Dosage and Administration: As physician directs. The Appliderm™ Filter/Applicator Unit removes any insoluble excipients from the compounded preparation and provides a convenient spill-proof container and topical application device which assures even, effi-

Continued on next page

Neutrogena—Cont.

cient coverage. The solution is applied directly to the skin by tilting the bottle and rubbing the Appliderm™ Applicator over the affected area.

Note: Laboratory and clinical evaluations necessary to determine the safety and efficacy of the preparations resulting from the addition of any drugs to Neutrogena® Vehicle/N® MILD have not been conducted. Neutrogena Corporation makes no claims regarding the safety or efficacy of extemporaneously prepared products utilizing Vehicle/N® MILD.

Precautions: Do not use near fire or flame due to alcohol content. Neutrogena® Vehicle/N® MILD contains substantial alcohol and is not suitable for use in acute dermatoses. Stinging may be noted if used on irritated or abraded skin. Avoid contact with eyes or eyelids. If the product accidentally comes in contact with eyes, rinse thoroughly with water and contact physician. For external use only. Keep out of reach of children.

Availability: 50 ml in plastic bottle with Appliderm™ Applicator.
NDC# 10812-9400-1
Patent Pending

Norcliff Thayer Inc.
ONE SCARSDALE ROAD
TUCKAHOE, NY 10707

A-200 Pyrinate® Liquid, Gel

A-200 Pyrinate® Liquid

Description: Active ingredients: pyrethrins 0.165%, piperonyl butoxide technical 2.00% (equivalent to 1.60% (butylcarbityl) (6-propylpiperonyl) ether and 0.40% related compounds), deodorized kerosene 5.00%. Inert ingredients 92.835%.

A-200 Pyrinate® Gel

Description: Active ingredients: pyrethrins 0.333%, piperonyl butoxide technical 4.00% (equivalent to 3.2% (butylcarbityl) (6-propylpiperonyl) ether and 0.8% related compounds), deodorized kerosene 5.333%. Inert ingredients 90.334%.

Actions: A-200 Pyrinate is an effective pediculicide for control of head lice (Pediculus humanus capitis), pubic lice (Phthirus pubis) and body lice (Pediculus humanus corporis), and their nits.

Indications: A-200 Pyrinate Liquid and Gel are indicated for the treatment of human pediculosis—head lice, body lice and pubic lice, and their eggs. A-200 Pyrinate Gel is specially formulated for pubic lice and head lice in children, where control of application is desirable.

Contraindications: A-200 Pyrinate is contraindicated in individuals hypersensitive to any of its ingredients or allergic to ragweed.

Precautions: A-200 Pyrinate is for external use only. It is harmful if swallowed or inhaled. It may be irritating to the eyes and mucous membranes. In case of accidental contact with eyes, they should be immediately flushed with water. If skin irritation or signs of infection are present, a physician should be consulted.

Administration and Dosage: Apply sufficient A-200 Pyrinate to completely "wet" the hair and scalp or skin of any infested area. Allow applicaton to remain no longer than 10 minutes. Wash and rinse with plenty of warm water. Remove dead lice and eggs from hair with fine comb. To restore body and luster to hair following scalp applications, follow with a good shampoo. If necessary, this treatment may be repeated, but should not exceed two applications within 24 hours.

In order to prevent reinfestation with lice, all clothing and bedding must be sterilized or treated concurrent with the application of this preparation.

How Supplied: A-200 Pyrinate Liquid in 2 and 4 fl. oz. bottles. A-200 Pyrinate Gel in 1 oz. tubes.

Literature Available: Patient literature available upon request.

[*Shown in Product Identification Section*]

ESOTÉRICA® MEDICATED FADE CREAM
Regular
Facial
Fortified with Sunscreen Scented
Fortified with Sunscreen Unscented

(See PDR For Nonprescription Drugs)

LIQUIPRIN®
(acetaminophen)

(See PDR For Nonprescription Drugs)

NATURE'S REMEDY® Laxative

(See PDR For Nonprescription Drugs)

NoSalt™
Salt Alternative

(See PDR For Nonprescription Drugs)

OXY WASH™ Antibacterial Skin Wash

(See PDR For Nonprescription Drugs)

OXY-5® LOTION
OXY-10® LOTION
Benzoyl Peroxide Lotion 5% and 10%

(See PDR For Nonprescription Drugs)

OXY-SCRUB®
Abradant Cleanser

(See PDR For Nonprescription Drugs)

TUMS® Antacid Tablets

(See PDR For Nonprescription Drugs)

Nordisk-USA
7315 WISCONSIN AVENUE
SUITE 851W
BETHESDA, MD 20814

PURIFIED PORK INSULIN PRODUCTS

INSULATARD™ NPH
U-100 Pork, Isophane purified pork insulin suspension.

WARNING: **ANY CHANGE OF INSULIN SHOULD BE MADE CAUTIOUSLY ONLY UNDER MEDICAL SUPERVISION. WHEN CHANGING TO PURIFIED PORK INSULIN FROM ANY OTHER INSULIN A DOSAGE ADJUSTMENT, IF ANY, IS LIKELY TO BE A REDUCTION TO AVOID HYPOGLYCEMIA. CHANGES IN PURITY, STRENGTH (U-40, U-80, U-100), BRAND (MANUFACTURER), TYPE (LENTE, NPH, REGULAR, ETC.) AND/OR SPECIES SOURCE (BEEF, PORK, BEEF/PORK) MAY RESULT IN THE NEED FOR A CHANGE IN DOSAGE. IT IS NOT POSSIBLE TO IDENTIFY WHICH PATIENTS WILL REQUIRE A REDUCTION IN DOSAGE TO AVOID HYPOGLYCEMIA WHEN USING THIS INSULIN. ADJUSTMENT MAY BE NEEDED WITH THE FIRST DOSE OR OVER A PERIOD OF SEVERAL WEEKS. (SEE DOSAGE ADJUSTMENT SECTION). BE AWARE OF THE POSSIBILITY OF SYMPTOMS OF EITHER HYPOGLYCEMIA OR HYPERGLYCEMIA. SEE SECTIONS ENTITLED INSULIN REACTION AND HYPERGLYCEMIA.**

Description: INSULATARD NPH is a suspension of protamine insulin crystals. It has a slower speed of action than VELOSULIN (Regular) and a shorter duration than Protamine Zinc Insulin. The effect on the blood sugar begins approximately 1½ hours after the injection and lasts up to approximately 24 hours, having its maximum effect between the 4th and 12th hour.

Directions: Shake vial carefully to obtain a uniformly cloudy suspension of the crystals. Avoid heavy foaming. Do not use a vial if the insulin remains clear after it has been shaken. Also do not use it if you see lumps that float or stick to the sides.

INSULATARD NPH can be mixed with any other Nordisk insulin preparation. In the mixture the different insulins will keep their original effect (stable mixtures).

Keep INSULATARD NPH in a cold place (refrigerator) at 2 degrees to 10 degrees C (35–50 degrees F), but do not let it freeze or be exposed to direct sunlight. Do not use the insulin after the expiration date stamped on the label.

Dosage Adjustment: Reductions in dosage resulting from the switchover to this purified pork insulin from any other insulin have been observed to be in the neighborhood of 10–20% initially to maintain control.

Adjustment may be needed either with the first dose or over a period of several weeks, and it is therefore recommended that the patient be monitored closely by a physician during the changeover and that dosage be adjusted downwards as necessary.

It is not possible to identify which patients will require a reduction in dose to avoid hypoglycemia when using purified pork insulins.

Be aware of the possibility of symptoms indicating the need for adjustment. See sections on Insulin Reaction or Hyperglycemia.

Use the Correct Syringe: INSULATARD NPH is available in the U-100 strength (100 units per ml). The patient must understand the markings on the syringe and use only a syringe marked for U-100.

Avoid contamination and possible infection by following these instructions:

Reusable syringes and needles must be sterile when used. The best method of sterilization is to boil the syringe, plunger and needle in water for 5 minutes. If this is not possible, as when travelling, the parts may be sterilized by immersion for at least 5 minutes in a sterilizing liquid like ethyl alcohol, 70%. Do not use bathing, rubbing or medicated alcohol for sterilization. Remove all liquid from the syringe by pushing the plunger in and out several times and leave it to dry if alcohol has been used for sterilization. To prepare the dose, clean the rubber cap with cotton dipped in alcohol such as ethyl alcohol, 70%. The rubber cap must never be removed. Air is drawn into the syringe corresponding in amount to the prescribed amount of insulin. The needle is plunged through the cap in a downward position and the vial and syringe then inverted so that the air may be pushed out of the syringe into the vial. The prescribed amount of insulin is drawn into the syringe, and this is best done by drawing up slightly more insulin than required and then pushing the piston back to the desired mark. In this way any air bubbles are forced out of the syringe. Withdraw the needle from the vial without changing the position of the plunger in the syringe and lay aside the syringe so that it will not come in contact with any object. Disinfect the skin with a cotton swab dipped in a suitable antiseptic, such as ethyl alcohol, 70%. Pinch up the skin that has been disinfected and push the needle at a right angle quickly into the tissue under the skin. Do not inject deeper into a muscle or a vein. Give each injection in a different place from the previous one. If you instruct the patient to mix two types of insulin in the syringe, air should be injected into each vial first.

Warning: Patients who have been directed to mix two types of insulin should be aware that insulin hypodermic syringes may vary in amount of space between the bottom line and the needle.

Because of this, the patient should not change:

1. The order of mixture prescribed, or
2. the model and brand of the syringe or needle.

Failure to heed this warning can result in a dosage error.

Insulin injections, a balanced diet, and regular exercise are required to secure proper control of diabetes. Urine should be tested regularly for sugar. Consistent presence of sugar in the urine indicates that diabetes is not properly controlled.

Adverse Reactions: Insulin allergy occurs very rarely, but when it does, it may cause a serious reaction including a general skin rash over the body, shortness of breath, fast pulse, sweating, and a drop in blood pressure.

In a very few diabetics, the skin where insulin has been injected may become red, swollen and itchy. This local reaction may occur if the injection is not properly made, if the skin is sensitive to the cleansing solution or if the patient is allergic to insulin.

Insulin Reaction: Insulin reaction (hypoglycemia) can occur if the patient takes too much insulin, misses a meal or exercises or works harder than normal. The symptoms, which usually come on suddenly, are hunger, dizziness, and sweating. Eating sugar or a sugar-sweetened product will normally correct the condition.

Hyperglycemia: Hyperglycemia can occur if the patient takes too little insulin, eats significantly more than usual, or develops a cold or other infection. The symptoms are thirst, frequent passing of urine, and in severe cases nausea and abdominal pain. These symptoms generally come on gradually.

How Supplied: 10 ml vials
100 units per ml.
NDC # 50445-200-01

MIXTARD®

U-100 Pork, Isophane purified pork insulin suspension and purified pork insulin injection

WARNING: ANY CHANGE OF INSULIN SHOULD BE MADE CAUTIOUSLY ONLY UNDER MEDICAL SUPERVISION. WHEN CHANGING TO PURIFIED PORK INSULIN FROM ANY OTHER INSULIN A DOSAGE ADJUSTMENT, IF ANY, IS LIKELY TO BE A REDUCTION TO AVOID HYPOGLYCEMIA. CHANGES IN PURITY, STRENGTH (U-40, U-80, U-100), BRAND (MANUFACTURER), TYPE (LENTE, NPH, REGULAR, ETC.) AND/OR SPECIES SOURCE (BEEF, PORK, BEEF/PORK) MAY RESULT IN THE NEED FOR A CHANGE IN DOSAGE. IT IS NOT POSSIBLE TO IDENTIFY WHICH PATIENTS WILL REQUIRE A REDUCTION IN DOSAGE TO AVOID HYPOGLYCEMIA WHEN USING THIS INSULIN. ADJUSTMENT MAY BE NEEDED WITH THE FIRST DOSE OR OVER A PERIOD OF SEVERAL WEEKS. (SEE DOSAGE ADJUSTMENT SECTION). BE AWARE OF THE POSSIBILITY OF SYMPTOMS OF EITHER HYPOGLYCEMIA OR HYPERGLYCEMIA. SEE SECTIONS ENTITLED INSULIN REACTION AND HYPERGLYCEMIA.

Description: MIXTARD is a standard mixture of 30% VELOSULIN (corresponding to Regular insulin) and 70% INSULATARD NPH. The content of VELOSULIN gives the preparation a rapid onset of effect on the blood sugar, approximately ½ hour after the injection. The content of INSULATARD NPH gives it a duration of up to 24 hours, depending on the size of the dose. The maximal effect lies between the 4th and the 8th hour after injection.

Directions: Shake vial carefully to obtain a uniformly cloudy suspension of the crystals. Avoid heavy foaming. Do not use a vial if the insulin remains clear after it has been shaken. Also do not use it if you see lumps that float or stick to the sides.

MIXTARD can be mixed with any other Nordisk insulin preparation. In the mixture the different insulins will keep their original effect (stable mixtures).

Keep MIXTARD in a cold place (refrigerator) at 2 degrees to 10 degrees C (35–50 degrees F), but do not let it freeze or be exposed to direct sunlight. Do not use the insulin after the expiration date stamped on the label.

Dosage Adjustment: Reductions in dosage resulting from the switchover to this purified pork insulin from any other insulin have been observed to be in the neighborhood of 10–20% initially to maintain control. Adjustment may be needed either with the first dose or over a period of several weeks, and it is therefore recommended that the patient be monitored closely by a physician during the changeover and that dosage be adjusted downwards as necessary.

It is not possible to identify which patients will require a reduction in dose to avoid hypoglycemia when using purified pork insulins.

Be aware of the possibility of symptoms indicating the need for adjustment. See sections on Insulin Reaction or Hyperglycemia.

Use the Correct Syringe: MIXTARD is available in the U-100 strength (100 units per ml). The patient must understand the markings on the syringe and use only a syringe marked for U-100.

Avoid contamination and possible infection by following these instructions:

Reusable syringes and needles must be sterile when used. The best method of sterilization is to boil the syringe, plunger and needle in water for 5 minutes. If this is not possible, as when travelling, the parts may be sterilized by immersion for at least 5 minutes in a sterilizing liquid like ethyl alcohol, 70%. Do not use bathing, rubbing or medicated alcohol for sterilization. Remove all liquid from the syringe by pushing the plunger in and out several times and leave it to dry if alcohol has been used for sterilization. To prepare the dose, clean the rubber cap with cotton dipped in alcohol such as ethyl alcohol, 70%. The rubber cap must never be removed. Air is drawn into the syringe corresponding in amount to the prescribed amount of insulin. The needle is plunged through the cap in a downward position and the vial and syringe then inverted so that the air may be pushed out of the syringe into the vial. The prescribed amount of insulin is drawn into the syringe, and this is best done by drawing up slightly more insulin than required and then pushing the piston back to the desired mark. In this way any air bubbles are forced out of the syringe. Withdraw the needle from the vial without changing the position of the plunger in the syringe and lay aside the syringe so that it will not come in contact with any object. Disinfect the skin with a cotton swab dipped in a suitable antiseptic, such as ethyl alcohol, 70%. Pinch up the skin that has been disinfected and push the needle at a right angle quickly into the tissue under the skin. Do not inject deeper into a muscle or a vein. Give each injection in a different place from the previous one. If you instruct the patient to mix two types of insulin in the syringe, air should be injected into each vial first.

Warning: Insulin injections, a balanced diet, and regular exercise are required to secure proper control of diabetes. Urine should be tested regularly for sugar. Consistent presence of sugar in the urine indicates that diabetes is not properly controlled.

Adverse Reactions: Insulin allergy occurs very rarely, but when it does, it may cause a serious reaction including a general skin rash over the body, shortness of breath, fast pulse, sweating, and a drop in blood pressure. In a very few diabetics, the skin where insulin has been injected may become red, swollen and itchy. This local reaction may occur if the injection is not properly made, if the skin is sensitive to the cleansing solution or if the patient is allergic to insulin.

Insulin Reaction: Insulin reaction (hypoglycemia) can occur if the patient takes too much insulin, misses a meal or exercises or works harder than normal. The symptoms, which usually come on suddenly, are hunger, dizziness, and sweating. Eating sugar or a sugar-sweetened product will normally correct the condition.

Hyperglycemia: Hyperglycemia can occur if the patient takes too little insulin, eats significantly more than usual, or develops a cold or other infection. The symptoms are thirst, frequent passing of urine, and in severe cases nausea and abdominal pain. These symptoms generally come on gradually.

How Supplied: 10 ml vials
100 units per ml.
NDC #50445-300-01

VELOSULIN™

U-100 Pork, Purified pork insulin injection

WARNING: ANY CHANGE OF INSULIN SHOULD BE MADE CAUTIOUSLY ONLY UNDER MEDICAL SUPERVISION. WHEN CHANGING TO PURIFIED PORK INSULIN FROM ANY OTHER INSULIN A DOSAGE ADJUSTMENT, IF ANY, IS LIKELY TO BE A REDUCTION TO AVOID HYPOGLYCEMIA. CHANGES IN PURITY, STRENGTH (U-40, U-80, U-100), BRAND (MANUFACTURER), TYPE (LENTE, NPH, REGULAR, ETC.) AND/OR SPECIES SOURCE (BEEF, PORK, BEEF/PORK) MAY RESULT IN THE NEED FOR A CHANGE IN DOSAGE. IT IS NOT POSSIBLE TO IDENTIFY WHICH PATIENTS WILL REQUIRE A REDUCTION IN DOSAGE TO AVOID HYPOGLYCEMIA WHEN USING THIS INSULIN. ADJUSTMENT MAY BE NEEDED WITH THE FIRST DOSE OR OVER A PERIOD OF SEVERAL WEEKS. (SEE DOSAGE ADJUSTMENT SECTION). BE AWARE OF THE POSSIBILITY OF SYMPTOMS OF EITHER HYPOGLYCEMIA OR HYPERGLYCEMIA. SEE SECTIONS ENTITLED INSULIN REACTION AND HYPERGLYCEMIA.

Description: VELOSULIN is a clear solution of insulin obtained from pork pancreas. It has a rapid onset of effect on the blood sugar, approximately ½ hour after the injection. The effect lasts up to approximately 8 hours with a maximal effect between the 1st and 3rd hour.

Directions: Do not use the preparation if the color has become other than water clear or if the liquid has become viscous. VELOSULIN can be mixed with any other Nordisk insulin preparation. In the mixture the different insulins will keep their original effect (stable mixtures).

Keep VELOSULIN in a cold place (refrigerator) at 2 degrees to 10 degrees C (35–50 degrees F), but do not let it freeze or be exposed to direct sunlight. Do not use the insulin after the expiration date stamped on the label.

Dosage Adjustment: Reductions in dosage resulting from the switchover to this purified pork insulin from any other insulin have been observed to be in the neighborhood of 10–20% initially to maintain control.

Adjustment may be needed either with the first dose or over a period of several weeks, and it is therefore recommended that the patient be monitored closely by a physician during the changeover and that dosage be adjusted downwards as necessary.

It is not possible to identify which patients will require a reduction in dose to avoid hypoglycemia when using purified pork insulins.

Be aware of the possibility of symptoms indicating the need for adjustment. See sections on Insulin Reaction or Hyperglycemia.

Use the Correct Syringe: VELOSULIN is available in the U-100 strength (100 units per

Continued on next page

Nordisk-USA—Cont.

ml). The patient must understand the markings on the syringe and use only a syringe marked for U-100.
Avoid contamination and possible infection by following these instructions:
Reusable syringes and needles must be sterile when used. The best method of sterilization is to boil the syringe, plunger and needle in water for 5 minutes. If this is not possible, as when travelling, the parts may be sterilized by immersion for at least 5 minutes in a sterilizing liquid like ethyl alcohol, 70%. Do not use bathing, rubbing or medicated alcohol for sterilization. Remove all liquid from the syringe by pushing the plunger in and out several times and leave it to dry if alcohol has been used for sterilization. To prepare the dose, clean the rubber cap with cotton dipped in alcohol such as ethyl alcohol, 70%. The rubber cap must never be removed. Air is drawn into the syringe corresponding in amount to the prescribed amount of insulin. The needle is plunged through the cap in a downward position and the vial and syringe then inverted so that the air may be pushed out of the syringe into the vial. The prescribed amount of insulin is drawn into the syringe, and this is best done by drawing up slightly more insulin than required and then pushing the piston back to the desired mark. In this way any air bubbles are forced out of the syringe. Withdraw the needle from the vial without changing the position of the plunger in the syringe and lay aside the syringe so that it will not come in contact with any object. Disinfect the skin with a cotton swab dipped in a suitable antiseptic, such as ethyl alcohol, 70%. Pinch up the skin that has been disinfected and push the needle at a right angle quickly into the tissue under the skin. Do not inject deeper into a muscle or vein. Give each injection in a different place from the previous one. If you instruct the patient to mix two types of insulin in the syringe, air should be injected into each vial first.
Warning: Patients who have been directed to mix two types of insulin should be aware that insulin hypodermic syringes may vary in amount of space between the bottom line and the needle.
Because of this, the patient should not change:
1. The order of mixture prescribed, or
2. The model and brand of the syringe or needle.

Failure to heed this warning can result in a dosage error.
Insulin injections, a balanced diet, and regular exercise are required to secure proper control of diabetes. Urine should be tested regularly for sugar. Consistent presence of sugar in the urine indicates that diabetes is not properly controlled.
Adverse Reactions: Insulin allergy occurs very rarely, but when it does, it may cause a serious reaction including a general skin rash over the body, shortness of breath, fast pulse, sweating, and a drop in blood pressure.
In a very few diabetics, the skin where insulin has been injected may become red, swollen and itchy. This local reaction may occur if the injection is not properly made, if the skin is sensitive to the cleansing solution or if the patient is allergic to insulin.
Insulin Reaction: Insulin reaction (hypoglycemia) can occur if the patient takes too much insulin, misses a meal or exercises or works harder than normal. The symptoms, which usually come on suddenly, are hunger, dizziness, and sweating. Eating sugar or a sugar-sweetened product will normally correct the condition.
Hyperglycemia: Hyperglycemia can occur if the patient takes too little insulin, eats significantly more than usual, or develops a cold or other infection. The symptoms are thirst, frequent passing of urine, and in severe cases nausea and abdominal pain. These symptoms generally come on gradually.
How Supplied: 10 ml vials
100 units per ml.
NDC # 50445-100-01

Norgine Laboratories, Inc.
420 LEXINGTON AVENUE
NEW YORK, NY 10170

ENZYPAN® Tablets

Composition: Each tablet contains pancreatin sufficient to digest in 2 hours time: 19 g. of protein, 43 g. of starch and 10 g. of fat; in addition it provides Ox Bile (des.), 0.056 g. and peptic potency equivalent to Pepsin 1-3,000, 9 mg.
Action and Uses: Releases the principal digestive enzymes consecutively from two specially constructed tablet sections. Valuable in digestive enzyme deficiencies leading to fat, protein or starch intolerance and such enzyme-deficiency-linked symptoms as fermentative or putrefactive dyspepsia, postprandial distress, epigastric fullness, flatulence, regurgitation.
Administration and Dosage: *Adults*—2 to 3 tablets during or after each meal. To be taken whole, with water.
How Supplied: Containers of 120, 500.

HEPP-IRON DROPS

Composition: Each ml. contains vitamin B_{12} (Cyanocobalamin) 25 mcg., iron ammonium citrate (equiv. to 20 mg. of iron) 120 mg., thiamine hydrochloride 10 mg., pyridoxine hydrochloride 2 mg., biotin 2.5 mcg.
Action and Uses: Hematinic; for iron-deficiency anemias.
Administration and Dosage: For use in iron deficiency anemias. Children 6 months to 5 years of age, 10 to 15 mg iron (0.5 to 0.7 ml.) daily, according to age and requirements; and for infants under 6 months of age, as directed by a physician. Dilute in some water or fruit juice.
How Supplied: 30 ml. bottles; dropper calibrated to 0.5 and 0.7 ml. doses.

MOVICOL® Granules

Composition: Gum Karaya and cortex rhamni frangulae in a pleasantly sweetened mixture.
Action and Uses: Treatment of constipation with natural mucilage (for bulk formation) and small amounts of well-aged frangula (for initial peristalsis). Especially in cardiovascular, hernial, rectal cases; diverticulosis; invalid, surgical, convalescent cases; geriatric patients; dieters; patients with sedentary habits. In bulk-producing capacity, 1 teaspoonful of Movicol equals 2 lbs. of consumed vegetables.
Administration and Dosage: *Adults*—1 or 2 heaped teaspoonfuls once or twice daily after the main meals, or on retiring. Dry granules are placed on the tongue in small amounts and, without chewing or crushing, swallowed with plenty of water. As bowel tone and rhythm are gradually restored, dosage may be reduced and ultimately discontinued.
Warning: Not to be used if abdominal pain, nausea or vomiting are present. Frequent or prolonged use may result in dependence on laxatives.
Contraindications: Intestinal obstruction, fecal impaction.
How Supplied: Containers of 200 and 500 grams.

MURIPSIN® Tablets

Composition: Each tablet contains: glutamic acid hydrochloride 500 mg.; pepsin 35 mg.; in a special base.*
Action and Uses: Gastric hydrochloric acid therapy in a solid tablet. Muripsin avoids corrosive unpleasantness and uncontrolled acid release; formulated with glutamic acid hydrochloride, it not only substitutes hydrochloric acid but also stimulates secretagogue action. Each tablet provides the equivalent of 15 minims of dilute hydrochloric acid. Useful in hydrochloric acid deficiencies, primary or secondary.
Administration and Dosage: For adults one to two tablets with each meal to be swallowed whole with water.
Contraindications: Hyperacidity or if peptic ulcers are present.
How Supplied: Containers of 100 and 500.
*U.S. Patent 2,958,627

NorthEast Unit-Dose & Repacking Co., Inc.
P.O. BOX 2896
LAUREL, MD 20708

CIRCUBID™ ℞
(ethaverine hydrochloride)
Capsules*

Description: Each capsule contains Ethaverine HCl 150 mg.
Actions: Ethaverine HCl acts directly on the smooth muscle cells without involving the autonomic nervous system or its receptors.
Indications: In peripheral and cerebral vascular insufficiency associated with arterial spasm, in spastic conditions of the gastro-intestinal and genitourinary tracts.
Contraindications: Contraindicated in the presence of complete atrioventricular dissociation.
Precautions: It should be administered with caution in patients with glaucoma. It should not be used in pregnant women or in women of childbearing age unless directed by a physician.
Adverse Reactions: Even though the incidence of side effects as reported in literature is very low, it is possible for a patient to evidence nausea, anorexia, abdominal distress, dryness of the throat, hypotension, flushing, sweating, vertigo, respiratory depression, cardiac depression, cardiac arrhythmia and headache. If these side effects occur, reduce dosage or discontinue medication.
Dosage: The usual adult dose is 300 mg. daily, one capsule every 12 hours. In more difficult cases the dosage may be increased to 600 mg. daily as determined by the physician. It is most effective given early in the course of the vascular disorder. Because of the chronic nature of the disease long term therapy is required.
How Supplied: Bottles of 100 NDC-50274-101-01 and 1000 NDC-50274-101-10.
* Manufactured to provide a prolonged therapeutic effect.

IDENTIFICATION PROBLEM?

Consult PDR's

Product Identification Section

where you'll find over 900

products pictured actual size

and in full color.

Norwich Eaton Pharmaceuticals, Inc.

Professional Products Group
(formerly Eaton Laboratories)
Consumer Products Group
(formerly Norwich Products)
NORWICH, NY 13815

Literature on Norwich Eaton products sent to physicians on request.

ALPHADERM® ℞
(1% hydrocortisone)
CREAM

The following text is based on official labeling in effect August 1, 1982.

Description: Contains hydrocortisone 1% in a powder-in-cream base incorporating a hypermolar solution of urea 10% (carbamide), purified water, sorbitol, polyoxyethylene fatty glyceride, starch, white petrolatum, triglycerides of saturated fatty acids, isopropyl myristate, and sorbitan monolaurate. The near neutral pH of the formulation is made possible by the stabilized delivery system in which urea is absorbed by a polysaccharide powder matrix. Alphaderm (1% hydrocortisone) Cream is hypoallergenic and contains no parabens or lanolin.

Action: Topical steroids are primarily effective because of their anti-inflammatory, antipruritic and vasocontrictive actions.

Indications: For relief of the inflammatory manifestations of corticosteroid-responsive dermatoses.

Contraindications: Topical steroids are contraindicated in those patients with a history of hypersensitivity to any of the components of the preparation.

Precautions: If irritation develops, the product should be discontinued and appropriate therapy instituted.

In the presence of an infection, the use of an appropriate antifungal or antibacterial agent should be instituted. If a favorable response does not occur promptly, the corticosteroid should be discontinued until the infection has been adequately controlled.

If extensive areas are treated or if the occlusive technique is used, there will be increased systemic absorption of the corticosteroid and suitable precautions should be taken, particularly in children and infants.

Although topical steroids have not been reported to have an adverse effect on human pregnancy, the safety of their use in pregnant women has not absolutely been established. In laboratory animals, increases in incidence of fetal abnormalities have been associated with exposure of gestating females to topical corticosteroids, in some cases at rather low dosage levels. Therefore, drugs of this class should not be used extensively on pregnant patients, in large amounts, or for prolonged periods of time.

The product is not for ophthalmic use.

Adverse Reactions: The following local adverse reactions have been reported with topical corticosteroids, especially under occlusive dressings:

1. Burning
2. Itching
3. Irritation
4. Dryness
5. Folliculitis
6. Hypertrichosis
7. Acneiform eruptions
8. Hypopigmentation
9. Perioral dermatitis
10. Allergic contact dermatitis
11. Maceration of the skin
12. Secondary infection
13. Skin atrophy
14. Striae
15. Miliaria

Dosage and Administration: Apply a small quantity of Alphaderm (1% hydrocortisone) Cream to affected areas twice daily.

How Supplied: Alphaderm (1% hydrocortisone) Cream is available in:

NDC 0149-0705-12 tubes of 30 grams
NDC 0149-0705-51 tubes of 100 grams

70512-P3

CHLORASEPTIC® LIQUID
(oral anesthetic, antiseptic)

Description: An alkaline solution containing phenol and sodium phenolate (total phenol 1.4%). In addition, Menthol Chloraseptic and Cherry Chloraseptic 1.5-oz Spray contain compressed nitrogen as a propellant.

Indications: Pleasant-tasting Chloraseptic is an antiseptic, anesthetic, deodorizing mouthwash and gargle. It is an alkaline solution designed specifically to maintain oral hygiene and to relieve local soreness and irritation without "caines." Chloraseptic may be used as a topical anesthetic while antibacterials are used systemically in the treatment of infection. Chloraseptic acts promptly, often providing effective surface anesthesia in minutes. It is a valuable adjunct for temporary relief of pain and discomfort and will reduce oral bacterial flora temporarily to improve oral hygiene.

Chloraseptic is indicated for prompt temporary relief of discomfort due to the following conditions: *Medical*—oropharyngitis and throat infections; acute tonsillitis; posttonsillectomy soreness; peritonsillar abscess; oropharyngeal manifestations of postnasal drip; throat and mouth dryness (smoker's cough); and before intubation (anti-gag) and after (for soreness); *Dental*—after oral surgery or extractions; aphthous ulcers and infectious stomatitis; Vincent's infection; gingivitis; preinjection topical anesthesia; insertion of immediate denture; pericoronitis; and x-rays and impressions (anti-gag).

Administration and Dosage: Chloraseptic Mouthwash and Gargle—*Irritated throat:* Advise patient to spray 5 times (children 6-12 years of age, 3 times) and swallow. May be used as a gargle. Repeat every 2 hours if necessary. *After oral surgery:* Advise patient to allow full-strength solution to run over affected areas for 15 seconds without swishing, then expel remainder. Repeat every 2 hours if necessary. Not for children under 6 years of age unless directed by a physician or dentist. *Adjunctive gingival therapy:* Rinse vigorously with full-strength solution for 15 seconds, working between teeth, then expel remainder. Repeat every 2 hours if necessary. *Daily deodorizing mouthwash and gargle:* Dilute with equal parts of water and rinse thoroughly, or spray full strength, then expel remainder.

Chloraseptic Spray: *Irritated throat:* Advise patient to spray throat about 2 seconds (children 6 to 12 years about 1 second) and swallow. Repeat every 2 hours if necessary. *After oral surgery:* Advise patient to spray affected area for 1 to 2 seconds, allow solution to remain for 15 seconds without swishing, then expel remainder. Repeat every 2 hours if necessary. *Adjunctive gingival therapy:* Spray affected area for about 2 seconds, swish for 15 seconds working between teeth, then expel remainder. Repeat every 2 hours if necessary. *Daily deodorizing spray:* Spray, rinse thoroughly, and expel remainder. Not for children under 6 years of age unless directed by a physician or dentist.

Consumer labeling contains the following caution statement:

Caution: Severe or persistent sore throat or sore throat accompanied by high fever, headache, nausea or vomiting may be serious. Consult your physician. If sore throat persists more than 2 days consult physician. Do not administer to children under 6 years unless directed by physician.

In addition, the 1.5 oz. nitrogen propelled spray contains the following statement:

Warning: AVOID SPRAYING IN EYES. CONTENTS UNDER PRESSURE. DO NOT PUNCTURE OR INCINERATE. (DO NOT BURN OR THROW IN FIRE, AS CAN WILL BURST.) DO NOT STORE AT TEMPERATURE ABOVE 120°F. (SUCH HIGH TEMPERATURES MAY CAUSE BURSTING.) KEEP OUT OF REACH OF CHILDREN.

To insure product quality, avoid excessive heat (over 104°F or 40°C). See bottom of can for expiration date and control number.

How Supplied: Available in menthol or cherry flavor—6 oz. size with sprayer, 12 oz. refill bottle, and 1.5 oz. nitrogen propelled spray. No prescription necessary.

CHLORASEPTIC® LOZENGES

Description: Each Chloraseptic Lozenge contains phenol, sodium phenolate (total phenol 32.5 mg).

Action and Uses: Chloraseptic Lozenges provide prompt temporary relief of discomfort due to mouth and gum irritations and of minor sore throat due to colds. They are anesthetic and antiseptic—and also may be used as a topical adjunct to systemic antibacterial therapy for severe cases. For prompt temporary relief of pain and discomfort associated with the following conditions: *Medical*—oropharyngitis and throat infections; acute tonsillitis; posttonsillectomy soreness; peritonsillar abscess; oropharyngeal manifestations of postnasal drip; and throat and mouth dryness (smoker's cough); *Dental*—after oral surgery; aphthous ulcers and infectious stomatitis; Vincent's infection; gingivitis; and pericoronitis.

Administration and Dosage: Adults: Dissolve 1 lozenge in the mouth every 2 hours; do not exceed 8 lozenges per day. Children 6-12 years: Dissolve 1 lozenge in the mouth every 3 hours; **do not exceed 4 lozenges per day.** Not for children under 6 unless directed by a physician or dentist.

Caution—Consult physician if sore throat is severe or lasts more than 2 days or is accompanied by high fever, headache, nausea or vomiting. Not for children under 6 unless directed by physician.

KEEP ALL MEDICINES OUT OF REACH OF CHILDREN.

Avoid excessive heat (over 104°F or 40°C).

How Supplied: Available in choice of menthol or cherry flavor—packages of 18 and 45 lozenges.

No prescription necessary.

CHILDREN'S CHLORASEPTIC® LOZENGES

Description: Each Children's Chloraseptic Lozenge contains 5 mg. benzocaine as anesthetic in a grape flavored base of sugar and corn syrup solids.

Action and Use: Children's Chloraseptic Lozenges provide prompt, temporary relief of minor sore throat pain which may accompany conditions such as tonsillitis, pharyngitis and in post tonsillectomy soreness, and discomfort of minor mouth and gum irritations.

Administration & Dosage: Allow one lozenge to dissolve slowly in the mouth. Repeat hourly if needed. Do not take more than 12 lozenges per day. Not for children under 3 unless directed by a physician.

In addition, consumer labeling carries the following statement:

Warning: Consult physician promptly if sore throat is severe or lasts more than 2 days or is accompanied by high fever, headache, nausea,

Continued on next page

Norwich Eaton—Cont.

or vomiting. Not for children under 3 years unless directed by physician.
Active ingredient: benzocaine (5 mg per lozenge).
STORE BELOW 86°F (30°C). PROTECT FROM MOISTURE.
KEEP ALL MEDICINES OUT OF REACH OF CHILDREN.
Packaging: Carton of 18 lozenges.

CHLORASEPTIC® COUGH CONTROL LOZENGES

Description: Each CHLORASEPTIC Cough Control Lozenge contains phenol and sodium phenolate (total phenol 32.5 mg), and a 10-mg therapeutic dose of dextromethorphan hydrobromide.
Action and Uses: CHLORASEPTIC Cough Control Lozenges provide fast relief of minor sore throat pain and control coughs due to colds. Each lozenge contains two active ingredients. One is the same agent contained in CHLORASEPTIC, a widely used medication for relief of minor sore throat pain. This ingredient acts as a local anesthetic stopping sore throat pain by temporarily blocking the nerve impulse transmission to the ninth cranial nerve. The second agent, dextromethorphan hydrobromide, a nonnarcotic antitussive, acts by selective suppression of the central cough mechanism. Dual-active CHLORASEPTIC Cough Control Lozenges provide temporary symptomatic relief of coughs and minor sore throat pain.
Administration and Dosage: Adults: Dissolve one lozenge slowly in mouth every two hours; do not exceed eight lozenges per day. Children 6 to 12 years: Dissolve one lozenge slowly in mouth every four hours; do not exceed four lozenges per day. Do not administer to children under 6 years of age unless directed by a physician.
Warning—Do not administer to children under 6 years of age unless directed by physician. Persistent cough may indicate the presence of a serious condition. Persons with a high fever or persistent cough should not use this preparation unless directed by physician. Consult physician promptly if sore throat is severe or lasts more than 2 days, or is accompanied by high fever, headache, nausea or vomiting. If pregnant or nursing, consult physician or pharmacist before taking this or any medicine.
KEEP ALL MEDICINES OUT OF REACH OF CHILDREN.
Avoid excessive heat (over 104°F or 40°C).
Packaging: Pocket-size box of 16 lozenges.

CHLORASEPTIC® GEL

Description: Chloraseptic Gel contains phenol, sodium phenolate (total phenol 1.4%) in a special adherent base.
Indications: For prompt, temporary relief of discomfort from minor mouth and gum irritations.
Warnings: If irritation or pain persists, discontinue use and consult physician or dentist. Do not administer to children under 6 years of age unless directed by a physician.
KEEP ALL MEDICINES OUT OF REACH OF CHILDREN.
Administration: Apply directly to the affected area. Repeat as necessary.
How Supplied: Chloraseptic Gel is available in ¼-oz tubes.

COMHIST® LA ℞

The following text is based on official labeling in effect August 1, 1982.
Description: Each yellow and clear capsule contains:
Chlorpheniramine maleate ....4 mg
Phenyltoloxamine citrate ....50 mg
Phenylephrine hydrochloride ....20 mg
in a special base to provide a prolonged therapeutic effect.
Actions: The antihistaminic agents chlorpheniramine maleate and phenyltoloxamine citrate suppress the histamine-mediated symptoms of allergic rhinitis, relieving sneezing, rhinorrhea, and itching of eyes, nose and throat. The vasoconstrictive action of phenylephrine hydrochloride decongests engorged mucous membranes of the respiratory tract.
Indications: COMHIST LA is indicated for the relief of rhinorrhea and congestion associated with seasonal and/or perennial allergic rhinitis and vasomotor rhinitis.
Contraindications: COMHIST LA is contraindicated in persons hypersensitive to any of its components. It should not be administered to nursing mothers, children under 12 years of age, persons with glaucoma, asthma, or severe hypertension, or persons taking monoamine oxidase inhibitors.
Usage in Pregnancy: Since the safety of COMHIST LA for use in pregnancy has not been established, potential benefits should be weighed against possible adverse effects.
Precautions: COMHIST LA should be used with caution in persons with prostatic hypertrophy, hypertension, cardiovascular disease, diabetes, thyroid disease, and peptic ulcer. The sedative effects of chlorpheniramine maleate and phenyltoloxamine citrate are additive to the CNS depressant effects of alcohol, hypnotics, sedatives, and tranquilizers. Because this drug may produce sedation, patients should be cautioned against engaging in activities requiring mental alertness, such as driving a car or operating machinery.
Adverse Reactions: Adverse reactions associated with use of COMHIST LA are sedation, excitation (especially in children), nervousness, insomnia, headache, dizziness, anorexia, dryness of the mouth, gastric irritation, urticaria, rash, hypotension, palpitations, blurred vision and urinary retention or frequency. Leukopenia, agranulocytosis, thrombocytopenia and convulsions rarely have been associated with the use of antihistamines.
Overdosage: Emesis may be induced by administering ipecac syrup. Since the effects of COMHIST LA may last 8 to 12 hours, treatment of overdosage directed toward supporting the patient and reversing the effects of the drug should be continued for at least that length of time. Saline cathartics may be useful in hastening the evacuation of unreleased medication.
Dosage: Adults and children over 12 years of age—1 capsule every 8 to 12 hours; not recommended for children under 12 years of age.
How Supplied:
Bottles of 100 **NDC** 0149-0446-01
Bottles of 500 **NDC** 0149-0446-05
Caution: Federal law prohibits dispensing without prescription.

44601-X1

COMHIST® LIQUID
decongestant/antihistaminic

Description: Each teaspoonful (5 ml) contains:
Chlorpheniramine maleate ....2 mg
Phenylephrine hydrochloride ....5 mg
Actions: The antihistaminic agent chlorpheniramine maleate suppresses the histamine-mediated symptoms of allergic rhinitis, relieving sneezing, rhinorrhea, and itching of eyes, nose and throat. The vasoconstrictive action of phenylephrine hydrochloride decongests engorged mucous membranes of the respiratory tract.
Indications: COMHIST LIQUID is indicated for the relief of rhinorrhea and congestion associated with seasonal and/or perennial allergic rhinitis and vasomotor rhinitis.
Overdosage: The treatment of overdosage should be directed toward supporting the patient and reversing the effects of the drug.
Professional Labeling: Dosage: Adults and children over 12 years—2 teaspoonfuls every 4 hours; children 6 to under 12 years—1 teaspoonful every 4 hours; children 3 to under 6 years—½ teaspoonful every 4 hours.
Note: Since COMHIST LIQUID is available without prescription, the following appears on the labeling: **Warnings:** This product should not be taken by children under 6 years, pregnant or nursing women, persons who have asthma, glaucoma, enlargement of the prostate gland, high blood pressure, heart disease, diabetes, thyroid disease, peptic ulcer, or persons presently taking a prescription antihypertensive or antidepressant drug containing an MAO inhibitor, except under the advice and supervision of a physician. May cause drowsiness. Avoid driving a motor vehicle, operating machinery, or drinking alcoholic beverages while taking this product. May cause excitability, especially in children. Do not exceed recommended dosage because nervousness, dizziness, or sleeplessness may occur. If symptoms do not improve within 7 days or are accompanied by high fever, consult a physician before continuing use.
How Supplied: NDC 0149-0442-16 oz. pint bottle

COMHIST® ℞
Baylor®

The following text is based on official labeling in effect August 1, 1982.
Description: Each scored, yellow tablet contains:
Chlorpheniramine maleate ....2 mg
Phenyltoloxamine citrate ....25 mg
Phenylephrine hydrochloride ....10 mg
Actions: The antihistaminic agents chlorpheniramine maleate and phenyltoloxamine citrate suppress the histamine-mediated symptoms of allergic rhinitis, relieving sneezing, rhinorrhea, and itching of eyes, nose and throat. The vasoconstrictive action of phenylephrine hydrochloride decongests engorged mucous membranes of the respiratory tract.
Indications: COMHIST is indicated for the relief of rhinorrhea and congestion associated with seasonal and/or perennial allergic rhinitis and vasomotor rhinitis.
Contraindications: COMHIST is contraindicated in persons hypersensitive to any of its components. It should not be administered to nursing mothers, children under 6 years of age, persons with glaucoma, asthma, or severe hypertension, or persons taking monoamine oxidase inhibitors.
Usage in Pregnancy: Since the safety of COMHIST for use in pregnancy has not been established, potential benefits should be weighed against possible adverse effects.
Precautions: COMHIST should be used with caution in persons with prostatic hypertrophy, hypertension, cardiovascular disease, diabetes, thyroid disease, and peptic ulcer. The sedative effects of chlorpheniramine maleate and phenyltoloxamine citrate are additive to the CNS depressant effects of alcohol, hypnotics, sedatives, and tranquilizers. Because this drug may produce sedation, patients should be cautioned against engaging in activities requiring mental alertness, such as driving a car or operating machinery.
Adverse Reactions: Adverse reactions associated with use of COMHIST are sedation, excitation (especially in children), nervousness, insomnia, headache, dizziness, anorexia, dryness of the mouth, gastric irritation, urticaria, rash, hypotension, palpitations, blurred vision and urinary retention or frequency. Leukopenia, agranulocytosis, thrombocytopenia and convulsions rarely have been associated with the use of antihistamines.

Overdosage: The treatment of overdosage should be directed toward supporting the patient and reversing the effects of the drug. Emesis may be induced by administering ipecac syrup.
Dosage: Adults and children over 12 years of age—1 or 2 tablets 3 times daily; children 6 to 12 years of age—1 tablet three times daily; not recommended for children under 6 years of age.
How Supplied: Bottles of 100 **NDC** 0149-0444-01
Caution: Federal law prohibits dispensing without prescription. 44401-P3

DANTRIUM® ℞
(dantrolene sodium)

The following text is based on official labeling in effect August 1, 1982.

Dantrium (dantrolene sodium) has a potential for hepatotoxicity, and should not be used in conditions other than those recommended. Symptomatic hepatitis (fatal and non-fatal) has been reported at various dose levels of the drug. The incidence reported in patients taking up to 400 mg/day is much lower than in those taking doses of 800 mg or more per day. Even sporadic short courses of these higher dose levels within a treatment regimen markedly increased the risk of serious hepatic injury. Liver dysfunction as evidenced by blood chemical abnormalities alone (liver enzyme elevations) have been observed in patients exposed to Dantrium for varying periods of time. Overt hepatitis has occurred at varying intervals after initiation of therapy, but has been most frequently observed between the third and twelfth month of therapy. The risk of hepatic injury appears to be greater in females, in patients over 35 years of age, and in patients taking other medication(s) in addition to Dantrium (dantrolene sodium). Dantrium should be used only in conjunction with appropriate monitoring of hepatic function including frequent determination of SGOT or SGPT. If no observable benefit is derived from the administration of Dantrium after a total of 45 days, therapy should be discontinued. The lowest possible effective dose for the individual patient should be prescribed.

Description: Dantrium is dantrolene sodium, chemically it is hydrated 1-[[[5-(4-nitrophenyl) -2-furanyl]methylene]amino]-2, 4-imidazolidinedione sodium salt. It is an orange powder, slightly soluble in water, but due to its slightly acidic nature the solubility increases somewhat in alkaline solution. The anhydrous salt has a molecular weight of 336. The hydrated salt contains approximately 15% water ($3\frac{1}{2}$ moles) and has a molecular weight of 399. The structural formula for the hydrated salt is:

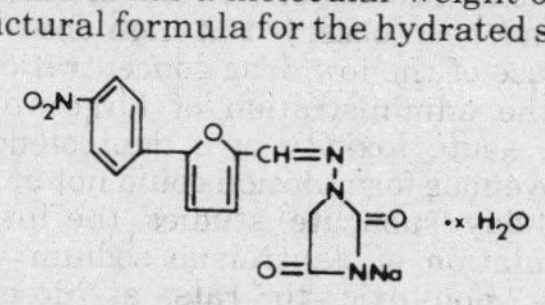

O_2N–C₆H₄–(furan)–CH=N–N(imidazolidinedione, =O, NNa, O=) · x H_2O

Dantrium (dantrolene sodium) is supplied in capsules of 25-mg, 50-mg, and 100-mg
Actions: In isolated nerve-muscle preparation, Dantrium (dantrolene sodium) has been shown to produce relaxation by affecting the contractile response of the skeletal muscle at a site beyond the myoneural junction, directly on the muscle itself. In skeletal muscle, Dantrium (dantrolene sodium) dissociates the excitation-contraction coupling, probably by interfering with the release of Ca^{++} from the sarcoplasmic reticulum. This effect appears to be more pronounced in fast muscle fibers as compared to slow ones, but generally affects both. A central nervous system effect occurs, with drowsiness, dizziness and generalized weakness occasionally present. Although Dantrium (dantrolene sodium) does not appear to directly affect the CNS, the extent of its indirect effect is unknown. The absorption of Dantrium (dantrolene sodium) after oral administration in humans is incomplete and slow but consistent, and dose-related blood levels are obtained. The duration and intensity of skeletal muscle relaxation is related to the dosage and blood levels. The mean biologic half-life of Dantrium (dantrolene sodium) in adults is 8.7 hours after a 100-mg dose. Specific metabolic pathways in the degradation and elimination of Dantrium (dantrolene sodium) in human subjects have been established. Metabolic patterns are similar in adults and children. In addition to the parent compound, dantrolene, which is found in measurable amounts in blood and urine, the major metabolites noted in body fluids are the 5-hydroxy analog and the acetamido analog. Since Dantrium (dantrolene sodium) is probably metabolized by hepatic microsomal enzymes, enhancement of its metabolism by other drugs is possible. However, neither phenobarbital nor diazepam appears to affect Dantrium (dantrolene sodium) metabolism.
Indications: Dantrium (dantrolene sodium) is indicated in controlling the manifestations of clinical spasticity resulting from upper motor neuron disorders (e.g. spinal cord injury, stroke, cerebral palsy, or multiple sclerosis). It is of particular benefit to the patient whose functional rehabilitation has been retarded by the sequelae of spasticity. Such patients must have presumably reversible spasticity where relief of spasticity will aid in restoring residual function. Dantrium (dantrolene sodium) is not indicated in the treatment of skeletal muscle spasm resulting from rheumatic disorders.
If improvement occurs, it will ordinarily occur within the dosage titration (see dosage and administration), and will be manifested by a decrease in the severity of spasticity and the ability to resume a daily function not quite attainable without Dantrium (dantrolene sodium).
Occasionally, subtle but meaningful improvement in spasticity may occur with Dantrium (dantrolene sodium) therapy. In such instances information regarding improvement should be solicited from the patient and those who are in constant daily contact and attendance with him. Brief withdrawal of Dantrium (dantrolene sodium) for a period of 2 to 4 days will frequently demonstrate exacerbation of the manifestations of spasticity and may serve to confirm a clinical impression.
A decision to continue the administration of Dantrium (dantrolene sodium) on a long-term basis is justified if introduction of the drug into the patient's regimen:

produces a significant reduction in painful and/or disabling spasticity such as clonus, or permits a significant reduction in the intensity and/or degree of nursing care required, or
rids the patient of any annoying manifestations of spasticity considered important by the patient himself.

Contraindications: Active hepatic disease, such as hepatitis and cirrhosis, is a contraindication for use of Dantrium (dantrolene sodium). Dantrium (dantrolene sodium) is contraindicated where spasticity is utilized to sustain upright posture and balance in locomotion or whenever spasticity is utilized to obtain or maintain increased function.
Warnings: It is important to recognize that fatal and non-fatal liver disorders of an idiosyncratic or hypersensitivity type may occur with Dantrium (dantrolene sodium) therapy.
At the start of Dantrium (dantrolene sodium) therapy, it is desirable to do liver function studies (SGOT, SGPT, alkaline phosphatase, total bilirubin) for a baseline or to establish whether there is pre-existing liver disease. If baseline liver abnormalities exist and are confirmed, there is a clear possibility that the potential for Dantrium (dantrolene sodium) hepatotoxicity could be enhanced, although such a possibility has not yet been established.
Liver function studies (e.g. SGOT or SGPT) should be performed at appropriate intervals during Dantrium (dantrolene sodium) therapy. If such studies reveal abnormal values, therapy should generally be discontinued. Only where benefits of the drug have been of major importance to the patient, should reinitiation or continuation of therapy be considered. Some patients have revealed a return to normal laboratory values in the face of continued therapy while others have not.
If symptoms compatible with hepatitis, accompanied by abnormalities in liver function tests or jaundice appear, Dantrium (dantrolene sodium) should be discontinued. If caused by Dantrium (dantrolene sodium) and detected early, the abnormalities in liver function characteristically have reverted to normal when the drug was discontinued.
Dantrium (dantrolene sodium) therapy has been reinstituted in a few patients who have developed clinical and/or laboratory evidence of hepatocellular injury. If such reinstitution of therapy is done, it should be attempted only in patients who clearly need Dantrium (dantrolene sodium) and only after previous symptoms and laboratory abnormalities have cleared. The patient should be hospitalized and the drug should be restarted in very small and gradually increasing doses. Laboratory monitoring should be frequent and the drug should be withdrawn immediately if there is any indication of recurrent liver involvement. Some patients have reacted with unmistakable signs of liver abnormality upon administration of a challenge dose, while others have not.
Dantrium (dantrolene sodium) should be used with particular caution in females and in patients over 35 years of age in view of apparent greater likelihood of drug-induced, potentially fatal, hepatocellular disease in these groups.
Long-term safety of Dantrium (dantrolene sodium) in humans has not been established. Chronic studies in rats, dogs and monkeys at dosages greater than 30 mg/kg/day showed growth or weight depression and signs of hepatopathy and possible occlusion nephropathy, all of which were reversible upon cessation of treatment. Sprague-Dawley female rats fed dantrolene sodium for 18 months at dosage levels of 15, 30 and 60 mg/kg/day showed an increased incidence of benign and malignant mammary tumors compared with concurrent controls and, at the highest dosage, an increase in the incidence of hepatic lymphangiomas and hepatic angiosarcomas. These effects were not seen in $2\frac{1}{2}$-year studies in Sprague-Dawley or Fischer 344 rats or in 2-year studies in mice of the HaM/ICR strain. Carcinogenicity in humans cannot be fully excluded, so that this possible risk of chronic administration must be weighed against the benefits of the drug (i.e., after a brief trial) for the individual patient.
Usage in Pregnancy: The safety of Dantrium (dantrolene sodium) for use in women who are or who may become pregnant has not been established. Dantrium (dantrolene sodium) should not be used in nursing mothers.
Usage in Children: The long-term safety of Dantrium (dantrolene sodium) in children under the age of 5 years has not been established. Because of the possibility that adverse effects of the drug could become apparent only after many years, a benefit-risk consideration of the long-term use of Dantrium (dantrolene sodium) is particularly important in pediatric patients.
Drug Interactions: While a definite drug interaction with estrogen therapy has not yet

Continued on next page

Norwich Eaton—Cont.

been established, caution should be observed if the two drugs are to be given concomitantly. Hepatotoxicity has occurred more often in women over 35 years of age receiving concomitant estrogen therapy.

Precautions: Dantrium (dantrolene sodium) should be used with caution in patients with impaired pulmonary function, particularly those with obstructive pulmonary disease, and in patients with severely impaired cardiac function due to myocardial disease. It should be used with caution in patients with a history of previous liver disease or dysfunction (See Warnings).

Patients should be cautioned against driving a motor vehicle or participating in hazardous occupations while taking Dantrium (dantrolene sodium). Caution should be exercised in the concomitant administration of tranquilizing agents.

Dantrium might possibly evoke a photosensitivity reaction; patients should be cautioned about exposure to sunlight while taking it.

Adverse Reactions: The most frequently occurring side effects of Dantrium have been drowsiness, dizziness, weakness, general malaise, fatigue, and diarrhea. These are generally transient, occurring early in treatment, and can often be obviated by beginning with a low dose and increasing dosage gradually until an optimal regimen is established. Diarrhea may be severe and may necessitate temporary withdrawal of Dantrium therapy. If diarrhea recurs upon readministration of Dantrium, therapy should probably be withdrawn permanently.

Other less frequent side effects, listed according to system, are:

Gastrointestinal: Constipation, GI bleeding, anorexia, swallowing difficulty, gastric irritation, abdominal cramps

Hepatobiliary: Hepatitis (See Warnings)

Neurologic: Speech disturbance, seizure, headache, light-headedness, visual disturbance, diplopia, alteration of taste, insomnia

Cardiovascular: Tachycardia, erratic blood pressure, phlebitis

Psychiatric: Mental depression, mental confusion, increased nervousness

Urogenital: Increased urinary frequency, crystalluria, hematuria, difficult erection, urinary incontinence and/or nocturia, difficult urination and/or urinary retention

Integumentary: Abnormal hair growth, acne-like rash, pruritus, urticaria, eczematoid eruption, sweating

Musculoskeletal: Myalgia, backache

Respiratory: Feeling of suffocation

Special Senses: Excessive tearing

Hypersensitivity: Pleural effusion with pericarditis

Other: Chills and fever

Dosage and Administration: Prior to the administration of Dantrium (dantrolene sodium) consideration should be given to the potential response to treatment. A decrease in spasticity sufficient to allow a daily function not otherwise attainable should be the therapeutic goal of treatment with Dantrium (dantrolene sodium). Refer to indications section for description of response to be anticipated.

It is important to establish a therapeutic goal (regain and maintain a specific function such as therapeutic exercise program, utilization of braces, transfer maneuvers, etc.) before beginning Dantrium (dantrolene sodium) therapy. Dosage should be increased until the maximum performance compatible with the dysfunction due to underlying disease is achieved. No further increase in dosage is then indicated.

Usual Dosage: It is important that the dosage be titrated and individualized for maximum effect. The lowest dose compatible with optimal reponse is recommended.

In view of the potential for liver damage in long-term Dantrium (dantrolene sodium) use, therapy should be stopped if benefits are not evident within 45 days.

Adults: Begin therapy with 25 mg once daily; increase to 25 mg two, three, or four times daily and then by increments of 25 mg up to as high as 100 mg two, three, or four times daily if necessary. As most patients will respond to a dose of 400 mg/day or less, rarely should doses higher than 400 mg/day be used. (See Box Warning.)

Each dosage level should be maintained for four to seven days to determine the patient's response. The dose should not be increased beyond, and may even have to be reduced to, the amount at which the patient received maximal benefit without adverse effects.

Children: A similar approach should be utilized starting with 0.5 mg/kg of body weight twice daily; this is increased to 0.5 mg/kg three or four times daily and then by increments of 0.5 mg/kg up to as high as 3.0 mg/kg two, three, or four times daily, if necessary. Doses higher than 100 mg four times daily should not be used in children.

Overdosage: For acute overdosage general supportive measures should be employed along with immediate gastric lavage.

Intravenous fluids should be administered in fairly large quantities to avert the possibility of crystalluria. An adequate airway should be maintained and artificial resuscitation equipment should be at hand. Electrocardiographic monitoring should be instituted, and the patient carefully observed. To date, no experience has been reported with dialysis; its value in Dantrium overdosage is not known.

How Supplied: Dantrium (dantrolene sodium) is available in:

25 mg: opaque, orange and light brown capsules.

NDC 0149-0030-05 bottles of 100

NDC 0149-0030-66 bottles of 500

NDC 0149-0030-77 hospital unit-dose strips in boxes of 100.

50 mg: opaque, orange and dark brown capsules.

NDC 0149-0031-05 bottles of 100.

100 mg: opaque, orange and light brown capsules.

NDC 0149-0033-05 bottles of 100

NDC 0149-0033-77 hospital unit-dose strips in boxes of 100.

Address medical inquiries to Norwich Eaton Pharmaceuticals Medical Department, Norwich, NY 13815.

03001-P3

DANTRIUM® ℞
(dantrolene sodium) INTRAVENOUS

The following text is based on official labeling in effect August 1, 1982.

Description: Dantrium Intravenous is a sterile, lyophilized formulation of dantrolene sodium, and in this form provides a preparation for intravenous use. Each 70 ml vial contains 20 mg dantrolene sodium, 3000 mg mannitol, and sufficient sodium hydroxide to yield a pH of approximately 9.5 when reconstituted with 60 ml sterile water for injection U.S.P. (without a bacteriostatic agent).

Dantrolene sodium is classified as a direct-acting skeletal muscle relaxant. Chemically, dantrolene sodium is hydrated 1-[[[5-(4-nitrophenyl)-2-furanyl]methylene]amino]-2, 4-imidazolidinedione sodium salt. The structural formula for the hydrated salt is:

O_2N — CH=NN — C=O, NNa, CH_2 — C=O $\cdot 3\tfrac{1}{2}H_2O$

The hydrated salt contains approximately 15% water ($3\frac{1}{2}$ moles) and has a molecular weight of 399. The anhydrous salt (dantrolene) has a molecular weight of 336.

Actions: Dantrolene sodium is a muscle relaxant acting specifically on skeletal muscle. It does not affect neuromuscular transmission nor does it have measurable effects on the electrically excitable surface membrane. Studies have shown that in the presence of dantrolene sodium, the responses of the muscle to caffeine are decreased or delayed.

In isolated muscle preparations, dantrolene sodium uncouples the excitation and contraction of skeletal muscle, probably by interfering with the release of calcium from the sarcoplasmic reticulum.

In the anesthetic-induced malignant hyperthermia syndrome, evidence points to an intrinsic abnormality of muscle tissue. In affected humans and swine, it has been postulated that "triggering agents" induce a sudden rise in myoplasmic calcium either by preventing the sarcoplasmic reticulum from accumulating calcium adequately, or by accelerating its release. This rise in myoplasmic calcium activates acute catabolic processes common to the malignant hyperthermia crisis.

Dantrolene sodium may prevent the increase in myoplasmic calcium and the acute catabolism within the muscle cell by interfering with the release of calcium from the sarcoplasmic reticulum to the myoplasm. Thus, the physiologic, metabolic, and biochemical changes associated with the crisis may be reversed or attenuated.

Specific metabolic pathways in the degradation and elimination of dantrolene sodium in humans have been established. Dantrolene is found in measurable amounts in blood and urine. In addition, its major metabolites in body fluids are the 5-hydroxy analog and the acetamido analog. Another metabolite with an unknown structure appears related to acetylamino-dantrolene. Dantrolene sodium may also undergo hydrolysis and subsequent oxidation forming nitrophenylfuroic acid.

Since dantrolene sodium is metabolized by the liver, enhancement of its metabolism by other drugs is possible. However, neither phenobarbital nor diazepam appears to affect dantrolene sodium metabolism.

The mean biologic half-life of dantrolene sodium after intravenous administration is about 5 hours. Based on assays of whole blood and plasma, slightly greater amounts of dantrolene are associated with red blood cells than with the plasma fraction of blood. Significant amounts of dantrolene are bound to plasma proteins, mostly albumin, and this binding is readily reversible. Binding to plasma protein is not significantly altered by diazepam, diphenylhydantoin, or phenylbutazone. Binding to plasma proteins is reduced by warfarin and clofibrate and increased by tolbutamide.

In animals, dantrolene sodium given intravenously has no appreciable effect on the cardiovascular system or on respiratory function. A transient inconsistent effect on smooth muscles has been observed at high doses.

Because of the low drug concentration requiring the administration of large volumes of fluid, acute toxicity of a dantrolene sodium intravenous formulation could not be assessed. In 14-day (subacute) studies, the intravenous formulation of dantrolene sodium was relatively non-toxic to rats at doses of 10 mg/kg/day and 20 mg/kg/day. While 10 mg/kg/day in dogs for 14 days evoked little toxicity, 20 mg/kg/day for 14 days caused hepatic changes of questionable biologic significance.

Indications: Dantrium Intravenous is indicated, along with appropriate supportive measures, for the management of the fulminant hypermetabolism of skeletal muscle characteristic of malignant hyperthermia crisis. It should be administered by intravenous injection as soon as the malignant hyperthermia reaction is recognized (i.e. tachycardia, tachypnea, central venous desaturation, hypercarbia, metabolic acidosis, skeletal muscle rigidity, increased utilization of anesthesia circuit carbon dioxide absorber, cyanosis and mottling of the skin, and, in many cases, fever).

Contraindications: None.

Warnings: *The use of Dantrium Intravenous in the management of malignant hyperthermia crisis is not a substitute for previously known supportive measures. These measures must be individualized, but it will usually be necessary to discontinue the suspect triggering agents, attend to increased oxygen requirements, manage the metabolic acidosis, institute cooling when necessary, attend to urinary output and monitor for electrolyte imbalance.*

Precautions:

a) Because of the high pH of the intravenous formulation of Dantrium, care must be taken to prevent extravasation of the intravenous solution into the surrounding tissues.

b) Pregnancy: The safety of Dantrium Intravenous in women who are or who may become pregnant has not been established; it should be given only when the potential benefits have been weighed against the possible risk to mother and child.

Adverse Reactions: The serious reactions reported with chronic oral Dantrium use have been hepatitis, seizures, and pleural effusion with pericarditis. Hypersensitivity with attendant skin reactions has been infrequently noted. None of the reactions reported in patients taking oral Dantrium have been reported in patients treated with short-term Dantrium Intravenous therapy for malignant hyperthermia.

Dosage and Administration: As soon as the malignant hyperthermia reaction is recognized, all anesthetic agents should be discontinued. Dantrium Intravenous should be administered by continuous rapid intravenous push beginning at a minimum dose of 1 mg/kg, and continuing until symptoms subside or the maximum cumulative dose of 10 mg/kg has been reached. If the physiologic and metabolic abnormalities reappear, the regimen may be repeated. It is important to note that administration of Dantrium Intravenous should be continuous until symptoms subside. The effective dose to reverse the crisis is directly dependent upon the individual's degree of susceptibility to malignant hyperthermia, the amount and time of exposure to the triggering agent, and the time elapsed between onset of the crisis and initiation of treatment.

Children's Dose: Experience to date indicates that the dose for children is the same as for adults.

Preoperatively: Dantrium (dantrolene sodium) Capsules are indicated preoperatively as possible protection against the development of a malignant hyperthermia crisis in individuals thought to be susceptible.

Oral administration of Dantrium Capsules: Administer 4 to 8 mg/kg/day of oral dantrolene in 3 or 4 divided doses for one or two days prior to surgery, with the last dose being given approximately 3 to 4 hours before scheduled surgery with a minimum of water.

This dosage usually will be associated with skeletal muscle weakness and sedation (sleepiness or drowsiness); adjustment can usually be made within the recommended dosage range to avoid incapacitation or excessive gastrointestinal irritation (including nausea and/or vomiting). See also the package insert for oral dantrolene sodium (Dantrium Capsules).

Post Crisis Follow-up: Dantrium (dantrolene sodium) Capsules should also be administered following a malignant hyperthermia crisis in doses to 4 to 8 mg/kg per day in four divided doses, for a one to three day period to prevent recurrence of the manifestations of malignant hyperthermia.

Preparations: Each vial of Dantrium Intravenous should be reconstituted by adding 60 ml of sterile water for injection U.S.P. (without a bacteriostatic agent), and the vial shaken until the solution is clear. The contents of the vial must be *protected from direct light* and *used within 6 hours* after reconstitution. Protect the reconstituted solutions from temperatures above 86°F (30°C) and below 59°F (15°C).

How Supplied: Dantrium Intravenous (NDC 0149-0734-01) is available in vials containing a sterile lyophilized mixture of 20 mg dantrolene sodium, 3000 mg mannitol, and sufficient sodium hydroxide to yield a pH of approximately 9.5 when reconstituted with 60 ml sterile water for injection U.S.P. (without a bacteriostatic agent).

Address medical inquiries to Norwich Eaton Pharmaceuticals, Inc., Medical Department, Norwich, NY 13815.

73401-P4

DUVOID® ℞

Bethanechol chloride—Oral

The following text is based on official labeling in effect August 1, 1982.

Description: Bethanechol chloride is an ester of a choline-like compound. The structural formula is:

$$\left[\begin{array}{l} CH_3CH{-}CH_2N^{+}(CH_3)_3 \\ \quad | \\ \quad O{-}CO{-}NH_2 \end{array}\right] Cl^{-}$$

Carbamate of (2-hydroxypropyl) trimethylammonium chloride

Actions: Bethanechol chloride acts principally by producing the effects of stimulation of the parasympathetic nervous system. It increases the tone of the detrusor urinae muscle, usually producing a contraction sufficiently strong to initiate micturition and empty the bladder. It stimulates gastric motility, increases gastric tone, and often restores impaired rhythmic peristalsis.

Stimulation of the parasympathetic nervous system releases acetylcholine at the nerve endings. When spontaneous stimulation is reduced and therapeutic intervention is required, acetylcholine can be given, but it is rapidly hydrolyzed by cholinesterase, and its effects are transient. Bethanechol chloride is not destroyed by cholinesterase and its effects are more prolonged than those of acetylcholine.

It has predominant muscarinic action and only feeble nicotinic action. Doses that stimulate micturition and defecation and increase peristalsis do not ordinarily stimulate ganglia or voluntary muscles. Therapeutic test doses in normal human subjects have little effect on heart rate, blood pressure, or peripheral circulation.

Indications: Acute postoperative and postpartum nonobstructive (functional) urinary retention, and neurogenic atony of the urinary bladder with retention.

Contraindications: Bethanechol chloride is contraindicated in the presence of mechanical obstruction of the gastrointestinal or urinary tracts, or in conditions where the integrity of the gastrointestinal or bladder wall is questionable. Also, it is contraindicated in spastic gastrointestinal disturbances, peptic ulcer, acute inflammatory conditions of the gastrointestinal tract, or peritonitis, or in marked vagotonia.

Other major contraindications to the use of bethanechol chloride are latent or active asthma, pregnancy, hyperthyroidism, and coronary occlusion. Additional contraindications are bradycardia, atrioventricular conduction defects, vasomotor instability, hypotension, hypertension, coronary artery disease, epilepsy, and parkinsonism.

Precautions: Special care and consideration are required when bethanechol chloride is administered to patients concomitantly being treated with other drugs with which pharmacologic interactions may occur. Examples of drugs with potentials for such interactions are: quinidine and procainamide, which may antagonize cholinergic effects; cholinergic drugs, particularly cholinesterase inhibitors, where additive effects may occur. When administered to patients receiving ganglionic blocking compounds a critical fall in blood pressure may occur which usually is preceded by severe abdominal symptoms.

In urinary retention, if the sphincter fails to relax as Duvoid (bethanechol chloride) contracts the bladder, urine may be forced up the ureter into the kidney pelvis. If there is bacteriuria, this may cause a reflux infection.

Adverse Reactions: Untoward effects are usually due to overdosage but occur infrequently with the oral administration of bethanechol chloride. Abdominal discomfort, salivation, flushing of the skin ("hot feeling") sweating, nausea and vomiting are early signs of overdosage. Asthmatic attacks, especially in asthmatic individuals may be precipitated. Substernal pressure or pain may occur, however, it is uncertain whether this is due to bronchoconstriction, or spasm of the esophagus. Myocardial hypoxia must be considered if a marked fall in blood pressure occurs.

Transient syncope with cardiac arrest, transient complete heart block, dyspnea, and orthostatic hypotension may be associated with large doses. Patients with hypertension may react to the drug with a precipitous fall in blood pressure. Short periods of atrial fibrillation have been observed in hyperthyroid individuals following the administration of cholinergic drugs. Also, involuntary defecation and urinary urgency may occur after large doses.

Atropine sulfate is a specific antidote. A dose of 0.6mg–1.2 mg (1/100 grain-1/50 grain), for intramuscular or intravenous administration should be readily available to counteract severe toxic cardiovascular or bronchoconstrictor responses to bethanechol chloride.

Dosage and Administration: Dosage must be individualized, depending on type and severity of the conditions to be treated.

The usual adult oral dose is administered with 10-mg, 25-mg, and 50-mg tablets 2, 3, or 4 times daily to a maximum dosage of 120 mg. The minimum effective dose is determined by giving 10 mg initially, and repeating with 25 mg, and then 50 mg at six hour intervals, until the desired response is obtained. The drug's effects appear within 60 to 90 minutes and persist for up to six hours. Individual doses should, therefore, be spaced at least six hours apart.

How Supplied: Duvoid (bethanechol chloride) is available in:

10-mg pale orange tablets coded "Eaton 045"
NDC 0149-0045-05 Unit-of-Use bottles of 100
NDC 0149-0045-77 hospital unit-dose strips in box of 100.

25-mg white tablets coded "Eaton 046"
NDC 0149-0046-05 Unit-of-Use bottles of 100
NDC 0149-0046-77 hospital unit-dose strips in box of 100.

50-mg tan tablets coded "Eaton 047"
NDC 0149-0047-05 Unit-of-Use bottles of 100
NDC 0149-0047-77 hospital unit-dose strips in box of 100.

Clinical Studies: Bethanechol chloride has been extensively used in the therapy of nonobstructive urinary retention. Although the dose of bethanechol chloride varies from individual to individual and depends upon the condition under therapy, oral doses of 10 mg to 30 mg given three or four times daily are often suggested.(1)

However, it has been reported that these doses are often inadequate in the treatment of nonobstructive urinary retention(2) and that the commonly used oral doses of 5 mg or 10 mg "achieves a purely placebo effect."(3) Even in those individuals considered to have detrusor super-sensitivity to bethanechol chloride an initial dose of 25 mg is suggested.(4) More re-

Continued on next page

Norwich Eaton—Cont.

cently it has been suggested that single oral doses of at least 50 mg, with total daily doses of 200 mg to 450 mg, may be necessary to meaningfully reduce residual urine volumes.(4–8)

The effects of oral and subcutaneous bethanechol chloride upon detrusor function have previously been evaluated by cystometry.(8,9) In general, the onset of subcutaneous dosage activity is more rapid and of shorter duration than oral medication.(8,9) In the comparison of oral and subcutaneous bethanechol chloride in patients with decompensated bladders, 5-mg subcutaneous drug produced maximum mean changes in cystometric pressure greater than did a single oral dose of 200 mg.(9)

Recently, the activity of 50-mg oral doses of Duvoid, Norwich Eaton brand of bethanechol chloride, was compared to that produced by 2 mg subcutaneous bethanechol chloride.(10) Both Duvoid (bethanechol chloride) and subcutaneous bethanechol chloride were associated with decreased bladder capacities and increased intravesical pressure. In addition, the 50-mg Duvoid (bethanechol chloride) dose appeared to cause little unwanted cholinergic activity in these individuals.

References (Clinical Studies):

1) Physicians' Desk Reference, ed. 31, Oradell, N.J.: Medical Economics Company, 1977; p 846—847, 1105.
2) Lapides J. Hodgson NB, Boyd RE, Shook EL, Lichtwardt JR. Further Observations on Pharmacologic Reactions of the Bladder. J Urol 79:707, 1958.
3) Kendall AR, Karafin L. Understanding and Rehabilitating the Atonic Neurogenic Bladder. Geriatrics 28:110, 1973.
4) Diokno AC, Koppenhoefer R. Bethanechol Chloride in Neurogenic Bladder Dysfunction. Urology 8:455, 1976.
5) Lapides J. Neurogenic Bladder: Principles of Treatment. Urol Clin North Am 1:81, 1974.
6) Smith DR. The Neurogenic Bladder. In General Urology, ed. 9, Los Altos, Cal.: Lange Medical Publications, 1976; p 315.
7) Bors E. Comarr AE. Disturbances of Micturition. In Neurological Urology: Baltimore, University Park Press, 1971; p 215.
8) Lapides J. Friend CR, Ajemian EP, Sonda LP. Comparison of Action of Oral and Parenteral Bethanechol Chloride upon the Urinary Bladder. Invest Urol 1:94, 1963.
9) Diokno AC, Lapides J. Action of Oral and Parenteral Bethanechol on Decompensated Bladder. Urology 10:23, 1977.
10) Data on file, Medical Department, Norwich Eaton Pharmaceuticals.

04505-P2

ENTEX® ℞

The following text is based on official labeling in effect August 1, 1982.

Description:
Each orange and white capsule contains:
Phenylephrine hydrochloride ....5 mg
Phenylpropanolamine hydrochloride ....45 mg
Guaifenesin ....200 mg

Actions: Phenylephrine hydrochloride and phenylpropanolamine hydrochloride are effective vasoconstrictors that decongest swollen mucous membranes of the respiratory tract. The expectorant guaifenesin enhances the flow of respiratory tract fluid, promotes ciliary action and facilitates removal of viscous, inspissated mucus. As a result, sinus, bronchial, and Eustachian tube drainage is improved, and dry, nonproductive coughs become more productive and less frequent.

Indications: ENTEX is indicated in respiratory conditions such as sinusitis, pharyngitis, bronchitis, and asthma, when these conditions are complicated by tenacious mucus and/or mucous plugs and congestion. ENTEX is also indicated as adjunctive therapy in serous otitis media and may be of value in avoiding secondary middle ear complications of nasopharyngeal congestion accompanying rhinitis.

Contraindications: ENTEX is contraindicated in individuals with known hypersensitivity to sympathomimetics, severe hypertension, or in patients receiving MAO inhibitors.

Usage in Pregnancy: Since the safety of ENTEX for use in pregnancy has not been established, potential benefits should be weighed against possible adverse effects. This product should not be used by nursing mothers.

Precautions: As with other sympathomimetic drugs, ENTEX should be used with caution in the presence of hypertension, hyperthyroidism, diabetes, heart disease, peripheral vascular disease, glaucoma, and prostatic hypertrophy.

Adverse Reactions: Possible adverse reactions include nervousness, insomnia, restlessness, headache, or gastric irritation. These reactions seldom, if ever, require discontinuation of therapy. Urinary retention may occur in patients with prostatic hypertrophy.

Overdosage: Treatment of overdosage should be directed toward supporting the patient and reversing the effects of the drug.

Dosage: Adults and children over 12—one capsule four times daily with food or fluid. Not recommended for children under 12 years.

How Supplied:
Bottles of 100 **NDC** 0149-0412-01
Bottles of 500 **NDC** 0149-0412-05

Caution: Federal law prohibits dispensing without prescription.

41201-P1

ENTEX® LIQUID ℞

The following text is based on official labeling in effect August 1, 1982.

Description:
Each 5 ml (one teaspoonful) contains:
Phenylephrine hydrochloride ....5 mg
Phenylpropanolamine hydrochloride .....20 mg
Guaifenesin ....100 mg
Alcohol 5%

Actions: Phenylephrine hydrochloride and phenylpropanolamine hydrochloride are effective vasoconstrictors that decongest swollen mucous membranes of the respiratory tract. The expectorant guaifenesin enhances the flow of respiratory tract fluid, promotes ciliary action and facilitates removal of viscous, inspissated mucus. As a result, sinus, bronchial, and Eustachian tube drainage is improved, and dry, nonproductive coughs become more productive and less frequent.

Indications: ENTEX LIQUID is indicated in respiratory conditions such as sinusitis, pharyngitis, bronchitis, and asthma, when these conditions are complicated by tenacious mucus and/or mucous plugs and congestion. ENTEX LIQUID is also indicated as adjunctive therapy in serous otitis media and may be of value in avoiding secondary middle ear complications of nasopharyngeal congestion accompanying rhinitis.

Contraindications: ENTEX LIQUID is contraindicated in individuals with known hypersensitivity to sympathomimetics, severe hypertension, or in patients receiving MAO inhibitors.

Usage in Pregnancy: Since the safety of ENTEX LIQUID for use in pregnancy has not been established, potential benefits should be weighed against possible adverse effects. This product should not be used in nursing mothers.

Precautions: As with other sympathomimetic drugs, ENTEX LIQUID should be used with caution in the presence of hypertension, hyperthyroidism, diabetes, heart disease, peripheral vascular disease, glaucoma, and prostatic hypertrophy.

Adverse Reactions: Possible adverse reactions to ENTEX LIQUID include nervousness, insomnia, restlessness, headache, nausea or gastric irritation. These reactions seldom, if ever, require discontinuation of therapy. Urinary retention may occur in patients with prostatic hypertrophy.

Overdosage: Treatment of overdosage should be directed toward supporting the patient and reversing the effects of the drug.

Dosage:
Children
2 to 4 years ....½ teaspoonful (2.5 ml) four times daily
4 to 6 years ....1 teaspoonful (5.0 ml) four times daily
6 to 12 years ....1½ teaspoonfuls (7.5 ml) four times daily
Over 12 years and adults ....2 teaspoonfuls (10.0 ml) four times daily

How Supplied: Pint bottles NDC 0149-0414-16

Caution: Federal law prohibits dispensing without prescription.

41401-P1

ENTEX® LA ℞

The following text is based on official labeling in effect August 1, 1982.

Description:
Each blue, scored, long-acting tablet contains:
Phenylpropanolamine hydrochloride ....75 mg
Guaifenesin ....400 mg
in a special base to provide a prolonged therapeutic effect.

Actions: Phenylpropanolamine hydrochloride is an effective vasoconstrictor that decongests swollen mucous membranes of the respiratory tract. The expectorant guaifenesin enhances the flow of respiratory tract fluid, promotes ciliary action and facilitates removal of viscous, inspissated mucus. As a result, sinus, bronchial, and Eustachian tube drainage is improved, and dry, nonproductive coughs become more productive and less frequent.

Indications: ENTEX LA is indicated in respiratory conditions such as sinusitis, pharyngitis, bronchitis, and asthma, when these conditions are complicated by tenacious mucus and/or mucous plugs and congestion. ENTEX LA is also indicated as adjunctive therapy in serous otitis media and may be of value in avoiding secondary middle ear complications of nasopharyngeal congestion accompanying rhinitis.

Contraindications: ENTEX LA is contraindicated in individuals with known hypersensitivity to sympathomimetics, severe hypertension, or in patients receiving MAO inhibitors.

Usage in Pregnancy: Since the safety of ENTEX LA for use in pregnancy has not been established, potential benefits should be weighed against possible adverse effects. This product should not be used by nursing mothers.

Precautions: DO NOT CRUSH OR CHEW ENTEX LA TABLETS BEFORE INGESTION. As with other sympathomimetic drugs, ENTEX LA should be used with caution in the presence of hypertension, hyperthyroidism, diabetes, heart disease, peripheral vascular disease, glaucoma, and prostatic hypertrophy.

Adverse Reactions: Possible adverse reactions include nervousness, insomnia, restlessness, or headache. These reactions seldom, if ever, require discontinuation of therapy. Urinary retention may occur in patients with prostatic hypertrophy.

Overdosage: Since the effects of ENTEX LA may last up to 12 hours, treatment of overdosage directed toward supporting the patient and reversing the effects of the drug should be continued for at least that length of time. Saline cathartics may be useful in hastening the evacuation of unreleased medication.

Dosage: Adults and children over 12—one tablet twice daily (every 12 hours). Not recommended for children under 12 years of age. Tablets may be broken in half for ease of ad-

ministration without affecting release of medication but not crushed or chewed.
How Supplied: **NDC** 0149-0436-01 bottles of 100 tablets.
Caution: Federal law prohibits dispensing without prescription.

43601-P1

FURACIN® (nitrofurazone) SOLUBLE DRESSING

℞

The following text is based on official labeling in effect August 1, 1982.
Description: Chemically, Furacin is nitrofurazone, 2-[(5-nitro-2-furanyl)methylene]hydrazinecarboxamide, with the following structure:

O_2N–[furan ring]–CH = NNHCONH$_2$

Furacin Soluble Dressing contains 0.2% nitrofurazone in Solubase® (a water-soluble base of polyethylene glycols 3350, 900, and 300).
The discoloration of this preparation by light does not indicate loss of efficacy.
Actions: Nitrofurazone is a synthetic nitrofuran with a broad antibacterial spectrum. It is bactericidal against most bacteria commonly causing surface infections, including many that have become antibiotic resistant.
It acts by inhibiting enzymes necessary for carbohydrate metabolism in bacteria. This action occurs in both the aerobic and anaerobic cycles of carbohydrate metabolism, explaining its bactericidal effect in aerobic, anaerobic, and facultative bacteria. Topically, it is without appreciable toxicity to human cells.
Indications: Furacin Soluble Dressing is a topical antibacterial agent indicated for adjunctive therapy of patients with second- and third-degree burns when bacterial resistance to other agents is a real or potential problem. It is also indicated in skin grafting where bacterial contamination may cause graft rejection and/or donor site infection particularly in hospitals with historical resistant-bacteria epidemics.
There is no known evidence of effectiveness of this product in the treatment of minor burns or surface bacterial infections involving wounds, cutaneous ulcers or the various pyodermas.
Contraindications: Known prior sensitization is a contraindication to the use of Furacin Soluble Dressing.
Warnings: Nitrofurazone has been shown to produce mammary tumors when fed at high doses to female Sprague-Dawley rats. The relevance of this to topical use in humans is unknown.
Furacin Soluble Dressing should be used with caution in patients with known or suspected renal impairment. The polyethylene glycols present in the base can be absorbed through denuded skin and may not be excreted normally by the compromised kidney. This may lead to symptoms of progressive renal impairment such as increased BUN, anion gap, and metabolic acidosis. (NOTE: Furacin Topical Cream does not contain polyethylene glycols.)
Usage in Pregnancy: Safe use of Furacin Soluble Dressing during pregnancy has not been established. Therefore, the drug is not recommended for the treatment of women of childbearing potential, unless the need for the therapeutic benefit of nitrofurazone is, in the attending physician's judgment, greater than the possible risk.
Precautions: Use of topical antimicrobials occasionally allows overgrowth of nonsusceptible organisms including fungi. If this occurs, or if irritation, sensitization or superinfection develop, treatment with Furacin Soluble Dressing should be discontinued and appropriate therapy instituted.
Adverse Reactions: Nitrofurazone has not been significantly toxic in man by topical application. In quantitative studies published in the period 1945–70, 206 instances of clinical skin reaction were reported out of 18,249 patients treated with nitrofurazone topical formulations, an overall incidence of 1.1 percent. The treatment of nitrofurazone sensitization is not distinctive; general measures commonly used for a variety of sensitization reactions are adequate, except for the rare instance of severe contact dermatitis in which steroid administration may be indicated.
Dosage and Administration:
BURNS: Apply directly to the lesion as with a spatula, or first place on gauze. Impregnated gauze may be used. Reapply once daily or once weekly, depending on the preferred dressing technique.
SKIN GRAFTS: The dressing is used both to prepare burns and other lesions for grafting, and postoperatively as a prophylactic measure. By rapid eradication of the infection, it can produce clean, firm granulation tissue. Because it is water-soluble and has negligible tissue toxicity, it does not intefere with successful takes. Flushing the gauze with sterile saline facilitates removal.
How Supplied: Furacin Soluble Dressing is available in:
NDC 0149-0704-12 tubes of 28 grams
NDC 0149-0704-11 tubes of 56 grams
NDC 0149-0704-51 jars of 135 grams
NDC 0149-0704-61 jars of 454 grams
NDC 0149-0704-90 jars of 5 pounds
Animal Toxicology: The oral administration of nitrofurazone for 7 days to rats at extremely high dosage levels of 240 mg/kg/day produced severe hepatorenal lesions whereas only renal changes were seen when the dosage level was reduced to 60 mg/kg/day for 60 days.
Dosage levels of 60 and 30 mg/kg/day shortened the time of appearance of the typical mammary gland tumor associated with older female rats. These tumors exhibited the same histological characteristics seen in the spontaneously occurring tumors and were seen only in the female animals. No mammary tumors were seen in rats treated with nitrofurazone orally for 1 year at levels of approximately 11 mg/kg/day. Spermatogenic arrest was noted in the male rats at dosage levels of 30 mg/kg/day and above.
Dogs treated orally with nitrofurazone for 400 days at levels of 11 mg/kg/day showed no toxic effects related to drug treatment. The single intravenous administration in dogs of 20, 35, or 75 mg/kg nitrofurazone produced clinical signs of lacrimation, salivation, emesis, diarrhea, excitation, weakness, ataxia and weight loss, whereas 100 mg/kg produced convulsions and death.
There was no evidence of toxicosis in rhesus monkeys treated with doses of nitrofurazone as high as 58 mg/kg/day for 10 weeks and 23 mg/kg/day for 63 weeks.
Finally, when 30 mg/kg of nitrofurazone was administered to pregnant rabbits once daily on days 7 through 15 of pregnancy there was a slight increase in the frequency of stillbirths, but no teratogenic effects were seen.
Preparation of Impregnated Gauze: Sterile gauze strips are placed in a tray and covered with Furacin Soluble Dressing. Repeat the procedure, adding several layers of gauze for each layer of Soluble Dressing. Sprinkling a little sterile water on each layer of dressing will minimize any color change from autoclaving. Cover the tray very loosely and autoclave at 121°C for 30 minutes at 15 to 20 pounds pressure.
To impregnate bandage rolls, place some Soluble Dressing in the bottom of a glass jar. Stand rolls on end. Place more Dressing on top.
Cover top of jar with aluminum foil. Autoclave at 121°C for 45 minutes at 15 to 20 pounds pressure.
Autoclaving more than once is not recommended.
For bacterial sensitivity tests: Furacin Sensi-Discs are available from BBL, Division of BioQuest.

70411-P6

FURADANTIN® (nitrofurantoin)

℞

The following text is based on official labeling in effect August 1, 1982.
Description: Furadantin is 1-[[(5-nitro-2-furanyl) methylene]amino]-2, 4-imidazolidinedione, a synthetic antimicrobial agent. It is a yellow, stable crystalline compound:

O_2N–[furan ring]–CH = N–N–C=O / NH / CH_2–C=O

Actions: Clinical Pharmacology: Orally administered Furadantin is readily absorbed and rapidly excreted in urine. During therapeutic drug dosage, only low blood concentrations are usually present. It is highly soluble in urine, to which it may impart a brown color. Following a therapeutic dose regimen (100 mg qid for 7 days) average urinary drug recoveries (0–24 hours) on day 1 and day 7 were 42.7% and 43.6%, respectively, for Furadantin.
Microbiology: Furadantin is an antibacterial agent for specific urinary tract infections. It is bacteriostatic in low concentrations (10 mcg/ml to 5 mcg/ml) and *in vitro* is considered to be bactericidal in higher concentrations. Its presumed mode of action is based upon its interference with several bacterial enzyme systems. Bacteria develop only a limited resistance to furan derivatives clinically. Furadantin is usually active against the following organisms *in vitro: Escherichia coli*, enterococci (e.g. *Streptococcus fecalis*) *Staphylococcus aureus*.
Note: Some strains of *Enterobacter* species and *Klebsiella* species are resistant to Furadantin. It is not active against most strains of *Proteus* species, and *Serratia* species. It has no activity against *Pseudomonas* species.
Susceptibility Tests—Quantitative methods that require measurement of zone diameters give the most precise estimates of antimicrobial susceptibility. One recommended procedure, (NCCLS, ASM-2)*, uses a disc containing 300 micrograms for testing susceptibility; interpretations correlate zone diameters of this disc test with MIC values for nitrofurantoin. Reports from the laboratory should be interpreted according to the following criteria:

Susceptible organisms produce zones of 17 mm or greater, indicating that the tested organism is likely to respond to therapy.
Organisms of intermediate susceptibility produce zones of 15 to 16 mm, indicating that the tested organism would be suceptible if high dosage is used.
Resistant organisms produce zones of 14 mm or less, indicating that other therapy should be selected.

A bacterial isolate may be considered susceptible if the MIC value for nitrofurantoin is not more than 25 micrograms per ml. Organisms are considered resistant if the MIC is not less than 100 micrograms per ml.
Indications: Furadantin is indicated for the treatment of urinary tract infections when due to susceptible strains of *E. coli*, enterococci, *S. aureus* (it is not indicated for the treatment of associated renal cortical or perinephric abscesses), and certain susceptible strains of *Klebsiella* species, *Enterobacter* species, and *Proteus* species.
Note: Specimens for culture and susceptibility testing should be obtained prior to and during drug administration.
Contraindications: Anuria, oliguria, or significant impairment of renal function (creatinine clearance under 40 ml per minute) are

Continued on next page

Norwich Eaton—Cont.

contraindications to therapy with this drug. Treatment of this type of patient carries an increased risk of toxicity because of impaired excretion of the drug. For the same reason, this drug is much less effective under these circumstances.
The drug is contraindicated in pregnant patients at term as well as in infants under one month of age because of the possibility of hemolytic anemia due to immature enzyme systems (glutathione instability).
The drug is also contraindicated in those patients with known hypersensitivity to Furadantin, Macrodantin® (nitrofurantoin macrocrystals), and other nitrofurantoin preparations.
Warnings: Acute, subacute and chronic pulmonary reactions have been observed in patients treated with nitrofurantoin products. If these reactions occur, the drug should be withdrawn and appropriate measures should be taken.
An insidious onset of pulmonary reactions (diffuse interstitial pneumonitis or pulmonary fibrosis, or both) in patients on long-term therapy warrants close monitoring of these patients.
There have been isolated reports giving pulmonary reactions as a contributing cause of death. (See Hypersensitivity reactions.)
Cases of hemolytic anemia of the primaquine sensitivity type have been induced by Furadantin. The hemolysis appears to be linked to a glucose-6-phosphate dehydrogenase deficiency in the red blood cells of the affected patients. This deficiency is found in 10 percent of Negroes and a small percentage of ethnic groups of Mediterranean and Near-Eastern origin. Any sign of hemolysis is an indication of to discontinue the drug. Hemolysis ceases when the drug is withdrawn.
Pseudomonas is the organism most commonly implicated in superinfections in patients treated with Furadantin.
Hepatitis, including chronic active hepatitis, has been observed rarely. Fatalities have been reported. The mechanism appears to be of an idiosyncratic hypersensitive type.
Precautions: Peripheral neuropathy may occur with Furandantin therapy; this may become severe or irreversible. Fatalities have been reported. Predisposing conditions such as renal impairment (creatinine clearance under 40 ml per minute), anemia, diabetes, electrolyte imbalance, vitamin B deficiency, and debilitating disease may enhance such occurrence.
Usage in Pregnancy: The safety of Furadantin during pregnancy and lactation has not been established. Use of this drug in women of childbearing potential requires that the anticipated benefit be weighed against the possible risks.
Adverse Reactions: Gastrointestinal reactions: Anorexia, nausea and emesis are the most frequent reactions; abdominal pain and diarrhea occur less frequently. These dose-related toxicity reactions can be minimized by reduction of dosage, especially in the female patient. Hepatitis occurs rarely.
Hypersensitivity reactions: Pulmonary sensitivity reactions may occur, which can be acute, subacute, or chronic.
Acute reactions are commonly manifested by fever, chills, cough, chest pain, dyspnea, pulmonary infiltration with consolidation or pleural effusion on x-ray, and eosinophilia. The acute reactions usually occur within the first week of treatment and are reversible with cessation of therapy. Resolution may be dramatic. In subacute reactions, fever and eosinophilia are observed less often. Recovery is somewhat slower, perhaps as long as several months. If the symptoms are not recognized as being drug related and nitrofurantoin is not withdrawn, symptoms may become more severe.
Chronic pulmonary reactions are more likely to occur in patients who have been on continuous nitrofurantoin therapy for six months or longer. The insidious onset of malaise, dyspnea on exertion, cough, and altered pulmonary function are common manifestations. Roentgenographic and histologic findings of diffuse interstitial pneumonitis or fibrosis, or both, are also common manifestations. Fever is rarely prominent.
The severity of these chronic pulmonary reactions and the degree of their resolution appear to be related to the duration of therapy after the first clinical signs appear. Pulmonary function may be permanently impaired even after cessation of nitrofurantoin therapy. This risk is greater when pulmonary reactions are not recognized early.
Dermatologic reactions: Maculopapular, erythematous, or eczematous eruption, pruritus, urticaria, and angioedema.
Other hypersensitivity reactions: Anaphylaxis, asthmatic attack in patients with history of asthma, cholestatic jaundice, hepatitis, including chronic active hepatitis, drug fever and arthralgia.
Hematologic reactions: Hemolytic anemia, granulocytopenia, leukopenia, eosinophilia, and megaloblastic anemia. Return of the blood picture to normal has followed cessation of therapy.
Neurological reactions: Peripheral neuropathy, headache, dizziness, nystagmus, and drowsiness.
Miscellaneous reactions: Transient alopecia. As with other antimicrobial agents, superinfections by resistant organisms may occur. With Furadantin, however, these are limited to the genitourinary tract because suppression or normal bacterial flora elsewhere in the body does not occur.
Dosage and Administration: DOSAGE—tablets and oral suspension:
Adults: 50–100 mg four times a day. **Children:** Should be calculated on the basis of 5–7 mg/kg of body weight per 24 hours to be given in divided doses four times a day (contraindicated under one month).

AVERAGE DOSE FOR CHILDREN
Furadantin (nitrofurantoin) Oral Suspension (5 mg/ml)

Body Weight		No. Teaspoonfuls
Pounds	**Kilograms**	**4 Times Daily**
15 to 26	7 to 11	½ (2.5 ml)
27 to 46	12 to 21	1 (5 ml)
47 to 68	22 to 30	1½ (7.5 ml)
69 to 91	31 to 41	2 (10 ml)

Administration: Furadantin may be given with food or milk to minimize gastric upset. Therapy should be continued for at least one week and for at least 3 days after sterility of the urine is obtained. Continued infection indicates the need for reevaluation.
If the drug is to be used for long-term suppressive therapy, reduction of dosage should be considered.
How Supplied: Furadantin is available in:
50-mg scored, yellow tablets coded "Eaton 036"
NDC 0149-0036-05 bottle of 100
NDC 0149-0036-66 bottle of 500
NDC 0149-0036-06 hospital unit-dose strips in box of 100
100-mg scored, yellow tablets coded "Eaton 037"
NDC 0149-0037-05 bottle of 100
NDC 0149-0037-66 bottle of 500
NDC 0149-0037-07 hospital unit-dose strips in box of 100
It should be dispensed in amber bottles.
Furadantin (nitrofurantoin) Oral Suspension is available in:
NDC 0149-0735-15 amber bottle of 60 ml
NDC 0149-0735-61 amber bottle of 470 ml
Avoid exposure to strong light which may darken the drug. It is stable in storage. It should be dispensed in amber bottles.
Furadantin 300 mcg Sensi-Discs for the laboratory detemination of bacterial sensitivity are available from BBL, division of BioQuest. For information on simple Furadantin assays in blood, serum, and urine, write or call the Medical Department. Literature sent to physicians on request.
Address medical inquires to Norwich Eaton Pharmaceuticals, Inc., Medical Department, Norwich, NY 13815.

03500-P3

* National Committee for Clinical Laboratory Standards. Approved Standard: ASM-2, Performance Standards for Antimicrobial Disc Susceptibility Tests, July, 1975.

FURACIN® TOPICAL CREAM ℞
(nitrofurazone)

The following text is based on official labeling in effect August 1, 1982.
Description: Chemically, Furacin is nitrofurazone, 2-[(5-nitro-2-furanyl)methylene]hydrazinecarbonxamide, with the following structure:

O_2N–[furan ring]–$CH = NNHCONH_2$

Furacin Topical Cream contains 0.2% Furacin in a watermiscible base consisting of glycerin, cetyl alcohol, mineral oil, an ethoxylated fatty alcohol, methylparaben, propylparaben, and water.
The discoloration of these preparations by light does not indicate loss of efficacy.
Actions: Nitrofurazone is a synthetic nitrofuran with a broad antibacterial spectrum. It is bactericidal against most bacteria commonly causing surface infections, including many that have become antibiotic resistant.
It acts by inhibiting enzymes necessary for carbohydrate metabolism in bacteria. This action occurs in both the aerobic and anaerobic cycles of carbohydrate metabolism, explaining its bactericidal effect in aerobic, anaerobic, and facultative bacteria. Topically, it is without appreciable toxicity to human cells.
Indications: Furacin is a topical antibacterial agent indicated for adjunctive therapy of patients with second- and third-degree burns when bacterial resistance to other agents is a real or potential problem.
It is also indicated in skin grafting where bacterial contamination may cause graft rejection and/or donor site infection particularly in hospitals with historical resistant-bacteria epidemics.
There is no known evidence of effectiveness of this product in the treatment of minor burns or surface bacterial infections involving wounds, cutaneous ulcers or the various pyodermas.
Contraindications: Known prior sensitization is a contraindication to the use of Furacin.
Warnings: Nitrofurazone has been shown to produce mammary tumors when fed at high doses to female Sprague-Dawley rats. The relevance of this to topical use in humans is unknown.
Usage in Pregnancy: Safe use of Furacin during pregnancy has not been established. Therefore, the drug is not recommended for the treatment of women of child-bearing potential, unless the need for the therapeutic benefit of nitrofurazone is, in the attending physician's judgment, greater than the possible risk.
Precautions: Use of topical antimicrobials occasionally allows overgrowth of nonsusceptible organisms including fungi. If this occurs, or if irritation, sensitization or superinfection develop, treatment with Furacin should be

discontinued and appropriate therapy instituted.

Adverse Reactions: Nitrofurazone has not been significantly toxic in man by topical application. In quantitative studies published in the period 1945–70, 206 instances of clinical skin reaction were reported out of 18,249 patients treated with nitrofurazone topical furmulations, an overall incidence of 1.1 percent. The treatment of nitrofurazone sensitization is not distinctive; general measures commonly used for a variety of sensitization reactions are adequate, except for the rare instance of severe contact dermatitis in which steroid administration may be indicated.

Dosage and Administration: **Furacin Soluble Dressing:** BURNS: Apply directly to the lesion as with a spatula, or first place on gauze. Impregnated gauze may be used. Reapply once daily or once weekly, depending on the preferred dressing technique.

SKIN GRAFTS: The dressing is used both to prepare burns and other lesions for grafting, and postoperatively as a prophylactic measure. By rapid eradication of the infection, it can produce clean, firm granulation tissue. Because it is water-soluble and has negligible tissue toxicity, it does not interfere with successful takes. Flushing the gauze with sterile saline facilitates removal.

Furacin Soluble Powder: Apply to the lesion directly from the shaker top vial or by means of a non-metallic powder insufflator such as DeVilbiss 119 or 288. To open vial, tear off aluminum top and lift off plastic cap.

Furacin Topical Cream: Apply directly to the lesion, or first place on gauze. Reapply once daily or every few days, depending on the usual dressing technique.

How Supplied: Furacin Soluble Dressing is available in:

NDC 0149-0704-12	tubes of 28 grams
NDC 0149-0704-11	tubes of 56 grams
NDC 0149-0704-51	jars of 135 grams
NDC 0149-0704-61	jars of 454 grams
NDC 0149-0704-90	jars of 5 pounds

Furacin Soluble Powder is available in:

NDC 0149-0723-11	shaker top vials of 14 grams

Furacin Topical Cream is available in:

NDC 0149-0777-15	tubes of 14 grams
NDC 0149-0777-12	tubes of 28 grams

Animal Toxicology: The oral administration of nitrofurazone for 7 days to rats at extremely high dosage levels of 240 mg/kg/day produced severe hepatorenal lesions whereas only renal changes were seen when the dosage level was reduced to 60 mg/kg/day for 60 days. Dosage levels of 60 and 30 mg/kg/day shortened the time of appearance of the typical mammary gland tumor associated with older female rats. These tumors exhibited the same histological characteristics seen in the spontaneously occurring tumors and were seen only in the female animals. No mammary tumors were seen in rats treated with nitrofurazone orally for 1 year at levels of approximately 11 mg/kg/day. Spermatogenic arrest was noted in the male rats at dosage levels of 30 mg/kg/day and above.

Dogs treated orally with nitrofurazone for 400 days at levels of 11 mg/kg/day showed no toxic effects related to drug treatment. The single intravenous administration in dogs of 20, 35, or 75 mg/kg nitrofurazone produced clinical signs of lacrimation, salivation, emesis, diarrhea, excitation, weakness, ataxia and weight loss, whereas 100 mg/kg produced convulsions and death.

There was no evidence of toxicosis in rhesus monkeys treated with doses of nitrofurazone as high as 58 mg/kg/day for 10 weeks and 23 mg/kg/day for 63 weeks.

Finally, when 30 mg/kg of nitrofurazone was administered to pregnant rabbits once daily on days 7 through 15 of pregnancy there was a slight increase in the frequency of stillbirths, but no teratogenic effects were seen.

Preparation of Impregnated Gauze: Sterile gauze strips are placed in a tray and covered with Furacin Soluble Dressing. Repeat the procedure, adding several layers of gauze for each layer of Soluble Dressing. Sprinkling a little sterile water on each layer of dressing will minimize any color change from autoclaving. Cover the tray very loosely and autoclave at 121°C for 30 minutes at 15 to 20 pounds pressure.

To impregnate bandage rolls, place some Soluble Dressing in the bottom of a glass jar. Stand rolls on end. Place more Dressing on top. Cover top of jar with aluminum foil. Autoclave at 121°C for 45 minutes at 15 to 20 pounds pressure.

Autoclaving more than once is not recommended.

For bacterial sensitivity tests: Furacin Sensi-Discs are available from BBL, Division of BioQuest.

70411-P4

IVADANTIN® ℞

(nitrofurantoin sodium)

STERILE—For Intravenous Use

The following text is based on official labeling in effect August 1, 1982.

Description: Ivadantin is a synthetic antibacterial agent for intravenous use. Each vial contains sufficient sterile powder to permit withdrawal, when reconstituted, of 180 mg (one adult dose) of nitrofurantoin, as the sodium salt:

O_2N–[furan]–CH=N–N–C=O, CH$_2$–C=O, N–Na

Actions: **Clinical Pharmacology:** Following intravenous administration of Ivadantin, nitrofurantoin is readily excreted in the urine. Under these conditions, about 45% of the drug dose is excreted unchanged in the urine. It is highly soluble in urine, to which it may impart a brown color. Usually, the blood drug levels present are low, and nitrofurantoin has a half-life of about 0.3 hours in whole blood.

Microbiology: Nitrofurantoin is an antibacterial agent for specific urinary tract infections. It is bacteriostatic in low concentrations (10 mcg/ml to 5 mcg/ml) and *in vitro* is considered to be bactericidal in higher concentrations. Its presumed mode of action is based upon its interference with several bacterial enzyme systems. Bacteria develop only a limited resistance to furan derivatives clinically.

Ivadantin is usually active against the following organisms *in vitro: Escherichia coli,* enterococci (e.g. *Streptococcus fecalis*), *Staphylococcus aureus.*

Note: Some strains of *Enterobacter* species and *Klebsiella* species are resistant to Ivadantin. It is not active against most strains of *Proteus* species, and *Serratia* species. It has no activity against *Pseudomonas* species.

Susceptibility Tests—Quantitative methods that require measurement of zone diameters give the most precise estimates of antimicrobial susceptibility. One recommended procedure, (NCCLS, ASM-2)*, uses a disc containing 300 micrograms for testing susceptibility; interpretations correlate zone diameters of this disc test with MIC values for nitrofurantoin. Reports from the laboratory should be interpreted according to the following criteria:

Susceptible organisms produce zones of 17 mm or greater, indicating that the tested organism is likely to respond to therapy.

Organisms of intermediate susceptibility produce zones of 15 to 16 mm, indicating that the tested organism would be susceptible if high dosage is used.

Resistant organisms produce zones of 14 mm or less, indicating that other therapy should be selected.

A bacterial isolate may be considered susceptible if the MIC value for nitrofurantoin is not more than 25 micrograms per ml. Organisms are considered resistant if the MIC is not less than 100 micrograms per ml.

Indications: Ivadantin should be used only in patients with clinically significant urinary tract infections when oral nitrofurantoin or nitrofurantoin macrocrystal therapy cannot be given.

Ivadantin is indicated for the treatment of urinary tract infections when due to susceptible strains of *E. coli,* enterococci, *S. aureus* (it is not indicated for the treatment of associated renal cortical or perinephric abscesses), and certain susceptible strains of *Klebsiella* species, *Enterobacter* species, and *Proteus* species.

Note: Specimens for culture and susceptibility testing should be obtained prior to and during drug administration.

Contraindications: Anuria, oliguria, or significant impairment of renal function (creatinine clearance under 40 ml per minute) are contraindications to therapy with this drug. Treatment of this type of patient carries an increased risk of toxicity because of impaired excretion of the drug. For the same reason, this drug is much less effective under these circumstances.

The drug is contraindicated in pregnant patients at term as well as in infants under one month of age because of the possibility of hemolytic anemia due to immature enzyme systems (glutathione instability).

The drug is also contraindicated in those patients with known hypersensitivity to Ivadantin, Macrodantin® (nitrofurantoin macrocrystals), Furadantin® (nitrofurantoin), and other nitrofurantoin preparations.

Warnings: Acute, subacute and chronic pulmonary reactions have been observed in patients treated with nitrofurantoin products. If these reactions occur, the drug should be withdrawn and appropriate measures should be taken.

An insidious onset of pulmonary reactions (diffuse interstitial pneumonitis or pulmonary fibrosis, or both) in patients on long-term therapy warrants close monitoring of these patients.

There have been isolated reports giving pulmonary reactions as a contributing cause of death. (See Hypersensitivity reactions.)

Cases of hemolytic anemia of the primaquine sensitivity type have been induced by nitrofurantoin. The hemolysis appears to be linked to a glucose-6-phosphate dehydrogenase deficiency in the red blood cells of the affected patients. This deficiency is found in 10 percent of Negroes and a small percentage of ethnic groups of Mediterranean and Near-Eastern origin. Any sign of hemolysis is an indication to discontinue the drug. Hemolysis ceases when the drug is withdrawn.

Pseudomonas is the organism most commonly implicated in superinfections in patients treated with nitrofurantoin.

Hepatitis, including chronic active hepatitis, has been observed rarely. Fatalities have been reported. The mechanism appears to be of an idiosyncratic hypersensitive type.

Precautions: Peripheral neuropathy may occur with nitrofurantoin therapy; this may become severe or irreversible. Fatalities have been reported. Predisposing conditions such as renal impairment (creatinine clearance under 40 ml per minute), anemia, diabetes, electrolyte imbalance, vitamin B deficiency, and debilitating disease may enhance such occurrence.

Usage in Pregnancy: The safety of nitrofurantoin during pregnancy and lactation has not been established. Use of the drug in women of childbearing potential requires that the an-

Continued on next page

Norwich Eaton—Cont.

ticipated benefit be weighed against the possible risks.

Usage in Children: Safety has not been established in children under 12 years.

Adverse Reactions: Gastrointestinal reactions: Anorexia, nausea, and emesis are the most frequent reactions and these are related to the drip speed; abdominal pain and diarrhea occur less frequently. Hepatitis occurs rarely.

Hypersensitivity Reactions: Pulmonary sensitivity reactions may occur which can be acute, subacute, or chronic.

Acute reactions are commonly manifested by fever, chills, cough, chest pain, dyspnea, pulmonary infiltration with consolidation or pleural effusion on x-ray, and eosinophilia. The acute reactions usually occur within the first week of treatment and are reversible with cessation of therapy. Resolution may be dramatic. In subacute reactions, fever and eosinophilia are observed less often. Recovery is somewhat slower, perhaps as long as several months. If the symptoms are not recognized as being drug related and nitrofurantoin is not withdrawn, symptoms may become more severe.

Chronic pulmonary reactions are more likely to occur in patients who have been on continuous nitrofurantoin therapy for six months or longer. The insidious onset of malaise, dyspnea on exertion, cough, and altered pulmonary function are common manifestations. Roentgenographic and histologic findings of diffuse interstitial pneumonitis or fibrosis, or both, are also common manifestations. Fever is rarely prominent.

The severity of these chronic pulmonary reactions and the degree of their resolution appear to be related to the duration of therapy after the first clinical signs appear. Pulmonary function may be permanently impaired even after cessation of nitrofurantoin therapy. This risk is greater when pulmonary reactions are not recognized early.

Dermatologic reactions: Maculopapular, erythematous, or eczematous eruption, pruritus, urticaria, and angioedema.

Other hypersensitivity reactions: Anaphylaxis, asthmatic attack in patients with history of asthma, cholestatic jaundice, hepatitis, including chronic active hepatitis, drug fever, and arthralgia.

Hematologic reactions: Hemolytic anemia, granulocytopenia, leukopenia, eosinophilia, and megaloblastic anemia. Return of the blood picture to normal has followed cessation of therapy.

Neurological reactions: Peripheral neuropathy, headache, dizziness, nystagmus, and drowsiness.

Miscellaneous reactions: Transient alopecia. As with other antimicrobial agents, superinfections by resistant organisms may occur. With nitrofurantoin, however, these are limited to the genitourinary tract because suppression of normal bacterial flora elsewhere in the body does not occur.

Dosage and Administration: Dosage: Patients weighing over 120 pounds: 180 mg of nitrofurantoin twice daily.

Patients weighing less than 120 pounds: 3 mg per pound of body weight per day in two equal doses.

Intravenous Administration: Dissolve just prior to use as follows: Add 20 ml of 5% dextrose injection, USP, or sterile water for injection, USP, to the vial of dry, sterile Ivadantin. To prepare the final solution, each ml of the initial dilution should be added to a minimum of 25 ml of parenteral fluid, e.g. 20 ml = 180 mg in at least 500 ml. (Do not use solutions containing methyl- and propyl-parabens, phenol or cresol as preservatives, since these compounds cause the Ivadantin to be precipitated out of solution.) Shake well to insure complete solution.

This final solution is to be given by intravenous drip at the rate of 50-60 drops (2-3 ml) per minute. The final solution should be used within 24 hours. It should be protected from ultraviolet light and excessive heat. Mixing other antibacterials in the same solution with nitrofurantoin sodium is not recommended. A list of known physical compatabilities will be supplied on request.

Therapy with peroral Macrodantin (nitrofurantoin macrocrystals) should replace the intravenous form when possible. The drug should be continued for at least one week and for at least three days after sterility of the urine is obtained. Continued infection indicates the need for reevaluation.

How Supplied: Sterile 20 ml vials containing one adult dose of sterile Ivadantin equivalent to 180 mg of nitrofurantoin.

Note: Mix just prior to use. Do not use intravenously without further dilution.

Furandantin (nitrofurantoin)/Macrodantin (nitrofurantoin macrocrystals) 300 mcg Sensi-Discs for the laboratory determination of bacterial sensitivity are available from BBL, Division of BioQuest. For information on simple Furadantin (nitrofurantoin) assays in blood, serum, and urine, write or call the Medical Department.

Literature sent to physicians on request.

78415-P2

* National Committee for Clinical Laboratory Standards. Approved Standard: ASM-2. Performance Standards for Antimicrobial Disc Susceptibility Tests, July, 1975.

LĀBID™ 250 mg ℞
(anhydrous theophylline)

The following text is based on official labeling in effect August 1, 1982.

Description: LāBID contains 250 mg anhydrous theophylline in a scored, long-acting, dye-free tablet. Theophylline is a white, odorless, crystalline powder, having a bitter taste, and is chemically related to theobromine and caffeine. LāBID has been specially formulated to provide therapeutic serum levels when administered every 12 hours, and minimizes the peaks and valleys of serum levels commonly found with shorter-acting theophylline products.

Clinical Pharmacology: The pharmacologic actions of theophylline include stimulation of respiration, augmentation of cardiac inotropy and chronotropy, relaxation of smooth muscles, including those in the bronchi and blood vessels (other than cerebral vessels) and diuresis. The main use of theophylline has been in the treatment of reversible airway obstruction. Theophylline is considered a potent medication for the control of chronic asthma. No development of tolerance occurs with chronic use of theophylline. The half-life is shortened with cigarette smoking and prolonged in alcoholism, reduced hepatic or renal function, congestive heart failure, and in patients receiving antibiotics such as lincomycin, clindamycin, troleandomycin, or erythromycin. High fever for prolonged periods and certain viral illnesses may decrease theophylline elimination. Newborn infants have extremely slow clearances and half-lives exceeding 24 hours.

Older adults with chronic obstructive pulmonary disease, any patients with cor pulmonale or other causes of heart failure, and patients with liver pathology may have much lower clearances with half-lives that exceed 24 hours. In comparative cross-over steady-state studies with immediate-release theophylline dosed at an average of 2.1 mg/K every 6 hours, LāBID 250 produced identical areas under curve when dosed at an average of 4.5 mg/K every 12 hours and adjusted for dosage difference. This confirms that LāBID 250 bio-availability dosed q12h is identical to liquid theophylline preparations dosed q6h. Data from the study also confirms a uniform and constant rate of absorption of theophylline from LāBID 250 in each subject. At steady-state, LāBID 250 provides adequate therapeutic theophylline levels. In single dose studies, LāBID 250 produces mean peak theophylline serum levels of 13.3 ± 4.6 mcg/ml at 4.9 ± 2.3 hours when dosed at an average of 7.9 mg/K.

Indications: For relief and/or prevention of symptoms from asthma and reversible bronchospasm associated with chronic bronchitis and emphysema.

Contraindications: LāBID is contraindicated in individuals who have shown hypersensitivity to any of its components or to xanthine derivatives.

Warnings: Status asthmaticus is a medical emergency. Optimal therapy frequently requires additional medication including corticosteroids when the patient is not rapidly responsive to bronchodilators. LāBID, as a long-acting theophylline, should not be used in status asthmaticus.

Since excessive theophylline doses may be associated with toxicity, periodic measurement of serum theophylline levels is recommended to assure maximal benefit without excessive risk. Incidence of toxicity increases at serum levels greater than 20 mcg/ml. Although early signs of theophylline toxicity, such as nausea and restlessness, are often seen, in some cases ventricular arrhythmias or seizures may be the first signs of toxicity.

Many patients who have excessive theophylline serum levels exhibit a tachycardia.

Theophylline preparations may worsen preexisting arrhythmias.

Usage in Pregnancy: Safe use in pregnancy has not been established relative to possible adverse effects on fetal development, but neither have adverse effects on fetal development been established. This is, unfortunately, true for most antiasthmatic medications. Therefore, use of theophylline in pregnant women should be balanced against the risk of uncontrolled asthma.

Precautions: DO NOT CRUSH OR CHEW LāBID 250 TABLETS BEFORE INGESTION.

Mean half-life in smokers is shorter than nonsmokers. Therefore, smokers may require larger doses of theophylline.

Theophylline should not be administered concurrently with other xanthine preparations.

Use with caution in patients with severe cardiac disease, severe hypoxemia, hypertension, hyperthyroidism, acute myocardial injury, cor pulmonale, congestive heart failure, liver disease, in the elderly (especially males), and in neonates. Great caution should be used in giving theophylline to patients with congestive heart failure. Such patients have shown markedly prolonged theophylline blood levels with theophylline persisting in serum for long periods following discontinuation of the drug.

Use theophylline cautiously in patients with a history of peptic ulcer.

Theophylline may occasionally act as a local gastrointestinal irritant, although G.I. symptoms are more commonly centrally mediated and associated with high serum concentration.

Adverse Reactions: The most consistent adverse reactions are due usually to overdose, and are:

Gastrointestinal: anorexia, nausea, vomiting, epigastric pain, hematemesis, diarrhea.

Central nervous system: headaches, irritability, restlessness, insomnia, reflex hyperexcitability, muscle twitching, clonic and tonic generalized convulsions.

Cardiovascular: palpitation, tachycardia, extrasystoles, flushing, hypotension, circulatory failure, ventricular arrhythmias.

Respiratory: tachypnea, respiratory arrest.

Renal: albuminuria, increased excretion of renal tubular cells and red blood cells; potentiation of diuresis.

Others: hyperglycemia, inappropriate ADH syndrome, fever, dehydration.

Drug Interactions:

Drug	Effect
Aminophylline with lithium carbonate	Increased excretion of lithium carbonate
Aminophylline with propranolol	Antagonism of propranolol effect
Theophylline with furosemide	Increased diuresis
Theophylline with hexamethonium	Decreased chronotropic effect
Theophylline with reserpine	Tachycardia
Theophylline with clindamycin, lincomycin, troleandomycin, or erythromycin	Increased theophylline blood levels
Theophylline with chlordiazepoxide	Chlordiazepoxide-induced fatty acid metabolism

Dosage and Administration: THE AVERAGE INITIAL ADULT DOSE IS ONE TO TWO LāBID 250 mg TABLETS EVERY 12 HOURS.

The recommended starting dose of LāBID for adolescents and adults is 6 mg per kg body weight every 12 hours based upon ideal body weight. If the desired relief is not achieved with this dose, and there are no systemic side effects (see Adverse Reactions), the dose may be increased by 1 mg per kg body weight every 2 days. With doses above 8 mg per kg every 12 hours, serum theophylline levels should be monitored.

Doses should be increased until therapeutic responses or side effects occur (higher doses may be necessary and well tolerated).

Occasional patients may require every 8 hours dosing.

THE AVERAGE INITIAL CHILDREN'S DOSE IS ONE-HALF TO ONE LāBID 250 mg TABLET EVERY 12 HOURS.

The recommended starting dose for children is 6 mg per kg body weight every 12 hours, and this dose can be increased by 1 mg per kg body weight every two days. With doses above 8 mg/kg every 12 hours, serum theophylline levels should be monitored.

Overdosage: Management

A. If potential overdose is established and seizure has not occurred:
  1) Induce vomiting.
  2) Administer activated charcoal.
  3) Administer a cathartic (this is particularly important if sustained release preparations have been taken).

B. If patient is having seizure:
  1) Establish an airway.
  2) Administer oxygen.
  3) Treat the seizure with intravenous diazepam 0.1 to 0.3 mg/kg up to 10 mg.
  4) Monitor vital signs, maintain blood pressure and provide adequate hydration.

C. Post-Seizure Coma:
  1) Maintain airway and oxygenation.
  2) Follow above recommendations to prevent absorption of drug, but intubation and lavage will have to be performed instead of inducing emesis, and the cathartic and charcoal will need to be introduced via a largebore gastric lavage tube.
  3) Continue to provide full supportive care and adequate hydration while waiting for drug to be metabolized. In general, the drug is metabolized sufficiently rapidly so as to not warrant consideration of dialysis.

How Supplied: LāBID 250 mg tablets are supplied in bottles of 100
NDC 0149-0402-01.

40201-P1

MACRODANTIN® ℞

(nitrofurantoin macrocrystals)
CAPSULES

The following text is based on official labeling in effect August 1, 1982.

Description: Macrodantin is a synthetic chemical of controlled crystal size. It is a stable, yellow crystalline compound. It is supplied in capsules containing 25 mg, 50 mg, and 100 mg.

1-[[(5-NITRO-2-FURANYL)METHYLENE] AMINO]-2. 4-IMIDAZOLIDINEDIONE

Actions: Clinical Pharmacology: Macrodantin is a larger crystal form of Furadantin® (nitrofurantoin). The absorption of Macrodantin is slower and its excretion somewhat less when compared to Furandantin. During therapeutic drug dosage, only low blood drug concentrations are usually present. A number of patients who cannot tolerate Furadantin (nitrofurantoin) Tablets are able to take Macrodantin Capsules without nausea. It is highly soluble in urine, to which it may impart a brown color. Following a therapeutic dose regimen (100 mg qid for 7 days) average urinary drug recoveries (0-24 hours) on day 1 and 7 were 37.9% and 35.0%, respectively, for Macrodantin.

Microbiology: Macrodantin is an antibacterial agent for specific urinary tract infections. It is bacteriostatic in low concentrations (10 mcg/ml to 5 mcg/ml) and *in vitro* is considered to be bactericidal in higher concentrations. Its presumed mode of action is based upon its interference with several bacterial enzyme systems. Bacteria develop only a limited resistance to furan derivatives clinically.

Macrodantin is usually active against the following organisms *in vitro: Escherichia coli,* enterococci (e.g. *Streptococcus fecalis), Staphylococcus aureus.*

Note: Some strains of *Enterobacter* species and *Klebsiella* species are resistant to Macrodantin. It is not active against most strains of *Proteus* species, and *Serratia* species. It has no activity against *Pseudomonas* species.

Susceptibility Tests—Quantitative methods that require measurement of zone diameters give the most precise estimates of antimicrobial susceptibility. One recommended procedure, (NCCLS, ASM-2)*, uses a disc containing 300 micrograms for testing susceptibility; interpretations correlate zone diameters of this disc test with MIC values for nitrofurantoin.

Reports from the laboratory should be interpreted according to the following criteria:

Susceptible organisms produce zones of 17 mm or greater, indicating that the tested organism is likely to respond to therapy.

Organisms of intermediate susceptibility produce zones of 15 to 16 mm, indicating that the tested organism would be susceptible if high dosage is used.

Resistant organisms produce zones of 14 mm or less, indicating that other therapy should be selected.

A bacterial isolate may be considered susceptible if the MIC value for nitrofurantoin is not more than 25 micrograms per ml. Organisms are considered resistant if the MIC is not less than 100 micrograms per ml.

Indications: Macrodantin is indicated for the treatment of urinary tract infections when due to susceptible strains of *E. coli,* enterococci, *S. aureus* (it is not indicated for the treatment of associated renal cortical or perinephric abscesses), and certain susceptible strains of *Klebsiella* species, *Enterobacter* species and *Proteus* species.

Note: Specimens for culture and susceptibility testing should be obtained prior to and during administration.

Contraindications: Anuria, oliguria, or significant impairment of renal function (creatinine clearance under 40 ml per minute) are contraindications to therapy with this drug. Treatment of this type of patient carries an increased risk of toxicity because of impaired excretion of the drug. For the same reason, this drug is much less effective under these circumstances.

The drug is contraindicated in pregnant patients at term as well as in infants under one month of age because of the possibility of hemolytic anemia due to immature enzyme systems (glutathione instability).

The drug is also contraindicated in those patients with known hypersensitivity to Macrodantin, Furadantin (nitrofurantoin), and other nitrofurantoin preparations.

Warnings: Acute, subacute and chronic pulmonary reactions have been observed in patients treated with nitrofurantoin products. If these reactions occur, the drug should be withdrawn and appropriate measures should be taken.

An insidious onset of pulmonary reactions (diffuse interstitial pneumonitis or pulmonary fibrosis, or both) in patients on long-term therapy warrants close monitoring of these patients.

There have been isolated reports giving pulmonary reactions as a contributing cause of death. (See Hypersensitivity reactions.)

Cases of hemolytic anemia of the primaquine sensitivity type have been induced by Macrodantin. The hemolysis appears to be linked to a glucose-6-phosphate dehydrogenase deficiency in the red blood cells of the affected patients. This deficiency is found in 10 percent of Negroes and a small percentage of ethnic groups of Mediterranean and Near-Eastern origin. Any sign of hemolysis is an indication to discontinue the drug. Hemolysis ceases when the drug is withdrawn.

Pseudomonas is the organism most commonly implicated in superinfections in patients treated with Macrodantin.

Hepatitis, including chronic active hepatitis, has been observed rarely. Fatalities have been reported. The mechanism appears to be of an idiosyncratic hypersensitive type.

Precautions: Peripheral neuropathy may occur with Macrodantin therapy; this may become severe or irreversible. Fatalities have been reported. Predisposing conditions such as renal impairment (creatinine clearance under 40 ml per minute), anemia, diabetes, electrolyte imbalance, vitamin B deficiency, and debilitating disease may enhance such occurrence.

Usage in Pregnancy: The safety of Macrodantin during pregnancy and lactation has not been established. Use of this drug in women of childbearing potential requires that the anticipated benefit be weighed against the possible risks.

Adverse Reactions: Gastrointestinal reactions: Anorexia, nausea and emesis are the most frequent reactions; abdominal pain and diarrhea occur less frequently. These dose-related toxicity reactions can be minimized by reduction of dosage, especially in the female patient. Hepatitis occurs rarely.

Hypersensitivity reactions: Pulmonary sensitivity reactions may occur, which can be acute, subacute, or chronic.

Acute reactions are commonly manifested by fever, chills, cough, chest pain, dyspnea, pulmonary infiltration with consolidation of pleural effusion on x-ray, and eosinophilia. The acute reactions usually occur within the first week of treatment and are reversible with cessation of therapy. Resolution may be dramatic. In subacute reactions, fever and eosinophilia are observed less often. Recovery is somewhat slower, perhaps as long as several months. If

Continued on next page

Norwich Eaton—Cont.

the symptoms are not recognized as being drug related and nitrofurantoin is not withdrawn, symptoms may become more severe.
Chronic pulmonary reactions are more likely to occur in patients who have been on continuous nitrofurantoin therapy for six months or longer. The insidious onset of malaise, dyspnea on exertion, cough, and altered pulmonary function are common manifestations. Roentgenographic ahd histologic findings of diffuse interstitial pneumonitis or fibrosis, or both, are also common manifestations. Fever is rarely prominent.
The severity of these chronic pulmonary reactions and the degree of their resolution appear to be related to the duration of therapy after the first clinical signs appear. Pulmonary function may be permanently impaired even after cessation of nitrofurantoin therapy. The risk is greater when pulmonary reactions are not recognized early.
Dermatologic reactions: Maculopapular, erythematous, or eczematous eruption, pruritus, urticaria and angioedema.
Other hypersensitivity reactions: Anaphylaxis, asthmatic attack in patients with history of asthma, cholestatic jaundice, hepatitis, including chronic active hepatitis, drug fever, and arthralgia.
Hematologic reactions: Hemolytic anemia, granulocytopenia, leukopenia, eosinophilia, and megaloblastic anemia. Return of the blood picture to normal has followed cessation of therapy.
Neurological reactions: Peripheral neuropathy, headache, dizziness, nystagmus, and drowsiness.
Miscellaneous reactions: Transient alopecia. As with other antimicrobial agents, superinfections by resistant organisms may occur. With Macrodantin, however, these are limited to the genitourinary tract because suppression of normal bacterial flora elsewhere in the body does not occur.
Dosage and Administration:
Dosage—Adults: 50–100 mg four times a day.
Children: Should be calculated on the basis of 5–7 mg/kg of body weight per 24 hours to be given in divided doses four times a day (contraindicated under one month).
Administration: Macrodantin may be given with food or milk to further minimize gastric upset.
Therapy should be continued for at least one week and for at least 3 days after sterility of the urine is obtained. Continued infection indicates the need for reevaluation.
If the drug is to be used for long-term suppressive therapy, a reduction of dosage should be considered.
How Supplied: Macrodantin is available in:
100-mg: opaque, yellow capsules:
NDC 0149-0009-01 bottle of 30
NDC 0149-0009-05 bottle of 100
NDC 0149-0009-66 bottle of 500
NDC 0149-0009-67 bottle of 1000
NDC 0149-0009-77 hospital unit-dose strips in box of 100
50-mg: opaque, yellow and white capsules:
NDC 0149-0008-01 bottle of 30
NDC 0149-0008-05 bottle of 100
NDC 0149-0008-66 bottle of 500
NDC 0149-0008-67 bottle of 1000
NDC 0149-0008-77 hospital unit-dose strips in box of 100
25-mg: opaque, white capsules:
NDC 0149-0007-05 bottle of 100
Furadantin (nitrofurantoin)/Macrodantin Sensi-Discs for the laboratory determination of bacterial sensitivity are available from BBL, Division of BioQuest. For information on simple nitrofurantoin assays in blood, serum, and urine, write or call the Medical Department. Literature sent to physicians on request.
Address medical inquiries to Norwich Eaton Pharmaceuticals, Inc. Medical Department, Norwich, NY 13815.

00700-P4

* National Committee for Clinical Laboratory Standards. Approved Standard: ASM-2. Performance Standards for Antimicrobial Disc Susceptibility Tests. July, 1975.

[*Shown in Product Identification Section*]

PEPTO-BISMOL® Liquid and Tablets

For upset stomach, indigestion and nausea. Controls common diarrhea.

Active Ingredient: Bismuth subsalicylate, 300 mg per tablet or 262 mg per 15 ml (tablespoon). Contains no sugar.
Indications: For indigestion—soothes irritated stomach with a protective coating action. For nausea brings fast, sure relief from distress of that queasy, nauseated feeling. For diarrhea, controls common diarrhea within 24 hours, without constipating, relieving gas pains and abdominal cramps.
Keep all medicines out of reach of children.
Caution: This product contains salicylates. If taken with aspirin and ringing of the ears occur, discontinue use. If pregnant, nursing or taking medicines for anticoagulation (thinning the blood), diabetes, or gout, consult physician or pharmacist before taking this product. If diarrhea is accompanied by high fever or continues more than 2 days, consult a physician.
Note: The beneficial medication may cause a temporary darkening of the stool and tongue.
Dosage Directions: LIQUID
Adults—2 tablespoonfuls.
Children—according to age:
10 to 14 years—4 teaspoonfuls
6 to 10 years—2 teaspoonfuls
3 to 6 years—1 teaspoonful
Repeat above dosage every ½ to 1 hour, if needed until 8 doses are taken.
TABLETS
Adults—2 Tablets
Children (6 to 10 years)—1 Tablet
Children (3 to 6 years)—½ Tablet
Chew or dissolve in mouth. Repeat every ½ to one hour as needed to maximum of 8 doses.
How Supplied: Pepto-Bismol is available in:
Liquid
NDC 0149-0039-04 bottle of 4 fl. oz.
NDC 0149-0039-08 bottle of 8 fl. oz.
NDC 0149-0039-42 bottle of 12 fl. oz.
NDC 0149-0039-16 bottle of 16 fl. oz.
Tablets
NDC 0149-0326-24 carton of 24 Tablets
NDC 0149-0326-42 carton of 42 Tablets
NDC 0149-0326-60 carton of 60 Tablets

SARENIN® ℞

(saralasin acetate)

(See Diagnostic Section.)

STANDARD VIVONEX®

Elemental Standard Diet/Soluble Powder

The following text is based on official labeling in effect August 1, 1982.
NUTRITIONAL INFORMATION AND USE INSTRUCTIONS
Standard Vivonex® is a patented, nutritionally complete elemental diet formulated for the nutritional management of patients with impaired digestion and/or malabsorption. Standard Vivonex has a chemically defined composition of all essential nutrients in simple, readily absorbable form: free amino acids, simple sugars, essential fatty acid, vitamins, minerals, and trace elements.
Composition: One 80-gram packet provides 300 Calories and 0.98 grams of available nitrogen with a caloric density of 1 Calorie per ml when diluted with water to a total volume of 300 ml:

	Amount per 80 g	Energy Distribution
Total energy	300 Calories	
Amino acids	6.56 g	8.2%
Carbohydrate	69.2 g	90.5%
Fat	0.435 g	1.3%
Linoleic acid	0.348 g	

Six 80-g packets of Standard Vivonex supply 5.88 grams of available nitrogen, 2.61 grams fat, 415 grams carbohydrate, and the following vitamins, minerals, and amino acids:

Vitamins, Minerals and Trace Elements	Per 6 Packets (480 Grams)	% U.S. RDA
Vitamin A	5000 IU	100
Vitamin D_2	400 IU	100
Vitamin E	30 IU	100
Vitamin C	60 mg	100
Folic Acid	0.4 mg	100
Thiamine	1.5 mg	100
Riboflavin	1.7 mg	100
Niacin	20 mg	100
Vitamin B_6	2 mg	100
Vitamin B_{12}	6 mcg	100
Biotin	0.3 mg	100
Pantothenic Acid	10 mg	100
Vitamin K_1	67 mcg	*
Choline	73.7 mg	*
Calcium	1 g	100
Phosphorus	1 g	100
Iodine	150 mcg	100
Iron	18 mg	100
Magnesium	400 mg	100
Copper	2 mg	100
Zinc	15 mg	100
Manganese	2.81 mg	*
Selenium†	0.150 mg	*
Molybdenum†	0.150 mg	*
Chromium†	0.050 mg	

* No U.S. RDA established
† Represents amounts of these metals added.

ESSENTIAL AMINO ACIDS	% Total Amino Acids
Isoleucine	4.55
Leucine	7.20
L-Lysine	5.41
Methionine	4.66
Phenylalanine	5.18
Threonine	4.55
Tryptophan	1.41
Valine	5.02
Total essential amino acids	37.98

NON-ESSENTIAL AMINO ACIDS	% Total Amino Acids
Alanine	4.85
Arginine	8.87
L-Aspartic Acid	10.35
L-Glutamine	17.07
Glycine	7.91
Histidine	2.21
Proline	6.48
Serine	3.34
L-Tyrosine	0.94
Total non-essential amino acids	62.02

ELECTROLYTES IN STANDARD VIVONEX
(one 80-gram packet diluted with water to total volume of 300 ml)

Cations	mEq/ 1000 ml	mg/80 g Packet	mg/6 Packets
Sodium	20.4	140.5	843.0
Potassium	30.0	351.5	2109.0
Calcium	27.7	166.7	1000.0
Magnesium	18.3	66.67	400.0
Manganese	0.0567	0.468	2.81
Iron	0.358	3.0	18.0
Copper	0.0350	0.333	2.0
Zinc	0.255	2.5	15.0
Selenium†	0.00211*	0.025	0.150
Molybdenum†	0.00174**	0.025	0.150

Chromium†	0.0016	0.008	0.050

*Calculated as Selenite
**Calculated as Molybdate
†Represents amounts of these metals added.

Anions	mEq/ 1000 ml	mg/80 g Packet	mg/6 Packets
Chloride	20.4	216.6	1300
Phosphate	54.0	166.6*	1000*
Acetate	18.7	331.8	1991
Iodide	0.00066	0.025	0.15

* Calculated as Phosphorus

In the standard dilution of 1 Calorie/ml, Standard Vivonex Unflavored has a pH of approximately 5.5 and an average osmolality of 550 mOsm/kg.

Actions and Uses: Standard Vivonex is a nutritionally complete, elemental diet that is rapidly utilized, since digestion is virtually obviated, and absorption can take place without the aid of peptidases. Standard Vivonex is absorbed within the first 100 cm of functional small intestine. It is essentially a no-residue diet. There is minimal stimulation of biliary, pancreatic, and intestinal secretions, because of its free L-amino acid nitrogen (protein) source, glucose oligosaccharide primary energy source, and low fat content. The low fat content also permits rapid gastric emptying and eliminates gastric residuals, thus minimizing the possibility of aspiration.

The balanced amino acid profile of Standard Vivonex insures optimum utilization and retention of its readily absorbed, elemental nitrogen source.

Standard Vivonex is useful in the dietary management of patients with impaired digestion and absorption which are secondary to a variety of diseases and disorders such as gastrointestinal disease, e.g. inflammatory bowel disease, cancer, intestinal atresia; condiions leading to partial function of the gastrointestinal tract, e.g. pancreatitis, fistula, partial obstruction, short-gut syndrome. Standard Vivonex is also useful in the dietary management of neonates and infants suffering from intractable diarrhea, as an aid in preparing the bowel for diagnostic and surgical procedures, and as a transition diet between parenteral and normal oral feeding. It is synthetically derived and contains no whole foodstuffs and therefore is hypoallergenic and well tolerated by patients with known food sensitivities. Standard Vivonex has been proven useful as an elimination diet for patients undergoing diagnosis of specific food allergens.

One packet diluted with 255 ml (8½ oz.) of water makes a single serving. Six packets of Standard Vivonex mixed thoroughly with 1530 ml of water provide a full day's supply for the average adult with 1800 Calories, 5.88 grams available nitrogen, 2.61 grams fat, and 415 grams carbohydrate. Standard Vivonex is a perishable liquid food when in solution. A full day's supply may be prepared at one time and stored in the refrigerator for up to 24 hours; shake the liquid briefly before serving. Do not leave at room temperature for more than 8 hours.

For oral use, Standard Vivonex must be flavored and served chilled over ice. Vivonex Flavor Packets were specifically developed for this purpose, although other flavoring agents may be used if their contribution to the elemental and nutritional qualities of the diet are kept in mind. Standard Vivonex should be sipped slowly, preferably with a straw, when served as a beverage. Initiate oral feeding with dilute solution, e.g. one packet diluted with 555 ml (18½ oz.), and gradually increase volume and concentration.

Oral feedings of elemental diets are sometimes met by poor patient acceptance because of taste and the lack of the usual appetite cues of normal meals. Varying the available flavors, serving chilled over ice and sipping through a straw, and educating and motivating the patient as to the therapeutic importance of this form of diet, are reportedly effective in improving patient acceptability.

Standard Vivonex may also be administered via feeding tube placed nasogastrically or into an esophagostomy, gastrostomy, or jejunostomy. Because of its homogeneity and low viscosity, as small as a 16 gauge catheter or #5 French feeding tube may be used to optimize patient tolerance. It is suggested that the diet be given at room temperature by continuous drip technique using the Vivonex Delivery System (**NDC** 0149-0050-10), a suitable infusion pump, or controller. At the 1 Calorie per ml dilution, Standard Vivonex supplies most of the daily fluid requirements. Additional fluids should be given when necessary to maintain adequate urine output.

During the first two days of use, Standard Vivonex may need to be over-diluted for the osmotically sensitive patient, gradually titrating up to full strength. The following administration schedule will facilitate GI adaptation, in most patients, within two days:

[See table above].

Hours	Strength	No. of Packets	Rate (ml/ hour)	Fluid Volume (ml)	Calories (Cal)	Nitrogen (g)
1–12	⅔	2	75	900	600	2
13–24	¾	3	100	1200	900	3
25–36	4/4	5	125	1500	1500	5
37–48	4/4	6	150	1800	1800	6

If diarrhea is encountered, revert one step to a more dilute solution, maintaining the patient at the last tolerated rate until free of symptoms for 8 hours. Then continue with progressive schedule until desired caloric/nitrogen intake is achieved.

Precautions: DO NOT ADMINISTER STANDARD VIVONEX PARENTERALLY.

Nausea, vomiting, abdominal cramps and distention, and diarrhea have been reported. Nausea is usually due to feeding rate, while diarrhea may also be caused by the diet concentration. If encountered, revert one step in the above administration schedule, and then continue slowly with a progressive schedule until desired caloric/nitrogen intake is achieved. Local water conditions have also been implicated in instances of diarrhea. Using deionized or distilled water in diet preparation, until patient tolerance with full strength diet is achieved, has been reported to be effective in this circumstance.

Aspiration is an uncommon complication with Standard Vivonex because of its low fat content. However, in patients suspected at risk, radiologically confirm the anatomic position of the feeding tube, elevate the head of the bed 30° while the patient is receiving diet intragastrically, and control the administration to 150 ml/hour or less, depending upon patient tolerance. Jejunal administration should also be considered.

Additional professional and technical information on all Vivonex products is available through your local Norwich Eaton Professional Products Group representative.

Supply Information: Standard Vivonex is available in cartons of six 80-g sealed packets for individual servings. Each packet provides 300 Calories in a total volume of 300 ml when mixed with 255 ml water.

Vivonex Flavor packets are available in Vanilla (**NDC** 0149-0054-02), Strawberry (**NDC** 0149-0056-02). Orange-Pineapple (**NDC** 0149-0058-02), and Lemon-Lime (**NDC** 0149-0057-02) flavors. The Vivonex Delivery System (**NDC** 0149-0050-10) is a disposable, gravity-drip tube feeding set with one liter capacity, complete with micro-drop cannula and connecting tubing.

HIGH NITROGEN VIVONEX®

Elemental High Nitrogen Diet/Soluble Powder

NUTRITIONAL INFORMATION AND USE INSTRUCTIONS

High Nitrogen Vivonex® is a patented, nutritionally complete, high nitrogen elemental diet formulated for the nutritional management of patients at risk for, or who are suffering from, protein/calorie malnutrition, or for patients with impaired digestion and/or malabsorption. High Nitrogen Vivonex has a chemically defined composition of all essential nutrients in simple, readily absorbable form: free amino acids, simple sugars, essential fatty acid, vitamins, minerals, and trace elements.

Composition: One 80-gram packet provides 300 Calories and 2 grams of available nitrogen with a caloric density of 1 Calorie per ml when diluted with water to a total volume of 300 ml:

	Amount per 80 g	Energy Distribution
Total energy	300 Calories	
Amino acids	13.31 g	17.7%
Carbohydrate	63.0 g	81.5%
Fat	0.261 g	0.78%
Linoleic acid	0.209 g	

Ten 80-g packets of High Nitrogen Vivonex supply 20.0 grams of available nitrogen, 2.61 grams fat. 630 grams carbohydrates, and the following vitamins, minerals, and amino acids:

Vitamins, Minerals and Trace Elements	Per 10 Packets (800 Grams)	% U.S. RDA
Vitamin A	5000 IU	100
Vitamin D_2	400 IU	100
Vitamin E	30 IU	100
Vitamin C	60 mg	100
Folic Acid	0.4 mg	100
Thiamine	1.5 mg	100
Riboflavin	1.7 mg	100
Niacin	20 mg	100
Vitamin B_1	2 mg	100
Vitamin B_{12}	6 mcg	100
Biotin	0.3 mg	100
Pantothenic Acid	10 mg	100
Vitamin K_1	67 mcg	*
Choline	73.7 mg	*
Calcium	1 g	100
Phosphorus	1 g	100
Iodine	150 mcg	100
Iron	18 mg	100
Magnesium	400 mg	100
Copper	2 mg	100
Zinc	15 mg	100
Manganese	2.81 mg	*
Selenium†	0.150 mg	*
Molybdenum†	0.150 mg	*
Chromium†	0.050 mg	*

*No U.S. RDA established.
†Represents amounts of these metals added.

ESSENTIAL AMINO ACIDS	% Total Amino Acids
Isoleucine	4.15
Leucine	6.57
L-Lysine	4.94
Methionine	4.58
Phenylalanine	7.10
Threonine	4.16
Tryptophan	1.28
Valine	4.58
Total essential amino acids	37.36

Continued on next page

Norwich Eaton—Cont.

NON-ESSENTIAL AMINO ACIDS	% Total Amino Acids
Alanine	5.18
Arginine	4.07
L-Aspartic Acid	11.06
L-Glutamine	18.22
Glycine	9.84
Histidine	2.36
Proline	6.92
Serine	4.15
L-Tyrosine	0.84
Total non-essential amino acids	62.64

ELECTROLYTES IN HIGH NITROGEN VIVONEX
(one 80-gram packet diluted with water to total volume of 300 ml)

Cations	mEq/ 1000 ml	mg/80 g Packet	mg/10 Packets
Sodium	23.0	158.6	1586.0
Potassium	30.0	351.9	3519.0
Calcium	16.6	100.0	1000.0
Magnesium	10.97	40.0	400.0
Manganese	0.0341	0.281	2.81
Iron	0.2148	1.8	18.0
Copper	0.02098	0.2	2.0
Zinc	0.153	1.5	15.0
Selenium†	0.00127*	0.015	0.150
Molybdenum†	0.00104**	0.015	0.150
Chromium†	0.001	0.005	0.050

*Calculated as Selenite
**Calculated as Molybdate
†Represents amounts of these metals added

Anions	mEq/ 1000 ml	mg/80 g Packet	mg/10 Packets
Chloride	23.1	244.6	2446.0
Phosphate	31.6	100.0*	1000.0*
Acetate	26.0	459.9	4599.3
Iodide	0.00039	0.015	0.15

* Calculated as Phosphorus

In the standard dilution of 1 Calorie/ml, High Nitrogen Vivonex Unflavored has a pH of approximately 5.0 and an average osmolality of 810 mOsm/kg.

Actions and Uses: High Nitrogen Vivonex is a nutritionally complete, high nitrogen elemental diet that is rapidly utilized, since digestion is virtually obviated, and absorption can take place without the aid of peptidases. High Nitrogen Vivonex is absorbed within the first 100 cm of functional small intestine. It is essentially a no-residue diet. There is minimal stimulation of biliary, pancreatic, and intestinal secretions, because of its free L-amino acid nitrogen (protein) source, glucose oligosaccharide primary energy source, and low fat content. The low fat content also permits rapid gastric emptying and eliminates gastric residuals, therefore minimizing the possibility of aspiration.

High Nitrogen Vivonex, by virtue of its balanced amino acid profile and nitrogen to Calorie ratio of 1:150, spares nitrogen for anabolic purposes and promotes efficient protein synthesis.

Day	Strength	No. of 80-g Packets	Approx. Rate (ml/hour)	Fluid Volume (ml)	Calories (Cal.)	Nitrogen (g)
Operation	1/4	1	50	1200	300	2
1	1/4	2	100	2400	600	4
2	1/2	4	100	2400	1200	8
3	1/2	4	100	2400	1200	8
4	3/4	6	100	2400	1800	12
5	4/4	8	100	2400	2400	16
6	4/4	10	125	3000	3000	20

High Nitrogen Vivonex is useful in the dietary management of patients with impaired digestion and absorption which are secondary to a variety of diseases and disorders such as gastrointestinal disease, e.g. inflammatory bowel disease, cancer, intestinal atresia; conditions leading to partial function of the gastrointestinal tract, e.g. pancreatitis, fistula, partial obstruction, short-gut syndrome; conditions causing increased metabolic needs, e.g. head and neck cancer, multiple trauma, severe burns and in the nutritional management of malnourished and cachectic patients. High Nitrogen Vivonex is also useful in the dietary management of neonates and infants suffering from intractable diarrhea, as an aid in preparing the bowel for diagnostic and surgical procedures, and as a transition diet between parenteral and normal oral feeding. High Nitrogen Vivonex has also been shown to be useful in obtaining positive protein balance and an earlier return to normal nutrition following major abdominal surgery by its administration during the immediate postoperative period. It is synthetically derived and contains no whole foodstuffs and therefore is hypoallergenic and well tolerated by patients with known food sensitivities.

One packet diluted with 255 ml (8½ oz.) of water makes a single serving. Ten packets of High Nitrogen Vivonex mixed thoroughly with 2550 ml of water provide the quantity of nutrients and energy required daily by the average catabolic adult. High Nitrogen Vivonex is a perishable liquid food when in solution. A full day's supply may be prepared at one time and stored in the refrigerator for up to 24 hours; shake the liquid briefly before serving. Do not leave at room temperature for more than 8 hours.

Oral Administration: For oral use, High Nitrogen Vivonex must be flavored and served chilled over ice. Vivonex Flavor Packets were specifically developed for this purpose, although other flavoring agents may be used if their contribution to the elemental and nutritional qualities of the diet are kept in mind. High Nitrogen Vivonex should be sippd slowly, preferably with a straw, when served as a beverage. Initiate oral feeding with dilute solution, e.g. one packet diluted with 555 ml (18½ oz.), and gradually increase volume and concentration.

Oral feedings of elemental diets are sometimes met by poor patient acceptance because of taste and the lack of the usual appetite cues of normal meals. Varying the available flavors, serving chilled over ice and sipping through a straw, and educating and motivating the patient as to the therapeutic importance of this form of diet, are reportedly effective in improving patient acceptability.

High Nitrogen Vivonex may also be administered via feeding tube placed nasogastrically, or into an esophagostomy, gastrostomy, or jejunostomy. Because of its homogeneity and low viscosity, as small as a 16 gauge catheter or #5 French feeding tube may be used to optimize patient tolerance. It is suggested that the diet be given at room temperature by continuous drip technique, either using the Vivonex Delivery System (**NDC** 0149-0050-10), or a suitable infusion pump. At the 1 Calorie per ml dilution, High Nitrogen Vivonex supplies most of the daily fluid requirements. Additional fluids should be given when necessary to maintain adequate urine output.

Gastric Administration: During the first few days of use, High Nitrogen Vivonex should be overdiluted, gradually titrating up to full strength. The following administration schedule will facilitate GI adaptation, in most patients, within four days:
[See table below].

Day	Strength	No. of 80-g Packets	Approx. Rate (ml/hour)	Fluid Volume (ml)	Calories (Cal.)	Nitrogen (g)
1	1/2	2	50	1200	600	4
2	1/2	3	75	1800	900	6
3	3/4	6	100	2400	1800	12
4	4/4	8	100	2400	2400	16
5	4/4	10	125	3000	3000	20

Jejunal Administration: Since intestinal adaptation varies by patient, the following administration schedule is offered as a general guideline for titration to full strength (1 Calorie/ml) High Nitrogen Vivonex:
[See table above].

In patients with severely compromised GI function, several days may be required to allow for adaptation to full strength diet. If diarrhea is encountered, revert one step to a more dilute solution, maintaining the patient at the last tolerated rate until free of symptoms for eight hours. Then continue with progressive schedule until desired caloric/nitrogen intake is achieved.

Precautions: DO NOT ADMINISTER HIGH NITROGEN VIVONEX PARENTERALLY.

Nausea, vomiting, abdominal cramps and distention, and diarrhea have been reported. Nausea is usually due to feeding rate, while diarrhea may also be caused by the diet concentration. If encountered, revert one step in the administration schedule, and then continue slowly with a progressive schedule until desired caloric/nitrogen intake is achieved. Local water conditions have also been implicated in instances of diarrhea. Using deionized or distilled water in diet preparation, until patient tolerence with full strength diet is achieved, has been reported effective in this circumstance.

Aspiration is an uncommon complication with High Nitrogen Vivonex because of its low fat content. However, in patients suspected at risk, radiologically confirm the anatomic position of the feeding tube, elevate the head of the bed 30° while the patient is receiving diet intragastrically, and control the administration to 150 ml/hour or less, depending upon patient tolerance. Jejunal administration should also be considered.

Additional professional and technical information on all Vivonex products is available through your local Norwich Eaton Professional Products Group representative.

Supply Information: For preparing a full day's supply, High Nitrogen Vivonex is available in cartons of ten 80-g sealed packets, each providing 300 Calories in a total volume of 300 ml when mixed with 255 ml water. Vivonex Flavor Packets are available in Vanilla (**NDC** 0149-0054-02), Strawberry (**NDC** 0149-0056-02), Orange-Pineapple (**NDC** 0149-0058-02) and Lemon-Lime (**NDC** 0149-0057-02) flavors. The Vivonex Delivery System is a disposable, gravity-drip tube feeding set with one liter capacity, complete with micro-drop cannula and connecting tubing.

VIVONEX® FLAVOR PACKETS NONNUTRITIVE
Exclusively for use with High Nitrogen Vivonex or Standard Vivonex.

Mixing Instructions: For normal dilution, place $8\frac{1}{2}$ ounces (255 ml) of water in a blender. Add contents of one 80-gram packet of **High Nitrogen Vivonex** or **Standard Vivonex** and one flavor packet. Blend at high speed until in solution. Flavor packets are readily dispersible and may also be added by stirring into the prepared unflavored diet solution. Serve well chilled.
See package insert enclosed in diet package for complete nutritional information and use instructions.
Storage: Store **Vivonex Flavor Packets** away from excessive heat. In normal dilution, **Vivonex** diets are perishable liquid foods, and refrigeration is necessary. No more than the amount for a single day should be prepared at one time.
Lemon-Lime Flavor
Contributes:
- Calories 8
- Protein ....0 gram
- Carbohydrate ....0.77 gram
- Fat ....0 gram
- Saccharin ....20 milligrams

Ingredients: Citric acid, dextrose, artificial flavor, saccharin and silicon dioxide.
Osmolality: Standard diet with flavor added—approximately 595 mOsm/kg; High Nitrogen diet with flavor added—approximately 855 mOsm/kg.
Orange-Pineapple Flavor
Contributes:
- Calories 8
- Protein ....0 gram
- Carbohydrate ....0.93 gram
- Fat ....0 gram
- Saccharin ....20 milligrams

Ingredients: Citric acid, dextrose, artificial flavor, saccharin, ethyl maltol, artificial color, silicon dioxide.
Osmolality: Standard diet with flavor added—approximately 595 mOsm/kg; High Nitrogen diet with flavor added—approximately 855 mOsm/kg.
Strawberry Flavor
Contributes:
- Calories 8
- Protein ....0 gram
- Carbohydrate ....1.71 gram
- Fat ....0 gram
- Saccharin ....20 milligrams

Ingredients: Dextrose, artificial flavor, citric acid, saccharin, silicon dioxide, artificial color.
Osmolality: Standard diet with flavor added—approximately 595 mOsm/kg; High Nitrogen diet with flavor added—approximately 855 mOsm/kg.
Artificial Vanilla Flavor
Nutritional Information: In addition to the nutritional values of **High Nitrogen Vivonex** and **Standard Vivonex**, each flavor packet contains the following:
- Calories 9
- Protein ....0 grams
- Carbohydrate ....2.2 grams
- Fat ....0 grams
- Saccharin ....0.020 grams

Ingredients: dextrose, artificial flavor, saccharin, silicon dioxide.
Osmolality: One Vanilla Flavor Packet in 300 ml of Standard Vivonex has an osmolality of approximately 600 mOsm/kg. One Vanilla Flavor Packet in 300 ml of High Nitrogen Vivonex has an osmolality of approximately 860 mOsm/kg.

VIVONEX® ACUTROL™ ℞
Enteral Feeding System

VIVONEX™ DECOMPRESSION TUBE ℞
Naso-esophago-gastric decompression tube

VIVONEX™ Delivery System ℞
Tube Feeding System

VIVONEX™ JEJUNOSTOMY KIT ℞
Needle catheter jejunostomy kit

VIVONEX™ MOSS* TUBE ℞
Naso-esophago-gastric decompression tube with duodenal feeding tube.
*TM of National Catheter Company

VIVONEX™ TUNGSTEN TIP TUBE ℞
Nasogastric/nasointestinal feeding tube

VIVONEX™ TUNGSTEN TIP STYLET TUBE ℞

OLC Laboratories, Inc.
99 N.W. MIAMI GARDENS DR.
MIAMI, FL 33169

TRYPTACIN
(brand of L.Tryptophan)
(See PDR for Nonprescription Drugs)

Obetrol Pharmaceuticals
(Division of Rexar Pharmacal Corp.)
396 ROCKAWAY AVE.
VALLEY STREAM, NY 11581

PRODUCT Number	PRODUCT
5432	**OBETROL-10** BLUE TABLETS ℞ Ⓒ Dextroamphetamine Sulfate 2.5mg. Dextroamphetamine Saccharate 2.5mg. Amphetamine Sulfate 2.5mg. Amphetamine Aspartate 2.5mg.
5433	**OBETROL-20** ℞ Ⓒ ORANGE TABLETS Dextroamphetamine Sulfate 5.0mg. Dextroamphetamine Saccharate 5.0mg. Amphetamine Sulfate 5.0mg. Amphetamine Aspartate 5.0mg.
5451	**DEXTROAMPHETAMINE SULFATE** 5mg. ℞ Ⓒ Scored Yellow Tablets
5452	**DEXTROAMPHETAMINE SULFATE** 10mg. ℞ Ⓒ Double Scored Yellow Tablets
5455	**METHAMPHETAMINE HYDROCHLORIDE** 5mg. ℞ Ⓒ Scored Pink Tablets
5456	**METHAMPHETAMINE HYDROCHLORIDE** 10mg. ℞ Ⓒ Double Scored Pink Tablets
5457	**X-TROZINE TABLETS** ℞ Ⓒ PHENDIMETRAZINE TARTRATE 35 mg. Colors: Blue; Green; Pink; Yellow
5463	**X-TROZINE CAPSULES** ℞ Ⓒ PHENDIMETRAZINE TARTRATE 35mg. Colors: Blue; Red/White; Blue/White
5462	**X-TROZINE LA-105** ℞ Ⓒ PHENDIMETRAZINE TARTRATE 105mg. Long Acting Capsules— Color: Brown/Clear
5468	**OBY-TRIM 30 CAPSULES** ℞ Ⓒ PHENTERMINE HYDROCHLORIDE 30mg. Colors: Black; Yellow; Brown/White

O'Neal, Jones & Feldman Pharmaceuticals
2510 METRO BLVD.
MARYLAND HEIGHTS MO 63043

A.C.T.H. "40" INJECTABLE ℞
Each ml. contains:
Adrenocorticotropic hormone ....40 unit
How Supplied: 5 ml. multiple dose vials.

A.C.T.H. "80" INJECTABLE ℞
Each ml. contains:
Adrenocorticotropic hormone ....80 unit
How Supplied: 5 ml. multiple dose vials.

ADENO INJECTION ℞
Each ml. contains:
Adenosine, 5 monophosphate ....25 mg.
How Supplied: 10 ml. multiple dose vials.

ANTILIRIUM ℞
(physostigmine salicylate)
Description: Antilirium injection is available in 2 ml ampules, each containing 2 mg of physostigmine salicylate.
Action: Antilirium (physostigmine salicylate) is a reversible anticholinesterase which effectively increases the concentration of acetylcholine at the sites of cholinergic transmission. The action of acetylcholine is normally very transient because of its hydrolysis by the enzyme, acetylcholinesterase. Antilirium inhibits the destructive action of acetylcholinesterase and thereby prolongs and exaggerates the effect of the acetylcholine. Antilirium contains a tertiary amine and easily penetrates the blood brain barrier, while an anticholinesterase, such as neostigmine, which has a quaternary ammonium ion, is not capable of crossing the barrier. Antilirium can reverse both central and perpheral anticholinergia. The anticholinergic syndrome has both central and peripheral signs and symptoms. Central toxic effects include anxiety, delirium, disorientation, hallucinations, hyperactivity, and seizures. Severe poisoning may produce coma, medullary paralysis and death. Perpheral toxicity is characterized by tachycardia, hyperpyrexia, mydriasis, vasodilatation, urinary retention, diminution of gastrointestinal motility, decrease of secretion in salivary and sweat glands, and loss of secretions in the pharynx, bronchi, and nasal passages.
Indications: To reverse the effects, toxic or otherwise, upon the central nervous system, caused by clinical or toxic dosages of drugs capable of producing the anticholinergic syndrome. It also has been reported that Antilirium (physostigmine) may antagonize the CNS-depressant effects of diazepam.
Contraindications: Antilirium should not be used in the presence of asthma, gangrene, diabetes, cardiovascular disease, mechanical obstruction of the intestines or urogenital tract or any vagotonic state, and in patients receiv-

Continued on next page

O'Neal, Jones & Feldman—Cont.

ing choline esters or depolarizing neuromuscular blocking agents (decamethonium, succinylcholine).

Warning: If excessive symptoms of salivation, emesis, urination and defecation occur, the use of Antilirium should be terminated. If excessive sweating or nausea occur, the dosage should be reduced. Intravenous administration should be at a slow, controlled rate, no more than 1 mg per minute (see dosage). Rapid administration can cause bradycardia, hypersalivation leading to respiratory difficulties and possibly convulsions.

An overdosage of Antilirium can cause a cholinergic crisis.

Precautions: Because of the possibility of hypersensitivity in an occasional patient, atropine sulfate injection should always be at hand since it is an antagonist and antidote for physostigmine.

Administration and Dosage: The usual adult dose of Antilirium is 0.5 to 2.0 mg intramuscularly or intravenously. Intravenous administration should be at a slow, controlled rate of no more than 1 mg per minute. It may be necessary to repeat dosages of 1 mg to 4 mg at intervals as life threatening signs such as arrhythmias, convulsions and deep coma recur. Physostigmine salicylate is rapidly metabolized (60 to 120 minutes) in the body.

PEDIATRIC DOSAGE: Should be reserved for life threatening situations only. Initially, no more than 0.5 mg by very slow intravenous injection, at least one minute duration. Dosage may be repeated at 5 to 10 minute intervals until a maximum dosage of 2 mg is attained.

IN ALL CASES OF POISONING, THE USUAL SUPPORTIVE MEASURES SHOULD BE UNDERTAKEN.

How Supplied: Ampules, 2 ml packed 12 per box, 1 mg per ml.

BANALG® HOSPITAL STRENGTH ARTHRITIC PAIN RELIEVER
BANALG® LINIMENT

(See PDR For Nonprescription Drugs)

BANCAP CAPSULES ℞
BANCAP c̄ CODEINE CAPSULES ℞

BANCAP CAPSULES

Each capsule contains:

Acetaminophen ....325 mg

Butalbital ....50 mg

(Warning: May be habit forming)

BANCAP c̄ CODEINE CAPSULES

Each capsule contains:

Acetaminophen ....325 mg

Butalbital ....50 mg

(Warning: May be habit forming)

Codeine phosphate ....30 mg

(Warning: May be habit forming)

How Supplied: Bottles of 100 and 500.

BANCAP HC CAPSULES ℞

Description:

Each hard gelatin capsule contains:

Hydrocodone Bitartrate ....5 mg

(WARNING: May be habit forming)

Acetaminophen ....500 mg

Acetaminophen is a nonopiate, non-salicylate analgesic and antipyretic which occurs as a white, odorless crystalline powder possessing a slightly bitter taste. Hydrocodone bitartrate is an opioid analgesic and antitussive and occurs as fine, white crystals or as a crystalline powder. It is affected by light.

Clinical Pharmacology: Hydrocodone is a semisynthetic narcotic analgesic and antitussive with multiple actions qualitatively similar to those of codeine. Most of these involve the central nervous system and smooth muscle. The precise mechanism of action of hydrocodone and other opiates is not known, although it is believed to relate to the existence of opiate receptors in the central nervous system. In additon to analgesia, narcotics may produce drowsiness, changes in mood and mental clouding.

Radioimmunoassay techniques have recently been developed for the analysis of hydrocodone in human plasma. after a 10 mg oral dose of hydrocodone bitartrate, a mean peak serum drug level of 23.6 ng/ml and an elimination half-life of 3.8 hours were found.

The analgesic action of acetaminophen involves peripheral and central influences, but the specific mechanism is as yet undetermined. Antipyretic activity is mediated through hypothalmic heat regulating centers. Acetaminophen inhibits prostaglandin synthetase. Therapeutic doses of acetaminophen have neglible effects on the cardiovascular or respiratory systems; however, toxic doses, may cause circulatory failure and rapid, shallow breathing. Acetaminophen is rapidly and almost completely absorbed from the gastrointestinal tract, producing maximum serum concentrations within 30 minutes to one hour. The plasma half-life in adults and children ranges from 0.90 hours to 3.25 hours with an average of approximately 2 hours. The drug distributes uniformly in most body fluids and is approximately 25% protein bound. Acetaminophen is conjugated in the liver, with less than 3% of the dose excreted unchanged in 24 hours. The primary metabolic pathway is conjugation to sulfate and glucuronide by-products. A minor oxidative pathway forms cysteine and mercapturic acid. These compounds are subsequently excreted by the kidneys into the urine.

Indications and Usage: For the relief of moderate to moderately severe pain.

Contraindications: Hypersensitivity to acetaminophen or hydrocodone.

Warnings: **Respiratory Depression:** At high doses or in sensitive patients, hydrocodone may produce dose-related respiratory depression by acting directly on brain stem respiratory centers. Hydrocodone also affects centers that control respiratory rhythm, and may produce irregular and periodic breathing.

Head Injury and Increased Intracranial Pressure: The respiratory depressant effects of narcotics and their capacity to elevate cerebrospinal fluid pressure may be markedly exaggerated in the presence of head injury, other intracranial lesions or a preexisting increase in intracranial pressure. Furthermore, narcotics produce adverse reactions which may obscure the clinical course of patients with head injuries.

Acute Abdominal Conditions: The administration of narcotics may obscure the diagnosis or clinical course of patients with acute abdominal conditions.

Precautions: **Special Risk Patients:** As with any narcotic analgesic agent, BANCAP HC Capsules should be used with caution in elderly or debilitated patients and those with severe impairment of hepatic or renal function, hypothyroidism, Addison's disease, prostatic hypertrophy or urethral stricture. The usual precautions should be observed and the possibility of respiratory depression should be kept in mind.

Information for Patients: BANCAP HC Capsules like all narcotics, may impair the mental and/or physical abilities required for the performance of potentially hazardous tasks such as driving a car or operating machinery; patients should be cautioned accordingly.

Cough Reflex: Hydrocodone suppresses the cough reflex; as with all narcotics, caution should be exercised when BANCAP HC Capsules are used postoperatively and in patients with pulmonary disease.

Drug Interactions: Patients receiving other narcotic analgesic, antipsychotics, antianxiety agents, or other CNS depressants (including alcohol) concommitantly with BANCAP HC Capsules may exhibit an additive CNS depression. When combined therapy is contemplated, the dose of one or both agents should be reduced.

The use of MAO inhibitors or tricyclic antidepressants with hydrocodone preparations may increase the effect of either the antidepressant or hydrocodone.

The concurrent use of anticholinergics with hydrocodone may produce paralytic ileus.

Usage in Pregnancy: Pregnancy Category C. Hydrocodone has been shown to be teratogenic in hamsters when given in doses 700 times the human dose. There are no adequate and well-controlled studies in pregnant women. BANCAP HC Capsules should be used during pregnancy only if the potential benefit justifies the potential risk to the fetus.

Nonteratogenic Effects: Babies born to mothers who have been taking opioids regularly prior to delivery will be physically dependent. The withdrawal signs include irritability and excessive crying, tremors, hyperactive reflexes, increased respiratory rate, increased stools, sneezing, yawning, vomiting, and fever. The intensity of the syndrome does not always correlate with the duration of maternal opiod use or dose. There is no consensus on the best method of managing withdrawal. Chlorpromazine 0.7 to 1.0 mg/kg q6h, and paregoric 2 to 4 drops/kg q4h, have been used to treat withdrawal symptoms in infants. The duration of therapy is 4 to 28 days, with the dosage decreased as tolerated.

Labor and Delivery: As with all narcotics, administration of BANCAP HC Capsules to the mother shortly before delivery may result in some degree of respiratory depression in the newborn, especially if higher doses are used.

Nursing Mothers: It is not known whether this drug is excreted in human milk. Because many drugs are excreted in human milk and because of the potential for serious adverse reactions in nursing infants from BANCAP HC Capsules, a decision should be made whether to discontinue nursing or to discontinue the drug, taking into account the importance of the drug to the mother.

Pediatric Use: Safety and effectiveness in children have not been established.

Adverse Reactions: Central Nervous System: Sedation, drowsiness, mental clouding, lethargy, impairment of mental and physical performance, anxiety, fear, dysphoria, dizziness, psychic dependence, mood changes.

Gastrointestinal System: Nausea and vomiting may occur; they are more frequent in ambulatory than in recumbent patients. The antiemetic phenothiazines are useful in suppressing these effects; however, some phenothiazine derivatives seem to be antianalgesic and to increase the amount of narcotic required to produce pain relief, while other phenothiazines reduce the amount of narcotic required to produce a given level of analgesia. Prolonged administration of BANCAP HC Capsules may produce constipation.

Genitourinary System: Ureteral spasm, spasm of vesical sphincters and urinary retention have been reported.

Respiratory Depression: BANCAP HC Capsules may produce dose-related respiratory depression by acting directly on brain stem respiratory centers. Hydrocodone also affects centers that control respiratory rhythm, and may produce irregular and periodic breathing. If significant respiratory depression occurs, it may be antagonized by the use of naloxone hydrochloride. Apply other supportive measures when indicated.

Drug-Abuse and Dependence: BANCAP HC Capsules are subject to the Federal Controlled Substance Act (Schedule III). Psychic dependence, physical dependence, and tolerance may develop upon repeated administration of narcotics; therefore, BANCAP HC Capsules should be prescribed and administered with caution. However, psychic dependence is un-

likely to develop when BANCAP HC Capsules are used for a short time for the treatment of pain.
Physical dependence, the condition in which continued administration of the drug is required to prevent the appearance of a withdrawal syndrome, assumes clinically significant proportions only after several weeks of continued narcotic use, although some mild degree of physical dependence may develop after a few days of narcotic therapy. Tolerance, in which increasingly large doses are required in order to produce the same degree of analgesia, is manifested initially by a shortened duration of analgesic effect, and subsequently by decreases in the intensity of analgesia. The rate of development of tolerance varies among patients.

Overdosage: Acetaminophen: Signs and Symptoms: Acetaminophen in massive overdosage may cause hepatic toxicity in some patients. In all cases of suspected overdose, immediately call your regional poison center or the Rocky Mountain Poison Center's toll-free number (800-525-5115) for assistance in diagnosis and for directions in the use of N-acetylcysteine as an antidote, a use currently restricted to investigational status.
In adults, hepatic toxicity has rarely been reported with acute overdoses of less than 10 grams and fatalities with less than 15 grams. Importantly, young children seem to be more resistant than adults to the hepatotoxic effect of an acetaminophen overdose. Despite this, the measures outlined below should be initiated in any adult or child suspected of having ingested an acetaminophen overdose.
Early symtoms following a potentially hepatotoxic overdose may include: nausea, vomiting, diaphoresis and general malaise. Clinical and laboratory evidence of hepatic toxicity may not be apparent until 48 to 72 hours post-ingestion.
Treatment: The stomach should be emptied promptly by lavage or by induction of emesis with syrup of ipecac. Patients' estimates of the quantity of a drug ingested are notoriously unreliable. Therefore, if an acetaminophen overdose is suspected, a serum acetaminophen assay should be obtained as early as possible, but no sooner than four hours following ingestion. Liver function studies should be obtained initially and repeated at 24-hour intervals.
The antidote, N-acetylcysteine, should be administered as early as possible, and within 16 hours of the overdose ingestion for optimal results. Following recovery, there are no residual, structural or functional hepatic abnormalities.
Hydrocodone: Signs and Symptoms: Serious overdose with hydrocodone is characterized by respiratory depression (a decrease in respiratory rate and Cortidal volume, Cheyne-Stokes respiration, cyanosis), extreme somnolence progressing to stupor or coma, skeletal muscle flaccidity, cold and clammy skin, and sometimes bradycardia and hypotension. In severe overdosage, apnea, circulatory collapse, cardiac arrest and death may occur.
Treatment: Primary attention should be given to the reestablishment of adequate respiratory exchange through provision of a patent airway and the institution of assisted or controlled ventilation. The narcotic antagonist, naloxone is a specific antidote against respiratory depression which may result from overdosage or unusual sensitivity to narcotics, including hydrocodone. Therefore, an appropriate dose of naloxone should be administered, preferably by the intravenous route, and simultaneously with efforts at respiratory resuscitation. Since the duration of action of hydrocodone may exceed that of the antagonist, the patient should be kept under continued surveillance and repeated doses of the antagonist should be administered as needed to maintain adequate respiration.
An antagonist should not be administered in the absence of clinically significant respiratory or cardiovascular depression. Oxygen, intravenous fluids, vasopressors and other supportive measures should be employed as indicated. Gastric emptying may be useful in removing unabsorbed drug.
Dosage and Administration: Dosage should be adjusted according to the severity of the pain and the response of the patient. However, it should be kept in mind that tolerance to hydrocodone can develop with continued use and that the incidence of untoward effects is closely related.
The usual dose is one capsule every six hours as needed for pain. If necessary, this dose may be repeated at four hour intervals. In cases of more severe pain, two capsules every six hours (up to 8 capsules in 24 hours) may be required.
How Supplied: Black and red capsules imprinted OJF 610.
Bottles of 100—NDC 0456-0610-01
Bottles of 500—NDC 0456-0610-02
Caution: Federal law prohibits dispensing without prescription.
Revised: MARCH 7, 1982

CETANE TIMED CAPSULES® OTC
(Ascorbic Acid U.S.P. 500 mg. - Timed Disintegrating)

Directions: One capsule daily as a dietary supplement.
How Supplied: Bottles of 100 and 1000.

CETANE INJECTION ℞
(Vitamin C)
Ascorbic Acid and Sodium Ascorbate with and without preservative

How Supplied:
30 ml. vial 500 mg/ml.
Ascorbic Acid without preservative
30 ml. vial 250 mg/ml.
Sodium Ascorbate with preservative
30 ml. vial 250 mg/ml.
Sodium Ascorbate without preservative

CONEX OTC
CONEX with CODEINE Ⓒ

Composition: CONEX: Each 5 ml contains:
Chlorpheniramine Maleate ....2 mg
Dextromethorphan ....7.5 mg
Phenylpropanolamine HC1 ....12.5 mg
CONEX WITH CODEINE: Each 5 ml contains:
Phenylpropanolamine HCl ....12.5 mg
Chlorpheniramine Maleate ....2 mg
Codeine Phosphate ....7.5 mg
(Warning: May be habit forming)
How Supplied: Bottles of 4 ounces.

DALALONE INJECTION ℞

Each ml. contains:
Dexamethasone Sodium Phosphate equivalent to Dexamethasone Phosphate ....4 mg.
How Supplied: 5 ml multiple dose vial.

DALALONE D.P. INJECTION ℞

Each ml. contains:
Dexamethasone Acetate, equivalent to Dexamethasone ....16 mg.
How Supplied: 5 ml. multiple dose vial.
1 ml. unit dose vial, Box of 5.

DALALONE I.L. INJECTION ℞

Each ml. contains:
Dexamethasone Acetate ....2 mg.
How Supplied: 5 ml. multiple dose vial.

DALALONE L.A. INJECTION ℞

Each ml. contains:
Dexamethasone Acetate equivalent to Dexamethasone ....8 mg
How Supplied: 5 ml multiple dose vial.

DALCAINE INJECTION ℞

Each ml. contains:
Lidocaine HCl 2% without preservative
How Supplied: 2 ml. unit dose vial (box of 10).

DEHIST ℞

Composition: Each **Capsule** contains:
Phenylephrine HCl ....15 mg
Phenylpropanolamine HCl ....30 mg
Chlorpheniramine Maleate ....8 mg
in a special base, providing timed release for the Chlorpheniramine Maleate and Phenypropanolamine HCl.
Injectable: Each ml contains:
Chlorpheniramine Maleate ....5.0 mg
Atropine Sulfate ....0.2 mg
How Supplied: Capsules, bottles of 30, 100 and 1000 (NDC-0456-1043).
Injectable, 10 ml multiple dose vial (NDC-0456-1049).

depMEDALONE "40" INJECTABLE ℞

Each ml. contains:
Methylprednisolone Acetate in aqueous suspension ....40 mg.
How Supplied: 5 ml. multiple dose vials.

depMEDALONE "80" INJECTABLE ℞

Each ml. contains:
Methylprednisolone Acetate in aqueous suspension ....80 mg.
How Supplied: 5 ml. multiple dose vials.

DURADYNE DHC TABLET Ⓒ ℞

Description: Each green, scored tablet contains:
Hydrocodone Bitartrate ....5 mg.
(WARNING: May be habit forming.)
Acetaminophen ....500 mg.
How Supplied: Bottles of 100 and 1000.

EFEROL INJECTION ℞

Each ml. contains:
dl-Alpha Tocopheryl Acetate....200 mg
How Supplied: 10 ml. multiple dose vial.

FEOSTAT Tablets OTC
FEOSTAT Suspension
FEOSTAT Drops
(Ferrous Fumarate)

FEOSTAT Tablets
Each chocolate-flavored chewable tablet contains:
Ferrous fumarate....100 mg.
(Elemental iron....33 mg.)
FEOSTAT Suspension
Each 5 cc. (teaspoonful) contains:
Ferrous fumarate....100 mg.
(Elemental iron....33 mg.)
FEOSTAT Drops
Each 12 drops (0.6 cc.) contains:
Ferrous fumarate....45 mg.
(Elemental iron....15 mg.)
How Supplied:
Tablets: Bottles of 100 and 1000.
Suspension: 8 ounce bottle.
Drops: 2 ounce bottle.

Continued on next page

O'Neal, Jones & Feldman—Cont.

HEPARIN SODIUM ℞
without preservatives

Each ml. contains:
Heparin Sodium (w/o pres.) ....1000 units
How Supplied: 5 ml. ampuls, Box 25

IODO-NIACIN® TABLETS ℞

Description: Each controlled action tablet contains:
Potassium Iodide ....135 mg
Niacinamide Hydroiodide ....25 mg
How Supplied: Bottles of 100 and 500.
[*Shown in Product Identification Section*]

NANDROBOLIC L.A. INJECTION ℞

Each ml. contains:
Nandrolone Decanoate ....100 mg.
How Supplied: 2 ml. multiple dose vial, boxes of 5.

OXYMYCIN INJECTION ℞

Each ml. contains:
Oxytetracycline ....50 mg.
How Supplied: 10 ml. multiple dose vial.

PEDAMETH® CAPSULE ℞
PEDAMETH® LIQUID ℞
(racemethionine)

Composition:
CAPSULES—200 mg. racemethionine.
LIQUID—75 mg. racemethionine per 5 cc. (teaspoon) in a fruit flavored base.
Indications:
Control of urine odor, dermatitis and ulcerations caused by ammoniacal urine in the incontinent adult patient.
Diaper rash caused by ammoniacal urine.
Contraindication: Do not administer to patients with history of liver disease as large doses of methionine may exaggerate the toxemia of the disease.
Precautions: It has been pointed out by Goldstein and in animal studies that excessive dosage of methionine, added alone to the diet over extended periods, may result in a weight gain below normal when protein intake is insufficient. Thus, it is essential that adequate protein intake be maintained during therapy and that recommended dosage not be exceeded. Methionine should not be administered on an empty stomach.
Dosage and Administration:
Capsules—Adults: one capsule three or four times a day after meals.
Liquid—Infants: 2 months to 6 months—one teaspoon (5 cc.) three times per day for 3-5 days. May be added to formula, milk or juice; 6 months to 14 months—one teaspoon (5 cc.) four times per day for 3-5 days. In severe cases it may be necessary to double the dosage the first two days of treatment.
How Supplied:
CAPSULES: Bottles of 50 and 500.
LIQUID: Pint Bottle.
[*Shown in Product Identification Section*]

ROGENIC INJECTION ℞

Each ml. contains:
Cyanocobalamin ....500 mcg
Peptonized Iron .... 20 mg
Liver (equiv. to Vit. B-12) .... 10 mcg
How Supplied: 10 ml multiple dose vial.

Products are cross-indexed by generic and chemical names in the **YELLOW SECTION**

Organon Pharmaceuticals
A Division of Organon Inc
375 MT. PLEASANT AVE.
WEST ORANGE, NJ 07052

COTAZYM® ℞
(Pancrelipase, USP)

COTAZYM-65B™ ℞

Description: Cotazym (Pancrelipase, USP) is a concentrate of pancreatic enzymes of porcine origin with standardized lipase activity.
Each capsule (regular or cherry flavored) contains:
Lipase—8,000 USP Units
Protease—30,000 USP Units
Amylase—30,000 USP Units
Precipitated calcium carbonate 25 mg.
Each regular packet contains:
Lipase—16,000 USP Units
Protease—60,000 USP Units
Amylase—60,000 USP Units
Precipitated calcium carbonate 50 mg.
Each cherry flavored packet contains:
Lipase—40,000 USP Units
Protease—150,000 USP Units
Amylase—150,000 USP Units
Precipitated calcium carbonate 50 mg.
Each Cotazym-65B capsule contains:
Lipase—8,000 USP Units
Protease—30,000 USP Units
Amylase—30,000 USP Units
Plus 65 mg mixed conjugated bile salts; cellulase 2 mg; Precipitated calcium carbonate 25 mg.

COTAZYM®

Indications and Usage: It is indicated in conditions where pancreatic enzymes are either absent or deficient with resultant inadequate fat digestion. Such conditions include but are not limited to chronic pancreatitis, pancreatectomy, cystic fibrosis and steatorrhea of diverse etiologies. Cotazym 65B is indicated where bile deficiencies coexist with the above conditions.
Contraindications: Known hypersensitivity to pork protein.
Precautions: In the event that capsules or packets are opened for any reason care should be taken so that powder is not inhaled or spilled on hands since it may prove irritating to the skin or mucous membranes.
Adverse Reactions: No adverse reactions have been reported. It should be noted, however, that extremely high doses of exogenous pancreatic enzymes have been associated with hyperuricosuria and hyperuricemia.
Dosage and Administration: One to three capsules or one to two packets just prior to each meal or snack or as directed by physician. Severe cases may require higher dosage and dietary adjustment.
Storage: Not to exceed 25°C. Dry place when opened.
Dispense: In tight container as defined in the USP.
Supplied: Cotazym capsules (regular) bottles of 100 and 500. NDC # 0052-0381-91, NDC # 0052-0381-95.
Cotazym capsules (cherry flavored) bottles of 100. NDC # 0052-0386-91.
Cotazym packets (regular) boxes of 250. NDC # 0052-0382-95.
Cotazym packets (cherry flavored) boxes of 100. NDC # 0052-0387-92.
Cotazym-65B, bottles of 100. NDC # 0052-0384-91.
[*Shown in Product Identification*]

COTAZYM-S™ ℞
Enteric coated spheres
(Pancrelipase USP)

Description: Cotazym-S contains enteric coated spheres of pancrelipase, a substance containing enzymes, principally lipase, with amylase and protease, obtained from the pancreas of the hog.
Each capsule contains:
Lipase—5,000 USP Units
Protease—20,000 USP Units
Amylase—20,000 USP Units

COTAZYM-S™

Clinical Pharmacology: Cotazym-S is protected against inactivation by gastric acidity, and active enzymes are released in the duodenum. The enzymes promote hydrolysis of fats into glycerol and fatty acids, protein into proteases and derived substances, and starch into dextrans and sugars.
Indications and Usage: Cotazym-S is indicated in conditions where pancreatic enzymes are either absent or deficient with resultant inadequate fat digestion. Such conditions include but are not limited to chronic pancreatitis, pancreatectomy, cystic fibrosis and steatorrhea of diverse etiologies.
Contraindications: Known hypersensitivity to pork protein.
Precautions: To maintain enteric coating integrity, do not chew or crush spheres.
Adverse Reactions: No adverse reactions have been reported. It should be noted, however, that extremely high doses of exogenous pancreatic enzymes have been associated with hyperuricosuria and hyperuricemia.
Dosage and Administration: One to two capsules with each meal or snack as directed by physician. Severe cases may require higher dosage and dietary adjustment. Cotazym-S capsules are usually easy to swallow, but in case of any difficulty, capsules may be opened and the spheres taken with liquids or soft foods which do not require chewing.
Storage: Not to exceed 25°C (77°F). Dry place when opened.
Dispense: In tight container as defined in the USP.
Supplied: Cotazym-S bottles of 100. NDC# 0052-0388-91.
[*Shown in Product Identification Section*]

DECA-DURABOLIN® ℞
(nandrolone decanoate injection USP)

Description: Deca-Durabolin is nandrolone decanoate injection, USP, a long-acting anabolic agent, dissolved in sesame oil for intramuscular injection. Chemically it is 19 nor-Δ^4-androstene-17 beta-ol-3-one-decanoate.
Action: Anabolic steroids are synthetic derivatives of testosterone. The action of Deca-Durabolin (nandrolone decanoate injection USP) is primarily anabolic (protein sparing). It promotes body tissue-building processes and reverses catabolic or tissue depleting processes. Nitrogen balance is improved with anabolic agents but only when there is sufficient intake of calories and protein. Whether this positive nitrogen balance is of primary benefit in the utilization of protein building dietary substances has not been established.
Certain clinical effects and adverse reactions demonstrate the androgenic properties of this class of drugs. The deletion of the CH3 group from the C-19-position has resulted in reduction of its androgenic properties and retention and enhancement of its anabolic, tissue-building properties. Thus it is possible to employ doses that provide significant anabolic effects without undesired androgenic effects. Complete dissociation of anabolic and androgenic effects has not been achieved. The actions of anabolic steroids are therefore similar to those of male sex hormones with the possibility of causing serious disturbances of growth and sexual development if given to young children. Anabolic steroids suppress the gonadotropic functions of the pituitary and may exert a direct effect upon the testis.

Indications:
Based on a review of this drug by the National Academy of Sciences, National Research Council and/or other information, FDA has classified the indication(s) as follows:
Probably Effective: As adjunctive therapy in senile and post-menopausal osteoporosis. Anabolic steroids are without value as primary therapy but may be of value as adjunctive therapy. Equal or greater consideration should be given to diet, calcium balance, physiotherapy and good general health-promoting measures.
Possibly Effective: In the treatment of those conditions in which a potent tissue-building or protein-sparing action is desired (eg. pre and post surgical care, burns), in the control of metastatic breast cancer and as adjuvant therapy of certain types of refractory anemia.
Final classification of the less than effective indications require further investigation.

Contraindications:
1. Male patients with carcinoma of the prostate or breast.
2. Carcinoma of the breast in some females.
3. Pregnancy because of masculinization of the fetus.
4. Nephrosis or the nephrotic phase of nephritis.

Warning: Anabolic steroids do not enhance athletic ability.
Precautions:
1. Hypercalcemia may develop both spontaneously and as a result of hormonal therapy in women with disseminated breast carcinoma. If it develops while on this agent, the drug should be stopped.
2. Caution is required in administering these agents to patients with cardiac, renal or hepatic disease. Edema may occur occasionally. Concomitant administration with adrenal steroids or ACTH may add to the edema.
3. If amenorrhea or menstrual irregularities develop the drug should be discontinued until the etiology is determined.
4. Anabolic steroids may increase sensitivity to oral anticoagulants. Dosage of the anticoagulant may have to be decreased in order to maintain the prothrombin time at the desired therapeutic level.
5. Anabolic steroids have been shown to alter glucose tolerance tests. Diabetics should be followed carefully and the insulin or oral hypoglycemic dosage adjusted accordingly.
6. Anabolic steroids should be used with caution in patients with benign prostatic hypertrophy.
7. Serum cholesterol may increase during therapy. Therefore, caution is required in administering these agents to patients with a history of myocardial infarction or coronary artery disease. Serial determinations of serum cholesterol should be made and therapy adjusted accordingly.

Adverse Reactions:
1. In Males
   a. Prepubertal
      1) Phallic enlargement
      2) Increased frequency of erections
   b. Post-pubertal
      1) Inhibition of testicular function and oligospermia
      2) Gynecomastia
2. In Females
   a. Hirsutism, male pattern baldness, deepening of the voice and clitoral enlargement. These changes are usually irreversible even after prompt discontinuance of therapy and are not prevented by concomitant use of estrogens.
   b. Menstrual irregularities
   c. Masculinization of the fetus.
3. In Both Sexes
   a. Nausea
   b. Increased or decreased libido
   c. Acne (especially in females and prepubertal males)
   d. Inhibition of gonadotropin secretion.
   e. Bleeding in patients on concomitant anticoagulant therapy.
   f. Premature closure of epiphysis in children.
4. Alterations in these clinical laboratory tests:
   a. The metyrapone test.
   b. Glucose tolerance test.
   c. The thyroid function tests: a decrease in the PBI, in thyroxine-binding capacity and radioactive iodine uptake.
   d. The electrolytes: retention of sodium, chlorides, water, potassium, phosphates and calcium.
   e. Liver function tests:
      1) Increased serum cholesterol.
      2) Suppression of clotting factors II, V, VII, AND X.
5. There have been rare reports of hepatocellular neoplasms and peliosis hepatis in association with long-term androgenic-anabolic steroid therapy.

Dosage and Administration: Deca-Durabolin (nandrolone decanoate injection USP) is intended for deep intramuscular injection into the gluteal muscle preferably. For general anabolic effects in adults, the average dosage recommended is 50 to 100 mg. every 3 to 4 weeks. For children from two to thirteen years of age, the average dose is 25 to 50 mg. every three to four weeks.
Higher doses may be required for the treatment of severe disease states such as metastatic breast cancer, refractory anemias, etc. The recommended dose is 100 to 200 mg. weekly based on therapeutic response, and consideration of the benefit-to-risk ratio.
Duration of therapy will depend on the response of the condition and the appearance of adverse reactions. If possible, therapy should be intermittent.
Deca-Durabolin should be regarded as adjunctive therapy and adequate quantities of nutrients should be consumed in order to obtain maximal therapeutic effects. When it is used in the treatment of refractory anemias, for example, adequate iron intake is required for a maximal response.

Supplied: Deca-Durabolin (in sterile sesame oil solution for intramuscular injection) is available in a potency of 50 mg./ml. with 10% benzyl alcohol (preservative):
1 ml. ampuls. NDC 0052-0696-14
2 ml. multiple dose vial. NDC 0052-0696-02
1 ml. prefilled Rediject® syringe. NDC 0052-0696-71
Also available in a potency of 100 mg./ml. with 10% benzyl alcohol (preservative):
2 ml. multiple dose vial. NDC 0052-0697-02
1 ml. prefilled Rediject® syringe. NDC 0052-0697-71
Also available in a potency of 200 mg/ml with 5% benzyl alcohol (preservative);
1 ml vial NDC 0052-0698-01
1 ml prefilled Rediject® syringe. NDC 0052-0698-71

DURABOLIN® ℞
(nandrolone phenpropionate injection, USP)

Description: Durabolin is nandrolone phenpropionate injection USP. Chemically it is 19 nor-Δ^4- androstene- 17β-ol-3-one-β-phenylpropionate.

Actions: Anabolic steroids are synthetic derivatives of testosterone. The action of Durabolin (nandrolone phenpropionate injection USP) is primarily anabolic (protein-sparing). It promotes body tissue-building processes and reverses catabolic or tissue depleting processes. Nitrogen balance is improved with anabolic agents but only when there is sufficient intake of calories and protein. Whether this positive nitrogen balance is of primary benefit in the utilization of protein building dietary substances has not been established.
Certain clinical effects and adverse reactions demonstrate the androgenic properties of this class of drugs. The deletion of the CH3 group from the C-19-position has resulted in reduction of its androgenic properties and retention and enhancement of its anabolic, tissue-building properties. Thus it is possible to employ doses that provide significant anabolic effects without undesired androgenic effects. Complete dissociation of anabolic and androgenic effects has not been achieved. The actions of anabolic steroids are therefore similar to those of male sex hormones with the possibility of causing serious disturbances of growth and sexual development if given to young children. Anabolic steroids suppress the gonadotropic functions of the pituitary and may exert a direct effect upon the testis.

Indications:
Based on a review of this drug by the National Academy of Sciences, National Research Council and/or other information, FDA has classified the indications as follows:
Effective: Control of metastatic breast cancer.
Probably Effective: As adjunctive therapy in senile and postmenopausal osteoporosis. Anabolic steroids are without value as primary therapy but may be of value as adjunctive therapy. Equal or greater consideration should be given to diet, calcium balance, physiotherapy and good health promoting measures.
Possibly Effective: For conditions in which a potent tissue building or protein sparing action is desired (eg., pre and post surgical care, burns), uremia and as adjuvant therapy of certain types of refractory anemia.
Final classification of the less than effective indications requires further investigation.

Contraindications:
1. Male patients with carcinoma of the prostate or breast.
2. Carcinoma of the breast in some females.
3. Pregnancy because of masculinization of the fetus.
4. Nephrosis or the nephrotic phase of nephritis.

Warning: Anabolic steroids do not enhance athletic ability.
Precautions:
1. Hypercalcemia may develop both spontaneously and as a result of hormonal therapy in women with disseminated breast carcinoma. If it develops while on this agent, the drug should be stopped.
2. Caution is required in administering these agents to patients with cardiac, renal or hepatic disease. Edema may occur occasionally. Concomitant administration with adrenal steroids or ACTH may add to the edema.
3. If amenorrhea or menstrual irregularities develop the drug should be discontinued until the etiology is determined.
4. Anabolic steroids may increase sensitivity to oral anticoagulants. Dosage of the anticoagulant may have to be decreased in order to maintain the prothrombin time at the desired therapeutic level.
5. Anabolic steroids have been shown to alter glucose tolerance tests. Diabetics should be followed carefully and the insu-

Continued on next page

Organon—Cont.

lin or oral hypoglycemic dosage adjusted accordingly.
6. Anabolic steroids should be used with caution in patients with benign prostatic hypertrophy.
7. Serum cholesterol may increase during therapy. Therefore, caution is required in administering these agents to patients with a history of myocardial infarction or coronary artery disease. Serial determinations of serum cholesterol should be made and therapy adjusted accordingly.

Adverse Reactions:

1. In Males
   a. Prepubertal.
      1) Phallic enlargement
      2) Increased frequency of erections
   b. Post-pubertal.
      1) Inhibition of testicular function and oligospermia
      2) Gynecomastia
2. In Females
   a. Hirsutism, male pattern baldness, deepening of the voice and clitoral enlargement. These changes are usually irreversible even after prompt discontinuance of therapy and are not prevented by concomitant use of estrogens.
   b. Menstrual irregularities.
   c. Masculinization of the fetus.
3. In Both Sexes
   a. Nausea.
   b. Increased or decreased libido.
   c. Acne (especially in females and prepubertal males).
   d. Inhibition of gonadotropin secretion.
   e. Bleeding in patients on concomitant anticoagulant therapy.
   f. Premature closure of epiphysis in children.
4. Alterations in these clinical laboratory tests:
   a. The metyrapone test.
   b. Glucose tolerance test.
   c. The thyroid function tests: a decrease in the PBI, in thyroxine-binding capacity and radioactive iodine uptake.
   d. The electrolytes: retention of sodium, chlorides, water, potassium, phosphates and calcium.
   e. Liver function tests:
      1) Increased serum cholesterol.
      2) Suppression of clotting factors II, V, VII, AND X.
5. There have been rare reports of hepatocellular neoplasms and peliosis hepatis in association with long-term androgenic-anabolic steroid therapy.

Dosage and Administration: Durabolin (nandrolone phenpropionate injection, USP) is intended for deep intramuscular injection into the gluteal muscle preferably. For general anabolic effects in adults the recommended dose is 25 to 50 mg. weekly. For children from two to thirteen years of age the recommended dose is 12.5 to 25 mg. every two to four weeks.
Higher doses may be required for the treatment of severe disease states such as metastatic breast cancer, refractory anemias, etc. The recommended dose is 50 to 100 mg. weekly based on therapeutic response and consideration of the benefit-to-risk ratio. Duration of therapy will depend on the response of the condition and the appearance of adverse reactions. If possible, therapy should be intermittent.
Durabolin should be regarded as adjunctive therapy and adequate quantities of nutrients should be consumed in order to obtain maximal therapeutic effects. When it is used in the treatment of refractory anemias, for example, adequate iron intake is required for a maximal response.

Supplied: Durabolin (in sterile seasame oil solution for intramuscular injection) is available in a potency of 25 mg/ml with 5% benzyl alcohol (preservative):
1 ml ampuls, box of 3. NDC 0052-0691-13
5 ml multiple dose vial NDC 0052-0691-05
Also available in a potency of 50 mg/ml with 10% benzyl alcohol (preservative):
2 ml multiple dose vial. NDC 0052-0695-02

HEXADROL® ℞
(dexamethasone tablets USP)

Description: Hexadrol (dexamethasone U.S.P.) is an analogue of prednisolone. Its spectrum of anti-inflammatory activity is similar to other corticosteroids but it is clinically effective in much lower doses. Unlike earlier corticosteroids it has the added advantage of lacking significant mineralocorticoid activity so that salt and water retention are rarely observed. Dexamethasone, $C_{22}H_{29}FO_5$, has a molecular weight of 392.47, its chemical name is Pregna-1, 4-diene-3, 20-dione, 9 fluoro-11, 17, 21-trihydroxy-16-methyl-(11 β, 16 α). It is white to practically white crystalline powder which is practically insoluble in water and melts at about 250°C (with decomposition).

Actions: Naturally occurring glucocorticoids (hydrocortisone and cortisone), which also have salt-retaining properties, are used as replacement therapy in adrenocortical deficiency states. Their synthetic analogs are primarily used for their potent anti-inflammatory effects in disorders of many organ systems. Glucocorticoids cause profound and varied metabolic effects. In addition, they modify the body's immune responses to diverse stimuli.

Indications:

1. Endocrine Disorders:
   Primary or secondary adrenocortical insufficiency (hydrocortisone or cortisone is the first choice; synthetic analogs may be used in conjunction with mineralocorticoids where applicable; in infancy mineralocorticoid supplementation is of particular importance).
   Congenital adrenal hyperplasia.
   Nonsuppurative thyroiditis.
   Hypercalcemia associated with cancer.
2. Rheumatic Disorders:
   As adjunctive therapy for short-term administration (to tide the patient over an acute episode or exacerbation) in:
   Psoriatic Arthritis.
   Rheumatoid arthritis including juvenile rheumatoid arthritis (selected cases may require low-dose maintenance therapy).
   Ankylosing spondylitis.
   Acute and subacute bursitis.
   Acute nonspecific tenosynovitis.
   Acute gouty arthritis.
   Post-traumatic osteoarthritis.
   Synovitis of osteoarthritis.
   Epicondylitis.
3. Collagen Diseases:
   During an exacerbation or as maintenance therapy in selected cases of:
   Systemic lupus erythematosus.
   Acute rheumatic carditis.
4. Dermatologic Diseases:
   Pemphigus.
   Bullous dermatitis herpetiformis.
   Severe erythema multiforme (Stevens-Johnson syndrome).
   Exfoliative dermatitis.
   Mycosis fungoides.
   Severe psoriasis.
   Severe seborrheic dermatitis.
5. Allergic States:
   Control of severe or incapacitating allergic conditions intractable to adequate trials of conventional treatment:
   Seasonal or perennial allergic rhinitis.
   Serum sickness.
   Bronchial asthma.
   Contact dermatitis.
   Atopic dermatitis.
   Drug hypersensitivity reactions.
6. Ophthalmic Diseases:
   Severe, acute and chronic allergic and inflammatory processes involving the eye and its adnexa such as:
   Allergic conjunctivitis.
   Keratitis.
   Allergic corneal marginal ulcers.
   Herpes zoster ophthalmicus.
   Iritis and iridocyclitis.
   Chorioretinitis.
   Anterior segment inflammation.
   Diffuse posterior uveitis and choroiditis.
   Optic neuritis.
   Sympathetic ophthalmia.
7. Respiratory Diseases:
   Symptomatic sarcoidosis.
   Loeffler's syndrome not manageable by other means.
   Berylliosis.
   Fulminating or disseminated pulmonary tuberculosis when concurrently accompanied by appropriate antituberculous chemotherapy.
   Aspiration pneumonitis.
8. Hematologic Disorders:
   Idiopathic thrombocytopenic purpura in adults.
   Secondary thrombocytopenia in adults.
   Acquired (autoimmune) hemolytic anemia.
   Erythroblastopenia (RBC anemia).
   Congenital (erythroid) hypoplastic anemia.
9. Neoplastic Diseases:
   For palliative management of:
   Leukemias and lymphomas in adults.
   Acute leukemia of childhood.
10. Edematous States:
   To induce a diuresis or remission of proteinuria in the nephrotic syndrome, without uremia, of the idiopathic type or that due to lupus erythematosus.
11. Gastrointestinal diseases:
   To tide the patient over a critical period of the disease in:
   Ulcerative colitis.
   Regional enteritis.
12. Nervous System:
   Acute exacerbations of multiple sclerosis.
13. Miscellaneous:
   Tuberculous meningitis with subarachnoid block or impending block when used concurrently with appropriate antituberculous chemotherapy.
   Trichinosis with neurologic or myocardial involvement.
   Diagnostic testing of adrenocortical hyperfunction.

Contraindications: Systemic fungal infections.

Warnings: In patients on corticosteroid therapy subjected to unusual stress, increased dosage of rapidly acting corticosteroids before, during, and after the stressful situation is indicated.
Corticosteroids may mask some signs of infection, and new infections may appear during their use. There may be decreased resistance and inability to localize infection when corticosteroids are used.
Prolonged use of corticosteroids may produce posterior subcapsular cataracts, glaucoma with possible damage to the optic nerves, and may enhance the establishment of secondary ocular infections due to fungi or viruses.

Usage in pregnancy: Since adequate human reproduction studies have not been done with corticosteroids, the use of these drugs in pregnancy, nursing mothers or women of childbearing potential requires that the possible benefits of the drug be weighed against the potential hazards to the mother and embryo or fetus. Infants born of mothers who have received substantial doses of corticosteroids during pregnancy, should be carefully observed for signs of hypoadrenalism. Average and large doses of hydrocortisone or cortisone can cause elevation of blood pressure, salt and water retention, and increased excretion of potassium. These effects are less likely to occur with the synthetic derivatives except when used in large doses. Dietary salt restriction and potassium supplementation may be necessary. All corticosteroids increase calcium excretion.

While on Corticosteroid Therapy Patients Should Not Be Vaccinated Against Smallpox. Other Immunization Procedures Should Not Be Undertaken in Patients Who are on Corticosteroids, Especially on High Dose, Because of Possible Hazards of Neurological Complications and a Lack of Antibody Response.

The use of Hexadrol in active tuberculosis should be restricted to those cases of fulminating or disseminated tuberculosis in which the corticosteroid is used for the management of the disease in conjunction with an appropriate antituberculous regimen.

If corticosteroids are indicated in patients with latent tuberculosis or tuberculin reactivity, close observation is necessary as reactivation of the disease may occur. During prolonged corticosteroid therapy, these patients should receive chemoprophylaxis.

Precautions: Drug-induced secondary adrenocortical insufficiency may be minimized by gradual reduction of dosage. This type of relative insufficiency may persist for months after discontinuation of therapy; therefore, in any situation of stress occurring during that period, hormone therapy should be reinstituted. Since mineralocorticoid secretion may be impaired, salt and/or a mineralocorticoid should be administered concurrently.

There is an enhanced effect of corticosteroids on patients with hypothyroidism and in those with cirrhosis.

Corticosteroids should be used cautiously in patients with ocular herpes simplex because of possible corneal perforation.

The lowest possible dose of corticosteroid should be used to control the condition under treatment, and when reduction in dosage is possible, the reduction should be gradual.

Psychic derangements may appear when corticosteroids are used, ranging from euphoria, insomnia, mood swings, personality changes, and severe depression, to frank psychotic manifestations. Also, existing emotional instability or psychotic tendencies may be aggravated by corticosteroids.

Aspirin should be used cautiously in conjunction with corticosteroids in hypoprothrombinemia.

Steroids should be used with caution in nonspecific ulcerative colitis, if there is a probability of impending perforation, abscess or other pyogenic infection; diverticulitis; fresh intestinal anastomoses; active or latent peptic ulcer; renal insufficiency; hypertension; osteoporosis; and myasthenia gravis.

Growth and development of infants and children on prolonged corticosteroid therapy should be carefully observed.

Although controlled clinical trials have shown corticosteroids to be effective in speeding the resolution of acute exacerbations of multiple sclerosis they do not show that they affect the ultimate outcome or natural history of the disease. The studies do show that relatively high doses of corticosteroids are necessary to demonstrate a significant effect. (See Dosage and Administration Section).

Since complications of treatment with glucocorticoids are dependent on the size of the dose and the duration of treatment a risk/benefit decision must be made in each individual case as to dose and duration of treatment and as to whether daily or intermittent therapy should be used.

Adverse Reactions:

Fluid and Electrolyte Disturbances.
- Sodium retention.
- Fluid retention.
- Congestive heart failure in susceptible patients.
- Potassium loss.
- Hypokalemic alkalosis.
- Hypertension.

Musculoskeletal.
- Muscle weakness.
- Steroid myopathy.
- Loss of muscle mass.
- Osteoporosis.
- Vertebral compression fractures.
- Aseptic necrosis of femoral and humeral heads.
- Pathologic fracture of long bones.

Gastrointestinal.
- Peptic ulcer with possible perforation and hemorrhage.
- Pancreatitis.
- Abdominal distention.
- Ulcerative esophagitis.

Dermatologic.
- Impaired wound healing.
- Thin fragile skin.
- Petechiae and ecchymoses.
- Facial erythema.
- Increased sweating.
- May suppress reactions to skin tests.

Neurological.
- Convulsions.
- Increased intracranial pressure with papilledema (pseudo-tumor cerebri) usually after treatment.
- Vertigo.
- Headache.

Endocrine.
- Menstrual irregularities.
- Development of Cushingoid state.
- Suppression of growth in children.
- Secondary adrenocortical and pituitary unresponsiveness, particularly in times of stress, as in trauma, surgery or illness.
- Decreased carbohydrate tolerance.
- Manifestations of latent diabetes mellitus.
- Increased requirements for insulin or oral hypoglycemic agents in diabetics.
- Posterior subcapsular cataracts.
- Increased intraocular pressure.
- Glaucoma.
- Exophthalmos.

Metabolic.
- Negative nitrogen balance due to protein catabolism.

Dosage and Administration: The initial dosage of Hexadrol (dexamethasone) may vary from 0.75 mg. to 9.0 mg. per day depending on the specific disease entity being treated. In situations of less severity lower doses will generally suffice while in selected patients higher initial doses may be required. The initial dosage should be maintained or adjusted until a satisfactory response is noted. If after a reasonable period of time there is a lack of satisfactory clinical response, Hexadrol (dexamethasone) should be discontinued and the patient transferred to other appropriate therapy. *IT SHOULD BE EMPHASIZED THAT DOSAGE REQUIREMENTS ARE VARIABLE AND MUST BE INDIVIDUALIZED ON THE BASIS OF THE DISEASE UNDER TREATMENT AND THE RESPONSE OF THE PATIENT.* After a favorable response is noted, the proper maintenance dosage should be determined by decreasing the initial drug dosage in small decrements at appropriate time intervals until the lowest dosage which will maintain an adequate clinical response is reached. It should be kept in mind that constant monitoring is needed in regard to drug dosage. Included in the situations which may make dosage adjustments necessary are changes in clinical status secondary to remissions or exacerbations in the disease process, the patient's individual drug responsiveness, and the effect of patient exposure to stressful situations not directly related to the disease entity under treatment; in this latter situation it may be necessary to increase the dosage of Hexadrol (dexamethasone) for a period of time consistent with the patient's condition. If after long-term therapy the drug is to be stopped, it is recommended that it be withdrawn gradually rather than abruptly.

In treatment of acute exacerbations of multiple sclerosis daily doses of 200 mg of prednisolone for a week followed by 80 mg every other day or 4–8 mg dexamethasone every other day for 1 month have been shown to be effective.

Patients currently being treated with other corticosteroids may be transferred conveniently to Hexadrol using the following dosage equivalents:

0.75 mg. dexamethasone equivalent to	25 mg. cortisone
	20 mg. hydrocortisone
	5 mg. prednisone or prednisolone
	4 mg. methylprednisolone
	4 mg. triamcinolone

How Supplied: Hexadrol (dexamethasone tablets, USP):

0.50 mg tablets (yellow, scored), bottles of 100 and 500; unit dose package of 100. NDC # 0052-0792-91, NDC # 0052-0792-95, NDC # 0052-0792-90.

0.75 mg tablets (white, scored), bottles of 100 and 500; unit dosage package of 100. NDC # 0052-0791-91, NDC # 0052-0791-95, NDC # 0052-0791-90.

1.5 mg tablets (peach, scored), bottles of 100; unit dose package of 100. NDC # 0052-0790-91, NDC # 0052-0790-90.

4.0 mg tablets (light green, scored), bottles of 100; unit dose package of 100. NDC # 0052-0798-91, NDC # 0052-0798-90.

Therapeutic Pack—package of six 1.5 mg and eight 0.75 mg tablets provides a one-week supply. NDC # 0052-0795-14.

[*Shown in Product Identification Section*]

HEXADROL® PHOSPHATE INJECTION ℞

(dexamethasone sodium phosphate injection USP)

Description: Hexadrol Phosphate Injection (dexamethasone sodium phosphate injection, USP) is a water-soluble inorganic ester of dexamethasone which produces a rapid response even when injected intramuscularly. Dexamethasone Sodium Phosphate, $C_{22}H_{28}FNa_2O_8P$, has a molecular weight of 516.41 and chemically is: Pregn-4-ene-3, 20-dione, 9-fluoro-11, 17-dihydroxy-16-methyl-21-(phosphonooxy)-, disodium salt, (11β, 16α)-. It occurs as a white to creamy white powder, is exceedingly hygroscopic, is soluble in water and its solutions have a pH between 7.5 and 10.5.

Actions: Naturally occurring glucocorticoids (hydrocortisone), which also have salt-retaining properties, are used as replacement therapy in adrenocortical deficiency states. Their synthetic analogs are primarily used for their potent anti-inflammatory effects in disorders of many organ systems.

Glucocorticoids cause profound and varied metabolic effects. In addition, they modify the body's immune responses to diverse stimuli.

Indications:

A. ***Intravenous or intramuscular administration.*** When oral therapy is not feasible and the strength, dosage form, and route of administration of the drug reasonably lend the preparation to the treatment of the condition, those products labeled for intravenous or intramuscular use are indicated as follows:

1. ***Endocrine disorders***

   Primary or secondary adrenocortical insufficiency (hydrocortisone or cortisone is the drug of choice; synthetic analogs may be used in conjunction with mineralocorticoids where applicable; in infancy, mineralocorticoid supplementation is of particular importance).

   Acute adrenocortical insufficiency (hydrocortisone or cortisone is the drug of

Continued on next page

Organon—Cont.

choice; mineralocorticoid supplementation may be necessary, particularly when synthetic analogs are used).
Preoperatively and in the event of serious trauma or illness, in patients with known adrenal insufficiency or when adrenocortical reserve is doubtful.
Shock unresponsive to conventional therapy if adrenocortical insufficiency exists or is suspected.
Congenital adrenal hyperplasia.
Nonsuppurative thyroiditis.
Hypercalcemia associated with cancer.

2. ***Rheumatic disorders.*** As adjunctive therapy for short-term administration (to tide the patient over an acute episode or exacerbation) in:
Post-traumatic osteoarthritis.
Synovitis of osteoarthritis.
Rheumatoid arthritis, including juvenile rheumatoid arthritis (selected cases may require low-dose maintenance therapy).
Acute and subacute bursitis.
Epicondylitis.
Acute nonspecific tenosynovitis.
Acute gouty arthritis.
Psoriatic arthritis.
Ankylosing spondylitis.
3. ***Collagen diseases.*** During an exacerbation or as maintenance therapy in selected cases of:
Systemic lupus erythematosus.
Acute rheumatic carditis.
4. ***Dermatologic diseases:***
Pemphigus.
Severe erythema multiforme (Stevens-Johnson syndrome).
Exfoliative dermatitis.
Bullous dermatitis herpetiformis.
Severe seborrheic dermatitis.
Severe psoriasis.
Mycosis fungoides.
5. ***Allergic states.*** Control of severe or incapacitating allergic conditions intractable to adequate trials of conventional treatment in:
Bronchial asthma.
Contact dermatitis.
Atopic dermatitis.
Serum sickness.
Seasonal or perennial allergic rhinitis.
Drug hypersensitivity reactions.
Urticarial transfusion reactions.
Acute noninfectious laryngeal edema (epinephrine is the drug of first choice).
6. ***Ophthalmic diseases.*** Severe acute and chronic allergic and inflammatory processes involving the eye, such as:
Herpes zoster ophthalmicus.
Iritis, iridocyclitis.
Chorioretinitis.
Diffuse posterior uveitis and choroiditis.
Optic neuritis.
Sympathetic ophthalmia.
Anterior segment inflammation.
Allergic conjunctivitis.
Allergic corneal marginal ulcers.
Keratitis.
7. ***Gastrointestinal diseases.*** To tide the patient over a critical period of disease in:
Ulcerative colitis (systemic therapy).
Regional enteritis (systemic therapy).
8. ***Respiratory diseases:***
Symptomatic sarcoidosis.
Berylliosis.
Fulminating or disseminated pulmonary tuberculosis when used concurrently with appropriate antituberculous chemotherapy.
Loeffler's syndrome not manageable by other means.
Aspiration pneumonitis.
9. ***Hematologic disorders:***
Acquired (autoimmune) hemolytic anemia.
Idiopathic thrombocytopenic purpura in adults (I.V. only; I.M. administration is contraindicated).
Secondary thrombocytopenia in adults.
Erythroblastopenia (RBC anemia).
Congenital (erythroid) hypoplastic anemia.
10. ***Neoplastic diseases.*** For palliative management of:
Leukemias and lymphomas in adults.
Acute leukemia of childhood.
11. ***Edematous state.*** To induce diuresis or remission of proteinuria in the nephrotic syndrome, without uremia, of the idiopathic type or that due to lupus erythematosus.
12. ***Nervous System.***
Acute exacerbations of multiple sclerosis.
13. ***Miscellaneous:***
Tuberculous meningitis with subarachnoid block or impending block when used concurrently with appropriate antituberculous chemotherapy.
Trichinosis with neurologic or myocardial involvement.
Diagnostic testing of adrenocortical hyperfunction.
Cerebral edema of diverse etiologies in conjunction with adequate neurological evaluation and management.

B. ***Intra-articular or soft tissue administration.*** When the strength and dosage form of the drug lend the preparation to the treatment of the condition, those products labeled for intra-articular or soft tissue administration are indicated as adjunctive therapy for short-term administration (to tide the patient over an acute episode or exacerbation) in:
Synovitis of osteoarthritis.
Rheumatoid arthritis.
Acute and subacute bursitis.
Acute gouty arthritis.
Epicondylitis.
Acute nonspecific tenosynovitis.
Post-traumatic osteoarthritis.

C. ***Intralesional administration.*** When the strength and dosage form of the drug lend the preparation to the treatment of the condition, those products labeled for intralesional administration are indicated for:
Keloids.
Localized hypertrophic, infiltrated, inflammatory lesions of: lichen planus, psoriatic plaques, granuloma annulare, and lichen simplex chronicus (neurodermatitis).
Discoid lupus erythematosus.
Necrobiosis lipodica diabeticorum.
Alopecia areata.
They also may be useful in cystic tumors of an aponeurosis or tendon (ganglia).

Contraindications: Systemic fungal infections.

Warnings: In patients on corticosteroid therapy subject to any unusual stress, increased dosage of rapidly acting corticosteroids before, during and after the stressful situation is indicated. Corticosteroids may mask some signs of infection, and new infections may appear during their use. There may be decreased resistance and inability to localize infection when corticosteroids are used.
Prolonged use of corticosteroids may produce posterior subcapsular cataracts, glaucoma with possible damage to the optic nerves, and may enhance the establishment of secondary ocular infections due to fungi or viruses.
Usage in Pregnancy. Since adequate human reproduction studies have not been done with corticosteroids, the use of these drugs in pregnancy, nursing mothers or women of childbearing potential requires that the possible benefits of the drug be weighed against the potential hazards to the mother and embryo or fetus. Infants born of mothers who have received substantial doses of corticosteroids during pregnancy should be carefully observed for signs of hypoadrenalism.
Average and large doses of cortisone or hydrocortisone can cause elevation of blood pressure, salt and water retention, and increased excretion of potassium. These effects are less likely to occur with the synthetic derivatives except when used in large doses. Patients with a stressed myocardium should be observed carefully and the drug administered slowly since premature ventricular contractions may occur with rapid administration. Dietary salt restriction and potassium supplementation may be necessary. All corticosteroids increase calcium excretion.
While on Corticosteroid Therapy Patients Should Not Be Vaccinated Against Smallpox. Other Immunization Procedures Should Not Be Undertaken in Patients Who Are on Corticosteroids, Especially in High Doses, Because of Possible Hazards of Neurological Complications and Lack of Antibody Response.
The use of Hexadrol Phosphate Injection in active tuberculosis should be restricted to those cases of fulminating or disseminated tuberculosis in which the corticosteroid is used for the management of the disease in conjunction with appropriate anti-tuberculous regimen.
If corticosteroids are indicated in patients with latent tuberculosis or tuberculin reactivity, close observation is necessary as reactivation of the disease may occur. During prolonged corticosteroid therapy, these patients should receive chemoprophylaxis.
Because rare instances of anaphylactoid reactions have occurred in patients receiving parenteral corticosteroid therapy, appropriate precautionary measures should be taken prior to administration, especially when the patient has a history of allergy to any drug.

Precautions: Drug-induced secondary adrenocortical insufficiency may be minimized by gradual reduction of dosage. This type of relative insufficiency may persist for months after discontinuation of therapy; therefore, in any situation of stress occurring during that period, hormone therapy should be reinstituted. Since mineralocorticoid secretion may be impaired, salt and/or a mineralocorticoid should be administered concurrently.
There is an enhanced effect of corticosteroids in patients with hypothyroidism and in those with cirrhosis.
Corticosteroids should be used cautiously in patients with ocular herpes simplex for fear of corneal perforation.
The lowest possible dose of corticosteroid should be used to control the condition under treatment, and when reduction in dosage is possible, the reduction must be gradual.
Psychic derangements may appear when corticosteroids are used ranging from euphoria, insomnia, mood swings, personality changes, and severe depression to frank psychotic manifestations. Also, existing emotional instability or psychotic tendencies may be aggravated by corticosteroids.
Aspirin should be used cautiously in conjunction with corticosteroids in hypoprothrombinemia.
Steroids should be used with caution in nonspecific ulcerative colitis, if there is a probability of impending perforation, abscess or other pyogenic infection, also in diverticulitis, fresh intestinal anastomoses, active or latent peptic ulcer, renal insufficiency, hypertension, osteoporosis, and myasthenia gravis.
Growth and development of infants and children on prolonged corticosteroid therapy should be carefully followed.
Intra-articular injection of a corticosteroid may produce systemic as well as local effects. Appropriate examination of any joint fluid present is necessary to exclude a septic process.

A marked increase in pain accompanied by local swelling, further restriction of joint motion, fever, and malaise are suggestive of septic arthritis. If this complication occurs and the diagnosis of sepsis is confirmed, appropriate antimicrobial therapy should be instituted.

Local injection of a steroid into a previously infected joint is to be avoided. Corticosteroids should not be injected into unstable joints.

Although controlled clinical trials have shown corticosteroids to be effective in speeding the resolution of acute exacerbations of multiple sclerosis they do not show that they affect the ultimate outcome or natural history of the disease. The studies do show that relatively high doses of corticosteroids are necessary to demonstrate a significant effect. (See Dosage and Administration Section).

Since complications of treatment with glucocorticoids are dependent on the size of the dose and the duration of treatment a risk/benefit decision must be made in each individual case as to dose and duration of treatment and as to whether daily or intermittent therapy should be used.

Adverse Reactions:

Fluid and electrolyte disturbances:
- Sodium retention
- Fluid retention
- Congestive heart failure in susceptible patients
- Potassium loss
- Hypokalemic alkalosis
- Hypertension

Musculoskeletal:
- Muscle weakness
- Steroid myopathy
- Loss of muscle mass
- Osteoporosis
- Vertebral compression fractures
- Aseptic necrosis of femoral and humeral heads
- Pathologic fracture of long bones

Gastrointestinal:
- Peptic ulcer with possible subsequent perforation and hemorrhage
- Pancreatitis
- Abdominal distention
- Ulcerative esophagitis

Dermatologic:
- Impaired wound healing
- Thin fragile skin
- Petechiae and ecchymoses
- Facial erythema
- Increased sweating
- May suppress reactions to skin tests

Neurological:
- Convulsions
- Increased intracranial pressure with papilledema (pseudotumor cerebri) usually after treatment
- Vertigo
- Headache

Endocrine:
- Menstrual irregularities
- Development of Cushingoid state
- Suppression of growth in children
- Secondary adrenocortical and pituitary unresponsiveness, particularly in times of stress, as in trauma, surgery, or illness
- Decreased carbohydrate tolerance
- Manifestations of latent diabetes mellitus
- Increased requirements for insulin or oral hypoglycemic agents in diabetics

Ophthalmic:
- Posterior subcapsular cataracts
- Increased intraocular pressure
- Glaucoma
- Exophthalmos

Metabolic:
- Negative nitrogen balance due to protein catabolism

Miscellaneous:
- Hyperpigmentation or hypopigmentation
- Subcutaneous and cutaneous atrophy
- Sterile abscess
- Postinjection flare, following intra-articular use
- Charcot-like arthropathy
- Itching, burning, tingling in the ano-genital region.

Dosage and Administration:

A. ***Intravenous or intramuscular administration.*** The initial dosage of Hexadrol Phosphate Injection (dexamethasone sodium phosphate injection, USP) may vary from 0.50 mg/day to 9.0 mg/day depending on the specific disease entity being treated. In situations of less severity, lower doses will generally suffice while in selected patients higher initial doses may be required. Usually the parenteral dosage ranges are one-third to one-half the oral dose given every 12 hours. However, in certain overwhelming, acute, life-threateing situations, administration in dosages exceeding the usual dosages may be justified and may be in multiples of the oral dosages.

For the treatment of unresponsive shock high pharmacologic doses of this product are currently recommended. Reported regimens range from 1 to 6 mg/kg of body weight as a single intravenous injection to 40 mg initially followed by repeat intravenous injection every 2 to 6 hours while shock persists.

For the treatment of cerebral edema in adults an initial intravenous dose of 10 mg. is recommended followed by 4 mg. intramuscularly every six hours until maximum response has been noted. This regimen may be continued for several days postoperatively in patients requiring brain surgery. Oral dexamethasone, 1 to 3 mg t.i.d., should be given as soon as possible and dosage tapered off over a period of five to seven days. Nonoperative cases may require continuous therapy to remain free of symptoms of increased intracranial pressure. The smallest effective dose should be used in children, preferably orally. This may approximate 0.2 mg/kg/24 hours in divided doses.

In treatment of acute exacerbations of multiple sclerosis daily doses of 200 mg of prednisolone for a week followed by 80 mg every other day or 4-8 mg dexamethasone every other day for 1 month have been shown to be effective.

The initial dosage should be maintained or adjusted until a satisfactory response is noted. If after a reasonable period of time there is a lack of satisfactory clinical response, Hexadrol Phosphate Injection should be discontinued and the patient transferred to other appropriate therapy. It Should Be Emphasized That Dosage Requirements Are Variable and Must Be Individualized on the Basis of the Disease Under Treatment and the Response of the Patient.

After a favorable response is noted, the proper maintenance dosage should be determined by decreasing the initial drug dosage in small decrements at appropriate time intervals until the lowest dosage which will maintain an adequate clinical response is reached. It should be kept in mind that constant monitoring is needed in regard to drug dosage. Included in the situations which may make dosage adjustments necessary are changes in clinical status secondary to remissions or exacerbations in the disease process, the patient's individual drug responsiveness and the effect of patient exposure to stressful situations not directly related to the disease entity under treatment; in this latter situation it may be necessary to increase the dosage of Hexadrol Phosphate Injection for a period of time consistent with the patient's condition. If after long-term therapy the drug is to be stopped, it is recommended that it be withdrawn gradually rather than abruptly.

B. ***Intra-articular, Soft Tissue and Intralesional Administration.*** The dose for intrasynovial administration is usually 2 to 4 mg. for large joints and 0.8 to 1 mg. for small joints. For soft tissue and bursal injections a dose of 2 to 4 mg. is recommended. Ganglia require a dose of 1 to 2 mg. A dose of 0.4 to 1 mg. is used for injection into tendon sheaths. Injection into intervertebral joints should not be attempted at any time and hip joint injection cannot be recommended as an office procedure. Intrasynovial and soft tissue injections should be employed only when affected areas are limited to 1 or 2 sites. It should be remembered that corticoids provide palliation only and that other conventional or curative methods of therapy should be employed when indicated.

Frequency of injection usually ranges from once every 3 to 5 days to once every 2 to 3 weeks. Frequent intra-articular injection may cause damage to joint tissue.

How Supplied—5-ml (4mg/ml) multiple dose vial NDC 0052-0796-05
- 5-ml (4mg/ml) multiple dose vial, box of 25 NDC 0052-0796-27
- 1-ml (4mg/ml) vial, box of 25 NDC 0052-0796-25
- 10-ml (10mg/ml) vial, (for intravenous use or intramuscular use only) NDC 0052-0797-10.
- 5-ml (20mg/ml) multiple dose vial (for intravenous or intramuscular use only) NDC 0052-0799-06
- 1-ml (4mg/ml) Prefilled Disposable Syringe, box of 25 NDC 0052-0796-26
- 5-ml (20mg/ml) Prefilled Disposable Syringe (for intravenous use) NDC 0052-0799-07
- 1-ml (10mg/ml) Prefilled Disposable Syringe, box of 25 NDC 0052-0797-26

Protect from bright light. Store at 15°-30°C (59°-86°F).

MAGNACAL®
Enteral Feeding Formula

(See PDR For Nonprescription Drugs)

MICROLIPID®
Modular Fat Supplement

(See PDR For Nonprescription Drugs)

PAVULON® ℞
(pancuronium bromide injection)

THIS DRUG SHOULD ONLY BE ADMINISTERED BY ADEQUATELY TRAINED INDIVIDUALS FAMILIAR WITH ITS ACTIONS, CHARACTERISTICS, AND HAZARDS.

Description: Pavulon (pancuronium bromide) is the aminosteroid 2 beta, 16 beta-dipiperidine-5 alpha-androstane-3 alpha, 17-beta-diol diacetate dimethobromide. It has the following structural formula:

Actions: Pavulon is a non-depolarizing neuromuscular blocking agent possessing all of the characteristic pharmacological actions of this class of drugs (curariform) on the myoneural junction.

Pavulon is approximately 5 times as potent as d-tubocurarine chloride.

Continued on next page

Organon—Cont.

The onset and duration of action of Pavulon is dose dependent. With the administration of 0.04 mg. per kg. the onset of action, as measured by a peripheral nerve stimulator, is usually within 45 seconds, and its peak effect is usually within 4½ minutes; recovery to 90% of control twitch height usually takes place in less than one hour. Larger doses, more suitable for endotracheal intubation, such as 0.08 mg. per kg. of Pavulon have an onset of action of about 30 seconds, and a peak effect within 3 minutes. Supplemental incremental doses of Pavulon, following the initial dose, slightly increase the magnitude of blockade, and significantly increase the duration of the blockade. Pavulon has little effect upon the circulatory system. The most frequently reported observation is a slight rise in pulse rate.
Human histamine assays, and clinical observations, as well as in *vivo* guinea pig testing, and in *vitro* mast cell testing, indicate that histamine release rarely, if ever, occurs.
Pavulon (pancuronium bromide) is antagonized by acetylcholine, anticholinesterases, and potassium ion. Its action is increased by inhalational anesthetics such as halothane, diethyl ether, enflurane and methoxyflurane, as well as quinine, magnesium salts, hypokalemia, some carcinomas, and certain antibiotics such as neomycin, streptomycin, kanamycin, gentamicin and bacitracin. The action of Pavulon may be altered by dehydration, electrolyte imbalance, acid-base imbalance, renal disease, and concomitant administration of other neuromuscular agents.
Pavulon has no known effect on consciousness, the pain threshold, or cerebration.
Indications: Pavulon is indicated as an adjunct to anesthesia to induce skeletal muscle relaxation. It may also be employed to facilitate the management of patients undergoing mechanical ventilation.
Contraindications: Pavulon is contraindicated in patients known to be hypersensitive to the drug or to the bromide ion.
Warnings: PAVULON SHOULD BE ADMINISTERED IN CAREFULLY ADJUSTED DOSAGE BY OR UNDER THE SUPERVISION OF EXPERIENCED CLINICIANS, WHO ARE FAMILIAR WITH ITS ACTIONS AND THE POSSIBLE COMPLICATIONS THAT MIGHT OCCUR FOLLOWING ITS USE. THE DRUG SHOULD NOT BE ADMINISTERED UNLESS FACILITIES FOR INTUBATION, ARTIFICIAL RESPIRATION, OXYGEN THERAPY, AND REVERSAL AGENTS ARE IMMEDIATELY AVAILABLE. THE CLINICIAN MUST BE PREPARED TO ASSIST OR CONTROL RESPIRATION.
In patients who are known to have myasthenia gravis small doses of Pavulon may have profound effects. A peripheral nerve stimulator is especially valuable in assessing the effects of Pavulon in such patients.
Usage in Pregnancy: The safe use of pancuronium bromide has not been established with respect to the possible adverse effects upon fetal development. Therefore, it should not be used in women of childbearing potential and particularly during early pregnancy unless in the judgment of the physician the potential benefits outweigh the unknown hazards.
Pavulon may be used in operative obstetrics (Cesarean section), but reversal of pancuronium may be unsatisfactory in patients receiving magnesium sulfate for toxemia of pregnancy, because magnesium salts enhance neuromuscular blockade. Dosage should usually be reduced, as indicated, in such cases.
Precautions: Although Pavulon has been used successfully in many patients with preexisting pulmonary, hepatic, or renal disease, caution should be exercised in these situations. This is particularly true of renal disease since a major portion of administered Pavulon is excreted unchanged in the urine.
Adverse Reactions: Neuromuscular: the most frequently noted adverse reactions consist primarily of an extension of the drug's pharmacological actions beyond the time period needed for surgery and anesthesia. This may vary from skeletal muscle weakness to profound and prolonged skeletal muscle relaxation resulting in respiratory insufficiency or apnea. Inadequate reversal of the neuromuscular blockade by anticholinesterase agents has also been observed with Pavulon (pancuronium bromide) as with all curariform drugs. These adverse reactions are managed by manual or mechanical ventilation until recovery is judged adequate.
Cardiovascular: A slight increase in pulse rate is frequently noted.
Gastrointestinal: Salivation is sometimes noted during very light anesthesia, especially if no anticholinergic premedication is used.
Skin: An occasional transient rash is noted accompanying the use of Pavulon.
Respiratory: One case of wheezing, responding to deepening of the inhalational anesthetic, has been reported.
Drug Interaction: The intensity of blockade and duration of action of Pavulon is increased in patients receiving potent volatile inhalational anesthetics such as halothane, diethyl ether, enflurane and methoxyflurane. No increase in intensity of blockade or duration of action of Pavulon is noted from the use of thiobarbiturates, narcotic analgesics, nitrous oxide, or droperidol.
Prior administration of succinylcholine, such as that used for endotracheal intubation, enhances the relaxant effect of Pavulon and the duration of action. If succinylcholine is used before Pavulon, the administration of Pavulon should be delayed until the succinylcholine shows signs of wearing off.
Dosage and Administration: Pavulon should be administered only by or under the supervision of experienced clincians. DOSAGE MUST BE INDIVIDUALIZED IN EACH CASE. The dosage information which follows has been derived from dose-response studies based on body weight and is intended to serve as a guide only. Since potent inhalational agents or prior administration of succinylcholine enhance the intensity of blockade and duration of Pavulon (see DRUG INTERACTION), these factors should be taken into consideration in selection of initial and incremental dosage.
In adults the initial intravenous dosage range is 0.04 to 0.1 mg. per kg. Later incremental doses starting at 0.01 mg. per kg. may be used. These increments slightly increase the magnitude of the blockade, and significantly increase the duration of blockade, because a significant number of myoneural junctions are still blocked when there is clinical need for more drug.
If Pavulon is used to provide skeletal muscle relaxation for endotracheal intubation, doses of 0.06 to 0.1 mg. per kg. are recommended. Conditions satisfactory for intubation are usually present within 2 to 3 minutes. The ability of the anesthetist to intubate with Pavulon (pancuronium bromide) improves with experience.
Dosage in Children: Dose response studies in children indicate that, with the exception of neonates, dosage requirements are the same as for adults. Neonates are especially sensitive to non-depolarizing neuromuscular blocking agents, such as Pavulon, (pancuronium bromide) during the first month of life. It is recommended that a test dose of 0.02 mg. per kg. be given first in this group to measure responsiveness.
Cesarean Section: The dosage to provide relaxation for intubation and operation is the same as for general surgical procedures. The dosage to provide relaxation, following usage of succinylcholine for intubation (see DRUG INTERACTION), is the same as for general surgical procedures.
Management of Prolonged Neuromuscular Blockade: Residual neuromuscular blockade beyond the time period needed for surgery and anesthesia may occur with Pavulon as with other neuromuscular blockers. This may be manifested by skeletal muscle weakness, decreased respiratory reserve, low tidal volume or apnea. A peripheral nerve stimulator may be used to assess the degree of residual neuromuscular blockade. Under such circumstances the primary treatment is manual or mechanical ventilation and maintenance of a patent airway until complete recovery of normal respiration is assured. Regonol (pyridostigmine bromide) or neostigmine, in conjunction with atropine, will usually antagonize the skeletal muscle relaxant action of Pavulon. These should be accompanied by or preceded by injection of atropine sulfate to minimize the incidence of cholinergic side effects, notably excessive secretions and bradycardia. Satisfactory reversal can be judged by adequacy of skeletal muscle tone, and by adequacy of respiration. A peripheral nerve stimulator may also be used to monitor restoration of twitch height. Failure of prompt reversal (within 30 minutes) may occur in the presence of extreme debilitation, carcinomatosis, and with concomitant use of certain broad spectrum antibiotics, or anesthetic agents and adjuncts which enhance neuromuscular blockade or cause respiratory depression of their own. Under such circumstances the management is the same as that of prolonged neuromuscular blockade; ventilation must be supported by artificial means until the patient has resumed control of his respiration. Prior to the use of reversal agents, reference to the specific package insert of the reversal agents should be made.
How Supplied:
2 ml. ampuls—2 mg./ml.—boxes of 25 NDC 0052-0444-26
5 ml. ampuls—2 mg./ml.—boxes of 25 NDC 0052-0444-25
10 ml. vials—1 mg./ml.—boxes of 25 NDC 0052-0443-25

PROPAC™
Modular Protein Supplement

(See PDR For Nonprescription Drugs)

REGONOL® ℞
(pyridostigmine bromide injection USP)

Description: Regonol (pyridostigmine bromide injection, USP) is an active cholinesterase inhibitor. Chemically, pyridostigmine bromide is 3-hydroxy-1-methylpyridinium bromide dimethylcarbamate. Its structural formula is:

$$\left[\text{CH}_3\text{-N}^+ \text{ pyridine ring, } \text{OCON(CH}_3)_2 \right] \text{Br}^-$$

Each ml. contains 5 mg. of pyridostigmine bromide compounded with 1% benzyl alcohol as the preservative. The pH is buffered with sodium citrate and citric acid and adjusted with sodium hydroxide if necessary.
Actions: Pyridostigmine bromide facilitates the transmission of impulses across the myoneural junction by inhibiting the destruction of acetylcholine by cholinesterase. Pyridostigmine is an analog of neostigmine but differs from it clinically by having fewer side effects. Currently available data indicate that pyridostigmine may have a significantly lower degree and incidence of bradycardia, salivation and gastrointestinal stimulation. Animal studies using the injectable form of pyridostigmine

and human studies using the oral preparation have indicated that pyridostigmine has a longer duration of action than does neostigmine measured under similar circumstances.
Indications: Pyridostigmine bromide is useful as a reversal agent or antagonist to nondepolarizing muscle relaxants.
Contraindications: Known hypersensitivity to anticholinesterase agents; intestinal and urinary obstructions of mechanical type.
Warnings: Pyridostigmine bromide should be used with particular caution in patients with bronchial asthma or cardiac dysrhythmias. Transient bradycardia may occur and be relieved by atropine sulfate. Atropine should also be used with caution in patients with cardiac dysrhythmias. When large doses of pyridostigmine bromide are administered, as during reversal of muscle relaxants, prior or simultaneous injection of atropine sulfate is advisable. Because of the possibility of hypersensitivity in an occasional patient, atropine and antishock medication should always be readily available.
When used as an antagonist to nondepolarizing muscle relaxants, adequate recovery of voluntary respiration and neuromuscular transmission must be obtained prior to discontinuation of respiratory assistance and there should be continuous patient observation. Satisfactory recovery may be defined by a combination of clinical judgement, respiratory measurements and observation of the effects of peripheral nerve stimulation. If there is any doubt concerning the adequacy of recovery from the effects of the nondepolarizing muscle relaxant, artificial ventilation should be continued until all doubt has been removed.
Use in Pregnancy—The safety of pyridostigmine bromide during pregnancy or lactation in humans has not been established. Therefore its use in women who are pregnant requires weighing the drug's potential benefits against its possible hazards to mother and child.
Adverse Reactions: The side effects of pyridostigmine bromide are most commonly related to overdosage and generally are of two varieties, muscarinic and nicotinic. Among those in the former group are nausea, vomiting, diarrhea, abdominal cramps, increased peristalsis, increased salivation, increased bronchial secretions, miosis and diaphoresis. Nicotinic side effects are comprised chiefly of muscle cramps, fasciculation and weakness. Muscarinic side effects can usually be counteracted by atropine. As with any compound containing the bromide radical, a skin rash may be seen in an occasional patient. Such reactions usually subside promptly upon discontinuance of the medication. Thrombophlebitis has been reported subsequent to intravenous administration.
Dosage and Administration: When pyridostigmine bromide is given intravenously to reverse the action of muscle relaxant drugs, it is recommended that atropine sulfate (0.6 to 1.2 mg.) or glycopyrrolate in equipotent doses be given intravenously immediately prior to or simultaneous with its administration. Side effects, notably excessive secretions and bradycardia are thereby minimized. Reversal dosages range from 0.1 - 0.25 mg/kg. Usually 10 to 20 mg. of pyridostigmine bromide will be sufficient for antagonism of the effects of the nondepolarizing muscle relaxants. Although full recovery may occur within 15 minutes in most patients, others may require a half hour or more. Satisfactory reversal can be evident by adequate voluntary respiration, respiratory measurements and use of a peripheral nerve stimulator device. It is recommended that the patient be well ventilated and a patent airway maintained until complete recovery of normal respiration is assured. Once satisfactory reversal has been attained, recurarization has not been reported.
Failure of pyridostigmine bromide to provide prompt (within 30 minutes) reversal may occur, e.g. in the presence of extreme debilitation, carcinomatosis, or with concomitant use of certain broad spectrum antibiotics or anesthetic agents, notably ether. Under these circumstances ventilation must be supported by artificial means until the patient has resumed control of his respiration.
How Supplied: Regonol is available in:
5 mg./ml.: 2 ml. ampuls—boxes of 25—NDC-0052-0460-02
5 ml. vials—boxes of 25—NDC-0052-0460-05
Protect from light.

RENU™
Isotonic Enteral Feeding Formula

(See PDR For Nonprescription Drugs)

SUMACAL®
Modular Carbohydrate Supplement

(See PDR For Nonprescription Drugs)

VITANEED®
Blenderized Enteral Feeding Formula

(See PDR For Nonprescription Drugs)

WIGRAINE® ℞

Description: Each Wigraine anti-migraine tablet and rectal suppository contains:

Ergotamine tartrate USP	1 mg
Caffeine USP	100 mg
Belladonna Alkaloids (levorotatory) (87.5% hyoscyamine and 12.5% atropine as sulfates)	0.1 mg
Phenacetin USP	130 mg

Wigraine tablets are uncoated and especially formulated to insure rapid disintegration and absorption. The suppositories contain the active ingredients in a synthetic cocoa butter base which melts rapidly at body temperature.
Clinical Pharmacology: Ergotamine tartrate is a natural amino acid ergot alkaloid exhibiting alpha adrenergic blocking and potent vasoconstricting activity. It is also a serotonin antagonist.
Caffeine is a cerebral vasoconstrictor which reduces cerebral blood flow. A synergistic effect is observed when it is combined with ergotamine tartrate, thereby providing a sound rationale for their use in treating migraine.
The anticholinergic and antiemetic alkaloids of belladonna provide relief in those individuals suffering from migraine induced nausea and vomiting. Suppositories are indicated if oral medication cannot be retained.
Phenacetin has analgesic and antipyretic properties similar to those of aspirin. It relieves pain of various types, including headache, thereby enhancing the vasoconstrictor effect.
Indications and Usage: Wigraine is indicated for the treatment of vascular headache such as migraine, migraine variants or histamine cephalalgia.
Contraindications: Peripheral vascular disease of any type, coronary heart disease, renal or hepatic disease, sepsis, pregnancy, hypertension or hypersensitivity to any of the ingredients.
Precautions: Wigraine tablets and suppositories are intended for the treatment of acute attacks and have no prophylactic value. Ergotamine is capable of producing all the signs and symptoms of ergotism. When prescribed in the correct dosage (see Dosage and Administration section) it is a safe and effective drug. Accordingly, care should be exercised to remain within the limits of recommended dosage.
Pregnancy Category C. Animal reproduction studies have not been conducted with Wigraine. It is also not known whether Wigraine can cause fetal harm when administered to a pregnant woman or can affect reproduction capacity. Wigraine should be given to a pregnant woman only if clearly needed.
Nursing Mothers. It is not known whether Wigraine is excreted in human milk. Because many drugs are excreted in human milk, caution should be exercised when Wigraine is administered to a nursing woman.
Adverse Reactions: Nausea, vomiting, weakness in the legs, muscle pains in the extremities, numbness and tingling in fingers and toes, precordial pain or distress, transient tachycardia or bradycardia, localized edema, itching or skin rash and drug fever. Chronic overdosage of phenacetin may produce methemoglobinemia, hemolytic anemia and so-called analgesic nephropathy. The primary renal lesion is papillary necrosis with secondary chronic interstitial nephritis.
Overdosage: In the unlikely event of an acute overdose of Wigraine toxic effects would be due primarily to the ergotamine and phenacetin components. Symptoms of acute overdosage of ergotamine include nausea, vomiting, diarrhea, severe thirst, tingling, itching and coldness of the skin, thready pulse, cyanosis of extremities, stupor, convulsions, coma and shock.
Adverse effects of acute overdosage of phenacetin include hepatic necrosis, renal tubular necrosis, hypoglycemic coma, hemolytic anemia and methemoglobinemia.
Treatment consists of complete removal of Wigraine by appropriate means (emesis of lavage) and symptomatic measures. These include maintenance of adequate pulmonary ventilation and peripheral circulation, control of convulsions, treatment of shock, etc. The use of anticoagulants and potent vasodilator drugs may be indicated.
Oral LD_{50} limits of the various components as outlined in NIOSH 1978 Registry of Toxic Effects of Chemical Substances, published by U.S. Department of Health, Education and Welfare are as follows: Ergotamine Tartrate IV LD_{50} in rats = 80mg/Kg, Caffeine IV LD_{50} in rats = 105mg/Kg, Belladonna Alkaloids (as atrophine) oral LD_{50} in rats = 622 mg/Kg, Phenacetin oral LD_{50} in rats = 1650mg/Kg.
Dosage and Administration: One or two Wigraine tablets or suppositories should be taken immediately upon the appearance of symptoms of headache, followed by one or two tablets or suppositories every 15 minutes until the pain subsides. No more than 6 Wigraine tablets or suppositories should be taken for one attack. If a patient requires more than one tablet or suppository to abort an attack, the initial dosage for the next attack of equal severity should be increased to obtain immediate relief. When possible, the patient should rest in a dark room for one hour after taking Wigraine tablets or suppositories to secure maximum effect. No more than 12 Wigraine tablets or suppositories should be administered during any seven day period.
How Supplied: Wigraine tablets are green and individually foil stripped and packaged in boxes of 20, NDC 0052-0541-20 and 100's NDC 0052-0541-91. Wigraine suppositories are individually foil wrapped and packaged in boxes of 12, NDC 0052-0546-12. Wigraine tablets should be stored at a maximum of 30°C (86°F) and the suppositories should be refrigerated at 2°–8°C (36°–46°F).
[*Shown in Product Identification Section*]

WIGRETTES® ℞
(ergotamine tartrate sublingual tablets)

Description: Each sublingual tablet contains 2.0 mg ergotamine tartrate.
Pharmacological Category: Vasoconstrictor, uterine stimulant, alpha adrenoreceptor antagonist.
Therapeutic Class: Anti-migraine.
Chemical Name: Ergotaman-3′, 6′, 18-trione, 12′ - hydroxy - 2′ - methyl - 5′ - (phenyl-methyl)-, (5′α,)-, [R-(R*,R*)] - 2,3 - dihydroxybutanedioate (2:1) tartrate

Continued on next page

Organon—Cont.

Structural Formula:

[Structural formula of ergotamine tartrate: $\left[\ldots\right]_2 \cdot H_2C_4H_4O_6$]

Clinical Pharmacology: The pharmacological properties of ergotamine are extremely complex; some of its actions are unrelated to each other, and even mutually antagonistic. The drug has partial agonist and/or antagonist activity against tryptaminergic, dopaminergic and alpha adrenergic receptors depending upon their site, and it is a highly active uterine stimulant. It causes constriction of peripheral and cranial blood vessels and produces depression of central vasomotor centers. The pain of a migraine attack is believed to be due to greatly increased amplitude of pulsations in the cranial arteries, especially the meningeal branches of the external carotid artery. Ergotamine reduces extracranial bloodflow, causes a decline in the amplitude of pulsation in the cranial arteries, and decreases hyperperfusion of the territory of the basilar artery. It does not reduce cerebral hemispheric blood flow. Long term usage has established the fact that ergotamine tartrate is effective in controlling up to 70% of acute migraine attacks, so that it is now considered specific for the treatment of this headache syndrome. Ergotamine produces constriction of both arteries and veins. In doses used in the treatment of vascular headaches, ergotamine usually produces only small increases in blood pressure, but it does increase peripheral resistance and decrease blood flow in various organs. Small doses of the drug increase the force and frequency of uterine contraction; larger doses increase the resting tone of the uterus also. The gravid uterus is particularly sensitive to these effects of ergotamine. Although specific teratogenic effects attributable to ergotamine have not been found, the fetus suffers if ergotamine is given to the mother. Retarded fetal growth and an increase in intrauterine death and resorption have been seen in animals. These are thought to result from ergotamine induced increases in uterine motility and vasoconstriction in the placental vascular bed.

The bioavailability of sublingually administered ergotamine has not been determined.

Ergotamine is metabolized by the liver largely undefined pathways, and 90% of the metabolites are excreted in the bile. The unmetabolized drug is erratically secreted in the saliva, and only traces of unmetabolized drug appear in the urine and feces. Ergotamine is secreted into breast milk. The elimination half-life of ergotamine from plasma is about 2 hours, but the drug may be stored in some tissues, which would account for its long lasting therapeutic and toxic actions.

Indications and Usage: Ergotamine tartrate is indicated as therapy to abort or prevent vascular headache, e.g., migraine, migraine variants, or so called "histaminic cephalalgia".

Contraindications: Ergotamine is contraindicated in peripheral vascular disease, (thromboangitis obliterans, luetic arteritis, severe arteriosclerosis, thrombophlebitis, Raynaud's disease), coronary heart disease, hypertension, impaired hepatic or renal function, severe pruritis, and sepsis. It is also contraindicated in patients who are hypersensitive to any of its components. Ergotamine may cause fetal harm when administered to a pregnant woman by virtue of its powerful uterine stimulant actions. It is contraindicated in women who are, or may become, pregnant.

Precautions:

General: Although signs and symptoms of ergotism rarely develop even after long term intermittent use of ergotamine, care should be exercised to remain within the limits of recommended dosage.

Drug Interactions: The effects of ergotamine tartrate may be potentiated by triacetyloleandomycin which inhibits the metabolism of ergotamine. The pressor effects of ergotamine and other vasoconstrictor drugs can combine to cause dangerous hypertension.

Carcinogenesis: No studies have been performed to investigate ergotamine tartrate for carcinogenic effects.

Pregnancy: Pregnancy Category X—See 'Contraindications' section.

Nursing Mothers: Ergotamine is secreted into human milk. It can reach the breast-fed infant by this route and exert pharmacologic effects in it. Caution should be exercised when ergotamine is administered to a nursing woman. Excessive dosing or prolonged administration of ergotamine may inhibit lactation.

Adverse Reactions: Nausea and vomiting occur in up to 10% of patients after ingestion of therapeutic doses of ergotamine. Weakness of the legs and pain in limb muscles are also frequent complaints. Numbness and tingling of the fingers and toes, precordial pain, transient changes in heart rate and localized edema and itching may also occur, particularly in patients who are sensitive to the drug.

Drug Abuse and Dependence: Patients who take ergotamine for extended periods of time may become dependent upon it and require progressively increasing doses for relief of vascular headaches, and for prevention of dysphoric effects which follow withdrawal of the drug.

Overdosage: Overdosage with ergotamine causes nausea, vomiting, weakness of the legs, pain in limb muscles, numbness and tingling of the fingers and toes, precordial pain, tachycardia or bradycardia, hypertension or hypotension and localized edema and itching together with signs and symptoms of ischemia due to vasoconstriction of peripheral arteries and arterioles. The feet and hands become cold, pale and numb. Muscle pain occurs while walking and later at rest also. Gangrene may ensue. Confusion, depression, drowsiness, and convulsions are occasional signs of ergotamine toxicity. Overdosage is particularly likely to occur in patients with sepsis or impaired renal or hepatic function. Patients with peripheral vascular disease are specially at risk of developing peripheral ischemia following treatment with ergotamine. Some cases of ergotamine poisoning have been reported in patients who have taken less than 5 mg of the drug. Usually, however, toxicity is seen at doses of ergotamine tartrate in excess of about 15 mg in 24 hours or 40 mg in a few days.

Treatment of ergotamine overdosage consists of withdrawal of the drug followed by symptomatic measures including attempts to maintain an adequate circulation in the affected parts. Anticoagulant drugs, low molecular weight dextran and potent vasodilator drugs may all be beneficial. Intravenous infusion of sodium nitroprusside has also been reported to be successful. Vasodilators must be used with special care in the presence of hypotension.

Nausea and vomiting may be relieved by atropine or antiemetic compounds of the phenothiazine group. Ergotamine is dialyzable.

Dosage and Administration: All efforts should be made to initiate therapy as soon as possible after the first symptoms of the attack are noted, since success is proportional to rapidity of treatment, lower dosages will be effective. At the first sign of an attack or to relieve symptoms after onset of an attack, one 2 mg tablet is placed under the tongue. Another tablet should be taken at half-hourly intervals thereafter, if necessary, but dosage must not exceed three tablets in any 24 hour period. Dosage should be limited to not more than five tablets (10 mg) in any one week.

How Supplied: Each Wigrettes® sublingual tablet (white) contains 2 mg of ergotamine tartrate. Wigrettes® are individually foiled, stripped and packaged in boxes of 24. NDC #0052-0547-24. Store at maximum of 30°C (86°F).

Ortho Diagnostic Systems Inc.

ROUTE 202
RARITAN, NEW JERSEY 08869

MICRhoGAM™ ℞

Rh_o (D) Immune Globulin (Human) Micro-Dose
For Intramuscular Use Only

Micro-Dose for use *only* after abortion or miscarriage up to 12 weeks gestation.

Description: MICRhoGAM Rh_o (D) Immune Globulin (Human), Micro-Dose, is a sterile, concentrated solution of specific immunoglobulin (IgG) containing anti-Rh_o (D). This product is prepared from fractionated human plasma (cold alcohol method) and may include immunoglobulin, which does not contain anti-Rh_o (D), derived from an intermediate plasma fraction prepared by other Bureau of Biologics licensed manufacturers. All plasma used in the manufacture of this product was tested for hepatitis B surface antigen and found to be non-reactive.

Active Ingredient

Anti-Rh_o (D) in 15% ± 1.5% serum globulin

Inactive Ingredients

15 mg/ml glycine (approximately)
2.9 mg/ml sodium chloride (approximately)
Preservative 0.01% thimerosal (mercury derivative)

Action: MICRhoGAM is used to prevent the formation of anti-Rh_o (D) in Rh_o (D) negative and D^u negative women who are exposed to the Rh_o (D) antigen at the time of abortion or miscarriage (up to 12 weeks gestation). The probable mechanism of action is the binding of passive antibody to antigen in the circulation, thereby preventing the stimulation of antigen sensitive cells and subsequent production of anti-Rh_o (D).

Indication: MICRhoGAM is indicated for the prevention of maternal Rh immunization following abortion or miscarriage up to 12 weeks gestation. The material should be administered to the Rh_o (D) negative, D^u negative woman as soon as possible after the spontaneous passage or surgical removal of the products of conception.

Clinical trials indicated that MICRhoGAM was effective when administered following abortions and in these trials the product was routinely injected within three (3) hours. However, if MICRhoGAM is not given within this time period, consideration should still be given to the administration of the product, since it was shown to be effective in a male volunteer study when given as long as 72 hours after the infusion of Rh_o (D) positive red cells.

FOR ABORTIONS OR MISCARRIAGES OCCURRING AFTER 12 WEEKS GESTATION, A STANDARD DOSE OF RhoGAM™ Rh_o (D) Immune Globulin (Human) IS INDICATED.

MICRhoGAM prophylaxis should be considered for every woman undergoing abortion or miscarriage up to 12 weeks gestation unless:

It has been proven that she is Rh_o (D) positive or D^u positive. [See direction circular such as that accompanying ORTHO™ Blood Grouping Serum Anti-D (Anti-Rh_o) for Slide and Modified Tube Tests.]

It has been proven that she is immunized to the Rh_o (D) antigen as demonstrated by the presence of anti-Rh_o (D) in her serum.
Or, it has been proven by Rh typing that the father and/or fetus is Rh negative.

Dosage: One vial of MICRhoGAM will suppress the immunogenic challenge of 2.5 ml of Rh_o (D) positive or D^u positive packed red blood cells (not whole blood), or the equivalent (5.0 ml) of whole blood in males. This dose will provide protection against maternal Rh isoimmunization for women undergoing abortion or miscarriage up to 12 weeks gestation.

Injection Control: After qualifying testing is performed, complete the injection control form included with the package of MICRhoGAM.

1. Separate the three-part form, remove the first copy and place it securely with the product.
2. The second copy should be retained in the laboratory for record.
3. Fold and place the card copy with the vial of MICRhoGAM, the direction circular and patient identification card.
4. Send the vial of MICRhoGAM, the direction circular and patient identification card to the patient's room for injection.
5. The empty vial of MICRhoGAM should be returned to the hospital or clinic laboratory with the card copy attached. The time of injection should be noted.

Injection Procedure

1. Verify the lot number of MICRhoGAM on the injection control form with the lot number printed on the vial of MICRhoGAM to be injected.
2. Establish complete patient identification.
3. Using a 1 ml capacity syringe and employing sterile technique, withdraw the entire contents of one vial of MICRhoGAM into the syringe.
4. Intramuscularly inject the entire contents of the vial into the post-abortion or post-miscarriage woman.
5. After injection, return the empty vial with its attached control form to the laboratory.

A patient identification card is included in the package for the physician's convenience and may be completed at his discretion.

INTRAMUSCULARLY INJECT THE ENTIRE CONTENTS OF ONE VIAL. DO NOT INJECT INTRAVENOUSLY.

Precautions: Reactions of Rh negative individuals given Rh_o (D) Immune Globulin (Human) are infrequent, of a mild nature and are mostly confined to the area of injection. A slight elevation of temperature has been noted in a small number of women who have received this material. Systemic reactions are rare and sensitization due to repeated injections of immune globulins is unusual. Immune Serum Globulin (Human) has not been reported to transmit hepatitis.

Packaging: MICRhoGAM is supplied in a package containing:

- one single-dose vial of MICRhoGAM
- direction circular
- patient injection control form
- patient identification card

MICRhoGAM is also supplied in a package containing:

- 50 single-dose vials of MICRhoGAM
- direction circular
- 50 patient injection control forms
- 50 patient identification cards

Storage: Store at 2° to 8°C. DO NOT FREEZE.

RhoGAM™ ℞

Rh_0 (D) Immune Globulin (Human)
For Intramuscular Use Only

Description: RhoGAM Rh_0(D) Immune Globulin (Human) is a sterile concentrated solution of specific immunoglobulin (IgG) containing anti-Rh_0(D) for intramuscular injection, prepared from fractionated human plasma (cold alcohol method). It may include immunoglobulin derived from a plasma fraction which does not contain anti-Rh_0(D) prepared by other licensed manufacturers. All plasma used in the manufacture of this product was tested for hepatitis B surface antigen by a licensed third generation test and found to be nonreactive.

Active Ingredient
Anti-Rh_0(D) in 15% ± 1.5% serum globulin

Inactive Ingredients
15 mg/ml glycine—approximately
2.9 mg/ml sodium chloride—approximately
Preservative: 0.01% thimerosal (mercury derivative)

Clinical Pharmacology: RhoGAM acts by suppressing the specific immune response of Rh negative individuals to Rh positive red blood cells. Exposure to Rh positive red blood cells can occur as a consequence of pregnancy, abortion or delivery or transfusion of an Rh negative recipient with Rh positive red blood cells. Prevention of isoimmunization by Rh positive red cells in susceptible females who may have Rh positive babies prevents hemolytic disease of the newborn. The injection of Rh_0(D) antibody to an Rh negative mother or to the Rh negative recipient of Rh positive red cells suppresses the antibody response and the formation of anti-Rh_0(D). The mechanism of action of RhoGAM is not fully understood; however, an immunostat hypothesis has been proposed.

The risk of isoimmunization is directly related to the number of Rh positive red cells to which the Rh negative individual is exposed. The risk was found to be three percent when 0.1 ml of fetal red blood cells are present in the mother and 65 percent when 5 ml are present.

Immunization of Rh negative women not previously exposed to Rh positive red cells occurs most frequently during the third stage of labor when fetal red cells enter the maternal circulation. However fetal-maternal hemorrhage has been noted as early as the second trimester of pregnancy and increases in size and frequency as gestation proceeds.

Clinical studies proved that administration of RhoGAM within 72 hours of delivery of a full-term infant reduced the incidence of Rh isoimmunization as a result of pregnancy from 12–13% to 1–2%. A lesser degree of protection is afforded if Rh antibody is administered beyond this time period. Data from Canada, Sweden and England indicate 1.5 to 1.8% of Rh negative women carrying Rh positive fetuses who are given Rh immune globulin postpartum may be immunized to Rh during the latter part of their pregnancies or following delivery. Bowman has reported that the incidence of immunization can be further reduced from approximately 1.6% to less than 0.1% by administering Rh immune globulin in two doses, one antepartum at 28 weeks gestation and another following delivery.

Abortion, either spontaneous or induced, and amniocentesis may cause fetal-maternal hemorrhage. The number of Rh negative women immunized to Rh has been reduced by administering Rh immune globulin following these procedures. Similarly, immunization resulting in the production of anti-Rh_0(D) following transfusion of Rh positive red cells to an Rh negative recipient may be prevented by administering Rh immune globulin.

Indications and Usage: RhoGAM is indicated for the prevention of isoimmunization in Rh negative individuals exposed to Rh positive red cells.

Pregnancy

1. RhoGAM is unequivocally indicated postpartum for an unsensitized Rh negative woman delivering an Rh_0(D) positive or D^u positive baby. If the Rh type of the baby cannot be determined, it should be presumed to be Rh positive. If RhoGAM is administered antepartum, it is essential that the mother receive another dose of RhoGAM after delivering an Rh_0(D) positive or D^u positive infant.
2. RhoGAM is indicated for an Rh negative woman after abortion or ectopic pregnancy unless the products of conception or the father are conclusively shown to be Rh negative.
3. Amniocentesis and other abdominal trauma resulting in fetal cells entering the maternal circulation are indications for RhoGAM.

Transfusion
RhoGAM may be indicated following transfusion of an Rh negative, premenopausal female with Rh positive red cells or whole blood, or components such as platelets or granulocytes prepared from Rh positive blood.

Contraindications: None known.

Warnings: Babies born of women given Rh immune globulin antepartum may have a weakly positive direct Coombs test at birth. Passively acquired anti-Rh_0(D) may be detected in maternal serum if antibody screening tests are performed subsequent to antepartum or postpartum administration of Rh immune globulin.

Precautions: The presence of fetal cells in a maternal blood sample or passive antibody given to the mother antepartum can affect the interpretation of laboratory tests to identify and monitor the candidate for RhoGAM. In case of doubt as to the patient's Rh type or immune status, RhoGAM should be administered.

Adverse Reactions: Reactions of Rh negative individuals given Rh immune globulin are infrequent, of a mild nature and mostly confined to the area of injection. An occasional patient may react more strongly both locally and generally. A slight elevation of temperature has been noted in a small number of postpartum women. There is no evidence that the safety of the fetus is jeopardized by the administration of RhoGAM antepartum.

Following mismatched transfusions and injection of several vials of RhoGAM, approximately five out of 22 subjects noted fever, myalgia and lethargy. Bilirubin levels of 0.4–6.8 mg% were observed in some of the treated subjects and one had splenomegaly. Systemic reactions are rare and sensitization due to repeated injection of immune globulins is unusual. Immune Serum Globulin (Human) prepared from plasma negative for HBsAg by third generation tests has not been reported to transmit hepatitis.

Dosage and Administration: One vial of RhoGAM will completely suppress the immune response to 15 ml of Rh positive red blood cells (packed cells, not whole blood).

Pregnancy

1. For postpartum prophylaxis, administer one vial of RhoGAM intramuscularly, preferably within three days of delivery. If an unusually large fetal-maternal hemorrhage is suspected, an approved laboratory procedure such as the Kleihauer-Betke technique should be used to estimate the volume of Rh positive red cells in the maternal circulation. The number of vials of RhoGAM to be given can be determined by dividing the volume of Rh positive red cells by 15.
2. For antepartum prophylaxis, one vial of RhoGAM is administered intramuscularly at approximately 28 weeks. This *must* be followed by another full dose (one vial) preferably within three days following delivery, if the infant is Rh positive.
3. Following amniocentesis, miscarriage, abortion, or ectopic pregnancy at or beyond the thirteenth week of gestation, it is recommended that one vial of RhoGAM be given. (If the products of conception are

Continued on next page

Ortho Diagnostics—Cont.

passed or removed prior to the thirteenth week of gestation, one vial of MICRhoGAM™ $Rh_0(D)$ Immune Globulin (Human) Micro-Dose may be used instead of RhoGAM.)

Transfusion

Rh Positive Red Cells to an Rh Negative Recipient

RhoGAM may be administered intramuscularly to prevent isoimmunization in eligible Rh negative premenopausal females who receive Rh positive red cells by transfusion, whether inadvertently or in association with leukocyte or platelet therapy. One vial protects against each 15 ml of transfused red cells.

How Supplied: RhoGAM is supplied in packages containing:

- one single-dose vial of RhoGAM
- package insert
- control form
- patient identification card

and

- 25 single-dose vials of RhoGAM
- package insert
- 25 control forms
- 25 patient identification cards

and

- 72 single-dose vials of RhoGAM
- package insert
- 75 control forms
- 75 patient identification cards

and

- one single-dose vial of RhoGAM
- package insert
- instructions for use of ancillary items
- one 3 ml MONOJECT® syringe with 22 gauge needle
- one 13 × 100 mm (7 ml) red top blood collection tube and sleeve
- one VENOJECT® 1½" 21 gauge blood collection needle
- two disposable PREPTIC® swabs
- injection record
- patient identification card
- patient information booklet (DS1-42)
- plastic bag
- label for patient's chart

Storage: Store at 2° to 8° C. DO NOT FREEZE.

Ortho Pharmaceutical Corporation
RARITAN, NJ 08869

ACI-JEL® Therapeutic Vaginal Jelly ℞

Description: ACI-JEL Vaginal Jelly is a bland, non-irritating, water-dispersible, buffered acid jelly for intravaginal use. ACI-JEL is classified as a Vaginal Therapeutic Jelly. ACI-JEL contains 2.279% glacial acetic acid ($C_2H_4O_2$), 0.025% oxyquinoline sulfate ($C_{18}H_{16}N_2O_6S$), 0.7% ricinoleic acid ($C_{18}H_{34}O_3$), 3% boric acid (H_3BO_3), and 5% glycerin ($C_3H_8O_3$) compounded with sodium carboxymethylcellulose, acacia, propylparaben, potassium hydroxide, stannous chloride, egg albumen, potassium bitartrate, perfume and purified water. ACI-JEL is formulated to pH 3.9–4.1.

Clinical Pharmacology: ACI-JEL acts to restore and maintain normal vaginal acidity through its buffer action.

Indications and Usage: ACI-JEL is indicated as adjunctive therapy in those cases where restoration and maintenance of vaginal acidity are desirable.

Contraindications: None known.

Warnings: No serious adverse reactions or potential safety hazards have been reported with the use of ACI-JEL.

Precautions: *General:* No special care is required for the safe and effective use of ACI-JEL. *Drug Interactions:* No incidence of drug interactions have been reported with concomitant use of ACI-JEL and any other medications. *Laboratory Tests:* The monitoring of vaginal acidity (pH) may be helpful in following the patient's response. (The normal vaginal pH has been shown to be in the range of 4.0 to 5.0.) *Carcinogenesis:* No long-term studies in animals have been performed to evaluate carcinogenic potential. *Pregnancy:* Pregnancy Category C. Animal reproduction studies have not been conducted with ACI-JEL. It is also not known whether ACI-JEL can cause fetal harm when administered to a pregnant woman or can affect reproduction capacity. ACI-JEL should be given to a pregnant woman only if clearly needed. *Nursing Mothers:* It is not known whether this drug is excreted in human milk. Because many drugs are excreted in human milk, caution should be exercised when ACI-JEL is administered to a nursing woman.

Adverse Reactions: No adverse reactions associated with use of the drug have been reported.

Dosage and Administration: The usual dose is one applicatorful, administered intravaginally, morning and evening. Duration of treatment may be determined by the patient's response to therapy.

How Supplied: 85g Tube with ORTHO® Measured-Dose Applicator.
NDC 0062-5420-77

CONCEPTROL® Birth Control Cream

(See PDR For Nonprescription Drugs)

CONCEPTROL® Contraceptive Gel Disposable

(See PDR For Nonprescription Drugs)

CONCEPTROL® SHIELDS®

(See PDR For Nonprescription Drugs)

CONCEPTROL® SUPREME®

(See PDR For Nonprescription Drugs)

DELFEN® Contraceptive Foam

(See PDR For Nonprescription Drugs)

DIENESTROL Cream ℞

(See ORTHO® Dienestrol Cream)

GYNOL II® Contraceptive Jelly

(See PDR For Nonprescription Drugs)

LIPPES LOOP® ℞
Intrauterine Device

Description: The LIPPES LOOP is made of polyethylene in the shape of a double S. Four different sizes are manufactured to allow for the variability in the size of the uterus. (See below.) A fine, double thread or "tail" made of polyethylene suture (monofilament) is attached to the lower end to facilitate removal. In addition, palpation of the tail through the cervix by the patient, or visualization by the physician, can assist in determining whether or not an undetected expulsion has occurred. A LIPPES LOOP comes prepackaged and sterilized with an introducer, together with an insertion tube in a polyethylene pouch. The insertion tube is equipped with a flange to aid in gauging the depth to which the insertion tube should be inserted through the cervical canal and into the uterine cavity. The four available sizes are as follows:

Loop A—22.5 mm. Blue thread. For nulliparous females.

Loop B—27.5 mm. WITH REDUCED RADII. Black thread. Suggested for women who have had premature pregnancy losses and multiparous females whose uteri sound out less than 6 cm.

Loop C—30 mm. WITH REDUCED RADII. Yellow thread. Suggested for use when Loop D is removed for bleeding or pain. The physician is advised to wait two to four weeks between removing a loop for bleeding and reinserting a second loop.

Loop D—30 mm. White thread. Suggested for use in women with one or more children.

Mode of Action or Principles of IUD Design: The exact mechanism of action of the LIPPES LOOP is not known. However, it is believed to interfere in some manner with nidation in the endometrium, probably through foreign body reaction in the uterus.

Indications and Usage: LIPPES LOOP is indicated for contraception.

Contraindications: IUD's should not be inserted when the following conditions exist:

1. Pregnancy or suspicion of pregnancy.
2. Abnormalities of the uterus resulting in distortion of the uterine cavity.
3. Pelvic inflammatory disease or a history of repeated pelvic inflammatory disease.
4. Postpartum endometritis or infected abortion in the past three months.
5. Known or suspected uterine or cervical malignancy including unresolved, abnormal "Pap" smear.
6. Genital bleeding of unknown etiology.
7. Cervicitis until infection is controlled.

Warnings:

1. Pregnancy. a. Long-term effects. Long-term effects on the offspring when pregnancy occurs with LIPPES LOOP in place are unknown.

b. Septic abortion. Reports have indicated an increased incidence of septic abortion associated in some instances with septicemia, septic shock, and death in patients becoming pregnant with an IUD in place. Most of these reports have been associated with the mid-trimester of pregnancy. In some cases, the initial symptoms have been insidious and not easily recognized. If pregnancy should occur with an IUD in place, the IUD should be removed if the string is visible or, if removal proves to be or would be difficult, termination of the pregnancy should be considered and offered the patient as an option, bearing in mind that the risks associated with an elective abortion increase with gestational age.

c. Continuation of pregnancy. If the patient chooses to continue the pregnancy, she must be warned of the increased risk of spontaneous abortion and of the increased risk of sepsis, including death, if the pregnancy continues with the IUD in place. The patient must be closely observed and she must be advised to report all abnormal symptoms, such as flu-like syndrome, fever, abdominal cramping and pain, bleeding, or vaginal discharge, immediately because generalized symptoms of septicemia may be insidious.

2. Ectopic pregnancy. a. A pregnancy that occurs with an IUD in place is more likely to be ectopic than a pregnancy occuring without an IUD in place. Accordingly, patients who become pregnant while using the IUD should be carefully evaluated for the possibility of an ectopic pregnancy.

b. Special attention should be directed to patients with delayed menses, slight metrorrhagia and/or unilateral pelvic pain, and to those patients who wish to terminate a pregnancy because of IUD failure, to determine whether ectopic pregnancy has occurred.

3. Pelvic Infection. An increased risk of pelvic infection has been reported with the IUD in place. Although the etiology of this risk is not understood, it has been suggested that the tail may act as a mechanism for the passage of vaginal bacteria into the uterus. This, at times, may result in the development of bilateral or unilateral tubo-ovarian abscesses or general peritonitis which may lead to hospitalization or surgery and infertility. Appropriate aerobic and anaerobic bacteriological studies should be done and antibiotic therapy initiated. The IUD should be removed and the continuing treatment reassessed based upon the results of culture and sensitivity tests.

Because of the increased risk of pelvic infection, the physician may wish each woman who has an IUD in place to have a periodic cervical vaginal "Pap" smear and pelvic exam. All "Pap" smears should include specific evaluation for actinomycosis.

4. Embedment. Partial penetration or lodging of the IUD in the endometrium can result in difficult removals.

5. Perforation. Partial or total perforation of the uterine wall or cervix may occur with the use of IUDs. The possibility of perforation must be kept in mind during insertion and at the time of any subsequent examination. If perforation occurs, the IUD should be removed. Adhesions, foreign body reactions, and intestinal obstruction may result if an IUD is left in the peritoneal cavity. There are a few reports that there has been migration after insertion apparently in the absence of perforation at insertion. In any event, it is possible for the IUD to perforate outside the uterus.

Precautions:

1. Patient counseling. Prior to insertion, the physician, nurse, or other trained health professional must provide the patient with the Patient Brochure. The patient should be given the opportunity to read the brochure and discuss fully any questions she may have concerning the IUD as well as other methods of contraception.

2. Patient evaluation and clinical considerations. a. A complete medical history should be obtained to determine conditions that might influence the selection of an IUD. Physical examination should include a pelvic examination, "Pap" smear, gonorrhea culture and, if indicated, appropriate tests for other forms of venereal disease. Papanicolaou smears should include specific evaluation for actinomycosis.

b. The uterus should be carefully sounded prior to insertion to determine the degree of patency of the endocervical canal and the internal os, and the direction and depth of the uterine cavity. In occasional cases, severe cervical stenosis may be encountered. Do not use excessive force to overcome this resistance.

c. The uterus should sound to a depth of 6 to 8 centimeters (cm). Insertion of an IUD into a uterine cavity measuring less than 6.5 cm by sounding may increase the incidence of expulsion, bleeding, pain and perforation.

d. The possibility of insertion in the presence of an existing undetermined pregnancy is reduced if insertion is performed during or shortly following a menstrual period. The IUD should not be inserted postpartum or postabortion until involution of the uterus is completed. The incidence of perforation and expulsion is greater if involution is not completed.

e. IUD's should be used with caution in those patients who have anemia or a history of menorrhagia or hypermenorrhea. Patients experiencing menorrhagia and/or metrorrhagia following IUD insertion may be at risk for the development of hypochromic microcytic anemia. Also, IUD's should be used with caution in patients receiving anticoagulants or having a coagulopathy.

f. Syncope, bradycardia, or other neurovascular episodes may occur during insertion or removal of IUD's, especially in patients with a previous disposition to these conditions.

g. Patients with valvular or congenital heart disease are more prone to develop subacute bacterial endocarditis than patients who do not have valvular or congenital heart disease. Use of an IUD in these patients may represent a potential source of septic emboli.

TABLE I

LIPPES LOOP Size	Number Woman/Months	Woman/Months of Use 1st Year After Insertion	Woman/Months of Use 2nd year After Insertion
A	13,453	8,751	4,702
B	12,463	9,660	2,803
C	50,775	31,032	19,743
D	121,566	72,046	49,520

h. Use of an IUD in those patients with cervicitis should be postponed until treatment has cured the infection (see CONTRAINDICATIONS Section).

i. Since an IUD may be expelled or displaced, patients should be reexamined and evaluated shortly after the first postinsertion menses, but definitely within three months after insertion. Thereafter, annual examination with appropriate medical and laboratory examination should be carried out.

j. The patient should be told that some bleeding and cramps may occur during the first few weeks after insertion, but if these symptoms continue or are severe, she should report them to her physician. The patient should be instructed on how to check to make certain that the thread still protrudes from the cervix, and she should be cautioned that there is no contraceptive protection if the IUD is expelled. She should be instructed to check the tail as often as possible, but at least after each menstrual period. The patient should be cautioned not to pull on the thread and displace the IUD. If partial expulsion occurs, removal is indicated and a new IUD may be inserted.

k. The use of medical diathermy (shortwave and microwave) in patients with metal-containing IUD's may cause heat injury to the surrounding tissue. Therefore, medical diathermy to the abdominal and sacral areas should not be used.

[LIPPES LOOP contains no metals. This section does not apply to LIPPES LOOP].

Adverse Reactions: These adverse reactions are not listed in any order of frequency or severity.

Reported adverse reactions include: endometritis, spontaneous abortion, septic abortion, septicemia, perforation of the uterus and cervix, embedment, migration resulting in partial or complete perforation, fragmentation of the IUD, pelvic infection (pelvic inflammatory disease), vaginitis, leukorrhea, cervical erosion, pregnancy, ectopic pregnancy, difficult removal, complete or partial expulsion of the IUD, intermenstrual spotting, prolongation of menstrual flow, anemia, pain and cramping, dysmenorrhea, backaches, dyspareunia, neurovascular episodes, including bradycardia and syncope secondary to insertion. Perforation into the abdomen has been followed by abdominal adhesions, intestinal penetration, intestinal obstruction, and cystic masses in the pelvis.

Directions For Use:

Preinsertion

1. It is imperative that sterile technique be maintained throughout the insertion procedure.

2. Perform a thorough pelvic examination to determine freedom from overt disease and to determine position and shape of the uterus. RULE OUT PREGNANCY AND OTHER CONTRAINDICATIONS.

3. With a speculum in place, gently insert a sterile sound to determine the depth and direction of the uterine canal. Be sure to determine the position of the uterus before insertion.

Occasionally a tenaculum is required if the uterine canal needs to be straightened. If a stenotic cervix must be dilated, use a sterile Hank's dilator rather than a Hegar's; dilation to a Hank's 16 to 18 should be sufficient.

Insertion

Caution: It is generally felt that perforations are caused at the time of insertion, although the perforation may not be detected until some time later. The position of the uterus should be determined during the preinsertion examination. Great care must be exercised during the preinsertion sounding and subsequent insertion. No attempt should be made to force the insertion. There are a few reports, however, that there has been migration after insertion apparently in the absence of perforation at insertion. In any event, it is possible for the IUD to perforate outside the uterus.

1. How to prepare the LIPPES LOOP Intrauterine Double-S inserter.

Using sterile gloves, hold tube in one hand and with the other draw LOOP into inserter by pulling the push rod. Continue to pull the push rod until all but the bulbous tip of the LOOP is entirely within the inserter. At this point, insure that both the flat surface of the bulbous tip and the inserter flange are in a horizontal plane.

Do this not more than one minute before insertion.

2. How to insert LIPPES LOOP Intrauterine Double-S.

Insert the loaded inserter gently through the endocervical canal, with the flange in a horizontal plane. DO NOT FORCE THE INSERTION. If resistance is encountered, do not proceed; perforation of the uterus may occur. If the flange makes contact with the cervix WITHOUT the inserter touching the fundal wall, withdraw ¼ inch before pressing the push rod to release the device in utero. Should the inserter touch the fundal wall BEFORE the flange makes contact, withdraw ½ inch prior to pressing the push rod to release the device in utero. With the inserter now in place, proceed, and WITHOUT UNDUE PRESSURE, push the rod slowly as far as it will go. LIPPES LOOP Intrauterine Double-S should now be in place. Withdraw the inserter tube and push rod from the cervical os until the tail is visible. Cut the tail leaving it as long as possible.

Time of Insertion

LIPPES LOOP Intrauterine Double-S should be inserted preferably the last one or two days of a normal menstrual period or the two days following the last day.

The expulsion and perforation rate may be increased when insertions are made before normal uterine involution occurs (usually four to six weeks postpartum or postabortion).

To Remove

To remove LIPPES LOOP Intrauterine Double-S, pull gently on the exposed tail. On those rare occasions that the tail is not available, the device should be carefully removed.

Clinical Studies: Different event rates have been recorded with the use of different IUD's. Inasmuch as these rates are usually derived from separate studies conducted by different investigators in several population groups, they cannot be compared with precision. Furthermore, event rates tend to be lower as clinical experience is expanded, possibly due to retention in the cinical study of those patients who accept the treatment regimen and do not discontinue due to adverse reactions or pregnancy. In clinical trials conducted by The Population Council with the LIPPES LOOP, use effectiveness was determined as follows for women, as tabulated by the life table method. (Rates are expressed as events per 100 women through 12 and 24 months of use.) This experience is based on 198,257 woman/months of use, including 121,489 woman/months of use

Continued on next page

Ortho Pharm.—Cont.

in first year after insertion, and 76,768 woman/months of use in second year after insertion. LIPPES LOOP Intrauterine Double-S devices are manufactured in four different sizes, and the figures given above represent the totals for the four sizes. The following table presents these figures individually for each size LOOP:
[See table on next preceding page].
Tables II–V below give the pregnancy expulsion, medical removal and continuation rates for each individual size LOOP.

TABLE II
LOOP A
(Annual Rates Per 100 Users)

	12 Months	24 Months (cumulative)
Pregnancy	5.3	9.7
Expulsion	23.9	27.7
Medical Removal	12.2	20.0
Continuation Rate	75.2	63.6

TABLE III
LOOP B
(Annual Rates Per 100 Users)

	12 Months	24 Months (cumulative)
Pregnancy	3.4	6.3
Expulsion	18.9	24.9
Medical Removal	15.1	23.8
Continuation Rate	74.6	59.2

TABLE IV
LOOP C
(Annual Rates Per 100 Users)

	12 Months	24 Months (cumulative)
Pregnancy	3.0	4.8
Expulsion	19.1	24.6
Medical Removal	14.3	22.1
Continuation Rate	76.5	62.8

TABLE V
LOOP D
(Annual Rates Per 100 Users)

	12 Months	24 Months (cumulative)
Pregnancy	2.7	4.2
Expulsion	12.7	16.0
Medical Removal	15.2	23.3
Continuation Rate	77.4	65.6

MASSE' ® Breast Cream

(See PDR For Nonprescription Drugs)

MONISTAT® 7 Vaginal Cream ℞
(miconazole nitrate 2%)

Description: MONISTAT 7 Vaginal Cream (miconazole nitrate 2%) is a water-miscible, white cream containing as the active ingredient, 2% miconazole nitrate, 1-[2,4-dichloro-β-(2,4-dichlorobenzyloxy) phenethyl] imidazole nitrate.
Actions: MONISTAT 7 Vaginal Cream exhibits fungicidal activity *in vitro* against species of the genus *Candida.* The pharmacologic mode of action is unknown.
Indications: MONISTAT 7 Vaginal Cream is indicated for the local treatment of vulvovaginal candidiasis (moniliasis). As MONISTAT 7 Vaginal Cream is effective only for candidal vulvovaginitis, the diagnosis should be confirmed by KOH smears and/or cultures. Other pathogens commonly associated with vulvovaginitis (Trichomonas and *Haemophilus vaginalis* [*Gardnerella*]) should be ruled out by appropriate laboratory methods.
MONISTAT 7 is effective in both pregnant and non-pregnant women, as well as in women taking oral contraceptives. (See PRECAUTIONS.)
Contraindications: Patients known to be hypersensitive to this drug.
Precautions:
General: Discontinue drug if sensitization or irritation is reported during use. Laboratory Tests: If there is a lack of response to MONISTAT 7, appropriate microbiological studies should be repeated to confirm the diagnosis and rule out other pathogens.
Pregnancy: Since MONISTAT is absorbed in small amounts from the human vagina, it should be used in the first trimester of pregnancy only when the physician considers it essential to the welfare of the patient.
Clinical studies, during which MONISTAT was used for 14 days, included 209 pregnant patients. Follow-up reports now available in 117 of these patients reveal no adverse effects or complications attributable to MONISTAT therapy in infants born to these women.
Adverse Reactions: During clinical studies with MONISTAT for a 14-day regimen, 39 of the 528 patients (7.4%) treated with MONISTAT reported complaints during therapy that were possibly drug-related. Most complaints were reported during the first week of therapy. Vulvovaginal burning, itching or irritation occurred in 6.6%, while other complaints such as vaginal burning, pelvic cramps, hives, skin rash and headache occurred rarely (each less than 0.2% patient incidence). The therapy-related dropout rate was 0.9%.
Clinical: Statistical analysis of randomized clinical trials, conducted to determine the shortest effective course of therapy with MONISTAT, demonstrates that a regimen of seven or more days has a cure rate equivalent to the 14-day regimen.
The graphic representation of this conclusion plots days of therapy versus cure rates. The solid line represents the mean therapeutic cure rate and the shaded area represents the 95% confidence interval.

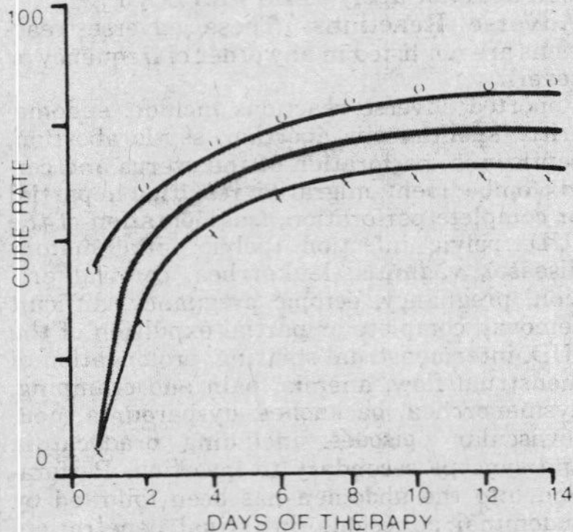

Dosage and Administration: One applicatorful is administered intravaginally once daily at bedtime for seven days. Course of therapy may be repeated after other pathogens have been ruled out by appropriate smears and cultures.
Supplied: MONISTAT 7 Vaginal Cream is available in 1.66 oz. (47 g) tubes with ORTHO® Measured-Dose Applicator.

MONISTAT® 7 Vaginal Suppositories ℞
(100 mg miconazole nitrate)

Description: MONISTAT 7 Vaginal Suppositories are water-miscible, white to off-white suppositories, each containing the antifungal agent, miconazole nitrate, 1-[2,4-dichloro-β-(2,4-dichloro-benzyloxy) phenethyl] imidazole nitrate, 100 mg, in a hydrogenated vegetable oil base. Miconazole nitrate for vaginal use is also available as MONISTAT 7 Vaginal Cream.
Clinical Pharmacology: Miconazole nitrate exhibits fungicidal activity *in vitro* against species of the genus *Candida.* The pharmacologic mode of action is unknown. Following intravaginal administration of MONISTAT 7 Vaginal Suppositories or MONISTAT 7 Vaginal Cream, small amounts are absorbed.
Administration of a single dose of MONISTAT 7 Vaginal Suppositories to healthy subjects resulted in a total recovery from the urine and feces of 0.85% (±0.43%) of the administered dose. For MONISTAT 7 Vaginal Cream the corresponding figure was 1.03% (±0.51%) of the administered dose.
Animal studies indicate that the drug crossed the placenta and doses above those used in humans result in embryo and feto-toxicity (80 mg/kg-orally) although this has not been reported in human subjects (see Precautions).
Indications and Usage: MONISTAT 7 Vaginal Suppositories are indicated for the local treatment of vulvovaginal candidiasis (moniliasis). Effectiveness in pregnancy has not been established. As MONISTAT 7 is effective only for candidal vulvovaginitis, the diagnosis should be confirmed by KOH smear and/or cultures. Other pathogens commonly associated with vulvovaginitis *(Trichomonas* and *Haemophilus vaginalis* [*Gardnerella*]) should be ruled out by appropriate laboratory methods.
Clinical: Statistical analyses of randomized clinical trials, conducted to determine the shortest effective course of therapy with miconazole nitrate vaginal cream and suppositories, demonstrate that a regimen of seven or more days had a cure rate equivalent to a 14-day regimen.
The graphic representation of this conclusion plots Days of Therapy versus Cure Rate for miconazole nitrate vaginal cream. (Results were similar with suppositories.) The solid line represents the mean therapeutic cure rate and the shaded area represents the 95% confidence interval.

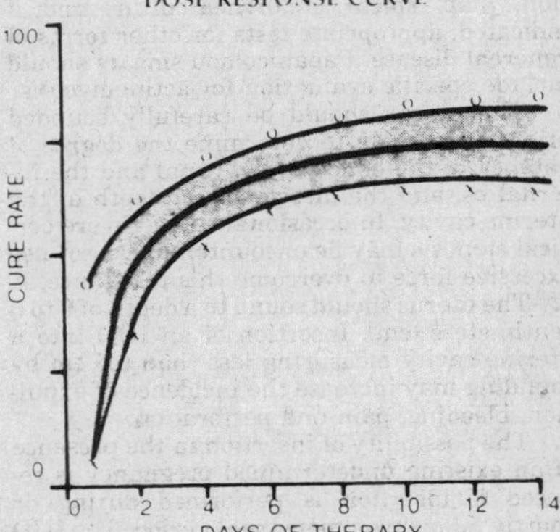

Contraindications: Patients known to be hypersensitive to this drug.
Precautions: General: Discontinue drug if sensitization or irritation is reported during use. Laboratory Tests: If there is a lack of response to MONISTAT 7, appropriate microbiological studies (standard KOH smear and/or cultures) should be repeated to confirm the diagnosis and rule out other pathogens.
Carcinogenesis, Mutagenesis, Impairment of Fertility: Long-term animal studies to determine carcinogenic potential have not been performed.
Fertility (reproduction): Oral administration of miconazole nitrate in rats has been reported to produce prolonged gestation. However, this effect was not observed in oral rabbit studies. In addition, signs of fetal and embryotoxicity were reported in rat and rabbit studies and dystocia in rat studies after oral doses at and above 80 mg/kg. Intravaginal administration did not produce these effects in rats.

Pregnancy: Since imidazoles are absorbed in small amounts from the human vagina, they should be used in the first trimester of pregnancy unless the physician considers it essential to the welfare of the patient.
Clinical studies, during which miconazole nitrate vaginal cream and suppositories were used for up to 14 days, were reported to include 487 pregnant patients. Follow-up reports available on 446 of these patients reveal no adverse effects or complications attributable to miconazole nitrate therapy in infants born to these women.
Nursing Mothers: It is not known whether miconazole nitrate is excreted in human milk. Because many drugs are excreted in human milk, caution should be exercised when miconazole nitrate is administered to a nursing woman.
Adverse Reactions: During clinical studies with miconazole nitrate cream for a 14-day regimen, 39 of the 528 patients (7.4%) treated with miconazole nitrate cream reported complaints during therapy that were possibly drug-related. Most complaints were reported during the first week of therapy. Vulvovaginal burning, itching or irritation occurred in 6.6%, while other complaints such as vaginal burning, pelvic cramps, hives, skin rash and headache occurred rarely (each less than 0.2% patient incidence). The therapy-related dropout rate was 0.9%.
During clinical studies with regimens which varied from 1 to 14 days, 1,057 patients were treated with miconazole nitrate suppositories. The incidence of vulvovaginal burning, itching or irritation was 0.5%, while complaints of skin rash occurred at only a 0.2% incidence.
Overdose: Overdosage of miconazole nitrate in humans has not been reported to date. In mice, rats, guinea pigs and dogs, the oral LD_{50} values were found to be 578.1, >640, 275.9 and >160 mg/kg, respectively.
Dosage and Administration: MONISTAT 7 Vaginal Suppositories: One suppository (100 mg miconazole nitrate) is inserted intravaginally once daily at bedtime for seven days. Before prescribing another course of therapy, the diagnosis should be reconfirmed by smears and/or cultures to rule out other pathogens.
How Supplied: MONISTAT 7 Vaginal Suppositories are available as 2.5g (100 mg miconazole nitrate) elliptically shaped white to off-white suppositories in packages of seven with a vaginal applicator. Store at 59°-86°F (13°-30°C).

ORTHO-CREME® Contraceptive Cream

(See PDR For Nonprescription Drugs)

ORTHO® Diaphragm Kit—ALL-FLEX® ℞

Action and Uses: The ALL-FLEX Diaphragm is a molded, buff-colored, latex vaginal diaphragm containing a distortion-free, dual spring-within-a-spring which provides unique arcing action no matter where compressed. Ideal not only where ordinary diaphragms are indicated but also in patients with mild cystocele, rectocele or retroversion. The diaphragm is used in conjunction with GYNOL II Contraceptive Jelly, ORTHO-GYNOL Contraceptive Jelly, or ORTHO-CREME Contraceptive Cream in conception control.
How Supplied: Available individually with tube of GYNOL II Contraceptive Jelly. Each diaphragm is contained in an attractive plastic compact. Sizes 55, 60, 65, 70, 75, 80, 85, 90, 95 mm.

ORTHO® Diaphragm Kit—Coil Spring ℞

Action and Uses: The ORTHO Diaphragm (coil spring) is a molded latex vaginal diaphragm. The rim encases a tension-adjusted cadmium-plated coil spring. The diaphragm is used in conjunction with GYNOL II Contraceptive Jelly, ORTHO-GYNOL Contraceptive Jelly or ORTHO-CREME Contraceptive Cream in conception control.
How Supplied: Available individually with tube of GYNOL II Contraceptive Jelly. Each diaphragm is contained in an attractive plastic compact. Sizes 50, 55, 60, 65, 70, 75, 80, 85, 90, 95, 100, 105 mm.

ORTHO® Diaphragm Kit—Flat Spring ℞

Action and Uses: The ORTHO-WHITE® Diaphragm is a molded pure white latex vaginal diaphragm containing a flat watch-type spring which allows compressibility in one plane only, thus facilitating insertion. The diaphragm is used in conjunction with GYNOL II Contraceptive Jelly, ORTHO-GYNOL Contraceptive Jelly, or ORTHO-CREME Contraceptive Cream in conception control.
How Supplied: Available individually with tube of GYNOL II Contraceptive Jelly. Each diaphragm is contained in an attractive plastic compact. Sizes 55, 60, 65, 70, 75, 80, 85, 90, 95 mm.

ORTHO® Dienestrol Cream ℞

1. ESTROGENS HAVE BEEN REPORTED TO INCREASE THE RISK OF ENDOMETRIAL CARCINOMA.
Three independent case control studies have shown an increased risk of endometrial cancer in postmenopausal women exposed to exogenous estrogens for prolonged periods.[1–3] This risk was independent of the other known risk factors for endometrial cancer. These studies are further supported by the finding that incidence rates of endometrial cancer have increased sharply since 1969 in eight different areas of the United States with population-based cancer reporting systems, an increase which may be related to the rapidly expanding use of estrogens during the last decade.[4]
The three case control studies reported that the risk of endometrial cancer in estrogen users was about 4.5 to 13.9 times greater than in nonusers. The risk appears to depend on both duration of treatment[1] and on estrogen dose.[3] In view of these findings, when estrogens are used for the treatment of menopausal symptoms, the lowest dose that will control symptoms should be utilized and medication should be discontinued as soon as possible. When prolonged treatment is medically indicated, the patient should be reassessed on at least a semiannual basis to determine the need for continued therapy. Although the evidence must be considered preliminary, one study suggests that cyclic administration of low doses of estrogen may carry less risk than continuous administration;[3] it therefore appears prudent to utilize such a regimen.
Close clinical surveillance of all women taking estrogens is important. In all cases of undiagnosed persistent or recurring abnormal vaginal bleeding, adequate diagnostic measures should be undertaken to rule out malignancy.
There is no evidence at present that "natural" estrogens are more or less hazardous than "synthetic" estrogens at equiestrogenic doses.
2. ESTROGENS SHOULD NOT BE USED DURING PREGNANCY
The use of female sex hormones, both estrogens and progestogens, during early pregnancy may seriously damage the offspring. It has been shown that females exposed *in utero* to diethylstilbestrol, a non-steroidal estrogen, have an increased risk of developing in later life a form of vaginal or cervical cancer that ordinarily is extremely rare.[5,6] This risk has been estimated as not greater than 4 per 1000 exposures.[7] Furthermore, a high percentage of such exposed women (from 30 to 90 percent) have been found to have vaginal adenosis,[8,13] epithelial changes of the vagina and cervix. Although these changes are histologically benign, it is not known whether they are precursors of malignancy. Although similar data are not available with the use of other estrogens, it cannot be presumed they would not induce similar changes.
Several reports suggest an association between intrauterine exposure to female sex hormones and congenital anomalies, including congenital heart defects and limb reduction defects.[13–16] One case control study[16] estimated a 4.7 fold increased risk of limb reduction defects in infants exposed in utero to sex hormones (oral contraceptives, hormone withdrawal tests for pregnancy, or attempted treatment for threatened abortion). Some of these exposures were very short and involved only a few days of treatment. The data suggest that the risk of limb reduction defects in exposed fetuses is somewhat less than 1 per 1000.
In the past, female sex hormones have been used during pregnancy in an attempt to treat threatened or habitual abortion. There is considerable evidence that estrogens are ineffective for these indications, and there is no evidence from well controlled studies that progestogens are effective for these uses.
If ORTHO Dienestrol Cream is used during pregnancy, or if the patient becomes pregnant while using this drug, she should be apprised of the potential risks to the fetus, and the advisability of pregnancy continuation.

Description:
ORTHO Dienestrol Cream
Cream for intravaginal use only
Active ingredient: Dienestrol 0.01%.
Compounded with: Glyceryl monostearate, peanut oil, glycerin, benzoic acid, glutamic acid, butylated hydroxyanisole, citric acid, sodium hydroxide and water.
Clinical Pharmacology: Systemic absorption and mode of action are undetermined.
Indications: ORTHO Dienestrol Cream is indicated in the treatment of atrophic vaginitis and kraurosis vulvae.
ORTHO DIENESTROL CREAM HAS NOT BEEN SHOWN TO BE EFFECTIVE FOR ANY PURPOSE DURING PREGNANCY AND ITS USE MAY CAUSE SEVERE HARM TO THE FETUS (*SEE* BOXED WARNING).
Contraindications: Estrogens should not be used in women with any of the following conditions:
1. Known or suspected cancer of the breast.
2. Known or suspected estrogen-dependent neoplasia.
3. Known or suspected pregnancy (*See* Boxed Warning).
4. Undiagnosed abnormal genital bleeding.
5. Active thrombophlebitis or thromboembolic disorders.
6. A past history of thrombophlebitis, thrombosis, or thromboembolic disorders associated with previous estrogen use.

Warnings:
1. *Induction of malignant neoplasms.* Long-term continuous administration of natural and synthetic estrogens in certain animal species increases the frequency of carcinomas of the breast, cervix, vagina, and liver. There is now evidence that estrogens increase the risk of carcinoma of the endometrium in humans. (*See* Boxed Warning.)

Continued on next page

Ortho Pharm.—Cont.

At the present time there is no satisfactory evidence that estrogens given to postmenopausal women increase the risk of cancer of the breast,[18] although a recent long-term followup of a single physician's practice has raised this possibility.[18a] Because of the animal data, there is a need for caution in prescribing estrogens for women with a strong family history of breast cancer or who have breast nodules, fibrocystic disease, or abnormal mammograms.

2. *Gall bladder disease.* A recent study has reported a 2 to 3-fold increase in the risk of surgically confirmed gall bladder disease in women receiving postmenopausal estrogens,[18] similar to the 2-fold increase previously noted in users of oral contraceptives.[19–24] In the case of oral contraceptives the increased risk appeared after two years of use.[24]

3. *Effects similar to those caused by estrogen-progestogen oral contraceptives.* There are several serious adverse effects of oral contraceptives, most of which have not, up to now, been documented as consequences of postmenopausal estrogen therapy. This may reflect the comparatively low doses of estrogen used in postmenopausal women. It would be expected that the larger doses of estrogen used to treat prostatic or breast cancer or postpartum breast engorgement are more likely to result in these adverse effects, and, in fact, it has been shown that there is an increased risk of thrombosis in men receiving estrogens for prostatic cancer and women for postpartum breast engorgement.[20–23]

a. *Thromboembolic disease.* It is now well established that users of oral contraceptives have an increased risk of various thromboembolic and thrombotic vascular diseases, such as thrombophlebitis, pulmonary embolism, stroke, and myocardial infarction.[24–31] Cases of retinal thrombosis, mesenteric thrombosis, and optic neuritis have been reported in oral contraceptive users. There is evidence that the risk of several of these adverse reactions is related to the dose of the drug.[32,33] An increased risk of postsurgery thromboembolic complications has also been reported in users of oral contraceptives.[34,35] If feasible, estrogen should be discontinued at least 4 weeks before surgery of the type associated with an increased risk of thromboembolism, or during periods of prolonged immobilization.

While an increased risk of thromboembolic and thrombotic disease in postmenopausal users of estrogens has not been found,[18–36] this does not rule out the possibility that such an increase may be present or that subgroups of women who have underlying risk factors or who are receiving relatively large doses of estrogens may have increased risk. Therefore estrogens should not be used in persons with active thrombophlebitis or thromboembolic disorders, and they should not be used (except in treatment of malignancy) in persons with a history of such disorders in association with estrogen use. They should be used with caution in patients with cerebral vascular or coronary artery disease and only for those in whom estrogens are clearly needed.

Large doses of estrogen (5 mg conjugated estrogens per day), comparable to those used to treat cancer of the prostate and breast, have been shown in a large prospective clinical trial in men to increase the risk of nonfatal myocardial infarction, pulmonary embolism and thrombophlebitis. When estrogen doses of this size are used, any of the thromboembolic and thrombotic adverse effects associated with oral contraceptive use should be considered a clear risk.

b. *Hepatic adenoma.* Benign hepatic adenomas appear to be associated with the use of oral contraceptives.[38–40] Although benign, and rare, these may rupture and may cause death through intra-abdominal hemorrhage. Such lesions have not yet been reported in association with other estrogen or progestogen preparations but should be considered in estrogen users having abdominal pain and tenderness, abdominal mass, or hypovolemic shock. Hepatocellular carcinoma has also been reported in women taking estrogen-containing oral contraceptives.[39] The relationship of this malignancy to these drugs is not known at this time.

c. *Elevated blood pressure.* Increased blood pressure is not uncommon in women using oral contraceptives. There is now a report that this may occur with use of estrogens in the menopause[41] and blood pressure should be monitored with estrogen use, especially if high doses are used.

d. *Glucose tolerance.* A worsening of glucose tolerance has been observed in a significant percentage of patients on estrogen-containing oral contraceptives. For this reason, diabetic patients should be carefully observed while receiving estrogen.

4. *Hypercalcemia.* Administration of estrogens may lead to severe hypercalcemia in patients with breast cancer and bone metastases. If this occurs, the drug should be stopped and appropriate measures taken to reduce the serum calcium level.

Precautions:

A. General Precautions.

1. A complete medical and family history should be taken prior to the initiation of any estrogen therapy. The pretreatment and periodic physical examinations should include special reference to blood pressure, breasts, abdomen, and pelvic organs, and should include a Papanicolaou smear. As a general rule, estrogen should not be prescribed for longer than one year without another physical examination being performed.

2. Fluid retention—Because estrogens may cause some degree of fluid retention, conditions which might be influenced by this factor such as epilepsy, migraine, and cardiac or renal dysfunction, require careful observation.

3. Certain patients may develop undesirable manifestations of excessive estrogenic stimulation, such as abnormal or excessive uterine bleeding, mastodynia, etc.

4. Oral contraceptives appear to be associated with an increased incidence of mental depression.[24] Although it is not clear whether this is due to the estrogenic or progestogenic component of the contraceptive, patients with a history of depression should be carefully observed.

5. Preexisting uterine leiomyomata may increase in size during estrogen use.

6. The pathologist should be advised of estrogen therapy when relevant specimens are submitted.

7. Patients with a past history of jaundice during pregnancy have an increased risk of recurrence of jaundice while receiving estrogen-containing oral contraceptive therapy. If jaundice develops in any patient receiving estrogen, the medication should be discontinued while the cause is investigated.

8. Estrogens may be poorly metabolized in patients with impaired liver function and they should be administered with caution in such patients.

9. Because estrogens influence the metabolism of calcium and phosphorus, they should be used with caution in patients with metabolic bone diseases that are associated with hypercalcemia or in patients with renal insufficiency.

10. Because of the effects of estrogens on epiphyseal closure, they should be used judiciously in young patients in whom bone growth is not complete.

11. Certain endocrine and liver function tests may be affected by estrogen-containing oral contraceptives. The following similar changes may be expected with larger doses of estrogen:

a. Increased sulfobromophthalein retention.

b. Increased prothrombin and factors VII, VIII, IX, and X; decreased antithrombin 3; increased norepinephrine-induced platelet aggregability.

c. Increased thyroid binding globulin (TBG) leading to increased circulating total thyroid hormone, as measured by PBI, T4 by column, or T4 by radioimmunoassay. Free T3 resin uptake is decreased, reflecting the elevated TBG; free T4 concentration is unaltered.

d. Impaired glucose tolerance.

e. Decreased pregnanediol excretion.

f. Reduced response to metyrapone test.

g. Reduced serum folate concentration.

h. Increased serum triglyceride and phospholipid concentration.

B. Information for the Patient. See text of Patient Package Information which is reproduced below.

C. Pregnancy Category X

See Contraindications and Boxed Warning.

D. Nursing Mothers. As a general principle, the administration of any drug to nursing mothers should be done only when clearly necessary since many drugs are excreted in human milk.

Adverse Reactions: (*See* Warnings regarding induction of neoplasia, adverse effects on the fetus, increased incidence of gall bladder disease, and adverse effects similar to those of oral contraceptives, including thromboembolism.) The following additional adverse reactions have been reported with estrogenic therapy, including oral contraceptives:

1. *Genitourinary system.*
Breakthrough bleeding, spotting, change in menstrual flow.
Dysmenorrhea.
Premenstrual-like syndrome.
Amenorrhea during and after treatment.
Increase in size of uterine fibromyomata.
Vaginal candidiasis.
Change in cervical eversion and in degree of cervical secretion.
Cystitis-like syndrome.

2. *Breasts.*
Tenderness, enlargement, secretion.

3. *Gastrointestinal.*
Nausea, vomiting.
Abdominal cramps, bloating.
Cholestatic jaundice.

4. *Skin.*
Chloasma or melasma which may persist when drug is discontinued.
Erythema multiforme.
Erythema nodosum.
Hemorrhagic eruption.
Loss of scalp hair.
Hirsutism.

5. *Eyes.*
Steepening of corneal curvature.
Intolerance to contact lenses.

6. *CNS.*
Headache, migraine, dizziness.
Mental depression.
Chorea.

7. *Miscellaneous.*
Increase or decrease in weight.
Reduced carbohydrate tolerance.
Aggravation of porphyria.
Edema.
Changes in libido.

Acute Overdosage: Numerous reports of ingestion of large doses of estrogen-containing oral contraceptives by young children indicate that serious ill effects do not occur. Overdosage of estrogen may cause nausea, and withdrawal bleeding may occur in females.

Dosage and Administration: *Given cyclically for short term use only:*

For treatment of atrophic vaginitis, or kraurosis vulvae associated with the menopause.

The lowest dose that will control symptoms should be chosen and medication should be discontinued as promptly as possible.

Attempts to discontinue or taper medication should be made at 3 to 6 month intervals.

The usual dosage range is one or two applicatorsful per day for one or two weeks, then gradually reduced to one half initial dosage for a similar period. A maintenance dosage of one applicatorful, one to three times a week, may be used after restoration of the vaginal mucosa has been achieved.

Treated patients with an intact uterus should be monitored closely for signs of endometrial cancer and appropriate diagnostic measures should be taken to rule out malignancy in the event of persistent or recurring abnormal vaginal bleeding.

Supplied: Available in 2.75 oz. (78g) tubes with or without ORTHO® Measured-Dose Applicator.

Physician References:

1. Ziel, H.K. and W.D. Finkle, "Increased Risk of Endometrial Carcinoma Among Users of Conjugated Estrogens," *New England Journal of Medicine,* 293:1167–1170, 1975.
2. Smith, D.C., R. Prentic, D.J. Thompson, and W.L. Hermann, "Association of Exogenous Estrogen and Endometrial Carcinoma," *New England Journal of Medicine,* 293:1164–1167, 1975.
3. Mack, T.M., M.C. Pike, B.E. Henderson, R.I. Pfeffer, V.R. Gerkins, M. Arthur, and S.E. Brown, "Estrogens and Endometrial Cancer in a Retirement Community," *New England Journal of Medicine,* 294:1267–1287, 1976.
4. Weiss, N.S., D.R. Szekely and D.F. Austin, "Increasing Incidence of Endometrial Cancer in the United States," *New England Journal of Medicine,* 294:1259–1262, 1976.
5. Herbst, A.L., H. Ulfelder and D.C. Poskanzer, "Adenocarcinoma of Vagina," *New England Journal of Medicine,* 284:878–881, 1971.
6. Greenwald, P., J. Barlow, P. Nasca, and W. Burnett, "Vaginal Cancer after Maternal Treatment with Synthetic Estrogens," *New England Journal of Medicine,* 285:390–392, 1971.
7. Lanier, A., K. Noller, D. Decker, L. Elveback, and L. Kurland, "Cancer and Stilbestrol. A Follow-up of 1719 Persons Exposed to Estrogens in Utero and Born 1943–1959," *Mayo Clinic Proceedings,* 48:793–799, 1973.
8. Herbst, A., R. Kurman, and R. Scully, "Vaginal and Cervical Abnormalities After Exposure to Stilbestrol In Utero," *Obstetrics and Gynecology,* 40:287–298, 1972.
9. Herbst, A., S. Robboy, G. Macdonald, and R. Scully, "The Effects of Local Progesterone on Stilbestrol-Associated Vaginal Adenosis," *American Journal of Obstetrics and Gynecology* 118:607–615, 1974.
10. Herbst, A., D. Poskanzer, S. Robboy, L. Friedlander, and R. Scully, "Prenatal Exposure to Stilbestrol, A Prospective Comparison of Exposed Female Offspring with Unexposed Controls," *New England Journal of Medicine,* 292:334–339, 1975.
11. Staffi, A., R. Mattingly, D. Foley, and W. Fetherston, "Clinical Diagnosis of Vaginal Adenosis," *Obstetrics and Gynecology,* 43:118–128, 1974.
12. Sherman, A.I., M. Goldrath, A. Berlin, V. Vakhariya, F. Banooni, W. Michaels, P. Goodman, S. Brown, "Cervical-Vaginal Adenosis After *In Utero* Exposure to Synthetic Estrogens," *Obstetrics and Gynecology,* 44:531–545, 1974.
13. Gal, I., B. Kirman, and J. Stern, "Hormone Pregnancy Tests and Congenital Malformation," *Nature,* 216:83, 1967.
14. Levy, E.P., A. Cohen, and F.C. Fraser, "Hormone Treatment During Pregnancy and Congenital Heart Defects," *Lancet,* 1:611, 1973.
15. Nora, J. and A. Nora, "Birth Defects and Oral Contraceptives," *Lancet,* 1:941–942, 1973.
16. Janerich, D.T., J.M. Piper, and D.M. Glebatis, "Oral Contraceptives and Congenital Limb-Reduction Defects," *New England Journal of Medicine,* 291:697–700, 1974.
17. "Estrogens for Oral or Parenteral Use," *Federal Register,* 40:8212, 1975.
18. Boston Collaborative Drug Surveillance Program, "Surgically Confirmed Gall Bladder Disease, Venous Thromboembolism and Breast Tumors in Relation to Post-Menopausal Estrogen Therapy," *New England Journal of Medicine,* 290:15–19, 1974.
18a. Hoover, R., L.A. Gray, Sr., P. Cole, and B. MacMahon, "Menopausal Estrogens and Breast Cancer," *New England Journal of Medicine,* 295:401–405, 1976.
19. Boston Collaborative Drug Surveillance Program, "Oral Contraceptives and Venous Thromboembolic Disease, Surgically Confirmed Gall Bladder Disease, and Breast Tumors," *Lancet* 1:1399–1404, 1973.
20. Daniel, D.G., H. Campbell, and A.C. Turnbull, "Puerperal Thromboembolism and Suppression of Lactation," *Lancet,* 2:287–289, 1967.
21. The Veterans Administration Cooperative Urological Research Group, "Carcinoma of the Prostate: Treatment Comparisons," *Journal of Urology,* 98:516–522, 1967.
22. Bailer, J.C., "Thromboembolism and Oestrogen Therapy," *Lancet,* 2:560, 1967.
23. Blackard, C., R. Doe, G. Mellinger, and D. Byar, "Incidence of Cardiovascular Disease and Death In Patients Receiving Diethylstilbestrol for Carcinoma of the Prostate," *Cancer,* 26:249–256, 1970.
24. Royal College of General Practitioners, "Oral Contraception and Thromboembolic Disease," *Journal of the Royal College of General Practitioners,* 13:267–279, 1967.
25. Inman, W.H.W. and M.P. Vessey, "Investigation of Deaths from Pulmonary, Coronary, and Cerebral Thrombosis and Embolism in Women of Child-Bearing Age," *British Medical Journal,* 2:193–199, 1968.
26. Vessey, M.P. and R. Doll, "Investigation of Relation Between Use of Oral Contraceptives and Thromboembolic Disease, A Further Report," *British Medical Journal,* 2:651–657, 1969.
27. Sartwell, P.E., A.T. Masi, F.G. Arthes, G.R. Greene, and H.E. Smith, "Thromboembolism and Oral Contraceptives: An Epidemiological Case Control Study," *American Journal of Epidemiology,* 90:365–380, 1969.
28. Collaborative Group for the Study of Stroke In Young Women, "Oral Contraception and Increased Risk of Cerebral Ischemia or Thrombosis," *New England Journal of Medicine,* 288:871–878, 1973.
29. Collaborative Group for the Study of Stroke in Young Women, "Oral Contraceptives and Stroke in Young Women: Associated Risk Factors," *Journal of the American Medical Association,* 231:718–722, 1975.
30. Mann, J.I. and W.H.W. Inman, "Oral Contraceptives and Death from Myocardial Infarction," *British Medical Journal,* 2:245–248, 1975.
31. Mann, J.I., M.P. Vessey, M. Thorogood, and R. Doll., "Myocardial Infarction in Young Women with Special Reference to Oral Contraceptive Practice," *British Medical Journal,* 2:241–245, 1975.
32. Inman, W.H.W., V.P. Vessey, B. Westerholm, and A. Engelund, "Thromboembolic Disease and the Steroidal Content of Oral Contraceptives," *British Medical Journal,* 2:203–209, 1970.
33. Stolley, P.D., J.A. Tonascia, M.S. Tockman, P.E. Sartwell, A.H. Rutledge, and M.P. Jacobs, "Thrombosis with Low-Estrogen Oral Contraceptives," *American Journal of Epidemiology,* 102:197–208, 1975.
34. Vessey, M.P., R. Doll, A.S. Fairbairn, and G. Glober, "Post-Operative Thromboembolism and the Use of the Oral Contraceptives," *British Medical Journal,* 3:123–126, 1970.
35. Greene, G.R. and P.E. Sartwell, "Oral Contraceptive Use in Patients with Thromboembolism Following Surgery, Trauma or Infection," *American Journal of Public Health,* 62:680–685, 1972.
36. Rosenberg, L., M.B. Armstrong and H. Jick, "Myocardial Infarction and Estrogen Therapy is Postmenopausal Women," *New England Journal of Medicine,* 294:1256–1259, 1976.
37. Coronary Drug Project Research Group, "The Coronary Drug Project: Initial Findings Leading to Modifications of Its Research Protocol, *Journal of the American Medical Association,* 214:1303–1313, 1970.
38. Baum, J., F. Holtz, J.J. Bookstein, and E.W. Klein, "Possible Association between Benign Hepatomas and Oral Contraceptives," *Lancet,* 2:926–928, 1973.
39. Mays, E.T., W.M. Christopherson, M.M. Mahr, and H.C. Williams, "Hepatic Changes in Young Women Ingesting Contraceptive Steroids, Hepatic Hemorrhage and Primary Hepatic Tumors." *Journal of the American Medical Association,* 235:730–782, 1976.
40. Edmondson, H.A., B. Henderson, and B. Benton, "Liver Cell Adenomas Associated with the Use of Oral Contraceptives," *New England Journal of Medicine,* 294:470–472, 1976.
41. Pfeffer, R.I. and S. Van Den Noore, "Estrogen Use and Stroke Risk in Postmenopausal Women," *American Journal of Epidemiology,* 103:445–456, 1976.

PATIENT INFORMATION ABOUT ESTROGENS

Estrogens are female hormones produced by the ovaries. The ovaries make several different kinds of estrogens. In addition, scientists have been able to make a variety of synthetic estrogens. As far as we know, all these synthetic estrogens have similar properties and therefore much the same usefulness, side effects, and risks. This leaflet is intended to help you understand what estrogens are used for, some of the risks involved in their use, and to help minimize these risks.

This leaflet includes important information about estrogens, but not all the information. If you want to know more, you can ask your doctor or pharmacist to let you read the package insert prepared for the doctor.

Uses of Estrogen: THERE IS NO PROPER USE OF ESTROGENS IN A PREGNANT WOMAN

Estrogens are prescribed by doctors for a number of purposes, including:

1. To provide estrogen during a period of adjustment when a woman's ovaries no longer produce it, in order to prevent certain uncomfortable symptoms of estrogen deficiency. (All women normally decrease the production of estrogens, generally between the ages of 45 and 55; this is called the menopause.)
2. To prevent symptoms of estrogen deficiency when a woman's ovaries have been removed surgically before the natural menopause.
3. To prevent pregnancy. (Estrogens are given along with a progestogen, another female hormone; these combinations are called oral contraceptives or birth control pills. Patient labeling is available to women taking oral contraceptives and they will not be discussed in this leaflet.)
4. To treat certain cancers in women and men.
5. To prevent painful swelling of the breasts after pregnancy in women who choose not to nurse their babies.

Estrogens in the Menopause: In the natural course of their lives, all women eventually experience a decrease in estrogen production. This usually occurs between ages 45 and 55 but may occur earlier or later. Sometimes the ovaries may need to be removed by an operation before natural menopause, producing a "surgical menopause."

When the amount of estrogen in the blood begins to decrease, many women may develop typical symptoms: Feelings of warmth in the

Continued on next page

Ortho Pharm.—Cont.

face, neck, and chest or sudden intense episodes of heat and sweating throughout the body (called "hot flashes" or "hot flushes"). These symptoms are sometimes very uncomfortable. A few women eventually develop changes in the vagina (called "atrophic vaginitis") which cause discomfort, especially during and after intercourse.

Estrogens can be prescribed to treat these symptoms of the menopause. It is estimated that considerably more than half of all women undergoing the menopause have only mild symptoms or no symptoms at all and therefore do not need estrogens. Other women may need estrogens for a few months, while their bodies adjust to lower estrogen levels. Sometimes the need will be for periods longer than six months. In an attempt to avoid over-stimulation of the uterus (womb), estrogens are usually given cyclically during each month of use, that is three weeks of pills followed by one week without pills.

Sometimes women experience nervous symptoms or depression during menopause. There is no evidence that estrogens are effective for such symptoms and they should not be used to treat them, although other treatment may be needed.

You may have heard that taking estrogens for long periods (years) after the menopause will keep your skin soft and supple and keep you feeling young. There is no evidence that this is so, however, and such long-term treatment carries important risks.

Estrogens to Prevent Swelling of the Breasts After Pregnancy: If you do not breast-feed your baby after delivery, your breasts may fill up with milk and become painful and engorged. This usually begins about three to four days after delivery and may last for a few days to up to a week or more. Sometimes the discomfort is severe, but usually it is not and can be controlled by pain-relieving drugs such as aspirin and by binding the breasts up tightly. Estrogens can be used to try to prevent the breasts from filling up. While this treatment is sometimes successful, in many cases the breasts fill up to some degree in spite of treatment. The dose of estrogens needed to prevent pain and swelling of the breasts is much larger than the dose needed to treat symptoms of the menopause and this may increase your chances of developing blood clots in the legs or lungs (see below). Therefore, it is important that you discuss the benefits and the risks of estrogen use with your doctor if you have decided not to breast-feed your baby.

Some of the Dangers of Estrogen:

1. *Cancer of the uterus.* If estrogens are used in the postmenopausal period for more than a year, there is an increased risk of *endometrial cancer* (cancer of the uterus). Women taking estrogens have roughly five to ten times as great a chance of getting this cancer as women who take no estrogens. To put this another way, while a postmenopausal woman not taking estrogens has one chance in 1,000 each year of getting cancer of the uterus, a woman taking estrogens has five to ten chances in 1,000 each year. For this reason *it is important to take estrogens only when you really need them.*

The risk of this cancer is greater the longer estrogens are used and also seems to be greater when larger doses are taken. For this reason *it is important to take the lowest dose of estrogen that will control symptoms and to take it only as long as it is needed.* If estrogens are needed for longer periods of time, your doctor will want to reevaluate your need for estrogens at least every six months.

Women using estrogens should report any irregular vaginal bleeding to their doctors; such bleeding may be of no importance, but it can be an early warning of cancer of the uterus. If you have undiagnosed vaginal bleeding, you should not use estrogens until a diagnosis is made and you are certain there is no cancer of the uterus. If you have had your uterus completely removed (total hysterectomy), there is no danger of developing cancer of the uterus.

2. *Other possible cancers.* Estrogens can cause development of other tumors in animals, such as tumors of the breast, cervix, vagina, or liver, when given for a long time. At present there is no good evidence that women using estrogen in the menopause have an increased risk of such tumors, but there is no way yet to be sure they do not; and one study raises the possibility that use of estrogens in the menopause may increase the risk of breast cancer many years later. This is a further reason to use estrogens only when clearly needed. While you are taking estrogens, it is important that you go to your doctor at least once a year for a physical examination. Also, if members of your family have had breast cancer or if you have breast nodules or abnormal mammograms (breast x-rays), your doctor may wish to carry out more frequent examinations of your breasts.

3. *Gall bladder disease.* Women who use estrogens after menopause are more likely to develop gall bladder disease needing surgery than women who do not use estrogens. Birth control pills have a similar effect.

4. *Abnormal blood clotting.* Oral contraceptives, some of which contain estrogens, increase the risk of blood clotting in various parts of the body. This can result in a stroke (if the clot is in the brain), a heart attack (clot in a blood vessel of the heart), or a pulmonary embolus (a clot which forms in the legs or pelvis, then breaks off and travels to the lungs). Any of these can be fatal. Blood clots may result in the loss of a limb, paralysis or loss of sight, depending on where the blood clot is formed or lodges if it breaks loose.

The larger doses of estrogen used to prevent swelling of the breasts after pregnancy have been reported to cause clotting in the legs and lungs.

It is recommended that if you have had any blood clotting disorders including clotting in the legs or lungs, or a heart attack or stroke, you should not use estrogens.

Special Warning About Pregnancy: You should not receive estrogen if you are pregnant. If this should occur, there is a greater than usual chance that the developing child will be born with a birth defect, although the possibility remains fairly small. A female child may have an increased risk of developing cancer of the vagina or cervix later in life (in the teens or twenties). Every possible effort should be made to avoid exposure to estrogens during pregnancy. If exposure occurs, see your doctor.

Some Other Effects of Estrogens: In addition to the serious known risks of estrogens described above, estrogens have the following side effects and potential risks:

1. *Nausea and vomiting.* The most common side effect of estrogen therapy is nausea. Vomiting is less common.
2. *Effects on breasts.* Estrogens may cause breast tenderness or enlargement and may cause the breasts to secrete a liquid.
3. *Effects on the uterus.* Estrogens may cause benign fibroid tumors of the uterus to get larger.

Some women will have menstrual bleeding when estrogens are stopped. But if the bleeding occurs on days you are still taking estrogens you should report this to your doctor.

4. *Effects on liver.* Women taking estrogens develop on rare occasions a tumor of the liver which can rupture and bleed into the abdomen. You should report any swelling or unusual pain or tenderness in the abdomen to your doctor immediately.

Women with a past history of jaundice (yellowing of the skin and white parts of the eyes) may get jaundice again during estrogen use.

5. *Other effects.* Estrogens may cause excess fluid to be retained in the body. This may make some conditions worse, such as epilepsy, migraine, heart disease, or kidney disease.

If any of the above occur, stop taking estrogens and call your doctor.

Summary: Estrogens have important uses, but they have serious risks as well. You must decide, with your doctor, whether the risks are acceptable to you in view of the benefits of treatment. Except where your doctor has prescribed estrogens for use in special cases of cancer of the breast or prostate, you should not use estrogens if you have cancer of the breast or uterus, are pregnant, have undiagnosed abnormal vaginal bleeding, blood clotting disorders including clotting in the legs or lungs, or have had a stroke, heart attack or angina.

You must understand that your doctor will require regular physical examinations while you are taking them and will try to discontinue the drug as soon as possible and use the smallest dose possible. You can help minimize the risk by being alert for signs of trouble including:

1. Abnormal bleeding from the vagina.
2. Pains in the calves or chest or sudden shortness of breath, or coughing blood (indicating possible clots in the legs, heart or lungs).
3. Severe headache, dizziness, faintness,, or changes in vision (indicating possible developing clots in the brain or eye).
4. Breast lumps (you should ask your doctor how to examine your own breasts).
5. Jaundice (yellowing of the skin).
6. Mental depression.
7. <u>Any</u> other unusual condition or problem.

Based on his or her assessment of your medical needs, your doctor has prescribed this drug for you. Do not give the drug to anyone else.

How Supplied: Available in 2.75 oz. (78g) tubes with or without ORTHO® Measured-Dose Applicator.

ORTHO® Disposable Applicator

(See PDR For Nonprescription Drugs)

ORTHO® Personal Lubricant

(See PDR For Nonprescription Drugs)

ORTHO-GYNOL® Contraceptive Jelly

(See PDR For Nonprescription Drugs)

ORTHO-NOVUM® Tablets ℞
and
MODICON® Tablets ℞
MICRONOR® ℞

Description:

ORTHO-NOVUM 10/11□21 Tablets are a combination oral contraceptive. Each white ORTHO-NOVUM 10/11□21 Tablet contains 0.5 mg of the progestational compound, norethindrone (17-hydroxy-19-nor-17α-pregn-4-en-20-yn-3-one), together with 0.035 mg of the estrogenic compound, ethinyl estradiol (19-nor-17α-pregna-1,3,5(10)-trien-20-yne-3,17-diol). Each peach ORTHO-NOVUM 10/11□21 Tablet contains 1 mg of the progestational compound, norethindrone (17-hydroxy-19-nor-17α-pregn-4-en-20-yn-3-one), together with 0.035 mg of the estrogenic compound, ethinyl estradiol (19-nor-17α-pregna-1,3,5(10)-trien-20-yne-3,17-diol).

ORTHO-NOVUM 10/11□28 Tablets are a combination oral contraceptive. Each white ORTHO-NOVUM 10/11□28 Tablet contains 0.5 mg of the progestational compound, norethindrone (17-hydroxy-19-nor-17α-pregn-4-en-20-yn-3-one), together with 0.035 mg of the estrogenic compound, ethinyl estradiol (19-nor-17α-pregna-1,3,5(10)-trien-20-yne-3,17-diol). Each peach ORTHO-NOVUM 10/11□28 Tablet contains 1 mg of the progestational compound, norethindrone (17-hydroxy-19-nor-17α-pregn-4-en-20-yn-3-one), together with 0.035 mg of the estrogenic compound, ethinyl estradiol (19-nor-17α-pregna-1,3,5(10)-trien-20-yne-3,17-diol). Each green tablet contains inert ingredients.

ORTHO-NOVUM 1/35□21 Tablets are a combination oral contraceptive. Each ORTHO-NOVUM 1/35□21 Tablet contains 1 mg of the progestational compound, norethindrone (17- hydroxy-19-nor-17α -pregn- 4 -en- 20-yn-3-one), together with 0.035 mg of the estrogenic compound, ethinyl estradiol (19-nor-17α-pregna-1,3,5(10)-trien-20-yne-3,17-diol).

ORTHO-NOVUM 1/35□28 Tablets are a combination oral contraceptive. Each peach ORTHO-NOVUM 1/35□28 Tablet contains 1 mg of the progestational compound, norethindrone (17-hydroxy-19-nor-17α-pregn-4-en-20-yn-3-one), together with 0.035 mg of the estrogenic compound ethinyl estradiol (19-nor-17α-pregna-1, 3, 5(10)-trien-20-yne-3, 17-diol). Each green tablet contains inert ingredients.

MODICON 21 Tablets are a combination oral contraceptive. Each MODICON 21 Tablet contains 0.5 mg of the progestational compound, norethindrone (17-hydroxy-19-nor-17α-pregn-4-en-20-yn-3-one), together with 0.035 mg of the estrogenic compound, ethinyl estradiol (19-nor-17α-pregna-1,3,5(10)-trien-20-yne-3,17-diol).

MODICON 28 Tablets are a combination oral contraceptive. Each white MODICON 28 Tablet contains 0.5 mg of the progestational compound, norethindrone (17-hydroxy-19-nor-17α-pregn-4-en-20-yn-3-one), together with 0.035 mg of the estrogenic compound, ethinyl estradiol (19-nor-17α-pregna-1,3,5(10)-trien-20-yne-3,17-diol). Each green tablet contains inert ingredients.

ORTHO-NOVUM 1/50□21 Tablets are a combination oral contraceptive. Each ORTHO-NOVUM 1/50□21 Tablet contains 1 mg of the progestational compound, norethindrone (17-hydroxy-19-nor- 17α -pregn-4-en-20-yn-3-one), together with 0.05 mg of the estrogenic compound, mestranol (3-methoxy-19-nor-17α-pregna-1,3,5(10)-trien-20-yn-17-ol).

ORTHO-NOVUM 1/50□28 Tablets are a combination oral contraceptive. Each yellow ORTHO-NOVUM 1/50□28 Tablet contains 1 mg of the progestational compound, norethindrone (17-hydroxy-19-nor-17α-pregn-4-en-20-yn-3-one), together with 0.05 mg of the estrogenic compound, mestranol (3-methoxy-19-nor-17α-pregna-1,3,5(10)-trien-20-yn-17-ol). Each green tablet contains inert ingredients.

ORTHO-NOVUM 1/80□21 Tablets are a combination oral contraceptive. Each ORTHO-NOVUM 1/80□21 Tablet contains 1 mg of the progestational compound, norethindrone (17-hydroxy-19-nor- 17α -pregn-4-en-20-yn-3-one), together with 0.08 mg of the estrogenic compound, mestranol (3-methoxy-19-nor-17α-pregna-1,3,5(10)-trien-20-yn-17-ol).

ORTHO-NOVUM 1/80□28 Tablets are a combination oral contraceptive. Each white ORTHO-NOVUM 1/80□28 Tablet contains 1 mg of the progestational compound, norethindrone (17-hydroxy-19-nor-17α-pregn-4-en-20-yn-3-one), together with 0.08 mg of the estrogenic compound, mestranol (3-methoxy-19-nor-17α-pregna-1,3,5(10)trien-20-yn-17-ol). Each green tablet contains inert ingredients.

ORTHO-NOVUM 2 mg□21 Tablets are a combination oral contraceptive. Each ORTHO-NOVUM 2 mg□21 Tablet contains 2 mg of the progestational compound, norethindrone (17- hydroxy-19-nor-17α -pregn- 4 -en- 20-yn-3-one), together with 0.10 mg of the estrogenic compound, mestranol (3-methoxy-19-nor-17α-pregna-1,3,5(10)-trien-20-yn-17-ol).

MICRONOR Tablets are a progestogen-only oral contraceptive. Each MICRONOR Tablet contains 0.35 mg of the progestational compound, norethindrone (17-hydroxy-19-nor-17α-pregn-4-en-20-yn-3-one), a synthetic progestogen.

Clinical Pharmacology Combination Oral Contraceptives Only: Combination oral contraceptives act primarily through the mechanism of gonadotropin suppression due to the estrogenic and progestational activity of the ingredients. Although the primary mechanism of action is inhibition of ovulation, alterations in the genital tract including changes in the cervical mucus (which increase the difficulty of sperm penetration) and the endometrium (which reduce the likelihood of implantation) may also contribute to contraceptive effectiveness.

Clinical Pharmacology Progestogen Oral Contraceptives: The primary mechanism through which MICRONOR prevents conception is not known, but progestogen-only contraceptives are known to alter the cervical mucus, exert a progestational effect on the endometrium, interfering with implantation, and, in some patients, suppress ovulation.

Indications and Usage: ORTHO-NOVUM 10/11□21, ORTHO-NOVUM 10/11□28, ORTHO-NOVUM 1/35□21, ORTHO-NOVUM 1/35□28, MODICON 21, MODICON 28, ORTHO-NOVUM 1/50□21, ORTHO-NOVUM 1/50□28, ORTHO-NOVUM 1/80□21, ORTHO-NOVUM 1/80□28, and MICRONOR are indicated for the prevention of pregnancy in women who elect to use oral contraceptives as a method of contraception.

ORTHO-NOVUM 2 mg□21 is indicated for the treatment of hypermenorrhea. ORTHO-NOVUM 2 mg□21 is indicated for the prevention of pregnancy in women who elect to use oral contraceptives as a method of contraception. (See first paragraph immediately following the opening WARNINGS statement.)

Oral contraceptives are highly effective. The pregnancy rate in women using conventional combination oral contraceptives (containing 35 mcg or more of ethinyl estradiol or 50 mcg or more of mestranol) is generally reported as less than one pregnancy per 100 woman-years of use. Slightly higher rates (somewhat more than one pregnancy per 100 woman-years of use) are reported for some combination products containing 35 mcg or less of ethinyl estradiol, and rates on the order of three pregnancies per 100 woman-years are reported for the progestogen-only oral contraceptives.

These rates are derived from separate studies conducted by different investigators in several population groups and cannot be compared precisely. Furthermore, pregnancy rates tend to be lower as clinical studies are continued, possibly due to selective retention in the longer studies of those patients who accept the treatment regimen and do not discontinue as a result of adverse reactions, pregnancy or other reasons.

The ORTHO-NOVUM 10/11□21 Tablet regimen consists of 10 white tablets followed by 11 peach tablets.

The ORTHO-NOVUM 10/11□28 Tablet regimen consists of 10 white tablets followed by 11 peach tablets and 7 green placebo tablets.

10 WHITE TABLETS

In clinical trials with a formulation containing 0.5 mg of norethindrone and 0.035 mg of ethinyl estradiol, 1,168 patients completed 16,345 cycles of use and a total of three pregnancies was reported. This represents a pregnancy rate of 0.22 per 100 woman-years.

11 PEACH TABLETS

In clinical trials with a formulation containing 1 mg norethindrone and 0.035 mg of ethinyl estradiol, 940 subjects completed 14,366 cycles of use. Two pregnancies were reported for a pregnancy rate of 0.17 per 100 woman-years.

The dropout rate for medical reasons, as observed in the clinical trials conducted with ORTHO-NOVUM 1/35 and MODICON, appears to be somewhat higher than observed with higher dose combination products. The dropout rate due to menstrual disorders and irregularities was also somewhat higher, dropouts being equally split between menstrual disorders and irregularities and other medical reasons attributable to the drug.

In clinical trials with ORTHO-NOVUM 1/35□21 and ORTHO-NOVUM 1/35□28, 940 subjects completed 14,366 cycles of use. Two pregnancies were reported for a pregnancy rate of 0.17 per 100 woman-years.

In clinical trials with MODICON and MODICON 28, 1,168 patients completed 16,345 cycles of use, and a total of three pregnancies was reported. This represents a pregnancy rate of 0.22 per 100 woman-years.

In clinical trials with ORTHO-NOVUM 1/50□21, 3,852 patients completed 45,937 cycles, and a total of 10 pregnancies was reported. This represents a pregnancy rate of 0.26 per 100 woman-years.

In clinical trials with ORTHO-NOVUM 1/50□28, 1,590 patients completed 7,330 cycles, and a total of three pregnancies was reported. This represents a pregnancy rate of 0.5 per 100 woman-years.

In clinical trials with ORTHO-NOVUM 1/80□21, and ORTHO-NOVUM 1/80□28, 3,464 patients completed 34,068 cycles, and a total of five pregnancies was reported. This represents a pregnancy rate of 0.18 per 100 woman-years.

In clinical trials with ORTHO-NOVUM 2 mg□20, 6,097 patients completed 121,233 cycles, and a total of 13 pregnancies was reported. This represents a pregnancy rate of 0.13 per 100 woman-years. In clinical trials with ORTHO-NOVUM 2 mg□21, 965 patients completed 3,743 cycles, and no pregnancies were reported. This represents a pregnancy rate of 0.0 per 100 woman-years.

In clinical trials with MICRONOR, 2,963 patients completed 25,901 cycles of therapy, and a total of 55 pregnancies was reported. This represents an average pregnancy rate of 2.54 per 100 woman-years.

A higher pregnancy rate of 3.72 was recorded in "fresh" patients (those who had never taken oral contraceptives prior to starting MICRONOR therapy) to a large extent because of incorrect tablet intake. This compares to the lower pregnancy rate of 1.95 recorded in "changeover" patients (those switched from other oral contraceptives).

This difference was found to be statistically significant. Furthermore, an even greater statistically significant difference in pregnancy rates between these two groups was found during the first six months of MICRONOR therapy. Therefore, it is especially important for "fresh" patients to strictly adhere to the regimen.

Table 1 gives ranges of pregnancy rates reported in the literature[1] for other means of contraception. The efficacy of these means of contraception (except the IUD) depends upon the degree of adherence to the method.

Table 1
Pregnancies Per 100 Woman-Years

IUD, less than 1–6;
Diaphragm with spermicidal product (creams or jellies), 2–20; Condom, 3–36; Aerosol foams, 2–29; Jellies and creams, 4–36; Periodic abstinence (rhythm) all types, less than 1–47;

1. Calendar method, 14–47;
2. Temperature method, 1–20;
3. Temperature method—intercourse only in postovulatory phase, less than 1–7;
4. Mucus method, 1–25;

No contraception, 60–80.

Dose-Related Risk of Thromboembolism From Oral Contraceptives: Two studies have shown a positive association between the dose of estrogens in oral contraceptives and the risk of thromboembolism.[2,3] For this reason, it is prudent and in keeping with good principles

Continued on next page

Ortho Pharm.—Cont.

of therapeutics to minimize exposure to estrogen. The oral contraceptive product prescribed for any given patient should be that product which contains the least amount of estrogen that is compatible with an acceptable pregnancy rate and patient acceptance. It is recommended that new acceptors of oral contraceptives be started on preparations containing .05 mg or less of estrogen.

Contraindications: Oral contraceptives should not be used in women with any of the following conditions:

1. Thrombophlebitis or thromboembolic disorders.
2. A past history of deep vein thrombophlebitis or thromboembolic disorders.
3. Cerebral vascular or coronary artery disease.
4. Known or suspected carcinoma of the breast.
5. Known or suspected estrogen-dependent neoplasia.
6. Undiagnosed, abnormal genital bleeding.
7. Oral contraceptive tablets may cause fetal harm when administered to a pregnant woman. Oral contraceptive tablets are contraindicated in women who are pregnant. If the patient becomes pregnant while taking this drug, the patient should be apprised of the potential hazard to the fetus (see WARNINGS, No. 5).
8. Benign or malignant liver tumor which developed during the use of oral contraceptives or other estrogen-containing products.

WARNINGS

Cigarette smoking increases the risk of serious cardiovascular side effects from oral contraceptive use. This risk increases with age and with heavy smoking (15 or more cigarettes per day) and is quite marked in women over 35 years of age. Women who use oral contraceptives should be strongly advised not to smoke.

The use of oral contraceptives is associated with increased risk of several serious conditions including thromboembolism, stroke, myocardial infarction, hepatic adenoma, gallbladder disease, hypertension. Practitioners prescribing oral contraceptives should be familiar with the following information relating to these risks.

ORTHO-NOVUM 2 mg□21 should only be used for contraception when lower dose formulations prove unacceptable.

1. THROMBOEMBOLIC DISORDERS AND OTHER VASCULAR PROBLEMS. An increased risk of thromboembolic and thrombotic disease associated with the use of oral contraceptives is well-established. Four principal studies in Great Britain[4,5,6,26] and three in the United States[7–10] have demonstrated an increased risk of fatal and nonfatal venous thromboembolism and stroke, both hemorrhagic and thrombotic. These studies estimate that users of oral contraceptives are 4 to 11 times more likely than nonusers to develop these diseases without evident cause (Tables 2,4). Overall excess mortality due to pulmonary embolism or stroke is on the order of 1.0 to 3.5 deaths annually per 100,000 users and increases with age (Table 3).

Table 2
Hospitalization Rates Due to Venous Thromboembolic Disease[6]

	Admissions annually per 100,000 women, age 20–44
Users of oral contraceptives	45
Nonusers	5

Table 3
Death Rates Due to Pulmonary Embolism or Cerebral Thrombosis[5]—Deaths Annually Per 100,000 Nonpregnant Women

	Age 20 to 34	Age 35 to 44
Users of oral contraceptives	1.5	3.9
Nonusers	.2	.5

Cerebrovascular Disorders: In a collaborative American study[9,10] of cerebrovascular disorders in women with and without predisposing causes, it was estimated that the risk of hemorrhagic stroke was 2.0 times greater in users than in nonusers and the risk of thrombotic stroke was 4.0 to 9.5 times greater in users than in nonusers (Table 4).

Table 4
Summary of Relative Risk of Thromboembolic Disorders and Other Vascular Problems in Oral Contraceptive Users Compared to Nonusers

	Relative risk, times greater
Idiopathic thromboembolic disease	4–11
Post surgery thromboembolic complications	4–6
Thrombotic stroke	4–9.5
Hemorrhagic stroke	2
Myocardial infarction	2–12

Myocardial Infarction: An increased risk of myocardial infarction associated with the use of oral contraceptives has been reported[11,12,13] confirming a previously suspected association (Tables 5 & 6). These studies, conducted in the United Kingdom, found, as expected, that the greater the number of underlying risk factors for coronary artery disease (cigarette smoking, hypertension, hypercholesterolemia, obesity, diabetes, history of preeclamptic toxemia), the higher the risk of developing myocardial infarction, regardless of whether the patient was an oral contraceptive user or not. Oral contraceptives, however, were found to be a clear additional risk factor.

The annual excess case rate (increased risk) of myocardial infarction (fatal and nonfatal) in oral contraceptive users was estimated to be approximately 7 cases per 100,000 women users in the 30–39 age group and 67 cases per 100,000 women users in the 40–44 age group.

In terms of relative risk, it has been estimated[52] that oral contraceptive users who do not smoke (smoking is considered a major predisposing condition to myocardial infarction) are about twice as likely to have a fatal myocardial infarction as nonusers who do not smoke. Oral contraceptive users who are also smokers have about a 5-fold increased risk of fatal infarction compared to users who do not smoke, but about a 10- to 12-fold increased risk compared to nonusers who do not smoke. Furthermore, the amount of smoking is also an important factor. In determining the importance of these relative risks, however, the baseline rates for various age groups, as shown in Table 5, must be given serious consideration.

The importance of other predisposing conditions mentioned above in determining relative and absolute risks have not as yet been quantified; it is quite likely that the same synergistic action exists, but perhaps to a lesser extent.

Table 5
Estimated Annual Mortality Rate Per 100,000 Women From Myocardial Infarction By Use Of Oral Contraceptives, Smoking Habits, And Age (in years)

	Myocardial Infarction			
	Women aged 30–39		Women aged 40–44	
Smoking habits	Users	Non-users	Users	Non-users
All smokers	10.2	2.6	62.0	15.9
Heavy[1]	13.0	5.1	78.7	31.3
Light	4.7	.9	28.6	5.7
Nonsmokers	1.8	1.2	10.7	7.4
Smokers and nonsmokers	5.4	1.9	32.8	11.7

[1]Heavy smoker: 15 or more cigarettes per day.
From Jain, A.K., Studies in Family Planning. 8:50, 1977.

[See table below].

Risk of dose: In an analysis of data derived from several national adverse reaction reporting systems,[2] British investigators concluded that the risk of thromboembolism including coronary thrombosis is directly related to the dose of estrogen used in oral contraceptives. Preparations containing 100 mcg or more of estrogen were associated with a higher risk of thromboembolism than those containing 50–80 mcg of estrogen. Their analysis did suggest, however, that the quantity of estrogen may not be the sole factor involved. This finding has been confirmed in the United States.[3] Careful epidemiological studies to determine the degree of thromboembolic risk associated with progestogen-only oral contraceptives have not been performed. Cases of thromboembolic disease have been reported in women using these products, and they should not be presumed to be free of excess risk.

The risk of thromboembolic and thrombotic disorders, in both users and nonusers of oral contraceptives, increases with age. Oral contraceptives are, however, an independent risk factor for these events.

Estimate of Excess Mortality From Circulatory Diseases: A large prospective study[53] carried out in the United Kingdom estimated the mortality rate per 100,000 women per year from diseases of the circulatory system for users and nonusers of oral contraceptives according to age, smoking habits, and duration of use. The overall excess death rate annually from circulatory diseases for oral contraceptive users was estimated to be 20 per 100,000 (ages 15–34—5/100,000; ages 35–44—33/100,000; ages 45–49—140/100,000), the risk being concentrated in older women, in those with a long duration of use and in cigarette smokers. It was not possible, however, to examine the interrelationships of age, smoking, and duration of use, nor to compare the effects of continuous versus intermittent use. Although the study showed a 10-fold increase in death due to circulatory diseases in users for five or more years, all of these deaths occurred in women 35 or older. Until larger numbers of women under 35 with continuous use for five or more years are available, it is not possible to assess the magnitude of the relative risk for this younger age group.

Another study published at the same time confirms a previously reported increase of mortality in pill users from cardiovascular disease.[54]

The available data from a variety of sources have been analyzed[14] to estimate the risk of death associated with various methods of contraception. The estimates of risk of death for

Table 6
Myocardial Infarction Rates in Users And Nonusers Of Oral Contraceptives in Britain[11,12,13]—Cases Annually Per 100,000 Women

	Nonfatal		Fatal	
	Age 30 to 39	Age 40 to 44	Age 30 to 39	Age 40 to 44
Users of oral contraceptives	5.6	56.9	5.4	32.0
Nonusers of oral contraceptives	2.1	9.9	1.9	12.0
Relative risk	2.7	5.7	2.8	2.8

each method include the combined risk of the contraceptive method (e.g., thromboembolic and thrombotic disease in the case of oral contraceptives) plus the risk attributable to pregnancy or abortion in the event of method failure. This latter risk varies with the effectiveness of the contraceptive method. The findings of this analysis are shown in Figure 1 below.[14]

The study concluded that the mortality associated with all methods of birth control is low and below that associated with childbirth, with the exception of oral contraceptives in women over 40 who smoke. (The rates given for pill only/smokers for each age group are for smokers as a class. For "heavy" smokers [more than 15 cigarettes a day], the rates given would be about double; for "light" smokers [less than 15 cigarettes a day], about 50 percent.)

The mortality associated with oral contraceptive use in nonsmokers over 40 is higher than with any other method of contraception in that age group.

The lowest mortality is associated with the condom or diaphragm backed up by early abortion.

The risk of thromboembolic and thrombotic disease associated with oral contraceptives increases with age after approximately age 30 and, for myocardial infarction, is further increased by hypertension, hypercholesterolemia, obesity, diabetes, or history of preeclamptic toxemia and especially by cigarette smoking. The risk of myocardial infarction in oral contraceptive users is substantially increased in women age 40 and over, especially those with other risk factors.

Based on the data currently available, the following chart gives a gross estimate of the risk of death from circulatory disorders associated with the use of oral contraceptives:

Smoking Habits and Other Predisposing Conditions—Risk Associated With Use Of Oral Contraceptives

Age	Below 30	30–39	40+
Heavy smokers	C	B	A
Light smokers	D	C	B
Nonsmokers (no predisposing conditions)	D	C,D	C
Nonsmokers (other predisposing conditions)	C	C,B	B,A

A—Use associated with very high risk.
B—Use associated with high risk.
C—Use associated with moderate risk.
D—Use associated with low risk.

The physician and the patient should be alert to the earliest manifestations of thromboembolic and thrombotic disorders (e.g., thrombophlebitis, pulmonary embolism, cerebrovascular insufficiency, coronary occlusion, retinal thrombosis, and mesenteric thrombosis). Should any of these occur or be suspected, the drug should be discontinued immediately.

A four- to six-fold increased risk of post surgery thromboembolic complications has been reported in oral contraceptives users.[15,16] If feasible, oral contraceptives should be discontinued at least four weeks before surgery of a type associated with an increased risk of thromboembolism or prolonged immobilization.

2. OCULAR LESIONS. There have been reports of neuro-ocular lesions such as optic neuritis or retinal thrombosis associated with the use of oral contraceptives. Discontinue oral contraceptive medication if there is unexplained, sudden or gradual, partial or complete loss of vision; onset of proptosis or diplopia; papilledema; or retinal vascular lesions and institute appropriate diagnostic and therapeutic measures.

3. CARCINOMA. Long-term continuous administration of either natural or synthetic estrogen in certain animal species increases the frequency of carcinoma of the breast, cervix, vagina, and liver. Certain synthetic progestogens, none currently contained in oral contraceptives, have been noted to increase the incidence of mammary nodules, benign and malignant, in dogs.

In humans, three case control studies have reported an increased risk of endometrial carcinoma associated with the prolonged use of exogenous estrogen in postmenopausal women.[17,18,19] One publication[20] reported on the first 21 cases submitted by physicians to a registry of cases of adenocarcinoma of the endometrium in women under 40 on oral contraceptives. Of the cases found in women without predisposing risk factors for adenocarcinoma of the endometrium (e.g., irregular bleeding at the time oral contraceptives were first given, polycystic ovaries), nearly all occurred in women who had used a sequential oral contraceptive. These products are no longer marketed. No evidence has been reported suggesting an increased risk of endometrial cancer in users of conventional combination or progestogen-only oral contraceptives.

Several studies[8,21–24] have found no increases in breast cancer in women taking oral contraceptives or estrogens. One study[25], however, while also noting no overall increased risk of breast cancer in women treated with oral contraceptives, found an excess risk in the subgroups of oral contraceptive users with documented benign breast disease. A reduced occurrence of benign breast tumors in users of oral contraceptives has been well-documented.[8,21,25,26,27]

In summary, there is at present no confirmed evidence from human studies of an increased risk of cancer associated with oral contraceptives. Close clinical surveillance of all women taking oral contraceptives is, nevertheless, essential. In all cases of undiagnosed persistent or recurrent abnormal vaginal bleeding, appropriate diagnostic measures should be taken to rule out malignancy. Women with a strong family history of breast cancer or who have breast nodules, fibrocystic disease or abnormal mammograms should be monitored with particular care if they elect to use oral contraceptives instead of other methods of contraception.

Figure 1. Estimated annual number of deaths associated with control of fertility and no control per 100,000 nonsterile women, by regimen of control and age of woman.

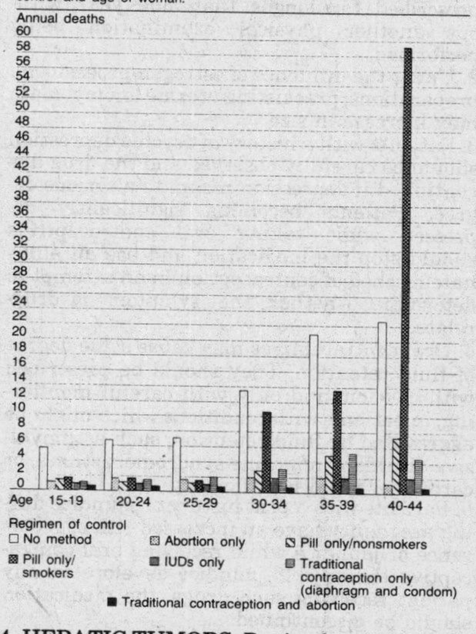

Annual deaths

Age 15-19 20-24 25-29 30-34 35-39 40-44

Regimen of control: No method; Abortion only; Pill only/nonsmokers; Pill only/smokers; IUDs only; Traditional contraception only (diaphragm and condom); Traditional contraception and abortion

4. HEPATIC TUMORS. Benign hepatic adenomas have been found to be associated with the use of oral contraceptives.[28,29,30,46] One study[46] showed that oral contraceptive formulations with high hormonal potency were associated with a higher risk than lower potency formulations and use of oral contraceptives with high hormonal potency and age over 30 years may further increase the woman's risk of hepatocellular adenoma. Although benign, hepatic adenomas may rupture and may cause death through intra-abdominal hemorrhage. This has been reported in short-term as well as long-term users of oral contraceptives. Two studies relate risk with duration of use of the contraceptive, the risk being much greater after four or more years of oral contraceptive use.[30,46] While hepatic adenoma is a rare lesion, it should be considered in women presenting abdominal pain and tenderness, abdominal mass or shock.

A few cases of hepatocellular carcinoma have been reported in women taking oral contraceptives. The relationship of these drugs to this type of malignancy is not known at this time.

5. USE IN OR IMMEDIATELY PRECEDING PREGNANCY, BIRTH DEFECTS IN OFFSPRING, AND MALIGNANCY IN FEMALE OFFSPRING. The use of female sex hormones—both estrogenic and progestational agents—during early pregnancy may seriously damage the offspring. It has been shown that females exposed in utero to diethylstilbestrol, a nonsteroidal estrogen, have an increased risk of developing in later life a form of vaginal or cervical cancer that is ordinarily extremely rare.[31,32] This risk has been estimated to be of the order of 1 to 4 in 1000 exposures.[33,47] Although there is no evidence at the present time that oral contraceptives further enhance the risk of developing this type of malignancy, such patients should be monitored with particular care if they elect to use oral contraceptives instead of other methods of contraception. Furthermore, a high percentage of such exposed women (from 30 to 90%) have been found to have epithelial changes of the vagina and cervix.[34–38] Although these changes are histologically benign, it is not known whether this condition is a precursor of vaginal malignancy. Male children so exposed may develop abnormalities of the urogenital tract.[48,49,50] Although similar data are not available with the use of other estrogens, it cannot be presumed that they would not induce similar changes.

An increased risk of congenital anomalies, including heart defects and limb defects, has been reported with the use of sex hormones, including oral contraceptives, in pregnancy.[39–42,51] One case control study[42] has estimated a 4.7-fold increase in risk of limb-reduction defects in infants exposed in utero to sex hormones (oral contraceptives, hormonal withdrawal tests for pregnancy or attempted treatment for threatened abortion). Some of these exposures were very short and involved only a few days of treatment. The data suggest that the risk of limb-reduction defects in exposed fetuses is somewhat less than one in 1,000 live births.

In the past, female sex hormones have been used during pregnancy in an attempt to treat threatened or habitual abortion. There is considerable evidence that estrogens are ineffective for these indications, and there is no evidence from well-controlled studies that progestogens are effective for these uses.

There is some evidence that triploidy and possibly other types of polyploidy are increased among abortuses from women who become pregnant soon after ceasing oral contraceptives.[43] Embryos with these anomalies are virtually always aborted spontaneously. Whether there is an overall increase in spontaneous abortion of pregnancies conceived soon after stopping oral contraceptives is unknown. It is recommended that for any patient who has missed two consecutive periods, pregnancy should be ruled out before continuing the contraceptive regimen. If the patient has not adhered to the prescribed schedule, the possibility of pregnancy should be considered at the

Continued on next page

Ortho Pharm.—Cont.

time of the first missed period (or after 45 days from the last menstrual period if the progestogen-only oral contraceptives are used), and further use of oral contraceptives should be withheld until pregnancy has been ruled out. If pregnancy is confirmed, the patient should be apprised of the potential risks to the fetus and the advisability of continuation of the pregnancy should be discussed in the light of these risks.
It is also recommended that women who discontinue oral contraceptives with the intent of becoming pregnant use an alternate form of contraception for a period of time before attempting to conceive. Many clinicians recommend three months although no precise information is available on which to base this recommendation.
The administration of progestogen-only or progestogen-estrogen combinations to induce withdrawal bleeding should not be used as a test of pregnancy.
6. GALLBLADDER DISEASE. Studies[8,23,26] report an increased risk of surgically confirmed gallbladder disease in users of oral contraceptives and estrogens. In one study, an increased risk appeared after two years of use and doubled after four or five years of use. In one of the other studies, an increased risk was apparent between six and twelve months of use.
7. CARBOHYDRATE AND LIPID METABOLIC EFFECTS. A decrease in glucose tolerance has been observed in a significant percentage of patients on oral contraceptives. For this reason, prediabetic and diabetic patients should be carefully observed while receiving oral contraceptives.
An increase in triglycerides and total phospholipids has been observed in patients receiving oral contraceptives.[44] The clinical significance of this finding remains to be defined.
8. ELEVATED BLOOD PRESSURE. An increase in blood pressure has been reported in patients receiving oral contraceptives.[26] In some women hypertension may occur within a few months of beginning oral contraceptive use. In the first year of use, the prevalence of women with hypertension is low in users and may be no higher than that of a comparable group of nonusers. The prevalence in users increases, however, with longer exposure, and in the fifth year of use is two and a half to three times the reported prevalence in the first year. Age is also strongly correlated with the development of hypertension in oral contraceptive users. Women who previously have had hypertension during pregnancy may be more likely to develop elevation of blood pressure when given oral contraceptives. Hypertension that develops as a result of taking oral contraceptives usually returns to normal after discontinuing the drug.
9. HEADACHE. The onset or exacerbation of migraine or development of headache of a new pattern which is recurrent, persistent, or severe, requires discontinuation of oral contraceptives and evaluation of the cause.
10. BLEEDING IRREGULARITIES. Breakthrough bleeding, spotting, and amenorrhea are frequent reasons for patients discontinuing oral contraceptives. In breakthrough bleeding, as in all cases of irregular bleeding from the vagina, nonfunctional causes should be borne in mind. In undiagnosed persistent or recurrent abnormal bleeding from the vagina, adequate diagnostic measures are indicated to rule out pregnancy or malignancy. If pathology has been excluded, time or a change to another formulation may solve the problem. Changing to an oral contraceptive with a higher estrogen content, while potentially useful in minimizing menstrual irregularity, should be done only if necessary since this may increase the risk of thromboembolic disease.

An alteration in menstrual patterns is likely to occur in women using progestogen-only oral contraceptives. The amount and duration of flow, cycle length, breakthrough bleeding, spotting and amenorrhea will probably be quite variable. Bleeding irregularities occur more frequently with the use of progestogen-only oral contraceptives than with the combinations and the dropout rate due to such conditions is higher.
Women with a past history of oligomenorrhea or secondary amenorrhea or young women without regular cycles may have a tendency to remain anovulatory or to become amenorrheic after dicontinuation of oral contraceptives. Women with these preexisting problems should be advised of this possibility and encouraged to use other contraceptive methods. Postuse anovulation, possibly prolonged, may also occur in women without previous irregularities.
11. ECTOPIC PREGNANCY. Ectopic as well as intrauterine pregnancy may occur in contraceptive failures. However, in progestogen-only oral contraceptive failures, the ratio of ectopic to intrauterine pregnancies is higher than in women who are not receiving oral contraceptives, since the drugs are more effective in preventing intrauterine than ectopic pregnancies.
12. BREAST FEEDING. Oral contraceptives given in the postpartum period may interfere with lactation. There may be a decrease in the quantity and quality of the breast milk. Furthermore, a small fraction of the hormonal agents in oral contraceptives has been identified in the milk of mothers receiving these drugs.[45] The effects, if any, on the breast-fed child have not been determined. If feasible, the use of oral contraceptives should be deferred until the infant has been weaned.

Precautions:

General

1. A complete medical and family history should be taken prior to the initiation of oral contraceptives. The pretreatment and periodic physical examinations should include special reference to blood pressure, breasts, abdomen and pelvic organs, including Papanicolaou smear and relevant laboratory tests. As a general rule, oral contraceptives should not be prescribed for longer than one year without another physical examination being performed.
2. Under the influence of estrogen-progestogen preparations, preexisting uterine leiomyomata may increase in size.
3. Patients with a history of psychic depression should be carefully observed and the drug discontinued if depression recurs to a serious degree. Patients becoming significantly depressed while taking oral contraceptives should stop the medication and use an alternate method of contraception in an attempt to determine whether the symptom is drug-related.
4. Oral contraceptives may cause some degree of fluid retention. They should be prescribed with caution, and only with careful monitoring, in patients with conditions which might be aggravated by fluid retention, such as convulsive disorders, migraine syndrome, asthma, or cardiac or renal insufficiency.
5. Patients with a past history of jaundice during pregnancy have an increased risk of recurrence of jaundice while receiving oral contraceptive therapy. If jaundice develops in any patient receiving such drugs, the medication should be discontinued.
6. Steroid hormones may be poorly metabolized in patients with impaired liver function and should be administered with caution in such patients.
7. Oral contraceptive users may have disturbances in normal tryptophan metabolism which may result in a relative pyridoxine deficiency. The clinical significance of this is yet to be determined.
8. Serum folate levels may be depressed by oral contraceptive therapy. Since the pregnant woman is predisposed to the development of folate deficiency and the incidence of folate deficiency increases with increasing gestation, it is possible that if a woman becomes pregnant shortly after stopping oral contraceptives, she may have a greater chance of developing folate deficiency and complications attributed to this deficiency.

Information for the Patient

(See Patient Labeling printed below.)

Drug Interactions: Reduced efficacy and increased incidence of breakthrough bleeding have been associated with concomitant use of rifampin. A similar association has been suggested with barbiturates, phenylbutazone, phenytoin sodium, ampicillin, and tetracycline.

Drug/Laboratory Test Interactions: The pathologist should be advised of oral contraceptive therapy when relevant specimens are submitted.
Certain endocrine and liver function tests and blood components may be affected by estrogen-containing oral contraceptives:

a. Increased sulfobromophthalein retention.
b. Increased prothrombin and factors VII, VIII, IX, and X; decreased antithrombin 3; increased norepinephrine-induced platelet aggregability.
c. Increased thyroid-binding globulin (TBG) leading to increased circulating total thyroid hormone, as measured by protein-bound iodine (PBI), T4 by column, or T4 by radioimmunoassay. Free T3 resin uptake is decreased, reflecting the elevated TBG, free T4 concentration is unaltered.
d. Decreased pregnanediol excretion.
e. Reduced response to metyrapone test.

Carcinogenesis, Mutagenesis, Impairment of Fertility: See WARNINGS section for information on carcinogenesis, mutagenesis and impairment of fertility.

Pregnancy: Pregnancy category X. See CONTRAINDICATIONS and WARNINGS.

Nursing Mothers: Because of the potential for tumorigenicity shown for oral contraceptives in animal and human studies, a decision should be made whether to discontinue the drug, taking into account the importance of the drug to the mother (see WARNINGS).

Adverse Reactions: An increased risk of the following serious adverse reactions has been associated with the use of oral contraceptives (see WARNINGS):

Thrombophlebitis. Hypertension.
Pulmonary embolism. Gallbladder disease.
Coronary thrombosis. Liver tumors.
Cerebral thrombosis. Congenital anomalies.
Cerebral hemorrhage.

There is evidence of an association between the following conditions and the use of oral contraceptives, although additional confirmatory studies are needed.

Mesenteric thrombosis.
Neuro-ocular lesion, e.g., retinal thrombosis and optic neuritis.

The following adverse reactions have been reported in patients receiving oral contraceptives and are believed to be drug-related:

Nausea and/or vomiting, usually the most common adverse reactions, occur in approximately 10 percent or less of patients during the first cycle. Other reactions, as a general rule, are seen much less frequently or only occasionally.
Gastrointestinal symptoms (such as abdominal cramps and bloating).
Breakthrough bleeding.
Spotting.
Change in menstrual flow.
Dysmenorrhea.
Amenorrhea during and after treatment.
Temporary infertility after discontinuance of treatment.

Edema.
Chloasma or melasma which may persist.
Breast changes: tenderness, enlargement, and secretion.
Change in weight (increase or decrease).
Change in cervical erosion and cervical secretion.
Possible diminution in lactation when given immediately postpartum.
Cholestatic jaundice.
Migraine.
Increase in size of uterine leiomyomata.
Rash (allergic).
Mental depression.
Reduced tolerance to carbohydrates.
Vaginal candidiasis.
Change in corneal curvature (steepening).
Intolerance to contact lenses.

The following adverse reactions have been reported in users of oral contraceptives, and the association has been neither confirmed nor refuted:

Premenstrual-like syndrome.
Cataracts.
Changes in libido.
Chorea.
Changes in appetite.
Cystitis-like syndrome.
Headache.
Nervousness.
Dizziness.
Hirsutism.
Loss of scalp hair.
Erythema multiforme.
Erythema nodosum.
Hemorrhagic eruption.
Vaginitis.
Porphyria.
Impaired renal function.

Overdosage: Serious ill effects have not been reported following acute ingestion of large doses of oral contraceptives by young children. Overdosage may cause nausea, and withdrawal bleeding may occur in females.

Dosage and Administration: To achieve maximum contraceptive effectiveness, ORTHO-NOVUM Tablets, MODICON Tablets and MICRONOR must be taken exactly as directed and at intervals not exceeding 24 hours.

21-DAY REGIMEN (Sunday Start)

When taking ORTHO-NOVUM 10/11□21, the first white tablet should be taken on the first Sunday after menstruation begins. If period begins on Sunday, the first white tablet is taken on that day. Tablets are taken as follows: One white tablet daily for 10 days, then one peach tablet daily for 11 days. For subsequent cycles, no tablets are taken for 7 days, then a white tablet is taken the next day (Sunday) etc. Contraceptives reliance should not be placed on these products until after the first 7 consecutive days of administration. The use of ORTHO-NOVUM 10/11□21 for contraception may be initiated postpartum. When the tablets are administered during the postpartum period, the increased risk of thromboembolic disease associated with the postpartum period must be considered. (See CONTRAINDICATIONS, WARNINGS, and PRECAUTIONS concerning thromboembolic disease.) The possibility of ovulation and conception prior to initiation of medication should be considered. If the patient misses more than one tablet, the patient should begin taking tablets again as soon as remembered and another method of contraception used for the balance of that tablet cycle.

21-DAY REGIMEN (21 days on, 7 days off)

The dosage of ORTHO-NOVUM 1/35□21, MODICON 21, ORTHO-NOVUM 1/50□21, ORTHO-NOVUM 1/80□21 and ORTHO-NOVUM 2 mg□21 for the initial cycle of therapy is one tablet administered daily from the 5th day through the 25th day of the menstrual cycle, counting the first day of menstrual flow as "Day 1." The use of these products for contraception may be initiated postpartum. When the tablets are administered during the postpartum period, the increased risk of thromboembolic disease associated with the postpartum period must be considered. (See CONTRAINDICATIONS, WARNINGS, and PRECAUTIONS concerning thromboembolic disease.) If ORTHO-NOVUM 1/35□21, MODICON 21, ORTHO-NOVUM 1/50□21, ORTHO-NOVUM 1/80□21, and ORTHO-NOVUM 2 mg□21 are first taken later than the fifth day of the first menstrual cycle of medication or postpartum, contraceptive reliance should not be placed on these products until after the first seven consecutive days of administration. For subsequent cycles, no tablets are taken for 7 days, then a new course is started of one tablet a day for 21 days. The dosage regimen then continues with 7 days of no medication, followed by 21 days of medication, instituting a three-weeks-on, one-week-off dosage regimen. The possibility of ovulation and conception prior to initiation of medication should be considered. If the patient misses more than one tablet, the patient should begin taking tablets again as soon as remembered and another method of contraception used for the balance of that tablet cycle.

ORTHO-NOVUM 2 mg□21: Following three months of treatment of hypermenorrhea, medication may be discontinued to determine the need for further therapy.

(See discussion of Dose-Related Risk of Thromboembolism from Oral Contraceptives.)

28-DAY REGIMEN (Sunday Start)

When taking ORTHO-NOVUM 10/11□28, the first white tablet should be taken on the first Sunday after menstruation begins. If period begins on Sunday, the first white tablet is taken on that day. Tablets are taken without interruption as follows: one white tablet daily for 10 days, one peach tablet daily for 11 days, then one green tablet daily for 7 days. After 28 tablets have been taken, a white tablet is then taken the next day (Sunday) etc.

When taking ORTHO-NOVUM 1/35□28, the first peach tablet should be taken on the first Sunday after mestruation begins. When taking MODICON 28 or ORTHO-NOVUM 1/80□28, the first white tablet should be taken on the first Sunday after menstruation begins. When taking ORTHO-NOVUM 1/50□28, the first yellow tablet should be taken on the first Sunday after menstruation begins. If period begins on Sunday, the first peach tablet, white tablet or yellow tablet is taken on that day. Tablets are taken without interruption as follows: One peach, white or yellow tablet daily for 21 days, then one green tablet daily for 7 days. After 28 tablets have been taken, a peach, white or yellow tablet is then taken the next day (Sunday) etc. Contraceptive reliance should not be placed on these products until after the first 7 consecutive days of administration.

The use of ORTHO-NOVUM 10/11□28, ORTHO-NOVUM 1/35□28, MODICON 28, ORTHO-NOVUM 1/50□28, and ORTHO-NOVUM 1/80□28 for contraception may be initiated postpartum. When the tablets are administered during the postpartum period, the increased risk of thromboembolic disease associated with the postpartum period must be considered. (See CONTRAINDICATIONS, WARNINGS, and PRECAUTIONS concerning thromboembolic disease.) The possibility of ovulation and conception prior to initiation of medication should be considered. If the patient misses more than one tablet, the patient should begin taking tablets again as soon as remembered and another method of contraception used for the balance of that tablet cycle.

MICRONOR (Continuous Regimen)

MICRONOR (norethindrone) is administered on a continuous daily dosage regimen starting on the first day of menstruation, i.e., one tablet each day, every day of the year. Tablets should be taken at the same time each day and continued daily. The patient should be advised that if prolonged bleeding occurs, she should consult her physician.

The use of MICRONOR for contraception may be initiated postpartum (see WARNINGS section). When MICRONOR is administered during the postpartum period, the increased risk of thromboembolic disease associated with the postpartum period must be considered. (See CONTRAINDICATIONS, WARNINGS, and PRECAUTIONS concerning thromboembolic disease.)

If the patient misses one tablet, MICRONOR should be discontinued immediately and a method of nonhormonal contraception should be used until menses has appeared or pregnancy has been excluded.

Alternatively, if the patient has taken the tablets correctly, and if menses does not appear when expected, a nonhormonal method of contraception should be substituted until an appropriate diagnostic procedure is performed to rule out pregnancy.

All Oral Contraceptives

Breakthrough bleeding, spotting, and amenorrhea are frequent reasons for patients discontinuing oral contraceptives. In breakthrough bleeding, as in all cases of irregular bleeding from the vagina, nonfunctional causes should be borne in mind. In undiagnosed persistent or recurrent abnormal bleeding from the vagina, adequate diagnostic measures are indicated to rule out pregnancy or malignancy. If pathology has been excluded, time or a change to another formulation may solve the problem. Changing to an oral contraceptive with a higher estrogen content, while potentially useful in minimizing menstrual irregularity, should be done only if necessary since this may increase the risk of thromboembolic disease.

Use of oral contraceptives in the event of a missed menstrual period:

1. If the patient has not adhered to the prescribed dosage regimen, the possibility of pregnancy should be considered after the first missed period (or after 45 days from the last menstrual period if the progestogen-only oral contraceptives are used) and oral contraceptives should be withheld until pregnancy has been ruled out.
2. If the patient has adhered to the prescribed regimen and misses two consecutive periods, pregnancy should be ruled out before continuing the contraceptive regimen.

How Supplied: ORTHO-NOVUM 10/11□21 Tablets are available in a DIALPAK* Tablet Dispenser containing 21 tablets. Each white tablet contains 0.5 mg of the progestational compound, norethindrone, together with a 0.035 mg of the estrogenic compound, ethinyl estradiol. Each peach tablet contains 1 mg of the progestational compound, norethindrone, together with 0.035 mg of the estrogenic compound, ethinyl estradiol. The white tablets are unscored with "Ortho" and "535" debossed on each side; the peach tablets are unscored with "Ortho" and "135" debossed on each side.

ORTHO-NOVUM 10/11□21 is available for clinic usage in a VERIDATE* Tablet Dispenser (unfilled) and VERIDATE Refills.

ORTHO-NOVUM 10/11□28 Tablets are available in a DIALPAK Tablet Dispenser containing 28 tablets. Each white tablet contains 0.5 mg of the progestational compound, norethindrone, together with 0.035 mg of the estrogenic compound, ethinyl estradiol. Each peach tablet contains 1 mg of the progestational compound, norethindrone, together with 0.035 mg of the estrogenic compound, ethinyl estradiol. Each green tablet contains inert ingredients. The white tablets are unscored with "Ortho" and "535" debossed on each side; the peach tablets are unscored with "Ortho" and "135" debossed on each side.

ORTHO-NOVUM 10/11□28 is available for clinic usage in VERIDATE Tablet Dispenser (unfilled) and VERIDATE Refills.

Continued on next page

Ortho Pharm.—Cont.

ORTHO-NOVUM 1/35□21 Tablets (as peach unscored tablets with "Ortho" and "135" debossed on each side) are available in a DIALPAK Tablet Dispenser containing 21 tablets. Each peach tablet contains 1 mg of the progestational compound, norethindrone, together with 0.035 mg of the estrogenic compound, ethinyl estradiol.

ORTHO-NOVUM 1/35□21 is available for clinic usage in a VERIDATE Tablet Dispenser (unfilled) and VERIDATE Refills.

ORTHO-NOVUM 1/35□28 Tablets (as peach unscored tablets with "Ortho" and "135" debossed on each side) are available in a DIALPAK Tablet Dispenser containing 28 tablets, 21 peach norethindrone with ethinyl estradiol tablets, and 7 green tablets containing inert ingredients. Each peach ORTHO-NOVUM 1/35□28 Tablet contains 1 mg of the progestational compound, norethindrone, together with 0.035 mg of the estrogenic compound, ethinyl estradiol.

ORTHO-NOVUM 1/35□28 is available for clinic usage in a VERIDATE Tablet Dispenser (unfilled) and VERIDATE Refills.

MODICON 21 Tablets (as white unscored tablets with "Ortho" and "535" debossed on each side) are available in a DIALPAK Tablet Dispenser containing 21 tablets. Each white tablet contains 0.5 mg of the progestational compound, norethindrone, together with 0.035 mg of the estrogenic compound, ethinyl estradiol.

MODICON 21 is available for clinic usage in a VERIDATE Tablet Dispenser (unfilled) and VERIDATE Refills.

MODICON 28 Tablets (as white unscored tablets with "Ortho" and "535" debossed on each side) are available in a DIALPAK Tablet Dispenser containing 28 tablets, 21 white norethindrone with ethinyl estradiol tablets and 7 green tablets containing inert ingredients. Each white MODICON 28 Tablet contains 0.5 mg of the progestational compound, norethindrone, together with 0.035 mg of the estrogenic compound, ethinyl estradiol.

MODICON 28 is available for clinic usage in a VERIDATE Tablet Dispenser (unfilled) and VERIDATE Refills.

ORTHO-NOVUM 1/50□21 Tablets (as yellow unscored tablets with "Ortho" and "150" debossed on each side) are available in a DIALPAK Tablet Dispenser containing 21 tablets and a dispensing unit which contains one DIALPAK and two refills of 21 tablets each. Each yellow ORTHO-NOVUM 1/50□21 Tablet contains 1 mg of the progestational compound, norethindrone, together with 0.05 mg of the estrogenic compound, mestranol.

ORTHO-NOVUM 1/50□21 is available for clinic usage in a VERIDATE Tablet Dispenser (unfilled) and VERIDATE Refills.

ORTHO-NOVUM 1/50□28 Tablets (as yellow unscored tablets with "Ortho" and "150" debossed on each side) are available in a DIALPAK Tablet Dispenser containing 28 tablets, 21 yellow norethindrone with mestranol tablets and 7 green tablets containing inert ingredients. Each yellow ORTHO-NOVUM 1/50□28 Tablet contains 1 mg of the progestational compound, norethindrone, together with 0.05 mg of the estrogenic compound, mestranol.

ORTHO-NOVUM 1/50□28 is available for clinic usage in a VERIDATE Tablet Dispenser (unfilled) and VERIDATE Refills.

ORTHO-NOVUM 1/80□21 Tablets (as white unscored tablets with "Ortho" and "1" debossed on each side) are available in a DIALPAK Tablet Dispenser containing 21 tablets and a dispensing unit which contains one DIALPAK and two refills of 21 tablets each. Each white ORTHO-NOVUM 1/80□21 Tablet contains 1 mg of the progestational compound, norethindrone, together with 0.08 mg of the estrogenic compound, mestranol.

ORTHO-NOVUM 1/80□21 is available for clinic usage in a VERIDATE Tablet Dispenser (unfilled) and VERIDATE Refills.

ORTHO-NOVUM 1/80□28 Tablets (as white unscored tablets with "Ortho" and "1" debossed on each side) are available in a DIALPAK Tablet Dispenser containing 28 tablets, 21 white norethindrone with mestranol tablets and 7 green tablets containing inert ingredients. Each white ORTHO-NOVUM 1/80□28 Tablet contains 1 mg of the progestational compound, norethindrone, together with 0.08 mg of the estrogenic compound, mestranol.

ORTHO-NOVUM 1/80□28 is available for clinic usage in a VERIDATE Tablet Dispenser (unfilled) and VERIDATE Refills.

ORTHO-NOVUM 2 mg□21 Tablets (as white unscored tablets with "Ortho" and "2" debossed on each side) are available in a DIALPAK Tablet Dispenser containing 21 tablets. Each white ORTHO-NOVUM 2 mg□21 Tablet contains 2 mg of the progestational compound, norethindrone, together with 0.10 mg of the estrogenic compound, mestranol.

MICRONOR Tablets (as lime unscored tablets with "Ortho" and "0.35" debossed on each side) are available in a DIALPAK Tablet Dispenser containing 28 tablets. Each lime MICRONOR Tablet contains 0.35 mg of the progestational compound norethindrone.

MICRONOR is available for clinic usage in a VERIDATE Tablet Dispenser (unfilled) and VERIDATE Refills.

References:

1."Population Reports," Series H, Number 2, May 1974; Series I, Number 1, June 1974; Series B, Number 2, January 1975; Series H, Number 3, 1975; Series H, Number 4, January 1976 (published by the Population Information Program, The George Washington University Medical Center, 2001 S. St. NW, Washington, D.C.). **2.** Inman, W.H.W., M.P. Vessey, B. Westerholm, and A. Engelund, "Thromboembolic disease and the steroidal content of oral contraceptives. A report to the Committee on Safety of Drugs," Brit Med J *2:*203–209, 1970. **3.** Stolley, P.D., J.A. Tonascia, M.S. Tockman, P.E. Sartwell, A.H. Rutledge, and M.P. Jacobs, "Thrombosis with low-estrogen oral contraceptives," Am J Epidemiol *102:*197–208, 1975. **4.** Royal College of General Practitioners, "Oral contraception and thromboembolic disease," J Coll Gen Pract *13:*267–279, 1967. **5.** Inman, W.H.W. and M.P. Vessey, "Investigation of deaths from pulmonary, coronary, and cerebral thrombosis and embolism in women of childbearing age," Brit Med J *2:*193–199, 1968. **6.** Vessey, M.P. and R. Doll, "Investigation of relation between use of oral contraceptives and thromboembolic disease. A further report," Brit Med J *2:*651–657, 1969. **7.** Sartwell, P.E., A.T. Masi, F.G. Arthes, G.R. Greene and H.E. Smith, "Thromboembolism and oral contraceptives: an epidemiological case control study," Am J Epidemiol *90:*365–380, 1969. **8.** Boston Collaborative Drug Surveillance Program, "Oral contraceptives and venous thromboembolic disease, surgically confirmed gall bladder disease and breast tumors," Lancet *1:*1399–1404, 1973. **9.** Collaborative Group for the Study of Stroke in Young Women, "Oral contraception and increased risk of cerebral ischemia or thrombosis," N Engl J Med *288:*871–878, 1973. **10.** Collaborative Group for the Study of Stroke in Young Women, "Oral contraceptives and strokes in young women: associated risk factors," JAMA *231:*718–722, 1975. **11.** Mann, J.I. and W.H.W. Inman, "Oral contraceptives and death from myocardial infarction," Brit Med J *2:*245–248, 1975. **12.** Mann, J.I., W.H.W. Inman, and M. Thorogood, "Oral contraceptive use in older women and fatal myocardial infarction," Brit Med J *2:*445–447, 1976. **13.** Mann. J.I., M.P. Vessey, M. Thorogood, and R. Doll, "Myocardial infarction in young women with special reference to oral contraceptive practice," Brit Med J *2:*241–245, 1975. **14.** Tietze, C., "New Estimate of Mortality Associated with Fertility Control," Family Planning Perspectives Vol. 9, No. 2, 74–76, 1977. **15.** Vessey, M.P., R. Doll, A.S. Fairbairn, and G. Glober, "Post-operative thromboembolism and the use of oral contraceptives," Brit Med J *3:*123–126, 1970. **16.** Greene, G.R., and P.E. Sartwell, "Oral contraceptive use in patients with thromboembolism following surgery, trauma, or infection," Am J Pub Health *62:*680–685, 1972. **17.** Smith, D.C., R. Prentice, D.J. Thompson, and W.L. Herrmann, "Association of exogenous estrogen and endometrial carcinoma," N Engl J Med *293:*1164–1167, 1975. **18.** Ziel, H.K. and W.D. Finkle, "Increased risk of endometrial carcinoma among users of conjugated estrogens," N Engl J Med *293:*1167–1170, 1975. **19.** Mack, T.N., M.C. Pike, B.E. Henderson, R.I. Pfeffer, V.R. Gerkins, M. Arthur, and S.E. Brown, "Estrogens and endometrial cancer in a retirement community," N Engl J Med *294:*1262–1267, 1976. **20.** Silverberg, S.G., and E.L. Makowski, "Endometrial carcinoma in young women taking oral contraceptive agents," Obstet Gynecol *46:*503–506, 1975. **21.** Vessey, M.P., R. Doll, and P.M. Sutton, "Oral contraceptives and breast neoplasia: a retrospective study," Brit Med J *3:*719–724, 1972. **22.** Vessey, M.P., R. Doll, and K. Jones, "Oral contraceptives and breast cancer. Progress report of an epidemiological study," Lancet *1:*941–943, 1975. **23.** Boston Collaborative Drug Surveillance Program, "Surgically confirmed gall bladder disease, venous thromboembolism and breast tumors in relation to postmenopausal estrogen therapy," N Engl J Med *290:*15–19, 1974. **24.** Arthes, F.G., P.E. Sartwell, and E.F. Lewison, "The Pill, estrogens, and the breast. Epidemiological aspects," Cancer *28:*1391–1394, 1971. **25.** Fasal, E., and R.S. Paffenbarger, "Oral contraceptives as related to cancer and benign lesions of the breast," J Natl Cancer Inst *55:*767–773, 1975. **26.** Royal College of General Practitioners, "Oral Contraceptives and Health," London, Pitman, 1974. **27.** Ory, H., P. Cole, B. MacMahon and R. Hoover, "Oral contraceptives and reduced risk of benign breast diseases," N Engl J Med *294:*419–422, 1976. **28.** Baum, J., F. Holtz, J.J. Bookstein, and E.W. Klein, "Possible association between benign hepatomas and oral contraceptives," Lancet *2:*926–928, 1973. **29.** Mays, E.T., W.M. Christopherson, M.M. Mahr, and H.C. Williams, "Hepatic changes in young women ingesting contraceptive steroids. Hepatic hemorrhage and primary hepatic tumors," JAMA *235:*730–732, 1976. **30.** Edmonsen, H.A., B. Henderson, and B. Benton, "Liver-cell adenomas associated with the use of oral contraceptives," N Engl J Med *294:*470–472, 1976. **31.** Herbst, A.L., H. Ulfelder, and D.C. Poskanzer, "Adenocarcinoma of the vagina," N Engl J Med *284:*878-881, 1971. **32.** Greenwald, P., J.J. Barlow, P.C. Nasca, and W. Burnett, "Vaginal cancer after maternal treatment with synthetic estrogens," N Engl J Med *285:*390–392, 1971. **33.** Lanier, A.P., K.L. Noller, D.G. Decker, L. Elveback, and L.T. Kurland, "Cancer and stilbestrol. A follow-up of 1719 persons exposed to estrogen in utero and born 1943–1959," Mayo Clinic Pro *48:*793–799, 1973. **34.** Herbst, A.L., R.J. Kurman, and R.E. Scully, "Vaginal and cervical abnormalities after exposure to stilbestrol in utero," Obstet Gynecol *40:*287–298, 1972. **35.** Herbst, A.L., S.J. Robboy, G.J. Macdonald, and R.E. Scully, "The effects of local progesterone on stilbestrol-associated vaginal adenosis," Am J Obstet Gynecol *118:*607–615, 1974. **36.** Herbst, A.L., D.C. Poskanzer, S.J. Robboy, L. Friedlander, and R.E. Scully, "Prenatal exposure to stilbestrol: a prospective comparison of exposed female offspring with unexposed controls," N Engl J Med *292:*334–339, 1975. **37.** Stafi, A., R.F. Mattingly, D.V. Foley, W. Fetherston, "Clinical diagnosis of vaginal adenosis," Obstet Gynecol *43:*118–128, 1974. **38.** Sherman, A.I., M. Goldrath, A. Berlin, V. Vakhariya, F. Banooni, W. Michaels, P. Goodman, and S. Brown, "Cervical-vaginal adenosis after in utero exposure to synthetic estrogens," Obstet Gynecol *44:*531–545, 1974. **39.** Gal, I., B. Kirman, and J. Stern, "Hormone pregnancy tests and congenital malformation," Nature *216:*83, 1967. **40.** Levy, E.P., A. Cohen, and F.C. Fraser, "Hormone treatment during pregnancy and congenital heart defects," Lancet *1:*611, 1973. **41.** Nora, J.J. and A.H. Nora, "Birth defects and oral contraceptives," Lancet *1:*941–942, 1973. **42.** Janerich, D.T., J.M. Piper, and D.M. Glebatis, "Oral contraceptives and congenital limb-reduction defects," N Engl J Med *291:*697–700, 1974. **43.** Carr, D.H., "Chromosome studies in selected spontaneous abortions: I. Conception after oral contraceptives," Canad Med Assoc J *103:*343–348, 1970. **44.** Wynn, V., J.W.H. Doar, and G.L. Mills, "Some effects of oral contraceptives on serum-lipid and lipoprotein levels," Lancet *2:*720–723, 1966. **45.** Laumas, K.R., P.K. Malkani, S. Bhatnagar, and V. Laumas, "Radioactivity in the breast milk of lactating women after oral administration of 3 H-norethynodrel," Amer J Obstet Gynecol *98:*411–413, 1967. **46.** Rooks, et al., JAMA *242:*644, 1979. **47.** Herbst, A.L., P. Cole, T. Colton, S.J. Robboy, R. E. Scully, "Age-incidence and Risk of Diethylstilbestrol-related Clear Cell Adenocarcinoma of the Vagina and Cervix," Am J Obstet Gynecol, *128:*43–50, 1977. **48.** Bibbo, M., M. Al-Naqeeb, I. Baccarini, W. Gill, M. Newton, K.M. Sleeper, M. Sonek, G.L. Wied, "Follow-up Study of Male and Female Offspring of DES-treated Mothers. A Preliminary Report," Jour of Repro Med, *15:*29–32, 1975. **49.** Gill, W.B., G.F.B. Schumacher, M. Bibbo, "Structural and Functional Abnormalities in the Sex Organs of Male Offspring of Mothers Treated with Diethylstilbestrol (DES)," Jour of Repro Med, *16:*147–153, 1976. **50.** Henderson, B.E., B. Senton, M. Cosgrove, J. Baptista, J. Aldrich, D. Townsend, W. Hart, T. Mack, "Urogenital Tract Abnormalities in Sons of Women Treated with Diethylstilbestrol," Pediatrics, *58:*505–507, 1976. **51.** Heinonen, O.P., D. Slone, R.R. Nonson, E.B. Hook, S. Shapiro, "Cardiovascular Birth Defects and Antenatal Exposure to Female Sex Hormones," N Engl J Med, *296:*67–70, 1977. **52.** Jain, A.K., "Mortality Risk Associated with the Use of Oral Contraceptives," Studies in Family Planning, *8:*50–54, 1977. **53.** Beral, V., "Mortality Among Oral Contraceptive Users," Lancet, *2:*727–731, 1977. **54.** Vessey, M.P., McPherson, K., and Johnson, B., "Mortality Among Women Participating in the Oxford/Family Planning Association Contraceptive Study," Lancet *2:*731–733, 1977.

Brief Summary Patient Package Insert

Cigarette smoking increases the risk of serious adverse effects on the heart and blood vessels from oral contraceptive use. This risk increases with age and with heavy smoking (15 or more cigarettes per day) and is quite marked in women over 35 years of age. Women who use oral contraceptives should not smoke.

Oral contraceptives taken as directed are about 99% effective in preventing pregnancy. (The mini-pill, however, is somewhat less effective.) Forgetting to take your pills increases the chance of pregnancy. Various drugs, such as antibiotics, may also decrease the effectiveness of oral contraceptives.

Women who have or have had clotting disorders, cancer of the breast or sex organs, unexplained vaginal bleeding, a stroke, heart attack, angina pectoris, or who suspect they may be pregnant should not use oral contraceptives.

Most side effects of the pill are not serious. The most common side effects are nausea, vomiting, bleeding between menstrual periods, weight gain, and breast tenderness. However, proper use of oral contraceptives requires that they be taken under your doctor's continuous supervision, because they can be associated with serious side effects which may be fatal. Fortunately, these occur very infrequently. The serious side effects are:

1. Blood clots in the legs, lungs, brain, heart or other organs and hemorrhage into the brain due to bursting of a blood vessel.
2. Liver tumors, which may rupture and cause severe bleeding.
3. Birth defects if the pill is taken while you are pregnant.
4. High blood pressure.
5. Gallbladder disease.

Some of the symptoms associated with these serious side effects are discussed in the detailed leaflet given you with your supply of pills. Notify your doctor if you notice any unusual physical disturbance while taking the pill.

The estrogen in oral contraceptives has been found to cause breast cancer and other cancers in certain animals. These findings suggest that oral contraceptives may also cause cancer in humans. However, studies to date in women taking currently marketed oral contraceptives have not confirmed that oral contraceptives cause cancer in humans.

The detailed leaflet describes more completely the benefits and risks or oral contraceptives. It also provides information on other forms of contraception. Read it carefully. If you have any questions, consult your doctor.

Caution: Oral contraceptives are of no value in the prevention or treatment of venereal disease.

Detailed Patient Labeling

What You Should Know About Oral Contraceptives: Oral contraceptives ("the pill") are the most effective way (except for sterilization) to prevent pregnancy. They are also convenient and, for most women, free of serious or unpleasant side effects. Oral contraceptives must always be taken under the continuous supervision of a physician.

The information in this leaflet under the headings "Who Should Not Use Oral Contraceptives," "The Dangers of Oral Contraceptives," and "How to Use Oral Contraceptives As Effectively As Possible, Once You Have Decided to Use Them" is also applicable when these drugs are used for other indications.

ORTHO-NOVUM 2 mg□21 may be prescribed for the treatment of hypermenorrhea.

It is important that any woman who considers using an oral contraceptive understand the risks involved. Although the oral contraceptives have important advantages over other methods of contraception, they have certain risks that no other method has. Only you can decide whether the advantages are worth these risks. This leaflet will tell you about the most important risks. It will explain how you can help your doctor prescribe the pill as safely as possible by telling him about yourself and being alert for the earliest signs of trouble. And it will tell you how to use the pill properly, so that it will be as effective as possible. There is more detailed information available in the leaflet prepared for doctors. Your pharmacist can show you a copy; you may need your doctor's help in understanding parts of it.

Who Should Not Use Oral Contraceptives:

A. If you have now, or have had in the past, any of the following conditions you should not use the pill:
   1. Heart attack or stroke.
   2. Clots in the legs or lungs.
   3. Angina pectoris.
   4. Known or suspected cancer of the breast or sex organs.
   5. Unusual vaginal bleeding that has not yet been diagnosed.

B. If you are pregnant or suspect that you are pregnant, do not use the pill.

C. Cigarette smoking increases the risk of serious adverse effects on the heart and blood vessels from oral contraceptive use. This risk increases with age and with heavy smoking (15 or more cigarettes per day) and is quite marked in women over 35 years of age. Women who use oral contraceptives should not smoke.

D. If you have scanty or irregular periods or are a young woman without a regular cycle, you should use another method of contraception because, if you use the pill, you may have difficulty becoming pregnant or may fail to have menstrual periods after discontinuing the pill.

Deciding To Use Oral Contraceptives: If you do not have any of the conditions listed above and are thinking about using oral contraceptives, to help you decide, you need information about the advantages and risks of oral contraceptives and of other contraceptive methods as well. This leaflet describes the advantages and risks of oral contraceptives. Except for sterilization, the IUD and abortion, which have their own exclusive risks, the only risks of other methods of contraception are those due to pregnancy should the method fail. Your doctor can answer questions you may have with respect to other methods of contraception. He can also answer any questions you may have after reading this leaflet on oral contraceptives.

1. What Oral Contraceptives Are and How They Work. Oral contraceptives are of two types. The most common, often simply called "the pill," is a combination of an estrogen and a progestogen, the two kinds of female hormones. The amount of estrogen and progestogen can vary, but the amount of estrogen is most important because both the effectiveness and some of the dangers of oral contraceptives are related to the amount of estrogen. This kind of oral contraceptive works principally by preventing release of an egg from the ovary. When the amount of estrogen is 50 micrograms or more, and the pill is taken as directed, oral contraceptives are more than 99% effective (i.e., there would be less than one pregnancy if 100 women used the pill for one year). Pills that contain 20 to 35 micrograms of estrogen vary slightly in effectiveness, ranging from 98% to more than 99% effective.

The second type of oral contraceptive, often called the "mini-pill," contains only a progestogen. It works in part by preventing release of an egg from the ovary but also by keeping sperm from reaching the egg and by making the uterus (womb) less receptive to any fertilized egg that reaches it. The mini-pill is less effective than the combination oral contraceptive, about 97% effective. In addition, the progestogen-only pill has a tendency to cause irregular bleeding which may be quite inconvenient, or cessation of bleeding entirely. The progestogen-only pill is used despite its lower effectiveness in the hope that it will prove not to have some of the serious side effects of the estrogen-containing pill (see below) but it is not yet certain that the mini-pill does in fact have fewer serious side effects. The discussion below, while based mainly on information about the combination pills, should be considered to apply as well to the mini-pill.

2. Other Nonsurgical Ways to Prevent Pregnancy. As this leaflet will explain, oral contraceptives have several serious risks. Other methods of contraception have lesser risks or none at all. They are also less effective than oral contraceptives, but, used properly, may be effective enough for many women. The follow-

Continued on next page

Ortho Pharm.—Cont.

ing table gives reported pregnancy rates (the number of women out of 100 who would become pregnant in one year) for these methods:

Pregnancies Per 100 Women Per Year

Intrauterine device (IUD), less than 1–6;
Diaphragm with spermicidal products (creams or jellies), 2–20;
Condom (rubber), 3–36; Aerosol foams, 2–29;
Jellies and creams, 4–36;
Periodic abstinence (rhythm) all types, less than 1–47;

1. Calendar method, 14–47;
2. Temperature method, 1–20;
3. Temperature method—intercourse only in postovulatory phase, less than 1–7;
4. Mucus method, 1–25;

No contraception, 60–80.

The figures (except for the IUD) vary widely because people differ in how well they use each method. Very faithful users of the various methods obtain very good results, except for users of the calendar method of periodic abstinence (rhythm). Except for the IUD, effective use of these methods requires somewhat more effort than simply taking a single pill every morning, but it is an effort that many couples undertake successfully. Your doctor can tell you a great deal more about these methods of contraception.

3. The Dangers of Oral Contraceptives.

a. *Circulatory disorders (abnormal blood clotting, heart attack, and stroke due to hemorrhage).* Blood clots (in various blood vessels of the body) are the most common of the serious side effects of oral contraceptives. A clot can result in a stroke (if the clot is in the brain), a heart attack (if the clot is in a blood vessel of the heart), or a pulmonary embolus (a clot which forms in the legs or pelvis, then breaks off and travels to the lungs). Any of these can be fatal. Clots also occur rarely in the blood vessels of the eye, resulting in blindness or impairment of vision in that eye. There is evidence that the risk of clotting increases with higher estrogen doses. It is therefore important to keep the dose of estrogen as low as possible, so long as the oral contraceptive used has an acceptable pregnancy rate and doesn't cause unacceptable changes in the menstrual pattern. Furthermore, cigarette smoking by oral contraceptive users increases the risk of serious adverse effects on the heart and blood vessels. This risk increases with age and with heavy smoking (15 or more cigarettes per day) and begins to become quite marked in women over 35 years of age. For this reason, women who use oral contraceptives should not smoke.

The risk of abnormal blood clotting increases with age in both users and nonusers of oral contraceptives, but the increased risk from the oral contraceptive appears to be present at all ages. For women aged 20 to 44 it is estimated that about 1 in 2,000 using oral contraceptives will be hospitalized each year because of abnormal clotting. Among nonusers in the same age group, about 1 in 20,000 would be hospitalized each year. For oral contraceptive users in general, it has been estimated that in women between the ages of 15 and 34 the risk of death due to a circulatory disorder is about 1 in 12,000 per year, whereas for nonusers the rate is about 1 in 50,000 per year. In the age group 35 to 44, the risk is estimated to be about 1 in 2,500 per year for oral contraceptive users and about 1 in 10,000 per year for nonusers.

Even without the pill the risk of having a heart attack increases with age and is also increased by such heart attack risk factors as high blood pressure, high cholesterol, obesity, diabetes, and cigarette smoking. Without any risk factors present, the use of oral contraceptives alone may double the risk of heart attack. However, the combination of cigarette smoking, especially heavy smoking, and oral contraceptive use greatly increases the risk of heart attack. Oral contraceptive users who smoke are about five times more likely to have a heart attack than users who do not smoke and about ten times more likely to have a heart attack than nonusers who do not smoke. It has been estimated that users between the ages of 30 and 39 who smoke have about a 1-in-10,000 chance each year of having a fatal heart attack compared to about a 1-in-50,000 chance in users who do not smoke, and about a 1-in-100,000 chance in nonusers who do not smoke. In the age group 40 to 44, the risk is about 1 in 1,700 per year for users who smoke compared to about 1 in 10,000 for users who do not smoke and to about one in 14,000 per year for nonusers who do not smoke. Heavy smoking (about 15 cigarettes or more a day) further increases the risk. If you do not smoke and have none of the other heart attack risk factors described above, you will have a smaller risk than listed. If you have several heart attack risk factors, the risk may be considerably greater than listed.

In addition to blood clotting disorders, it has been estimated that women taking oral contraceptives are twice as likely as nonusers to have a stroke due to rupture of a blood vessel in the brain.

One report suggests that the risk of circulatory diseases appears to increase the longer you are on the pill.

b. *Formation of tumors.* Studies have found that when certain animals are given the female sex hormone estrogen, which is an ingredient of oral contraceptives, continuously for long periods, cancers may develop in the breast, cervix, vagina, and liver.

These findings suggest that oral contraceptives may cause cancer in humans. However, studies to date in women taking currently marketed oral contraceptives have not confirmed that oral contraceptives cause cancer in humans. Several studies have found no increase in breast cancer in users, although one study suggested oral contraceptives might cause an increase in breast cancer in women who already have benign breast disease (e.g., cysts).

Women with a strong family history of breast cancer or who have breast nodules, fibrocystic disease, or abnormal mammograms or who were exposed to DES (diethylstilbestrol), an estrogen, during their mother's pregnancy must be followed very closely by their doctors if they choose to use oral contraceptives instead of another method of contraception. Many studies have shown that women taking oral contraceptives have less risk of getting benign breast disease than those who have not used oral contraceptives. Recently, strong evidence has emerged that estrogens (one component of oral contraceptives), when given for periods of more than one year to women after the menopause, increase the risk of cancer of the uterus (womb). There is also some evidence that a kind of oral contraceptive which is no longer marketed, the sequential oral contraceptive, may increase the risk of cancer of the uterus. There remains no evidence, however, that the oral contraceptives now available increase the risk of this cancer.

Oral contraceptives do cause, although rarely, a benign (nonmalignant) tumor of the liver. These tumors do not spread, but they may rupture and cause internal bleeding, which may be fatal. A few cases of cancer of the liver have been reported in women using oral contraceptives, but it is not yet known whether the drug caused them.

c. *Dangers to a developing child if oral contraceptives are used in or immediately preceding pregnancy.* Oral contraceptives should not be taken by pregnant women because they may damage the developing child. An increased risk of birth defects, including heart defects and limb defects, has been associated with the use of sex hormones, including oral contraceptives, in pregnancy. In addition, the developing female child whose mother has received DES (diethylstilbestrol), an estrogen, during pregnancy has a risk of getting cancer of the vagina or cervix in her teens or young adulthood. This risk is estimated to be about 1 to 4 in 1000 exposures. Abnormalities of the urinary and sex organs have been reported in male offspring so exposed. It is possible that other estrogens, such as the estrogens in oral contraceptives, could have the same effect in the child if the mother takes them during pregnancy.

If you stop taking oral contraceptives to become pregnant, your doctor may recommend that you use another method of contraception for a short while, for example three months. The reason for this is that there is evidence from studies in women who have had "miscarriages" soon after stopping the pill, that the lost fetuses are more likely to be abnormal. Whether there is an overall increase in "miscarriage" in women who become pregnant soon after stopping the pill as compared with women who do not use the pill is not known, but is possible that there may be. If, however, you do become pregnant soon after stopping oral contraceptives, and do not have a miscarriage, there does not appear to be evidence that the baby has an increased risk of being abnormal.

d. *Gallbladder disease.* Women who use oral contraceptives have a greater risk than nonusers of having gallbladder disease requiring surgery. The increased risk may first appear within one year of use and may double after four or five years of use.

e. *Other side effects of oral contraceptives.* Some women using oral contraceptives experience unpleasant side effects. Some of these may be temporary. Your breasts may feel tender, nausea and vomiting may occur, you may gain or lose weight, and your ankles may swell. A spotty darkening of the skin, particularly of the face, is possible and may persist. You may notice unexpected vaginal bleeding or changes in your menstrual period. Irregular bleeding is frequently seen when using the mini-pill or combination oral contraceptives containing less than 50 micrograms of estrogen.

More serious side effects include worsening of migraine, asthma, epilepsy, and kidney or heart disease because of a tendency for water to be retained in the body when oral contraceptives are used. Other side effects are growth of preexisting fibroid tumors of the uterus; mental depression; and liver problems with jaundice (yellowing of the skin). Your doctor may find that levels of sugar and fatty substances in your blood are elevated; the long-term effects of these changes are not known. Some women develop high blood pressure while taking oral contraceptives, which ordinarily returns to the original levels when the oral contraceptive is stopped.

Other reactions, although not proved to be caused by oral contraceptives, are occasionally reported. These include more frequent urination and some discomfort when urinating, kidney disease, nervousness, dizziness, some loss of scalp hair, an increase in body hair, an increase or decrease in sex drive, appetite changes, cataracts, and a need for a change in contact lens prescription or inability to use contact lenses.

After you stop using oral contraceptives there may be a delay before you are able to become pregnant or before you resume having menstrual periods. This is especially true of women who had irregular menstrual cycles prior to the use of oral contraceptives. As discussed previously, your doctor may recommend that you wait a short while after stopping the pill before you try to become pregnant. During this time, use another form of contraception. You should consult your physician before resuming use of oral contraceptives after childbirth, especially if you plan to nurse your baby. Drugs in oral contraceptives are known to appear in the milk, and the long-range effect on infants is not known at this time. Furthermore, oral contraceptives may cause a decrease in your milk supply as well as in the quality of the milk.

4. Comparison of the Risks of Oral Contraceptives and Other Contraceptive Methods. The many studies on the risks and effectiveness of oral contraceptives and other methods of contraception have been analyzed to estimate the risk of death associated with various methods of contraception. This risk has two parts: (a) the risk of the method itself (e.g., the risk that oral contraceptives will cause death due to abnormal clotting), and (b) the risk of death due to pregnancy or abortion in the event the method fails. The results of this analysis are shown in the bar graph (Figure 1). The height of the bars is the number of deaths per 100,000 women each year. There are six sets of bars, each set referring to a specific age group of women. Within each set of bars there is a single bar for each of the different contraceptive methods. For oral contraceptives, there are two bars—one for smokers and the other for nonsmokers. The analysis is based on present knowledge and new information could, of course, alter it. The analysis shows that the risk of death from all methods of birth control is low and below that associated with childbirth, except for oral contraceptives in women over 40 who smoke. It shows that the lowest risk of death is associated with the condom or diaphragm (traditional contraception) backed up by early abortion in case of failure of the condom or diaphragm to prevent pregnancy. Also, at any age the risk of death (due to unexpected pregnancy) from the use of traditional contraception, even without a backup of abortion, is generally the same as or less than that from use of oral contraceptives.

How To Use Oral Contraceptives As Effectively As Possible, Once You Have Decided To Use Them:

1. What to Tell your Doctor.

You can make use of the pill as effectively as possible by telling your doctor if you have any of the following:

a. Conditions that mean you should not use oral contraceptives:

Clots in the legs or lungs.
Clots in the legs or lungs in the past.
A stroke, heart attack, or angina pectoris.
Known or suspected cancer of the breast or sex organs.
Unusual vaginal bleeding that has not yet been diagnosed.
Known or suspected pregnancy.

b. Conditions that your doctor will want to watch closely or which might cause him to suggest another method of contraception:

A family history of breast cancer.
Breast nodules, fibrocystic disease of the breast, or an abnormal mammogram.

Diabetes.	Heart or kidney disease.
High blood pressure.	Epilepsy.
High cholesterol.	Mental depression.
Cigarette smoking.	Fibroid tumors of the uterus.
Migraine headaches.	Gallbladder disease.

c. Once you are using oral contraceptives, you should be alert for signs of a serious adverse effect and call your doctor if they occur:

Sharp pain in the chest, coughing blood, or sudden shortness of breath (indicating possible clots in the lungs).
Pain in the calf (possible clot in the leg).
Crushing chest pain or heaviness (indicating possible heart attack).
Sudden severe headache or vomiting, dizziness or fainting, disturbance of vision or speech or weakness or numbness in an arm or leg (indicating a possible stroke).
Sudden partial or complete loss of vision (indicating a possible clot in the eye).
Breast lumps (you should ask your doctor to show you how to examine your own breasts).
Severe pain in the abdomen (indicating a possible ruptured tumor of the liver).
Severe depression.
Yellowing of the skin (jaundice).

2. How to Take the Pill So That it is Most Effective.

Reduced effectiveness and an increased incidence of breakthrough bleeding have been associated with the use of oral contraceptives with antibiotics such as rifampicin, ampicillin, and tetracycline or with certain other drugs, such as barbiturates, phenylbutazone or phenytoin sodium. You should use an additional means of contraception during any cycle in which any of these drugs are taken.

To achieve maximum contraceptive effectiveness, ORTHO-NOVUM, MODICON, and MICRONOR must be taken exactly as directed and at intervals not exceeding 24 hours.

ORTHO-NOVUM 10/11—Sunday-Start Package

21-Day Regimen: The first white tablet should be taken on the first Sunday after the menstrual period begins. If period begins on Sunday, begin taking tablets that day. Take one white tablet at the same time each day for 10 consecutive days, then take one peach tablet daily for 11 days. During the FIRST cycle, it is important that you use another method of birth control until you have taken a white tablet daily for seven consecutive days. After taking your last peach tablet, wait for seven days during which time a menstrual period usually occurs. After the seven-day waiting period, on Sunday, start taking a white tablet each day for the next 10 days, then a peach tablet for the next 11 days, thus using a three-week-on, one-week-off regimen.

28-Day Regimen: The first white tablet should be taken on the first Sunday after the menstrual period begins. If period begins on Sunday, begin taking tablets that day. Take one white tablet at the same time each day for 10 consecutive days, take one peach tablet daily for 11 days, then take one green tablet daily for 7 days, during which time your period usually occurs. During the FIRST cycle, it is important that you use another method of birth control until you have taken a white tablet daily for seven consecutive days. After 28 tablets have been taken, (last green tablet will always be taken on a Saturday) take the first tablet (white) from your next package the following day (Sunday) whether or not you are still menstruating. With the 28-day regimen, pills are taken every day of the year.

ORTHO-NOVUM 1/35, MODICON, ORTHO-NOVUM 1/50, ORTHO-NOVUM 1/80 and ORTHO-NOVUM 2 mg

21-day Regimen: Counting the first day of menstrual flow as "Day 1," take one tablet daily from the 5th through the 25th day of the menstrual cycle. If the first tablet is taken later than the 5th day of the menstrual cycle or postpartum, contraceptive reliance should not be placed on ORTHO-NOVUM or MODICON until after the first seven consecutive days of administration. Take a tablet the same time each day, preferably at bedtime, for 21 days, then wait for 7 days during which time a menstrual period usually occurs. Following this 7-day waiting period, start taking a tablet each day for the next 21 days, thus using a three-weeks-on, one-week-off dosage regimen.

When ORTHO-NOVUM 2 mg□21 Tablets are used for the treatment of hypermenorrhea, your physician will discuss the regimen with you.

ORTHO-NOVUM 1/35, MODICON, ORTHO-NOVUM 1/50 and ORTHO-NOVUM 1/80.

28-Day Regimen: The first white, yellow or peach tablet should be taken on the first Sunday after the menstrual period begins. If period begins on Sunday, begin taking tablets that day. Take one white, yellow or peach tablet at the same time each day for 21 consecutive days, then take one green tablet daily for 7 days during which time your menstrual period usually occurs. During the FIRST cycle, it is important that you use another method of birth control until you have taken a white, yellow or peach tablet daily for seven consecutive days. After 28 tablets have been taken, (last green tablet will always be taken on a Saturday) take the first tablet (white, yellow or peach) from your next package the following day (Sunday) whether or not you are still menstruating. With the 28-day regimen, pills are taken every day of the year.

Continuous Regimen (MICRONOR): The first MICRONOR Tablet should be taken on the first day of the menstrual period.

Take one tablet at the same time each day without interruption for as long as contraceptive protection is desired.

The effectiveness of progestogen-only oral contraceptives, such as MICRONOR, is lower than that of the combination estrogen oral contraceptives containing both estrogen and progestogen. If 100 women utilized an estrogen-containing oral contraceptive for a period of one year, generally less than one pregnancy would be expected to occur; however, if MICRONOR had been utilized, approximately three pregnancies might occur.

Women who participated in the clinical studies with MICRONOR and who had not taken other oral contraceptives before starting MICRONOR had a higher pregnancy rate (four women out of 100), particularly during the first six months of therapy, and to a large extent because they did not take their tablets correctly.

Of course, if you don't take your tablets as directed, or forget to take them every day, the chance you may become pregnant is naturally greater.

MICRONOR (norethindrone) will probably cause some changes in your menstrual pattern. Your cycle, that is the time between menstrual periods, will vary. For example, you might have a 28-day cycle, followed by a 17-day cycle, followed by a 35-day cycle, etc. This is common with MICRONOR.

While using MICRONOR, your period may be longer or shorter than before. If bleeding lasts more than eight days, be sure to let your doctor know.

At times there may be no menstrual period after a cycle of pills. Therefore, if you miss one menstrual period but have taken the pills *exactly as you were supposed to,* continue as usual into the next cycle. If you have not taken them correctly and miss a menstrual period, or if you are taking mini-pills and it is 45 days or more from the start of your last menstrual period, you may be pregnant and should stop taking oral contraceptives until your doctor determines whether or not you are pregnant. Until you can get to your doctor, use another form of contraception. If two consecutive menstrual periods are missed, you should stop taking pills until it is determined whether you are pregnant. If you do become pregnant while using oral contraceptives, you should discuss the risks to the developing child with your doctor.

3. Periodic Examination.

Your doctor will take a complete medical and family history before prescribing oral contraceptives. At that time and about once a year thereafter, he will generally examine your blood pessure, breasts, abdomen, and pelvic organs (including a Papanicolaou smear, i.e., test for cancer).

Summary: Oral contraceptives are the most effective method, except sterilization, for preventing pregnancy. Other methods, when used

Continued on next page

Ortho Pharm.—Cont.

conscientiously, are also very effective and have fewer risks.
Women who use oral contraceptives should not smoke.
In addition, if you have certain conditions or have had these conditions in the past, you should not use oral contraceptives because the risk is too great. These conditions are listed in the booklet. If you do not have these conditions and decide to use the "pill," please read the booklet carefully so that you can use the "pill."

Based on his or her assessment of your medical needs, your doctor has prescribed this drug for you. Do not give the drug to anyone else.

SULTRIN® Triple Sulfa Cream and Vaginal Tablets ℞

Composition: SULTRIN Cream contains sulfathiazole 3.42%, sulfacetamide 2.86%, sulfabenzamide 3.7% and urea 0.64%, compounded with glyceryl monostearate, cetyl alcohol 2%, stearic acid, cholesterol, lanolin, lecithin, peanut oil, propylparaben, propylene glycol, diethylaminoethyl stearamide, phosphoric acid, methylparaben and water.
Composition: Each SULTRIN Tablet contains sulfathiazole 172.5 mg, sulfacetamide 143.75 mg, and sulfabenzamide 184.0 mg, compounded with urea, lactose, guar gum, starch and magnesium stearate.
Indications: SULTRIN Cream and SULTRIN Tablets are indicated for treatment of *Haemophilus vaginalis* (*Gardnerella*) vaginitis.
Contraindications: Sulfonamide sensitivity and kidney disease.
Dosage: SULTRIN Cream. One applicatorful intravaginally twice daily for 4 to 6 days. The dosage may then be reduced one-half to one-quarter.
SULTRIN Vaginal Tablets. 1 tablet intravaginally before retiring and again in the morning for 10 days. This course may be repeated if necessary.
Packaging: Cream — 78 g tubes with the ORTHO® Measured-Dose Applicator.
Vaginal Tablets—Package of 20 foil-wrapped tablets with vaginal applicator.

Ortho Pharmaceutical Corporation
DERMATOLOGICAL DIVISION
ROUTE 202
RARITAN, NJ 08869

CLODERM® ℞
(clocortolone pivalate)
Cream 0.1%
For Topical Use Only

Description: CLODERM Cream 0.1% contains the medium potency topical corticosteroid, clocortolone pivalate, in a specially formulated water-washable emollient cream base consisting of purified water, white petrolatum, mineral oil, stearyl alcohol, polyoxyl 40 stearate, carbomer 934P, edetate disodium, sodium hydroxide, with methylparaben and propylparaben as preservatives.
Chemically, clocortolone pivalate is 9-chloro-6α-fluoro-11β, 21-dihydroxy-16α-methylpregna-1,4-diene-3,20-dione 21-pivalate.
Clinical Pharmacology: Topical corticosteroids share anti-inflammatory, anti-pruritic and vasoconstrictive actions.
The mechanism of anti-inflammatory activity of the topical corticosteroids is unclear. Various laboratory methods, including vasoconstrictor assays, are used to compare and predict potencies and/or clinical efficacies of the topical corticosteroids. There is some evidence to suggest that a recognizable correlation exists between vasoconstrictor potency and therapeutic efficacy in man.
Pharmacokinetics: The extent of percutaneous absorption of topical corticosteroids is determined by many factors including the vehicle, the integrity of the epidermal barrier, and the use of occlusive dressings.
Topical corticosteroids can be absorbed from normal intact skin. Inflammation and/or other disease processes in the skin increase percutaneous absorption. Occlusive dressings substantially increase the percutaneous absorption of topical corticosteroids. Thus, occlusive dressings may be a valuable therapeutic adjunct for treatment of resistant dermatoses. (See *DOSAGE AND ADMINISTRATION*).
Once absorbed through the skin, topical corticosteroids are handled through pharmacokinetic pathways similar to systemically administered corticosteroids. Corticosteroids are bound to plasma proteins in varying degrees. Corticosteroids are metabolized primarily in the liver and are then excreted by the kidneys. Some of the topical corticosteroids and their metabolites are also excreted into the bile.
Indications and Usage: Topical corticosteroids are indicated for the relief of the inflammatory and pruritic manifestations of corticosteroid-responsive dermatoses.
Contraindications: Topical corticosteroids are contraindicated in those patients with a history of hypersensitivity to any of the components of the preparation.
Precautions
General: Systemic absorption of topical corticosteroids has produced reversible hypothalamic-pituitary-adrenal (HPA) axis suppression, manifestations of Cushing's syndrome, hyperglycemia, and glucosuria in some patients.
Conditions which augment systemic absorption include the application of the more potent steroids, use over large surface areas, prolonged use, and the addition of occlusive dressings.
Therefore, patients receiving a large dose of a potent topical steroid applied to a large surface area or under an occlusive dressing should be evaluated periodically for evidence of HPA axis suppression by using the urinary free cortisol and ACTH stimulation tests. If HPA axis suppression is noted, an attempt should be made to withdraw the drug, to reduce the frequency of application, or to substitute a less potent steroid.
Recovery of HPA axis function is generally prompt and complete upon discontinuation of the drug. Infrequently, signs and symptoms of steroid withdrawal may occur, requiring supplemental systemic corticosteroids.
Children may absorb proportionally larger amounts of topical corticosteroids and thus be more susceptible to systemic toxicity (See *PRECAUTIONS—Pediatric Use*).
If irritation develops, topical corticosteroids should be discontinued and appropriate therapy instituted.
In the presence of dermatological infections, the use of an appropriate antifungal or antibacterial agent should be instituted. If a favorable response does not occur promptly, the corticosteroid should be discontinued until the infection has been adequately controlled.
Information for the Patient: Patients using topical corticosteroids should receive the following information and instructions:

1. This medication is to be used as directed by the physician. It is for external use only. Avoid contact with the eyes.
2. Patients should be advised not to use this medication for any disorder other than for which it was prescribed.
3. The treated skin area should not be bandaged or otherwise covered or wrapped as to be occlusive unless directed by the physician.
4. Patients should report any signs of local adverse reactions especially under occlusive dressing.
5. Parents of pediatric patients should be advised not to use tight-fitting diapers or plastic pants on a child being treated in the diaper area, as these garments may constitute occlusive dressings.

Laboratory Tests: The following tests may be helpful in evaluating the HPA axis suppression:
Urinary free cortisol test
ACTH stimulation test
Carcinogenesis, Mutagenesis, and Impairment of Fertility: Long-term animal studies have not been performed to evaluate the carcinogenic potential or the effect on fertility of topical corticosteroids.
Studies to determine mutagenicity with prednisolone and hydrocortisone have revealed negative results.
Pregnancy Category C: Corticosteroids are generally teratogenic in laboratory animals when administered systemically at relatively low dosage levels. The more potent corticosteroids have been shown to be teratogenic after dermal application in laboratory animals. There are no adequate and well-controlled studies in pregnant women on teratogenic effects from topically applied corticosteroids. Therefore, topical corticosteroids should be used during pregnancy only if the potential benefit justifies the potential risk to the fetus. Drugs of this class should not be used extensively on pregnant patients, in large amounts, or for prolonged periods of time.
Nursing Mothers: It is not known whether topical administration of corticosteroids could result in sufficient systemic absorption to produce detectable quantities in breast milk. Systemically administered corticosteroids are secreted into breast milk in quantities *not* likely to have a deleterious effect on the infant. Nevertheless, caution should be exercised when topical corticosteroids are administered to a nursing woman.
Pediatric Use: Pediatric patients may demonstrate greater susceptibility to topical corticosteroid-induced HPA axis suppression and Cushing's syndrome than mature patients because of a larger skin surface area to body weight ratio.
Hypothalamic-pituitary-adrenal (HPA) axis suppression, Cushing's syndrome, and intracranial hypertension have been reported in children receiving topical corticosteroids. Manifestations of adrenal suppression in children include linear growth retardation, delayed weight gain, low plasma cortisol levels, and absence of response to ACTH stimulation. Manifestations of intracranial hypertension include bulging fontanelles, headaches, and bilateral papilledema.
Administration of topical corticosteroids to children should be limited to the least amount compatible with an effective therapeutic regimen. Chronic corticosteroid therapy may interfere with the growth and development of children.
Adverse Reactions: The following local adverse reactions are reported infrequently with topical corticosteroids, but may occur more frequently with the use of occlusive dressings. These reactions are listed in an approximate decreasing order of occurrence:
Burning
Itching
Irritation
Dryness
Folliculitis
Hypertrichosis
Acneiform eruptions
Hypopigmentation
Perioral dermatitis
Allergic contact dermatitis
Maceration of the skin
Secondary infection
Skin atrophy

Striae
Miliaria

Overdosage: Topically applied corticosteroids can be absorbed in sufficient amounts to produce systemic effects (see *PRECAUTIONS*).

Dosage and Administration: Topical corticosteroids are generally applied to the affected area as a thin film from one to four times daily depending on the severity of the condition.

Occlusive dressings may be used for the management of psoriasis or recalcitrant conditions.

If an infection develops, the use of occlusive dressings should be discontinued and appropriate antimicrobial therapy instituted.

How Supplied: CLODERM (clocortolone pivalate) Cream 0.1% is supplied in tubes containing 15 grams and 45 grams.

Store CLODERM Cream between 59° and 86°F. Avoid freezing.

GRIFULVIN V® ℞

(griseofulvin microsize)
Tablets/Suspension

Description: Griseofulvin microsize is an antibiotic derived from a species of *Penicillium.*

Actions: GRIFULVIN V (griseofulvin microsize) acts systemically to inhibit the growth of Trichophyton, Microsporum and Epidermophyton genera of fungi. Fungistatic amounts are deposited in the keratin, which is gradually exfoliated and replaced by noninfected tissue. Griseofulvin absorption from the gastrointestinal tract varies considerably among individuals, mainly because of insolubility of the drug in aqueous media of the upper G.I. tract. The peak serum level found in fasting adults given 0.5 gm. occurs at about four hours and ranges between 0.5 and 2.0 mcg./ml.

It should be noted that some individuals are consistently "poor absorbers" and tend to attain lower blood levels at all times. This may explain unsatisfactory therapeutic results in some patients. Better blood levels can probably be attained in most patients if the tablets are administered after a meal with a high fat content.

Indications: Major indications for GRIFULVIN V griseofulvin microsize are:

Tinea capitis (ringworm of the scalp)
Tinea corporis (ringworm of the body)
Tinea pedis (athlete's foot)
Tinea unguium (onychomycosis; ringworm of the nails)
Tinea cruris (ringworm of the thigh)
Tinea barbae (barber's itch)

GRIFULVIN V (griseofulvin microsize) inhibits the growth of those genera of fungi that commonly cause ringworm infections of the hair, skin, and nails, such as:

Trichophyton rubrum
Trichophyton tonsurans
Trichophyton mentagrophytes
Trichophyton interdigitalis
Trichophyton verrucosum
Trichophyton sulphureum
Trichophyton schoenleini
Microsporum audouini
Microsporum canis
Microsporum gypseum
Epidermophyton floccosum
Trichophyton megnini
Trichophyton gallinae
Trichophyton crateriform

Note: Prior to therapy, the type of fungi responsible for the infection should be indentified. The use of the drug is not justified in minor or trivial infections which will respond to topical antifungal agents alone.

It is *not* effective in:

Bacterial infections
Candidiasis (Moniliasis)
Histoplasmosis
Actinomycosis
Sporotrichosis
Chromoblastomycosis
Coccidioidomycosis
North American Blastomycosis
Cryptococcosis (Torulosis)
Tinea versicolor
Nocardiosis

Contraindications: This drug is contraindicated in patients with porphyria, hepatocellular failure, and in individuals with a history of hypersensitivity to griseofulvin.

Warnings:

Usage in Pregnancy: Safe use of GRIFULVIN V (griseofulvin microsize) in pregnancy has not been established.

Prophylactic Usage: Safety and efficacy of prophylactic use of this drug has not been established.

Chronic feeding of griseofulvin, at levels ranging from 0.5-2.5% of the diet, resulted in the development of liver tumors in several strains of mice, particularly in males. Smaller particle sizes result in an enhanced effect. Lower oral dosage levels have not been tested. Subcutaneous administration of relatively small doses of griseofulvin once a week during the first three weeks of life has also been reported to induce hepatomata in mice. Although studies in other animal species have not yielded evidence of tumorigenicity, these studies were not of adequate design to form a basis for conclusions in this regard.

In subacute toxicity studies, orally administered griseofulvin produced hepatocellar necrosis in mice, but this has not been seen in other species. Disturbances in porphyrin metabolism have been reported in griseofulvin-treated laboratory animals. Griseofulvin has been reported to have a colchicine-like effect on mitosis and cocarcinogenicity with methylcholanthrene in cutaneous tumor induction in laboratory animals.

Reports of animal studies in the Soviet literature state that a griseofulvin preparation was found to be embryotoxic and teratogenic on oral administration to pregnant Wistar rats. Rat reproduction studies done thus far in the United States and Great Britain have been inconclusive in this regard, and additional animal reproduction studies are underway. Pups with abnormalities have been reported in the litters of a few bitches treated with griseofulvin.

Suppression of spermatogenesis has been reported to occur in rats but investigation in man failed to confirm this.

Precautions: Patients on prolonged therapy with any potent medication should be under close observation. Periodic monitoring or organ system function, including renal, hepatic and hemopoietic, should be done.

Since griseofulvin is derived from species of penicillin, the possibility of cross sensitivity with penicillin exists; however, known penicillin-sensitive patients have been treated without difficulty.

Since a photosensitivity reaction is occasionally associated with griseofulvin therapy, patients should be warned to avoid exposure to intense natural or artificial sunlight. Should a photosensitivity reaction occur, lupus erythematosus may be aggravated.

Patients on warfarin-type anticoagulant therapy may require dosage adjustment of the anticoagulant during and after griseofulvin therapy. Concomitant use of barbiturates usually depresses griseofulvin activity and may necessitate raising the dosage.

Adverse Reactions: When adverse reactions occur, they are most commonly of the hypersensitivity type such as skin rashes, urticaria and rarely, angioneurotic edema, and may necessitate withdrawal of therapy and appropriate countermeasures. Paresthesias of the hands and feet have been reported rarely after extended therapy. Other side effects reported occasionally are oral thrush, nausea, vomiting, epigastric distress, diarrhea; headache, fatigue, dizziness, insomnia, mental confusion and impairment of performance of routine activities.

Proteinuria and leukopenia have been reported rarely. Administration of the drug should be discontinued if granulocytopenia occurs.

When rare, serious reactions occur with griseofulvin, they are usually associated with high dosages, long periods of therapy, or both.

Dosage and Administration: Accurate diagnosis of the infecting organism is essential. Identification should be made either by direct microscopic examination of a mounting of infected tissue in a solution of potassium hydroxide or by culture on an appropriate medium. Medication must be continued until the infecting organism is completely eradicated as indicated by appropriate clinical or laboratory examination. Representative treatment periods are tinea capitis, 4 to 6 weeks; tinea corporis, 2 to 4 weeks; tinea pedis, 4 to 8 weeks; tinea unguium—depending on rate of growth—fingernails, at least 4 months; toenails, at least 6 months.

General measures in regard to hygiene should be observed to control sources of infection or reinfection. Concommitant use of appropriate topical agents is usually required, particularly in treatment of tinea pedis since in some forms of athlete's foot, yeasts and bacteria may be involved. Griseofulvin will not eradicate the bacterial or monilial infection.

Adults: A daily dose of 500 mg. will give a satisfactory response in most patients with tinea corporis, tinea cruris, and tinea capitis. For those fungus infections more difficult to eradicate such as tinea pedis and tinea unguium, a daily dose of 1.0 gram is recommended.

Children: Approximately 5 mg. per pound of body weight per day is an effective dose for most children. On this basis the following dosage schedule for children is suggested:

Children weighing 30 to 50 pounds—125 mg. to 250 mg. daily.
Children weighing over 50 pounds—250 mg. to 500 mg. daily.

How Supplied: GRIFULVIN V (griseofulvin microsize) 250 mg. Tablets in bottles of 100 (white, scored, imprinted "ORTHO").

GRIFULVIN V (griseofulvin microsize) 500 mg. Tablets in bottles of 100 and 500 (white, scored, imprinted "ORTHO").

Dispense GRIFULVIN V tablets in well-closed container as defined in the official compendia.

GRIFULVIN V (griseofulvin microsize) Suspension 125 mg. per 5 cc. in bottles of 4 fl. oz.

Dispense GRIFULVIN V suspension in tight, light-resistant container as defined in the official compendia.

MECLAN® ℞

(meclocycline sulfosalicylate)
Cream 1%

Description: MECLAN (meclocycline sulfosalicylate) Cream 1% is a homogeneous smooth yellow cream, each gram of which contains meclocycline sulfosalicylate equivalent to 10 mg. of meclocycline activity in an aqueous cream vehicle consisting of glyceryl stearate, propylene glycol stearate, caprylic/capric triglyceride, paraffin, trihydroxystearin, polysorbate 40, sorbitol solution, propyl gallate, sorbic acid, sodium formaldehyde sulfoxylate, perfume, and water. The vehicle is pharmaceutically compatible with both oil- and water-based systems.

Chemically meclocycline sulfosalicylate is [4S-(4α, 4aα, 5α, 5aα, 12aα)]-7-chloro-4-(dimethylamino) - 1, 4,4a,5,5a,6,11,12a-octahydro-3,5,10, 12,12a-pentahydroxy-6-methylene-1, 11- dioxo-2-naphthacenecarboxamide 5-sulfosalicylate.

Actions (Clinical Pharmacology): The mode of action of MECLAN Cream in the treat-

Continued on next page

Ortho Derm.—Cont.

ment of acne is not fully understood. However, it appears that meclocycline possesses a localized effect, since it is not absorbed through the skin in sufficient quantities to be detected systemically. In subtotal body inunction studies, up to 40 times the average treatment dose was applied to 20 human subjects daily for 28 days. No measurable amounts of meclocycline appeared in the blood (0.1 microgram/ml. level of detectability) or urine (0.02 microgram/ml. level of detectability).

Indication: MECLAN Cream (meclocycline sulfosalicylate) is indicated for topical application in the treatment of acne vulgaris.

Contraindications: MECLAN is contraindicated in persons who have shown hypersensitivity to any of its ingredients or to any of the other tetracyclines.

Warnings: Although no absorption has been demonstrated by 28-day inunction studies in humans, the possibility exists that significant percutaneous absorption may result from prolonged use. Therefore, caution is advised in administering MECLAN (meclocycline sulfosalicylate) to persons with hepatic or renal dysfunction.

Precautions: This drug is for external use only and should be kept out of the eyes, nose, and mouth. It should be used with caution by patients who are sensitive to formaldehyde.

Pregnancy: Pregnancy Category B. Reproduction studies have been performed in rats and rabbits at oral doses up to 1000 times the human dose (assuming the human dose to be one gram of cream per day) and have revealed no evidence of impaired fertility or harm to the fetus due to meclocycline sulfosalicylate. There was, however, a slight delay in ossification in rabbits when meclocycline was applied topically. There are no adequate and well-controlled studies in pregnant women. Because animal reproduction studies are not always predictive of human response, this drug should be used during pregnancy only if clearly needed.

Nursing Mothers: It is not known whether this drug is excreted in human milk. Because many drugs are excreted in human milk, caution should be exercised when meclocycline sulfosalicylate is administered to a nursing woman.

Adverse Reactions: MECLAN is well tolerated by the skin. In the clinical trials there was one report of acute contact dermatitis. There were isolated reports of skin irritation. Temporary follicular staining may occur with excessive application. Patch testing has demonstrated no photosensitivity or contact allergy potential.

Dosage and Administration: It is recommended that MECLAN be applied to the affected area twice daily, morning and evening. Less frequent application may be used depending on patient response. Excessive use of MECLAN Cream may cause staining of some fabrics.

How Supplied: MECLAN (meclocycline sulfosalicylate) Cream 1% is supplied in 20 gram and 45 gram sealed tubes.

MONISTAT-DERM™ ℞

(miconazole nitrate 2%)
Cream and Lotion
For Topical Use Only

Description: MONISTAT-DERM (miconazole nitrate 2%) Cream and Lotion each contain miconazole nitrate* 2%, formulated into a water-miscible base consisting of pegoxol 7 stearate, peglicol 5 oleate, mineral oil, benzoic acid, and butylated hydroxyanisole.

*Chemical name: 1-[2,4-dichloro-β-{(2,4-dichlorobenzyl)oxy} phenethyl] imidazole mononitrate.

Actions: Miconazole nitrate is a synthetic antifungal agent which inhibits the growth of the common dermatophytes, *Trichophyton rubrum, Trichophyton mentagrophytes,* and *Epidermophyton floccosum,* the yeast-like fungus. *Candida albicans,* and the organism responsible for tinea versicolor *(Malassezia furfur).*

Indications: For topical application in the treatment of tinea pedis (athlete's foot), tinea cruris, and tinea corporis caused by *Trichophyton rubrum, Trichophyton mentagrophytes,* and *Epidermophyton floccosum,* in the treatment of cutaneous candidiasis (moniliasis), and in the treatment of tinea versicolor.

Contraindications: MONISTAT-DERM (miconazole nitrate 2%) Cream and Lotion have no known contraindications.

Precautions: If a reaction suggesting sensitivity or chemical irritation should occur, use of the medication should be discontinued.
For external use only. Avoid introduction of MONISTAT-DERM Cream and Lotion into the eyes.

Adverse Reactions: There have been isolated reports of irritation, burning, and maceration associated with application of MONISTAT-DERM.

Dosage and Administration: Sufficient MONISTAT-DERM Cream should be applied to cover affected areas twice daily (morning and evening) in patients with tinea pedis, tinea cruris, tinea corporis, and cutaneous candidiasis, and once daily in patients with tinea versicolor. It is preferable to use MONISTAT-DERM Lotion in intertriginous areas; if the cream is used, it should be applied sparingly and smoothed in well to avoid maceration effects.
Early relief of symptoms (2 to 3 days) is experienced by the majority of patients and clinical improvement may be seen fairly soon after treatment is begun; however, *Candida* infections and tinea cruris and corporis should be treated for two weeks and tinea pedis for one month in order to reduce the possibility of recurrence. If a patient shows no clinical improvement after a month of treatment, the diagnosis should be redetermined. Patients with tinea versicolor usually exhibit clinical and mycological clearing after two weeks of treatment.

How Supplied: MONISTAT-DERM (miconazole nitrate 2%) Cream containing miconazole nitrate at 2% strength is supplied in 15 g., 1 oz. and 3 oz. tubes. MONISTAT-DERM (miconazole nitrate 2%) Lotion containing miconazole nitrate at 2% w/w strength is supplied in polyethylene squeeze bottles in quantities of 30 ml. and 60 ml.

PERSA–GEL® 5% & 10% ℞

(benzoyl peroxide)
acetone-base gel

PERSA-GEL W 5% & 10%

(benzoyl peroxide)
water-base gel

Description: PERSA-GEL and PERSA-GEL W 5% and 10% (benzoyl peroxide 5% and 10%) are topical gel preparations for use in the treatment of acne vulgaris. Benzoyl peroxide is an oxidizing agent which possesses antibacterial properties and is classified as a keratolytic.
PERSA-GEL contains benzoyl peroxide 5% or 10% as the active ingredient in a gel base containing acetone, carbomer 940, trolamine, sodium lauryl sulfate, propylene glycol and purified water.
PERSA-GEL W contains benzoyl peroxide 5% or 10% as the active ingredient containing purified water, carbomer, sodium hydroxide, hydroxypropyl methylcellulose 2906, and laureth 4.

Clinical Pharmacology: The mechanism of action of benzoyl peroxide has not been determined but may be related to its antibacterial activity against **Propionibacterium acnes** and its ability to cause drying and peeling. Benzoyl peroxide reduces the concentration of free fatty acids in the sebum. Little is known about the percutaneous penetration, metabolism, and excretion of benzoyl peroxide, although it is likely that benzoic acid is a major metabolite. There is no evidence of systemic toxicity caused by benzoyl peroxide in humans.

Indications and Usage: These products are indicated for the topical treatment of acne vulgaris.

Contraindications: These products are contraindicated in patients with a history of hypersensitivity to any of the components of the preparations.

Precautions: General: For external use only. If severe irritation develops, discontinue use and institute appropriate therapy. After the reaction clears, treatment may often be resumed with less frequent application. This preparation should not be used in or near the eyes or on mucous membranes.

Information for Patients: Avoid contact with eyes, eyelids, lips and mucous membranes. If accidental contact occurs, rinse with water. May bleach hair and colored fabrics. If excessive irritation develops, discontinue use and consult your physician.

Carcinogenesis, Mutagenesis, Impairment of Fertility: There is no evidence in the published literature that benzoyl peroxide is carcinogenic, mutagenic or that it impairs fertility.

Pregnancy: Pregnancy Category C: Animal reproduction studies have not been conducted with benzoyl peroxide. It is also not known whether benzoyl peroxide can cause fetal harm when administered to a pregnant woman or can affect reproduction capacity. Benzoyl peroxide should be used by a pregnant woman only if clearly needed. There are no data available on the effect of benzoyl peroxide on the growth, development and functional maturation of the unborn child.

Nursing Mothers: It is not known whether this drug is excreted in human milk. Because many drugs are excreted in human milk, caution should be exercised when benzoyl peroxide is administered to a nursing woman.

Pediatric Use: Safety and effectiveness in children have not been established.

Adverse Reactions: Allergic contact dermatitis has been reported with topical benzoyl peroxide therapy.

Dosage and Administration: PERSA-GEL or PERSA-GEL W 5% or 10% should be applied once or twice daily to affected areas after washing with a mild cleanser and water. The degree of drying and peeling can be adjusted by modification of the dosage schedule.

How Supplied:
PERSA-GEL 5%, 1.5 oz. tubes
(**NDC** 0062-8610-31)
PERSA-GEL 5%, 3 oz. tubes
(**NDC** 0062-8610-03)
PERSA-GEL 10%, 1.5 oz. tubes
(**NDC** 0062-8600-31)
PERSA-GEL 10%, 3 oz. tubes
(**NDC** 0062-8600-03)
PERSA-GEL W 5% 1.5 oz. tubes
(**NDC** 0062-8630-31)
PERSA-GEL W 5% 3.0 oz. tubes
(**NDC** 0062-8630-03)
PERSA-GEL W 10% 1.5 oz. tubes
(**NDC** 0062-8620-31)
PERSA-GEL W 10% 3.0 oz. tubes
(**NDC** 0062-8620-03)
Store at controlled room temperature (59°–86°F).

PURPOSE® Dry Skin Cream

(See PDR For Nonprescription Drugs)

PURPOSE® Shampoo

(See PDR For Nonprescription Drugs)

PURPOSE® Soap

(See PDR For Nonprescription Drugs)

RETIN-A®
(tretinoin)
Cream•Gel•Liquid ℞

Description: RETIN-A (tretinoin) acne treatment is available in gel, cream and liquid vehicles. RETIN-A (tretinoin) Gel contains tretinoin (retinoic acid; vitamin A acid) in either of two strengths, 0.025% or 0.01% by weight, in a gel vehicle of butylated hydroxytoluene, hydroxypropyl cellulose, and alcohol 90% w/w. RETIN-A (tretinoin) Cream contains tretinoin in either of two strengths, 0.1% or 0.05% by weight, in a hydrophilic cream vehicle of stearic acid, isopropyl myristate, polyoxyl 40 stearate, stearyl alcohol, xanthan gum, sorbic acid, and butylated hydroxytoluene. RETIN-A (tretinoin) Liquid contains tretinoin 0.05% by weight, polyethylene glycol 400, butylated hydroxytoluene, and alcohol 55%.

Indications: RETIN-A is indicated for topical application in the treatment of acne vulgaris, primarily grades I, II, and III in which comedones, papules, and pustules predominate. It is not effective in most cases of severe pustular and deep cystic nodular varieties (acne conglobata).

Contraindications: Use of the product should be discontinued if hypersensitivity to any of the ingredients is noted.

Warnings: Recent studies in hairless albino mice suggest that tretinoin may accelerate the tumorigenic potential of ultraviolet radiation. Although the significance to man is not clear, patients should avoid or minimize exposure to sun.

Concomitant topical medication should be used with caution because of possible interaction with tretinoin. Particular caution should be exercised in using preparations containing peeling agents (such as sulfur, resorcinol, benzoyl peroxide, or salicylic acid) with RETIN-A. It also is advisable to "rest" a patient's skin until the effects of peeling agents subside before use of RETIN-A is begun.

Exposure to sunlight, including sunlamps, should be minimized during the use of RETIN-A, and patients with sunburn should be advised not to use the product until fully recovered because of heightened susceptibility to sunlight as a result of the use of tretinoin. Patients who may be required to have considerable sun exposure due to occupation and those with inherent sensitivity to the sun should exercise particular caution. Use of sunscreen products and protective clothing over treated areas may be prudent when exposure cannot be avoided. Weather extremes, such as wind or cold, also may be irritating to patients under treatment with tretinoin.

RETIN-A (tretinoin) acne treatment should be kept away from the eyes, the mouth, angles of the nose, and mucous membranes. Topical use may induce severe local erythema and peeling at the site of application. If the degree of local irritation warrants, patients should be directed to use the medication less frequently, discontinue use temporarily, or discontinue use altogether. Tretinoin has been reported to cause severe irritation on eczematous skin and should be used with utmost caution in patients with this condition.

Precaution: Medicated or abrasive soaps and cleansers, soaps and cosmetics that have a strong drying effect, and products with high concentrations of alcohol, astringents, spices, or lime should be used with caution because of possible interaction with tretinoin.

If medication is applied excessively, no more rapid or better results will be obtained and marked redness, peeling, or discomfort may occur.

Adverse Reactions: The skin of certain sensitive individuals may become excessively red, edematous, blistered, or crusted. If these effects occur, the medication should either be discontinued until the integrity of the skin is restored, or the medication should be adjusted to a level the patient can tolerate. True contact allergy to topical tretinoin is rarely encountered. Temporary hyper- or hypopigmentation has been reported with repeated application of RETIN-A. Some individuals have been reported to have heightened susceptibility to sunlight while under treatment with RETIN-A. To date, all adverse effects of RETIN-A have been reversible upon discontinuance of therapy (see Dosage and Administration Section).

Dosage and Administration: RETIN-A Gel, Cream or Liquid should be applied once a day, before retiring, to the skin where acne lesions appear, using enough to cover the entire affected area lightly. Liquid: The liquid may be applied using a fingertip, gauze pad, or cotton swab. If gauze or cotton is employed, care should be taken not to oversaturate it to the extent that the liquid would run into areas where treatment is not intended. Gel: Excessive application results in "pilling" of the gel, which minimizes the likelihood of overapplication by the patient.

Application may cause a transitory feeling of warmth or slight stinging. In cases where it has been necessary to temporarily discontinue therapy or to reduce the frequency of application, therapy may be resumed or frequency of application increased when the patients become able to tolerate the treatment.

It should be noted that just as some patients require less frequent applications or other dosage forms, others may respond better to more frequent applications of tretinoin. Alterations of vehicle, drug concentration, or dose frequency should be closely monitored by careful observation of the clinical therapeutic response and skin tolerance.

During the early weeks of therapy, an *apparent* exacerbation of inflammatory lesions may occur. This is due to the action of the medication on deep, previously unseen lesions and should not be considered a reason to discontinue therapy.

Therapeutic results should be noticed after two to three weeks, but more than six weeks of therapy may be required before definite beneficial effects are seen. Once the acne lesions have responded satisfactorily, it may be possible to maintain the improvement with less frequent applications, or other dosage forms.

Patients treated with RETIN-A tretinoin acne treatment may use cosmetics, but the areas to be treated should be cleansed thoroughly before the medication is applied.

How Supplied: RETIN-A (tretinoin) is supplied as:

1. A 0.025% Gel in tubes of 15 grams and 45 grams, and 0.01% Gel in tubes of 15 grams and 45 grams.
2. A 0.1% Cream in tubes of 20 grams, and 0.05% Cream in tubes of 20 grams and 45 grams.
3. A 0.05% Liquid in amber bottles containing 28 ml.

Important Notice

Before prescribing or administering

any product described in

PHYSICIANS' DESK REFERENCE

always consult the PDR Supplement for

possible new or revised information.

Parke-Davis

Division of Warner-Lambert Company
201 TABOR ROAD
MORRIS PLAINS, NEW JERSEY 07950

Parke-Davis

Div Warner-Lambert Inc
SANTURCE, PR 00911

PARCODE®
(Parke-Davis Accurate Recognition Code)

Code Number	Product Name
001	**Peritrate® Tablets** Each tablet contains 20 mg pentaerythritol tetranitrate.
002-003	*Unassigned*
004	**Peritrate® SA Sustained Action Tablets** Each tablet contains 80 mg pentaerythritol tetranitrate (20 mg in the immediate release layer and 60 mg in the sustained release base).
005-006	*Unassigned*
007	**Dilantin® Infatabs®** Each tablet contains 50 mg phenytoin sodium, USP.
008	**Peritrate® Tablets** Each tablet contains 40 mg pentaerythritol tetranitrate.
009	*Unassigned*
010	**Chlorpromazine Hydrochloride Tablets, USP (Promapar®)** Each tablet contains 10 mg chlorpromazine hydrochloride, USP.
011-012	*Unassigned*
013	**Peritrate® Tablets** Each tablet contains 10 mg pentaerythritol tetranitrate.
014-024	*Unassigned*
025	**Chlorpromazine Hydrochloride Tablets, USP (Promapar®)** Each tablet contains 25 mg chlorpromazine hydrochloride, USP.
026-033	*Unassigned*
034	**Gelusil® Tablets** Each tablet contains 200 mg aluminum hydroxide, 200 mg magnesium hydroxide, and 25 mg simethicone.
035-036	*Unassigned*
037	**Ferrous Sulfate Filmseals®, USP (325 mg)**
038-042	*Unassigned*
043	**Gelusil-II® Tablets** Each tablet contains 400 mg aluminum hydroxide, 400 mg magnesium hydroxide, and 30 mg simethicone.
044	*Unassigned*
045	**Gelusil-M® Tablets** Each tablet contains 300 mg aluminum hydroxide, 400 mg magnesium hydroxide, and 25 mg simethicone.

This product information was prepared in August, 1982. On these and other Parke-Davis Products, information may be obtained by addressing PARKE-DAVIS, Division of Warner-Lambert Company, Morris Plains, New Jersey 07950.

Continued on next page

Parke-Davis—Cont.

046-
049 *Unassigned*
050 **Chlorpromazine Hydrochloride Tablets, USP (Promapar®)**
Each tablet contains 50 mg chlorpromazine hydrochloride, USP.
051-
054 *Unassigned*
055 **Cascara Sagrada Extract Filmseal®**
Each film-coated tablet contains 325 mg (5 grains) cascara sagrada extract.
056-
099 *Unassigned*
100 **Chlorpromazine Hydrochloride Tablets, USP (Promapar®)**
Each tablet contains 100 mg chlorpromazine hydrochloride, USP.
101 **Sinubid® Tablets**
Each tablet contains 300 mg acetaminophen, 300 mg phenacetin, 100 mg phenylpropanolamine hydrochloride, and 66 mg phenyltoloxamine citrate.
102-
110 *Unassigned*
111 **Ergostat® Sublingual Tablets**
Each tablet contains 2 mg ergotamine tartrate.
112-
165 *Unassigned*
166 **Mandelamine® Tablets**
Each tablet contains 0.5 gram methenamine mandelate, USP.
167 **Mandelamine® Tablets**
Each tablet contains 1.0 gram methenamine mandelate, USP.
168-
179 *Unassigned*
180 **Pyridium® Tablets**
Each tablet contains 200 mg phenazopyridine hydrochloride, USP.
181 **Pyridium® Tablets**
Each tablet contains 200 mg phenazopyridine hydrochloride, USP.
182 **Pyridium® Plus Tablets**
Each tablet contains 150 mg phenazopyridine hydrochloride (Pyridium®), 0.3 mg hyoscyamine hydrobromide, and 15 mg butabarbital.
183-
199 *Unassigned*
200 **Brondecon® Tablets**
Each tablet contains 200 mg oxtriphylline and 100 mg guaifenesin.
201 **Chlorpromazine Hydrochloride Tablets, USP (Promapar®)**
Each tablet contains 200 mg chlorpromazine hydrochloride, USP.
202 **Procan® SR Tablets, 250 mg**
Each sustained-release tablet contains 250 mg procainamide hydrochloride.
203 *Unassigned*
204 **Procan® SR Tablets, 500 mg**
Each sustained-release tablet contains 500 mg procainamide hydrochloride.
205 **Procan® SR Tablets, 750 mg**
Each sustained-release tablet contains 750 mg procainamide hydrochloride.
206-
209 *Unassigned*
210 **Choledyl® Tablets**
Each tablet contains 100 mg oxtriphylline, USP.
211 **Choledyl® Tablets**
Each tablet contains 200 mg oxtriphylline, USP.
212 **Natafort® Filmseal®**
Each tablet represents vitamin A (acetate), (1.8 mg) 6,000 IU; vitamin D (ergocalciferol), (10 mcg) 400 IU; folic acid, 1 mg; vitamin B_1 (thiamine mononitrate), 3 mg; vitamin B_2 (riboflavin), 2 mg; vitamin B_6 (pyridoxine hydrochloride), 15 mg; vitamin B_{12} (cyanocobalamin), crystalline, 6 mcg; vitamin C (ascorbic acid), 120 mg; nicotinamide (niacinamide), 20 mg; vitamin E (*dl*-alpha tocopheryl acetate), (30 mg) 30 IU; calcium (as calcium carbonate), 350 mg; magnesium (as magnesium oxide), 100 mg; iodine (as potassium iodide), 0.15 mg; iron (as ferrous fumarate), 65 mg; zinc (as zinc oxide), 25 mg; and docusate sodium, 50 mg.
213 *Unassigned*
214 **Choledyl® SA Tablets**
Each sustained-action tablet contains 400 mg oxtriphylline, USP.
215-
220 *Unassigned*
221 **Choledyl® SA Tablets**
Each sustained-action tablet contains 600 mg oxtriphylline, USP.
222-
229 *Unassigned*
230 **Tedral® Tablets**
Each tablet contains 130 mg theophylline, 24 mg ephedrine hydrochloride, and 8 mg phenobarbital.
231 **Tedral® SA Tablets**
Each sustained-action tablet contains 180 mg anhydrous theophylline (90 mg in the immediate release layer and 90 mg in the sustained-release layer); 48 mg ephedrine hydrochloride (16 mg in the immediate release layer and 32 mg in the sustained-release layer); 25 mg phenobarbital in the immediate release layer.
232-
236 *Unassigned*
237 **Zarontin® Capsules**
Each capsule contains 250 mg ethosuximide, USP.
238 **Tedral-25® Tablets**
Each tablet contains 130 mg theophylline, 24 mg ephedrine hydrochloride, and 25 mg butabarbital.
239 *Unassigned*
240 **Abdol® with Minerals Capsules**
241-
246 *Unassigned*
247 **D-S-S Capsules**
Each capsule contains 100 mg docusate sodium.
248 **D-S-S Plus Capsules**
Each capsule contains 100 mg docusate sodium and 30 mg casanthranol.
249-
250 *Unassigned*
251 **Proloid® Tablets**
Each tablet contains ½ grain thyroglobulin, USP.
252 **Proloid® Tablets**
Each tablet contains 1 grain thyroglobulin, USP.
253 **Proloid® Tablets**
Each tablet contains 1½ grains thyroglobulin, USP.
254 **Proloid® Tablets**
Each tablet contains 3 grains thyroglobulin, USP.
255-
256 *Unassigned*
257 **Proloid® Tablets**
Each tablet contains 2 grains thyroglobulin, USP.
258-
259 *Unassigned*
260 **Euthroid®-½ Tablets**
Each tablet contains ½ grain liotrix.
261 **Euthroid®-1 Tablets**
Each tablet contains 1 grain liotrix.
262 **Euthroid®-2 Tablets**
Each tablet contains 2 grains liotrix.
263 **Euthroid®-3 Tablets**
Each tablet contains 3 grains liotrix.
264-
267 *Unassigned*
268 **Meclomen® Capsules**
Each capsule contains 50 mg meclofenamate sodium.
269 **Meclomen® Capsules**
Each capsule contains 100 mg meclofenamate sodium.
270 **Nardil® Tablets**
Each tablet contains 15 mg phenelzine sulfate, USP.
271 **Amitriptyline Hydrochloride Tablets**
Each tablet contains 100 mg amitriptyline hydrochloride, USP.
272 **Amitriptyline Hydrochloride Tablets**
Each tablet contains 10 mg amitriptyline hydrochloride, USP.
273 **Amitriptyline Hydrochloride Tablets**
Each tablet contains 25 mg amitriptyline hydrochloride, USP.
274 **Amitriptyline Hydrochloride Tablets**
Each tablet contains 50 mg amitriptyline hydrochloride, USP.
275 **Amitriptyline Hydrochloride Tablets**
Each tablet contains 75 mg amitriptyline hydrochloride, USP.
276 **Ⓒ Centrax® Tablets**
Each tablet contains 10 mg prazepam.
277 *Unassigned*
278 **Amitriptyline Hydrochloride Tablets**
Each tablet contains 150 mg amitriptyline hydrochloride, USP.
279-
300 *Unassigned*
301 **Papase® Tablets**
Each tablet contains proteolytic enzymes extracted from *Carica papaya*.
302-
319 *Unassigned*
320 **Parsidol® Tablets**
Each tablet contains 10 mg ethosuximide hydrochloride.
321 **Parsidol® Tablets**
Each tablet contains 50 mg ethosuximide hydrochloride.
322-
334 *Unassigned*
335 **Myadec® Tablets**
Each tablet represents vitamin A 10,000 IU; vitamin D 400 IU; vitamin E 30 IU; vitamin C 250 mg; folic acid 0.4 mg; thiamine 10 mg; riboflavin 10 mg; niacin 100 mg; vitamin B_6 5 mg; vitamin B_{12} 6 mcg; pantothenic acid 20 mg; iodine 150 mcg; iron 20 mg; magnesium 100 mg; copper 2 mg; zinc 20 mg; manganese 1.25 mg.
336 *Unassigned*
337 **Eldec® Kapseals®**
Each capsule represents vitamin A (acetate), (0.5 mg) 1,667 IU; vitamin C (ascorbic acid), 66.7 mg; vitamin B_1 (thiamine mononitrate), 10 mg; vitamin B_2 (riboflavin), 0.87 mg; vitamin B_6 (pyridoxine hydrochloride), 0.67 mg; nicotinamide (niacinamide), 16.7 mg; *dl*-panthenol, 10 mg; ferrous sulfate, dried, 16.7 mg; iodine (as potassium iodide), 0.05 mg; calcium carbonate, 66.7 mg; vitamin E (*dl*-alpha tocopheryl acetate), (10 mg) 10 IU; vitamin B_{12} (cyanocobalamin), 2 mcg; folic acid, 0.33 mg. The Kapseal is a Dark Blue No. 1 capsule with Light Blue opaque band.
338-
361 *Unassigned*
362 **Dilantin® Kapseals®**
Each Kapseal contains 100 mg extended phenytoin sodium, USP. The Kapseal is a No. 3 capsule with Orange band. (The Orange band on White capsule is a trademark registered in the US Patent Office.)

363-
364 *Unassigned*
365 **Dilantin® Kapseals®**
Each Kapseal contains 30 mg extended phenytoin sodium, USP. The Kapseal is a No. 4 capsule with Pink opaque band.
366-
367 *Unassigned*
368 **Taka-Combex® Kapseals®**
Each Kapseal represents Taka-Diastase® (*Aspergillus oryzae* enzymes), 2½ grains; thiamine mononitrate, 10 mg; riboflavin, 10 mg; pyridoxine hydrochloride, 0.5 mg; cyanocobalamin, 1 mcg; niacinamide, 10 mg; *dl*-panthenol, 6 mg; ascorbic acid, 30 mg; liver concentrate, 0.34 g. The Kapseal is a Brown No. 1 capsule with Yellow opaque band.
369-
370 *Unassigned*
371 **Abdec® Kapseals®**
Each Kapseal represents vitamin A (acetate) (3 mg), 10,000 IU; ergocalciferol, (10 mcg) 400 IU; ascorbic acid, 75 mg; thiamine mononitrate, 5 mg; riboflavin, 3 mg; pyridoxine hydrochloride, 1.5 mg; cyanocobalamin, 2 mcg; niacinamide, 25 mg; *dl*-panthenol, 10 mg; *dl*-alpha tocopheryl acetate (5 mg), 5 IU. The Kapseal is a Garnet No. 3 capsule with Black band.
372 *Unassigned*
373 **Benadryl® Kapseals®**
Each Kapseal contains 50 mg diphenhydramine hydrochloride. The Kapseal is a Pink No. 4 capsule with White opaque band. (The White band on Pink capsule is a trademark registered in the US Patent Office.)
374 *Unassigned*
375 **Dilantin® with Phenobarbital (¼ grain) Kapseals®**
Each Kapseal contains Dilantin (phenytoin sodium), 100 mg; phenobarbital, 16 mg (¼ grain). The Kapseal is a No. 3 capsule with Garnet band.
376-
377 *Unassigned*
378 **Benadryl® with Ephedrine Sulfate Kapseals ®**
Each Kapseal contains Benadryl (diphenhydramine hydrochloride), 50 mg; ephedrine sulfate, 25 mg. The Kapseal is a Pink No. 4 capsule with Dark Blue band.
379 **Chloromycetin® Kapseals®**
Each Kapseal contains 250 mg chloramphenicol. The Kapseal is a White opaque No. 2 capsule with Gray opaque band. (The Gray band on White capsule is a trademark registered in the US Patent Office.)
380-
381 *Unassigned*
382 **Geriplex® Kapseals®**
Each Kapseal represents vitamin A (acetate), (1.5 mg) 5,000 IU; ascorbic acid,* 50 mg; thiamine mononitrate, 5 mg; riboflavin, 5 mg; cyanocobalamin, 2 mcg; choline dihydrogen citrate, 20 mg; niacinamide, 15 mg; *dl*-alpha tocopheryl acetate, (5 mg), 5 IU; ferrous sulfate,† 30 mg; copper sulfate, 4 mg; manganese sulfate (monohydrate), 4 mg; zinc sulfate, 2 mg; calcium phosphate, dibasic (anhydrous), 200 mg. The Kapseal is a Blue No. 1 capsule with Yellow opaque band.

---

*Supplied as sodium ascorbate.
†Supplied as dried ferrous sulfate equivalent to the labeled amount of ferrous sulfate.

383-
388 *Unassigned*
389 **Ambodryl® Hydrochloride Kapseals®**
Each Kapseal contains 25 mg bromodiphenhydramine hydrochloride, USP. The Kapseal is a Pink Tint No. 4 capsule with Pink band.
390 **Natabec® Kapseals®**
Each Kapseal represents vitamin A (acetate), 4,000 IU; vitamin D (ergocalciferol), 400 IU; vitamin C (ascorbic acid), 50 mg; vitamin B, (as thiamine mononitrate; vitamin B_1), 3.0 mg; riboflavin (vitamin B_2), 2.0 mg; nicotinamide (niacinamide), 10 mg; vitamin B_6 (pyridoxine hydrochloride), 3 mg; vitamin B_{12}, crystalline (cyanocobalamin), 5 mcg; calcium carbonate, 600 mg; ferrous sulfate, 150 mg.
391-
392 *Unassigned*
393 **Milontin® Kapseals®**
Each Kapseal contains 500 mg phensuximide, USP. The Kapseal is a Light Orange No. 0 capsule with Orange band.
394-
401 *Unassigned*
402 **Amcill® Capsules, 250 mg**
Each capsule contains ampicillin trihydrate equivalent to 250 mg ampicillin.
403 *Unassigned*
404 **Amcill® Capsules, 500 mg**
Each capsule contains ampicillin trihydrate equivalent to 500 mg ampicillin.
405-
406 *Unassigned*
407 **Tetracycline Hydrochloride Capsules, USP, 250 mg (Cyclopar®)**
Each capsule contains 250 mg tetracycline hydrochloride, USP.
408-
419 *Unassigned*
420 **Quinine Sulfate Capsules, USP**
Each capsule contains 0.325 g (5 grains) quinine sulfate.
421-
436 *Unassigned*
437 **Estrovis® Tablets**
Each tablet contains 100 mcg quinestrol.
438-
470 *Unassigned*
471 **Benadryl® Capsules**
Each capsule contains 25 mg diphenhydramine hydrochloride.
472-
489 *Unassigned*
490 **Easprin™ Enteric Coated Tablets**
Each tablet contains 15 grains (975 mg) aspirin, USP.
491-
502 *Unassigned*
503 **Panteric® Filmseals®**
Each film-coated tablet contains 5 grains (0.325 g) pancreatin, triple strength.
504-
524 *Unassigned*
525 **Celontin® Kapseals®**
Each Kapseal contains 300 mg methsuximide, USP. The Kapseal is a Yellow Tint No. 2 capsule with Orange band.
526-
528 *Unassigned*
529 **Humatin® Capsules**
Each capsule contains paromomycin sulfate, USP, equivalent to 250 mg paromomycin.
530 *Unassigned*
531 **Dilantin® with Phenobarbital (½ grain) Kapseals®**
Each Kapseal contains Dilantin (phenytoin sodium), 100 mg; phenobarbital, 32 mg (½ grain). The Kapseal is a No. 3 capsule with Black band.
532 *Unassigned*
533 **Calcium Lactate Tablets, USP**
Each tablet contains 325 mg calcium lactate.
534 **Natabec® with Fluoride Kapseals®**
Each Kapseal represents vitamin A (acetate) (1.2 mg), 4,000 IU*; vitamin D (ergocalciferol) (10 mcg), 400 IU; vitamin C (ascorbic acid), 50 mg; thiamine mononitrate (vitamin B_1), 3 mg; riboflavin (vitamin B_2), 2.0 mg; nicotinamide (niacinamide), 20 mg; vitamin B_6 (pyridoxine hydrochloride), 3 mg; vitamin B_{12}, crystalline (cyanocobalamin), 5 mcg; ferrous sulfate, 150 mg; calcium carbonate, 600 mg; sodium fluoride, 2.2 mg.

---

*international units
The Kapseal is a Pastel Pink No. 0 capsule with Ruby Red opaque band.
535-
536 *Unassigned*
537 **Celontin® (Half Strength) Kapseals®**
Each Kapseal contains 150 mg methsuximide, USP. The Kapseal is a Yellow Tint No. 4 capsule with Brown opaque band.
538-
539 *Unassigned*
540 **Ponstel® Kapseals®**
Each Kapseal contains 250 mg mefenamic acid. The Kapseal is an Ivory opaque No. 1 capsule with Light Blue opaque band. The blue band on ivory capsule combination is a Parke-Davis trademark.
541 **Natabec-FA® Kapseals®**
Each Kapseal represents vitamin A (acetate), (1.2 mg) 4,000 IU; ergocalciferol (10 mcg), 400 IU; ascorbic acid, 50 mg; thiamine mononitrate, 3 mg; riboflavin, 2 mg; pyridoxine hydrochloride, 3 mg; cyanocobalamin, 5 mcg; folic acid, 0.1 mg; niacinamide, 20 mg; calcium carbonate, 600 mg; ferrous sulfate,* 150 mg.

---

*Supplied as dried ferrous sulfate equivalent to the labeled amount of ferrous sulfate.
The Kapseal is a Pink Tint opaque No. 0 capsule with White opaque band.
542-
543 *Unassigned*
544 **Geriplex-FS® Kapseals®**
Each Kapseal represents vitamin A (acetate) (1.5 mg), 5,000 IU; ascorbic acid,* 50 mg; thiamine mononitrate, 5 mg; riboflavin, 5 mg; cyanocobalamin, 2 mcg; choline dihydrogen citrate, 20 mg; niacinamide, 15 mg; *dl*-alpha tocopheryl acetate (5 mg), 5 IU; iron,† 6 mg; copper sulfate, 4 mg; manganese sulfate (monohydrate), 4 mg; zinc sulfate, 2 mg; calcium phosphate, dibasic (anhydrous), 200 mg; Taka-Diastase® (*aspergillus oryzae enzymes*); 2½ gr; docusate sodium, 100 mg.

---

*Supplied as sodium ascorbate.
†Supplied as 30 mg dried ferrous sulfate.
The Kapseal is a Blue No. 0 capsule with White opaque band.
545-
546 *Unassigned*
547 **Natabec ℞® Kapseals®**
Each Kapseal represents vitamin A (acetate) (1.2 mg), 4,000 IU; ergocalcif-

Continued on next page

This product information was prepared in August, 1982. On these and other Parke-Davis Products, information may be obtained by addressing PARKE-DAVIS, Division of Warner-Lambert Company, Morris Plains, New Jersey 07950.

Parke-Davis—Cont.

erol, (10 mcg) 400 IU; ascorbic acid, 50 mg; thiamine mononitrate, 3 mg; riboflavin, 2 mg; pyridoxine hydrochloride, 3 mg; cyanocobalamin, 5 mcg; niacinamide, 10 mg; folic acid, 1 mg; calcium carbonate, precipitated, 600 mg; ferrous sulfate,* 150 mg.

*Supplied as dried ferrous sulfate equivalent to the labeled amount of ferrous sulfate.

The Kapseal is a Blue opaque No. 0 capsule with Pink opaque band. The banded capsule is a Warner-Lambert trademark registered in the US Patent Office.

548-
549 *Unassigned*

550 **Thera-Combex H-P® Kapseals®**
Each Kapseal contains: ascorbic acid, 500 mg; thiamine mononitrate, 25 mg; riboflavin, 15 mg; pyridoxine hydrochloride, 10 mg; cyanocobalamin, 5 mcg; niacinamide, 100 mg; *dl*-panthenol, 20 mg.
The Kapseal is a Brown No. 0 capsule with Green opaque band.

551 *Unassigned*

552 **ⒸCentrax® Capsules**
Each capsule contains 5 mg prazepam.

553 **ⒸCentrax® Capsules**
Each capsule contains 10 mg prazepam.

554 **ⒸCentrax® Capsules**
Each capsule contains 20 mg prazepam.

555-
603 *Unassigned*

604 **Calcium Lactate Tablets, USP**
Each tablet contains 650 mg (10 grains) calcium lactate.

605 *Unassigned*

606 **Aspirin Tablets, USP (White)**
Each tablet contains 325 mg (5 grains) aspirin.

607 **ⒸPhenobarbital Tablets, USP**
Each tablet contains 60 mg (1 grain) phenobarbital.

608-
617 *Unassigned*

618 **Placebo tablet in Norlestrin [28] 1/50.**

619-
621 *Unassigned*

622 **Ferrous Fumarate Tablets**
Each tablet contains 75 mg ferrous fumarate, USP.

623-
633 *Unassigned*

634 **ⒸAcetaminophen with Codeine Phosphate Tablets, No. 2**
Each tablet contains 300 mg acetaminophen and 15 mg (¼ grain) codeine phosphate.

635 **ⒸAcetaminophen with Codeine Phosphate Tablets, No. 3**
Each tablet contains 300 mg acetaminophen and 30 mg (½ grain) codeine phosphate.

636 **Betapar® Tablets**
Each scored, light green tablet contains 4 mg meprednisone, USP.

637 **ⒸAcetaminophen with Codeine Phosphate Tablets, No. 4**
Each tablet contains 300 mg acetaminophen and 60 mg (1 grain) codeine phosphate.

638 **Tabron® Filmseal®**
Each film-coated tablet represents ferrous fumarate, 304.2 mg (represents 100 mg of elemental iron); ascorbic acid, 500 mg; thiamine mononitrate, 6 mg; riboflavin, 6 mg; pyridoxine hydrochloride, 5 mg; cyanocobalamin, 25 mcg; folic acid, 1 mg; niacinamide, 30 mg; calcium pantothenate, 10 mg; *dl*-alpha tocopheryl acetate (30 mg), 30 IU; docusate sodium, 50 mg.

639 *Unassigned*

640 **Acetaminophen Tablets, USP (Tapar®)**
Each tablet contains 325 mg (5 grains) acetaminophen, USP.

641-
646 *Unassigned*

647 **ⒸMeprobamate Tablets, USP**
Each tablet contains 400 mg meprobamate, USP.

648 **Penicillin V Potassium Tablets, USP, 250 mg (Penapar VK®)**
Each tablet contains penicillin V potassium equivalent to 250 mg (400,000 units) penicillin V.

649-
668 *Unassigned*

669 **Lopid® Capsules**
Each capsule contains 300 mg gemfibrozil.

670-
671 *Unassigned*

672 **Erythromycin Stearate Filmseals (Erypar®)**
Each Filmseal® contains 250 mg erythromycin as erythromycin stearate.

673 **Penicillin V Potassium Tablets, USP, 500 mg (Penapar VK®)**
Each tablet contains penicillin V potassium equivalent to 500 mg (800,000 units) penicillin V.

674-
678 *Unassigned*

679 **Aspirin Compound Tablets, White**
Each tablet contains aspirin, 3½ grains; phenacetin, 2½ grains; caffeine, ½ grain.

680-
691 *Unassigned*

692 **ⒸPropoxyphene Hydrochloride Capsules, USP**
Each capsule contains 65 mg propoxyphene hydrochloride.

693 *Unassigned*

694 **ⒸPropoxyphene Compound 65, Capsules**
Each capsule contains 65 mg propoxyphene hydrochloride, 227 mg aspirin, 162 mg phenacetin, and 32.4 mg caffeine.

695 *Unassigned*

696 **ERYC® Capsules**
Each capsule contains 250 mg erythromycin, USP.

697 **Tetracycline Hydrochloride Capsules, USP, 500 mg (Cyclopar® 500)**
Each capsule contains 500 mg tetracycline hydrochloride, USP.

698 **ⒸPhenobarbital Tablets, USP**
Each tablet contains 100 mg (1½ grains) phenobarbital.

699 **ⒸPhenobarbital Tablets, USP**
Each tablet contains 15 mg (¼ grain) phenobarbital.

700 **ⒸPhenobarbital Tablets, USP**
Each tablet contains 30 mg (½ grain) phenobarbital.

701 *Unassigned*

702 **Hydrochlorothiazide Tablets, USP (Thiuretic®)**
Each tablet contains 25 mg hydrochlorothiazide.

703-
709 *Unassigned*

710 **Hydrochlorothiazide Tablets, USP (Thiuretic®)**
Each tablet contains 50 mg hydrochlorothiazide.

711-
724 *Unassigned*

725 **ⒸAspirin with Codeine Phosphate Tablets, No. 2**
Each tablet contains codeine phosphate, ¼ grain; aspirin, 325 mg.

726 **ⒸAspirin with Codeine Phosphate Tablets, No. 3**
Each tablet contains codeine phosphate, ½ grain; aspirin, 325 mg.

727 **ⒸAspirin with Codeine Phosphate Tablets, No. 4**
Each tablet contains codeine phosphate, 1 grain; aspirin, 325 mg.

728-
729 *Unassigned*

730 **Amoxicillin Capsules (Utimox®), USP, 250 mg**
Each capsule contains 250 mg amoxicillin.

731 **Amoxicillin Capsules (Utimox®), USP, 500 mg**
Each capsule contains 500 mg amoxicillin.

732 -
746 *Unassigned*

747 **Povan® Filmseal®**
Each film-coated tablet contains pyrvinium pamoate equivalent to 50 mg pyrvinium.

748 **Paladac® with Minerals Tablets**
Each tablet represents *vitamins:* vitamin A (acetate), (1.2 mg) 4,000 IU; ergocalciferol, (10 mcg) 400 units; ascorbic acid,* 50 mg; thiamine mononitrate, 3 mg; riboflavin, 3 mg; pyridoxine hydrochloride, 1 mg; cyanocobalamin, 5 mcg; niacinamide, 20 mg; pantothenic acid (as the calcium salt), 5 mg; *dl*-alpha tocopheryl acetate (10 mg), 10 IU. *Minerals*†: calcium, 23 mg; iron, 5 mg; phosphorus, 17 mg; iodine, 0.05 mg; potassium, 2.5 mg; magnesium, 1 mg.

*Supplied partly as sodium ascorbate.
†Supplied as calcium phosphate dibasic, ferric phosphate, potassium iodide, potassium sulfate, and magnesium oxide.

749-
771 *Unassigned*

772 **Tolbutamide Tablets**
Each tablet contains 500 mg tolbutamide, USP.

773-
791 *Unassigned*

792 **ⒸAspirin Compound with Codeine Phosphate Tablets, No. 2**
Each tablet contains codeine phosphate, ¼ grain; aspirin, 3½ grains; phenacetin, 2½ grains; caffeine, ½ grain.

793 **ⒸAspirin Compound with Codeine Phosphate Tablets, No. 3**
Each tablet contains codeine phosphate, ½ grain; aspirin, 3½ grains; phenacetin, 2½ grains; caffeine, ½ grain.

794-
799 *Unassigned*

800 **ⒸChlordiazepoxide Hydrochloride Capsules, USP**
Each capsule contains 5 mg chlordiazepoxide hydrochloride.

801 **ⒸChlordiazepoxide Hydrochloride Capsules, USP**
Each capsule contains 10 mg chlordiazepoxide hydrochloride.

802 **ⒸChlordiazepoxide Hydrochloride Capsules, USP**
Each capsule contains 25 mg chlordiazepoxide hydrochloride.

803-
848 *Unassigned*

849 **Quinidine Sulfate Tablets, USP**
Each tablet contains 3 grains (200 mg) quinidine sulfate.

850 **Duraquin® (quinidine gluconate) Tablets, 330 mg**
Each scored, white, sustained-release tablet contains 330 mg quinidine gluconate.

851-
881 *Unassigned*
882 **Norlutin® Tablets**
Each tablet contains 5 mg norethindrone, USP.
883-
900 *Unassigned*
901 **Norlestrin® 2.5/50 Tablets**
Each tablet contains norethindrone acetate, 2.5 mg; ethinyl estradiol, 50 mcg.
902-
903 *Unassigned*
904 **Norlestrin® 1/50 Tablets**
Each tablet contains norethindrone acetate, 1 mg; ethinyl estradiol, 50 mcg.
905-
914 *Unassigned*
915 **Loestrin® 1/20 Tablets**
Each tablet contains norethindrone acetate, 1 mg; ethinyl estradiol, 20 mcg.
916 **Loestrin® 1.5/30 Tablets**
Each tablet contains norethindrone acetate, 1.5 mg; ethinyl estradiol, 30 mcg.
917 *Unassigned*
918 **Norlutate® Tablets**
Each tablet contains 5 mg norethindrone acetate.
919 **Erythromycin Stearate Filmseals (Erypar®)**
Each Filmseal® contains 500 mg erythromycin as erythromycin stearate.
920-
924 *Unassigned*
925 **Renoquid® Tablets**
Each tablet contains 250 mg sulfacytine.
926-
931 *Unassigned*
932 **©Meprobamate Tablets, USP**
Each tablet contains 200 mg meprobamate.
933-
999 *Unassigned*

ADRENALIN® CHLORIDE SOLUTION ℞
(Epinephrine Injection, USP), 1:1000

Description: A sterile solution intended for subcutaneous or intramuscular injection. When diluted, it may also be administered intracardially or intravenously. Each milliliter contains 1 mg Adrenalin (epinephrine) as the hydrochloride dissolved in Water for Injection, USP, with sodium chloride added for isotonicity. The ampoules contain not more than 0.1% sodium bisulfite as an antioxidant, and the air in the ampoule has been displaced by nitrogen. The Steri-Vials® contain 0.5% Chloretone® (chlorobutanol) (chloroform derivative) as a preservative and not more than 0.15% sodium bisulfite as an antioxidant. Epinephrine is the active principle of the adrenal medulla, chemically described as (−)-3,4-Dihydroxy-α-[(methylamino) methyl] benzyl alcohol.

Clinical Pharmacology: Adrenalin (epinephrine) is a sympathomimetic drug. It activates an adrenergic receptive mechanism on effector cells and imitates all actions of the sympathetic nervous system except those on the arteries of the face and sweat glands. Epinephrine acts on both alpha and beta receptors and is the most potent alpha receptor activator.

Indications and Usage: In general, the most common uses of epinephrine are to relieve respiratory distress due to bronchospasm, to provide rapid relief of hypersensitivity reactions to drugs and other allergens, and to prolong the action of infiltration anesthetics. Its cardiac effects may be of use in restoring cardiac rhythm in cardiac arrest due to various causes, but it is not used in cardiac failure or in hemorrhagic, traumatic, or cardiogenic shock. Epinephrine is used as a hemostatic agent. It is also used in treating mucosal congestion of hay fever, rhinitis, and acute sinusitis; to relieve bronchial asthmatic paroxysms; in syncope due to complete heart block or carotid sinus hypersensitivity; for symptomatic relief of serum sickness, urticaria, angioneurotic edema; for resuscitation in cardiac arrest following anesthetic accidents; in simple (open angle) glaucoma; for relaxation of uterine musculature and to inhibit uterine contractions. Epinephrine Injection can be utilized to prolong the action of intraspinal and local anesthetics (see Contraindications).

Contraindications: Epinephrine is contraindicated in narrow angle (congestive) glaucoma, shock, during general anesthesia with halogenated hydrocarbons or cyclopropane and in individuals with organic brain damage. Epinephrine is also contraindicated with local anesthesia of certain areas, eg, fingers, toes, because of the danger of vasoconstriction producing sloughing of tissue; in labor because it may delay the second stage; in cardiac dilatation and coronary insufficiency.

Warnings: Administer with caution to elderly people; to those with cardiovascular disease, hypertension, diabetes or hyperthyroidism; in psychoneurotic individuals, and in pregnancy.

Patients with long-standing bronchial asthma and emphysema who have developed degenerative heart disease should be administered the drug with extreme caution.

Overdosage or inadvertent intravenous injection of epinephrine may cause cerebrovascular hemorrhage resulting from the sharp rise in blood pressure.

Fatalities may also result from pulmonary edema because of the peripheral constriction and cardiac stimulation produced. Rapidly acting vasodilators such as nitrites, or alpha blocking agents may counteract the marked pressor effects of epinephrine.

Precautions:

General: Adrenalin (epinephrine injection) should be protected from exposure to light. Do not remove ampoules or syringes from carton until ready to use. The solution should not be used if it is brown in color or contains a precipitate.

Epinephrine is readily destroyed by alkalies and oxidizing agents. In the latter category are oxygen, chlorine, bromine, iodine, permanganates, chromates, nitrites and salts of easily reducible metals, especially iron.

Drug Interactions: Use of epinephrine with excessive doses of digitalis, mercurial diuretics, or other drugs that sensitize the heart to arrhythmias is not recommended. Anginal pain may be induced when coronary insufficiency is present.

The effects of epinephrine may be potentiated by tricyclic antidepressants; certain antihistamines, eg, diphenhydramine, tripelennamine, d-chlorpheniramine; and sodium l-thyroxine.

Usage in Pregnancy: Pregnancy Category C. Adrenalin (epinephrine) has been shown to be teratogenic in rats when given in doses about 25 times the human dose. There are no adequate and well controlled studies in pregnant women. Adrenalin should be used during pregnancy only if the potential benefit justifies the potential risk to the fetus.

Adverse Reactions: Transient and minor side effects of anxiety, headache, fear and palpitations often occur with therapeutic doses, especially in hyperthyroid individuals. Repeated local injections can result in necrosis at sites of injection from vascular constriction. "Epinephrine-fastness" can occur with prolonged use.

Dosage and Administration: Subcutaneously or intramuscularly—0.2 to 1 ml (mg). Start with a small dose and increase if required.

Note: The subcutaneous is the preferred route of administration. If given intramuscularly, injection into the buttocks should be avoided.

For bronchial asthma and certain allergic manifestations, eg, angioedema, urticaria, serum sickness, anaphylactic shock, use epinephrine subcutaneously. For bronchial asthma in pediatric patients, administer 0.01 mg/kg or 0.3 mg/m^2 to a maximum of 0.5 mg subcutaneously, repeated every four hours if required.

For cardiac resuscitation—A dose of 0.5 ml (0.5 mg) diluted to 10 ml with sodium chloride injection can be administered intravenously or intracardially to restore myocardial contractility. External cardiac massage should follow intracardial administration to permit the drug to enter coronary circulation. The drug should be used secondarily to unsuccessful attempts with physical or electromechanical methods.

Ophthalmologic use (for producing conjunctival decongestion, to control hemorrhage, produce mydriasis and reduce intraocular pressure)—use a concentration of 1:10,000 (0.1 mg/ml) to 1:1,000 (1 mg/ml).

Intraspinal use (Amp 88)—Usual dose is 0.2 to 0.4 ml (0.2 to 0.4 mg) added to anesthetic spinal fluid mixture (may prolong anesthetic action by limiting absorption). For use with local anesthetic—Epinephrine 1:100,000 (0.01 mg/ml) to 1:20,000 (0.05 mg/ml) is the usual concentration employed with local anesthetics.

How Supplied:

N 0071-4188-03 (Amp 88) Sterile solution containing 1 mg Adrenalin (epinephrine) as the hydrochloride in each 1-ml ampoule (1:1000). For intramuscular or subcutaneous use. When diluted, it may also be administered intracardially, intravenously, or intraspinally. Supplied in packages of ten.

N 0071-4011-13 (S.V. 11) Sterile solution containing 1 mg Adrenalin (epinephrine) as the hydrochloride (1:1000). For intramuscular or subcutaneous use. When diluted, it may also be administered intracardially or intravenously. Supplied in a 30 ml Steri-Vial® (rubber-diaphragm-capped vial.)

4188G040

AGORAL® PLAIN
AGORAL® RASPBERRY
AGORAL® MARSHMALLOW

Description: Each tablespoonful (15 ml) of Agoral Plain (white) contains 4.2 grams mineral oil in a thoroughly homogenized emulsion with agar, tragacanth, acacia, egg albumin, glycerin and water.

Each tablespoonful (15 ml) of Agoral Raspberry (pink) or of Agoral Marshmallow (white) contains 4.2 grams mineral oil and 0.2 grams phenolphthalein in a thoroughly homogenized emulsion with agar, tragacanth, acacia, egg albumin, glycerin and water.

Actions: Agoral, containing mineral oil, facilitates defecation by lubricating the fecal mass and softening the stool. More effective than nonemulsified oil in penetrating the feces, Agoral thereby greatly reduces the possibility of oil leakage at the anal sphincter. Phenolphthalein gently stimulates motor activity of the lower intestinal tract. Agoral's combined lubricating-softening and peristaltic actions can help to restore a normal pattern of evacuation.

Indications: Relief of constipation. Agoral may be especially required when straining at stool is a hazard, as in hernia, cardiac, or hypertensive patients; during convalescence from surgery; before and after surgery for hemorrhoids or other painful anorectal disor-

Continued on next page

This product information was prepared in August, 1982. On these and other Parke-Davis Products, information may be obtained by addressing PARKE-DAVIS, Division of Warner-Lambert Company, Morris Plains, New Jersey 07950.

Parke-Davis—Cont.

ders; for obstetrical patients; for patients confined to bed.
The management of chronic constipation should also include attention to fluid intake, diet and bowel habits.
Contraindications: Sensitivity to phenolphthalein.
Dosage and Management:
(Taken at bedtime, laxation may be expected the next morning.)

	Adults	Children over 6 years
Agoral Plain (without phenolphthalein)	1 to 2 tablespoonfuls	2 to 4 teaspoonfuls
Agoral Raspberry	½ to 1 tablespoonful	1 to 2 teaspoonfuls
Agoral Marshmallow	½ to 1 tablespoonful	1 to 2 teaspoonfuls
	Take at bedtime only, unless other time is advised by physician.	

Agoral may be taken alone or in milk, water, fruit juice, or any miscible food.
Expectant or nursing mothers, bedridden or aged patients, young children or infants should use only on advice of physician.
Supplied: Agoral Plain (without phenolphthalein), plastic bottles of 16 fl oz (N 0071-2071-23). Agoral (raspberry flavor), plastic bottles of 16 fl oz (N 0071-2072-23). Agoral (marshmallow flavor), plastic bottles of 8 fl oz (N 0071-2070-20) and 16 fl oz (N 0071-2070-23).

AMCILL® ℞

(ampicillin, USP) as the trihydrate
Ampicillin Capsules, USP—250 mg and 500 mg
Ampicillin for Oral Suspension, USP 125 mg/5 ml and 250 mg/5 ml

Description: Ampicillin is a semisynthetic penicillin derived from the basic penicillin nucleus, 6-aminopenicillanic acid.
Actions: Microbiology: *In vitro* studies have shown sensitivity of the following microorganisms to ampicillin:
Gram Positive: Alpha- and beta-hemolytic streptococci, *Diplococcus pneumoniae*, staphylococci (nonpenicillinase-producing), *Bacillus anthracis, Clostridia* spp, *Corynebacterium xerose*, and most strains of enterococci.
The drug does not resist destruction by penicillinase, hence is not effective against penicillin G-resistant staphylococci.
Gram Negative: *Haemophilus influenzae, Neisseria gonorrhoeae, N meningitidis, Proteus mirabilis*, and many strains of *Salmonella* (including *S typhosa*), *Shigella* spp, and *Escherichia coli*.
Testing for Susceptibility: The invading organism should be cultured and its sensitivity demonstrated as a guide to therapy. If the Kirby-Bauer method of disc sensitivity is used, a 10-mcg ampicillin disc should be used to determine the relative *in vitro* susceptibility.
Human Pharmacology: Ampicillin is stable in the presence of gastric acid and is well-absorbed from the gastrointestinal tract. It diffuses readily into most body tissues and fluids. However, penetration into the cerebrospinal fluid and brain occurs only with meningeal inflammation. Ampicillin is excreted largely unchanged in the urine. Its excretion can be delayed by concurrent administration of probenecid. Ampicillin is the least serum bound of all the penicillins, averaging 20% compared to 60% to 90% for other penicillins. Average peak blood serum levels of approximately 3 mcg/ml are attained in approximately two hours following a 500-mg dose of ampicillin in the capsule form. A dose of 250 mg ampicillin, as the oral suspension, produces average blood serum levels of approximately 2 mcg/ml within one and one-half hours.
Indications: Ampicillin is indicated primarily in the treatment of infections caused by susceptible strains of the following microorganisms: *Shigella, Salmonella* (including *S typhosa), E coli, H influenzae, P mirabilis*, and *N gonorrhoeae*. Ampicillin may also be indicated in certain infections caused by susceptible gram positive organisms: penicillin G-sensitive staphylococci, streptococci, pneumococci, and enterococci.
Bacteriology studies to determine the causative organisms and their sensitivity to ampicillin should be performed. Therapy may be instituted prior to the results of sensitivity testing.
Contraindication: Ampicillin is contraindicated in patients with a history of a hypersensitivity reaction to the penicillins.
Warning: Serious and occasionally fatal hypersensitivity (anaphylactic) reactions have been reported in patients on penicillin therapy. Although anaphylaxis is more frequent following parenteral therapy, it has occurred in patients on oral penicillins. These reactions are more apt to occur in individuals with a history of sensitivity to multiple allergens.
There have been reports of individuals with a history of penicillin hypersensitivity who experienced severe reactions when treated with cephalosporins. Before therapy with any penicillin, careful inquiry should be made concerning previous hypersensitivity reactions to penicillins, cephalosporins, or other allergens. Serious anaphylactoid reactions require immediate emergency treatment with epinephrine. Oxygen, intravenous steroids, and airway management, including intubation, should also be administered as indicated.
Usage in Pregnancy: Safety for use in pregnancy has not been established.
Precautions: As with any potent drug, periodic assessment of renal, hepatic, and hematopoietic functions should be made during prolonged therapy.
The possibility of superinfections with mycotic or bacterial pathogens should be kept in mind during therapy. If superinfections occur, appropriate therapy should be instituted.
Adverse Reactions: As with other penicillins, it may be expected that untoward reactions will be essentially limited to sensitivity phenomena. They are more likely to occur in individuals who have previously demonstrated hypersensitivity to penicillins and in those with a history of allergy, asthma, hay fever, or urticaria.
The following adverse reactions have been reported as associated with the use of ampicillin.
Gastrointestinal—Glossitis, stomatitis, black "hairy" tongue, nausea, vomiting, enterocolitis, pseudomembranous colitis, and diarrhea have been reported. (These reactions are usually associated with oral dosage forms.)
Hypersensitivity Reactions—Erythematous maculopapular rashes have been reported fairly frequently. Urticaria, erythema multiforme, and an occasional case of exfoliative dermatitis have been reported. Anaphylaxis is the most serious reaction experienced and has usually been associated with the parenteral dosage form.
NOTE: Urticaria, other skin rashes, and serum sickness-like reactions may be controlled with antihistamines and, if necessary, systemic corticosteroids. Whenever such reactions occur, ampicillin should be discontinued unless, in the opinion of the physician, the condition being treated is life-threatening and amenable only to ampicillin therapy. Serious anaphylactic reactions require the immediate use of epinephrine, oxygen, and intravenous steroids.
Liver—A moderate rise in serum glutamic oxaloacetic transaminase (SGOT) has been noted, particularly in infants, but the significance of this finding is unknown.
Hemic and Lymphatic Systems—Anemia, thrombocytopenia, thrombocytopenic purpura, eosinophilia, leukopenia, and agranulocytosis have been reported during therapy with the penicillins. These reactions are usually reversible on discontinuation of therapy and are believed to be hypersensitivity phenomena.
Other—Since infectious mononucleosis is viral in origin, ampicillin should not be used in the treatment. A high percentage of patients with mononucleosis who received ampicillin developed a skin rash.
Dosage and Administration:
Infections of the respiratory tract and soft tissues
Patients weighing 20 kg (44 lb) or more: 250 mg every six hours
Patients weighing less than 20 kg (44 lb): 50 mg/kg/day in equally divided doses at 6- or 8-hour intervals
Infections of the gastrointestinal and genitourinary tracts
Patients weighing 20 kg (44 lb) or more: 500 mg every six hours
Patients weighing less than 20 kg (44 lb): 100 mg/kg/day in equally divided doses at 6- or 8-hour intervals
In the treatment of chronic urinary tract and intestinal infections, frequent bacteriologic and clinical appraisal is necessary. Smaller doses than those recommended above should not be used. Higher doses should be used for stubborn or severe infections. In stubborn infections, therapy may be required for several weeks. It may be necessary to continue clinical and/or bacteriologic follow-up for several months after cessation of therapy.
Urethritis in males or females due to *N gonorrhoeae:*
3.5 grams with 1 gram probenecid, administered simultaneously.
In the treatment of complications of gonorrheal urethritis, such as prostatitis and epididymitis, prolonged and intensive therapy is recommended. Cases of gonorrhea with a suspected primary lesion of syphilis should have darkfield examinations before receiving treatment. In all other cases where concomitant syphilis is suspected, monthly serologic tests should be made for a minimum of four months.
Treatment of all infections should be continued for a minimum of 48 to 72 hours beyond the time that the patient becomes asymptomatic or evidence of bacterial eradication has been obtained. A minimum of ten days treatment is recommended for any infection caused by Group A beta-hemolytic streptococci to help prevent the occurrence of acute rheumatic fever or acute glomerulonephritis.
Directions For Dispensing Oral Suspensions
Prepare suspension at time of dispensing. For ease in preparation, add water to the bottle in two portions, and shake well after each addition.
125 MG/5 ML
Add a total of 88 ml to the 100-ml package and 173 ml to the 200-ml package. This will provide 100 and 200 ml of suspension. Each 5 ml (teaspoonful) will contain ampicillin trihydrate equivalent to 125 mg ampicillin. The reconstituted suspension is stable for 14 days under refrigeration.
250 MG/5 ML
Add a total of 70 ml to the 100-ml package and 140 ml to the 200-ml package. This will provide 100 and 200 ml of suspension. Each 5 ml (teaspoonful) will contain ampicillin trihydrate equivalent to 250 mg ampicillin. The reconstituted suspension is stable for 14 days under refrigeration.
How Supplied:
N 0071-0402 (Capsule 402)—Amcill Capsules, 250 mg. Each capsule contains ampicillin trihydrate equivalent to 250 mg ampicillin. Bottles of 100 and 500, and unit-dose packages of 100 (10 strips of 10 capsules each).
N 0071-0404 (Capsule 404)—Amcill Capsules, 500 mg. Each capsule contains ampicillin tri-

hydrate equivalent to 500 mg ampicillin. Bottles of 100 and 500, and unit-dose packages of 100 (10 strips of 10 capsules each).

[Shown in Product Identification Section]

N 0071-2301—Amcill for Oral Suspension 125 mg/5 ml. Each 5 ml of reconstituted suspension contains ampicillin trihydrate equivalent to 125 mg ampicillin. Available in 100-ml and 200-ml individual bottles and packs of six.

N 0071-2302—Amcill for Oral Suspension 250 mg/5 ml. Each 5 ml of reconstituted suspension contains ampicillin trihydrate equivalent to 250 mg ampicillin. Available in 100-ml and 200-ml individual bottles and packs of six.

AHFS 8:12.16 **7000G092**

Amcill products are manufactured by John D. Copanos Inc., Baltimore, MD 21225 and distributed by Parke-Davis, Morris Plains, NJ 07950.

AMITRIPTYLINE HYDROCHLORIDE ℞
Tablets USP
(Amitril®)

Description: Amitriptyline HCl, a dibenzocycloheptadiene derivative, is a white, crystalline compound that is readily soluble in water.

It is designated chemically as 5-(3-dimethylaminopropylidene)-dibenzo [a,d][1,4] cycloheptadiene hydrochloride. The molecular weight is 313.87. The empirical formula is $C_{20}H_{23}N \cdot HCl$.

Clinical Pharmacology: Amitriptyline HCl is an antidepressant with sedative effects. Its mechanism of action in man is not known. It is not a monoamine oxidase inhibitor and it does not act primarily by stimulation of the central nervous system.

Amitriptyline inhibits the membrane pump mechanism responsible for reuptake of norepinephrine and serotonin into adrenergic and serotonergic neurons. Pharmacologically this action may potentiate or prolong neuronal activity since reuptake of these biogenic amines is important physiologically in terminating its transmitting activity. This interference with reuptake of norepinephrine and/or serotonin is believed by some to underlie the antidepressant activity of amitriptyline.

Indications and Usage: For the relief of symptoms of depression. Endogenous depression is more likely to be alleviated than are other depressive states.

Contraindications: Amitriptyline HCl is contraindicated in patients who have shown prior hypersensitivity to it. It should not be given concomitantly with a monoamine oxidase inhibitor. Hyperpyretic crises, severe convulsions, and deaths have occurred in patients receiving tricyclic antidepressant and monoamine oxidase inhibiting drugs simultaneously. When it is desired to replace a monoamine oxidase inhibitor with amitriptyline, a minimum of 14 days should be allowed to elapse after the former is discontinued. Amitriptyline HCl should then be initiated cautiously with gradual increase in dosage until optimum response is achieved.

This drug is not recommended for use during the acute recovery phase following myocardial infarction.

Warnings: Amitriptyline HCl may block the antihypertensive action of guanethidine or similarly acting compounds. It should be used with caution in patients with a history of seizures and because of its atropine-like action, in patients with a history of urinary retention, angle-closure glaucoma, or increased intraocular pressure. In patients with angle-closure glaucoma, even average doses may precipitate an attack.

Patients with cardiovascular disorders should be watched closely. Tricyclic antidepressant drugs, including amitriptyline, particularly when given in high doses, have been reported to produce arrhythmias, sinus tachycardia, and prolongation of the conduction time. Myocardial infarction and stroke have been reported with drugs of this class.

Close supervision is required when amitriptyline is given to hyperthyroid patients or those receiving thyroid medication.

This drug may impair mental and/or physical abilities required for performance of hazardous tasks, such as operating machinery or driving a motor vehicle.

Amitriptyline may enhance the response to alcohol and the effects of barbiturates and other CNS depressants. In patients who may use alcohol excessively, it should be borne in mind that the potentiation may increase the danger inherent in any suicide attempt or overdosage.

Usage in Pregnancy—Safe use of amitriptyline during pregnancy and lactation has not been established; therefore, in administering the drug to pregnant patients, nursing mothers, or women who may become pregnant, the possible benefits must be weighed against the possible hazards to mother and child.

Animal reproduction studies have been inconclusive and clinical experience has been limited.

Usage in Children—In view of the lack of experience in children, the drug is not recommended at the present time for patients under 12 years of age.

Precautions: Schizophrenic patients may develop increased symptoms of psychosis; patients with paranoid symptomatology may have an exaggeration of such symptoms; manic depressive patients may experience a shift to the manic phase.

In these circumstances the dose of amitriptyline may be reduced or a major tranquilizer such as perphenazine may be administered concurrently.

When this drug is given with anticholinergic agents or sympathomimetic drugs, including epinephrine combined with local anesthetics, close supervision and careful adjustment of dosages are required.

Paralytic ileus may occur in patients taking tricyclic antidepressants in combination with anticholinergic-type drugs.

Caution is advised if patients receive large doses of ethchlorvynol concurrently. Transient delirium has been reported in patients who were treated with one gram of ethchlorvynol and 75 to 150 mg of amitriptyline.

The possibility of suicide in depressed patients remains until significant remission occurs. Potentially suicidal patients should not have access to large quantities of this drug. Prescriptions should be written for the smallest amount feasible.

Concurrent administration of amitriptyline and electroshock therapy may increase the hazards associated with such therapy. Such treatment should be limited to patients for whom it is essential.

Discontinue the drug several days before elective surgery if possible.

Both elevation and lowering of blood sugar levels have been reported.

Amitriptyline should be used with caution in patients with impaired liver function.

Adverse Reactions:

Note: Included in the listing which follows are a few adverse reactions which have not been reported with this specific drug. However, pharmacological similarities among the tricyclic antidepressant drugs require that each of the reactions be considered when amitriptyline is administered.

Cardiovascular: Hypotension, hypertension, tachycardia, palpitation, myocardial infarction, arrhythmias, heart block, stroke.

CNS and Neuromuscular: Confusional states, disturbed concentration; disorientation; delusions; hallucinations; excitement; anxiety; restlessness; insomnia; nightmares; numbness, tingling, and paresthesias of the extremities; peripheral neuropathy; incoordination; ataxia; tremors; seizures; alteration in EEG patterns; extrapyramidal symptoms; tinnitus; syndrome of inappropriate ADH (antidiuretic hormone) secretion.

Anticholinergic: Dry mouth, blurred vision, disturbance of accommodation, constipation, paralytic ileus, urinary retention, dilatation of urinary tract.

Allergic: Skin rash, urticaria, photo-sensitization, edema of face and tongue.

Hematologic: Bone marrow depression including agranulocytosis, leukopenia, eosinophilia, purpura, thrombocytopenia.

Gastrointestinal: Nausea, epigastric distress, vomiting, anorexia, stomatitis, peculiar taste, diarrhea, parotid swelling, black tongue. Rarely hepatitis (including altered liver function and jaundice).

Endocrine: Testicular swelling and gynecomastia in the male, breast enlargement and galactorrhea in the female, increased or decreased libido, elevation and lowering of blood sugar levels.

Other: Dizziness, weakness, fatigue, headache, weight gain or loss, increased perspiration, urinary frequency, mydriasis, drowsiness, alopecia.

Withdrawal Symptoms: Abrupt cessation of treatment after prolonged administration may produce nausea, headache and malaise. These are not indicative of addiction.

Overdosage:

Manifestations—High doses may cause temporary confusion, disturbed concentration, or transient visual hallucinations. Overdosage may cause drowsiness; hypothermia; tachycardia and other arrhythmic abnormalities, such as bundle branch block; ECG evidence of impaired conduction; congestive heart failure; dilated pupils; convulsions; severe hypotension; stupor; and coma. Other symptoms may be agitation, hyperactive reflexes, muscle rigidity, vomiting, hyperpyrexia, or any of those listed under ADVERSE REACTIONS.

All patients suspected of having taken an overdosage should be admitted to a hospital as soon as possible.

Treatment is symptomatic and supportive. Empty the stomach as quickly as possible by emesis followed by gastric lavage upon arrival at the hospital. Following gastric lavage, activated charcoal may be administered. Twenty to 30 g of activated charcoal may be given every four to six hours during the first 24 to 48 hours after ingestion. An ECG should be taken and close monitoring of cardiac function instituted if there is any sign of abnormality. Maintain an open airway and adequate fluid intake; regulate body temperature.

The intravenous administration of 1–3 mg of physostigmine salicylate has been reported to reverse the symptoms of tricyclic antidepressant poisoning. Because physostigmine is rapidly metabolized, the dosage of physostigmine should be repeated as required particularly if life threatening signs such as arrhythmias, convulsions, and deep coma recur or persist after the initial dosage of physostigmine. Because physostigmine itself may be toxic, it is not recommended for routine use.

Standard measures should be used to manage circulatory shock and metabolic acidosis. Cardiac arrhythmias may be treated with neostigmine, pyridostigmine, or propranolol. Should cardiac failure occur, the use of digitalis should be considered. Close monitoring of cardiac function for not less than five days is advisable.

Continued on next page

This product information was prepared in August, 1982. On these and other Parke-Davis Products, information may be obtained by addressing PARKE-DAVIS, Division of Warner-Lambert Company, Morris Plains, New Jersey 07950.

Parke-Davis—Cont.

Anticonvulsants may be given to control convulsions. Amitriptyline increases the CNS depressant action, but not the anticonvulsant action of barbiturates; therefore, an inhalation anesthetic, diazepam, or paraldehyde is recommended for control of convulsions.
Dialysis is of no value because of low plasma concentrations of the drug.
Since overdosage is often deliberate, patients may attempt suicide by other means during the recovery phase.
Deaths by deliberate or accidental overdosage have occurred with this class of drugs.

Dosage and Administration:

Oral Dosage:—Dosage should be initiated at a low level and increased gradually, noting carefully the clinical response and any evidence of intolerance.

Initial Dosage for Adults—Twenty-five mg three times a day usually is satisfactory for outpatients. If necessary this may be increased to a total of 150 mg a day. Increases are made preferably in the late afternoon and/or bedtime doses. A sedative effect may be apparent before the antidepressant effect is noted, but an adequate therapeutic effect may take as long as 30 days to develop.
An alternative method of initiating therapy in outpatients is to begin with 50 to 100 mg amitriptyline HCl at bedtime. This may be increased by 25 to 50 mg as necessary in the bedtime dose to a total of 150 mg per day.
Hospitalized patients may require 100 mg a day initially. This can be increased gradually to 200 mg a day if necessary. A small number of hospitalized patients may need as much as 300 mg a day.

Adolescent and Elderly Patients—In general, lower dosages are recommended for these patients. Ten mg three times a day with 20 mg at bedtime may be satisfactory in adolescent and elderly patients who do not tolerate higher doses.

Maintenance—The usual maintenance dose is 25 mg two to four times a day. In some patients 10 mg four times a day is sufficient. When satisfactory improvement has been reached, dosage should be reduced to the lowest amount that will maintain relief of symptoms. It is appropriate to continue maintenance therapy three months or longer to lessen the possibility of relapse.

Usage in Children—In view of the lack of experience in children, this drug is not recommended at the present time for patients under 12 years of age.

How Supplied: Amitriptyline HCl tablets are supplied as film-coated tablets as follows:
N 0071-0272 10 mg (tan, P-D 272), in bottles of 100 and unit-dose packages of 100 (10 strips of 10 tablets each).
N 0071-0273 25 mg (coral, P-D 273), in bottles of 100 and 1000 and unit-dose packages of 100 (10 strips of 10 tablets each).
N 0071-0274 50 mg (blue/purple, P-D 274), in bottles of 100 and 1000 and unit-dose packages of 100 (10 strips of 10 tablets each).
N 0071-0275 75 mg (green, P-D 275), in bottles of 100.
N 0071-0271 100 mg (brown/mustard, P-D 271), in bottles of 100 and unit-dose packages of 100 (10 strips of 10 tablets each).
N 0071-0278 150 mg (orange, P-D 278), in bottles of 100.

Store at controlled room temperature between 59°–86°F [15°–30°C].

6000G032

AMOXICILLIN ℞

(Utimox®)
Amoxicillin Capsules, USP—250 and 500 mg
Amoxicillin for Oral Suspension, USP—125 mg/5 ml and 250 mg/5 ml

Description: Amoxicillin is a semisynthetic penicillin, an analogue of ampicillin, with a broad spectrum of bactericidal activity against many gram-positive and gram-negative microorganisms. Chemically, it is D-(-)-α-amino-*p*-hydroxybenzyl penicillin trihydrate.

Actions:

Pharmacology
Amoxicillin is stable in the presence of gastric acid and may be given with no regard for food. It is rapidly absorbed after oral administration. It diffuses readily into most body tissues and fluids, with the exception of brain and spinal fluid, except when meninges are inflamed. The half-life of amoxicillin is 1 hour. Most of the amoxicillin is excreted unchanged in the urine; its excretion can be delayed by concurrent administration of probenecid. Amoxicillin is not highly protein-bound. In blood serum, amoxicillin is approximately 20% protein-bound as compared to 60% for penicillin G.
Orally administered doses of 250 mg and 500 mg amoxicillin capsules result in average peak blood levels, one to two hours after administration, in the range of 3.5 mcg/ml to 5.0 mcg/ml, and 5.5 mcg/ml to 7.5 mcg/ml, respectively.
Orally administered doses of amoxicillin suspension 125 mg/5 ml and 250 mg/5 ml result in average peak blood levels, one to two hours after administration, in the range of 1.5 mcg/ml to 3.0 mcg/ml, and 3.5 mcg/ml to 5.0 mcg/ml, respectively.
Detectable serum levels are observed up to 8 hours after an orally administered dose of amoxicillin. Approximately 60% of an orally administered dose of amoxicillin is excreted in the urine within six to eight hours.

Microbiology
Amoxicillin is similar to ampicillin in its bactericidal action against susceptible organisms during the stage of active multiplication. It acts through the inhibition of biosynthesis of cell wall mucopeptide. *In vitro* studies have demonstrated the susceptibility of most strains of the following gram-positive bacteria: alpha- and beta-hemolytic streptococci, *Diplococcus pneumoniae*, nonpenicillinase-producing staphylococci, and *Streptococcus faecalis.* Amoxicillin is active *in vitro* against many strains of *Haemophilus influenzae, Neisseria gonorrhoeae, Escherichia coli,* and *Proteus mirabilis.* Because it does not resist destruction by penicillinase, the drug is not effective against penicillinase-producing bacteria, particularly resistant staphylococci. All strains of *Pseudomonas* and most strains of *Klebsiella* and *Enterobacter* are resistant.

Disc Susceptibility Tests
Quantitative methods that require measurement of zone diameters give the most precise estimates of antibiotic susceptibility. One such procedure* has been recommended for use with discs for testing susceptibility to ampicillin class antibiotics. Interpretations correlate diameters of the disc test with MIC values for amoxicillin. With this procedure, a report from the laboratory of "susceptible" indicates that the infecting organism is likely to respond to therapy. A report of "resistant" indicates that the infecting organism is not likely to respond to therapy. A report of "intermediate susceptibility" suggests that the organism would be susceptible if high dosage is used, or if the infection is confined to tissues and fluids (eg, urine), in which high antibiotic levels are attained.

Indications: Amoxicillin is indicated in the treatment of infections due to susceptible strains of the following.
Gram-negative organisms—*H influenzae, E coli, P mirabilis,* and *N gonorrhoeae*
Gram-positive organisms—Streptococci (including *Str faecalis), D pneumoniae,* and nonpenicillinase-producing staphylococci
Therapy may be instituted prior to obtaining results from bacteriological and susceptibility studies to determine the causative organisms and their susceptibility to amoxicillin.
Indicated surgical procedures should be performed.

Contraindication: The use of this drug is contraindicated in individuals with a history of an allergic reaction to the penicillins.

Warnings: SERIOUS AND OCCASIONALLY FATAL HYPERSENSITIVITY (ANAPHYLACTOID) REACTIONS HAVE BEEN REPORTED IN PATIENTS ON PENICILLIN THERAPY. ALTHOUGH ANAPHYLAXIS IS MORE FREQUENT FOLLOWING PARENTERAL THERAPY, IT HAS OCCURRED IN PATIENTS ON ORAL PENICILLINS. THESE REACTIONS ARE MORE APT TO OCCUR IN INDIVIDUALS WITH A HISTORY OF SENSITIVITY TO MULTIPLE ALLERGENS.
THERE HAVE BEEN REPORTS OF INDIVIDUALS WITH A HISTORY OF PENICILLIN HYPERSENSITIVITY WHO HAVE EXPERIENCED SEVERE REACTIONS WHEN TREATED WITH CEPHALOSPORINS. BEFORE THERAPY WITH ANY PENICILLIN, CAREFUL INQUIRY SHOULD BE MADE CONCERNING PREVIOUS HYPERSENSITIVITY REACTIONS TO PENICILLINS, CEPHALOSPORINS, AND OTHER ALLERGENS. IF AN ALLERGIC REACTION OCCURS, APPROPRIATE THERAPY SHOULD BE INSTITUTED AND DISCONTINUANCE OF AMOXICILLIN THERAPY CONSIDERED.
SERIOUS ANAPHYLACTOID REACTIONS REQUIRE IMMEDIATE EMERGENCY TREATMENT WITH EPINEPHRINE. OXYGEN, INTRAVENOUS STEROIDS, AND AIRWAY MANAGEMENT, INCLUDING INTUBATION, SHOULD ALSO BE ADMINISTERED AS INDICATED.
Usage in Pregnancy—Safety for use in pregnancy has not been established.

Precautions: As with any potent drug, periodic assessment of renal, hepatic, and hematopoietic functions should be made during prolonged therapy.
The possibility of superinfections with mycotic or bacterial pathogens should be kept in mind during therapy. If superinfections occur (usually involving *Enterobacter, Pseudomonas,* or *Candida),* the drug should be discontinued and/or appropriate therapy instituted.

Adverse Reactions: As with other penicillins, it may be expected that untoward reactions will be essentially limited to sensitivity phenomena. They are more likely to occur in individuals who have previously demonstrated hypersensitivity to penicillins and in those with a history of allergy, asthma, hay fever, or urticaria.
The following adverse reactions have been reported as associated with the use of penicillins.
Gastrointestinal—Nausea, vomiting, and diarrhea
Hypersensitivity Reactions—Erythematous maculopapular rashes and urticaria have been reported.
Note—Urticaria, other skin rashes, and serum sickness-like reactions may be controlled with antihistamines and, if necessary, systemic corticosteroids. Whenever such reactions occur, amoxicillin should be discontinued unless, in the opinion of the physician, the condition being treated is life-threatening and amenable only to amoxicillin therapy.
Liver—A moderate rise in serum glutamic oxaloacetic transaminase (SGOT) has been noted, but the significance of this finding is unknown.
Hemic and Lymphatic Systems—Anemia, thrombocytopenia, thrombocytopenic purpura, eosinophilia, leukopenia, and agranulocytosis have been reported during therapy with the penicillins. These reactions are usu-

ally reversible on discontinuation of therapy and are believed to be hypersensitivity phenomena.

Dosage and Administration: Infections of the ear, nose, and throat due to streptococci, pneumococci, nonpenicillinase-producing staphylococci, and *H influenzae:*

Infections of the genitourinary tract due to *E coli, P mirabilis,* and *Str faecalis:*

Infections of the skin and soft tissues due to streptococci, susceptible staphylococci, and *E coli:*

Usual Dosage:

Adults: 250 mg every 8 hours

Children: 20 mg/kg/day in divided doses every 8 hours.

Children weighing 20 kg or more should be dosed according to the adult recommendations.

In severe infections or those caused by less susceptible organisms: 500 mg every 8 hours for adults, and 40 mg/kg/day in divided doses every 8 hours for children may be needed.

Infections of the lower respiratory tract due to streptococci, pneumococci, nonpenicillinase-producing staphylococci, and *H influenzae:*

Usual Dosage:

Adults: 500 mg every 8 hours

Children: 40/kg/day in divided doses every 8 hours

Children weighing 20 kg or more should be dosed according to the adult recommendations.

Gonorrhea, acute, uncomplicated anogenital and urethral infections due to *N gonorrhoeae:* (males and females) 3 grams as a single dose.

Cases of gonorrhea with a suspected lesion of syphilis should have darkfield examinations before receiving amoxicillin and monthly serological tests for a minimum of four months.

Larger doses may be required for stubborn or severe infections.

The children's dosage is intended for individuals whose weight will not cause a dosage to be calculated greater than that recommended for adults.

It should be recognized that in the treatment of chronic urinary tract infections, frequent bacteriological and clinical appraisals are necessary. Smaller doses than those recommended above should not be used. Even higher doses may be needed at times. In stubborn infections, therapy may be required for several weeks. It may be necessary to continue clinical and/or bacteriological follow-up for several months after cessation of therapy. Except for gonorrhea, treatment should be continued for a minimum of 48 to 72 hours beyond the time that the patient becomes asymptomatic or evidence of bacterial eradication has been obtained.

It is recommended that there be at least 10 days' treatment for any infection caused by hemolytic streptococci to prevent the occurrence of acute rheumatic fever or glomerulonephritis.

After reconstitution, the required amount of suspension should be placed directly on the child's tongue for swallowing. Alternate means of administration are to add the required amount of suspension to formula, milk, fruit juice, water, ginger ale, or cold drinks. These preparations should then be taken immediately. To be certain the child is receiving full dosage, such preparations should be consumed in entirety.

Directions for Preparing Oral Suspension: Prepare suspension at the time of dispensing. For ease of preparation, add water to the bottle in two portions and shake well after each addition. Each teaspoonful (5 ml) will contain 125 mg or 250 mg amoxicillin.

Product	Bottle Size	Amount of Water Required for Reconstitution
125 mg/5 ml	80 ml	70 ml
	100 ml	87 ml
	150 ml	130 ml
	200 ml	170 ml
250 mg/5 ml	80 ml	56 ml
	100 ml	70 ml
	150 ml	105 ml
	200 ml	140 ml

NOTE: SHAKE THE ORAL SUSPENSION WELL BEFORE USING.

Keep bottle tightly closed. The reconstituted suspension is stable for 14 days under refrigeration.

How Supplied:

Amoxicillin Capsules are supplied as:

N 0071-0730-24 250 mg—Bottles of 100
N 0071-0730-30 250 mg—Bottles of 500
N 0071-0730-40 250 mg—Unit dose packages of 100 (10 strips of 10)

Each capsule contains amoxicillin trihydrate equivalent to 250 mg amoxicillin.

N 0071-0731-24 500 mg—Bottles of 100
N 0071-0731-40 500 mg—Unit dose packages of 100 (10 strips of 10)

Each capsule contains amoxicillin trihydrate equivalent to 500 mg amoxicillin.

[*Shown in Product Identification Section*]

Amoxicillin for Oral Suspension is supplied as:

N 0071-2500-16 125 mg/5 ml—80 ml individual bottles and packs of six.
N 0071-2500-17 125 mg/5 ml—100 ml individual bottles and packs of six.
N 0071-2500-18 125 mg/5 ml—150 ml individual bottles and packs of six.
N 0071-2500-20 125 mg/5 ml—200 ml individual bottles and packs of six.

When reconstituted according to directions, each 5 ml of reconstituted suspension contains amoxicillin trihydrate equivalent to 125 mg amoxicillin.

N 0071-2501-16 250 mg/5 ml—80 ml individual bottles and packs of six.
N 0071-2501-17 250 mg/5 ml—100 ml individual bottles and packs of six.
N 0071-2501-18 250 mg/5 ml—150 ml individual bottles and packs of six.
N 0071-2501-20 250 mg/5 ml—200 ml individual bottles and packs of six.

When reconstituted according to directions, each 5 ml of reconstituted suspension contains amoxicillin trihydrate equivalent to 250 mg amoxicillin.

* Bauer, A.W., Kirby, W.M.M., Sherris, J.C., and Turck, M.: Antibiotic Testing by a Standardized Single Disc Method, *Am. J. Clin. Pathol.*, 45:493, 1966; Standardized Disc Susceptibility Test, *FEDERAL REGISTER* 37:20527-29, 1972.

Manufactured by John D. Copanos Inc., Baltimore, MD 21225 and distributed by Parke-Davis, Morris Plains, NJ 07950.

AHFS: 8:12.16 **7000G083**

ANUSOL® Suppositories/Ointment

Description:

	Anusol Suppositories each contains	Anusol Ointment each gram
Bismuth subgallate	2.25%	—
Bismuth Resorcin Compound	1.75%	—
Benzyl Benzoate	1.2 %	12 mg
Peruvian Balsam	1.8 %	18 mg
Zinc Oxide	11.0 %	110 mg
Analgine™ (pramoxine hydrochloride)	—	10 mg
	Also contains the following inactive ingredients: dibasic calcium phosphate and certified coloring in a hydrogenated vegetable oil base.	Also contains the following inactive ingredients: dibasic calcium phosphate and kaolin in a liquid petrolatum-cocoa butter-polyethylene wax base containing glyceryl monooleate and glyceryl stearate.

Actions: Anusol Suppositories and Anusol Ointment help to relieve pain, itching and discomfort arising from irritated anorectal tissues. They have a soothing, lubricant action on mucous membranes.

Analgine (pramoxine hydrochloride) in Anusol Ointment is a rapidly acting local anesthetic for the skin and mucous membranes of the anus and rectum. Analgine is also chemically distinct from procaine, cocaine, and dibucaine and can often be used in the patient previously sensitized to other surface anesthetics. Surface analgesia lasts for several hours.

Indications: Anusol Suppositories and Anusol Ointment are adjunctive therapy for the symptomatic relief of pain and discomfort in: external and internal hemorrhoids, proctitis, papillitis, cryptitis, anal fissures, incomplete fistulas, and relief of local pain and discomfort following anorectal surgery.

Anusol Ointment is also indicated for pruritus ani.

Contraindications: Anusol Suppositories and Anusol Ointment are contraindicated in those patients with a history of hypersensitivity to any of the components of the preparations.

Precautions: Symptomatic relief should not delay definitive diagnoses or treatment.

If irritation develops, these preparations should be discontinued. These preparations are not for ophthalmic use.

Adverse Reactions: Upon application of Anusol Ointment which contains Analgine, a patient may occasionally experience burning, especially if the anoderm is not intact. Sensitivity reactions have been rare; discontinue medication if suspected.

Dosage and Administration: Anusol Suppositories—Adults: Remove foil wrapper and insert suppository into the anus. Insert one suppository in the morning and one at bedtime, and one immediately following each evacuation.

Anusol Ointment—Adults: After gentle bathing and drying of the anal area, remove tube cap and apply freely to the exterior surface and gently rub in. Ointment should be applied every 3 or 4 hours, or, when necessary, every 2 hours.

NOTE: If staining from either of the above products occurs, the stain may be removed from fabric by hand or machine washing with household detergent.

How Supplied: Anusol Suppositories—boxes of 12 (N 0071-1088-07), 24 (N 0071-1088-13) and 48 (N 0071-1088-18) in silver foil strips.

[*Shown in Product Identification Section*]

Anusol Ointment—one-ounce tubes (N 0071-3075-13) with plastic applicator.

Store between 15°–30° C (59°–86° F).

ANUSOL–HC® SUPPOSITORIES ℞
Hemorrhoidal Suppositories

ANUSOL–HC® CREAM ℞
Rectal Cream
with Hydrocortisone Acetate

Description:

	Anusol-HC Suppositories each contains	Anusol-HC Cream each gram
Hydrocortisone Acetate	10.0 mg	5.0 mg
Bismuth Subgallate	2.25%	22.5 mg

Continued on next page

This product information was prepared in August, 1982. On these and other Parke-Davis Products, information may be obtained by addressing PARKE-DAVIS, Division of Warner-Lambert Company, Morris Plains, New Jersey 07950.

Parke-Davis—Cont.

Bismuth Resorcin Compound	1.75%	17.5 mg
Benzyl Benzoate	1.2 %	12.0 mg
Peruvian Balsam	1.8 %	18.0 mg
Zinc Oxide	11.0 %	110.0 mg
	Also contains the following inactive ingredients: dibasic calcium phosphate and certified coloring in a hydrogenated vegetable oil base.	Also contains the following inactive ingredients: propylene glycol, propylparaben, methylparaben, polysorbate 60 and sorbitan monostearate in a water-miscible base of mineral oil, glyceryl monostearate and water.

Actions: Anusol-HC Suppositories and Anusol-HC Cream help to relieve pain, itching and discomfort arising from irritated anorectal tissues. These preparations have a soothing, lubricant action on mucous membranes, and the antiinflammatory action of hydrocortisone acetate in Anusol-HC helps to reduce hyperemia and swelling.

The hydrocortisone acetate in Anusol-HC is primarily effective because of its antiinflammatory, antipruritic and vasoconstrictive actions.

Indications: Anusol-HC Suppositories and Anusol-HC Cream are adjunctive therapy for the symptomatic relief of pain and discomfort in: external and internal hemorrhoids, proctitis, papillitis, cryptitis, anal fissures, incomplete fistulas and relief of local pain and discomfort following anorectal surgery.

Anusol-HC Cream is also indicated for pruritus ani.

Anusol-HC is especially indicated when inflammation is present. After acute symptoms subside, most patients can be maintained on regular Anusol® Suppositories or Ointment.

Contraindications: Anusol-HC Suppositories and Anusol-HC Cream are contraindicated in those patients with a history of hypersensitivity to any of the components of the preparations.

Warnings: The safe use of topical steroids during pregnancy has not been fully established. Therefore, during pregnancy, they should not be used unnecessarily on extensive areas, in large amounts, or for prolonged periods of time.

Precautions: Symptomatic relief should not delay definitive diagnoses or treatment.

If irritation develops, Anusol-HC Suppositories and Anusol-HC Cream should be discontinued and appropriate therapy instituted.

In the presence of an infection the use of an appropriate antifungal or antibacterial agent should be instituted. If a favorable response does not occur promptly, the corticosteroid should be discontinued until the infection has been adequately controlled.

Care should be taken when using the corticosteroid hydrocortisone acetate in children and infants.

Anusol-HC is not for ophthalmic use.

Dosage and Administration: Anusol-HC Suppositories—Adults: Remove foil wrapper and insert suppository into the anus. Insert one suppository in the morning and one at bedtime, for 3 to 6 days or until inflammation subsides. Then maintain patient comfort with regular Anusol Suppositories.

Anusol-HC Cream—Adults: After gentle bathing and drying of the anal area, remove tube cap and apply to the exterior surface and gently rub in. For internal use, attach the plastic applicator and insert into the anus by applying gentle continuous pressure. Then squeeze the tube to deliver medication. Cream should be applied 3 or 4 times a day for 3 to 6 days until inflammation subsides. Then maintain patient comfort with regular Anusol Ointment.

NOTE: If staining from either of the above products occurs, the stain may be removed from fabric by hand or machine washing with household detergent.

How Supplied: Anusol-HC Suppositories—boxes of 12 (N 0071-1089-07) and boxes of 24 (N 0071-1089-13); in silver foil strips.

[*Shown in Product Identification Section*]

Anusol-HC Cream—one-ounce tube (N 0071-3090-13); with plastic applicator.

Store between 15°–30° C (59°–86° F).

[*Shown in Product Identification Section*]

1089 G 010

APLISOL® ℞

(tuberculin purified protein derivative, diluted)
Stabilized Solution

For complete product information, consult Diagnostic Products Information Section.

APLITEST® ℞

(tuberculin purified protein derivative)
Multiple-Puncture Device

For complete product information, consult Diagnostic Products Information Section.

BENADRYL® ℞

(diphenhydramine hydrochloride, USP)
Kapseals®
Capsules
Elixir
Parenteral

Description: Benadryl (diphenhydramine hydrochloride) is 2-(diphenylmethoxy)-N, N-dimethylethylamine hydrochloride, and occurs as a white, crystalline powder, and is freely soluble in water and alcohol.

Actions: Diphenhydramine hydrochloride is an antihistamine with anticholinergic (drying) and sedative side effects. Antihistamines appear to compete with histamine for cell receptor sites on effector cells.

Indications: ***Oral:*** Benadryl in the oral form is effective for the following indications.

Antihistaminic: For perennial and seasonal (hay fever) allergic rhinitis; vasomotor rhinitis, allergic conjunctivitis due to inhalant allergens and foods: mild, uncomplicated allergic skin manifestations of urticaria and angioedema; amelioration of allergic reactions to blood or plasma, dermatographism; as therapy for anaphylactic reactions *adjunctive* to epinephrine and other standard measures after the acute manifestations have been controlled

Motion sickness: For active and prophylactic treatment of motion sickness

Antiparkinsonism: For parkinsonism (including drug-induced extrapyramidal reactions) in the elderly unable to tolerate more potent agents; mild cases of parkinsonism (including drug-induced) in other age groups; in other cases of parkinsonism (including drug-induced) in combination with centrally acting anticholinergic agents

Parenteral: Benadryl in the injectable form is effective for the following conditions when Benadryl in the oral form is impractical.

Antihistaminic: For amelioration of allergic reactions to blood or plasma; in anaphylaxis as an adjunct to epinephrine and other standard measures after the acute symptoms have been controlled; and for other uncomplicated allergic conditions of the immediate type when oral therapy is impossible or contraindicated.

Motion Sickness: For active treatment of motion sickness

Antiparkinsonism: For use in parkinsonism when oral therapy is impossible or contraindicated, as follows: parkinsonism in the elderly who are unable to tolerate more potent agents, mild cases of parkinsonism in other age groups, and in other cases of parkinsonism in combination with centrally acting anticholinergic agents.

Contraindications: ***Oral and Parenteral:***

Use in Newborn or Premature Infants: This drug should *not* be used in newborn or premature infants.

Use in Nursing Mothers: Because of the higher risk of antihistamines for infants generally and for newborns and prematures in particular, antihistamine therapy is contraindicated in nursing mothers.

Use in Lower Respiratory Disease: Antihistamines *should NOT* be used to treat lower respiratory tract symptoms, including asthma.

Antihistamines are also contraindicated in the following conditions.

Hypersensitivity to diphenhydramine hydrochloride and other antihistamines of similar chemical structure

Monoamine oxidase inhibitor therapy (See Drug Interactions section.)

Warnings: ***Oral and Parenteral:*** Antihistamines should be used with considerable caution in patients with narrow-angle glaucoma, stenosing peptic ulcer, pyloroduodenal obstruction, symptomatic prostatic hypertrophy, or bladder-neck obstruction.

Use in Children: In infants and children, especially, antihistamines in *overdosage* may cause hallucinations, convulsions, or death.

As in adults, antihistamines may diminish mental alertness in children. In the young child, particularly, they may produce excitation.

Use in Pregnancy: Experience with this drug in pregnant women is inadequate to determine whether there exists a potential for harm to the developing fetus.

Use With CNS Depressants: Diphenhydramine hydrochloride has additive effects with alcohol and other CNS depressants (hypnotics, sedatives, tranquilizers, etc).

Use in Activities Requiring Mental Alertness: Patients should be warned about engaging in activities requiring mental alertness, such as driving a car or operating appliances, machinery, etc.

Use in the Elderly (approximately 60 years or older): Antihistamines are more likely to cause dizziness, sedation, and hypotension in elderly patients.

Precautions: ***Oral and Parenteral:*** Diphenhydramine hydrochloride has an atropine-like action and, therefore, should be used with caution in patients with a history of bronchial asthma, increased intraocular pressure, hyperthyroidism, cardiovascular disease, or hypertension.

Drug Interactions: ***Oral and Parenteral:*** MAO inhibitors prolong and intensify the anticholinergic (drying) effects of antihistamines.

Adverse Reactions: ***Oral and Parenteral:*** The most frequent adverse reactions are underscored.

1. *General:* Urticaria, drug rash, anaphylactic shock, photosensitivity, excessive perspiration, chills, dryness of mouth, nose, and throat
2. *Cardiovascular System:* Hypotension, headache, palpitations, tachycardia, extrasystoles
3. *Hematologic System:* Hemolytic anemia, thrombocytopenia, agranulocytosis
4. *Nervous System:* <u>Sedation, sleepiness, dizziness, disturbed coordination,</u> fatigue, confusion, restlessness, excitation, nervousness, tremor, irritability, insomnia, euphoria, paresthesia, blurred vision, diplopia, vertigo, tinnitus, acute labyrinthitis, hysteria, neuritis, convulsions
5. *GI System:* <u>Epigastric distress</u>, anorexia, nausea, vomiting, diarrhea, constipation
6. *GU System:* Urinary frequency, difficult urination, urinary retention, early menses
7. *Respiratory System:* <u>Thickening of bronchial secretions</u>, tightness of chest and wheezing, nasal stuffiness

Overdosage: ***Oral and Parenteral:*** Antihistamine overdosage reactions may vary from central nervous system depression to stimulation. Stimulation is particularly likely in children. Atropine-like signs and symptoms—dry mouth; fixed, dilated pupils; flushing—and gastrointestinal symptoms may also occur.

If vomiting has not occurred spontaneously, the patient should be induced to vomit. This is best done by having the patient drink a glass of water or milk, after which the patient should be made to gag. Precautions against aspiration must be taken, especially in infants and children.

If vomiting is unsuccessful, gastric lavage is indicated within 3 hours after ingestion and even later if large amounts of milk or cream were given beforehand. Isotonic or ½ isotonic saline is the lavage solution of choice.

Saline cathartics, as milk of magnesia, by osmosis draw water into the bowel and therefore are valuable for their action in rapid dilution of bowel content.

Stimulants should *not* be used.

Vasopressors may be used to treat hypotension.

Dosage and Administration: ***Oral and Parenteral:***

DOSAGE SHOULD BE INDIVIDUALIZED ACCORDING TO THE NEEDS AND THE RESPONSE OF THE PATIENT.

Oral:

A single oral dose of diphenhydramine hydrochloride is quickly absorbed, with maximum activity occurring in approximately one hour. The duration of activity following an average dose of Benadryl (diphenhydramine hydrochloride) is from four to six hours.

ADULTS: 25 to 50 mg three or four times daily

CHILDREN (over 20 lb): 12.5 to 25 mg three to four times daily. Maximum daily dosage not to exceed 300 mg. For physicians who wish to calculate the dose on the basis of body weight or surface area, the recommended dosage is 5 mg/kg/24 hours or 150 mg/m^2/24 hours.

The basis for determining the most effective dosage regimen will be the response of the patient to medication and the condition under treatment.

In motion sickness, full dosage is recommended for prophylactic use, the first dose to be given 30 minutes before exposure to motion and similar doses before meals and upon retiring for the duration of exposure.

Parenteral: Benadryl in the injectable form is indicated when the oral form is impractical.

CHILDREN: 5 mg/kg/24 hours or 150 mg/m^2/24 hours. Maximum daily dosage is 300 mg. Divide into four doses, administered intravenously or deeply intramuscularly.

ADULTS: 10 to 50 mg intravenously or deeply intramuscularly; 100 mg if required; maximum daily dosage is 400 mg.

How Supplied:

Benadryl is supplied in the oral form as:

N 0071-0373-24—Bottle of 100
N 0071-0373-32—Bottle of 1000
N 0071-0373-40—Unit dose (10/10's)

Each capsule contains 50 mg diphenhydramine hydrochloride.

N 0071-0471-24—Bottle of 100
N 0071-0471-32—Bottle of 1000
N 0071-0471-40—Unit dose (10/10's)

Each capsule contains 25 mg diphenhydramine hydrochloride. **0373G010**

[*Shown in Product Identification Section*]

Benadryl is also supplied in the following oral dosage form:

Elixir
N 0071-2220-17—4-oz bottle
N 0071-2220-23—Pint bottle
N 0071-2220-32—Gallon bottle
N 0071-2220-40—Unit-dose (5 ml× 100)

Each 5 ml of elixir contains 12.5 mg diphenhydramine hydrochloride with 14% alcohol.

2220 G 300

Benadryl in parenteral form is supplied as:

N 0071-4015-10 (10-ml vial)
N 0071-4015-13 (30-ml vial)

Sterile solution for parenteral use containing 10 mg diphenhydramine hydrochloride in each milliliter of solution with 0.1 mg/ml benzethonium chloride as a germicidal agent. Supplied in multiple-dose vials (Steri-Vials®).

N 0071-4402-10 (10-ml vial)

Sterile solution for parenteral use containing 50 mg diphenhydramine hydrochloride in each milliliter of solution with 0.1 mg/ml benzethonium chloride as a germicidal agent. Supplied in multiple-dose vials.

N 0071-4259-03 1-ml ampoule

Sterile solution for parenteral use containing 50 mg diphenhydramine hydrochloride. Supplied in packages of 10.

N 0071-4259-40 (individual cartons)
N 0071-4259-41 (2 trays of 5 syringes each)

Sterile solution for parenteral use containing 50 mg diphenhydramine hydrochloride in a 1-ml disposable syringe. (Steri-Dose®). Supplied in packages of ten.

The pH of the solutions for parenteral use have been adjusted with either sodium hydroxide or hydrochloric acid. **4259G010**

BENYLIN® Cough Syrup — OTC

Description: Each teaspoonful (5 ml) contains Benadryl® (diphenhydramine hydrochloride), 12.5 mg. Alcohol, 5%.

Indications: For the temporary relief of cough due to minor throat and bronchial irritation as may occur with the common cold or with inhaled irritants.

Warnings: May cause marked drowsiness. Keep this and all drugs out of the reach of children. In case of accidental overdosage, seek professional assistance or contact a poison control center immediately. Do not give to children under 6 years of age except under the advice and supervision of a physician. May cause excitability, especially in children. Do not take this product for persistent or chronic cough such as occurs with smoking, asthma, emphysema, or when cough is accompanied by excessive secretions, or if you have epilepsy, glaucoma, or difficulty in urination due to enlargement of the prostate gland except under the advice and supervision of a physician.

Caution: Avoid driving a motor vehicle or operating heavy machinery, or drinking alcoholic beverages. A persistent cough may be a sign of a serious condition. If cough persists for more than one week, tends to recur, or is accompanied by high fever, rash, or persistent headache, consult a physician. If pregnant or nursing, consult your physician before taking this or any medicine.

Directions: Adults—two teaspoonfuls every four hours, not to exceed twelve teaspoonfuls in twenty-four hours; Children (6 to under 12 years), one teaspoonful every four hours not to exceed six teaspoonfuls in twenty-four hours; or as directed by a physician. Your physician should be contacted for the recommended dosage for children 2 to under 6 years. Do not give to children under 2 years except under the advice and supervision of a physician.

How Supplied: N 0071-2195-Benylin Cough Syrup is supplied in 4-oz, 1-pt, 1-gal bottles, and unit-dose bottles of 5 ml and 10 ml.

Store below 30°C (86°F).

Protect from freezing.

BENYLIN DM® Cough Syrup

(See PDR For Nonprescription Drugs)

BRONDECON® — ℞

oxtriphylline and guaifenesin

Description: Each tablet contains 200 mg oxtriphylline and 100 mg guaifenesin. Each 5 ml teaspoonful of elixir contains 100 mg oxtriphylline and 50 mg guaifenesin; alcohol 20%.

NOTE: 100 mg oxtriphylline is equivalent to 64 mg anhydrous theophylline.

Actions: Brondecon, a bronchodilator and expectorant, helps to relieve symptoms of bronchospasm as well as obstruction caused by viscid mucus in the bronchioles.

Oxtriphylline, the choline salt of theophylline, is a xanthine bronchodilating agent. Compared to aminophylline, oxtriphylline is less irritating to the gastric mucosa, better absorbed from the gastrointestinal tract, more stable and more soluble. The expectorant component of Brondecon is guaifenesin, which tends to increase the secretion and decrease the viscosity of fluids of the respiratory tract. These physiologic fluids help to lubricate the inflamed mucous membranes of the bronchi and also help the patient to expel viscid mucus thus making cough more productive.

Indications: Brondecon is an adjunct in the management of bronchitis, bronchial asthma, asthmatic bronchitis, pulmonary emphysema, and similar chronic obstructive lung disease. It is indicated when both relaxation of bronchospasm and expectorant action are desirable.

Precautions: Concurrent use of other xanthine preparations may lead to adverse reactions, particularly CNS stimulation in children.

Adverse Reactions: Gastric distress and, occasionally, palpitation and CNS stimulation have been reported.

Dosage: Tablets—over 12 years of age: one tablet, 4 times a day.

Elixir—over 12 years of age: two teaspoonfuls, 4 times a day; from 2 to 12 years: one teaspoonful per 60 lb body weight, 4 times a day.

Above recommendations are averages. Dosage should be individualized.

Supplied: Salmon-pink tablets in bottles of 100 (N 0071-0200-24). Elixir, dark red, cherry-flavored in 237 ml (8 fl oz) (N 0071-2201-20) and 474 ml (16 fl oz) (N 0071-2201-23) bottles.

Store between 15° and 30°C (59° and 86°F).

[*Shown in Product Identification Section*]

0200 G 010

CALADRYL® Cream
CALADRYL® Lotion

Description: *Caladryl Lotion*—A drying, antihistaminic, calamine-Benadryl® lotion containing calamine; 1% Benadryl (diphenhydramine hydrochloride); camphor; and 2% alcohol

Caladryl Cream—a drying, antihistaminic, calamine-Benadryl cream containing 1% Benadryl (diphenhydramine hydrochloride) and camphor

Indications: For relief of itching due to mild poison ivy or oak, insect bites, or other minor skin irritations, and soothing relief of mild sunburn.

Warnings: Should not be applied to blistered, raw, or oozing areas of the skin. Discontinue use if burning sensation or rash develops or condition persists. Remove by washing with soap and water. Use on extensive areas of the skin or for longer than seven days only as directed by a physician.

Caution: Keep away from eyes or other mucous membranes.

FOR EXTERNAL USE ONLY

Keep this and all drugs out of the reach of children. In case of accidental ingestion, seek pro-

Continued on next page

This product information was prepared in August, 1982. On these and other Parke-Davis Products, information may be obtained by addressing PARKE-DAVIS, Division of Warner-Lambert Company, Morris Plains, New Jersey 07950.

Parke-Davis—Cont.

fessional assistance or contact a Poison Control Center immediately.
Directions: Caladryl Cream—Apply topically three or four times daily. Cleanse skin with soap and water and dry area before each application.
Caladryl Lotion—SHAKE WELL. Apply topically three or four times daily. Cleanse skin with soap and water and dry area before each application.
How Supplied: N 0071-3226-14: Caladryl Cream; 1½-oz tubes
N 0071-3181: Caladryl Lotion—2½-oz (75 ml) squeeze bottles and 6-oz bottles.

CALADRYL® HYDROCORTISONE ½% CREAM
CALADRYL® HYDROCORTISONE ½% LOTION

Description: An antipruritic containing as the active ingredient hydrocortisone acetate equivalent to ½% hydrocortisone.
Indications: For the temporary relief of minor skin irritations, itching, and rashes due to: eczema, dermatitis, insect bites, poison ivy, poison oak, poison sumac, soaps, detergents, cosmetics, jewelry, and itchy genital and anal areas.
Warnings: For external use only. Avoid contact with the eyes. If condition worsens or if symptoms persist for more than 7 days, discontinue use and consult a physician. Do not use on children under 2 years of age except under the advice and supervision of a physician. Keep this and all drugs out of the reach of children. In case of accidental ingestion, seek professional assistance or contact a Poison Control Center immediately.
Store at room temperature.
Directions: For adults and children 2 years of age and older: Apply to affected area 3 to 4 times daily. For children under 2 years of age there is no recommended dosage except under the advice and supervision of a physician.
How Supplied: N 0071-3030-11 Caladryl Hydrocortisone ½% Cream—½ oz (15 g) tubes
N 0071-3002-13 Caladryl Hydrocortisone ½% Lotion—1 fl oz (30 ml) bottles

CELONTIN® KAPSEALS® ℞
(methsuximide capsules, USP)

Description: Celontin (methsuximide) is an anticonvulsant succinimide, chemically designated as N,2-Dimethyl-2-phenylsuccinimide.
Action: Methsuximide suppresses the paroxysmal three-cycle-per-second spike and wave activity associated with lapses of consciousness which is common in absence (petit mal) seizures. The frequency of epileptiform attacks is reduced, apparently by depression of the motor cortex and elevation of the threshold of the central nervous system to convulsive stimuli.
Indication: Celontin is indicated for the control of absence (petit mal) seizures that are refractory to other drugs.
Contraindication: Methsuximide should not be used in patients with a history of hypersensitivity to succinimides.
Warnings: Blood dyscrasias, including some with fatal outcome, have been reported to be associated with the use of succinimides; therefore, periodic blood counts should be performed.
It has been reported that succinimides have produced morphological and functional changes in animal liver. For this reason, methsuximide should be administered with extreme caution to patients with known liver or renal disease. Periodic urinalysis and liver function studies are advised for all patients receiving the drug.
Cases of systemic lupus erythematosus have been reported with the use of succinimides. The physician should be alert to this possibility.
Usage in Pregnancy: The effects of Celontin in human pregnancy and nursing infants are unknown.
Recent reports suggest an association between the use of anticonvulsant drugs by women with epilepsy and an elevated incidence of birth defects in children born to these women. Data are more extensive with respect to phenytoin and phenobarbital, but these are also the most commonly prescribed anticonvulsants; less systematic or anecdotal reports suggest a possible similar association with the use of all known anticonvulsant drugs.
The reports suggesting an elevated incidence of birth defects in children of drug-treated epileptic women cannot be regarded as adequate to prove a definite cause-and-effect relationship. There are intrinsic methodologic problems in obtaining adequate data on drug teratogenicity in humans; the possibility also exists that other factors, eg, genetic factors or the epileptic condition itself, may be more important than drug therapy in leading to birth defects. The great majority of mothers on anticonvulsant medication deliver normal infants. It is important to note that anticonvulsant drugs should not be discontinued in patients in whom the drug is administered to prevent major seizures because of the strong possibility of precipitating status epilepticus with attendant hypoxia and threat to life. In individual cases where the severity and frequency of the seizure disorder are such that the removal of medication does not pose a serious threat to the patient, discontinuation of the drug may be considered prior to and during pregnancy, although it cannot be said with any confidence that even minor seizures do not pose some hazard to the developing embryo or fetus.
The prescribing physician will wish to weigh these considerations in treating or counseling epileptic women of childbearing potential.
Hazardous Activities: Methsuximide may impair the mental and/or physical abilities required for the performance of potentially hazardous tasks, such as driving a motor vehicle or other such activity requiring alertness; therefore, the patient should be cautioned accordingly.
Precautions: It is recommended that the physician withdraw the drug slowly on the appearance of unusual depression, aggressiveness, or other behavioral alterations.
As with other anticonvulsants, it is important to proceed slowly when increasing or decreasing dosage, as well as when adding or eliminating other medication. Abrupt withdrawal of anticonvulsant medication may precipitate absence (petit mal) status.
Methsuximide, when used alone in mixed types of epilepsy, may increase the frequency of grand mal seizures in some patients.
Adverse Reactions: Gastrointestinal System: Gastrointestinal symptoms occur frequently and have included nausea or vomiting, anorexia, diarrhea, weight loss, epigastric and abdominal pain, and constipation.
Hemopoietic System: Hemopoietic complications associated with the administration of methsuximide have included eosinophilia, leukopenia, monocytosis, and pancytopenia.
Nervous System: Neurologic and sensory reactions reported during therapy with methsuximide have included drowsiness, ataxia or dizziness, irritability and nervousness, headache, blurred vision, photophobia, hiccups, and insomnia. Drowsiness, ataxia, and dizziness have been the most frequent side effects noted. Psychologic abnormalities have included confusion, instability, mental slowness, depression, hypochondriacal behavior, and aggressiveness. There have been rare reports of psychosis, suicidal behavior, and auditory hallucinations.
Integumentary System: Dermatologic manifestations which have occurred with the administration of methsuximide have included urticaria, Stevens-Johnson syndrome, and pruritic erythematous rashes.
Other: Miscellaneous reactions reported include periorbital edema and hyperemia.
Dosage and Administration: Optimum dosage of Celontin must be determined by trial. A suggested dosage schedule is 300 mg per day for the first week. If required, dosage may be increased thereafter at weekly intervals by 300 mg per day for the three weeks following to a daily dosage of 1.2 g. Because therapeutic effect and tolerance vary among patients, therapy with Celontin must be individualized according to the response of each patient. Optimal dosage is that amount of Celontin which is barely sufficient to control seizures so that side effects may be kept to a minimum. The smaller capsule (150 mg) facilitates administration to small children.
Celontin may be administered in combination with other anticonvulsants when other forms of epilepsy coexist with absence (petit mal.)
How Supplied:
N 0071-0525-24 (P-D 525)—Celontin Kapseals, each containing 300 mg methsuximide; bottles of 100.
N 0071-0537-24 (P-D 537)—Celontin Kapseals, Half Strength, each containing 150 mg methsuximide, bottles of 100.

0537G010

[Shown in Product Identification Section]

CENTRAX® ℂ ℞
(prazepam)*

* Product of Warner-Lambert Inc.

Description: Centrax (prazepam) is a benzodiazepine derivative. Chemically, prazepam is 7-chloro-1-(cyclopropylmethyl)-1, 3-dihydro-5-phenyl-2H-1, 4-benzodiazepin-2-one, and has a molecular weight of 324.8.
Clinical Pharmacology: Studies in normal subjects have shown that Centrax (prazepam) has depressant effects on the central nervous system. Oral administration of single doses as high as 60 mg and of divided doses up to 100 mg three times a day (300 mg total daily dosage) were without toxic effects.
Single, oral doses of Centrax (prazepam) in normal subjects produced average peak blood levels of the major metabolite norprazepam at 6 hours postadministration, with significant amounts still present after 48 hours. Prazepam was slowly absorbed over a prolonged period; rather constant blood levels were maintained on multiple-dose schedules; and excretion was prolonged. The mean half-life of norprazepam measured in subjects given 10 mg prazepam three times a day for one week was 63 (± 15 SD) hours before and 70 (± 10 SD) hours after multiple dosing—a nonsignificant difference. Human metabolism studies showed that prior to elimination from the body, prazepam is metabolized in large part to 3-hydroxyprazepam and oxazepam.
Indications: Centrax is indicated for the management of anxiety disorders or for the short-term relief of the symptoms of anxiety. Anxiety or tension associated with the stress of everyday life usually does not require treatment with an anxiolytic.
The effectiveness of Centrax in long-term use, that is, more than 4 months, has not been assessed by systematic clinical studies. The physician should periodically reassess the usefulness of the drug for the individual patient.
Contraindications: Centrax (prazepam) is contraindicated in patients with a known hypersensitivity to the drug and in those with acute narrow-angle glaucoma.
Warnings: Centrax (prazepam) is not recommended in psychotic states and in those psychiatric disorders in which anxiety is not a prominent feature.

Patients taking Centrax should be cautioned against engaging in hazardous occupations requiring mental alertness, such as operating dangerous machinery including motor vehicles.

Because Centrax has a central nervous system depressant effect, patients should be advised against the simultaneous use of other CNS-depressant drugs, including phenothiazines, narcotics, barbiturates, MAO inhibitors, and other antidepressants. The effects of alcohol may also be increased with prazepam.

Physical and Psychological Dependence: Withdrawal symptoms similar in character to those noted with barbiturates and alcohol have occurred following abrupt discontinuance of benzodiazepine drugs. These symptoms include convulsions, tremor, abdominal and muscle cramps, vomiting and sweating. Addiction-prone individuals, such as drug addicts and alcoholics, should be under careful surveillance when receiving benzodiazepines because of the predisposition of such patients to habituation and dependence.

Withdrawal symptoms have also been reported following abrupt discontinuance of benzodiazepines taken continuously at therapeutic levels for several months.

Precautions: *Usage in Pregnancy and Lactation:* An increased risk of congenital malformations associated with the use of minor tranquilizers (chlordiazepoxide, diazepam, and meprobamate) during the first trimester of pregnancy has been suggested in several studies. Prazepam, a benzodiazepine derivative, has not been studied adequately to determine whether it, too, may be associated with an increased risk of fetal abnormality. Because use of these drugs is rarely a matter of urgency, their use during this period should almost always be avoided. The possibility that a woman of childbearing potential may be pregnant at the time of institution of therapy should be considered. Patients should be advised that if they become pregnant during therapy or intend to become pregnant, they should communicate with their physicians about the desirability of discontinuing the drug. In view of their molecular size, prazepam and its metabolites are probably excreted in human milk. Therefore, this drug should not be given to nursing mothers.

In those patients in whom a degree of depression accompanies the anxiety, suicidal tendencies may be present and protective measures may be required. The least amount of drug that is feasible should be available to the patient at any one time.

Patients taking Centrax (prazepam) for prolonged periods should have blood counts and liver function tests periodically. The usual precautions in treating patients with impaired renal or hepatic functions should also be observed. Hepatomegaly and cholestasis were observed in chronic toxicity studies in rats and dogs.

In elderly or debilitated patients, the initial dose should be small, and increments should be made gradually, in accordance with the response of the patient, to preclude ataxia or excessive sedation.

Pediatric Use: Safety and effectiveness in patients below the age of 18 have not been established.

Adverse Reactions: The side effects most frequently reported during double-blind, placebo-controlled trials employing a typical 30-mg divided total daily dosage and the percent incidence in the prazepam group were fatigue (11.6%), dizziness (8.7%), weakness (7.7%), drowsiness (6.8%), lightheadedness (6.8%), and ataxia (5.0%). Less frequently reported were headache, confusion, tremor, vivid dreams, slurred speech, palpitation, stimulation, dry mouth, diaphoresis, and various gastrointestinal complaints. Other side effects included pruritus, transient skin rashes, swelling of feet, joint pains, various genitourinary complaints, blurred vision, and syncope. Single, nightly dose, controlled trials of variable dosages showed a dose-related incidence of these same side effects. Transient and reversible aberrations of liver function tests have been reported, as have been slight decreases in blood pressure and increases in body weight.

These findings are characteristic of benzodiazepine drugs.

Overdosage: As in the management of overdosage with any drug, it should be borne in mind that multiple agents may have been taken.

Vomiting should be induced if it has not occurred spontaneously. Immediate gastric lavage is also recommended. General supportive care, including frequent monitoring of vital signs and close observation of the patient, is indicated. Hypotension, though unlikely, may be controlled with Levophed® (levarterenol bitartrate), or Aramine® (metaraminol bitartrate).

Dosage and Administration: Centrax (prazepam) is administered orally in divided doses. The usual daily dose is 30 mg. The dose should be adjusted gradually within the range of 20 mg to 60 mg daily in accordance with the response of the patient. In elderly or debilitated patients it is advisable to initiate treatment at a divided daily dose of 10 mg to 15 mg (see Precautions).

Centrax may also be administered as a single, daily dose at bedtime. The recommended starting nightly dose is 20 mg. The response of the patient to several days' treatment will permit the physician to adjust the dose upwards or, occasionally, downwards to maximize antianxiety effect with a minimum of daytime drowsiness. The optimum dosage will usually range from 20 mg to 40 mg.

Drug Interactions: If Centrax (prazepam) is to be combined with other drugs acting on the central nervous system, careful consideration should be given to the pharmacology of the agents to be employed. The actions of the benzodiazepines may be potentiated by barbiturates, narcotics, phenothiazines, monoamine oxidase inhibitors, or other antidepressants.

If Centrax (prazepam) is used to treat anxiety associated with somatic disease states, careful attention must be paid to possible drug interaction with concomitant medication.

How Supplied:

Centrax 5 mg—Each capsule contains 5 mg prazepam. Available in bottles of 100 (N 0071-0552-24), and 500 (N 0071-0552-30). Centrax 10 mg—Each capsule contains 10 mg prazepam. Available in bottles of 100 (N 0071-0553-24), and 500 (N 0071-0553-30). Centrax 20 mg—Each capsule contains 20 mg prazepam. Available in bottles of 100 (N 0071-0554-24). Also supplied as Centrax Tablets (prazepam tablets, USP) 10 mg light blue, scored tablets in bottles of 100 (N 0071-0276-24) and unit dose (N 0071-0276-40).

0552G012

[Shown in Product Identification Section]

CHLOROMYCETIN® CREAM, 1% ℞
(chloramphenicol cream)

Description: Each gram of Chloromycetin Cream, 1%, contains 10 mg chloramphenicol with 0.1% propylparaben in a water-miscible ointment base of liquid petrolatum, cetyl alcohol, sodium lauryl sulfate, sodium phosphate buffer, and water.

Clinical Pharmacology: Chloramphenicol is a broad-spectrum antibiotic originally isolated from *Streptomyces venezuelae.* It is primarily bacteriostatic and acts by inhibition of protein synthesis by interfering with the transfer of activated amino acids from soluble RNA to ribosomes. Development of resistance to chloramphenicol can be regarded as minimal for staphylococci and many other species of bacteria.

Indications and Usage: Chloromycetin (chloramphenicol) Cream, 1%, is indicated for the treatment of superficial skin infections caused by bacteria susceptible to chloramphenicol. Deeper cutaneous infections should be treated with appropriate systemic antibiotics.

Contraindication: This product is contraindicated in persons sensitive to any of its components.

Warnings: Bone marrow hypoplasia, including aplastic anemia and death, has been reported following the local application of chloramphenicol.

Precautions: The prolonged use of antibiotics may occasionally result in overgrowth of nonsusceptible organisms, including fungi. If new infections appear during medication, the drug should be discontinued and appropriate measures should be taken.

In all except very superficial infections, the topical use of chloramphenicol should be supplemented by appropriate systemic medication.

Adverse Reactions: Signs of local irritation with subjective symptoms of itching or burning, angioneurotic edema, urticaria, vesicular and maculopapular dermatitis have been reported in patients sensitive to chloramphenicol and are causes for discontinuing the medication. Similar sensitivity reactions to other materials in topical preparations may also occur. Blood dyscrasias have been reported in association with the use of chloramphenicol (See WARNINGS).

Dosage and Administration: Apply to the infected area three or four times daily after cleansing.

How Supplied:

N 0071-3166-13 (Ointment 66)

Chloromycetin Cream (chloramphenicol cream), 1%, is supplied in 1-oz tubes.

AHFS 84:04.04 3166 G 011

KAPSEALS®/CAPSULES CHLOROMYCETIN® ℞
(chloramphenicol capsules, USP)

WARNING

Serious and fatal blood dyscrasias (aplastic anemia, hypoplastic anemia, thrombocytopenia, and granulocytopenia) are known to occur after the administration of chloramphenicol. In addition, there have been reports of aplastic anemia attributed to chloramphenicol which later terminated in leukemia. Blood dyscrasias have occurred after both short-term and prolonged therapy with this drug. Chloramphenicol must not be used when less potentially dangerous agents will be effective, as described in the Indications section. *It must not be used in the treatment of trivial infections or where it is not indicated, as in colds, influenza, infections of the throat; or as a prophylactic agent to prevent bacterial infections.*

Precautions: It is essential that adequate blood studies be made during treatment with the drug. While blood studies may detect early peripheral blood changes, such as leukopenia, reticulocytopenia, or granulocytopenia, before they become irreversible, such studies cannot be relied on to detect bone marrow depression prior to development of aplastic anemia. To facilitate appropriate studies and observa-

Continued on next page

This product information was prepared in August, 1982. On these and other Parke-Davis Products, information may be obtained by addressing PARKE-DAVIS, Division of Warner-Lambert Company, Morris Plains, New Jersey 07950.

Parke-Davis—Cont.

tion during therapy, it is desirable that patients be hospitalized.

Description: Chloramphenicol is an antibiotic that is clinically useful for, *and should be reserved for,* serious infections caused by organisms susceptible to its antimicrobial effects when less potentially hazardous therapeutic agents are ineffective or contraindicated. Sensitivity testing is essential to determine its indicated use, but may be performed concurrently with therapy initiated on clinical impression that one of the indicated conditions exists (see Indications section).

Actions and Pharmacology: *In vitro* chloramphenicol exerts mainly a bacteriostatic effect on a wide range of gram-negative and gram-positive bacteria and is active *in vitro* against rickettsiae, the lymphogranuloma psittacosis group, and *Vibrio cholerae.* It is particularly active against *Salmonella typhi* and *Hemophilus influenzae.* The mode of action is through interference or inhibition of protein synthesis in intact cells and in cell-free systems.

Chloramphenicol administered orally is absorbed rapidly from the intestinal tract. In controlled studies in adult volunteers using the recommended dosage of 50 mg/kg/day, a dosage of 1 g every 6 hours for 8 doses was given. Using the microbiological assay method, the average peak serum level was 11.2 mcg/ml one hour after the first dose. A cumulative effect gave a peak rise to 18.4 mcg/ml after the fifth dose of 1 g. Mean serum levels ranged from 8 to 14 mcg/ml over the 48-hour period. Total urinary excretion of chloramphenicol in these studies ranged from a low of 68% to a high of 99% over a three-day period. From 8 to 12% of the antibiotic excreted is in the form of free chloramphenicol; the remainder consists of microbiologically inactive metabolites, principally the conjugate with glucuronic acid. Since the glucuronide is excreted rapidly, most chloramphenicol detected in the blood is in the microbiologically active free form. Despite the small proportion of unchanged drug excreted in the urine, the concentration of free chloramphenicol is relatively high, amounting to several hundred mcg/ml in patients receiving divided doses of 50 mg/kg/day. Small amounts of active drug are found in bile and feces. Chloramphenicol diffuses rapidly, but its distribution is not uniform. Highest concentrations are found in liver and kidney, and lowest concentrations are found in brain and cerebrospinal fluid. Chloramphenicol enters cerebrospinal fluid even in the absence of meningeal inflammation, appearing in concentrations about half of those found in the blood. Measurable levels are also detected in pleural and in ascitic fluids, saliva, milk, and in the aqueous and vitreous humors. Transport across the placental barrier occurs with somewhat lower concentration in cord blood of newborn infants than in maternal blood.

Indications: **In accord with the concepts in the warning box and this indications section, chloramphenicol must be used only in those serious infections for which less potentially dangerous drugs are ineffective or contraindicated. However, chloramphenicol may be chosen to initiate antibiotic therapy on the clinical impression that one of the conditions below is believed to be present; *in vitro* sensitivity tests should be performed concurrently so that the drug may be discontinued as soon as possible if less potentially dangerous agents are indicated by such tests. The decision to continue use of chloramphenicol rather than another antibiotic when both are suggested by *in vitro* studies to be effective against a specific pathogen should be based upon severity of the infection, susceptibility of the pathogen to the various antimicrobial drugs, efficacy of the various drugs in the infection, and the important additional concepts contained in the Warning Box above:**

1. Acute infections caused by *Salmonella typhi*

Chloramphenicol is a drug of choice.* It is not recommended for the routine treatment of the typhoid carrier state.

2. Serious infections caused by susceptible strains in accordance with the concepts expressed above:

a. *Salmonella* species
b. *H influenzae,* specifically meningeal infections
c. Rickettsia
d. Lymphogranuloma-psittacosis group
e. Various gram-negative bacteria causing bacteremia, meningitis, or other serious gram-negative infections
f. Other susceptible organisms which have been demonstrated to be resistant to all other appropriate antimicrobial agents.

3. Cystic fibrosis regimens

Contraindications: Chloramphenicol is contraindicated in individuals with a history of previous hypersensitivity and/or toxic reaction to it. *It must not be used in the treatment of trivial infections or where it is not indicated, as in colds, influenza, infections of the throat; or as a prophylactic agent to prevent bacterial infections.*

* In the treatment of typhoid fever, some authorities recommend that chloramphenicol be administered at therapeutic levels for 8 to 10 days after the patient has become afebrile to lessen the possibility of relapse.

Precautions: 1. Baseline blood studies should be followed by periodic blood studies approximately every two days during therapy. The drug should be discontinued upon appearance of reticulocytopenia, leukopenia, thrombocytopenia, anemia, or any other blood study findings attributable to chloramphenicol. However, it should be noted that such studies do not exclude the possible later appearance of the irreversible type of bone marrow depression.

2. Repeated courses of the drug should be avoided if at all possible. Treatment should not be continued longer than required to produce a cure with little or no risk of relapse of the disease.

3. Concurrent therapy with other drugs that may cause bone marrow depression should be avoided.

4. Excessive blood levels may result from administration of the recommended dose to patients with impaired liver or kidney function, including that due to immature metabolic processes in the infant. The dosage should be adjusted accordingly or, preferably, the blood concentration should be determined at appropriate intervals.

5. There are no studies to establish the safety of this drug in pregnancy.

6. Since chloramphenicol readily crosses the placental barrier, caution in use of the drug is particularly important during pregnancy at term or during labor because of potential toxic effects on the fetus ("gray syndrome").

7. Precaution should be used in therapy of premature and full-term infants to avoid "gray syndrome" toxicity. (See Adverse Reactions.) Serum drug levels should be carefully followed during therapy of the newborn infant.

8. Precaution should be used in therapy during lactation because of the possibility of toxic effects on the nursing infant.

9. The use of this antibiotic, as with other antibiotics, may result in an overgrowth of nonsusceptible organisms, including fungi. If infections caused by nonsusceptible organisms appear during therapy, appropriate measures should be taken.

Adverse Reactions:

1. Blood Dyscrasias

The most serious adverse effect of chloramphenicol is bone marrow depression. Serious and fatal blood dyscrasias (aplastic anemia, hypoplastic anemia, thrombocytopenia, and granulocytopenia) are known to occur after the administration of chloramphenicol. An irreversible type of marrow depression leading to aplastic anemia with a high rate of mortality is characterized by the appearance weeks or months after therapy of bone marrow aplasia or hypoplasia. Peripherally, pancytopenia is most often observed, but in a small number of cases only one or two of the three major cell types (erythrocytes, leukocytes, platelets) may be depressed.

A reversible type of bone marrow depression, which is dose-related, may occur. This type of marrow depression is characterized by vacuolization of the erythroid cells, reduction of reticulocytes, and leukopenia, and responds promptly to the withdrawal of chloramphenicol.

An exact determination of the risk of serious and fatal blood dyscrasias is not possible because of lack of accurate information regarding (1) the size of the population at risk, (2) the total number of drug-associated dyscrasias, and (3) the total number of nondrug-associated dyscrasias.

In a report to the California State Assembly by the California Medical Association and the State Department of Public Health in January 1967, the risk of fatal aplastic anemia was estimated at 1:24,200 to 1:40,500 based on two dosage levels.

There have been reports of aplastic anemia attributed to chloramphenicol which later terminated in leukemia.

Paroxysmal nocturnal hemoglobinuria has also been reported.

2. Gastrointestinal Reactions

Nausea, vomiting, glossitis and stomatitis, diarrhea, and enterocolitis may occur in low incidence.

3. Neurotoxic Reactions

Headache, mild depression, mental confusion, and delirium have been described in patients receiving chloramphenicol. Optic and peripheral neuritis have been reported, usually following long-term therapy. If this occurs, the drug should be promptly withdrawn.

4. Hypersensitivity Reactions

Fever, macular and vesicular rashes, angioedema, urticaria, and anaphylaxis may occur. Herxheimer reactions have occurred during therapy for typhoid fever.

5. "Gray Syndrome"

Toxic reactions including fatalities have occurred in the premature and newborn; the signs and symptoms associated with these reactions have been referred to as the "gray syndrome". One case of "gray syndrome" has been reported in an infant born to a mother having received chloramphenicol during labor. One case has been reported in a 3-month-old infant. The following summarizes the clinical and laboratory studies that have been made on these patients:

(a) In most cases, therapy with chloramphenicol had been instituted within the first 48 hours of life.
(b) Symptoms first appeared after 3 to 4 days of continued treatment with high doses of chloramphenicol.
(c) The symptoms appeared in the following order:
  (1) abdominal distention with or without emesis;
  (2) progressive pallid cyanosis;
  (3) vasomotor collapse, frequently accompanied by irregular respiration;
  (4) death within a few hours of onset of these symptoms.
(d) The progression of symptoms from onset to exitus was accelerated with higher dose schedules.

(e) Preliminary blood serum level studies revealed unusually high concentrations of chloramphenicol (over 90 mcg/ml after repeated doses).

(f) Termination of therapy upon early evidence of the associated symptomatology frequently reversed the process with complete recovery.

Dosage and Administration:

Dosage Recommendations For Oral Chloramphenicol Preparations

The majority of microorganisms susceptible to chloramphenicol will respond to a concentration between 5 and 20 mcg/ml. The desired concentration of active drug in blood should fall within this range over most of the treatment period. Dosage of 50 mg/kg/day divided into 4 doses at intervals of 6 hours will usually achieve and sustain levels of this magnitude. Except in certain circumstances (eg, premature and newborn infants and individuals with impairment of hepatic or renal function), lower doses may not achieve these concentrations. Chloramphenicol, like other potent drugs, should be prescribed at recommended doses known to have therapeutic activity. Close observation of the patient should be maintained and in the event of any adverse reactions, dosage should be reduced or the drug discontinued, if other factors in the clinical situation permit.

Adults

Adults should receive 50 mg/kg/day (approximately one 250-mg capsule per each 10 lbs body weight) in divided doses at 6-hour intervals. In exceptional cases, patients with infections due to moderately resistant organisms may require increased dosage up to 100 mg/kg/day to achieve blood levels inhibiting the pathogen, but these high doses should be decreased as soon as possible. Adults with impairment of hepatic or renal function or both may have reduced ability to metabolize and excrete the drug. In instances of impaired metabolic processes, dosages should be adjusted accordingly. (See discussion under Newborn Infants.) Precise control of concentration of the drug in the blood should be carefully followed in patients with impaired metabolic processes by the available microtechniques (information available on request).

Children

Dosage of 50 mg/kg/day divided into 4 doses at 6-hour intervals yields blood levels in the range effective against most susceptible organisms. Severe infections (eg, bacteremia or meningitis), especially when adequate cerebrospinal fluid concentrations are desired, may require dosage up to 100 mg/kg/day; however, it is recommended that dosage be reduced to 50 mg/kg/day as soon as possible. Children with impaired liver or kidney function may retain excessive amounts of the drug.

Newborn Infants

(See section titled "Gray Syndrome" under Adverse Reactions.)

A total of 25 mg/kg/day in 4 equal doses at 6-hour intervals usually produces and maintains concentrations in blood and tissues adequate to control most infections for which the drug is indicated. Increased dosage in these individuals, demanded by severe infections, should be given only to maintain the blood concentration within a therapeutically effective range. After the first two weeks of life, full-term infants ordinarily may receive up to a total of 50 mg/kg/day equally divided into 4 doses at 6-hour intervals. **These dosage recommendations are extremely important because blood concentration in all premature infants and full-term infants under two weeks of age differs from that of other infants.** This difference is due to variations in the maturity of the metabolic functions of the liver and the kidneys.

When these functions are immature (or seriously impaired in adults), high concentrations of the drug are found which tend to increase with succeeding doses.

Infants and Children with Immature Metabolic Processes

In young infants and other children in whom immature metabolic functions are suspected, a dose of 25 mg/kg/day will usually produce therapeutic concentrations of the drug in the blood. In this group particularly, the concentration of the drug in the blood should be carefully following by microtechniques. (Information available on request.)

How Supplied:

Kapseals No. 379, Chloromycetin (Chloramphenicol Capsules), each contain 250 mg chloramphenicol.

N 0071-0379-09 Bottles of 16.

N 0071-0379-24 Bottles of 100.

N 0071-0379-40 Unit dose packages of 100 (10/10's).

[Shown in Product Identification Section]

AHFS 8:12.08 **0379G100**

Chloromycetin, brand of chloramphenicol. Reg. US Pat Off

Storage: Store at a room temperature below 86°F(30°C). Protect from moisture and excessive heat.

CHLOROMYCETIN® OPHTHALMIC OINTMENT, 1% ℞

(chloramphenicol ophthalmic ointment, USP)

Description: Each gram of Chloromycetin Ophthalmic Ointment, 1%, contains 10 mg chloramphenicol in a special base of liquid petrolatum and polyethylene. It contains no preservatives. Sterile ointment.

Clinical Pharmacology: Chloramphenicol is a broad-spectrum antibiotic originally isolated from *Streptomyces venezuelae.* It is primarily bacteriostatic and acts by inhibition of protein synthesis by interfering with the transfer of activated amino acids from soluble RNA to ribosomes. It has been noted that chloramphenicol is found in measurable amounts in the aqueous humor following local application to the eye. Development of resistance to chloramphenicol can be regarded as minimal for staphylococci and many other species of bacteria.

Indications and Usage: Chloromycetin (chloramphenicol) Ophthalmic Ointment, 1%, is indicated for the treatment of superficial ocular infections involving the conjunctiva and/or cornea caused by chloramphenicol-susceptible organisms. Bacteriological studies should be performed to determine the causative organisms and their sensitivity to chloramphenicol.

Contraindication: This product is contraindicated in persons sensitive to any of its components.

Warnings: Bone marrow hypoplasia including aplastic anemia and death has been reported following the local application of chloramphenicol.

Precautions: The prolonged use of antibiotics may occasionally result in overgrowth of nonsusceptible organisms, including fungi. If new infections appear during medication, the drug should be discontinued and appropriate measures should be taken.

In all except very superficial infections, the topical use of chloramphenicol should be supplemented by appropriate systemic medication.

Adverse Reactions: Blood dyscrasias have been reported in association with the use of chloramphenicol. (see Warnings).

Dosage and Administration: A small amount of ointment placed in the lower conjunctival sac every three hours, or more frequently if deemed advisable by the prescribing physician. Administration should be continued day and night for the first 48 hours, after which the interval between applications may be increased. Treatment should be continued for at least 48 hours after the eye appears normal.

How Supplied:

N 0071-3070-07 (Stock 18-70-139)

Chloromycetin (chloramphenicol) Ophthalmic Ointment, 1% is supplied, sterile, in ophthalmic ointment tubes of 3.5 grams.

Chloromycetin, brand of chloramphenicol. Reg US Pat Off

AHFS 52:04.04 **3070G020**

CHLOROMYCETIN® OTIC ℞

(chloramphenicol otic)

Description: Each milliliter of Chloromycetin Otic contains 5 mg (0.5%) chloramphenicol in propylene glycol. Sterile.

Clinical Pharmacology: Chloramphenicol is a broad-spectrum antibiotic originally isolated from *Streptomyces venezuelae.* It is primarily bacteriostatic and acts by inhibition of protein synthesis by interfering with the transfer of activated amino acids from soluble RNA to ribosomes. Development of resistance to chloramphenicol can be regarded as minimal for staphylococci and many other species of bacteria.

Indications and Usage: Chloromycetin (chloramphenicol) Otic is indicated for the treatment of superficial infections of the external auditory canal caused by susceptible strains of various gram-positive and gram-negative organisms including:

Staphylococcus aureus, Escherichia coli, Hemophilus influenzae, Pseudomonas aeruginosa, Aerobacter aerogenes, Klebsiella pneumoniae, and *Proteus* species.

Deeper infections should be treated with appropriate systemic antibiotics.

Contraindication: This product is contraindicated in persons sensitive to any of its components.

Warnings: Bone marrow hypoplasia, including aplastic anemia and death, has been reported following the local application of chloramphenicol.

Precautions: The prolonged use of antibiotics may occasionally result in overgrowth of nonsusceptible organisms, including fungi. If new infections appear during medication, the drug should be discontinued and appropriate measures should be taken.

In all except very superficial infections, the topical use of chloramphenicol should be supplemented by appropriate systemic medication.

Adverse Reactions: Signs of local irritation, with subjective symptoms of itching or burning, angioneurotic edema, urticaria, vesicular and maculopapular dermatitis, have been reported in patients sensitive to chloramphenicol and are causes for discontinuing the medication. Similar sensitivity reactions to other materials in topical preparations may also occur. Blood dyscrasias have been reported in association with the use of chloramphenicol (See WARNINGS).

Dosage and Administration: Instill 2 or 3 drops into the ear three times daily.

How Supplied: N 0071-3313-35—Chloromycetin (chloramphenicol) Otic is supplied in 15-ml vials with droppers.

AHFS 52:04.04 **3313G021**

121 870600/21

Continued on next page

This product information was prepared in August, 1982. On these and other Parke-Davis Products, information may be obtained by addressing PARKE-DAVIS, Division of Warner-Lambert Company, Morris Plains, New Jersey 07950.

Parke-Davis—Cont.

ORAL SUSPENSION
CHLOROMYCETIN® PALMITATE ℞
(chloramphenicol palmitate oral suspension)

WARNING

Serious and fatal blood dyscrasias (aplastic anemia, hypoplastic anemia, thrombocytopenia, and granulocytopenia) are known to occur after the administration of chloramphenicol. In addition, there have been reports of aplastic anemia attributed to chloramphenicol which later terminated in leukemia. Blood dyscrasias have occurred after both short-term and prolonged therapy with this drug. Chloramphenicol must not be used when less potentially dangerous agents will be effective, as described in the Indications section. ***It must not be used in the treatment of trivial infections or where it is not indicated, as in colds, influenza, infections of the throat; or as a prophylactic agent to prevent bacterial infections.***

Precautions: It is essential that adequate blood studies be made during treatment with the drug. While blood studies may detect early peripheral blood changes, such as leukopenia, reticulocytopenia, or granulocytopenia, before they become irreversible, such studies cannot be relied on to detect bone marrow depression prior to development of aplastic anemia. To facilitate appropriate studies and observation during therapy, it is desirable that patients be hospitalized.

Description: Chloramphenicol is an antibiotic that is clinically useful for, *and should be reserved for,* serious infections caused by organisms susceptible to its antimicrobial effects when less potentially hazardous therapeutic agents are ineffective or contraindicated. Sensitivity testing is essential to determine its indicated use, but may be performed concurrently with therapy initiated on clinical impression that one of the indicated conditions exists (see Indications section).

Actions and Pharmacology: *In vitro* chloramphenicol exerts mainly a bacteriostatic effect on a wide range of gram-negative and gram-positive bacteria and is active *in vitro* against rickettsiae, the lymphogranuloma-psittacosis group and *Vibrio cholerae.* It is particularly active against *Salmonella typhi* and *Hemophilus influenzae.* The mode of action is through interference or inhibition of protein synthesis in intact cells and in cell-free systems.

Chloramphenicol administered orally is absorbed rapidly from the intestinal tract. In controlled studies in adult volunteers using the recommended dosage of 50 mg/kg/day, a dosage of 1 g every 6 hours for 8 doses was given. Using the microbiological assay method, the average peak serum level was 11.2 mcg/ml one hour after the first dose.

A cumulative effect gave a peak rise to 18.4 mcg/ml after the fifth dose of 1 g. Mean serum levels ranged from 8 to 14 mcg/ml over the 48-hour period. Total urinary excretion of chloramphenicol in these studies ranged from a low of 68% to a high of 99% over a three-day period. From 8% to 12% of the antibiotic excreted is in the form of free chloramphenicol; the remainder consists of microbiologically inactive metabolites, principally the conjugate with glucuronic acid. Since the glucuronide is excreted rapidly, most chloramphenicol detected in the blood is in the microbiologically active free form. Despite the small proportion of unchanged drug excreted in the urine, the concentration of free chloramphenicol is relatively high, amounting to several hundred mcg/ml in patients receiving divided doses of 50 mg/kg/day. Small amounts of active drug are found in bile and feces. Chloramphenicol diffuses rapidly, but its distribution is not uniform. Highest concentrations are found in liver and kidney, and lowest concentrations are found in brain and cerebrospinal fluid. Chloramphenicol enters cerebrospinal fluid even in the absence of meningeal inflammation, appearing in concentrations about half of those found in the blood. Measurable levels are also detected in pleural and in ascitic fluids, saliva, milk and in the aqueous and vitreous humors. Transport across the placental barrier occurs with somewhat lower concentration in cord blood of newborn infants than in maternal blood.

Indications: In accord with the concepts in the Warning Box and this Indications section, chloramphenicol must be used only in those serious infections for which less potentially dangerous drugs are ineffective or contraindicated. However, chloramphenicol may be chosen to initiate antibiotic therapy on the clinical impression that one of the conditions below is believed to be present; *in vitro* sensitivity tests should be performed concurrently so that the drug may be discontinued as soon as possible if less potentially dangerous agents are indicated by such tests. The decision to continue use of chloramphenicol rather than another antibiotic when both are suggested by *in vitro* studies to be effective against a specific pathogen should be based upon severity of the infection, susceptibility of the pathogen to the various antimicrobial drugs, efficacy of the various drugs in the infection, and the important additional concepts contained in the Warning Box above.

1. Acute infections caused by *Salmonella typhi*

Chloramphenicol is a drug of choice.* It is not recommended for the routine treatment of the typhoid carrier state.

2. Serious infections caused by susceptible strains in accordance with the concepts expressed above:

a. Salmonella species
b. *H influenzae,* specifically meningeal infections
c. Rickettsia
d. Lymphogranuloma-psittacosis group
e. Various gram-negative bacteria causing bacteremia, meningitis or other serious gram-negative infections
f. Other susceptible organisms which have been demonstrated to be resistant to all other appropriate antimicrobial agents.

3. Cystic fibrosis regimens

---

* In the treatment of typhoid fever some authorities recommend that chloramphenicol be administered at therapeutic levels for 8 to 10 days after the patient has become afebrile to lessen the possibility of relapse.

Contraindications: Chloramphenicol is contraindicated in individuals with a history of previous hypersensitivity and/or toxic reaction to it. *It must not be used in the treatment of trivial infections or where it is not indicated, as in colds, influenza, infections of the throat; or as a prophylactic agent to prevent bacterial infections.*

Precautions:

1. Baseline blood studies should be followed by periodic blood studies approximately every two days during therapy. The drug should be discontinued upon appearance of reticulocytopenia, leukopenia, thrombocytopenia, anemia, or any other blood study findings attributable to chloramphenicol. However, it should be noted that such studies do not exclude the possible later appearance of the irreversible type of bone marrow depression.
2. Repeated courses of the drug should be avoided if at all possible. Treatment should not be continued longer than required to produce a cure with little or no risk of relapse of the disease.
3. Concurrent therapy with other drugs that may cause bone marrow depression should be avoided.
4. Excessive blood levels may result from administration of the recommended dose to patients with impaired liver or kidney function, including that due to immature metabolic processes in the infant. The dosage should be adjusted accordingly or, preferably, the blood concentration should be determined at appropriate intervals.
5. There are no studies to establish the safety of this drug in pregnancy.
6. Since chloramphenicol readily crosses the placental barrier, caution in use of the drug is particularly important during pregnancy at term or during labor because of potential toxic effects on the fetus (gray syndrome).
7. Precaution should be used in therapy of premature and full-term infants to avoid "gray syndrome" toxicity. (See "Adverse Reactions.") Serum drug levels should be carefully followed during therapy of the newborn infant.
8. Precaution should be used in therapy during lactation because of the possibility of toxic effects on the nursing infant.
9. The use of this antibiotic, as with other antibiotics, may result in an overgrowth of nonsusceptible organisms, including fungi. If infections caused by nonsusceptible organisms appear during therapy, appropriate measures should be taken.

Adverse Reactions:

1. Blood Dyscrasias

The most serious adverse effect of chloramphenicol is bone marrow depression. Serious and fatal blood dyscrasias (aplastic anemia, hypoplastic anemia, thrombocytopenia, and granulocytopenia) are known to occur after the administration of chloramphenicol. An irreversible type of marrow depression leading to aplastic anemia with a high rate of mortality is characterized by the appearance weeks or months after therapy of bone marrow aplasia or hypoplasia. Peripherally, pancytopenia is most often observed, but in a small number of cases only one or two of the three major cell types (erythrocytes, leukocytes, platelets) may be depressed.

A reversible type of bone marrow depression, which is dose related, may occur. This type of marrow depression is characterized by vacuolization of the erythroid cells, reduction of reticulocytes and leukopenia, and responds promptly to the withdrawal of chloramphenicol.

An exact determination of the risk of serious and fatal blood dyscrasias is not possible because of lack of accurate information regarding 1) the size of the population at risk, 2) the total number of drug-associated dyscrasias, and 3) the total number of nondrug associated dyscrasias.

In a report to the California State Assembly by the California Medical Association and the State Department of Public Health in January 1967, the risk of fatal aplastic anemia was estimated at 1:24,200 to 1:40,500 based on two dosage levels.

There have been reports of aplastic anemia attributed to chloramphenicol which later terminated in leukemia.

Paroxysmal nocturnal hemoglobinuria has also been reported.

2. Gastrointestinal Reactions

Nausea, vomiting, glossitis and stomatitis, diarrhea and enterocolitis may occur in low incidence.

3. Neurotoxic Reactions

Headache, mild depression, mental confusion and delirium have been described in patients receiving chloramphenicol. Optic and peripheral neuritis have been reported, usually following long-term therapy. If this occurs, the drug should be promptly withdrawn.

4. Hypersensitivity Reactions
Fever, macular and vesicular rashes, angioedema, urticaria and anaphylaxis may occur. Herxheimer reactions have occurred during therapy for typhoid fever.

5. "Gray Syndrome"
Toxic reactions including fatalities have occurred in the premature and newborn, the signs and symptoms associated with these reactions have been referred to as the gray syndrome. One case of gray syndrome has been reported in an infant born to a mother having received chloramphenicol during labor. One case has been reported in a 3-month-old infant. The following summarizes the clinical and laboratory studies that have been made on these patients.

(a) In most cases therapy with chloramphenicol had been instituted within the first 48 hours of life.

(b) Symptoms first appeared after 3 to 4 days of continued treatment with high doses of chloramphenicol

(c) The symptoms appeared in the following order:

1) abdominal distention with or without emesis;
2) progressive pallid cyanosis;
3) vasomotor collapse, frequently accompanied by irregular respiration;
4) death within a few hours of onset of these symptoms.

(d) The progression of symptoms from onset to exitus was accelerated with higher dose schedules.

(e) Preliminary blood serum level studies revealed unusually high concentrations of chloramphenicol (over 90 mcg/ml after repeated doses).

(f) Termination of therapy upon early evidence of the associated symptomatology frequently reversed the process with complete recovery.

Dosage and Administration:

Dosage Recommendations
The majority of microorganisms susceptible to chloramphenicol will respond to a concentration between 5 and 20 mcg/ml. The desired concentration of active drug in blood should fall within this range over most of the treatment period. Dosage of 50 mg/kg/day divided into 4 doses at intervals of 6 hours will usually achieve and sustain levels of this magnitude.
Except in certain circumstances (eg. premature and newborn infants and individuals with impairment of hepatic or renal function) lower doses may not achieve these concentrations. Chloramphenicol, like other potent drugs, should be prescribed at recommended doses known to have therapeutic activity. Close observation of the patient should be maintained and in the event of any adverse reactions, dosage should be reduced or the drug discontinued, if other factors in the clinical situation permit.

Adults
Adults should receive 50 mg/kg/day in divided doses at 6-hour intervals. In exceptional cases patients with infections due to moderately resistant organisms may require increased dosage up to 100 mg/kg/day to achieve blood levels inhibiting the pathogen, but these high doses should be decreased as soon as possible. Adults with impairment of hepatic or renal function or both may have reduced ability to metabolize and excrete the drug. In instances of impaired metabolic processes, dosages should be adjusted accordingly. (See discussion under Newborn Infants.) Precise control of concentration of the drug in the blood should be carefully followed in patients with impaired metabolic processes by the available microtechniques (information available on request).

Children
Dosage of 50 mg/kg/day divided into 4 doses at 6-hour intervals yields blood levels in the range effective against most susceptible organisms. Severe infections (eg. bacteremia or meningitis), especially when adequate cerebrospinal fluid concentrations are desired, may require dosage up to 100 mg/kg/day; however, it is recommended that dosage be reduced to 50 mg/kg/day as soon as possible. Children with impaired liver or kidney function may retain excessive amounts of the drug.

Newborn Infants
(See section titled "Gray Syndrome" under Adverse Reactions.)
A total of 25 mg/kg/day in 4 equal doses at 6-hour intervals usually produces and maintains concentrations in blood and tissues adequate to control most infections for which the drug is indicated. Increased dosage in these individuals, demanded by severe infections, should be given only to maintain the blood concentration within a therapeutically effective range. After the first two weeks of life, full-term infants ordinarily may receive up to a total of 50 mg/kg/day equally divided into 4 doses at 6-hour intervals. *These dosage recommendations are extremely important because blood concentration in all premature infants and full-term infants under two weeks of age differs from that of other infants.* This difference is due to variations in the maturity of the metabolic functions of the liver and the kidneys.
When these functions are immature (or seriously impaired in adults), high concentrations of the drug are found which tend to increase with succeeding doses.

Infants and Children with Immature Metabolic Processes
In young infants and other children in whom immature metabolic functions are suspected, a dose of 25 mg/kg/day will usually produce therapeutic concentrations of the drug in the blood. In this group particularly, the concentration of the drug in the blood should be carefully followed by microtechniques. (Information available on request.)

How Supplied:
N 0071-2310-15
Oral Suspension Chloromycetin (chloramphenicol) Palmitate, each 5 ml contains chloramphenicol palmitate equivalent to 150 mg chloramphenicol with 0.5% sodium benzoate as preservative, in bottles of 60 ml.
Chloramphenicol Palmitate is hydrolyzed to chloramphenicol before absorption. Resulting blood concentration is similar to that produced by the oral administration of chloramphenicol.

Chloromycetin, brand of chloramphenicol. Reg. US Pat Off

2310G040

CHLOROMYCETIN® SODIUM SUCCINATE ℞

(sterile chloramphenicol sodium succinate, USP)
FOR INTRAVENOUS ADMINISTRATION

WARNING
Serious and fatal blood dyscrasias (aplastic anemia, hypoplastic anemia, thrombocytopenia, and granulocytopenia) are known to occur after the administration of chloramphenicol. In addition, there have been reports of aplastic anemia attributed to chloramphenicol which later terminated in leukemia. Blood dyscrasias have occurred after both short-term and prolonged therapy with this drug. Chloramphenicol must not be used when less potentially dangerous agents will be effective, as described in the Indications section. *It must not be used in the treatment of trivial infections or where it is not indicated, as in colds, influenza, infections of the throat; or as a prophylactic agent to prevent bacterial infections.*

Precautions: It is essential that adequate blood studies be made during treatment with the drug. While blood studies may detect early peripheral blood changes, such as leukopenia, reticulocytopenia, or granulocytopenia, before they become irreversible, such studies cannot be relied on to detect bone marrow depression prior to development of aplastic anemia. To facilitate appropriate studies and observation during therapy, it is desirable that patients be hospitalized.

IMPORTANT CONSIDERATIONS IN PRESCRIBING INJECTABLE CHLORAMPHENICOL SODIUM SUCCINATE
CHLORAMPHENICOL SODIUM SUCCINATE IS INTENDED FOR INTRAVENOUS USE ONLY. IT HAS BEEN DEMONSTRATED TO BE INEFFECTIVE WHEN GIVEN INTRAMUSCULARLY.

1. Chloramphenicol sodium succinate must be hydrolyzed to its microbiologically active form and there is a lag in achieving adequate blood levels compared with the base given intravenously.
2. The oral form of chloramphenicol is readily absorbed and adequate blood levels are achieved and maintained on the recommended dosage.
3. Patients started on intravenous chloramphenicol sodium succinate should be changed to the oral form as soon as practicable.

Description: Chloramphenicol is an antibiotic that is clinically useful for, *and should be reserved for,* serious infections caused by organisms susceptible to its antimicrobial effects when less potentially hazardous therapeutic agents are ineffective or contraindicated. Sensitivity testing is essential to determine its indicated use, but may be performed concurrently with therapy initiated on clinical impression that one of the indicated conditions exists (see Indications section).
Each gram (10 ml of a 10% solution) of chloramphenicol sodium succinate contains approximately 52 mg (2.25 mEq) of sodium.

Actions and Pharmacology: *In vitro* chloramphenicol exerts mainly a bacteriostatic effect on a wide range of gram-negative and gram-positive bacteria and is active *in vitro* against rickettsiae, the lymphogranuloma-psittacosis group, and *Vibrio cholerae.* It is particularly active against *Salmonella typhi* and *Hemophilus influenzae.* The mode of action is through interference or inhibition of protein synthesis in intact cells and in cell-free systems.
Chloramphenicol administered orally is absorbed rapidly from the intestinal tract. In controlled studies in adult volunteers using the recommended dosage of 50 mg/kg/day, a dosage of 1 g every 6 hours for 8 doses was given. Using the microbiological assay method, the average peak serum level was 11.2 mcg/ml one hour after the first dose. A cumulative effect gave a peak rise to 18.4 mcg/ml after the fifth dose of 1 g. Mean serum levels ranged from 8 to 14 mcg/ml over the 48-hour period. Total urinary excretion of chloramphenicol in these studies ranged from a low of 68% to a high of 99% over a three-day period. From 8 to 12% of the antibiotic excreted is in the form of free chloramphenicol; the remainder consists of microbiologically inactive metabolites, principally the conjugate with glucuronic acid. Since the glucuronide is excreted rapidly, most chlo-

Continued on next page

This product information was prepared in August, 1982. On these and other Parke-Davis Products, information may be obtained by addressing PARKE-DAVIS, Division of Warner-Lambert Company, Morris Plains, New Jersey 07950.

Parke-Davis—Cont.

ramphenicol detected in the blood is in the microbiologically active free form. Despite the small proportion of unchanged drug excreted in the urine, the concentration of free chloramphenicol is relatively high, amounting to several hundred mcg/ml in patients receiving divided doses of 50 mg/kg/day. Small amounts of active drug are found in bile and feces. Chloramphenicol diffuses rapidly, but its distribution is not uniform. Highest concentrations are found in liver and kidney, and lowest concentrations are found in brain and cerebrospinal fluid. Chloramphenicol enters cerebrospinal fluid even in the absence of meningeal inflammation, appearing in concentrations about half of those found in the blood. Measurable levels are also detected in pleural and in ascitic fluids, saliva, milk, and in the aqueous and vitreous humors. Transport across the placental barrier occurs with somewhat lower concentration in cord blood of newborn infants than in maternal blood.

Indications: In accord with the concepts in the warning box and this Indications section, chloramphenicol must be used only in those serious infections for which less potentially dangerous drugs are ineffective or contraindicated. However, chloramphenicol may be chosen to initiate antibiotic therapy on the clinical impression that one of the conditions below is believed to be present; *in vitro* sensitivity tests should be performed concurrently so that the drug may be discontinued as soon as possible if less potentially dangerous agents are indicated by such tests. The decision to continue use of chloramphenicol rather than another antibiotic when both are suggested by *in vitro* studies to be effective against a specific pathogen should be based upon severity of the infection, susceptibility of the pathogen to the various antimicrobial drugs, efficacy of the various drugs in the infection, and the important additional concepts contained in the Warning Box above:

1. Acute infections caused by *S typhi**

It is not recommended for the routine treatment of the typhoid carrier state.

2. Serious infections caused by susceptible strains in accordance with the concepts expressed above:

a. *Salmonella* species
b. *H influenzae,* specifically meningeal infections
c. Rickettsia
d. Lymphogranuloma-psittacosis group
e. Various gram-negative bacteria causing bacteremia, meningitis, or other serious gram-negative infections
f. Other susceptible organisms which have been demonstrated to be resistant to all other appropriate antimicrobial agents.

3. Cystic fibrosis regimens

*In the treatment of typhoid fever, some authorities recommend that chloramphenicol be administered at therapeutic levels for 8 to 10 days after the patient has become afebrile to lessen the possibility of relapse.

Contraindications: Chloramphenicol is contraindicated in individuals with a history of previous hypersensitivity and/or toxic reaction to it. *It must not be used in the treatment of trivial infections or where it is not indicated, as in colds, influenza, infections of the throat; or as a prophylactic agent to prevent bacterial infection.*

Precautions:

1. Baseline blood studies should be followed by periodic blood studies approximately every two days during therapy. The drug should be discontinued upon appearance of reticulocytopenia, leukopenia, thrombocytopenia, anemia, or any other blood study findings attributable to chloramphenicol. However, it should be noted that such studies do not exclude the possible later appearance of the irreversible type of bone marrow depression.

2. Repeated courses of the drug should be avoided if at all possible. Treatment should not be continued longer than required to produce a cure with little or no risk of relapse of the disease.

3. Concurrent therapy with other drugs that may cause bone marrow depression should be avoided.

4. Excessive blood levels may result from administration of the recommended dosage to patients with impaired liver or kidney function, including that due to immature metabolic processes in the infant. The dosage should be adjusted accordingly or, preferably, the blood concentration should be determined at appropriate intervals.

5. There are no studies to establish the safety of this drug in pregnancy.

6. Since chloramphenicol readily crosses the placental barrier, caution in use of the drug is particularly important during pregnancy at term or during labor because of potential toxic effects on the fetus (gray syndrome).

7. Precaution should be used in therapy of premature and full-term infants to avoid gray syndrome toxicity (see Adverse Reactions). Serum drug levels should be carefully followed during therapy of the newborn infant.

8. Precaution should be used in therapy during lactation because of the possibility of toxic effects on the nursing infant.

9. The use of this antibiotic, as with other antibiotics, may result in an overgrowth of nonsusceptible organisms, including fungi. If infections caused by nonsusceptible organisms appear during therapy, appropriate measures should be taken.

Adverse Reactions:

1. Blood Dyscrasias

The most serious adverse effect of chloramphenicol is bone marrow depression. Serious and fatal blood dyscrasias (aplastic anemia, hypoplastic anemia, thrombocytopenia, and granulocytopenia) are known to occur after the administration of chloramphenicol. An irreversible type of marrow depression leading to aplastic anemia with a high rate of mortality is characterized by the appearance weeks or months after therapy of bone marrow aplasia or hypoplasia. Peripherally, pancytopenia is most often observed, but in a small number of cases only one or two of the three major cell types (erythrocytes, leukocytes, platelets) may be depressed.

A reversible type of bone marrow depression, which is dose-related, may occur. This type of marrow depression is characterized by vacuolization of the erythroid cells, reduction of reticulocytes, and leukopenia, and responds promptly to the withdrawal of chloramphenicol.

An exact determination of the risk of serious and fatal blood dyscrasias is not possible because of lack of accurate information regarding (1) the size of the population at risk, (2) the total number of drug-associated dyscrasias, and (3) the total number of nondrug-associated dyscrasias.

In a report to the California State Assembly by the California Medical Association and the State Department of Public Health in January 1967, the risk of fatal aplastic anemia was estimated at 1:24,200 to 1:40,500 based on two dosage levels.

There have been reports of aplastic anemia attributed to chloramphenicol which later terminated in leukemia.

Paroxysmal nocturnal hemoglobinuria has also been reported.

2. Gastrointestinal Reactions

Nausea, vomiting, glossitis and stomatitis, diarrhea, and enterocolitis may occur in low incidence.

3. Neurotoxic Reactions

Headache, mild depression, mental confusion, and delirium have been described in patients receiving chloramphenicol. Optic and peripheral neuritis have been reported, usually following long-term therapy. If this occurs, the drug should be promptly withdrawn.

4. Hypersensitivity Reactions

Fever, macular and vesicular rashes, angioedema, urticaria, and anaphylaxis may occur. Herxheimer reactions have occurred during therapy for typhoid fever.

5. "Gray Syndrome"

Toxic reactions including fatalities have occurred in the premature and newborn; the signs and symptoms associated with these reactions have been referred to as the gray syndrome. One case of gray syndrome has been reported in an infant born to a mother having received chloramphenicol during labor. One case has been reported in a 3-month-old infant. The following summarizes the clinical and laboratory studies that have been made on these patients:

a) In most cases, therapy with chloramphenicol had been instituted within the first 48 hours of life.
b) Symptoms first appeared after 3 to 4 days of continued treatment with high doses of chloramphenicol.
c) The symptoms appeared in the following order:
   (1) abdominal distention with or without emesis;
   (2) progressive pallid cyanosis;
   (3) vasomotor collapse, frequently accompanied by irregular respiration;
   (4) death within a few hours of onset of these symptoms.
d) The progression of symptoms from onset to exitus was accelerated with higher dose schedules.
e) Preliminary blood serum level studies revealed unusually high concentrations of chloramphenicol (over 90 mcg/ml after repeated doses).
f) Termination of therapy upon early evidence of the associated symptomatology frequently reversed the process with complete recovery.

Administration: Chloramphenicol, like other potent drugs, should be prescribed at recommended doses known to have therapeutic activity. Administration of 50 mg/kg/day in divided doses will produce blood levels of the magnitude to which the majority of susceptible microorganisms will respond.

As soon as feasible, an oral dosage form of chloramphenicol should be substituted for the intravenous form because adequate blood levels are achieved with chloramphenicol by mouth.

The following method of administration is recommended:

Intravenously as a 10% (100 mg/ml) solution to be injected over at least a one-minute interval. This is prepared by the addition of 10 ml of an aqueous diluent, such as water for injection or 5% dextrose injection.

Dosage:

Adults

Adults should receive 50 mg/kg/day in divided doses at 6-hour intervals. In exceptional cases, patients with infections due to moderately resistant organisms may require increased dosage up to 100 mg/kg/day to achieve blood levels inhibiting the pathogen, but these high doses should be decreased as soon as possible. Adults with impairment of hepatic or renal function or both may have reduced ability to metabolize and excrete the drug. In instances of impaired metabolic processes, dosages should be adjusted accordingly. (See discussion under Newborn Infants.) Precise control of concentration of the drug in the blood should be carefully followed in patients with impaired metabolic processes by the available microtechniques (information available on request).

Children

Dosage of 50 mg/kg/day divided into 4 doses at 6-hour intervals yields blood levels in the range effective against most susceptible organisms. Severe infections (eg, bacteremia or meningitis), especially when adequate cerebrospinal fluid concentrations are desired, may require dosage up to 100 mg/kg/day; however, it is recommended that dosage be reduced to 50 mg/kg/day as soon as possible. Children with impaired liver or kidney function may retain excessive amounts of the drug.

Newborn Infants

(See section titled Gray Syndrome under Adverse Reactions.)

A total of 25 mg/kg/day in 4 equal doses at 6-hour intervals usually produces and maintains concentrations in blood and tissues adequate to control most infections for which the drug is indicated. Increased dosage in these individuals, demanded by severe infections, should be given only to maintain the blood concentration within a therapeutically effective range. After the first two weeks of life, full-term infants ordinarily may receive up to a total of 50 mg/kg/day equally divided into 4 doses at 6-hour intervals. *These dosage recommendations are extremely important because blood concentration in all premature infants and full-term infants under two weeks of age differs from that of other infants.* This difference is due to variations in the maturity of the metabolic functions of the liver and the kidneys.

When these functions are immature (or seriously impaired in adults), high concentrations of the drug are found which tend to increase with succeeding doses.

Infants and Children with Immature Metabolic Processes

In young infants and other children in whom immature metabolic functions are suspected, a dose of 25 mg/kg/day will usually produce therapeutic concentrations of the drug in the blood. In this group particularly, the concentration of the drug in the blood should be carefully followed by microtechniques. (Information available on request.)

How Supplied: N 0071-4057-03[06]—(Steri-Vial® No. 57) Chloromycetin Sodium Succinate (Chloramphenicol Sodium Succinate for Injection, USP) is freeze-dried in the vial and supplied in Steri-Vials (rubber diaphragm-capped vials). When reconstituted as directed, each vial contains a sterile solution equivalent to 100 mg of chloramphenicol per milliliter (1 g/10 ml). Available in packages of 10 vials.

Chloromycetin, brand of chloramphenicol, Reg US Pat Off

AHFS 8:12.08 **121 865000/YE**

CHLOROMYXIN™ ℞

(chloramphenicol-polymyxin ophthalmic ointment)

Description: Each gram of Chloromyxin (chloramphenicol-polymyxin ophthalmic ointment) contains 10 mg (1%) chloramphenicol and 10,000 units polymyxin B (as the sulfate) in a special base of liquid petrolatum and polyethylene. Sterile.

Clinical Pharmacology: Chloramphenicol is a broad-spectrum antibiotic originally isolated from *Streptomyces venezuelae.* It is primarily bacteriostatic and acts by inhibition of protein synthesis by interfering with the transfer of activated amino acids from soluble RNA to ribosomes. It has been noted that chloramphenicol is found in measurable amounts in the aqueous humor following local application to the eye. Development of resistance to chloramphenicol can be regarded as minimal for staphylococci and many other species of bacteria.

Polymyxin B sulfate is one of a group of basic polypeptide antibiotics derived from *B polymyxa (B aerosporus)* and has a bactericidal action against almost all gram-negative bacilli except the *Proteus* group. Polymyxins increase the permeability of bacterial cell wall membranes. All gram-positive bacteria, fungi, and the gram-negative cocci, *Neisseria gonorrhoeae* and *N meningitidis,* are resistant.

Indications and Usage: Chloromyxin (chloramphenicol-polymyxin ophthalmic ointment) is indicated for the treatment of superficial ocular infections involving the conjunctiva and/or cornea caused by chloramphenicol- and/or polymyxin-susceptible organisms.

Contraindication: This product is contraindicated in persons sensitive to any of its components.

Warnings: Bone marrow hypoplasia, including aplastic anemia and death, has been reported following the local application of chloramphenicol.

Precautions: The prolonged use of antibiotics may occasionally result in overgrowth of nonsusceptible organisms, including fungi. If new infections appear during medication, the drug should be discontinued and appropriate measures should be taken.

In all except very superficial infections, the topical use of chloramphenicol should be supplemented by appropriate systemic medication.

Adverse Reactions: Blood dyscrasias have been reported in association with the use of chloramphenicol (See WARNINGS).

Dosage and Administration: A small amount of ointment placed in the lower conjunctival sac every three hours, or more frequently if deemed advisable by the prescribing physician. Administration should be continued day and night for the first 48 hours, after which the interval between applications may be increased. Treatment should be continued for at least 48 hours after the eye appears normal.

Total dosage of polymyxin, systemic and ophthalmic, exceeding 2.5 mg (25,000 units)/kg/day should be avoided.

How Supplied: N 0071-3082-07 Chloromyxin (chloramphenicol-polymyxin ophthalmic ointment) is supplied sterile in ophthalmic ointment tubes of 3.5 g.

AHFS 52:04.04

3082G020
121 870450/ZJ

CHOLEDYL® ℞

Tablets/Elixir
(oxtriphylline, USP)

Description: Each partially enteric coated tablet contains 200 mg or 100 mg oxtriphylline. Each 5 ml teaspoonful of the elixir contains 100 mg oxtriphylline; alcohol 20%.

NOTE: 100 mg oxtriphylline is equivalent to 64 mg anhydrous theophylline.

Actions: Choledyl (oxtriphylline) is a xanthine bronchodilator—the choline salt of theophylline. Choledyl, compared to aminophylline, is less irritating to the gastric mucosa, more readily absorbed from the gastrointestinal tract, more stable and more soluble.

Like other xanthines, oxtriphylline is known to increase vital capacity which has been impaired by bronchospasm and air-trapping. Development of tolerance has been reported infrequently, and therefore Choledyl is useful for long-term therapy of bronchospasm.

Indications: Choledyl (oxtriphylline) is indicated for relief of acute bronchial asthma and for reversible bronchospasm associated with chronic bronchitis and emphysema.

Warning: Use in pregnancy—animal studies revealed no evidence of teratogenic potential. Safety in human pregnancy has not been established; use during lactation or in patients who are or who may become pregnant requires that the potential benefits of the drug be weighed against its possible hazards to the mother and child.

Precautions: Concurrent use of other xanthine-containing preparations may lead to adverse reactions, particularly CNS stimulation in children.

Adverse Reactions: Gastric distress and, occasionally, palpitation and CNS stimulation have been reported.

Dosage:

Tablets—Adults: 200 mg, 4 times a day.

Elixir—Adults: 200 mg (two teaspoonfuls or 10 ml), 4 times a day; Children (2 to 12): 100 mg (one teaspoonful or 5 ml) per 60 lb body weight, 4 times a day.

Above recommendations are averages. Dosage should be individualized.

Supplied: N 0071-0211—Choledyl 200 mg, yellow, partially enteric coated tablets in bottles of 100, 1000, and unit dose packages (10 x 10 strips);

N 0071-0210-24 Choledyl 100 mg, red partially enteric coated tablets in bottles of 100;

N 0071-2215-23 Choledyl elixir, sherry-flavored in bottles of 16 fl oz (1 pint) 474 ml.

Store between 59° and 86°F (15° and 30°C).

Toxicity:

Oxtriphylline, aminophylline and caffeine appear to be more toxic to newborn than to adult rats. No teratogenic effects have been seen.

[*Shown in Product Identification Section*]

0210 G 010

CHOLEDYL® PEDIATRIC SYRUP ℞

(oxtriphylline)

Description: Choledyl (oxtriphylline) is a xanthine bronchodilator—the choline salt of theophylline.

Each 5 ml of Choledyl Pediatric Syrup contains 50 mg oxtriphylline (equivalent to 32 mg of anhydrous theophylline).

Clinical Pharmacology: Theophylline directly relaxes the smooth muscle of the bronchial airways and pulmonary blood vessels, thus acting mainly as a bronchodilator, pulmonary vasodilator and smooth muscle relaxant. The drug also possesses other actions typical of the xanthine derivatives: coronary vasodilator, diuretic, cardiac stimulant, cerebral stimulant and skeletal muscle stimulant. The actions of theophylline may be mediated through inhibition of phosphodiesterase and a resultant increase in intracellular cyclic AMP which could mediate smooth muscle relaxation. At concentrations higher than attained *in vivo,* theophylline also inhibits the release of histamine by mast cells.

Theophylline has been shown to react additively with beta agonists that increase intracellular cyclic AMP through the stimulation of adenyl cyclase (isoproterenol).

Apparently, the development of tolerance does not occur with chronic use of theophylline.

Theophylline Elimination Characteristics

	Theophylline Clearance Rates (mean ± S.D.)	Half-life Average (mean ± S.D.)
Children (over 6 months of age)	1.45 ± .58 ml/kg/min	3.7 ± 1.1 hours
Adult non-smokers with uncomplicated asthma	.65 ± .19 ml/kg/min	8.7 ± 2.2 hours

Continued on next page

This product information was prepared in August, 1982. On these and other Parke-Davis Products, information may be obtained by addressing PARKE-DAVIS, Division of Warner-Lambert Company, Morris Plains, New Jersey 07950.

Parke-Davis—Cont.

The half-life is shortened with cigarette smoking. The half-life is prolonged in alcoholism, reduced hepatic or renal function, congestive heart failure, and in patients receiving antibiotics such as TAO (troleandomycin), erythromycin and clindamycin. High fever for prolonged periods may decrease theophylline elimination.

(See table on preceding page)

Newborn infants have extremely slow clearances and half-lives exceeding 24 hours, which approach those seen for older children after about 3–6 months.

The half-life of theophylline is prolonged in patients with congestive heart failure, in those with reduced hepatic or renal function, and in alcoholism. The half-life of theophylline may also be prolonged by concurrent use of various drugs such as phenobarbital, and certain antibiotics, including troleandomycin, erythromycin, and lincomycin.

Theophylline half-life is shortened in cigarette smokers (1 to 2 packs/day) as compared to nonsmokers. The increase in theophylline clearance caused by smoking is probably the result of induction of drug metabolizing enzymes that do not readily normalize after cessation of smoking. It appears that between 3 months and 2 years may be necessary for normalization of the effect of smoking on theophylline pharmacokinetics.

Actions: Choledyl (oxtriphylline), the choline salt of theophylline, effects significant improvement in pulmonary function parameters which have been impaired by bronchospasm. It is more soluble than either aminophylline or theophylline.

Indications: Choledyl (oxtriphylline) is indicated for relief of acute and chronic bronchial asthma and for reversible bronchospasm associated with chronic bronchitis and emphysema.

Contraindications: Choledyl is contraindicated in individuals who have shown hypersensitivity to theophylline or to Choledyl (oxtriphylline) or any of its components.

Warnings: Status asthmaticus is a medical emergency. Optimal therapy frequently requires additional medication including corticosteroids when the patient is not rapidly responsive to bronchodilators.

Excessive theophylline doses may be associated with toxicity, and serum theophylline levels are recommended to assure maximal benefit without excessive risk; incidence of toxicity increases at levels greater than 20 mcg theophylline/ml. Morphine, curare, and stilbamidine should be used with caution in patients with airflow obstruction since they stimulate histamine release and can induce asthmatic attacks. These drugs may also suppress respiration leading to respiratory failure. Alternative drugs should be chosen whenever possible.

There is excellent correlation between high blood levels of theophylline resulting from conventional doses and associated clinical manifestations of toxicity in patients with liver dysfunction or chronic obstructive lung disease.

There is excellent correlation between high serum levels of theophylline (over 20 mcg/ml) and the clinical manifestations of toxicity. Careful reduction of dosage and monitoring of serum levels are especially important in patients manifesting a decrease in total body theophylline clearance rate, including those with generalized debility, acute hypoxia, cardiac decompensation, hepatic dysfunction, or renal failure. Dosage reduction may also be necessary in patients who are older than 55 years of age, particularly males.

Serious toxic effects may occur suddenly and are not invariably preceded by minor adverse effects such as nausea, vomiting, and restlessness. Convulsions, tachycardia, or ventricular arrhythmias may be the first sign of toxicity. Children have a marked sensitivity to the CNS stimulant action of theophylline. Serious toxic effects, including fatalities have been reported in children as well as adults.

Theophylline products may worsen pre-existing arrhythmias.

Precautions: General: Mean half-life in smokers is shorter than nonsmokers. Therefore, smokers may require larger doses of theophylline. Theophylline should not be administered concurrently with other xanthine medications or with xanthine-containing beverages or foods. Use with caution in patients with severe cardiac disease, severe hypoxemia, hypertension, hyperthyroidism, acute myocardial injury, cor pulmonale, congestive heart failure, or liver disease, and in the elderly (especially males) and in neonates. Great caution should especially be used in giving theophylline to patients in congestive heart failure. Such patients have shown markedly prolonged theophylline blood level curves with theophylline persisting in serum for long periods following discontinuation of the drug.

Use theophylline cautiously in patients with a history of peptic ulcer. Theophylline may occasionally act as a local irritant to the G.I. tract although gastrointestinal symptoms are more commonly central and associated with serum theophylline concentrations over 20 mcg/ml.

Drug Interactions: Theophylline-containing preparations have exhibited interaction with the following drugs:

Drug	Effect
Lithium carbonate	Increased excretion of lithium carbonate.
Propranolol	Antagonism of propranolol effect.
Furosemide	Increased furosemide diuresis.
Hexamethonium	Decreased hexamethonium-induced chronotropic effect.
Reserpine	Reserpine-induced tachycardia.
Chlordiazepoxide	Chlordiazepoxide-induced fatty acid mobilization.
Troleandomycin erythromycin or lincomycin	Increased theophylline plasma levels.

Usage in Pregnancy: Safe use of Choledyl (oxtriphylline) in pregnancy and lactation has not been established relative to possible adverse effects on fetal or neonatal development. Therefore Choledyl (oxtriphylline) should not be used in patients who are pregnant or who may become pregnant, or during lactation unless, in the judgment of the physician, the potential benefits outweigh the possible hazards.

Adverse Reactions: The most consistent adverse reactions are usually due to overdose and are:

1. Gastrointestinal: nausea, vomiting, epigastric pain, hematemesis, diarrhea.
2. Central nervous system: headaches, irritability, restlessness, insomnia, reflex hyperexcitability, muscle twitching, clonic and tonic generalized convulsions.
3. Cardiovascular: palpitation, tachycardia, extrasystoles, flushing, hypotension, circulatory failure, life-threatening ventricular arrhythmias.
4. Respiratory: tachypnea.
5. Renal: albuminuria, increased excretion of renal tubular cells and red blood cells, diuresis.
6. Others: hyperglycemia and inappropriate antidiuretic hormone (ADH) syndrome.

Dosage and Administration: Therapeutic serum levels associated with optimal likelihood of benefit and minimal risk of toxicity are considered to be between 10 mcg/ml and 20 mcg/ml. Levels above 20 mcg/ml may produce toxic effects. There is great variation from patient to patient in dosage needed in order to achieve a therapeutic blood level because of variable rates of elimination. Because of this wide variation from patient to patient and the relatively narrow therapeutic blood level range, dosage must be individualized; monitoring of theophylline serum levels is highly recommended.

Dosage should be calculated on the basis of lean (ideal) body weight—mg/kg. Theophylline does not distribute into fatty tissue.

Giving theophylline with food may prevent the rare case of stomach irritation, and although absorption may be slower, it is still complete. When rapidly absorbed products such as solutions are used, dosing to maintain "around the clock" blood levels generally requires administration every 6 hours to obtain the greatest efficacy for use in children; dosing intervals up to 8 hours may be satisfactory for adults because of their slower elimination. Children and adults requiring higher than average doses may benefit from products with slower absorption. This may allow longer dosing intervals and/or less fluctuation in serum concentration over a dosing interval during chronic therapy.

In patients receiving concurrent bronchodilator therapy, eg, beta agonists, downward adjustment of Choledyl (oxtriphylline) dosage is necessary.

(See table above)

CHOLEDYL (OXTRIPHYLLINE) DOSAGE FOR PATIENT POPULATION

Acute Symptoms of Asthma Requiring Rapid Theophyllinization:

I. *Not currently receiving theophylline products:*

GROUP	ORAL LOADING DOSE CHOLEDYL	MAINTENANCE DOSE FOR NEXT 12 HOURS CHOLEDYL	MAINTENANCE DOSE BEYOND 12 HOURS CHOLEDYL
1. Children 6 months to 9 years	9.4 mg/kg *(6 mg/kg)	6.2 mg/kg q4 hrs *(4 mg/kg q4 hrs)	6.2 mg/kg q6 hrs *(4 mg/kg q6 hrs)
2. Children age 9–16 and young adult smokers	9.4 mg/kg *(6 mg/kg)	4.7 mg/kg q4 hrs *(3 mg/kg q4 hrs)	4.7 mg/kg q6 hrs *(3 mg/kg q6 hrs)
3. Otherwise healthy nonsmoking adults	9.4 mg/kg *(6 mg/kg)	4.7 mg/kg q6 hrs *(3 mg/kg q6 hrs)	4.7 mg/kg q8 hrs *(3 mg/kg q8 hrs)
4. Older patients and patients with cor pulmonale	9.4 mg/kg *(6 mg/kg)	3.1 mg/kg q6 hrs *(2 mg/kg q6 hrs)	3.1 mg/kg q8 hrs *(2 mg/kg q8 hrs)
5. Patients with congestive heart failure, liver failure	9.4 mg/kg *(6 mg/kg)	3.1 mg/kg q8 hrs *(2 mg/kg q8 hrs)	1.6–3.1 mg/kg q12 hrs *(1–2 mg/kg q12 hrs)

*Anhydrous theophylline indicated in ( )

II. *Those currently receiving theophylline products:*

Determine where possible, the time, amount, route of administration and form of the patient's last dose.

The loading dose for theophylline will be based on the principle that each 0.8 mg/kg of Chole-

Approximate Choledyl Pediatric Syrup Dosage (administered every 6 hours)

Body Weight lbs.	Kg.	<9 years Initial Dose 6.2 mg/kg	<9 years Max. Dose 9.4 mg/kg	9–12 years Initial Dose 6.2 mg/kg	9–12 years Max. Dose 7.8 mg/kg	12–16 years Initial Dose 6.2 mg/kg	12–16 years Max. Dose 7 mg/kg	>16 years Initial Dose 6.2 mg/kg	>16 years Max. Dose 5
18	8	1 tsp	1½ tsp	—	—	—	—	—	—
36	16	2 tsp	3 tsp	2 tsp	2½ tsp	—	—	—	—
54	24	3 tsp*	4½ tsp	3 tsp*	3½ tsp	3 tsp*	3½ tsp	—	—
72	32	3 tsp*	6 tsp	3 tsp*	5 tsp	3 tsp*	4½ tsp	—	—
90	40	3 tsp*	7 tsp**	3 tsp*	6 tsp	3 tsp*	5½ tsp	3 tsp*	3 tsp
108	48	3 tsp*	7 tsp**	3 tsp*	7 tsp**	3 tsp*	6½ tsp	3 tsp*	4 tsp
								3 tsp*	5 tsp

NOTE: The initial dosage may be increased in approximately 25 percent increments at 2 to 3 day intervals as clinically indicated and tolerated until the maximum dosage is reached.
1 mg Choledyl (oxtriphylline) = 0.64 mg anhydrous theophylline
*Initial Dosage should not exceed 625 mg/day Choledyl (400 mg/day theophylline)
**Maximum Dosage should not exceed 1400 mg/day Choledyl (900 mg/day theophylline)

dyl (oxtriphylline) (0.5 mg/kg of theophylline) administered as a loading dose will result in a 1 mcg/ml increase in serum theophylline concentration. Ideally, then, the loading dose should be deferred if a serum theophylline concentration can be rapidly obtained. If this is not possible, the clinician must exercise his judgment in selecting a dose based on the potential for benefit and risk. When there is sufficient respiratory distress to warrant a small risk, 4 mg/kg Choledyl (oxtriphylline) (2.5 mg/kg of theophylline) is likely to increase the serum concentration when administered as a loading dose in rapidly absorbed form by only about 5 mcg/ml. If the patient is not already experiencing theophylline toxicity, this is unlikely to result in dangerous adverse effects.

Following the decision regarding loading dose in this group of patients, the subsequent maintenance dosage recommendations are the same as those described above.

To achieve optimal therapeutic theophylline dosage, monitoring of serum theophylline concentrations is recommended. However, it is not always possible or practical to obtain a serum theophylline level.

Patients should be closely monitored for signs of toxicity. The present data suggest that the above dosage recommendations will achieve therapeutic serum concentrations with minimal risk of toxicity for most patients. However, some risk of toxic serum concentration is still present.

Adverse reactions to theophylline often occur when serum theophylline levels exceed 20 mcg/ml.

Chronic Asthma

Theophyllinization is a treatment of first choice for the management of chronic asthma (to prevent symptoms and maintain patent airways). Slow clinical titration is generally preferred to assure acceptance and safety of the medication.

	Choledyl (oxtriphylline)
Initial dose:	25 mg*/kg/day or 625 mg/day (whichever is lower) in 3 to 4 divided doses at 6–8 hour intervals.
Increased dose:	The above dosage may be increased in approximately 25 percent increments at 2 to 3 day intervals so long as no intolerance is observed until the maximum, indicated below, is reached.
*25 mg Choledyl	= 16 mg anhydrous theophylline

Maximum dose of Choledyl Pediatric Syrup without measurement of serum theophylline concentration:

Not to exceed the following: (WARNING: DO NOT ATTEMPT TO MAINTAIN ANY DOSE THAT IS NOT TOLERATED)

Age <9 years	—37.5 mg/kg/day **(24 mg/kg/day)
Age 9–12 years	—31 mg/kg/day **(20 mg/kg/day)
Age 12–16 years	—28 mg/kg/day **(18 mg/kg/day)
Age >16 years	—20 mg/kg/day or 1400 mg/day (WHICHEVER IS LESS) **(13 mg/kg/day or 900 mg/day) (WHICHEVER IS LESS)

NOTE: Use ideal body weight for obese patients.

**anhydrous theophylline indicated in ()

To assist in determining dosage of Choledyl Pediatric Syrup in chronic asthma the above information has been summarized in the Approximate Choledyl Pediatric Syrup Dosage table. (See table top right)

Measurement of serum theophylline concentration during chronic therapy

If the above maximum dosages are to be maintained or exceeded, serum theophylline measurement is recommended. This should be obtained at the approximate time of peak absorption (1 to 1½ hours after dosing) during chronic therapy. It is important that the patient will have missed *no* doses during the previous 48 hours and that dosing intervals will have been reasonably typical, with no added doses during that period of time.

DOSAGE ADJUSTMENT BASED ON SERUM THEOPHYLLINE MEASUREMENTS IF THE ABOVE INSTRUCTIONS HAVE NOT BEEN FOLLOWED MAY RESULT IN RISK OF TOXICITY TO THE PATIENT.

Caution should be exercised for younger children who cannot complain of minor side effects. Older adults, those with cor pulmonale, congestive heart failure, and/or liver disease, may have unusually low dosage requirements and thus may experience toxicity at the maximal dosage recommended above.

It is important that no patient be maintained on any dosage that he is not tolerating. In instructing patients to increase dosage according to the schedule above, they should be instructed to not take a subsequent dose if apparent side effects occur and to resume therapy at a lower dose once adverse effects have disappeared.

Overdosage: Serious toxic effects due to overdosage may occur suddenly and are not invariably preceded by minor adverse effects. Therefore, careful observation of the patient and prompt institution of appropriate therapeutic measures are essential in all cases of overdosage. All patients suspected of overdosage should be hospitalized.

Signs and symptoms of overdosage are related primarily to the cardiovascular, gastrointestinal, and central nervous systems.

Cardiovascular symptoms include precordial pain, tachycardia, ventricular and other arrhythmias; also varying degrees of hypotension including in extreme cases, severe shock, cardiovascular collapse and death.

Gastrointestinal symptoms include abdominal pain, nausea, persistent vomiting, and hematemesis.

Central nervous system symptoms include headache, dizziness, restlessness, irritability, tremors, hyperactivity, and agitation followed, in severe cases, by convulsions, drowsiness, coma and death.

Treatment of overdosage should be directed toward minimizing absorption and supporting vital functions.

In the alert patient emesis should be induced, followed by appropriate additional measures, as listed below. In the obtunded patient, the airway should be secured immediately by means of an endotracheal tube with cuff inflated. After the airway has been secured, lavage should be carried out, and activated charcoal slurry and a cathartic should be administered.

CNS stimulation may be controlled with diazepam, 0.1–0.3 mg/kg intravenously in children, and 10 mg intravenously in adults. Respiration should be supported by appropriate means.

Hypotension and shock should be treated with appropriate fluid replacement, avoiding the use of vasopressors, if possible. Additional supportive measures should be carried out as required.

Serial serum theophylline levels are of value in following the patient's course and in guiding further management.

Forced diuresis is of no value because of the small amount of theophylline excreted unchanged by the kidney. There has been a single report of survival with the use of an activated charcoal column (hemoperfusion) in massive theophylline overdosage.

How Supplied:

N 0071-2217-23—Choledyl Pediatric Syrup, 50 mg oxtriphylline/5 ml (equivalent to 32 mg anhydrous theophylline), is supplied as a vanilla-mint flavored syrup in bottles of 16 fl oz (474 ml).

2217G051

CHOLEDYL® SA ℞

(Oxtriphylline)

Sustained Action

Description: Choledyl (oxtriphylline) is a xanthine bronchodilator—the choline salt of theophylline.

Each film-coated Choledyl SA tablet contains 400 mg or 600 mg oxtriphylline (equivalent to 256 mg or 384 mg anhydrous theophylline, respectively).

Each tablet of Choledyl SA contains oxtriphylline in a tablet matrix specially designed for the prolonged release of the drug in the gastrointestinal tract. Following release of the drug, the expended wax tablet matrix, which is not absorbed, may be detected in the stool.

Clinical Pharmacology: Choledyl (oxtriphylline), the choline salt of theophylline, effects significant improvement in pulmonary function parameters which have been impaired by bronchospasm. It is more soluble than either aminophylline or theophylline. Film-coated Choledyl SA tablets are less irritating to the gastric mucosa than aminophylline.

Choledyl SA tablets have been formulated to provide therapeutic serum levels when administered every 12 hours and minimize the peaks and valleys of serum levels commonly found with shorter acting theophylline products.

The sustained action characteristic of Choledyl SA tablets has been demonstrated in studies in human subjects. Single and multiple dose studies have shown equivalent steady-state theophylline plasma levels of Choledyl SA tablets given every 12 hours when compared with an

Continued on next page

This product information was prepared in August, 1982. On these and other Parke-Davis Products, information may be obtained by addressing PARKE-DAVIS, Division of Warner-Lambert Company, Morris Plains, New Jersey 07950.

Parke-Davis—Cont.

equal total daily dose of (the nonsustained action) Choledyl Elixir given every six hours.
Theophylline directly relaxes the smooth muscle of the bronchial airways and pulmonary blood vessels, thus acting mainly as a bronchodilator, pulmonary vasodilator and smooth muscle relaxant. The drug also possesses other actions typical of the xanthine derivatives: coronary vasodilator, diuretic, cardiac stimulant, cerebral stimulant and skeletal muscle stimulant. The actions of theophylline may be mediated through inhibition of phosphodiesterase and a resultant increase in intracellular cyclic AMP which could mediate smooth muscle relaxation. At concentrations higher than attained *in vivo,* theophylline also inhibits the release of histamine by mast cells.
Theophylline has been shown to react synergistically with beta agonists that increase intracellular cyclic AMP through the stimulation of adenyl cyclase (isoproterenol).
Apparently, the development of tolerance does not occur with chronic use of theophylline.
The half-life is shortened with cigarette smoking. The half-life is prolonged in alcoholism, reduced hepatic or renal function, congestive heart failure, and in patients receiving antibiotics such as TAO (troleandomycin), erythromycin and clindamycin. High fever for prolonged periods may decrease theophylline elimination.

Theophylline Elimination Characteristics

	Theophylline Clearance Rates (mean ± S.D.)	Half-Life Average (mean ± S.D.)
Children (over 6 months of age)	1.45 ± .58 ml/kg/min	3.7 ± 1.1 hours
Adult non-smokers with uncomplicated asthma	.65 ± .19 ml/kg/min	8.7 ±2.2 hours

Newborn infants have extremely slow clearance and half-lives exceeding 24 hours, which approach those seen for older children after about 3–6 months.
Older adults with chronic obstructive pulmonary disease, and patients with cor pulmonale or other causes of heart failure, and patients with liver pathology may have much lower clearances with half-lives that may exceed 24 hours.
The half-life of theophylline is prolonged in patients with congestive heart failure, in those with reduced hepatic or renal function, and in alcoholism. The half-life of theophylline may also be prolonged by concurrent use of various drugs such as phenobarbital, and certain antibiotics, including troleandomycin, erythromycin, and lincomycin.
Theophylline half-life is shortened in cigarette smokers (1 to 2 packs/day) as compared to nonsmokers. The increase in theophylline clearance caused by smoking is probably the result of induction of drug metabolizing enzymes that do not readily normalize after cessation of smoking. It appears that between 3 months and 2 years may be necessary for normalization of the effect of smoking on theophylline pharmacokinetics.
Indications: Choledyl (oxtriphylline) is indicated for relief of acute and chronic bronchial asthma and for reversible bronchospasm associated with chronic bronchitis and emphysema.
Contraindications: Choledyl is contraindicated in individuals who have shown hypersensitivity to theophylline or to Choledyl (oxtriphylline) or any of its components.
Warnings: Status asthmaticus is a medical emergency. Optimal therapy frequently requires additional medication including corticosteroids when the patient is not rapidly responsive to bronchodilators.
Excessive theophylline doses may be associated with toxicity, and serum theophylline levels are recommended to assure maximal benefit without excessive risk; incidence of toxicity increases at levels greater than 20 mcg theophylline/ml. Morphine, curare, and stilbamidine should be used with caution in patients with airflow obstruction since they stimulate histamine release and can induce asthmatic attacks. These drugs may also suppress respiration leading to respiratory failure. Alternative drugs should be chosen whenever possible.
There is an excellent correlation between high blood levels of theophylline resulting from conventional doses and associated clinical manifestations of toxicity in patients with liver dysfunction or chronic obstructive lung disease.
There is excellent correlation between high serum levels of theophylline (over 20 mcg/ml) and the clinical manifestations of toxicity. Careful reduction of dosage and monitoring of serum levels are especially important in patients manifesting a decrease in total body theophylline clearance rate, including those with generalized debility, acute hypoxia, cardiac decompensation, hepatic dysfunction, or renal failure. Dosage reduction may also be necessary in patients who are older than 55 years of age, particularly males.
Serious toxic effects may occur suddenly and are not invariably preceded by minor adverse effects such as nausea, vomiting, and restlessness. Convulsions, tachycardia, or ventricular arrhythmias may be the first sign of toxicity.
Children have a marked sensitivity to the CNS stimulant action of theophylline. Serious toxic effects, including fatalities have been reported in children as well as adults.
Theophylline products may worsen pre-existing arrhythmias.
Usage in Pregnancy: Safe use of Choledyl (oxtriphylline) in pregnancy and lactation has not been established relative to possible adverse effects on fetal or neonatal development. Therefore Choledyl (oxtriphylline) should not be used in patients who are pregnant or who may become pregnant, or during lactation unless, in the judgment of the physician, the potential benefits outweigh the possible hazards.
Precautions: Mean half-life in smokers is shorter than nonsmokers, therefore, smokers may require larger doses of theophylline. Theophylline should not be administered concurrently with other xanthine medications or with xanthine-containing beverages or foods.
Use with caution in patients with severe cardiac disease, severe hypoxemia, hypertension, hyperthyroidism, acute myocardial injury, cor pulmonale, congestive heart failure, or liver disease, and in the elderly (especially males) and in neonates. Great caution should especially be used in giving theophylline to patients in congestive heart failure. Such patients have shown markedly prolonged theophylline blood level curves with theophylline persisting in serum for long periods following discontinuation of the drug.
Use theophylline cautiously in patients with a history of peptic ulcer. Theophylline may occasionally act as a local irritant to the GI tract although gastrointestinal symptoms are more commonly central and associated with serum theophylline concentrations over 20 mcg/ml.
Adverse Reactions: The most consistent adverse reactions are usually due to overdose and are:
1. Gastrointestinal: nausea, vomiting, epigastric pain, hematemesis, diarrhea.
2. Central nervous system: headaches, irritability, restlessness, insomnia, reflex hyperexcitability, muscle twitching, clonic and tonic generalized convulsions.
3. Cardiovascular: palpitation, tachycardia, extrasystoles, flushing, hypotension, circulatory failure, life-threatening ventricular arrhythmias.
4. Respiratory: tachypnea.
5. Renal: albuminuria, increased excretion of renal tubular cells and red blood cells, diuresis.
6. Others: hyperglycemia and inappropriate antidiuretic hormone (ADH) syndrome.

Drug Interactions: Theophylline-containing preparations have exhibited interaction with the following drugs:

Drug	Effect
Lithium carbonate	Increased excretion of lithium carbonate.
Propranolol	Antagonism of propranolol effect.
Furosemide	Increased furosemide diuresis.
Hexamethonium	Decreased hexamethonium-induced chronotropic effect
Reserpine	Reserpine-induced tachycardia.
Chlordiazepoxide	Chlordiazepoxide-induced fatty acid mobilization.
Troleandomycin, erythromycin or lincomycin	Increased theophyline plasma levels.

Dosage and Administration: Therapy should be initiated and daily dosage requirements established utilizing a nonsustained-action form of Choledyl (oxtriphylline) (eg, Choledyl Tablets, Elixir).
If the total daily maintenance dosage requirement of the Choledyl (oxtriphylline) nonsustained preparation is established at approximately 1200 mg, Choledyl SA 600 mg Sustained Action Tablets, one every 12 hours, may be substituted to provide smoother steady-state theophylline levels and the convenience of bid dosage. Similarly, if the total daily maintenance dosage is established at approximately 800 mg, Choledyl SA 400 mg Sustained Action Tablets, one every 12 hours, may be substituted.
Therapeutic serum levels associated with optimal likelihood of benefit and minimal risk of toxicity are considered to be between 10 mcg/ml and 20 mcg/ml. Levels above 20 mcg/ml may produce toxic effects.
There is great variation from patient to patient in dosage needed in order to achieve a therapeutic blood level because of variable rates of elimination. Because of this wide variation from patient to patient and the relatively narrow therapeutic blood level range, dosage must be individualized; monitoring of theophylline serum levels is highly recommended.
Dosage should be calculated on the basis of lean (ideal) body weight—mg/kg. Theophylline does not distribute into fatty tissue.
Giving Choledyl (oxtriphylline) with food may prevent the rare case of stomach irritation, and although absorption may be slower, it is still complete.
When rapidly absorbed products such as solutions are used, dosing to maintain "around the clock" blood levels generally requires administration every 6 hours to obtain the greatest efficacy for use in children, dosing intervals up to 8 hours may be satisfactory for adults because of their slower elimination. Children and adults requiring higher than average doses may benefit from products with slower absorption. This may allow longer dosing intervals and/or less fluctuation in serum concentration over a dosing interval during chronic therapy.
In patients receiving concurrent bronchodilator therapy, eg, beta agonists, downward adjustment of Choledyl (oxtriphylline) dosage is necessary.

The following dosage information relates to initiation and titration of daily dosage requirements utilizing a nonsustained action form of Choledyl (eg Choledyl Tabs, Elixir).
[See table right].

II. *Those currently receiving theophylline products:*
Determine where possible, the time, amount, route of administration and form of the patient's last dose.
The loading dose for theophylline will be based on the principle that each 0.8 mg/kg of Choledyl (oxtriphylline) (0.5 mg/kg of theophylline) administered as a loading dose will result in a 1 mcg/ml increase in serum theophylline concentration. Ideally, then, the loading dose should be deferred if a serum theophylline concentration can be rapidly obtained. If this is not possible, the clinician must exercise his judgment in selecting a dose based on the potential for benefit and risk. When there is sufficient respiratory distress to warrant a small risk, 4 mg/kg Choledyl (oxtriphylline) (2.5 mg/kg of theophylline) is likely to increase the serum concentration when administered as a loading dose in rapidly absorbed form by only about 5 mcg/ml. If the patient is not already experiencing theophylline toxicity, this is unlikely to result in dangerous adverse effect.
Following the decision regarding loading dose in this group of patients, the subsequent maintenance dosage recommendations are the same as those described above.
To achieve optimal therapeutic theophylline dosage, monitoring of serum theophylline concentrations is recommended. However, it is not always possible or practical to obtain a serum theophylline level.
Patients should be closely monitored for signs of toxicity. The present data suggests that the above dosage recommendations will achieve therapeutic serum concentrations with minimal risk of toxicity for most patients. However, some risk of toxic serum concentrations is still present.
Adverse reactions to theophylline often occur when serum theophylline levels exceed 20 mcg/ml.

Chronic Asthma
Theophyllinization is a treatment of first choice for the management of chronic asthma (to prevent symptoms and maintain patent airways). Slow clinical titration is generally preferred to assure acceptance and safety of the medication.
[See table below].

Maximum dose of Choledyl (oxtriphylline) without measurement of serum theophylline concentration:
Not to exceed the following: (WARNING: DO NOT ATTEMPT TO MAINTAIN ANY DOSE THAT IS NOT TOLERATED)

Age <9 years	—37.5 mg/kg/day **(24 mg/kg/day)
Age 9–12 years	—31 mg/kg/day **(20 mg/kg/day)
Age 12–16 years	—28 mg/kg/day **(18 mg/kg/day)
Age >16 years	—20 mg/kg/day or 1400 mg/day (WHICHEVER IS LESS) **(13 mg/kg/day or 900 mg/day) (WHICHEVER IS LESS)

Note: Use ideal body weight for obese patients.
**anhydrous theophylline indicated in ( )

CHOLEDYL (OXTRIPHYLLINE) DOSAGE FOR PATIENT POPULATION

Acute Symptoms of Asthma Requiring Rapid Theophyllinization:
1. *Not currently receiving theophylline products:*

GROUP	ORAL LOADING DOSE CHOLEDYL	MAINTENANCE DOSE FOR NEXT 12 HOURS CHOLEDYL	MAINTENANCE DOSE BEYOND 12 HOURS CHOLEDYL
1. Children 6 months to 9 years	9.4 mg/kg *(6 mg/kg)	6.2 mg/kg q4 hrs *(4 mg/kg q4 hrs)	6.2 mg/kg q6 hrs *(4 mg/kg q6 hrs)
2. Children age 9–16 and young adult smokers	9.4 mg/kg *(6 mg/kg)	4.7 mg/kg q4 hrs *(3 mg/kg q4 hrs)	4.7 mg/kg q6 hrs *(3 mg/kg q6 hrs)
3. Otherwise healthy nonsmoking adults	9.4 mg/kg *(6 mg/kg)	4.7 mg/kg q6 hrs *(3 mg/kg q6 hrs)	4.7 mg/kg q8 hrs *3 mg/kg q8 hrs)
4. Older patients and patients with cor pulmonale	9.4 mg/kg *(6 mg/kg)	3.1 mg/kg q6 hrs *(2 mg/kg q6 hrs)	3.1 mg/kg q8 hrs *(2 mg/kg q8 hrs)
5. Patients with congestive heart failure, liver failure	9.4 mg/kg *(6 mg/kg)	3.1 mg/kg q8 hrs *(2 mg/kg q8 hrs)	1.6–3.1 mg/kg q12 hrs *(1–2 mg/kg q12 hrs)

*Anhydrous theophylline indicated in ( )

If the total daily maintenance dosage requirement of the Choledyl (oxtriphylline) nonsustained preparation is established at approximately 1200 mg, Choledyl SA 600 mg Sustained Action Tablets, one every 12 hours, may be substituted to provide smoother steady-state theophylline levels and the convenience of bid dosage. Similarly, if the total daily maintenance dosage is established at approximately 800 mg, Choledyl SA 400 mg Sustained Action Tablets, one every 12 hours, may be substituted.

Measurement of serum theophylline concentration during chronic therapy
If the above maximum dosages are to be maintained or exceeded, serum theophylline measurement is recommended. This should be obtained at the approximate time of peak absorption (1 to 2 hours after dosing) during chronic therapy. It is important that the patient will have missed *no* doses during the previous 48 hours and that dosing intervals will have been reasonably typical, with no added doses during that period of time.

DOSAGE ADJUSTMENT BASED ON SERUM THEOPHYLLINE MEASUREMENTS IF THE ABOVE INSTRUCTIONS HAVE NOT BEEN FOLLOWED MAY RESULT IN RISK OF TOXICITY TO THE PATIENT.

Caution should be exercised for younger children who cannot complain of minor side effects. Older adults, those with cor pulmonale, congestive heart failure, and/or liver disease, may have unusually low dosage requirements and thus may experience toxicity at the maximal dosage recommended above.
It is important that no patient be maintained on any dosage that he is not tolerating. In instructing patients to increase dosage according to the schedule above, they should be instructed to not take a subsequent dose if apparent side effects occur and to resume therapy at a lower dose once adverse effects have disappeared.

Overdosage: Serious toxic effects due to overdosage may occur suddenly and are not invariably preceded by minor adverse effects. Therefore, careful observation of the patient and prompt institution of appropriate therapeutic measures are essential in all cases of overdosage. All patients suspected of overdosage should be hospitalized.

Signs and symptoms of overdosage are related primarily to the cardiovascular, gastrointestinal, and central nervous systems.
Cardiovascular symptoms include precordial pain, tachycardia, ventricular and other arrhythmias; also varying degrees of hypotension including, in extreme cases, severe shock, cardiovascular collapse and death.
Gastrointestinal symptoms include abdominal pain, nausea, persistent vomiting, and hematemesis.
Central nervous system symptoms include headache, dizziness, restlessness, irritability, tremors, hyperactivity, and agitation followed, in severe cases, by convulsions, drowsiness, coma and death.

Treatment of overdosage should be directed toward minimizing absorption and supporting vital functions.
In the alert patient emesis should be induced, followed by appropriate additional measures, as listed below.
In the obtunded patient, the airway should be secured immediately by means of an endotracheal tube with cuff inflated. After the airway has been secured, lavage should be carried out, and activated charcoal slurry and a cathartic should be administered.
CNS stimulation may be controlled with diazepam, 0.1–0.3 mg/kg intravenously in children, and 10 mg intravenously in adults. Respiration should be supported by appropriate means. Hypotension and shock should be treated with appropriate fluid replacement, avoiding the use of vasopressors, if possible. Additional supportive measures should be carried out as required.
Serial serum theophylline levels are of value in following the patient's course and in guiding further management.
Forced diuresis is of no value because of the small amount of theophylline excreted unchanged by the kidney. There has been a single report of survival with the use of an activated charcoal column (hemoperfusion) in massive theophylline overdosage.

Continued on next page

	Choledyl (oxtriphylline)
Initial dose:	25 mg*/kg/day or 625 mg/day (whichever is lower) in 3 to 4 divided doses at 6–8 hour intervals.
Increased dose:	The above dosage may be increased in approximately 25 percent increments at 2 to 3 day intervals so long as no intolerance is observed until the maximum indicated below is reached.

*25 mg Choledyl = 16 mg anhydrous theophylline

This product information was prepared in August, 1982. On these and other Parke-Davis Products, information may be obtained by addressing PARKE-DAVIS, Division of Warner-Lambert Company, Morris Plains, New Jersey 07950.

Parke-Davis—Cont.

How Supplied:
Choledyl SA 400 mg—each sustained action tablet contains 400 mg oxtriphylline. Available as pink film-coated tablets in bottles of 100 (N 0071-0214-24), and unit-dose 100's (N 0071-0214-40).
Choledyl SA 600 mg—each sustained action tablet contains 600 mg oxtriphylline. Available as tan film-coated tablets in bottles of 100 (N 0071-0221-24), and unit-dose 100's (N 0071-0221-40).
[*Shown in Product Identification Section*]

COLY-MYCIN® M PARENTERAL ℞
(sterile colistimethate sodium, USP)
for intramuscular and intravenous use

Description: Coly-Mycin M Parenteral (sterile colistimethate sodium) contains the sodium salt of colistimethate. Colistimethate sodium is a polypeptide antibiotic with an approximate molecular weight of 1750; the empirical formula is $C_{58}H_{105}N_{16}Na_5O_{28}S_5$.

Clinical Pharmacology:

Microbiology
Coly-Mycin M Parenteral has bactericidal activity against the following gram-negative bacilli: *Enterobacter aerogenes, Escherichia coli, Klebsiella pneumoniae*, and *Pseudomonas aeruginosa*.

Human Pharmacology
Typical serum and urine levels following a single 150 mg dose of Coly-Mycin M Parenteral IM or IV in normal adult subjects are shown in Figure 1.

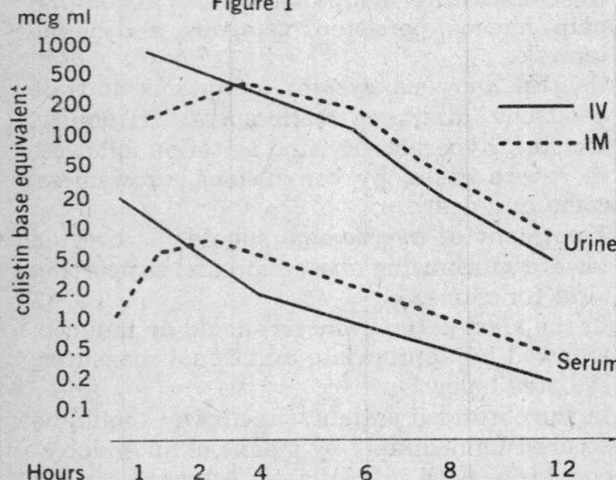

Figure 1. Urine and serum values in adults following parenteral (IM or IV) administration of Coly-Mycin M Parenteral

Higher serum levels were obtained at 10 minutes following IV administration. Serum concentration declined with a half-life of 2-3 hours following either intravenous or intramuscular administration in adults and children, including premature infants.
Colistimethate sodium is transferred across the placental barrier, and blood levels of about 1 mcg/ml are obtained in the fetus following intravenous administration to the mother.
Average urine levels ranged from about 270 mcg/ml at 2 hours to about 15 mcg/ml at 8 hours after intravenous administration and from about 200 to about 25 mcg/ml during a similar period following intramuscular administration.

Indications and Usage: Coly-Mycin M Parenteral (sterile colistimethate sodium) is indicated for the treatment of acute or chronic infections due to sensitive strains of certain gram-negative bacilli. It is particularly indicated when the infection is caused by sensitive strains of ***Pseudomonas aeruginosa.*** This antibiotic is not indicated for infections due to *Proteus* or *Neisseria*. Coly-Mycin M Parenteral has proven clinically effective in treatment of infections due to the following gram-negative organisms: ***Enterobacter aerogenes, Escherichia coli, Klebsiella pneumoniae,*** and ***Pseudomonas aeruginosa.***
Pending results of appropriate bacteriologic cultures and sensitivity tests, Coly-Mycin M Parenteral may be used to initiate therapy in serious infections that are suspected to be due to gram-negative organisms.

Contraindications: The use of Coly-Mycin M Parenteral is contraindicated for patients with a history of sensitivity to the drug.

Warning: Maximum daily dose should not exceed 5 mg/kg/day (2.3 mg/lb) with normal renal function.
Transient neurological disturbances may occur. These include circumoral paresthesias or numbness, tingling or formication of the extremities, generalized pruritus, vertigo, dizziness, and slurring of speech. For these reasons, patients should be warned not to drive vehicles or use hazardous machinery while on therapy. Reduction of dosage may alleviate symptoms. Therapy need not be discontinued, but such patients should be observed with particular care. Overdosage can result in renal insufficiency, muscle weakness and apnea. See PRECAUTIONS for use concomitantly with curariform drugs, and DOSAGE and ADMINISTRATION Section for use in renal impairment.

Precautions: Since Coly-Mycin M Parenteral (sterile colistimethate sodium) is eliminated mainly by renal excretion, it should be used with caution when the possibility of impaired renal function exists. The decline in renal function with advanced age should be considered.
When actual renal impairment is present, Coly-Mycin M Parenteral may be used, but the greatest caution should be exercised and the dosage should be reduced in proportion to the extent of the impairment. Administration of amounts of Coly-Mycin M Parenteral in excess of renal excretory capacity will lead to high serum levels and can result in further impairment of renal function, initiating a cycle which, if not recognized, can lead to acute renal insufficiency, renal shutdown and further concentration of the antibiotic to toxic levels in the body. At this point, interference of nerve transmission at neuromuscular junctions may occur and result in muscle weakness and apnea.
Easily recognized signs indicating the development of impaired renal function are diminishing urine output, rising BUN and serum creatinine. If present, therapy with Coly-Mycin M Parenteral (sterile colistimethate sodium) should be discontinued immediately.
If a life-threatening situation exists, therapy may be reinstated at a lower dosage after blood levels have fallen.
Certain other antibiotics (kanamycin, streptomycin, dihydrostreptomycin, polymyxin, neomycin) have also been reported to interfere with the nerve transmission at the neuromuscular junction. Based on this reported activity, they should not be given concomitantly with Coly-Mycin M Parenteral except with the greatest caution. The antibiotics with a gram-positive antimicrobial spectrum, e.g., penicillin, tetracycline, sodium cephalothin, have not been reported to interfere with nerve transmission and, accordingly, would not be expected to potentiate this activity of Coly-Mycin M Parenteral.
Other drugs, including curariform muscle relaxants (ether, tubocurarine, succinylcholine, gallamine, decamethonium and sodium citrate), potentiate the neuromuscular blocking effect and should be used with extreme caution in patients being treated with Coly-Mycin M Parenteral.
If apnea occurs, it may be treated with assisted respiration, oxygen, and calcium chloride injections.

Use in Pregnancy: The safety of colistimethate sodium during human pregnancy has not been established.

Adverse Reactions: Respiratory arrest has been reported following intramuscular administration of colistimethate sodium. Impaired renal function increases the possibility of apnea and neuromuscular blockade following administration of colistimethate sodium. This has been generally due to failure to follow recommended guidelines, usually overdosage, failure to reduce dose commensurate with degree of renal impairment, and/or concomitant use of other antibiotics or drugs with neuromuscular blocking potential.
A decrease in urine output or increase in blood urea nitrogen or serum creatinine can be interpreted as signs of nephrotoxicity, which is probably a dose-dependent effect of colistimethate sodium. These manifestations of nephrotoxicity are reversible following discontinuation of the antibiotic.
Increases of blood urea nitrogen have been reported for patients receiving Coly-Mycin M Parenteral (sterile colistimethate sodium) at dose levels of 1.6-5 mg/kg per day. The BUN values returned to normal following cessation of Coly-Mycin M Parenteral administration.
Paresthesia, tingling of the extremities or tingling of the tongue and generalized itching or urticaria have been reported by patients who received Coly-Mycin M Parenteral by intravenous or intramuscular injection. In addition, the following adverse reactions have been reported for colistimethate sodium: drug fever and gastrointestinal upset, vertigo, and slurring of speech. The subjective symptoms reported by the adult may not be manifest in infants or young children, thus requiring close attention to renal function.

Dosage and Administration:
Important: Coly-Mycin M Parenteral (sterile colistimethate sodium) is supplied in vials containing colistimethate sodium equivalent to 150 mg colistin base activity per vial.
Reconstitution: The *150-mg* vial should be reconstituted with *2.0 ml* Sterile Water for Injection USP. The reconstituted solution provides colistimethate sodium at a concentration of 75 mg/ml.
During reconstitution swirl *gently* to avoid frothing.
Dosage: *Adults and children—intravenous or intramuscular administration*—Coly-Mycin M Parenteral should be given in 2 to 4 divided doses at dose levels of 2.5 to 5 mg/kg per day for patients with normal renal function, depending on the severity of the infection.
The daily dose should be reduced in the presence of any renal impairment, which can often be anticipated from the history.
Modifications of dosage in the presence of renal impairment are presented in Table 1.
[See table on next page].

INTRAVENOUS ADMINISTRATION

1. Direct Intermittent Administration — slowly inject one-half of the total daily dose over a period of 3 to 5 minutes every 12 hours.
2. Continuous Infusion — slowly inject one-half the total daily dose over 3 to 5 minutes. Add the remaining half of the total daily dose of Coly-Mycin M Parenteral to one of the following: 0.9% NaCl; 5% dextrose in 0.9% NaCl; 5% dextrose in water; 5% dextrose in 0.45% NaCl; 5% dextrose in 0.225% NaCl; lactated Ringer's solution, or 10% invert sugar solution. There are not sufficient data to recommend usage of Coly-Mycin M Parenteral with other drugs or with other than the above listed infusion solutions.

Administer by slow intravenous infusion starting 1 to 2 hours after the initial dose at a rate of 5-6 mg/hr in the presence of normal renal function. In the presence of impaired renal function, reduce the infusion rate depending on the degree of renal impairment.

The choice of intravenous solution and the volume to be employed are dictated by the requirements of fluid and electrolyte management.

Any infusion solution containing colistimethate sodium should be freshly prepared and used for no longer than 24 hours.

How Supplied: Coly-Mycin M Parenteral (sterile colistimethate sodium) is supplied in vials containing colistimethate sodium (150 mg colistin base equivalent per vial) as a white to slightly yellow lyophilized cake and is available as one vial per carton (N 0071-4145-01) or as 50 vials per carton (N 0071-4145-01[19]).

STORE AT CONTROLLED ROOM TEMPERATURE (15° to 30°C) (59° to 86°F).

STORE RECONSTITUTED SOLUTION IN REFRIGERATOR (2° to 8°C) (36° to 46°F) OR AT CONTROLLED ROOM TEMPERATURE (15° to 30°C) (59° to 86°F), and use within 7 days.

Toxicology and Animal Pharmacology:

Acute Toxicity: The intravenous LD_{50} was 41.5 mg/kg in the dog and 739 mg/kg in the mouse; intramuscular toxicity was 42 mg/kg in the dog and 267 mg/kg in the mouse.

Subacute Toxicity: In albino rabbits and beagle dogs, IV doses of 5, 10 and 20 mg/kg/day for 28 days resulted in elevated blood urea nitrogen in the dog (10 mg/kg/day dose group) and in both 20 mg/kg dose groups.

Clinical Studies: Clinically, Coly-Mycin M Parenteral (sterile colistimethate sodium) has been of particular therapeutic value in acute and chronic urinary tract infections caused by sensitive strains of *Pseudomonas aeruginosa*. Colistimethate sodium is clinically effective in the treatment of infections due to other sensitive gram-negative pathogenic bacilli that have become resistant to broad-spectrum antibiotics.

Colistimethate sodium has been used to treat bacteriuria and overt urinary infections in pregnant women during the third trimester. However, in view of the evidence of possible embryotoxic and teratogenic effects of colistimethate sodium in pregnant rabbits, caution should be exercised in use of this drug in women of childbearing potential.

4145G011

Table 1

SUGGESTED MODIFICATION OF DOSAGE SCHEDULES OF COLY-MYCIN M PARENTERAL (STERILE COLISTIMETHATE SODIUM) FOR ADULTS WITH IMPAIRED RENAL FUNCTION

RENAL FUNCTION	Normal	DEGREE OF IMPAIRMENT Mild	Moderate	Considerable
Plasma creatinine, (mg/100 ml)	0.7–1.2	1.3–1.5	1.6–2.5	2.6–4.0
Urea clearance, % of normal	80–100	40–70	25–40	10–25
DOSAGE				
Unit dose of Coly-Mycin M, mg	100–150	75–115	66–150	100–150
Frequency, times/day	4 to 2	2	2 or 1	every 36 hr
Total daily dose, mg	300	150–230	133–150	100
Approximate daily dose, mg/kg/day	5.0	2.5–3.8	2.5	1.5

Note: The suggested unit dose is 2.5–5 mg/kg; however, the time INTERVAL between injections should be increased in the presence of impaired renal function.

COLY-MYCIN® S FOR ORAL SUSPENSION ℞

(colistin sulfate for oral suspension, USP)
FOR ORAL USE ONLY

Description: Coly-Mycin S For Oral Suspension (colistin sulfate for oral suspension) contains the sulfate salt of colistin, a polypeptide antibiotic with a molecular weight of approximately 1170. The empirical formula of colistin is $C_{53}H_{100}N_{16}O_{13}$.

Clinical Pharmacology: Colistin sulfate has *in vitro* bactericidal activity against most gram-negative enteric pathogens, especially enteropathogenic *E. coli* and *Shigella* (but not *Proteus*). In infants and children, it has effectively controlled acute infections of the intestinal tract due to these pathogens. Susceptible strains of *E. coli* and *Shigella in vitro* or *in vivo* rarely develop resistance to colistin sulfate. Cross resistance to polymyxin B sulfate does exist, but cross resistance to broad spectrum antibiotics has not been encountered.

Indications and Usage: Diarrhea in infants and children, caused by susceptible strains of enteropathogenic *E. coli*.

Gastroenteritis due to *Shigella* organisms. Clinical response may vary due to the absence of tissue levels in the bowel wall.

Contraindications: Known hypersensitivity to the drug.

Warnings: Although colistin sulfate is not absorbed systemically in measurable amounts, it is assumed that slight absorption may occur. Therefore, in the presence of azotemia or, if dosages above the recommended range are used, a potential for possible renal toxicity exists.

With prolonged usage, suppression of intestinal bacterial flora may occur. There may be a resultant overgrowth of organisms (such as *Proteus*); appropriate therapy should be initiated immediately.

Precautions: Renal function should be assessed prior to initiation of therapy.

Adverse Reactions: Within the recommended dosage range, none reported.

Dosage and Administration: The usual dosage of colistin sulfate is 5–15 mg/kg/day (2.3–6.9 mg/pound/day) given in three divided doses. Higher doses may be necessary. Each 5 ml of suspension contains the equivalent of 25 mg colistin sulfate. A 10-pound infant would require 23–69 mg of colistin sulfate or approximately ⅓ to 1 teaspoon three times a day. A 50-pound patient would require 115–340 mg colistin sulfate or approximately 1½ to 4½ teaspoons three times a day.

Preparation: Coly-Mycin S For Oral Suspension (colistin sulfate for oral suspension) is a dry powder which is reconstituted with 37 ml of distilled water. To reconstitute, slowly add one half of the diluent, replace the cap and shake well. Add the remaining diluent and repeat shaking. Volume after reconstitution is 60 ml. When reconstituted, Coly-Mycin S Oral Suspension is a chocolate-flavored mixture, each 5 ml teaspoonful containing the equivalent of 25 mg of colistin base. Reconstituted Coly-Mycin S Oral Suspension is stable for two weeks when kept below 15°C (59°F).

Supplied: Bottles containing colistin sulfate equivalent to 300 mg colistin base (N 0071-2142-15).

Before reconstitution store between 15° and 30°C (59° and 86°F).

2142 G 010

COLY-MYCIN® S OTIC ℞

with Neomycin and Hydrocortisone
(colistin sulfate—neomycin sulfate—thonzonium bromide—hydrocortisone acetate otic suspension)

Description: Coly-Mycin S Otic with Neomycin and Hydrocortisone (colistin sulfate-neomycin sulfate-thonzonium bromide-hydrocortisone acetate otic suspension) is a sterile aqueous suspension containing in each ml: Colistin base activity, 3 mg (as the sulfate); Neomycin base activity, 3.3 mg (as the sulfate); Hydrocortisone acetate, 10 mg (1%); Thonzonium bromide, 0.5 mg (0.05%); Polysorbate 80, acetic acid, and sodium acetate in a buffered aqueous vehicle. Thimerosal (mercury derivative), 0.002%, added as a preservative. It is a non-viscous liquid, buffered at pH 5, for instillation into the canal of the external ear or direct application to the affected aural skin.

Clinical Pharmacology:

1. Colistin sulfate—an antibiotic with bactericidal action against most gram-negative organisms, notably *Pseudomonas aeruginosa, E. coli.*, and *Klebsiella-Aerobacter.*
2. Neomycin sulfate—a broad-spectrum antibiotic, bactericidal to many pathogens, notably *Staph aureus* and *Proteus* sp.
3. Hydrocortisone acetate—a corticosteroid that controls inflammation, edema, pruritus and other dermal reactions.
4. Thonzonium bromide—a surface-active agent that promotes tissue contact by dispersion and penetration of the cellular debris and exudate.

Indications and Usage: For the treatment of superficial bacterial infections of the external auditory canal, caused by organisms susceptible to the action of the antibiotics; and for the treatment of infections of mastoidectomy and fenestration cavities, caused by organisms susceptible to the antibiotics.

Contraindications: This product is contraindicated in those individuals who have shown hypersensitivity to any of its components, and in herpes simplex, vaccinia and varicella.

Warnings: As with other antibiotic preparations, prolonged treatment may result in overgrowth of nonsusceptible organisms and fungi. If the infection is not improved after one week, cultures and susceptibility tests should be repeated to verify the identity of the organism and to determine whether therapy should be changed.

Patients who prefer to warm the medication before using should be cautioned against heat-

Continued on next page

This product information was prepared in August, 1982. On these and other Parke-Davis Products, information may be obtained by addressing PARKE-DAVIS, Division of Warner-Lambert Company, Morris Plains, New Jersey 07950.

Parke-Davis—Cont.

ing the solution above body temperature, in order to avoid loss of potency.

Precautions: General: If sensitization or irritation occurs, medication should be discontinued promptly.

This drug should be used with care in cases of perforated eardrum and in longstanding cases of chronic otitis media because of the possibility of ototoxicity caused by neomycin.

Treatment should not be continued for longer than ten days.

Allergic cross-reactions may occur which could prevent the use of any or all of the following antibiotics for the treatment of future infections: kanamycin, paromomycin, streptomycin, and possibly gentamicin.

Adverse Reactions: Neomycin is a not uncommon cutaneous sensitizer. There are articles in the current literature that indicate an increase in the prevalence of persons sensitive to neomycin.

Dosage and Administration: The external auditory canal should be thoroughly cleansed and dried with a sterile cotton applicator.

For adults, 4 drops of the suspension should be instilled into the affected ear 3 or 4 times daily. For infants and children, 3 drops are suggested because of the smaller capacity of the ear canal.

The patient should lie with the affected ear upward and then the drops should be instilled. This position should be maintained for 5 minutes to facilitate penetration of the drops into the ear canal. Repeat, if necessary, for the opposite ear.

If preferred, a cotton wick may be inserted into the canal and then the cotton may be saturated with the solution. This wick should be kept moist by adding further solution every 4 hours. The wick should be replaced at least once every 24 hours.

How Supplied:

Coly-Mycin S Otic is supplied as:

N 0071-3141-08—5 ml bottle

N 0071-3141-10—10 ml bottle

Each ml contains: Colistin sulfate equivalent to 3 mg of colistin base, Neomycin sulfate equivalent to 3.3 mg neomycin base, Hydrocortisone acetate 10 mg (1%), Thonzonium bromide 0.5 mg (0.05%), and Polysorbate 80 in an aqueous vehicle buffered with acetic acid and sodium acetate. Thimerosal (mercury derivative) 0.002% added as a preservative.

Shake well before using.

Store at controlled room temperature 15°–30°C (59°–86°F). Stable for 18 months at room temperature; prolonged exposure to higher temperatures should be avoided.

3141G032
121 888150/32

KAPSEALS®
DILANTIN® ℞
(Extended Phenytoin Sodium Capsules, USP)

Description: Phenytoin Sodium is an antiepileptic drug. Phenytoin sodium is related to the barbiturates in chemical structure, but has a five-membered ring. The chemical name is sodium 5,5-diphenyl-2,4-imidazolidinedione.

Each Dilantin—*Extended Phenytoin Sodium Capsule* USP contains 30 mg or 100 mg phenytoin sodium. Product *in vivo* performance is characterized by a slow and extended rate of absorption with peak blood concentrations expected in 4 to 12 hours as contrasted to *Prompt Phenytoin Sodium Capsules* USP with a rapid rate of absorption with peak blood concentration expected in 1 ½ to 3 hours.

Clinical Pharmacology: Phenytoin is an antiepileptic drug which can be useful in the treatment of epilepsy. The primary site of action appears to be *the motor cortex* where spread of seizure activity is inhibited. Possibly by promoting sodium efflux from neurons, phenytoin tends to *stabilize* the threshold against hyperexcitability caused by excessive stimulation or environmental changes capable of reducing membrane sodium gradient. This includes the reduction of posttetanic potentiation at synapses. Loss of posttetanic potentiation prevents cortical seizure foci from detonating adjacent cortical areas. Phenytoin reduces the maximal activity of brain stem centers responsible for the tonic phase of tonic-clonic (grand mal) seizures.

The plasma half-life in man after oral administration of phenytoin averages 22 hours, with a range of 7 to 42 hours. Steady-state therapeutic levels are achieved 7 to 10 days after initiation of therapy with recommended doses of 300 mg/day.

Optimum control without clinical signs of toxicity occurs more often with serum levels between 10 and 20 mcg/ml, although some mild cases of tonic-clonic (grand mal) epilepsy may be controlled with lower serum levels of phenytoin.

In most patients maintained at a steady dosage, stable phenytoin serum levels are achieved. There may be wide interpatient variability in phenytoin serum levels with equivalent dosages. Patients with unusually low levels may be noncompliant or hypermetabolizers of phenytoin. Unusually high levels result from liver disease, congenital enzyme deficiency or drug interactions which result in metabolic interference. The patient with large variations in phenytoin plasma levels, despite standard doses, presents a difficult clinical problem. Serum level determinations in such patients may be particularly helpful.

Most of the drug is excreted in the bile as inactive metabolites which are then reabsorbed from the intestinal tract and excreted in the urine. Urinary excretion of phenytoin and its metabolites occurs partly with glomerular filtration but more importantly, by tubular secretion. Because phenytoin is hydroxylated in the liver by an enzyme system which is saturable, small incremental doses may produce very substantial increases in serum levels, when these are in the upper range. The steady-state level may be double or triple from an increase in dosage of 10% or more, resulting in toxicity.

Indications and Usage: Dilantin is indicated for the control of tonic-clonic and psychomotor (grand mal and temporal lobe) seizures and prevention and treatment of seizures occurring during or following neurosurgery.

Phenytoin serum level determinations may be necessary for optimal dosage adjustments (see Dosage and Administration).

Contraindications: Phenytoin is contraindicated in those patients who are hypersensitive to phenytoin or other hydantoins.

Warnings: Abrupt withdrawal of phenytoin in epileptic patients may precipitate status epilepticus. When, in the judgment of the clinician, the need for dosage reduction, discontinuation, or substitution of alternative antiepileptic medication arises, this should be done gradually. However, in the event of an allergic or hypersensitivity reaction, rapid substitution of alternative therapy may be necessary. In this case, alternative therapy should be an antiepileptic drug not belonging to the hydantoin chemical class.

There have been a number of reports suggesting a relationship between phenytoin and the development of lymphadenopathy (local or generalized) including benign lymph node hyperplasia, pseudolymphoma, lymphoma, and Hodgkin's Disease.

Although a cause and effect relationship has not been established, the occurrence of lymphadenopathy indicates the need to differentiate such a condition from other types of lymph node pathology. Lymph node involvement may occur with or without symptoms and signs resembling serum sickness eg, fever, rash and liver involvement.

In all cases of lymphadenopathy, follow-up observation for an extended period is indicated and every effort should be made to achieve seizure control using alternative antiepileptic drugs.

Acute alcoholic intake may increase phenytoin serum levels while chronic alcoholic use may decrease serum levels.

Usage in Pregnancy:

A number of reports suggests an association between the use of antiepileptic drugs by women with epilepsy and a higher incidence of birth defects in children born to these women. Data are more extensive with respect to phenytoin and phenobarbital, but these are also the most commonly prescribed antiepileptic drugs; less systematic or anecdotal reports suggest a possible similar association with the use of all known antiepileptic drugs.

The reports suggesting a higher incidence of birth defects in children of drug-treated epileptic women cannot be regarded as adequate to prove a definite cause and effect relationship. There are intrinsic methodologic problems in obtaining adequate data on drug teratogenicity in humans; genetic factors or the epileptic condition itself may be more important than drug therapy in leading to birth defects. The great majority of the mothers on antiepileptic medication deliver normal infants. It is important to note that antiepileptic drugs should not be discontinued in patients in whom the drug is administered to prevent major seizures, because of the strong possibility of precipitating status epilepticus with attendant hypoxia and threat to life. In individual cases where the severity and frequency of the seizure disorder are such that the removal of medication does not pose a serious threat to the patient, discontinuation of the drug may be considered prior to and during pregnancy, although it cannot be said with any confidence that even minor seizures do not pose some hazards to the developing embryo or fetus. The prescribing physician will wish to weigh these considerations in treating and counseling epileptic women of childbearing potential.

In addition to the reports of increased incidence of congenital malformation, such as cleft lip/palate and heart malformations in children of women receiving phenytoin and other antiepileptic drugs, there have more recently been reports of a fetal hydantoin syndrome. This consists of prenatal growth deficiency, microcephaly and mental deficiency in children born to mothers who have received phenytoin, barbiturates, alcohol, or trimethadione. However, these features are all interrelated and are frequently associated with intrauterine growth retardation from other causes.

There have been isolated reports of malignancies, including neuroblastoma, in children whose mothers received phenytoin during pregnancy.

An increase in seizure frequency during pregnancy occurs in a high proportion of patients, because of altered phenytoin absorption or metabolism. Periodic measurement of serum phenytoin levels is particularly valuable in the management of a pregnant epileptic patient as a guide to an appropriate adjustment of dosage. However, postpartum restoration of the original dosage will probably be indicated.

Neonatal coagulation defects have been reported within the first 24 hours in babies born to epileptic mothers receiving phenobarbital and/or phenytoin. Vitamin K_1 has been shown to prevent or correct this defect and has been recommended to be given to the mother before delivery and the neonate after birth.

Precautions:

General:

The liver is the chief site of biotransformation of phenytoin; patients with impaired liver function, elderly patients, or those who are gravely ill may show early signs of toxicity.

A small percentage of individuals who have been treated with phenytoin have been shown to metabolize the drug slowly. Slow metabolism may be due to limited enzyme availability and lack of induction; it appears to be genetically determined.

Phenytoin should be discontinued if a skin rash appears (see "Warnings" section regarding drug discontinuation). If the rash is exfoliative, purpuric, or bullous or if lupus erythematosus or Stevens-Johnson syndrome is suspected, use of the drug should not be resumed. (See Adverse Reactions.) If the rash is of a milder type (measles-like or scarlatiniform), therapy may be resumed after the rash has completely disappeared. If the rash recurs upon reinstitution of therapy, further phenytoin medication is contraindicated.

Hyperglycemia, resulting from the drug's inhibitory effects on insulin release, has been reported. Phenytoin may also raise the serum glucose level in diabetic patients.

Osteomalacia has been associated with phenytoin therapy and is considered to be due to phenytoin's interference with Vitamin D metabolism.

Phenytoin is not indicated for seizures due to hypoglycemic or other causes. Appropriate diagnostic procedures should be performed as indicated.

Phenytoin is not effective for absence (petit mal) seizures. If tonic-clonic (grand-mal) and absence (petit mal) seizures are present, combined drug therapy is needed.

Information for Patients:

Patients taking phenytoin should be advised of the importance of adhering strictly to the prescribed dosage regimen, and of informing the physician of any clinical condition in which it is not possible to take the drug orally as prescribed, eg, surgery, etc.

Patients should also be cautioned on the use of other drugs or alcoholic beverages without first seeking the physician's advice.

The importance of good dental hygiene should be stressed in order to minimize the development of gingival hyperplasia and its complications.

Laboratory Tests:

Phenytoin serum level determinations may be necessary to achieve optimal dosage adjustments.

Drug Interactions:

1. Drugs which may *increase* phenytoin serum levels include: tolbutamide, chloramphenicol, dicumarol, disulfiram, isoniazid, chlordane, phenylbutazone, acute alcohol intake, aminosalicylic acid, chlordiazepoxide HCl, chlorpromazine, diazepam, estrogens, ethosuximide, halothane, methylphenidate, prochlorperazine, sulfaphenazole.
2. Drugs which may *decrease* phenytoin serum levels include: carbamazepine, chronic alcohol abuse, reserpine. Molindon Hydrochloride contains calcium ions which interfere with the absorption of phenytoin.
3. Drugs which may either increase or decrease phenytoin serum levels include: phenobarbital, valproic acid, and sodium valproate. Similarly, the effect of phenytoin on phenobarbital, valproic acid and sodium valproate serum levels is unpredictable.
4. Although not a true drug interaction, tricyclic antidepressants may precipitate seizures in susceptible patients and phenytoin dosage may need to be adjusted.
5. Drugs whose efficacy is impaired by phenytoin include: corticosteroids, coumarin anticoagulants, oral contraceptives, quinidine, and vitamin D.

Serum level determinations are especially helpful when possible drug interactions are suspected.

Drug/Laboratory Test Interactions:

Phenytoin may cause decreased serum levels of protein-bound iodine (PBI). It may also produce lower than normal values for dexamethasone or metyrapone tests. Phenytoin may cause raised serum levels of glucose, alkaline phosphatase, and gamma glutamyl transpeptidase (GGT).

Carcinogenesis:

See 'Warnings' section for information on carcinogenesis.

Pregnancy:

See Warnings

Nursing Mothers:

Infant breast feeding is not recommended for women taking this drug because phenytoin appears to be secreted in low concentrations in human milk.

Adverse Reactions:

Central Nervous System: The most common manifestations encountered with phenytoin therapy are referable to this system and are usually dose-related. These include nystagmus, ataxia, slurred speech, and mental confusion. Dizziness, insomnia, transient nervousness, motor twitchings, and headaches have also been observed. There have also been rare reports of phenytoin induced dyskinesias, including chorea, dystonia, tremor and asterixis, similar to those induced by phenothiazine and other neuroleptic drugs.

Gastrointestinal System: Nausea, vomiting and constipation.

Integumentary System: Dermatological manifestations sometimes accompanied by fever have included scarlatiniform or morbilliform rashes. A morbilliform rash (measles-like) is the most common; other types of dermatitis are seen more rarely. Other more serious forms which may be fatal have included bullous, exfoliative or purpuric dermatitis, lupus erythematosus, and Stevens-Johnson syndrome (see Precautions).

Hemopoietic System: Hemopoietic complications, some fatal, have occasionally been reported in association with administration of phenytoin. These have included thrombocytopenia, leukopenia, granulocytopenia, agranulocytosis, and pancytopenia. While macrocytosis and megaloblastic anemia have occurred, these conditions usually respond to folic acid therapy. Lymphadenopathy including benign lymph node hyperplasia, pseudolymphoma, lymphoma, and Hodgkin's Disease have been reported (see Warnings).

Connective Tissue System: Coarsening of the facial features, enlargement of the lips, gingival hyperplasia, hirsutism, and Peyronie's Disease.

Other: Systemic lupus erythematosus, periarteritis nodosa, toxic hepatitis, liver damage, and immuno-globulin abnormalities may occur.

Overdosage: The lethal dose in children is not known. The lethal dose in adults is estimated to be 2 to 5 grams. The initial symptoms are nystagmus, ataxia, and dysarthria. Other signs are tremor, hyperflexia, lethargy, slurred speech, nausea, vomiting. The patient may become comatose and hypertensive. Death is due to respiratory and circulatory depression.

There are marked variations among individuals with respect to phenytoin plasma levels where toxicity may occur. Nystagmus, on lateral gaze, usually appears at 20 mcg/ml, ataxia at 30 mcg/ml, dysarthria and lethargy appear when the plasma concentration is over 40 mcg/ml, but as high a concentration as 50 mcg/ml has been reported without evidence of toxicity. As much as 25 times the therapeutic dose has been taken to result in a serum concentration over 100 mcg/ml with complete recovery.

Treatment:

Treatment is nonspecific since there is no known antidote.

The adequacy of the respiratory and circulatory systems should be carefully observed and appropriate supportive measures employed. Hemodialysis can be considered since phenytoin is not completely bound to plasma proteins. Total exchange transfusion has been used in the treatment of severe intoxication in children.

In acute overdosage the possibility of other CNS depressants, including alcohol, should be borne in mind.

Dosage and Administration:

*Serum concentrations should be monitored in changing from Extended Phenytoin Sodium Capsules USP (Dilantin) to Prompt Phenytoin Sodium Capsules USP.

General:

Dosage should be individualized to provide maximum benefit. In some cases serum blood level determinations may be necessary for optimal dosage adjustments—the clinically effective serum level is usually 10-20 mcg/ml. With recommended dosage, a period of seven to ten days may be required to achieve steady-state blood levels with phenytoin and changes in dosage (increase or decrease) should not be carried out at intervals shorter than seven to ten days.

Adult Dosage:

Divided Daily Dosage

Patients who have received no previous treatment may be started on one 100 mg Dilantin (Extended Phenytoin Sodium Capsule) three times daily and the dosage then adjusted to suit individual requirements. For most adults, the satisfactory maintenance dosage will be one capsule three to four times a day. An increase up to two capsules three times a day may be made, if necessary.

Once-a-Day Dosage:

In adults, if seizure control is established with divided doses of three 100 mg Dilantin capsules daily, once-a-day dosage with 300 mg of extended phenytoin sodium capsules may be considered. Studies comparing divided doses of 300 mg with a single daily dose of this quantity indicated absorption, peak plasma levels, biologic half-life, difference between peak and minimum values, and urinary recovery were equivalent. Once-a-day dosage offers a convenience to the individual patient or to nursing personnel for institutionalized patients and is intended to be used only for patients requiring this amount of drug daily. A major problem in motivating noncompliant patients may also be lessened when the patient can take this drug once a day. However, patients should be cautioned not to miss a dose, inadvertently.

Only extended phenytoin sodium capsules are recommended for once-a-day dosing. Inherent differences in dissolution characteristics and resultant absorption rates of phenytoin due to different manufacturing procedures and/or dosage forms preclude such recommendation for other phenytoin products. When a change in the dosage form or brand is prescribed, careful monitoring of phenytoin serum levels should be carried out.

Loading Dose:

Some authorities have advocated use of an oral loading dose of phenytoin in adults who require rapid steady-state serum levels and where intravenous administration is not desirable. This dosing regimen should be reserved for patients in a clinic or hospital setting where phenytoin serum levels can be closely monitored. Patients with a history of renal or liver disease should not receive the oral loading regimen.

Initially, one gram of phenytoin capsules is divided into 3 doses (400 mg, 300 mg, 300 mg) and administered at two-hourly intervals. Normal maintenance dosage is then instituted 24

Continued on next page

This product information was prepared in August, 1982. On these and other Parke-Davis Products, information may be obtained by addressing PARKE-DAVIS, Division of Warner-Lambert Company, Morris Plains, New Jersey 07950.

Parke-Davis—Cont.

hours after the loading dose, with frequent serum level determinations.

Pediatric Dosage:
Initially, 5 mg/kg/day in two or three equally divided doses, with subsequent dosage individualized to a maximum of 300 mg daily. A recommended daily maintenance dosage is usually 4 to 8 mg/kg. Children over 6 years old may require the minimum adult dose (300 mg/day).

How Supplied:
N 0071-0362 (Kapseal 362)—Dilantin 100 mg; in 100's, 1,000's and unit dose 100's.
N 0071-0365 (Kapseal 365)—Dilantin 30 mg; in 100's, 1,000's and unit dose 100's.
[*Shown in Product Identification Section*]

Also available as:
N 0071-2214—Dilantin-125® Suspension 125 mg phenytoin/5 ml with a maximum alcohol content not greater than 0.6 percent, available in 8-oz bottles and individual unit dose foil pouches which deliver 5 ml (125 mg phenytoin). The minimum sales unit is 100 pouches.
N 0071-2315—Dilantin-30® Pediatric Suspension 30 mg phenytoin/5 ml with a maximum alcohol content not greater than 0.6 percent; available in 8-oz bottles and individual unit dose foil pouches which deliver 5 ml (30 mg phenytoin). The minimum sales unit is 100 pouches.
N 0071-0375 (Kapseal 375)—Dilantin with Phenobarbital each contain 100 mg phenytoin sodium with 16 mg (1/4 gr) phenobarbital; in 100's and 1,000's.
N 0071-0531 (Kapseal 531)—Dilantin with Phenobarbital each contain 100 mg phenytoin sodium with 32 mg (1/2 gr) phenobarbital; in 100's, 1,000's and unit dose 100's.
N 0071-0007 (Tablet 7)—Dilantin Infatabs® each contain 50 mg phenytoin, 100's and unit dose 100's.

For Parenteral Use:
N 0071-4488-05 (Ampoule 1488)—Dilantin ready-mixed solution containing 50 mg phenytoin sodium per milliliter is supplied in 2-ml ampoules. Packages of ten.
N 0071-4488-41 (Steri-Dose® 4488)—Dilantin ready-mixed solution containing 50 mg phenytoin sodium per milliliter is supplied in a 2-ml sterile disposable syringe (22 gauge × 1 1/4 inch needle). Packages of ten individually cartoned syringes.
N 0071-4475-35 (Ampoule 1475)—Dilantin ready-mixed solution containing 50 mg phenytoin sodium per milliliter is supplied in 5-ml ampoules with one 6-ml sterile disposable syringe (22 gauge × 1 1/4 inch needle). Packages of ten.
N 0071-4475-08 (Ampoule 1475)—Dilantin ready-mixed solution containing 50 mg phenytoin sodium per milliliter is supplied in packages of ten 5-ml ampoules without syringes.
Store below 30°C (86°F). Protect from light and moisture.

0362G020
121 882400/20

INFATABS®
DILANTIN® ℞
(Phenytoin Tablets, USP)

NOT FOR ONCE A DAY DOSING

Description: Dilantin is an antiepileptic drug.
Dilantin (phenytoin) is related to the barbiturates in chemical structure, but has a five-membered ring. The chemical name is 5,5-diphenyl-2,4-imidazolidinedione.
Each Dilantin Infatab, for oral administration, contains 50 mg phenytoin.

Clinical Pharmacology: Phenytoin is an antiepileptic drug which can be useful in the treatment of epilepsy. The primary site of action appears to be the motor cortex where spread of seizure activity is inhibited. Possibly by promoting sodium efflux from neurons, phenytoin tends to stabilize the threshold against hyperexcitability caused by excessive stimulation or environmental changes capable of reducing membrane sodium gradient. This includes the reduction of posttetanic potentiation at synapses. Loss of posttetanic potentiation prevents cortical seizure foci from detonating adjacent cortical areas. Phenytoin reduces the maximal activity of brain stem centers responsible for the tonic phase of tonic-clonic (grand mal) seizures.
Clinical studies using Dilantin Infatabs have shown an average plasma half-life of 14 hours with a range of 7 to 29 hours. Steady-state therapeutic levels are achieved 7 to 10 days after initiation of therapy with recommended doses of 300 mg/day.
Optimum control without clinical signs of toxicity occurs more often with serum levels between 10 and 20 mcg/ml, although some mild cases of tonic-clonic (grand mal) epilepsy may be controlled with lower-serum levels of phenytoin.
In most patients maintained at a steady dosage, stable phenytoin serum levels are achieved. There may be wide interpatient variability in phenytoin serum levels with equivalent dosages. Patients with unusually low levels may be noncompliant or hypermetabolizers of phenytoin. Unusually high levels result from liver disease, congenital enzyme deficiency or drug interactions which result in metabolic interference. The patient with large variations in phenytoin plasma levels, despite standard doses, presents a difficult clinical problem. Serum level determinations in such patients may be particularly helpful.
Most of the drug is excreted in the bile as inactive metabolites which are then reabsorbed from the intestinal tract and excreted in the urine. Urinary excretion of phenytoin and its metabolites occurs partly with glomerular filtration but more importantly, by tubular secretion. Because phenytoin is hydroxylated in the liver by an enzyme system which is saturable, small incremental doses may produce very substantial increases in serum levels, when these are in the upper range. The steady-state level may be double or triple from an increase in dosage of 10% or more, resulting in toxicity.
Clinical studies show that chewed and unchewed Dilantin Infatabs are bioequivalent, yield approximately equivalent plasma levels, and are more rapidly absorbed than 100-mg Dilantin Kapseals.®

Indications and Usage: Dilantin Infatabs (Phenytoin Tablets, USP) are indicated for the control of tonic-clonic and psychomotor (grand mal and temporal lobe) seizures and prevention and treatment of seizures occurring during or following neurosurgery. Phenytoin serum level determinations may be necessary for optimal dosage adjustments (see Dosage and Administration).

Contraindications: Phenytoin is contraindicated in those patients who are hypersensitive to phenytoin or other hydantoins.

Warnings: Abrupt withdrawal of phenytoin in epileptic patients may precipitate status epilepticus. When, in the judgment of the clinician, the need for dosage reduction, discontinuation, or substitution of alternative antiepileptic medication arises, this should be done gradually. However, in the event of an allergic or hypersensitivity reaction, rapid substitution of alternative therapy may be necessary. In this case, alternative therapy should be an antiepileptic drug not belonging to the hydantoin chemical class.
There have been a number of reports suggesting a relationship between phenytoin and the development of lymphadenopathy (local or generalized) including benign lymph node hyperplasia, pseudolymphoma, lymphoma, and Hodgkin's Disease. Although a cause and effect relationship has not been established, the occurrence of lymphadenopathy indicates the need to differentiate such a condition from other types of lymph node pathology. Lymph node involvement may occur with or without symptoms and signs resembling serum sickness eg, fever, rash and liver involvement. In all cases of lymphadenopathy, follow-up observation for an extended period is indicated and every effort should be made to achieve seizure control using alternative antiepileptic drugs.
Acute alcoholic intake may increase phenytoin serum levels while chronic alcoholic use may decrease serum levels.

Usage in Pregnancy
A number of reports suggest an association between the use of antiepileptic drugs by women with epilepsy and a higher incidence of birth defects in children born to these women. Data are more extensive with respect to phenytoin and phenobarbital, but these are also the most commonly prescribed antiepileptic drugs; less systematic or anecdotal reports suggest a possible similar association with the use of all known antiepileptic drugs.
The reports suggesting a higher incidence of birth defects in children of drug-treated epileptic women cannot be regarded as adequate to prove a definite cause and effect relationship. There are intrinsic methodologic problems in obtaining adequate data on drug teratogenicity in humans: genetic factors or the epileptic condition itself, may be more important than drug therapy in leading to birth defects. The great majority of mothers on antiepileptic medication deliver normal infants. It is important to note that antiepileptic drugs should not be discontinued in patients in whom the drug is administered to prevent major seizures, because of the strong possibility of precipitating status epilepticus with attendant hypoxia and threat to life. In individual cases where the severity and frequency of the seizure disorder are such that the removal of medication does not pose a serious threat to the patient, discontinuation of the drug may be considered prior to and during pregnancy, although it cannot be said with any confidence that even minor seizures do not pose some hazard to the developing embryo or fetus. The prescribing physician will wish to weigh these considerations in treating or counseling epileptic women of childbearing potential.
In addition to the reports of increased incidence of congenital malformations, such as cleft lip/palate and heart malformations in children of women receiving phenytoin and other antiepileptic drugs, there have more recently been reports of a fetal hydantoin syndrome. This consists of prenatal growth deficiency, microcephaly and mental deficiency in children born to mothers who have received phenytoin, barbiturates, alcohol, or trimethadione. However, these features are all interrelated and are frequently associated with intrauterine growth retardation from other causes.
There have been isolated reports of malignancies, including neuroblastoma, in children whose mothers received phenytoin during pregnancy.
An increase in seizure frequency during pregnancy occurs in a high proportion of patients, because of altered phenytoin absorption or metabolism. Periodic measurement of serum phenytoin levels is particularly valuable in the management of a pregnant epileptic patient as a guide to an appropriate adjustment of dosage. However, postpartum restoration of the original dosage will probably be indicated.
Neonatal coagulation defects have been reported within the first 24 hours in babies born to epileptic mothers receiving phenobarbital and/or phenytoin. Vitamin K has been shown to prevent or correct this defect and has been recommended to be given to the mother before delivery and to the neonate after birth.

Precautions:

General
The liver is the chief site of biotransformation of phenytoin; patients with impaired liver

function, elderly patients, or those who are gravely ill may show early signs of toxicity.
A small percentage of individuals who have been treated with phenytoin have been shown to metabolize the drug slowly. Slow metabolism may be due to limited enzyme availability and lack of induction; it appears to be genetically determined.
Phenytoin should be discontinued if a skin rash appears (see "Warnings" section regarding drug discontinuation). If the rash is exfoliative, purpuric, or bullous or if lupus erythematosus or Stevens-Johnson syndrome is suspected, use of the drug should not be resumed, (see Adverse Reactions). If the rash is of a milder type (measles-like or scarlatiniform), therapy may be resumed after the rash has completely disappeared. If the rash recurs upon reinstitution of therapy, further phenytoin medication is contraindicated.
Hyperglycemia, resulting from the drug's inhibitory effects on insulin release, has been reported. Phenytoin may also raise the serum glucose level in diabetic patients.
Osteomalacia has been associated with phenytoin therapy and is considered to be due to phenytoin's interference with Vitamin D metabolism.
Phenytoin is not indicated for seizures due to hypoglycemic or other causes. Appropriate diagnostic procedures should be performed as indicated.
Phenytoin is not effective for absence (petit mal) seizures. If tonic-clonic (grand-mal) and absence (petit mal) seizures are present, combined drug therapy is needed.

Information for Patients
Patients taking phenytoin should be advised of the importance of adhering strictly to the prescribed dosage regimen, and of informing the physician of any clinical condition in which it is not possible to take the drug orally as prescribed, eg, surgery, etc.
Patients should also be cautioned on the use of other drugs or alcoholic beverages without first seeking the physician's advice.
The importance of good dental hygiene should be stressed in order to minimize the development of gingival hyperplasia and its complications.

Laboratory Tests
Phenytoin serum level determinations may be necessary to achieve optimal dosage adjustments.

Drug Interactions
1. Drugs which may <u>increase</u> phenytoin serum levels include: tolbutamide, chloramphenicol, dicumarol, disulfiram, isoniazid, chlordane, phenylbutazone, acute alcohol intake, aminosalicylic acid, chlordiazepoxide HCl, chlorpromazine, diazepam, estrogens, ethosuximide, halothane, methylphenidate, prochlorperazine, sulfaphenazole.
2. Drugs which may <u>decrease</u> phenytoin serum levels include: carbamazepine, chronic alcohol abuse, reserpine. Molindon Hydrochloride contains calcium ions which interfere with the absorption of phenytoin.
3. Drugs which may either increase or decrease phenytoin serum levels include: Phenobarbital, valproic acid, and sodium valproate. Similarly, the effect of phenytoin on phenobarbital, valproic acid and sodium valproate serum levels is unpredictable.
4. Although not a true drug interaction, tricyclic antidepressants may precipitate seizures in susceptible patients and phenytoin dosage may need to be adjusted.
5. Drugs whose efficacy is impaired by phenytoin include: corticosteroids, coumarin anticoagulants, oral contraceptives, quinidine, and vitamin D.
Serum level determinations are especially helpful when possible drug interactions are suspected.

Drug/Laboratory Test Interactions
Phenytoin may cause decreased serum levels of protein-bound iodine (PBI). It may also produce lower than normal values for dexamethasone or metyrapone tests. Phenytoin may cause raised serum levels of glucose, alkaline phosphatase, and gamma glutamyl transpeptidase (GGT).

Carcinogenesis
See 'Warnings' section for information on carcinogenesis.

Pregnancy
See Warnings

Nursing Mothers
Infant breast-feeding is not recommended for women taking this drug because phenytoin appears to be secreted in low concentrations in human milk.

Adverse Reactions:
Central Nervous System: The most common manifestations encountered with phenytoin therapy are referable to this system and are usually dose-related. These include nystagmus, ataxia, slurred speech, and mental confusion. Dizziness, insomnia, transient nervousness, motor twitchings, and headache have also been observed.
There have also been rare reports of phenytoin induced dyskinesias, including chorea, dystonia, tremor and asterixis, similar to those induced by phenothiazine and other neuroleptic drugs.
Gastrointestinal System: Nausea, vomiting, and constipation.
Integumentary System: Dermatological manifestations sometimes accompanied by fever have included scarlatiniform or morbilliform rashes. A morbilliform rash (measles-like) is the most common; other types of dermatitis are seen more rarely. Other more serious forms which may be fatal have included bullous, exfoliative or purpuric dermatitis, lupus erythematosus, and Stevens-Johnson syndrome (see Precautions).
Hemopoietic System: Hemopoietic complications, some fatal, have occasionally been reported in association with administration of phenytoin. These have included thrombocytopenia, leukopenia, granulocytopenia, agranulocytosis, and pancytopenia. While macrocytosis and megaloblastic anemia have occurred, these conditions usually respond to folic acid therapy. Lymphadenopathy including benign lymph node hyperplasia, pseudolymphoma, lymphoma, and Hodgkin's Disease have been reported (see Warnings).
Connective Tissue System: Coarsening of the facial features, enlargement of the lips, gingival hyperplasia, hirsutism, and Peyronie's Disease.
Other: Systemic lupus erythematosus, periarteritis nodosa, toxic hepatitis, liver damage, and immunoglobulin abnormalities may occur.

Overdosage: The lethal dose in children is not known. The lethal dose in adults is estimated to be 2 to 5 grams. The initial symptoms are nystagmus, ataxia, and dysarthria. Other signs are tremor, hyperflexia, lethargy, slurred speech, nausea, vomiting. The patient may become comatose and hypertensive. Death is due to respiratory and circulatory depression.
There are marked variations among individuals with respect to phenytoin plasma levels where toxicity may occur. Nystagmus on lateral gaze usually appears at 20 mcg/ml, ataxia at 30 mcg/ml, dysarthria and lethargy appear when the plasma concentration is over 40 mcg/ml, but as high a concentration as 50 mcg/ml has been reported without evidence of toxicity. As much as 25 times the therapeutic dose has been taken to result in a serum concentration over 100 mcg/ml with complete recovery.

Treatment
Treatment is nonspecific since there is no known antidote.
The adequacy of the respiratory and circulatory systems should be carefully observed and appropriate supportive measures employed. Hemodialysis can be considered since phenytoin is not completely bound to plasma proteins. Total exchange transfusion has been used in the treatment of severe intoxication in children.
In acute overdosage the possibility of other CNS depressants, including alcohol, should be borne in mind.

Dosage and Administration: When given in equal doses, Dilantin Infatabs yield higher plasma levels than Dilantin Kapseals.® For this reason, care should be taken when switching a patient from one dosage form to the other.

General
Not for once a day dosing.
Dosage should be individualized to provide maximum benefit. In some cases, serum blood level determinations may be necessary for optimal dosage adjustments—the clinically effective serum level is usually 10–20 mcg/ml. With recommended dosage, a period of seven to ten days may be required to achieve steady-state blood levels with phenytoin and changes in dosage (increase or decrease) should not be carried out at intervals shorter than seven to ten days.
Dilantin Infatabs can be either chewed thoroughly before being swallowed or swallowed whole.

Adult Dosage
Patients who have received no previous treatment may be started on two Infatabs three times daily, and the dose is then adjusted to suit individual requirements. For most adults, the satisfactory maintenance dosage will be six to eight Infatabs daily; an increase to twelve Infatabs daily may be made, if necessary.

Pediatric Dosage
Initially, 5 mg/kg/day in two or three equally divided doses, with subsequent dosage individualized to a maximum of 300 mg daily. A recommended daily maintenance dosage is usually 4 to 8 mg/kg. Children over 6 years old may require the minimum adult dose (300 mg/day). If the daily dosage cannot be divided equally, the larger dose should be given before retiring.

How Supplied:
Dilantin Infatabs are supplied as:
N 0071-0007-24—Bottle of 100.
N 0071-0007-40—Unit dose (10/10's).
Each tablet contains 50 mg phenytoin.
[*Shown in Product Identification Section*]
Store at controlled room temperature (59°–86°F).
Protect from moisture.
Dilantin is also supplied in the following forms:
N 0071-0362-24—Bottle of 100.
N 0071-0362-32—Bottle of 1000.
N 0071-0362-40—Unit dose (10/10's).
Each capsule contains 100 mg phenytoin sodium.
N 0071-0365-24—Bottle of 100.
N 0071-0365-32—Bottle of 1000.
N 0071-0365-40—Unit dose (10/10's).
Each capsule contains 30 mg phenytoin sodium.
N 0071-2214-20—8 oz bottle.
N 0071-2214-40—Unit dose pouches (5 ml × 100).
Each 5 ml of suspension contains 125 mg phenytoin with a maximum alcohol content not greater than 0.6 percent.
N 0071-2315-20—8 oz bottle.
N 0071-2315-40—Unit dose pouches (5 ml × 100).

Continued on next page

This product information was prepared in August, 1982. On these and other Parke-Davis Products, information may be obtained by addressing PARKE-DAVIS, Division of Warner-Lambert Company, Morris Plains, New Jersey 07950.

Parke-Davis—Cont.

Each 5 ml of suspension contains 30 mg phenytoin with a maximum alcohol content not greater than 0.6 percent.
N 0071-0375-24—Bottle of 100.
N 0071-0375-32—Bottle of 1000.
Each capsule contains phenytoin sodium 100 mg and phenobarbital 16 mg (1/4 gr).
N 0071-0531-24—Bottle of 100.
N 0071-0531-32—Bottle of 1000.
N 0071-0531-40—Unit dose (10/10's).
Each capsule contains phenytoin sodium 100 mg and phenobarbital 32 mg (1/2 gr).
N 0071-4488-05—2-ml ampoules.
A sterile solution for parenteral use containing 50 mg phenytoin sodium per ml. Supplied in packages of ten.
N 0071-4488-41—2-ml prefilled syringes.
A sterile solution for parenteral use containing 50 mg phenytoin sodium per ml in an individually cartoned disposable syringe (22 gauge × 1 1/4 inch needle). Supplied in packages of ten.
N 0071-4475-35—5-ml ampoules with syringes.
A sterile solution for parenteral use containing 50 mg phenytoin sodium per ml. One 6-ml sterile disposable syringe (22 gauge ×1 1/4 inch needle). Supplied in packages of ten.
N 0071-4475-08—5-ml ampoules.
A sterile solution for parenteral use containing 50 mg phenytoin sodium per ml. Supplied in packages of ten.

0007G041

Parenteral DILANTIN® ℞
(Phenytoin Sodium Injection)

> **IMPORTANT NOTE**
> This drug must be administered slowly. Do not exceed 50 mg per minute intravenously.

Description: Ampoule Dilantin (phenytoin sodium injection) is a ready-mixed solution of phenytoin sodium in a vehicle containing 40% propylene glycol and 10% alcohol in water for injection, adjusted to pH 12 with sodium hydroxide. Phenytoin sodium is related to the barbiturates in chemical structure, but has a five-membered ring. The chemical name is sodium 5,5-diphenyl-2,4-imidazolidinedione.

Clinical Pharmacology: Phenytoin is an anticonvulsant which may be useful in the treatment of status epilepticus of the grand mal type. The primary site of action appears to be the motor cortex where spread of seizure activity is inhibited. Possibly by promoting sodium efflux from neurons, phenytoin tends to stabilize the threshold against hyperexcitability caused by excessive stimulation or environmental changes capable of reducing membrane sodium gradient. This includes the reduction of posttetanic potentiation at synapses. Loss of posttetanic potentiation prevents cortical seizure foci from detonating adjacent cortical areas. Phenytoin reduces the maximal activity of brain stem centers responsible for the tonic phase of grand mal seizures.

A fall in plasma levels may occur when patients are changed from oral to intramuscular administration. The drop is caused by slower absorption, as compared to oral administration, due to the poor water solubility of phenytoin. Intravenous administration is the preferred route for producing rapid therapeutic serum levels.

There are occasions when intramuscular administration may be required, ie, postoperatively, in comatose patients, for GI upsets. During these periods, a sufficient dose must be administered intramuscularly to maintain the plasma level within the therapeutic range. Where oral dosage is resumed following intramuscular usage, the oral dose should be properly adjusted to compensate for the slow, continuing IM absorption to avoid toxic symptoms.

Patients stabilized on a daily oral regimen of Dilantin experience a drop in peak blood levels to 50–60 percent of stable levels if crossed over to an equal dose administered intramuscularly. However, the intramuscular depot of poorly soluble material is eventually absorbed, as determined by urinary excretion of 5-(p-hydroxyphenyl)-5-phenylhydantoin (HPPH), the principal metabolite, as well as the total amount of drug eventually appearing in the blood.

A short-term (one week) study indicates that patients do not experience the expected drop in blood levels when crossed over to the intramuscular route, if the Dilantin IM dose is increased by 50 percent over the previously established oral dose. To avoid drug cumulation due to absorption from the muscle depots, it is recommended that for the first week back on oral Dilantin, the dose be reduced to half of the original oral dose (one-third of the IM dose). Experience for periods greater than one week is lacking and blood level monitoring is recommended. For administration of Dilantin in patients who cannot take oral medication for periods greater than a week gastric intubation may be considered.

Indications: Parenteral Dilantin is indicated for the control of status epilepticus of the grand mal type, and prevention and treatment of seizures occurring during neurosurgery.

Contraindications: Phenytoin is contraindicated in patients with a history of hypersensitivity to hydantoin products.

Because of its effect on ventricular automaticity, phenytoin is contraindicated in sinus bradycardia, sino-atrial block, second and third degree A-V block, and patients with Adams-Stokes syndrome.

Warnings:

Intravenous administration should not exceed 50 mg per minute.

Phenytoin sodium injection is not indicated in seizures due to hypoglycemia or other causes which may be immediately identified and corrected.

Appropriate diagnostic procedures should be performed as indicated.

Phenytoin metabolism may be significantly altered by the concomitant use of other drugs, such as:

a. Barbiturates may enhance the rate of metabolism of phenytoin. This effect, however, is variable and unpredictable. It has been reported that in some patients the concomitant administration of carbamazepine resulted in an increased rate of phenytoin metabolism.

b. Coumarin anticoagulants, disulfiram, phenylbutazone, and sulfaphenazole may inhibit the metabolism of phenytoin, resulting in signs of phenytoin toxicity. The effect of dicumarol in inhibiting the metabolism of phenytoin in the liver has been well documented.

c. Isoniazid inhibits the metabolism of phenytoin so that with combined therapy patients who are slow acetylators may suffer from phenytoin intoxication.

d. Tricyclic antidepressants in high doses may precipitate seizures and the dosage of phenytoin may have to be adjusted.

The results of certain clinical laboratory tests, eg, metyrapone, 1-mg dexamethasone, and protein-bound iodine, may be altered if the patient has been receiving phenytoin.

Phenytoin should be used with caution in patients with hypotension and severe myocardial insufficiency.

The intramuscular route is not recommended for the treatment of status epilepticus since blood levels of phenytoin in the therapeutic range cannot be readily achieved with doses and methods of administration ordinarily employed.

Usage in Pregnancy: The effects of Dilantin in human pregnancy and nursing infants are unknown.

Recent reports suggest an association between the use of anticonvulsant drugs by women with epilepsy and an elevated incidence of birth defects in children born to these women. Data are more extensive with respect to phenytoin and phenobarbital, but these are also the most commonly prescribed anticonvulsants; less systematic or anecdotal reports suggest a possible similar association with the use of all known anticonvulsant drugs.

The reports suggesting an elevated incidence of birth defects in children of drug-treated epileptic women cannot be regarded as adequate to prove a definite cause and effect relationship. There are intrinsic methodologic problems in obtaining adequate data on drug teratogenicity in humans; the possibility also exists that other factors, eg, genetic factors or the epileptic condition itself, may be more important than drug therapy in leading to birth defects. The great majority of mothers on anticonvulsant medication deliver normal infants. It is important to note that anticonvulsant drugs should not be discontinued in patients in whom the drug is administered to prevent major seizures because of the strong possibility of precipitating status epilepticus with attendant hypoxia and threat to life. In individual cases where the severity and frequency of the seizure disorder are such that the removal of medication does not pose a serious threat to the patient, discontinuation of the drug may be considered prior to and during pregnancy, although it cannot be said with any confidence that even minor seizures do not pose some hazard to the developing embryo or fetus.

The prescribing physician will wish to weigh these considerations in treating or counseling epileptic women of child-bearing potential.

Precautions: The addition of Dilantin solution to intravenous infusion is not recommended due to lack of solubility and resultant precipitation.

The liver is the site of biotransformation. Patients with impaired liver function, elderly patients, or those who are gravely ill may show early toxicity.

A small percentage of individuals who have been treated with phenytoin have been shown to metabolize the drug slowly. Slow metabolism may be due to limited enzyme availability and lack of induction; it appears to be genetically determined.

Drugs that control grand mal are not effective against petit mal seizures. Therefore, if both conditions are present, combined drug therapy is needed.

Each injection of intravenous Dilantin should be followed by an injection of sterile saline through the same needle or intravenous catheter to avoid local venous irritation due to the alkalinity of the solution. Continuous infusion should be avoided.

Hyperglycemia, resulting from the drug's inhibitory effect on insulin release, has been reported. Phenytoin may also raise the blood sugar level in persons already suffering from hyperglycemia.

Adverse Reactions: The most notable signs of toxicity associated with the intravenous use of this drug are cardiovascular collapse and/or central nervous system depression. Hypotension does occur when the drug is administered rapidly by the intravenous route. The *rate* of administration is very important; it should not exceed 50 mg per minute. At this rate, toxicity should be minimized.

Severe cardiotoxic reactions and fatalities have been reported with atrial and ventricular conduction depression and ventricular fibrillation. Severe complications are most commonly encountered in elderly or gravely ill patients.

Parenteral Dilantin sometimes causes drowsiness, nystagmus, circumoral tingling, vertigo, nausea and rarely vomiting. When these effects are observed, the plasma concentration is usually above 20 mcg/ml which is just above the usual therapeutic plasma concentration. Administration of this drug has produced an elevation in plasma glucose concentration.

Dosage and Administration: The addition of Dilantin solution to intravenous infusion is not recommended due to lack of solubility and resultant precipitation.

Not to exceed 50 mg per minute, intravenously. There is a relatively small margin between full therapeutic effect and minimally toxic doses of this drug.

The solution is suitable for use as long as it remains free of haziness and precipitate. Upon refrigeration or freezing a precipitate might form; this will dissolve again after the solution is allowed to stand at room temperature. The product is still suitable for use. Only a clear solution should be used. A faint yellow coloration may develop, however, this has no effect on the potency of the solution.

In the treatment of status epilepticus, the intravenous route is preferred because of the delay in absorption of phenytoin when administered intramuscularly.

Status Epilepticus:

Intravenously: 150 to 250 mg administered slowly, then 100 to 150 mg 30 minutes later if necessary. Higher doses may be required to control seizures. Dosage for children is usually determined according to weight in proportion to the dosage for a 150-pound adult. Pediatric dosage may also be calculated on the basis of 250 mg per square meter of body surface.

If the state of the patient is such that immobilization of an extremity is impossible due to convulsions, or veins are inaccessible, medication can be given intramuscularly during the attack.

If administration of phenytoin does not terminate the seizure, the clinician may consider the use of other anticonvulsants, intravenous barbiturates, general anesthesia, or other measures.

Neurosurgery: Prophylactic dosage—100 to 200 mg (2 to 4 ml) intramuscularly at approximately 4-hour intervals during surgery and continued during the postoperative period.

When intramuscular administration is required for a patient previously stabilized orally, compensating dosage adjustments are necessary to maintain therapeutic plasma levels. An intramuscular dose 50% greater than the oral dose is necessary to maintain these levels. When returned to oral administration, the dose should be reduced by 50% of the original oral dose for one week to prevent excessive plasma levels due to sustained release from intramuscular tissue sites.

If the patient requires more than a week of IM Dilantin, alternative routes should be explored, such as gastric intubation. For time periods less than one week, the patient shifted back from IM administration should receive one half the original oral dose for the same period of time the patient received IM Dilantin. Monitoring plasma levels would help prevent a fall into the subtherapeutic range. Serum blood level determinations are especially helpful when possible drug interactions are suspected.

Overdosage: The mean lethal dose in adults is estimated to be 2 to 5 grams. The cardinal initial symptoms are nystagmus, ataxia and dysarthria. The patient then becomes comatose, pupils unresponsive and hypotension occurs. Death is due to respiratory depression and apnea. Treatment is nonspecific since there is no known antidote. If the gag reflex is absent, the airway should be supported. Oxygen, vasopressors and assisted ventilation may be necessary for central nervous system, respiratory and cardiovascular depression.

Finally, hemodialysis can be considered since phenytoin is not completely bound to plasma proteins. Total exchange transfusion has been utilized in the treatment of severe intoxication in children.

How Supplied:

N 0071-4488-05 (Ampoule 1488) Dilantin ready-mixed solution containing 50 mg phenytoin sodium per milliliter is supplied in 2-ml ampoules. Packages of ten.

N 0071-4488-41 (Steri-Dose® 4488) Dilantin ready-mixed solution containing 50 mg phenytoin sodium per milliliter is supplied in a 2-ml sterile disposable syringe (22 gauge x 1¼ inch needle). Packages of ten individually cartoned syringes.

N 0071-4475-35 (Ampoule 1475) Dilantin ready-mixed solution containing 50 mg phenytoin sodium per milliliter is supplied in 5-ml ampoules with one 6-ml sterile disposable syringe (22 gauge x 1¼ inch needle). Packages of ten.

N 0071-4475-08 (Ampoule 1475) Dilantin ready-mixed solution containing 50 mg phenytoin sodium per milliliter is supplied in packages of ten 5-ml ampoules without syringes.

AHFS Category 28:12 **YC**

DILANTIN-30® PEDIATRIC/ DILANTIN-125® ℞

(Phenytoin Oral Suspension, USP)

Description: Dilantin (phenytoin) is related to the barbiturates in chemical structure, but has a five-membered ring. The chemical name is 5,5-diphenyl-2,4 imidazolidinedione.

Action: Phenytoin is an anticonvulsant drug which can be useful in the treatment of epilepsy. The primary site of action appears to be the motor cortex where spread of seizure activity is inhibited. Possibly by promoting sodium efflux from neurons, phenytoin tends to stabilize the threshold against hyperexcitability caused by excessive stimulation or environmental changes capable of reducing membrane sodium gradient. This includes the reduction of posttetanic potentiation at synapses. Loss of posttetanic potentiation prevents cortical seizure foci from detonating adjacent cortical areas. Phenytoin reduces the maximal activity of brain stem centers responsible for the tonic phase of grand mal seizures.

Indications: Dilantin (phenytoin) is indicated for the control of grand mal and psychomotor seizures.

Contraindication: Dilantin is contraindicated in those patients with a history of hypersensitivity to hydantoin products.

Warnings: Abrupt withdrawal of phenytoin in epileptic patients may precipitate status epilepticus. When in the judgment of the clinician the need for dosage reduction, discontinuation, or substitution of alternative anticonvulsant medication arises, this should be done gradually. In the event of an allergic or hypersensitivity reaction, more rapid substitution of alternative therapy may be necessary. In this case, alternative therapy should be an anticonvulsant not belonging to the hydantoin chemical class. Phenytoin is not indicated in seizures due to hypoglycemia or other causes which may be immediately identified and corrected. Appropriate diagnostic procedures should be performed as indicated.

Phenytoin metabolism may be significantly altered by the concomitant use of other drugs such as:

a. Barbiturates may enhance the rate of metabolism of phenytoin. This effect, however, is variable and unpredictable. It has been reported that in some patients the concomitant administration of carbamazepine resulted in an increased rate of phenytoin metabolism.

b. Coumarin anticoagulants, disulfiram, phenylbutazone, and sulfaphenazole may inhibit the metabolism of phenytoin, resulting in increased serum levels of the drug. This may lead to an increased incidence of nystagmus, ataxia, or other toxic signs. The effect of dicumarol in inhibiting the metabolism of phenytoin in the liver has been well documented.

c. Isoniazid inhibits the metabolism of phenytoin so that with combined therapy, patients who are slow acetylators may suffer from phenytoin intoxication.

d. Tricyclic antidepressants in high doses may precipitate seizures, and the dosage of phenytoin may have to be adjusted accordingly.

Phenytoin may interfere with the metyrapone and the 1-mg dexamethasone tests. It may also suppress the protein-bound iodine. However, this has not been associated with any clinical signs of hypothyroidism, the T-3 is normal.

Usage in Pregnancy: The effects of Dilantin (phenytoin) in human pregnancy and nursing infants are unknown.

Recent reports suggest an association between the use of anticonvulsant drugs by women with epilepsy and an elevated incidence of birth defects in children born to these women. Data are more extensive with respect to phenytoin and phenobarbital, but these are also the most commonly prescribed anticonvulsants; less systematic or anecdotal reports suggest a possible similar association with the use of all known anticonvulsant drugs.

The reports suggesting an elevated incidence of birth defects in children of drug-treated epileptic women cannot be regarded as adequate to prove a definite cause and effect relationship. There are intrinsic methodologic problems in obtaining adequate data on drug teratogenicity in humans; the possibility also exists that other factors, eg, genetic factors or the epileptic condition itself, may be more important than drug therapy in leading to birth defects. The great majority of mothers on anticonvulsant medication deliver normal infants. It is important to note that anticonvulsant drugs should not be discontinued in patients in whom the drug is administered to prevent major seizures because of the strong possibility of precipitating status epilepticus with attendant hypoxia and threat to life. In individual cases where the severity and frequency of the seizure disorder are such that the removal of medication does not pose a serious threat to the patient, discontinuation of the drug may be considered prior to and during pregnancy, although it cannot be said with any confidence that even minor seizures do not pose some hazard to the developing embryo or fetus.

The prescribing physician will wish to weigh these considerations in treating or counseling epileptic women of childbearing potential.

Precautions: The liver is the chief site of biotransformation of phenytoin; patients with impaired liver function may show early signs of toxicity. Elderly patients or those who are gravely ill may show early signs of toxicity.

A small percentage of individuals who have been treated with phenytoin have been shown to metabolize the drug slowly. Slow metabolism may be due to limited enzyme availability and lack of induction; it appears to be genetically determined.

Phenytoin has been associated with reversible lymph node hyperplasia. If lymph node enlargement occurs in patients on phenytoin, every effort should be made to substitute another anticonvulsant drug or drug combination.

Drugs that control grand mal are not effective for petit mal seizures. Therefore, if both condi-

Continued on next page

This product information was prepared in August, 1982. On these and other Parke-Davis Products, information may be obtained by addressing PARKE-DAVIS, Division of Warner-Lambert Company, Morris Plains, New Jersey 07950.

Parke-Davis—Cont.

tions are present, combined drug therapy is needed.

The phenytoin should be discontinued if a skin rash appears (see Warnings section regarding drug discontinuation). If the rash is exfoliative, purpuric, or bullous, use of the drug should not be resumed. If the rash is a milder type (measles-like or scarlatiniform), therapy may be resumed after the rash has completely disappeared. If the rash recurs upon reinstitution of therapy, further phenytoin medication is contraindicated.

Osteomalacia has been associated with anticonvulsant therapy, including phenytoin.

Hyperglycemia, resulting from the drug's inhibitory effect on insulin release, has been reported. Phenytoin may also raise the blood sugar level in persons already suffering from hyperglycemia.

Adverse Reactions:

Central Nervous System: The most common manifestations encountered with phenytoin therapy are referable to this system. These include nystagmus, ataxia, slurred speech, and mental confusion. Dizziness, insomnia, transient nervousness, motor twitchings, and headache have also been observed. These side effects may disappear with continuing therapy at a reduced dosage level.

Gastrointestinal System: Phenytoin may cause nausea, vomiting, and constipation. Administration of the drug with or immediately after meals may help prevent gastrointestinal discomfort.

Integumentary System: Dermatological manifestations sometimes accompanied by fever have included scarlatiniform or morbilliform rashes. A morbilliform rash (measles-like) is the most common; other types of dermatitis are seen more rarely. Rashes are more frequent in children and young adults. Other more serious forms which may be fatal have included bullous, exfoliative, or purpuric dermatitis, lupus erythematosus, and Stevens-Johnson syndrome.

Hemopoietic System: Hemopoietic complications, some fatal, have occasionally been reported in association with administration of phenytoin. These have included thrombocytopenia, leukopenia, granulocytopenia, agranulocytosis, and pancytopenia. While macrocytosis and megaloblastic anemia have occurred, these conditions usually respond to folic acid therapy. The occasional occurrence of lymphadenopathy indicates the need to differentiate such a condition from other lymph gland pathology.

Other: Gingival hyperplasia occurs frequently; this incidence may be reduced by good oral hygiene including gum massage, frequent brushing and appropriate dental care. Polyarthropathy and hirsutism occur occasionally. Hyperglycemia has been reported. Toxic hepatitis, liver damage, and periarteritis nodosa may occur and can be fatal.

Dosage and Administration: Dosage should be individualized to provide maximum benefit. In some cases, serum blood level determinations may be necessary for optimal dosage adjustments—the clinically effective serum level is usually 10–20 mcg/ml. Serum blood level determinations are especially helpful when possible drug interactions are suspected. With recommended dosage, a period of seven to ten days may be required to achieve therapeutic blood levels with Dilantin (phenytoin).

Adult Dose: Patients who have received no previous treatment may be started on one teaspoonful of Dilantin-125 Suspension three times daily, and the dose then adjusted to suit individual requirements. An increase to five teaspoonfuls daily may be made, if necessary.

Pediatric Dose: Initially, 5 mg/kg/day in two or three equally divided doses, with subsequent dosage individualized to a maximum of 300 mg daily. A recommended daily maintenance dosage is usually 4 to 8 mg/kg. Children over 6 years may require the minimum adult dose (300 mg/day).

Management of Overdosage: The mean lethal dose in adults is estimated to be 2 to 5 grams. The cardinal initial symptoms are nystagmus, ataxia, and dysarthria. The patient then becomes comatose, the pupils are unresponsive and hypotension occurs. Death is due to respiratory depression and apnea.

Treatment is nonspecific since there is no known antidote. First, the stomach should be emptied. If the gag reflex is absent, the airway should be supported. Oxygen, vasopressors, and assisted ventilation may be necessary for central nervous system, respiratory, and cardiovascular depression. Finally, hemodialysis can be considered since phenytoin is not completely bound to plasma proteins. Total exchange transfusion has been utilized in the treatment of severe intoxication in children.

How Supplied:

N 0071-2214—Dilantin-125® Suspension (phenytoin oral suspension, USP), 125 mg phenytoin/5 ml with a maximum alcohol content not greater than 0.6 percent; available in 8-oz bottles and individual unit dose foil pouches which deliver 5 ml (125 mg phenytoin). The minimum sales unit is 100 pouches.

N 0071-2315—Dilantin-30® Pediatric Suspension (phenytoin oral suspension, USP), 30 mg phenytoin/5 ml with a maximum alcohol content not greater than 0.6 percent, available in 8-oz bottles and individual unit dose foil pouches which deliver 5 ml (30 mg phenytoin). The minimum sales unit is 100 pouches.

Also available as:

N 0071-0362 (Kapseal® 362)—Dilantin (extended phenytoin sodium capsules, USP) 100 mg; in 100's, 1000's and unit dose 100's.

N 0071-0365 (Kapseal 365)—Dilantin (extended phenytoin sodium capsules, USP) 30 mg. in 100's, 1000's and unit dose 100's.

N 0071-0375 (Kapseal 375)—Dilantin with Phenobarbital each contain 100 mg phenytoin sodium with 16 mg (¼ gr) phenobarbital; in 100's and 1000's.

N 0071-0531 (Kapseal 531)—Dilantin with Phenobarbital each contain 100 mg phenytoin sodium with 32 mg (½ gr) phenobarbital; in 100's, 1000's and unit dose 100's.

N 0071-0007 (Tablet 7)—Dilantin Infatabs® (phenytoin tablets, USP) each contain 50 mg phenytoin; 100's and unit dose 100's.

For Parenteral Use:

N 0071-4488-05 (Ampoule 1488)—Dilantin ready-mixed solution containing 50 mg phenytoin sodium per milliliter is supplied in 2-ml ampoules. Packages of ten.

N 0071-4475-35 (Ampoule 1475)—Dilantin (phenytoin sodium injection) ready-mixed solution containing 50 mg phenytoin sodium per milliliter is supplied in 5-ml ampoules with one 6-ml sterile disposable syringe (22 gauge x 1¼ inch needle). Packages of ten.

N 0071-4475-08 (Ampoule 1475)—Dilantin ready-mixed solution containing 50 mg phenytoin sodium per milliliter is supplied in packages of ten 5-ml ampoules without syringes.

N 0071-4488-41 (Steri-Dose® 4488)—Dilantin ready-mixed solution containing 50 mg phenytoin sodium per milliliter is supplied in a 2-ml sterile disposable syringe (22 gauge x 1¼ inch needle). Packages of ten individually cartoned syringes.

2214G100

DOPASTAT™ ℞

Brand of
(Dopamine Hydrochloride)

Description: Dopamine hydrochloride is 3,4 dihydroxyphenethylamine hydrochloride, a naturally-occurring biochemical catecholamine precursor of norepinephrine.

Dopamine hydrochloride is a white, odorless crystalline powder, freely soluble in water and soluble in alcohol. It is sensitive to light, alkalis, iron salts and oxidizing agents.

Each milliliter of the clear, practically colorless, sterile, pyrogen-free dopamine hydrochloride injection contains 40 mg of dopamine hydrochloride (equivalent to 32.31 mg of dopamine base) in Water for Injection, USP, containing 1% sodium bisulfite as a preservative.

Actions: Dopamine hydrochloride exerts an inotropic effect on the myocardium resulting in an increased cardiac output. Dopamine hydrochloride produces less increase in myocardial oxygen consumption than isoproterenol and its use is usually not associated with a tachyarrhythmia. Clinical studies indicate that dopamine hydrochloride usually increases systolic and pulse pressure with either no effect or a slight increase in diastolic pressure. Total peripheral resistance at low and intermediate therapeutic doses is usually unchanged. Blood flow to peripheral vascular beds may decrease while mesenteric flow increases. Dopamine hydrochloride has also been reported to dilate the renal vasculature presumptively by activation of a "dopaminergic" receptor. This action is accompanied by increases in glomerular filtration rate, renal blood flow, and sodium excretion. An increase in urinary output produced by dopamine is usually not associated with a decrease in osmolality of the urine.

Indications: Dopamine hydrochloride is indicated for the correction of hemodynamic imbalances present in the shock syndrome due to myocardial infarctions, trauma, endotoxic septicemia, open heart surgery, renal failure, and chronic cardiac decompensation as in congestive failure.

Where appropriate, restoration of blood volume with a suitable plasma expander or whole blood should be instituted or completed prior to administration of dopamine hydrochloride.

Patients most likely to respond adequately to dopamine hydrochloride are those in whom physiological parameters, such as urine flow, myocardial function, and blood pressure, have not undergone profound deterioration. Multiclinic trials indicate that the shorter the time interval between onset of signs and symptoms and initiation of therapy with volume correction and dopamine hydrochloride, the better the prognosis.

Poor Perfusion of Vital Organs—Urine flow appears to be one of the better diagnostic signs by which adequacy of vital organ perfusion can be monitored. Nevertheless, the physician should also observe the patient for signs of reversal of confusion or comatose condition. Loss of pallor, increase in toe temperature, and/or adequacy of nail bed capillary filling may also be used as indices of adequate dosage. Clinical studies have shown that when dopamine hydrochloride is administered before urine flow has diminished to levels approximately 0.3 ml/minute, prognosis is more favorable. Nevertheless, in a number of oliguric or anuric patients, administration of dopamine hydrochloride has resulted in an increase in urine flow which in some cases reached normal levels. Dopamine hydrochloride may also increase urine flow in patients whose output is within normal limits and thus may be of value in reducing the degree of pre-existing fluid accumulation. It should be noted that at doses above those optimal for the individual patient, urine flow may decrease, necessitating reduction of dosage. Concurrent administration of dopamine hydrochloride and diuretic agents may produce an additive or potentiating effect.

Low Cardiac Output—Increased cardiac output is related to dopamine hydrochloride's direct inotropic effect on the myocardium. Increased cardiac output at low or moderate doses appears to be related to a favorable prognosis. Increase in cardiac output has been associated with either static or decreased systemic vascular resistance (SVR). Static or decreased

SVR associated with low or moderate movements in cardiac output is believed to be a reflection of differential effects on specific vascular beds with increased resistance in peripheral beds (eg, femoral) and concomitant decreases in mesenteric and renal vascular beds. Redistribution of blood flow parellels these changes so that an increase in cardiac output is accompanied by an increase in mesenteric and renal blood flow. In many instances the renal fraction of the total cardiac output has been found to increase. Increase in cardiac output produced by dopamine hydrochloride is not associated with substantial decreases in systemic vascular resistance as may occur with isoproterenol.

Hypotension—Hypotension due to inadequate cardiac output can be managed by administration of low to moderate doses of dopamine hydrochloride, which have little effect on SVR. At high therapeutic doses, dopamine hydrochloride's alpha adrenergic activity becomes more prominent and thus may correct hypotension due to diminished SVR. As in the case of other circulatory decompensation states, prognosis is better in patients whose blood pressure and urine flow have not undergone profound deterioration. Therefore, it is suggested that the physician administer dopamine hydrochloride as soon as a definite trend toward decreased systolic and diastolic pressure becomes evident.

Contraindications: Dopamine hydrochloride should not be used in patients with pheochromocytoma.

Warnings: Dopamine hydrochloride should not be administered in the presence of uncorrected tachyarrhythmias or ventricular fibrillation.

Do NOT add dopamine hydrochloride to any alkaline solution, since the drug is inactivated in alkaline solution.

Patients who have been treated with monoamine oxidase (MAO) inhibitors prior to the administration of dopamine hydrochloride will require substantially reduced dosage. Dopamine is metabolized by MAO, and inhibition of this enzyme prolongs and potentiates the effect of dopamine hydrochloride. The starting dose in such patients should be reduced to at least one-tenth (1/10) of the usual dose.

Usage in Pregnancy—Animal studies have revealed no evidence of teratogenic effects from dopamine hydrochloride. In one study, administration of dopamine hydrochloride to pregnant rats resulted in a decreased survival rate of the newborn and a potential for cataract formation in the survivors. The drug may be used in pregnant women when, in the judgment of the physician, the expected benefits outweigh the potential risk to the fetus.

Usage in Children—The safety and efficacy of this drug in children has not been established. Dopamine hydrochloride has been used in a limited number of pediatric patients but such use has been inadequate to fully define proper dosage and limitations for use. Further studies are in progress.

Precautions:

Avoid Hypovolemia—Prior to treatment with dopamine hydrochloride, hypovolemia should be fully corrected, if possible, with either whole blood or plasma as indicated.

Decreased Pulse Pressure—If a disproportionate rise in the diastolic pressure (ie, a marked decrease in the pulse pressure) is observed in patients receiving dopamine hydrochloride, the infusion rate should be decreased and the patient observed carefully for further evidence of predominant vasoconstrictor activity, unless such an effect is desired.

Extravasation—Dopamine hydrochloride should be infused into a large vein whenever possible to prevent the possibility of extravasation into tissue adjacent to the infusion site. Extravasation may cause necrosis and sloughing of surrounding tissue. Large veins of the antecubital fossa are preferred to veins in the dorsum of the hand or ankle. Less suitable infusion sites should be used only if the patient's condition requires immediate attention. The physician should switch to more suitable sites as rapidly as possible. The infusion site should be continuously monitored for free flow.

Occlusive Vascular Disease—Patients with a history of occlusive vascular disease (for example, atherosclerosis, arterial embolism, Raynaud's disease, cold injury, diabetic endarteritis, and Buerger's disease) should be closely monitored for any changes in color or temperature of the skin in the extremities. If a change in skin color or temperature occurs and is thought to be the result of compromised circulation to the extremities, the benefits of continued dopamine hydrochloride infusion should be weighed against the risk of possible necrosis. This condition may be reversed by either decreasing or discontinuing the rate of infusion.

IMPORTANT

Antidote for Peripheral Ischemia: To prevent sloughing and necrosis in ischemic areas, the area should be infiltrated as soon as possible with 10 to 15 ml of Saline solution containing from 5 to 10 mg of Regitine® (brand of phenotolamine), an adrenergic blocking agent. A syringe with a fine hypodermic needle should be used, and the solution liberally infiltrated throughout the ischemic area. Sympathetic blockade with phentolamine causes immediate and conspicuous local hyperemic changes if the area is infiltrated within 12 hours. Therefore, *phentolamine should be given as soon as possible* after the extravasation is noted.

Avoid Cyclopropane or Halogenated Hydrocarbon Anesthetics—Cyclopropane or halogenated hydrocarbon anesthetics increase cardiac autonomic irritability and therefore may sensitize the myocardium to the action of certain intravenously administered catecholamines. This interaction appears to be related both to pressor activity and to beta adrenergic stimulating properties of these catecholamines. Therefore, as with certain other catecholamines, and because of the theoretical arrhythmogenic potential, dopamine hydrochloride should be used with EXTREME CAUTION in patients inhaling cyclopropane or halogenated hydrocarbon anesthetics.

Careful Monitoring Required—Close monitoring of the following indices—urine flow, cardiac output and blood pressure—during dopamine hydrochloride infusion is necessary as in the case of any adrenergic agent.

Adverse Reactions: The most frequent adverse reactions observed in clinical evaluation of dopamine hydrochloride included ectopic beats, nausea, vomiting, tachycardia, anginal pain, palpitation, dyspnea, headache, hypotension, and vasoconstriction. Other adverse reactions which have been reported infrequently were aberrant conduction, bradycardia, piloerection, widened QRS complex, azotemia, and elevated blood pressure.

Dosage and Administration:

WARNING: This is a potent drug. It must be diluted before administration to patient.

Suggested Dilution—Transfer contents of one ampoule (5 ml containing 200 mg dopamine hydrochloride) by aseptic technique to either a 250 ml or 500 ml bottle of one of the following sterile intravenous solutions:

1. Sodium Chloride Injection, USP
2. Dextrose 5% Injection, USP
3. Dextrose (5%) and Sodium Chloride (0.9%) Injection, USP
4. 5% Dextrose in 0.45% Sodium Chloride Solution
5. Dextrose (5%) in Lactated Ringer's Solution
6. Sodium Lactate (1/6 Molar) Injection, USP
7. Lactated Ringer's Injection, USP

Dopamine hydrochloride has been found to be stable for a minimum of 24 hours after dilution in the sterile intravenous solutions listed above. However, as with all intravenous admixtures, dilution should be made just prior to administration.

Do NOT add dopamine hydrochloride injection to 5% Sodium Bicarbonate or other alkaline intravenous solutions, since the drug is inactivated in alkaline solution.

Rate of Administration—Dopamine hydrochloride, after dilution, is administered intravenously through a suitable intravenous catheter or needle. An IV drip chamber or other suitable metering device is essential for controlling the rate of flow in drops/minute. Each patient must be individually titrated to the desired hemodynamic and/or renal response with dopamine hydrochloride. In titrating to the desired increase in systolic blood pressure, the optimum dosage rate for renal response may be exceeded, thus necessitating a reduction in rate after the hemodynamic condition is stabilized.

Administration at rates greater than 50 mcg/kg/minute have safely been used in advanced circulatory decompensation states. If unnecessary fluid expansion is of concern, adjustment of drug concentration may be preferred over increasing the flow rate of a less concentrated dilution.

Suggested Regimen:

1. When appropriate, increase blood volume with whole blood or plasma until central venous pressure is 10 to 15 cm. H_2O or pulmonary wedge pressure is 14-18 mm Hg.
2. Begin administration of diluted solution at doses of 2-5 mcg/kg/minute dopamine hydrochloride in patients who are likely to respond to modest increments of heart force and renal perfusion.

In more seriously ill patients, begin administration of diluted solution at doses of 5 mcg/kg/minute dopamine hydrochloride and increase gradually using 5-10 mcg/kg/minute increments up to 20-50 mcg/kg/minute as needed. If doses of dopamine hydrochloride in excess of 50 mcg/kg/minute are required, it is suggested that urine output be checked frequently. Should urine flow begin to decrease in the absence of hypotension, reduction of dopamine hydrochloride dosage should be considered. Multiclinic trials have shown that more than 50% of the patients were satisfactorily maintained on doses of dopamine hydrochloride less than 20 mcg/kg/minute. In patients who do not respond to these doses with adequate arterial pressures or urine flow, additional increments of dopamine hydrochloride may be employed in an effort to produce an appropriate arterial pressure and central perfusion.

3. Treatment of all patients requires constant evaluation of therapy in terms of the blood volume, augmentation of myocardial contractility, and distribution of peripheral perfusion. Dosage of dopamine hydrochloride should be adjusted according to the patient's response, with particular attention to diminution of established urine flow rate, increasing tachycardia or development of new dysrhythmias as indices for decreasing or temporarily suspending the dosage.

Continued on next page

This product information was prepared in August, 1982. On these and other Parke-Davis Products, information may be obtained by addressing PARKE-DAVIS, Division of Warner-Lambert Company, Morris Plains, New Jersey 07950.

Parke-Davis—Cont.

4. As with all potent intravenously administered drugs, care should be taken to control the rate of administration so as to avoid inadvertent administration of a bolus of drug.

Overdosage: In case of accidental overdosage, as evidenced by excessive blood pressure elevation, reduce rate of administration or temporarily discontinue dopamine hydrochloride until patient's condition stabilizes. Since dopamine hydrochloride's duration of action is quite short, no additional remedial measures are usually necessary. If these measures fail to stabilize the patient's condition, use of the short acting alpha adrenergic blocking agent phentolamine should be considered.

How Supplied:
Dopamine hydrochloride is supplied as:
N 0071-4210-08—5-ml ampoules. Each ml contains 40 mg dopamine hydrochloride (equivalent to 32.31 mg dopamine base). Supplied as packages of ten individually cartoned 5-ml ampoules.

4210G041

DURAQUIN® ℞
(quinidine gluconate tablets)
SUSTAINED RELEASE

Description: Quinidine gluconate is the gluconate of an alkaloid which may be obtained from various species of Cinchona and their hybrids, from *Remijia pedunculata* Fluckiger (Fam. Rubiaceae), or prepared from quinine. Quinidine gluconate contains, on the dry basis, not less than 99% of $C_{20}H_{24}N_2O_2 \cdot C_6H_{12}O_7$ (520.58). Quinidine is chemically described as 6-methoxy-alpha- (5-vinyl-2 quinuclidinyl) -4 quinolinemethanol and is the dextrorotatory isomer of quinine. Each 330-mg sustained-release tablet, representing 206 mg of quinidine base, is equivalent to 248 mg of quinidine sulfate.

Actions: The antiarrhythmic activity consists of two actions: (a) prolongation of effective refractory period of the atrial or ventricular muscle which leads to termination of arrhythymia; (b) decrease in excitability of ectopic foci of the heart. In addition, quinidine blocks vagal innervation and facilitates conduction in the atrial-ventricular junction.

Clinical Pharmacology: In clinical studies, single doses of Duraquin produced a mean maximum plasma level at 2 hours which was maintained for 12 hours. This broad plateau indicates slow, continuous absorption from the gastrointestinal tract.

In multiple-dose studies, administration of Duraquin tablets, 660 mg every 12 hours, produced steady state (equilibrium) plasma levels shortly after 24 hours. The average quinidine plasma levels (Cramer and Isaksson assay[1]) were 0.81 mcg/ml and the mean peak levels were 1.16 mcg/ml in a group of normal male subjects weighing 75 kg. Following the last dose at steady state, quinidine plasma levels decreased at an approximate rate of 50% in 10 hours. This compares to the expected plasma half-life of 6.3 hours for quinidine sulfate tablets, USP.

Therapeutic and toxic effects coordinate better with plasma levels than with dosage. While therapeutic levels of 3 to 6 mcg/ml with a range of 1.5 to 9 mcg/ml have been reported, these values are based on peak plasma levels determined by the less specific Edgar and Sokolow assay.[2] This procedure yields quinidine levels averaging 22% higher than the Cramer and Isaksson assay. Plasma levels vary considerably in patients receiving identical doses. Therefore, it is advisable to adjust the dosage by monitoring plasma quinidine levels.

Indications: Duraquin tablets are indicated for the prevention of premature atrial, nodal, or ventricular contractions. They are also indicated for the maintenance of normal sinus rhythm following spontaneous reversion or electrical conversion of atrial, nodal, or ventricular tachycardia, atrial flutter and fibrillation (either paroxysmal or chronic).

Contraindications:
1. History of hypersensitivity to quinidine manifested by thrombocytopenia, skin eruption, febrile reactions, etc.
2. Complete A-V block
3. Complete bundle branch block or other severe intraventricular conduction defects exhibiting marked QRS widening or bizarre complexes
4. Myasthenia gravis
5. Arrhythmias associated with digitalis toxicity

Warnings:
1. (a) In the treatment of atrial fibrillation with rapid ventricular response, ventricular rate should be controlled with digitalis glycosides *prior* to administration of quinidine.
(b) In the treatment of atrial flutter with quinidine, reversion to sinus rhythm may be preceded by progressive reduction in the degree of A-V block to a 1:1 ratio resulting in an extremely high ventricular rate. This potential hazard may be reduced by digitalization prior to administration of quinidine.

Recent reports have described increased, potentially toxic, digoxin plasma levels when quinidine is administered concurrently. When concurrent use is necessary, digoxin dosage should be reduced and plasma concentration should be monitored and patients observed closely for digitalis intoxication.

2. Quinidine cardiotoxicity may be manifested by increased PR and QT intervals, 50% widening of QRS, and/or ventricular ectopic beats or tachycardia. Appearance of these toxic signs during quinidine administration mandates immediate discontinuation of the drug, and/or close clinical and electrocardiographic monitoring. Note: Quinidine effect is enhanced by potassium and reduced in the presence of hypokalemia.
3. "Quinidine Syncope" may occur as a complication of long-term therapy. It is manifested by sudden loss of consciousness and ventricular arrhythmias with bizarre QRS complexes. This syndrome does not appear to be related to dose or plasma levels but occurs more often with prolonged QT intervals.
4. Because quinidine antagonizes the effect of vagal excitation upon the atrium and the A-V node, the administration of parasympathomimetic drugs (choline esters) or the use of any other procedure to enhance vagal activity may fail to terminate paroxysmal supraventricular tachycardia in patients receiving quinidine.
5. Quinidine should be used with extreme caution in: a) the presence of incomplete A-V block, since a complete block and asystole may result. Quinidine may cause unpredictable abnormalities of rhythm in digitalized hearts. Therefore, it should be used with caution in the presence of digitalis intoxication. (See 1.(b) above).
b) Partial bundle branch block.
c) Severe congestive heart failure and hypotensive states due to the depressant effects of quinidine on myocardial contractility and arterial pressure.
d) Poor renal function, especially renal tubular acidosis, because of the potential accumulation of quinidine in plasma leading to toxic concentrations.

Precautions:
1. Test Dose
A preliminary test dose of a single tablet of quinidine *sulfate* should be administered prior to the initiation of the sustained release gluconate to determine whether the patient has an idiosyncrasy to the quinidine molecule.
2. Hypersensitivity
During the first weeks of therapy; hypersensitivity to quinidine, although rare, should be considered (eg, angioedema, purpura, acute asthmatic episode, vascular collapse).
3. Long-Term Therapy
Periodic blood counts and liver and kidney function tests should be performed during long-term therapy and the drug should be discontinued if blood dyscrasias or signs of hepatic or renal disorders occur.
4. Large Doses
ECG monitoring and determination of plasma quinidine levels are recommended when doses greater than 2.5 g/day are administered.
5. Usage in Pregnancy
The use of quinidine, in pregnancy, should be reserved only for those cases where the benefits outweigh the possible hazards to the patient and fetus.
6. Nursing Mothers
The drug should be used with extreme caution in nursing mothers because the drug is excreted in breast milk.
7. General
In patients exhibiting asthma, muscle weakness, and infection with fever *prior* to quinidine administration, hypersensitivity reactions to the drug may be masked.

Drug Interactions:
1. Caution should be used when quinidine and its analogs are administered concurrently with coumarin anticoagulants. This combination may reduce prothrombin levels and cause bleeding.
2. Quinidine, a weak base, may have its half-life prolonged in patients who are concurrently taking drugs that can alkalize the urine, such as thiazide diuretics, sodium bicarbonate, and carbonic anhydrase inhibitors. Quinidine and drugs which alkalize the urine should be used together cautiously.
3. Quinidine exhibits a distinct anticholinergic activity in the myocardial tissues. An additive vagolytic effect may be seen when quinidine and drugs having anticholinergic blocking activity are used together. Drugs having cholinergic activity may be antagonized by quinidine.
4. Quinidine and other antiarrhythmic agents may produce additive cardiac depressant effects when administered together.
5. Quinidine interaction with cardiac glycosides (digoxin); See Warnings.
6. Antacids may delay absorption of quinidine but appear unlikely to cause incomplete absorption.
7. Phenobarbital and phenytoin may reduce plasma half-life of quinidine by 50%.
8. Quinidine may potentiate the neuromuscular blocking effect in ventilatory depression of patients receiving decamethonium, tubocurare, or succinylcholine.

Adverse Reactions: Symptoms of cinchonism (ringing in the ears, headache, disturbed vision) may appear in sensitive patients after a single dose of the drug.

Gastrointestinal: The most common side effects encountered with quinidine are referable to this system. Diarrhea frequently occurs, but it rarely necessitates withdrawal of the drug. Nausea, vomiting, and abdominal pain also occur. Some of these effects may be minimized by administering the drug with meals.

Cardiovascular: Widening of QRS complex, cardiac asystole, ventricular ectopic beats, idioventricular rhythms including ventricular tachycardias and fibrillation; paradoxical tachycardia, arterial embolism and hypotension.

Hematologic: acute hemolytic anemia, hypoprothrombinemia, thrombocytopenic purpura, agranulocytosis.

CNS: headache, fever, vertigo, apprehension, excitement, confusion, delirium and syncope, disturbed hearing (tinnitus, decreased auditory acuity), disturbed vision (mydriasis, blurred vision, disturbed color perception, photophobia, diplopia, night blindness, scotomata); optic neuritis.

Dermatologic: cutaneous flushing with intense pruritus.

Hypersensitivity reactions: angioedema, acute asthmatic episode, vascular collapse, respiratory arrest.

Dosage and Administration: Dosage should be titrated to give the desired clinical effect, e.g., elimination of paroxysmal rhythm or reduction in premature contractions (See Clinical Pharmacology). This will often require prolonged ambulatory ECG monitoring, as hour-to-hour variability renders brief ECG recordings unreliable. When doses larger than 2.5g/day are used, quinidine blood levels should be monitored, if possible, and serial ECGs should be followed (See Warnings and Precautions).

For prevention of premature contractions and maintenance of normal sinus rhythm following spontaneous reversion or electrical conversion, the usual dosage is from 330 mg to 660 mg every eight hours, most patients requiring the higher dosage.

In elderly patients, and in patients in the lower end of the normal weight range, plasma quinidine determinations should be considered. Dosage adjustments may be required.

Overdosage: Cardiotoxic effects of quinidine may be reversed in part by molar sodium lactate; the hypotension may be reversed by vasoconstrictors and by catecholamines (since the vasodilation is partly due to alpha-adrenergic blockade).

How Supplied: N 0071-0850 (P-D 850) Duraquin (quinidine gluconate tablets) 330-mg tablets are supplied in bottles of 100 and in unit-dose packages of 100 (10 strips of 10 tablets each).

0850G010

---

[1] Cramer, G. and Isaksson, B. Quantitative Determination of Quinidine in Plasma, Scandinavian J. Clin. & Lab Investigation 15, 553, 1963.

[2] Edgar, A.L. and Sokolow, M. Experiences with the Photofluorometric Determination of Quinidine in Blood J. Lab Clin. Med. 36, 478, 1950.

[Shown in Product Identification Section]

EASPRIN™
(Aspirin Tablets, USP)
Enteric Coated Tablets

Description: Easprin (Aspirin Tablets, USP) enteric coated tablets contain 15 grains (975 mg) aspirin for oral administration. The enteric coating is designed to prevent the release of aspirin in the stomach and thereby reduce gastric irritation and total occult blood loss. The pharmacologic effects of aspirin include analgesia, antipyresis, antiinflammatory activity, and antirheumatic activity.

Clinical Pharmacology: Aspirin is a salicylate that has demonstrated antiinflammatory, analgesic, antipyretic, and antirheumatic activity.

Aspirin's mode of action as an antiinflammatory and antirheumatic agent may be due to inhibition of synthesis and release of prostaglandins.

Aspirin appears to produce analgesia by virtue of both a peripheral and CNS effect. Peripherally, aspirin acts by inhibiting the synthesis and release of prostaglandins. Acting centrally, it would appear to produce analgesia at a hypothalamic site in the brain, although the mode of action is not known.

Aspirin also acts on the hypothalamus to produce antipyresis; heat dissipation is increased as a result of vasodilation and increased peripheral blood flow. Aspirin's antipyretic activity may also be related to inhibition of synthesis and release of prostaglandins.

In a crossover study, Easprin at a dose of one tablet (15 grains) three times a day produced an average fecal blood loss of 1.36 ml per day. Uncoated aspirin at a dosage of three 5 grain tablets given three times a day caused an averge fecal blood loss of 2.90 ml per day.

Easprin Tablets are enteric coated. This coating acts to prevent the release of aspirin in the stomach but permits the tablet to dissolve with resultant absorption in the upper portion of the small intestine. This reduces any gastric irritation that may occur with uncoated aspirin but does delay the onset of action. Aspirin is rapidly hydrolyzed primarily in the liver to salicylic acid, which is conjugated with glycine (forming salicyluric acid) and glucuronic acid and excreted largely in the urine. As a result of the rapid hydrolysis, plasma concentrations of aspirin are always low and rarely exceed 20 mcg/ml at ordinary therapeutic doses. The peak salicylate level for uncoated aspirin occurs in about 2 hours; however with enteric coated aspirin tablets this is delayed. A direct correlation between salicylate plasma levels and clinical analgesic effectiveness has not been definitely established, but effective analgesia is usually achieved at plasma levels of 15 to 30 mg per 100 ml. Effective antiinflammatory activity is usually achieved at salicylate plasma levels of 20 to 30 mg per 100 ml. There is also poor correlation between toxic symptoms and plasma salicylate concentrations, but most patients exhibit symptoms of salicylism at plasma salicylate levels of 35 mg per 100 ml. The plasma half-life for aspirin is approximately 15 minutes; that for salicylate lengthens as the dose increases: Doses of 300 to 650 mg have a half-life of 3.1 to 3.2 hours; with doses of 1 gram, the half-life is increased to 5 hours and with 2 grams it is increased to about 9 hours.

Salicylates are excreted mainly by the kidney. Studies in man indicate that salicylate is excreted in the urine as free salicylic acid (10%), salicyluric acid (75%), salicylic phenolic (10%), and acyl (5%) glucuronides and gentisic acid.

Indications and Usage: Easprin is indicated in patients who need the higher 15 grain dose of aspirin in the long-term palliative treatment of mild to moderate pain and inflammation of arthritic and other inflammatory conditions.

Contraindications: Easprin should not be used in patients who have previously exhibited hypersensitivity to aspirin and/or nonsteroidal antiinflammatory agents.

Easprin should not be given to patients with a recent history of gastrointestinal bleeding or in patients with bleeding disorders (eg, hemophilia).

Warnings: Easprin Tablets should be used with caution when anticoagulants are prescribed concurrently, for aspirin may depress the concentration of prothrombin in plasma and thereby increase bleeding time. Large doses of salicylates have a hypoglycemic action and may enhance the effect of the oral hypoglycemics. Consequently, they should not be given concomitantly; if however, this is necessary, the dosage of the hypoglycemic agent must be reduced while the salicylate is given. This hypoglycemic action may also affect the insulin requirements of diabetics.

Although salicylates in large doses are uricosuric agents, smaller amounts may decrease the uricosuric effects of probenecid, sulfinpyrazone, and phenylbutazone.

Precautions:

General: Easprin Tablets should be administered with caution to patients with asthma, nasal polyps, or nasal allergies.

In patients receiving large doses of aspirin and /or prolonged therapy, mild salicylate intoxication (salicylism) may develop that may be reversed by reduction in dosage.

Although the fecal blood loss with Easprin is less than that with uncoated aspirin tablets, Easprin Tablets should be administered with caution to patients with a history of gastric distress, ulcer, or bleeding problems. Occult gastrointestinal bleeding occurs in many patients but is not correlated with gastric distress. The amount of blood lost is usually insignificant clinically, but with prolonged administration, it may result in iron deficiency anemia.

Sodium excretion produced by spironolactone may be decreased in the presence of salicylates.

Salicylates can produce changes in thyroid function tests.

Salicylates should be used with caution in patients with severe hepatic damage, preexisting hypoprothrombinemia, or Vitamin K deficiency, and in those undergoing surgery.

Drug Interactions:

Anticoagulants: See Warnings

Hypoglycemic Agents: See Warnings.

Uricosuric Agents: Aspirin may decrease the effects of probenecid, sulfinpyrazone, and phenylbutazone.

Spironolactone: See above.

Alcohol: Has a synergistic effect with aspirin in causing gastrointestinal bleeding.

Corticosteroids: Concomitant administration with aspirin may increase the risk of gastrointestinal ulceration.

Pyrazolone Derivatives (phenylbutazone, oxyphenbutazone, and possibly dipyrone): Concomitant administration with aspirin may increase the risk of gastrointestinal ulceration.

Nonsteroidal Antiinflammatory Agents: Aspirin is contraindicated in patients who are hypersensitive to nonsteroidal antiinflammatory agents.

Urinary Alkalinizers: Decrease aspirin effectiveness by increasing the rate of salicylate renal excretion.

Phenobarbital: Decreases aspirin effectiveness by enzyme induction.

Propranolol: May decrease aspirin's antiinflammatory action by competing for the same receptors.

Antacids: Easprin should not be given concurrently with antacids, since an increase in the pH of the stomach may affect the enteric coating of the tablets.

Usage in Pregnancy: Aspirin does not appear to have any teratogenic effects. However, it has been reported that adverse effects were increased in the mother and fetus following chronic ingestion of aspirin. Prolonged pregnancy and labor with increased bleeding before and after delivery, as well as decreased birth weight and increased rate of stillbirth were correlated with high blood salicylate levels. Because of possible adverse effects on the neonate and the potential for increased maternal blood loss, aspirin should be avoided during the last three months of pregnancy.

Adverse Reactions:

Gastrointestinal: Dyspepsia, nausea, vomiting, diarrhea, gastrointestinal bleeding, and /or ulceration.

Ear: Tinnitus, vertigo, reversible hearing loss.

Hematologic: Prolongation of bleeding time, leukopenia, thrombocytopenia, purpura, decreased plasma iron concentration and shortened erythrocyte survival time.

Dermatologic and Hypersensitivity: Urticaria, angioedema, pruritus, various skin eruptions, asthma, and anaphylaxis.

Miscellaneous: Acute reversible hepatotoxicity, mental confusion, drowsiness, sweating,

Continued on next page

This product information was prepared in August, 1982. On these and other Parke-Davis Products, information may be obtained by addressing PARKE-DAVIS, Division of Warner-Lambert Company, Morris Plains, New Jersey 07950.

Parke-Davis—Cont.

dizziness, headache, fever, thirst, and dimness of vision.

Overdosage:
Overdosage of 200 to 500 mg/kg is in the fatal range. Early symptoms are CNS stimulation with vomiting, hyperpnea, hyperactivity, and possibly convulsions. This progresses quickly to depression, coma, respiratory failure, and collapse. These symptoms are accompanied by severe electrolyte disturbances.
In the treatment of salicylate overdosage, intensive supportive therapy should be instituted immediately. Plasma salicylate levels should be measured in order to determine the severity of the poisoning and to provide a guide for therapy. Emptying of the stomach should be accomplished as soon as possible with ipecac syrup unless the patient is depressed. In depressed patients use airway protected gastric lavage. Delay absorption with activated charcoal and give a saline cathartic. Proceed according to Standard Reference Procedures for Salicylate Intoxication.

Dosage and Administration:
Usual Adult Dosage: One tablet 3 to 4 times daily.
If necessary, dosage may be increased until relief is obtained, but dosage should be maintained slightly below that which produces tinnitus. Plasma salicylate levels may also be helpful in determining proper dosage (see Clinical Pharmacology section).

How Supplied: Easprin enteric coated tablets each containing 15 grains (975 mg) aspirin are available:
N 0071-0490-24—Bottles of 100
Storage: Store at controlled room temperature 59° to 86°F (15° to 30°C).

0490G010

ELASE® ℞
(fibrinolysin and desoxyribonuclease, combined [bovine])
ELASE OINTMENT ℞
(fibrinolysin and desoxyribonuclease, combined [bovine], ointment)
ELASE–CHLOROMYCETIN® OINTMENT ℞
(fibrinolysin and desoxyribonuclease, combined [bovine], with chloramphenicol ointment)

Description: Elase is a combination of two lytic enzymes, fibrinolysin and desoxyribonuclease, supplied as a lyophilized powder and in an ointment base of liquid petrolatum and polyethylene. The fibrinolysin component is derived from bovine plasma and the desoxyribonuclease is isolated in a purified form from bovine pancreas. The fibrinolysin used in the combination is activated by chloroform.
Elase-Chloromycetin Ointment: Elase-Chloromycetin Ointment contains two lytic enzymes, fibrinolysin and desoxyribonuclease, combined with chloramphenicol in an ointment base.
Chloramphenicol is a broad-spectrum antibiotic originally isolated from *Streptomyces venezuelae.* It is therapeutically active against a wide variety of susceptible organisms, both gram-positive and gram-negative. Chemically, chloramphenicol may be identified as D(-)-*threo*-1-*p*-nitrophenyl -2 -dichloroacetamido-1, 3-propanediol.

Action: Combination of these two enzymes is based on the observation that purulent exudates consist largely of fibrinous material and nucleoprotein. Desoxyribonuclease attacks the desoxyribonucleic acid (DNA) and fibrinolysin attacks principally fibrin of blood clots and fibrinous exudates.
The activity of desoxyribonuclease is limited principally to the production of large polynucleotides, which are less likely to be absorbed than the more diffusible protein fractions liberated by certain enzyme preparations obtained from bacteria. The fibrinolytic action of Elase and of the enzymes in Elase Ointment and Elase-Chloromycetin Ointment is directed mainly against denatured proteins, such as those found in devitalized tissue, while protein elements of living cells remain relatively unaffected.
Elase, Elase Ointment, and Elase-Chloromycetin Ointment are combinations of active enzymes. This is an important consideration in treating patients suffering from lesions resulting from impaired circulation.
The enzymatic action of Elase helps to produce clean surfaces and thus supports healing in a variety of exudative lesions.
Elase-Chloromycetin Ointment:
Chloramphenicol is a broad-spectrum antibiotic that is primarily bacteriostatic and acts by inhibition of protein synthesis by interfering with the transfer of activated amino acids from soluble RNA to ribosomes. Development of resistance to chloramphenicol can be regarded as minimal for staphylococci and many other species of bacteria.
The action of Elase-Chloromycetin helps to produce clean surfaces and thus supports healing in a variety of exudative lesions.

Indications: Elase and Elase Ointment are indicated for topical use as debriding agents in a variety of inflammatory and infected lesions. These include: (1) general surgical wounds; (2) ulcerative lesions—trophic, decubitus, stasis, arteriosclerotic; (3) second- and third-degree burns; (4) circumcision and episiotomy. Elase and Elase Ointment are used intravaginally in: (1) cervicitis—benign, postpartum, and postconization, and (2) vaginitis. Elase is used as an irrigating agent in the following conditions: (1) infected wounds—abscesses, fistulae, and sinus tracts; (2) otorhinolaryngologic wounds; (3) superficial hematomas (except when the hematoma is adjacent to or within adipose tissue).
Elase-Chloromycetin Ointment:
Elase-Chloromycetin Ointment is indicated for use in the treatment of infected lesions, such as burns, ulcers, and wounds where the actions of both a debriding agent and a topical antibiotic are desired. This dual-purpose approach is especially useful in the treatment of infections caused by organisms that utilize a process of fibrin deposition as protective device (ie, coagulase and the staphylococcus). Appropriate measures should be taken to determine the susceptibility of the pathogen to chloramphenicol.

Contraindications: These products (Elase, Elase Ointment, Elase-Chloromycetin Ointment) are contraindicated in individuals with a history of hypersensitivity reactions to any of their components. Elase is not recommended for parenteral use because the bovine fibrinolysin may be antigenic.

Warnings: ***Elase-Chloromycetin Ointment:***
Bone marrow hypoplasia, including aplastic anemia and death, has been reported following the local application of chloramphenicol.

Precautions: ***Elase-Chloromycetin Ointment:***
The prolonged use of antibiotics may occasionally result in overgrowth of nonsusceptible organisms, including fungi. If new infections appear during medication, the drug should be discontinued and appropriate measures should be taken.
In all except very superficial infections, the topical use of chloramphenicol should be supplemented by appropriate systemic medication.
Elase, Elase Ointment, Elase-Chloromycetin Ointment: The usual precautions against allergic reactions should be observed, particularly in persons with a history of sensitivity to materials of bovine origin or to mercury compounds.
Elase: To be maximally effective, Elase solutions must be freshly prepared before use. The loss in activity is reduced by refrigeration; however, even when stored in a refrigerator, the solution should not be used 24 hours or more after reconstitution.

Adverse Reactions: Side effects attributable to the enzymes have not been a problem at the dose and for the indications recommended herein. With higher concentrations, side effects have been minimal, consisting of local hyperemia.
Chills and fever attributable to antigenic action of profibrinolysin activators of bacterial origin are not a problem with Elase, Elase Ointment, or Elase-Chloromycetin Ointment.
Elase-Chloromycetin Ointment: Signs of local irritation, with subjective symptoms of itching or burning, angioneurotic edema, urticaria, vesicular and maculopapular dermatitis have been reported in patients sensitive to chloramphenicol and are causes for discontinuing the medication. Similar sensitivity reactions to other materials in topical preparations may also occur. Blood dyscrasias have been associated with the use of chloramphenicol.

Preparation of Elase Solution: The contents of each vial may be reconstituted with 10 ml of isotonic sodium chloride solution. Higher or lower concentrations can be prepared if desired by varying the amount of the diluent.

Dosage and Administration: Since the conditions for which Elase and Elase Ointment and Elase-Chloromycetin Ointment are helpful vary considerably in severity, dosage must be adjusted to the individual case; however, the following general recommendations can be made.
Successful use of enzymatic debridement depends on several factors: (1) dense, dry eschar, if present, should be removed surgically before enzymatic debridement is attempted; (2) the enzyme must be in constant contact with the substrate; (3) accumulated necrotic debris must be periodically removed; (4) the enzyme must be replenished at least once daily; and (5) secondary closure or skin grafting must be employed as soon as possible after optimal debridement has been attained. It is further essential that wound-dressing techniques be performed carefully under aseptic conditions and that appropriate systemically acting antibiotics be administered concomitantly if, in the opinion of the physician, they are indicated.
General Topical Uses: ***Elase Ointment:*** Local application should be repeated at intervals for as long as enzyme action is desired. After application Elase Ointment becomes rapidly and progressively less active and is probably exhausted for practical purposes at the end of 24 hours. A recommended procedure for application of Elase Ointment follows.

1. Clean the wound with water, peroxide, or normal saline and dry area gently. If there is a dense, dry eschar present, it should be removed surgically before applying Elase.
2. Apply a *thin* layer of Elase Ointment.
3. Cover with petrolatum gauze or another type of nonadhering dressing.
4. Change the dressing at least ONCE a day, preferably two or three times daily. Frequency of application is more important than the amount of Elase used. Flush away the necrotic debris and fibrinous exudates with saline, peroxide, or warm water so that newly applied ointment can be in direct contact with the substrate.

Elase: Local application should be repeated at intervals for as long as enzyme action is desired. Elase solution may be applied topically as a liquid, spray, or wet dressing. Application of a gentle spray of the solution can be accomplished by using a conventional atomizer. After application, Elase, especially in solution, becomes rapidly and progressively less active and is probably exhausted for practical purposes at the end of 24 hours. The dry material for solution is stable at room temperature through the expiration date printed on the package. A recommended procedure for application of a solution of Elase using a Wet-to-Dry method follows.

1. Mix one vial of Elase powder with 10 to 50 ml of saline and saturate strips of fine-mesh gauze or an unfolded sterile gauze sponge with the Elase solution.
2. Pack ulcerated area with the Elase-saturated gauze, making sure the gauze remains in contact with the necrotic substrate (if the lesion is covered with a heavy eschar, it must be removed surgically before wet-to-dry debridement is begun).
3. ALLOW GAUZE TO DRY IN CONTACT WITH THE ULCERATED LESION (approximately six to eight hours). As the gauze dries, the necrotic tissues slough and become enmeshed in the gauze.
4. Remove dried gauze. This mechanically debrides the area. Repeat wet-to-dry procedure three or four times daily, since frequent dressing changes greatly enhance results. After two, three, or four days, the area becomes clean and starts to fill in with granulation tissue.

Intravaginal use: ***Elase Ointment:*** In mild to moderate vaginitis and cervicitis, 5 ml of Elase Ointment should be deposited deep in the vagina once nightly at bedtime for approximately five applications, or until the entire contents of one 30-g tube has been used. The patient should be checked by her physician to determine possible need for further therapy. In more severe cervicitis and vaginitis, some physicians prefer to initiate therapy with an application of Elase (fibrinolysin and desoxyribonuclease, combined, [bovine]) in solution. See Elase package insert.

Elase: In severe cervicitis and vaginitis, the physician may instill 10 ml of the solution intravaginally, wait one or two minutes for the enzyme to disperse and then insert a cotton tampon in the vaginal canal. The tampon should be removed the next day. Continuing therapy should then be instituted with Elase Ointment (fibrinolysin and desoxyribonuclease, combined [bovine] ointment). See Elase Ointment package insert.

Abscesses, empyema cavities, fistulae, sinus tracts or subcutaneous hematomas: Despite the contraindication against parenteral use, Elase has been used in irrigating these specific conditions. The Elase solution should be drained and replaced at intervals of six to ten hours to reduce the amount of by-product accumulation and minimize loss of enzyme activity. Traces of blood in the discharge usually indicate active filling in of the cavity.

How Supplied:
ELASE (fibrinolysin and desoxyribonuclease, combined [bovine])
N 0071-4256-01 Elase—lyophilized powder for solution
Elase is supplied in rubber diaphragm-capped vials of 30-ml capacity containing 25 units (Loomis) of fibrinolysin and 15,000 units (modified Christensen method) of desoxyribonuclease with 0.1 mg thimerosal (mercury derivative).
This product also contains sodium chloride and sucrose as incidental ingredients.

121 876350/ZF

ELASE OINTMENT (fibrinolysin and desoxyribonuclease, combined [bovine], ointment)
N 0071-4279-10 Elase Ointment, 10 g.
The 10-g tube contains 10 units of fibrinolysin and 6,666 units of desoxyribonuclease with 0.04 mg thimerosal (mercury derivative) in a special ointment base of liquid petrolatum and polyethylene.
N 0071-4279-13 Elase Ointment, 30 g.
The 30-g tube contains 30 units of fibrinolysin and 20,000 units of desoxyribonuclease with 0.12 mg thimerosal (mercury derivative) in a special ointment base of liquid petrolatum and polyethylene. For gynecologic use, six disposable vaginal applicators (V-Applicator*) as a separate package are available for this tube when required to facilitate administration of the proper dose.
These products also contain sodium chloride and sucrose as incidental ingredients.

121 855100/ZF

ELASE-CHLOROMYCETIN OINTMENT (fibrinolysin and desoxyribonuclease, combined [bovine], with chloramphenicol ointment)
Elase-Chloromycetin (fibrinolysin-desoxyribonuclease-chloramphenicol) is supplied in 30-g and 10-g ointment tubes. The 10-g tubes have an elongated nozzle to facilitate the application to surface lesions.
The 30-g tubes contain 30 units (Loomis) of fibrinolysin (bovine) and 20,000 units** of desoxyribonuclease with 0.12 mg thimerosal (mercury derivative) (as a preservative) and 0.3 g† chloramphenicol in a special ointment base of liquid petrolatum and polyethylene.
The 10-g tubes contain 10 units (Loomis) of fibrinolysin (bovine) and 6,666 units** of desoxyribonuclease with 0.04 mg thimerosal (mercury derivative) (as a preservative) and 0.1 g† chloramphenicol in a special ointment base of liquid petrolatum and polyethylene.
The ointment contains sodium chloride and sucrose used in its manufacture.
*Trademark
**Modified Christensen method.
†10 mg chloramphenicol per gram, or 1%.

121 863300/ZD

ELDEC® KAPSEALS® ℞

Composition: Each capsule contains vitamin A (acetate), 1,667 IU; vitamin C (ascorbic acid), 66.7 mg; vitamin B_1 (thiamine mononitrate), 10 mg; vitamin B_2 (riboflavin), 0.87 mg; vitamin B_6 (pyridoxine hydrochloride), 0.67 mg; nicotinamide (niacinamide), 16.7 mg; *dl*-panthenol, 10 mg; ferrous sulfate, dried, 16.7 mg; iodine (as potassium iodide), 0.05 mg; calcium carbonate, precipitated, 66.7 mg; vitamin E (*dl*-alpha tocopheryl acetate), (10 mg) 10 IU; vitamin B_{12} (cyanocobalamin), 2 mcg; folic acid, 0.33 mg.
Action and Uses: For certain vitamin and mineral deficiencies.
Caution—Folic acid in doses above 0.1 mg daily may obscure pernicious anemia in that hematologic remission can occur while neurological manifestations remain progressive.
Dosage: The usual dosage of Eldec is one capsule three times a day.
How Supplied: N 0071-0337-24 Eldec (Kapseal 398), bottles of 100. Parcode® No. 337; new ID code imprint, formerly 398—no formula change.
[*Shown in Product Identification Section*]

ERGOSTAT® ℞
(ergotamine tartrate tablets)
Sublingual Tablets

Description: Each sublingual tablet contains 2 mg ergotamine tartrate.
Action: Ergotamine is an alpha-adrenergic blocking agent with a direct stimulating effect on the smooth muscle of peripheral and cranial blood vessels and produces depression of central vasomotor centers. Ergostat also has the properties of a serotonin antagonist.
Ergostat (ergotamine tartrate tablets) exerts a direct effect on cranial blood vessels, causing vasoconstriction, with concomitant decrease in the pulsations probably responsible for migraine and other vascular headache symptoms. Ergostat is thus generally considered to be a specific agent for therapy in this condition.
Because ergotamine is a nonnarcotic, it avoids the dangers inherent with repeated use of narcotics in the treatment of frequent migraine attacks.
Indications: Vascular headaches, such as migraine and cluster headache (histaminic cephalalgia)
Precautions: Avoid prolonged administration or dosage in excess of that recommended because of the danger of ergotism and gangrene.
Contraindications: Contraindicated in sepsis, occlusive vascular disease (thromboangiitis obliterans, luetic arteritis, severe arteriosclerosis, coronary artery disease, thrombophlebitis, Raynaud's disease), hepatic disease, renal disease, severe pruritus, hypertension, and pregnancy; hypersensitivity to ergot alkaloids
Adverse Reactions: When prescribed in correct dosage, in the absence of contraindications, ergotamine is a safe and useful drug; few serious complications have been reported from its use in the migraine syndrome. Unpleasant side effects which may occur include nausea and vomiting, diarrhea, weakness in the legs, muscle pains in the extremities, numbness and tingling of fingers and toes, precordial distress and pain, and transient tachycardia or bradycardia. Localized edema and itching may occur in the rare sensitive patient. Side effects are usually not such as to necessitate interruption of therapy.
Dosage and Administration: All efforts should be made to initiate therapy as soon as possible after the first symptoms of the attack are noted, because success is proportional to rapidity of treatment, and lower dosages will be effective. At the first sign of an attack, or to relieve the symptoms of the full-blown attack, one sublingual tablet (2 mg) is placed under the tongue. Another sublingual tablet (2 mg) should be placed under the tongue at half-hour intervals thereafter, if necessary, for a total of three tablets (6 mg). Dosage must not exceed three tablets (6 mg) in any 24-hour period. Limit dosage to not more than five tablets (10 mg) in any one week.
How Supplied: N 0071-0111-13 — Ergostat (ergotamine tartrate tablets) Sublingual Tablets, 2 mg, each in an individual foil pouch with two strips of 12 pouches packaged in a plastic vial.
AHFS 12:16 **YB**
[*Shown in Product Identification Section*]

ERYC® ℞
(Erythromycin Capsules, USP)

Description: ERYC Capsules contain enteric-coated pellets of erythromycin base for oral administration. Erythromycin is produced by a strain of *Streptomyces erythraeus* and belongs to the macrolide group of antibiotics. It is basic and readily forms salts with acids, but it is the base which is microbiologically active. Each ERYC Capsule contains 250 milligrams of erythromycin base. Erythromycin base is 14-Ethyl-7, 12, 13-trihydroxy-3, 5, 7, 9, 11, 13-hexamethyl- 2, 10- dioxo-6-[(3, 4, 6-trideoxy-3-(dimethylamino) -*β*-D*xylo*-hexapyranosyl)oxy] oxacyclotetradec-4-yl 2, 6-dideoxy-3-C-methyl-3-O-methyl-*α*L-*ribo*-hexopyranoside.
Clinical Pharmacology: Orally administered erythromycin base and its salts are readily absorbed in the microbiologically active form. Inter-individual variations in the absorption of erythromycin are, however, observed, and some patients do not achieve acceptable serum levels. Erythromycin is largely bound to plasma proteins, and the freely dissociating bound fraction after administration of erythromycin base represents 90% of the total erythromycin absorbed. After absorption erythromycin diffuses readily into most body fluids. In the absence of meningeal inflammation, low concentrations are normally achieved in the spinal fluid but the passage of the drug across the blood-brain barrier increases in meningitis. Erythromycin is excreted in breast

Continued on next page

This product information was prepared in August, 1982. On these and other Parke-Davis Products, information may be obtained by addressing PARKE-DAVIS, Division of Warner-Lambert Company, Morris Plains, New Jersey 07950.

Parke-Davis—Cont.

milk. The drug crosses the placental barrier but fetal plasma levels are low.

In the presence of normal hepatic function erythromycin is concentrated in the liver and is excreted in the bile; the effect of hepatic dysfunction on biliary excretion of erythromycin is not known. After oral administration less than 5% of the administered dose can be recovered in the active form in the urine.

The enteric coating of pellets in ERYC Capsules protects the erythromycin base from inactivation by gastric acidity. Because of their small size and enteric coating, the pellets readily pass intact from the stomach to the small intestine and dissolve efficiently to allow absorption of erythromycin in a uniform manner. After administration of a single dose of a 250 mg ERYC capsule, peak serum levels in the range of 1.13 to 1.68 mcg/ml are attained in approximately 3 hours and decline to 0.30-0.42 mcg/ml in 6 hours. Optimal conditions for stability in the presence of gastric secretion and for complete absorption are attained when ERYC is taken on an empty stomach.

Microbiology Erythromycin acts by inhibition of protein synthesis by binding 50 S ribosomal subunits of susceptible organisms. It does not affect nucleic acid synthesis. Antagonism has been demonstrated between clindamycin and erythromycin. Resistance to erythromycin by some strains of *Haemophilus influenzae* and staphylococci has been demonstrated. Specimens should be obtained for culture and susceptibility testing.

Erythromycin is usually active against the following organisms in *vitro* and in clinical infections:

Streptococcus pyogenes
Alpha hemolytic streptococci (viridans group)
Staphylococcus aureus (Resistant organisms may emerge during treatment.)
Streptococcus pneumoniae
Mycoplasma pneumoniae (Eaton's Agent)
Haemophilus influenzae (Many strains are resistant to erythromycin alone, but are susceptible to erythromycin and sulfonamides together.)
Treponema pallidum
Corynebacterium diphtheriae
Corynebacterium minutissimum
Entamoeba histolytica
Listeria monocytogenes
Neisseria gonorrhoeae
Bordetella pertussis
Legionella pneumophila (agent of Legionnaires' Disease)

Susceptibility Testing Quantitative methods that require measurement of zone diameters give the most precise estimates of antibiotic susceptibility. One such standardized single disc procedure has been recommended for use with discs to test susceptibility to erythromycin.[1] Interpretation involves correlation of the zone diameters obtained in the disc test with minimum inhibitory concentration (MIC) values for erythromycin.

Reports from the laboratory giving results of the standardized single-disc susceptibility test using a 15 mcg erythromycin disc should be interpreted according to the following criteria:

Susceptible organisms produce zones of 18 mm or greater indicating that the tested organism is likely to respond to therapy.

Resistant organisms produce zones of 13 mm or less, indicating that other therapy should be selected.

Organisms of intermediate susceptibility produce zones of 14 to 17 mm. The "intermediate" category provides a "buffer zone" which should prevent small uncontrolled technical factors from causing major discrepancies in interpretations, thus when a zone diameter falls within the "intermediate" range, the results may be considered equivocal. If alternate drugs are not available, confirmation by dilution tests may be indicated.

A bacterial isolate may be considered susceptible if the MIC value[2] (minimal inhibitory concentration) for erythromycin is not more than 2 mcg/ml. Organisms are considered resistant if the MIC is 8 mcg/ml or higher.

Indications and Usage:

ERYC is indicated in children and adults for the treatment of the following conditions:

Upper respiratory tract infections of mild to moderate degree caused by *Streptococcus pyogenes* (group A beta hemolytic streptococci); *Streptococcus pneumoniae (Diplococcus pneumoniae): Haemophilus influenzae* (when used concomitantly with adequate doses of sulfonamides, since not all strains of *H influenzae* are susceptible at the erythromycin concentrations ordinarily achieved). (See appropriate sulfonamide labeling for prescribing information.)

Lower respiratory tract infections of mild to moderate severity caused by *Streptococcus pyogenes* (group A beta hemolytic streptococci): *Streptococcus pneumoniae (Diplococcus pneumoniae).*

Respiratory tract infections due to *Mycoplasma pneumoniae (Eaton's agent).*

Pertussis (whooping cough) caused by *Bordetella pertussis.* Erythromycin is effective in eliminating the organism from the nasopharynx of infected individuals, rendering them noninfectious. Some clinical studies suggest that erythromycin may be helpful in the prophylaxis of pertussis in exposed susceptible individuals.

Diphtheria—As an adjunct to antitoxin in infections due to *Corynebacterium diphtheriae,* to prevent establishment of carriers and to eradicate the organism in carriers.

Erythrasma—In the treatment of infections due to *Corynebacterium minutissimum.*

Intestinal amebiasis caused by *Entamoeba histolytica* (oral erythromycins only). Extraenteric amebiasis requires treatment with other agents.

Infections due to *Listeria monocytogenes.*

Skin and soft tissue infections of mild to moderate severity caused by *Streptococcus pyogenes* and *Staphylococcus aureus* (Resistant staphylococci may emerge during treatment.)

Primary syphilis caused by *Treponema pallidum.* Erythromycin (oral forms only) is an alternate choice of treatment for primary syphilis in patients allergic to the penicillins. In treatment of primary syphilis, spinal fluid should be examined before treatment and as part of the follow-up after therapy.

The use of erythromycin for the treatment of *in utero* syphilis is not recommended (See CLINICAL PHARMACOLOGY).

Legionnaires' disease caused by *Legionella pneumophila.*

Although no controlled clinical efficacy studies have been conducted, *in vitro* and limited preliminary clinical data suggest that erythromycin may be effective in treating Legionnaires' disease.

Therapy with erythromycin should be monitored by bacteriological studies and by clinical response (See CLINICAL PHARMACOLOGY—Microbiology).

Injectable benzathine penicillin G is considered by the American Heart Association to be the drug of choice in the treatment and prevention of streptococcal pharyngitis and in long-term prophylaxis of rheumatic fever.

When oral medication is preferred for treatment of the above conditions, penicillin G, V, or erythromycin are alternate drugs of choice.

Although no controlled clinical efficacy trials have been conducted, erythromycin has been suggested by the American Heart Association and the American Dental Association for use in a regimen for prophylaxis against bacterial endocarditis in patients allergic to penicillin who have congenital and/or rheumatic or other acquired valvular heart disease when they undergo dental procedures and surgical procedures of the upper respiratory tract.[3] (Erythromycin is not suitable prior to genitourinary surgery where the organisms likely to lead to bacteremia are gram-negative bacilli or the enterococcal group of streptococci).

NOTE: When selecting antibiotics for the prevention of bacterial endocarditis the physician or dentist should read the full joint 1977 statement of the American Heart Association and the American Dental Association.[3]

Contraindication: ERYC is contraindicated in patients with known hypersensitivity to this antibiotic.

Warning: There have been a few reports of hepatic dysfunction, with or without jaundice, occurring in patients receiving erythromycin ethylsuccinate, base, and stearate products.

Precautions: Caution should be exercised when erythromycin is administered to patients with impaired hepatic function (see CLINICAL PHARMACOLOGY and WARNING).

Erythromycin use in patients who are receiving high doses of theophylline may be associated with an increase in serum theophylline levels and potential theophylline toxicity. In case of theophylline toxicity and/or elevated serum theophylline levels, the dose of theophylline should be reduced while the patient is receiving concomitant erythromycin therapy.

Erythromycin interferes with the fluorometric determination of urinary catecholamines.

Prolonged or repeated use of erythromycin may result in an overgrowth of nonsusceptible bacteria or fungi. If superinfection occurs, erythromycin should be discontinued and appropriate therapy instituted.

When indicated, incision and drainage or other surgical procedures should be performed in conjunction with antibiotic therapy.

Pregnancy Category B—Reproduction studies have been performed in rats, mice and rabbits using erythromycin and its various salts and esters, at doses which were several times multiples of the usual human dose. No evidence of impaired fertility or harm to the fetus that appeared related to erythromycin was reported in these studies. There are, however, no adequate and well-controlled studies in pregnant women. Because animal reproduction studies are not always predictive of human response, this drug should be used during pregnancy only if clearly needed.

Labor and Delivery—The effect of ERYC on labor and delivery is unknown.

Nursing Mothers—Erythromycin is excreted in milk (see CLINICAL PHARMACOLOGY).

Pediatric Use—See INDICATIONS AND USAGE and DOSAGE AND ADMINISTRATION.

Adverse Reactions: The most frequent side effects of oral erythromycin preparations are gastrointestinal and are dose-related. They include nausea, vomiting, abdominal pain, diarrhea and anorexia. Symptoms of hepatic dysfunction and/or abnormal liver function test results may occur (see WARNING).

Mild allergic reactions such as rashes with or without pruritus, urticaria, bullous fixed eruptions, and eczema have been reported with erythromycin. Serious allergic reactions, including anaphylaxis have been reported.

A few cases of transient deafness have been reported with high doses of erythromycin.

Dosage and Administration: Optimum and uniform serum levels of erythromycin are obtained when ERYC Capsules are administered one hour before meals or in the fasting state.

ADULTS: The usual dose is 250 mg every 6 hours taken one hour before meals. If twice-a-day dosage is desired, the recommended dose is 500 mg every 12 hours. Dosage may be increased up to 4 grams per day, accord-

ing to the severity of infection. Twice-a-day dosing is not recommended when doses larger than 1 gram daily are administered.
CHILDREN: Age, weight, and severity of the infection are important factors in determining the proper dosage. The usual dosage is 30 to 50 mg/kg/day in divided doses. For the treatment of more severe infections, this dose may be doubled.

Streptococcal infections: A therapeutic dosage of oral erythromycin should be administered for at least 10 days. For continuous prophylaxis against recurrences of streptococcal infections in persons with a history of rheumatic heart disease, the dose is 250 mg twice a day.
For the prevention of bacterial endocarditis in penicillin-allergic patients with valvular heart disease who are to undergo dental procedures or surgical procedures of the upper respiratory tract, the adult dose is 1.0 grams orally (20 mg/kg for children) one and one-half to 2 hours prior to the procedure and then 500 mg (10 mg/kg for children) orally every 6 hours for 8 doses.[3] (See INDICATIONS AND USAGE).

Primary syphilis: 30-40 grams given in divided doses over a period of 10-15 days.

Intestinal amebiasis: 250 mg four times daily for 10 to 14 days for adults; 30 to 50 mg/kg/day in divided doses for 10 to 14 days for children.

Legionnaires' Disease: Although optimal doses have not been established, doses utilized in reported clinical data were those recommended above (1 to 4 grams daily in divided doses).

Pertussis: Although optimum dosage and duration of therapy have not been established, doses of erythromycin utilized in reported clinical studies were 40-50 mg/kg/day, given in divided doses for 5 to 14 days.

How Supplied:
ERYC (Capsule 696), clear and orange opaque capsules, each containing 250 mg erythromycin as enteric coated pellets, are available as follows:
N 0071-0696-24 Bottles of 100
N 0071-0696-30 Bottles of 500
N 0071-0696-40 Unit dose package of 100 (10 strips of 10 capsules each).

Storage Conditions: Store at a room temperature below 30°C (86°F). Protect from moisture and light.

References:

1. Approved Standard ASM-2 "Performance Standards for Anti-microbial Disc Susceptibility Test." National Committee for Clinical Laboratory Standards. 771 East Lancaster Avenue, Villanova. PA 19085.
2. Ericson, H.M. and Sherris, J.C.: "Antibiotic Sensitivity Testing Report of an International Collaborative Study." *Acta Pathologica et Microbiologica Scandinavica.* Section B. Supp. 217, 1971, pp. 1-90.
3. Am. Heart Assoc. and Am. Dental Assoc. "Prevention of Bacterial Endocarditis." *Circulation.*" Vol. 56, No. 1, July, 1977. 139A-143A.

[*Shown in Product Identification Section*]

0696G011

ERYTHROMYCIN STEARATE TABLETS, USP ℞

(Erypar®)

Description: Erythromycin is produced by a strain of *Streptomyces erythraeus* and belongs to the macrolide group of antibiotics. It is basic and readily forms salts with acids. The base, the stearate salt, and the esters are poorly soluble in water, and are suitable for oral administration.
The film-coated tablets contain 250 mg or 500 mg of erythromycin as erythromycin stearate, USP. Each tablet is buffered with sodium citrate.

Clinical Pharmacology: The mode of action of erythromycin is by inhibition of protein synthesis without affecting nucleic acid synthesis. Resistance to erythromycin of some strains of *Hemophilus influenzae* and staphylococci has been demonstrated. Culture and susceptibility testing should be done. If the Kirby-Bauer method of disc susceptibility is used, a 15-mcg erythromycin disc should give a zone diameter of at least 18 mm when tested against an erythromycin-susceptible organism.
Orally administered erythromycin is readily absorbed by most patients, especially on an empty stomach, but patient variation is observed.
After absorption, erythromycin diffuses readily into most body fluids. In the absence of meningeal inflammation, low concentrations are normally achieved in the spinal fluid, but passage of the drug across the blood-brain barrier increases in meningitis. In the presence of normal hepatic function, erythromycin is concentrated in the liver and excreted in the bile; the effect of hepatic dysfunction on excretion of erythromycin by the liver into the bile is not known. After oral administration, less than 5 percent of the activity of the administered dose can be recovered in the urine.
Erythromycin crosses the placental barrier but fetal plasma levels are generally low.

Indications and Usage: *Streptococcus pyogenes* (Group A beta-hemolytic *Streptococcus*): Upper and lower respiratory tract, skin, and soft-tissue infections of mild to moderate severity
Injectable benzathine penicillin G is considered by the American Heart Association to be the drug of choice in the treatment and prevention of streptococcal pharyngitis and in the long-term prophylaxis of rheumatic fever.
When oral medication is preferred for treatment of streptococcal pharyngitis, penicillin G, V, or erythromycin are alternate drugs of choice.
When oral medication is given, the importance of strict adherence by the patient to the prescribed dosage regimen must be stressed. A therapeutic dose should be administered for at least 10 days.
Although no controlled clinical efficacy trials have been conducted, oral erythromycin has been suggested by the American Heart Association and American Dental Association for use in a regimen for prophylaxis against bacterial endocarditis in patients hypersensitive to penicillin who have congenital heart disease or rheumatic or other acquired valvular heart disease when they undergo dental procedures and surgical procedures of the upper respiratory tract.[1] Erythromycin is not suitable prior to genitourinary or gastrointestinal tract surgery.
Note: When selecting antibiotics for the prevention of bacterial endocarditis, the physician or dentist should read the full joint statement of the American Heart Association and the American Dental Association.[1]
Staphylococcus aureus: Acute infections of skin and soft tissue of mild to moderate severity. Resistant organisms may emerge during treatment.
Diplococcus pneumoniae: Upper respiratory tract infections (eg, otitis media, pharyngitis) and lower respiratory tract infections (eg, pneumonia) of mild to moderate degree
Mycoplasma pneumoniae (Eaton agent, PPLO): In the treatment of primary atypical pneumonia, when due to this organism
Treponema pallidum: Erythromycin is an alternate choice of treatment for primary syphilis in patients allergic to the penicillins. In treatment of primary syphilis, spinal fluid examinations should be done before treatment and as part of follow-up after therapy.
Corynebacterium diphtheriae and *C minutissimum:* As an adjunct to antitoxin, to prevent establishment of carriers, and to eradicate the organism in carriers
In the treatment of erythrasma
Entamoeba histolytica: In the treatment of intestinal amebiasis only. Extra-enteric amebiasis requires treatment with other agents.
Listeria monocytogenes: Infections due to this organism
Legionnaires' Disease: Although no controlled clinical efficacy studies have been conducted, *in vitro* and limited preliminary clinical data suggest that erythromycin may be effective in treating Legionnaires' Disease.

Contraindication: Erythromycin is contraindicated in patients with known hypersensitivity to this antibiotic.

Precautions: Erythromycin is principally excreted by the liver. Caution should be exercised in administering the antibiotic to patients with impaired hepatic function. There have been reports of hepatic dysfunction, with or without jaundice, occurring in patients receiving oral erythromycin products.
Recent data from studies of erythromycin reveal that its use in patients who are receiving high doses of theophylline may be associated with an increase of serum theophylline levels and potential theophylline toxicity. In case of theophylline toxicity and/or elevated serum theophylline levels, the dose of theophylline should be reduced while the patient is receiving concomitant erythromycin therapy.
Surgical procedures should be performed when indicated.

Usage during pregnancy and lactation: The safety of erythromycin for use during pregnancy has not been established.
Erythromycin crosses the placental barrier. Erythromycin also appears in breast milk.

Adverse Reactions: The most frequent side effects of oral erythromycin preparations are gastrointestinal, such as abdominal cramping and discomfort, and are dose-related. Nausea, vomiting, and diarrhea occur infrequently with usual oral doses.
During prolonged or repeated therapy, there is a possibility of overgrowth of nonsusceptible bacteria or fungi. If such infections occur, the drug should be discontinued and appropriate therapy instituted.
Mild allergic reactions, such as urticaria and other skin rashes, have occurred. Serious allergic reactions, including anaphylaxis, have been reported.

Dosage and Administration: Optimum blood levels are obtained when doses are given on an empty stomach.
Adults: 250 mg every six hours is the usual dose; or 500 mg every 12 hours, one hour before meals. Dosage may be increased up to 4 grams per day according to the severity of the infection.
Children: Age, weight, and severity of the infection are important factors in determining the proper dosage: 30 to 50 mg/kg/day, in divided doses, is the usual dose. For more severe infections, this dosage may be doubled.
If dosage is desired on a twice-a-day schedule in either adults or children, one half of the total daily dose may be given every 12 hours, one hour before meals.
In the treatment of streptococcal infections, a therapeutic dosage of erythromycin should be administered for at least 10 days. In continuous *prophylaxis* of streptococcal infections in persons with a history of rheumatic heart disease, the dose is 250 mg twice a day.
For prophylaxis against bacterial endocarditis[1] in patients with congenital heart disease or rheumatic or other acquired valvular heart disease when undergoing dental procedures or surgical procedures of the upper respiratory tract, give 1.0 gm (20 mg/kg for children) orally

Continued on next page

This product information was prepared in August, 1982. On these and other Parke-Davis Products, information may be obtained by addressing PARKE-DAVIS, Division of Warner-Lambert Company, Morris Plains, New Jersey 07950.

Parke-Davis—Cont.

1½-2 hours before the procedure, and then 500 mg (10 mg/kg for children) orally every 6 hours for 8 doses.
For treatment of primary syphilis: 30 to 40 grams given in divided doses over a period of 10 to 15 days.
For dysenteric amebiasis: Adults: 250 mg four times daily for 10 to 14 days. Children: 30 to 50 mg/kg/day in divided doses for 10 to 14 days.
For treatment of Legionnaires' Disease: Although optimal doses have not been established, doses utilized in reported clinical data were those recommended above (1 to 4 grams erythromycin stearate daily in divided doses).
How Supplied:
Erythromycin Stearate Tablets, USP are supplied as:
N 0071-0672-24—bottle of 100
N 0071-0672-30—bottle of 500
N 0071-0672-40—unit dose (10/10's)
Each film-coated tablet contains 250 mg erythromycin as erythromycin stearate.
N 0071-0919-24—bottle of 100
Each film-coated tablet contains 500 mg erythromycin as erythromycin stearate.
AHFS 8:12.12 **0672G010**
[*Shown in Product Identification Section*]
Reference:
1. American Heart Association. Prevention of bacterial endocarditis. *Circulation.* 56:139A-143A 1977.

ESTROVIS® ℞
(Quinestrol tablets, USP)*

*Product of Warner-Lambert Inc

Warning:
1. Estrogens Have Been Reported to Increase the Risk of Endometrial Carcinoma.
Three independent case control studies have shown an increased risk of endometrial cancer in postmenopausal women exposed to exogenous estrogens for prolonged periods.[1–3] This risk was independent of the other known risk factors for endometrial cancer. These studies are further supported by the finding that incidence rates of endometrial cancer have increased sharply since 1969 in eight different areas of the United States with population-based cancer reporting systems, an increase which may be related to the rapidly expanding use of estrogens during the last decade.[4]
The three case control studies reported that the risk of endometrial cancer in estrogen users was about 4.5 to 13.9 times greater than in nonusers. The risk appears to depend on both duration of treatment[1] and on estrogen dose.[3] In view of these findings, when estrogens are used for the treatment of menopausal symptoms, the lowest dose that will control symptoms should be utilized and medication should be discontinued as soon as possible. When prolonged treatment is medically indicated, the patient should be reassessed on at least a semiannual basis to determine the need for continued therapy. Although the evidence must be considered preliminary, one study suggests that cyclic administration of low doses of estrogen may carry less risk than continuous administration.[3] Therefore, while it appears prudent to utilize such a regimen with other orally administered estrogens, Estrovis may be administered, following a seven-day priming schedule, on a once weekly maintenance dosage beginning two weeks after the start of treatment.
Close clinical surveillance of all women taking estrogens is important. In all cases of undiagnosed persistent or recurring abnormal vaginal bleeding, adequate diagnostic measures should be undertaken to rule out malignancy.
There is no evidence at present that "natural" estrogens are more or less hazardous than "synthetic" estrogens at equiestrogenic doses.
2. Estrogens Should not be Used During Pregnancy.
The use of female sex hormones, both estrogens and progestogens, during early pregnancy may seriously damage the offspring. It has been shown that females exposed *in utero* to diethylstilbestrol, a nonsteroidal estrogen, have an increased risk of developing in later life a form of vaginal or cervical cancer that is ordinarily extremely rare.[5–6] This risk has been estimated as not greater than 4 per 1,000 exposures.[7] Furthermore, a high percentage of such exposed women (from 30 to 90%) have been found to have vaginal adenosis,[8–12] epithelial changes of the vagina and cervix. Although these changes are histologically benign, it is not known whether they are precursors of malignancy. Although similar data are not available with the use of other estrogens, it cannot be presumed they would not induce similar changes.
Several reports suggest an association between intrauterine exposure to female sex hormones and congenital anomalies, including congenital heart defects and limb- reduction defects.[13–16] One case control study[16] estimated a 4.7-fold increased risk of limb-reduction defects in infants exposed *in utero* to sex hormones (oral contraceptives, hormone withdrawal tests for pregnancy, or attempted treatment for threatened abortion). Some of these exposures were very short and involved only a few days of treatment. The data suggest that the risk of limb-reduction defects in exposed fetuses is somewhat less than 1 per 1,000.
In the past, female sex hormones have been used during pregnancy in an attempt to treat threatened or habitual abortion. There is considerable evidence that estrogens are ineffective for these indications, and there is no evidence from well-controlled studies that progestogens are effective for these uses.
If Estrovis (quinestrol) is used during pregnancy, or if the patient becomes pregnant while taking this drug, she should be apprised of the potential risks to the fetus and the advisability of pregnancy continuation.

Description: Estrovis (quinestrol) is available as a 100-mcg oral tablet. It is an estrogen. Estrovis (quinestrol) is the 3-cyclopentylether of ethinyl estradiol. The chemical name is 3-cyclopentyloxy-17α-ethynylestra-1, 3, 5 (10)-trien-17β-ol.
It is a white, essentially odorless powder, insoluble in water and soluble in alcohol, chloroform, and ether.
Clinical Pharmacology: Estrovis (quinestrol) is an orally effective estrogen as judged by conventional assay procedures employing vagina and uterine end-points in mice, rats and rabbits.
The estrogenic effects of Estrovis have been demonstrated in clinical studies by its effects on the endometrium, maturation of the vaginal epithelium, thinning of cervical mucus, suppression of pituitary gonadotropin, inhibition of ovulation, and prevention of postpartum breast discomfort.
Indications: Estrovis (quinestrol) is indicated in the treatment of:
1. Moderate to severe vasomotor symptoms associated with the menopause. (There is no evidence that estrogens are effective for nervous symptoms or depression which might occur during menopause, and they should not be used to treat these conditions.)
2. Atrophic vaginitis
3. Kraurosis vulvae
4. Female hypogonadism
5. Female castration
6. Primary ovarian failure

Estrovis (Quinestrol) Has Not Been Shown to be Effective for any Purpose during Pregnancy and Its Use May Cause Severe Harm to the Fetus (See Boxed Warning).
Contraindications: Estrogens should not be used in women (or men) with any of the following conditions:
1. Known or suspected cancer of the breast except in appropriately selected patients being treated for metastatic disease
2. Known or suspected estrogen-dependent neoplasia
3. Known or suspected pregnancy (See Boxed Warning)
4. Undiagnosed abnormal genital bleeding
5. Active thrombophlebitis or thromboembolic disorders
6. A past history of thrombophlebitis, thrombosis, or thromboembolic disorders associated with previous estrogen use (except when used in treatment of breast or prostatic malignancy)

Warnings:
1. *Induction of malignant neoplasms.* Long-term continuous administration of natural and synthetic estrogens in certain animal species increases the frequency of carcinomas of the breast, cervix, vagina, and liver. There is now evidence that estrogens increase the risk of carcinoma of the endometrium in humans. (See Boxed Warning.)
At the present time, there is no satisfactory evidence that estrogens given to postmenopausal women increase the risk of cancer of the breast,[18] although a recent long-term follow up of a single physician's practice has raised this possibility.[18a] Because of the animal data, there is a need for caution in prescribing estrogens for women with a strong family history of breast cancer or who have breast nodules, fibrocystic disease, or abnormal mammograms.
2. *Gallbladder disease.* A recent study has reported a 2- to 3-fold increase in the risk of surgically confirmed gallbladder disease in women receiving postmenopausal estrogens,[18] similar to the 2-fold increase previously noted in users of oral contraceptives.[19–24] In the case of oral contraceptives, the increased risk appeared after two years of use.[24]
3. *Effects similar to those caused by estrogen-progestogen oral contraceptives.* There are several serious adverse effects of oral contraceptives, most of which have not, up to now, been documented as consequences of postmenopausal estrogen therapy. This may reflect the comparatively low doses of estrogen used in postmenopausal women. It would be expected that the larger doses of estrogen used to treat prostatic or breast cancer or postpartum breast engorgement are more likely to result in these adverse effects, and, in fact, it has been shown that there is an increased risk of thrombosis in men receiving estrogens for prostatic cancer and women for postpartum breast engorgement.[20–23]
a. *Thromboembolic disease.* It is now well established that users of oral contraceptives have an increased risk of various thromboembolic and thrombotic vascular diseases, such as thrombophlebitis, pulmonary embolism, stroke, and myocardial infarction.[24–31] Cases of retinal thrombosis, mesenteric thrombosis, and optic neuritis have been reported in oral contraceptive users. There is evidence that the risk of several of these adverse reactions is related to the dose of the drug.[32,33] An increased risk of postsurgery thromboembolic complications has also been reported in users of oral contraceptives.[34,35] If feasible, estrogen should be discontinued at least 4 weeks before surgery

of the type associated with an increased risk of thromboembolism, or during periods of prolonged immobilization.

While an increased rate of thromboembolic and thrombotic disease in postmenopausal users of estrogens has not been found,[18,36] this does not rule out the possibility that such an increase may be present or that subgroups of women who have underlying risk factors or who are receiving relatively large doses of estrogens may have increased risk. Therefore, estrogens should not be used in persons with active thrombophlebitis or thromboembolic disorders, and they should not be used (except in treatment of malignancy) in persons with a history of such disorders in association with estrogen use. They should be used with caution in patients with cerebral vascular or coronary artery disease and only for those in whom estrogens are clearly needed.

Large doses of estrogen (5 mg conjugated estrogens per day), comparable to those used to treat cancer of the prostate and breast, have been shown in a large prospective clinical trial in men[37] to increase the risk of nonfatal myocardial infarction, pulmonary embolism, and thrombophlebitis. When estrogen doses of this size are used, any of the thromboembolic and thrombotic adverse effects associated with oral contraceptive use should be considered a clear risk.

b. *Hepatic adenoma.* Benign hepatic adenomas appear to be associated with the use of oral contraceptives.[38–40] Although benign, and rare, these may rupture and may cause death through intra-abdominal hemorrhage. Such lesions have not yet been reported in association with other estrogen or progestogen preparations but should be considered in estrogen users having abdominal pain and tenderness, abdominal mass, or hypovolemic shock. Hepatocellular carcinoma has also been reported in women taking estrogen-containing oral contraceptives.[39] The relationship of this malignancy to these drugs is not known at this time.

c. *Elevated blood pressure.* Increased blood pressure is not uncommon in women using oral contraceptives. There is now a report that this may occur with use of estrogens in the menopause[11] and blood pressure should be monitored with estrogen use, especially if high doses are used.

d. *Glucose tolerance.* A worsening of glucose tolerance has been observed in a significant percentage of patients on estrogen-containing oral contraceptives. For this reason, diabetic patients should be carefully observed while receiving estrogen.

4. *Hypercalcemia.* Administration of estrogens may lead to severe hypercalcemia in patients with breast cancer and bone metastases. If this occurs, the drug should be stopped and appropriate measures taken to reduce the serum calcium level.

Precautions:

A. General Precautions

1. A complete medical and family history should be taken prior to the initiation of any estrogen therapy. The pretreatment and periodic physical examinations should include special reference to blood pressure, abdomen, and pelvic organs, and should include a Papanicolaou smear. As a general rule, estrogen should not be prescribed for longer than one year without another physical examination being performed.

2. Fluid retention—Because estrogens may cause some degree of fluid retention, conditions which might be influenced by this factor, such as epilepsy, migraine, and cardiac or renal dysfunction, require careful observation.

3. Certain patients may develop undesirable manifestations of excessive estrogenic stimulation, such as abnormal or excessive uterine bleeding, mastodynia, etc.

4. Oral contraceptives appear to be associated with an increased incidence of mental depression.[24] Although it is not clear whether this is due to the estrogenic or progestogenic component of the contraceptive, patients with a history of depression should be carefully observed.

5. Preexisting uterine leiomyomata may increase in size during estrogen use.

6. The pathologist should be advised of estrogen therapy when relevant specimens are submitted.

7. Patients with a past history of jaundice during pregnancy have an increased risk of recurrence of jaundice while receiving estrogen-containing oral contraceptive therapy. If jaundice develops in any patient receiving estrogen, the medication should be discontinued while the cause is investigated.

8. Estrogens may be poorly metabolized in patients with impaired liver function and they should be administered with caution in such patients.

9. Because estrogens influence the metabolism of calcium and phosphorus, they should be used with caution in patients with metabolic bone diseases that are associated with hypercalcemia or in patients with renal insufficiency.

10. Because of the effects of estrogens on epiphyseal closure, they should be used judiciously in young patients in whom bone growth is not complete.

11. Certain endocrine and liver function tests may be affected by estrogen-containing oral contraceptives. The following similar changes may be expected with larger doses of estrogen:

a. Increased sulfobromophthalein retention.

b. Increased prothrombin and factors VII, VIII, IX, and X; decreased antithrombin 3; increased norepinephrine-induced platelet aggregability.

c. Increased thyroid binding globulin (TBG) leading to increased circulating total thyroid hormone, as measured by PHI, T4 by column, or T4 by radioimmunoassay. Free T3 resin uptake is decreased, reflecting the elevated TBG; free T4 concentration is unaltered.

d. Impaired glucose tolerance.

e. Decreased pregnanediol excretion.

f. Reduced response to metyrapone test.

g. Reduced serum folate concentration.

h. Increased serum triglyceride and phospholipid concentration.

B. Information for the patient. See text of Patient Package Insert.

C. Pregnancy. See Contraindications and Boxed Warning.

D. Nursing Mothers. As a general principle, the administration of any drug to nursing mothers should be done only when clearly necessary because many drugs are excreted in human milk.

Adverse Reactions: (See Warnings regarding induction of neoplasia, adverse effects on the fetus, increased incidence of gallbladder disease, and adverse effects similar to those of oral contraceptives, including thromboembolism.) The following additional adverse reactions have been reported with estrogenic therapy, including oral contraceptives:

1. *Genitourinary system.*
Breakthrough bleeding, spotting, change in menstrual flow
Dysmenorrhea
Premenstrual-like syndrome
Amenorrhea during and after treatment
Increase in size of uterine fibromyomata
Vaginal candidiasis
Change in cervical eversion and in degree of cervical secretion
Cystitis-like syndrome

2. *Breasts.*
Tenderness, enlargement, secretion

3. *Gastrointestinal.*
Nausea, vomiting
Abdominal cramps, bloating
Cholestatic jaundice

4. *Skin.*
Chloasma or melasma which may persist when drug is discontinued
Erythema multiforme
Erythema nodosum
Hemorrhagic eruption
Loss of scalp hair
Hirsutism

5. *Eyes.*
Steepening of corneal curvature
Intolerance to contact lenses

6. *CNS.*
Headache, migraine, dizziness
Mental depression
Chorea

7. *Miscellaneous.*
Increase or decrease in weight
Reduced carbohydrate tolerance
Aggravation of porphyria
Edema
Changes in libido

Acute Overdosage: Numerous reports of ingestion of large doses of estrogen-containing oral contraceptives by young children indicate that serious ill effects do not occur. Overdosage of estrogen may cause nausea, and withdrawal bleeding may occur in females.

Dosage and Administration: For treatment of moderate to severe vasomotor symptoms associated with the menopause, and for atrophic vaginitis, kraurosis vulvae, female hypogonadism, female castration, and primary ovarian failure.

One Estrovis (quinestrol) 100-mcg tablet once daily for seven days, followed by one 100-mcg tablet weekly as a maintenance schedule, commencing two weeks after inception of treatment. The dosage may be increased to 200 mcg weekly if the therapeutic response is not that which may be desirable or considered optimal. The lowest maintenance dose that will control symptoms should be chosen and medication should be discontinued as promptly as possible. Attempts to discontinue or taper medication should be made at three- to six-month intervals.

Treated patients with an intact uterus should be monitored closely for signs of endometrial cancer and appropriate diagnostic measures should be taken to rule out malignancy in the event of persistent or recurring abnormal vaginal bleeding.

How Supplied: N 0071-0437-24 (P-D 437) Estrovis (quinestrol) 100-mcg tablets are supplied in bottles of 100.

0437G023

Physician References:

1. Ziel, H.K. and W.D. Finkle, "Increased Risk of Endometrial Carcinoma Among Users of Conjugated Estrogens." *New England Journal of Medicine,* 293:1167–1170, 1975.

2. Smith, D.C., R. Prentic, D.J. Thompson, and W.L. Hermann, "Association of Exogenous Estrogen and Endometrial Carcinoma." *New England Journal of Medicine,* 293:1164–1167, 1975.

3. Mack, T.M., M.C. Pike, B.E. Henderson, R.I. Pfeffer, V.R. Gerkins, M. Arthur, and S.E. Brown, "Estrogens and Endometrial Cancer in a Retirement Community." *New England Journal of Medicine,* 294:1262–1267, 1976.

4. Weiss, N.D., D.R. Szekely and D.F. Austin, "Increasing Incidence of Endometrial Cancer in the United States." *New England Journal of Medicine,* 294:1259–1262, 1976.

5. Herbst, A.L., H. Ulfelder and D.C. Poskanzer, "Adenocarcinoma of Vagina." *New England Journal of Medicine,* 284:878–881, 1971.

Continued on next page

This product information was prepared in August, 1982. On these and other Parke-Davis Products, information may be obtained by addressing PARKE-DAVIS, Division of Warner-Lambert Company, Morris Plains, New Jersey 07950.

Parke-Davis—Cont.

6. Greenwald, P., J. Barlow, P. Nasca, and W. Burnett, "Vaginal Cancer after Maternal Treatment with Synthetic Estrogens." *New England Journal of Medicine,* 285:390–392, 1971.
7. Lanier, A., K. Noller, D. Decker, L. Elveback, and L. Kurland, "Cancer and Stilbestrol, A Follow-Up of 1719 Persons Exposed to Estrogens in *Utero* and Born 1943–1959." *Mayo Clinic Proceedings,* 48:793–799, 1973.
8. Herbst, A., R. Kurman, and R. Scully, "Vaginal and Cervical Abnormalities After Exposure to Stilbestrol in Utero." *Obstetrics and Gynecology,* 40:287–298, 1972.
9. Herbst, A., S. Robboy, G. Macdonald, and R. Scully, "The Effects of Local Progesterone on Stilbestrol-Associated Vaginal Adenosis." *American Journal of Obstetrics and Gynecology,* 118:607–615, 1974.
10. Herbst, A., D. Poskanzer, S. Robboy, L. Friedlander, and R. Scully, "Prenatal Exposure to Stilbestrol, A Prospective Comparison of Exposed Female Offspring with Unexpected Controls." *New England Journal of Medicine,* 292:334–339, 1975.
11. Stafl, A., R. Mattingly, D. Foley, and W. Fetherston, "Clinical Diagnosis of Vaginal Adenosis." *Obstetrics and Gynecology,* 43:118–128, 1974.
12. Sherman, A.I., M. Goldrath, A. Berlin, V. Vakhariya, F. Banooni, W. Michaels, P. Goodman, S. Brown, "Cervical-Vaginal Adenosis After *In Utero* Exposure to Synthetic Estrogens," *Obstetrics and Gynecology,* 44:531–545, 1974.
13. Gal, I., B. Kirman, and J. Stern, "Hormone Pregnancy Tests and Congenital Malformation," *Nature,* 216:83, 1967.
14. Levy, E.P., A. Cohen, and F.C. Fraser, "Hormone Treatment During Pregnancy and Congenital Heart Defects," *Lancet,* 1:611, 1973.
15. Nora, J. and A. Nora, "Birth Defects and Oral Contraceptives," *Lancet,* 1:941–942, 1973.
16. Janerich, D.T., J.M. Piper, and D.M. Glebatis, "Oral Contraceptives and Congenital Limb-Reduction Defects," *New England Journal of Medicine,* 291:697–700, 1974.
17. "Estrogens for Oral or Parenteral Use," *Federal Register,* 40:8212, 1975.
18. Boston Collaborative Drug Surveillance Program "Surgically Confirmed Gallbladder Disease, Venous Thromboembolism and Breast Tumors in Relation to Post-Menopausal Estrogen Therapy," *New England Journal of Medicine,* 210:15–19, 1974.
18a. Hoover, R., L.A. Gray, Sr., P. Cole, and B. MacMahon, "Menopausal Estrogens and Breast Cancer." *New England Journal of Medicine,* 295:401–405, 1976.
19. Boston Collaborative Drug Surveillance Program, "Oral Contraceptives and Venous Thromboembolic Disease, Surgically Confirmed Gallbladder Disease, and Breast Tumors," *Lancet,* 1:1399–1404, 1973.
20. Daniel, D.G., H. Campbell, and A.C. Turnbull, "Puerperal Thromboembolism and Suppression of Lactation." *Lancet,* 2:287–289, 1967.
21. The Veterans Administration Cooperative Urological Research Group, "Carcinoma of the Prostate: Treatment Comparisons," *Journal of Urology,* 98:516–522, 1967.
22. Ballar, J.C., "Thromboembolism and Oestrogen Therapy," *Lancet,* 2, 560. 1967.
23. Blackard, C., R. Doe, G. Mellinger, and D. Byar, "Incidence of Cardiovascular Disease and Death in Patients Receiving Diethylstilbestrol for Carcinoma of the Prostate," *Cancer,* 26:249–256, 1970.
24. Royal College of General Practitioners, "Oral Contraception and Thromboembolic Disease," *Journal of the Royal College of General Practitioners,* 13, 267–279, 1967.
25. Inman, W.H.W. and M.P. Vessey, "Investigation of Deaths from Pulmonary, Coronary, and Cerebral Thrombosis and Embolism in Women of Child-Bearing Age." *British Medical Journal,* 2:193–199, 1968.
26. Vessey, M.P. and R. Doll, "Investigation of Relation Between Use of Oral Contraceptives and Thromboembolic Disease, A Further Report," *British Medical Journal,* 2:651–657, 1969.
27. Sartwell, P.E., A.T. Masi, F.G. Arthes, G.R. Greene and H.E. Smith, "Thromboembolism and Oral Contraceptives: An Epidemiological Case Control Study." *American Journal of Epidemiology,* 90:365–380, 1969.
28. Collaborative Group for the Study of Stroke in Young Women, "Oral Contraception and Increased Risk of Cerebral Ischemia or Thrombosis," *New England Journal of Medicine,* 288:871–878, 1973.
29. Collaborative Group for the Study of Stroke in Young Women: "Oral Contraceptives and Stroke in Young Women: Associated Risk Factors," 231:718–722, 1975. *Journal of the American Medical Assoc.* 231:718–722, 1975.
30. Mann, J.I. and W.H.W. Inman, "Oral Contraceptives and Death from Myocardial Infarction," *British Medical Journal,* 2:245–248, 1975.
31. Mann, J.I., M.P. Vessey, M. Thorogood, and R. Doll, "Myocardial Infarction in Young Women with Special Reference to Oral Contraceptive Practice," *British Medical Journal,* 2:241–245, 1975.
32. Inman, W.H.W., M.P. Vessey, B. Westerholm, and A. Engelund. "Thromboembolic Disease and the Steroidal Content of Oral Contraceptives," *British Medical Journal,* 2:203–209, 1970.
33. Stolley, P.D., J.A. Tonascia, M.S. Tockman, P.E. Sartwell, A.H. Rutledge, and M.P. Jacobs, "Thrombosis with Low-Estrogen Oral Contraceptives," *American Journal of Epidemiology,* 102:197–208, 1975.
34. Vessey, M.P., R. Doll, A.S. Fairbairn, and G. Glober, "Post-Operative Thromboembolism and the use of the Oral Contraceptives," *British Medical Journal,* 3:123–126, 1970.
35. Greene, G.R. and P.E. Sartwell, "Oral Contraceptive Use in Patients with Thromboembolism Following Surgery, Trauma or Infection," *American Journal of Public Health,* 62:680–685, 1972.
36. Rosenberg, L., M.B. Armstrong and H. Jick "Myocardial Infarction and Estrogen Therapy in Post-menopausal Women," *New England Journal of Medicine,* 294:1256–1259, 1976.
37. Coronary Drug Project Research Group, "The Coronary Drug Project: Initial Findings Leading to Modifications of Its Research Protocol," *Journal of the American Medical Association,* 214:1303–1313, 1970.
38. Baum, J., F. Holtz, J.J. Bookstein, and E.W. Klein, "Possible Association between Benign Hepatomas and Oral Contraceptives," *Lancet,* 2:926–928, 1973.
39. Mays, E.T., W.M. Christopherson, M.M. Mahr, and H.C. Williams, "Hepatic Changes in Young Women Ingesting Contraceptive Steroids, Hepatic Hemorrhage and Primary Hepatic Tumors," *Journal of the American Medical Association,* 235:780–782, 1976.
40. Edmondson, H.A., B. Henderson, and B. Benton, "Liver Cell Adenomas Association with the Use of Oral Contraceptives," *New England Journal of Medicine,* 294:470–472, 1976.
41. Pfeffer, A.I. and S. Van Den Noore, "Estrogen use and Stroke Risk in Post-menopausal Women," *American Journal of Epidemiology,* 103:545–546, 1976.

[*Shown in Product Identification Section*]

EUTHROID® ℞
(liotrix tablets, USP)*

*Product of Warner-Lambert Inc

Description: Euthroid is synthetic microcrystalline levothyroxine sodium (T_4) USP and synthetic microcrystalline liothyronine sodium (T_3) USP combined in a constant 4:1 ratio.

Clinical Pharmacology: Euthroid provides replacement therapy for the thyroactive material normally supplied by the human thyroid. The normal thyroid gland produces and stores thyroglobulin, the active components of which are two metabolically active hormones: levothyroxine and liothyronine. Euthroid (liotrix) provides a combination of these hormones in purified, synthetic form, supplied in a constant 4:1 ratio in order to simulate as closely as possible the physiologic and metabolic effects of normal endogenous thyroid secretions.

In contrast with the individual synthetic, metabolically active hormones, Euthroid will usually produce normal results for PBI, T_3, and other thyroid function tests—consistent with clinical progress—when persons with endogenous thyroid deficiencies are made euthyroid. Liothyronine sodium (T_3) acts more rapidly and for a shorter period of time than preparations of biological origin. Customarily, its use as a single agent produces inappropriately decreased PBI values. Levothyroxine sodium (T_4), on the other hand, is more tightly bound by plasma protein fractions and is somewhat slower acting than liothyronine sodium (T_3); its use as a single agent tends to produce inappropriately elevated PBI values. Euthroid, with its unvarying 4:1 ratio of T_4/T_3, permits interpretation of appropriate laboratory tests consistent with the total clinical status of the patient.

Indications and Usage: Euthroid provides thyroid replacement therapy in all conditions of inadequate production of thyroid hormones, namely:

1) Hypothyroidism, including cretinism and myxedema.
2) Simple (nontoxic) goiter.
3) Subacute or chronic thyroiditis including Hashimoto's disease.
4) Prevention of goiter in hyperthyroid patients undergoing treatment with thiouracil derivatives.
5) Usage in patients who may manifest intolerance to thyroid products of animal origin.

Contraindications: Acute myocardial infarction, adrenal insufficiency, hypersensitivity to any component of this drug.

Warnings:

> Drugs with thyroid hormone activity, alone or together with other therapeutic agents, have been used for the treatment of obesity. In euthyroid patients, doses within the range of daily hormonal requirements are ineffective for weight reduction. Larger doses may produce serious or even life-threatening manifestations of toxicity, particularly when given in association with sympathomimetic amines such as those used for their anorectic effects.

Liotrix should not be used in the presence of cardiovascular disease unless thyroid replacement therapy is clearly indicated. If the latter exists, low doses should be instituted (Euthroid-½ or Euthroid-1) and increased by the same amount in increments at 2-week intervals. This demands careful clinical judgment. Morphologic hypogonadism and nephroses should be ruled out and adrenal deficiency due to hypopituitarism corrected before liotrix therapy is started.

If hypothyroidism and adrenal insufficiency exist concomitantly, cortisone or similar steroids should be given at dose levels sufficient to correct the adrenal insufficiency before at-

tempting replacement therapy with thyroid hormones.
Likewise, the possibility of alterations in the prothrombin time must be considered and closely monitored in patients on anticoagulant therapy.
Myxedematous patients are very sensitive to thyroid hormones, and dosage should be started at a very low level and increased gradually.
Surgery: Euthroid-treated patients with coronary artery disease should be carefully observed during surgery, since the possibility of precipitating cardiac arrhythmias may be greater in patients treated with thyroid hormones.
Precautions: Hypothyroid patients are especially sensitive to thyroid preparations, and those with severe hypothyroidism may be unusually so.
Initiation of thyroid replacement therapy in patients with diabetes must be carefully monitored because of potential fluctuation in daily insulin or oral hypoglycemic requirements.
As with all thyroid preparations, this drug will alter the results of thyroid function tests.
Euthroid-½, -1, -3 contain FD&C yellow No. 5 (tartrazine) which may cause allergic-type reactions (including bronchial asthma) in certain susceptible individuals. Although the overall incidence of FD&C yellow No. 5 (tartrazine) sensitivity in the population is low, it is frequently seen in patients who also have aspirin hypersensitivity.
Drug Interactions: The possibility of alterations in the prothrombin time must be considered and closely monitored in patients on anticoagulant therapy.
Adverse Reactions: Overdosage or too rapid increase in dosage of thyroid preparations can produce signs and symptoms of hyperthyroidism, such as menstrual irregularities, nervousness, cardiac arrhythmias, and angina pectoris.
Overdosage:
Symptoms: Headache, instability, nervousness, sweating, tachycardia, and unusual bowel motility. Angina pectoris or congestive heart failure may be induced or aggravated. Shock may develop. Massive overdosage may result in symptoms resembling thyroid storm; chronic excessive dosage will produce the signs and symptoms of hyperthyroidism.
Treatment: Shock—Supportive measures should be utilized. Treatment of unrecognized adrenal insufficiency should be considered.
Dosage and Administration: Initial dosage should be low and gradually increased at 2-week intervals until the desired clinical response is obtained.
Laboratory criteria of euthyroidism include a PBI of 3.5 to 8 mcg; T_3, T_4, and BEI tests are useful.
For most patients, a single daily dose of Euthroid-1, -2, or -3 will maintain euthyroidism. Transfer of a patient from a maintenance dose of another thyroid preparation to Euthroid can usually be effected smoothly. See table for initiating therapy or converting from other thyroid preparations.
[See table above].
Dosage for cretinism or severe hypothyroidism in children is the same as for adults with myxedema. Eventual maintenance dosage in the growing child may be higher than in the adult.
Supplied: Square monogrammed tablets of four potencies, each identified by a different color (see table).
Euthroid-½ is supplied as N 0710-0260-24—Bottles of 100.
Euthroid-1 is supplied as N 0710-0261-24—Bottles of 100. N 0710-0261-32—Bottles of 1000.
Euthroid-2 is supplied as: N 0710-0262-24—Bottles of 100.
Euthroid-3 is supplied as: N 0710-0263-24—Bottles of 100.

Euthroid (liotrix tablets, USP)			Approximate Equivalents: Natural	Synthetic	
Tablet	T_4*/T_3**	Color	Thyroid USP	T_4*	T_3**
	mcg				
Euthroid-½	(30/7.5)	pale orange	½ grain	.05 mg	12.5 mcg
Euthroid-1	(60/15)	light brown	1 grain	.1 mg	25.0 mcg
Euthroid-2	(120/30)	violet	2 grains	.2 mg	50.0 mcg
Euthroid-3	(180/45)	gray	3 grains	.3 mg	75.0 mcg

*T_4=levothyroxine sodium (*l*-thyroxine) **T_3=liothyronine sodium (*l*-triiodothyronine)

STORE BETWEEN 59° and 86°F (15° and 30°C).
Licensed under U.S. Patent 2,823,164
[*Shown in Product Identification Section*]
0260 G 021

FLUOGEN® ℞
(influenza virus vaccine)

The formulation of influenza virus vaccine for use during each season is established by the Bureau of Biologics, Food and Drug Administration, Public Health Service. For information regarding the current formulation, please refer to the product package insert, contact your Parke-Davis representative, or call (201) 540-2000.

FUROSEMIDE INJECTION, USP ℞
(10 mg/ml)

Warning: Furosemide is a potent diuretic which, if given in excessive amounts, can lead to a profound diuresis with water and electrolyte depletion. Therefore, careful medical supervision is required and dose and dose schedule have to be adjusted to the individual patient's needs. (See under "DOSAGE AND ADMINISTRATION.")
Description: Furosemide is an anthranilic acid derivative. It is a white to slightly yellow, odorless, crystalline powder. It is practically insoluble in water; freely soluble in acetone, in dimethylformamide, and in solutions of alkali hydroxides; soluble in methanol; sparingly soluble in alcohol; slightly soluble in ether; very slightly soluble in chloroform. Chemically it is 4-chloro-N-furfuryl-5-sulfamoyl-anthranilic acid.
Actions: Investigations into the mode of action of furosemide have utilized micropuncture studies in rats, stop flow experiments in dogs and various clearance studies in both humans and experimental animals. It has been demonstrated that furosemide inhibits primarily the reabsorption of sodium and chloride not only in the proximal and distal tubules but also in the loop of Henle. The high degree of efficacy is largely due to this unique site of action. The action of the distal tubule is independent of any inhibitory effect on carbonic anhydrase and aldosterone.
The onset of diuresis following intravenous administration is within 5 minutes and somewhat later after intramuscular administration. The peak effect occurs within the first half hour. The duration of diuretic effect is approximately 2 hours.
Indications: Parenteral therapy should be reserved for patients unable to take oral medication or for patients in emergency clinical situations.
Furosemide is indicated for the treatment of edema associated with congestive heart failure, cirrhosis of the liver, and renal disease, including the nephrotic syndrome. Furosemide is particularly useful when an agent with greater diuretic potential than that of those commonly employed is desired.
Furosemide is indicated as adjunctive therapy in acute pulmonary edema. The intravenous administration of furosemide is indicated when a rapid onset of diuresis is desired, eg, in acute pulmonary edema.
If gastrointestinal absorption is impaired or oral medication is not practical for any reason, furosemide is indicated by the intravenous or intramuscular route. Parenteral use should be replaced with oral furosemide as soon as practical.
Contraindications: Furosemide is contraindicated in anuria. It is contraindicated in patients with a history of hypersensitivity to this compound.
Warnings: Excessive diuresis may result in dehydration and reduction in blood volume with circulatory collapse and with the possibility of vascular thrombosis and embolism, particularly in elderly patients. Excessive loss of potassium in patients receiving digitalis glycosides may precipitate digitalis toxicity. Care should also be exercised in patients receiving potassium-depleting steroids.
Frequent serum electrolyte, CO_2 and BUN determinations should be performed during the first few months of therapy and periodically thereafter, and abnormalities corrected or the drug temporarily withdrawn.
In patients with hepatic cirrhosis and ascites, initiation of therapy with furosemide is best carried out in the hospital. In hepatic coma and in states of electrolyte depletion, therapy should not be instituted until the basic condition is improved. Sudden alterations of fluid and electrolyte balance in patients with cirrhosis may precipitate hepatic coma; therefore, strict observation is necessary during the period of diuresis. Supplemental potassium chloride and, if required, an aldosterone antagonist are helpful in preventing hypokalemia and metabolic alkalosis.
If increasing azotemia and oliguria occur during treatment of severe progressive renal disease, the drug should be discontinued.
As with many other drugs, patients should be observed regularly for the possible occurrence of blood dyscrasias, liver damage, or other idiosyncratic reactions.
Patients with known sulfonamide sensitivity may show allergic reactions to furosemide.
Furosemide may add to or potentiate the therapeutic effect of other antihypertensive drugs. Potentiation occurs with ganglionic or peripheral adrenergic blocking drugs.
The possibility exists of exacerbation or activation of systemic lupus erythematosus.
Furosemide appears in breast milk. If use of the drug is deemed essential, the patient should stop nursing.
Parenterally administered furosemide may increase the ototoxic potential of aminoglyco-

Continued on next page

This product information was prepared in August, 1982. On these and other Parke-Davis Products, information may be obtained by addressing PARKE-DAVIS, Division of Warner-Lambert Company, Morris Plains, New Jersey 07950.

Parke-Davis—Cont.

side antibiotics. Especially in the presence of impaired renal function, the use of parenterally administered furosemide in patients to whom aminoglycoside antibiotics are also being given should be avoided, except in life-threatening situations.
Cases of tinnitus and reversible hearing impairments have been reported. There have also been some reports of cases in which irreversible hearing impairment occurred. Usually, ototoxicity has been reported when furosemide was injected rapidly in patients with severe impairment of renal function at doses exceeding several times the usual recommended dose and in whom other drugs known to be ototoxic were given. If the physician elects to use high dose parenteral therapy in patients with severely impaired renal function, controlled intravenous infusion is advisable [for adults, an infusion rate not exceeding 4 mg furosemide per minute has been used].

Precautions: As with any effective diuretic, electrolyte depletion may occur during therapy with furosemide, especially in patients receiving higher doses and a restricted salt intake. Periodic determinations of serum electrolytes to detect possible imbalance should be performed at appropriate intervals.
All patients receiving furosemide therapy should be observed for signs of fluid or electrolyte imbalance: namely, hyponatremia, hypochloremic alkalosis and hypokalemia. Serum and urine electrolyte determinations are particularly important when the patient is vomiting excessively or receiving parenteral fluids. Medication such as digitalis may also influence serum electrolytes. Warning signs, irrespective of cause, are dryness of mouth, thirst, weakness, lethargy, drowsiness, restlessness, muscle pains or cramps, muscular fatigue, hypotension, oliguria, tachycardia, arrhythmia and gastrointestinal disturbances such as nausea and vomiting.
Hypokalemia may develop with furosemide as with any other potent diuretic, especially with brisk diuresis, when cirrhosis is present, or during concomitant use of corticosteroids or ACTH.
Interference with adequate oral electrolyte intake will also contribute to hypokalemia. Digitalis therapy may exaggerate metabolic effects of hypokalemia, especially with reference to myocardial activity.
Asymptomatic hyperuricemia can occur and gout may rarely be precipitated.
Periodic checks on urine and blood glucose should be made in diabetics and even those suspected of latent diabetes when receiving furosemide. Increases in blood glucose and alterations in glucose tolerance tests with abnormalities of the fasting and 2-hour postprandial sugar have been observed, and rare cases of precipitation of diabetes mellitus have been reported.
Furosemide may lower serum calcium levels, and rare cases of tetany have been reported. Accordingly, periodic serum calcium levels should be obtained.
Reversible elevations of BUN may be seen. These have been observed in association with dehydration, which should be avoided, particularly in patients with renal insufficiency.
Patients receiving high doses of salicylates, as in rheumatic disease, in conjunction with furosemide may experience salicylate toxicity at lower doses because of competitive renal excretory sites.
Furosemide has a tendency to antagonize the skeletal muscle relaxing effect of tubocurarine and may potentiate the action of succinylcholine.
Lithium generally should not be given with diuretics because they reduce its renal clearance and add a high risk of lithium toxicity.
It has been reported in the literature that diuretics such as furosemide may enhance the nephrotoxicity of cephaloridine. Therefore, furosemide and cephaloridine should not be administered simultaneously.
Furosemide may decrease arterial responsiveness to norepinephrine. This diminution is not sufficient to preclude effectiveness of the pressor agent for therapeutic use.

Pregnancy:
Pregnancy Category C. Furosemide has been shown to cause unexplained maternal deaths and abortions in rabbits at 2, 4 and 8 times the human dose. There are no adequate and well-controlled studies in pregnant women. Furosemide should be used during pregnancy only if the potential benefit justifies the potential risk to the fetus.
The effects of furosemide on embryonic and fetal development and on pregnant dams were studied in mice, rats and rabbits.
Furosemide caused unexplained maternal deaths and abortions in the rabbit when 50 mg/kg (4 times the maximal recommended human dose of 600 mg per day) was administered between days 12 and 17 of gestation. In a previous study the lowest dose of only 25 mg/kg (2 times the maximal recommended human dose of 600 mg per day) caused maternal deaths and abortions. In a third study, none of the pregnant rabbits survived a dose of 100 mg/kg. Data from the above studies indicate fetal lethality that can precede maternal deaths.
The results of the mouse study and one of the three rabbit studies also showed an increased incidence of hydronephrosis (distention of the renal pelvis and, in some cases, of the ureters) in fetuses derived from treated dams as compared to the incidence in fetuses from the control group.

Adverse Reactions:
Gastrointestinal System Reactions
1. anorexia
2. oral and gastric irritation
3. nausea
4. vomiting
5. cramping
6. diarrhea
7. constipation
8. jaundice (intrahepatic cholestatic jaundice)
9. pancreatitis

Central Nervous System Reactions
1. dizziness
2. vertigo
3. paresthesias
4. headache
5. xanthopsia
6. blurred vision
7. tinnitus and hearing loss

Hematologic Reactions
1. anemia
2. leukopenia
3. agranulocytosis (rare)
4. thrombocytopenia
5. aplastic anemia (rare)

Dermatologic-Hypersensitivity Reactions
1. purpura
2. photosensitivity
3. rash
4. uticaria
5. necrotizing angiitis (vasculitis, cutaneous vasculitis)
6. exfoliative dermatitis
7. erythema multiforme
8. pruritus

Cardiovascular Reactions
Orthostatic hypotension may occur and be aggravated by alcohol, barbiturates or narcotics.

Other
1. hyperglycemia
2. glycosuria
3. hyperuricemia
4. muscle spasm
5. weakness
6. restlessness
7. urinary bladder spasm
8. thrombophlebitis
9. transient pain at the injection site following intramuscular injection

Whenever adverse reactions are moderate or severe, furosemide dosage should be reduced or therapy withdrawn.

Dosage and Administration:
Adults—Parenteral therapy should be reserved for patients for whom oral medication is not practical or in emergency situations where prompt diuresis is desired. Parenteral therapy should be replaced by oral therapy as soon as this is practical for continued mobilization of edema.
Edema The usual initial dose of furosemide is 20 to 40 mg given as a single dose, injected intramuscularly or intravenously. The intravenous injection should be given slowly (1 to 2 minutes). Ordinarily, a prompt diuresis ensues. Depending on the patient's response, a second dose can be administered 2 hours after the first dose or later.
If the diuretic response with a single dose of 20 to 40 mg is not satisfactory, increase this dose by increments of 20 mg not sooner than 2 hours after the previous dose until the desired diuretic effect has been obtained. This individually determined single dose should then be given once or twice daily.
If the physician elects to use high dose parenteral therapy it should be administered as a controlled infusion at a rate not exceeding 4 mg/min. Furosemide Injection, USP is a mildly buffered alkaline solution which should not be mixed with acidic solutions of pH below 5.5. To prepare infusion solutions, isotonic saline and lactated Ringer's injection and 5% dextrose injection have been used after pH has been adjusted when necessary.
Therapy should be individualized according to patient response. This therapy should be titrated to gain maximal therapeutic response as well as the minimal dose possible to maintain that therapeutic response. Close medical supervision is necessary.
Acute Pulmonary Edema The usual initial dose of furosemide is 40 mg injected intravenously. The injection should be given slowly (1 to 2 minutes). If 40 mg furosemide does not produce a satisfactory response within 1 hour, the dose may be increased to 80 mg given intravenously (over 1 to 2 minutes).
If deemed necessary, additional therapy (eg, digitalis, oxygen) can be administered concomitantly.
Infants and Children—Parenteral therapy should be reserved for patients for whom oral medication is not practical or in emergency situations where prompt diuresis is desired. Parenteral therapy should be replaced by oral therapy as soon as this is practical for continued mobilization of edema.
The usual initial dose of furosemide, injected intravenously or intramuscularly, in infants and children is 1 mg/kg body weight and should be given slowly under close medical supervision. If the diuretic response after the initial dose is not satisfactory, dosage may be increased by 1 mg/kg not sooner than 2 hours after the previous dose, until the desired diuretic effect has been obtained. Doses greater than 6 mg/kg body weight are not recommended.

How Supplied: Furosemide Injection, USP is supplied as a sterile solution for parenteral use as follows:
N 0071-4143-05 2 ml amber ampoule, carton of 10 ampoules
N 0071-4143-08 4 ml amber ampoule, carton of 10 ampoules
N 0071-4143-10 10 ml amber ampoule, carton of 10 ampoules
Each milliliter of solution contains 10 mg furosemide, with sodium chloride for isotonicity and sodium hydroxide to make the solution slightly alkaline.

Store at controlled room temperature, 15°-30°C (59°-86°F). Do not use if solution is discolored.

4143G010

GELUSIL®

Antacid-Anti-gas
Liquid/Tablets

Each teaspoonful (5 ml) or tablet contains:
200 mg aluminum hydroxide
200 mg magnesium hydroxide
25 mg simethicone

Advantages:

- High acid-neutralizing capacity
- Low sodium content
- Simethicone for antiflatulent activity
- Good taste for better patient compliance
- Fast dissolution of chewed tablets for prompt relief

Indications: Gelusil, a carefully balanced combination of two widely used antacids and the antiflatulent simethicone, is effective for the relief of symptoms associated with heartburn, sour stomach and acid indigestion with gas. Gelusil provides symptomatic relief of hyperacidity associated with the diagnosis of peptic ulcer, gastritis, peptic esophagitis, gastric hyperacidity and hiatal hernia, and it alleviates or relieves the symptoms of gas and postoperative gas pain.

Actions and Uses: The proven neutralizing power of aluminum hydroxide and of magnesium hydroxide combine to give Gelusil dependable antacid action without the acid rebound sometimes associated with calcium carbonate.

The pleasant peppermint-flavored taste of Gelusil Liquid and Tablets encourages patient acceptance of, and compliance with, recommended antacid-anti-gas regimens.

Gelusil Tablets are easy to chew and are specifically formulated to dissolve readily, providing prompt onset of action and reliable relief of symptoms.

Gelusil is appropriate whenever there is a need for well-accepted, effective antacid-anti-gas therapy.

Dosage and Administration: Two or more teaspoonfuls or tablets one hour after meals and at bedtime, or as directed by a physician. Tablets should be chewed.

The following information is provided to facilitate treatment:

Gelusil	LIQUID	TABLETS
Acid-neutralizing capacity	24 mEq/ 10 ml	22 mEq/ 2 tabs
Sodium	0.7 mg/ 5 ml	0.8 mg/ tab
Lactose	0	0

Warnings: Do not take more than 12 tablets or teaspoonfuls in a 24-hour period, or use this maximum dosage for more than 2 weeks, or use this product if you have kidney disease, except under the advice and supervision of a physician.

Keep this and all drugs out of the reach of children.

Drug Interaction Precaution: Do not take this product if you are presently taking a prescription antibiotic drug containing any form of tetracycline.

All aluminum-containing antacids, including Gelusil, may prevent proper absorption of tetracycline.

How Supplied:

N 0071-2036—**Liquid**—In plastic bottles of 6 fl oz and 12 fl oz.

N 0071-0034—**Tablets**—White, embossed Gelusil P-D 034—individual strips of 10 in boxes of 50, 100 and 1000; 165 tablets loose-packed in plastic bottles.

[Shown in Product Identification Section]

GELUSIL-M®

Antacid-Anti-gas
Liquid/Tablets

Each teaspoonful (5 ml) or tablet contains:
300 mg aluminum hydroxide
200 mg magnesium hydroxide
25 mg simethicone

Advantages:

- High acid-neutralizing capacity
- Low sodium content
- Simethicone for antiflatulent activity
- Good taste for better patient compliance
- Fast dissolution of chewed tablets for prompt relief

Indications: Gelusil-M, a carefully balanced combination of two widely used antacids and the antiflatulent simethicone, is effective for the relief of symptoms associated with heartburn, sour stomach, and acid indigestion with gas. Gelusil-M provides symptomatic relief of hyperacidity associated with the diagnosis of peptic ulcer, gastritis, peptic esophagitis, gastric hyperacidity and hiatal hernia, and it alleviates or relieves the symptoms of gas and postoperative gas pain.

Actions and Uses: The proven neutralizing power of aluminum hydroxide and magnesium hydroxide combine to give Gelusil-M dependable antacid action without the acid rebound sometimes associated with calcium carbonate.

The pleasant spearmint-flavored taste of Gelusil-M Liquid and Tablets encourages patient acceptance of, and compliance with, recommended antacid-anti-gas regimens.

Gelusil-M Tablets are easy to chew and are specifically formulated to dissolve readily providing prompt onset of action and reliable relief of symptoms.

Gelusil-M is appropriate whenever there is a need for well-accepted, effective antacid-antigas therapy.

Dosage and Administration: Two or more teaspoonfuls or tablets one hour after meals and at bedtime, or as directed by a physician. Tablets should be chewed.

The following information is provided to facilitate treatment:

Gelusil-M	LIQUID	TABLETS
Acid-neutralizing capacity	30 mEq/ 10 ml	25 mEq/ 2 tabs
Sodium	1.2 mg/ 5 ml	1.3 mg/ tab
Lactose	0	0

Warnings: Do not take more than 10 teaspoonfuls or tablets in a 24-hour period, or use this maximum dosage for more than 2 weeks, or use this product if you have kidney disease, except under the advice and supervision of a physician.

Keep this and all drugs out of the reach of children.

Drug Interaction Precaution: Do not take this product if you are presently taking a prescription antibiotic drug containing any form of tetracycline.

All aluminum-containing antacids, including Gelusil-M, may prevent proper absorption of tetracycline.

How Supplied:

N 0071-2043- **Liquid**—In plastic bottles of 12 fl oz.

N 0071-0045-**Tablets**—White, embossed P-D 045—individual strips of 10 in boxes of 100.

GELUSIL-II®

Antacid-Anti-gas
Liquid/Tablets
High Potency

Each teaspoonful (5 ml) or tablet contains:
400 mg aluminum hydroxide
400 mg magnesium hydroxide
30 mg simethicone

Advantages:

- High acid-neutralizing capacity
- Low sodium content
- Simethicone for antiflatulent activity
- Good taste for better patient compliance
- Fast dissolution of chewed tablets for prompt relief
- Double strength antacid

Indications: Gelusil-II, a carefully balanced, high-potency combination of two widely used antacids and the antiflatulent simethicone, is effective for the relief of symptoms associated with heartburn, sour stomach and acid indigestion with gas. Gelusil-II provides symptomatic relief of hyperacidity associated with the diagnosis of peptic ulcer, gastritis, peptic esophagitis, gastric hyperacidity and hiatal hernia, and it alleviates or relieves the symptoms of gas and postoperative gas pain.

Actions and Uses: The proven neutralizing power of aluminum hydroxide and magnesium hydroxide combine to give Gelusil-II dependable antacid action without the acid rebound sometimes associated with calcium carbonate. The higher potency of Gelusil-II is achieved by greater concentration of antacid ingredients per dosage unit.

The pleasant taste of Gelusil-II Liquid (citrus-flavored) and Tablets (orange-flavored) encourages patient acceptance of, and compliance with, recommended antacid-anti-gas regimens.

Gelusil-II Tablets are easy to chew and are specifically formulated to dissolve readily, providing prompt onset of action and reliable relief of symptoms.

Gelusil-II is appropriate whenever there is a need for well-accepted, effective antacid-antigas therapy.

Dosage and Administration: Two or more teaspoonfuls or tablets one hour after meals and at bedtime, or as directed by a physician. Tablets should be chewed.

The following information is provided to facilitate treatment:

Gelusil-II	LIQUID	TABLETS
Acid-neutralizing capacity	48 mEq/ 10 ml	42 mEq/ 2 tabs
Sodium	1.3 mg/ 5 ml	2.1 mg/ tab
Lactose	0	0

Warnings: Do not take more than 8 tablets or teaspoonfuls in a 24-hour period, or use this maximum dosage for more than 2 weeks, or use this product if you have kidney disease, except under the advice and supervision of a physician.

Keep this and all drugs out of the reach of children.

Drug Interaction Precaution: Do not take this product if you are presently taking a prescription antibiotic containing any form of tetracycline.

All aluminum-containing antacids, including Gelusil-II, may prevent proper absorption of tetracycline.

How Supplied:

N 0071-0042-**Liquid**—In plastic bottles of 12 fl oz.

N 0071-0043-**Tablets**—Double-layered white/orange, embossed W/C 043 or P-D 043 - individual strips of 10 in boxes of 80.

[Shown in Product Identification Section]

Continued on next page

This product information was prepared in August, 1982. On these and other Parke-Davis Products, information may be obtained by addressing PARKE-DAVIS, Division of Warner-Lambert Company, Morris Plains, New Jersey 07950.

Parke-Davis—Cont.

GENERICS

The following is a list of the generic names of all Parke-Davis solid-oral product forms which are marketed under the generic name or a trade name.

0634- Ⓒ Acetaminophen with Codeine Phosphate Tablets, No. 2
0635- Ⓒ Acetaminophen with Codeine Phosphate Tablets, No. 3
0637- Ⓒ Acetaminophen with Codeine Phosphate Tablets, No. 4
0640- Acetaminophen Tablets, USP (Tapar®), 325 mg
0272- Amitriptyline Hydrochloride Tablets, USP (Amitril®), 10 mg
0273- Amitriptyline Hydrochloride Tablets, USP (Amitril®), 25 mg
0274- Amitriptyline Hydrochloride Tablets, USP (Amitril®), 50 mg
0275- Amitriptyline Hydrochloride Tablets, USP (Amitril®), 75 mg
0271- Amitriptyline Hydrochloride Tablets, USP (Amitril®), 100 mg
0278- Amitriptyline Hydrochloride Tablets, USP (Amitril®), 150 mg
0730- Amoxicillin (Utimox®) Capsules, 250 mg
0731- Amoxicillin (Utimox®) Capsules, 500 mg
0402- Ampicillin Capsules, USP (Amcill® Capsules), 250 mg
0404- Ampicillin Capsules, USP (Amcill® Capsules), 500 mg
0606- Aspirin Tablets, USP, 325 mg
0679- Aspirin Compound Tablets
0792- Ⓒ Aspirin Compound with Codeine Phosphate Tablets No. 2
0793- Ⓒ Aspirin Compound with Codeine Phosphate Tablets No. 3
0389- Bromodiphenhydramine Hydrochloride Capsules, USP (Ambodryl® Kapseals®), 25 mg
0533- Calcium Lactate Tablets, USP, 325 mg
0604- Calcium Lactate Tablets, USP, 650 mg
0055- Cascara Tablets, USP (Cascara Sagrada Extract Filmseal®), 325 mg
0379- Chloramphenicol Capsules, USP (Chloromycetin® Kapseals), 250 mg
0800- Ⓒ Chlordiazepoxide Hydrochloride Capsules, USP, 5 mg
0801- Ⓒ Chlordiazepoxide Hydrochloride Capsules, USP, 10 mg
0802- Ⓒ Chlordiazepoxide Hydrochloride Capsules, USP, 25 mg
0010- Chlorpromazine Hydrochloride Tablets, USP (Promapar®), 10 mg
0025 Chlorpromazine Hydrochloride Tablets, USP, 25 mg
0050- Chlorpromazine Hydrochloride Tablets, USP, 50 mg
0100- Chlorpromazine Hydrochloride Tablets, USP, 100 mg
0201- Chlorpromazine Hydrochloride Tablets, USP, 200 mg
0471- Diphenhydramine Hydrochloride Capsules, USP (Benadryl®), 25 mg
0373- Diphenhydramine Hydrochloride Capsules, USP (Benadryl® Kapseals), 50 mg
0247- Docusate Sodium Capsules, USP (DSS Capsules), 100 mg
0248- Docusate Sodium with Casanthranol Capsules (DSS Plus Capsules)
0111- Ergotamine Tartrate Tablets (Ergostat® Sublingual Tablets), 2 mg
0672- Erythromycin Stearate Tablets, USP (Erypar® Filmseal), 250 mg
0919- Erythromycin Stearate Tablets, USP (Erypar® Filmseal), 500 mg
0237- Ethosuximide Capsules, USP (Zarontin® Capsules), 250 mg
0037- Ferrous Sulfate Filmseal, 325 mg
0702- Hydrochlorothiazide Tablets, USP (Thiuretic®), 25 mg
0710- Hydrochlorothiazide Tablets, USP (Thiuretic®), 50 mg
0268- Meclofenamate Sodium (Meclomen®) Capsules, 50 mg
0269- Meclofenamate Sodium (Meclomen) Capsules, 100 mg
0540- Mefenamic Acid (Ponstel® Kapseals), 250 mg
0636- Meprednisone Tablets, USP (Betapar® Tablets), 4 mg
0932- Ⓒ Meprobamate Tablets, USP, 200 mg
0647- Ⓒ Meprobamate Tablets, USP, 400 mg
0525- Methsuximide Capsules, USP (Celontin® Kapseals), 300 mg
0537- Methsuximide Capsules, USP (Celontin® Kapseals), 150 mg
1460- Nitroglycerin Tablets, USP (Nitrostat® Sublingual Tablets), 0.15 mg
1469- Nitroglycerin Tablets, USP (Nitrostat® Sublingual Tablets), 0.3 mg
1470- Nitroglycerin Tablets, USP (Nitrostat® Sublingual Tablets), 0.4 mg
1471- Nitroglycerin Tablets, USP (Nitrostat® Sublingual Tablets), 0.6 mg
0882- Norethindrone Tablets, USP (Norlutin® Tablets), 5 mg
0918- Norethindrone Acetate Tablets, USP (Norlutate® Tablets), 5 mg
0210- Oxtriphylline (Choledyl) Tablets, USP, 100 mg
0211- Oxtriphylline (Choledyl) Tablets, USP, 200 mg
0503- Pancreatin Tablets, USP (Panteric® Filmseal), 325 mg
0529- Paromomycin Sulfate Capsules, USP (Humatin® Capsules), 250 mg
0648- Penicillin V Potassium Tablets, USP (Penapar VK®), 250 mg
0673- Penicillin V Potassium Tablets, USP (Penapar VK®), 500 mg
0699- Ⓒ Phenobarbital Tablets, USP, 15 mg
0700- Ⓒ Phenobarbital Tablets, USP, 30 mg
0607- Ⓒ Phenobarbital Tablets, USP, 60 mg
0698- Ⓒ Phenobarbital Tablets, USP, 100 mg
0393- Phensuximide Capsules, USP (Milontin® Kapseals), 500 mg
0007- Phenytoin Tablets, USP (Dilantin® Infatabs®), 50 mg
0362- Phenytoin Sodium, Extended, Capsules, USP (Dilantin® Kapseals), 100 mg
0365- Phenytoin Sodium, Extended, Capsules, USP (Dilantin® Kapseals), 30 mg
0552- Ⓒ Prazepam (Centrax®) Capsules, 5 mg
0553- Ⓒ Prazepam (Centrax®) Capsules, 10 mg
0554 Ⓒ Prazepam (Centrax®) Capsules, 20 mg
0276- Ⓒ Prazepam (Centrax®) Tablets, 10 mg
0202 Procainamide Hydrochloride Tablets, Sustained Release (Procan® SR), 250 mg
0204 Procainamide Hydrochloride Tablets, Sustained Release (Procan® SR), 500 mg
0205 Procainamide Hydrochloride Tablets, Sustained Release (Procan® SR), 750 mg
0692- Ⓒ Propoxyphene Hydrochloride Capsules, USP, 65 mg
0694- Ⓒ Propoxyphene Compound 65, Capsules
0747- Pyrvinium Pamoate Tablets, USP (Povan® Filmseal), 50 mg
0437- Quinestrol tablets (Estrovis® Tablets), 100 mcg
0850- Quinidine Gluconate Tablets, Sustained Release, (Duraquin® Tablets), 330 mg
0849- Quinidine Sulfate Tablets, USP, 200 mg
0420- Quinine Sulfate Capsules, USP, 325 mg
0925- Sulfacytine Tablets (Renoquid® Tablets), 250 mg
0407- Tetracycline Hydrochloride Capsules, USP (Cyclopar®), 250 mg
0697- Tetracycline Hydrochloride Capsules, USP (Cyclopar® 500), 500 mg
0251- Thyroglobulin Tablets (Proloid®), ½ grain
0252- Thyroglobulin Tablets (Proloid®), 1 grain
0253- Thyroglobulin Tablets (Proloid®), 1½ grains
0257- Thyroglobulin Tablets (Proloid®), 2 grains
0254- Thyroglobulin Tablets (Proloid®), 3 grains

GERIPLEX®

Geriatric Vitamin-Mineral Formula

Composition: Each Kapseal represents:

Vitamins:

Vitamin A (acetate)	(1.5 mg) 5,000 IU*
Vitamin C (ascorbic acid)†	50 mg
Vitamin B_1 (thiamine mononitrate)	5 mg
Vitamin B_2 (riboflavin)	5 mg
Vitamin B_{12}, crystalline (cyanocobalamin)	2 mcg
Choline dihydrogen citrate	20 mg
Nicotinamide (niacinamide)	15 mg
Vitamin E (*dl*-alpha tocopheryl acetate, 5 mg)	5 IU*

Minerals and Enzymes:

Ferrous sulfate‡	30 mg
Copper sulfate	4 mg
Manganese sulfate (monohydrate)	4 mg
Zinc sulfate	2 mg
Calcium phosphate, dibasic (anhydrous)	200 mg
Taka-Diastase® (aspergillus oryzae enzymes)	2½ gr

* International Units
†Supplied as sodium ascorbate
‡Supplied as dried ferrous sulfate equivalent to the labeled amount of ferrous sulfate or 6 mg elemental iron

Action and Uses: A preparation containing vitamins and minerals for middle-aged and older individuals.

Administration and Dosage: Usual dosage—one capsule daily, with or immediately after a meal.

How Supplied: N 0071-0382-24—Bottles of 100. Parcode® No. 382.

GERIPLEX-FS® KAPSEALS®

Composition: Each Kapseal represents:

Vitamin A (acetate)	(1.5 mg) 5,000 IU*
Vitamin C (ascorbic acid)†	50 mg
Vitamin B_1 (thiamine mononitrate)	5 mg
Vitamin B_2 (riboflavin)	5 mg
Vitamin B_{12}, crystalline (cyanocobalamin)	2 mcg
Choline dihydrogen citrate	20 mg
Nicotinamide (niacinamide)	15 mg
Vitamin E (*dl*-alpha tocopheryl acetate, 5 mg)	5 IU*
Iron‡	30 mg
Copper sulfate	4 mg
Manganese sulfate (monohydrate)	4 mg
Zinc sulfate	2 mg
Calcium phosphate, dibasic (anhydrous)	200 mg
Taka-Diastase® (aspergillus oryzae enzymes)	2½ gr
Docusate sodium	100 mg

* International Units
†Supplied as sodium ascorbate
‡Supplied as 30 mg dried ferrous sulfate

Action and Uses: A preparation containing vitamins, minerals, and a fecal softener for middle-aged and older individuals. The fecal softening agent, docusate sodium, acts to soften stools and make bowel movements easier.

Administration and Dosage: USUAL DOSAGE—One capsule daily, with or immediately after a meal.

How Supplied: N 0071-0544-24—Bottles of 100. Parcode® No. 544.

[*Shown in Product Identification Section*]

GERIPLEX-FS® LIQUID

Geriatric Vitamin Formula with Iron and a Fecal Softener

Composition: Each 30 ml represents vitamin B_1 (thiamine hydrochloride), 1.2 mg; vitamin B_2 (as riboflavin-5′-phosphate sodium), 1.7 mg; vitamin B_6 (pyridoxine hydrochloride), 1 mg; vitamin B_{12} (cyanocobalamin) crystalline, 5 mcg; niacinamide, 15 mg; iron (as ferric ammonium citrate, green), 15 mg; Pluronic® F-68,* 200 mg; alcohol, 18%.

Administration and Dosage: USUAL ADULT DOSAGE—Two tablespoonfuls (30 ml) daily or as recommended by the physician.

How Supplied: N 0071-2454-23—16-oz bottles.

*Pluronic is a registered trademark of BASF Wyandotte Corporation for polymers of ethylene oxide and propylene oxide.

HYDROCHLOROTHIAZIDE TABLETS, USP ℞

(Thiuretic®)

Description: Hydrochlorothiazide is a member of the benzothiadiazine (thiazide) family of drugs, closely related to chlorothiazide. Its chemical name is 6-chloro-3,4-dihydro-*2H*-1,2,4-benzothiadiazine-7-sulfonamide 1,1-dioxide.
Hydrochlorothiazide is a white, or practically white, crystalline compound which is slightly soluble in water and soluble in alcohol.
Clinically, hydrochlorothiazide is a diuretic-antihypertensive agent, available in 25 mg and 50 mg strength tablets for oral administration.

Clinical Pharmacology: The diuretic and saluretic effects of hydrochlorothiazide result from a drug-induced inhibition of the renal tubular reabsorption of electrolytes. The excretion of sodium and chloride is greatly enhanced. Potassium excretion is also enhanced to a variable degree, as it is with the other thiazides. Although urinary excretion of bicarbonate is increased slightly, there is usually no significant change in urinary pH. Hydrochlorothiazide has a per mg natriuretic activity approximately 10 times that of the prototype thiazide, chlorothiazide. At maximal therapeutic dosages, all thiazides are approximately equal in their diuretic/natriuretic effects.
There is significant natriuresis and diuresis within two hours after administration of a single oral dose of hydrochlorothiazide. These effects reach a peak in about six hours and persist for about 12 hours following oral administration of a single dose.
Like other benzothiadiazines, hydrochlorothiazide also has antihypertensive properties, and may be used for this purpose either alone or to enhance the antihypertensive action of other drugs. The mechanism by which the benzothiadiazines, including hydrochlorothiazide, produce a reduction of elevated blood pressure is not known. However, sodium depletion appears to be involved.
Hydrochlorothiazide is readily absorbed from the gastrointestinal tract and is excreted unchanged by the kidneys. Excretion of the drug is essentially complete within 24 hours.

Indications and Usage: Hydrochlorothiazide is indicated in the management of hypertension either as the sole therapeutic agent or to enhance the effectiveness of other antihypertensive drugs in the more severe forms of hypertension.
Hydrochlorothiazide is indicated as adjunctive therapy in edema associated with congestive heart failure, hepatic cirrhosis, and corticosteroid and estrogen therapy.
Hydrochlorothiazide has also been found useful in edema due to various forms of renal dysfunction such as the nephrotic syndrome, acute glomerulonephritis, and chronic renal failure.

Usage in Pregnancy: The routine use of diuretics in an otherwise healthy pregnant woman is inappropriate and exposes mother and fetus to unnecessary hazard. Diuretics do not prevent development of toxemia of pregnancy, and there is no satisfactory evidence that they are useful in the treatment of developed toxemia.
Edema during pregnancy may arise from pathological causes or from the physiological and mechanical consequences of pregnancy. Thiazides are indicated in pregnancy when edema is due to pathological causes, just as they are in the absence of pregnancy (however, see PRECAUTIONS below). Dependent edema in pregnancy, resulting from restriction of venous return by the expanded uterus, is properly treated through elevation of the lower extremities and use of support hose; use of diuretics to lower intravascular volume in this case is illogical and unnecessary. There is hypervolemia during normal pregnancy which is harmful to neither the fetus nor the mother (in the absence of cardiovascular disease), but which is associated with edema, including generalized edema, in the majority of pregnant women. If this edema produces discomfort, increased recumbency will often provide relief. In rare instances, this edema may cause extreme discomfort which is not relieved by rest. In these cases, a short course of diuretics may provide relief and may be appropriate.

Contraindications: Anuria.
Hypersensitivity to this or other sulfonamide-derived drugs.

Warnings: Thiazides should be used with caution in patients with renal disease or significant impairment of renal function. In patients with renal disease, thiazides may precipitate azotemia. Cumulative effects of the drug may develop in patients with impaired renal function.
Thiazides should be used with caution in patients with impaired hepatic function or progressive liver disease, since minor alterations of fluid and electrolyte balance may precipitate hepatic coma.
Thiazides may add to or potentiate the action of other antihypertensive drugs. Potentiation occurs with ganglionic or peripheral adrenergic blocking drugs.
Sensitivity reactions may occur in patients with a history of allergy or bronchial asthma.
The possibility of exacerbation or activation of systemic lupus erythematosus has been reported.

Precautions: Periodic determinations of serum electrolytes should be performed at appropriate intervals for the purpose of detecting possible electrolyte imbalances. All patients receiving thiazide therapy should be observed for clinical signs of fluid or electrolyte imbalance, namely, hyponatremia, hypochloremic alkalosis, and hypokalemia. Serum and urine electrolyte determinations are particularly important when a patient is vomiting excessively or receiving parenteral fluids. Warning signs of electrolyte imbalance include dryness of mouth, thirst, weakness, lethargy, drowsiness, restlessness, muscle pains or cramps, muscular fatigue, hypotension, oliguria, tachycardia, and gastrointestinal disturbances such as nausea and vomiting.
Hypokalemia may develop with thiazides as with any other potent diuretic, especially when brisk diuresis occurs, severe cirrhosis is present, or when corticosteroids or ACTH are given concomitantly. Interference with the adequate oral intake of electrolytes will also contribute to the possible development of hypokalemia. Potassium depletion, even of a mild degree, resulting from thiazide use may sensitize a patient to the effects of cardiac glycosides such as digitalis.
Any chloride deficit is generally mild and usually does not require specific treatment except under extraordinary circumstances (as in liver disease or renal disease). Dilutional hyponatremia may occur in edematous patients in hot weather; appropriate therapy is water restriction rather than administration of salt except in rare instances where the hyponatremia is life threatening.
In actual salt depletion, appropriate replacement is the therapy of choice.
Hyperuricemia may occur or frank gout may be precipitated in certain patients receiving thiazide therapy.
Insulin requirements in diabetic patients may be increased, decreased or unchanged. Latent diabetes mellitus may become manifest during thiazide administration.
Thiazide drugs may increase the responsiveness to tubocurarine.
The antihypertensive effects of the drug may be enhanced in the postsympathectomy patient.
Thiazides may decrease arterial responsiveness to norepinephrine. This diminution is not sufficient to preclude effectiveness of the pressor agent for therapeutic use.
If progressive renal impairment becomes evident as indicated by a rising nonprotein nitrogen or blood urea nitrogen, a careful reappraisal of therapy is necessary with consideration given to withholding or discontinuing diuretic therapy.
Thiazides may decrease serum PBI levels without signs of thyroid disturbance.
Thiazides have been reported, on rare occasions, to have elevated serum calcium to hyper-

Continued on next page

This product information was prepared in August, 1982. On these and other Parke-Davis Products, information may be obtained by addressing PARKE-DAVIS, Division of Warner-Lambert Company, Morris Plains, New Jersey 07950.

Parke-Davis—Cont.

calcemic levels. The serum calcium levels have returned to normal when the medication has been stopped. This phenomenon may be related to the ability of the thiazide diuretics to lower the amount of calcium excreted in the urine.

Usage in Pregnancy: Thiazides cross the placental barrier and appear in cord blood. The use of thiazides in pregnant women requires that the anticipated benefit be weighed against possible hazards to the fetus. These hazards include fetal or neonatal jaundice, thrombocytopenia, and possible other adverse reactions that have occurred in the adults. (Also see INDICATIONS AND USAGE, above.)

Nursing Mothers: Thiazides appear in breast milk. If use of the drug is deemed essential, the patient should stop nursing.

Adverse Reactions:

A. ***Gastrointestinal System***

1. anorexia
2. gastric irritation
3. nausea
4. vomiting
5. cramping
6. diarrhea
7. constipation
8. jaundice (intrahepatic cholestatic jaundice)
9. pancreatitis

B. ***Central Nervous System***

1. dizziness
2. vertigo
3. paresthesias
4. headache
5. xanthopsia

C. ***Hematologic***

1. leukopenia
2. agranulocytosis
3. thrombocytopenia
4. aplastic anemia

D. ***Dermatologic-Hypersensitivity***

1. purpura
2. photosensitivity
3. rash
4. urticaria
5. necrotizing angiitis (vasculitis) (cutaneous vasculitis)

E. ***Cardiovascular***

Orthostatic hypotension may occur and may be aggravated by alcohol, barbiturates, or narcotics.

F. ***Other***

1. hyperglycemia
2. glycosuria
3. hypercalcemia
4. hyperuricemia
5. muscle spasm
6. weakness
7. restlessness
8. severe fluid and electrolyte derangements (rarely)

Whenever adverse reactions are moderate or severe, thiazide dosage should be reduced or therapy withdrawn.

Overdosage: Symptoms of overdosage include electrolyte imbalance and signs of potassium deficiency such as confusion, dizziness, muscular weakness and gastrointestinal disturbances. General supportive measures including replacement of fluids and electrolytes may be indicated in treatment of overdosage.

Dosage and Administration: Hydrochlorothiazide is administered orally. Therapy should be individualized according to the patient's requirements and response. The response of the patient depends on factors such as the nature and degree of the disease, state of hydration, cardiac output, physical activity, diet, and concurrent administration of other drugs. Therapy should be titrated to attain the maximum therapeutic effect at minimum dosage.

Adult Dose: For the management of edema, the usual initial adult dosage is 25 to 200 mg daily given in 1 to 3 doses. When nonedematous weight is attained, a maintenance dosage of 25 to 100 mg daily or intermittently may be instituted. Occasionally, up to 200 mg daily is required in refractory patients.

For the management of hypertension, the usual initial adult dosage is 50 to 100 mg daily, given in 2 divided doses. The dosage may be increased if necessary to a maximum of 200 mg daily, given in 2 divided doses. Maintenance dosage is determined by the patient's blood pressure and usually ranges from 25 to 100 mg daily in a single dose.

When therapy is prolonged or large doses are used, particular attention should be given to the patient's electrolyte status. Supplemental potassium may be required.

In the treatment of hypertension, hydrochlorothiazide may be employed either alone or concurrently with other antihypertensive drugs. Combined therapy may provide adequate control of hypertension with lower dosage of the component drugs and fewer or less severe side effects.

For treatment of moderate to severe hypertension, supplemental use of other more potent antihypertensive agents may be indicated.

When other antihypertensive agents are to be added to the regimen, this should be accomplished gradually. Additional potent antihypertensive agents should be given at only half the usual dose since their effect is potentiated by pretreatment with hydrochlorothiazide.

Pediatric Dose: The usual pediatric dosage is 1 mg hydrochlorothiazide per pound of body weight per day, given in 2 divided doses. Infants younger than 6 months of age may require up to 1.5 mg per pound per day in 2 divided doses.

How Supplied: Hydrochlorothiazide Tablets, USP, 25 mg (white, round, scored, coded P-D 702) are available in bottles of 100 (N 0071-0702-24).

Hydrochlorothiazide Tablets, USP, 50 mg (white, round, scored, coded P-D 710) are available in bottles of 100 (N 0071-0710-24), bottles of 1000 (N 0071-0710-32), and unit dose packages of 100 (N 0071-0710-40).

0702G011

KETALAR® ℞

(Ketamine Hydrochloride Injection, USP)

SPECIAL NOTE

EMERGENCE REACTIONS HAVE OCCURRED IN APPROXIMATELY 12 PERCENT OF PATIENTS.

THE PSYCHOLOGICAL MANIFESTATIONS VARY IN SEVERITY BETWEEN PLEASANT DREAM-LIKE STATES, VIVID IMAGERY, HALLUCINATIONS, AND EMERGENCE DELIRIUM. IN SOME CASES THESE STATES HAVE BEEN ACCOMPANIED BY CONFUSION, EXCITEMENT, AND IRRATIONAL BEHAVIOR WHICH A FEW PATIENTS RECALL AS AN UNPLEASANT EXPERIENCE. THE DURATION ORDINARILY IS NO MORE THAN A FEW HOURS; IN A FEW CASES, HOWEVER, RECURRENCES HAVE TAKEN PLACE UP TO 24 HOURS POSTOPERATIVELY. NO RESIDUAL PSYCHOLOGICAL EFFECTS ARE KNOWN TO HAVE RESULTED FROM USE OF KETALAR.

THE INCIDENCE OF THESE EMERGENCE PHENOMENA IS LEAST IN THE YOUNG (15 YEARS OF AGE OR LESS) AND ELDERLY (OVER 65 YEARS OF AGE) PATIENT. ALSO, THEY ARE LESS FREQUENT WHEN THE DRUG IS GIVEN INTRAMUSCULARLY AND THE INCIDENCE IS REDUCED AS EXPERIENCE WITH THE DRUG IS GAINED.

THE INCIDENCE OF PSYCHOLOGICAL MANIFESTATIONS DURING EMERGENCE, PARTICULARLY DREAM-LIKE OBSERVATIONS AND EMERGENCE DELIRIUM, MAY BE REDUCED BY USING LOWER RECOMMENDED DOSAGES OF KETALAR IN CONJUNCTION WITH INTRAVENOUS DIAZEPAM DURING INDUCTION AND MAINTENANCE OF ANESTHESIA. (See Dosage and Administration.) ALSO, THESE REACTIONS MAY BE REDUCED IF VERBAL, TACTILE AND VISUAL STIMULATION OF THE PATIENT IS MINIMIZED DURING THE RECOVERY PERIOD. THIS DOES NOT PRECLUDE THE MONITORING OF VITAL SIGNS.

IN ORDER TO TERMINATE A SEVERE EMERGENCE REACTION THE USE OF A SMALL HYPNOTIC DOSE OF A SHORT-ACTING OR ULTRASHORT-ACTING BARBITURATE MAY BE REQUIRED.

WHEN KETALAR IS USED ON AN OUTPATIENT BASIS, THE PATIENT SHOULD NOT BE RELEASED UNTIL RECOVERY FROM ANESTHESIA IS COMPLETE AND THEN SHOULD BE ACCOMPANIED BY A RESPONSIBLE ADULT.

Description: Ketalar is a nonbarbiturate anesthetic, chemically designated *dl* 2-(o-chlorophenyl)-2-(methylamino) cyclohexanone hydrochloride. It is formulated as a slightly acid (pH 3.5-5.5) sterile solution for intravenous or intramuscular injection in concentrations containing the equivalent of either 10, 50 or 100 mg ketamine base per milliliter and contains not more than 0.1 mg/ml Phemerol® (benzethonium chloride) added as a preservative. The 10 mg/ml solution has been made isotonic with sodium chloride.

Clinical Pharmacology: Ketalar is a rapid-acting general anesthetic producing an anesthetic state characterized by profound analgesia, normal pharyngeal-laryngeal reflexes, normal or slightly enhanced skeletal muscle tone, cardiovascular and respiratory stimulation, and occasionally a transient and minimal respiratory depression.

A patent airway is maintained partly by virtue of unimpaired pharyngeal and laryngeal reflexes. (See Warnings and Precautions.)

The biotransformation of Ketalar includes N-dealkylation (metabolite I), hydroxylation of the cyclohexone ring (metabolites III and IV), conjugation with glucuronic acid and dehydration of the hydroxylated metabolites to form the cyclohexene derivative (metabolite II).

Following intravenous administration, the ketamine concentration has an initial slope (alpha phase) lasting about 45 minutes with a half-life of 10 to 15 minutes. This first phase corresponds clinically to the anesthetic effect of the drug. The anesthetic action is terminated by a combination of redistribution from the CNS to slower equilibrating peripheral tissues and by hepatic biotransformation to metabolite I. This metabolite is about ⅓ as active as ketamine in reducing halothane requirements (MAC) of the rat. The later half-life of ketamine (beta phase) is 2.5 hours.

The anesthetic state produced by Ketalar has been termed "dissociative anesthesia" in that it appears to selectively interrupt association pathways of the brain before producing somesthetic sensory blockade. It may selectively depress the thalamoneocortical system before significantly obtunding the more ancient cerebral centers and pathways (reticular-activating and limbic systems).

Elevation of blood pressure begins shortly after injection, reaches a maximum within a few minutes and usually returns to preanesthetic values within 15 minutes after injection. In the majority of cases, the systolic and diastolic blood pressure peaks from 10% to 50% above preanesthetic levels shortly after induction of anesthesia, but the elevation can be higher or longer in individual cases (see Contraindications).

Ketamine has a wide margin of safety; several instances of unintentional administration of overdoses of Ketalar (up to ten times that usu-

ally required) have been followed by prolonged but complete recovery.
Ketalar has been studied in over 12,000 operative and diagnostic procedures, involving over 10,000 patients from 105 separate studies. During the course of these studies Ketalar was administered as the sole agent, as induction for other general agents, or to supplement low-potency agents.
Specific areas of application have included the following:
1. debridement, painful dressings, and skin grafting in burn patients, as well as other superficial surgical procedures.
2. neurodiagnostic procedures such as pneumoencephalograms, ventriculograms, myelograms, and lumbar punctures. See also Precaution concerning increased intracranial pressure.
3. diagnostic and operative procedures of the eye, ear, nose, and mouth, including dental extractions.
4. diagnostic and operative procedures of the pharynx, larynx, or bronchial tree. NOTE: Muscle relaxants, with proper attention to respiration, may be required (see Precautions).
5. sigmoidoscopy and minor surgery of the anus and rectum, and circumcision.
6. extraperitoneal procedures used in gynecology such as dilatation and curettage.
7. orthopedic procedures such as closed reductions, manipulations, femoral pinning, amputations, and biopsies.
8. as an anesthetic in poor-risk patients with depression of vital functions.
9. in procedures where the intramuscular route of administration is preferred.
10. in cardiac catheterization procedures.
In these studies, the anesthesia was rated either "excellent" or "good" by the anesthesiologist and the surgeon at 90% and 93%, respectively; rated "fair" at 6% and 4%, respectively; and rated "poor" at 4% and 3%, respectively. In a second method of evaluation, the anesthesia was rated "adequate" in at least 90%, and "inadequate" in 10% or less of the procedures.

Indications and Usage: Ketalar is indicated as the sole anesthetic agent for diagnostic and surgical procedures that do not require skeletal muscle relaxation. Ketalar is best suited for short procedures but it can be used, with additional doses, for longer procedures.
Ketalar is indicated for the induction of anesthesia prior to the administration of other general anesthetic agents.
Ketalar is indicated to supplement low-potency agents, such as nitrous oxide.
Specific areas of application are described in the Clinical Pharmacology section.

Contraindications: Ketamine hydrochloride is contraindicated in those in whom a significant elevation of blood pressure would constitute a serious hazard and in those who have shown hypersensitivity to the drug.

Warnings: Cardiac function should be continually monitored during the procedure in patients found to have hypertension or cardiac decompensation.
Postoperative confusional states may occur during the recovery period. (See Special Note.)
Respiratory depression may occur with overdosage or too rapid a rate of administration of Ketalar, in which case supportive ventilation should be employed. Mechanical support of respiration is preferred to administration of analeptics.

Precautions:

General

Ketalar should be used by or under the direction of physicians experienced in administering general anesthetics and in maintenance of an airway and in the control of respiration.
Because pharyngeal and laryngeal reflexes are usually active, Ketalar should not be used alone in surgery or diagnostic procedures of the pharynx, larynx, or bronchial tree. Mechanical stimulation of the pharynx should be avoided, whenever possible, if Ketalar is used alone. Muscle relaxants, with proper attention to respiration, may be required in both of these instances.
Resuscitative equipment should be ready for use.
The incidence of emergence reactions may be reduced if verbal and tactile stimulation of the patient is minimized during the recovery period. This does not preclude the monitoring of vital signs (see Special Note).
The intravenous dose should be administered over a period of 60 seconds. More rapid administration may result in respiratory depression or apnea and enhanced pressor response.
In surgical procedures involving visceral pain pathways, Ketalar should be supplemented with an agent which obtunds visceral pain.
Use with caution in the chronic alcoholic and the acutely alcohol-intoxicated patient.
An increase in cerebrospinal fluid pressure has been reported following administration of ketamine hydrochloride. Use with extreme caution in patients with preanesthetic elevated cerebrospinal fluid pressure.

Information for Patients

As appropriate, especially in cases where early discharge is possible, the duration of Ketalar and other drugs employed during the conduct of anesthesia should be considered. The patients should be cautioned that driving an automobile, operating hazardous machinery or engaging in hazardous activities should not be undertaken for 24 hours or more (depending upon the dosage of Ketalar and consideration of other drugs employed) after anesthesia.

Drug Interactions

Prolonged recovery time may occur if barbiturates and/or narcotics are used concurrently with Ketalar.
Ketalar is clinically compatible with the commonly used general and local anesthetic agents when an adequate respiratory exchange is maintained.

Usage in Pregnancy

Since the safe use in pregnancy, including obstetrics (either vaginal or abdominal delivery), has not been established, such use is not recommended (see Animal Reproduction).

Adverse Reactions:

Cardiovascular: Blood pressure and pulse rate are frequently elevated following administration of Ketalar alone. However, hypotension and bradycardia have been observed. Arrhythmia has also occurred.
Respiration: Although respiration is frequently stimulated, severe depression of respiration or apnea may occur following rapid intravenous administration of high doses of Ketalar. Laryngospasms and other forms of airway obstruction have occurred during Ketalar anesthesia.
Eye: Diplopia and nystagmus have been noted following Ketalar administration.
It also may cause a slight elevation in intraocular pressure measurement.
Psychological: (See Special Note).
Neurological: In some patients, enhanced skeletal muscle tone may be manifested by tonic and clonic movements sometimes resembling seizures (see Dosage and Administration).
Gastrointestinal: Anorexia, nausea and vomiting have been observed; however this is not usually severe and allows the great majority of patients to take liquids by mouth shortly after regaining consciousness (see Dosage and Administration).
General: Local pain and exanthema at the injection site have infrequently been reported. Transient erythema and/or morbilliform rash have also been reported.

Overdosage: Respiratory depression may occur with overdosage or too rapid a rate of administration of Ketalar, in which case supportive ventilation should be employed. Mechanical support of respiration is preferred to administration of analeptics.

Dosage and Administration:

Note: Barbiturates and Ketalar, being chemically incompatible because of precipitate formation, *should not* be injected from the same syringe.
If the Ketalar dose is augmented with diazepam, the two drugs must be given separately. Do not mix Ketalar and diazepam in syringe or infusion flask. For additional information on the use of diazepam, refer to the Warnings and Dosage and Administration Sections of the diazepam insert.

Preoperative Preparations:

1. While vomiting has been reported following Ketalar administration, some airway protection may be afforded because of active laryngeal-pharyngeal reflexes. However, since aspiration may occur with Ketalar and since protective reflexes may also be diminished by supplementary anesthetics and muscle relaxants, the possibility of aspiration must be considered. Ketalar is recommended for use in the patient whose stomach is not empty when, in the judgment of the practitioner, the benefits of the drug outweigh the possible risks.
2. Atropine, scopolamine, or another drying agent should be given at an appropriate interval prior to induction.

Onset and Duration:

Because of rapid induction following the initial intravenous injection, the patient should be in a supported position during administration.
The onset of action of Ketalar is rapid; an intravenous dose of 2 mg/kg (1 mg/lb) of body weight usually produces surgical anesthesia within 30 seconds after injection, with the anesthetic effect usually lasting five to ten minutes. If a longer effect is desired, additional increments can be administered intravenously or intramuscularly to maintain anesthesia without producing significant cumulative effects.
Intramuscular doses, from experience primarily in children, in a range of 9 to 13 mg/kg (4 to 6 mg/lb) usually produce surgical anesthesia within 3 to 4 minutes following injection, with the anesthetic effect usually lasting 12 to 25 minutes.

Dosage:

As with other general anesthetic agents, the individual response to Ketalar is somewhat varied depending on the dose, route of administration, and age of patient, so that dosage recommendation cannot be absolutely fixed. The drug should be titrated against the patient's requirements.

Induction:

Intravenous Route: The initial dose of Ketalar administered intravenously may range from 1 mg/kg to 4.5 mg/kg (0.5 to 2 mg/lb). The average amount required to produce five to ten minutes of surgical anesthesia has been 2 mg/kg (1 mg/lb).
Alternatively, in adult patients an induction dose of 1.0 mg to 2.0 mg/kg intravenous ketamine at a rate of 0.5 mg/kg/min may be used for induction of anesthesia. In addition, diazepam in 2 mg to 5 mg doses, administered in a separate syringe over 60 seconds, may be used. In most cases, 15.0 mg of intravenous diazepam *or less* will suffice. The incidence of psychological manifestations during emergence, particularly dream-like observations and emergence delirium, may be reduced by this induction dosage program.
Note: The 100 mg/ml concentration of Ketalar *should not* be injected intravenously with-

Continued on next page

This product information was prepared in August, 1982. On these and other Parke-Davis Products, information may be obtained by addressing PARKE-DAVIS, Division of Warner-Lambert Company, Morris Plains, New Jersey 07950.

Parke-Davis—Cont.

out proper dilution. It is recommended the drug be diluted with an equal volume of either Sterile Water for Injection, USP, Normal Saline, or 5% Dextrose in Water.

Rate of Administration: It is recommended that Ketalar be administered slowly (over a period of 60 seconds). More rapid administration may result in respiratory depression and enhanced pressor response.

Intramuscular Route: The initial dose of Ketalar administered intramuscularly may range from 6.5 to 13 mg/kg (3 to 6 mg/lb). A dose of 10 mg/kg (5 mg/lb) will usually produce 12 to 25 minutes of surgical anesthesia.

Maintenance of Anesthesia:

The maintenance dose should be adjusted according to the patient's anesthetic needs and whether an additional anesthetic agent is employed.

Increments of one-half to the full induction dose may be repeated as needed for maintenance of anesthesia. However, it should be noted that purposeless and tonic-clonic movements of extremities may occur during the course of anesthesia. These movements do not imply a light plane and are not indicative of the need for additional doses of the anesthetic. It should be recognized that the larger the total dose of Ketalar administered, the longer will be the time to complete recovery.

Adult patients induced with Ketalar augmented with intravenous diazepam may be maintained on Ketalar given by slow microdrip infusion technique at a dose of 0.1 to 0.5 mg/minute, augmented with diazepam 2 to 5 mg administered intravenously as needed. In many cases 20 mg *or less* of intravenous diazepam total for combined induction and maintenance will suffice. However, slightly more diazepam may be required depending on the nature and duration of the operation, physical status of the patient, and other factors. The incidence of psychological manifestations during emergence, particularly dream-like observations and emergence delirium, may be reduced by this maintenance dosage program.

Dilution: To prepare a dilute solution containing 1 mg of ketamine per ml, aseptically transfer 10 ml (50 mg per ml Steri-Vial) or 5 ml (100 mg per ml Steri-Vial) to 500 ml of 5% Dextrose Injection, USP or Sodium Chloride (0.9%) Injection, USP (Normal Saline) and mix well. The resultant solution will contain 1 mg of ketamine per ml.

The fluid requirements of the patient and duration of anesthesia must be considered when selecting the appropriate dilution of Ketalar. If fluid restriction is required, Ketalar can be added to a 250 ml infusion as described above to provide a Ketalar concentration of 2 mg/ml. Ketalar Steri-Vials, 10 mg/ml are not recommended for dilution.

Supplementary Agents:

Ketalar is clinically compatible with the commonly used general and local anesthetic agents when an adequate respiratory exchange is maintained.

The regimen of a reduced dose of Ketalar supplemented with diazepam can be used to produce balanced anesthesia by combination with other agents such as nitrous oxide and oxygen.

How Supplied: Ketalar is supplied as the hydrochloride in concentrations equivalent to ketamine base.

N 0071-4581-15—Each 50-ml vial contains 10 mg/ml. Supplied in cartons of 10.

N 0071-4581-13—Each 25-ml vial contains 10 mg/ml. Supplied in cartons of 10.

N 0071-4581-12—Each 20-ml vial contains 10 mg/ml. Supplied in cartons of 10.

N 0071-4582-10—Each 10-ml vial contains 50 mg/ml. Supplied in cartons of 10.

N 0071-4585-08—Each 5-ml vial contains 100 mg/ml. Supplied in cartons of 10.

Animal Pharmacology and Toxicology:

Toxicity: The acute toxicity of Ketalar has been studied in several species. In mature mice and rats, the intraperitoneal LD_{50} values are approximately 100 times the average human intravenous dose and approximately 20 times the average human intramuscular dose. A slightly higher acute toxicity observed in neonatal rats was not sufficiently elevated to suggest an increased hazard when used in children. Daily intravenous injections in rats of five times the average human intravenous dose and intramuscular injections in dogs at four times the average human intramuscular dose demonstrated excellent tolerance for as long as 6 weeks. Similarly, twice weekly anesthetic sessions of one, three, or six hours' duration in monkeys over a four-to six-week period were well tolerated.

Interaction With Other Drugs Commonly Used For Preanesthetic Medication: Large doses (three or more times the equivalent effective human dose) of morphine, meperidine, and atropine increased the depth and prolonged the duration of anesthesia produced by a standard anesthetizing dose of Ketalar in Rhesus monkeys. The prolonged duration was not of sufficient magnitude to contraindicate the use of these drugs for preanesthetic medication in human clinical trials.

Blood Pressure: Blood pressure responses to Ketalar vary with the laboratory species and experimental conditions. Blood pressure is increased in normotensive and renal hypertensive rats with and without adrenalectomy and under pentobarbital anesthesia.

Intravenous Ketalar produces a fall in arterial blood pressure in the Rhesus monkey and a rise in arterial blood pressure in the dog. In this respect the dog mimics the cardiovascular effect observed in man. The pressor response to Ketalar injected into intact, unanesthetized dogs is accompanied by a tachycardia, rise in cardiac output and a fall in total peripheral resistance. It causes a fall in perfusion pressure following a large dose injected into an artificially perfused vascular bed (dog hindquarters), and it has little or no potentiating effect upon vasoconstriction responses of epinephrine or norepinephrine. The pressor response to Ketalar is reduced or blocked by chlorpromazine (central depressant and peripheral α-adrenergic blockade), by β-adrenergic blockade, and by ganglionic blockade. The tachycardia and increase in myocardial contractile force seen in intact animals does not appear in isolated hearts (Langendorff) at a concentration of 0.1 mg of Ketalar nor in Starling dog heart-lung preparations at a Ketalar concentration of 50 mg/kg of HLP. These observations support the hypothesis that the hypertension produced by Ketalar is due to selective activation of central cardiac stimulating mechanisms leading to an increase in cardiac output. The dog myocardium is not sensitized to epinephrine and Ketalar appears to have a weak antiarrhythmic activity.

Metabolic Disposition: Ketalar is rapidly absorbed following parenteral administration. Animal experiments indicated that Ketalar was rapidly distributed into body tissues, with relatively high concentrations appearing in body fat, liver, lung, and brain; lower concentrations were found in the heart, skeletal muscle, and blood plasma. Placental transfer of the drug was found to occur in pregnant dogs and monkeys. No significant degree of binding to serum albumin was found with Ketalar.

Balance studies in rats, dogs, and monkeys resulted in the recovery of 85% to 95% of the dose in the urine, mainly in the form of degradation products. Small amounts of drug were also excreted in the bile and feces. Balance studies with tritium-labeled Ketalar in human subjects (1 mg/lb given intravenously) resulted in the mean recovery of 91% of the dose in the urine and 3% in the feces. Peak plasma levels averaged about 0.75 μg/ml, and CSF levels were about 0.2 μg/ml, 1 hour after dosing.

Ketalar undergoes N-demethylation and hydroxylation of the cyclohexanone ring, with the formation of water-soluble conjugates which are excreted in the urine. Further oxidation also occurs with the formation of a cyclohexanone derivative. The unconjugated N-demethylated metabolite was found to be less than one-sixth as potent as Ketalar. The unconjugated demethyl cyclohexanone derivative was found to be less than one-tenth as potent as Ketalar. Repeated doses of Ketalar administered to animals did not produce any detectable increase in microsomal enzyme activity.

Reproduction: Male and female rats, when given five times the average human intravenous dose of Ketalar for three consecutive days about one week before mating, had a reproductive performance equivalent to that of saline-injected controls. When given to pregnant rats and rabbits intramuscularly at twice the average human intramuscular dose during the respective periods of organogenesis, the litter characteristics were equivalent to those of saline-injected controls. A small group of rabbits was given a single large dose (six times the average human dose) of Ketalar on Day 6 of pregnancy to simulate the effect of an excessive clinical dose around the period of nidation. The outcome of pregnancy was equivalent in control and treated groups.

To determine the effect of Ketalar on the perinatal and postnatal period, pregnant rats were given twice the average human intramuscular dose during Days 18 to 21 of pregnancy. Litter characteristics at birth and through the weaning period were equivalent to those of the control animals. There was a slight increase in incidence of delayed parturition by one day in treated dams of this group. Three groups each of mated beagle bitches were given 2.5 times the average human intramuscular dose twice weekly for the three weeks of the first, second, and third trimesters of pregnancy, respectively, without the development of adverse effects in the pups.

121 866700/30

LOESTRIN® 21 1/20 ℞

(Each white tablet contains 1 mg norethindrone acetate and 20 mcg ethinyl estradiol.)

LOESTRIN® 21 1.5/30 ℞

(Each green tablet contains 1.5 mg norethindrone acetate and 30 mcg ethinyl estradiol.)

LOESTRIN® Fe 1/20 ℞

(Each white tablet contains 1 mg norethindrone acetate and 20 mcg ethinyl estradiol. Each brown tablet contains 75 mg ferrous fumarate, USP.)

LOESTRIN® Fe 1.5/30 ℞

(Each green tablet contains 1.5 mg norethindrone acetate and 30 mcg ethinyl estradiol. Each brown tablet contains 75 mg ferrous fumarate, USP)

Each white tablet contains: norethindrone acetate (17 alpha-ethinyl-19-nortestosterone acetate), 1 mg; ethinyl estradiol (17 alpha-ethinyl-1,3,5(10)-estratriene-3,17 beta-diol), 20 mcg.

Each green tablet contains: norethindrone acetate (17 alpha-ethinyl-19-nortestosterone acetate). 1.5 mg; ethinyl estradiol (17 alpha-ethinyl-1,3,5(10)-estratriene-3, 17 beta-diol), 30 mcg.

Each brown tablet contains 75 mg ferrous fumarate, USP.

Description: Loestrin is a progestogen-estrogen combination.

Loestrin **Fe** 1/20 and 1.5/30 provides a continuous dosage regimen consisting of 21 oral con-

	Myocardial infarction			
	Women aged 30–39		Women aged 40–44	
Smoking habits	Users	Nonusers	Users	Nonusers
All smokers	10.2	2.6	62.0	15.9
Heavy*	13.0	5.1	78.7	31.3
Light	4.7	0.9	28.6	5.7
Nonsmokers	1.8	1.2	10.7	7.4
Smokers and nonsmokers	5.4	1.9	32.8	11.7

*Heavy smoker: 15 or more cigarettes per day. From Jain, A.K., Studies in Family Planning 8:50, 1977.

traceptive tablets and seven ferrous fumarate tablets. The ferrous fumarate tablets are present to facilitate ease of drug administration via a 28-day regimen and are not intended to serve any therapeutic purpose.

Clinical Pharmacology: Combination oral contraceptives act primarily through the mechanism of gonadotropin suppression due to the estrogenic and progestational activity of the ingredients. Although the primary mechanism of action is inhibition of ovulation, alterations in the genital tract, including changes in the cervical mucus (which increase the difficulty of sperm penetration) and the endometrium (which reduce the likelihood of implantation) may also contribute to contraceptive effectiveness.

Indications and Usage: Loestrin is indicated for the prevention of pregnancy in women who elect to use oral contraceptives as a method of contraception.

Oral contraceptives are highly effective. The pregnancy rate in women using conventional combination oral contraceptives (containing 35 mcg or more of ethinyl estradiol or 50 mcg or more of mestranol) is generally reported as less than one pregnancy per 100 women-years of use. Slightly higher rates (somewhat more than one pregnancy per 100 woman-years of use) are reported for some combination products containing 35 mcg or less of ethinyl estradiol, and rates on the order of three pregnancies per 100 woman-years are reported for the progestogen-only oral contraceptives.

These rates are derived from separate studies conducted by different investigators in several population groups and cannot be compared precisely. Furthermore, pregnancy rates tend to be lower as clinical studies are continued, possibly due to selective retention in the longer studies of those patients who accept the treatment regimen and do not discontinue as a result of adverse reactions, pregnancy, or other reasons.

In clinical trials with Loestrin 1/20, 1,431 patients completed 15,899 cycles and a total of 10 pregnancies were reported. This represents a pregnancy rate of 0.75 per 100 woman-years based upon data that include the cases where patients failed to comply with the dosage regimen. The pregnancy rate in patients who adhered to the dosage regimen was 0.30 per 100 woman-years (four pregnancies in these trials).

In clinical trials with Loestrin 1.5/30, 1,289 patients completed 17,139 cycles and a total of 7 pregnancies were reported. This represents a pregnancy rate of 0.49 per 100 woman-years based upon data that include the cases where patients failed to comply with the dosage regimen. The pregnancy rate in patients who adhered to the dosage regimen was 0.07 per 100 woman-years (one pregnancy in these trials).

Table 1 gives ranges of pregnancy rates reported in the literature[1] for other means of contraception. The efficacy of these means of contraception (except the IUD) depends upon the degree of adherence to the method.

Table 1 Pregnancies per 100 Woman-Years

IUD, less than 1–6; Diaphragm with spermicidal products (creams or jellies), 2–20; Condom, 3–36; Aerosol foams, 2–29; Jellies and creams, 4–36; Periodic abstinence (rhythm) all types less than 1–47; *1. Calendar method, 14–47; 2. Temperature method, 1–20; 3. Temperature method—intercourse only in post-ovulatory phase, less than 1–7; 4. Mucus method, 1–25;* No contraception, 60–80.

Dose-Related Risk of Thromboembolism from Oral Contraceptives

Two studies have shown a positive association between the dose of estrogens in oral contraceptives and the risk of thromboembolism.[2,3] For this reason, it is prudent and in keeping with good principles of therapeutics to minimize exposure to estrogen. The oral contraceptive product prescribed for any given patient should be that product which contains the least amount of estrogen that is compatible with an acceptable pregnancy rate and patient acceptance. It is recommended that new acceptors of oral contraceptives be started on preparations containing 0.05 mg or less of estrogen.

Contraindications: Oral contraceptives should not be used in women with any of the following conditions.

1. Thrombophlebitis or thromboembolic disorders
2. A past history of deep vein thrombophlebitis or thromboembolic disorders.
3. Cerebral vascular or coronary artery disease
4. Known or suspected carcinoma of the breast
5. Known or suspected estrogen-dependent neoplasia
6. Undiagnosed abnormal genital bleeding
7. Known or suspected pregnancy (see Warning No. 5)
8. Benign or malignant liver tumor which developed during the use of oral contraceptives or other estrogen-containing products.

Warnings:

Cigarette smoking increases the risk of serious cardiovascular side effects from oral contraceptive use. This risk increases with age and with heavy smoking (15 or more cigarettes per day) and is quite marked in women over 35 years of age. Women who use oral contraceptives should be strongly advised not to smoke. The use of oral contraceptives is associated with increased risk of several serious conditions including thromboembolism, stroke, myocardial infarction, hepatic adenoma, gallbladder disease, and hypertension. Practitioners prescribing oral contraceptives should be familiar with the following information relating to these risks.

1. *Thromboembolic Disorders and Other Vascular Problems.* An increased risk of thromboembolic and thrombotic disease associated with the use of oral contraceptives is well established. Three principal studies in Great Britain[4–6] and three in the United States[7–10] have demonstrated an increased risk of fatal and nonfatal venous thromboembolism and stroke, both hemorrhagic and thrombotic. These studies estimate that users of oral contraceptives are 4 to 11 times more likely than nonusers to develop these diseases without evident cause (Table 2).

Cerebrovascular Disorders

In a collaborative American study[9,10] of cerebrovascular disorders in women with and without predisposing causes, it was estimated that the risk of hemorrhagic stroke was 2.0 times greater in users than nonusers and the risk of thrombotic stroke was 4 to 9.5 times greater in users than in nonusers (Table 2).

Table 2

Summary of relative risk of thromboembolic disorders and other vascular problems in oral contraceptive users compared to nonusers

	Relative risk, times greater
Idiopathic thromboembolic disease	4–11
Postsurgery thromboembolic complications	4–6
Thrombotic stroke	4–9.5
Hemorrhagic stroke	2
Myocardial infarction	2–12

Myocardial Infarction

An increased risk of myocardial infarction associated with the use of oral contraceptives has been reported[11–13] confirming a previously suspected association. These studies, conducted in the United Kingdom, found, as expected, that the greater the number of underlying risk factors for coronary artery disease (cigarette smoking, hypertension, hypercholesterolemia, obesity, diabetes, history of preeclamptic toxemia) the higher the risk of developing myocardial infarction, regardless of whether the patient was an oral contraceptive user or not. Oral contraceptives, however, were found to be a clear additional risk factor.

In terms of relative risk, it has been estimated[52] that oral contraceptive users who do not smoke (smoking is considered a major predisposing condition to myocardial infarction) are about twice as likely to have a fatal myocardial infarction as nonusers who do not smoke. Oral contraceptive users who are also smokers have about a 5-fold increased risk of fatal infarction compared to users who do not smoke, but about a 10- to 12-fold increased risk compared to nonusers who do not smoke. Furthermore, the amount of smoking is also an important factor. In determining the importance of these relative risks, however, the baseline rates for various age groups, as shown in Table 3, must be given serious consideration. The importance of other predisposing conditions mentioned above in determining relative and absolute risks has not as yet been quantified; it is quite likely that the same synergistic action exists, but perhaps to a lesser extent.

Table 3

Estimated annual mortality rate per 100,000 women from myocardial infarction by use of oral contraceptives, smoking habits, and age (in years)

[See table above].

Risk of Dose

In an analysis of data derived from several national adverse reaction reporting systems,[2] British investigators concluded that the risk of thromboembolism, including coronary thrombosis, is directly related to the dose of estrogen used in oral contraceptives. Preparations containing 100 mcg or more of estrogen were associated with a higher risk of thromboembolism than those containing 50 to 80 mcg of estrogen. Their analysis did suggest, however, that the quantity of estrogen may not be the sole factor involved. This finding has been confirmed in the United States. Careful epidemiological

Continued on next page

This product information was prepared in August, 1982. On these and other Parke-Davis Products, information may be obtained by addressing PARKE-DAVIS, Division of Warner-Lambert Company, Morris Plains, New Jersey 07950.

Parke-Davis—Cont.

studies to determine the degree of thromboembolic risk associated with progestogen-only oral contraceptives have not been performed. Cases of thromboembolic disease have been reported in women using these products, and they should not be presumed to be free of excess risk.

Estimate of Excess Mortality from Circulatory Diseases

A large prospective study [53] carried out in the U.K. estimated the mortality rate per 100,000 women per year from diseases of the circulatory system for users and nonusers of oral contraceptives according to age, smoking habits, and duration of use. The overall excess death rate annually from circulatory diseases for oral contraceptive users was estimated to be 20 per 100,000 (ages 15 to 34—5/100,000; ages 35 to 44— 33/100,000; ages 45 to 49—140/100,000), the risk being concentrated in older women, in those with a long duration of use, and in cigarette smokers. It was not possible, however, to examine the interrelationships of age, smoking, and duration of use, nor to compare the effects of continuous versus intermittent use. Although the study showed a 10-fold increase in death due to circulatory diseases in users for 5 or more years, all of these deaths occurred in women 35 or older. Until larger numbers of women under 35 with continuous use for 5 or more years are available, it is not possible to assess the magnitude of the relative risk for this younger age group.

The available data from a variety of sources have been analyzed[14] to estimate the risk of death associated with various methods of contraception. The estimates of risk of death for each method include the combined risk of the contraceptive method (eg, thromboembolic and thrombotic disease in the case of oral contraceptives) plus the risk attributable to pregnancy or abortion in the event of method failure. This latter risk varies with the effectiveness of the contraceptive method. The findings of this analysis are shown in Figure 1 which follows.[14] The study concluded that the mortality associated with all methods of birth control is low and below that associated with childbirth, with the exception of oral contraceptives in women over 40 who smoke. (The rates given for pill only/smokers for each age group are for smokers as a class. For "heavy" smokers [more than 15 cigarettes a day] the rates given would be about double, for "light" smokers [less than 15 cigarettes a day] about 50 percent.) The lowest mortality is associated with the condom or diaphragm backed up by early abortion.

[See bar graph below].

The risk of thromboembolic and thrombotic disease associated with oral contraceptives increases with age after approximately age 30 and, for myocardial infarction, is further increased by hypertension, hypercholesterolemia, obesity, diabetes, or history of preeclamptic toxemia and especially by cigarette smoking.

Based on the data currently available, the following chart gives a gross estimate of the risk of death from circulatory disorders associated with the use of oral contraceptives.

Smoking Habits and Other Predisposing Conditions—Risk Associated with Use of Oral Contraceptives

Age	Below 30	30–39	40+
Heavy smokers	C	B	A
Light smokers	D	C	B
Nonsmokers (no predisposing conditions)	D	C,D	C
Nonsmokers (other predisposing conditions)	C	C,B	B,A

A—Use associated with very high risk
B—Use associated with high risk
C—Use associated with moderate risk
D—Use associated with low risk

The physician and the patient should be alert to the earliest manifestations of thromboembolic and thrombotic disorders (eg, thrombophlebitis, pulmonary embolism, cerebrovascular insufficiency, coronary occlusion, retinal thrombosis, and mesenteric thrombosis). Should any of these occur or be suspected, the drug should be discontinued immediately.

A four- to six-fold increased risk of postsurgery thromboembolic complications has been reported in oral contraceptive users.[15,16] If feasible, oral contraceptives should be discontinued at least 4 weeks before surgery of a type associated with an increased risk of thromboembolism or prolonged immobilization.

2. *Ocular Lesions.* There have been reports of neuro-ocular lesions, such as optic neuritis or retinal thrombosis, associated with the use of oral contraceptives. Discontinue oral contraceptive medication if there is unexplained, sudden or gradual, partial or complete loss of vision; onset of proptosis or diplopia; papilledema; or retinal vascular lesions and institute appropriate diagnostic and therapeutic measures.

3. *Carcinoma.* Long-term continuous administration of either natural or synthetic estrogen in certain animal species increases the frequency of carcinoma of the breast, cervix, vagina, and liver. Certain synthetic progestogens, none currently contained in oral contraceptives, have been noted to increase the incidence of mammary nodules, benign and malignant, in dogs.

In humans, three case control studies have reported an increased risk of endometrial carcinoma associated with the prolonged use of exogenous estrogen in post-menopausal women.[17–19] One publication[20] reported on the first 21 cases submitted by physicians to a registry of cases of adenocarcinoma of the endometrium in women under 40 on oral contraceptives. Of the cases found in women without predisposing risk factors for adenocarcinoma of the endometrium (eg, irregular bleeding at the time oral contraceptives were first given, polycystic ovaries), nearly all occurred in women who had used a sequential oral contraceptive. These products are no longer marketed. No evidence has been reported suggesting an increased risk of endometrial cancer in users of conventional-combination or progestogen-only oral contraceptives.

Several studies[8,21–24] have found no increase in breast cancer in women taking oral contraceptives or estrogens. One study,[25] however, while also noting no overall increased risk of breast cancer in women treated with oral contraceptives, found an excess risk in the subgroups of oral contraceptive users with documented benign breast disease. A reduced occurrence of benign breast tumors in users of oral contraceptives has been well-documented.[8,21,25–27]

In summary, there is at present no confirmed evidence from human studies of an increased risk of cancer associated with oral contracep-

Figure 1. Estimated annual number of deaths associated with control of fertility and no control per 100,000 nonsterile women, by regimen of control and age of woman.

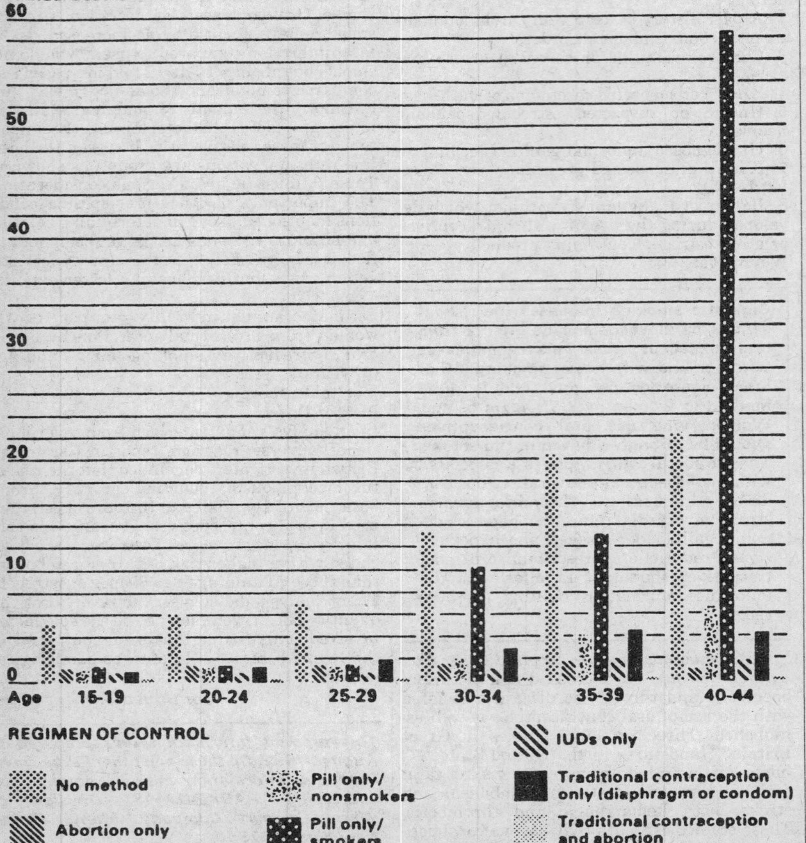

tives. Close clinical surveillance of all women taking oral contraceptives is, nevertheless, essential. In all cases of undiagnosed persistent or recurrent abnormal vaginal bleeding, appropriate diagnostic measures should be taken to rule out malignancy. Women with a strong family history of breast cancer or who have breast nodules, fibrocystic disease, or abnormal mammograms, should be monitored with particular care if they elect to use oral contraceptives instead of other methods of contraception.

4. *Hepatic Tumors.* Benign hepatic adenomas have been found to be associated with the use of oral contraceptives.[28–30,46] One study[46] showed that oral contraceptive formulations with high hormonal potency were associated with a higher risk than lower potency formulations. Although benign, hepatic adenomas may rupture and may cause death through intra-abdominal hemorrhage. This has been reported in short-term as well as long-term users of oral contraceptives. Two studies relate risk with duration of use of the contraceptive, the risk being much greater after 4 or more years of oral contraceptive use.[30,46] While hepatic adenoma is a rare lesion, it should be considered in women presenting abdominal pain and tenderness, abdominal mass or shock.

A few cases of hepatocellular carcinoma have been reported in women taking oral contraceptives. The relationship of these drugs to this type of malignancy is not known at this time.

5. *Use in or Immediately Preceding Pregnancy, Birth Defects in Offspring, and Malignancy in Female Offspring.* The use of female sex hormones—both estrogenic and progestational agents—during early pregnancy may seriously damage the offspring. It has been shown that females exposed *in utero* to diethylstilbestrol, a nonsteroidal estrogen, have an increased risk of developing in later life a form of vaginal or cervical cancer that is ordinarily extremely rare.[31,32] This risk has been estimated to be of the order of 1 in 1,000 exposures or less.[33,47] Although there is no evidence at the present time that oral contraceptives further enhance the risk of developing this type of malignancy, such patients should be monitored with particular care if they elect to use oral contraceptives instead of other methods of contraception. Furthermore, a high percentage of such exposed women (from 30% to 90%) have been found to have epithelial changes of the vagina and cervix.[34–38]Although these changes are histologically benign, it is not known whether this condition is a precursor of vaginal malignancy. Male children so exposed may develop abnormalities of the urogenital tract.[48–50] Although similar data are not available with the use of other estrogens, it cannot be presumed that they would not induce similar changes.

An increased risk of congenital anomalies, including heart defects and limb defects, has been reported with the use of sex hormones, including oral contraceptives, in pregnancy.[39–42,51] One case control study[42] has estimated a 4.7-fold increase in risk of limb-reduction defectes in infants exposed *in utero* to sex hormones (oral contraceptives, hormonal withdrawal tests for pregnancy or attempted treatment for threatened abortion). Some of these exposures were very short and involved only a few days of treatment. The data suggest that the risk of limb-reduction defects in exposed fetuses is somewhat less than 1 in 1,000 live births.

In the past, female sex hormones have been used during pregnancy in an attempt to treat threatened or habitual abortion. There is considerable evidence that estrogens are ineffective for these indications, and there is no evidence from well-controlled studies that progestogens are effective for these uses.

There is some evidence that triploidy and possibly other types of polyploidy are increased among abortuses from women who become pregnant soon after ceasing oral contraceptives.[43] Embryos with these anomalies are virtually always aborted spontaneously. Whether there is an overall increase in spontaneous abortion of pregnancies conceived soon after stopping oral contraceptives is unknown.

It is recommended that for any patient who has missed two consecutive periods, pregnancy should be ruled out before continuing the contraceptive regimen. If the patient has not adhered to the prescribed schedule, the possibility of pregnancy should be considered at the time of the first missed period, and further use of oral contraceptives should be withheld until pregnancy has been ruled out. If pregnancy is confirmed, the patient should be apprised of the potential risks to the fetus and the advisability of continuation of the pregnancy should be discussed in the light of these risks.

It is also recommended that women who discontinue oral contraceptives with the intent of becoming pregnant use an alternate form of contraception for a period of time before attempting to conceive. Many clinicians recommend 3 months although no precise information is available on which to base this recommendation.

The administration of progestogen-only or progestogen-estrogen combinations to induce withdrawal bleeding should not be used as a test of pregnancy.

6. *Gallbladder Disease.* Studies[8,23,26] report an increased risk of surgically confirmed gallbladder disease in users of oral contraceptives and estrogens. In one study, an increased risk appeared after 2 years of use and doubled after 4 or 5 years of use. In one of the other studies, an increased risk was apparent between 6 and 12 months of use.

7. *Carbohydrate and Lipid Metabolic Effects.* A decrease in glucose tolerance has been observed in a significant percentage of patients on oral contraceptives. For this reason, prediabetic and diabetic patients should be carefully observed while receiving oral contraceptives. An increase in triglycerides and total phospholipids has been observed in patients receiving oral contraceptives.[44] The clinical significance of this finding remains to be defined.

8. *Elevated Blood Pressure.* An increase in blood pressure has been reported in patients receiving oral contraceptives.[26] In some women, hypertension may occur within a few months of beginning oral contraceptive use. In the first year of use, the prevalence of women with hypertension is low in users and may be no higher than that of a comparable group of nonusers. The prevalance in users increases, however, with longer exposure, and in the fifth year of use is two and a half to three times the reported prevalence in the first year. Age is also strongly correlated with the development of hypertension in oral contraceptive users. Women who previously have had hypertension during pregnancy may be more likely to develop elevation of blood pressure when given oral contraceptives. Hypertension that develops as a result of taking oral contraceptives usually returns to normal after discontinuing the drug.

9. *Headache.* The onset or exacerbation of migraine or development of headache of a new pattern which is recurrent, persistent, or severe, requires discontinuation of oral contraceptives and evaluation of the cause.

10. *Bleeding Irregularities.* Breakthrough bleeding, spotting and amenorrhea are frequent reasons for patients discontinuing oral contraceptives. In breakthrough bleeding, as in all cases of irregular bleeding from the vagina, nonfunctional causes should be borne in mind. In undiagnosed persistent or recurrent abnormal bleeding from the vagina, adequate diagnostic measures are indicated to rule out pregnancy or malignancy. If pathology has been excluded, time or a change to another formulation may solve the problem. Changing to an oral contraceptive with a higher estrogen content, while potentially useful in minimizing menstrual irregularity, should be done only if necessary since this may increase the risk of thromboembolic disease.

Women with a past history of oligomenorrhea or secondary amenorrhea or young women without regular cycles may have a tendency to remain anovulatory or to become amenorrheic after discontinuation of oral contraceptives. Women with these preexisting problems should be advised of this possibility and encouraged to use other contraceptive methods. Post-use anovulation, possibly prolonged, may also occur in women without previous irregularities.

11. *Ectopic Pregnancy.* Ectopic as well as intrauterine pregnancy may occur in contraceptive failures. However, in progestogen-only oral contraceptive failures, the ratio of ectopic to intrauterine pregnancies is higher than in women who are not receiving oral contraceptives, since the drugs are more effective in preventing intrauterine than ectopic pregnancies.

12. *Breast-Feeding.* Oral contraceptives given in the postpartum period may interfere with lactation. There may be a decrease in the quantity and quality of the breast milk. Furthermore, a small fraction of the hormonal agents in oral contraceptives has been identified in the milk of mothers receiving these drugs.[45] The effects, if any, on the breast-fed child have not been determined. If feasible, the use of oral contraceptives should be deferred until the infant has been weaned.

Precautions:

General

1. A complete medical and family history should be taken prior to the initiation of oral contraceptives. The pretreatment and periodic physical examinations should include special reference to blood pressure, breasts, abdomen and pelvic organs, including Papanicolaou smear and relevant laboratory tests. As a general rule, oral contraceptives should not be prescribed for longer than 1 year without another physical examination being performed.
2. Under the influence of estrogen-progestogen preparations preexisting uterine leiomyomata may increase in size.
3. Patients with a history of psychic depression should be carefully observed and the drug discontinued if depression recurs to a serious degree. Patients becoming significantly depressed while taking oral contraceptives should stop the medication and use an alternate method of contraception in an attempt to determine whether the symptom is drug related.
4. Oral contraceptives may cause some degree of fluid retention. They should be prescribed with caution, and only with careful monitoring, in patients with conditions which might be aggravated by fluid retention, such as convulsive disorders, migraine syndrome, asthma, or cardiac or renal insufficiency.
5. Patients with a past history of jaundice during pregnancy have an increased risk of recurrence of jaundice while receiving oral contraceptive therapy. If jaundice develops in any patient receiving such drugs, the medication should be discontinued.
6. Steroid hormones may be poorly metabolized in patients with impaired liver function and should be administered with caution in such patients.
7. Oral contraceptive users may have disturbances in normal tryptophan metabolism which may result in a relative pyridoxine deficiency.

Continued on next page

This product information was prepared in August, 1982. On these and other Parke-Davis Products, information may be obtained by addressing PARKE-DAVIS, Division of Warner-Lambert Company, Morris Plains, New Jersey 07950.

Parke-Davis—Cont.

The clinical significance of this is yet to be determined.

8. Serum folate levels may be depressed by oral contraceptive therapy. Since the pregnant woman is predisposed to the development of folate deficiency and the incidence of folate deficiency increases with increasing gestation, it is possible that if a woman becomes pregnant shortly after stopping oral contraceptives, she may have a greater chance of developing folate deficiency and complications attributed to this deficiency.

9. The pathologist should be advised of oral contraceptive therapy when relevant specimens are submitted.

10. Certain endocrine and liver function tests and blood components may be affected by estrogen-containing oral contraceptives:

a. Increased sulfobromophthalein retention

b. Increased prothrombin and factors VII, VIII, IX, and X; decreased antithrombin 3; increased norepinephrine-induced platelet aggregability

c. Increased thyroid binding globulin (TBG) leading to increased circulating total thyroid hormone, as measured by protein-bound iodine (PBI), T4 by column, or T4 by radioimmunoassay. Free T3 resin uptake is decreased, reflecting the elevated TBG, free T4 concentration is unaltered

d. Decreased pregnanediol excretion

e. Reduced response to metyrapone test

Information For The Patient: See Patient Labeling printed following the reference section.

Drug Interactions: Reduced efficacy and increased incidence of breakthrough bleeding have been associated with concomitant use of rifampin. A similar association has been suggested with barbiturates, phenylbutazone, phenytoin sodium, tetracycline, and ampicillin.

Carcinogenesis: See Warnings section for information on the carcinogenic potential of oral contraceptives.

Pregnancy: Pregnancy category X. See Contraindications and Warnings.

Nursing Mothers: See Warnings.

Adverse Reactions: An increased risk of the following serious adverse reactions has been associated with the use of oral contraceptives (see Warnings):

Thrombophlebitis
Pulmonary embolism
Coronary thrombosis
Cerebral thrombosis
Cerebral hemorrhage
Hypertension
Gallbladder disease
Benign hepatomas
Congenital anomalies

There is evidence of an association between the following conditions and the use of oral contraceptives, although additional confirmatory studies are needed:

Mesenteric thrombosis
Neuro-ocular lesions, eg, retinal thrombosis and optic neuritis

The following adverse reactions have been reported in patients receivng oral contraceptives and are believed to be drug related:

Nausea and/or vomiting, usually the most common adverse reactions, occur in approximately 10 percent or less of patients during the first cycle. Other reactions, as a general rule, are seen much less frequently or only occasionally:

Gastrointestinal symptoms (such as abdominal cramps and bloating)
Breakthrough bleeding
Spotting
Change in menstrual flow
Dysmenorrhea
Amenorrhea during and after treatment
Temporary infertility after discontinuance of treatment
Edema
Chloasma or melasma which may persist
Breast changes: tenderness, enlargement and secretion
Change in weight (increase or decrease)
Change in cervical erosion and cervical secretion
Possible diminution in lactation when given immediately postpartum
Cholestatic jaundice
Migraine
Increase in size of uterine leiomyomata
Rash (allergic)
Mental depression
Reduced tolerance to carbohydrates
Vaginal candidiasis
Change in corneal curvature (steepening)
Intolerance to contact lenses

The following adverse reactions have been reported in users of oral contraceptives, and the association has been neither confirmed nor refuted:

Premenstrual-like syndrome
Cataracts
Changes in libido
Chorea
Changes in appetite
Cystitis-like syndrome
Headache
Nervousness
Dizziness
Hirsutism
Loss of scalp hair
Erythema multiforme
Erythema nodosum
Hemorrhagic eruption
Vaginitis
Porphyria

Acute Overdose: Serious ill effects have not been reported following acute ingestion of large doses of oral contraceptives by young children. Overdosage may cause nausea, and withdrawal bleeding may occur in females.

Dosage and Administration For 21-Day Dosage Regimen: To achieve maximum contraceptive effectiveness, Loestrin must be taken exactly as directed and at intervals not exceeding 24 hours. Loestrin **21** provides the patient with a convenient tablet schedule of "3 weeks on—1 week off."

The first day of menstrual flow is considered Day 1. Initially, the patient begins taking tablets on Day 5 and takes one tablet daily for 21 days. She then takes no tablets for seven days. After the seven days during which no tablets are taken, the patient begins a new course of one tablet daily for 21 days. Each course of tablets will begin on the same day of the week as the first course. Likewise, the interval of no tablets will always start on the same day of the week.

Tablets should be taken regularly with a meal or at bedtime. It should be stressed that efficacy of medication depends on strict adherence to the dosage schedule.

Special Notes on Administration

Menstruation usually begins two or three days, but may begin as late as the fourth or fifth day after discontinuing medication. Because of the relatively low estrogenic content, Loestrin is not a good cyclic regulator. There are patients whose inherent hormone balance will require larger amounts of estrogen to achieve cyclic regularity than that contained in Loestrin. These patients experience altered bleeding patterns, which do not conform to treatment schedules, while taking Loestrin tablets. However, it is important that patients adhere to the dosage schedule regardless of when bleeding occurs.

The occurrence of altered bleeding is highest in Cycle 1. The majority of patients will have seven days or less of total bleeding during the 28-day cycle (including both withdrawal bleeding and breakthrough bleeding and spotting). Should irregular bleeding occur, patients should be reassured and instructed to continue taking the tablets as directed. If by the third cycle the irregular patterns are unacceptable, consideration should be given to changing the medication to a product with a higher estrogen content (Norlestrin® *1/50 or Norlestrin 2.5/50). The physician should be alert to the fact that the irregular bleeding patterns could mask bleeding from organic causes, and appropriate diagnostic measures should be taken if the bleeding persists or continues after changing to a higher estrogen-content product.

If a patient forgets to take one or more tablets, the following is suggested. If one tablet is missed, take it as soon as remembered, or take two tablets the next day. If two consecutive tablets are missed, take two tablets daily for the next two days, then resume the regular schedule. While there is little likelihood of pregnancy occurring if the patient misses only one or two tablets, the possibility of pregnancy increases with each successive day that tablets are missed. *However if the patient is taking* Loestrin **21** 1/20, *in addition to taking two white tablets a day for two days the patient should use an additional means of contraception for seven consecutive days.* If three consecutive tablets are missed, begin a new compact of tablets starting seven days after the last tablet was taken. The patient should use an alternate means of contraception, other than oral tablets, until the start of the next menstrual period.

The possibility of ovulation occurring increases with each successive day that scheduled tablets are missed. While there is little likelihood of ovulation occurring if only one tablet is missed, the possibility of spotting or bleeding is increased. This is particularly likely to occur if two or more consecutive tablets are missed.

*Norlestrin (Norethindrone Acetate and Ethinyl Estradiol Tablets, USP)

Dosage and Administration For 28-Day Dosage Regimen: To achieve maximum contraceptive effectiveness, Loestrin must be taken exactly as directed and at intervals not exceeding 24 hours.

Loestrin **Fe** provides a continuous administration regimen consisting of 21 *light-colored* tablets of Loestrin and 7 brown tablets of ferrous fumarate. There is no need for the patient to count days between cycles because there are no "off-tablet days."

The dosage schedule is one *light-colored* tablet daily for 21 days, starting initially on Day 5 of the menstrual cycle, followed without interruption by one brown tablet daily for 7 days. The first day of menstrual flow is considered Day 1. Upon completion of this first course of tablets, a second course of tablets is started without interruption. All subsequent courses also are taken without interruption.

Tablets should be taken regularly with a meal or at bedtime. It should be stressed that efficacy of medication depends on strict adherence to the dosage schedule.

Special Notes on Administration

Menstruation usually begins two or three days, but may begin as late as the fourth or fifth day, after the brown tablets have been started. Because of the relatively low estrogenic content, Loestrin is not a good cyclic regulator. There are patients whose inherent hormone balance will require larger amounts of estrogen to achieve cyclic regularity than that contained in Loestrin. These patients experience altered bleeding patterns, which do not conform to treatment schedules, while taking the *light-colored* Loestrin tablets. However, it is important that patients adhere to the dosage schedule regardless of when bleeding occurs.

The occurrence of altered bleeding is highest in Cycle 1. The majority of patients will have seven days or less of total bleeding during the

28-day cycle (including both withdrawal bleeding and breakthrough bleeding and spotting). Should irregular bleeding occur, patients should be reassured and instructed to continue taking the tablets as directed. If by the third cycle the irregular patterns are unacceptable, consideration should be given to changing the medication to a product with a higher estrogen content (Norlestrin *1/50 or Norlestrin 2.5/50). The physician should be alert to the fact that the irregular bleeding patterns could mask bleeding from organic causes, and appropriate diagnostic measures should be taken if the bleeding persists or continues after changing to a higher estrogen-content product.

If a patient forgets to take one or more *light-colored* tablets, the following is suggested. If one *light-colored* tablet is missed, take it as soon as remembered, or take two *light-colored* tablets the next day. If two consecutive *light-colored* tablets are missed, take two *light-colored* tablets daily for the next two days, then resume the regular schedule. While there is little likelihood of pregnancy occurring if the patient misses only one or two *light-colored* tablets, the possibility of pregnancy increases with each successive day that *light-colored* tablets are missed. *However, if the patient is taking* Loestrin **Fe** 1/20, *in addition to taking two* white *tablets a day for two days, the patient should use an additional means of contraception for seven consecutive days.* If three consecutive *light-colored* tablets are missed, begin a new compact of tablets, starting seven days after the last *light-colored* tablet was taken. The patient should use an alternate means of contraception, other than oral tablets, until the start of the next menstrual period.

The possibility of ovulation occurring increases with each successive day that scheduled *light-colored* tablets are missed. While there is little likelihood of ovulation occurring if only one *light-colored* tablet is missed, the possibility of spotting or bleeding is increased. This is particularly likely to occur if two or more consecutive *light-colored* tablets are missed.

If one or more brown tablets are missed, the *light-colored* tablets should be started no later than the eighth day after the last *light-colored* tablet was taken. The possibility of conception occurring is not increased if brown tablets are missed.

*Norlestrin (Norethindrone Acetate and Ethinyl Estradiol Tablets, USP)

Use of oral contraceptives in the event of a missed menstrual period:

1. If the patient has not adhered to the prescribed dosage regimen, the possibility of pregnancy should be considered after the first missed period and oral contraceptives should be withheld until pregnancy has been ruled out.
2. If the patient has adhered to the prescribed regimen and misses two consecutive periods, pregnancy should be ruled out before continuing the contraceptive regimen.

After several months on treatment, bleeding may be reduced to a point of virtual absence. This reduced flow may occur as a result of medication, in which event it is not indicative of pregnancy.

How Supplied:

Loestrin **21** 1/20 is available in compacts each containing 21 tablets. Each tablet contains 1 mg of norethindrone acetate and 20 mcg of ethinyl estradiol. Available in packages of five compacts and packages of five refills.

Loestrin **Fe** 1/20 is available in compacts each containing 21 white tablets and 7 brown tablets. Each white tablet contains 1 mg of norethindrone acetate and 20 mcg of ethinyl estradiol. Each brown tablet contains 75 mg ferrous fumarate, USP. Available in packages of five compacts and packages of five refills.

Loestrin **21** 1.5/30 is available in compacts each containing 21 tablets. Each tablet contains 1.5 mg of norethindrone acetate and 30 mcg of ethinyl estradiol. Available in packages of five compacts and packages of five refills.

Loestrin **Fe** 1.5/30 is available in compacts each containing 21 green tablets and 7 brown tablets. Each green tablet contains 1.5 mg of norethindrone acetate and 30 mcg of ethinyl estradiol. Each brown tablet contains 75 mg ferrous fumarate, USP. Available in packages of five compacts and packages of five refills.

References:

1. "*Population Reports*," Series H, Number 2, May 1974; Series 1, Number 1, June 1974; Series B, Number 2, January 1975; Series H, Number 3, 1975; Series H, Number 4, January 1976 (published by the Population Information Program, The George Washington University Medical Center, 2001 S. St. NW., Washington, D.C.)
2. Inman, W. H. W., M. P. Vessey, B. Westerholm, and A. Engelund. "Thromboembolic disease and the steroidal content of oral contraceptives. A report to the Committee on Safety of Drugs," *Brit Med J* 2:203–209, 1970.
3. Stolley, P.D., J. A. Tonascia, M. S. Tockman, P. E. Sartwell, A. H. Rutledge, and M. P. Jacobs, "Thrombosis with low-estrogen oral contraceptives," *Am J Epidemiol* 102: 197–208, 1975.
4. Royal College of General Practitioners, "Oral contraception and thromboembolic disease," *J Coll Gen Pract* 13:267–279, 1967.
5. Inman, W. H. W. and M. P. Vessey, "Investigation of deaths from pulmonary, coronary and cerebral thrombosis and embolism in women of childbearing age," *Brit Med. J* 2-193–199, 1968.
6. Vessey, M. P. and R. Doll, "Investigation of relation between use of oral contraceptives and thromboembolic disease. A further report," *Brit Med J* 2:651–657, 1969.
7. Sartwell, P. E., A. T. Masi, F. G. Arthes, G. R. Greene, and H. E. Smith, "Thromboembolism and oral contraceptives an epidemiological case control study," *Am J Epidemiol* 90:365–380, 1969.
8. Boston Collaborative Drug Surveillance Program. "Oral contraceptives and venous thromboembolic disease, surgically confirmed gallbladder disease and breast tumors," *Lancet* 1:1399–1404, 1973.
9. Collaborative Group for the Study of Stroke in Young Women, "Oral contraception and increased risk of cerebral ischemia or thrombosis," *N Engl J Med* 288:871–878, 1973.
10. Collaborative Group for the Study of Stroke in Young Women, "Oral contraceptives and stroke in young women: associated risk factors," *JAMA* 231:718–722, 1975.
11. Mann, J. I., and W. H. W. Inman, "Oral contraceptives and death from myocardial infarction," *Brit Med J* 2:245–248, 1975.
12. Mann, J. I., W. H. W. Inman, and M. Thorogood, "Oral contraceptive use in older women and fatal myocardial infarction," *Bit Med J* 2:445–447, 1976.
13. Mann, J. I., M. P. Vessey, M. Thorogood and R. Doll, "Myocardial infarction in young women with special reference to oral contraceptive practice," *Brit Med J* 2:241–245, 1975.
14. Tietze, C., "New Estimates of Mortality Associated with Fertility Control," *Family Planning Perspectives,* 9:74–76, 1977.
15. Vessey, M. P., R. Doll, A. S. Fairbairn, and G. Glober, "Post-operative thromboembolism and the use of oral contraceptives," *Brit Med J* 3:123–126, 1970.
16. Greene, G. R., P. E. Sartwell, "Oral contraceptive use in patients with thromboembolism following surgery, trauma or infection," *Am J Pub Health* 62:680–685, 1972.
17. Smith, D. C., R. Prentice, D. J. Thompson and W. L. Herrmann, "Association of exogenous estrogen and endometrial carcinoma," *N Engl J Med* 293:1164–1167, 1975.
18. Ziel, H. K., and W. D. Finkle, "Increased risk of endometrial carcinoma among users of conjugated estrogens," *N Engl J Med* 293: 1167–1170, 1975.
19. Mack, T. N., M. C. Pike, B. E. Henderson, R. I. Pfeffer, V. R. Gerkins, M. Arthur and S. E. Brown, "Estrogens and endometrial cancer in a retirement community," *N Engl J Med* 294: 1262–1267, 1976.
20. Silverberg, S. G., and E. L. Makowski, "Endometrial carcinoma in young women taking oral contraceptive agents," *Obstet Gynecol* 46:503–506, 1975.
21. Vessey, M. P., R. Doll, and P. M. Sutton, "Oral contraceptives and breast neoplasia: a retrospective study," *Brit Med J* 3:719–724, 1972.
22. Vessey, M. P., R. Doll, and K. Jones, "Oral contraceptives and breast cancer. Progress report of an epidemiological study," *Lancet* 1:941–943, 1975.
23. Boston Collaborative Drug Surveillance Program, "Surgically confirmed gallbladder disease, venous thromboembolism and breast tumors in relation to postmenopausal estrogen therapy," *N Engl J Med* 290:14–19, 1974.
24. Arthes, F. G., P. E. Sartwell, and E. F. Lewison, "The pill, estrogens, and the breast, Epidemiologic aspects," *Cancer* 28:1391–1394, 1971.
25. Fasal, E., and R. S. Paffenbarger, "Oral contraceptives as related to cancer and benign lesions of the breast." *J Natl Cancer Inst* 55:767–773, 1975.
26. Royal College of General Practitioners, "Oral Contraceptives and Health," London, Pitman, 1974.
27. Ory, H., P. Cole, B. MacMahon, and R. Hoover, "Oral contraceptives and reduced risk of benign breast diseases," *N Engl J Med* 294:419–422, 1976.
28. Baum, J., F. Holtz, J. J. Bookstein, and E. W. Klein, "Possible association between benign hepatomas and oral contraceptives," *Lancet* 2:926–928, 1973.
29. Mays, E. T., W. M. Christopherson, M. M. Mahr, and H. C. Williams, "Hepatic changes in young women ingesting contraceptive steroids. Hepatic hemorrhage and primary hepatic tumors," *JAMA* 235:730–732, 1976.
30. Edmondson, H. A., B. Henderson, and B. Benton, "Liver-cell adenomas associated with use of oral contraceptives," *N Engl J Med* 294:470–472, 1976.
31. Herbst, A. L., H. Ulfelder, and D. C. Poskanzer, "Adenocarcinoma of the vagina," *N Engl J Med* 284:878–881, 1971.
32. Greenwald, P., J. J. Barlow, P. C. Nasca and W. Burnett, "Vaginal cancer after maternal treatment with synthetic estrogens," *N Engl J Med* 285:390–392, 1971.
33. Lanier, A. P., K. L. Noller, D. G. Decker, L. Elveback, and L. T. Kurland, "Cancer and stilbestrol. A follow-up of 1719 persons exposed to estrogens in utero and born 1943–1959," *Mayo Clin Pro* 48:793–799, 1973.
34. Herbst, A. L., R. J. Kurman, and R. E. Scully, "Vaginal and cervical abnormalities after exposure to stilbestrol in utero," *Obstet Gynecol* 40:287–298, 1972.
35. Herbst, A. L., S. J. Robboy, G. J. Macdonald, and R. E. Scully, "The effects of local progesterone on stilbestrol-associated vaginal adenosis," *Am J. Obstet Gynecol* 118:607–615, 1974.
36. Herbst, A. L., D. C. Poskanzer, S. J. Robboy, L. Friedlander, and R. E. Scully, "Prenatal exposure to stilbestrol: a prospective comparison of exposed female offspring with unexposed controls," *N Engl J Med* 292:334–339, 1975.

Continued on next page

This product information was prepared in August, 1982. On these and other Parke-Davis Products, information may be obtained by addressing PARKE-DAVIS, Division of Warner-Lambert Company, Morris Plains, New Jersey 07950.

Parke-Davis—Cont.

37. Stafl, A., R. F. Mattingly, D. V. Foley, W. Fetherston, "Clinical diagnosis of vaginal adenosis," *Obstet Gynecol* 43:118–128, 1974.
38. Sherman, A. I., M. Goldrath, A. Berlin, V. Vakhariya, F. Banooni, W. Michaels, P. Goodman, and S. Brown, "Cervical-vaginal adenosis after in utero exposure to synthetic estrogens," *Obstet Gynecol* 44:531–545, 1974.
39. Gal, I., B. Kirman, and J. Stern, "Hormone pregnancy tests and congenital malformation," *Nature* 216:83, 1967.
40. Levy, E. P., A. Cohen, and F. C. Fraser, "Hormone treatment during pregnancy and congenital heart defects," *Lancet* 1:611, 1973.
41. Nora, J. J., and A. H. Nora, "Birth defects and oral contraceptives," *Lancet* 1:941–942, 1973.
42. Janerich, D. T., J. M. Piper, and D. M. Glebatis, "Oral contraceptives and congenital limb-reduction defects," *N Engl J Med* 291:697–700, 1974.
43. Carr, D. H., "Chromosome studies in selected spontaneous abortions: I. Conception after oral contraceptives," *Canad Med Assoc J* 103:343–348, 1970.
44. Wynn, V., J. W. H. Doar, and G. L. Mills, "Some effects of oral contraceptives on serum-lipid and lipoprotein levels," *Lancet* 2:720–723, 1966.
45. Laumas, K. R., P. K. Malkani, S. Bhatnagar, and V. Laumas, "Radioactivity in the breast milk of lactating women after oral administration of 3 H-norethynodrel," *Amer J Obstet Gynecol* 98:411–413, 1967.
46. Center for Disease Control, "Increased Risk of Hepatocellular Adenoma in Women with Long-term use of Oral Contraceptives," *Morbidity and Mortality Weekly Report* 26:293–294, 1977.
47. Herbst, A. L., P. Cole, T. Colton, S. J. Robboy, R. E. Scully, "Age-incidence and Risk of Diethylstilbestrol-related Clear Cell Adenocarcinoma of the Vagina and Cervix," *Am J. Obstet Cynecol* 128:43–50, 1977.
48. Bibbo, M., M. Al-Naqeeb, I. Baccarini, W. Gill, M. Newton, K. M. Sleeper, M. Sonek, G. L. Wied, "Follow-Up Study of Male and Female Offspring of DES-treated Mothers. A Preliminary Report," *Jour of Repro Med* 15:29–32, 1975.
49. Gill, W. B., G. F. B. Schumacher, M. Bibbo, "Structural and Functional Abnormalities in the Sex Organs of Male Offpsring of Mothers Treated with Diethylstilbestrol (DES)," *Jour of Repro Med* 16:147–153, 1976.
50. Henderson, B. E., B. Benton, M. Cosgrove, J. Baptista, J. Aldrich, D. Townsend, W. Hart, T. Mack, "Urogenital Tract Abnormalities in Sons of Women Treated with Diethylstilbestrol," *Pediatrics* 58:505–507, 1976.
51. Heinonen, O. P., D. Slone, R. R. Nonson, E. B. Hook, S. Shapiro, "Cardiovascular Birth Defects and Antenatal Exposure to Female Sex Hormones," *N Engl J Med* 296:67–70, 1977.
52. Jain, A. K., "Mortality Risk Associated with the Use of Oral Contraceptives," *Studies in Family Planning* 8:50–54, 1977.
53. Beral, V., "Mortality Among Oral Contraceptive Users," *Lancet* 2:727–731, 1977.

The patient labeling for oral contraceptive drug products is set forth below:

Brief Summary Patient Package Insert

> Cigarette smoking increases the risk of serious adverse effects on the heart and blood vessels from oral contraceptive use. This risk increases with age and with heavy smoking (15 or more cigarettes per day) and is quite marked in women over 35 years of age. Women who use oral contraceptives should not smoke.

Oral contraceptives taken as directed are about 99% effective in preventing pregnancy. (The mini-pill, however is somewhat less effective.) Forgetting to take your pills increases the chance of pregnancy. Various drugs, such as antibiotics, may also decrease the effectiveness of oral contraceptives.

Women who have or have had clotting disorders, cancer of the breast or sex organs, unexplained vaginal bleeding, a stroke, heart attack, angina pectoris, or who suspect they may be pregnant should not use oral contraceptives.

Most side effects of the pill are not serious. The most common side effects are nausea, vomiting, bleeding between menstrual periods, weight gain, and breast tenderness. However, proper use of oral contraceptives requires that they be taken under your doctor's continuous supervision, because they can be associated with serious side effects which may be fatal. Fortunately, these occur very infrequently.

The serious side effects are:

1. Blood clots in the legs, lungs, brain, heart or other organs and hemorrhage into the brain due to bursting of a blood vessel
2. Liver tumors, which may rupture and cause severe bleeding
3. Birth defects if the pill is taken while you are pregnant
4. High blood pressure
5. Gallbladder disease

The symptoms associated with these serious side effects are discussed in the detailed leaflet given you with your supply of pills. Notify your doctor if you notice any unusual physical disturbance while taking the pill.

The estrogen in oral contraceptives has been found to cause breast cancer and other cancers in certain animals. These findings suggest that oral contraceptives may also cause cancer in humans. However, studies to date in women taking currently marketed oral contraceptives have not confirmed that oral contraceptives cause cancer in humans.

The detailed leaflet describes more completely the benefits and risks of oral contraceptives. It also provides information on other forms of contraception. Read it carefully. If you have any questions, consult your doctor.

Caution: Oral contraceptives are of no value in the prevention or treatment of venereal disease.

Detailed Patient Labeling

What You Should Know About Oral Contraceptives

Oral contraceptives ("the pill") are the most effective way (except for sterilization) to prevent pregnancy . They are also convenient and, for most women, free of serious or unpleasant side effects. Oral contraceptives must always be taken under the continuous supervision of a physician.

It is important that any woman who considers using an oral contraceptive understand the risks involved. Although the oral contraceptives have important advantages over other methods of contraception, they have certain risks that no other method has. Only you can decide whether the advantages are worth these risks. This leaflet will tell you about the most important risks. It will explain how you can help your doctor prescribe the pill as safely as possible by telling him about yourself and being alert for the earliest signs of trouble. And it will tell you how to use the pill properly, so that it will be as effective as possible. There is more detailed information available in the leaflet prepared for doctors. Your pharmacist can show you a copy; you may need your doctor's help in understanding parts of it.

Who Should Not Use Oral Contraceptives

A. If you have any of the following conditions you should not use the pill:

1. Clots in the legs or lungs
2. Angina pectoris
3. Known or suspected cancer of the breast or sex organs
4. Unusual vaginal bleeding that has not yet been diagnosed
5. Known or suspected pregnancy

B. If you have had any of the following conditions you should not use the pill:

1. Heart attack or stroke
2. Clots in the legs or lungs

> C. Cigarette smoking increases the risk of serious adverse effects on the heart and blood vessels from oral contraceptive use. This risk increases with age and with heavy smoking (15 or more cigarettes per day) and is quite marked in women over 35 years of age. Women who use oral contraceptives should not smoke.

D. If you have scanty or irregular periods or are a young woman without a regular cycle, you should use another method of contraception because, if you use the pill, you may have difficulty becoming pregnant or may fail to have menstrual periods after discontinuing the pill.

Deciding To Use Oral Contraceptives

If you do not have any of the conditions listed above and are thinking about using oral contraceptives, to help you decide, you need information about the advantages and risks of oral contraceptives and of other contraceptive methods as well. This leaflet describes the advantages and risks of oral contraceptives. Except for sterilization, the IUD and abortion, which have their own exclusive risks, the only risks of other methods of contraception are those due to pregnancy should the method fail. Your doctor can answer questions you may have with respect to other methods of contraception. He can also answer any questions you may have after reading this leaflet on oral contraceptives.

1. What Oral Contraceptives Are and How They Work. Oral contraceptives are of two types. The most common, often simply called "the pill," is a combination of an estrogen and a progestogen, the two kinds of female hormones. The amount of estrogen and progestogen can vary, but the amount of estrogen is most important because both the effectiveness and some of the dangers of oral contraceptives are related to the amount of estrogen. This kind of oral contraceptive works principally by preventing release of an egg from the ovary. When the amount of estrogen is 50 micrograms or more, and the pill is taken as directed, oral contraceptives are more than 99% effective (ie, there would be less than one pregnancy if 100 women used the pill for 1 year). Pills that contain 20 to 35 micrograms of estrogen vary slightly in effectiveness, ranging from 98% to more than 99% effective. Norlestrin was shown in clinical trials to be more than 99% effective.

The second type of oral contraceptive, often called the "mini-pill," contains only a progestogen. It works in part by preventing release of an egg from the ovary but also by keeping sperm from reaching the egg and by making the uterus (womb) less receptive to any fertilized egg that reaches it. The mini-pill is less effective than the combination oral contraceptive, about 97% effective.

In addition, the progestogen-only pill has a tendency to cause irregular bleeding which may be quite inconvenient, or cessation of bleeding entirely. The progestogen-only pill is used despite its lower effectiveness in the hope that it will prove not to have some of the serious side effects of the estrogen-containing pill (which follows) but it is not yet certain that the mini-pill does in fact have fewer serious side effects. The discussion which follows, while based mainly on information about the combination pills, should be considered to apply, as well, to the mini-pill.

2. Other Nonsurgical Ways to Prevent Pregnancy. As this leaflet will explain, oral contraceptives have several serious risks. Other methods of contraception have lesser risks or

none at all. They are also less effective than oral contraceptives but, used properly, may be effective enough for many women. The following gives reported pregnancy rates (the number of women out of 100 who would become pregnant in 1 year) for these methods:

Pregnancies Per 100 Women Per Year

Intrauterine device (IUD), less than 1-6; Diaphragm with spermicidal products (creams or jellies), 2-20; Condom (rubber), 3-36; Aerosol foams, 2-29; Jellies and creams, 4-36; Periodic abstinence (rhythm) all types, less than 1-47; *1. Calendar method, 14-47; 2. Temperature method, 1-20; 3. Temperature method—intercourse only in post-ovulatory phase, less than 1-7; 4. Mucus method, 1-25;* No contraception, 60-80.

The figures (except for the IUD) vary widely because people differ in how well they use each method. Very faithful users of the various methods obtain very good results except for users of the calendar method of periodic abstinence (rhythm). Except for the IUD, effective use of these methods requires somewhat more effort than simply taking a single pill every morning, but it is an effort that many couples undertake successfully. Your doctor can tell you a great deal more about these methods of contraception.

3. The Dangers of Oral Contraceptives.

a. *Circulatory disorders (abnormal blood clotting and stroke due to hemorrhage).* Blood clots (in various blood vessels of the body) are the most common of the serious side effects of oral contraceptives. A clot can result in a stroke (if the clot is in the brain), a heart attack (if the clot is in a blood vessel of the heart), or a pulmonary embolus (a clot which forms in the legs or pelvis, then breaks off and travels to the lungs). Any of these can be fatal. Clots also occur rarely in the blood vessels of the eye, resulting in blindness or impairment of vision in that eye. There is evidence that the risk of clotting increases with higher estrogen doses. It is, therefore, important to keep the dose of estrogen as low as possible, so long as the oral contraceptive used has an acceptable pregnancy rate and doesn't cause unacceptable changes in the menstrual pattern. Furthermore, cigarette smoking by oral contraceptive users increases the risk of serious adverse effects on the heart and blood vessels. This risk increases with age and with heavy smoking (15 or more cigarettes per day) and begins to become quite marked in women over 35 years of age. For this reason, women who use oral contraceptives should not smoke.

The risk of abnormal clotting increases with age in both users and nonusers of oral contraceptives, but the increased risk from the contraceptives appears to be present at all ages. For oral contraceptive users in general, it has been estimated that in women between the ages of 15 and 34 the risk of death due to a circulatory disorder is about 1 in 12,000 per year, whereas for nonusers the rate is about 1 in 50,000 per year. In the age group 35 to 44, the risk is estimated to be about 1 in 2,500 per year for oral contraceptive users and about 1 in 10,000 per year for nonusers.

Even without the pill the risk of having a heart attack increases with age and is also increased by such heart attack risk factors as high blood pressure, high cholesterol, obesity, diabetes, and cigarette smoking. Without any risk factors present, the use of oral contraceptives alone may double the risk of heart attack. However, the combination of cigarette smoking, especially heavy smoking, and oral contraceptive use greatly increases the risk of heart attack. Oral contraceptive users who smoke are about 5 times more likely to have a heart attack than users who do not smoke and about 10 times more likely to have a heart attack than nonusers who do not smoke. It has been estimated that users between the ages of 30 and 39 who smoke have about a 1 in 10,000 chance each year of having a fatal heart attack compared to about a 1 in 50,000 chance in users who do not smoke, and about a 1 in 100,000 chance in nonusers who do not smoke. In the age group 40 to 44, the risk is about 1 in 1,700 per year for users who smoke compared to about 1 in 10,000 for users who do not smoke and to about 1 in 14,000 per year for nonusers who do not smoke. Heavy smoking (about 15 cigarettes or more a day) further increases the risk. If you do not smoke and have none of the other heart attack risk factors described above, you will have a smaller risk than listed. If you have several heart attack risk factors, the risk may be considerably greater than listed.

In addition to blood-clotting disorders, it has been estimated that women taking oral contraceptives are twice as likely as nonusers to have a stroke due to rupture of a blood vessel in the brain.

b. *Formation of tumors.* Studies have found that when certain animals are given the female sex hormone estrogen, which is an ingredient of oral contraceptives, continuously for long periods, cancers may develop in the breast, cervix, vagina, and liver.

These findings suggest that oral contraceptives may cause cancer in humans. However, studies to date in women taking currently marketed oral contraceptives have not confirmed that oral contraceptives cause cancer in humans. Several studies have found no increase in breast cancer in users, although one study suggested oral contraceptives might cause an increase in breast cancer in women who already have benign breast disease (eg, cysts).

Women with a strong family history of breast cancer or who have breast nodules, fibrocystic disease, or abnormal mammograms or who were exposed to DES (diethylstilbestrol), an estrogen, during their mother's pregnancy must be followed very closely by their doctors if they choose to use oral contraceptives instead of another method of contraception. Many studies have shown that women taking oral contraceptives have less risk of getting benign breast disease than those who have not used oral contraceptives. Recently, strong evidence has emerged that estrogens (one component of oral contraceptives), when given for periods of more than one year to women after the menopause, increase the risk of cancer of the uterus (womb). There is also some evidence that a kind of oral contraceptive which is no longer marketed, the sequential oral contraceptive, may increase the risk of cancer of the uterus. There remains no evidence, however, that the oral contraceptives now available increase the risk of this cancer.

Oral contraceptives do cause, although rarely, a benign (nonmalignant) tumor of the liver. These tumors do not spread, but they may rupture and cause internal bleeding, which may be fatal. A few cases of cancer of the liver have been reported in women using oral contraceptives, but it is not yet known whether the drug caused them.

c. *Dangers to a developing child if oral contraceptives are used in or immediately preceding pregnancy.* Oral contraceptives should not be taken by pregnant women because they may damage the developing child. An increased risk of birth defects, including heart defects and limb defects, has been associated with the use of sex hormones, including oral contraceptives, in pregnancy. In addition, the developing female child whose mother has received DES (diethylstilbestrol), an estrogen, during pregnancy has a risk of getting cancer of the vagina or cervix in her teens or young adulthood. This risk is estimated to be about 1 in 1,000 exposures or less. Abnormalities of the urinary and sex organs have been reported in male offspring so exposed. It is possible that other estrogens, such as the estrogens in oral contraceptives, could have the same effect in the child if the mother takes them during pregnancy.

If you stop taking oral contraceptives to become pregnant, your doctor may recommend that you use another method of contraception for a short while. The reason for this is that there is evidence from studies in women who have had "miscarriages" soon after stopping the pill, that the lost fetuses are more likely to be abnormal. Whether there is an overall increase in "miscarriage" in women who become pregnant soon after stopping the pill, as compared with women who do not use the pill, is not known, but it is possible that there may be. If, however, you do become pregnant soon after stopping oral contraceptives, and do not have a miscarriage, there is no evidence that the baby has an increased risk of being abnormal.

d. *Gallbladder disease.* Women who use oral contraceptives have a greater risk than nonusers of having gallbladder disease requiring surgery. The increased risk may first appear within 1 year of use and may double after 4 or 5 years of use.

e. *Other side effects of oral contraceptives.* Some women using oral contraceptives experience unpleasant side effects that are not dangerous and are not likely to damage their health. Some of these may be temporary. Your breasts may feel tender, nausea and vomiting may occur, you may gain or lose weight, and your ankles may swell. A spotty darkening of the skin, particularly of the face, is possible and may persist. You may notice unexpected vaginal bleeding or changes in your menstrual period. Irregular bleeding is frequently seen when using the mini-pill or combination oral contraceptives containing less than 50 micrograms of estrogen.

More serious side effects include worsening of migraine, asthma, epilepsy, and kidney or heart disease because of a tendency for water to be retained in the body when oral contraceptives are used. Other side effects are growth of preexisting fibroid tumors of the uterus, mental depression, and liver problems with jaundice (yellowing of the skin). Your doctor may find that levels of sugar and fatty substances in your blood are elevated; the long-term effects of these changes are not known. Some women develop high blood pressure while taking oral contraceptives, which ordinarily returns to the original levels when the oral contraceptive is stopped.

Other reactions, although not proved to be caused by oral contraceptives, are occasionally reported. These include more frequent urination and some discomfort when urinating, nervousness, dizziness, some loss of scalp hair, an increase in body hair, an increase or decrease in sex drive, appetite changes, cataracts, and a need for a change in contact lens prescription or inability to use contact lenses.

After you stop using oral contraceptives there may be a delay before you are able to become pregnant or before you resume having menstrual periods. This is especially true of women who had irregular menstrual cycles prior to the use of oral contraceptives. As discussed previously, your doctor may recommend that you wait a short while after stopping the pill before you try to become pregnant. During this time, use another form of contraception. You should consult your physican before resuming use of oral contraceptives after childbirth, especially if you plan to nurse your baby. Drugs in oral contraceptives are known to appear in the milk, and the long-range effect on infants is not known at this time. Furthermore, oral con-

Continued on next page

This product information was prepared in August, 1982. On these and other Parke-Davis Products, information may be obtained by addressing PARKE-DAVIS, Division of Warner-Lambert Company, Morris Plains, New Jersey 07950.

Parke-Davis—Cont.

traceptives may cause a decrease in your milk supply as well as in the quality of the milk.

4. Comparison of the Risks of Oral Contraceptives and Other Contraceptive Methods. The many studies on the risks and effectiveness of oral contraceptives and other methods of contraception have been analyzed to estimate the risk of death associated with various methods of contraception. This risk has two parts: (a) the risk of the method itself (eg, the risk that oral contraceptives will cause death due to abnormal clotting); and (b) the risk of death due to pregnancy or abortion in the event the method fails. The results of this analysis are shown in the following bar graph. The height of the bars is the number of deaths per 100,000 women each year. There are six sets of bars, each set referring to a specific age group of women. Within each set of bars, there is a single bar for each of the different contraceptive methods. For oral contraceptives, there are two bars—one for smokers and the other for nonsmokers. The analysis is based on present knowledge and new information could, of course, alter it. The analysis shows that the risk of death from all methods of birth control is low and below that associated with childbirth, except for oral contraceptives in women over 40 who smoke. It shows that the lowest risk of death is associated with the condom or diaphragm (traditional contraception) backed up by early abortion in case of failure of the condom or diaphragm to prevent pregnancy. Also, at any age the risk of death (due to unexpected pregnancy) from the use of traditional contraception, even without a backup of abortion, is generally the same as or less than that from use of oral contraceptives.

[See bar graph below].

How to Use Oral Contraceptives As Safely and Effectively As Possible, Once You Have Decided to Use Them

1. What to Tell your Doctor.

You can make use of the pill as safely as possible, by telling your doctor if you have any of the following:

a. Conditions that mean you should not use oral contraceptives:

Clots in the legs or lungs
Clots in the legs or lungs in the past
A stroke, heart attack, or angina pectoris
Known or suspected cancer of the breast or sex organs
Unusual vaginal bleeding that has not yet been diagnosed
Known or suspected pregnancy

b. Conditions that your doctor will want to watch closely or which might cause him to suggest another method of contraception:

A family history of breast cancer
Breast nodules, fibrocystic disease of the breast, or an abnormal mammogram
Diabetes
High blood pressure
High cholesterol
Cigarette smoking
Migraine headaches
Heart or kidney disease
Epilepsy
Mental depression
Fibroid tumors of the uterus
Gallbladder disease

c. Once you are using oral contraceptives, you should be alert for signs of a serious adverse effect and call your doctor if they occur:

Sharp pain in the chest, coughing blood, or sudden shortness of breath (indicating possible clots in the lungs)
Pain in the calf (possible clot in the leg)
Crushing chest pain or heaviness (indicating possible heart attack)
Sudden severe headache or vomiting, dizziness or fainting, disturbance of vision or speech, or weakness or numbness in an arm or leg (indicating a possible stroke)
Sudden partial or complete loss of vision (indicating a possible clot in the eye)
Breast lumps (you should ask your doctor to show you how to examine your own breasts)
Severe pain in the abdomen (indicating a possible ruptured tumor of the liver)
Severe depression
Yellowing of the skin (jaundice)

2. How to Take the Pill So That It Is Most Effective.

Reduced effectiveness and an increased incidence of breakthrough bleeding have been associated with the use of oral contraceptives with antibiotics such as rifampin, ampicillin, and tetracycline or with certain other drugs, such as barbiturates, phenylbutazone or phenytoin sodium. You should use an additional means of contraception during any cycle in which any of these drugs are taken.

Directions For 21-Day Dosage Regimen

a. The first day of your period is Day 1. On the fifth day (Day 5), start taking one tablet daily, beginning with the tablet in the upper left corner of the Petipac. In the space provided, write the day you start. To remove a tablet, press down on it with your thumb or finger. The tablet will drop through a hole in the bottom of the Petipac. Do not press on the tablet with your thumbnail or fingernail, or any other sharp object.

If your period begins on:	Start taking tablets on:
Sunday	Thursday
Monday	Friday
Tuesday	Saturday
Wednesday	Sunday
Thursday	Monday
Friday	Tuesday
Saturday	Wednesday

b. Continue to take one tablet daily until all the tablets have been taken.

c. After you have taken all 21 tablets, stop and don't take any tablets for the next seven days. You should have a menstrual period one to three days after you stop taking tablets; sometimes, it may take a day or so longer.

d. After seven days, during which you take no tablets, put a new refill in your Petipac and begin a new course of tablets, taking one tablet daily for 21 days. You will always start each new course of 21 tablets on the same day of the week. Likewise, the interval of no tablets will always start on the same day of the week.

e. If spotting should occur at an unexpected time, continue to take your tablets as directed. Spotting is usually temporary and without significance. However, if bleeding should occur at an unexpected time, consult your physician. Call your physician regarding any problem or change in your general health that may concern you.

f. If you forget to take a tablet, take it as soon as you remember, even if it is the next day.

Figure 1. Estimated annual number of deaths associated with control of fertility and no control per 100,000 nonsterile women, by regimen of control and age of woman.

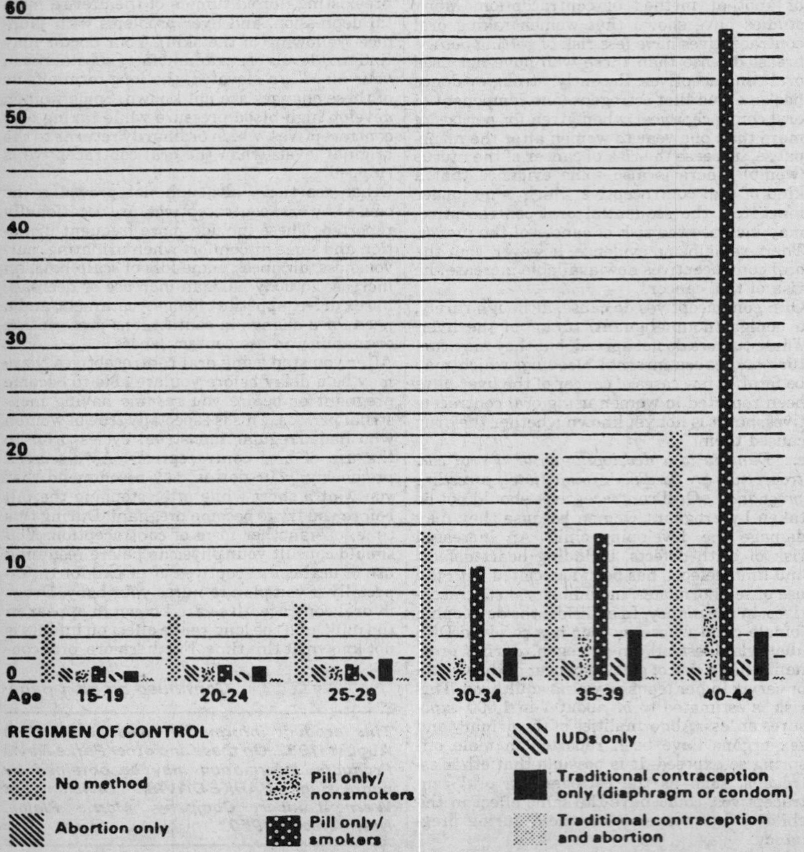

Then take the next scheduled tablet at the usual time. If you miss two consecutive tablets, take two tablets daily for the next two days. Then resume the regular schedule. While there is little likelihood of pregnancy occurring if you miss only one or two tablets, the possibility of pregnancy increases with each successive day that tablets are missed. *However, if you are taking* Loestrin **21** 1/20, *in addition to taking two white tablets a day for two days, you should use an additional means of contraception for seven consecutive days.* If you miss three consecutive tablets, discard any tablets remaining and begin a new course of tablets, starting seven days after the last tablet was taken, even if you are still menstruating. You should use an alternate means of contraception, other than oral tablets, until the start of your next menstrual period.

Remembering to take tablets according to schedule is stressed because of its importance in providing you the greatest degree of protection.

Directions For 28-Day Dosage Regimen

a. The first day of your period is Day 1. On the fifth day (Day 5), start taking one *light-colored* tablet daily, beginning with the tablet in the upper left corner of the Petipac. In the space provided, write the day you start. Take all the tablets in the top row first, followed by the second row, and so on. To remove a tablet, press down on it with your thumb or finger. The tablet will drop through a hole in the bottom of the Petipac. Do not press on the tablet with your thumbnail or fingernail, or any other sharp object.

If your period begins on:	Start taking tablets on:
Sunday	Thursday
Monday	Friday
Tuesday	Saturday
Wednesday	Sunday
Thursday	Monday
Friday	Tuesday
Saturday	Wednesday

b. On the day after taking the last *light-colored* tablet, begin taking one *brown* tablet daily until all the tablets have been taken.

c. When the last tablet has been taken, put a new refill in your Petipac and, without interruption, begin a new course of tablets by taking the *light-colored* tablets first, followed by the *brown* tablets. There should never be a day when you are not taking a tablet.

d. Continue taking *light-colored* tablets without interruption whether or not your period has occurred or is still in progress. Your period will usually occur during the time you are taking *brown* tablets.

e. If spotting should occur at an unexpected time, continue to take your tablets as directed. Spotting is usually temporary and without significance. However, if bleeding should occur at an unexpected time, consult your physician. Call your physician regarding any problem or change in your general health that may concern you.

f. If you forget to take a *light-colored* tablet, take it as soon as you remember, even if it is the next day. Then take the next scheduled *light-colored* tablet at the usual time. If you miss two consecutive *light-colored* tablets, take two *light-colored* tablets daily for the next two days. Then resume the regular schedule. While there is little likelihood of pregnancy occurring if you miss only one or two tablets, the possibility of pregnancy increases with each successive day that tablets are missed. *However, if you are taking* Loestrin **Fe** 1/20, *in addition to taking two white tablets a day for two days, you should use an additional means of contraception for seven consecutive days.* If you miss three consecutive *light-colored* tablets discard any tablets remaining and begin a new course of tablets, starting seven days after the last *light-colored* tablet was taken, even if you are still menstruating. You should use an alternate means of contraception, other than oral tablets, until the start of your next menstrual period.

g. If you miss one or more *brown* tablets discard the remainder and begin a new course of tablets no later than the eighth day after you took the last *light-colored* tablet. Under no circumstances should you substitute a *brown* tablet for a *light-colored* one, or take any *brown* tablet before you have taken all the *light-colored* tablets, unless your physician advises you to do so. Remembering to take tablets according to schedule is stressed because of its importance in providing you the greatest degree of protection.

Missed Menstrual Periods For Both Dosage Regimens: At times there may be no menstrual period after a cycle of pills. Therefore, if you miss one menstrual period but have taken the pills *exactly as your were supposed to,* continue as usual into the next cycle. If you have not taken the pills correctly and miss a menstrual period, *you may be pregnant* and should stop taking oral contraceptives until your doctor determines whether or not you are pregnant. Until you can get to your doctor, use another form of contraception. If two consecutive menstrual periods are missed, you should stop taking pills until it is determined whether you are pregnant. If you do become pregnant while using oral contraceptives, you should discuss the risks to the developing child with your doctor.

Periodic Examination

Your doctor will take a complete medical and family history before prescribing oral contraceptives. At that time and about once a year thereafter, he will generally examine your blood pressure, breasts, abdomen, and pelvic organs (including a Papanicolaou smear, ie, test for cancer).

Summary: Oral contraceptives are the most effective method, except sterilization, for preventing pregnancy. Other methods, when used conscientiously, are also very effective and have fewer risks. The serious risks of oral contraceptives are uncommon and the "pill" is a very convenient method of preventing pregnancy.

If you have certain conditions or have had these conditions in the past, you should not use oral contraceptives because the risk is too great. These conditions are listed in this leaflet. If you do not have these conditions, and decide to use the "pill," please read this leaflet carefully so that you can use the "pill" most safely and effectively.

Based on his or her assessment of your medical needs, your doctor has prescribed this drug for you. Do not give this drug to anyone else.

0913G150

[*Shown in Product Identification Section*]

LOPID® ℞
(gemfibrozil)
Capsules

Description: LOPID (gemfibrozil) is a lipid regulating agent. It is available as capsules for oral administration. Each capsule contains 300 mg gemfibrozil. The chemical name is 5-(2,5-dimethylphenoxy)-2,2-dimethylpentanoic acid. The empirical formula is $C_{15}H_{22}O_3$ and the molecular weight is 250.35; the solubility in water and acid is 0.0019% and in dilute base it is greater than 1%. The melting point is 58°-61°C. Gemfibrozil is a white solid which is stable under ordinary conditions.

Clinical Pharmacology: LOPID is a lipid regulating agent which lowers elevated serum lipids primarily by decreasing serum triglyceride with a variable reduction in total serum cholesterol. These decreases occur primarily in the very low density lipoprotein (VLDL) fraction and less frequently in the low density lipoprotein (LDL) fraction. In addition, LOPID may increase the high density lipoprotein (HDL) cholesterol fraction, an action considered of possible benefit to inhibition of the atherosclerotic process. The mechanism of action has not been definitively established. In man, LOPID has been shown to inhibit peripheral lipolysis and to decrease the hepatic extraction of free fatty acids, thus reducing hepatic triglyceride production. LOPID also inhibits synthesis of VLDL carrier apoprotein, leading to a decrease in VLDL production.

Animal studies suggest that LOPID may, in addition to elevating HDL cholesterol, reduce incorporation of long-chain fatty acids into newly formed triglycerides, accelerate turnover and removal of cholesterol from the liver, and increase excretion of cholesterol in the feces.

LOPID is well absorbed from the gastrointestinal tract after oral administration. Peak plasma levels occur in one to two hours with a plasma half-life of 1.5 hours following single doses and 1.3 hours following multiple doses. Plasma levels appear proportional to dose and do not demonstrate accumulation across time following multiple doses.

LOPID mainly undergoes oxidation of a ring methyl group to successively form a hydroxymethyl and a carboxyl metabolite. Approximately seventy percent of the administered human dose is excreted in the urine, primarily as unchanged gemfibrozil. Six percent of the dose is accounted for in the feces. In a large, controlled multicenter trial of 427 patients, lipid and lipoprotein changes from average baseline (%) by hyperlipoproteinemic (HLP) type are summarized below for those patients receiving gemfibrozil, 1200 mg/day, at the end of 12 weeks.

[See table above].

HLP Type	TRIGLYCERIDE	CHOLESTEROL				RATIO:
		Total	VLDL	LDL	HDL	HDL Cholesterol / Total Cholesterol
IIa	−44%	−4.2%	−44.3%	−5.8%	+24.6%	+33%
IIb	−45%	−8.6%	−45.0%	−6.4%	+19.5%	+34%
IV	−40%	−1.8%	−40.8%	+14.6%	+17.4%	+23%

Indications and Usage: Drug therapy should not be used for the routine treatment of elevated blood lipids for the prevention of coronary heart disease. Dietary therapy specific for the type of hyperlipidemia is the initial treatment of choice. Excess body weight and excess alcoholic intake may be important factors in hypertriglyceridemia and should be addressed prior to any drug therapy. Physical exercise can be an important ancillary measure.

Continued on next page

This product information was prepared in August, 1982. On these and other Parke-Davis Products, information may be obtained by addressing PARKE-DAVIS, Division of Warner-Lambert Company, Morris Plains, New Jersey 07950.

Parke-Davis—Cont.

Contributory diseases such as hypothyroidism or diabetes mellitus should be looked for and adequately treated. The use of drugs should be considered only when reasonable attempts have been made to obtain satisfactory results with nondrug methods. If the decision is to use drugs, the patient should be instructed that this does not reduce the importance of adhering to diet.
Because of chemical, pharmacological, and clinical similarities between gemfibrozil and clofibrate, and the adverse findings with clofibrate in two large clinical studies (see Warnings), use of gemfibrozil should be restricted to the following indications. LOPID may be considered for the treatment of adult patients with very high serum triglyceride levels (type IV hyperlipidemia) who present a risk of abdominal pain and pancreatitis and who do not respond adequately to a determined dietary effort to control them. Patients with triglyceride levels in excess of 750 mg per deciliter are likely to present such risk. LOPID (gemfibrozil) has little effect on elevated cholesterol levels in most subjects. A minority of subjects show a more pronounced response. However, it must be understood that there is no evidence that use of any lipid-altering drug will be beneficial in preventing death from coronary heart disease (See WARNINGS). Therefore, the physician should be very selective and confine gemfibrozil treatment to patients with clearly defined risk due to severe hypercholesterolemia (eg, individuals with familial hypercholesterolemia starting in childhood) who inadequately respond to appropriate diet and more effective cholesterol-lowering drugs.
LOPID is not useful for the hypertriglyceridemia of Type I hyperlipidemia.
The biochemical response to gemfibrozil is variable, and it is not always possible to predict from the lipoprotein type or other factors which patients will obtain favorable results. It is essential that lipid levels be assessed and that the drug be discontinued after three months in any patient in whom lipids do not show significant improvement.
The effect of drug-induced reduction of serum cholesterol or triglyceride levels or elevation of HDL cholesterol levels on morbidity or mortality due to coronary heart disease has not been established. Several years may be required before ongoing long-term investigations will resolve this question.

Contraindications:
1. Hepatic or severe renal dysfunction, including primary biliary cirrhosis.
2. Preexisting gallbladder disease. (See Warnings).
3. Hypersensitivity to gemfibrozil.

Warnings:
1. Because of chemical, pharmacological, and clinical similarities between gemfibrozil and clofibrate, the adverse findings with clofibrate in two large clinical studies may also apply to gemfibrozil. In the first of those studies, the Coronary Drug Project, 1000 subjects with previous myocardial infarction were treated for five years with clofibrate. There was no difference in mortality between the clofibrate-treated subjects and 3000 placebo-treated subjects, but twice as many clofibrate-treated subjects developed cholelithiasis and cholecystitis requiring surgery. In the other study, conducted by the World Health Organization, 5000 subjects without known coronary heart disease were treated with clofibrate for five years and followed one year beyond. There was a statistically significant 36% higher total mortality in the clofibrate-treated than in a comparable placebo-treated control group. The excess mortality was due to noncardiovascular causes, including malignancy, postcholecystectomy complications, and pancreatitis. The higher risk of clofibrate-treated subjects for gallbladder disease was confirmed.
2. Long-Term Toxicity and Animal Tumorigenicity Studies: Long-term studies have been conducted in rats and mice at one and ten times the human dose. The incidence of benign liver nodules and liver carcinomas was significantly increased in high dose male rats. The incidence of liver carcinomas increased also in low dose males, but this increase was not statistically significant (p greater than 0.05). There were no statistically significant differences from controls in the incidence of liver tumors in female rats, and in male and female mice. Electron microscopy studies have demonstrated a florid hepatic peroxisome proliferation following LOPID administration to the male rat. Similar changes have not been found in the human liver.
Male rats had a dose-related increase of benign Leydig cell tumors. Subcapsular bilateral cataracts occurred in 10%, and unilateral in 6.3% of the high dose males.
3. Since a reduction of mortality from coronary artery disease has not been demonstrated and liver and interstitial cell testicular tumors were increased in male rats, LOPID should be administered only to those patients described in the Indications and Usage Section. If a significant serum lipid response is not obtained, LOPID should be discontinued.
4. Cholelithiasis—LOPID may increase cholesterol excretion into the bile leading to cholelithiasis. If cholelithiasis is suspected gallbladder studies are indicated. LOPID therapy should be discontinued if gallstones are found.
5. Concomitant Anticoagulants—Caution should be exercised when anticoagulants are given in conjunction with LOPID. The dosage of the anticoagulant should be reduced to maintain the prothrombin time at the desired level to prevent bleeding complications. Frequent prothrombin determinations are advisable until it has been definitely determined that the prothrombin level has stabilized.

Precautions:
1. **Initial Therapy**—Before instituting LOPID (gemfibrozil) therapy, every attempt should be made to control serum lipids with appropriate diet, exercise, weight loss in obese patients, and other medical problems such as diabetes mellitus and hypothyroidism.
2. **Continued Therapy**—Pretreatment laboratory studies should be performed to ensure that patients have abnormal levels of serum lipids. Periodic determinations of serum lipids should be obtained during LOPID administration. The drug should be withdrawn after three months if the lipid response is inadequate.
3. **Seasonal Variation of Lipid Levels**—LOPID is not expected to alter seasonal variations of higher serum lipid values in midwinter and late summer or the lower values in fall and spring.
4. **Impairment of Fertility**—Administration of approximately three and ten times the human dose to male rats for 10 weeks resulted in a dose-related decrease of fertility. Subsequent studies demonstrated that this effect was reversed after a drug-free period of about eight weeks, and it was not transmitted to their offspring.
5. **Pregnancy Category B**—Reproduction studies have been performed in the rat at doses 3 and 9 times the human dose, and in the rabbit at 2 and 6.7 times the human dose. These studies have revealed no evidence of impaired fertility in females or harm to the fetus due to LOPID. Minor fetotoxicity was manifested by reduced birth rates observed at the high dose levels. No significant malformations were found among almost 400 offspring from 36 litters of rats and 100 fetuses from 22 litters of rabbits.
There are no studies in pregnant women. In view of the fact that LOPID is tumorigenic in male rats, the use of LOPID in pregnancy should be reserved for those patients where the benefit clearly outweighs the possible risk to the patient or fetus.
6. **Nursing Mothers**—Because of the potential for tumorigenicity shown for gemfibrozil in male rats, a decision should be made whether to discontinue nursing or discontinue the drug, taking into account the importance of the drug to the mother.
7. **Hematologic Changes**—Mild hemoglobin, hematocrit and white blood cell decreases have been observed in occasional patients following initiation of LOPID therapy. However, these levels stabilize during long-term administration. Therefore, periodic blood counts are recommended during the first 12 months of LOPID administration.
8. **Liver Function**—Abnormal liver function tests have been observed occasionally during LOPID administration, including elevations of SGOT, SGPT, LDH, and alkaline phosphatase. These are usually reversible when LOPID is discontinued. Therefore periodic liver function studies are recommended and LOPID therapy should be terminated if abnormalities persist.
9. **Cardiac Arrhythmias**—Although no clinically significant abnormalities occurred that could be attributed to LOPID, the possibility exists that such abnormalities may occur.
10. **Use in Children**—Safety and efficacy in children have not been established.

Adverse Reactions: In controlled clinical trials of 805 patients, including 245 who received LOPID for at least one year, the most frequently reported adverse reactions associated with LOPID involved the gastrointestinal system. In decreasing order of frequency, these were abdominal pain (6.0%), epigastric pain (4.9%), diarrhea (4.8%), nausea (4.0%), vomiting (1.6%), and flatulence (1.1%). Other adverse reactions where the probability of a causal relationship to LOPID therapy exists are listed by system.
Integumentary: rash, dermatitis, pruritus, urticaria
Central Nervous System: headache, dizziness, blurred vision
Musculoskeletal: painful extremities
Hematopoietic: anemia, eosinophilia, leukopenia
Other reactions have been reported under conditions where a causal relationship is difficult to establish, thus the physician should be alert to these occurrences. Reports of viral and bacterial infections (common cold, cough, and urinary tract infections) were more common in gemfibrozil than in placebo-treated patients.
Other reactions were:
Gastrointestinal: dry mouth, constipation, anorexia, gas pain, dyspepsia
Musculoskeletal: back pain, arthralgia, muscle cramps, myalgia, swollen joints
Central Nervous System: vertigo, insomnia, paresthesia, tinnitus
Clinical Laboratory: hypokalemia, liver function abnormalities (increased SGOT, SGPT, LDH, CPK, alkaline phosphatase)
Miscellaneous: fatigue, malaise, syncope

Dosage and Administration: The recommended dose for adults is 1200 mg administered in two divided doses 30 minutes before the morning and evening meal. Some patients will experience therapeutic effects on 900 mg/day; a few may require 1500 mg/day for satisfactory results.

Drug Interactions: CAUTION SHOULD BE EXERCISED WHEN ANTICOAGULANTS ARE GIVEN IN CONJUNCTION WITH LOPID (GEMFIBROZIL). THE DOSAGE OF THE ANTICOAGULANT SHOULD BE REDUCED TO MAINTAIN THE PROTHROMBIN TIME AT THE DESIRED LEVEL TO PREVENT BLEEDING COMPLICATIONS. FREQUENT PROTHROMBIN DETERMINATIONS ARE ADVISABLE UNTIL IT HAS BEEN DEFINITELY DETERMINED THAT THE PROTHROMBIN LEVEL HAS STABILIZED.

Management of Overdosage: While there has been no reported case of overdosage, symptomatic supportive measures should be taken should it occur.

How Supplied:
N 0071-0669-24 (Capsule 669) LOPID Capsules, each containing 300 mg gemfibrozil, are available in 100's.
Parcode® No. 669.

Storage: Store below 30°C (86°F).

0669G011

[*Shown in Product Identification Section*]

MANDELAMINE® TABLETS ℞
(methenamine mandelate tablets, USP)

MANDELAMINE SUSPENSION FORTE, 500 mg/5ml ℞

MANDELAMINE SUSPENSION, 250 mg/5ml ℞
(methenamine mandelate oral suspension, USP)

MANDELAMINE GRANULES ℞
(methenamine mandelate)

Description: Mandelamine, a urinary antibacterial agent, is the chemical combination of mandelic acid with methenamine. Mandelamine is available as film-coated tablets, suspension, and granules.

Actions: Mandelamine is readily absorbed but remains essentially inactive until it is excreted by the kidney and concentrated in the urine. An acid urine is essential for antibacterial action with maximum efficacy occurring at pH 5.5 or less. In an acid urine, mandelic acid exerts its antibacterial action and also contributes to the acidification of the urine. Mandelic acid is excreted by both glomerular filtration and tubular excretion. The methenamine component, in an acid urine, is hydrolyzed to ammonia and to the bactericidal agent formaldehyde. There is equally effective antibacterial activity against both gram-positive and gram-negative organisms, since the antibacterial action of mandelic acid and formaldehyde is nonspecific. There are reports that Mandelamine is ineffective in some infections with *Proteus vulgaris* and urea-splitting strains of *Pseudomonas aeruginosa* and *A aerogenes.* Since urea-splitting strains may raise the pH of the urine, particular attention to supplementary acidification is required. However, results in any single case will depend to a large extent on the underlying pathology and the overall management.

Rationale: *Prophylactic use*—Urine is a good culture medium for many urinary pathogens. Inoculation by a few organisms (relapse or reinfection) may lead to bacteriuria in susceptible individuals. Thus, the rationale of management in recurring urinary tract infection (bacteriuria) is to change the urine from a growth-supporting to a growth-inhibiting medium. There is a growing body of evidence that long-term administration of Mandelamine can prevent the recurrence of bacteriuria in patients with chronic pyelonephritis.

Therapeutic use—Mandelamine helps to sterilize the urine and, in some situations in which underlying pathologic conditions prevent sterilization by any means, it can help to suppress the bacteriuria. Mandelamine should not be used alone for acute infections with parenchymal involvement causing systemic symptoms such as chills and fever. A thorough diagnostic investigation as a part of the overall management of the urinary tract infection should accompany the use of Mandelamine.

Indications: Mandelamine is indicated for the suppression or elimination of bacteriuria associated with pyelonephritis, cystitis, and other chronic urinary tract infections; also for infected residual urine sometimes accompanying neurologic diseases. When used as recommended, Mandelamine is particularly suitable for long-term therapy because of its safety and because resistance to the nonspecific bactericidal action of formaldehyde does not develop. Pathogens resistant to other antibacterial agents may respond to Mandelamine because of the nonspecific effect of formaldehyde formed in an acid urine.

Contraindication: Renal insufficiency.

Precautions: Dysuria may occur (usually at higher than recommended dosage). This can be controlled by reducing the dosage and the acidification. When urine acidification is contraindicated or unattainable (as with some urea-splitting bacteria), the drug is not recommended.

To avoid inducing lipid pneumonia, administer Mandelamine Suspension Forte and Mandelamine Suspension with care to elderly, debilitated or otherwise susceptible patients.

Adverse Reactions: An occasional patient may experience gastrointestinal disturbance or a generalized skin rash.

Dosage and Management: The average adult dosage is 4 grams daily given as 1.0 gram after each meal and at bedtime. Children 6 to 12 should receive half the adult dose and children under 6 years of age should receive 250 mg per 30 lb body weight, four times daily. [See accompanying Mandelamine Dosage Chart].

Since an acid urine is essential for antibacterial activity with maximum efficacy occurring at pH 5.5 or below, restriction of alkalinizing foods and medication is thus desirable. If testing of urine pH reveals the need, supplemental acidification should be given.

MANDELAMINE
(methenamine mandelate)
DOSAGE CHART

	Adults	Children
Tablets and Granules		
	1 tablet q.i.d.	—
1.0 gram	1 packet granules* q.i.d.	—
	2 tablets q.i.d.	(Ages 6–12) 1 tablet q.i.d.
0.5 gram	—	(Ages 6–12) 1 packet granules* q.i.d.
0.25 gram	—	(Age under 6) 1 tablet per 30 lb body weight q.i.d.
Suspension Forte†		
500 mg/5 ml teaspoonful	2 teaspoonfuls (10 ml) q.i.d.	(Ages 6–12) 1 teaspoonful (5 ml) q.i.d.
Suspension†		
250 mg/5 ml teaspoonful	—	(Age under 6) 1 teaspoonful (5 ml) per 30 lb body weight q.i.d.

*Contents of packet to be dissolved in 2–4 oz water immediately before using.
†Suspensions are in vegetable oil. Shake well before using.

How Supplied:
1-gram Tablets P-D 167: purple, film coated, in bottles of 100 (N 0071-0167-24) and 1000 (N 0071-0167-32; also unit dose in 10 x 10 strips (N 0071-0167-40). 0.5-gram Tablets P-D 166; brown, film coated, in bottles of 100 (N 0071-0166-24) and 1000 (N 0071-0166-32); also unit dose in 10 x 10 strips (N 0071-0166-40).
Granules: orange flavored, in individual packets of 1 gram, cartons of 56 (N 0071-2176-03[19]), and individual packets of 0.5 gram, cartons of 56 (N 0071-2177-02[19]).
Suspension Forte: pink, cherry flavored in bottles of 8 fl oz (N 0071-2174-20) and 16 fl oz (N 0071-2174-23). U.S. Patent No. 3,077,438.
Suspension: Cream colored, coconut flavored in bottles of 16 fl oz (N 0071-2173-23).
STORE BETWEEN 15°–30°C (59°–86°F).

[*Shown in Product Identification Section*]

0166 G 030 (3/80)

MECLOMEN® ℞
(meclofenamate sodium)*

*Product of Warner-Lambert Inc

Description: Meclomen (meclofenamate sodium) is N-(2, 6-dichloro-m-tolyl) anthranilic acid, sodium salt, monohydrate. It is an anti-inflammatory drug for oral administration. Meclomen capsules contain 50 or 100 mg meclofenamic acid as the sodium salt.
It is a white powder with a melting point 287 to 291 C, molecular weight 336.15, and water solubility greater than 250 mg/ml.

Clinical Pharmacology: Meclomen is a nonsteroidal agent which has demonstrated antiinflammatory, analgesic, and antipyretic activity in laboratory animals. The mode of action, like that of other nonsteroidal antiinflammatory agents, is not known. Therapeutic action does not result from pituitary-adrenal stimulation. In animal studies, Meclomen was found to inhibit prostaglandin synthesis and to compete for binding at the prostaglandin receptor site. These properties may be responsible for the antiinflammatory action of Meclomen. There is no evidence that Meclomen alters the course of the underlying disease.

Following a single oral dose to normal human volunteers, peak plasma levels occurred in 0.5 to 1 hour, with a half-life of 2 hours (3.3 hours following multiple doses). Plasma levels are proportional to dose. There is no evidence of accumulation of drug. Urinary and fecel excretion of tritium-labeled Meclomen account for 80 to 102% of the total dose, with about two thirds appearing in urine and one third in feces. Most of the urinary excretion occurs as the glucuronide conjugates of the metabolites, with only small amounts of free drug recovered.

In several human isotope studies, Meclomen, at a dosage of 300 mg/day, produced a fecal blood loss of 1 to 2 ml per day, and 2 to 3 ml per day at 400 mg/day. Aspirin, at a dosage of 3.6 g/day, caused a fecal blood loss of 6 ml per day.
In a multiple-dose, one-week study in normal human volunteers, Meclomen had little or no effect on collagen-induced platelet aggregation, platelet count, or bleeding time. In comparison, aspirin suppressed collagen-induced platelet aggregation and increased bleeding time. The concomitant administration of antacids (aluminum and magnesium hydroxides) does not interfere with absorption of Meclomen.

Controlled clinical trials comparing Meclomen with aspirin demonstrated comparable efficacy in rheumatoid arthritis. The Meclomen-treated patients had fewer reactions involving the special senses, specifically tinnitus, but more gastrointestinal reactions, specifically diarrhea.

Continued on next page

This product information was prepared in August, 1982. On these and other Parke-Davis Products, information may be obtained by addressing PARKE-DAVIS, Division of Warner-Lambert Company, Morris Plains, New Jersey 07950.

Parke-Davis—Cont.

The incidence of patients who discontinued therapy due to adverse reactions was similar for both the Meclomen- and aspirin-treated groups.

The improvement with Meclomen reported by patients and the reduction of the disease activity, as evaluated by both physicians and patients with rheumatoid arthritis, are associated with a significant reduction in number of tender joints, severity of tenderness, and duration of morning stiffness.

The improvement, reported by patients and as evaluated by physicians, in patients treated with Meclomen for osteoarthritis is associated with a significant reduction in night pain, pain on walking, degree of starting pain, and pain on passive motion. The function of knee joints also improved significantly.

Meclomen has been used in combination with gold salts or corticosteroids in patients with rheumatoid arthritis. Studies have demonstrated that Meclomen contributes to the improvement of patients' conditions while maintained on gold salts or corticosteroids. Data are inadequate to demonstrate that Meclomen in combination with salicylates produces greater improvement than that achieved with Meclomen alone.

Indications and Usage: Meclomen is indicated for relief of the signs and symptoms of acute and chronic rheumatoid arthritis and osteoarthritis. Meclomen is not recommended as the initial drug for treatment because of gastrointestinal side effects, including diarrhea which is sometimes severe. Selection of Meclomen requires a careful assessment of the benefit/risk ratio. (See Precautions, Warnings, and Adverse Reactions sections.)

The safety and effectiveness of Meclomen have not been established in those patients with rheumatoid arthritis who are designated by the American Rheumatism Association as Functional Class IV (incapacitated, largely or wholly bedridden, or confined to a wheelchair, little or no self-care).

Meclomen is not recommended in children because adequate studies to demonstrate safety and efficacy have not been carried out.

Contraindications: Meclomen should not be used in patients who have previously exhibited hypersensitivity to it.

Because the potential exists for cross sensitivity to aspirin or other nonsteroidal antiinflammatory drugs, Meclomen should not be given to patients in whom these drugs induce symptoms of bronchospasm, allergic rhinitis, or urticaria.

Warnings: In patients with a history of upper gastrointestinal tract disease, Meclomen should be given under close supervision and only after consulting the Adverse Reactions section. Peptic ulceration and gastrointestinal bleeding, sometimes severe, including one fatality, have been reported in patients receiving Meclomen.

Diarrhea, gastrointestinal irritation, and abdominal pain may be associated with Meclomen therapy. Dosage reduction or temporarily stopping the drug have generally controlled these symptoms. (See Adverse Reactions and Dosage and Administration sections.)

Precautions:

General

Patients receiving nonsteroidal antiinflammatory agents, such as Meclomen, should be evaluated periodically to insure that the drug is still necessary and well tolerated. (See other Precautions, Warnings, and Adverse Reactions.)

Decreases in hemoglobin and/or hematocrit levels have occurred in approximately one of six patients, but rarely required discontinuation of Meclomen therapy. The clinical data revealed no evidence of increased chronic blood loss, bone-marrow suppression, or hemolysis to account for the decreases in hemoglobin or hematocrit levels. Patients who are receiving long-term Meclomen therapy should have hemoglobin and hematocrit values determined if anemia is suspected on clinical grounds.

Ophthalmic examinations performed prior to and following extended Meclomen use have not shown drug-related changes. However, because of adverse eye findings in animal studies with other nonsteroidal antiinflammatory drugs, ophthalmologic studies should be carried out if any visual symptoms should develop during Meclomen administration.

When Meclomen is used in combination with steroid therapy, any reduction in steroid dosage should be gradual to avoid the possible complications of sudden steroid withdrawal.

Information for Patients

Patients should be advised that nausea, vomiting, diarrhea, and abdominal pain have been associated with the use of Meclomen. The patient should be made aware of a possible drug connection and accordingly should consider discontinuing the drug and contacting his or her physician if any of these conditions are severe.

Meclomen may be taken with meals or milk to control gastrointestinal complaints. Concomitant administration of an antacid (specifically, aluminum and magnesium hydroxides) does not interfere with the absorption of the drug.

Laboratory Tests

Patients receiving long-term Meclomen therapy should have hemoglobin and hematocrit values determined if signs or symptoms of anemia occur.

Low white blood cell counts were rarely observed in clinical trials. These low counts were transient and usually returned to normal while the patient continued on Meclomen therapy. Persistent leukopenia, granulocytopenia, or thrombocytopenia warrant further clinical evaluation and may require discontinuation of the drug.

When abnormal blood chemistry values are obtained, follow-up studies are indicated. Elevations of serum transaminase levels and of alkaline phosphatase levels occurred in approximately 4% of patients. An occasional patient had elevations of serum creatinine or BUN levels.

Drug Interactions:

1. ***Warfarin***

Meclomen enhances the effect of warfarin. Therefore, when Meclomen is given to a patient receiving warfarin, the dosage of warfarin should be reduced to prevent excessive prolongation of the prothrombin time.

2. ***Aspirin***

Concurrent administration of aspirin may lower Meclomen plasma levels, possibly by competing for protein-binding sites. The urinary excretion of Meclomen is unaffected by aspirin, indicating no change in Meclomen absorption. Meclomen does not affect serum salicylate levels. Greater fecal blood loss results from concomitant administration of both drugs than from either drug alone.

3. ***Propoxyphene***

The concurrent administration of propoxyphene hydrochloride does not affect the bioavailability of Meclomen.

4. ***Antacids***

Concomitant administration of aluminum and magnesium hydroxides does not interfere with absorption of Meclomen.

Carcinogenesis

An 18-month study in rats revealed no evidence of carcinogenicity.

Usage in Pregnancy: Meclomen, like aspirin and other nonsteroidal antiinflammatory drugs, causes fetotoxicity, minor skeletal malformations, eg, supernumerary ribs, and delayed ossification in rodent reproduction trials, but no major teratogenicity. Similarly, it prolongs gestation and interferes with parturition and with normal development of young before weaning. Meclomen is not recommended for use during pregnancy, particularly in the 1st and 3rd trimesters based on these animal findings. There are, however, no adequate and well-controlled studies in pregnant women.

Usage in Nursing Mothers: It is not known whether Meclomen is excreted in human milk. Because of the effects on suckling rodents and the fact that many drugs are excreted in human milk, Meclomen is not recommended for nursing women.

Pediatric Use: Safety and effectiveness in children below the age of 14 have not been established.

Adverse Reactions

Incidence Greater than 1%

The following adverse reactions were observed in clinical trials and included observations from more than 2,700 patients, 594 of whom are treated for one year and 248 for at least two years.

Gastrointestinal

The most frequently reported adverse reactions associated with Meclomen involve the gastrointestinal system. In controlled studies of up to six months' duration, these disturbances occurred in the following decreasing order of frequency with the approximate incidences in parentheses: diarrhea (10-33%), nausea with or without vomiting (11%), other gastrointestinal disorders (10%), and abdominal pain.* In long-term uncontrolled studies of up to four years' duration, one third of the patients had at least one episode of diarrhea some time during Meclomen therapy.

In approximately 4% of the patients in controlled studies, diarrhea was severe enough to require discontinuation of Meclomen. The occurrence of diarrhea is dose related, generally subsides with dose reduction, and clears with termination of therapy. The incidence of diarrhea in patients with osteoarthritis is generally lower than that reported in patients with rheumatoid arthritis.

Other reactions less frequently reported were pyrosis,* flatulence,* anorexia, constipation, stomatitis, and peptic ulcer. The majority of the patients with peptic ulcer had either a history of ulcer disease or were receiving concomitant antiinflammatory drugs, including corticosteroids which are known to produce peptic ulceration.

Cardiovascular

edema

Integumentary

rash,* urticaria, pruritus

Central Nervous System

headache,* dizziness*

Special Senses

tinnitus

*Incidence between 3% and 9%. Those reactions occurring in 1 to 3% of patients are not marked with an asterisk.

Incidence Less than 1%.

Probably Causally Related

The following adverse reactions were reported less frequently than 1% during controlled clinical trials and through voluntary reports since marketing. The probability of a causal relationship exists between the drug and these adverse reactions.

Gastrointestinal: Bleeding with or without obvious ulcer formation

Renal: Renal failure.

Hematologic: Neutropenia, thrombocytopenic purpura

Dermatologic: Erythema multiforme, Stevens-Johnson syndrome

Incidence Less than 1%

Causal Relationship Unknown

Other reactions have been reported but under conditions where a causal relationship could not be established. However, in these rarely reported events, that possibility cannot be excluded. Therefore, these observations are listed to alert physicians.

Cardiovascular
palpitations
Central Nervous System
malaise, fatigue, paresthesia, insomnia, depression
Special Senses
blurred vision, taste disturbances
Renal
nocturia

Overdosage: Although dosages up to 600 mg/day of Meclomen have been given, no specific information is available on the management of acute massive overdosage. Should accidental overdosage occur, the stomach should be emptied by inducing emesis or by careful gastric lavage, followed by the administration of activated charcoal. Laboratory studies with a related compound indicate that Meclomen should be adsorbed from the gastrointestinal tract by activated charcoal. Vital functions should be monitored and supported. Because meclofenamate and its metabolites are largely in tissue compartments and are strongly bound by plasma proteins, hemodialysis and peritoneal dialysis may be of little value.

Dosage and Administration:
Usual Dosage
For rheumatoid arthritis and osteoarthritis, including acute exacerbations of chronic disease, the dosage is 200 to 400 mg per day, administered in three or four equal doses.
Therapy should be initiated at the lower dosage, then increased as necessary to improve clinical response. The dosage sould be individually adjusted for each patient depending on the severity of the symptoms and the clinical response. The daily dosage should not exceed 400 mg per day. The smallest dosage of Meclomen that yields clinical control should be employed. Although improvement may be seen in some patients in a few days, two to three weeks of treatment may be required to obtain the optimum therapeutic benefit.
After a satisfactory response has been achieved, the dosage should be adjusted as required. A lower dosage may suffice for long-term administration.
If gastrointestinal complaints occur, see WARNINGS and PRECAUTIONS. Meclomen may be administered with meals or with milk. If intolerance occurs, the dosage may need to be reduced. Therapy should be terminated if any severe adverse reactions occur.

How Supplied:
(Capsule 268) Meclomen capsules, each containing meclofenamate sodium monohydrate equivalent to 50 mg meclofenamic acid, are available:
N 0071-0268-24—bottles of 100
N 0071-0268-40—Uni/Use® 100s (10 × 10)
(Capsule 269) Meclomen capsules, each containing meclofenamate sodium monohydrate equivalent to 100 mg meclofenamic acid, are available:
N 0071-0269-24—bottles of 100
N 0071-0269-30—bottles of 500
N 0071-0269-40—Uni/Use 100s (10 x 10)

Storage: Store at room temperature below 30°C (86°F). Protect from moisture and light.

0268G031
121 886900/31

[*Shown in Product Identification Section*]

MILONTIN® ℞
(phensuximide, USP)

Description: Milontin (phensuximide) is an anticonvulsant succinimide, chemically designated as N-methyl-2-phenylsuccinimide.

Action: Phensuximide suppresses the paroxysmal three-cycle-per-second spike and wave activity associated with lapses of consciousness which is common in absence (petit mal) seizures. The frequency of epileptiform attacks is reduced, apparently by depression of the motor cortex and elevation of the threshold of the central nervous system to convulsive stimuli.

Indication: Milontin is indicated for the control of absence (petit mal) seizures.

Contraindication: Phensuximide should not be used in patients with a history of hypersensitivity to succinimides.

Warnings: Blood dyscrasias, including some with fatal outcome, have been reported to be associated with the use of succinimides; therefore, periodic blood counts should be performed.
It has been reported that succinimides have produced morphological and functional changes in animal liver. For this reason, phensuximide should be administered with extreme caution to patients with known liver or renal diseases. Periodic urinalysis and liver function studies are advised for all patients receiving the drug.
Cases of systemic lupus erythematosus have been reported with the use of succinimides. The physician should be alert to this possibility.

Usage in pregnancy: The effects of Milontin in human pregnancy and nursing infants are unknown.
Recent reports suggest an association between the use of anticonvulsant drugs by women with epilepsy and an elevated incidence of birth defects in children born to these women. Data is more extensive with respect to phenytoin and phenobarbital, but these are also the most commonly prescribed anticonvulsants; less systematic or anecdotal reports suggest a possible similar association with the use of all known anticonvulsant drugs.
The reports suggesting an elevated incidence of birth defects in children of drug-treated epileptic women cannot be regarded as adequate to prove a definite cause-and-effect relationship. There are intrinsic methodologic problems in obtaining adequate data on drug teratogenicity in humans; the possibility also exists that other factors, eg, genetic factors or the epileptic condition itself, may be more important than drug therapy in leading to birth defects. The great majority of mothers on anticonvulsant medication deliver normal infants. It is important to note that anticonvulsant drugs should not be discontinued in patients in whom the drug is administered to prevent major seizures because of the strong possibility of precipitating status epilepticus with attendant hypoxia and threat to life. In individual cases where the severity and frequency of the seizure disorder are such that the removal of medication does not pose a serious threat to the patient, discontinuation of the drug may be considered prior to and during pregnancy, although it cannot be said with any confidence that even minor seizures do not pose some hazard to the developing embryo or fetus.
The prescribing physician will wish to weigh these considerations in treating or counseling epileptic women of childbearing potential.

Hazardous activities: Phensuximide may impair the mental and/or physical abilities required for the performance of potentially hazardous tasks, such as driving a motor vehicle or other such activity requiring alertness; therefore, the patient should be cautioned accordingly.

Precautions: Phensuximide, when used alone in mixed types of epilepsy, may increase the frequency of grand mal seizures in some patients.
As with other anticonvulsants, it is important to proceed slowly when increasing or decreasing dosage, as well as when adding or eliminating other medication. Abrupt withdrawal of anticonvulsant medication may precipitate absence (petit mal) status.

Adverse Reactions:
Gastrointestinal System: Gastrointestinal symptoms, such as nausea, vomiting, and anorexia, occur frequently, but may be the result of overdosage.
Nervous System: Neurologic and sensory reactions reported during therapy with phensuximide have included drowsiness, dizziness, ataxia, headache, dreamlike state, and lethargy. Side effects, such as drowsiness and dizziness, may be relieved by a reduction in total dosage.
Integumentary System: Dermatologic manifestations reported to be associated with the administration of phensuximide have included pruritus, skin eruptions, erythema multiforme, and erythematous rashes.
Genitourinary System: Genitourinary complications which have been reported include urinary frequency, renal damage, and hematuria.
Hemopoietic System: Hemopoietic complications associated with the administration of phensuximide include granulocytopenia, transient leukopenia, and pancytopenia.
Other: Miscellaneous reactions reported have been alopecia and muscular weakness.

Dosage and Administration: Milontin (phensuximide capsules, USP) is administered by the oral route in doses of 500 mg to 1 g two or three times daily. As with other anticonvulsant medication, the dosage should be adjusted to suit individual requirements. The total dosage, irrespective of age, may, therefore, vary between 1 and 3 g per day, the average being 1.5 g.
Milontin may be administered in combination with other anticonvulsants when other forms of epilepsy coexist with absence (petit mal).

How Supplied:
N 0071-0393-24 (Kapseal® 393)—Milontin Kapseals, each containing 0.5 g phensuximide; bottles of 100.

0393G010

[*Shown in Product Identification Section*]

MYADEC®

Each tablet represents:		% of US Recommended Daily Allowances (US RDA)
Vitamins		
Vitamin A	10,000 IU*	200%
Vitamin D	400 IU	100%
Vitamin E	30 IU	100%
Vitamin C	250 mg	417%
Folic Acid	0.4 mg	100%
Thiamine	10 mg	667%
Riboflavin	10 mg	588%
Niacin†	100 mg	500%
Vitamin B_6	5 mg	250%
Vitamin B_{12}	6 mcg	100%
Pantothenic Acid	20 mg	200%
Minerals		
Iodine	150 mcg	100%
Iron	20 mg	111%
Magnesium	100 mg	25%
Copper	2 mg	100%
Zinc	20 mg	133%
Manganese	1.25 mg	‡

Ingredients: Sodium ascorbate, magnesium oxide, niacinamide, microcrystalline cellulose, ferrous fumarate, zinc sulfate monohydrate, ascorbic acid, gelatin, hydroxypropyl methylcellulose, vitamin E acetate, polyvinylpyrrolidone, calcium pantothenate, FD and C yellow no 6 lake, silicon dioxide, riboflavin, thiamine mononitrate, polyethylene glycol 3350, magnesium stearate, pyridoxine hydrochloride, cupric sulfate anhydrous, sugar, vitamin A, manganese sulfate monohydrate, titanium dioxide, FD and C blue no 2 lake, FD and C red no 3 lake, ethylcellulose, methylparaben, candelilla

Continued on next page

This product information was prepared in August, 1982. On these and other Parke-Davis Products, information may be obtained by addressing PARKE-DAVIS, Division of Warner-Lambert Company, Morris Plains, New Jersey 07950.

Parke-Davis—Cont.

wax, citric acid anhydrous, hydroxypropyl cellulose, polysorbate 80, folic acid, vanillin, potassium iodide, propylparaben, vitamin D_2, vitamin B_{12}.

* International Units
† Supplied as niacinamide
‡ No US Recommended Daily Allowance (US RDA) has been established for this nutrient.

Actions and Uses: High-potency vitamin supplement with minerals for adults.
Dosage: One tablet daily with a full meal.
How Supplied: N 0071-0335. In bottles of 130 and 250 and unit-dose packages of 100 (10 strips of 10 tablets).

NARDIL® ℞
(phenelzine sulfate tablets, USP)

Description: Nardil (phenelzine sulfate) is a potent inhibitor of monoamine oxidase (MAO). Chemically, it is a hydrazine derivative, phenethylhydrazine sulfate.
Actions: Monoamine oxidase is a complex enzyme system, widely distributed throughout the body. Drugs that inhibit monoamine oxidase in the laboratory are associated with a number of clinical effects. Thus, it is unknown whether MAO inhibition *per se*, other pharmacologic actions, or an interaction of both is responsible for the clinical effects observed. Therefore, the physician should become familiar with all the effects produced by drugs of this class.
Indications: Nardil (phenelzine sulfate) has been found to be effective in depressed patients clinically characterized as "atypical," "nonendogenous," or "neurotic." These patients often have mixed anxiety and depression and phobic or hypochondriacal features. There is less conclusive evidence of its usefulness with severely depressed patients with endogenous features.
Nardil should rarely be the first antidepressant drug used. Rather, it is more suitable for use with patients who have failed to respond to the drugs more commonly used for these conditions.
Nardil has had considerable use in combination with dibenzazepine derivatives in treatment-resistant patients without a significant incidence of serious side effects.
Contraindications: Nardil (phenelzine sulfate) is contraindicated in patients with known sensitivity to the drug, pheochromocytoma, congestive heart failure, a history of liver disease, or abnormal liver function tests. (See WARNINGS for other conditions.)
The potentiation of sympathomimetic substances by MAO inhibitors may result in hypertensive crises (See WARNINGS); therefore, patients taking Nardil (phenelzine sulfate) should not be given **sympathomimetic drugs** (including methyl dopa, L-dopa, dopamine, and tryptamine-containing substances as well as epinephrine and norepinephrine); or foods with a high concentration of tryptamine-containing substances or **tyramine** (pods of broad beans, aged cheeses, beer, wines, pickled herring, yogurt, liver, yeast extract). Excessive amounts of caffeine and chocolate can also cause hypertensive reactions.
Nardil (phenelzine sulfate) should not be used in combination with some CNS depressants such as alcohol and narcotics (e.g., meperidine); death has been reported in patients who have received meperidine and Nardil concomitantly. Nardil should not be administered together with or in rapid succession to other MAO inhibitors because HYPERTENSIVE CRISES and convulsive seizures, fever, marked sweating, excitation, delirium, tremor, coma, and circulatory collapse may occur.

List of MAO Inhibitors

Generic Name	Trademark
pargyline hydrochloride	Eutonyl® (Abbott Laboratories)
pargyline hydrochloride and methyclothiazide	Eutron® (Abbott Laboratories)
furazolidone	Furoxone® (Eaton Laboratories)
isocarboxazid	Marplan® (Roche Laboratories)
procarbazine	Matulane® (Roche)
tranylcypromine	Parnate® (Smith Kline & French Laboratories)

Patients taking Nardil (phenelzine sulfate) should not undergo elective surgery requiring general anesthesia. Also, they should not be given cocaine or local anesthesia containing sympathomimetic vasoconstrictors. The possible combined hypotensive effects of Nardil and spinal anesthesia should be kept in mind. Nardil (phenelzine sulfate) should be discontinued at least 10 days prior to elective surgery.
IMPORTANT
Warnings: The most serious reactions to Nardil (phenelzine sulfate) involve changes in blood pressure.
Hypertensive Crises: The most important reaction associated with Nardil (phenelzine sulfate) administration is the occurrence of hypertensive crises, which have sometimes been fatal.
These crises are characterized by some or all of the following symptoms: occipital headache which may radiate frontally, palpitation, neck stiffness or soreness, nausea, vomiting, sweating (sometimes with fever and sometimes with cold, clammy skin), dilated pupils, and photophobia. Either tachycardia or bradycardia may be present and can be associated with constricting chest pain.
NOTE: Intracranial bleeding has been reported in association with the increase in blood pressure.
Blood pressure should be observed frequently to detect evidence of any pressor response in all patients receiving Nardil (phenelzine sulfate). Therapy should be discontinued immediately upon the occurrence of palpitation or frequent headaches during therapy.
Recommended treatment in hypertensive crisis: If a hypertensive crisis occurs, Nardil (phenelzine sulfate) should be discontinued immediately and therapy to lower blood pressure should be instituted immediately. On the basis of present evidence, phentolamine is recommended. (The dosage reported for phentolamine is 5 mg intravenously.) Care should be taken to administer this drug slowly in order to avoid producing an excessive hypotensive effect. Fever should be managed by means of external cooling.
Warning to the patient: All patients should be warned against eating foods with high tyramine content (aged cheeses, wines, beer, pickled herring, broad bean pods, yogurt, liver, yeast extract); any high protein food that is aged or has undergone breakdown by putrefaction process to improve flavor is suspect of being able to produce a hypertensive crisis in patients taking MAO inhibitors; against drinking alcoholic beverages and against self-medication with certain proprietary agents such as cold, hay fever or reducing preparations while undergoing Nardil (phenelzine sulfate) therapy. Beverages containing caffeine may be used in moderation.
Patients should be instructed to report promptly the occurrence of headache or other unusual symptoms.
Concomitant Use with Tricyclic (Dibenzazepine) Derivatives
If the decision is made to administer Nardil concurrently with other antidepressant drugs, or within less than 10 days after discontinuation of antidepressant therapy, the patient should be cautioned by the physician regarding the possibility of adverse drug interaction.

List of Tricyclic (dibenzazepine derivative) Drugs

Generic Name	Trademark
nortriptyline hydrochloride	Aventyl® (Eli Lilly & Co.)
amitriptyline hydrochloride	Amitril® (Parke-Davis)
amitriptyline hydrochloride	Elavil® (Merck Sharp & Dohme)
amitriptyline hydrochloride	Endep® (Roche Laboratories)
perphenazine & amitriptyline hydrochloride	Etrafon® (Schering Corporation)
perphenazine & amitriptyline hydrochloride	Triavil® (Merck Sharp & Dohme)
desipramine hydrochloride	Norpramin® (Merrell-National)
desipramine hydrochloride	Pertofrane® (USV)
imipramine hydrochloride	Tofranil® (Geigy)
doxepin	Adapin® (Pennwalt)
doxepin	Sinequan® (Pfizer)

Nardil (phenelzine sulfate) should be used with caution in combination with antihypertensive drugs, including thiazide diuretics, since hypotension may result. MAO inhibitors including Nardil are contraindicated in patients receiving guanethidine.
Use in Pregnancy: The safe use of Nardil (phenelzine sulfate) during pregnancy or lactation has not been established. The potential benefit of this drug, if used during pregnancy, lactation, or in women of childbearing age, should be weighed against the possible hazard to the mother or fetus.
Doses of Nardil in pregnant mice well exceeding the maximum recommended human dose have caused a significant decrease in the number of viable offspring per mouse. In addition, the growth of young dogs and rats has been retarded by doses exceeding the maximum human dose.
Use in Children: Nardil (phenelzine sulfate) is not recommended for patients under 16 years of age since there are no controlled studies of safety in this age group.
Nardil, as with other hydrazine derivatives, has been reported to induce pulmonary and vascular tumors in an uncontrolled lifetime study in mice.
Precautions: In depressed patients, the possibility of suicide should always be considered and adequate precautions taken. It is recommended that careful observations of patients undergoing Nardil (phenelzine sulfate) treatment be maintained until control of depression is achieved. If necessary, additional measures (ECT, hospitalization, etc.) should be instituted.
All patients undergoing treatment with Nardil should be closely followed for symptoms of postural hypotension. Hypotensive side effects have occurred in hypertensive as well as normal and hypotensive patients. Blood pressure usually returns to pretreatment levels rapidly when the drug is discontinued or the dosage is reduced.
Because the effect of Nardil (phenelzine sulfate) on the convulsive threshold may be variable, adequate precautions should be taken when treating epileptic patients.
Of the more severe side effects that have been reported with any consistency, hypomania has been the most common. This reaction has been largely limited to patients in whom disorders characterized by hyperkinetic symptoms coexist with, but are obscured by, depressive affect; hypomania usually appeared as depression improved. If agitation is present, it may be increased with Nardil (phenelzine sulfate). Hypomania and agitation have also been reported at

higher than recommended doses, or following long-term therapy.
Nardil may cause excessive stimulation in schizophrenic patients; in manic-depressive states it may result in a swing from a depressive to a manic phase.
MAO inhibitors, including Nardil (phenelzine sulfate), potentiate hexobarbital hypnosis in animals. Therefore, barbiturates should be given at a reduced dose with Nardil.
MAO inhibitors inhibit the destruction of serotonin and norepinephrine, which are believed to be released from tissue stores by rauwolfia alkaloids. Accordingly, caution should be exercised when rauwolfia is used concomitantly with an MAO inhibitor, including Nardil (phenelzine sulfate).
There is conflicting evidence as to whether or not MAO inhibitors affect glucose metabolism or potentiate hypoglycemic agents. This should be kept in mind if Nardil is administered in diabetics.
Adverse Reactions: Nardil (phenelzine sulfate) is a potent inhibitor of monoamine oxidase. Because this enzyme is widely distributed throughout the body, diverse pharmacologic effects can be expected to occur. When they occur, such effects tend to be mild or moderate in severity (see below), often subside as treatment continues, and can be minimized by adjusting dosage; rarely is it necessary to institute counteracting measures or to discontinue Nardil. Common side effects include dizziness, constipation, dry mouth, postural hypotension, drowsiness, weakness and fatigue, edema, gastrointestinal disturbances, tremors, twitching, and hyperreflexia.
Less common mild to moderate side effects, some of which have been reported in a single patient or by a single physician, include blurred vision, glaucoma, sweating, skin rash, jitteriness, palilalia, urinary retention, euphoria, nystagmus, sexual disturbances and hypernatremia.
Although reported less frequently, and sometimes only once, additional severe side effects have included ataxia, shock-like coma, edema of the glottis, transient respiratory and cardiovascular depression following ECT, leukopenia, toxic delirium, reversible jaundice, manic reaction, convulsions, acute anxiety reaction and precipitation of schizophrenia. To date, fatal progressive necrotizing hepatocellular damage has been reported in a very few patients.
Dosage and Administration: *Initial dose*—the usual starting dose of Nardil (phenelzine sulfate) is one tablet (15 mg) three times a day.
Early phase treatment: dosage should be increased to at least 60 mg per day at a fairly rapid pace consistent with patient tolerance. It may be necessary to increase dosage up to 90 mg per day to obtain sufficient MAO inhibition. Many patients do not show a clinical response until treatment at 60 mg has been continued for at least 4 weeks.
Maintenance dose—after maximum benefit from Nardil is achieved, dosage should be reduced slowly over several weeks. Maintenance dose may be as low as 1 tablet, 15 mg, a day or every other day, and should be continued for as long as is required.
Overdosage: Accidental or intentional overdosage with any medication is possible and may be somewhat more common in patients who are depressed. Mild overdoses of Nardil (phenelzine sulfate) are characterized by the appearance of drowsiness, followed by dizziness, ataxia, and irritability. With the usual supportive measures and no specific treatment, complete recovery from mild overdoses usually occurs within 3 to 4 days.
There are no data on the average lethal dose in man.
In severe overdosage of Nardil the initial manifestation is faintness, with hypotension and, occasionally, precordial pain and intense headache. Should hypotension require the use of vasopressors it should be remembered that they are potentiated by Nardil (phenelzine sulfate). Hyperactivity and marked agitation may occur. The skin may be cool and clammy with profuse perspiration; coma, seizures, and signs of peripheral circulatory collapse may also occur. In some cases trismus and opisthotonos may be observed, the pulse may become fast and irregular, and respiration may become shallow. Treatment is largely symptomatic and may vary from patient to patient. Measures generally recommended to counteract overdosage of MAO inhibitors should be followed; mainly, these include bed rest, maintenance of hydration and electrolyte balance, avoidance of CNS stimulants, and, when necessary, use of an intravenous phenothiazine.
How Supplied: Tablets—each orange-coated tablet bears the P-D 270 monogram and contains phenelzine sulfate equivalent to 15 mg of phenelzine base; bottles of 100 (N 0071-0270-24).
Store Between 15° and 30°C (59° and 86°F).
[*Shown in Product Identification Section*]
0270 G 020

NATABEC® KAPSEALS®

Each capsule represents:

Vitamins	
Vitamin A	4,000 IU*
Vitamin D	400 IU
Vitamin C (ascorbic acid)	50 mg
Thiamine (vitamin B_1)	3 mg
Riboflavin (vitamin B_2)	2.0 mg
Nicotinamide +	10 mg
Vitamin B_6	3 mg
Vitamin B_{12}	5 mcg
Minerals	
Precipitated Calcium Carbonate	600 mg
Dried Ferrous Sulfate	150 mg

*IU = International Units
+Supplied as niacinamide
Action and Uses: A multivitamin and mineral supplement for use during pregnancy and lactation
Dosage: One capsule daily, or as directed by physician
How Supplied: N 0071-0390-24. In bottles of 100, Parcode® 390
The color combination of the banded capsule is a Warner-Lambert trademark.
[*Shown in Product Identification Section*]

NATABEC Rx® KAPSEALS® ℞

Vitamin and Mineral Formula Containing Folic Acid

Each Kapseal Represents:

Vitamin A (acetate)	4,000 units
Vitamin D (ergocalciferol)	400 units
Vitamin C (ascorbic acid)	50 mg
Vitamin B_1 (thiamine mononitrate)	3 mg
Vitamin B_2 (riboflavin)	2 mg
Vitamin B_6 (pyridoxine hydrochloride)	3 mg
Vitamin B_{12} (cyanocobalamin) crystalline	5 mcg
Nicotinamide (niacinamide)	10 mg
Folic acid	1 mg
Calcium carbonate, precipitated	600 mg
Ferrous sulfate*	150 mg

* Supplied as dried ferrous sulfate equivalent to the labeled amount of ferrous sulfate.
Action and Uses: Vitamin and mineral formula containing 1 mg folic acid for use during pregnancy and lactation
Caution—Folic acid in doses above 0.1 mg daily may obscure pernicious anemia in that hematologic remission can occur while neurological manifestations remain progressive.
Dosage: One capsule daily or as directed by the physician.
How Supplied: N 0071-0547-24—bottles of 100.
The pink band on blue capsule is a Warner-Lambert trademark registered in the US Patent Office.
[*Shown in Product Identification Section*]

NATAFORT® FILMSEAL® ℞

Each tablet represents:

Vitamin A (acetate)	6,000 IU*
Vitamin D (ergocalciferol)	400 IU
Vitamin C (ascorbic acid)	120 mg
Thiamine (vitamin B_1) (thiamine mononitrate)	3 mg
Riboflavin (vitamin B_2)(riboflavin)	2 mg
Vitamin B_6 (pyridoxine HCl)	15 mg
Vitamin B_{12} (cyanocobalamin) crystalline	6 mcg
Folic acid	1 mg
Nicotinamide (niacinamide)	20 mg
Vitamin E (*dl* alpha tocopheryl acetate)	30 IU
Calcium†	350 mg
Iodine†	0.15 mg
Iron†	65 mg
Magnesium†	100 mg
Zinc†	25 mg
Docusate sodium	50 mg

* IU = International Units
† The minerals are supplied as calcium carbonate, magnesium oxide, potassium iodide, ferrous fumarate, and zinc oxide.
Indications: Comprehensive prenatal vitamin and mineral formula including 1 mg of folic acid to prevent megaloblastic anemia of pregnancy.
Caution—Folic acid in doses above 0.1 mg daily may obscure pernicious anemia in that hematologic remission can occur while neurological manifestations remain progessive.
Usual Dosage: One tablet daily.
How Supplied: N 0071-0212-24 bottles of 100.

NITROSTAT® ℞

(nitroglycerin tablets, USP)

Description: Nitrostat is a stabilized sublingual nitroglycerin tablet manufactured by a patented process* which prevents the migration of nitroglycerin by adding the nonvolatile fixing agent, polyethylene glycol 4000. This stabilized formulation has been shown to be more stable and more uniform than conventional molded tablets.
Action: Nitroglycerin relaxes smooth muscles. This relaxation produces a vasodilatory effect principally on the systemic venous system with some effect on the arterioles. The mechanism of action for relieving anginal episodes is related to this vasodilatory effect.
Nitroglycerin is rapidly absorbed following sublingual administration. Its onset of action is approximately one to three minutes. Significant pharmacologic effects are present for 30 to 60 minutes following administration by the above route.
Indications: Nitroglycerin is indicated for the prophylaxis, treatment and management of patients with angina pectoris.
Contraindications: Sublingual nitroglycerin therapy is contraindicated in patients with early myocardial infarction, severe anemia, increased intracranial pressure, and

Continued on next page

This product information was prepared in August, 1982. On these and other Parke-Davis Products, information may be obtained by addressing PARKE-DAVIS, Division of Warner-Lambert Company, Morris Plains, New Jersey 07950.

Parke-Davis—Cont.

those with a known hypersensitivity to nitroglycerin.

Precautions: Only the smallest dose required for effective relief of the acute anginal attack should be used. Excessive use may lead to the development of tolerance. Nitrostat tablets are intended for sublingual or buccal administration and should not be swallowed. The drug should be discontinued if blurring of vision or drying of the mouth occurs. Excessive dosage of nitroglycerin may produce severe headaches.

Adverse Reactions: Transient headache may occur immediately after use. Vertigo, weakness, palpitation, and other manifestations of postural hypotension may develop occasionally, particularly in erect, immobile patients. Syncope due to nitrate vasodilation has been reported. Alcohol may accentuate the cerebral ischemia symptoms.

Method of Administration: One tablet should be dissolved under the tongue or in the buccal pouch at the first sign of an acute anginal attack. The dose may be repeated approximately every five minutes until relief is obtained. Nitrostat may be used prophylactically five to ten minutes prior to engaging in activities which might precipitate an acute attack.

How Supplied: Nitrostat is supplied in four strengths in bottles containing 100 tablets each, with color-coded labels, and in color-coded Patient Convenience Packages of four bottles of 25 tablets each.

N 0071-0568—0.15 mg (1/400 grain)
N 0071-0569—0.3 mg (1/200 grain)
N 0071-0570—0.4 mg (1/150 grain)
N 0071-0571—0.6 mg (1/100 grain)
AHFS 24:12 **0568 G 060 (4-80)**

[*Shown in Product Identification Section*]

NITROSTAT® IV ℞
(Nitroglycerin for Infusion)

NOT FOR DIRECT INTRAVENOUS INJECTION. NITROSTAT IV IS A CONCENTRATED, POTENT DRUG WHICH MUST BE DILUTED IN DEXTROSE (5%) INJECTION, USP OR SODIUM CHLORIDE (0.9%) INJECTION, USP PRIOR TO ITS INFUSION. THE CONTAINER AND ADMINISTRATION SET USED FOR INFUSION MAY AFFECT THE AMOUNT OF INTRAVENOUS NITROGLYCERIN DELIVERED TO THE PATIENT. (SEE WARNINGS AND DOSAGE AND ADMINISTRATION SECTIONS.)

CAUTION: SEVERAL PREPARATIONS OF NITROGLYCERIN FOR INJECTION ARE AVAILABLE. THEY DIFFER IN CONCENTRATION AND/OR VOLUME PER VIAL. WHEN SWITCHING FROM ONE PRODUCT TO ANOTHER, ATTENTION MUST BE PAID TO THE DILUTION AND DOSAGE AND ADMINISTRATION INSTRUCTIONS.

Description: Nitrostat IV is a clear, practically colorless additive solution for intravenous infusion after dilution. Each milliliter contains 0.8 mg nitroglycerin, with citric acid and sodium citrate as buffers, and 5% alcohol in Water for Injection, USP.

The solution is sterile, nonpyrogenic, and nonexplosive. Intravenous nitroglycerin, an organic nitrate, is a vasodilator. The chemical name for nitroglycerin is 1,2,3 propanetriol trinitrate and its chemical structure is:

$$\begin{array}{c} H_2C-O-NO_2 \\ | \\ HC-O-NO_2 \\ | \\ H_2C-O-NO_2 \end{array}$$

Clinical Pharmacology: Relaxation of vascular smooth muscle is the principal pharmacologic action of intravenous nitroglycerin. Although venous effects predominate, nitroglycerin produces, in a dose-related manner, dilation of both arterial and venous beds. Dilation of the postcapillary vessels, including large veins, promotes peripheral pooling of blood and decreases venous return to the heart, reducing left ventricular end-diastolic pressure (preload). Arteriolar relaxation reduces systemic vascular resistance and arterial pressure (afterload). Myocardial oxygen consumption or demand (as measured by the pressure-rate product, tension-time index and stroke-work index) is decreased by both the arterial and venous effects of nitroglycerin, and a more favorable supply-demand ratio can be achieved.

Therapeutic doses of intravenous nitroglycerin reduce systolic, diastolic and mean arterial blood pressure. Effective coronary perfusion pressure is usually maintained, but can be compromised if blood pressure falls excessively or increased heart rate decreases diastolic filling time.

Elevated central venous and pulmonary capillary wedge pressures, pulmonary vascular resistance and systemic vascular resistance are also reduced by nitroglycerin therapy. Heart rate is usually slightly increased, presumably a reflex response to the fall in blood pressure. Cardiac index may be increased, decreased, or unchanged. Patients with elevated left ventricular filling pressure and systemic vascular resistance values in conjunction with a depressed cardiac index are likely to experience an improvement in cardiac index. On the other hand, when filling pressures and cardiac index are normal, cardiac index may be slightly reduced by intravenous nitroglycerin.

Nitroglycerin is widely distributed in the body with an apparent volume of distribution of approximately 200 liters in adult male subjects, and is rapidly metabolized to dinitrates and mononitrates, with a short half-life, estimated at 1 to 4 minutes. This results in a low plasma concentration after intravenous infusion. At plasma concentrations of between 50 and 500 ng/ml, the binding of nitroglycerin to plasma proteins is approximately 60%, while that of 1,2 dinitroglycerin and 1,3 dinitroglycerin is 60% and 30% respectively. The activity and half-life of 1,2 dinitroglycerin and 1,3 dinitroglycerin are not well characterized. The mononitrate is not active.

Indications and Usage:

Nitrostat IV is indicated for:

1. *Control of blood pressure in perioperative hypertension,* ie, hypertension associated with surgical procedures, especially cardiovascular procedures, such as the hypertension seen during intratracheal intubation, anesthesia, skin incision, sternotomy, cardiac bypass, and in the immediate postsurgical period.
2. *Congestive Heart Failure Associated with Acute Myocardial Infarction.*
3. *Treatment of Angina Pectoris* in patients who have not responded to recommended doses of organic nitrates and/or a beta blocker.
4. *Production of controlled hypotension during surgical procedures.*

Contraindications:

Nitrostat IV should not be administered to individuals with:

1. A known hypersensitivity to nitroglycerin or a known idiosyncratic reaction to organic nitrates.
2. Hypotension or uncorrected hypovolemia, as the use of Nitrostat IV in such states could produce severe hypotension or shock.
3. Increased intracranial pressure (eg, head trauma or cerebral hemorrhage).
4. Constrictive pericarditis and pericardial tamponade.

Warnings:

1. Nitroglycerin readily migrates into many plastics. To avoid absorption of nitroglycerin into plastic parenteral solution containers, the dilution and storage of nitroglycerin for intravenous infusion should be made only in glass parenteral solution bottles.
2. Some filters also absorb nitroglycerin; they should be avoided if possible.
3. Forty to 80% of the total amount of nitroglycerin in the final diluted solution for infusion is absorbed by the polyvinyl chloride (PVC) tubing of the intravenous administration sets currently in general use. The higher rates of absorption occur when flow rates are low, nitroglycerin concentrations are high, and tubing is long. Although the rate of loss is highest during the early phase of administration (when flow rates are lowest), the loss is neither constant nor self-limiting; consequently no simple calculation or correction can be performed to convert the theoretical infusion rate (based on the concentration of the infusion solution) to the actual delivery rate.

Because of this problem, Parke-Davis, Division of Warner-Lambert Company has developed a nonabsorbing infusion set, Nitrostat IV intravenous infusion set, in which the loss of nitroglycerin is minimal (less than 5%). The Nitrostat IV intravenous infusion set or a similar infusion set is recommended for infusions of intravenous nitroglycerin.

Dosage instructions must be followed with care. It should be noted that when these infusion sets are used, the calculated dose will be delivered to the patient because the loss of nitroglycerin due to absorption in standard PVC tubing will be kept to a minimum. Note that the dosages commonly used in published studies utilized general-use PVC infusion sets and recommended doses based on this experience are too high if the new infusion sets are used.

Precautions: Nitrostat IV should be used with caution in patients who have severe hepatic or renal disease.

Excessive hypotension, especially for prolonged periods of time, must be avoided because of possible deleterious effects on the brain, heart, liver, and kidney from poor perfusion and the attendant risk of ischemia, thrombosis, and altered function of these organs. Paradoxical bradycardia and increased angina pectoris may accompany nitroglycerin-induced hypotension. Patients with normal or low pulmonary capillary wedge pressure are especially sensitive to the hypotensive effects of intravenous nitroglycerin. If pulmonary capillary wedge pressure is being monitored, it will be noted that a fall in wedge pressure precedes the onset of arterial hypotension, and the pulmonary capillary wedge pressure is thus a useful guide to safe titration of the drug.

Carcinogenesis, Mutagenesis, Impairment of Fertility:

No long-term studies in animals were performed to evaluate the carcinogenic potential of nitroglycerin.

Pregnancy:

Category C: Animal reproduction studies have not been conducted with nitroglycerin. It is also not known whether nitroglycerin can cause fetal harm when administered to a pregnant woman or can affect reproduction capacity. Nitroglycerin should be given to a pregnant woman only if clearly needed.

Nursing Mother:

It is not known whether nitroglycerin is excreted in human milk. Because many drugs are excreted in human milk, caution should be exercised when intravenous nitroglycerin is administered to a nursing woman.

Pediatric Use:

The safety and effectiveness of nitroglycerin in children have not been established.

Adverse Reactions: The most frequent adverse reaction in patients treated with nitroglycerin is headache, which occurs in approximately 2% of patients. Other adverse reactions occurring in less than 1% of patients are the following: tachycardia, nausea, vomiting, apprehension, restlessness, muscle twitching,

retrosternal discomfort, palpitations, dizziness and abdominal pain.
The following additional adverse reactions have been reported with the oral and/or topical use of nitroglycerin: cutaneous flushing, weakness, and occasionally drug rash or exfoliative dermatitis.

Overdosage: Accidental overdosage of nitroglycerin may result in severe hypotension and reflex tachycardia which can be treated by elevating the legs and decreasing or temporarily terminating the infusion until the patient's condition stabilizes. Since the duration of the hemodynamic effects following nitroglycerin administration is quite short, additional corrective measures are usually not required. However, if further therapy is indicated, administration of an intravenous alpha adrenergic agonist (eg, methoxamine or phenylephrine) should be considered.

Dosage and Administration:

NOT FOR DIRECT INTRAVENOUS INJECTION
NITROSTAT IV IS A CONCENTRATED, POTENT DRUG WHICH MUST BE DILUTED IN DEXTROSE (5%) INJECTION, USP OR SODIUM CHLORIDE (0.9%) INJECTION, USP PRIOR TO ITS INFUSION.
NITROSTAT IV SHOULD NOT BE ADMIXED WITH OTHER DRUGS.

Dilution: It is important to consider the fluid requirements of the patient as well as the expected duration of infusion in selecting the appropriate dilution of nitroglycerin.
Solution Preparation for an Infusion Pump (60 microdrops = 1 ml)

Aseptically transfer 10 ml (8 mg nitroglycerin) of Nitrostat IV into a *glass,* IV bottle containing 250 ml of 5% Dextrose Injection, USP or 0.9% Sodium Chloride Injection, USP and mix well. The resultant solution will contain approximately 30 mcg/ml of nitroglycerin and is stable for at least 96 hours at controlled room temperature (15° to 30° C) or under refrigeration.

RATE OF ADMINISTRATION
(microdrops per minute or milliliters per hour)

Desired Dose (mcg/min)	10 ml in 250 ml = 30 mcg/ml (approx) Microdrops Per Minute	ml/hour
5	10	10
10	20	20
15	30	30
20	40	40
30	60	60
40	80	80
50	100	100

The tables below contain dosage information if a higher concentration of nitroglycerin or a longer duration of infusion is desired. Aseptically transfer the required volume from the ampoules to 250 ml of either 5% Dextrose Injection, USP or 0.9% Sodium Chloride Injection, USP.

If the concentration is adjusted, it is imperative to flush or replace the Nitrostat IV infusion set before a new concentration is utilized. The dead space of the set is approximately 15 ml and, depending on the flow rate, it could take from 9 minutes to 3 hours for the new concentration to reach the patient if the set were not flushed or replaced.

RATE OF ADMINISTRATION
(microdrops per minute or milliliters per hour)

Desired Dose (mcg/min)	20 ml in 250 ml = 60 mcg/ml (approx) Microdrops Per Minute	ml/hour
5	5	5
10	10	10
15	15	15
20	20	20
30	30	30
40	40	40
50	50	50
60	60	60
80	80	80
100	100	100

Desired Dose (mcg/min)	30 ml in 250 ml = 85 mcg/ml (approx) Microdrops Per Minute	ml/hour
5	3	3.529
10	7	7.058
15	10	10.588
20	14	14.117
30	21	21.176
40	28	28.235
50	35	35.294
60	42	42.352
80	56	56.47
100	70	70.588

Dosage: *IMPORTANT NOTICE:* Dosage is affected by the type of container used as well as the type of infusion set used (See Warnings). Although the usual starting adult dose range reported in clinical studies was 25 mcg/min or more, those studies used *PVC TUBING. The use of nonabsorbing tubing will result in the need to use reduced doses.*
The recommended dosage when using the nonabsorbing Nitrostat IV Intravenous Infusion Set should initially be 5 mcg/min delivered through an infusion pump capable of exact and constant delivery of the drug. Subsequent titration must be adjusted to the clinical situation, with dose increments becoming more cautious as partial response is seen. Initial titration should be 5 mcg/min increments, with increases every 3 to 5 minutes until some response is noted. If no response is seen at 20 mcg/min, increments of 10 and later 20 mcg/min can be used. Once a partial blood pressure response is observed, the dose increase should be reduced and the interval between increments should be lengthened. Patients with normal or low left ventricular filling pressure or pulmonary capillary wedge pressure (eg, angina patients without other complications) may be hypersensitive to the effects of nitroglycerin and may respond fully to doses as small as 5 mcg/min. These patients require especially careful titration and monitoring.
There is no fixed optimum dose of nitroglycerin. Due to variations in the responsiveness of individual patients to the drug, each patient must be titrated to the desired level of hemodynamic function. Therefore, continuous monitoring of physiologic parameters (blood pressure and heart rate in all patients, other measurements such as pulmonary capillary wedge pressure, as appropriate) MUST BE PERFORMED to achieve the correct dose. Adequate systemic blood pressure and coronary perfusion pressure must be maintained.

Directions For Preparing Nitrostat IV Infusion Set:

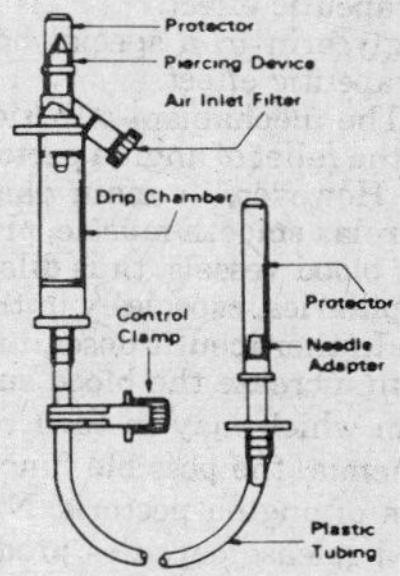

Caution—The fluid path and areas under the protectors of the intravenous infusion set are sterile. Do not use if damaged or if end protectors are not in place.

1. Position control clamp 6 to 8 inches from the needle adapter end of set, then close clamp. (To close clamp, rotate screw stem clockwise.)
2. With IV solution bottle in the upright position,
   a) remove plastic protector from the piercing device,
   b) THRUST the piercing device STRAIGHT DOWN through the CENTER of the target area in the rubber stopper (push straight down, do not twist).
   c) squeeze drip chamber and hold.
3. Invert the bottle and suspend from suitable stand.
4. Release pressure from drip chamber.
5. Remove needle adapter protector by pulling straight off (do not twist off).
If required, place needle on needle adapter. Hold this end of the tubing above the level of the nitroglycerin solution in the bottle. Loosen the control clamp and allow the solution to run into and to fill the tubing and needle. Displace the air in the entire injection set by raising or lowering the intravenous needle end of tubing until all the air bubbles are expelled.
(NOTE: Drip chamber should not be completely filled.)
6. Attach the infusion set to a suitable mechanical infusion control device.
7. Tighten control clamp and proceed with venipuncture or connect to needle.
8. Adjust infusion control device for precise measurement of flow rate.

How Supplied:
N 0071-4572-35 Nitrostat IV Infusion Kit containing one 10-ml ampoule of Nitrostat IV, 8 mg (0.8 mg/ml) and one disposable intravenous infusion set.
N 0071-4572-10 Carton of 10 ×10-ml ampoules of Nitrostat IV.
Store at controlled room temperature 15°–30° C (59°–86° F).

4572G020

NITROSTAT® SR Capsules ℞
(Nitroglycerin Capsules)
Sustained Release

Description: Each Nitrostat SR capsule contains:
2.5 mg nitroglycerin in a special base for prolonged therapeutic effect.

Continued on next page

This product information was prepared in August, 1982. On these and other Parke-Davis Products, information may be obtained by addressing PARKE-DAVIS, Division of Warner-Lambert Company, Morris Plains, New Jersey 07950.

Parke-Davis—Cont.

6.5 mg nitroglycerin in a special base for prolonged therapeutic effect.
9 mg nitroglycerin in a special base for prolonged therapeutic effect.
Actions: The mechanism of action of nitroglycerin in the relief of angina pectoris is not as yet known. However, its main pharmacologic action is to relax smooth muscle, principally in the smaller blood vessels, thus dilating arterioles and capillaries, especially in the coronary circulation. In therapeutic doses, nitroglycerin is thought to increase the blood supply to the myocardium which may in turn relieve myocardial ischemia, the possible functional basis for the pain of angina pectoris. Nitroglycerin in sustained release capsules produces a prolonged action for 8 to 12 hours.

Indication
Based on a review of this drug by the National Academy of Sciences—National Research Council and/or other information, FDA has classified the indication as follows.
"Possibly" effective: For the management, prophylaxis or treatment of anginal attacks.
Final classification of the less-than-effective indication requires further investigation.

Contraindications: Acute or recent myocardial infarction, severe anemia, closed-angle glaucoma, postural hypotension, increased intracranial pressure and idiosyncrasy to the drug.
Warnings: Capsules must be swallowed. FOR ORAL, NOT SUBLINGUAL USE. Nitrostat SR Capsules are not intended for immediate relief of anginal attacks.

Precautions: Intraocular pressure may be increased; therefore, caution is required in administering to patients with glaucoma. Tolerance to this drug and cross-tolerance to other organic nitrites and nitrates may occur. If blurring of vision, dryness of mouth or lack of benefit occurs, the drug should be discontinued.

Adverse Reactions: Severe and persistent headaches, cutaneous flushing, dizziness and weakness. Occasionally, drug rash or exfoliative dermatitis, and nausea and vomiting may occur; these responses may disappear with a decrease in dosage. Adverse effects are enhanced by ingestion of alcohol, which appears to increase absorption from the gastrointestinal tract.

Dosage and Administration: Administer the smallest effective dose 2 or 3 times daily, at 8- to 12-hour intervals, unless clinical response suggests a different regimen. Discontinue if not effective.

How Supplied:
Nitrostat SR 2.5 mg Capsules are available in bottles of 60 and 100 capsules.
Nitrostat SR 6.5 mg Capsules are available in bottles of 60 and 100 capsules.
Nitrostat SR 9 mg Capsules are available in bottles of 60 capsules.
Storage: Store at a controlled room temperature (59° to 86°F). Dispense only in the original unopened container.

0883G010

NORLESTRIN® 21 1/50 ℞
(Each tablet contains 1 mg norethindrone acetate and 50 mcg ethinyl estradiol.)

NORLESTRIN® 21 2.5/50 ℞
(Each tablet contains 2.5 mg norethindrone acetate and 50 mcg ethinyl estradiol.)

NORLESTRIN® Fe 1/50 ℞
(Each yellow tablet contains 1 mg norethindrone acetate and 50 mcg ethinyl estradiol. Each brown tablet contains 75 mg ferrous fumarate, USP.)

NORLESTRIN® Fe 2.5/50 ℞
(Each pink tablet contains 2.5 mg norethindrone acetate and 50 mcg ethinyl estradiol. Each brown tablet contains 75 mg ferrous fumarate, USP.)

NORLESTRIN® 28 1/50 ℞
(Each yellow tablet contains 1 mg norethindrone acetate and 50 mcg ethinyl estradiol. Each white tablet is inert.)

Each yellow tablet contains: norethindrone acetate (17 alpha-ethinyl-19-nortestosterone acetate), 1 mg; ethinyl estradiol (17 alpha-ethinyl-1,3,5(10)-estratriene-3, 17 beta-diol), 50 mcg.
Each pink tablet contains: norethindrone acetate (17 alpha-ethinyl-19-nortestosterone acetate). 2.5 mg; ethinyl estradiol (17 alpha-ethinyl-1,3,5(10)-estratriene-3, 17 beta-diol), 50 mcg.
Each brown tablet contains 75 mg ferrous fumarate, USP.
Each white tablet is inert.
Description: Norlestrin is a progestogen-estrogen combination.
Norlestrin **Fe** 1/50 and 2.5/50 provides a continuous dosage regimen consisting of 21 oral contraceptive tablets and seven ferrous fumarate tablets. The ferrous fumarate tablets are present to facilitate ease of drug administration via a 28-day regimen and are not intended to serve any therapeutic purpose.
Norlestrin **28** 1/50 provides a continuous dosage regimen consisting of 21 oral contraceptive tablets and 7 inert tablets.
Clinical Pharmacology: Combination oral contraceptives act primarily through the mechanism of gonadotropin suppression due to the estrogenic and progestational activity of the ingredients. Although the primary mechanism of action is inhibition of ovulation, alterations in the genital tract, including changes in the cervical mucus (which increase the difficulty of sperm penetration) and the endometrium (which reduce the likelihood of implantation) may also contribute to contraceptive effectiveness.
Indications and Usage: Norlestrin is indicated for the prevention of pregnancy in women who elect to use oral contraceptives as a method of contraception.
Oral contraceptives are highly effective. The pregnancy rate in women using conventional combination oral contraceptives (containing 35 mcg or more of ethinyl estradiol or 50 mcg or more of mestranol) is generally reported as less than one pregnancy per 100 woman-years of use. Slightly higher rates (somewhat more than 1 pregnancy per 100 woman-years of use) are reported for some combination products containing 35 mcg or less of ethinyl estradiol, and rates on the order of 3 pregnancies per 100 woman-years are reported for the progestogen-only oral contraceptives.
These rates are derived from separate studies conducted by different investigators in several population groups and cannot be compared precisely. Furthermore, pregnancy rates tend to be lower as clinical studies are continued, possibly due to selective retention in the longer studies of those patients who accept the treatment regimen and do not discontinue as a result of adverse reactions, pregnancy, or other reasons.

In clinical trials with Norlestrin 1/50, 1,156 patients completed 25,983 cycles and a total of one pregnancy was reported. This represents a pregnancy rate of 0.05 per 100 woman-years. In clinical trials with Norlestrin 2.5/50, 3,829 patients completed 96,388 cycles and a total of 18 pregnancies were reported. This represents a pregnancy rate of 0.22 per 100 woman-years based upon data that include the cases where patients failed to comply with the dosage regimen. The pregnancy rate in patients who adhered to the dosage regimen was 0.02 per 100 woman-years (two pregnancies in these trials).
Table 1 gives ranges of pregnancy rates reported in the literature[1] for other means of contraception. The efficacy of these means of contraception (except the IUD) depends upon the degree of adherence to the method.
Table 1 Pregnancies per 100 Woman-Years
IUD, less than 1–6; Diaphragm with spermicidal products (creams or jellies), 2–20; Condom, 3–36; Aerosol foams, 2–29; Jellies and creams, 4–36; Periodic abstinence (rhythm) all types, less than 1–47; *1. Calendar method, 14–47; 2. Temperature method, 1–20; 3. Temperature method—intercourse only in post-ovulatory phase, less than 1–7; 4. Mucus method, 1–25;* No contraception, 60–80.
Dose-Related Risk of Thromboembolism from Oral Contraceptives
Two studies have shown a positive association between the dose of estrogens in oral contraceptives and the risk of thromboembolism.[2,3] For this reason, it is prudent and in keeping with good principles of therapeutics to minimize exposure to estrogen. The oral contraceptive product prescribed for any given patient should be that product which contains the least amount of estrogen that is compatible with an acceptable pregnancy rate and patient acceptance. It is recommended that new acceptors of oral contraceptives be started on preparations containing 0.05 mg or less of estrogen.
Contraindications: Oral contraceptives should not be used in women with any of the following conditions.
1. Thrombophlebitis or thromboembolic disorders
2. A past history of deep vein thrombophlebitis or thromboembolic disorders
3. Cerebral vascular or coronary artery disease
4. Known or suspected carcinoma of the breast
5. Known or suspected estrogen-dependent neoplasia
6. Undiagnosed abnormal genital bleeding
7. Known or suspected pregnancy (see Warning No. 5)
8. Benign or malignant liver tumor which developed during the use of oral contraceptives or other estrogen-containing products.
Warnings:

Cigarette smoking increases the risk of serious cardiovascular side effects from oral contraceptive use. This risk increases with age and with heavy smoking (15 or more cigarettes per day) and is quite marked in women over 35 years of age. Women who use oral contraceptives should be strongly advised not to smoke.
The use of oral contraceptives is associated with increased risk of several serious conditions including thromboembolism, stroke, myocardial infarction, hepatic adenoma, gallbladder disease, and hypertension. Practitioners prescribing oral contraceptives should be familiar with the following information relating to these risks.

1. *Thromboembolic Disorders and Other Vascular Problems.* An increased risk of thromboembolic and thrombotic disease associated with the use of oral contraceptives is well established. Three principal studies in Great Britain[4–6] and three in the United States[7–10] have demonstrated an increased risk of fatal

Myocardial infarction

Smoking habits	Women aged 30–39		Women aged 40–44	
	Users	Nonusers	Users	Nonusers
All smokers	10.2	2.6	62.0	15.9
Heavy*	13.0	5.1	78.7	31.3
Light	4.7	0.9	28.6	5.7
Nonsmokers	1.8	1.2	10.7	7.4
Smokers and nonsmokers	5.4	1.9	32.8	11.7

*Heavy smoker: 15 or more cigarettes per day. From Jain, A.K., Studies in Family Planning 8:50, 1977.

and nonfatal venous thromboembolism and stroke, both hemorrhagic and thrombotic. These studies estimate that users of oral contraceptives are 4 to 11 times more likely than nonusers to develop these diseases without evident cause (Table 2).

Cerebrovascular Disorders

In a collaborative American study[9,10] of cerebrovascular disorders in women with and without predisposing causes, it was estimated that the risk of hemorrhagic stroke was 2.0 times greater in users than nonusers and the risk of thrombotic stroke was 4 to 9.5 times greater in users than in nonusers (Table 2).

Table 2

Summary of relative risk of thromboembolic disorders and other vascular problems in oral contraceptive users compared to nonusers

	Relative risk, times greater
Idiopathic thromboembolic disease	4–11
Postsurgery thromboembolic complications	4–6
Thrombotic stroke	4–9.5
Hemorrhagic stroke	2
Myocardial infarction	2–12

Myocardial Infarction

An increased risk of myocardial infarction associated with the use of oral contraceptives has been reported[11–13] confirming a previously suspected association. These studies, conducted in the United Kingdom, found, as expected, that the greater the number of underlying risk factors for coronary artery disease (cigarette smoking, hypertension, hypercholesterolemia, obesity, diabetes, history of preeclamptic toxemia) the higher the risk of developing myocardial infarction, regardless of whether the patient was an oral contraceptive user or not. Oral contraceptives, however, were found to be a clear additional risk factor.

In terms of relative risk, it has been estimated[52] that oral contraceptive users who do not smoke (smoking is considered a major predisposing condition to myocardial infarction) are about twice as likely to have a fatal myocardial infarction as nonusers who do not smoke. Oral contraceptive users who are also smokers have about a 5-fold increased risk of fatal infarction compared to users who do not smoke, but about a 10- to 12-fold increased risk compared to nonusers who do not smoke. Furthermore, the amount of smoking is also an important factor. In determining the importance of these relative risks, however, the baseline rates for various age groups, as shown in Table 3, must be given serious consideration. The importance of other predisposing conditions mentioned above in determining relative and absolute risks has not yet been quantified; it is quite likely that the same synergistic action exists, but perhaps to a lesser extent.

Table 3

Estimated annual mortality rate per 100,000 women from myocardial infarction by use of oral contraceptives, smoking habits, and age (in years)

[See table above].

Risk of Dose

In an analysis of data derived from several national adverse reaction reporting systems,[2] British investigators concluded that the risk of thromboembolism, including coronary thrombosis, is directly related to the dose of estrogen used in oral contraceptives. Preparations containing 100 mcg or more of estrogen were associated with a higher risk of thromboembolism than those containing 50 to 80 mcg of estrogen. Their analysis did suggest, however, that the quantity of estrogen may not be the sole factor involved. This finding has been confirmed in the United States. Careful epidemiological studies to determine the degree of thromboembolic risk associated with progestogen-only oral contraceptives have not been performed. Cases of thromboembolic disease have been reported in women using these products, and they should not be presumed to be free of excess risk.

Estimate of Excess Mortality from Circulatory Diseases

A large prospective study [53] carried out in the U.K. estimated the mortality rate per 100,000 women per year from diseases of the circulatory system for users and nonusers of oral contraceptives according to age, smoking habits, and duration of use. The overall excess death rate annually from circulatory diseases for oral contraceptive users was estimated to be 20 per 100,000 (ages 15 to 34—5/100,000; ages 35 to 44—33/100,000; ages 45 to 49—140/100,000), the risk being concentrated in older women, in those with a long duration of use, and in cigarette smokers. It was not possible, however, to examine the interrelationships of age, smoking, and duration of use, nor to compare the effects of continuous versus intermittent use. Although the study showed a 10-fold increase in death due to circulatory diseases in users for 5 or more years, all of these deaths occurred in women 35 or older. Until larger numbers of women under 35 with continuous use for 5 or more years are available, it is not possible to assess the magnitude of the relative risk for this younger age group.

The available data from a variety of sources have been analyzed[14] to estimate the risk of death associated with various methods of contraception. The estimates of risk of death for each method include the combined risk of the contraceptive method (eg, thromboembolic and thrombotic disease in the case of oral contraceptives) plus the risk attributable to pregnancy or abortion in the event of method failure. This latter risk varies with the effectiveness of the contraceptive method. The findings of this analysis are shown in Figure 1 which follows.[14] The study concluded that the mortality associated with all methods of birth control is low and below that associated with childbirth, with the exception of oral contraceptives in women over 40 who smoke. (The rates given for pill only/smokers for each age group are for smokers as a class. For "heavy" smokers [more than 15 cigarettes a day] the rates given would be about double, for "light" smokers [less than 15 cigarettes a day] about 50 percent.) The lowest mortality is associated with the condom or diaphragm backed up by early abortion.

[See bar graph on next page].

The risk of thromboembolic and thrombotic disease associated with oral contraceptives increases with age after approximately age 30 and, for myocardial infarction, is further increased by hypertension, hypercholesterolemia, obesity, diabetes, or history of preeclamptic toxemia and especially by cigarette smoking.

Based on the data currently available, the following chart gives a gross estimate of the risk of death from circulatory disorders associated with the use of oral contraceptives.

Smoking Habits and Other Predisposing Conditions—Risk Associated with Use of Oral Contraceptives

Age:	Below 30	30–39	40+
Heavy smokers	C	B	A
Light smokers	D	C	B
Nonsmokers (no predisposing conditions)	D	C,D	C
Nonsmokers (other predisposing conditions)	C	C,B	B,A

A—Use associated with very high risk
B—Use associated with high risk
C—Use associated with moderate risk
D—Use associated with low risk

The physician and the patient should be alert to the earliest manifestations of thromboembolic and thrombotic disorders (eg, thrombophlebitis, pulmonary embolism, cerebrovascular insufficiency, coronary occlusion, retinal thrombosis, and mesenteric thrombosis). Should any of these occur or be suspected, the drug should be discontinued immediately.

A four- to six-fold increased risk of postsurgery thromboembolic complications has been reported in oral contraceptive users.[15,16] If feasible, oral contraceptives should be discontinued at least 4 weeks before surgery of a type associated with an increased risk of thromboembolism or prolonged immobilization.

2. *Ocular Lesions.* There have been reports of neuro-ocular lesions, such as optic neuritis or retinal thrombosis, associated with the use of oral contraceptives. Discontinue oral contraceptive medication if there is unexplained, sudden or gradual, partial or complete loss of vision; onset of proptosis or diplopia; papilledema; or retinal vascular lesions and institute appropriate diagnostic and therapeutic measures.

3. *Carcinoma.* Long-term continuous administration of either natural or synthetic estrogen in certain animal species increases the frequency of carcinoma of the breast, cervix, vagina, and liver. Certain synthetic progestogens, none currently contained in oral contraceptives, have been noted to increase the incidence of mammary nodules, benign and malignant, in dogs.

In humans, three case control studies have reported an increased risk of endometrial carcinoma associated with the prolonged use of exogenous estrogen in post-menopausal women.[17–19] One publication[20] reported on the first 21 cases submitted by physicians to a registry of cases of adenocarcinoma of the endometrium in women under 40 on oral contraceptives. Of the cases found in women without predisposing risk factors for adenocarcinoma of the endometrium (eg, irregular bleeding at the time oral contraceptives were first given,

Continued on next page

This product information was prepared in August, 1982. On these and other Parke-Davis Products, information may be obtained by addressing PARKE-DAVIS, Division of Warner-Lambert Company, Morris Plains, New Jersey 07950.

Parke-Davis—Cont.

polycystic ovaries), nearly all occurred in women who had used a sequential oral contraceptive. These products are no longer marketed. No evidence has been reported suggesting an increased risk of endometrial cancer in users of conventional-combination or progestogen-only oral contraceptives.

Several studies[8,21–24] have found no increase in breast cancer in women taking oral contraceptives or estrogens. One study,[25] however, while also noting no overall increased risk of breast cancer in women treated with oral contraceptives, found an excess risk in the subgroups of oral contraceptive users with documented benign breast disease. A reduced occurrence of benign breast tumors in users of oral contraceptives has been well-documented.[8,21,25–27]

In summary, there is at present no confirmed evidence from human studies of an increased risk of cancer associated with oral contraceptives. Close clinical surveillance of all women taking oral contraceptives is, nevertheless, essential. In all cases of undiagnosed persistent or recurrent abnormal vaginal bleeding, appropriate diagnostic measures should be taken to rule out malignancy. Women with a strong family history of breast cancer or who have breast nodules, fibrocystic disease, or abnormal mammograms, should be monitored with particular care if they elect to use oral contraceptives instead of other methods of contraception.

4. *Hepatic Tumors.* Benign hepatic adenomas have been found to be associated with the use of oral contraceptives.[28–30,46] One study[46] showed that oral contraceptive formulations with high hormonal potency were associated with a higher risk than lower potency formulations. Although benign, hepatic adenomas may rupture and may cause death through intraabdominal hemorrhage. This has been reported in short-term as well as long-term users of oral contraceptives. Two studies relate risk with duration of use of the contraceptive, the risk being much greater after 4 or more years of oral contraceptive use.[30,46] While hepatic adenoma is a rare lesion, it should be considered in women presenting abdominal pain and tenderness, abdominal mass or shock.

A few cases of hepatocellular carcinoma have been reported in women taking oral contraceptives. The relationship of these drugs to this type of malignancy is not known at this time.

5. *Use in or Immediately Preceding Pregnancy, Birth Defects in Offspring, and Malignancy in Female Offspring.* The use of female sex hormones—both estrogenic and progestational agents—during early pregnancy may seriously damage the offspring. It has been shown that females exposed *in utero* to diethylstilbestrol, a nonsteroidal estrogen, have an increased risk of developing in later life a form of vaginal or cervical cancer that is ordinarily extremely rare.[31,32] This risk has been estimated to be of the order of 1 in 1,000 exposures or less.[33,47] Although there is no evidence at the present time that oral contraceptives further enhance the risk of developing this type of malignancy, such patients should be monitored with particular care if they elect to use oral contraceptives instead of other methods of contraception. Furthermore, a high percentage of such exposed women (from 30% to 90%) have been found to have epithelial changes of the vagina and cervix.[34–38] Although these changes are histologically benign, it is not known whether this condition is a precursor of vaginal malignancy. Male children so exposed may develop abnormalities of the urogenital tract.[48–50] Although similar data are not available with the use of other estrogens, it cannot be presumed that they would not induce similar changes.

An increased risk of congenital anomalies, including heart defects and limb defects, has been reported with the use of sex hormones, including oral contraceptives, in pregnancy.[39–42,51] One case control study[42] has estimated a 4.7-fold increase in risk of limb-reduction defects in infants exposed *in utero* to sex hormones (oral contraceptives, hormonal withdrawal tests for pregnancy or attempted treatment for threatened abortion). Some of these exposures were very short and involved only a few days of treatment. The data suggest that the risk of limb-reduction defects in exposed fetuses is somewhat less than 1 in 1,000 live births.

In the past, female sex hormones have been used during pregnancy in an attempt to treat threatened or habitual abortion. There is considerable evidence that estrogens are ineffective for these indications, and there is no evidence from well-controlled studies that progestogens are effective for these uses.

There is some evidence that triploidy and possibly other types of polyploidy are increased among abortuses from women who become pregnant soon after ceasing oral contraceptives.[43] Embryos with these anomalies are virtually always aborted spontaneously. Whether there is an overall increase in spontaneous abortion of pregnancies conceived soon after stopping oral contraceptives is unknown.

It is recommended that for any patient who has missed two consecutive periods, pregnancy should be ruled out before continuing the contraceptive regimen. If the patient has not adhered to the prescribed schedule, the possibility of pregnancy should be considered at the time of the first missed period, and further use of oral contraceptives should be withheld until pregnancy has been ruled out. If pregnancy is confirmed, the patient should be apprised of the potential risks to the fetus and the advisability of continuation of the pregnancy should be discussed in the light of these risks.

It is also recommended that women who discontinue oral contraceptives with the intent of becoming pregnant use an alternate form of contraception for a period of time before attempting to conceive. Many clinicians recommend 3 months although no precise information is available on which to base this recommendation.

The administration of progestogen-only or progestogen-estrogen combinations to induce withdrawal bleeding should not be used as a test of pregnancy.

6. *Gallbladder Disease.* Studies[8,23,26] report an increased risk of surgically confirmed gallbladder disease in users of oral contraceptives and estrogens. In one study, an increased risk appeared after 2 years of use and doubled after 4 or 5 years of use. In one of the other studies, an increased risk was apparent between 6 and 12 months of use.

7. *Carbohydrate and Lipid Metabolic Effects.* A decrease in glucose tolerance has been observed in a significant percentage of patients on oral contraceptives. For this reason, prediabetic and diabetic patients should be carefully observed while receiving oral contraceptives.

An increase in triglycerides and total phospholipids has been observed in patients receiving oral contraceptives.[44] The clinical significance of this finding remains to be defined.

8. *Elevated Blood Pressure.* An increase in blood pressure has been reported in patients receiving oral contraceptives.[26] In some

Figure 1. Estimated annual number of deaths associated with control of fertility and no control per 100,000 nonsterile women, by regimen of control and age of woman.

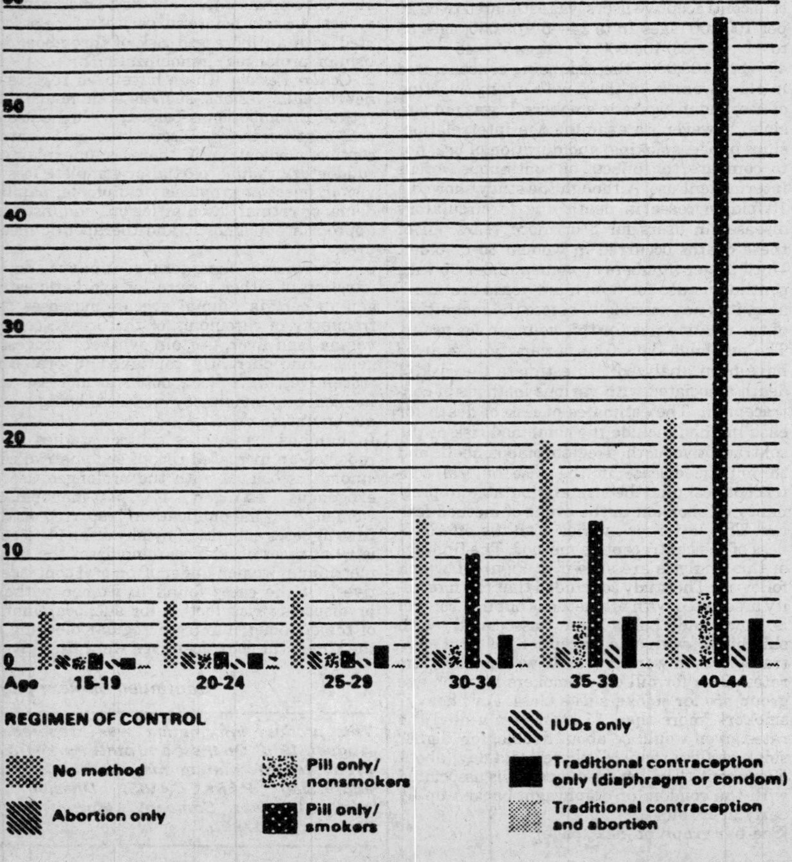

women, hypertension may occur within a few months of beginning oral contraceptive use. In the first year of use, the prevalence of women with hypertension is low in users and may be no higher than that of a comparable group of nonusers. The prevalence in users increases, however, with longer exposure, and in the fifth year of use is two and a half to three times the reported prevalence in the first year. Age is also strongly correlated with the development of hypertension in oral contraceptive users. Women who previously have had hypertension during pregnancy may be more likely to develop elevation of blood pressure when given oral contraceptives. Hypertension that develops as a result of taking oral contraceptives usually returns to normal after discontinuing the drug.

9. *Headache.* The onset or exacerbation of migraine or development of headache of a new pattern which is recurrent, persistent, or severe, requires discontinuation of oral contraceptives and evaluation of the cause.

10. *Bleeding Irregularities.* Breakthrough bleeding, spotting and amenorrhea are frequent reasons for patients discontinuing oral contraceptives. In breakthrough bleeding, as in all cases of irregular bleeding from the vagina, nonfunctional causes should be borne in mind. In undiagnosed persistent or recurrent abnormal bleeding from the vagina, adequate diagnostic measures are indicated to rule out pregnancy or malignancy. If pathology has been excluded, time or a change to another formulation may solve the problem. Changing to an oral contraceptive with a higher estrogen content, while potentially useful in minimizing menstrual irregularity, should be done only if necessary since this may increase the risk of thromboembolic disease.

Women with a past history of oligomenorrhea or secondary amenorrhea or young women without regular cycles may have a tendency to remain anovulatory or to become amenorrheic after discontinuation of oral contraceptives. Women with these preexisting problems should be advised of this possibility and encouraged to use other contraceptive methods. Post-use anovulation, possibly prolonged, may also occur in women without previous irregularities.

11. *Ectopic Pregnancy.* Ectopic as well as intrauterine pregnancy may occur in contraceptive failures. However, in progestogen-only oral contraceptive failures, the ratio of ectopic to intrauterine pregnancies is higher than in women who are not receiving oral contraceptives, since the drugs are more effective in preventing intrauterine than ectopic pregnancies.

12. *Breast-Feeding.* Oral contraceptives given in the postpartum period may interfere with lactation. There may be a decrease in the quantity and quality of the breast milk. Furthermore, a small fraction of the hormonal agents in oral contraceptives has been identified in the milk of mothers receiving these drugs.[45] The effects, if any, on the breast-fed child have not been determined. If feasible, the use of oral contraceptives should be deferred until the infant has been weaned.

Precautions:

General

1. A complete medical and family history should be taken prior to the initiation of oral contraceptives. The pretreatment and periodic physical examinations should include special reference to blood pressure, breasts, abdomen and pelvic organs, including Papanicolaou smear and relevant laboratory tests. As a general rule, oral contraceptives should not be prescribed for longer than 1 year without another physical examination being performed.

2. Under the influence of estrogen-progestogen preparations preexisting uterine leiomyomata may increase in size.

3. Patients with a history of psychic depression should be carefully observed and the drug discontinued if depression recurs to a serious degree. Patients becoming significantly depressed while taking oral contraceptives should stop the medication and use an alternate method of contraception in an attempt to determine whether the symptom is drug related.

4. Oral contraceptives may cause some degree of fluid retention. They should be prescribed with caution, and only with careful monitoring, in patients with conditions which might be aggravated by fluid retention, such as convulsive disorders, migraine syndrome, asthma, or cardiac or renal insufficiency.

5. Patients with a past history of jaundice during pregnancy have an increased risk of recurrence of jaundice while receiving oral contraceptive therapy. If jaundice develops in any patient receiving such drugs, the medication should be discontinued.

6. Steroid hormones may be poorly metabolized in patients with impaired liver function and should be administered with caution in such patients.

7. Oral contraceptive users may have disturbances in normal tryptophan metabolism which may result in a relative pyridoxine deficiency. The clinical significance of this is yet to be determined.

8. Serum folate levels may be depressed by oral contraceptive therapy. Since the pregnant woman is predisposed to the development of folate deficiency and the incidence of folate deficiency increases with increasing gestation, it is possible that if a woman becomes pregnant shortly after stopping oral contraceptives, she may have a greater chance of developing folate deficiency and complications attributed to this deficiency.

9. The pathologist should be advised of oral contraceptive therapy when relevant specimens are submitted.

10. Certain endocrine and liver function tests and blood components may be affected by estrogen-containing oral contraceptives:

a. Increased sulfobromophthalein retention

b. Increased prothrombin and factors VII, VIII, IX, and X; decreased antithrombin 3; increased norepinephrine-induced platelet aggregability

c. Increased thyroid binding globulin (TBG) leading to increased circulating total thyroid hormone, as measured by protein-bound iodine (PBI), T4 by column, or T4 by radioimmunoassay. Free T3 resin uptake is decreased, reflecting the elevated TBG, free T4 concentration is unaltered

d. Decreased pregnanediol excretion

e. Reduced response to metyrapone test

Information For The Patient: See Patient Labeling printed following the reference section.

Drug Interactions: Reduced efficacy and increased incidence of breakthrough bleeding have been associated with concomitant use of rifampin. A similar association has been suggested with barbiturates, phenylbutazone, phenytoin sodium, tetracycline, and ampicillin.

Carcinogenesis: See Warnings section for information on the carcinogenic potential of oral contraceptives.

Pregnancy: Pregnancy category X. See Contraindications and Warnings.

Nursing Mothers: See Warnings.

Adverse Reactions: An increased risk of the following serious adverse reactions has been associated with the use of oral contraceptives (see Warnings):

- Thrombophlebitis
- Pulmonary embolism
- Coronary thrombosis
- Cerebral thrombosis
- Cerebral hemorrhage
- Hypertension
- Gallbladder disease
- Benign hepatomas
- Congenital anomalies

There is evidence of an association between the following conditions and the use of oral contraceptives, although additional confirmatory studies are needed:

- Mesenteric thrombosis
- Neuro-ocular lesions, eg, retinal thrombosis and optic neuritis

The following adverse reactions have been reported in patients receiving oral contraceptives and are believed to be drug related:

Nausea and/or vomiting, usually the most common adverse reactions, occur in approximately 10 percent or less of patients during the first cycle. Other reactions, as a general rule, are seen much less frequently or only occasionally.

- Gastrointestinal symptoms (such as abdominal cramps and bloating)
- Breakthrough bleeding
- Spotting
- Change in menstrual flow
- Dysmenorrhea
- Amenorrhea during and after treatment
- Temporary infertility after discontinuance of treatment
- Edema
- Chloasma or melasma which may persist
- Breast changes: tenderness, enlargement and secretion
- Change in weight (increase or decrease)
- Change in cervical erosion and cervical secretion
- Possible diminution in lactation when given immediately postpartum
- Cholestatic jaundice
- Migraine
- Increase in size of uterine leiomyomata
- Rash (allergic)
- Mental depression
- Reduced tolerance to carbohydrates
- Vaginal candidiasis
- Change in corneal curvature (steepening)
- Intolerance to contact lenses

The following adverse reactions have been reported in users of oral contraceptives, and the association has been neither confirmed nor refuted:

- Premenstrual-like syndrome
- Cataracts
- Changes in libido
- Chorea
- Changes in appetite
- Cystitis-like syndrome
- Headache
- Nervousness
- Dizziness
- Hirsutism
- Loss of scalp hair
- Erythema multiforme
- Erythema nodosum
- Hemorrhagic eruption
- Vaginitis
- Porphyria

Acute Overdose: Serious ill effects have not been reported following acute ingestion of large doses of oral contraceptives by young children. Overdosage may cause nausea, and withdrawal bleeding may occur in females.

Dosage and Administration For 21-Day Dosage Regimen: To achieve maximum contraceptive effectiveness, Norlestrin must be taken exactly as directed and at intervals not exceeding 24 hours. Norlestrin **21** provides the patient with a convenient tablet schedule of "3 weeks on—1 week off."

The first day of menstrual flow is considered Day 1. Initially, the patient begins taking tablets on Day 5 and takes one tablet daily for 21 days. She then takes no tablets for seven days.

Continued on next page

This product information was prepared in August, 1982. On these and other Parke-Davis Products, information may be obtained by addressing PARKE-DAVIS, Division of Warner-Lambert Company, Morris Plains, New Jersey 07950.

Parke-Davis—Cont.

After the seven days during which no tablets are taken, the patient begins a new course of one tablet daily for 21 days. Each course of tablets will begin on the same day of the week as the first course. Likewise, the interval of no tablets will always start on the same day of the week.
Tablets should be taken regularly with a meal or at bedtime. It should be stressed that efficacy of medication depends on strict adherence to the dosage schedule.

Special Notes on Administration

Menstruation usually begins two or three days, but may begin as late as the fourth or fifth day, after discontinuing medication.
If spotting occurs while on the usual regimen of one tablet daily, the patient should continue medication without interruption.
If a patient forgets to take one or more tablets, the following is suggested: If one tablet is missed, take it as soon as remembered, or take two tablets the next day. If two consecutive tablets are missed, take two tablets daily for the next two days, then resume the regular schedule. If three consecutive tablets are missed, begin a new compact of tablets, starting seven days after the last tablet was taken.
The possibility of ovulation occurring increases with each successive day that scheduled tablets are missed. When three consecutive tablets are missed the patient should use an alternate means of contraception, other than oral tablets, until the start of the next menstrual period.
While there is little likelihood of ovulation occurring if only one tablet is missed, the possibility of spotting or bleeding is increased. This is particularly likely to occur if two or more consecutive tablets are missed.
In the rare case of bleeding which resembles menstruation, the patient should be advised to discontinue medication and then begin taking tablets from a new compact on the fifth day (Day 5). Persistent bleeding which is not controlled by this method indicates the need for reexamination of the patient at which time nonfunctional causes should be borne in mind.

Dosage and Administration For 28-Day Dosage Regimen: To achieve maximum contraceptive effectiveness, Norlestrin must be taken exactly as directed and at intervals not exceeding 24 hours.
Norlestrin **Fe** and **28** provides a continuous administration regimen consisting of 21 *light-colored* tablets of Norlestrin and 7 brown tablets of ferrous fumarate or 7 white inert tablets. There is no need for the patient to count days between cycles because there are no "off-tablet days."
The dosage schedule is one *light-colored* tablet daily for 21 days, starting initially on Day 5 of the menstrual cycle, followed without interruption by one brown or white tablet daily for 7 days. The first day of menstrual flow is considered Day 1. Upon completion of this first course of tablets, a second course of tablets is started without interruption. All subsequent courses also are taken without interruption.
Tablets should be taken regularly with a meal or at bedtime. It should be stressed that efficacy of medication depends on strict adherence to the dosage schedule.

Special Notes on Administration

Menstruation usually begins two or three days, but may begin as late as the fourth or fifth day, after the brown or white tablets have been started. In any event, the next course of tablets should be started without interruption. There should never be a day when the patient is not taking a tablet.
If spotting occurs while the patient is taking *light-colored* tablets, continue medication without interruption.
If a patient forgets to take one or more *light-colored* tablets, the following is suggested: If one *light-colored* tablet is missed, take it as soon as remembered, or take two *light-colored* tablets the next day. If two consecutive *light-colored* tablets are missed, take two *light-colored* tablets daily for the next two days, then resume the regular schedule. If three consecutive *light-colored* tablets are missed, begin a new compact of tablets, starting seven days after the last *light-colored* tablet was taken.
The possibility of ovulation occurring increases with each successive day that scheduled *light-colored* tablets are missed. When three consecutive *light-colored* tablets are missed, the patient should use an alternate means of contraception, other than oral tablets, until the start of the next menstrual period.
While there is little likelihood of ovulation occurring if only one *light-colored* tablet is missed, the possibility of spotting or bleeding is increased. This is particularly likely to occur if two or more consecutive *light-colored* tablets are missed.
If one or more brown or white tablets are missed, the *light-colored* tablets should be started no later than the eighth day after the last *light-colored* tablet was taken. The possibility of conception occurring is not increased if brown or white tablets are missed.
In the rare case of bleeding which resembles menstruation, the patient should be advised to discontinue medication and then begin taking tablets from a new compact on the fifth day (Day 5). Persistent bleeding which is not controlled by this method indicates the need for reexamination of the patient, at which time nonfunctional causes should be borne in mind.

Use of oral contraceptives in the event of a missed menstrual period:

1. If the patient has not adhered to the prescribed dosage regimen, the possibility of pregnancy should be considered after the first missed period and oral contraceptives should be withheld until pregnancy has been ruled out.
2. If the patient has adhered to the prescribed regimen and misses two consecutive periods, pregnancy should be ruled out before continuing the contraceptive regimen.

After several months on treatment, bleeding may be reduced to a point of virtual absence. This reduced flow may occur as a result of medication, in which event it is not indicative of pregnancy.

How Supplied:

Norlestrin **21** 1/50 is available in compacts each containing 21 tablets. Each tablet contains 1 mg of norethindrone acetate and 50 mcg of ethinyl estradiol. Available in packages of five compacts and packages of five refills.
Norlestrin **21** 2.5/50 is available in compacts each containing 21 tablets. Each tablet contains 2.5 mg of norethindrone acetate and 50 mcg of ethinyl estradiol. Available in packages of five compacts and packages of five refills.
Norlestrin **Fe** 1/50 is available in compacts each containing 21 yellow tablets and 7 brown tablets. Each yellow tablet contains 1 mg of norethindrone acetate and 50 mcg of ethinyl estradiol. Each brown tablet contains 75 mg ferrous fumarate, USP. Available in packages of five compacts and packages of five refills.
Norlestrin **Fe** 2.5/50 is available in compacts each containing 21 pink tablets and 7 brown tablets. Each pink tablet contains 2.5 mg of norethindrone acetate and 50 mcg of ethinyl estradiol. Each brown tablet contains 75 mg ferrous fumarate, USP. Available in packages of five compacts and packages of five refills.
Norlestrin **28** 1/50 is available in compacts each containing 21 yellow tablets and 7 white inert tablets. Each yellow tablet contains 1 mg of norethindrone acetate and 50 mcg of ethinyl estradiol. Available in packages of five compacts and packages of five refills.

References:

1. "*Population Reports,*" Series H, Number 2, May 1974; Series 1, Number 1, June 1974; Series B, Number 2, January 1975; Series H, Number 3, 1975; Series H, Number 4, January 1976 (published by the Population Information Program, The George Washington University Medical Center, 2001 S. St. NW., Washington, D.C.)
2. Inman, W. H. W., M. P. Vessey, B. Westerholm, and A. Engelund. "Thromboembolic disease and the steroidal content of oral contraceptives. A report to the Committee on Safety of Drugs," *Brit Med J* 2:203–209, 1970.
3. Stolley, P.D., J. A. Tonascia, M. S. Tockman, P. E. Sartwell, A. H. Rutledge, and M. P. Jacobs, "Thrombosis with low-estrogen oral contraceptives," *Am J Epidemiol* 102: 197–208, 1975.
4. Royal College of General Practitioners, "Oral contraception and thromboembolic disease," *J Coll Gen Pract* 13:267–279, 1967.
5. Inman, W. H. W. and M. P. Vessey, "Investigation of deaths from pulmonary, coronary and cerebral thrombosis and embolism in women of childbearing age," *Brit Med. J* 2-193–199, 1968.
6. Vessey, M. P. and R. Doll, "Investigation of relation between use of oral contraceptives and thromboembolic disease. A further report," *Brit Med J* 2:651–657, 1969.
7. Sartwell, P. E., A. T. Masi, F. G. Arthes, G. R. Greene, and H. E. Smith, "Thromboembolism and oral contraceptives an epidemiological case control study," *Am J Epidemiol* 90:365–380, 1969.
8. Boston Collaborative Drug Surveillance Program. "Oral contraceptives and venous thromboembolic disease, surgically confirmed gallbladder disease and breast tumors," *Lancet* 1:1399–1404, 1973.
9. Collaborative Group for the Study of Stroke in Young Women, "Oral contraception and increased risk of cerebral ischemia or thrombosis," *N Engl J Med* 288:871–878, 1973.
10. Collaborative Group for the Study of Stroke in Young Women, "Oral contraceptives and stroke in young women: associated risk factors," *JAMA* 231:718–722, 1975.
11. Mann, J. I., and W. H. W. Inman, "Oral contraceptives and death from myocardial infarction," *Brit Med J* 2:245–248, 1975.
12. Mann, J. I., W. H. W. Inman, and M. Thorogood, "Oral contraceptive use in older women and fatal myocardial infarction," *Bit Med J* 2:445–447, 1976.
13. Mann, J. I., M. P. Vessey, M. Thorogood and R. Doll, "Myocardial infarction in young women with special reference to oral contraceptive practice," *Brit Med J* 2:241–245, 1975.
14. Tietze, C., "New Estimates of Mortality Associated with Fertility Control," *Family Planning Perspectives,* 9:74–76, 1977.
15. Vessey, M. P., R. Doll, A. S. Fairbairn, and G. Glober, "Post-operative thromboembolism and the use of oral contraceptives," *Brit Med J* 3:123–126, 1970.
16. Greene, G. R., P. E. Sartwell, "Oral contraceptive use in patients with thromboembolism following surgery, trauma or infection," *Am J Pub Health* 62:680–685, 1972.
17. Smith, D. C., R. Prentice, D. J. Thompson and W. L. Herrmann, "Association of exogenous estrogen and endometrial carcinoma," *N Engl J Med* 293:1164–1167, 1975.
18. Ziel, H. K., and W. D. Finkle, "Increased risk of endometrial carcinoma among users of conjugated estrogens," *N Engl J Med* 293: 1167–1170, 1975.
19. Mack, T. N., M. C. Pike, B. E. Henderson, R. I. Pfeffer, V. R. Gerkins, M. Arthur and S. E. Brown, "Estrogens and endometrial cancer in a retirement community," *N Engl J Med* 294: 1262–1267, 1976.
20. Silverberg, S. G., and E. L. Makowski, "Endometrial carcinoma in young women taking oral contraceptive agents," *Obstet Gynecol* 46:503–506, 1975.

21. Vessey, M. P., R. Doll, and P. M. Sutton, "Oral contraceptives and breast neoplasia: a retrospective study," *Brit Med J* 3:719–724, 1972.
22. Vessey, M. P., R. Doll, and K. Jones, "Oral contraceptives and breast cancer. Progress report of an epidemiological study," *Lancet* 1:941–943, 1975.
23. Boston Collaborative Drug Surveillance Program, "Surgically confirmed gallbladder disease, venous thromboembolism and breast tumors in relation to postmenopausal estrogen therapy," *N Engl J Med* 290:14–19, 1974.
24. Arthes, F. G., P. E. Sartwell, and E. F. Lewison, "The pill, estrogens, and the breast, Epidemiologic aspects," *Cancer* 28:1391–1394, 1971.
25. Fasal, E., and R. S. Paffenbarger, "Oral contraceptives as related to cancer and benign lesions of the breast." *J Natl Cancer Inst* 55:767–773, 1975.
26. Royal College of General Practitioners, "Oral Contraceptives and Health," London, Pitman, 1974.
27. Ory, H., P. Cole, B. MacMahon, and R. Hoover, "Oral contraceptives and reduced risk of benign breast diseases," *N Engl J Med* 294:419–422, 1976.
28. Baum, J., F. Holtz, J. J. Bookstein, and E. W. Klein, "Possible association between benign hepatomas and oral contraceptives," *Lancet* 2:926–928, 1973.
29. Mays, E. T., W. M. Christopherson, M. M. Mahr, and H. C. Williams, "Hepatic changes in young women ingesting contraceptive steroids. Hepatic hemorrhage and primary hepatic tumors," *JAMA* 235:730–732, 1976.
30. Edmondson, H. A., B. Henderson, and B. Benton, "Liver-cell adenomas associated with use of oral contraceptives," *N Engl J Med* 294:470–472, 1976.
31. Herbst, A. L., H. Ulfelder, and D. C. Poskanzer, "Adenocarcinoma of the vagina," *N Engl J Med* 284:878–881, 1971.
32. Greenwald, P., J. J. Barlow, P. C. Nasca and W. Burnett, "Vaginal cancer after maternal treatment with synthetic estrogens," *N Engl J Med* 285: 390–392, 1971.
33. Lanier, A. P., K. L. Noller, D. G. Decker, L. Elveback, and L. T. Kurland, "Cancer and stilbestrol. A follow-up of 1719 persons exposed to estrogens in utero and born 1943–1959," *Mayo Clin Pro* 48:793–799, 1973.
34. Herbst, A. L., R. J. Kurman, and R. E. Scully, "Vaginal and cervical abnormalities after exposure to stilbestrol in utero," *Obstet Gynecol* 40:287–298, 1972.
35. Herbst, A. L., S. J. Robboy, G. J. Macdonald, and R. E. Scully, "The effects of local progesterone on stilbestrol-associated vaginal adenosis," *Am J. Obstet Gynecol* 118:607–615, 1974.
36. Herbst, A. L., D. C. Poskanzer, S. J. Robboy, L. Friedlander, and R. E. Scully, "Prenatal exposure to stilbestrol: a prospective comparison of exposed female offspring with unexposed controls," *N Engl J Med* 292:334–339, 1975.
37. Stafl, A., R. F. Mattingly, D. V. Foley, W. Fetherston, "Clinical diagnosis of vaginal adenosis," *Obstet Gynecol* 43:118–128, 1974.
38. Sherman, A. I., M. Goldrath, A. Berlin, V. Vakhariya, F. Banooni, W. Michaels, P. Goodman, and S. Brown, "Cervical-vaginal adenosis after in utero exposure to synthetic estrogens," *Obstet Gynecol* 44:531–545, 1974.
39. Gal, I., B. Kirman, and J. Stern, "Hormone pregnancy tests and congenital malformation," *Nature* 216:83, 1967.
40. Levy, E. P., A. Cohen, and F. C. Fraser, "Hormone treatment during pregnancy and congenital heart defects," *Lancet* 1:611, 1973.
41. Nora, J. J., and A. H. Nora, "Birth defects and oral contraceptives," *Lancet* 1:941–942, 1973.
42. Janerich, D. T., J. M. Piper, and D. M. Glebatis, "Oral contraceptives and congenital limb-reduction defects," *N Engl J Med* 291:697–700, 1974.
43. Carr, D. H., "Chromosome studies in selected spontaneous abortions: I. Conception after oral contraceptives," *Canad Med Assoc J* 103:343–348, 1970.
44. Wynn, V., J. W. H. Doar, and G. L. Mills, "Some effects of oral contraceptives on serum-lipid and lipoprotein levels," *Lancet* 2:720–723, 1966.
45. Laumas, K. R., P. K. Malkani, S. Bhatnagar, and V. Laumas, "Radioactivity in the breast milk of lactating women after oral administration of 3 H-norethynodrel," *Amer J Obstet Gynecol* 98:411–413, 1967.
46. Center for Disease Control, "Increased Risk of Hepatocellular Adenoma in Women with Long-term use of Oral Contraceptives," *Morbidity and Mortality Weekly Report* 26:293–294, 1977.
47. Herbst, A. L., P. Cole, T. Colton, S. J. Robboy, R. E. Scully, "Age-incidence and Risk of Diethylstilbestrol-related Clear Cell Adenocarcinoma of the Vagina and Cervix," *Am J. Obstet Cynecol* 128:43–50, 1977.
48. Bibbo, M., M. Al-Naqeeb, I. Baccarini, W. Gill, M. Newton, K. M. Sleeper, M. Sonek, G. L. Wied, "Follow-Up Study of Male and Female Offspring of DES-treated Mothers. A Preliminary Report," *Jour of Repro Med* 15:29–32, 1975.
49. Gill, W. B., G. F. B. Schumacher, M. Bibbo, "Structural and Functional Abnormalities in the Sex Organs of Male Offspring of Mothers Treated with Diethylstilbestrol (DES)," *Jour of Repro Med* 16:147–153, 1976.
50. Henderson, B. E., B. Benton, M. Cosgrove, J. Baptista, J. Aldrich, D. Townsend, W. Hart, T. Mack, "Urogenital Tract Abnormalities in Sons of Women Treated with Diethylstilbestrol," *Pediatrics* 58:505–507, 1976.
51. Heinonen, O. P., D. Slone, R. R. Nonson, E. B. Hook, S. Shapiro, "Cardiovascular Birth Defects and Antenatal Exposure to Female Sex Hormones," *N Engl J Med* 296:67–70, 1977.
52. Jain, A. K., "Mortality Risk Associated with the Use of Oral Contraceptives," *Studies in Family Planning* 8:50–54, 1977.
53. Beral, V., "Mortality Among Oral Contraceptive Users," *Lancet* 2:727–731, 1977.

The patient labeling for oral contraceptive drug products is set forth below:

Brief Summary Patient Package Insert

> Cigarette smoking increases the risk of serious adverse effects on the heart and blood vessels from oral contraceptive use. This risk increases with age and with heavy smoking (15 or more cigarettes per day) and is quite marked in women over 35 years of age. Women who use oral contraceptives should not smoke.

Oral contraceptives taken as directed are about 99% effective in preventing pregnancy. (The mini-pill, however is somewhat less effective.) Forgetting to take your pills increases the chance of pregnancy. Various drugs, such as antibiotics, may also decrease the effectiveness of oral contraceptives.

Women who have or have had clotting disorders, cancer of the breast or sex organs, unexplained vaginal bleeding, a stroke, heart attack, angina pectoris, or who suspect they may be pregnant should not use oral contraceptives.

Most side effects of the pill are not serious. The most common side effects are nausea, vomiting, bleeding between menstrual periods, weight gain, and breast tenderness. However, proper use of oral contraceptives requires that they be taken under your doctor's continuous supervision, because they can be associated with serious side effects which may be fatal. Fortunately, these occur very infrequently.

The serious side effects are:

1. Blood clots in the legs, lungs, brain, heart or other organs and hemorrhage into the brain due to bursting of a blood vessel
2. Liver tumors, which may rupture and cause severe bleeding
3. Birth defects if the pill is taken while you are pregnant
4. High blood pressure
5. Gallbladder disease

The symptoms associated with these serious side effects are discussed in the detailed leaflet given you with your supply of pills. Notify your doctor if you notice any unusual physical disturbance while taking the pill.

The estrogen in oral contraceptives has been found to cause breast cancer and other cancers in certain animals. These findings suggest that oral contraceptives may also cause cancer in humans. However, studies to date in women taking currently marketed oral contraceptives have not confirmed that oral contraceptives cause cancer in humans.

The detailed leaflet describes more completely the benefits and risks of oral contraceptives. It also provides information on other forms of contraception. Read it carefully. If you have any questions, consult your doctor.

Caution: Oral contraceptives are of no value in the prevention or treatment of venereal disease.

Detailed Patient Labeling

What You Should Know About Oral Contraceptives

Oral contraceptives ("the pill") are the most effective way (except for sterilization) to prevent pregnancy. They are also convenient and, for most women, free of serious or unpleasant side effects. Oral contraceptives must always be taken under the continuous supervision of a physician.

It is important that any woman who considers using an oral contraceptive understand the risks involved. Although the oral contraceptives have important advantages over other methods of contraception, they have certain risks that no other method has. Only you can decide whether the advantages are worth these risks. This leaflet will tell you about the most important risks. It will explain how you can help your doctor prescribe the pill as safely as possible by telling him about yourself and being alert for the earliest signs of trouble. And it will tell you how to use the pill properly, so that it will be as effective as possible. There is more detailed information available in the leaflet prepared for doctors. Your pharmacist can show you a copy; you may need your doctor's help in understanding parts of it.

Who Should Not Use Oral Contraceptives

A. If you have any of the following conditions you should not use the pill:

1. Clots in the legs or lungs
2. Angina pectoris
3. Known or suspected cancer of the breast or sex organs
4. Unusual vaginal bleeding that has not yet been diagnosed
5. Known or suspected pregnancy

B. If you have had any of the following conditions you should not use the pill:

1. Heart attack or stroke
2. Clots in the legs or lungs

> C. Cigarette smoking increases the risk of serious adverse effects on the heart and blood vessels from oral contraceptive use. This risk increases with age and with heavy smoking (15 or more cigarettes per day) and is quite marked in women over 35

Continued on next page

This product information was prepared in August, 1982. On these and other Parke-Davis Products, information may be obtained by addressing PARKE-DAVIS, Division of Warner-Lambert Company, Morris Plains, New Jersey 07950.

Parke-Davis—Cont.

years of age. Women who use oral contraceptives should not smoke.

D. If you have scanty or irregular periods or are a young woman without a regular cycle, you should use another method of contraception because, if you use the pill, you may have difficulty becoming pregnant or may fail to have menstrual periods after discontinuing the pill.

Deciding To Use Oral Contraceptives

If you do not have any of the conditions listed above and are thinking about using oral contraceptives, to help you decide, you need information about the advantages and risks of oral contraceptives and of other contraceptive methods as well. This leaflet describes the advantages and risks of oral contraceptives. Except for sterilization, the IUD and abortion, which have their own exclusive risks, the only risks of other methods of contraception are those due to pregnancy should the method fail. Your doctor can answer questions you may have with respect to other methods of contraception. He can also answer any questions you may have after reading this leaflet on oral contraceptives.

1. What Oral Contraceptives Are and How They Work. Oral contraceptives are of two types. The most common, often simply called "the pill," is a combination of an estrogen and a progestogen, the two kinds of female hormones. The amount of estrogen and progestogen can vary, but the amount of estrogen is most important because both the effectiveness and some of the dangers of oral contraceptives are related to the amount of estrogen. This kind of oral contraceptive works principally by preventing release of an egg from the ovary. When the amount of estrogen is 50 micrograms or more, and the pill is taken as directed, oral contraceptives are more than 99% effective (ie, there would be less than one pregnancy if 100 women used the pill for 1 year). Pills that contain 20 to 35 micrograms of estrogen vary slightly in effectiveness, ranging from 98% to more than 99% effective. Norlestrin was shown in clinical trials to be more than 99% effective.

The second type of oral contraceptive, often called the "mini-pill," contains only a progestogen. It works in part by preventing release of an egg from the ovary but also by keeping sperm from reaching the egg and by making the uterus (womb) less receptive to any fertilized egg that reaches it. The mini-pill is less effective than the combination oral contraceptive, about 97% effective.

In addition, the progestogen-only pill has a tendency to cause irregular bleeding which may be quite inconvenient, or cessation of bleeding entirely. The progestogen-only pill is used despite its lower effectiveness in the hope that it will prove not to have some of the serious side effects of the estrogen-containing pill (which follows) but it is not yet certain that the mini-pill does in fact have fewer serious side effects. The discussion which follows, while based mainly on information about the combination pills, should be considered to apply, as well, to the mini-pill.

2. Other Nonsurgical Ways to Prevent Pregnancy. As this leaflet will explain, oral contraceptives have several serious risks. Other methods of contraception have lesser risks or none at all. They are also less effective than oral contraceptives but, used properly, may be effective enough for many women. The following gives reported pregnancy rates (the number of women out of 100 who would become pregnant in 1 year) for these methods:

Pregnancies Per 100 Women Per Year

Intrauterine device (IUD), less than 1-6; Diaphragm with spermicidal products (creams or jellies), 2-20; Condom (rubber), 3-36; Aerosol foams, 2-29; Jellies and creams, 4-36; Periodic abstinence (rhythm) all types, less than 1-47; 1. *Calendar method, 14-47; 2. Temperature method, 1-20; 3. Temperature method—intercourse only in post-ovulatory phase, less than 1-7; 4. Mucus method, 1-25;* No contraception, 60-80.

The figures (except for the IUD) vary widely because people differ in how well they use each method. Very faithful users of the various methods obtain very good results except for users of the calendar method of periodic abstinence (rhythm). Except for the IUD, effective use of these methods requires somewhat more effort than simply taking a single pill every morning, but it is an effort that many couples undertake successfully. Your doctor can tell you a great deal more about these methods of contraception.

3. The Dangers of Oral Contraceptives.

a. *Circulatory disorders (abnormal blood clotting and stroke due to hemorrhage).* Blood clots (in various blood vessels of the body) are the most common of the serious side effects of oral contraceptives. A clot can result in a stroke (if the clot is in the brain), a heart attack (if the clot is in a blood vessel of the heart), or a pulmonary embolus (a clot which forms in the legs or pelvis, then breaks off and travels to the lungs). Any of these can be fatal. Clots also occur rarely in the blood vessels of the eye, resulting in blindness or impairment of vision in that eye. There is evidence that the risk of clotting increases with higher estrogen doses. It is, therefore, important to keep the dose of estrogen as low as possible, so long as the oral contraceptive used has an acceptable pregnancy rate and doesn't cause unacceptable changes in the menstrual pattern. Furthermore, cigarette smoking by oral contraceptive users increases the risk of serious adverse effects on the heart and blood vessels. This risk increases with age and with heavy smoking (15 or more cigarettes per day) and begins to become quite marked in women over 35 years of age. For this reason, women who use oral contraceptives should not smoke.

The risk of abnormal clotting increases with age in both users and nonusers of oral contraceptives, but the increased risk from the contraceptives appears to be present at all ages. For oral contraceptive users in general, it has been estimated that in women between the ages of 15 and 34 the risk of death due to a circulatory disorder is about 1 in 12,000 per year, whereas for nonusers the rate is about 1 in 50,000 per year. In the age group 35 to 44, the risk is estimated to be about 1 in 2,500 per year for oral contraceptive users and about 1 in 10,000 per year for nonusers.

Even without the pill the risk of having a heart attack increases with age and is also increased by such heart attack risk factors as high blood pressure, high cholesterol, obesity, diabetes, and cigarette smoking. Without any risk factors present, the use of oral contraceptives alone may double the risk of heart attack. However, the combination of cigarette smoking, especially heavy smoking, and oral contraceptive use greatly increases the risk of heart attack. Oral contraceptive users who smoke are about 5 times more likely to have a heart attack than users who do not smoke and about 10 times more likely to have a heart attack than nonusers who do not smoke. It has been estimated that users between the ages of 30 and 39 who smoke have about a 1 in 10,000 chance each year of having a fatal heart attack compared to about a 1 in 50,000 chance in users who do not smoke, and about a 1 in 100,000 chance in nonusers who do not smoke. In the age group 40 to 44, the risk is about 1 in 1,700 per year for users who smoke compared to about 1 in 10,000 for users who do not smoke and to about 1 in 14,000 per year for nonusers who do not smoke. Heavy smoking (about 15 cigarettes or more a day) further increases the risk. If you do not smoke and have none of the other heart attack risk factors described above, you will have a smaller risk than listed. If you have several heart attack risk factors, the risk may be considerably greater than listed.

In addition to blood-clotting disorders, it has been estimated that women taking oral contraceptives are twice as likely as nonusers to have a stroke due to rupture of a blood vessel in the brain.

b. *Formation of tumors.* Studies have found that when certain animals are given the female sex hormone estrogen, which is an ingredient of oral contraceptives, continuously for long periods, cancers may develop in the breast, cervix, vagina, and liver.

These findings suggest that oral contraceptives may cause cancer in humans. However, studies to date in women taking currently marketed oral contraceptives have not confirmed that oral contraceptives cause cancer in humans. Several studies have found no increase in breast cancer in users, although one study suggested oral contraceptives might cause an increase in breast cancer in women who already have benign breast disease (eg, cysts).

Women with a strong family history of breast cancer or who have breast nodules, fibrocystic disease, or abnormal mammograms or who were exposed to DES (diethylstilbestrol), an estrogen, during their mother's pregnancy must be followed very closely by their doctors if they choose to use oral contraceptives instead of another method of contraception. Many studies have shown that women taking oral contraceptives have less risk of getting benign breast disease than those who have not used oral contraceptives. Recently, strong evidence has emerged that estrogens (one component of oral contraceptives), when given for periods of more than one year to women after the menopause, increase the risk of cancer of the uterus (womb). There is also some evidence that a kind of oral contraceptive which is no longer marketed, the sequential oral contraceptive, may increase the risk of cancer of the uterus. There remains no evidence, however, that the oral contraceptives now available increase the risk of this cancer.

Oral contraceptives do cause, although rarely, a benign (nonmalignant) tumor of the liver. These tumors do not spread, but they may rupture and cause internal bleeding, which may be fatal. A few cases of cancer of the liver have been reported in women using oral contraceptives, but it is not yet known whether the drug caused them.

c. *Dangers to a developing child if oral contraceptives are used in or immediately preceding pregnancy.* Oral contraceptives should not be taken by pregnant women because they may damage the developing child. An increased risk of birth defects, including heart defects and limb defects, has been associated with the use of sex hormones, including oral contraceptives, in pregnancy. In addition, the developing female child whose mother has received DES (diethylstilbestrol), an estrogen, during pregnancy has a risk of getting cancer of the vagina or cervix in her teens or young adulthood. This risk is estimated to be about 1 in 1,000 exposures or less. Abnormalities of the urinary and sex organs have been reported in male offspring so exposed. It is possible that other estrogens, such as the estrogens in oral contraceptives, could have the same effect in the child if the mother takes them during pregnancy.

If you stop taking oral contraceptives to become pregnant, your doctor may recommend that you use another method of contraception for a short while. The reason for this is that there is evidence from studies in women who have had "miscarriages" soon after stopping the pill, that the lost fetuses are more likely to be abnormal. Whether there is an overall increase in "miscarriage" in women who become pregnant soon after stopping the pill, as compared with women who do not use the pill, is not known, but it is possible that there may be. If, however, you do become pregnant soon after stopping oral contraceptives, and do not have a miscarriage, there is no evidence that the baby has an increased risk of being abnormal.

d. *Gallbladder disease.* Women who use oral contraceptives have a greater risk than nonusers of having gallbladder disease requiring surgery. The increased risk may first appear within 1 year of use and may double after 4 or 5 years of use.

e. *Other side effects of oral contraceptives.* Some women using oral contraceptives experience unpleasant side effects that are not dangerous and are not likely to damage their health. Some of these may be temporary. Your breasts may feel tender, nausea and vomiting may occur, you may gain or lose weight, and your ankles may swell. A spotty darkening of the skin, particularly of the face, is possible and may persist. You may notice unexpected vaginal bleeding or changes in your menstrual period. Irregular bleeding is frequently seen when using the mini-pill or combination oral contraceptives containing less than 50 micrograms of estrogen.

More serious side effects include worsening of migraine, asthma, epilepsy, and kidney or heart disease because of a tendency for water to be retained in the body when oral contraceptives are used. Other side effects are growth of preexisting fibroid tumors of the uterus, mental depression, and liver problems with jaundice (yellowing of the skin). Your doctor may find that levels of sugar and fatty substances in your blood are elevated; the long-term effects of these changes are not known. Some women develop high blood pressure while taking oral contraceptives, which ordinarily returns to the original levels when the oral contraceptive is stopped.

Other reactions, although not proved to be caused by oral contraceptives, are occasionally reported. These include more frequent urination and some discomfort when urinating, nervousness, dizziness, some loss of scalp hair, an increase in body hair, an increase or decrease in sex drive, appetite changes, cataracts, and a need for a change in contact lens prescription or inability to use contact lenses.

After you stop using oral contraceptives there may be a delay before you are able to become pregnant or before you resume having menstrual periods. This is especially true of women who had irregular menstrual cycles prior to the use of oral contraceptives. As discussed previously, your doctor may recommend that you wait a short while after stopping the pill before you try to become pregnant. During this time, use another form of contraception. You should consult your physician before resuming use of oral contraceptives after childbirth, especially if you plan to nurse your baby. Drugs in oral contraceptives are known to appear in the milk, and the long-range effect on infants is not known at this time. Furthermore, oral contraceptives may cause a decrease in your milk supply as well as in the quality of the milk.

4. Comparison of the Risks of Oral Contraceptives and Other Contraceptive Methods. The many studies on the risks and effectiveness of oral contraceptives and other methods of contraception have been analyzed to estimate the risk of death associated with various methods of contraception. This risk has two parts: (a) the risk of the method itself (eg, the risk that oral contraceptives will cause death due to abnormal clotting); and (b) the risk of death due to pregnancy or abortion in the event the method fails. The results of this analysis are shown in the following bar graph. The height of the bars is the number of deaths per 100,000 women each year. There are six sets of bars, each set referring to a specific age group of women. Within each set of bars, there is a single bar for each of the different contraceptive methods. For oral contraceptives, there are two bars—one for smokers and the other for nonsmokers. The analysis is based on present knowledge and new information could, of course, alter it. The analysis shows that the risk of death from all methods of birth control is low and below that associated with childbirth, except for oral contraceptives in women over 40 who smoke. It shows that the lowest risk of death is associated with the condom or diaphragm (traditional contraception) backed up by early abortion in case of failure of the condom or diaphragm to prevent pregnancy. Also, at any age the risk of death (due to unexpected pregnancy) from the use of traditional contraception, even without a backup of abortion, is generally the same as or less than that from use of oral contraceptives.

[See bar graph above].

Figure 1. Estimated annual number of deaths associated with control of fertility and no control per 100,000 nonsterile women, by regimen of control and age of woman.

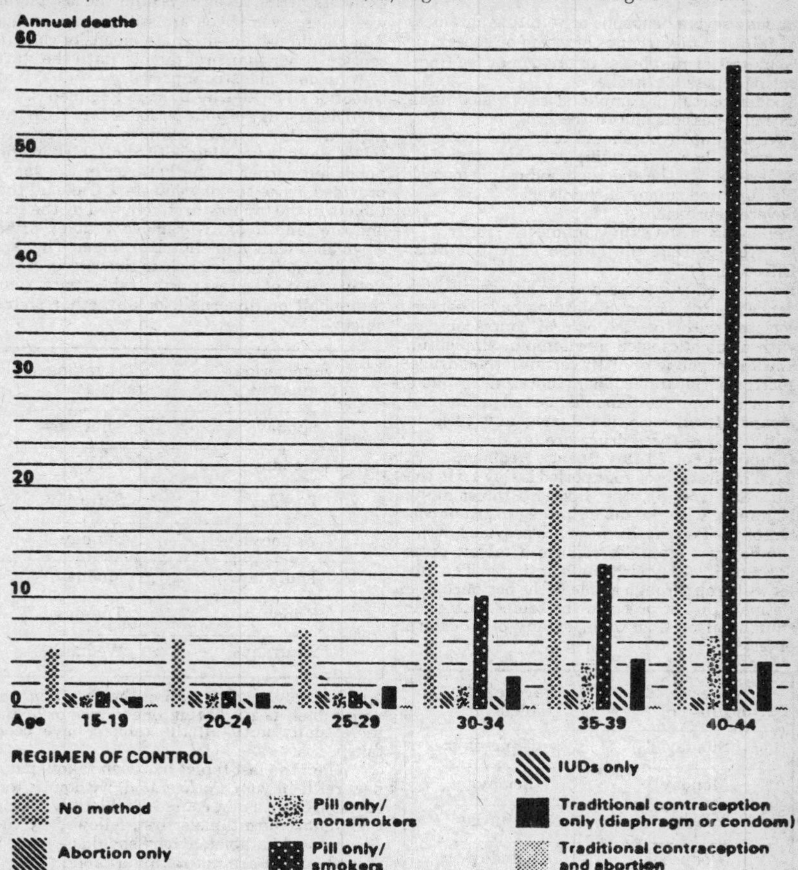

How to Use Oral Contraceptives As Safely and Effectively As Possible, Once You Have Decided to Use Them

1. What to Tell your Doctor.

You can make use of the pill as safely as possible, by telling your doctor if you have any of the following:

a. Conditions that mean you should not use oral contraceptives:

Clots in the legs or lungs
Clots in the legs or lungs in the past
A stroke, heart attack, or angina pectoris
Known or suspected cancer of the breast or sex organs
Unusual vaginal bleeding that has not yet been diagnosed
Known or suspected pregnancy

b. Conditions that your doctor will want to watch closely or which might cause him to suggest another method of contraception:

A family history of breast cancer
Breast nodules, fibrocystic disease of the breast, or an abnormal mammogram
Diabetes
High blood pressure
High cholesterol
Cigarette smoking
Migraine headaches
Heart or kidney disease
Epilepsy
Mental depression
Fibroid tumors of the uterus
Gallbladder disease

c. Once you are using oral contraceptives, you should be alert for signs of a serious adverse effect and call your doctor if they occur:

Sharp pain in the chest, coughing blood, or sudden shortness of breath (indicating possible clots in the lungs)
Pain in the calf (possible clot in the leg)
Crushing chest pain or heaviness (indicating possible heart attack)

Continued on next page

This product information was prepared in August, 1982. On these and other Parke-Davis Products, information may be obtained by addressing PARKE-DAVIS, Division of Warner-Lambert Company, Morris Plains, New Jersey 07950.

Parke-Davis—Cont.

Sudden severe headache or vomiting, dizziness or fainting, disturbance of vision or speech, or weakness or numbness in an arm or leg (indicating a possible stroke)
Sudden partial or complete loss of vision (indicating a possible clot in the eye)
Breast lumps (you should ask your doctor to show you how to examine your own breasts)
Severe pain in the abdomen (indicating a possible ruptured tumor of the liver)
Severe depression
Yellowing of the skin (jaundice)
2. How to Take the Pill So That It Is Most Effective.
Reduced effectiveness and an increased incidence of breakthrough bleeding have been associated with the use of oral contraceptives with antibiotics such as rifampin, ampicillin, and tetracycline or with certain other drugs, such as barbiturates, phenylbutazone or phenytoin sodium. You should use an additional means of contraception during any cycle in which any of these drugs are taken.

Directions For 21-Day Dosage Regimen
a. The first day of your period is Day 1. On the fifth day (Day 5), start taking a tablet daily, beginning with the tablet in the upper left corner of the Petipac. In the space provided, write the day you start. To remove a tablet, press down on it with your thumb or finger. The tablet will drop through a hole in the bottom of the Petipac. Do not press on the tablet with your thumbnail or fingernail, or any other sharp object.

If your period begins on:	Start taking tablets on:
Sunday	Thursday
Monday	Friday
Tuesday	Saturday
Wednesday	Sunday
Thursday	Monday
Friday	Tuesday
Saturday	Wednesday

b. Continue to take one tablet daily until all the tablets have been taken.
c. After you have taken all 21 tablets, stop and don't take any tablets for the next seven days. You should have a menstrual period one to three days after you stop taking tablets; sometimes, it may take a day or so longer.
d. After seven days, during which you take no tablets, put a new refill in your Petipac and begin a new course of tablets, taking one tablet daily for 21 days. You will always start each new course of 21 tablets on the same day of the week. Likewise, the interval of no tablets will always start on the same day of the week.
e. If spotting should occur at an unexpected time, continue to take your tablets as directed. Spotting is usually temporary and without significance. However, if bleeding should occur at an unexpected time, consult your physician. Call your physician regarding any problem or change in your general health that may concern you.
f. If you forget to take a tablet, take it as soon as you remember, even if it is the next day. Then take the next scheduled tablet at the usual time. If you miss two consecutive tablets, take two tablets daily for the next two days. Then resume the regular schedule. While there is little likelihood of pregnancy occurring if you miss only one or two tablets, the possibility of pregnancy increases with each successive day that tablets are missed. If you miss three consecutive tablets, discard any tablets remaining and begin a new course of tablets, starting seven days after the last tablet was taken, even if you are still menstruating. You should use an alternate means of contraception, other than oral tablets, until the start of your next menstrual period.

Directions For 28-Day Dosage Regimen
a. The first day of your period is Day 1. On the fifth day (Day 5), start taking one *light-colored* tablet daily, beginning with the tablet in the upper left corner of the Petipac. In the space provided, write the day you start. Take all the tablets in the top row first, followed by the second row, and so on. To remove a tablet, press down on it with your thumb or finger. The tablet will drop through a hole in the bottom of the Petipac. Do not press on the tablet with your thumbnail or fingernail, or any other sharp object.

If your period begins on:	Start taking tablets on:
Sunday	Thursday
Monday	Friday
Tuesday	Saturday
Wednesday	Sunday
Thursday	Monday
Friday	Tuesday
Saturday	Wednesday

b. On the day after taking the last *light-colored* tablet, begin taking one *brown* or *white* tablet daily until all the tablets have been taken.
c. When the last tablet has been taken, put a new refill in your Petipac and, without interruption, begin a new course of tablets by taking the *light-colored* tablets first, followed by the *brown* or *white* tablets. There should never be a day when you are not taking a tablet.
d. Continue taking *light-colored* tablets without interruption whether or not your period has occurred or is still in progress. Your period will usually occur during the time you are taking *brown* or *white* tablets.
e. If spotting should occur at an unexpected time, continue to take your tablets as directed. Spotting is usually temporary and without significance. However, if bleeding should occur at an unexpected time, consult your physician. Call your physician regarding any problem or change in your general health that may concern you.
f. If you forget to take a *light-colored* tablet, take it as soon as you remember, even if it is the next day. Then take the next scheduled *light-colored* tablet at the usual time. If you miss two consecutive *light-colored* tablets, take two *light-colored* tablets daily for the next two days. Then resume the regular schedule. While there is little likelihood of pregnancy occurring if you miss only one or two *light-colored* tablets, the possibility of pregnancy increases with each successive day that scheduled *light-colored* tablets are missed. If you miss three consecutive *light-colored* tablets, discard any tablets remaining and begin a new course of tablets, starting seven days after the last *light-colored* tablet was taken, even if you are still menstruating. You should use an alternate means of contraception, other than oral tablets, until the start of your next menstrual period.
g. If you miss one or more *brown* or *white* tablets discard the remainder and begin a new course of tablets no later than the eighth day after you took the last *light-colored* tablet. Under no circumstances should you substitute a *brown* or *white* tablet for a *light-colored* one, or take any *brown* or *white* tablets before you have taken all the *light-colored* tablets, unless your physician advises you to do so.

Missed Menstrual Period For Both Dosage Regimens: At times there may be no menstrual period after a cycle of pills. Therefore, if you miss one menstrual period but have taken the pills *exactly as your were supposed to,* continue as usual into the next cycle. If you have not taken the pills correctly and miss a menstrual period, *you may be pregnant* and should stop taking oral contraceptives until your doctor determines whether or not you are pregnant. Until you can get to your doctor, use another form of contraception. If two consecutive menstrual periods are missed, you should stop taking pills until it is determined whether you are pregnant. If you do become pregnant while using oral contraceptives, you should discuss the risks to the developing child with your doctor.

Periodic Examination
Your doctor will take a complete medical and family history before prescribing oral contraceptives. At that time and about once a year thereafter, he will generally examine your blood pressure, breasts, abdomen, and pelvic organs (including a Papanicolaou smear, ie, test for cancer).

Summary: Oral contraceptives are the most effective method, except sterilization, for preventing pregnancy. Other methods, when used conscientiously, are also very effective and have fewer risks. The serious risks of oral contraceptives are uncommon and the "pill" is a very convenient method of preventing pregnancy.
If you have certain conditions or have had these conditions in the past, you should not use oral contraceptives because the risk is too great. These conditions are listed in this leaflet. If you do not have these conditions, and decide to use the "pill," please read this leaflet carefully so that you can use the "pill" most safely and effectively.
Based on his or her assessment of your medical needs, your doctor has prescribed this drug for you. Do not give this drug to anyone else.

0907G130

[*Shown in Product Identification Section*]

NORLUTIN® ℞
(norethindrone tablets, USP)*
NORLUTATE® ℞
(norethindrone acetate tablets, USP)*

*Product of Warner-Lambert Inc

WARNING
THE USE OF PROGESTATIONAL AGENTS DURING THE FIRST FOUR MONTHS OF PREGNANCY IS NOT RECOMMENDED.
Progestational agents have been used beginning with the first trimester of pregnancy in an attempt to prevent habitual abortion or to treat threatened abortion. There is no adequate evidence that such use is effective and there is evidence of potential harm to the fetus when such drugs are given during the first four months of pregnancy. Furthermore, in the vast majority of women, the cause of abortion is a defective ovum, which progestational agents could not be expected to influence. In addition, the use of progestational agents, with their uterine-relaxant properties, in patients with fertilized defective ova may cause a delay in spontaneous abortion. Therefore, the use of such drugs during the first four months of pregnancy is not recommended.
Several reports suggest an association between intrauterine exposure to female sex hormones and congenital anomalies, including congenital heart defects and limb reduction defects.[1–5] One study[4] estimated

a 4.7 fold increased risk of limb reduction defects in infants exposed *in utero* to sex hormones (oral contraceptives, hormone withdrawal test for pregnancy, or attempted treatment for threatened abortion). Some of these exposures were very short and involved only a few days of treatment. The data suggest that the risk of limb reduction defects in exposed fetuses is somewhat less than 1 in 1,000.
If the patient is exposed to Norlutin or Norlutate during the first four months of pregnancy or if she becomes pregnant while taking either of these drugs, she should be apprised of the potential risk to the fetus.

Description: Norlutin is the 17 alpha-ethinyl derivative of 19-nortestosterone. It is a purified crystalline compound that provides orally potent progestational action. The use of norethindrone is indicated in those clinical conditions associated with a deficiency in the secretion of progesterone.
Norlutate is the acetic acid ester of norethindrone, which is the 17 alpha-ethinyl derivative of 19-nortestosterone. The use of norethindrone acetate is indicated in those clinical conditions associated with a deficiency in the secretion of progesterone.
Norethindrone acetate differs from norethindrone only in potency; the acetate is approximately twice as potent.
Actions: Transforms proliferative endometrium into secretory endometrium
Inhibits (at the usual dosage range) the secretion of pituitary gonadotropins, which in turn prevents follicular maturation and ovulation.
May also demonstrate some estrogenic, anabolic, or androgenic activity but should not be relied upon.
Indications: Norlutin and Norlutate are indicated in amenorrhea; in abnormal uterine bleeding due to hormonal imbalance in the absence of organic pathology, such as submucous fibroids or uterine cancer; and in endometriosis.
Contraindications:
1. Thrombophlebitis, thromboembolic disorders, cerebral apoplexy, or patients with a past history of these conditions
2. Known or suspected carcinoma of the breast
3. Undiagnosed vaginal bleeding
4. Missed abortion
5. As a diagnostic test for pregnancy

Warnings:
1. Discontinue medication pending examination if there is a sudden partial or complete loss of vision, or if there is sudden onset of proptosis, diplopia, or migraine. If examination reveals papilledema or retinal vascular lesions, medication should be withdrawn.
2. Detectable amounts of progestogens have been identified in the milk of mothers receiving them. The effect of this on the nursing infant has not been determined.
3. Because of the occasional occurrence of thrombophlebitis and pulmonary embolism in patients taking progestogens, the physician should be alert to the earliest manifestations of the disease.
4. Masculinization of the female fetus has occurred when progestogens have been used in pregnant women.
5. Some beagle dogs treated with medroxyprogesterone acetate developed mammary nodules. Although nodules occasionally appeared in control animals, they were intermittent in nature, whereas nodules in treated animals were larger and more numerous, and persisted. There is no general agreement as to whether the nodules are benign or malignant. Their significance with respect to humans has not been established.

Precautions:
1. The pretreatment physical examination should include special reference to breasts and pelvic organs, as well as a Papanicolaou smear.
2. Because this drug may cause some degree of fluid retention, conditions which might be influenced by this factor, such as epilepsy, migraine, asthma, cardiac or renal dysfunction, require careful observation.
3. In cases of breakthrough bleeding, as in all cases of irregular bleeding per vaginam, nonfunctional causes should be borne in mind. In cases of undiagnosed vaginal bleeding, adequate diagnostic measures are indicated.
4. Patients who have a history of psychic depression should be carefully observed and the drug discontinued if the depression recurs to a serious degree.
5. Any possible influence of prolonged progestogen therapy on pituitary, ovarian, adrenal, hepatic, or uterine functions awaits further study.
6. A decrease in glucose tolerance has been observed in a small percentage of patients on estrogen-progestogen combination drugs. The mechanism of this decrease is obscure. For this reason, diabetic patients should be carefully observed while receiving progestogen therapy.
7. The age of the patient constitutes no absolute limiting factor, although treatment with progestogens may mask the onset of the climacteric.
8. The pathologist should be advised of progestogen therapy when relevant specimens are submitted.
9. Steroid hormones are metabolized by the liver, therefore, these drugs should be administered with caution in patients with impaired liver function.
10. Information for the Patient. See text of Patient Package Insert which is printed following references.

Adverse Reactions: The following adverse reactions have been observed in women taking progestogens.
1. Breakthrough bleeding
2. Spotting
3. Change in menstrual flow
4. Amenorrhea
5. Edema
6. Changes in weight (increase or decrease)
7. Changes in cervical erosion and cervical secretions
8. Cholestatic jaundice
9. Rash (allergic) with and without pruritus
10. Melasma or chloasma
11. Mental depression

The following laboratory result may be altered by the use of progestogens:
Pregnanediol determination.
In addition, the following laboratory results may be altered by the concomitant use of estrogens with progestogens.
1. Hepatic function
2. Coagulation tests: increase in prothrombin, factors VII, VIII, IX, and X
3. Increase in PBI, BEI, and a decrease in T3 uptake
4. Metyrapone test

A statistically significant association has been demonstrated between use of estrogen-progestogen combination drugs and the following serious adverse reactions: thrombophlebitis; pulmonary embolism, and cerebral thrombosis and embolism. For this reason, patients on progestogen therapy should be carefully observed.
Although available evidence is suggestive of an association, such a relationship has been neither confirmed nor refuted for the following serious adverse reactions:
Neuro-ocular lesions, eg, retinal thrombosis and optic neuritis.
The following adverse reactions have been observed in patients receiving estrogen-progestogen combination drugs.
1. Rise in blood pressure in susceptible individuals
2. Premenstrual-like syndrome
3. Changes in libido
4. Changes in appetite
5. Cystitis-like syndrome
6. Headache
7. Nervousness
8. Dizziness
9. Fatigue
10. Backache
11. Hirsutism
12. Loss of scalp hair
13. Erythema multiforme
14. Erythema nodosum
15. Hemorrhagic eruption
16. Itching

In view of these observations, patients on progestogen therapy should be carefully observed for their occurrence.

Dosage and Administration: Norlutin (norethindrone tablets, USP): *Therapy with Norlutin must be adapted to the specific indications and therapeutic response of the individual patient.*
This dosage schedule assumes the interval between menses to be 28 days.
Amenorrhea, abnormal uterine bleeding due to hormonal imbalance in the absence of organic pathology: 5 to 20 mg Norlutin starting with the fifth day of the menstrual cycle and ending on the 25th day.
Endometriosis: Initial daily dosage of 10 mg Norlutin for two weeks with increments of 5 mg per day of Norlutin every two weeks until 30 mg per day of Norlutin is reached. Therapy may be held at this level for from six to nine months or until annoying breakthrough bleeding demands temporary termination.
Norlutate (norethindrone acetate tablets, USP): *Therapy with Norlutate must be adapted to the specific indications and therapeutic response of the individual patient.*
This dosage schedule assumes the interval between menses to be 28 days.
Amenorrhea, abnormal uterine bleeding due to hormonal imbalance in the absence of organic pathology: 2.5 to 10 mg Norlutate starting with the fifth day of the menstrual cycle and ending on the 25th day.
Endometriosis: Initial daily dosage of 5 mg Norlutate for two weeks, with increments of 2.5 mg per day of Norlutate every two weeks until 15 mg per day of Norlutate is reached. Therapy may be held at this level for from six to nine months or until annoying breakthrough bleeding demands temporary termination.
How Supplied: N 0710-0882-19 (Tablet 882)—Norlutin is supplied as 5-mg scored tablets in bottles of 50. **0882G010**
[*Shown in Product Identification Section*]
N 0710-0918-50 (Tablet 918)—Norlutate is supplied as 5-mg scored tablets in bottles of 50.
AHFS 68:32 **0918 G 040**
[*Shown in Product Identification Section*]

PATIENT LABELING FOR PROGESTOGENS
WARNING FOR WOMEN
There is an increased risk of birth defects in children whose mothers take these drugs during the first four months of pregnancy.
Norlutin and Norlutate are similar to the progesterone hormones naturally produced by the body. Progesterone and progesterone-like drugs are used to treat menstrual disorders, to

Continued on next page

This product information was prepared in August, 1982. On these and other Parke-Davis Products, information may be obtained by addressing PARKE-DAVIS, Division of Warner-Lambert Company, Morris Plains, New Jersey 07950.

Parke-Davis—Cont.

test if the body is producing certain hormones, and to treat some forms of cancer in women. These drugs have been used as a test for pregnancy but such use is no longer considered safe because of possible damage to a developing baby. Also, more rapid methods for testing for pregnancy are now available.
These drugs have also been used to prevent miscarriage in the first few months of pregnancy. No adequate evidence is available to show that they are effective for this purpose and there is evidence of an increased risk of birth defects, such as heart or limb defects, if these drugs are taken during the first four months of pregnancy. Furthermore, most cases of early miscarriage are due to causes which could not be helped by these drugs.
The exact risk of taking these drugs early in pregnancy and having a baby with a birth defect is not known. However, one study found that babies born to women who had taken sex hormones (such as progesterone-like drugs) during the first three months of pregnancy were 4 to 5 times more likely to have abnormalities of the arms or legs than if their mothers had not taken such drugs. Some of these women had taken these drugs for only a few days. The chance that an infant whose mother had taken this drug will have this type of defect is about 1 in 1,000.
If you take Norlutin or Norlutate and later find you were pregnant when you took it, be sure to discuss this with your doctor as soon as possible.

OPHTHOCHLOR® ℞
(chloramphenicol ophthalmic solution) 0.5%

Description: Ophthochlor Ophthalmic Solution, 0.5%, is a sterile, buffered solution containing 0.5% (5 mg/ml) of chloramphenicol. It contains no preservatives.
Clinical Pharmacology: Chloramphenicol is a broad-spectrum antibiotic originally isolated from *Streptomyces venezuelae.* It is primarily bacteriostatic and acts by inhibition of protein synthesis by interfering with the transfer of activated amino acids from soluble RNA to ribosomes. It has been noted that chloramphenicol is found in measurable amounts in the aqueous humor following local application to the eye. Development of resistance to chloramphenicol can be regarded as minimal for staphylococci and many other species of bacteria.
Indications and Usage: Ophthochlor (chloramphenicol ophthalmic solution), 0.5%, is indicated for the treatment of superficial ocular infections involving the conjunctiva and/or cornea caused by chloramphenicol-susceptible organisms. Bacteriological studies should be performed to determine the causative organisms and their sensitivity to chloramphenicol.
Contraindication: This product is contraindicated in persons sensitive to any of its components.
Warnings: Bone marrow hypoplasia, including aplastic anemia and death, has been reported following the local application of chloramphenicol.
Precautions: The prolonged use of antibiotics may occasionally result in overgrowth of nonsusceptible organisms, including fungi. If new infections appear during medication, the drug should be discontinued and appropriate measures should be taken. In all except very superficial infections, the topical use of chloramphenicol should be supplemented by appropriate systemic medication.
Adverse Reactions: Blood dyscrasias have been reported in association with the use of chloramphenicol (See WARNINGS).
Dosage and Administration: Two drops applied to the affected eye every three hours, or more frequently if deemed advisable by the prescribing physician. Administration should be continued day and night for the first 48 hours, after which the interval between applications may be increased. Treatment should be continued for at least 48 hours after the eye appears normal.
How Supplied: N 0071-3395-11—15-ml bottles—Ophthochlor Ophthalmic Solution, 0.5%, is supplied in plastic dropper bottles and contains no preservatives. Each ml contains 5 mg chloramphenicol in a boric acid-sodium borate buffer solution. Sodium hydroxide may have been added for adjustment of pH. To protect it from light, the solution should be dispensed in the carton. This product should be stored in a refrigerator until dispensed. Discard solution within 21 days from date dispensed.
AHFS 52:04.04 **3395G010**
[*Shown in Product Identification Section*]

OPHTHOCORT® ℞
(Chloramphenicol-Polymyxin-Hydrocortisone Acetate Ophthalmic Ointment)

Description: Ophthocort® (Chloramphenicol-Polymyxin-Hydrocortisone Acetate Ophthalmic Ointment) is a sterile antibiotic/antiinflammatory ointment for ophthalmic administration. Each gram of Ophthocort contains 10 mg chloramphenicol, 10,000 units polymyxin B (as the sulfate), and 5 mg hydrocortisone acetate in a special base of liquid petrolatum and polyethylene. It contains no preservatives.
Clinical Pharmacology: Corticoids suppress the inflammatory response to a variety of agents and they probably delay or slow healing. Since corticoids may inhibit the body's defense mechanism against infection, a concomitant antimicrobial drug may be used when this inhibition is considered to be clinically significant in a particular case.
The antiinfective components in this combination are included to provide action against specific organisms susceptible to them. Chloramphenicol is considered active against a wide spectrum of gram-negative and gram-positive organisms such as *Escherichia coli, Haemophilus influenzae, Staphylococcus aureus, Streptococcus hemolyticus,* and *Moraxella lacunata* (Morax-Axenfeld bacillus). Development of resistance to chloramphenicol can be regarded as minimal for staphylococci and many other species of bacteria. Chloramphenicol is primarily bacteriostatic and acts by inhibition of protein synthesis by interfering with the transfer of activated amino acids from soluble RNA to ribosomes. It has been noted that chloramphenicol is found in measurable amounts in the aqueous humor following local application to the eye.
Polymyxin B sulfate has a bactericidal action against almost all gram-negative bacilli except the Proteus group. All gram-positive bacteria, fungi, and the gram-negative cocci, *N gonorrhoeae* and *N meningitidis,* are resistant.
When a decision to administer both a corticoid and an antimicrobial is made, the administration of such drugs in combination has the advantage of greater patient compliance and convenience, with the added assurance that the appropriate dosage of both drugs is administered, plus assured compatibility of ingredients when both types of drug are in the same formulation and, particularly, that the correct volume of drug is delivered and retained.
The relative potency of corticosteroids depends on the molecular structure, concentration, and release from the vehicle.
Indications and Usage: For steroid-responsive inflammatory ocular conditions for which a corticosteroid is indicated and where bacterial infection or a risk of bacterial ocular infection exists.
Ocular steroids are indicated in inflammatory conditions of the palpebral and bulbar conjunctiva, cornea, and anterior segment of the globe where the inherent risk of steroid use in certain infective conjunctivitides is accepted to obtain a diminution in edema and inflammation. They are also indicated in chronic anterior uveitis and corneal injury from chemical radiation, thermal burns, or penetration of foreign bodies.
The use of a combination drug with an antiinfective component is indicated where the risk of infection is high or where there is an experience that potentially dangerous numbers of bacteria will be present in the eye.
The particular antiinfective drugs in this product are active against the following common bacterial eye pathogens.
Staphylococcus aureus
Streptococci, including *Streptococcus pneumoniae*
Escherichia coli
Hemophilus influenzae
Klebsiella/Enterobacter species
Neisseria species
Pseudomonas aeruginosa
The product does not provide adequate coverage against:
Serratia marcescens
Contraindications: Epithelial herpes simplex keratitis (dendritic keratitis), vaccinia, varicella, and many other viral diseases of the cornea and conjunctiva. Mycobacterial infection of the eye. Fungal diseases of ocular structures. Hypersensitivity to a component of the medication. (Hypersensitivity to the antibiotic component occurs at a higher rate than for other components.)
The use of these combinations is always contraindicated after uncomplicated removal of a corneal foreign body.
Warnings: Bone marrow hypoplasia including aplastic anemia and death has been reported following the local application of chloramphenicol.
Prolonged use of steroids may result in glaucoma, with damage to the optic nerve, defects in visual acuity and fields of vision, and posterior subcapsular cataract formation. Prolonged use may suppress the host response and thus increase the hazard of secondary ocular infections. In those diseases causing thinning of the cornea or sclera, perforations have been known to occur with the use of topical steroids. In acute purulent conditions of the eye, steroids may mask infection or enhance existing infection. If these products are used for 10 days or longer, intraocular pressure should be routinely monitored even though it may be difficult in children and uncooperative patients.
Employment of steroid medication in the treatment of herpes simplex requires great caution.
Precautions: The initial prescription and renewal of the medication order beyond 8 grams should be made by a physician only after examination of the patient with the aid of magnification, such as slit lamp biomicroscopy and, where appropriate, fluorescein staining.
The possibility of persistent fungal infections of the cornea should be considered after prolonged steroid dosing.
The prolonged use of antibiotics may occasionally result in overgrowth of nonsusceptible organisms, including fungi. If new infections appear during medication, the drug should be discontinued and appropriate measures should be taken.
In all except very superficial infections the topical use of chloramphenicol should be supplemented by appropriate systemic medication.
Adverse Reactions: There have been reports of punctate staining of the cornea following intensive treatment (every one to two hours during the waking day) of corneal ulcers with Ophthocort. In each reported case, the staining has disappeared after discontinuation of the medication.
Blood dyscrasias have been reported in association with the use of chloramphenicol. (See WARNINGS.)

Adverse reactions have occurred with steroid /antiinfective combination drugs which can be attributed to the steroid component, the antiinfective component, or the combination. Exact incidence figures are not available since no denominator of treated patients is available.
Reactions occurring most often from the presence of the antiinfective ingredient are allergic sensitizations. The reactions due to the steroid component in decreasing order of frequency are: elevation of intraocular pressure (IOP) with possible development of glaucoma, and infrequent optic nerve damage; posterior subcapsular cataract formation; and delayed wound healing.
Secondary Infection: The development of secondary infection has occurred after use of combinations containing steroids and antimicrobials. Fungal infections of the cornea are particularly prone to develop coincidentally with long-term applications of steroid. The possibility of fungal invasion must be considered in any persistent corneal ulceration where steroid treatment has been used.
Secondary bacterial ocular infection following suppression of host responses also occurs.
Dosage and Administration: Application of a small amount of ointment, placed in the lower conjunctival sac, is made to the affected eye every three hours, or more frequently if deemed advisable by the prescribing physician. Administration should be continued day and night for the first 48 hours, after which the interval between applications may be increased. Treatment should be continued for at least 48 hours after the eye appears normal.
Not more than 8 grams should be prescribed initially and the prescription should not be refilled without further evaluation as outlined in Precautions above.
How Supplied: N 0071-3079-07 Ophthocort (chloramphenicol-polymyxin-hydrocortisone acetate ophthalmic ointment): Each gram of ointment contains 10 mg chloramphenicol, 10,000 units polymyxin B (as the sulfate), and 5 mg hydrocortisone acetate in a special base of liquid petrolatum and polyethylene. Supplied in 3.5 g tubes.

3079G010
121 887800/10

PAPASE® ℞

(proteolytic enzymes extracted from *Carica papaya*)

Description: Each tablet of Papase contains proteolytic enzymes extracted from *Carica papaya;* the tablet is standardized to 10,000 Warner-Lambert Units of enzyme activity. Tablets may be administered orally or buccally.
Actions: Papase is an anti-inflammatory agent standardized to provide optimal therapeutic activity.

Indications
Based on a review of this drug by the National Academy of Sciences—National Research Council and/or other information, FDA has classified the indications as follows:
"Possibly" effective for relieving symptomatology related to episiotomy.
Final classification of the less-than-effective indications requires further investigation.

Contraindications: Concomitant use with anticoagulants is the only known contraindication. However, it is not recommended in generalized or systemic infections, or in severe disorders of blood clotting, or in patients with a prior allergic reaction to Papase or papain.
Warning—Use in Pregnancy: Safe use of this drug in pregnancy has not been established.
Precautions: This drug should be used with caution in patients with severe renal or hepatic disease.
Adverse Reactions: The incidence of side effects is low. The following reactions have been described: nausea, vomiting, diarrhea, dizziness, pruritus, rash, and urticaria. To date, buccal ulceration has not been observed in patients, even those receiving Papase (proteolytic enzymes extracted from *Carica papaya*) for prolonged periods. An occasional patient, however, has experienced a mild, local tingling at the site of buccal absorption; this sensation usually subsided when the tablet was moved.
Dosage and Administration: Usual Prophylactic Dosage—Two tablets, 1 or 2 hours before episiotomy.
Usual Therapeutic Dosage—Two tablets 4 times a day for at least five days.
Tablets may be administered buccally or orally, swallowed with water, or chewed.
Supplied: Green peppermint-flavored tablets (with desiccant) in bottles of 100 (N 0071-0301-24) and 1000 (N 0071-0301-32).
Standardization — Since anti-inflammatory action is related to proteolytic enzyme activity, Papase has been specially prepared and carefully standardized on this basis. The method used is a milk-clotting assay,[1] the results of which are expressed in Warner-Lambert Units. One Warner-Lambert Unit is that quantity of proteolytic enzymes extracted from *Carica papaya* which, under the conditions specified in the method of assay, will clot 2.64 microliters of milk substrate in 2 minutes at 40° C.
Store between 15° and 30°C (59° and 86°F).
Reference: 1. Hinkle ET Jr, Alford, AC: *Ann. New York Acad. Sc. 54*(2):208, 1951.

[*Shown in Product Identification Section*]

0301 G 010

PARSIDOL® ℞

(Ethopropazine Hydrochloride Tablets, USP)

Description: Parsidol, an orally effective antiparkinsonism drug, is a phenothiazine derivative. The chemical name is: 10H-Phenothiazine-10-ethanamine, N,N-diethyl-α-methyl-,monohydrochloride.
Actions: Among a wide variety of pharmacologic effects, Parsidol exerts significant anticholinergic (para-sympatholytic) actions. Although its specific mode of action in parkinsonism is unknown, it exerts a marked influence upon the neuromuscular symptoms of the disease. Most of the symptoms of parkinsonism —rigidity, spasms, tremors, sialorrhea, oculogyric crises, and festination—will respond to therapy with this drug. Parsidol is one of the drugs effective against tremor; in certain instances, however, rigidity may respond better to treatment than tremor. It is highly effective given alone or in combination with other drugs such as atropine, stramonium, dextroamphetamine, and antihistamines. Combination therapy with appropriate agents increases its efficacy in the control of specific symptoms in extreme cases, e.g., atropine plus Parsidol in refractory oculogyric crises. Unlike other phenothiazine derivatives, Parsidol does not potentiate central nervous system depressants nor does it have an antiemetic action.
Indications: Parsidol is effective as an adjunct in the therapy of all forms of parkinsonism (postencephalitic, idiopathic, and arteriosclerotic). Although chemically a phenothiazine derivative, Parsidol is distinct from other drugs of its class and is useful in the control of extrapyramidal disorders due to central nervous system drugs such as reserpine and phenothiazines.
Contraindications: Glaucoma or prostatic hypertrophy. Hypersensitivity.
Warning: Safety of use during pregnancy and lactation has not been established. This drug should not be used in pregnant patients unless the expected benefits outweigh the potential risk. Patients receiving this drug should be cautioned against hazardous activities requiring complete mental alertness, such as operating machinery or driving a motor vehicle.
Precautions: Use with caution in patients for whom anticholinergic action would be undesirable. Because chronic use may predispose elderly persons toward glaucoma, older patients should be checked periodically for glaucoma.
Antiparkinsonism agents, when used to treat extrapyramidal reactions resulting from phenothiazines or reserpine in patients with mental disorders, may exacerbate mental symptoms and precipitate a toxic psychosis.
Permanent extrapyramidal symptoms have been described with prolonged phenothiazine therapy. The possibility that ethopropazine might mask the development of these symptoms has not been investigated.
Adverse Reactions: The most common side effects reported to occur with Parsidol are drowsiness and cerebral reaction (this latter effect has been described as fogginess, inability to think, lassitude, forgetfulness and confusion). Additional side effects (dryness of mouth, nausea, vomiting, blurring of vision and diplopia, constipation, and urinary retention—signs of the drug's anticholinergic effects) are rarely severe and either disappear as the drug is continued, or diminish when the dose is reduced. Less commonly observed side effects include epigastric discomfort, muscular cramping, paresthesia, a sensation of heaviness of the limbs, skin rash and, following high dosages, mild, transient hypotension. Although Parsidol is different from other drugs of the phenothiazine class, the following side effects are theoretically possible with its use: EEG slowing, seizures, ECG abnormalities (e.g., tachycardia), rare hematologic reactions (agranulocytosis, pancytopenia, purpura), certain endocrinologic disturbances, jaundice, pigmentation of the cornea, lens, retina, or skin, and visual hallucinations.
Dosage: Initial dosage is usually 50 mg once or twice a day, increase gradually if necessary. Patients with mild-to-moderate symptoms are frequently controlled with 100 to 400 mg daily. Severe cases may require further gradual increase to 500 to 600 mg or more daily.
How Supplied:
Parsidol Tablets are supplied as:
N 0071-0320-24 10 mg (white) bottles of 100
N 0071-0321-24 50 mg (white, scored) bottles of 100

0320G010

[*Shown in Product Identification Section*]

PENICILLIN V POTASSIUM, USP ℞

(Penapar VK®)

Description: Penicillin V is the phenoxymethyl analog of penicillin G.
Action and Pharmacology: Penicillin V exerts a bactericidal action against penicillin-sensitive microorganisms during the stage of active multiplication. It acts through the inhibition of biosynthesis of cell wall mucopeptide. It is not active against the penicillinase-producing bacteria, which include many strains of staphylococci. The drug exerts high *in vitro* activity against staphylococci (except penicillinase-producing strains), streptococci (groups A, C, G, H, L, and M), and pneumococci. Other organisms sensitive *in vitro* to penicillin V are *Corynebacterium diphtheriae, Bacillus anthra-*

Continued on next page

This product information was prepared in August, 1982. On these and other Parke-Davis Products, information may be obtained by addressing PARKE-DAVIS, Division of Warner-Lambert Company, Morris Plains, New Jersey 07950.

Parke-Davis—Cont.

cis, Clostridia, *Actinomyces bovis, Streptobacillus moniliformis, Listeria monocytogenes*, Leptospira, and *N gonorrhoeae. Treponema pallidum* is extremely sensitive.

Penicillin V has the distinct advantage over penicillin G in resistance to inactivation by gastric acid. It may be given with meals; however, blood levels are slightly higher when the drug is given on an empty stomach. Average blood levels are two to five times higher than the levels following the same dose of oral penicillin G and also show much less individual variation.

Once absorbed, penicillin V is about 80% bound to serum protein. Tissue levels are highest in the kidneys, with lesser amounts in the liver, skin, and intestines. Small amounts are found in all other body tissues and the cerebrospinal fluid. The drug is excreted as rapidly as it is absorbed in individuals with normal kidney function; however, recovery of the drug from the urine indicates that only about 25% of the dose given is absorbed. In neonates, young infants, and individuals with impaired kidney function, excretion is considerably delayed.

Indications: Penicillin V is indicated in the treatment of mild to moderately severe infections due to penicillin G-sensitive microorganisms that are sensitive to the low serum levels common to this particular dosage form. Therapy should be guided by bacteriologic studies (including sensitivity tests) and by clinical response.

NOTE: Severe pneumonia, empyema, bacteremia, pericarditis, meningitis, and arthritis should not be treated with penicillin V during the acute stage.

Indicated surgical procedures should be performed.

The following infections will usually respond to adequate dosage of penicillin V:

Streptococcal infections (without bacteremia); mild to moderate infections of the upper respiratory tract, scarlet fever, and mild erysipelas

NOTE: Streptococci in groups A, C, G, H, L, and M are very sensitive to penicillin. Other groups, including group D (enterococcus), are resistant.

Pneumococcal infections. Mild to moderately severe infections of the respiratory tract

Staphylococcal infections—penicillin G-sensitive; mild infections of the skin and soft tissues.

NOTE: Reports indicate an increasing number of strains of staphylococci resistant to penicillin G, emphasizing the need for culture and sensitivity studies in treating suspected staphylococcal infections.

Fusospirochetosis (Vincent's gingivitis and pharyngitis); mild to moderately severe infections of the oropharynx usually respond to therapy with oral penicillin.

NOTE: Necessary dental care should be accomplished in infections involving the gum tissue.

Medical conditions in which oral penicillin therapy is indicated as prophylaxis:

For the prevention of recurrence following rheumatic fever and/or chorea: prophylaxis with oral penicillin on a continuing basis has proved effective in preventing recurrence of these conditions.

Although no controlled clinical efficacy studies have been conducted, penicillin V has been suggested by the American Heart Association and the American Dental Association for use as part of a parenteral-oral regimen and as an alternative oral regimen for prophylaxis against bacterial endocarditis in patients with congenital heart disease or rheumatic or other acquired valvular heart disease when they undergo dental procedures and surgical procedures of the respiratory tract.[1] Since it may happen that *alpha* hemolytic streptococci relatively resistant to penicillin may be found when patients are receiving continuous oral penicillin for secondary prevention of rheumatic fever, prophylactic agents other than penicillin may be chosen for these patients and prescribed in addition to their continuous rheumatic fever prophylactic regimen. Oral penicillin should not be used as adjunctive prophylaxis for genitourinary instrumentation or surgery, lower intestinal tract surgery, sigmoidoscopy, and childbirth.

NOTE: When selecting antibiotics for the prevention of bacterial endocarditis, the physician or dentist should read the full joint statement of the American Heart Association and the American Dental Association.[1]

Contraindications: A previous hypersensitivity reaction to any penicillin is a contraindication.

Warning: Serious and occasionally fatal hypersensitivity (anaphylactoid) reactions have been reported in patients on penicillin therapy. Although anaphylaxis is more frequent following parenteral therapy, it has occurred in patients on oral penicillins. These reactions are more apt to occur in individuals with a history of sensitivity to multiple allergens.

There have been well-documented reports of individuals with a history of penicillin hypersensitivity reactions who have experienced severe hypersensitivity reactions when treated with a cephalosporin. Before therapy with a penicillin, careful inquiry should be made concerning previous hypersensitivity reactions to penicillins, cephalosporins, and other allergens. If an allergic reaction occurs, the drug should be discontinued and the patient treated with the usual agents, eg, pressor amines, antihistamines, and corticosteroids.

Precautions: Penicillin should be used with caution in individuals with histories of significant allergies and/or asthma.

The oral route of administration should not be relied upon in patients with severe illness, or with nausea, vomiting, gastric dilatation, cardiospasm, or intestinal hypermotility.

Occasional patients will not absorb therapeutic amounts of orally administered penicillin.

In streptococcal infections, therapy must be sufficient to eliminate the organism (ten days minimum); otherwise, the sequelae of streptococcal disease may occur. Cultures should be taken following completion of treatment to determine whether streptococci have been eradicated.

Prolonged use of antibiotics may promote the overgrowth of nonsusceptible organisms, including fungi. Should superinfection occur, appropriate measures should be taken.

Adverse Reactions: Although the incidence of reactions to oral penicillins has been reported with much less frequency than following parenteral therapy, it should be remembered that all degrees of hypersensitivity, including fatal anaphylaxis, have been reported with oral penicillin.

The most common reactions to oral penicillin are nausea, vomiting, epigastric distress, diarrhea, and black hairy tongue. The hypersensitivity reactions reported are skin eruptions (maculopapular to exfoliative dermatitis), urticaria and other serum sickness reactions, laryngeal edema, and anaphylaxis. Fever and eosinophilia may frequently be the only reaction observed. Hemolytic anemia, leukopenia, thrombocytopenia, neuropathy, and nephropathy are infrequent reactions and usually associated with high doses of parenteral penicillin.

Dosage and Administration: The dosage of penicillin V should be determined according to the sensitivity of the causative microorganisms and the severity of the infection, and adjusted to the clinical response of the patient.

The usual dosage recommendations for adults and children 12 years and over are as follows.

Streptococcal infections—mild to moderately severe—of the upper respiratory tract and including scarlet fever and erysipelas: 125 to 250 mg (200,000 to 400,000 units) every six to eight hours for ten days

Pneumococcal infections—mild to moderately severe—of the respiratory tract, including otitis media: 250 mg (400,000 units) every six hours until the patient has been afebrile for at least two days

Staphylococcal infections—mild infections of skin and soft tissue (culture and sensitivity tests should be performed): 250 mg (400,000 units) every six to eight hours

Fusospirochetosis (Vincent's infection) of the oropharynx—mild to moderately severe infections: 250 mg (400,000 units) every six to eight hours

For the prevention of recurrence following rheumatic fever and/or chorea: 125 mg (200,000 units) twice daily on a continuing basis.

NOTE: Therapy for children under 12 years of age is calculated on the basis of body weight. For infants and small children, the suggested dosage is 15 to 56 mg (25,000 to 90,000 units) per kg per day in three to six divided doses.

For prophylaxis against bacterial endocarditis[1] in patients with congenital heart disease or rheumatic or other acquired valvular heart disease when undergoing dental procedures or surgical procedures of the upper respiratory tract, one of two regimens may be selected:

(1) For the oral regimen, give 2.0 gm of penicillin V (1.0 gm for children under 60 lbs) ½ to 1 hour before the procedure, and then, 500 mg (250 mg for children under 60 lbs) every 6 hours for 8 doses; or

(2) For the combined parenteral-oral regimen give one million units of aqueous crystalline penicillin G (30,000 units/kg in children) intramuscularly mixed with 600,000 units procaine penicillin G (600,000 units for children) ½ to 1 hour before the procedure, and then oral penicillin V, 500 mg for adults or 250 mg for children under 60 lbs, every 6 hours for 8 doses. Doses for children should not exceed recommendations for adults for a single dose or for a 24 hour period.

How Supplied:

Penicillin V Tablets are supplied as:

N 0071-0648-24 250 mg—Bottle of 100.
N 0071-0648-32 250 mg—Bottle of 1000.
N 0071-0648-40 250 mg—Unit dose Package of 100 (10 strips of 10).

Each tablet contains penicillin V potassium equivalent to 250 mg (400,000 units) penicillin V.

N 0071-0673-24 500 mg—Bottle of 100.
N 0071-0673-30 500 mg—Bottle of 500.

Each tablet contains penicillin V potassium equivalent to 500 mg (800,000 units) penicillin V.

[*Shown in Product Identification Section*]

Penicillin V For Oral Solution is supplied as:

N 0071-2449-17 125 mg/5 ml—100 ml individual bottles and packs of six.
N 0071-2449-20 125 mg/5 ml—200 ml individual bottles and packs of six.

When reconstituted according to directions, each 5 ml contains penicillin V potassium equivalent to 125 mg (200,000 units) penicillin V.

N 0071-2506-17 250 mg/5 ml—100 ml individual bottles and packs of six.
N 0071-2506-20 250 mg/5 ml—200 ml individual bottles and packs of six.

When reconstituted according to directions, each 5 ml contains penicillin V potassium equivalent to 250 mg (400,000 units) penicillin V.

Reference:

1. American Heart Association: Prevention of bacterial endocarditis. *Circulation* 56: 139A-143A, 1977.

Manufactured by John D. Copanos Inc., Baltimore, MD 21225 and distributed by Parke-Davis, Warner-Lambert Co, Morris Plains, NJ 07950

AHFS 8:12.16 **7000 G 103**

PERITRATE® SA ℞
(pentaerythritol tetranitrate tablets)
Sustained Action*

PERITRATE® ℞
(pentaerythritol tetranitrate tablets, USP)*
*Product of Warner-Lambert Inc

Description: Peritrate SA Sustained Action 80 mg: each tablet contains pentaerythritol tetranitrate 80 mg (20 mg in the immediate release layer and 60 mg in sustained release base).
Peritrate 40 mg: each tablet contains pentaerythritol tetranitrate 40 mg.
Peritrate 20 mg: each tablet contains pentaerythritol tetranitrate 20 mg.
Peritrate 10 mg: each tablet contains pentaerythritol tetranitrate 10 mg.
Pentaerythritol tetranitrate is a nitric acid ester of a tetrahydric alcohol (pentaerythritol).
Actions: The exact cause of angina pectoris (that is, the pain associated with coronary artery disease) remains obscure, despite the numerous and often conflicting hypotheses concerning its pathophysiology. Therapy at the present time, therefore, remains essentially empirical. Customarily, clinical improvement has been measured by: reduction in (1) number, intensity and duration of angina pectoris attacks and (2) necessity for glyceryl trinitrate intake for prevention or relief of anginal attacks. Peritrate SA (pentaerythritol tetranitrate) Sustained Action and Peritrate (pentaerythritol tetranitrate) have been reported in clinical usage to reduce in number and severity the incidence of angina pectoris attacks, with concomitant reduction in glyceryl trinitrate intake.
In the evaluation of Peritrate and Peritrate SA in angina pectoris, clinical improvement has been customarily measured subjectively by: reduction in number and severity of attacks and necessity for glyceryl trinitrate intake for prevention or abortion of anginal attacks. Individual patterns of angina pectoris differ widely as does the symptomatic response to antianginal agents such as pentaerythritol tetranitrate. The published literature contains both favorable and unfavorable clinical reports. In conjunction with total management of the patient with angina pectoris, Peritrate and Peritrate SA have been accepted as safe for prolonged administration and widely regarded as useful.

Indications
Based on a review of this drug by the National Academy of Sciences—National Research Council and/or other information, FDA has classified the indications as follows:
"Possibly" effective: Peritrate is indicated for the relief of angina pectoris (pain associated with coronary artery disease). It is not intended to abort the acute anginal episode but is widely regarded as useful in the prophylactic treatment of angina pectoris.
Final classification of the less-than-effective indications requires further investigation.

Contraindications: Peritrate SA and Peritrate are contraindicated in patients who have a history of sensitivity to the drug.
Warnings: Data supporting the use of Peritrate or Peritrate SA during the early days of the acute phase of myocardial infarction (the period during which clinical and laboratory findings are unstable) are insufficient to establish safety.
This drug can act as a physiological antagonist to norepinephrine, acetylcholine, histamine, and many other agents.
Precautions: Should be used with caution in patients who have glaucoma. Tolerance to this drug and cross-tolerance to other nitrites and nitrates may occur.
Adverse Reactions: Side effects reported to date have been predominantly related to rash (which requires discontinuation of medication) and headache and gastrointestinal distress, which are usually mild and transient with continuation of medication. In some cases severe persistent headaches may occur. In addition, the following adverse reactions to nitrates such as pentaerythritol tetranitrate have been reported in the literature:
(a) Cutaneous vasodilatation with flushing.
(b) Transient episodes of dizziness and weakness, as well as other signs of cerebral ischemia associated with postural hypotension, may occasionally develop.
(c) An occasional individual exhibits marked sensitivity to the hypotensive effects of nitrite and severe responses (nausea, vomiting, weakness, restlessness, pallor, perspiration and collapse) can occur, even with the usual therapeutic doses. Alcohol may enhance this effect.

Dosage: Peritrate may be administered in individualized doses up to 160 mg a day. Dosage can be initiated at one 10 mg or 20 mg tablet q.i.d. and titrated upward to 40 mg (two 20 mg tablets or one 40 mg tablet) q.i.d. one-half hour before or one hour after meals and at bedtime. Tablets can be chewed or swallowed whole. Alternatively, Peritrate SA can be administered on a convenient b.i.d. (on an empty stomach) dosage schedule. One tablet immediately on arising and 1 tablet 12 hours later. Tablets should not be chewed.
Supplied:
Peritrate SA Sustained Action 80 mg—double layer, biconvex, dark green/light green tablets in bottles of 100 (N 0710-0004-24) and 1000 (N 0710-0004-32).
[*Shown in Product Identification Section*]
Also in unit dose package of 10 × 10 strips (N 0710-0004-40).
Peritrate 40 mg—coral scored tablets in bottles of 100 (N 0710-0008-24).
[*Shown in Product Identification Section*]
Peritrate 20 mg—light green, scored tablets in bottles of 100 (N 0710-0001-24) and 1000 (N 0710-0001-32).
[*Shown in Product Identification Section*]
Also in unit dose package of 10 × 10 strips (N 0710-0001-40).
Peritrate 10 mg—light green, unscored tablets in bottles of 100 (N 0710-0013-24) and 1000 (N 0710-0013-32).
[*Shown in Product Identification Section*]
Animal Pharmacology: In a series of carefully designed studies in pigs, Peritrate was administered for 48 hours before an artificially induced occlusion of a major coronary artery and for seven days thereafter. The pigs were sacrificed at various intervals for periods up to six weeks. The result showed a significantly larger number of survivors in the drug-treated group. Damage to myocardial tissue in the drug-treated survivors was less extensive than in the untreated group. Studies in dogs subjected to oligemic shock through progressive bleeding have demonstrated that Peritrate is vasoactive at the postarteriolar level, producing increased blood flow and better tissue perfusion. These animal experiments cannot be translated to the drug's actions in humans.
0004G010/0001G010

PITOCIN® ℞
(oxytocin injection, USP) synthetic

IMPORTANT NOTICE
Pitocin is not indicated for the elective induction of labor because available data and information are inadequate to define the benefits-to-risks considerations in the use of the drug product. Elective induction of labor is defined as the initiation of labor in an individual with a term pregnancy who is free of medical indications for the initiation of labor.

Description: Pitocin (oxytocin injection, USP) is a sterile, aqueous solution of synthetic oxytocic hormone standardized to contain 10 units/ml and containing 0.5% Chloretone® (chlorobutanol) (chloroform derivative) as a preservative, with the acidity adjusted with acetic acid. The drug is prepared synthetically to avoid possible contamination with vasopressin (ADH) and its antidiuretic and cardiovascular effects. However, the physician should be cognizant of the fact that even highly purified synthetic oxytocin contains inherent pressor-antidiuretic properties which may become manifest following administration of large doses (see Precautions).
Action: Uterine motility is controlled by a variety of biochemical and regulatory processes. Oxytocin appears to act primarily on uterine myofibril activity by increasing the permeability of the cell membranes to sodium ions, thus augmenting the number of contracting myofibrils, and thereby enabling the uterus to produce the necessary number of contractions. The effect depends on the uterine threshold of excitability. The sensitivity of the uterus to oxytocin increases gradually during gestation; then increases sharply before parturition.
Indications: Antepartum: Pitocin is indicated for the initiation or improvement of uterine contractions, where this is desirable and considered suitable, for the following purposes: induction of labor in patients with a medical indication for the initiation of labor, such as mild preeclampsia at or near term, when delivery is in the best interest of mother and fetus or when membranes are prematurely ruptured and delivery is indicated; stimulation or reinforcement of labor, as in selected cases of uterine inertia; as adjunctive therapy in the management of incomplete or inevitable abortion. In the first trimester, curettage is generally considered primary therapy. In second trimester abortion, oxytocin infusion will often be successful in emptying the uterus. Other means of therapy, however, may be required in such cases.
Postpartum: Pitocin is indicated to produce uterine contractions during the third stage of labor and to control postpartum bleeding or hemorrhage.
Contraindications: Pitocin is contraindicated in any of the following conditions: significant cephalopelvic disproportion; unfavorable fetal positions or presentations which are undeliverable without conversion prior to delivery (as, for example, transverse lies); in obstetrical emergencies where the benefit-to-risk ratio for either the fetus or the mother favors surgical intervention; in cases of fetal distress where delivery is not imminent; prolonged use in uterine inertia or severe toxemia; hypertonic uterine patterns; patients with hypersensitivity to the drug; induction or augmentation of labor in those cases where vaginal delivery is contraindicated, such as invasive cervical carcinoma, cord presentation or prolapse, total placentia previa, and vasa previa.
Warnings: Pitocin, when given for induction or stimulation of labor, must be administered only by the intravenous route and with adequate medical supervision in a hospital.

Continued on next page

This product information was prepared in August, 1982. On these and other Parke-Davis Products, information may be obtained by addressing PARKE-DAVIS, Division of Warner-Lambert Company, Morris Plains, New Jersey 07950.

Parke-Davis—Cont.

Precautions:
1. All patients receiving intravenous oxytocin must be under continuous observation by trained personnel with a thorough knowledge of the drug and qualified to identify complications. A physician qualified to manage any complications should be immediately available.
2. When properly administered, oxytocin should stimulate uterine contractions comparable to those seen in normal labor. Overstimulation of the uterus by improper administration can be hazardous to both mother and fetus. Even with proper administration and adequate supervision, hypertonic contractions can occur in patients whose uteri are hypersensitive to oxytocin. This fact must be considered by the physician in exercising judgment regarding patient selection.
3. Except in unusual circumstances, oxytocin should not be administered in the following conditions: fetal distress, partial placenta previa, prematurity, borderline cephalopelvic disproportion, and in any conditions where there is a predisposition for uterine rupture, such as previous major surgery on the cervix or uterus including cesarean section, overdistention of the uterus, grand multiparity, or past history of uterine sepsis or of traumatic delivery. Because of the variability of the combinations of factors which may be present in the conditions listed above, the definition of "unusual circumstances" must be left to the judgment of the physician. The decision can only be made by carefully weighing the potential benefits which oxytocin can provide in a given case against rare but definite potential for the drug to produce hypertonicity or tetanic spasm.
4. Maternal deaths due to hypertensive episodes, subarachnoid hemorrhage, rupture of the uterus, and fetal deaths due to various causes have been reported associated with the use of parenteral oxytocic drugs for induction of labor or for augmentation in the first and second stages of labor.
5. Oxytocin has been shown to have an intrinsic antidiuretic effect, acting to increase water reabsorption from the glomerular filtrate. Consideration should, therefore, be given to the possibility of water intoxication, particularly when oxytocin is administered continuously by infusion and the patient is receiving fluids by mouth.
6. When oxytocin is used for induction or reinforcement of already existent labor, patients should be carefully selected. Pelvic adequacy must be considered and maternal and fetal conditions evaluated before use of the drug.

Adverse Reactions: Fetal bradycardia, anaphylactic reaction, postpartum hemorrhage, cardiac arrhythmia, and pelvic hematoma have been reported.

Excessive dosage or hypersensitivity to the drug may result in uterine hypertonicity, spasm, tetanic contraction, or rupture.

Side effects that may also occur during spontaneous labor, such as nausea, vomiting, and premature ventricular contractions, have been noted occasionally with oxytocin.

A fatality due to afibrinogenemia has been reported, naming oxytocin injection as a possible cause. The possibility of increased blood loss and afibrinogenemia should be kept in mind when administering the drug.

Severe water intoxication with convulsions and coma has occurred, associated with a slow oxytocin infusion over a 24-hour period. Maternal death due to oxytocin-induced water intoxication has been reported.

Dosage and Administration: Dosage of oxytocin is determined by uterine response. The following dosage information is based upon the various regimens and indications in general use.

A. Induction or Stimulation of Labor

Intravenous infusion (drip method) is the only acceptable method of parenteral administration for the induction or stimulation of labor. Accurate control of the rate of infusion flow is essential. An infusion pump or other such device and at least external electronic monitoring are necessary for the safe administration of oxytocin for the induction or stimulation of labor. If uterine contractions become too powerful, the infusion can be abruptly stopped, and oxytocic stimulation of the uterine musculature will soon wane.
1. An intravenous infusion of non-oxytocin containing solution should be started. (Physiologic electrolyte solution should be used.)
2. To prepare the standard solution for infusion, the contents of one 1-ml ampoule is combined aseptically with 1,000 ml of 0.9% aqueous sodium chloride solution or other nonhydrating diluent. The combined solution (1 ml=10 milliunits) is rotated in the infusion bottle to insure thorough mixing. Add the container with dilute oxytocic solution to the system through use of a constant infusion pump.
3. The initial dose should be 1 to 2 mU/minute. At 15 to 30 minute intervals, the dose should be gradually increased in increments of 1 to 2 mU/minute until the desired contraction pattern has been established, which should be comparable to that seen in normal labor.
4. The fetal heart rate, resting uterine tone, and the frequency, duration, and force of contractions should be monitored.
5. The oxytocin infusion should be discontinued immediately in the event of uterine hyperactivity or fetal distress. Oxygen should be administered to the mother. The mother and the fetus must be evaluated by the responsible physician.

B. Control of Postpartum Uterine Bleeding

1. Intravenous Infusion (Drip Method)

To control postpartum bleeding, 10 to 40 units of oxytocin may be added to 1,000 ml of 5% dextrose injection and run at a rate necessary to control uterine atony.

Intramuscular Administration

1 ml (10 units) of oxytocin can be given after delivery of the placenta.

C. Treatment of Incomplete or Inevitable Abortion:

Intravenous infusion with physiologic saline solution, 500 ml, or 5% dextrose in physiologic saline solution to which 10 units of Pitocin have been added should be infused at a rate of 10 to 20 milliunits (20 to 40 drops) per minute.

How Supplied: N 0071-4160-02 (Ampoule 163)
Contains 5 units in a 0.5-ml ampoule, packages of ten
N 0071-4160-03 (Ampoule 160)
Contains 10 units in a 1-ml ampoule, packages of ten
N 0071-4160-40 (Steri-Dose® syringe 1489)
Contains 10 units in a 1-ml sterile disposable syringe, packages of ten
N 0071-4160-10 (Steri-Vial® 1541)
Contains 10 units per milliliter in a 10-ml Steri-Vial (multiple dose vial)
AHFS 76:00 **121 858950/60**
4160 G060

PITRESSIN™ ℞

(vasopressin injection, USP)
synthetic

Description: Pitressin (vasopressin injection) is a sterile, aqueous solution of synthetic vasopressin (8-arginine vasopressin) of the posterior pituitary gland. It is substantially free from the oxytocic principle and is standardized to contain 20 pressor units/ml. The solution contains 0.5% Chloretone® (chlorobutanol) (chloroform derivative) as a preservative. The acidity of the solution is adjusted with acetic acid.

Action: The antidiuretic action of vasopressin is ascribed to increasing reabsorption of water by the renal tubules.

Vasopressin can cause contraction of smooth muscle of the gastrointestinal tract and of all parts of the vascular bed, especially the capillaries, small arterioles and venules, with less effect on the smooth musculature of the large veins. The direct effect on the contractile elements is neither antagonized by adrenergic blocking agents nor prevented by vascular denervation.

Contraindication: Anaphylaxis or hypersensitivity to the drug or its components.

Indications: Pitressin is indicated for prevention and treatment of postoperative abdominal distention, in abdominal roentgenography to dispel interfering gas shadows, and in diabetes insipidus.

Warnings: This drug should not be used in patients with vascular disease, especially disease of the coronary arteries, except with extreme caution. In such patients, even small doses may precipitate anginal pain, and with larger doses, the possibility of myocardial infarction should be considered.

Vasopressin may produce water intoxication. The early signs of drowsiness, listlessness, and headaches should be recognized to prevent terminal coma and convulsions.

Precautions: Vasopressin should be used cautiously in the presence of epilepsy, migraine, asthma, heart failure, or any state in which a rapid addition to extracellular water may produce hazard for an already overburdened system.

Chronic nephritis with nitrogen retention contraindicates the use of vasopressin until reasonable nitrogen blood levels have been attained.

Adverse Reactions: Local or systemic allergic reactions may occur in hypersensitive individuals. The following side effects have been reported following the administration of vasopressin: tremor, sweating, vertigo, circumoral pallor, "pounding" in head, abdominal cramps, passage of gas, nausea, vomiting, urticaria, bronchial constriction. Anaphylaxis (cardiac arrest and/or shock) has been observed shortly after injection of vasopressin.

Dosage and Administration: Pitressin may be administered subcutaneously or intramuscularly.

Ten units of Pitressin (0.5 ml) will usually elicit full physiologic response in adult patients; 5 units will be adequate in many cases. Pitressin should be given intramuscularly at three- or four-hour intervals as needed. The dosage should be proportionately reduced for children. (For an additional discussion of dosage, consult the sections below).

When determining the dose of Pitressin for a given case, the following should be kept in mind.

It is particularly desirable to give a dose not much larger than is just sufficient to elicit the desired physiologic response. Excessive doses may cause undesirable side actions—blanching of the skin, abdominal cramps, nausea—which, though not serious, may be alarming to the patient. Spontaneous recovery from such side actions occurs in a few minutes. It has been found that one or two glasses of water given at the time Pitressin is administered reduces such symptoms.

Abdominal Distention: In the average postoperative adult patient, give 5 units (0.25 ml) initially; increase to 10 units (0.5 ml) at subsequent injections if necessary. It is recommended that Pitressin be given intramuscularly and that injections be repeated at three- or four-hour intervals as required. Dosage to be reduced proportionately for children.

Pitressin used in this manner will frequently prevent, or relieve, postoperative distention. These recommendations apply also to distention complicating pneumonia or other acute toxemias.

Abdominal Roentgenography: For the average case, two injections of 10 units each (0.5 ml) are suggested. These should be given two hours and one half hour, respectively, before films are exposed. Many roentgenologists advise giving an enema prior to the first dose of Pitressin.

Diabetes Insipidus: Pitressin may be given by injection or administered intranasally on cotton pledgets, by nasal spray, or by dropper. The dose by injection is 5 to 10 units (0.25 to 0.5 ml) repeated two or three times daily as needed. When Pitressin is administered intranasally by spray or on pledgets, the dosage and interval between treatments must be determined for each patient.

How Supplied: *Pitressin (vasopressin injection, USP) synthetic is supplied in ampoules as follows.*

N 0071-4200-02
0.5 ml (10 pressor units). Packages of 10
N 0071-4200-03
1 ml (20 pressor units). Packages of 10

Note: When ordering Pitressin Ampoules, Synthetic, be sure to state whether the 10- or 20-unit is desired. **121 885550/YG**

PITRESSIN® TANNATE IN OIL ℞
(vasopressin tannate)
FOR INTRAMUSCULAR USE ONLY

Description: Pitressin Tannate (vasopressin tannate) is a water-insoluble chemical compound of vasopressin, the pressor fraction of the posterior lobe of the pituitary gland, and tannic acid.

Action: The antidiuretic action of vasopressin tannate is ascribed to increasing reabsorption of water by the renal tubules.

Vasopressin can cause contraction of smooth muscle of the gastrointestinal tract and of all parts of the vascular bed, especially the capillaries, small arterioles, and venules, with less effect on the smooth musculature of the large veins. These effects are ordinarily not seen to a significant degree with recommended antidiuretic doses of vasopressin tannate. The direct effect on the contractile elements is neither antagonized by adrenergic blocking agents nor prevented by vascular denervation.

Indications: Pitressin Tannate in Oil is indicated for the control or prevention of the symptoms and complications of diabetes insipidus due to a deficiency of endogenous posterior pituitary antidiuretic hormone.

Contraindication: Anaphylaxis or hypersensitivity to the drug or its components.

Warnings:

This preparation should never be administered intravenously.

This drug should not be used in patients with vascular disease, especially disease of the coronary arteries, except with extreme caution. In such patients, even small doses may precipitate anginal pain.

Vasopressin may produce water intoxication. The early signs of drowsiness, listlessness, and headaches should be recognized to prevent terminal coma and convulsions.

Precautions: Vasopressin should be used cautiously in the presence of epilepsy, migraine, asthma, heart failure, or any state in which a rapid addition to extracellular water may produce hazard for an already overburdened system.

Chronic nephritis with nitrogen retention contraindicates the use of vasopressin until reasonable nitrogen blood levels have been attained.

Adverse Reactions: Local or systemic allergic reactions may occur in hypersensitive individuals. The following side effects have been reported following the administration of vasopressin: tremor, sweating, vertigo, circumoral pallor, "pounding" in head, abdominal cramps, passage of gas, nausea, vomiting, urticaria, bronchial constriction, anaphylaxis, cardiac arrest.

Dosage and Administration: Intramuscular —0.3 to 1 ml repeated as required. The duration of action varies with the patient and his condition, and may be as prolonged as 48 to 96 hours.

How Supplied:

N 0071-4302-03 (Ampoule 302)

Pitressin Tannate in Oil is supplied as a suspension containing 5 pressor units per ml in peanut oil, in 1-ml ampoules, packages of 10.

AHFS 68:28 **4302G040**
121 864700/40

PONSTEL® ℞
(mefenamic acid)

Description: Ponstel (mefenamic acid) is N-(2,3-xylyl)-anthranilic acid. It is an analgesic agent for oral administration. Ponstel is available in capsules containing 250 mg of mefenamic acid.

It is a white powder with a melting point of 230–231° C, molecular weight 241.28, and water solubility of 0.004% at pH 7.1.

Clinical Pharmacology: Ponstel is a nonsteroidal agent with demonstrated antiinflammatory, analgesic, and antipyretic activity in laboratory animals.[1,2] The mode of action is not known. In animal studies, Ponstel was found to inhibit prostaglandin synthesis and to compete for binding at the prostaglandin receptor site.[3] Pharmacologic studies show Ponstel did not relieve morphine abstinence signs in abstinent, morphine-habituated monkeys.[1]

Following a single 1-gram oral dose, peak plasma levels of 10 µg/ml occurred in 2 to 4 hours with a half-life of 2 hours. Following multiple doses, plasma levels are proportional to dose with no evidence of drug accumulation. One gram of Ponstel given four times daily produces peak blood levels of 20 µg/ml by the second day of administration.[4]

Following a single dose, sixty-seven percent of the total dose is excreted in the urine as unchanged drug or as one of two metabolites. Twenty to twenty-five percent of the dose is excreted in the feces during the first three days.[4]

In controlled, double-blind, clinical trials, Ponstel was evaluated for the treatment of primary spasmodic dysmenorrhea. The parameters used in determining efficacy included pain assessment by both patient and investigator; the need for concurrent analgesic medication; and evaluation of change in frequency and severity of symptoms characteristic of spasmodic dysmenorrhea. Patients received either Ponstel, 500 mg (2 capsules) as an initial dose and 250 mg every 6 hours, or placebo at onset of bleeding or of pain, whichever began first. After three menstrual cycles, patients were crossed over to the alternate treatment for an additional three cycles. Ponstel was significantly superior to placebo in all parameters, and both treatments (drug and placebo) were equally tolerated.

Indications and Usage: Ponstel is indicated for the relief of moderate pain[5] when therapy will not exceed one week. Ponstel is also indicated for the treatment of primary dysmenorrhea.[5,6]

Studies in children under 14 years of age have been inadequate to evaluate the safety and effectiveness of Ponstel.

Contraindications: Ponstel should not be used in patients who have previously exhibited hypersensitivity to it.

Because the potential exists for cross-sensitivity to aspirin or other nonsteroidal antiinflammatory drugs, Ponstel should not be given to patients in whom these drugs induce symptoms of bronchospasm, allergic rhinitis, or urticaria.

Ponstel is contraindicated in patients with active ulceration or chronic inflammation of either the upper or lower gastrointestinal tract.

Ponstel should be avoided in patients with preexisting renal disease.

Warnings: In patients with a history of ulceration or chronic inflammation of the upper or lower gastrointestinal tract, Ponstel should be given under close supervision and only after consulting the Adverse Reactions Section.

If diarrhea occurs, the dosage should be reduced or temporarily suspended (see Adverse Reactions and Dosage and Administration). Certain patients who develop diarrhea may be unable to tolerate the drug because of recurrence of the symptoms on subsequent exposure.

Precautions: If rash occurs, administration of the drug should be stopped.

A false-positive reaction for urinary bile, using the diazo tablet test, may result after mefenamic acid administration. If biliuria is suspected, other diagnostic procedures, such as the Harrison spot test, should be performed.

In chronic animal toxicity studies of Ponstel at doses 7 to 28 times the recommended human dose, rats had minor microscopic renal papillary necrosis, dogs had edema and blunting of the renal papilla, and monkeys had renal papillary edema.[5] Normal human volunteers had mild BUN elevations with prolonged administration at greater than therapeutic doses.[5] The significance of these findings is unknown. However, since Ponstel is eliminated primarily through the kidneys,[4] the drug should not be administered to patients with significantly impaired renal function.

Information for Patients: Patients should be advised that if rash, diarrhea or other digestive problems arise, they should stop the drug and consult their physician.

Patients in whom aspirin or other nonsteroidal antiinflammatory drugs induce symptoms of bronchospasm, allergic rhinitis, or urticaria should be made aware that the potential exists for cross-sensitivity to Ponstel.

The long-term effects, if any, of intermittent Ponstel therapy for dysmenorrhea are not known. Women on such therapy should consult their physician if they should decide to become pregnant.

Drug Interactions: Ponstel may prolong prothrombin time.[5] Therefore, when the drug is administered to patients receiving oral anticoagulant drugs, frequent monitoring of prothrombin time is necessary.

Use in Pregnancy: Pregnancy Category C. Reproduction studies have been performed in rats, rabbits and dogs. Rats given up to 10 times the human dose showed decreased fertility, delay in parturition, and a decreased rate of survival to weaning. Rabbits at 2.5 times the human dose showed an increase in the number of resorptions. There were no fetal anomalies observed in these studies nor in dogs at up to 10 times the human dose.[5]

There are no adequate and well-controlled studies in pregnant women. Because animal reproduction studies are not always predictive of human response, this drug should be used only if clearly needed.

The use of Ponstel in late pregnancy is not recommended because of the effects on the fetal cardiovascular system of drugs of this class.

Nursing Mothers: Trace amounts of Ponstel may be present in breast milk and transmitted to the nursing infant[7]; thus Ponstel should not be taken by the nursing mother because of the effects on the infant cardiovascular system of drugs of this class.

Continued on next page

This product information was prepared in August, 1982. On these and other Parke-Davis Products, information may be obtained by addressing PARKE-DAVIS, Division of Warner-Lambert Company, Morris Plains, New Jersey 07950.

Parke-Davis—Cont.

Use in Children: Safety and effectiveness in children below the age of 14 have not been established.

Adverse Reactions:

Gastrointestinal: The most frequently reported adverse reactions associated with the use of Ponstel involve the gastrointestinal tract. In controlled studies for up to eight months, the following disturbances were reported in decreasing order of frequency: diarrhea (approximately 5% of patients), nausea with or without vomiting, other gastrointestinal symptoms, and abdominal pain.

In certain patients, the diarrhea was of sufficient severity to require discontinuation of medication. The occurrence of the diarrhea is usually dose related, generally subsides on reduction of dosage, and rapidly disappears on termination of therapy.

Other gastrointestinal reactions less frequently reported were anorexia, pyrosis, flatulence, and constipation.

Gastrointestinal ulceration with and without hemorrhage has been reported.

Hematopoietic: Cases of autoimmune hemolytic anemia have been associated with the continuous administration of Ponstel for 12 months or longer. In such cases the Coombs test results are positive with evidence of both accelerated RBC production and RBC destruction. The process is reversible upon termination of Ponstel administration.

Decreases in hematocrit have been noted in 2–5% of patients and primarily in those who have received prolonged therapy. Leukopenia, eosinophilia, thrombocytopenic purpura, agranulocytosis, pancytopenia, and bone marrow hypoplasia have also been reported on occasion.

Nervous System: Drowsiness, dizziness, nervousness, headache, blurred vision, and insomnia have occurred.

Integumentary: Urticaria, rash, and facial edema have been reported.

Renal: As with other nonsteroidal antiinflammatory agents, renal failure, including papillary necrosis, has been reported. In elderly patients renal failure has occurred after taking Ponstel for 2–6 weeks. The renal damage may not be completely reversible. Hematuria and dysuria have also been reported with Ponstel.

Other: Eye irritation, ear pain, perspiration, mild hepatic toxicity, and increased need for insulin in a diabetic have been reported. There have been rare reports of palpitation, dyspnea, and reversible loss of color vision.

Overdosage: Although doses up to 6000 mg/day have been given, no specific information is available on the management of acute massive overdosage.

Should accidental overdosage occur, the stomach should be emptied by inducing emesis or by careful gastric lavage followed by the administration of activated charcoal.[8] Laboratory studies indicate that Ponstel should be adsorbed from the gastrointestinal tract by activated charcoal.[4] Vital functions should be monitored and supported. Because mefenamic acid and its metabolities are firmly bound to plasma proteins, hemodialysis and peritoneal dialysis may be of little value.[4]

Dosage and Administration: Administration is by the oral route, preferably with food. The recommended regimen in acute pain for adults and children over 14 years of age is 500 mg as an initial dose followed by 250 mg every six hours as needed, usually not to exceed one week.[5]

For the treatment of primary dysmenorrhea, the recommended dosage is 500 mg as an initial dose followed by 250 mg every 6 hours, starting with the onset of bleeding and associated symptoms. Clinical studies indicate that effective treatment can be initiated with the start of menses and should not be necessary for more than 2 to 3 days.[6]

How Supplied: N 0710-0540-24 (P-D 540) Ponstel (mefenamic acid) is available as 250 mg capsules in bottles of 100.

References:

1. Winder CV, et al: Antiinflammatory, antipyretic and antinociceptive properties of N-(2,3-xylyl) anthranilic acid (mefenamic acid). *J Pharmacol Exp Ther* 138: 405–413, 1962.
2. Wax J, et al: Comparative activities, tolerances and safety of nonsteroidal antiinflammatory agents in rats. *J Pharmacol Exp Ther* 192: 172–178, 1975.
3. Ferreira SH, Vane JR: Aspirin and prostaglandins, in *The Prostaglandins,* Ramwell PW Ed, Plenum Press, NY, vol. 2, 1974, pp 1–47.
4. Glazko AJ: Experimental observations of flufenamic, mefenamic, and meclofenamic acids. Part III. Metabolic disposition, in *Fenamates in Medicine.* A Symposium, London 1966; *Annals of Physical Medicine,* supplement, pp 23–36, 1967.
5. Data on file, Medical Affairs Dept, Parke-Davis.
6. Budoff PW: Use of mefenamic acid in the treatment of primary dysmenorrhea. *JAMA* 241: 2713–2716, 1979.
7. Buchanan RA, et al: The breast milk excretion of mefenamic acid. *Curr Ther Res* 10:592, 1968.
8. Corby DG, Decker WJ: Management of acute poisoning with activated charcoal. *Pediatrics* 54:324, 1974.

Direct Medical Inquiries to: Parke-Davis
Div of Warner-Lambert Inc, 201 Tabor Road
Morris Plains, NJ 07950
Att: Medical Affairs Department

0540G012

POVAN® FILMSEAL® ℞

(pyrvinium pamoate tablets, USP)*

*Product of Warner-Lambert Inc

Description: Pyrvinium pamoate, a cyanine dye, is 6-dimethylamino-2-(2-[2, 5-dimethyl-1-phenyl-3-pyrrolyl] - vinyl) -1- methylquinolinium as the pamoate. It is a deep red crystalline powder which is stable to heat, light, and air, and is practically insoluble in water.

Actions: Pyrvinium pamoate appears to exert its anthelmintic effect by preventing the parasite from using exogenous carbohydrates. The parasite's endogenous reserves are depleted, and it dies. Povan is not appreciably absorbed from the gastrointestinal tract.

Indication: Povan is indicated for the treatment of enterobiasis.

Warnings: No animal or human reproduction studies have been performed. Therefore, the use of this drug during pregnancy requires that the potential benefits be weighed against its possible hazards to the mother and fetus.

Precautions: To forestall undue concern and help avoid accidental staining, patients and parents should be advised of the staining properties of Povan. Tablets should be swallowed whole to avoid staining of teeth. Parents and patients should be informed that pyrvinium pamoate will color the stool a bright red. This is not harmful to the patient. If emesis occurs, the vomitus will probably be colored red and will stain most materials.

Adverse Reactions: Nausea, vomiting, cramping, diarrhea, and hypersensitivity reactions (photosensitization and other allergic reactions) have been reported. The gastrointestinal reactions occur more often in older children and adults who have received large doses. Emesis is more frequently seen with Povan Suspension than with Povan Filmseals.

Dosage and Administration: For control of pinworm infections in children and adults, Povan is administered orally in a single dose of 5 mg pyrvinium per kilogram body weight. If necessary, the dose may be repeated in two or three weeks.

Pinworm infection can pass easily from person to person by transfer of eggs through direct contact, handling contaminated objects, and breathing airborne eggs in dust. Therefore, if an infection is detected in any member of a family or institution group, treatment of all members should be considered for complete parasite eradication.

Dosage may be conveniently determined by referring to the Table.

Povan (pyrvinium pamoate): Dosage Table

BODY WEIGHT lb	kg	DOSAGE (Number of Tablets)
154*	70	7
143	65	7
132	60	6
121	55	6
110	50	5
99	45	5
88	40	4
77	35	4
66	30	3
55	25	3
44	20	2
33	15	2

*Because the gastrointestinal tract of adults does not appreciably increase in size with increased weight gain, the dosage for adults need not exceed that recommended for a patient weighing 154 lb. A single dose of seven tablets should be adequate for patients who weigh more than 154 lb.

How Supplied:

N 0710-0747-19 (Tablet 747)—Each Povan Filmseal contains pyrvinium pamoate equivalent to 50 mg pyrvinium. Supplied in bottles of 50.

[*Shown in Product Identification Section*]

NSN: 6505-00-890-1093

AHFS 8:08 **0747 G 050**

PROCAN® SR ℞

(procainamide hydrochloride tablets)
SUSTAINED RELEASE

> The prolonged administration of procainamide often leads to the development of a positive antinuclear antibody (ANA) test with or without symptoms of lupus erythematosus-like syndrome. If a positive ANA titer develops, the benefit/risk ratio related to continued procainamide therapy should be assessed. This may necessitate consideration of alternative antiarrhythmic therapy.

Description: Procan SR is an antiarrhythmic drug. Each tablet of Procan SR contains procainamide hydrochloride in a tablet matrix specially designed for the prolonged release of the drug in the gastrointestinal tract. Following release of the drug, the expended wax tablet matrix, which is not absorbed, may be detected in the stool. Procan SR is available for oral administration as green, film-coated tablets containing 250 mg procainamide hydrochloride; as yellow, scored, film-coated tablets containing 500 mg procainamide hydrochloride; and as orange scored film-coated tablets containing 750 mg procainamide hydrochloride.

Procainamide hydrochloride is the amide analogue of procaine hydrochloride. The chemical name is 4-amino-N-[2-(diethylamino)ethyl]benzamide monohydrochloride.

Clinical Pharmacology: Procainamide depresses the excitability of cardiac muscle to electrical stimulation, and slows conduction in the atrium, the bundle of His, and the ventricle. The refractory period of the atrium is considerably more prolonged than that of the ventricle. Contractility of the heart is usually not affected nor is cardiac output decreased to any extent unless myocardial damage exists. In the absence of any arrhythmia, the heart rate may occasionally be accelerated by conventional doses, suggesting that the drug possesses anticholinergic properties. Larger doses can induce atrioventricular block and ventricular extrasystoles which may proceed to ventricular fibrillation. These effects on the myocardium are reflected in the electrocardiogram; a widening of the QRS complex occurs most consistently; less regularly, the P-R and Q-T intervals are prolonged; and the QRS and T waves show some decrease in voltage.

The sustained-release characteristic of Procan SR tablets has been demonstrated in studies in human subjects. A multiple-dose study has shown equivalent steady-state plasma levels of Procan SR tablets given every six hours when compared with an equal total daily dose of Pronestyl® (procainamide hydrochloride capsules, E.R. Squibb and Sons) given every three hours.

Procainamide is less readily hydrolyzed than procaine, and plasma levels decline slowly—about 10% to 20% per hour for standard dosage forms of procainamide. The drug is excreted primarily in the urine, about 10% as free and conjugated p-aminobenzoic acid and about 60% in the unchanged form. The fate of the remainder is unknown.

Indications and Usage: Oral procainamide is indicated in the treatment of premature ventricular contractions and ventricular tachycardia, atrial fibrillation, and paroxysmal atrial tachycardia.

Contraindications: It has been suggested that procainamide be contraindicated in patients with myasthenia gravis. Hypersensitivity to the drug is an absolute contraindication; in this connection, cross-sensitivity to procaine and related drugs must be borne in mind. Procainamide should not be administered to patients with complete atrioventricular heart block. Procainamide is also contraindicated in cases of second degree and third degree A-V block unless an electrical pacemaker is operative.

Precautions:

General—During administration of the drug, evidence of untoward myocardial responses should be carefully watched for in all patients. In the presence of an abnormal myocardium, procainamide may at times produce untoward responses. In atrial fibrillation or flutter, the ventricular rate may increase suddenly as the atrial rate is slowed. Adequate digitalization reduces, but does not abolish, this danger. If myocardial damage exists, ventricular tachysystole is particularly hazardous. Correction of atrial fibrillation, with resultant forceful contractions of the atrium, may cause a dislodgement of mural thrombi and produce an embolic episode. However, it has been suggested that in a patient who is already discharging emboli, procainamide is more likely to stop than to aggravate the process.

Attempts to adjust the heart rate in a patient who has developed ventricular tachycardia during an occlusive coronary episode should be carried out with extreme caution. Caution is also required in marked disturbances of atrioventricular conduction such as A-V block, bundle branch block, or severe digitalis intoxication, where the use of procainamide may result in additional depression of conduction and ventricular asystole or fibrillation.

Because patients with severe organic heart disease and ventricular tachycardia may also have complete heart block, which is difficult to diagnose under these circumstances, this complication should always be kept in mind when treating ventricular arrhythmias with procainamide. If the ventricular rate is significantly slowed by procainamide without attainment of regular atrioventricular conduction, the drug should be stopped and the patient reevaluated since asystole may result under these circumstances.

In patients receiving normal dosage, but who have both liver and kidney disease, symptoms of overdosage (principally ventricular tachycardia and severe hypotension) may occur due to drug accumulation.

Instances of a syndrome resembling lupus erythematosus have been reported in connection with maintenance procainamide therapy. The mechanism of this syndrome is uncertain. Polyarthralgia, arthritis, and pleuritic pain are common symptoms; to a lesser extent fever, myalgia, skin lesions, pleural effusion, and pericarditis may occur. Rare cases of thrombocytopenia or Coombs-positive hemolytic anemia have been reported which may be related to this syndrome.

Laboratory Tests—Patients receiving procainamide for extended periods of time, or in whom symptoms suggestive of a lupus-like reaction appear, should have antinuclear antibody titers measured at regular intervals.

The drug should be discontinued if there is a rising titer (antinuclear antibody) or clinical symptoms of LE appear. The LE syndrome may be reversible upon discontinuation of the drug. If discontinuation of the drug does not cause remission of the symptoms, steroid therapy may be effective. If the syndrome develops in a patient with recurrent life-threatening arrhythmias not controllable by other antiarrhythmic agents, steroid suppressive therapy may be used concomitantly with procainamide. It is recommended that tests for lupus erythematosus be carried out at regular intervals in patients receiving maintenance procainamide therapy.

Routine blood counts are advisable during maintenance procainamide therapy.

Adverse Reactions: Agranulocytosis has occasionally followed the repeated use of the drug, and deaths have occurred. Therefore, routine blood counts are advisable during maintenance procainamide therapy. The patient should be instructed to report any soreness of the mouth, throat or gums, unexplained fever, or any symptoms of upper respiratory tract infection. If any of these should occur, and leucocyte counts indicate cellular depression, procainamide therapy should be discontinued and appropriate treatment should be instituted immediately.

Hypersensitivity reactions, such as angioneurotic edema and maculopapular rash have also occurred.

A syndrome resembling lupus erythematosus has been reported (see PRECAUTIONS).

Hypotension following oral administration is rare.

Large oral doses of procainamide may sometimes produce anorexia, nausea, urticaria, and/or pruritus.

Reactions consisting of fever and chills have also been reported, including a case with fever and chills plus nausea, vomiting, abdominal pain, acute hepatomegaly, and a rise in serum glutamic oxaloacetic transaminase following single doses of the drug. Bitter taste, diarrhea, weakness, mental depression, giddiness, and psychosis with hallucinations have been reported. The possibility of such untoward effects should be borne in mind.

Dosage and Administration: Procan SR tablets are a sustained-release product form. The duration of action of procainamide hydrochloride supplied in this sustained-release product form allows dosing at intervals of every six hours instead of the more frequent every-three-hour dosing interval required for standard preparations of oral procainamide hydrochloride. The convenient six-hour dosing schedule may encourage patient compliance.

Ventricular tachycardia—Treatment with standard procainamide hydrochloride is recommended until the tachycardia is interrupted or the limit of tolerance is reached. Maintenance may then be continued with Procan SR.

The suggested dosage is as follows. An initial dose of 1 g of standard procainamide hydrochloride followed thereafter by a total daily dose of 50 mg/kg of body weight given at three-hour intervals. The suggested oral dosage for premature ventricular contractions is 50 mg/kg of body weight daily given in divided doses at three-hour intervals.

The suggested maintenance dosage of Procan SR is 50 mg/kg of body weight daily given in divided doses at six-hour intervals.

Although the dosage for each patient must be determined on an individual basis, the following may be used as a guide for providing the total daily dosage: patients weighing less than 55 kg (120 lb), 0.5 g every six hours; patients weighing between 55 and 91 kg (120 and 200 lb) 0.75 g every six hours; and patients weighing over 91 kg (200 lb), 1 g every six hours.

Atrial fibrillation and paroxysmal atrial tachycardia.

Treatment with standard procainamide hydrochloride is recommended until the arrhythmia is interrupted or the limit of tolerance is reached. Maintenance may then be continued with Procan SR.

The suggested dosage is as follows. An initial dose of 1.25 g of standard procainamide hydrochloride may be followed in one hour by 0.75 g if there have been no electrocardiographic changes. Standard procainamide hydrochloride may then be given at a dose of 0.5 g to 1 g every two hours until interruption of the arrhythmia or the tolerance limit is reached.

The suggested maintenance dosage for Procan SR is 1 g every six hours.

If procainamide therapy is continued for appreciable periods, electrocardiograms should be made occasionally to determine the need for the drug.

How Supplied:

Procan SR 250 mg (green, film-coated tablets, P-D 202) is available in bottles of 100 (N 0071-0202-24) and in unit-dose packages of 100 (10 strips of 10 tablets each) (N 0071-0202-40). Each sustained-release tablet contains 250 mg procainamide hydrochloride.

Procan SR 500 mg (yellow, scored, film-coated tablets, P-D 204) is available in bottles of 100 (N 0071-0204-24) and in unit-dose packages of 100 (10 strips of 10 tablets each) (N 0071-0204-40). Each sustained-release tablet contains 500 mg procainamide hydrochloride.

Procan SR 750 mg (orange scored film-coated tablets, P-D 205) is available in bottles of 100 (N 0071-0205-24) and in unit-dose packages of 100 (10 strips of 10 tablets each) (N 0071-0205-40). Each sustained-release tablet contains 750 mg procainamide hydrochloride.

Storage—Protect from moisture. Store bottles below 30°C(86°F). Store unit-dose packages at controlled room temperature, 15°–30°C (59°–86°F).

0202G011

PROLOID® ℞

(thyroglobulin tablets, USP)*

*Product of Warner-Lambert Inc

Description: Proloid is obtained from a purified extract of hog thyroid. It contains the known calorigenically active components, levothyroxine (T_4) and liothyronine (T_3).

Chromatographic analysis to standardize the levothyroxine and liothyronine content of Pro-

Continued on next page

This product information was prepared in August, 1982. On these and other Parke-Davis Products, information may be obtained by addressing PARKE-DAVIS, Division of Warner-Lambert Company, Morris Plains, New Jersey 07950.

Parke-Davis—Cont.

loid is routinely employed. See instructions for use.

Proloid is stable when stored at room temperature.

Actions: The actions of the thyroid hormone(s) involve the maturation and proper function of such organ systems as the endocrine, nervous, skeletal, reproductive, and gastrointestinal. The calorigenic and other actions of thyroid hormone(s) are instrumental in maintaining the normal functional capacity of tissues in organ systems throughout the body.

Indications: Proloid is thyroid replacement therapy for conditions of inadequate endogenous thyroid production: e.g., cretinism and myxedema. Replacement therapy will be effective only in manifestations of hypothyroidism. In simple (nontoxic) goiter, Proloid may be tried therapeutically, in nonemergency situations, in an attempt to reduce the size of such goiters.

Contraindication: Thyroid preparations are contraindicated in the presence of uncorrected adrenal insufficiency.

Warnings:

> Drugs with thyroid hormone activity, alone or together with other therapeutic agents, have been used for the treatment of obesity. In euthyroid patients, doses within the range of daily hormonal requirements are ineffective for weight reduction. Larger doses may produce serious or even life-threatening manifestations of toxicity, particularly when given in association with sympathomimetic amines such as those used for their anorectic effects.

Thyroglobulin should not be used in the presence of cardiovascular disease unless thyroid-replacement therapy is clearly indicated. If the latter exists, low doses should be instituted beginning at 0.5 to 1.0 grain (approximately 32 to 65 mg) and increased by the same amount in increments at two-week intervals. This demands careful clinical judgment.

Morphologic hypogonadism and nephroses should be ruled out before the drug is administered. If hypopituitarism is present, the adrenal deficiency must be corrected prior to starting the drug.

Myxedematous patients are very sensitive to thyroid and dosage should be started at a very low level and increased gradually.

Precaution: As with all thyroid preparations this drug will alter results of thyroid function tests.

Adverse Reactions: Overdosage or too rapid increase in dosage may result in signs and symptoms of hyperthyroidism, such as menstrual irregularities, nervousness, cardiac arrhythmias, and angina pectoris.

Dosage and Administration: Optimal dosage of Proloid is usually determined by the patient's clinical response. Confirmatory tests include BMR, $T_3{}^{131}I$ resin sponge uptake, $T_3{}^{131}I$ red cell uptake, Thyro Binding Index (TBI), and Achilles Tendon Reflex Test. Clinical experience has shown that a normal PBI (3.5-8 mcg/100 ml) will be obtained in patients made clinically euthyroid when the content of T_4 and T_3 is adequate. Dosage should be started in small amounts and increased gradually with increments at intervals of one to two weeks. Usual maintenance dose is 0.5 to 3.0 grains (approximately 32 to 200 mg) daily.

Instructions for Use: The following conversion table lists the approximate equivalents of other thyroid preparations to Proloid when changing medication from desiccated thyroid, T_4 (levothyroxine sodium), T_3 (liothyronine sodium), or T_4/T_3 (liotrix). (See table below)

In changing from Thyroid USP to Proloid substitute the equivalent dose of Proloid. Each patient may still require fine adjustment of dosage because the equivalents are only estimates.

Overdosage: Symptoms: Headache, instability, nervousness, sweating, tachycardia, with unusual bowel motility. Angina pectoris or congestive heart failure may be induced or aggravated. Shock may develop. Massive overdosage may result in symptoms resembling thyroid storm. Chronic excessive dosage will produce the signs and symptoms of hyperthyroidism.

(Treatment: In shock, supportive measures should be utilized. Treatment of unrecognized adrenal insufficiency should be considered.)

[See table above].

Store at controlled room temperature 15°–30°C (59°–86°F).

[Shown in Product Identification Section]

0250G011

How Supplied:

Proloid tablets are supplied

N 0710-0251-24	½ grain (32 mg)		Bottles of 100
N 0710-0251-32	½ grain (32 mg)		Bottles of 1000
N 0710-0252-24	1 grain (65 mg)	Scored	Bottles of 100
N 0710-0252-32	1 grain (65 mg)	Scored	Bottles of 1000
N 0710-0253-24	1½ grain (100 mg)		Bottles of 100
N 0710-0253-32	1½ grain (100 mg)		Bottles of 1000
N 0710-0257-24	2 grain (130 mg)	Scored	Bottles of 100
N 0710-0254-24	3 grain (200 mg)		Bottles of 100
N 0710-0254-32	3 grain (200 mg)		Bottles of 1000

Tablets are gray and uncoated.

Conversion Table

Dose of Proloid (thyroglobulin) grain	mg	Dose of Desiccated Thyroid grain	Dose of T_4 (levothyroxine sodium) mg	Dose of T_3 (liothyronine sodium) mcg	Dose of liotrix (T_4/T_3)
1	(65)	1	0.1	25	#1 (60 mcg/15 mcg)
2	(130)	2	0.2	50	#2 (120 mcg/30 mcg)
3	(200)	3	0.3	75	#3 (180 mcg/45 mcg)
4	(260)	4	0.4	100	
5	(325)	5	0.5	125	

PYRIDIUM® ℞

(phenazopyridine HCl tablets, USP)*

*Product of Warner-Lambert Inc

Description: Pyridium (phenozopyridine HCl) is a urinary tract analgesic agent, chemically designated 2.6-Pyridinediamine, 3-(phenylazo), monohydrochloride.

Actions: Pyridium (phenazopyridine HCl) is excreted in the urine where it exerts a topical analgesic effect on the mucosa of the urinary tract. This action helps to relieve pain, burning, urgency and frequency. Since Pyridium (phenazopyridine HCl) is an analgesic, it should be used only for relief of symptoms. It is, however, compatible with antibacterial therapy and can help to relieve pain and discomfort during the interval before antibacterial therapy controls the infection.

Indications: Symptomatic relief of pain, burning, urgency, frequency, and other discomforts arising from irritation of the lower urinary tract mucosa. These symptoms may result from infection, trauma, surgery, endoscopic procedures, or passage of sounds or catheters. Its topical, analgesic action may reduce or eliminate the need for systemic analgesics or narcotics. The use of Pyridium (phenazopyridine HCl) for symptomatic relief should not delay definitive diagnosis and treatment.

Contraindications: Renal insufficiency. A yellowish tinge of the skin or sclerae may indicate accumulation due to impaired renal excretion and the need to discontinue therapy.

Adverse Reactions: Occasional gastrointestinal disturbance. Methemoglobinemia, hemolytic anemia, renal and hepatic toxicity have been described, usually at overdose levels (see Overdosage section).

Dosage and Management: 200 mg tablets: Average adult dosage is one tablet 3 times a day after meals. 100 mg tablets: Average adult dosage is two tablets 3 times a day after meals. Note: Patients should be told that Pyridium (phenazopyridine HCl) produces a reddish-orange discoloration of the urine.

Overdosage: Exceeding the recommended dose in patients with good renal function or administering the usual dose to patients with impaired renal function (common in elderly patients), may lead to increased serum levels and toxic reactions. Methemoglobinemia generally follows a massive, acute overdose. Methylene blue, 1 to 2 mg/kg body weight intravenously, or ascorbic acid 100 to 200 mg given orally should cause prompt reduction of the methemoglobinemia and disappearance of the cyanosis which is an aid in diagnosis. Oxidative Heinz body hemolytic anemia may also occur, and "bite cells" (degmacytes) may be present in a chronic overdosage situation. Red blood cell G-6-PD deficiency may predispose to hemolysis. Renal and hepatic impairment and occasional failure, usually due to hypersensitivity, may also occur.

Supplied: N 0710-0180—Pyridium Tablets, 100 mg, are supplied in bottles of 100 and 1,000, and in unit-dose packages of 100 (10 strips of 10 tablets).

N 0710-0181—Pyridium Tablets, 200 mg, are supplied in bottles of 100, 1000, and in unit-dose packages of 100 (10 strips of 10 tablets).

STORE BETWEEN 15°–30°C (59°–86°F).

[Shown in Product Identification Section]

0180 G 010

PYRIDIUM® PLUS Tablets ℞

This product was formerly named Dolonil®; there are no changes in the formula.*

*Product of Warner-Lambert Inc

Description: Each tablet contains 150 mg phenazopyridine hydrochloride (Pyridium®); 0.3 mg hyoscyamine hydrobromide; 15 mg butabarbital (may be habit forming).

Actions: Relieves lower urinary symptoms of pain, frequency, urgency, burning and dysuria arising from inflammation of the urothelium, the mucosal lining of the lower urinary tract. Lower urinary tract pain can cause reflex spasm of the detrusor. Pain and spasm are often aggravated by apprehension to promote a pain-spasm-apprehension cycle. Each of the three pharmacologic components of Pyridium Plus acts against a phase of this cycle.

Phenazopyridine hydrochloride (Pyridium), excreted in the urine, is a topical analgesic to relieve pain and discomfort.

Hyoscyamine hydrobromide, a parasympatholytic, acts to relieve detrusor muscle spasm. Butabarbital, a short-to-intermediate-acting sedative, helps to allay associated anxiety and apprehension.

Indications: Pyridium Plus is indicated for the symptomatic relief of pain, burning, frequency, urgency, and dysuria, particularly when accompanied by detrusor muscle spasm and apprehension. These symptoms may arise from infection, trauma, surgery, endoscopic procedures, or passage of sounds or catheters. Pyridium Plus therapy does not interfere with antibacterial therapy and can help to relieve symptoms of pain and discomfort before definitive treatment is effective. The use of Pyridium Plus for symptomatic relief should not delay definitive diagnosis and treatment. In the absence of infection, Pyridium Plus may be the only medication required.

Contraindications: Renal or hepatic insufficiency; glaucoma; bladder neck obstruction; porphyria; sensitivity to any component. A yellowish tinge of the skin or sclerae may indicate accumulation due to impaired renal excretion of phenazopyridine (Pyridium) and the need to discontinue therapy.

Warning: BUTABARBITAL MAY BE HABIT-FORMING

Drowsiness or dizziness may occur. Patients should be instructed to use caution in driving or operating machinery.

Precautions: Patients should be told that Pyridium Plus produces a reddish-orange discoloration of the urine.

Adverse Reactions: Methemoglobinemia, hemolytic anemia, and renal and hepatic toxicity have been described for phenazopyridine, usually at overdosage levels (see Overdosage Section).

Hyoscyamine hydrobromide is an atropinic drug that may produce adverse effects characteristic of this class of drugs. Dry mouth, drowsiness, or dizziness is noted in more than one third of patients (and may occur in half of the patients of older age groups). Other atropine-like effects, such as blurred vision, may occur. There may be occasional gastrointestinal disturbances.

Butabarbital is a short- to intermediate-acting barbiturate which has the potential for adverse reactions attributable to barbiturates.

Dosage: Adult Dosage—One tablet four times a day (after meals and at bedtime).

Overdosage: Pyridium Plus is a combination of three active drugs and overdosage can be expected to show the effects related to each ingredient. Management includes the usual measures to empty the stomach by emesis or gavage, administration of a charcoal slurry, and supportive measures as needed.

Toxicity and management suggestions relating to the individual ingredients are as follows.

Phenazopyridine Hydrochloride (Pyridium): Exceeding the recommended dosage in patients with good renal function or administering the usual dosage to patients with impaired renal function (common in elderly patients) may lead to increased serum levels and toxic reactions. Methemoglobinemia generally follows a massive, acute overdose. Methylene blue, 1 to 2 mg/kg body weight intravenously, or ascorbic acid, 100 to 200 mg given orally, should cause prompt reduction of the methemoglobinemia and disappearance of cyanosis which is an aid in diagnosis. Oxidative Heinz body hemolytic anemia may also occur, and "bite cells" (degmacytes) may be present in a chronic overdosage situation. Red blood cell G-6-PD deficiency may predispose to hemolysis. Renal and hepatic impairment and occasional failure, usually due to hypersensitivity, may also occur.

Hyoscyamine Hydrobromide: Overdosage of hyoscyamine, a form of atropine, will cause dilated pupils; blurred vision; rapid pulse; increased intraocular tension; hot, dry, red skin; dry mouth; disorientation; delirium; fever; convulsions; and coma. As an antidote, physostigmine salicylate may be given IV slowly. Dilute 1 mg in 5 mg of saline and use 1 ml of this dilution in children. Repeat every five minutes as needed up to a total of 2 mg in children, or 6 mg in adults, every 30 minutes.

Butabarbital: This drug may produce sedation and respiratory depression progressing to coma, depending on the amount ingested. General and supportive measures should be instituted.

How Supplied: N 0710-0182-24. Bottles of 100. Tablets are dark maroon and square.

0182G060

[*Shown in Product Identification Section*]

SINUBID® ℞

Description: Each Sinubid tablet contains:

acetaminophen	300 mg
phenacetin	300 mg
phenylpropanolamine hydrochloride	100 mg
phenyltoloxamine citrate	66 mg

Actions: Sinubid is designed to provide symptomatic relief of coryza and nasal congestion when given twice a day (every 12 hours). Sinubid can provide symptomatic relief of headache, fever, and other symptoms associated with mucosal congestion (nasopharyngeal), general malaise, and irritability associated with the common cold, allergic and vasomotor disorders, sinusitis, and rhinitis.

Sinubid contains two analgesic-antipyretics (acetaminophen and phenacetin) to relieve the pain of sinus headache and nasal congestion. These analgesic-antipyretics are rapidly absorbed and as effective as aspirin in raising the pain threshold but have the advantage of causing little or no gastric irritation. Sinubid, because it contains no salicylates, can be used by patients who are allergic to aspirin.

Decongestion of the nasopharyngeal mucosa is provided by phenylpropanolamine hydrochloride, a sympathomimetic amine which provides symptomatic relief. Because its vasoconstrictor activity is similar to that of ephedrine, but less likely to cause CNS stimulation, Sinubid may eliminate the need for topical decongestants.

Phenyltoloxamine citrate is a mild antihistamine which may provide symptomatic relief of seasonal and perennial allergic rhinitis, vasomotor rhinitis, nasal and sinus symptoms of sinusitis, and adjunctive therapy for bacterial sinusitis in uncomplicated upper respiratory infections.

Indications: Sinubid is indicated for the rapid, prolonged, symptomatic relief of nasal congestion in sinus or other frontal headache; allergic and vasomotor manifestations of upper respiratory disorders such as sinusitis, allergic rhinitis, vasomotor rhinitis, coryza; facial pain and "pressure" of acute and chronic sinusitis; and for the relief of accompanying fever. Sinubid is indicated only for intermittent treatment of the above noted acute symptoms.

Contraindications: This compound should not be used in patients whose oversensitivity to small doses of sympathomimetic amines produces sleeplessness, dizziness, lightheadedness, weakness, tremulousness, or cardiac arrhythmias. The drug is contraindicated in any patient hypersensitive to any of the ingredients of the formulation.

Warnings: Instruct patients not to drive or operate machinery if drowsiness occurs. Individuals should not ingest alcoholic beverages, monoamine oxidase inhibitors, or barbiturates while taking this medication.

Precautions: Individuals with high blood pressure, heart disease, diabetes mellitus, chronic renal disease, or thyroid disease should use only as directed by a physician. Excessive or prolonged use of phenacetin-containing products should be avoided.

Usage in Pregnancy: Since there is no adequate experience in pregnant women who have received this drug, safety in pregnancy has not been established. This drug should not be used in nursing mothers.

Adverse Reactions: The following adverse reactions have been reported for each of the individual or combinations of ingredients: *Acetaminophen*—urticaria, epigastric distress, dizziness, and palpitation. *Phenacetin*—cyanosis with methemoglobinemia, hemolytic anemia, dyspnea, headache, vascular collapse, and kidney damage from prolonged use. *Phenylpropanolamine HCl*—anxiety, restlessness, tension, insomnia, tremor, weakness, headache, vertigo, sweating, arrhythmia, nausea, and vomiting. *Phenyltoloxamine Citrate*—urticaria, drowsiness, disturbed coordination, inability to concentrate, dizziness, insomnia, tremors, nervousness, palpitation, convulsions, muscular weakness, gastric distress, diarrhea, intestinal cramps, blurred vision, hypotension, urinary retention, dryness of mouth, throat and nose.

Dosage:

Adults: One tablet twice daily (every 12 hours).

Children (6-12 years of age): One-half tablet twice daily (every 12 hours).

Tablets should not be chewed.

Supplied: Sinubid (P-D 101, formerly imprinted W/C 100) is an ellipsoid, bi-layered (light pink/pink), scored tablet, supplied in bottles of 100 (N 0071-0101-24).

STORE BETWEEN 15° and 30°C (59° and 86°F).

[*Shown in Product Identification Section*]

0101 G 020

SURITAL® Ⓒ ℞
(thiamylal sodium for injection, USP)

Description: Surital (thiamylal sodium for injection, USP) is sodium-5-allyl-5-(1-methylbutyl)-2-thiobarbiturate.

Actions: Thiamylal sodium is a rapid, ultra-short-acting barbiturate, intravenous, anesthetic agent.

Indications: Surital is indicated for induction of anesthesia, for supplementing other anesthetic agents, as intravenous anesthesia for short surgical procedures with minimal painful stimuli, or as an agent for inducing a hypnotic state.

Contraindications: Thiamylal sodium is contraindicated when general anesthesia is contraindicated, in patients with latent or manifest porphyria, or in patients with a known hypersensitivity to barbiturates.

Warnings: RESUSCITATIVE EQUIPMENT AND DRUGS SHOULD BE IMMEDIATELY AVAILABLE. This drug should be administered by persons qualified in the use of intravenous anesthetics.

Repeated and continuous infusion may cause cumulative effects resulting in prolonged somnolence, and respiratory and circulatory depression.

Usage in pregnancy: Safe use of thiamylal sodium has not been established with respect to adverse effects upon fetal development. Therefore, thiamylal sodium should not be used in women of childbearing potential, and particularly during early pregnancy, unless, in the judgment of the physician, the expected benefits outweigh the potential hazards.

Precautions: Respiratory depression, apnea, or hypotension may occur due to variations in tolerance from individual to individual or to physical status of patient. Caution should be exercised in debilitated patients, or those with impaired function of respiratory, circulatory, renal, hepatic, and endocrine systems.

Thiamylal sodium should be used with extreme caution in patients in status asthmaticus.

Continued on next page

This product information was prepared in August, 1982. On these and other Parke-Davis Products, information may be obtained by addressing PARKE-DAVIS, Division of Warner-Lambert Company, Morris Plains, New Jersey 07950.

Parke-Davis—Cont.

Extravascular injection may cause pain, swelling, ulceration, and necrosis. Intra-arterial injection is dangerous and may produce gangrene of an extremity.

Adverse Reactions: The following adverse reactions have been reported: circulatory depression, thrombophlebitis, pain at injection site, and respiratory depression, including apnea, laryngospasm, bronchospasm, salivation, hiccups, emergence delirium, headache, injury to nerves adjacent to injection site, skin rashes, urticaria, nausea, and emesis.

Dosage and Administration: The dosage is individualized according to the patient's response.

A 2.5% solution is recommended for induction of anesthesia as well as for maintenance by intermittent intravenous injection. A dilute solution (0.3%) may be used by continuous drip for maintenance. The rate of injection during induction should be approximately 1 ml of 2.5% solution every five seconds; an initial injection of 3 to 6 ml of 2.5% solution is generally sufficient to produce short periods of surgical anesthesia.

Sterile Water for Injection is the preferred solvent for preparing Surital (thiamylal sodium for injection, USP) solutions. Initially, Surital solutions are clear, but they may become cloudy on aging. Thiamylal sodium cannot be reconstituted with Ringer's Solution or solutions containing bacteriostatic or buffer agents, because they may tend to cause precipitation. In preparing dilute solutions for continuous drip maintenance, either 5% dextrose or isotonic sodium chloride should be used instead of sterile water for injection to avoid extreme hypotonicity. Dextrose solutions are occasionally sufficiently acid, however, to cause precipitation. Injection of air into the solution should be avoided because this may hasten the development of cloudiness.

Solutions of atropine sulfate, *d*-tubocurarine, or succinylcholine may be given concurrently with Surital, but they should not be mixed prior to administration.

Thiamylal sodium solutions should be prepared under aseptic conditions. Solutions cannot be heated for sterilization. The solutions should be stored in a refrigerator and used within six days. If kept at room temperature, the solution should be used within 24 hours. Only clear solutions should be used; discard if cloudiness or precipitate form. Refrigeration of the reconstituted Surital contributes to the maintenance of a clear solution

[See table below].

How Supplied: Surital is supplied as follows.
N 0071-4064-03 (35-64-25)
1 g, in packages of 25 (Steri-Vial® 64)
N 0071-4122-08 (35-122-10)
5 g, in packages of 10 (Steri-Vial 122)
N 0071-4123-10 (35-123-10)
10 g, in packages of 10 (Steri-Vial 123)

AHFS 28:24 **YC**

TABRON® FILMSEAL® ℞

Each tablet represents:

Ferrous fumarate .... 304.2 mg
(represents 100 mg of elemental iron)
Vitamin C (ascorbic acid) .... 500 mg
Vitamin B_1 (thiamine mononitrate) .... 6 mg
Vitamin B_2 (riboflavin) .... 6 mg
Vitamin B_6 (pyridoxine hydrochloride) .... 5 mg
Vitamin B_{12} (cyanocobalamin), crystalline .... 25 mcg
Folic acid .... 1 mg
Nicotinamide (niacinamide) .... 30 mg
Calcium pantothenate .... 10 mg
Vitamin E (*dl*-alpha tocopheryl acetate) .... (30 mg) 30 IU
Docusate sodium .... 50 mg

Caution—Folic acid in doses above 0.1 mg daily may obscure pernicious anemia in that hematologic remission can occur while neurological manifestations remain progressive.

Indications: Tabron is a hematinic for the treatment of iron-deficiency anemia and folate deficiency.

Dosage: Usual adult dose: One tablet per day.

How Supplied: N 0071-0638—Bottles of 100 and unit-dose packages of 100 (ten 10s). Parcode® No. 638

[*Shown in Product Identification Section*]

TEDRAL®* TEDRAL® SA* TEDRAL-25®* TEDRAL® EXPECTORANT** TEDRAL® SUSPENSION** TEDRAL® ELIXIR**

*Product of Warner-Lambert Inc
** Manufactured by Warner-Lambert Co; distributed by Warner-Lambert Inc

Caution: Federal law prohibits dispensing Tedral SA, Tedral-25, or Tedral Expectorant without prescription.

Description:

Tedral: each tablet contains 130 mg theophylline, 24 mg ephedrine hydrochloride, and 8 mg phenobarbital.

Tedral SA: each tablet contains 180 mg anhydrous theophylline (90 mg in the immediate release layer and 90 mg in the sustained release layer); 48 mg ephedrine hydrochloride (16 mg in the immediate release layer and 32 mg in the sustained release layer); 25 mg phenobarbital in the immediate release layer.

Tedral-25: each tablet contains 130 mg theophylline, 24 mg ephedrine hydrochloride, and 25 mg butabarbital.

Tedral Expectorant: each tablet contains 130 mg theophylline, 24 mg ephedrine hydrochloride, 8 mg phenobarbital, and 100 mg guaifenesin.

Tedral Suspension: each 5 ml teaspoonful of suspension contains 65 mg theophylline, 12 mg ephedrine hydrochloride, and 4 mg phenobarbital.

Tedral Elixir: each 5 ml teaspoonful contains 32.5 mg theophylline, 6 mg ephedrine hydrochloride, and 2 mg phenobarbital; the alcohol content is 15%.

Actions: Tedral combines theophylline and ephedrine—widely accepted oral bronchodilators, with differing modes of action—with the sedative phenobarbital.

From experimental evidence,[1] it appears that a combination of a sympathomimetic and methylxanthine is more effective than either drug alone in inhibiting the release of bronchoconstricting mediators (histamine and slow-reacting substance of anaphylaxis) produced by antigen-antibody (IgE) interaction on sensitive cells. The β-adrenergic stimulation by the sympathomimetics produces cyclic 3′5′-adenosine monophosphate (cAMP), and the degradation of cAMP by the specific enzyme phosphodiesterase is inhibited by methylxanthines. Thus, at present, the principal action of the Tedral formulations in the relief or prevention of bronchoconstriction appears to be involved with the cAMP system.

Phenobarbital is incorporated to counteract possible stimulation by ephedrine and to provide a mild, long-acting sedative for the apprehensive asthmatic patient.

Tedral SA provides sustained as well as immediate bronchodilation for the asthmatic patient, with the convenience of b.i.d. dosage.

The nervous or apprehensive asthmatic patient can benefit from butabarbital in **Tedral-25.** This formulation can also be useful in the occasional patient who is unduly sensitive to ephedrine.

Tedral Expectorant combines Tedral with guaifenesin which helps to increase the volume and decrease the viscosity of fluids of the respiratory tract. By aiding lubrication of the mucous membranes of the bronchi, Tedral Expectorant helps the patient to cough up viscid mucus.

Tedral Suspension and **Tedral Elixir** are convenient formulations for children and other persons who may have difficulty in swallowing tablets.

Indications: Tedral, Tedral SA, Tedral-25, Tedral Expectorant, Tedral Suspension and **Tedral Elixir** are indicated for the symptomatic relief of bronchial asthma, asthmatic bronchitis, and other bronchospastic disorders. They may also be used prophylactically to abort or minimize asthmatic attacks and are of value in managing occasional, seasonal or perennial asthma.

Tedral SA (Sustained Action) offers the convenience of b.i.d. dosage.

Tedral-25 is indicated when there is excessive nervousness, apprehension or sensitivity to ephedrine.

Tedral Expectorant is indicated only when both relaxation of bronchospasm and expectoration are desired.

Tedral Suspension and **Tedral Elixir** are convenient for persons who may have difficulty in swallowing tablets.

These Tedral formulations are adjuncts in the total management of the asthmatic patient. Acute or severe asthmatic attacks may necessitate supplemental therapy with others drugs by inhalation or other parenteral routes.

Contraindications: Sensitivity to any of the ingredients; porphyria.

Warnings: Drowsiness may occur. Phenobarbital and butabarbital may be habit-forming.

Precautions: Use with caution in the presence of cardiovascular disease, severe hypertension, hyperthyroidism, prostatic hypertrophy, or glaucoma.

Adverse Reactions: Mild epigastric distress, palpitation, tremulousness, insomnia, difficulty of micturition, and CNS stimulation have been reported.

Dosage and Administration:

Tedral
Adults—One or two tablets every 4 hours.
Children—(Over 60 lb) one-half the adult dose.

Tedral SA
Adults—One tablet on arising and one tablet 12 hours later. Tablets should not be chewed.
Children—Not established for children under 12.

Tedral-25
Adults—One tablet every 4 hours.
Children—(6-12) one-half the adult dose.

Tedral Expectorant
Adults—One or two tablets 4 times a day.
Children—Not established for children under 12.

PREPARING SURITAL SOLUTIONS

Surital (g)	Amount of solvent required (in ml) for percentage solutions shown								
	0.2%	0.3%	0.4%	2%	2.5%	3%	4%	5%	10%
1	500	333	250	50	40	33.3	25	20	10
5	2,500	1,670	1,250	250	200	167	125	100	50
10	5,000	3,333	2,500	500	400	333	250	200	100

Tedral Suspension
Adults—Two to four teaspoonfuls every 4 hours.
Children—One teaspoonful per 60 lb body weight, every 4–6 hours. Should be given to children under 2 years of age only with extreme caution.
SHAKE BOTTLE WELL.
Tedral Elixir
Children—One teaspoonful per 30 lb body weight, every 4–6 hours. Should be given to children under 2 years of age only with extreme caution.
Adults—One to two tablespoonfuls every four hours.
How Supplied:
Tedral is supplied as white, uncoated, scored tablets in bottles of 24 (N 0710-0230-13), 100 (N 0710-0230-24), 1000 (N 0710-0230-32) and unit dose (10/10)(N 0710-0230-40).
Tedral SA is supplied as double-layered, uncoated, coral/mottled white tablets in bottles of 100 (N 0710-0231-24), 1000 (N 0710-0231-32) and unit dose (10/10)(N 0710-0231-40).
Tedral-25 is supplied as salmon-pink, uncoated scored tablets in bottles of 100 (N 0710-0238-24).
Tedral Expectorant is supplied as white tablets in bottles of 100 (N 0710-0239-24).
Tedral Suspension is supplied as a yellow, licorice-flavored suspension in bottles of 8 fl oz (237 ml)(N 0710-2237-20) and in bottles of 16 fl oz (474 ml)(N 0710-2237-23).
Tedral Elixir is supplied as a dark red, cherry-flavored elixir in bottles of 16 fl oz (474 ml)(N 0710-2242-23).
Reference:
1. Koopman WJ, Orange RP, Austen KF: *J. Immunol.* 105: 1096, November 1970.
[*Shown in Product Identification Section*]

TETRACYCLINE HCl CAPSULES, USP ℞
Cyclopar®/Cyclopar® 500

Description: Tetracycline hydrochloride capsules, USP, contain the broad-spectrum antibiotic, tetracycline hydrochloride. Tetracycline hydrochloride is a yellow, odorless, crystalline powder with the chemical formula $C_{22}H_{24}N_2O_8 \cdot HCl$.
Actions: The tetracyclines are primarily bacteriostatic and are thought to exert their antimicrobial effect by the inhibition of protein synthesis. Tetracyclines are active against a wide range of gram-negative and gram-positive organisms.
The drugs in the tetracycline class have closely similar antimicrobial spectra, and cross-resistance among them is common. Microorganisms may be considered susceptible if the MIC (minimum inhibitory concentration) is not more than 4.0 mcg/ml, and intermediate if the MIC is 4.0 to 12.5 mcg/ml.
Susceptibility plate testing: A tetracycline disc may be used to determine microbial susceptibility to drugs in the tetracycline class. If the Kirby-Bauer method of disc susceptibility testing is used, a 30-mcg tetracycline disc should give a zone of at least 19 mm when tested against a tetracycline-susceptible bacterial strain.
Tetracyclines are readily absorbed and are bound to plasma proteins in varying degrees. They are concentrated by the liver in the bile and excreted in the urine and feces at high concentrations and in a biologically active form.
Indications: Tetracycline is indicated in infections caused by the following microorganisms.
Rickettsiae (Rocky Mountain spotted fever, typhus fever and the typhus group, Q fever, rickettsialpox, and tick fevers)
Mycoplasma pneumoniae (PPLO, Eaton agent)
Agents of psittacosis and ornithosis
Agents of lymphogranuloma venereum and granuloma inguinale
The spirochetal agent of relapsing fever (*Borrelia recurrentis)*
The following gram-negative microorganisms:
Haemophilus ducreyi (chancroid)
Pasteurella pestis and *Pasteurella tularensis*
Bartonella bacilliformis
Bacteroides species
Vibrio comma and *Vibrio fetus*
Brucella species (in conjunction with streptomycin)
Because many strains of the following groups of microorganisms have been shown to be resistant to tetracyclines, culture and susceptibility testing is recommended.
Tetracycline is indicated for treatment of infections caused by the following gram-negative microorganisms when bacteriologic testing indicates appropriate susceptibility to the drug.
Escherichia coli
Enterobacter aerogenes (formerly *Aerobacter aerogenes)*
Shigella species
Mima species and *Herellea* species
Haemophilus influenzae (respiratory infections)
Klebsiella species (respiratory and urinary infections)
Tetracycline is indicated for treatment of infections caused by the following gram-positive microorganisms when bacteriologic testing indicates appropriate susceptibility to the drug.
Streptococcus species:
Up to 44 percent of strains of *Streptococcus pyogenes* and 74 percent of *Streptococcus faecalis* have been found to be resistant to tetracycline drugs. Therefore, tetracyclines should not be used for streptococcal disease unless the organism has been demonstrated to be sensitive.
For upper respiratory infections due to group A beta-hemolytic streptococci, penicillin is the usual drug of choice, including prophylaxis of rheumatic fever.
Diplococcus pneumoniae
Staphylococcus aureus
Skin and soft-tissue infections. Tetracyclines are not the drugs of choice in the treatment of any type of staphylococcal infection.
When penicillin is contraindicated, tetracyclines are alternative drugs in the treatment of infections due to:
Neisseria gonorrhoeae,
Treponema pallidum and *Treponema pertenue* (syphilis and yaws),
Listeria monocytogenes,
Clostridium species,
Bacillus anthracis,
Fusobacterium fusiforme (Vincent's infection),
Actinomyces species.
In acute intestinal amebiasis, the tetracyclines may be a useful adjunct to amebicides.
In severe acne, the tetracyclines may be useful adjunctive therapy.
Tetracyclines are indicated in the treatment of trachoma, although the infectious agent is not always eliminated, as judged by immunofluorescence.
Inclusion conjunctivitis may be treated with oral tetracyclines or with a combination of oral and topical agents.
Contraindication: This drug is contraindicated in persons who have shown hypersensitivity to any of the tetracyclines.
Warnings: THE USE OF DRUGS OF THE TETRACYCLINE CLASS DURING TOOTH DEVELOPMENT (LAST HALF OF PREGNANCY, INFANCY, AND CHILDHOOD TO THE AGE OF 8 YEARS) MAY CAUSE PERMANENT DISCOLORATION OF THE TEETH (YELLOW-GRAY-BROWN). This adverse reaction is more common during long-term use of the drugs but has been observed following repeated short-term courses. Enamel hypoplasia has also been reported. TETRACYCLINE DRUGS, THEREFORE, SHOULD NOT BE USED IN THIS AGE GROUP UNLESS OTHER DRUGS ARE NOT LIKELY TO BE EFFECTIVE OR ARE CONTRAINDICATED.
If renal impairment exists, even usual oral or parenteral doses may lead to excessive systemic accumulation of the drug and possible liver toxicity. Under such conditions, lower than usual total doses are indicated and, if therapy is prolonged, serum level determinations of the drug may be advisable.
Photosensitivity manifested by an exaggerated sunburn reaction has been observed in some individuals taking tetracyclines. Patients apt to be exposed to direct sunlight or ultraviolet light should be advised that this reaction can occur with tetracycline drugs, and treatment should be discontinued at the first evidence of skin erythema.
The antianabolic action of the tetracyclines may cause an increase in BUN. While this is not a problem in those with normal renal function, in patients with significantly impaired function, higher serum levels of tetracycline may lead to azotemia, hyperphosphatemia, and acidosis.
Usage in pregnancy. (See above Warnings about use during tooth development).
Results of animal studies indicate that tetracyclines cross the placenta, are found in fetal tissues, and can have toxic effects on the developing fetus (often related to retardation of skeletal development.) Evidence of embryotoxicity has also been noted in animals treated early in pregnancy.
Usage in newborns, infants, and children. (See above Warnings about use during tooth development.)
All tetracyclines form a stable calcium complex in any bone-forming tissue. A decrease in the fibula growth rate has been observed in prematures given oral tetracycline in doses of 25 mg/kg every 6 hours. This reaction was shown to be reversible when the drug was discontinued.
Tetracyclines are present in the milk of lactating women who are taking a drug in this class.
Precautions: As with other antibiotic preparations, use of this drug may result in overgrowth of nonsusceptible organisms, including fungi. If superinfection occurs, the antibiotic should be discontinued and appropriate therapy instituted.
In venereal diseases when coexistent syphilis is suspected, darkfield examination should be done before treatment is started and the blood serology repeated monthly for at least four months.
Because tetracyclines have been shown to depress plasma prothrombin activity, patients who are on anticoagulant therapy may require downward adjustment of their anticoagulant dosage.
In long-term therapy, periodic laboratory evaluation of organ systems, including hematopoietic, renal, and hepatic studies, should be performed.
All infections due to Group A beta-hemolytic streptococci should be treated for at least 10 days.
Since bacteriostatic drugs may interfere with the bactericidal action of penicillin, it is advisable to avoid giving tetracycline in conjunction with penicillin.

Continued on next page

This product information was prepared in August, 1982. On these and other Parke-Davis Products, information may be obtained by addressing PARKE-DAVIS, Division of Warner-Lambert Company, Morris Plains, New Jersey 07950.

Parke-Davis—Cont.

Adverse Reactions: Gastrointestinal: anorexia, nausea, vomiting, diarrhea, glossitis, dysphagia, enterocolitis, and inflammatory lesions (with monilial overgrowth) in the anogenital region. These reactions have been caused by both the oral and parenteral administration of tetracyclines.
Skin: maculopapular and erythematous rashes. Exfoliative dermatitis has been reported but is uncommon. Photosensitivity is discussed above. (See Warnings.)
Renal toxicity: rise in BUN has been reported and is apparently dose-related. (See Warnings.)
Hypersensitivity reactions: urticaria, angioneurotic edema, anaphylaxis, anaphylactoid purpura, pericarditis, and exacerbation of systemic lupus erythematosus
Bulging fontanels have been reported in young infants following full therapeutic dosage. This sign disappeared rapidly when the drug was discontinued.
Blood: hemolytic anemia, thrombocytopenia, neutropenia, and eosinophilia have been reported.
When given over prolonged periods, tetracyclines have been reported to produce brown-black microscopic discoloration of thyroid glands. No abnormalities of thyroid function studies are known to occur.
Dosage and Administration: Therapy should be continued for at least 24 to 48 hours after symptoms and fever have subsided.
Concomitant therapy: Antacids containing aluminum, calcium, or magnesium impair absorption and should not be given to patients taking oral tetracycline.
Food and some dairy products also interfere with absorption. Oral forms of tetracycline should be given 1 hour before or 2 hours after meals. Pediatric oral dosage forms should not be given with milk formulas and should be given at least 1 hour prior to feeding.
In patients with renal impairment (See Warnings.): Total dosage should be decreased by reduction of recommended individual doses and/or by extending time intervals between doses.
In the treatment of streptococcal infections, a therapeutic dose of tetracycline should be administered for at least 10 days.
Adults: Usual daily dosage, 1 to 2 grams divided in two or four equal doses, depending on the severity of the infection.
For children above eight years of age: Usual daily dosage, 10 to 20 mg (25 to 50 mg/kg) per pound of body weight divided in four equal doses.
For treatment of brucellosis, 500 mg tetracycline four times daily for three weeks should be accompanied by streptomycin, 1 gram, intramuscularly twice daily the first week and once daily the second week.
For treatment of syphilis, a total of 30 to 40 grams in equally divided doses over a period of 10 to 15 days should be given. Close follow-up, including laboratory tests, is recommended.
For the treatment of acute gonococcal urethritis, a single, initial dose of 1.5 grams followed by 0.5 grams every 4 to 6 hours for 4 to 6 days should be given. Female patients may require more prolonged therapy.
How Supplied:
Tetracycline hydrochloride capsules, USP (Cyclopar)
N 0071-0407-24 250 mg Bottles of 100.
N 0071-0407-32 250 mg Bottles of 1000.
Each capsule contains 250 mg tetracycline hydrochloride.
Tetracycline hydrochloride capsules, USP (Cyclopar 500)
N 0071-0697-24 500 mg Bottles of 100.
Each capsule contains 500 mg tetracycline hydrochloride.
AHFS 8:12.24 **0407G100**
[*Shown in Product Identification Section*]

THERA-COMBEX H-P®
High-Potency Vitamin B Complex with 500 mg Vitamin C

Composition: Each Kapseal contains:

Ascorbic acid (vitamin C)	500 mg
Thiamine (vitamin B_1) mononitrate	25 mg
Riboflavin (vitamin B_2)	15 mg
Pyridoxine hydrochloride (vitamin B_6)	10 mg
Vitamin B_{12} (cyanocobalamin)	5 mcg
Niacinamide	100 mg
dl-Panthenol	20 mg

Uses: For the prevention or treatment of vitamin B complex and vitamin C deficiencies.
Dosage: One or two capsules daily
How Supplied: N 0071-0550-24—Bottles of 100. Parcode® No. 550
[*Shown in Product Identification Section*]

THROMBOSTAT™ ℞
(Thrombin, USP) Bovine Origin

Thrombostat must not be injected! Apply on the surface of bleeding tissue as a solution or powder.
Description: Thrombostat (thrombin, USP) is a protein substance produced through a conversion reaction in which prothrombin of bovine origin is activated by tissue thromboplastin in the presence of calcium chloride. It is supplied as a sterile powder that has been freeze-dried in the final container. Also contained in this preparation are calcium chloride, sodium chloride, aminoacetic acid (glycine) and Phemerol® (benzethonium chloride). Glycine is included to make the dried product friable and more readily soluble, and benzethonium chloride as a preservative as follows: 0.4 mg per 1000 unit vial, 0.1 mg per 5000 unit vial, 0.2 mg per 10,000 unit vial, and 0.4 mg per 20,000 unit vial.
A 5 ml, 10 ml, or 20 ml vial of Isotonic Saline is enclosed to be used as a diluent with the 5 ml, 5000 US (NIH) unit; 10 ml, 10,000 US (NIH) unit; or 20 ml, 20,000 US (NIH) unit vial, respectively, of Thrombostat.
Isotonic Saline is a sterile, isotonic solution of sodium chloride in water for injection, USP. It contains Phemerol® (benzethonium chloride) 0.02 mg per ml as a preservative. (See Dosage and Administration for additional information on diluents which may be used.)
This product is prepared under rigid assay control. A US (NIH) unit is defined as the amount required to clot 1 ml of standardized fibrinogen solution in 15 seconds. Approximately 2 US (NIH) units are required to clot 1 ml of oxalated human plasma in the same period of time.
Action: Thrombostat requires no intermediate physiological agent for its action. It clots the fibrinogen of the blood directly. **Failure to clot blood occurs in the rare case where the primary clotting defect is the absence of fibrinogen itself.** The speed with which thrombin clots blood is dependent upon its concentration. For example, the contents of a 5000 US (NIH) unit vial of Thrombostat dissolved in 5 ml of saline diluent is capable of clotting an equal volume of blood in less than a second, or 1000 ml in less than a minute.
Indications: Thrombostat (thrombin, USP) is indicated as an aid in hemostasis wherever oozing blood from capillaries and small venules is accessible.
In various types of surgery solutions of Thrombostat may be used in conjunction with absorbable gelatin sponge, USP for hemostasis.
Contraindication: Thrombostat is contraindicated in persons known to be sensitive to any of its components and/or to material of bovine origin.
Warning: Because of its action in the clotting mechanism, Thrombostat must not be injected or otherwise allowed to enter large blood vessels. Extensive intravascular clotting and even death may result. Thrombostat is an antigenic substance and has caused sensitivity and allergic reactions when injected into animals.
Precautions: Consult the absorbable gelatin sponge product labeling for complete information for use prior to utilizing the thrombin-saturated sponge procedure.
Adverse Reactions: An allergic type reaction following the use of Thrombostat for treatment of epistaxis has been reported. Febrile reactions have also been observed following the use of Thrombostat in certain surgical procedures but no cause-effect relationship has been established.
Dosage and Administration: Solutions of Thrombostat may be prepared in sterile distilled water or isotonic saline. The intended use determines the strength of the solution to prepare. For general use in plastic surgery, dental extractions, skin grafting, neurosurgery, etc., solutions containing approximately 100 units per ml are frequently used. For this, 10 ml of diluent added to the 1000 unit package is suitable. Where bleeding is profuse, as from cut surfaces of liver and spleen, concentrations as high as 1000 to 2000 units per ml may be required. For this the 5000 unit vial dissolved in 5 ml or 2.5 ml respectively, of the diluent supplied in the package is convenient. Intermediate strengths to suit the needs of the case may be prepared by selecting the proper strength package and dissolving the contents in an appropriate volume of diluent. In many situations, it may be advantageous to use Thrombostat in dry form on oozing surfaces.
Caution: Solutions should be used the day they are prepared. If several hours are to elapse, the solution should be refrigerated, preferably frozen, and not used after 48 hours.
The following techniques are suggested for the topical application of Thrombostat.

1. The recipient surface should be sponged (not wiped) free of blood before Thrombostat is applied.
2. A spray may be used or the surface may be flooded using a sterile syringe and small gauge needle. The most effective hemostasis results when the Thrombostat mixes freely with the blood as soon as it reaches the surface.
3. In instances where Thrombostat in dry form is needed, the vial is opened by removing the metal ring by grasping the edge where it is scored and tearing, using sterile pliers. The rubber-diaphragm cap may be easily removed and the dried Thrombostat is then broken up into a powder by means of a sterile glass rod or other suitable sterile instrument.
4. Sponging of treated surfaces should be avoided in order that the clot remain securely in place.

Thrombostat may be used in conjunction with absorbable gelatin sponge, USP as follows:

1. Prepare Thrombostat solution of the desired strength.
2. Immerse sponge strips of the desired size in the Thrombostat solution. Knead the sponge strips vigorously with moistened fingers to remove trapped air, thereby facilitating saturation of the sponge.
3. Apply saturated sponge to bleeding area. Hold in place for 10 to 15 seconds with a pledget of cotton or a small gauze sponge.

How Supplied: Thrombostat is supplied as:
N 0071-4173-35—Package contains one 5000 US (NIH) unit vial of Thrombostat and one 5 ml vial of Isotonic Saline Diluent with Phemerol, 0.02 mg per ml, as a preservative.
N 0071-4176-35—Package contains one 10,000 US (NIH) unit vial of Thrombostat and one 10 ml vial of Isotonic Saline Diluent with Phemerol, 0.02 mg per ml, as a preservative.
N 0071-4177-01—Package contains one 1000 US (NIH) unit vial of Thrombostat.
N 0071-4180-35—Package contains one 20,000 US (NIH) unit vial of Thrombostat and one 20

ml vial of Isotonic Saline Diluent with Phemerol, 0.02 mg per ml, as a preservative.

121 861950/12
4173G012

TUCKS®

Pre-Moistened Hemorrhoidal/Vaginal Pads

Indications: Temporarily relieve external discomfort of simple hemorrhoids.
—Soothe, cool, and comfort itching, burning, and irritation of sensitive rectal and outer vaginal areas.
—As a compress, to help relieve discomfort from rectal/vaginal surgical stitches.
—Effective hygienic wipe to cleanse rectal area of irritation-causing residue.
—Solution buffered to help prevent further irritation.

Directions: For external use only. Use as a wipe following bowel movement, during menstruation, or after napkin or tampon change. Or, as a compress, apply to affected area 10 to 15 minutes as needed. Change compresses every 5 minutes.

Warning: In case of rectal bleeding, consult physician promptly. In case of continued irritation, discontinue use and consult a physician. Keep this and all medication out of the reach of children. In case of accidental ingestion seek professional assistance or contact a Poison Control Center immediately.

Contains: Soft pads pre-moistened with a solution containing 50% Witch Hazel, 10% Glycerin USP, Purified Water USP deionized q.s., Methylparaben USP 0.1% and Benzalkonium Chloride USP 0.003% as preservatives. Buffered to acid pH.

Store between 59° and 86°F.

How Supplied: Jars of 40 and 100. Also available as Tucks Take-Alongs®, individual, foil-wrapped, nonwoven wipes, 12 packets per box Tucks—N 0071-1703.
Tucks Take-Alongs—N 0071-1704-01

TUCKS® OINTMENT, CREAM

Composition: Tucks Ointment and Cream contain a specially formulated aqueous phase of 50% witch hazel (hamamelis water). Both have an acid pH, pleasant odor, and are nonstaining.
Both non-staining Tucks Ointment and Tucks Cream exert a temporary soothing, cooling, mildly astringent effect on such superficial irritations as simple hemorrhoids, vaginal and rectal area itch, post episiotomy discomfort and anorectal surgical wounds. Neither the Ointment or Cream contain steroids or skin sensitizing "caine" type topical anesthetics.

Warning: Symptomatic relief should not delay definitive diagnosis and treatment. If itching or irritation continues, discontinue use and consult physician. In case of rectal bleeding, consult physician promptly.

Dosage and Administration: Apply locally three or four times daily. Applicator provided for rectal instillation.

How Supplied: Tucks Ointment and Tucks Cream (water-washable) in 40-g tubes with rectal applicators
Tucks Ointment—N 0071-3021-14
Tucks Cream—N 0071-3022-14 **7000G070**

UTICORT® ℞

(betamethasone benzoate)
Cream, 0.025%
Gel, 0.025%
Lotion, 0.025%
Ointment, 0.025%

For external use only
Caution: Federal law prohibits dispensing without prescription.

Description: Uticort Gel/Cream/Ointment /Lotion contain the active fluorinated corticosteroid compound betamethasone benzoate, the 17-benzoate ester of betamethasone, having the chemical formula of 9-fluoro-11β, 17, 21-trihydroxy-16β-methylpregna-1, 4-diene-3, 20-dione 17-benzoate.
Each gram of 0.025% Gel contains 0.25 mg of betamethasone benzoate in a specially formulated gel base consisting of 13.8% (w/w) alcohol, carboxyvinyl polymer, propylene glycol, disodium edetate, diisopropanolamine and purified water. The gel is self-liquefying, clear, greaseless and nonstaining. The active ingredient is completely solubilized and remains in the clear film without crystallization after evaporation of volatile substances.
Each gram of 0.025% Cream contains 0.25 mg of betamethasone benzoate in a water-washable emollient cream base consisting of cetyl alcohol, glyceryl stearate, light mineral oil, propylene glycol, disodium monooleamidosulfosuccinate, citric acid and purified water.
Each gram of 0.025% Ointment contains 0.25 mg of betamethasone benzoate in an emollient ointment base of light mineral oil, glyceryl stearate, food starch-modified and polyethylene.
In this formulation the active ingredient is micronized to provide uniform distribution and optimal activity.
Each gram of 0.025% Lotion contains 0.25 mg of betamethasone benzoate in a water miscible, oil- and fat-free vehicle consisting of cetyl alcohol, stearyl alcohol, propylene glycol, sodium lauryl sulfate, purified water, and propyl-, butyl-, and methylparabens as preservatives.

Clinical Pharmacology: Topical corticosteroids share antiinflammatory, antipruritic and vasoconstrictive actions.
The mechanism of antiinflammatory activity of the topical corticosteroids is unclear. Various laboratory methods, including vasoconstrictor assays, are used to compare and predict potencies and/or clinical efficacies of the topical corticosteroids. There is some evidence to suggest that a recognizable correlation exists between vasoconstrictor potency and therapeutic efficacy in man.

Pharmacokinetics
The extent of percutaneous absorption of topical corticosteroids is determined by many factors including the vehicle, the integrity of the epidermal barrier, and the use of occlusive dressings.
Topical corticosteroids can be absorbed from normal intact skin. Inflammation and/or other disease processes in the skin increase percutaneous absorption.
Occlusive dressings substantially increase the percutaneous absorption of topical corticosteroids. Thus, occlusive dressings may be a valuable therapeutic adjunct for treatment of resistant dermatoses (See *DOSAGE AND ADMINISTRATION*.)

Once absorbed through the skin, topical corticosteroids are handled through pharmacokinetic pathways similar to systemically administered corticosteroids. Corticosteroids are bound to plasma proteins in varying degrees. Corticosteroids are metabolized primarily in the liver and are then excreted by the kidneys. Some of the topical corticosteroids and their metabolites are also excreted into the bile.

Indications and Usage: Topical corticosteroids are indicated for the relief of the inflammatory and pruritic manifestations of corticosteroid-responsive dermatoses.

Contraindications: Topical corticosteroids are contraindicated in those patients with a history of hypersensitivity to any of the components of the preparation.

Precautions:
General
Systemic absorption of topical corticosteroids has produced reversible hypothalamic-pituitary-adrenal (HPA) axis suppression, manifestations of Cushing's syndrome, hyperglycemia and glucosuria in some patients.
Conditions which augment systemic absorption include the application of the more potent steroids, use over large surface areas, prolonged use, and the addition of occlusive dressings.
Therefore, patients receiving a large dose of a potent topical steroid applied to a large surface area or under an occlusive dressing should be evaluated periodically for evidence of HPA axis suppression by using the urinary free cortisol and ACTH stimulation tests. If HPA axis suppression is noted, an attempt should be made to withdraw the drug, to reduce the frequency of application, or to substitute a less potent steroid.
Recovery of HPA axis function is generally prompt and complete upon discontinuation of the drug. Infrequently, signs and symptoms of steroid withdrawal may occur, requiring supplemental systemic corticosteroids.
Children may absorb proportionally larger amounts of topical corticosteroids and thus be more susceptible to systemic toxicity (See *PRECAUTIONS—Pediatric Use*).
If irritation develops, topical corticosteroids should be discontinued and appropriate therapy instituted.
In the presence of dermatological infections, the use of an appropriate antifungal or antibacterial agent should be instituted. If a favorable response does not occur promptly, the corticosteroid should be discontinued until the infection has been adequately controlled.

Information for the Patient
Patients using topical corticosteroids should receive the following information and instructions:
1. This medication is to be used as directed by the physician. It is for external use only. Avoid contact with the eyes.
2. Patients should be advised not to use this medication for any disorder other than for which it was prescribed.
3. The treated skin area should not be bandaged or otherwise covered or wrapped as to be occlusive unless directed by the physician.
4. Patients should report any signs of local adverse reactions especially under occlusive dressing.
5. Parents of pediatric patients should be advised not to use tight-fitting diapers or plastic pants on a child being treated in the diaper area, as these garments may constitute occlusive dressings.

Laboratory Tests
The following tests may be helpful in evaluating the HPA axis suppression:
Urinary free cortisol test
ACTH stimulation test

Carcinogenesis, Mutagenesis, and Impairment of Fertility
Long-term animal studies have not been performed to evaluate the carcinogenic potential or the effect on fertility of topical corticosteroids.
Studies to determine mutagenicity with prednisolone and hydrocortisone have revealed negative results.

Continued on next page

This product information was prepared in August, 1982. On these and other Parke-Davis Products, information may be obtained by addressing PARKE-DAVIS, Division of Warner-Lambert Company, Morris Plains, New Jersey 07950.

Parke-Davis—Cont.

Pregnancy Category C
Corticosteroids are generally teratogenic in laboratory animals when administered systemically at relatively low dosage levels. The more potent corticosteroids have been shown to be teratogenic after dermal application in laboratory animals. There are no adequate and well-controlled studies in pregnant women on teratogenic effects from topically applied corticosteroids. Therefore, topical corticosteroids should be used during pregnancy only if the potential benefit justifies the potential risk to the fetus. Drugs of this class should not be used extensively on pregnant patients, in large amounts, or for prolonged periods of time.
Nursing Mothers
It is not known whether topical administration of corticosteroids could result in sufficient systemic absorption to produce detectable quantities in breast milk. Systemically administered corticosteroids are secreted into breast milk in quantities *not* likely to have a deleterious effect on the infant. Nevertheless, caution should be exercised when topical corticosteroids are administered to a nursing woman.
Pediatric Use
Pediatric patients may demonstrate greater susceptibility to topical corticosteroid-induced HPA axis suppression and Cushing's syndrome than mature patients because of a larger skin surface area to body weight ratio.
Hypothalamic-pituitary-adrenal (HPA) axis suppression, Cushing's syndrome, and intracranial hypertension have been reported in children receiving topical corticosteroids. Manifestations of adrenal suppression in children include linear growth retardation, delayed weight gain, low plasma cortisol levels, and absence of response to ACTH stimulation. Manifestations of intracranial hypertension include bulging fontanelles, headaches, and bilateral papilledema.
Administration of topical corticosteroids to children should be limited to the least amount compatible with an effective therapeutic regimen. Chronic corticosteroid therapy may interfere with the growth and development of children.
Uticort (Betamethasone Benzoate) Gel/Cream/Ointment/Lotion are not for ophthalmic use.
Adverse Reactions: The following local adverse reactions are reported infrequently with topical corticosteroids, but may occur more frequently with the use of occlusive dressings. These reactions are listed in an approximate decreasing order of occurrence.

Burning
Itching
Irritation
Dryness
Folliculitis
Hypertrichosis
Acneiform eruptions
Hypopigmentation
Perioral dermatitis
Allergic contact dermatitis
Maceration of the skin
Secondary infection
Skin atrophy
Striae
Miliaria

Overdosage: Topically applied corticosteroids can be absorbed in sufficient amounts to produce systemic effects (See *PRECAUTIONS*).
Dosage and Administration: Topical corticosteroids are generally applied to the affected area as a thin film from two to four times daily depending on the severity of the condition.
Occlusive dressings may be used for the management of psoriasis or recalcitrant conditions.
If an infection develops, the use of occlusive dressings should be discontinued and appropriate antimicrobial therapy instituted.
How Supplied:
Uticort Gel 0.025% is supplied as:
N 0071-3025-11—15 gram tube
N 0071-3025-15—60 gram tube
Each gram of Uticort Gel contains 0.25 mg of betamethasone benzoate
Uticort Cream 0.025% is supplied as:
N 0071-3027-11—15 gram tube
N 0071-3027-15—60 gram tube
Each gram of Uticort Cream contains 0.25 mg of betamethasone benzoate
Uticort Ointment 0.025% is supplied as:
N 0071-3026-11—15 gram tube
N 0071-3026-15—60 gram tube
Each gram of Uticort Ointment contains 0.25 mg of betamethasone benzoate
Uticort Lotion 0.025% is supplied as:
N 0071-3029-11—15 ml plastic bottle
N 0071-3029-15—60 ml plastic bottle
US Patent Nos. 3,529,060 and 3,749,773
Store between 59°–86° F.

3026G010

VIRA–A® ℞
(vidarabine for infusion)

Description: Vira-A is the trade name for vidarabine (also known as adenine arabinoside and Ara-A), an antiviral drug. Vira-A is a purine nucleoside obtained from fermentation cultures of *Streptomyces antibioticus.* Each milliliter of sterile suspension contains 200 milligrams of vidarabine monohydrate equivalent to 187.4 milligrams of vidarabine. Each milliliter contains 0.1 milligrams Phemerol® (benzethonium chloride) as a preservative; sodium phosphate, USP, 1.8 milligrams, and sodium biphosphate, USP, 4.8 milligrams, as buffering agents. Hydrochloric acid may have been added to adjust pH. Vira-A is a white, crystalline solid with this empirical formula: $C_{10}H_{13}N_5O_4.H_2O$. The molecular weight is 285.2; the solubility is 0.45 mg/ml at 25 C; and the melting point ranges from 260 to 270 C. The chemical name is 9-β-D-arabinofuranosyladenine monohydrate.
Clinical Pharmacology: Following intravenous administration, Vira-A is rapidly deaminated into arabinosylhypoxanthine (Ara-Hx), the principal metabolite, which is promptly distributed into the tissues. Peak Ara-Hx and Ara-A plasma levels ranging from 3 to 6 μg/ml and 0.2 to 0.4 μg/ml, respectively, are attained after slow intravenous infusion of Vira-A doses of 10 mg/kg of body weight. These levels reflect the rate of infusion and show no accumulation across time. The mean half-life of Ara-Hx is 3.3 hours. Ara-Hx penetrates into the cerebrospinal fluid (CSF) to give a CSF/plasma ratio of approximately 1:3.
Excretion of Vira-A is principally via the kidneys. Urinary excretion is constant over 24 hours. Forty-one to 53% of the daily dose is recovered in the urine as Ara-Hx with 1 to 3% appearing as the parent compound. There is no evidence of fecal excretion of drug or metabolites. In patients with impaired renal function Ara-Hx may accumulate in the plasma and reach levels several-fold higher than those described above.
Vira-A possesses *in vitro* and *in vivo* antiviral activity against *Herpesvirus* simplex (Herpes simplex virus) types 1 and 2.
The antiviral mechanism of action has not yet been established. The drug is converted into nucleotides which appear to be involved with the inhibition of viral replication. In KB cells infected with Herpes simplex virus type 1, Vira-A inhibits viral DNA synthesis. Vira-A is rapidly deaminated to Ara-Hx, the principal metabolite, in cell cultures, laboratory animals, and humans.
Ara-Hx also possesses *in vitro* antiviral activity but this activity is significantly less than the activity of Vira-A.
Indications and Usage: Vira-A is indicated in the treatment of Herpes simplex virus encephalitis. Controlled studies indicated that Vira-A therapy will reduce the mortality caused by Herpes simplex virus encephalitis from 70 to 28% 30 days following onset. In a larger uncontrolled study of 75 patients with biopsy-proven herpes simplex encephalitis, the mortality 6 months from onset was 39%, similar to 44% in the initial controlled study at 6 months.
Morbidity from both studies one year after onset was: normal 53%, moderately debilitated 29%, and severely damaged 18%. Vira-A does not appear to alter morbidity and resulting serious neurological sequelae in the comatose patient. Therefore early diagnosis and treatment are essential.
Herpes simplex virus encephalitis should be suspected in patients with a history of an acute febrile encephalopathy associated with disordered mentation, altered level of consciousness and focal cerebral signs.
Studies which may support the suspected diagnosis include examination of cerebrospinal fluid and localization of an intra-cerebral lesion by brain scan, electroencephalography or computerized axial tomography (CAT).
Brain biopsy is required in order to confirm the etiological diagnosis by means of viral isolation in cell cultures.
Detection of Herpes simplex virus in the biopsied brain tissue can also be reliably done by specific fluorescent antibody techniques. Detection of Herpes virus-like particles by electron microscopy or detection of intranuclear inclusions by histopathologic techniques only provides a presumptive diagnosis.
Contraindications: Vira-A is contraindicated in patients who develop hypersensitivity reactions to it.
Warnings: Vira-A should not be administered by the intramuscular or subcutaneous route because of its low solubility and poor absorption.
There are no reports available to indicate that Vira-A for infusion is effective in the management of encephalitis due to varicella-zoster or vaccinia viruses. Vira-A is not effective against infections caused by adenovirus or RNA viruses. It is also not effective against bacterial or fungal infections. There are no data to support efficacy of Vira-A against cytomegalovirus, vaccinia virus, or smallpox virus.
Precautions:
General—Treatment should be discontinued in the patient with a brain biopsy negative for Herpes simplex virus in cell culture.
Special care should be exercised when administering Vira-A to patients susceptible to fluid overloading or cerebral edema. Examples are patients with CNS infections and impaired renal function.
Patients with impaired renal function, such as post-operative renal transplant recipients, may have a slower rate of renal excretion of Ara-Hx. Therefore, the dose of Vira-A may need to be adjusted according to the severity of impairment. These patients should be carefully monitored.
Patients with impaired liver function should also be observed for possible adverse effects.
Although clear evidence of adverse experience in humans from simultaneous Vira-A and allopurinol administration has not been reported, laboratory studies indicate that allopurinol may interfere with Vira-A metabolism. Therefore, caution is recommended when administering Vira-A to patients receiving allopurinol.
Laboratory Tests—Appropriate hematologic tests are recommended during Vira-A administration since hemoglobin, hematocrit, white blood cells, and platelets may be depressed during therapy.
Some degree of immunocompetence must be present in order for Vira-A to achieve clinical response.
Carcinogenesis—Chronic parenteral (IM) studies of vidarabine have been conducted in mice and rats.

In the mouse study, there was a statistically significant increase in liver tumor incidence among the vidarabine-treated females. In the same study, some vidarabine-treated male mice developed kidney neoplasia. No renal tumors were found in the vehicle-treated control mice or the vidarabine-treated female mice.

In the rat study, intestinal, testicular, and thyroid neoplasia occurred with greater frequency among the vidarabine-treated animals than in the vehicle-treated controls. The increases in thyroid adenoma incidence in the high-dose (50 mg/kg) males and the low-dose (30 mg/kg) females were statistically significant.

Hepatic megalocytosis, associated with vidarabine treatment, has been found in short- and long-term rodent (rat and mouse) studies. It is not clear whether or not this represents a preneoplastic change.

Mutagenesis—Results of *in vitro* experiments indicate that vidarabine can be incorporated into mammalian DNA and can induce mutation in mammalian cells (mouse L5178Y cell line). Thus far, *in vivo* studies have not been as conclusive, but there is some evidence (dominant lethal assay in mice) that vidarabine may be capable of producing mutagenic effects in male germ cells.

It has also been reported that vidarabine causes chromosome breaks and gaps when added to human leukocytes *in vitro*. While the significance of these effects in terms of mutagenicity is not fully understood, there is a well-known correlation between the ability of various agents to produce such effects and their ability to produce heritable genetic damage.

Pregnancy Category C—Vira-A given parenterally is teratogenic in rats and rabbits. Doses of 5 mg/kg or higher given intramuscularly to pregnant rabbits during organogenesis induced fetal abnormalities. Doses of 3 mg/kg or less did not induce teratogenic changes in pregnant rabbits. Vira-A doses ranging from 30 to 250 mg/kg were given intramuscularly to pregnant rats during organogenesis; signs of maternal toxicity were induced at doses of 100 mg/kg or higher and frank fetal anomalies were found at doses of 150 to 250 mg/kg.

A safe dose for the human embryo or fetus has not been established.

There are no adequate and well controlled studies in pregnant women. Vira-A should be used during pregnancy only if the potential benefit justifies the potential risk to the fetus.

Nursing Mothers—It is not known whether Vira-A is excreted in human milk. Because many drugs are excreted in human milk and because of the potential tumorigenicity shown for Vira-A in animal studies, a decision should be made whether to discontinue nursing or to discontinue the drug, taking into account the importance of the drug to the mother.

Adverse Reactions: The principal adverse reactions involve the gastrointestinal tract and are anorexia, nausea, vomiting, and diarrhea. These reactions are mild to moderate, and seldom require termination of Vira-A therapy.

CNS disturbances have been reported at therapeutic doses. These are tremor, dizziness, hallucinations, confusion, psychosis, and ataxia.

Hematologic clinical laboratory changes noted in controlled and uncontrolled studies were a decrease in hemoglobin or hematocrit, white blood cell count, and platelet count. SGOT elevations were also observed. Other changes occasionally observed were decreases in reticulocyte count and elevated total bilirubin.

Other symptoms which have been reported are weight loss, malaise, pruritus, rash, hematemesis, and pain at the injection site.

Overdosage: Acute massive overdose of the intravenous form has been reported without any serious evidence of adverse effect. Because of the low solubility of Vira-A, acute water overloading would pose a greater threat to the patient than Vira-A. Doses of Vira-A over 20 mg/kg/day can produce bone marrow depression with concomitant thrombocytopenia and leukopenia. If a massive overdose of the intravenous form occurs, hematologic, liver, and renal functions should be carefully monitored.

Dosage and Administration: CAUTION—THE CONTENTS OF THE VIAL MUST BE DILUTED IN AN APPROPRIATE INTRAVENOUS SOLUTION PRIOR TO ADMINISTRATION. RAPID OR BOLUS INJECTION MUST BE AVOIDED.

Dosage—Herpes simplex virus encephalitis—15 mg/kg/day for 10 days.

Method of Preparation—Each 5-ml vial contains 1 gram of Vira-A (200 mg per ml of suspension). The solubility of Vira-A in intravenous infusion fluids is limited. Each one mg of Vira-A requires 2.22 ml of intravenous infusion fluid for complete solubilization. Therefore, each one liter of intravenous infusion fluid will solubilize a maximum of 450 mg of Vira-A.

Any appropriate intravenous solution is suitable for use as a diluent *EXCEPT* biologic or colloidal fluids (e.g., blood products, protein solutions, etc.).

Shake the Vira-A vial well to obtain a homogeneous suspension before measuring and transferring.

Prepare the Vira-A solution for intravenous administration by aseptically transferring the proper dose of Vira-A into an appropriate intravenous infusion fluid. The intravenous infusion fluid used to prepare the Vira-A solution should be prewarmed to 35 ° to 40°C (95° to 100°F) to facilitate solution of the drug following its transference. Depending on the dose to be given, more than one liter of intravenous infusion fluid may be required. Thoroughly agitate the prepared admixture until *completely* clear. Complete solubilization of the drug, as indicated by a completely clear solution, is ascertained by careful visual inspection. Final filtration with an in-line membrane filter (0.45 μ pore size or smaller) is necessary. Dilution should be made just prior to administration and used at least within 48 hours. Subsequent agitation, shaking, or inversion of the bottle is unnecessary once the drug is completely in solution. DO NOT REFRIGERATE THE DILUTION.

Administration—Using aseptic technique, slowly infuse the total daily dose by intravenous infusion (prepared as discussed above) at a constant rate over a 12- to 24-hour period.

How Supplied:

N 0071-4150-08 (Steri-Vial® 4150) Vira-A (Vidarabine for Infusion), a sterile suspension containing 200 mg/ml, is supplied in 5 ml Steri-Vials; packages of 10.

Animal Pharmacology and Toxicity:

Acute Toxicity: The intraperitoneal LD_{50} for Vira-A ranged from 3,890 to 4,500 mg/kg in mice, and from 2,239 to 2,512 mg/kg in rats, suggesting a low order of toxicity to a single parenteral dose. Hepatic megalocytosis was observed in rats after single, intraperitoneal injections at doses near and exceeding the LD_{50} value. The hepatic megalocytosis appeared to regress completely over several months. Acute intravenous LD_{50} values could not be obtained because of the limited solubility of Vira-A.

Subacute Toxicity: Rats, dogs, and monkeys have been given daily intramuscular injections of Vira-A as a 20% suspension for 28 days. These animal species showed dose related decreases in hemoglobin, hematocrit, and lymphocytes. Bone marrow depression was also observed in monkeys. Except for localized, injection-site injury and weight gain inhibition or loss, rats tolerated daily doses up to 150 mg/kg, and dogs tolerated daily doses up to 50 mg/kg. Megalocytosis was not seen in the rats dosed by the intramuscular route for 28 days. Rhesus monkeys were particularly sensitive to Vira-A. Daily intramuscular doses of 15 mg/kg were tolerable, but doses of 25 mg/kg or higher induced progressively severe clinical signs of CNS toxicity. Three monkeys given slow intravenous infusions of Vira-A in solution at a dose of 15 mg/kg daily for 28 days had no significant adverse reactions.

4150G020
121 886700/20

VIRA–A® ℞

(vidarabine ophthalmic ointment, USP), 3%

Description: VIRA-A is the trade name for vidarabine (also known as adenine arabinoside and Ara-A), an antiviral drug for the topical treatment of epithelial keratitis caused by Herpes simplex virus. The chemical name is 9-β-D-arabinofuranosyladenine. Each gram of the ophthalmic ointment contains 30 mg of vidarabine monohydrate equivalent to 28.11 mg of vidarabine in a sterile, inert, petrolatum base.

Clinical Pharmacology: Vira-A is a purine nucleoside obtained from fermentation cultures of *Streptomyces antibioticus*. Vira-A possesses *in vitro* and *in vivo* antiviral activity against Herpes simplex types 1 and 2, Varicella-Zoster, and Vaccinia viruses. Except for Rhabdovirus and Oncornavirus, Vira-A does not display *in vitro* antiviral activity against other RNA or DNA viruses, including Adenovirus.

The antiviral mechanism of action has not been established. Vira-A appears to interfere with the early steps of viral DNA synthesis. Vira-A is rapidly deaminated to arabinosylhypoxanthine (Ara-Hx), the principal metabolite. Ara-Hx also possesses *in vitro* antiviral activity but this activity is less than that of Vira-A. Because of the low solubility of Vira-A, trace amounts of both Vira-A and Ara-Hx can be detected in the aqueous humor only if there is an epithelial defect in the cornea. If the cornea is normal, only trace amounts of Ara-Hx can be recovered from the aqueous humor.

Systemic absorption of Vira-A should not be expected to occur following ocular administration and swallowing lacrimal secretions. In laboratory animals, Vira-A is rapidly deaminated in the gastrointestinal tract to Ara-Hx. In contrast to topical idoxuridine, Vira-A demonstrated less cellular toxicity in the regenerating corneal epithelium in the rabbit.

Indications and Usage: Vira-A Ophthalmic Ointment, 3%, is indicated for the treatment of acute keratoconjunctivitis and recurrent epithelial keratitis due to Herpes simplex virus types 1 and 2. It is also effective in superficial keratitis caused by Herpes simplex virus which has not responded to topical idoxuridine or when toxic or hypersensitivity reactions to idoxuridine have occurred. The effectiveness of Vira-A Ophthalmic Ointment, 3%, against stromal keratitis and uveitis due to Herpes simplex virus has not been established.

The clinical diagnosis of keratitis caused by Herpes simplex virus is usually established by the presence of typical dendritic or geographic lesions on slit-lamp examination.

In controlled and uncontrolled clinical trials, an average of seven and nine days of continuous Vira-A Ophthalmic Ointment, 3%, therapy was required to achieve corneal re-epithelialization. In the controlled trials, 70 of 81 subjects (86%) re-epithelialized at the end of three weeks of therapy. In the uncontrolled trials, 101 of 142 subjects (71%) re-epithelialized at the end of three weeks. Seventy-five percent of the subjects in these uncontrolled

Continued on next page

This product information was prepared in August, 1982. On these and other Parke-Davis Products, information may be obtained by addressing PARKE-DAVIS, Division of Warner-Lambert Company, Morris Plains, New Jersey 07950.

Parke-Davis—Cont.

trials had either not healed previously or had developed hypersensitivity to topical idoxuridine therapy.

The following topical antibiotics: gentamicin, erythromycin, and chloramphenicol; or topical steroids: prednisolone or dexamethasone, have been administered concurrently with Vira-A Ophthalmic Ointment, 3%, without an increase in adverse reactions.

Contraindication: Vira-A Ophthalmic Ointment, 3%, is contraindicated in patients who develop hypersensitivity reactions to it.

Warnings: Normally, corticosteroids alone are contraindicated in Herpes simplex virus infections of the eye. If Vira-A Ophthalmic Ointment, 3%, is administered concurrently with topical corticosteroid therapy, corticosteroid-induced ocular side effects must be considered. These include corticosteroid-induced glaucoma or cataract formation and progression of a bacterial or viral infection.

Vira-A is not effective against RNA virus or adenoviral ocular infections. It is also not effective against bacterial, fungal, or chlamydial infections of the cornea or nonviral trophic ulcers.

Although viral resistance to VIRA-A has not been observed, this possibility may exist.

Precautions:

General—The diagnosis of keratoconjunctivitis due to Herpes simples virus should be established clinically prior to prescribing VIRA-A Ophthalmic Ointment, 3%.

Patients should be forewarned that VIRA-A Ophthalmic Ointment, 3%, like any ophthalmic ointment, may produce a temporary visual haze.

Carcinogenesis—Chronic parenteral (IM) studies of vidarabine have been conducted in mice and rats.

In the mouse study, there was a statistically significant increase in liver tumor incidence among the vidarabine-treated females. In the same study some vidarabine-treated male mice developed kidney neoplasia. No renal tumors were found in the vehicle-treated control mice or the vidarabine-treated female mice.

In the rat study, intestinal, testicular, and thyroid neoplasia occurred with greater frequency among the vidarabine-treated animals than in the vehicle-treated controls. The increases in thyroid adenoma incidence in the high dose (50 mg/kg) males and the low dose (30 mg/kg) females were statistically significant.

Hepatic megalocytosis, associated with vidarabine treatment, has been found in short- and long-term rodent (rat and mouse) studies. It is not clear whether or not this represents a preneoplastic change.

The recommended frequency and duration of administration should not be exceeded (See Dosage and Administration).

Mutagenesis—Results of *in vitro* experiments indicate that vidarabine can be incorporated into mammalian DNA and can induce mutation in mammalian cells (mouse L5178Y cell line). Thus far, *in vivo* studies have not been as conclusive, but there is some evidence (dominant lethal assay in mice) that vidarabine may be capable of producing mutagenic effects in male germ cells.

It has also been reported that vidarabine causes chromosome breaks and gaps when added to human leukocytes *in vitro*. While the significance of these effects in terms of mutagenicity is not fully understood, there is a well-known correlation between the ability of various agents to produce such effects and their ability to produce heritable genetic damage.

Pregnancy Category C—VIRA-A parenterally is teratogenic in rats and rabbits. Ten percent VIRA-A ointment applied to 10% of the body surface during organogenesis induced fetal abnormalities in rabbits. When 10% VIRA-A ointment was applied to 2% to 3% of the body surface of rabbits, no fetal abnormalities were found. This dose greatly exceeds the total recommended ophthalmic dose in humans. The possibility of embryonic or fetal damage in pregnant women receiving VIRA-A Ophthalmic Ointment, 3%, is remote. The topical ophthalmic dose is small, and the drug relatively insoluble. Its ocular penetration is very low. However, a safe dose for a human embryo or fetus has not been established. There are no adequate and well controlled studies in pregnant women. VIRA-A should be used during pregnancy only if the potential benefit justifies the potential risk to the fetus.

Nursing Mothers—It is not known whether VIRA-A is secreted in human milk. Because many drugs are excreted in human milk and because of the potential for tumorigenicity shown for VIRA-A in animal studies, a decision should be made whether to discontinue nursing or to discontinue the drug, taking into account the importance of the drug to the mother. However, breast milk excretion is unlikely because VIRA-A is rapidly deaminated in the gastrointestinal tract.

Adverse Reactions: Lacrimation, foreign body sensation, conjunctival injection, burning, irritation, superficial punctate keratitis, pain, photophobia, punctal occlusion, and sensitivity have been reported with VIRA-A Ophthalmic Ointment, 3%. The following have also been reported but appear disease-related: uveitis, stromal edema, secondary glaucoma, trophic defects, corneal vascularization, and hyphema.

Overdosage: Acute massive overdosage by oral ingestion of the ophthalmic ointment has not occurred. However, the rapid deamination to arabinosylhypoxanthine should preclude any difficulty. The oral LD_{50} for vidarabine is greater than 5020 mg/kg in mice and rats. No untoward effects should result from ingestion of the entire contents of a tube.

Overdosage by ocular instillation is unlikely because any excess should be quickly expelled from the conjunctival sac. Too frequent administration should be avoided.

Dosage and Administration: Administer approximately one half inch of VIRA-A Ophthalmic Ointment, 3%, into the lower conjunctival sac five times daily at three-hour intervals.

If there are no signs of improvement after 7 days, or complete re-epithelialization has not occurred by 21 days, other forms of therapy should be considered. Some severe cases may require longer treatment.

After re-epithelialization has occurred, treatment for an additional seven days at a reduced dosage (such as twice daily) is recommended in order to prevent recurrence.

How Supplied: N 0071-3677-07 (Stock 18-1677-139)

VIRA-A Ophthalmic Ointment, 3%, is supplied sterile in ophthalmic ointment tubes of 3.5 g. The base is a 60:40 mixture of solid and liquid petrolatum.

3677G020
121 880400/20

[*Shown in Product Identification Section*]

ZARONTIN® ℞
(ethosuximide, USP)
Capsules

Description: Zarontin (ethosuximide) is an anticonvulsant succinimide, chemically designated as alpha-ethyl-alpha-methyl-succinimide.

Action: Ethosuximide suppresses the paroxysmal three-cycle-per-second spike and wave activity associated with lapses of consciousness which is common in absence (petit mal) seizures. The frequency of epileptiform attacks is reduced, apparently by depression of the motor cortex and elevation of the threshold of the central nervous system to convulsive stimuli.

Indication: Zarontin is indicated for the control of absence (petit mal) epilepsy.

Contraindication: Ethosuximide should not be used in patients with a history of hypersensitivity to succinimides.

Warnings: Blood dyscrasias, including some with fatal outcome, have been reported to be associated with the use of ethosuximide; therefore, periodic blood counts should be performed.

Ethosuximide is capable of producing morphological and functional changes in the animal liver. In humans, abnormal liver and renal function studies have been reported.

Ethosuximide should be administered with extreme caution to patients with known liver or renal diseases. Periodic urinalysis and liver function studies are advised for all patients receiving the drug.

Cases of systemic lupus erythematosus have been reported with the use of ethosuximide. The physician should be alert to this possibility.

Usage in Pregnancy: The effects of Zarontin in human pregnancy and nursing infants are unknown.

Recent reports suggest an association between the use of anticonvulsant drugs by women with epilepsy and an elevated incidence of birth defects in children born to these women. Data are more extensive with respect to phenytoin and phenobarbital, but these are also the most commonly prescribed anticonvulsants. Less systematic or anecdotal reports suggest a possible similar association with the use of all known anticonvulsant drugs.

The reports suggesting an elevated incidence of birth defects in children of drug-treated epileptic women cannot be regarded as adequate to prove a definite cause-and-effect relationship. There are intrinsic methodologic problems in obtaining adequate data on drug teratogenicity in humans. The possibility also exists that other factors, eg, genetic factors or the epileptic condition itself, may be more important than drug therapy in leading to birth defects. The great majority of mothers on anticonvulsant medication deliver normal infants. It is important to note that anticonvulsant drugs should not be discontinued in patients in whom the drug is administered to prevent major seizures because of the strong possibility of precipitating status epilepticus with attendant hypoxia and threat to life. In individual cases where the severity and frequency of the seizure disorder are such that the removal of medication does not pose a serious threat to the patient, discontinuation of the drug may be considered prior to and during pregnancy, although it cannot be said with any confidence that even minor seizures do not pose some hazard to the developing embryo or fetus.

The prescribing physician will wish to weigh these considerations in treating or counseling epileptic women of childbearing potential.

Hazardous Activities: Ethosuximide may impair the mental and/or physical abilities required for the performance of potentially hazardous tasks, such as driving a motor vehicle or other such activity requiring alertness; therefore, the patient should be cautioned accordingly.

Precautions: Ethosuximide, when used alone in mixed types of epilepsy, may increase the frequency of grand mal seizures in some patients.

As with other anticonvulsants, it is important to proceed slowly when increasing or decreasing dosage, as well as when adding or eliminating other medication. Abrupt withdrawal of anticonvulsant medication may precipitate absence (petit mal) status.

Adverse Reactions:

Gastrointestinal System: Gastrointestinal symptoms occur frequently and include anorexia, vague gastric upset, nausea and vomiting, cramps, epigastric and abdominal pain, weight loss, and diarrhea.

Hemopoietic System: Hemopoietic complications associated with the administration of ethosuximide have included leukopenia, agranulocytosis, pancytopenia, aplastic anemia, and eosinophilia.
Nervous System: Neurologic and sensory reactions reported during therapy with ethosuximide have included drowsiness, headache, dizziness, euphoria, hiccups, irritability, hyperactivity, lethargy, fatigue, and ataxia. Psychiatric or psychological aberrations associated with ethosuximide administration have included disturbances of sleep, night terrors, inability to concentrate, and aggressiveness. These effects may be noted particularly in patients who have previously exhibited psychological abnormalities. There have been rare reports of paranoid psychosis, increased libido, and increased state of depression with overt suicidal intentions.
Integumentary System: Dermatologic manifestations which have occurred with the administration of ethosuximide have included urticaria, Stevens-Johnson syndrome, systemic lupus erythematosus, and pruritic erythematous rashes.
Miscellaneous: Other reactions reported have included myopia, vaginal bleeding, swelling of the tongue, gum hypertrophy, and hirsutism.

Dosage and Administration:
Zarontin Capsules (ethosuximide capsules, USP): Zarontin is administered by the oral route. The initial dose for patients 3 to 6 years of age is one capsule (250 mg) per day; for patients 6 years of age and older, 2 capsules (500 mg) per day. The dose thereafter must be individualized according to the patient's response. Dosage should be increased by small increments. One useful method is to increase the daily dose by 250 mg every four to seven days until control is achieved with minimal side effects. Dosages exceeding 1.5 g daily, in divided doses, should be administered only under the strictest supervision of the physician. The *optimal* dose for most children is 20 mg/kg/day. This dose has given average plasma levels within the accepted therapeutic range of 40 to 100 mcg/ml. Subsequent dose schedules can be based on effectiveness and plasma level determinations.
Zarontin may be administered in combination with other anticonvulsants when other forms of epilepsy coexist with absence (petit mal). The *optimal* dosage for most children is 20 mg/kg/day.

How Supplied:
N 0071-0237-24 Bottle of 100. Each capsule contains 250 mg ethosuximide.

0237G020

[*Shown in Product Identification Section*]

ZARONTIN® ℞
(ethosuximide)
Syrup

Description: Zarontin (ethosuximide) is an anticonvulsant succinimide, chemically designated as alpha-ethyl-alpha-methyl-succinimide.
Each teaspoonful (5 ml), for oral administration, contains 250 mg ethosuximide in a raspberry flavored base.
Clinical Pharmacology: Ethosuximide suppresses the paroxysmal three cycle per second spike and wave activity associated with lapses of consciousness which is common in absence (petit mal) seizures. The frequency of epileptiform attacks is reduced, apparently by depression of the motor cortex and elevation of the threshold of the central nervous system to convulsive stimuli.
Indication and Usage: Zarontin is indicated for the control of absence (petit mal) epilepsy.
Contraindication: Ethosuximide should not be used in patients with a history of hypersensitivity to succinimides.
Warnings: Blood dyscrasias, including some with fatal outcome, have been reported to be associated with the use of ethosuximide; therefore, periodic blood counts should be performed. Ethosuximide is capable of producing morphological and functional changes in the animal liver. In humans, abnormal liver and renal function studies have been reported.
Ethosuximide should be administered with extreme caution to patients with known liver or renal disease. Periodic urinalysis and liver function studies are advised for all patients receiving the drug.
Cases of systemic lupus erythematosus have been reported with the use of ethosuximide. The physician should be alert to this possibility.
Hazardous Activities: Ethosuximide may impair the mental and/or physical abilities required for the performance of potentially hazardous tasks, such as driving a motor vehicle or other such activity requiring alertness; therefore, the patient should be cautioned accordingly.
Usage in Pregnancy: The effects of Zarontin in human pregnancy and nursing infants are unknown.
Recent reports suggest an association between the use of anticonvulsant drugs by women with epilepsy and an elevated incidence of birth defects in children born to these women. Data are more extensive with respect to phenytoin and phenobarbital, but these are also the most commonly prescribed anticonvulsants; less systematic or anecdotal reports suggest a possible similar association with the use of all known anticonvulsant drugs.
The reports suggesting an elevated incidence of birth defects in children of drug-treated epileptic women cannot be regarded as adequate to prove a definite cause and effect relationship. There are intrinsic methodologic problems in obtaining adequate data on drug teratogenicity in humans; the possibility also exists that other factors, eg. genetic factors or the epileptic condition itself, may be more important than drug therapy in leading to birth defects. The great majority of mothers on anticonvulsant medication deliver normal infants. It is important to note that anticonvulsant drugs should not be discontinued in patients in whom the drug is administered to prevent major seizures because of the strong possibility of precipitating status epilepticus with attendant hypoxia and threat to life. In individual cases where the severity and frequency of the seizure disorder are such that the removal of medication does not pose a serious threat to the patient, discontinuation of the drug may be considered prior to and during pregnancy, although it cannot be said with any confidence that even minor seizures do not pose some hazard to the developing embryo or fetus.
The prescribing physician will wish to weigh these considerations in treating or counseling epileptic women of childbearing potential.

Precautions:
General: Ethosuximide, when used alone in mixed types of epilepsy, may increase the frequency of grand mal seizures in some patients. As with other anticonvulsants, it is important to proceed slowly when increasing or decreasing dosage, as well as when adding or eliminating other medication. Abrupt withdrawal of anticonvulsant medication may precipitate absence (petit mal) status.
Information for Patient: Ethosuximide may impair the mental and/or physical abilities required for the performance of potentially hazardous tasks such as driving a motor vehicle or other such activity requiring alertness; therefore, the patient should be cautioned accordingly.
Pregnancy: See WARNINGS

Adverse Reactions:
Gastrointestinal System: Gastrointestinal symptoms occur frequently and include anorexia, vague gastric upset, nausea and vomiting, cramps, epigastric and abdominal pain, weight loss, and diarrhea.
Hemopoietic System: Hemopoietic complications associated with the administration of ethosuximide have included leukopenia, agranulocytosis, pancytopenia, aplastic anemia, and eosinophilia.
Nervous System: Neurologic and sensory reactions reported during therapy with ethosuximide have included drowsiness, headache, dizziness, euphoria, hiccups, irritability, hyperactivity, lethargy, fatigue, and ataxia. Psychiatric or psychological aberrations associated with ethosuximide administration have included disturbances of sleep, night terrors, inability to concentrate, and aggressiveness. These effects may be noted particularly in patients who have previously exhibited psychological abnormalities. There have been rare reports of paranoid psychosis, increased libido, and increased state of depression with overt suicidal intentions.
Integumentary System: Dermatologic manifestations which have occurred with the administration of ethosuximide have included urticaria, Stevens-Johnson syndrome, systemic lupus erythematosus, and pruritic erythematous rashes.
Miscellaneous: Other reactions reported have included myopia, vaginal bleeding, swelling of the tongue, gum hypertrophy, and hirsutism.
Dosage and Administration: Zarontin is administered by the oral route. The *initial* dose for patients 3 to 6 years of age is one teaspoonful (250 mg) per day; for patients 6 years of age and older, 2 teaspoonfuls (500 mg) per day. The dose thereafter must be individualized according to the patient's response. Dosage should be increased by small increments. One useful method is to increase the daily dose by 250 mg every four to seven days until control is achieved with minimal side effects. Dosages exceeding 1.5 g daily, in divided doses, should be administered only under the strictest supervision of the physician. The *optimal* dose for most children is 20 mg/kg/day. This dose has given average plasma levels within the accepted therapeutic range of 40 to 100 mcg/ml. Subsequent dose schedules can be based on effectiveness and plasma level determinations.
Zarontin may be administered in combination with other anticonvulsants when other forms of epilepsy coexist with absence (petit mal). The optimal dose for most children is 20 mg/kg/day.

How Supplied:
Zarontin is supplied as:
N0071-2418-23–1 pint bottles. Each 5 ml of syrup contains 250 mg ethosuximide in a raspberry flavored base. Store below 30°C (86°F). Protect from freezing and light.
Zarontin is also supplied in the following form:
N0071-0237-24–Bottle of 100. Each capsule contains 250 mg ethosuximide. Store below 30°C (86°F).

2418G021

ZIRADRYL® Lotion

Description: A zinc oxide-Benadryl lotion of 2% Benadryl® (diphenhydramine hydrochloride) and 2% zinc oxide; contains 2% alcohol.
Indications: For relief of itching in ivy or oak poisoning.
Warning: Should not be applied to extensive, or raw, oozing areas, or for a prolonged time, except as directed by a physician. Hyper-

Continued on next page

This product information was prepared in August, 1982. On these and other Parke-Davis Products, information may be obtained by addressing PARKE-DAVIS, Division of Warner-Lambert Company, Morris Plains, New Jersey 07950.

Parke-Davis—Cont.

sensitivity to any of the components may occur.
Caution: Do not use in the eyes. If the condition for which this preparation is used persists or if a rash or irritation develops, discontinue use and consult a physician. *FOR EXTERNAL USE ONLY*
Directions: *SHAKE WELL*
For relief of itching, cleanse affected area and apply generously three or four times daily. Temporary stinging sensation may follow application. Discontinue use if stinging persists. Easily removed with water.
How Supplied: N 0071-3224-19—6-oz bottles

Pedinol Pharmacal Inc.
110 BELL STREET
W. BABYLON, NY 11704

BREEZEE MIST FOOT POWDER OTC

Composition: Aluminum Chlorhydroxide, Menthol, Undecylenic Acid.
Indications: Topical treatment for hyperhidrosis, bromidrosis and tinea pedis (athlete's foot).
How Supplied: 4 oz. aerosol can.

CASTELLANI PAINT ℞

Composition: Basic Fushsin, Phenol, Resorcinol, Acetone, Alcohol.
Indications: Topical antifungal agent for macerations and ulcerations.
Precautions: If irritation or sensitivity develops, discontinue treatment and consult podiatrist or physician.
Administration: Apply to affected areas once or twice a day.
How Supplied: 1 oz. and 1 pt. plastic bottle. Colorless (without basic fushsin), 1 pt. plastic bottle.

FUNGOID CREME and SOLUTION ℞

Composition: Cetyl Pyridinium Chloride, Triacetin, Chloroxylenol, Vanishing Creme Base
Indications: Topical treatment for fungus, yeast and bacterial infections of the skin.
Precautions: If irritation or sensitivity develops, discontinue treatment and consult podiatrist or physician.
Administration: Apply to affected areas three times a day.
How Supplied: 1 oz. plastic tube; 15cc plastic bottle with controlled dropper.

FUNGOID TINCTURE ℞

Composition: Cetyl Pyridinium Chloride, Triacetin, Chloroxylenol.
Indications: Topical treatment for ringworm infections of the nails, tinea unguium (onychomycosis).
Precautions: If irritation or sensitivity develops, discontinue treatment and consult podiatrist or physician.
Administration: Apply to affected nails twice a day.
How Supplied: 1 oz. bottle with brush applicator, 1 pt. bottle.

HYDRISALIC GEL ℞

Composition: Salicyclic Acid 6%, Isopropanol, Propylene Glycol, Hydroxypropyl Cellulose.
Indications: Topical treatment for hyperkeratotic skin.
Precautions: Use should be limited to children under 12 years of age. If irritation or sensitivity develops, discontinue treatment and consult podiatrist or physician.
Administration: Apply to affected area in the evening. Wash hands thoroughly following application. The medication is washed off the following morning.
How Supplied: 1 oz. plastic tubes.

HYDRISEA LOTION OTC

Composition: Dead Sea Salts Concentrate 8%, Coloring Agent.
Indications: Topical treatment for scaly, dry skin.
Precautions: If irritation or sensitivity develops, discontinue treatment and consult podiatrist or physician.
Administration: Apply twice daily.
How Supplied: 4 oz. plastic bottle.

HYDRISINOL CREME AND LOTION OTC

Composition: Sulfonated Hydrogenated Castor Oil, N.F. IX, Hydrogenated Vegetable Oil.
Indications: Topical emollient to soften dry, cracked, calloused skin.
Administration: Apply as needed.
How Supplied: 4 oz. and 1 lb. jars; 8 oz. plastic bottle.

OSTI-DERM LOTION OTC

Composition: Liquified Phenol, Glycerin, Zinc Oxide, Magnesium Carbonate, Aluminum Acetate Solution (Burow's Solution), Camphor Water, in a Hydrated Aluminum Silicate Gel.
Indications: Topical treatment for bromidrosis, hyperhidrosis, decubitus ulcers, blisters, itching, poison ivy and dermatitis.
Precautions: Check skin sensitivity to phenol. If irritation or sensitivity develops, discontinue treatment and consult podiatrist or physician.
Administration: Apply 2–3 times a day.
How Supplied: 45cc plastic tube.

PEDI-BATH SALTS OTC

Composition: Colloidal Sulphur, Sodium, Magnesium Sulphate, Potassium Iodide, Sodium Chloride, Sodium Bicarb., Pine Needle Oil.
Indications: Topical foot bath; soak for tired aching feet.
Dosage and Administration: Two capsful in a foot bath.
How Supplied: 6 oz. plastic bottle.

PEDI-BORO SOAKS PAKS OTC

Composition: Aluminum Sulfate, Calcium Acetate, Coloring Agent.
Actions: A soothing astringent wet dressing of a modified Burow's Solution, buffered.
Dosage and Administration: Dissolve 1 or 2 paks in a pint of water. Prepare fresh daily.
How Supplied: Box of 12 and Box of 100.

PEDI-CORT V CREME ℞

Composition: Hydrocortisone 1%, Iodochlorhydroxyquin 3%.
Indications: Topical anti-inflammatory antifungal, antibacterial, antipruritic creme for the skin.
Contraindications: Hypersensitivity to any of the ingredients. Not for use in the presence of tuberculosis, vaccinia, varicella or other viral skin conditions.
Precautions: Observe all precautions for using a steroid preparation. If irritation or sensitivity develops, discontinue treatment and consult podiatrist or physician.
Administration: Apply 1–3 times a day.
How Supplied: 20 gm. tubes.

PEDI-DRI FOOT POWDER ℞

Composition: Aluminum Chlorhydroxide, Menthol, Zinc Undecylenate, Formaldehyde.
Indications: Topical treatment for hyperhidrosis, bromidrosis and tinea pedis (athlete's foot).
Precautions: Check for skin sensitivity to formaldehyde. If irritation or sensitivity develops, discontinue treatment and consult podiatrist or physician.
Administration: Apply twice a day.
How Supplied: 2 oz. plastic bottle.

PEDI-VIT A CREME OTC

Composition: Vitamin A.
Indications: Topical treatment for irritated, dry, sensitive skin.
Administration: Apply daily as needed.
How Supplied: 2 oz. jar and 1 lb. jar.

SALACTIC FILM ℞

Composition: Salicyclic Acid 16.7% U.S.P., Lactic Acid 16.7% U.S.P., Flexible Collodian U.S.P., Coloring Agent.
Indications: Topical treatment as a keratolytic agent for removal of verrucae.
Contraindications: Diabetics or patients with impaired blood circulation. Do not use on moles, birthmarks or warts with hair growing from them.
Precautions: Highly flammable. Keep bottle tightly capped when not in use. If irritation or sensitivity develops, discontinue treatment and consult podiatrist or physician.
Administration: Apply once daily as directed.
How Supplied: ½ oz. bottle with brush applicator.

UREACIN-10 Lotion OTC
UREACIN-20, UREACIN-40 Creme

Composition: Urea 10%, Urea 20% and 40%, Vegetable Oil Base.
Indications: Ureacin-10 Lotion, Ureacin-20 Creme is a topical treatment for rough, dry, cracked, calloused skin. Ureacin-40 Creme is indicated for the treatment of nail destruction and dissolution.
Precautions: If irritation or sensitivity develops, discontinue treatment and consult podiatrist or physician.
Administration: Rub in gently two or three times a day to affected area. Ureacin-40 Creme to be applied to diseased nail surface by podiatrist or physician only.
How Supplied: 8 oz. plastic bottle, 3 oz. plastic tube, 1 oz. jar.

For further product information please contact Pedinol Pharmacal Inc.

Pennwalt Corp.
Prescription Division
ROCHESTER, NY 14623

ADAPIN® ℞
(doxepin HCl)

Description: **Adapin (doxepin HCl)** is an isomeric mixture of N,N-dimethyldibenz(b,e) oxepin-$\Delta^{11(6H)}$,γ-propylamine hydrochloride.
Actions: Adapin has a variety of pharmacological actions with its predominant action on the central nervous system. While its mechanism of action is not known, studies have demonstrated that it is neither a monoamine oxidase inhibitor nor a primary stimulant of the central nervous system.
In a large series of patients systematically observed for withdrawal symptoms, none were reported—a finding which is consistent with the virtual absence of euphoria as a side effect and the lack of addictive potential characteristic of this type of chemical compound.
Indications: In controlled clinical evaluations, Adapin has shown marked antianxiety and significant antidepressant effects. Adapin

has been found to be well tolerated even in elderly patients.
Adapin is indicated for the treatment of patients with:

1. Psychoneurotic anxiety and/or depressive reactions.
2. Mixed symptoms of anxiety and depression.
3. Anxiety and/or depression associated with alcoholism.
4. Anxiety associated with organic disease.
5. Psychotic depressive disorders including involutional depression and manic-depressive reactions.

Target symptoms of psychoneurosis that respond particularly well to Adapin include: anxiety, tension, depression, somatic symptoms and concerns, insomnia, guilt, lack of energy, fear, apprehension and worry.
Because Adapin provides antidepressant as well as antianxiety effects, it is of particular value in patients in whom anxiety masks depression. Patients who have not responded to other antianxiety or antidepressant drugs may benefit from Adapin.
Contraindications: Because Adapin has an anticholinergic effect, it is contraindicated in patients with glaucoma or a tendency toward urinary retention.
Use of Adapin is contraindicated in patients who have been found hypersensitive to it.
Warnings: *Usage in Pregnancy:* Adapin has not been evaluated in pregnant patients. Therefore, it should not be used during pregnancy unless, in the judgment of the physician, it is essential to the welfare of the patient.
In animal reproduction studies of Adapin, gross and microscopic examination of the offspring gave no evidence of drug-related teratogenic effect. Following doses of up to 25 mg./kg./day for 8 to 9 months, no changes were observed in the number of live births, litter size, or lactation. A decreased rate of conception was observed when male rats were given 25 mg./kg./day for prolonged periods —an effect which has occurred with other psychotropic drugs and has been attributed to drug effect on the central and/or autonomic nervous systems.
Usage in Children: The use of Adapin in children under 12 years of age is not recommended, because safe conditions for its use have not been established.
MAO Inhibitors: Serious side effects and even death have been reported following the concomitant use of certain drugs with MAO inhibitors. Therefore, MAO inhibitors should be discontinued at least two weeks prior to the cautious initiation of therapy with Adapin (doxepin HCl). The exact length of time may vary and is dependent upon the particular MAO inhibitor being used, the length of time it has been administered, and the dosage involved.
Alcohol: In patients who may use alcohol excessively, it should be borne in mind that the potentiation may increase the danger inherent in any suicide attempt or overdosage.
Precautions: Drowsiness may occur with Adapin (doxepin HCl); therefore, patients should be warned of its possible occurrence and cautioned against driving a motor vehicle or operating hazardous machinery while taking the drug.
Patients should also be cautioned that the effects of alcoholic beverages may be increased.
Since suicide is an inherent risk in depressed patients and remains a risk through the initial phases of improvement, depressed patients should be closely supervised.
Although Adapin has shown effective tranquilizing activity, the possibility of activating or unmasking latent psychotic symptoms should be kept in mind.
Compounds structurally related to Adapin can block the effects of guanethidine and similarly acting compounds. However, at the usual clinical dosages, 75 mg. to 150 mg. per day, Adapin has been given concomitantly with guanethidine without blocking its antihypertensive effect. But at dosages of 300 mg. per day or higher, Adapin has exerted a significant blocking effect.
Adapin, like other structurally related psychotropic drugs, potentiates norepinephrine response in animals. But this effect has not been observed with Adapin in humans, which is in accord with the low incidence of tachycardia reported clinically.
This product contains FD&C Yellow No. 5 (tartrazine) which may cause allergic-type reactions (including bronchial asthma) in certain susceptible individuals. Although the overall incidence of FD&C Yellow No. 5 (tartrazine) sensitivity in the general population is low, it is frequently seen in patients who also have aspirin hypersensitivity.
Adverse Reactions: *Anticholinergic Effects:* Dry mouth, blurred vision and constipation have been reported. These are usually mild, and often subside as therapy is continued or dosage reduced.
Central Nervous System Effects: Drowsiness has been observed. It usually occurs early in the course of therapy and tends to subside as therapy continues. (See Dosage and Administration section.)
Cardiovascular Effects: Tachycardia and hypotension have been reported infrequently.
Other infrequently reported adverse effects include extrapyramidal symptoms, gastrointestinal reactions, secretory effects (such as increased sweating), weakness, dizziness, fatigue, weight gain, edema, paresthesias, flushing, chills, tinnitus, photophobia, decreased libido, rash, and pruritus.
Dosage and Administration: *In most patients with mild to moderate anxiety and/or depression:* A starting dose of 25 mg. t.i.d. is recommended. Decrease or increase the dosage at appropriate intervals according to individual response. Usual optimum dosage is 75 mg. to 150 mg. per day. As an alternate regimen the total daily dosage, up to 150 mg., may be given at bedtime without loss of effectiveness. In some patients with mild symptomatology or emotional symptoms accompanying organic disease, dosage as low as 25 mg. to 50 mg. per day has provided effective control.
In more severe anxiety and/or depression: 50 mg. t.i.d. may be required to start—if necessary, gradually increase to 300 mg. per day. Additional effectiveness is rarely obtained by exceeding 300 mg. per day.
Although optimal antidepressant response may not be evident for two to three weeks, antianxiety activity is rapidly apparent.
Overdosage: Symptoms—An increase of any of the reported adverse reactions, primarily excessive sedation and anticholinergic effects such as blurred vision and dry mouth. Other effects may be: pronounced tachycardia, hypotension and extrapyramidal symptoms. Treatment—Essentially symptomatic; supportive therapy in the case of hypotension and excessive sedation.
How Supplied: Each capsule contains doxepin, as the hydrochloride, 10 mg. (NDC 0018-0356), 25 mg. (NDC 0018-0357), 50 mg. (NDC 0018-0358), 75 mg. (NDC 0018-0361) and 100 mg (NDC 0018-0359) capsules in bottles of 100, and 1000.

Rev 6/80

[*Shown in Product Identification Section*]

INFALYTE™
Oral Electrolyte Replenisher Powder

The remarkable success of the diarrheal-disease program of the World Health Organization (WHO) has demonstrated that, even in the presence of vomiting which often accompanies diarrhea, oral rehydration therapy with a standard glucose-electrolyte solution is the most simple and effective way to:

1. restore water and electrolyte losses in patients of all ages, including newborns, with mild to moderate dehydration caused by acute diarrhea—and—
2. compensate for the losses during continuing diarrhea.

The sodium content of the oral rehydration solution recommended by WHO is designed to replace the large sodium losses seen in cholera. Physicians in developed countries where cholera rarely occurs have been hesitant to use the WHO formula feeling it might cause hypernatremia in patients with milder types of diarrhea. Infalyte contains 45% less sodium chloride than the WHO formula. Therefore, the sodium content of Infalyte in solution (50 mEq/L) is more in keeping with the fecal sodium losses which occur in mild to moderate diarrhea thereby reducing the possibility of inducing hypernatremia while retaining the effectiveness of the WHO formulation.[1]
In addition to its safety, simplicity and effectiveness, oral rehydration and maintenance with Infalyte in solution is less expensive and more comfortable for the patient than intravenous therapy. Since intravenous therapy usually requires hospitalization, oral rehydration could eliminate this additional expense and inconvenience in many cases.
In cases of severe dehydration requiring intravenous therapy, once the patient's blood pressure and pulse rate have stabilized and the estimated dehydration reduced to 5 to 8%, the patient may be switched from intravenous to oral replacement therapy for the completion of rehydration.

[1]Santosham M, Daum RS, Dillman L, et al: Oral rehydration therapy of infantile diarrhea. N Engl J Med 306: 1070-6, 1982.

Indications: When diluted as directed, Infalyte provides a solution suitable for oral administration to restore water and elelectrolytes lost in patients of all ages, including newborns, with mild to moderate dehydration due to acute diarrhea of mild to moderate severity. It is also indicated to maintain hydration and electrolyte balance as long as diarrhea continues.
Ingredients: D-glucose, sodium bicarbonate, potassium chloride and sodium chloride.

Composition of the Solution Made with Infalyte™

Ingredient	mEq/liter	mmol/liter
Sodium	50	50
Potassium	20	20
Chloride	40	40
Bicarbonate	30	30
Glucose	111	111

Osmolarity (mOsm/liter) 251
Each liter provides 77 calories

Preparation of Solution: Dissolve contents of packet in 1 quart (32 fl. oz. or 960 ml) of drinking water. Prepared solution should be covered, refrigerated and used within 24 hours.
Therapy:
Dosage Information for Infants and Young Children
(NOTE: Breast feeding may be continued during rehydration and maintenance therapy with Infalyte in solution even in the presence of vomiting.)
See appropriate column of the following table for the approximate volume of Infalyte in solution to be given. Lesser amounts would be needed by those also receiving breast milk.
Recommended Total Daily Intake of Infalyte in Solution for Infants and Young Children to:
(A) Replace fluid and electrolyte deficit in mild to moderate dehydration due to diarrhea of mild to moderate severity.

Continued on next page

Pennwalt—Cont.

(B) Maintain fluid and electrolyte balance during continuing diarrhea:
[See table below].

1. It is recommended that no food or other liquids (except for breast feeding as noted above) be given during the first eight hours of rehydration therapy with Infalyte in solution. Infalyte in solution should be offered at frequent intervals.
2. After eight hours of Infalyte therapy, food may be offered even if diarrhea has not stopped. For those not being breast fed, cow's milk or commercial lactose-containing products prepared from cow's milk should not be given.
Instead, a soy-based, lactose-free formula diluted 1 to 1 with water may be given.
Those capable of eating should be offered such things as rice cereal mixed with water, pureed fruit such as applesauce or bananas mixed with water, etc.
3. When diarrhea stops, discontinue Infalyte therapy. Avoid cow's milk and other lactose-containing liquids for the next 24 hours at which time the normal diet may be resumed.

Dosage Information for Older Children and Adults

See appropriate column of table below for approximate volume of Infalyte™ in solution to be given.

Recommended Total Daily Intake of Infalyte in solution for Older Children and Adults to:

(A) Replace fluid and electrolyte deficit in mild to moderate dehydration due to diarrhea of mild to moderate severity.
(B) Maintain fluid and electrolyte balance during continuing diarrhea.
[See table above right].

1. It is recommended that no food or other liquids be given during the first eight hours of rehydration therapy with Infalyte in solution. Infalyte in solution should be taken at frequent intervals.
2. After eight hours of Infalyte therapy, age-appropriate food may be offered even if the diarrhea has not stopped. Cow's milk should be avoided until the diarrhea has stopped for 24 hours.
3. When diarrhea stops discontinue Infalyte therapy and resume normal diet.

501-Z-404-100M **8/82**

	(A) Replacement to Correct Dehydration	(B) Maintenance to Prevent Dehydration
Children 4 to 12 years old	Approximate amount 2 to 3 quarts	Approximate amount 1 to 2 quarts
Older children and adults	3 to 4 quarts	2 to 3 quarts

Body Weight		(A) Replacement to Correct Dehydration	(B) Maintenance to Prevent Dehydration
lb	kg	Approximate fl. oz.	Approximate fl. oz.
5	2.3	14	8
10	4.5	22	14
15	6.8	30	19
20	9.1	37	23
25	11.4	44	27
30	13.6	50	31
35	15.9	56	35
40	18.2	61	38

IONAMIN® ©

(phentermine resin)

Description: Ionamin '15' and Ionamin '30' contain 15 mg. and 30 mg. respectively of phentermine as the cationic exchange resin complex. Phentermine is α, α-dimethyl phenylethylamine (phenyl-tertiary-butylamine).

Actions: Ionamin is a sympathomimetic amine with pharmacologic activity similar to the prototype drug of this class used in obesity, amphetamine (d- and d*l*-amphetamine). Actions include central nervous system stimulation and elevation of blood pressure. Tachyphylaxis and tolerance have been demonstrated with all drugs of this class in which these phenomena have been looked for.

Drugs of this class used in obesity are commonly known as "anorectics" or "anorexigenics." It has not been established, however, that the action of such drugs in treating obesity is primarily one of appetite suppression. Other central nervous system actions, or metabolic effects may be involved.

Adult obese subjects instructed in dietary management and treated with "anorectic" drugs, lose more weight on the average than those treated with placebo and diet, as determined in relatively short-term clinical trials.

The magnitude of increased weight loss of drug-treated patients over placebo-treated patients is only a fraction of a pound a week. The rate of weight loss is greatest in the first weeks of therapy for both drug and placebo subjects and tends to decrease in succeeding weeks. The possible origins of the increased weight loss due to the various drug effects are not established. The amount of weight loss associated with the use of an "anorectic" drug varies from trial to trial, and the increased weight loss appears to be related in part to variables other than the drugs prescribed, such as the physician-investigator, the population treated, and the diet prescribed. Studies do not permit conclusions as to the relative importance of the drug and non-drug factors on weight loss.

The natural history of obesity is measured in years, whereas the studies cited are restricted to a few weeks or months duration; thus, the total impact of drug-induced weight loss over that of diet alone must be considered clinically limited.

The bioavailability of Ionamin has been studied in humans in which blood levels of phentermine were measured by a gas-chromatography method. Blood levels obtained with the 15 mg. and 30 mg. resin complex formulations indicated slower absorption with a reduced but prolonged peak concentration and without a significant difference in prolongation of blood levels when compared with the same doses of phentermine hydrochloride. The clinical significance of these differences is not known. In clinical trials establishing the efficacy of Ionamin, a single daily dose produced an effect comparable to that produced by other regimens of "anorectic" drug therapy.

Indication: Ionamin is indicated in the management of exogenous obesity as a short-term (a few weeks) adjunct in a regimen of weight reduction based on caloric restriction. The limited usefulness of agents of this class (see ACTIONS) should be measured against possible risk factors inherent in their use such as those described below.

Contraindications: Advanced arteriosclerosis, symptomatic cardiovascular disease, moderate to severe hypertension, hyperthyroidism, known hypersensitivity, or idiosyncrasy to the sympathomimetic amines, glaucoma.

Agitated states.

Patients with a history of drug abuse.

During or within 14 days following the administration of monoamine oxidase inhibitors (hypertensive crises may result).

Warnings: If tolerance to the "anorectic" effect develops, the recommended dose should not be exceeded in an attempt to increase the effect: rather, the drug should be discontinued. Ionamin may impair the ability of the patient to engage in potentially hazardous activities such as operating machinery or driving a motor vehicle; the patient should therefore be cautioned accordingly.

When using CNS active agents, consideration must always be given to the possibility of adverse interactions with alcohol.

Drug Dependence: Ionamin is related chemically and pharmacologically to amphetamine (d- and d*l*- amphetamine) and other stimulant drugs that have been extensively abused. The possibility of abuse of Ionamin should be kept in mind when evaluating the desirability of including a drug as part of a weight reduction program. Abuse of amphetamine (d- and d*l*-amphetamine) and related drugs may be associated with intense psychological dependence and severe social dysfunction. There are reports of patients who have increased the dosage of some of these drugs to many times that recommended. Abrupt cessation following prolonged high dosage administration results in extreme fatigue and mental depression; changes are also noted on the sleep EEG. Manifestations of chronic intoxication with anorectic drugs include severe dermatoses, marked insomnia, irritability, hyperactivity, and personality changes. The most severe manifestation of chronic intoxications is psychosis, often clinically indistinguishable from schizophrenia.

Usage in Pregnancy: Safe use in pregnancy has not been established. Use of Ionamin by women who are or may become pregnant requires that the potential benefit be weighed against the possible hazard to mother and infant.

Usage in Children: Ionamin is not recommended for use in children under 12 years of age.

Precautions: Caution is to be exercised in prescribing Ionamin for patients with even mild hypertension. Insulin requirements in diabetes mellitus may be altered in association with the use of Ionamin and the concomitant dietary regimen.

Ionamin may decrease the hypotensive effect of guanethidine.

The least amount feasible should be prescribed or dispensed at one time in order to minimize the possibility of overdosage.

Adverse Reactions:

Cardiovascular: Palpitation, tachycardia, elevation of blood pressure.

Central Nervous System: Overstimulation, restlessness, dizziness, insomnia, euphoria, dysphoria, tremor, headache; rarely psychotic episodes at recommended doses with some drugs in this class.

Gastrointestinal: Dryness of the mouth, unpleasant taste, diarrhea, constipation, other gastrointestinal disturbances.

Allergic: Urticaria.

Endocrine: Impotence, changes in libido.

Dosage and Administration: One capsule daily, before breakfast or 10–14 hours before retiring. For individuals exhibiting greater drug responsiveness, Ionamin '15' will usually suffice. Ionamin '30' is recommended for less responsive patients. Ionamin is not recommended for use in children under 12 years of age.

Overdosage: Manifestations of acute overdosage may include restlessness, tremor, hyperreflexia, rapid respiration, confusion, assaultiveness, hallucinations, panic states.
Fatigue and depression usually follow the central stimulation.
Cardiovascular effects include arrhythmias, hypertension, or hypotension and circulatory collapse. Gastrointestinal symptoms include nausea, vomiting, diarrhea, and abdominal cramps. Overdosage of pharmacologically similar compounds has resulted in fatal poisoning, usually terminating in convulsions and coma.
Management of acute Ionamin intoxication is largely symptomatic and includes lavage and sedation with a barbiturate. Experience with hemodialysis or peritoneal dialysis is inadequate to permit recommendation in this regard. Intravenous phentolamine (Regitine) has been suggested on pharmacologic grounds for possible acute, severe hypertension, if this complicates overdosage.

How Supplied: Two strengths: Ionamin (phentermine resin) 15 mg. (NDC 0018-0903) yellow and gray capsules; Ionamin (phentermine resin) 30 mg. (NDC 0018-0904) yellow capsules. Available on prescription only. Stock bottles of 100 and 400. Rev 7/80

[*Shown in Product Identification Section*]

KOLYUM® LIQUID/KOLYUM® POWDER ℞

(potassium gluconate and potassium chloride)

Description: Potassium Supplement
Each tablespoonful (15 ml) of Kolyum Liquid or 5 g packet of Kolyum Powder provides 20 mEq potassium ion and 3.4 mEq chloride ion in a palatable sugar-free cherry-flavored vehicle. These mEq quantities are derived from the presence of potassium gluconate 3.9g and potassium chloride 0.25g. The blandness of the potassium gluconate and the presence of sorbitol in the formulation permit a high level of gastrointestinal tolerance.

Clinical Pharmacology: Potassium ion is the principal intracellular cation of most body tissues. Potassium ions participate in a number of essential physiological processes including the maintenance of intracellular tonicity, the transmission of nerve impulses, the contraction of cardiac, skeletal and smooth muscle, and the maintenance of normal renal function.
Potassium depletion may occur whenever the rate of potassium loss through renal excretion and/or loss from the gastrointestinal tract exceeds the rate of potassium intake. Such depletion usually develops slowly as a consequence of prolonged therapy with oral diuretics, primary or secondary hyperaldosteronism, diabetic ketoacidosis, severe diarrhea, or inadequate replacement of potassium in patients on prolonged parenteral nutrition. Potassium depletion due to these causes is usually accompanied by a concomitant deficiency of chloride and is manifested by hypokalemia and metabolic alkalosis. Potassium depletion may produce weakness, fatigue, disturbances of cardiac rhythm (primarily ectopic beats), prominent U-waves in the electrocardiogram and in advanced cases, flaccid paralysis and/or impaired ability to concentrate urine.
Potassium depletion associated with metabolic alkalosis is managed by correcting the fundamental causes of the deficiency whenever possible and administering supplemental potassium chloride, in the form of high potassium food, or a potassium salt supplement.

Indications and Usage: Kolyum is indicated for the prevention and treatment of hypokalemia which may occur secondary to diuretic or corticosteroid administration. Kolyum may be used in the treatment of cardiac arrhythmias due to digitalis intoxication. In hypokalemic states, especially in patients on salt-free diets, hypochloremic alkalosis may occur; treatment may then require chloride in addition to potassium supplementation. Kolyum provides 3.4 mEq of chloride per dose and therefore it may be used as an adjunct to the treatment of hypochloremic alkalosis.

Contraindications: Hyperkalemia from any cause, severe renal impairment with oliguria or azotemia, untreated Addison's disease, adynamia episodica hereditaria (periodic paralysis, hyperkalemic type), acute dehydration, heat cramps, and patients receiving a potassium-sparing diuretic.

Warnings:
Hyperkalemia
In patients with impaired mechanisms for excreting potassium, the administration of potassium salts can produce hyperkalemia and cardiac arrest. This occurs most commonly if one of these patients is given potassium by the intravenous route, but may also occur if potassium is given orally. Potentially fatal hyperkalemia can develop rapidly and be asymptomatic.
The use of potassium salts in patients with chronic renal disease, or any other condition which impairs potassium excretion, requires particularly careful monitoring of the serum potassium concentration and appropriate dosage adjustment.
Digitalis Intoxication
In the event that digitalis intoxication causes A-V block, potassium salts should not be given. In this situation potassium may potentiate the effect of digitalis on the conduction system, thus further depressing A-V conduction and ventricular responsiveness and inducing more dangerous arrhythmias.
Interaction with Potassium-Sparing Diuretics
Hypokalemia should not be treated by the concomitant administration of potassium salts and potassium-sparing diuretic (e.g., spironolactone or triamterene), since the simultaneous administration of these agents can produce severe hyperkalemia.
Metabolic acidosis
Hypokalemia in patients with metabolic acidosis should be treated with an alkalinizing potassium salt such as potassium bicarbonate, potassium citrate, or potassium acetate.

Precautions: The treatment of potassium depletion, particularly in the presence of cardiac disease, renal disease, or acidosis, requires careful attention to acid-base balance and appropriate monitoring of serum electrolytes, the electrocardiogram, and the clinical status of the patient. In interpreting the serum potassium level, the physician should bear in mind that acute alkalosis per se can produce hypokalemia even in the absence of a deficit in total body potassium, while acute acidosis per se can increase the serum potassium into the normal range even in the presence of a reduced total body potassium. Potassium supplements must be administered with caution, since the amount of the deficiency and the daily intake are not accurately known. Extreme caution should be exercised in patients receiving aldosterone antagonists since potassium intoxication may occur.

Adverse Reactions: The most common adverse reactions to oral potassium salts are nausea, vomiting, abdominal discomfort, and diarrhea. These symptoms, due to irritation of the gastrointestinal tract, are best managed by additional dilution, administration with meals or reducing the dose. One of the most severe adverse effects is hyperkalemia (see Contraindications, Warnings and Overdosage).

Overdosage: Potassium intoxication may result from overdose of potassium or from ordinary therapeutic doses as in the conditions stated in "Contraindications". It is important to recognize that hyperkalemia is usually asymptomatic and may be manifested only by an increased serum potassium concentration and a clinical picture of A-V block (characteristic electrocardiograph changes may include peaking of T-waves, loss of P-wave, depression of S-T segment and prolongation of the QT interval). The symptoms and signs of potassium intoxication include paresthesias and weakness of the extremities, flaccid paralysis, listlessness, mental confusion, hypotension, cardiac arrhythmias and heart block. Hyperkalemia, when detected, must be treated immediately because lethal levels can be reached in a few hours.
Treatment of Hyperkalemia
1) Dextrose solution, 10% or 25%, containing 10 units of crystalline insulin per 20 g dextrose, given i.v. in a dose of 300-500 ml in one hour.
2) Absorption and exchange of potassium ions using cation exchange resins, orally and as retention enema. (Caution: Ammonium cycle exchange resins should not be used in patients with hepatic cirrhosis.)
3) Hemodialysis and peritoneal dialysis.
4) Ingestion of potassium-containing foods and medication should be stopped.
5) Transition from the hyperkalemic state to one of hypokalemia should be guarded against, especially in patients taking digitalis, as hypokalemia increases sensitivity to digitalis.

Dosage: The usual adult dose of Kolyum Liquid is one tablespoonful (15 ml) in 30 ml (one fluid ounce) or more of water twice daily. The usual adult dose of Kolyum Powder is one packet (5 g) dissolved in 3–4 fluid ounces of cool water twice daily.
This daily dose of Kolyum Liquid or Kolyum Powder supplies 40 mEq of potassium ion, the approximate daily requirement, as well as 6.7 mEq of chloride ion. Deviations from this recommendation may be indicated; as no average total daily dose can be defined, the response of the patient to the dose of the drug must be assessed clinically. Larger doses may be required, but should be administered under close supervision because of the possibility of potassium intoxication.

How Supplied:
Kolyum Liquid
Stock bottles of 1 pint and 1 gallon (NDC-0018-0858).
Dispense in amber glass bottles. **Store at room temperature.**
Kolyum Powder
Cartons of 30, 5 g packets (NDC-0018-0604).
Dispense in original packet to keep product moisture-free. **Store at room temperature.**
Kolyum Liquid and Powder are available on prescription only.
Rev. 5/21/81

NESACAINE® ℞

(Chloroprocaine Hydrochloride)
INJECTION
Multidose vials with preservative

NESACAINE®–CE ℞

(Chloroprocaine Hydrochloride)
INJECTION
Single dose vials without preservative

Description: The active ingredient in Nesacaine and Nesacaine-CE is chloroprocaine hydrochloride (β -diethylaminoethyl-2-chloro-4-aminobenzoate hydrochloride).
It is incompatible with caustic alkalis and their carbonates, soaps, silver salts, iodine, and iodides.
Nesacaine, supplied in multidose vials, contains methylparaben as a preservative and should not be used for caudal or epidural anesthesia.
Nesacaine-CE, is supplied in single-dose vials. It contains no preservative, hence, any unused portion should be discarded.
While Nesacaine and Nesacaine-CE are sterile solutions, the vials may be autoclaved for ter-

Continued on next page

Pennwalt—Cont.

minal sterilization with no significant decrease in potency. Sterilization of vials with ethylene oxide is not recommended, since absorption through the closure may occur.

As with other anesthetics having a free aromatic amino group, Nesacaine and Nesacaine-CE solutions are slightly photosensitive and may become discolored after prolonged exposure to light. It is recommended that these vials be stored in the original outer containers, protected from direct sunlight. Discolored solution should not be administered. If exposed to low temperatures, Nesacaine (chloroprocaine hydrochloride) and Nesacaine-CE may deposit crystals of chloroprocaine hydrochloride, which will redissolve with shaking when returned to room temperature. The product should not be used if it contains undissolved material.

Clinical Pharmacology: The parenteral administration of Nesacaine and Nesacaine-CE stabilizes the neuronal membrane and prevents the initiation and transmission of nerve impulses, thereby effecting local anesthetic action. The onset of action is rapid (usually within 6 to 12 minutes) and the duration of anesthesia is up to 60 minutes depending upon the amount used, and the route of administration.

Chloroprocaine is rapidly hydrolyzed in plasma by pseudocholinesterase. The hydrolysis of chloroprocaine results in the production of 2-chloro-4-aminobenzoic acid and β-diethylaminoethanol. Solutions of Nesacaine and Nesacaine-CE do not injure nervous tissue and are not irritating to other tissues in the concentrations recommended.

Indications:

Nesacaine, in multidose vials with preservative is indicated for the production of local anesthesia by infiltration and regional nerve block. It is not to be used for caudal or epidural anesthesia.

Nesacaine-CE, in single dose vials without preservative, is indicated for the production of local anesthesia by infiltration and regional nerve block, including caudal and epidural blocks.

Contraindications: Nesacaine and Nesacaine-CE are contraindicated in patients hypersensitive (allergic) to drugs of the PABA ester group.

Although central nervous system disease is generally considered a contraindication to caudal or epidural nerve block, it is not a contraindication to peripheral nerve block. Pathologic changes of the vertebral column may make epidural puncture impossible or inadvisable.

Warnings: RESUSCITATIVE EQUIPMENT AND DRUGS SHOULD BE IMMEDIATELY AVAILABLE WHEN ANY LOCAL ANESTHETIC IS USED.

NESACAINE (Chloroprocaine Hydrochloride) INJECTION contains a preservative and should not be used for caudal or epidural anesthesia. As NESACAINE-CE contains no preservative, discard unused drug remaining in vial after initial use. Equipment and drugs necessary for the treatment of inadvertent intravascular injection, intrathecal injection, or excessive dosage should be immediately available.

Usage in Pregnancy: Safe use of chloroprocaine hydrochloride has not been established with respect to adverse effects upon fetal development. This fact should be carefully considered before administering this drug to women of childbearing potential, particularly during early pregnancy. This does not preclude the use of the drug at term for obstetrical analgesia. Adverse effects on the fetus, course of labor, or delivery have rarely been observed when proper dosage and proper technique have been employed.

There are no data concerning use of chloroprocaine for obstetrical paracervical block when toxemia of pregnancy is present or when fetal distress or prematurity is anticipated in advance of the block; such use is, therefore, not recommended.

The following information should be considered by clinicians who select chloroprocaine for obstetrical paracervical block anesthesia: 1. Fetal bradycardia (generally a heart rate of less than 120 per minute for more than 2 minutes) has been noted by electronic monitoring in about 5% to 10% of the cases (various studies) where initial total doses of 120 mg to 400 mg of chloroprocaine were employed. The incidence of bradycardia, within this dose range, might not be dose related. 2. Fetal acidosis has not been demonstrated by blood gas monitoring around the time of bradycardia or afterwards. These data are limited and are generally restricted to non-toxemic cases where fetal distress or prematurity was not anticipated in advance of the block. 3. No intact chloroprocaine, and only trace quantities of a hydrolysis product, 2-chloro-4-aminobenzoic acid, have been demonstrated in umbilical cord arterial or venous plasma following properly administered paracervical block with chloroprocaine. 4. The role of drug factors and non-drug factors associated with fetal bradycardia following paracervical block are unexplained at this time.

In obstetrics, if vasoconstrictor drugs are used either to correct hypotension or are added to the local anesthetic solution, the obstetrician should be warned that some oxytocic drugs may cause severe persistent hypertension and even rupture of a cerebral blood vessel may occur during the postpartum period.

Solutions containing vasoconstrictors, particularly epinephrine and norepinephrine, should be used with extreme caution in patients receiving certain antidepressants, such as MAO inhibitors and tricyclic compounds, since severe prolonged hypertension may occur.

Precautions: The safety and effectiveness of chloroprocaine hydrochloride injections depend upon proper dosage, correct technique, adequate precautions and readiness for emergencies.

The lowest dosage that results in effective anesthesia should be used to avoid high plasma levels and serious undesirable systemic side effects. Tolerance varies with the status of the patient. Debilitated patients, elderly patients, acutely ill patients, and children should be given reduced doses commensurate with their age and physical status.

Solutions containing vasoconstrictors should be used cautiously in the presence of disease which may adversely affect the patient's cardiovascular system.

INJECTIONS SHOULD ALWAYS BE MADE SLOWLY AND WITH FREQUENT ASPIRATIONS TO AVOID INADVERTENT RAPID INTRAVASCULAR ADMINISTRATION WHICH CAN PRODUCE SYSTEMIC TOXICITY.

Chloroprocaine hydrochloride should be employed cautiously in persons with known drug allergies or sensitivities.

The decision whether or not to use local anesthesia in the following conditions depends on the physician's appraisal of the advantages as opposed to the risk:

Injection of solutions containing epinephrine in areas where the blood supply is limited (i.e., ears, nose, digits, etc.) or when peripheral vascular disease is present.

Serious cardiac arrhythmias may occur if preparations containing a vasopressor are employed in patients during or following the administration of chloroform, halothane, cyclopropane, trichloroethylene, or other related agents.

Adverse Reactions:

Systemic

Systemic adverse reactions result from high plasma levels due to rapid absorption, inadvertent intravascular injection or excessive dosage. Hypersensitivity, idiosyncrasy, or diminished tolerance (as in patients with plasma cholinesterase deficiency) are other causes of reactions. Reactions due to overdosage (high plasma levels) are systemic and involve the central nervous system and the cardiovascular system.

Central nervous system reactions: These are characterized by excitation and/or depression. Restlessness, anxiety, dizziness, blurred vision or tremors may occur, possibly proceeding to convulsions. However, excitement may be transient or absent, with depression the first manifestation of an adverse reaction. This may quickly be followed by drowsiness merging into unconsciousness and respiratory arrest.

Cardiovascular system reactions: High systemic doses cause depression of the myocardium manifested by an initial episode of hypotension and bradycardia, and even cardiac arrest.

Treatment of systemic reactions: Treatment of a patient with toxic manifestations consists of assuring and maintaining a patent airway and supporting ventilation with oxygen and assisted or controlled ventilation (respiration) as required. This usually will be sufficient in the management of most reactions. Should a convulsion persist despite ventilatory therapy, small increments of anticonvulsive agents may be given intravenously, such as a benzodiazepine (e.g., diazepam), or ultra-short acting barbiturate (e.g. thiopental or thiamylal) or a short-acting barbiturate (e.g. pentobarbital or secobarbital). Cardiovascular depression may require circulatory assistance with intravenous fluids and/or vasopressors (e.g. ephedrine) as dictated by the clinical situation. Allergic reactions are rare and may occur as a result of sensitivity to chloroprocaine or to methylparaben used as a preservative and are characterized by cutaneous lesions, urticaria, edema and anaphylactoid type symptomatology. These allergic reactions should be managed by conventional means. The detection of potential sensitivity by skin testing is of limited value.

Neurologic

In the practice of epidural block, occasional inadvertent penetration of the subarachnoid space by the catheter may occur. The subsequent reactions depend on the amount of drug administered subdurally and may include, among others, spinal block of varying magnitude, loss of bowel and bladder control, loss of perineal sensation and sexual function. Persistent neurological deficit of some lower spinal segments with slow recovery (several months) has been reported in rare instances. (See DOSAGE AND ADMINISTRATION, CAUDAL AND EPIDURAL BLOCK)

Dosage and Administration: The lowest dose needed to provide effective anesthesia should be administered. As with all local anesthetics, the dosage depends upon the area to be anesthetized, vascularity of the tissues, number of neuronal segments to be blocked, individual tolerance and the technique emloyed. For specific techniques and procedures, refer to standard textbooks.

The maximum single recommended doses of chloroprocaine hydrochloride are: without epinephine, 800 mg; with epinephrine (1:200,000), 1000 mg. The recommended dosage is based on requirements for the average adult and should be reduced for elderly or debilitated patients and children.

Preparation of Epinephrine Solutions—To prepare a 1 to 200,000 epinephrine-chloroprocaine hydrochloride solution add 0.15 ml of a 1 to 1,000 epinephrine injection U.S.P. to 30 ml of Nesacaine-CE.

As a guide for some routine procedures, suggested doses are given below:

1. Infiltration and Nerve Block: Nesacaine or Nesacaine-CE
(Chloroprocaine Hydrochloride) INJECTION
Local Infiltration
Quantity depends on the concentration of the solution, the site to be infiltrated, and the discretion of the operator.

Nerve Blocks	Volume	Concentration
Mandibular	2–3 ml	2%
Infraorbital	0.5–1 ml	2%
Brachial Plexus	30–40 ml	2%
Digital (without epinephrine)	3–4 ml	1%
Obstetrical		
Pudendal Block	10 ml each side	2%
Paracervical Block (see WARNINGS section)	3 ml per each of 4 sites	1%

2. Caudal and Epidural Block: Nesacaine-CE (Chloroprocaine Hydrochloride) Injection
For caudal anesthesia the initial dose is 15 to 25 ml of a 2% or 3% solution. Repeated doses may be given at 40 to 60 minute intervals.
For epidural anesthesia in the lumbar and sacral regions 2.0 to 2.5 ml per segment of a 2% or 3% solution can be used. The usual total volume of Nesacaine-CE is from 15 to 25 ml. Repeated doses 2 to 6 ml less than the original dose may be given at 40 to 50 minute intervals.
In order to guard against possible adverse reactions resulting from inadvertent penetration of the subarachnoid space, the following procedures are recommended.

1. Use of an adequate (in the case of Nesacaine-CE, approximately 3 ml of 3% or 5 ml of 2%) test dose prior to induction of complete block. This test dose should be repeated if the patient is moved in such a fashion as to have displaced the epidural catheter. At least 5 minutes should elapse after each test dose prior to proceeding further.
2. Injection of a large, single therapeutic dose through a catheter should be avoided; instead, repeated fractional doses are advocated.
3. In the event of the known injection of a large volume of Nesacaine-CE into the subarachnoid space, an appropriate amount of cerebrospinal fluid (such as 10 ml) should be withdrawn through the catheter or by separate lumbar puncture.

How Supplied: NESACAINE (Chloroprocaine Hydrochloride) INJECTION is supplied as follows:
1% solution in 30 ml multiple dose vials, 12 vials per package.
Each ml contains 10 mg of Chloroprocaine Hydrochloride, 0.6% sodium chloride and 0.2% sodium bisulfite in water for injection, with methylparaben 0.1% added as preservative and hydrochloric acid to adjust pH.
2% solution in 30 ml multiple dose vials, 12 vials per package.
Each ml contains 20 mg of Chloroprocaine Hydrochloride, 0.4% sodium chloride and 0.2% sodium bisulfite in water for injection, with methylparaben 0.1% added as preservative and hydrochloric acid to adjust pH.
NESACAINE-CE (Chloroprocaine Hydrochloride) INJECTION is supplied as follows:
2% solution in 30 ml single dose vials, packaged 12 vials per package.
Each ml contains 20 mg of Chloroprocaine Hydrochloride, 0.4% sodium chloride and 0.2% sodium bisulfite in water for injection, and hydrochloric acid to adjust pH.
3% solution in 30 ml single dose vials, packaged 12 vials per package.
Each ml contains 30 mg of Chloroprocaine Hydrochloride, 0.2% sodium chloride and 0.2% sodium bisulfite in water for injection, and hydrochloric acid to adjust pH.
Rev 12/80

Antitussive
TUSSIONEX® ©
(Resin Complexes of Hydrocodone and Phenyltoloxamine)

TUSSIONEX® Capsules, Suspension and Tablets
Composition: Each capsule, teaspoonful (5 ml.) or tablet contains 5 mg. hydrocodone (*Warning:* may be habit-forming), and 10 mg. phenyltoloxamine as cationic resin complexes.
Effects: An effective antitussive which acts for approximately 12 hours.
Dosage: *Adults:* 1 teaspoonful (5 ml.), capsule or tablet every 8-12 hours. May be adjusted to individual requirements. *Children:* Under 1 year: ¼ teaspoonful every 12 hours. From 1-5 years: ½ teaspoonful every 12 hours. Over 5 years: 1 teaspoonful every 12 hours.
Side Effects: Negligible, but when encountered may include mild constipation, nausea, facial pruritus, drowsiness, which disappear with adjustment of dose or discontinuance of treatment.
Precaution: In young children the respiratory center is especially susceptible to the depressant action of narcotic cough suppressants. Benefit to risk ratio should be carefully considered especially in children with respiratory embarrassment. Estimation of dosage relative to the age and weight of the child is of great importance.
Overdosage: Immediately evacuate the stomach. Respiratory depression, if any, can be counteracted by respiratory stimulants. Convulsions, sometimes seen in children, can be controlled by intravenous administration of short-acting barbiturates. Hypothermia can be controlled by the usual supportive methods.
How Supplied: Tussionex Suspension, neutral in taste, golden color; 16 oz. and 900 ml. bottles. Tussionex Tablets, light brown, scored; bottles of 100. Tussionex Capsules, green and white; bottles of 50. A prescription for 2 oz. of the Suspension, or 12 Capsules or Tablets, constitutes a 6 day supply in the average case.
Rev 11/79

Diuretic, Antihypertensive
ZAROXOLYN® ℞
(Metolazone)

Each ZAROXOLYN Tablet contains 2½, 5, or 10 mg of metolazone.
Description: ZAROXOLYN (metolazone) has the molecular formula $C_{16}H_{16}ClN_3O_3S$ and a molecular weight of 365.84 and its chemical name is 7-chloro-1,2,3,4-tetrahydro-2-methyl-4-oxo-3-o-tolyl-6-quinazolinesulfonamide.
Metolazone is only sparingly soluble in water, but more soluble in plasma, blood, alkali, and organic solvents.
Actions: ZAROXOLYN (metolazone) is a diuretic/saluretic/antihypertensive drug. The action of ZAROXOLYN results in an interference with the renal tubular mechanism of electrolyte reabsorption. The mechanism of this action is unknown. ZAROXOLYN acts primarily to inhibit sodium reabsorption at the cortical diluting site and in the proximal convoluted tubule. Sodium and chloride ions are excreted in approximately equivalent amounts. The increased delivery of sodium to the distal tubular exchange site may result in increased potassium excretion.
DRUG INTERACTION STUDIES: In animals pretreated with ZAROXOLYN, the drug did not alter the characteristic effect of heparin on clotting time nor protamine antagonism; dicumarol on prothrombin time nor Vitamin K antagonism; the response of guanethidine, reserpine and hydralazine to cardiovascular parameters nor the pressor response of the subsequent dose of norepinephrine.
ZAROXOLYN and furosemide, administered concurrently have produced marked diuresis in some patients where edema or ascites was refractory to treatment with maximum recommended doses of these or other diuretics administered alone. The mechanism of this interaction is not known.
In clinical usage, ZAROXOLYN does not inhibit carbonic anhydrase. Its proximal action has been evidenced in humans by increased excretion of phosphate and magnesium ions, by markedly increased fractional excretion of sodium in patients with severely compromised glomerular filtration, and in animals by the results of micropuncture studies. Decrease in calcium ion excretion has not been noted.
At maximum therapeutic dosage ZAROXOLYN is approximately equal to thiazide diuretics in its diuretic potency. However, ZAROXOLYN may produce diuresis in patients with glomerular filtration rates below 20 ml/min.
When ZAROXOLYN is given, diuresis and saluresis usually begin within one hour and persist for 12 to 24 hours depending on dosage. Maximum effect occurs about two hours after administration. At the higher recommended dosages, effect may be prolonged beyond 24 hours. *A single daily dose is recommended.* For most patients the duration of effect can be varied by adjusting the daily dose.
The prolonged duration of action of ZAROXOLYN is attributed to protein-binding and enterohepatic recycling. A small amount of ZAROXOLYN is metabolized and the fraction so changed is nontoxic. The primary route of excretion is renal.
The mechanism whereby diuretics function in the control of hypertension is unknown; both renal and extra-renal actions may be involved. An antihypertensive effect may be seen as early as three to four days after ZAROXOLYN has been started. Administration for three to four weeks, however, is usually required for optimum antihypertensive effect.
Indications: ZAROXOLYN (metolazone) is indicated in the management of hypertension either as the sole therapeutic agent or to enhance the effectiveness of other antihypertensive drugs in the more severe forms of hypertension.
ZAROXOLYN (metolazone) is indicated for the treatment of salt and water retention including
—edema accompanying congestive heart failure
—edema accompanying renal diseases, including the nephrotic syndrome, and states of diminished renal function

Usage in Pregnancy
The routine use of diuretics in an otherwise healthy woman is inappropriate and exposes mother and fetus to unnecessary hazard. Diuretics do not prevent development of toxemia of pregnancy, and there is no satisfactory evidence that they are useful in the treatment of developed toxemia.
Edema during pregnancy may arise from pathological causes or from the physiologic and mechanical consequences of pregnancy. ZAROXOLYN is indicated in pregnancy when edema is due to pathologic causes, just as it is in the absence of pregnancy (however, see Warnings, below). Dependent edema in pregnancy, resulting from restriction of venous return by the expanded uterus, is properly treated through elevation of the lower extremities and use of support hose; use of diuretics to lower intravascular volume in this case is illogical and unnecessary. There is hypervolemia during normal pregnancy which is harmful to neither the fetus nor the mother (in the absence of cardiovascular disease), but which is associated with edema, including generalized edema, in the majority of pregnant women. If this edema produces discomfort, increased recumbency will often provide relief. In rare instances, this edema may cause extreme discomfort which is not relieved by rest. In these

Continued on next page

Pennwalt—Cont.

cases, a short course of diuretics may provide relief and may be appropriate.

Contraindications: Anuria.

Hepatic coma or pre-coma; known allergy or hypersensitivity to ZAROXOLYN (metolazone).

Warnings: While not reported to date, cross-allergy theoretically may occur when ZAROXOLYN (metolazone) is given to patients known to be allergic to sulfonamide-derived drugs, thiazides, or quinethazone.

Hypokalemia may occur, with consequent weakness, cramps, and cardiac dysrhythmias. Hypokalemia is a particular hazard in digitalized patients; dangerous or fatal arrhythmias may be precipitated.

Azotemia and hyperuricemia may be noted or precipitated during the administration of ZAROXOLYN. (Infrequently, gouty attacks have been reported in persons with history of gout.)

If azotemia and oliguria worsen during treatment of patients with severe renal disease, ZAROXOLYN should be discontinued.

Until additional data have been obtained, ZAROXOLYN is not recommended for patients in the pediatric age group.

Unusually large or prolonged effects on volume and electrolytes may result when ZAROXOLYN and furosemide are administered concurrently. It is recommended that concurrent administration of these diuretics for treatment of resistant edema be started under hospital conditions in order to provide for adequate monitoring.

When ZAROXOLYN is used with other antihypertensive drugs, particular care must be taken, especially during initial therapy. Dosage of other antihypertensive agents, especially the ganglionic blockers, should be reduced.

ZAROXOLYN may be given with a potassium-sparing diuretic when indicated. In this circumstance, diuresis may be potentiated and dosages should be reduced. Potassium retention and hyperkalemia may result; the serum potassium should be determined frequently. Potassium supplementation is contraindicated when a potassium-sparing diuretic is given.

Usage in Pregnancy

ZAROXOLYN crosses the placental barrier and appears in cord blood. The use of ZAROXOLYN in pregnant women requires that the anticipated benefit be weighed against possible hazards to the fetus. These hazards include fetal or neonatal jaundice, thrombocytopenia, and possibly other adverse reactions which have occurred in the adult.

Nursing Mothers

ZAROXOLYN appears in breast milk. If use of the drug is deemed essential, the patient should stop nursing.

Precautions: Periodic determination of serum electrolytes to detect possible electrolyte imbalance should be performed at appropriate intervals. Blood urea nitrogen, uric acid, and glucose levels should be assessed at intervals during diuretic therapy.

All patients receiving ZAROXOLYN (metolazone) therapy should be observed for clinical signs of fluid and/or electrolyte imbalance; namely, hyponatremia, hypochloremic alkalosis, and hypokalemia. Serum and urine electrolyte determinations are particularly important when the patient is vomiting excessively or receiving parenteral fluids. Medication such as digitalis may also influence serum electrolytes. Warning signs, irrespective of cause, are: dryness of mouth, thirst, weakness, lethargy, drowsiness, restlessness, muscle pains or cramps, muscular fatigue, hypotension, oliguria, tachycardia, and gastrointestinal disturbances such as nausea and vomiting.

The serum potassium should be determined at regular intervals, and potassium supplementation instituted whenever indicated. Hypokalemia will be more common in association with intensive or prolonged diuretic therapy, with concomitant steroid or ACTH therapy, and with inadequate electrolyte intake.

While not reported to date for ZAROXOLYN, related diuretics have increased responsiveness to tubocurarine and decreased arterial responsiveness to norepinephrine. Accordingly, it may be advisable to discontinue ZAROXOLYN three days before elective surgery.

Caution should be observed when administering ZAROXOLYN to hyperuricemic or gouty patients. ZAROXOLYN exerts minimal effects on glucose metabolism; insulin requirements may be affected in diabetics, and hyperglycemia and glycosuria may occur in patients with latent diabetes.

Chloride deficit and hypochloremic alkalosis may occur. In patients with severe edema accompanying cardiac failure or renal disease, a low-salt syndrome may be produced; hot weather and a low-salt diet will contribute.

Caution should be observed when administering ZAROXOLYN to patients with severely impaired renal function. As most of the drug is excreted by the renal route, cumulative effects may be seen in this circumstance.

Orthostatic hypotension may occur, this may be potentiated by alcohol, barbiturates, narcotics, or concurrent therapy with other antihypertensive drugs.

While not reported for ZAROXOLYN, use of other diuretics has been associated on rare occasions with pathological changes in the parathyroid glands and with hypercalcemia. This possibility should be kept in mind with clinical use of ZAROXOLYN.

Adverse Reactions: Adverse reactions encountered during therapy with potent medications should be considered in two groups: those that represent extensions of the expected pharmacologic actions of the drug, and those which are pharmacologically unexpected, idiosyncratic, specially toxic, due to allergy or hypersensitivity, or due to unexplained causes.

For ZAROXOLYN (metolazone), adverse reactions constituting extensions of the expected pharmacologic actions of this potent diuretic/saluretic/antihypertensive drug may include:

Gastrointestinal reactions: constipation.

Central nervous system reactions: syncope, dizziness, drowsiness.

Cardiovascular reactions: orthostatic hypotension, excessive volume depletion, hemoconcentration, venous thrombosis.

Other reactions: dryness of the mouth, symptomatic and asymptomatic hypokalemia, hyponatremia, hypochloremia; hypochloremic alkalosis, hypophosphatemia, hyperuricemia, hyperglycemia, glycosuria, increase in BUN or creatinine, fatigue, muscle cramps or spasm, weakness, restlessness sometimes resulting in insomnia.

In the second classification, adverse reactions to ZAROXOLYN may include:

Gastrointestinal reactions: nausea, vomiting, anorexia, diarrhea, abdominal bloating, epigastric distress, intrahepatic cholestatic jaundice, hepatitis.

Central nervous system reactions: vertigo, headache, paresthesias.

Hematologic reactions: leukopenia, aplastic anemia.

Dermatologic-hypersensitivity reactions: urticaria and other skin rashes, purpura, necrotizing angiitis (cutaneous vasculitis).

Cardiovascular reactions: palpitation, chest pain, transient blurred vision.

Other reactions: chills, acute gouty attacks.

Adverse reactions which have occurred with other diuretics, but which have not been reported to date for ZAROXOLYN (metolazone), include: pancreatitis, xanthopsia, agranulocytosis, thrombocytopenia, and photosensitivity. These reactions should be considered as possible occurrences with clinical usage of ZAROXOLYN. Whenever adverse reactions are moderate or severe, ZAROXOLYN dosage should be reduced or therapy withdrawn.

Dosage and Administration: Therapy should be individualized according to patient response. Programs of therapy with ZAROXOLYN (metolazone) should be titrated to gain a maximal initial therapeutic response, and to determine the minimal dose possible to maintain that therapeutic response.

ZAROXOLYN is a potent drug with a prolonged, 12-to-24-hour duration of action. When an initially-desired therapeutic effect has been obtained, it is ordinarily advisable to reduce the dosage of ZAROXOLYN to a lower maintenance level. The time interval required for the initial higher-dosage regimen may vary from days in edematous states to three or four weeks in the treatment of elevated blood pressure.

The daily dosage depends on the severity of each patient's condition, his sodium intake, and his responsiveness. Therefore, dosage adjustment is usually necessary during the course of therapy. A decision to reduce the daily dosage of ZAROXOLYN from a higher induction level to a lower maintenance level should be based on the results of thorough clinical and laboratory evaluations. If antihypertensive drugs or diuretics are given concurrently with ZAROXOLYN, careful dosage adjustment may be necessary.

Usual single daily dosage schedules

Suitable initial dosages will usually fall in the ranges given:

Edema of cardiac failure: ZAROXOLYN 5–10 mg. once daily

Edema of renal disease: ZAROXOLYN 5–20 mg. once daily

Mild to moderate essential hypertension:
ZAROXOLYN 2½–5 mg. once daily

For patients with congestive cardiac failure who tend to experience paroxysmal nocturnal dyspnea, it is usually advisable to employ a dosage near the upper end of the range, to ensure prolongation of diuresis and saluresis for a full 24-hour period.

How Supplied: ZAROXOLYN (metolazone) is provided as: pink 2½ mg tablets, blue 5 mg tablets, and yellow 10 mg tablets; in package sizes of 100, 500, 1000 and unit-dose strip packages of 100 (10 × 10's).

Rev 6/82

[*Shown in Product Identification Section*]

Persōn & Covey, Inc.

616 ALLEN AVENUE
GLENDALE, CA 91201

A.C.N® **OTC**
Water-miscible Vitamin A, C, and Niacinamide Tablets

(See PDR For Nonprescription Drugs)

DHS* Conditioning Rinse **OTC**

(See PDR For Nonprescription Drugs)

DHS* Shampoo **OTC**
Dermatological Hair and Scalp Shampoo

(See PDR For Nonprescription Drugs)

DHS* Tar Shampoo **OTC**
Dermatological Hair and Scalp Shampoo

(See PDR For Nonprescription Drugs)

DHS* Zinc Dandruff Shampoo **OTC**

(See PDR For Nonprescription Drugs)

*TM

DRYSOL™ ℞

A Solution of:
Aluminum Chloride (Hexahydrate) 20% w/v in Anhydrous Ethyl Alcohol (S.D. Alcohol 40) 93% v/v.

Indication: An aid in the management of hyperhidrosis.

Directions: Apply Drysol™ to the affected area once a day, only at bedtime. To help prevent irritation, the area should be completely dry prior to application. Do not apply Drysol to broken, irritated or recently shaved skin.

For Maximum Effect: Your doctor may instruct you to cover the treated area with saran wrap held in place by a snug fitting "T" or body shirt, mitten or sock. (Never hold saran in place with tape.) Wash the treated area the following morning. Excessive sweating may be stopped after two or more treatments. Thereafter, apply Drysol™ once or twice weekly or as needed.

Notice: Drysol™ will probably produce a burning or prickling sensation. Keep cap tightly closed when not in use to prevent evaporation.

Warning: For external use only. Keep out of the reach of children. Avoid contact with the eyes. If irritation or sensitization occurs, discontinue use or consult with a physician. Drysol™ may be harmful to certain fabrics.

Package: 37.5 cc polyethylene bottle. NDC 0096-0707-37.
35 cc bottle with convenient Dab-O-Matic™ applicator head. NDC 0096-0707-35.

Assembly Instructions: (For 35cc Dab-O-Matic™ bottle only.) Remove and discard original cap. Push special Dab-O-Matic applicator into bottle opening using the white cap as a holder. Screw cap down to seat applicator.

Patient instruction sheets are available upon request.

ENISYL* 500 Tablets OTC
ENISYL* 334 Tablets
Lysine Hydrochloride

(See PDR For Nonprescription Drugs)
*TM

SOLBAR® OTC
Dioxybenzone and Oxybenzone Cream, U.S.P. PABA FREE

(See PDR For Nonprescription Drugs)

SOLBAR® PLUS 15 OTC
Sun Protectant Cream

(See PDR For Nonprescription Drugs)

XERAC® OTC
(alcohol gel)

(See PDR For Nonprescription Drugs)

XERAC AC* ℞
Aluminum Chloride Hexahydrate in Anhydrous Ethanol

CAUTION: FEDERAL LAW PROHIBITS DISPENSING WITHOUT PRESCRIPTION.

Description: A solution of Aluminum Chloride (Hexahydrate) 6.25% (w/v) in Anhydrous Ethyl Alcohol (S.D. Alcohol 40) 96% (v/v).

Indication: For topical application as an antiperspirant (anhidrotic).

Directions: Apply Xerac AC* to the axillae at bedtime or as directed by physician. Application of Xerac AC is facilitated by the special swab applicator head of the Xerac AC dispenser. To help prevent irritation, the area should be completely dry prior to application. Do not apply Xerac AC to broken or irritated skin. Keep container tightly closed.

Adverse Reactions: Transient stinging or itching may occur. It is not evidence of contact sensitivity and may be prevented or reduced by applying Xerac AC* only to skin which is completely dry or by removing the solution with soap and water.

Warning: For External Use Only. Some users of this product will experience skin irritation. If this occurs, discontinue use. Avoid contact with the eyes. This product may be harmful to certain fabrics. Keep the container tightly closed when not in use to prevent evaporation. Keep this and all medication out of the reach of children.

Assembly Instructions: Remove and discard original cap. Push special Dab-O-Matic™ applicator into bottle opening using the white cap as a holder. Screw cap down to seat applicator.

How Supplied: Xerac AC*—35 cc bottle with special swab applicator head.
NDC 0096-0709-35.
*TM

XERAC BP5™ ℞
XERAC BP10™ ℞
(benzoyl peroxide hydrogel*)

Composition: Xerac BP5™ contains 5% Benzoyl Peroxide, Laureth-4, Carbomer-934, Triethanolamine, Disodium EDTA and Purified Water.
Xerac BP10™ contains 10% Benzoyl Peroxide, Laureth-4, Carbomer-934, Triethanolamine, Disodium EDTA and Purified Water.

Indication: A topical aid in the management of acne.

Actions: Provides the drying and desquamation necessary in the topical treatment of acne.

Administration and Dosage: After washing affected area, rub Xerac BP™ into affected area once or twice daily. The desired degree of drying and peeling may be regulated by increasing or decreasing the dosage schedule.

Contraindication: Should not be used by individuals known to be sensitive to any ingredient of Xerac BP™.

Precautions: For external use only. Avoid contact with the eyes, eyelids and mucous membranes. Keep all medication out of the reach of children. May bleach colored fabrics. If excessive irritation develops, discontinue use and consult physician.

How Supplied: 45 g (1.5 oz.) and 90 g (3 oz.) plastic tubes.
45 g tubes
Xerac BP5™ - NDC 0096-0790-45
Xerac BP10™ - NDC 0096-0791-45
90 g tubes
Xerac BP5™ - NDC 0096-0790-90
Xerac BP10™ - NDC 0096-0791-90
*TM

Pfipharmecs Division

PFIZER INC.
235 EAST 42ND STREET
NEW YORK, NY 10017

Pfipharmecs is a division of Pfizer Inc. which provides economical distribution of a line of time honored antibiotics and certain over-the-counter products to retail and hospital pharmacists. These products include those listed here. Full color identification photographs of the solid oral dosage forms and key injectable antibiotic products listed here can be found in the Product Identification Section.

PRODUCT IDENTIFICATION CODES

To provide quick and positive identification of Pfipharmecs Division products, we have imprinted the product identification number of the National Drug Code on tablets and capsules.

In order that you may quickly identify a product by its code number, we have compiled below a numerical list of code numbers of prescription products with their corresponding product names.

Product Identification Code	NUMERICAL PRODUCT INDEX Product
015	Tetracyn (tetracycline HCl) 250 mg capsules
016	Tetracyn (tetracycline HCl) 500 mg capsules
023	Isoject Pfizerpen-AS Aqueous Suspension (penicillin G procaine) 1,200,000 units/2 ml
024	Pfizer-E (erythromycin stearate) 250 mg tablets
028	Pfizer-E (erythromycin stearate) 500 mg tablets
029	Tetrastatin (tetracycline HCl & nystatin) 250 mg capsules
041	Neobiotic (neomycin sulfate) 500 mg tablets
046	Pfizerpen G (penicillin G potassium) 200,000 units tablets
047	Pfizerpen G (penicillin G potassium) 250,000 units tablets
048	Pfizerpen G (penicillin G potassium) 400,000 units tablets
051	Pfizerpen for Injection (penicillin G potassium) 1,000,000 units/vial
052	Pfizerpen for Injection (penicillin G potassium) 5,000,000 units/vial
053	Pfizerpen for Injection (penicillin G potassium) 20,000,000 units/vial
054	Pfizerpen-AS Aqueous Suspension (pencillin G procaine) 3,000,000 units/vial
069	Terra-Cortril Topical Ointment (oxytetracycline HCl and hydrocortisone)
072	Terramycin (oxytetracycline HCl) capsules 125 mg
073	Terramycin (oxytetracycline HCl) capsules 250 mg.
075	Terramycin Intramuscular Injection (oxytetracycline) 50 mg/ml, 10 ml
080	Terramycin Ophthalmic Ointment with Polymyxin B Sulfate (oxytetracycline HCl with polymyxin B sulfate)
082	Terramycin (calcium oxytetracycline) syrup 2 oz. and 1 pint
084	Terramycin (oxytetracycline) film-coated tablets 250 mg
088	Terrastatin (oxytetracycline with Nystatin) capsules 250 mg
104	Pfizerpen G (penicillin G potassium) 800,000 units tablets
105	Pfizerpen VK (penicillin V potassium) 250 mg tablets
106	Pfizerpen VK (penicillin V potassium) 500 mg tablets
300	Pfizerpen-A (ampicillin) 250 mg capsules
310	Pfizerpen-A (ampicillin) 500 mg capsules
335	Sterane (prednisolone) 5 mg tablets
526	Isoject Vistaril Intramuscular Solution (hydroxyzine HCl) 25 mg/ml, 1 ml
525	Steraject Vistaril Intramuscular Solution, Cartridges (hydroxyzine HCl) 25 mg/ml
527	Isoject Vistaril Intramuscular Solution (hydroxyzine HCl) 50 mg/ml, 1 ml
527	Steraject Vistaril Intramuscular Solution, Cartridges (hydroxyzine HCl) 50 mg/ml

Continued on next page

Pfipharmecs—Cont.

528	**Isoject Vistaril Intramuscualr Solution (hydroxyzine HCl) 100 mg/ml, 1 ml**
528	**Steraject Vistaril Intramuscular Solution, Cartridges (hydroxyzine HCl) 100 mg/ml, 2 ml**
545	**Vistaril Intramuscular Solution (hydroxyzine HCl) 25 mg/ml**
545	**Vistaril Intramuscular Solution Unit-Dose Vials (hydroxyzine HCl) 25 mg/ml**
546	**Vistaril Intramuscular Solution (hydroxyzine HCl) 50 mg/ml**
546	**Vistaril Intramuscular Solution Unit-Dose Vials (hydroxyzine HCl) 50 mg/ml, 75 mg/1.5 ml, 100 mg/2 ml**
640	**Antiminth (pyrantel pamoate) 60 ml oral suspension (50 mg of pyrantel base/ml)**
1643	**Isoject Permapen Aqueous Suspension (penicillin G benzathine) 1,200,000 units/2 ml**

ANTIMINTH® ℞
(pyrantel pamoate)
ORAL SUSPENSION

Actions: Antiminth has demonstrated anthelmintic activity against *Enterobius vermicularis* (pinworm) and *Ascaris Lumbricoides* (common roundworm). The anthelmintic action is probably due to the neuromuscular blocking property of the drug.
Antiminth is partially absorbed after an oral dose. Plasma levels of unchanged drug are low. Peak levels (0.05–0.13 μg.ml.) are reached in 1–3 hours. Quantities greater than 50% of administered drug are excreted in feces as the unchanged form, whereas only 7% or less of the dose is found in urine as the unchanged form of the drug and its metabolites.
Indications: For the treatment of ascariasis (common roundworm infection) and enterobiasis (pinworm infection).
Warnings:
Usage in Pregnancy
Reproduction studies have been performed in animals and there was no evidence of propensity for harm to the fetus. The relevance to the human is not known.
There is no experience in pregnant women who have received this drug.
This drug has not been extensively studied in children under two years; therefore, in the treatment of children under the age of two years, the relative benefit/risk should be considered.
Precautions: Minor transient elevations of SGOT have occurred in a small percentage of patients. Therefore, this drug should be used with caution in patients with pre-existing liver dysfunction.
Adverse Reactions: The most frequently encountered adverse reactions are related to the gastrointestinal system.
Gastrointestinal and hepatic reactions: anorexia, nausea, vomiting, gastralgia, abdominal cramps, diarrhea and tenesmus, transient elevation of SGOT.
CNS reactions: headache, dizziness, drowsiness, and insomnia.
Skin reactions: rashes.
Dosage and Administration:
Children and Adults
Antiminth Oral Suspension (50 mg. of pyrantel base/ml.) should be administered in a single dose of 11 mg. of pyrantel base per kg. of body weight (or 5 mg./lb.); maximum total dose 1 gram. This corresponds to a simplified dosage regimen of 1 ml. of Antiminth per 10 lb. of body weight. (One teaspoonful = 5 ml.)
Antiminth (pyrantel pamoate) Oral Suspension may be administered without regard to ingestion of food or time of day, and purging is not necessary prior to, during, or after therapy. It may be taken with milk or fruit juices.
How Supplied: Antiminth Oral Suspension is available as a pleasant tasting caramel flavored suspension which contains the equivalent of 50 mg. pyrantel base per ml., supplied in 60 ml. bottles.
[*Shown in Product Identification Section*]

BACITRACIN TOPICAL OINTMENT

How Supplied: Each gram contains 500 units of Bacitracin. Available in ½ ounce tubes sold in cartons of twelve. A prescription is not required.

BONINE®
(meclizine hydrochloride)
Chewable Tablets

Actions: BONINE is an antihistamine which shows marked protective activity against nebulized histamine and lethal doses of intravenously injected histamine in guinea pigs. It has a marked effect in blocking the vasodepressor response to histamine, but only a slight blocking action against acetylcholine. Its activity is relatively weak in inhibiting the spasmogenic action of histamine on isolated guinea pig ileum.
Indications: BONINE is effective in the management of nausea, vomiting and dizziness associated with motion sickness.
Contraindications: Meclizine HCl is contraindicated in individuals who have shown a previous hypersensitivity to it.
Warnings: Since drowsiness may, on occasion, occur with the use of this drug, patients should be warned of this possibility and cautioned against driving a car or operating dangerous machinery.
Patients should avoid alcoholic beverages while taking this drug. Due to its potential anticholinergic action, this drug should be used with caution in patients with asthma, glaucoma, or enlargement of the prostate gland.
Usage in Children:
Clinical studies establishing safety and effectiveness in children have not been done; therefore, usage is not recommended in children under 12 years of age.
Usage in Pregnancy:
Meclizine, or any other medication, should be used during pregnancy only if clearly necessary.
Adverse Reactions: Drowsiness, dry mouth, and on rare occasions, blurred vision have been reported.
Dosage and Administration: For motion sickness 1 or 2 tablets of BONINE should be taken one hour prior to embarkation against motion sickness. Therefore, the dose may be repeated every 24 hours for the duration of the journey.
How Supplied: BONINE (meclizine HCl) is available in convenient packets of 8 chewable tablets of 25 mg. meclizine HCl.
[*Shown in Product Identification Section*]

CORTRIL® ℞
(hydrocortisone)
Topical Ointment

How Supplied: Topical Ointment 1.0%: ½ oz. (14.2 Gm.) tube containing 10 mg./Gm. of hydrocortisone.

CORYBAN®-D CAPSULES
Decongestant Cold Capsules

Composition: Each capsule contains:
Caffeine U.S.P. ....30 mg.
Chlorpheniramine maleate U.S.P. ....2 mg.
Phenylpropanolamine HCl ....25 mg.
How Supplied: In bottles of 24, light and dark blue capsules.

CORYBAN®-D COUGH SYRUP
With Decongestant
(Sugar and Saccharin Free Formula)

Composition: Each 5 ml (1 teaspoonful) contains:
Dextromethorphan HBr U.S.P. ....7.5 mg.
Guaifenesin ....50 mg.
Phenylephrine HCl ....5 mg.
Acetaminophen ....120 mg.
Alcohol* 7.5%
* Small loss unavoidable
How Supplied: Coryban-D Cough Syrup is available in 4-ounce dripless spout bottles. Sorbitol, which is contained in this product, is a nutritive, carbohydrate sweetening agent which is metabolized more slowly than sugar.

LI-BAN™ Spray
Lice Control Spray

THIS PRODUCT IS NOT FOR USE ON HUMANS OR ANIMALS

Active Ingredient:

(5-Benzyl-3-Furyl) methyl 2, 2-dimethyl-3-(2-methylpropenyl) cyclopropanecarboxylate	0.500%
Related Compounds	0.068%
Aromatic petroleum hydrocarbons	0.664%
Inert Ingredients	98.768%
	100.000%

Actions: A highly active synthetic pyrethroid for the control of lice and louse eggs on garments, bedding, furniture and other inanimate objects.
Warnings: Avoid contamination of feed and foodstuffs. Cover or remove fishbowls. HARMFUL IF SWALLOWED. This product is not for use on humans or animals. If lice infestations should occur on humans, consult either your physician or pharmacist for a product for use on humans.
Physical and Chemical Hazards: Contents under pressure. Do not use or store near heat or open flame. Do not puncture or incinerate container. Exposure to temperatures above 130° F may cause bursting.
Direction For Use: It is a violation of Federal law to use this product in a manner inconsistent with its labeling.
Shake well before each use. Remove protective cap. Aim spray opening away from person. Push button to spray. CAUTION! Avoid spraying in eyes. Avoid breathing spray mist. Avoid contact with skin. In case of contact wash immediately with soap and water. Vacate room after treatment and ventilate before reoccupying.
To kill lice and louse eggs: Spray in an inconspicuous area to test for possible staining or discoloration. Inspect again after drying, then proceed to spray entire area to be treated.
Hold container upright with nozzle away from you. Depress valve and spray from a distance of 8 to 10 inches.
Spray each square foot for 3 seconds. Spray only those garments, parts of bedding, including mattresses and furniture that cannot be either laundered or dry cleaned.
Allow all sprayed articles to dry thoroughly before use. Repeat treatment as necessary.
Buyer assumes all risks of use, storage or handling of this material not in strict accordance with direction given herewith.

DISPOSAL OF CONTAINER
Wrap container and dispose of in trash. Do not incinerate.
How Supplied: 5 ounce aerosol can.

NEOBIOTIC® TABLETS ℞
(neomycin sulfate)

How Supplied: Available in 500 mg. white tablets, in bottles of 100. Identification code #041.

PERMAPEN® *Isoject*® ℞
(penicillin G benzathine)
in Aqueous Suspension
1,200,000 units
For Intramuscular Use Only

STORE BETWEEN 2°–8°C. (36°–46°F.)
SHAKE WELL BEFORE USING

Description: Permapen (penicillin G benzathine) is a repository penicillin compound which provides blood levels for long periods following its intramuscular injection. This property is the result of its extremely low solubility in water. Chemically, this compound is dibenzylethylenediamine dipenicillin G.
Actions and Pharmacology: Penicillin G exerts a bactericidal action against penicillin-sensitive microorganisms during the stage of active multiplication. It acts through the inhibition of biosynthesis of cell wall mucopeptide. It is not active against the penicillinase-producing bacteria, which includes many strains of staphylococci. Penicillin G exerts high in vitro activity against staphylococci (except penicillinase-producing strains), streptococci (groups A, C, G, H, L and M), and pneumococci. Other organisms sensitive to penicillin G are: *Corynebacterium diphtheriae, Bacillus anthracts,* Clostridia, *Actinomyces bovis, Streptobacillus moniliformis, Listeria monocytogenes,* and Leptospira. *Treponema pallidum* is extremely sensitive to the bactericidal action of penicillin G.
Intramuscular penicillin G benzathine is absorbed very slowly into the blood stream from the intramuscular site and converted by hydrolysis to penicillin G. This combination of hydrolysis and slow absorption results in blood serum levels much lower than other parenteral penicillins.
Approximately 60% of penicillin G is bound to serum protein. The drug is distributed throughout the body tissues in widely varying amounts. Highest levels are found in the kidneys with lesser amounts in the liver, skin and intestines. Penicillin G penetrates into all other tissues and the spinal fluid to a lesser degree. With normal kidney function the drug is excreted rapidly by tubular excretion. In neonates and young infants and in individuals with impaired kidney function, excretion is considerably delayed.
Indications: Intramuscular penicillin G benzathine is indicated in the treatment of infections due to penicillin G-sensitive microorganisms that are susceptible to the low and very prolonged serum levels common to this particular dosage form. Therapy should be guided by bacteriological studies (including sensitivity tests) and by clinical response.
The following infections will usually respond to adequate dosage of intramuscular penicillin G benzathine.
Streptococcal infections (Group A—without bacteremia). Mild to moderate infections of the upper respiratory tract (pharyngitis).
Venereal infections—Syphilis, yaws, bejel and pinta.
Medical Conditions in Which Penicillin G Benzathine Therapy Is Indicated as Prophylaxis:
Rheumatic fever and/or chorea—Prophylaxis with penicillin G benzathine has proven effective in preventing recurrence of these conditions. It has also been used as followup prophylactic therapy for rheumatic heart disease and acute glomerulonephritis.

Contraindications: A history of a previous hypersensitivity reaction to any of the penicillins is a contraindication.
Warning: Serious and occasionally fatal hypersensitivity (anaphylactoid) reactions have been reported in patients on penicillin therapy. Although anaphylaxis is more frequent following parenteral therapy it has occurred in patients on oral penicillins. These reactions are more apt to occur in individuals with a history of sensitivity to multiple allergens.
There have been well documented reports of individuals with a history of penicillin hypersensitivity reactions who have experienced severe hypersensitivity reactions when treated with a cephalosporin. Before therapy with a penicillin, careful inquiry should be made concerning previous hypersensitivity reactions to penicillins, cephalosporins, and other allergens. If an allergic reaction occurs, the drug should be discontinued and the patient treated with the usual agents, e.g., pressor amines, antihistamines and corticosteroids.
Precautions: Penicillin should be used with caution in individuals with histories of significant allergies and/or asthma.
In intramuscular therapy, care should be taken to avoid accidental intravenous administration.
As with all intramuscular preparations, penicillin G benzathine should be injected well within the body of a relatively large muscle. ADULTS: The preferred sites are the upper outer quadrant of the buttock, (i.e., gluteus maximus), and the mid-lateral thigh. CHILDREN: It is recommended that intramuscular injections be given preferably in the mid-lateral muscles of the thigh. In infants and small children the periphery of the upper outer quadrant of the gluteal region should only be used when necessary, such as in burn patients, in order to minimize the possibility of damage to the sciatic nerve.
The deltoid area should be used only if well developed such as in certain adults and older children, and then only with caution to avoid radial nerve injury. Intramuscular injections should not be made into the lower and mid-third of the upper arm. As with all intramuscular injections, aspiration is necessary to help avoid inadvertent injection into a blood vessel. Irritation at the site of injection may occur. In addition, subcutaneous and fat-layer injections should be avoided since they may cause pain and induration. If these occur, they may be relieved by the application of an ice pack.
In streptococcal infections, therapy must be sufficient to eliminate the organism; otherwise the sequelae of streptococcal disease may occur. Cultures should be taken following completion of treatment to determine whether streptococci have been eradicated.
Prolonged use of antibiotics may promote the overgrowth of nonsusceptible organisms, including fungi. Should superinfection occur, appropriate measures should be taken.
Adverse Reactions: The hypersensitivity reactions reported are skin eruptions (maculopapular to exfoliative dermatitis), urticaria and other serum sickness reactions, laryngeal edema and anaphylaxis. Fever and eosinophilia may frequently be the only reaction observed. Hemolytic anemia, leucopenia, thrombocytopenia, neuropathy and nephropathy are infrequent reactions and usually associated with high doses of parenteral penicillin.
Administration and Dosage:
Pediatric Dosage Schedules: In children under 12 years of age, dosage should be adjusted in accordance with the age and weight of the child and the severity of the infection.
Under 2 years of age, the dose may be divided between the two buttocks if necessary.
Streptococcal infections (group A) pharyngitis—A single injection of—900,000 units for older children; 1,200,000 units for adults.

Venereal infections—
Syphilis—Primary, secondary and latent—2.4 million units (1 dose).
Late Syphilis (tertiary and neurosyphilis)—3 million units at 7 day intervals for a total of 6–9 million units.
Congenital Syphilis—under 2 years of age—50,000 units/kg body weight; age 2–12 years—adjust dosage based on adult dosage schedule.
Yaws, Bejel and Pinta—1.2 million units (1 injection).
Prophylaxis—for rheumatic fever and glomerulonephritis.
Following an acute attack, penicillin G benzathine (parenteral) may be given in doses of 1,200,000 units once a month or 600,000 units every 2 weeks.
How Supplied: Permapen (penicillin G benzathine) Aqueous Suspension is supplied in ISOJECT syringe filled with 1 or 2 ml. ISOJECT is a pre-filled disposable syringe unit with a 20-gauge, 1¼ inch needle. Each ml contains: 600,000 units penicillin G benzathine; 0.006 g sodium citrate; 0.003 g polyvinylpyrrolidone; 0.010 g lecithin, and 0.003 g sodium carboxymethylcellulose. Preservatives: methylparaben 0.09%; propylparaben 0.01%.
[*Shown in Product Identification Section*]

PFIZER-E® ℞
(erythromycin stearate)
Film Coated Tablets

Indications: *Streptococcus pyogenes* (Group A beta hemolytic streptococcus): Upper and lower respiratory tract, skin, and soft tissue infections of mild to moderate severity.
Injectable benzathine penicillin G is considered by the American Heart Association to be the drug of choice in the treatment and prevention of streptococcal pharyngitis and in long term prophylaxis of rheumatic fever.
When oral medication is preferred for treatment of the above conditions, penicillin G, V, or erythromycin are alternate drugs of choice. When oral medication is given, the importance of strict adherence by the patient to the prescribed dosage regimen must be stressed. A therapeutic dose should be administered for at least 10 days.
Alpha-hemolytic streptococci (viridans group): Short term prophylaxis of bacterial endocarditis prior to dental or other operative procedures in patients with a history of rheumatic fever or congenital heart disease who are hypersensitive to penicillin. (Erythromycin is not suitable prior to genitourinary surgery where the organisms likely to lead to bacteremia are gram-negative bacilli or the enterococcus group of streptococci.)
Staphylococcus aureus: Acute infections of skin and soft tissue of mild to moderate severity. Resistant organisms may emerge during treatment.
Diplococcus pneumoniae: Upper respiratory tract infections (e.g. otitis media, pharyngitis) and lower respiratory tract infections (e.g. pneumonia) of mild to moderate degree.
Mycoplasma pneumoniae (Eaton agent, PPLO): For respiratory infections due to this organism.
Hemophilus influenzae: For upper respiratory tract infections of mild to moderate severity when used concomitantly with adequate doses of sulfonamides. Not all strains of this organism are susceptible at the erythromycin concentrations ordinarily achieved. (See appropriate sulfonamide labeling for prescribing information.)
Treponema pallidum: Erythromycin is an alternate choice of treatment for primary syphilis in patients allergic to the penicillins. In treatment of primary syphilis, spinal fluid examinations should be done before treatment and as part of follow-up after therapy.

Continued on next page

Pfipharmecs—Cont.

Corynebacterium diphtheriae and *C. minutissimum:* As an adjunct to antitoxin, to prevent establishment of carriers, and to eradicate the organism in carriers.
In the treatment of erythrasma.
Entamoeba histolytica: In the treatment of intestinal amebiasis only. Extra-enteric amebiasis requires treatment with other agents.
Listeria monocytogenes: Infections due to this organism.
Neisseria gonorrhoeae: Erythromycin lactobionate for injection-I.V. in conjunction with erythromycin stearate orally, as an alternative drug in treatment of acute pelvic inflammatory disease caused by *N. gonorrhoeae* in female patients with a history of sensitivity to penicillin. Before treatment of gonorrhea, patients who are suspected of also having syphilis should have a microscopic examination for *T. pallidum* (by immunofluorescence or dark field) before receiving erythromycin, and monthly serologic tests for a minimum of 4 months.
Legionnaires' Disease: Although no controlled clinical efficacy studies have been conducted, *in vitro* and limited preliminary clinical data suggest that erythromycin may be effective in treating Legionnaires' Disease.
Contraindications: Erythromycin is contraindicated in patients with known hypersensitivity to this antibiotic.
Warnings: Usage in pregnancy: Safety for use in pregnancy has not been established.
Precautions: Erythromycin is principally excreted by the liver. Caution should be exercised in administering the antibiotic to patients with impaired hepatic function. There have been reports of hepatic dysfunction, with or without jaundice, occurring in patients receiving oral erythromycin products.
Recent data from studies of erythromycin reveal that its use in patients who are receiving high doses of theophylline may be associated with an increase of serum theophylline levels and potential theophylline toxicity. In case of theophylline toxicity and/or elevated serum theophylline levels, the dose of theophylline should be reduced while the patient is receiving concomitant erythromycin therapy.
Surgical procedures should be performed when indicated.
Adverse Reactions: The most frequent side effects of oral erythromycin preparations are gastrointestinal, such as abdominal cramping and discomfort, and are dose-related. Nausea, vomiting, and diarrhea occur infrequently with usual oral doses.
During prolonged or repeated therapy, there is a possibility of overgrowth of nosusceptible bacteria or fungi. If such infections occur, the drug should be discontinued and appropriate therapy instituted.
Mild allergic reactions such as urticaria and other skin rashes have occurred. Serious allergic reactions, including anaphylaxis, have been reported.
Dosage and Administration: Optimum blood levels are obtained when doses are given on an empty stomach.
Adults: 250 mg every six hours is the usual dose; or 500 mg every 12 hours one hour before meals. Dosage may be increased up to 4 or more grams per day according to the severity of the infection.
Children: Age, weight, and severity of the infection are important factors in determining the proper dosage. 30–50 mg/kg/day, in divided doses, is the usual dose. For more severe infections this dose may be doubled.
When dosage is desired on a twice-a-day schedule in either adults or children, one-half of the total daily dose may be given every 12 hours, one hour before meals.
In the treatment of streptococcal infections, a therapeutic dosage of erythromycin should be administered for at least 10 days. In continuous *prophylaxis* of streptococcal infections in persons with a history of rheumatic heart disease, the dose is 250 mg twice a day.
When used prior to surgery to prevent endocarditis (see *Alpha-hemolytic streptococci*), a recommended schedule for adults is: 500 mg before the procedure and 250 mg every 6 hours for 4 doses after the procedure. For small children: 30 to 50 mg/kg/day divided into three or four evenly spaced doses.
For treatment of primary syphilis: 30–40 grams given in divided doses over a period of 10–15 days.
For treatment of acute pelvic inflammatory disease caused by *N. gonorrhoeae:* 500 mg erythromycin lactobionate for injection-I.V. every 6 hours for 3 days, followed by 250 mg erythromycin stearate every 6 hours for 7 days.
For intestinal amebiasis: Adults: 250 mg four times daily for 10 to 14 days. Children: 30–50 mg/kg/day in divided doses for 10 to 14 days.
For treatment of Legionnaires' Disease: Although optimal doses have not been established, daily doses of erythromycin stearate utilized in reported clinical data were 1 to 4 grams in divided doses.
How Supplied: Pfizer-E (erythromycin stearate) Film Coated Tablets, 250 mg. Each tablet contains erythromycin stearate equivalent to 250 mg erythromycin.
Bottles of 100's.
Unit Dose package of 100's.
Pfizer-E (erythromycin stearate) Film Coated Tablets, 500 mg. Each tablet contains erythromycin stearate equivalent to 500 mg erythromycin.
Bottles of 100's.

Buffered PFIZERPEN® (penicillin G potassium) for Injection ℞

Description: Buffered Pfizerpen (penicillin G potassium) for Injection is a sterile, pyrogen-free powder which is stable for 36 months when stored at room temperature.
Each million units contains approximately 6.8 milligrams of sodium (0.3 mEq.) and 65.6 milligrams of potassium (1.68 mEq.).
Actions and Pharmacology: Penicillin G exerts a bactericidal action against penicillin-sensitive microorganisms during the stage of active multiplication. It acts through the inhibition of biosynthesis of cell wall mucopeptide. It is not active against the penicillinase-producing bacteria, which include many strains of staphylococci. Penicillin G exerts high *in vitro* activity against staphylococci (except penicillinase-producing strains), streptococci (groups A, C, G, H, L, and M) and pneumococci. Other organisms sensitive to penicillin G are *N. gonorrhoeae, Corynebacterium diphtheriae, Bacillus anthracis,* Clostridia, *Actinomyces bovis, Streptobacillus moniliformis, Listeria monocytogenes* and Leptospira. *Treponema pallidum* is extremely sensitive to the bactericidal action of penicillin G. Some species of gram-negative bacilli are sensitive to moderate to high concentrations of the drug obtained with intravenous administration. These include most strains of *Escherichia coli,* all strains of *Proteus mirabilis,* Salmonella and Shigella and some strains of *Aerobacter aerogenes* and *Alcaligenes fecalis.*
Sensitivity Plate Testing: If the Kirby-Bauer method of disc sensitivity is used, a 10 unit penicillin disc should give a zone greater than 28 mm when tested against a penicillin-sensitive bacterial strain.
Aqueous penicillin G is rapidly absorbed following both intramuscular and subcutaneous injection. Approximately 60 percent of the total dose of 300,000 units is excreted in the urine within this 5-hour period. For this reason high and frequent doses are required to maintain the elevated serum levels desirable in treating certain severe infections in individuals with normal kidney function. In neonates and young infants and in individuals with impaired kidney function, excretion is considerably delayed.
Indications: Aqueous penicillin G (parenteral) is indicated in the therapy of severe infections caused by penicillin G-sensitive microorganisms when rapid and high penicillinemia is required. Therapy should be guided by bacteriological studies (including sensitivity tests) and by clinical response.
The following infections will usually respond to adequate dosage of aqueous penicillin G (parenteral):

Streptococcal infections.

NOTE: Streptococci in groups A, C, H, G, L, and M are very sensitive to penicillin G. Some group D organisms are sensitive to the high serum levels obtained with aqueous penicillin G.
Aqueous penicillin (parenteral) is the penicillin dosage form of choice for bacteremia, empyema, severe pneumonia, pericarditis, endocarditis, meningitis and other severe infections caused by sensitive strains of the gram-positive species listed above.

Pneumococcal infections.

Staphylococcal infections—penicillin G sensitive.

Other infections:

Anthrax.
Actinomycosis.
Clostridial infections (including tetanus).
Diphtheria (to prevent carrier state).
Erysipeloid (*Erysipelothrix insidiosa*) endocarditis.
Fusospirochetal infections—severe infections of the oropharynx (Vincent's), lower respiratory tract and genital area due to *Fusobacterium fusiformisans* spirochetes.
Gram-negative bacillary infections (bateremias)—(*E. coli, A. aero genes, A. faecalis,* Salmonella, Shigella and *P. mirabilis*).
Listeria infections (*Listeria monocytogenes*).
Meningitis and endocarditis.
Pasteurella infections (*Pasteurella multocida*).
Bacteremia and meningitis.
Rat-bite fever (*Spirillum minus* or *Streptobacillus moniliformis*).
Gonorrheal endocarditis and arthritis (*N. gonorrhoeae*).
Syphilis (*T. pallidum*) including congenital syphilis.
Meningococcic meningitis.

Although no controlled clinical efficacy studies have been conducted, aqueous crystalline penicillin G for injection and penicillin G procaine suspension have been suggested by the American Heart Association and the American Dental Association for use as part of a combined parenteral-oral regimen for prophylaxis against bacterial endocarditis in patients with congenital heart disease or rheumatic, or other acquired valvular heart disease when they undergo dental procedures and surgical procedures of the upper respiratory tract.[1] Since it may happen that *alpha* hemolytic streptococci relatively resistant to penicillin may be found when patients are receiving continuous oral penicillin for secondary prevention of rheumatic fever, prophylactic agents other than penicillin may be chosen for these patients and prescribed in addition to their continuous rheumatic fever prophylactic regimen.
NOTE: When selecting antibiotics for the prevention of bacterial endocarditis the physician or dentist should read the full joint statement of the American Heart Association and the American Dental Association.[1]
Contraindications: A history of a previous hypersensitivity reaction to any of the penicillins is a contraindication.

Warnings: Serious and occasionally fatal hypersensitivity (anaphylactoid) reactions have been reported in patients on penicillin therapy. Although anaphylaxis is more frequent following parenteral therapy it has occurred in patients on oral penicillins. These reactions are more apt to occur in individuals with a history of sensitivity to multiple allergens.

There have been well documented reports of individuals with a history of penicillin hypersensitivity reactions who have experienced severe hypersensitivity reactions when treated with a cephalosporin. Before therapy with a penicillin, careful inquiry should be made concerning previous hypersensitivity reactions to penicillins, cephalosporins, and other allergens. If an allergic reaction occurs, the drug should be discontinued and the patient treated with the usual agents, e.g., pressor amines, antihistamines, and corticosteroids.

Precautions: Penicillin should be used with caution in individuals with histories of significant allergies and/or asthma.

In streptococcal infections, therapy must be sufficient to eliminate the organism (10 days minimum) otherwise the sequelae of streptococcal disease may occur. Cultures should be taken following the completion of treatment to determine whether streptococci have been eradicated.

Aqueous penicillin G by the intravenous route in high doses (above 10 million units), should be administered slowly because of the adverse effects of electrolyte imbalance from either the potassium or sodium content of the penicillin. The patient's renal, cardiac and vascular status should be evaluated and if impairment of function is suspected or known to exist a reduction in the total dosage should be considered. Frequent evaluation of electrolyte balance, renal and hematopoietic function is recommended during therapy when high doses of intravenous aqueous penicillin G are used.

Prolonged use of antibiotics may promote overgrowth of non-susceptible organisms, including fungi. Should superinfection occur, appropriate measures should be taken. Indwelling intravenous catheters encourage superinfections and should be avoided whenever possible.

Therapy of susceptible infections should be accompanied by any indicated surgical procedures.

Adverse Reactions: Penicillin is a substance of low toxicity but does have a significant index of sensitization. The following hypersensitivity reactions have been reported: skin rashes ranging from maculopapular eruptions to exfoliative dermatitis: urticaria and reactions resembling serum sickness, including chills, fever, edema, arthralgia and prostration. Severe and occasionally fatal anaphylaxis has occurred (see "Warnings").

Hemolytic anemia, leucopenia, thrombocytopenia, nephropathy, and neuropathy are rarely observed adverse reactions and are usually associated with high intravenous dosage.

Patients given continuous intravenous therapy with penicillin G potassium in high dosage (10 million to 100 million units daily) may suffer severe or even fatal potassium poisoning, particularly if renal insufficiency is present. Hyperreflexia, convulsions and coma may be indicative of this syndrome.

Cardiac arrhythmias and cardiac arrest may also occur. (High dosage of penicillin G sodium may result in congestive heart failure due to high sodium intake.)

The Jarisch-Herxheimer reaction has been reported in patients treated for syphilis.

Administration and Dosage: *Severe infections due to Susceptible Strains of Streptococci, Pneumococci and Staphylococci*—bacteremia, pneumonia, endocarditis, pericarditis, empyema, meningitis and other severe infections—a minimum of 5 million units daily.

Syphilis—Aqueous penicillin G may be used in the treatment of acquired and congenital syphilis, but because of the necessity of frequent dosage, hospitalization is recommended. Dosage and duration of therapy will be determined by age of patient and stage of the disease.

Gonorrheal endocarditis—a minimum of 5 million units daily.

Meningococcic meningitis—1–2 million units intramuscularly every 2 hours, or continuous I.V. drip of 20–30 million units/day.

Actinomycosis—1–6 million units/day for cervico-facial cases; 10–20 million units/day for thoracic and abdominal disease.

Clostridial infections—20 million units/day; penicillin is adjunctive therapy to antitoxin.

Fusospirochetal infections—severe infections of oropharynx, lower respiratory tract and genital area—5–10 million units/day.

Rat-bite fever (*Spirillum minus* or *Streptobacillus moniliformis*)—12–15 million units/day for 3–4 weeks.

Listeria infections (*Listeria monocytogenes*).

Neonates—500,000 to 1 million units/day.

Adults with meningitis—15–20 million units/day for 2 weeks.

Adults with endocarditis—15–20 million units/day for 4 weeks.

Pasteurella infections (*Pasteurella multocida*).

Bacteremia and meningitis—4–6 million units/day for 2 weeks.

Erysipeloid (*Erysipelothrix insidiosa*).

Endocarditis—2–20 million units/day for 4–6 weeks.

Gram-negative bacillary infections (*E. coli, A. aerogenes, A. faecalis,* Salmonella, Shigella and *Proteus mirabilis*).

Bacteremia—20–80 million units/day.

Diphtheria (carrier state)—300,000–400,000 units of penicillin/day in divided doses for 10–12 days.

Anthrax—a minimum of 5 million units of penicillin/day in divided doses until cure is effected.

For prophylaxis against bacterial endocarditis[1] in patients with congenital heart disease or rheumatic, or other acquired valvular heart disease when undergoing dental procedures or surgical procedures of the upper respiratory tract, use a combined parenteral-oral regimen. One million units of aqueous crystalline penicillin G (30,000 units/kg in children) intramuscularly mixed with 600,000 units procaine penicillin G (600,000 units for children) should be given one-half to one hour before the procedure. Oral penicillin V (phenoxymethyl penicillin), 500 mg for adults or 250 mg for children less than 60 lb, should be given every 6 hours for 8 doses. Doses for children should not exceed recommendations for adults for a single dose or for a 24 hour period.

The following table shows the amount of solvent required for solution of various concentrations.

[See table above].

Desired Concentration (units/ml)	Approx. Volume (ml) 1,000,000 units	Solvent for Vial of 5,000,000 units	Infusion Only 20,000,000 units
50,000	19.6	...	...
100,000	9.6	...	...
250,000	3.6	18.2	74.2
500,000	1.6	8.2	32.4
750,000	...	4.8	...
1,000,000	...	3.2	11.5

When the required volume of solvent is greater than the capacity of the vial, the penicillin can be dissolved by first injecting only a portion of the solvent into the vial, then withdrawing the resultant solution and combining it with the remainder of the solvent in a larger sterile container.

Buffered Pfizerpen (penicillin G potassium) for Injection is highly water soluble. It may be dissolved in small amounts of Water for Injection, or Sterile Isotonic Sodium Chloride Solution for Parenteral Use. All solutions should be stored in a refrigerator. When refrigerated, penicillin solutions may be stored for seven days without significant loss of potency.

Buffered Pfizerpen (penicillin G potassium) for Injection may be given intramuscularly or by continuous intravenous drip for dosages of 500,000, 1,000,000, or 5,000,000 units. It is also suitable for intrapleural, intraarticular, and other local instillations.

THE 20,000,000 UNIT DOSAGE MAY BE ADMINISTERED BY INTRAVENOUS INFUSION ONLY.

(1) Intramuscular Injection: Keep total volume of injection small. The intramuscular route is the preferred route of administration. Solutions containing up to 100,000 units of penicillin per ml of diluent may be used with a minimum of discomfort. Greater concentration of penicillin G per ml is physically possible and may be employed where therapy demands. When large dosages are required, it may be advisable to administer aqueous solutions of penicillin by means of continuous intravenous drip.

(2) Continuous Intravenous Drip: Determine the volume of fluid and rate of its administration required by the patient in a 24-hour period in the usual manner for fluid therapy, and add the appropriate daily dosage of penicillin to this fluid. For example, if an adult patient requires 2 liters of fluid in 24 hours and a daily dosage of 10 million units of penicillin, add 5 million units to 1 liter and adjust the rate of flow so that the liter will be infused in 12 hours.

(3) Intrapleural or Other Local Infusion: If fluid is aspirated, give infusion in a volume equal to ¼ or ½ the amount of fluid aspirated, otherwise, prepare as for intramuscular injection.

(4) Intrathecal Use: The intrathecal use of penicillin in meningitis must be highly individualized. It should be employed only with full consideration of the possible irritating effects of penicillin when used by this route. The preferred route of therapy in bacterial meningitides is intravenous, supplemental by intramuscular injection.

How Supplied: Buffered Pfizerpen (penicillin G potassium) for Injection is available in vials containing respectively 1,000,000, 5,000,000, and 20,000,000 units of dry powder for reconstitution; buffered with sodium citrate and citric acid to an optimum pH.

Each million units contains approximately 6.8 milligrams of sodium (0.3 mEq.) and 65.6 milligrams of potassium (1.68 mEq.).

Reference:

1. American Heart Association. 1977. Prevention of bacterial endocarditis. Circulation. **56**:139A–143A.

PFIZERPEN-A® •

(ampicillin)

CAPSULES 250 mg and 500 mg
for ORAL SUSPENSION 125 mg/5 ml and 250 mg/5 ml

℞

Indications: Pfizerpen-A is indicated in the treatment of infections due to susceptible strains of the following:

gram-negative organisms—*Shigellae, Salmonellae* (including *S. typhosa*), *H. influenzae, E. coli* and *P. mirabilis, N. gonorrhoeae,* and *N. meningitidis;*

Continued on next page

Pfipharmecs—Cont.

gram-positive organisms—Streptococci, *D. pneumoniae*, and nonpenicillinase-producing staphylococci.

Because of its wide spectrum and bactericidal action, it may be useful in instituting therapy; however, bacteriological studies to determine the causative organisms and their sensitivity to ampicillin should be performed.

Indicated surgical procedures should be performed.

Contraindications: The use of this drug is contraindicated in individuals with a history of an allergic reaction to any of the penicillins.

Warnings:

SERIOUS AND OCCASIONALLY FATAL HYPERSENSITIVITY (ANAPHYLACTOID) REACTIONS HAVE BEEN REPORTED IN PATIENTS ON PENICILLIN THERAPY. ALTHOUGH ANAPHYLAXIS IS MORE FREQUENT FOLLOWING PARENTERAL THERAPY, IT HAS OCCURRED IN PATIENTS ON ORAL PENICILLINS. THESE REACTIONS ARE MORE APT TO OCCUR IN INDIVIDUALS WITH A HISTORY OF PENICILLIN HYPERSENSITIVITY AND/OR HYPERSENSITIVITY REACTIONS TO MULTIPLE ALLERGENS. THERE HAVE BEEN REPORTS OF INDIVIDUALS WITH A HISTORY OF PENICILLIN HYPERSENSITIVITY WHO HAVE EXPERIENCED SEVERE REACTIONS WHEN TREATED WITH CEPHALOSPORINS. BEFORE THERAPY WITH A PENICILLIN, CAREFUL INQUIRY SHOULD BE MADE CONCERNING PREVIOUS HYPERSENSITIVITY REACTIONS TO PENICILLINS, CEPHALOSPORINS, AND OTHER ALLERGENS. IF AN ALLERGIC REACTION OCCURS, THE DRUG SHOULD BE DISCONTINUED AND THE APPROPRIATE THERAPY INSTITUTED.

SERIOUS ANAPHYLACTOID REACTIONS REQUIRE IMMEDIATE EMERGENCY TREATMENT WITH EPINEPHRINE, OXYGEN, INTRAVENOUS STEROIDS, AND AIRWAY MANAGEMENT, INCLUDING INTUBATION, SHOULD ALSO BE ADMINISTERED AS INDICATED.

Usage in Pregnancy:

Safety for use in pregnancy has not been established.

Precautions: As with any antibiotic preparation, constant observations for signs of overgrowth of nonsusceptible organisms, including fungi, are essential. Should superinfection occur (usually involving Aerobacter, Pseudomonas, or Candida), the drug should be discontinued and/or appropriate therapy instituted. As with any other potent agent, it is advisable to check periodically for organ-system dysfunction during prolonged therapy; this includes renal, hepatic, and hematropoietic systems. This is particularly important in prematures, neonates and other infants.

Adverse Reactions: As with other penicillins, it may be expected that untoward reactions will be essentially limited to sensitivity phenomena. They are more likely to occur in individuals who have previously demonstrated hypersensitivity to pencillins and in those with a history of allergy, asthma, hay fever, or urticaria. The following adverse reactions have been reported as associated with the use of ampicillin.

Gastrointestinal—glossitis, stomatitis, black "hairy" tongue, nausea, vomiting, enterocolitis, pseudomembranous colitis and diarrhea. (These reactions are usually associated with oral dosage forms.)

Hypersensitivity reactions—An erythematous maculopapular rash has been reported fairly frequently. Urticaria and erythema multiforme have been reported occasionally. A few cases of exfoliative dermatitis have been reported. Anaphylaxis is the most serious reaction experienced and has usually been associated with the parenteral dosage form.

Note: Urticaria, other skin rashes, and serum sickness-like reactions may be controlled with antihistamines and, if necessary, systemic corticosteroids. Whenever such reactions occur, ampicillin should be discontinued, unless in the opinion of the physician, the condition being treated is life-threatening and amenable only to ampicillin therapy.

Liver—A moderate rise in serum glutamic oxaloacetic transaminase (SGOT) has been noted, particularly in infants, but the significance of this finding is unknown.

Hemic and Lymphatic Systems—Anemia, thrombocytopenia, thrombocytopenic purpura, eosinophilia, leukopenia, and agranulocytosis have been reported during therapy with the penicillins. These reactions are usualy reversible on discontinuation of therapy and are believed to be sensitivity reactions.

Dosage: *Infections of the ear, nose, throat, and lower respiratory tract* due to streptococci, pneumococci, and nonpenicillinase-producing staphylococci, and also those infections of *the upper and lower respiratory tract due to H. influenzae:*

Adults—250 mg every 6 hours.
Children—50/mg/kg/day in divided doses every 6 or 8 hours.

Infections of the genitourinary tract caused by sensitive gram-negative and gram-positive bacteria:

Adults—500 mg every 6 hours. Larger doses may be required for severe infections.
Children—100 mg/kg/day in divided doses every 6 hours.

Uncomplicated urethritis due to N. gonorrhoeae:

Adult males and females—3.5 grams single oral dose administered simultaneously with 1.0 gram of probenecid.

Cases of gonorrhea with a suspected lesion of syphilis should have dark field examinations before receiving ampicillin, and monthly serological tests for a minimum of 4 months.

Infections of the gastrointestinal tract:

Adults—500 mg every 6 hours.
Children—100 mg/kg/day in divided doses every 6 hours.

Larger doses may be required for stubborn or severe infections. The children's dosage is intended for individuals whose weight will not cause a dosage to be calculated greater than that recommended for adults. Children weighing more than 20 kg should be dosed accordingly to the adult recommendations.

It should be recognized that in the treatment of chronic urinary tract and intestinal infections, frequent bacteriological and clinical appraisals are necessary. Smaller doses than those recommended above should not be used. Even higher doses may be needed at times. In stubborn infections, therapy may be required for several weeks. It may be necessary to continue clinical and/or bacteriological follow-up for several months after cessation of therapy.

Treatment should be continued for a minimum of 48 to 72 hours beyond the time that the patient becomes asymptomatic or evidence of bacterial eradication has been obtained. It is recommended that there be at least 10 days treatment for any infection caused by hemolytic streptococci, to help prevent the occurrence of acute rheumatic fever or glomerulonephritis.

Directions for Mixing Oral Suspension: Prepare suspension at time of dispensing as follows: Add 66 ml of water to the 100 ml package and 132 ml of water to the 200 ml package. Shake vigorously. This will provide 100 and 200 ml of suspension, respectively. Each teaspoonful (5 ml) will contain 125 mg or 250 mg ampicillin. SHAKE WELL BEFORE USING. Keep bottle tightly closed. The reconstituted suspension is stable for 7 days at room temperature (70°F) or 14 days under refrigeration (40°F).

How Supplied: Pfizerpen-A (ampicillin) Capsules: Ampicillin trihydrate equivalent to 250 mg or 500 mg ampicillin per capsule.

250 mg: bottles of 100 and 500.
500 mg: bottles of 100.

Pfizerpen-A (ampicillin) for Oral Suspension. Each 5 ml of reconstituted suspension contains ampicillin trihydrate equivalent to 125 mg or 250 mg ampicillin.

125 mg/5 ml: bottles of 100 ml, 150 ml and 200 ml.
250 mg/5 ml: bottles of 100 ml, 150 ml and 200 ml.

***Pfizer formerly distributed Ampicillin manufactured by Beecham Laboratories under the trademark Pen A. Pfizerpen-A Capsules and Oral Suspension are currently manufactured by Pfizer Inc.**

[*Shown in Product Identification Section*]

PFIZERPEN®-AS ℞

(penicillin G procaine)
in Aqueous Suspension
For Intramuscular Use Only

Description: Pfizerpen-AS (penicillin G procaine) is a highly potent antibacterial agent effective against a wide variety of pathogenic organisms. It is an equimolecular compound of procaine and penicillin G in aqueous suspension for intramuscular administration.

Actions and Pharmacology: Penicillin G exerts a bactericidal action against penicillin-sensivitive micoorganisms during the stage of active multiplication. It acts through the inhibition of biosynthesis of cell wall mucopeptide. It is not active against the penicillinase-producing bacteria, which include many strains of staphylococci. Penicillin G exerts high in vitro activity against staphylococci (except penicillinase-producing strains), streptococci (groups A.C.G.H.L. and M.) and pneumococci. Other organisms sensitive to penicillin G are *N. gonorrhoeae, Corvnebacterium diphtheriae, Bacillus anthracis,* Clostrida, *Actinomyces bovis, Streptobacillus moniliformis, Listera monocytogenes* and Leptospira. *Treponemia pallidum* is extremely sensitive to the bactericidal action of penicillin G.

Sensitivity plate testing: If the Kirby-Bauer method of disc sensitivity is used, a 10-unit penicillin disc should give a zone greater than 28 mm when tested against a penicillin-sensitive bacterial strain.

Penicillin G procaine is an equimolecular compound of procaine and penicillin G administered intramuscularly as a suspension. It dissolves slowly at the site of injection, giving a plateau type of blood level at about 4 hours which falls slowly over a period of the next 15-20 hours.

Approximately 60% of penicillin G is bound to serum protein. The drug is distributed throughout the body tissues in widely varying amounts. Highest levels are found in the kidneys with lesser amounts in the liver, skin and intestines. Penicillin G penetrates into all other tissues to a lesser degree with a very small level found in the cerebrospinal fluid. With normal kidney function the drug is excreted rapidly by tubular excretion. In neonates and young infants and in individuals with impaired kidney functions, excretion is considerably delayed. Approximately 60-90% of a dose of parenteral penicillin G is excreted in the urine within 24-36 hours.

Indications: Penicillin G procaine is indicated in the treatment of moderately severe infections due to penicillin G-sensitive microorganisms that are sensitive to the low and persistent serum levels common to this paritcular dosage form. Therapy should be guided by bacteriological studies (including sensitivity tests) and by clinical response.

NOTE: When high sustained serum levels are required, aqueous penicillin G either IM or IV should be used.

The following infections will usually respond to adequate dosages of intramuscular penicillin G procaine.

Streptococcal infections: Group A (without bacteremia). Moderately severe to severe infections of the upper respiratory tract (including middle ear infections—otitis media), skin and soft tissue infections, scarlet fever, and erysipelas.

NOTE: Streptococci in groups A.C.H.G.L. and M are very sensitive to penicillin G. Other groups, including group D (enterococcus) are resistant. Aqueous penicillin is recommended for streptococcal infections with bacteremia.

Pneumococcal infections: Moderately severe infections of the respiratory tract (including middled ear infections—otitis media).

NOTE: Severe pneumonia, empyema, bacteremia, pericarditis, meningitis, peritonitis, and purulent or septic arthritis of pneumococcal etiology are better treated with aqueous penicillin G during the acute stage.

Staphylococcal infections: penicillin G-sensitive. Moderately severe infections of the skin and soft tissues.

NOTE: Reports indicate an increasing number of strains of staphylococci resistant to penicillin G emphasizing the need for culture and sensitivity studies in treating suspected staphylococcal infections.

Indicated surgical procedures should be performed.

Fusospirochetosis (Vincent's gingivitis and pharyngitis). Moderately severe infections of the oropharynx respond to therapy with penicillin G procaine.

NOTE: Necessary dental care should be accomplished in infections involving the gum tissue.

Treponema pallidum (syphilis): all stages.

N. gonorrhoeae; acute and chronic (without bacteremia).

Yaws, Bejel, Pinta.

C. diphtheriae— penicillin G procaine as an adjunct to antitoxin for prevention of the carrier stage.

Anthrax.

Streptobacillus monoliformis and *Spirillum minus* infections (rat bite fever).

Erysipeloid.

Subacute bacterial endocarditis (group A streptococcus) only in extremely sensitive infections.

Prophylaxis Against Bacterial Endocarditis— Penicillin G procaine may be given to patients with congential and/or rheumatic heart lesions who are to undergo dental or upper respiratory tract surgery or instrumentation. Prophylaxis should be instituted the day of the procedure and continued for 2 or more days following.

NOTE: Since patients who have a past history of rheumatic fever and are receiving continuous prophylaxis may harbor increased numbers of penicillin-resistant organisms, use of another prophylactic anti-infective agent should be considered. If penicillin is to be used in these patients at surgery, the regular rheumatic fever program should be interrupted 1 week prior to the contemplated surgery. At the time of surgery, penicillin may be reinstituted as a prophylactic measure against the hazards of surgically induced bacteremia.

Contraindications: A previous hypersensitivity reaction to any penicillin or procaine is a contraindication.

Warnings: Serious and occasionally fatal hypersensitivity (anaphylactoid) reactions have been reported in patients on penicillin therapy. Although anaphylaxis is more frequent following parenteral therapy it has occurred in patients on oral penicillins. These reactions are more apt to occur in individuals with a history of sensitivity to multiple allergens.

There have been well documented reports of individuals with a history of penicillin hypersensitivity reactions who have experienced severe hypersensitivity reactions when treated with a cephalosporin. Before therapy with a penicillin, careful inquiry should be made concerning previous hypersensitivity reactions to penicillins, cephalosporins, and other allergens. If an allergic reaction occurs, the drug should be discontinued and the patient treated with the usual agents *e.g.,* pressor amines, antihistamines and corticosteroids.

Immediate toxic reactions to procaine may occur in some individuals, particularly when a large single dose is administered in the treatment of gonorrhea (4.8 million units). These reactions may be manifested by mental disturbances including anxiety, confusion, agitation, depression, weakness, seizures, hallucinations, combativeness, and expressed "fear of impending death". The reactions noted in carefully controlled studies occurred in approximately one in 500 patients treated for gonorrhea. Reactions are transient, lasting from 15-30 minutes.

Precautions: Penicillin should be used with caution in individuals with histories of significant allergies and/or asthma.

In intramuscular therapy, care should be taken to avoid accidental intravenous administration.

As with all intramuscular preparations, Pfizerpen-AS (penicillin G procaine) should be injected well within the body of a relatively large muscle. ADULTS: The preferred site is the upper outer quadrant of the buttock, (i.e., gluteus maximus), or the mid-lateral thigh. CHILDREN: It is recommended that intramuscular injections be given preferably in the mid-lateral muscles of the thigh. In infants and small children the periphery of the upper outer quadrant of the gluteal region should only be used when necessary, such as in burn patients, in order to minimize the possibility of damage to the sciatic nerve.

The deltoid area should be used only if well developed such as in certain adults and older children, and then only with caution to avoid radial nerve injury. Intramuscular injections should not be made into the lower and mid-third of the upper arm. As with all intramuscualr injections, aspiration is necessary to help avoid inadvertent injection into a blood vessel.

In suspected staphylococcal infections, proper laboratory studies, including sensitivity tests, should be performed.

A small percentage of patients are sensitive to procaine. If there is a history of sensitivity make the usual test: Inject intradermally 0.1 ml of a 1 to 2 percent procaine solution. Development of an erythema, wheal, flare or eruption indicates procaine sensitivity. Sensitivity should be treated by the usual methods, including barbiturates, and penicillin G procaine preparations should not be used. Antihistamines appear beneficial in treatment of procaine reactions.

The use of antibiotics may result in overgrowth of nonsusceptible organisms. Constant observation of the patient is essential. If new infections due to bacteria or fungi appear during therapy, the drug should be discontinued and appropriate measures taken. Whenever allergic reactions occur, penicillin should be withdrawn unless, in the opinion of the physician, the condition being treated is life threatening and amenable only to penicillin therapy.

In prolonged therapy with penicillin, and particularly with high dosage schedules, periodic evaluation of the renal and hematopoietic systems are recommended.

When treating gonococcal infections in which primary or secondary syphilis may be suspected, proper diagnostic procedures, including dark field examinations should be done. In all cases in which concomitant syphilis is suspected, monthly serological tests should be made for at least four months.

Adverse Reactions: Penicillin is a substance of low toxicity, but does possess a significant index of sensitization. The following hypersensitivity reactions associated with use of penicillin have been reported: skin rashes, ranging from maculopapular eruptions to exfoliative dermatitis; urticaria; serum sickness-like reactions, including chills, fever, edema, arthralgia and prostration. Severe and often fatal anaphylaxis has been reported (see "Warnings"). As with other treatments for syphilis, the Jarisch-Herxheimer reaction has been reported.

Procaine toxicity manifestations have been reported (see Warnings). Procaine hypersensitivity reactions have not been reported with this drug.

Administration and Dosage:

Pediatric Dosage Schedules: In children under 3 months of age, the absorption of aqueous penicillin G produces such high and sustained levels that penicillin G procaine dosage forms offer no advantages and are usually unnecessary.

In children under 12 years of age, dosage should be adjusted in accordance with the age and weight of the child and the severity of the infection.

Under 2 years of age, the dose may be divided between the two buttocks if necessary.

Penicillin G procaine (aqueous) is for intramuscular injection only.

Recommended dosage for penicillin G procaine aqueous:

Pneumonia (pneumococcal), moderately severe (uncomplicated): 600,000-1,000,000 units daily.

Streptococcal infections (group A), moderately severe to severe tonsillitis, erysipelas, scarlet fever, upper respiratory tract, skin and soft tissue: 600,000-1,000,000 units daily for 10 day minimum.

Staphylococcal infections, moderately severe to severe: 600,000-1,000,000 units daily.

Bacterial endocarditis (group A streptococci) only in extremely sensitive infections: 600,000-1,000,000 units daily.

To prevent bacterial endocarditis in patients with rheumatic or congenital heart lesions who are to undergo dental or upper respiratory tract surgery or instrumentation:

600,000 units penicillin G procaine aqueous the day of the procedure.

600,000 units aqueous penicillin G 1-2 hours before surgery.

600,000 units penicillin G procaine aqueous daily for 2 days following surgery.

Syphilis

Primary, secondary and latent with a negative spinal fluid in adults and children over 12 years of age: 600,000 units daily for 8 days—total 4,800,000 units.

Late (tertiary, neurosyphilis and latent syphilis with positive spinal fluid examination or no spinal fluid examination): 600,000 units daily for 10-15 days—total 6-9 million units.

Congenital syphilis (early and late) under 70 lb. body weight 50,000 units/kg/day for 10 days.

Yaws, Bejel, and Pinta—Treatment as syphilis in corresponding stage of disease.

Gonorrheal infections (uncomplicated): Men or women—4.8 million units intramuscularly divided into at least two doses and injected at different sites at one visit, together with 1 gram of oral probenecid, preferably given at least 30 minutes prior to the injection.

NOTE: gonorrheal endocarditis should be treated intensively with aqueous penicillin G.

Diphtheria-adjunctive therapy with antitoxin:

300,000-600,000 units daily.

Diphtheria carrier state—300,000 units daily for 10 days.

Anthrax-cutaneous: 600,000-1,000,000 units/day.

Vincent's infection (fusospirochetosis): 600,000-1,000,000 units/day.

Continued on next page

Pfipharmecs—Cont.

Erysipeloid: 600,000-1,000,000 units/day.
Streptobacillus moniliformis and spirillum minus (rat bite fever). 600,000-1,000,000 units/day.

How Supplied: Pfizerpen-AS (penicillin G procaine) in Aqueous Suspension is supplied in 10 ml vials (3,000,000 units). Each ml contains 300,000 units penicillin G procaine; and as w/v: 0.8% Sodium citrate; 0.15% sodium carboxymethylcellulose; 25% of sorbitol solution U.S.P.; 0.06% polyvinylpyrrolidone, and 0.6% lecithin.
Preservatives: 0.103% methylparaben; 0.011% propylparaben.
Pfizerpen-AS (penicillin G procaine) in Aqueous Suspension ISOJECT disposable syringes are available in the following sizes:
1.0 ml (600,000 units); and 2.0 ml (1,200,000 units)
Each ml contains: 600,000 units of penicillin G procaine; 0.005 gram sodium citrate; 0.01 gram urea; 0.0025 gram sodium carboxymethycellulose; 0.0008 gram methylcellulose; 0.01 gram polyvinylpyrrolidone; 0.006 gram lecithin; 0.00015 gram butylparaben; 0.005 gram sodium formaldehyde sulfoxylate, sodium hydroxide to adjust to optimum pH, in water for injection.
[*Shown in Product Identification Section*]

PFIZERPEN®-AS ℞
(penicillin G procaine)
Isoject®
in Aqueous Suspension
1,200,000 units
For Intramuscular Use Only

STORE BETWEEN 2°-8°C (36°-46°F)
SHAKE WELL BEFORE USING

Description: Pfizerpen-AS (penicillin G procaine) is a highly potent antibacterial agent effective against a wide variety of pathogenic organisms. It is an equimolecular compound of procaine and penicillin G in aqueous suspension for intramuscular administration.

Actions and Pharmacology: Penicillin G exerts a bactericidal action against penicillin-sensitive microorganisms during the stage of active multiplication. It acts through the inhibition of biosynthesis of cell wall mucopeptide. It is not active against the penicillinase-producing bacteria, which include many strains of staphylococci. Penicillin G exerts high *in vitro* activity against staphylococci (except penicillinase-producing strains) streptococci (groups A, C, G, H, I, and M) and pneumococci. Other organisms sensitive to penicillin G are *N. gonorrhoeae, Corynebacterium diphtheriae, Bacillus anthracis,* Clostridia, *Actimomyces bovis, Streptobacillus moniliformis, Listeria monocytogenes* and Leptospira. *Treponema pallidum* is extremely sensitive to the bactericidal action of penicillin G.
Sensitivity plate testing: If the Kirby-Bauer method of disc sensitivity is used, a 10-unit penicillin disc should give a zone greater than 28 mm when tested against a penicillin-sensitive bacterial strain.
Penicillin G procaine is an equimolecular compound of procaine and penicillin G administrered intramuscularly as a suspension. It dissolves slowly at the site of injection, giving a plateau type of blood level at about 4 hours which falls slowly over a period of the next 15–20 hours.
Approximately 60% of penicillin G is bound to serum protein. The drug is distributed throughout the body tissues in widely varying amounts. Highest levels are found in the kidneys with lesser amounts in the liver, skin and intestines. Penicillin G penetrates into all other tissues to a lesser degree with a very small level found in the cerebrospinal fluid. With normal kidney function the drug is excreted rapidly by tubular excretion. In neonates and young infants and in individuals with impaired kidney functions, excretion is considerably delayed. Approximately 60–90% of a dose of parenteral penicillin G is excreted in the urine within 24–36 hours.

Indications: Penicillin G procaine is indicated in the treatment of moderately severe infections due to penicillin G-sensitive microorganisms that are sensitive to the low and persistent serum levels common to this particular dosage form. Therapy should be guided by bacteriological studies (including sensitivity tests) and by clinical response.
NOTE: When high sustained serum levels are required aqueous penicillin G either IM or IV should be used.
The following infections will usually respond to adequate dosages of intramuscular penicillin G procaine.
Streptococcal infections Group A (without bacteremia). Moderately severe to severe infections of the upper repiratory tract (including middle ear infections—otitis media), skin and soft tissue infections, scarlet fever, and erysipelas.
NOTE: Streptococci in groups A, C, H, G, L, and M are very sensitive to penicillin G. Other groups, including group D (enterococcus) are resistant. Adqueous penicillin is recommended for streptococcal infections with bactermia.
Pneumococcal infections: Moderately severe infections of the respiratory tract (including middle ear infections—otitis media).
NOTE: Severe pneumonia, empyema, bacteremia, pericarditis, meningitis, peritonitis, and purulent or septic arthritis of pneumococcal etiology are better treated with aqueous penicillin G during the acute stage.
Staphylococcal infections—penicillin G-sensitive. Moderately severe infections of the skin and soft tissues.
NOTE: Reports indicate an increasing number of strains of staphylococci resistant to penicillin G emphasizing the need for culture and sensitivity studies in treating suspected staphylococcal infections.
Indicated surgical procedures should be performed.
Fusospirochetosis (Vincent's gingivitis and pharyngitis). Moderately severe infections of the oropharynx respond to therapy with penicillin G procaine.
NOTE: Necessary dental care should be accomplished in infections involving the gum tissue.
Treponema pallidum (syphilis); all stages.
N. gonorrhoeae: acute and chronic (without bacteremia).
Yaws, Bejel, Pinta.
C. diphtheriae—penicillin G procaine as an adjunct to antitoxin for prevention of the carrier stage.
Anthrax.
Steptobacillus moniliformis and *Spirillum minus* infections (rat bite fever).
Erysipeloid.
Subacute bacterial endocarditis (group A streptococcus) only in extremely sensitive infections.
Prophylaxis Against Bacterial Endocarditis—Although no controlled clinical efficacy studies have been conducted, aqueous crystalline penicillin G for injection and penicillin G procaine suspension have been suggested by the American Heart Association and the American Dental Association for use as part of a combined parenteral-oral regimen for prophylaxis against bacterial endocarditis in patients with congenital heart disease or rheumatic, or other acquired valvular heart disease when they undergo dental procedures and surgical procedures of the upper respiratory tract.[1] Since it may happen that *alpha* hemolytic streptococci relatively resistant to penicillin may be found when patients are receiving continuous oral penicillin for secondary prevention of rheumatic fever, prophylactic agents other than penicillin may be chosen for these patients and prescribed in addition to their continuous rheumatic fever prophylactic regimen.
NOTE: When selecting antibiotics for the prevention of bacterial endocarditis the physician or dentist should read the full joint statement of the American Heart Association and the American Dental Association.[1]

Contraindications: A previous hypersensitivity reaction to any penicillin or procaine is a contraindication.

Warnings: Serious and occasionally fatal hypersensitivity (anaphylactoid) reactions have been reported in patients on penicillin therapy. Although anaphylaxis is more frequent following parenteral therapy it has occurred in patients on oral penicillins. These reactions are more apt to occur in individuals with a history of sensitivity to multiple allergens.
There have been well documented reports of individuals with a history of penicillin hypersensitivity reactions who have experienced severe hypersensitivity reactions when treated with a cephalosporin. Before therapy with a penicillin, careful inquiry should be made concerning previous hypesensitivity reactions to penicillins, cephalosporins, and other allergens. If an allergic reaction occurs, the drug should be discontinued and the patient treated with the usual agents, e.g., pressor amines, antihistamines, and corticosteroids.
Immediate toxic reactions to procaine may occur in some individuals, particularly when a large single dose is administered in the treatment of gonorrhea (4.8 million units). These reactions may be mainfested by mental disturbances including anxiety, confusion, agitation, depression, weakness, seizures, hallucinations, combativeness, and expressed "fear of impending death." The reactions noted in carefully controlled studies occurred in approximately one in 500 patients treated for gonorrhea. Reactions are transient, lasting from 15–30 minutes.

Precautions: Penicillin should be used with caution in individuals with histories of significant allergies and/or asthma.
In intramuscular therapy, care should be taken to avoid accidental intravenous administration.
As with all intramuscular preparations, Pfizerpen-AS (penicillin G procaine) should be injected well within the body of a relatively large muscle. ADULTS: The preferred sites are the upper outer quadrant of the buttock, (i.e., gluteus maximus) and the mid-lateral thigh. CHILDREN: It is recommended that intramuscular injections be given preferably in the midlateral muscles of the thigh. In infants and small children the periphery of the upper outer quadrant of the gluteal region should only be used when necessary, such as in burn patients, in order to minimize the possibility of damage to the sciatic nerve.
The deltoid area should be used only if well developed such as in certain adults and older children, and then only with caution to avoid radial nerve injury. Intramuscular injections should not be made into the lower and mid-third of the upper arm. As with all intramuscular injections, aspiration is necessary to help avoid inadvertent injection into a blood vessel.
In suspected staphylococcal infections, proper laboratory studies, including sensitivity tests should be performed.
A small percentage of patients are sensitive to procaine. If there is a history of sensitivity make the usual test: Inject intradermally 0.1 ml of a 1 to 2 percent procaine solution. Development of an erythema, wheal, flare or eruption indicates procaine sensitivity. Sensitivity should be treated by the usual methods, including barbiturates, and penicillin G procain preparations should not be used. Antihistamines appear beneficial in treatment of procaine reactions.
The use of antibiotics may result in overgrowth of nonsusceptible organisms. Constant obser-

vation of the patient is essential. If new infections due to bacteria or fungi appear during therapy, the drug should be discontinued and appropriate measures taken. Whenever allergic reactions occur, penicillin should be withdrawn unless, in the opinion of the physician, the condition being treated is life threatening and amenable only to penicillin therapy.

In prolonged therapy with penicillin, and particularly with high dosage schedules, periodic evaluation of the renal and hematopoietic systems are recommended.

When treating gonococcal infections in which primary or secondary syphilis may be suspected, proper diagnostic procedures, including dark field examinations should be done. In all cases in which concomitant syphilis is suspected, monthly serological tests should be made for at least four months.

Adverse Reactions: Penicillin is a substance of low toxicity, but does possess a significant index of sensitization. The following hypersensitivity reactions associated with use of pencillin have been reported: skin rashes, ranging from maculopapular eruptions to exfoliative dermatitis; urticaria; serum sickness-like reactions, including chills, fever, edema, arthralgia and prostration. Severe and often fatal anaphylaxis has been reported (see "Warnings"). As with other treatments for syphilis, the Jarisch Herxheimer reaction has been reported.

Procaine toxicity manifestations have been reported (see "Warnings"). Procaine hypersensitivity reactions have not been reported with this drug.

Administration and Dosage:

Pediatric Dosage Schedules: In children under 3 months of age, the absorption of aqueous penicillin G produces such high and sustained levels that penicillin G procaine dosage forms offer no advantages and are usually unnecessary.

In children under 12 years of age, dosage should be adjusted in accordance with the age and weight of the child and the severity of the infection.

Under 2 years of age, the dose may be divided between the two buttocks if necessary.

Penicillin G procaine (aqueous) is for intramuscular injection only.

Recommended dosage for penicillin G procaine aqueous:

Pneumonia (pneumococcal), moderately severe (uncomplicated): 600,000—1,000,000 units daily.

Streptococcal infections (group A), moderately severe to severe tonsillitis, erysipelas, scarlet fever, upper respiratory tract, skin and soft tissue: 600,000—1,000,000 units daily for 10 day minimum.

Staphylococcal infections, moderately severe to severe: 600,000—1,000,000 units daily.

Bacterial endocarditis (group A streptococci) only in extremely sensitive infections: 600,000—1,000,000 units daily.

For prophylaxis against bacterial endocarditis in patients with congenital heart disease or rheumatic, or other acquired valvular heart disease when undergoing dental procedures or surgical procedures of the upper respiratory tract, use a combined parenteral-oral regimen. One millions units of aqueous crystalline penicillin G (30,000 units/kg in children) intramuscularly mixed with 600,000 units procaine penicillin G (600,000 units for children) should be given one-half to one hour before the procedure. Oral penicillin V (phenoxymethyl penicillin). 500 mg for adults or 250 mg for children less than 60 lb. should be given every 6 hours for 8 doses. Doses for children should not exceed recommendations for adults for a single dose or for a 24 hour period.

Syphilis—

Primary, secondary and latent with a negative spinal fluid in adults and children over 12 years of age: 600,000 units daily for 8 days—total 4,800,000 units.

Late (tertiary, neurosyphilis and latent syphilis with positive spinal fluid examination or no spinal fluid examination): 600,000 units daily for 10-15 days—total 6-9 million units.

Congenital syphilis (early and late): 50,000 units/kg per day for a minimum of 10 days.

Yaws, Bejel, and Pinta-Treatment as syphilis in corresponding stage of disease.

Gonorrheal infectons (uncomplicated): Men or Women—4.8 million units intramuscularly divided into at least two doses and injected at different sites at one visit, together with 1 gram of oral probenecid, preferably given at least 30 minutes prior to the injection.

NOTE: Gonorrheal endocarditis should be treated intensively with aqueous penicillin G.

Diptheria—adjunctive therapy with antitoxin: 300,000-600,000 units daily.

Diptheria carrier state—300,000 units daily for 10 days.

Anthrax-cutaneous: 600,000-1,000,000 units/day.

Vincent's infection (fusospirochetosis): 600,000-1,000,000 units/day.

Erysipeloid: 600,000-1,000,000 units/day.

Streptobacillus moniliformis and spirillum minus (rat bite fever): 600,000-1,000,000 units/day.

How Supplied: Pfizerpen-AS (penicillin G procaine) in Aqueous Suspension is supplied in 10 ml vials (3,000,000 units). Each ml contains 300,000 units pencillin G procaine; and as w/v: 0.8% sodium citrate; 0.15% sodium carboxymethylcellulose; 25% of sorbitol solution U.S.P.: 0.06% polyvinylpyrrolidone, and 0.6% lecithin.

Preservatives: 0.13% methylparaben: 0.011% propylparaben.

Pfizerpen-AS (penicillin G procaine) in Aqueous Suspension is available in 2.0 ml (1,200,000 units) ISOJECT disposable syringes.

Each ml contains: 600,000 units of penicillin G procaine; 0.005 gram sodium citrate; 0.01 gram urea; 0.0025 gram sodium carboxymethylcellulose; 0.0008 gram methylcellulose; 0.01 gram polyvinylpyrrolidone; 0.006 gram lecithin; 0.00015 gram butylparaben; 0.005 gram sodium formaldehyde sulfoxylate, sodium hydroxide to adjust to optimum pH, in water for injection.

Reference:

1. American Heart Association. 1977. Prevention of bacterial endocarditis. Circulation. 56:139A-143A.

[*Shown in Product Indentification Section*]

PFIZERPEN G® (penicillin G potassium) TABLETS BUFFERED FOR ORAL ADMINISTRATION ℞

Indications: Oral penicillin G is indicated in the treatment of mild to moderately severe infections due to penicillin G-sensitive microorganisms that are sensitive to the low serum levels common to this particular dosage form. Therapy should be guided by bacteriological studies (including sensitivity tests) and by clinical response.

NOTE: Severe pneumonia, empyema, bacteremia, pericarditis, meningitis, and purulent or septic arthritis should not be treated with oral penicillin during the acute stage.

Indicated surgical procedures should be performed.

The following infections will usually respond to adequate dosage of oral penicillin G.

1. *Streptococcal infections* (Group A) (without bacteremia). Mild to moderate infections of the upper respiratory tract (including middle ear infections—otitis media), skin and soft tissue infections, scarlet fever, and mild erysipelas.

NOTE: Streptococci in groups A, C, H, G, L, and M are very sensitive to penicillin G. Other groups, including group D (enterococcus) are resistant.

2. *Pneumococcal infections.* Mild to moderately severe infections of the respiratory tract (including middle ear infections—otitis media).

3. *Staphylococcal infections.* Penicillin G sensitive. Mild infections of the skin and soft tissues.

NOTE: Reports indicate an increasing number of strains of staphylococci resistant to penicillin G, emphasizing the need for culture and sensitivity studies in treating suspected staphylococcal infections.

4. *Fusospirochetosis* (Vincent's gingivitis and pharyngitis)—Mild to moderately severe infections of the oropharynx usually respond to therapy with oral penicillin G.

NOTE: Necessary dental care should be accomplished in infections involving the gum tissue.

5. *Oral penicillin G therapy is indicated as prophylaxis for the prevention of recurrence following rheumatic fever and/or chorea.* Prophylaxis with oral penicillin G on a continuing basis has proven effective in preventing recurrence of these conditions.

Contraindications: A previous hypersensitivity reaction to any penicillin is a contraindication.

Warnings: Serious and occasionally fatal hypersensitivity (anaphylactoid) reactions have been reported in patients on penicillin therapy. Although anaphylaxis is more frequent following parenteral therapy it has occurred in patients on oral penicillins. These reactions are more apt to occur in individuals with a history of sensitivity to multiple allergens.

There have been well documented reports of individuals with a history of penicillin hypersensitivity reactions who have experienced severe hypersensitivity reactions when treated with a cephalosporin. Before therapy with a penicillin, careful inquiry should be made concerning previous hypersensitivity reactions to penicillins, cephalosporins, and other allergens. If an allergic reaction occurs, the drug should be discontinued and the patient treated with the usual agents e.g., pressor amines, antihistamines and corticosteroids.

Precautions: Penicillin should be used with caution in individuals with histories of significant allergies and/or asthma.

The oral route of administration should not be relied upon in patients with severe illness, or with nausea, vomiting, gastric dilatation, cardiospasm or intestinal hypermotility.

Occasional patients will not absorb therapeutic amounts of orally administered penicillin.

In streptococcal infections, therapy must be sufficient to eliminate the organism (10 days minimum); otherwise the sequelae of streptococcal disease may occur. Cultures should be taken following completion of treatment to determine whether streptococci have been eradicated.

Prolonged use of antibiotics may promote the overgrowth of nonsusceptible organisms, including fungi. Should superinfection occur, appropriate measures should be taken.

Adverse Reactions: Although the incidence of reactions to oral penicillins has been reported with much less frequency than following parenteral therapy, it should be remembered that all degrees of hypersensitivity including fatal anaphylaxis, have been reported with oral penicillin.

The most common reactions to oral penicillin are nausea, vomiting, epigastric distress, diarrhea, and black hairy tongue. The hypersensitivity reactions reported are skin eruptions (maculopapular to exfoliative dermatitis), urticaria and other serum sickness reactions, laryngeal edema and anaphylaxis. Fever and eosinophilia may frequently be the only reaction observed. Hemolytic anemia, leukopenia, thrombocytopenia, neuropathy, and nephrop-

Continued on next page

Pfipharmecs—Cont.

athy are infrequent reactions and usually associated with high doses of parenteral penicillin.

Dosage and Administration: The dosage of penicillin G (oral) should be determined according to the sensitivity of the causative microorganism and the severity of infection, and adjusted to the clinical response of the patient. Oral penicillin G should be given at least 1 hour before or 2 hours after meals.

The usual dosage recommendation for adults and children 12 years and over is as follows:

Streptococcal infections—Mild to moderately severe—of the upper respiratory tract and including scarlet fever and mild erysipelas.

200,000–250,000 units q. 6–8 hours for 10 days for mild infections.

400,000–500,000 units q. 8 hours for 10 days for moderately severe infections; alternatively, 500 mg (800,000 units) may be given b.i.d.

Pneumococcal infections—Mild to moderately severe—of the respiratory tract, including otitis media.

400,000–500,000 units q. 6 hours until the patient has been afebrile for at least 2 days.

Staphylococcal infections—Mild infections of skin and soft tissue (culture and sensitivity tests should be performed).

200,000–500,000 units q. 6–8 hours until infection is cured.

Fusospirochetosis (Vincent's infection) of the oropharynx—Mild to moderately severe infections.

400,000–500,000 units q. 6–8 hours.

For the prevention of recurrence following rheumatic fever and/or chorea:

200,000–250,000 units twice daily on a continuing basis.

NOTE: Therapy for children under 12 years of age is calculated on the basis of body weight. For infants and small children the suggested dose is 25,000 to 90,000 units per kg per day in 3 to 6 divided doses.

How Supplied: Pfizerpen G (penicillin G potassium) Tablets, buffered with calcium carbonate, for oral administration are available in the following forms and quantities:

200,000 units—bottles of 100 and 500 tablets.
250,000 units—bottles of 100 tablets.
400,000 units—bottles of 100 and 1000 tablets.
800,000 units—bottles of 100 tablets.

Tablets are white, and are scored for easy calibration of dosage.

[*Shown in Product Identification Section*]

PFIZERPEN VK® ℞
(penicillin V potassium)
Tablets and Powder For Oral Solution

Indications: Penicillin V potassium is indicated in the treatment of mild to moderately severe infections due to penicillin G-sensitive microorganisms that are sensitive to the low serum levels common to this particular dosage form. Therapy should be guided by bacteriological studies (including sensitivity tests) and by clinical response.

NOTE: Severe pneumonia, empyema, bacteremia, pericarditis, meningitis, and arthritis should not be treated with penicillin V during the acute stage.

Indicated surgical procedures should be performed.

The following infections will usually respond to adequate dosage of penicillin V:

Streptococcal infections (without bacteremia). Mild to moderate infections of the upper respiratory tract, scarlet fever, and mild erysipelas.

NOTE: Streptococci in groups A, C, G, H, L, and M are very sensitive to penicillin. Other groups, including group D (enterococcus) are resistant.

Pneumococcal infections. Mild to moderately severe infections of the respiratory tract.

Staphylococcal infections—penicillin G-sensitive. Mild infections of the skin and soft tissues.

NOTE: Reports indicate an increasing number of strains of staphylococci resistant to penicillin G, emphasizing the need for culture and sensitivity studies in treating suspected staphylococcal infections.

Fusospirochetosis (Vincent's gingivitis and pharyngitis). Mild to moderately severe infections of the oropharynx usually respond to therapy with oral penicillin.

NOTE: Necessary dental care should be accomplished in infections involving the gum tissue.

Medical conditions in which oral penicillin therapy is indicated as prophylaxis:

For the prevention of recurrence following rheumatic fever and/or chorea. Prophylaxis with oral penicillin on a continuing basis has proven effective in preventing recurrence of these conditions.

To prevent bacterial endocarditis in patients with congenital and/or rheumatic heart lesions in patients to undergo dental procedures or minor upper respiratory tract surgery or instrumentation. Prophylaxis should be instituted the day of the procedure and for 2 or more days following. Patients who have a past history of rheumatic fever and are receiving continuous prophylaxis may harbor increased numbers of penicillin-resistant organisms; use of another prophylactic anti-infective agent should be considered. If penicillin is to be used in these patients at surgery, the regular rheumatic fever program should be interrupted 1 week prior to the contemplated surgery. At the time of surgery, penicillin may be reinstituted as a prophylactic measure against the hazards of surgically induced bacteremia.

NOTE: Oral penicillin should not be used as adjunctive prophylaxis for genitourinary instrumentation or surgery, lower intestinal tract surgery, sigmoidoscopy, and childbirth.

Contraindications: A previous hypersensitivity reaction to any penicillin is a contraindication.

Warnings: Serious and occasionally fatal hypersensitivity (anaphylactoid) reactions have been reported in patients on penicillin therapy. Although anaphylaxis is more frequent following parenteral therapy it has occurred in patients on oral penicillins. These reactions are more apt to occur in individuals with a history of sensitivity to multiple allergens.

There have been well documented reports of individuals with a history of penicillin hypersensitivity reactions who have experienced severe hypersensitivity reactions when treated with a cephalosporin. Before therapy with a penicillin, careful inquiry should be made concerning previous hypersensitivity reactions to penicillins, cephalosporins, and other allergens. If an allergic reaction occurs, the drug should be discontinued and the patient treated with the usual agents e.g., pressor amines, antihistamines, and corticosteroids.

Precautions: Penicillin should be used with caution in individuals with histories of significant allergies and/or asthma.

The oral route of administration should not be relied upon in patients with severe illness, or with nausea, vomiting, gastric dilatation, cardiospasm, or intestinal hypermotility.

Occasional patients will not absorb therapeutic amounts of orally administered penicillin.

In streptococcal infections, therapy must be sufficient to eliminate the organism (10 days minimum); otherwise the sequelae of streptococcal disease may occur. Cultures should be taken following completion of treatment to determine whether streptococci have been eradicated.

Prolonged use of antibiotics may promote the overgrowth of nonsusceptible organisms, including fungi. Should superinfection occur, appropriate measures should be taken.

Adverse Reactions: Although the incidence of reactions to oral penicillins has been reported with much less frequency than following parenteral therapy, it should be remembered that all degrees of hypersensitivity including fatal anaphylaxis, have been reported with oral penicillin.

The most common reactions to oral penicillin are nausea, vomiting, epigastric distress, diarrhea, and black hairy tongue. The hypersensitivity reactions reported are skin eruptions (maculopapular to exfoliative dermatitis), urticaria and other serum sickness reactions, laryngeal edema, and anaphylaxis. Fever and eosinophilia may frequently be the only reaction observed. Hemolytic anemia, leukopenia, thrombocytopenia, neuropathy, and nephropathy are infrequent reactions and usually associated with high doses of parenteral penicillin.

Administration and Dosage: The dosage of penicillin V should be determined according to the sensitivity of the causative microorganisms and the severity of infection, and adjusted to the clinical response of the patient.

The usual dosage recommendations for adults and children 12 years and over are as follows:

Streptococcal infections—mild to moderately severe—of the upper respiratory tract and including scarlet fever and erysipelas: 200,000 to 500,000 units every 6 to 8 hours for 10 days.

Pneumococcal infections—mild to moderately severe—of the respiratory tract, including otitis media; 400,000 to 500,000 units every 6 hours until the patient has been afebrile for at least 2 days.

Staphylococcal infections—mild infections of skin and soft tissue (culture and sensitivity tests should be performed): 400,000 to 500,000 units every 6 to 8 hours.

Fusospirochetosis (Vincent's infection) of the oropharynx—mild to moderately severe infections: 400,000 to 500,000 units every 6 to 8 hours.

For the prevention of recurrence following rheumatic fever and/or chorea: 200,000 to 250,000 units twice daily on a continuing basis.

To prevent bacterial endocarditis in patients with rheumatic or congenital heart lesions who are to undergo dental or upper respiratory tract surgery or instrumentation: 500,000 units given the day of the procedure, 500,000 aqueous penicillin G I.M. units 1 hour before the procedure, and 500,000 units every 6 hours for 2 days.

NOTE: Therapy for children under 12 years of age is calculated on the basis of body weight. For infants and small children the suggested dose is 25,000 to 90,000 units per kg. per day in three to six divided doses.

How Supplied: Pfizerpen VK (penicillin V potassium) for Oral Solution. Each 5 ml of reconstituted solution contains penicillin V potassium equivalent to 125 or 250 mg penicillin V.

125 mg (200,000 units): bottles of 100 ml, 150 ml, and 200 ml

250 mg (400,000 units): bottles of 100 ml, 150 ml, and 200 ml

Pfizerpen VK (penicillin V potassium) tablets. Each tablet contains penicillin V potassium equivalent to 250 mg (400,000 units) or 500 mg (800,000 units) penicillin V.

250 mg (400,000 units): bottles of 100 and 1000.
500 mg (800,000 units): bottles of 100.

[*Shown in Product Identification Section*]

Directions for Reconstituting Oral Solutions: Prepare the formulation at the time of dispensing. For ease in preparation, tap bottle lightly to loosen powder, add water to the bottle in two portions and shake well after each addition. The reconstituted solutions are stable for 14 days under refrigeration.

125 mg/5 ml

Add 60 ml water to the 100 ml package, 90 ml water to the 150 ml package, and 120 ml water to the 200 ml package. This will provide 100 ml, 150 ml, and 200 ml of solution respectively. Each 5 ml (teaspoonful) will contain penicillin

V potassium equivalent to 125 mg of penicillin V.

250 mg/5 ml

Add 60 ml water to the 100 ml package, 90 ml water to the 150 ml package, and 120 ml water to the 200 ml package. This will provide 100 ml, 150 ml, and 200 ml of solution respectively. Each 5 ml (teaspoonful) will contain penicillin V potassium equivalent to 250 mg of penicillin V.

RID™
Liquid Pediculicide

Description: Rid is a liquid pediculicide whose active ingredients are: pyrethrins 0.3%, piperonyl butoxide, technical 3.00%, equivalent to 2.4% (butylcarbityl) (6-propylpiperonyl) ether and to 0.6% related compounds, petroleum distillate 1.20% and benzyl alcohol 2.4%. Inert ingredients 93.1%.

Actions: RID kills head lice (Pediculus humanus capitis), body lice (Pediculus humanus humanus), and pubic or crab lice (Phthirus pubis), and their eggs on contact.

The pyrethrins act as a contact poison and affect the parasite's nervous system, resulting in paralysis and death. The efficacy of the pyrethrins is enhanced by the synergist, piperonyl butoxide.

Indications: RID is indicated for the treatment of infestations of head lice, body lice and pubic (crab) lice and their eggs.

Warning: RID should be used with caution by ragweed sensitized persons.

Precautions: This product is for external use only. It is harmful if swallowed. It should not be inhaled. It should be kept out of the eyes and contact with mucous membranes should be avoided. If accidental contact with eyes occurs, flush immediately with water. In case of infection or skin irritation, discontinue use and consult a physician. Consult a physician if infestation of eyebrows or eyelashes occurs. Avoid contamination of feed or foodstuffs. Do not reuse container. Destroy when empty.

Do not transport or store below 32°F (0°C).

Dosage and Administration: (1) Apply RID undiluted to hair and scalp or to any other infested area until entirely wet. Do not use on eyelashes or eyebrows. (2) Allow RID to remain on area for 10 minutes but no longer. (3) Wash thoroughly with warm water and soap or shampoo. (4) Dead lice and eggs may require removal with fine-toothed comb provided. A second application should be made in 7 to 10 days to kill any newly hatched lice. Do not exceed two consecutive applications within 24 hours.

Since lice infestations are spread by contact, each family member should be examined carefully. If infested, he or she should be treated promptly to avoid spread or reinfestation of previously treated individuals. Contaminated clothing and other articles, such as hats, etc. should be dry cleaned, boiled or otherwise treated until decontaminated to prevent reinfestation or spread.

How Supplied: In 2 and 4 fl. oz. bottles. Fine-toothed comb to aid in removal of dead lice and nits and patient instruction booklet are included in each package of RID.

[*Shown in Product Identification Section*]

STERANE® TABLETS ℞
(prednisolone)
For Oral Administration

How Supplied: Sterane (prednisolone) is supplied in 5 mg tablets, bottles of 100 and 500.

TERRA-CORTRIL® ℞
Terramycin® (oxytetracycline HCl)–
Cortril® (hydrocortisone)
TOPICAL OINTMENT
Not for Ophthalmic Use

Description: Terra-Cortril Topical Ointment contains Terramycin (oxytetracycline HCl) equivalent to 30 mg oxytetracycline per gram of ointment, and 1.0% (10 mg/g Cortril (hydrocortisone) in a petrolatum base. Oxytetracycline is a product of the metabolism of *Streptomyces rimosus* and is one of the family of tetracycline antibiotics. Chemically, hydrocortisone is 11β, 17α, 21-trihydroxy-pregn-4-ene-3, 20-dione. The empirical formula is $C_{21}H_{30}O_5$ and the molecular weight is 362.

Actions: Terra-Cortril Topical Ointment contains both the anti-infective activity of Terramycin and the anti-inflammatory activity of Cortril.

Terramycin is a potent broad-spectrum antibiotic which is useful topically for prevention or treatment of superficial cutaneous infections due to a variety of pyogenic bacteria, both gram-positive and gram-negative.

Cortril is primarily effective because of its anti-inflammatory, anti-pruritic, and vasoconstrictive actions.

In the treatment of superficial infections of the skin amenable to Terramycin therapy, the anti-inflammatory action of the Cortril in this ointment will afford prompt symptomatic relief while the Terramycin is acting against the causative organisms.

Where topical therapy with Cortril is of value, the added presence of Terramycin will serve to prevent or eradicate secondary bacterial complications. Since varying degrees of bacterial infection frequently complicate those skin conditions for which Cortril topical therapy is indicated, this combined preparation may offer therapeutic advantages over the use of Cortril alone.

Terra-Cortril Topical Ointment is thus useful in the treatment of skin conditions in which antibacterial and anti-inflammatory effects are desired.

In the allergic dermatoses, the inciting allergens in the food or environment should be determined and eliminated. Patch tests, intradermal tests or other suitable procedures should be employed to determine the allergens. In patients with widespread dermatitits, oral therapy with Cortril may be advisable.

Supplemental therapy with oral Terramycin is advisable in the treatment of severe infections or those which may become systemic.

Indications

Based on a review of Terra-Cortril Topical Ointment by the National Academy of Sciences—National Research Council and/or other information, the FDA has classified the indications as follows:

"Possibly" effective:

Cutaneous Infections: including superficial pyogenic infections, pyoderma, pustular dermatitis, and infections associated with minor burns or wounds (under close supervision).

Atopic Dermatitis: including allergic eczema, both disseminated and circumscribed neurodermatitis, pruritus with lichenification, eczematoid dermatitis, food eczema, and infantile eczema.

Contact Dermatitis: due to plants, drugs, cosmetics, clothing material, and miscellaneous substances.

Nonspecific Pruritus of the anus, vulva, and scrotum.

Final classification of these indications requires further investigation.

Contraindications:

1. Acute herpes simplex, vaccinia and varicella.
2. Tuberculosis. } of the skin
3. Fungal diseases. } of the skin
4. Hypersensitivity to any of the components of the drug.

Precautions: If irritation develops, the product should be discontinued and appropriate therapy instituted.

The use of Terramycin® (oxytetracycline HCl) and other antibiotics may result in an overgrowth of resistant organisms—particularly Monilia and staphylococci. Constant observation of the patient for this possibility is essential. If new infections due to nonsusceptible bacteria or fungi appear during therapy, appropriate measures should be taken.

If a favorable response does not occur promptly, the corticosteroid should be discontinued until the infection has been adequately controlled.

If extensive areas are treated or if the occlusive technique is used there will be increased systematic absorption of the corticosteroid and suitable precautions should be taken, particularly in children and infants.

Although topical steroids have not been reported to have an adverse affect on human pregnancy, the safety of their use in pregnant women has not absolutely been established. In laboratory animals, increases in incidence of fetal abnormalities have been associated with exposure of gestating females to topical corticosteroids, in some cases at rather low dosage levels. Therefore, drugs of this class should not be used extensively on pregnant patients, in large amounts, or for prolonged periods of time.

The product is not for ophthalmic use.

Adverse Reactions: Cortril® (hydrocortisone) and Terramycin (oxytetracycline HCl) are well tolerated by the epithelial tissues and may be used topically with minimal untoward effects. Allergic reactions may occur occasionally, but are rare.

The following local adverse reactions have been reported with topical corticosteroids, especially under occlusive dressings.

1. Burning
2. Itching
3. Irritation
4. Dryness
5. Folliculitis
6. Hypertrichosis
7. Acneiform eruptions
8. Hypopigmentation
9. Perioral dermatitis
10. Allergic Contact Dermatitis
11. Maceration of the skin
12. Secondary infection
13. Skin atrophy
14. Striae
15. Miliaria

The use of Terra-Cortril Topical Ointment should be discontinued if such reactions occur.

Dosage: After thorough cleansing of the affected skin areas, a small amount of the ointment should be applied gently. Applications should be made two to four times daily. When actual infection is present, the ointment may be applied on sterile gauze and, by this means, kept in continuous contact with the affected area. Care should be taken not to discontinue therapy too soon after the initial response has been obtained.

Supply: Terra-Cortril Topical Ointment is supplied in ½ oz (14.2 g) tubes.

The active ingredients are incorporated in mineral oil and petrolatum.

[*Shown in Product Identification Section*]

Continued on next page

Pfipharmecs—Cont.

TERRAMYCIN® ℞
Capsules
(oxytetracycline HCl)
Syrup
(calcium oxytetracycline)
Film-coated Tablets
(oxytetracycline)

Description: Oxytetracycline is a product of the metabolism of *Streptomyces rimosus* and is one of the family of tetracycline antibiotics.
Oxytetracycline diffuses readily through the placenta into the fetal circulation, into the pleural fluid and, under some circumstances, into the cerebrospinal fluid. It appears to be concentrated in the hepatic system and excreted in the bile, so that it appears in the feces, as well as in the urine, in a biologically active form.
Actions: Oxytetracycline is primarily bacteriostatic and is thought to exert its antimicrobial effect by the inhibition of protein synthesis. Oxytetracycline is active against a wide range of gram-negative and gram-positive organisms. The drugs in the tetracycline class have closely similar antimicrobial spectra, and cross-resistance among them is common. Microorganisms may be considered susceptible if the M.I.C. (minimum inhibitory concentration) is not more than 4.0 mcg/ml and intermediate if the M.I.C. is 4.0 to 12.5 mcg/ml.
Susceptibility plate testing: A tetracycline disc may be used to determine microbial susceptiblity to drugs in the tetracycline class. If the Kirby-Bauer method of disc susceptibility testing is used, a 30 mcg tetracycline disc should give a zone of at least 19 mm when tested against a tetracycline-susceptible bacterial strain.
Tetracyclines are readily absorbed and are bound to plasma proteins in varying degree. They are concentrated by the liver in the bile and excreted in the urine and feces at high concentrations and in a biologically active form.
Indications: Oxytetracycline is indicated in infections caused by the following microorganisms:
Rickettsiae (Rocky Mountain spotted fever, typhus fever and the typhus group, Q fever, rickettsialpox and tick fevers),
Mycoplasma pneumoniae (PPLO, Eaton Agent),
Agents of psittacosis and ornithosis,
Agents of lymphogranuloma venereum and granuloma inguinale,
The spirochetal agent of relapsing fever *(Borrelia recurrentis)*.
The following gram-negative microorganisms:
Haemophilus ducreyi (chancroid),
Pasteurella pestis and *Pasteurella tularensis*,
Bartonella bacilliformis,
Bacteroides species,
Vibrio comma and *Vibrio fetus*,
Brucella species (in conjunction with streptomycin).
Because many strains of the following groups of microorganisms have been shown to be resistant to tetracyclines, culture and susceptibility testing are recommended.
Oxytetracycline is indicated for treatment of infections caused by the following gram-negative microorganisms, when bacteriologic testing indicates appropriate susceptibility to the drug:
Escherichia coli,
Enterobacter aerogenes (formerly *Aerobacter aerogenes*),
Shigella species,
Mima species and *Herellea* species,
Haemophilus influenzae (respiratory infections),
Klebsiella species (respiratory and urinary infections).
Oxytetracycline is indicated for treatment of infections caused by the following gram-positive microorganisms when bacteriologic testing indicates appropriate susceptibility to the drug:
Streptococcus species:
Up to 44 percent of strains of *Streptococcus pyogenes* and 74 percent of *Streptococcus faecalis* have been found to be resistant to tetracycline drugs. Therefore, tetracyclines should not be used for streptococcal disease unless the organism has been demonstrated to be sensitive.
For upper respiratory infections due to Group A beta-hemolytic streptococci, penicillin is the usual drug of choice, including prophylaxis of rheumatic fever.
Diplococcus pneumoniae,
Staphylococcus aureus, skin and soft tissue infections. Oxytetracycline is not the drug of choice in the treatment of any type of staphylococcal infections.
When penicillin is contraindicated, tetracyclines are alternative drugs in the treatment of infections due to:
Neisseria gonorrhoeae
In acute intestinal amebiasis, the tetracyclines may be a useful adjunct to amebicides.
In severe acne, the tetracyclines may be useful adjunctive therapy. (This indication is for the oral use only, not for I.M. or I.V.)
Tetracyclines are indicated in the treatment of trachoma, although the infectious agent is not always eliminated, as judged by immunofluorescence.
Inclusion conjunctivitis may be treated with oral tetracyclines or with a combination of oral and topical agents.
Contraindications: This drug is contraindicated in persons who have shown hypersensitivity to any of the tetracyclines.
Warnings: THE USE OF DRUGS OF THE TETRACYCLINE CLASS DURING TOOTH DEVELOPMENT (LAST HALF OF PREGNANCY, INFANCY, AND CHILDHOOD TO THE AGE OF 8 YEARS) MAY CAUSE PERMANENT DISCOLORATION OF THE TEETH (YELLOW-GRAY-BROWN). This adverse reaction is more common during long term use of the drugs but has been observed following repeated short term courses. Enamel hypoplasia has also been reported. *TETRACYCLINE DRUGS, THEREFORE, SHOULD NOT BE USED IN THIS AGE GROUP UNLESS OTHER DRUGS ARE NOT LIKELY TO BE EFFECTIVE OR ARE CONTRAINDICATED.*
When the need for intensive treatment outweighs its potential dangers (mostly during pregnancy or in individuals with known or suspected renal or liver impairment), it is advisable to perform renal and liver function tests before and during therapy. Also, tetracycline serum concentrations should be followed.
If renal impairment exists, even usual oral or parenteral doses may lead to excessive systemic accumulation of the drug and possible liver toxicity. Under such conditions, lower than usual total doses are indicated, and if therapy is prolonged, serum level determinations of the drug may be advisable. This hazard is of particular importance in the parenteral administration of tetracyclines to pregnant or postpartum patients with pyelonephritis.
When used under these circumstances, the blood level should not exceed 15 mcg/ml and liver function tests should be made at frequent intervals. Other potentially hepatotoxic drugs should not be prescribed concomitantly.
Photosensitivity manifested by an exaggerated sunburn reaction has been observed in some individuals taking tetracyclines. Patients apt to be exposed to direct sunlight or ultraviolet light should be advised that this reaction can occur with tetracycline drugs, and treatment should be discontinued at the first evidence of skin erythema.
The antianabolic action of the tetracyclines may cause an increase in BUN. While this is not a problem in those with normal renal function, in patients with significantly impaired function, higher serum levels of tetracycline may lead to azotemia, hyperphosphatemia, and acidosis.
Usage in pregnancy. (See above "Warnings" about use during tooth development.)
Results of animal studies indicate that tetracyclines cross the placenta, are found in fetal tissues and can have toxic effects on the developing fetus (often related to retardation of skeletal development). Evidence of embryotoxicity has also been noted in animals treated early in pregnancy.
Usage in newborns, infants, and children. (See above "Warnings" about use during tooth development.)
All tetracyclines form a stable calcium complex in any bone forming tissue. A decrease in the fibula growth rate has been observed in prematures given oral tetracycline in doses of 25 mg/kg every 6 hours. This reaction was shown to be reversible when the drug was discontinued.
Tetracyclines are present in the milk of lactating women who are taking a drug in this class.
Precautions: As with other antibiotic preparations, use of this drug may result in overgrowth of nonsusceptible organisms, including fungi. If superinfection occurs, the antibiotic should be discontinued and appropriate therapy instituted.
In venereal diseases when coexistent syphilis is suspected, a dark field examination should be done before treatment is started and the blood serology repeated monthly for at least 4 months.
Because tetracyclines have been shown to depress plasma prothrombin activity, patients who are on anticoagulant therapy may require downward adjustment of their anticoagulant dosage.
In long term therapy, periodic laboratory evaluation of organ systems, including hematopoietic, renal and hepatic studies should be performed.
All infections due to Group A beta-hemolytic streptococci should be treated for at least 10 days.
Since bacteriostatic drugs may interfere with the bactericidal action of penicillin, it is advisable to avoid giving tetracycline in conjunction with penicillin.
Adverse Reactions: Gastrointestinal: anorexia, nausea, vomiting, diarrhea, glossitis, dysphagia, enterocolitis, and inflammatory lesions (with monilial overgrowth) in the anogenital region. These reactions have been caused by both the oral and parenteral administration of tetracyclines. Rare instances of esophagitis and esophageal ulcerations have been reported in patients receiving capsule and tablet forms of drugs in the tetracycline class. Most of these patients took medications immediately before going to bed. (See Dosage and Administration.)
Skin: maculopapular and erythematous rashes. Exfoliative dermatitis has been reported but is uncommon. Photosensitivity is discussed above. (See "Warnings.")
Renal toxicity: Rise in BUN has been reported and is apparently dose related. (See "Warnings.")
Hypersensitivity reactions: Urticaria, angioneurotic edema, anaphylaxis, axaphylactoid purpura, pericarditis and exacerbation of systemic lupus erythematosus.
Bulging fontanels in infants and benign intracranial hypertension in adults have been reported in individuals receiving full therapeutic dosages. These conditions disappeared rapidly when the drug was discontinued.
Blood: Hemolytic anemia, thrombocytopenia, neutropenia and eosinophilia have been reported.
When given over prolonged periods, tetracyclines have been reported to produce brown-black microscopic discoloration of thyroid glands. No abnormalities of thyroid function studies are known to occur.

Dosage and Administration:

Oral: Capsules and Syrup only:

Adults: Usual daily dose, 1–2 g divided in four equal doses, depending on the severity of the infection.

Film-coated Tablets only:

Adults: A dosage schedule providing 2 tablets initially, then 1 tablet every six hours, is the usual average dose. In severe infections a larger dose (2 to 4 grams daily) may be indicated.

The total daily dose should be administered in four equal portions given at six hour intervals.

All Oral Forms:

For children above eight years of age: Usual daily dose, 10–20 mg per pound (25–50 mg/kg) of body weight divided in four equal doses.

Therapy should be continued for at least 24–48 hours after symptoms and fever have subsided.

For treatment of brucellosis, 500 mg oxytetracycline four times daily for 3 weeks should be accompanied by streptomycin, 1 gram intramuscularly twice daily the first week, and once daily the second week.

For treatment of uncomplicated gonorrhea, when penicillin is contraindicated, tetracycline may be used for the treatment of both males and females in the following dividend dosage schedule: 1.5 grams initially followed by 0.5 gram q.i.d. for a total of 9.0 grams.

For treatment of syphilis, a total of 30–40 grams in equally divided doses over a period of 10–15 days should be given. Close follow-up, including laboratory tests, is recommended.

Administration of adequate amounts of fluid along with capsule and tablet forms of drugs in the tetracycline class is recommended to wash down the drugs and reduce the risk of esophageal irritation and ulceration. (See Adverse Reactions.)

Concomitant therapy: Antacids containing aluminum, calcium, or magnesium impair absorption and should not be given to patients taking oral tetracyclines.

Food and some dairy products also interfere with absorption. Oral forms of tetracyclines should be given 1 hours before or 2 hours after meals. Pediatric oral dosage forms should not be given with milk formulas and should be given at least 1 hour prior to feeding.

In patients with renal impairment: (See "Warnings.") Total dosage should be decreased by reduction of recommended individual doses and/or by extending time intervals between doses.

In the treatment of streptococcal infections, a therapeutic dose of oxytetracycline should be administered for at least 10 days.

How Supplied:

Oral: Terramycin (oxytetracycline HCl) Capsules are available as opaque, yellow, hard gelatin capsules which contain either oxytetracycline HCl equivalent to 250 mg of oxytetracycline, and glucosamine hydrochloride (imprinted with code number 073): bottles of 16, 100, and 500; or oxytetracycline HCl equivalent to 125 mg of oxytetracycline, and glucosamine hydrochloride (imprinted with code number 072): bottles of 100.

Terramycin (calcium oxytetracycline) Syrup is available as a preconstituted fruit-flavored aqueous suspension. Each teaspoonful (5 ml) contains calcium oxytetracycline equivalent to 125 mg of oxytetracycline, and N-acetylglucosamine: bottles of 2 oz. and 1 pint.

Terramycin (oxytetracycline) Tablets are available as:

250 mg film-coated tablets (imprinted with code number 084): bottles of 100.

[*Capsules Shown in Product Identification Section*]

(Capsules & Syrup)	60-0755-00-6
(Film-coated Tablets)	23-1127-00-2

contents per ml (w/v)

Ingredient	2 ml Single Dose Ampules and isoject		10 ml/Vial Multidose
	100 mg/2 ml	250 mg/2 ml	50 mg/ml 10 ml (5 × 2 ml Doses)
oxytetracycline	50 mg	25 mg	50 mg
lidocaine	2.0%	2.0%	2.0%
magnesium chloride hexahydrate	2.5%	6.0%	2.5%
sodium formaldehyde sulfoxylate	0.5%	0.5%	0.3%
α-monothioglycerol	—	—	1.0%
monoethanolamine	approx. 1.7%	approx. 4.2%	approx. 2.6%
citric acid	—	—	1.0%
propyl gallate	—	—	0.02%
propylene glycol	75.2%	67.0%	74.1%
water	18.8%	16.8%	18.5%

TERRAMYCIN® ℞

(oxytetracycline)
INTRAMUSCULAR SOLUTION*
FOR INTRAMUSCULAR USE ONLY
contains 2% lidocaine

Description: Oxytetracycline is a product of the metabolism of *Streptomyces rimosus* and is one of the family of tetracycline antibiotics.

Oxytetracycline diffuses readily through the placenta into the fetal circulation, into the pleural fluid and, under some circumstances, into the cerebrospinal fluid. It appears to be concentrated in the hepatic system and excreted in the bile, so that it appears in the feces, as well as in the urine, in a biologically active form.

Composition:

[See table above].

Actions: Oxytetracycline is primarily bacteriostatic and is thought to exert its antimicrobial effect by the inhibition of protein synthesis. Oxytetracycline is active against a wide range of gram-negative and gram-positive organisms.

The drugs in the tetracycline class have closely similar antimicrobial spectra, and cross resistance among them is common. Microorganisms may be considered susceptible if the M.I.C. (minimum inhibitory concentration) is not more than 4.0 mcg/ml and intermediate if the M.I.C. is 4.0 to 12.5 mcg/ml.

Susceptibility plate testing: A tetracycline disc may be used to determine microbial susceptibility to drugs in the tetracycline class. If the Kirby-Bauer method of disc susceptibility testing is used, a 30 mcg tetracycline disc should give a zone of at least 19 mm when tested against an oxytetracycline-susceptible bacterial strain.

Tetracyclines are readily absorbed and are bound to plasma proteins in varying degree. They are concentrated by the liver in the bile and excreted in the urine and feces at high concentrations and in a biologically active form.

Indications: Oxytetracycline is indicated in infections caused by the following microorganisms:

Rickettsiae (Rocky Mountain spotted fever, typhus fever and the typhus group, Q fever, rickettsialpox and tick fevers).

Mycoplasma pneumoniae (PPLO, Eaton agent),
Agents of psittacosis and ornithosis,
Agents of lymphogranuloma venereum and granuloma inguinale,
The spirochetal agent of relapsing fever (*Borrelia recurrentis*).

The following gram-negative microorganisms:
Haemophilus ducreyi (chancroid),
Pasteurella pestis and *Pasteurella tularensis,*
Bartonella bacilliformis,
Bacteroides species,
Vibrio comma and *Vibrio fetus,*
Brucella species (in conjunction with streptomycin).

Because many strains of the following groups of microorganisms have been shown to be resistant to tetracyclines, culture and susceptibility testing are recommended.

Oxytetracycline is indicated for treatment of infections caused by the following gram-negative microorganisms, when bacteriologic testing indicates appropriate susceptibility to the drug:
Escherichia coli,
Enterobacter aerogenes (formerly *Aerobacter aerogenes),*
Shigella species,
Mima species and *Herellea* species,
Haemophilus influenzae (respiratory infections),
Klebsiella species (respiratory and urinary infections).

Oxytetracycline is indicated for treatment of infections caused by the following gram-positive microorganisms when bacteriologic testing indicates appropriate susceptibility to the drug: Streptococcus species;

Up to 44 percent of strains of *Streptococcus pyogenes* and 74 percent of *Streptococcus faecalis* have been found to be resistant to tetracycline drugs. Therefore, tetracyclines should not be used for streptococcal disease unless the organism has been demonstrated to be sensitive.

For upper respiratory infections due to Group A beta-hemolytic streptococci, penicillin is the usual drug of choice, including prophylaxis of rheumatic fever.

Diplococcus pneumoniae,
Staphylococcus aureus, skin and soft tissue infections. Oxytetracycline is not the drug of choice in the treatment of any type of staphylococcal infections.

When penicillin is contraindicated, tetracyclines are alternative drugs in the treatment of infections due to:
Neisseria gonorrhoeae,
Treponema pallidum and *Treponema pertenue* (syphilis and yaws),
Listeria monocytogenes,
Clostridium species,
Bacillus anthracis,
Fusobacterium fusiforme (Vincent's infection),
Actinomyces species.

In acute intestinal amebiasis, the tetracyclines may be a useful adjunct to amebicides.

Tetracyclines are indicated in the treatment of trachoma, although the infectious agent is not always eliminated, as judged by immunofluorescence.

Inclusion conjunctivitis may be treated with oral tetracyclines or with a combination of oral and topical agents.

Contraindications: This drug is contraindicated in persons who have shown hypersensitivity to any of the tetracyclines.

Warnings: THE USE OF TETRACYCLINES DURING TOOTH DEVELOPMENT (LAST HALF OF PREGNANCY, INFANCY, AND

Continued on next page

Pfipharmecs—Cont.

CHILDHOOD TO THE AGE OF 8 YEARS) MAY CAUSE PERMANENT DISCOLORATION OF THE TEETH (YELLOW-GRAY-BROWN).

This adverse reaction is more common during long term use of the drugs but has been observed following repeated short term courses. Enamel hypoplasia has also been reported. *TETRACYCLINES, THEREFORE, SHOULD NOT BE USED IN THIS AGE GROUP UNLESS OTHER DRUGS ARE NOT LIKELY TO BE EFFECTIVE OR ARE CONTRAINDICATED.*

If renal impairment exists, even usual oral or parenteral doses may lead to excessive systemic accumulation of the drug and possible liver toxicity. Under such conditions, lower than usual total doses are indicated and, if therapy is prolonged, serum level determinations of the drug may be advisable. This hazard is of particular importance in the parenteral administration of tetracyclines to pregnant or postpartum patients with pyelonephritis. When used under these circumstances, the blood level should not exceed 15 mcg/ml and liver function tests should be made at frequent intervals. Other potentially hepatotoxic drugs should not be prescribed concomitantly.

(In the presence of renal dysfunction, particularly in pregnancy, intravenous tetracycline therapy in daily doses exceeding 2 grams has been associated with deaths due to liver failure.)

Photosensitivity manifested by an exaggerated sunburn reaction has been observed in some individuals taking tetracyclnes. Patients apt to be exposed to direct sunlight or ultraviolet light should be advised that this reaction can occur with tetracycline drugs, and treatment should be discontinued at the first evidence of skin erythema.

The antianabolic action of the tetracyclines may cause an increase in BUN. While this is not a problem in those with normal renal function, in patients with significantly impaired function, higher serum levels of this drug may lead to azotemia, hyperphosphatemia, and acidosis.

Usage in pregnancy. (See above "Warnings" about use during tooth development.)

Results of animal studies indicate that tetracyclines cross the placenta, are found in fetal tissues and can have toxic effects on the developing fetus (often related to retardation of skeletal development). Evidence of embryotoxicity has also been noted in animals treated early in pregnancy.

Usage in newborns, infants, and children. (See above "Warnings" about use during tooth deveopment).

All tetracyclines form a stable calcium complex in any bone-forming tissue. A decrease in the fibula growth rate has been observed in prematures given oral tetracyclne in doses of 25 mg/kg every 6 hours. This reaction was shown to be reversible when the drug was discontinued.

Tetracyclines are present in the milk of lactating women who are taking a drug in this class.

Precautions: As with all intramuscular preparations, Terramycin (oxytetracycline) Intramuscular Solution should be injected well within the body of a relatively large muscle. ADULTS: The preferred sites are the upper outer quadrant of the buttock, (i.e., gluteus maximus), and the mid-lateral thigh. CHILDREN: It is recommended that intramuscular injections be given preferably in the mid-lateral muscles of the thigh. In infants and small children the periphery of the upper outer quadrant of the gluteal region should be used only when necessary, such as in burn patients, in order to minimize the possibility of damage to the sciatic nerve. The deltoid area should be used only if well developed such as in certain adults and older children, and then only with caution to avoid radial nerve injury. Intramuscular injections should not be made into the lower and mid-thirds of the upper arm. As with all intramuscular injections, aspiration is necessary to help avoid inadvertent injection into a blood vessel.

As with other antibiotic preparations, use of this drug may result in overgrowth of nonsusceptible organisms, including fungi. If superinfection occurs, the antibiotic should be discontinued and appropriate therapy instituted.

In venereal diseases when coexistent syphilis is suspected, a dark field examination should be done before treatment is started and the blood serology repeated monthly for at least 4 months.

Because tetracyclines have been shown to depress plasma prothrombin activity, patients who are on anticoagulant therapy may require downward adjustment of their anticoagulant dosage.

In long term terapy, periodic laboratory evaluation of organ systems, including hematopoietic, renal and hepatic studies should be performed.

All infections due to Group A beta-hemolytic streptococci should be treated for at least 10 days.

Since bacteriostatic drugs may interfere with the bactericidal action of penicillin, it is advisable to avoid giving tetracycline in conjunction with penicillin.

Adverse Reactions: Local irritation may be present after intramuscular injection. The injection should be deep, with care taken not to injure the sciatic nerve nor inject intravascularly.

Gastrointestinal: anorexia, nausea, vomiting, diarrhea, glossitis, dyphagia, enterocolitis, and inflammatory lesions (with monilial overgrowth) in the anogenital region. These reactions have been caused by both the oral and parenteral administration of tetracyclines.

Skin: maculopapular and erythematous rashes. Exfoliative dermatitis has been reported but is uncommon. Photosensitivity is discussed above. (See "Warnings").

Renal toxicity: Rise in BUN has been reported and is apparently dose related. (See "Warnings").

Hypersensitivity reactions: Urticaria, angioneurotic edema, anaphylaxis, anaphylactoid purpura, pericarditis, and exacerbation of systemic lupus erythematosus.

Bulging fontanels in infants and benign intracranial hypertension in adults have been reported in individuals receiving full therapeutic dosages. These conditions disappeared rapidly when the drug was discontinued.

Blood: Hemolytic anemia, thrombocytopenia, neutropenia, and eosinophilia have been reported.

When given over prolonged periods, tetracyclines have been reported to produce brown-black microscopic discoloration of thyroid glands. No abnormalities of thyroid function studies are known to occur.

Dosage and Administration:

Intramuscular Administration:

Adults: The usual daily dose is 250 mg administered once every 24 hours or 300 mg given in divided doses at 8 to 12 hour intervals.

For children above eight years of age: 15–25 mg/kg body weight up to a maximum of 250 mg per single daily injection. Dosage may be divided and given at 8 to 12 hour intervals.

Intramuscular therapy should be reserved for situations in which oral therapy is not feasible. The intramuscular administration of oxytetracycline produces lower blood levels than oral administration in the recommended dosages. Patients placed on intramuscular oxytetracycline should be changed to the oral dosage form as soon as possible. If rapid, high blood levels are needed, oxytetracycline should be administered intravenously.

In patients with renal impairment: (See "Warnings") Total dosage should be decreased by reduction of recommended individual doses and/or by extending time intervals between doses.

How Supplied: Terramycin (oxytetracycline) Intramuscular Solution is available as follows:

Potency of 250 mg/2 ml—in 2 ml pre-scored glass ampules, packages of 5 and 100.

2 ml Isoject® disposable syringe, packages of 10.

Potency of 100 mg/2 ml in 2 ml pre-scored glass ampules, packages of 5 and 100.

2 ml Isoject® disposable syringe, packages of 10.

Potency of 50 mg/ml in 10 ml multiple dose vials, packages of 5.

*U.S. Pat. Nos. 3,017,323 and 3,026,248

[Shown in Product Identification Section]

TERRAMYCIN® OINTMENT

(oxytetracycline hydrochloride topical ointment with polymyxin B sulfate)

How Supplied: Each gram contains oxytetracycline hydrochloride equivalent to 30 mg. of oxytetracycline; and also 10,000 units of polymyxin B sulfate.

Available in ½ ounce and one ounce tubes, both sizes sold in cartons of twelve. A prescription is *not* required.

TERRAMYCIN® ℞

(oxytetracycline HCl with polymyxin B sulfate)
OPHTHALMIC OINTMENT
STERILE

Description: Each gram of sterile ointment contains oxytetracycline HCl equivalent to 5 mg oxytetracycline, 10,000 units of polymyxin B sulfate, white petrolatum, and liquid petrolatum.

Actions: Terramycin® (oxytetracycline HCl) is a widely used antibiotic with clinically proved activity against gram-positive and gram-negative bacteria, rickettsiae, spirochetes, large viruses, and certain protozoa.

Polymyxin B Sulfate, one of a group of related antibiotics derived from *Bacillus polymyxa*, is rapidly bactericidal. This action is exclusively against gram-negative organisms. It is particularly effective against *Pseudomonas aeruginosa (B. pyocyaneus)* and Koch-Weeks bacillus, frequently found in local infections of the eye.

There is thus made available a particularly effective antimicrobial combination of the broad-spectrum antibiotic Terramycin as well as polymyxin B sulfate against primarily causative or secondarily infecting organisms.

Indications: The sterile preparation. Terramycin with Polymyxin B Sulfate Ophthalmic Ointment, is indicated for the treatment of superficial ocular infections involving the conjunctiva and/or cornea caused by Terramycin with Polymyxin B Sulfate-susceptible organisms.

It may be administered topically alone, or as an adjunct to systemic therapy.

It is effective in infections caused by susceptible strains of staphylococci, streptococci, pneumococci, *Hemophilus influenzae, Pseudomonas aeruginosa*, Koch-Weeks bacillus, and *Proteus.*

Contraindications: This drug is contraindicated in individuals who have shown hypersensitivity to any of its components.

Precautions: As with all antibiotic preparations, use of this drug may result in overgrowth of nonsusceptible organisms, including fungi. If super-infection occurs, the antibiotic should be discontinued and appropriate specific therapy should be instituted.

Adverse Reactions: Terramycin with Polymyxin B Sulfate Ophthalmic Ointment is well tolerated by the epithelial membranes and other tissues of the eye. Allergic or inflammatory reactions due to individual hypersensitivity are rare.

Dosage and Administration: Approximately ½ inch of the ointment is squeezed from the tube onto the lower lid of the affected eye two to four times daily.

The patient should be instructed to avoid contamination of the tip of the tube when applying the ointment.

How Supplied: Terramycin with Polymyxin B Sulfate Ophthalmic Ointment is supplied in ⅛ oz., (3.5 g) tubes.

[*Shown in Product Identification Section*]

TETRACYN® ℞
(tetracycline hydrochloride)
CAPSULES

Indications: Tetracycline is indicated in infections caused by the following microorganisms:

Rickettsiae: Rocky Mountain spotted fever, typhus fever and the typhus group, Q fever, rickettsialpox and tick fevers.

Mycoplasma pneumoniae (PPLO, Eaton agent),

Agents of psittacosis and ornithosis,

Agents of lymphogranuloma venereum and granuloma inguinale,

The spirochetal agent of relapsing fever *(Borrelia recurrentis).*

The following gram-negative microorganisms:

Haemophilus ducreyi (chancroid),

Pasteurella pestis and *Pasteurella tularensis,*

Bartonella bacilliformis,

Bacteroides species,

Vibrio comma and *Vibrio fetus,*

Brucella species (in conjunction with streptomycin).

Because many strains of the following groups of microorganisms have been shown to be resistant to tetracyclines, culture and susceptibility testing are recommended.

Tetracycline is indicated for treatment of infections caused by the following gram-negative microorganisms, when bacteriologic testing indicates appropriate susceptibility to the drug.

Escherichia coli,

Enterobacter aerogenes (formerly *Aerobacter aerogenes*),

Shigella species,

Mima species and *Herellea* species,

Haemophilus influenzae (respiratory infections),

Klebsiella species (respiratory and urinary infections).

Tetracycline is indicated for treatment of infections caused by the following gram-positive microorganisms when bacteriologic testing indicates appropriate susceptibility to the drug:

Streptococcus species:

Up to 44 percent of strains of *Streptococcus pyogenes* and 74 percent of *Streptococcus faecalis* have been found to be resistant to tetracycline drugs. Therefore, tetracyclines should not be used for streptococcal disease unless the organism has been demonstrated to be sensitive.

For upper respiratory infections due to Group A beta-hemolytic streptococci, penicillin is the usual drug of choice, including prophylaxis of rheumatic fever.

Diplococcus pneumoniae,

Staphylococcus aureus, skin and soft tissue infections. Tetracyclines are not the drugs of choice in the treatment of any type of staphylococcal infections.

When penicillin is contraindicated, tetracyclines are alternative drugs in the treatment of infections due to:

Neisseria gonorrhoeae,

Treponema pallidum and *Treponema pertenue* (syphilis and yaws),

Listeria monocytogenes,

Clostridium species,

Bacillus anthracis,

Fusobacterium fusiforme (Vincent's infection),

Actinomyces species.

In acute intestinal amebiasis, the tetracyclines may be a useful adjunct to amebicides.

In severe acne, the tetracyclines may be useful adjunctive therapy.

Tetracyclines are indicated in the treatment of trachoma, although the infectious agent is not always eliminated, as judged by immunofluorescence.

Inclusion conjunctivitis may be treated with oral tetracyclines or with a combination of oral and topical agents.

Contraindications: This drug is contraindicated in persons who have shown hypersensitivity to any of the tetracyclines.

Warnings: THE USE OF DRUGS OF THE TETRACYCLINE CLASS DURING TOOTH DEVELOPMENT (LAST HALF OF PREGNANCY, INFANCY, AND CHILDHOOD TO THE AGE OF 8 YEARS) MAY CAUSE PERMANENT DISCOLORATION OF THE TEETH (YELLOW-GRAY-BROWN). This adverse reaction is more common during long term use of the drugs but has been observed following repeated short term courses. Enamel hypoplasia has also been reported. *TETRACYCLINE DRUGS, THEREFORE, SHOULD NOT BE USED IN THIS AGE GROUP UNLESS OTHER DRUGS ARE NOT LIKELY TO BE EFFECTIVE OR ARE CONTRAINDICATED.*

If renal impairment exists, even usual oral or parenteral doses may lead to excessive systemic accumulation of the drug and possible liver toxicity. Under such conditions, lower than usual total doses are indicated and, if therapy is prolonged, serum level determinations of the drug may be advisable.

Photosensitivity manifested by an exaggerated sunburn reaction has been observed in some individuals taking tetracyclines. Patients apt to be exposed to direct sunlight or ultraviolet light should be advised that this reaction can occur with tetracycline drugs, and treatment should be discontinued at the first evidence of skin erythema.

The antianabolic action of the tetracyclines may cause an increase in BUN. While this is not a problem in those with normal renal function, in patients with significantly impaired function, higher serum levels of tetracycline may lead to azotemia, hyperphosphatemia, and acidosis.

Usage in pregnancy. (See above "Warnings" about use during tooth development.)

Results of animal studies indicate that tetracyclines cross the placenta, are found in fetal tissues and can have toxic effects on the developing fetus (often related to retardation of skeletal development). Evidence of embryotoxicity has also been noted in animals treated early in pregnancy.

Usage in newborns, infants, and children. (See above "Warnings" about use during tooth development.)

All tetracyclines form a stable calcium complex in any bone-forming tissue. A decrease in the fibula growth rate has been observed in prematures given oral tetracycline in doses of 25 mg/kg every 6 hours. This reaction was shown to be reversible when the drug was discontinued.

Tetracyclines are present in the milk of lactating women who are taking a drug in this class.

Precautions: As with other antibiotic preparations, use of this drug may result in overgrowth of nonsusceptible organisms, including fungi. If superinfection occurs, the antibiotic should be discontinued and appropriate therapy instituted.

In venereal diseases when coexistent syphilis is suspected, a dark field examination should be done before treatment is started and the blood serology repeated monthly for at least 4 months.

Because tetracyclines have been shown to depress plasma prothrombin activity, patients who are on anticoagulant therapy may require downward adjustment of their anticoagulant dosage.

In long term therapy, periodic laboratory evaluation of organ systems, including hematopoietic, renal and hepatic studies should be performed.

All infections due to Group A beta-hemolytic streptococci should be treated for at least 10 days.

Since bacteriostatic drugs may interfere with the bactericidal action of penicillin, it is advisable to avoid giving tetracycline in conjunction with penicillin.

Adverse Reactions: Gastrointestinal: anorexia, nausea, vomiting, diarrhea, glossitis, dysphagia, enterocolitis, and inflammatory lesions (with monilial overgrowth) in the anogenital region. These reactions have been caused by both the oral and parenteral administration of tetracyclines. Rare instances of esophagitis and esophageal ulcerations have been reported in patients receiving capsule forms of drugs in the tetracycline class. Most of these patients took medications immediately before going to bed. (See Dosage and Administration.)

Skin: maculopapular and erythematous rashes. Exfoliative dermatitis has been reported but is uncommon. Photosensitivity is discussed above. (See "Warnings").

Renal toxicity: Rise in BUN has been reported and is apparently dose related. (See "Warnings").

Hypersensitivity reactions: urticaria, angioneurotic edema, anaphylaxis, anaphylactoid purpura, pericarditis, and exacerbation of systemic lupus erythematosus.

Bulging fontanels in infants and benign intracranial hypertension in adults have been reported in individuals receiving full therapeutic dosages. These conditions disappeared rapidly when the drug was discontinued.

Blood: Hemolytic anemia, thrombocytopenia, neutropenia, and eosinophilia have been reported.

When given over prolonged periods, tetracyclines have been reported to produce brown-black microscopic discoloration of thyroid glands. No abnormalities of thyroid function studies are known to occur.

Dosage and Administration: Therapy should be continued for at least 24–48 hours after symptoms and fever have subsided.

Administration of adequate amounts of fluid along with capsule forms of drugs in the tetracycline class is recommended to wash down the drugs and reduce the risk of esophageal irritation and ulceration. (See Adverse Reactions.)

Concomitant therapy: Antacids containing aluminum, calcium, or magnesium impair absorption and should not be given to patients taking oral tetracycline. Food and some dairy products also interfere with absorption. Oral forms of tetracycline should be given one hour before or two hours after meals. Pediatric oral dosage forms should not be given with milk formulas and should be given at least one hour prior to feeding.

In patients with renal impairment (See "Warnings") total dosage should be decreased by reduction of recommended individual doses and/or by extending time intervals between doses.

In the treatment of streptococcal infections, a therapeutic dose of tetracycline should be administered for at least 10 days. The dosage required to produce optimum therapeutic response will vary from one patient to another depending upon the severity of the infection, the degree of susceptibility of the organism, and the response of the individual.

The suggested minimum adult dosage for tetracycline is 1 gram daily in divided doses given as 500 mg twice a day or 250 mg four times a day. Higher doses, such as 500 mg four times daily, may be required for severe infections or

Continued on next page

Pfipharmecs—Cont.

for those infections which do not respond to the smaller dose.

For children above eight years of age: Usual daily dose, 10–20 mg per pound (25–50 mg/kg) of body weight divided in four equal doses.

A gram a day in two divided doses of 500 mg each, has been found effective in certain types of skin infections.

For treatment of brucellosis, 500 mg tetracycline four times daily for three weeks should be accompanied by streptomycin, one gram intramuscularly twice daily the first week and once daily the second week.

For treatment of uncomplicated gonorrhea, when penicillin is contraindicated, tetracycline may be used for the treatment of both males and females in the following divided dosage schedule: 1.5 grams initially, followed by 0.5 gram q.i.d. for a total of 9.0 grams.

For treatment of syphilis, a total of 30 to 40 grams in equally divided doses over a period of 10–15 days should be given. Close follow-up, including laboratory tests, is recommended.

How Supplied: Tetracyn (tetracycline HCl) Capsules, available in opaque, black and white, hard gelatin capsules contain 250 mg of tetracycline HCl: bottles of 100, 1000.

Tetracyn® 500 (tetracycline HCl) Capsules, available in opaque, black and blue, hard gelatin capsules contain 500 mg of tetracycline HCl: bottles of 100.

[*Shown in Product Identification Section*]

TETRASTATIN® ℞
tetracycline HCl 250 mg
nystatin 250,000 units
CAPSULES

Actions: Tetracyn® (tetracycline HCl) is a crystalline antibiotic which possesses potent antimicrobial activity. It is well tolerated and effective in the treatment of many diseases caused by gram-positive or gram-negative bacteria.

Nystatin is an antibiotic with activity against a number of fungi, including *Candida albicans* (Monilia). It adds significant prophylaxis against overgrowth or superinfection by such fungi.

Indications

Based on a review of this drug by the National Academy of Sciences-National Research Council and/or other information, FDA has classified the indications as follows:

"Lacking substantial evidence of effectiveness as a fixed combination":

Tetrastatin is indicated in a wide variety of infections caused by susceptible bacteria. Tetracyn (tetracycline HCl) is very rapidly absorbed, diffuses readily into tissues to combat infection, and is well tolerated. Nystatin, the first available antifungal antibiotic, has been used successfully as a prophylactic agent for the suppression of *Candida albicans* and as a therapeutic agent in the management of active monilial infections.

The following have been clinically established as indications for the use of Tetracyn (tetracycline HCl):

RESPIRATORY TRACT INFECTIONS: Pneumococcal pneumonia; other types of bacterial pneumonia; bronchopneumonia; pertussis; follicular tonsillitis; acute bronchitis; otitis media; mastoiditis, and a number of upper respiratory infections.

GENITOURINARY INFECTIONS: Acute and chronic urinary infections such as cystitis; urethritis; pyelonephritis; ureteritis; and prostatitis; caused by susceptible staphylococci, streptococci, A. aerogenes, E. coli, and some mixed infections; gonorrhea.

INFECTIONS OF THE NERVOUS SYSTEM: Bacterial meningitis caused by the meningococcus, H. influenzae and other susceptible organisms, as well as bacterial infections localized elsewhere in the nervous system.

SURGICAL INFECTIONS: Peritonitis, acute bacterial cholecystitis, infected wounds and incisions, serious soft tissue infections, and osteomyelitis.

In the treatment of staphylococcal infections, indicated surgical procedures should be carried out in all cases.

INFECTIONS IN OBSTETRICS AND GYNECOLOGY: Puerperal infection, salpingo-oöphoritis, pelvic inflammatory disease, and infection resulting from incomplete abortion.

OTHER INFECTIONS: Eye infections, gastrointestinal infections, and skin infections caused by susceptible bacteria; rickettsial infections such as Rocky Mountain spotted fever and epidemic typhus; certain infections with large viruses such as lymphogranuloma venereum and psittacosis; brucellosis and bartonellosis; bacillary dysentery; acute intestinal amebic infections; septicemia, and subacute bacterial endocarditis due to susceptible organisms. It is usually not possible to predict with certainty which patients may develop clinical moniliasis as a result of broad-spectrum antibiotic therapy. However, the added protection afforded by Tetrastatin against monilial superinfection of intestinal origin is especially important for patients who are most likely to be susceptible to the overgrowth of *Candida albicans.* Among such patients are those requiring high or prolonged antibiotic dosage; debilitated or elderly patients; diabetics; infants; patients receiving concomitant cortisone or related steriod therapy; patients who have developed a monilial complication on previous broad-spectrum therapy; and women, particularly during pregnancy.

Final classification of the less than effective indications requires further investigation. Clinical studies to substantiate the efficacy of Tetrastatin are ongoing. Completion of these ongoing studies will provide data for final classification of these indications.

Contraindications: This drug is contraindicated in individuals who have shown hypesensitivity to any of its components.

Warnings: Tetracycline may form a stable calcium complex in any bone forming tissue with no serious harmful effects reported thus far in humans. However, use of tetracycline during tooth development (last trimester of pregnancy, neonatal period and early childhood) may cause discoloration of the teeth (yellow-grey-brownish). This effect occurs mostly during long term use of the drug but it has also been observed in usual short treatment courses.

If renal impairment exists even usual doses may lead to excessive accumulation of the drug and possible liver toxicity. Under such conditions, lower than usual doses are indicated and if therapy is prolonged, tetracycline serum level determinations may be advisable.

Certain hypersensitive individuals may develop a photodynamic reaction precipitated by a direct exposure to natural or artificial sunlight during the use of this drug. This reaction is usually of the photoallergic type which may also be produced by other tetracycline derivatives. Individuals with a history of photosensitivity reactions should be instructed to avoid direct exposure to natural or artificial sunlight while under treatment with this or other tetracycline drugs, and treatment should be discontinued at first evidence of skin discomfort.

NOTE: Tetracyn (tetracycline HCl) has been rarely implicated as the causative agent of photosensitivity.

Precautions: If a superimposed infection which may be caused by resistant organisms is observed, the antibiotic should be discontinued and a therapeutic trial of other antibiotics as indicated by susceptibility testing may be indicated.

Increased intracranial pressure with bulging fontanelles has been observed occasionally in infants receiving therapeutic doses of tetracycline. Although the mechanism for this phenomenon is unknown, the signs and symptoms have disappeared rapidly upon cessation of treatment with no sequelae.

In long term therapy with this as with other potent drugs, periodic laboratory evaluation of organ systems, including hematopoietic, renal and hepatic studies should be accomplished.

When treating gonorrhea in which lesions of primary or secondary syphilis are suspected, proper diagnostic procedures including dark field examinations, should be followed. In other cases in which concomitant syphilis is suspected, monthly serological tests should be made for at least four months.

Adverse Reactions: Glossitis, stomatitis, proctitis, nausea, diarrhea, vaginitis and dermatitis as well as reactions of an allergic nature may occur but are rare. If adverse reactions occur or individual idiosyncrasy or allergy occurs, discontinue medication. Rare instances of esophagitis and esophageal ulcerations have been reported in patients receiving capsule forms of drugs in the tetracycline class. Most of these patients took medications immediately before going to bed. (See Dosage and Administration.)

With tetracycline therapy bulging fontanels in infants and benign intracranial hypertension in adults have been reported in individuals receiving full therapeutic dosages. These conditions disappeared rapidly when the drug was discontinued.

Elevation of SGOT or SGPT values or elevated BUN have been reported with the use of tetracyclines, the significance of which is not known at this time. Anemia, neutropenia, and eosinophilia have been reported with the use of tetracyclines.

Dosage and Administration: The dosage of Tetrastatin required to produce optimum therapeutic response will vary from one patient to another depending upon the severity of the infection, the degree of susceptibility of the organism, and the response of the individual to treatment. In the average adult the suggested daily dose should be 1 to 2 g of tetracycline HCl divided into four equal parts (250 mg to 500 mg q.i.d. or 1 to 2 capsules of Tetrastatin q.i.d.). Higher daily doses may be required for severe infections or for those patients who do not respond rapidly to lower dosage. Therapy should continue for at least 24 to 48 hours after symptoms and fever have subsided. When used in streptococcal infections therapy should continue for ten days to prevent the possible development of rheumatic fever or glomerulonephritis.

In subacute bacterial endocarditis, therapy 6 to 8 weeks should be maintained. A rest period may be given at the end of these periods of treatment and therapy again begun if the specific infectious agent can still be demonstrated.

When using Tetracyn (tetracycline HCl) in the treatment of brucellosis, the course of therapy should be three weeks and supplemented with intramuscular injections of streptomycin in a dosage of 1 g twice daily the first week, and 1 g daily the second and third weeks.

The recommended dosage of Tetrastatin as indicated above is the same as that for Tetracyn (tetracycline HCl). Because of the diminished possibility of fungal overgrowth it may be anticipated that gastrointestinal disturbances should be minimized.

Administration of adequate amounts of fluid along with capsule forms of drugs in the tetracycline class is recommended to wash down the drugs and reduce the risk of esophageal irritation and ulceration. (See Adverse Reactions.)

To aid absorption of the drug, it should be given at least one hour before or two hours after eating. Tetracycline should not be given with milk formulas or calcium-containing foods. Aluminum hydroxide gel and similar substances when given with antibiotics have been shown to decrease absorption and are contraindicated.

How Supplied: Tetrastatin Capsules are available in opaque, black and pink, hard gelatin capsules; each capsule contains 250 mg of tetracycline HCl and 250,000 units of nystatin: bottles of 100.

VISTARIL® ℞
(hydroxyzine hydrochloride)
Intramuscular Solution
For Intramuscular Use Only

Chemistry: Hydroxyzine hydrochloride is designated chemically as 1-(p-chlorobenzhydryl) 4-[2-(2-hydroxyethoxy) ethyl] piperazine dihydrochloride.

Actions: VISTARIL (hydroxyzine hydrochloride) is unrelated chemically to phenothiazine, reserpine, and meprobamate. Hydroxyzine has demonstrated its clinical effectiveness in the chemotherapeutic aspect of the total management of neuroses and emotional disturbances manifested by anxiety, tension, agitation, apprehension or confusion.

Hydroxyzine has been shown clinically to be a rapid-acting true ataraxic with a wide margin of safety. It induces a calming effect in anxious, tense, psychoneurotic adults and also in anxious, hyperkinetic children without impairing mental alertness. It is not a cortical depressant, but its action may be due to a suppression of activity in certain key regions of the subcortical area of the central nervous system.

Primary skeletal muscle relaxation has been demonstrated experimentally.

Hydroxyzine has been shown experimentally to have antispasmodic properties, apparently mediated through interference with the mechanism that reponds to spasmogenic agents such as serotonin, acetylcholine, and histamine.

Antihistaminic effects have been demonstrated experimentally and confirmed clinically

An antiemetic effect, both by the apomorphine test and the veriloid test, has been demonstrated. Pharmacological and clinical studies indicate that hydroxyzine in therapeutic dosage does not increase gastric secretion or acidity and in most cases provides mild antisecretory benefits.

Indications: The total management of anxiety, tension, and psychomotor agitation in conditions of emotional stress requires in most instances a combined approach of psychotherapy and chemotherapy. Hydroxyzine has been found to be particularly useful for this latter phrase of therapy in its ability to render the disturbed patient more amenable to psychotherapy in long term treatment of the psychoneurotic and psychotic, although it should not be used as the sole treatment of psychosis or of clearly demonstrated cases of depression.

Hydroxyzine is also useful in alleviating the manifestations of anxiety and tension as in the preparation for dental procedures and in acute emotional problems. It has also been recommended for the management of anxiety associated with organic disturbances and as adjunctive therapy in alcoholism and allergic conditions with strong emotional overlay, such as in asthma, chronic urticaria, and pruritus.

VISTARIL (hydroxyzine hydrochloride) Intramuscular Solution is useful in treating the following types of patients when intramuscular administration is indicated:

1. The acutely disturbed or hysterical patient.
2. The acute or chronic alcoholic with anxiety withdrawal symptoms or delirium tremens.
3. As pre- and postoperative and pre- and postpartum adjunctive medication to permit reduction in narcotic dosage, allay anxiety and control emesis.

VISTARIL (hydroxyzine hydrochloride) has also demonstrated effectiveness in controlling nausea and vomiting, excluding nausea and vomiting of pregnancy. (See Contraindications.)

In prepartum states, the reduction in narcotic requirement effected by hydroxyzine is of particular benefit to both mother and neonate.

Hydroxyzine benefits the cardiac patient by its ability to allay the associated anxiety and apprehension attendant to certain types of heart disease. Hydroxyzine is not known to interfere with the action of digitalis in any way and may be used concurrently with this agent.

The effectiveness of hydroxyzine in long term use, that is, more than 4 months, has not been assessed by systematic clinical studies. The physician should reassess periodically the usefulness of the drug for the individual patient.

Contraindications: Hydroxyzine hydrochloride intramuscular solution is intended only for intramuscular administration and should not, under any circumstances, be injected subcutaneously, intra-arterially, or intravenously.

This drug is contraindicated for patients who have shown a previous hypersensitivity to it.

Hydroxyzine, when administered to the pregnant mouse, rat, and rabbit, induced fetal abnormalities in the rat at doses substantially above the human therapeutic range. Clinical data in human beings are inadequate to establish safety in early pregnancy. Until such data are available, hydroxyzine is contraindicated in early pregnancy.

Precautions: THE POTENTIATING ACTION OF HYDROXYZINE MUST BE CONSIDERED WHEN THE DRUG IS USED IN CONJUNCTION WITH CENTRAL NERVOUS SYSTEM DEPRESSANTS SUCH AS NARCOTICS, BARBITURATES, AND ALCOHOL. Therefore when central nervous system depressants are administered concomitantly with hydroxyzine their dosage should be reduced up to 50 per cent. The efficacy of hydroxyzine as adjunctive pre- and postoperative sedative medication has also been well established, especially as regards its ability to allay anxiety, control emesis, and reduce the amount of narcotic required.

HYDROXYZINE MAY POTENTIATE NARCOTICS AND BARBITURATES, so their use in preanesthetic adjunctive therapy should be modified on an individual basis. Atropine and other belladonna alkaloids are not affected by the drug.

When hydroxyzine is used preoperatively or prepartum, narcotic requirements may be reduced as much as 50 per cent. Thus, when 50 mg of VISTARIL (hydroxyzine hydrochloride) Intramuscular Solution is employed, meperidine dosage may be reduced from 100 mg to 50 mg. The administration of meperidine may result in severe hypotension in the postoperative patient or any individual whose ability to maintain blood pressure has been compromised by a depleted blood volume. Meperidine should be used with great caution and in reduced dosage in patients who are receiving other pre- and/or postoperative medications and in whom there is a risk of respiratory depression, hypotension, and profound sedation or coma occurring. Before using any medications concomitant with hydroxyzine, the manufacturer's prescribing information should be read carefully.

Since drowsiness may occur with the use of this drug, patients should be warned of this possibility and cautioned against driving a car or operating dangerous machinery while taking this drug.

As with all intramuscular preparations, VISTARIL Intramuscular Solution should be injected well within the body of a relatively large muscle. Inadvertent subcutaneous injection may result in significant tissue damage.

ADULTS: The preferred site is the upper outer quadrant of the buttock, (i.e., gluteus maximus), or the mid-lateral thigh.

CHILDREN: It is recommended that intramuscular injections be given preferably in the mid-lateral muscles of the thigh. In infants and small children the periphery of the upper outer quadrant of the gluteal region should be used only when necessary, such as in burn patients, in order to minimize the possibility of damage to the sciatic nerve.

The deltoid area should be used only if well developed such as in certain adults and older children, and then only with caution to avoid radial nerve injury. Intramuscular injections should not be made into the lower and mid-third of the upper arm. As with all intramuscular injections, aspiration is necessary to help avoid inadvertent injection into a blood vessel.

Adverse Reactions: Therapeutic doses of hydroxyzine seldom produce impairment of mental alertness. However, drowsiness may occur; if so, it is usually transitory and may disappear in a few days of continued therapy or upon reduction of the dose. Dryness of the mouth may be encountered at higher doses. Extensive clinical use has substantiated the absence of toxic effects on the liver or bone marrow when administered in the recommended doses for over four years of uninterrupted therapy. The absence of adverse effects has been further demonstrated in experimental studies in which excessively high doses were administered.

Involuntary motor activity, including rare instances of tremor and convulsions, has been reported, usually with doses considerably higher than those recommended. Continuous therapy with over one gram per day has been employed in some patients without these effects having been encountered.

Dosage and Administration: The recommended dosages for VISTARIL (hydroxyzine hydrochloride) Intramuscular Solution are:

For adult psychiatric and emotional emergencies, including acute alcoholism.	I.M.: 50–100 mg stat., and q. 4–6h., p.r.n.
Nausea and vomiting excluding nausea and vomiting of pregnancy.	Adults: 25–100 mg I.M. Children: 0.5 mg/lb. body weight I.M.
Pre- and postoperative adjunctive medication.	Adults: 25–100 mg I.M. Children: 0.5 mg/lb. body weight I.M.
Pre- and postpartum adjunctive therapy.	25–100 mg I.M.

As with all potent medications, the dosage should be adjusted according to the patient's response to therapy.

FOR ADDITIONAL INFORMATION ON THE ADMINISTRATION AND SITE OF SELECTION SEE PRECAUTIONS SECTION. NOTE: VISTARIL (hydroxyzine hydrochloride) Intramuscular Solution may be administered without further dilution.

Patients may be started on intramuscular therapy when indicated. They should be maintained on oral therapy whenever this route is practicable.

Supply: Vistaril IM is an aqueous solution containing either 25 mg or 50 mg hydroxyzine HCl per ml, 0.9% benzyl alcohol and sodium hydroxide to adjust to optimum pH.

Multi-Dose Vials
25 mg per ml, 10 ml vials
50 mg per ml, 10 ml vials

Unit Dose Vials: Packages of 10 vials
25 mg per vial, 1 ml fill

Continued on next page

Pfipharmecs—Cont.

50 mg per vial, 1 ml fill
75 mg per vial, 1.5 ml fill
100 mg per vial, 2 ml fill
Isojects: Packages of 10 Isojects
25 mg per Isoject, 1 ml fill
50 mg per Isoject, 1 ml fill
100 mg per Isoject, 2 ml fill
Steraject® Cartridges: Packages of 10 cartridges
25 mg per Steraject, 1 ml fill
50 mg per Steraject, 1 ml fill
100 mg per Steraject, 2 ml fill

WART-OFF™ OTC

Active Ingredient: Salicylic Acid, U.S.P., 17%, in Flexible Collodion, U.S.P. Wart-Off™ Solution contains approx. 20.5% Alcohol and 54.2% Ether—small losses are unavoidable.
Indications: Removal of Warts
Warnings: Keep this and all medications out of reach of children to avoid accidental poisoning.
Flammable—Do not use near fire or flame. For external use only. In case of accidental ingestion, contact a physician or a Poison Control Center immediately. Do not use near eyes or on mucous membranes. Diabetics or other people with impaired circulation should not use Wart-Off™. Do not use on moles, birthmarks or unusual warts with hair growing from them. If wart persists, see your physician. If pain should develop, consult your physician. **Do not apply to surrounding skin.**
Dosage and Administration: Instructions For Use: Read warning and enclosed instructional brochure. Do not apply to surrounding skin. Make sure that surrounding skin is protected from accidental application. Apply Wart-Off™ to warts only. Before applying, soak affected area in hot water for several minutes. If any tissue has been loosened, remove by rubbing surface of wart gently with special brush enclosed in Wart-Off™ package. Dry thoroughly. Warts are contagious, so don't share your towel. Apply once or twice daily. Using plastic applicator attached to cap, apply one drop at a time until entire wart is covered. Lightly cover with small adhesive bandage. Replace cap tightly. This treatment may be used daily for three to four weeks if necessary.
How Supplied: 0.5 fluid ounce bottle with pinpoint plastic applicator, special cleaning brush and instructional brochure.
[*Shown in Product Identification Section*]

Pfizer Laboratories Division

PFIZER INC.
235 EAST 42ND STREET
NEW YORK, NY 10017

Full prescribing information for all Pfizer Laboratories products is available from your Pfizer Laboratories representative.

Product Identification Codes

To provide quick and positive identification of Pfizer Laboratories Division products, we have imprinted the product identification number of the National Drug Code on most tablets and capsules.
In order that you may quickly identify a product by its code number, we have compiled below a numerical list of code numbers with their corresponding product names. We are also listing the code numbers by alphabetical order of products.

NUMERICAL PRODUCT INDEX

Product Identification Code	Product
072 & 073	Terramycin® (Oxytetracycline HCl) Capsules (see Pfipharmecs listing.)
084	Terramycin® (Oxytetracycline) Film Coated Tablets (See Pfipharmecs listing.)
094	Vibramycin® Hyclate (Doxycycline Hyclate) Capsules 50 mg.
095	Vibramycin® Hyclate (Doxycycline Hyclate) Capsules 100 mg.
099	Vibra-Tabs® (Doxycycline Hyclate) Film Coated Tablets 100 mg.
180	Vistrax® 5 (Oxyphencyclimine HCl 5 mg. and Hydroxyzine HCl 25 mg.) Tablets
181	Vistrax® 10 (Oxyphencyclimine HCl 10 mg. and Hydroxyzine HCl 25 mg.) Tablets
201	Bonine® (Meclizine HCl) Chewable Tablets 25 mg.
260	Procardia® (Nifedipine) Capsules 10 mg.
322	Feldene® (Piroxicam) Capsules 10 mg.
323	Feldene® (Piroxicam) Capsules 20 mg.
375	Renese® (Polythiazide) Tablets 1 mg.
376	Renese® (Polythiazide) Tablets 2 mg.
377	Renese® (Polythiazide) Tablets 4 mg.
393	Diabinese® (Chlorpropamide) Tablets 100 mg.
394	Diabinese® (Chlorpropamide) Tablets 250 mg.
430	Minizide® 1 Capsules (1 mg. Prazosin HCl and 0.5 mg. Polythiazide)
431	Minipress® (Prazosin HCl) Capsules 1 mg.
432	Minizide® 2 Capsules (2 mg. Prazosin HCl and 0.5 mg. Polythiazide)
436	Minizide® 5 Capsules (5 mg. Prazosin HCl and 0.5 mg. Polythiazide)
437	Minipress® (Prazosin HCl) Capsules 2 mg.
438	Minipress® (Prazosin HCl) Capsules 5 mg.
441	Moderil® (Rescinnamine) Tablets 0.25 mg.
442	Moderil® (Rescinnamine) Tablets 0.5 mg.
446	Renese®-R (Polythiazide 2.0 mg. and Reserpine 0.25 mg.) Tablets
534-539	Sinequan® (Doxepin HCl) Capsules (See Roerig listing.)
541	Vistaril® (Hydroxyzine Pamoate) Capsules 25 mg.
542	Vistaril® (Hydroxyzine Pamoate) Capsules 50 mg.
543	Vistaril® (Hydroxyzine Pamoate) Capsules 100 mg.

ALPHABETICAL PRODUCT INDEX

Product	Product Identification Code
Bonine® (Meclizine HCl) Chewable Tablets 25 mg.	201
Diabinese® (Chlorpropamide) Tablets 100 mg.	393
Diabinese® (Chlorpropamide) Tablets 250 mg.	394
Feldene® (Piroxicam) Capsules 10 mg.	322
Feldene® (Piroxicam) Capsules 20 mg.	323
Minipress® (Prazosin HCl) Capsules 1 mg.	431
Minipress® (Prazosin HCl) Capsules 2 mg.	437
Minipress® (Prazosin HCl) Capsules 5 mg.	438
Minizide® 1 Capsules (1 mg. Prazosin HCl and 0.5 mg. Polythiazide)	430
Minizide® 2 Capsules (2 mg. Prazosin HCl and 0.5 mg. Polythiazide)	432
Minizide® 5 Capsules (5 mg. Prazosin HCl and 0.5 mg. Polythiazide)	436
Moderil® (Rescinnamine) Tablets 0.25 mg.	441
Moderil® (Rescinnamine) Tablets 0.5 mg.	442
Procardia® (Nifedipine) Capsules 10 mg.	260
Renese® (Polythiazide) Tablets 1 mg.	375
Renese® (Polythiazide) Tablets 2 mg.	376
Renese® (Polythiazide) Tablets 4 mg.	377
Renese®-R (Polythiazide 2.0 mg. and Reserpine 0.25 mg.) Tablets	446
Sinequan® (Doxepin HCl) Capsules (See Roerig listing.)	534-539
Terramycin® (Oxytetracycline HCl) Capsules (See Pfipharmecs listing.)	072 & 073
Terramycin® (Oxytetracycline) Film Coated Tablets (See Pfipharmecs listing.)	084
Vibramycin® Hyclate (Doxycycline Hyclate) Capsules 50 mg.	094
Vibramycin® Hyclate (Doxycycline Hyclate) Capsules 100 mg.	095
Vibra-Tabs® (Doxycycline Hyclate) Film Coated Tablets 100 mg.	099
Vistaril® (Hydroxyzine Pamoate) Capsules 25 mg.	541
Vistaril® (Hydroxyzine Pamoate) Capsules 50 mg.	542
Vistaril® (Hydroxyzine Pamoate) Capsules 100 mg.	543
Vistrax® 5 (Oxyphencyclimine HCl 5 mg. and Hydroxyzine HCl 25 mg.) Tablets	180
Vistrax® 10 (Oxyphencyclimine HCl 10 mg. and Hydroxyzine HCl 25 mg.) Tablets	181

BONINE® OTC
(meclizine hydrochloride)
Chewable Tablets

Description: Chemically, BONINE (meclizine HCl) is 1-(*p*-chloro-α-phenylbenzyl)-4-(*m*-methylbenzyl) piperazine dihydrochloride monohydrate.
Actions: BONINE is an antihistamine which shows marked protective activity against nebulized histamine and lethal doses of intravenously injected histamine in guinea pigs. It has a marked effect in blocking the vasodepressor response to histamine, but only a slight blocking action against acetylcholine. Its activity is relatively weak in inhibiting the spasmogenic action of histamine on isolated guinea pig ileum.
Antihistamines have been observed to have both stimulant and depressant effects on the CNS, but no clear explanation exists in regard to their diverse central actions. The site and mode of their central action is unknown.
Indications: BONINE is effective in the management of nausea, vomiting and dizziness associated with motion sickness.
Contraindications: Meclizine HCl is contraindicated in individuals who have shown a previous hypersensitivity to it.
Warnings: Since drowsiness may, on occasion, occur with the use of this drug, patients should be warned of this possibility and cautioned against driving a car or operating dangerous machinery.
Patients should avoid alcoholic beverages while taking this drug. Due to its potential anticholinergic action, this drug should be used with caution in patients with asthma, glaucoma, or enlargement of the prostate gland.
Usage in Children:
Clinical studies establishing safety and effectiveness in children have not been done; therefore, usage is not recommended in children under 12 years of age.
Usage in Pregnancy:
Pregnancy Category B. Reproduction studies in rats have shown cleft palates at 25–50 times the human dose. Epidemiological studies in pregnant women, however, do not indicate that

meclizine increases the risk of abnormalities when administered during pregnancy. Despite the animal findings, it would appear that the possibility of fetal harm is remote. Nevertheless, meclizine, or any other medication, should be used during pregnancy only if clearly necessary.

Adverse Reactions: Drowsiness, dry mouth, and on rare occasions, blurred vision have been reported.

Dosage and Administration: The initial dose of 25–50 mg. of BONINE should be taken one hour prior to embarkation for protection against motion sickness. Thereafter, the dose may be repeated every 24 hours for the duration of the journey.

How Supplied: BONINE (meclizine HCl) is supplied as 25 mg. scored chewable tablets (imprinted with code number 201) (bottles of 100 and 500). (60-1464-37-6)

Literature Available: Yes.

DIABINESE®
(chlorpropamide)
Tablets ℞

Actions: DIABINESE (chlorpropamide) IS AN ORAL HYPOGLYCEMIC AGENT. IT IS NOT AN ORAL INSULIN, THOUGH THE PRECISE MECHANISM OF ACTION IS NOT COMPLETELY UNDERSTOOD.

DIABINESE was discovered and synthesized by researchers of Pfizer Inc. It was evaluated thoroughly in a broad clinical program, and these studies have shown it to be a potent, active, oral hypoglycemic agent, valuable in the treatment of selected diabetic patients. It is generally used alone to control the mild to moderately severe maturity-onset, stable diabetic. While chlorpropamide is a sulfonamide derivative, it is devoid of antibacterial activity.

A method developed by chemists at Pfizer Inc. (description available on request) permits the easy measurement of the drug in blood. Chlorpropamide does not interfere with the usual tests to detect albumin in the urine.

DIABINESE is absorbed rapidly from the gastrointestinal tract. Within one hour after a single oral dose, it is readily detectable in the blood, and the level reaches a maximum within two to four hours. It undergoes metabolism in humans and it is excreted in the urine as unchanged drug and as hydroxylated or hydrolyzed metabolites. The biological half-life of chlorpropamide averages about 36 hours. Within 96 hours, 80–90% of a single oral dose is excreted in the urine. However, long-term administration of therapeutic doses does not result in undue accumulation in the blood, since absorption and excretion rates become stabilized in about 5 to 7 days after the initiation of therapy.

DIABINESE exerts a hypoglycemic effect in normal humans within one hour, becoming maximal at 3 to 6 hours and persisting for at least 24 hours. The potency of chlorpropamide is approximately six times that of tolbutamide. Some experimental results suggest that its increased effectiveness may be the result of slower excretion and absence of significant deactivation.

The mode of action of chlorpropamide is believed to be that of stimulation of synthesis and release of endogenous insulin.

There is now evidence that improvement in pancreatic beta cell function, with consequent improvement in glucose tolerance, may occur with prolonged administration of chlorpropamide. Accordingly, in individuals with asymptomatic diabetes mellitus, principally manifested by an abnormal glucose tolerance, continuous use of chlorpropamide may result in "normalization" of their tolerance to glucose.

Indications: DIABINESE is indicated in uncomplicated diabetes mellitus of the stable, mild or moderately severe, non-ketotic, maturity-onset type, which cannot be completely controlled by diet alone. It can often be used in patients of this type in place of insulin. It may also prove effective in controlling certain patients who have shown an inadequate response or true primary or secondary failure to other sulfonylurea agents. In patients requiring high doses or frequent administration of another oral agent, control may be facilitated through its use.

Patient selection: The most likely patient for therapy is one in whom diabetes is of the maturity-onset (adult) type, stable, and not controllable by dietary regulation alone. A past history of diabetic coma does not necessarily preclude successful therapeutic control with DIABINESE. A trial period may be indicated in certain patients who might be expected to respond to this type of medication, but failed in initial trials with tolbutamide or subsequently after having been on other sulfonylureas for variable periods of time, or in patients whose diabetic control with tolbutamide is not as good as the physician would think best for his patient. DIABINESE may provide effective and improved control of the diabetes. The final evaluation of response in patients who qualify as candidates for DIABINESE is a therapeutic trial for a period of at least seven days. During the trial period, the absence of ketonuria together with a satisfactory reduction of glycosuria and hyperglycemia, or maintenance of previously satisfactory control, indicates that the patient is responsive and amenable to control with the drug. However, the development of ketonuria within 24 hours after withdrawal of insulin usually will be indicative of a poor response. The patient is considered nonresponsive if he fails to achieve satisfactory lowering of blood sugar levels or fails to obtain objective or subjective clinical improvement and if he develops ketonuria or glycosuria. Insulin is indicated for the therapy of such patients.

Contraindications: Use of DIABINESE is not indicated in patients having:

1. Juvenile or growth-onset diabetes mellitus.
2. Severe or unstable "brittle" diabetes.
3. Diabetes complicated by ketosis and acidosis, diabetic coma, major surgery, severe infection, or severe trauma.

DIABINESE is contraindicated during pregnancy. Safe conditions for the use of DIABINESE in pregnancy have not been established, and serious consideration should be given to the potential hazard of its use in women of the childbearing age who may become pregnant.

DIABINESE is contraindicated in patients with serious impairment of hepatic, renal, or thyroid function. Pseudo-diabetes with azotemia due to chronic renal disease has been misdiagnosed as diabetes mellitus.

Precautions: Since animal studies suggest that the action of barbiturates may be prolonged by therapy with chlorpropamide, barbiturates should be employed with caution. Similarly, studies showing an exaggerated hypoglycemic effect of chlorpropamide in adrenalectomized animals suggest cautious use in patients with Addison's disease. In some patients, a disulfiram-like reaction may be produced by the ingestion of alcohol.

Caution should be exercised when antibacterial sulfonamides, phenylbutazone, salicylates, probenecid, dicoumarol, or MAO inhibitors are administered concomitantly with chlorpropamide as hypoglycemia resultant from either potentiation or accumulation of sulfonylureas has been reported.

During the first six weeks of therapy, the physician should be in contact with the patient at least once a week. During this initial period, the patient must be observed for evidence of occasional drug reactions as described in the ADVERSE REACTIONS section. Because of the possibility of the following manifestations of hypersensitivity the patient should be instructed to report immediately to his physician if he does not feel as well as usual, or notes any pruritus, rash, jaundice, dark urine, light colored stools, low-grade fever, sore throat or diarrhea. As with all drugs, careful attention must be given to weigh the therapeutic advantages against the nature and incidence of side effects.

During the period of transition to DIABINESE (chlorpropamide), the patient's urine should be tested for sugar and acetone at least three times daily and the results reviewed by the physician at least once a week. Frequent laboratory determinations of liver function should also be seriously considered. Although transient minor alterations, particularly of cephalin flocculation, thymol turbidity, and serum alkaline phosphatase levels are not unusual and are probably of no clinical significance, a progressive rise in the alkaline phosphatase value should alert the physician to the possibility of incipient biliary stasis and jaundice, and chlorpropamide therapy should be promptly discontinued. After the initial six weeks of therapy, subsequent patient-physician contacts may be at less frequent intervals, the exact frequency dependent on the judgment of the physician.

The drug should be used as an adjunct to, not a substitute for, dietary regulation, for this remains the primary consideration of diabetic management. It does not alter the need to educate the patient to such standard prophylactic and therapeutic measures as weight and exercise control, proper hygiene, and prompt care of intercurrent infection.

Alcohol and decreased diet may lead to hypoglycemia, ketosis, coma and death. Thiazides, on the other hand, have been shown to suppress insulin secretion, and therefore will contribute to hyperglycemia.

Warnings: DIABINESE SHOULD NOT BE USED IN JUVENILE DIABETES OR IN DIABETES COMPLICATED BY ACIDOSIS, COMA, SEVERE INFECTION, MAJOR SURGICAL PROCEDURES, OR SEVERE TRAUMA. HERE, INSULIN IS INDISPENSABLE.

Although DIABINESE given alone has controlled some patients with mild maturity-onset diabetes of the stable type during the stress of mild infection or minor surgery, insulin therapy is generally essential during intercurrent complications (for example, ketoacidosis, severe trauma, major surgical procedures, severe infections, severe diarrhea, nausea and vomiting, etc.). The severity of the diabetes, the nature of the complication, and availability of laboratory facilities determine whether therapy with chlorpropamide can be continued or should be withdrawn while insulin is being used.

IN CASES OF ACCIDENTAL INGESTION BY CHILDREN, DUE NOTE SHOULD BE TAKEN OF THE FACT THAT 3–5 DAYS ARE REQUIRED FOR COMPLETE ELIMINATION OF CHLORPROPAMIDE FROM THE BODY, AND THE PATIENT SHOULD BE KEPT UNDER CLOSE OBSERVATION FOR THIS PERIOD OF TIME DESPITE APPARENT RECOVERY.

Since insulin still remains the standard therapy for patients during periods of stress or complication, the patient on chlorpropamide must be instructed in the use of insulin. The patient must also be alerted to the early detection and prompt treatment of hypoglycemia since this complication, although less frequent, may develop on sulfonylurea therapy as well as on insulin therapy. HYPOGLYCEMIA IF IT OCCURS, MAY BE PROLONGED. (See section on ADVERSE REACTIONS.)

During the initial period of therapy with chlorpropamide, hypoglycemic reactions may occasionally occur, particularly during the transi-

Continued on next page

Pfizer—Cont.

tion from insulin to the oral drug. Hypoglycemia within 24 hours after withdrawal of the intermediate or long-acting types of insulin will usually prove to be the result of insulin carry-over and not primarily due to the effect of chlorpropamide.

Adverse Reactions: The majority of the side effects have been dose-related, transient, and have responded to dose reduction or withdrawal of the medication. However, clinical experience thus far has shown that, as with other sulfonylureas, some side effects associated with hypersensitivity may be severe and deaths have been reported in some instances.

Chlorpropamide has a somewhat higher reported incidence of side effects than tolbutamide.

Certain untoward reactions associated with idiosyncrasy or hypersensitivity have occurred, including jaundice, skin eruptions rarely progressing to erythema multiforme and exfoliative dermatitis, and probably depression of formed elements of the blood, show no direct relationship to the size of the dose. They occur characteristically during the first six weeks of therapy. With a few exceptions, these manifestations have been mild and readily reversible on the withdrawal of the drug.

The more severe manifestations may require other therapeutic measures, including corticosteroid therapy. DIABINESE (chlorpropamide) should be discontinued promptly when the development of sensitivity is suspected.

Jaundice has been reported, and is usually promptly reversible on discontinuance of therapy. On the basis of considerable histopathologic evidence, the jaundice is cholangiolitic and results primarily from intracanalicular biliary stasis rather than hepatocellular degeneration. The alkaline phosphatase which frequently shows serial and progressive elevation in these patients is of particular diagnostic value. THE OCCURRENCE OF PROGRESSIVE ELEVATION SHOULD SUGGEST THE POSSIBILITY OF INCIPIENT JAUNDICE AND CONSTITUTES AN INDICATION FOR WITHDRAWAL OF THE DRUG.

In contrast, transient alterations of certain liver function tests seen occasionally following institution of sulfonylurea therapy, appear to be of no clinical significance.

Skin rash may be either the only manifestation of sensitivity, or occur in association with jaundice, frequently preceding it. Low grade fever and eosinophilia may also occur in association with, or preceding the development of clinical jaundice. Rarely, severe diarrhea, sometimes accompanied by bleeding into the lower bowel and due to nonspecific proctocolitis, has been associated with other hypersensitivity manifestations, particularly jaundice, skin rash, or both. The occurrence, singly or together, of any of these hypersensitivity manifestations, should constitute an indication for prompt termination of the drug, and such other therapeutic measures as are dictated by the circumstances should be instituted.

Leukopenia, thrombocytopenia and mild anemia, which occur occasionally, are generally benign and revert to normal, following cessation of the drug. Leukopenia of mild degree, and not associated with a shift in the differential count, may be transient and frequently reverts to normal even while the drug is continued.

Cases of aplastic anemia and agranulocytosis, generally similar to blood dyscrasias associated with other sulfonylureas have been reported. Lymphocytosis appears to be of no clinical significance.

Dose-related side effects previously mentioned are generally transient and not of a serious nature and would include anorexia, nausea, vomiting, and epigastric discomfort as evidence of gastrointestinal intolerance, and various vague neurologic symptoms, particularly weakness and paresthesias. These manifestations are generally a direct function of dosage and were reported much more frequently during the early clinical history of the drug when some clinicians employed relatively high doses. These side effects are reversible on reduction of the daily dosage, or if necessary, by withdrawal of the medication.

Administration of the total daily drug requirement in two doses rather than one is sometimes an effective measure for alleviating symptoms of gastrointestinal intolerance.

Hypoglycemia, although not a true side effect, but rather an exaggeration of the expected therapeutic action, may be the result of dosage in excess of the patient's immediate requirements, as is the case with any hypoglycemic agent. Since the development of hypoglycemia is a function of many factors including diet, this effect is at times seen in patients on the usual recommended dosage. It is readily controlled by administration of glucose. Its occurrence is an obvious indication for immediate re-evaluation and adjustment of the insulin or chlorpropamide dosage.

BECAUSE OF THE PROLONGED HYPOGLYCEMIC ACTION OF DIABINESE, PATIENTS WHO BECOME HYPOGLYCEMIC DURING THERAPY WITH THIS DRUG REQUIRE CLOSE SUPERVISION FOR A MINIMUM PERIOD OF 3 TO 5 DAYS, during which time frequent feedings or glucose administration are essential. The anorectic patient or the profoundly hypoglycemic patient should be hospitalized.

Rare cases of phototoxic reactions have been reported.

Edema associated with hyponatremia has been infrequently reported with DIABINESE therapy. This is thought to occur by potentiation of available ADH with subsequent water retention. The condition is usually readily reversible upon discontinuation of medication.

Dosage: The total daily dosage is generally taken at a single time each morning with breakfast. Occasionally cases of gastrointestinal intolerance may be relieved by dividing the daily dosage. A LOADING OR PRIMING DOSE IS NOT NECESSARY AND SHOULD NOT BE USED.

Initial Therapy: 1. The mild to moderately severe, middle-aged, stable diabetic patient should be started on 250 mg daily. Because the geriatric diabetic patient appears to be more sensitive to the hypoglycemic effect of sulfonylurea drugs, older patients should be started on smaller amounts of DIABINESE, in the range of 100 to 125 mg daily.

2. No transition period is necessary when transferring patients from other oral hypoglycemic agents to DIABINESE. The other agent may be discontinued abruptly and chlorpropamide started at once. In prescribing chlorpropamide, due consideration must be given to its greater potency.

3. The large majority of mild to moderately severe middle-aged, stable diabetic patients receiving insulin can be placed directly on the oral drug and their insulin abruptly discontinued. For patients requiring more than 40 units of insulin daily, therapy with DIABINESE may be initiated with a 50 per cent reduction in insulin for the first few days, with subsequent further reductions dependent upon the response.

During the insulin withdrawal period, the patient should test his urine for sugar and ketone bodies at least three times daily and report the results frequently to his physician. If they are abnormal, the physician should be notified immediately. In some cases, it may be advisable to consider hospitalization during the transition period.

Five to seven days after the initial therapy, the blood level of chlorpropamide reaches a plateau. Dosage may subsequently be adjusted upward or downward by increments of not more than 50 to 125 mg at intervals of three to five days to obtain optimal control. More frequent adjustments are usually undesirable.

Maintenance Therapy: Most moderately severe, middle-aged stable diabetic patients are controlled by approximately 250 mg daily. Many investigators have found that some milder diabetics do well on daily doses of 100 mg or less. Many of the more severe diabetics may require 500 mg daily for adequate control. PATIENTS WHO DO NOT RESPOND COMPLETELY TO 500 MG DAILY WILL USUALLY NOT RESPOND TO HIGHER DOSES. Maintenance doses above 750 mg daily should be avoided.

Supply: DIABINESE (chlorpropamide) Tablets:

250 mg: Blue "D"-shaped, scored tablets (imprinted with code #394)—bottles of 100's, 250's, 1000's, and Unit-Dose packages of 100.

100 mg: Blue "D"-shaped, scored tablets (imprinted with code #393)—bottles of 100's, 500's, and Unit-Dose packages of 100.

(69-2141-37-4)

Literature Available: Yes.

[*Shown in Product Identification Section*]

FELDENE® ℞
(piroxicam)
CAPSULES
For Oral Use

Description: FELDENE (piroxicam) is 4-Hydroxy-2-methyl-*N*-2-pyridinyl -2*H*-1,2- benzothiazine-3-carboxamide 1,1-dioxide, an oxicam. Members of the oxicam family are not carboxylic acids, but they are acidic by virtue of the enolic 4-hydroxy substituent. FELDENE occurs as a white crystalline solid, sparingly soluble in water, dilute acid and most organic solvents. It is slightly soluble in alcohols and in aqueous alkaline solution. It exhibits a weakly acidic 4-hydroxy proton (pKa 5.1) and a weakly basic pyridyl nitrogen (pKa 1.8).

Clinical Pharmacology: FELDENE has shown anti-inflammatory, analgesic and antipyretic properties in animals. Edema, erythema, tissue proliferation, fever, and pain can all be inhibited in laboratory animals by the administration of FELDENE. It is effective regardless of the etiology of the inflammation. The mode of action of FELDENE is not fully established at this time. However, a common mechanism for the above effects may exist in the ability of FELDENE to inhibit the biosynthesis of prostaglandins, known mediators of inflammation.

It is established that FELDENE does not act by stimulating the pituitary-adrenal axis.

FELDENE is well absorbed following oral administration. Drug plasma concentrations are proportional for 10 and 20 mg doses, generally peak within three to five hours after medication, and subsequently decline with a mean half-life of 50 hours (range of 30 to 86 hours, although values outside of this range have been encountered).

This prolonged half-life results in the maintenance of relatively stable plasma concentrations throughout the day on once daily doses and to significant drug accumulation upon multiple dosing. A single 20 mg dose generally produces peak piroxicam plasma levels of 1.5 to 2 mcg/ml, while maximum drug plasma concentrations, after repeated daily ingestion of 20 mg FELDENE, usually stabilize at 3–8 mcg/ml. Most patients approximate steady state plasma levels within 7 to 12 days. Higher levels, which approximate steady state at two to three weeks, have been observed in patients in whom longer plasma half-lives of piroxicam occurred.

FELDENE and its biotransformation products are excreted in urine and feces, with about twice as much appearing in the urine as the feces. Metabolism occurs by hydroxylation at the 5 position of the pyridyl side chain and conjugation of this product; by cyclodehydration; and by a sequence of reactions involving hydrolysis of the amide linkage, decarboxylation, ring contraction, and N-demethylation. Less than 5% of the daily dose is excreted unchanged.

Concurrent administration of aspirin (3900 mg/day) and FELDENE (20 mg/day), resulted in a reduction of plasma levels of piroxicam to about 80% of their normal values. The use of FELDENE in conjunction with aspirin is not recommended because data are inadequate to demonstrate that the combination produces greater improvement than that achieved with aspirin alone and the potential for adverse reactions is increased. Concomitant administration of antacids had no effect on FELDENE plasma levels. The effects of impaired renal function or hepatic disease on plasma levels have not been established.

FELDENE, like salicylates and other nonsteroidal anti-inflammatory agents, is associated with symptoms of gastrointestinal tract irritation (see ADVERSE REACTIONS). However, in a study utilizing ^{51}Cr-tagged red blood cells, 20 mg of FELDENE administered as a single dose for four days did not result in a significant increase in fecal blood loss and did not detectably affect the gastric mucosa. In the same study a total daily dose of 3900 mg of aspirin, i.e., 972 mg q.i.d., caused a significant increase in fecal blood loss and mucosal lesions as demonstrated by gastroscopy.

In controlled clinical trials, the effectiveness of FELDENE (piroxicam) has been established for both acute exacerbations and long-term management of rheumatoid arthritis and osteoarthritis.

The therapeutic effects of FELDENE are evident early in the treatment of both diseases with a progressive increase in response over several (8–12) weeks. Efficacy is seen in terms of pain relief and, when present, subsidence of inflammation.

Doses of 20 mg/day FELDENE display a therapeutic effect comparable to therapeutic doses of aspirin, with a lower incidence of minor gastrointestinal effects and tinnitus.

FELDENE has been administered concomitantly with fixed doses of gold and corticosteroids. The existence of a "steroid-sparing" effect has not been adequately studied to date.

Indications and Usage: FELDENE is indicated for acute or long-term use in the relief of signs and symptoms of the following:

1. osteoarthritis
2. rheumatoid arthritis

Dosage recommendations for use in children have not been established.

Contraindications: FELDENE should not be used in patients who have previously exhibited hypersensitivity to it, or in individuals with the syndrome comprised of bronchospasm, nasal polyps, and angioedema precipitated by aspirin or other nonsteroidal anti-inflammatory drugs.

Warnings: Peptic ulceration, perforation, and G.I. bleeding—sometimes severe, and, in rare instances fatal—have been reported with patients receiving FELDENE. If FELDENE must be given to patients with a history of upper gastrointestinal tract disease, the patient should be under close supervision (see ADVERSE REACTIONS). In controlled clinical trials, incidence of peptic ulceration with the maximum recommended FELDENE capsule dose of 20 mg per day was 0.8%. The use of doses higher than the recommended dose is associated with an increase in the incidence of gastrointestinal irritation and ulcers.

Precautions: As with other anti-inflammatory agents, long-term administration to animals results in renal papillary necrosis and related pathology in rats, mice, and dogs.

As with other drugs that inhibit prostaglandin biosynthetase, reversible elevations of BUN have been reported in clinical studies with FELDENE. The effect is thought to result from inhibition of renal prostaglandin synthesis resulting in a change in medullary and deep cortical blood flow with an attendant effect on renal function. Because of the extensive renal excretion of piroxicam, patients with impaired renal function should be carefully monitored.

Although other nonsteroidal anti-inflammatory drugs do not have the same direct effects on platelets that aspirin does, all drugs inhibiting prostaglandin biosynthesis do interfere with platelet function to some degree; therefore, patients who may be adversely affected by such an action should be carefully observed when FELDENE (piroxicam) is administered.

Because of reports of adverse eye findings with nonsteroidal anti-inflammatory agents, it is recommended that patients who develop visual complaints during treatment with FELDENE have ophthalmic evaluation.

As with other nonsteroidal anti-inflammatory drugs, borderline elevations of one or more liver tests may occur in up to 15% of patients. These abnormalities may progress, may remain essentially unchanged, or may be transient with continued therapy. The SGPT (ALT) test is probably the most sensitive indicator of liver dysfunction. Meaningful (3 times the upper limit of normal) elevations of SGPT or SGOT (AST) occurred in controlled clinical trials in less than 1% of patients. A patient with symptoms and/or signs suggesting liver dysfunction, or in whom an abnormal liver test has occurred, should be evaluated for evidence of the development of more severe hepatic reaction while on therapy with FELDENE. Severe hepatic reactions, including jaundice and cases of fatal hepatitis, have been reported with other nonsteroidal anti-inflammatory drugs. Although such reactions are rare, if abnormal liver tests persist or worsen, if clinical signs and symptoms consistent with liver disease develop, or if systemic manifestations occur (e.g. eosinophilia, rash, etc.), FELDENE should be discontinued. (See also ADVERSE REACTIONS.)

Less than 1.0% of patients receiving FELDENE have shown reversible elevation of one or more liver function parameters. While concurrent aspirin may have been involved in some of these changes, a relationship to FELDENE could not be excluded. Studies in patients with impaired liver function have not been done.

Although at the recommended dose of 20 mg/day of FELDENE increased fecal blood loss due to gastrointestinal irritation did not occur (see CLINICAL PHARMACOLOGY), in about 4% of the patients treated with FELDENE alone or concomitantly with aspirin, reductions in hemoglobin and hematocrit values were observed. Therefore, these values should be determined if signs or symptoms of anemia occur.

Peripheral edema has been observed in approximately 2% of the patients treated with FELDENE. Therefore, as with other nonsteroidal anti-inflammatory drugs, FELDENE should be used with caution in patients with compromised cardiac function, hypertension or other conditions predisposing to fluid retention.

Drug Interactions: FELDENE is highly protein bound, and, therefore, might be expected to displace other protein-bound drugs. Although *in vitro* studies have shown this not to occur with dicoumarol, physicians should closely monitor patients for a change in dosage requirements when administering FELDENE to patients on coumarin-type anticoagulants and other highly protein-bound drugs.

Plasma levels of piroxicam are depressed to approximately 80% of their normal values when FELDENE is administered in conjunction with aspirin (3900 mg/day), but concomitant administration of antacids has no effect on piroxicam plasma levels (see CLINICAL PHARMACOLOGY).

Carcinogenesis, Chronic Animal Toxicity and Impairment of Fertility

Subacute and chronic toxicity studies have been carried out in rats, mice, dogs, and monkeys.

The pathology most often seen was that characteristically associated with the animal toxicology of anti-inflammatory agents; renal papillary necrosis (see PRECAUTIONS) and gastrointestinal lesions.

In classical studies in laboratory animals piroxicam did not show any teratogenic potential.

Reproductive studies revealed no impairment of fertility in animals.

Pregnancy and Nursing Mothers

Like other drugs which inhibit the synthesis and release of prostaglandins, piroxicam increased the incidence of dystocia and delayed parturition in pregnant animals when piroxicam administration was continued late into pregnancy. Gastrointestinal tract toxicity was increased in pregnant females in the last trimester of pregnancy compared to nonpregnant females or females in earlier trimesters of pregnancy.

FELDENE is not recommended for use in nursing mothers or in pregnant women because of the animal findings and since safety for such use has not been established in humans.

Use in Children

Dosage recommendations and indications for use in children have not been established.

Adverse Reactions: The incidence of adverse reactions to piroxicam is based on clinical trials involving approximately 2300 patients, about 400 of whom were treated for more than one year and 170 for more than two years. About 30% of all patients receiving daily doses of 20 mg of FELDENE experienced side effects. Gastrointestinal symptoms were the most prominent side effects—occurring in approximately 20% of the patients, which in most instances did not interfere with the course of therapy. Of the patients experiencing gastrointestinal side effects, approximately 5% discontinued therapy with an overall incidence of peptic ulceration of about 1%.

Other than the gastrointestinal symptoms, edema, dizziness, headache, changes in hematological parameters, and rash have been reported in a small percentage of patients. Routine ophthalmoscopy and slit-lamp examinations have revealed no evidence of ocular changes in 205 patients followed from 3 to 24 months while on therapy.

Adverse reactions are listed below by body system for all patients in clinical trials with FELDENE (piroxicam) at doses of 20 mg/day.

Incidence Greater than 1% The following adverse reactions occurred more frequently than 1 in 100.

Gastrointestinal: stomatitis, anorexia, epigastric distress*, nausea*, constipation, abdominal discomfort, flatulence, diarrhea, abdominal pain, and indigestion.

Hematological: decreases in hemoglobin* and hematocrit* (see PRECAUTIONS), leucopenia, eosinophilia.

Urogenital: BUN elevations (see PRECAUTIONS)

Central Nervous System: dizziness, somnolence, vertigo

Special Senses: tinnitus

Body as a Whole: headache, malaise

Cardiovascular/Respiratory: edema (see PRECAUTIONS)

Dermatologic: pruritus, rash

*Reactions occurring in 3% to 6% of patients treated with FELDENE.

Incidence Less Than 1% (Causal Relationship Probable)

Continued on next page

Pfizer—Cont.

The following adverse reactions occurred less frequently than 1 in 100. The probability exists that there is a causal relationship between FELDENE and these reactions.

Gastrointestinal: liver function abnormalities (see PRECAUTIONS), vomiting, hematemesis, melena, gastrointestinal bleeding, perforation and ulceration, and dry mouth.

Hematological: thrombocytopenia

Dermatologic: sweating, erythema, bruising, desquamation, erythema multiforme, toxic epidermal necrolysis, Stevens-Johnson syndrome, photoallergic skin reactions.

Special Senses: swollen eyes, blurred vision, eye irritations

Body as a Whole: pain (colic)

Cardiovascular/Respiratory: hypertension (see PRECAUTIONS)

Urogenital: hematuria

Metabolic: hypoglycemia, weight increase, weight decrease

Central Nervous System: depression, insomnia, nervousness

Incidence Less Than 1% (Causal Relationship Unknown)

Other adverse reactions were reported with a frequency of less than 1 in 100, but a causal relationship between FELDENE and the reaction could not be determined.

Cardiovascular/Respiratory: palpitations, dyspnea

Central Nervous System: akathisia

Urogenital System: dysuria

Hematological: aplastic anaemia

Overdosage: In the event treatment for overdosage is required the long plasma half-life (see CLINICAL PHARMACOLOGY) of piroxicam should be considered. The absence of experience with acute overdosage precludes characterization of sequelae and recommendation of specific antidotal efficacy at this time. It is reasonable to assume, however, that the standard measures of gastric evacuation and general supportive therapy would apply.

Administration and Dosage:

Rheumatoid Arthritis, Osteoarthritis

It is recommended that FELDENE therapy be initiated and maintained at a single daily dose of 20 mg. If desired the daily dose may be divided. Because of the long half-life of FELDENE, steady-state blood levels are not reached for 7–12 days. Therefore although the therapeutic effects of FELDENE are evident early in treatment, there is a progressive increase in response over several weeks and the effect of therapy should not be assessed for two weeks.

Dosage recommendations and indications for use in children have not been established.

How Supplied: FELDENE Capsules for oral administration

Bottles of 100: 10 mg (NDC 0069-3220-66) maroon and blue #322
20 mg (NDC 0069-3230-66) maroon #323

Bottles of 500: 20 mg (NDC 0069-3230-73) maroon #323

Unit dose packages of 100: 20 mg (NDC 0069-3230-41) maroon #323

© 1982, PFIZER INC. 65-4100-76-3

Literature Available: Yes.

[*Shown in Product Identification Section*]

MINIPRESS® CAPSULES ℞

(prazosin hydrochloride)

For Oral Use

Description: MINIPRESS (prazosin hydrochloride), a quinazoline derivative, is the first of a new chemical class of antihypertensives. It is the hydrochloride salt of 1-(4-amino-6,7-dimethoxy-2-quinazolinyl)-4-(2-furoyl) piperazine.

It is a white, crystalline substance, slightly soluble in water and isotonic saline and has a molecular weight of 419.87. Each 1 mg capsule of MINIPRESS (prazosin hydrochloride) contains drug equivalent to 1 mg free base.

Actions: The exact mechanism of the hypotensive action of prazosin is unknown. Prazosin causes a decrease in total peripheral resistance and was originally thought to have a direct relaxant action on vascular smooth muscle. Recent animal studies, however, have suggested that the vasodilator effect of prazosin is also related to blockade of postsynaptic *alpha*-adrenoceptors. The results of dog forelimb experiments demonstrate that the peripheral vasodilator effect of prazosin is confined mainly to the level of the resistance vessels (arterioles). Unlike conventional *alpha*-blockers, the antihypertensive action of prazosin is usually not accompanied by a reflex tachycardia. Tolerance has not been observed to develop in long term therapy.

Hemodynamic studies have been carried out in man following acute single dose administration and during the course of long term maintenance therapy. The results confirm that the therapeutic effect is a fall in blood pressure unaccompanied by a clinically significant change in cardiac output, heart rate, renal blood flow and glomerular filtration rate. There is no measurable negative chronotropic effect.

In clinical studies to date, MINIPRESS (prazosin hydrochloride) has not increased plasma renin activity.

In man, blood pressure is lowered in both the supine and standing positions. This effect is most pronounced on the diastolic blood pressure.

Following oral administration, human plasma concentrations reach a peak at about three hours with a plasma half-life of two to three hours. The drug is highly bound to plasma protein. Bioavailability studies have demonstrated that the total absorption relative to the drug in a 20% alcoholic solution is 90%, resulting in peak levels approximately 65% of that of the drug in solution. Animal studies indicate that MINIPRESS (prazosin hydrochloride) is extensively metabolized, primarily by demethylation and conjugation, and excreted mainly via bile and feces. Less extensive human studies suggest similar metabolism and excretion in man.

MINIPRESS (prazosin hydrochloride) has been administered without any adverse drug interaction in limited clinical experience to date with the following: (1) cardiac glycosides—digitalis and digoxin; (2) hypoglycemics—insulin, chlorpropamide, phenformin, tolazamide, and tolbutamide; (3) tranquilizers and sedatives—chlordiazepoxide, diazepam, and phenobarbital; (4) antigout—allopurinol, colchicine, and probenecid; (5) antiarrhythmics — procainamide, propranolol (see WARNINGS however), and quinidine; and (6) analgesics, antipyretics and anti-inflammatories — propoxyphene, aspirin, indomethacin, and phenylbutazone.

Indications: MINIPRESS (prazosin hydrochloride) is indicated in the treatment of hypertension. As an antihypertensive drug, it is mild to moderate in activity. It can be used as the initial agent or it may be employed in a general treatment program in conjunction with a diuretic and/or other antihypertensive drugs as needed for proper patient response.

Warnings: **MINIPRESS (prazosin hydrochloride) may cause syncope with sudden loss of consciousness. In most cases this is believed to be due to an excessive postural hypotensive effect, although occasionally the syncopal episode has been preceded by a bout of severe tachycardia with heart rates of 120–160 beats per minute. Syncopal episodes have usually occurred within 30 to 90 minutes of the initial dose of the drug; occasionally they have been reported in association with rapid dosage increases or the introduction of another antihypertensive drug into the regimen of a patient taking high doses of MINIPRESS (prazosin hydrochloride). The incidence of syncopal episodes is approximately 1% in patients given an initial dose of 2 mg or greater. Clinical trials conducted during the investigational phase of this drug suggest that syncopal episodes can be minimized by limiting the initial dose of the drug to 1 mg, by subsequently increasing the dosage slowly, and by introducing any additional antihypertensive drugs into the patient's regimen with caution (see DOSAGE AND ADMINISTRATION). Hypotension may develop in patients given MINIPRESS who are also receiving a beta-blocker such as propranolol.**

If syncope occurs, the patient should be placed in the recumbent position and treated supportively as necessary. This adverse effect is self-limiting and in most cases does not recur after the initial period of therapy or during subsequent dose titration.

Patients should always be started on the 1 mg capsules of MINIPRESS (prazosin hydrochloride). The 2 and 5 mg capsules are not indicated for initial therapy.

More common than loss of consciousness are the symptoms often associated with lowering of the blood pressure, namely, dizziness and lightheadedness. The patient should be cautioned about these possible adverse effects and advised what measures to take should they develop. The patient should also be cautioned to avoid situations where injury could result should syncope occur during the initiation of MINIPRESS (prazosin hydrochloride) therapy.

Usage in Pregnancy:

Although no teratogenic effects were seen in animal testing, the safety of MINIPRESS (prazosin hydrochloride) in pregnancy has not been established. MINIPRESS (prazosin hydrochloride) is not recommended in pregnant women unless the potential benefit outweighs potential risk to mother and fetus.

Usage in Children:

No clinical experience is available with the use of MINIPRESS (prazosin hydrochloride) in children.

Adverse Reactions: The most common reactions associated with MINIPRESS (prazosin hydrochloride) therapy are: dizziness 10.3%, headache 7.8%, drowsiness 7.6%, lack of energy 6.9%, weakness 6.5%, palpitations 5.3%, and nausea 4.9%. In most instances side effects have disappeared with continued therapy or have been tolerated with no decrease in dose of drug.

The following reactions have been associated with MINIPRESS (prazosin hydrochloride), some of them rarely. (In some instances exact causal relationships have not been established).

Gastrointestinal: vomiting, diarrhea, constipation, abdominal discomfort and/or pain.

Cardiovascular: edema, dyspnea, syncope, tachycardia.

Central Nervous System: nervousness, vertigo, depression, paresthesia.

Dermatologic: rash, pruritus, alopecia, lichen planus.

Genitourinary: urinary frequency, incontinence, impotence, priapism.

EENT: blurred vision, reddened sclera, epistaxis, tinnitus, dry mouth, nasal congestion.

Other: diaphoresis.

Single reports of pigmentary mottling and serous retinopathy, and a few reports of cataract development or disappearance have been reported. In these instances, the exact causal relationship has not been established because the baseline observations were frequently inadequate.

In more specific slit-lamp and funduscopic studies, which included adequate baseline examinations, no drug-related abnormal ophthalmological findings have been reported.

Dosage and Administration: The dose of MINIPRESS (prazosin hydrochloride) should be adjusted according to the patient's individual blood pressure response. The following is a guide to its administration:

Initial Dose:

1 mg two or three times a day. (See Warnings.)

Maintenance Dose:

Dosage may be slowly increased to a total daily dose of 20 mg given in divided doses. The therapeutic dosages most commonly employed have ranged from 6 mg to 15 mg daily given in divided doses. Doses higher than 20 mg usually do not increase efficacy, however a few patients may benefit from further increases up to a daily dose of 40 mg given in divided doses. After initial titration some patients can be maintained adequately on a twice daily dosage regimen.

Use With Other Drugs:

When adding a diuretic or other antihypertensive agent, the dose of MINIPRESS (prazosin hydrochloride) should be reduced to 1 mg or 2 mg three times a day and retitration then carried out.

Overdosage: Accidental ingestion of at least 50 mg of MINIPRESS (prazosin hydrochloride) in a two year old child resulted in profound drowsiness and depressed reflexes. No decrease in blood pressure was noted. Recovery was uneventful.

Should overdosage lead to hypotension, support of the cardiovascular system is of first importance. Restoration of blood pressure and normalization of heart rate may be accomplished by keeping the patient in the supine position. If this measure is inadequate, shock should first be treated with volume expanders. If necessary, vasopressors should then be used. Renal function should be monitored and supported as needed. Laboratory data indicate MINIPRESS (prazosin hydrochloride) is not dialysable because it is protein bound.

Toxicology: Testicular changes, necrosis and atrophy have occurred at 25 mg/kg/day (60 times the usual maximum recommended dose of 20 mg per day in humans) in long term (one year or more) studies in rats and dogs. No testicular changes were seen in rats or dogs at the 10 mg/kg/day level (24 times the usual maximum recommended dose of 20 mg per day in humans). In view of the testicular changes observed in animals, 105 patients on long term MINIPRESS (prazosin hydrochloride) therapy were monitored for 17-ketosteroid excretion and no changes indicating a drug effect were observed. In addition, 27 males on MINIPRESS (prazosin hydrochloride) alone for up to 51 months did not demonstrate changes in sperm morphology suggestive of drug effect.

How Supplied: MINIPRESS (prazosin hydrochloride) is available in 1 mg (white #431), 2 mg (pink and white #437) capsules in bottles of 250, 1000, and unit dose institutional packages of 100 (10 × 10's); and 5 mg (blue and white #438) capsules in bottles of 250, 500 and unit dose institutional packages of 100 (10 × 10's).

69-2318-37-6

Literature Available—Yes.

[*Shown in Product Identification Section*]

MINIZIDE® CAPSULES ℞

(prazosin hydrochloride/polythiazide)

FOR ORAL ADMINISTRATION

This fixed combination drug is not indicated for initial therapy of hypertension. Hypertension requires therapy titrated to the individual patient. If the fixed combination represents the dose so determined, its use may be more convenient in patient management. The treatment of hypertension is not static, but must be re-evaluated as conditions in each patient warrant.

Description: MINIZIDE is a combination of MINIPRESS® (prazosin hydrochloride) plus RENESE® (polythiazide).

MINIPRESS (prazosin hydrochloride), a quinazoline derivative, is the first of a new chemical class of antihypertensives. It is the hydrochloride salt of 1-(4-amino-6,7-dimethoxy-2-quinazolinyl)-4-(2-furoyl) piperazine.

It is a white, crystalline substance, slightly soluble in water and isotonic saline, and has a molecular weight of 419.87. Each 1 mg capsule of MINIPRESS (prazosin hydrochloride) contains drug equivalent to 1 mg free base.

RENESE (polythiazide) is an orally effective, nonmercurial diuretic, saluretic, and antihypertensive agent.

It is designated chemically as 2-methyl-3,4-dihydro-3 (2,2,2-trifluoroethylthiomethyl)-6-chloro-7-sulfamyl 1,2,4-benzothiadiazine 1,1 dioxide.

It is a white, crystalline substance insoluble in water, but readily soluble in alkaline solution.

Clinical Pharmacology:

MINIZIDE (prazosin hydrochloride/polythiazide)

Minizide produces a more pronounced antihypertensive response than occurs after either prazosin hydrochloride or polythiazide alone in equivalent doses.

MINIPRESS (prazosin hydrochloride)

The exact mechanism of the hypotensive action of prazosin is unknown. Prazosin causes a decrease in total peripheral resistance and was originally thought to have a direct relaxant action on vascular smooth muscle. Recent animal studies, however, have suggested that the vasodilator effect of prazosin is also related to blockade of postsynaptic *alpha*-adrenoceptors. The results of dog forelimb experiments demonstrate that the peripheral vasodilator effect of prazosin is confined mainly to the level of the resistance vessels (arterioles). Unlike conventional *alpha*-blockers, the antihypertensive action of prazosin is usually not accompanied by a reflex tachycardia. Tolerance has not been observed to develop in long term therapy.

Hemodynamic studies have been carried out in man following acute single dose administration and during the course of long term maintenance therapy. The results confirm that the therapeutic effect is a fall in blood pressure unaccompanied by a clinically significant change in cardiac output, heart rate, renal blood flow, and glomerular filtration rate. There is no measurable negative chronotropic effect.

In clinical studies to date, MINIPRESS has not increased plasma renin activity.

In man, blood pressure is lowered in both the supine and standing positions. This effect is most pronounced on the diastolic blood pressure.

Following oral administration, human plasma concentrations reach a peak at about three hours with a plasma half-life of two to three hours. The drug is highly bound to plasma protein. Bioavailability studies have demonstrated that the total absorption relative to the drug in a 20% alcoholic solution is 90%, resulting in peak levels approximately 65% of that of the drug in solution. Animal studies indicate that MINIPRESS is extensively metabolized, primarily by demethylation and conjugation, and excreted mainly via bile and feces. Less extensive human studies suggest similar metabolism and excretion in man.

MINIPRESS has been administered without any adverse drug interaction in limited clinical experience to date with the following: (1) cardiac glycosides—digitalis and digoxin; (2) hypoglycemics—insulin, chlorpropamide, phenformin, tolazamide, and tolbutamide; (3) tranquilizers and sedatives—chlordiazepoxide, diazepam, and phenobarbital; (4) antigout — allopurinol, colchicine, and probenecid; (5) antiarrhythmics — procainamide, propranolol (see WARNINGS however), and quinidine; and (6) analgesics, antipyretics and anti-inflammatories—propoxyphene, aspirin, indomethacin, and phenylbutazone.

RENESE (polythiazide)

RENESE is a member of the benzothiadiazine (thiazide) family of diuretic/antihypertensive agents. Its mechanism of action results in an interference with the renal tubular mechanism of electrolyte reabsorption. At maximal therapeutic dosage all thiazides are approximately equal in their diuretic potency. The mechanism whereby thiazides function in the control of hypertension is unknown. Renese is well absorbed, giving peak human plasma concentrations about 5 hours after oral administration. Drug is removed slowly thereafter with a plasma elimination half-life of approximately 27 hours. One fifth of the drug is recovered unchanged in human urine; the remainder is cleared via feces and as metabolites. Animal studies indicate metabolism occurs by rupture of the thiadiazine ring and loss of the side chain.

Indications and Usage: MINIZIDE is indicated in the treatment of hypertension. (See box warning.)

Contraindications: RENESE (polythiazide) is contraindicated in patients with anuria, and in patients known to be sensitive to thiazides or to other sulfonamide derivatives.

Warnings:

MINIPRESS (prazosin hydrochloride)

MINIPRESS may cause syncope with sudden loss of consciousness. In most cases this is believed to be due to an excessive postural hypotensive effect, although occasionally the syncopal episode has been preceded by a bout of severe tachycardia with heart rates of 120–160 beats per minute. Syncopal episodes have usually occurred within 30 to 90 minutes of the initial dose of the drug; occasionally they have been reported in association with rapid dosage increases or the introduction of another antihypertensive drug into the regimen of a patient taking high doses of MINIPRESS. The incidence of syncopal episodes is approximately 1% in patients given an initial dose of 2 mg or greater. Clinical trials conducted during the investigational phase of this drug suggest that syncopal episodes can be minimized by limiting the initial dose of the drug to 1 mg, by subsequently increasing the dosage slowly, and by introducing any additional antihypertensive drugs into the patient's regimen with caution (see DOSAGE AND ADMINISTRATION). Hypotension may develop in patients given MINIPRESS who are also receiving a beta-blocker such as propranolol.

If syncope occurs, the patient should be placed in the recumbent position and treated supportively as necessary. This adverse effect is self-limiting and in most cases does not recur after the initial period of therapy or during subsequent dose titration.

Patients should always be started on the 1 mg capsules of MINIPRESS (prazosin hydrochloride). The 2 and 5 mg capsules are not indicated for initial therapy.

Continued on next page

Pfizer—Cont.

More common than loss of consciousness are the symptoms often associated with lowering of the blood pressure, namely, dizziness and lightheadedness. The patient should be cautioned about these possible adverse effects and advised what measures to take should they develop. The patient should also be cautioned to avoid situations where injury could result should syncope occur during the initiation of MINIPRESS therapy.

RENESE (polythiazide)

RENESE should be used with caution in severe renal disease. In patients with renal disease, thiazides may precipitate azotemia. Cumulative effects of the drug may develop in patients with impaired renal function.

Thiazides should be used with caution in patients with impaired hepatic function or progressive liver disease, since minor alterations of fluid and electrolyte balance may precipitate hepatic coma.

Sensitivity reactions may occur in patients with a history of allergy or bronchial asthma.

The possibility of exacerbation or activation of systemic lupus erythematosus has been reported.

Thiazides may be additive or potentiative of the action of other antihypertensive drugs.

Potentiation occurs with ganglionic or peripheral adrenergic blocking drugs.

Periodic determinations of serum electrolytes to detect possible electrolyte imbalance should be performed at appropriate intervals.

All patients receiving thiazide therapy should be observed for clinical signs of fluid or electrolyte imbalance, namely, hyponatremia, hypochloremic alkalosis, and hypokalemia. Serum and urine electrolyte determinations are particularly important when the patient is vomiting excessively or receiving parenteral fluids. Medications such as digitalis may also influence serum electrolytes. Warning signs, irrespective of cause, are: dryness of mouth, thirst, weakness, lethargy, drowsiness, restlessness, muscle pains or cramps, muscular fatigue, hypotension, oliguria, tachycardia, and gastrointestinal disturbances such as nausea and vomiting.

Hypokalemia may develop with thiazides as with any potent diuretic, especially with brisk diuresis, when severe cirrhosis is present, or during concomitant use of corticosteroids or ACTH.

Interference with adequate oral electrolyte intake will also contribute to hypokalemia. Digitalis therapy may exaggerate the metabolic effects of hypokalemia, especially with reference to myocardial activity.

Any chloride deficit is generally mild and usually does not require specific treatment except under extraordinary circumstances (as in hepatic or renal disease). Dilutional hyponatremia may occur in edematous patients in hot weather; appropriate therapy is water restriction rather than administration of salt, except in rare instances when the hyponatremia is life-threatening. In actual salt depletion, appropriate replacement is the therapy of choice.

Hyperuricemia may occur or frank gout may be precipitated in certain patients receiving thiazide therapy.

Insulin requirements in diabetic patients may be either increased, decreased, or unchanged. Latent diabetes mellitus may become manifest during thiazide administration.

Thiazide drugs may increase responsiveness to tubocurarine.

The antihypertensive effects of the drug may be enhanced in the post-sympathectomy patient.

Thiazides may decrease arterial responsiveness to norepinephrine. This diminution is not sufficient to preclude effectiveness of the pressor agent for therapeutic use.

If progressive renal impairment becomes evident, as indicated by a rising nonprotein nitrogen or blood urea nitrogen, a careful reappraisal of therapy is necessary with consideration given to withholding or discontinuing diuretic therapy.

Thiazides may decrease serum protein-bound iodine levels without signs of thyroid disturbance.

Precautions:

Carcinogenesis, Mutagenesis, Impairment of Fertility: No carcinogenic or mutagenic studies have been conducted with MINIZIDE. However, no carcinogenic potential was demonstrated in 18 month studies in rats with either MINIPRESS or RENESE at dose levels more than 100 times the usual maximum human doses. MINIPRESS was not mutagenic in *in vivo* genetic toxicology studies.

MINIZIDE produced no impairment of fertility in male or female rats at 50 and 25 mg/kg/day of MINIPRESS and RENESE respectively. In chronic studies (one year or more) of MINIPRESS in rats and dogs, testicular changes consisting of atrophy and necrosis occurred at 25 mg/kg/day (60 times the usual maximum recommended human dose). No testicular changes were seen in rats or dogs at 10 mg/kg/day (24 times the usual maximum recommended human dose). In view of the testicular changes observed in animals, 105 patients on long term MINIPRESS therapy were monitored for 17-ketosteroid excretion and no changes indicating a drug effect were observed. In addition, 27 males on MINIPRESS alone for up to 51 months did not have changes in sperm morphology suggestive of drug effect.

Use in Pregnancy: Pregnancy Category C. MINIZIDE was not teratogenic in either rats or rabbits when administered in oral doses more than 100 times the usual maximum human dose. Studies in rats indicated that the combination of RENESE (40 times the usual maximum recommended human dose) and MINIPRESS (8 times the usual maximum recommended human dose) caused a greater number of stillbirths, a more prolonged gestation, and a decreased survival of pups to weaning than that caused by MINIPRESS alone. There are no adequate and well controlled studies in pregnant women. Therefore, MINIZIDE should be used in pregnancy only if the potential benefit justifies the potential risk to the fetus.

Nursing Mothers: It is not known whether MINIPRESS or RENESE are excreted in human milk. Thiazides appear in breast milk. Thus, if use of the drug is deemed essential the patient should stop nursing.

Pediatric Use: Safety and effectiveness in children has not been established.

Adverse Reactions:

MINIPRESS (prazosin hydrochloride)

The most common reactions associated with MINIPRESS therapy are: dizziness 10.3%, headache 7.8%, drowsiness 7.6%, lack of energy 6.9%, weakness 6.5%, palpitations 5.3%, and nausea 4.9%. In most instances side effects have disappeared with continued therapy or have been tolerated with no decrease in dose of drug.

The following reactions have been associated with MINIPRESS, some of them rarely. (In some instances exact causal relationships have not been established.)

Gastrointestinal: vomiting, diarrhea, constipation, abdominal discomfort and/or pain.

Cardiovascular: edema, dyspnea, syncope, tachycardia.

Central Nervous System: nervousness, vertigo, depression, paresthesia.

Dermatologic: rash, pruritus, alopecia, lichen planus.

Genitourinary: urinary frequency, incontinence, impotence, priapism.

EENT: blurred vision, reddened sclera, epistaxis, tinnitus, dry mouth, nasal congestion.

Other: diaphoresis.

Single reports of pigmentary mottling and serous retinopathy, and a few reports of cataract development or disappearance have been reported. In these instances, the exact causal relationship has not been established because the baseline observations were frequently inadequate.

In more specific slit-lamp and funduscopic studies, which included adequate baseline examinations, no drug-related abnormal ophthalmological findings have been reported.

RENESE (polythiazide)

Gastrointestinal: anorexia, gastric irritation, nausea, vomiting, cramping, diarrhea, constipation, jaundice (intrahepatic cholestatic jaundice), pancreatitis.

Central Nervous System: dizziness, vertigo, paresthesia, headache, xanthopsia.

Hematologic: leukopenia, agranulocytosis, thrombocytopenia, aplastic anemia.

Dermatologic: purpura, photosensitivity, rash, urticaria, necrotizing angiitis, (vasculitis) (cutaneous vasculitis).

Cardiovascular: Orthostatic hypotension may occur and be aggravated by alcohol, barbiturates, or narcotics.

Other: hyperglycemia, glycosuria, hyperuricemia, muscle spasm, weakness, restlessness.

Overdosage:

MINIPRESS (prazosin hydrochloride)

Accidental ingestion of at least 50 mg of MINIPRESS in a two year old child resulted in profound drowsiness and depressed reflexes. No decrease in blood pressure was noted. Recovery was uneventful.

Should overdosage lead to hypotension, support of the cardiovascular system is of first importance. Restoration of blood pressure and normalization of heart rate may be accomplished by keeping the patient in the supine position. If this measure is inadequate, shock should first be treated with volume expanders. If necessary, vasopressors should then be used. Renal function should be monitored and supported as needed. Laboratory data indicate that MINIPRESS is not dialysable because it is protein bound.

RENESE (polythiazide)

Should overdosage with RENESE occur, electrolyte balance and adequate hydration should be maintained. Gastric lavage is recommended, followed by supportive treatment. Where necessary, this may include intravenous dextrose and saline with potassium and other electrolyte therapy, administered with caution as indicated by laboratory testing at appropriate intervals.

Dosage and Administration:

MINIZIDE (prazosin hydrochloride/ polythiazide)

Dosage: as determined by individual titration of MINIPRESS (prazosin hydrochloride) and RENESE (polythiazide). (See box warning.)

Usual MINIZIDE dosage is one capsule two or three times daily, the strength depending upon individual requirement following titration.

The following is a general guide to the administration of the individual components of MINIZIDE:

MINIPRESS (prazosin hydrochloride)

Initial Dose: 1 mg two or three times a day. (See Warnings.)

Maintenance Dose: Dosage may be slowly increased to a total daily dose of 20 mg given in divided doses. The therapeutic dosages most commonly employed have ranged from 6 mg to 15 mg daily given in divided doses. Doses higher than 20 mg usually do not increase efficacy, however a few patients may benefit from further increases up to a daily dose of 40 mg given in divided doses. After initial titration some patients can be maintained adequately on a twice daily dosage regimen.

Use With Other Drugs: When adding a diuretic or other antihypertensive agent, the dose of MINIPRESS should be reduced to 1 mg or 2 mg three times a day and retitration then carried out.

RENESE (polythiazide)
The usual dose of Renese for antihypertensive therapy is 2 to 4 mg daily.

How Supplied: [See table right].

69-2463-37-1

Literature Available: Yes.
[*Shown in Product Identification Section*]

MINIZIDE CAPSULES
prozosin HCl/polythiazide
How Supplied:

STRENGTH	COMPONENTS	COLOR	CAPSULE CODE	PKG. SIZE
MINIZIDE 1	1 mg prazosin + 0.5 mg polythiazide	Blue-Green	430	100's
MINIZIDE 2	2 mg prazosin + 0.5 mg polythiazide	Blue-Green/Pink	432	100's
MINIZIDE 5	5 mg prazosin + 0.5 mg polythiazide	Blue-Green/Blue	436	100's

MODERIL®
(rescinnamine)
TABLETS ℞

Description: Rescinnamine is a pure crystalline alkaloid that has been identified chemically as the 3,4,5-trimethoxycinnamic acid ester of methyl reserpate. Pure rescinnamine occurs as white, needle-shaped crystals that are readily absorbed when ingested.
Moderil is available as oval, scored salmon tablets providing 0.5 mg. of crystalline rescinnamine or as oval, scored yellow tablets providing 0.25 mg. of crystalline rescinnamine.

Actions: Rescinnamine probably produces its antihypertensive effects through depletion of tissue stores of catecholamines (epinephrine and norepinephrine) from peripheral sites. By contrast, its sedative and tranquilizing properties are thought to be related to depletion of 5-hydroxytryptamine from the brain.
Rescinnamine is characterized by slow onset of action and sustained effect. Both its cardiovascular and central nervous system effects may persist following withdrawal of the drug.

Indications: Indicated in the treatment of mild essential hypertension.

Contraindications: Do not use in patients with known hypersensitivity, mental depression—especially with suicidal tendencies, active peptic ulcer, and ulcerative colitis. It is also contraindicated in patients receiving electroconvulsive therapy.

Warnings: Extreme caution should be exercised in treating patients with a history of mental depression. Discontinue the drug at the first sign of despondency, early morning insomnia, loss of appetite, impotence, or self-depreciation. Drug-induced depression may persist for several months after drug withdrawal and may be severe enough to result in suicide.

Usage in pregnancy: The safety of rescinnamine for use during pregnancy or lactation has not been established. Therefore, the drug should be used in pregnant patients or in women of child-bearing potential only when, in the judgment of the physician, its use is deemed essential to the welfare of the patient. Increased respiratory secretions, nasal congestion, cyanosis, and anorexia may occur in infants born to rescinnamine-treated mothers, since this preparation is known to cross the placental barrier, appearing in cord blood and breast milk.

Precautions: Because Rauwolfia preparations increase gastrointestinal motility and secretion, this drug should be used cautiously in patients with a history of peptic ulcer, ulcerative colitis, or gallstones where biliary colic may be precipitated.
Caution should be exercised when treating hypertensive patients with renal insufficiency since they adjust poorly to lowered blood pressure levels.
Use rescinnamine cautiously with digitalis and quinidine since cardiac arrhythmias have occurred with Rauwolfia preparations.
Preoperative withdrawal of rescinnamine does not assure that circulatory instability will not occur. It is important that the anesthesiologist be aware of the patient's drug intake and consider this in the over-all management, since hypotension has occurred in patients receiving Rauwolfia preparations. Anticholinergic and/or adrenergic drugs (metaraminol, norepinephrine) have been employed to treat adverse vagocirculatory effects.

Adverse Reactions: Rauwolfia preparations have caused gastrointestinal reactions including hypersecretion, nausea and vomiting, anorexia, and diarrhea; cardiovascular reactions including angina-like symptoms, arrhythmias particularly when used concurrently with digitalis or quinidine, and bradycardia; and central nervous system reactions including drowsiness, depression, nervousness, paradoxical anxiety, nightmares, rare parkinsonian syndrome, C.N.S. sensitization manifested by dull sensorium, deafness, glaucoma, uveitis, and optic atrophy. Nasal congestion is a frequent complaint; and pruritus, rash, dryness of mouth, dizziness, headache, dyspnea, purpura, impotence or decreased libido, dysuria, muscular aches, conjunctival injection, and weight gain have been reported. Extrapyramidal tract symptoms have also occurred. These reactions are usually reversible and disappear when the drug is discontinued.
Water retention with edema in patients with hypertensive vascular disease may occur rarely, but the condition generally clears with cessation of therapy, or with the administration of a diuretic agent.

Dosage and Administration: For adults the average initial dose is 0.5 mg. orally, twice daily. Increase dosage gradually, if necessary. Maintenance doses may vary from 0.25 mg. to 0.5 mg. daily. Higher doses should be used cautiously because serious mental depression and other side effects may be increased considerably.
Concomitant use of rescinnamine and ganglionic blocking agents, guanethidine, veratrum, hydralazine, methyldopa, chlorthalidone, or thiazides necessitates careful titration of dosage with each agent.

Supply:
0.25 mg. tablets, oval, scored, yellow (imprinted with code number 441): bottles of 100.
0.5 mg. tablets, oval, scored, salmon (imprinted with code number 442): bottles of 100.

(60-0695-00-7)

[*Shown in Product Identification Section*]

PROCARDIA®
(nifedipine)
CAPSULES ℞
For Oral Use

Description: PROCARDIA (nifedipine) is an antianginal drug belonging to a new class of pharmacological agents, the calcium channel blockers. Nifedipine is 3,5-pyridinedicarboxylic acid, 1,4-dihydro-2,6-dimethyl-4-(2-nitrophenyl)-, dimethyl ester, $C_{17}H_{18}N_2O_6$.
Nifedipine is a yellow crystalline substance, practically insoluble in water but soluble in ethanol. It has a molecular weight of 346.3. PROCARDIA CAPSULES are formulated as soft gelatin capsules for oral administration each containing 10 mg nifedipine.

Clinical Pharmacology: PROCARDIA (nifedipine) is a calcium ion influx inhibitor (slow channel blocker or calcium ion antagonist) and inhibits the transmembrane influx of calcium ions into cardiac muscle and smooth muscle. The contractile processes of cardiac muscle and vascular smooth muscle are dependent upon the movement of extracellular calcium ions into these cells through specific ion channels. PROCARDIA selectively inhibits calcium ion influx across the cell membrane of cardiac muscle and vascular smooth muscle without changing serum calcium concentrations.

Mechanism of Action
The precise means by which this inhibition relieves angina has not been fully determined, but includes at least the following two mechanisms:

1) Relaxation and prevention of coronary artery spasm
PROCARDIA dilates the main coronary arteries and coronary arterioles, both in normal and ischemic regions, and is a potent inhibitor of coronary artery spasm, whether spontaneous or ergonovine-induced. This property increases myocardial oxygen delivery in patients with coronary artery spasm, and is responsible for the effectiveness of PROCARDIA in vasospastic (Prinzmetal's or variant) angina. Whether this effect plays any role in classical angina is not clear, but studies of exercise tolerance have not shown an increase in the maximum exercise rate-pressure product, a widely accepted measure of oxygen utilization. This suggests that, in general, relief of spasm or dilation of coronary arteries is not an important factor in classical angina.

2) Reduction of oxygen utilization
PROCARDIA regularly reduces arterial pressure at rest and at a given level of exercise by dilating peripheral arterioles and reducing the total peripheral resistance (afterload) against which the heart works. This unloading of the heart reduces myocardial energy consumption and oxygen requirements and probably accounts for the effectiveness of PROCARDIA in chronic stable angina.

Pharmacokinetics and Metabolism
PROCARDIA is rapidly and fully absorbed after oral administration. The drug is detectable in serum 10 minutes after oral administration, and peak blood levels occur in approximately 30 minutes. It is highly bound by serum proteins. PROCARDIA is extensively converted to inactive metabolites and approximately 80 percent of PROCARDIA and metabolites are eliminated via the kidneys. The half-life of nifedipine in plasma is approximately two hours. There is no information on the effects of renal or hepatic impairment on excretion or metabolism of PROCARDIA.

Hemodynamics
Like other slow channel blockers, PROCARDIA exerts a negative inotropic effect on isolated myocardial tissue. This is rarely, if ever, seen in intact animals or man, probably because of reflex responses to its vasodilating effects. In man, PROCARDIA causes decreased peripheral vascular resistance and a fall in systolic and diastolic pressure, usually modest (5-10mm Hg systolic), but sometimes larger. There is usually a small increase in heart rate, a reflex response to vasodilation. Measurements of cardiac function in patients with normal ventricular function have generally found

Continued on next page

Pfizer—Cont.

a small increase in cardiac index without major effects on ejection fraction, left ventricular end diastolic pressure (LVEDP) or volume (LVEDV). In patients with impaired ventricular function, most acute studies have shown some increase in ejection fraction and reduction in left ventricular filling pressure.

Electrophysiologic Effects

Although like other members of its class, PROCARDIA decreases sinoatrial node function and atrioventricular conduction in isolated myocardial preparations, such effects have not been seen in studies in intact animals or in man. In formal electrophysiologic studies, predominantly in patients with normal conduction systems, PROCARDIA has had no tendency to prolong atrioventricular conduction, prolong sinus node recovery time, or slow sinus rate.

Indications and Usage:

I. Vasospastic Angina

PROCARDIA (nifedipine) is indicated for the management of vasospastic angina confirmed by any of the following criteria: 1) classical pattern of angina at rest accompanied by ST segment elevation, 2) angina or coronary artery spasm provoked by ergonovine, or 3) angiographically demonstrated coronary artery spasm. In those patients who have had angiography, the presence of significant fixed obstructive disease is not incompatible with the diagnosis of vasospastic angina, provided that the above criteria are satisfied. PROCARDIA may also be used where the clinical presentation suggests a possible vasospastic component but where vasospasm has not been confirmed, e.g., where pain has a variable threshold on exertion or in unstable angina where electrocardiographic findings are compatible with intermittent vasospasm, or when angina is refractory to nitrates and/or adequate doses of beta blockers.

II. Chronic Stable Angina (Classical Effort-Associated Angina)

PROCARDIA is indicated for the management of chronic stable angina (effort-associated angina) without evidence of vasospasm in patients who remain symptomatic despite adequate doses of beta blockers and/or organic nitrates or who cannot tolerate those agents.

In chronic stable angina (effort-associated angina) PROCARDIA has been effective in controlled trials of up to eight weeks duration in reducing angina frequency and increasing exercise tolerance, but confirmation of sustained effectiveness and evaluation of long term safety in these patients are incomplete.

Controlled studies in small numbers of patients suggest concomitant use of PROCARDIA and beta blocking agents may be beneficial in patients with chronic stable angina, but available information is not sufficient to predict with confidence the effects of concurrent treatment, especially in patients with compromised left ventricular function or cardiac conduction abnormalities. When introducing such concomitant therapy, care must be taken to monitor blood pressure closely since severe hypotension can occur from the combined effects of the drugs. (See Warnings.)

Contraindications: Known hypersensitivity reaction to PROCARDIA.

Warnings:

Excessive Hypotension

Although in most patients, the hypotensive effect of PROCARDIA is modest and well tolerated, occasional patients have had excessive and poorly tolerated hypotension. These responses have usually occurred during initial titration or at the time of subsequent upward dosage adjustment, and may be more likely in patients on concomitant beta blockers.

Severe hypotension and/or increased fluid volume requirements have been reported in patients receiving PROCARDIA together with a beta blocking agent who underwent coronary artery bypass surgery using high dose fentanyl anesthesia. The interaction with high dose fentanyl appears to be due to the combination of PROCARDIA and a beta blocker, but the possibility that it may occur with PROCARDIA alone, with low doses of fentanyl, in other surgical procedures, or with other narcotic analgesics cannot be ruled out. In PROCARDIA treated patients where surgery using high dose fentanyl anesthesia is contemplated, the physician should be aware of these potential problems and, if the patient's condition permits, sufficient time (at least 36 hours) should be allowed for PROCARDIA to be washed out of the body prior to surgery.

Increased Angina

Occasional patients have developed well documented increased frequency, duration or severity of angina on starting PROCARDIA or at the time of dosage increases. The mechanism of this response is not established but could result from decreased coronary perfusion associated with decreased diastolic pressure with increased heart rate, or from increased demand resulting from increased heart rate alone.

Beta Blocker Withdrawal

Patients recently withdrawn from beta blockers may develop a withdrawal syndrome with increased angina, probably related to increased sensitivity to catecholamines. Initiation of PROCARDIA treatment will not prevent this occurrence and might be expected to exacerbate it by provoking reflex catecholamine release. There have been occasional reports of increased angina in a setting of beta blocker withdrawal and PROCARDIA initiation. It is important to taper beta blockers if possible, rather than stopping them abruptly before beginning PROCARDIA.

Congestive Heart Failure

Rarely, patients, usually receiving a beta blocker, have developed heart failure after beginning PROCARDIA. Patients with tight aortic stenosis may be at greater risk for such an event, as the unloading effect of PROCARDIA would be expected to be of less benefit to these patients, owing to their fixed impedance to flow across the aortic valve.

Precautions:

General: Hypotension: Because PROCARDIA decreases peripheral vascular resistance, careful monitoring of blood pressure during the initial administration and titration of PROCARDIA is suggested. Close observation is especially recommended for patients already taking medications that are known to lower blood pressure. See Warnings.

Peripheral edema: Mild to moderate peripheral edema, typically associated with arterial vasodilation and not due to left ventricular dysfunction, occurs in about one in ten patients treated with PROCARDIA. This edema occurs primarily in the lower extremities and usually responds to diuretic therapy. With patients whose angina is complicated by congestive heart failure, care should be taken to differentiate this peripheral edema from the effects of increasing left ventricular dysfunction.

Drug interactions: Beta-adrenergic blocking agents: See Indications and Warnings. Experience in over 1400 patients in a non-comparative clinical trial has shown that concomitant administration of PROCARDIA and beta-blocking agents is usually well tolerated, but there have been occasional literature reports suggesting that the combination may increase the likelihood of congestive heart failure, severe hypotension or exacerbation of angina.

Long acting nitrates: PROCARDIA may be safely co-administered with nitrates, but there have been no controlled studies to evaluate the antianginal effectiveness of this combination.

Digitalis: Administration of PROCARDIA with digoxin increased digoxin levels in nine of twelve normal volunteers. The average increase was 45%. Another investigator found no increase in digoxin levels in thirteen patients with coronary artery disease. In an uncontrolled study of over two hundred patients with congestive heart failure during which digoxin blood levels were not measured, digitalis toxicity was not observed. Since there have been isolated reports of patients with elevated digoxin levels, it is recommended that digoxin levels be monitored when initiating, adjusting, and discontinuing PROCARDIA to avoid possible over- to under-digitalization.

Carcinogenesis, mutagenesis, impairment of fertility: Nifedipine was administered orally to rats for two years and was not shown to be carcinogenic. When given to rats prior to mating, nifedipine caused reduced fertility at a dose approximately 30 times the maximum recommended human dose. *In vivo* mutagenicity studies were negative.

Pregnancy: Pregnancy category C. Nifedipine has been shown to be teratogenic in rats when given in doses 30 times the maximum recommended human dose. Nifedipine was embryotoxic (increased fetal resorptions, decreased fetal weight, increased stunted forms, increased fetal deaths, decreased neonatal survival) in rats, mice and rabbits at doses of from 3 to 10 times the maximum recommended human dose. In pregnant monkeys, doses ⅔ and twice the maximum recommended human dose resulted in small placentas and underdeveloped chorionic villi. In rats doses three times maximum human dose and higher caused prolongation of pregnancy. There are no adequate and well controlled studies in pregnant women. PROCARDIA should be used during pregnancy only if the potential benefit justifies the potential risk to the fetus.

Adverse Reactions: In multiple-dose U.S. and foreign controlled studies in which adverse reactions were reported spontaneously, adverse effects were frequent but generally not serious and rarely required discontinuation of therapy or dosage adjustment. Most were expected consequences of the vasodilator effects of PROCARDIA.

Adverse Effect	PROCARDIA (%) (N = 226)	Placebo (%) (N = 235)
Dizziness, lightheadedness, giddiness	27	15
Flushing, heat sensation	25	8
Headache	23	20
Weakness	12	10
Nausea, heartburn	11	8
Muscle cramps, tremor	8	3
Peripheral edema	7	1
Nervousness, mood changes	7	4
Palpitation	7	5
Dyspnea, cough, wheezing	6	3
Nasal congestion, sore throat	6	8

There is also a large uncontrolled experience in over 2100 patients in the United States. Most of the patients had vasospastic or resistant angina pectoris, and about half had concomitant treatment with beta-adrenergic blocking agents. The most common adverse events were the same ones seen in the controlled trials, with dizziness or lightheadedness, peripheral edema, nausea, weakness, headache and flushing each occurring in about 10 per cent of patients, transient hypotension in about 5 per cent, palpitation in about 2 per cent and syncope in about 0.5 per cent. Syncopal episodes did not recur with reduction in the dose of PROCARDIA or concomitant antianginal medication. Very rarely, introduction of PROCARDIA therapy was associated with an increase in anginal pain, possibly due to associated hypotension.

Several of these side effects appear to be dose related. Peripheral edema occurred in about one in 25 patients at doses less than 60 mg per day and in about one patient in eight at 120 mg per day or more. Transient hypotension, generally of mild to moderate severity and seldom requiring discontinuation of therapy, occurred in one of 50 patients at less than 60 mg per day and in one of 20 patients at 120 mg per day or more.

In addition, 2 percent or fewer of patients reported the following:

Respiratory: Nasal and chest congestion, shortness of breath

Gastrointestinal: Diarrhea, constipation, cramps, flatulence

Musculoskeletal: Inflammation, joint stiffness, muscle cramps

CNS: Shakiness, nervousness, jitteriness, sleep disturbances, blurred vision, difficulties in balance

Other: Dermatitis, pruritus, urticaria, fever, sweating, chills, sexual difficulties.

In addition, more serious adverse events were observed, not readily distinguishable from the natural history of the disease in these patients. It remains possible, however, that some or many of these events were drug related. Myocardial infarction occurred in about 4% of patients and congestive heart failure or pulmonary edema in about 2%. Ventricular arrhythmias or conduction disturbances each occurred in fewer than 0.5% of patients.

In a subgroup of over 1000 patients receiving PROCARDIA with concomitant beta blocker therapy, the pattern and incidence of adverse experiences was not different from that of the entire group of PROCARDIA treated patients (see **Precautions**).

In a subgroup of patients with a diagnosis of congestive heart failure as well as angina, dizziness or lightheadedness, peripheral edema, headache or flushing each occurred in one in eight patients. Hypotension occurred in about one in 20 patients. Syncope occurred in approximately one patient in 250. Myocardial infarction or symptoms of congestive heart failure each occurred in about one patient in 15. Atrial or ventricular dysrhythmias each occurred in about one patient in 150.

Laboratory tests: Rare, mild to moderate, transient elevations of enzymes such as alkaline phosphatase, CPK, LDH, SGOT, and SGPT have been noted, and a single incident of significantly elevated transaminases and alkaline phosphatase was seen in a patient with a history of gall bladder disease after about eleven months of nifedipine therapy. The relationship to PROCARDIA therapy is uncertain. These laboratory abnormalities have rarely been associated with clinical symptoms. Cholestasis, possibly due to PROCARDIA therapy, has been reported twice in the extensive world literature.

Overdosage: Although there is no well documented experience with PROCARDIA overdosage, available data suggest that gross overdosage could result in excessive peripheral vasodilation with subsequent marked and probably prolonged systemic hypotension. Clinically significant hypotension due to PROCARDIA overdosage calls for active cardiovascular support including monitoring of cardiac and respiratory function, elevation of extremities, and attention to circulating fluid volume and urine output. A vasoconstrictor (such as norepinephrine) may be helpful in restoring vascular tone and blood pressure, provided that there is no contraindication to its use. Clearance of PROCARDIA would be expected to be prolonged in patients with impaired liver function. Since PROCARDIA is highly protein-bound, dialysis is not likely to be of benefit.

Dosage and Administration: The dosage of PROCARDIA needed to suppress angina and that can be tolerated by the patient must be established by titration. Excessive doses can result in hypotension.

The starting dose is one 10 mg capsule, swallowed whole, 3 times/day. The usual effective dose range is 10–20 mg three times daily. Some patients, especially those with evidence of coronary artery spasm, respond only to higher doses, more frequent administration, or both. In such patients, doses of 20–30 mg three or four times daily may be effective. Doses above 120 mg daily are rarely necessary. More than 180 mg per day is not recommended.

In most cases, PROCARDIA titration should proceed over a 7–14 day period so that the physician can assess the response to each dose level and monitor the blood pressure before proceeding to higher doses.

If symptoms so warrant, titration may proceed more rapidly provided that the patient is assessed frequently. Based on the patient's physical activity level, attack frequency, and sublingual nitroglycerin consumption, the dose of PROCARDIA may be increased from 10 mg tid to 20 mg tid and then to 30 mg tid over a three-day period.

In hospitalized patients under close observation, the dose may be increased in 10 mg increments over four to six-hour periods as required to control pain and arrhythmias due to ischemia. A single dose should rarely exceed 30 mg.

No "rebound effect" has been observed upon discontinuation of PROCARDIA. However, if discontinuation of PROCARDIA is necessary, sound clinical practice suggests that the dosage should be decreased gradually with close physician supervision.

Co-Administration with Other Antianginal Drugs

Sublingual nitroglycerin may be taken as required for the control of acute manifestations of angina, particularly during PROCARDIA titration. See **Precautions, Drug Interactions,** for information on co-administration of PROCARDIA with beta blockers or long acting nitrates.

How Supplied: Each orange, soft gelatin PROCARDIA CAPSULE (code #260) contains 10 mg of nifedipine. PROCARDIA Capsules are supplied in bottles of 100 (NDC 0069-2600-66), 300 (NDC 0069-2600-72), and unit dose (10 × 10) (NDC 0069-2600-41).

The capsules should be protected from light and moisture and stored at controlled room temperature 59° to 77°F (15° to 25°C) in the manufacturer's original container.

© 1982, PFIZER INC. 65-4052-00-7

Literature Available: Yes

[*Shown in Product Identification Section*]

RENESE® ℞
(polythiazide)
TABLETS
for Oral Administration

Description: Renese is designated generically as polythiazide, and chemically as 2-methyl-3, 4-dihydro-3-(2,2,2-trifluoroethylthiomethyl)-6-chloro-7-sulfamyl 1,2,4-benzothiadiazine 1,1 dioxide. It is a white crystalline substance, insoluble in water but readily soluble in alkaline solution.

Action: The mechanism of action results in an interference with the renal tubular mechanism of electrolyte reabsorption. At maximal therapeutic dosage all thiazides are approximately equal in their diuretic potency. The mechanism whereby thiazides function in the control of hypertension is unknown.

Indications: Renese is indicated as adjunctive therapy in edema associated with congestive heart failure, hepatic cirrhosis, and corticosteroid and estrogen therapy.

Renese has also been found useful in edema due to various forms of renal dysfunction as: Nephrotic syndrome; Acute glomerulonephritis; and Chronic renal failure.

Renese is indicated in the management of hypertension either as the sole therapeutic agent or to enhance the effectiveness of other antihypertensive drugs in the more severe forms of hypertension.

Usage in Pregnancy: The routine use of diuretics in an otherwise healthy woman is inappropriate and exposes mother and fetus to unnecessary hazard. Diuretics do not prevent development of toxemia of pregnancy, and there is no satisfactory evidence that they are useful in the treatment of developed toxemia.

Edema during pregnancy may arise from pathological causes or from the physiologic and mechanical consequences of pregnancy. Thiazides are indicated in pregnancy when edema is due to pathologic causes, just as they are in the absence of pregnancy (however, see Warnings, below). Dependent edema in pregnancy, resulting from restriction of venous return by the expanded uterus, is properly treated through elevation of the lower extremities and use of support hose; use of diuretics to lower intravascular volume in this case is illogical and unnecessary. There is hypervolemia during normal pregnancy which is harmful to neither the fetus nor the mother (in the absence of cardiovascular disease), but which is associated with edema, including generalized edema, in the majority of pregnant women. If this edema produces discomfort, increased recumbency will often provide relief. In rare instances, this edema may cause extreme discomfort which is not relieved by rest. In these cases, a short course of diuretics may provide relief and may be appropriate.

Contraindications: Anuria. Hypersensitivity to this or other sulfonamide derived drugs.

Warnings: Thiazides should be used with caution in severe renal disease. In patients with renal disease, thiazides may precipitate azotemia. Cumulative effects of the drug may develop in patients with impaired renal function.

Thiazides should be used with caution in patients with impaired hepatic function or progressive liver disease, since minor alterations of fluid and electrolyte balance may precipitate hepatic coma.

Thiazides may add to or potentiate the action of other antihypertensive drugs. Potentiation occurs with ganglionic or peripheral adrenergic blocking drugs.

Sensitivity reactions may occur in patients with a history of allergy or bronchial asthma. The possibility of exacerbation or activation of systemic lupus erythematosus has been reported.

Usage in pregnancy. Thiazides cross the placental barrier and appear in cord blood. The use of thiazides in pregnant women requires that the anticipated benefit be weighed against possible hazards to the fetus. These hazards include fetal or neonatal jaundice, thrombocytopenia, and possibly other adverse reactions which have occurred in the adult.

Nursing Mothers. Thiazides appear in breast milk. If use of the drug is deemed essential, the patient should stop nursing.

Precautions: Periodic determination of serum electrolytes to detect possible electrolyte imbalance should be performed at appropriate intervals.

All patients receiving thiazide therapy should be observed for clinical signs of fluid or electrolyte imbalance; namely, hyponatremia, hypochloremic alkalosis, and hypokalemia. Serum and urine electrolyte determinations are particularly important when the patient is vomiting excessively or receiving parenteral fluids. Medication such as digitalis may also influence serum electrolytes. Warning signs, irrespective of cause, are: dryness of mouth, thirst, weakness, lethargy, drowsiness, restlessness, muscle pains or cramps, muscular fatigue, hypotension, oliguria, tachycardia, and gastrointestinal disturbances such as nausea and vomiting.

Hypokalemia may develop with thiazides as with any other potent diuretic, especially with brisk diuresis, when severe cirrhosis is present, or during concomitant use of corticosteroids or ACTH.

Continued on next page

Pfizer—Cont.

Interference with adequate oral electrolyte intake will also contribute to hypokalemia. Digitalis therapy may exaggerate metabolic effects of hypokalemia especially with reference to myocardial activity.
Any chloride deficit is generally mild and usually does not require specific treatment except under extraordinary circumstances (as in liver disease or renal disease). Dilutional hyponatremia may occur in edematous patients in hot weather; appropriate therapy is water restriction, rather than administration of salt except in rare instances when the hyponatremia is life threatening. In actual salt depletion, appropriate replacement is the therapy of choice.
Hyperuricemia may occur or frank gout may be precipitated in certain patients receiving thiazide therapy.
Insulin requirements in diabetic patients may be increased, decreased, or unchanged. Latent diabetes mellitus may become manifest during thiazide administration.
Thiazide drugs may increase the responsiveness to tubocurarine.
The antihypertensive effects of the drug may be enhanced in the postsympathectomy patient.
Thiazides may decrease arterial responsiveness to norepinephrine. This diminution is not sufficient to preclude effectiveness of the pressor agent for therapeutic use.
If progressive renal impairment becomes evident, as indicated by a rising nonprotein nitrogen or blood urea nitrogen, a careful reappraisal of therapy is necessary with consideration given to withholding or discontinuing diuretic therapy.
Thiazides may decrease serum PBI levels without signs of thyroid disturbance.

Adverse Reactions:

A. GASTROINTESTINAL SYSTEM REACTIONS
1. anorexia
2. gastric irritation
3. nausea
4. vomiting
5. cramping
6. diarrhea
7. constipation
8. jaundice (intrahepatic cholestatic jaundice)
9. pancreatitis

B. CENTRAL NERVOUS SYSTEM REACTIONS
1. dizziness
2. vertigo
3. paresthesias
4. headache
5. xanthopsia

C. HEMATOLOGIC REACTIONS
1. leukopenia
2. agranulocytosis
3. thrombocytopenia
4. aplastic anemia

D. DERMATOLOGIC–HYPERSENSITIVITY REACTIONS
1. purpura
2. photosensitivity
3. rash
4. urticaria
5. necrotizing angiitis (vasculitis) (cutaneous vasculitis)

E. CARDIOVASCULAR REACTION
Orthostatic hypotension may occur and may be aggravated by alcohol, barbiturates or narcotics.

F. OTHER
1. hyperglycemia
2. glycosuria
3. hyperuricemia
4. muscle spasm
5. weakness
6. restlessness

Whenever adverse reactions are moderate or severe, thiazide dosage should be reduced or therapy withdrawn.

Dosage and Administration: Therapy should be individualized according to patient response. This therapy should be titrated to gain maximal therapeutic response as well as the minimal dose possible to maintain that therapeutic response. The usual dosage of Renese tablets for diuretic therapy is 1 to 4 mg daily, and for antihypertensive therapy is 2 to 4 mg daily.

How Supplied: RENESE (polythiazide) Tablets are available as:
1 mg white, scored tablets (imprinted with code number 375) in bottles of 100 and 1000.
2 mg yellow, scored tablets (imprinted with code number 376) in bottles of 100 and 1000.
4 mg white, scored tablets (imprinted with code number 377) in bottles of 100 and 1000.
(60-1116-00-2)

Literature Available: Yes.
[*Shown in Product Identification Section*]

RENESE®-R ℞
polythiazide/reserpine

> **Warning**
> This fixed combination drug is not indicated for initial therapy of hypertension. Hypertension requires therapy titrated to the individual patient. If the fixed combination represents the dosage so determined, its use may be more convenient in patient management. The treatment of hypertension is not static, but must be reevaluated as conditions in each patient warrant.

RENESE-R tablets combine polythiazide and reserpine, two antihypertensive agents with complementary properties. Each blue, scored tablet of RENESE-R provides:
Renese (polythiazide) .... 2.0 mg
Reserpine .... 0.25 mg

Actions: RENESE (polythiazide) is a member of the benzothiadiazine (thiazide) family of diuretic/antihypertensive agents. RENESE (polythiazide) alone has demonstrated clinical effectiveness in lowering elevated blood pressure in patients without visible edema as well as in edematous hypertensive patients. This antihypertensive action probably comes about through depletion of sodium and fluid accumulation in the blood vessel wall.
RENESE (polythiazide) is 2-methyl-3,4-dihydro-3 (2,2,2-trifluoroethylthiomethyl)-6-chloro-7-sulfamyl 1,2,4-benzothiadiazine 1,1 dioxide.
Reserpine, an alkaloid of Rauwolfia serpentina has several complementary actions of benefit to the hypertensive patient, including a calming effect and a slowing of the pulse rate. Its ultimate effect in lowering blood pressure is thought to be due to vasodilatation unaccompanied by reduction in cardiac performance, probably as a result of depletion of norepinephrine from tissue receptor sites.
Since polythiazide reduces or eliminates the sodium and fluid retention frequently associated with hypertension, it enhances the efficacy of reserpine in lowering elevated blood pressure. RENESE-R often has been found to be more effective than equivalent doses of either agent alone. Both the cardiovascular and central nervous system effects may persist following withdrawal of the drug.

Indications: Hypertension (see box warning).

Contraindications:

A. Related to polythiazide:
1. Advanced renal or hepatic failure.
2. Hypersensitivity to this or other sulfonamide derivatives.

B. Related to reserpine:
1. Demonstrated hypersensitivity.
2. Mental depression.
3. Demonstrated peptic ulcer or ulcerative colitis.

Warnings: Serum electrolyte determinations are especially indicated for patients with severe derangement of metabolic processes, e.g., surgery, vomiting, or parenteral fluid therapy. Electrolyte imbalance may be caused by certain diseases such as cirrhosis, or it may result from drug therapy, such as therapy with corticosteroids. Patients with cirrhosis who are continually receiving RENESE-R should be observed carefully for the development of hepatic precoma or coma. Indications of impending hepatic failure are tremor, confusion, drowsiness, and hepatic fetor.
Thiazides may precipitate kidney failure and uremia in patients with pre-existing renal pathology and impaired renal function.
Available information tends to implicate all oral dosage forms of potassium salts ingested in solid form with or without thiazides in the etiology of nonspecific, small bowel lesions consisting of ulceration with or without stenosis, causing obstruction, hemorrhage and perforation, and frequently requiring surgery. Deaths due to these complications have been reported.
All oral dosage forms of potassium salts ingested in solid form should be used only when adequate dietary supplementation is not practical and should be discontinued immediately if abdominal pain, distention, nausea, vomiting or gastrointestinal bleeding occur.
RENESE-R does not itself contain enteric-coated potassium.
Electroshock therapy should not be given within one week of cessation of reserpine.

Usage in Pregnancy and the Childbearing Age. Since thiazides appear in breast milk, the usage of polythiazide is contraindicated in nursing mothers. Thiazides cross the placental barrier and appear in cord blood. The safety of reserpine for use during pregnancy or lactation has not been established. When polythiazide and reserpine are used in women of childbearing age, the potential benefits of this drug combination should be weighed against the possible hazards to the fetus. The hazards include fetal or neonatal jaundice, thrombocytopenia, and possibly other adverse reactions which have occurred in the adult.

Precautions: Since all diuretic agents may reduce serum levels of sodium, chloride, and potassium, especially with brisk diuresis or when used concurrently with steroids, patients should be observed regularly for early signs of fluid or electrolyte imbalance and serum electrolyte studies should be performed periodically. Warning signs of possible electrolyte imbalance irrespective of cause include fatigue, muscle cramps, gastrointestinal disturbances, lethargy, oliguria, and tachycardia. In extreme cases, hypotension, shock, and coma may develop. Frequently, serum electrolyte levels do not correlate with signs or symptoms of electrolyte imbalance. Unduly restricted salt intake as well as concurrent administration of digitalis may exaggerate metabolic effects of hypokalemia. A favorable ratio of potassium to sodium excretion lessens the possibility of hypokalemia. However, should this occur or be suspected, foods with a high potassium content (bananas, apricots, citrus fruits, prune juice, etc.) should be given. When necessary, oral potassium supplements may be administered. If other antihypertensive agents are used concurrently, lower than usual doses of RENESE-R and of the other agents should be considered.
Like other thiazide diuretics, polythiazide may cause a rise in serum uric acid levels with or without overt symptoms of gout. Thiazides are known to disturb glucose tolerance in some individuals, even when there is no history of glucose intolerance or diabetes in the individual or his family. Likewise, thiazides may decrease PBI levels without signs of thyroid disturbances.
Thiazide drugs may augment the paralyzing actions of tubocurarine, and may decrease the arterial responsiveness to norepinephrine. Extra precautions may be necessary in patients who may require these drugs or their derivatives, as in surgery. The antihypertensive effects of the drug may be enhanced in the postsympathectomy patient.

Reserpine: Since reserpine may increase gastric acid secretion, it should be used cautiously in patients with a history of peptic ulcer or ulcerative colitis. Extreme caution is needed in patients with a history of mental depression, and reserpine should be discontinued at the first sign of depressive symptoms. Parkinsonism and confusion have been encountered, particularly in psychiatric patients, and constitute an indication for withdrawal of the drug. Caution should be exercised when treating patients with impairment of renal function, as lowered blood pressure may result in further decompensation and embarrassment of function. Reserpine should be used cautiously with digitalis or quinidine as the concurrent use may enhance the appearance of arrhythmias. Discontinue the drug one to two weeks prior to elective surgery since an unexpected degree of hypotension and bradycardia have been reported in patients receiving anesthetic agents concurrently with reserpine, probably due to a reduced responsiveness to norepinephrine. For emergency surgical procedures vagal blocking agents may be given parenterally to prevent or reverse hypotension and/or bradycardia. Reserpine may cause increased appetite and weight gain in some patients.

Adverse Reactions: Polythiazide: Side effects such as nausea, vertigo, weakness, paresthesias, and fatigue occur but seldom require cessation of therapy. Most of these can be overcome by reducing the dose or taking measures to improve electrolyte imbalance. Maculopapular skin rash has been reported, as has reversible cholestatic jaundice. Leukopenia (neutropenia) and purpura, with or without thrombocytopenia, have been reported rarely, and agranulocytosis and aplastic anemia have been reported with the older thiazides but not as yet with the newer compounds such as polythiazide. Pancreatitis, photosensitivity reactions, gastrointestinal disturbances, headache, xanthopsia, necrotizing angiitis, orthostatic hypotension, and dizziness have all been reported following the use of the benzothiadiazine class of diuretics.

Reserpine: Gastrointestinal reactions include hypersecretion, nausea and vomiting, anorexia, and diarrhea. Cardiovascular reactions reported include angina-like symptoms, arrhythmias—particularly when used concurrently with digitalis or quinidine, flushing of the skin, and bradycardia. Central nervous system reactions range from drowsiness, depression, nervousness, paradoxical anxiety, nightmares, and a rare Parkinsonian syndrome to C.N.S. sensitization manifested by deafness, glaucoma, uveitis, and optic atrophy. Nasal congestion is a frequent complaint, and pruritus, rash, dryness of mouth, dizziness, headache, purpura, impotence or decreased libido, and miosis have been reported with use of this drug. These reactions are usually reversible and disappear when the drug is discontinued.

Dosage: As determined by individual titration (see box warning).

Initial dosages of the combination should conform to those dosages of the individual components established during titration.

Maintenance dosages range from ½ tablet to 2 tablets daily. Dosage of other antihypertensive agents, particularly ganglionic blockers, that are used concomitantly should be reduced.

Supply: RENESE-R tablets (2 mg polythiazide-0.25 mg reserpine) are available as blue, scored tablets (imprinted with code number 446) in bottles of 100 and 1,000.

(60-1200-00-7)

Literature Available: Yes.

[*Shown in Product Identification Section*]

SINEQUAN® ℞

(doxepin HCl)
Capsules
Oral Concentrate

Sinequan® (doxepin HCl) is manufactured and distributed by Roerig, a division of Pfizer Pharmaceuticals. Please refer to Roerig PRODUCT INFORMATION and PRODUCT IDENTIFICATION sections for complete information.

TERRAMYCIN® ℞

Capsules
(oxytetracycline HCl)
Syrup
(calcium oxytetracycline)
Film-coated Tablets
(oxytetracycline)

Terramycin® is manufactured by Pfizer Pharmaceuticals and distributed by the Pfipharmecs Division. Please refer to Pfipharmecs PRODUCT INFORMATION for a full product description. Terramycin® (oxytetracycline HCl) Capsules appear under Pfipharmecs in the PRODUCT IDENTIFICATION section.

VIBRAMYCIN® Hyclate ℞

(doxycycline hyclate)
CAPSULES
VIBRA-TABS®
(doxycycline hyclate)
FILM COATED TABLETS
VIBRAMYCIN® Calcium
(doxycycline calcium oral suspension)
SYRUP
VIBRAMYCIN® Monohydrate
(doxycycline monohydrate)
FOR ORAL SUSPENSION

Description: Vibramycin is a broad-spectrum antibiotic synthetically derived from oxytetracycline, and is available as Vibramycin Monohydrate (doxycycline monohydrate), Vibramycin Hyclate and Vibra-Tabs (doxycycline hydrochloride hemiethanolate hemihydrate), and Vibramycin Calcium (doxycycline calcium). The chemical designation of this light-yellow crystalline powder is alpha-6-deoxy-5-oxytetracycline. Doxycycline has a high degree of lipoid solubility and a low affinity for calcium binding. It is highly stable in normal human serum. Doxycycline will not degrade into an epianhydro form.

Actions: Doxycycline is primarily bacteriostatic and is thought to exert its antimicrobial effect by the inhibition of protein synthesis. Doxycycline is active against a wide range of gram-positive and gram-negative organisms. The drugs in the tetracycline class have closely similar antimicrobial spectra, and cross resistance among them is common. Microorganisms may be considered susceptible if the M.I.C. (minimum inhibitory concentration) is less than 4.0 mcg/ml and intermediate if the M.I.C. is 4.0 to 12.5 mcg/ml.

Susceptibility plate testing: If the Kirby-Bauer method of disc susceptibility testing is used, a 30 mcg doxycycline disc should give a zone of at least 16 mm when tested against a doxycycline-susceptible bacterial strain. A tetracycline disc may be used to determine microbial susceptibility. If the Kirby-Bauer method of disc susceptibility testing is used, a 30 mcg tetracycline disc should give a zone of at least 19 mm when tested against a tetracycline-susceptible bacterial strain.

Tetracyclines are readily absorbed and are bound to plasma proteins in varying degree. They are concentrated by the liver in the bile, and excreted in the urine and feces at high concentrations and in a biologically active form.

Doxycycline is virtually completely absorbed after oral administration.

Following a 200 mg dose, normal adult volunteers averaged peak serum levels of 2.6 mcg/ml of doxycycline at 2 hours decreasing to 1.45 mcg/ml at 24 hours. Excretion of doxycycline by the kidney is about 40%/72 hours in individuals with normal function (creatinine clearance about 75 ml/min.). This percentage excretion may fall as low as 1–5%/72 hours in individuals with severe renal insufficiency (creatinine clearance below 10 ml/min.). Studies have shown no significant difference in serum half-life of doxycycline (range 18–22 hours) in individuals with normal and severely impaired renal function.

Hemodialysis does not alter serum half-life.

Indications: Doxycycline is indicated in infections caused by the following microorganisms:

Rickettsiae: Rocky Mountain spotted fever, typhus fever and the typhus group, Q fever, rickettsialpox, and tick fevers.

Mycoplasma pneumoniae (PPLO, Eaton agent),

Agents of psittacosis and ornithosis,

Agents of lymphogranuloma venereum and granuloma inguinale,

The spirochetal agent of relapsing fever (*Borrelia recurrentis*).

The following gram-negative microorganisms:

Haemophilus ducreyi (chancroid),

Pasteurella pestis, and *Pasteurella tularensis*,

Bartonella bacilliformis,

Bacteroides species,

Vibrio comma and *Vibrio fetus*,

Brucella species (in conjunction with streptomycin).

Because many strains of the following groups of microorganisms have been shown to be resistant to tetracyclines, culture and susceptibility testing are recommended.

Doxycycline is indicated for treatment of infections caused by the following gram-negative microorganisms, when bacteriologic testing indicates appropriate susceptibility to the drug:

Escherichia coli,

Enterobacter aerogenes (formerly *Aerobacter aerogenes*),

Shigella species,

Mima species and *Herellea* species,

Haemophilus influenzae (respiratory infections),

Klebsiella species (respiratory and urinary infections).

Doxycycline is indicated for treatment of infections caused by the following gram-positive microorganisms when bacteriologic testing indicates appropriate susceptibility to the drug:

Streptococcus species:

Up to 44 percent of strains of *Streptococcus pyogenes* and 74 percent of *Streptococcus faecalis* have been found to be resistant to tetracycline drugs. Therefore, tetracyclines should not be used for streptococcal disease unless the organism has been demonstrated to be sensitive.

For upper respiratory infections due to group A beta-hemolytic streptococci, penicillin is the usual drug of choice, including prophylaxis of rheumatic fever.

Diplococcus pneumoniae,

Staphylococcus aureus, respiratory, skin and soft-tissue infections. Tetracyclines are not the drug of choice in the treatment of any type of staphylococcal infection.

When penicillin is contraindicated, doxycycline is an alternative drug in the treatment of infections due to:

Neisseria gonorrhoeae,

Treponema pallidum and *Treponema pertenue* (syphilis and yaws),

Listeria monocytogenes,

Clostridium species,

Bacillus anthracis,

Fusobacterium fusiforme (Vincent's infection),

Actinomyces species.

In acute intestinal amebiasis doxycycline may be a useful adjunct to amebicides.

In severe acne doxycycline may be useful adjunctive therapy.

Doxycycline is indicated in the treatment of trachoma, although the infectious agent is not always eliminated, as judged by immunofluorescence.

Inclusion conjunctivitis may be treated with oral doxycycline alone, or with a combination of topical agents.

Continued on next page

Pfizer—Cont.

Contraindications: This drug is contraindicated in persons who have shown hypersensitivity to any of the tetracyclines.

Warnings: THE USE OF DRUGS OF THE TETRACYCLINE CLASS DURING TOOTH DEVELOPMENT (LAST HALF OF PREGNANCY, INFANCY AND CHILDHOOD TO THE AGE OF 8 YEARS) MAY CAUSE PERMANENT DISCOLORATION OF THE TEETH (YELLOW-GRAY-BROWN). This adverse reaction is more common during long term use of the drugs but has been observed following repeated short term courses. Enamel hypoplasia has also been reported. *TETRACYCLINE DRUGS, THEREFORE, SHOULD NOT BE USED IN THIS AGE GROUP UNLESS OTHER DRUGS ARE NOT LIKELY TO BE EFFECTIVE OR ARE CONTRAINDICATED.*

Photosensitivity manifested by an exaggerated sunburn reaction has been observed in some individuals taking tetracyclines. Patients apt to be exposed to direct sunlight or ultraviolet light should be advised that this reaction can occur with tetracycline drugs, and treatment should be discontinued at the first evidence of skin erythema.

The antianabolic action of the tetracyclines may cause an increase in BUN. Studies to date indicate that this does not occur with the use of doxycycline in patients with impaired renal function.

Usage in Pregnancy: (See above "Warnings" about use during tooth development.)

Results of animal studies indicate that tetracyclines cross the placenta, are found in fetal tissues, and can have toxic effects on the developing fetus (often related to retardation of skeletal development). Evidence of embryotoxicity has also been noted in animals treated early in pregnancy.

Usage in Newborns, Infants, and Children: (See above "Warnings" about use during tooth development.)

As with other tetracyclines, doxycycline forms a stable calcium complex in any bone-forming tissue. A decrease in the fibula growth rate has been observed in prematures given oral tetracycline in doses of 25 mg/kg every six hours. This reaction was shown to be reversible when the drug was discontinued.

Tetracyclines are present in the milk of lactating women who are taking a drug in this class.

Precautions: As with other antibiotic preparations, use of this drug may result in overgrowth of nonsusceptible organisms, including fungi. If superinfection occurs, the antibiotic should be discontinued and appropriate therapy should be instituted.

In venereal disease when coexistent syphilis is suspected, a dark field examination should be done before treatment is started and the blood serology repeated monthly for at least four months.

Because the tetracyclines have been shown to depress plasma prothrombin activity, patients who are on anticoagulant therapy may require downward adjustment of their anticoagulant dosage.

In long term therapy, periodic laboratory evaluation of organ systems, including hematopoietic, renal, and hepatic studies should be performed.

All infections due to group A beta-hemolytic streptococci should be treated for at least 10 days.

Since bacteriostatic drugs may interfere with the bactericidal action of penicillin, it is advisable to avoid giving tetracycline in conjunction with penicillin.

Adverse Reactions: Due to oral doxycycline's virtually complete absorption, side effects of the lower bowel, particularly diarrhea, have been infrequent. The following adverse reactions have been observed in patients receiving tetracyclines:

Gastrointestinal: anorexia, nausea, vomiting, diarrhea, glossitis, dysphagia, enterocolitis, and inflammatory lesions (with monilial overgrowth) in the anogenital region. These reactions have been caused by both the oral and parenteral administration of tetracyclines. Rare instances of esophagitis and esophageal ulcerations have been reported in patients receiving capsule and tablet forms of drugs in the tetracycline class. Most of these patients took medications immediately before going to bed. (See Dosage and Administration.)

Skin: maculopapular and erythematous rashes. Exfoliative dermatitis has been reported but is uncommon. Photosensitivity is discussed above (see "Warnings").

Renal toxicity: Rise in BUN has been reported and is apparently dose related. (See "Warnings.")

Hypersensitivity reactions: urticaria, angioneurotic edema, anaphylaxis, anaphylactoid purpura, pericarditis, and exacerbation of systemic lupus erythematosus.

Bulging fontanels in infants and benign intracranial hypertension in adults have been reported in individuals receiving full therapeutic dosages. These conditions disappeared rapidly when the drug was discontinued.

Blood: Hemolytic anemia, thrombocytopenia, neutropenia, and eosinophilia have been reported with tetracyclines.

When given over prolonged periods, tetracyclines have been reported to produce brown-black microscopic discoloration of thyroid glands. No abnormalities of thyroid function studies are known to occur.

Dosage and Administration: THE USUAL DOSAGE AND FREQUENCY OF ADMINISTRATION OF DOXYCYCLINE DIFFERS FROM THAT OF THE OTHER TETRACYCLINES. EXCEEDING THE RECOMMENDED DOSAGE MAY RESULT IN AN INCREASED INCIDENCE OF SIDE EFFECTS.

Adults: The usual dose of oral doxycycline is 200 mg on the first day of treatment (administered 100 mg every 12 hours) followed by a maintenance dose of 100 mg/day. The maintenance dose may be administered as a single dose or as 50 mg every 12 hours. In the management of more severe infections (particularly chronic infections of the urinary tract), 100 mg every 12 hours is recommended.

For children above eight years of age: The recommended dosage schedule for children weighing 100 pounds or less is 2 mg/lb. of body weight divided into two doses on the first day of treatment, followed by 1 mg/lb. of body weight given as a single daily dose or divided into two doses, on subsequent days. For more severe infections up to 2 mg/lb. of body weight may be used. For children over 100 lbs. the usual adult dose should be used.

Acute gonococcal infections: 200 mg stat. and 100 mg at bedtime, the first day, followed by 100 mg b.i.d. for 3 days.

As an alternate single visit dose, administer 300 mg stat followed in one hour by a second 300 mg dose. The dose may be administered with food, including milk or carbonated beverage, as required.

Primary and secondary syphilis: 300 mg a day in divided doses for at least 10 days.

The therapeutic antibacterial serum activity will usually persist for 24 hours following recommended dosage.

When used in streptococcal infections, therapy should be continued for 10 days.

Administration of adequate amounts of fluid along with capsule and tablet forms of drugs in the tetracycline class is recommended to wash down the drugs and reduce the risk of esophageal irritation and ulceration. (See Adverse Reactions.)

If gastric irritation occurs, it is recommended that doxycycline be given with food or milk. The absorption of doxycycline is not markedly influenced by simultaneous ingestion of food or milk.

Concomitant therapy: Antacids containing aluminum, calcium, or magnesium impair absorption and should not be given to patients taking oral doxycycline.

Studies to date have indicated that administration of doxycycline at the usual recommended doses does not lead to excessive accumulation of the antibiotic in patients with renal impairment.

How Supplied: Vibramycin Hyclate (doxycycline hyclate) is available in capsules containing doxycycline hyclate equivalent to:

50 mg doxycycline (imprinted with code number 094)
bottles of 50
unit-dose pack of 100 (10 x 10's)
X-pack of 50 (5 x 10's)

100 mg doxycycline (imprinted with code number 095)
bottles of 50 and 500
unit-dose pack of 100 (10 x 10's)
V-pack of 25 (5 x 5's)
Nine-Paks (10 x 9's)

Vibra-Tabs (doxycycline hyclate) is available in film coated tablets (imprinted with code number 099) containing doxycycline hyclate equivalent to:

100 mg of doxycycline
bottles of 50 and 500
unit-dose pack of 100 (10 x 10's)

Vibramycin Calcium Syrup (doxycycline calcium oral suspension) is available as a raspberry-apple flavored oral suspension. Each teaspoonful (5 ml) contains doxycycline calcium equivalent to 50 mg of doxycycline: bottles of 1 oz. (30 ml) and 1 Pint (473 ml).

Vibramycin Monohydrate (doxycycline monohydrate) for Oral Suspension is available as a pleasant tasting, raspberry flavored, dry powder for oral suspension. When reconstituted, each teaspoonful (5 ml) contains doxycycline monohydrate equivalent to 25 mg of doxycycline: 2 oz. (60 ml) bottles.

60-1680-00-5

Literature Available: Yes.

[*Shown in Product Identification Section*]

VIBRAMYCIN® Hyclate ℞
(doxycycline hyclate for injection)
INTRAVENOUS
For Intravenous Use Only

Description: Vibramycin (doxycycline hyclate for injection) Intravenous is a broad-spectrum antibiotic synthetically derived from oxytetracycline, and is available as Vibramycin Hyclate (doxycycline hydrochloride hemiethanolate hemihydrate). The chemical designation of this light-yellow crystalline powder is alpha-6-deoxy-5-oxytetracycline. Doxycycline has a high degree of lipoid solubility and a low affinity for calcium binding. It is highly stable in normal human serum.

Actions: Doxycycline is primarily bacteriostatic and thought to exert its antimicrobial effect by the inhibition of protein synthesis. Doxycycline is active against a wide range of gram-positive and gram-negative organisms.

The drugs in the tetracycline class have closely similar antimicrobial spectra and cross resistance among them is common. Microorganisms may be considered susceptible to doxycycline (likely to respond to doxycycline therapy) if the minimum inhibitory concentration (M.I.C.) is not more than 4.0 mcg/ml. Microorganisms may be considered intermediate (harboring partial resistance) if the M.I.C. is 4.0 to 12.5 mcg/ml and resistant (not likely to respond to therapy) if the M.I.C. is greater than 12.5 mcg/ml.

Susceptibility plate testing: If the Kirby-Bauer method of disc susceptibility testing is used, a 30 mcg doxycycline disc should give a zone of at least 16 mm when tested against a doxycycline-susceptible bacterial strain. A tetracycline disc may be used to determine microbial susceptibility. If the Kirby-Bauer method of disc susceptibility testing is used, a 30 mcg tetracycline disc should give a zone of at least 19 mm when tested against a tetracycline-susceptible bacterial strain.

Tetracyclines are readily absorbed and are bound to plasma proteins in varying degree. They are concentrated by the liver in the bile, and excreted in the urine and feces at high concentrations and in a biologically active form.

Following a single 100 mg dose administered in a concentration of 0.4 mg/ml in a one-hour infusion, normal adult volunteers average a peak of 2.5 mcg/ml, while 200 mg of a concentration of 0.4 mg/ml administered over two hours averaged a peak of 3.6 mcg/ml.

Excretion of doxycycline by the kidney is about 40 percent/72 hours in individuals with normal function (creatinine clearance about 75 ml/min.). This percentage excretion may fall as low as 1-5 percent/72 hours in individuals with severe renal insufficiency (creatinine clearance below 10 ml/min.). Studies have shown no significant difference in serum half-life of doxycycline (range 18-22 hours) in individuals with normal and severely impaired renal function.

Hemodialysis does not alter this serum half-life of doxycycline.

Indications: Doxycycline is indicated in infections caused by the following microorganisms:

Rickettsiae (Rocky Mountain spotted fever, typhus fever, and the typhus group, Q fever, rickettsialpox and tick fevers).

Mycoplasma pneumoniae (PPLO, Eaton Agent).

Agents of psittacosis and ornithosis.

Agents of lymphogranuloma venereum and granuloma inguinale.

The spirochetal agent of relapsing fever *(Borrelia recurrentis)*.

The following gram-negative microorganisms:

Haemophilus ducreyi (chancroid),
Pasteurella pestis and *Pasteurella tularensis,*
Bartonella bacilliformis,
Bacteroides species,
Vibrio comma and *Vibrio fetus,*
Brucella species (in conjunction with streptomycin).

Because many strains of the following groups of microorganisms have been shown to be resistant to tetracyclines, culture and susceptibility testing are recommended.

Doxycycline is indicated for treatment of infections caused by the following gram-negative microorganisms when bacteriologic testing indicates appropriate susceptibility to the drug:

Escherichia coli,
Enterobacter aerogenes (formerly *Aerobacter aerogenes),*
Shigella species,
Mima species and *Herellea* species,
Haemophilus influenzae (respiratory infections),
Klebsiella species (respiratory and urinary infections).

Doxycycline is indicated for treatment of infections caused by the following gram-positive microorganisms when bacteriologic testing indicates appropriate susceptibility to the drug:

Streptococcus species:

Up to 44 percent of strains of *Streptococcus pyogenes* and 74 percent of *Streptococcus faecalis* have been found to be resistant to tetracycline drugs. Therefore, tetracyclines should not be used for streptococcal disease unless the organism has been demonstrated to be sensitive.

For upper respiratory infections due to group A beta-hemolytic streptococci, penicillin is the usual drug of choice, including prophylaxis of rheumatic fever.

Diplococcus pneumoniae,
Staphylococcus aureus, respiratory, skin and soft tissue infections. Tetracyclines are not the drugs of choice in the treatment of any type of staphylococcal infections.

When penicillin is contraindicated, doxycycline is an alternative drug in the treatment of infections due to:

Neisseria gonorrhoeae and *N. meningitidis,*
Treponema pallidum and *Treponema pertenue* (syphilis and yaws),
Listeria monocytogenes,
Clostridium species,
Bacillus anthracis,
Fusobacterium fusiforme (Vincent's infection),
Actinomyces species.

In acute intestinal amebiasis, doxycycline may be a useful adjunct to amebicides.

Doxycycline is indicated in the treatment of trachoma, although the infectious agent is not always eliminated, as judged by immunofluorescence.

Contraindications: This drug is contraindicated in persons who have shown hypersensitivity to any of the tetracyclines.

Warnings: THE USE OF DRUGS OF THE TETRACYCLINE CLASS DURING TOOTH DEVELOPMENT (LAST HALF OF PREGNANCY, INFANCY AND CHILDHOOD TO THE AGE OF 8 YEARS) MAY CAUSE PERMANENT DISCOLORATION OF THE TEETH (YELLOW-GRAY-BROWN). This adverse reaction is more common during long-term use of the drugs but has been observed following repeated short-term courses. Enamel hypoplasia has also been reported. *TETRACYCLINE DRUGS, THEREFORE, SHOULD NOT BE USED IN THIS AGE GROUP UNLESS OTHER DRUGS ARE NOT LIKELY TO BE EFFECTIVE OR ARE CONTRAINDICATED.*

Photosensitivity manifested by an exaggerated sunburn reaction has been observed in some individuals taking tetracyclines. Patients apt to be exposed to direct sunlight or ultraviolet light should be advised that this reaction can occur with tetracycline drugs, and treatment should be discontinued at the first evidence of skin erythema.

The antianabolic action of the tetracyclines may cause an increase in BUN. Studies to date indicate that this does not occur with the use of doxycycline in patients with impaired renal function.

Usage in Pregnancy

(See above "Warnings" about use during tooth development.)

Vibramycin (doxycycline hyclate for injection) Intravenous has not been studied in pregnant patients. It should not be used in pregnant women unless, in the judgement of the physician, it is essential for the welfare of the patient.

Results of animal studies indicate that tetracyclines cross the placenta, are found in fetal tissues and can have toxic effects on the developing fetus (often related to retardation of skeletal development). Evidence of embryotoxicity has also been noted in animals treated early in pregnancy.

Usage in Children

The use of Vibramycin Intravenous in children under 8 years is not recommended because safe conditions for its use have not been established.

(See above "Warnings" about use during tooth development.)

As with other tetracyclines, doxycycline forms a stable calcium complex in any bone-forming tissue. A decrease in the fibula growth rate has been observed in prematures given oral tetracycline in doses of 25 mg/kg every 6 hours. This reaction was shown to be reversible when the drug was discontinued.

Tetracyclines are present in the milk of lactating women who are taking a drug in this class.

Precautions: As with other antibiotic preparations, use of this drug may result in overgrowth of nonsusceptible organisms, including fungi. If superinfection occurs, the antibiotic should be discontinued and appropriate therapy instituted.

In venereal diseases when coexistent syphilis is suspected, a dark field examination should be done before treatment is started and the blood serology repeated monthly for at least 4 months.

Because tetracyclines have been shown to depress plasma prothrombin activity, patients who are on anticoagulant therapy may require downward adjustment of their anticoagulant dosage.

In long-term therapy, periodic laboratory evaluation of organ systems, including hematopoietic, renal, and hepatic studies should be performed.

All infections due to group A beta-hemolytic streptococci should be treated for at least 10 days.

Since bacteriostatic drugs may interfere with the bactericidal action of penicillin, it is advisable to avoid giving tetracycline in conjunction with penicillin.

Adverse Reactions: Gastrointestinal: anorexia, nausea, vomiting, diarrhea, glossitis, dysphagia, enterocolitis, and inflammatory lesions (with monilial overgrowth) in the anogenital region. These reactions have been caused by both the oral and parenteral administration of tetracyclines.

Skin: maculopapular and erythematous rashes. Exfoliative dermatitis has been reported but is uncommon. Photosensitivity is discussed above. (See "Warnings.")

Renal toxicity: Rise in BUN has been reported and is apparently dose related. (See "Warnings.")

Hypersensitivity reactions: urticaria, angioneurotic edema, anaphylaxis, anaphylactoid purpura, pericarditis and exacerbation of systemic lupus erythematosus.

Bulging fontanels in infants and benign intracranial hypertension in adults have been reported in individuals receiving full therapeutic dosages. These conditions disappeared rapidly when the drug was discontinued.

Blood: Hemolytic anemia, thrombocytopenia, neutropenia and eosinophilia have been reported.

When given over prolonged periods, tetracyclines have been reported to produce brown-black microscopic discoloration of thyroid glands. No abnormalities of thyroid function studies are known to occur.

Dosage and Administration: Note: Rapid administration is to be avoided. Parenteral therapy is indicated only when oral therapy is not indicated. Oral therapy should be instituted as soon as possible. If intravenous therapy is given over prolonged periods of time, thrombophlebitis may result.

THE USUAL DOSAGE AND FREQUENCY OF ADMINISTRATION OF VIBRAMYCIN I.V. (100-200 MG/DAY) DIFFERS FROM THAT OF THE OTHER TETRACYCLINES (1-2 G/DAY). EXCEEDING THE RECOMMENDED DOSAGE MAY RESULT IN AN INCREASED INCIDENCE OF SIDE EFFECTS.

Studies to date have indicated that Vibramycin at the usual recommended doses does not lead to excessive accumulation of the antibiotic in patients with renal impairment.

Adults: The usual dosage of Vibramycin (doxycycline hyclate for injection) I.V. is 200 mg on the first day of treatment administered in one or two infusions. Subsequent daily dosage is 100 to 200 mg depending upon the severity of infection, with 200 mg administered in one or two infusions.

In the treatment of primary and secondary syphilis, the recommended dosage is 300 mg daily for at least 10 days.

For children above eight years of age: The recommended dosage schedule for children

Continued on next page

Pfizer—Cont.

weighing 100 pounds or less is 2 mg/lb. of body weight on the first day of treatment, administered in one or two infusions. Subsequent daily dosage is 1 to 2 mg/lb. of body weight given as one or two infusions, depending on the severity of the infection. For children over 100 pounds the usual adult dose should be used. (See "Warning" Section for Usage in Children.)

General: The duration of infusion may vary with the dose (100 to 200 mg per day), but is usually one to four hours. A recommended minimum infusion time for 100 mg of a 0.5 mg/ml solution is one hour. Therapy should be continued for at least 24-48 hours after symptoms and fever have subsided. The therapeutic antibacterial serum activity will usually persist for 24 hours following recommended dosage.

Intravenous solutions should not be injected intramuscularly or subcutaneously. Caution should be taken to avoid the inadvertent introduction of the intravenous solution into the adjacent soft tissue.

Preparation of Solution: To prepare a solution containing 10 mg/ml, the contents of the vial should be reconstituted with 10 ml (for the 100 mg/vial container) or 20 ml (for the 200 mg/vial container) of Sterile Water for Injection or any of the ten intravenous infusion solutions listed below. Each 100 mg of Vibramycin (i.e., withdraw entire solution from the 100 mg vial) is further diluted with 100 ml to 1000 ml of the intravenous solutions listed below. Each 200 mg of Vibramycin (i.e., withdraw entire solution from the 200 mg vial) is further diluted with 200 ml to 2000 ml of the following intravenous solutions:

1. Sodium Chloride Injection, USP
2. 5% Dextrose Injection, USP
3. Ringer's Injection, USP
4. Invert Sugar, 10% in Water
5. Lactated Ringer's Injection, USP
6. Dextrose 5% in Lactated Ringer's
7. Normosol-M® in D5-W (Abbott)
8. Normosol-R® in D5-W (Abbott)
9. Plasma-Lyte® 56 in 5% Dextrose (Travenol)
10. Plasma-Lyte® 148 in 5% Dextrose (Travenol)

This will result in desired concentrations of 0.1 to 1.0 mg/ml. Concentrations lower than 0.1 mg/ml or higher than 1.0 mg/ml are not recommended.

Stability:

When diluted with Sodium Chloride Injection, USP, or 5% Dextrose Injection, USP, or Ringer's Injection, USP, or Invert Sugar, 10% in Water, or Normosol-M® in D5-W (Abbott), or Normosol-R® in D5-W (Abbott), or Plasma-Lyte® 56 in 5% Dextrose (Travenol), or Plasma-Lyte® 148 in 5% Dextrose (Travenol), infusion of the solution (ca. 1.0 mg/ml) or lower concentrations (not less than 0.1 mg/ml) must be completed within 12 hours after reconstitution to ensure adequate stability. During infusion, the solution must be protected from direct sunlight. Reconstituted solutions (1.0 to 0.1 mg/ml) may also be stored up to 72 hours prior to start of infusion, if refrigerated and protected from sunlight and artificial light. Again, infusion must then be completed within 12 hours. Solutions must be used within these time periods or discarded.

When diluted with Lactated Ringer's Injection, USP, or Dextrose 5% in Lactated Ringer's, infusion of the solution (ca. 1.0 mg/ml) or lower concentrations (not less than 0.1 mg/ml) must be completed within six hours after reconstitution to ensure adequate stability. During infusion, the solution must be protected from direct sunlight. Solutions must be used within this time period or discarded.

Solutions of Vibramycin (doxycycline hyclate for injection) at a concentration of 10 mg/ml in Sterile Water for Injection, when frozen immediately after reconstitution are stable for 8 weeks when stored at −20°C. If the product is warmed, care should be taken to avoid heating it after the thawing is complete. Once thawed the solution should not be refrozen.

How Supplied: Vibramycin (doxycycline hyclate for injection) Intravenous is available as a sterile powder in a vial containing doxycycline hyclate equivalent to 100 mg of doxycycline with 480 mg of ascorbic acid, packages of 5; and in individually packaged vials containing doxycycline hyclate equivalent to 200 mg of doxycycline with 960 mg of ascorbic acid.

(60-1940-00-8)

Literature Available: Yes.

VISTARIL® ℞

(hydroxyzine pamoate)
Capsules and Oral Suspension

Description: Hydroxyzine pamoate is designated chemically as 1-(p-chlorobenzhydryl) 4-[2-(2-hydroxyethoxy) ethyl] diethylenediamine salt of 1,1'- methylene bis (2 hydroxy-3-naphthalene carboxylic acid).

Clinical Pharmacology: Vistaril (hydroxyzine pamoate) is unrelated chemically to the phenothiazines, reserpine, meprobamate, or the benzodiazepines.

Vistaril is not a cortical depressant, but its action may be due to a suppression of activity in certain key regions of the subcortical area of the central nervous system. Primary skeletal muscle relaxation has been demonstrated experimentally. Bronchodilator activity, and antihistaminic and analgesic effects have been demonstrated experimentally and confirmed clinically. An antiemetic effect, both by the apomorphine test and the veriloid test, has been demonstrated. Pharmacological and clinical studies indicate that hydroxyzine in therapeutic dosage does not increase gastric secretion or acidity and in most cases has mild antisecretory activity. Hydroxyzine is rapidly absorbed from the gastrointestinal tract and Vistaril's clinical effects are usually noted within 15 to 30 minutes after oral administration.

Indications: For symptomatic relief of anxiety and tension associated with psychoneurosis and as an adjunct in organic disease states in which anxiety is manifested.

Useful in the management of pruritus due to allergic conditions such as chronic urticaria and atopic and contact dermatoses, and in histamine-mediated pruritus.

As a sedative when used as premedication and following general anesthesia, **Hydroxyzine may potentiate meperidine (Demerol®) and barbiturates,** so their use in pre-anesthetic adjunctive therapy should be modified on an individual basis. Atropine and other belladonna alkaloids are not affected by the drug. Hydroxyzine is not known to interfere with the action of digitalis in any way and it may be used concurrently with this agent.

The effectiveness of hydroxyzine as an antianxiety agent for long term use, that is more than 4 months, has not been assessed by systematic clinical studies. The physician should reassess periodically the usefulness of the drug for the individual patient.

Contraindications: Hydroxyzine, when administered to the pregnant mouse, rat, and rabbit, induced fetal abnormalities in the rat and mouse at doses substantially above the human therapeutic range. Clinical data in human beings are inadequate to establish safety in early pregnancy. Until such data are available, hydroxyzine is contraindicated in early pregnancy.

Hydroxyzine pamoate is contraindicated for patients who have shown a previous hypersensitivity to it.

Warnings: **Nursing Mothers:** It is not known whether this drug is excreted in human milk. Since many drugs are so excreted, hydroxyzine should not be given to nursing mothers.

Precautions: THE POTENTIATING ACTION OF HYDROXYZINE MUST BE CONSIDERED WHEN THE DRUG IS USED IN CONJUNCTION WITH CENTRAL NERVOUS SYSTEM DEPRESSANTS SUCH AS NARCOTICS, NON-NARCOTIC ANALGESICS AND BARBITURATES. Therefore, when central nervous system depressants are administered concomitantly with hydroxyzine their dosage should be reduced. Since drowsiness may occur with use of the drug, patients should be warned of this possibility and cautioned against driving a car or operating dangerous machinery while taking Vistaril (hydroxyzine pamoate). Patients should be advised against the simultaneous use of other CNS depressant drugs, and cautioned that the effect of alcohol may be increased.

Adverse Reactions: Side effects reported with the administration of Vistaril are usually mild and transitory in nature.

Anticholinergic: Dry mouth.

Central Nervous System: Drowsiness is usually transitory and may disappear in a few days of continued therapy or upon reduction of the dose. Involuntary motor activity including rare instances of tremor and convulsions has been reported, usually with doses considerably higher than those recommended. Clinically significant respiratory depression has not been reported at recommended doses.

Overdosage: The most common manifestation of overdosage of Vistaril is hypersedation. As in the management of overdosage with any drug, it should be borne in mind that multiple agents may have been taken.

If vomiting has not occurred spontaneously, it should be induced. Immediate gastric lavage is also recommended. General supportive care, including frequent monitoring of the vital signs and close observation of the patient, is indicated. Hypotension, though unlikely, may be controlled with intravenous fluids and Levophed® (levarterenol) or Aramine® (metaraminol). Do not use epinephrine as Vistaril counteracts its pressor action. Caffeine and Sodium Benzoate Injection, U.S.P., may be used to counteract central nervous system depressant effects.

There is no specific antidote. It is doubtful that hemodialysis would be of any value in the treatment of overdosage with hydroxyzine. However, if other agents such as barbiturates have been ingested concomitantly, hemodialysis may be indicated. There is no practical method to quantitate hydroxyzine in body fluids or tissue after its ingestion or administration.

Dosage: For symptomatic relief of anxiety and tension associated with psychoneurosis and as an adjunct in organic disease states in which anxiety is manifested: in adults, 50–100 mg q.i.d.; children under 6 years, 50 mg daily in divided doses and over 6 years, 50–100 mg daily in divided doses.

For use in the management of pruritus due to allergic conditions such as chronic urticaria and atopic and contact dermatoses, and in histamine-mediated pruritus: in adults, 25 mg t.i.d. or q.i.d.; children under 6 years, 50 mg daily in divided doses and over 6 years, 50–100 mg daily in divided doses.

As a sedative when used as a premedication and following general anesthesia: 50–100 mg in adults, and 0.6 mg/kg in children.

When treatment is initiated by the intramuscular route of administration, subsequent doses may be administered orally.

As with all medications, the dosage should be adjusted according to the patient's response to therapy.

Supply:

Vistaril Capsules (hydroxyzine pamoate equivalent to hydroxyzine hydrochloride)

25 mg: 100's and 500's, and unit dose (10 × 10's)—two-tone green capsules (imprinted with code number 541).
50 mg: 100's and 500's, and unit dose (10 × 10's)—green and white capsules (imprinted with code number 542).
100 mg: 100's and 500's, and unit dose (10 × 10's)—green and gray capsules (imprinted with code number 543).

Vistaril Oral Suspension (hydroxyzine pamoate equivalent to 25 mg hydroxyzine hydrochloride per teaspoonful-5 ml): 1 pint bottles and 4 ounce (120 ml) bottles in packages of 4.
Bibliography: Available on request.
(60-0846-00-9)
[*Shown in Product Identification Section*]

VISTARIL® ℞
(hydroxyzine hydrochloride)
Intramuscular Solution
For Intramuscular Use Only

Vistaril® Intramuscular Solution is manufactured by Pfizer Pharmaceuticals and distributed by the Pfipharmecs Division. Please refer to Pfipharmecs PRODUCT INFORMATION for a full product description of Vistaril® Intramuscular Solution.

VISTRAX® TABLETS ℞
(oxyphencyclimine HCl and hydroxyzine HCl)

Composition: ***Each Vistrax 5 tablet contains:***
oxyphencyclimine HCl ....5 mg
hydroxyzine HCl ....25 mg
Each Vistrax 10 tablet contains:
oxyphencyclimine HCl ....10 mg
hydroxyzine HCl ....25 mg

Description: Vistrax is a combination of oxyphencyclimine HCl and hydroxyzine HCl. Oxyphencyclimine HCl is a crystalline substance designated chemically as: (1,4,5,6-tetrahydro-1-methyl-2-pyrimidinyl) methyl alpha-phenylcyclohexaneglycolate monohydrochloride.
Hydroxyzine HCl is designated chemically as: 2-[2- [4- (p-chloro-alpha-phenylbenzyl) -1-piperazinyl] ethoxy] ethanol dihydrochloride.
Actions: Oxyphencyclimine HCl provides long acting suppression of gastric secretion through its anticholinergic action. The mechanism of this action is the inhibition of acetylcholine at postganglionic cholinergic sites in structures innervated by postganglionic parasympathetic nerves and on smooth muscle not so innervated but responsive to acetylcholine. Hydroxyzine HCl has been shown clinically to be an effective antianxiety agent. It induces a calming effect in anxious, tense individuals without impairing mental alertness. It is not a cortical depressant, but its action may be due to a suppression of activity in certain key regions of the subcortical area of the central nervous system.

Indications
Based on a review of this drug by the National Academy of Sciences—National Research Council and/or other information, FDA has classified the indications as follows:
Possibly Effective: As adjunctive therapy in peptic ulcer; irritable bowel syndrome (irritable colon, spastic colon, mucous colitis, functional gastrointestinal disorders); functional diarrhea; drug induced diarrhea; ulcerative colitis, and urinary bladder spasm and ureteral spasm (i.e., smooth muscle spasm).
Final classification of these less than effective indications requires further investigation.

Contraindications: Because of its anticholinergic activity, Vistrax is contraindicated in the presence of glaucoma, obstructive uropathy (i.e. bladder neck obstruction due to prostatic hypertrophy), obstructive disease of the gastrointestinal tract (as in achalasia, pyloroduodenal stenosis, etc.); paralytic ileus; intestinal atony of the elderly or debilitated patient; unstable cardiovascular status in acute hemorrhage; severe ulcerative colitis; toxic megacolon complicating ulcerative colitis; myasthenia gravis.
Warnings: Hydroxyzine, when administered to the pregnant mouse, rat, and rabbit, induced fetal abnormalities in the rat at doses substantially above the human therapeutic range. Clinical data in human beings are inadequate to establish safety in early pregnancy. Until such data are available, hydroxyzine-containing drugs are not advised in early pregnancy. In the presence of a high environmental temperature, heat prostration can occur with drug use (fever and heatstroke due to decreased sweating).
Diarrhea may be an early symptom of incomplete intestinal obstruction, especially in patients with ileostomy or colostomy. In this instance treatment with this drug would be inappropriate and possibly harmful.
Vistrax may produce drowsiness or blurred vision. In this event, the patient should be warned not to engage in activities requiring mental alertness such as operating a motor vehicle or other machinery, or perform hazardous work while taking this drug.
Precautions: Anticholinergics should be used with caution in patients with:
autonomic neuropathy,
hepatic or renal disease,
ulcerative colitis—(Large doses may suppress intestinal motility to the point of producing a paralytic ileus and the use of this drug may precipitate or aggravate the serious complication of toxic megacolon.),
hyperthyroidism, coronary heart disease, congestive heart failure, cardiac arrhythmias, hypertension and nonobstructing prostatic hypertrophy; hiatal hernia associated with reflux esophagitis, since anticholinergic drugs may aggravate this condition.
It should be noted that the use of anticholinergic drugs in the treatment of gastric ulcer may produce a delay in gastric emptying time and may complicate such therapy (antral stasis).
The use of this drug in the presence of complication of biliary tract disease should not be relied upon.
Tachycardia should be thoroughly investigated before giving anticholinergic (atropine-like) drugs since they may increase the heart rate.
With overdosage, a curare-like action may occur.
Adverse Reactions: As with other anticholinergics, oxyphencyclimine HCl produces certain effects which may be physiologic or toxic depending upon the individual patient's response. The physician must delineate these.
Adverse reactions may include xerostomia; urinary hesitancy and retention; blurred vision and tachycardia; palpitations; mydriasis; dilatation of the pupil; cycloplegia, increased ocular tension; loss of taste; headaches; nervousness; drowsiness; weakness; dizziness; insomnia; nausea; vomiting; impotence; suppression of lactation; constipation; bloated feeling; severe allergic reaction or drug idiosyncrasies including anaphylaxis, urticaria and other dermal manifestation; some degree of mental confusion and/or excitement especially in elderly persons.
Decreased sweating is another adverse reaction that may occur. It should be noted that adrenergic innervation of the eccrine sweat glands on the palms and soles makes complete control of sweating impossible. An end point of complete anhidrosis cannot occur because large doses of drug would be required, and this would produce severe side effects from parasympathetic paralysis.
Side effects which occasionally occur with hydroxyzine HCl are drowsiness, xerostomia, and, at extremely high doses, involuntary motor activity, all of which may be controlled by reduction of the dosage or discontinuation of the medication.
Dosage and Administration: The recommended adult dose is usually one Vistrax 5 or one Vistrax 10 tablet two times a day or three times a day, depending on individual response. Proper diet and antacids should be used where indicated as concomitant therapy. The safe use of Vistrax in children has not been established; therefore, the drug should not be used in children.
Drug Interactions: The potentiating action of hydroxyzine must be considered when the drug is used in combination with central nervous system depressants.
How Supplied: Vistrax 5 is available as white scored tablets (imprinted with code number 180) in bottles of 100. Vistrax 10 is available as black and white scored tablets (imprinted with code number 181) in bottles of 100. (60-2258-00-1)
Literature Available: Yes.
[*Shown in Product Identification Section*]

Pharmacia Laboratories

Division of Pharmacia Inc.
800 CENTENNIAL AVENUE
PISCATAWAY, NJ 08854

AZULFIDINE® (sulfasalazine USP) ℞
Tablets
AZULFIDINE® (sulfasalazine USP) ℞
EN-tabs®
AZULFIDINE® (sulfasalazine USP) ℞
Oral Suspension

Description: AZULFIDINE Tablets contain sulfasalazine U.S.P., 500 mg/tablet. AZULFIDINE EN-tabs contain sulfasalazine U.S.P., 500 mg/enteric-coated tablet. AZULFIDINE EN-tabs are film coated with cellulose acetate phthalate to prevent disintegration of the tablet in the stomach and thus reduce possible irritation of the gastric mucosa. Cellulose acetate phthalate coatings disintegrate due to the hydrolytic effect of the intestinal esterases, even when the intestinal contents are acid.
AZULFIDINE Oral Suspension is an aqueous solution of sulfasalazine U.S.P. (250 mg/5 ml) with microcrystalline cellulose, Xanthan Gum, polysorbate 80, sodium benzoate, sucrose, and flavor.
Sulfasalazine is synthesized by the diazotization of sulfapyridine and the coupling of the diazonium salt with salicylic acid. Further processing results in a bright orange colored substance that chemically is designated: 5-[p-(2-Pyridylsulfamoyl) phenyl] azo] salicylic acid. Reductive splitting of the azo linkage yields sulfapyridine and 5-aminosalicylic acid.
Actions: After oral administration, AZULFIDINE is partially absorbed and extensively metabolized, as described below.
About one-third of a given dose of sulfasalazine (SS) is absorbed from the small intestine. The remaining two-thirds pass to the colon where the compound is split (presumably by intestinal bacteria) into its components, 5-aminosalicylic acid (5-ASA) and sulfapyridine (SP). Most of the SP thus liberated is absorbed, whereas only about one-third of the 5-ASA is absorbed, the remainder being excreted in the feces. The distribution, metabolism and excretion of SS and its two components are as follows:
AZULFIDINE Tablets:
Sulfasalazine (SS): Detectable serum concentrations of SS have been found in healthy sub-

Continued on next page

Pharmacia—Cont.

jects within 90 minutes after the ingestion of a single 2 g dose of AZULFIDINE Tablets. Maximum concentrations of SS occur between 1.5 and 6 hours, with the mean peak concentrations (14 mcg/ml) occurring at 3 hours. Small amounts of SS are excreted unchanged in the urine.

Sulfapyridine (SP): Following absorption and distribution, SP is acetylated and hydroxylated in the liver, and then conjugated with glucuronic acid. After ingestion of a single 2 g dose of AZULFIDINE Tablets by healthy subjects, SP and its various metabolites appear in the serum within 3 to 6 hours. Maximum concentrations of total SP occur between 6 and 24 hours, with the mean peak concentration (21 mcg/ml) occurring at 12 hours. The total recovery of SS and its SP metabolites from the urine of healthy subjects 3 days after the administration of a single 2 g dose of AZULFIDINE Tablets averaged 91%.

Mean serum concentrations of total SP, i.e., SP + its metabolites, tend to be significantly greater in patients with a slow acetylator phenotype than in those with a fast acetylator phenotype. SP serum concentrations greater than 50 mcg/ml appear to be associated with adverse reactions.

5-Aminosalicylic Acid (5-ASA): The serum concentration of 5-ASA in patients with ulcerative colitis was found to range from 0 to 4 mcg/ml, and to exist mainly in the form of free 5-ASA. The urinary recovery of this compound was mostly in the acetylated form.

AZULFIDINE EN-tabs

Sulfasalazine (SS): Detectable serum concentrations of SS have been found in healthy subjects within 90 minutes after the ingestion of a single 2 g dose of AZULFIDINE EN-tabs. Maximum concentrations of SS occur between 3 and 12 hours, with the mean peak concentrations (6 mcg/ml) occurring at 6 hours. Small amounts of SS are excreted unchanged in the urine.

Sulfapyridine (SP): Following absorption and distribution, SP is acetylated and hydroxylated in the liver, and then conjugated with glucuronic acid. After ingestion of a single 2 g dose of AZULFIDINE EN-tabs by healthy subjects, peak concentrations of SP and its various metabolites appear in the serum between 12 and 24 hours, with the peak concentration (13 mcg/ml) occurring at 12 and lasting until 24 hours. The total recovery of SS and its SP metabolites from the urine of healthy subjects 3 days after the administration of a single 2 g dose of AZULFIDINE EN-tabs averaged 81%.

Mean serum concentrations of total SP, i.e., SP + its metabolites, tend to be significantly greater in patients with a slow acetylator phenotype than in those with a fast acetylator phenotype. SP serum concentrations greater than 50 mcg/ml appear to be associated with adverse reactions.

5-Aminosalicylic Acid (5-ASA): The serum concentration of 5-ASA in patients with ulcerative colitis was found to range from 0 to 4 mcg/ml: and to exist mainly in the form of free 5-ASA. The urinary recovery of this compound was mostly in the acetylated form.

AZULFIDINE Oral Suspension

Sulfasalazine (SS): Detectable serum concentrations of SS have been found in healthy subjects within 90 minutes after the injestion of a single 2 g dose of AZULFIDINE Oral Suspension.

Maximum concentrations of SS occur between 1.5 and 6 hours, with the mean peak concentration (20 mcg/ml) occurring at 3 hours. Small amounts of SS are excreted unchanged in the urine.

Sulfapyridine (SP): Following absorption and distribution, SP is acetylated and hydroxylated in the liver, and then conjugated with glucuronic acid. After ingestion of a single 2 g dose of AZULFIDINE Oral Suspension by healthy subjects, SP and its various metabolites appear in the serum within 3 to 6 hours. Maximum concentrations of total SP occur between 9 and 24 hours with the mean peak concentration (19 mcg/ml) occurring at 12 hours. The total recovery of SS and its SP metabolites from the urine of healthy subjects 3 days after the administration of a single 2 g dose of AZULFIDINE Oral Suspension averaged 75%.

Mean serum concentrations of total SP, i.e., SP + its metabolites, tend to be significantly greater in patients with a slow acetylator phenotype than in those with a fast acetylator phenotype. SP serum concentrations greater than 50 mcg/ml appear to be associated with adverse reactions.

5-Aminosalicylic Acid (5-ASA): The serum concentrations of 5-ASA in normal subjects was found to range from 0 to 4 mcg/ml, and to exist mainly in the form of free 5-ASA. The urinary recovery of this compound was mostly in the acetylated form.

The mode of action of AZULFIDINE is still under investigation. It may be related to the immunosuppressant properties that have been observed in animal and in vitro models, to its affinity for connective tissue, and/or to the relatively high concentration it reaches in serous fluids, the liver and intestinal wall, as demonstrated in autoradiographic studies in animals. AZULFIDINE has also been described as a highly efficient vehicle for carrying its principal metabolites, SP and 5-ASA, to the colon, where a local action for both of them has been postulated.

Indications: AZULFIDINE is indicated in the treatment of mild to moderate ulcerative colitis, and as adjunctive therapy in severe ulcerative colitis.

AZULFIDINE EN-tabs are particularly indicated in patients who cannot take the regular AZULFIDINE tablet because of gastrointestinal intolerance, and in whom there is evidence that this intolerance is not primarily due to high blood levels of sulfapyridine and its metabolites, e.g. patients experiencing nausea, vomiting, etc., when taking the first few doses of the drug or patients in whom a reduction in dosage does not alleviate the gastrointestinal side effects.

Contraindications: Hypersensitivity to sulfonamides or salicylates. In infants under 2 years. Intestinal and urinary obstruction. Patients with porphyria should not receive sulfonamides, as these drugs have been reported to precipitate an acute attack.

Warnings:

Use in pregnancy: Teratology studies have been performed with AZULFIDINE in rats and rabbits at doses up to 6 times the maximum recommended human dose and have revealed no evidence of harm to the developing fetus. There are, however, no adequate and well-controlled studies in pregnant women.

Because animal reproduction studies are not always predictive of human response, this drug should be used during pregnancy only if clearly needed.

Nursing mothers: Sulfonamides are excreted in the milk. In the newborn, they compete with bilirubin for binding sites on the plasma proteins and may thus cause kernicterus. Insignificant amounts of uncleaved sulfasalazine have been found in milk, whereas the sulfapyridine levels in milk are about 30-60 percent of those in the serum. Sulfapyridine has been shown to have a poor bilirubin-displacing capacity.

Impairment of fertility: Oligospermia and infertility have been described in men treated with AZULFIDINE. Withdrawal of the drug appears to reverse these effects.

Other warnings: Only after critical appraisal should AZULFIDINE be used in patients with hepatic or renal damage or blood dyscrasias. Deaths associated with the administration of AZULFIDINE have been reported from hypersensitivity reactions, agranulocytosis, aplastic anemia, other blood dyscrasias, renal and liver damage, irreversible neuromuscular and CNS changes, and fibrosing alveolitis. The presence of clinical signs such as sore throat, fever, pallor, purpura, or jaundice may be indications of serious blood disorders. Complete blood counts as well as urinalysis with careful microscopic examination should be done frequently in patients receiving AZULFIDINE.

Precautions: AZULFIDINE should be given with caution to patients with severe allergy or bronchial asthma. Adequate fluid intake must be maintained in order to prevent crystalluria and stone formation. Patients with glucose-6-phosphate dehydrogenase deficiency should be observed closely for signs of hemolytic anemia. This reaction is frequently dose related. If toxic or hypersensitivity reactions occur, the drug should be discontinued immediately.

Isolated instances have been reported when AZULFIDINE EN-tabs have passed undisintegrated. This may be due to a lack of intestinal esterases in these patients (see description). If this is observed, the administration of AZULFIDINE EN-tabs should be discontinued immediately.

Adverse Reactions: Adverse reactions have been observed in 5 to 55% of patients included in clinical studies reported in the literature. Experience suggests that with daily dosage of 4 g or more adverse reactions tend to increase. The most common adverse reactions associated with AZULFIDINE therapy are anorexia, nausea, vomiting, and gastric distress. The following adverse reactions have been reported to occur during therapy with AZULFIDINE.

Blood dyscrasias: Agranulocytosis, aplastic anemia, thrombocytopenia, leukopenia, hemolytic anemia. Heinz Body anemia, megaloblastic (macrocytic) anemia, purpura, hypoprothrombinemia, "cyanosis" and methemoglobinemia.

Hypersensitivity reactions: Generalized skin eruptions, erythema multiforme (Stevens-Johnson syndrome), parapsoriasis varioliformis acuta (Mucha-Haberman syndrome), exfoliative dermatitis, epidermal necrolysis (Lyell's syndrome) with corneal damage, pruritus, urticaria, photosensitization, anaphylaxis, serum sickness syndrome, chills, drug fever, periorbital edema, conjunctival and scleral injection, arthralgia; transient pulmonary changes with eosinophilia and decreased pulmonary function; allergic myocarditis; polyarteritis nodosa, L.E. syndrome, and hepatitis with immune complexes. Incidents of alopecia have also been reported.

Gastrointestinal reactions: Anorexia, nausea, emesis, abdominal pains, diarrhea, bloody diarrhea, impaired folic acid and digoxin absorption, stomatitis, pancreatitis, and hepatitis.

CNS reactions: Headache, vertigo, tinnitus, hearing loss, peripheral neuropathy, transient lesions of posterior spinal column, transverse myelitis, ataxia, convulsions, insomnia, mental depression, hallucinations and drowsiness.

Renal reactions: Crystalluria, hematuria, proteinuria, and nephrotic syndrome. Toxic nephrosis with oliguria and anuria.

The sulfonamides bear certain chemical similarities to some goitrogens, diuretics, (acetazolamide and the thiazides), and oral hypoglycemic agents. Goiter production, diuresis, and hypoglycemia have occurred rarely in patients receiving sulfonamides. Cross-sensitivity may exist with these agents.

Rats appear to be especially susceptible to the goitrogenic effects of sulfonamides and long-term administration has produced thyroid malignancies in this species.

AZULFIDINE produces an orange-yellow color when the urine is alkaline. Similar discoloration of the skin has also been reported.

Treatment of Overdosage and Sensitivity Reactions:
Overdosage: Gastric lavage or emesis plus catharsis as indicated. Alkalinize urine. If kidney function is normal, force fluids. If anuria is present, restrict fluids and salt, and treat for renal failure. Catheterization of the ureters may be indicated for complete renal blockage by crystals. For agranulocytosis discontinue the drug immediately, hospitalize the patient and institute appropriate therapy.
Sensitivity reactions: Discontinue treatment immediately. Urticaria, other skin rashes, and serum sickness-like reactions may be controlled with antihistamines and, if necessary, systemic corticosteriods.
Dosage and Administration: Dosage should be adjusted to each individual's response and tolerance. The drug should be given in evenly divided doses over each 24-hour period; intervals between nighttime doses should not exceed 8 hours, with administration after meals recommended when feasible. Experience suggests that with daily dosages of 4 g or more adverse reactions tend to increase; hence patients receiving these dosages should be carefully observed for the appearance of adverse effects.
Usual Dosage:
AZULFIDINE Tablets and AZULFIDINE EN-tabs
Initial therapy: Adults: 3-4 g daily in evenly divided doses. In some cases it is advisable to initiate therapy with a small dosage, e.g. 1-2 g daily, to lessen adverse gastrointestinal effects. If daily doses up to 8 g are required to achieve desired effects, the increased risk of toxicity should be kept in mind. Children: 40-60 mg per kg body weight in each 24-hour period, divided into 3-6 doses.
Maintenance therapy: Adults: 2 g daily. Children: 30 mg per kg body weight in each 24-hour period, divided into 4 doses. Response to therapy and adjustment of dosage should be determined by periodic examination. It is often necessary to continue medication, even when clinical symptoms, including diarrhea, have been controlled. When endoscopic examination confirms satisfactory improvement, dosage is reduced to a maintenance level. If diarrhea recurs, dosage should be increased to previous effective levels.
If symptoms of gastric intolerance (anorexia, nausea, vomiting, etc.) occur after the first few doses of AZULFIDINE, they are probably due to mucosal irritation, and may be alleviated by distributing the total daily dose more evenly over the day or by giving enteric-coated EN-tabs. If such symptoms occur after the first few days of treatment with AZULFIDINE, they are probably due to increased serum levels of total sulfapyridine, and may be alleviated by halving the dose and subsequently increasing it gradually over several days. If symptoms continue, the drug should be stopped for 5-7 days, then reinstituted at a lower daily dose.
AZULFIDINE Oral Suspension
[Each 5 ml (one teaspoonful) contains 250 mg of sulfasalazine.]
Initial Therapy:
Adults: 3-4 g daily in evenly divided doses. In some cases it is advisable to initiate therapy with a smaller dosage, e.g. 1-2 g daily, to lessen adverse gastrointestinal effects. If daily doses up to 8 g are required to achieve desired effects, the increased risk of toxicity should be kept in mind.
Children: 40-60 mg per kg body weight in each 24-hour period, divided into 3-6 doses.
Maintenance Therapy:
Adults: 2 g daily.
Children: 30 mg per kg body weight in each 24-hour period, divided into 4 doses.
Response to therapy and adjustment of dosage should be determined by periodic examination. It is often necessary to continue medication, even when clinical symptoms including diarrhea, have been controlled. When endoscopic examination confirms satisfactory improvement, dosage is reduced to a maintenance level. If diarrhea recurs, dosage should be increased to previous effective levels.
How Supplied:
AZULFIDINE Tablets 500 mg 100's — NDC No. 0016-0101-01
AZULFIDINE Tablets 500 mg 500's — NDC No. 0016-0101-05
AZULFIDINE Unit Dose Tablets
500 mg 100's — NDC No. 0016-0101-11
AZULFIDINE Unit Dose Tablets
500 mg 1000's — NDC No. 0016-0101-10
AZULFIDINE EN-tabs 500 mg 100's — NDC No. 0016-0102-01
AZULFIDINE EN-tabs 500 mg 500's — NDC No. 0016-0102-05
AZULFIDINE Oral Suspension 250 mg/5 ml — 1 Pint (473 ml) — NDC No. 0016-0103-06
Store at Room Temperature (15°-30°C/59°-86°F)
Avoid Freezing
Shake Well Before Using
Revised Oct. 1981.
[*Shown in Product Identification Section*]

HEALON® ℞
(sodium hyaluronate)

Description: HEALON is a sterile, nonpyrogenic, viscoelastic preparation of a highly purified, noninflammatory, high molecular weight fraction of sodium hyaluronate.
HEALON contains 10 mg/ml of sodium hyaluronate, dissolved in physiological sodium chloride-phosphate buffer (pH 7.0-7.5). This high molecular weight polymer is made up of repeating disaccharide units of N-acetylglucosamine and sodium glucuronate linked by $\beta 1$–3 and $\beta 1$–4 glycosidic bonds.
Characteristics: Sodium hyaluronate is a physiological substance that is widely distributed in the extracellular matrix of connective tissues in both animals and man. For example, it is present in the vitreous and aqueous humor of the eye, the synovial fluid, the skin and the umbilical cord. Sodium hyaluronates prepared from various human and animal tissues are not chemically different from each other.
HEALON is a specific fraction of sodium hyaluronate developed as an ophthalmo- surgical aid for use in anterior segment and vitreous procedures. It is specific in that:
1. It has a high molecular weight;
2. It is reported to be nonantigenic[1,7];
3. It does not cause inflammatory[2]or foreign body reactions.
4. It has a high viscosity.

Furthermore, the 1% solution of HEALON is transparent, is reported to remain in the anterior chamber for less than 6 days, [3] protects corneal endothelial tissues[4,5] and other ocular structures, and may decrease the chances for formation of adhesions and synechia.[6] HEALON does not interefere with epithelialization and normal wound healing.
Uses: The principal intended use of HEALON is as an opthalmo-surgical aid in various anterior segment procedures, such as intra- and extra-capsular cataract surgery, intraocular lens (IOL) implantation, keratoplasty, and glaucoma surgery. It has also been used successfully as a vitreous replacement after vitrectomy and retinal detachment surgery.
In surgical procedures in the anterior segment of the eye, instillation of HEALON serves to maintain a deep anterior chamber during surgery, allowing for more efficient manipulation with less trauma to the corneal endothelium and other surrounding tissues.
Furthermore, its viscoelasticity helps to push back the vitreous face and prevent formation of a postoperative flat chamber.
Contraindications: At present there are no known contraindications to the use of HEALON when used as recommended.
Precautions: Those normally associated with the surgical procedure being performed. Postoperative intraocular pressure may be elevated as a result of pre-existing glaucoma and by operative procedures and sequelae thereto, including enzymatic zonulysis, absence of an iridectomy, trauma to filtration structures, and by blood and lenticular remnants in the anterior chamber. Since the exact role of these factors is difficult to predict in any individual case, the following precautions are recommended:
— Don't overfill the anterior chamber with HEALON (except in glaucoma surgery—see Application section).
— Remove some of the HEALON by irrigation and/or aspiration at the close of surgery (except in glaucoma surgery—see Application section).
— Carefully monitor intraocular pressure, especially during the immediate postoperative period. If significant rises are observed, treat with appropriate therapy.

When air is used in conjunction with HEALON, care should be taken to avoid trapping the air behind the iris.
Because HEALON is a highly purified fraction extracted from avian tissues and is known to contain minute amounts of protein, the physician should be aware of potential risks of the type that can occur with the injection of any biological material.
Adverse Reactions: HEALON has been extremely well tolerated after injection into human eyes. A transient rise of intraocular pressure postoperatively has been reported in some cases.
Rarely, postoperative inflammatory reactions (iritis, hypopyon) have been reported. Their relationship to HEALON has not been established.
Applications: Cataract surgery—IOL implantation
A sufficient amount of HEALON is slowly and carefully introduced (using a cannula or needle) into the anterior chamber.
Injection of HEALON can be performed either before or after delivery of the lens. Injection prior to lens delivery will, however, have the additional advantage of protecting the corneal endothelium from possible damage arising from the removal of the cataractous lens.[5] HEALON may also be used to coat surgical instruments and the IOL prior to insertion.
Additional HEALON can be injected during surgery to replace any HEALON lost during surgical manipulation (see Precautions section).
Glaucoma filtration surgery: In conjunction with the performance of the trabeculectomy, HEALON is injected slowly and carefully through a corneal paracentesis to reconstitute the anterior chamber. Further injection of HEALON can be continued to allow it to extrude into the subconjunctival filtration site through and around the sutured outer scleral flap.
Corneal transplant surgery: After removal of the corneal button, the anterior chamber is filled with HEALON. The donor graft can then be placed on top of the bed of HEALON and sutured in place. Additional HEALON may be injected to replace the HEALON lost as a result of surgical manipulation (see Precaution section).
How Supplied: HEALON is a sterile, nonpyrogenic, viscoelastic preparation supplied in disposable glass syringes, delivering 0.75 ml or 0.4 ml sodium hyaluronate (10 mg/ml) dissolved in physiological sodium chloride-phosphate buffer (pH 7.0-7.5). Each ml of HEALON contains 10 mg of sodium hyaluronate, 8.5 mg of sodium chloride, 0.28 mg of disodium hydrogen phosphate dihydrate, 0.04 mg of sodium dihydrogen phosphate hydrate and q.s. water for injection U.S.P. HEALON syringes are terminally sterilized and aseptically packaged.

Continued on next page

Pharmacia—Cont.

Refrigerated HEALON should be allowed to attain room temperature (approximately 30 minutes) prior to use.
For intraocular use.
Store at 2–8°C.
Protect from freezing.
Protect from light.
References: See Full Product Information.
Caution: Federal law restricts this device to sale by or on the order of a physician.
Revised June 1981

HYSKON® Hysteroscopy Fluid ℞
32% (W/V) dextran 70 in dextrose

Description: HYSKON Hysteroscopy Fluid is a clear, viscid, sterile, non-pyrogenic solution of dextran 70 (32% W/V) in dextrose (10% W/V). Dextran 70 is that fraction of dextran, a branched polysaccharide composed of glucose units, having a weight average molecular weight of 70,000. The fluid is electrolyte-free and non-conductive. At room temperature HYSKON Hysteroscopy Fluid has a viscosity of 220 cS.
HYSKON has a tendency to crystalize when subjected to temperature variations or when stored for long periods. If flakes of dextran are present, heat at 100°–110° C until complete dissolution is achieved.
Indications: HYSKON Hysteroscopy Fluid is indicated for use with the hysteroscope as an aid in distending the uterine cavity and in irrigating and visualizing its surfaces.
Contraindications: HYSKON Hysteroscopy Fluid should not be instilled in patients known to be hypersensitive to dextran. All other contraindications are those relative to the hysteroscopic procedure itself, such as pregnancy, endometrial carcinoma, etc.
Warnings: It is not known to what extent systemic absorption of dextran 70 occurs from the uterine and peritoneal cavities. Because of the possibility that absorption can occur, the physician should familiarize himself with the systemic effects of this drug. The most alarming are severe, sometimes fatal anaphylactoid reactions, which are quite rare. Other noteworthy effects include plasma volume expansion and transient prolongation of bleeding time.
Adverse Reactions: The physician should be mindful of the fact that adverse reactions are known to occur with the administration of dextran 70. Such reactions, some of which have also been reported with the use of HYSKON, have included: allergic phenomena (generalized itching, macular rash, anaphylactoid reactions, urticaria, nasal congestion, wheezing, tightness of chest and mild hypotension), nausea, vomiting, fever and joint pains.
Dosage and Administration: The amount of HYSKON Hysteroscopy Fluid required per patient depends on a number of factors, such as the type and length of the diagnostic procedure, whether or not manipulation or surgery is performed, etc. Most often, however, the amount of HYSKON instilled into the uterus will be between 50 and 100 milliliters.
HYSKON should be introduced into the uterine cavity through the cannula of a hysteroscope under low pressure (approximately 100 mm Hg) until the uterus is sufficiently distended to permit adequate visualization. During the hysteroscopic examination, HYSKON should be infused at a rate that keeps the cavity suitably distended. To avoid injection of the fluid into the tissues of the uterus and parametria and to avoid having unnecessary amounts of the fluid pass into the peritoneal cavity and backwards along the side of the hysteroscope, infusion pressures greater than 150 mm Hg should not be used.
How Supplied: HYSKON Hysteroscopy Fluid (32% W/V dextran 70 in 10% W/V dextrose) is available as a sterile, nonpyrogenic solution in 100 ml bottles packed 12 to a carton..................................NDC No. 0016-0231-61.
and 250 ml bottles packed 6 to a carton.........
....NDC No. 0016-0231-62
Keep from cold during transportation.
Caution: Federal law restricts this device to sale by or on the order of a physician.
Revised February 1982

MACRODEX® ℞
(Plasma Volume Expander)

6% Dextran 70 in 5% Dextrose Injection. 500 ml.
6% Dextran 70 in 0.9% Sodium Chloride Injection. 500 ml.

RHEOMACRODEX® ℞
(low molecular weight dextran)

10% Dextran 40 in 5% Dextrose Injection. 500 ml.
10% Dextran 40 in 0.9% Sodium Chloride Injection. 500 ml.

The following products which are manufactured by KabiVitrum AB, Stockholm, Sweden, are distributed in the U.S.A. by Pharmacia under license from KabiVitrum AB.
We will be pleased to answer all inquiries and send full prescribing information upon request.

CRESCORMON® ℞
somatropin
Sterile powder 4 IU/vial

How Supplied:
Crescormon® is supplied as a 4 IU (approx. 2 mg) vial of lyophilized, sterile somatropin; no preservative is included. Each vial of Crescormon is accompanied by a 2 ml sterile ampule of Sodium Chloride Injection. Each carrier carton contains ten combined packages of Crescormon and Sodium Chloride Injection.
NDC No: 00016-8050-1
Revision date Jan. 1982

KABIKINASE® ℞
(Streptokinase)

How Supplied: KABIKINASE® (streptokinase) is supplied as a lyophilized powder in 5 ml vials containing 250,000, 600,000, or 750,000 IU per vial of purified streptokinase, and shipped in cartons containing 10 vials.
In each vial there is a 10% overfill above that stated on the label. Each vial also contains 11.0 mg of Sodium L-Glutamate per 100,000 IU of streptokinase and 14.5 mg of Albumin Human per 100,000 IU of streptokinase as stabilizers.
250,000 IU **NDC** 00016-8025-2
600,000 IU **NDC** 00016-8026-2
750,000 IU **NDC** 00016-8027-2

SECRETIN-KABI ℞
secretin

How Supplied: Secretin-Kabi is supplied as a lyophilized sterile powder in 10 ml vials containing 75 CU. Each box contains 5 vials Secretin-Kabi 75 CU. Secretin-Kabi 75 CU should be stored at −20°C. (freezer). However, the biological activity of Secretin-Kabi will not be significantly decreased by storage at 25°C or below for up to 3 weeks. Expiration date is marked on the label.
NDC 00016-075-05
Revision date Jan. 1982

Products are cross-indexed by generic and chemical names in the

YELLOW SECTION

Pharmacraft Division
PENNWALT CORPORATION
755 JEFFERSON ROAD
ROCHESTER, NY 14623

ALLEREST® Tablets, Childrens Chewable Tablets and Headache Strength Tablets

(See PDR For Nonprescription Drugs)

ALLEREST® Timed Release Allergy Capsules

(See PDR For Nonprescription Drugs)

CaldeCORT®
Hydrocortisone Multi-Purpose Anti-Itch Cream, Spray, Ointment and Towlettes

(See PDR For Nonprescription Drugs)

CALDESENE® Medicated Ointment

(See PDR For Nonprescription Drugs)

CALDESENE® Medicated Baby Powder

(See PDR For Nonprescription Drugs)

CRUEX®
Antifungal Cream

(See PDR For Nonprescription Drugs)

CRUEX®
Antifungal Powder

(See PDR For Nonprescription Drugs)

DESENEX® Antifungal Products

(See PDR For Nonprescription Drugs)

DESENEX® Antifungal Spray Powder

(See PDR For Nonprescription Drugs)

SINAREST® Tablets

(See PDR For Nonprescription Drugs)

Wm. P. Poythress & Co. Incorporated
16 N. 22nd ST.
POST OFFICE BOX 26946
RICHMOND, VA 23261

ANTROCOL® ℞
TABLETS AND CAPSULES

Composition: Each tablet or capsule contains atropine sulfate, 0.195 mg.; phenobarbital, 16 mg. (Warning: may be habit-forming); blended for even absorption.
Action and Uses: Antrocol provides the prompt and predictable antispasmodic and antisecretory actions of atropine, blended for mild sedation. In peptic ulcer the ratio of stronger than usual parasympatholytic to sedative activity in Antrocol permits effective lowering of the gastric acid titer without exceeding optimal mild continuous sedation. In addition to the treatment of peptic ulcer, Antrocol is useful in correcting many digestive disturbances and is also effective in preventing recurrence of ulcer.
Dosage: 2 to 8 tablets or capsules per day as indicated. Functional gastro-intestinal spasms: One tablet or capsule after each meal. Peptic Ulcer: To obtain the desired antisecretory effect, dosage up to 8 tablets or capsules per day. Prophylactic: One tablet or capsule after the morning and evening meal is usually sufficient to help prevent recurrence of ulcer.

Side Effects: Toxic levels of atropine may produce flushing, dryness of mouth, cycloplegia, tachycardia and urinary retention.
Precautions: Use cautiously in prostatic hypertrophy. Do not use in glaucoma.
How Supplid: Tablets in bottles of 100, 500. Capsules in bottles of 100, 500.
[*Shown in Product Identification Section*]

ANTROCOL® ELIXIR ℞

A Sugar-free Antisecretory—Sedative

Composition: Each 1 cc contains atropine sulate 0.039 mg., phenobarbital (Warning: may be habit-forming) 3 mg., and 20% alcohol (v/v) in a citrus flavored—artifically colored elixir.
Caution: Federal law prohibits dispensing without prescription.
Actions and Uses: Antrocol Elixir provides the prompt and predictable antispasmodic and antisecretory action of the belladonna alkaloid, atropine, in a stronger than usual ratio with phenobarbital, permitting effective spasmolysis without exceeding optimal mild sedation. Antrocol Elixir is indicated for the symptomatic relief of colic, pylorospasm and a wide range of functional gastrointestinal disturbances. In peptic ulcer the ratio of stronger than usual parasympatholytic to sedative activity in Antrocol permits effective lowering of the gastric acid titer without exceeding optimal mild continuous sedation.
Contraindicated in glaucoma.
Dosage (average): 0.5 cc for each 15 lbs of body weight. 5 cc (1 teaspoonful) is the average adult dose. May be repeated 3 to 4 times daily.
Suggested Average Pediatric Dosage:
(Clark's Rule)

Weight of Child	Dosage
15 lbs.	0.5 cc (10 drops)
30 lbs.	1 cc (20 drops)
45 lbs.	1.5 cc (30 drops)
60 lbs.	2 cc
90 lbs.	3 cc

Side Effects: Toxic levels of atropine may produce flushing, dryness of the mouth, cycloplegia, tachycardia and urinary retention.
Precautions: Use cautiously in prostatic hypertrophy. Do not use in glaucoma.
How Supplied: 1 pint and 1 fl. oz. (30 cc) dropper bottles in individual printed cartons with individually wrapped droppers calibrated from 0.5 cc to 1 cc.

BENSULFOID® ℞

Composition: Issued in 130 mg. tablets and in powder form, Bensulfoid is a fusion, 33% by weight, of a highly reactive sulfur onto colloidal bentonite. The particles of Bensulfoid (300 mesh) consist of tiny disks of bentonite on which sulfur is adsorbed on the laminar structure. The distinctive manufacturing process of Bensulfoid produces a finely-divided physical complex, colloidal in nature, which possesses the gelforming and adsorbing properties of bentonite. This is accomplished by fusing one part of precipitated sulfur, U.S.P., with two parts of bentonite, U.S.P., in an electrically heated blending reactor. The resulting sulfur-coated bentonite particles are as finely divided as bentonite, and they retain all of the physical properties of bentonite. In addition, the chemical reactivity of the sulfur is increased many times. In contrast to bentonite, which has a pH of 9, the pH of Bensulfoid is close to neutral, and its adsorption is based on its finely divided state rather than on ion exchange.
Action and Uses: Bensulfoid has many physical properties that are useful in prescription compounding. When combined with oral medications Bensulfoid acts as a dispersing agent and carrier for the active drugs. Its affinity for neutral drug molecules in aqueous mixtures is greater than that of bentonite, but it readily releases these drugs to physiologically absorbing surfaces. This promotes more even drug absorption. When taken orally the sulfur exerts practically no pharmacological effect in the recommended dosage. It is absorbed as sulfide and oxidized to sulfate. Its sulfur is converted into soluble sulfides 40 times faster than precipitated sulfur. Topical prescriptions should not contain more than 8.5% Bensulfoid and its use should be discontinued if skin irritation develops.
How Supplied: Powder, 1-ounce bottles. Tablets, bottles of 100. Each tablet contains 130 mg. of Bensulfoid.

BENSULFOID® LOTION

(See PDR For Nonprescription Drugs)

LODRANE 130 TABLETS ℞
LODRANE 260 TABLETS ℞

(theophylline anhydrous)

Description: Lodrane 130 and Lodrane 260: Each tablet contains 130 mg. or 260 mg. of theophylline anhydrous in a sustained release bead formulation.
Indications: For relief and/or prevention of symptoms from asthma and reversible bronchospasm associated with chronic bronchitis and emphysema.
Contraindications: In individuals who have shown hypersensitivity to any of its components.
Warnings: Status asthmaticus is a medical emergency. Optimal therapy frequently requires additional medication including corticosteroids when the patient is not rapidly responsive to bronchodilators.
Excessive theophylline doses may be associated with toxicity thus serum theophylline levels are recommended to assure maximal benefit without excessive risk. Incidence of toxicity increases at levels greater than 20 mcg/ml. Morphine, curare, and stilbamidine should be used with caution in patients with airflow obstruction since they stimulate histamine release and can induce asthmatic attacks. They may also suppress respiration leading to respiratory failure. Alternative drugs should be chosen whenever possible.
There is an excellent correlation between high blood levels of theophylline resulting from conventional doses and associated clinical manifestations of toxicity in (1) patients with lowered body plasma clearances (due to transient cardiac decomposition), (2) patients with liver dysfunction or chronic obstructive lung disease, (3) patients who are older than 55 years of age, particularly males.
There are often no early signs of less serious theophylline toxicity such as nausea and restlessness, which may appear in up to 50 percent of patients prior to onset of convulsions. Ventricular arrhythmias or seizures may be the first signs of toxicity.
Usage in Pregnancy: Safe use in pregnancy has not been established relative to possible adverse effects on fetal development, but neither have adverse effects on fetal development been established. This is, unfortunately, true for most antiasthmatic medications. Therefore, use of theophylline in pregnant women should be balanced against the risk of uncontrolled asthma.
Precautions: Mean half-life in smokers is shorter than non-smokers, therefore, smokers may require larger doses of theophylline. Theophylline should not be administered concurrently with other xanthine medications. Use with caution in patients with severe cardiac disease, severe hypoxemia, hypertension, hyperthyroidism, acute myocardial injury, cor pulmonale, congestive heart failure, liver disease, and in the elderly (especially males) and neonates. Great caution should especially be used in giving theophylline to patients in congestive heart failure. Such patients have shown markedly prolonged theophylline blood level curves with theophylline persisting in serum for long periods following discontinuation of the drug.
Use theophylline cautiously in patients with history of peptic ulcer. Theophylline may occasionally act as a local irritant to G.I. tract although gastrointestinal symptoms are more commonly central and associated with serum concentrations over 20 mcg/ml.
Adverse Reactions: The most consistent adverse reactions are usually due to overdose and are:

1. Gastrointestinal: nausea, vomiting, epigastric pain, hematemesis, diarrhea.
2. Central nervous system: headaches, irritability, restlessness, insomnia, reflex hyperexcitability, muscle twitching, clonic and tonic generalized convulsions.
3. Cardiovascular: palpitation, tachycardia, extra systoles, flushing, hypotension, circulatory failure, life threatening ventricular arrhythmias.
4. Respiratory: tachypnea.
5. Renal: albuminuria, increased excretion of renal tubular potentiation or diuresis, and red blood cells.
6. Others: hyperglycemia and inappropriate ADH syndrome.

Dosage and Administration: Therapeutic serum levels associated with optimal likelihood for benefit and minimal risk of toxicity are considered to be between 10 mcg/ml and 20 mcg/ml. Levels above 20 mcg/ml may produce toxic effects. There is great variation from patient to patient in dosage needed in order to achieve a therapeutic blood level because of variable rates of elimination. Because of this wide variation from patient to patient, and the relatively narrow therapeutic blood level range, dosage must be individualized and monitoring of theophylline serum levels is highly recommended.
Dosage should be calculated on the basis of lean (ideal) body weight where mg/kg doses are stated. Theophylline does not distribute into fatty tissue.
Giving theophylline with food may prevent the rare case of stomach irritation; and though absorption may be slower, it is still complete. When rapidly absorbed products such as solutions are used, dosing to maintain "around the clock" blood levels generally requires administration every 6 hours to obtain the greatest efficacy for clinical use in children; dosing intervals up to 8 hours may be satisfactory for adults because of their slower elimination. Children, and adults requiring higher than average doses, may benefit from products with slower absorption which may allow longer dosing intervals and/or less fluctuation in serum concentration over a dosing interval during chronic therapy.
[See table on next page].
The loading dose for theophylline will be based on the principle that each .5 mg/kg of theophylline administered as a loading dose will result in a 1 mcg/ml increase in serum theophylline concentration. Ideally, then, the loading dose should be deferred if a serum theophylline concentration can be rapidly obtained. If this is not possible, the clinician must exercise his judgment in selecting a dose based on the potential for benefit and risk. When there is sufficient respiratory distress to warrant a small risk, 2.5 mg/kg of theophylline is likely to increase the serum concentration when administered as a loading dose in rapidly absorbed form by only about 5 mcg/ml. If the patient is not already experiencing theophylline toxicity, this is unlikely to result in dangerous adverse effects.
Subsequent to the modified decision regarding loading dose in this group of patients, the sub-

Continued on next page

Poythress—Cont.

sequent maintenance dosage recommendations are the same as those described above.
Comments: To achieve optimal therpeutic theophylline dosage, it is recommended to monitor serum theophylline concentrations. However, it is not always possible or practical to obtain a serum theophylline level.
Patients should be closely monitored for signs of toxicity. The present data suggest that the above dosage recommendations will achieve therapeutic serum concentrations with minimal risk of toxicity for most patients. However, some risk of toxic serum concentrations is still present.
Adverse reactions to theophylline often occur when serum theophylline levels exceed 20 mcg/ml.
Chronic Asthma:
Theophyllinization is a treatment of first choice for the management of chronic asthma (to prevent symptoms and maintain patent airways). Slow clinical titration is generally preferred to assure acceptance and safety of the medication.
Initial dose: 60 mg/kg/day or 400 mg/day (whichever is lower) in 3–4 divided doses at 6–8 hour intervals. (520 mg/day in 1–2 divided doses at 12 hour intervals for sustained release formulations).
Increased dose: The above dosage may be increased in approximately 25 percent increments at 2–3 day intervals so long as no intolerance is observed, until the maximum indicated below is reached.
Maximum dose without measurement of serum concentrations: Not to exceed the following: (WARNING: DO NOT ATTEMPT TO MAINTAIN ANY DOSE THAT IS NOT TOLERATED)
Age 9 years—24 mg/kg/day
Age 9–12 years—20 mg/kg/day
Age 12–16 years—18 mg/kg/day
Age 16 years—13 mg/kg/day
or 900 mg/day (WHICHEVER IS LESS)
Note: Use ideal body weight for obese patients.
Measurement of serum theophylline concentration during chronic therapy:
If the above maximum doses are to be maintained or exceeded, serum theophylline measurement is recommended. This should be obtained at the approximate time of peak absorption during chronic therapy for the product (1–2 hours for liquids, 3–5 hours for sustained release preparations). It is important that the patient will have missed no doses during the previous 48 hours and that dosing intervals will have been reasonably typical with no added doses during that period of time. DOSAGE ADJUSTMENT BASED ON SERUM THEOPHYLLINE MEASUREMENTS WHEN THESE INSTRUCTIONS HAVE NOT BEEN FOLLOWED MAY RESULT IN RECOMMENDATIONS THAT PRESENT RISK OF TOXICITY TO THE PATIENT.

How Supplied: Lodrane 130 Tablets and Lodrane 260 Tablets. Supplied in bottles of 100 and 1000 tablets.
[*Shown in Product Identification Section*]

MUDRANE® Tablets ℞

Composition: Each tablet contains potassium iodide, 195 mg.; aminophylline (anhydrous), 130 mg.; phenobarbital, 8 mg. (Warning: may be habit-forming); ephedrine HCl, 16 mg.
Indications: A bronchodilator-mucolytic, Mudrane gives prompt symptomatic relief in bronchial asthma, emphysema and asthmatic bronchitis. Mudrane dilates the bronchi, liquefies the mucus plugs. The stability of Mudrane has been achieved without coating the potassium iodide; thus all the components in the fast-disintegrating tablet begin their actions promptly. The phenobarbital in slight excess of ephedrine minimizes the side-effect of nervousness. Mudrane is buffered for gastric tolerance.
Contraindications: *Aminophylline/theopylline* is contraindicated in the presence of severe cardiac arrhythmias in patients with massive myocardial damage. *Ephedrine* is contraindicated in the presence of severe heart disease, severe hypertension and in hyperthyroidism. *Phenobarbital* is contraindicated in porphyria and in patients with known phenobarbital sensitivity. *Potassium iodide* is contraindicated in pregnancy (to protect the fetus against possible iodide-induced depression of thyroid activity), in tuberculosis (produces gumma dissolution), and in acne; also, in the presence of known iodide sensitivity.
Precautions: *Aminophylline/theophylline* should be avoided in patients with massive myocardial damage and/or severe cardiac arrhythmias, and severe agitation. *Ephedrine* should be used with caution in the presence of severe cardiac disease, particularly arrhythmias and angina pectoris, it should be avoided in hyperthyroidism and severe hypertension. *Phenobarbial* may be habit-forming. Avoid overdosage. *Potassium iodide:* Discontinue in the presence of skin rash, swelling of the eyelids, or severe frontal headache. Long use may cause goiter.
Adverse Reactions: *Aminophylline/theophylline* may cause cardiac arrhythmias and aggravate severe myocardial disease; may cause headaches and tachycardia; vomiting and dizziness are not uncommon. *Ephedrine* may cause nervousness, tachycardia, extrasystole and ventricular arrhythmias in patients hypersensitive to CNS stimulation. Also, ephedrine may cause urinary retention, especially in the presence of partial prostatic obstruction. Psychoneurosis may be aggravated. Pre-existing anginal pain will be aggravated. *Phenobarbital* may produce severe skin rash; avoid overdosage; may be habit-forming. *Potassium iodide* may cause nausea; over very long period of use, iodides may cause goiter. Discontinue if patient developes skin rash, eye irritation, eyelid swelling or severe frontal headache.

DOSAGE FOR PATIENT POPULATION

Acute Symptoms of Asthma Requiring Rapid Theophyllinization:
I. Not currently receiving theophylline products

GROUP	ORAL LOADING DOSE (THEOPHYLLINE)	MAINTENANCE DOSE FOR NEXT 12 HOURS (THEOPHYLLINE)	MAINTENANCE DOSE BEYOND 12 HOURS (THEOPHYLLINE)
1. Children 6 months to 9 years	6 mg/kg	4 mg/kg q4h	4 mg/kg q6h
2. Children age 9–16 and smoking young adults	6 mg/kg	3 mg/kg q4h	3 mg/kg q6h
3. Otherwise healthy	6 mg/kg	3 mg/kg q6h	3 mg/kg q8h
4. Older adults and patients with cor pulmonale	6 mg/kg	2 mg/kg q6h	2 mg/kg q8h
5. Patients with congestive heart failure, liver failure	6 mg/kg	2 mg/kg q8h	1–2 mg/kg q12h

II. Those currently receiving theophylline products: Determine, where possible, the time, amount, route of administration and form of the patient's last dose.

Dosage: One tablet with full glass of water, 3 or 4 times daily, as required. Divide tablet for child's dose.
How Supplied: Mudrane Yellow scored tablets in bottles or 100 and 1,000.
[*Shown in Product Identification Section*]

MUDRANE®-2 TABLETS ℞

Composition: Each tablet contains potassium iodide 195 mg. aminophylline (anhydrous) 130 mg.
Indications: When ephedrine is too exciting or contraindicated, Mudrane-2 gives prompt symptomatic relief in asthma, emphysema and asthmatic bronchitis through its bronchodilator-mucolytic actions. The stability of Mudrane-2 has been achieved without coating the potassium iodide; thus the components in the fast disintegrating tablet begin their actions promptly.
Contraindications: Precautions: Adverse Reactions: See under Mudrane tablets above, as listed for aminophylline/theophylline and potassium iodide.
Dosage: One tablet with full glass of water, 3 or 4 times daily.
How Supplied: White scored tablets in bottles of 100.
[*Shown in Product Identification Section*]

MUDRANE® GG TABLETS ℞

Compositions: Each tablet contains aminophylline (anhydrous), 130 mg.; ephedrine HCl, 16mg.; phenobarbital, 8 mg. (Warning: may be habit-forming); Guaifenesin, 100 mg.
Indications: Same as Mudrane, EXCEPT Guaifenesin, 100 mg. replaces potassium iodide as a mucolytic-expectorant. Mudrane GG should be prescribed when acne or tuberculosis co-exist, during pregnancy, or when iodide intolerance is present. In emphysema, requiring constant Mudrane therapy, Mudrane GG may be substituted every fourth week to reduce the possibility of iodide sensitivity.
Contraindications: Precautions: Adverse Reactions: See under Mudrane tablets above as listed for aminophylline/theophylline, ephedrine HCl, and phenobarbital.
Dosage: One tablet with full glass of water, 3 or 4 times daily.
How Supplied: Yellow, mottled, GG embossed tablets in bottles of 100 and 1,000
[*Shown in Product Identification Section*]

MUDRANE® GG-2 TABLETS ℞

Composition: Each tablet contains aminophylline (anhydrous), 130 mg.; Guaifenesin, 100 mg.
Indications: When ephedrine is too exciting or contraindicated, Mudrane GG-2 gives prompt symptomatic relief in asthma, emphysema and asthmatic bronchitis through its bronchodilator-mucolytic actions.
Contraindications: Precautions: Adverse Reactions: See under Mudrane tablets above, as listed for aminophylline/theophylline.
Dosage: One tablet with full glass of water, 3 or 4 times daily.
How Supplied: Green, mottled, GG embossed tablets in bottles of 100.
[*Shown in Product Identification Section*]

MUDRANE® GG ELIXIR ℞

Composition: Each 5 ml teaspoonful contains theophylline, 20 mg.; ephedrine HCl, 4 mg.; phenobarbital 2.5 mg. (Warning: may be habit-forming); Guaifenesin, 26 mg. The theophylline in the Elixir is in solution. (The theophylline in the tablet is supplied by aminophylline for prompt solubility from the rapid-disintegrating, uncoated tablet. Preserved with 0.1% paraben. Contains 20% alcohol.
Indications: Mudrane GG Elixir is a sugar-free bronchodilator-mucolytic especially for-

mulated for pediatric use. Mudrane GG Elixir supplies the active ingredients of Mudrane GG tablets for the relief of asthma and asthmatic bronchitis.
Contraindications: Precautions: Adverse Reactions: See under Mudrane tablets above, as listed for aminophylline/theophylline, ephedrine HCl, and phenobarbital.
Dosage: Children, 1 ml for each 10 lbs. of body weight; one teaspoonful for 50 lb. child. May be repeated 3 or 4 times daily. Adult, one tablespoonful, 3 or 4 times daily. All doses should be followed with water.
How Supplied: A red liquid in pints and one-half gallon bottles.

PANALGESIC

Composition: Methyl salicylate, 55%; aspirin, 5%; menthol and camphor, 2%; emollient oils, 20%; alcohol, 18% by weight.
Action and Uses: Panalgesic, an external application for relief of superficial aches and pains, supplies salicylates in the proper environment for maximum skin absorption, producing counterirritation, analgesia,local anesthesia, and asepsis. Panalgesic lessens the discomfort of muscular fatigue, and of trauma, and increases the blood level of salicylate by dermal absorption.
Method of Application: Apply externally to affected area with a gentle massage 3 or 4 times daily.
Warning: Do not use otherwise than as directed. Keep out of reach of children to avoid accidental poisoning. Discontinue use if excessive irritation of the skin develops. Avoid getting into eyes or on mucous membrane.
How Supplied: 4-ounce; 1-pint; one-half gallon bottles.

SOLFOTON® TABLETS, CAPSULES, AND S/C (SUGAR-COATED) TABLETS ©

Composition: Each tablet or capsule contains phenobarbital, 16 mg. (Warning: may be habit-forming). Blended for even absorption.
Action and Uses: Solfoton is safe for maintaining mild continuous sedation over long periods. No bizarre physical or psychic states nor reduced effectiveness have been noted following prolonged use. The mild continuous sedation of Solfoton therapy will help in creating empathy with the patient preparatory to outlining a health plan. Solfoton is the ideal clinical approach to frequently encountered mild chronic anxiety states—it subtly blunts and normalizes the hyper-reactive CNS to environmental stimuli.
Administration and Dosage: One tablet or capsule at 6-hour intervals will usually maintain sedation at the threshold of calmness.
Side Effects: Identical to those of 16 mg. phenobarbital.
How Supplied: Uncoated tablets: bottles of 100, 500, 5,000. Tablets S./C: bottles 100, 500. Capsules: bottles 100, 500.
[*Shown in Product Identification Section*]

TROCINATE ℞
(Thiphenamil hydrochloride)

Description: Trocinate, chemically, is 2-diethylaminoethyldiphenylthioacetate hydrochloride. Trocinate may be dispensed only upon the prescription of a physician. Trocinate is manufactured by Wm. P. Poythress and Company, Incorporated, Richmond, Virginia, and has been marketed since 1950.
Actions: Trocinate is a potent antispasmodic and smooth muscle relaxant that acts like papaverine on smooth muscle. Trocinate exerts a strong local anesthetic effect on contact with mucous membranes.

INDICATIONS
Trocinate is indicated for relief of smooth muscle spasm.
In Gastroenterology: for relief of pain and discomfort due to smooth muscle spasm associated with spastic colitis, irritable colon, mucous colitis, acute enterocolitis, and functional gastrointestinal disorders.
LIMITATIONS OF EFFECTIVENESS
On the basis of the opinions of the National Academy of Science and National Research Council Committees and other information, the Food and Drug Administration considers this drug to be limited in its effectiveness, as follows:
Probably effective, as follows: May be useful in the irritable bowel syndrome (irritable colon, spastic colon, mucous colitis, acute enterocolitis, and functional gastrointestinal disorders); and in neurogenic bowel disturbances (including the splenic flexure syndrome and neurogenic colon).
To be effective the dosage must be titrated to the individual patient's needs.

Contraindications: Trocinate is contraindicated in obstructive uropathy (for example, bladder neck obstruction due to prostatic hypertrophy); obstructive disease of the gastrointestinal tract (as in achalasia, paralytic ileus, pyloroduodenal stenosis, etc.); intestinal atony of elderly or debilitated patient; severe ulcerative colitis; toxic megacolon complicating ulcerative colitis; myasthenia gravis.
Warnings: Use in Pregnancy—The safety of the use of Trocinate during pregnancy has not been established.
Diarrhea may be an early symptom of incomplete intestinal obstruction, especially in patients with ileostomy or colostomy. In this instance treatment with this drug may be inappropriate and possibly harmful.
Dosage and Administration: Adult: Initially, 400 milligrams. May be repeated four hours later. Trocinate acts very promptly and, when effective, relieves discomfort with two to four doses. Relief may usually be maintained with reduced frequency of dosage.
The safety and efficacy of Trocinate in children has not been determined, and Trocinate should not be administered to children.
Management of Overdosage: In twenty years of usage of Trocinate, side-effects have been so very infrequent that no typical symptoms and physical signs of overdosage have become known. Skin rash, mild hypotension and colicky abdominal pain when observed have rapidly disappeared with stoppage of the drug.
How Supplied:
400 mg. branded, pink sugar-coated tablets
Bottles of 25's........................NDC 95-0029-26
Bottles of 100's......................NDC 95-0029-01
100 mg. branded, pink sugar-coated tablets
Bottles of 100's......................NDC 95-0028-01
Bottles of 500's......................NDC 95-0028-05
[*Shown in Product Identification Section*]

URO-PHOSPHATE TABLETS ℞
(Methenamine, sodium acid phosphate)

Protect from Heat. Store at room temperature 60°–75°F

Description: Uro-Phosphate, a urinary antibacterial agent, is the combination of methenamine 300 mg. and sodium acid phosphate 500 mg. supplied in a white sugar-coated tablet.
Actions: Methenamine is readily absorbed from the gastrointestinal tract but remains essentially inactive until concentrated and excreted by the kidney in an acid urine where hydrolysation produces antibacterial formaldehyde. An acid urine is essential for the conversion of methenamine to antibacterial formaldehyde with the maximum efficacy occurring at pH 5.5 or less. Methenamine alone may be ineffective in some infections with Proteus vulgaris and urea-splitting strains of Pseudomonas aeruginosa and A. aerogenes as they may raise the pH of the urine inhibiting formaldehyde formation. Sodium acid phosphate, a natural urine acidifier, generally provides urine pH at an acid level conducive to formaldehyde production. Results in any individual case will depend on dosage, underlying pathology and overall management.
Indications: Uro-Phosphate (methenamine and sodium acid phosphate) is indicated for suppressive or prophylactic treatment of chronic bacteriuria associated with pyelonephritis, cystitis, significant residual urine accompanying some neurological diseases and with prolonged bladder catheterization. The safety and nonspecific bacteriacidal effect of formaldehyde does not lead to bacterial resistance to Uro-Phosphate.
Contraindications: Renal insufficiency, severe dehydration or acidosis. Methenamine preparations should not be given patients taking sulfonamides since formaldehyde may form an insoluble precipitate with some sulfonamides in urine.
Warning: Safe use in pregnancy is not established.
Precautions: Large doses of methenamine (8 grams daily for 3 to 4 weeks) have caused bladder irritation, painful and frequent micturition, albuminures and gross hematuria. Care should be taken to maintain an acid pH of the urine especially when treating infections due to urea-splitting pathogens such as Proteus and strains of Pseudomonas.
Adverse Reactions: Minor adverse reactions have been reported in fewer than 3.5% of patients treated. These reactions have included nausea, upset stomach, dysuria and rash.
Dosage and Administration: 1 or 2 tablets at 4 to 6 hour intervals is usually sufficient to maintain proper urine acidity. Two tablets on retiring will maintain comfort and lessen frequency when residual urine is present.
How Supplied: White sugar-coated tablets:
Bottles of 100's NDC 0095-0031-01
Bottles of 1000's NDC 0095-0031-10
Mfd. for Wm. P. Poythress Co., Inc., Richmond, Virginia 23261 by ICN Pharmaceuticals, Inc., Cincinnati, Ohio 45213
[*Shown in Product Identification Section*]

Procter & Gamble
P. O. BOX 171
CINCINNATI, OH 45201

DIDRONEL® ℞
(etidronate disodium)

Description: DIDRONEL tablets contain 200 mg of etidronate disodium, the disodium salt of (1-hydroxyethylidene) diphosphonic acid, for oral administration. This compound, also known as EHDP, regulates bone metabolism. It is a white powder, highly soluble in water, with a molecular weight of 250 and the following structural formula:

```
        ONa   OH   ONa
        |     |    |
   HO — P  —  C  — P — OH
        ↓     |    ↓
        O     CH3  O
```

Clinical Pharmacology: DIDRONEL acts primarily on bone. It can inhibit the formation, growth and dissolution of hydroxyapatite crystals and their amorphous percursors by chemisorption to calcium phosphate surfaces. Inhibition of crystal resorption occurs at lower doses than are required to inhibit crystal growth. Both effects increase as the dose increases.

Continued on next page

Procter & Gamble—Cont.

DIDRONEL is not metabolized. Absorption averages about 1% of an oral dose of 5 mg/kg body weight/day. This increases to about 2.5% at 10 mg/kg/day and 6% at 20 mg/kg/day. Most of the absorbed drug is cleared from the blood within 6 hours. Within 24 hours about half of the absorbed dose is excreted in the urine. The remainder is chemicaly adsorbed to bone, especially to areas of elevated osteogenesis, and is slowly eliminated. Unabsorbed drug is excreted intact in the feces.

DIDRONEL therapy does not adversely affect serum levels of parathyroid hormone or calcium. Hyperphosphatemia has been observed in DIDRONEL patients, usually in association with doses of 10–20 mg/kg/day. No adverse effects have been traced to this, and it is not a contraindication for therapy. It is apparently due to drug-related increased tubular reabsorption of phosphate by the kidney. Serum phosphate levels generally return to normal 2–4 weeks post-therapy.

PAGET'S DISEASE

Paget's disease of bone (osteitis deformans) is an idiopathic, progressive disease characterized by abnormal and accelerated bone metabolism in one or more bones. Signs and symptoms may include bone pain and/or deformity, neurologic disorders, elevated cardiac output and other vascular disorders, and increased serum alkaline phosphatase and/or urinary hydroxyproline levels. Bone fractures are common in patients with Paget's disease.

DIDRONEL slows accelerated bone turnover (resorption and accretion) in pagetic lesions and, to a lesser extent, in normal bone. This has been demonstrated histologically, scintigraphically, biochemically, and through calcium kinetic and balance studies. Reduced bone turnover is often accompanied by symptomatic improvement, including reduced bone pain. Also, the incidence of pagetic fractures may be reduced, and elevated cardiac output and other vascular disorders may be improved by DIDRONEL therapy.

HETEROTOPIC OSSIFICATION

Heterotopic ossification, also referred to as myositis ossificans (circumscripta, progressiva or traumatica), ectopic calcification, periarticular ossification, or paraosteoarthropathy, is characterized by metaplastic osteogenesis. It usually presents with signs of localized inflammation or pain, elevated skin temperature, and redness. When tissues near joints are involved, functional loss may also be present.

Heterotopic ossification may occur for no known reason as in myositis ossificans progressiva or may follow a wide variety of surgical, occupational, and sports trauma (e.g., hip arthroplasty, spinal cord injury, head injury, burns and severe thigh bruises). Heterotropic ossification has also been observed in non-traumatic conditions (e.g., infections of the central nervous system, peripheral neuropathy, tetanus, biliary cirrhosis, Peyronie's disease, as well as in association with a variety of benign and malignant neoplasms).

Clinical trials have demonstrated the efficacy of Didronel in heterotropic ossification following total hip replacement, or due to spinal cord injury.

—*Heterotopic ossification complicating total hip replacement* typically develops radiographically 3–8 weeks post-operatively in the pericapsular area of the affected hip joint. The overall incidence is about 50%; about one-third of these cases are clinically significant.

—*Heterotopic ossification due to spinal cord injury* typically develops radiographically 1–4 months after injury. It occurs below the level of injury, usually at major joints. The overall incidence is about 40%; about one-half of these cases are clinically significant.

DIDRONEL chemisorbs to calcium hydroxyapatite crystals and their amorphous precursors, blocking the aggregation, growth and mineralization of these crystals. This is thought to be the mechanism by which DIDRONEL prevents or retards heterotopic ossification. There is no evidence DIDRONEL affects mature heterotopic bone.

Indications and Usage:

PAGET'S DISEASE

DIDRONEL is indicated for the treatment of symptomatic Paget's disease of bone.

DIDRONEL therapy usually arrests or significantly impedes the disease process as evidenced by:

—Symptomatic relief, including decreased pain and/or increased mobility (experienced by 3 out of 5 patients).

—Reductions in serum alkaline phosphatase and urinary hydroxyproline levels (30% or more in 4 out of 5 patients).

—Histomorphometry showing reduced numbers of osteoclasts and osteoblasts, and more lamellar bone formation.

—Bone scans showing reduced radionuclide uptake at pagetic lesions.

In addition, reductions in pagetically elevated cardiac output and skin temperature have been observed in some patients. Also, the incidence of pagetic fractures may be reduced when DIDRONEL is administered intermittently over a period of years.

In many patients, the disease process will be suppressed for a period of at least one year following cessation of therapy. The upper limit of this period has not been determined.

DIDRONEL's effects have not been studied in patients with asymptomatic Paget's disease. However, DIDRONEL treatment of such patients may be warranted if extensive involvement threatens irreversible neurologic damage, major joints, or major weight-bearing bones.

HETEROTOPIC OSSIFICATION

DIDRONEL is indicated in the prevention and treatment of heterotopic ossification following total hip replacement or due to spinal cord injury.

DIDRONEL reduces the incidence of clinically important heterotopic bone by about two-thirds. Among those patients who form heterotopic bone, DIDRONEL retards the progression of immature lesions and reduces the severity by at least half. Follow-up data (at least nine months post-therapy) suggest these benefits persist.

In total hip replacement patients, DIDRONEL does not promote loosening of the prosthesis or impede trochanteric reattachment.

In spinal cord injury patients, DIDRONEL does not inhibit fracture healing or stabilization of the spine.

Contraindications: None known.

Warnings: ***In Paget's patients*** the response to therapy may be of slow onset and continue for months after DIDRONEL therapy is discontinued. Dosage should not be increased prematurely. A 90-day drug-free interval should be provided between courses of therapy.

Heterotopic ossification: No specific warnings.

Precautions:

General. Patients should maintain an adequate nutritional status, particularly an adequate intake of calcium and vitamin D.

Therapy has been withheld from some patients with enterocolitis since diarrhea may be experienced, particularly at higher doses.

DIDRONEL is not metabolized and is excreted intact via the kidney. There is no experience to specifically guide treatment in patients with impaired renal function. DIDRONEL dosage should be reduced when reductions in glomerular filtration rates are present. Patients with renal impairment should be closely monitored.

DIDRONEL suppresses bone turnover, and may retard mineralization of osteoid laid down during the bone accretion process. These effects are dose and time dependent. Osteoid, which may accumulate noticeably at doses of 10–20 mg/kg/day, mineralizes normally post-therapy. In patients with fractures, especially of long bones, it may be advisable to delay or interrupt treatment until callus is evident.

Carcinogenesis. Long-term studies in rats have indicated that DIDRONEL is not carcinogenic.

Pregnancy: Teratogenic Effects. Pregnancy Category B.

Reproduction/teratology studies performed in rats and rabbits at doses up to five times the maximum human dose by the intended route of administration have revealed no evidence of impaired fertility or harm to the fetus due to DIDRONEL. At doses of twenty-two times the maximum human dose, a decrease in live fetuses were observed in rats. The only incidence of malformations occurred in rats at exaggerated doses following parenteral administration and were skeletal in nature. These malformations were deemed the result of the pharmacological action of the drug. There are no adequate, well-controlled studies in pregnant women. Because animal reproduction studies are not always predictive of human response, this drug should be used during pregnancy only if clearly needed.

Nursing Mothers. It is not known whether this drug is excreted in human milk. Because many drugs are excreted in human milk, caution should be exercised when DIDRONEL is administered to a nursing woman.

Pediatric Use. Safety and effectiveness in children have not been established.

Adverse Reactions: The incidence of gastrointestinal complaints (diarrhea, nausea) is the same for DIDRONEL at 5 mg/kg/day as for placebo, about 1 patient in 15. At 10–20 mg/kg/day the incidence may increase to 2 or 3 in 10. These complaints are often alleviated by dividing the total daily dose.

In Paget's patients increased or recurrent bone pain at pagetic sites, and/or the onset of pain at previously asymptomatic sites has been reported. At 5 mg/kg/day about 1 patient in 10 (versus 1 in 15 in the placebo group) report these phenomena. At higher doses the incidence rises to about 2 in 10. When therapy continues, pain resolves in some patients but persists in others.

Heterotopic ossification: No specific adverse reactions.

Overdosage: While there is no experience with acute overdosage, it is theoretically possible that enough DIDRONEL could be taken to result in hypocalcemia.

Dosage and Administration: DIDRONEL should be taken as a single, oral dose. However, should gastrointestinal discomfort occur, the dose may be divided. To maximize absorption, patients should avoid taking the following items within two hours of dosing:

—Food, especially those high in calcium, such as milk or milk products.

—Vitamins with mineral supplements or antacids which are high in metals such as calcium, iron, magnesium or aluminum.

PAGET'S DISEASE

Initial Treatment Regimens:

5–10 mg/kg/day, not to exceed 6 months, or

11–20 mg/kg/day, not to exceed 3 months.

The recommended initial dose is 5 mg/kg/day for a period not to exceed six months. Doses above 10 mg/kg/day should be reserved for when 1) lower doses are ineffective or 2) there is an overriding need to suppress rapid bone turnover (especially when irreversible neurologic damage is possible) or reduce elevated cardiac output. Doses in excess of 20 mg/kg/day are not recommended.

Retreatment Guidelines. Retreatment should be initiated only after: 1) a DIDRONEL-free period of at least 90 days and 2) there is biochemical, symptomatic or other evidence of active disease process. It is advisable to monitor patients every 3–6 months although some patients may go drug free for extended periods. Retreatment regimens are the same as for initial treatment. For most patients the original dose will be adequate for retreatment. If not, consideration should be given to increasing the dose within the recommended guidelines.

HETEROTOPIC OSSIFICATION

The following treatment regimens have been shown to be effective:

—*Total Hip Replacement Patients: 20 mg/kg/day for 1 month before and 3 months after surgery (4 months total).*

—*Spinal Cord Injured Patients: 20 mg/kg/day for 2 weeks followed by 10 mg/kg/day for 10 weeks (12 weeks total). DIDRONEL therapy should begin as soon as medically feasible following the injury, preferably prior to evidence of heterotopic ossification.*

Retreatment has not been studied.

How Supplied: Rectangular white 200 mg tablets with "P&G" on one face and "402" on the other, in bottles of 60.

Revised 7/82

Made in U.S.A. for PROCTOR & GAMBLE, Cincinnati, Ohio 45202 by KV Pharmaceutical Company, St. Louis, MO 63144

[*Shown in Product Identification Section*]

HEAD & SHOULDERS®

Antidandruff Shampoo

(See PDR For Nonprescription Drugs)

TOPICYCLINE® ℞

(tetracycline hydrochloride for topical solution)

Description: TOPICYCLINE is a topical antibiotic preparation containing 2.2 mg of tetracycline hydrochloride per ml as the active ingredient, as well as 4-epitetracycline hydrochloride and sodium bisulfite in an aqueous base of 40% ethanol, citric acid and n-decyl methyl sulfoxide.

Tetracycline is 4-(dimethylamino)-1,4,4a,5,5a, 6, 11, 12a-octahydro-3, 6, 10, 12, 12a-pentahydroxy-6-methyl-1, 11-dioxo-2-naphthacenecarboxamide, the structural formula of which is:

OH O OH OH O CONH₂ 10 11 12 1 2 9 8 7 6 5 4 3 OH HO CH₃ N(CH₃)₂

Clinical Pharmacology: TOPICYCLINE delivers tetracycline to the pilosebaceous apparatus and the adjacent tissues. TOPICYCLINE reduces inflammatory acne lesions, but its mode of action is not fully understood.

In clinical studies, use of TOPICYCLINE on the face and neck twice daily delivered to the skin an average dose of 2.9 mg of tetracycline hydrochloride per day. Patients who used the medication twice daily on other acne-involved areas in addition to the face and neck applied an average dose of 4.8 mg of tetracycline hydrochloride per day.

TOPICYCLINE has been formulated such that the recrystallization properties of the tetracyclines on the skin greatly reduce or eliminate the yellow color often associated with topical tetracycline.

Indications and Usage: TOPICYCLINE is indicated in the treatment of acne vulgaris.

Contraindications: TOPICYCLINE is contraindicated in persons who have shown hypersensitivity to any of its ingredients or to any of the other tetracyclines.

Precautions: This drug is for external use only and care should be taken to keep it out of the eyes, nose, and mouth.

A two-year dermal study in mice has been performed with TOPICYCLINE and indicates there is no carcinogenic potential with this drug.

Pregnancy Category B. Reproduction studies have been performed in rats and rabbits at doses of up to 246 times the human dose (assuming the human dose to be 1.3 ml/40kg/day) and have revealed no evidence of impaired fertility or harm to the fetus from TOPICYCLINE. There are, however, no adequate and well-controlled studies in pregnant women. Because animal reproduction studies are not always predictive of human response, this drug should be used during pregnancy only if clearly needed.

It is not known whether tetracycline or any other component of TOPICYCLINE administered in this topical form, is excreted in human milk. Because many drugs are excreted in human milk, caution should be exercised when TOPICYCLINE is administered to a nursing woman.

Safety and effectiveness in children below the age of eleven have not been established.

Adverse Reactions: Among the 838 patients treated with TOPICYCLINE under normal usage conditions during clinical evaluation, there was one instance of severe dermatitis requiring systemic steroid therapy.

About one-third of patients are likely to experience a stinging or burning sensation upon application of TOPICYCLINE. The sensation ordinarily lasts no more than a few minutes, and does not occur at every application. There has been no indication that patients experience sufficient discomfort to reduce the frequency of use or to discontinue use of the product.

The kinds of side effects often associated with oral or parenteral administration of tetracyclines (e.g., various gastrointestinal complaints, vaginitis, hematologic abnormalities, manifestations of systemic hypersensitivity reactions, and dental and skeletal disorders) have not been observed with TOPICYCLINE. Because of TOPICYCLINE's topical form of administration, it is highly unlikely that such side effects will occur from its use.

Dosage and Administration: It is recommended that TOPICYCLINE be applied generously twice-daily to the entire affected area (not just to individual lesions) until the skin is thoroughly wet. Instructions to the patient for proper application are provided on the TOPICYCLINE bottle label. Patients may continue their normal use of cosmetics.

Concomitant use with benzoyl peroxide or oral tetracycline has been reported without observed problems.

How Supplied: TOPICYCLINE is supplied in a single carton containing a powder and a liquid which must be combined prior to using. Complete instructions for mixing are provided on the carton.

Once combined, the TOPICYCLINE bottle contains 70 ml of medication. This constitutes about an eight-week supply for treating the face and neck, or about a four-week supply for treating the face, neck and additional acne-involved areas. Differences in individual usage habits will result in variation from these averages.

TOPICYCLINE should be kept at controlled room temperature or below.

Caution: Federal law prohibits dispensing without prescription.

NDC 37000-401-03

Made in U.S.A. for PROCTER & GAMBLE, Cincinnati, Ohio 45202 by Taylor Pharmacal, Decatur, Illinois 62525. A product of Procter & Gamble research. U.S. patent 3527864 and Patent pending.

[*Shown in Product Identification Section*]

The Purdue Frederick Company

100 CONNECTICUT AVENUE NORWALK, CT 06856

BETADINE® AEROSOL SPRAY

(povidone-iodine)

Topical Antiseptic Germicide

The nitrogen pressurized spray is easy to apply over large areas; eliminates the use of a contact applicator on the tender site. Also used for pre- and postoperative prepping of operative site, treatment of burns, including third-degree burns, decubitus and stasis ulcers, as a spray on the skin to be covered with a cast, and as a general topical microbicide.

BETADINE Aerosol Spray is film-forming and may be applied with or without bandages.

Administration: Spray the affected area thoroughly as needed. The improved actuator permits spraying from any angle.

How Supplied: Aerosol, nitrogen propelled, 3 fl. oz. bottle.

BETADINE® DOUCHE

(povidone-iodine)

A pleasantly scented solution, BETADINE DOUCHE is clinically effective in the treatment of vaginitis. Also effective as a cleansing douche.

Advantages: Low surface tension, with uniform wetting action to assist penetration into vaginal crypts and crevices. Active in the presence of blood, pus, or vaginal secretions. Virtually nonirritating to vaginal mucosa. Will not stain skin or natural fabrics.

Directions for Use: As a Therapeutic Douche: Two (2) tablespoonfuls to a quart of lukewarm water once daily. As a Routine Cleansing Douche: One (1) tablespoonful to a quart of lukewarm water once or twice per week.

How Supplied: 1 oz., 8 oz., 1 gallon plastic bottles. Disposable ½ oz. (1 tablespoonful) packettes.

Also Available: BETADINE Douche Kit and **Disposable** BETADINE Medicated Douche.

BETADINE® HĒLAFOAM® SOLUTION

(povidone-iodine)

Topical Antiseptic Microbicide

Description: BETADINE Hēlafoam Solution is a unique, broad-spectrum microbicidal foam which helps prevent infection in burns and wounds. The light, protective foam may be applied directly from canister to burn site. BETADINE Hēlafoam Solution adheres to the site of the burn wound with virtually no run-off.

Action and Uses: For use as a microbicide of choice for disinfection of wounds and for antiseptic treatment of lacerations, abrasions, and first-, second- and third-degree burns. For use as a prophylactic anti-infective agent in hospital and office procedures, including postoperative application to incisions to protect against possible infection. BETADINE Hēlafoam Solution may be bandaged or covered with gauze.

By helping to control bacterial proliferation, BETADINE Hēlafoam Solution aids in prevention of partial-thickness burns progressing to full-thickness burns. A lower incidence of burn wound sepsis may help reduce the need for grafting or permit earlier grafting and shorten hospital stay.

Dosage and Administration: Shake well. Hold can upright and firmly press release button on top of can. Apply directly to treatment site, spreading gently with sterile-gloved hand or with sterile tongue-depressor. Alternative methods of application are to dispense directly

Continued on next page

Purdue Frederick—Cont.

onto sterile-gloved hand and apply gently over the treatment site; or onto sterile gauze and cover the wound thoroughly with the impregnated gauze. Apply BETADINE Hēlafoam Solution liberally, as needed.
Warning: Contents under pressure. Do not puncture or incinerate. Do not expose to temperatures above 120° Fahrenheit. Store at controlled room temperature (59°–86°F).
Supplied: Aerosol, 9 oz. (250 gm.) canister.

BETADINE® OINTMENT
(povidone-iodine)

Action: BETADINE Ointment, in a water-soluble base, is a topical agent active against organisms commonly encountered in skin and wound infections. BETADINE Ointment kills gram-positive and gram-negative bacteria (including antibiotic-resistant strains). fungi, viruses, protozoa and yeasts.
The broad-spectrum activity of BETADINE Ointment provides microbicidal action against most commonly occurring skin bacteria. Its range of antibacterial activity encompasses many bacteria—including antibiotic-resistant forms.
The active ingredient in BETADINE Ointment substantially retains the broad-spectrum germicidal activity of iodine without the undesirable features or disadvantages of iodine. BETADINE Ointment is virtually nonirritating, does not block air from reaching the site of application, and washes easily off skin and natural fabrics. The site to which BETADINE Ointment is applied can be bandaged.
Indications: Therapeutically, BETADINE Ointment may be used as an adjunct to systemic therapy where indicated; for primary or secondary topical infections caused by iodine-susceptible organisms such as, infected burns, infected surgical incisions, infected decubitus or stasis ulcers, pyodermas, secondarily infected dermatoses, and infected traumatic lesions.
Prophylactically: BETADINE Ointment may be used to prevent microbial contamination in burns, incisions and other topical lesions; for degerming skin in hyperalimentation, catheter care, the umbilical area or circumcision. The use of BETADINE Ointment for abrasions, minor cuts, and wounds, may prevent the development of infections and permit wound healing.
Administration: Apply directly to affected area as needed. May be bandaged.
Supplied: $\frac{1}{32}$ oz. and $\frac{1}{8}$ oz. packettes; 1 oz. tubes; 16 oz. (1 lb.) and 5 lbs.

BETADINE® SKIN CLEANSER
(povidone-iodine)

BETADINE Skin Cleanser is a sudsing antiseptic liquid cleanser. It essentially retains the broad microbicidal spectrum of iodine, yet virtually without the undesirable features associated with iodine. BETADINE Skin Cleanser kills gram-positive and gram-negative bacteria (including antibiotic-resistant strains), fungi, viruses, protozoa and yeasts. It forms rich golden lather; virtually nonirritating; nonstaining to skin and natural fabrics.
Indications: BETADINE Skin Cleanser aids in degerming the skin of patients with common pathogens, including *Staphylococcus aureus.* To help prevent the recurrence of acute inflammatory skin infections caused by iodine-susceptible pyogenic bacteria. In pyodermas, as a topical adjunct to systemic antimicrobial therapy. To help prevent spread of infection in acne pimples. Also kills three organisms often associated with acne vulgaris: *Staph. epidermidis, Corynebacterium acnes* and Pityrosporon.
Directions for Use: Wet the skin and apply a sufficient amount of Skin Cleanser to work up a rich golden lather. Allow lather to remain about 3 minutes. Then rinse. Repeat 2-3 times a day or as needed.
Caution: In rare instances of local sensitivity, discontinue use by the individual.
How Supplied: 1 fl. oz. and 4 fl. oz. plastic bottles.
Note: Blue stains on starched linen will wash off with soap and water.

BETADINE® SOLUTION
(povidone-iodine)
Topical Antiseptic Microbicide

Action and Uses: For preoperative prepping of operative site, including the vagina, and as a general topical microbicide for: disinfection of wounds; emergency treatment of lacerations and abrasions; second– and third–degree burns; as a prophylactic anti-infective agent in hospital and office procedures, including post-operative application to incisions to help prevent infection; trichomonal, monilial, and nonspecific infectious vaginitis; oral moniliasis (thrush); bacterial and mycotic skin infections; decubitus and stasis ulcers; preoperatively, in the mouth and throat, as a swab. BETADINE Solution is microbicidal, and not merely bacteriostatic. It *kills* gram-positive and gram-negative bacteria (including antibiotic-resistant strains), fungi, viruses, protozoa and yeasts.
Administration: Apply full strength as often as needed as a paint, spray, or wet soak. May be bandaged. In preoperative prepping, avoid "pooling" beneath the patient.
How Supplied: $\frac{1}{2}$ oz., 8 oz., 16 oz. (1 pt.), 32 oz. (1 qt.) and 1 gal. plastic bottles and 1 oz. packettes.
Also Available: BETADINE® Solution Swab Aid® Pads for degerming small areas of skin or mucous membranes prior to injections, aspirations, catheterization and surgery; boxes of 100 packettes. Also: disposable BETADINE Solution Swabsticks, in packettes of 1's and 3's.

BETADINE® SURGICAL SCRUB
(povidone-iodine)
Topical Antiseptic Germicide

Action and Uses: An antiseptic, germicidal, sudsing skin cleanser for pre- and postoperative scrubbing or washing by hospital operating room personnel; for preoperative use on patients; and general use as an antiseptic germicide in physician's office. Forms rich, golden lather, virtually nonirritating; nonstaining to skin and natural fabrics.
Caution: In rare instance of local irritation or sensitivity, discontinue use by individual.
Directions for Use:
A. For Preoperative Washing by Operating Personnel
1. Wet hands and forearms with water. Pour about 5 cc. (1 teaspoonful) of BETADINE Surgical Scrub on the palm of the hand and spread over both hands and forearms. Without adding more water, rub the Scrub thoroughly over all areas for about five minutes. Use a brush if desired. Clean thoroughly under fingernails. Add a little water and develop copious suds. Rinse thoroughly under running water.
2. Complete the wash by scrubbing with another 5 cc. of BETADINE Surgical Scrub in the same way.

B. For Preoperative Use on Patients
After the skin area is shaved, wet it with water. Apply BETADINE Surgical Scrub (1 cc. is sufficient to cover an area of 20-30 square inches), develop lather and scrub thoroughly for about five minutes. Rinse off by aid of sterile gauze saturated with water. The area may then be painted with BETADINE Solution or sprayed with BETADINE Aerosol Spray and allowed to dry.

C. For use in the Physician's Office
Use for washing whenever a germicidal detergent is required. For maximum degerming of the hands proceed as under (A). To prepare the patient's skin proceed as under (B).
Note: Blue stains on starched linen will wash off with soap and water.
Supplied: 16 oz. (1 pint) plastic bottle with and without pump, 32 oz. (1 quart) and 1 gal. plastic bottles, and $\frac{1}{2}$ oz. packettes.

BETADINE® Viscous Formula
Antiseptic Gauze Pad
(povidone-iodine)

Description: BETADINE Viscous Formula Antiseptic Gauze Pads are available both as 3″ × 9″ or as 5″ × 9″ gauze pads impregnated with BETADINE Solution (povidone-iodine) in a viscous base that is formulated to remain moist for an extended period of time.
Actions: The active ingredient in BETADINE Viscous Formula Antiseptic Gauze Pad kills both gram-positive and gram-negative bacteria (including antibiotic-resistant strains), viruses, fungi, protozoa and yeasts. It is rapidly effective against *Staphylococcus aureus.* It is microbicidal, not merely bacteriostatic. . . and maintains its activity in the presence of blood, pus and serum.
Uses: AS A TOPICAL MICROBICIDAL DRESSING
To help prevent topical infection; for disinfection of wounds; for antiseptic treatment of lacerations, abrasions and first-, second- and third-degree burns; for use as a prophylactic anti-infective agent in hospital and office procedures; for postoperative application to incisions to help protect against possible infection; for antiseptic treatment of cutaneous ulcers.
Directions for use: To open, separate seam in either corner of packette and peel down. Remove the gauze pad and apply directly to affected area. Gauze pad may be bandaged.
Supplied: 3″ × 9″ in boxes of 12, 5″ × 9″ in boxes of 12.
Also Available: BETADINE® Antiseptic Gauze Pad, impregnated with BETADINE Solution in a water-soluble base of polyethylene glycols.

CARDIOQUIN® TABLETS ℞
(quinidine polygalacturonate)

Description: Each scored CARDIOQUIN Tablet contains 275 mg quinidine polygalacturonate equivalent in quinidine content to 3 grains (200 mg) of quinidine sulfate.
Actions: The quinidine component slows conduction time, prolongs the refractory period, and depresses the excitability of heart muscle. Polygalacturonate slows ionization of the drug and protects the gastrointestinal tract by its demulcent effect.[1–3]
Indications: CARDIOQUIN Tablets are indicated as maintenance therapy after spontaneous and electrical conversion of atrial tachycardia, flutter or fibrillation and in the treatment of:
- Premature atrial and ventricular contractions.
- Paroxysmal atrial tachycardia.
- Paroxysmal A-V junctional rhythm.
- Atrial flutter.
- Paroxysmal atrial fibrillation.
- Established atrial fibrillation when therapy is appropriate.
- Paroxysmal ventricular tachycardia when not associated with complete heartblock.

Contraindications:
1. History of hypersensitivity to quinidine manifested by thrombocytopenia, skin eruptions, febrile reactions, etc.
2. Complete A-V block.
3. Complete bundle branch block or other severe intraventricular conduction defects

exhibiting marked QRS widening or bizarre complexes.
4. Myasthenia gravis.
5. Arrhythmias associated with digitalis toxicity.

Warnings:

1. In the treatment of atrial fibrillation with rapid ventricular response, ventricular rate should be controlled with digitalis glycosides *prior* to administration of quinidine.

2. In the treatment of atrial flutter with quinidine, reversion to sinus rhythm may be preceded by progressive reduction in the degree of A-V block to a 1:1 ratio resulting in an extremely high ventricular rate. This potential hazard may be reduced by digitalization prior to administration of quinidine.

Recent reports have described increased, potentially toxic, digoxin plasma levels when quinidine is administered concurrently. When concurrent use is necessary, digoxin dosage should be reduced and plasma concentration should be monitored and patients observed closely for digitalis intoxication.

3. Quinidine cardiotoxicity may be manifested by increased P-R and Q-T intervals, 50% widening of QRS, and/or ventricular ectopic beats or tachycardia. Appearance of these toxic signs during quinidine administration mandates immediate discontinuation of the drug, and/or close clinical and electrocardiographic monitoring. Note: Quinidine effect is enhanced by potassium and reduced in the presence of hypokalemia.

4. Quinidine syncope may occur as a complication of long-term therapy. It is manifested by sudden loss of consciousness and by ventricular arrhythmias with bizarre QRS complexes. This syndrome does not appear to be related to dose or plasma levels but occurs more often with prolonged Q-T intervals.

5. Because quinidine antagonizes the effect of vagal excitation upon the atrium and the A-V note, the administration of parasympathomimetic drugs (choline esters) or the use of any other procedure to enhance vagal activity may fail to terminate paroxysmal supraventricular tachycardia in patients receiving quinidine.

6. Quinidine should be used with extreme caution in:

a) The presence of incomplete A-V block, since a complete block and asystole may result.

b) Quinidine may cause unpredictable abnormalities of rhythm in digitalized hearts. Therefore, it should be used with caution in the presence of digitalis intoxication (see 2 above).

c) Partial bundle branch block.

d) Severe congestive heart failure and hypotensive states due to the depressant effects of quinidine on myocardial contractility and arterial pressure.

e) Poor renal function, especially renal tubular acidosis, because of the potential accumulation of quinidine in plasma leading to toxic concentrations.

Precautions:

1. Test Dose—A preliminary test dose of a single tablet of quinidine *sulfate* should be administered prior to the initiation of treatment with CARDIOQUIN Tablets to determine whether the patient has an idiosyncrasy to the quinidine molecule.

2. Hypersensitivity—During the first weeks of therapy, hypersensitivity to quinidine, although rare, should be considered (e.g., angioedema, purpura, acute asthmatic episode, vascular collapse).

3. Long-Term Therapy— Periodic blood counts and liver and kidney function tests should be performed during long-term therapy, and the drug should be discontinued if blood dyscrasias or signs of hepatic or renal disorders occur.

4. Large Doses—ECG monitoring and determination of plasma quinidine levels are recommended when doses greater than 2.5 g/day are administered.

5. Usage in Pregnancy—The use of quinidine in pregnancy should be reserved only for those cases where the benefits outweigh the possible hazards to the patient and fetus.

6. Nursing Mothers—The drug should be used with extreme caution in nursing mothers because the drug is excreted in breast milk.

7. General—In patients exhibiting asthma, muscle weakness and infection with fever *prior* to quinidine administration, hypersensitivity reactions to the drug may be masked.

Drug Interactions:

1. Caution should be used when quinidine and its analogs are administered concurrently with coumarin anticoagulants. This combination may reduce prothrombin levels and cause bleeding.

2. Quinidine, a weak base, may have its half-life prolonged in patients who are concurrently taking drugs that can alkalize the urine, such as thiazide diuretics, sodium bicarbonate, and carbonic anhydrase inhibitors. Quinidine and drugs which alkalize the urine should be used together cautiously.

3. Quinidine exhibits a distinct anticholinergic activity in the myocardial tissues. An additive vagolytic effect may be seen when quinidine and drugs having anticholinergic blocking activity are used together. Drugs having cholinergic activity may be antagonized by quinidine.

4. Quinidine and other antiarrhythmic agents may produce additive cardiac depressant effects when administered together.

5. Quinidine interaction with cardiac glycosides (digoxin). See **Warnings.**

6. Antacids may delay absorption of quinidine but appear unlikely to cause incomplete absorption.

7. Phenobarbital and phenytoin may reduce plasma half-life of quinidine by 50%.

8. Quinidine may potentiate the neuromuscular blocking effect in ventilatory depression of patients receiving decamethonium, tubocurare or succinylcholine.

Adverse Reactions: Symptoms of cinchonism (ringing in the ears, headache, disturbed vision) may appear in sensitive patients after a single dose of the drug.

Gastrointestinal: The most common side-effects encountered with quinidine are referable to this system. Diarrhea frequently occurs, but it rarely necessitates withdrawal of the drug. Nausea, vomiting and abdominal pain also occur. Some of these effects may be minimized by administering the drug with meals.

Cardiovascular: Widening of QRS complex, cardiac asystole, ventricular ectopic beats, idioventricular rhythms including ventricular tachycardias and fibrillation; paradoxical tachycardia, arterial embolism and hypotension.

Hematologic: acute hemolytic anemia, hypoprothrombinemia, thrombocytopenic purpura, agranulocytosis.

CNS: headache, fever, vertigo, apprehension, excitement, confusion, delirium and syncope, disturbed hearing (tinnitus, decreased auditory acuity), disturbed vision (mydriasis, blurred vision, disturbed color perception, photophobia, diplopia, night blindness, scotomata); optic neuritis.

Dermatologic: Cutaneous flushing with intense pruritus.

Hypersensitivity Reactions: Angioedema, acute asthmatic episode, vascular collapse, respiratory arrest, hepatic dysfunction.

Dosage and Administration:

Each CARDIOQUIN Tablet contains 275 mg quinidine polygalacturonate, equivalent to a 3-grain tablet of quinidine sulfate. Dosage must be adjusted to individual patient's needs, both for conversion and maintenance. An initial dose of 1 to 3 tablets may be used to terminate arrhythmia, and may be repeated in 3-4 hours. If normal sinus rhythm is not restored after 3 or 4 equal doses, the dose may be increased by ½ to 1 tablet (137.5 to 275 mg) and administered three to four times before any further dosage increase. For maintenance, one tablet may be used two or three times a day; generally, one tablet morning and night will be adequate.

Overdosage: Cardiotoxic effects of quinidine may be reversed in part by molar sodium lactate; the hypotension may be reversed by vasoconstrictors and by catecholamines (since vasodilation is partly due to alpha-adrenergic blockage).

Supplied: Uncoated, scored tablets in bottles of 100.

References:

1. Schwartz, G.: *Angiology* 10:115 (Apr.) 1959.
2. Tricot, R., Nogrette, P.: *Presse med.* 68:1085 (June 4) 1960.
3. Shaftel, N., Halpern, A.: *Am. J. Med. Sci.* 236:184 (Aug.) 1958.

CERUMENEX® DROPS ℞

(triethanolamine polypeptide oleate-condensate)

A UNIQUE CERUMENOLYTIC AGENT FOR EFFECTIVE AND EASY REMOVAL OF EARWAX

Composition: CERUMENEX Drops contain (10%) Triethanolamine polypeptide oleate-condensate in propylene glycol with chlorbutanol (0.5%), for effective, convenient cerumenolytic action and easy removal of earwax.

Among its properties are:

1. Aqueous-miscible solution—low surface tension and optimal viscosity.
2. Slightly acid pH range to approximate surface of normal ear canal.
3. Hygroscopic — helps absorb aqueous transudates.
4. Antiseptic protection against contamination.

Advantages:

- USUALLY EFFECTIVE WITH A SINGLE 15-30 MINUTE TREATMENT.
- EXCELLENT RESULTS REPORTED IN OVER 90% OF ABOUT 2,700 ADULT AND PEDIATRIC PATIENTS.
- HELPS AVOID PAINFUL INSTRUMENTATION.
- SIMPLE AND EASY TO ADMINISTER.

Action: CERUMENEX Drops are specifically designed as a cerumenolytic agent, to emulsify and disperse excess or impacted earwax for easier removal without painful instrumentation. They are usually effective with a single 15-30 minute treatment, and are simple and easy to administer (See Dosage and Administration).

Indications:

- REMOVAL OF CERUMEN.
- REMOVAL OF IMPACTED CERUMEN PRIOR TO EAR EXAMINATION.
- REMOVAL OF IMPACTED CERUMEN PRIOR TO OTOLOGIC THERAPY.
- REMOVAL OF IMPACTED CERUMEN PRIOR TO AUDIOMETRY.

Contraindications:

- A history of a previous untoward reaction to CERUMENEX Drops.
- A positive patch test (see "Precautions").
- Knowledge or suspicion of a perforated eardrum or otitis media may be considered as a relative contraindication.

Precautions:

It is recommended that the following precautions be observed in prescribing and administration of this agent:

1. Extreme caution is indicated in patients with demonstrable dermatologic idiosyncrasies or with history of allergic reactions in general.
2. In case of doubt, a patch test should be performed by placing a drop of CERUMENEX Drops on the flexor surface of the

Continued on next page

Purdue Frederick—Cont.

arm or forearm and covering it with a small Band-Aid® strip. The results are read and interpreted after 24 hours. Positive reaction indicates the probability of an allergic reaction following instillation in the ear.

3. Exposure of the ear canal to the CERUMENEX Drops should be limited to 15-30 minutes.
4. Patients must be instructed not to exceed the time of exposure, nor to use the medication more frequently than directed by the physician.
5. When administering CERUMENEX Drops, care must be taken to avoid undue exposure of the periaural skin during the instillation and the flushing out of the medication. If the medication comes in contact with the skin, the area should be washed with soap and water. Use of proper technique (see Dosage and Administration) will help avoid such undue exposure.
6. Although introduction of CERUMENEX Drops (triethanolamine polypeptide oleate-condensate) into the middle ear of animals with surgically perforated drums or into patients with ruptured drums has been accomplished without untoward reactions, the use of this medication should be avoided in the presence of underlying disease in the middle ear (otitis media, perforated drum) and it should be used only with caution in certain types of external otitis.
7. Patients should be advised to discontinue the use of the medication in case of a possible reaction and to consult their physician promptly.

Adverse Reactions:
Clinical Reactions of Possible Allergic Origin
Localized dermatitis reactions were reported in about 1% of 2,700 patients treated, ranging from a very mild erythema and pruritus of the external canal to a severe eczematoid reaction involving the external ear and periauricular tissue, generally with duration of 2-10 days. In all cases, complete and uneventful resolution occurred without residual sequelae, sometimes without supplemental therapy. Such therapy may consist of only symptomatic relief in mild cases and may include anti-inflammatory agents when indicated. Thus, while reactions of a possible allergic origin may occur, their incidence is minimal and usually not disproportionate to other commonly used dermatologic agents.

Dosage and Administration:

1. Fill ear canal with CERUMENEX Drops with the patient's head tilted at a 45° angle.
2. Insert cotton plug and allow to remain 15-30 minutes.
3. Then gently flush ear with lukewarm water, using soft rubber syringe (avoid excessive pressure). Avoid undue exposure of large skin areas to the drug. If a second application is necessary in unusually hard impactions, the procedure may be repeated.

How Supplied: 6 ml and 12 ml bottles with cellophane wrapped blunt-end dropper.

[*Shown in Product Identification Section*]

FIBERMED®
High-Fiber Supplements

Description: FIBERMED High-Fiber Supplements provide a measured quantity of natural dietary fiber with precision in a palatable, ready-to-eat form. Each FIBERMED Supplement contains 5.0 grams of dietary fiber—supplied by corn, wheat and oats.

FIBERMED overcomes problems associated with other fiber-containing products—problems such as variable fiber content, inconvenience and monotonous taste. FIBERMED Supplements are exceptional among high-fiber products because of their convenience and good taste, qualities which encourage good compliance.

Two FIBERMED High-Fiber Supplements a day help provide the supplementary bulk patients may need in their diet to avoid constipation. Many individuals can increase their fiber intake by as much as 50% or more simply by eating two FIBERMED Supplements each day.

Ready-to-eat FIBERMED Supplements can be eaten anytime, anyplace. Unlike most high-fiber foods or powdered bulks, FIBERMED requires no preparation and no mixing. They can be eaten with milk, coffee, tea, juice, soup or fruit; or dunked in a beverage. As with any healthful diet, drinking adequate fluids is important.

FIBERMED Supplements are satisfying (only 60 calories per supplement) and help reduce the desire for snacks and desserts that are highly caloric.

Ingredients: Corn Bran, Brown Sugar, Wheat Flour, Corn Starch, Wheat Bran, Oat Flakes, Corn Germ Meal, Vegetable Shortening (Partially Hydrogenated Soybean Oil), Sodium Bicarbonate, Vanilla Flavor, Peanut Butter Flavor, Ammonium Bicarbonate, Baking Acid, Sodium Propionate, Salt and Citric Acid.

Nutrition Information Per Serving:

Serving Size	1 supplement
Servings per package	14
Calories	60
Protein	1 g
Carbohydrate	14 g*
Fat	2 g

Percentage of U.S. Recommended Daily Allowances (% U.S. RDA):

Riboflavin (Vitamin B_2)	2
Niacin	2
Iron	4

Contains less than 2% of the U.S. RDA of Protein, Vitamin A, Vitamin C, Thiamine and Calcium.

*Includes 4.6 g of simple carbohydrates (brown sugar) and 9.4 g of complex carbohydrates.

Usage: Dietary fiber, as contained in FIBERMED, increases the softness and size of stools and regulates the time required for food wastes to travel through the gastrointestinal tract.

Because of its influence on gastrointestinal function, dietary fiber may be beneficial in disorders related to the consistency of stools and to gastrointestinal transit time. Diverticular disease, hiatus hernia, hemorrhoids and irritable bowel syndrome are among such disorders involving digestive functions that a diet high in fiber can benefit. (This data is presented solely as background information on the effect of fiber on gastrointestinal function.)

FIBERMED Supplements are indicated when it is desirable to regulate gastrointestinal transit time and to increase stool weight. Because of their taste and convenience, FIBERMED Supplements are the product of choice to significantly increase intake of dietary fiber in uniform amounts.

Two FIBERMED Supplements a day provide a high level of dietary fiber—10 grams—more dietary fiber than a serving of high-fiber cereal.

Directions: Usually two FIBERMED Supplements per day.

Supplied: FIBERMED Supplements are supplied in boxes of 14 and institutional packs of 288. For most individuals, 14 is a week's supply.

[*Shown in Product Identification Section*]

PHYLLOCONTIN® TABLETS ℞
(aminophylline, hydrous)
225 mg*
***Controlled release, equivalent to 178 mg anhydrous theophylline**

Description: Phyllocontin Tablets are scored, yellowish-white, with a slight ammoniacal odor and bitter taste. The active ingredient of Phyllocontin Tablets is aminophylline USP in the dihydrate form, a compound containing 79% anhydrous theophylline ($C_7H_8N_4O_2$) and 14% anhydrous ethylenediamine ($C_2H_8N_2$). The structural formula of aminophylline hydrous is:

[theophylline structure]$_2$ · CH_2NH_2–CH_2NH_2 · $2H_2O$ MW = 456.46

Clinical Pharmacology: Theophylline directly relaxes the smooth muscle of the bronchial airways and pulmonary blood vessels. The drug also produces other actions typical of the xanthine derivatives: coronary vasodilation, diuresis, and cardiac, cerebral and skeletal muscle stimulation. These actions may be mediated through inhibition of phosphodiesterase and a resultant increase in intracellular cyclic AMP. Apparently no development of tolerance occurs with chronic use of aminophylline.

In vitro, theophylline, the active moiety in aminophylline, has been shown to act synergistically with beta agonists that increase intracellular cyclic AMP through the stimulation of adenyl cyclase, but synergism has not been demonstrated in patient studies. More data are needed to determine if theophylline and beta agonists have a clinically important additive effect *in vivo*.

Pharmacokinetics: The half-life of theophylline or aminophylline is prolonged in patients suffering from chronic alcoholism, impaired hepatic or renal function, or congestive heart failure, and in patients receiving macrolide antibiotics and cimetidine. Older adults (over age 55) and patients with chronic obstructive pulmonary disease, with or without cor pulmonale, may also have much slower clearance rates; in these individuals the theophylline half-life may exceed 24 hours. High fever for prolonged periods may reduce the rate of theophylline elimination.

Newborns and neonates have extremely slow clearance rates compared to older infants (over 6 months) and children, and may also have a theophylline half-life of over 24 hours.

The half-life of theophylline in smokers averages 4 to 5 hours contrasted with 7 to 9 hours in nonsmokers. Theophylline pharmacokinetics may not return to normal until 3 months to 2 years after the cessation of smoking.

Indications: Phyllocontin Tablets are indicated for relief and/or prevention of symptoms from asthma and reversible bronchospasm associated with chronic bronchitis and emphysema.

Contraindications: In individuals who have shown hypersensitivity to its components, including ethylenediamine.

Warnings: Phyllocontin Tablets 225 mg are not recommended for children under the age of 6.

Status asthmaticus is a medical emergency.

Defined as that degree of bronchospasm which is not rapidly responsive to usual doses of conventional bronchodilators, status asthmaticus optimally requires parenterally administered drugs under closed medical supervision, preferably in an intensive care setting.

Excessive aminophylline doses may be associated with toxicity, and determination of serum theophylline levels is recommended to assure maximal benefit without excessive risk. Do not attempt to maintain any dose that is not tolerated. The incidence of toxicity increases at serum levels greater than 20 mcg/ml. Reduced theophylline clearance may result in increased serum levels and potential toxicity in patients: (1) with impaired renal or liver function, (2) over 55 years of age, particularly males and those with chronic lung disease, (3) with cardiac failure, (4) requiring macrolide antibiotics or cimetidine, and (5) in neonates. Theophylline clearance may be decreased during active influenza infection or after immunization for influenza.

Less serious signs of theophylline toxicity, i.e. nausea and restlessness, may appear in up to 50% of patients. Unfortunately however, serious side effects such as ventricular arrhythmias, convulsions or even death may appear as the first sign of toxicity without any previous warning. Stated differently: serious toxicity is not reliably preceded by less severe side effects.

Many patients who require theophylline or aminophylline may exhibit tachycardia due to their underlying disease process, so that the cause/effect relationship to elevated serum theophylline concentrations may not be appreciated.

Theophylline and aminophylline products may cause dysrhythmia and/or worsen pre-existing arrhythmias.

Precautions—General: Theophylline half-life is shorter in smokers than in nonsmokers. Therefore, smokers may require larger or more frequent doses. Morphine and curare should be used with caution in patients with airway obstruction as they may suppress respiration and stimulate histamine release. Alternative drugs should be used when possible. Theophylline or aminophylline should not be administered concurrently with other xanthine medications. Use with caution in patients with severe cardiac disease, severe hypoxemia, hypertension, hyperthyroidism, acute myocardial injury, cor pulmonale, congestive heart failure, or liver disease, in the elderly (especially males) and in neonates. In particular, great caution should be used in giving theophylline to patients with congestive heart failure. Frequently, such patients have markedly prolonged theophylline serum levels with theophylline persisting in serum for long periods following discontinuation of the drug.

Use theophylline or aminophylline cautiously in patients with history of peptic ulcer. Theophylline may occasionally act as a local irritant to the G.I. tract, although gastrointestinal symptoms are more commonly centrally mediated and associated with serum drug concentrations over 20 mcg/ml.

Information for Patients: The physician should reinforce the importance of taking only the prescribed dose at the prescribed time interval between doses. If necessary, taking the drug with food will help avoid local irritation of the G.I. tract. Scored tablets may be broken in half but not crushed or chewed.

Drug Interactions: Toxic synergism with ephedrine has been documented and may occur with other sympathomimetic bronchodilators. In addition, the following drug interactions have been demonstrated:

Drug: Aminophylline with lithium carbonate
Effect: Increased excretion of lithium carbonate

Drug: Aminophylline with propranolol
Effect: Antagonism of propranolol effect

Drug: Theophylline with cimetidine
Effect: Increased theophylline blood levels

Drug: Theophylline with troleandomycin and erythromycin
Effect: Increased theophylline blood levels

Drug—Laboratory Test Interactions: When plasma levels of theophylline are measured by spectrophotometric methods, coffee, tea, cola beverages, chocolate and acetaminophen may cause falsely high values.

Carcinogenesis, Mutagenesis, and Impairment of Fertility: Long-term animal studies have not been performed to evaluate the carcinogenic potential, mutagenic potential or the effect on fertility of xanthine compounds.

Pregnancy: Category C—Animal reproduction studies have not been conducted with theophylline or aminophylline. It is not known whether theophylline can cause fetal harm when administered to a pregnant woman or can affect reproduction capacity. Xanthines should be given to a pregnant woman only if clearly needed.

Nursing Mothers: It has been reported that theophylline distributes readily into breast milk and may cause adverse effects in the infant. Caution must be used if prescribing xanthines to a mother who is nursing, taking into account the risks and benefits of this therapy.

Pediatric Use: This drug is not recommended for children under six (6) years of age.

Adverse Reactions: The most consistent adverse reactions are usually due to overdose and are:

1. Gastrointestinal: nausea, vomiting, epigastric pain, hematemesis, diarrhea.
2. Central Nervous System: headaches, irritability, restlessness, insomnia, reflex hyperexcitability, muscle twitching, clonic and tonic generalized convulsions.
3. Cardiovascular: palpitation, tachycardia, extrasystoles, flushing, hypotension, circulatory failure, ventricular arrhythmias.
4. Respiratory: tachypnea.
5. Renal: albuminuria, increased excretion of renal tubular and red blood cells, potentiation of diuresis.
6. Others: hyperglycemia and inappropriate ADH syndrome; rash (consider ethylenediamine).

Management of Overdosage:

1. If potential oral overdose is established and seizure has not occurred:
   A. Induce vomiting.
   B. Administer a cathartic. This is particularly important with sustained release drugs.
   C. Administer activated charcoal.
2. If patient is having a seizure:
   A. Establish an airway.
   B. Administer oxygen.
   C. Treat the seizure with intravenous diazepam, 0.1 to 0.3 mg/kg up to 10 mg.
   D. Monitor vital signs, maintain blood pressure and provide adequate hydration.
3. Post-Seizure Coma:
   A. Maintain airway and oxygenation.
   B. If a result of oral mediction, follow above recommendations to prevent absorption of the drug, but intubation and lavage will have to be performed instead of inducing emesis, and the cathartic and charcoal will need to be introduced via a large bore gastric lavage tube.
   C. Continue to provide full supportive care and adequate hydration while waiting for the drug to be metabolized. In general, the drug is metabolized sufficiently rapidly so as not to warrant consideration of dialysis. However, if serum levels exceed 50 mcg/ml, charcoal hemoperfusion may be indicated.

DOSAGE ADJUSTMENT WITH SERUM THEOPHYLLINE MEASUREMENT CONTROL

If serum theophylline is:	mcg/ml	
Within normal limits	10 to 20	Maintain dose if tolerated.[1]
Too high	25 to 30	Skip next dose and decrease subsequent doses by about 25%.
	Over 30	Skip next two doses and decrease subsequent doses by 50%. Recheck serum theophylline.
Too low	7.5 to 10	Increase dose by about 25%.[1,2]
	5 to 7.5	Increase dose by about 25% to the nearest dose increment and recheck serum theophylline for guidance in further dosage adjustment. (Another increase will probably be needed, but this provides a safety check.)

[1] Recheck serum theophylline concentration at 6- and 12-month intervals. Finer adjustments in dosage may be needed for some patients.

[2] Dividing the daily dose into 3 doses administered at 8-hour intervals may be indicated if symptoms occur repeatedly at the end of a dosing interval.

Dosage Guidelines: In chronic therapy, theophylline as found in Phyllocontin Tablets is a treatment of first choice for the management of chronic asthma and other obstructive pulmonary diseases to prevent symptoms and maintain patent airways. Monitoring clinical response and determining serum theophylline, when appropriate, minimizes risk of toxicity due to overdosing. Slow clinical titration is generally preferred to assure acceptance and safety of the medication.

There is a great variation from patient to patient in the dosage needed to achieve a therapeutic blood level because of variable rates of elimination. Because of these wide variations from patient to patient, dosage must be individualized and monitoring of therapeutic response and/or theophylline serum levels is highly recommended. However, it is not always possible or practical to obtain a serum theophylline level. When serum theophylline levels are not measured, patients should be closely monitored for signs of toxicity and the total daily dose of Phyllocontin Tablets should not exceed the "Maximum Dose Without Measurement of Serum Concentration" shown below.

When measurement of serum theophylline levels has revealed the need to prescribe higher dosages, the patient's serum theophylline levels should be monitored as part of an ongoing management program.

Dosage and Administration: Therapeutic serum theophylline levels associated with optimal likelihood for benefit and minimal risk of toxicity for most patients are considered to be between 10 mcg/ml and 20 mcg/ml.

The usual initial dose of Phyllocontin Tablets is one to two 225 mg tablets twice daily. In young patients, smokers, and others exhibiting rapid theophylline clearance, serum levels may indicate a need for dosing every 8 hours.

After 2 to 3 days, if the desired response is not achieved with the usual initial dose and there are no adverse reactions, the dose may be increased to the following "Maximum Dose Without Measurement of Serum Concentration." (See table below)

If the increased dose is tolerated but the therapeutic response is not satisfactory, serum theophylline levels should be determined about 4 hours after the last dose, and dosage may be adjusted according to "Dosage Adjustment With Serum Theophylline Measurement Control." (See table above)

Measurement of Serum Theophylline Concentration during Chronic Therapy: Serum theopylline measurement is recommended to determine whether it falls within the therapeutic range. This should be obtained at the approximate time of peak absorption during chronic therapy, which is 3 to 5 hours after the last dose of Phyllocontin Tablets. It is important that the patient will have missed *no* doses during the previous 72 hours and that dosing intervals will have been reasonably typical with no added doses during that period of time. Dosage adjustment based on serum theophylline measurements when these instructions have not been followed may result in risk of toxicity to the patient.

Note: It is important that patients be maintained on a dosage which is therapeutically effective and tolerated. In instructing patients to increase dosage to achieve efficacy, caution must be given *not* to take a subsequent dose if apparent side effects occur and to resume therapy at a lower dose once adverse effects have disappeared.

Caution: Federal law prohibits dispensing without prescription.

How Supplied: Phyllocontin (aminophylline, hydrous) 225 mg scored Controlled Release Tablets are supplied in bottles of 100.

U.S. Patent Numbers 3965256 and 4235870
12/28/82

PRIODERM® LOTION ℞
(0.5% malathion)

Description: A pleasantly scented, clear liquid containing 0.5% malathion in 78% isopropyl alcohol, terpineol, dipentene and pine needle oil.

Clinical Pharmacology: Malathion is lousicidal and ovicidal *in vitro.* Louse eggs succumb to 3 seconds of exposure to 0.062% malathion in acetone and lice to about 0.003%, respectively. Resistance to malathion could not be induced.

Human safety studies included a 21-day cumulative irritancy and others undertaken to determine the potential for contact sensitization, phototoxicity, and photo-contact sensitization. Application of Prioderm Lotion showed no evidence of sensitization and a very low level of irritation.

Indications and Usage: Prioderm Lotion is indicated for the treatment of head lice and their ova.

Contraindications: Prioderm Lotion should not be used by individuals with known sensitivity to Prioderm Lotion or to any of its components.

MAXIMUM DOSE WITHOUT MEASUREMENT OF SERUM CONCENTRATION

Not to exceed the following:

Age Range (years)	Phyllocontin 225 mg	Anhydrous theophylline, equivalents
Age 6 to 9 years	30 mg/kg/day	24 mg/kg/day
Age 9 to 12 years	25 mg/kg/day	20 mg/kg/day
Age 12 to 16 years	23 mg/kg/day	18 mg/kg/day
Age > 16 years	17 mg/kg/day or 1100 mg (whichever is less)	13 mg/kg/day or 900 mg (whichever is less)

A total daily dose of up to 17 mg/kg/day in divided doses (not to exceed 4 Phyllocontin Tablets per day) may be allowable without measurement of serum concentration.

Dosage should be calculated on the basis of lean (ideal) body weight when mg/kg doses are used. Theophylline does not distribute into fatty tissue.

Purdue Frederick—Cont.

> WARNING: PRIODERM LOTION CONTAINS FLAMMABLE ALCOHOL. THE LOTION AND WET HAIR SHOULD NOT BE EXPOSED TO OPEN FLAME OR ELECTRIC HEAT, INCLUDING HAIR DRYERS. DO NOT SMOKE WHILE APPLYING LOTION, OR WHILE HAIR IS WET. ALLOW HAIR TO DRY NATURALLY AND UNCOVERED AFTER APPLICATION.

Precautions: If accidentally placed in the eye, flush immediately with water.

Carcinogenesis, Mutagenesis and Fertility—Malathion is neither carcinogenic in male or female F344 rats after 2 years feeding with up to 4000 ppm (0.4%) nor is it tumorigenic in Osborn-Mendel rats or B6C3F1 mice after a similar feeding for 80 weeks with 8,000 ppm (0.8%) and 16,000 ppm (1.6%), respectively. Tests for mutagenicity have not been conducted.

Pregnancy Category B—There was no evidence of teratogenicity in studies utilizing single i.p. injections of malathion at 600 and 900 mg/kg in pregnant rats or oral dosing with up to 300 mg/kg on days 6 through 15 of gestation. A reproduction study in rats failed to show any gross fetal abnormalities attributable to feeding malathion up to 2,500 ppm in the diet during a three-generation evaluation period. These studies employed at least 50 to 70 times the adult human topical dose. Because animal reproduction studies are not always predictive of human response, this drug should be used during pregnancy only if clearly needed.

Nursing Mothers—In a study of percutaneous absorption of malathion in an acetone solution, malathion was reported to be absorbed through human skin only to the extent of 8% of the applied dose. However, percutaneous absorption from the Prioderm Lotion formulation has not been studied and it is not known whether malathion is excreted in human milk. Because many drugs are excreted in human milk, caution should be exercised when Prioderm Lotion is administered to the nursing mother.

Adverse Reactions: Irritation of the scalp has been reported.

Overdosage: Consideration should be given as part of the treatment program to the high concentration of isopropyl alcohol in the vehicle.

Malathion, although a weaker cholinesterase inhibitor and therefore safer than other organophosphates, may be expected to exhibit the same symptoms of cholinesterase depletion after accidental ingestion orally. Vomiting should be induced promptly or the stomach lavaged with 5% sodium bicarbonate solution. Severe respiratory distress is the major and most serious symptom of organophosphate poisoning requiring artifical respiration and large doses of i.m. or i.v. atropine. The usual starting dose of atropine is 1 to 4 mg with supplementation hourly, as needed, to counteract the symptoms of cholinesterase depletion. Repeat analyses of serum and RBC cholinesterase assist in establishing the diagnosis and formulating a long-range prognosis.

Dosage and Administration: 1) Sprinkle Prioderm Lotion on **DRY** hair and rub gently until the hair and scalp are thoroughly wet. Pay special attention to the back of the head and neck. 2) Allow to dry naturally—use no heat and leave uncovered. 3) After 8-12 hours, the hair should be shampooed. 4) Rinse and use a fine-toothed comb to remove dead lice and eggs. 5) If required, repeat with second application of Prioderm Lotion in 7 to 9 days.

Further treatment is generally not necessary. Other family members should be evaluated to determine if infested and if so, receive treatment.

Caution: Federal law prohibits dispensing without a prescription.

How Supplied: Prioderm Lotion (0.5% malathion) in bottles of 2 fl. oz. (59 ml).

SENOKOT® SYRUP
(standardized extract of senna fruit)

Action and Uses: For relief of functional constipation and whenever gentle laxation is indicated. A deliciously flavored liquid laxative, predictably and reliably effective.

Contraindications: Acute surgical abdomen.

Administration and Dosage: Preferably at bedtime. Adults: 2 to 3 tsp. (maximum—3 tsp. b.i.d.). For older, debilitated, and OB/GYN patients, the physician may consider prescribing ½ the initial adult dose. Children 5-15 years: 1 to 2 tsp. (maximum—2 tsp. b.i.d.). 1-5 years: ½ to 1 tsp. (maximum—1 tsp. b.i.d.). 1 month to 1 year: ¼ to ½ tsp. (maximum—½ tsp. b.i.d.). If comfortable evacuation is not achieved by the second day, decrease or increase daily dosage (up to maximum) by one half the starting dose until optimum dose for evacuation is established.

How Supplied: Bottles of 2 and 8 fl. oz.

SENOKOT® TABLETS/GRANULES
(standardized senna concentrate)

Action and Uses: Indicated for relief of functional constipation (chronic or occasional). SENOKOT Tablets/Granules contain a natural vegetable derivative, purified and standardized for uniform action. The current theory of the mechanism of action is that glycosides are transported to the colon, where they are changed to aglycones that stimulate Auerbach's plexus to induce peristalsis. This virtually colon-specific action is gentle, effective and predictable, usually inducing comfortable evacuation of well-formed stool within 8-10 hours. Found effective even in many previously intractable cases of functional constipation, SENOKOT preparations may aid in rehabilitation of the constipated patient by facilitating regular elimination. At proper dosage levels, SENOKOT preparations are virtually free of adverse reactions (such as loose stools or abdominal discomfort) and enjoy high patient acceptance. Numerous and extensive clinical studies show their high degree of effectiveness in varieties of functional constipation: chronic, geriatric, antepartum and postpartum, drug-induced, pediatric, as well as in functional constipation concurrent with heart disease or anorectal surgery.

Contraindications: Acute surgical abdomen.

Administration and Dosage: Preferably at bedtime. GRANULES (deliciously cocoa-flavored): Adults: 1 level tsp. (maximum—2 level tsp. b.i.d.). For older, debilitated, and OB/GYN patients, the physician may consider prescribing ½ the initial adult dose. Children above 60 lb.: ½ level tsp. (maximum—1 level tsp. b.i.d.). TABLETS: Adults: 2 tablets (maximum—4 tablets b.i.d.). For older, debilitated, and OB/-GYN patients, the physician may consider prescribing ½ the initial dose. Children above 60 lb.: 1 tablet (maximum—2 tablets b.i.d.). To meet individual requirements, if comfortable bowel movement is not achieved by the second day, decrease or increase daily by ½ level tsp. or 1 tablet (up to maximum) until optimal dose for evacuation is established.

How Supplied: Granules: 2, 6, and 12 oz. plastic canisters. Tablets: Box of 20, bottles of 50 and 100.

SENOKOT Tablets Unit Strip Packs in boxes of 100 tablets; each tablet individually sealed in see-through pockets.

SENOKOT®-S Tablets
(standardized senna concentrate and docusate sodium)
Natural Laxative/Stool Softener Combination

Action and Uses: SENOKOT-S Tablets are designed to relieve both aspects of functional constipation—bowel inertia and hard, dry stools. They provide a natural neuroperistaltic stimulant combined with a classic stool softener: standardized senna concentrate gently stimulates Auerbach's plexus in the colonic wall, while docusate sodium softens the stool for smoother and easier evacuation. This coordinated dual action of the two ingredients results in colon-specific, predictable laxative effect, usually in 8–10 hours. Administering the tablets at bedtime allows the patient an uninterrupted night's sleep, with a comfortable evacuation in the morning. Flexibility of dosage permits fine adjustment to individual requirements. At proper dosage levels, SENOKOT-S Tablets are virtually free from side effects. SENOKOT-S Tablets are highly suitable for relief of postsurgical and postpartum constipation, and effectively counteract drug-induced constipation. They facilitate regular elimination in impaction-prone and elderly patients, and are indicated in the presence of cardiovascular disease where straining must be avoided, as well as in the presence of hemorrhoids and anorectal disease.

Contraindications: Acute surgical abdomen.

Administration and Dosage: (preferably at bedtime) Recommended Initial Dosage: ADULTS—2 tablets (maximum dosage—4 tablets b.i.d.); CHILDREN (above 60 lbs.)—1 tablet (maximum dosage—2 tablets b.i.d.). For older or debilitated patients, the physician may consider prescribing half the initial adult dose. To meet individual requirements, if comfortable bowel movement is not achieved by the second day, dosage may be decreased or increased by 1 tablet, up to maximum, until the most effective dose is established.

Supplied: Bottles of 30 and 60 Tablets.

TRILISATE® TABLETS/LIQUID ℞
(choline magnesium trisalicylate)
500 mg or 750 mg
salicylate content

Description: TRILISATE Tablets/Liquid are non-steroidal, anti-inflammatory preparations combining choline salicylate and magnesium salicylate in mixtures which are freely soluble in water.

TRILISATE Tablets are available in scored, pale pink 500 mg tablets and scored, off-white 750 mg tablets. Trilisate Liquid is a cherry-cordial flavored liquid providing 500 mg salicylate content per teaspoonful (5 ml) for oral administration.

Each 500 mg tablet contains 293 mg of choline salicylate combined with 362 mg of magnesium salicylate to provide 500 mg salicylate content. Each 750 mg tablet contains 440 mg of choline salicylate combined with 544 mg of magnesium salicylate to provide 750 mg salicylate content. TRILISATE Liquid contains 293 mg of choline salicylate combined with 362 mg of magnesium salicylate to provide 500 mg salicylate per teaspoonful (5 ml) in a clear amber, cherry-cordial flavored vehicle.

Clinical Pharmacology: TRILISATE Tablets/Liquid contain salicylate with anti-inflammatory, analgesic, and antipyretic action. On ingestion of TRILISATE Tablets/Liquid, the salicylate moiety is absorbed rapidly and reaches peak blood levels within an average of one to two hours after single doses of the tablets or liquid. The primary route of excretion is renal: the excretion products are chiefly the glycine and glucuronide conjugates. The bioequivalence of TRILISATE Liquid and Tablets 500 mg/750 mg has been established. With the tablets, a steady-state condition is usually reached after 4 to 5 doses, and the half-life of elimination, on repeated administration of the tablets, is 9 to 17 hours. This permits a maintenance dosage schedule of once or twice daily. Unlike aspirin and certain other non-steroidal anti-inflammatory agents, such as arylpropionic acid derivatives and arylacetic acid derivatives, choline magnesium trisalicylate, at therapeutic dosage levels, does not affect platelet aggregation, as shown in in-vitro and in-vivo studies.

Indications and Usage: Salicylates are considered the base therapy of choice in the arthritides; and TRILISATE preparations are indicated for the relief of the signs and symptoms of rheumatoid arthritis, osteoarthritis and other arthritides. TRILISATE Tablets or Liquid are indicated in the long-term management of these diseases and especially in the acute flare of rheumatoid arthritis. TRILISATE Tablets or Liquid are also indicated for the treatment of acute painful shoulder.

TRILISATE preparations are effective and generally well tolerated, and are logical choices whenever salicylate treatment is indicated. They are particularly suitable when a once-a-day or b.i.d. dosage regimen is important to patient compliance; when gastrointestinal intolerance to aspirin is encountered; when gastrointestinal microbleeding or hematologic effects of aspirin are considered a patient hazard; and when interference (or the risk of interference) with normal platelet function by aspirin or by propionic acid derivatives is considered to be clinically undesirable. Use of TRILISATE Liquid is appropriate when a liquid dosage form is preferred, as in the elderly patient.

The efficacy of TRILISATE preparations has not been studied in those patients who are designated by the American Rheumatism Association as belonging in Functional Class IV (incapacitated, largely or wholly bedridden or confined to a wheelchair, with little or no self-care).

Contraindications: Patients who are hypersensitive to non-acetylated salicylates should not take TRILISATE Tablets or Liquid.

Precautions: Like other salicylates, TRILISATE preparations should be used with caution in patients with chronic renal insufficiency or with active erosive gastritis or peptic ulcer.

Reports indicate that when acetylated salicylates are given with steroids, the butazones, or alcohol, the risk of gastrointestinal ulceration is increased. Caution should be exercised in patients requiring coumarin or indandione anticoagulants, or heparin.

While salicylates are not known to be associated with teratogenic potential in man, the usual care should be exercised in the administration of any drug during pregnancy. Because of the possible inhibition of prostaglandin with high doses of salicylates, the use of TRILISATE (choline magnesium trisalicylate) preparations immediately prior to the onset of labor is not recommended. TRILISATE Tablets or Liquid are presently not recommended for children under twelve years.

Adverse Reactions: Choline magnesium trisalicylate is generally well tolerated at recommended dosage ranges, and has been shown to be particularly well tolerated by the gastrointestinal system. Salicylism and/or salicylate intoxication may occur with large doses or with extended therapy.

Tinnitus may be regarded as a therapeutic guide. Should it develop, reduction of dosage is recommended.

Dosage: The recommended initial daily dosage for rheumatoid arthritis, osteoarthritis, the more severe arthritides, and acute painful shoulder is 2000 mg to 3000 mg daily in divided doses (b.i.d.) or single dose (q.d.).

Based on patient response or salicylate blood levels, dosage may be adjusted to achieve optimum therapeutic effect. Salicylate blood levels should be in the range of 15 to 30 mg/100 ml for anti-inflammatory effect and 5 to 15 mg/100 ml for analgesia and antipyrexia.

Each 500 mg tablet or teaspoonful is equivalent in salicylate content to 10 gr of aspirin and each 750 mg tablet to 15 gr of aspirin.

If the physician prefers, the recommended daily dosage may be administered on a t.i.d. schedule.

As with other therapeutic agents, individual dosage adjustment is advisable, and a number of patients may require higher or lower dosages than those recommended. Certain patients require 2–3 weeks therapy for optimal effect.

TRILISATE Liquid may be mixed with fruit juices just before drinking.

Caution: Federal law prohibits dispensing without a prescription.

How Supplied: 500 mg TRILISATE Tablets (pale pink, scored) in bottles of 100 tablets. 750 mg TRILISATE Tablets (off-white, scored) in bottles of 100 tablets.

[*Shown in Product Identification Section*]

TRILISATE Liquid in bottles of 8 fl. oz. (237 ml).

U.S. Patent Numbers 3759980 and 4067974

Reed & Carnrick
1 NEW ENGLAND AVENUE
PISCATAWAY, NJ 08854

ALPHOSYL®
Lotion, Cream

Description: Special crude coal tar extract 5.0% and allantoin 1.7% in synergistic combination in a greaseless, stainless vanishing cream base.

Actions: In the treatment of psoriasis and other chronic dermatoses with itching, scaling and erythema.

Precautions: ALPHOSYL is safe for use as directed. However, if irritation and/or redness occurs, discontinue use and consult physician. Alphosyl is for external use only; avoid contact with the eyes.

Directions for use: SHAKE WELL BEFORE USING.

1.) Apply ALPHOSYL Lotion to affected areas two to four times daily, morning and night, massaging thoroughly into the lesions.

2.) For persistent, long term cases, with heavy scaling and crusting, a hot daily bath is recommended to soften and facilitate removal of scales, prior to applying ALPHOSYL Lotion.

3.) MAINTENANCE THERAPY: Once the condition is under control, ALPHOSYL Lotion should be applied 2 to 3 times weekly to help prevent recurrence. Treatments may be repeated as directed by physician.

How Supplied: ALPHOSYL Lotion 8 fl. oz.; ALPHOSYL Cream 2 oz. tube.

ALSO AVAILABLE as ALPHOSYL-HC Lotion (0.5% hydrocortisone) in 4 oz. bottles and ALPHOSYL-HC Cream (0.5% hydrocortisone) in 30 g tubes, on prescription.

CORTIFOAM® ℞
(hydrocortisone acetate) 10%

Description: Contains hydrocortisone acetate 10% as the sole active ingredient in 20 g of a foam containing propylene glycol, ethoxylated stearyl alcohol, polyoxyethylene-10-stearyl ether, cetyl alcohol, methylparaben and propylparaben, trolamine, water and inert propellants, dichlorodifluoromethane and dichlorotetrafluoroethane.

Each application delivers approximately 900 mg of foam containing 80 mg of hydrocortisone (90 mg of hydrocortisone acetate).

Clinical Pharmacology: CORTIFOAM provides effective topical administration of an anti-inflammatory corticosteroid as adjunctive therapy of ulcerative proctitis.

Indications: CORTIFOAM is indicated as adjunctive therapy in the topical treatment of ulcerative proctitis of the distal portion of the rectum in patients who cannot retain hydrocortisone or other corticosteroid enemas. Direct observations of methylene blue-containing foam have shown staining about 10 centimeters into the rectum.

Contraindications: Local contraindications to the use of intrarectal steroids include obstruction, abscess, perforation, peritonitis, fresh intestinal anastomoses, extensive fistulas and sinus tracts. Tuberculosis (active, latent or questionably healed), ocular herpes simplex and acute psychosis are usually considered absolute contraindications to the use of corticosteroids. Relative contraindications include active peptic ulcer, acute glomerulonephritis, myasthenia gravis, osteoporosis, diverticulitis, thrombophlebitis, psychic disturbances, pregnancy, diabetes, hyperthyroidism, acute coronary disease, hypertension, limited cardiac reserve, and local or systemic infections, including fungal or exanthematous diseases. Where these conditions exist, the expected benefits from steroid therapy must be weighed against the risks involved in its use. Pregnancy is a relative contraindication to corticosteroids, particularly during third trimester. If corticosteroids must be administered in pregnancy, watch newborn infant closely for signs of hypoadrenalism, and administer appropriate therapy if needed.

Warning: Do not insert any part of the aerosol container into the anus. Contents of the container are under pressure, but not flammable. Do not burn or puncture the aerosol container. Store at room temperature but not over 120° F. Because CORTIFOAM is not expelled, systemic hydrocortisone absorption may be greater from CORTIFOAM than from corticosteroid enema formulations. If there is no evidence of clinical or proctologic improvement within two or three weeks after starting CORTIFOAM therapy, or if the patient's condition worsens, discontinue the drug.

Precautions: Steroid therapy should be administered with caution in patients with severe ulcerative disease because these patients are predisposed to perforation of the bowel wall. Where surgery is imminent, it is hazardous to wait more than a few days for a satisfactory response to medical treatment. General precautions common to all corticosteroid therapy should be observed during treatment with CORTIFOAM. These include gradual withdrawal of therapy to allow for possible adrenal insufficiency and awareness to possible growth suppression in children. Patients should be kept under close observation, for, as with all drugs, rare individuals may react unfavorably under certain conditions. If severe reactions or idiosyncrasies occur, steroids should be discontinued immediately and appropriate measures instituted. Do not employ in immediate or early postoperative period following ileorectostomy.

Adverse Reactions: Corticosteroid therapy may produce side effects which include moon face, fluid retention, excessive appetite and weight gain, abnormal fat deposits, mental symptoms, hypertrichosis, acne, ecchymosis, increased sweating, pigmentation, dry scaly skin, thinning scalp hair, thrombophlebitis, decreased resistance to infection, negative nitrogen balance with delayed bone and wound healing, menstrual disorders, neuropathy, peptic ulcer, decreased glucose tolerance, hypopotassemia, adrenal insufficiency, necrotizing angiitis, hypertension, pancreatitis and increased intraocular pressure. In children, suppression of growth may occur. Increased intracranial pressure may occur and possibly acount for headache, insomnia and fatigue. Subcapsular cataracts may result from prolonged usage. Long-term use of all corticosteroids results in catabolic effects characterized by negative protein and calcium balance. Osteoporosis, spontaneous fractures and aseptic necrosis of the hip and humerus may occur as part of this catabolic phenomenon. Where hypopotasse-

Continued on next page

Reed & Carnrick—Cont.

mia and other symptoms associated with fluid and electrolyte imbalance call for potassium supplementation and salt poor or salt-free diets, these may be instituted and are compatible with diet requirements for ulcerative proctitis.
Administration and Dosage: Usual dose is one applicatorful once or twice daily for two or three weeks, and every second day thereafter, administered rectally. The patient directions packaged with the applicator describe how to use the aerosol container and applicator. Satisfactory response usually occurs within five to seven days marked by a decrease in symptoms. Symptomatic improvement in ulcerative proctitis should not be used as the sole criterion for evaluating efficacy. Sigmoidoscopy is also recommended to judge dosage adjustment, duration of therapy and rate of improvement.
Directions For Use: 1) Shake foam container vigorously before use. Hold container upright and insert into opening of the tip of the applicator. Be sure applicator plunger is drawn all the way out. Container must be held upright to obtain proper flow of medication 2) To fill, press down slowly on container cap. When foam reaches fill line in the applicator, it is ready for use. Caution: The aerosol container should never be inserted directly into the anus. 3) Remove applicator from container. Allow some foam to remain on the applicator tip. Hold applicator by barrel and gently insert tip into the anus. With applicator in place, push plunger in order to expel foam, then withdraw applicator. (Applicator parts should be pulled apart for thorough cleaning with warm water.)
How Supplied: CORTIFOAM is supplied in an aerosol container with a special rectal applicator. Each applicator delivers approximately 900 mg of foam containing approximately 80 mg of hydrocortisone as 90 mg of hydrocortisone acetate. The aerosol container will deliver a minimum of 14 applications.
Literature Available: Patient information available on request.

[*Shown in Product Identification Section*]

DILATRATE-® SR ℞
[isosorbide dinitrate]
Sustained Release Capsules 40 mg

Description: DILATRATE-SR (isosorbide dinitrate) provides up to 12 hours of continuous vasodilatation.
Actions: The basic action is that of all nitrates, the relaxation of smooth muscle. How this relates to its clinical usefulness in the treatment of angina pectoris (pain of coronary artery disease) is not clear, since the exact cause of this pain is also obscure.
The objective of therapy is a decrease in the frequency and severity of attacks of angina pectoris and a decrease in the need to use nitroglycerin. This is the only practical way to judge the effects of therapy, especially since there is a wide variation in symptomatic response to treatment.

Indications:
Based on a review of this drug by the National Academy of Sciences-National Research Council and/or other information, FDA has classified the indications as follows:
"Possibly" effective: When taken by the oral route, is indicated for the relief of angina pectoris (pain of coronary artery disease). It is not intended to abort the acute anginal episode, but is widely regarded in the prophylactic treatment of angina pectoris.
Final classification of the less-than-effective indication requires further investigation.

Contraindications: Idiosyncracy to this drug.
Warnings: Data supporting the use of nitrates and nitrites during the early days of the acute phase of myocardial infarction (the period during which clinical and laboratory findings are unstable) are insufficient to establish safety.
Precautions:
1. Tolerance to this drug, and cross-tolerance to other nitrates or nitrites may occur.
2. In patients with functional or organic gastrointestinal hypermotility or malabsorption syndrome it is suggested that either the 5 mg or 10 mg oral tablets or 2.5 mg or 5 mg sublingual tablets be the preferred therapy.

Adverse Reactions:
1. Cutaneous vasodilation with flushing.
2. Headache is common and may be severe and persistent.
3. Transient episodes of dizziness and weakness, as well as other signs of cerebral ischemia associated with postural hypotension, may occasionally develop.
4. This drug can act as a physiological antagonist to norepinephrine, acetylcholine, histamine, and many other agents.
5. An occasional individual exhibits marked sensitivity to the hypotensive effects of nitrite, and severe responses (nausea, vomiting, weakness, restlessness, pallor, perspiration and collapse) can occur even with the usual therapeutic dose. Alcohol may enhance this effect.
6. Drug rash and/or exfoliative dermatitis may occasionally occur.

Dosage and Administration:
Initiating Therapy: In starting patients on isosorbide dinitrate, it is necessary to adjust the dosage until the smallest effective dose is determined.
Occasionally, severe hypotensive responses may occur with this dosage form.
DILATRATE-SR 40 mg Sustained Release Capsules: Average dose is one capsule orally, every 6 to 12 hrs. according to need.
It is recommended that DILATRATE-SR be taken on an empty stomach. If vascular headache cannot be effectively controlled by ordinary measures, dosages may be taken with meals to minimize this side effect.
How Supplied: Bottles of 100 (flesh cap and colorless body) capsules.
Storage: Store at controlled room temperature 15–30°C (59–86°F) in a dry place.
Warning: Keep out of reach of children.

[*Shown in Product Identification Section*]

EPIFOAM™ ℞
(hydrocortisone acetate) 1%

Description: A topical steroid foam containing hydrocortisone acetate 1%
Inactive ingredients: Pramoxine HCl, propylene glycol, cetyl alcohol, PEG-100 stearate, glyceryl stearate, laureth-23, polyoxyl-40 stearate, methylparaben, propylparaben, trolamine or hydrochloric acid to adjust pH, purified water, butane and propane propellant (inert).
Actions: Topical steroids are primarily effective because of their anti-inflammatory, antipruritic and vasoconstrictive actions.
Indications: For relief of the inflammatory manifestations of corticosteroid-responsive dermatoses.
Contraindications: Topical steroids are contraindicated in those patients with a history of hypersensitivity to any of the components of the preparation.
Precautions: If irritation develops, the product should be discontinued and appropriate therapy instituted.
In the presence of an infection, the use of appropriate antifungal or antibacterial agents should be instituted. If a favorable response does not occur promptly, the corticosteroid should be discontinued until the infection has been adequately controlled.
If extensive areas are treated or if the occlusive technique is used, the possibility exists of increased systemic absorption of the corticosteroid and suitable precautions should be taken, particularly in children and infants. Although topical steroids have not been reported to have any adverse effect on human pregnancy, the safety of their use in pregnant women has not absolutely been established. In laboratory animals, increases in incidence of fetal abnormalities have been associated with exposure of gestating females to topical corticosteroids, in some cases at rather low dosage levels. Therefore, drugs of this class should not be used extensively on pregnant patients, in large amounts, or for prolonged periods of time.
The product is not for ophthalmic use.
Adverse Reactions: The following local adverse reactions have been reported with topical corticosteroids: burning, itching, irritation, dryness, folliculitis, hypertrichosis, acneiform eruptions, hypopigmentation, allergic contact dermatitis, maceration of the skin, secondary infection, skin atrophy, striae and miliaria.
Dosage and Administration: Apply to affected areas 3 or 4 times daily. Transfer the medication to a pad and apply gently, or apply the foam directly. Refer to the enclosed "Directions for Use".
How Supplied: Available in 10 g pressurized cans.

[*Shown in Product Identification Section*]

KWELL® Cream ℞
(lindane) 1%

Description: Active ingredient lindane 1%. Inert ingredients: 99% in a non-greasy pleasantly scented water-dispersible cream, containing stearic acid, lanolin, glycerin, 2-amino-2-methyl-1-propanol, perfume and purified water.
Actions and Indications: KWELL Cream is an ectoparasiticide and ovacide indicated for the treatment of patients with Sarcoptes scabiei (scabies), as well as infestations of Pediculus capitis (head lice), Phthirus pubis (crab lice), and their ova.
Contraindications: KWELL Cream is contraindicated for individuals with known sensitivity to the product or to any of its components.
Warning: KWELL CREAM SHOULD BE USED WITH CAUTION, ESPECIALLY ON INFANTS, CHILDREN AND PREGNANT WOMEN. LINDANE PENETRATES HUMAN SKIN AND HAS THE POTENTIAL FOR CNS TOXICITY. STUDIES INDICATE THAT POTENTIAL TOXIC EFFECTS OF TOPICALLY APPLIED LINDANE ARE GREATER IN THE YOUNG. Seizures have been reported after the use of lindane, but a cause and effect relationship has not been established.
Simultaneous application of creams, ointments or oils may enhance the percutaneous absorption of lindane.
Precautions: If accidental ingestion occurs, prompt gastric lavage will rid the body of large amounts of the toxicant. However, since oils favor absorption, saline cathartics for intestinal evacuation should be given rather than oil laxatives. If central nervous system manifestations occur, they can be antagonized by the administration of pentobarbital or phenobarbital.
If accidental contact with the eyes occurs, flush with water. If irritation or sensitization occurs, discontinue use and consult a physician.
Adverse Reactions: Eczematous eruptions due to irritation from this product have been reported.

ADMINISTRATION
CAUTION: USE ONLY AS DIRECTED. DO NOT EXCEED RECOMMENDED DOSAGE.
NOTE: PLEASE READ CAREFULLY.

Directions for Use:
Pediculosis capitis (head lice)—KWELL Shampoo is the most convenient dosage form but the lotion and cream are also effective.
Apply a sufficient quantity to cover only the affected and adjacent hairy areas. The cream should be rubbed into scalp and hair, and left in place for 8–12 hours followed by a thorough washing (shower or bath.)
Retreatment is usually not necessary. Demonstrable living lice after 7 days indicate that retreatment is necessary.
Pediculosis pubis (crab lice)—Apply a sufficient quantity to cover thinly the hair and skin of the pubic area, and if infested the thighs, trunk, and axillary regions. The medication should be rubbed into the skin and hair, and left in place for 8–12 hours followed by a thorough washing (shower or bath).
Retreatment is usually not necessary. Demonstrable living lice after 7 days indicate that retreatment is necessary. Sexual contacts should be treated simultaneously.
Scabies (Sarcoptes scabiei)—The cream should be applied to dry skin in a thin layer and rubbed in thoroughly. If crusted lesions are present, a warm bath preceding the medication is helpful. If a warm bath is used, allow the skin to dry and cool before applying the cream. Usually one ounce is sufficient for an adult. A total body application should be made from the neck down. Scabies rarely affects the head of children or adults but may occur in infants. The cream should be left on for 8–12 hours and should then be removed by a thorough washing (shower or bath).
ONE APPLICATION IS USUALLY CURATIVE.
Many patients exhibit persistent pruritus after treatment; this is rarely a sign of treatment failure and is not an indication for retreatment, unless living mites can be demonstrated.
How Supplied: KWELL Cream in tubes of 2 oz (57G) and jars of 16 oz (454G).
Literature Available: Patient information and instruction pads with directions for use available on request.

KWELL® Lotion (lindane) 1% ℞

Description: Active ingredient lindane 1%. Inert ingredients: 99% in a non-greasy, pleasantly scented base, containing glyceryl monostearate, cetyl alcohol, stearic acid, trolamine, 2-amino-2-methyl-1-propanol, butyl p-hydroxybenzoate, methyl p-hydroxy-benzoate, Irish moss extract, perfume and purified water.
Actions and Indications: KWELL Lotion is an ectoparasiticide and ovacide indicated for the treatment of patients with Sarcoptes scabiei (scabies), as well as infestations of Pediculus capitis (head lice), Phthirus pubis (crab lice), and their ova.
Contraindications: KWELL Lotion is contraindicated for individuals with known sensitivity to the product or to any of its components.
Warning: KWELL LOTION SHOULD BE USED WITH CAUTION, ESPECIALLY ON INFANTS, CHILDREN AND PREGNANT WOMEN. LINDANE PENETRATES HUMAN SKIN AND HAS THE POTENTIAL FOR CNS TOXICITY. STUDIES INDICATE THAT POTENTIAL TOXIC EFFECTS OF TOPICALLY APPLIED LINDANE ARE GREATER IN THE YOUNG. Seizures have been reported after the use of lindane, but a cause and effect relationship has not been established.
Simultaneous application of creams, ointments or oils may enhance the percutaneous absorption of lindane.
Precautions: If accidental ingestion occurs, prompt gastric lavage will rid the body of large amounts of the toxicant. However, since oils favor absorption, saline cathartics for intestinal evacuation should be given rather than oil laxatives. If central nervous system manifestations occur, they can be antagonized by the administration of pentobarbital or phenobarbital.
If accidental contact with the eyes occurs, flush with water. If irritation or sensitization occurs, discontinue use and consult a physician.
Adverse Reactions: Eczematous eruptions due to irritation from this product have been reported.

ADMINISTRATION
CAUTION: USE ONLY AS DIRECTED. DO NOT EXCEED RECOMMENDED DOSAGE.
NOTE: PLEASE READ CAREFULLY.

Directions For Use:
Pediculosis capitis (head lice)—KWELL Shampoo is the most convenient dosage form but the lotion and cream are also effective.
Apply a sufficient quantity to cover only the affected and adjacent hairy areas. The lotion should be rubbed into scalp and hair, and left in place for 8–12 hours followed by a thorough washing (shower or bath).
Retreatment is usually not necessary. Demonstrable living lice after 7 days indicate that retreatment is necessary.
Pediculosis pubis (crab lice)—Apply a sufficient quantity to cover thinly the hair and skin of the pubic area, and if infested, the thighs, trunk, and axillary regions. The medication should be rubbed into the skin and hair and left in place for 8–12 hours followed by a thorough washing (shower or bath).
Retreatment is usually not necessary. Demonstrable living lice after 7 days indicate that retreatment is necessary. Sexual contacts should be treated simultaneously.
Scabies (Sarcoptes scabiei)—The lotion should be applied to dry skin in a thin layer and rubbed in thoroughly. If crusted lesions are present, a warm bath preceding the medication is helpful. If a warm bath is used, allow the skin to dry and cool before applying the lotion. Usually one ounce is sufficient for an adult. A total body application should be made from the neck down. Scabies rarely affects the head of children or adults but may occur in infants. The lotion should be left on for 8–12 hours and should then be removed by a thorough washing (shower or bath). ONE APPLICATION IS USUALLY CURATIVE.
Many patients exhibit persistent pruritus after treatment; this is rarely a sign of treatment failure and is not an indication for retreatment, unless living mites can be demonstrated.
How Supplied: KWELL Lotion in bottles of 2 fl. oz (59ml), 16 fl. oz (472ml) and 1 gallon (3.8 L).
Literature Available: Patient information and instruction pads with directions for use available on request.

KWELL® Shampoo (lindane) 1% ℞

Description: Active ingredient lindane 1%. Inert ingredients: 99% in a cosmetically pleasant shampoo base, containing polyoxyethylene sorbitan monostearate, TEA-lauryl sulfate, acetone and purified water.
Actions and Indications: KWELL Shampoo is an ectoparasiticide and ovicide indicated for the treatment of infestations of Pediculus capitis (head lice), Phthirus pubis (crab lice), and their nits.
Contraindications: KWELL Shampoo is contraindicated for individuals with known sensitivity to the product or to any of its components.
Warning: KWELL SHAMPOO SHOULD BE USED WITH CAUTION, ESPECIALLY ON INFANTS, CHILDREN AND PREGNANT WOMEN. LINDANE PENETRATES HUMAN SKIN AND HAS THE POTENTIAL FOR CNS TOXICITY. STUDIES INDICATE THAT POTENTIAL TOXIC EFFECTS OF TOPICALLY APPLIED LINDANE ARE GREATER IN THE YOUNG. Seizures have been reported after the use of lindane, but a cause and effect relationship has not been established.
Simultaneous application of creams, ointments or oils may enhance the percutaneous absorption of lindane.
Precautions: If accidental ingestion occurs, prompt gastric lavage will rid the body of large amounts of the toxicant. However, since oils favor absorption, saline cathartics for intestinal evacuation should be given rather than oil laxatives. If central nervous system manifestations occur, they can be antagonized by the administration of pentobarbital, or phenobarbital.
If accidental contact with the eyes occurs, flush with water. If irritation or sensitization occurs, discontinue use and consult a physician.
Adverse Reactions: Eczematous eruptions due to irritation from this product have been reported.

ADMINISTRATION
CAUTION: USE ONLY AS DIRECTED. DO NOT EXCEED RECOMMENDED DOSAGE.
NOTE: PLEASE READ CAREFULLY

Directions For Use:
Pediculosis capitis (head lice)—1) Apply a sufficient quantity of the shampoo to thoroughly wet the hair and skin of the infested and adjacent hairy areas. 2) Work thoroughly into the hair and allow to remain in place 4 minutes. 3) Add small quantities of water until a good lather forms. 4) Rinse thoroughly. Towel briskly. When the hair is dry, any remaining nits or nit shells may be removed by fine-tooth combing or with tweezers.
Retreatment is usually not necessary. Demonstrable living lice after 7 days indicate that retreatment is necessary.
Pediculosis pubis (crab lice)—1) Apply a sufficient quantity of the shampoo to thoroughly wet the hair and skin of the infested and adjacent, hairy areas. 2) Work thoroughly into the hair and allow to remain in place 4 minutes. 3) Add small quantities of water until a good lather forms. 4) Rinse thoroughly. Towel briskly. When the hair is dry, any remaining nits or nit shells may be removed by fine tooth combing or tweezers. 5) Sexual contacts should be examined and treated if necessary.
Retreatment is usually not necessary. Demonstrable living lice after 7 days indicate that retreatment is required. Sexual contacts should be treated simultaneously.
NOTE: KWELL Shampoo is intended only for head lice and crab lice infestations and should not be used as a routine shampoo. For other ectoparasitic infestations, such as scabies, the use of KWELL Cream or KWELL Lotion is recommended.
How Supplied: KWELL Shampoo in bottles of 2 fl. oz (59ml), 16 fl. oz (472ml) and 1 gallon (3.8L).
Literature Available: Patient information and instruction pads with directions for use available on request.

PHAZYME® Tablets

Description: A pink coated two-phase tablet. The outer layer releases in the stomach: specially activated simethicone 20 mg. The enteric coated core releases in the small intestine: pancreatic enzymes (protease 3,000 USP units, lipase 240 USP units, amylase 2,000 USP units), and specially activated simethicone 40 mg.
Actions: PHAZYME is the only dual approach to the problem of gastrointestinal gas. Simethicone minimizes gas formation and re-

Continued on next page

Reed & Carnrick—Cont.

lieves gas entrapment in both the stomach and the lower G.I. tract. This action combats pain, due to gastrointestinal gas. Pancreatic enzymes enhance the normal digestive process and help to reduce gas formation. Also, for relief of gas distress associated with other functional or organic conditions such as: diverticulitis, spastic colitis, hyperacidity, post-cholecystectomy syndrome and chronic cholecystitis.
Indications: PHAZYME is indicated for the relief of occasional or chronic pain caused by gas entrapped in the stomach or in the lower gastrointestinal tract—resulting from aerophagia, postoperative distention, dyspepsia and food intolerance.
Contraindications: A known sensitivity to any ingredient.
Dosage: One or two tablets with each meal and at bedtime or as required.
How Supplied: Pink coated two-phase tablet in bottles of 50, 100, and 1,000.
[*Shown in Product Identification Section*]

PHAZYME®-95 Tablets

Description: A red coated two-phase tablet with the highest dose of simethicone available in a single tablet. The outer layer releases in the stomach: specially activated simethicone 25 mg. The enteric coated core releases in the small intestine: pancreatic enzymes (protease 6,000 USP units, lipase 480 USP units, amylase 4,000 USP units), and specially activated simethicone 70 mg.
Actions: PHAZYME is the only dual approach to the problem of gastrointestinal gas. Simethicone minimizes gas formation and relieves gas entrapment in both the stomach and the lower G.I. tract. This action combats pain due to gastrointestinal gas. Pancreatic enzymes enhance the normal digestive process and help to reduce gas formation. Also, for relief of gas distress associated with other functional or organic conditions such as: diverticulitis, spastic colitis, hyperacidity, post-cholecystectomy syndrome and chronic cholecystitis.
Indications: PHAZYME-95 is indicated for the relief of acute severe lower intestinal pain due to gas—resulting from aerophagia, postoperative distention, dyspepsia and food intolerance.
Contraindications: A known sensitivity to any ingredient.
Dosage: One tablet with each meal and at bedtime, or as required.
How Supplied: Red coated two-phase tablets, in bottles of 100.
[*Shown in Product Identification Section*]

PHAZYME®-PB Tablets ℂ ℞

Description: A yellow coated two-phase tablet. The outer layer releases in the stomach: specially activated simethicone 20 mg and phenobarbital 15 mg, (WARNING: MAY BE HABIT FORMING). The enteric coated core releases in the small intestine: pancreatic enzymes (protease 3,000 USP units, lipase 240 USP units, amylase 2,000 USP units), and specially activated simethicone 40 mg.
Actions: PHAZYME-PB provides the same advantages of the PHAZYME formula (minimizes gas formation, relieves gas entrapment) and in addition, supplies the calming benefits of phenobarbital to control the emotional component of gastrointestinal gas pain. Also, for relief of gas distress associated with other functional or organic conditions such as: diverticulitis, spastic colitis, hyperacidity, post-cholecystectomy syndrome and chronic cholecystitis.
Indications: PHAZYME-PB is indicated for gas pain associated with anxiety-resulting in aerophagia, post-operative distention, dyspepsia and food intolerance.
Contraindications: Known sensitivity to barbiturates or to any ingredient.
Warning: May be habit forming.
Precautions: Excessive use may produce drowsiness.
Dosage: One or two tablets with each meal and at bedtime or as required.
How Supplied: Yellow coated two-phase tablets in bottles of 100 and 1000.
[*Shown in Product Identification Section*]

proctoFoam®/non-steroid
(pramoxine HCl 1%)

Description: proctoFoam is a foam for anal and perianal use containing pramoxine hydrochloride 1%, in a water-miscible mucoadhesive foam base of mineral oil.
Actions: proctoFoam is an anesthetic mucoadhesive foam which medicates the anorectal mucosa, and provides prompt temporary relief from itching and pain. Its lubricating action helps make bowel evacuations more comfortable.
Indications: Prompt, temporary relief of anorectal inflammation, pruritus and pain associated with hemorrhoids, proctitis, cryptitis, fissures, postoperative pain and pruritus ani.
Contraindications: Contraindicated in persons hypersensitive to any of the ingredients.
Warning: Not for prolonged use. Do not use more than four consecutive weeks. If redness, pain, irritation or swelling persists or rectal bleeding occurs, discontinue use and consult a physician. Keep this and all medicines out of the reach of children.
Caution: Do not insert any part of the aerosol container into the anus. Contents of the container are under pressure, but not flammable. Do not burn or puncture the aerosol container. Store at room temperature, not over 120° F.
Dosage:
One applicatorful two or three times daily and after bowel evacuation.

1. To fill—Shake foam container vigorously before use. Hold container upright and insert into opening of applicator tip. With applicator drawn out all the way, press down on container cap. When foam reaches fill line in the applicator, it is ready to use.

CAUTION: The aerosol container should never be inserted directly into the anus.

2. To administer—Separate applicator from container. Hold applicator by barrel and gently insert tip into the anus. With applicator in place, push plunger in order to expel foam, then withdraw applicator. (Applicator parts should be pulled apart for thorough cleaning with warm water.)

Note: To relieve itching place some foam on a tissue and apply externally.
How Supplied: Available in 15 g aerosol container, with special plastic applicator. The aerosol supplies approximately 18 applications.
Literature Available: Instruction pads with directions for use available upon request.
[*Shown in Product Identification Section*]

PROCTOFOAM®-HC ℞
(hydrocortisone acetate) 1%

Description: PROCTOFOAM-HC contains as active ingredient: Hydrocortisone acetate 1% in a hydrophilic base containing: pramoxine hydrochloride, propylene glycol, ethoxylated cetyl and stearyl alcohol, polyoxyethylene-10-stearyl ether, cetyl alcohol, methylparaben, propylparaben, trolamine, purified water; propellant (inert) dichlorodifluoromethane and dichlorotetrafluoroethane.
Actions: Topical steroids are primarily effective because of their anti-inflammatory, antipruritic and vasoconstrictive actions.
Indications: For relief of the inflammatory manifestations of corticosteroid-responsive dermatoses of the anogenital area.
Contraindications: Topical steroids are contraindicated in those patients with a history of sensitivity to any of the components of the preparation.
Precautions: If irritation develops, the product should be discontinued and appropriate therapy instituted.
In the presence of an infection, the use of appropriate antifungal or antibacterial agents should be instituted. If a favorable response does not occur promptly, the corticosteroid should be discontinued until the infection has been adequately controlled.
If extensive areas are treated or if the occlusive technique is used, the possibility exists of increased systemic absorption of the corticosteroid and suitable precautions should be taken particularly in children and infants.
Although topical steroids have not been reported to have an adverse effect on human pregnancy, the safety of their use in pregnant women has not absolutely been established. In laboratory animals, increases in incidence of fetal abnormalities have been associated with exposure of gestating females to topical corticosteroids, in some cases at rather low dosage levels. Therefore, drugs of this class should not be used extensively on pregnant patients, in large amounts, or for prolonged periods of time.
This product is not for ophthalmic use.
Adverse Reactions: The following local adverse reactions have been reported with topical corticosteroids, especially under occlusive dressings: burning, itching, irritation, dryness, folliculitis, hypertrichosis, acneiform eruptions, hypopigmentation, allergic contact dermatitis, maceration of the skin, secondary infection, skin atrophy, striae, and miliaria.
Dosage and Administration: Apply to affected areas 3 or 4 times daily. Use the applicator supplied for rectal application. For perianal use, transfer a small quantity to a tissue and apply gently.
1.) Shake foam container vigorously before use. Hold container upright and insert into opening of the tip of the applicator. Be sure applicator plunger is drawn all the way out. CONTAINER MUST BE HELD UPRIGHT TO OBTAIN PROPER FLOW OF MEDICATION.
2.) To fill, press down slowly on container cap. When foam reaches fill line in the applicator, it is ready for use. Caution: The aerosol container should never be inserted directly into the anus.
3.) Remove applicator from container. Allow some foam to remain on the applicator tip. Hold applicator by barrel and gently insert tip into the anus. With applicator in place, push plunger in order to expel foam, then withdraw applicator. (Applicator parts should be pulled apart for thorough cleaning with warm water.)
(See accompanying illustration)

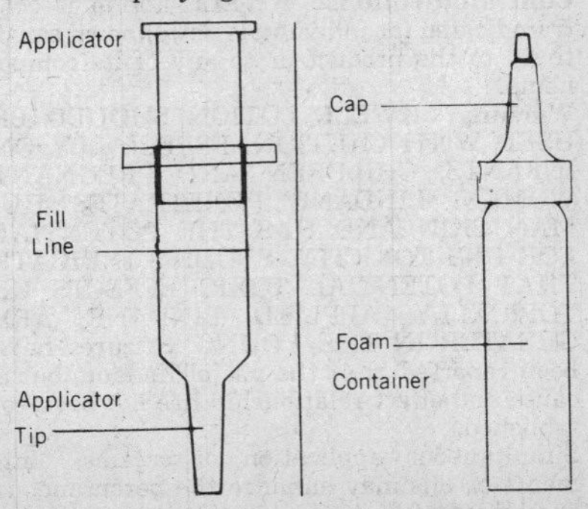

How Supplied: In aerosol container containing 10 g, with special rectal applicator. The aerosol supplies approximately 18 applications.

Literature Available: Instruction pads with directions for use available upon request.

[Shown in Product Identification Section]

PROXIGEL® Oral Cleanser
(carbamide peroxide 11%)

Description: PROXIGEL is a cleansing aid for minor oral inflammations. Active ingredient: Carbamide peroxide 11% in a water free gel base.

Actions: PROXIGEL releases oxygen on contact with mouth tissues to provide cleansing effects. Unlike liquid preparations, PROXIGEL Oral Cleanser's unique viscous base adheres to affected areas for longer oxygenating and debriding action.

Indications: PROXIGEL is recommended for recurrent aphthous ulcerations (canker sores) and relief of minor inflammation of gums and other surfaces of the mouth and lips. PROXIGEL is also useful as adjunctive therapy in gingivitis, periodontitis, stomatitis, Vincent's infection and denture irritation. PROXIGEL helps to inhibit odor causing bacteria and helps soothe painful tissues.

Precautions: If condition persists or worsens, or irritation develops, discontinue use.

Dosage and Administration: Do not dilute. Use 4 times a day, or as directed. Apply directly with or without nozzle. Gently massage medication with finger or swab on affected area. Do not drink or rinse for 5 minutes. Always replace cap on nozzle after use. Store in cool place between 46° and 59°F (8° and 15 °C) or in a refrigerator.

How Supplied: Plastic tubes 1.2 oz. with special applicator top and guard cap.

R&C SPRAY™ Lice Control Insecticide

Description: Active ingredients: 3-Phenoxybenzyl d-cis and trans 2,2-dimethyl-3-(2-methylpropenyl)

cyclopropanecarboxylate	0.382%
Other Isomers	0.018%
Petroleum Distillates	4.255%
Inert Ingredients:	95.345%
	100.000%

Actions: R&C SPRAY is specially formulated to kill lice and their nits on inanimate objects.

Indications: R&C SPRAY is recommended for use only on bedding, mattresses, furniture and other objects infested or possibly infested with lice which cannot be laundered or dry cleaned.

Warnings: Contents under pressure. Do not use or store near heat or open flame. Do not puncture or incinerate container. Exposure to temperatures above 130°F may cause bursting. It is a violation of Federal law to use this product in a manner inconsistent with its labeling. NOT FOR USE ON HUMANS OR ANIMALS.

Caution: Avoid spraying in eyes. Avoid breathing spray mist. Avoid contact with the skin. In case of contact, wash immediately with soap and water. Harmful if swallowed. Vacate room after treatment and ventilate before reoccupying. Avoid contamination of feed and foodstuffs.

Remove pets, birds and cover fish aquariums before spraying.

Directions: SHAKE WELL BEFORE AND OCCASIONALLY DURING USE. Spray on an inconspicuous area to test for possible staining or discoloration. Inspect after drying, then proceed to spray entire area to be treated.

Hold container upright with nozzle away from you. Depress valve and spray from a distance of 8 to 10 inches. Spray each square foot for about three seconds. For mattresses, furniture, or similar objects (that cannot be laundered or dry cleaned): Spray thoroughly. Do not use article until spray is dry. Repeat treatment as necessary. Do not use in commercial food processing, preparation, storage or serving areas.

How Supplied: In 5 oz. aerosol container.

EPA REG NO	36232-2
EPA EST NO	(C) 11598-CT-1
	(D) 11525-RI-1
	(E) 5590-IL-1

TRICHOTINE® Powder Vaginal Douche

Description: A detergent, mucolytic, vaginal douche containing sodium lauryl sulfate, sodium perborate, sodium chloride, and aromatics.

Actions: Low surface tension enables TRICHOTINE to penetrate the rugal folds, remove mucous, debris, and vaginal discharge thereby making treatment of vaginitis more effective. TRICHOTINE deodorizes and affords prompt relief from itching and burning.

Indications: TRICHOTINE helps to establish a normal healthy mucosa as an adjunct in therapy of vaginitis. It may also be used in postmenstrual, postcoital or routine vaginal cleansing.

Contraindications: None reported.

Warning: For routine use, do not use more than twice weekly. May be used more frequently in concomitant use for treatment of vaginitis. Discontinue use if irritation develops.

Precautions: Use only in fresh solution—never use dry.

Side Effects: None reported.

Directions For Use: Dissolve one tablespoonful to each quart of warm water and mix thoroughly.

How Supplied: 5 oz., 12 oz., and 20 oz.

Literature Available: Instructions for the use of TRICHOTINE available in pads of 50 sheets.

TRICHOTINE® Liquid Vaginal Douche

Description: A detergent, mucolytic, vaginal douche containing sodium lauryl sulfate, sodium borate, with alcohol (SDA 23A) 8% and aromatics.

Actions: (See TRICHOTINE Powder above).

Indications: (See TRICHOTINE Powder above).

Contraindications: None reported.

Warning: For routine use, do not use more than twice weekly. May be used more frequently in concomitant use for treatment of vaginitis. Discontinue use if irritation develops.

Precautions: Use only fresh solution. Do not use full strength.

Side Effects: None reported.

Directions For Use: Two capfuls mixed well to each quart of warm water.

How Supplied: 4 and 8 fl. oz. plastic bottles.

Literature Available: Instructions for the use of TRICHOTINE are available in pads of 50 sheets.

TRICHOTINE®-D Disposable Vaginal Douche

Description: A detergent, mucolytic, vaginal douche containing trisodium EDTA, sodium lauryl sulfate, and sodium phosphate, premeasured in a disposable bag. Designed to be used once and thrown away to avoid the risk of infection from an improperly cleaned nozzle or syringe.

Actions: (See TRICHOTINE Powder above)

Indications: (See TRICHOTINE Powder above)

Contraindications: None reported.

Warning: For routine use, do not use more than twice weekly. May be used more frequently in concomitant use for treatment of vaginitis. Discontinue use if irritation develops.

Precautions: For one time use only, do not refill.

Side Effects: None reported.

Directions for Use: Hold bag in an upright position to avoid loss of premeasured powder, and remove foil cover from neck of bag. Fill with water up to the "Fill Line" (12 oz.). Screw the nozzle on the neck of the bag until locked tightly into position. Dispose of unit after use.

How Supplied: Twin Pack - Consisting of two disposable douche units, each containing premeasured powder which holds 12 oz. when filled with water. Each unit is individually sealed in a sanitary wrapper.

Literature Available: Instructions for the use of TRICHOTINE-D are available in pads of 50 sheets.

Reid-Provident Laboratories Inc.

Executive Offices
640 TENTH STREET, N.W.
ATLANTA, GA 30318
Scientific Affairs and Manufacturing
25 FIFTH ST., N.W.
ATLANTA, GA 30308

CALINATE®-FA ℞

Prenatal dietary supplement containing:

Ascorbic Acid (As Sodium Ascorbate)	50 mg.
Niacinamide	20 mg.
d-panthenol	1 mg.
Iron (From Ferrous Fumarate)	60 mg.
Iodine (From Potassium Iodide)	0.02 mg.
Manganese (From Manganese Oxide)	0.2 mg.
Magnesium (From Magnesium Oxide)	0.2 mg.
Zinc (From Zinc Oxide)	0.1 mg.
Copper (From Cupric Oxide)	0.15 mg.
Calcium (Calcium Carbonate 625 mg.)	250 mg.
Vitamin A (Palmitate)	4000 USP Units
Vitamin D_2 (Calciferol)	400 USP Units
Thiamine Mononitrate (Vitamin B_1)	3 mg.
Riboflavin (Vitamin B_2)	3 mg.
Pyridoxine HCl (Vitamin B_6)	5 mg.
Cyanocobalamin (Vitamin B_{12})	1 mcg.
Folic Acid	1 mg.

Indications: Prenatal dietary supplement.

Precautions: Folic acid may obscure pernicious anemia in that hematologic remission can occur while neurological manifestations remain progressive.

Usual Dosage: One tablet daily before a meal, or as directed by physician.

Caution: Federal law prohibits dispensing without prescription.

How Supplied:
NDC 0063-1139-06 bottles of 100
NDC 0063-1139-09 bottles of 1000

[Shown in Product Identification Section]

ESTRATAB® ℞
Esterified Estrogens
0.3 mg., 0.625 mg. 1.25 mg. 2.5 mg.

How Supplied:

NDC 0063-1014-06	0.3 mg. Bottles of 100
NDC 0063-1022-06	0.625 mg. Bottles of 100
NDC 0063-1022-09	0.625 mg. Bottles of 1000
NDC 0063-1024-06	1.25 mg. Bottles of 100
NDC 0063-1024-09	1.25 mg. Bottles of 1000
NDC 0063-1025-06	2.5 mg. Bottles of 100
NDC 0063-1025-09	2.5 mg. Bottles of 1000

[Shown in Product Identification Section]

ESTRATEST® ℞
ESTRATEST® H.S. (Half-Strength) ℞
Androgen-Estrogen Therapy

Description:
ESTRATEST® Oral Tablets
Each dark green tablet contains:

Continued on next page

Reid-Provident—Cont.

Esterified Estrogens, U.S.P. ....1.25 mg
Methyltestosterone, U.S.P. ....2.5 mg
ESTRATEST® H.S. (Half-Strength) Oral Tablets
Each light green tablet contains:
Esterified Estrogens, U.S.P. ....0.625 mg
Methyltestosterone, U.S.P. ....1.25 mg

How Supplied:
Estratest® NDC 0063-1026-06 bottles of 100
NDC 0063-1026-09 bottles of 1000
Estratest® H.S. NDC 0063-1023-06 bottles of 100
[Shown in Product Identificaion Section]

HISTALET® Syrup ℞
HISTALET® DM Syrup
HISTALET® X Syrup
HISTALET® X Tablets
HISTALET® FORTE Tablets
for oral use only

[See table below].
Histalet® Forte Tablets:
Each tablet contains:
Phenylephrine HCl ....10 mg.
Phenylpropanolamine HCl ....50 mg.
Pyrilamine Maleate ....25 mg.
Chlorpheniramine Maleate ....4 mg.

Indications: The Histalets® are indicated for the Common Cold, Nasal Congestion, Acute Upper Respiratory Infections, Sinusitis, Hay Fever or Upper Respiratory Allergies, Seasonal and Perennial Allergic Rhinitis, Vasomotor Rhinitis, Rhinorrhea, Allergic Asthma, Non Productive and Productive Cough, Acute Bronchitis, Croup, Emphysema, Tracheobronchitis and Influenza. Decongestants have been used for many years to relieve eustachian tube congestion associated with acute eustachian salpingitis, aerotitis media, acute otitis media and serous otitis media.

Contraindications: Contraindicated in patients with severe hypertension, severe coronary artery disease, hyperthyroidism, and in patients on MAO inhibitor therapy. Patient idiosyncrasy to adrenergic agents may be manifested by insomnia, dizziness, weakness, tremor or arrhythmias.

Nursing Mothers: Pseudoephedrine is contraindicated in nursing mothers because of the higher than usual risk for infants from sympathomimetic amines.

Hypersensitivity: This drug is contraindicated in patients with hypersensitivity or idiosyncrasy to sympathomimetic amines or antihistamines & dextromethorphan.

Precautions: Pseudoephedrine should be used with caution in patients with diabetes, hypertension, cardiovascular disease and hyper-reactivity to ephedrine. The antihistaminic agent may cause drowsiness and ambulatory patients who operate machinery or motor vehicles should be cautioned accordingly.

Warnings: Should be used judiciously and sparingly in patients with hypertension, diabetes mellitus, ischemic heart disease, increased intraocular pressure, and prostatic hypertrophy, See, however, **Contraindications**. Sympathomimetics may produce central nervous stimulation with convulsions or cardiovascular collapse with accompanying hypotension.

Do not exceed recommended dosage.

Usage in Pregnancy: The safety of pseudoephedrine for use during pregnancy has not been established.

Use in Elderly: The elderly (60 years and older) are more likely to have adverse reactions to sympathomimetics. Overdosage of sympathomimetics in this age group may cause hallucinations, convulsions, CNS depression, and death.

Dosage: Histalet® Syrup, Histalet® DM Syrup and Histalet® X Syrup—ADULTS—2 teaspoonfuls 4 times daily, CHILDREN (6–12)—1 teaspoonful 4 times daily, CHILDREN (2–6)—½ teaspoonful 4 times daily, CHILDREN (under 2)—only as directed by physician.

DO NOT EXCEED 4 DOSES IN 24 HOUR PERIOD

Histalet® X Tablets—ADULTS—1 tablet, 2–3 times daily, CHILDREN (6—12)—½ tablet 2–3 times daily.

Histalet® Forte Tablets—ADULTS—1 tablet, 2–3 times daily, CHILDREN (6–12)—½ tablet 2–3 times daily.

Do not exceed recommended dosage.

How Supplied:
Histalet® Syrup NDC 0063-1035-12, pint bottles
Histalet® DM Syrup NDC 0063-1037-12, pint bottles
Histalet® X Syrup NDC 0063-1045-12, pint bottles
Histalet® X Tablets NDC 0063-1046-06, bottles of 100 tablets
Histalet® Forte Tablets NDC 0063-1039-06 bottles of 100 tablets
NDC 0063-1039-07 bottles of 250 tablets
[Shown in Product Identification Section]

MELFIAT® CIII
Phendimetrazine Tartrate 35 mg tablets

How Supplied:
NDC 0063-1079-06 Bottles of 100
NDC 0063-1079-09 Bottles of 1000
[Shown in Product Identification Section]

MELFIAT®-105 CIII ℞
UNICELLES®
(phendimetrazine tartrate)
105 mg.
Slow Release Capsules

Description: Chemical name: Phendimetrazine Tartrate (+) 3, 4 Dimethyl-2-phenylmorpholine tartrate. Phendimetrazine Tartrate is a white, odorless powder with a bitter taste. It is soluble in water, methanol and ethanol. It has a molecular weight of 341. The capsule is manufactured in a special base which is designed for prolonged release.

Clinical Pharmacology: Phendimetrazine Tartrate is a sympathomimetic amine with pharmacologic activity similar to the prototype of drugs of this class used in obesity, the amphetamines. Actions include central nervous system stimulation and elevation of blood pressure. Tachyphylaxis and tolerance have been demonstrated with all drugs of this class in which these phenomena have been looked for.

Drugs of this class used in obesity are commonly known as "anorectics" or "anorexigenics". It has not been established, however, that the action of such drugs in treating obesity is primarily one of appetite suppression. Other central nervous system actions, or metabolic effects, may be involved, for example. Adult obese subjects instructed in dietary management and treated with "anorectic" drugs, lose more weight on the average than those treated with placebo and diet, as determined in relatively short-term clinical trials.

The magnitude of increased weight loss of drug-treated patients over placebo-treated patients is only a fraction of a pound a week. The rate of weight loss is greatest in the first weeks of therapy for both drug and placebo subjects and tends to decrease in succeeding weeks. The possible origins of the increased weight loss due to the various drug effects are not established. The amount of weight loss associated with the use of an "anorectic" drug varies from trial to trial, and the increased weight loss appears to be related in part to variables other than the drug prescribed, such as the physician-investigator, the population treated, and the diet prescribed. Studies do not permit conclusions as to the relative importance of the drug and non-drug factors on weight loss.

The natural history of obesity is measured in years, whereas the studies cited are restricted to a few weeks duration; thus, the total impact of drug-induced weight loss over that of diet alone must be considered clinically limited.

The active drug, 105 mg. of Phendimetrazine Tartrate in each capsule of this special timed release dosage form approximates the action of three 35 mg. non-timed doses taken at four hour intervals.

The major route of elimination is via the kidneys where most of the drug and metabolites are excreted. Some of the drug is metabolized to Phenmetrazine and also Phendimetrazine-N-oxide.

The average half-life of elimination when studied under controlled conditions is about 3.7 hours for both the timed and non-timed forms. The absorption half-life of the drug from conventional non-timed 35 mg. phendimetrazine tablets is appreciably more rapid than the absorption rate of the drug from the timed release formulation.

Indications and Usage: MELFIAT-105 (Phendimetrazine Tartrate) is indicated in the management of exogenous obesity as a short term adjunct (a few weeks) in a regimen of weight reduction based on caloric restriction. The limited usefulness of agents of this class (see CLINICAL PHARMACOLOGY) should be measured against possible risk factors inherent in their use such as those described below.

Contraindications: Advanced arteriosclerosis, symptomatic cardiovascular disease, moderate to severe hypertension, hyperthyroidism, known hypersensitivity, or idiosyncrasy to the sympathomimetic amines, glaucoma.

Agitated states.

Patients with a history of drug abuse.

During or within 14 days following the administration of monoamine oxidase inhibitors, (hypertensive crises may result).

Warnings: Tolerance to the anorectic effect usually develops within a few weeks. When this occurs, the recommended dose should not be exceeded in an attempt to increase the effect; rather, the drug should be discontinued. Phendimetrazine Tartrate may impair the ability of the patient to engage in potentially hazardous activities such as operating machinery or driving a motor vehicle; the patient should therefore be cautioned accordingly.

Drug Dependence: Phendimetrazine Tartrate is related chemically and pharmacologically to the amphetamines. Amphetamines and related stimulant drugs have been extensively abused, and the possibility of abuse of Phendimetrazine Tartrate should be kept in mind when evaluating the desirability of including a drug as part of a weight reduction program. Abuse of amphetamines and related drugs may be associated with intense psychological dependence and severe social dysfunc-

DOSAGE SCHEDULE FOR HISTALET® FAMILY

Formula:	Per 5 ml:			Per tab
	Histalet® Syrup	Histalet® DM Syrup	Histalet® X Syrup	Histalet® X Tablets
Pseudoephedrine HCl	45 mg	45 mg	45 mg	120 mg
Chlorpheniramine Maleate	3 mg	3 mg	3 mg	8 mg
Dextromethorphan HBr		15 mg		
Guaifenesin			200 mg	200 mg

tion. There are reports of patients who have increased the dosage to many times that recommended. Abrupt cessation following prolonged high dosage administration results in extreme fatigue and mental depression; changes are also noted on the sleep EEG. Manifestations of chronic intoxication with anorectic drugs include severe dermatoses, marked insomnia, irritability, hyperactivity, and personality changes. The most severe manifestation of chronic intoxications is psychosis, often clinically indistinguishable from schizophrenia.

Usage in Pregnancy: The safety of phendimetrazine tartrate in pregnancy and lactation has not been established. Therefore, Phendimetrazine Tartrate should not be taken by women who are or may become pregnant.

Usage in Children: Phendimetrazine Tartrate is not recommended for use in children under 12 years of age.

Precaution: Caution is to be exercised in prescribing Phendimetrazine Tartrate for patients with even mild hypertension.

Insulin requirements in diabetes mellitus may be altered in association with the use of Phendimetrazine Tartrate and the concomitant dietary regimen. Phendimetrazine Tartrate may decrease the hypotensive effect of guanethidine. The least amount feasible should be prescribed or dispensed at one time in order to minimize the possibility of overdosage.

Adverse Reactions: Cardiovascular: Palpitation, tachycardia, elevation of blood pressure.

Central Nervous System: Overstimulation, restlessness, dizziness, insomnia, euphoria, dysphoria, tremor, headache; rarely psychotic episodes at recommended doses.

Gastrointestinal: Dryness of the mouth, unpleasant taste, diarrhea, constipation, other gastrointestinal disturbances.

Allergic: Urticaria.

Endocrine: Impotence, changes in libido.

Overdosage: Manifestations of acute overdosage with Phendimetrazine Tartrate include restlessness, tremor, hyperreflexia, rapid respiration, confusion, assaultiveness, hallucinations, panic states.

Fatigue and depression usually follow the central stimulation.

Cardiovascular effects include arrhythmias, hypertension or hypotension and circulatory collapse. Gastrointestinal symptoms include nausea, vomiting, diarrhea, and abdominal cramps. Fatal poisoning usually terminates in convulsions and coma. Management of acute Phendimetrazine Tartrate intoxication is largely symptomatic and includes lavage and sedation with a barbiturate. Experience with hemodialysis or peritoneal dialysis is inadequate to permit recommendation in this regard. Acidification of the urine increases Phendimetrazine Tartrate excretion. Intravenous phentolamine (Regitine) has been suggested for possible acute, severe hypertension, if this complicates Phendimetrazine Tartrate overdosage.

Dosage and Administration: Since MELFIAT-105 (Phendimetrazine Tartrate 105 mg.) is a slow release dosage form, limit to one slow release capsule in the morning.

MELFIAT-105 (Phendimetrazine Tartrate) is not recommended for use in children under 12 years of age.

How Supplied: Each orange and clear slow release capsule contains 105 mg. Phendimetrazine Tartrate in bottles of 100 (NDC 0063-1082-06).

Caution: Federal law prohibits dispensing without prescription.

[*Shown in Product Identification Section*]

Each tablet contains:	ZENATE	% U.S. RDA Pregnant or Lactating Women
VITAMINS:		
A (as palmitate)	5,000I.U.	62.5
D (as calciferol)	400I.U.	100
E (as dl-alpha tocopheryl acetate)	30I.U.	100
C (ascorbic acid)	80mg.	133
Folic Acid	1mg.	125
Thiamine (as thiamine mononitrate Vitamin B_1)	3mg.	176
Riboflavin (Vitamin B_2)	3mg.	150
Niacin (as niacinamide)	20mg.	100
B_6 (as pyridoxine hydrochloride)	10mg.	400
B_{12} (cyanocobalamin)	12mcg.	150
MINERALS:		
Calcium (from 833mg. calcium carbonate)	300mg.	23
Iodine (from 230mcg. potassium iodide)	175mcg.	117
Iron (from 198mg. ferrous fumarate)	65mg.	361
Magnesium (from 173mg. magnesium oxide)	100mg.	22
Zinc (from 25mg. zinc oxide)	20mg.	133
SURFACTANT:		
Docusate Sodium USP (DSS)	50mg.	

P-V-TUSSIN® SYRUP ℞
P-V-TUSSIN® TABLETS

Antitussive-Antihistamine-Expectorant Liquid and Tablets

Description: Each teaspoonful (5 ml) of P-V-TUSSIN® Syrup contains: Hydrocodone Bitartrate 2.5 mg (WARNING: May be habit forming), Phenylephrine HCl 5 mg, Pyrilamine Maleate 6 mg, Chlorpheniramine Maleate 2 mg, Phenindamine Tartrate 5 mg, Ammonium Chloride 50 mg; Alcohol 5%

Each Scored P-V-TUSSIN® Tablet contains: Hydrocodone Bitartrate 5 mg (WARNING: May be habit forming), Phenindamine Tartrate 25 mg, Guaifenesin 200 mg.

Indications and Usage: For the symptomatic relief of cough and nasal congestion due to common cold, upper respiratory tract congestion associated with the common cold, influenza, bronchitis and sinusitis.

Contraindications: P-V-TUSSIN® Syrup and Tablets is contraindicated in patients with a known hypersensitivity to hydrocodone bitartrate, phenylephrine HCl, pyrilamine maleate, chlorpheniramine maleate, phenindamine tartrate, ammonium chloride, or guaifenesin.

Warning: Hydrocodone should be prescribed and administered with the same degree of caution as all oral medications containing a narcotic analgesic.

Precautions: General Precautions—Use with caution in the presence of hypertension, cardiovascular disease, hyperthyroidism, or diabetes.

Information for Patients—Patients should be cautioned against driving a car or engaging in mechanical operations which require alertness, until it is known that they do not respond to the drug by becoming drowsy or dizzy.

Drug Interactions—Hydrocodone may potentiate the effects of other narcotics, general anesthetics, tranquilizers, sedatives and hypnotics, tricyclic antidepressants, MAO inhibitors, alcohol and other CNS depressants.

Adverse Reactions: Adverse reactions, when they occur, include sedation, nausea, vomiting and constipation.

Drug Abuse and Dependence: Controlled Substance—P-V-Tussin® is a schedule III drug. Dependence—Continued use of hydrocodone may result in true addiction.

Dosage and Administration:

P-V-Tussin® Syrup:

Adults, 2 teaspoonfuls every 4 to 6 hours

Children 6 to 12, 1 teaspoonful every 4 to 6 hours

Children 3 to 6, ½ to 1 teaspoonful every 4 to 6 hours.

Children 1 to 3, ½ teaspoonful every 4 to 6 hours.

Dose for children should not be repeated more than 4 times in a 24 hour period.

P-V-Tussin® Tablets:

Adults and children over 12, 1 tablet 4 times daily or as directed by physician. Children 6 to 12, ½ tablet 4 times daily. Should be taken after meals and at bedtime, not less than 4 hours apart. Do not exceed the recommended dosage.

Caution: Federal law prohibits dispensing without prescription.

How Supplied:

P-V-Tussin® Syrup

NDC 0063-1087-12, pint bottles

NDC 0063-1087-13, gallon bottles

P-V-Tussin® Tablets

NDC 0063-1088-06, bottles of 100 tablets

[*Shown in Product Identification Section*]

UNIPRES® ℞

Formula: Each tablet contains:

Hydralazine Hydrochloride .... 25 mg.
Hydrochlorothiazide .... 15 mg.
Reserpine .... 0.1 mg.

How Supplied:

NDC 0063-1132-06 Bottles of 100

NDC 0063-1132-09 Bottles of 1000

[*Shown in Product Identification Section*]

ZENATE PRENATAL TABLETS ℞

(Film Coated)

Description: [See table above].

Clinical Advantages: Each tablet contains iron that is specifically formulated to minimize gastric irritation. DSS is added as a stool softener to minimize any associated constipation.

Indications and Uses: Vitamin-mineral dietary adjunct in nutritional stress associated with pregnancy and lactation.

Zenate is a phosphorous free[1] vitamin-mineral dietary supplement with surfactant, specifically formulated for use during pregnancy and lactation. All ingredients covered by a warning or caution for usage in pregnancy have been formulated so as not to exceed maximum recommended strengths. The formulation includes essential vitamins and minerals, including 300 mg. of elemental calcium, 65 mg. of elemental iron and 20 mg. of elemental zinc. Zenate also offers 1 mg. of folic acid to aid in the prevention of megaloblastic anemia.

Precautions: Folic Acid in doses above 0.1 mg. daily may obscure pernicious anemia in that hematologic remission can occur while neurological manifestations remain progressive. Periodic laboratory studies are considered essential and are recommended. Allergic sensitization has been reported following both oral and parenteral administration of Folic Acid.

Dosage and Administration: As a dietary adjunct in nutritional stress associated with

Continued on next page

Reid-Provident—Cont.

pregnancy and lactation. One tablet daily before the first meal, or as directed by physician.
How Supplied: Bottles of 100 baby blue film coated tablets.
NDC 0063-1145-06.
Caution: Federal Law Prohibits Dispensing Without Prescription.
Reference: 1. Pitkin, R.M.: Vitamins and Minerals in Pregnancy. *Clinics in Perinatology,* 2:221–232, 1975.
[*Shown in the Product Identification Section*]

Reid-Provident Laboratories, Inc.
DIRECT DIVISION
640 TENTH ST., N.W.
ATLANTA, GA 30318

AQUATAG® ℞
(benzthiazide tablets, USP)

How Supplied:
25 mg. scored tablets:
NDC 0063-1231-06 Bottles of 100
NDC 0063-1231-09 Bottles of 1000
50 mg. scored tablets:
NDC 0063-1234-06 Bottles of 100
NDC 0063-1234-09 Bottles of 1000

BACARATE® TABLETS Ⓒ ℞
(phendimetrazine tartrate)
35 mg.

How Supplied:
NDC 0063-1654-06 Bottles of 100
NDC 0063-1654-09 Bottles of 1000
[*Shown in Product Identification Section*]

ESCOT® CAPSULES

Description: Each capsule contains:
Bismuth Aluminate ....100 mg.
Aluminum Hydroxide
Coprecipitate 130 mg.
Magnesium Carbonate
Magnesium Trisilicate ....160 mg.
How Supplied:
NDC 0063-2510-06 Bottles of 100

NEOTEP® GRANUCAPS* ℞

Description: Each red and clear Granucap* contains:
Chlorpheniramine Maleate ....9 mg.
Phenylephrine Hydrochloride ....21 mg.
How Supplied:
NDC 0063-2832-06 Bottles of 100
NDC 0063-2832-09 Bottles of 1000
*Granucap—T.M. Reg.

QUINITE™ TABLETS ℞

Each tablet contains:
Quinine sulfate ....260mg.
How Supplied:
NDC 0063-1623-06 Bottles of 100
NDC 0063-1623-08 Bottles of 500

SPRX-105 Ⓒ ℞
(phendimetrazine tartrate)
105mg.
Slow Release Capsules

Description: Chemical name: Phendimetrazine Tartrate (+) 3, 4 Dimethyl-2-phenyl-morpholine tartrate. Phendimetrazine Tartrate is a white, odorless powder with a bitter taste. It is soluble in water, methanol and ethanol. It has a molecular weight of 341. The capsule is manufactured in a special base which is designed for prolonged release.
Clinical Pharmacology: Phendimetrazine Tartrate is a sympathomimetic amine with pharmacologic activity similar to the prototype of drugs of this class used in obesity, the amphetamines. Actions include central nervous system stimulation and elevation of blood pressure. Tachyphylaxis and tolerance have been demonstrated with all drugs of this class in which these phenomena have been looked for.
Drugs of this class used in obesity are commonly known as "anorectics" or "anorexigenics". It has not been established, however, that the action of such drugs in treating obesity is primarily one of appetite suppression. Other central nervous system actions, or metabolic effects, may be involved, for example. Adult obese subjects instructed in dietary management and treated with "anorectic" drugs, lose more weight on the average than those treated with placebo and diet, as determined in relatively short-term clinical trials.
The magnitude of increased weight loss of drug-treated patients over placebo-treated patients is only a fraction of a pound a week. The rate of weight loss is greatest in the first weeks of therapy for both drug and placebo subjects and tends to decrease in succeeding weeks. The possible origins of the increased weight loss due to the various drug effects are not established. The amount of weight loss associated with the use of an "anorectic" drug varies from trial to trial, and the increased weight loss appears to be related in part to variables other than the drug prescribed, such as the physician-investigator, the population treated, and the diet prescribed. Studies do not permit conclusions as to the relative importance of the drug and non-drug factors on weight loss.
The natural history of obesity is measured in years, whereas the studies cited are restricted to a few weeks duration; thus, the total impact of drug-induced weight loss over that of diet alone must be considered clinically limited.
The active drug, 105mg. of Phendimetrazine Tartrate in each capsule of this special timed release dosage form approximates the action of three 35mg. non-timed doses taken at four hour intervals.
The major route of elimination is via the kidneys where most of the drug and metabolites are excreted. Some of the drug is metabolized to Phenmetrazine and also Phendimetrazine-N-oxide.
The average half-life of elimination when studied under controlled conditions is about 3.7 hours for both the timed and non-timed forms. The absorption half-life of the drug from conventional non-timed 35mg. phendimetrazine tablets is appreciably more rapid than the absorption rate of the drug from the timed release formulation.
Indications and Usage: SPRX-105 (Phendimetrazine Tartrate) is indicated in the management of exogenous obesity as a short term adjunct (a few weeks) in a regimen of weight reduction based on caloric restriction. The limited usefulness of agents of this class (see CLINICAL PHARMACOLOGY) should be measured against possible risk factors inherent in their use such as those described below.
Contraindications: Advanced arteriosclerosis, symptomatic cardiovascular disease, moderate to severe hypertension, hyperthyroidism, known hypersensitivity, or idiosyncrasy to the sympathomimetic amines, glaucoma.
Agitated states.
Patients with a history of drug abuse.
During or within 14 days following the administration of monoamine oxidase inhibitors, (hypertensive crises may result).
Warnings: Tolerance to the anorectic effect usually develops within a few weeks. When this occurs, the recommended dose should not be exceeded in an attempt to increase the effect; rather, the drug should be discontinued. Phendimetrazine Tartrate may impair the ability of the patient to engage in potentially hazardous activities such as operating machinery or driving a motor vehicle; the patient should therefore be cautioned accordingly.
Drug Dependence: Phendimetrazine Tartrate is related chemically and pharmacologically to the amphetamines. Amphetamines and related stimulant drugs have been extensively abused, and the possibility of abuse of Phendimetrazine Tartrate should be kept in mind when evaluating the desirability of including a drug as part of a weight reduction program. Abuse of amphetamines and related drugs may be associated with intense psychological dependence and severe social dysfunction. There are reports of patients who have increased the dosage to many times that recommended. Abrupt cessation following prolonged high dosage administration results in extreme fatigue and mental depression; changes are also noted on the sleep EEG. Manifestations of chronic intoxication with anorectic drugs include severe dermatoses, marked insomnia, irritability, hyperactivity, and personality changes. The most severe manifestation of chronic intoxications is psychosis, often clinically indistinguishable from schizophrenia.
Usage in Pregnancy: The safety of phendimetrazine tartrate in pregnancy and lactation has not been established. Therefore, Phendimetrazine Tartrate should not be taken by women who are or may become pregnant.
Usage in Children: Phendimetrazine tartrate is not recommended for use in children under 12 years of age.
Precaution: Caution is to be exercised in prescribing Phendimetrazine Tartrate for patients with even mild hypertension.
Insulin requirements in diabetes mellitus may be altered in association with the use of Phendimetrazine Tartrate and the concomitant dietary regimen. Phendimetrazine Tartrate may decrease the hypotensive effect of guanethidine. The least amount feasible should be prescribed or dispensed at one time in order to minimize the possibility of overdosage.
Adverse Reactions: Cardiovascular: Palpitation, tachycardia, elevation of blood pressure.
Central Nervous System: Overstimulation, restlessness, dizziness, insomnia, euphoria, dysphoria, tremor, headache; rarely psychotic episodes at recommended doses.
Gastrointestinal: Dryness of the mouth, unpleasant taste, diarrhea, constipation, other gastrointestinal disturbances.
Allergic: Urticaria.
Endocrine: Impotence, changes in libido.
Overdosage: Manifestations of acute overdosage with Phendimetrazine Tartrate include restlessness, tremor, hyperreflexia, rapid respiration, confusion, assaultiveness, hallucinations, panic states.
Fatigue and depression usually follow the central stimulation.
Cardiovascular effects include arrhythmias, hypertension or hypotension and circulatory collapse. Gastrointestinal symptoms include nausea, vomiting, diarrhea, and abdominal cramps. Fatal poisoning usually terminates in convulsions and coma. Management of acute Phendimetrazine Tartrate intoxication is largely symptomatic and includes lavage and sedation with a barbiturate. Experience with hemodialysis or peritoneal dialysis is inadequate to permit recommendation in this regard. Acidification of the urine increases Phendimetrazine Tartrate excretion. Intravenous phentolamine (Regitine) has been suggested for possible acute, severe hypertension, if this complicates Phendimetrazine Tartrate overdosage.
Dosage and Administration: Since SPRX-105 (Phendimetrazine Tartrate 105mg.) is a slow release dosage form, limit to one slow release capsule in the morning.
SPRX-105 (Phendimetrazine Tartrate) is not recommended for use in children under 12 years of age.
How Supplied: Each brown and clear slow release capsule contains 105mg. Phendimetra-

zine Tartrate in bottles of 28, 100, 500 and 1000.
Caution: Federal law prohibits dispensing without prescription.
[*Shown in Product Identification Section*]

SULADYNE® TABLETS ℞
(sulfamethizole, sulfadiazine, phenazopyridine HCl)

Description: Each maroon-colored tablet contains: sulfamethizole, 125 mg.; sulfadiazine, 125 mg.; phenazopyridine hydrochloride, 75 mg.
How Supplied:
NDC 0063-1725-06 Bottles of 100

UNPROCO® CAPSULES ℞

Description: Each capsule contains:
Guaifenesin ....200 mg.
Dextromethorphan HBr .... 30 mg.
How Supplied:
NDC 0063-2805-06 Bottles of 100
NDC 0063-2805-08 Bottles of 500

X-OTAG® S.R. TABLETS ℞

Description: Each yellow tablet contains:
Orphenadrine Citrate ....100 mg.
How Supplied:
NDC 0063-1261-07 Bottles of 250.
NDC 0063-1261-08 Bottles of 500.
[*Shown in Product Identification Section*]

Research Industries Corporation

Pharmaceutical Division
1847 WEST 2300 SOUTH
SALT LAKE CITY, UTAH 84119

RIMSO®-50 ℞
(brand of dimethyl sulfoxide)

Description:
RIMSO®-50, brand of dimethyl sulfoxide (DMSO)
50% w/w Aqueous Solution for intravesical instillation
Each ml contains 0.54 gm dimethyl sulfoxide
STERILE AND PYROGEN-FREE
Intravesical instillation for the treatment of interstitial cystitis
NOT FOR I.M. OR I.V. INJECTION
Caution: Federal law prohibits dispensing without a prescription
The active component of RIMSO®-50 is dimethyl sulfoxide which has the empirical formula C_2H_6OS.
Dimethyl sulfoxide is a clear, colorless and essentially odorless liquid which is miscible with water and most organic solvents. Other physical characteristics include: molecular weight 78.13, melting point 18.4°C, and a specific gravity of 1.1014.
Clinical Pharmacology: Dimethyl sulfoxide is metabolized in man by oxidation to dimethyl sulfone or by reduction to dimethyl sulfide. Dimethyl sulfoxide and dimethyl sulfone are excreted in the urine and feces. Dimethyl sulfide is eliminated through the breath and skin and is responsible for the characteristic odor from patients on dimethyl sulfoxide medication. Dimethyl sulfone can persist in serum for longer than two weeks after a single intravesical instillation. No residual accumulation of dimethyl sulfoxide has occurred in man or lower animals who have received treatment for protracted periods of time. Following topical application, dimethyl sulfoxide is absorbed and generally distributed in the tissues and body fluids.
Indications and Usage: RIMSO®-50 (dimethyl sulfoxide) is indicated for the symptomatic relief of patients with interstitial cystitis. RIMSO®-50 has not been approved as being safe and effective for any other indication. There is no clinical evidence of effectiveness of dimethyl sulfoxide in the treatment of bacterial infections of the urinary tract.
Contraindications: None known.
Warnings: Dimethyl sulfoxide can initiate the liberation of histamine and there has been an occasional hypersensitivity reaction with topical administration of dimethyl sulfoxide. This hypersensitivity has been reported in one patient receiving intravesical RIMSO®-50. The physician should be cognizant of this possibility in prescribing RIMSO®-50. If anaphylactoid symptoms develop, appropriate therapy should be instituted.
Precautions: Changes in the refractive index and lens opacities have been seen in monkeys, dogs and rabbits given high doses of dimethyl sulfoxide chronically. Since lens changes were noted in animals, full eye evaluations, including slit lamp examinations are recommended prior to and periodically during treatment.
Approximately every six months patients receiving dimethyl sulfoxide should have a biochemical screening, particularly liver and renal function tests, and complete blood count.
Intravesical instillation of RIMSO®-50 may be harmful to patients with urinary tract malignancy because of dimethyl sulfoxide-induced vasodilation.
Some data indicate that dimethyl sulfoxide potentiates other concomitantly administered medications.
Pregnancy Category C. Dimethyl sulfoxide caused teratogenic responses in hamsters, rats and mice when administered intraperitoneally at high doses (2.5–12 gm/kg). Oral or topical doses of dimethyl sulfoxide did not cause problems of reproduction in rats, mice and hamsters. Topical doses (5 gm/kg first two days, then 2.5 gm/kg–last eight days) produced terata in rabbits, but in another study, topical doses of 1.1 gm/kg days 3 through 16 of gestation failed to produce any abnormalities. There are no adequate and well controlled studies in pregnant women. Dimethyl sulfoxide should be used during pregnancy only if the potential benefit justifies the potential risk to the fetus.
It is not known whether this drug is excreted in human milk. Because many drugs are excreted in human milk, caution should be exercised when dimethyl sulfoxide is administered to a nursing woman.
Safety and effectiveness in children have not been established.
Information available to be given to the patient is reprinted at the end of this text.
Adverse Reactions: A garlic-like taste may be noted by the patient within a few minutes after instillation of RIMSO®-50 (dimethyl sulfoxide). This taste may last several hours and because of the presence of metabolites an odor on the breath and skin may remain for 72 hours.
Transient chemical cystitis has been noted following instillation of dimethyl sulfoxide.
The patient may experience moderately severe discomfort on administration. Usually this becomes less prominent with repeated administration.
Drug Abuse and Dependence: None known.
Overdosage: The oral LD_{50} of dimethyl sulfoxide in the dog is greater than 10 gm/kg. It is improbable that this dosage level could be obtained with intravesical instillation of RIMSO®–50 in the patient.
In case of accidental oral ingestion, specific measures should be taken to induce emesis. Additional measures which may be considered are gastric lavage, activated charcoal and forced diuresis.
Dosage and Administration: Instillation of 50 ml of RIMSO®–50 (dimethyl sulfoxide) directly into the bladder may be accomplished by catheter or asepto syringe and allowed to remain for 15 minutes. Application of an analgesic lubricant gel such as lidocaine jelly to the urethra is suggested prior to insertion of the catheter to avoid spasm. The medication is expelled by spontaneous voiding. It is recommended that the treatment be repeated every two weeks until maximum symptomatic relief is obtained. Thereafter, time intervals between therapy may be increased appropriately.
Administration of oral analgesic medication or suppositories containing belladonna and opium prior to the instillation of RIMSO®-50 can reduce bladder spasm.
In patients with severe interstitial cystitis with very sensitive bladders, the initial treatment, and possibly the second and third (depending on patient response) should be done under anesthesia. (Saddle block has been suggested).
How Supplied:
Bottles contain 50 ml of sterile and pyrogen-free RIMSO®-50 (50% w/w dimethyl sulfoxide aqueous solution).
Dimethyl sulfoxide is clear and colorless
Protect from strong light
Store at room temperature (59° to 86°F) (15° to 30°C)
Do not autoclave
NDC #0433-0433-05
For additional information concerning RIMSO®-50, contact the Pharmaceutical Division, Research Industries Corporation, Salt Lake City, Utah

RIMSO®-50 is manufactured by Tera Pharmaceuticals, Inc., Buena Park, California, for the Pharmaceutical Division, Research Industries Corp., Salt Lake City, Utah.

INFORMATION FOR PATIENTS

RIMSO®-50 is a sterile solution of 50% dimethyl sulfoxide and 50% water that has been approved by the U.S. Food and Drug Administration for use in the symptomatic relief of patients with interstitial cystitis.
RIMSO®-50 will be instilled in the bladder on an in-patient or out-patient basis, which will be determined by your physician.
Some data indicate that dimethyl sulfoxide could change the effectiveness of any medication(s) that you may be presently receiving. Be sure to mention the names and dosage of all medications you are taking to your physician before a RIMSO®-50 instillation.
A garlic-like taste may be noted by the patient within a few minutes after instillation of RIMSO®-50 (dimethyl sulfoxide). This taste may last several hours. An odor on the breath and skin may be present and remain for up to 72 hours.
Some patients may experience discomfort on administration of the drug. Usually this becomes less prominent with repeated administration.
If you are pregnant or nursing, ask your physician about the advisability of using RIMSO®-50.
Some eye changes have been observed in animals treated with DMSO in large doses for prolonged periods. Therefore your doctor may want you to have eye evaluations, including slit-lamp examinations prior to and periodically during treatment.

RIMSO®–100 OTC
(brand of sterile and pyrogen-free dimethyl sulfoxide)
Cryopreservative Solution

Description: RIMSO-100 meets the following specifications:
Quantitative composition: Not less than 99.0% dimethyl sulfoxide, water content — maximum 0.5%
Dimethyl sulfoxide is a clear, colorless and essentially odorless liquid which is miscible with water and most organic solvents. Empirical formula C_2H_6OS, molecular weight 78.13,

Continued on next page

Research Industries—Cont.

melting point 65.12° F (18.4° C), specific gravity 1.100
Storage: Store at 68° to 86° F (20° to 30° C)
Protect from strong light.
Warning: Combustible at high temperatures
Do not autoclave
Not for injection
Do not use unless solution is clear
How Supplied: RIMSO-100 is available in 10 ml ampules, 70 ml multi-dose bottles, and 70 ml screw-top bottles.
For additional information concerning RIMSO-100, contact the Pharmaceutical Division, Research Industries Corporation, Salt Lake City, Utah, 84119. (801) 972-5500
RIMSO-100 is manufactured by Tera Pharmaceuticals, Inc., Buena Park, California, for the Pharmaceutical Division, Research Industries Corporation, Salt Lake City, Utah, 84119.

Rho Mu Corporation

Subsidiary of Richardson-Vicks Inc.
10 WESTPORT ROAD
WILTON, CT 06897

PERCOGESIC®
Analgesic Tablets

Description: Each tablet contains:
Acetaminophen ....325 mg
Phenyltoloxamine citrate ....30 mg
Indications: For relief of mild to moderate pain of simple headache; for temporary relief of such pain and discomfort associated with muscle and joint soreness, neuralgia, sinusitis, minor menstrual cramps, the common cold or grippe, toothache and minor aches and pains of rheumatism and arthritis.
Warning: If arthritic or rheumatic pain persist for more than 10 days; if redness or swelling is present; or in arthritic or rheumatic conditions affecting children under 12 years of age, consult a physician immediately. When used for temporary, symptomatic relief of colds, if relief does not occur in 3 days, discontinue use and consult physician. This preparation may cause drowsiness. Do not drive or operate machinery while taking this medication. Do not administer to children under 6 years of age or exceed recommended dosage unless directed by a physician. Keep this and all drugs out of reach of children. In case of overdosage, seek professional assistance or contact a poison control center immediately. Do not use for more than 10 days unless directed by a physician.
Administration and Dosage:
ADULTS (12 years and over)—1 or 2 tablets every four hours. Maximum daily dose—8 tablets
CHILDREN (6-12 years)—one-half adult dose. Maximum daily dose—4 tablets
How Supplied: Child-resistant sealed packets of 24 tablets and bottles of 50 and 90 tablets.

Riker Laboratories, Inc.

19901 NORDHOFF ST.
NORTHRIDGE, CA 91324

[See table below].

ALU-TAB® Tablets and ALU-CAP® Capsules

Description: Each green Alu-Tab "swallow" tablet contains 600 mg. of aluminum hydroxide dried gel. Each red and green Alu-Cap capsule contains 475 mg. of aluminum hydroxide dried gel.
Actions: Antacid actions include neutralization of gastric hyperacidity and mild astringent and absorbent properties. Aluminum hydroxide dried gel increases phosphate excretion in the bowel by the formation of nonabsorbable salts.*
Indications: Treatment in uncomplicated peptic ulcer and gastric hyperacidity.
Precautions: Aluminum hydroxide is essentially a nontoxic compound. If constipation occurs, medication should be discontinued and a physician should be consulted. Aluminum hydroxide must be given with care to patients who have recently suffered massive upper gastrointestinal hemorrhage. Do not give this product to any patient presently taking a prescription antibiotic drug containing any form of tetracycline.
Dosage and Administration: Two Alu-Tab "swallow" tablets three times a day or as prescribed by physician. Two Alu-Cap capsules three times a day and one at bedtime, or as prescribed by physician.
How Supplied: Bottles of 250 green film-coated Alu-Tab "swallow" tablets (NDC **0089-0107-25**). Bottles of 100 red and green Alu-Cap capsules (NDC **0089-0106-10**).
*Goodman, L.S., and Gilman, A.: *The Pharmacological Basis of Therapeutics,* 4th ed., London, The Macmillan Co., 1970, p. 1005.

CALCIUM DISODIUM VERSENATE* ℞
(calcium disodium edetate injection, U.S.P.) Injection

WARNING
Calcium Disodium Edetate is capable of producing toxic and potentially fatal effects. The dosage schedule should be followed and at no time should the recommended daily dose be exceeded. In lead encephalopathy avoid rapid infusion; intramuscular route is preferred.

Description: Calcium Disodium Versenate Injection (Calcium Disodium Edetate Injection, U.S.P.) is a sterile concentrated solution (20%) containing 200 mg. of calcium disodium edetate per ml. for intravenous infusion or intramuscular injection.
Clinical Pharmacology: The calcium in calcium disodium edetate is readily displaced by heavy metals, such as lead, to form stable complexes. Following parenteral injection, the chelate formed is excreted in the urine, with 50 percent appearing in the first hour after administration.
Indications and Usage: Calcium disodium edetate is indicated for the reduction of blood levels and depot stores of lead in lead poisoning (acute and chronic) and lead encephalopathy.
Contraindications: Calcium disodium edetate should not be given during periods of anuria.
Warnings: See box warning above.
Usage in pregnancy: The safe use of calcium disodium edetate has not been established with respect to possible adverse effects upon fetal development. Therefore, it should not be used in women of child-bearing potential and particularly during early pregnancy unless, in the judgment of the physician, the potential benefits outweigh the possible hazards.
Precautions: Severe acute lead poisoning by itself may cause proteinuria and microscopic hematuria. Calcium disodium edetate may produce the same signs of renal damage. Routine urinalysis should be done daily during each course of therapy to determine whether the proteinuria and hematuria is improving or the evidence of renal tubular injury is getting worse. The presence of large renal epithelial cells or increasing numbers of red blood cells in the urinary sediment or greater proteinuria call for immediate stopping of calcium disodium edetate administration. Evidence of renal impairment should be looked for by periodic blood urea nitrogen determinations before and during each course of therapy. The patient should also be monitored for irregularities of cardiac rhythm.
Adverse Reactions: The principal toxic effect is renal tubular necrosis.
Dosage and Administration: Calcium disodium edetate is equally effective whether administered intravenously, subcutaneously or intramuscularly. Because of convenience in administration and greater safety in treating symptomatic children, many physicians experienced in the treatment of lead poisoning pre-

The following Riker products are available in Military and Veterans Administration depots:

Military Depot Items	National Stock Number
Circanol® Tablets 1 mg. 100's	6505-01-017-1626
Disalcid® Tablets 500's	6505-01-067-2750
Duo-Medihaler® (aerosol) w/adapter 22.5 ml.	6505-00-071-7861
Lipo-Hepin® (heparin sodium injection, U.S.P. aqueous)	
1,000 U/ml. 10 ml. vial	6505-00-153-9740
10,000 U/ml. 5 ml. vial	6505-00-584-2914
20,000 U/ml. 2 ml. vial	6505-00-579-8432
Medihaler-Iso® (aerosol) w/adapter 15 ml.	6505-00-023-6481
Medihaler-Iso® (aerosol) w/adapter 22.5 ml.	6505-00-014-8486
Norflex® Tablets 100's	6505-00-138-8462
Norgesic® Tablets 500's	6505-00-952-6762
Norgesic® Forte Tablets 500's	6505-01-029-9116
Tepanil® Ten-tab® (controlled-release tablet) 75 mg. 100's	6505-00-082-2684
Urex® Tablets 100's	6505-00-126-3207

Veterans Administration Depot Items	National Stock Number
Alu-Cap® Capsules 100's	6505-00-166-7844
Disalcid® Tablets 500's	6505-01-067-2750A
Duo-Medihaler® (aerosol) w/adapter 22.5 ml.	6505-00-071-7861A
Lipo Hepin®/BL (heparin sodium injection, U.S.P. aqueous) (Derived from beef lung)	
1000 U/ml. 10 ml. vial	6505-00-088-6747
1000 U/ml. 30 ml. vial	6505-01-030-3253
10,000 U/ml. 4 ml. vial	6505-00-584-2916
Medihaler-Iso® (aerosol) w/adapter 22.5 ml.	6505-00-014-8486A
Norflex® Tablets 100's	6505-00-138-8462A
Norgesic® Tablets 500's	6505-00-952-6762A
Norgesic® Forte Tablets 500's	6505-01-029-9116A
Theolair™ Tablets 125 mg. 250's	6505-01-075-8307A
Theolair™ Tablets 250 mg. 250's	6505-01-075-8308A
Thedlair™-SR Tablets 250 mg. 100's	6505-01-094-1613A
Urex® Tablets 500's	6505-00-443-4501

fer the intramuscular route which is recommended in patients with either overt or incipient lead encephalopathy. Rapid intravenous infusions may be lethal by suddenly increasing intracranial pressure in this group of patients with cerebral edema.

Note: In patients with lead encephalopathy and increased intracranial pressure, excess fluids must be avoided. In such case a 20 percent solution of calcium disodium edetate is mixed with procaine to give a final concentration of 0.5 percent of procaine in the mixture which is administered intramuscularly.

Acutely ill individuals may be dehydrated from vomiting. Since calcium disodium edetate is excreted almost exclusively in the urine, it is very important to establish urine flow by intravenous infusion before the first dose of the chelating agent is given. Once urine flow is established further intravenous fluid is restricted to basal water and electrolyte requirements. Administration of calcium disodium edetate should be stopped whenever there is cessation of urine flow in order to avoid unduly high tissue levels of the drug.

Intravenous Administration: Dilute the 5 ml. (1 gram, 20% solution) from an ampule with 250-500 ml. of Solution Isotonic Sodium Chloride, USP, or sterile 5% dextrose solution in water. In asymptomatic adults, administer this diluted solution over a period of at least one hour. Such doses may be administered twice daily for periods up to 5 days. The therapy should then be interrupted for 2 days and followed by an additional 5 days of treatment, if indicated.

In mildy affected or asymptomatic individuals the dosage of 50 mg./kg. per day should not be exceeded.

In symptomatic adults, fluids should be kept to basal levels and the time of administration increased to two hours. A second daily infusion is to be given six or more hours after the first.

Intramuscular Administration: This is the route of choice for children. The dosage should not exceed 0.5 gram per 30 pounds of body weight twice daily (total, 1.0 gram/30 lbs./day). This is equivalent to 35 mg./kg. twice daily (total, approx. 75 mg./kg./day). In mild cases a dose of 50 mg./kg. per day should not be exceeded. For young children the total daily dose may be given in divided doses every 8 or 12 hours for 3 to 5 days. A second course may be given after a rest period of 4 or more days. Procaine to produce a concentration of 0.5% should be added to minimize pain at injection site. (1 ml. of 1% procaine solution for each ml. of concentrated Calcium Disodium Versenate solution, or crystalline procaine may be used to reduce volume.)

Regardless of method of administration, doses larger than those recommended should not be undertaken.

Lead Encephalopathy: This condition is relatively rare in adults but is quite common in children in whom the mortality rate has been high. Recent reports by Chisolm and by Coffin et al who employed a combination of BAL and calcium disodium edetate, suggest that this may be the preferred treatment, although calcium disodium edetate alone has been used over a longer period of time. Each group administered calcium disodium edetate intramuscularly concurrently with BAL in separate deep I.M. sites. Procaine was added to the 20% solution of calcium disodium edetate to give a procaine concentration of 0.5%. In the studies of Coffin and Chisolm, 125 children with acute lead encephalopathy have been treated with this combined therapy with only one death.

How Supplied: Calcium Disodium Versenate Injection, 5 ml. ampules containing 200 mg. of calcium disodium edetate per ml., boxes containing 6 ampules.
(NDC **0089-0510-06**).

*Registered trademark of the Dow Chemical Company

CAL·SUP™
Calcium Supplement 300 mg

Composition: Each tablet contains 750 mg calcium carbonate (equivalent to 300 mg elemental calcium) with glycine.

Indications: For use in the prevention of calcium deficiency when needed or recommended by a physician.

Dosage and Administration: Take three or four tablets daily, or as directed by your physician. Chew, swallow or melt in the mouth.

Three tablets daily provide:

Quantity	U.S. RDA†	
Calcium 900 mg	90%*	69%**

Four tablets daily provide:

Quantity	U.S. RDA†	
Calcium 1200 mg	120%*	92%**

† U.S. recommended daily allowance
* For adults and children 12 or more years of age
** For pregnant and lactating women

How Supplied: Bottles of 100 white tablets (NDC **0089-0110-10**).

CIRCANOL® ℞
(ergoloid mesylates)
TABLETS FOR SUBLINGUAL ADMINISTRATION

Description: Each white, round, sublingual 0.5 mg tablet contains dihydroergocornine 0.167 mg, dihydroergocristine 0.167 mg and dihydroergocryptine 0.167 mg (dihydro-alpha-ergocryptine and dihydro-beta-ergocryptine in the proportion of 2:1) as the methanesulfonates (mesylates), representing a total of 0.5 mg.

Each white, oval, sublingual 1.0 mg tablet contains dihydroergocornine 0.333 mg, dihydroergocristine 0.333 mg and dihydroergocryptine 0.333 mg (dihydro-alpha-ergocryptine and dihydro-beta-ergocryptine in the proportion of 2:1) as the methanesulfonates (mesylates), representing a total of 1.0 mg.

How Supplied: Circanol (ergoloid mesylates) sublingual tablets are supplied as 0.5 mg white round tablets in bottles of 100 (NDC **0089-0121-10**) and 1,000 (NDC **0089-0121-80**) and 1.0 mg white oval tablets in bottles of 1,000 (NDC **0089-0123-80**) and 100 (NDC **0089-0123-10**).

[*Shown in Product Identification Section*]

DEANER® ℞
and
DEANER®-250
(deanol acetamidobenzoate)

Description: Each tablet contains 250 mg., 100 mg. or 25 mg. of deanol (2-dimethylaminoethanol) as the para-acetamidobenzoic acid salt.

Pharmacology: The concept that deanol is a precursor of acetylcholine which affects the central nervous system is supported by evidence derived from biochemical and pharmacologic studies. Studies with Carbon 14-labeled deanol indicate that it crosses the blood-brain barrier and probably is converted intracellulary to acetylcholine. It does not depress the appetite or cause jitteriness, as does amphetamine. Deanol does not affect the BMR, blood pressure, or pulse rate, and is not an MAO inhibitor.

The toxicity of deanol is very low. Laboratory tests and clinical, pathological and histopathological examinations have disclosed no harmful changes attributable to the drug.

Indications:
Based on a review of this drug by the National Academy of Sciences—National Research Council and/or other information, FDA has classified the indications as follows:
"Possibly" effective:
1. Learning problems—learning in deficit of that usually associated with apparent level of intelligence, including I.Q. Reading difficulties. Shortened attention span.
2. Behavior problems—hyperkinetic behavior problem syndrome characterized by distractibility, motor disinhibition, dissociation, and perseveration.
3. Or, as more frequently encountered, hyperkinetic behavior and learning disorders incorporating varying combinations of both of the above. Under-achievers. Reading and speech difficulties. Impaired motor coordination. Hyperactive, impulsive/compulsive behavior, often described as asocial, antisocial, delinquent, stimulus-governed.
Final classification of the less than effective indications requires further investigation.

Contraindications: No absolute contraindications are known. Grand mal epilepsy and mixed epilepsy with a grand mal component are relative contraindications.

Side Actions: Neither sensitization nor serious side effects have been reported with DEANER (deanol acetamidobenzoate). Mild overstimulation and the following minor side actions, if encountered, usually disappear with continued treatment or with reduction in dosage: dull occipital headache early in therapy; constipation; tenseness in neck, masseter and quadriceps muscles; insomnia; pruritus; transient rash. Rarely postural hypotension occurs.

Administration and Dosage: Starting dose: 500 mg. daily. If satisfactory improvement occurs, the maintenance dosage will vary from 250 to 500 mg. daily. The maintenance dosage should be adjusted to the needs of the individual patient.

How Supplied: Deaner-250: 250 mg. scored, white, capsule shaped, film coated tablets in bottles of 50 (NDC **0089-0135-05**); Deaner: 100 mg. scored, pink, round tablets in bottles of 50 (NDC **0089-0137-05**) and 25 mg. scored, white, round tablets in bottles of 100 (NDC **0089-0131-10**).

DISALCID® ℞
(salsalate)
Tablets and Capsules

Description: DISALCID (salsalate) is a nonsteroidal anti-inflammatory agent for oral administration. Chemically, salsalate (salicylsalicylic acid or 2-hydroxy-benzoic acid, 2-carboxyphenyl ester) is a dimer of salicylic acid.

Each round, aqua, film coated DISALCID tablet contains 500 mg salsalate. Each aqua and white DISALCID capsule contains 500 mg salsalate. Each capsule-shaped aqua, scored, film coated DISALCID tablet contains 750 mg salsalate.

Clinical Pharmacology: DISALCID is insoluble in acid gastric fluids (<0.1 mg/ml at pH 1.0), but readily soluble in the small intestine where it is partially hydrolyzed to two molecules of salicylic acid. A significant portion of the parent compound is absorbed unchanged and undergoes rapid esterase hydrolysis in the body; its half-life is about one hour. About 13% is excreted through the kidneys as a glucuronide conjugate of the parent compound, the remainder as salicylic acid and its metabolites. Thus, the amount of salicylic acid available from DISALCID is about 15% less than from aspirin, when the two drugs are administered on a salicylic acid molar equivalent basis (3.6 g salsalate/5 g aspirin). Salicylic acid

Continued on next page

Riker—Cont.

biotransformation is saturated at anti-inflammatory doses of DISALCID. Such capacity-limited biotransformation results in an increase in the half-life of salicylic acid from 3.5 to 16 or more hours. Thus, dosing with DISALCID twice a day will satisfactorily maintain blood levels within the desired therapeutic range (10-30 mg/100 ml) throughout the 12-hour intervals. Therapeutic blood levels continue for up to 16 hours after the last dose. The parent compound does not show capacity-limited biotransformation, nor does it accumulate in the plasma on multiple dosing. Food slows the absorption of all salicylates including DISALCID.

The mode of anti-inflammatory action of DISALCID and other nonsteroidal anti-inflammatory drugs remains unclear. Although salicylic acid (the primary metabolite of DISALCID) is a weak inhibitor of prostaglandin synthesis *in vitro*, it has been shown to inhibit prostaglandin synthesis *in vivo* as potently as aspirin and indomethacin. However, unlike aspirin, DISALCID does not inhibit platelet aggregation.[1] The usefulness of salicylic acid, the active *in vivo* product of DISALCID, in the treatment of arthritic disorders has been established.[2,3] In contrast to aspirin and the other nonsteroidal anti-inflammatory drugs, DISALCID does not cause gastrointestinal blood loss.[4]

Indications and Usage: DISALCID is indicated for relief of the signs and symptoms of rheumatoid arthritis, osteoarthritis and related rheumatic disorders.

DISALCID can safely be given to aspirin-sensitive patients (and those sensitive to tartrazine, FD&C Yellow No. 5), since it does not induce asthma in such patients.[5]

Contraindications: DISALCID is contraindicated in patients hypersensitive to salsalate.

Warnings: See "PRECAUTIONS".

Precautions:

General Precautions:

Patients on long-term treatment with DISALCID should be warned not to take other salicylates so as to avoid potentially toxic concentrations. Great care should be exercised when DISALCID is prescribed in the presence of chronic renal insufficiency. Protein binding of salicylic acid can be influenced by nutritional status, competitive binding of other drugs, and fluctuations in serum proteins caused by disease (rheumatoid arthritis, etc.).

Laboratory Tests:

Plasma salicylic acid concentrations should be periodically monitored during long-term treatment with DISALCID to aid maintenance of therapeutically effective levels: 10 to 30 mg/100 ml. Toxic manifestations are not usually seen until plasma concentrations exceed 30 mg/100 ml (see OVERDOSAGE). Urinary pH should also be regularly monitored: sudden acidification, as from pH 6.5 to 5.5, can double the plasma level, resulting in toxicity.

Drug Interactions:

Salicylates antagonize the uricosuric action of drugs used to treat gout. Aspirin and other salicylate drugs will be additive to DISALCID and may increase plasma concentrations of salicylic acid to toxic levels. Drugs and foods that raise urine pH will increase renal clearance and urinary excretion of salicylic acid, thus lowering plasma levels; acidifying drugs or foods will decrease urinary excretion and increase plasma levels. Salicylates may competitively displace anticoagulant drugs from plasma protein binding sites and thereby predispose to systemic bleeding. Salicylates may enhance the hypoglycemic effect of oral antidiabetic drugs of the sulfonylurea class. Salicylate competes with a number of drugs for protein binding sites, notably penicillin, thiopental, thyroxine, triiodothyronine, phenytoin, sulfinpyrazone, naproxen, warfarin, methotrexate, and possibly corticosteroids.

Drug/Laboratory Test Interactions:

Salicylate competes with thyroid hormone for binding to plasma proteins, which may be reflected in a depressed plasma T_4 value in some patients; thyroid function and basal metabolism are unaffected.

Carcinogenesis:

No long-term animal studies have been performed with DISALCID to evaluate its carcinogenic potential; however, several such studies using aspirin and other salicylates have failed to demonstrate any association of these agents with cancerous cell changes.

Use in Pregnancy:

Pregnancy Category C: Salsalate and salicylic acid have been shown to be teratogenic and embryocidal in rats when given in doses 4-5 times the usual human dose. These effects were not observed at doses twice as great as the usual human dose. There are no adequate and well-controlled studies in pregnant women. DISALCID should be used during pregnancy only if the potential benefit justifies the potential risk to the fetus.

Labor and Delivery:

There exist no adequate and well-controlled studies in pregnant women. Although adverse effects on mother or infant have not been reported with DISALCID use during labor, caution is advised when anti-inflammatory dosage is involved. However, other salicylates have been associated with prolonged gestation and labor, maternal and neonatal bleeding sequelae, potentiation of narcotic and barbiturate effects (respiratory or cardiac arrest in the mother), delivery problems and stillbirth.

Nursing Mothers:

It is not known whether salsalate per se is excreted in human milk; salicylic acid, the primary metabolite of DISALCID, has been shown to appear in human milk in concentrations approximating the maternal blood level. Thus the infant of a mother on DISALCID therapy might ingest in mother's milk 30-80% as much salicylate per Kg body weight as the mother is taking. Accordingly, caution should be exercised when DISALCID is administered to a nursing woman.

Pediatric Use:

Safety and effectiveness in children have not been established.

Adverse Reactions:

Auditory system: Tinnitus and temporary hearing loss can occur. Tinnitus probably represents blood salicylic acid levels reaching or exceeding the upper limit of the therapeutic range. It is therefore a helpful guide to dose titration. Temporary hearing loss disappears gradually upon discontinuation of the drug.

Gastrointestinal system: Nausea, dyspepsia and heartburn occur occasionally.

Drug Abuse and Dependence: Drug abuse and dependence have not been reported with DISALCID.

Overdosage: No deaths after overdosage have been reported for DISALCID. Death has followed ingestion of 10-30 g of other salicylates in adults, but much larger amounts have been ingested without fatal outcome.

The oral LD_{50} for DISALCID in rats is approximately 2000 mg/kg (sixty times the recommended maximum single dose for adults).

Symptoms: The usual symptoms of salicylism—tinnitus, vertigo, headache, confusion, drowsiness, sweating, hyperventilation, vomiting and diarrhea—will occur. More severe intoxication will lead to disruption of electrolyte balance and blood pH, and hyperthermia and dehydration.

Treatment: Further absorption of DISALCID from the G.I. tract should be prevented by emesis (syrup of ipecac) and, if necessary, by gastric lavage.

Fluid and electrolyte imbalance should be corrected by the administration of appropriate I.V. therapy. Adequate renal function should be maintained. Hemodialysis or peritoneal dialysis may be required in extreme cases.

Dosage and Administration:

Adults: the usual dosage is 3000 mg daily, given in divided doses as follows: 1) Two doses of two 750 mg tablets; 2) two doses of three 500 mg tablets/capsules; or 3) three doses of two 500 mg tablets/capsules. Dosage should be adjusted depending on individual response. Alleviation of symptoms is gradual, and full benefits may not be evident for 3-4 days, when plasma salicylate levels have achieved steady state. There is no evidence for development of tissue tolerance (tachyphlaxis), but salicylate therapy may induce increased activity of metabolizing liver enzymes, causing a greater rate of salicyluric acid production and excretion, with a resultant increase in dosage requirement for maintenance of therapeutic serum salicylate levels.

Children: DISALCID has not been evaluated in children. No dosage recommendations can, therefore, be made.

How Supplied:

750 mg tablets in bottles of 100 (NDC 0089-0151-10)

500 mg tablets in bottles of 100 (NDC 0089-0149-10)

500 mg tablets in bottles of 500 (NDC 0089-0149-50)

500 mg capsules in bottles of 100 (NDC 0089-0148-10)

References:

1. Estes D, Kaplan K: Lack of Platelet Effect With the Aspirin Analog, Salsalate. Arthritis and Rheumatism, 23, 1303, 1980.
2. Dick C, Dick PH, Nuki G, et al: Effect of Anti-inflammatory Drug Therapy on Clearance of ^{133}Xe from Knee Joints of Patients with Rheumatoid Arthritis. British Med. J. *3*:278–280, 1969.
3. Dick WC, Grayson MF, Woodburn A, et al: Indices of inflammatory activity. Ann. of the Rheum. Dis. *29*:643–648, 1970.
4. Cohen A: Fecal Blood Loss and Plasma Salicylate Study of Salicylsalicylic Acid and Aspirin. J. Clin. Pharmacol. *19*:242–247, 1979.
5. Simon MR, Salberg DJ, Muller BF, et al: Lack of Adverse Reactions to Salsalate in Asthmatic Subjects. Data on file, Medical Department, Riker Laboratories, Inc.

[*Shown in Product Identification Section*]

DISIPAL® ℞
(orphenadrine hydrochloride)
TABLETS

Description: Each tablet contains 50 mg. orphenadrine hydrochloride (2-dimethylaminoethyl 2-methylbenzhydryl ether hydrochloride).

Actions: In the laboratory, DISIPAL (orphenadrine hydrochloride) demonstrates parasympatholytic and antitremor activity, as well as clinically unimportant degrees of antihistaminic and local anesthetic actions. The drug acts centrally, producing effective relaxation of muscle spasm. DISIPAL (orphenadrine hydrochloride) has greater parasympatholytic and antitremor activity than its chemical relative, diphenhydramine. An outstanding difference between orphenadrine and diphenhydramine is the absence of a soporific action.

Chronic toxicity studies, in rats and dogs, have shown no gross or microscopic evidence of drug induced pathology. The daily oral dosage was 20 milligrams per kilogram for the dog and 75 milligrams per kilogram for the rats. No abnormalities of the blood or urine were produced during a six month period of continuous medication.

Indications: DISIPAL (orphenadrine hydrochloride) is effective for use as an adjunct in the therapy of all forms of parkinsonism (postencephalitic, arteriosclerotic, idiopathic).

Contraindications: Contraindications are due to the anticholinergic action of orphenadrine. DISIPAL (orphenadrine hydrochloride) should not be used in patients with glaucoma, pyloric or duodenal obstruction, stenosing peptic ulcers, prostatic hypertrophy or obstructions at the bladder neck, achalasia (megaesophagus) and myasthenia gravis. DISIPAL (orphenadrine hydrochloride) should be used with caution in patients with tachycardia. Since mental confusion, anxiety and tremors have been reported in patients receiving orphenadrine and propoxyphene concurrently, it is recommended that DISIPAL not be given in combination with propoxyphene (Darvon®).

Warning:

Use in pregnancy: Since safety of the use of this preparation in pregnancy, during lactation, or in the child-bearing age has not been established, use of the drug in such patients requires that the potential benefits of the drug be weighed against its possible hazard to the mother and child.

Adverse Reactions: Side effects of DISIPAL (orphenadrine hydrochloride) are mainly due to the mild anticholinergic action of orphenadrine and are usually associated with higher dosage. Dryness of the mouth is the first side effect to appear. When the daily dose is increased, possible side actions include: tachycardia, palpitation, urinary hesitancy or retention, blurred vision, dilatation of the pupil, increased ocular tension, weakness, nausea, vomiting, headache, dizziness, constipation and drowsiness and rarely, urticaria and other dermatoses. Infrequently, an elderly patient may experience some degree of mental confusion. These mild side effects can usually be eliminated by reduction in dosage. Two cases of aplastic anemia associated with orphenadrine citrate have been reported. No causal relationship has been established, and no reports were received in connection with the use of DISIPAL.

Dosage and Administration: Usual dosage, one tablet (50 mg.) three times daily. In combination with other agents and in the treatment of Parkinson's syndrome, smaller doses often suffice. Doses up to 250 mg. daily have been used without the occurrence of disagreeable side effects.

How Supplied: Bottles of 100 (NDC **0089-0161-10**), and 500 tablets (NDC **0089-0161-50**).

DUO-MEDIHALER® ℞

(isoproterenol hydrochloride, phenylephrine bitartrate)

Description: Duo-Medihaler (isoproterenol hydrochloride and phenylephrine bitartrate) is an aerosol device which delivers micronized particles of isoproterenol hydrochloride and phenylephrine bitartrate suspended in an inert mixture of sorbitan trioleate, cetylpyridinium chloride with fluorochlorohydrocarbons as propellants. This drug-propellant system is contained in a hermetically sealed metal vial. Each valve actuation releases a uniform aerosolized dose of 0.16 mg isoproterenol hydrochloride (equivalent to 0.137 mg of isoproterenol base) and 0.24 mg phenylephrine bitartrate (equivalent to 0.126 mg of phenylephrine base).

Actions: Duo-Medihaler provides rapid and prolonged symptomatic relief of dyspnea resulting from bronchospasm and congestion and edema of the respiratory mucosa. Isoproterenol acts almost exclusively by stimulating beta adrenergic receptors within the tracheobronchial tree. The main action of isoproterenol is to prevent and relieve bronchoconstriction. Phenylephrine is a powerful alpha-receptor stimulant and as such produces vasoconstriction which is of considerable value in reducing edema and congestion of the bronchiolar vascular beds. It is believed that phenylephrine is synergistic with isoproterenol through its vasoconstricting and mild bronchodilatory actions. This reduces bronchiolar blood flow, thereby decreasing the engorgement of the bronchiolar tree and slowing the systemic absorption of the isoproterenol, as well as adding further bronchodilatation.

Indications: Duo-Medihaler is indicated for the treatment of bronchospasm associated with acute and chronic bronchial asthma, pulmonary emphysema, bronchitis, and bronchiectasis.

Contraindications: Known hypersensitivity to either agent constitutes a contraindication to the use of this drug. Isoproterenol preparations are generally contraindicated in patients with pre-existing cardiac arrhythmias associated with tachycardia because the cardiac stimulant effect of the drug may aggravate such disorders.

Warnings: Excessive use of an adrenergic aerosol should be discouraged, as it may lose its effectiveness. Occasional patients have been reported to develop severe paradoxical airway resistance with repeated, excessive use of isoproterenol inhalation preparations. The cause of this refractory state is unknown. It is advisable that in such instances the use of this preparation be discontinued immediately and alternative therapy instituted, since in the reported cases the patients did not respond to other forms of therapy until the drug was withdrawn.

Deaths have been reported following excessive use of isoproterenol inhalation preparations and the exact cause is unknown. Cardiac arrest was noted in several instances.

Precautions: Isoproterenol should not be administered with epinephrine, since both drugs are direct cardiac stimulants and their combined effects may produce serious arrhythmias. If desired, these drugs may be alternated, provided an interval of at least four hours has elapsed.

Although there has been no evidence of teratogenic effects with these drugs, use of any drug in pregnancy, lactation, or in women of childbearing age requires that the potential benefit of the drug be weighed against its possible hazard to the mother and child.

Duo-Medihaler should be used with caution in patients with cardiovascular disorders including coronary insufficiency, diabetes, or hyperthyroidism, and in persons sensitive to sympathomimetic amines.

Adverse Reactions: Overdosage with isoproterenol can produce palpitation, tachycardia, tremulousness, flushing, anginal-type pain, nausea, dizziness, weakness and sweating, while overdosage with phenylephrine can induce cardiac irregularities, central nervous system disturbances and reflex bradycardia. The individual patient's sensitivity to either drug would dictate the overdosage signs. However, there is reason to believe the overdosage effects of either drug are antagonized by the other drug in the mixture.

Dosage and Administration: The recommended dose for the relief of dyspnea in the acute episode is 1 to 2 inhalations. Start with one inhalation. If no relief is evident after 2 to 5 minutes, a second inhalation may be taken. For daily maintenance, use 1 to 2 inhalations 4 to 6 times daily or as directed by the physician. No more than two inhalations should be taken at any one time, or more than 6 inhalations in any one hour during a 24-hour period, unless advised by physician.

How Supplied:

For long-term use:

Initial Rx: Duo-Medihaler with adapter (450 doses, 22.5 ml.) NDC **0089-0732-21**.

Refill: Duo-Medihaler refill vial (450 doses, 22.5 ml.) NDC **0089-0732-11**.

For patients with less frequent need:

Initial Rx: Duo-Medihaler with adapter (300 doses, 15 ml.) NDC **0089-0735-21**.

Refill: Duo-Medihaler refill (300 doses, 15 ml.) NDC **0089-0735-11**.

ESTOMUL-M®

Liquid/Tablets

Description:

Estomul-M® Liquid—

Each tablespoon (15 ml.) contains:

Aluminum hydroxide }Co-Precipitate 918 mg.
Magnesium carbonate

Estomul-M® Tablet—

Each tablet contains:

Aluminum hydroxide }Co-Precipitate 500 mg.
Magnesium carbonate

Magnesium oxide 45 mg.

How Supplied:

Estomul-M® Liquid—Bottles of 12 fluid ounces (NDC **0089-0921-12**).

Estomul-M® Tablets—Bottles of 100 tablets (NDC **0089-0193-10**).

LIPO-HEPIN® ℞

(heparin sodium injection, U.S.P.) Aqueous DERIVED FROM PORCINE INTESTINAL MUCOSA

Description: Heparin Sodium Injection, USP is a sterile solution of heparin sodium derived from animal tissues (i.e. porcine intestinal mucosa, or bovine lung tissue) standardized for use as an anticoagulant, in water for injection with 0.9% benzyl alcohol as a preservative and sodium chloride to make solutions under 10,000 U/ml isotonic. The potency is determined by biological assay using a USP reference standard based upon units of heparin activity per milligram.

How Supplied:

Lipo-Hepin® (heparin sodium injection, U.S.P.) derived from porcine intestinal mucosa is available in single-dose ampules, vials, and disposable syringes, and in multiple-dose vials for subcutaneous or intravenous injection. [See table above].

Preservative: Benzyl alcohol 0.9%. Sodium chloride added to 1,000; 2,000 and 5,000 units per ml. concentrations to make solutions isotonic.

MULTIPLE-DOSE VIALS

NATIONAL DRUG CODE NO.	VIAL CONTENT	POTENCY: U.S.P. UNITS PER ML.
0089-0 410-01	10 ml	1,000
0089-0 415-01	10 ml	5,000
0089-0 425-01	5 ml	10,000
0089-0 435-01	5 ml	20,000
0089-0 445-01	5 ml	40,000

SYRINGES

NATIONAL DRUG CODE NO.	SYRINGES TO DELIVER	POTENCY: U.S.P. Units per 0.5 ML.
0089-0 464-10	0.5 ml	5,000

Continued on next page

Riker—Cont.

MEDIHALER-EPI®
(epinephrine bitartrate)
FOR TEMPORARY RELIEF FROM ACUTE PAROXYSMS OF BRONCHIAL ASTHMA.

FOR ORAL INHALATION THERAPY ONLY

Each inhalation delivers 0.3 mg epinephrine bitartrate equivalent to 0.16 mg of epinephrine base.
How Supplied: 15 ml. size: Available as a combination package (vial with oral adapter) or as a refill (vial only).

MEDIHALER ERGOTAMINE® ℞
(ergotamine tartrate)

Description: Medihaler Ergotamine (ergotamine tartrate) is an aerosol device which contains a fine particle suspension of 9.0 mg. ergotamine tartrate per ml. in an inert, nontoxic aerosol vehicle. Each depression of the valve delivers a measured dose of 0.36 mg. to the patient.
Action: Ergotamine exerts a constrictor action upon the cranial vessels.
Indications: As therapy to abort vascular headache, e.g., migraine, migraine variants, or so-called "histaminic cephalalgia."
Contraindications: Ergotamine tartrate should not be used in the presence of coronary artery disease, peripheral vascular disease, hypertension, impaired renal or hepatic function, infectious states or malnutrition.
Ergotamine tartrate is contraindicated in patients with a history of hypersensitivity reactions.
Pregnancy: Ergotamine tartrate is contraindicated in pregnancy.
Warnings: Patients who are being treated with Medihaler Ergotamine should be informed adequately of the symptoms of ergotism. Close medical supervision by the physician is recommended so that he may react appropriately should signs of ergotism develop. Six inhalations per day, if continued daily, entail the risk of vasospastic complications. Avoid prolonged administration or in excess of the recommended dosage because of the danger of ergotism and gangrene.
Pediatric Patients: Since there is no experience in children who have received this drug, safety and efficacy in children have not been established.
Nursing Mothers: Whether ergotamine tartrate is excreted in mothers' milk is not known. As a general rule, nursing should not be undertaken while a patient is on a drug (since many drugs are excreted in human milk).
Adverse Reactions: Ergotamine tartrate may cause nausea and vomiting. Patients with headaches may become nauseated and drug induced distress may be difficult to evaluate.
Ergotamine in large doses raises arterial pressure, produces coronary vasoconstriction and slows the heart both by direct action and its effect on the vagus. Under this condition, ergotamine also has oxytocic and spasmolytic properties. The above conditions are seen as a consequence of overdosage and may be manifested at the dosage recommended for control of headaches.
Vasoconstrictive complications, at times of a serious nature, may occur. These include pulselessness, weakness, muscle pains and paresthesias of the extremities and precordial distress and pain. Although these effects occur most commonly with long term therapy at relatively high doses, they have also been reported with short term or normal doses. Other adverse effects include transient tachycardia or bradycardia, nausea, vomiting, localized edema and itching.
Dosage and Administration:
Adults: A single inhalation at the first sign of headache or prodrome. Repeat this procedure in 5 minutes if relief is not obtained. Space any additional inhalations at no less than 5-minute intervals. No more than 6 inhalations should be administered in any 24-hour period, and no more than 15 in a one week period.
Children: A recommended dose for children has not been determined.
Directions For Use: Before each use, remove dust cap and shake Medihaler.

1. Breathe out fully and place mouthpiece well into the mouth, aimed at the back of the throat.
2. As you begin to breathe in deeply, press the vial firmly down into the adapter with the index finger. This releases one dose.
3. Release pressure on vial and remove unit from mouth. Hold the breath as long as possible, then breathe out slowly.

How Supplied: Metal vial (2.5 ml.) and adapter. Each depression of the valve delivers 0.36 mg. ergotamine tartrate. (NDC **0089-0762-21**).

MEDIHALER-ISO® ℞
(isoproterenol sulfate)

Description: Medihaler-Iso (isoproterenol sulfate) is an aerosol device which contains a fine particle suspension of 2.0 mg. per ml. isoproterenol sulfate in an inert propellant consisting of sorbitan trioleate and fluorochlorohydrocarbons. Each depression of the valve delivers a measured dose of 0.08 mg. to the patient.
Actions: Isoproterenol is a short-acting sympathomimetic drug. It produces pharmacologic response in the cardiovascular system and on the smooth muscles of the bronchial tree. The drug will prevent or overcome histamine-induced asthma in both experimental animals and man, and is effective when used prophylactically. It is one of the most potent bronchodilators known and can be used in patients who do not respond to the bronchodilating action of epinephrine. Isoproterenol has a cardioaccelerating effect, but its vaso-constricting action is less pronounced than that of epinephrine. Therapeutic doses may produce a slight increase in systolic blood pressure, but a slight decrease in diastolic. Larger doses may cause peripheral vasodilatation in the renal, mesenteric and femoral beds, and some patients respond with a decrease in diastolic, but no change in systolic pressure. Such effects are usually of very short duration.
Indications: For the treatment of bronchospasm associated with acute and chronic bronchial asthma, pulmonary emphysema, bronchitis, and bronchiectasis.
Contraindications: Use of isoproterenol in patients with pre-existing cardiac arrhythmias associated with tachycardia is contraindicated because the cardiac stimulant effects of the drug may aggravate such disorders.
Warnings: Excessive use of an adrenergic aerosol should be discouraged, as it may lose its effectiveness.
Occasional patients have been reported to develop severe paradoxical airway resistance with repeated, excessive use of isoproterenol inhalation preparations. The cause of this refractory state is unknown. It is advisable that in such instances the use of this preparation be discontinued immediately and alternative therapy instituted, since in the reported cases the patients did not respond to other forms of therapy until the drug was withdrawn.
Deaths have been reported following excessive use of isoproterenol inhalation preparations and the exact cause is unknown. Cardiac arrest was noted in several instances.
Precautions: Isoproterenol and epinephrine may be used interchangeably if the patient becomes unresponsive to one or the other but should not be used concurrently. If desired, these drugs may be alternated, provided an interval of at least four hours has elapsed.
As with all sympathomimetic drugs, isoproterenol should be used with great caution in the presence of cardiovascular disorders, including coronary insufficiency, hypertension, hyperthyroidism and diabetes, or when there is a sensitivity to sympathomimetic amines.
Although there has been no evidence of teratogenic effects with this drug, use of any drug in pregnancy, lactation, or in women of childbearing age requires that the potential benefit of the drug be weighed against its possible hazard to the mother and child.
Adverse Reactions: Only a small percentage of patients experience any side effects following oral inhalation of aerosolized isoproterenol. Overdosage may produce tachycardia with resultant coronary insufficiency, palpitations, vertigo, nausea, tremors, headache, insomnia, central excitation, and blood pressure changes. These reactions are similar to those produced by other sympathomimetic agents.
Dosage and Administration: The usual dose for the relief of dyspnea in the acute episode is 1 to 2 inhalations. Start with one inhalation. If no relief is evident after 2 to 5 minutes, a second inhalation may be taken. For daily maintenance, use 1 to 2 inhalations 4 to 6 times daily or as directed by the physician. The physician should be careful to instruct the patient in the proper technique of administration so that the number of inhalations per treatment and the frequency of retreatment may be titrated to the patient's response.
No more than two inhalations should be taken at any one time, nor more than six inhalations in any one hour during a 24-hour period unless advised by the physician.
How Supplied:
Medihaler-Iso (isoproterenol sulfate) with oral adapter (300 doses 15 ml.) NDC **0089-0785-21**.
Medihaler-Iso (isoproterenol sulfate) refill vial only (300 doses 15 ml.) NDC **0089-0785-11**.
Medihaler-Iso (isoproterenol sulfate) with oral adapter (450 doses 22.5 ml.) NDC **0089-0782-21**.
Medihaler-Iso (isoproterenol sulfate) refill vial only (450 doses 22.5 ml.) NDC **0089-0782-11**.

NORFLEX® ℞
(orphenadrine citrate)
Tablets and Injectable

Description: Orphenadrine citrate is the citrate salt of orphenadrine (2-dimethylaminoethyl 2-methylbenzhydryl ether citrate). It occurs as a white, crystalline powder having a bitter taste. It is practically odorless; sparingly soluble in water, slightly soluble in alcohol.
Actions: The mode of therapeutic action has not been clearly identified, but may be related to its analgesic properties. Orphenadrine citrate also possesses anti-cholinergic actions.
Indications: Orphenadrine citrate is indicated as an adjunct to rest, physical therapy, and other measures for the relief of discomfort associated with acute painful musculo skeletal conditions. The mode of action of the drug has not been clearly identified, but may be related to its analgesic properties. Orphenadrine citrate does not directly relax tense skeletal muscles in man.
Contraindications: Contraindicated in patients with glaucoma, pyloric or duodenal obstruction, stenosing peptic ulcers, prostatic hypertrophy or obstruction of the bladder neck, cardio-spasm (megaesophagus) and myasthenia gravis.
Contraindicated in patients who have demonstrated a previous hypersensitivity to the drug.
Warnings: Some patients may experience transient episodes of lightheadedness, dizziness or syncope. Norflex may impair the ability of the patient to engage in potentially hazardous activities such as operating machinery or driving a motor vehicle; ambulatory patients should therefore be cautioned accordingly.

Usage in Pregnancy: Safe use of orphenadrine has not been established with respect to adverse effects upon fetal development. Therefore, Norflex should be used in women of childbearing potential and particularly during early pregnancy only when in the judgment of the physician the potential benefits outweigh the possible hazards.

Usage in Children: Safety and effectiveness in children have not been established; therefore, this drug is not recommended for use in the pediatric age group.

Precautions: Confusion, anxiety and tremors have been reported in few patients receiving propoxyphene and orphenadrine concomitantly. As these symptoms may be simply due to an additive effect, reduction of dosage and/or discontinuation of one or both agents is recommended in such cases.

Orphenadrine citrate should be used with caution in patients with tachycardia, cardiac decompensation, coronary insufficiency, cardiac arrhythmias.

Safety of continuous long-term therapy with orphenadrine has not been established. Therefore, if orphenadrine is prescribed for prolonged use, periodic monitoring of blood, urine and liver function values is recommended.

Adverse Reactions: Adverse effects of orphenadrine are mainly due to the mild anticholinergic action of orphenadrine, and are usually associated with higher dosage. Dryness of the mouth is usually the first adverse effect to appear. When the daily dose is increased, possible adverse effects include: tachycardia, palpitation, urinary hesitancy or retention, blurred vision, dilatation of pupils, increased ocular tension, weakness, nausea, vomiting, headache, dizziness, constipation, drowsiness, hypersensitivity reactions, pruritus, hallucinations, agitation, tremor, gastric irritation, and rarely urticaria and other dermatoses. Infrequently, an elderly patient may experience some degree of mental confusion. These adverse reactions can usually be eliminated by reduction in dosage. Very rare cases of aplastic anemia associated with the use of orphenadrine tablets have been reported. No causal relationship has been established.

Rare instances of anaphylactic reaction have been reported associated with the intramuscular injection of Norflex injectable.

Dosage and Administration:

TABLETS: Adults—Two tablets per day; one in the morning and one in the evening.

INJECTABLE: Adults—One 2 ml. ampul (60 mg.) intravenously or intramuscularly; may be repeated every 12 hours. Relief may be maintained by 1 Norflex Tablet twice daily.

How Supplied:

TABLETS: Bottles of 100 (NDC **0089-0221-10**) and 500 (NDC **0089-0221-50**), each tablet containing 100 mg. of orphenadrine citrate.

INJECTABLE: Boxes of 6 (NDC **0089-0540-06**) and 50 (NDC **0089-0540-50**) 2 ml. ampuls, each ampul containing 60 mg. of orphenadrine citrate in aqueous solution, made isotonic with sodium chloride.

[*100 mg. Tablet Shown in Product Identification Section*]

NORGESIC® and NORGESIC® FORTE ℞

Actions: Orphenadrine citrate is a centrally acting (brain stem) compound which in animals selectively blocks facilitatory functions of the reticular formation. Orphenadrine does not produce myoneural block, nor does it affect crossed extensor reflexes. Orphenadrine prevents nicotine-induced convulsions but not those produced by strychnine.

Chronic administration of Norgesic to dogs and rats has revealed no drug-related toxicity. No blood or urine changes were observed, nor were there any macroscopic or microscopic pathological changes detected. Extensive experience with combinations containing aspirin and caffeine has established them as safe agents. The addition of orphenadrine citrate does not alter the toxicity of aspirin and caffeine.

The mode of therapeutic action of orphenadrine has not been clearly identified, but may be related to its analgesic properties. Orphenadrine citrate also possesses anti-cholinergic actions.

Indications:

1. Symptomatic relief of mild to moderate pain of acute musculo-skeletal disorders.
2. The orphenadrine component is indicated as an adjunct to rest, physical therapy, and other measures for the relief of discomfort associated with acute painful musculoskeletal conditions.

   The mode of action of orphenadrine has not been clearly identified, but may be related to its analgesic properties. Norgesic and Norgesic Forte do not directly relax tense skeletal muscles in man.

Contraindications: Because of the mild anticholinergic effect of orphenadrine, Norgesic or Norgesic Forte should not be used in patients with glaucoma, pyloric or duodenal obstruction, achalasia, prostatic hypertrophy or obstructions at the bladder neck. Norgesic or Norgesic Forte is also contraindicated in patients with myasthenia gravis and in patients known to be sensitive to aspirin or caffeine.

The drug is contraindicated in patients who have demonstrated a previous hypersensitivity to the drug.

Warnings: Norgesic Forte may impair the ability of the patient to engage in potentially hazardous activities such as operating machinery or driving a motor vehicle; ambulatory patients should therefore be cautioned accordingly.

Salicylates should be used with extreme caution in the presence of peptic ulcers and coagulation abnormalities.

Usage in Pregnancy:

Since safety of the use of this preparation in pregnancy, during lactation, or in the childbearing age has not been established, use of the drug in such patients requires that the potential benefits of the drug be weighed against its possible hazard to the mother and child.

Usage in Children:

The safe and effective use of this drug in children has not been established. Usage of this drug in children under 12 years of age is not recommended.

Precautions: Confusion, anxiety and tremors have been reported in few patients receiving propoxyphene and orphenadrine concomitantly. As these symptoms may be simply due to an additive effect, reduction of dosage and/or discontinuation of one or both agents is recommended in such cases.

Safety of continuous long term therapy with Norgesic Forte has not been established; therefore, if Norgesic Forte is prescribed for prolonged use, periodic monitoring of blood, urine and liver function values is recommended.

Adverse Reactions: Side effects of Norgesic or Norgesic Forte are those seen with aspirin and caffeine or those usually associated with mild anticholinergic agents. These may include tachycardia, palpitation, urinary hesitancy or retention, dry mouth, blurred vision, dilatation of the pupil, increased intraocular tension, weakness, nausea, vomiting, headache, dizziness, constipation, drowsiness, and rarely, urticaria and other dermatoses. Infrequently an elderly patient may experience some degree of confusion. Mild central excitation and occasional hallucinations may be observed. These mild side effects can usually be eliminated by reduction in dosage. One case of aplastic anemia associated with the use of Norgesic has been reported. No causal relationship has been established. Rare G.I. hemorrhage due to aspirin content may be associated with the administration of Norgesic or Norgesic Forte. Some patients may experience transient episodes of light-headedness, dizziness or syncope.

Dosage and Administration:

Norgesic: Adults 1 to 2 tablets 3 to 4 times daily.

Norgesic Forte: Adults ½ to 1 tablet 3 to 4 times daily.

How Supplied: Norgesic tablets can be identified by their three layers colored light green, white and yellow. Each round tablet contains orphenadrine citrate (2-dimethylaminoethyl 2-methylbenzhydryl ether citrate) 25 mg., aspirin 385 mg., and caffeine 30 mg.

Norgesic Forte tablets are exactly twice the strength of Norgesic. They are identified by their scored capsule shape and by their three layers colored light green, white and yellow. Each capsule shaped tablet contains orphenadrine citrate 50 mg., aspirin 770 mg., and caffeine 60 mg.

Norgesic: Bottles of 100 (NDC **0089-0231-10**) and 500 tablets (NDC **0089-0231-50**).

Norgesic Forte: Bottles of 100 tablets (NDC **0089-0233-10**) and 500 tablets (NDC **0089-0233-50**).

[*Shown in Product Identification Section*]

RAUWILOID® ℞

(alseroxylon)
tablets

Description: Each tablet contains 2 mg. of the alseroxylon fraction of Rauwolfia serpentina, equivalent to not less than 0.15 mg. and not more than 0.20 mg. reserpine-rescinnamine group alkaloids expressed as reserpine.

How Supplied: Bottles of 100 (NDC **0089-0265-10**) and 1000 (NDC **0089-0265-80**) tablets.

Concentrated Solution

SODIUM VERSENATE ℞

(disodium edetate injection U.S.P.)
For preparing intravenous infusions only

Description: Solution Sodium Versenate (Riker) is a sterile aqueous 20 percent solution of the disodium salt of ethylenediaminetetraacetic acid containing one gram of anhydrous disodium edetate per five milliliters. At a pH of 7 there are 2.4 equivalents of sodium per mole of edetate.

How Supplied: 15 ml. ampuls containing 3 Gm. disodium edetate in boxes of 5 (NDC **0089-0572-05**) to be diluted before administration.

TEPANIL® Ⓒ ℞

(diethylpropion hydrochloride, N.F.)

TEPANIL® TEN-TAB® Ⓒ ℞

(controlled release tablet)

Description: Diethylpropion hydrochloride, a sympathomimetic agent, is 1-phenyl-2-diethylamino-1-propanone hydrochloride.

In Tepanil Ten-tab tablets, diethylpropion hydrochloride is dispersed in a hydrophilic matrix. On exposure to water the diethylpropion hydrochloride is released at a relatively uniform rate as a result of slow hydration of the matrix. The result is controlled release of the anorexic agent.

Actions: Tepanil is a sympathomimetic amine with some pharmacologic activity similar to that of the prototype drugs of this class used in obesity, the amphetamines. Actions include some central nervous system stimulation and elevation of blood pressure. Tolerance has been demonstrated with all drugs of this class in which these phenomena have been looked for.

Drugs of this class used in obesity are commonly known as "anorectics" or "anorexigenics." It has not been established, however, that the action of such drugs in treating obesity is primarily one of appetite suppression. Other

Continued on next page

Riker—Cont.

central nervous system actions, or metabolic effects may be involved, for example.

Adult obese subjects instructed in dietary management and treated with "anorectic" drugs lose more weight on the average than those treated with placebo and diet, as determined in relatively short-term clinical trials. The magnitude of increased weight loss of drug-treated patients over placebo-treated patients is some fraction of a pound a week. However, some patients lose more weight than this and some lose less. The rate of weight loss is greatest in the first weeks of therapy for both drug and placebo subjects and tends to decrease in succeeding weeks. The possible origins of the increased weight loss due to the various drug effects are not established. The amount of weight loss associated with the use of an "anorectic" drug varies from trial to trial, and the increased weight loss appears to be related in part to variables other than the drug prescribed, such as the physician-investigator, the population treated, and the diet prescribed. Studies do not permit conclusions as to the relative importance of the drug and non-drug factors on weight loss.

The natural history of obesity is measured in years, whereas most studies cited are restricted to a few weeks duration; thus, the total impact of drug-induced weight loss over that of diet alone must be considered clinically limited.

The controlled-release characteristics of Tepanil Ten-tab have been demonstrated by studies in humans in which plasma levels of diethylpropion-related material were measured by phosphorescence analysis. Plasma levels obtained with the 75 mg. Ten-tab formulation administered once daily indicated a more gradual release than the standard formulation. The formulation has not been shown superior in effectiveness to the same dosage of the standard, noncontrolled-release formulation.

Indication: Tepanil and Tepanil Ten-tab are indicated in the management of exogenous obesity as a short-term adjunct (a few weeks) in a regimen of weight reduction based on caloric restriction. The limited usefulness of agents of this class (see ACTIONS) should be measured against possible risk factors inherent in their use such as those described below.

Contraindications: Advanced arteriosclerosis, hyperthyroidism, known hypersensitivity, or idiosyncrasy to the sympathomimetic amines, glaucoma.

Agitated states.

Patients with a history of drug abuse.

During or within 14 days following the administration of monoamine oxidase inhibitors; (hypertensive crises may result).

Warnings: If tolerance develops, the recommended dose should not be exceeded in an attempt to increase the effect; rather, the drug should be discontinued. Tepanil may impair the ability of the patient to engage in potentially hazardous activities such as operating machinery or driving a motor vehicle; the patient should therefore be cautioned accordingly.

Drug Dependence: Tepanil has some chemical and pharmacologic similarities to the amphetamines and other related stimulant drugs that have been extensively abused. There are occasional reports of subjects dependent on amphetamine later chronically abusing diethylpropion. The possibility of abuse should be kept in mind when evaluating the desirability of including a drug as part of a weight reduction program. Abuse of amphetamines and related drugs may be associated with varying degrees of psychologic dependence and social dysfunction which, in the case of certain drugs, may be severe. There are reports of patients who have increased the dosage to many times that recommended.

Abrupt cessation following prolonged high dosage administration results in extreme fatigue and mental depression; changes are also noted on the sleep EEG. Manifestations of chronic intoxication with anorectic drugs include severe dermatoses, marked insomnia, irritability, hyperactivity, and personality changes. The most severe manifestation of chronic intoxications is psychosis, often clinically indistinguishable from schizophrenia.

Use in Pregnancy: Although rat and human reproductive studies have not indicated adverse effects, the use of Tepanil by women who are pregnant or may become pregnant requires that the potential benefits be weighed against the potential risks.

Use in Children: Tepanil is not recommended for use in children under 12 years of age.

The possibility of an interaction with alcohol should be considered.

Precautions: Caution is to be exercised in prescribing Tepanil for patients with hypertension or with symptomatic cardiovascular disease, including arrhythmias. Tepanil should not be administered to patients with severe hypertension. Insulin requirements in diabetes mellitus may be altered in association with the use of Tepanil and the concomitant dietary regimen.

Tepanil may decrease the hypotensive effect of guanethidine.

The least amount feasible should be prescribed or dispensed at one time in order to minimize the possibility of overdosage.

Reports suggest that Tepanil may increase convulsions in some epileptics. Therefore, epileptics receiving Tepanil should be carefully monitored. Titration of dose or discontinuance of Tepanil may be necessary.

Adverse Reactions: Cardiovascular: Palpitation, tachycardia, elevation of blood pressure, precordial pain, arrhythmia. One published report described T-wave changes in the ECG of a healthy young male after ingestion of diethylpropion hydrochloride.

Central Nervous System: Overstimulation, nervousness, restlessness, dizziness, jitteriness, insomnia, anxiety, euphoria, depression, dysphoria, tremor, headache; rarely psychotic episodes at recommended doses. In a few epileptics an increase in convulsive episodes has been reported.

Gastrointestinal: Dryness of the mouth, unpleasant taste, nausea, vomiting, abdominal discomfort, diarrhea, constipation, other gastrointestinal disturbances.

Allergic: Urticaria, rash, ecchymosis, erythema.

Endocrine: Impotence, changes in libido, menstrual upset.

Hematopoietic System: Bone marrow depression, agranulocytosis, leukopenia.

Miscellaneous: A variety of miscellaneous adverse reactions has been reported by physicians. These include complaints such as dyspnea, hair loss, muscle pain, dysuria, and polyuria.

Dosage and Administration: Tepanil (diethylpropion hydrochloride):

One 25 mg. tablet three times daily, one hour before meals, and in midevening if desired to overcome night hunger.

Tepanil Ten-tab (diethylpropion hydrochloride) controlled-release:

One 75 mg. tablet daily, swallowed whole, in midmorning.

Tepanil is not recommended for use in children under 12 years of age.

Overdosage: Manifestations of acute overdosage include restlessness, tremor, hyperreflexia, rapid respiration, confusion, assaultiveness, hallucinations, panic states. Fatigue and depression usually follow the central stimulation.

Cardiovascular effects include arrhythmias, hypertension or hypotension and circulatory collapse. Gastrointestinal symptoms include nausea, vomiting, diarrhea, and abdominal cramps. Overdose of pharmacologically similar compounds has resulted in fatal poisoning, usually terminating in convulsions and coma.

Management of acute Tepanil intoxication is largely symptomatic and includes lavage and sedation with a barbiturate. Experience with hemodialysis or peritoneal dialysis is inadequate to permit recommendation in this regard. Intravenous phentolamine (Regitine®) has been suggested on pharmacologic grounds for possible acute, severe hypertension, if this complicates Tepanil overdosage.

How Supplied: Tepanil 25 mg.: bottles of 100 (NDC **0089-0351-10**) and 1000 (NDC **0089-0351-80**) white tablets. Tepanil Ten-tab 75 mg.: bottles of 30 (NDC **0089-0353-03**), 100 (NDC **0089-0353-10**), and 250 (NDC **0089-0353-25**) white tablets.

[*Shown in Product Identification Section*]

THEOLAIR™ ℞
(theophylline)
TABLETS
THEOLAIR™ ℞
LIQUID
THEOLAIR™–SR ℞
TABLETS

Description: THEOLAIR™ brand theophylline products are oral bronchodilators. Chemically, theophylline is 3,7-Dihydro-1,3-dimethyl-1*H*-purine-2,6-dione.

THEOLAIR Tablets contain 125 mg or 250 mg anhydrous theophylline.

THEOLAIR Liquid contains 80 mg theophylline per 15 ml (tablespoonful) in a nonalcoholic solution.

THEOLAIR-SR Tablets contain 250 mg or 500 mg anhydrous theophylline, in a sustained-release formulation.

Clinical Pharmacology: Theophylline directly relaxes the smooth muscle of the bronchial airways and pulmonary blood vessels, thus acting mainly as a bronchodilator and smooth muscle relaxant. The drug also has other actions typical of the xanthine derivatives: coronary vasodilation; diuresis; cardiac, cerebral, and skeletal muscle stimulation. The actions of theophylline may be mediated through inhibition of phosphodiesterase and a resultant increase in intracellular cyclic AMP which could mediate smooth muscle relaxation. At concentrations higher than those attained in vivo, theophylline also inhibits the release of histamine by mast cells.

In vitro, theophylline has been shown to act synergistically with beta agonists (isoproterenol) that increase intracellular cyclic AMP through the stimulation of adenyl cyclase, but synergism has not been demonstrated in patients. More data are needed to determine if

THEOPHYLLINE ELIMINATION CHARACTERISTICS

	Theophylline Clearance Rates (mean + SD)	Half-Life Average (mean + SD)
Children (over 6 months of age)	1.45 ± 0.58 ml/kg/min	3.7 ± 1.1 hrs
Adult non-smokers with uncomplicated asthma	0.65 ± 0.19 ml/kg/min	8.7 ± 2.2 hrs

theophylline and beta agonists have a clinically important additive effect in vivo.
Development of tolerance is not known to occur with chronic use of theophylline.
The half-life of theophylline is shortened in patients who smoke. The half-life is prolonged in patients with alcoholism, reduced hepatic or renal function, or congestive heart failure and in patients receiving cimetidine or antibiotics such as troleandomycin (TAO), and erythromycin. High fever for prolonged periods may reduce the rate of theophylline elimination. Administration of influenza vaccine and infection with influenza virus have been associated with an impaired rate of theophylline elimination and consequent increases in serum theophylline levels, sometimes with toxic symptoms. High carbohydrate, low protein diets prolong theophylline half-life, whereas high protein, low carbohydrate diets shorten the half-life.
(See table on preceding page)
Newborn infants have extremely slow theophylline clearance rates; the half-life in such infants may exceed 24 hours. Not until three to six months of age do these rates approach those seen in older children.
Older adults with chronic obstructive pulmonary disease, patients with cor pulmonale or other causes of heart failure, and patients with liver pathology may have much slower clearance rates; half-life of theophylline may exceed 24 hours in these patients.
The half-life of theophylline in smokers (one to two packs/day) averaged four to five hours among various studies, much shorter than the half-life in nonsmokers, which averaged about seven to nine hours. The increase in theophylline clearance caused by smoking is probably the result of induction of drug-metabolizing enzymes that do not readily normalize after cessation of smoking. it appears that between three months and two years may be necessary for normalization of the effect of smoking on theophylline pharmacokinetics.
Theophylline is completely absorbed from THEOLAIR Tablets and Liquid, and from THEOLAIR-SR Tablets. The time of peak absorption occurs at one to two hours after dosing with THEOLAIR Tablets and Liquid, and at four to six hours after dosing with THEOLAIR-SR Tablets. Multiple-dose studies in patients have shown that THEOLAIR-SR Tablets given q 12 hrs maintain therapeutic levels similar to those after the same daily dose of THEOLAIR Tablets and Liquid given q 6 hrs.
Food may slow the absorption of theophylline from THEOLAIR Tablets and Liquid, and from THEOLAIR-SR Tablets. However, absorption is still complete.
THEOLAIR-SR Tablets may be broken in half. Neither the rate nor the extent of absorption is changed.

Indications and Usage: For relief or prevention of symptoms of asthma and reversible bronchospasm associated with chronic bronchitis and emphysema. Theophylline is the drug of choice for control of chronic asthma, to prevent bronchospasm.

Contraindications: These products are contraindicated in individuals who are hypersensitive to any of their components, or to other xanthine derivatives, eg, aminophylline, theobromine, caffeine.

Warnings: Status asthmaticus is a medical emergency. Optimal therapy frequently requires additional medication including corticosteroids when the patient does not rapidly respond to bronchodilators.
Excessive theophylline doses may be associated with toxicity. The determination of serum theophylline levels is recommended to assure maximal benefit without excessive risk. Incidence of toxicity increases at serum theophylline levels greater than 20 mcg/ml. Morphine, curare, and stilbamidine should be used with caution in patients with airflow obstruction because they stimulate histamine release; these drugs may also suppress respiration leading to respiratory failure. Alternative drugs should be chosen whenever possible.
There is a direct and consistent correlation between high blood levels of theophylline resulting from conventional doses and associated clinical manifestations of toxicity in (1) patients with lowered body plasma clearances (due to transient cardiac decompensation), (2) patients with liver dysfunction or chronic obstructive lung disease, (3) patients who are older than 55 years of age, particularly men.
Less serious signs of theophylline toxicity such as nausea and restlessness may appear in up to 50% of patients. However, serious side effects such as ventricular arrhythmias and convulsions may appear without warning as the first signs of toxicity.
Many patients who have higher theophylline serum levels exhibit tachycardia.
Theophylline may worsen preexisting arrhythmias.

Precautions:

General Precautions:
Mean half-life in smokers is shorter than in nonsmokers; therefore smokers may require larger doses of theophylline. Theophylline should not be administered concurrently with other xanthine medications. Use with caution in patients with severe cardiac disease, severe hypoxemia, hypertension, hyperthyroidism, acute myocardial injury, cor pulmonale, congestive heart failure, or liver disease; in the elderly (especially men); and in neonates. In particular, great caution should be used in giving theophylline to patients with congestive heart failure. Frequently, such patients have markedly prolonged theophylline serum levels that can persist for long periods following discontinuation of the drug.
Use theophylline cautiously in patients with a history of peptic ulcer. Theophylline may occasionally act as a local irritant to the G.I. tract, although gastrointestinal symptoms are more commonly centrally mediated and associated with serum drug concentrations over 20 mcg/ml.

Information For Patients:
If nausea, vomiting, restlessness, irregular heartbeat, or convulsions occur, contact a physician immediately.
Take only the amount of drug that has been prescribed. Do not take a larger dose, or take the drug more often, or for a longer time than recommended.
Do not take other medicines unless under the advice of a physician, especially those for pulmonary disorders.
Avoid drinking large amounts of coffee, tea, cocoa, or cola, or eating large quantities of chocolate while taking this medicine, since these foods may increase the side effects of theophylline.

Laboratory Tests:
Serum levels of theophylline should be monitored periodically to maintain optimum levels of 10 to 20 mcg/ml. The incidence of toxicity increases sharply above this range. For such measurements, serum should be obtained one to two hours after administration of THEOLAIR Tablets and Liquid or four to six hours after THEOLAIR-SR Tablets. Patient compliance with the prescribed THEOLAIR regimen should have been good for the 48 hours preceding serum collection, (ie, no missed doses), otherwise any increase in dosage based on serum theophylline level may increase the risk of toxicity. Because of the narrow range for therapeutic serum levels and great within-patient and between-patient variation in dosage necessary to produce and maintain such levels, measurement of serum theophylline is advised for individualization of dosage, both initially and during maintenance therapy. Serum level monitoring is especially recommended when theophylline products are expected to be administered chronically. Certain patients may have slow elimination rates due to underlying conditions (see Clinical Pharmacology, Warnings and General Precautions sections); in such patients, conventional doses may produce high serum levels and associated signs of toxicity.

Drug Interactions:
Drug/Drug—Toxic synergism with ephedrine has been documented and may occur with some other sympathomimetic bronchodilators. The administration of theophylline and sympathomimetic drugs concurrently is of particular concern in patients with cardiac arrhythmias. The following table lists drugs known to interact with theophylline and the effects of their concomitant use.
[See table below].

DRUG	EFFECT
Theophylline with furosemide	Increased diuresis
Theophylline with hexamethonium	Decreased hexamethonium-induced chronotropic effect
Theophylline with reserpine	Reserpine-induced tachycardia
Theophylline with cimetidine	Increased theophylline blood levels
Theophylline with troleandomycin or erythromycin	Increased theophylline blood levels
Theophylline with allopurinol	Increased theophylline blood levels
Theophylline with propranolol	Decreased propranolol activity
Theophylline with lithium carbonate	Increased excretion of lithium

Drug/Food—Food may slow the absorption of theophylline, however absorption of the drug is still complete. Patients who eat high carbohydrate, low protein foods can have slower theophylline elimination rates and thus a possibility of higher plasma levels. Conversely, those who eat high protein, low carbohydrate foods can have higher rates and lower theophylline levels.
Drug/Laboratory Test Interactions—Theophylline therapy can falsely increase the results of tests for erythrocyte sedimentation rate, serum uric acid, bilirubin, plasma free fatty acids, and urinary catecholamines. Uptake of ^{131}I can be decreased.

Carcinogenesis, Mutagenesis, Impairment of Fertility:
No long-term study of theophylline has been performed to evaluate carcinogenic potential. Chromosomal breakage has been observed in cultures of human cells exposed to theophylline at concentrations 25 times the maximum therapeutic blood level. Testicular atrophy and impaired spermatogenesis have been reported in rats fed theophylline at levels approximating 250 to 500 mg/kg per day, approximately 15 to 30 times the daily dosage in adults.

Pregnancy Category C:
Theophylline has been shown to be teratogenic in mice when given in doses 15 times the human dose. There are no adequate and well-controlled studies in pregnant women. Theophylline should be used during pregnancy only if the potential benefit justifies the potential risk to the fetus. The danger of uncontrolled asthma in the pregnant woman should be considered.
Nonteratogenic Effects—Theophylline has been detected in umbilical cord serum, and jitteriness and tachycardia have been reported in neonates whose mothers received theophylline prior to delivery.

Nursing Mothers:
Theophylline is present in breast milk, but data indicate that concentrations potentially toxic to a nursing infant should not normally occur. One infant was irritable on days the

Continued on next page

Riker—Cont.

mother took aminophylline. Concentration of theophylline in breast milk parallels that in the mother's serum or saliva and, thus, it is recommended that the mother nurse her infant just before she takes theophylline, when maternal levels are expected to be the lowest.

Pediatric Use:
Safety and effectiveness of theophylline in children below the age of six months have not been established.

Adverse Reactions: The most consistent adverse reactions are usually due to overdose and are:

Gastrointestinal: nausea, vomiting, epigastric pain, hematemesis, diarrhea.

Central nervous system: headaches, irritability, restlessness, insomnia, reflex hyperexcitability, muscle twitching, clonic and tonic generalized convulsions.

Cardiovascular: palpitation, tachycardia, extra systoles, flushing, hypotension, circulatory failure, life threatening ventricular arrhythmias.

Respiratory: tachypnea.

Renal: albuminuria, increased excretion of renal tubular and red blood cells, potentiation of diuresis.

Others: hyperglycemia and inappropriate ADH syndrome.

Drug Abuse and Dependance: Drug abuse and dependance have not been reported with theophylline.

Overdosage:
Management:

A. If potential overdose is established and seizure has not occurred:
   1. Induce vomiting.
   2. Administer a cathartic (this is particularly important if a sustained-release preparation of theophylline, THEOLAIR-SR Tablets, has been taken.)
   3. Administer activated charcoal.

B. If patient is having a seizure:
   1. Establish an airway.
   2. Administer oxygen.
   3. Treat the seizure with intravenous diazepam, 0.1 to 0.3 mg/kg up to a maximum dose of 10 mg.
   4. Monitor vital signs, maintain blood pressure, and provide adequate hydration.

C. Post-seizure coma:
   1. Maintain airway and oxygenation.
   2. Follow above recommendations to prevent absorption of drug, but intubation and lavage will have to be performed instead of inducing emesis, and the cathartic and charcoal will need to be introduced via a large-bore gastric lavage tube.
   3. Continue to provide full supportive care and adequate hydration while waiting for drug to be metabolized. In general, the drug is metabolized sufficiently rapidly so that dialysis is not required.

D. General:
   Serum theophylline should be monitored until the level is less than 20 mcg/ml.
   Electrolyte balance and hydration should be maintained by intravenous fluids.
   If hypotension is not corrected by intravenous fluids, vasopressor drugs may be administered cautiously. (Caution: Sympathomimetic drugs may precipitate cardiac arrhythmia.)
   Theophylline is dialyzable. However, in patients with very high serum theophylline levels and severe intoxication, charcoal hemoperfusion may be employed. This procedure is very effective in removing theophylline from the blood, and is to be preferred over peritoneal dialysis or hemodialysis.

The oral LD_{50} of theophylline in mice is 415 mg/kg and in rats is 470 mg/kg.

Dosage and Administration: Therapeutic serum levels associated with optimal likelihood for benefit and minimal risk of toxicity are generally considered to be between 10 and 20 mcg/ml. Levels above 20 mcg/ml may produce toxic effects. There is great variation from patient to patient in dosage needed to achieve a therapeutic blood level because of variable rates of elimination. Because of this wide interpatient variation and the relatively narrow therapeutic blood level range, dosage must be individualized. Periodic monitoring of theophylline serum levels is highly recommended. Dosage should be calculated on the basis of lean (ideal) body weight where doses are stated in milligrams per kilogram. Theophylline does not distribute into fatty tissue.

Giving theophylline with food may prevent the rare case of stomach irritation; and though absorption may be slower, it is still complete. When theophylline products are used which are rapidly absorbed (THEOLAIR Liquid, THEOLAIR Tablets), dosing to maintain "around-the-clock" blood levels generally requires administration every 6 hours to obtain the greatest efficacy in children; dosing intervals up to 8 hours may be satisfactory for adults because they eliminate theophylline more slowly. Children, and adults with higher than average rates of elimination, may benefit from products with more sustained absorption (THEOLAIR-SR Tablets) which allow longer dosing intervals and/or less fluctuation in serum concentration over a dosing interval during chronic therapy. THEOLAIR-SR Tablets should be taken every 12 hours in adults and most children. Some children with higher-than-average rates of elimination may require more frequent dosing. **THEOLAIR-SR Tablets may be broken in half but should not be chewed or crushed.**

ACUTE SYMPTOMS OF ASTHMA REQUIRING RAPID THEOPHYLLINIZATION:

Patients Not Currently Receiving Theophylline Products:

For patients of all ages, give an oral loading dose of 6 mg/kg regular (not sustained release) theophylline (THEOLAIR Tablets or THEOLAIR Liquid).

Patients Currently Receiving Theophylline Products:

Determine (where possible) the time, amount, route of administration and form of the patient's last dose.

The loading dose for theophylline will be based on the principle that each 0.5 mg/kg administered as a loading dose will result in a 1.0 mcg/ml increase in serum theophylline concentration. Ideally, then, the loading dose should be deferred if a serum theophylline concentration can be obtained rapidly. If this is not possible, the clinician must exercise his judgement in selecting a dose based on the potential for benefit and risk. When there is sufficient respiratory distress to warrant a small risk, 2.5 mg/kg of theophylline administered as a loading dose in a rapidly absorbed form is likely to increase the serum concentration by approximately 5 mcg/ml. If the patient is not experiencing theophylline toxicity, this is unlikely to result in dangerous adverse effects.

CHRONIC ASTHMA (NOT REQUIRING RAPID THEOPHYLLINIZATION):

Theophylline administration is a treatment of first choice for the management of chronic asthma (to prevent symptoms and maintain patent airways). Slow clinical titration is generally preferred to assure acceptance and safety of the medications. Refer to Convenient Dosing Guide. **WARNING: DO NOT ATTEMPT TO MAINTAIN ANY DOSE THAT IS NOT TOLERATED.**

The table shown below provides simplified guidelines for theophylline maintenance therapy using THEOLAIR Tablets and THEOLAIR-SR Tablets for four major categories of **patients three years old and older**, grouped by age and weight. Dosage adjustments should be made as needed to accomodate the tolerance and requirements for optimal benefit of individual patients. Use lean (ideal) body weight for obese patients.

[See table below].

Patients six months to three years of age (≤ 14 kg body weight) should be given a maximum of 4 mg/kg q 4 hrs as the appropriate volume of THEOLAIR Liquid (see table below).

THEOLAIR Liquid

½ tblsp	= 40 mg	2 tblsp	= 160 mg
1 tblsp	= 80 mg	2½ tblsp	= 200 mg
1½ tblsp	= 120 mg	3 tblsp	= 240 mg

How Supplied:

THEOLAIR Tablets:

125 mg tablets—Bottles of 100 (NDC 0089-0342-10) and boxes of 250 unit-dose, aluminum foil, non-child-resistant strips (NDC **0089-0342-26**). Each round, white, scored tablet imprinted with "RIKER" on one side and "342" on the other.

250 mg tablets—Bottles of 100 (NDC **0089-0344-10**) and boxes of 250 unit-dose, aluminum foil, non-child-resistant strips (NDC **0089-0960-16**). Each capsule-shaped, white, scored tablet imprinted with "RIKER" on one side and "THEOLAIR 250" on the other.

STORE BELOW 30 C (86 F).

THEOLAIR Liquid:

1 pint (NDC 0089-0960-16)

CONVENIENT DOSING GUIDE FOR MAINTENANCE THERAPY

			Q 6 HRS			Q 12 HRS**		
AGE (YRS)	WEIGHT (LBS)	RECOMMENDED MAXIMUM DAILY DOSE*	MG PER DOSE	NO. OF TABLETS	TABLET SIZE	MG PER DOSE	NO. OF TABLETS	TABLET SIZE
3–6	30–45 (14–20 kg)	24 mg/kg	62.5	½	THEOLAIR 125	125	½	THEOLAIR-SR 250
7–9	46–65 (21–30 kg)	24 mg/kg	125	1	THEOLAIR 125	250	1	THEOLAIR-SR 250
10–16	66–120 (30–55 kg)	18–20 mg/kg	187.5	1½	THEOLAIR 125	375	1½	THEOLAIR-SR 250
>16	121–155 (55–70 kg)	13 mg/kg	250	1	THEOLAIR 250	500 500	2 1	THEOLAIR-SR 250 THEOLAIR-SR 500

*Doses exceeding these recommendations or >1000 mg/day require monitoring of serum theophylline levels.

**Some patients, especially small children, may require dosing at 8-hour intervals (one third of total daily dose) to maintain control of symptoms.

STORE BETWEEN 15–30 C (59–86 F).

THEOLAIR-SR Tablets:

250 mg sustained-release tablets—Bottles of 100 (NDC **0089-0345-10**) and bottles of 250 (NDC **0089-0345-25**). Each round, white, scored tablet imprinted with "RIKER" on one side and "SR 250" on the other.

500 mg sustained-release tablets—Bottles of 100 (NDC **0089-0347-10**) and bottles of 250 (NDC **0089-0347-25**). Each capsule-shaped, white, scored tablet imprinted on one side with "RIKER" and "SR-500" on the other.

STORE BELOW 30 C (86 F).

[Shown in Product Identification Section]

THEOLAIR™–PLUS TABLETS AND LIQUID ℞

Description: Theolair-Plus contains anhydrous theophylline and guaifenesin and is available in two tablet strengths and as a pleasant tasting liquid.

Theolair-Plus 125—containing 125 mg of theophylline and 100 mg of quaifenesin.

Theolair-Plus 250—containing 250 mg of theophylline and 200 mg of guaifenesin.

Theolair-Plus Liquid—containing 125 mg of theophylline and 100 mg of guaifenesin per 15 ml.

Theophylline, a xanthine compound, is a white, odorless crystalline powder, having a bitter taste.

Guaifenesin, a guaiacol compound, is a white to slightly yellow crystalline powder with a bitter, aromatic taste.

How Supplied:

THEOLAIR-PLUS 125 tablets: Bottles of 100 (NDC 0089-0348-10).

THEOLAIR-PLUS 250 tablets: Bottles of 100 (NDC 0089-0349-10).

[Shown in Product Identification Section]

THEOLAIR-PLUS LIQUID—1 pint (NDC 0089-0962-16)

Ulo® (chlophedianol hydrochloride) Syrup ℞

Description: The active ingredient in ULO is 2-Chloro-α-[2-(dimethylamino) ethyl]benzhydrol hydrochloride.

How Supplied: ULO Syrup, bottles of 12 fluid ounces containing 25 mg per 5 ml (1 teaspoonful) of chlophedianol hydrochloride. (NDC **0089-0971-12**).

UREX® (methenamine hippurate) ℞

Description: Urex (methenamine hippurate) is the hippuric acid salt of methenamine (hexamethylenetetramine).

Actions: Urex (methenamine hippurate) is active against a broad spectrum of both gram-positive and gram-negative urinary tract pathogens. It is readily absorbed and excreted. It exerts its antibacterial activity when excreted by the kidney and concentrated in the urine where it dissociates to hippuric acid and methenamine. In an acid urine some of the methenamine component is hydrolyzed to ammonia and the bactericidal agent formaldehyde.

Indications: Urex is indicated for the suppression or elimination of bacteriuria associated with acute, chronic and recurrent infections of the urinary tract, especially when long term therapy is indicated.

Contraindications: Urex (methenamine hippurate) is contraindicated in patients with renal insufficiency, severe hepatic insufficiency or severe dehydration. It also is contraindicated as the sole therapeutic agent in acute parenchymal infections causing systemic symptoms.

Warning: Use in pregnancy: In early pregnancy the safe use of "Urex" is not established. In the last trimester, safety is suggested, but not definitely proven.

Precautions:

1. Large doses of methenamine (8 grams daily for 3 to 4 weeks) have caused bladder irritation, painful and frequent micturition, albuminuria and gross hematuria.
2. Care should be taken to maintain an acid pH of the urine especially when treating infections due to urea-splitting organisms such as Proteus and strains of Pseudomonas.
3. In a few instances in one study, the serum transaminase levels showed a mild elevation during treatment which returned to normal while the patients were still receiving Urex. Because of this one report, it is recommended that liver function studies be performed periodically on patients receiving the drug, especially those with liver dysfunction.

Adverse Reactions: Minor adverse reactions have been reported in fewer than 3.5% of patients treated. These reactions have included: nausea, "upset stomach," dysuria and rash.

Dosage and Administration: One tablet (1.0 Gm.) twice daily for adults and children over 12 years of age. One-half to one tablet (0.5 to 1.0 Gm.) twice daily for children 6-12 years of age. The antibacterial activity of Urex is greater in acid urine. Therefore, restriction of alkalinizing foods and medications is desirable. If necessary, as indicated by urinary pH and clinical response, supplemental acidification of the urine may be instituted. As is the case with all urinary tract infections, the efficacy of therapy should be monitored by repeated urine cultures.

How Supplied: One gram scored, white tablets, bottles of 100 (NDC **0089-0371-10**) and 500 (NDC **0089-0371-50**).

Animal Pharmacology and Toxicology: Up to 600 mg./kg. of Urex in a single dose were administered intravenously to dogs and rats without toxic effects being observed. Chronic oral administration of 50-200 mg./kg./day to dogs and 800-6400 mg./kg./day to rats produced gastric and bladder irritation with some hemorrhagic sites and ulceration observed at autopsy.

Urex was administered to rats at a dose of 800 mg./kg./day as part of a study of teratogenicity. Urex did not prevent conception, increase fetal death rate or produce teratogenesis. Studies in rabbits at dosage levels producing no toxicity in the parent animals (100-113 mg./kg./day) revealed no prevention of conception, no increase in fetal death rate, no embryopathy and no teratogenicity. At a higher dose of 800 mg./kg./day (20 times the recommended human dose) most of the pregnant rabbits died. However, the two that survived bore viable normal young.

Amounts of Urex equivalent to twice the recommended human dose were administered to rats for twelve months and monkeys for six months without producing any adverse effects.

Clinical Studies: Within one-half hour after ingestion of a single one gram dose of Urex, antibacterial activity is demonstrable in the urine. Urine shows continuous antibacterial activity when Urex is administered at the recommended dosage schedule of one gram twice daily. Over 90% of methenamine moiety is excreted in the urine within 24 hours after administration of a single one gram dose. Similarly, the hippurate moiety is rapidly absorbed and excreted, and it reaches the urine by both tubular secretion and glomerular filtration. This may be of importance in older patients or those with some degree of renal impairment.

Urex is effective clinically against most common urinary tract pathogens. It has demonstrable antibacterial activity in vitro against Escherichia coli, Micrococcus pyogenes, Enterobacter aerogenes, Pseudomonas aeruginosa, and Proteus vulgaris at pH 5.0-6.8. The minimal inhibitory concentrations are significantly lower in more acidic media; therefore, the efficacy of Urex can be increased by acidification of urine.

Using the gradient plate technique of Szybalski no resistant bacterial strains were found to have developed when Urex was tested against both gram-positive and gram-negative pathogens, including Streptococcus fecalis, Proteus vulgaris, Micrococcus pyogenes, Aerobacter aerogenes and Escherichia coli.

The efficacy of Urex at the recommended dose has been established in clinical trials involving approximately 400 patients. Objective measurement of efficacy (reversal of positive cultures) has demonstrated the therapeutic effectiveness of Urex in a wide variety of urinary tract infections. Symptomatic relief was usually reported within 24-72 hours followed by culture reversal in the majority of patients monitored. Studies in children 6-12 years of age have shown similar results. Of 50 children monitored with serial urine cultures, eradication of the infecting organism was achieved in 34 (68%).

Hematologic studies were carried out in over 20% of all patients involved in the clinical trials. There was no instance of significant drug-related alteration of hemograms, blood urea nitrogen, serum creatinine, serum transaminase levels or liver profiles. Gastroscopic examination of 20 patients who received a single one gram dose of Urex revealed no mucosal irritation attributable to the drug.

[Shown in Product Identification Section]

The Robertson/Taylor Co.

A division of Intra-Medic Formulations, Inc.
135 E. OAKLAND PARK BLVD.
FORT LAUDERDALE, FL 33334

MEDI–TEC 90 Therapeutic Conditioner with Strengthening Agents

Composition: A concentrated liquid, lanolin free conditioning formula applied through the hair immediately following a thorough cleansing with Medi-Tec 90 Therapeutice shampoo and Scalp Cleanser to condition and protect the hair shaft. Contains: Deionized water, Stearalkonium, Chloride, Panthenol, Biotin, Niacin, Octoxynol-9, Quartemium-15, fragrance, FD&C yellow #5, FD&C blue #1.

Actions and Usage: Medi-Tec 90 Therapeutic Conditioner with strengthening agents is a comprehensive, protective conditioning treatment that completes the total Medi-Tec 90 hair and scalp therapeutic program.

Specifically developed for dermotologists to recommend in cases where severe thinning of the scalp and excess hairfallout can be treated with the direct application of Medi-Tec 90 Formulations.

How Supplied:

240 ml. Medi-Tec 90™ Therapeutic Conditioner with strengthening agents, NDC-51729-4290-08.

480 ml. Medi-Tec 90™ Therapeutic Conditioner with strengthening agents, NDC-51729-4290-16.

MEDI–TEC 90 Therapeutic Scalp Stimulant with Strengthening Agents

Composition: A spray which is applied liberally onto the scalp 2 to 3 times daily. Before using Medi-Tec 90 Therapeutic Scalp Stimulant, cleanse hair and scalp daily (evening or morning) with lanolin free shampoo or Medi-Tec 90 Therapeutic Shampoo and Scalp Cleanser with strengthening agents. Contains:

Continued on next page

Robertson/Taylor—Cont.

Deionized water, Polysorbate 60, Biotin, Panthenol, Niacin, Acetamide MEA.
Actions and Usage: Medi-Tec 90 Scalp Stimulant: An odorless, greaseless surfactant containing non-chemical vasodilators, proteins, and vitamin H along with a base formulation whose efficacy as a complete baldness treatment is now under study.
Specifically developed for dermotologists to recommend in cases where severe thinning of the scalp and excess hair fallout can be treated with the direct application of Medi-Tec 90 Formulations.
How Supplied:
240 ml. Medi-Tec 90™ Therapeutic Scalp Stimulant with strengthening agents, NDC-51729-4490-08.
480 ml. Medi-Tec 90™ Therapeutic Scalp Stimulant with strengthening agents, NDC-51729-4490-16.

MEDI-TEC 90 Therapeutic Shampoo and Scalp Cleanser with Strengthening Agents

Composition: A mild liquid surfactant which is liberally applied to the hair and scalp. Contains: Deionized water, Sodium Lauryl Sulfate, Lauramide DEA, Acetamide MEA, Polysorbate 20, Panthenol, Biotin, Niacin, Quarterium-15, fragrance, FD&C blue #1.
Actions and Usage: An effective lanolin free surfactant to be used alone or in conjunction with all Medi-Tec 90 Formulations. Medi-Tec 90 Therapeutic Shampoo and Scalp Cleanser cleans away debris and sebum while gently stimulating the scalp with non-chemical vasodilators.
Specifically developed for dermotologists to recommend in cases where severe thinning of the scalp and excess hair fallout can be treated with the direct application of Medi-Tec 90 Formulations.
How Supplied:
240 ml. Medi-Tec 90™ Therapeutic Shampoo and Scalp Cleanser with strengthening agents, NDC-51729-4390-08.
480 ml. Medi-Tec 90™ Therapeutic Shampoo and Scalp Cleanser with strengthening agents, NDC-51729-4390-16.

A. H. Robins Company
PHARMACEUTICAL DIVISION
1407 CUMMINGS DRIVE
RICHMOND, VA 23220

ALLBEE® WITH C CAPSULES

One capsule daily provides:

	Percentage of U.S. Recommended Daily Allowance (U.S. RDA)	
Vitamin C	500	300.0 mg
Thiamine (Vitamin B_1)	1000	15.0 mg
Riboflavin (Vitamin B_2)	600	10.2 mg
Niacin	250	50.0 mg
Vitamin B_6	250	5.0 mg
Pantothenic Acid	100	10.0 mg

Ingredients: Ascorbic Acid; Gelatin; Niacinamide; Lactose; Corn Starch; Thiamine Mononitrate; Calcium Pantothenate; Riboflavin; Magnesium Stearate; Pyridoxine Hydrochloride; Light Mineral Oil; FD&C Yellow No. 5; Vanillin; Artificial Color.
Action and Uses: Allbee with C is a high potency formulation of B and C vitamins. Its components have important roles in general nutrition, healing of wounds, and prevention of hemorrhage. It is recommended for deficiencies of B-vitamins and ascorbic acid in conditions such as febrile diseases, chronic or acute infections, burns, fractures, surgery, toxic conditions, physiologic stress, alcoholism, prolonged exposure to high temperature, geriatrics, gastritis, peptic ulcer, and colitis; and in conditions involving special diets and weight-reduction diets.
In dentistry, Allbee with C is recommended for deficiencies of B-vitamins and ascorbic acid in conditions such as herpetic stomatitis, aphthous stomatitis, cheilosis, herpangina, gingivitis.
Precaution: This product contains FD&C Yellow No. 5 (tartrazine) which may cause allergic-type reactions (including bronchial asthma) in certain susceptible individuals. Although the overall incidence of FD&C Yellow No. 5 (tartrazine) sensitivity in the general population is low, it is frequently seen in patients who have aspirin hypersensitivity.
Dosage: The recommended OTC dosage for adults and children twelve or more years of age, other than pregnant or lactating women, is one capsule daily. Under the direction and supervision of a physician, the dose and frequency of administration may be increased in accordance with the patient's requirements.
How Supplied: Yellow and green capsules, monogrammed AHR and 0674, in bottles of 30 (NDC 0031-0674-56), 100 (NDC 0031-0674-63), 1,000 capsules (NDC 0031-0674-74) and in Dis-Co® Unit Dose Packs of 100 (NDC 0031-0674-64).

[*Shown in Product Identification Section*]

ALLBEE® C-800 TABLETS
ALLBEE® C-800 plus Iron tablets

(See PDR For Nonprescription Drugs)

ALLBEE-T® TABLETS

One tablet daily provides:

	Percentage of U.S. Recommended Daily Allowance (U.S. RDA)	
Vitamin C	833	500.0 mg
Thiamine (Vitamin B_1)	1033	15.5 mg
Riboflavin (Vitamin B_2)	588	10.0 mg
Niacin	500	100.0 mg
Vitamin B_6	410	8.2 mg
Vitamin B_{12}	83	5.0 mcg
Pantothenic Acid	230	23.0 mg

Ingredients: Sodium Ascorbate; Desiccated Liver; Lactose; Niacinamide; Hydroxypropyl Methylcellulose; Calcium Pantothenate; Stearic Acid; Povidone; Thiamine Mononitrate; Artificial Color; Propylene Glycol; Riboflavin; Pyridoxine Hydrochloride; Vanillin; Gelatin; Cyanocobalamin.
Actions and Uses: Allbee-T is a high potency, therapeutic formulation of the important B-complex vitamins with Vitamin C.
Allbee-T is indicated for the management of vitamin deficiency states involving one or more B-vitamins or Vitamin C, as in the following:
1. Conditions characterized by an increased requirement for B-complex vitamins and vitamin C, such as severe burns, fractures, surgical procedures, febrile illnesses, hyperthyroidism, acute and chronic infections and alcoholism.
2. Conditions in which the intake and/or absorption of the water-soluble vitamins may be impaired, such as gastritis, colitis, peptic ulcer disease, malabsorption syndromes, weight reduction and other therapeutic diets.
3. Conditions characterized by oral lesions such as cheilosis, gingivitis, and stomatitis where deficiencies of water-soluble vitamins may exist.
Precaution: Not intended for the treatment of pernicious anemia.
Dosage: The recommended OTC dosage for adults and children twelve or more years of age, other than pregnant or lactating women, is one tablet daily. Under the direction and supervision of a physician, the dose and frequency of administration may be increased in accordance with the patient's requirements.
How Supplied: Orange, capsule-shaped, film-coated tablets engraved AHR in bottles of 100 (NDC 0031-0688-63) and 500 (NDC 0031-0688-70).

[*Shown in Product Identification Section*]

DIMACOL® CAPSULES
DIMACOL® LIQUID

Composition: Each capsule or 5 ml (one teaspoonful) contains:

Guaifenesin, USP	100 mg
Pseudoephedrine Hydrochloride, USP	30 mg
Dextromethorphan Hydrobromide, USP	15 mg
Liquid: Alcohol	4.75%

Actions: Dimacol helps reduce nasal congestion and suppresses cough associated with the common cold and other upper respiratory disorders.
Guaifenesin enhances the output of lower respiratory tract fluid. The enhanced flow of less viscid secretions promotes ciliary action, and facilitates the removal of inspissated mucus. As a result, dry unproductive coughs become more productive and less frequent. *Pseudoephedrine hydrochloride* is an orally effective nasal decongestant. Through its vasoconstrictor action, pseudoephedrine gently but promptly reduces edema and congestion of nasal passages. *Dextromethorphan hydrobromide* is a synthetic, non-narcotic cough suppressant. The antitussive effectiveness of dextromethorphan has been demonstrated in both animal and clinical studies, and the incidence of toxic effects has been remarkably low.
Indications: Dimacol is indicated for the management of cough accompanied by nasal mucosal congestion and edema, and nasal hypersecretion, associated with the common cold, upper respiratory infection and sinusitis.
Contraindications: Hypersensitivity to any of the ingredients. Dimacol should not be administered to patients receiving MAO inhibitors.
Precautions: Administer with caution in the presence of hypertension, heart disease, peripheral vascular disease, diabetes or hyperthyroidism.
Note: Guaifenesin has been shown to produce a color interference with certain clinical laboratory determinations of 5-hydroxyindoleacetic acid (5-HIAA) and vanilmandelic acid (VMA).
Adverse Reactions: The following adverse reactions may possibly occur: nausea, vomiting, dry mouth, nervousness, insomnia.
Dosage and Administration: Adults and children over 12 years of age, one capsule or one teaspoonful (5 ml) three times a day.
Children 6 to 12 years, ½ teaspoonful 3 times a day. Children under 6 years of age, as directed by a physician.
How Supplied: Orange and green capsules in bottles of 100 (NDC 0031-1650-63), and 500 (NDC 0031-1650-70) and consumer packages of 12 (NDC 0031-1650-46) and 24 (NDC 0031-1650-54) (individually packaged).
Orange colored, chocolate flavored liquid in bottles of one pint (NDC 0031-1660-25).

[*Shown in Product Identification Section*]

DIMETANE EXTENTABS® ℞
brand of Brompheniramine Maleate, USP
8 mg and 12 mg

Actions: Brompheniramine maleate is an antihistamine, with anticholinergic (drying) and sedative side effects. Antihistamines appear to compete with histamine for cell receptor sites on effector cells.
Indications: Perennial and seasonal allergic rhinitis; vasomotor rhinitis; allergic conjuncti-

vitis due to inhalant allergens and foods; mild, uncomplicated allergic skin manifestations of urticaria and angioedema; amelioration of allergic reactions to blood or plasma; dermatographism; as therapy for anaphylactic reactions ***adjunctive*** to epinephrine and other standard measures after the acute manifestations have been controlled.

Contraindications: Use in children six years of age and under. This drug should not be used in children six years of age and under.

Use in Nursing Mothers. Because of the higher risk of antihistamines for infants generally and for newborns and prematures in particular, antihistamine therapy is contraindicated in nursing mothers.

Use in Lower Respiratory Disease. Antihistamines **should NOT** be used to treat lower respiratory tract symptoms including asthma.

Antihistamines are also contraindicated in the following conditions: hypersensitivity to brompheniramine maleate and other antihistamines of similar chemical structure; monoamine oxidase inhibitor therapy (see Drug Interaction section).

Warnings: Antihistamines should be used with considerable caution in patients with: narrow angle glaucoma; stenosing peptic ulcer; pyloroduodenal obstruction; symptomatic prostatic hypertrophy; bladder neck obstruction.

Use in Children. In infants and children, especially, antihistamines in **overdosage** may cause hallucinations, convulsions, or death.

As in adults, antihistamines may diminish mental alertness in children. In the young child, particularly, they may produce excitation.

Use in Pregnancy. Experience with this drug in pregnant women is inadequate to determine whether there exists a potential for harm to the developing fetus.

Use with CNS Depressants. Dimetane has additive effects with alcohol and other CNS depressants (hypnotics, sedatives, tranquilizers, etc.)

Use in Activities Requiring Mental Alertness. Patients should be warned about engaging in activities requiring mental alertness, such as driving a car or operating appliances, machinery, etc.

Use in the Elderly (approximately 60 years or older). Antihistamines are more likely to cause dizziness, sedation, and hypotension in elderly patients.

Precautions: As with other antihistamines, Dimetane has an atropine-like action, and, therefore, should be used with caution in patients with: history of bronchial asthma; increased intraocular pressure; hyperthyroidism; cardiovascular disease; hypertension.

Drug Interactions: MAO inhibitors prolong and intensify the anticholinergic (drying) effects of antihistamines.

Adverse Reactions: The most frequent adverse reactions are italicized:

General: Urticaria, drug rash, anaphylactic shock, photosensitivity, excessive perspiration, chills, dryness of mouth, nose, and throat.

Cardiovascular System: Hypotension, headache, palpitations, tachycardia, extrasystoles.

Hematologic System: Hemolytic anemia, thrombocytopenia, agranulocytosis.

Nervous System: Sedation, sleepiness, dizziness, disturbed coordination, fatigue, confusion, restlessness, excitation, nervousness, tremor, irritability, insomnia, euphoria, paresthesias, blurred vision, diplopia, vertigo, tinnitus, acute labyrinthitis, hysteria, neuritis, convulsions.

G.I. System: Epigastric distress, anorexia, nausea, vomiting, diarrhea, constipation.

G.U. System: Urinary frequency, difficult urination, urinary retention, early menses.

Respiratory System: Thickening of bronchial secretions, tightness of chest and wheezing, nasal stuffiness.

Overdosage: Antihistamine overdosage reactions may vary from central nervous system depression to stimulation. Stimulation is particularly likely in children. Atropine-like signs and symptoms—dry mouth; fixed, dilated pupils; flushing; and gastrointestinal symptoms may also occur.

If vomiting has not occurred spotaneously, the patient should be induced to vomit. This is best done by having him drink a glass of water or milk after which he should be made to gag. Precautions against aspiration must be taken, especially in infants and children.

If vomiting is unsuccessful, gastric lavage is indicated within 3 hours after ingestion and even later if large amounts of milk or cream were given beforehand. Isotonic and ½ isotonic saline is the lavage solution of choice.

NOTE: Extentabs will not be dissolved during the process of lavage, and the tubes ordinarily employed in lavage are not large enough in diameter to remove Extentabs.

Saline cathartics, as milk of magnesia, by osmosis draw water into the bowel and therefore, are valuable for their action in rapid dilution of bowel content.

Stimulants should **not** be used.

Vasopressors may be used to treat hypotension.

Dosage and Administration: DOSAGE SHOULD BE INDIVIDUALIZED ACCORDING TO THE NEEDS AND THE RESPONSE OF THE PATIENTS.

Adults: One Extentab (8 or 12 mg) every eight to twelve hours or twice daily.

Children over six. One Extentab (8 or 12 mg) every twelve hours.

How Supplied: Extentabs, 8 mg are available as Persian rose-colored, coated tablets, in bottles of 100 (NDC 0031-1868-63) and 500 (NDC 0031-1868-70).

Extentabs, 12 mg are available as peach-colored, coated tablets, in bottles of 100 (NDC 0031-1843-63) and 500 (NDC 0031-1843-70).

[*Shown in Product Identification Section*]

DIMETANE®

brand of Brompheniramine Maleate, USP
Tablets—4 mg
Elixir—2 mg/5 ml
Alcohol, 3%

Actions: Brompheniramine maleate is an antihistamine, with anticholinergic (drying) and sedative side effects. Antihistamines appear to compete with histamine for cell receptor sites on effector cells.

Indications: For effective, temporary relief of hay fever/upper respiratory allergy symptoms: itchy, watery eyes; sneezing; itching nose or throat.

Contraindications: ***Use in Newborn or Premature Infants.*** This drug should **not** be used in newborn or premature infants.

Use in Nursing Mothers. Because of the higher risk of antihistamines for infants generally and for newborns and prematures in particular, antihistamine therapy is contraindicated in nursing mothers.

Use in Lower Respiratory Disease. Antihistamines **should NOT** be used to treat lower respiratory tract symptoms including asthma.

This drug is also contraindicated in the following conditions: hypersensitivity to brompheniramine maleate and other antihistamines of similar chemical structure; monoamine oxidase inhibitor therapy (see Drug Interaction section).

Warnings: Antihistamines should be used with considerable caution in patients with: narrow angle glaucoma; stenosing peptic ulcer; pyloroduodenal obstruction; symptomatic prostatic hypertrophy; bladder neck obstruction.

Use in Children. In infants and children, especially, antihistamines in **overdosage** may cause hallucinations, convulsions, or death.

As in adults, antihistamines may diminish mental alertness in children. In the young child, particularly, they may produce excitation.

Use in Pregnancy. Experience with this drug in pregnant women is inadequate to determine whether there exists a potential for harm to the developing fetus.

Use with CNS Depressants. Dimetane has additive effects with alcohol and other CNS depressants (hypnotics, sedatives, tranquilizers, etc.).

Use in Activities Requiring Mental Alertness. Patients should be warned about engaging in activities requiring mental alertness, such as driving a car or operating appliances, machinery, etc.

Use in the Elderly (approximately 60 years or older). Antihistamines are more likely to cause dizziness, sedation, and hypotension in elderly patients.

Precautions: As with other antihistamines, Dimetane has an atropine-like action and, therefore, should be used with caution in patients with: history of bronchial asthma; increased intraocular pressure; hyperthyroidism; cardiovascular disease; hypertension.

Drug Interactions: MAO inhibitors prolong and intensify the anticholinergic (drying) effects of antihistamines.

Adverse Reactions: The most frequent adverse reactions are italicized:

General: Urticaria, drug rash, anaphylactic shock, photosensitivity, excessive perspiration, chills, dryness of mouth, nose, and throat.

Cardiovascular System: Hypotension, headache, palpitations, tachycardia, extrasystoles.

Hematologic System: Hemolytic anemia, thrombocytopenia, agranulocytosis.

Nervous System: Sedation, sleepiness, dizziness, disturbed coordination, fatigue, confusion, restlessness, excitation, nervousness, tremor, irritability, insomnia, euphoria, paresthesias, blurred vision, diplopia, vertigo, tinnitus, acute labyrinthitis, hysteria, neuritis, convulsions.

G.I. System: Epigastric distress, anorexia, nausea, vomiting, diarrhea, constipation.

G.U. System: Urinary frequency, difficult urination, urinary retention, early menses.

Respiratory System: Thickening of bronchial secretions, tightness of chest and wheezing, nasal stuffiness.

Overdosage: Antihistamine overdosage reactions may vary from central nervous system depression to stimulation. Stimulation is particularly likely in children. Atropine-like signs and symptoms—dry mouth; fixed, dilated pupils; flushing; and gastrointestinal symptoms may also occur.

If vomiting has not occurred spontaneously, the patient should be induced to vomit. This is best done by having him drink a glass of water or milk after which he should be made to gag. Precautions against aspiration must be taken, especially in infants and children.

If vomiting is unsuccessful, gastric lavage is indicated within 3 hours after ingestion and even later if large amounts of milk or cream were given beforehand. Isotonic and ½ isotonic saline is the lavage solution of choice.

Saline cathartics, such as milk of magnesia, by osmosis draw water into the bowel and therefore, are valuable for their action in rapid dilution of bowel content.

Continued on next page

Prescribing information on A. H. Robins products listed here is based on official labeling in effect August 1, 1982, with Indications, Contraindications, Warnings, Precautions, Adverse Reactions, and Dosage stated in full.

Robins—Cont.

Stimulants should **not** be used.

Vasopressors may be used to treat hypotension.

Dosage and Administration: The recommended OTC dosage is:

Adults and children 12 years of age and over: 1 tablet or 2 teaspoonfuls every four to six hours, not to exceed 6 tablets or 12 teaspoonfuls in 24 hours.

Children 6 to under 12 years: ½ tablet or 1 teaspoonful every four to six hours, not to exceed 3 tablets or 6 teaspoonfuls in 24 hours.

Children under 6 years: use as directed by a physician.

Under physician supervision, children 2 to under 6 years: ½ teaspoonful every four to six hours, not to exceed 3 teaspoonfuls in 24 hours.

How Supplied: 4 mg tablets are available as peach-colored, compressed, scored tablets in cartons of 24 individually packaged blister units (NDC 0031-1857-54), and in bottles of 100 (NDC 0031-1857-63) and 500 (NDC 0031-1857-70). 2 mg per 5 ml peach-colored liquid is available in bottles of 4 fl. oz. (NDC 0031-1807-12), 1 pint (NDC 0031-1807-25) and 1 gallon (NDC 0031-1807-29).

[*Shown in Product Identification Section*]

DIMETANE® DECONGESTANT ELIXIR
DIMETANE® DECONGESTANT TABLETS

(See PDR For Nonprescription Drugs)

DIMETAPP® ELIXIR ℞

Each 5 ml (1 teaspoonful) contains:
Brompheniramine Maleate, USP.............4 mg
Phenylephrine Hydrochloride, USP.........5 mg
Phenylpropanolamine
Hydrochloride, USP...............................5 mg
Alcohol, 2.3%

Actions: Dimetapp effectively reduces excessive nasopharyngeal secretions and diminishes inflammatory mucosal edema and congestion in the upper respiratory tract.

The antihistaminic action of brompheniramine maleate reduces or abolishes the allergic response of nasal tissue. It is complemented by the mild vasoconstrictor action of phenylephrine hydrochloride and phenylpropanolamine hydrochloride which provide a nasal decongestant effect.

Indications

Based on a review of this drug by the National Academy of Sciences—National Research Council and/or other information, FDA has classified the following indications as "probably effective" for Dimetapp Elixir: The symptomatic treatment of seasonal and perennial allergic rhinitis and vasomotor rhinitis; and "lacking substantial evidence of effectiveness as a fixed combination" for the following indications: Symptomatic relief of allergic manifestations of upper respiratory illnesses, acute sinusitis, nasal congestion, and otitis.

Final classification of the less-than-effective indications requires further investigation.

Contraindications: Hypersensitivity to antihistamines of the same chemical class. Dimetapp is contraindicated during pregnancy and in concurrent MAO inhibitor therapy. Because of its drying and thickening effect on the lower respiratory secretions, Dimetapp is not recommended in the treatment of bronchial asthma.

Warnings: ***Use in children.*** In infants and children particularly, antihistamines in overdosage may produce convulsions and death.

Precautions: Administer with care to patients with cardiac or peripheral vascular diseases or hypertension. Until the patient's response has been determined, he should be cautioned against engaging in operations requiring alertness such as driving an automobile, operating machinery, etc. Patients receiving antihistamines should be warned against possible additive effects with CNS depressants such as alcohol, hypnotics, sedatives, tranquilizers, etc.

Adverse Reactions: Adverse reactions to Dimetapp may include hypersensitivity reactions such as rash, urticaria, leukopenia, agranulocytosis and thrombocytopenia; drowsiness, lassitude, giddiness, dryness of the mucous membranes, tightness of the chest, thickening of bronchial secretions, urinary frequency and dysuria, palpitation, hypotension/hypertension, headache, faintness, dizziness, tinnitus, incoordination, visual disturbances, mydriasis, CNS depressant and (less often) stimulant effect, increased irritability or excitement, anorexia, nausea, vomiting, diarrhea, constipation, and epigastric distress.

Dosage and Administration: Adults—1 to 2 teaspoonfuls 3 or 4 times daily.

Children (4 to 12 years)—1 teaspoonful 3 or 4 times daily; (2 to 4 years)—¾ teaspoonful 3 or 4 times daily; (7 months to 2 years)—½ teaspoonful 3 or 4 times daily; (1 to 6 months)—¼ teaspoonful 3 or 4 times daily.

How Supplied: Grape flavored Elixir in 4 fl. oz. (NDC 0031-2224-12), pints (NDC 0031-2224-25), gallons (NDC 0031-2224-29), and 5 ml Dis-Co® Unit Dose Packs (10 × 10s) (NDC 0031-2224-23).

DIMETAPP EXTENTABS® ℞

Each Extentab contains:
Brompheniramine Maleate, USP...........12 mg
Phenylephrine Hydrochloride, USP.......15 mg
Phenylpropanolamine
Hydrochloride, USP...............................15 mg

Extentabs provide a continuous release of medication which affords effects for ten to twelve hours.

Actions: Dimetapp Extentabs effectively reduce excessive nasopharyngeal secretions and diminish inflammatory mucosal edema and congestion in the upper respiratory tract. The antihistaminic action of brompheniramine maleate reduces or abolishes the allergic response of nasal tissue. It is complemented by the mild vasoconstrictor action of phenylephrine hydrochloride and phenylpropanolamine hydrochloride which provide a nasal decongestant effect.

Indications

Based on a review of this drug by the National Academy of Sciences—National Research Council and/or other information, FDA has classified the following indications as "lacking substantial evidence of effectiveness as a fixed combination" for Dimetapp Extentabs: For the symptomatic treatment of seasonal and perennial allergic rhinitis and vasomotor rhinitis, allergic manifestations of upper respiratory illnesses, acute sinusitis, nasal congestion, and otitis.

Final classification of the less-than-effective indications requires further investigation.

Contraindications: Hypersensitivity to antihistamines of the same chemical class. Dimetapp Extentabs are contraindicated during pregnancy and in children under 12 years of age. Because of its drying and thickening effect on the lower respiratory secretions, Dimetapp is not recommended in the treatment of bronchial asthma. Also, Dimetapp Extentabs are contraindicated in concurrent MAO inhibitor therapy.

Warnings: ***Use in Children.*** In infants and children particularly, antihistamines in overdosage may produce convulsions and death.

Precautions: Administer with care to patients with cardiac or peripheral vascular diseases or hypertension. Until the patient's response has been determined, he should be cautioned against engaging in operations requiring alertness such as driving an automobile, operating machinery, etc. Patients receiving antihistamines should be warned against possible additive effects with CNS depressants such as alcohol, hypnotics, sedatives, tranquilizers, etc.

Adverse Reactions: Adverse reactions to Dimetapp Extentabs may include hypersensitivity reactions such as rash, urticaria, leukopenia, agranulocytosis and thrombocytopenia; drowsiness, lassitude, giddiness, dryness of the mucous membranes, tightness of the chest, thickening of bronchial secretions, urinary frequency and dysuria, palpitation, hypotension/hypertension, headache, faintness, dizziness, tinnitus, incoordination, visual disturbances, mydriasis, CNS depressant and (less often) stimulant effect, increased irritability or excitement, anorexia, nausea, vomiting, diarrhea, constipation, and epigastric distress.

Dosage and Administration: Adults and Children 12 years and over. One Extentab morning and evening. If indicated, one Extentab every 8 hours may be given.

How Supplied: Light blue Extentabs monogrammed AHR and Dimetapp in bottles of 100 (NDC 0031-2274-63), 500 (NDC 0031-2274-70) and Dis-Co® unit dose packs of 100 (NDC 0031-2274-64).

[*Shown in Product Identification Section*]

DONNAGEL®
DONNAGEL®-PG Ⓒ

Composition: *Donnagel:* Each 30 ml (one fluid ounce) contains Kaolin, USP (90 gr.) 6.0 g., Pectin, USP (2 gr.) 142.8 mg., Hyoscyamine Sulfate, USP 0.1037 mg., Atropine Sulfate, USP 0.0194 mg., Scopolamine Hydrobromide, USP 0.0065 mg., Sodium Benzoate, NF (preservative) 60 mg., alcohol 3.8 per cent.

Donnagel-PG: Each 30 ml (one fluid ounce) contains the basic Donnagel formula plus powdered opium, USP (equivalent to paregoric 6 ml.) 24 mg. (Warning: may be habit forming), alcohol 5.0 per cent.

Description: Donnagel combines the adsorbent and detoxifying effects of kaolin and pectin with the antispasmodic efficacy of the natural belladonna alkaloids. The latter, present in a specific, fixed ratio, help control hypermotility and hypersecretion in the gastrointestinal tract.

Indications: Donnagel is indicated in the treatment of diarrhea.

Donnagel-PG contains a paregoric equivalent for more complete symptomatic control of acute, non-specific diarrheas. This combination of drugs affords a more complete approach for stopping diarrhea and relieving tenesmus and pain. The belladonna alkaloids partly antagonize the occasional cramping effect of opium upon the colon.

Contraindications: Glaucoma, advanced renal or hepatic disease or hypersensitivity to any of the ingredients.

Precautions: As with all preparations containing belladonna alkaloids, the Donnagel formulations must be administered cautiously to patients with incipient glaucoma or urinary bladder neck obstruction as in prostatic hypertrophy.

Adverse Reactions: Blurred vision, dry mouth, difficult urination or flushing and dryness of the skin may occur at higher dosage levels, rarely at the usual dose.

Dosage and Administration: (Donnagel and Donnagel-PG). *Adults*—Two tablespoonfuls (one fl. oz.) initially, followed by 1 tablespoonful every 3 hours.

Children over 6 years of age—Two teaspoonfuls initially and 1 or 2 teaspoonfuls every 3 hours thereafter.

Pediatric Dosage Recommendations:

Body Weight	Dosage
10 lb.	30 minims or ½ teaspoonful
20 lb.	1 teaspoonful
30 lb. and over	1-2 teaspoonfuls

To be dosed every 3 hours, not to exceed 4 doses in a 24-hour period.

How Supplied: Donnagel (light green, aromatic suspension) in 4 fl. oz. (NDC 0031-3016-12) and pint (NDC 0031-3016-25). Donnagel-PG (light yellow, banana-flavored suspension) in 6 fl. oz. (NDC 0031-3083-15) and pint (NDC 0031-3083-25).

DONNATAL® TABLETS ℞
DONNATAL® CAPSULES ℞
DONNATAL® ELIXIR ℞

Description: Each Donnatal tablet, capsule or 5 ml (teaspoonful) of elixir (23% alcohol) contains:

Phenobarbital, USP (¼ gr) ....16.2 mg
(Warning: May be habit forming)
Hyoscyamine Sulfate, USP ....0.1037 mg
Atropine Sulfate, USP ....0.0194 mg
Scopolamine Hydrobromide, USP ..0.0065 mg

Actions: This drug combination provides natural belladonna alkaloids in a specific, fixed ratio combined with phenobarbital to provide peripheral anticholinergic/antispasmodic action and mild sedation.

Indications

Based on a review of this drug by the National Academy of Sciences—National Research Council and/or other information, FDA has classified the following indications as "possibly" effective:

For use as adjunctive therapy in the treatment of irritable bowel syndrome (irritable colon, spastic colon, mucous colitis) and acute enterocolitis.

May also be useful as adjunctive thrapy in the treatment of duodenal ulcer. IT HAS NOT BEEN SHOWN CONCLUSIVELY WHETHER ANTICHOLINERGIC/ANTISPASMODIC DRUGS AID IN THE HEALING OF A DUODENAL ULCER, DECREASE THE RATE OF RECURRENCES OR PREVENT COMPLICATIONS.

Contraindications: Glaucoma, obstructive uropathy (for example, bladder neck obstruction due to prostatic hypertrophy); obstructive disease of the gastrointestinal tract (as in achalasia, pyloroduodenal stenosis, etc.); paralytic ileus, intestinal atony of the elderly or debilitated patient; unstable cardiovascular status in acute hemorrhage; severe ulcerative colitis especially if complicated by toxic megacolon; myasthenia gravis; hiatal hernia associated with reflux esophagitis.

Donnatal is contraindicated in patients with known hypersensitivity to any of the ingredients. Phenobarbital is contraindicated in acute intermittent porphyria and in those patients in whom phenobarbital produces restlessness and/or excitement.

Warnings: In the presence of a high environmental temperature, heat prostration can occur with belladonna alkaloids (fever and heatstroke due to decreased sweating).

Diarrhea may be an early symptom of incomplete intestinal obstruction, especially in patients with ileostomy or colostomy. In this instance treatment with this drug would be inapproprite and possibly harmful.

Donnatal may produce drowsiness or blurred vision. The patient should be warned, should these occur, not to engage in activities requiring mental alertness, such as operating a motor vehicle or other machinery, and not to perform hazardous work.

Phenobarbital may decrease the effect of anticoagulants, and necessitate larger doses of the anticoagulant for optimal effect. When the phenobarbital is discontinued, the dose of the anticoagulant may have to be decreased.

Phenobarbital may be habit forming and should not be administered to individuals known to be addiction prone or to those with a history of physical and/or psychological dependence upon drugs.

Since barbiturates are metabolized in the liver, they should be used with caution and initial doses should be small in patients with hepatic dysfunction.

Precautions: Use with caution in patients with: autonomic neuropathy, hepatic or renal disease, hyperthyroidism, coronary heart disease, congestive heart failure, cardiac arrhythmias, tachycardia, and hypertension.

Belladonna alkaloids may produce a delay in gastric emptying (antral stasis) which would complicate the management of gastric ulcer.

Theoretically, with overdosage, a curare-like action may occur.

Carcinogenesis, mutagenesis. Long-term studies in animals have not been performed to evaluate carcinogenic potential.

Pregnancy Category C. Animal reproduction studies have not been conducted with Donnatal. It is not known whether Donnatal can cause fetal harm when adminnistered to a pregnant woman or can affect reproduction capacity. Donnatal should be given to a pregnant woman only if clearly needed.

Nursing mothers. It is not known whether this drug is excreted in human milk. Because many drugs are excreted in human milk, caution should be exercised when Donnatal is administered to a nursing mother.

Adverse Reactions: Adverse reactions may include xerostomia; urinary hesitancy and retention; blurred vision; tachycardia; palpitation; mydriasis; cycloplegia; increased ocular tension; loss of taste sense, headache, nervousness; drowsiness; weakness; dizziness; insomnia; nausea vomiting; impotence; suppression of lactation; constipation; bloated feeling; musculoskeletal pain; severe allergic reaction or drug idiosyncrasies, including anaphylaxis, urticaria and other dermal manifestations; and decreased sweating. Elderly patients may react with symptoms of excitement, agitation, drowsiness, and other untoward manifestations to even small doses of the drug.

Phenobarbital may produce excitement in some patients, rather than a sedative effect. In patients habituated to barbiturates, abrupt withdrawal may produce delirium or convulsions.

Dosage and Administration: The dosage of Donnatal should be adjusted to the needs of the individual patient to assure symptomatic control with a minimum of adverse effects.

Donnatal Tablets or Capsules. Adults: One or two Donnatal tablets or capsules three or four times a day according to condition and severity of symptoms.

Donnatal Elixir. Adults: One or two teaspoonfuls of elixir three or four times a day according to conditions and severity of symptoms.

Children (Elixir)—may be dosed every 4 or 6 hours.:

Body Weight	Starting Dosage q4h	Starting Dosage q6h
10 lb (4.5 kg)	0.5 ml	0.75 ml
20 lb (9.1 kg)	1.0 ml	1.5 ml
30 lb (13.6 kg)	1.5 ml	2.0 ml
50 lb (22.7 kg)	½ tsp	¾ tsp
75 lb (34.0 kg)	¾ tsp	1 tsp
100 lb (45.4 kg)	1 tsp	1½ tsp

Overdosage: The signs and symptoms of overdose are headache, nausea, vomiting, blurred vision, dilated pupils, hot and dry skin, dizziness, dryness of the mouth, difficulty in swallowing, CNS stimulation. Treatment should consist of gastric lavage, emetics, and activated charcoal. If indicated, parenteral cholinergic agents such as physostigmine or bethanechol chloride, should be added.

How Supplied: *Donnatal Tablets.* white, compressed, embossed "R" on one side, scored and engraved 4250 on the reverse side; in bottles of 100 (NDC 0031-4250-63), 1000 (NDC 0031-4250-74) and Dis-Co® Unit Dose Packs of 100 (NDC 0031-4250-64).

Donnatal Capsules. Green and white, monogrammed "AHR" and "4207"; in bottles of 100 (NDC 0031-4207-63) and 1000 (NDC 0031-4207-74).

Donnatal Elixir. Green citrus flavored, in 4 fl. oz. (NDC 0031-4221-12), pints (NDC 0031-4221-25), gallons (NDC 0031-4221-29) and 5 ml Dis-Co® Unit Dose Packs (4 × 25s) (NDC 0031-4221-13).

Store at controlled room temperature, between 15°C and 30°C (59°F and 86°F).

Dispense in tight, light-resistant container.

[*Shown in Product Identification Section*]

DONNATAL EXTENTABS® ℞

Description: Each Donnatal Extentab contains:

Phenobarbital, USP (¾gr) ....48.6 mg
(Warning: May be habit forming)
Hyoscyamine Sulfate, USP ....0.3111 mg
Atropine Sulfate, USP ....0.0582 mg
Scopolamine Hydrobromide, USP ....0.0195 mg

Each Donnatal Extentab contains the equivalent of three Donnatal tablets. The Extentab is designed to release the ingredients gradually to provide effects for up to twelve (12) hours.

Actions: Donnatal provides natural belladonna alkaloids in a specific, fixed ratio combined with phenobarbital to provide peripheral anticholinergic/antispasmodic action and mild sedation.

Indications

Based on a review of this drug by the National Academy of Sciences—National Research Council and/or other information, FDA has classified the following indications as "possibly" effective:

For use as adjunctive therapy in the treatment of irritable bowel syndrome (irritable colon, spastic colon, mucous colitis) and acute enterocolitis.

May also be useful as adjunctive therapy in the treatment of duodenal ulcer. IT HAS NOT BEEN SHOWN CONCLUSIVELY WHETHER ANTICHOLINERGIC/ANTISPASMODIC DRUGS AID IN THE HEALING OF A DUODENAL ULCER, DECREASE THE RATE OF RECURRENCES OR PREVENT COMPLICATIONS.

Contraindications: Glaucoma, obstructive uropathy (for example, bladder neck obstruction due to prostatic hypertrophy); obstructive disease of the gastrointestinal tract (as in achalasia, pyloroduodenal stenosis, etc.); paralytic ileus, intestinal atony of the elderly or debilitated patient; unstable cardiovascular status in acute hemorrhage; severe ulcerative colitis especially if complicated by toxic megacolon; myasthenia gravis, hiatal hernia associated with reflux esophagitis.

Donnatal is contraindicated in patients with known hypersensitivity to any of the ingredi-

Continued on next page

Prescribing information on A. H. Robins products listed here is based on official labeling in effect August 1, 1982, with Indications, Contraindications, Warnings, Precautions, Adverse Reactions, and Dosage stated in full.

Robins—Cont.

ents. Phenobarbital is contraindicated in acute intermittent porphyria and in those patients in whom phenobarbital produces restlessness and/or excitement.
Warnings: In the presence of a high environmental temperature, heat prostration can occur with belladonna alkaloids (fever and heatstroke due to decrease sweating).
Diarrhea may be an early symptom of incomplete intestinal obstruction, especially in patients with ileostomy or colostomy. In this instance treatment with this drug would be inappropriate and possibly harmful.
Donnatal may produce drowsiness or blurred vision. The patient should be warned, should these occur, not to engage in activities requiring mental alertness, such as operating a motor vehicle or other machinery, and not to perform hazardous work.
Phenobarbital may decrease the effect of anticoagulants and necessitate larger doses of the anticoagulant for optimal effect. When the phenobarbital is discontinued, the dose of the anticoagulant may have to be decreased.
Phenobarbital may be habit forming and should not be administered to individuals known to be addiction prone or to those with a history of physical and/or psychological dependence upon drugs.
Since barbiturates are metabolized in the liver, they should be used with caution and initial doses should be small in patients with hepatic dysfunction.
Precautions: Use with caution in patients with: autonomic neuropathy, hepatic or renal disease, hyperthyroidism, coronary heart disease, congestive heart failure, cardiac arrhythmias, tachycardia, and hypertension.
Belladonna alkaloids may produce a delay in gastric emptying (antral stasis) which would complicate the management of gastric ulcer.
Theoretically, with overdosage, a curare-like action may occur.
Carcinogenesis, mutagenesis. Long-term studies in animals have not been performed to evaluate carcinogenic potential.
Pregnancy Category C. Animal reproduction studies have not been conducted with Donnatal. It is not known whether Donnatal can cause fetal harm when administered to a pregnant woman or can affect reproduction capacity. Donnatal should be given to a pregnant woman only if clearly needed.
Nursing mothers. It is not known whether this drug is excreted in human milk. Because many drugs are excreted in human milk, caution should be exercised when Donnatal is administered to a nursing mother.
Adverse Reactions. Adverse reactions may include xerostomia; urinary hesitancy and retention; blurred vision; tachycardia; palpitation; mydriasis; cycloplegia; increased ocular tension; loss of taste sense; headache; nervousness; drowsiness; weakness; dizziness; insomnia; nausea; vomiting; impotence; suppression of lactation; constipation; bloated feeling, musculoskeletal pain; severe allergic reaction or drug idiosyncrasies, including anaphylaxis, urticaria and other dermal manifestations; and decreased sweating. Elderly patients may react with symptoms of excitement, agitation, drowsiness, and other untoward manifestations to even small doses of the drug.
Phenobarbital may produce excitement in some patients, rather than a sedative effect. In patients habituated to barbiturates, abrupt withdrawal may produce delirium or convulsions.
Dosage and Administration: The dosage of Donnatal Extentabs should be adjusted to the needs of the individual patient to assure symptomatic control with a minimum of adverse reactions. The usual dose is one Extentab every twelve (12) hours. If indicated, one Extentab every eight (8) hours may be given.
Overdosage: The signs and symptoms of overdose are headache, nausea, vomiting, blurred vision, dilated pupils; hot and dry skin, dizziness, dryness of the mouth, difficulty in swallowing, CNS stimulation. Treatment should consist of gastric lavage, emetics, and activated charcoal. If indicated, parenteral cholinergic agents such as physostigmine or bethanechol chloride should be added.
How Supplied: Pale green, coated tablets, monogrammed AHR and Donnatal Extentab in bottles of 100 (NDC 0031-4235-63) and 500 (NDC 0031-4235-70); and Dis-Co® Unit Dose Packs of 100 (NDC 0031-4235-64).
Store at controlled room temperature, between 15°C and 30°C (59°F and 86°F).
Dispense in well-closed, light-resistant container.

[*Shown in Product Identification Section*]

DONNAZYME® TABLETS ℞

Description: Donnazyme tablets are available for oral administration. Each tablet contains:

Pancreatin, USP equivalent	300 mg
Pepsin	150 mg
Bile Salts	150 mg
Hyoscyamine Sulfate, USP	0.0518 mg
Atropine Sulfate, USP	0.0097 mg
Scopolamine Hydrobromide, USP	0.0033 mg
Phenobarbital USP (1/8 gr)	8.1 mg

(Warning: may be habit forming)
The combination of anticholinergic/antispasmodic/sedative components with natural digestive enzymes plus bile salts makes it useful for symptomatic relief of functional G.I. disorders.
Clinical Pharmacology: The outer layer of Donnazyme tablets is gastric-soluble and contains the belladonna alkaloids, phenobarbital and pepsin. These ingredients rapidly become available for absorption as the tablet begins disintegrating in the stomach. The pepsin supplements the stomach's digestive secretions by aiding the breakdown of proteins into proteoses and peptones. Spasmolysis and sedation are produced as the belladonna alkaloids and phenobarbital are absorbed.
The core of the tablet contains pancreatin and bile salts. It is designed to disintegrate in the alkaline medium of the duodenum where it releases the active enzyme components of pancreatin (trypsin, amylase and lipase), along with the bile salts. Trypsin breaks down larger protein fractions into peptides; amylase converts starch into maltose; lipase splits fat into fatty acids and glycerin; and bile salts enhance the fat-splitting action of the lipase and aid in the emulsification of fats and the absorption of fatty acids.
Indications and Usage: Donnazyme is indicated for the relief of symptoms associated with "nervous indigestion" and other functional G.I. disorders in the absence of organic pathology. Some of these conditions are chronic pancreatitis, chronic gastritis, postcholecystectomy syndrome, and chronic billary disorders. Donnazyme may prove especially useful in patients with decreased digestive enzyme secretory activity, which is frequently suspect in older patients with visceral complaints.
Contraindications: Glaucoma, obstructive uropathy (for example, bladder neck obstruction due to prostatic hypertrophy); obstructive disease of the gastrointestinal tract (as in achalasia, pyloroduodenal stenosis, etc.); paralytic ileus, intestinal atony of the elderly or debilitated patient, unstable cardiovascular status in acute hemorrhage, severe ulcerative colitis especially if complicated by toxic megacolon; myasthenia gravis; hiatal hernia associated with reflux esophagitis.
Donnazyme is contraindicated in patients with known hypersensitivity to any of the ingredients. Phenobarbital is contraindicated in acute intermittent porphyria and in those patients in whom phenobarbital produces restlessness and/or excitement.
Warnings: In the presence of a high environmental temperature, heat prostration can occur with belladonna alkaloids (fever and heatstroke due to decreased sweating).
Diarrhea may be an early symptom of incomplete intestinal obstruction, especially in patients with ileostomy or colostomy. In this instance, treatment with this drug would be inappropriate and possibly harmful.
Donnazyme may produce drowsiness or blurred vision. The patient should be warned, should these occur, not to engage in activities requiring mental alertness, such as operating a motor vehicle or other machinery, and not to perform hazardous work.
Phenobarbital may decrease the effect of anticoagulants and necessitate larger doses of the anticoagulant for optimal effect. When the phenobarbital is discontinued, the dose of the anticoagulant may have to be decreased.
Phenobarbital may be habit forming and should not be administered to individuals known to be addiction prone or to those with a history of physical and/or psychological dependence upon drugs.
Since barbiturates are metabolized in the liver, they should be used with caution and initial small doses in patients with hepatic dysfunction.
Precautions: ***General.*** Use with caution in patients with autonomic neuropathy, hepatic or renal disease, hyperthyroidism, coronary heart disease, congestive heart failure, cardiac arrhythmias, tachycardia, and hypertension.
Belladonna alkaloids may produce a delay in gastric emptying (antral stasis) which would complicate the management of gastric ulcer.
Theoretically, with overdosage, a curare-like action may occur.
Carcinogenesis, mutagenesis: Long-term studies in animals have not been performed to evaluate carcinogenic potential.
Pregnancy Category C. Animal reproduction studies have not been conducted with Donnazyme. It is not known whether Donnazyme can cause fetal harm when administered to a pregnant woman or can affect reproduction capacity. Donnazyme should be given to a pregnant woman only if clearly needed.
Nursing mothers: It is not known whether this drug is excreted in human milk. Because many drugs are excreted in human milk, caution should be exercised when Donnazyme is administered to a nursing mother.
Pediatric Use: Safety and effectiveness in children have not been established.
Adverse Reactions: Adverse reactions may include xerostomia; urinary hesitancy and retention; blurred vision; tachycardia; palpitation; mydriasis; cycloplegia; increased ocular tension; loss of taste sense; headache; nervousness; drowsiness; weakness, dizziness, insomnia; nausea; vomiting; impotence; suppression of lactation; constipation; bloated feeling; musculoskeletal pain; severe allergic reaction or drug idiosyncrasies, including "anaphylaxis, urticaria and other dermal manifestations; and decreased sweating." Elderly patients may react with symptoms of excitement, agitation, drowsiness, and other untoward manifestations to even small doses of the drug.
Phenobarbital may produce excitement in some patients, rather than a sedative effect. In patients habituated to barbiturates, abrupt withdrawal may produce delirium or convulsions.
Overdosage. The signs and symptoms of overdose are headache, nausea, vomiting, blurred vision, dilated pupils, hot and dry skin, dizziness, dryness of the mouth, difficulty in swallowing, CNS stimulation. Treatment should consist of gastric lavage, emetics, and

activated charcoal. If indicated, parenteral cholinergic agents, such as physostigmine or bethanechol chloride, should be added.

Dosage and Administration: Adult dosage: Two tablets after each meal.

How Supplied: Kelly green tablets in bottles of 100 (NDC 0031-4649-63) and 500 (NDC 0031-4649-70). Store at controlled room temperature, between 15°C and 30°C (59°F and 86°F). Dispense in tight container.

[*Shown in Product Identification Section*]

DOPRAM® INJECTABLE ℞

brand of Doxapram Hydrochloride Injection, USP

Composition: Each 1 ml contains:
Doxapram Hydrochloride, USP.............20 mg.
Water for Injection, USP ....q.s.
Chlorobutanol, NF (as preservative)........0.5%

Actions: Doxapram hydrochloride produces respiratory stimulation mediated through the peripheral carotid chemoreceptors. As the dosage level is increased, the central respiratory centers in the medulla are stimulated with progressive stimulation of other parts of the brain and spinal cord.

The onset of respiratory stimulation following the recommended single intravenous injection of doxapram hydrochloride usually occurs in 20–40 seconds with peak effect at 1–2 minutes. The duration of effect may vary from 5–12 minutes.

The respiratory stimulant action is manifested by an increase in tidal volume associated with a slight increase in respiratory rate.

A pressor response may result following doxapram administration. Provided there is no impairment of cardiac function, the pressor effect is more marked in hypovolemic than in normovolemic states. The pressor response is due to the improved cardiac output rather than peripheral vasoconstriction. Following doxapram administration an increased release of catecholamines has been noted.

Although opiate induced respiratory depression is antagonized by doxapram, the analgesic effect is not affected.

Indications:

1. ***Post-anesthesia.***
   a. When the possibility of airway obstruction and/or hypoxia have been eliminated, doxapram may be used to stimulate respiration in patients with drug-induced post-anesthesia respiratory depression or apnea other than that due to muscle relaxant drugs.
   b. To pharmacologically stimulate deep breathing in the so-called "stir-up" regimen in the postoperative patient. (Simultaneous administration of oxygen is desirable.)
2. ***Drug-induced central nervous system depression.***
   Exercising care to prevent vomiting and aspiration, doxapram may be used to stimulate respiration, hasten arousal, and to encourage the return of laryngopharyngeal reflexes in patients with mild to moderate respiratory and CNS depression due to drug overdosage.
3. ***Chronic pulmonary disease associated with acute hypercapnia.***
   Doxaram is indicated as a temporary measure in hospitalized patients with acute respiratory insufficiency superimposed on chronic obstructive pulmonary disease. Its use should be for a short period of time (approximately 2 hours) as an aid in the prevention of elevation of arterial CO_2 tension during the administration of oxygen. It should not be used in conjuction with mechanical ventilation. The adequacy of ventilation MUST be assessed by measurements of arterial blood gases as well as careful monitoring of the cardiovascular indices.

Contraindications:

1. ***General Contraindications.***
   Doxapram is not recommended in the following conditions: epilepsy and other convulsive states; incompetence of the ventilatory mechanism due to muscle paresis, flail chest, pneumothorax, airway obstruction, and extreme dyspnea; severe hypertension and cerebrovascular accidents; hypersensitivity to doxapram; evidence of head injury.
2. ***Contraindications in pulmonary disease.***
   Doxapram is not recommended in the following conditions: strongly suspected or confirmed pulmonary embolism, pneumothorax, acute bronchial asthma, respiratory failure due to neuromuscular disorders, and in restrictive respiratory diseases such as pulmonary fibrosis.
3. ***Contraindications in cardiovascular disease.***
   Doxapram is not recommended in the following conditions: coronary artery disease, frank uncompensated heart failure.

Warnings:

1. ***Warning in post-anesthetic use.***
   a. Doxapram is neither an antagonist to muscle relaxant drugs nor a specific narcotic antagonist. Adequacy of airway and oxygenation must be assured prior to doxapram administration.
   b. Doxapram should be administered with great care and only under close supervision to patients with cerebral edema, history of bronchial asthma, severe tachycardia, cardiac arrhythmia, cardiac disease, hyperthyroidism, or pheochromocytoma.
   c. Since narcosis may recur after stimulation with doxapram, care should be taken to maintain close observation until the patient has been fully alert for ½ to 1 hour.
2. ***Warning in drug-induced CNS and respiratory depression.***
   Doxapram alone may not stimulate adequate spontaneous breathing or provide sufficient arousal in patients who are ***severely*** depressed either due to respiratory failure or to CNS depressant drugs, but should be used as an adjunct to establish supportive measures and resuscitative techniques.
3. ***Warning in chronic obstructive pulmonary disease.***
   a. In an attempt to lower pCO_2, the rate of infusion of doxapram should not be increased in severely ill patients because of the associated increased work in breathing.
   b. Doxapram should not be used in conjunction with mechanical ventilation.
4. ***Warning in pregnancy.***
   Clinically the safe use of doxapram in pregnancy has not been established. The physician must weigh the need against possible risks in using the drug in pregnant patients or in women of childbearing potential.
5. ***Warning in children 12 years of age and under.***
   Doxapram is not recommended for use in patients 12 years of age or under because studies to adequately evaluate its safety and efficacy have not been performed.

Precautions:

1. ***General precautions.***
   a. An adequate airway is essential.
   b. Recommended dosages of doxapram should be employed and maximum total dosages should not be exceeded. In order to avoid side effects, it is advisable to use the minimum effective dosage.
   c. Monitoring of the blood pressure and deep tendon reflexes is recommended to prevent overdosage.
   d. Vascular extravasation or use of a single injection site over an extended period should be avoided since either may lead to thrombophlebitis or local skin irritation.
   e. Rapid infusion may result in hemolysis.
   f. Lowered pCO_2 induced by hyperventilation produces cerebral vasoconstriction and slowing of the cerebral circulation. This should be taken into consideration on an individual basis.
   g. Intravenous short-acting barbiturates, oxygen and resuscitative equipment should be readily available to manage overdosage manifested by excessive central nervous system stimulation. Slow administration of the drug, careful observation of the patient during administration and for some time subsequently, are advisable. These precautions are to assure that the protective reflexes have been restored and to prevent possible posthyperventilation hypoventilation.
   h. Doxapram should be administered cautiously to patients receiving sympathomimetic or monoamine oxidase inhibiting drugs, since an additive pressor effect may occur.
   i. Blood pressure increases are generally modest but significant increases have been noted in some patients. Because of this doxapram is not recommended for use in severe hypertension (see Contraindications).
   j. If sudden hypotension or dyspnea develops, doxapram should be stopped.
2. ***Precautions in post-anesthetic use.***
   a. In patients who have received muscle relaxants, doxapram may temporarily mask the residual effects of muscle relaxant drugs.
   b. Since an increase in epinephrine release has been noted with doxapram, it is recommended that initiation of therapy be delayed for at least 10 minutes following the discontinuance of anesthetics known to sensitize the myocardium to catecholamines, such as halothane, cyclopropane and enflurane.
   c. The same consideration to pre-existing disease states should be exercised as in non-anesthetized individuals. See Contraindications and Warnings covering use in hypertension, asthma, disturbances of respiratory mechanics including airway obstruction, CNS disorders including increased cerebrospinal fluid pressure, convulsive disorders, acute agitation, and profound metabolic disorders.
3. ***Precautions in chronic obstructive pulmonary disease.***
   a. Arrhythmias seen in some patients in acute respiratory failure secondary to chronic obstructive pulmonary disease are probably the result of hypoxia. Doxapram should be used with caution in these patients.
   b. Arterial blood gases should be drawn prior to the initiation of doxapram infusion and oxygen administration, then at least every ½ hour. Doxapram administration does not diminish the need for careful monitoring of the patient or the need for supplemental oxygen in patients with acute respiratory failure. Doxapram should be stopped if the arterial blood gases deteriorate, and mechanical ventilation initiated.

Adverse Reactions: The following adverse reactions have been reported:

1. ***Central and autonomic nervous systems.***
   Headache, dizziness, apprehension, disorientation, pupillary dilatation, hyperactivity, involuntary movements, convulsions, muscle spasticity, increased deep tendon reflexes, clonus, bilateral Babinski; pyrexia,

Continued on next page

Prescribing information on A. H. Robins products listed here is based on official labeling in effect August 1, 1982, with Indications, Contraindications, Warnings, Precautions, Adverse Reactions, and Dosage stated in full.

Robins—Cont.

flushing, sweating; pruritus and paresthesia such as a feeling of warmth, burning, or hot sensation especially in the area of genitalia and perineum.

2. ***Respiratory***
Cough, dyspnea, tachypnea, laryngospasm, bronchospasm, hiccough, and rebound hypoventilation.
3. ***Cardiovascular.***
Phlebitis, variations in heart rate, lowered T-waves, arrhythmias, chest pain, tightness in chest. A mild to moderate increase in blood pressure is commonly noted. The elevation in blood pressure may be of concern only in hypertensive patients. (See Contraindications.)
4. ***Gastrointestinal.***
Nausea, vomiting, diarrhea, desire to defecate.
5. ***Genitourinary.***
Urinary retention, stimulation of urinary bladder with spontaneous voiding.
6. ***Laboratory determinations.***
A decrease in hemoglobin, hematocrit, or red blood cell count has been observed in postoperative patients. In the presence of preexisting leukopenia, a further decrease in WBC has been observed following anesthesia and treatment with doxapram hydrochloride. Elevation of BUN and albuminuria have also been observed. As some of the patients cited above had received multiple drugs concomitantly, a cause and effect relationship could not be determined.

Dosage and Administration:

1. Doxapram hydrochloride is compatible with 5% and 10% dextrose in water or normal saline. ADMIXTURE OF DOXAPRAM WITH ALKALINE SOLUTIONS SUCH AS 2.5% THIOPENTAL SODIUM OR BICARBONATE WILL RESULT IN PRECIPITATION.
2. ***In post-anesthetic use.***
   a. By i.v. injection (see Table I. Dosage for post-anesthetic use—I.V.)

[See table below].

   b. By infusion. The solution is prepared by adding 250 mg of doxapram (12.5 ml) to 250 ml of dextrose or saline solution. The infusion is initiated at a rate of approximately 5 mg/minute until a satisfactory respiratory response is observed, and maintained at a rate of 1–3 mg/minute. The rate of infusion should be adjusted to sustain the desired level of respiratory stimulation with a minimum of side effects. The recommended total dosage by infusion is 4 mg/kg (2.0 mg/lb), not to exceed 3 grams.
3. ***In the management of drug-induced CNS depression.***
(See Table II. Dosage for drug-induced CNS depression.)

[See table above].

METHOD ONE
Using Single and/or Repeat Single I.V. ***Injections.***

Table II. Dopram Injectable Dosage for drug-induced CNS depression.

Level of Depression	METHOD ONE Priming dose single/repeat i.v. injection mg/kg	mg/lb	METHOD TWO Rate of intermittent i.v. infusion mg/kg/hr	mg/lb/hr
Mild*	1.0	0.5	1.0–2.0	0.5–1.0
Moderate†	2.0	1.0	2.0–3.0	1.0–1.5

*Mild Depression
Class 0: Asleep, but can be aroused and can answer questions.
Class 1: Comatose, will withdraw from painful stimuli, reflexes intact.

†Moderate Depression
Class 2: Comatose, will not withdraw from painful stimuli, reflexes intact.
Class 3: Comatose, reflexes absent, no depression of circulation or respiration.

a. Give priming dose of 1.0 mg/lb (2.0 mg/kg) body weight and repeat in 5 minutes.
b. Repeat same dose q1–2h until patient wakens. Watch for relapse into unconsciousness or development of respiratory depression, since Dopram does not affect the metabolism of CNS-depressant drugs.
c. If relapse occurs, resume 1–2 hourly injections until arousal is sustained, or total maximum daily dose (3 grams) is given. Allow patient to sleep until 24 hours have elapsed from first injection of Dopram, using assisted or automatic respiration if necessary.
d. Repeat procedure until patient breathes spontaneously and sustains desired level of consciousness, or until maximum dosage (3 grams) is given.
e. Repetitive doses should be administered only to patients who have shown response to the initial dose.
f. Failure to respond appropriately indicates the need for neurologic evaluation for a possible central nervous system source of sustained coma.

METHOD TWO
By Intermittent I.V. ***Infusion.***

a. Give priming dose as in Method One.
b. If patient wakens, watch for relapse; if no response, continue general supportive treatment for 1–2 hours and repeat Dopram. If some respiratory stimulation occurs, prepare I.V. infusion by adding 250 mg of Dopram (12.5 ml) to 250 ml of saline or dextrose solution. Deliver at rate of 1–3 mg/min (60–180 ml/hr) according to size of patient and depth of coma. Discontinue Dopram if patient begins to waken or at end of 2 hours.
c. Continue supportive treatment for ½ to 2 hours and repeat Step b.
d. Do not exceed 3 grams.

4. ***Chronic obstructive pulmonary disease associated with acute hypercapnia.***
   a. One vial of doxapram (400 mg) should be mixed with 180 ml of the intravenous solution (concentration of 2.0 mg/ml). The infusion should be started at 1–2 mg/minute (½–1 ml/minute); if indicated, increase to a maximum of 3 mg/minute. Arterial blood gases should be determined prior to the onset of doxapram's administration and at least every half hour during the two hours of infusion to insure against the insidious development of CO_2-RETENTION AND ACIDOSIS. Alteration of oxygen concentration or flow rate may necessitate adjustment in the rate of doxapram infusion.
   b. Predictable blood gas patterns are more readily established with a continuous infusion of doxapram. If the blood gases show evidence of deterioration, the infusion of doxapram should be discontinued.
   c. ADDITIONAL INFUSIONS BEYOND THE SINGLE MAXIMUM TWO HOUR ADMINISTRATION PERIOD ARE NOT RECOMMENDED.

Table I. Dopram Injectable Dosage for post-anesthetic use—I.V.

I.V. Administration	Recommended dosage mg/kg	mg/lb	Maximum dose per single injection mg/kg	mg/lb	Maximum total dose mg/kg	mg/lb
Single Injection	0.5–1.0	0.25–0.5	1.5	0.70	1.5	0.70
Repeat Injections (5 min. intervals)	0.5–1.0	0.25–0.5	1.5	0.70	2.0	1.0
Infusion	0.5–1.0	0.25–0.5	—	—	4.0	2.0

Overdosage: Excessive pressor effect, tachycardia, skeletal muscle hyperactivity, and enhanced deep tendon reflexes may be early signs of overdosage. Therefore, the blood pressure, pulse rate, and deep tendon reflexes should be evaluated periodically and the dosage or infusion rate adjusted accordingly. Convulsive seizures are unlikely at recommended dosages, but intravenous anticonvulsants, oxygen, and resuscitative equipment should be available.

How Supplied: Dopram Injectable (doxapram hydrochloride injection) is available in 20 ml multiple dose vials containing 20 mg of doxapram hydrochloride per ml, 20 mg/ml, with chlorobutanol 0.5% as the preservative (NDC 0031-4849-83).

Additional literature available upon request.
Manufactured for Pharmaceutical Division, A. H. Robins Company, Richmond, Virginia 23220 by Elkins-Sinn, Inc., Cherry Hill, New Jersey 08034, a subsidiary of A. H. Robins Co.

ENTOZYME® TABLETS ℞

Description: Entozyme tablets are available for oral administration. Each tablet contains:
Pancreatin, USP equivalent ....300 mg
Pepsin ....250 mg
Bile salts ....150 mg
Natural Digestive Enzymes

Construction: Entozyme is a specially constructed tablet. The outer layer dissolves in the stomach and releases pepsin. The "inner tablet" is protected by an enteric coating that disintegrates in the alkaline medium of the small intestine and releases pancreatin and bile salts, thus preserving the digestive potency of the pancreatin as it passes through the stomach.

Clinical Pharmacology: Entozyme should be considered a form of nutritional therapy since it is made up of naturally-occurring digestive enzymes. Entozyme enhances proteolysis by its peptic and tryptic activity, carbohydrate digestion by amylolytic activity, and fat emulsification and transport by lipolytic activity and the action of the bile salts. The components of six Entozyme tablets will digest 60 grams of fat, 48 grams of protein and 48 grams of carbohydrate, amounts of food that yield nearly 1,000 calories (one-third to one-half the daily caloric intake for many patients).

Indications and Usage: Entozyme is indicated for the relief of steatorrhea, pyrosis, flatulence, and belching associated with incomplete digestion of food due to a deficiency of digestive enzymes.

By effectively supplementing the patient's secretion of digestive enzymes, Entozyme promotes more complete digestion of carbohydrates, proteins and fats.

Contraindications: Biliary tract obstruction or hypersensitivity to any of the ingredients.

Warnings: Do not administer to patients who are allergic to pork products.

Precautions: *Carcinogenesis, mutagenesis.* Long-term studies in animals have not been performed to evaluate carcinogenic potential.

Pregnancy Category C. Animal reproduction studies have not been conducted with Entozyme. It is not known whether Entozyme can cause fetal harm when administered to a pregnant woman or can affect reproduction capacity. Entozyme should be given to a pregnant woman only if clearly needed.

Nursing mothers. It is not known whether this drug is excreted in human milk. Because many drugs are excreted in human milk, caution should be exercised when Entozyme is administered to a nursing woman.

Pediatric Use. Safety and effectiveness in children have not been established.

Adverse Reactions: Skin rash is the most freqently reported adverse reaction to Entozyme, and appears to be associated with hypersensitivity to pork protein in the pancreatin. At high doses, a laxative effect may occur.

Overdosage: Excessive dosage may produce a laxative effect. Systemic toxicity does not occur.

Dosage and Administration: Two tablets with each meal and 1 or 2 tablets with each snack. The dose may be increased as necessary to achieve adequate digestion. Entozyme tablets should be swallowed whole and not crushed or chewed.

How Supplied: White coated tablets, monogrammed "AHR" and 5049 in bottles of 100 (NDC 0031-5049-63) and 500 (NDC 0031-5049-70).

Store at controlled room temperature, between 15°C and 30°C (59°F and 86°F). Dispense in tight container.

[*Shown in Product Identification Section*]

EXNA® TABLETS ℞

brand of Benzthiazide Tablets, USP

Description: Each round, yellow scored Exna tablet contains benzthiazide 50 mg.

Action: The mechanism of action results in an interference with the renal tubular mechanism of electrolyte reabsorption. At maximal therapeutic dosage all thiazides are approximately equal in their diuretic potency. The mechanism whereby thiazides function in the control of hypertension is unknown.

Indications: Exna (benzthiazide) is indicated as adjunctive therapy in edema associated with congestive heart failure, hepatic cirrhosis and corticosteroid and estrogen therapy.

Exna has also been found useful in edema due to various forms of renal dysfunction as: nephrotic syndrome; acute glomerulonephritis; and chronic renal failure.

Exna is indicated in the management of hypertension either as the sole therapeutic agent or to enhance the effectiveness of other antihypertensive drugs in the more severe forms of hypertension.

Usage in Pregnancy. The routine use of diuretics in an otherwise healthy woman is inappropriate and exposes mother and fetus to unnecessary hazard. Diuretics do not prevent development of toxemia of pregnancy, and there is no satisfactory evidence that they are useful in the treatment of developed toxemia.

Edema during pregnancy may arise from pathological causes or from the physiologic and mechanical consequences of pregnancy. Thiazides are indicated in pregnancy when edema is due to pathologic causes, just as they are in the absence of pregnancy (however, see Warnings). Dependent edema in pregnancy, resulting from restriction of venous return by the expanded uterus, is properly treated through elevation of the lower extremities and use of support hose; use of diuretics to lower intravascular volume in this case is illogical and unnecessary. There is hypervolemia during normal pregnancy which is harmful to neither the fetus nor the mother (in the absence of cardiovascular disease), but which is associated with edema, including generalized edema, in the majority of pregnant women. If this edema produces discomfort, increased recumbency will often provide relief. In rare instances, this edema may cause extreme discomfort which is not relieved by rest. In these cases, a short course of diuretics may provide relief and may be appropriate.

Contraindications: Anuria. Hypersensitivity to this or other sulfonamide derived drugs.

Warnings: Thiazides should be used with caution in severe renal disease. In patients with renal disease, thiazides may precipitate azotemia. Cumulative effects of the drug may develop in patients with impaired renal function.

Thiazides should be used with caution in patients with impaired hepatic function or progressive liver disease, since minor alterations of fluid and electrolyte balance may precipitate hepatic coma.

Thiazides may add to or potentiate the action of other antihypertensive drugs. Potentiation occurs with ganglionic or peripheral adrenergic blocking drugs.

Sensitivity reactions may occur in patients with a history of allergy or bronchial asthma.

The possibility of exacerbation or activation of systemic lupus erythematosus has been reported.

Usage in Pregnancy: Thiazides cross the placental barrier and appear in cord blood. The use of thiazides in pregnant women requires that the anticipated benefit be weighed against possible hazards to the fetus. These hazards include fetal or neonatal jaundice, thrombocytopenia, and possibly other adverse reactions which have occurred in the adult.

Nursing Mothers. Thiazides appear in breast milk. If use of the drug is deemed essential, the patient should stop nursing.

Precautions: Periodic determination of serum electrolytes to detect possible electrolyte imbalance should be performed at appropriate intervals.

All patients receiving thiazide therapy should be observed for clinical signs of fluid or electrolyte imbalance; namely, hyponatremia, hypochloremic alkalosis, and hypokalemia. Serum and urine electrolyte determinations are particularly important when the patient is vomiting excessively or receiving parenteral fluids. Medication such as digitalis may also influence serum electrolytes. Warning signs, irrespective of cause, are: dryness of mouth, thirst, weakness, lethargy, drowsiness, restlessness, muscle pains or cramps, muscular fatigue, hypotension, oliguria, tachycardia, and gastrointestinal disturbances such as nausea and vomiting.

Hypokalemia may develop with thiazides as with any other potent diuretic especially with brisk diuresis, when severe cirrhosis is present or during concomitant use of corticosteroids or ACTH.

Interference with adequate oral electrolyte intake will also contribute to hypokalemia. Digitalis therapy may exaggerate metabolic effects of hypokalemia especially with reference to myocardial activity.

Any chloride deficit is generally mild and usually does not require specific treatment except under extraordinary circumstances (as in liver disease or renal disease). Dilutional hyponatremia may occur in edematous patients in hot weather; appropriate therapy is water restriction, rather than administration of salt except in rare instances when the hyponatremia is life threatening. In actual salt depletion, appropriate replacement is the therapy of choice.

Hyperuricemia may occur or frank gout may be precipitated in certain patients receiving thiazide therapy.

Insulin requirements in diabetic patients may be increased, decreased, or unchanged. Latent diabetes mellitus may become manifest during thiazide administration.

Thiazide drugs may increase the responsiveness to tubocurarine.

The antihypertensive effects of the drug may be enhanced in the postsympathectomy patient.

Thiazides may decrease arterial responsiveness to norepinephrine. This diminution is not sufficient to preclude effectiveness of the pressor agent for therapeutic use.

If progressive renal impairment becomes evident, as indicated by a rising nonprotein nitrogen or blood urea nitrogen, a careful reappraisal of therapy is necessary with consideration given to withholding or discontinuing diuretic therapy.

Thiazides may decrease serum PBI levels without signs of thyroid disturbance.

This product contains FD&C Yellow No. 5 (tartrazine) which may cause allergic-type reactions (including bronchial asthma) in certain susceptible individuals. Although the overall incidence of FD&C Yellow No. 5 (tartrazine) sensitivity in the general population is low, it is frequently seen in patients who have aspirin hypersensitivity.

Adverse Reactions: ***Gastrointestinal System Reaction:*** anorexia; gastric irritation; nausea; vomiting, cramping; diarrhea; constipation; jaundice (intrahepatic cholestatic jaundice); pancreatitis.

Central Nervous System Reactions: dizziness; vertigo; parasthesias; headache; xanthopsia.

Hematologic Reactions: leukopenia, agranulocytosis; thrombocytopenia; aplastic anemia.

Dermatologic-Hypersensitivity Reactions: purpura; photosensitivity; rash; urticaria; necrotizing angiitis (vasculitis) (cutaneous vasculitis).

Cardiovascular Reaction: Orthostatic hypotension may occur and may be aggravated by alcohol, barbiturates or narcotics.

Other: hyperglycemia; glycosuria; hyperuricemia; muscle spasm; weakness; restlessness.

Whenever adverse reactions are moderate or severe, thiazide dosage should be reduced or therapy withdrawn.

Dosage and Administration: Therapy should be individualized according to patient response. This therapy should be titrated to gain maximal therapeutic response as well as the minimal dose possible to maintain that therapeutic response.

	Diuretic	Antihypertensive
Benzthiazide	50 to 200 mg	50 to 200 mg

Continued on next page

Prescribing information on A. H. Robins products listed here is based on official labeling in effect August 1, 1982, with Indications, Contraindications, Warnings, Precautions, Adverse Reactions, and Dosage stated in full.

Robins—Cont.

Edema: ***Initiation of diuresis:*** 50 to 200 mg daily should be used for several days, or until dry weight is attained. With 100 mg or more daily, it is generally preferable to administer benzthiazide in two doses, following morning and evening meals.
Maintenance of diuresis: 50 to 150 mg daily depending upon the patient's response. To maintain effectiveness, reduction to minimal effective dosage should be gradual.
Hypertension: *Initiation of antihypertensive therapy:* 50 to 100 mg daily is the average dose. It may be given in two doses of 25 mg or 50 mg each after breakfast and after lunch. This dosage may be continued until a therapeutic drop in blood pressure occurs.
Maintenance of antihypertensive therapy: Dosage should be adjusted according to the patient response, either upward to as much as 50 mg q.i.d., or downward to the minimal effective dosage level.
How Supplied: Exna (benzthiazide) is supplied in 50 mg yellow, scored tablets, packaged in bottles of 100 (NDC 0031-5449-63).
[*Shown in Product Identification Section*]

MICRO-K EXTENCAPS® ℞
brand of Potassium Chloride

Description: Micro-K Extencaps are hard gelatin capsules, each containing 600 mg of dispersible small crystalline particles of potassium chloride (equivalent to 8 mEq K). Each particle is microencapsulated with a polymeric coating which allows for controlled release of potassium and chloride ions over an eight- to ten-hour period. The dispersibility of the microcapsules and the controlled release of ions are intended to minimize the likelihood of high localized concentrations of potassium chloride and resultant mucosal ulceration within the gastrointestinal tract.
The polymeric coating forming the microcapsules functions as a water-permeable membrane. Fluids pass through the membrane and gradually dissolve the potassium chloride within the microcapsules. The resulting potassium chloride solution slowly diffuses outward through the membrane.
Actions: Potassium ion is the principal intracellular cation of most body tissues. Potassium ions participate in a number of essential physiological processes, including the maintenance of intracellular tonicity, the transmission of nerve impulses, the contraction of cardiac, skeletal, and smooth muscle and the maintenance of normal renal function.
Potassium depletion may occur whenever the rate of potassium loss through renal excretion and/or loss from the gastrointestinal tract exceeds the rate of potassium intake. Such depletion usually develops slowly as a consequence of prolonged therapy with oral diuretics, primary or secondary hyperaldosteronism, diabetic ketoacidosis, severe diarrhea, or inadequate replacement of potassium in patients on prolonged parenteral nutrition. Potassium depletion due to these causes is usually accompanied by a concomitant deficiency of chloride and is manifested by hypokalemia and metabolic alkalosis. Potassium depletion may produce weakness, fatigue, disturbances of cardiac rhythm (primarily ectopic beats), prominent U-waves in the electrocardiogram, and in advanced cases, flaccid paralysis and/or impaired ability to concentrate urine.
Potassium depletion associated with metabolic alkalosis is managed by correcting the fundamental causes of the deficiency whenever possible and administering supplemental potassium chloride, in the form of high potassium food or potassium chloride solution, capsules or tablets. In rare circumstances (e.g., patients with renal tubular acidosis) potassium depletion may be associated with metabolic acidosis and hyperchloremia. In such patients potassium replacement should be accomplished with potassium salts other than the chloride, such as potassium bicarbonate, potassium citrate, or potassium acetate.
INDICATIONS: BECAUSE OF REPORTS OF INTESTINAL AND GASTRIC ULCERATION AND BLEEDING WITH SLOW-RELEASE POTASSIUM CHLORIDE PREPARATIONS, THESE DRUGS SHOULD BE RESERVED FOR THOSE PATIENTS WHO CANNOT TOLERATE OR REFUSE TO TAKE LIQUID OR EFFERVESCENT POTASSIUM PREPARATIONS OR FOR PATIENTS IN WHOM THERE IS A PROBLEM OF COMPLIANCE WITH THESE PREPARATIONS.
1. For therapeutic use in patients with hypokalemia with or without metabolic alkalosis; in digitalis intoxication and in patients with hypokalemic familial periodic paralysis.
2. For prevention of potassium depletion when the dietary intake of potassium is inadequate in the following conditions: patients receiving digitalis and diuretics for congestive heart failure; hepatic cirrhosis with ascites; states of aldosterone excess with normal renal function; potassium-losing nephropathy, and certain diarrheal states.
3. The use of potassium salts in patients receiving diuretics for uncomplicated essential hypertension is often unnecessary when such patients have a normal dietary pattern. Serum potassium should be checked periodically, however, and, if hypokalemia occurs, dietary supplementation with potassium-containing foods may be adequate to control milder cases. In more severe cases, supplementation with potassium salts may be indicated.
Contraindications: Potassium supplements are contraindicated in patients with hyperkalemia since a further increase in serum potassium concentration in such patients can produce cardiac arrest. Hyperkalemia may complicate any of the following conditions: chronic renal failure, systemic acidosis such as diabetic acidosis, acute dehydration, extensive tissue breakdown as in severe burns, adrenal insufficiency, or the administration of a potassium-sparing diuretic (e.g., spironolactone, triamterene).
Wax-matrix potassium chloride preparations have produced esophageal ulceration in certain cardiac patients with esophageal compression due to an enlarged left atrium.
All solid dosage forms of potassium supplements are contraindicated in any patient in whom there is cause for arrest or delay in tablet passage through the gastrointestinal tract. In these instances, potassium supplementation should be with a liquid preparation.
Warnings: *Hyperkalemia.* In patients with impaired mechanisms for excreting potassium, the administration of potassium salts can produce hyperkalemia and cardiac arrest. This occurs most commonly in patients given potassium by the intravenous route but may also occur in patients given potassium orally. Potentially fatal hyperkalemia can develop rapidly and be asymptomatic.
The use of potassium salts in patients with chronic renal disease, or any other condition which impairs potassium excretion, requires particularly careful monitoring of the serum potassium concentration and appropriate dosage adjustments.
Interaction with Potassium-Sparing Diuretics. Hypokalemia should not be treated by the concomitant administration of potassium salts and a potassium-sparing diuretic (e.g., spironolactone or triamterene), since the simultaneous administration of these agents can produce severe hyperkalemia.
Gastrointestinal lesions. Potassium chloride tablets have produced stenotic and/or ulcerative lesions of the small bowel and deaths, in addition to upper gastrointestinal bleeding. These lesions are caused by a high localized concentration of potassium ion in the region of a rapidly dissolving tablet which injures the bowel wall and thereby produces obstruction, hemorrhage, or perforation.
Micro-K Extencaps contain microcapsules which disperse upon dissolution of the hard gelatin capsule. The microcapsules are formulated to provide a controlled release of potassium chloride. The dispersibility of the microcapsules and the controlled release of ions from the microcapsules are intended to minimize the possibility of a high local concentration near the gastrointestinal mucosa and the ability of the KCl to cause stenosis or ulceration. Other means of accomplishing this (e.g., incorporation of KCl into a wax matrix) have reduced the frequency of such lesions to less than one per 100,000 patient years (compared to 40–50 per 100,000 patient years with enteric-coated KCl), but have not eliminated them. The frequency of GI lesions with Micro-K Extencaps is, at present, unknown. Micro-K Extencaps should be discontinued immediately and the possibility of bowel obstruction or perforation considered if severe vomiting, abdominal pain, distention, or gastrointestinal bleeding occurs.
Metabolic Acidosis. Hypokalemia in patients with metabolic *acidosis* should be treated with an alkalinizing potassium salt such as potassium bicarbonate, potassium citrate, or potassium acetate.
Precautions: The diagnosis of potassium depletion is ordinarily made by demonstrating hypokalemia in a patient with a clinical history suggesting some cause for potassium depletion. In interpreting the serum potassium level, the physician should bear in mind that acute alkalosis per se can produce hypokalemia in the absence of a deficit in total body potassium, while acute acidosis per se can increase the serum potassium concentration into the normal range even in the presence of a reduced total body potassium. The treatment of potassium depletion, particularly in the presence of cardiac disease, renal disease, or acidosis, requires careful attention to acid-base balance and appropriate monitoring of serum electrolytes, the electrocardiogram, and the clinical status of the patient.
Adverse Reactions: The most common adverse reactions to oral potassium salts are nausea, vomiting, abdominal discomfort, and diarrhea. These symptoms are due to irritation of the gastrointestinal tract and may be minimized by taking the dose with meals or by reducing the dose.
Intestinal bleeding, ulceration, perforation and obstruction have been reported in patients treated with solid dosage forms of potassium salts and may occur with Micro-K Extencaps (see Contraindications and Warnings).
One of the most severe adverse effects of potassium supplementation is hyperkalemia (see Contraindications, Warnings, and Overdosage).
Skin rash has been reported rarely with potassium preparations.
Overdosage: The administration of oral potassium salts to persons with normal excretory mechanisms for potassium rarely causes serious hyperkalemia. However, if excretory mechanisms are impaired or if potassium is administered too rapidly intravenously, potentially fatal hyperkalemia can result (see Contraindications and Warnings). It is important to recognize that hyperkalemia is usually asymptomatic and may be manifested only by an increased serum potassium concentration and characteristic electrocardiogram changes (peaking of T-waves, loss of P-wave, depression of S-T segment, and prolongation of the QT interval). Late manifestations include muscle paralysis and cardiovascular collapse from cardiac arrest.
Treatment measures for hyperkalemia include the following: (1) elimination of foods and medications containing potassium and of potassium-sparing diuretics; (2) intravenous adminis-

tration of 300 to 500 ml/hr of 10% dextrose solution containing 10–20 units of insulin per 1,000 ml; (3) correction of acidosis, if present, with intravenous sodium bicarbonate; (4) use of exchange resins, hemodialysis, or peritoneal dialysis.

In treating hyperkalemia, it should be recalled that in patients who have been stabilized on digitalis, too rapid a lowering of the serum potassium concentration can produce digitalis toxicity.

Dosage and Administration: The usual dietary intake of potassium by the average adult is 40 to 80 mEq per day. Potassium depletion sufficient to cause hypokalemia usually requires the loss of 200 or more mEq of potassium from the total body store.

Dosage must be adjusted to the individual needs of each patient, but typically is in the range of 2 to 3 Micro-K Extencaps per day (16 to 24 mEq K) for the prevention of hypokalemia and 5 to 12 Micro-K Extencaps (40 to 96 mEq K) or more per day for the treatment of potassium depletion. If more than 2 Micro-K Extencaps are prescribed per day, the total daily dosage should be divided into two or more separate doses.

How Supplied: Pale orange capsules (Extencaps), each containing 600 mg microencapsulated potassium chloride (equivalent to 8 mEq K) in bottles of 100 (NDC 0031-5720-63), and 500 (NDC 0031-5720-70) and Dis-Co® unit dose packs of 100 (NDC 0031-5720-64).

Animal Toxicology: The ulcerogenic potential of microencapsulated KCl was studied in anesthetized cats by direct applications on exteriorized gastric mucosa. The microcapsules of KCl were found to be non-ulcerogenic and significantly less irritating than wax-matrix tablets and 20% solution of KCl.

In groups of monkeys (up to 8 monkeys per group) receiving different formulations of potassium chloride at equivalent daily dosage (2400 mg KCl) for four and one-half days, Micro-K Extencaps showed no tendency to cause intestinal ulceration (similar to liquid KCl and a wax-matrix preparation but in contrast to an enteric-coated KCl tablet) and minimal gastric irritation (less than a wax-matrix preparation).

U.S. Patent No. 4,259,315

[Shown in Product Identification Section]

MITROLAN® TABLETS

brand of Calcium Polycarbophil

Each chewable tablet contains:
Calcium Polycarbophil (equivalent to 500 mg Polycarbophil, USP)

Actions: Mitrolan (calcium polycarbophil) is a hydrophilic agent. As a bulk laxative, Mitrolan retains free water within the lumen of the intestine, and indirectly opposes dehydrating forces of the bowel, promoting well-formed stools. In diarrhea, when the intestinal mucosa is incapable of absorbing water at normal rates, Mitrolan absorbs free fecal water, forming a gel and producing formed stools. Thus, in both diarrhea and constipation, the drug works by restoring a more normal moisture level and providing bulk in the patient's intestinal tract.

Indications: For the treatment of constipation or diarrhea, associated with conditions such as irritable bowel syndrome and diverticulosis. Also for the treatment of acute non-specific diarrhea. Restores normal stool consistency by regulating its water and bulk content.

Contraindications: As with all hydrophilic bulking agents, calcium polycarbophil should not be used in patients with signs of gastrointestinal obstruction.

Adverse Reactions: Abdominal fullness may be noted occasionally. An adjustment of the dosage schedule with smaller doses given more frequently but spaced evenly throughout the day may provide relief of this symptom during continued use of Mitrolan.

Drug Interaction: Antacids containing aluminum, calcium or magnesium impair absorption of tetracycline. Although Mitrolan is not an antacid, it releases free calcium after ingestion and should not be used by any patient who is taking a prescription antibiotic drug containing any form of tetracycline.

Directions of Use:

CHEW TABLETS BEFORE SWALLOWING.

Recommended dosage for OTC use: Adults—Chew and swallow 2 tablets 4 times a day, or as needed. Do not exceed 12 tablets in a 24-hour period. Children (6 to under 12 years)—Chew and swallow 1 tablet 3 times a day, or as needed. Do not exceed 6 tablets in a 24-hour period. Children (3 to under 6 years)—Chew and swallow 1 tablet 2 times a day, or as needed. Do not exceed 3 tablets in a 24-hour period.

For episodes of severe diarrhea, the dose may be repeated every ½ hour, but do not exceed the maximum daily dosage.

Dosage may be adjusted according to individual response.

When using as a laxative, patient should drink a full glass (8 fl. oz.) of water or other liquid with each dose.

Sodium Content: Less than 0.02 mEq (0.46 mg) per tablet.

How Supplied: ***Chewable Tablets***—cartons of 36 individually packaged blister units (NDC 0031-1535-57), and bottles of 100 (NDC 0031-1535-63).

[Shown in Product Identification Section]

PABALATE® TABLETS

Description: Pabalate® tablets are intended for oral administration.

Each enteric-coated tablet contains:
Sodium Salicylate, USP ....0.3 g
Sodium Adminobenzoate ....0.3 g

Clinical Pharmacology: Sodium salicylate is a mild analgesic with antiinflammatory and antipyretic activity. Compared to aspirin, sodium salicylate has substantially less effect on platelet adhesiveness. In large doses, however, it has a hypoprothrombinemic effect. Sodium salicylate in conventional dosage form dissolves in the stomach and is absorbed as unionized salicylic acid. However, in Pabalate, the enteric coating delays release of the salicylate until the tablet reaches the alkaline medium of the intestine. After absorption, salicylic acid is extensively bound to plasma protein, and the bound portion is in equilibrium with the free salicylate in the plasma. The action of sodium aminobenzoate in this formulation has not been established.

Indications: Pabalate tablets are indicated for the temporary relief of mild to moderate pain.

Contraindications: Hypersensitivity to any of the ingredients. Presence of an active ulcer, hypoprothrombinemia, Vitamin K deficiency, severe hepatic or renal damage, or hemophilia. This product is not recommended for persons on a sodium-restricted diet.

Precautions:

General: Treatment with salicylates may interfere with blood clotting; therefore, salicylate therapy should be stopped at least one week prior to surgery.

Drug Interaction: This product contains sodium aminobenzoate, the aminobenzoic acid portion of which inhibits the bacteriostatic action of sulfonamides when the two are present concurrently.

Carcinogenesis, mutagenesis: Long-term studies in animals have not been performed to evaluate carcinogenic potential.

Pregnancy Category C: Animal reproduction studies have not been conducted with Pabalate.

Safe use of Pabalate has not been established with regard to possible adverse effects upon fetal development. Therefore, Pabalate should not be used in women who are or may become pregnant and particularly during early pregnancy unless in the judgment of the physician the potential benefits outweigh the possible hazards.

Nursing Mothers: Salicylates appear in human milk in moderate amounts. They can produce a bleeding tendency by decreasing the amount of prothrombin in the infant's blood. As a general rule, nursing should not be undertaken while a patient is on this drug.

Pediatric Use: Safety and effectiveness in children below the age of 12 years have not been established.

Adverse Reactions: The most frequent adverse reactions to products such as Pabalate which contain salicylates are nausea and gastrointestinal upset. Fine rash with or without pruritus and urticaria occus less frequently. The occasional occurrence of mild salicylism (diarrhea, tinnitus, dizziness) may require an adjustment in dosage.

Overdosage: Mild chronic overdosage, termed salicylism, may cause symptoms such as tinnitus, nausea, headache, hyperventilation, dizziness, drowsiness, mental confusion, dimness of vision, sweating, thirst and occasionally diarrhea. Withdrawal of salicylates and supportive therapy may be sufficient treatment.

A more severe degree of salicylate intoxication may occur with acute massive overdosage or the chronic administration of more moderate overdoses, especially in infants and children. CNS effects are more pronounced and may progress to dilirium, hallucinations, gereralized convulsions and coma. A variety of cutaneous lesions may be observed.

A most important feature of salicylate intoxication is a disturbance of acid-base balance and plasma electrolytes. Careful monitoring of these laboratory parameters along with plasma glucose concentration is essential. The type and quantity of repair solutions used will depend upon interpretation of the laboratory data. Bicarbonate solution should be administered IV in order to produce alkaline diuresis. Correction of hypoglycemia and ketosis by the administration of glucose is essential.

Since hyperthermia and dehydration are immediate threats to life, external sponging and the administration of adequate quantities of IV fluids are important first steps to correct these conditions and maintain adequate renal function.

If hemorrhagic phenomena (petechiae, thrombocytopenia) occur, whole blood transfusions and vitamin K may be necessary.

The gastrointestinal tract should be emptied either by emesis or purging to remove undissolved tablets in cases of acute ingestion of a large single dose. Since enteric coated tablets do not disintegrate in the stomach, they cannot be removed by lavage.

Rapid and immediate removal of salicylate from the body by alkaline diuresis is essential. In more severe cases, extrarenal measures such as peritoneal dialysis, hemodialysis, hemoperfusion or exchange transfusion may be required.

Dosage and Administration: The average adult dose is two tablets every 4 hours. Due to the enteric coating, tablets should not be taken within one hour of ingesting milk or antacids.

How Supplied: Yellow, enteric-coated tablets, monogrammed AHR and 5816 in bottles of 100 (NDC 0031-5816-63) and 500 (NDC 0031-5816-70).

Continued on next page

Prescribing information on A. H. Robins products listed here is based on official labeling in effect August 1, 1982, with Indications, Contraindications, Warnings, Precautions, Adverse Reactions, and Dosage stated in full.

Robins—Cont.

Store at Controlled Room Temperature, Between 15°C and 30°C (59°F and 86°F).
[*Shown in Product Identification section*]

PABALATE®–SF TABLETS ℞

Description: Pabalate®-SF tablets are intended for oral administration.
Each enteric-coated tablet contains:
Potassium Salicylate ....0.3 g
Potassium Aminobenzoate ....0.3 g
Potassium content per tablet:
131.5 mg (3.4 mEq)
Clinical Pharmacology: Potassium salicylate is a mild analgesic with antiinflammatory and antipyretic activity. Compared to aspirin, potassium salicylate has substantially less effect on platelet adhesiveness. In large doses, however, it has a hypoprothrombinemic effect. Potassium salicylate in conventional dosage form dissolves in the stomach and is absorbed as un-ionized salicylic acid. However, in Pabalate-SF, the enteric coating delays release of the salicylate until the tablet reaches the alkaline medium of the intestine. After absorption, salicylic acid is extensively bound to plasma protein, and the bound portion is in equilibrium with the free salicylate in the plasma. The action of potassium aminobenzoate in this formulation has not been established.
Indications: Pabalate-SF tablets are indicated for the temporary relief of mild to moderate pain complicated by conditions in which the restriction of sodium intake may be desirable, such as: congestive heart failure, essential hypertension and glomerulonephritis.
Contraindications: Hypersensitivity to any of the ingredients. Presence of an active ulcer, hypoprothrombinemia, Vitamin K deficiency, severe hepatic or renal damage, hemophilia, or hyperkalemia. Do not administer to patients who are receiving a potassium-sparing diuretic.
Warnings: There have been several reports, published and unpublished, concerning nonspecific small bowel lesions consisting of stenosis with or without ulceration, associated with the administration of enteric-coated thiazides with potassium salts. These lesions may occur with enteric-coated potassium tablets alone or when they are used with nonenteric-coated thiazides, or certain other oral diuretics.
These small bowel lesions have caused obstruction, hemorrhage, and perforation. Surgery was frequently required and deaths have occurred.
Based on a large survey of physicians and hospitals, both American and foreign, the incidence of these lesions is low, and a causal relationship in man has not been definitely established.
Available information tends to implicate enteric-coated potassium salts although lesions of this type also occur spontaneously. Therefore, coated potassium-containing formulations should be administered only when indicated, and should be discontinued immediately if abdominal pain, distension, nausea, vomiting, or gastrointestinal bleeding occur.
When prescribing Pabalate-SF for patients who are receiving concurrent potassium supplementation (e.g., to replace potassium excreted during thiazide therapy), it should be kept in mind that each Pabalate-SF tablet contains 131.5 mg (3.4 mEq) of potassium. A decrease in supplemental potassium dosage should be considered in order to avoid hyperkalemia.
The use of potassium salts in patients with chronic renal disease, or any other condition which impairs potassium excretion, requires particularly careful monitoring of the serum potassium concentration and appropriate dosage adjustment.
Precautions: ***General:*** Treatment with salicylates may interfere with blood clotting; therefore, salicylate therapy should be stopped at least one week prior to surgery.
Drug Interaction: This product contains aminobenzoic acid which inhibits the bacteriostatic action of sulfonamides when the two are administered concurrently.
Carcinogenesis, mutagenesis: Long-term studies in animals have not been performed to evaluate carcinogenic potential.
Pregnancy Category C: Animal reproduction studies have not been conducted with Pabalate-SF.
Safe use of Pabalate-SF has not been established with regard to possible adverse effects upon fetal development. Therefore, Pabalate-SF should not be used in women who are or may become pregnant and particularly during early pregnancy unless in the judgment of the physician the potential benefits outweigh the possible hazards.
Nursing Mothers: Salicylates appear in human milk in moderate amounts. They can produce a bleeding tendency by decreasing the amount of prothrombin in the infant's blood. As a general rule, nursing should not be undertaken while a patient is on this drug.
Pediatric Use: Safety and effectiveness in children below the age of 12 have not been established.
Adverse Reactions: Hyperkalemia is a potential adverse effect (see Contraindications and Warnings). The most frequent adverse reactions to products such as Pabalate-SF which contain potassium and/or salicylates are nausea and gastrointestinal upset. Fine rash with or without pruritus and urticaria occur less frequently. The occasional occurrence of mild salicylism may require adjustment in dosage.
Overdosage: Overdose may cause symptoms of hyperkalemia and/or salicylate intoxication. Mild chronic overdosage, termed salicylism, may cause symptoms such as tinnitus, nausea, headache, hyperventilation, dizziness, drowsiness, mental confusion, dimness of vision, sweating, thirst, and occasionally diarrhea. Withdrawal of salicylates and supportive therapy may be sufficient treatment.
A more severe degree of salicylate intoxication may occur with acute massive overdosage or the chronic administration of more moderate overdoses, especially in infants and children. CNS effects are more pronounced and may progress to dilirium, hallucinations, generalized convulsions and coma. A variety of cutaneous lesions may be observed.
A most important feature of salicylate intoxication is a disturbance of acid-base balance and plasma electrolytes. Careful monitoring of these laboratory parameters along with plasma glucose concentration is essential. The type and quantity of repair solutions used will depend upon interpretation of the laboratory data. Bicarbonate solution should be administered IV in order to produce alkaline diuresis. Correction of hypoglycemia and ketosis by the administration of glucose is essential.
Since hyperthermia and dehydration are immediate treats to life, external sponging and the administration of adequate quantities of IV fluids are important first steps to correct these conditions and maintain adequate renal function.
If hemorrhagic phenomena (petechiae, thrombocytopenia) occur, whole blood transfusions and vitamin K may be necessary.
The gastrointestinal tract should be emptied either by emesis or purging to remove undissolved tablets in cases of acute ingestion of a large single dose. Since enteric-coated tablets do not disintegrate in the stomach, they cannot be removed by lavage.
Rapid and immediate removal of salicylate from the body by alkaline diuresis is essential. In more severe cases, extrarenal measures such as peritoneal dialysis, hemodialysis, hemoperfusion or exchange transfusion may be required.
Dosage and Administration: The average adult dose is two tablets every 4 hours. Due to the enteric coating, tablets should not be taken within one hour of ingesting milk or antacids.
How Supplied: Persian rose, enteric-coated tablets, monogrammed AHR and 5883 in bottles of 100 (NDC 0031-5883-63) and 500 (NDC 0031-5883-70).
Store at Controlled Room Temperature, Between 15°C and 30°C (59°F and 86°F).
Dispense in well-closed container.
[*Shown in Product Identification Section*]

PHENAPHEN® WITH CODEINE NO. 2 ℞ ©

Codeine Phosphate, USP ....15 mg
(Warning: May be habit forming)
Acetaminophen, USP ....325 mg

PHENAPHEN® WITH CODEINE NO. 3 ℞ ©

Codeine Phosphate, USP ....30 mg
(Warning: May be habit forming)
Acetaminophen, USP ....325 mg

PHENAPHEN® WITH CODEINE NO. 4 ℞ ©

Codeine Phosphate, USP ....60 mg
(Warning: May be habit forming)
Acetaminophen, USP ....325 mg

Description: Acetaminophen occurs as a white, odorless, crystalline powder possessing a slightly bitter taste. Codeine is an alkaloid, obtained from opium or prepared from morphine by methylation. Codeine occurs as colorless or white crystals, effloresces slowly in dry air and is affected by light.
Actions: Acetaminophen is a non-opiate, non-salicylate analgesic and antipyretic. Codeine is an opiate analgesic and antitussive. Codeine retains at least one-half of its analgesic activity when administered orally.
Indications and Usage: Phenaphen with Codeine No. 2 is indicated for the relief of mild to moderately severe pain.
Phenaphen with Codeine No. 3 is indicated for the relief of mild to moderately severe pain.
Phenaphen with Codeine No. 4 is indicated for the relief of moderate to moderately severe pain.
Contraindications: Hypersensitivity to acetaminophen or codeine.
Warnings: ***Drug dependence.*** Codeine can produce drug dependence of the morphine type, and, therefore, has the potential for being abused. Psychic dependence, physical dependence and tolerance may develop upon repeated administration of this drug and it should be prescribed and administered with the same degree of caution appropriate to the use of other oral narcotic medications. These acetaminophen with codeine dosage forms are subject to the Federal Controlled Substances Act (Schedule III).
Precautions: ***General:***
Head injury and increased intracranial pressure. The respiratory depressant effects of narcotics and their capacity to elevate cerebrospinal fluid pressure may be markedly exaggerated in the presence of head injury, other intracranial lesions or a pre-existing increase in intracranial pressure. Furthermore, narcotics produce adverse reactions which may obscure the clinical course of patients with head injuries.
Acute abdominal condition. The administration of products containing codeine or other narcotics may obscure the diagnosis or clinical course in patients with acute abdominal conditions.
Special risk patients. Acetaminophen with codeine should be given with caution to certain patients such as the elderly or debilitated, and those with severe impairment of hepatic or renal function, hypothyroidism, Addison's dis-

ease, and prostatic hypertrophy or urethral stricture.

Information for Patients. Codeine may impair the mental and/or physical abilities required for the performance of potentially hazardous tasks such as driving a car or operating machinery. The patient taking this drug should be cautioned accordingly.

Drug Interactions. Patients receiving other narcotic analgesics, antipsychotics, antianxiety agents, or other CNS depressants (including alcohol) concomitantly with acetaminophen and codeine may exhibit additive CNS depression due to codeine component. When such therapy is contemplated, the dose of one or both agents should be reduced.

The use of monoamine oxidase inhibitors or tricyclic antidepressants with codeine preparations may increase the effect of either the antidepressant or codeine.

The concurrent use of anticholinergics with codeine may produce paralytic use.

Usage in Pregnancy. Safe use in pregnancy has not been established relative to possible adverse effects on fetal development. Therefore, acetaminophen and codeine should not be used in pregnant women unless, in the judgment of the physician, the potential benefits outweigh the possible hazards.

Nursing Mothers. It is not known whether the components of this drug are excreted in human milk. Because many drugs are excreted in human milk, caution should be exercised when acetaminophen with codeine is administered to a nursing woman.

Adverse Reactions: The most frequently observed adverse reactions include lightheadedness, dizziness, sedation; shortness of breath, nausea and vomiting. These effects seem to be more prominent in ambulatory than in nonambulatory patients, and some of these adverse reactions may be alleviated if the patient lies down.

Other adverse reactions include euphoria, dysphoria, constipation and pruritus. At higher doses, codeine has most of the disadvantages of morphine including respiratory depression.

Overdosage:

Acetaminophen:

Signs and Symptoms: Acetaminophen in massive overdosage may cause hepatic toxicity in some patients. In all cases of suspected overdose, immediately call your regional poison center or the Rocky Mountain Poison Center's toll-free number (800-525-6115) for assistance in diagnosis and for directions in the use of N-acetylcysteine as an antidote, a use currently restricted to investigational status.

In adults, hepatic toxicity has rarely been reported with acute overdoses of less than 10 grams and fatalities with less than 15 grams. Importantly, young children seem to be more resistant than adults to the hepatotoxic effect of an acetaminophen overdose. Despite this, the measures outlined below should be initiated in any adult or child suspected of having ingested an acetaminophen overdose.

Early symptoms following a potentially hepatotoxic overdose may include nausea, vomiting, diaphoresis and general malaise. Clinical and laboratory evidence of hepatic toxicity may not be apparent until 48 to 72 hours post-ingestion.

Treatment: The stomach should be emptied promptly by lavage or by induction of emesis with syrup of ipecac. Patient's estimates of the quantity of a drug ingested are notoriously unreliable. Therefore, if an acetaminophen overdose is suspected, a serum acetaminophen assay should be obtained as early as possible, but no sooner than four hours following ingestion. Liver function studies should be obtained initially and repeated at 24-hour intervals.

The antidote, N-acetylcysteine, should be administered as early as possible, and within 16 hours of the overdose ingestion for optimal results. Following recovery, there are no residual, structural or functional hepatic abnormalities.

Codeine:

Signs and Symptoms: Serious overdose with codeine is characterized by respiratory depression (a decrease in respiratory rate and/or tidal volume. Cheyne-Stokes respiration, cyanosis), extreme somnolence progressing to stupor or coma, skeletal muscle flaccidity, cold and clammy skin, and sometimes bradycardia and hypotension. In severe overdosage, apnea, circulatory collapse, cardiac arrest and death may occur.

Treatment: Primary attention should be given to the reestablishment of adequate respiratory exchange through provision of a patent airway and the institution of assisted or controlled ventilation. The narcotic antagonist naloxone is a specific antidote against respiratory depression which may result from overdosage or unusual sensitivity to narcotics, including codeine. Therefore, an appropriate dose of naloxone (see package insert) should be administered, preferably by the intravenous route, and simultaneously with efforts at respiratory resuscitation. Since the duration of action of codeine may exceed that of the antagonist, the patient should be kept under continued surveillance and repeated doses of the antagonist should be administered as needed to maintain adequate respiration.

An antagonist should not be administered in the absence of clinically significant respiratory or cardiovascular depression. Oxygen, intravenous fluids, vasopressors and other supportive measures should be employed as indicated.

Gastric emptying may be useful in removing unabsorbed drug.

Dosage and Administration: Dosage should be adjusted according to severity of pain and response of the patient. However, it should be kept in mind that tolerance to codeine can develop with continued use and that the incidence of untoward effects is dose related. This product is inappropriate even in high doses for severe or intractable pain. Adult doses of codeine higher than 60 mg fail to give commensurate relief of pain but merely prolong analgesia and are associated with an appreciably increased incidence of undesirable side effects. Equivalently high doses in children would have similar effects. The usual adult dose for Phenaphen with Codeine No. 2 and Phenaphen with Codeine No. 3 is one or two capsules every 4 hours as required. The usual adult dose for Phenaphen with Codeine No. 4 is one capsule every 4 hours as required.

How Supplied: Phenaphen with Codeine No. 2, black and yellow capsules in bottles of 100 (NDC 0031-6242-63) and 500 (NDC 0031-6242-70) and Dis-Co® Unit Dose Packs (4 × 25's) (6242-61).

Phenaphen with Codeine No. 3, black and green capsules in bottles of 100 (NDC 0031-6257-63) and 500 (NDC 0031-6257-70) and Dis-Co® Unit Dose Packs (4 × 25's) (6257-61) and (40 × 25's) (6257-72).

Phenaphen with Codeine No. 4, green and white capsules in bottles of 100 (NDC 0031-6274-63) and 500 (NDC 0031-6274-70) and Dis-Co® Unit Dose Packs (4 × 25's) (6274-61).

Store at controlled room temperature, between 15°C and 30°C (59°F and 86°F).

Dispense capsules in well-closed container.

Also available without codeine as Phenaphen® Capsules containing 325 mg of acetaminophen.

[Shown in Product Identification Section]

PHENAPHEN®-650 WITH CODEINE TABLETS ℞ Ⓒ

Description:

Each Phenaphen®-650 with Codeine tablet contains:

Codeine Phosphate, USP .... 30 mg
(Warning: May be habit forming)
Acetaminophen, USP .... 650 mg

Acetaminophen occurs as a white, odorless, crystalline powder possessing a slightly bitter taste. Codeine is an alkaloid, obtained from opium or prepared from morphine by methylation. Codeine occurs as colorless or white crystals, effloresces slowly in dry air and is affected by light.

Actions: Acetaminophen is a non-opiate, non-salicylate analgesic and antipyretic. Codeine is an opiate analgesic and antitussive. Codeine retains at least one-half of its analgesic activity when administered orally.

Indications and Usage: Phenaphen-650 with Codeine is indicated for the relief of mild to moderately severe pain.

Contraindications: Hypersensitivity to acetaminophen or codeine.

Warnings: ***Drug dependence.*** Codeine can produce drug dependence of the morphine type, and, therefore, has the potential for being abused. Psychic dependence, physical dependence and tolerance may develop upon repeated administration of this drug and it should be prescribed and administered with the same degree of caution appropriate to the use of other oral narcotic medications. This acetaminophen with codeine dosage form is subject to the Federal Controlled Substances Act (Schedule III).

Precautions: ***General:***

Head Injury and increased intracranial pressure. The respiratory depressant effects of narcotics and their capacity to elevate cerebrospinal fluid pressure may be markedly exaggerated in the presence of head injury, other intracranial lesions or a pre-existing increase in intracranial pressure. Furthermore, narcotics product adverse reactions which may obscure the clinical course of patients with head injuries.

Acute abdominal conditions. The administration of products containing codeine or other narcotics may obscure the diagnosis or clinical course in patients with acute abdominal conditions.

Special risk patients. Acetaminophen with codeine should be given with caution to certain patients such as the elderly or debilitated, and those with severe impairment of hepatic or renal function, hypothyroidism, Addison's disease, and prostatic hypertrophy or urethral stricture.

Information for Patients. Codeine may impair the mental and/or physical abilities required for the performance of potentially hazardous tasks such as driving a car or operating machinery. The patient taking this drug should be cautioned accordingly.

Drug Interactions. Patients receiving other narcotic analgesics, antipsychotics, antianxiety agents, or other CNS depressants (including alcohol) concomitantly with acetaminophen and codeine may exhibit additive CNS depression due to the codeine component. When such therapy is contemplated, the dose of one or both agents should be reduced.

The use of monoamine oxidase inhibitors or tricyclic antidepressants with codeine preparations may increase the effect of either the antidepressant or codeine.

The concurrent use of anticholinergics with codeine may produce paralytic ileus.

Usage in Pregnancy. Safe use in pregnancy has not been established relative to possible

Continued on next page

Prescribing information on A. H. Robins products listed here is based on official labeling in effect August 1, 1982, with Indications, Contraindications, Warnings, Precautions, Adverse Reactions, and Dosage stated in full.

Robins—Cont.

adverse effects on fetal development. Therefore, acetaminophen and codeine should not be used in pregnant women unless, in the judgment of the physician, the potential benefits outweigh the possible hazards.

Nursing Mothers. It is not known whether the components of this drug are excreted in human milk. Because many drugs are excreted in human milk, caution should be exercised when acetaminophen with codeine is administered to a nursing woman.

Adverse Reactions. The most frequently observed adverse reactions include lightheadedness, dizziness, sedation; shortness of breath, nausea and vomiting. These effects seem to be more prominent in ambulatory than in nonambulatory patients, and some of these adverse reactions may be alleviated if the patient lies down.

Other adverse reactions include euphoria, dysphoria, constipation and pruritus. At higher doses, codeine has most of the disadvantages of morphine including respiratory depression.

Overdosage:

Acetaminophen:

Signs and Symptoms: Acetaminophen in massive overdosage may cause hepatic toxicity in some patients. In all cases of suspected overdose, immediately call your regional poison center or the Rocky Mountain Poison Center's toll-free number (800-525-6115) for assistance in diagnosis and for directions in the use of N-acetylcysteine as an antidote, a use currently restricted to investigational status.

In adults, hepatic toxicity has rarely been reported with acute overdoses of less than 10 grams and fatalities with less than 15 grams. Importantly, young children seem to be more resistant than adults to the hepatotoxic effect of an acetaminophen overdose. Despite this, the measures outlined below should be initiated in any adult or child suspected of having ingested an acetaminophen overdose.

Early symptoms following a potentially hepatotoxic overdose may include: nausea, vomiting, diaphoresis and general malaise. Clinical and laboratory evidence of hepatic toxicity may not be apparent until 48 to 72 hours post-ingestion.

Treatment: The stomach should be emptied promptly by lavage or by induction of emesis with syrup of ipecac. Patient's estimates of the quantity of a drug ingested are notoriously unreliable. Therefore, if an acetaminophen overdose is suspected, a serum acetaminophen assay should be obtained as early as possible, but no sooner than four hours following ingestion. Liver function studies should be obtained initially and repeated at 24-hour intervals.

The antidote, N-acetylcysteine, should be administered as early as possible, and within 16 hours of the overdose ingestion for optimal results. Following recovery, there are no residual, structural or functional hepatic abnormalities.

Codeine:

Signs and Symptoms: Serious overdose with codeine is characterized by respiratory depression (a decrease in respiratory rate and/or tidal volume, Cheyne-Stokes respiration, cyanosis), extreme somnolence progressing to stupor or coma, skeletal muscle flaccidity, cold and clammy skin, and sometimes bradycardia and hypotension. In severe overdosage, apnea, circulatory collapse, cardiac arrest and death may occur.

Treatment: Primary attention should be given to the reestablishment of adequate respiratory exchange through provision of a patent airway and the institution of assisted or controlled ventilation. The narcotic antagonist naloxone is a specific antidote against respiratory depression which may result from overdosage or unusual sensitivity to narcotics, including codeine. Therefore, an appropriate dose of naloxone (see package insert) should be administered, preferably by the intravenous route, and simultaneously with efforts at respiratory resuscitation. Since the duration of action of codeine may exceed that of the antagonist, the patient should be kept under continued surveillance and repeated doses of the antagonist should be administered as needed to maintain adequate respiration.

An antagonist should not be administered in the absence of clinically significant respiratory or cardiovascular depression. Oxygen, intravenous fluids, vasopressors and other supportive measures should be employed as indicated.

Gastric emptying may be useful in removing unabsorbed drug.

Dosage and Administration: Dosage should be adjusted according to severity of pain and response of the patient. However, it should be kept in mind that tolerance to codeine can develop with continued use and that the incidence of untoward effects is dose related. This product is inappropriate even in high doses for severe or intractable pain. Adult doses of codeine higher than 60 mg fail to give commensurate relief of pain but merely prolong analgesia and are associated with an appreciably increased incidence of undesirable side effects. Equivalently high doses in children would have similar effects. The usual adult dose for Phenaphen-650 with Codeine is one tablet every four hours as required.

How Supplied: *Phenaphen-650 with Codeine* is available as a scored, white, capsule-shaped compressed tablet, engraved AHR and 6251 in bottles of 50 (NDC 0031-6251-60) and Dis-Co® Unit Dose Packs (4 × 25's) (6251-61).

Store at controlled room temperature, between 15°C and 30°C (59°F and 86°F).

Dispense tablets in well-closed container.

[*Shown in Product Identification Section*]

PONDIMIN® TABLETS ℞ Ⓒ

brand of fenfluramine hydrochloride
Tablets—20 mg

Description: Pondimin (fenfluramine hydrochloride) is an anorectic drug, available in orange, scored, compressed tablets for oral administration. Each tablet contains fenfluramine hydrochloride 20 mg.

Pondimin is a phenethylamine with the chemical name, N-ethyl-α-methyl-m-(trifluoromethyl) phenethylamine hydrochloride.

Clinical Pharmacology: Fenfluramine is a sympathomimetic amine, the pharmacologic activity of which differs somewhat from that of the prototype drugs of this class used in obesity, the amphetamines, in appearing to produce more central nervous system depression than stimulation.

The mechanism of action of Pondimin is unclear but may be related to brain levels (or turnover rates) of serotonin or to increased glucose utilization. The antiappetite effects of Pondimin are suppressed by serotonin-blocking drugs and by drugs that lower brain levels of the amine. Furthermore, decreased serotonin levels produced by selective brain lesions suppress the action of Pondimin.

In a study of 20 normal males, fenfluramine increased glucose utilization, resulting in decreased blood glucose levels. Experimental work in animals suggested that increased glucose utilization activated the satiety center and decreased the activity of the feeding center. Perhaps by this mechanism Pondimin inhibits appetite. The relationship between glucose utilization and serotonin has not been clarified.

Fenfluramine is well-absorbed from the gastrointestinal tract, and a maximal anorectic effect is generally seen after 2 to 4 hours. In man, fenfluramine is de-ethylated to norfenfluramine which is subsequently oxidized to m-trifluoromethyl benzoic acid and excreted as the glycine conjugate, m-trifluoromethylhippuric acid. Other compunds found in the urine include unchanged fenfluramine and norfenfluramine.

The rate of excretion of fenfluramine is pH dependent, with much smaller amounts appearing in an alkaline than in an acid urine. The half-life of fenfluramine is said to be about 20 hours, compared with 5 hours for amphetamines; however, if urinary excretion is rapid and the pH maintained in the acidic range (below pH 5), half-life can be reduced to 11 hours. Fenfluramine and norfenfluramine reach steady state concentrations in plasma within 3 to 4 days following chronic dosage.

The greatest weight loss is seen in those patients who maintain the highest levels of Pondimin. A 2-to-3-kg weight loss over 6 weeks is associated with a plasma level of 0.1 mcg/ml (or 10 mcg/100 ml).

Fenfluramine is widely distributed in almost all body tissues. It is soluble in lipids and crosses the blood-brain barrier. Fenfluramine crosses the placenta readily in monkeys.

Indications and Usage: Pondimin is indicated in the management of exogenous obesity as a short-term (a few weeks) adjunct in a regimen of weight reduction based on caloric restriction.

Drugs of this class used in obesity are commonly known as "anorectics" by "anorexigenics." It has not been established, however, that the action of such drug in treating obesity is primarily one of appetite suppression. Other central nervous system actions or metabolic effects may be involved.

Adult obese subjects instructed in dietary management and treated with "anorectic" drugs, lose more weight on the average than those treated with placebo and diet, as determined in relatively short-term trials.

The average magnitude of increased weight loss of drug-treated patients over placebo-treated is only a fraction of a pound a week. The rate of weight loss is greatest in the first weeks of therapy for both drug and placebo subjects and tends to decrease in succeeding weeks. The possible origins of the increased weight loss due to the various drug effects are not established. The average amount of weight loss associated with the use of an "anorectic" drug varies from trial to trial, and the increased weight loss appears to be related in part to variables other than the drug, prescribed such as the physician-investigator, the population treated and the diet prescribed. Studies do not permit conclusions as to the relative importance of the drug and non-drug factors on weight loss.

The natural history of obesity is measured in years, whereas the studies cited are restricted to a few weeks duration; thus, the total impact of drug-induced weight loss over that of diet alone must be considered clinically limited.

Contraindications: Fenfluramine is contraindicated in patients with glaucoma or with hypersensitivity to fenfluramine or other sympathomimetic amines. Do not administer fenfluramine during or within 14 days following the administration of monoamine oxidase inhibitors, since hypertensive crises may result. Patients with a history of drug abuse should not receive the drug.

Do not administer fenfluramine to patients with alcoholism since psychiatric symptoms (paranoia, depression, psychosis) have been reported in a few such patients who had been administered this drug.

A fatal cardiac arrest has been reported shortly after the induction of anesthesia in a patient who had been taking fenfluramine prior to surgery. Fenfluramine may have a catecholamine-depleting effect when administered for prolonged periods of time; therefore, potent anesthetic agents should be administered with caution to patients taking fenfluramine. If general anesthesia cannot be avoided, full cardiac monitoring and facilities for instant resuscitative measures are a minimum necessity.

Warnings: When tolerance to the "anorectic" effect develops, the maximum recommended dose should not be exceeded in an attempt to increase the effect; rather, the drug should be discontinued.

Precautions: ***General.*** Fenfluramine differs in its pharmacological profile from other "anorectic" drugs with which the prescribing practitioner may be familiar. Correspondingly, there are possible adverse effects not associated with other "anorectics"; such effects include those of diarrhea, sedation, and depression. The possibility of these effects should be weighed against the possible advantage of decreased central nervous system stimulation and/or abuse potential.

Use only with caution in hypertension, with monitoring of blood pressure, since evidence is insufficient to rule out a possible adverse effect on blood pressure in some hypertensive patients. The drug is not recommended in severely hypertensive patients. The drug is not recommended for patients with symptomatic cardiovascular disease including arrhythmias.

Information for Patients. Fenfluramine may impair the ability of the patient to engage in potentially hazardous activities such as operating machinery or driving a motor vehicle (see "Adverse Reactions"); the patient should be cautioned accordingly.

Drug Interactions. Fenfluramine may increase slightly the effect of antihypertensive drugs, e.g., guanethidine, methyldopa, reserpine.

Other CNS depressant drugs should be used with caution in patients taking fenfluramine, since the effects may be additive.

Carcinogenesis, Mutagenesis. No carcinogenic studies or mutagenic studies have been undertaken with this drug.

Teratogenic Effects and Fertility Impairment: Pregnancy Category C. Pondimin was shown to produce a questionable embryotoxic effect in rats and a reduced conception rate when given in a dose of 20 times the human dose. However, additional reproduction studies in rats, rabbits, mice, and monkeys at doses up to, respectively, 5 times, 20 times, 1 time, and 5 times the human dose yielded negative results.

There are no adequate and well-controlled studies in pregnant women. Pondimin should be used during pregnancy only if the potential benefit justifies the potential risk to the fetus.

Labor and Delivery. The effect of fenfluramine during labor or delivery on the mother and the fetus is unknown. The effect on later growth, development, and functional maturation of the child is unknown.

Nursing Mothers. It is not known whether this drug is excreted in human milk. Because many drugs are excreted in human milk, caution should be exercised when fenfluramine is administered to a nursing mother.

Pediatric Use. Safety and effectiveness in children below the age of 12 have not been established.

Adverse Reactions: The most common adverse reactions of fenfluramine are drowsiness, diarrhea, and dry mouth. Less frequent adverse reactions reported in association with fenfluramine are:

Central nervous system. Dizziness, confusion; incoordination; headache; elevated mood; depression; anxiety, nervousness, or tension; insomnia; weakness or fatigue; increased or decreased libido; agitation, dysarthria.

Gastrointestinal. Constipation; abdominal pain; nausea.

Autonomic. Sweating; chills; blurred vision.

Genitourinary. Dysuria; urinary frequency.

Cardiovascular. Palpitation; hypotension; hypertension; fainting.

Skin. Rash; urticaria; burning sensation.

Miscellaneous. Eye irritation; myalgia; fever; chest pain; bad taste.

Drug Abuse and Dependence: Pondimin (fenfluramine hydrochloride) is a controlled substance in Schedule IV. Fenfluramine is related chemically to the amphetamines, although it differs somewhat pharmacologically. The amphetamines and related stimulant drugs have been extensively abused and can produce tolerance and severe psychological dependence, as well as other adverse organic and mental changes. In this regard, there has been a report of abuse of fenfluramine by subjects with a history of abuse of other drugs. Abuse of 80 to 400 milligrams of the drug has been reported to be associated with euphoria, derealization, and perceptual changes. Fenfluramine did not produce signs of dependence in animals and appears to produce sedation more often than CNS stimulation at therapeutic doses. Its abuse potential appears qualitatively different from that of amphetamines. The possibility that fenfluramine may induce dependence should be kept in mind when evaluating the desirability of including the drug in the weight reduction programs of individual patients.

Overdosage: ***Signs and Symptoms:*** Only limited data have been reported concerning clinical effects and management of overdosage of fenfluramine.

Agitation and drowsiness, confusion, flushing, tremor (or shivering), fever, sweating, abdominal pain, hyperventilation, and dilated nonreactive pupils seem frequent in fenfluramine overdosage. Reflexes may be either exaggerated or depressed and some patients may have rotary nystagmus. Tachycardia may be present, but blood pressure may be normal or only slightly elevated. Convulsions, coma, and ventricular extrasystoles, culminating in ventricular fibrillation, and cardiac arrest, may occur at higher dosages.

Human Toxicity. Less than 5 mg/kg are toxic to humans. Five-ten mg/kg may produce coma and convulsions. Reported single overdoses have ranged from 300 to 2000 mg; the lowest reported fatal dose was a few hundred mg in a small child, and the highest reported nonfatal dose was 1800 mg in an adult. Most deaths were apparently due to respiratory failure and cardiac arrest.

Toxic effects will appear within 30 to 60 minutes and may progress rapidly to potentially fatal complications in 90 to 240 minutes. Symptoms may persist for extended periods depending upon the dose ingested.

Management. After overdosage, only a small percentage of the drug is excreted in the urine. Forced acid diuresis has been recommended only in extreme cases in which the patient survives the early hours of intoxication but fails to show decisive improvement from other measures. Hemodialysis and peritoneal dialysis are of theoretical advantage but have not been used clinically.

Reportedly the treatment of fenfluramine intoxication should include:

- ***Gastric lavage*** (but not drug-induced emesis because the patient may become unconscious at a very early stage.)
- In the event that gastric lavage is not feasible due to trismus, consult an anesthesiologist for endotracheal intubation after administration of muscle relaxants; only then gastric evacuation should be tried.
- Administration of activated charcoal after emesis or lavage may reduce absorption of drug.
- ***Monitoring of vital functions.*** If necessary, mechanical respiration, defibrillation, or "cardioversion" should be instituted.
- ***Drug therapy.*** Diazepam or phenobarbital for convulsions or muscular hyperactivity. In the presence of extreme trachycardia; propranolol; in the presence of ventricular extrasystoles; lidocaine; in the presence of hyperpyrexia; chlorpromazine.

Since fenfluramine has been shown to have a slight lowering effect on blood sugar in some patients, the theoretical possibility of hypoglycemia should be borne in mind although this effect has not been reported in cases of clinical overdosage.

Dosage and Administration: Therapy with fenfluramine should be initiated at a dosage of one 20-mg tablet 3 times daily before meals, but thereafter the dosage should be adjusted to the need and response of the patient. Depending on the degree of effectiveness and side effects, the dosage may be increased at weekly intervals by 1 tablet daily until a *maximum* dosage of 2 tablets 3 times daily is attained. In patients in whom the initial dosage is not well tolerated, dosage may be reduced to 2 tablets daily and thereafter gradually increased in order to minimize the chance of side effects.

How Supplied: Pondimin is available in 20-mg orange, scored, compressed tablets monogrammed AHR and 6447, in bottles of 100 (NDC 0031-6447-63) and 500 (NDC 0031-6447-70).

Store at controlled room temperature between 15°C and 30°C (59°F and 86°F).

Dispense in well-closed container.

[*Shown in Product Identification Section*]

QUINIDEX EXTENTABS® ℞

brand of Quinidine Sulfate, USP

Composition: Each Extentab (extended action tablet) contains 300 mg. Quinidine Sulfate, USP.

Description: Quinidex Extentabs (quinidine sulfate) are constructed to release one-third of their alkaloidal salt, quinidine sulfate (100 mg), on reaching the stomach, to begin absorption in the upper intestinal tract. The remaining two-thirds of the active drug (200 mg) is evenly distributed throughout a homogeneous core which slowly dissolves as it moves along the intestinal tract, releasing the quinidine sulfate for continuous absorption over an 8-12 hour period.

Action: The action of quinidine in preventing aberrant cardiac rhythms of atrial and ventricular origin resides in its ability to (a) depress excitability of cardiac muscle, (b) slow the rate of spontaneous rhythm, (c) decrease vagal tone, and (d) prolong conduction and effective refractory period.

Indications: Quinidex Extentabs are indicated in the treatment of:

Premature atrial and ventricular contractions.
Paroxysmal atrial tachycardia.
Paroxysmal A-V junctional rhythm.
Atrial flutter.
Paroxysmal atrial fibrillation.
Established atrial fibrillation when therapy is appropriate.
Paroxysmal ventricular tachycardia when not associated with complete heartblock.
Maintenance therapy after electrical conversion of atrial fibrillation and/or flutter.

Contraindications: Intraventricular conduction defects. A-V block. Idiosyncrasy or hypersensitivity.

Aberrant impulses and abnormal rhythms due to escape mechanisms should not be treated with quinidine.

Warning: In the treatment of atrial flutter, reversion to sinus rhythm may be preceded by a progressive reduction in the degree of A-V

Continued on next page

Prescribing information on A. H. Robins products listed here is based on official labeling in effect August 1, 1982, with Indications, Contraindications, Warnings, Precautions, Adverse Reactions, and Dosage stated in full.

Robins—Cont.

block to a 1:1 ratio and resulting extremely rapid ventricular rate.

Precautions: All the precautions applying to regular quinidine therapy apply to the Extentab form. Use with care in patients with severe congestive failure, renal insufficiency or with digitalis intoxication.

Patients should be carefully observed for signs of toxicity: e.g., (1) allergy or idiosyncrasy, such as febrile reactions, skin eruptions, and thrombocytopenia (extremely rare); (2) "cinchonism," such as tinnitus, blurred vision, dizziness, lightheadedness, and tremor, (3) G-I symptoms (nausea, vomiting, diarrhea, and colic); (4) cardiotoxic effects such as ventricular extrasystoles occurring at a rate of one or more every 6 normal beats, an increase of the QRS complex of 50% or more, a complete A-V block, or ventricular tachycardia.

NOTE: The development of "cinchonism" is not usually sufficient reason for terminating quinidine therapy. G-I symptoms can also be minimized by giving the drug with food.

Adverse Reactions: Cases of quinidine-induced hypoprothrombinemic hemorrhage in patients on chronic anticoagulant drug therapy have been reported.

Dosage: Two Quinidex Extentabs every 8 to 12 hours.

How Supplied: White sugar-coated Extentabs monogrammed Quinidex and AHR in bottles of 100 (NDC 0031-6649-63) and 250 (NDC 0031-6649-67).

[*Shown in Product Identification Section*]

REGLAN® ℞
(Metoclopramide Hydrochloride)
Tablets and Injectable

Description: Reglan (metoclopramide hydrochloride) is available in both oral and parenteral forms.

Reglan Tablets are white, round, compressed tablets engraved Reglan and AHR on one side and scored on the opposite side.

Each tablet contains:
Metoclopramide base **10 mg**
(as the monohydrochloride monohydrate)

Reglan Injectable is a clear, colorless, sterile solution with a pH of 2.5–5.0; for intravenous or intramuscular administration.

Each **2** ml ampul contains:
Metoclopramide base **10 mg**
(as the monohydrochloride monohydrate)
Sodium Metabisulfite, NF 2.96 mg, Sodium Chloride, USP 14 mg, Water for Injection, USP q.s.

Each **10** ml ampul contains:
Metoclopramide base **50 mg**
(as the monohydrochloride monohydrate)
Sodium Metabisulfite, NF 14.8 mg, Sodium Chloride, USP 70 mg, Water for Injection, USP q.s.

Metoclopramide hydrochloride is a white crystalline, odorless substance, freely soluble in water. Chemically, it is 4-amino-5-chloro-N-[2-(diethylamino)ethyl]-2-methoxy benzamide monohydrochloride monohydrate. Molecular weight 354.3.

Clinical Pharmacology: Metoclopramide stimulates motility of the upper gastrointestinal tract without stimulating gastric, biliary, or pancreatic secretions. Its mode of action is unclear. It seems to sensitize tissues to the action of acetylcholine. The effect of metoclopramide on motility is not dependent on intact vagal innervation, but it can be abolished by anticholinergic drugs.

Metoclopramide increases the tone and amplitude of gastric (especially antral) contractions, relaxes the pyloric sphincter and the duodenal bulb, and increases peristalsis of the duodenum and jejunum resulting in accelerated gastric emptying and intestinal transit. It increases the resting tone of the lower esophageal sphincter. It has little, if any, effect on the motility of the colon or gallbladder.

Like the phenothiazines and related drugs, which are also dopamine antagonists, metoclopramide produces sedation and may produce extrapyramidal reactions, although these are comparatively rare (See Warnings). Metoclopramide inhibits the central and peripheral effects of apomorphine, induces release of prolactin and causes a transient increase in circulating aldosterone levels.

The onset of pharmacological action of metoclopramide is 1 to 3 minutes following an intravenous dose, 10 to 15 minutes following intramuscular administration, and 30 to 60 minutes following an oral dose; pharmacological effects persist for 1 to 2 hours.

Approximately 85% of the radioactivity of an orally administered radioactive dose appears in the urine within 72 hours. Of the 85% eliminated in the urine, about half was present as free or conjugated metoclopramide.

Indications and Usage: ***Diabetic, gastroparesis (diabetic gastric stasis).*** Reglan (metoclopramide hydrochloride) is indicated for the relief of symptoms associated with acute and recurrent diabetic gastric stasis. The usual manifestations of delayed gastric emptying (e.g., nausea, vomiting, heartburn, persistent fullness after meals and anorexia) appear to respond to Reglan within different time intervals. Significant relief of nausea occurs early and continues to improve over a three-week period. Relief of vomiting and anorexia may precede the relief of abdominal fullness by one week or more.

Prevention of emesis induced by cisplatin (alone or in combination). Reglan Injectable is indicated for the prophylaxis of vomiting associated with cisplatin cancer chemotherapy.

Small bowel intubation. Reglan Injectable may be used to facilitate small bowel intubation in adults and children in whom the tube does not pass the pylorus with conventional maneuvers.

Radiological examination. Reglan Injectable may be used to stimulate gastric emptying and intestinal transit of barium in cases where delayed emptying interferes with radiological examination of the stomach and/or small intestine.

Contraindications: Metoclopramide should not be used whenever stimulation of gastrointestinal motility might be dangerous, e.g., in the presence of gastrointestinal hemorrhage, mechanical obstruction, or perforation.

Metoclopramide is contraindicated in patients with pheochromocytoma because the drug may cause a hypertensive crisis, probably due to release of catecholamines from the tumor. Such hypertensive crises may be controlled by phentolamine.

Meloclopramide is contraindicated in patients with known sensitivity or intolerance to the drug.

Metoclopramide should not be used in epileptics or patients receiving other drugs which are likely to cause extrapyramidal reactions, since the frequency and severity of seizures or extrapyramidal reactions may be increased.

Warnings: Extrapyramidal symptoms occur in approximately 1 in 500 patients treated with metoclopramide. These occur more frequently in children and young adults and are even more frequent at the higher doses used in prophylaxis of vomiting due to cancer chemotherapy. If extrapyramidal symptoms should occur, inject 50 mg Benadryl® (diphenhydramine hydrochloride) intramuscularly, and EPS will subside. These most often consist of feelings of restlessness; occasionally they may include involuntary movements of limbs and facial grimacing; rarely, torticollis, oculogyric crisis, rhythmic protrusion of tongue, bulbar type of speech or trismus. One dystonic reaction resembling tetanus has been reported, as have rare persistent dyskinesias.

Precautions: ***General.*** Patients should be cautioned about engaging in activities requiring mental alertness for a few hours after the drug has been administered.

Intubation and Radiology. Intravenous injections of metoclopramide should be made slowly over a 1- to 2-minute period, since a transient but intense feeling of anxiety and restlessness, followed by drowsiness, may occur with rapid administration.

Vomiting prophylaxis (cancer chemotherapy). Intravenous administration of Reglan Injectable diluted in one of the following large volume parenteral solutions should be made slowly over a period of not less than 15 minutes: Dextrose-5% in Water, Sodium Chloride Injection, Dextrose-5% in 0.45% Sodium Chloride, Ringer's Injection, Lactated Ringer's Injection. Dilutions should be protected from light after preparation.

Drug Interaction. The effects of metoclopramide on gastrointestinal motility are antagonized by anticholinergic drugs and narcotic analgesics. Additive sedative effects can occur when metoclopramide is given with alcohol, sedatives, hypnotics, narcotics or tranquilizers. Absorption of drugs from the stomach may be diminished (e.g., digoxin) by metoclopramide, whereas absorption of drugs from the small bowel may be accelerated (e.g., acetaminophen, tetracycline, levodopa, ethanol).

Gastroparesis (gastric stasis) may be responsible for poor diabetic control in some patients. Exogenously administered insulin may begin to act before food has left the stomach and lead to hypoglycemia.

Because the action of metoclopramide will influence the delivery of food to the intestines and thus the rate of absorption, insulin dosage or timing of dosage may require adjustment.

Carcinogensis, Mutagenesis.

Metoclopramide elevates prolactin levels and the elevation persists during chronic administration. Tissue culture experiments indicate that approximately one-third of human breast cancers are prolactin-dependent *in vitro*, a factor of potential importance if the prescription of metoclopramide is contemplated in a patient with previously detected breast cancer. Although disturbances such as galactorrhea, amenorrhea, gynecomastia, and impotence have been reported with prolactin-elevating drugs, the clinical significance of elevated serum prolactin levels is unknown for most patients. An increase in mammary neoplasms has been found in rodents after chronic administration of prolactin-stimulating neuroleptic drugs. Neither clinical studies nor epideminologic studies conducted to date, however, have shown an association between chronic administration of these drugs and mammary tumorigenesis; the available evidence is too limited to be conclusive at this time.

Pregnancy Category B. Reproduction studies performed in rats, mice, and rabbits by the i.v., i.m., s.c. and oral routes at maximum levels ranging from 12 to 250 times the human dose have demonstrated no impairment of fertility or significant harm to the fetus due to metoclopramide. There are, however, no adequate and well-controlled studies in pregnant women. Because animal reproduction studies are not always predictive of human response, this drug should be used during pregnancy only if clearly needed.

Nursing Mothers. It is not known whether this drug is excreted in human milk. Because many drugs are excreted in human milk, caution should be exercised when metoclopramide is administered to a nursing mother.

Adverse Reactions: The most frequent adverse reactions to metoclopramide are restlessness, drowsiness, fatigue and lassitude, which occur in approximately ten percent of patients. Less frequently, insomnia, headache, dizziness, nausea, or bowel disturbances may occur. (See Warnings and Precautions sections).

A single instance of supraventricular tachycardia following intramuscular administration has been reported.

Overdosage: Symptoms of overdosage may

include drowsiness, disorientation and extrapyramidal reactions. Anticholinergic or antiparkinson drugs or antihistamines with anticholinergic properties may be helpful in controlling the extrapyramidal reactions. Symptoms are self-limiting and usually disappear within 24 hours.

Dosage and Administration: ***For the relief of symptoms associated with diabetic gastroparesis (diabetic gastric stasis):*** If patients have severe symptoms with nausea and vomiting and oral administration would be difficult, treatment should begin with Reglan Injectable (IM or IV) 10 mg 30 minutes before each meal and at bedtime until symptoms subside sufficiently to allow oral administration. In patients who can tolerate oral Reglan, administer 1 tablet 30 minutes before each meal and at bedtime (4 doses daily) for 2-8 weeks, depending on response and the likelihood of continued well-being upon drug discontinuation. Since diabetic gastric stasis is frequently recurrent, Reglan therapy should be reinstituted at the earliest manifestation.

For the prevention of emesis induced by cisplatin (alone or in combination): Reglan Injectable should be diluted in 50 ml of a large volume parenteral solution (Dextrose-5% in water, Sodium Chloride Injection, Dextrose-5% in 0.45% Sodium Chloride, Ringer's Injection or Lactated Ringer's Injection). Intravenous infusions should be made slowly over a period of not less than 15 minutes, 30 minutes before beginning cisplatin and repeated every 2 hours for two doses, then every 3 hours for three doses.

The initial two doses should be 2 mg/kg. If vomiting is suppressed, a 1 mg/kg dose can be tried.

If extrapyramidal symptoms should occur, inject 50 mg Benadryl® (diphenhydramine hydrochloride) intramuscularly, and EPS will subside.

To facilitate small bowel intubation: If the tube has not passed the pylorus with conventional maneuvers in 10 minutes, a single dose (undiluted) may be administered slowly by the intravenous route over a 1- to 2-minute period. The recommended single dose is: Adults—10 mg metoclopramide base (2 ml). Children (6–14 years of age)—2.5 to 5 mg metoclopramide base (0.5 to 1 ml); (under 6 years of age)—0.1 mg/kg metoclopramide base.

To aid in radiological examinations: In patients where delayed gastric emptying interferes with radiological examination of the stomach and/or small intestine, a single dose may be administered slowly by the intravenous route over a 1- to 2-minute period.

For dosage, see intubation, above.

Parenteral drug products should be inspected visually for particulate matter and discoloration prior to administration, whenever solution and container permit.

How Supplied: Each white, round, scored, compressed Reglan® Tablet contains 10 mg metoclopramide base (as the monohydrochloride monohydrate). Available in bottles of 100 (NDC 0031-6701-63), and 500 tablets (NDC 0031-6701-70) and Dis-Co® Unit Dose Packs of 100 tablets (NDC 0031-6701-64). Dispense tablets in tight container.

Each **2** ml ampul of Reglan® Injectable contains 10 mg metoclopramide base (as the monohydrochloride monohydrate). Available in cartons of 5 (NDC 0031-6702-90) and 25 ampuls (NDC 0031-6702-95).

Each **10** ml ampul of Reglan® Injectable contains 50 mg metoclopramide base (as the monohydrochloride monohydrate). Available in cartons of 25 ampuls (NDC 0031-6702-94).

Store ampuls in carton until used. Do not store open ampul for later use.

Dilutions may be stored for up to 48 hours after preparation if protected from light. Dilutions also should be protected from light during infusion.

TABLETS AND INJECTABLE SHOULD BE STORED AT CONTROLLED ROOM TEMPERATURE BETWEEN 15°C and 30°C (59°F and 86°F).

Reglan Injectable is manufactured for Pharmaceutical Division, A. H. Robins Company, Richmond, Virginia 23220 by Elkins-Sinn, Inc., Cherry Hill, NJ 08034, a subsidiary of A. H. Robins.

[*Shown in Product Identification Section*]

ROBAXIN® INJECTABLE ℞
brand of Methocarbamol Injection, USP

Description: Robaxin Injectable is a parenteral dosage form.

Each ml contains:
Methocarbamol, USP **100 mg**; Polyethylene Glycol 300, NF 0.5 ml; Water for Injection, USP q. s. pH adjusted, when necessary, with hydrochloric acid and/or sodium hydroxide.

AFTER MIXING WITH I. V. INFUSION FLUIDS, **DO NOT REFRIGERATE.**

Actions: The mechanism of action of methocarbamol in humans has not been established, but may be due to general central nervous system depression. It has no direct action on the contractile mechanism of striated muscle, the motor end plate or the nerve fiber.

Indications: The injectable form of methocarbamol is indicated as an adjunct to rest, physical therapy, and other measures for the relief of discomfort associated with acute, painful musculoskeletal conditions. The mode of action of this drug has not been clearly identified, but may be related to its sedative properties. Methocarbamol does not directly relax tense skeletal muscles in man.

Contraindications: Robaxin Injectable should not be administered to patients with known or suspected renal pathology. This caution is necessary because of the presence of polyethylene glycol 300 in the vehicle.

A much larger amount of polyethylene glycol 300 than is present in recommended doses of Robaxin Injectable is known to have increased pre-existing acidosis and urea retention in patients with renal impairment. Although the amount present in this preparation is well within the limits of safety, caution dictates this contraindication.

Robaxin Injectable is contraindicated in patients hypersensitive to any of the ingredients.

Warnings: Since methocarbamol may possess a general central nervous system depressant effect, patients receiving Robaxin Injectable (methocarbamol injection) should be cautioned about combined effects with alcohol and other CNS depressants.

Safe use of Robaxin Injectable has not been established with regard to possible adverse effects upon fetal development. Therefore, Robaxin Injectable should not be used in women who are or may become pregnant and particularly during early pregnancy unless in the judgment of the physician the potential benefits outweigh the possible hazards.

Precautions: As with other agents administered either intravenously or intramuscularly, careful supervision of dose and rate of injection should be observed. Rate of injection should not exceed 3 ml per minute—i.e., one 10 ml vial in approximately three minutes. Since Robaxin Injectable is hypertonic, vascular extravasation must be avoided. A recumbent position will reduce the likelihood of side reactions.

Blood aspirated into the syringe does not mix with the hypertonic solution. This phenomenon occurs with many other intravenous preparations. The blood may be safely injected with the methocarbamol, or the injection may be stopped when the plunger reaches the blood, whichever the physician prefers.

The total dosage should not exceed 30 ml (three vials) a day for more than three consecutive days except in the treatment of tetanus.

Caution should be observed in using the injectable form in suspected or known epileptic patients.

Safety and effectiveness in children below the age of 12 years have not been established except in tetanus. See special directions for use in tetanus.

It is not known whether this drug is secreted in human milk. As a general rule, nursing should not be undertaken while a patient is on a drug since many drugs are excreted in human milk.

Methocarbamol may cause a color interference in certain screening tests for 5-hydroxyindoleacetic acid (5-HIAA) and vanilmandelic acid (VMA).

Adverse Reactions: Dizziness, light-headedness, drowsiness, vertigo, fainting, syncope, hypotension, gastrointestinal upset, metallic taste, thrombophlebitis, sloughing at the site of injection, pain at the site of injection, anaphylactic reaction, urticaria, pruritus, rash, conjunctivitis with nasal congestion, flushing, nystagmus, diplopia, mild muscular incoordination, bradycardia, blurred vision, headache, fever. In most cases of syncope there was spontaneous recovery. In others, epinephrine, injectable steroids and/or injectable antihistamines were employed to hasten recovery. Certain of these complaints may have been due to an overly rapid rate of intravenous injection. The onset of convulsive seizures during intravenous administration has been reported, including instances in known epileptics. The psychic trauma of the procedure may have been a contributing factor. Although several observers have reported success in terminating epileptiform seizures with Robaxin Injectable, its administration to patients with epilepsy is not recommended.

Dosage and Administration:

For Intravenous and Intramuscular Use Only.

Total adult dosage should not exceed 30 ml (3 vials) a day for more than 3 consecutive days except in the treatment of tetanus. A like course may be repeated after a lapse of 48 hours if the condition persists. Dosage and frequency of injection should be based on the severity of the condition being treated and therapeutic response noted.

For the relief of symptoms of moderate degree, 10 ml (one vial) may be adequate. Ordinarily this injection need not be repeated, as the administration of the oral form will usually sustain the relief initiated by the injection. For the severest cases or in postoperative conditions in which oral administration is not feasible, 20 to 30 ml (two to three vials) may be required.

Directions For Intravenous Use:

Robaxin Injectable may be administered undiluted directly into the vein at a *maximum rate of three ml per minute.* It may also be added to an intravenous drip of Sodium Chloride Injection (Sterile Isotonic Sodium Chloride Solution for Parenteral Use) or five per cent Dextrose Injection (Sterile 5 per cent Dextrose Solution); one vial given as a single dose should not be diluted to more than 250 ml for I.V. infusion. Care should be exercised to avoid vascular extravasation of this hypertonic solution which may result in thrombophlebitis. It is preferable that the patient be in a recumbent position during and for at least 10 to 15 minutes following the injection.

Directions For Intramuscular Use:

When the intramuscular route is indicated, not more than five ml (one-half vial) should be injected into each gluteal region. The injections may be repeated at eight hour intervals, if necessary. When satisfactory relief of symptoms is achieved, it can usually be maintained with tablets.

Prescribing information on A. H. Robins products listed here is based on official labeling in effect August 1, 1982, with Indications, Contraindications, Warnings, Precautions, Adverse Reactions, and Dosage stated in full.

Continued on next page

Robins—Cont.

NOT RECOMMENDED FOR SUBCUTANEOUS ADMINISTRATION.

Special Directions For Use in Tetanus: There is clinical evidence which suggests that methocarbamol may have a beneficial effect in the control of the neuromuscular manifestations of tetanus. It does not, however, replace the usual procedure of debridement, tetanus antitoxin, penicillin, tracheotomy, attention to fluid balance, and supportive care. Robaxin Injectable should be added to the regimen as soon as possible.

For adults: Inject one or two vials directly into the tubing of the previously inserted indwelling needle. An additional 10 ml or 20 ml may be added to the infusion bottle so that a total of up to 30 ml (three vials) is given as the initial dose (note Precautions). This procedure should be repeated every six hours until conditions allow for the insertion of a nasogastric tube. Crushed Robaxin (methocarbamol) tablets suspended in water or saline may then be given through this tube. Total daily oral doses up to 24 grams may be required as judged by patient response.

For children: A minimum initial dose of 15 mg/kg is recommended. This dosage may be repeated every six hours as indicated. The maintenance dosage may be given by injection into the tubing or by I.V. infusion with an appropriate quantity of fluid. See directions for I.V. use.

How Supplied: Robaxin Injectable—10 ml single dose vials in packages of 5 (NDC 0031-7409-87) and 25 (NDC 0031-7409-94).

Manufactured for Pharmaceutical Division, A. H. Robins Company, Richmond, Virginia 23220 by Elkins-Sinn, Inc., Cherry Hill, New Jersey 08034, a subsidiary of A. H. Robins Co.

ROBAXIN® TABLETS ℞
brand of Methocarbamol Tablets, USP
500 mg per tablet

ROBAXIN®-750 TABLETS
brand of Methocarbamol Tablets, USP ℞
750 mg per tablet

Actions: The mechanism of action of methocarbamol in humans has not been established, but may be due to general central nervous system depression. It has no direct action on the contractile mechanism of striated muscle, the motor end plate or the nerve fiber.

Indications: Robaxin (methocarbamol) is indicated as an adjunct to rest, physical therapy, and other measures for the relief of discomforts associated with acute, painful musculoskeletal conditions. The mode of action of this drug has not been clearly identified, but may be related to its sedative properties. Methocarbamol does not directly relax tense skeletal muscles in man.

Contraindications: Robaxin is contraindicated in patients hypersensitive to any of the ingredients.

Warnings: Since methocarbamol may possess a general central nervous system depressant effect, patients receiving Robaxin/Robaxin-750 (methocarbamol tablets) should be cautioned about combined effects with alcohol and other CNS depressants.

Safe use of methocarbamol has not been established with regard to possible adverse effects upon fetal development. Therefore, methocarbamal tablets should not be used in women who are or may become pregnant and particularly during early pregnancy unless in the judgment of the physician the potential benefits outweigh the possible hazards.

Precautions: Safety and effectiveness in children below the age of 12 years have not been established.

It is not known whether this drug is secreted in human milk. As a general rule, nursing should not be undertaken while a patient is on a drug since many drugs are excreted in human milk. Methocarbamol may cause a color interference in certain screening tests for 5-hydroxyindoleacetic acid (5-HIAA) and vanilmandelic acid (VMA).

Adverse Reactions: Lightheadedness, dizziness, drowsiness, nausea, allergic manifestations such as urticaria, pruritus, rash, conjunctivitis with nasal congestion, blurred vision, headache, fever.

Dosage and Administration: Robaxin (methocarbamol), 500 mg.—Adults: initial dosage, 3 tablets q.i.d.; maintenance dosage, 2 tablets q.i.d.

Robaxin-750 (methocarbamol), 750 mg—Adults: initial dosage, 2 tablets q.i.d.; maintenance dosage, 1 tablet q.4h. or 2 tablets t.i.d. Six grams a day are recommended for the first 48 to 72 hours of treatment. (For severe conditions 8 grams a day may be administered.) Thereafter, the dosage can usually be reduced to approximately 4 grams a day.

How Supplied: Robaxin—white, scored tablets monogrammed AHR and Robaxin in bottles of 100 (NDC 0031-7429-63), 500 (NDC 0031-7429-70), and Dis-Co® unit dose packs of 100 (NDC 0031-7429-64).

Robaxin-750—white capsule-shaped tablets monogrammed Robaxin 750 on one side, AHR on the reverse side in bottles of 100 (NDC 0031-7449-63), 500 (NDC 0031-7449-70), and Dis-Co® unit dose packs of 100 (NDC 0031-7449-64).

[*Shown in Product Identification Section*]

ROBAXISAL® TABLETS ℞

Description: For oral administration, Robaxisal is available as a pink and white laminated tablet containing:

Methocarbamol, USP ....400 mg
Aspirin, USP..325 mg

Actions: Robaxisal provides a double approach to the management of discomforts associated with musculoskeletal disorders.

Methocarbamol. The mechanism of action of methocarbamol in humans has not been established, but may be due to general central nervous system depression. It has no direct action on the contractile mechanism of striated muscle, the motor end plate or the nerve fiber.

Aspirin. Aspirin is a mild analgesic with anti-inflammatory and antipyretic activity.

Indications: Robaxisal is indicated as an adjunct to rest, physical therapy, and other measures for the relief of discomfort associated with acute, painful musculoskeletal conditions. The mode of action of methocarbamol has not been clearly identified but may be related to its sedative properties. Methocarbamol does not directly relax tense skeletal muscles in man.

Contraindications: Hypersensitivity to methocarbamol or aspirin.

Warnings: Since methocarbamol may possess a general central nervous system depressant effect, patients receiving Robaxisal should be cautioned about combined effects with alcohol and other CNS depressants.

Precautions: Products containing aspirin should be administered with caution to patients with gastritis or peptic ulceration, or those receiving hypoprothrombinemic anticoagulants.

Methocarbomal may cause a color interference in certain screening tests for 5-hydroxyindoleacetic acid (5-HIAA) and vanilmandelic acid (VMA).

Pregnancy. Safe use of Robaxisal has not been established with regard to possible adverse effects upon fetal development. Therefore, Robaxisal should not be used in women who are or may become pregnant and particularly during early pregnancy unless in the judgment of the physician the potential benefits outweigh the possible hazards.

Nursing Mothers. It is not known whether methocarbamol is secreted in human milk; however, aspirin does appear in human milk in moderate amounts. It can produce a bleeding tendency either by interfering with the function of the infant's platelets or by decreasing the amount of prothrombin in the blood. The risk is minimal if the mother takes the aspirin just after nursing and if the infant has an adequate store of vitamin K.

As a general rule, nursing should not be undertaken while a patient is on a drug.

Pediatric Use. Safety and effectiveness in children 12 years of age and below have not been established.

Use in Activities Requiring Mental Alertness. Robaxisal may rarely cause drowsiness. Until the patient's response has been determined, he should be cautioned against the operation of motor vehicles or dangerous machinery.

Adverse Reactions: The most frequent adverse reaction to methocarbamol is dizziness or lightheadedness and nausea. This occurs in about one in 20–25 patients. Less frequent reactions are drowsiness, blurred vision, headache, fever, allergic manifestations such as urticaria, pruritus, and rash.

Adverse reactions that have been associated with the use of aspirin include: nausea and other gastrointestinal discomfort, gastritis, gastric erosion, vomiting, constipation, diarrhea, angio-edema, asthma, rash, pruritus, urticaria.

Gastrointestinal discomfort may be minimized by taking Robaxisal with food.

Dosage and Administration: Adults and children over 12 years of age: Two tablets four times daily. Three tablets four times daily may be used in severe conditions for one to three days in patients who are able to tolerate salicylates. These dosage recommendations provide respectively 3.2 and 4.8 grams of methocarbamol per day.

Overdosage: Toxicity due to overdosage of methocarbomal is unlikely; however, acute overdosage of aspirin may cause symptoms of salicylate intoxication.

Treatment of Overdosage. Supportive therapy for 24 hours, as methocarbamol is excreted within that time. If salicylate intoxication occurs, especially in children, the hyperpnea may be controlled with sodium bicarbonate. Judicious use of 5% CO_2 with 95% O_2 may be of benefit. Abnormal electrolyte patterns should be corrected with appropriate fluid therapy.

How Supplied: Robaxisal® is supplied as pink and white laminated, compressed tablets monogrammed AHR and Robaxisal in bottles of 100 (NDC 0031-7469-63), 500 (NDC 0031-7469-70) and Dis-Co® Unit Dose Packs of 100 (NDC 0031-7469-64).

[*Shown in Product Identification Section*]

ROBICILLIN VK ℞
brand of
Penicillin V Potassium, USP
for oral use

Description: Penicillin V is the phenoxymethyl analog of penicillin G. The chemical formula is $C_{16}H_{18}N_2O_5S$.

Action and Pharmacology: Penicillin V exerts a bactericidal action against penicillin sensitive microorganisms during the stage of active multiplication. It acts through the inhibition of biosynthesis of cell wall mucopeptide. It is not active against the penicillinase producing bacteria, which include many strains of staphylococci. The drug exerts high in vitro activity against staphylococci (except penicillinase-producing strains), streptococci (groups A, C, G, H, L, and M) and pneumococci. Other organisms sensitive in vitro to penicillin V are **Corynebacterium diphtheriae, Bacillus anthracis,** Clostridia, **Actinomyces bovis, Streptobacillus moniliformis, Listeria monocytogenes,** Leptospira and **N. gonorrhoeae. Treponema pallidum** is extremely sensitive.

Penicillin V has the distinct advantage over penicillin G in resistance to inactivation by gastric acid. It may be given with meals; however, blood levels are slightly higher when the drug is given on an empty stomach. Average blood levels are two to five times higher than the levels following the same dose of oral penicillin G and also show much less individual variation.

Once absorbed, penicillin V is about 80% bound to serum protein. Tissue levels are highest in the kidneys, with lesser amounts in the liver, skin and intestines. Small amounts are found in all other body tissues and the cerebrospinal fluid. The drug is excreted as rapidly as it is absorbed in individuals with normal kidney function; however, recovery of the drug from the urine indicates that only about 25% of the dose given is absorbed. In neonates, young infants and individuals with impaired kidney function, excretion is considerably delayed.

Indications: Penicillin V is indicated in the treatment of mild to moderately severe infections due to penicillin-G sensitive microorganisms that are sensitive to the low serum levels common to this particular dosage form. Therapy should be guided by bacteriological studies (including sensitivity tests) and by clinical response.

Note: Severe pneumonia, empyema, bacteremia, pericarditis, meningitis, and arthritis should not be treated with penicillin V during the acute stage.

Indicated surgical procedures should be performed.

The following infections will usually respond to adequate dosage of Penicillin V:

Streptococcal infections (without bacteremia). Mild to moderate infections of the upper respiratory tract, scarlet fever, and mild erysipelas.

Note: Streptococci in groups A, C, G, H, L, and M are very sensitive to penicillin. Other groups, including group D (enterococcus) are resistant.

Pneumococcal infections. Mild to moderately severe infections of the respiratory tract.

Staphylococcal infections—penicillin G sensitive. Mild infections of the skin and soft tissues.

Note: Reports indicate an increasing number of strains of staphylococci resistant to penicillin G, emphasizing the need for culture and sensitivity studies in treating suspected staphylococcal infections.

Fusospirochetosis (Vincent's gingivitis and pharyngitis)—Mild to moderately severe infections of the oropharynx usually respond to therapy with oral penicillin.

Note: Necessary dental care should be accomplished in infections involving the gum tissue.

Medical conditions in which oral penicillin therapy is indicated as prophylaxis:

For the prevention of recurrence following rheumatic fever and/or chorea: Prophylaxis with oral penicillin on a continuing basis has proven effective in preventing recurrence of these conditions.

Although no controlled clinical efficacy studies have been conducted, penicillin V has been suggested by the American Heart Association and the American Dental Association for use as part of a parenteral-oral regimen and as an alternative oral regimen for prophylaxis against bacterial endocarditis in patients with congenital and/or rheumatic or other acquired valvular heart disease when they undergo dental procedures and surgical procedures of the respiratory tract.[1] Since it may happen that *alpha* hemolytic streptococci relatively resistant to penicillin may be found when patients are receiving continuous oral penicillin for secondary prevention of rheumatic fever, prophylactic agents other than penicillin may be chosen for these patients and prescribed in addition to their continuous rheumatic fever prophylactic regimen. Oral penicillin should not be used as adjunctive prophylaxis for genitourinary instrumentation or surgery, lower intestinal tract surgery, sigmoidoscopy, and childbirth.

Note: When selecting antibiotics, for the prevention of bacterial endocarditis, the physician or dentist should read the full joint statement of the American Heart Association and the American Dental Association.[1]

Contraindications: A previous hypersensitivity reaction to any penicillin is a contraindication.

Warnings: Serious and occasionally fatal hypersensitivity (anaphylactoid) reactions have been reported in patients on penicillin therapy. Although anaphylaxis is more frequent following parenteral therapy it has occurred in patients on oral penicillins. These reactions are more apt to occur in individuals with a history of sensitivity to multiple allergens.

There have been well documented reports of individuals with a history of penicillin hypersensitivity reactions who have experienced severe hypersensitivity reactions when treated with a cephalosporin. Before therapy with a penicillin, careful inquiry should be made concerning previous hypersensitivity reactions to penicillins, cephalosporins, and other allergens. If an allergic reaction occurs, the drug should be discontinued and the patient treated with the usual agents e.g., pressor amines, antihistamines and corticosteroids.

Precautions: Penicillin should be used with caution in individuals with histories of significant allergies and/or asthma.

The oral route of administration should not be relied upon in patients with severe illness, or with nausea, vomiting, gastric dilatation, cardiospasm or intestinal hypermotility.

Occasionally patients will not absorb therapeutic amounts of orally administered penicillin.

In streptococcal infections, therapy must be sufficient to eliminate the organism (10 days minimum); otherwise the sequelae of streptococcal disease may occur. Cultures should be taken following completion of treatment to determine whether streptococci have been eradicated.

Prolonged use of antibiotics may promote the overgrowth of non-susceptible organisms, including fungi. Should superinfection occur, appropriate measures should be taken.

Adverse Reactions: Although the incidence of reactions to oral penicillins has been reported with much less frequency than following parenteral therapy, it should be remembered that all degrees of hypersensitivity including fatal anaphylaxis, have been reported with oral penicillin.

The most common reactions to oral penicillin are nausea, vomiting, epigastric distress, diarrhea, and black hairy tongue. The hypersensitivity reactions reported are skin eruptions (maculo-papular to exfoliative dermatitis), urticaria and other serum sickness reactions, laryngeal edema and anaphylaxis. Fever and eosinophilia may frequently be the only reaction observed. Hemolytic anemia, leucopenia, thrombocytopenia, neuropathy, and nephropathy are infrequent reactions and usually associated with high doses of parenteral penicillin.

Administration and Dosage: The dosage of penicillin V should be determined according to the sensitivity of the causative microorganisms and the severity of infection, and adjusted to the clinical response of the patient.

The usual dosage recommendations for adults and children 12 years and over are as follows:

Streptococcal infections—mild to moderately severe—of the upper respiratory tract and including scarlet fever, and mild erysipelas; 125 mg (200,000 units) every 6–8 hours for 10 days for mild infections; 250–500 mg (400,000–800,000 units) every 8 hours for 10 days for moderately severe infections.

Pneumococcal infections—mild to moderately severe—of the respiratory tract, including otitis media: 250–500 mg (400,000–800,000 units) every 6 hours until the patient has been afebrile for at least 2 days.

Staphylococcal infections—mild infections of skin and soft tissue (culture and sensitivity tests should be performed): 250–500 mg (400,000–800,000 units) every 6-8 hours.

Fusospirochetosis (Vincent's infection) of the oropharynx. Mild to moderately severe infections: 250mg (400,000 units) every 6-8 hours.

For the prevention of recurrence following rheumatic fever and/or chorea: 125 mg (200,000 units) twice daily on a continuing basis.

For prophylaxis against bacterial endocarditis[1] in patients with rheumatic, congenital or other acquired valvular heart disease when undergoing dental procedures or surgical procedures of the upper respiratory tract, one of two regimens may be selected:

1. For the oral regimen, give 2.0 Gm of penicillin V (1.0 Gm for children under 60 lbs) ½ to 1 hour before the procedure, and then, 500 mg (250 mg for children under 60 lbs) every 6 hours for 8 doses; or
2. For the combined parenteral-oral regimen, give one million units of aqueous crystalline penicillin G (30,000 units/kg in children) intramuscularly mixed with 600,000 units procaine penicillin G (600,000 units for children) ½ to 1 hour before the procedure, and then oral penicillin V, 500 mg (250 mg for children less than 60 lbs) every 6 hours for 8 doses. Doses for children should not exceed recommendations for adults for a single dose or for a 24-hour period.

Note: Therapy for children under 12 years of age is calculated on the basis of body weight. For infants and small children the suggested dose is 25,000 to 90,000 units per kg per day in three to six divided doses.

How Supplied:

Penicillin V Potassium for Oral Solution, USP 125 mg (200,000 Units) per 5 ml in bottles of 100 ml (NDC 0031-8205-09) and 200 ml (NDC 0031-8205-10).

250 mg (400,000 Units) per 5 ml in bottles of 100 ml (NDC 0031-8207-09) and 200 ml (NDC 0031-8207-10).

Penicillin V Potassium Tablets, U.S.P.

250 mg. (400,000 Units)—bottles of 100 (NDC 0031-8217-63) and 1,000 tablets (NDC 0031-8217-74).

500 mg. (800,000 Units)—bottles of 100 (NDC 0031-8227-63) and 500 tablets (NDC 0031-8227-70).

[1] American Heart Association. 1977. Prevention of bacterial endocarditis. Circulation. 56:139A-143A.

Manufactured for Pharmaceutical Division, A. H. Robins Inc. INC. Richmond, Virginia 23220 by Biocraft Laboratories, Inc., Elmwood Park, New Jersey 07407.

[*Shown in Product Identification Section*]

ROBIMYCIN ROBITABS® ℞

brand of Erythromycin Tablets, USP enteric-coated

250 mg erythromycin base

Description: Erythromycin is produced by a strain of ***Streptomyces erythraeus*** and belongs to the macrolide group of antibiotics. It is basic and readily forms salts with acids. The base, the stearate salt, and the esters are poorly soluble in water and are suitable for oral administration. Robimycin Robitabs®, brand of Erythromycin Tablets, USP (enteric-coated), are specially coated to protect the antibiotic from the inactivating effects of gastric acidity and to permit efficient absorption in the small intestine.

Actions: The mode of action of erythromycin is inhibition of protein synthesis without affecting nucleic acid synthesis. Resistance to erythromycin of some strains of ***Haemophilus***

Continued on next page

Prescribing information on A. H. Robins products listed here is based on official labeling in effect August 1, 1982, with Indications, Contraindications, Warnings, Precautions, Adverse Reactions, and Dosage stated in full.

Robins—Cont.

influenzae and staphylococci has been demonstrated. Culture and susceptibility testing should be done. If the Kirby-Bauer method of disc susceptibility is used, a 15 mcg erythromycin disc should give a zone diameter of at least 18 mm when tested against an erythromycin susceptible organism.

Robimycin Robitabs®, brand of erythromycin Tablets, USP (enteric-coated), are absorbed either when administered with meals or when given between meals on an empty stomach. However, absorption may be temporarily delayed by the presence of food. Some interpatient variability in absorption of orally-administered erythromycin has been observed.

After absorption, erythromycin diffuses readily into most body fluids. In the absence of meningeal inflammation, low concentrations are normally achieved in the spinal fluid but passage of the drug across the blood-brain barrier increases in meningitis. In the presence of normal hepatic function, erythromycin is concentrated in the liver and excreted in the bile; the effect of hepatic dysfunction on excretion of erythromycin by the liver into the bile is not known. After oral administration, less than 5 percent of the activity of the administered dose can be recovered in the urine.

Erythromycin crosses the placental barrier but fetal plasma levels are low.

Indications: Robimycin is indicated in the treatment of infections due to the following microorganisms:

Streptococcus pyogenes (Group A beta hemolytic streptococcus): For upper and lower respiratory tract, skin, and soft tissue infections of mild to moderate severity.

Injectable benzathine penicillin G is considered by the American Heart Association to be the drug of choice in the treatment and prevention of streptococcal pharyngitis and in long-term prophylaxis of rheumatic fever.

When oral medication is preferred for treatment of the above conditions, penicillin G, V, or erythromycin are alternate drugs of choice.

When oral medication is given, the importance of strict adherence by the patient to the prescribed dosage regimen must be stressed. A therapeutic dose should be administered for at least 10 days.

Alpha-hemolytic streptococci (viridans group): Although no controlled clinical efficacy trials have been conducted, oral erythromycin has been suggested by the American Heart Association and the American Dental Association for use in a regimen for prophylaxis of bacterial endocarditis in patients hypersensitive to penicillin who have congenital and/or rheumatic or other acquired valvular heat disease when they undergo dental procedures and surgical procedures of the upper respiratory tract.[1] Erythromycin is not suitable prior to genitourinary or gastrointestinal tract surgery.

NOTE: When selecting antibiotics for the prevention of bacterial endocarditis, the physician or dentist should read the full joint statement of the American Heart Association and the American Dental Association.[1]

Staphylococcus aureus: For acute infections of skin and soft tissue of mild to moderate severity. Resistant organisms may emerge during treatment.

Streptococcus pneumoniae (Diplococcus pneumoniae): For upper respiratory tract infections (e.g., Otitis media, pharyngitis) and lower respiratory tract infections (e.g., pneumonia) of mild to moderate degree.

Mycoplasma pneumoniae (Eaton agent, PPLO): For respiratory infections due to this organism.

Hemophilus influenzae: For upper respiratory tract infections of mild to moderate severity when used concomitantly with adequate doses of sulfonamides. Not all strains of this organism are susceptible at the erythromycin concentrations ordinarily achieved (see appropriate sulfonamide labeling for prescribing information).

Treponema pallidum: Erythromycin (oral forms only) is an alternate choice of treatment for primary syphilis in patients allergic to the penicillins. In treatment of primary syphilis, spinal fluid examinations should be done before treatment and as part of followup after therapy.

Corynebacterium diphtheriae and C. *minutissimum:* As an adjunct to antitoxin, to prevent establishment of carriers, and to eradicate the organism in carriers.

In the treatment of erythrasma.

Entamoeba histolytica: In the treatment of intestinal amebiasis only. Extraenteric amebiasis requires treatment with other agents.

Listeria monocytogenes: Infections due to this organism.

Neisseria gonorrhoeae: Erythromycin lactobionate for injection in conjunction with erythromycin stearate or base orally, as an alternative drug in treatment of acute pelvic inflammatory disease caused by ***N. gonorrhoeae*** in female patients with a history of sensitivity to penicillin. Before treatment of gonorrhea, patients who are suspected of also having syphilis should have a microscopic examination for ***T. pallidum*** (by immunofluorescence or darkfield) before receiving erythromycin, and monthly serologic tests for a minimum of 4 months.

Legionnaires' Disease: Although no controlled clinical efficacy studies have been conducted, *in vitro* and limited preliminary clinical data suggest that erythromycin may be effective in treating Legionnaires' Disease.

Contraindications: Erythromycin is contraindicated in patients with known hypersensitivity to this antibiotic.

Warnings: Usage in pregnancy: Safety for use in pregnancy has not been established.

Precautions: Erythromycin is principally excreted by the liver. Caution should be exercised in administering the antibiotic to patients with impaired hepatic function.

There have been reports of hepatic dysfunction, with or without jaundice, occurring in patients receiving oral erythromycin products. Although the majority of these cases have been associated with erythromycin estolate, there have been some reports of hepatic dysfunctions in conjunction with the erythromycin base, stearate an ethylsuccinate.

Recent data from studies of erythromycin reveal that its use in patients who are receiving high doses of theophylline may be associated with an increase of serum theophylline levels and potential theophylline toxicity. In case of theophylline toxicity and/or elevated serum theophylline levels, the dose of theophylline should be reduced while the patient is receiving concomitant erythromycin therapy.

Surgical procedures should be performed when indicated.

Adverse Reactions: The most frequent side effects of erythromycin preparations are gastrointestinal, such as abdominal cramping and discomfort, and are dose-related. Nausea, vomiting, and diarrhea occur infrequently with usual oral doses.

During prolonged or repeated therapy, there is a possibility of overgrowth of nonsusceptible bacteria or fungi. If such infections occur, the drug should be discontinued and appropriate therapy instituted.

Mild allergic reactions such as urticaria and other skin rashes have occurred. Serious allergic reactions, including anaphylaxis have been reported.

Dosage and Administration: Robimycin Robitabs®, brand of Erythromycin Tables, USP (enteric-coated), may be administered orally without regard to meals, i.e., with meals or on an emply stomach.

Adults: 250 mg every 6 hours is the usual dose. Dosage may be increased up to 4 or more grams per day according to the severity of the infection.

Children: Age, weight, and severity of the infection are important factors in determining the proper dosage. 30–50 mg/kg/day, in divided doses, is the usual dose. For more severe infections this dose may be doubled.

If dosage is desired on a twice-a-day schedule in either adults or children, one-half of the total daily dose may be given every 12 hours. Twice-a-day dosing is not recommended when doses larger than 1 gram daily are administered.

In the treatment of streptococcal infections, a therapeutic dosage of erythromycin should be administered for at least 10 days. In continuous ***prophylaxis*** of streptococcal infections in persons with a history of rheumatic heart disease, the dose is 250 mg twice a day.

For prophylaxis of bacterial endocarditis[1] in patients with rheumatic, congenital, or other acquired valvular heat disease when undergoing dental procedures or surgical procedures of the upper respiratory tract, give 1.0 Gm (20 mg/kg for children) orally 1½-2 hours before the procedure, and then 500 mg (10 mg/kg for children) orally every 6 hours for 8 doses.

For treatment of primary syphilis: 30–40 grams given in divided doses over a period of 10–15 days.

For treatment of acute pelvic inflammatory disease caused by N. gonorrhoeae: After initial treatment with erythromycin lactobionate for injection (500 mg every 6 hours for 3 days), the oral dosage recommendation is 250 mg every 6 hours for 7 days.

For dysenteric amebiasis: 250 mg four times daily for 10 to 14 days, for adults; 30–50 mg/kg/day in divided doses for 10 to 14 days, for children.

For treatment of Legionnaires' Disease: Although optimal doses have not been established, doses utilized in reported clinical data were those recommended above (1 to 4 grams erythromycin base daily in divided doses).

How Supplied: Robimycin Robitabs®, brand of Erythromycin Tablets, USP (enteric-coated), 250 mg (pale green, round) are available in bottles of 100 (NDC 0031-8317-63) and 500 (NDC 0031-8317-70).

[1]American Heart Association. 1977. Prevention of bacterial endocarditis. Circulation. 56:139A-143A.

[*Shown in Product Identification Section*]

ROBINUL® TABLETS ℞
ROBINUL® FORTE TABLETS ℞
brand of Glycopyrrolate Tablets, USP

Description: Robinul and Robinul Forte tablets contain the synthetic anticholinergic, glycopyrrolate. Glycopyrrolate is a quaternary ammonium compound with the following chemical name: 3-[(cyclopentyhydroxyphenylacetyl)oxy]-1,1-dimethylpyrrolidinium bromide.

Robinul tablets are scored, compressed pink tablets engraved AHR and 7824. Each tablet contains:

Glycopyrrolate, USP....................................1 mg

Robinul Forte tablets are scored, compressed pink tablets engraved $\frac{AHR}{2}$ on one side and 7840 on the reverse side. Each tablet contains:

Glycopyrrolate, USP....................................2 mg

Actions: Glycopyrrolate, like other anticholinergic (antimuscarinic) agents, inhibits the action of acetylcholine on structures innervated by postganglionic cholinergic nerves and on smooth muscles that respond to acetylcholine but lack cholinergic innervation. These peripheral cholinergic receptors are present in the autonomic effector cells of smooth muscle, cardiac muscle, the sinoatrial node, the atrioventricular node, exocrine glands, and, to a limited degree, in the autonomic ganglia. Thus, it diminishes the volume and free acidity of gastric secretions and controls excessive

pharyngeal, tracheal, and bronchial secretions.
Glycopyrrolate antagonizes muscarinic symptoms (e.g., bronchorrhea, bronchospasm, bradycardia, and intestinal hypermotility) induced by cholinergic drugs such as the anticholinesterases.
The highly polar quaternary ammonium group of glycopyrrolate limits its passage across lipid membranes, such as the blood-brain barrier, in contrast to atropine sulfate and scopolamine hydrobromide, which are non-polar tertiary amines which penetrate lipid barriers easily.
Indications: For use as adjunctive therapy in the treatment of peptic ulcer.
Contraindications: Glaucoma; obstructive uropathy (for example, bladder neck obstruction due to prostatic hypertrophy); obstructive disease of the gastrointestinal tract (as in achalasia, pyloroduodenal stenosis, etc.); paralytic ileus; intestinal atony of the elderly or debilitated patient; unstable cardiovascular status in acute hemorrhage; severe ulcerative colitis; toxic megacolon complicating ulcerative colitis; myasthenia gravis. Robinul (glycopyrrolate) tablets are contraindicated in those patients with a hypersensitivity to glycopyrrolate.
Warnings: In the presence of a high environmental temperature, heat prostration (fever and heat stroke due to decreased sweating) can occur with use of Robinul.
Diarrhea may be an early symptom of incomplete intestinal obstruction, especially in patients with ileostomy or colostomy. In this instance treatment with this drug would be inappropriate and possibly harmful.
Robinul (glycopyrrolate) may produce drowsiness or blurred vision. In this event, the patient should be warned not to engage in activities requiring mental alertness such as operating a motor vehicle or other machinery, or performing hazardous work while taking this drug.
Theoretically, with overdosage a curare-like action may occur, i.e., neuromuscular blockade leading to muscular weakness and possible paralysis.
Pregnancy. The safety of this drug during pregnancy has not been established. The use of any drug during pregnancy requires that the potential benefits of the drug be weighed against possible hazards to mother and child. Reproduction studies in rats revealed no teratogenic effects from glycopyrrolate; however, the potent anticholinergic action of this agent resulted in diminished rates of conception and of survival at weaning, in a dose-related manner. Other studies in dogs suggest that this may be due to diminished seminal secretion which is evident at high doses of glycopyrrolate. Information on possible adverse effects in the pregnant female is limited to uncontrolled data derived from marketing experience. Such experience has revealed no reports of teratogenic or other fetus-damaging potential. No controlled studies to establish the safety of the drug in pregnancy have been performed.
Nursing Mothers. It is not known whether this drug is secreted in human milk. As a general rule, nursing should not be undertaken while a patient is on a drug since many drugs are excreted in human milk.
Pediatric Use. Since there is no adequate experience in children who have received this drug, safety and efficacy in children have not been established.
Precautions: Use Robinul with caution in the elderly and in all patients with:

- Autonomic neuropathy.
- Hepatic or renal disease.
- Ulcerative colitis—large doses may suppress intestinal motility to the point of producing a paralytic ileus and for this reason may precipitate or aggravate "toxic megacolon," a serious complication of the disease.
- Hyperthyroidism, coronary heart disease, congestive heart failure, cardiac tachyarrhythmias, tachycardia, hypertension and prostatic hypertrophy.
- Hiatal hernia associated with reflux esophagitis, since anticholinergic drugs may aggravate this condition.

Adverse Reactions: Anticholinergics produce certain effects, most of which are extensions of their fundamental pharmacological actions. Adverse reactions to anticholinergics in general may include xerostomia; decreased sweating; urinary hesitancy and retention; blurred vision; tachycardia, palpitations; dilatation of the pupil; cycloplegia; increased ocular tension; loss of taste; headaches; nervousness; mental confusion; drowsiness; weakness; dizziness; insomnia; nausea; vomiting; constipation; bloated feeling; impotence; suppression of lactation; severe allergic reaction or drug idiosyncrasies including anaphylaxis; urticaria and other dermal manifestations.
Robinul (glycopyrrolate) is chemically a quaternary ammonium compound; hence, its passage across lipid membranes, such as the blood-brain barrier, is limited in contrast to atropine sulfate and scopolamine hydrobromide. For this reason the occurrence of CNS related side effects is lower, in comparison to their incidence following administration of anticholinergics which are chemically tertiary amines that can cross this barrier readily.
Overdosage: The symptoms of overdosage of glycopyrrolate are peripheral in nature rather than central.
1. To guard against further absorption of the drug—use gastric lavage, cathartics and/or enemas.
2. To combat peripheral anticholinergic effects (residual mydriasis, dry mouth, etc.) —utilize a quaternary ammonium anticholinesterase, such as neostigmine methylsulfate.
3. To combat hypotension—use pressor amines (norepinephrine, metaraminol) i.v.; and supportive care.
4. To combat respiratory depression—administer oxygen; utilize a respiratory stimulant such as Dopram® i.v.; artificial respiration.

Dosage and Administration: ***The dosage of Robinul or Robinul Forte should be adjusted to the needs of the individual patient to assure symptomatic control with a minimum of adverse reactions. The presently recommended maximum daily dosage of glycopyrrolate is 8 mg.***
Robinul (glycopyrrolate, 1 mg) tablets. The recommended initial dosage of Robinul for adults is one tablet three times daily (in the morning, early afternoon, and at bedtime). Some patients may require two tablets at bedtime to assure overnight control of symptoms. For maintenance, a dosage of one tablet twice a day is frequently adequate.
Robinul Forte (glycopyrrolate, 2 mg) tablets. The recommended dosage of Robinul Forte for adults is one tablet two or three times daily at equally spaced intervals.
Robinul tablets are not recommended for use in children under the age of 12 years.
Drug Interactions: There are no known drug interactions.
How Supplied: Robinul (glycopyrrolate, 1 mg) tablets in bottles of 100 (NDC 0031-7824-63) and 500 (NDC 0031-7824-70).
Robinul Forte (glycopyrrolate, 2 mg) tablets in bottles of 100 (NDC 0031-7840-63) and 500 (NDC 0031-7840-70).

[*Shown in Product Identification Section*]

ROBINUL® INJECTABLE ℞
brand of Glycopyrrolate Injection, USP

Description: Robinul (glycopyrrolate) is a synthetic anticholinergic agent. Each 1 ml contains:

Glycopyrrolate, USP ....0.2 mg
Water for Injection, USP ....q.s.
Benzyl Alcohol, NF (preservative) 0.9%

pH adjusted, when necessary, with hydrochloric acid and/or sodium hydroxide.
For Intramuscular or Intravenous administration.
Unlike atropine, glycopyrrolate is completely ionized at physiological pH values.
Robinul Injectable is a clear, colorless, sterile liquid; pH 2.0–3.0.
Clinical Pharmacology: Glycopyrrolate, like other anticholinergic (antimuscarinic) agents, inhibts the action of acetylcholine on structures innervated by postganglionic cholinergic nerves and on smooth muscles that respond to acetylcholine but lack cholinergic innervation. These peripheral cholinergic receptors are present in the autonomic effector cells of smooth muscle, cardiac muscle, the sinoatrial node, the atrioventricular node, exocrine glands, and, to a limited degree, in the autonomic ganglia. Thus, it dimishes the volume and free acidity of gastric secretions and controls excessive pharyngeal, tracheal, and bronchial secretions.
Glycopyrrolate antagonizes muscarinic symptoms (e.g., bronchorrhea, bronchospasm, bradycardia, and intestinal hypermotility) induced by cholinergic drugs such as the anticholinesterases.
The highly polar quaternary ammonium group of glycopyrrolate limits its passage across lipid membranes, such as the blood-brain barrier, in contrast to atropine sulfate and scopolamine hydrobromide, which are non-polar tertiary amines which penetrate lipid barriers easily.
Peak effects occur approximately 30 to 45 minutes after intramuscular administration. The vagal blocking effects persist for 2 to 3 hours and the antisialagogue effects persist up to 7 hours, periods longer than for atropine. With intravenous injection, the onset of action is generally evident within one minute.
Indications and Usage:
In Anesthesia: Robinul (glycopyrrolate) Injectable is indicated for use as a preoperative antimuscarinic to reduce salivary, tracheobronchial, and pharyngeal secretions; to reduce the volume and free acidity of gastric secretions; and, to block cardiac vagal inhibitory reflexes during induction of anesthesia and intubation. When indicated, Robinul Injectable may be used intraoperatively to counteract drug-induced or vagal traction reflexes with the associated arrhythmias. Glycopyrrolate protects against the peripheral muscarinic effects (e.g., bradycardia and excessive secretions) of cholinergic agents such as neostigmine and pyridostigmine given to reverse the neuromuscular blockade due to nondepolarizing muscle relaxants.
In Peptic Ulcer: For use in adults as adjunctive therapy for the treatment of peptic ulcer when rapid anticholinergic effect is desired or when oral medication is not tolerated.
Contraindications: Known hypersensitivity to glycopyrrolate.
In addition, in the management of ***peptic ulcer*** patients, because of the longer duration of therapy, Robinul Injectable may be contraindicated in patients with concurrent glaucoma; obstructive uropathy (for example, bladder neck obstruction due to prostatic hypertrophy); obstructive disease of the gastrointestinal tract (as in achalasia, pyloroduodenal stenosis, etc.); paralytic ileus, intestinal atony of

Continued on next page

Prescribing information on A. H. Robins products listed here is based on official labeling in effect August 1, 1982, with Indications, Contraindications, Warnings, Precautions, Adverse Reactions, and Dosage stated in full.

Robins—Cont.

the elderly or debilitated patient; unstable cardiovascular status in acute hemorrhage; severe ulcerative colitis; toxic megacolon complicating ulcerative colitis; myasthenia gravis.

Warnings: This drug should be used with great caution, if at all, in patients with glaucoma or asthma.

In the ambulatory patient. Robinul (glycopyrrolate) may produce drowsiness or blurred vision. The patient should be cautioned regarding activities requiring mental alertness such as operating a motor vehicle or other machinery or performing hazardous work while taking this drug.

In addition, in the presence of a high environmental temperature, heat prostration (fever and heat stroke due to decreased sweating) can occur with use of Robinul (glycopyrrolate).

Diarrhea may be an early symptom of incomplete intestinal obstruction, expecially in patients with ileostomy or colostomy. In this instance treatment with Robinul (glycopyrrolate) would be inappropriate and possibly harmful.

Precautions: ***General.***

Investigate any tachycardia before giving glycopyrrolate since an increase in the heart rate may occur.

Use with caution in patients with: coronary artery disease; congestive heart failure; cardiac arrhythmias; hypertension; hyperthyroidism.

In managing ulcer patients, use Robinul with caution in the elderly and in all patients with autonomic neuropathy, hepatic or renal disease, ulcerative colitis or hiatal hernia, since anticholinergic drugs may aggravate these conditions.

With overdosage, a curare-like action may occur.

Drug Interactions. The intravenous administration of any anticholinergic in the presence of cyclopropane anesthesia can result in ventricular arrhythmias; therefore, caution should be observed if Robinul (glycopyrrolate) Injectable is used during cyclopropane anesthesia. If the drug is given in small incremental doses of 0.1 mg or less, the likelihood of producing ventricular arrhythmias is reduced.

Carcinogenesis, mutagenesis, impairment of fertility. Long-term studies in animals have not been performed to evaluate carcinogenic potential. In the teratology studies, diminished rates of conception and of survival at weaning were observed in rats, in a dose-related manner. Studies in dogs suggest that this may be due to diminished seminal secretion which is evident at high doses of glycopyrrolate.

Pregnancy Category B. Reproduction studies have been performed in rats and rabbits up to 1000 times the human dose and have revealed no teratogenic effects from glycopyrrolate. There are, however, no adequate and well-controlled studies in pregnant women. Because animal reproduction studies are not always predictive of human response, this drug should be used during pregnancy only if clearly needed.

Nursing Mothers. It is not known whether this drug is excreted in human milk. Because many drugs are excreted in human milk, caution should be exercised when Robinul is administered to a nursing woman.

Pediatric Use. Safety and effectiveness in children below the age of 12 years have not been established for the management of peptic ulcer.

Adverse Reactions: Anticholinergics produce certain effects, most of which are extensions of their pharmacologic actions. Adverse reactions to anticholinergics in general may include dry mouth; urinary hesitancy and retention; blurred vision due to mydriasis; increased ocular tension; tachycardia; palpitation; decreased sweating; loss of taste; headache; nervousness; drowsiness; weakness; dizziness; insomnia; nausea; vomiting; impotence; suppression of lactation; constipation; bloated feeling; severe allergic reaction or drug idiosyncrasies incuding anaphylaxis; urticaria and other dermal manifestations; some degree of mental confusion and/or excitement, especially in elderly persons.

Robinul is chemically a quaternary ammonium compound; hence, its passage across lipid membranes, such as the blood-brain barrier is limited in contrast to atropine sulfate and scopolamine hydrobromide. For this reason the occurrence of CNS related side effects is lower, in comparison to their incidence following administration of anticholinergics which are chemically tertiary amines that can cross this barrier readily.

Overdosage: To combat peripheral anticholinergic effects, a quaternary ammonium anticholinesterase such as neostigmine methylsulfate (which does not cross the blood-brain barrier) may be given intravenously in increments of 0.25 mg in adults. This dosage may be repeated every five to ten minutes until anticholinergic over-activity is reversed or up to a maximum of 2.5 mg. Proportionately smaller doses should be used in children. Indication for repetitive doses of neostigmine should be based on close monitoring of the decrease in heart rate and the return of bowel sounds.

In the unlikely event that CNS symptoms (excitement, restlessness, convulsions, psychotic behavior) occur, physostigmine (which does cross the blood-brain barrier) should be used. Physostigmine 0.5 to 2 mg should be slowly administered intravenously and repeated as necessary up to a total of 5 mg in adults. Proportionately smaller doses should be used in children.

Fever should be treated symptomatically. In the event of a curare-like effect on respiratory muscles, artificial respiration should be instituted and maintained until effective respiratory action returns.

Dosage and Administration: Robinul (glycopyrrolate) Injectable may be administered intramuscularly, or intravenously, without dilution, in the following indications:

Adults: ***Preanesthetic Medication.*** The recommended dose of Robinul (glycopyrrolate) Injectable is 0.002 mg (0.01 ml) per pound of body weight by intramuscular injection, given 30 to 60 minutes prior to the anticipated time of induction of anesthesia or at the time the preanesthetic narcotic and/or sedative are administered.

Intraoperative Medication. Robinul (glycopyrrolate) Injectable may be used during surgery to counteract drug induced or vagal traction reflexes with the associated arrhythmias (e.g., bradycardia). It should be administered intravenously as single doses of 0.1 mg (0.5 ml) and repeated, as needed, at intervals of 2–3 minutes. The usual attempts should be made to determine the etiology of the arrhythmia, and the surgical or anesthetic manipulations necessary to correct parasympathetic imbalance should be performed.

Reversal of Neuromuscular Blockade. The recommended dose of Robinul (glycopyrrolate) Injectable is 0.2 mg (1.0 ml) for each 1.0 mg of neostigmine or 5.0 mg of pyridostigmine. In order to minimize the appearance of cardiac side effects, the drugs may be administered simultaneously by intravenous injection and may be mixed in the same syringe.

Children: ***Preanesthetic Medication.*** The recommended dose of Robinul (glycopyrrolate) Injectable in children to 12 years of age is 0.002 mg (0.01 ml) per pound of body weight intramuscularly, given 30 to 60 minutes prior to the anticipated time of induction of anesthesia or at the time the preanesthetic narcotic and/or sedative are administered.

Children under 2 years of age may require up to 0.004 mg (0.02 ml) per pound of body weight.

Intraoperative Medication. Because of the long duration of action of Robinul (glycopyrrolate) if used as preanesthetic medication, additional Robinul (glycopyrrolate) Injectable for anticholinergic effect intraoperatively is rarely needed; in the event it is required the recommended pediatric dose is 0.002 mg (0.01 ml) per pound of body weight intravenously, not to exceed 0.1 mg (0.5 ml) in a single dose which may be repeated, as needed, at intervals of 2–3 minutes. The usual attempts should be made to determine the etiology of the arrhythmia, and the surgical or anesthetic manipulations necessary to correct parasympathetic imbalance should be performed.

Reversal of Neuromuscular Blockade. The recommended pediatric dose of Robinul (glycopyrrolate) Injectable is 0.2 mg (1.0 ml) for each 1.0 mg of neostigmine or 5.0 mg of pyridostigmine. In order to minimize the appearance of cardiac side effects, the drugs may be administered simultaneously by intravenous injection and may be mixed in the same syringe.

Adults: ***Peptic Ulcer.*** The usual recommended dose of Robinul Injectable is 0.1 mg (0.5 ml) administered at 4-hour intervals, 3 or 4 times daily intravenously or intramuscularly. Where more profound effect is required, 0.2 mg (1.0 ml) may be given. Some patients may need only a single dose, and frequency of administration should be dictated by patient response up to a maximum of four times daily.

Robinul Injectable is not recommended for peptic ulcers in children under 12 years of age. (See Precautions.)

NOTE: Parenteral drug products should be inspected visually for particulate matter and discoloration prior to administration whenever solution and container permit.

Admixture Compatibilities. Robinul (glycopyrrolate) Injectable is compatible for mixing and injection with the following injectable dosage forms: 5% and 10% glucose in water or saline; atropine sulfate, USP; Antilirium® (physostigmine salicylate); Benadryl® (diphenhydramine HCl); codeine phosphate, USP; Emete-Con® (benzquinamide HCl); hydromorphone HCl, USP; Inapsine® (droperidol); Innovar® (droperidol and fentabyl citrate); Largon® (propiomazine HCl); Levo-Dromoran® (levorphanol tartrate); lidocaine, USP; Mepergan® (meperidine and promethazine HCls); meperidine HCl, USP; Mestinon®/Regonol® (pyridostigmine bromide); morphine sulfate, USP; Nisentil® (alphaprodine HCl); Nubain® (nalbuphine HCl); Numorphan® (oxymorphone HCl); Pantopon® (opium alkaloids HCls); procaine HCl, USP; promethazine HCl, USP; Prostigmin® (neostigmine methylsulfate, USP); scopolamine HBr, USP; Sparine® (promazine HCl); Stadol® (butorphanol tartrate); Sublimaze® (fentanyl citrate); Talwin® (pentazocine lactate); Tigan® (trimethobenzamide HCl); Vesprin® (triflupromazine HCl); and Vistaril® (hydroxyzine HCl). Robinul Injectable may be administered via the tubing of a running infusion of physiological saline or lactated Ringer's solution.

Since the stability of glycopyrrolate is questionable above a pH of 6.0, do *not* combine Robinul Injectable in the same syringe with Brevital® (methohexital Na); Chloromycetin® (chloramphenicol Na succinate); Dramamine® (dimenhydrinate); Nembutal® (pentobarbital Na); Pentothal® (thiopental Na); Seconal® (secobarbital Na); sodium bicarbonate (Abbott); or Valium® (diazepam). A gas will evolve or a precipitate may form. Mixing with Decadron® (dexamethazone Na phosphate) or a buffered solution of lactated Ringer's solution will result in a pH higher than 6.0. Mixing chlorpromazine HCl, USP, or Compazine® (prochlorperazine) with other agents in a syringe is not recommended by the manufacturer, although the mixture with Robinul Injectable is physically compatible.

How Supplied: Robinul (glycopyrrolate) Injectable, 0.2 mg/ml, is available in 1 ml single dose vials packaged in 5's (NDC 0031-7890-87), and 25's (NDC 0031-7890-11), 2 ml single dose vials packaged in 25's (NDC 0031-7890-95), 5 ml multiple dose vials packaged individually (NDC 0031-7890-93) and in 25's (NDC 0031-7890-06), and 20 ml (NDC 0031-7890-83) multiple dose vials.

Store at controlled room temperature, between 15°C and 30°C (59°F and 86°F).

Manufactured for Pharmaceutical Division, A. H. Robins Company, Richmond, Virginia 23220 by Elkins-Sinn, Inc., Cherry Hill, NJ 08034, a subsidiary of A. H. Robins Co.

ROBITET® '250' ℞
hydrochloride Robicaps†
(Tetracycline Hydrochloride Capsules, USP)

ROBITET® '500' ℞
hydrochloride Robicaps
(Tetracycline Hydrochloride Capsules, USP)

Description: Tetracycline is a broad-spectrum antibiotic prepared from the cultures of certain streptomyces species. Robitet '250' Robicaps are pink and brown hard gelatin capsules each containing 250 mg tetracycline hydrochloride.

Robitet '500' Robicaps are cream and brown hard gelatin capsules each containing 500 mg tetracycline hydrochloride.

Actions: The tetracyclines are primarily bacteriostatic and are thought to exert their antimicrobial effect by the inhibition of protein synthesis. Tetracyclines are active against a wide range of gram-negative and gram-positive organisms.

The drugs in the tetracycline class have closely similar antimicrobial spectra, and cross-resistance among them is common. Micro-organisms may be considered susceptible if the MIC (minimum inhibitory concentration) is not more than 4.0 mcg./ml. and intermediate if the MIC is 4.0 to 12.5 mcg./ml.

Susceptibility plate testing: A tetracycline disc may be used to determine microbial susceptibility to drugs in the tetracycline class. If the Kirby-Bauer method of disc susceptibility testing is used, a 30 mcg. tetracycline disc should give a zone of at least 19 mm. when tested against a tetracycline-susceptible bacterial strain.

Tetracyclines are readily absorbed and are bound to plasma proteins in varying degree. They are concentrated by the liver in the bile and excreted in the urine and feces at high concentrations and in a biologically active form.

Indications: Tetracycline is indicated in infections caused by the following microorganisms: Rickettsiae (Rocky Mountain spotted fever, typhus fever and the typhus group, Q fever, rickettsialpox and tick fevers), *Mycoplasma pneumoniae* (PPLO, Eaton Agent), Agents of psittacosis and ornithosis, Agents of lymphogranuloma venereum and granuloma inguinale, The spirochetal agent of relapsing fever *(Borrelia recurrentis)*.

The following gram-negative micro-organisms: *Haemophilus ducreyi* (chancroid), *Pasteurella pestis* and *Pasteurella tularensis, Bartonella bacilliformis, Bacteroides* species, *Vibrio comma* and *Vibrio fetus, Brucella* species (in conjunction with streptomycin).

Because many strains of the following groups of micro-organisms have been shown to be resistant to tetracyclines, culture and susceptibility testing are recommended.

Tetracycline is indicated for treatment of infections caused by the following gram-negative micro-organisms, when bacteriologic testing indicates appropriate susceptibility to the drug: *Escherichia coli, Enterobacter aerogenes* (formerly *Aerobacter aerogenes), Shigella* species, *Mima* species and *Herellea* species, *Haemophilus influenzae* (respiratory infections), *Klebsiella* species (respiratory and urinary infections).

Tetracycline is indicated for treatment of infections caused by the following gram-positive micro-organisms when bacteriologic testing indicates appropriate susceptibility to the drug: Streptococcus species: Up to 44 percent of strains of *Streptococcus pyogenes* and 74 percent of *Streptococcus faecalis* have been found to be resistant to tetracycline drugs. Therefore, tetracyclines should not be used for streptococcal disease unless the organism has been demonstrated to be sensitive. For upper respiratory infections due to group A beta-hemolytic streptococci, penicillin is the usual drug of choice, including prophylaxis of rheumatic fever.

Diplococcus pneumoniae, Staphylococcus aureus, skin and soft tissue infections. Tetracyclines are not the drugs of choice in the treatment of any type of staphylococcal infections.

When penicillin is contraindicated, tetracyclines are alternative drugs in the treatment of infections due to: *Neisseria gonorrhoeae, Treponema pallidum* and *Treponema pertenue* (syphilis and yaws), *Listeria monocytogenes, Clostridium* species, *Bacillus anthracis, Fusobacterium fusiforme* (Vincent's infection), *Actinomyces* species.

In acute intestinal amebiasis, the tetracyclines may be a useful adjunct to amebicides.

In severe acne, the tetracyclines may be useful adjunctive therapy.

Tetracyclines are indicated in the treatment of trachoma, although the infectious agent is not always eliminated, as judged by immunofluorescence.

Inclusion conjunctivitis may be treated with oral tetracyclines or with a combination of oral and topical agents.

Contraindication: This drug is contraindicated in persons who have shown hypersensitivity to any of the tetracyclines.

Warnings: THE USE OF DRUGS OF THE TETRACYCLINE CLASS DURING TOOTH DEVELOPMENT (LAST HALF OF PREGNANCY, INFANCY AND CHILDHOOD TO THE AGE OF 8 YEARS) MAY CAUSE PERMANENT DISCOLORATION OF THE TEETH (YELLOW-GRAY-BROWN). This adverse reaction is more common during long-term use of the drugs but has been observed following repeated short-term courses. Enamel hypoplasia has also been reported. TETRACYCLINE DRUGS, THEREFORE, SHOULD NOT BE USED IN THIS AGE GROUP UNLESS OTHER DRUGS ARE NOT LIKELY TO BE EFFECTIVE OR ARE CONTRAINDICATED.

If renal impairment exists, even usual oral or parenteral doses may lead to excessive systemic accumulation of the drug and possible liver toxicity. Under such conditions, lower than usual total doses are indicated and, if therapy is prolonged, serum level determinations of the drug may be advisable.

Photosensitivity manifested by an exaggerated sunburn reaction has been observed in some individuals taking tetracyclines. Patients apt to be exposed to direct sunlight or ultraviolet light should be advised that this reaction can occur with tetracycline drugs, and treatment should be discontinued at the first evidence of skin erythema.

The anti-anabolic action of the tetracyclines may cause an increase in BUN. While this is not a problem in those with normal renal function, in patients with significantly impaired function, higher serum levels of tetracycline may lead to azotemia, hyperphosphatemia, and acidosis.

Usage in pregnancy. (See above "Warnings" about use during tooth development.)

Results of animal studies indicate that tetracyclines cross the placenta, are found in fetal tissues and can have toxic effects on the developing fetus (often related to retardation of skeletal development). Evidence of embryotoxicity has also been noted in animals treated early in pregnancy.

Usage in newborns, infants, and children. (See above "Warnings" about use during tooth development.)

All tetracyclines form a stable calcium complex in any bone forming tissue. A decrease in the fibula growth rate has been observed in prematures given oral tetracycline in doses of 25 mg./kg. every 6 hours. This reaction was shown to be reversible when the drug was discontinued.

Tetracyclines are present in the milk of lactating women who are taking a drug in this class.

Precautions: As with other antibiotic preparations, use of this drug may result in overgrowth of nonsusceptible organisms, including fungi. If superinfection occurs, the antibiotic should be discontinued and appropriate therapy instituted.

In venereal diseases when coexistent syphilis is suspected, darkfield examination should be done before treatment is started and the blood serology repeated monthly for at least 4 months.

Because tetracyclines have been shown to depress plasma prothrombin activity, patients who are on anticoagulant therapy may require downward adjustment of their anticoagulant dosage.

In long-term therapy, periodic laboratory evaluation of organ systems, including hematopoietic, renal and hepatic studies should be performed.

All infections due to Group A beta-hemolytic streptococci should be treated for at least 10 days.

Since bacteriostatic drugs may interfere with the bactericidal action of penicillin, it is advisable to avoid giving tetracycline in conjunction with penicillin.

Adverse Reactions: Gastrointestinal: Anorexia, nausea, vomiting, diarrhea, glossitis, dysphagia, enterocolitis, and inflammatory lesions (with monilial overgrowth) in the anogenital region. These reactions have been caused by both the oral and parenteral administration of tetracyclines.

Skin: maculopapular and erythematous rashes. Exfoliative dermatitis has been reported but is uncommon. Photosensitivity is discussed above. (See "Warnings.")

Renal toxicity: Rise in BUN has been reported and is apparently dose related. (See "Warnings.")

Hypersensitivity reactions: urticaria, angioneurotic edema, anaphylaxis, anaphylactoid purpura, pericarditis and exacerbation of systemic lupus erythematosis.

Bulging fontanels have been reported in young infants following full therapeutic dosage. This sign disappeared rapidly when the drug was discontinued.

Blood: Hemolytic anemia, thrombocytopenia, neutropenia and eosinophilia have been reported.

When given over prolonged periods, tetracyclines have been reported to produce brown-black microscopic discoloration of thyroid glands. No abnormalities of thyroid function studies are known to occur.

Dosage and Administration: Therapy should be continued for at least 24-48 hours after symptoms and fever have subsided.

Concomitant therapy: Antacids containing aluminum, calcium, or magnesium impair absorption and should not be given to patients taking oral tetracycline.

Continued on next page

Prescribing information on A. H. Robins products listed here is based on official labeling in effect August 1, 1982, with Indications, Contraindications, Warnings, Precautions, Adverse Reactions, and Dosage stated in full.

Robins—Cont.

Food and some dairy products also interfere with absorption. Oral forms of tetracycline should be given 1 hour before or 2 hours after meals. Pediatric oral dosage forms should not be given with milk formulas and should be given at least 1 hour prior to feeding.
In patients with renal impairment: (See "Warnings.") Total dosage should be decreased by reduction of recommended individual doses and/or by extending time intervals between doses.
In the treatment of streptococcal infections, a therapeutic dose of tetracycline should be administered for at least 10 days.
ADULTS: Usual daily dose, 1-2 Gm. divided in two or four equal doses, depending on the severity of the infection.
FOR CHILDREN ABOVE EIGHT YEARS OF AGE: Usual daily dose, 10-20 mg. per pound (25-50 mg./kg.) of body weight divided in four equal doses.
For treatment of brucellosis, 500 mg. tetracycline four times daily for 3 weeks should be accompanied by streptomycin. 1 gram intramuscularly twice daily the first week, and once daily the second week.
For treatment of syphilis, a total of 30-40 grams in equally divided doses over a period of 10-15 days should be given. Close followup, including laboratory tests, is recommended.
Treatment of uncomplicated gonorrhea: When penicillin is contraindicated, tetracycline may be used for the treatment of both males and females in the following divided dosage schedule: 1.5 grams initially followed by 0.5 grams q.i.d. for a total of 9.0 grams.
How Supplied: Robitet Robicaps® (Tetracycline Hydrochloride Capsules, USP), 250 mg in bottles of 100 (NDC 0031-8417-63) and 1000 (NDC 0031-8417-74); 500 mg in bottles of 100 (NDC 0031-8427-63) and 500 (NDC 00311-8427-70).

†**Robicaps® is A. H. Robins' registered trademark for capsules.**

[*Shown in Product Identification Section*]

ROBITUSSIN®
ROBITUSSIN-CF®
ROBITUSSIN-DM®
ROBITUSSIN-PE®

(See PDR For Nonprescription Drugs)

ROBITUSSIN A-C® ©

Robitussin and codeine.
Each 5 ml (1 teaspoonful) contains:
Guaifenesin, USP ....100 mg
Codeine Phosphate, USP ....10 mg
(Warning: May be habit forming)
Alcohol 3.5 per cent
In a palatable, aromatic syrup
Actions: Robitussin A-C combines the expectorant, guaifenesin, with the cough suppressant, codeine. Guaifenesin enhances the output of lower respiratory tract fluid (RTF). The enhanced flow of less viscid secretions promotes ciliary action, and facilitates the removal of inspissated mucus. As a result, dry, unproductive coughs become more productive and less frequent.
Codeine phosphate is favored for its efficacy in low dosage. Robitussin A-C is especially useful when concurrent expectorant and cough suppressant actions are desired.
Indications: Robitussin A-C is useful in combating coughs associated with the common cold, bronchitis, laryngitis, tracheitis, pharyngitis, pertussis, influenza, and measles.
Contraindications: Hypersensitivity to any of the ingredients.
Warnings: Use this product with caution in children under 2 years or in children taking another drug. Prescribe cautiously for patients with persistent or chronic cough such as comes with smoking, asthma, emphysema, or where cough is accompanied by excessive secretions. In patients with chronic pulmonary disease or shortness of breath, this product should be administered with caution. This product may cause or aggravate constipation.
Note: Guaifenesin has been shown to produce a color interference with certain clinical laboratory determinations of 5-hydroxyindoleacetic acid (5-HIAA) and vanillylmandelic acid (VMA).
Adverse Reactions: Rarely, nausea, gastrointestinal upset, constipation, and drowsiness may occur. No serious side effects from guaifenesin have been reported.
Dosage: Adults and children 12 years of age and over: 2 teaspoonfuls every four hours, not to exceed 12 teaspoonfuls in a 24 hour period; children 6 to under 12 years: 1 teaspoonful every four hours, not to exceed 6 teaspoonfuls in a 24 hour period; children 2 to under 6 years: ½ teaspoonful every four hours, not to exceed 3 teaspoonfuls in a 24 hour period; children under 2 years: use as directed by physician.
How Supplied: Bottles of 2 ounces (NDC 0031-8674-05), 4 ounces (NDC 0031-8674-12), one pint (NDC 0031-8674-25), and one gallon (NDC 0031-8674-29).

ROBITUSSIN® -DAC ©

Each 5 ml (1 teaspoonful) contains:
Guaifenesin, USP ....100 mg
Pseudoephedrine
Hydrochloride, USP .... 30 mg
Codeine Phosphate, USP .... 10 mg
(Warning: May be habit forming)
In a palatable, aromatic syrup
Alcohol 1.4 per cent
Indications: For the temporary relief of cough and nasal congestion as may occur with the common cold or with inhaled irritants.
Contains the expectorant, guaifenesin, which relieves irritated membranes in the respiratory passageways by preventing dryness through increased mucus flow. The nasal decongestant, pseudoephedrine, reduces the swelling of nasal passages. The antitussive, codeine, calms the cough control center and relieves coughing.
Contraindications: Hypersensitivity to any of the ingredients, marked hypertension, hyperthyroidism, or in patients who are receiving MAO inhibitors or antihypertensive medication.
Warnings: Use this product with caution in children under 2 years or in children taking another drug. Prescribe cautiously for patients with persistent or chronic cough such as comes with smoking, asthma, emphysema, or where cough is accompanied by excessive secretions. Caution should be taken in administering this drug to patients with high blood pressure, heart disease or diabetes. In patients with chronic pulmonary disease or shortness of breath, this product should be administered with caution. As with all products containing sympathomimetic amines, use with caution in patients with prostatic hypertrophy or glaucoma. Do not exceed recommended dosage because at higher doses nervousness, dizziness or sleeplessness may occur. May cause or aggravate constipation.
Note: Guaifenesin has been shown to produce a color interference with certain clinical laboratory determinations of 5-hydroxyindoleacetic acid (5-HIAA) and vanillylmandelic acid (VMA).
Adverse Reactions: Agitation, dizziness, insomnia, palpitations or nausea may occur. In such instances, reduction in frequency and/or quantity of dose is indicated.
Recommended Dosage: Adults and children 12 years of age and over: 1 or 2 teaspoonfuls every four hours, not to exceed 8 teaspoonfuls in a 24-hour period; children 6 to under 12 years: 1 teaspoonful every four hours, not to exceed 4 teaspoonfuls in a 24-hour period; children 2 to under 6 years: ½ teaspoonful every four hours, not to exceed 2 teaspoonfuls in a 24-hour period; children under 2 years: use as directed by physician.
How Supplied: Robitussin-DAC is available in pints (NDC 0031-8680-25).

Z-BEC®

One tablet daily provides:

Vitamin Composition	Percentage of U.S. Recommended Daily Allowance (U.S. RDA)	
Vitamin E	150	45.0 I.U.
Vitamin C	1000	600.0 mg
Thiamine (Vitamin B_1)	1000	15.0 mg
Riboflavin (Vitamin B_2)	600	10.2 mg
Niacin	500	100.0 mg
Vitamin B_6	500	10.0 mg
Vitamin B_{12}	100	6.0 mcg
Pantothenic Acid	250	25.0 mg
Mineral Composition		
Zinc	150	22.5 mg*

*22.5 mg zinc (equivalent to zinc content in 100 mg Zinc Sulfate, USP)
Ingredients: Niacinamide Ascorbate; Ascorbic Acid; Microcrystalline Cellulose; Zinc Sulfate; Vitamin E Acetate; Hydrolyzed Protein; Calcium Pantothenate; Modified Starch; Hydroxypropyl Methylcellulose; Thiamine Mononitrate; Stearic Acid; Pyridoxine Hydrochloride; Riboflavin; Silicon Dioxide; Polysorbate 20; Magnesium Stearate; Lactose; Povidone; Propylene Glycol; Artificial Color; Vanillin; Hydroxypropyl Cellulose; Gelatin; Sorbic Acid; Sodium Benzoate; Cyanocobalamin.
Actions and Uses: Z-BEC is a high potency formulation. Its components have important roles in general nutrition, healing of wounds, and prevention of hemorrhage. It is recommended for deficiencies of these components in conditions such as febrile diseases, chronic or acute infections, burns, fractures, surgery, leg ulcers, toxic conditions, physiologic stress, alcoholism, prolonged exposure to high temperature, geriatrics, gastritis, peptic ulcer, and colitis; and in conditions involving special diets and weight-reduction diets.
In dentistry, Z-BEC is recommended for deficiencies of its components in conditions such as herpetic stomatitis, aphthous stomatitis, cheilosis, herpangina and gingivitis.
Precaution: Not intended for the treatment of pernicious anemia.
Dosage: The recommended OTC dosage for adults and children twelve or more years of age, other than pregnant or lactating women, is one tablet daily with food or after meals. Under the direction and supervision of a physician, the dose and frequency of administration may be increased in accordance with the patient's requirements.
How Supplied: Green film-coated, capsule-shaped tablets in bottles of 60 (NDC 0031-0689-62), 500 (NDC 0031-0689-70) and DisCo® Unit Dose Packs of 100 (NDC 0031-0689-64).

[*Shown in Product Identification Section*]

Products are cross-indexed by

generic and chemical names

in the

YELLOW SECTION

Roche Laboratories
Division of Hoffmann-La Roche Inc.
NUTLEY, NJ 07110

ACCUTANE® ℞
(isotretinoin/Roche)
CAPSULES

The following text is complete prescribing information based on official labeling in effect Dec. 1, 1982.

Description: Accutane (isotretinoin/Roche), a retinoid which inhibits sebaceous gland function and keratinization, is available in 10-mg and 40-mg soft gelatin capsules for oral administration. Chemically, isotretinoin is 13-*cis*-retinoic acid and is related to both retinoic acid and retinol (vitamin A). It is a yellow-orange to orange crystalline powder with a molecular weight of 300.44.

Clinical Pharmacology: The exact mechanism of action of Accutane is unknown.

Cystic Acne: Clinical improvement in cystic acne patients occurs in association with a reduction in sebum secretion. The decrease in sebum secretion is temporary and is related to the dose and duration of treatment with Accutane, and reflects a reduction in sebaceous gland size and an inhibition of sebaceous gland differentiation.[1]

Clinical Pharmacokinetics: The pharmacokinetic profile of isotretinoin is predictable and can be described using linear pharmacokinetic theory.

After oral administration of 80 mg (two 40-mg capsules), peak plasma concentrations ranged from 167 to 459 ng/ml (mean 256 ng/ml) and mean time to peak was 3.2 hours in normal volunteers, while in acne patients peak concentrations ranged from 98 to 535 ng/ml (mean 262 ng/ml) with a mean time to peak of 2.9 hours. The drug is 99.9% bound in human plasma almost exclusively to albumin. The terminal elimination half-life of isotretinoin ranged from 10 to 20 hours in volunteers and patients. Following an 80-mg liquid suspension oral dose of ^{14}C-isotretinoin, ^{14}C-activity in blood declined with a half-life of 90 hours. Relatively equal amounts of radioactivity were recovered in the urine and feces with 65% to 83% of the dose recovered.

The major identified metabolite in blood and urine is 4-*oxo*-isotretinoin. Tretinoin and 4-*oxo*-tretinoin were also observed. The terminal elimination of 4-*oxo*-isotretinoin is formation rate limited and therefore the apparent half-life of the 4-*oxo*-metabolite is similar to isotretinoin following Accutane administration. After two 40-mg capsules of isotretinoin, maximum concentrations of the metabolite of 87 to 399 ng/ml occurred at 6 to 20 hours. The blood concentration of the major metabolite generally exceeded that of isotretinoin after six hours.

The mean $\pm$ SD minimum steady-state blood concentration of isotretinoin was 160 $\pm$ 19 ng/ml in ten patients receiving 40-mg *b.i.d.* doses. After single and multiple doses, the mean ratio of areas under the blood concentration:time curves of 4-*oxo*-isotretinoin to isotretinoin was 3 to 3.5.

Tissue Distribution in Animals: Tissue distribution of ^{14}C-isotretinoin in rats after oral dosing revealed high concentrations of radioactivity in many tissues after 15 minutes, with a maximum in one hour, and declining to nondetectable levels by 24 hours in most tissues. After seven days, however, low levels of radioactivity were detected in the liver, ureter, adrenal, ovary and lacrimal gland.

Indications and Usage: *Cystic Acne:* Accutane is indicated for the treatment of severe recalcitrant cystic acne, and a single course of therapy has been shown to result in complete and prolonged remission of disease in many patients.[1–3] If a second course of therapy is needed, it should not be initiated until at least eight weeks after completion of the first course, since experience has shown that patients may continue to improve while off drug. Because of significant adverse effects associated with its use, Accutane should be reserved for patients with severe cystic acne who are unresponsive to conventional therapy, including systemic antibiotics.

Contraindications: Teratogenicity was observed in rats at a dose of isotretinoin of 150 mg/kg/day. In rabbits a dose of 10 mg/kg/day was teratogenic and embryotoxic, and induced abortion. There are no adequate and well-controlled studies in pregnant women.

Because teratogenicity has been observed in animals given isotretinoin, patients who are pregnant or intend to become pregnant while undergoing treatment should not receive Accutane. Women of childbearing potential should not be given Accutane unless an effective form of contraception is used, and they should be fully counseled on the potential risks to the fetus should they become pregnant while undergoing treatment. Should pregnancy occur during treatment, the physician and patient should discuss the desirability of continuing the pregnancy.

Accutane should not be given to patients who are sensitive to parabens, which are used as preservatives in the formulation.

Warnings: Although no abnormalities of the human fetus have been reported thus far, animal studies with retinoids suggest that teratogenic effects may occur. It is recommended that contraception be continued for one month or until a normal menstrual period has occurred following discontinuation of Accutane therapy.

Blood lipid determinations should be performed before Accutane is given and then at intervals until the lipid response to Accutane is established, which usually occurs within four weeks. (See PRECAUTIONS.)

Approximately 25% of patients receiving Accutane experienced an elevation in plasma triglycerides. Approximately 15% developed a decrease in high density lipoproteins and about 7% showed an increase in cholesterol levels. These effects on triglycerides, HDL and cholesterol were reversible upon cessation of Accutane therapy.

Patients with increased tendency to develop hypertriglyceridemia include those with diabetes mellitus, obesity, increased alcohol intake and familial history.

The consequences of hypertriglyceridemia are not well understood, but may increase the patient's cardiovascular risk status. Therefore, every attempt should be made to control significant triglyceride elevation.

Some patients have been able to reverse triglyceride elevation by reduction in weight, restriction of dietary fat and alcohol, and reduction in dose while continuing Accutane.[4]

An obese male patient with Darier's disease developed elevated triglycerides and subsequent eruptive xanthomas.[5]

The erythrocyte sedimentation rate was elevated in 40% of patients receiving Accutane, while 13% of patients developed high platelet counts.

Cheilitis was reported in 90% of the patients and conjunctivitis was noted in about 38% of the patients receiving Accutane. Musculoskeletal symptoms were recorded in about 16% of patients. In clinical trials of disorders of keratinization, five patients treated for over two years showed skeletal abnormalities. These five included hyperostosis with spine degeneration in three adult patients, and two children who showed x-ray findings suggestive of possible premature closure of the epiphysis. Increases in alkaline phosphatase and SGOT were seen in 14% and 11% of patients, respectively.

In rats given isotretinoin at dosages of 32 and 8 mg/kg/day for 39 or 78 weeks, serum alkaline phosphatase was elevated but did not remain elevated when these dosages were given for 104 weeks. Serum alkaline phosphatase was also elevated in dogs given 60 to 120 mg/kg/day of isotretinoin for approximately one year.

In rats given isotretinoin at a dosage of 32 mg/kg/day for approximately 15 weeks, long bone fracture has been observed.

In rats given 32 or 8 mg/kg/day of isotretinoin for 18 months or longer, the incidences of focal calcification, fibrosis and inflammation of the myocardium, calcification of coronary, pulmonary and mesenteric arteries and metastatic calcification of the gastric mucosa were greater than in control rats of similar age. Focal endocardial and myocardial calcifications associated with calcification of the coronary arteries were observed in two dogs after approximately six to seven months of treatment with isotretinoin at a dosage of 60 to 120 mg/kg/day.

In dogs given isotretinoin chronically at a dosage of 60 mg/kg/day, corneal ulcers and corneal opacities were encountered at a higher incidence than in control dogs. In general, these ocular changes tended to revert toward normal when treatment with isotretinoin was stopped, but did not completely clear during the observation period. In Accutane studies to date, of 72 patients who had normal pretreatment ophthalmological examinations, five developed corneal opacities while on Accutane (all five patients had a disorder of keratinization and none were cystic acne patients).

Precautions: *Information for Patients:* Because of the relationship of Accutane to vitamin A, patients should be advised against taking vitamin supplements containing vitamin A to avoid additive toxic effects.

Women of childbearing potential should be instructed to use an effective form of contraception when Accutane therapy is required. (See CONTRAINDICATIONS and WARNINGS.)

As may be seen with healing cystic acne lesions, an occasional exaggerated healing response, manifested by exuberant granulation tissue with crusting, has also been reported in patients on therapy with Accutane.

Laboratory Tests: The incidence of hypertriglyceridemia is 1 patient in 4 on Accutane therapy. Pretreatment and follow-up blood lipids should be obtained under fasting conditions. After consumption of alcohol at least 36 hours should elapse before these determinations are made. It is recommended that these tests be performed at weekly or biweekly intervals until the lipid response to Accutane is established.

Carcinogenesis, Mutagenesis, Impairment of Fertility: In Fischer 344 rats given isotretinoin at dosages of 32 or 8 mg/kg/day for greater than 18 months, there was an increased incidence of pheochromocytoma. The incidence of adrenal medullary hyperplasia was also increased at the higher dosage. The relatively high level of spontaneous pheochromocytomas occurring in the Fischer 344 rat makes it a poor model for study of this tumor, since the increase in adrenal medullary proliferative lesions following chronic treatment with relatively high dosages of isotretinoin may be an accentuation of a genetic predisposition in the Fischer 344 rat, and its relevance to the human population is not clear. In addition, a decreased incidence of liver adenomas, liver angiomas and leukemia was noted at the dose levels of 8 and 32 mg/kg/day.

No mutagenesis was noted in the Ames test at concentrations up to 2 mg/plate.

No adverse effects on gonadal function, fertility, conception rate, gestation or parturition were observed at dose levels of 2, 8 or 32 mg/kg/day in male and female rats.

In dogs, testicular atrophy was noted after treatment with isotretinoin for approximately

Continued on next page

Roche Labs.—Cont.

30 weeks at dosages of 60 or 20 mg/kg/day. In general, there was microscopic evidence for appreciable depression of spermatogenesis but some sperm were observed in all testes examined and in no instance were completely atrophic tubules seen. In studies in 66 human males, 30 of whom were patients with cystic acne, no significant changes were noted in the count or motility of spermatozoa in the ejaculate. Studies further evaluating this in humans are being conducted.

Pregnancy: Category X. See "CONTRAINDICATIONS" section.

Nursing Mothers: It is not known whether this drug is excreted in human milk. Because of the potential for adverse effects, nursing mothers should not receive Accutane.

Adverse Reactions: *Clinical*: The percentages of adverse reactions listed below reflect the total experience in Accutane studies, including investigational studies of disorders of keratinization, with the exception of those pertaining to dry skin and mucous membranes. These latter reflect the experience only in patients with cystic acne because reactions relating to dryness are more commonly recognized as adverse reactions in this disease. Included in this category are dry skin, pruritus, epistaxis, dry nose and dry mouth, which may be seen in up to 80% of cystic acne patients.

The most frequent adverse reaction to Accutane is cheilitis, which occurs in over 90% of patients. A less frequent reaction was conjunctivitis (about two patients in five).

Approximately 16% of patients treated with Accutane developed musculoskeletal symptoms during treatment. In general, these were mild to moderate and rarely required discontinuation of the drug. These symptoms cleared rapidly with discontinuation of Accutane.

In less than one patient in ten—rash, temporary thinning of hair.

In approximately one patient in twenty— peeling of palms and soles, skin infections, nonspecific urogenital findings, nonspecific gastrointestinal symptoms, fatigue, headache and increased susceptibility to sunburn.

The following reactions have been reported in less than 1% of patients and may bear no relationship to therapy—changes in skin pigment (hypo- and hyperpigmentation), urticaria, bruising, disseminated herpes simplex, edema, hair problems (other than thinning), respiratory infections, mild gastrointestinal bleeding, weight loss, paresthesias, dizziness and abnormal menses.

In Accutane studies to date, of 72 patients who had normal pretreatment ophthalmological examinations, five developed corneal opacities while on Accutane (all five patients had a disorder of keratinization and none were cystic acne patients).

Laboratory: Accutane therapy induces change in serum lipids in a significant number of treated subjects. Approximately 25% of patients had elevation of plasma triglycerides. Five out of 135 patients treated for cystic acne and 32 out of 298 total subjects treated for all diagnoses showed an elevation of triglycerides above 500 mg percent. About 16% of patients showed a mild to moderate decrease in serum high density lipoprotein (HDL) levels while receiving treatment with Accutane and about 7% of patients experienced minimal elevations of serum cholesterol during treatment. Abnormalities of serum triglycerides, HDL and cholesterol were reversible upon cessation of Accutane therapy. Approximately 40% of patients receiving Accutane developed elevated sedimentation rates, often from elevated baseline values.

From one in ten to one in five patients showed decreases in red blood cell parameters and white blood cell counts, elevated platelet counts, white cells in the urine, increased alkaline phosphatase, SGOT or SGPT.

Less than one in ten patients showed proteinuria, red blood cells in the urine or elevated fasting blood sugar.

Dose Relationship and Duration: Most adverse reactions appear to be dose related, with the more pronounced effects occurring at doses above 1.0 mg/kg/day. Adverse reactions seen in cystic acne patients were reversible when therapy was discontinued.

Overdosage: The oral LD_{50} of isotretinoin is greater than 4000 mg/kg in rats and mice and is approximately 1960 mg/kg in rabbits. There has been no experience with acute overdosage in human beings.

Dosage and Administration: In general, the initial dose of Accutane should be individualized according to the patient's weight and severity of the disease. After two or more weeks of treatment, the dose should be adjusted according to the appearance of clinical side effects and the response of the disease.

The recommended course of therapy is one to two mg/kg, given in two divided doses daily for fifteen to twenty weeks. If the total cyst count has been reduced by more than 70% prior to this time period, the drug may be discontinued. After a period of two months off therapy, and if warranted by persistent severe cystic acne, a second course of therapy may be initiated. Patients whose disease is primarily manifest on the chest and back instead of the face, as well as patients who weigh more than 70 kg, may require doses at the higher end of the range.

ACCUTANE DOSING BY BODY WEIGHT

Body Weight kilograms	pounds	Total Mg/Day 1 mg/kg	2 mg/kg
40	88	40	80
50	110	50	100
60	132	60	120
70	154	70	140
80	176	80	160
90	198	90	180
100	220	100	200

How Supplied: Soft gelatin capsules, 10 mg (light pink), imprinted ACCUTANE 10 ROCHE; bottles of 100 (NDC-0004-0155-01).

Soft gelatin capsules, 40 mg (yellow), imprinted ACCUTANE 40 ROCHE; bottles of 100 (NDC-0004-0156-01).

References:

1. Peck, GL, Olsen, TG, Yoder, FW, Strauss, JS, Downing, DT, Pandya, M, Butkus, D, Arnaud-Battandier, J: Prolonged remissions of cystic and conglobate acne with 13-*cis*-retinoic acid. *N Engl J Med 300*:329–333, 1979. 2. Farrell, LN, Strauss, JS, Stranieri, AM: The treatment of severe cystic acne with 13-*cis*-retinoic acid. Evaluation of sebum production and the clinical response in a multiple-dose trial. *J Am Acad Dermatol 3*:602–611, 1980. 3. Jones, H, Blanc, D, Cunliffe, WJ: 13-*cis*-retinoic acid and acne. *Lancet 2*:1048–1049, 1980. 4. Katz, RA, Jorgensen, H, Nigra, TP: Elevation of serum triglyceride levels from oral isotretinoin in disorders of keratinization. *Arch Dermatol 116*:1369–1372, 1980. 5. Dicken, CH, Connolly, SM: Eruptive xanthomas associated with isotretinoin (13-*cis*-retinoic acid). *Arch Dermatol 116*:951–952, 1980.

(Shown in Product Identification Section)

ALURATE® ELIXIR Ⓒ
(aprobarbital/Roche)

The following text is complete prescribing information based on official labeling in effect August 1, 1982.

The following sections contain information specifically applicable to Alurate as well as information pertinent to other barbiturates. The information pertinent to other barbiturates should be considered when administering Alurate.

Description: Alurate (aprobarbital/Roche) is an intermediate-acting barbiturate which is used as a sedative-hypnotic. As with other barbiturates, it acts as a CNS depressant. Alurate is available for oral administration as a red elixir providing 40 mg of aprobarbital per teaspoonful (5 ml) in a vehicle containing 20 percent alcohol. Chemically, aprobarbital is 5-allyl-5-isopropylbarbituric acid. It is a bitter, white crystalline powder with an empirical formula of $C_{10}H_{14}N_2O_3$ and a molecular weight of 210.23.

Clinical Pharmacology: Barbiturates are capable of producing all levels of CNS mood alteration from excitation to mild sedation, hypnosis and deep coma. Overdosage can produce death. In high enough therapeutic doses, barbiturates induce anesthesia.

Barbiturates depress the sensory cortex, decrease motor activity, alter cerebellar function and produce drowsiness, sedation and hypnosis.

Barbiturate-induced sleep differs from physiological sleep. Sleep laboratory studies have demonstrated that barbiturates reduce the amount of time spent in the rapid eye movement (REM) phase of sleep or dreaming stage. Also, Stages III and IV sleep are decreased. Patients may experience markedly increased dreaming, nightmares and/or insomnia if barbiturates are prescribed for a period of time and then abruptly withdrawn. It is recommended that dosage be reduced gradually over a period of 5 or 6 days to lessen REM rebound and disturbed sleep (for example, decrease the dose from 3 to 2 doses a day for 1 week).

In studies, secobarbital sodium and pentobarbital sodium have been found to lose most of their effectiveness for both inducing and maintaining sleep by the end of 2 weeks of continued drug administration, even with the use of multiple doses. Other barbiturates might also be expected to lose their effectiveness for inducing and maintaining sleep after about 2 weeks. Therefore, as sleep medications, the barbiturates are of limited value beyond short-term use.

Barbiturates have little analgesic action at subanesthetic doses. Rather, they may increase the reaction to painful stimuli. All barbiturates exhibit anticonvulsant activity in anesthetic doses; however, only phenobarbital, mephobarbital and metharbital are effective as oral anticonvulsants in subhypnotic doses.

Barbiturates are respiratory depressants; the degree of depression is dose-dependent. With hypnotic doses, respiratory depression produced by barbiturates is similar to that which occurs during physiologic sleep. Hypnotic doses also cause a slight decrease in blood pressure and heart rate.

Studies in laboratory animals have shown that barbiturates cause reduction in the tone and contractility of the uterus, ureters and urinary bladder. However, concentrations of the drugs required to produce this effect in humans are not reached with sedative-hypnotic doses.

Barbiturates do not impair normal hepatic function, but have been shown to induce liver microsomal enzymes, thus altering the metabolism of certain other drugs. (See Precautions — Drug Interactions section.)

Pharmacokinetics: Barbiturates are absorbed in varying degrees following oral administration. The onset of action for oral barbiturate administration varies from 20 to 60 minutes. Duration of action, which is related to the rate at which the barbiturates are redistributed throughout the body, varies among persons and in the same person from time to time. Aprobarbital, which is an intermediate-acting barbiturate, has a duration of action ranging from 6 to 8 hours.

Barbiturates are weak acids that are absorbed and rapidly distributed to all tissues and fluids, with high concentrations in the brain, liver and kidneys. Lipid solubility of the barbiturates is the dominant factor in their distribution throughout the body. Barbiturates are bound to plasma and tissue proteins to a varying degree, with the degree of binding increasing directly as a function of lipid solubility. Aprobarbital is approximately 20 percent plasma protein-bound.

The half-life of aprobarbital ranges from 14 to 34 hours with a mean half-life of 24 hours.

Barbiturates are metabolized primarily by the hepatic microsomal enzyme system; the metabolic products are excreted in the urine and, less commonly, in the feces. Approximately 13 to 24 percent of aprobarbital is eliminated unchanged in the urine. The inactive metabolites of the barbiturates are excreted as conjugates of glucuronic acid.

Indications and Usage: Alurate is indicated for sedation and induction of sleep, on a short-term basis, in conditions requiring a sedative-hypnotic.

Contraindications: Barbiturates are contraindicated in patients with known barbiturate sensitivity. Barbiturates are also contraindicated in patients with a history of manifest or latent porphyria.

Warnings: *Habit forming:* Barbiturates may be habit forming. Tolerance and psychological and physical dependence may occur with continued use. (See Drug Abuse and Dependence section.) Patients who have a psychological dependence on barbiturates may increase the dosage or decrease the dosage interval without consulting a physician and may subsequently develop a physical dependence. To minimize the possibility of overdosage or the development of dependence, the quantity of sedative-hypnotic barbiturates prescribed or dispensed should be limited to the amount required between appointments. Abrupt cessation after prolonged use may result in withdrawal symptoms, including delirium, convulsions and possibly death.

Barbiturates should be withdrawn gradually from any patient known to be taking excessive doses over long periods of time.

Acute or chronic pain: Caution should be exercised when barbiturates are administered to patients with acute or chronic pain, because paradoxical excitement may be induced or important symptoms may be masked.

Use in pregnancy: Barbiturates can cause fetal damage when administered to a pregnant woman. Retrospective case-controlled studies have suggested a connection between maternal consumption of barbiturates and a higher than expected incidence of fetal abnormalities. Following oral administration, barbiturates readily cross the placental barrier and are distributed throughout the placenta and fetal tissues, with highest concentrations found in the liver and brain.

Withdrawal symptoms occur in infants born to mothers who receive barbiturates throughout the last trimester of pregnancy. (See Drug Abuse and Dependence section.) If this drug is used during pregnancy, or if the patient becomes pregnant while taking this drug, the patient should be apprised of the potential hazard to the fetus.

Synergistic effects: The concomitant use of alcohol or other CNS depressants may produce additive CNS-depressant effects.

Precautions: *General:* Barbiturates may be habit forming. Tolerance and psychological and physical dependence may occur with continued use. (See Drug Abuse and Dependence section.) Barbiturates should be administered with caution, if at all, to patients who are mentally depressed, have suicidal tendencies, or a history of drug abuse. Elderly or debilitated patients may react to barbiturates with marked excitement, depression and confusion. In some persons, barbiturates repeatedly produce excitement rather than depression. In patients with hepatic damage, barbiturates should be administered with caution, and initially in reduced doses. Barbiturates should not be administered to patients showing the premonitory signs of hepatic coma.

Information for Patients: The use of barbiturates carries with it an associated risk of psychological and/or physical dependence. The patient should be warned against increasing the dose of the drug without consulting a physician.

Barbiturates may impair mental and/or physical abilities required for the performance of potentially hazardous tasks, such as driving a car or operating machinery.

Alcohol should not be consumed while taking barbiturates. Concurrent use of barbiturates with other CNS depressants (*e.g.,* alcohol, narcotics, tranquilizers, antihistamines) may result in additional CNS depressant effects.

Laboratory Tests: Prolonged therapy with barbiturates should be accompanied by periodic laboratory evaluation of organ systems, including hematopoietic, renal and hepatic systems.

Drug Interactions: Most reports of clinically significant drug interactions occurring with the barbiturates have involved phenobarbital. However, the application of these data to other barbiturates appears valid and warrants serial blood level determinations of the relevant drugs when there are multiple therapies.

1. *Anticoagulants.* Phenobarbital lowers the plasma levels of dicumarol (name previously used: bishydroxycoumarin) and causes a decrease in anticoagulant activity as measured by the prothrombin time. Barbiturates can induce hepatic microsomal enzymes resulting in increased metabolism of and decreased anticoagulant response to oral anticoagulants (*e.g.,* warfarin, acenocoumarol, dicumarol and phenprocoumon). Patients stabilized on anticoagulant therapy may require dosage adjustments if barbiturates are added to or withdrawn from their dosage regimen.

2. *Corticosteroids.* Barbiturates appear to enhance the metabolism of exogenous corticosteroids, probably through the induction of hepatic microsomal enzymes. Patients stabilized on corticosteroid therapy may require dosage adjustments if barbiturates are added to or withdrawn from their dosage regimen.

3. *Griseofulvin.* Phenobarbital appears to interfere with the absorption of orally administered griseofulvin, thus decreasing its blood level. This effect on therapeutic response has not been established; however, it would be preferable to avoid concomitant administration of these drugs.

4. *Doxycycline.* Phenobarbital has been shown to shorten the half-life of doxycycline for as long as two weeks after discontinuance of the barbiturate therapy. This action is probably the result of induction of hepatic microsomal enzymes that metabolize the antibiotic. If phenobarbital and doxycycline are administered concurrently, the clinical response to doxycycline should be monitored closely.

5. *Phenytoin, sodium valproate, valproic acid.* The effect of barbiturates on the metabolism of phenytoin appears to be variable. Some investigators report an accelerating effect, while others report no effect. Because the effect is not predictable, phenytoin and barbiturate blood levels should be monitored more frequently if these drugs are given concurrently. Sodium valproate and valproic acid appear to decrease barbiturate metabolism; therefore, barbiturate blood levels should be monitored and appropriate dosage adjustments made.

6. *Central nervous system depressants.* The concomitant use of other central nervous system depressants, including other sedatives or hypnotics, antihistamines, tranquilizers or alcohol, may produce additive effects.

7. *Monoamine oxidase inhibitors (MAOI).* MAOI prolong the effects of barbiturates, probably because metabolism of the barbiturates is inhibited.

8. *Estradiol, estrone, progesterone and other steroidal hormones.* Pretreatment with or concurrent administration of phenobarbital may decrease the effect of estradiol by increasing its metabolism. There have been reports of patients treated with antiepileptic drugs (*e.g.,* phenobarbital) who became pregnant while taking oral contraceptives. An alternate contraceptive method might be suggested to women taking phenobarbital.

Carcinogenesis: 1. Animal data. Phenobarbital sodium is carcinogenic in mice and rats after lifetime administration. In mice, it produced benign and malignant liver cell tumors. In rats, benign liver cell tumors were observed very late in life.

2. Human data. In a 29-year epidemiological study of 9136 patients who were treated on an anticonvulsant protocol which included phenobarbital sodium, results indicated a higher than normal incidence of hepatic carcinoma. Previously, some of these patients were treated with Thorotrast, a drug which is known to produce hepatic carcinomas. Thus, this study did not provide sufficient evidence that phenobarbital sodium is carcinogenic in humans.

A retrospective study of 84 children with brain tumors matched to 73 normal controls and 78 cancer controls (malignant disease other than brain tumors) suggested an association between exposure to barbiturates prenatally and an increased incidence of brain tumors.

Pregnancy: 1. Teratogenic Effects. Pregnancy Category D. See Warnings section.

2. Nonteratogenic Effects. Reports of infants suffering from long-term barbiturate exposure *in utero* include the acute withdrawal syndrome of seizures and hyperirritability from birth. A delayed onset of the symptoms may be seen for up to 14 days. (See Drug Abuse and Dependence section.)

Labor and Delivery: Hypnotic doses of barbiturates do not appear to significantly impair uterine activity during labor. Full anesthetic doses of barbiturates decrease the force and frequency of uterine contractions. Administration of sedative-hypnotic barbiturates to the mother during labor may result in respiratory depression in the newborn.

Premature infants are particularly susceptible to the depressant effects of barbiturates. If barbiturates are used during labor and delivery, resuscitation equipment should be available.

Data are not currently available to evaluate the effect of these barbiturates when forceps delivery or other intervention is necessary. Also, data are not available to determine the effect of these barbiturates on the later growth, development and functional maturation of the child.

Nursing mothers: Small amounts of barbiturates are excreted in the human milk. Because of the potential for serious adverse reactions in nursing infants from barbiturates, a decision should be made whether to discontinue nursing or to discontinue the drug, taking into account the importance of the drug to the mother.

Pediatric use: Safety and effectiveness in children have not been established.

Adverse Reactions: The following adverse reactions have been reported following the use of Alurate in an incidence of less than 1 in 100 patients.

Nervous system: Dizziness, nervousness.

Digestive system: Nausea and vomiting.

Other reported reactions: Headache, hypersensitivity reactions (skin rashes) and purpura.

Although the following adverse reactions have not been reported with Alurate, they have been compiled from surveillance of thousands of hospitalized patients receiving barbiturates and should be considered when administering Alurate:

More than 1 in 100 patients. The most common adverse reaction estimated to occur at a rate of 1 to 3 patients per 100 is:

Continued on next page

Roche Labs.—Cont.

Nervous system: Somnolence.
Less than 1 in 100 patients. Adverse reactions estimated to occur at a rate of less than 1 in 100 patients are listed below, grouped by organ system and by decreasing order of occurrence:
Nervous system: Agitation, confusion, hyperkinesia, ataxia, CNS depression, nightmares, psychiatric disturbances, hallucinations, insomnia, anxiety, thinking abnormality.
Respiratory system: Hypoventilation, apnea.
Cardiovascular system: Bradycardia, hypotension, syncope.
Digestive system: Constipation.
Other reported reactions: Hypersensitivity reactions (angioedema, exfoliative dermatitis), fever, liver damage, megaloblastic anemia following chronic phenobarbital use.

Drug Abuse and Dependence: Alurate is subject to Class III control under the Federal Controlled Substances Act.
Barbiturates may be habit forming. Tolerance, psychological dependence and physical dependence may occur especially following prolonged use of high doses of barbiturates. Daily administration in excess of 400 mg of pentobarbital or secobarbital for approximately 90 days is likely to produce some degree of physical dependence. A dosage of from 600 to 800 mg taken for at least 35 days is sufficient to produce withdrawal seizures. The average daily dose for the barbiturate addict is usually about 1.5 grams. As tolerance to barbiturates develops, the amount needed to maintain the same level of intoxication increases; tolerance to fatal dosage, however, does not increase more than twofold. As this occurs, the margin between an intoxicating dosage and fatal dosage becomes smaller.
Symptoms of acute intoxication with barbiturates include unsteady gait, slurred speech and sustained nystagmus. Mental signs of chronic intoxication include confusion, poor judgment, irritability, insomnia and somatic complaints.
Symptoms of barbiturate dependence are similar to those of chronic alcoholism. If an individual appears to be intoxicated with alcohol to a degree that is radically disproportionate to the amount of alcohol in his or her blood, the use of barbiturates should be suspected. The lethal dose of a barbiturate is far less if alcohol is also ingested.
The symptoms of barbiturate withdrawal can be severe and may cause death. Minor withdrawal symptoms may appear 8 to 12 hours after the last dose of a barbiturate. These symptoms usually appear in the following order: anxiety, muscle twitching, tremor of hands or fingers, progressive weakness, dizziness, distortion in visual perception, nausea, vomiting, insomnia and orthostatic hypotension. Major withdrawal symptoms (convulsions and delirium) may occur within 16 hours and last up to 5 days after abrupt cessation of these drugs. Intensity of withdrawal symptoms gradually declines over a period of approximately 15 days. Individuals susceptible to barbiturate abuse and dependence include alcoholics and opiate abusers, as well as other sedative-hypnotic and amphetamine abusers.
Drug dependence to barbiturates arises from repeated administration of a barbiturate or an agent with barbiturate-like effect on a continuous basis, generally in amounts exceeding therapeutic dosage levels. The characteristics of drug dependence to barbiturates include: (a) a strong desire or need to continue taking the drug; (b) a tendency to increase the dose; (c) a psychic dependence on the effects of the drug related to subjective and individual appreciation of those effects; and (d) a physical dependence on the effects of the drug requiring its presence for maintenance of homeostasis and resulting in a definite, characteristic and self-limited abstinence syndrome when the drug is withdrawn.
Treatment of barbiturate dependence consists of cautious and gradual withdrawal of the drug. Barbiturate-dependent patients can be withdrawn by using a number of different withdrawal regimens. In all cases withdrawal takes an extended period of time. One method involves substituting 30 mg of phenobarbital for each 100 mg of the short-acting barbiturate which the patient has been taking. The total daily amount of phenobarbital is then administered in 4 divided doses, not to exceed 600 mg daily. Should signs of withdrawal occur on the first day of treatment, a loading dose of 200 mg of phenobarbital may be administered IM, and the daily oral dosage increased. After stabilization with phenobarbital is achieved, the total daily dose of phenobarbital is decreased by 30 mg a day as long as withdrawal is proceeding smoothly. An alternative method of treatment is to decrease the daily dosage of the barbiturate which the patient has been taking by 10 percent/day, if tolerated by the patient.
Infants physically dependent on barbiturates may be given phenobarbital 3 to 10 mg/kg/day. After withdrawal symptoms (hyperactivity, disturbed sleep, tremors, hyperreflexia) are relieved, the dosage of phenobarbital should be gradually decreased and completely withdrawn over a 2-week period.

Overdosage: The toxic dose of barbiturates varies considerably. In general, an oral dose of 1 gram of most barbiturates produces serious poisoning in an adult. Death commonly occurs after ingestion of 2 to 10 grams of barbiturate. Barbiturate intoxication may be confused with alcoholism, bromide intoxication and with various neurological disorders.
Acute overdosage with barbiturates is manifested by CNS and respiratory depression which may progress to Cheyne-Stokes respiration, areflexia, constriction of the pupils to a slight degree (though in severe poisoning they may show paralytic dilation), oliguria, tachycardia, hypotension, lowered body temperature and coma. Typical shock syndrome (apnea, circulatory collapse, respiratory arrest and death) may occur.
In extreme overdose, all electrical activity in the brain may cease, in which case the EEG may be "flat," which does not necessarily indicate clinical death. This effect is fully reversible unless hypoxic damage occurs. Consideration should be given to the possibility of barbiturate intoxication even in situations that appear to involve trauma.
Complications such as pneumonia, pulmonary edema, cardiac arrhythmias, congestive heart failure and renal failure may occur. Uremia may increase CNS sensitivity to barbiturates if renal function is impaired. Differential diagnosis should include hypoglycemia, head trauma, cerebrovascular accidents, convulsive states and diabetic coma. Blood levels from acute overdosage for some barbiturates are listed in the accompanying table.
[See table below].
Treatment of overdosage is mainly supportive and consists of the following:
1. Maintenance of an adequate airway, with assisted respiration and oxygen administration as necessary.
2. Monitoring of vital signs and fluid balance.
3. If the patient is conscious and has not lost the gag reflex, emesis may be induced with ipecac. Care should be taken to prevent pulmonary aspiration of vomitus. After completion of vomiting, 30 grams activated charcoal, in a glass of water, may be administered.
4. If emesis is contraindicated, gastric lavage may be performed with a cuffed endotracheal tube in place with the patient in the face down position. Activated charcoal may be left in the emptied stomach and a saline cathartic administered.
5. Fluid therapy and other standard treatment for shock, if needed.
6. If renal function is normal, forced diuresis may aid in the elimination of the barbiturate. *Alkalinization of the urine increases renal excretion of some barbiturates, especially* phenobarbital, *aprobarbital* and mephobarbital (which is metabolized to phenobarbital).
7. Although not recommended as a routine procedure, hemodialysis may be used in severe barbiturate intoxication or if the patient is anuric or in shock.
8. Patient should be rolled from side to side every 30 minutes.
9. Antibiotics should be given if pneumonia is suspected.
10. Appropriate nursing care to prevent hypostatic pneumonia, decubiti, aspiration and other complications in patients with altered states of consciousness.

Dosage and Administration: *Usual Adult Dosage:* As a sedative, one 5-ml teaspoonful (40 mg) three times daily; for mild insomnia, one to two 5-ml teaspoonfuls before retiring; for pronounced insomnia, two to four 5-ml teaspoonfuls before retiring.
Special Patient Population: Dosage should be reduced in the elderly or debilitated because these patients may be more sensitive to barbiturates. Dosage should be reduced for patients with impaired renal function or hepatic disease.

How Supplied: Elixir (red) providing 40 mg of aprobarbital/Roche per 5 ml in a vehicle containing 20 percent alcohol — bottles of 16 oz (1 pint) (NDC 0004-1000-28).

Concentration of Barbiturate in the Blood Versus Degree of CNS Depression

Barbiturate	Onset/ duration	Degree of depression in nontolerant persons*				
		1	2	3	4	5
		Barbiturate blood levels in ppm (mcg/ml)				
Pentobarbital	Fast/short	≤2	0.5 to 3	10 to 15	12 to 25	15 to 40
Secobarbital	Fast/short	≤2	0.5 to 5	10 to 15	15 to 25	15 to 40
Amobarbital	Intermediate/ intermediate	≤3	2 to 10	30 to 40	30 to 60	40 to 80
Butabarbital	Intermediate/ intermediate	≤5	3 to 25	40 to 60	50 to 80	60 to 100
Phenobarbital	Slow/long	≤10	5 to 40	50 to 80	70 to 120	100 to 200

*Categories of degree of depression in nontolerant persons:
1. Under the influence and appreciably impaired for purposes of driving a motor vehicle or performing tasks requiring alertness and unimpaired judgment and reaction time.
2. Sedated, therapeutic range, calm, relaxed, and easily aroused.
3. Comatose, difficult to arouse, significant depression of respiration.
4. Compatible with death in aged or ill persons or in presence of obstructed airway, other toxic agents, or exposure to cold.
5. Usual lethal level, the upper end of the range includes those who received some supportive treatment.

ANCOBON® ℞
(flucytosine/Roche)

The following text is complete prescribing information based on official labeling in effect August 1, 1982.

> WARNING
> Use with extreme caution in patients with impaired renal function. Close monitoring of hematologic, renal and hepatic status of all patients is essential. These instructions should be thoroughly reviewed before administration of Ancobon.

Description: Flucytosine, an antifungal agent, is a fluorinated pyrimidine chemically related to fluorouracil and floxuridine. Chemically, it is 5-fluorocytosine, a white to off-white crystalline powder, with a molecular weight of 129.1.

Actions: Flucytosine has *in vitro* and *in vivo* activity against Candida and Cryptococcus. The exact mode of action against these fungi is not known. Ancobon is not metabolized significantly when given orally to man.

SUSCEPTIBILITY:

Cryptococcus: Most strains initially isolated from clinical material have shown flucytosine minimal inhibitory concentrations (MIC's) ranging from .46 to 7.8 mcg/ml. Any isolate with an MIC greater than 12.5 mcg/ml is considered resistant. *In vitro* resistance has developed in originally susceptible strains during therapy. It is recommended that clinical cultures for susceptibility testing be taken initially and at weekly intervals during therapy. The initial culture should be reserved as a reference in susceptibility testing of subsequent isolates.

Candida: As high as 40 to 50 percent of the pretreatment clinical isolates of Candida have been reported to be resistant to flucytosine. It is recommended that susceptibility studies be performed as early as possible and be repeated during therapy. An MIC value greater than 100 mcg/ml is considered resistant.

Interference with *in vitro* activity of flucytosine occurs in complex or semisynthetic media. In order to rely upon the recommended *in vitro* interpretations of susceptibility, it is essential that the broth medium and the testing procedure used be that described by Shadomy.[1]

Indications: Ancobon is indicated only in the treatment of serious infections caused by susceptible strains of Candida and/or Cryptococcus. Candida: septicemia, endocarditis and urinary system infections have been effectively treated with flucytosine. Limited trials in pulmonary infections justify the use of flucytosine. Cryptococcus: meningitis and pulmonary infections have been treated effectively. Studies in septicemias and urinary tract infections are limited, but good responses have been reported.

Contraindications: Patients with a known hypersensitivity to the drug.

Warnings: Ancobon must be given with extreme caution to patients with impaired renal function. Since Ancobon is excreted primarily by the kidneys, renal impairment may lead to accumulation of the drug. Assays for blood levels of Ancobon should be done in order to determine the adequacy of renal excretion in such patients.[1]

Ancobon must be given with extreme caution to patients with bone marrow depression. Patients may be more prone to depression of bone marrow function if they: 1) have a hematologic disease, 2) are being treated with radiation or drugs which depress bone marrow, or 3) have a history of treatment with such drugs or radiation. Frequent monitoring of hepatic function and of the hematopoietic system is indicated during therapy.

Usage in Pregnancy: Safe use of Ancobon in pregnancy has not been established. NOTE: Teratogenic effects have been seen in rats which metabolize flucytosine to fluorouracil. Use of Ancobon in pregnancy, lactation and in women of childbearing age requires that the potential benefits of therapy be weighed against its possible hazards.

Precautions: Before therapy with Ancobon is instituted, the hematologic and renal status of the patient should be determined (see WARNINGS), and close monitoring of the patient is essential. Liver enzyme levels (alkaline phosphatase, SGOT, SGPT) should be determined at frequent intervals during therapy, as indicated.

Adverse Reactions: Nausea, vomiting, diarrhea, rash, anemia, leukopenia, thrombopenia, and elevation of hepatic enzymes, BUN and creatinine have been reported. Less frequently reported were confusion, hallucinations, headache, sedation and vertigo.

Dosage and Administration: The usual dosage is 50 to 150 mg/kg/day at 6-hour intervals. Nausea or vomiting may be reduced or avoided if the capsules are given a few at a time over a 15-minute period. If the BUN or the serum creatinine is elevated, or if there are other signs of renal impairment, the initial dose should be at the lower level (see WARNINGS).

How Supplied: Capsules, containing 250 mg flucytosine/Roche, green and gray; containing 500 mg flucytosine/Roche, white and gray; bottles of 100.

Reference:

1. Shadomy, S.: *Appl. Microbiol., 17*:871, 1969.

[*Shown in Product Identification Section*]

ARFONAD® ℞
(trimethaphan camsylate/Roche)
Ampuls

The following text is complete prescribing information based on official labeling in effect August 1, 1982.

Description: A thiophanium derivative, Arfonad is a vasodepressor agent used for inducing controlled hypotension. Chemically, trimethaphan camsylate is (+)-1,3-dibenzyldecahydro-2-oxoimidazo [4, 5-c] thieno [1,2-a]-thiolium 2-oxo-10-bornanesulfonate. It has a molecular weight of 596.80.

Arfonad is stable under refrigeration; it should not be frozen, to avoid ampul breakage which may result from ice formation. Each 10-ml ampul contains 500 mg trimethaphan camsylate/Roche compounded with 0.013% sodium acetate and pH adjusted to approximately 5.2 with hydrochloric acid.

Actions: Arfonad is primarily a ganglionic blocking agent. It blocks transmission in autonomic ganglia without producing any preceding or concomitant change in the membrane potentials of the ganglion cells. It does not modify the conduction of impulses in the preganglionic or postganglionic neurones and does not prevent the release of acetylcholine by preganglionic impulses. Arfonad produces ganglionic blockade by occupying receptor sites on the ganglion cells and by stabilizing the postsynaptic membranes against the action of acetylcholine liberated from the presynaptic nerve endings.

In addition to ganglionic blocking, Arfonad may also exert a direct peripheral vasodilator effect. By inducing vasodilation, it causes pooling of blood in the dependent periphery and the splanchnic system. The vasodilation results in a lowering of the blood pressure. Arfonad liberates histamine.

Indications: Arfonad is indicated for the production of controlled hypotension during surgery; for the short term (acute) control of blood pressure in hypertensive emergencies; in the emergency treatment of pulmonary edema in patients with pulmonary hypertension associated with systemic hypertension.

Contraindications: Arfonad is contraindicated in those conditions where hypotension may subject the patient to undue risk, e.g., uncorrected anemia, hypovolemia, shock (both incipient and frank), asphyxia, or uncorrected respiratory insufficiency. Inadequate availability of fluids and inability to replace blood for technical reasons may also constitute contraindications.

Warnings: Arfonad is a powerful hypotensive drug and should always be diluted before use.

It is recommended that the use of Arfonad to produce hypotension in surgical or medical indications be limited to physicians with proper training in this technique. Adequate facilities, equipment and personnel should be available for vigilant monitoring of the circulation since Arfonad is an extremely potent hypotensive agent. Adequate oxygenation must be assured throughout the treatment period, especially in regard to coronary and cerebral circulation.

Arfonad should be used with extreme caution in patients with arteriosclerosis, cardiac disease, hepatic or renal disease, degenerative disease of the central nervous system, Addison's disease, diabetes and patients who are under treatment with steroids.

Usage in Pregnancy: Induced hypotension may have serious consequences upon the fetus.

Precautions: Arfonad should be used with care in patients who have been receiving antihypertensive drugs, since an additive hypotensive effect may occur. It should be used with caution with anesthetic agents, especially spinal anesthetics, which themselves may produce hypotension. Also, use with great caution in the elderly or debilitated, or in children. Because Arfonad liberates histamine, it should be used with caution in allergic individuals. Concomitant therapy with other drugs can modify materially the dose of Arfonad necessary to achieve the desired response.

Diuretic agents may enhance markedly the responses evoked by ganglionic-blocking drugs. NOTE: Pupillary dilation does not necessarily indicate anoxia or the depth of anesthesia, since Arfonad appears to have a specific effect on the pupil.

Some animal studies indicate that aggressive dosage administration may result in respiratory arrest. Rare cases of respiratory arrest in humans have been reported, although a causal relationship has not been established. It is recommended that the patient's respiratory status be monitored closely, particularly if large doses of Arfonad are used.

Dosage and Administration: Arfonad must always be diluted and administered by intravenous infusion. Solutions should be freshly prepared and any unused portions discarded. For this purpose a 0.1 per cent (1 mg/ml) concentration of Arfonad in 5% Dextrose Injection USP should be employed. Use of other diluents is not recommended, since experience with them has not been reported. The infusion fluid used for administration of Arfonad should not be employed as a vehicle for the simultaneous administration of any other drugs. One (1) ampul of Arfonad—10 ml, 50 mg/ml—should be diluted to 500 ml. Since individual response varies, the rate of administration must be adjusted to the requirements of each patient.

The patient should be positioned so as to avoid cerebral anoxia and, when used in surgery, adequate anesthesia established. Intravenous drip with Arfonad is started at an average rate of 3 to 4 ml (3 to 4 mg) per minute (see chart below). The rate of administration is then adjusted to maintain the desired level of hypotension. Since there is a marked variation of individual response, **frequent blood pressure determinations are essential to maintain**

Continued on next page

Roche Labs.—Cont.

proper control. Rates from as low as 0.3 ml (0.3 mg) per minute to rates exceeding 6 ml (6 mg) per minute have been found necessary in the experience of clinical investigators of Arfonad.

0.1% (1 mg/ml) CONCENTRATION OF ARFONAD

Delivery System Drops/ml	Drops/Min to Obtain 3–4 ml (3–4 mg) Arfonad
10	30–40
15	45–60
60	180–240

For surgical use, administration of Arfonad should be stopped prior to wound closure in order to permit blood pressure to return to normal. A systolic pressure of 100 mm will usually be attained within 10 minutes after stopping Arfonad.

Overdosage: Vasopressor agents may be used to correct undesirable low pressures during surgery or to effect a more rapid return to normotensive levels. Phenylephrine HCl or mephentermine sulfate should be tried initially and nonepinephrine should be reserved for refractory cases.

How Supplied: Ampuls, 10 ml, boxes of 10.

AZO GANTANOL® ℞

The following text is complete prescribing information based on official labeling in effect August 1, 1982.

Composition: Each tablet contains 0.5 Gm sulfamethoxazole/Roche and 100 mg phenazopyridine hydrochloride.

Description: Azo Gantanol combines the antibacterial effectiveness of sulfamethoxazole/Roche (Gantanol®) with the local urinary analgesic activity of phenazopyridine hydrochloride.

Gantanol (sulfamethoxazole/Roche) is an intermediate-dosage sulfonamide. Sulfamethoxazole is an almost white, odorless, tasteless compound. Chemically, it is N^1-(5-methyl-3-isoxazolyl) sulfanilamide.

Phenazopyridine hydrochloride is a urinary analgesic. Chemically, it is 3-phenylazo-2,6-diaminopyridine hydrochloride.

Sulfonamides exist in the blood as free, conjugated (acetylated and possibly other forms) and protein-bound forms. The "free" form is considered to be the therapeutically active form. It has been shown that approximately 70 per cent of Gantanol is protein bound in the blood;[1] of the unbound portion 80 to 90 per cent is in the nonacetylated form.[2,3] Excretion of sulfonamides is chiefly by the kidneys with glomerular filtration as the primary mechanism.

Actions: The systemic sulfonamides are bacteriostatic agents. The spectrum of activity is similar for all. Sulfonamides competitively inhibit bacterial synthesis of folic acid (pteroylglutamic acid) from para-aminobenzoic acid. Resistant strains are capable of utilizing folic acid precursors or preformed folic acid.

Phenazopyridine hydrochloride has a specific analgesic effect in the urinary tract, promptly relieving pain and burning.

Indications: In adults, urinary tract infections complicated by pain (primarily pyelonephritis, pyelitis and cystitis) due to susceptible organisms (usually *E. coli, Klebsiella-Aerobacter, Staphylococcus aureus, Proteus mirabilis,* and, less frequently, *Proteus vulgaris)* in the absence of obstructive uropathy or foreign bodies.

Important note. In vitro sulfonamide sensitivity tests are not always reliable. The test must be carefully coordinated with bacteriologic and clinical response. When the patient is already taking sulfonamides, follow-up cultures should have aminobenzoic acid added to the culture media.

Currently, the increasing frequency of resistant organisms is a limitation of the usefulness of antibacterial agents including the sulfonamides.

Wide variation in blood levels may result with identical doses. Blood levels should be measured in patients receiving sulfonamides for serious infections. Free sulfonamide blood levels of 5 to 15 mg per 100 ml may be considered therapeutically effective for most infections, with blood levels of 12 to 15 mg per 100 ml optimal for serious infections; 20 mg per 100 ml should be the maximum total sulfonamide level, as adverse reactions occur more frequently above this level.

Contraindications: Children below age 12. Hypersensitivity to sulfonamides. Pregnancy at term and during the nursing period, because sulfonamides pass the placenta and are excreted in the milk and may cause kernicterus. Because Azo Gantanol contains phenazopyridine hydrochloride it is contraindicated in glomerulonephritis, severe hepatitis, uremia, and pyelonephritis of pregnancy with gastrointestinal disturbances.

Warnings: *Usage in Pregnancy:* The safe use of sulfonamides in pregnancy has not been established. The teratogenicity potential of most sulfonamides has not been thoroughly investigated in either animals or humans. However, a significant increase in the incidence of cleft palate and other bony abnormalities of offspring has been observed when certain sulfonamides of the short, intermediate and long-acting types were given to pregnant rats and mice at high oral doses (7 to 25 times the human therapeutic dose).

Deaths associated with the administration of sulfonamides have been reported from hypersensitivity reactions, agranulocytosis, aplastic anemia and other blood dyscrasias.

The presence of clinical signs such as sore throat, fever, pallor, purpura or jaundice may be early indications of serious blood disorders. Complete blood counts should be done frequently in patients receiving sulfonamides.

The frequency of renal complications is considerably lower in patients receiving the more soluble sulfonamides. Urinalysis with careful microscopic examination should be obtained frequently in patients receiving sulfonamides.

Precautions: Sulfonamides should be given with caution to patients with impaired renal or hepatic function and to those with severe allergy or bronchial asthma. In glucose-6-phosphate dehydrogenase-deficient individuals, hemolysis may occur. This reaction is frequently dose-related. Adequate fluid intake must be maintained in order to prevent crystalluria and stone formation.

Adverse Reactions: *Blood dyscrasias:* Agranulocytosis, aplastic anemia, thrombocytopenia, leukopenia, hemolytic anemia, purpura, hypoprothrombinemia and methemoglobinemia.

Allergic reactions: Erythema multiforme (Stevens-Johnson syndrome), generalized skin eruptions, epidermal necrolysis, urticaria, serum sickness, pruritus, exfoliative dermatitis, anaphylactoid reactions, periorbital edema, conjunctival and scleral injection, photosensitization, arthralgia and allergic myocarditis.

Gastrointestinal reactions: Nausea, emesis, abdominal pains, hepatitis, diarrhea, anorexia, pancreatitis and stomatitis.

C.N.S. reactions: Headache, peripheral neuritis, mental depression, convulsions, ataxia, hallucinations, tinnitus, vertigo and insomnia.

Miscellaneous reactions: Drug fever, chills, and toxic nephrosis with oliguria and anuria. Polyarteritis nodosa and L.E. phenomenon have occurred.

The sulfonamides bear certain chemical similarities to some goitrogens, diuretics (acetazolamide and the thiazides) and oral hypoglycemic agents. Goiter production, diuresis and hypoglycemia have occurred rarely in patients receiving sulfonamides. Cross-sensitivity may exist with these agents.

Dosage and Administration: Azo Gantanol is intended for the acute, painful phase of urinary tract infections. The usual dosage in adults is 4 tablets initially followed by 2 tablets morning and evening for up to 3 days. If pain persists, causes other than infection should be sought. After relief of pain has been obtained, continued treatment of the infection with Gantanol (sulfamethoxazole/Roche) may be considered.

NOTE: Patients should be told that the orange-red dye (phenazopyridine HCl) will color the urine soon after ingestion of the medication.

How Supplied: Tablets, red, film-coated, each containing 0.5 Gm sulfamethoxazole/Roche and 100 mg phenazopyridine HCl—bottles of 100 and 500.

References:

1. Struller, T.: *Antibiot. Chemother., 14:* 179, 1968.
2. Boger, W. P., and Gavin, J. J.: *Antibiotics and Chemother., 10*:572, 1960.
3. Brandman, O., and Engelberg, R.: *Curr. Therap. Res., 2*:364, 1960.

[*Shown in Product Identification Section*]

AZO GANTRISIN® ℞

The following text is complete prescribing information based on official labeling in effect August 1, 1982.

Description: Azo Gantrisin is a combination containing 0.5 Gm of the antibacterial sulfisoxazole/Roche and 50 mg of the urinary analgesic phenazopyridine hydrochloride per tablet for oral administration.

Gantrisin® (sulfisoxazole/Roche), a rapid-acting sulfonamide, is N^1-(3,4-dimethyl-5-isoxazolyl)sulfanilamide. It is a white to slightly yellowish, odorless, slighty bitter, crystalline powder which is soluble in alcohol and very slightly soluble in water. Sulfisoxazole has an empirical formula of $C_{11}H_{13}N_3O_3S$, and a molecular weight of 267.30.

Phenazopyridine hydrochloride, a local urinary analgesic, is 2,6-diamino-3-(phenylazo)-pyridine monohydrochloride. It is a light or dark red to dark violet, odorless, slightly bitter, crystalline powder with an empirical formula of $C_{11}H_{11}N_5 \cdot HCl$, and a molecular weight of 249.70.

Clinical Pharmacology: An oral dose of sulfisoxazole is rapidly and completely absorbed. Sulfonamides are present in the blood as free, conjugated (acetylated and possibly other forms) and protein-bound forms. The amount present as "free" drug is considered to be the therapeutically active form. Approximately 85% of a dose of sulfisoxazole is bound to plasma proteins.

Following a single 2.0-Gm dose of sulfisoxazole, the mean time of peak plasma concentration was 2.5 hours; the mean peak plasma concentration was 169 μg/ml, ranging from 127 to 211 μg/ml. Of the 97% of the original dose excreted in the urine within 0 to 48 hours, 52% was free sulfisoxazole and 45% was the metabolite N^4-acetyl sulfisoxazole. The mean elimination half-life was 5.8 hours, ranging from 4.6 to 7.8 hours.

Sulfonamides are excreted primarily by the kidneys through glomerular filtration. The drug diffuses across the placenta into the fetus and crosses the blood-brain barrier.

Phenazopyridine hydrochloride has a specific local analgesic effect in the urinary tract, promptly relieving pain and burning. No pharmacokinetic data are available on this drug.

Microbiology: The systemic sulfonamides are bacteriostatic agents. The spectrum of activity is similar for all. Sulfonamides competitively inhibit bacterial synthesis of folic acid (pteroylglutamic acid) from *para*-aminobenzoic acid. Resistant strains are capable of utilizing folic acid precursors or preformed folic acid.

Indications: Azo Gantrisin is indicated for the treatment of adults with urinary tract infections complicated by pain (primarily pyelonephritis, pyelitis and cystitis) due to susceptible organisms (usually *E. coli, Klebsiella-Enterobacter, Staphylococcus aureus, Proteus mirabilis* and, less frequently, *Proteus vulgaris)* in the absence of obstructive uropathy or foreign bodies.

Important Note: In vitro sensitivity tests for sulfonamides are not always reliable, and must be carefully coordinated with bacteriologic and clinical response. When the patient is already taking sulfonamides, follow-up cultures should have aminobenzoic acid added to the culture media.

Currently, the increasing frequency of resistant organisms is a limitation of the usefulness of antibacterial agents, including the sulfonamides.

Wide variation in blood levels may result with identical doses of a sulfonamide. Blood levels should be measured in patients receiving these drugs for serious infections. Free sulfonamide blood levels of 5 to 15 mg/100 ml may be considered therapeutically effective for most infections, with blood levels of 12 to 15 mg/100 ml being optimal for serious infections. The maximum sulfonamide level should be 20 mg/100 ml, since adverse reactions occur more frequently above this concentration.

Contraindications: Azo Gantrisin is contraindicated in patients with a known sensitivity to either of its components; in children younger than 12 years; and in pregnancy *at term* and during the nursing period, because sulfonamides pass the placenta and are excreted in the milk and may cause kernicterus.

Azo Gantrisin, because it contains phenazopyridine hydrochloride, is also contraindicated in glomerulonephritis, severe hepatitis, uremia, and pyelonephritis of pregnancy with gastrointestinal disturbances.

Warnings: Sulfonamides are bacteriostatic and resistance is frequent in organisms responsible for common infections. Sulfa drugs will not eradicate group A streptococci and have not been demonstrated, in these infections, to prevent sequelae such as rheumatic fever and glomerulonephritis.

Deaths associated with the administration of sulfonamides have been reported from hypersensitivity reactions, agranulocytosis, aplastic anemia and other blood dyscrasias.

The presence of clinical signs such as sore throat, fever, pallor, purpura or jaundice may be early indications of serious blood disorders. Blood counts and renal function tests are recommended during treatment.

Precautions: *General:* Sulfonamides should be given with caution to patients with impaired renal or hepatic function and to those with severe allergy or bronchial asthma. In glucose-6-phosphate dehydrogenase-deficient individuals, hemolysis may occur; this reaction is frequently dose-related.

The frequency of renal complications is considerably lower in patients receiving the more soluble sulfonamides. Adequate fluid intake must be maintained in order to prevent crystalluria and stone formation.

Information for Patients: Patients should maintain an adequate fluid intake. Patients should also be told that soon after ingestion of this medication, the phenazopyridine HCl component will produce reddish-orange discoloration of the urine.

Laboratory Tests: Urinalysis with careful microscopic examination should be performed at least once a week for patients receiving sulfonamides. Blood counts should be performed regularly in patients receiving sulfonamide therapy for longer than two weeks. Blood levels of a sulfonamide should be measured in patients receiving these drugs for serious infection (see INDICATIONS section).

Drug Interactions: It has been reported that some sulfonamides may displace oral anticoagulants from plasma protein binding sites and thereby increase the anticoagulant effect. Sulfonamides can also displace methotrexate from plasma protein binding sites.

Drug/Laboratory Test Interactions: Both components of Azo Gantrisin have been reported to affect results of liver function tests in isolated cases of hepatitis.

Carcinogenesis, Mutagenesis, Impairment of Fertility:

Carcinogenesis: Azo Gantrisin has not undergone adequate trials relating to carcinogenicity; however, each component has been evaluated separately. Sulfisoxazole was not carcinogenic in either sex in rats given 400 mg/kg/day or in mice given 2000 mg/kg/day.

In a carcinogenicity study of phenazopyridine, a dosage of approximately 375 mg/kg/day (65 times the human therapeutic dose) produced adenocarcinomas of the colon in rats of either sex. A dosage of approximately 180 mg/kg/day (31 times the human therapeutic dose) was not carcinogenic in male mice, but this dosage did produce hepatocellular adenomas and carcinomas in female mice. Considering the recommended three-day course of therapy for Azo Gantrisin, these findings are not considered to be clinically relevant.

Mutagenesis: There are no studies available that evaluate the mutagenic potential of Azo Gantrisin or either of its components.

Impairment of Fertility: Azo Gantrisin has not undergone adequate trials relating to impairment of fertility; each component, however, has been studied in laboratory animals. In a reproduction study of rats given 800 mg/kg/day sulfisoxazole, no effects were observed regarding mating behavior, conception rate or fertility index (percent pregnant). No effects on fertility were demonstrated in a two-litter reproduction study of rats given 50 mg/kg/day phenazopyridine.

Pregnancy:

Teratogenic Effects: Pregnancy Category C. Each component of Azo Gantrisin has been evaluated in reproduction studies in laboratory animals. At dosages of 800 mg/kg/day, sulfisoxazole was not teratogenic in either rats or rabbits, and had no perinatal or postnatal effects in rats. However, in two other teratogenicity studies, cleft palates developed in both rats and mice after administration of 500 to 1000 mg/kg/day sulfisoxazole (8 to 16 times the therapeutic dose for an individual weighing 143 lbs). In regard to phenazopyridine, no congenital malformations developed in rats given 50 mg/kg/day.

There are no adequate or well-controlled studies of Azo Gantrisin in either laboratory animals or in pregnant women. It is not known whether Azo Gantrisin can cause fetal harm when administered to a pregnant woman or can affect reproduction capacity. Azo Gantrisin should be used during pregnancy only if the potential benefit justifies the potential risk to the fetus.

Nonteratogenic Effects: See **Contraindications** section.

Nursing Mothers: See **Contraindications** section.

Pediatric Use: See **Contraindications** section.

Adverse Reactions: Included in the listing that follows are adverse reactions that have not been reported with this specific drug; however, the pharmacologic similarities among the sulfonamides require that each of the reactions be considered with Azo Gantrisin administration.

Allergic: Anaphylaxis, generalized allergic reactions, angioneurotic edema, arteritis and vasculitis, myocarditis, serum sickness, conjunctival and scleral injection. In addition, periarteritis nodosa and systemic lupus erythematosus have been reported.

Cardiovascular: Tachycardia, palpitations, syncope and cyanosis.

Dermatologic: Rash, urticaria, pruritus, erythema multiforme, Stevens-Johnson syndrome, toxic epidermal necrolysis, exfoliative dermatitis and photosensitivity.

Endocrine: The sulfonamides bear certain chemical similarities to some goitrogens, diuretics (acetazolamide and the thiazides) and oral hypoglycemic agents. Cross-sensitivity may exist with these agents. Goiter production, diuresis and hypoglycemia have occurred rarely in patients receiving sulfonamides.

Gastrointestinal: Nausea, emesis, abdominal pain, anorexia, diarrhea, glossitis, stomatitis, flatulence, salivary gland enlargement, G.I. hemorrhage, pseudomembranous enterocolitis, melena and pancreatitis. Hepatic dysfunction and jaundice have also been reported following the use of sulfonamides.

Genitourinary: Crystalluria, hematuria, BUN and creatinine elevation, nephritis and toxic nephrosis with oliguria and anuria. Acute renal failure and urinary retention have also been reported.

Hematologic: Leukopenia, agranulocytosis, aplastic anemia, thrombocytopenia, purpura, hemolytic anemia, anemia, eosinophilia, clotting disorders including hypoprothrombinemia and hypofibrinogenemia, sulfhemoglobinemia and methemoglobinemia.

Musculoskeletal: Arthralgia, chest pain and myalgia.

Neurologic: Headache, dizziness, peripheral neuritis, paresthesia, convulsions, tinnitus, vertigo, ataxia and intracranial hypertension.

Psychiatric: Psychosis, hallucinations, disorientation, depression and anxiety.

Miscellaneous: Edema (including periorbital), pyrexia, drowsiness, weakness, fatigue, lassitude, rigors, flushing, hearing loss, insomnia and pneumonitis.

Overdosage: Signs and symptoms of overdosage with Azo Gantrisin include anorexia, colic, nausea, vomiting, dizziness, drowsiness, and even unconsciousness. Pyrexia, hematuria and crystalluria may be noted. Blood dyscrasias and jaundice are potential late manifestations of overdosage.

General principles of treatment include instituting gastric lavage or emesis; forcing oral fluids; and administering intravenous fluids if urine output is low and renal function is normal. The patient should be monitored with blood counts and appropriate blood chemistries, including electrolytes. If the patient becomes cyanotic, the possibility of methemoglobinemia should be considered and, if present, the condition should be treated appropriately with intravenous 1% methylene blue. If a significant blood dyscrasia or jaundice occurs, specific therapy should be instituted for these complications.

The oral LD_{50} of Azo Gantrisin in mice is 4317 mg/kg.

Dosage and Administration: Azo Gantrisin is intended for the acute, painful phase of urinary tract infections. The recommended dosage in adults is 4 to 6 tablets initially, followed by 2 tablets four times daily for up to three days. If pain persists, causes other than infection should be sought. After relief of pain has been otained, continued treatment of the infection with Gantrisin® (sulfisoxazole/Roche) may be considered.

How Supplied: Each red, film-coated tablet contains 0.5 Gm sulfisoxazole/Roche and 50 mg phenazopyridine HCl. Azo Gantrisin is available in bottles of 100 tablets (NDC-0004-0012-01) and 500 tablets (NDC-0004-0012-14). Imprint on tablets: AZO GANTRISIN® ROCHE.

[*Shown in Product Identification Section*]

Continued on next page

Roche Labs.—Cont.

BACTRIM™ I.V. INFUSION ℞
(trimethoprim and sulfamethoxazole/Roche)

The following text is complete prescribing information based on official labeling in effect August 1, 1982.

Description: Bactrim I.V. Infusion, a sterile solution for intravenous infusion only, is a synthetic antibacterial combination product. Each 5 ml contains 80 mg trimethoprim (16 mg/ml) and 400 mg sulfamethoxazole (80 mg/ml) compounded with 40% propylene glycol, 10% ethyl alcohol and 0.3% diethanolamine; 1% benzyl alcohol and 0.1% sodium metabisulfite as preservatives; water for injection; and pH adjusted to approximately 10 with sodium hydroxide.

Trimethoprim is 2,4-diamino-5-(3,4,5-trimethoxybenzyl)pyrimidine. It is a white to light yellow, odorless, bitter compound with a molecular weight of 290.3.

Sulfamethoxazole is N^1-(5-methyl-3-isoxazolyl)sulfanilamide. It is an almost white in color, odorless, tasteless compound with a molecular weight of 253.28.

Clinical Pharmacology: Following a one-hour intravenous infusion of a single dose of 160 mg trimethoprim plus 800 mg sulfamethoxazole to 11 patients whose weight ranged from 105 lb to 165 lb (mean, 143 lb), the mean plasma concentrations of trimethoprim and sulfamethoxazole were 3.4 ± 0.3 μg/ml and 46.3 ± 2.7 μg/ml, respectively. Following repeated intravenous administration of the same dose at eight-hour intervals, the mean plasma concentrations just prior to and immediately after each infusion at steady state were 5.6 ± 0.6 μg/ml and 8.8 ± 0.9 μg/ml for trimethoprim and 70.6 ± 7.3 μg/ml and 105.6 ± 10.9 μg/ml for sulfamethoxazole. The mean plasma half-life was 11.3 ± 0.7 hours for trimethoprim and 12.8 ± 1.8 hours for sulfamethoxazole. All of these 11 patients had normal renal function, and their ages ranged from 17 to 78 years (median, 60 years).[1]

Pharmacokinetic studies in children and adults suggest an age-dependent half-life of trimethoprim, as indicated in the following table.[2]

Age (years)	No. of Patients	Mean TMP Half-life (hours)
<1	2	7.67
1-10	9	5.49
10-20	5	8.19
20-63	6	12.82

Sulfamethoxazole exists in the blood as free, conjugated and protein-bound forms; trimethoprim is present as free and protein-bound and metabolized forms. The free forms are considered to be the therapeutically active forms. Approximately 44 percent of trimethoprim and 70 percent of sulfamethoxazole are protein-bound in blood. The presence of 10 mg percent sulfamethoxazole in plasma decreases the protein binding of trimethoprim to an insignificant degree; trimethoprim does not influence the protein binding of sulfamethoxazole.

Excretion of Bactrim is chiefly by the kidneys through both glomerular filtration and tubular secretion. Urine concentrations of both sulfamethoxazole and trimethoprim are considerably higher than are concentrations in the blood. When administered together as in Bactrim, neither sulfamethoxazole nor trimethoprim affects the urinary excretion pattern of the other.

Microbiology:

Sulfamethoxazole inhibits bacterial synthesis of dihydrofolic acid by competing with *para*-aminobenzoic acid. Trimethoprim blocks the production of tetrahydrofolic acid from dihydrofolic acid by binding to and reversibly inhibiting the required enzyme, dihydrofolate reductase. Thus, Bactrim blocks two consecutive steps in the biosynthesis of nucleic acids and proteins essential to many bacteria.

In vitro studies have shown that bacterial resistance develops more slowly with Bactrim than with trimethoprim or sulfamethoxazole alone.

In vitro serial dilution tests have shown that the spectrum of antibacterial activity of Bactrim includes common bacterial pathogens with the exception of *Pseudomonas aeruginosa.* The following organisms are usually susceptible: *Escherichia coli, Klebsiella-Enterobacter, Proteus mirabilis,* indole-positive *Proteus* species, *Haemophilus influenzae* (including ampicillin-resistant strains), *Streptococcus pneumoniae, Shigella flexneri* and *Shigella sonnei.* It should be noted, however, that there are little clinical data on the use of intravenous Bactrim in serious systemic infections due to *H. influenzae* and *S. pneumoniae.*

(See table above)

REPRESENTATIVE MINIMUM INHIBITORY CONCENTRATION VALUES FOR BACTRIM-SUSCEPTIBLE ORGANISMS (MIC—μg/ml)

Bacteria	Trimethoprim alone	Sulfamethoxazole alone	TMP/SMX (1:20) TMP	SMX
Escherichia coli	0.05 – 1.5	1.0 – 245	0.05 – 0.5	0.95 – 9.5
Proteus spp. indole positive	0.5 – 5.0	7.35 – 300	0.05 – 1.5	0.95 – 28.5
Proteus mirabilis	0.5 – 1.5	7.35 – 30	0.05 – 0.15	0.95 – 2.85
Klebsiella-Enterobacter	0.15 – 5.0	2.45 – 245	0.05 – 1.5	0.95 – 28.5
Haemophilus influenzae	0.15 – 1.5	2.85 – 95	0.015 – 0.15	0.285 – 2.85
Streptococcus pneumoniae	0.15 – 1.5	7.35 – 24.5	0.05 – 0.15	0.95 – 2.85
Shigella flexneri	<0.01 – 0.04	<0.16 – >320	<0.002 – 0.03	0.04 – 0.625
Shigella sonnei	0.02 – 0.03	0.625 – >320	0.004 – 0.06	0.08 – 1.25

The recommended quantitative disc susceptibility method may be used for estimating the susceptibility of bacteria to Bactrim.[3,4] With this procedure, a report from the laboratory of "Susceptible to trimethoprim-sulfamethoxazole" indicates that the infection is likely to respond to therapy with Bactrim. If the infection is confined to the urine, a report of "Intermediate susceptibility to trimethoprim-sulfamethoxazole" also indicates that the infection is likely to respond. A report of "Resistant to trimethoprim-sulfamethoxazole" indicates that the infection is unlikely to respond to therapy with Bactrim.

Indications and Usage:

PNEUMOCYSTIS CARINII PNEUMONITIS: Bactrim I.V. Infusion is indicated in the treatment of *Pneumocystis carinii* pneumonitis in children and adults.

SHIGELLOSIS: Bactrim I.V. Infusion is indicated in the treatment of enteritis caused by susceptible strains of *Shigella flexneri* and *Shigella sonnei* in children and adults.

URINARY TRACT INFECTIONS: Bactrim I.V. Infusion is indicated in the treatment of severe or complicated urinary tract infections due to susceptible strains of *Escherichia coli, Klebsiella-Enterobacter* and *Proteus* species when oral administration of Bactrim is not feasible and when the organism is not susceptible to single agent antibacterials effective in the urinary tract.

Although appropriate culture and susceptibility studies should be performed, therapy may be started while awaiting the results of these studies.

Contraindications: Hypersensitivity to trimethoprim or sulfonamides. Documented megaloblastic anemia due to folate deficiency.

Pregnancy at term and during the nursing period, because sulfonamides pass the placenta and are excreted in the milk and may cause kernicterus.

Infants less than two months of age.

Warnings: BACTRIM I.V. INFUSION SHOULD NOT BE USED IN THE TREATMENT OF STREPTOCOCCAL PHARYNGITIS. Clinical studies have documented that patients with group A β-hemolytic streptococcal tonsillopharyngitis have a greater incidence of bacteriologic failure when treated with Bactrim than do those patients treated with penicillin, as evidenced by failure to eradicate this organism from the tonsillopharyngeal area.

Deaths associated with the administration of sulfonamides have been reported from hypersensitivity reactions, agranulocytosis, aplastic anemia and other blood dyscrasias. Experience with trimethoprim alone is much more limited, but it has been reported to interfere with hematopoiesis in occasional patients. In elderly patients concurrently receiving certain diuretics, primarily thiazides, an increased incidence of thrombopenia with purpura has been reported.

The presence of clinical signs such as sore throat, fever, pallor, purpura or jaundice may be early indications of serious blood disorders.

Precautions:

i) *General:* Bactrim should be given with caution to patients with impaired renal or hepatic function, to those with possible folate deficiency and to those with severe allergy or bronchial asthma. In glucose-6-phosphate dehydrogenase-deficient individuals, hemolysis may occur. This reaction is frequently dose-related. Adequate fluid intake must be maintained in order to prevent crystalluria and stone formation.

Local irritation and inflammation due to extravascular infiltration of the infusion have been observed. If these occur, the infusion should be discontinued and restarted at another site.

ii) *Laboratory tests:* Appropriate culture and susceptibility studies should be performed before and throughout treatment. Complete blood counts should be done frequently in patients receiving Bactrim. If a significant reduction in the count of any formed blood element is noted, Bactrim should be discontinued. Urinalyses with careful microscopic examination and renal function tests should be performed during therapy, particularly for those patients with impaired renal function.

iii) *Drug interactions:* It has been reported that Bactrim may prolong the prothrombin time in patients who are receiving the anticoagulant warfarin. This interaction should be kept in mind when Bactrim is given to patients already on anticoagulant therapy, and the coagulation time should be reassessed.

iv) *Carcinogenesis, mutagenesis, impairment of fertility:*

Carcinogenesis: Long-term studies in animals to evaluate carcinogenic potential have not been conducted with Bactrim I.V. Infusion.

Mutagenesis: Bacterial mutagenic studies have not been performed with sulfamethoxazole and trimethoprim in combination. Trimethoprim was demonstrated to be non-mutagenic in the Ames assay. No chromosomal damage was observed in human leukocytes cultured *in vitro* with sulfamethoxazole and trimethoprim alone or in combination; the concentrations used exceeded blood levels of these compounds following therapy with Bactrim. Observations of leukocytes obtained from patients treated with Bactrim revealed no chromosomal abnormalities.

Impairment of Fertility: Bactrim I.V. Infusion has not been studied in animals for evidence of impairment of fertility. However, studies in rats at oral dosages as high as 70 mg/kg trimethoprim plus 350 mg/kg sulfamethoxazole daily showed no adverse effects on fertility or general reproductive performance.

v) *Pregnancy:* Teratogenic Effects: Pregnancy Category C. In rats, oral doses of 533 mg/kg sulfamethoxazole or 200 mg/kg trimethoprim produced teratological effects manifested mainly as cleft palates. The highest dose which did not cause cleft palates in rats was 512 mg/kg sulfamethoxazole or 192 mg/kg trimethoprim when administered separately. In two studies in rats, no teratology was observed when 512 mg/kg of sulfamethoxazole was used in combination with 128 mg/kg of trimethoprim. However, in one study, cleft palates were observed in one litter out of nine when 355 mg/kg of sulfamethoxazole was used in combination with 88 mg/kg of trimethoprim.

In some rabbit studies, an overall increase in fetal loss (dead and resorbed and malformed conceptuses) was associated with doses of trimethoprim six times the human therapeutic dose.

While there are no large, well-controlled studies on the use of trimethoprim plus sulfamethoxazole in pregnant women, Brumfitt and Pursell[5] reported the outcome of 186 pregnancies during which the mother received either placebo or oral trimethoprim in combination with sulfamethoxazole.

The incidence of congenital abnormalities was 4.5% (3 of 66) in those who received placebo and 3.3% (4 of 120) in those receiving trimethoprim plus sulfamethoxazole. There were no abnormalities in the 10 children whose mothers received the drug during the first trimester. In a separate survey, Brumfitt and Pursell also found no congenital abnormalities in 35 children whose mothers had received oral trimethoprim plus sulfamethoxazole at the time of conception or shortly thereafter.

Because trimethoprim plus sulfamethoxazole may interfere with folic acid metabolism, Bactrim I.V. Infusion should be used during pregnancy only if the potential benefit justifies the potential risk to the fetus.

Nonteratogenic Effects: See "CONTRAINDICATIONS" section.

vi) *Nursing mothers:* See "CONTRAINDICATIONS" section.

Adverse Reactions: The most frequently reported adverse reactions to Bactrim I.V. Infusion are nausea and vomiting, thrombocytopenia and rash. These occur in less than one-twentieth of patients. Local reaction, pain and slight irritation on I.V. administration are infrequent; thrombophlebitis has been observed rarely.

For completeness, all major reactions to sulfonamides and to trimethoprim are included below, even though they may not have been reported with Bactrim I.V. Infusion.

Allergic Reactions: Generalized skin eruptions, pruritus, urticaria, erythema multiforme, Stevens-Johnson syndrome, epidermal necrolysis, serum sickness, exfoliative dermatitis, anaphylactoid reactions, periorbital edema, conjunctival and scleral injection, photosensitization, arthralgia and allergic myocarditis.

Blood Dyscrasias: Megaloblastic anemia, hemolytic anemia, purpura, thrombocytopenia, leukopenia, agranulocytosis, aplastic anemia, hypoprothrombinemia and methemoglobinemia.

Gastrointestinal Reactions: Glossitis, stomatitis, nausea, emesis, abdominal pains, hepatitis, diarrhea, pseudomembranous colitis and pancreatitis.

C.N.S. Reactions: Headache, peripheral neuritis, mental depression, ataxia, convulsions, hallucinations, tinnitus, vertigo, insomnia, apathy, fatigue, muscle weakness and nervousness.

Miscellaneous Reactions: Drug fever, chills, and toxic nephrosis with oliguria and anuria. Periarteritis nodosa and L.E. phenomenon have occurred.

The sulfonamides bear certain chemical similarities to some goitrogens, diuretics (acetazolamide and the thiazides) and oral hypoglycemic agents. Cross-sensitivity may exist with these agents. Diuresis and hypoglycemia have occurred rarely in patients receiving sulfonamides.

Overdosage: Since there has been no extensive experience in humans with single doses of Bactrim I.V. Infusion in excess of 25 ml (400 mg trimethoprim and 2000 mg sulfamethoxazole), the maximum tolerated dose in humans is unknown.

Use of Bactrim I.V. Infusion at high doses and/or for extended periods of time may cause bone marrow depression manifested as thrombocytopenia, leukopenia and/or megaloblastic anemia. If signs of bone marrow depression occur, the patient should be given leucovorin 3 to 6 mg intramuscularly daily for three days, or as required to restore normal hematopoiesis.

Peritoneal dialysis is not effective and hemodialysis is only moderately effective in eliminating trimethoprim and sulfamethoxazole.

The Bactrim I.V. Infusion LD_{50} in mice is 700 mg/kg or 7.3 ml/kg; in rats and rabbits the LD_{50} is >500 mg/kg or >5.2 ml/kg. The vehicle produced the same LD_{50} in each of these species as the active drug.

The signs and symptoms noted in mice, rats and rabbits with Bactrim I.V. Infusion or its vehicle at the high I.V. doses used in acute toxicity studies included ataxia, decreased motor activity, loss of righting reflex, tremors or convulsions, and/or respiratory depression.

Dosage and Administration: CONTRAINDICATED IN INFANTS LESS THAN TWO MONTHS OF AGE. CAUTION—BACTRIM I.V. INFUSION MUST BE DILUTED IN 5% DEXTROSE IN WATER SOLUTION PRIOR TO ADMINISTRATION. DO NOT MIX BACTRIM I.V. INFUSION WITH OTHER DRUGS OR SOLUTIONS. RAPID INFUSION OR BOLUS INJECTION MUST BE AVOIDED.

Dosage:

Children and Adults:

Pneumocystis carinii Pneumonitis: Total daily dose is 15 to 20 mg/kg (based on the trimethoprim component), given in three or four equally divided doses q 6 to 8 hours for up to 14 days. One investigator noted that a total daily dose of 10 to 15 mg/kg was sufficient in ten adult patients with normal renal function.[6]

Severe Urinary Tract Infections and Shigellosis: Total daily dose is 8 to 10 mg/kg (based on the trimethoprim component), given in two to four equally divided doses q 6, 8 or 12 hours for up to 14 days for severe urinary tract infections and five days for shigellosis.

For Patients with Impaired Renal Function: When renal function is impaired, a reduced dosage should be employed using the following table:

Creatinine Clearance (ml/min)	Recommended Dosage Regimen
Above 30	Usual standard regimen
15-30	½ the usual regimen
Below 15	Use not recommended

Method of Preparation: Bactrim I.V. Infusion must be diluted. Each 5 ml should be added to 125 ml of 5% dextrose in water. After diluting with 5% dextrose in water, the solution should not be refrigerated and should be used within six hours. If upon visual inspection there is cloudiness or evidence of precipitation after mixing, the solution should be discarded and a fresh solution prepared.

The following infusion sets have been tested and found satisfactory: unit-dose glass containers (McGaw Laboratories, Cutter Laboratories, Inc., and Abbott Laboratories); unit-dose plastic containers (Viaflex from Travenol Laboratories and Accumed from McGaw Laboratories). No other systems have been tested and therefore no others can be recommended.

Dilution: EACH 5 ML OF BACTRIM I.V. INFUSION SHOULD BE ADDED TO 125 ML OF 5% DEXTROSE IN WATER.

NOTE: IN THOSE INSTANCES WHERE FLUID RESTRICTION IS DESIRABLE, each 5 ml may be added to 75 ml of 5% dextrose in water. Under these circumstances the solution should be mixed just prior to use and should be administered within two hours. If upon visual inspection there is cloudiness or evidence of crystallization after mixing, the solution should be discarded and a fresh solution prepared.

DO NOT MIX BACTRIM I.V. INFUSION – 5% DEXTROSE IN WATER WITH OTHER DRUGS OR SOLUTIONS.

Administration: The solution should be given by intravenous drip over a period of 60 to 90 minutes. Rapid infusion or bolus injection must be avoided. Bactrim I.V. Infusion should not be used intramuscularly.

How Supplied: 5-ml *ampuls*, containing 80 mg trimethoprim (16 mg/ml) and 400 mg sulfamethoxazole (80 mg/ml) for infusion with 5% dextrose in water. Boxes of 10 (NDC-0004-1943-06).

5-ml *vials*, containing 80 mg trimethoprim (16 mg/ml) and 400 mg sulfamethoxazole (80 mg/ml) for infusion with 5% dextrose in water. Boxes of 10 (NDC-0004-1956-01).

STORE AT ROOM TEMPERATURE (15° – 30°C or 59° – 86°F). DO NOT REFRIGERATE.

Bactrim is also available as *DS (double strength) Tablets*, containing 160 mg trimethoprim and 800 mg sulfamethoxazole—bottles of 100 and 500; Tel-E-Dose® packages of 100; Prescription Paks of 20.

Tablets, containing 80 mg trimethoprim and 400 mg sulfamethoxazole—bottles of 100 and 500; Tel-E-Dose® packages of 100; Prescription Paks of 40.

Pediatric Suspension, containing 40 mg trimethoprim and 200 mg sulfamethoxazole per teaspoonful (5 ml); cherry flavored—bottles of 100 ml and 16 oz (1 pint).

Suspension, containing 40 mg trimethoprim and 200 mg sulfamethoxazole per teaspoonful (5 ml); fruit-licorice flavored—bottles of 16 oz (1 pint).

REFERENCES:

1. Grose WE, Bodey GP, Loo TL: Clinical Pharmacology of Intravenously Administered Trimethoprim-Sulfamethoxazole. *Antimicrob Agents Chemother 15*:447-451, Mar 1979.

Continued on next page

Roche Labs.—Cont.

2. Siber GR, Gorham C, Durbin W, Lesko L, Levin MJ: Pharmacology of Intravenous Trimethoprim-Sulfamethoxazole in Children and Adults. *Current Chemotherapy and Infectious Diseases,* American Society for Microbiology, Washington, D.C., 1980, Vol. 1, pp. 691-692.
3. Bauer AW, Kirby WMM, Sherris JC, Turck M: Antibiotic Susceptibility Testing by a Standardized Single Disk Method. *Am J Clin Pathol 45*:493-496, Apr 1966.
4. Approved Standard ASM-2 Performance Standards for Antimicrobial Disc Susceptibility Test: National Committee for Clinical Laboratory Standards, 771 East Lancaster Avenue, Villanova, Pennsylvania 19085.
5. Brumfitt W and Pursell R: Trimethoprim/Sulfamethoxazole in the Treatment of Bacteriuria in Women. *J Infect Dis 128*(Suppl): S657-S663, Nov 1973.
6. Winston DJ, Lau WK, Gale RP, Young LS: Trimethoprim-Sulfamethoxazole for the Treatment of *Pneumocystis carinii* pneumonia. *Ann Intern Med 92*:762-769, June 1980.

BACTRIM™ ℞

(trimethoprim and sulfamethoxazole/Roche)
Tablets, Suspension,
Pediatric Suspension,
DS (double strength) Tablets

The following text is complete prescribing information based on official labeling in effect August 1, 1982.

Description: Bactrim is a synthetic antibacterial combination product, available in DS (double strength), notched, capsule-shaped, white tablets, each containing 160 mg trimethoprim and 800 mg sulfamethoxazole; in scored, light-green tablets, each containing 80 mg trimethoprim and 400 mg sulfamethoxazole; as a pink, cherry-flavored pediatric suspension and as a pink, fruit-licorice flavored suspension, both forms containing in each teaspoonful (5 ml) 40 mg trimethoprim and 200 mg sulfamethoxazole, compounded with 0.3% alcohol.

Trimethoprim is 2,4-diamino-5-(3,4,5-trimethoxybenzyl) pyrimidine. It is a white to light yellow, odorless, bitter compound with a molecular weight of 290.3.

Sulfamethoxazole is N^1-(5-methyl-3-isoxazolyl)sulfanilamide. It is an almost white in color, odorless, tasteless compound with a molecular weight of 253.28.

Actions: *Clinical Pharmacology:* Bactrim is rapidly absorbed following oral administration. The blood levels of trimethoprim and sulfamethoxazole are similar to those achieved when each component is given alone. Peak blood levels for the individual components occur one to four hours after oral administration. The half-lives of sulfamethoxazole (10 hours) and trimethoprim (8 to 10 hours) are relatively the same regardless of whether these compounds are administered as individual components or as Bactrim. Detectable amounts of trimethoprim and sulfamethoxazole are present in the blood 24 hours after drug administration. Free sulfamethoxazole and trimethoprim blood levels are proportionately dose-dependent. On repeated administration, the steady-state ratio of trimethoprim to sulfamethoxazole levels in the blood is about 1:20.

Sulfamethoxazole exists in the blood as free, conjugated and protein-bound forms; trimethoprim is present as free, protein-bound and metabolized forms. The free forms are considered to be the therapeutically active forms. Approximately 44 percent of trimethoprim and 70 percent of sulfamethoxazole are protein-bound in the blood. The presence of 10 mg percent sulfamethoxazole in plasma decreases the protein binding of trimethoprim to an insignificant degree; trimethoprim does not influence the protein binding of sulfamethoxazole.

Excretion of Bactrim is chiefly by the kidneys through both glomerular filtration and tubular secretion. Urine concentrations of both sulfamethoxazole and trimethoprim are considerably higher than are the concentrations in the blood. When administered together as in Bactrim, neither sulfamethoxazole nor trimethoprim affects the urinary excretion pattern of the other.

Microbiology: Sulfamethoxazole inhibits bacterial synthesis of dihydrofolic acid by competing with *para*-aminobenzoic acid. Trimethoprim blocks the production of tetrahydrofolic acid from dihydrofolic acid by binding to and reversibly inhibiting the required enzyme, dihydrofolate reductase. Thus, Bactrim blocks two consecutive steps in the biosynthesis of nucleic acids and proteins essential to many bacteria.

In vitro studies have shown that bacterial resistance develops more slowly with Bactrim than with trimethoprim or sulfamethoxazole alone.

In vitro serial dilution tests have shown that the spectrum of antibacterial activity of Bactrim includes the common urinary tract pathogens with the exception of *Pseudomonas aeruginosa.* The following organisms are usually susceptible: *Escherichia coli, Klebsiella-Enterobacter, Proteus mirabilis* and indole-positive proteus species.

In addition, the usual spectrum of antimicrobial activity of Bactrim includes the following bacterial pathogens isolated from middle ear exudate and from bronchial secretions: *Haemophilus influenzae,* including ampicillin-resistant strains, and *Streptococcus pneumoniae. Shigella flexneri* and *Shigella sonnei* are also usually susceptible.

[See table below].

The recommended quantitative disc susceptibility method (*Federal Register, 37:*20527–20529, 1972; Bauer AW, Kirby WMM, Sherris JC, Turck M: Antibiotic Susceptibility Testing by a Standardized Single Disc Method, *Am J Clin Pathol, 45:*493–496, 1966) may be used for estimating the susceptibility of bacteria to Bactrim. With this procedure, a report from the laboratory of "Susceptible to trimethoprim-sulfamethoxazole" indicates that the infection is likely to respond to therapy with Bactrim. If the infection is confined to the urine, a report of "Intermediate susceptibility to trimethoprim-sulfamethoxazole" also indicates that the infection is likely to respond. A report of "Resistant to trimethoprim-sulfamethoxazole" indicates that the infection is unlikely to respond to therapy with Bactrim.

Indications and Usage:

URINARY TRACT INFECTIONS: For the treatment of urinary tract infections due to susceptible strains of the following organisms: *Escherichia coli, Klebsiella-Enterobacter, Proteus mirabilis, Proteus vulgaris* and *Proteus morganii.* It is recommended that initial episodes of uncomplicated urinary tract infections be treated with a single effective antibacterial agent rather than the combination.

Note: Currently, the increasing frequency of resistant organisms is a limitation of the usefulness of all antibacterial agents, especially in the treatment of these urinary tract infections.

ACUTE OTITIS MEDIA: For the treatment of acute otitis media in children due to susceptible strains of *Haemophilus influenzae* or *Streptococcus pneumoniae* when in the judgment of the physician Bactrim offers some advantage over the use of other antimicrobial agents. To date, there are limited data on the safety of repeated use of Bactrim in children under two years of age. Bactrim is not indicated for prophylactic or prolonged administration in otitis media at any age.

ACUTE EXACERBATIONS OF CHRONIC BRONCHITIS IN ADULTS: For the treatment of acute exacerbations of chronic bronchitis due to susceptible strains of *Haemophilus influenzae* or *Streptococcus pneumoniae* when in the judgment of the physician Bactrim offers some advantage over the use of a single antimicrobial agent.

SHIGELLOSIS: For the treatment of enteritis caused by susceptible strains of *Shigella flexneri* and *Shigella sonnei* when antibacterial therapy is indicated.

***PNEUMOCYSTIS CARINII* PNEUMONITIS: Bactrim is also indicated in the treatment of documented *Pneumocystis carinii* pneumonitis.**

Contraindications: Hypersensitivity to trimethoprim or sulfonamides. Patients with documented megaloblastic anemia due to folate deficiency. Pregnancy at term and during the nursing period because sulfonamides pass the placenta and are excreted in the milk and may cause kernicterus. Infants less than two months of age.

Warnings: BACTRIM SHOULD NOT BE USED IN THE TREATMENT OF STREPTOCOCCAL PHARYNGITIS. Clinical studies have documented that patients with group A β-hemolytic streptococcal tonsillopharyngitis have a greater incidence of bacteriologic failure when treated with Bactrim than do those patients treated with penicillin, as evidenced by failure to eradicate this organism from the tonsillopharyngeal area.

REPRESENTATIVE MINIMUM INHIBITORY CONCENTRATION VALUES FOR BACTRIM-SUSCEPTIBLE ORGANISMS
(MIC—mcg/ml)

Bacteria	Trimethoprim Alone	Sulfamethoxazole Alone	TMP/SMX (1:20) TMP	SMX
Escherichia coli	0.05 – 1.5	1.0 – 245	0.05 – 0.5	0.95 – 9.5
Proteus spp. indole positive	0.5 – 5.0	7.35 – 300	0.05 – 1.5	0.95 – 28.5
Proteus mirabilis	0.5 – 1.5	7.35 – 30	0.05 – 0.15	0.95 – 2.85
Klebsiella-Enterobacter	0.15 – 5.0	2.45 – 245	0.05 – 1.5	0.95 – 28.5
Haemophilus influenzae	0.15 – 1.5	2.85 – 95	0.015 – 0.15	0.285 – 2.85
Streptococcus pneumoniae	0.15 – 1.5	7.35 – 24.5	0.05 – 0.15	0.95 – 2.85
Shigella flexneri	<0.01 – 0.04	<0.16 – >320	<0.002 – 0.03	0.04 – 0.625
Shigella sonnei	0.02 – 0.03	0.625 – >320	0.004 – 0.06	0.08 – 1.25

Each Berocca® tablet contains:	Quantity	U.S. RDA—Adults and children 4 or more years of age	U.S. RDA—Pregnant or lactating women
Vitamin C (ascorbic acid)	500 mg	60 mg	60 mg
Vitamin B_1 (as thiamine mononitrate)	15 mg	1.5 mg	1.7 mg
Vitamin B_2 (riboflavin)	15 mg	1.7 mg	2 mg
Niacin (as niacinamide)	100 mg	20 mg	20 mg
Vitamin B_6 (as pyridoxine HCl)	4 mg	2 mg	2.5 mg
Pantothenic acid (as calcium *d*-pantothenate)	18 mg	10 mg	10 mg
Folic acid	0.5 mg	0.4 mg	0.8 mg
Vitamin B_{12} (cyanocobalamin)	5 mcg	6 mcg	8 mcg

Deaths associated with the administration of sulfonamides have been reported from hypersensitivity reactions, agranulocytosis, aplastic anemia and other blood dyscrasias. Experience with trimethoprim alone is much more limited, but it has been reported to interfere with hematopoiesis in occasional patients. In elderly patients concurrently receiving certain diuretics, primarily thiazides, an increased incidence of thrombopenia with purpura has been reported.

The presence of clinical signs such as sore throat, fever, pallor, purpura or jaundice may be early indications of serious blood disorders. Complete blood counts should be done frequently in patients receiving Bactrim. If a significant reduction in the count of any formed blood element is noted, Bactrim should be discontinued.

Precautions: *General:* Bactrim should be given with caution to patients with impaired renal or hepatic function, to those with possible folate deficiency and to those with severe allergy or bronchial asthma. In glucose-6-phosphate dehydrogenase-deficient individuals, hemolysis may occur. This reaction is frequently dose-related. Adequate fluid intake must be maintained in order to prevent crystalluria and stone formation. Urinalyses with careful microscopic examination and renal function tests should be performed during therapy, particularly for those patients with impaired renal function.

It has been reported that Bactrim may prolong the prothrombin time of patients who are receiving the anticoagulant warfarin. This interaction should be kept in mind when Bactrim is given to patients already on anticoagulant therapy, and the coagulation time should be reassessed.

Pregnancy: Teratogenic Effects: Pregnancy Category C. In rats, doses of 533 mg/kg sulfamethoxazole or 200 mg/kg trimethoprim produced teratological effects manifested mainly as cleft palates. The highest dose which did not cause cleft palates in rats was 512 mg/kg sulfamethoxazole or 192 mg/kg trimethoprim when administered separately. In two studies in rats, no teratology was observed when 512 mg/kg of sulfamethoxazole was used in combination with 128 mg/kg of trimethoprim. In one study, however, cleft palates were observed in one litter out of 9 when 355 mg/kg of sulfamethoxazole was used in combination with 88 mg/kg of trimethoprim.

In some rabbit studies, an overall increase in fetal loss (dead and resorbed and malformed conceptuses) was associated with doses of trimethoprim 6 times the human therapeutic dose.

While there are no large well-controlled studies on the use of trimethoprim plus sulfamethoxazole in pregnant women, Brumfitt and Pursell (Trimethoprim/Sulfamethoxazole in the Treatment of Bacteriuria in Women. *J Infect Dis 128* (Suppl): S657-S663, 1973) reported the outcome of 186 pregnancies during which the mother received either placebo or trimethoprim in combination with sulfamethoxazole. The incidence of congenital abnormalities was 4.5% (3 of 66) in those who received placebo and 3.3% (4 of 120) in those receiving trimethoprim plus sulfamethoxazole. There were no abnormalities in the 10 children whose mothers received the drug during the first trimester. In a separate survey, Brumfitt and Pursell also found no congenital abnormalities in 35 children whose mothers had received trimethoprim plus sulfamethoxazole at the time of conception or shortly thereafter.

Because trimethoprim plus sulfamethoxazole may interfere with folic acid metabolism, Bactrim should be used during pregnancy only if the potential benefit justifies the potential risk to the fetus.

Nonteratogenic Effects: See "Contraindications" section.

Nursing Mothers: See "Contraindications" section.

Adverse Reactions: For completeness, all major reactions to sulfonamides and to trimethoprim are included below, even though they may not have been reported with Bactrim.

Blood dyscrasias: Agranulocytosis, aplastic anemia, megaloblastic anemia, thrombopenia, leukopenia, hemolytic anemia, purpura, hypoprothrombinemia and methemoglobinemia.

Allergic reactions: Erythema multiforme, Stevens-Johnson syndrome, generalized skin eruptions, epidermal necrolysis, urticaria, serum sickness, pruritus, exfoliative dermatitis, anaphylactoid reactions, periorbital edema, conjunctival and scleral injection, photosensitization, arthralgia and allergic myocarditis.

Gastrointestinal reactions: Glossitis, stomatitis, nausea, emesis, abdominal pains, hepatitis, diarrhea, pseudomembranous colitis and pancreatitis.

C.N.S. reactions: Headache, peripheral neuritis, mental depression, convulsions, ataxia, hallucinations, tinnitus, vertigo, insomnia, apathy, fatigue, muscle weakness and nervousness.

Miscellaneous reactions: Drug fever, chills, and toxic nephrosis with oliguria and anuria. Periarteritis nodosa and L. E. phenomenon have occurred.

The sulfonamides bear certain chemical similarities to some goitrogens, diuretics (acetazolamide and the thiazides) and oral hypoglycemic agents. Goiter production, diuresis and hypoglycemia have occurred rarely in patients receiving sulfonamides. Cross-sensitivity may exist with these agents. Rats appear to be especially susceptible to the goitrogenic effects of sulfonamides, and long-term administration has produced thyroid malignancies in the species.

Dosage and Administration: Not recommended for use in infants less than two months of age.

URINARY TRACT INFECTIONS AND SHIGELLOSIS IN ADULTS AND CHILDREN, AND ACUTE OTITIS MEDIA IN CHILDREN:

Adults: The usual adult dosage in the treatment of urinary tract infections is one Bactrium DS (double strength) tablet, two Bactrim tablets or four teaspoonfuls (20 ml) of Bactrim Pediatric Suspension or Bactrim Suspension every 12 hours for 10 to 14 days. An identical daily dosge is used for 5 days in the treatment of shigellosis.

Children: The recommended dose for children with urinary tract infections or acute otitis media is 8 mg/kg trimethoprim and 40 mg/kg sulfamethoxazole per 24 hours, given in two divided doses every 12 hours for 10 days. An identical daily dosage is used for 5 days in the treatment of shigellosis. The following table is a guideline for the attainment of this dosage:

Children two months of age or older:

Weight lb	Weight kg	Dose—every 12 hours Teaspoonfuls	Tablets
22	10	1 teasp. (5 ml)	—
44	20	2 teasp. (10 ml)	1 tablet
66	30	3 teasp. (15 ml)	1½ tablets
88	40	4 teasp. (20 ml)	2 tablets or 1 DS tablet

For patients with renal impairment:

Creatinine Clearance (ml/min)	Recommended Dosage Regimen
Above 30	Usual standard regimen
15–30	½ the usual regimen
Below 15	Use not recommended

ACUTE EXACERBATIONS OF CHRONIC BRONCHITIS IN ADULTS:

The usual adult dosage in the treatment of acute exacerbations of chronic bronchitis is one Bactrim DS (double strength) tablet, two Bactrim tablets or four teaspoonfuls (20 ml) of Bactrim Pediatric Suspension or Bactrim Suspension every 12 hours for 14 days.

PNEUMOCYSTIS CARINII PNEUMONITIS:

The recommended dosage for patients with *Pneumocystis carinii* pneumonitis is 20 mg/kg trimethoprim and 100 mg/kg sulfamethoxazole per 24 hours given in equally divided doses every 6 hours for 14 days. The following table is a guideline for the attainment of this dosage in children:

Weight lb	Weight kg	Dose—every six hours Teaspoonfuls	Tablets
18	8	1 teasp. (5 ml)	—
35	16	2 teasp. (10 ml)	1 tablet
53	24	3 teasp. (15 ml)	1½ tablets
70	32	4 teasp. (20 ml)	2 tablets or 1 DS tablet

How Supplied: *DS (double strength) Tablets,* containing 160 mg trimethoprim and 800 mg sulfamethoxazole—bottles of 100 and 500; Tel-E-Dose® packages of 100; Prescription Paks of 20.

Tablets, containing 80 mg trimethoprim and 400 mg sulfamethoxazole—bottles of 100 and 500; Tel-E-Dose® packages of 100; Prescription Paks of 40.

Pediatric Suspension, containing 40 mg trimethoprim and 200 mg sulfamethoxazole per teaspoonful (5 ml); cherry flavored—bottles of 100 ml and 16 oz (1 pint).

Suspension, containing 40 mg trimethoprim and 200 mg sulfamethoxazole per teaspoonful (5 ml); fruit-licorice flavored—bottles of 16 oz (1 pint).

[*Shown in Product Identification Section*]

BEROCCA® TABLETS ℞

The following text is complete prescribing information based on official labeling in effect August 1, 1982.

[See table above].

Description: Berocca is a prescription-only oral multivitamin tablet specially formulated for prophylactic or therapeutic nutritional supplementation in conditions requiring water-soluble vitamins.

Continued on next page

Roche Labs.—Cont.

Berocca tablets supply *therapeutic* levels of ascorbic acid, vitamins B_1, B_2, B_6, niacin and pantothenic acid and a *supplemental* level of vitamin B_{12}. Berocca tablets also supply a supplemental level of folic acid for pregnant or lactating women and a therapeutic level for adults and children four or more years of age.

Clinical Pharmacology: Vitamins are essential for normal metabolic functions including hematopoiesis. The B-complex vitamins are necessary for the conversion of carbohydrate, protein and fat into tissue and energy. Ascorbic acid (C) is involved in collagen formation and tissue repair.

The water-soluble vitamins (B-complex and C) are not significantly stored by the body; excess quantities are excreted in the urine. They must be replenished regularly through diet or other means to maintain essential tissue levels. Thus, these vitamins are rapidly depleted in conditions interfering with their intake or absorption.

Indications and Usage: Berocca is indicated for supportive nutritional supplementation in conditions in which water-soluble vitamins are required prophylactically or therapeutically. These include:

Conditions causing depletion, or reduced absorption or bioavailability of water-soluble vitamins—

Gastrointestinal disorders, chronic alcoholism, febrile illnesses, prolonged or wasting diseases, hyperthyroidism or poorly controlled diabetes.

Conditions resulting in increased needs for water-soluble vitamins—

Pregnancy, severe burns, recovery from surgery.

Contraindications: Berocca is contraindicated in patients known to be hypersensitive to any of its components.

Warnings: Berocca is not intended for treatment of pernicious anemia or other megaloblastic anemias where vitamin B_{12} is deficient. Neurologic involvement may develop or progress, despite temporary remission of anemia, in patients with vitamin B_{12} deficiency who receive supplemental folic acid and who are inadequately treated with B_{12}.

Precautions: *General:* Certain conditions listed above may require additional nutritional supplementation. During pregnancy, for instance, supplementation with fat-soluble vitamins and minerals may be required according to the dietary habits of the individual. Berocca is not intended for treatment of severe specific deficiencies.

Information for the Patient: Because toxic reactions have been reported with injudicious use of certain vitamins, urge patients to follow your specific instructions regarding dosage regimen. As with any medication, advise patients to keep Berocca out of reach of children.

Drug and Treatment Interactions: As little as 5 mg pyridoxine daily can decrease the efficacy of levodopa in the treatment of parkinsonism. Therefore, Berocca is not recommended for patients undergoing such therapy.

Adverse Reactions: Adverse reactions have been reported with specific vitamins, but generally at levels substantially higher than those in Berocca. However, allergic and idiosyncratic reactions are possible at lower levels.

Dosage and Administration: Usual adult dosage: one tablet daily.

Berocca is available on prescription only.

How Supplied: Light green, capsule-shaped tablets—bottles of 100 (NDC 0004-0020-01) and 500 (NDC 0004-0020-14).

Imprint on tablets: BEROCCA®
ROCHE

[*Shown in Product Identification Section*]

BEROCCA® PLUS TABLETS ℞

The following text is complete prescribing information based on official labeling in effect August 1, 1982.

[See table below].

Description: Berocca Plus is a prescription-only oral multivitamin/mineral tablet specially formulated for prophylactic or therapeutic nutritional supplementation in physiologically stressful conditions.

Berocca Plus supplies: *therapeutic* levels of water-soluble vitamins (ascorbic acid and all B-complex vitamins except biotin); *supplemental* levels of biotin, fat-soluble vitamins (A and E) and minerals (iron, chromium, manganese, copper and zinc); plus magnesium.

Clinical Pharmacology: Vitamins and minerals are essential for normal metabolic functions including hematopoiesis. The B-complex vitamins are necessary for the conversion of carbohydrate, protein and fat into tissue and energy. Ascorbic acid is involved in tissue repair and collagen formation. Vitamin A is necessary for proper functioning of the retina; it appears to be essential to the integrity of epithelial cells. Vitamin E is an antioxidant which preserves essential cellular constituents. Magnesium is a structural component of body tissues; iron, chromium, manganese, copper and zinc serve as catalysts in enzyme systems which perform vital cellular functions.

Water-soluble vitamins (B-complex and C) are not significantly stored by the body and must be replaced continually to maintain essential tissue levels; excess quantities are excreted in urine. These vitamins are rapidly depleted in conditions interfering with their intake or absorption. Berocca Plus supplies therapeutic levels of vitamin C and all B-complex vitamins (except biotin).

Fat-soluble vitamins and several trace minerals, however, can accumulate in the body and do not need replacement as frequently. Therefore, Berocca Plus supplies more conservative levels of vitamins A and E and various essential minerals.

Specifically, Berocca Plus contains an adequate level of vitamin B_6 (25 mg) to normalize the tryptophan metabolism disturbance which has been associated with the use of estrogenic oral contraceptives or other estrogen therapy. It provides zinc (22.5 mg) which facilitates wound healing, the level of folic acid (0.8 mg) recommended during pregnancy, and ascorbic acid (500 mg) which has been demonstrated to improve the absorption of inorganic iron.

Indications: Berocca Plus is indicated for prophylactic or therapeutic nutritional supplementation in physiologically stressful conditions. These include:

Conditions causing depletion, or reduced absorption or bioavailability of essential vitamins and minerals—

Inadequate intake due to highly restricted or unbalanced diets such as those frequently associated with anorexic conditions and other states of severe malnutrition.

Gastrointestinal disorders, chronic alcoholism, chronic or acute infections (especially those involving febrile illness), prolonged or wasting disease, congestive heart failure, hyperthyroidism, poorly controlled diabetes or other physiologic stress.

Also, patients on estrogenic oral contraceptives or other estrogen therapy, antibacterials which affect intestinal microflora, or other interfering drugs.

Certain conditions resulting from severe B-vitamin or ascorbic acid deficiency—

Cheilosis, gingivitis, stomatitis and certain other classic water-soluble vitamin deficiency syndromes.

Conditions resulting in increased needs for essential vitamins and minerals—

Recovery from surgery or trauma involving severe burns, fractures or other extensive tissue damage.

Also, pregnant women and those with heavy menstrual bleeding.

Contraindications: Berocca Plus is contraindicated in patients hypersensitive to any of its components.

Warnings: Not intended for treatment of pernicious anemia or other megaloblastic anemias where vitamin B_{12} is deficient. Neurologic involvement may develop or progress, despite temporary remission of anemia, in patients with vitamin B_{12} deficiency who receive supplemental folic acid and who are inadequately treated with B_{12}.

Precautions: *General:* Certain conditions listed above may require additional nutritional supplementation. During pregnancy, for instance, supplementation with vitamin D and calcium may be required according to the dietary habits of the individual. Berocca Plus is not intended for treatment of severe specific deficiencies.

Information for the Patient: Because toxic reactions have been reported with injudicious use of certain vitamins and minerals, urge patients to follow your specific instructions regarding dosage regimen. Advise patients to keep Berocca Plus out of reach of children.

Drug and Treatment Interactions: As litte as 5 mg pyridoxine daily can decrease the efficacy of levodopa in the treatment of parkinsonism. Therefore, Berocca Plus is not recommended for patients undergoing such therapy.

Adverse Reactions: Adverse reactions have been reported with specific vitamins and min-

Each Berocca® Plus tablet contains:	Quantity	U.S. RDA—Adults and children 4 or more years of age	U.S. RDA—Pregnant or lactating women
Fat-Soluble Vitamins			
Vitamin A (as vitamin A acetate)	5000 IU	5000 IU	8000 IU
Vitamin E (as *dl*-alpha tocopheryl acetate)	30 IU	30 IU	30 IU
Water-Soluble Vitamins			
Vitamin C (ascorbic acid)	500 mg	60 mg	60 mg
Vitamin B_1 (as thiamine mononitrate)	20 mg	1.5 mg	1.7 mg
Vitamin B_2 (riboflavin)	20 mg	1.7 mg	2 mg
Niacin (as niacinamide)	100 mg	20 mg	20 mg
Vitamin B_6 (as pyridoxine HCl)	25 mg	2 mg	2.5 mg
Biotin	0.15 mg	0.30 mg	0.30 mg
Pantothenic acid (as calcium pantothenate)	25 mg	10 mg	10 mg
Folic acid	0.8 mg	0.4 mg	0.8 mg
Vitamin B_{12} (cyanocobalamin)	50 mcg	6 mcg	8 mcg
Minerals			
Iron (as ferrous fumarate)	27 mg	18 mg	18 mg
Chromium (as chromium nitrate)	0.1 mg	0.05–0.2 mg*	
Magnesium (as magnesium oxide)	50 mg	400 mg	450 mg
Manganese (as manganese dioxide)	5 mg	2.5–5 mg*	
Copper (as cupric oxide)	3 mg	2 mg	2 mg
Zinc (as zinc oxide)	22.5 mg	15 mg	15 mg

*Not established. Estimated by NAS/NRC as safe and adequate daily dietary intake for adults.

erals, but generally at levels substantially higher than those in Berocca Plus. However, allergic and idiosyncratic reactions are possible at lower levels. Iron, even at the usual recommended levels, has been associated with gastrointestinal intolerance in some patients.
Dosage and Administration: Usual adult dosage: one tablet daily. Not recommended for children. *Berocca Plus is available on prescription only.*
How Supplied: Golden yellow, capsule-shaped tablets—bottles of 100.
Imprint on tablets: (front) BEROCCA PLUS; (back) ROCHE.
[*Shown in Product Identification Section*]

BEROCCA®-C BEROCCA®-C 500 ℞

The following text is complete prescribing information based on official labeling in effect August 1, 1982.
Description: Berocca-C provides generous amounts of six important B-complex vitamins plus an ample dose of vitamin C (ascorbic acid) in readily absorbable form.
Each 2 ml of Berocca-C contains:

Thiamine HCl (B_1)	10 mg
Riboflavin (B_2) (as riboflavin 5′-phosphate sodium)	10 mg
Niacinamide	80 mg
Pyridoxine HCl (B_6)	20 mg
Dexpanthenol (equivalent to 23.2 mg calcium pantothenate)	20 mg
d-biotin	0.2 mg
Ascorbic acid (C)	100 mg

compounded with 1% benzyl alcohol as preservative and pH adjusted with sodium hydroxide (to approximately 4.2 with the vial, 5.1 with the ampul).
Berocca-C 500 is a duplex package containing one 2-ml ampul of Berocca-C and a separate 2-ml ampul of 400 mg of Vitamin C Sodium Injectable compounded with 0.2% parabens (methyl and propyl) as preservatives, and pH adjusted to 5.5—7.0 with sodium bicarbonate. When the contents of both ampuls are aspirated into the same syringe, the resulting solution (4 ml) will contain equal amounts of the vitamins listed above, with the exception of vitamin C which increases to 500 mg.
Note: the formula of Berocca-C contains a soluble form of riboflavin which permits use of a larger dose and minimizes pain upon injection. While this form of riboflavin causes darkening of the solution which may intensify on prolonged storage, this in no way affects the safety and therapeutic efficacy of the preparation. Berocca-C is ready for immediate use, is stable for at least 18 months and need not be refrigerated.
Indications: Disorders requiring parenteral administration of water-soluble vitamins. Pre- and postoperative treatment; when requirements are increased, as in fever, severe burns, increased metabolism, hyperthyroidism, pregnancy; gastrointestinal disorders interfering with intake or absorption of water-soluble vitamins; prolonged or wasting diseases; alcoholism. In addition to these states indicated above, Berocca-C 500 is particularly useful in severe burns, shock, trauma or other instances when the need for vitamin C is increased out of proportion to that for other vitamins.
Precautions: Occasional sensitivity to thiamine hydrochloride has been reported. When not diluted with infusion fluids, Berocca-C should be injected SLOWLY. Intramuscular administration may cause transient pain.
Side Effects: Occasional hypersensitivity reactions to thiamine hydrochloride have been encountered, principally after repeated intravenous injections of concentrated solutions. Consequently, if the patient has previously received thiamine, subsequent injections should be given with care, and administration discontinued if untoward reactions develop. Pain on intramuscular injection has rarely been reported.
Dosage and Administration: Berocca-C is preferably administered by addition to parenteral infusion fluids—amino acids, glucose solutions, physiologic saline or electrolyte replacement fluids. From 2 ml to 20 ml of Berocca-C per liter of infusion fluid may be added to such solutions.
The contents of a duplex package of Berocca-C 500 (1 ampul of Berocca-C and 1 ampul of Vitamin C Sodium Injectable) should be aspirated into the same syringe—preferably shortly before administration. This preparation may then be added to parenteral infusion fluids—amino acids, glucose solutions, physiologic saline or electrolyte replacement fluids. Four ml of Berocca-C 500 per liter of infusion fluid are usually adequate. If desired, further amounts of vitamin C may be added to such solutions.
A dose of no more than 2 ml of Berocca-C or 4 ml of Berocca-C 500 may also be given undiluted by SLOW intravenous or intramuscular injection. Intravenous injection is usually preferable, since intramuscular administration may cause temporary pain.
Berocca-C may be administered until it is possible to replace it with oral vitamin supplementation.
How Supplied: Berocca-C ampuls: 2 ml, boxes of 10. Vials: 20 ml, boxes of 1. Berocca-C 500 Duplex Package: Contains one 2-ml ampul of Berocca-C and one 2-ml ampul containing 400 mg ascorbic acid—boxes of 10.

BEROCCA®-WS INJECTABLE ℞

Water-Soluble Vitamins for Intramuscular Use

The following text is complete prescribing information based on official labeling in effect August 1, 1982.
Description: Berocca-WS is a sterile injectable solution of nine water-soluble vitamins for intramuscular use. Each duplex package contains Solution 1 and Solution 2 in either ampuls or vials. When the contents of both containers are combined, 2 ml of the resulting parenteral multivitamin solution will provide eight B-complex vitamins and vitamin C at levels recommended by the American Medical Association.*
**Multivitamin Preparations for Parenteral Use: A Statement by the Nutrition Advisory Group.* American Medical Association Department of Foods and Nutrition, 1975. *JPEN 3:*258–269, Jul-Aug 1979.
Each ml of Berocca-WS Solution 1 provides:

Thiamine hydrochloride (B_1)	3	mg
d-Biotin	60	mcg
Riboflavin (as riboflavin 5′-phosphate sodium) (B_2)	3.6	mg
Niacinamide	40	mg
Pyridoxine hydrochloride (B_6)	4	mg
d-Panthenol	15	mg
Ascorbic acid (C)	100	mg

compounded with propylene glycol 40%, gentisic acid ethanolamide 2%, disodium edetate 0.01%, and benzyl alcohol 1% as stabilizers and preservatives; and sodium hydroxide to adjust pH to approximately 5.
Each ml of Berocca-WS Solution 2 provides:

Cyanocobalamin (B_{12})	5	mcg
Folic acid	400	mcg

compounded with gentisic acid ethanolamide 2%, disodium edetate 0.01%, sodium citrate 0.2% and benzyl alcohol 1% as stabilizers and preservatives; and sodium hydroxide and citric acid to adjust pH to approximately 6.
Clinical Pharmacology· Vitamins are essential for maintenance of normal metabolic functions including hematopoiesis. The water-soluble vitamins play vital roles in the conversion of carbohydrate, protein and fat into tissue and energy. *Thiamine (B_1)* acts as a coenzyme in carbohydrate metabolism. *Riboflavin (B_2)* functions as a coenzyme in the electron transport system associated with conversion of tissue oxidations into usable energy. *Niacin* serves as a coenzyme in oxidation-reduction reactions in tissue respiration. *Pyridoxine hydrochloride (B_6)* is essential for the metabolism of amino acids. *Pantothenic acid* functions as a coenzyme in various metabolic acetylation reactions and *biotin* in specific carboxylation reactions in lipid metabolism. *Folic acid* and *cyanocobalamin (B_{12})* are metabolically interrelated. They are essential to nucleic acid synthesis and normal maturation of red blood cells. *Ascorbic acid (C)* performs a vital function in the process of cellular respiration, and is involved in both carbohydrate and amino acid metabolism. It is essential for collagen formation and tissue repair.
The water-soluble vitamins (B-complex and C) are not significantly stored by the body; excess quantities are excreted in the urine. They must be replenished regularly through diet or other means to maintain essential tissue levels. Thus these vitamins are rapidly depleted in conditions interfering with their intake or absorption. Parenteral administration of water-soluble vitamins rapidly restores tissue levels.
Indications: Berocca-WS is indicated for adults and children 11 years of age or older for conditions in which (1) intake or absorption of the water-soluble vitamins is inadequate and oral intake must be supplemented; or (2) there is a known or suspected serious depletion of the water-soluble vitamins and immediate treatment by the intramuscular route is advisable. Conditions which may require parenteral administration of water-soluble vitamins may include disorders which can affect oral intake, gastrointestinal absorption or utilization. For example: comatose states, persistent vomiting, prolonged fever, severe infectious diseases, major surgery, extensive burns, fractures and other traumas, chronic alcoholism, diarrhea, achlorhydria or liver disease.
The physician should not await the development of clinical signs of vitamin deficiency before initiating therapy as there are few specific or pathognomonic signs of early vitamin deficiencies.
Contraindications: Berocca-WS is contraindicated in patients known to be hypersensitive to any of its components.
Warnings: Allergic reactions may occur in patients hypersensitive to the components of Berocca-WS.
Patients who have early Leber's disease (hereditary optic nerve atrophy) have been found to suffer severe, acute optic atrophy when treated with vitamin B_{12}. Pyridoxine can decrease the efficacy of levodopa in the treatment of patients with parkinsonism. Folic acid may alter patient response to methotrexate therapy. These facts should be considered before prescribing Berocca-WS for such patients. Folic acid in doses above 0.1 mg daily may obscure pernicious anemia. Berocca-WS is not intended for treatment of pernicious anemia or other megaloblastic anemias where vitamin B_{12} is deficient. Neurologic involvement may develop or progress, despite temporary remission of anemia, in patients with vitamin B_{12} deficiency who receive supplemental folic acid and who are inadequately treated with B_{12}. This product should not be used as primary treatment for specific vitamin deficiencies such as beriberi, pellagra, scurvy, and riboflavin or pyridoxine deficiency.
The possibility of injury to the sciatic nerve should be kept in mind when administering vitamins intramuscularly.
Precautions: Transient pain may be experienced upon intramuscular injection. Injections should be made into a large muscle mass to insure rapid absorption and to minimize pain.

Continued on next page

Roche Labs.—Cont.

Most antibiotics, methotrexate and pyrimethamine invalidate diagnostic microbiological blood assays for folic acid and cyanocobalamin. Safety and effectiveness in children under the age of 11 have not been established.

Adverse Reactions: Allergic sensitization has been reported following parenteral administration of folic acid and thiamine.

Dosage and Administration: For intramuscular use. The recommended daily dose is 2 ml of reconstituted Berocca-WS (1 ml of Solution 1 and 1 ml of Solution 2).

Note: Berocca-WS contains a soluble form of riboflavin which permits use of a large dose and minimizes pain on injection. This form of riboflavin may result in darkening of the solution, and the color change is intensified on prolonged storage. However, the darkening of the solution in no way affects the safety and therapeutic efficacy of the preparation.

Parenteral drug products should be inspected visually for particulate matter prior to administration, whenever solution and container permit.

Important: Directions For Reconstitution and Storage:

Ampuls: To prepare solution for a single dose injection, mix 1 ml of Berocca-WS Solution 1 with 1 ml of Berocca-WS Solution 2. Reconstituted product is ready for administration.

Multiple dose vials: To prepare solution for 10 doses, add 10 ml of Berocca-WS Solution 2 to 10 ml of Berocca-WS Solution 1 (20 ml vial, 10 ml fill). Reconstituted product is ready for administration of single doses of 2 ml.

Store unreconstituted product in refrigerator (2°–8° C, 36°–46° F). PROTECT FROM LIGHT. DO NOT STORE AT ROOM TEMPERATURE. Store reconstituted (mixed) product for no longer than 14 days in refrigerator (2°–8° C, 36°–46° F). PROTECT FROM LIGHT.

How Supplied: *Ampuls:* Duplex packages, each containing a 1-ml ampul of Solution 1 and a 1-ml ampul of Solution 2; boxes of 25.

Vials: Duplex packages, each containing a 20-ml vial (10-ml fill) of Solution 1 and a 10-ml vial (10-ml fill) of Solution 2; boxes of 1.

CLONOPIN® ℭ
(clonazepam/Roche)

The following text is complete prescribing information based on official labeling in effect August 1, 1982.

Description: Chemically, clonazepam is 5-(2-chlorophenyl) -1, 3-dihydro-7-nitro-2H-1,4-benzodiazepin-2-one. It is a light yellow crystalline powder. It has a molecular weight of 315.7.

Actions: In laboratory animals, Clonopin exhibits several pharmacologic properties which are characteristic of the benzodiazepine class of drugs. Convulsions produced in rodents by pentylenetetrazol or electrical stimulation are antagonized, as are convulsions produced by photic stimulation in susceptible baboons. A taming effect in aggressive primates, muscle weakness and hypnosis are likewise produced by Clonopin. In humans it is capable of suppressing the spike and wave discharge in absence seizures (petit mal) and decreasing the frequency, amplitude, duration and spread of discharge in minor motor seizures.

Single oral dose administration of Clonopin to humans gave maximum blood levels of drug, in most cases, within one to two hours. The half-life of the parent compound varied from approximately 18 to 50 hours, and the major route of excretion was in the urine. In humans, five metabolites have been identified. In general, the biotransformation of clonazepam followed two pathways: oxidative hydroxylation at the C-3 position and reduction of the 7-nitro function to form 7-amino and/or 7-acetyl-amino derivatives.

Indications: Clonopin is useful alone or as an adjunct in the treatment of the Lennox-Gastaut syndrome (petit mal variant), akinetic and myoclonic seizures. In patients with absence seizures (petit mal) who have failed to respond to succinimides, Clonopin may be useful.

In some studies, up to 30% of patients have shown a loss of anticonvulsant activity, often within three months of administration. In some cases, dosage adjustment may reestablish efficacy.

Contraindications: Clonopin should not be used in patients with a history of sensitivity to benzodiazepines, nor in patients with clinical or biochemical evidence of significant liver disease. It may be used in patients with open angle glaucoma who are receiving appropriate therapy, but is contraindicated in acute narrow angle glaucoma.

Warnings: Since Clonopin produces CNS depression, patients receiving this drug should be cautioned against engaging in hazardous occupations requiring mental alertness, such as operating machinery or driving a motor vehicle. They should also be warned about the concomitant use of alcohol or other CNS-depressant drugs during Clonopin therapy (see Drug Interactions).

Usage in Pregnancy: The effects of Clonopin in human pregnancy and nursing infants are unknown.

Recent reports suggest an association between the use of anticonvulsant drugs by women with epilepsy and an elevated incidence of birth defects in children born to these women. Data are more extensive with respect to diphenylhydantoin and phenobarbital, but these are also the most commonly prescribed anticonvulsants; less systematic or anecdotal reports suggest a possible similar association with the use of all known anticonvulsant drugs.

The reports suggesting an elevated incidence of birth defects in children of drug-treated epileptic women cannot be regarded as adequate to prove a definite cause and effect relationship. There are intrinsic methodologic problems in obtaining adequate data on drug teratogenicity in humans; the possibility also exists that other factors, *e.g.*, genetic factors or the epileptic condition itself, may be more important than drug therapy in leading to birth defects. The great majority of mothers on anticonvulsant medication deliver normal infants. It is important to note that anticonvulsant drugs should not be discontinued in patients in whom the drug is administered to prevent seizures because of the strong possibility of precipitating status epilepticus with attendant hypoxia and threat to life. In individual cases where the severity and frequency of the seizure disorder are such that the removal of medication does not pose a serious threat to the patient, discontinuation of the drug may be considered prior to and during pregnancy, although it cannot be said with any confidence that even mild seizures do not pose some hazards to the developing embryo or fetus.

These considerations should be weighed in treating or counseling epileptic women of childbearing potential.

Use of Clonopin in women of childbearing potential should be considered only when the clinical situation warrants the risk. Mothers receiving Clonopin should not breast feed their infants.

In a two-generation reproduction study with Clonopin given orally to rats at 10 or 100 mg/kg/day, there was a decrease in the number of pregnancies and a decrease in the number of offspring surviving until weaning. When Clonopin was administered orally to pregnant rabbits at 0.2, 1.0, 5.0 or 10.0 mg/kg/day, a nondose-related incidence of cleft palates, open eyelids, fused sternebrae and limb defects was observed at the 0.2 and 5.0 mg/kg/day levels. Nearly all of the malformations were seen from one dam in each of the affected dosages.

Usage in Children: Because of the possibility that adverse effects on physical or mental development could become apparent only after many years, a benefit-risk consideration of the long-term use of Clonopin is important in pediatric patients.

Physical and Psychological Dependence: Withdrawal symptoms similar in character to those noted with barbiturates and alcohol have occurred following abrupt discontinuance of benzodiazepine drugs. These symptoms include convulsions, tremor, abdominal and muscle cramps, vomiting and sweating. Addiction-prone individuals, such as drug addicts or alcoholics, should be under careful surveillance when receiving benzodiazepines because of the predisposition of such patients to habituation and dependence.

Precautions: When used in patients in whom several different types of seizure disorders coexist, Clonopin may increase the incidence or precipitate the onset of generalized tonic-clonic seizures (grand mal). This may require the addition of appropriate anticonvulsants or an increase in their dosages. The concomitant use of valproic acid and clonazepam may produce absence status.

Periodic blood counts and liver function tests are advisable during long-term therapy with Clonopin.

The abrupt withdrawal of Clonopin, particularly in those patients on long-term, high-dose therapy, may precipitate status epilepticus. Therefore, when discontinuing Clonopin, gradual withdrawal is essential. While Clonopin is being gradually withdrawn, the simultaneous substitution of another anticonvulsant may be indicated. Metabolites of Clonopin are excreted by the kidneys; to avoid their excess accumulation, caution should be exercised in the administration of the drug to patients with impaired renal function.

Clonopin may produce an increase in salivation. This should be considered before giving the drug to patients who have difficulty handling secretions. Because of this and the possibility of respiratory depression, Clonopin should be used with caution in patients with chronic respiratory diseases.

Adverse Reactions: The most frequently occurring side effects of Clonopin are referable to CNS depression. Experience to date has shown that drowsiness has occurred in approximately 50% of patients and ataxia in approximately 30%. In some cases, these may diminish with time; behavior problems have been noted in approximately 25% of patients. Others, listed by system, are:

Neurologic: Abnormal eye movements, aphonia, choreiform movements, coma, diplopia, dysarthria, dysdiadochokinesis, "glassy-eyed" appearance, headache, hemiparesis, hypotonia, nystagmus, respiratory depression, slurred speech, tremor, vertigo.

Psychiatric: Confusion, depression, forgetfulness, hallucinations, hysteria, increased libido, insomnia, psychosis, suicidal attempt (the behavior effects are more likely to occur in patients with a history of psychiatric disturbances).

Respiratory: Chest congestion, rhinorrhea, shortness of breath, hypersecretion in upper respiratory passages.

Cardiovascular: Palpitations.

Dermatologic: Hair loss, hirsutism, skin rash, ankle and facial edema.

Gastrointestinal: Anorexia, coated tongue, constipation, diarrhea, dry mouth, encopresis, gastritis, hepatomegaly, increased appetite, nausea, sore gums.

Genitourinary: Dysuria, enuresis, nocturia, urinary retention.

Musculoskeletal: Muscle weakness, pains.

Miscellaneous: Dehydration, general deterioration, fever, lymphadenopathy, weight loss or gain.

Hematopoietic: Anemia, leukopenia, thrombocytopenia, eosinophilia.

Hepatic: Transient elevations of serum transaminases and alkaline phosphatase.

Drug Interactions: The CNS-depressant action of the benzodiazepine class of drugs may be potentiated by alcohol, narcotics, barbiturates, nonbarbiturate hypnotics, antianxiety agents, the phenothiazines, thioxanthene and butyrophenone classes of antipsychotic agents, monoamine oxidase inhibitors and the tricyclic antidepressants, and by other anticonvulsant drugs.

Overdosage: Symptoms of Clonopin overdosage, like those produced by other CNS depressants, include somnolence, confusion, coma and diminished reflexes. Treatment includes monitoring of respiration, pulse and blood pressure, general supportive measures and immediate gastric lavage. Intravenous fluids should be administered and an adequate airway maintained. Hypotension may be combated by the use of levarterenol or metaraminol. Methylphenidate or caffeine and sodium benzoate may be given to combat CNS depression. Dialysis is of no known value.

Dosage and Administration: *Infants and Children:* Clonopin is administered orally. In order to minimize drowsiness, the initial dose for infants and children (up to 10 years of age or 30 kg of body weight) should be between 0.01 to 0.03 mg/kg/day but not to exceed 0.05 mg/kg/day given in two or three divided doses. Dosage should be increased by no more than 0.25 to 0.5 mg every third day until a daily maintenance dose of 0.1 to 0.2 mg/kg of body weight has been reached unless seizures are controlled or side effects preclude further increase. Whenever possible, the daily dose should be divided into three equal doses. If doses are not equally divided, the largest dose should be given before retiring.

Adults: The initial dose for adults should not exceed 1.5 mg/day divided into three doses. Dosage may be increased in increments of 0.5 to 1 mg every three days until seizures are adequately controlled or until side effects preclude any further increase. Maintenance dosage must be individualized for each patient depending upon response. Maximum recommended daily dose is 20 mg.

The use of multiple anticonvulsants may result in an increase of depressant adverse effects. This should be considered before adding Clonopin to an existing anticonvulsant regimen.

How Supplied: Scored tablets—0.5 mg, orange; 1 mg, blue; 2 mg, white—Prescription Paks of 100.

[*Shown in Product Identification Section*]

EFUDEX® ℞
(fluorouracil/Roche)

The following text is complete prescribing information based on official labeling in effect August 1, 1982.

Description: Efudex solutions and cream are topical preparations containing the fluorinated pyrimidine 5-fluorouracil, an antineoplastic antimetabolite.

Efudex Solution consists of 2% or 5% fluorouracil/Roche on a weight/weight basis, compounded with propylene glycol, tris(hydroxymethyl)aminomethane, hydroxypropyl cellulose, parabens (methyl and propyl) and disodium edetate.

Efudex Cream contains 5% fluorouracil/Roche in a vanishing cream base consisting of white petrolatum, stearyl alcohol, propylene glycol, polysorbate 60 and parabens (methyl and propyl).

Actions: There is evidence that the metabolism of fluorouracil in the anabolic pathway blocks the methylation reaction of deoxyuridylic acid to thymidylic acid. In this fashion fluorouracil interferes with the synthesis of deoxyribonucleic acid (DNA) and to a lesser extent inhibits the formation of ribonucleic acid (RNA). Since DNA and RNA are essential for cell division and growth, the effect of fluorouracil may be to create a thymine deficiency which provokes unbalanced growth and death of the cell. The effects of DNA and RNA deprivation are most marked on those cells which grow more rapidly and which take up fluorouracil at a more rapid pace. The catabolic metabolism of fluorouracil results in degradative products (e.g., CO_2, urea, α-fluoro-β-alanine) which are inactive.

Studies in man with topical application of ^{14}C-labeled Efudex demonstrated insignificant absorption as measured by ^{14}C content of plasma, urine and respiratory CO_2.

Indications: Efudex is recommended for the topical treatment of multiple actinic or solar keratoses. In the 5% strength it is also useful in the treatment of superficial basal cell carcinomas, when conventional methods are impractical, such as with multiple lesions or difficult treatment sites. The diagnosis should be established prior to treatment, since this new method has not been proven effective in other types of basal cell carcinomas. With isolated, easily accessible lesions, conventional techniques are preferred since success with such lesions is almost 100% with these methods. The success rate with Efudex cream and solution is approximately 93%. This 93% success rate is based on 113 lesions in 54 patients. Twenty-five lesions treated with the solution produced one failure and 88 lesions treated with the cream produced 7 failures.

Contraindications: Efudex is contraindicated in patients with known hypersensitivity to any of its components.

Warnings: If an occlusive dressing is used, there may be an increase in the incidence of inflammatory reactions in the adjacent normal skin. A porous gauze dressing may be applied for cosmetic reasons without increase in reaction.

Prolonged exposure to ultraviolet rays should be avoided while under treatment with Efudex because the intensity of the reaction may be increased.

Usage in Pregnancy: Safety for use in pregnancy has not been established.

Precautions: If Efudex is applied with the fingers, the hands should be washed immediately afterward. Efudex should be applied with care near the eyes, nose and mouth. Solar keratoses which do not respond should be biopsied to confirm the diagnosis. Patients should be forewarned that the reaction in the treated areas may be unsightly during therapy, and, in some cases, for several weeks following cessation of therapy.

Follow-up biopsies should be performed as indicated in the management of superficial basal cell carcinoma.

Adverse Reactions: The most frequently encountered local reactions are pain, pruritus, hyperpigmentation and burning at the site of application. Other local reactions include dermatitis, scarring, soreness, tenderness, suppuration, scaling and swelling.

Also reported are insomnia, stomatitis, irritability, medicinal taste, photosensitivity, lacrimation and telangiectasia, although a causal relationship is remote.

Laboratory abnormalities reported are leukocytosis, thrombocytopenia, toxic granulation and eosinophilia.

Dosage and Administration: When Efudex is applied to a lesion, a response occurs with the following sequence: erythema, usually followed by vesiculation, erosion, ulceration, necrosis and epithelization.

Actinic or solar keratosis: Apply cream or solution twice daily in an amount sufficient to cover the lesions. Medication should be continued until the inflammatory response reaches the erosion, necrosis and ulceration stage, at which time use of the drug should be terminated. The usual duration of therapy is from two to four weeks. Complete healing of the lesions may not be evident for one to two months following cessation of Efudex therapy.

Superficial basal cell carcinomas: **Only the 5% strength is recommended.** Apply cream or solution twice daily in an amount sufficient to cover the lesions. Treatment should be continued for at least three to six weeks. Therapy may be required for as long as 10 to 12 weeks before the lesions are obliterated. As in any neoplastic condition, the patient should be followed for a reasonable period of time to determine if a cure has been obtained.

How Supplied: Efudex Solution, 10-ml drop dispensers—containing 2% or 5% fluorouracil/Roche on a weight/weight basis, compounded with propylene glycol, tris(hydroxymethyl)aminomethane, hydroxypropyl cellulose, parabens (methyl and propyl) and disodium edetate.

Efudex Cream, 25-Gm tubes—containing 5% fluorouracil/Roche in a vanishing cream base consisting of white petrolatum, stearyl alcohol, propylene glycol, polysorbate 60 and parabens (methyl and propyl).

EMCYT® ℞
(estramustine phosphate sodium/Roche)
CAPSULES

The following text is complete prescribing information based on official labeling in effect August 1, 1982.

Description: Estramustine phosphate sodium, an antineoplastic agent, is an off-white powder readily soluble in water. Emcyt is available as white opaque capsules, each containing estramustine phosphate sodium equivalent to 140 mg estramustine phosphate, for oral administration.

Chemically, estramustine phosphate sodium is estra-1,3,5(10)-triene-3,17β-diol-3[bis-(2-chloroethyl)carbamate] 17-(dihydrogen phosphate), disodium salt. It is also referred to as estradiol 3-bis(2-chloroethyl)carbamate 17-(dihydrogen phosphate), disodium salt.

Estramustine phosphate sodium has an empiric formula of $C_{23}H_{30}Cl_2NNa_2O_6P$ and a calculated molecular weight of 582.4.

Clinical Pharmacology: Estramustine phosphate is a molecule combining estradiol and nornitrogen mustard by a carbamate link. The molecule is phosphorylated to make it water soluble.

Estramustine phosphate taken orally is readily dephosphorylated during absorption, and the major metabolites in plasma are estramustine, the estrone analog, estradiol and estrone.

Prolonged treatment with estramustine phosphate produces elevated total plasma concentrations of estradiol that fall within ranges similar to the elevated estradiol levels found in prostatic cancer patients given conventional estradiol therapy. Estrogenic effects, as demonstrated by changes in circulating levels of steroids and pituitary hormones, are similar in patients treated with either estramustine phosphate or conventional estradiol.

The metabolic urinary patterns of the estradiol moiety of estramustine phosphate and estradiol itself are very similar, although the metabolites derived from estramustine phosphate are excreted at a slower rate.

Indications and Usage: Emcyt is indicated in the palliative treatment of patients with metastatic and/or progressive carcinoma of the prostate.

Contraindications: Emcyt should not be used in patients with any of the following conditions:

1) Known hypersensitivity to either estradiol or to nitrogen mustard.
2) Active thrombophlebitis or thromboembolic disorders, except in those cases where the actual tumor mass is the cause of the thromboembolic phenomenon and the phy-

Continued on next page

Roche Labs.—Cont.

sician feels the benefits of therapy may outweigh the risks.

Warnings: It has been shown that there is an increased risk of thrombosis, including nonfatal myocardial infarction, in men receiving estrogens for prostatic cancer. Emcyt should be used with caution in patients with a history of thrombophlebitis, thrombosis or thromboembolic disorders, especially if they were associated with estrogen therapy. Caution should also be used in patients with cerebral vascular or coronary artery disease.
Glucose Tolerance—Because glucose tolerance may be decreased, diabetic patients should be carefully observed while receiving Emcyt.
Elevated Blood Pressure—Because hypertension may occur, blood pressure should be monitored periodically.

Precautions: *General:* Fluid Retention—Exacerbation of preexisting or incipient peripheral edema or congestive heart disease has been seen in some patients receiving Emcyt therapy. Other conditions which might be influenced by fluid retention, such as epilepsy, migraine or renal dysfunction, require careful observation.
Emcyt may be poorly metabolized in patients with impaired liver function and should be administered with caution in such patients.
Because Emcyt may influence the metabolism of calcium and phosphorus, it should be used with caution in patients with metabolic bone diseases that are associated with hypercalcemia or in patients with renal insufficiency.
Information for the Patient: Because of the possibility of mutagenic effects, patients should be advised to use contraceptive measures.
Laboratory Tests: Certain endocrine and liver function tests may be affected by estrogen-containing drugs. Abnormalities of hepatic enzymes and of bilirubin have occurred in patients receiving Emcyt, but have seldom been severe enough to require cessation of therapy. Such tests should be done at appropriate intervals during therapy and repeated after the drug has been withdrawn for two months.
Carcinogenesis, Mutagenesis, Impairment of Fertility: Long-term continuous administration of estrogens in certain animal species increases the frequency of carcinomas of the breast and liver. Compounds structurally similar to Emcyt are carcinogenic in mice. Carcinogenic studies of Emcyt have not been conducted in man. Although testing by the Ames method failed to demonstrate mutagenicity for estramustine phosphate sodium, it is known that both estradiol and nitrogen mustard are mutagenic. For this reason and because some patients who had been impotent while on estrogen therapy have regained potency while taking Emcyt, the patient should be advised to use contraceptive measures.

Adverse Reactions: In a randomized, double-blind trial comparing therapy with Emcyt in 93 patients (11.5 to 15.9 mg/kg/day) or diethylstilbestrol (DES) in 93 patients (3.0 mg/day), the following adverse effects were reported:

	EMCYT n=93	DES n=93
CARDIOVASCULAR–RESPIRATORY		
Cardiac Arrest	0	2
Cerebrovascular Accident	2	0
Myocardial Infarction	3	1
Thrombophlebitis	3	7
Pulmonary Emboli	2	5
Congestive Heart Failure	3	2
Edema	19	17
Dyspnea	11	3
Leg Cramps	8	11
Upper Respiratory Discharge	1	1
Hoarseness	1	0
GASTROINTESTINAL		
Nausea	15	8
Diarrhea	12	11
Minor Gastrointestinal Upset	11	6
Anorexia	4	3
Flatulence	2	0
Vomiting	1	1
Gastrointestinal Bleeding	1	0
Burning Throat	1	0
Thirst	1	0
INTEGUMENTARY		
Rash	1	4
Pruritus	2	2
Dry Skin	2	0
Pigment Changes	0	3
Easy Bruising	3	0
Flushing	1	0
Night Sweats	0	1
Fingertip—Peeling Skin	1	0
Thinning Hair	1	1
BREAST CHANGES		
Tenderness	66	64
Enlargement		
Mild	60	54
Moderate	10	16
Marked	0	5
MISCELLANEOUS		
Lethargy Alone	4	3
Depression	0	2
Emotional Lability	2	0
Insomnia	3	0
Headache	1	1
Anxiety	1	0
Chest Pain	1	1
Hot Flashes	0	1
Pain in Eyes	0	1
Tearing of Eyes	1	1
Tinnitus	0	1
LABORATORY ABNORMALITIES		
Hematologic		
Leukopenia	4	2
Thrombopenia	1	2
Hepatic		
Bilirubin Alone	1	5
Bilirubin and LDH	0	1
Bilirubin and SGOT	2	1
Bilirubin, LDH and SGOT	2	0
LDH and/or SGOT	31	28
Miscellaneous		
Hypercalcemia—Transient	0	1

Overdosage: Although there has been no experience with overdosage to date, it is reasonable to expect that such episodes may produce pronounced manifestations of the known adverse reactions. In the event of overdosage, the gastric contents should be evacuated by gastric lavage and symptomatic therapy should be initiated. Hematologic and hepatic parameters should be monitored for at least six weeks after overdosage of Emcyt.

Dosage and Administration: The recommended daily dose is 14 mg per kg of body weight (*i.e.*, one 140 mg capsule for each 10 kg or 22 lb of body weight), given in 3 or 4 divided doses. Most patients in studies in the United States have been treated at a dosage range of 10 to 16 mg per kg per day.
Patients should be treated for 30 to 90 days before the physician determines the possible benefits of continued therapy. Therapy should be continued as long as the favorable response lasts. Some patients have been maintained on therapy for more than three years at doses ranging from 10 to 16 mg per kg of body weight per day.

How Supplied: White opaque capsules, each containing estramustine phosphate sodium equivalent to 140 mg estramustine phosphate—bottles of 100 (NDC 0004-0132-02).

Note: Emcyt should be stored in the refrigerator at 36° to 46°F (2° to 8°C).

[*Shown in Product Identification Section*]

ENDEP® ℞

(amitriptyline HCl/Roche)
TABLETS

The following text is complete prescribing information based on official labeling in effect August 1, 1982.

Description: Endep (amitriptyline HCl/Roche), a tricyclic antidepressant, is available as 10-mg, 25-mg, 50-mg, 75-mg, 100-mg and 150-mg tablets for oral administration.
Amitriptyline HCl, a dibenzocycloheptadiene derivative, is a white crystalline compound that is readily soluble in water. It is designated chemically as 10, 11-dihydro-*N,N*-dimethyl-5*H*-dibenzo[*a,d*]-cycloheptene- $\Delta^{5,\gamma}$-propylamine hydrochloride. The molecular weight is 313.87. The empirical formula is $C_{20}H_{23}N \cdot HCL$.

Clinical Pharmacology: Endep is an antidepressant with sedative effects. Its mechanism of action in man is not known. It is not a monoamine oxidase inhibitor, and it does not act primarily by stimulation of the central nervous system.
Amitriptyline inhibits the membrane pump mechanism responsible for uptake of norepinephrine and serotonin in adrenergic and serotonergic neurons. Pharmacologically this action may potentiate or prolong neuronal activity, since reuptake of these biogenic amines is important physiologically in terminating its transmitting activity. This interference with reuptake of norepinephrine and/or serotonin is believed by some to underlie the antidepressant activity of amitriptyline.
Amitriptyline undergoes extensive metabolism primarily through N-demethylation to nortriptyline, an active metabolite, followed by extensive hydroxylation to their respective 10-hydroxy metabolites which are eliminated as glucuronide conjugates.
Following a single oral dose of 75 mg of amitriptyline HCl, the mean maximum plasma concentrations of 39.4 ng/ml of amitriptyline and 16.1 ng/ml of nortriptyline were reached in approximately 4 and 10 hours, respectively. The average minimum steady-state plasma concentrations in patients receiving 50 mg of amitriptyline HCl, three times a day for an average of 32 days, were 81 ng/ml for amitriptyline, 71 ng/ml for nortriptyline, 12 ng/ml for 10-hydroxyamitriptyline, 91 ng/ml for conjugated 10-hydroxyamitriptyline, 82 ng/ml for 10-hydroxynortriptyline and 176 ng/ml for conjugated 10-hydroxynortriptyline. Steady-state plasma concentrations are usually reached by day 14. The mean apparent half-life of elimination of amitriptyline is 22.4 hours and the apparent half-life of elimination of nortriptyline is 26.0 hours. Amitriptyline is approximately 96% bound to plasma proteins. Amitriptyline has been shown to cross the blood-brain barrier in cats, mice and rats. It has also been shown to pass the placental barrier and to enter fetal circulation in mice after intramuscular and intravenous administration. Amitriptyline is excreted in human breast milk.

Indications and Usage: Endep is indicated for the relief of symptoms of depression. Endogenous depression is more likely to be alleviated than are other depressive states.

Contraindications: Endep is contraindicated in patients who have shown prior hypersensitivity to this agent; cross-sensitivity to other tricyclic antidepressants can occur.
Endep is not recommended for use during the acute recovery phase following myocardial infarction.
Endep should not be given concomitantly with a monoamine oxidase inhibitor. Hyperpyretic crises, severe convulsions and deaths have occurred in patients receiving tricyclic antidepressant and monoamine oxidase inhibiting drugs simultaneously. When it is desired to replace a monoamine oxidase inhibitor with Endep, a minimum of 14 days should be allowed to elapse after the former is discontin-

ued. Endep should then be initiated cautiously with gradual increase in dosage until optimum response is achieved.

Warnings: Endep should be used with caution in patients with a history of seizures and, because of its atropine-like action, in patients with a history of urinary retention, angle-closure glaucoma or increased intraocular pressure.

In patients with angle-closure glaucoma, even average doses may precipitate an attack.

Patients with cardiovascular disorders should be watched closely. Tricyclic antidepressant drugs, including Endep, particularly when given in high doses, have been reported to produce arrhythmias, sinus tachycardia and prolongation of the conduction time. Myocardial infarction and stroke have been reported with drugs of this class.

Close supervision is required when Endep is given to hyperthyroid patients or those receiving thyroid medication.

Amitriptyline HCl may enhance the response to alcohol and the effects of barbiturates and other CNS depressants. In patients who may use alcohol excessively, it should be borne in mind that the potentiation may increase the danger inherent in any suicide attempt or overdosage.

Precautions: *General:* Schizophrenic patients may develop increased symptoms of psychosis; patients with paranoid symptomatology may have an exaggeration of such symptoms; manic depressive patients may experience a shift to the manic phase. In these circumstances, the dose of Endep may be reduced or a major tranquilizer such as perphenazine may be administered concurrently.

The possibility of suicide in depressed patients remains during treatment and until significant remission occurs. Potentially suicidal patients should not have access to large quantities of this drug. Prescriptions should be written for the smallest amount feasible.

Concurrent administration of Endep and electroshock therapy may increase the hazards associated with such therapy. Such treatment should be limited to patients for whom it is essential.

Amitriptyline HCl should be used with caution in patients with impaired liver function.

Both elevation and lowering of blood sugar levels have been reported.

The drug should be discontinued several days before elective surgery, if possible.

Information for Patients: Patients should be cautioned about engaging in hazardous occupations requiring complete mental alertness such as operating machinery or driving a motor vehicle after ingesting the drug.

Patients receiving amitriptyline HCl should also be cautioned about the possible combined effects with alcohol, barbiturates and other CNS depressants.

Drug Interactions: MAO inhibitors—see CONTRAINDICATIONS section. Thyroid medications; alcohol, barbiturates and other CNS depressants—see WARNINGS section.

Endep may block the antihypertensive action of guanethidine or similarly acting compounds.

When Endep is given with anticholinergic agents or sympathomimetic drugs, including epinephrine combined with local anesthetics, close supervision and careful adjustment of dosages are required.

Paralytic ileus may occur in patients taking tricyclic antidepressants in combination with anticholinergic-type drugs.

Caution is advised if patients receive large doses of ethchlorvynol concurrently. Transient delirium has been reported in patients who were treated with one gram of ethchlorvynol and 75 to 150 mg of amitriptyline HCl.

Carcinogenesis, Mutagenesis, Impairment of Fertility: Carcinogenesis: Amitriptyline HCl has not been adequately studied in animals to permit an evaluation of its carcinogenic potential. However, in a study during which relatively small numbers of rats received amitriptyline HCl as a dietary admixture at dosages up to 100 mg/kg/day for 78 weeks, no increase in the incidence of any tumor was reported.

Mutagenesis: Amitriptyline HCl was tested in a bacterial mutagenesis assay (Ames test) in the presence and absence of activating enzymes. No evidence for mutagenicity was found using *Salmonella* tester strains TA 1535, TA 100, TA 98 and TA 1537 at concentrations up to 5000 mcg/plate.

Impairment of Fertility: Amitriptyline HCl was studied in a Segment I fertility and general reproduction study in rats at dosages up to 20 mg/kg/day. There were no adverse effects on fertility, fetal growth and development, litter size, pup survival or pup growth. Similarly, no adverse effects were reported in a rat litter test in which amitriptyline HCl was administered at dosages up to 20 mg/kg/day.

Pregnancy: Teratogenic Effects: Pregnancy Category C. Animal reproduction studies have been inconclusive, and clinical experience has been limited. Amitriptyline HCl was tested in rats and in rabbits for teratogenic potential at dosages up to 20 mg/kg/day. Although stunting and increased neonatal mortality were observed in rabbits, there was no evidence for teratogenicity in either rats or rabbits. In a brief report, amitriptyline HCl was shown to be teratogenic in the hamster at dosages up to 100 mg/kg administered intraperitoneally on day 8 of gestation. In a more detailed study, amitriptyline HCl was shown to produce malformations in the rabbit at dosages of 15 to 60 mg/kg/day and in the mouse at dosages of 14 to 56 mg/kg/day. In another study, amitriptyline HCl was shown to be teratogenic in JBT/Jd and JBT/Ju strains of mice at dosages of 60 to 65 mg/kg, respectively; these dosages are near the litter LD_{50}. The dosages which were teratogenic in animals ranged from 10.5 to 70 times the maximum recommended adult maintenance dosage of 100 mg/day of Endep and from 3.5 to 23 times the maximum recommended initial dosage for hospitalized patients (300 mg/day).

There are no adequate or well-controlled studies of Endep in pregnant women. Endep should be used during pregnancy only if the potential benefit justifies the potential risk to the fetus.

Nonteratogenic Effects: Amitriptyline HCl was tested in rats in a Segment II study at dosages up to 20 mg/kg/day. No significant adverse effects were observed in the peri- or postnatal development and growth of pups.

Nursing Mothers: Amitriptyline and its metabolite, nortriptyline, are excreted in breast milk. Because of the potential for serious adverse reactions from Endep in nursing infants, a decision should be made whether to discontinue nursing or to discontinue the drug, taking into account the importance of the drug to the mother.

Pediatric Use: Safety and effectiveness in children below the age of 12 have not been established.

Adverse Reactions: *Note:* Included in this listing which follows are a few adverse reactions which have not been reported with this specific drug. However, pharmacological similarities among the tricyclic antidepressant drugs require that each of the reactions be considered when Endep is administered.

Cardiovascular: Hypotension, hypertension, tachycardia, palpitation, myocardial infarction, arrhythmias, heart block, stroke.

CNS and Neuromuscular: Confusional states; disturbed concentration; disorientation; delusions; hallucinations; excitement; anxiety; restlessness; insomnia; nightmares; numbness; tingling and paresthesias of the extremities; peripheral neuropathy; incoordination; ataxia; tremors; seizures; alteration in EEG patterns; extrapyramidal symptoms; tinnitus; syndrome of inappropriate ADH (antidiuretic hormone) secretion.

Anticholinergic: Dry mouth, blurred vision, disturbance of accommodation, constipation, paralytic ileus, urinary retention, dilatation of urinary tract.

Allergic: Skin rash, urticaria, photosensitization, edema of face and tongue.

Hematologic: Bone marrow depression including agranulocytosis, leukopenia, eosinophilia, purpura, thrombocytopenia.

Gastrointestinal: Nausea, epigastric distress, vomiting, anorexia, stomatitis, peculiar taste, diarrhea, parotid swelling, black tongue. Rarely, hepatitis (including altered liver function and jaundice).

Endocrine: Testicular swelling and gynecomastia in the male, breast enlargement and galactorrhea in the female, increased or decreased libido, elevation and lowering of blood sugar levels.

Other: Dizziness, weakness, fatigue, headache, weight gain or loss, increased perspiration, urinary frequency, mydriasis, drowsiness, alopecia.

Withdrawal Symptoms: Abrupt cessation of treatment after prolonged administration may produce nausea, headache and malaise. These are not indicative of addiction.

Overdosage: *Manifestations:* High doses may cause temporary confusion, disturbed concentration or transient visual hallucinations. Overdosage may cause drowsiness; hypothermia; tachycardia and other arrhythmic abnormalities, such as bundle branch block; ECG evidence of impaired conduction; congestive heart failure; dilated pupils; convulsions; severe hypotension; stupor and coma. Other symptoms may be agitation, hyperactive reflexes, muscle rigidity, vomiting, hyperpyrexia or any of those listed in the ADVERSE REACTIONS section.

Treatment: **All patients suspected of having taken an overdosage should be admitted to a hospital as soon as possible.** Treatment is symptomatic and supportive. Empty the stomach as quickly as possible by emesis followed by gastric lavage upon arrival at the hospital. Following gastric lavage, activated charcoal may be administered. Twenty to 30 Gm of activated charcoal may be given every four to six hours during the first 24 to 48 hours after ingestion. An ECG should be taken and close monitoring of cardiac function instituted if there is any sign of abnormality. Maintain an open airway and adequate fluid intake; regulate body temperature.

The intravenous administration of 1 to 3 mg of physostigmine salicylate has been reported to reverse the symptoms of tricyclic antidepressant poisoning. Because physostigmine is rapidly metabolized, the dosage of physostigmine should be repeated as required, particularly if life-threatening signs such as arrhythmias, convulsions and deep coma recur or persist after the initial dosage of physostigmine. Because physostigmine itself may be toxic, it is not recommended for routine use.

Standard measures should be used to manage circulatory shock and metabolic acidosis. Cardiac arrhythmias may be treated with neostigmine, pyridostigmine or propranolol. Should cardiac failure occur, the use of digitalis should be considered. Close monitoring of cardiac function for not less than five days is advisable.

Anticonvulsants may be given to control convulsions. Amitriptyline increases the CNS depressant action but not the anticonvulsant action of barbiturates; therefore, an inhalation anesthetic, diazepam or paraldehyde is recommended for control of convulsions.

Dialysis is of no value because of low plasma concentrations of the drug.

Since overdosage is often deliberate, patients may attempt suicide by other means during the recovery phase.

Continued on next page

Roche Labs.—Cont.

Deaths by deliberate or accidental overdosage have occurred with this class of drugs.
The acute oral toxicity of amitriptyline HCl is as follows:

Species	LD_{50}± S.E. (mg/kg)
Mouse	260 ± 16
Rat	617 ± 50
Rabbit	446 ± 32
Dog	≈ 290

Dosage and Administration: *Oral Dosage:* Dosage should be initiated at a low level and increased gradually, noting carefully the clinical response and any evidence of intolerance.
Initial Dosage for Adults: Twenty-five mg 3 times a day usually is satisfactory for outpatients. If necessary, this may be increased to a total of 150 mg a day. Increases are made preferably in the late afternoon and/or bedtime doses. A sedative effect may be apparent before the antidepressant effect is noted, but an adequate therapeutic effect may take as long as 30 days to develop.
An alternative method of initiating therapy in outpatients is to begin with 50 to 100 mg amitriptyline HCl at bedtime. This may be increased by 25 to 50 mg as necessary in the bedtime dose to a total of 150 mg per day.
Hospitalized patients may require 100 mg a day initially. This can be increased gradually to 200 mg a day if necessary. A small number of hospitalized patients may need as much as 300 mg a day.
Adolescent and Elderly Patients: In general, lower dosages are recommended for these patients. Ten mg 3 times a day with 20 mg at bedtime may be satisfactory in adolescent and elderly patients who do not tolerate higher dosages.
Maintenance: The usual maintenance dosage of amitriptyline HCl is 50 to 100 mg per day. In some patients 40 mg per day is sufficient. For maintenance therapy the total daily dosage may be given in a single dose preferably at bedtime. When satisfactory improvement has been reached, dosage should be reduced to the lowest amount that will maintain relief of symptoms. It is appropriate to continue maintenance therapy 3 months or longer to lessen the possibility of relapse.
Usage in Children: In view of the lack of experience in children, this drug is not recommended at the present time for patients under 12 years of age.
How Supplied: 10-mg tablets, orange, round, film-coated, scored—bottles of 100 (NDC 0004-0106-01) and 500 (NDC 0004-0106-14); Tel-E-Dose® packages of 100 (NDC 0004-0106-49); Prescription Paks of 60 (NDC 0004-0106-59). Imprint on tablets: ROCHE 106.
25-mg tablets, orange, round, film-coated, scored—bottles of 100 (NDC 0004-0107-01) and 500 (NDC 0004-0107-14); Tel-E-Dose® packages of 100 (NDC 0004-0107-49); Prescription Paks of 60 (NDC 0004-0107-59). Imprint on tablets: ROCHE 107.
50-mg tablets, orange, round, film-coated, scored—bottles of 100 (NDC 0004-0109-01) and 500 (NDC 0004-0109-14); Tel-E-Dose® packages of 100 (NDC 0004-0109-49); Prescription Paks of 60 (NDC 0004-0109-59). Imprint on tablets: ROCHE 109.
75-mg tablets, yellow, round, film-coated, scored—bottles of 100 (NDC 0004-0114-01); Tel-E-Dose® packages of 100 (NDC 0004-0114-49); Prescription Paks of 30 (NDC 0004-0114-57). Imprint on tablets: ROCHE 114.
100-mg tablets, peach, round, film-coated, scored—bottles of 100 (NDC 0004-0116-01); Tel-E-Dose® packages of 100 (NDC 0004-0116-49); Prescription Paks of 30 (NDC 0004-0116-57). Imprint on tablets: ROCHE 116.
150-mg tablets, salmon, round, film-coated, scored—bottles of 100 (NDC 0004-0124-01); Tel-E-Dose® packages of 100 (NDC 0004-0124-49); Prescription Paks of 30 (NDC 0004-0124-57). Imprint on tablets: ENDEP 150 ROCHE.
[*Shown in Product Identification Section*]

FANSIDAR® ℞
(sulfadoxine and pyrimethamine/Roche) TABLETS

The following text is complete prescribing information based on official labeling in effect August 1, 1982.
Description: Fansidar is an antimalarial agent, each tablet containing 500 mg N^1-(5,6-dimethoxy-4-pyrimidinyl) sulfanilamide (sulfadoxine) and 25 mg 2,4-diamino-5-(p-chlorophenyl)-6-ethylpyrimidine (pyrimethamine).
Clinical Pharmacology: Fansidar is an antimalarial agent which acts by reciprocal potentiation of its two components, achieved by a sequential blockade of two enzymes involved in the biosynthesis of folinic acid within the parasites.
Both the sulfadoxine and the pyrimethamine of Fansidar are absorbed orally and are excreted mainly by the kidney. Following a single tablet administration, sulfadoxine peak plasma concentrations of 51 to 76 mcg/ml were achieved in 2.5 to 6 hours and the pyrimethamine peak plasma concentrations of 0.13 to 0.4 mcg/ml were achieved in 1.5 to 8 hours. The apparent half-life of elimination of sulfadoxine ranged from 100 to 231 hours with a mean of 169 hours, whereas pyrimethamine half-lives ranged from 54 to 148 hours with a mean of 111 hours. Both drugs appear in breast milk of nursing mothers.
Fansidar is effective against certain plasmodia strains that are resistant to chloroquine. Fansidar susceptibility of plasmodia may vary by locations and time.
Fansidar is compatible with other antimalarial drugs, particularly quinine, and with antibiotics. It does not interfere with antidiabetic agents.
Indications and Usage: Fansidar is indicated for the treatment of malaria due to susceptible strains of plasmodia. The drug is also indicated for prophylaxis using a weekly or biweekly regimen.
Contraindications: Hypersensitivity to pyrimethamine or sulfonamides. Patients with documented megaloblastic anemia due to folate deficiency. Infants less than two months of age. Pregnancy at term and during the nursing period because sulfonamides pass the placenta and are excreted in the milk and may cause kernicterus.
Warnings: Deaths associated with the administration of sulfonamides have been reported from hypersensitivity reactions, agranulocytosis, aplastic anemia and other blood dyscrasias. Fansidar prophylaxis should be discontinued if a significant reduction in the count of any formed blood element is noted or at the occurrence of active bacterial or fungal infections. Fansidar prophylactic regimen has been reported to cause leukopenia during a treatment of two months or longer. This leukopenia is generally mild and reversible.
Precautions:
1. *General:* Fansidar should be given with caution to patients with impaired renal or hepatic function, to those with possible folate deficiency and to those with severe allergy or bronchial asthma. As with some sulfonamide drugs, in glucose-6-phosphate dehydrogenase-deficient individuals, hemolysis may occur. Urinalysis with microscopic examination and renal function tests should be performed during therapy of those patients who have impaired renal function.
2. *Information for the patient:* Adequate fluid intake must be maintained in order to prevent crystalluria and stone formation.
The patient should be warned that the appearance of sore throat, fever, pallor, purpura, jaundice or glossitis may be early indications of serious disorders which require prophylactic treatment to be stopped and medical treatment to be sought.
Females should be cautioned against becoming pregnant and should not breast feed their infants during Fansidar therapy or prophylactic treatment.
Patients should be warned to keep Fansidar out of reach of children.
3. *Laboratory tests:* Periodic blood counts and analysis of urine for crystalluria are desirable during prolonged prophylaxis.
4. *Drug interactions:* Antifolic drugs such as sulfonamides or trimethoprim-sulfamethoxazole combinations should not be used while the patient is receiving Fansidar for antimalarial prophylaxis.
If signs of folic acid deficiency develop, Fansidar should be discontinued. Folinic acid (leucovorin) may be administered in doses of 3 mg to 9 mg intramuscularly daily, for 3 days or longer, for depressed platelet or white blood cell counts in patients with drug-induced folic acid deficiency when recovery is too slow.
5. *Carcinogenesis, mutagenesis, impairment of fertility:* Pyrimethamine was not found carcinogenic in female mice or in male and female rats. The carcinogenic potential of pyrimethamine in male mice could not be assessed from the study because of markedly reduced lifespan. Pyrimethamine was found to be mutagenic in laboratory animals and also in human bone marrow following 3 or 4 consecutive daily doses totaling 200 mg to 300 mg. Pyrimethamine was not found mutagenic in the Ames test.
6. *Pregnancy:* Teratogenic effects: Pregnancy Category C. Fansidar has been shown to be teratogenic in rats when given in weekly doses approximately 12 times the weekly human prophylactic dose. Teratology studies with pyrimethamine plus sulfadoxine (1:20) in rats showed the minimum oral teratogenic dose to be approximately 0.9 mg/kg pyrimethamine plus 18 mg/kg sulfadoxine. In rabbits, no teratogenic effects were noted at oral doses as high as 20 mg/kg pyrimethamine plus 400 mg/kg sulfadoxine.
There are no adequate and well-controlled studies in pregnant women.
Because pyrimethamine plus sulfadoxine may interfere with folic acid metabolism, Fansidar therapy should be used during pregnancy only if the potential benefit justifies the potential risk to the fetus.
Nonteratogenic effects: See "CONTRAINDICATIONS" section.
7. *Nursing mothers:* See "CONTRAINDICATIONS" section.
8. *Pediatric use:* Fansidar should not be given to infants less than two months of age because of inadequate development of the glucuronide-forming enzyme system.
Adverse Reactions: For completeness, all major reactions to sulfonamides and to pyrimethamine are included below, even though they may not have been reported with Fansidar.
Blood dyscrasias: Agranulocytosis, aplastic anemia, megaloblastic anemia, thrombopenia, leukopenia, hemolytic anemia, purpura, hypoprothrombinemia and methemoglobinemia.
Allergic reactions: Erythema multiforme, Stevens-Johnson syndrome, generalized skin eruptions, epidermal necrolysis, urticaria, serum sickness, pruritus, exfoliative dermatitis, anaphylactoid reactions, periorbital edema, conjunctival and scleral injection, photosensitization, arthralgia and allergic myocarditis.
Gastrointestinal reactions: Glossitis, stomatitis, nausea, emesis, abdominal pains, hepatitis, diarrhea and pancreatitis.
C.N.S. reactions: Headache, peripheral neuritis, mental depression, convulsions, ataxia, hallucinations, tinnitus, vertigo, insomnia, apathy, fatigue, muscle weakness and nervousness.

Miscellaneous reactions: Drug fever, chills, and toxic nephrosis with oliguria and anuria. Periarteritis nodosa and L. E. phenomenon have occurred.

The sulfonamides bear certain chemical similarities to some goitrogens, diuretics (acetazolamide and the thiazides) and oral hypoglycemic agents. Diuresis and hypoglycemia have occurred rarely in patients receiving sulfonamides. Cross-sensitivity may exist with these agents. Rats appear to be especially susceptible to the goitrogenic effects of sulfonamides, and long-term administration has produced thyroid malignancies in the species.

Overdosage: Acute intoxication may be manifested by anorexia, vomiting and central nervous system stimulation (including convulsions), followed by megaloblastic anemia, leukopenia, thrombocytopenia, glossitis and crystalluria. In acute intoxication, emesis and gastric lavage followed by purges may be of benefit. The patient should be adequately hydrated to prevent renal damage. The renal and hematopoietic systems should be monitored for at least one month after an overdosage. If the patient is having convulsions, the use of a parenteral barbiturate is indicated. For depressed platelet or white blood cell counts, folinic acid (leucovorin) should be administered in a dosage of 3 mg to 9 mg intramuscularly daily for 3 days or longer.

Dosage and Administration:

(a) *Curative treatment of acute malaria*

For the treatment of acute attacks with a single dose of Fansidar, the following number of tablets is used either in sequence with quinine or primaquine, or alone:

Adults	2 to 3 tablets
9 to 14 years	2 tablets
4 to 8 years	1 tablet
Under 4 years	½ tablet

For acute attacks of malaria due to *Plasmodium vivax* and *Plasmodium malaria,* a single dose of Fansidar followed by primaquine for two weeks has been used to prevent relapse.

(b) *Prophylaxis management*

For malaria prophylaxis, Fansidar may be used alone. The first dose of Fansidar should be taken one or two days before departure to an endemic area; administration should be continued during the stay and for four to six weeks after return, and should be followed by a regimen of primaquine.

	Once Weekly	Once Every Two Weeks
Adults	1 tablet	2 tablets
9 to 14 years	¾ tablet	1½ tablets
4 to 8 years	½ tablet	1 tablet
Under 4 years	¼ tablet	½ tablet

How Supplied: Scored tablets, containing 500 mg sulfadoxine and 25 mg pyrimethamine—boxes of 25 (NDC-0004-0161-03).

[*Shown in Product Identification Section*]

FLUOROURACIL ℞
(5-fluorouracil/Roche)
INJECTABLE

The following text is complete prescribing information based on official labeling in effect August 1, 1982.

> WARNING
>
> It is recommended that FLUOROURACIL be given only by or under the supervision of a qualified physician who is experienced in cancer chemotherapy and who is well versed in the use of potent antimetabolites. Because of the possibility of severe toxic reactions, it is recommended that patients be hospitalized at least during the initial course of therapy.
>
> These instructions should be thoroughly reviewed before administration of Fluorouracil.

Description: FLUOROURACIL Roche (5-fluorouracil) is a fluorinated pyrimidine belonging to the category of antimetabolites. Fluorouracil resembles the natural uracil molecule in structure, except that a hydrogen atom has been replaced by a fluorine atom in the 5 position.

Actions: There is evidence that the metabolism of fluorouracil in the anabolic pathway blocks the methylation reaction of deoxyuridylic acid to thymidylic acid. In this fashion 5-fluorouracil interferes with the synthesis of deoxyribonucleic acid (DNA) and to a lesser extent inhibits the formation of ribonucleic acid (RNA). Since DNA and RNA are essential for cell division and growth, the effect of fluorouracil may be to create a thymine deficiency which provokes unbalanced growth and death of the cell. The effects of DNA and RNA deprivation are most marked on those cells which grow more rapidly and which take up fluorouracil at a more rapid pace. The catabolic metabolism of fluorouracil results in degradative products (e.g., CO_2, urea, α-fluoro-β-alanine) which are inactive. Following an intravenous injection, no intact drug can be detected in the plasma after three hours. Approximately 15 percent is excreted intact in the urine in six hours, of which over 90 percent is excreted in the first hour. Of the injected intravenous dose 60 to 80 percent is excreted as respiratory CO_2 in 8 to 12 hours.

Indications: Fluorouracil is effective in the palliative management of carcinoma of the colon, rectum, breast, stomach and pancreas in patients who are considered incurable by surgery or other means.

Contraindications: Fluorouracil therapy is contraindicated for patients in a poor nutritional state, those with depressed bone marrow function or those with potentially serious infections.

Warnings: THE DAILY DOSE OF FLUOROURACIL IS NOT TO EXCEED 800 MG. IT IS RECOMMENDED THAT PATIENTS BE HOSPITALIZED DURING THEIR FIRST COURSE OF TREATMENT.

Fluorouracil should be used with extreme caution in poor risk patients with a history of high-dose pelvic irradiation, previous use of alkylating agents or who have a widespread involvement of bone marrow by metastatic tumors or impaired hepatic or renal function. The drug is not intended as an adjuvant to surgery. Although severe toxicity is more likely in poor risk patients, fatalities may be encountered occasionally even in patients in relatively good condition.

Usage in Pregnancy: Safe use of Fluorouracil has not been established with respect to adverse effects on fetal development. Therefore, this drug should not be used during pregnancy, particularly in the first trimester, unless in the judgment of the physician the potential benefits to the patient outweigh the hazards.

Because the risk of mutagenesis has not been evaluated, such possible effects on males and females must be considered.

Combination Therapy: Any form of therapy which adds to the stress of the patient, interferes with nutrition or depresses bone marrow function will increase the toxicity of Fluorouracil.

Precautions: Fluorouracil is a highly toxic drug with a narrow margin of safety. Therefore, patients should be carefully supervised, since therapeutic response is unlikely to occur without some evidence of toxicity. Patients should be informed of expected toxic effects, particularly oral manifestations. White blood counts with differential are recommended before each dose. Severe hematological toxicity, gastrointestinal hemorrhage and even death may result from the use of Fluorouracil despite meticulous selection of patients and careful adjustment of dosage.

Therapy is to be discontinued promptly whenever one of the following signs of toxicity appears:

Stomatitis or *esophagopharyngitis,* At the first visible sign.

Leukopenia (WBC under 3500), or a *rapidly falling white blood count.*

Vomiting, Intractable.

Diarrhea, Frequent bowel movements or watery stools.

Gastrointestinal ulceration and bleeding.

Thrombocytopenia, Platelets under 100,000.

Hemorrhage from any site.

Adverse Reactions: Stomatitis and esophagopharyngitis (which may lead to sloughing and ulceration), diarrhea, anorexia, nausea and emesis are commonly seen during therapy.

Leukopenia usually follows every course of adequate therapy with Fluorouracil. The lowest white blood cell counts are commonly observed between the 9th and 14th days after the first course of treatment, although uncommonly the maximal depression may be delayed for as long as 20 days. By the 30th day the count has usually returned to the normal range.

Alopecia and dermatitis may be seen in a substantial number of cases. Patients should be alerted to the possibility of alopecia as a result of therapy and should be informed that it is a transient effect. The dermatitis most often seen is a pruritic maculopapular rash usually appearing on the extremities and less frequently on the trunk. It is generally reversible and usually responsive to symptomatic treatment. Dry skin and fissuring have also been noted. Photosensitivity, as manifested by erythema or increased pigmentation of the skin, has been observed on occasion. Also noted were photophobia, lacrimation, epistaxis, euphoria, acute cerebellar syndrome (which may persist following discontinuation of treatment) and nail changes, including loss of nails. Myocardial ischemia has also been reported.

Dosage and Administration: *General Instructions:* Administration of Fluorouracil Injectable should be done only intravenously, using care to avoid extravasation. No dilution is required.

All dosages are based on the patient's actual weight. However, the estimated lean body mass (dry weight) is used if the patient is obese or if there has been a spurious weight gain due to edema, ascites or other forms of abnormal fluid retention.

It is recommended that prior to treatment each patient be carefully evaluated in order to estimate as accurately as possible the optimum initial dosage of Fluorouracil.

Dosage: Twelve mg/kg are given intravenously once daily for four successive days. The daily dose should not be more than 800 mg. *If no toxicity is observed,* 6 mg/kg are given on the 6th, 8th, 10th and 12th days unless toxicity occurs. No therapy is given on the 5th, 7th, 9th or 11th days. *Therapy is to be discontinued at the end of the 12th day, even if no toxicity has become apparent.* (See CONTRAINDICATIONS and WARNINGS.)

Poor risk patients or those who are not in adequate nutritional state (see CONTRAINDICATIONS and WARNINGS) should receive 6 mg/kg/day for three days. *If no toxicity is observed,* 3 mg/kg may be given on the 5th, 7th and 9th days *unless toxicity occurs.* No therapy is given on the 4th, 6th or 8th days. The daily dose should not exceed 400 mg.

A sequence of injections on either schedule constitutes a "course of therapy."

Maintenance Therapy: In instances where toxicity has not been a problem, it is recommended that therapy be continued using either of the following schedules:

Continued on next page

Roche Labs.—Cont.

1. Repeat dosage of first course every 30 days after the last day of the previous course of treatment.
2. When toxic signs resulting from the initial course of therapy have subsided, administer a maintenance dosage of 10 to 15 mg/kg/week as a single dose. Do not exceed 1 Gm per week.

The amount of the drug to be used should take into account the patient's reaction to the previous course and should be adjusted accordingly. Some patients have received from 9 to 45 courses of treatment during periods which ranged from 12 to 60 months.

How Supplied: *Injectable:* 10-ml ampuls (for intravenous use) containing 500 mg 5-fluorouracil in a colorless to faint yellow aqueous solution, with pH adjusted to approximately 9.0 with sodium hydroxide. Boxes of 10.
Note: Although Fluorouracil ampul solution may discolor slightly during storage, the potency and safety are not adversely affected.
Store at room temperature (59° to 86°F). Protect from light. If a precipitate occurs due to exposure to low temperatures, resolubilize by heating to 140°F with vigorous shaking; allow to cool to body temperature before using.

FUDR ℞
(floxuridine/Roche)

The following text is complete prescribing information based on official labeling in effect August 1, 1982.

FOR INTRA-ARTERIAL INFUSION ONLY

WARNING
It is recommended that FUDR be given only by or under the supervision of a qualified physician who is experienced in cancer chemotherapy and intra-arterial drug therapy.
Because of the possibility of severe toxic reactions, all patients should be hospitalized for initiation of treatment.

Description: Floxuridine is a fluorinated pyrimidine belonging to the category of antimetabolites. It is a white to off-white odorless solid, soluble in alcohol and freely soluble in water. The 2% aqueous solution has a pH of 4.0 to 5.5. Chemically, floxuridine is 2′-deoxy-5-fluorouridine with a molecular weight of 246.19.

Actions: When FUDR is given by intra-arterial injection it is apparently rapidly catabolized to 5-fluorouracil. Thus, rapid injection of FUDR produces the same toxic and antimetabolic effects as does 5-fluorouracil. The primary effect is to interfere with the synthesis of deoxyribonucleic acid (DNA) and to a lesser extent inhibit the formation of ribonucleic acid (RNA). However, when FUDR is given by continuous intra-arterial infusion its direct anabolism to FUDR-monophosphate is enhanced, thus increasing the inhibition of DNA.

Indications: FUDR is effective in the palliative management of gastrointestinal adenocarcinoma metastatic to the liver, when given by continuous regional intra-arterial infusion in carefully selected patients who are considered incurable by surgery or other means. Patients with known disease extending beyond an area capable of infusion via a single artery should, except in unusual circumstances, be considered for systemic therapy with other chemotherapeutic agents.

Contraindications: FUDR therapy is contraindicated for patients in a poor nutritional state, those with depressed bone marrow function, or those with potentially serious infections.

Warnings: IT IS IMPERATIVE THAT ALL PATIENTS BE HOSPITALIZED FOR INITIATION OF TREATMENT.
FUDR should be used with extreme caution in poor risk patients with impaired hepatic or renal function or a history of high-dose pelvic irradiation or previous use of alkylating agents. The drug is not intended as an adjuvant to surgery.
Usage in Pregnancy: Safe use of FUDR has not been established with respect to adverse effects on fetal development. Therefore, this drug should not be used during pregnancy, particularly in the first trimester, unless in the judgment of the physician the potential benefits to the patient outweigh the hazards.
Because teratogenicity and mutagenicity have been demonstrated in animals, such possible effects on men and women must be considered.
Combination Therapy: Any form of therapy which adds to the stress of the patient, interferes with nutrition, or depresses bone marrow function will increase the toxicity of FUDR (floxuridine).
Therapy is to be discontinued promptly whenever one of the following signs of toxicity appears:
Stomatitis or esophagopharyngitis, At the first visible sign.
Leukopenia (WBC under 3500), or a rapidly falling white blood count.
Vomiting, Intractable.
Diarrhea, Frequent bowel movements or watery stools.
Gastrointestinal ulceration and bleeding.
Thrombocytopenia, Platelets under 100,000.
Hemorrhage from any site.

Precautions: FUDR is potentially a highly toxic drug with a narrow margin of safety. Therefore, patients should be carefully supervised since therapeutic response is unlikely to occur without some evidence of toxicity. Patients should be informed of expected toxic effects, particularly oral manifestations. Careful monitoring of the white blood count and platelet count is recommended. Severe hematological toxicity, gastrointestinal hemorrhage and even death may result from the use of FUDR despite meticulous selection of patients and careful adjustment of dosage. Although severe toxicity is more likely in poor risk patients, fatalities may be encountered occasionally even in patients in relatively good condition.

Adverse Reactions: The adverse reactions to the arterial infusion of FUDR are generally related to the drug-infused area and can be grouped under the following categories: functional gastrointestinal, mucosal gastrointestinal, hematologic, dermatologic, miscellaneous clinical reactions, laboratory abnormalities and procedural complications of regional arterial infusion.
The more common adverse reactions are nausea, vomiting, diarrhea, enteritis, stomatitis and localized erythema. The more common laboratory abnormalities are anemia, leukopenia, and elevations of alkaline phosphatase, serum transaminase, serum bilirubin and lactic dehydrogenase.
Other adverse reactions are:
Functional gastrointestinal: anorexia, cramps and pain.
Mucosal gastrointestinal: duodenal ulcer, duodenitis, gastritis, gastroenteritis, glossitis and pharyngitis.
Dermatological: alopecia, dermatitis, nonspecific skin toxicity and rash.
Other clinical reactions: fever, lethargy, malaise, and weakness.
Laboratory abnormalities: BSP, prothrombin, total proteins, sedimentation rate and thrombopenia.
Procedural complications of regional arterial infusion: arterial aneurysm, arterial ischemia, arterial thrombosis, bleeding at catheter site, catheter blocked, displaced or leaking, embolism, fibromyositis, infection at catheter site, abscesses and thrombophlebitis.

Dosage and Administration: The recommended therapeutic dose schedule of FUDR by continuous arterial infusion is 0.1 to 0.6 mg/kg/day. The higher dose ranges (0.4 to 0.6 mg) are usually employed for hepatic artery infusion because the liver metabolizes the drug, thus reducing the potential for systemic toxicity. Therapy can be given until adverse reactions appear. When these side effects have subsided, therapy may be resumed. The patient should be maintained on therapy as long as response to FUDR continues. The administration of FUDR is best achieved with the use of an appropriate pump to overcome pressure in large arteries and to ensure a uniform rate of infusion.

How Supplied: 500 mg FUDR (floxuridine/Roche) sterile powder, in a 5-ml vial. This is reconstituted with 5 ml sterile water. Reconstituted vials should be stored under refrigeration (36° to 46°F.) for not more than two weeks.

Clinical Studies: In 349 evaluable patients treated with continuous arterial infusion of FUDR, 144 obtained significant objective response associated with clinical benefit for at least one month, and an additional 14 patients had objective and subjective benefits for at least one year.

GANTANOL® ℞
(sulfamethoxazole/Roche)
TABLETS • SUSPENSION •
DS (double strength) TABLETS

The following text is complete prescribing information based on official labeling in effect August 1, 1982.

Description: Gantanol is an intermediate-dosage sulfonamide. Sulfamethoxazole is an almost white, odorless, tasteless compound. Chemically, it is N^1-(5-methyl-3-isoxazolyl)-sulfanilamide.
In a single dose study using two grams of drug, levels of free sulfamethoxazole achieved in the plasma with the tablet and suspension dosage forms were compared in a group of 19 normal subjects. There was no significant difference between the plasma levels obtained with the two dosage forms. The mean concentration of free sulfamethoxazole in plasma after administration of tablets was:

1½ hours	8.38 mg%
3 hours	12.08 mg%
6 hours	9.82 mg%
9 hours	7.9 mg%
12 hours	6.45 mg%

Administration of Gantanol at the adult recommended dosage of 2 Gm initially followed by 1 Gm every 12 hours for 4 days produced average blood concentrations of 5.8 mg% total sulfonamide and 5.1 mg% free sulfonamide 6 hours following the last dose.
Sulfonamides exist in the blood as free, conjugated (acetylated and possibly other forms) and protein-bound forms. The "free" form is considered to be the therapeutically active form. It has been shown that approximately 70 per cent of Gantanol is protein bound in the blood; of the unbound portion 80 to 90 per cent is in the nonacetylated form. Excretion of sulfonamides is chiefly by the kidneys with glomerular filtration as the primary mechanism.

Actions: The systemic sulfonamides are bacteriostatic agents. The spectrum of activity is similar for all. Sulfonamides competitively inhibit bacterial synthesis of folic acid (pteroylglutamic acid) from para-aminobenzoic acid. Resistant strains are capable of utilizing folic acid precursors or preformed folic acid.

Indications: Acute, recurrent or chronic urinary tract infections (primarily pyelonephritis, pyelitis and cystitis) due to susceptible organisms (usually *E. coli, Klebsiella-Aerobacter,* staphylococcus, *Proteus mirabilis,* and, less frequently, *Proteus vulgaris)* in the absence of obstructive uropathy or foreign bodies.

Meningococcal meningitis prophylaxis when sulfonamide-sensitive group A strains are known to prevail in family groups or larger closed populations. (The prophylactic usefulness of sulfonamides when group B or C infections are prevalent is not proven and in closed population groups may be harmful.)
In acute otitis media due to *Haemophilus influenzae* when used concomitantly with adequate doses of penicillin.
Trachoma. Inclusion conjunctivitis. Nocardiosis. Chancroid. Toxoplasmosis as adjunctive therapy with pyrimethamine. Malaria due to chloroquine-resistant strains of *Plasmodium falciparum,* when used as adjunctive therapy.
Important note. *In vitro* sulfonamide sensitivity tests are not always reliable. The test must be carefully coordinated with bacteriologic and clinical response. When the patient is already taking sulfonamides, follow-up cultures should have aminobenzoic acid added to the culture media.
Currently, the increasing frequency of resistant organisms is a limitation of the usefulness of antibacterial agents including the sulfonamides, especially in the treatment of chronic and recurrent urinary tract infections.
Wide variation in blood levels may result with identical doses. Blood levels should be measured in patients receiving sulfonamides for serious infections. Free sulfonamide blood levels of 5 to 15 mg per 100 ml may be considered therapeutically effective for most infections, with blood levels of 12 to 15 mg per 100 ml optimal for serious infections; 20 mg per 100 ml should be the maximum total sulfonamide level, as adverse reactions occur more frequently above this level.
Contraindications: Hypersensitivity to sulfonamides. Infants less than 2 months of age (except in the treatment of congenital toxoplasmosis as adjunctive therapy with pyrimethamine). Pregnancy at term and during the nursing period, because sulfonamides pass the placenta and are excreted in the milk and may cause kernicterus.
Warnings: *Usage in Pregnancy:* The safe use of sulfonamides in pregnancy has not been established. The teratogenicity potential of most sulfonamides has not been thoroughly investigated in either animals or humans. However, a significant increase in the incidence of cleft palate and other bony abnormalities of offspring has been observed when certain sulfonamides of the short, intermediate and long-acting types were given to pregnant rats and mice at high oral doses (7 to 25 times the human therapeutic dose).
The sulfonamides should not be used for the treatment of Group A beta-hemolytic streptococcal infections. In an established infection, they will not eradicate the streptococcus, and therefore will not prevent sequelae such as rheumatic fever and glomerulonephritis.
Deaths associated with the administration of sulfonamides have been reported from hypersensitivity reactions, agranulocytosis, aplastic anemia and other blood dyscrasias.
The presence of clinical signs such as sore throat, fever, pallor, purpura or jaundice may be early indications of serious blood disorders. Complete blood counts should be done frequently in patients receiving sulfonamides.
The frequency of renal complications is considerably lower in patients receiving the more soluble sulfonamides. Urinalysis with careful microscopic examination should be obtained frequently in patients receiving sulfonamides. At the present time there are insufficient clinical data on prolonged or recurrent therapy in chronic renal diseases of children under 6 years.
Precautions: Sulfonamides should be given with caution to patients with impaired renal or hepatic function and to those with severe allergy or bronchial asthma. In glucose-6-phosphate dehydrogenase-deficient individuals, hemolysis may occur. This reaction is frequently dose-related. Adequate fluid intake must be maintained in order to prevent crystalluria and stone formation.
Adverse Reactions: *Blood dyscrasias:* Agranulocytosis, aplastic anemia, thrombocytopenia, leukopenia, hemolytic anemia, purpura, hypoprothrombinemia and methemoglobinemia.
Allergic reactions: Erythema multiforme (Stevens-Johnson syndrome), generalized skin eruptions, epidermal necrolysis, urticaria, serum sickness, pruritus, exfoliative dermatitis, anaphylactoid reactions, periorbital edema, conjunctival and scleral injection, photosensitization, arthralgia and allergic myocarditis.
Gastrointestinal reactions: Nausea, emesis, abdominal pains, hepatitis, diarrhea, anorexia, pancreatitis and stomatitis.
C.N.S. reactions: Headache, peripheral neuritis, mental depression, convulsions, ataxia, hallucinations, tinnitus, vertigo and insomnia.
Miscellaneous reactions: Drug fever, chills, and toxic nephrosis with oliguria and anuria. Periarteritis nodosa and L.E. phenomenon have occurred.
The sulfonamides bear certain chemical similarities to some goitrogens, diuretics (acetazolamide and the thiazides) and oral hypoglycemic agents. Goiter production, diuresis and hypoglycemia have occurred rarely in patients receiving sulfonamides. Cross-sensitivity may exist with these agents.
Rats appear to be especially susceptible to the goitrogenic effects of sulfonamides, and long-term administration has produced thyroid malignancies in the species.
Dosage and Administration: Systemic sulfonamides are contraindicated in infants under 2 months of age, except in the treatment of congenital toxoplasmosis as adjunctive therapy with pyrimethamine.
The usual dosage schedule is as follows:

Children

Infants (2 Months or Older) and Children	Initial Dose (50-60 mg/kg)	Dose Morning and Evening Daily Thereafter (25-30 mg/kg)
20 lbs	1 tablet or 1 teasp. (0.5 Gm)	½ tablet or ½ teasp. (0.25 Gm)
40 lbs	2 tablets or 2 teasp. (1 Gm)	1 tablet or 1 teasp. (0.5 Gm)
60 lbs	3 tablets or 3 teasp. (1.5 Gm)	1½ tablets or 1½ teasp. (0.75 Gm)
80 lbs	2 DS (double strength) tablets or 4 tablets or 4 teasp. (2 Gm)	1 DS (double strength) tablet or 2 tablets or 2 teasp. (1 Gm)

The maximum dose for children should not exceed 75 mg/kg/24 hours.

Adults

Mild to Moderate Infections	2 DS (double strength) tablets or 4 tablets or 4 teasp. (2 Gm)	1 DS (double strength) tablet or 2 tablets or 2 teasp. (1 Gm)

Note: One teaspoonful equals 5 ml.
Severe Infections: 2 DS (double strength) tablets, or 4 tablets, or 4 teasp. (2 Gm) initially, followed by 1 DS (double strength) tablet, or 2 tablets, or 2 teasp. (1 Gm) three times daily thereafter.
How Supplied: DS (double strength) tablets, light orange, scored, each containing 1 Gm sulfamethoxazole/Roche—bottles of 100; Tel-E-Dose® packages of 100.
Tablets, green, scored, each containing 0.5 Gm sulfamethoxazole/Roche—bottles of 100 and 500; Tel-E-Dose® packages of 100.
Suspension, 10%, 0.5 Gm sulfamethoxazole/Roche per teaspoonful (5 ml), cherry-flavored—bottles of 16 oz (1 pint).
[*Shown in Product Identification Section*]

GANTRISIN® ℞
(sulfisoxazole diolamine/Roche)
OPHTHALMIC SOLUTION
OPHTHALMIC OINTMENT

The following text is complete prescribing information based on official labeling in effect August 1, 1982.
Description: GANTRISIN Ophthalmic Ointment and Solution are sulfonamide preparations specifically for topical ophthalmic use. The solution is a sterile, isotonic preparation containing 4% (40 mg/ml) sulfisoxazole/Roche in the form of the diolamine salt and phenylmercuric nitrate 1:100,000 added as a preservative. It has a physiologic pH, and does not cause significant stinging or burning on application. The ointment is a sterile preparation containing 4% sulfisoxazole in the form of the diolamine salt compounded with white petrolatum, mineral oil and phenylmercuric nitrate 1:50,000 added as a preservative. Both dosage forms are stable at room temperature and do not require refrigeration.
Actions: Sulfonamides exert a bacteriostatic effect against a wide range of gram-positive and gram-negative microorganisms by restricting, through competition with para-aminobenzoic acid, the synthesis of folic acid which bacteria require for growth.
Indications: For the treatment of conjunctivitis, corneal ulcer, and other superficial ocular infections due to susceptible microorganisms, and as an adjunct in systemic sulfonamide therapy of trachoma.
Contraindications: Hypersensitivity to sulfonamide preparations.
Precautions: Gantrisin Ophthalmic Solution and Ointment are incompatible with silver preparations. Ophthalmic ointments may retard corneal healing. Nonsusceptible organisms, including fungi, may proliferate with the use of these preparations. Sulfonamides are inactivated by the para-aminobenzoic acid present in purulent exudates. Should undesirable reactions occur, discontinue administration immediately.
Dosage and Administration: Solution: Instill two to three drops in the eye three or more times daily. Care should be taken not to touch dropper tip to any surface, as contamination of solution may result. Ointment: Instill small amount in the lower conjunctival sac one to three times daily and at bedtime.
How Supplied: Solution: ½-oz bottles with dropper. Ointment: ⅛-oz tubes.

GANTRISIN® ℞
(sulfisoxazole/Roche) Tablets
GANTRISIN® ℞
(acetyl sulfisoxazole/Roche)
Pediatric Suspension and Syrup
LIPO GANTRISIN® ℞
(acetyl sulfisoxazole/Roche)
GANTRISIN® ℞
(sulfisoxazole diolamine/Roche)
Injectable

The following text is complete prescribing information based on official labeling in effect August 1, 1982.
Description: Sulfisoxazole is a white to slightly yellowish, odorless, slightly bitter, crystalline powder. It is soluble in alcohol and very slightly soluble in water. Chemically, it is N^1-(3,4-dimethyl-5-isoxazolyl)sulfanilamide.
Acetyl sulfisoxazole, the tasteless form of sulfisoxazole, is N^1-acetyl sulfisoxazole and must be differentiated from the N^4-acetyl sulfisoxazole which is a metabolite of sulfisoxazole. The in-

Continued on next page

Roche Labs.—Cont.

jectable form is the 2,2′-iminodiethanol salt of N^1-(3,4-dimethyl-5-isoxazolyl)sulfanilamide.

N^1-acetyl sulfisoxazole is believed to be metabolized to sulfisoxazole by digestive enzymes in the gastrointestinal tract and this enzymatic splitting is presumed responsible for the delayed absorption and attainment of blood levels.[1] With continued administration of N^1-acetyl sulfisoxazole, blood levels approximate those of sulfisoxazole.[1]

Sulfonamides exist in the blood as free, conjugated (acetylated and possibly other forms) and protein-bound forms. The "free" form is considered to be the therapeutically active form.

The concentrations of free and total sulfonamide in the blood with oral doses of 1 Gm sulfisoxazole every 4 hours have been reported as 5.85 mg% and 9.17 mg% respectively, at 24 hours.[2] In adults, doses of 3 Gm of the N^1-acetyl sulfisoxazole every 4 hours produced average blood levels of 8.7 mg%.[3]

With Lipo Gantrisin (acetyl sulfisoxazole/Roche in lipid emulsion), administration of 100 mg/kg every 12 hours produced mean blood levels of free sulfonamide ranging between 8.8 and 16.6 mg% over a 24-hour period; continued administration yielded mean levels of between 11.7 and 16.8 mg% free sulfonamide.[4]

With a dosage schedule of 2 Gm intravenously every 8 hours, average blood levels of 11.7 mg/100 ml free and 16.7 mg/100 ml total were obtained.[2] With subcutaneous injection of 200 mg/kg sulfisoxazole, the average blood level at 12 hours was 10.4 mg% and at 24 hours, 7.1 mg%.[5] With single intramuscular dosage of 2 Gm, the plasma levels peaked from 1 to 4 hours, with average levels of 13.8 mg% of free sulfisoxazole[6] and 16.0 mg% total sulfisoxazole[7] obtained at 2 hours.

Approximately 85% of sulfisoxazole is protein bound in the blood;[8] of the unbound portion 65 to 72% is in the nonacetylated form.[1]

In normal subjects cerebrospinal fluid levels of sulfisoxazole have been reported to range from 8 to 57% of blood levels.[3,9] Higher cerebrospinal fluid levels are found in patients with inflamed meninges.[9]

Excretion of sulfonamides is chiefly by the kidneys with glomerular filtration as the primary mechanism.

Actions: The systemic sulfonamides are bacteriostatic agents. The spectrum of activity is similar for all. Sulfonamides competitively inhibit bacterial synthesis of folic acid (pteroylglutamic acid) from para-aminobenzoic acid. Resistant strains are capable of utilizing folic acid precursors or preformed folic acid.

Indications: Injectable sulfonamides should be used only when oral administration is impractical. Gantrisin is indicated for acute, recurrent or chronic urinary tract infections (primarily cystitis, pyelitis and pyelonephritis) due to susceptible organisms (usually *E. coli, Klebsiella-Aerobacter*, staphylococcus, *Proteus mirabilis*, and, less frequently, *Proteus vulgaris)* in the absence of obstructive uropathy or foreign bodies.

Meningococcal meningitis where the organism has been demonstrated to be susceptible. *Haemophilus influenzae* meningitis as adjunctive therapy with parenteral streptomycin.

Meningococcal meningitis prophylaxis when sulfonamide-sensitive group A strains are known to prevail in family groups or larger closed populations. (The prophylactic usefulness of sulfonamides when group B or C infections are prevalent is not proven and in closed population groups may be harmful.)

In acute otitis media due to *Haemophilus influenzae* when used concomitantly with adequate doses of penicillin or erythromycin (see appropriate erythromycin labeling for prescribing information).

Trachoma. Inclusion conjunctivitis. Nocardiosis. Chancroid. Toxoplasmosis as adjunctive therapy with pyrimethamine. Malaria due to chloroquine-resistant strains of *Plasmodium falciparum*, when used as adjunctive therapy.

Important note. In vitro sulfonamide sensitivity tests are not always reliable. The test must be carefully coordinated with bacteriologic and clinical response. When the patient is already taking sulfonamides, follow-up cultures should have aminobenzoic acid added to the culture media.

Currently, the increasing frequency of resistant organisms is a limitation of the usefulness of antibacterial agents including the sulfonamides, especially in the treatment of chronic and recurrent urinary tract infections.

Wide variation in blood levels may result with identical doses. Blood levels should be measured in patients receiving sulfonamides for serious infections. Free sulfonamide blood levels of 5 to 15 mg per 100 ml may be considered therapeutically effective for most infections, with blood levels of 12 to 15 mg per 100 ml optimal for serious infections; 20 mg per 100 ml should be the maximum total sulfonamide level, as adverse reactions occur more frequently above this level.

Contraindications: Hypersensitivity to sulfonamides. Infants less than 2 months of age (except in the treatment of congenital toxoplasmosis as adjunctive therapy with pyrimethamine). Pregnancy at term and during the nursing period, because sulfonamides pass the placenta and are excreted in the milk and may cause kernicterus.

Warnings: *Usage in Pregnancy:* The safe use of sulfonamides in pregnancy has not been established. The teratogenicity potential of most sulfonamides has not been thoroughly investigated in either animals or humans. However, a significant increase in the incidence of cleft palate and other bony abnormalities of offspring has been observed when certain sulfonamides of the short, intermediate and long-acting types were given to pregnant rats and mice at high oral doses (7 to 25 times the human therapeutic dose).

The sulfonamides should not be used for the treatment of Group A beta-hemolytic streptococcal infections. In an established infection, they will not eradicate the streptococcus, and therefore will not prevent sequelae such as rheumatic fever and glomerulonephritis.

Deaths associated with the administration of sulfonamides have been reported from hypersensitivity reactions, agranulocytosis, aplastic anemia and other blood dyscrasias.

The presence of clinical signs such as sore throat, fever, pallor, purpura or jaundice may be early indications of serious blood disorders. Complete blood counts should be done frequently in patients receiving sulfonamides.

The frequency of renal complications is considerably lower in patients receiving the more soluble sulfonamides. Urinalysis with careful microscopic examination should be obtained frequently in patients receiving sulfonamides.

Occasional severe systemic reactions may follow rapid intravenous administration.

Precautions: Sulfonamides should be given with caution to patients with impaired renal or hepatic function and to those with severe allergy or bronchial asthma. In glucose-6-phosphate dehydrogenase-deficient individuals, hemolysis may occur. This reaction is frequently dose-related. Adequate fluid intake must be maintained in order to prevent crystalluria and stone formation.

Adverse Reactions: *Blood dyscrasias:* Agranulocytosis, aplastic anemia, thrombocytopenia, leukopenia, hemolytic anemia, purpura, hypoprothrombinemia and methemoglobinemia.

Allergic reactions: Erythema multiforme (Stevens-Johnson syndrome), generalized skin eruptions, epidermal necrolysis, urticaria, serum sickness, pruritus, exfoliative dermatitis, anaphylactoid reactions, periorbital edema, conjunctival and scleral injection, photosensitization, arthralgia and allergic myocarditis.

Gastrointestinal reactions: Nausea, emesis, abdominal pains, hepatitis, diarrhea, anorexia, pancreatitis and stomatitis.

C.N.S. reactions: Headache, peripheral neuritis, mental depression, convulsions, ataxia, hallucinations, tinnitus, vertigo and insomnia.

Miscellaneous reactions: Drug fever, chills and toxic nephrosis with oliguria and anuria. Periarteritis nodosa and L.E. phenomenon have occurred. Local reaction may occur with intramuscular injection.

The sulfonamides bear certain chemical similarities to some goitrogens, diuretics (acetazolamide and the thiazides) and oral hypoglycemic agents. Goiter production, diuresis and hypoglycemia have occurred rarely in patients receiving sulfonamides. Cross-sensitivity may exist with these agents.

Rats appear to be especially susceptible to the goitrogenic effects of sulfonamides, and long-term administration has produced thyroid malignancies in the species.

Dosage and Administration: Systemic sulfonamides are contraindicated in infants under 2 months of age, except in the treatment of congenital toxoplasmosis as adjunctive therapy with pyrimethamine. Injectable sulfonamides should be used only when oral administration is impractical.

TABLETS, PEDIATRIC SUSPENSION AND SYRUP (0.5 Gm sulfisoxazole per tablet or the equivalent in each 5-ml teaspoonful of the suspension or syrup)—

Usual dose for infants over 2 months of age and children:

Initial dose: One-half of the 24-hour dose.

Maintenance dose: 150 mg/kg/24 hours or 4 Gm/M^2/24 hours—dose to be divided into 4 to 6 doses/24 hours with maximum of 6 Gm/24 hours.

Usual adult dose:

Initial dose: 2 to 4 Gm.

Maintenance dose: 4 to 8 Gm/24 hours, divided into 4 to 6 doses/24 hours.

LIPO GANTRISIN (containing the equivalent of 1 Gm sulfisoxazole in each 5-ml teaspoonful)—

Usual dose for infants over 2 months of age and children:

Initial dose: 60 to 75 mg/kg.

Maintenance dose: 60 to 75 mg/kg twice daily. The maximum dose should not exceed 6 Gm/24 hours.

Usual adult dose:

4 to 5 Gm every twelve hours.

INJECTABLE: For subcutaneous and intravenous administration the 40% solution must be diluted to a concentration of 5% (combine a 5-ml ampul with 35 ml of water for injection USP). Administration of the drug in combination with parenteral fluids is not recommended. The use of diluents other than water for injection USP may cause precipitation.

Injectable Gantrisin may be given intramuscularly without dilution.

Usual dose for infants over 2 months of age, children and adults:

Initial dose: One-half of the 24-hour dose.

Maintenance dose: 100 mg/kg/24 hours or 2.25 Gm/M^2/24 hours, administered in a 5% solution—

a. Subcutaneous administration, divided into 3 doses/24 hours.

b. Intravenous administration, divided into 4 doses/24 hours. (Administer by slow injection or intravenous drip.)

For example—give 1 ml/kg of 5% solution as an initial dose. This should be followed by 0.50 ml/kg of 5% solution four times daily for intravenous administration or 0.66 ml/kg t.i.d. for subcutaneous administration.

c. Intramuscular administration, divided into 2 or 3 doses/24 hours. Up to 10 ml can be given, but not more than 5 ml in any one site. For children, the volume given intramuscularly in any one site should be correspondingly less than in adults.

How Supplied: *Tablets,* containing 0.5 Gm sulfisoxazole/Roche, white, scored—bottles of 100, 500 and 1000; drums of 5000; Tel-E-Dose® packages of 100; Prescription Paks of 100.

Pediatric Suspension, containing, in each teaspoonful (5 ml), the equivalent of approximately 0.5 Gm sulfisoxazole in the form of acetyl sulfisoxazole/Roche; raspberry flavored—bottles of 4 oz and 16 oz (1 pint).

Syrup, containing, in each teaspoonful (5 ml), the equivalent of approximately 0.5 Gm sulfisoxazole in the form of acetyl sulfisoxazole/Roche; chocolate flavored—bottles of 16 oz (1 pint).

Lipo Gantrisin — the long-acting form—containing, in each teaspoonful (5 ml), the equivalent of 1 Gm sulfisoxazole in the form of acetyl sulfisoxazole/Roche in a homogenized mixture containing a readily digestible vegetable oil; vanilla-mint flavored—bottles of 16 oz (1 pint).

Injectable, 5-ml ampuls, containing 2 Gm sulfisoxazole/Roche in the form of the diolamine salt. Each ml of solution contains 400 mg sulfisoxazole/Roche in the form of the diolamine salt compounded with 2 mg sodium metabisulfite. Packages of 10.

References:

1. Randall, L.O., *et al: Antibiot Chemother 4:*877-885, Aug. 1954.
2. Svec, F.A., Rhodes, P.S., Rohr, J.H.: *Arch Intern Med 85:*83-90, Jan. 1950.
3. Flake, R.E., *et al: J Lab Clin Med 44:*582-588, Oct. 1954.
4. Krugman, S.: *Ann NY Acad Sci 69:*399-403, Aug. 1957.
5. Price, P.C., Hansen, A.E.: *Texas Rep Biol Med 9:*764-769, Winter 1951.
6. Kaplan, S.A., *et al: J Pharm Sci 61:*773-778, May 1972.
7. Data on file, Hoffmann-La Roche Inc., Nutley, N.J.
8. Struller, T.: *Antibiot Chemother 14:*179-215, 1968.
9. Sarnoff, S.J.: *Proc Soc Exp Biol Med 68:*23-26, May 1948.

[*Shown in Product Identification Section*]

KONAKION® ℞
(phytonadione/Roche)
INJECTABLE
FOR INTRAMUSCULAR USE ONLY

The following text is complete prescribing information based on official labeling in effect August 1, 1982.

Description: Konakion is an essentially clear, aqueous dispersion of vitamin K_1, available for injection by the intramuscular route only. Slight opalescence may occur in the 10 mg ampuls. However, this does not affect the potency, safety or usefulness of the preparation.

The ingredients are as follows: *0.5-ml ampuls:* Each 0.5 ml contains 1 mg phytonadione (vitamin K_1) compounded with 10 mg polysorbate 80, 0.45% phenol as preservative, 10.4 mg propylene glycol, 0.17 mg sodium acetate and 0.00002 ml glacial acetic acid.

1-ml ampuls: Each ml contains 10 mg phytonadione (vitamin K_1) compounded with 40 mg polysorbate 80, 20.7 mg propylene glycol, 0.8 mg sodium acetate and 0.00006 ml glacial acetic acid.

Actions: Konakion possesses the same type and degree of activity as does naturally occurring vitamin K, which is necessary for the synthesis in the liver of prothrombin (factor II), proconvertin (factor VII), plasma thromboplastin component (factor IX), and Stuart factor (factor X).

The prothrombin test is sensitive to the levels of factors II, VII and X. The mechanism by which vitamin K promotes formation of these clotting factors in the liver is not known.

The action of the aqueous dispersion when administered parenterally is generally detectable within an hour or two, and hemorrhage is usually controlled within 3 to 6 hours. A normal prothrombin level may often be obtained in 12 to 14 hours.

In the prophylaxis and treatment of hemorrhagic disease of the newborn, Konakion has demonstrated a greater margin of safety than that of the water-soluble vitamin K analogs.

Indications:

- anticoagulant-induced prothrombin deficiency;
- prophylaxis and therapy of hemorrhagic disease of the newborn;
- hypoprothrombinemia due to oral antibacterial therapy;
- hypoprothrombinemia secondary to factors limiting absorption or synthesis of vitamin K, *e.g.,* obstructive jaundice, biliary fistula, sprue, ulcerative colitis, celiac disease, intestinal resection, cystic fibrosis of the pancreas and regional enteritis;
- other drug-induced hypoprothrombinemia (such as that due to salicylates) where it is definitely shown that the result is due to interference with vitamin K metabolism.

Contraindications: Parenteral use in persons who are hypersensitive to the drug.

Warnings: Konakion promotes the synthesis of prothrombin by the liver and does not directly counteract the effects of the oral anticoagulants; it takes up to two hours for vitamin K to promote prothrombin synthesis. Fresh plasma or blood transfusions may be required for severe blood loss or lack of response to vitamin K. Phytonadione will not counteract the anticoagulant action of heparin.

When vitamin K_1 is used to correct excessive anticoagulant-induced hypoprothrombinemia, anticoagulant therapy still being indicated, the patient is again faced with the clotting hazards existing prior to starting the anticoagulant therapy. Phytonadione is not a clotting agent, but over-zealous therapy with vitamin K may restore conditions which originally permitted thromboembolic phenomena. Dosage, therefore, should be kept as low as possible, and prothrombin time should be checked regularly as clinical conditions indicate.

Repeated large doses of vitamin K are not warranted in liver disease if the response to initial use of the vitamin is unsatisfactory (Koller test). Failure to respond to vitamin K may indicate the presence of a coagulation defect or that the condition being treated is unresponsive to vitamin K.

Effects on reproduction have not been studied in animals. There is no adequate information on whether this drug may affect fertility in human males or females or have a teratogenic potential or other adverse effects on the fetus.

Precautions: Store in a dark place and protect from light at all times.

Temporary resistance to prothrombin-depressing anticoagulants may result, especially when larger doses of phytonadione are used. If relatively large doses have been employed, it may be necessary when reinstituting anticoagulant therapy to use somewhat larger doses of the prothrombin-depressing anticoagulant or to use one which acts on a different principle, such as heparin.

Adverse Reactions: Pain, swelling and tenderness at the injection site have occurred rarely. The possibility of allergic sensitivity, including an anaphylactoid reaction, should be kept in mind.

Although Konakion has a greater margin of safety than the water-soluble vitamin K analogs, hyperbilirubinemia has been reported in the newborn, particularly in prematures when used at 5 to 10 times the recommended dosage. This effect, with its possibility of attendant kernicterus, should be borne in mind if such dosages are deemed necessary.

Dosage and Administration: The human minimum daily requirements for vitamin K have not been established officially. Minimal daily requirements have been estimated at 1 to 5 micrograms per kilogram of body weight for infants and 0.03 micrograms per kilogram for adults. The dietary abundance of vitamin K satisfies the requirements normally except for the neonatal period of 5 to 8 days.

INFANTS

Neonatal hemorrhage due to hypoprothrombinemia:
- *Prophylactic*—1 to 2 mg intramuscularly, immediately after birth.
- *Control*—1 to 2 mg intramuscularly, daily.

ADULTS

Hypoprothrombinemia due to:
- *Anticoagulant therapy* (except of heparin type)—5 to 10 mg I.M. initially; up to 20 mg, if necessary.
- *Antibacterial therapy*—5 to 20 mg I.M.
- *Factors limiting absorption or synthesis*—2 to 20 mg I.M.
- *Other drugs* (*e.g.,* salicylates)—2 to 20 mg I.M.

In older children and adults, injection of Konakion should be in the upper outer quadrant of the buttocks. In infants and young children, the anterolateral aspect of the thighs or the deltoid region is preferred so that danger of sciatic nerve injury is avoided.

Storage: Konakion is stable in the air, but is photosensitive, decomposing with loss of potency on exposure to light. Therefore, it should be stored in a dark place and protected from light at all times. Konakion need not be refrigerated. Store at 59° to 86°F.

How Supplied: Ampuls, 0.5 ml (boxes of 10). Ampuls, 1 ml (boxes of 10).

LAROBEC® TABLETS ℞

The following text is complete prescribing information based on official labeling in effect August 1, 1982.

Each Larobec® tablet contains:	Quantity	U.S. RDA—Adults and children 4 or more years of age
Water-Soluble Vitamins		
Vitamin C (ascorbic acid)	500 mg	60 mg
Vitamin B_1 (as thiamine mononitrate)	15 mg	1.5 mg
Vitamin B_2 (riboflavin)	15 mg	1.7 mg
Niacin (as niacinamide)	100 mg	20 mg
Pantothenic acid (as calcium *d*-pantothenate)	18 mg	10 mg
Folic acid	0.5 mg	0.4 mg
Vitamin B_{12} (cyanocobalamin)	5 mcg	6 mcg

Description: Larobec is a prescription-only oral multivitamin tablet specially formulated for patients who require prophylactic or therapeutic nutritional supplementation of water-soluble vitamins and are receiving levodopa therapy for Parkinson's disease and syndrome. Larobec provides *therapeutic* levels of ascorbic acid, vitamins B_1, B_2, niacin, pantothenic acid and folic acid and a *supplemental* level of vitamin B_{12} *without* pyridoxine (vitamin B_6), which has been reported to reduce the clinical benefits of levodopa therapy.

Clinical Pharmacology: Vitamins are essential for maintenance of normal metabolic functions including hematopoiesis. The water-soluble vitamins play vital roles in the conversion of carbohydrate, protein and fat into tissue and energy. *Thiamine (B_1)* acts as a coenzyme in carbohydrate metabolism. *Riboflavin (B_2)* functions as a coenzyme in the electron transport system associated with conversion of tissue oxidations into usable energy. *Niacin*

Continued on next page

Roche Labs.—Cont.

serves as a coenzyme in oxidation-reduction reactions in tissue respiration. *Pantothenic acid* functions as a coenzyme in various metabolic acetylation reactions. *Folic acid* and *cyanocobalamin (B_{12})* are metabolically interrelated. They are essential to nucleic acid synthesis and normal maturation of red blood cells. *Ascorbic acid (C)* performs a vital function in the process of cellular respiration, and is involved in both carbohydrate and amino acid metabolism. It is essential for collagen formation and tissue repair.

The water-soluble vitamins (B-complex and C) are not significantly stored by the body; excess quantities are excreted in the urine. They must be replenished regularly through diet or other means to maintain essential tissue levels. Thus these vitamins are rapidly depleted in conditions interfering with their intake or absorption.

Indications and Usage: Larobec is indicated for supportive nutritional supplementation when a water-soluble vitamin formulation (without pyridoxine) is required prophylactically or therapeutically in patients who are undergoing treatment with levodopa.

Contraindications: Larobec is contraindicated in patients known to be hypersensitive to any of its components.

Warnings: Administration of vitamin B_6 may be required if signs of pyridoxine deficiency develop. Folic acid in doses above 0.1 mg daily may obscure pernicious anemia. Larobec is not intended for treatment of pernicious anemia or other megaloblastic anemias where vitamin B_{12} is deficient. Neurologic involvement may develop or progress, despite temporary remission of anemia, in patients with vitamin B_{12} deficiency who receive supplemental folic acid and who are inadequately treated with B_{12}.

Precautions: *General:* Certain patients may require additional nutritional supplementation with fat-soluble vitamins and minerals according to the dietary habits of the individual. Larobec is not intended for treatment of severe specific vitamin deficiencies.

Information for the Patient: Because toxic reactions have been reported with injudicious use of certain vitamins, urge patients to follow your specific instructions regarding dosage regimen. As with any medication, advise patients to keep Larobec out of reach of children.

Adverse Reactions: Adverse reactions have been reported with specific vitamins, but generally at levels substantially higher than those in Larobec. However, allergic and idiosyncratic reactions are possible at lower levels.

Dosage and Administration: Usual adult dosage: one tablet daily.

Larobec is available on prescription only.

How Supplied: Orange-colored, capsule-shaped tablets—bottles of 100 (NDC 0004-0073-01).

Imprint on tablets: LAROBEC®
ROCHE

[*Shown in Product Identification Section*]

LARODOPA® ℞
(levodopa/Roche)

The following text is complete prescribing information based on official labeling in effect August 1, 1982.

In order to reduce the high incidence of adverse reactions, it is necessary to individualize the therapy and to gradually increase the dosage to the desired therapeutic level.

Description: Chemically, levodopa is (−)-3-(3,4-dihydroxyphenyl)-*L*-alanine. It is a colorless, crystalline compound, slightly soluble in water and insoluble in alcohol, with a molecular weight of 197.2.

Actions: Evidence indicates that the symptoms of Parkinson's disease are related to depletion of striatal dopamine. Since dopamine apparently does not cross the blood-brain barrier, its administration is ineffective in the treatment of Parkinson's disease. However, levodopa, the levo-rotatory isomer of dihydroxyphenylalanine (dopa) which is the metabolic precursor of dopamine, does cross the blood-brain barrier. Presumably it is converted into dopamine in the basal ganglia. This is generally thought to be the mechanism whereby oral levodopa acts in relieving the symptoms of Parkinson's disease.

The major urinary metabolites of levodopa in man appear to be dopamine and homovanillic acid (HVA). In 24-hour urine samples, HVA accounts for 13 to 42 percent of the ingested dose of levodopa.

Indications: Larodopa is indicated in the treatment of idiopathic Parkinson's disease (Paralysis Agitans), postencephalitic parkinsonism, symptomatic parkinsonism which may follow injury to the nervous system by carbon monoxide intoxication, and manganese intoxication. It is indicated in those elderly patients believed to develop parkinsonism in association with cerebral arteriosclerosis.

Contraindications: Monoamine oxidase (MAO) inhibitors and Larodopa should not be given concomitantly and these inhibitors must be discontinued two weeks prior to initiating therapy with Larodopa. Larodopa is contraindicated in patients with known hypersensitivity to the drug and in narrow angle glaucoma. Because levodopa may activate a malignant melanoma, it should not be used in patients with suspicious, undiagnosed skin lesions or a history of melanoma.

Warnings: Larodopa should be administered cautiously to patients with severe cardiovascular or pulmonary disease, bronchial asthma, renal, hepatic or endocrine disease.

Care should be exercised in administering Larodopa to patients with a history of myocardial infarction who have residual atrial, nodal or ventricular arrhythmias. If Larodopa is necessary in this type of patient, it should be used in a facility with a coronary care unit or an intensive care unit.

One must be on the alert for the possibility of upper gastrointestinal hemorrhage in those patients with a past history of active peptic ulcer disease.

All patients should be carefully observed for the development of depression with concomitant suicidal tendencies. Psychotic patients should be treated with caution.

Pyridoxine hydrochloride (vitamin B_6) in oral doses of 10 to 25 mg rapidly reverses the toxic and therapeutic effects of Larodopa. This should be considered before recommending vitamin preparations containing pyridoxine hydrochloride (vitamin B_6).

Usage in Pregnancy: The safety of Larodopa in women who are or who may become pregnant has not been established; hence it should be given only when the potential benefits have been weighed against possible hazards to mother and child. Studies in rodents have shown that levodopa at dosages in excess of 200 mg/kg/day has an adverse effect on fetal and postnatal growth and viability.

Larodopa should not be used in nursing mothers.

Usage in Children: The safety of Larodopa under the age of 12 has not been established.

Precautions: Periodic evaluations of hepatic, hematopoietic, cardiovascular and renal function are recommended during extended therapy in all patients.

Patients with chronic wide angle glaucoma may be treated cautiously with Larodopa, provided the intraocular pressure is well controlled and the patient monitored carefully for changes in intraocular pressure during therapy.

Postural hypotensive episodes have been reported as adverse reactions. Therefore, Larodopa should be administered to patients on antihypertensive drug cautiously (for patients receiving pargyline, see note on MAO inhibitors contraindications), and it may be necessary to adjust the dosage of the antihypertensive drugs.

Adverse Reactions: The most serious adverse reactions associated with the administration of Larodopa having frequent occurrences are: adventitious movements such as choreiform and/or dystonic movements. Other serious adverse reactions with a lower incidence are: cardiac irregularities and/or palpitations, orthostatic hypotensive episodes, bradykinetic episodes (the "on-off" phenomena), mental changes including paranoid ideation and psychotic episodes, depression with or without the development of suicidal tendencies, dementia, and urinary retention.

Rarely, gastrointestinal bleeding, development of duodenal ulcer, hypertension, phlebitis, hemolytic anemia, agranulocytosis, and convulsions have been observed. (The causal relationship between convulsions and Larodopa has not been established.)

Adverse reactions of a less serious nature having a relatively frequent occurrence are the following: anorexia, nausea and vomiting with or without abdominal pain and distress, dry mouth, dysphagia, sialorrhea, ataxia, increased hand tremor, headache, dizziness, numbness, weakness and faintness, bruxism, confusion, insomnia, nightmares, hallucinations and delusions, agitation and anxiety, malaise, fatigue and euphoria. Occurring with a lesser order of frequency are the following: muscle twitching and blepharospasm (which may be taken as an early sign of overdosage; consideration of dosage reduction may be made at this time), trismus, burning sensation of the tongue, bitter taste, diarrhea, constipation, flatulence, flushing, skin rash, increased sweating, bizarre breathing patterns, urinary incontinence, diplopia, blurred vision, dilated pupils, hot flashes, weight gain or loss, dark sweat and/or urine.

Rarely, oculogyric crises, sense of stimulation, hiccups, development of edema, loss of hair, hoarseness, priapism and activation of latent Horner's syndrome have been observed.

Elevations of blood urea nitrogen, SGOT, SGPT, LDH, bilirubin, alkaline phosphatase or protein-bound iodine have been reported; and the significance of this is not known. Occasional reductions in WBC, hemoglobin, and hematocrit have been noted.

Leukopenia has occurred and requires cessation, at least temporarily, of Larodopa administration. The Coombs test has occasionally become positive during extended therapy. Elevations of uric acid have been noted when colorimetric method was used but not when uricase method was used.

Overdosage: For acute overdosage general supportive measures should be employed, along with immediate gastric lavage. Intravenous fluids should be administered judiciously and an adequate airway maintained.

Electrocardiographic monitoring should be instituted and the patient carefully observed for the possible development of arrhythmias; if required, appropriate antiarrhythmic therapy should be given. Consideration should be given to the possibility of multiple drug ingestion by the patient. To date, no experience has been reported with dialysis; hence its value in Larodopa overdosage is not known. Although pyridoxine hydrochloride (vitamin B_6) has been reported to reverse the antiparkinson effects of Larodopa, its usefulness in the management of acute overdosage has not been established.

Dosage and Administration: The optimal daily dose of Larodopa, *i.e.*, the dose producing maximal improvement with tolerated side effects, must be determined and *carefully titrated for each individual patient.* The usual initial dosage is 0.5 to 1 Gm daily, divided in two or more doses with food.

The total daily dosage is then increased gradually in increments not more than 0.75 Gm every three to seven days as tolerated. The usual optimal therapeutic *dosage should not exceed 8 Gm.* The exceptional patient may carefully be given more than 8 Gms as required. In some patients, a significant therapeutic response may not be obtained until six months of treatment.

In the event general anesthesia is required, Larodopa therapy may be continued as long as the patient is able to take fluids and medication by mouth. If therapy is temporarily interrupted, the usual daily dosage may be administered as soon as the patient is able to take oral medication. Whenever therapy has been interrupted for longer periods, dosage should again be adjusted gradually; however, in many cases the patient can be rapidly titrated to his previous therapeutic dosage.

How Supplied: Tablets, pink, scored, each containing levodopa/Roche 0.1 Gm, bottles of 100; 0.25 Gm or 0.5 Gm—bottles of 100 and 500. Capsules, each containing levodopa/Roche 0.1 Gm (pink and scarlet)—bottles of 100; 0.25 Gm (pink and beige) or 0.5 Gm (pink)—bottles of 100 and 500.

[*Shown in Product Identification Section*]

LAROTID® ℞
(amoxicillin/Roche)
CAPSULES and
FOR ORAL SUSPENSION

The following text is complete prescribing information based on official labeling in effect August 1, 1982.

Description: Larotid (amoxicillin/Roche) is a semi-synthetic antibiotic, an analog of ampicillin, with a broad spectrum of bactericidal activity against many gram-positive and gram-negative microorganisms. Chemically, amoxicillin is D-(−)-α-amino-p-hydroxybenzyl penicillin trihydrate.

Actions:

Pharmacology: Amoxicillin is stable in the presence of gastric acid and may be given without regard to meals. It is rapidly absorbed after oral administration. It diffuses readily into most body tissues and fluids, with the exception of brain and spinal fluid, except when meninges are inflamed. The half-life of amoxicillin is 61.3 minutes. Most of the amoxicillin is excreted unchanged in the urine; its excretion can be delayed by concurrent administration of probenecid. Amoxicillin is not highly protein-bound. In blood serum, amoxicillin is approximately 20 percent protein-bound, as compared with 60 percent for penicillin-G.

Orally administered doses of 250 mg and 500 mg amoxicillin capsules result in average peak blood levels one to two hours after administration in the range of 3.5 mcg/ml to 5 mcg/ml and 5.5 mcg/ml to 7.5 mcg/ml, respectively.

Orally administered doses of amoxicillin suspension 125 mg/5 ml and 250 mg/5 ml result in average peak blood levels one to two hours after administration in the range of 1.5 mcg/ml to 3 mcg/ml and 3.5 mcg/ml to 5 mcg/ml, respectively.

Detectable serum levels are observed up to eight hours after an orally administered dose of amoxicillin. Approximately 60 percent of an orally administered dose of amoxicillin is excreted in the urine within six to eight hours. Following a 1-Gm dose and utilizing a special skin window technique to determine levels of the antibiotic, it was noted that therapeutic levels were found in the interstitial fluid.

Microbiology: Larotid is similar to ampicillin in its bactericidal action against susceptible organisms during the stage of active multiplication. It acts through the inhibition of biosynthesis of cell wall mucopeptide. *In vitro* studies have demonstrated the susceptibility of most strains of the following gram-positive bacteria: alpha- and beta-hemolytic streptococci, *Diplococcus pneumoniae,* nonpenicillinase-producing staphylococci, and *Streptococcus faecalis.* It is active *in vitro* against many strains of *Hemophilus influenzae, Neisseria gonorrhoeae, Escherichia coli* and *Proteus mirabilis.* Because it does not resist destruction by penicillinase, it is *not* effective against penicillinase-producing bacteria, particularly resistant staphylococci. All strains of Pseudomonas and most strains of Klebsiella and Enterobacter are resistant.

Disc Susceptibility Tests: Quantitative methods that require measurement of zone diameters give the most precise estimates of antibiotic susceptibility. One such procedure[1] has been recommended for use with discs for testing susceptibility to ampicillin class antibiotics. Interpretations correlate diameters of the disc test with MIC values for amoxicillin. With this procedure, a report from the laboratory of "susceptible" indicates that the infecting organism is likely to respond to therapy. A report of "resistant" indicates that the infecting organism is not likely to respond to therapy. A report of "intermediate susceptibility" suggests that the organism would be susceptible if high dosage is used, or if the infection is confined to tissues and fluids (*e.g.,* urine), in which high antibiotic levels are attained.

Indications: Larotid is indicated in the treatment of infections due to susceptible strains of the following:

Gram-negative organisms: *H. influenzae, E. coli, P. mirabilis* and *N. gonorrhoeae.*

Gram-positive organisms: Streptococci (including *Streptococcus faecalis*), *D. pneumoniae* and nonpenicillinase-producing staphylococci.

Therapy may be instituted prior to obtaining results from bacteriological and susceptibility studies to determine the causative organisms and their susceptibility to amoxicillin.

Indicated surgical procedures should be performed.

Contraindications: The use of this drug is contraindicated in individuals with a history of an allergic reaction to the penicillins.

WARNINGS: SERIOUS AND OCCASIONALLY FATAL HYPERSENSITIVITY (ANAPHYLACTOID) REACTIONS HAVE BEEN REPORTED IN PATIENTS ON PENICILLIN THERAPY. ALTHOUGH ANAPHYLAXIS IS MORE FREQUENT FOLLOWING PARENTERAL THERAPY, IT HAS OCCURRED IN PATIENTS ON ORAL PENICILLINS. THESE REACTIONS ARE MORE LIKELY TO OCCUR IN INDIVIDUALS WITH A HISTORY OF SENSITIVITY TO MULTIPLE ALLERGENS. THERE HAVE BEEN REPORTS OF INDIVIDUALS WITH A HISTORY OF PENICILLIN HYPERSENSITIVITY WHO HAVE EXPERIENCED SEVERE REACTIONS WHEN TREATED WITH CEPHALOSPORINS. BEFORE THERAPY WITH ANY PENICILLIN, CAREFUL INQUIRY SHOULD BE MADE CONCERNING PREVIOUS HYPERSENSITIVITY REACTIONS TO PENICILLINS, CEPHALOSPORINS OR OTHER ALLERGENS. IF AN ALLERGIC REACTION OCCURS, APPROPRIATE THERAPY SHOULD BE INSTITUTED AND DISCONTINUANCE OF AMOXICILLIN THERAPY CONSIDERED. **SERIOUS ANAPHYLACTOID REACTIONS REQUIRE IMMEDIATE EMERGENCY TREATMENT WITH EPINEPHRINE. OXYGEN, INTRAVENOUS STEROIDS AND AIRWAY MANAGEMENT, INCLUDING INTUBATION, SHOULD ALSO BE ADMINISTERED AS INDICATED.**

Usage in Pregnancy: Safety for use in pregnancy has not been established.

Precautions: As with any potent drug, periodic assessment of renal, hepatic and hematopoietic function should be made during prolonged therapy.

The possibility of superinfections with mycotic or bacterial pathogens should be kept in mind during therapy. If superinfections occur (usually involving Enterobacter, Pseudomonas or Candida), the drug should be discontinued and/or appropriate therapy instituted.

Adverse Reactions: As with other penicillins, it may be expected that untoward reactions will be essentially limited to sensitivity phenomena. They are more likely to occur in individuals who have previously demonstrated hypersensitivity to penicillins and in those with a history of allergy, asthma, hay fever or urticaria. The following adverse reactions have been reported as associated with the use of the penicillins:

Gastrointestinal: Nausea, vomiting and diarrhea.

Hypersensitivity Reactions: Erythematous maculopapular rashes and urticaria have been reported.

NOTE: Urticaria, other skin rashes and serum sickness-like reactions may be controlled with antihistamines and, if necessary, systemic corticosteroids. Whenever such reactions occur, amoxicillin should be discontinued, unless, in the opinion of the physician, the condition being treated is life-threatening and amenable only to amoxicillin therapy.

Liver: A moderate rise in serum glutamic oxaloacetic transaminase (SGOT) has been noted, but the significance of this finding is unknown.

Hemic and Lymphatic Systems: Anemia, thrombocytopenia, thrombocytopenic purpura, eosinophilia, leukopenia and agranulocytosis have been reported during therapy with the penicillins. These reactions are usually reversible on discontinuation of therapy and are believed to be hypersensitivity phenomena.

Dosage and Administration: The dosages listed below are those usually recommended. The children's dosage is intended for individuals whose weight will not cause a dosage to be calculated greater than that recommended for adults.

Infections of the ear, nose and throat due to streptococci, pneumococci, nonpenicillinase-producing staphylococci and *H. influenzae;* infections of the genitourinary tract due to *E. coli, Proteus mirabilis* and *Streptococcus faecalis;* infections of the skin and soft tissues due to streptococci, susceptible staphylococci and *E. coli:*

USUAL DOSAGE:

Adults: 250 mg every 8 hours.

Children: 20 mg/kg/day in divided doses every 8 hours.

Children weighing 20 kg or more should be dosed according to the adult recommendations.

In severe infections or those caused by less susceptible organisms:

500 mg every 8 hours for adults and 40 mg/kg/day in divided doses every 8 hours for children may be needed.

Infections of the lower respiratory tract due to streptococci, pneumococci, nonpenicillinase-producing staphylococci and *H. influenzae:*

USUAL DOSAGE:

Adults: 500 mg every 8 hours.

Children: 40 mg/kg/day in divided doses every 8 hours.

Children weighing 20 kg or more should be dosed according to the adult recommendations.

Gonorrhea, acute uncomplicated anogenital and urethral infections due to *N. gonorrhoeae* (males and females):

USUAL DOSAGE:

Adults: 3 grams as a single oral dose.

Prepubertal children: 50 mg/kg amoxicillin combined with 25 mg/kg probenecid as a single dose.

Continued on next page

Roche Labs.—Cont.

Note: Since probenecid is contraindicated in children under 2 years, this regimen should not be used in these cases.
Cases of gonorrhea with a suspected lesion of syphilis should have dark-field examinations before receiving amoxicillin and monthly serological tests for a minimum of four months.

It should be recognized that in the treatment of chronic urinary tract infections, frequent bacteriological and clinical appraisals are necessary. Smaller doses than those recommended above should not be used. Even higher doses may be needed at times. In stubborn infections, therapy may be required for several weeks. It may be necessary to continue clinical and/or bacteriological follow-up for several months after cessation of therapy. Except for gonorrhea, treatment should be continued for a minimum of 48 to 72 hours beyond the time that the patient becomes asymptomatic or evidence of bacterial eradication has been obtained. It is recommended that there be at least 10 days' treatment for any infection caused by hemolytic streptococci to prevent the occurrence of acute rheumatic fever or glomerulonephritis.

Dosage and Administration of Pediatric Drops: Usual dosage for all indications except infections of the lower respiratory tract:

Under 6 kg (13 lbs): 0.5 ml every 8 hours.
6–8 kg (13–18 lbs): 1 ml every 8 hours.

Infections of the lower respiratory tract:

Under 6 kg (13 lbs): 1 ml every 8 hours.
6–8 kg (13–18 lbs): 2 ml every 8 hours.

Children weighing more than 8 kg (18 lbs) should receive the appropriate dose of the oral suspension 125 mg or 250 mg/5 ml.

After reconstitution, the required amount of suspension should be placed directly on the child's tongue for swallowing. Alternate means of administration are to add the required amount of suspension to formula, milk, fruit juice, water, ginger ale or cold drinks. These preparations should then be taken immediately. To be certain the child is receiving full dosage, such preparations should be consumed in entirety.

Directions for Mixing Oral Suspension: Prepare suspension at time of dispensing as follows: Add the required amount of water (see table below) to the bottle. For ease of preparation, add water in two portions. Shake well after each addition of water. Each teaspoonful (5 ml) will contain 125 mg or 250 mg amoxicillin.

Bottle Size	Amount of Water Required for Reconstitution
80 ml	53 ml
100 ml	66 ml
150 ml	100 ml

Directions for Mixing Pediatric Drops: Add 11 ml of water to the bottle and shake vigorously. Each ml of suspension will contain 50 mg amoxicillin.

NOTE: SHAKE WELL BEFORE USING.

Keep bottle tightly closed. Any unused portion of the reconstituted suspension must be discarded after 14 days. Refrigeration is preferable, but not required.

How Supplied: *Capsules,* containing 250 mg amoxicillin as the trihydrate, beige and brown—bottles of 100 and 500; containing 500 mg amoxicillin as the trihydrate, beige—bottles of 50 and 500; both strengths also supplied in Tel-E-Dose® packages of 100; and in Prescription Paks of 18, available singly and in trays of 10.

Oral suspension: Each 5 ml of reconstituted suspension contains 125 mg or 250 mg amoxicillin as the trihydrate—bottles of 80 ml, 100 ml and 150 ml. Tel-E-Dose® packages of 10; when reconstituted with 5 ml of water, each dose will contain 125 mg or 250 mg amoxicillin as the trihydrate.

Pediatric drops for oral suspension: Each ml of reconstituted suspension contains 50 mg amoxicillin as the trihydrate—bottles of 15 ml.

Reference:

1. Bauer, A. W., *et al.:* Antibiotic Susceptibility Testing by a Standardized Single Disc Method, *Am. J. Clin. Pathol., 45:*493-496, 1966. Standardized Disc Susceptibility Test, *Fed. Reg., 37:*20527-20529, 1972.

[*Shown in Product Identification Section*]

LEVO-DROMORAN® Ⓒ

(levorphanol tartrate/Roche)
Ampuls • Vials • Tablets

The following text is complete prescribing information based on official labeling in effect August 1, 1982.

Action: Levo-Dromoran (levorphanol tartrate/Roche) is a highly potent synthetic analgesic with properties and actions similar to those of morphine. It produces a degree of analgesia at least equal to that of morphine and greater than that of meperidine at far smaller doses than either. It is longer acting than either; from 6 to 8 hours of pain relief can be expected with Levo-Dromoran whether given orally or by injection. It is almost as effective orally as it is parenterally. Its safety margin is about equal to that of morphine, but it is less likely to produce nausea, vomiting and constipation.

Indications: Levo-Dromoran is recommended whenever a narcotic-analgesic is required. It is recommended for the relief of pain whether moderate or severe. For example, it may be used in alleviating pain due to biliary and renal colic, myocardial infarction, and severe trauma; intractable pain due to cancer and other tumors; and for postoperative pain relief. Used preoperatively, it allays apprehension, provides prolonged analgesia, reduces thiopental requirements and shortens recovery-room time. Levo-Dromoran is compatible with a wide range of anesthetic agents. It is a useful supplement to nitrous oxide-oxygen anesthesia. It has been given by slow intravenous injection for special indications.

Contraindications: As with the use of morphine, Levo-Dromoran is contraindicated in acute alcoholism, bronchial asthma, increased intracranial pressure, respiratory depression and anoxia.

Warning: May be habit forming. Levo-Dromoran is a narcotic with an addiction liability similar to that of morphine, and for this reason the same precautions should be taken in administering the drug as with morphine. As with all narcotics, Levo-Dromoran should be used in early pregnancy only when expected benefits outweigh risks.

Precautions: To prevent or to counteract narcotic-induced respiratory depression (particularly in parturients and neonates, or during nitrous oxide-oxygen anesthesia with narcotic supplementation), Levo-Dromoran combined with Lorfan® (levallorphan tartrate/Roche) —a narcotic antagonist —is recommended. In appropriate combination [1 part Lorfan to 10 parts Levo-Dromoran] respiratory depression is usually prevented without significantly reducing the pain relief provided by Levo-Dromoran. Lorfan usually acts within 1 minute and its action lasts for 2 to 5 hours.

Adverse Reactions: As is true with the use of any narcotic-analgesic, nausea, emesis and dizziness are not uncommon in the ambulatory patient. Respiratory depression, hypotension, urinary retention and various cardiac arrhythmias have been infrequently reported following the use of Levo-Dromoran, primarily in surgical patients. Occasional allergic reactions in the form of skin rash or urticaria have been reported. Pruritus or sweating are rarely observed.

Dosage and Administration: Good medical practice dictates that the dose of any narcotic-analgesic be appropriate to the degree of pain to be relieved. This is especially important during the postoperative period because (a) residual CNS-depressant effects of anesthetic agents may still be present, and (b) later, gradual lessening of pain may not warrant full narcotizing doses. The average adult dose is 2 mg orally or subcutaneously. The dosage may be increased to 3 mg, if necessary. When Levo-Dromoran is used in combination with the narcotic antagonist Lorfan, the following dosage ratio is recommended: Levo-Dromoran/Lorfan (subcutaneous or I.V.)—10:1 [*e.g.,* 2 mg Levo-Dromoran and 0.2 mg Lorfan].

Antidote for Overdosage: In the event of overdosage of the narcotic, Lorfan is a quick and effective antidote. When the narcotic dosage is of unknown magnitude, Lorfan 1 mg intravenously is usually adequate. If required, one or two additional 0.5 mg doses may be given at 3-minute intervals.

How Supplied: *Ampuls,* 1 ml (boxes of 10). Each ml of solution contains 2 mg levorphanol tartrate/Roche (WARNING: May be habit forming) compounded with 0.2% parabens (methyl and propyl) as preservatives, and sodium hydroxide to adjust pH to approximately 4.3.

Multiple Dose Vials, 10 ml, 2 mg/ml (boxes of 1). Each ml of solution contains 2 mg levorphanol tartrate/Roche (WARNING: May be habit forming) compounded with 0.45% phenol as preservative, and sodium hydroxide to adjust pH to approximately 4.3.

Oral Tablets, 2 mg, scored (bottles of 100). Each tablet contains 2 mg levorphanol tartrate/Roche (WARNING: May be habit forming). Narcotic order required.

[*Shown in Product Identification Section*]

LORFAN® ℞

(levallorphan tartrate/Roche)
ampuls • vials

The following text is complete prescribing information based on official labeling in effect August 1, 1982.

Description: Chemically, levallorphan tartrate is (−)-*N*-allyl-3-hydroxymorphinan tartrate. It is chemically related to levorphanol tartrate from which it differs in the replacement of the methyl group on the nitrogen atom by an allyl group. Levallorphan tartrate is a white or practically white, odorless, crystalline powder; it is soluble in water and sparingly soluble in alcohol.

Each ml contains 1 mg levallorphan tartrate/Roche. The pH is adjusted to approximately 4.3 with sodium hydroxide. The solution in ampuls is compounded with 0.2% methyl and propyl parabens and that in vials is compounded with 0.45% phenol as preservatives.

Actions: Lorfan acts as a narcotic antagonist in the presence of a strong narcotic effect. If used in the absence of such a narcotic effect, Lorfan may cause respiratory depression and other undesirable effects.

Indications: For use in the treatment of significant narcotic-induced respiratory depression.

Contraindications: Mild respiratory depression. Narcotic addicts in whom it may produce withdrawal symptoms.

Warnings: Lorfan is ineffective against respiratory depression due to barbiturates, anesthetics, other nonnarcotic agents or pathologic causes, and may increase it.

Precautions: If used in the absence of a narcotic, Lorfan may cause respiratory depression. Artificial respiration with oxygen and other supportive measures should be employed in conjunction with Lorfan in the treatment of significant narcotic-induced respiratory depression. Lorfan does not counteract mild respiratory depression and may increase it. Repeated doses of Lorfan result in decreasing effectiveness and may eventually produce respiratory depression equal to or greater than that produced by narcotics.

Adverse Reactions: Dysphoria, miosis, pseudoptosis, lethargy, dizziness, drowsiness, gastric upset and sweating. Pallor, nausea and a sense of heaviness in the limbs may occur.

In high dosage Lorfan may produce psychotomimetic manifestations such as weird dreams, visual hallucinations, disorientation and feelings of unreality.

In *asphyxia neonatorum,* irritability and a tendency to increased crying may occur.

Dosage and Administration: Administration of Lorfan should be accompanied by the use of other resuscitative measures, such as oxygen or artificial respiration.

Adults: To reverse respiratory depression from narcotic overdosage—1 mg Lorfan intravenously; may be followed, if required, by one or two additional doses of 0.5 mg at 10 to 15 minute intervals. The initial dose should not exceed 1 mg if there is doubt as to whether a narcotic produced the respiratory depression. The total dose should not exceed 3 mg. This regimen may also be employed to overcome narcotic-induced respiratory depression in the parturient woman.

Neonates: To decrease respiratory depression secondary to narcotic administration to the mother, inject 0.05 to 0.1 mg Lorfan (approximately one-tenth the adult dose) into the umbilical cord vein immediately after delivery. If this vein cannot be used, injection may be made intramuscularly or subcutaneously.

Overdosage: Assisted respiration, including a patent airway, the administration of oxygen, and other supportive measures, should be used.

How Supplied: Ampuls, 1 ml, boxes of 10; vials, 10 ml. Each ml contains 1 mg levallorphan tartrate/Roche.

MARPLAN® TABLETS ℞

(isocarboxazid/Roche)

The following text is complete prescribing information based on official labeling in effect August 1, 1982.

Description: Marplan (isocarboxazid/Roche) is an amine-oxidase inhibitor. Chemically, isocarboxazid is 5-methyl-3-isoxazolecarboxylic acid 2-benzylhydrazide.

Isocarboxazid is a colorless, crystalline substance with very little taste.

Actions: Isocarboxazid, a potent inhibitor of amine-oxidase, exhibits antidepressant activity. *In vivo* and *in vitro* studies demonstrated inhibition of amine-oxidase in the brain, heart and liver.

The oral LD_{50} in mice was 171 mg/kg and in rats, 270 mg/kg. In rats administered 120 mg/kg daily for 6 weeks, isocarboxazid produced a reduction of growth rate and appetite. In chronic tolerance studies of 24 weeks duration, hyperexcitability and depression of growth rate occurred in male rats given oral doses of 5 mg/kg/day and in both sexes of this species given 10 mg/kg/day orally. The relevance of these findings to the clinical use of Marplan is not known. No hematologic changes were observed.

Dogs given 15 mg/kg/day for 2 weeks showed emetic effects and a slight lowering of hemoglobin and hematocrit. No adverse effects were noted, however, at doses of 10 mg/kg/day for 6 weeks. Given as successively increasing daily oral doses to a dog, isocarboxazid was tolerated up to 40 mg/kg.

Monkeys given 20 mg/kg/day orally for 2 weeks tolerated the drug with no apparent adverse effects.

Reproduction studies were carried out in rats given 0.5 and 5 mg/kg/day of isocarboxazid as a dietary mixture for 10 weeks prior to mating and continuing through two mating cycles to the weaning of the second litter. The parent animals remained in good condition throughout the test period. Litters of the treated groups compared favorably with those of the controls. No evidence of teratogenic effects was seen in any of the young.

INDICATIONS: Based on a review of this drug by the National Academy of Sciences—National Research Council and/or other information, FDA has classified the indications as follows:

"Probably" effective for the treatment of depressed patients who are refractory to tricyclic antidepressants or electroconvulsive therapy and depressed patients in whom tricyclic antidepressants are contraindicated.

Final classification of the less-than-effective indications requires further investigation.

Careful selection of candidates for Marplan—with due regard to the symptomatology of the patient and to the properties of the compound—will result in more effective therapy. Complete review of the package insert is advised before initiating treatment.

Contraindications: Marplan is contraindicated in patients with known hypersensitivity to the drug, severe impairment of liver or renal function, congestive heart failure or pheochromocytoma.

The potentiation of sympathomimetic substances by MAO inhibitors may result in *hypertensive crisis;* therefore, patients taking Marplan should not be given *sympathomimetic drugs* (including amphetamines, methyldopa, levodopa, dopamine, and tryptophan as well as epinephrine and norepinephrine) nor *foods with a high concentration of tryptophan* (broad beans) or *tyramine* (cheese, beers, wines, pickled herring, chicken livers, yeast extract). Excessive amounts of caffeine can also cause hypertensive reactions.

These hypertensive crises can be fatal, due to circulatory collapse or intracranial bleeding. Hypertensive crises are characterized by some or all of the following symptoms: occipital headache which may radiate frontally, neck stiffness or soreness, nausea, vomiting, photophobia, dilated pupils, sweating (sometimes with fever and sometimes with cold, clammy skin) and palpitations. Either tachycardia or bradycardia may be present, and can be associated with constricting chest pain. These crises usually occur within several hours after the ingestion of a contraindicated substance. Marplan should be discontinued immediately upon the occurrence of palpitations or frequent headaches.

Recommended treatment in hypertensive crisis: Marplan should be discontinued and therapy to lower blood pressure should be started immediately. A successful method of treatment is with an alpha-adrenergic blocking agent such as phentolamine, 5 mg, I.V., or pentolinium, 3 mg, subcutaneously. These drugs should be administered slowly to avoid excessive hypotension. Fever should be managed by external cooling.

Marplan should not be administered together with or immediately following other MAO inhibitors or dibenzazepines. Such combinations can produce hypertensive crisis, fever, marked sweating, excitation, delirium, tremor, twitching, convulsions, coma, and circulatory collapse. At least 10 days should elapse between the discontinuation of Marplan and the institution of another antidepressant, or the discontinuation of another MAO inhibitor and the institution of Marplan.

Some other amine-oxidase inhibitors commonly used in this country include: pargyline HCl, phenelzine sulfate and tranylcypromine. Some antidepressants (dibenzazepine derivatives) commonly used in this country include amitriptyline HCl, desipramine HCl, imipramine HCl, nortriptyline HCl and protriptyline HCl.

Patients taking Marplan should not undergo elective surgery requiring general anesthesia. Should spinal anesthesia be essential, consideration should be given to possible combined hypotensive effects of Marplan and the blocking agent. Also, they should not be given cocaine or local anesthetic solutions containing sympathomimetic vasoconstrictors. Marplan should be discontinued at least 10 days prior to elective surgery.

Marplan should not be used in combination with CNS depressants such as narcotics and ethanol (see PRECAUTIONS for barbiturates). Circulatory collapse and death have been reported from the combination of amine-oxidase inhibitors and a single dose of meperidine.

Warnings: Because the most serious reactions to Marplan relate to effects on blood pressure, it is not advisable to use this drug in elderly or debilitated patients or in the presence of hypertension, cardiovascular or cerebrovascular disease. Patients with severe or frequent headaches should not be considered as candidates for therapy with Marplan because headaches during therapy may be the first symptom of a hypertensive reaction to the drug.

Marplan should be used with caution in combination with antihypertensive drugs including thiazide diuretics since hypotension may result.

In patients who may be suicidal risks, no single form of treatment, such as Marplan, electroshock or other therapy, should be relied on as a sole therapeutic measure. The strictest supervision, and preferably hospitalization, are advised.

Warning to patient: All patients taking Marplan should be warned against self-medication with proprietary cold, hay fever or reducing preparations, since most of these contain sympathomimetic agents. They should be warned against eating the foods previously mentioned that contain high concentrations of tyramine or tryptophan. Beverages containing caffeine should be used in moderation. Patients should be instructed to report promptly the occurrence of headache or other unusual symptoms.

Use in Children: Marplan is not recommended for use in patients under 16 years of age since there are no controlled studies of safety or efficacy in this group.

Use in Pregnancy: Safe use of Marplan during pregnancy or lactation has not yet been established. Before prescribing Marplan in pregnancy, lactation, or in women of childbearing age, the potential benefit of the drug should be weighed against its possible hazard to mother and child. (See ACTIONS.)

Precautions: Concomitant use of Marplan and other psychotropic agents is not recommended because of possible potentiating effects and decreased margin of safety. This is especially true in patients who may subject themselves to an overdosage of drugs. If combination therapy is indicated, careful consideration should be given to the pharmacology of all agents to be employed. The effects of Marplan may persist for a substantial period after discontinuation of the drug, and this should be borne in mind when another drug is prescribed following Marplan. To avoid potentiation, the physician wishing to terminate treatment with Marplan and begin therapy with another agent should allow for an interval of 10 days.

Marplan should be used cautiously in hyperactive or agitated patients, as well as schizophrenic patients, because it may cause excessive stimulation. Characteristically, in manic-depressive states there may be a tendency for patients to swing from a depressive to a manic phase. If such a swing should occur during Marplan therapy, brief discontinuation of the drug, followed by resumption of therapy at a reduced dosage, is advised.

Continued on next page

Roche Labs.—Cont.

Clinical evidence indicates only a low incidence of altered liver function or jaundice in patients treated with Marplan. It is difficult to differentiate most cases of drug-induced hepatocellular jaundice from viral hepatitis since they are histopathologically and biochemically indistinguishable. Moreover, many of the clinical signs and symptoms are identical. While some of the few cases of jaundice reported during Marplan therapy may have been drug-induced, the reaction is rare. Nevertheless, Marplan is an amine-oxidase inhibitor and, as with the use of all these agents, it is advisable to watch for hepatic complications. It is suggested that periodic liver function tests, such as bilirubins, alkaline phosphatase or transaminases, be performed during Marplan therapy; use of the drug should be discontinued at the first sign of hepatic dysfunction or jaundice. In patients with impaired renal function, Marplan should be used cautiously to prevent accumulation.

Marplan appears to have varying effects in epileptic patients; while some have a decrease in frequency of seizures, others have more seizures. Appropriate consideration must be given to the latter possibility if Marplan is prescribed for such patients.

All patients taking Marplan should be watched for symptoms of postural hypotension. If such hypotension occurs, the dose should be reduced or the drug discontinued.

Since the MAO inhibitors, including Marplan potentiate hexobarbital hypnosis in animals, the dose of barbiturates if given concomitantly should be reduced.

Since the MAO inhibitors inhibit the destruction of serotonin, which is believed to be released from tissue stores by rauwolfia alkaloids, caution should be exercised when these drugs are used together.

There is conflicting evidence as to whether MAO inhibitors affect glucose metabolism or potentiate hypoglycemic agents. This should be considered if Marplan is used in diabetics.

Adverse Reactions: Marplan is a potent therapeutic agent with a relatively low incidence of adverse reactions. Since Marplan affects many enzyme systems of the body, a variety of side effects may be anticipated. The most frequently noted have been orthostatic hypotension, associated in some patients with falling, disturbances in cardiac rate and rhythm, complaints of dizziness and vertigo, constipation, headache, overactivity, hyperreflexia, tremors and muscle twitching, mania, hypomania, jitteriness, confusion and memory impairment, insomnia, peripheral edema, weakness, fatigue, dryness of the mouth, blurred vision, hyperhidrosis, anorexia and body weight changes, gastrointestinal disturbances, and minor sensitivity reactions such as skin rashes. Isolated cases of akathisia, ataxia, black tongue, coma, dysuria, euphoria, hematologic changes, incontinence, neuritis, photosensitivity, sexual disturbances, spider telangiectases and urinary retention have been reported. These side effects sometimes necessitate discontinuation of therapy. In rare instances, hallucinations have been reported with high dosages, but they have disappeared upon reduction of dosage or discontinuation of therapy. Toxic amblyopia was reported in one psychiatric patient who had received isocarboxazid for about a year; no causal relationship to isocarboxazid was established.

Dosage and Administration: As with other potent drugs, for maximum therapeutic effect the dosage of Marplan must be individually adjusted on the basis of careful observation of the patient. The usual starting dose is 30 mg daily, to be given in single or divided doses. Marplan has a cumulative effect; therefore, as soon as clinical improvement is observed, the dosage should be reduced to a maintenance level of 10 to 20 mg daily (or less). Since daily doses larger than 30 mg may cause an increase in the incidence or severity of side effects, it is recommended that this dosage generally not be exceeded. Many patients may show a favorable response to Marplan therapy within a week or less; however, since Marplan acts by directly affecting enzyme metabolism, a beneficial effect may not be seen in some patients for three or four weeks. If no response is obtained by then, continued administration is unlikely to help.

Management of Overdosage: The lethal dose of Marplan in man is not known. There has been one report of a fatality in a patient who ingested 400 mg of Marplan together with an unspecified amount of another drug. Major overdosage may be evidenced by symptoms such as tachycardia, hypotension, coma, convulsions, respiratory depression, sluggish reflexes, pyrexia and diaphoresis; these signs may persist for 8 to 14 days. General supportive measures should be employed, along with immediate gastric lavage or emetics. If the latter are given, the danger of aspiration must be borne in mind. An adequate airway should be maintained, with supplemental oxygen if necessary. The mechanism by which amine-oxidase inhibitors produce hypotension is not fully understood, but there is evidence that these agents block the vascular bed response. Thus it is suggested that plasma may be of value in the management of this hypotension. Administration of pressor amines such as Levophed® (levarterenol bitartrate) may be of limited value (note that their effects may be potentiated by Marplan). Continue treatment for several days until homeostasis is restored. Liver function studies are recommended during the 4 to 6 weeks after recovery, as well as at the time of overdosage. As with the management of intentional overdosage with any drug, it should be borne in mind that multiple agents may have been ingested.

How Supplied: Tablets, 10 mg isocarboxazid/Roche each, peach-colored, scored—bottles of 100.

[*Shown in Product Identification Section*]

MATULANE® ℞
(procarbazine hydrochloride/Roche)

The following text is complete prescribing information based on official labeling in effect August 1, 1982.

> **WARNING**
> **It is recommended that MATULANE be given only by or under the supervision of a physician experienced in the use of potent antineoplastic drugs. Adequate clinical and laboratory facilities should be available to patients for proper monitoring of treatment.**
> ***The enclosed instructions should be thoroughly reviewed before administration of MATULANE.***

Description: Matulane (procarbazine hydrochloride/Roche) has demonstrated an antineoplastic effect against Hodgkin's disease. The mode of cytotoxic action of Matulane has not yet been clearly defined; however, there is evidence that the drug may act by inhibition of protein, RNA and DNA synthesis. No cross-resistance with other chemotherapeutic agents, radiotherapy or steroids has been demonstrated.

Clinical studies, in which the duration of response is at least a month, show an over-all response rate of approximately 50 per cent. This includes both objective regression of disease and associated clinical benefit. These observations have been made in patients who have had prior treatment with radiotherapy and other antineoplastic agents.

The number of patients with malignant diseases other than Hodgkin's disease who have received Matulane therapy is inadequate at this time for any definitive statement regarding efficacy. Therefore, the use of this drug should be limited to Hodgkin's disease.

Chemistry: Procarbazine hydrochloride is *N*-isopropyl-*α*- (2-methylhydrazino) -*p*-toluamide monohydrochloride. It is a white to pale yellow crystalline substance, soluble but unstable in water or aqueous solutions. The molecular weight is 257.76.

Actions: In laboratory studies, procarbazine hydrochloride produced a variety of biologic effects. Among these have been immunosuppression, teratogenesis, carcinogenesis, cytotoxicity with mitotic suppression and chromatin derangement, and an antineoplastic effect against a spectrum of transplanted tumors in mice and rats. The major drug toxicities in acute and chronic animal studies were hematologic with granulocyte depression, thrombocyte depression and anemia. Reticuloendothelial system lymphocytic depletion, marrow cell depression, testicular atrophy and mucous membrane ulceration were further evidence of *in vivo* cytotoxicity.

Distribution of the drug in body fluids, studied in dog and man, showed rapid equilibration between plasma and cerebrospinal fluid after oral administration. Pharmacological studies indicated excellent gastrointestinal absorption. The major portion of drug was excreted in the urine as N-isopropylterephthalamic acid with approximately 25 to 42 per cent appearing during the first 24 hours after administration.

Leukemia and pulmonary tumors in mice, and mammary adenocarcinomas in rats, have been observed subsequent to procarbazine hydrochloride administration in high doses. The oral LD_{50} of procarbazine hydrochloride in mice and rats was determined to be 1320 $\pm$ 66 mg/kg and 785 $\pm$ 34 mg/kg respectively. In rabbits the oral LD_{50} was 147 $\pm$ 11.5 mg/kg.

Indication: Matulane is recommended for the palliative management of generalized Hodgkin's disease and in those patients who have become resistant to other forms of therapy. Although prolongation of survival time may not be evident, amelioration of the disease symptoms and regression of tumors have been demonstrated frequently. The drug should be used as an adjunct to standard modalities of therapy.

Contraindications: Matulane is contraindicated in patients with 1) known hypersensitivity to the drug, or 2) inadequate marrow reserve as demonstrated by bone marrow aspiration. Due consideration of this possible state should be given to each patient who has leukopenia, thrombocytopenia or anemia.

Warnings: To minimize CNS depression and possible synergism, barbiturates, antihistamines, narcotics, hypotensive agents or phenothiazines should be used with caution. Ethyl alcohol should not be used since there may be an Antabuse (disulfiram)-like reaction. Because Matulane exhibits some amine oxidase inhibitory activity, sympathomimetic drugs, tricyclic antidepressant drugs (*e.g.,* amitriptyline HCl, imipramine HCl), and other drugs and foods with known high tyramine content, such as ripe cheese and bananas, should be avoided. A further phenomenon of toxicity common to many hydrazine derivatives is hemolysis and the appearance of Heinz-Ehrlich inclusion bodies in erythrocytes.

Use In Pregnancy: Teratogenicity has been reported in animals. Use of any drug in pregnancy, lactation or in women of childbearing age requires that the potential benefit of the drug be weighed against its possible hazard to mother and child.

Precautions: Undue toxicity may occur if Matulane is used in patients with known impairment of renal and/or hepatic function.

When appropriate, hospitalization for the initial course of treatment should be considered. If radiation or a chemotherapeutic agent known to have marrow-depressant activity has been used, an interval of one month or longer without such therapy is recommended before starting treatment with Matulane. The length of this interval may also be determined by evidence of bone marrow recovery based on successive bone marrow studies.

Adverse Reactions: Leukopenia, anemia and thrombopenia occur frequently. Nausea and vomiting are the most commonly reported side effects. Other less frequent gastrointestinal complaints include anorexia, stomatitis, dry mouth, dysphagia, diarrhea and constipation. Pain, including myalgia and arthralgia, chills and fever, sweating, weakness, fatigue, lethargy and drowsiness are often noted. Intercurrent infections, effusion, edema, cough, and pneumonitis have been reported. Bleeding tendencies such as petechiae, purpura, epistaxis, hemoptysis, hematemesis and melena have not been rare. Dermatitis, pruritus, herpes, hyperpigmentation, flushing, alopecia and jaundice have also been noted. Paresthesias and neuropathies, headache, dizziness, depression, apprehension, nervousness, insomnia, nightmares, hallucinations, falling, unsteadiness, ataxia, footdrop, decreased reflexes, tremors, coma, confusion and convulsions have been less common. Hoarseness, tachycardia, retinal hemorrhage, nystagmus, photophobia, photosensitivity, genitourinary symptoms, hypotension and fainting have been rare. Isolated instances of diplopia, inability to focus, papilledema, altered hearing and slurred speech have occurred. Coincidental onset of leukemia during Matulane therapy has been reported in rare instances.

Dosage and Administration:

General Instructions: Baseline laboratory data should be obtained prior to initiation of therapy. The hematologic status as indicated by hemoglobin, hematocrit, white blood count (WBC), differential, reticulocytes and platelets should be monitored closely—at least every 3 or 4 days. Bone marrow depression often occurs 2 to 8 weeks after the start of treatment. If leukopenia occurs, hospitalization of the patient may be needed for appropriate treatment to prevent systemic infection.

Hepatic and renal evaluation are indicated prior to beginning therapy. Urinalysis, transaminase, alkaline phosphatase and blood urea nitrogen should be repeated at least weekly.

Prompt cessation of therapy is recommended if any one of the following occurs:

Central nervous system signs or symptoms such as paresthesias, neuropathies or confusion.

Leukopenia (white blood count under 4000).

Thrombocytopenia (platelets under 100,000).

Hypersensitivity reaction.

Stomatitis—The first small ulceration or persistent spot soreness around the oral cavity is a signal for cessation of therapy.

Diarrhea—Frequent bowel movements or watery stools.

Hemorrhage or bleeding tendencies.

Therapy may be resumed, at the discretion of the physician, after toxic side effects have cleared on clinical evaluation and appropriate laboratory studies. Adjustment to a lower dosage schedule is recommended.

Dosage:

General Instructions: All dosages are based on the patient's actual weight. However, the estimated lean body mass (dry weight) is used if the patient is obese or if there has been a spurious weight gain due to edema, ascites or other forms of abnormal fluid retention.

Adults—To minimize nausea and vomiting experienced by a high percentage of patients beginning Matulane therapy, single or divided doses of 2 to 4 mg/kg/day (to the nearest 50 mg) for the first week are recommended. Daily dosage should then be maintained at 4 to 6 mg/kg/day until the white blood count falls below 4000 per cmm or the platelets fall below 100,000 per cmm or until maximum response is obtained. Upon evidence of hematologic toxicity the drug should be discontinued until there has been satisfactory recovery. Treatment may then be resumed at 1 to 2 mg/kg/day. When maximum response is obtained, the dose may be maintained at 1 to 2 mg/kg/day.

Children—Use of Matulane in children has been quite limited. Very close clinical monitoring is mandatory. Undue toxicity, evidenced by tremors, coma and convulsions, has occurred in a few cases. Dosage, therefore, must be highly individualized. The following dosage schedule is provided as a guideline only.

50 mg daily is recommended for the first week. Daily dosage should then be maintained at 100 mg per square meter of body surface (to the nearest 50 mg) until leukopenia or thrombocytopenia occurs or maximum response is obtained. Upon evidence of hematologic toxicity the drug should be discontinued until there has been satisfactory recovery. Treatment may then be resumed at 50 mg per day. When maximum response is attained, the dose may be maintained at 50 mg daily.

How Supplied: *Capsules:* containing the equivalent of 50 mg procarbazine as the hydrochloride, ivory; bottles of 100.

[*Shown in Product Identification Section*]

MENRIUM® 5-2 ℞

Each tablet contains 5 mg chlordiazepoxide and 0.2 mg water-soluble esterified estrogens.

MENRIUM® 5-4

Each tablet contains 5 mg chlordiazepoxide and 0.4 mg water-soluble esterified estrogens.

MENRIUM® 10-4

Each tablet contains 10 mg chlordiazepoxide and 0.4 mg water-soluble esterified estrogens.

The following text is complete prescribing information based on official labeling in effect August 1, 1982.

Since estrogens are a component of Menrium, please note:

1. ESTROGENS HAVE BEEN REPORTED TO INCREASE THE RISK OF ENDOMETRIAL CARCINOMA.

Three independent case control studies have shown an increased risk of endometrial cancer in postmenopausal women exposed to exogenous estrogens for prolonged periods.[1–3] This risk was independent of the other known risk factors for endometrial cancer. These studies are further supported by the finding that incidence rates of endometrial cancer have increased sharply since 1969 in eight different areas of the United States with population-based cancer reporting systems, an increase which may be related to the rapidly expanding use of estrogens during the last decade.[4] The three case control studies reported that the risk of endometrial cancer in estrogen users was about 4.5 to 13.9 times greater than in nonusers. The risk appears to depend on both duration of treatment[1] and on estrogen dose.[3] In view of these findings, when estrogens are used for the treatment of menopausal symptoms, the lowest dose that will control symptoms should be utilized and medication should be discontinued as soon as possible. When prolonged treatment is medically indicated, the patient should be reassessed on at least a semiannual basis to determine the need for continued therapy. Although the evidence must be considered preliminary, one study suggests that cyclic administration of low doses of estrogen may carry less risk than continuous administration;[3] it therefore appears prudent to utilize such a regimen.

Close clinical surveillance of all women taking estrogens is important. In all cases of undiagnosed persistent or recurring abnormal vaginal bleeding, adequate diagnostic measures should be undertaken to rule out malignancy.

There is no evidence at present that "natural" estrogens are more or less hazardous than "synthetic" estrogens at equiestrogenic doses.

2. ESTROGENS SHOULD NOT BE USED DURING PREGNANCY

The use of female sex hormones, both estrogens and progestogens, during early pregnancy may seriously damage the offspring. It has been shown that females exposed in utero to diethylstilbestrol, a non-steroidal estrogen, have an increased risk of developing, in later life, a form of vaginal or cervical cancer that is ordinarily extremely rare.[5,6] This risk has been estimated as not greater than 4 per 1000 exposures.[7] Furthermore, a high percentage of such exposed women (from 30 to 90 percent) have been found to have vaginal adenosis,[8–12] epithelial changes of the vagina and cervix. Although these changes are histologically benign, it is not known whether they are precursors of malignancy. Although similar data are not available with the use of other estrogens, it cannot be presumed they would not induce similar changes.

Several reports suggest an association between intrauterine exposure to female sex hormones and congenital anomalies, including congenital heart defects and limb reduction defects.[13–16] One case control study[16] estimated a 4.7 fold increased risk of limb reduction defects in infants exposed in utero to sex hormones (oral contraceptives, hormone withdrawal tests for pregnancy, or attempted treatment for threatened abortion). Some of these exposures were very short and involved only a few days of treatment. The data suggest that the risk of limb reduction defects in exposed fetuses is somewhat less than 1 per 1,000. In the past, female sex hormones have been used during pregnancy in an attempt to treat threatened or habitual abortion. There is considerable evidence that estrogens are ineffective for these indications, and there is no evidence from well-controlled studies that progestogens are effective for these uses.

If Menrium is used during pregnancy, or if the patient becomes pregnant while taking this drug, she should be apprised of the potential risks to the fetus, and the advisability of pregnancy continuation.

Description: Menrium affords in a single formulation the psychotropic action of Librium® (chlordiazepoxide/Roche) and hormonal replacement in the form of water-soluble esterified estrogens (expressed in terms of sodium estrone sulfate) to provide comprehensive management of the menopausal syndrome or the climacteric.

Librium (chlordiazepoxide/Roche) is a versatile therapeutic agent of proven value for the relief of anxiety and tension. It is indicated when anxiety, tension or apprehension are significant components of the clinical profile. It is among the safer of the effective psychopharmacologic compounds.

Chlordiazepoxide is 7-chloro-2-methylamino-5-phenyl-3H-1, 4-benzodiazepine 4-oxide. It is a slightly yellow, crystalline material and is insoluble in water. The molecular weight is 299.75.

Water-soluble esterified estrogens provide hormonal replacement in the menopausal patient, the need for which is widely recog-

Continued on next page

Roche Labs.—Cont.

nized and accepted. Esterified estrogens is a mixture of the sodium salts of the sulfate esters of the estrogenic substances, principally estrone, that are of the type excreted by pregnant mares. It is a white-to buff-colored, amorphous powder, odorless or having a slight, characteristic odor.

Clinical Pharmacology: The estrogenic component of Menrium is water-soluble esterified estrogens—steroidal compounds—which occur naturally. The action of this substance is substantially equal to the action of both conjugated estrogens, also naturally occurring, and synthetic estrogenic substances.

Menopausal changes, such as atrophic changes of the genital tract and breasts due to a slow decline in estrogen secretion, may be reversed by substitution therapy with estrogenic substances.

Estrogens are, in general, completely absorbed following oral administration. Estrogens are detoxified by the liver, and excretion occurs by way of the urine and the feces.

Librium (chlordiazepoxide HCl/Roche) has anti-anxiety and sedative actions. The drug has been studied extensively in many species of animals and these studies are suggestive of action on the limbic system of the brain, which recent evidence indicates is involved in emotional responses. However, the precise mechanism of action in man is not known. The drug blocks EEG arousal from stimulation of the brain stem reticular formation. The mean ±S.E. plasma peak time is 1.4 (±0.3) hours, and the half-life ranges between 7.1 to 19.8 hours with a mean ±S.E. half-life of 12.0 (±0.7) hours. After the drug is discontinued, plasma levels are usually at the lowest quantitatively detectable amounts by 48–72 hours. Chlordiazepoxide HCl is excreted in urine with 1% or less unchanged and 12 to 34% recoverable as conjugates.

Indications: Menrium is indicated in the management of the manifestations generally associated with the menopausal syndrome—anxiety and tension, vasomotor complaints and hormonal deficiency states.

MENRIUM HAS NOT BEEN SHOWN TO BE EFFECTIVE FOR ANY PURPOSE DURING PREGNANCY AND ITS USE MAY CAUSE SEVERE HARM TO THE FETUS (SEE BOXED WARNING).

Contraindications: Menrium is contraindicated in patients with known hypersensitivity to chlordiazepoxide and/or esterified estrogens.

Estrogens should not be used in women (or men) with any of the following conditions:

1. Known or suspected cancer of the breast except in appropriately selected patients being treated for metastatic disease.
2. Known or suspected estrogen-dependent neoplasia.
3. Known or suspected pregnancy. (See Boxed Warning.)
4. Undiagnosed abnormal genital bleeding.
5. Active thrombophlebitis or thromboembolic disorders.
6. A past history of thrombophlebitis, thrombosis, or thromboembolic disorders associated with previous estrogen use.

Warnings:

1. *Induction of malignant neoplasms.* Long term continuous administration of natural and synthetic estrogens in certain animal species increases the frequency of carcinomas of the breast, cervix, vagina, and liver. There is now evidence that estrogens increase the risk of carcinoma of the endometrium in humans. (See Boxed Warning.)

At the present time there is no satisfactory evidence that estrogens given to postmenopausal women increase the risk of cancer of the breast,[17] although a recent long-term followup of a single physician's practice has raised this possibility.[18] Because of the animal data, there is a need for caution in prescribing estrogens for women with a strong family history of breast cancer or who have breast nodules, fibrocystic disease, or abnormal mammograms.

2. *Gall bladder disease.* A recent study has reported a 2- to 3-fold increase in the risk of surgically confirmed gall bladder disease in women receiving postmenopausal estrogens,[17] similar to the 2-fold increase previously noted in users of oral contraceptives.[19,24] In the case of oral contraceptives the increased risk appeared after two years of use.[24]

3. *Effects similar to those caused by estrogen-progestogen oral contraceptives.* There are several serious adverse effects of oral contraceptives, most of which have not, up to now, been documented as consequences of postmenopausal estrogen therapy. This may reflect the comparatively low doses of estrogen used in postmenopausal women. It would be expected that the larger doses of estrogen used to treat prostatic or breast cancer or postpartum breast engorgement are more likely to result in these adverse effects, and, in fact, it has been shown that there is an increased risk of thrombosis in men receiving estrogens for prostatic cancer and women for postpartum breast engorgement.[20–23]

a. *Thromboembolic disease.* It is now well established that users of oral contraceptives have an increased risk of various thromboembolic and thrombotic vascular diseases, such as thrombophlebitis, pulmonary embolism, stroke, and myocardial infarction.[24–31] Cases of retinal thrombosis, mesenteric thrombosis, and optic neuritis have been reported in oral contraceptive users. There is evidence that the risk of several of these adverse reactions is related to the dose of the drug.[32,33] An increased risk of postsurgery thromboembolic complications has also been reported in users of oral contraceptives.[34,35] If feasible, estrogen should be discontinued at least 4 weeks before surgery of the type associated with an increased risk of thromboembolism, or during periods of prolonged immobilization.

While an increased rate of thromboembolic and thrombotic disease in postmenopausal users of estrogens has not been found,[17,36] this does not rule out the possibility that such an increase may be present or that subgroups of women who have underlying risk factors or who are receiving relatively large doses of estrogens may have increased risk. Therefore, estrogens should not be used in persons with active thrombophlebitis or thromboembolic disorders, and they should not be used in persons with a history of such disorders in association with estrogen use. They should be used with caution in patients with cerebral vascular or coronary artery disease and only for those in whom estrogens are clearly needed.

Large doses of estrogen (5 mg conjugated estrogens per day), comparable to those used to treat cancer of the prostate and breast, have been shown in a large prospective clinical trial in men[37] to increase the risk of nonfatal myocardial infarction, pulmonary embolism and thrombophlebitis. When estrogen doses of this size are used, any of the thromboembolic and thrombotic adverse effects associated with oral contraceptive use should be considered a clear risk.

b. *Hepatic adenoma.* Benign hepatic adenomas appear to be associated with the use of oral contraceptives.[38–40] Although benign, and rare, these may rupture and may cause death through intra-abdominal hemorrhage. Such lesions have not yet been reported in association with other estrogen or progestogen preparations but should be considered in estrogen users having abdominal pain and tenderness, abdominal mass, or hypovolemic shock. Hepatocellular carcinoma has also been reported in women taking estrogen-containing oral contraceptives.[39] The relationship of this malignancy to these drugs is not known at this time.

c. *Elevated blood pressure.* Increased blood pressure is not uncommon in women using oral contraceptives. There is now a report that this may occur with the use of estrogens in the menopause[41] and blood pressure should be monitored with estrogen use, especially if high doses are used.

d. *Glucose tolerance.* A worsening of glucose tolerance has been observed in a significant percentage of patients on estrogen-containing oral contraceptives. For this reason, diabetic patients should be carefully observed while receiving estrogen.

4. *Hypercalcemia.* Administration of estrogens may lead to severe hypercalcemia in patients with breast cancer and bone metastases. If this occurs, the drug should be stopped and appropriate measures taken to reduce the serum calcium level.

As in the case of other preparations containing CNS-acting drugs, patients receiving Menrium should be cautioned about possible combined effects with alcohol and other CNS depressants. Other causes of manifestations of the menopausal syndrome, such as pregnancy, should be excluded. As is true of all preparations containing CNS-acting drugs, patients receiving Menrium should be cautioned against hazardous occupations requiring complete mental alertness such as operating machinery or driving a motor vehicle.

Physical and Psychological Dependence: Withdrawal symptoms have not been observed in more than 1300 subjects during clinical trials with Menrium. Physical and psychological dependence have rarely been reported in persons taking recommended doses of Librium (chlordiazepoxide/Roche). However, caution must be exercised in administering Librium to individuals known to be addiction-prone or those whose history suggests they may increase the dosage on their own initiative. Withdrawal symptoms following discontinuation of chlordiazepoxide hydrochloride have been reported. These symptoms (including convulsions) are similar to those seen with barbiturates.

Precautions:

A. General Precautions.

1. A complete medical and family history should be taken prior to the initiation of any estrogen therapy. The pretreatment and periodic physical examinations should include special reference to blood pressure, breasts, abdomen, and pelvic organs, and should include a Papanicolaou smear. As a general rule, estrogen should not be prescribed for longer than one year without another physical examination being performed.
2. Fluid retention—Because estrogens may cause some degree of fluid retention, conditions which might be influenced by this factor such as epilepsy, migraine, and cardiac or renal dysfunction, require careful observation.
3. Certain patients may develop undesirable manifestations of excessive estrogenic stimulation, such as abnormal or excessive uterine bleeding, mastodynia, etc.
4. Oral contraceptives appear to be associated with an increased incidence of mental depression.[24] Although it is not clear whether this is due to the estrogenic or progestogenic component of the contraceptive, patients with a history of depression should be carefully observed.
5. Preexisting uterine leiomyomata may increase in size during estrogen use.
6. The pathologist should be advised of estrogen therapy when relevant specimens are submitted.
7. Patients with a past history of jaundice during pregnancy have an increased risk of recurrence of jaundice while receiving estrogen-containing oral contraceptive therapy. If jaundice develops in any patient receiving es-

trogen, the medication should be discontinued while the cause is investigated.

8. Estrogens may be poorly metabolized in patients with impaired liver function and they should be administered with caution in such patients.

9. Because estrogens influence the metabolism of calcium and phosphorus, they should be used with caution in patients with metabolic bone diseases that are associated with hypercalcemia or in patients with renal insufficiency.

10. Because of the effects of estrogens on epiphyseal closure, they should be used judiciously in young patients in whom bone growth is not complete.

11. Certain endocrine and liver function tests may be affected by estrogen-containing oral contraceptives. The following similar changes may be expected with larger doses of estrogen:

a. Increased sulfobromophthalein retention.
b. Increased prothrombin and factors VII, VIII, IX, and X; decreased antithrombin 3; increased norepinephrine-induced platelet aggregability.
c. Increased thyroid binding globulin (TBG) leading to increased circulating total thyroid hormone, as measured by PBI, T4 by column, or T4 by radioimmunoassay. Free T3 resin uptake is decreased, reflecting the elevated TBG; free T4 concentration is unaltered.
d. Impaired glucose tolerance.
e. Decreased pregnanediol excretion.
f. Reduced response to metyrapone test.
g. Reduced serum folate concentration.
h. Increased serum triglyceride and phospholipid concentration.

B. Information for the Patient.

See Text of Patient Package Insert which follows below.

WHAT YOU SHOULD KNOW ABOUT ESTROGENS

Estrogens are female hormones produced by the ovaries. The ovaries make several different kinds of estrogens. In addition, scientists have been able to make a variety of synthetic estrogens. As far as we know, all these estrogens have similar properties and therefore much the same usefulness, side effects, and risks. This leaflet is intended to help you understand what estrogens are used for, the risks involved in their use, and how to use them as safely as possible.

This leaflet includes the most important information about estrogens, but not all the information. If you want to know more, you can ask your doctor or pharmacist to let you read the package insert prepared for the doctor.

Uses of Estrogen: Estrogens are prescribed by doctors for a number of purposes, including:

1. To provide estrogen during a period of adjustment when a woman's ovaries no longer produce it, in order to prevent certain uncomfortable symptoms of estrogen deficiency. (All women normally stop producing estrogens, generally between the ages of 45 and 55; this is called the menopause.)
2. To prevent symptoms of estrogen deficiency when a woman's ovaries have been removed surgically before the natural menopause.
3. To prevent pregnancy. (Estrogens are given along with a progestogen, another female hormone; these combinations are called oral contraceptives or birth control pills. Patient labeling is available to women taking oral contraceptives and they will not be discussed in this leaflet.)
4. To treat certain cancers in women and men.
5. To prevent painful swelling of the breasts after pregnancy in women who choose not to nurse their babies.

THERE IS NO PROPER USE OF ESTROGENS IN A PREGNANT WOMAN.

Estrogens in the Menopause: In the natural course of their lives, all women eventually experience a decrease in estrogen production. This usually occurs between ages 45 and 55 but may occur earlier or later. Sometimes the ovaries may need to be removed before natural menopause by an operation, producing a "surgical menopause."

When the amount of estrogen in the blood begins to decrease, many women may develop typical symptoms: Feelings of warmth in the face, neck, and chest or sudden intense episodes of heat and sweating throughout the body (called "hot flashes" or "hot flushes"). These symptoms are sometimes very uncomfortable. A few women eventually develop changes in the vagina (called "atrophic vaginitis") which cause discomfort, especially during and after intercourse.

Estrogens can be prescribed to treat these symptoms of the menopause. It is estimated that considerably more than half of all women undergoing the menopause have only mild symptoms or no symptoms at all and therefore do not need estrogens. Other woman may need estrogens for a few months, while their bodies adjust to lower estrogen levels. Sometimes the need will be for periods longer than six months. In an attempt to avoid overstimulation of the uterus (womb), estrogens are usually given cyclically during each month of use, that is three weeks of pills followed by one week without pills.

Sometimes women experience nervous symptoms or depression during menopause. There is no evidence that estrogens are effective for such symptoms and they should not be used to treat them, although other treatment may be needed.

You may have heard that taking estrogens for long periods (years) after the menopause will keep your skin soft and supple and keep you feeling young. There is no evidence that this is so, however, and such long-term treatment carries important risks.

Estrogens to Prevent Swelling of the Breasts After Pregnancy: If you do not breast feed your baby after delivery, your breasts may fill up with milk and become painful and engorged. This usually begins about 3 to 4 days after delivery and may last for a few days to up to a week or more. Sometimes the discomfort is severe, but usually it is not and can be controlled by pain relieving drugs such as aspirin and by binding the breasts up tightly. Estrogens can be used to try to prevent the breasts from filling up. While this treatment is sometimes successful, in many cases the breasts fill up to some degree in spite of treatment. The dose of estrogens needed to prevent pain and swelling of the breasts is much larger than the dose needed to treat symptoms of the menopause and this may increase your chances of developing blood clots in the legs or lungs (see below). Therefore, it is important that you discuss the benefits and the risks of estrogen use with your doctor if you have decided not to breast feed your baby.

The Dangers of Estrogens:

1. *Cancer of the uterus.* If estrogens are used in the postmenopausal period for more than a year, there is an increased risk of *endometrial cancer* (cancer of the uterus). Women taking estrogens have roughly 5 to 10 times as great a chance of getting this cancer as women who take no estrogens. To put this another way, while a postmenopausal woman not taking estrogens has 1 chance in 1,000 each year of getting cancer of the uterus, a woman taking estrogens has 5 to 10 chances in 1,000 each year. For this reason *it is important to take estrogens only when you really need them.*

The risk of this cancer is greater the longer estrogens are used and also seems to be greater when larger doses are taken. For this reason *it is important to take the lowest dose of estrogen that will control symptoms and to take it only as long as it is needed.* If estrogens are needed for longer periods of time, your doctor will want to reevaluate your need for estrogens at least every six months.

Women using estrogens should report any irregular vaginal bleeding to their doctors; such bleeding may be of no importance, but it can be an early warning of cancer of the uterus. If you have undiagnosed vaginal bleeding, you should not use estrogens until a diagnosis is made and you are certain there is no cancer of the uterus.

If you have had your uterus completely removed (total hysterectomy), there is no danger of developing cancer of the uterus.

2. *Other possible cancers.* Estrogens can cause development of other tumors in animals, such as tumors of the breast, cervix, vagina, or liver, when given for a long time. At present there is no good evidence that women using estrogen in the menopause have an increased risk of such tumors, but there is no way yet to be sure they do not; and one study raises the possibility that use of estrogens in the menopause may increase the risk of breast cancer many years later. This is a further reason to use estrogens only when clearly needed. While you are taking estrogens, it is important that you go to your doctor at least once a year for a physical examination. Also, if members of your family have had breast cancer or if you have breast nodules or abnormal mammograms (breast x-rays), your doctor may wish to carry out more frequent examinations of your breasts.

3. *Gall bladder disease.* Women who use estrogens after menopause are more likely to develop gall bladder disease needing surgery as women who do not use estrogens. Birth control pills have a similar effect.

4. *Abnormal blood clotting.* Oral contraceptives increase the risk of blood clotting in various parts of the body. This can result in a stroke (if the clot is in the brain), a heart attack (clot in a blood vessel of the heart), or a pulmonary embolus (a clot which forms in the legs or pelvis, then breaks off and travels to the lungs). Any of these can be fatal.

At this time use of estrogens in the menopause is not known to cause such blood clotting, but this has not been fully studied and there could still prove to be such a risk. It is recommended that if you have had clotting in the legs or lungs or a heart attack or stroke while you were using estrogens or birth control pills, you should not use estrogens (unless they are being used to treat cancer of the breast or prostate). If you have had a stroke or heart attack or if you have angina pectoris, estrogens should be used with great caution and only if clearly needed (for example, if you have severe symptoms of the menopause).

The larger doses of estrogen used to prevent swelling of the breasts after pregnancy have been reported to cause clotting in the legs and lungs.

Special Warning About Pregnancy: You should not receive estrogen if you are pregnant. If this should occur, there is a greater than usual chance that the developing child will be born with a birth defect, although the possibility remains fairly small. A female child may have an increased risk of developing cancer of the vagina or cervix later in life (in the teens or twenties). Every possible effort should be made to avoid exposure to estrogens during pregnancy. If exposure occurs, see your doctor.

Other Effects of Estrogens: In addition to the serious known risks of estrogens described above, estrogens have the following side effects and potential risks:

1. *Nausea and vomiting.* The most common side effect of estrogen therapy is nausea. Vomiting is less common.
2. *Effects on breasts.* Estrogens may cause breast tenderness or enlargement and may cause the breasts to secrete a liquid. These effects are not dangerous.

Continued on next page

Roche Labs.—Cont.

3. *Effects on the uterus.* Estrogens may cause benign fibroid tumors of the uterus to get larger.
Some women will have menstrual bleeding when estrogens are stopped. But if the bleeding occurs on days you are still taking estrogens you should report this to your doctor.
4. *Effects on liver.* Women taking oral contraceptives develop on rare occasions a tumor of the liver which can rupture and bleed into the abdomen. So far, these tumors have not been reported in women using estrogens in the menopause, but you should report any swelling or unusual pain or tenderness in the abdomen to your doctor immediately.
Women with a past history of jaundice (yellowing of the skin and white parts of the eyes) may get jaundice again during estrogen use. If this occurs, stop taking estrogens and see your doctor.
5. *Other effects.* Estrogens may cause excess fluid to be retained in the body. This may make some conditions worse, such as epilepsy, migraine, heart disease, or kidney disease.
Summary: Estrogens have important uses, but they have serious risks as well. You must decide, with your doctor, whether the risks are acceptable to you in view of the benefits of treatment. Except where your doctor has prescribed estrogens for use in special cases of cancer of the breast or prostate, you should not use estrogens if you have cancer of the breast or uterus, are pregnant, have undiagnosed abnormal vaginal bleeding, clotting in the legs or lungs, or have had a stroke, heart attack or angina, or clotting in the legs or lungs in the past while you were taking estrogens.
You can use estrogens as safely as possible by understanding that your doctor will require regular physical examinations while you are taking them and will try to discontinue the drug as soon as possible and use the smallest dose possible. Be alert for signs of trouble including:
1. Abnormal bleeding from the vagina.
2. Pains in the calves or chest or sudden shortness of breath, or coughing blood (indicating possible clots in the legs, heart, or lungs).
3. Severe headache, dizziness, faintness, or changes in vision (indicating possible developing clots in the brain or eye).
4. Breast lumps (you should ask your doctor how to examine your own breasts).
5. Jaundice (yellowing of the skin).
6. Mental depression.
Based on his or her assessment of your medical needs, your doctor has prescribed this drug for you. Do not give the drug to anyone else.

C. Pregnancy: See Contraindications and Box Warning.
D. Nursing Mothers: As a general principle, the administration of any drug to nursing mothers should be done only when clearly necessary since many drugs are excreted in human milk.
In elderly and debilitated patients, it is recommended that the dosage be limited to the smallest effective amount to preclude the development of ataxia or oversedation (10 mg chlordiazepoxide or less per day initially, to be increased gradually as needed and tolerated). In general, the concomitant administration of Menrium and other psychotropic agents is not recommended. If such combination therapy seems indicated, careful consideration should be given to the pharmacology of the agents to be employed—particularly when the known potentiating compounds such as the MAO inhibitors and phenothiazines are to be used. The usual precautions in treating patients with impaired renal or hepatic function should be observed.
Paradoxical reactions to chlordiazepoxide, e.g., excitement, stimulation and acute rage, have been reported in psychiatric patients and should be watched for during Menrium therapy. The usual precautions are indicated when chlordiazepoxide is used in the treatment of anxiety states where there is any evidence of impending depression; it should be borne in mind that suicidal tendencies may be present and protective measures may be necessary.
Although clinical studies have not established a cause and effect relationship, physicians should be aware that variable effects on blood coagulation have been reported very rarely in patients receiving oral anticoagulants and Librium (chlordiazepoxide/Roche).
Adverse Reactions: No side effects or manifestations not seen with either compound alone have been reported with the administration of Menrium. However, since Menrium contains chlordiazepoxide and water-soluble esterified estrogens, the possibility of untoward effects which may be seen with either of these two compounds cannot be excluded.
(See Warnings regarding induction of neoplasia, adverse effects on the fetus, increased incidence of gall bladder disease, and adverse effects similar to those of oral contraceptives, including thromboembolism.) The following additional adverse reactions have been reported with estrogenic therapy, including oral contraceptives:
1. *Genitourinary system.*
Breakthrough bleeding, spotting, change in menstrual flow.
Dysmenorrhea.
Premenstrual-like syndrome.
Amenorrhea during and after treatment.
Increase in size of uterine fibromyomata.
Vaginal candidiasis.
Change in cervical eversion and in degree of cervical secretion.
Cystitis-like syndrome.
2. *Breasts.*
Tenderness, enlargement, secretion.
3. *Gastrointestinal.*
Nausea, vomiting.
Abdominal cramps, bloating.
Cholestatic jaundice.
4. *Skin.*
Chloasma or melasma which may persist when drug is discontinued.
Erythema multiforme.
Erythema nodosum.
Hemorrhagic eruption.
Loss of scalp hair.
Hirsutism.
5. *Eyes.*
Steepening of corneal curvature.
Intolerance to contact lenses.
6. *CNS.*
Headache, migraine, dizziness.
Mental depression.
Chorea.
7. *Miscellaneous.*
Increase or decrease in weight.
Reduced carbohydrate tolerance.
Aggravation of porphyria.
Edema.
Changes in libido.
When chlordiazepoxide has been used alone the necessity of discontinuing therapy because of undesirable effects has been rare. Drowsiness, ataxia and confusion have been reported in some patients—particularly the elderly and debilitated. While these effects can be avoided in almost all instances by proper dosage adjustment, they have occasionally been observed at the lower dosage ranges. In a few instances syncope has been reported.
Other adverse reactions reported during therapy include isolated instances of skin eruptions, edema, minor menstrual irregularities, nausea and constipation, extrapyramidal symptoms, as well as increased and decreased libido. Such side effects have been infrequent and are generally controlled with reduction of dosage. Changes in EEG patterns (low-voltage fast activity) have been observed in patients during and after Librium (chlordiazepoxide/Roche) treatment.
Blood dyscrasias, including agranulocytosis, jaundice and hepatic dysfunction have occasionally been reported during therapy. When Librium treatment is protracted, periodic blood counts and liver function tests are advisable.
Management of Overdosage: Numerous reports of ingestion of large doses of estrogen-containing oral contraceptives by young children indicate that serious ill effects do not occur. Overdosage of estrogen may cause nausea, and withdrawal bleeding may occur in females. Manifestations of Librium (chlordiazepoxide/Roche) overdosage include somnolence, confusion, coma and diminished reflexes. Respiration, pulse and blood pressure should be monitored, as in all cases of drug overdosage, although, in general, these effects have been minimal following Librium overdosage. General supportive measures should be employed, along with immediate gastric lavage. Intravenous fluids should be administered and an adequate airway maintained. Hypotension may be combated by the use of Levophed® (levarterenol) or Aramine (metaraminol). Dialysis is of limited value. There have been occasional reports of excitation in patients following chlordiazepoxide overdosage; if this occurs barbiturates should not be used. As with the management of intentional overdosage with any drug, it should be borne in mind that multiple agents may have been ingested.
Dosage: The lowest dose that will control symptoms should be chosen and medication should be discontinued as promptly as possible.
MENRIUM 5-2—for the majority of patients with the menopausal syndrome or the climacteric having anxiety and tension and hormonal deficiency states requiring estrogen replacement—One tablet, t.i.d.
MENRIUM 5-4—for patients with the menopausal syndrome or the climacteric with anxiety and tension and more severe vasomotor manifestations—One tablet, t.i.d.
MENRIUM 10-4—for patients with the menopausal syndrome or the climacteric with pronounced anxiety and tension and marked vasomotor complaints—One tablet, t.i.d.
Therapy should be continued for 21-day courses, followed by one-week rest periods. While these dosage schedules will prove generally satisfactory, individual adjustment of dosage is desirable, since some patients may obtain satisfactory relief with as little as one tablet daily of Menrium 5-2.
Treated patients with an intact uterus should be monitored closely for signs of endometrial cancer and appropriate diagnostic measures should be taken to rule out malignancy in the event of persistent or recurring abnormal vaginal bleeding.
How Supplied: Menrium 5-2, light green tablets—each tablet contains 5 mg chlordiazepoxide and 0.2 mg water-soluble esterified estrogens—bottles of 100; Menrium 5-4, dark green tablets—each tablet contains 5 mg chlordiazepoxide and 0.4 mg water-soluble esterified estrogens—bottles of 100; Menrium 10-4, purple tablets—each tablet contains 10 mg chlordiazepoxide and 0.4 mg water-soluble esterified estrogens—bottles of 100.

Physician References:

1. Ziel HK, Finkel WD: *N Engl J Med 293*:1167–1170, 1975
2. Smith DC, *et al: N Engl J Med 293*:1164–1167, 1975
3. Mack TM, *et al: N Engl J Med 294*:1262–1267, 1976
4. Weiss NS, Szekely DR, Austin DF: *N Engl J Med 294*:1259–1262, 1976
5. Herbst AL, Ulfelder H, Poskanzer DC: *N Engl J Med 284*:878–881, 1971
6. Greenwald P, *et al: N Engl J Med 285*:390–392, 1971

7. Lanier A, *et al: Mayo Clin Proc 48*:793–799, 1973
8. Herbst A, Kurman R, Scully R: *Obstet Gynecol 40*:287–298, 1972
9. Herbst A, *et al: Am J Obstet Gynecol 118*:607–615, 1974
10. Herbst, A, *et al: N Engl J Med 292*:334–339, 1975
11. Stafl A, *et al: Obstet Gynecol 43*:118–128, 1974
12. Sherman AI, *et al: Obstet Gynecol 44*:531–545, 1974
13. Gal I, Kirman B, Stern J: *Nature 216*:83, 1967
14. Levy EP, Cohen A, Fraser FC: *Lancet 1*:611, 1973
15. Nora J, Nora A: *Lancet 1*:941–942, 1973
16. Janerich DT, Piper JM, Glebatis DM: *N Engl J Med 291*:697–700, 1974
17. Boston Collaborative Drug Surveillance Program: *N Engl J Med 290*:15–19, 1974
18. Hoover R, *et al: N Engl J Med 295*:401–405, 1976
19. Boston Collaborative Drug Surveillance Program: *Lancet 1*:1399–1404, 1973
20. Daniel DG, Campbell H, Turnbull AC: *Lancet 2*:287–289, 1967
21. The Veterans Administration Cooperative Urological Research Group: *J Urol 98*:516–522, 1967
22. Bailar JC: *Lancet 2*:560, 1967
23. Blackard C, *et al: Cancer 26*:249–256, 1970
24. Royal College of General Practitioners: *J Coll Gen Pract 13*:267–279, 1967
25. Inman WHW, Vessey MP: *Br Med J 2*:193–199, 1968
26. Vessey MP, Doll R: *Br Med J 2*:651–657, 1969
27. Sartwell PE, *et al: Am J Epidemiol 90*:365–380, 1969
28. Collaborative Group for the Study of Stroke in Young Women: *N Engl J Med 288*:871–878, 1973
29. Collaborative Group for the Study of Stroke in Young Women: *JAMA 231*:718–722, 1975
30. Mann JI, Inman WHW: *Br Med J 2*:245–248, 1975
31. Mann JI, *et al: Br Med J 2*:241–245, 1975
32. Inman WHW, *et al: Br Med J 2*:203–209, 1970
33. Stolley PD, *et al: Am J Epidemiol 102*:197–208, 1975
34. Vessey MP, *et al: Br Med J 3*:123–126, 1970
35. Greene GR, Sartwell PE: *Am J Public Health 62*:680–685, 1972
36. Rosenberg L, Armstrong MB, Jick H: *N Engl J Med 294*:1256–1259, 1976
37. Coronary Drug Project Research Group: *JAMA 214*:1303–1313, 1970
38. Baum J, *et al: Lancet 2*:926–928, 1973
39. Mays ET, *et al: JAMA 235*:730–732, 1976
40. Edmondson HA, Henderson B, Benton B: *N Engl J Med 294*:470–472, 1976
41. Pfeffer RI, Van Den Noort S: *Am J Epidemiol 103*:445–456, 1976

[*Shown in Product Identification Section*]

MESTINON® INJECTABLE ℞
(pyridostigmine bromide/Roche)

The following text is complete prescribing information based on official labeling in effect August 1, 1982.

Description: Mestinon Injectable is an active cholinesterase inhibitor. Chemically, pyridostigmine bromide is 3-hydroxy-1-methylpyridinium bromide dimethylcarbamate.

Each ml contains 5 mg pyridostigmine bromide/Roche compounded with 0.2% parabens (methyl and propyl) as preservatives, 0.02% sodium citrate and pH adjusted to approximately 5.0 with citric acid and, if necessary, sodium hydroxide.

Actions: Mestinon facilitates the transmission of impulses across the myoneural junction by inhibiting the destruction of acetylcholine by cholinesterase. Pyridostigmine is an analog of neostigmine (Prostigmin®) but differs from it clinically by having fewer side effects. Currently available data indicate that pyridostigmine may have a significantly lower degree and incidence of bradycardia, salivation and gastrointestinal stimulation. Animal studies using the injectable form of pyridostigmine and human studies using the oral preparation have indicated that pyridostigmine has a longer duration of action than does neostigmine measured under similar circumstances.

Indications: Mestinon Injectable is useful in the treatment of myasthenia gravis and as a reversal agent or antagonist to nondepolarizing muscle relaxants such as curariform drugs and gallamine triethiodide.

Contraindications: Known hypersensitivity to anticholinesterase agents; intestinal and urinary obstructions of mechanical type.

Warnings: Mestinon Injectable should be used with particular caution in patients with bronchial asthma or cardiac dysrhythmias. Transient bradycardia may occur and be relieved by atropine sulfate. Atropine should also be used with caution in patients with cardiac dysrhythmias. When large doses of Mestinon are administered, as during reversal of muscle relaxants, the prior or simultaneous injection of atropine sulfate is advisable. Because of the possibility of hypersensitivity in an occasional patient, atropine and antishock medication should always be readily available.

As is true of all cholinergic drugs, overdosage of Mestinon may result in cholinergic crisis, a state characterized by increasing muscle weakness which, through involvement of the muscles of respiration, may lead to death. Myasthenic crisis due to an increase in the severity of the disease is also accompanied by extreme muscle weakness and thus may be difficult to distinguish from cholinergic crisis on a symptomatic basis. Such differentiation is extremely important, since increases in doses of Mestinon or other drugs in this class in the presence of cholinergic crisis or of a refractory or "insensitive" state could have grave consequences. Osserman and Genkins[1] indicate that the two types of crisis may be differentiated by the use of Tensilon® (edrophonium chloride) as well as by clinical judgment. The treatment of the two conditions obviously differs radically. Whereas the presence of *myasthenic crisis* requires more intensive anticholinesterase therapy, *cholinergic crisis,* according to Osserman and Genkins,[1] calls for the prompt withdrawal of all drugs of this type. The immediate use of atropine in cholinergic crisis is also recommended. A syringe containing 1 mg of atropine sulfate should be immediately available to be given in aliquots intravenously to counteract severe cholinergic reactions.

Atropine may also be used to abolish or obtund gastrointestinal side effects or other muscarinic reactions; but such use, by masking signs of overdosage, can lead to inadvertent induction of cholinergic crisis.

For detailed information on the management of patients with myasthenia gravis, the physician is referred to one of the excellent reviews such as those by Osserman and Genkins,[2] Grob[3] or Schwab.[4,5]

When used as an antagonist to nondepolarizing muscle relaxants, adequate recovery of voluntary respiration and neuromuscular transmission must be obtained prior to discontinuation of respiratory assistance and there should be continuous patient observation. Satisfactory recovery may be defined by a combination of clinical judgment, respiratory measurements and observation of the effects of peripheral nerve stimulation. If there is any doubt concerning the adequacy of recovery from the effects of the nondepolarizing muscle relaxant, artificial ventilation should be continued until all doubt has been removed.

Usage in Pregnancy: The safety of Mestinon during pregnancy or lactation in humans has not been established. Therefore, use of Mestinon in women who may become pregnant requires weighing the drug's potential benefits against its possible hazards to mother and child.

Adverse Reactions: The side effects of Mestinon are most commonly related to overdosage and generally are of two varieties, muscarinic and nicotinic. Among those in the former group are nausea, vomiting, diarrhea, abdominal cramps, increased peristalsis, increased salivation, increased bronchial secretions, miosis and diaphoresis. Nicotinic side effects are comprised chiefly of muscle cramps, fasciculation and weakness. Muscarinic side effects can usually be counteracted by atropine, but for reasons shown in the preceding section the expedient is not without danger. As with any compound containing the bromide radical, a skin rash may be seen in an occasional patient. Such reactions usually subside promptly upon discontinuance of the medication. Thrombophlebitis has been reported subsequent to intravenous administration.

Dosage and Administration:

For Myasthenia Gravis—To supplement oral dosage, pre- and postoperatively, during labor and postpartum, during myasthenic crisis, or whenever oral therapy is impractical, approximately 1/30th of the oral dose of Mestinon may be given parenterally, either by intramuscular or *very slow* intravenous injection. *The patient must be closely observed for cholinergic reactions, particularly if the intravenous route is used.*

For details regarding the management of myasthenic patients who are to undergo major surgical procedures, see the article by Foldes.[6]

Neonates of myasthenic mothers may have transient difficulty in swallowing, sucking and breathing. Injectable Mestinon may be indicated—by symptomatology and use of the Tensilon® (edrophonium chloride) test—until Mestinon Syrup can be taken. To date the world literature consists of less than 100 neonate patients.[7] Of these only 5 were treated with injectable pyridostigmine, with the vast majority of the remaining neonates receiving neostigmine. Dosage requirements of Mestinon Injectable are minute, ranging from 0.05 mg to 0.15 mg/kg of body weight given intramuscularly. It is important to differentiate between cholinergic and myasthenic crises in neonates. (See WARNINGS.)

Mestinon given parenterally one hour before completion of second stage labor enables patients to have adequate strength during labor and provides protection to infants in the immediate postnatal state. For further information on the use of Mestinon Injectable in neonates of myasthenic mothers, see the article by Namba.[7]

NOTE: For information on a diagnostic test for myasthenia gravis, and on the evaluation and stabilization of therapy, please see product information on Tensilon® (edrophonium chloride/Roche).

For Reversal of Nondepolarizing Muscle Relaxants: When Mestinon Injectable is given intravenously to reverse the action of muscle relaxant drugs, it is recommended that atropine sulfate (0.6 to 1.2 mg) also be given intravenously immediately prior to the Mestinon. Side effects, notably excessive secretions and bradycardia, are thereby minimized. Usually 10 or 20 mg of Mestinon will be sufficient for antagonism of the effects of the nondepolarizing muscle relaxants. Although full recovery may occur within 15 minutes in most patients, others may require a half hour or more. Satisfactory reversal can be evident by adequate voluntary respiration, respiratory measurements and use of a peripheral nerve stimulator device. It is recommended that the patient be well ventilated and a patent airway maintained until complete recovery of normal respiration is as-

Continued on next page

Roche Labs.—Cont.

sured. Once satisfactory reversal has been attained, recurarization has not been reported. For additional information on the use of Mestinon for antagonism of nondepolarizing muscle relaxants see the article by Katz[8] and McNall.[9]

Failure of Mestinon Injectable to provide prompt (within 30 minutes) reversal may occur, *e.g.,* in the presence of extreme debilitation, carcinomatosis, or with concomitant use of certain broad spectrum antibiotics or anesthetic agents, notably ether. Under these circumstances ventilation must be supported by artificial means until the patient has resumed control of his respiration.

How Supplied: Mestinon is available in 2-ml ampuls (boxes of 10).

References:

1. K. E. Osserman and G. Genkins, *J.A.M.A. 183:*97, 1963.
2. K. E. Osserman and G. Genkins, *New York State J. Med., 61:*2076, 1961.
3. D. Grob, *Arch. Intern. Med., 108:*615, 1961.
4. R. S. Schwab, *New Eng. J. Med., 268:*596, 1963.
5. R. S. Schwab, *New Eng. J. Med., 268:*717, 1963.
6. F. F. Foldes and P. McNall, *Anesthesiology, 23:*837, 1962.
7. T. Namba *et al., Pediatrics, 45:*488, 1970.
8. R. L. Katz, *Anesthesiology, 28:*528, 1967.
9. P. McNall *et al., Anesthesia and Analgesia, 48:*1026, 1969.

MESTINON® ℞

(pyridostigmine bromide/Roche)
TABLETS and SYRUP
TIMESPAN® TABLETS

The following text is complete prescribing information based on official labeling in effect August 1, 1982.

Description: Mestinon is an orally active cholinesterase inhibitor. Chemically, pyridostigmine bromide is 3-hydroxy-1-methylpyridinium bromide dimethylcarbamate.

Actions: Mestinon inhibits the destruction of acetylcholine by cholinesterase and thereby permits freer transmission of nerve impulses across the neuromuscular junction. Pyridostigmine is an analog of neostigmine (Prostigmin®), but differs from it in certain clinically significant respects; for example, pyridostigmine is characterized by a longer duration of action and fewer gastrointestinal side effects.

Indication: Mestinon is useful in the treatment of myasthenia gravis.

Contraindications: Mestinon is contraindicated in mechanical intestinal or urinary obstruction, and particular caution should be used in its administration to patients with bronchial asthma. Care should be observed in the use of atropine for counteracting side effects, as discussed below.

Warnings: Although failure of patients to show clinical improvement may reflect underdosage, it can also be indicative of overdosage. As is true of all cholinergic drugs, overdosage of Mestinon may result in cholinergic crisis, a state characterized by increasing muscle weakness which, through involvement of the muscles of respiration, may lead to death. Myasthenic crisis due to an increase in the severity of the disease is also accompanied by extreme muscle weakness, and thus may be difficult to distinguish from cholinergic crisis on a symptomatic basis. Such differentiation is extremely important, since increases in doses of Mestinon or other drugs of this class in the presence of cholinergic crisis or of a refractory or "insensitive" state could have grave consequences. Osserman and Genkins[1] indicate that the differential diagnosis of the two types of crisis may require the use of Tensilon® (edrophonium chloride/Roche) as well as clinical judgment. The treatment of the two conditions obviously differs radically. Whereas the presence of myasthenic crisis suggests the need for more intensive anticholinesterase therapy, the diagnosis of cholinergic crisis, according to Osserman and Genkins,[1] calls for the prompt *withdrawal* of all drugs of this type. The immediate use of atropine in cholinergic crisis is also recommended.

Atropine may also be used to abolish or obtund gastrointestinal side effects or other muscarinic reactions; but such use, by masking signs of overdosage, can lead to inadvertent induction of cholinergic crisis.

For detailed information on the management of patients with myasthenia gravis, the physician is referred to one of the excellent reviews such as those by Osserman and Genkins,[2] Grob[3] or Schwab.[4,5]

Usage in Pregnancy: The safety of Mestinon during pregnancy or lactation in humans has not been established. Therefore, use of Mestinon in women who may become pregnant requires weighing the drug's potential benefits against its possible hazards to mother and child.

Adverse Reactions: The side effects of Mestinon are most commonly related to overdosage and generally are of two varieties, muscarinic and nicotinic. Among those in the former group are nausea, vomiting, diarrhea, abdominal cramps, increased peristalsis, increased salivation, increased bronchial secretions, miosis and diaphoresis. Nicotinic side effects are comprised chiefly of muscle cramps, fasciculation and weakness. Muscarinic side effects can usually be counteracted by atropine, but for reasons shown in the preceding section the expedient is not without danger. As with any compound containing the bromide radical, a skin rash may be seen in an occasional patient. Such reactions usually subside promptly upon discontinuance of the medication.

Dosage and Administration: Mestinon is available in three dosage forms:

Syrup—raspberry-flavored, containing 60 mg pyridostigmine bromide per teaspoonful (5 ml). This form permits accurate dosage adjustment for children and "brittle" myasthenic patients who require fractions of 60-mg doses. It is more easily swallowed, especially in the morning, by patients with bulbar involvement.

Conventional tablets—each containing 60 mg pyridostigmine bromide.

Timespan tablets—each containing 180 mg pyridostigmine bromide. This form provides uniformly slow release, hence prolonged duration of drug action; it facilitates control of myasthenic symptoms with fewer individual doses daily. The immediate effect of a 180-mg Timespan tablet is about equal to that of a 60-mg conventional tablet; however, its duration of effectiveness, although varying in individual patients, averages 2½ times that of a 60-mg dose.

Dosage: The size and frequency of the dosage must be adjusted to the needs of the individual patient.

Syrup and conventional tablets—The average dose is ten 60-mg tablets or ten 5-ml teaspoonfuls daily, spaced to provide maximum relief when maximum strength is needed. In severe cases as many as 25 tablets or teaspoonfuls a day may be required, while in mild cases one to six tablets or teaspoonfuls a day may suffice.

Timespan tablets—One to three 180-mg tablets, once or twice daily, will usually be sufficient to control symptoms; however, the needs of certain individuals may vary markedly from this average. The interval between doses should be at least six hours. For optimum control, it may be necessary to use the more rapidly acting regular tablets or syrup in conjunction with Timespan therapy.

Note: For information on a diagnostic test for myasthenia gravis, and for the evaluation and stabilization of therapy, please see product literature on Tensilon® (edrophonium chloride/Roche).

How Supplied: *Syrup,* 60 mg pyridostigmine bromide per teaspoonful (5 ml) and 5% alcohol—bottles of 16 fluid ounces (1 pint).

Tablets, scored, 60 mg pyridostigmine bromide each—bottles of 100 and 500.

Timespan tablets, scored, 180 mg pyridostigmine bromide each—bottles of 100.

Note: Because of the hygroscopic nature of the Timespan tablets, mottling may occur. This does not affect their efficacy.

References:

1. K. E. Osserman and G. Genkins, *J.A.M.A., 183:*97, 1963.
2. K. E. Osserman and G. Genkins, *New York State J. Med., 61:*2076, 1961.
3. D. Grob, *Arch. Int. Med., 108:*615, 1961.
4. R. S. Schwab, *New England J. Med., 268:*596, 1963.
5. R. S. Schwab, *New England J. Med., 268:*717, 1963.

[*Shown in Product Identification Section*]

NIPRIDE® ℞

(sodium nitroprusside/Roche)

The following text is complete prescribing information based on official labeling in effect August 1, 1982.

Nipride is only to be used as an infusion with sterile 5% dextrose in water. Not for direct injection.
Nipride should be used only when the necessary facilities and equipment for continuous monitoring of blood pressure are available.
If at infusion rates of up to 10 μg/kg/minute, an adequate reduction of blood pressure is not obtained within ten minutes, administration of Nipride should be terminated.
The instructions included herein should be reviewed thoroughly before administration of Nipride.

Description: Nipride (sodium nitroprusside/Roche) in injectable form contains the equivalent of 50 mg of sodium nitroprusside dihydrate (sodium nitrosylpentacyanoferrate [III]) in a 5-ml amber-colored, rubber-stoppered vial. Chemically, sodium nitroprusside is $Na_2Fe(CN)_5NO \cdot 2H_2O$. It is a reddish-brown powder which is soluble in water. In aqueous solution, it is photosensitive and should be protected from light.

Actions: Nipride is a potent, immediate acting, intravenous hypotensive agent. This action is probably due to the nitroso (NO) group. Its effect is almost immediate and ends when the IV infusion is stopped. Generally, Nipride is rapidly metabolized to cyanide and subsequently converted to thiocyanate through the mediation of a hepatic enzyme, rhodanase. The rate of conversion from cyanide to thiocyanate is dependent on the availability of sulfur, usually thiosulfate. The hypotensive effect is augmented by ganglionic blocking agents, volatile liquid anesthetics (such as halothane and enflurane) and by most other circulatory depressants.

The hypotensive effects of Nipride are caused by peripheral vasodilatation as a result of a direct action on the blood vessels, independent of autonomic innervation. No relaxation is seen in the smooth muscle of the uterus or duodenum *in situ* in animals.

Indications: Nipride is indicated for the immediate reduction of blood pressure of patients in hypertensive crises. Concomitant oral antihypertensive medication should be started while the hypertensive emergency is being brought under control with Nipride. There is no contraindication in using Nipride simultaneously with oral antihypertensive medications.

Nipride is also indicated for producing controlled hypotension during anesthesia in order to reduce bleeding in surgical procedures where surgeon and anesthesiologist deem it appropriate.

Contraindications: Nipride should not be used in the treatment of compensatory hypertension, *e.g.*, arteriovenous shunt or coarctation of the aorta.

The use of Nipride to produce controlled hypotension during surgery is contraindicated in patients with known inadequate cerebral circulation. Nipride is not intended for use during emergency surgery in moribund patients (A.S.A. Class 5E).

Warnings:

If excessive amounts of Nipride are used and/or sulfur—usually thiosulfate—supplies are depleted, cyanide toxicity can occur. (See OVERDOSAGE.)

If sodium nitroprusside infusion is to be extended, particularly if renal impairment is present, close attention should be given to not exceeding the recommended maximum infusion rate of 10 micrograms/kg/min. If in the course of therapy increased tolerance to the drug (as shown by the need for higher infusion rate) develops, it is essential to monitor blood acid-base balance, as metabolic acidosis is the earliest and most reliable evidence of cyanide toxicity. If signs of metabolic acidosis appear, Nipride should be discontinued and an alternate drug administered.

Serum thiocyanate levels do not reflect cyanide toxicity. However, serum thiocyanate levels should be monitored daily if treatment is to be extended, especially in patients with renal dysfunction. Thiocyanate accumulation and toxicity may manifest itself as tinnitus, blurred vision, delirium.

Since cyanide is converted into thiocyanate through the mediation of a hepatic enzyme, rhodanase, Nipride should be used with caution in patients with hepatic insufficiency.

Since thiocyanate inhibits both the uptake and binding of iodine, caution should be exercised in using Nipride in patients with hypothyroidism or severe renal impairment.

The following Warnings apply to use of Nipride for controlled hypotension during anesthesia:

1. Tolerance to blood loss, anemia and hypovolemia may be diminished. If possible, preexisting anemia and hypovolemia should be corrected prior to employing controlled hypotension.
2. Hypotensive anesthetic techniques may alter pulmonary ventilation perfusion ratio. Patients intolerant of additional dead air space at ordinary oxygen partial pressure may benefit from higher oxygen partial pressure.
3. Extreme caution should be exercised in patients who are especially poor surgical risks (A.S.A. Class 4 and 4E).

Nipride is only to be used as an infusion with sterile 5% dextrose in water. Not for direct injection.

Infusion rates greater than 10 μg/kg/minute are rarely required. If, at this rate, an adequate reduction in blood pressure is not obtained within 10 minutes, administration of Nipride should be stopped.

Hypertensive patients are more sensitive to the intravenous effect of sodium nitroprusside than are normotensive subjects. Patients who are receiving concomitant antihypertensive medications are more sensitive to the hypotensive effect of sodium nitroprusside and the dosage of Nipride should be adjusted accordingly.

Usage in Pregnancy: The safety of Nipride in women who are or who may become pregnant has not been established; hence, it should be given only when the potential benefits have been weighed against possible hazard to mother and child.

Precautions: Adequate facilities, equipment and personnel should be available for frequent and vigilant monitoring of blood pressure, since the hypotensive effect of Nipride occurs rapidly. When the infusion is slowed or stopped, blood pressure usually begins to rise immediately and returns to pretreatment levels within one to ten minutes. It should be used with caution and initially in low doses in elderly patients, since they may be more sensitive to the hypotensive effects of the drug. Young, vigorous males may require somewhat larger than ordinary doses of sodium nitroprusside for hypotensive anesthesia; however, the infusion rate of 10 μg/kg/minute should not be exceeded. Deepening of anesthesia, if indicated, might permit satisfactory conditions to exist within the recommended dosage range.

Because of the rapid onset of action and potency of Nipride, it should preferably be administered with the use of an infusion pump, micro-drip regulator, or any similar device that would allow precise measurement of the flow rate.

Once dissolved in solution, Nipride tends to deteriorate in the presence of light. Therefore, it should be protected from light by wrapping the container of the prepared solution with aluminum foil or other opaque materials. Solutions of Nipride should not be kept or used longer than twenty-four hours, while protected from light.

Nipride in aqueous solution yields the nitroprusside ion which reacts with even minute quantities of a wide variety of inorganic and organic substances to form usually highly colored reaction products (blue, green or dark red). If this occurs the infusion should be replaced.

Adverse Reactions: Nausea, retching, diaphoresis, apprehension, headache, restlessness, muscle twitching, retrosternal discomfort, palpitations, dizziness and abdominal pain have been noted with too rapid reduction in blood pressure, but these symptoms rapidly disappeared with slowing of the rate of the infusion or temporary discontinuation of infusion and did not reappear with continued slower rate of administration. Irritation at the infusion site may occur.

One case of hypothyroidism following prolonged therapy with intravenous sodium nitroprusside has been reported. A patient with severe hypertension with uremia received 3900 mg of sodium nitroprusside intravenously over a period of 21 days. This is one of the longest reported intravenous uses of this agent. There was no tachyphylaxis, but the patient developed evidence of hypothyroidism, together with retention of thiocyanate (9.5 mg/100 ml). With peritoneal dialysis the thiocyanate level diminished and the signs of hypothyroidism subsided.

Dosage and Administration: The contents of a 50-mg Nipride vial should be dissolved in 2 to 3 ml of dextrose in water. No other diluent should be used. Depending on the desired concentration, all of the prepared stock solution should be diluted in 250 to 1000 ml of 5 percent dextrose in water and promptly wrapped in aluminum foil or other opaque materials affording protection from light. Both the stock solution and the infusion solution should be freshly prepared and any unused portion discarded. The freshly prepared solution for infusion has a very faint brownish tint. If it is highly colored, it should be discarded (see PRECAUTIONS). *Once prepared, the solution should not be kept or used longer than 24 hours, while protected from light. The infusion fluid used for the administration of Nipride should not be employed as a vehicle for simultaneous administration of any other drug.*

In patients who are not receiving antihypertensive drugs, the average dose of Nipride for both adults and children is 3 μg/kg/minute (range of 0.5 to 10 μg/kg/minute). Usually, at 3 μg/kg/minute, blood pressure can be lowered by about 30 to 40 percent below the pretreatment diastolic levels and maintained. In hypertensive patients receiving concomitant antihypertensive medications, smaller doses are required. In order to avoid excessive levels of thiocyanate and lessen the possibility of a precipitous drop in blood pressure, infusion rates greater than 10 μg/kg/minute should rarely be used. If, at this rate, an adequate reduction of blood pressure is not obtained within 10 minutes, administration of Nipride should be stopped.

1 Vial (50 mg) Nipride in 1000 ml 5% DW (50 μg/ml)
1 Vial (50 mg) Nipride in 500 ml 5% DW (100 μg/ml)
1 Vial (50 mg) Nipride in 250 ml 5% DW (200 μg/ml)

Dose	μg/kg/min
Average	3
Range	0.5 to 10

The intravenous infusion of Nipride should be administered by an infusion pump, micro-drip regulator or any similar device that will allow precise measurement of the flow rate. Care should be taken to avoid extravasation. The rate of administration should be adjusted to maintain the desired antihypertensive or hypotensive effect, as determined by frequent blood pressure determinations. It is recommended that the blood pressure should not be allowed to drop at a too rapid rate and the systolic pressure not be lowered below 60 mmHg. In hypertensive emergencies Nipride infusion may be continued until the patient can safely be treated with oral antihypertensive medications alone.

How Supplied: Nipride injectable is supplied in 5-ml amber-colored vials containing the equivalent of 50 mg sodium nitroprusside dihydrate for reconstitution with dextrose in water—boxes of 1.

Human Pharmacology: Sodium nitroprusside administered intravenously to hypertensive and normotensive patients produced a marked lowering of the arterial blood pressure, slight increase in heart rate, a mild decrease in cardiac output and a moderate diminution in calculated total peripheral vascular resistance.

The decrease in calculated total peripheral vascular resistance suggests arteriolar vasodilatation. The decreases in cardiac and stroke index noted may be due to the peripheral vascular pooling of blood.

In hypertensive patients, moderate depressor doses induce renal vasodilatation roughly equivalent to the decrease in pressure without an appreciable increase in renal blood flow or a decrease in glomerular filtration.

In normotensive subjects, acute reduction of mean arterial pressure to 60 to 75 mmHg by infusion of sodium nitroprusside caused a significant increase in renin activity of renal venous plasma in correlation with the degree of reduction in pressure. Renal response to reduction in pressure was more striking in renovascular hypertensive patients, with significant increase in renin release occurring from the involved kidney at mean arterial pressures ranging from 90 to 137 mmHg. Furthermore, the magnitude of renin release from the involved kidney was significantly greater when compared with that in normotensive subjects, while in the contralateral, uninvolved kidney, no significant release of renin was detected during the reduction of pressure.

Overdosage: The first signs of sodium nitroprusside overdosage are those of profound hypotension. As with instances of depletion of thiosulfate supplies, overdosage may lead to cyanide toxicity. Metabolic acidosis and in-

Continued on next page

Roche Labs.—Cont.

creasing tolerance to the drug are early indications of overdosage. These may be associated with or followed by dyspnea, headache, vomiting, dizziness, ataxia and loss of consciousness. Sodium nitroprusside should then be immediately discontinued. Other signs of cyanide poisoning are coma, imperceptible pulse, absent reflexes, widely dilated pupils, pink color, distant heart sounds, and shallow breathing. Oxygen alone will not provide relief. Nitrites should be administered to induce methemoglobin formation. Methemoglobin, in turn, combines with cyanide bound to cytochrome oxidase to liberate cytochrome oxidase and form a non-toxic complex, cyanmethemoglobin. Cyanide then gradually dissociates from the latter and is converted by administration of thiosulfate to sodium thiocyanate in the presence of rhodanase.

Treatment: In cases of massive overdosage when signs of cyanide toxicity are present use the following regimen:

1. Discontinue administration of Nipride.
2. Administer amyl nitrite inhalations for 15 to 30 seconds each minute until 3% sodium nitrite solution can be prepared for I.V. administration.
3. Sodium nitrite 3% solution should be injected intravenously at a rate not exceeding 2.5 to 5.0 ml/minute up to a total dose of 10 to 15 ml with careful monitoring of the blood pressure.
4. Following the above steps, inject sodium thiosulfate intravenously, 12.5 Gm in 50 ml of 5% dextrose in water over a ten-minute period.
5. Since signs of overdosage may reappear, the patient must be observed for several hours.
6. If signs of overdosage reappear, sodium nitrite and sodium thiosulfate injections are repeated in one-half of the above doses.
7. During the administration of nitrites and later when thiocyanate formation is taking place, blood pressure may drop but can be corrected with vasopressor agents.

NISENTIL® Ⓒ II

(alphaprodine HCl/Roche)
INJECTABLE

The following text is complete prescribing information based on official labeling in effect August 1, 1982.

WARNINGS

- **Nisentil should be used with great caution and in reduced dosage in patients who are receiving other narcotic analgesics, general anesthetics, tranquilizers (including phenothiazines), sedative-hypnotics (including barbiturates), tricyclic antidepressants, MAO inhibitors and other CNS depressants, including alcohol. The depressant effects of Nisentil are potentiated in the presence of such drugs. *Fatalities, severe cerebral damage, respiratory depression, hypotension and profound sedation or coma may result.***
- **The DOSAGE AND ADMINISTRATION section should be strictly adhered to and careful attention should be given to the OVERDOSAGE section, particularly for treatment of respiratory depression.**
- **Nisentil should be used only when resuscitative equipment and personnel trained in such use are immediately available.**
- **Narcan (naloxone hydrochloride) should be immediately available when Nisentil use is contemplated. If clinically necessary, narcotic reversal with an agent such as Narcan should be performed following procedures in which Nisentil has been administered and the patient closely monitored by trained personnel familiar with such use. (See manufacturer's product information for full details of use.)**
- **Nisentil should be administered by intravenous, subcutaneous or submucosal routes only. (See DOSAGE AND ADMINISTRATION section.) Nisentil should *never* be administered intramuscularly because absorption is too unpredictable.**

Description: Nisentil (alphaprodine hydrochloride/Roche), a synthetic narcotic analgesic, is a sterile aqueous solution for intravenous, subcutaneous or submucosal administration.

Alphaprodine hydrochloride, a white powder which is freely soluble in water, has a calculated molecular weight of 297.82. Chemically, alphaprodine hydrochloride, a piperidine derivative, is (±)-1,3-dimethyl-4-phenyl-4-piperidinol propionate (ester) hydrochloride.

Clinical Pharmacology: Nisentil is a rapid-acting narcotic analgesic with a short duration of action. Except for its more rapid onset and shorter duration of analgesic action, the pharmacologic properties of Nisentil are similar to those of morphine or meperidine. Also, Nisentil is more potent than meperidine. Nisentil acts principally on the central nervous system and on organs composed of smooth muscle. Nisentil is metabolized and probably detoxified by the liver. There is evidence that Nisentil enters the fetal circulation.

In man, the half-life of Nisentil has been reported to be 131 minutes following intravenous administration.

The onset of action following intravenous administration is 1 to 2 minutes; the duration of analgesic action is 30 to 90 minutes. Subcutaneous administration provides analgesic effects usually within 10 minutes (ranging from 2 to 30 minutes). The duration of action following subcutaneous administration of Nisentil lasts from 1 hour to over 2 hours, depending upon the dosage administered, as compared to the duration of action of meperidine, which is 2 to 4 hours.

Indications and Usage: Nisentil is indicated for obstetric analgesia; for urologic examinations and procedures—particularly cystoscopy; preoperatively in major surgery; in minor surgery where rapid analgesia of brief duration is desirable—particularly in children requiring analgesia during dental procedures. Nisentil is indicated in children only for analgesia during dental procedures.

Contraindications: Nisentil is contraindicated in patients with a known hypersensitivity to this drug or to other opiates.

Warnings: (See WARNINGS box.) *Drug Dependence. Nisentil may be habit forming.* Nisentil can produce drug dependence of the morphine type and has the potential for being abused. Psychological and physical dependence and tolerance may develop upon repeated administration of Nisentil; it should be prescribed and administered with the same degree of caution appropriate to the use of morphine.

Intravenous Use: When Nisentil is given intravenously, special attention should be given to the possibility of respiratory depression. Such depression is especially likely in patients with pulmonary disease and in the elderly or debilitated. The patient should be lying down when the drug is administered, and Narcan (naloxone hydrochloride), a narcotic antagonist, and facilities for assisted or controlled respiration should be immediately available.

Hypotensive Effects: The administration of Nisentil may result in severe hypotension in the postoperative patient or in any individual whose ability to maintain blood pressure has been compromised by a depleted blood volume or by the administration of drugs, such as the phenothiazines or certain anesthetics. Narcotics may produce orthostatic hypotension in ambulatory patients.

Head Injury: The respiratory depressant effects of Nisentil may be markedly exaggerated in the presence of head injury or other intracranial lesions. Furthermore, narcotics produce adverse reactions which may obscure the clinical course of patients with head injuries. In such patients, Nisentil must be used with extreme caution and only if its use is deemed essential.

Asthma and Other Respiratory Conditions: Nisentil should be used with extreme caution in patients with bronchial asthma, chronic obstructive pulmonary disease or *cor pulmonale*. Similarly, it should be used with extreme caution in patients having a decreased respiratory reserve or with preexisting respiratory depression, hypoxia or hypercapnia. In such patients, usual therapeutic doses of narcotics may decrease respiratory drive while simultaneously increasing airway resistance to the point of apnea.

Chronic Pain: Nisentil should not be used for relief of chronic pain because its short duration of action would require more frequent administration and might increase the possibility of physical dependence.

Precautions: *General:* The administration of Nisentil or other narcotics may obscure the diagnosis or clinical course in patients with acute abdominal conditions. Nisentil should be administered with caution and the initial dose should be reduced in patients who are elderly or debilitated, and in those patients with acute alcoholism, severe CNS depression, delirium tremens, severe impairment of hepatic or renal function, hypothyroidism, Addison's disease, toxic psychosis and prostatic hypertrophy or urethral stricture.

Nisentil should be used with caution in patients with atrial flutter and other supraventricular tachycardias because of a possible vagolytic action which may produce a significant increase in the ventricular response rate. Nisentil may aggravate preexisting convulsions in patients with convulsive disorders. If dosage is escalated substantially above recommended levels because of tolerance development, convulsions may occur in individuals without a history of convulsive disorders.

Information for Patients: When Nisentil is administered to ambulatory patients, they should be cautioned against engaging in hazardous occupations requiring complete mental alertness such as operating machinery or driving a motor vehicle following drug administration.

Drug Interactions: (See WARNINGS box.)

Carcinogenesis, Mutagenesis, Impairment of Fertility: There have been no studies performed with Nisentil to permit an evaluation of its carcinogenic or mutagenic potential. Studies have not been performed to determine the effect of Nisentil on fertility or reproduction.

Pregnancy: Teratogenic Effects: Pregnancy Category C. There are no adequate or well-controlled studies of Nisentil in either laboratory animals or in pregnant women. While the safety and efficacy of Nisentil as an analgesic agent in obstetrics have been established, it is not known whether the drug can cause fetal harm when administered earlier in pregnancy. Nisentil should be used prior to the labor period only if it is clearly needed.

Nonteratogenic Effects: Animal studies have demonstrated that Nisentil depresses fetal respiratory movement and maternal respiratory rate in the rabbit and that it depresses both fetal and maternal cerebral oxygen availability in the guinea pig. (Also see *Labor and Delivery* section.)

Labor and Delivery: When used as an obstetric analgesic, Nisentil passes into the fetal circulation, which may produce depression of respiration and physiologic functions in the newborn. Narcan Neonatal should be used to reverse respiratory depression in the newborn. Resuscitation may be required. (See OVERDOSAGE section.) It has been reported that Nisentil may shorten the duration of labor; however, other studies have reported that Nisentil does not decrease the duration of labor. One study showed that in 9.6% of patients, Nisentil interfered with the mechanism of labor by decreasing the frequency and duration of uterine contractions. A possible explanation of this occurrence is that the drug was administered too early in labor. There are no long-term follow-up studies available on the growth, development and functional maturation of the child.

Nursing Mothers: It is not known whether alphaprodine is excreted in human milk. Because many drugs are excreted in human milk, caution should be exercised when alphaprodine is administered to a nursing woman.

Pediatric Use: Use of Nisentil in children for indications other than pediatric dentistry cannot be recommended because safety and effectiveness have not been established.

Adverse Reactions: Note: Included in this listing are adverse reactions which have not been reported with this specific drug; however, the pharmacologic similarities among the narcotics require that each of the reactions be considered with Nisentil administration.

Deaths and cerebral damage have been reported, especially when Nisentil has been given concomitantly with other CNS depressants. (See WARNINGS box.)

The major hazard of Nisentil administration, as with other narcotic analgesics, is respiratory depression which has led to respiratory arrest. This has also been reported following the administration of Nisentil preoperatively and during labor. The severity of respiratory depression may warrant active measures, particularly in neonatal situations. It is recommended that Narcan (naloxone hydrochloride) be administered in such cases. (See OVERDOSAGE section.) Circulatory depression, shock and cardiac arrest have also been reported following the administration of narcotic analgesics.

Other adverse reactions include:

Neurologic: Pinpoint pupils, visual disturbances, coma, sedation, dizziness, lightheadedness, headache, tremors, uncoordinated muscle movements.

Psychiatric: Euphoria, dysphoria, weakness, agitation, disorientation, confusion, hallucinations.

Cardiovascular: Hypotension, collapse, tachycardia, bradycardia, palpitation, syncope, phlebitis.

Dermatologic: Rash, urticaria (both local and generalized), pruritus, wheal and flare over the vein with intravenous injection.

Gastrointestinal: Nausea, emesis, constipation, dry mouth, biliary tract spasm.

Genitourinary: Urinary retention.

Miscellaneous: Diaphoresis, flushing, pain at the site of injection, allergic and anaphylactoid reactions, local tissue irritation and induration following subcutaneous injection.

Drug Abuse and Dependence: Nisentil is subject to Schedule II control under the Federal Controlled Substances Act of 1970. A narcotic order is required. This drug can produce drug dependence of the morphine type, and therefore has the potential for being abused. Psychological and physical dependence and tolerance may develop upon repeated administration of Nisentil, and consequently the same precautions should be taken in administering the drug as with morphine.

Overdosage: Serious overdosage with Nisentil is characterized by respiratory depression (a decrease in respiratory rate and/or tidal volume, Cheyne-Stokes respiration, cyanosis), extreme somnolence progressing to stupor or coma, skeletal muscle flaccidity, cold and clammy skin, and sometimes bradycardia and hypotension. In severe overdosage, apnea, circulatory collapse, cardiac arrest and death may occur. The triad of coma, pinpoint pupils and depressed respiration strongly suggests opioid poisoning.

Primary attention should be given to the reestablishment of adequate respiratory exchange through provision of a patent airway and through the institution of assisted or controlled ventilation. The narcotic antagonist Narcan (naloxone hydrochloride) is a specific antidote against respiratory depression resulting from narcotic overdosage or unusual sensitivity to narcotics. An appropriate dose of this antagonist should be administered simultaneously, preferably by the intravenous route, with efforts at respiratory resuscitation.

Oxygen, intravenous fluids, vasopressors and other supportive measures should be employed if needed.

Management of Respiratory Depression in Neonates: As in the case of adults, primary attention should be given to the reestablishment of adequate respiratory exchange through provision of a patent airway and through the institution of assisted or controlled ventilation. Administer Narcan (naloxone hydrochloride) at an initial dose of 0.01 mg/kg body weight by I.M., I.V., or S.C. routes. This dose may be repeated at 2- to 3-minute intervals, if necessary, until adequate narcotic reversal is accomplished. Oxygen, intravenous fluids, vasopressors or other supportive measures should be employed.

Note: The administration of the usual dose of a narcotic antagonist will precipitate an acute withdrawal syndrome in patients physically dependent on narcotics. The severity of this syndrome will depend on the degree of physical dependence and the dose of the antagonist administered.

The use of narcotic antagonists in such patients should be avoided if possible. If a narcotic antagonist must be used in physically-dependent patients to treat serious respiratory depression, the antagonist should be administered with extreme care using only $\frac{1}{5}$ to $\frac{1}{10}$ the usual initial dose.

Death, cerebral damage and respiratory arrest have been reported when Nisentil has been administered within recommended dosages but concomitantly with other CNS depressants or administered intramuscularly. (See WARNINGS box.) Death and cerebral damage have been reported in children administered $2\frac{1}{2}$ to $7\frac{1}{2}$ times the recommended dosage of Nisentil.

The acute toxicity of Nisentil is as follows:

Species	Route	LD_{50} (mg/kg)
Mouse	I.V.	51.5 ± 4.0
Rat	I.V.	25.0 ± 6.8
	S.C.	50.0 ± 17.7
	P.O.	90.0 ± 18.7
Rabbit	I.V.	22.0 ± 2.9
Dog	I.V.	36.2 ± 18.3

Dosage and Administration: The dosages suggested are the usual amounts employed in adults; however, as with any other narcotic analgesic, good medical practice dictates the use of the minimal effective dose. If dosage is escalated substantially above recommended levels because of tolerance development, convulsions may occur. *The usual dosage is in the range of 0.4 to 0.6 mg/kg intravenously or 0.4 to 1.2 mg/kg subcutaneously.* Initially, the lower dosage range is recommended in order to evaluate the patient's response. Thus, *the initial intravenous dose should not exceed 30 mg, nor should the initial subcutaneous dose exceed 60 mg.* The total dose administered by any route should not be more than 240 mg in 24 hours. Whenever this drug is given intravenously, a narcotic antagonist and facilities for resuscitation should be available.

Subcutaneous administration provides analgesic effects usually within 10 minutes, lasting from 1 to over 2 hours. If required, an additional $\frac{1}{4}$ dose may be given 30 minutes after the initial dose. The *intravenous* route is recommended when more rapid onset (1 to 2 minutes) and shorter duration ($\frac{1}{2}$ to $1\frac{1}{2}$ hours) of action are desired. An additional amount of $\frac{1}{4}$ the initial dose may be injected after 15 minutes, if required.

Obstetrics: Initially, 40 to 60 mg subcutaneously after cervical dilation has begun, repeated as required at two-hour intervals. Nisentil may be combined with scopolamine or atropine, and may be used in conjunction with nerve block or inhalation anesthesia as required. (See WARNINGS box on use with CNS depressants.)

Urologic Procedures, e.g., Cystoscopy: Initially, 20 to 30 mg intravenously.

Preoperatively in Major Surgery: Initially, 20 to 40 mg subcutaneously or 10 to 20 mg intravenously.

Minor Surgery: Initially, 40 mg subcutaneously or 20 mg intravenously.

Pediatric Dentistry: The usual recommended dose is 0.3 to 0.6 mg/kg by submucosal route only. If clinically necessary, narcotic reversal with an agent such as Narcan (naloxone hydrochloride) should be performed following procedures in which Nisentil has been administered and the patient closely monitored by trained personnel familiar with such use. (See manufacturer's product information for full details of use.) **Nisentil should be used with great caution and in reduced dosage in pediatric dental patients who are receiving other narcotic analgesics, general anesthetics, tranquilizers (including phenothiazines), sedative-hypnotics (including barbiturates), tricyclic antidepressants, MAO inhibitors and other CNS depressants. The depressant effects of Nisentil are potentiated in the presence of such drugs. Fatalities, severe cerebral damage, respiratory depression, hypotension and profound sedation or coma may result.** *Use of Nisentil in children for indications other than pediatric dentistry cannot be recommended due to limited experience.*

Parenteral drug products should be inspected visually for particulate matter and discoloration prior to administration, whenever possible.

How Supplied: Nisentil is supplied in:

1-ml ampuls—each ml contains 40 mg/ml alphaprodine hydrochloride compounded with 0.0875% citric acid and sodium citrate to adjust pH to approximately 4.6—boxes of 10 (NDC 0004-1915-06).

10-ml vials—each ml contains 60 mg/ml alphaprodine hydrochloride compounded with 0.45% phenol as preservative, 0.0875% citric acid and sodium citrate to adjust pH to approximately 4.6 (NDC 0004-1917-06).

Narcotic order required.

NOLUDAR® 300 Ⓒ
(methyprylon/Roche)
CAPSULES

NOLUDAR® Ⓒ
(methyprylon/Roche)
TABLETS

The following text is complete prescribing information based on official labeling in effect August 1, 1982.

Description: Noludar (methyprylon/Roche), a hypnotic, is available in three dosage forms for oral use: capsules containing 300 mg of methyprylon (Noludar® 300), tablets containing 200 mg of methyprylon and tablets containing 50 mg of methyprylon.

Chemically, methyprylon, a piperidine derivative, is 3,3-diethyl-5-methyl-2,4-piperidinedione. Methyprylon is a white crystalline powder, freely soluble in water, with a molecular weight of 183.25.

Clinical Pharmacology: In animal studies, methyprylon has been shown to increase the threshold of the arousal centers in the brain-

Continued on next page

Roche Labs.—Cont.

stem. In humans, when taken at bedtime, Noludar usually induces sleep within 45 minutes and provides sleep for 5 to 8 hours.

Methyprylon is rapidly absorbed following oral administration and is approximately 60% bound to plasma proteins. Mean peak plasma concentrations of methyprylon in six subjects following a single 650-mg dose occurred at one to two hours postadministration at concentrations of 5.7 to 10.0 mcg/ml. The concentrations declined to 3.3 to 7.9 mcg/ml at 4 hours. Trace amounts of the dihydro-metabolite were detected in the one- to four-hour plasma specimens. Following administration of 400 mg of Noludar, less than 1% of the dose was recovered as intact drug and approximately 23% as identified metabolites in the 0- to 72-hour urine specimens. Identified metabolites include the dihydro-metabolite, the 6-oxo, the 5-hydroxymethyl and the 5-carboxyl derivatives. Methyprylon is metabolized by two pathways: dehydrogenation with subsequent oxidation to form the alcohol and corresponding acid, and oxidation to form 6-oxymethyprylon. Therapeutic blood concentrations are approximately 1 mg%. Serum concentrations in excess of 30 mg/l are generally consistent with unconsciousness in the acutely poisoned patient.

Indications and Usage: Noludar is indicated for use as a hypnotic. In the sleep laboratory it has been objectively determined that Noludar is effective for at least 7 consecutive nights of drug administration. Since insomnia is often transient and intermittent, the prolonged use of hypnotics is usually not indicated and should only be undertaken concomitantly with appropriate evaluation of the patient.

Contraindications: Noludar is contraindicated in patients with known hypersensitivity to the drug.

Warnings: *Synergistic effects:* The concomitant use of alcohol or other CNS depressants may produce additive CNS depressant effects.

Precautions: *General:* Total daily intake should not exceed 400 mg, as greater amounts do not significantly increase hypnotic effects. Caution should be exercised in treating patients with impaired renal or hepatic function. In view of isolated reports associating methyprylon with exacerbation of porphyria, caution should be exercised in prescribing methyprylon to patients suffering from this disease.

Information for patients: Patients receiving Noludar should be cautioned about possible combined effects with alcohol and other CNS depressants. Since Noludar is an effective hypnotic agent, patients should also be cautioned against engaging in hazardous occupations requiring complete mental alertness, such as operating machinery or driving a motor vehicle shortly after ingesting the drug.

Laboratory tests: If Noludar is used repeatedly or over prolonged periods of time, periodic blood counts should be made.

Drug interactions: Noludar stimulates the hepatic microsomal enzyme system. (Also see WARNINGS section.)

Carcinogenesis, mutagenesis, impairment of fertility: Studies sufficient to evaluate the carcinogenic or mutagenic potential of Noludar have not been performed. Noludar had no adverse effects on the reproductive process in rats when administered at dose levels of 5 and 50 mg/kg/day.

Pregnancy: Teratogenic effects: Pregnancy Category B. Reproduction studies have been performed in rats and in rabbits at doses up to approximately 9 times the maximum recommended human dose and have revealed no evidence of teratogenic effects on the fetus due to Noludar. There are, however, no adequate or well-controlled studies in pregnant women. Because animal reproduction studies are not always predictive of human response, this drug should be used in pregnancy only if clearly needed.

Nonteratogenic effects: At a dose of 50 mg/kg/day, Noludar caused an increased incidence of resorptions in the rabbit.

Nursing mothers: It is not known whether this drug is excreted in human milk. Because many drugs are excreted in human milk, caution should be exercised when Noludar is administered to a nursing woman.

Pediatric use: Safety and effectiveness in children below the age of 12 have not been established.

Adverse Reactions: *Neurologic:* Convulsions, hallucinations, ataxia, EEG changes, pyrexia, morning drowsiness, headache, dizziness, vertigo.

Psychiatric: Acute brain syndrome and confusion (particularly in elderly patients), paradoxical excitation, anxiety, depression, nightmares, dreaming.

Hematologic: Aplastic anemia, thrombocytopenic purpura, neutropenia.

Cardiovascular: Hypotension, syncope.

Ophthalmic: Diplopia, blurred vision.

Gastrointestinal: Esophagitis, vomiting, nausea, diarrhea, constipation.

Allergic: Generalized allergic reactions.

Dermatologic: Pruritus, rash.

Miscellaneous: Hangover effect.

Drug Abuse and Dependence: Noludar is subject to Schedule III control under the Federal Controlled Substances Act of 1970. Physical and psychological dependence have been reported in patients receiving Noludar therapy. Withdrawal symptoms, when they occur, tend to resemble those associated with the withdrawal of barbiturates and should be treated in a similar fashion. Caution must be exercised in administering Noludar to individuals known to be addiction-prone or to those whose history suggests that they may increase the dosage on their own initiative. As with all hypnotic agents, good medical practice suggests the desirability of limiting repeated prescriptions without adequate medical supervision.

Overdosage: Manifestations of Noludar overdosage include somnolence, confusion, coma, shock, constricted pupils, respiratory depression, hypotension, tachycardia, edema and hepatic dysfunction. Blood concentrations of methyprylon associated with serious toxic symptoms in humans have been reported to range from 3 to 6 mg%. Blood concentrations of methyprylon that have been reported to cause death range from 5.3 to 114 mg%. A fatality occurred after ingestion of 6 grams of the drug. Respiration, pulse and blood pressure should be monitored, as in all cases of drug overdosage. General supportive measures should be employed, along with immediate gastric lavage with precautions to prevent pulmonary aspiration. Appropriate intravenous fluids should be administered and an adequate airway maintained. Hypotension may be combated by the use of Levophed® (norepinephrine bitartrate), Aramine (metaraminol bitartrate) or other accepted antihypotensive measures. Several reports clearly indicate that hemodialysis is of value. Therefore, its use should be considered, especially in those cases where supportive measures are failing and adequate urinary output cannot be maintained. There have been occasional reports of excitation and convulsions in patients following methyprylon overdosage, almost invariably during the recovery phase. Should these occur, barbiturates may be used, but only with great caution. As with the management of intentional overdosage of any drug, it should be borne in mind that multiple agents may have been ingested.

The acute toxicity of Noludar is as follows:

Species	Route	$LD_{50} \pm$ S.E. (mg/kg)
Mouse	P.O.	1000 ± 45
Rat	P.O.	400 ± 32
Rabbit	P.O.	340 ± 78

Dosage and Administration: The dosage should be individualized for maximum beneficial effects. The usual adult dosage is one capsule (300 mg) or one or two tablets of 200 mg (200 or 400 mg) before retiring.

Noludar is not recommended for use in children under 12 years of age. In children over 12 years, the effective dosage of Noludar varies greatly and, therefore, should also be individualized. Treatment may be initiated with one 50-mg tablet at bedtime, and increased up to 200 mg, if required.

How Supplied: Noludar is available as amethyst and white 300-mg capsules in bottles of 100 (NDC 0004-0019-01) and in bottles of 500 (NDC 0004-0019-14); as 50-mg white, scored tablets in bottles of 100 (NDC 0004-0016-01); and as 200-mg white, scored tablets in bottles of 100 (NDC 0004-0017-01). Imprints on all dosage forms of Noludar are as follows: Noludar 300—NOLUDAR® 300 Roche; Noludar 50-mg tablets—ROCHE 16; Noludar 200-mg tablets—ROCHE 17.

[*Shown in Product Identification Section*]

PANTOPON® Ⓒ

(hydrochlorides of opium alkaloids/Roche)

The following text is complete prescribing information based on official labeling in effect August 1, 1982.

Description: Pantopon (hydrochlorides of opium alkaloids), a narcotic analgesic, is a sterile injectable preparation for intramuscular and subcutaneous administration. It contains all the alkaloids of opium in a highly purified form free from inert matter and in approximately the same proportions as they occur in nature.

Hydrochlorides of opium alkaloids is a yellowish-gray powder which is freely soluble in water. The approximate composition of Pantopon is as follows: anhydrous morphine — 50 percent, and bases of secondary opium alkaloids — 29.9 to 34.2 percent. One part of Pantopon is equivalent to five parts of opium, U.S.P.

One ml of Pantopon contains 20 mg hydrochlorides of opium alkaloids compounded with 6% alcohol, 136 mg glycerin, 0.2% parabens (methyl and propyl) as preservatives, and either acetic acid, sodium hydroxide, or both, as necessary to adjust pH to approximately 3.3.

Clinical Pharmacology: The action of Pantopon is essentially that of opium. Pantopon, therefore, exhibits not only the action of morphine but also the actions of codeine, papaverine and other alkaloids present in opium. The other alkaloids in Pantopon enhance the sedative and analgesic effects of morphine and tend to minimize its undesirable side effects. Pharmacokinetic data on Pantopon are not available, however, data are available on morphine, the major component of Pantopon.

Morphine acts as an agonist interacting with stereospecific receptors in the brain and other tissues; the receptor sites are distributed throughout the CNS and are present in highest concentrations in the limbic system, thalamus, striatum, hypothalamus, midbrain and spinal cord. Morphine is well absorbed after subcutaneous and intramuscular administration. When therapeutic concentrations of morphine are present in plasma, approximately one-third of the drug is protein bound. Unbound morphine accumulates in parenchyma tissues (such as lung, liver, kidney and spleen) and skeletal muscle; however, 24 hours following the last dose, concentrations of the drug in these tissues are quite low.

The half-life of morphine in plasma is about 2.5 to 3 hours in young adults; in older patients, the half-life may be more prolonged. The major metabolic pathway for the drug is conjugation with glucuronic acid and the major route of elimination is through glomerular filtration. Ninety percent of the total excretion takes place during the first 24 hours after administration, although traces of the drug are detectable in the urine for well over 48 hours. About 7 to 10% of administered morphine eventually appears in the feces.

Indications and Usage: Pantopon is indicated in conditions in which the analgesic, sedative-hypnotic or narcotic effect of an opiate is needed. It is recommended for the relief of severe pain in place of morphine.

Contraindications: Pantopon is contraindicated in patients with a known hypersensitivity to this drug or to other opiates.

Warnings: *Drug Dependence. Pantopon may be habit forming.* Pantopon can produce drug dependence of the morphine type and has the potential for being abused. Psychological and physical dependence and tolerance may develop upon repeated administration of Pantopon; it should be prescribed and administered with the same degree of caution appropriate to the use of morphine.

Intravenous Use: Pantopon should not be administered intravenously. Rapid intravenous injection of narcotic analgesics increases the incidence of adverse reactions; severe respiratory depression, apnea, hypotension, peripheral circulatory collapse and cardiac arrest have occurred.

Interaction with Other Central Nervous System Depressants: Pantopon should be used with great caution and in reduced dosage in patients who are concurrently receiving other narcotic analgesics, general anesthetics, tranquilizers (including phenothiazines), sedative-hypnotics (including barbiturates), tricyclic antidepressants, MAO inhibitors and other CNS depressants, including alcohol. Respiratory depression, hypotension and profound sedation or coma may result.

Hypotensive Effects: The administration of Pantopon may result in severe hypotension in the postoperative patient or in any individual whose ability to maintain blood pressure has been compromised by a depleted blood volume or by the administration of drugs, such as phenothiazines or certain anesthetics.

Head Injury: The respiratory depressant effects of Pantopon may be markedly exaggerated in the presence of head injury or other intracranial lesions. Furthermore, narcotics produce adverse reactions which may obscure the clinical course of patients with head injuries. In such patients Pantopon must be used with extreme caution and only if its use is deemed essential.

Asthma and Other Respiratory Conditions: Pantopon should be used with extreme caution in patients with bronchial asthma, chronic obstructive pulmonary disease or *cor pulmonale.* Similarly, it should be used with extreme caution in patients having a decreased respiratory reserve or with pre-existing respiratory depression, hypoxia or hypercapnia. In such patients, usual therapeutic doses of narcotics may decrease respiratory drive while simultaneously increasing airway resistance to the point of apnea.

Precautions: *General:* The administration of Pantopon or other narcotics may obscure the diagnosis or clinical course in patients with acute abdominal conditions. Pantopon should be administered with caution and the initial dose should be reduced in patients who are elderly or debilitated and in those patients with severe impairment of hepatic or renal function, hypothyroidism, Addison's disease, toxic psychosis, and prostatic hypertrophy or urethral stricture.

Information for Patients: In the unlikely event that Pantopon would be administered to ambulatory patients, they should be cautioned that Pantopon may impair the mental and/or physical abilities required for the performance of potentially hazardous tasks such as driving a car or operating machinery.

Drug Interactions: See WARNINGS section.

Carcinogenesis, mutagenesis, impairment of fertility: There have been no studies performed with Pantopon to permit an evaluation of its carcinogenic or mutagenic potential. Studies have not been performed to determine the effect of Pantopon on fertility and reproduction.

Pregnancy:

Teratogenic Effects. Pregnancy Category C. Animal studies have demonstrated the teratogenicity of morphine, the major component of Pantopon, in rats, mice and hamsters.

There are no adequate or well-controlled studies of Pantopon in either laboratory animals or in pregnant women. It is also not known whether Pantopon can cause fetal harm when administered to a pregnant woman or if it can affect reproductive capacity. Pantopon should be used during pregnancy only if the potential benefit justifies the potential risk to the fetus.

Nursing Mothers: It has been reported that morphine is excreted in human milk in microgram amounts. Because of the potential for serious adverse reactions from Pantopon in nursing infants, a decision should be made whether to discontinue nursing or to discontinue the drug, taking into account the importance of the drug to the mother.

Pediatric Use: Safety and effectiveness in children have not been established.

Adverse Reactions:

Note: Included in this listing are adverse reactions which have not been reported with this specific drug; however, the pharmacologic similarities among the narcotics require that each of the reactions be considered with Pantopon administration.

Neurologic: Respiratory depression and arrest, pinpoint pupils, visual disturbances, coma, sedation, dizziness, headache, tremors, uncoordinated muscle movements. Inadvertent injection in close proximity to a nerve may result in a sensory-motor paralysis which is usually, though not always, transitory.

Psychiatric: Delirium, euphoria, dysphoria, weakness, agitation, hallucinations.

Cardiovascular: Hypotension, collapse, tachycardia, bradycardia, palpitation.

Dermatologic: Rash, urticaria (local and generalized), pruritus.

Gastrointestinal: Nausea, emesis, constipation, dry mouth, biliary tract spasm.

Genitourinary: Urinary retention.

Miscellaneous: Diaphoresis, flushing, pain at the site of injection, anaphylactoid reactions.

Drug Abuse and Dependence: Pantopon is subject to Schedule II control under the Federal Controlled Substances Act of 1970. This drug can produce drug dependence of the morphine type and, therefore, has the potential for being abused. Psychological and physical dependence and tolerance may develop upon repeated administration of Pantopon, and consequently the same precautions should be taken in administering the drug as with morphine. A narcotic order is required.

Overdosage: Serious overdosage with Pantopon is characterized by respiratory depression (a decrease in respiratory rate and/or tidal volume, Cheyne-Stokes respiration, cyanosis), extreme somnolence progressing to stupor or coma, skeletal muscle flaccidity, cold and clammy skin, and sometimes bradycardia and hypotension. In severe overdosage, apnea, circulatory collapse, cardiac arrest and death may occur. The triad of coma, pinpoint pupils and depressed respiration strongly suggests opioid poisoning.

Primary attention should be given to the reestablishment of adequate respiratory exchange through provision of a patent airway and through the institution of assisted or controlled ventilation. The narcotic antagonist, naloxone hydrochloride (Narcan), is a specific antidote against respiratory depression resulting from narcotic overdosage or unusual sensitivity to narcotics. An appropriate dose of this antagonist should be administered, preferably by the intravenous route, simultaneously with efforts at respiratory resuscitation. Levallorphan tartrate (Lorfan®) is also a narcotic antagonist which may be used in these cases. Administration is by the intravenous route, in an initial dose of 1 mg; followed at 10 to 15 minute intervals by additional doses of 0.5 mg as needed.

An antagonist should not be administered in the absence of clinically significant respiratory or cardiovascular depression.

Oxygen, intravenous fluids, vasopressors and other supportive measures should be employed if needed.

Note: The administration of the usual dose of a narcotic antagonist will precipitate an acute withdrawal syndrome in patients physically dependent on narcotics. The severity of this syndrome will depend on the degree of physical dependence and the dose of the antagonist administered. The use of narcotic antagonists in such patients should be avoided if possible. If a narcotic antagonist must be used in physically dependent patients to treat serious respiratory depression, the antagonist should be administered with extreme care using only one-fifth to one-tenth the usual initial dose.

The intravenous LD_{50} of Pantopon in mice is 96 to 99 mg/kg.

Dosage and Administration: One-third grain (20 mg) of Pantopon with a morphine content of 1/6 grain (10 mg) is therapeutically equivalent to and is usually administered where 1/4 grain (15 mg) of morphine is indicated.

Usual Adult Dosage:

5 to 20 mg (1/12 to 1/3 grain) approximately every 4 to 5 hours according to the individual needs and severity of pain. Administer only by intramuscular or subcutaneous injection.

Parenteral drug products should be inspected visually for particulate matter and discoloration prior to administration, whenever solution and container permit.

How Supplied: Pantopon is supplied in 1-ml ampuls each containing 20 mg (1/3 grain) hydrochlorides of opium alkaloids/Roche — boxes of 10 (NDC 0004-1918-06).

PROSTIGMIN® ℞

(neostigmine methylsulfate/Roche)
INJECTABLE

The following text is complete prescribing information based on official labeling in effect August 1, 1982.

Description: Prostigmin (neostigmine methylsulfate/Roche) Injectable, an anticholinesterase agent, is a sterile aqueous solution intended for intramuscular, intravenous or subcutaneous administration.

Prostigmin Injectable is available in the following concentrations:

Prostigmin 1:2000 Ampuls— each ml contains 0.5 mg neostigmine methylsulfate compounded with 0.2% parabens (methyl and propyl) as preservatives and sodium hydroxide to adjust pH to approximately 5.9.

Prostigmin 1:4000 Ampuls— each ml contains 0.25 mg neostigmine methylsulfate compounded with 0.2% parabens (methyl and propyl) as preservatives and sodium hydroxide to adjust pH to approximately 5.9.

Prostigmin 1:1000 Multiple Dose Vials— each ml contains 1 mg neostigmine methylsulfate compounded with 0.45% phenol as preservative, 0.2 mg sodium acetate, and acetic acid and sodium hydroxide to adjust pH to approximately 5.9.

Prostigmin 1:2000 Multiple Dose Vials— each ml contains 0.5 mg neostigmine methylsulfate compounded with 0.45% phenol as preservative, 0.2 mg sodium acetate, and acetic acid and sodium hydroxide to adjust pH to approximately 5.9.

Continued on next page

Roche Labs.—Cont.

Chemically, neostigmine methylsulfate is (*m*-hydroxyphenyl)trimethylammonium methylsulfate dimethylcarbamate. It has a molecular weight of 334.39.

Clinical Pharmacology: Neostigmine inhibits the hydrolysis of acetylcholine by competing with acetylcholine for attachment to acetylcholinesterase at sites of cholinergic transmission. It enhances cholinergic action by facilitating the transmission of impulses across neuromuscular junctions. It also has a direct cholinomimetic effect on skeletal muscle and possibly on autonomic ganglion cells and neurons of the central nervous system. Neostigmine undergoes hydrolysis by cholinesterase and is also metabolized by microsomal enzymes in the liver. Protein binding to human serum albumin ranges from 15 to 25 percent. Following intramuscular administration, neostigmine is rapidly absorbed and eliminated. In a study of five patients with myasthenia gravis, peak plasma levels were observed at 30 minutes, and the half-life ranged from 51 to 90 minutes. Approximately 80 percent of the drug was eliminated in urine within 24 hours; approximately 50 percent as the unchanged drug, and 30 percent as metabolites. Following intravenous administration, plasma half-life ranges from 47 to 60 minutes have been reported with a mean half-life of 53 minutes.

The clinical effects of neostigmine usually begin within 20 to 30 minutes after intramuscular injection and last from 2.5 to 4 hours.

Indications and Usage: Prostigmin is indicated for:

— the symptomatic control of myasthenia gravis when oral therapy is impractical.

— the prevention and treatment of postoperative distention and urinary retention after mechanical obstruction has been excluded.

— reversal of effects of nondepolarizing neuromuscular blocking agents (*e.g.*, tubocurarine, metocurine, gallamine, or pancuronium) after surgery.

Contraindications: Prostigmin is contraindicated in patients with known hypersensitivity to the drug. It is also contraindicated in patients with peritonitis or mechanical obstruction of the intestinal or urinary tract.

Warnings: Prostigmin should be used with caution in patients with epilepsy, bronchial asthma, bradycardia, recent coronary occlusion, vagotonia, hyperthyroidism, cardiac arrhythmias or peptic ulcer. When large doses of Prostigmin are administered, the prior or simultaneous injection of atropine sulfate may be advisable. Separate syringes should be used for the Prostigmin and atropine. Because of the possibility of hypersensitivity in an occasional patient, atropine and antishock medication should always be readily available.

Precautions: *General:* It is important to differentiate between myasthenic crisis and cholinergic crisis caused by overdosage of Prostigmin. Both conditions result in extreme muscle weakness but require radically different treatment. (See OVERDOSAGE section.)

Drug Interactions: Prostigmin does not antagonize, and may in fact prolong, the Phase I block of *depolarizing* muscle relaxants such as succinylcholine or decamethonium. Certain antibiotics, especially neomycin, streptomycin and kanamycin, have a mild but definite nondepolarizing blocking action which may accentuate neuromuscular block. These antibiotics should be used in the myasthenic patient only where definitely indicated, and then careful adjustment should be made of the anticholinesterase dosage. Local and some general anesthetics, antiarrhythmic agents and other drugs that interfere with neuromuscular transmission should be used cautiously, if at all, in patients with myasthenia gravis; the dose of Prostigmin may have to be increased accordingly.

Carcinogenesis, Mutagenesis and Impairment of Fertility: There have been no studies with Prostigmin which would permit an evaluation of its carcinogenic or mutagenic potential. Studies on the effect of Prostigmin on fertility and reproduction have not been performed.

Pregnancy:

Teratogenic Effects: Pregnancy Category C. There are no adequate or well-controlled studies of Prostigmin in either laboratory animals or in pregnant women. It is not known whether Prostigmin can cause fetal harm when administered to a pregnant woman or can affect reproductive capacity. Prostigmin should be given to a pregnant woman only if clearly needed.

Nonteratogenic Effects: Anticholinesterase drugs may cause uterine irritability and induce premature labor when given intravenously to pregnant women near term.

Nursing Mothers: It is not known whether Prostigmin is excreted in human milk. Because many drugs are excreted in human milk and because of the potential for serious adverse reactions from Prostigmin in nursing infants, a decision should be made whether to discontinue nursing or to discontinue the drug, taking into account the importance of the drug to the mother.

Pediatric Use: Safety and effectiveness in children have not been established.

Adverse Reactions: Side effects are generally due to an exaggeration of pharmacological effects of which salivation and fasciculation are the most common. Bowel cramps and diarrhea may also occur.

The following additional adverse reactions have been reported following the use of either neostigmine bromide or neostigmine methylsulfate:

Allergic: Allergic reactions and anaphylaxis.

Neurologic: Dizziness, convulsions, loss of consciousness, drowsiness, headache, dysarthria, miosis and visual changes.

Cardiovascular: Cardiac arrhythmias (including bradycardia, tachycardia, A-V block and nodal rhythm) and nonspecific EKG changes have been reported, as well as cardiac arrest, syncope and hypotension. These have been predominantly noted following the use of the injectable form of Prostigmin.

Respiratory: Increased oral, pharyngeal and bronchial secretions, dyspnea, respiratory depression, respiratory arrest and bronchospasm.

Dermatologic: Rash and urticaria.

Gastrointestinal: Nausea, emesis, flatulence and increased peristalsis.

Genitourinary: Urinary frequency.

Musculoskeletal: Muscle cramps and spasms, arthralgia.

Miscellaneous: Diaphoresis, flushing and weakness.

Overdosage: Overdosage of Prostigmin can cause cholinergic crisis, which is characterized by increasing muscle weakness, and through involvement of the muscles of respiration, may result in death. Myasthenic crisis, due to an increase in the severity of the disease, is also accompanied by extreme muscle weakness and may be difficult to distinguish from cholinergic crisis on a symptomatic basis. However, such differentiation is extremely important because increases in the dose of Prostigmin or other drugs in this class, in the presence of cholinergic crisis or of a refractory or "insensitive" state, could have grave consequences. The two types of crises may be differentiated by the use of Tensilon® (edrophonium chloride/Roche) as well as by clinical judgment.

Treatment of the two conditions differs radically. Whereas the presence of *myasthenic crisis* requires more intensive anticholinesterase therapy, *cholinergic crisis* calls for the prompt withdrawal of all drugs of this type. The immediate use of atropine in cholinergic crisis is also recommended.

Atropine may also be used to abolish or minimize gastrointestinal side effects or other muscarinic reactions; but such use, by masking signs of overdose, can lead to inadvertent induction of cholinergic crisis.

The LD_{50} of neostigmine methylsulfate in mice is 0.3 ± 0.02 mg/kg intravenously, 0.54 ± 0.03 mg/kg subcutaneously, and 0.395 ± 0.025 mg/kg intramuscularly; in rats the LD_{50} is 0.315 ± 0.019 mg/kg intravenously, 0.445 ± 0.032 mg/kg subcutaneously, and 0.423 ± 0.032 mg/kg intramuscularly.

Dosage and Administration: *Symptomatic control of myasthenia gravis:* One ml of the 1:2000 solution (0.5 mg) subcutaneously or intramuscularly. Subsequent doses should be based on the individual patient's response. In most patients, however, oral treatment with Prostigmin (neostigmine bromide) tablets, 15 mg each, is adequate for control of symptoms.

Prevention of postoperative distention and urinary retention: One ml of the 1:4000 solution (0.25 mg) subcutaneously or intramuscularly as soon as possible after operation; repeat every 4 to 6 hours for two or three days.

Treatment of postoperative distention: One ml of the 1:2000 solution (0.5 mg) subcutaneously or intramuscularly, as required.

Treatment of urinary retention: One ml of the 1:2000 solution (0.5 mg) subcutaneously or intramuscularly. If urination does not occur within an hour, the patient should be catheterized. After the patient has voided, or the bladder has been emptied, continue the 0.5 mg injections every three hours for at least 5 injections.

Reversal of Effects of Nondepolarizing Neuromuscular Blocking Agents: When Prostigmin is administered intravenously, it is recommended that atropine sulfate (0.6 to 1.2 mg) also be given intravenously using separate syringes. Some authorities have recommended that the atropine be injected several minutes before the Prostigmin rather than concomitantly. The usual dose is 0.5 to 2 mg Prostigmin given by *slow* intravenous injection, repeated as required. Only in exceptional cases should the total dose of Prostigmin exceed 5 mg. It is recommended that the patient be well ventilated and a patent airway maintained until complete recovery of normal respiration is assured. The optimum time for administration of the drug is during hyperventilation when the carbon dioxide level of the blood is low. It should never be administered in the presence of high concentrations of halothane or cyclopropane. In cardiac cases and severely ill patients, it is advisable to titrate the exact dose of Prostigmin required, using a peripheral nerve stimulator device. In the presence of bradycardia, the pulse rate should be increased to about 80/minute with atropine before administering Prostigmin.

Parenteral drug products should be inspected visually for particulate matter and discoloration prior to administration, whenever solution and container permit.

How Supplied:

Prostigmin 1:2000 (0.5 mg neostigmine methylsulfate/ml), 1-ml ampuls — boxes of 10 (NDC 0004-1919-06).

Prostigmin 1:4000 (0.25 mg neostigmine methylsulfate/ml), 1-ml ampuls — boxes of 10 (NDC 0004-1920-06).

Prostigmin 1:1000 (1 mg neostigmine methylsulfate/ml), 10-ml multiple dose vials — (NDC 0004-1921-06).

Prostigmin 1:2000 (0.5 mg neostigmine methylsulfate/ml), 10-ml multiple dose vials — (NDC 0004-1922-06).

PROSTIGMIN® ℞
(neostigmine bromide/Roche)
TABLETS

The following text is complete prescribing information based on official labeling in effect August 1, 1982.

Description: Prostigmin (neostigmine bromide/Roche), an anticholinesterase agent, is available for oral administration in 15-mg tablets. Chemically, neostigmine bromide is (*m*-hydroxyphenyl)trimethylammonium bromide dimethylcarbamate. It is a white, crystalline, bitter powder, soluble 1:1 in water, with a molecular weight of 303.20.

Clinical Pharmacology: Neostigmine inhibits the hydrolysis of acetylcholine by competing with acetylcholine for attachment to acetylcholinesterase at sites of cholinergic transmission. It enhances cholinergic action by facilitating the transmission of impulses across neuromuscular junctions. It also has a direct cholinomimetic effect on skeletal muscle and possibly on autonomic ganglion cells and neurons of the central nervous system. Neostigmine undergoes hydrolysis by cholinesterase and is also metabolized by microsomal enzymes in the liver. Protein binding to human serum albumin ranges from 15 to 25 percent. Neostigmine bromide is poorly absorbed from the gastrointestinal tract following oral administration. As a rule, 15 mg of neostigmine bromide orally is equivalent to 0.5 mg of neostigmine methylsulfate parenterally, due to poor absorption of the tablet from the intestinal tract. In a study in fasting myasthenic patients, the extent of absorption was estimated to be 1 to 2 percent of the ingested 30-mg single oral dose. Peak concentrations in plasma occurred 1 to 2 hours following drug ingestion, with considerable individual variations. The half-life ranged from 42 to 60 minutes with a mean half-life of 52 minutes.

Indications and Usage: Prostigmin is indicated for the symptomatic treatment of myasthenia gravis. Its greatest usefulness is in prolonged therapy where no difficulty in swallowing is present. In acute myasthenic crisis where difficulty in breathing and swallowing is present, the parenteral form (neostigmine methylsulfate) should be used. The patient can be transferred to the oral form as soon as it can be tolerated.

Contraindications: Prostigmin is contraindicated in patients with known hypersensitivity to the drug. Because of the presence of the bromide ion, it should not be used in patients with a previous history of reaction to bromides. It is contraindicated in patients with peritonitis or mechanical obstruction of the intestinal or urinary tract.

Warnings: Prostigmin should be used with caution in patients with epilepsy, bronchial asthma, bradycardia, recent coronary occlusion, vagotonia, hyperthyroidism, cardiac arrhythmias or peptic ulcer. As a rule, 15 mg of neostigmine bromide orally is equivalent to 0.5 mg of neostigmine methylsulfate parenterally, due to poor absorption of the tablet from the intestinal tract. Large doses should be avoided in situations where there might be an increased absorption rate from the intestinal tract. It should be used with caution when coadministered with anticholinergic drugs, in order to avoid reduction of intestinal motility.

Precautions: *General:* It is important to differentiate between myasthenic crisis and cholinergic crisis caused by overdosage of Prostigmin. Both conditions result in extreme muscle weakness but require radically different treatment. (See OVERDOSAGE section.)

Drug Interactions: Certain antibiotics, especially neomycin, streptomycin and kanamycin, have a mild but definite nondepolarizing blocking action which may accentuate neuromuscular block. These antibiotics should be used in the myasthenic patient only where definitely indicated, and then careful adjustment should be made of adjunctive anticholinesterase dosage.

Local and some general anesthetics, antiarrhythmic agents and other drugs that interfere with neuromuscular transmission should be used cautiously, if at all, in patients with myasthenia gravis; the dose of Prostigmin may have to be increased accordingly.

Carcinogenesis, Mutagenesis and Impairment of Fertility: There have been no studies with Prostigmin which would permit an evaluation of its carcinogenic or mutagenic potential. Studies on the effect of Prostigmin on fertility and reproduction have not been performed.

Pregnancy:

Teratogenic Effects: Pregnancy Category C. There are no adequate or well-controlled studies of Prostigmin in either laboratory animals or in pregnant women. It is not known whether Prostigmin can cause fetal harm when administered to a pregnant woman or can affect reproductive capacity. Prostigmin should be given to a pregnant woman only if clearly needed.

Nonteratogenic Effects: Anticholinesterase drugs may cause uterine irritability and induce premature labor when given intravenously to pregnant women near term.

Nursing Mothers: It is not known whether Prostigmin is excreted in human milk. Because many drugs are excreted in human milk and because of the potential for serious adverse reactions from Prostigmin in nursing infants, a decision should be made whether to discontinue nursing or to discontinue the drug, taking into account the importance of the drug to the mother.

Pediatric Use: Safety and effectiveness in children have not been established.

Adverse Reactions: Side effects are generally due to an exaggeration of pharmacological effects of which salivation and fasciculation are the most common. Bowel cramps and diarrhea may also occur.

The following additional adverse reactions have been reported following the use of either neostigmine bromide or neostigmine methylsulfate:

Allergic: Allergic reactions and anaphylaxis.

Neurologic: Dizziness, convulsions, loss of consciousness, drowsiness, headache, dysarthria, miosis and visual changes.

Cardiovascular: Cardiac arrhythmias (including bradycardia, tachycardia, A-V block and nodal rhythm) and nonspecific EKG changes have been reported, as well as cardiac arrest, syncope and hypotension. These have been predominantly noted following the use of the injectable form of Prostigmin.

Respiratory: Increased oral, pharyngeal and bronchial secretions, and dyspnea. Respiratory depression, respiratory arrest and bronchospasm have been reported following the use of the injectable form of Prostigmin.

Dermatologic: Rash and urticaria.

Gastrointestinal: Nausea, emesis, flatulence and increased peristalsis.

Genitourinary: Urinary frequency.

Musculoskeletal: Muscle cramps and spasms, arthralgia.

Miscellaneous: Diaphoresis, flushing and weakness.

Overdosage: Overdosage of Prostigmin can cause cholinergic crisis, which is characterized by increasing muscle weakness, and through involvement of the muscles of respiration, may result in death. Myasthenic crisis, due to an increase in the severity of the disease, is also accompanied by extreme muscle weakness and may be difficult to distinguish from cholinergic crisis on a symptomatic basis. However, such differentiation is extremely important because increases in the dose of Prostigmin or other drugs in this class, in the presence of cholinergic crisis or of a refractory or "insensitive" state, could have grave consequences. The two types of crises may be differentiated by the use of Tensilon® (edrophonium chloride/Roche) as well as by clinical judgment.

Treatment of the two conditions differs radically. Whereas the presence of *myasthenic crisis* requires more intensive anticholinesterase therapy, *cholinergic crisis* calls for the prompt withdrawal of all drugs of this type. The immediate use of atropine in cholinergic crisis is also recommended. Atropine may also be used to abolish or minimize gastrointestinal side effects or other muscarinic reactions; but such use, by masking signs of overdosage, can lead to inadvertent induction of cholinergic crisis. The LD_{50} of neostigmine methylsulfate in mice is 0.3 $\pm$ 0.02 mg/kg intravenously, 0.54 $\pm$ 0.03 mg/kg subcutaneously, and 0.395 $\pm$ 0.025 mg/kg intramuscularly; in rats the LD_{50} is 0.315 $\pm$ 0.019 mg/kg intravenously, 0.445 $\pm$ 0.032 mg/kg subcutaneously, and 0.423 $\pm$ 0.032 mg/kg intramuscularly.

Dosage and Administration: The onset of action of Prostigmin given orally is slower than when given parenterally, but the duration of action is longer and the intensity of action more uniform. Dosage requirements for optimal results vary from 15 mg to 375 mg per day. In some instances it may be necessary to exceed these dosages, but the possibility of cholinergic crisis must be recognized. The average dose is 10 tablets (150 mg) administered over a 24-hour period. The interval between doses is of paramount importance. The dosage schedule should be adjusted for each patient and changed as the need arises. Frequently, therapy is required day and night. Larger portions of the total daily dose may be given at times when the patient is more prone to fatigue (afternoon, mealtimes, etc.). The patient should be encouraged to keep a daily record of his or her condition to assist the physician in determining an optimal therapeutic regimen.

How Supplied: Scored, white tablets containing 15 mg neostigmine bromide — bottles of 100 (NDC 0004-0035-01) and 1000 (NDC 0004-0035-13). Imprint on tablets: Roche 35.

[*Shown in Product Identification Section*]

QUARZAN® ℞
(clidinium bromide/Roche)
CAPSULES

The following text is complete prescribing information based on official labeling in effect August 1, 1982.

Description: Clidinium bromide is 3-hydroxy-1-methylquinuclidinium bromide benzilate. A white or nearly white crystalline compound, it is soluble in water and has a calculated molecular weight of 432.36.

Clidinium bromide is a quaternary ammonium compound with anticholinergic and antispasmodic activity. Quarzan is available as green and red opaque capsules each containing 2.5 mg clidinium bromide, and green and grey opaque capsules each containing 5 mg clidinium bromide.

Actions: Quarzan inhibits gastrointestinal motility and diminishes gastric acid secretion. Its anticholinergic activity approximates that of atropine sulfate and propantheline bromide.

Indications: Quarzan is effective as adjunctive therapy in peptic ulcer disease. **Quarzan has not been shown to be effective in contributing to the healing of peptic ulcer, decreasing the rate of recurrence or preventing complications.**

Contraindications: Known hypersensitivity to clidinium bromide or to other anticholinergic drugs, glaucoma, obstructive uropathy (for example, bladder neck obstruction due to prostatic hypertrophy), obstructive disease of the gastrointestinal tract (for example, pyloroduodenal stenosis), paralytic ileus, intestinal atony of the elderly or debilitated patient, unstable cardiovascular status in acute hemorrhage, severe ulcerative colitis, toxic megacolon complicating ulcerative colitis, myasthenia gravis.

Warnings: Quarzan may produce drowsiness or blurred vision. The patient should be cautioned regarding activities requiring mental alertness such as operating a motor vehicle or other machinery or performing hazardous

Continued on next page

Roche Labs.—Cont.

work while taking this drug. In the presence of high environmental temperature, heat prostration (fever and heat stroke) may occur with the use of anticholinergics due to decreased sweating. Diarrhea may be an early symptom of incomplete intestinal obstruction, especially in patients with ileostomy or colostomy. Use of anticholinergics in patients with suspected intestinal obstruction would be inappropriate and possibly harmful. With overdosage, a curare-like action may occur, *i.e.*, neuromuscular blockade leading to muscular weakness and possible paralysis.

Usage in Pregnancy: No controlled studies in humans have been performed to establish the safety of the drug in pregnancy. Uncontrolled data derived from clinical usage have failed to show abnormalities attributable to its use. Reproduction studies in rats have failed to show any impaired fertility or abnormality in the fetuses that might be associated with the use of Quarzan. Use of any drug in pregnancy or in women of childbearing potential requires that the pontential benefit of the drug be weighed against the possible hazards to mother and fetus.

Nursing Mothers: As with all anticholinergic drugs, Quarzan may be secreted in human milk and may inhibit lactation. As a general rule, nursing should not be undertaken while a patient is on Quarzan, or the drug should not be used by nursing mothers.

Pediatric Use: Since there is no adequate experience in children who have received this drug, safety and efficacy in children have not been established.

Precautions: Use Quarzan with caution in the elderly and in all patients with autonomic neuropathy, hepatic or renal disease, ulcerative colitis—large doses may suppress intestinal motility to the point of producing a paralytic ileus and for this reason precipitate or aggravate "toxic megacolon," a serious complication of the disease; hyperthyroidism; coronary heart disease; congestive heart failure; cardiac tachy-arrhythmias; tachycardia; hypertension; prostatic hypertrophy; hiatal hernia associated with reflux esophagitis, since anticholinergic drugs may aggravate this condition.

Adverse Reactions: As with other anticholinergic drugs, the most frequently reported adverse effects are dryness of mouth, blurring of vision, urinary hesitancy and constipation. Other adverse effects reported with the use of anticholinergic drugs include decreased sweating, urinary retention, tachycardia, palpitations, dilatation of the pupils, cycloplegia, increased ocular tension, loss of taste, headaches, nervousness, mental confusion, drowsiness, weakness, dizziness, insomnia, nausea, vomiting, bloated feeling, impotence, suppression of lactation and severe allergic reactions or drug idiosyncrasies including anaphylaxis, urticaria and other dermal manifestations.

Overdosage: The symptoms of overdosage with Quarzan progress from an intensification of the usual side effects to CNS disturbances (from restlessness and excitement to psychotic behavior), circulatory changes (flushing, tachycardia, fall in blood pressure, circulatory failure), respiratory failure, paralysis and coma. Treatment should consist of: *General measures*—(1) gastric lavage, (2) maintenance of adequate airway, using artificial respiration if needed, (3) administration of i.v. fluids, and (4) for fever: alcohol sponging or ice packs.

Specific measures—(1) Antidotes: physostigmine (Antilirium) 0.5 to 2 mg, i.v., repeated as needed up to a total of 5 mg; or pilocarpine, 5 mg, s.c. at intervals until mouth is moist; neostigmine may also be useful. (2) Against excitement: sodium pentothal 2% may be given i.v. or chloral hydrate (100 to 200 ml, 2% solution) *rectally.* (3) Against hypotension and circulatory collapse: levarterenol (Levophed®) or metaraminol (Aramine) infusions. (4) Against CNS depression: caffeine and sodium benzoate. The usefulness of dialysis is not known.

Dosage and Administration: For maximum efficacy, dosage should be individualized according to severity of symptoms and occurrence of side effects. The usual dosage is 2.5 to 5 mg three or four times daily before meals and at bedtime. Dosage in excess of 20 mg daily is usually not required to obtain maximum effectiveness. For the aged or debilitated, one 2.5-mg capsule three times daily before meals is recommended. The desired pharmacological effect of the drug is unlikely to be attained without occasional side effects.

Drug Interactions: No specific drug interactions are known.

How Supplied: Opaque capsules, 2.5 mg, green and red; 5 mg, green and grey—bottles of 100.

[*Shown in Product Identification Section*]

ROCALTROL® ℞
(calcitriol/Roche)
CAPSULES

The following text is complete prescribing information based on official labeling in effect November 1982.

Description: Calcitriol is a colorless, crystalline compound which occurs naturally in humans. It has a calculated molecular weight of 416.65 and is soluble in organic solvents but relatively insoluble in water. Chemically, calcitriol is 9,10-seco(5Z,7E)-5,7,10(19)-cholestatriene-1α,3β, 25-triol.

The other names frequently used for calcitriol are 1,25-dihydroxycholecalciferol, 1,25-hydroxyvitamin D_3, 1,25-DHCC, 1,25$(OH)_2D_3$ and 1, 25-diOHC.

Rocaltrol is synthetically manufactured calcitriol and is available as soft gelatin capsules for oral administration in the following strengths: 0.25 mcg (light orange, oval) and 0.5 mcg (dark orange, oblong).

Clinical Pharmacology: The natural supply of vitamin D in man mainly depends on the ultraviolet rays of the sun for conversion of 7-dehydrocholesterol to vitamin D_3 (cholecalciferol). It is now known that vitamin D_3 must be metabolically activated in the liver and the kidney before it is fully active on its target tissues. The initial transformation is catalyzed by a vitamin D_3-25-hydroxylase enzyme (25-OHase) present in the liver, and the product of this reaction is 25-hydroxy-vitamin D_3 [25-$(OH)D_3$]. The latter undergoes hydroxylation in the mitochondria of kidney tissue, and this reaction is activated by the renal 25-hydroxyvitamin D_3-1α-hydroxylase (alpha-OHase) to produce 1,25-$(OH)_2D_3$ (calcitriol), the active form of vitamin D_3.

The two known sites of action of calcitriol are intestine and bone, but additional evidence suggests that it also acts on the kidney and the parathyroid gland. It is the most active known form of vitamin D_3 in stimulating intestinal calcium transport. In acutely uremic rats calcitriol has been shown to stimulate intestinal calcium absorption. It has been suggested that a vitamin D-resistant state exists in uremic patients because of the failure of the kidney to adequately convert precursors to the active compound, calcitriol.

Calcitriol when administered is rapidly absorbed from the intestine. After an oral dose of tritiated calcitriol, the peak concentration of radioactivity in the serum was reported after 4 hours. Vitamin D metabolites are known to be transported in blood, bound to specific plasma proteins. The pharmacologic activity of an administered dose of calcitriol is about 3 to 5 days. Two metabolic pathways for calcitriol seem to have been identified; conversion to 1,24,25-$(OH)_3D_3$ and to an unknown substance with a loss of a side chain at C26 or C27 position.

Indications and Usage: Rocaltrol is indicated in the management of hypocalcemia in patients undergoing chronic renal dialysis. In studies to date, it has been shown to reduce elevated parathyroid hormone levels in some of these patients.

It is also indicated in the management of hypocalcemia and its clinical manifestations in patients with postsurgical hypoparathyroidism, idiopathic hypoparathyroidism, and pseudohypoparathyroidism.

Contraindications: Rocaltrol should not be given to patients with hypercalcemia or evidence of vitamin D toxicity.

Warnings: Since Rocaltrol is the most potent metabolite of vitamin D available, pharmacologic doses of vitamin D and its derivatives should be withheld during Rocaltrol treatment to avoid possible additive effects and hypercalcemia.

Aluminum carbonate or hydroxide gel should be used to control serum phosphate levels in patients undergoing dialysis.

Magnesium-containing antacid and Rocaltrol should not be used concomitantly in patients on chronic renal dialysis, because such use may lead to the development of hypermagnesemia.

Overdosage of any form of vitamin D is dangerous (see also OVERDOSAGE). Progressive hypercalcemia due to overdosage of vitamin D and its metabolites may be so severe as to require emergency attention. Chronic hypercalcemia can lead to generalized vascular calcification, nephrocalcinosis and other soft-tissue calcification. **The serum calcium times phosphate (Ca × P) product should not be allowed to exceed 70.** Radiographic evaluation of suspect anatomical regions may be useful in the early detection of this condition.

Precautions:

i) *General:* Excessive dosage of Rocaltrol induces hypercalcemia and in some instances hypercalciuria; therefore, early in treatment during dosage adjustment, serum calcium should be determined twice weekly. A fall in serum alkaline phosphatase levels usually antedates the appearance of hypercalcemia and may be an indication of impending hypercalcemia. Should hypercalcemia develop, the drug should be discontinued immediately. Rocaltrol should be given cautiously to patients on digitalis, because hypercalcemia in such patients may precipitate cardiac arrhythmias.

   In patients with normal renal function, chronic hypercalcemia may be associated with an increase in serum creatinine. While this is usually reversible, it is important in such patients to pay careful attention to those factors which may lead to hypercalcemia. Rocaltrol therapy should always be started at the lowest possible dose and should not be increased without careful monitoring of the serum calcium. An estimate of daily dietary calcium intake should be made and the intake adjusted when indicated.

   Patients with normal renal function taking Rocaltrol should avoid dehydration. Adequate fluid intake should be maintained.

ii) *Information for the patient:* The patient and his or her parents or spouse should be informed about compliance with dosage instructions, adherence to instructions about diet and calcium supplementation and avoidance of the use of unapproved nonprescription drugs. Patients should also be carefully informed about the symptoms of hypercalcemia (see ADVERSE REACTIONS).

iii) *Essential laboratory tests:* Serum calcium, phosphorus, magnesium and alkaline phosphatase and 24-hour urinary calcium and phosphorus should be determined periodically. During the initial phase of the medication, serum calcium should be determined more frequently (twice weekly).

iv) *Drug Interactions:* Cholestyramine has been reported to reduce intestinal absorption of fat soluble vitamins; as such it may impair intestinal absorption of Rocaltrol.

v) *Carcinogenesis, mutagenesis, impairment of fertility:* Long-term studies in animals have not been completed to evaluate the carcinogenic potential of Rocaltrol. There was no evidence of mutagenicity as studied by the Ames Method. No significant effects of Rocaltrol on fertility and/or general reproductive performances were reported.

vi) *Use in pregnancy:* Rocaltrol has been found to be teratogenic in rabbits when given in doses 4 and 15 times the dose recommended for human use. All 15 fetuses in 3 litters at these doses showed external and skeletal abnormalities. However, none of the other 23 litters (156 fetuses) showed significant abnormalities compared with controls. Teratology studies in rats showed no evidence of teratogenic potential. There are no studies in pregnant women.

vii) *Nursing mothers:* It is not known whether this drug is excreted in human milk. As a general rule, nursing should not be undertaken while a patient is on a drug, since many drugs are excreted in human milk.

viii) *Pediatric use:* Safety and efficacy of Rocaltrol in children undergoing dialysis have not been established.

Adverse Reactions: Since Rocaltrol is believed to be the active hormone which exerts vitamin D activity in the body, adverse effects are, in general, similar to those encountered with excessive vitamin D intake. The early and late signs and symptoms of vitamin D intoxication associated with hypercalcemia include:

a. *Early:* Weakness, headache, somnolence, nausea, vomiting, dry mouth, constipation, muscle pain, bone pain and metallic taste.

b. *Late:* Polyuria, polydipsia, anorexia, weight loss, nocturia, conjunctivitis (calcific), pancreatitis, photophobia, rhinorrhea, pruritus, hyperthermia, decreased libido, elevated BUN, albuminuria, hypercholesterolemia, elevated SGOT and SGPT, ectopic calcification, hypertension, cardiac arrhythmias and, rarely, overt psychosis.

In clinical studies of hypoparathyroidism and pseudohypoparathyroidism, hypercalcemia was noted on at least one occasion in about 1 in 3 patients and hypercalciuria in about 1 in 7. Elevated serum creatinine levels were observed in about 1 in 6 patients (approximately one half of whom had normal levels at baseline).

One case of erythema multiforme was confirmed by rechallenge.

Overdosage: Administration of Rocaltrol to patients in excess of their daily requirements can cause hypercalcemia, hypercalciuria and hyperphosphatemia. High intake of calcium and phosphate concomitant with Rocaltrol may lead to similar abnormalities. High levels of calcium in the dialysate bath may contribute to the hypercalcemia.

Treatment of Hypercalcemia and Overdosage in Patients on Hemodialysis: General treatment of hypercalcemia (greater than 1 mg/dl above the upper limit of the normal range) consists of immediate discontinuation of Rocaltrol therapy, institution of a low calcium diet and withdrawal of calcium supplements. Serum calcium levels should be determined daily until normocalcemia ensues. Hypercalcemia frequently resolves in two to seven days. When serum calcium levels have returned to within normal limits, Rocaltrol therapy may be reinstituted at a dose of 0.25 mcg/day less than prior therapy. Serum calcium levels should be obtained at least twice weekly after all dosage changes and subsequent dosage titration. Persistent or markedly elevated serum calcium levels may be corrected by dialysis against a calcium-free dialysate.

Treatment of Accidental Overdosage of Rocaltrol: The treatment of acute accidental overdosage of Rocaltrol should consist of general supportive measures. If drug ingestion is discovered within a relatively short time, induction of emesis or gastric lavage may be of benefit in preventing further absorption. If the drug has passed through the stomach, the administration of mineral oil may promote its fecal elimination. Serial serum electrolyte determinations (especially calcium ion), rate of urinary calcium excretion and assessment of electrocardiographic abnormalities due to hypercalcemia should be obtained. Such monitoring is critical in patients receiving digitalis. Discontinuation of supplemental calcium and a low calcium diet are also indicated in accidental overdosage. Due to the relatively short duration of the pharmacological action of calcitriol, further measures are probably unnecessary. Should, however, persistent and markedly elevated serum calcium levels occur, there are a variety of therapeutic alternatives which may be considered, depending on the patient's underlying condition. These include the use of drugs such as phosphates and corticosteroids as well as measures to induce an appropriate forced diuresis. The use of peritoneal dialysis against a calcium-free dialysate has also been reported.

Dosage and Administration: The optimal daily dose of Rocaltrol must be carefully determined for each patient.

The effectiveness of Rocaltrol therapy is predicated on the assumption that each patient is receiving an adequate daily intake of calcium. The RDA for calcium in adults is 1000 mg. To ensure that each patient receives an adequate daily intake of calcium, the physician should either prescribe a calcium supplement or instruct the patient in proper dietary measures.

Dialysis patients:

The recommended initial dose of Rocaltrol is 0.25 mcg/day. If a satisfactory response in the biochemical parameters and clinical manifestations of the disease state is not observed, dosage may be increased by 0.25 mcg/day at four- to eight-week intervals. During this titration period, serum calcium levels should be obtained at least twice weekly, and if hypercalcemia is noted, the drug should be immediately discontinued until normocalcemia ensues.

Patients with normal or only slightly reduced serum calcium levels may respond to Rocaltrol doses of 0.25 mcg every other day. Most patients undergoing hemodialysis respond to doses between 0.5 and 1 mcg/day.

Hypoparathyroidism:

The recommended initial dose of Rocaltrol is 0.25 mcg/day given in the morning. If a satisfactory response in the biochemical parameters and clinical manifestations of the disease is not observed, the dose may be increased at two- to four-week intervals. During the dosage titration period, serum calcium levels should be obtained at least twice weekly and, if hypercalcemia is noted, Rocaltrol should be immediately discontinued until normocalcemia ensues. Careful consideration should also be given to lowering the dietary calcium intake. Most adult patients and pediatric patients aged 6 years and older have responded to dosages in the range of 0.5 to 2 mcg daily. Pediatric patients in the 1- to 5-year age group with hypoparathyroidism have usually been given 0.25 to 0.75 mcg daily. The number of treated patients with pseudohypoparathyroidism less than 6 years of age is too small to make dosage recommendations.

How Supplied: 0.25 mcg calcitriol/Roche in soft gelatin, light orange, oval capsules, imprinted (front) HLR, (back) 143; bottles of 30 and 100.

0.5 mcg calcitriol/Roche in soft gelatin, dark orange, oblong capsules, imprinted (front) ROCHE, (back) 144; bottles of 100.

Rocaltrol should be protected from heat and light.

[*Shown in Product Identification Section*]

RONIACOL® ℞

(nicotinyl alcohol/Roche)
TIMESPAN® TABLETS
TABLETS
ELIXIR

The following text is complete prescribing information based on official labeling in effect August 1, 1982.

Description: Roniacol (nicotinyl alcohol/Roche) is a well-tolerated vasodilator which is available in three dosage forms: Timespan Tablets, each providing 150 mg nicotinyl alcohol in the form of the tartrate salt in a sustained-release form; scored Tablets, each containing 50 mg nicotinyl alcohol in the form of the tartrate salt; and port-wine flavored Elixir, containing 50 mg nicotinyl alcohol per teaspoonful (5 ml).

Properties: Roniacol acts selectively by relaxing the musculature of peripheral blood vessels. In the management of conditions associated with deficient circulation, its action is smooth and gradual in onset. When administered in the sustained-release Timespan Tablet, increased blood flow is provided for up to 12 hours with a single dose. Patients usually do not develop tolerance on prolonged medication. The Timespan Tablet releases some of the drug immediately and the remainder continuously over a period of approximately twelve hours, thus increasing the blood flow in ischemic extremities for 10 to 12 hours by specific dilation of peripheral vessels.

INDICATIONS:

Based on a review of this drug by the National Academy of Sciences—National Research Council and/or other information, FDA has classified the indications as follows:

"Possibly" effective: In conditions associated with deficient circulation; *e.g.,* peripheral vascular disease, vascular spasm, varicose ulcers, decubital ulcers, chilblains, Meniere's syndrome and vertigo.

Final classification of the less-than-effective indications requires further investigation.

Caution: Roche Laboratories endorses the principle of caution in the administration of any therapeutic agent to pregnant patients.

Side Effects: Transient flushing, gastric disturbances, minor skin rashes and allergies may occur in some patients, seldom requiring discontinuation of the drug.

Dosage: *Timespan Tablets*—one or two tablets morning and night. *Tablets*—one or two tablets 3 times daily. *Elixir*—one or two teaspoonfuls 3 times daily.

How Supplied: *Timespan Tablets,* containing 150 mg nicotinyl alcohol in the form of the tartrate salt—bottles of 100 and 500. *Tablets,* containing 50 mg nicotinyl alcohol in the form of the tartrate salt—scored, bottles of 100 and 500. *Elixir,* containing 50 mg nicotinyl alcohol per teaspoonful (5 ml) —bottles of 16 oz.

[*Shown in Product Identification Section*]

SOLATENE® ℞

(beta-carotene/Roche)
capsules

The following text is complete prescribing information based on official labeling in effect August 1, 1982.

Description: Solatene (beta-carotene), precursor of vitamin A, is supplied in 30-mg capsules for oral administration. Beta-carotene is a carotenoid pigment occurring naturally in

Continued on next page

Roche Labs.—Cont.

green and yellow vegetables. Chemically, beta-carotene has the empirical formula $C_{40}H_{56}$ and a calculated molecular weight of 536.85. Trans-beta-carotene is a red, crystalline compound which is insoluble in water.

Clinical Pharmacology: Beta-carotene, a pro-vitamin A, belongs to the class of carotenoid pigments. In terms of its vitamin activity, 6 μg of dietary beta-carotene is considered equivalent to 1 μg of vitamin A (retinol). Bioavailability of beta-carotene depends on the presence of fat in the diet to act as a carrier, and bile in the intestinal tract for its absorption. Beta-carotene is metabolized, primarily in the intestine, to vitamin A at a rate of approximately 50% to 60% of normal dietary intake and falls off rapidly as intake goes up. In humans, an appreciable amount of unchanged beta-carotene is absorbed and stored in various tissues, especially the depot fat. Small amounts may be converted to vitamin A in the liver. The vitamin A derived from beta-carotene follows the same metabolic pathway as that from dietary sources. The major route of elimination is fecal excretion. Excessive ingestion of carotenes is not harmful, but it may cause yellow coloration of the skin, which disappears upon reduction or cessation of intake.

Indications and Usage: Solatene is used to reduce the severity of photosensitivity reactions in patients with erythropoietic protoporphyria (EPP).

Contraindications: Solatene is contraindicated in patients with known hypersensitivity to the drug.

Warnings: Solatene has not been shown to be effective as a sunscreen.

Precautions: *General:* Solatene should be used with caution in patients with impaired renal or hepatic function because safe use in the presence of these conditions has not been established.

Information for Patients: Patients receiving Solatene should be advised against taking supplementary vitamin A since Solatene administration will fulfill normal vitamin A requirements. They should be cautioned to continue sun protection, and forewarned that their skin may appear slightly yellow while receiving Solatene.

Carcinogenesis, Mutagenesis, Impairment of Fertility: Long-term studies in animals to determine carcinogenesis have not been completed. *In vitro* and *in vivo* studies to evaluate mutagenic potential were negative. No effects on fertility in male rats were observed at doses as high as 500 mg/kg/day (100 times the recommended human dose).

Pregnancy: Teratogenic Effects: Pregnancy Category C. Beta-carotene has been shown to be fetotoxic (*i.e.,* cause an increase in resorption rate), but not teratogenic when given to rats at doses 300 to 400 times the maximum recommended human dose. No such fetotoxicity was observed at 75 times the maximum recommended human dose or less. A three-generation reproduction study in rats receiving beta-carotene at a dietary concentration of 0.1% (1000 ppm) has revealed no evidence of impaired fertility or effect on the fetus. There are no adequate and well-controlled studies in pregnant women. Solatene should be used during pregnancy only if the potential benefit justifies the potential risk to the fetus.

Nursing Mothers: It is not known whether this drug is excreted in human milk. Because many drugs are excreted in human milk, caution should be exercised when Solatene is administered to a nursing mother.

Adverse Reactions: Some patients may have occasional loose stools while taking Solatene. This reaction is sporadic and may not require discontinuance of medication. Other reactions which have been reported rarely are ecchymoses and arthralgia.

Overdosage: There are no reported cases of overdosage. The oral LD_{50} of beta-carotene (suspended in 5% gum acacia solution) in mice and rats is greater than 20,000 mg/kg. No lethality was observed in mice following administration of 30-mg beadlet capsules (ground and suspended in 5% gum acacia) at a dose of 1200 mg/kg beta-carotene.

Dosage and Administration: Solatene may be administered either as a single daily dose or in divided doses, preferably with meals.

Usage in Children: The usual dosage for children under 14 is 30 to 150 mg (1 to 5 capsules) per day. Capsules may be opened and the contents mixed in orange juice or tomato juice to aid administration.

Usage in Adults: The usual adult dosage is 30 to 300 mg (1 to 10 capsules) per day.

Dosage should be adjusted depending on the severity of the symptoms and the response of the patient. Several weeks of therapy are necessary to accumulate enough Solatene in the skin to exert its effect. Patients should be instructed not to increase exposure to sunlight until they appear carotenemic (first seen as yellowness of palms and soles). This usually occurs after two to six weeks of therapy. Exposure to the sun may then be increased gradually. The protective effect is not total and each patient should establish his or her own limits of exposure.

How Supplied: Solatene is available in blue and green capsules, each containing 30 mg of beta-carotene—bottles of 100 (NDC 0004-0115-01). Imprint on capsules: SOLATENE ROCHE.

[*Shown in Product Identification Section*]

SYNKAYVITE® ℞

(menadiol sodium diphosphate/Roche)
Injectable

The following text is complete prescribing information based on official labeling in effect August 1, 1982.

Description: Menadiol sodium diphosphate is a synthetic, water-soluble vitamin-K analog. Chemically, it is 2-methyl-1,4-naphthalenediol bis (dihydrogen phosphate) tetrasodium salt. The composition is as follows: *1 ml ampuls, 5 mg/ml:* Each ml contains 5 mg menadiol sodium diphosphate/Roche compounded with 2.5 mg sodium metabisulfite, 0.45% phenol as preservative, 0.4% sodium chloride for isotonicity and pH adjusted to approximately 8.0 with sodium hydroxide.

1 ml ampuls, 10 mg/ml: Each ml contains 10 mg menadiol sodium diphosphate/Roche compounded with 2.5 mg sodium metabisulfite, 0.45% phenol as preservative, 0.4% sodium chloride for isotonicity and pH adjusted to approximately 8.0 with sodium hydroxide.

2 ml ampuls, 75 mg/2 ml: Each 2 ml contains 75 mg menadiol sodium diphosphate/Roche compounded with 5 mg sodium metabisulfite, 0.45% phenol as preservative, 0.4% sodium chloride for isotonicity and pH adjusted to approximately 8.0 with sodium hydroxide.

Actions: Synkayvite is a synthetic water-soluble derivative of menadione (vitamin K_3) to which it is converted *in vivo.* Its potency is approximately one-half that of menadione. Vitamin K is necessary for the synthesis in the liver of prothrombin (factor II), proconvertin (factor VII), thromboplastin (factor IX) and Stuart factor (factor X). The prothrombin test is sensitive to the levels of factors II, VII and X. The mechanism by which vitamin K promotes formation of these clotting factors in the liver is not known. The action of Synkayvite is generally detectable within an hour or two.

Indications: Synkayvite is indicated in the treatment of hypoprothrombinemia secondary to factors limiting absorption or synthesis of vitamin K, *e.g.,* obstructive jaundice, biliary fistula, sprue, ulcerative colitis, celiac disease, intestinal resection, cystic fibrosis of the pancreas, regional enteritis and antibacterial therapy.

It is also indicated in hypoprothrombinemia secondary to administration of salicylates.

May also be used as a liver function test, although newer methods are available.

Contraindications: Vitamin K, or any of its synthetic analogs, should not be administered to the mother during the last few weeks of pregnancy as a prophylactic measure against physiologic hypoprothrombinemia or hemorrhagic disease of the newborn.

Warnings: In the prophylaxis and treatment of hemorrhagic disease of the newborn, the water-soluble vitamin K analogs are not as safe as Konakion® (phytonadione/Roche).

Synkayvite will not counteract the anticoagulant action of heparin.

Usage in Pregnancy: Effects on reproduction have not been studied in animals. There is no adequate information on whether this drug may affect fertility in human males or females or have a teratogenic potential or other adverse effect on the fetus.

Precautions: Temporary resistance to prothrombin-depressing anticoagulants may result, especially when larger doses of Synkayvite are used. If relatively large doses have been employed, it may be necessary when reinstituting anticoagulant therapy to use larger doses of the prothrombin-depressing anticoagulant, or to use one which acts on a different principle, such as heparin.

Since the liver is the site of metabolic synthesis of prothrombin, hypoprothrombinemia resulting from hepatocellular damage is not corrected by administration of vitamin K. Repeated large doses of vitamin K are not warranted in liver disease if the response to initial use of the vitamin is unsatisfactory (Koller Test). Failure to respond to vitamin K may indicate the presence of a coagulation defect or that the condition being treated is unresponsive to vitamin K.

Adverse Reactions: In adults, bromsulfalein retention and prolongation of prothrombin time have been reported after maximum doses of vitamin K analogs. In infants (particularly premature babies), excessive doses of vitamin K analogs may cause increased bilirubinemia in the first few days of life. This, in turn, may result in kernicterus, which may lead to brain damage or even death. Immaturity is apparently an important factor in the appearance of toxic reactions to vitamin K analogs as full term and larger premature infants demonstrate greater tolerance than smaller premature infants.

Menadione can induce erythrocyte hemolysis in persons having a genetic deficiency of glucose-6-phosphate dehydrogenase in their red blood cells.

In patients with severe hepatic disease, large doses of menadione may further depress liver function.

Occasional allergic reactions, such as skin rash and urticaria, have been reported.

Dosage and Administration: The minimum daily requirements for vitamin K in humans have not been established officially. Minimal daily requirements have been estimated at 1 to 5 micrograms per kilogram for infants and 0.03 micrograms per kilogram for adults. The dietary abundance of vitamin K normally satisfies the requirements except for the neonatal period of 5 to 8 days.

Synkayvite may be injected subcutaneously, intramuscularly or intravenously. The response after intravenous administration may be more prompt, but more sustained action follows intramuscular or subcutaneous use. The usual recommended dosages are given in the accompanying chart.

[See table on next page].

Storage: Synkayvite need not be refrigerated. Store at room temperature (59° to 86°F).

How Supplied: 1-ml ampuls (5 mg/ml); 1-ml ampuls (10 mg/ml); and 2-ml ampuls (75 mg/2 ml)—boxes of 10.

USUAL RECOMMENDED DOSAGES FOR SYNKAYVITE INJECTABLE

	ADULTS	CHILDREN
For treatment of hypoprothrombinemia	5 to 15 mg once or twice daily	5 to 10 mg once or twice daily
For liver function test	75 mg intravenously	

SYNKAYVITE® ℞
(menadiol sodium diphosphate/Roche)
Tablets

The following text is complete prescribing information based on official labeling in effect August 1, 1982.

Description: Menadiol sodium diphosphate is a synthetic, water-soluble vitamin-K analog. Chemically, it is 2-methyl-1,4-naphthalenediol bis (dihydrogen phosphate) tetrasodium salt.

Actions: Synkayvite is a synthetic, water-soluble derivative of menadione (vitamin K_3) to which it is converted *in vivo*. Its potency is approximately one-half that of menadione. Vitamin K is necessary for the synthesis in the liver of prothrombin (factor II), proconvertin (factor VII), thromboplastin (factor IX) and Stuart factor (factor X). The prothrombin test is sensitive to the levels of factors II, VII and X. The mechanism by which vitamin K promotes formation of these clotting factors in the liver is not known.

Indications: Vitamin K deficiency secondary to the administration of antibacterial therapy.
Hypoprothrombinemia secondary to obstructive jaundice and biliary fistulas.
Hypoprothrombinemia secondary to administration of salicylates.

Contraindications: Vitamin K, or any of its synthetic analogs, should not be administered to the mother during the last few weeks of pregnancy as a prophylactic measure against physiologic hypoprothrombinemia or hemorrhagic disease of the newborn.

Warnings: Synkayvite will not counteract the anticoagulant action of heparin.
Usage in Pregnancy: Effects on reproduction have not been studied in animals. There is no adequate information on whether this drug may affect fertility in human males or females or have a teratogenic potential or other adverse effect on the fetus.

Precautions: Temporary resistance to prothrombin-depressing anticoagulants may result, especially when larger doses of Synkayvite are used. If relatively large doses have been employed, it may be necessary when reinstituting anticoagulant therapy to use somewhat larger doses of the prothrombin-depressing anticoagulant or to use one which acts on a different principle, such as heparin.
Since the liver is the site of metabolic synthesis of prothrombin, hypoprothrombinemia resulting from hepatocellular damage is not corrected by administration of vitamin K. Repeated large doses of vitamin K are not warranted in liver disease if the response to initial use of the vitamin is unsatisfactory (Koller Test). Failure to respond to vitamin K may indicate the presence of a coagulation defect or that the condition being treated is unresponsive to vitamin K.

Adverse Reactions: Bromsulfalein retention and prolongation of prothrombin time have been reported after maximum doses of vitamin K analogs.
Menadione can induce erythrocyte hemolysis in persons having a genetic deficiency of glucose-6-phosphate dehydrogenase in their red blood cells.
In patients with severe hepatic disease, large doses of menadione may further depress liver function.
Occasional allergic reactions, such as skin rash and urticaria, have been reported. There have also been minor instances of gastric upset.

Dosage and Administration: The minimum daily requirements for vitamin K in humans have not been established officially. Minimal daily requirements have been estimated as 0.03 micrograms per kilogram for adults. The dietary abundance of vitamin K normally satisfies the requirements except for the neonatal period of 5 to 8 days.

For hypoprothrombinemia secondary to obstructive jaundice and biliary fistulas. . . 5 mg daily
For hypoprothrombinemia secondary to the administration of antibacterials or salicylates. . . 5 to 10 mg daily

How Supplied: Tablets, 5 mg menadiol sodium diphosphate/Roche each—bottles of 100.
[*Shown in Product Identification Section*]

TARACTAN® TABLETS ℞
(chlorprothixene/Roche)
TARACTAN® CONCENTRATE ℞
(chlorprothixene lactate and HCl/Roche)
TARACTAN® AMPULS ℞
(chlorprothixene HCl/Roche)

The following text is complete prescribing information based on official labeling in effect August 1, 1982.

Description: Tablets—each containing 10 mg, 25 mg, 50 mg or 100 mg chlorprothixene. Concentrate—100 mg/5 ml as the lactate and hydrochloride, fruit flavored. Ampuls—25 mg/2 ml as the hydrochloride, with 0.2% parabens (methyl and propyl) added as preservatives and pH adjusted to approximately 3.4 with HCl.
Taractan is a thioxanthene derivative. Chemically, it is the alpha isomer of 2-chloro-*N,N*-dimethylthioxanthene-Δ^9, γ-propylamine. In chemical structure chlorprothixene resembles the phenothiazines; however, in place of the nitrogen (N) in the phenothiazine ring, chlorprothixene carries a carbon atom with a double bond to a side chain.

Actions: EEG changes following the injection of Taractan into cats suggest that it acts on the brain stem. Effects demonstrated were the synchronization of the EEG tracings during rest, a shortening of cortical activation obtained by stimulation of the reticular formation, and modifications of elicited potentials.

Indications: Taractan is indicated for the management of manifestations of psychotic disorders. Taractan has not been shown effective in the management of behavioral complications in patients with mental retardation.

Contraindications: Circulatory collapse, comatose states due to central depressant drugs (alcohol, hypnotics, opiates, etc.) and known sensitivity to the drug are contraindications.

Warnings: *Usage in Pregnancy:* The safety of Taractan during pregnancy or lactation in humans has not been established. Therefore, use of Taractan in women who may become pregnant requires weighing the drug's potential benefits against its possible hazards to mother and child. For the results of reproductive and teratogenic studies in rats and rabbits see ANIMAL PHARMACOLOGY AND TOXICOLOGY.
This drug may impair the mental and/or physical abilities required for the performance of hazardous tasks such as operating machinery or driving a motor vehicle; therefore, the patient should be cautioned accordingly.
As in the case of other CNS-acting drugs, patients receiving Taractan should be cautioned about possible combined effects with alcohol.
The safety and efficacy of Taractan have not been established for oral administration in children under age 6 or for parenteral use in those under age 12.

Precautions: Because of its structural similarity to the phenothiazines, all of the precautions associated with phenothiazine therapy should be considered when patients receive Taractan.
Therefore, Taractan should be used with caution in patients who:

—are receiving barbiturates or narcotics, because of additive effects of central nervous system depressants. The dosage of the narcotic or barbiturate should be reduced when given concomitantly with Taractan.
—are receiving atropine or related drugs, because of additive anticholinergic effects.
—have a history of epilepsy. When necessary, Taractan may be used concomitantly with anticonvulsant drugs. However, use of Taractan may lower the convulsive threshold; therefore, an adequate dosage of the anticonvulsant should be maintained.
—are exposed to extreme heat or phosphorous insecticides.
—have cardiovascular disease.
—have respiratory impairment due to acute pulmonary infections or chronic respiratory disorders such as severe asthma or emphysema.

The concurrent use of Taractan and electroshock treatment should be reserved for those patients for whom it is essential, but the hazards may be increased.
Taractan may augment or interfere with the absorption, metabolism or therapeutic activity of other psychotropic drugs and vice versa.
The appearance of signs of blood dyscrasias requires immediate discontinuance of the drug and the institution of appropriate therapy.
The possibility of liver damage, variations in thyroid function, pigmentary retinopathy, lenticular or corneal deposits and development of irreversible dyskinesias should be kept in mind when patients are on prolonged therapy.
When used in the treatment of agitated states accompanying depression, the usual precautions indicated with such patients are necessary, particularly the recognition that a suicidal tendency may be present and protective measures necessary.
Taractan tablets contain FD&C Yellow No. 5 (tartrazine) which may cause allergic-type reactions (including bronchial asthma) in certain susceptible individuals. Although the overall incidence of FD&C Yellow No. 5 (tartrazine) sensitivity in the general population is low, it is frequently seen in patients who also have aspirin hypersensitivity.
Abrupt Withdrawal: Taractan is not known to produce physical dependence. However, gastritis, nausea and vomiting, dizziness and tremulousness have been reported following abrupt cessation of high-dose therapy.
Neuroleptic drugs elevate prolactin levels; the elevation persists during chronic administration. Tissue culture experiments indicate that approximately one-third of human breast cancers are prolactin-dependent *in vitro*, a factor of potential importance if the prescription of these drugs is contemplated in a patient with a previously detected breast cancer. Although disturbances such as galactorrhea, amenorrhea, gynecomastia and impotence have been reported, the clinical significance of elevated serum prolactin levels is unknown for most patients. An increase in mammary neoplasms has been found in rodents after chronic administration of neuroleptic drugs. Neither clinical studies nor epidemiologic studies conducted to date, however, have shown an association between chronic administration of these drugs and mammary tumorigenesis; the available

Continued on next page

Roche Labs.—Cont.

evidence is considered too limited to be conclusive at this time.

Adverse Reactions: Not all of the following adverse reactions have been reported with Taractan; however, pharmacological similarities to the various phenothiazine derivatives require that each be considered.

Note: *Sudden death* has occasionally been reported in patients who have received phenothiazines. In some cases death was apparently due to cardiac arrest, in others the cause appeared to be asphyxia due to failure of the cough reflex. In some patients the cause could not be determined nor could it be established that death was due to the phenothiazine.

Drowsiness: May occur particularly during the first or second week, after which it generally disappears. If troublesome, dosage may be lowered.

Jaundice: Incidence is low. It usually occurs between the second and fourth weeks and is regarded as a sensitivity reaction. The clinical picture resembles infectious hepatitis with laboratory features of obstructive jaundice. It is usually reversible; however, chronic jaundice has been reported.

Hematological Disorders: Agranulocytosis, eosinophilia, leukopenia, hemolytic anemia, thrombocytopenic purpura and pancytopenia.

Agranulocytosis: Most cases have occurred between the fourth and tenth weeks of therapy. Patients should be watched closely during that period for the sudden appearance of sore throat or other signs of infection. If white blood count and differential show significant cellular depression, discontinue the drug and start appropriate therapy. However, a slightly lowered white count is not in itself an indication to discontinue the drug.

Cardiovascular: Postural hypotension, tachycardia (especially with sudden marked increase in dosage), bradycardia, cardiac arrest, faintness and dizziness. Occasionally the hypotensive effect may produce a shock-like condition. In the event a vasoconstrictor is required, levarterenol and phenylephrine are the most suitable. Other pressor agents, including epinephrine, should not be used, as a paradoxical further lowering of the blood pressure may ensue.

ECG changes, nonspecific, usually reversible, have been observed in some patients receiving phenothiazine tranquilizers. Their relationship to myocardial damage has not been confirmed.

CNS Effects: Neuromuscular (Extrapyramidal) Reactions: These are usually dosage-related and take three forms: (1) pseudoparkinsonism, (2) akathisia (motor restlessness) and (3) dystonias. Dystonias include spasms of the neck muscles, extensor rigidity of back muscles, carpopedal spasm, eyes rolled back, convulsions, trismus and swallowing difficulties. These resemble serious neurological disorders but usually subside within 48 hours. Management of the extrapyramidal symptoms, depending upon the type and severity, includes sedation, injectable diphenhydramine and the use of antiparkinsonism agents. In rare instances, persistent dyskinesias usually involving the face, tongue and jaw have been reported to last months, even years, particularly in elderly patients with previous brain damage.

Hyperreflexia has been reported in the newborn when a phenothiazine was used during pregnancy.

Adverse Behavioral Effects: Paradoxical exacerbation of psychotic symptoms.

Other CNS Effects: Cerebral edema. Abnormality of cerebrospinal fluid proteins. Convulsive seizures, particularly in patients with EEG abnormalities or a history of such disorders. Hyperpyrexia.

Allergic Reactions: Urticaria, itching, erythema, photosensitivity (avoid undue exposure to the sun), eczema. Severe reactions including exfoliative dermatitis (rare); contact dermatitis in nursing personnel administering the drug; asthma, laryngeal edema, angioneurotic edema, anaphylactoid reactions.

Endocrine Disorders: Lactation and moderate breast engorgement in females and gynecomastia in males on large doses, changes in libido, false-positive pregnancy tests, amenorrhea, hyperglycemia, hypoglycemia, glycosuria.

Autonomic Reactions: Dry mouth, nasal congestion, constipation, adynamic ileus, myosis, mydriasis, urinary retention.

Special Considerations in Long-Term Therapy: After prolonged administration of high doses, pigmentation of the skin has occurred chiefly in the exposed areas, especially in females on large doses. Ocular changes consisting of deposition of fine particulate matter in the cornea and lens, progressing in more severe cases to star-shaped lenticular opacities; epithelial keratopathies; pigmentary retinopathy.

Persistent Tardive Dyskinesia: As with all antipsychotic agents, tardive dyskinesia may appear in some patients on long-term therapy or may occur after drug therapy has been discontinued. The risk seems to be greater in elderly patients on high-dose therapy, especially females. The symptoms are persistent and in some patients appear to be irreversible. The syndrome is characterized by rhythmical involuntary movements of the tongue, face, mouth, or jaw (*e.g.,* protrusion of tongue, puffing of cheeks, puckering of mouth, chewing movements). Sometimes these may be accompanied by involuntary movements of extremities.

There is no known effective treatment for tardive dyskinesia; antiparkinsonism agents usually do not alleviate the symptoms of this syndrome. It is suggested that all antipsychotic agents be discontinued if these symptoms appear. Should it be necessary to reinstitute treatment, or increase the dosage of the agent, or switch to a different antipsychotic agent, the syndrome may be masked.

It has been reported that fine vermicular movements of the tongue may be an early sign of the syndrome and if the medication is stopped at that time the syndrome may not develop.

Other Adverse Reactions: Enlargement of the parotid gland; increases in appetite and weight; peripheral edema.

The occurrence of a systemic lupus erythematosus-like syndrome has been related to phenothiazine therapy.

Dosage and Administration: Dosage should be individually adjusted according to diagnosis and severity of the condition. In general, small doses should be used initially, and increased to the optimal effective level as rapidly as possible based on therapeutic response. When higher dosage is required, greater sedation may be encountered; therefore, patients should be closely supervised. Lethargy and drowsiness are readily controlled by dosage reduction. Initially, lower doses (10 to 25 mg three or four times daily) should be used for elderly or debilitated patients.

For convenience in prescribing and dispensing, all recommended dosages are expressed as strengths of the active moiety, chlorprothixene.

Taractan may be administered orally as tablets or concentrate. The concentrate, containing 100 mg of the drug per 5 ml teaspoonful, is pleasantly flavored and may be administered alone or in milk, water, fruit juices, coffee and carbonated beverages.

Oral	**Average Daily Dose**
Adults:	Initially, 25 to 50 mg three or four times daily; to be increased as needed. Dosages exceeding 600 mg daily are rarely required.
Children (over 6 years of age):	10 to 25 mg three or four times daily.
Parenteral	
Not to be used in children under the age of 12.	25 to 50 mg I.M. up to three or four times daily.

Pain or induration at the site of injection is minimal. Since postural hypotension may occur in some patients, injection should be given with the patient seated or recumbent. If hypotension does occur, recovery is usually spontaneous; however, the patient should be observed until symptoms of weakness or dizziness pass. As soon as the acutely agitated patient is brought under control, oral medication should be instituted. The changeover should be made gradually, with oral and parenteral doses being given alternately on the same day, then oral doses only, adjusted to the required maintenance level.

Overdosage: Taractan can be fatal in overdosage in the range of 2.5 to 4 Gm or above. Manifestations of overdosage are drowsiness, coma, respiratory depression, hypotension (which may appear after a delay of several hours and may persist for two to three days), tachycardia, pyrexia and constricted pupils. Convulsions, hyperactivity and hematuria may be seen in the recovery period.

Treatment is essentially symptomatic. Early gastric lavage is recommended, along with supportive measures such as I.V. fluids and the maintenance of an adequate airway. Severe hypotension usually responds to the use of levarterenol or metaraminol. Should coma be prolonged, caffeine and sodium benzoate, or ethamivan may be used, but the possibility must be borne in mind that these may lead to a convulsive episode. Should convulsions occur, the judicious use of sodium amytal is recommended. **Epinephrine must not be used in these patients.**

How Supplied: Tablets—10 mg, 25 mg, 50 mg or 100 mg chlorprothixene—bottles of 100 and 500.

Concentrate—containing, in each teaspoonful, chlorprothixene 100 mg base (as the lactate and hydrochloride)—bottles of 16 fluid ounces (1 pint).

Ampuls—containing chlorprothixene 25 mg/2 ml as the hydrochloride—boxes of 10.

Animal Pharmacology and Toxicology: In mice, the oral LD_{50} of the two oral dosage forms of chlorprothixene were 350 ± 27 mg/kg (as the 2 per cent concentrate) and 220 ± 24 mg/kg (as the tablet form ground and suspended in 5 per cent gum acacia). For the injectable form the intramuscular LD_{50} in mice was greater than 125 mg/kg.

Reproduction Studies: Reproductive and teratological studies in rats and rabbits were performed at levels of 12 and 24 mg/kg. In the rats, a decreased conception rate and an increased incidence of stillborns was noted at both levels. An increased number of resorptions was noted only at the high dose level. There was a decrease in the number of implantation sites at both doses. The number of live fetuses per litter and the mean fetal body weights were reduced slightly at 12 mg/kg and more so at 24 mg/kg. No teratological effects were observed. No deleterious effects on reproduction were seen in rabbits nor were any teratological findings noted.

[*Shown in Product Identification Section*]

TEL-E-DOSE®

Tel-E-Dose is a unit package designed by Roche for convenience in dispensing medications in the hospital and nursing home. Each unit, sealed against contamination and moisture, is clearly identified by product name and strength and carries the control number and expiration date.

Currently available in this package form are the following products: Bactrim™ (80 mg trimethoprim and 400 mg sulfamethoxazole) tablets; Bactrim™ DS (160 mg trimethoprim and 800 mg sulfamethoxazole) tablets; Endep® (amitriptyline HCl) tablets, 10 mg, 25 mg, 50 mg, 75 mg, 100 mg, 150 mg; Gantanol® (sulfamethoxazole) tablets, 0.5 Gm; Gantanol® DS (sulfamethoxazole) tablets, 1 Gm; Gantrisin® (sulfisoxazole) tablets, 0.5 Gm; Larotid® (amoxicillin) capsules, 250 mg, 500 mg; Larotid® (amoxicillin) oral suspension, 125 mg and 250 mg; Trimpex® (trimethoprim) tablets, 100 mg.

TENSILON® ℞

(edrophonium chloride/Roche)
Injectable Solution
ampuls • vials

The following text is complete prescribing information based on official labeling in effect August 1, 1982.

Description: Tensilon is a short and rapid-acting cholinergic drug. Chemically, edrophonium chloride is ethyl (*m*-hydroxyphenyl)-dimethylammonium chloride.

10-ml vials: Each ml contains, in a sterile solution, 10 mg edrophonium chloride/Roche compounded with 0.45% phenol and 0.2% sodium sulfite as preservatives, buffered with sodium citrate and citric acid, and pH adjusted to approximately 5.4.

1-ml ampuls: Each ml contains, in a sterile solution, 10 mg edrophonium chloride/Roche compounded with 0.2% sodium sulfite, buffered with sodium citrate and citric acid, and pH adjusted to approximately 5.4.

Actions: Tensilon is an anticholinesterase drug. Its pharmacological action is due primarily to the inhibition or inactivation of acetylcholinesterase at sites of cholinergic transmission. Its effect is manifest within 30 to 60 seconds after injection and lasts an average of 10 minutes.

Indications: Tensilon is recommended for the differential diagnosis of myasthenia gravis and as an adjunct in the evaluation of treatment requirements in this disease. It may also be used for evaluating emergency treatment in myasthenic crises. Because of its brief duration of action, it is not recommended for maintenance therapy in myasthenia gravis.

Tensilon is also useful whenever a curare antagonist is needed to reverse the neuromuscular block produced by curare, tubocurarine, gallamine triethiodide or dimethyl-tubocurarine. It is *not* effective against decamethonium bromide and succinylcholine chloride. It may be used adjunctively in the treatment of respiratory depression caused by curare overdosage.

Contraindications: Known hypersensitivity to anticholinesterase agents; intestinal and urinary obstructions of mechanical type.

Warnings: Whenever anticholinesterase drugs are used for testing, a syringe containing 1 mg of atropine sulfate should be immediately available to be given in aliquots intravenously to counteract severe cholinergic reactions which may occur in the hypersensitive individual, whether he is normal or myasthenic. Tensilon should be used with caution in patients with bronchial asthma or cardiac dysrhythmias. The transient bradycardia which sometimes occurs can be relieved by atropine sulfate. Isolated instances of cardiac and respiratory arrest following administration of Tensilon have been reported. It is postulated that these are vagotonic effects.

Usage in Pregnancy: The safety of Tensilon during pregnancy or lactation in humans has not been established. Therefore, use of Tensilon in women who may become pregnant requires weighing the drug's potential benefits against its possible hazards to mother and child.

Responses to Tensilon in Myasthenic and Nonmyasthenic Individuals

	Myasthenic*	Adequate**	Cholinergic***
Muscle Strength . . . (ptosis, diplopia, dysphonia, dysphagia, dysarthria, respiration, limb strength)	Increased	No change	Decreased
Fasciculations . . . (orbicularis oculi, facial muscles, limb muscles)	Absent	Present or absent	Present or absent
Side reactions . . . (lacrimination, diaphoresis, salivation, abdominal cramps, nausea, vomiting, diarrhea)	Absent	Minimal	Severe

*Myasthenic Response—occurs in untreated myasthenics and may serve to establish diagnosis; in patients under treatment, indicates that therapy is inadequate.

**Adequate Response—observed in treated patients when therapy is stabilized; a typical response in normal individuals. In addition to this response in nonmyasthenics, the phenomenon of forced lid closure is often observed in psychoneurotics.[1]

***Cholinergic Response—seen in myasthenics who have been overtreated with anticholinesterase drugs.

Precautions: Patients may develop "anticholinesterase insensitivity" for brief or prolonged periods. During these periods the patients should be carefully monitored and may need respiratory assistance. Dosages of anticholinesterase drugs should be reduced or withheld until patients again become sensitive to them.

Adverse Reactions: Careful observation should be made for severe cholinergic reactions in the hyperreactive individual. The myasthenic patient in crisis who is being tested with Tensilon should be observed for bradycardia or cardiac standstill and cholinergic reactions if an overdose is given. The following reactions common to anticholinesterase agents may occur, although not all of these reactions have been reported with the administration of Tensilon, probably because of its short duration of action and limited indications: **Eye:** Increased lacrimation, pupillary constriction, spasm of accommodation, diplopia, conjunctival hyperemia. **CNS:** Convulsions, dysarthria, dysphonia, dysphagia. **Respiratory:** Increased tracheobronchial secretions, laryngospasm, bronchiolar constriction, paralysis of muscles of respiration, central respiratory paralysis. **Cardiac:** Arrhythmias (especially bradycardia), fall in cardiac output leading to hypotension. **G.I.:** Increased salivary, gastric and intestinal secretion, nausea, vomiting, increased peristalsis, diarrhea, abdominal cramps. **Skeletal Muscle:** Weakness, fasciculations. **Miscellaneous:** Increased urinary frequency and incontinence, diaphoresis.

Dosage and Administration: *Tensilon Test in the Differential Diagnosis of Myasthenia Gravis:*[1-8]

Intravenous Dosage (Adults): A tuberculin syringe containing 1 ml (10 mg) of Tensilon is prepared with an intravenous needle, and 0.2 ml (2 mg) is injected intravenously within 15 to 30 seconds. The needle is left *in situ*. *Only* if no reaction occurs after 45 seconds is the remaining 0.8 ml (8 mg) injected. If a cholinergic reaction (muscarinic side effects, skeletal muscle fasciculations and increased muscle weakness) occurs after injection of 0.2 ml (2 mg), the test is discontinued and atropine sulfate 0.4 mg to 0.5 mg is administered intravenously. After one-half hour the test may be repeated.

Intramuscular Dosage (Adults): In adults with inaccessible veins, dosage for intramuscular injection is 1 ml (10 mg) of Tensilon. Subjects who demonstrate hyperreactivity to this injection (cholinergic reaction), should be retested after one-half hour with 0.2 ml (2 mg) of Tensilon intramuscularly to rule out false-negative reactions.

Dosage (Children): The intravenous testing dose of Tensilon in children weighing up to 75 lbs is 0.1 ml (1 mg); above this weight, the dose is 0.2 ml (2 mg). If there is no response after 45 seconds, it may be titrated up to 0.5 ml (5 mg) in children under 75 lbs, given in increments of 0.1 ml (1 mg) every 30 to 45 seconds and up to 1 ml (10 mg) in heavier children. In infants, the recommended dose is 0.05 ml (0.5 mg). Because of technical difficulty with intravenous injection in children, the intramuscular route may be used. In children weighing up to 75 lbs, 0.2 ml (2 mg) is injected intramuscularly. In children weighing more than 75 lbs, 0.5 ml (5 mg) is injected intramuscularly. All signs which would appear with the intravenous test appear with the intramuscular test except that there is a delay of two to ten minutes before a reaction is noted.

Tensilon Test for Evaluation of Treatment Requirements in Myasthenia Gravis: The recommended dose is 0.1 ml to 0.2 ml (1 mg to 2 mg) of Tensilon, administered intravenously one hour after oral intake of the drug being used in treatment.[1-5] Response will be myasthenic in the undertreated patient, adequate in the controlled patient, and cholinergic in the overtreated patient. Responses to Tensilon in myasthenic and nonmyasthenic individuals are summarized in the accompanying chart.[2] [See table above].

Tensilon Test in Crisis: The term *crisis* is applied to the myasthenic whenever severe respiratory distress with objective ventilatory inadequacy occurs and the response to medication is not predictable. This state may be secondary to a sudden increase in severity of myasthenia gravis (myasthenic crisis), or to overtreatment with anticholinesterase drugs (cholinergic crisis).

When a patient is apneic, controlled ventilation must be secured immediately in order to avoid cardiac arrest and irreversible central nervous system damage. No attempt is made to test with Tensilon until respiratory exchange is adequate. *Dosage used at this time is most important:* If the patient is cholinergic, Tensilon will cause increased oropharyngeal secretions and further weakness in the muscles of respiration. If the crisis is myasthenic, the test clearly improves respiration and the patient can be treated with longer-acting intravenous anticholinesterase medication. When the test is performed, there should not be more than 0.2 ml (2 mg) Tensilon in the syringe. An intravenous dose of 0.1 ml (1 mg) is given initially. The patient's heart action is carefully observed. If, after an interval of one minute, this dose does not further impair the patient, the remaining 0.1 ml (1 mg) can be injected. If no clear improvement of respiration occurs after 0.2 ml (2 mg) dose, it is usually wisest to discontinue all anticholinesterase drug therapy and secure controlled ventilation by tracheostomy with assisted respiration.[5]

For Use as a Curare Antagonist: Tensilon should be administered by intravenous injection in 1 ml (10 mg) doses given slowly over a period of 30 to 45 seconds so that the onset of cholinergic reaction can be detected. This dosage may be repeated whenever necessary. The maximal dose for any one patient should be 4 ml (40 mg). Because of its brief effect, Tensilon

Continued on next page

Roche Labs.—Cont.

should not be given prior to the administration of curare, tubocurarine, gallamine triethiodide or dimethyl-tubocurarine; it should be used at the time when its effect is needed. When given to counteract curare overdosage, the effect of each dose on the respiration should be carefully observed before it is repeated, and assisted ventilation should always be employed.

Drug Interactions: Care should be given when administering this drug to patients with symptoms of myasthenic weakness who are also on anticholinesterase drugs. Since symptoms of anticholinesterase overdose (cholinergic crisis) may mimic underdosage (myasthenic weakness), their condition may be worsened by the use of this drug. (See OVERDOSAGE section for treatment.)

Overdosage: With drugs of this type, muscarine-like symptoms (nausea, vomiting, diarrhea, sweating, increased bronchial and salivary secretions and bradycardia) often appear with overdosage (cholinergic crisis). An important complication that can arise is obstruction of the airway by bronchial secretions. These may be managed with suction (especially if tracheostomy has been performed) and by the use of atropine. Many experts have advocated a wide range of dosages of atropine *(for Tensilon, see atropine dosage below)*, but if there are copious secretions, up to 1.2 mg intravenously may be given initially and repeated every 20 minutes until secretions are controlled. Signs of atropine overdosage such as dry mouth, flush and tachycardia should be avoided as tenacious secretions and bronchial plugs may form. A total dose of atropine of 5 to 10 mg or even more may be required. The following steps should be taken in the management of overdosage of Tensilon:

1. Adequate respiratory exchange should be maintained by assuring an open airway, and the use of assisted respiration augmented by oxygen.
2. Cardiac function should be monitored until complete stabilization has been achieved.
3. Atropine sulfate in doses of 0.4 to 0.5 mg should be administered intravenously. This may be repeated every 3 to 10 minutes. Because of the short duration of action of Tensilon the total dose required will seldom exceed 2 mg.
4. Pralidoxime chloride (a cholinesterase reactivator) may be given intravenously at the rate of 50 to 100 mg per minute; usually the total dose does not exceed 1000 mg. Extreme caution should be exercised in the use of pralidoxime chloride when the cholinergic symptoms are induced by double-bond phosphorous anticholinesterase drugs.[9]
5. If convulsions or shock is present, appropriate measures should be instituted.

How Supplied: *Multiple Dose Vials,* 10 ml. *Ampuls,* 1 ml, boxes of 10.

References:

1. Osserman, K.E. and Kaplan, L.I., *J.A.M.A., 150:*265, 1952.
2. Osserman, K.E., Kaplan, L.I. and Besson, G., *J. Mt. Sinai Hosp., 20:*165, 1953.
3. Osserman, K.E. and Kaplan, L.I., *Arch. Neurol. & Psychiat., 70:*385, 1953.
4. Osserman, K.E. and Teng, P., *J.A.M.A., 160:*153, 1956.
5. Osserman, K.E. and Genkins, G., *Ann. N.Y. Acad. Sci., 135:*312, 1966.
6. Tether, J.E., Second International Symposium Proceedings, Myasthenia Gravis, 1961, p. 444.
7. Tether, J.E., in H.F. Conn: *Current Therapy 1960,* Philadelphia, W. B. Saunders Company, p. 551.
8. Tether, J.E., in H.F. Conn: *Current Therapy 1965,* Philadelphia, W. B. Saunders Company, p. 556.
9. Grob, D. and Johns, R.J., *J.A.M.A., 166:*1855, 1958.

TRIMPEX® ℞

(trimethoprim)
TABLETS

The following text is complete prescribing information based on official labeling in effect August 1, 1982.

Description: Trimpex (trimethoprim) is a synthetic antibacterial, available in scored white tablets, each containing 100 mg trimethoprim. Trimethoprim is 2,4-diamino-5-(3,4,5-trimethoxybenzyl) pyrimidine. It is a white to light yellow, odorless, bitter compound with a molecular weight of 290.3.

Clinical Pharmacology: Trimethoprim is rapidly absorbed following oral administration. Mean peak serum levels of approximately 1.0 mcg/ml occur 1 to 4 hours after oral administration of a single 100 mg dose. The half-life of trimethoprim is 8 to 10 hours.

Trimethoprim exists in the blood as free, protein-bound and metabolized forms. Approximately 44% of trimethoprim is protein-bound in the blood. The free form is considered to be the therapeutically active form.

Excretion of trimethoprim is chiefly by the kidneys through glomerular filtration and tubular secretion. Urine concentrations of trimethoprim are considerably higher than are the concentrations in the blood. Trimethoprim urine levels, after a single oral dose of 100 mg, ranged from 30 to 160 mcg/ml during the 0 to 4 hour period and declined to approximately 18 to 91 mcg/ml during the 8 to 24 hour period. After oral administration, 50% to 60% of trimethoprim is excreted in the urine within 24 hours, approximately 80% of this being unmetabolized trimethoprim.

Microbiology: Trimpex blocks the production of tetrahydrofolic acid from dihydrofolic acid by binding to and reversibly inhibiting the enzyme dihydrofolate reductase. This binding is very much stronger for the bacterial enzyme than for the corresponding mammalian enzyme. Thus, Trimpex selectively interferes with bacterial biosynthesis of nucleic acids and proteins.

In vitro serial dilution tests have shown that the spectrum of antibacterial activity of Trimpex includes the common urinary tract pathogens with the exception of *Pseudomonas aeruginosa.*

Representative Minimum Inhibitory Concentrations For Trimethoprim-Susceptible Organisms

Bacteria	Trimethoprim MIC —mcg/ml (Range)
Escherichia coli	0.05—1.5
Proteus mirabilis	0.5—1.5
Klebsiella pneumoniae	0.5—5.0
Enterobacter species	0.5—5.0

The recommended quantitative disc susceptibility method[1,2] may be used for estimating the susceptibility of bacteria to Trimpex. Reports from the laboratory giving results of the standardized test using the 5 mcg trimethoprim disc should be interpreted according to the following criteria:

Organisms producing zones of 16 mm or greater are classified as susceptible whereas those producing zones of 11 to 15 mm are classified as having intermediate susceptibility.

A report from the laboratory of "Susceptible to trimethoprim" or "Intermediate susceptibility to trimethoprim" indicates that the infection is likely to respond when, as in uncomplicated urinary tract infections, effective therapy is dependent upon the urine concentration of trimethoprim.

Organisms producing zones of 10 mm or less are reported as resistant, indicating that other therapy should be selected.

Dilution methods for determining susceptibility are also used, and results are reported as the minimum drug concentration inhibiting microbial growth (MIC).[3]

If the MIC is 8 mcg per ml or less, the microorganism is considered "susceptible." If the MIC is 16 mcg per ml or greater, the microorganism is considered "resistant."

Normal vaginal and fecal flora are the source of most pathogens causing urinary tract infections. It is therefore relevant to consider the suppressive effect of trimethoprim in these sites.

Concentrations of trimethoprim in vaginal secretions are consistently greater than those found simultaneously in the serum, being typically 1.6 times the concentration of simultaneously obtained serum samples. Sufficient trimethoprim is excreted in the feces to markedly reduce or eliminate trimethoprim-susceptible organisms from the fecal flora.

The dominant fecal organisms (non-*Enterobacteriaceae), Bacteroides* spp. and *Lactobacillus* spp., are not susceptible to trimethoprim levels obtained with the recommended dosage.

Indications and Usage: For the treatment of initial episodes of uncomplicated urinary tract infections due to susceptible strains of the following organisms: *Escherichia coli, Proteus mirabilis, Klebsiella pneumoniae* and *Enterobacter* species.

Cultures and susceptibility tests should be performed to determine the susceptibility of the bacteria to trimethoprim. Therapy may be initiated prior to obtaining the results of these tests.

Contraindications: Trimpex is contraindicated in individuals hypersensitive to trimethoprim and in those with documented megaloblastic anemia due to folate deficiency.

Warnings: Experience with trimethoprim alone is limited, but it has been reported rarely to interfere with hematopoiesis, especially when administered in large doses and/or for prolonged periods.

The presence of clinical signs such as sore throat, fever, pallor or purpura may be early indications of serious blood disorders. Complete blood count should be obtained if any of these signs are noted in a patient receiving trimethoprim and the drug discontinued if a significant reduction in the count of any formed blood element is found.

Precautions: *General:* Trimethoprim should be given with caution to patients with possible folate deficiency. Folates may be administered concomitantly without interfering with the antibacterial action of trimethoprim. Trimethoprim should also be given with caution to patients with impaired renal or hepatic function.

Pregnancy: Teratogenic Effects: Pregnancy Category C. Trimethoprim has been shown to be teratogenic in the rat when given in doses 40 times the human dose. In some rabbit studies, the overall increase in fetal loss (dead and resorbed and malformed conceptuses) was associated with doses 6 times the human therapeutic dose. While there are no large well-controlled studies on the use of trimethoprim in pregnant women, Brumfitt and Pursell[4] reported the outcome of 186 pregnancies during which the mother received either placebo or trimethoprim in combination with sulfamethoxazole. The incidence of congenital abnormalities was 4.5% (3 of 66) in those who received placebo and 3.3% (4 of 120) in those receiving trimethoprim plus sulfamethoxazole. There were no abnormalities in the 10 children whose mothers received the drug during the first trimester. In a separate survey, Brumfitt and Pursell also found no congenital abnormalities in 35 children whose mothers had received trimethoprim plus sulfamethoxazole at the time of conception or shortly thereafter.

Because trimethoprim may interfere with folic acid metabolism, Trimpex should be used during pregnancy only if the potential benefit justifies the potential risk to the fetus.

Nursing Mothers: Trimethoprim is excreted in human milk. Because trimethoprim may interfere with folic acid metabolism, caution should be exercised when Trimpex is administered to a nursing woman.

Pediatric Use: The safety of trimethoprim in infants under two months of age has not been demonstrated. The effectiveness of trimethoprim has not been established in children under 12 years of age.

Adverse Reactions: The adverse effects encountered most often with trimethoprim were rash and pruritus. Other adverse effects reported involved the gastrointestinal and hematopoietic systems.

Dermatologic Reactions: Rash, pruritus and exfoliative dermatitis. At the recommended dose of 100 mg b.i.d., the incidence of rash is 2.9%. In clinical studies which employed high doses of Trimpex, an elevated incidence of rash was noted. These rashes were maculopapular, morbilliform, pruritic and generally mild to moderate, appearing 7 to 14 days after the initiation of therapy.

Gastrointestinal Reactions: Epigastric distress, nausea, vomiting and glossitis.

Hematologic Reactions: Thrombocytopenia, leukopenia, neutropenia, megaloblastic anemia and methemoglobinemia.

Miscellaneous Reactions: Fever, elevation of serum transaminase and bilirubin, and increases in BUN and serum creatinine levels.

Overdosage:

Acute: Signs of acute overdosage with trimethoprim may appear following ingestion of 1 gram or more of the drug and include nausea, vomiting, dizziness, headaches, mental depression, confusion and bone marrow depression (see CHRONIC OVERDOSAGE). Treatment consists of gastric lavage and general supportive measures. Acidification of the urine will increase renal elimination of trimethoprim. Peritoneal dialysis is not effective and hemodialysis only moderately effective in eliminating the drug.

Chronic: Use of trimethoprim at high doses and/or for extended periods of time may cause bone marrow depression manifested as thrombocytopenia, leukopenia and/or megaloblastic anemia. If signs of bone marrow depression occur, trimethoprim should be discontinued and the patient should be given leucovorin, 3 to 6 mg intramuscularly daily for three days, or as required to restore normal hematopoiesis.

Dosage and Administration: The usual oral adult dosage is 100 mg of Trimpex every 12 hours for 10 days.

The use of trimethoprim in patients with a creatinine clearance of less than 15 ml/min is not recommended. For patients with a creatinine clearance of 15 to 30 ml/min, the dose should be 50 mg every 12 hours.

The effectiveness of trimethoprim has not been established in children under 12 years of age.

How Supplied: Tablets, containing 100 mg trimethoprim—bottles of 100; Tel-E-Dose® packages of 100; and Prescription Paks of 20.

References:

1. Bauer AW, Kirby WMM, Sherris JC, Turck M: Antibiotic Susceptibility Testing by Standardized Single Disk Method, *Am J Clin Path 45*:493–496, 1966.

2. Approved Standard ASM-2 Performance Standards for Antimicrobial Disc Susceptibility Test; National Committee for Clinical Laboratory Standards, 771 East Lancaster Avenue, Villanova, Pennsylvania 19085.

3. Ericsson HM, Sherris JC: "Antibiotic Sensitivity Testing. Report of an International Collaborative Study." Acta Pathologica et Microbiologica Scandinavica, Section B, Suppl. 217, 1971, pp. 1–90.

4. Brumfitt W, Pursell R: Trimethoprim/Sulfamethoxazole in the Treatment of Bacteriuria in Women. *J Inf Dis 128* Suppl: S657–S663, 1973.

[*Shown in Product Identification Section*]

VALIUM® Injectable ©
(diazepam/Roche)

The following text is complete prescribing information based on official labeling in effect August 1, 1982.

Description: Each ml contains 5 mg diazepam/Roche compounded with 40% propylene glycol, 10% ethyl alcohol, 5% sodium benzoate and benzoic acid as buffers, and 1.5% benzyl alcohol as preservative.

Diazepam is a benzodiazepine derivative developed through original Roche research. Chemically, diazepam is 7-chloro-1,3-dihydro-1-methyl-5-phenyl-2H-1, 4-benzodiazepin-2-one. It is a colorless crystalline compound, insoluble in water and has a molecular weight of 284.74.

Actions: In animals, diazepam appears to act on parts of the limbic system, the thalamus and hypothalamus, and induces calming effects. Diazepam, unlike chlorpromazine and reserpine, has no demonstrable peripheral autonomic blocking action, nor does it produce extrapyramidal side effects; however, animals treated with diazepam do have a transient ataxia at higher doses. Diazepam was found to have transient cardiovascular depressor effects in dogs. Long-term experiments in rats revealed no disturbances of endocrine function. Injections into animals have produced localized irritation of tissue surrounding injection sites and some thickening of veins after intravenous use.

Indications: Valium is indicated for the management of anxiety disorders or for the short-term relief of the symptoms of anxiety. Anxiety or tension associated with the stress of everyday life usually does not require treatment with an anxiolytic.

In acute alcohol withdrawal, Valium may be useful in the symptomatic relief of acute agitation, tremor, impending or acute delirium tremens and hallucinosis.

As an adjunct prior to endoscopic procedures if apprehension, anxiety or acute stress reactions are present, and to diminish the patient's recall of the procedures. (See WARNINGS.)

Valium is a useful adjunct for the relief of skeletal muscle spasm due to reflex spasm to local pathology (such as inflammation of the muscles or joints, or secondary to trauma); spasticity caused by upper motor neuron disorders (such as cerebral palsy and paraplegia); athetosis; stiff-man syndrome; and tetanus.

Injectable Valium is a useful adjunct in status epilepticus and severe recurrent convulsive seizures.

Valium is a useful premedication (the I.M. route is preferred) for relief of anxiety and tension in patients who are to undergo surgical procedures. Intravenously, prior to cardioversion for the relief of anxiety and tension and to diminish the patient's recall of the procedure.

Contraindications: Injectable Valium is contraindicated in patients with a known hypersensitivity to this drug; acute narrow angle glaucoma; and open angle glaucoma unless patients are receiving appropriate therapy.

Warnings: *When used intravenously, the following procedures should be undertaken to reduce the possibility of venous thrombosis, phlebitis, local irritation, swelling, and, rarely, vascular impairment: the solution should be injected slowly, taking at least one minute for each 5 mg (1 ml) given; do not use small veins, such as those on the dorsum of the hand or wrist; extreme care should be taken to avoid intra-arterial administration or extravasation.*

Do not mix or dilute Valium with other solutions or drugs in syringe or infusion flask. If it is not feasible to administer Valium directly I.V., it may be injected slowly through the infusion tubing as close as possible to the vein insertion.

Extreme care must be used in administering Injectable Valium, particularly by the I.V. route, to the elderly, to very ill patients and to those with limited pulmonary reserve because of the possibility that apnea and/ or cardiac arrest may occur. Concomitant use of barbiturates, alcohol or other central nervous system depressants increases depression with increased risk of apnea. Resuscitative equipment including that necessary to support respiration should be readily available.

When Valium is used with a narcotic analgesic, the dosage of the narcotic should be reduced by at least one-third and administered in small increments. In some cases the use of a narcotic may not be necessary.

Injectable Valium should not be administered to patients in shock, coma, or in acute alcoholic intoxication with depression of vital signs. As is true of most CNS-acting drugs, patients receiving Valium should be cautioned against engaging in hazardous occupations requiring complete mental alertness, such as operating machinery or driving a motor vehicle.

Tonic status epilepticus has been precipitated in patients treated with I.V. Valium for petit mal status or petit mal variant status.

Physical and Psychological Dependence: Withdrawal symptoms (similar in character to those noted with barbiturates and alcohol) have occurred following abrupt discontinuance of diazepam (convulsions, tremor, abdominal and muscle cramps, vomiting and sweating). These were usually limited to those patients who had received excessive doses over an extended period of time. Although infrequently seen, milder withdrawal symptoms have also been reported following abrupt discontinuance of benzodiazepines taken continuously, generally at higher therapeutic levels, for at least several months. Consequently, after extended therapy, abrupt discontinuation should generally be avoided and a gradual tapering in dosage followed. Particularly addiction-prone individuals (such as drug addicts or alcoholics) should be under careful surveillance when receiving diazepam or other psychotropic agents because of the predisposition of such patients to habituation and dependence.

***Usage in Pregnancy:* An increased risk of congenital malformations associated with the use of minor tranquilizers (diazepam, meprobamate and chlordiazepoxide) during the first trimester of pregnancy has been suggested in several studies. Because use of these drugs is rarely a matter of urgency, their use during this period should almost always be avoided. The possibility that a woman of childbearing potential may be pregnant at the time of institution of therapy should be considered. Patients should be advised that if they become pregnant during therapy or intend to become pregnant they should communicate with their physicians about the desirability of discontinuing the drug.**

In humans, measurable amounts of diazepam were found in maternal and cord blood, indicating placental transfer of the drug. Until additional information is available, Valium Injectable is not recommended for obstetrical use.

Use in Children: Efficacy and safety of parenteral Valium has not been established in the neonate (30 days or less of age).

Prolonged central nervous system depression has been observed in neonates, apparently due to inability to biotransform Valium into inactive metabolites.

In pediatric use, in order to obtain maximal clinical effect with the minimum amount of drug and thus to reduce the risk of hazardous

Continued on next page

Roche Labs.—Cont.

side effects, such as apnea or prolonged periods of somnolence, it is recommended that the drug be given slowly over a three-minute period in a dosage not to exceed 0.25 mg/kg. After an interval of 15 to 30 minutes the initial dosage can be safely repeated. If, however, relief of symptoms is not obtained after a third administration, adjunctive therapy appropriate to the condition being treated is recommended.

Precautions: Although seizures may be brought under control promptly, a significant proportion of patients experience a return to seizure activity, presumably due to the short-lived effect of Valium after I.V. administration. The physician should be prepared to re-administer the drug. However, Valium is not recommended for maintenance, and once seizures are brought under control, consideration should be given to the administration of agents useful in longer term control of seizures.

If Valium is to be combined with other psychotropic agents or anticonvulsant drugs, careful consideration should be given to the pharmacology of the agents to be employed—particularly with known compounds which may potentiate the action of Valium, such as phenothiazines, narcotics, barbiturates, MAO inhibitors and other antidepressants. In highly anxious patients with evidence of accompanying depression, particularly those who may have suicidal tendencies, protective measures may be necessary. The usual precautions in treating patients with impaired hepatic function should be observed. Metabolites of Valium are excreted by the kidney; to avoid their excess accumulation, caution should be exercised in the administration to patients with compromised kidney function.

Since an increase in cough reflex and laryngospasm may occur with peroral endoscopic procedures, the use of a topical anesthetic agent and the availability of necessary countermeasures are recommended.

Until additional information is available, injectable diazepam is not recommended for obstetrical use.

Injectable Valium has produced hypotension or muscular weakness in some patients particularly when used with narcotics, barbiturates or alcohol.

Lower doses (usually 2 mg to 5 mg) should be used for elderly and debilitated patients.

The clearance of Valium and certain other benzodiazepines can be delayed in association with Tagamet (cimetidine) administration. The clinical significance of this is unclear.

Adverse Reactions: Side effects most commonly reported were drowsiness, fatigue and ataxia; venous thrombosis and phlebitis at the site of injection. Other adverse reactions less frequently reported include: *CNS:* confusion, depression, dysarthria, headache, hypoactivity, slurred speech, syncope, tremor, vertigo. *G.I.:* constipation, nausea. *G.U.:* incontinence, changes in libido, urinary retention. *Cardiovascular:* bradycardia, cardiovascular collapse, hypotension. *EENT:* blurred vision, diplopia, nystagmus. *Skin:* urticaria, skin rash. *Other:* hiccups, changes in salivation, neutropenia, jaundice. Paradoxical reactions such as acute hyperexcited states, anxiety, hallucinations, increased muscle spasticity, insomnia, rage, sleep disturbances and stimulation have been reported; should these occur, use of the drug should be discontinued. Minor changes in EEG patterns, usually low-voltage fast activity, have been observed in patients during and after Valium therapy and are of no known significance.

In peroral endoscopic procedures, coughing, depressed respiration, dyspnea, hyperventilation, laryngospasm and pain in throat or chest have been reported.

Because of isolated reports of neutropenia and jaundice, periodic blood counts and liver function tests are advisable during long-term therapy.

Dosage and Administration: Dosage should be individualized for maximum beneficial effect. The usual recommended dose in older children and adults ranges from 2 mg to 20 mg I.M. or I.V., depending on the indication and its severity. In some conditions, e.g., tetanus, larger doses may be required. (See dosage for specific indications.) In acute conditions the injection may be repeated within one hour although an interval of 3 to 4 hours is usually satisfactory. Lower doses (usually 2 mg to 5 mg) and slow increase in dosage should be used for elderly or debilitated patients and when other sedative drugs are administered. (See WARNINGS and ADVERSE REACTIONS.)

For dosage in infants above the age of 30 days and children, see the specific indications below. When intravenous use is indicated, facilities for respiratory assistance should be readily available.

Intramuscular: Injectable Valium should be injected deeply into the muscle.

Intravenous use: (See WARNINGS, particularly for use in children.) The solution should be injected slowly, taking at least one minute for each 5 mg (1 ml) given. Do not use small veins, such as those on the dorsum of the hand or wrist. Extreme care should be taken to avoid intra-arterial administration or extravasation. Do not mix or dilute Valium with other solutions or drugs in syringe or infusion flask. If it is not feasible to administer Valium directly I.V., it may be injected slowly through the infusion tubing as close as possible to the vein insertion.

[See table on next page].

Once the acute symptomatology has been properly controlled with Injectable Valium, the patient may be placed on oral therapy with Valium if further treatment is required.

Management of Overdosage:

Manifestations of Valium overdosage include somnolence, confusion, coma, and diminished reflexes. Respiration, pulse and blood pressure should be monitored, as in all cases of drug overdosage, although, in general, these effects have been minimal. General supportive measures should be employed, along with intravenous fluids, and an adequate airway maintained. Hypotension may be combated by the use of Levophed® (levarterenol) or Aramine (metaraminol). Dialysis is of limited value.

How Supplied: Ampuls, 2 ml, boxes of 10; Vials, 10 ml, boxes of 1; Tel-E-Ject® (disposable syringes), 2 ml, boxes of 10.

Animal Pharmacology: Oral LD_{50} of diazepam is 720 mg/kg in mice and 1240 mg/kg in rats. Intraperitoneal administration of 400 mg/kg to a monkey resulted in death on the sixth day.

Reproduction Studies: A series of rat reproduction studies was performed with diazepam in oral doses of 1, 10, 80 and 100 mg/kg given for periods ranging from 60–228 days prior to mating. At 100 mg/kg there was a decrease in the number of pregnancies and surviving offspring in these rats. These effects may be attributable to prolonged sedative activity, resulting in lack of interest in mating and lessened maternal nursing and care of the young. Neonatal survival of rats at doses lower than 100 mg/kg was within normal limits. Several neonates, both controls and experimentals, in these rat reproduction studies showed skeletal or other defects. Further studies in rats at doses up to and including 80 mg/kg/day did not reveal significant teratological effects on the offspring. Rabbits were maintained on doses of 1, 2, 5 and 8 mg/kg from day 6 through day 18 of gestation. No adverse effects on reproduction and no teratological changes were noted.

[*Shown in Product Identification Section*]

VALRELEASE™ Ⓒ

(diazepam/Roche)

CAPSULES

A slow-release dosage form of Valium® (diazepam/Roche)

The following text is complete prescribing information based on official labeling in effect August 1, 1982.

Description: Diazepam is a benzodiazepine derivative developed through original Roche research. Chemically, diazepam is 7-chloro-1,3-dihydro-1-methyl-5-phenyl-2*H*-1,4-benzodiazepin-2-one. It is a colorless crystalline compound, insoluble in water and has a molecular weight of 284.74.

Valrelease capsules provide the actions of Valium® (diazepam/Roche) in a slow-release dosage form.

Pharmacology: In animals, diazepam appears to act on parts of the limbic system, the thalamus and hypothalamus, and induces calming effects. Diazepam, unlike chlorpromazine and reserpine, has no demonstrable peripheral autonomic blocking action, nor does it produce extrapyramidal side effects; however, animals treated with diazepam do have a transient ataxia at higher doses. Diazepam was found to have transient cardiovascular depressor effects in dogs. Long-term experiments in rats revealed no disturbances of endocrine function.

Oral LD_{50} of diazepam is 720 mg/kg in mice and 1240 mg/kg in rats. Intraperitoneal administration of 400 mg/kg to a monkey resulted in death on the sixth day.

Reproduction Studies: A series of rat reproduction studies was performed with diazepam in oral doses of 1, 10, 80 and 100 mg/kg. At 100 mg/kg there was a decrease in the number of pregnancies and surviving offspring in these rats. Neonatal survival of rats at doses lower than 100 mg/kg was within normal limits. Several neonates in these rat reproduction studies showed skeletal or other defects. Further studies in rats at doses up to and including 80 mg/kg/day did not reveal teratological effects on the offspring.

In humans, measurable blood levels of diazepam were obtained in maternal and cord blood, indicating placental transfer of the drug.

The administration of one 15-mg Valrelease capsule results in blood levels of diazepam over a 24-hour period which are comparable to those of 5-mg Valium tablets given three times daily.

The mean time to maximum plasma diazepam concentrations after administration of 15-mg Valrelease capsules to eleven fasted subjects was 5.3 hours. The harmonic mean half-life of diazepam was 36 hours. The range of average minimum steady-state plasma diazepam concentrations during once daily administration of 15-mg Valrelease capsules to eleven normal subjects was 196 to 341 ng/ml.

Indications: Valrelease is indicated for the management of anxiety disorders or for the short-term relief of the symptoms of anxiety. Anxiety or tension associated with the stress of everyday life usually does not require treatment with an anxiolytic.

In acute alcohol withdrawal, Valrelease may be useful in the symptomatic relief of acute agitation, tremor, impending or acute delirium tremens and hallucinosis.

Valrelease is a useful adjunct for the relief of skeletal muscle spasm due to reflex spasm to local pathology (such as inflammation of the muscles or joints, or secondary to trauma); spasticity caused by upper motor neuron disorders (such as cerebral palsy and paraplegia); athetosis; and stiff-man syndrome.

RECOMMENDED DOSAGE FOR INJECTABLE VALIUM® (diazepam/Roche)

	USUAL ADULT DOSAGE	DOSAGE RANGE IN CHILDREN (I.V. administration should be made slowly)
Moderate Anxiety Disorders and Symptoms of Anxiety	2 mg to 5 mg, I.M. or I.V. Repeat in 3 to 4 hours, if necessary.	
Severe Anxiety Disorders and Symptoms of Anxiety	5 mg to 10 mg, I.M. or I.V. Repeat in 3 to 4 hours, if necessary.	
Acute Alcohol Withdrawal: As an aid in symptomatic relief of acute agitation, tremor, impending or acute delirium tremens and hallucinosis.	10 mg, I.M. or I.V. initially, then 5 mg to 10 mg in 3 to 4 hours, if necessary.	
Endoscopic Procedures: Adjunctively, if apprehension, anxiety or acute stress reactions are present prior to endoscopic procedures. Dosage of narcotics should be reduced by at least a third and in some cases may be omitted. See *Precautions* for peroral procedures.	Titrate I.V. dosage to desired sedative response, such as slurring of speech, with slow administration immediately prior to the procedure. Generally 10 mg or less is adequate, but up to 20 mg I.V. may be given, particularly when concomitant narcotics are omitted. If I.V. cannot be used, 5 mg to 10 mg I.M. approximately 30 minutes prior to the procedure.	
Muscle Spasm: Associated with local pathology, cerebral palsy, athetosis, stiff-man syndrome or tetanus.	5 mg to 10 mg, I.M. or I.V. initially, then 5 mg to 10 mg in 3 to 4 hours, if necessary. For tetanus, larger doses may be required.	For tetanus in infants over 30 days of age, 1 mg to 2 mg I.M. or I.V., slowly, repeated every 3 to 4 hours as necessary. In children 5 years or older, 5 mg to 10 mg repeated every 3 to 4 hours may be required to control tetanus spasms. Respiratory assistance should be available.
Status Epilepticus and Severe Recurrent Convulsive Seizures: In the convulsing patient, the I.V. route is by far preferred. This injection should be administered slowly. However, if I.V. administration is impossible, the I.M. route may be used.	5 mg to 10 mg initially (I.V. preferred). This injection may be repeated if necessary at 10 to 15 minute intervals up to a maximum dose of 30 mg. If necessary, therapy with Valium (diazepam) may be repeated in 2 to 4 hours; however, residual active metabolites may persist, and readministration should be made with this consideration. Extreme caution must be exercised with individuals with chronic lung disease or unstable cardiovascular status.	Infants over 30 days of age and children under 5 years, 0.2 mg to 0.5 mg slowly every 2 to 5 minutes up to a maximum of 5 mg (I.V. preferred). Children 5 years or older, 1 mg every 2 to 5 minutes up to a maximum of 10 mg (slow I.V. administration preferred). Repeat in 2 to 4 hours if necessary. EEG monitoring of the seizure may be helpful.
Preoperative Medication: To relieve anxiety and tension. (If atropine, scopolamine or other premedications are desired, they must be administered in separate syringes.)	10 mg, I.M. (preferred route), before surgery.	
Cardioversion: To relieve anxiety and tension and to reduce recall of procedure.	5 mg to 15 mg, IV., within 5 to 10 minutes prior to the procedure.	

Valrelease may be used adjunctively in convulsive disorders, although it has not proved useful as the sole therapy.

The effectiveness of diazepam in long-term use, that is, more than 4 months, has not been assessed by systematic clinical studies. The physician should periodically reassess the usefulness of the drug for the individual patient.

Contraindications: Valrelease is contraindicated in patients with a known hypersensitivity to this drug and, because of lack of sufficient clinical experience, in children under 6 months of age. It may be used in patients with open angle glaucoma who are receiving appropriate therapy, but is contraindicated in acute narrow angle glaucoma.

Warnings: Valrelease is not of value in the treatment of psychotic patients and should not be employed in lieu of appropriate treatment.

As is true of most preparations containing CNS-acting drugs, patients receiving Valrelease should be cautioned against engaging in hazardous occupations requiring complete mental alertness such as operating machinery or driving a motor vehicle.

As with other agents which have anticonvulsant activity, when Valrelease is used as an adjunct in treating convulsive disorders, the possibility of an increase in the frequency and/or severity of grand mal seizures may require an increase in the dosage of standard anticonvulsant medication. Abrupt withdrawal of Valrelease in such cases may also be associated with a temporary increase in the frequency and/or severity of seizures.

Since Valrelease has a central nervous system depressant effect, patients should be advised against the simultaneous ingestion of alcohol and other CNS-depressant drugs during Valrelease therapy.

Physical and Psychological Dependence: Withdrawal symptoms (similar in character to those noted with barbiturates and alcohol) have occurred following abrupt discontinuance of diazepam (convulsions, tremor, abdominal and muscle cramps, vomiting and sweating). These were usually limited to those patients who had received excessive doses over an extended period of time. Although infrequently seen, milder withdrawal symptoms have also been reported following abrupt discontinuance of benzodiazepines taken continuously, generally at higher therapeutic levels, for at least several months. Consequently, after extended therapy, abrupt discontinuation should be generally avoided and a gradual tapering in dosage followed. Particularly addiction-prone individuals (such as drug addicts or alcoholics) should be under careful surveillance when receiving diazepam or other psychotropic agents because of the predisposition of such patients to habituation and dependence.

Usage in Pregnancy: **An increased risk of congenital malformations associated with the use of minor tranquilizers (diazepam, meprobamate and chlordiazepoxide) during the first trimester of pregnancy has been suggested in several studies. Because use of these drugs is rarely a matter of urgency, their use during this period should almost always be avoided. The possibility that a woman of childbearing potential may be pregnant at the time of institution of therapy should be considered. Patients should be advised that if they become pregnant during therapy or intend to become pregnant they should communicate with their physicians about the desirability of discontinuing the drug.**

Management of Overdosage: Manifestations of diazepam overdosage include somnolence, confusion, coma and diminished reflexes. Respiration, pulse and blood pressure should be monitored, as in all cases of drug overdosage, although, in general, these effects have been minimal following overdosage. General supportive measures should be employed, along with immediate gastric lavage. Intravenous

Roche Labs.—Cont.

fluids should be administered and an adequate airway maintained. Hypotension may be combated by the use of Levophed® (levarterenol) or Aramine (metaraminol). Dialysis is of limited value. As with the management of intentional overdosage with any drug, it should be borne in mind that multiple agents may have been ingested.

Precautions: If Valrelease is to be combined with other psychotropic agents or anticonvulsant drugs, careful consideration should be given to the pharmacology of the agents to be employed—particularly with known compounds which may potentiate the action of diazepam, such as phenothiazines, narcotics, barbiturates, MAO inhibitors and other antidepressants. The usual precautions are indicated for severely depressed patients or those in whom there is any evidence of latent depression; particularly the recognition that suicidal tendencies may be present and protective measures may be necessary. The usual precautions in treating patients with impaired renal or hepatic function should be observed.

In elderly and debilitated patients, it is recommended that the dosage be limited to the smallest effective amount to preclude the development of ataxia or oversedation (2 mg to 2½ mg once or twice daily, initially, to be increased gradually as needed and tolerated).

The clearance of Valium and certain other benzodiazepines can be delayed in association with Tagamet (cimetidine) administration. The clinical significance of this is unclear.

Adverse Reactions: Side effects most commonly reported were drowsiness, fatigue and ataxia. Infrequently encountered were confusion, constipation, depression, diplopia, dysarthria, headache, hypotension, incontinence, jaundice, changes in libido, nausea, changes in salivation, skin rash, slurred speech, tremor, urinary retention, vertigo and blurred vision. Paradoxical reactions such as acute hyperexcited states, anxiety, hallucinations, increased muscle spasticity, insomnia, rage, sleep disturbances and stimulation have been reported; should these occur, use of the drug should be discontinued.

Because of isolated reports of neutropenia and jaundice, periodic blood counts and liver function tests are advisable during long-term therapy. Minor changes in EEG patterns, usually low-voltage fast activity, have been observed in patients during and after diazepam therapy and are of no known significance.

Dosage and Administration: Dosage should be individualized for maximum beneficial effect. While the usual daily dosages given below will meet the needs of most patients, there will be some who may require higher doses. In such cases dosage should be increased cautiously to avoid adverse effects.

Whenever oral Valium® (diazepam/Roche), 5 mg t.i.d., would be considered the appropriate dosage, one 15-mg Valrelease capsule daily may be used.

Note: If 1 mg or 2½ mg is the desired dose, scored Valium (diazepam/Roche) tablets should be used.

Valrelease 15-mg capsules are recommended for elderly or debilitated patients and children only when it has been determined that 5 mg oral Valium t.i.d. is the optimal daily dose. Oral Valium is not recommended for children under 6 months of age.

Adults:	USUAL DAILY DOSE
Management of Anxiety Disorders and Relief of Symptoms of Anxiety.	Depending upon severity of symptoms—1 or 2 (15 to 30 mg) capsules once daily
Symptomatic Relief in Acute Alcohol Withdrawal	2 capsules (30 mg) the first 24 hours, followed by 1 capsule (15 mg) daily as needed.
Adjunctively for Relief of Skeletal Muscle Spasm.	1 or 2 capsules (15 to 30 mg) once daily
Adjunctively in Convulsive Disorders.	1 or 2 capsules (15 to 30 mg) once daily

How Supplied: For oral administration, Valrelease (diazepam/Roche) capsules—15 mg (yellow and blue)—bottles of 100; Prescription Paks of 30.

[*Shown in Product Identification Section*]

VI-PENTA® F CHEWABLES ℞

The following text is complete prescribing information based on official labeling in effect August 1, 1982.

Description: Vi-Penta F Chewables is a prescription-only chewable multivitamin tablet containing eleven vitamins and dietary fluoride. Vi-Penta F Chewables is specially formulated to provide daily nutritional support and aid in the prevention of tooth decay in children three years of age and older. Each fruit-flavored tablet contains less than one calorie and will not interfere with the appetite.

Each chewable tablet contains:

Fat-Soluble Vitamins	
Vitamin A (as vitamin A acetate)	5000 IU
Vitamin D_2 (ergocalciferol)	400 IU
Vitamin E (as *dl*-alpha-tocopheryl acetate)	2 IU
Water-Soluble Vitamins	
Vitamin C (as ascorbic acid and sodium ascorbate)	60 mg
Vitamin B_1 (as thiamine mononitrate)	1.2 mg
Vitamin B_2 (riboflavin)	1.5 mg
Niacin (as niacinamide)	10 mg
Vitamin B_6 (as pyridoxine HCl)	1 mg
d-biotin	40 mcg
Pantothenic acid (as calcium *d*-pantothenate)	9 mg
Vitamin B_{12} (cyanocobalamin)	3 mcg
Trace Elements	
Fluoride (as sodium fluoride)	1 mg

Clinical Pharmacology: Vitamins are necessary for maintenance of normal metabolic functions including hematopoiesis. *Vitamin A* is necessary for proper functioning of the retina; it appears to be essential to the integrity of epithelial cells. *Vitamin D* is necessary for the absorption of calcium and for the proper development and maintenance of bone structure. *Vitamin E* is an antioxidant which preserves essential cellular constituents, including those of the red blood cell. It also serves as protection against lipid peroxidation.

The water-soluble vitamins play vital roles in the conversion of carbohydrate, protein and fat into tissue and energy. *Thiamine (B_1)* acts as a coenzyme in carbohydrate metabolism. *Riboflavin (B_2)* functions as a coenzyme in the electron transport system associated with conversion of tissue oxidations into usable energy. *Niacin* serves as a coenzyme in oxidation-reduction reactions in tissue respiration. *Pyridoxine (B_6)* is essential for the metabolism of amino acids. *Pantothenic acid* functions as a coenzyme in various metabolic acetylation reactions and *biotin* in specific carboxylation reactions in lipid metabolism. *Cyanocobalamin (B_{12})* is essential to nucleic acid synthesis and normal maturation of red blood cells. *Ascorbic acid (C)* performs a vital function in the process of cellular respiration, and is involved in both carbohydrate and amino acid metabolism. It is essential for collagen formation and tissue repair.

Fluorine is an essential trace element that renders the dentine and enamel of teeth more resistant to acid.

There is ample evidence that the fluoridation of drinking water leads to a substantial decrease in the incidence of dental caries in childhood. This effect is greatest when fluoride is ingested during the first 9 to 10 years of life when teeth are developing. However, in areas where drinking water is devoid of natural or artificially controlled fluoride, or where fluoridation is not feasible, a single daily dose of fluoride as a dietary supplement is recommended as an effective substitute.

Recognizing the merits of dietary fluoride supplements, the Council on Dental Therapeutics of the American Dental Association strongly urges: "*Such administration should be consistent and continuous over long periods of time if substantial benefit is to be anticipated.*"

Indications and Usage: Vi-Penta F Chewable Tablets are indicated for supportive nutritional supplementation and as an aid in the prevention of tooth decay in children three years of age and older who reside in areas where the fluoride content of drinking water is known to be less than 0.7 parts per million.

Contraindications: Vi-Penta F Chewables is contraindicated in patients known to be hypersensitive to any of its components.

Warnings: This preparation should not be used in areas where the fluoride content of drinking water is known to be 0.7 parts per million or greater. The recommended dose of Vi-Penta F Chewables should not be exceeded, since dental fluorosis may result from continued ingestion of excessive amounts of fluoride.

Precautions: *General:* Certain patients may require nutritional supplementation with folic acid as well as other nutrients according to the dietary needs of the individual. Vi-Penta F Chewables is not intended for treatment of pernicious anemia or other severe specific vitamin deficiencies.

Information for the Patient: Because dental fluorosis may result from continued ingestion of excessive amounts of fluoride and toxic reactions have been reported with injudicious use of certain vitamins, urge patients to follow your specific instructions regarding dosage regimen. As with any medication, advise patients to keep Vi-Penta F Chewables out of reach of children.

Adverse Reactions: Adverse reactions have been reported with specific vitamins, but generally at levels substantially higher than those in Vi-Penta F Chewables. However, allergic and idiosyncratic reactions are possible at lower levels.

Dosage and Administration: Usual dosage for children three years of age and over: one tablet daily, chewed or crushed.

Vi-Penta F Chewables is available on prescription only.

How Supplied: Green, yellow, pink, purple and orange shield-shaped, biconvex tablets, engraved ROCHE 51—bottles of 100 chewable tablets (NDC 0004-0051-01).

[*Shown in Product Identification Section*]

VI-PENTA® F INFANT DROPS ℞

The following text is complete prescribing information based on official labeling in effect August 1, 1982.

Description: Vi-Penta F Infant Drops is a prescription-only liquid multivitamin preparation containing ascorbic acid, dietary fluoride and fat-soluble vitamins A, D and E. It is specially formulated to provide daily nutritional support and aid in the prevention of tooth decay in infants from birth. Vi-Penta F Infant Drops is a fruit-flavored, liquid preparation in an aqueous nonalcoholic vehicle that may be administered by dropping directly on the tongue or mixing with liquids or food.

Each 0.6 ml provides:

Fat-Soluble Vitamins	
Vitamin A (as vitamin A palmitate)	5000 IU
Vitamin D_2 (ergocalciferol)	400 IU
Vitamin E (as *dl*-alpha-tocopheryl acetate)	2 IU
Water-Soluble Vitamins	
Vitamin C (ascorbic acid)	50 mg
Trace Elements	
Fluoride (as sodium fluoride)	0.5 mg

Clinical Pharmacology: Vitamins are necessary for maintenance of normal metabolic functions including hematopoiesis. *Vitamin A* is necessary for proper functioning of the retina; it appears to be essential to the integrity of epithelial cells. *Vitamin D* is necessary for the absorption of calcium and for the proper development and maintenance of bone structure. *Vitamin E* is an antioxidant which preserves essential cellular constituents, including those of the red blood cell. It also serves as protection against lipid peroxidation. *Vitamin C* performs a vital function in the process of cellular respiration, and is involved in both carbohydrate and amino acid metabolism. It is essential for collagen formation and tissue repair. *Fluorine* is an essential trace element that renders the dentine and enamel of teeth more resistant to acid.

There is ample evidence that the fluoridation of drinking water leads to a substantial decrease in the incidence of dental caries in childhood. This effect is greatest when fluoride is ingested during the first 9 to 10 years of life when teeth are developing. However, in areas where drinking water is devoid of natural or artificially controlled fluoride, or where fluoridation is not feasible, a single daily dose of fluoride as a dietary supplement is recommended as an effective substitute.

Recognizing the merits of dietary fluoride supplements, the Council on Dental Therapeutics of the American Dental Association strongly urges: "*Such administration should be consistent and continuous over long periods of time if substantial benefit is to be anticipated.*"

Indications and Usage: Vi-Penta F Infant Drops is indicated for supportive nutritional supplementation and as an aid in the prevention of tooth decay in infants from birth who reside in areas where the fluoride content of drinking water is known to be less than 0.7 parts per million.

Contraindications: Vi-Penta F Infant Drops is contraindicated in patients known to be hypersensitive to any of its components.

Warnings: This preparation should not be used in areas where the fluoride content of drinking water is known to be 0.7 parts per million or greater. The recommended dose of Vi-Penta F Infant Drops should not be exceeded, since dental fluorosis may result from continued ingestion of excessive amounts of fluoride.

Precautions: *General:* Certain patients may require nutritional supplementation with the B-complex vitamins as well as other nutrients according to the dietary needs of the individual. Vi-Penta F Infant Drops is not intended for treatment of severe specific vitamin deficiencies.

Information for the Patient: Because dental fluorosis may result from continued ingestion of excessive amounts of fluoride and toxic reactions have been reported with injudicious use of certain vitamins, urge patients to follow your specific instructions regarding dosage regimen. As with any medication, advise patients to keep Vi-Penta F Infant Drops out of reach of children. Vi-Penta F Infant Drops should be stored under refrigeration.

Adverse Reactions: Adverse reactions have been reported with specific vitamins, but generally at levels substantially higher than those in Vi-Penta F Infant Drops. However, allergic and idiosyncratic reactions are possible at lower levels.

Dosage and Administration: Usual dosage for infants from birth: 0.6 ml daily, as measured by the dropper. Vi-Penta F Infant Drops may be administered by dropping directly on the tongue or mixing with liquids or food.

Vi-Penta F Infant Drops is available on prescription only.

How Supplied: Fruit-flavored liquid in bottle of 30 ml, packaged with a calibrated dropper (NDC 0004-1012-23).

NOTE TO THE PHARMACIST: Vi-Penta F Infant Drops should be dispensed in the original special plastic containers, since contact with glass leads to instability and precipitation. Preparation should be stored under refrigeration.

VI-PENTA® F MULTIVITAMIN DROPS ℞

The following text is complete prescribing information based on official labeling in effect August 1, 1982.

Description: Vi-Penta F Multivitamin Drops is a prescription-only liquid multivitamin preparation containing ten vitamins and dietary fluoride. It is specially formulated to provide daily nutritional support and aid in the prevention of tooth decay in infants and children. Vi-Penta F Multivitamin Drops is a fruit-flavored, liquid preparation in an aqueous nonalcoholic vehicle that may be administered by dropping directly on the tongue or mixing with liquids or food.

Each 0.6 ml provides:

Fat-Soluble Vitamins	
Vitamin A (as vitamin A palmitate)	5000 IU
Vitamin D_2 (ergocalciferol)	400 IU
Vitamin E (as *dl*-alpha-tocopheryl acetate)	2 IU
Water-Soluble Vitamins	
Vitamin C (ascorbic acid)	50 mg
Vitamin B_1 (as thiamine HCl)	1 mg
Vitamin B_2 (as riboflavin-5′-phosphate sodium)	1 mg
Niacin (as niacinamide)	10 mg
Vitamin B_6 (as pyridoxine HCl)	0.8 mg
d-Biotin	30 mcg
Pantothenic acid (as *d*-panthenol)	10 mg
Trace Elements	
Fluoride (as sodium fluoride)	0.5 mg

Clinical Pharmacology: Vitamins are necessary for maintenance of normal metabolic functions including hematopoiesis. *Vitamin A* is necessary for proper functioning of the retina; it appears to be essential to the integrity of epithelial cells. *Vitamin D* is necessary for the absorption of calcium and for the proper development and maintenance of bone structure. *Vitamin E* is an antioxidant which preserves essential cellular constituents, including those of the red blood cell. It also serves as protection against lipid peroxidation.

The water-soluble vitamins play vital roles in the conversion of carbohydrate, protein and fat into tissue and energy. *Thiamine (B_1)* acts as a coenzyme in carbohydrate metabolism. *Riboflavin (B_2)* functions as a coenzyme in the electron transport system associated with conversion of tissue oxidations into usable energy. *Niacin* serves as a coenzyme in oxidation-reduction reactions in tissue respiration. *Pyridoxine (B_6)* is essential for the metabolism of amino acids. *Pantothenic acid* functions as a coenzyme in various metabolic acetylation reactions and *biotin* in specific carboxylation reactions in lipid metabolism. *Ascorbic acid (C)* performs a vital function in the process of cellular respiration, and is involved in both carbohydrate and amino acid metabolism. It is essential for collagen formation and tissue repair.

Fluorine is an essential trace element that renders the dentine and enamel of teeth more resistant to acid.

There is ample evidence that the fluoridation of drinking water leads to a substantial decrease in the incidence of dental caries in childhood. This effect is greatest when fluoride is ingested during the first 9 to 10 years of life when teeth are developing. However, in areas were drinking water is devoid of natural or artificially controlled fluoride, or where fluoridation is not feasible, a single daily dose of fluoride as a dietary supplement is recommended as an effective substitute.

Recognizing the merits of dietary fluoride supplements, the Council on Dental Therapeutics of the American Dental Association strongly urges: "*Such administration should be consistent and continuous over long periods of time if substantial benefit is to be anticipated.*"

Indications and Usage: Vi-Penta F Multivitamin Drops is indicated for supportive nutritional supplementation and as an aid in the prevention of tooth decay in infants and children who reside in areas where the fluoride content of drinking water is known to be less than 0.7 parts per million.

Contraindications: Vi-Penta F Multivitamin Drops is contraindicated in patients known to be hypersensitive to any of its components.

Warnings: This preparation should not be used in areas where the fluoride content of drinking water is known to be 0.7 parts per million or greater. The recommended dose of Vi-Penta F Multivitamin Drops should not be exceeded, since dental fluorosis may result from continued ingestion of excessive amounts of fluoride.

Precautions: *General:* Certain patients may require nutritional supplementation with folic acid and vitamin B_{12} as well as other nutrients according to the dietary needs of the individual. Vi-Penta F Multivitamin Drops is not intended for treatment of severe specific vitamin deficiencies.

Information for the Patient: Because dental fluorosis may result from continued ingestion of excessive amounts of fluoride and toxic reactions have been reported with injudicious use of certain vitamins, urge patients to follow your specific instructions regarding dosage regimen. As with any medication, advise patients to keep Vi-Penta F Multivitamin drops out of reach of children. Vi-Penta F Multivitamin Drops should be stored under refrigeration.

Adverse Reactions: Adverse reactions have been reported with specific vitamins, but generally at levels substantially higher than those in Vi-Penta F Multivitamin Drops. However, allergic and idiosyncratic reactions are possible at lower levels.

Dosage and Administration: Usual dosage for infants and children: 0.6 ml daily, as measured by the dropper. Vi-Penta F Multivitamin Drops may be administered by dropping directly on the tongue or mixing with liquids or food.

Vi-Penta F Multivitamin Drops is available on prescription only.

How Supplied: Fruit-flavored liquid in bottles of 30 ml, packaged with a calibrated dropper (NDC 0004-1014-23).

NOTE TO THE PHARMACIST: Vi-Penta F Multivitamin Drops should be dispensed in the original special plastic containers, since contact with glass leads to instability and precipitation. Preparation should be stored under refrigeration.

VI-PENTA® INFANT DROPS
VI-PENTA® MULTIVITAMIN DROPS

The following text is complete prescribing information based on official labeling in effect August 1, 1982.

Composition: Vi-Penta Infant Drops and Vi-Penta Multivitamin Drops are designed to fill the vitamin needs of specific age groups. (See Composition Table next page)

Action and Uses: Vi-Penta Drops are water miscible and can be mixed with food or infant formula, or placed directly on the tongue.

Vi-Penta Infant Drops—a selective formula for prevention of vitamin deficiencies in infants and young children. *Vi-Penta Multivitamin Drops*—a comprehensive formula for daily nutritional support in adults as well as children of all ages. It is an especially convenient dosage form when a small volume liquid vitamin supplement is desired, such as to supplement the diets of those patients with conditions which

Continued on next page

Roche Labs.—Cont.

permanently or temporarily impair their ability to swallow, chew or consume normal amounts and/or kinds of food.

Dosage: The average daily dose is 0.6 cc; therapeutic doses should be given according to the needs of the patient.

How Supplied: Vi-Penta Infant Drops and Vi-Penta Multivitamin Drops—fruit flavored, 50-cc bottles packaged with calibrated dropper.

Vi-Penta Composition Table

Each 0.6 cc of Vi-Penta Infant Drops Provides:		% minimum daily requirements (MDR) Infants (under 1 year)	Young Children (1–6 years)
Vitamin A (as the palmitate)	5000 U.S.P. Units	333%	166%
Vitamin D_2	400 U.S.P. Units	100%	100%
Vitamin C	50 mg	500%	250%
Vitamin E (as *dl-α*-tocopheryl acetate)	2 Int. Units	*	*

Each 0.6 cc of Vi-Penta Multivitamin Drops provides:		% minimum daily requirements (MDR) Infants (under 1 year)	Children (1–6 years)	Children (6–12 years)
Vitamin A (as the palmitate)	5000 U.S.P. Units	333%	166%	166%
Vitamin D_2	400 U.S.P. Units	100%	100%	100%
Vitamin C	50 mg	500%	250%	250%
Vitamin B_1 (as hydrochloride)	1 mg	400%	200%	133%
Vitamin B_2 (as riboflavin-5′-phosphate sodium)	1 mg	166%	111%	111%
Vitamin B_6	1 mg	*	*	*
Vitamin E (as *dl-α*-tocopheryl acetate)	2 Int. Units	*	*	*
d-Biotin	30 mcg	†	†	†
Niacinamide	10 mg	*	200%	133%
D-Panthenol (equiv. to 11.6 mg Calcium pantothenate)	10 mg	†	†	†

*MDR for these vitamins has not been determined.
†The need for these vitamins in human nutrition has not been established.

Roche Products Inc.
MANATI, PUERTO RICO 00701

DALMANE® Ⓒ
(flurazepam hydrochloride/Roche)
Capsules

The following text is complete prescribing information based on official labeling in effect August 1, 1982.

Description: Flurazepam hydrochloride is chemically 7-chloro-1-[2-(diethylamino)ethyl]-5-(*o*-fluorophenyl) - 1,3-dihydro -2*H*-1,4-benzodiazepin-2-one dihydrochloride. It is a pale yellow, crystalline compound, freely soluble in U.S.P. alcohol and very soluble in water. It has a molecular weight of 460.826.

Clinical Pharmacology: Flurazepam hydrochloride is rapidly absorbed from the G.I. tract. Flurazepam is rapidly metabolized and is excreted primarily in the urine. Following a single oral dose, peak flurazepam plasma concentrations ranging from 0.5 to 4.0 ng/ml occur at 30 to 60 minutes post-dosing. The harmonic mean apparent half-life of flurazepam is 2.3 hours. The blood level profile of flurazepam and its major metabolites was determined in man following the oral administration of 30 mg daily for 2 weeks. The N_1-hydroxyethyl-flurazepam was measurable only during the early hours after a 30 mg dose and was not detectable after 24 hours. The major metabolite in blood was N_1-desalkyl-flurazepam, which reached steady-state (plateau) levels after 7 to 10 days of dosing, at levels approximately five- to sixfold greater than the 24-hour levels observed on Day 1. The half-life of elimination of N_1-desalkyl-flurazepam ranged from 47 to 100 hours. The major urinary metabolite is conjugated N_1-hydroxyethyl-flurazepam which accounts for 22 to 55 percent of the dose. Less than 1% of the dose is excreted in the urine as N_1-desalkyl-flurazepam.

This pharmacokinetic profile may be responsible for the clinical observation that flurazepam is increasingly effective on the second or third night of consecutive use and that for one or two nights after the drug is discontinued both sleep latency and total wake time may still be decreased.

Indications: Dalmane is a hypnotic agent useful for the treatment of insomnia characterized by difficulty in falling asleep, frequent nocturnal awakenings, and/or early morning awakening. Dalmane can be used effectively in patients with recurring insomnia or poor sleeping habits, and in acute or chronic medical situations requiring restful sleep. Sleep laboratory studies have objectively determined that Dalmane is effective for at least 28 consecutive nights of drug administration. Since insomnia is often transient and intermittent, short-term use is usually sufficient. Prolonged use of hypnotics is usually not indicated and should only be undertaken concomitantly with appropriate evaluation of the patient.

Contraindications: Dalmane is contraindicated in patients with known hypersensitivity to the drug.

Usage in Pregnancy: Benzodiazepines may cause fetal damage when administered during pregnancy. An increased risk of congenital malformations associated with the use of diazepam and chlordiazepoxide during the first trimester of pregnancy has been suggested in several studies.

Dalmane is contraindicated in pregnant women. Symptoms of neonatal depression have been reported; a neonate whose mother received 30 mg of Dalmane nightly for insomnia during the 10 days prior to delivery appeared hypotonic and inactive during the first four days of life. Serum levels of N_1-desalkyl-flurazepam in the infant indicated transplacental circulation and implicate this long-acting metabolite in this case. If there is a likelihood of the patient becoming pregnant while receiving flurazepam, she should be warned of the potential risks to the fetus. Patients should be instructed to discontinue the drug prior to becoming pregnant. The possibility that a woman of childbearing potential may be pregnant at the time of institution of therapy should be considered.

Warnings: Patients receiving Dalmane should be cautioned about possible combined effects with alcohol and other CNS depressants. Also, caution patients that an additive effect may occur if alcoholic beverages are consumed during the day following the use of Dalmane for nighttime sedation. The potential for this interaction continues for several days following discontinuance of flurazepam, until serum levels of psychoactive metabolites have declined.

Patients should also be cautioned about engaging in hazardous occupations requiring complete mental alertness such as operating machinery or driving a motor vehicle after ingesting the drug, including potential impairment of the performance of such activities which may occur the day following ingestion of Dalmane.

Usage in Children: Clinical investigations of Dalmane have not been carried out in children. Therefore, the drug is not currently recommended for use in persons under 15 years of age.

Physical and Psychological Dependence: Physical and psychological dependence have not been reported or observed in persons taking recommended doses of Dalmane. Withdrawal symptoms have been reported following abrupt discontinuance of anxiolytic benzodiazepines taken continuously, generally at higher therapeutic levels, for at least several months. These have not been specifically reported for Dalmane. However, if it is determined that a patient has been taking Dalmane for a prolonged period of time, particularly at excessive doses, abrupt discontinuation should generally be avoided and a gradual tapering of dosage followed. Also, as with any hypnotic, caution must be exercised in administering Dalmane to individuals known to be addiction-prone or those whose history suggests they may increase the dosage on their own initiative.

Precautions: Since the risk of the development of oversedation, dizziness, confusion and/or ataxia increases substantially with larger doses in elderly and debilitated patients, it is recommended that in such patients the dosage be limited to 15 mg. If Dalmane is to be combined with other drugs having known hypnotic properties or CNS-depressant effects, due consideration should be given to potential additive effects.

The usual precautions are indicated for severely depressed patients or those in whom there is any evidence of latent depression; particularly the recognition that suicidal tendencies may be present and protective measures may be necessary.

The usual precautions should be observed in patients with impaired renal or hepatic function and chronic pulmonary insufficiency.

Adverse Reactions: Dizziness, drowsiness, light-headedness, staggering, ataxia and falling have occurred, particularly in elderly or debilitated persons. Severe sedation, lethargy, disorientation and coma, probably indicative of drug intolerance or overdosage, have been reported.

Also reported were headache, heartburn, upset stomach, nausea, vomiting, diarrhea, constipation, gastrointestinal pain, nervousness, talkativeness, apprehension, irritability, weakness, palpitations, chest pains, body and joint pains and genitourinary complaints. There have also been rare occurrences of leukopenia, granulocytopenia, sweating, flushes, difficulty in focusing, blurred vision, burning eyes, faintness, hypotension, shortness of breath, pruritus, skin rash, dry mouth, bitter taste, excessive salivation, anorexia, euphoria, depression, slurred speech, confusion, restlessness, hallucinations, and elevated SGOT, SGPT, total and direct bilirubins, and alkaline phosphatase. Paradoxical reactions, *e.g.*, excitement, stimulation and hyperactivity, have also been reported in rare instances.

Dosage and Administration: Dosage should be individualized for maximal beneficial effects. The usual adult dosage is 30 mg before retiring. In some patients, 15 mg may suffice. In elderly and/or debilitated patients, 15 mg is usually sufficient for a therapeutic response and it is therefore recommended that therapy be initiated with this dosage.

Overdosage: Manifestations of Dalmane overdosage include somnolence, confusion and coma. Respiration, pulse and blood pressure should be monitored as in all cases of drug overdosage. General supportive measures should be employed, along with immediate gastric lavage. Intravenous fluids should be administered and an adequate airway maintained. Hypotension and CNS depression may be combated by judicious use of appropriate therapeutic agents. The value of dialysis has not been determined. If excitation occurs in patients following Dalmane overdosage, barbiturates should not be used. As with the management of intentional overdosage with any drug, it should be borne in mind that multiple agents may have been ingested.

How Supplied: Dalmane (flurazepam hydrochloride/Roche) capsules—15 mg, orange and ivory; 30 mg, red and ivory—bottles of 100 and 500; Tel-E-Dose® packages of 100, available in trays of 4 reverse-numbered boxes of 25, and in boxes containing 10 strips of 10; Prescription Paks of 30, available in trays of 10.

[*Shown in Product Identification Section*]

LIBRAX®

℞

The following text is complete prescribing information based on official labeling in effect August 1, 1982.

Composition: Each capsule contains 5 mg chlordiazepoxide hydrochloride (Librium®) and 2.5 mg clidinium bromide (Quarzan®).

Description: Librax combines in a single capsule formulation the antianxiety action of Librium (chlordiazepoxide hydrochloride/Roche) and the anticholinergic/spasmolytic effects of Quarzan (clidinium bromide/Roche), both exclusive developments of Roche research.

Librium (chlordiazepoxide hydrochloride/Roche) is a versatile therapeutic agent of proven value for the relief of anxiety and tension. It is indicated when anxiety, tension or apprehension are significant components of the clinical profile. It is among the safer of the effective psychopharmacologic compounds.

Chlordiazepoxide hydrochloride is 7-chloro-2-methylamino-5-phenyl- 3 H -1, 4-benzodiazepine 4-oxide hydrochloride. A colorless, crystalline substance, it is soluble in water. It is unstable in solution and the powder must be protected from light. The molecular weight is 336.22.

Quarzan (clidinium bromide/Roche) is a synthetic anticholinergic agent which has been shown in experimental and clinical studies to have a pronounced antispasmodic and antisecretory effect on the gastrointestinal tract.

Animal Pharmacology: Chlordiazepoxide hydrochloride has been studied extensively in many species of animals and these studies are suggestive of action on the limbic system of the brain,[1,2,3] which recent evidence indicates is involved in emotional responses.[4,5]

Hostile monkeys were made tame by oral drug doses which did not cause sedation. Chlordiazepoxide hydrochloride revealed a "taming" action with the elimination of fear and aggression.[6] The taming effect of chlordiazepoxide hydrochloride was further demonstrated in rats made vicious by lesions in the septal area of the brain. The drug dosage which effectively blocked the vicious reaction was well below the dose which caused sedation in these animals.[6]

The oral LD_{50} of single doses of chlordiazepoxide hydrochloride, calculated according to the method of Miller and Tainter,[7] is 720 ± 51 mg/kg as determined in mice observed over a period of five days following dosage.

Clidinium bromide is an effective anticholinergic agent with activity approximating that of atropine sulfate against acetylcholine-induced spasms in isolated intestinal strips. On oral administration in mice it proved an effective antisialagogue in preventing pilocarpine-induced salivation. Spontaneous intestinal motility in both rats and dogs is reduced following oral dosing with 0.1 to 0.25 mg/kg. Potent cholinergic ganglionic blocking effects (vagal) are produced with intravenous usage in anesthetized dogs.

Oral doses of 2.5 mg/kg to dogs produced signs of nasal dryness and slight pupillary dilation. In two other species, monkeys and rabbits, doses of 5 mg/kg, p.o., given three times daily for 5 days did not produce apparent secretory or visual changes.

The oral LD_{50} of single doses of clidinium bromide is 860±57 mg/kg as determined in mice observed over a period of 5 days following dosage; the calculations were made according to the method of Miller and Tainter.[7]

Effects on Reproduction: Reproduction studies in rats fed chlordiazepoxide hydrochloride, 10, 20 and 80 mg/kg daily, and bred through one or two matings showed no congenital anomalies, nor were there adverse effects on lactation of the dams or growth of the newborn. However, in another study at 100 mg/kg daily there was noted a significant decrease in the fertilization rate and a marked decrease in the viability and body weight of offspring which may be attributable to sedative activity, thus resulting in lack of interest in mating and lessened maternal nursing and care of the young.[8,9] One neonate in each of the first and second matings in the rat reproduction study at the 100 mg/kg dose exhibited major skeletal defects. Further studies are in progress to determine the significance of these findings.

Two series of reproduction experiments with clidinium bromide were carried out in rats, employing dosages of 2.5 and 10 mg/kg daily in each experiment. In the first experiment clidinium bromide was administered for a 9-week interval prior to mating; no untoward effect on fertilization or gestation was noted. The offspring were taken by caesarean section and did not show a significant incidence of congenital anomalies when compared to control animals. In the second experiment adult animals were given clidinium bromide for ten days prior to and through two mating cycles. No significant effects were observed on fertility, gestation, viability of offspring or lactation, as compared to control animals, nor was there a significant incidence of congenital anomalies in the offspring derived from these experiments.

A reproduction study of Librax was carried out in rats through two successive matings. Oral daily doses were administered in two concentrations: 2.5 mg/kg chlordiazepoxide hydrochloride with 1.25 mg/kg clidinium bromide, or 25 mg/kg chlordiazepoxide hydrochloride with 12.5 mg/kg clidinium bromide. In the first mating no significant differences were noted between the control or the treated groups, with the exception of a slight decrease in the number of animals surviving during lactation among those receiving the highest dosage. As with all anticholinergic drugs, an inhibiting effect on lactation may occur. In the second mating similar results were obtained except for a slight decrease in the number of pregnant females and in the percentage of offspring surviving until weaning. No congenital anomalies were observed in both matings in either the control or treated groups. Additional animal reproduction studies are in progress.

Indications: Based on a review of this drug by the National Academy of Sciences—National Research Council and/or other information, FDA has classified the indications as follows:

"Possibly" effective: as adjunctive therapy in the treatment of peptic ulcer and in the treatment of the irritable bowel syndrome (irritable colon, spastic colon, mucous colitis) and acute enterocolitis.

Final classification of the less-than-effective indications requires further investigation.

Contraindications: Librax is contraindicated in the presence of glaucoma (since the anticholinergic component may produce some degree of mydriasis) and in patients with prostatic hypertrophy and benign bladder neck obstruction. It is contraindicated in patients with known hypersensitivity to chlordiazepoxide hydrochloride and/or clidinium bromide.

Warnings: As in the case of other preparations containing CNS-acting drugs, patients receiving Librax should be cautioned about possible combined effects with alcohol and other CNS depressants. For the same reason, they should be cautioned against hazardous occupations requiring complete mental alertness such as operating machinery or driving a motor vehicle.

Physical and Psychological Dependence: Physical and psychological dependence have rarely been reported in persons taking recommended doses of Librium (chlordiazepoxide hydrochloride/Roche). However, caution must be exercised in administering Librium to individuals known to be addiction-prone or those whose history suggests they may increase the dosage on their own initiative. Withdrawal symptoms following discontinuation of chlordiazepoxide hydrochloride have been reported.[10] These symptoms (including convulsions) are similar to those seen with barbiturates.

***Usage in Pregnancy:* An increased risk of congenital malformations associated with the use of minor tranquilizers (chlordiazepoxide, diazepam and meprobamate) during the first trimester of pregnancy has been suggested in several studies. Because use of these drugs is rarely a matter of urgency, their use during this period should almost always be avoided. The possibility that a woman of childbearing potential may be pregnant at the time of institution of therapy should be considered. Patients should be advised that if they become pregnant during therapy or intend to become pregnant they should communicate with their physicians about the desirability of discontinuing the drug.**

As with all anticholinergic drugs, an inhibiting effect on lactation may occur. (See Animal Pharmacology.)

Management of Overdosage: Manifestations of Librium (chlordiazepoxide hydrochloride/Roche) overdosage include somnolence, confusion, coma and diminished reflexes. Respiration, pulse and blood pressure should be monitored, as in all cases of drug overdosage, although, in general, these effects have been minimal following Librium overdosage.

While the signs and symptoms of Librax overdosage may be produced by either of its components, usually such symptoms will be overshadowed by the anticholinergic actions of Quarzan (clidinium bromide/Roche). The symptoms of overdosage of Quarzan are excessive dryness of mouth, blurring of vision, urinary hesitancy and constipation.

General supportive measures should be employed, along with immediate gastric lavage. Administer physostigmine (Antilirium) 0.5 to 2 mg at a rate of no more than 1 mg per minute. This may be repeated in 1 to 4 mg doses if arrhythmias, convulsions or deep coma recur. Intravenous fluids should be administered and an adequate airway maintained. Hypotension may be combated by the use of Levophed® (levarterenol) or Aramine (metaraminol). Ritalin (methylphenidate) or caffeine and sodium benzoate may be given to combat CNS-depressive effects. Dialysis is of limited value. Should excitation occur, barbiturates should not be used. As with the management of intentional

Continued on next page

Roche Products—Cont.

overdosage with any drug, it should be borne in mind that multiple agents may have been ingested.

Precautions: In elderly and debilitated patients, it is recommended that the dosage be limited to the smallest effective amount to preclude the development of ataxia, oversedation, or confusion (not more than two Librax capsules per day initially, to be increased gradually as needed and tolerated). In general, the concomitant administration of Librax and other psychotropic agents is not recommended. If such combination therapy seems indicated, careful consideration should be given to the pharmacology of the agents to be employed—particularly when the known potentiating compounds such as the MAO inhibitors and phenothiazines are to be used. The usual precautions in treating patients with impaired renal or hepatic function should be observed. Paradoxical reactions to chlordiazepoxide hydrochloride, *e.g.*, excitement, stimulation and acute rage, have been reported in psychiatric patients and should be watched for during Librax therapy. The usual precautions are indicated when chlordiazepoxide hydrochloride is used in the treatment of anxiety states where there is any evidence of impending depression; it should be borne in mind that suicidal tendencies may be present and protective measures may be necessary. Although clinical studies have not established a cause and effect relationship, physicians should be aware that variable effects on blood coagulation have been reported very rarely in patients receiving oral anticoagulants and Librium.

Adverse Reactions:[11] No side effects or manifestations not seen with either compound alone have been reported with the administration of Librax. However, since Librax contains chlordiazepoxide hydrochloride and clidinium bromide, the possibility of untoward effects which may be seen with either of these two compounds cannot be excluded.

When chlordiazepoxide hydrochloride has been used alone the necessity of discontinuing therapy because of undesirable effects has been rare.[12] Drowsiness,[13] ataxia[14] and confusion[9] have been reported in some patients—particularly the elderly and debilitated.[9] While these effects can be avoided in almost all instances by proper dosage adjustment, they have occasionally been observed at the lower dosage ranges. In a few instances syncope has been reported.[15]

Other adverse reactions reported during therapy with Librium (chlordiazepoxide hydrochloride/Roche) include isolated instances of skin eruptions,[13] edema,[16] minor menstrual irregularities,[13] nausea and constipation,[17] extrapyramidal symptoms,[9] as well as increased and decreased libido. Such side effects have been infrequent and are generally controlled with reduction of dosage. Changes in EEG patterns (low-voltage fast activity) have been observed in patients during and after Librium treatment.[18]

Blood dyscrasias,[11] including agranulocytosis,[19] jaundice and hepatic dysfunction[20] have occasionally been reported during therapy with Librium. When Librium treatment is protracted, periodic blood counts and liver function tests are advisable.

Adverse effects reported with use of *Librax* are those typical of anticholinergic agents, *i.e.*, dryness of the mouth, blurring of vision, urinary hesitancy and constipation. Constipation has occurred most often when Librax therapy has been combined with other spasmolytic agents and/or a low residue diet.

Dosage: Because of the varied individual responses to tranquilizers and anticholinergics, the optimum dosage of Librax varies with the diagnosis and response of the individual patient. The dosage, therefore, should be individualized for maximum beneficial effects. The usual maintenance dose is 1 or 2 capsules, 3 or 4 times a day administered before meals and at bedtime.

How Supplied: Librax is available in green capsules, each containing 5 mg chlordiazepoxide hydrochloride (Librium®) and 2.5 mg clidinium bromide (Quarzan®)—bottles of 100 and 500; Tel-E-Dose® packages of 100; Prescription Paks of 50.

References:

1. Schallek, W., *et al:* Arch. Int. Pharmacodyn. *149*:467-483, 1964.
2. Himwich, H. E., *et al:* J. Neuropsych. *3* (Suppl. 1):S15-S26, August 1962.
3. Morillo, A., *et al:* Psychopharmacologia *3* (No. 5):386-394, 1962.
4. MacLean, P. D.: Psychosomatic Med. *17*:355-366, September 1955.
5. Morgan, C. T.: Physiological Psychology, 3rd Ed.; New York, McGraw-Hill, 1965.
6. Randall, L. O. *et al:* J. Pharm. Exper. Therap. *129*:163-171, June 1960.
7. Miller, L. C. and Tainter, M. C.: Proc. Soc. Exp. Biol. Med. 57:261, 1944.
8. Zbinden, G., *et al:* Toxicology and Applied Pharmacology *3*:619-637, November 1961.
9. Data on file, Hoffmann-La Roche Inc., Nutley, New Jersey.
10. Hollister, L. E., *et al:* Psychopharmacologia *2*:63-68, 1961.
11. Bibliography and References available on request from Roche Laboratories.
12. Rickels, K. *et al:* Med. Times *93*:238-245, March 1965.
13. Tobin, J. M. *et al:* J. Amer. Med. Assoc. *174*:1242-1249, November 1960.
14. Jenner, F. A., *et al:* J. Ment. Sci. *107*:575-582, May 1961.
15. Robinson, R. C. V.: Dis. Nerv. System *21*:43-45, March 1960.
16. Rose, J. T.: Amer. J. Psychiat. *120*:899-900, March 1964.
17. Hines, L. R.: Curr. Therap. Res. *2*:227-236, June 1960.
18. Gibbs, F. A. and Gibbs, E. L.: J. Neuropsych., 3 (Suppl. 1):S73-S78, August 1962.
19. Kaelbling, R., *et al:* J. Amer. Med. Assoc. *174*:1863-1865, December 1960.
20. Cacioppo, J., *et al:* Amer. J. Psychiat. *117*:1040-1041, May 1961.

[*Shown in Product Identification Section*]

LIBRIUM® CAPSULES Ⓒ
(chlordiazepoxide HCl/Roche)

LIBRITABS® Ⓒ
(chlordiazepoxide/Roche)

The following text is complete prescribing information based on official labeling in effect August 1, 1982.

Description: Librium (the original chlordiazepoxide HCl) and Libritabs (the original chlordiazepoxide), prototypes for the benzodiazepine compounds, were synthesized and developed at Hoffmann-La Roche Inc. They are versatile therapeutic agents of proven value for the relief of anxiety, and are among the safer of the effective psychopharmacologic compounds available, as demonstrated by extensive clinical evidence.

Chlordiazepoxide hydrochloride is 7-chloro-2-(methylamino)-5-phenyl-3H-1,4-benzodiazepine 4-oxide hydrochloride. A white to practically white crystalline substance, it is soluble in water. It is unstable in solution and the powder must be protected from light. The molecular weight is 336.22.

Chlordiazepoxide is 7-chloro-2-(methylamino)-5-phenyl-3H-1,4-benzodiazepine 4-oxide. A yellow crystalline substance, it is insoluble in water. The powder must be protected from light. The molecular weight is 299.76.

Actions: Librium (chlordiazepoxide HCl/Roche) and Libritabs (chlordiazepoxide/Roche) have antianxiety, sedative, appetite-stimulating and weak analgesic actions. The precise mechanism of action is not known. The drugs block EEG arousal from stimulation of the brain stem reticular formation. It takes several hours for peak blood levels to be reached and the half-life of the drugs is between 24 and 48 hours. After Librium or Libritabs is discontinued plasma levels decline slowly over a period of several days. Chlordiazepoxide is excreted in the urine, with 1 to 2% unchanged and 3 to 6% as a conjugate.

Indications: Librium and Libritabs are indicated for the management of anxiety disorders or for the short-term relief of symptoms of anxiety, withdrawal symptoms of acute alcoholism, and preoperative apprehension and anxiety. Anxiety or tension associated with the stress of everyday life usually does not require treatment with an anxiolytic.

The effectiveness of Librium or Libritabs in long-term use, that is, more than 4 months, has not been assessed by systematic clinical studies. The physician should periodically reassess the usefulness of the drug for the individual patient.

Contraindications: Librium and Libritabs are contraindicated in patients with known hypersensitivity to the drug.

Warnings: Chlordiazepoxide HCl and chlordiazepoxide may impair the mental and/or physical abilities required for the performance of potentially hazardous tasks such as driving a vehicle or operating machinery. Similarly, they may impair mental alertness in children. The concomitant use of alcohol or other central nervous system depressants may have an additive effect. PATIENTS SHOULD BE WARNED ACCORDINGLY.

Physical and Psychological Dependence: Physical and psychological dependence have rarely been reported in persons taking recommended doses of chlordiazepoxide HCl or chlordiazepoxide. However, caution must be exercised in administering chlordiazepoxide HCl or chlordiazepoxide to individuals known to be addiction-prone or those whose histories suggest they may increase the dosage on their own initiative. Withdrawal symptoms following abrupt discontinuation of chlordiazepoxide HCl or chlordiazepoxide have been reported in patients receiving excessive doses over extended periods of time. These symptoms (including convulsions) are similar to those seen with barbiturates. Although infrequently seen, milder withdrawal symptoms have also been reported following abrupt discontinuance of benzodiazepines taken continuously, generally at higher therapeutic levels, for at least several months. Consequently, after extended therapy, abrupt discontinuation should generally be avoided and a gradual tapering in dosage followed.

Usage in Pregnancy: An increased risk of congenital malformations associated with the use of minor tranquilizers (chlordiazepoxide, diazepam and meprobamate) during the first trimester of pregnancy has been suggested in several studies. Because use of these drugs is rarely a matter of urgency, their use during this period should almost always be avoided. The possibility that a woman of childbearing potential may be pregnant at the time of institution of therapy should be considered. Patients should be advised that if they become pregnant during therapy or intend to become pregnant they should communicate with their physicians about the desirability of discontinuing the drug.

Precautions: In elderly and debilitated patients, it is recommended that the dosage be limited to the smallest effective amount to preclude the development of ataxia or oversedation (10 mg or less per day initially, to be increased gradually as needed and tolerated). In general, the concomitant administration of Librium or Libritabs and other psychotropic agents is not recommended. If such combination therapy seems indicated, careful consideration should be given to the pharmacology of the agents to be employed — particularly when the known potentiating compounds such as the MAO inhibitors and phenothiazines are to be used. The usual precautions in treating patients with impaired renal or hepatic function should be observed.

Paradoxical reactions, *e.g.,* excitement, stimulation and acute rage, have been reported in psychiatric patients and in hyperactive aggressive children, and should be watched for during Librium or Libritabs therapy. The usual precautions are indicated when Librium or Libritabs is used in the treatment of anxiety states where there is any evidence of impending depression; it should be borne in mind that suicidal tendencies may be present and protective measures may be necessary. Although clinical studies have not established a cause and effect relationship, physicians should be aware that variable effects on blood coagulation have been reported very rarely in patients receiving oral anticoagulants and Librium or Libritabs. In view of isolated reports associating chlordiazepoxide HCl and chlordiazepoxide with exacerbation of porphyria, caution should be exercised in prescribing these agents to patients suffering from this disease.

Adverse Reactions: The necessity of discontinuing therapy because of undesirable effects has been rare. Drowsiness, ataxia and confusion have been reported in some patients — particularly the elderly and debilitated. While these effects can be avoided in almost all instances by proper dosage adjustment, they have occasionally been observed at the lower dosage ranges. In a few instances syncope has been reported.

Other adverse reactions reported during therapy include isolated instances of skin eruptions, edema, minor menstrual irregularities, nausea and constipation, extrapyramidal symptoms, as well as increased and decreased libido. Such side effects have been infrequent and are generally controlled with reduction of dosage. Changes in EEG patterns (low-voltage fast activity) have been observed in patients during and after Librium or Libritabs treatment.

Blood dyscrasias (including agranulocytosis), jaundice and hepatic dysfunction have occasionally been reported during therapy. When Librium or Libritabs treatment is protracted, periodic blood counts and liver function tests are advisable.

Dosage and Administration: Because of the wide range of clinical indications for Librium and Libritabs, the optimum dosage varies with the diagnosis and response of the individual patient. The dosage, therefore, should be individualized for maximum beneficial effects.

ADULTS	Usual Daily Dose
Relief of mild and moderate anxiety disorders and symptoms of anxiety	5 mg or 10 mg, 3 or 4 times daily
Relief of severe anxiety disorders and symptoms of anxiety	20 mg or 25 mg, 3 or 4 times daily
Geriatric patients, or in the presence of debilitating disease	5 mg, 2 to 4 times daily

Preoperative apprehension and anxiety: On days preceding surgery, 5 to 10 mg orally, 3 or 4 times daily. If used as preoperative medication, 50 to 100 mg I.M.* one hour prior to surgery.

CHILDREN	Usual Daily Dose
Because of the varied response of children to CNS-acting drugs, therapy should be initiated with the lowest dose and increased as required.	5 mg, 2 to 4 times daily (may be increased in some children to 10 mg, 2 or 3 times daily)
Since clinical experience in children under 6 years of age is limited, the use of the drug in this age group is not recommended.	

For the relief of withdrawal symptoms of acute alcoholism, the parenteral form* is usually used initially. If the drug is administered orally, the suggested initial dose is 50 to 100 mg, to be followed by repeated doses as needed until agitation is controlled — up to 300 mg per day. Dosage should then be reduced to maintenance levels.

* See package insert for injectable Librium (chlordiazepoxide HCl/Roche).

Management of Overdosage: Manifestations of Librium or Libritabs overdosage include somnolence, confusion, coma and diminished reflexes. Respiration, pulse and blood pressure should be monitored, as in all cases of drug overdosage, although, in general, these effects have been minimal following Librium or Libritabs overdosage. General supportive measures should be employed, along with immediate gastric lavage. Intravenous fluids should be administered and an adequate airway maintained. Hypotension may be combated by the use of Levophed® (levarterenol) or Aramine (metaraminol). Dialysis is of limited value. There have been occasional reports of excitation in patients following chlordiazepoxide HCl or chlordiazepoxide overdosage; if this occurs barbiturates should not be used. As with the management of intentional overdosage with any drug, it should be borne in mind that multiple agents may have been ingested.

How Supplied: Librium (chlordiazepoxide HCl/Roche) capsules — 5 mg, green and yellow; 10 mg, green and black; 25 mg, green and white — bottles of 100 and 500; Tel-E-Dose® packages of 100, available in trays of 4 reverse-numbered boxes of 25, and in boxes containing 10 strips of 10; Prescription Paks of 50.

Libritabs (chlordiazepoxide/Roche) tablets — 5 mg, 10 mg or 25 mg, green — bottles of 100 and 500.

[*Shown in Product Identification Section*]

LIBRIUM® INJECTABLE (chlordiazepoxide HCl/Roche) Ⓒ

Librium Injectable is manufactured by Hoffmann-La Roche Inc., Nutley, N.J. 07110 and distributed by Roche Products Inc., Manati, P.R. 00701.

The following text is complete prescribing information based on official labeling in effect August 1, 1982.

Description: Librium is a versatile therapeutic agent of proven value for the relief of anxiety and tension.

Librium is the first of a new class, unrelated chemically and pharmacologically to other types of tranquilizers. Librium promptly relieves anxiety and is among the safer of the effective psychopharmacologic compounds available.

Chlordiazepoxide HCl is 7-chloro-2-methylamino-5-phenyl-3H-1,4-benzodiazepine 4-oxide hydrochloride. A colorless, crystalline substance, it is soluble in water. It is unstable in solution and the powder must be protected from light. The molecular weight is 336.22.

Animal Pharmacology: The drug has been studied extensively in many species of animals and these studies are suggestive of action on the limbic system of the brain, which recent evidence indicates is involved in emotional responses.

Hostile monkeys were made tame by oral drug doses which did not cause sedation. Librium revealed a "taming" action with the elimination of fear and aggression. The taming effect of Librium was further demonstrated in rats made vicious by lesions in the septal area of the brain. The drug dosage which effectively blocked the vicious reaction was well below the dose which caused sedation in these animals.

The LD_{50} of parenterally administered chlordiazepoxide HCl was determined in mice (72 hours) and rats (5 days), and calculated according to the method of Miller and Tainter, with the following results: mice, I.V., 123 $\pm$ 12 mg/kg; mice, I.M., 366 $\pm$ 7 mg/kg; rats, I.V., 120 $\pm$ 7 mg/kg; rats, I.M., $>$160 mg/kg.

Effects on Reproduction: Reproduction studies in rats fed 10, 20 and 80 mg/kg daily and bred through one or two matings showed no congenital anomalies, nor were there adverse effects on lactation of the dams or growth of the newborn. However, in another study at 100 mg/kg daily there was noted a significant decrease in the fertilization rate and a marked decrease in the viability and body weight of offspring which may be attributable to sedative activity, thus resulting in lack of interest in mating and lessened maternal nursing and care of the young. One neonate in each of the first and second matings in the rat reproduction study at the 100 mg/kg dose exhibited major skeletal defects. Further studies are in progress to determine the significance of these findings.

Indications: Injectable Librium is indicated for the management of anxiety disorders or for the short-term relief of symptoms of anxiety, withdrawal symptoms of acute alcoholism, and preoperative apprehension and anxiety. Anxiety or tension associated with the stress of everyday life usually does not require treatment with an anxiolytic.

Contraindications: Librium is contraindicated in patients with known hypersensitivity to the drug.

Warnings: As in the case of other CNS-acting drugs, patients receiving Librium should be cautioned about possible combined effects with alcohol and other CNS depressants.

As is true of all preparations containing CNS-acting drugs, patients receiving Librium should be cautioned against hazardous occupations requiring complete mental alertness such as operating machinery or driving a motor vehicle.

Physical and Psychological Dependence: Physical and psychological dependence have rarely been reported in persons taking recommended doses of Librium. However, caution must be exercised in administering Librium to individuals known to be addiction-prone or those whose history suggests they may increase the dosage on their own initiative. Withdrawal symptoms following abrupt discontinuation of chlordiazepoxide HCl have been reported in patients receiving excessive doses over extended periods of time. These symptoms (including convulsions) are similar to those seen with barbiturates. Although infrequently seen, milder withdrawal symptoms have also been reported following abrupt discontinuance of benzodiazepines taken continuously, generally at higher therapeutic levels, for at least several months. Consequently, after extended therapy, abrupt discontinuation should generally be avoided and a gradual tapering in dosage followed.

***Usage in Pregnancy:* An increased risk of congenital malformations associated with the use of minor tranquilizers (chlordiazepoxide, diazepam and meprobamate) during the first trimester of pregnancy has been suggested in several studies. Because use of these drugs is rarely a matter of urgency, their use during this period should almost always be avoided. The possibility that a woman of childbearing potential may be pregnant at the time of institution of therapy should be considered. Patients should be advised that if they become pregnant during therapy or intend to become pregnant they should**

Continued on next page

Roche Products—Cont.

communicate with their physicians about the desirability of discontinuing the drug.

Management of Overdosage: Manifestations of Librium overdosage include somnolence, confusion, coma and diminished reflexes. Respiration, pulse and blood pressure should be monitored, as in all cases of drug overdosage, although, in general, these effects have been minimal following Librium overdosage. General supportive measures should be employed, along with immediate gastric lavage. Intravenous fluids should be administered and an adequate airway maintained. Hypotension may be combated by the use of Levophed® (levarterenol) or Aramine (metaraminol). Dialysis is of limited value. There have been occasional reports of excitation in patients following Librium overdosage; if this occurs barbiturates should not be used. As with the management of intentional overdosage with any drug, it should be borne in mind that multiple agents may have been ingested.

Precautions: Injectable Librium (intramuscular or intravenous) is indicated primarily in acute states, and patients receiving this form of therapy should be kept under observation, preferably in bed, for a period of up to three hours. Ambulatory patients should not be permitted to operate a vehicle following an injection. Injectable Librium should not be given to patients in shock or comatose states. Reduced dosage (usually 25 to 50 mg) should be used for elderly or debilitated patients, and for children age twelve or older. In general, the concomitant administration of Librium and other psychotropic agents is not recommended. If such combination therapy seems indicated, careful consideration should be given to the pharmacology of the agents to be employed—particularly when the known potentiating compounds such as the MAO inhibitors and phenothiazines are to be used. The usual precautions in treating patients with impaired renal or hepatic function should be observed.

Paradoxical reactions, *e.g.,* excitement, stimulation and acute rage, have been reported in psychiatric patients and in hyperactive aggressive children, and should be watched for during Librium therapy. The usual precautions are indicated when Librium is used in the treatment of anxiety states where there is any evidence of impending depression; it should be borne in mind that suicidal tendencies may be present and protective measures may be necessary. Although clinical studies have not established a cause and effect relationship, physicians should be aware that variable effects on blood coagulation have been reported very rarely in patients receiving oral anticoagulants and Librium. In view of isolated reports associating chlordiazepoxide with exacerbation of porphyria, caution should be exercised in prescribing chlordiazepoxide to patients suffering from this disease.

Adverse Reactions: The necessity of discontinuing therapy because of undersirable effects has been rare. Drowsiness, ataxia and confusion are more commonly seen in the elderly and debilitated.

Other adverse reactions reported during therapy include isolated instances of syncope, hypotension, tachycardia, skin eruptions, edema, minor menstrual irregularities, nausea and constipation, extrapyramidal symptoms, blurred vision, as well as increased and decreased libido. Such side effects have been infrequent and are generally controlled with reduction of dosage. Similarly, hypotension associated with spinal anesthesia has occurred. Pain following intramuscular injection has been reported. Changes in EEG patterns (low-voltage fast activity) have been observed in patients during and after Librium treatment. Blood dyscrasias (including agranulocytosis), jaundice and hepatic dysfunction, have occasionally been reported during therapy. When Librium treatment is protracted, periodic blood counts and liver function tests are advisable.

Preparation and Administration of Solutions: Solutions of Librium for intramuscular or intravenous use should be prepared aseptically. Sterilization by heating should not be attempted.

Intramuscular: Add 2 ml of *Special Intramuscular Diluent* to contents of 5-ml dry-filled amber ampul of Librium Sterile Powder (100 mg). Avoid excessive pressure in injecting this special diluent into the ampul containing the powder since bubbles will form on the surface of the solution. Agitate gently until completely dissolved. Solution should be prepared immediately before administration. Any unused solution should be discarded. Deep intramuscular injection should be given *slowly* into the upper outer quadrant of the gluteus muscle.

Caution: Although the Librium preparation made with the intramuscular diluent has been given intravenously without untoward effects, such administration is not recommended because of the air bubbles which form when the intramuscular diluent is added to the Librium powder. Do not use diluent solution if it is opalescent or hazy.

Intravenous: In most cases, intramuscular injection is the preferred route of administration of Injectable Librium since beneficial effects are usually seen within 15 to 30 minutes. When, in the judgment of the physician, even more rapid action is mandatory, Injectable Librium may be administered intravenously. A suitable solution for intravenous administration may be prepared as follows: Add 5 ml of *sterile physiological saline* or *sterile water for injection* to contents of 5-ml dry-filled amber ampul of Librium Sterile Powder (100 mg). Agitate gently until thoroughly dissolved. Solution should be prepared immediately before administration. Any unused portion should be discarded. *Intravenous injection should be given slowly over a one-minute period.*

Caution: Librium solution made with physiological saline or sterile water for injection should not be given intramuscularly because of pain on injection.

Dosage: Dosage should be individualized according to the diagnosis and the response of the patient. While 300 mg may be given during a 6-hour period, this dose should not be exceeded in any 24-hour period.

INDICATION	ADULT DOSAGE*
Withdrawal Symptoms of Acute Alcoholism	50 to 100 mg I.M. or I.V. initially; repeat in 2 to 4 hours, if necessary
Acute or Severe Anxiety Disorders or Symptoms of Anxiety	50 to 100 mg I.M. or I.V. initially; then 25 to 50 mg 3 or 4 times daily, if necessary
Preoperative Apprehension and Anxiety	50 to 100 mg I.M. one hour prior to surgery

* Lower doses (usually 25 to 50 mg) should be used for elderly or debilitated patients, and for older children. Since clinical experience in children under 12 years of age is limited, the use of the drug in this age group is not recommended.

In most cases, acute symptoms may be rapidly controlled by parenteral administration so that subsequent treatment, if necessary, may be given orally. (See package insert for Oral Librium.)

How Supplied: For Parenteral Administration: Ampuls—Duplex package consisting of a 5-ml dry-filled ampul containing 100 mg chlordiazepoxide HCl in dry crystalline form, and a 2-ml ampul of Special Intramuscular Diluent (for intramuscular administration) compounded with 1.5% benzyl alcohol, 4% polysorbate 80, 20% propylene glycol, 1.6% maleic acid and sodium hydroxide to adjust pH to approximately 3.0. Boxes of 10.

Caution: Before preparing solution for intramuscular or intravenous administration, please read instructions for PREPARATION AND ADMINISTRATION OF SOLUTIONS.

LIMBITROL® TABLETS Ⓒ

LIMBITROL 10–25

Each tablet contains 10 mg chlordiazepoxide and 25 mg amitriptyline in the form of the hydrochloride salt.

LIMBITROL 5–12.5

Each tablet contains 5 mg chlordiazepoxide and 12.5 mg amitriptyline in the form of the hydrochloride salt.

The following text is complete prescribing information based on official labeling in effect August 1, 1982.

Description: Limbitrol combines in a tablet for oral administration, chlordiazepoxide, an agent for the relief of anxiety and tension, and amitriptyline, an antidepressant.

Chlordiazepoxide is a benzodiazepine with the formula 7-chloro-2-(methylamino)-5-phenyl-3*H*-1,4-benzodiazepine 4-oxide. It is a slightly yellow crystalline material and is insoluble in water. The molecular weight is 299.76.

Amitriptyline is a dibenzocycloheptadiene derivative. The formula is 10,11-dihydro-*N,N*-dimethyl-5H-dibenzo [a, d] cycloheptene-$\Delta^{5,\gamma}$-propylamine hydrochloride. It is a white or practically white crystalline compound that is freely soluble in water. The molecular weight is 313.87.

Actions: Both components of Limbitrol exert their action in the central nervous system. Extensive studies with chlordiazepoxide in many animal species suggest action in the limbic system. Recent evidence indicates that the limbic system is involved in emotional response. Taming action was observed in some species. The mechanism of action of amitriptyline in man is not known, but the drug appears to interfere with the reuptake of norepinephrine into adrenergic nerve endings. This action may prolong the sympathetic activity of biogenic amines.

Indications: Limbitrol is indicated for the treatment of patients with moderate to severe depression associated with moderate to severe anxiety.

The therapeutic response to Limbitrol occurs earlier and with fewer treatment failures than when either amitriptyline or chlordiazepoxide is used alone.

Symptoms likely to respond in the first week of treatment include: insomnia, feelings of guilt or worthlessness, agitation, psychic and somatic anxiety, suicidal ideation and anorexia.

Contraindications: Limbitrol is contraindicated in patients with hypersensitivity to either benzodiazepines or tricyclic antidepressants. It should not be given concomitantly with a monoamine oxidase inhibitor. Hyperpyretic crises, severe convulsions and deaths have occurred in patients receiving a tricyclic antidepressant and a monoamine oxidase inhibitor simultaneously. When it is desired to replace a monoamine oxidase inhibitor with Limbitrol, a minimum of 14 days should be allowed to elapse after the former is discontinued. Limbitrol should then be initiated cautiously with gradual increase in dosage until optimum response is achieved.

This drug is contraindicated during the acute recovery phase following myocardial infarction.

Warnings: Because of the atropine-like action of the amitriptyline component, great care should be used in treating patients with a history of urinary retention or angle-closure glaucoma. In patients with glaucoma, even average doses may precipitate an attack. Severe constipation may occur in patients taking tricyclic antidepressants in combination with anticholinergic-type drugs.

Patients with cardiovascular disorders should be watched closely. Tricyclic antidepressant drugs, particularly when given in high doses, have been reported to produce arrhythmias, sinus tachycardia and prolongation of conduction time. Myocardial infarction and stroke have been reported in patients receiving drugs of this class.

Because of the sedative effects of Limbitrol, patients should be cautioned about combined effects with alcohol or other CNS depressants. The additive effects may produce a harmful level of sedation and CNS depression.

Patients receiving Limbitrol should be cautioned against engaging in hazardous occupations requiring complete mental alertness, such as operating machinery or driving a motor vehicle.

Usage in Pregnancy: Safe use of Limbitrol during pregnancy and lactation has not been established. Because of the chlordiazepoxide component, please note the following:

An increased risk of congenital malformations associated with the use of minor tranquilizers (chlordiazepoxide, diazepam and meprobamate) during the first trimester of pregnancy has been suggested in several studies. Because use of these drugs is rarely a matter of urgency, their use during this period should almost always be avoided. The possibility that a woman of childbearing potential may be pregnant at the time of institution of therapy should be considered. Patients should be advised that if they become pregnant during therapy or intend to become pregnant they should communicate with their physicians about the desirability of discontinuing the drug.

Physical and Psychological Dependence: Experience with Limbitrol is as yet too limited to reasonably assess the combination's potential for physical and psychological dependence. However, since physical and psychological dependence to chlordiazepoxide have been reported rarely, caution must be exercised in administering Limbitrol to individuals known to be addiction-prone or to those whose history suggests they may increase the dosage on their own initiative.

In the so far limited experience with Limbitrol withdrawal symtoms have not been reported. However, withdrawal symptoms following abrupt cessation of prolonged therapy with either component alone have been reported. With amitriptyline, these have been noted to consist of nausea, headache and malaise; for chlordiazepoxide, the symptoms (including convulsions) are similar to those seen with barbiturates.

Precautions: *General:* Use with caution in patients with a history of seizures.

Close supervision is required when Limbitrol is given to hyperthyroid patients or those on thyroid medication.

The usual precautions should be observed when treating patients with impaired renal or hepatic function.

Patients with suicidal ideation should not have easy access to large quantities of the drug. The possibility of suicide in depressed patients remains until significant remission occurs.

Essential Laboratory Tests: Patients on prolonged treatment should have periodic liver function tests and blood counts.

Drug and Treatment Interactions: Because of its amitriptyline component, Limbitrol may block the antihypertensive action of guanethidine or compounds with a similar mechanism of action.

The effects of concomitant administration of Limbitrol and other psychotropic drugs have not been evaluated. Sedative effects may be additive.

The drug should be discontinued several days before elective surgery.

Concurrent administration of ECT and Limbitrol should be limited to those patients for whom it is essential.

Pregnancy: See WARNINGS section.

Nursing Mothers: It is not known whether this drug is excreted in human milk. As a general rule, nursing should not be undertaken while a patient is on a drug, since many drugs are excreted in human milk.

Pediatric Use: Safety and effectiveness in children below the age of 12 years have not been established.

Elderly Patients: In elderly and debilitated patients it is recommended that dosage be limited to the smallest effective amount to preclude the development of ataxia, oversedation, confusion or anticholinergic effects.

Adverse Reactions: Adverse reactions to Limbitrol are those associated with the use of either component alone. Most frequently reported were drowsiness, dry mouth, constipation, blurred vision, dizziness and bloating. Other side effects occurring less commonly included vivid dreams, impotence, tremor, confusion and nasal congestion. Many symptoms common to the depressive state, such as anorexia, fatigue, weakness, restlessness and lethargy, have been reported as side effects of treatment with both Limbitrol and amitriptyline.

Granulocytopenia, jaundice and hepatic dysfunction of uncertain etiology have also been observed rarely with Limbitrol. When treatment with Limbitrol is prolonged, periodic blood counts and liver function tests are advisable.

Note: Included in the listing which follows are adverse reactions which have not been reported with Limbitrol. However, they are included because they have been reported during therapy with one or both of the components or closely related drugs.

Cardiovascular: Hypotension, hypertension, tachycardia, palpitations, myocardial infarction, arrhythmias, heart block, stroke.

Psychiatric: Euphoria, apprehension, poor concentration, delusions, hallucinations, hypomania and increased or decreased libido.

Neurologic: Incoordination, ataxia, numbness, tingling and paresthesias of the extremities, extrapyramidal symptoms, syncope, changes in EEG patterns.

Anticholinergic: Disturbance of accommodation, paralytic ileus, urinary retention, dilatation of urinary tract.

Allergic: Skin rash, urticaria, photosensitization, edema of face and tongue, pruritus.

Hematologic: Bone marrow depression including agranulocytosis, eosinophilia, purpura, thrombocytopenia.

Gastrointestinal: Nausea, epigastric distress, vomiting, anorexia, stomatitis, peculiar taste, diarrhea, black tongue.

Endocrine: Testicular swelling and gynecomastia in the male, breast enlargement, galactorrhea and minor menstrual irregularities in the female and elevation and lowering of blood sugar levels.

Other: Headache, weight gain or loss, increased perspiration, urinary frequency, mydriasis, jaundice, alopecia, parotid swelling.

Overdosage: There has been limited experience with Limbitrol overdosage *per se;* the manifestations of overdosage and recommendations for treatment are based on clinical experience with its components. Primary concern should be with the dangers associated with amitriptyline overdosage. Deaths by deliberate or accidental overdosage have occurred with this class of drugs.

All patients suspected of having an overdosage of Limbitrol should be admitted to a hospital as soon as possible.

Manifestations: High doses may cause drowsiness, temporary confusion, disturbed concentration or transient visual hallucinations. Overdosage may cause hypothermia, tachycardia and other arrhythmias, ECG evidence of impaired conduction (such as bundle branch block), congestive heart failure, dilated pupils, convulsions, severe hypotension, stupor and coma. Other symptoms may be agitation, hyperactive reflexes, muscle rigidity, vomiting, hyperpyrexia or any of those listed under Adverse Reactions.

Treatment: Empty the stomach as quickly as possible by emesis or lavage. In the comatose patient a cuff endotracheal tube should be placed in position prior to either of these measures. The instillation of activated charcoal into the stomach also should be considered. If the patient is stuporous but responds to stimuli, only close observation and nursing care may be required. It is essential to maintain an adequate airway and fluid intake. Body temperature should be watched closely and appropriate measures taken should deviations occur.

The intramuscular or slow intravenous administration of 1 to 3 mg in adults (or 0.5 mg in children) of physostigmine salicylate (Antilirium)[1–3] has been reported to reverse the manifestations of amitriptyline overdosage. Because of its relatively short half-life, additional doses may be needed at intervals of 30 minutes to 2 hours.

Convulsions may be treated by the use of an inhalation anesthetic rather than the use of barbiturates. Cardiac monitoring is advisable, and the cautious use of digitalis or other antiarrhythmic agents should be considered if serious cardiovascular abnormalities occur. Serum potassium levels should be monitored and kept within normal limits by the use of appropriate I.V. fluids. Standard measures including oxygen, I.V. fluids, plasma expanders and corticosteroids may be used to control circulatory shock.

Dialysis is unlikely to be of value, as it has not proven useful in overdosages of either amitriptyline or chlordiazepoxide. Since many suicidal attempts involve multiple drugs including barbiturates, the possibility of dialysis being beneficial for removal of other drugs should not be overlooked.

Treatment should be continued for at least 48 hours, along with cardiac monitoring in patients who do not respond to therapy promptly. Since relapses are frequent, patients should be hospitalized until their conditions remain stable without physostigmine for at least 24 hours.

Since overdosage is often deliberate, patients may attempt suicide by other means during the recovery phase.

References:

1. Granacher RP, Baldessarini RJ: Physostigmine: Its use in acute anticholinergic syndrome with antidepressant and antiparkinson drugs. *Arch Gen Psychiatry 32*:375–380, March 1975.

2. Burks JS, Walker JE, Rumack BH, Ott JE: Tricyclic antidepressant poisoning: Reversal of coma, choreoathetosis, and myoclonus by physostigmine. *JAMA 230*:1405–1407, Dec. 9, 1974.

3. Snyder BD, Blonde L, McWhirter WR: Reversal of amitriptyline intoxication by physostigmine. *JAMA 230*:1433–1434, Dec. 9, 1974.

Dosage and Administration: Optimum dosage varies with the severity of the symptoms and the response of the individual patient. When a satisfactory response is obtained, dosage should be reduced to the smallest amount needed to maintain the remission. The larger portion of the total daily dose may be taken at bedtime. In some patients, a single dose at bedtime may be sufficient. In general, lower dosages are recommended for elderly patients.

Limbitrol 10–25 is recommended in an initial dosage of three or four tablets daily in divided doses; this may be increased to six tablets daily

Continued on next page

Roche Products—Cont.

as required. Some patients respond to smaller doses and can be maintained on two tablets daily.
Limbitrol 5–12.5 in an initial dosage of three or four tablets daily in divided doses may be satisfactory in patients who do not tolerate higher doses.
How Supplied: White, film-coated tablets, each containing 10 mg chlordiazepoxide and 25 mg amitriptyline (as the hydrochloride salt) and blue, film-coated tablets, each containing 5 mg chlordiazepoxide and 12.5 mg amitriptyline (as the hydrochloride salt)—bottles of 100 and 500; Tel-E-Dose® packages of 100; Prescription Paks of 50.
[*Shown in Product Identification Section*]

TEL-E-DOSE®

Tel-E-Dose is a unit package designed by Roche for convenience in dispensing medications in the hospital and nursing home. Each unit, sealed against contamination and moisture, is clearly identified by product name and strength and carries the control number and expiration date.
Currently available in this package form are the following products: Dalmane® (flurazepam HCl) capsules, 15 mg, 30 mg; Librax® (5 mg chlordiazepoxide HCl and 2.5 mg clidinium Br) capsules; Librium® (chlordiazepoxide HCl) capsules, 5 mg, 10 mg, 25 mg; Limbitrol® (chlordiazepoxide and amitriptyline HCl) tablets, 10–25, 5–12.5; Valium® (diazepam) tablets, 2 mg, 5 mg, 10 mg.

VALIUM® TABLETS Ⓒ
(diazepam/Roche)

The following text is complete prescribing information based on official labeling in effect August 1, 1982.
Description: Valium (diazepam/Roche) is a benzodiazepine derivative developed through original Roche research. Chemically, diazepam is 7- chloro - 1,3 - dihydro - 1 - methyl - 5 - phenyl - 2H-1,4-benzodiazepin-2-one. It is a colorless crystalline compound, insoluble in water and has a molecular weight of 284.74.
Pharmacology: In animals Valium appears to act on parts of the limbic system, the thalamus and hypothalamus, and induces calming effects. Valium, unlike chlorpromazine and reserpine, has no demonstrable peripheral autonomic blocking action, nor does it produce extrapyramidal side effects; however, animals treated with Valium do have a transient ataxia at higher doses. Valium was found to have transient cardiovascular depressor effects in dogs. Long-term experiments in rats revealed no disturbances of endocrine function.
Oral LD_{50} of diazepam is 720 mg/kg in mice and 1240 mg/kg in rats. Intraperitoneal administration of 400 mg/kg to a monkey resulted in death on the sixth day.
Reproduction Studies: A series of rat reproduction studies was performed with diazepam in oral doses of 1, 10, 80 and 100 mg/kg. At 100 mg/kg there was a decrease in the number of pregnancies and surviving offspring in these rats. Neonatal survival of rats at doses lower than 100 mg/kg was within normal limits. Several neonates in these rat reproduction studies showed skeletal or other defects. Further studies in rats at doses up to and including 80 mg/kg/day did not reveal teratological effects on the offspring.
In humans, measurable blood levels of Valium were obtained in maternal and cord blood, indicating placental transfer of the drug.
Indications: Valium is indicated for the management of anxiety disorders or for the short-term relief of the symptoms of anxiety. Anxiety or tension associated with the stress of everyday life usually does not require treatment with an anxiolytic.
In acute alcohol withdrawal, Valium may be useful in the symptomatic relief of acute agitation, tremor, impending or acute delirium tremens and hallucinosis.
Valium is a useful adjunct for the relief of skeletal muscle spasm due to reflex spasm to local pathology (such as inflammation of the muscles or joints, or secondary to trauma); spasticity caused by upper motor neuron disorders (such as cerebral palsy and paraplegia); athetosis; and stiff-man syndrome.
Oral Valium may be used adjunctively in convulsive disorders, although it has not proved useful as the sole therapy.
The effectiveness of Valium in long-term use, that is, more than 4 months, has not been assessed by systematic clinical studies. The physician should periodically reassess the usefulness of the drug for the individual patient.
Contraindications: Valium is contraindicated in patients with a known hypersensitivity to this drug and, because of lack of sufficient clinical experience, in children under 6 months of age. It may be used in patients with open angle glaucoma who are receiving appropriate therapy, but is contraindicated in acute narrow angle glaucoma.
Warnings: Valium is not of value in the treatment of psychotic patients and should not be employed in lieu of appropriate treatment. As is true of most preparations containing CNS-acting drugs, patients receiving Valium should be cautioned against engaging in hazardous occupations requiring complete mental alertness such as operating machinery or driving a motor vehicle.
As with other agents which have anticonvulsant activity, when Valium is used as an adjunct in treating convulsive disorders, the possibility of an increase in the frequency and/or severity of grand mal seizures may require an increase in the dosage of standard anticonvulsant medication. Abrupt withdrawal of Valium in such cases may also be associated with a temporary increase in the frequency and/or severity of seizures.
Since Valium has a central nervous system depressant effect, patients should be advised against the simultaneous ingestion of alcohol and other CNS-depressant drugs during Valium therapy.
Physical and Psychological Dependence: Withdrawal symptoms (similar in character to those noted with barbiturates and alcohol) have occurred following abrupt discontinuance of diazepam (convulsions, tremor, abdominal and muscle cramps, vomiting and sweating). These were usually limited to those patients who had received excessive doses over an extended period of time. Although infrequently seen, milder withdrawal symptoms have also been reported following abrupt discontinuance of benzodiazepines taken continuously, generally at higher therapeutic levels, for at least several months. Consequently, after extended therapy, abrupt discontinuation should generally be avoided and a gradual tapering in dosage followed. Particularly addiction-prone individuals (such as drug addicts or alcoholics) should be under careful surveillance when receiving diazepam or other psychotropic agents because of the predisposition of such patients to habituation and dependence.
***Usage in Pregnancy:* An increased risk of congenital malformations associated with the use of minor tranquilizers (diazepam, meprobamate and chlordiazepoxide) during the first trimester of pregnancy has been suggested in several studies. Because use of these drugs is rarely a matter of urgency, their use during this period should almost always be avoided. The possibility that a woman of childbearing potential may be pregnant at the time of institution of therapy should be considered. Patients should be advised that if they become pregnant during therapy or intend to become pregnant they should communicate with their physicians about the desirability of discontinuing the drug.**
Management of Overdosage: Manifestations of Valium overdosage include somnolence, confusion, coma and diminished reflexes. Respiration, pulse and blood pressure should be monitored, as in all cases of drug overdosage, although, in general, these effects have been minimal following overdosage. General supportive measures should be employed, along with immediate gastric lavage. Intravenous fluids should be administered and an adequate airway maintained. Hypotension may be combated by the use of Levophed® (levarterenol) or Aramine (metaraminol). Dialysis is of limited value. As with the management of intentional overdosage with any drug, it should be borne in mind that multiple agents may have been ingested.

Precautions: If Valium is to be combined with other psychotropic agents or anticonvulsant drugs, careful consideration should be given to the pharmacology of the agents to be employed—particularly with known compounds which may potentiate the action of Valium, such as phenothiazines, narcotics, barbiturates, MAO inhibitors and other antidepressants. The usual precautions are indicated for severely depressed patients or those in whom there is any evidence of latent depression; particularly the recognition that suicidal tendencies may be present and protective measures may be necessary. The usual precautions in treating patients with impaired renal or hepatic function should be observed.
In elderly and debilitated patients, it is recommended that the dosage be limited to the smallest effective amount to preclude the development of ataxia or oversedation (2 mg to 2½ mg once or twice daily, initially, to be increased gradually as needed and tolerated).
The clearance of Valium and certain other benzodiazepines can be delayed in association with Tagamet (cimetidine) administration. The clinical significance of this is unclear.

Adverse Reactions: Side effects most commonly reported were drowsiness, fatigue and ataxia. Infrequently encountered were confusion, constipation, depression, diplopia, dysarthria, headache, hypotension, incontinence, jaundice, changes in libido, nausea, changes in salivation, skin rash, slurred speech, tremor, urinary retention, vertigo and blurred vision. Paradoxical reactions such as acute hyperexcited states, anxiety, hallucinations, increased muscle spasticity, insomnia, rage, sleep disturbances and stimulation have been reported; should these occur, use of the drug should be discontinued.
Because of isolated reports of neutropenia and jaundice, periodic blood counts and liver function tests are advisable during long-term therapy. Minor changes in EEG patterns, usually low-voltage fast activity, have been observed in patients during and after Valium therapy and are of no known significance.

Dosage and Administration: Dosage should be individualized for maximum beneficial effect. While the usual daily dosages given below will meet the needs of most patients, there will be some who may require higher doses. In such cases dosage should be increased cautiously to avoid adverse effects.

	USUAL DAILY DOSE
Adults:	
Management of Anxiety Disorders and Relief of Symptoms of Anxiety	Depending upon severity of symptoms —2 mg to 10 mg, 2 to 4 times daily

Symptomatic Relief in Acute Alcohol Withdrawal.	10 mg, 3 or 4 times during the first 24 hours, reducing to 5 mg, 3 or 4 times daily as needed
Adjunctively for Relief of Skeletal Muscle Spasm.	2 mg to 10 mg, 3 or 4 times daily
Adjunctively in Convulsive Disorders.	2 mg to 10 mg, 2 to 4 times daily
Geriatric Patients, or in the presence of debilitating disease.	2 mg to 2½ mg, 1 or 2 times daily initially; increase gradually as needed and tolerated
Children: Because of varied responses to CNS-acting drugs, initiate therapy with lowest dose and increase as required. Not for use in children under 6 months.	1 mg to 2½ mg, 3 or 4 times daily initially; increase gradually as needed and tolerated

How Supplied: For oral administration, Valium scored tablets—2 mg, white; 5 mg, yellow; 10 mg, blue—bottles of 100* and 500;* Prescription Paks of 50, available in trays of 10.* Tel-E-Dose® packages of 100, available in trays of 4 reverse-numbered boxes of 25,† and in boxes containing 10 strips of 10.†

* Supplied by Roche Products Inc., Manati, Puerto Rico 00701

† Supplied by Roche Laboratories, Division of Hoffmann-La Roche Inc., Nutley, New Jersey 07110

[*Shown in Product Identification Section*]

Roerig

A division of Pfizer Pharmaceuticals
235 EAST 42nd STREET
NEW YORK, NY 10017

Product Identification Codes

To provide quick and positive identification of Roerig Division products, we have imprinted the product identification number of the National Drug Code on most tablets and capsules. In order that you may quickly identify a product by its code number, we have compiled below a numerical list of code numbers with their corresponding product names. We are also listing the code numbers by alphabetical order of products.

Numerical Listing

Product Ident. Number	Product
035	**Spectrobid® (bacampicillin HCl) Tablets, 400 mg., equivalent to 280 mg. ampicillin**
092	**Urobiotic®-250 (oxytetracycline HCl 250 mg. with sulfamethizole 250 mg. and phenazopyridine 50 mg.) Capsules**
143	**Geocillin® (carbenicillin indanyl sodium) Tablets, equivalent to 382 mg. carbenicillin**
159	**TAO® (troleandomycin) Capsules, 250 mg.**
210	**Antivert® (meclizine HCl) Tablets, 12.5 mg.**
211	**Antivert® /25 (meclizine HCl) Tablets, 25 mg.**
212	**Antivert® /25 (meclizine HCl) Chewable Tablets**
220	**Sustaire® (theophylline [anhydrous]) Tablets, 100 mg.**
221	**Sustaire® (theophylline [anhydrous]) Tablets, 300 mg.**
254	**Marax® (ephedrine sulfate, 25 mg; theophylline, 130 mg; and Atarax® [hydroxyzine HCl], 10 mg) Tablets**
294	**Cartrax® 10 (hydroxyzine HCl & pentaerythritol tetranitrate) Tablets**
295	**Cartrax® 20 (hydroxyzine HCl & pentaerythritol tetranitrate) Tablets**
504	**Heptuna® plus (iron plus vitamins and minerals), Capsules.**
534	**Sinequan® (doxepin HCl) Capsules 10 mg.**
535	**Sinequan® (doxepin HCl) Capsules 25 mg.**
536	**Sinequan® (doxepin HCl) Capsules 50 mg.**
537	**Sinequan® (doxepin HCl) Capsules 150 mg.**
538	**Sinequan® (doxepin HCl) Casules 100 mg.**
539	**Sinequan® (doxepin HCl) Capsules 75 mg.**
560	**Atarax® (hydroxyzine HCl) Tablets, 10 mg.**
561	**Atarax® (hydroxyzine HCl) Tablets, 25 mg.**
562	**Atarax® (hydroxyzine HCl) Tablets, 50 mg.**
563	**Atarax® (hydroxyzine HCl) Tablets, 100 mg.**
571	**Navane® (thiothixene) Capsules, 1 mg.**
572	**Navane® (thiothixene) Capsules, 2 mg.**
573	**Navane® (thiothixene) Capsules, 5 mg.**
574	**Navane® (thiothixene) Capsules, 10 mg.**
577	**Navane® (thiothixene) Capsules, 20 mg.**

Alphabetical Listing

Prod. Ident. Number	Product
210	**Antivert® (meclizine HCl) Tablets, 12.5 mg.**
211	**Antivert® /25 (meclizine HCl) Tablets, 25 mg.**
212	**Antivert® /25 (meclizine HCl) Chewable Tablets**
560	**Atarax® (hydroxyzine HCl) Tablets, 10 mg.**
561	**Atarax® (hydroxyzine HCl) Tablets, 25 mg.**
562	**Atarax® (hydroxyzine HCl) Tablets, 50 mg.**
563	**Atarax® (hydroxyzine HCl) Tablets, 100 mg.**
294	**Cartrax® 10 (hydroxyzine HCl & pentaerythritol tetranitrate) Tablets**
295	**Cartrax® 20 (hydroxyzine HCl & pentaerythritol tetranitrate) Tablets**
143	**Geocillin® (carbenicillin indanyl sodium) Tablets equivalent to 382 mg. carbenicillin**
504	**Heptuna® plus (iron plus vitamins and minerals), Capsules.**
254	**Marax® (ephedrine sulfate, 25 mg; theophylline, 130 mg; and Atarax® [hydroxyzine HCl], 10 mg) Tablets**
571	**Navane® (thiothixene) Capsules, 1 mg.**
572	**Navane® (thiothixene) Capsules, 2 mg.**
573	**Navane® (thiothixene) Capsules, 5 mg.**
574	**Navane® (thiothixene) Capsules, 10 mg.**
577	**Navane® (thiothixene) Capsules, 20 mg.**
534	**Sinequan® (doxepin HCl) Capsules 10 mg.**
535	**Sinequan® (doxepin HCl) Capsules 25 mg.**
536	**Sinequan® (doxepin HCl) Capsules 50 mg.**
539	**Sinequan® (doxepin HCl) Capsules 75 mg.**
538	**Sinequan® (doxepin HCl) Capsules 100 mg.**
537	**Sinequan® (doxepin HCl) Capsules 150 mg.**
035	**Spectrobid® (bacampicillin HCl) Tablets, 400 mg., equivalent to 280 mg. ampicillin**
220	**Sustaire® (theophylline [anhydrous]) Tablets, 100 mg.**
221	**Sustaire® (theophylline [anhydrous]) Tablets, 300 mg.**
159	**TAO® (troleandomycin) Capsules, 250 mg.**
092	**Urobiotic®-250 (oxytetracycline HCl 250 mg. with sulfamethizole 250 mg. and phenazopyridine 50 mg.) Capsules**

ANTIVERT® TABLETS ℞
(12.5 mg. meclizine HCl)

ANTIVERT®/25 TABLETS ℞
(25 mg. meclizine HCl)

ANTIVERT®/25 CHEWABLE TABLETS ℞
(25 mg. meclizine HCl)

Description: Chemically, Antivert (meclizine HCl) is 1-(*p*-chloro-α-phenylbenzyl)-4-(*m*-methylbenzyl) piperazine dihydrochloride monohydrate.

Actions: Antivert is an antihistamine which shows marked protective activity against nebulized histamine and lethal doses of intravenously injected histamine in guinea pigs. It has a marked effect in blocking the vasodepressor response to histamine, but only a slight blocking action against acetylcholine. Its activity is relatively weak in inhibiting the spasmogenic action of histamine on isolated guinea pig ileum.

INDICATIONS

Based on a review of this drug by the National Academy of Sciences-National Research Council and/or other information, FDA has classified the indications as follows:

Effective: Management of nausea and vomiting, and dizziness associated with motion sickness.

Possibly Effective: Management of vertigo associated with diseases affecting the vestibular system.

Final classification of the less than effective indications requires further investigation.

Contraindications: Meclizine HCl is contraindicated in individuals who have shown a previous hypersensitivity to it.

Warnings: Since drowsiness may, on occasion, occur with use of this drug, patients should be warned of this possibility and cautioned against driving a car or operating dangerous machinery.

Patients should avoid alcoholic beverages while taking the drug. Due to its potential anticholinergic action, this drug should be used with caution in patients with asthma, glaucoma, or enlargement of the prostate gland.

USAGE IN CHILDREN:

Clinical studies establishing safety and effectiveness in children have not been done; therefore, usage is not recommended in children under 12 years of age.

Continued on next page

Roerig—Cont.

USAGE IN PREGNANCY:
Pregnancy Category B. Reproduction studies in rats have shown cleft palates at 25–50 times the human dose. Epidemiological studies in pregnant women, however, do not indicate that meclizine increases the risk of abnormalities when administered during pregnancy. Despite the animal findings, it would appear that the possibility of fetal harm is remote. Nevertheless, meclizine, or any other medication, should be used during pregnancy only if clearly necessary.

Adverse Reactions: Drowsiness, dry mouth and, on rare occasions, blurred vision have been reported.

Dosage and Administration:
Vertigo:
For the control of vertigo associated with diseases affecting the vestibular system, the recommended dose is 25 to 100 mg. daily, in divided dosage, depending upon clinical response.
Motion Sickness:
The initial dose of 25 to 50 mg. of Antivert should be taken one hour prior to embarkation for protection against motion sickness. Thereafter, the dose may be repeated every 24 hours for the duration of the journey.

How Supplied:
Antivert—12.5 mg. tablets: Bottles of 100, 1000 and unit dose 100's.
Antivert/25—25 mg. tablets: Bottles of 100, 1000 and unit dose 100's.
Antivert/25 Chewable Tablets—25 mg. pink scored tablets: Bottles of 100 and 500.
[*Shown in Product Identification Section*]

ATARAX® ℞
(hydroxyzine hydrochloride)
TABLETS AND SYRUP

Description: Hydroxyzine hydrochloride is designated chemically as 1-(p-chlorobenzhydryl) 4-[2-(2-hydroxyethoxy)-ethyl] piperazine dihydrochloride.

Clinical Pharmacology: Atarax is unrelated chemically to the phenothiazines, reserpine, meprobamate, or the benzodiazepines. Atarax is not a cortical depressant, but its action may be due to a suppression of activity in certain key regions of the subcortical area of the central nervous system. Primary skeletal muscle relaxation has been demonstrated experimentally. Bronchodilator activity, and antihistaminic and analgesic effects have been demonstrated experimentally and confirmed clinically. An antiemetic effect, both by the apomorphine test and the veriloid test, has been demonstrated. Pharmacological and clinical studies indicate that hydroxyzine in therapeutic dosage does not increase gastric secretion or acidity and in most cases has mild antisecretory activity. Hydroxyzine is rapidly absorbed from the gastrointestinal tract and Atarax's clinical effects are usually noted within 15 to 30 minutes after oral administration.

Indications: For symptomatic relief of anxiety and tension associated with psychoneurosis and as an adjunct in organic disease states in which anxiety is manifested.
Useful in the management of pruritus due to allergic conditions such as chronic urticaria and atopic and contact dermatoses, and in histamine-mediated pruritus.
As a sedative when used as premedication and following general anesthesia. **Hydroxyzine may potentiate meperidine (Demerol®) and barbiturates,** so their use in pre-anesthetic adjunctive therapy should be modified on an individual basis. Atropine and other belladonna alkaloids are not affected by the drug. Hydroxyzine is not known to interfere with the action of digitalis in any way and it may be used concurrently with this agent.
The effectiveness of hydroxyzine as an antianxiety agent for long term use, that is more than 4 months, has not been assessed by systematic clinical studies. The physician should reassess periodically the usefulness of the drug for the individual patient.

Contraindications: Hydroxyzine, when administered to the pregnant mouse, rat, and rabbit, induced fetal abnormalities in the rat and mouse at doses substantially above the human therapeutic range. Clinical data in human beings are inadequate to establish safety in early pregnancy. Until such data are available, hydroxyzine is contraindicated in early pregnancy.
Hydroxyzine is contraindicated for patients who have shown a previous hypersensitivity to it.

Warnings:
Nursing Mothers: It is not known whether this drug is excreted in human milk. Since many drugs are so excreted, hydroxyzine should not be given to nursing mothers.

Precautions: THE POTENTIATING ACTION OF HYDROXYZINE MUST BE CONSIDERED WHEN THE DRUG IS USED IN CONJUNCTION WITH CENTRAL NERVOUS SYSTEM DEPRESSANTS SUCH AS NARCOTICS, NON-NARCOTIC ANALGESICS AND BARBITURATES. Therefore when central nervous system depressants are administered concomitantly with hydroxyzine their dosage should be reduced.
Since drowsiness may occur with use of this drug, patients should be warned of this possibility and cautioned against driving a car or operating dangerous machinery while taking Atarax. Patients should be advised against the simultaneous use of other CNS depressant drugs, and cautioned that the effect of alcohol may be increased.

Adverse Reactions: Side effects reported with the administration of Atarax (hydroxyzine hydrochloride) are usually mild and transitory in nature.
Anticholinergic: Dry mouth.
Central Nervous System: Drowsiness is usually transitory and may disappear in a few days of continued therapy or upon reduction of the dose. Involuntary motor activity including rare instances of tremor and convulsions have been reported, usually with doses considerably higher than those recommended. Clinically significant respiratory depression has not been reported at recommended doses.

Overdosage: The most common manifestation of Atarax overdosage is hypersedation. As in the management of overdosage with any drug, it should be borne in mind that multiple agents may have been taken.
If vomiting has not occurred spontaneously, it should be induced. Immediate gastric lavage is also recommended. General supportive care, including frequent monitoring of the vital signs and close observation of the patient, is indicated. Hypotension, though unlikely, may be controlled with intravenous fluids and Levophed® (levarterenol), or Aramine® (metaraminol). Do not use epinephrine as Atarax counteracts its pressor action. Caffeine and Sodium Benzoate Injection, U.S.P., may be used to counteract central nervous system depressant effects.
There is no specific antidote. It is doubtful that hemodialysis would be of any value in the treatment of overdosage with hydroxyzine. However, if other agents such as barbiturates have been ingested concomitantly, hemodialysis may be indicated. There is no practical method to quantitate hydroxyzine in body fluids or tissue after its ingestion or administration.

Dosage: For symptomatic relief of anxiety and tension associated with psychoneurosis and as an adjunct in organic disease states in which anxiety is manifested: in adults, 50–100 mg q.i.d.: children under 6 years, 50 mg daily in divided doses and over 6 years, 50–100 mg daily in divided doses.
For use in the management of pruritus due to allergic conditions such as chronic urticaria and atopic and contact dermatoses, and in histamine-mediated pruritus: in adults, 25 mg t.i.d. or q.i.d.; children under 6 years, 50 mg daily in divided doses and over 6 years, 50–100 mg daily in divided doses.
As a sedative when used as a premedication and following general anesthesia: 50–100 mg in adults, and 0.6 mg/kg in children.
When treatment is initiated by the intramuscular route of administration, subsequent doses may be administered orally.
As with all medications, the dosage should be adjusted according to the patient's response to therapy.

Supply:
Atarax Tablets
10 mg: 100's (NDC 0049-5600-66), 500's (NDC 0049-5600-73), Unit Dose 10 × 10's (NDC 0049-5600-41), and Unit of Use 40's (NDC 0049-5600-43)—orange tablets
25 mg: 100's (NDC 0049-5610-66), 500's (NDC 0049-5610-73), Unit Dose 10 × 10's (NDC 0049-5610-41), and Unit of Use 40's (NDC 0049-5610-43)—green tablets
50 mg: 100's (NDC 0049-5620-66), 500's (NDC 0049-5620-73), and Unit Dose 10 × 10's (NDC 0049-5620-41)—yellow tablets
Atarax 100 Tablets
100 mg: 100's (NDC 0049-5630-66), and Unit Dose 10 × 10's (NDC 0049-5630-41)—red tablets
Atarax Syrup
10 mg per teaspoon (5 ml): 1 pint bottles (NDC 0049-5590-15)
Alcohol Content—Ethyl Alcohol—0.5% v/v
Bibliography: Available on request.
[*Shown in Product Identification Section*]

CARTRAX® ℞
(pentaerythritol tetranitrate and hydroxyzine hydrochloride)
TABLETS
For Oral Administration

Description: CARTRAX is a combination of pentaerythritol tetranitrate and hydroxyzine HCl. Pentaerythritol tetranitrate is a nitric acid ester of a tetrahydric alcohol. The chemical formula is 2,2-bisdihydroxymethyl-1,3-propanediol tetranitrate.
Hydroxyzine HCl is designated chemically as 1-(p-chlorobenzhydryl)-4-(2-(2-hydroxyethoxy)-ethyl) piperazine dihydrochloride.

Actions: Pentaerythritol tetranitrate is a slow acting organic nitrate with a vasodilator action.
Hydroxyzine HCl has been shown clinically to be an effective antianxiety agent. It is not a cortical depressant, but its action may be due to a suppression of activity in certain key regions of the subcortical area of the central nervous system.

Indications
Based on a review of this drug by the National Academy of Sciences-National Research Council and/or other information, the FDA has classified the indications as follows:
Possibly Effective: For the management or treatment of:
1. Angina Pectoris,
2. Angina Decubitus,
3. Precordial Pain,
4. Status Anginosus.

Final classification of these less than effective indications requires further investigation.

Contraindications: This drug is contraindicated in individuals who are hypersensitive to it or any of its components.

Hydroxyzine, when administered to the pregnant mouse, rat, and rabbit induced fetal abnormalities in the rat at doses substantially above the human therapeutic range. Clinical data in human beings are inadequate to establish safety in early pregnancy. Until such data are available, hydroxyzine is contraindicated in early pregnancy.

Precautions: Due to the Atarax® (hydroxyzine HCl) component, mild transient drowsiness may occur. Patients should be warned of the possibility and cautioned against driving an automobile or operating dangerous machinery while taking this drug.

Like all nitrates PETN may increase intraocular pressure; therefore caution is required in administering this drug to patients with glaucoma. Tolerance to this drug, and cross tolerance to other nitrates and nitrites may occur.

THE POTENTIATING ACTION OF HYDROXYZINE HYDROCHLORIDE, ALTHOUGH MILD, MUST BE TAKEN INTO CONSIDERATION WHEN THE DRUG IS USED IN CONJUNCTION WITH CENTRAL NERVOUS SYSTEM DEPRESSANTS; AND WHEN OTHER CENTRAL NERVOUS SYSTEM DEPRESSANTS ARE ADMINISTERED CONCOMITANTLY WITH HYDROXYZINE THEIR DOSAGE SHOULD BE REDUCED.

Caution should be observed in patients with anemia; however, anemia to date is not considered to be a contraindication to its use.

Adverse Reactions: Cutaneous vasodilatation with flushing may occur and transient episodes of dizziness and weakness as well as other signs of cerebral ischemia and postural hypotension may occur. Side effects of PETN are the same as those of other nitrates, except that these appear to be relatively infrequent and methemoglobinemia has not been demonstrated following prolonged use. Headache is common and may be severe and persistent. Nausea, occasionally observed, tends to disappear after four or five days' medication. This drug can act as a physiologic antagonist to norepinephrine, acetylcholine, histamine, and many other agents. An occasional individual exhibits marked sensitivity to the hypotensive effects of nitrite and severe responses (nausea, vomiting, weakness, restlessness, pallor and collapse) can occur even with usual therapeutic dose. Alcohol may enhance this effect.

Drug rash and/or exfoliative dermatitis may occur.

The amount of Atarax (hydroxyzine hydrochloride) present in CARTRAX has not resulted in disturbing side effects. When used alone specifically as a tranquilizer in the normal dosage range (25 to 50 mg. three or four times a day), side effects are infrequent; even at these higher doses, no serious side effects have been reported and confirmed to date. Those which do occasionally occur are drowsiness, xerostomia and, at extremely high doses, involuntary motor activity including rare instances of tremor and convulsions, all of which may be controlled by reduction of the dosage or discontinuation of the medication. With the relatively low dose of Atarax in CARTRAX, these effects are not likely to occur.

Dosage: CARTRAX is initially administered orally in usual beginning doses of 1 or 2 tablets three to four times daily of the CARTRAX-10 (yellow) tablet.

For dosage flexibility CARTRAX-20 (pink) tablets may be utilized at a level of 1 tablet three to four times a day.

The tablets should be administered before meals for optimal effects.

Dosage schedules should be arranged on an individual basis, with particular attention given to the aged or debilitated patient, with the physician observing the patient for a decrease in the incidence and severity of anginal attacks, improved exercise tolerance, improved electrocardiographic status, and decreased need for nitroglycerin.

How Supplied:
CARTRAX-10: hydroxyzine hydrochloride 10 mg. combined with PETN 10 mg. (yellow tablet).
CARTRAX-20: hydroxyzine hydrochloride 10 mg. combined with PETN 20 mg. (pink tablet).
Both forms are packaged in bottles of 100 tablets.

EMETE-CON®
(benzquinamide hydrochloride) ℞
For Intramuscular and Intravenous Use

Description: Benzquinamide is a non-amine-depleting benzoquinolizine derivative, chemically unrelated to the phenothiazines and to other antiemetics.

Chemically, Emete-con (benzquinamide hydrochloride) is N,N-diethyl-1,3,4,6,7,11b-hexahydro-2-hydroxy-9, 10-dimethoxy- 2H -benzo-[a]quinolizine-3-carboxamide acetate hydrochloride. The empirical formula is $C_{22}H_{32}N_2O_5 \cdot HCl$ and the molecular weight is 441.

Emete-con for injection contains benzquinamide hydrochloride equivalent to 50 mg/vial of benzquinamide. When reconstituted with 2.2 ml of proper diluent, each vial yields 2 ml of a solution containing benzquinamide hydrochloride equivalent to 25 mg/ml of benzquinamide. When reconstituted this product maintains its potency for 14 days at room temperature.

Actions: Benzquinamide HCl exhibited antiemetic, antihistaminic, mild anticholinergic and sedative action in animals. Studies conducted in dogs and human volunteers have demonstrated suppression of apomorphine-induced vomiting; however, relevance to clinical efficacy has not been established. The mechanism of action in humans is unknown. The onset of antiemetic activity in humans usually occurs within 15 minutes.

Benzquinamide metabolism has been studied in animals and in man. In both species, 5-10% of an administered dose is excreted unchanged in the urine. The remaining drug undergoes metabolic transformation in the liver by at least three pathways to a spectrum of metabolites which are excreted in the urine and in the bile, from which the more polar metabolites are not reabsorbed but are excreted in the feces. The half-life in plasma of Emete-con is about 40 minutes. More than 95% of an administered dose was excreted within 72 hours in animal studies using C14-labeled benzquinamide. In blood, benzquinamide is about 58% bound to plasma protein.

Indications: Emete-con is indicated for the prevention and treatment of nausea and vomiting associated with anesthesia and surgery. Since the incidence of postoperative and post-anesthetic vomiting has decreased with the adoption of modern techniques and agents, the prophylactic use of Emete-con should be restricted to those patients in whom emesis would endanger the results of surgery or result in harm to the patient.

Contraindications: Emete-con is contraindicated in individuals who have demonstrated hypersensitivity to the drug.

Warnings:

Use in Pregnancy
No teratogenic effects of benzquinamide were demonstrated in reproduction studies in chick embryos, mice, rats and rabbits. The relevance of these data to the human is not known. However, safe use of this drug in pregnancy has not been established and its use in pregnancy is not recommended.

Use in Children
As the data available at present are insufficient to establish proper dosage in children, the use of Emete-con in children is not recommended.

Intravenous use
Sudden increase in blood pressure and transient arrhythmias (premature ventricular and auricular contractions) have been reported following intravenous administration of benzquinamide. Until a more predictable pattern of the effect of intravenous benzquinamide has been established, the intramuscular route of administration is considered preferable. The intravenous route of administration should be restricted to patients without cardiovascular disease and receiving no pre-anesthetic and/or concomitant cardiovascular drugs.

If patients receiving pressor agents or epinephrine-like drugs are also given benzquinamide, the latter should be given in fractions of the normal dose. Blood pressure should be monitored. Safeguards against hypertensive reactions are particularly important in hypertensive patients.

Precautions: Benzquinamide, like other antiemetics, may mask signs of overdosage of toxic drugs or may obscure diagnosis of such conditions as intestinal obstruction and brain tumor.

Adverse Reactions: The following adverse reactions have been reported in subjects who have received benzquinamide. However, drowsiness appears to be the most common reaction. One case of pronounced allergic reaction has been encountered, characterized by pyrexia and urticaria.

System Affected
Autonomic Nervous System: Dry mouth, shivering, sweating, hiccoughs, flushing, salivation, blurred vision.
Cardiovascular System: Hypertension, hypotension, dizziness, atrial fibrillation, premature auricular and ventricular contractions. Hypertensive episodes have occurred after IM and IV administration.
Central Nervous System: Drowsiness, insomnia, restlessness, headache, excitement, nervousness.
Gastrointestinal System: Anorexia, nausea.
Musculoskeletal System: Twitching, shaking/tremors, weakness.
Skin: Hives/rash.
Other Systems: Fatigue, shaking chills, increased temperature.

Dosage and Administration:
Intramuscular: 50 mg (0.5 mg/kg–1.0 mg/kg) First dose may be repeated in one hour with subsequent doses every 3-4 hours, as necessary. The precautions applicable to all intramuscular injections should be observed. Emete-con should be injected well within the mass of a larger muscle. The deltoid area should be used only if well developed. Injections should not be made into the lower and mid-thirds of the upper arm. Aspiration of the syringe should be carried out to avoid inadvertent intravascular injection.

Therapeutic blood levels and demonstrable antiemetic activity appear within fifteen minutes of intramuscular administration. When the objective of therapy is the prevention of nausea and vomiting, intramuscular administration is recommended at least fifteen minutes prior to emergence from anesthesia.

Intravenous: 25 mg (0.2 mg/kg–0.4 mg/kg as a single dose) administered slowly (1 ml per 0.5 to 1 minute). Subsequent doses should be given intramuscularly.

The intravenous route of administration should be restricted to patients without cardiovascular disease (See WARNINGS). If it is necessary to use Emete-con intravenously in elderly or debilitated patients, benzquinamide should be administered cautiously and the lower dose range is recommended.

This preparation must be initially reconstituted with 2.2 ml of Sterile Water for Injection, Bacteriostatic Water for Injection with benzyl alcohol or with methylparaben and propylparaben. This procedure yields 2 ml of a solution equivalent to 25 mg benzquinamide/ml, which maintains its potency for 14 days at room temperature.

Continued on next page

Roerig—Cont.

Overdosage:
Manifestations: On the basis of acute animal toxicology studies, gross Emete-con overdosage in humans might be expected to manifest itself as a combination of Central Nervous System stimulant and depressant effects. This speculation is derived from experimental studies in which intravenous doses of benzquinamide, at least 150 times the human therapeutic dose, were administered to dogs.
Treatment: There is no specific antidote for Emete-con overdosage. General supportive measures should be instituted, as indicated. Atropine may be helpful. Although there has been no direct experience with dialysis, it is not likely to be of value, since benzquinamide is extensively bound to plasma protein.
How Supplied: Emete-con for IM/IV use is available in a vial containing benzquinamide HCl equivalent to 50 mg of benzquinamide in packages of 10 vials.
Caution: Federal law prohibits dispensing without prescription.

GEOCILLIN® ℞
(carbenicillin indanyl sodium)
TABLETS
For Oral Use

Description: Geocillin (carbenicillin indanyl sodium), a semisynthetic penicillin, is the sodium salt of the indanyl ester of Geopen® (carbenicillin disodium). Geocillin is acid stable and well absorbed following oral administration.
Actions:
Microbiology
The antibacterial activity of Geocillin is due to its rapid conversion to carbenicillin by hydrolysis. Though Geocillin provides substantial *in vitro* activity against a variety of both gram-positive and gram-negative microorganisms, the most important aspect of its profile is in its antipseudomonal and antiproteus activity. Because of the high urine levels obtained following administration, Geocillin has demonstrated clinical efficacy in urinary infections due to susceptible strains of:
Escherichia coli
Proteus mirabilis
Proteus morgani
Proteus rettgeri
Proteus vulgaris
Pseudomonas
Enterobacter
Enterococci
In addition, *in vitro* data, not substantiated by clinical studies, indicate the following pathogens to be usually susceptible to Geocillin:

DRUG	DOSE	Mean Urine Concentration of Carbenicillin mcg/ml Hours After Initial Dose 0–3	3–6	6–24
Geocillin	1 tablet q.6 hr.	1130	352	292
Geocillin	2 tablets q.6 hr.	1428	789	809

Mean serum concentrations of carbenicillin in this study for these dosages are:

DRUG	DOSE	Mean Serum Concentration mcg/ml Hours After Initial Dose ½	1	2	4	6	24	25	26	28
Geocillin	1 tablet q.6 hr.	5.1	6.5	3.2	1.9	0.0	0.4	8.8	5.4	0.4
Geocillin	2 tablets q.6 hr.	6.1	9.6	7.9	2.6	0.4	0.8	13.2	12.8	3.8

Staphylococcus (non-penicillinase producing)
Streptococcus
Most *Klebsiella* species are often resistant to the action of Geocillin. Some strains of *Pseudomonas* have developed resistance to carbenicillin.
Susceptibility Testing
Geopen (carbenicillin disodium) Susceptibility Powder or 100 mcg. Geopen Susceptibility Discs may be used to determine microbial susceptibility to Geocillin.
Interpretations:
[See table below].
Interpretations of susceptible, intermediate, and resistant correlate zone size diameters with MIC values. A laboratory report of "susceptible" indicates that the suspected causative microorganism most likely will respond to therapy with carbenicillin. A laboratory report of "resistant" indicates that the infecting microorganism most likely will not respond to therapy. A laboratory report of "intermediate" indicates that the microorganism is most likely susceptible if a high dosage of carbenicillin is used, or if the infection is such that high levels of carbenicillin may be attained as in urine.
Pharmacology
Geocillin is acid stable and well absorbed following oral administration. After absorption, Geocillin is rapidly hydrolyzed to carbenicillin, which is primarily excreted in the urine. In a study utilizing volunteers with normal renal function, the following mean urine levels of carbenicillin were achieved:
[See table above].
Indications: Geocillin (carbenicillin indanyl sodium) is indicated in the treatment of acute and chronic infections of the upper and lower urinary tract and in asymptomatic bacteriuria due to susceptible strains of the following organisms:
Escherichia coli
Proteus mirabilis
Proteus morgani
Proteus rettgeri
Proteus vulgaris
Pseudomonas
Enterobacter
Enterococci
Geocillin is also indicated in the treatment of prostatitis due to susceptible strains of the following organisms:
Escherichia coli
Enterococcus *(S. faecalis)*
Proteus mirabilis
Enterobacter sp.
WHEN HIGH RAPID BLOOD AND URINE LEVELS OF ANTIBIOTIC ARE INDICATED, THERAPY WITH GEOPEN (CARBENICILLIN DISODIUM) SHOULD BE INITIATED BY PARENTERAL ADMINISTRATION FOLLOWED, AT THE PHYSICIAN'S DISCRETION, BY ORAL THERAPY.
NOTE: Susceptibility testing should be performed prior to and during the course of therapy to detect the possible emergence of resistant organisms which may develop.
Contraindications: Geocillin is ordinarily contraindicated in patients who have a known penicillin allergy.
Warnings: Serious and occasionally fatal hypersensitivity (anaphylactic) reactions have been reported in patients on oral penicillin therapy. These reactions are more apt to occur in individuals with a history of sensitivity to multiple allergens.
There have been reports of individuals with a history of penicillin hypersensitivity who have experienced severe hypersensitivity reactions when treated with a cephalosporin, and vice versa. Therefore, before therapy with a penicillin, careful inquiry should be made concerning previous hypersensitivity reactions to penicillins, cephalosporins, and other allergens.
SERIOUS ANAPHYLACTOID REACTIONS REQUIRE IMMEDIATE EMERGENCY TREATMENT WITH EPINEPHRINE. OXYGEN, INTRAVENOUS STEROIDS AND AIRWAY MANAGEMENT, INCLUDING INTUBATION, SHOULD ALSO BE ADMINISTERED AS INDICATED.
Usage in Children: Since only limited clinical data is available to date in children, the safety of Geocillin administration in this age group has not yet been established.
Usage in Pregnancy: Safety for use in pregnancy has not been established.
Precautions: Periodic assessment of organ system function including renal, hepatic and hematopoietic systems is recommended during prolonged therapy.

	Susceptible	Intermediate	Resistant
Pseudomonas aeruginosa and Enterococci			
Inhibition Zone	17 mm or greater*	16 mm–14 mm	13 mm or less
MIC	125 mcg/ml or less	greater than 125 mcg/ml less than 250 mcg/ml	250 mcg/ml or greater
Escherichia coli, Proteus species, and Enterobacter.			
Inhibition Zone	23 mm or greater	22 mm–18 mm	17 mm or less
MIC	15 mcg/ml or less	greater than 20 mcg/ml less than 40 mcg/ml	greater than 40 mcg/ml

*Zone diameter interpretations apply only to results obtained by the Bauer, Kirby, Sherris and Turck method of Susceptibility Testing Am. J. Clin. Path. 45:493, 1966.

Long term use of Geocillin may result in the overgrowth of nonsensitive organisms. If superinfection occurs during therapy, appropriate measures should be taken.

Since carbenicillin is excreted by the kidney, patients with severe renal impairment (creatinine clearance of less than 10 ml/min.) will not achieve therapeutic urine levels of carbenicillin.

Adverse Reactions: The following adverse reactions may occur during therapy with Geocillin:

Gastrointestinal Disturbances: Nausea, vomiting, and diarrhea.

Hypersensitivity Reactions: Skin rashes, urticaria, or pruritus have been reported infrequently.

Blood, Hepatic and Renal Studies: As with other penicillins, anemia, thrombocytopenia, leukopenia, neutropenia, and eosinophilia may occur.

Mild SGOT elevations have been observed following Geocillin administration.

Other reactions that have been reported are flatulence, dry mouth, furry tongue, vaginitis, and abdominal cramps.

Dosage and Administration:

Geocillin is available as a coated tablet, to be administered orally.

Usual Adult Dose

URINARY TRACT INFECTIONS	
Escherichia coli, Proteus species, and *Enterobacter*	1-2 tablets 4 times daily
Pseudomonas and Enterococci	2 tablets 4 times daily
PROSTATITIS	
Escherichia coli, Proteus mirabilis, Enterobacter and Enterococcus	2 tablets 4 times daily

How Supplied: Geocillin is available as film-coated tablets in bottles of 100's, and unit-dose packages of 100 (10 × 10s). Each tablet contains carbenicillin indanyl sodium equivalent to 382 mg of carbenicillin.

[*Shown in Product Identification Section*]

GEOPEN® ℞

sterile carbenicillin disodium
For Intramuscular and Intravenous Use

Description: Geopen (carbenicillin disodium) is a new semisynthetic injectable penicillin. Geopen is a benzylpenicillin derivative with substitution by an ionizable functional group in the alpha position.

Actions:

Microbiology

Though Geopen has substantial *in vitro* activity against a variety of both gram-positive and gram-negative microorganisms the most important aspect of its profile is in its antipseudomonal and antiproteus effect.

Organisms found to be susceptible to Geopen *in vitro* include the following:
Staphylococcus aureus
(Non-penicillinase producing)
Staphylococcus albus
Diplococcus pneumoniae
Beta-hemolytic Streptococci
Streptococcus faecalis
Hemophilus influenzae
Neisseria species
Enterobacter species
Proteus mirabilis
Proteus morgani
Proteus rettgeri
Proteus vulgaris
Escherichia coli
Salmonella species
Pseudomonas aeruginosa
Anaerobic bacteria, including:
Bacteroides species
Peptostreptococcus species
Peptococcus species
Clostridium species
Fusobacterium species

In vitro synergism between Geopen and gentamicin sulfate in certain strains of *Pseudomonas aeruginosa* has been demonstrated.

Geopen is not stable in the presence of penicillinase.

Most *Klebsiella* species are resistant to the action of Geopen.

Some of the newly emerging pathogenic strains of such microorganisms as *Herellea, Mima, Citrobacter* and *Serratia* have shown susceptibility to Geopen.

Some strains of *Pseudomonas* have developed resistance to Geopen fairly rapidly.

Pharmacology

Geopen is not absorbed orally, hence, it must be administered by the intramuscular or intravenous routes.

Following intramuscular injection, peak blood levels are obtained within 1–2 hours. The administration of probenecid results in somewhat higher and more prolonged serum levels as noted in the table above.

CARBENICILLIN BLOOD LEVELS AND URINARY EXCRETION

Dosage	ROUTE	SERUM LEVELS mcg/ml								Urinary excretion of administered dose
		¼ hr.	½ hr.	1 hr.	2 hr.	3 hr.	4 hr.	6 hr.	8 hr.	0–9 hours
500 mg.	IM	8	10	13	9.8	6.5	3.2	0	—	85%
1000 mg.	IM	—	13	18	15	12	7.5	1.7	0.7	74.6%*
2000 mg.	IM	26	38	47	37	25	15	5.9	1.2	79%
1000 mg.	IV	71	45	31	14	8.2	3	0	—	73%
1000 mg. +	IV									
1 Gm. probenecid	Oral	72	55	40	26	17	12	6.5	2.0	74%

*0–24 hr. collection

The **MIC** for many strains of *Pseudomonas* and *Bacteroides fragilis* is relatively high; serum levels of 100 mcg./ml. or greater are required. However, the low degree of toxicity of carbenicillin permits the use of doses large enough to achieve adequate levels for these strains.

Other susceptible organisms usually require serum levels in the range of 10-25 mcg/ml.

Geopen is not highly bound to serum proteins and is excreted unchanged in high concentrations in the urine. After a 0.5 to 2 grams I.M. dose, a urine concentration of 1,000 to 5,000 mcg/ml may be achieved.

Indications: Geopen is primarily indicated in the treatment of infections due to susceptible *Pseudomonas aeruginosa, Proteus* species (particularly indole positive strains) and certain strains of *Escherichia coli.*

By virtue of the very high urinary levels achieved, Geopen is particularly effective in urinary tract infections due to one or more of the above mentioned organisms.

Clinical studies have demonstrated the effectiveness of Geopen in the following infections when due to these organisms:

1. Severe systemic infections and septicemia including meningitis due to *Hemophilus influenzae* and *Streptococcus pneumoniae.* Although Geopen possesses *in vitro* activity against many ampicillin-resistant *H. influenzae,* clinical data are insufficient to recommend its use for treatment of meningitis due to ampicillin-resistant strains.
2. Genitourinary tract infections including those due to *Neisseria gonorrhoeae, Enterobacter* and *Streptococcus faecalis* (enterococcus).
3. Acute and chronic respiratory infections. Though clinical improvement has been shown, bacteriologic cures cannot be expected in patients with chronic respiratory disease and cystic fibrosis.
4. Soft tissue infections.

Geopen is also indicated in the treatment of the following infections due to susceptible anaerobic bacteria:

1. Septicemia.
2. Lower respiratory tract infections such as empyema, anaerobic pneumonitis and lung abscess.
3. Intra-abdominal infections such as peritonitis and intra-abdominal abscess. (Typically resulting from anaerobic organisms resident in the normal gastrointestinal tract.)
4. Infections of the female pelvis and genital tract such as endometritis, pelvic inflammatory disease, pelvic abscess and salpingitis.
5. Skin and soft tissue infections.

Although Geopen (carbenicillin disodium) is indicated primarily in gram-negative infections, its activity against gram-positive organisms should be kept in mind when both gram-positive and gram-negative organisms are isolated (see Actions).

In the treatment of infections due to certain susceptible strains of *Pseudomonas aeruginosa,* clinical efficacy may be enhanced by the use of combined therapy with Geopen (carbenicillin disodium) and gentamicin sulfate in full therapeutic dosages. For additional prescribing information, see the gentamicin sulfate package insert.

NOTE: During therapy, sensitivity testing should be repeated frequently to detect the possible emergence of resistant organisms which may develop, particularly if a suboptimal dose regimen is used.

Contraindications: Geopen is ordinarily contraindicated in patients who have a known penicillin allergy.

Warnings: Serious and occasional fatal hypersensitivity (anaphylactic) reactions have been reported in patients on penicillin therapy. These reactions are more apt to occur in individuals with a history of sensitivity to multiple allergens.

Patients with renal impairment should be observed for bleeding manifestations. Such patients should be dosed strictly according to recommendations (see Dosage and Administration section). If bleeding manifestations appear, the antibiotic should be discontinued and appropriate therapy be instituted.

There have been reports of individuals with a history of penicillin hypersensitivity reactions who have experienced severe hypersensitivity reactions when treated with a cephalosporin. Before therapy with a penicillin, careful inquiry should be made concerning previous hypersensitivity reactions to penicillins, cephalosporins, and other allergens. If an allergic reaction occurs, appropriate therapy should be instituted and discontinuance of carbenicillin therapy considered, unless, in the opinion of

Continued on next page

Roerig—Cont.

the physician the condition being treated is life threatening and amenable only to carbenicillin therapy. The usual agents (antihistamines, pressor amines and corticosteroids) should be readily available.

SERIOUS ANAPHYLACTOID REACTIONS REQUIRE IMMEDIATE EMERGENCY TREATMENT WITH EPINEPHRINE. OXYGEN AND INTRAVENOUS CORTICOSTEROIDS SHOULD ALSO BE ADMINISTERED AS INDICATED.

Usage in Pregnancy
Safety for use in pregnancy has not been established.

Precautions: While Geopen exhibits the characteristic low toxicity of the penicillin group of antibiotics, as with any other potent agent, it is advisable to check periodically for organ system dysfunction, including renal, hepatic and hematopoietic systems, during prolonged therapy.

Emergence of resistant organisms, such as *Klebsiella spp.*, and *Serratia spp.*, which may cause superinfection, should be kept in mind.

Geopen is a disodium salt of carboxybenzylpenicillin and hence each gram of Geopen contains 4.7 mEq. of sodium. In patients where sodium restriction is necessary, such as cardiac patients, periodic electrolyte determinations and monitoring of cardiac status should be made.

In a few patients receiving high doses of Geopen, hypokalemia has been reported. Periodic serum potassium determinations should be made and corrective measures should be implemented when necessary.

As with any penicillin preparation, an allergic response, including anaphylaxis, may occur particularly in a hypersensitive individual.

Cases of gonorrhea with a suspected primary lesion of syphilis should have dark field examinations before treatment. In all other cases where concomitant syphilis is suspected, monthly serological tests should be made for a minimum of 4 months.

Adverse Reactions: The following adverse reactions may occur:

Hypersensitivity reactions: Skin rashes, pruritus, urticaria, drug fever, and anaphylactic reactions.

Gastrointestinal disturbances: Nausea

Hemic and Lymphatic Systems: As with other penicillins, anemia, thrombocytopenia, leukopenia, neutropenia, and eosinophilia may occur.

Blood, Hepatic and Renal Studies: As with other semisynthetic penicillins, SGOT and SGPT elevations have been observed after Geopen administration (particularly in children). In all studies to date, no clinical manifestations of hepatic or renal disorders have been demonstrated.

CNS: As with other penicillins, convulsions or neuromuscular irritability could occur with excessively high serum levels.

Other: Pain at the site of injection after intramuscular and intravenous administration has been reported but is rarely accompanied by induration.

Several uremic patients receiving high doses (24 grams/day) have developed hemorrhagic manifestations associated with abnormalities of coagulation tests such as clotting time and prothrombin time. On withdrawal of the antibiotic, the bleeding ceased. The exact relationship of these findings to carbenicillin therapy is not clear.

Vein Irritation and Phlebitis have been reported occasionally, particularly when undiluted solution was directly injected into the vein.

Dosage and Administration:
[See table right].

NEONATES: In the neonate, for severe systemic infections (sepsis) due to susceptible

Dosage and Administration: Indication: Clinical experience indicates that in serious urinary tract and systemic infections intravenous therapy in the higher doses should be used. The recommended maximum dose is 40 g per day. Intramuscular injections should not exceed 2 g per injection.

ADULTS:	*Pseudomonas*	*Proteus and E. coli*	*Enterobacter and S. faecalis*	*Anaerobes*	*H. influenzae and S. pneumoniae*
Urinary Tract Infections Serious	200 mg/kg/day by I.V. drip	200 mg/kg/day by I.V. drip	200 mg/kg/day by I.V. drip		
Uncomplicated	1–2 g I.M. or I.V. every 6 hours	1–2 g I.M. or I.V. every 6 hours	1–2 g I.M. or I.V. every 6 hours		
Severe Systemic Infections Septicemia Respiratory Infections Soft Tissue Infections	400–500 mg/kg/day (30–40 grams) I.V. in divided doses or continuously	300–400 mg/kg/day (20–30 grams) I.V. in divided doses or continuously		400–500 mg/kg/day (30–40 grams) I.V. in divided doses or continuously	
Infections complicated by renal insufficiency (Creatinine clearance less than 5 ml/min)		2 g. I.V.(1) every 8–12 hours			

ADULTS:	*Pseudomonas*	*Proteus and E. coli*	*Enterobacter and S. faecalis*	*Anaerobes*	*H. influenzae and S. pneumoniae*
Meningitis					400-500 mg/kg day (30-40 grams) I.V. in divided doses or continuously
During peritoneal dialysis		2 g I.V. every 6 hours			
During hemodialysis		2 g I.V. every 4 hours			

(1) The serum half-life of Geopen in patients with severe renal failure is 12.5 hours. As a consequence 2 grams of Geopen administered intravenously to these patients every 8–12 hours will give Geopen serum levels of approximately 100 mcg/ml, a level notably free of any untoward effects while adequate for treatment of a majority of the infections amenable to Geopen therapy.

Treatment of gonorrhea(2); acute uncomplicated ano-genital and urethral infections due to *N. gonorrhoeae.*

SINGLE 4 g I.M. injection, divided between 2 sites.

(2) Probenecid in a dosage of 1 gram may be administered orally about 30 minutes prior to the I.M. treatment of acute gonorrhoeal infections. For complete information and dosage of probenecid, refer to manufacturer's product information.

CHILDREN:	*Pseudomonas*	*Proteus and E. coli*	*Enterobacter and S. faecalis*	*Anaerobes*	*H. influenzae and S. pneumoniae*
Urinary Tract Infections	50–200 mg/kg/day in divided doses every 4–6 hours I.M. or I.V.	50–100 mg/kg/day in divided doses every 4–6 hours I.M. or I.V.	50–200 mg/kg/day in divided doses every 4–6 hours I.M. or I.V.		
Severe Systemic Infections Septicemia Respiratory Infections Soft Tissue Infections	400–500 mg/kg/day I.V. in divided doses or by continuous drip	300–400 mg/kg/day I.M. or I.V. in divided doses		400–500 mg/kg/day I.V. in divided doses or by continuous drip	
Infections complicated by renal insufficiency (Creatinine clearance less than 5 ml/min)		Clinical data is insufficient to recommend an optimum dose			
Meningitis					400-500 mg/kg day in divided doses or by continuous drip

strains of *Pseudomonas, Proteus,* and *E. coli, H. influenzae* and *S. pneumoniae*, the following Geopen (carbenicillin disodium) dosages may be given I.M. or by fifteen (15) minute I.V. infusion:

Infants under 2000 g body weight.
Initial dose: 100 mg/kg.
Subsequent doses during first week: 75 mg/kg./8 hrs (225 mg/kg./day)
After 7 days of age: 100 mg/kg./6 hrs (400 mg/kg./day)

Infants over 2000 g body weight.
Initial dose: 100 mg/kg.
Subsequent doses during first 3 days: 75 mg/kg./6 hrs (300 mg/kg./day)
After 3 days of age: 100 mg/kg./6 hrs (400 mg/kg./day)

NOTE: This dosage schedule should give maximum serum levels of approximately 150-175 mcg/ml and minimum levels of approximately 50-75 mcg/ml of Geopen.

Gentamicin may be used concurrently with carbenicillin for initial therapy until results of culture and susceptibility studies are known. Seriously ill patients should receive the higher doses. GEOPEN has proved to be useful in infections in which protective mechanisms are impaired, such as in acute leukemia and during therapy with immunosuppressive or oncolytic drugs.

Intramuscular Use

As with all intramuscular preparations, Geopen (carbenicillin disodium) should be injected well within the body of a relatively large muscle.

Adults: The preferred site is the upper outer quadrant of the buttock (i.e., gluteus maximus), or the mid-lateral thigh.

Children: It is recommended that intramuscular injections be given preferably in the midlateral muscles of the thigh. In infants and small children the periphery of the upper outer quadrant of the gluteal region should be used only when necessary, such as in burn patients, in order to minimize the possibility of damage to the sciatic nerve.

The deltoid area should be used only if well developed such as in certain adults and older children, and then only with caution to avoid radial nerve injury. Intramuscular injections should not be made into the lower and mid-third of the upper arm. As with all intramuscular injections, aspiration is necessary to help avoid inadvertent injection into a blood vessel.

Intravenous Use

As with all intravenous administrations, particular attention should be directed to insure that the drug is injected only into a vein (including aspiration and proper anatomical site selection) to avoid either intra-arterial injection or extravasation.

Preparation of Solution:

For Intramuscular Use—The 1 g vial should be reconstituted with 2.0 ml. of Sterile Water for Injection. In order to facilitate reconstitution, up to 3.6 ml. of Sterile Water for Injection can be used.

Amount of Diluent to be added to the 1 g Vial	Volume to be Withdrawn for a 1 g Dose
2.0 ml	2.5 ml
2.5 ml	3.0 ml
3.6 ml	4.0 ml

The 2 g vial should be reconstituted with 4.0 ml. of Sterile Water for Injection. In order to facilitate reconstitution, up to 7.2 ml. of Sterile Water for Injection can be used.

Amount of Diluent to be added to the 2 g Vial	Volume to be Withdrawn for a 1 g Dose
4.0 ml	2.5 ml
5.0 ml	3.0 ml
7.2 ml	4.0 ml

The 5 g vial should be reconstituted with 7 ml. of Sterile Water for Injection. In order to facilitate reconstitution, up to 17 ml. of Sterile Water for Injection can be used.

Amount of Diluent to be added to the 5 g Vial	Volume to be Withdrawn for a 1 g Dose
7.0 ml	2.0 ml
9.5 ml	2.5 ml
12.0 ml	3.0 ml
17.0 ml	4.0 ml

After reconstitution, no significant loss of potency occurs for 24 hours at room temperature, and for 72 hours if refrigerated. Any of these unused solutions should be discarded.

For Direct Intravenous Injection—Following reconstitution, each gram should be further diluted by no less than 5 ml of Sterile Water for Injection. In order to avoid vein irritation, the solution should be administered as slowly as possible.

For Intravenous Infusion—Following reconstitution according to directions, Geopen (carbenicillin disodium) may be added to the desired volume of usual intravenous infusion solutions.

WHEN USING THE 2 g, 5 g, AND 10 g PIGGYBACK UNITS OR BULK PHARMACY PACK FOR. . .

Intravenous Use

As with all intravenous administrations, particular attention should be directed to insure that the drug is injected only into a vein (including aspiration and proper anatomical site selection) to avoid either intra-arterial injection or extravasation.

For Direct Intravenous Injection

The 2 gram vial should be reconstituted with a minimum of 20 ml. Sterile Water for Injection.

Amount of Diluent	Concentration of Solution
100 ml	1 g/50 ml
50 ml	1 g/25 ml
20 ml	1 g/10 ml

The 5 gram vial should be reconstituted with a minimum of 50 ml. of Sterile Water for Injection.

Amount of Diluent	Concentration of Solution
100 ml	1 g/20 ml
50 ml	1 g/10 ml

The 10 gram vial should be reconstituted with a minimum of 95 ml of Sterile Water for Injection.

Amount of Diluent	Concentration of Solution
95 ml	1 g/10 ml

In order to avoid vein irritation, the solution should be administered as slowly as possible. A dilution of 1 g/20 ml or more will further reduce the incidence of vein irritation.

After reconstitution, no significant loss of potency occurs for 24 hours at room temperature and for 72 hours if refrigerated. Any of these unused solutions should be discarded.

Bulk Pharmacy Package

The 30 gram vial should be reconstituted by adding 80 ml of water in two separate 40 ml aliquots. Add 40 ml, shake 25 seconds and add the last 40 ml aliquot and shake for final solution. The resulting solution will contain 300 mg/ml of carbenicillin. Transfer recommended dosage to appropriate intravenous infusion solution.

Reconstituted bulk solution should not be used for direct infusion.

After reconstitution, no significant loss of potency occurs for 24 hours at room temperature and for 72 hours if refrigerated. Any of these unused solutions should be discarded.

For Continuous Intravenous Infusion

After reconstitution as directed, Geopen (carbenicillin disodium) may be added to the desired volume of usual intravenous infusion solutions.

Studies of Geopen at concentrations of 10 mg/ml and 100 mg/ml in the following intravenous infusion diluents indicate no significant loss of potency when stored at room temperature and under refrigeration (5°C) for the time periods stated:

(See table above)

Intravenous Solution	*Stability* Room Temperature	*Stability* Refrigerated
Sterile water for injection	72 hours	14 days
Sodium chloride injection, USP	72 hours	14 days
Dextrose injection, USP (5%)	72 hours	14 days
Ringer's injection, USP	72 hours	14 days
Dextrose 5% with 0.255% sodium chloride	24 hours	3 days
Lactated Ringer's injection, USP	24 hours	3 days
5% dextrose with electrolyte #48	24 hours	3 days
5% Levugen (fructose) with electrolyte #75	24 hours	3 days
Invert sugar 10% in water	24 hours	3 days
Dextrose 5% and 0.45% sodium chloride, USP	24 hours	3 days
5% alcohol, 5% dextrose in water	24 hours	3 days
5% alcohol, 5% dextrose in 0.9% sodium chloride	24 hours	3 days
5% dextrose in alcohol	24 hours	3 days
Maintenance electrolyte solution (electrolyte #75)	24 hours	3 days
Pediatric maintenance electrolyte solution (electrolyte #48)	24 hours	3 days

Discard any unused solutions after the time periods outlined above.

It is recommended that Geopen and gentamicin sulfate not be mixed together in the same IV solution due to the gradual inactivation of gentamicin sulfate under these circumstances. The therapeutic effect of the two drugs remains unimpaired when administered separately.

For Intramuscular Use Only:

Geopen for intramuscular injection ONLY may be diluted with one of the following:

1. 0.5% Lidocaine Hydrochloride (without epinephrine).
2. Bacteriostatic Water containing 0.9% Benzyl Alcohol.

For reconstitution of Geopen with these diluents for intramuscular use ONLY, follow the directions for the amount of diluent in the **PREPARATION OF SOLUTION, For Intramuscular Use section.**

Geopen may be diluted with these solutions and stored for 24 hours at room temperature or for 72 hours when refrigerated. Discard unused solutions stored longer than these time periods.

For full product information, refer to the package insert for Lidocaine Hydrochloride (without epinephrine).

How Supplied: Geopen is available in 1 g, 2 g, and 5 g vials for intramuscular/intravenous use.

Geopen is available in 2 g, 5 g, 10 g Piggyback Units, and 30 g Bulk Pharmacy Pack for intravenous use.

HEPTUNA® PLUS CAPSULES ℞

(Hard Gelatin)

Fortified Oral Hematopoietic Formulation

Each capsule contains:

HEMATOPOIETIC FACTORS

Ferrous Sulfate, dried, U.S.P. (provides 100 mg of elemental iron) ...311 mg

Continued on next page

Roerig—Cont.

Desiccated Liver (undefatted) ....50 mg
Vitamin B_{12}, cobalamin concentrate NF (as Stablets®) ....5 mcg
With intrinsic factor concentrate (non-inhibitory) ....25 mg

VITAMINS

B_1 (thiamine mononitrate, U.S.P.) ....3.1 mg
B_2 (riboflavin, U.S.P.) ....2 mg
B_6 (pyridoxine hydrochloride, U.S.P.) ..1.6 mg
Vitamin C (from sodium ascorbate) ....150 mg
Niacin (niacinamide, U.S.P.) ....15 mg
Pantothenic Acid (calcium pantothenate, U.S.P.) ....0.9 mg

MINERALS

Copper (from copper sulfate) ....1 mg
Molybdenum (from sodium molybdate) ....0.2 mg
Calcium (from dibasic calcium phosphate) ....37.4 mg
Iodine (from potassium iodide) ....0.05 mg
Manganese (from manganese sulfate) ....0.033 mg
Magnesium (from magnesium sulfate) ...2 mg
Phosphorus (from dibasic calcium phosphate) ....29 mg
Potassium (from potassium sulfate) .....1.7 mg
Stablets® U.S. Pat. No. 2.830.933

Indications: Heptuna Plus is a multicomponent preparation effective in the treatment of those anemias amenable to oral hematinic therapy. These include pernicious anemia and other megaloblastic anemias, and also iron deficiency anemia. Heptuna Plus also contains balanced amounts of vitamin B complex, vitamin C, and minerals as nutritional supplements.

Clinical Pharmacology:

Hematopoietic Factors

Vitamin B_{12}: Exogenous sources of B_{12} are required for normal growth and maintenance of normal erythropoiesis as well as nucleo-protein synthesis, myelin synthesis, and cell reproduction. Vitamin B_{12} is irregularly absorbed from the intact gastrointestinal tract. Free vitamin B_{12} is bound to intrinsic factor which is normally secreted by the gastric mucosal tissue, and acts as a carrier protein for active transport through the gastrointestinal tract. This normal active transport system is usually saturated by 1.5 to 3 mg of vitamin B_{12}. Under conditions of functional or anatomical derangements of the stomach or ileum, where secretion of intrinsic factor is abnormally low, absorption of vitamin B_{12} will proceed poorly, if at all. Megaloblastic anemias may develop after gastrectomy, in Addinsonian permicious anemia, and in fish tapeworm (*Diphyllobothrium latum*) infection; treatment to free the host of competing bacteria and parasites is required. Other causes of B_{12}deficiency are strict vegetarianism, surgical compromise of gastric or ileum activity, gastric atrophy due to multiple sclerosis or iron deficiency or malabsorption syndromes of various etiologies; in this last case parenteral therapy or oral therapy with massive doses of vitamin B_{12} may be necessary for successful treatment. The megaloblastic anemias of malabsorption syndromes may be due to a deficiency of folate—which is not contained in Heptuna Plus, as well as to B_{12} deficiency, and combined therapy may be warranted.

Desiccated Liver: Desiccated Liver is an extract of mammalian livers used in Heptuna Plus as a source of naturally occurring riboflavin, nicotinic acid, and choline as a nutritional supplement. Desiccated liver (undefatted) 50 mg. provides approximately 2.5 mcg riboflavin, 12.5 mcg nicotinic acid, and 0.5 mg choline.

Ferrous Sulfate: As compared to other sources of iron, ferrous sufate provides the highest amounts of elemental iron for utilization in patients with hypochronic anemias. Iron is a constituent of hemoglobin and its administration usually corrects erythropoietic abnormalities, and may reverse esophageal and gastrointestinal tissue changes associated with iron deficiency.

Approximately 25% of an orally administered dose of ferrous sulfate will be utilizable iron. The primary sites of iron absorption are the duodenum, the jejunum, the stomach, and the proximal portion of the ileum. The ferrous species of iron is the most readily absorbed fraction. While the exact mechanism of absorption is not known, the absorption, metabolism, and excretion of iron appear to be related to body requirements for this mineral. The excretion of iron as ferritin is by way of epithelial cells sloughed from the skin and gastrointestinal tract. There may be trace losses in bile, and cell-free sweat.

Vitamins

Vitamin C: It is known that an acidic environment favors the maintenance of iron in the ferrous state, retards formation of insoluble complexes of iron with food or other substrates, and will thus promote gastric absorption of ferrous iron. The vitamin C content of Heptuna Plus, in addition to contributing to the overall acidic environment of gastric fluids, may also be useful as a supplement to deficiency states. Prolonged and severe vitamin C deficiency is associated with an anemia which is usually hypochronic but occasionally megaloblastic. Vitamin C is also utilized in intracellular reactions such as conversion of folic acid and carbohydrate synthesis.

Vitamin B Complex (B_1, B_2, B_6, Niacin, Pantothenic Acid): These are provided in Heptuna Plus as nutritional supplements. Vitamin B complex is essential for the metabolism of carbohydrates and protein. Administration of these water-soluble vitamins may be useful in deficiency states associated with febrile diseases, severe burns, gastrointestinal disorders interfering with absorption of these vitamins, in prolonged or wasting diseases, or in nutritional deficiency.

One capsule of Heptuna Plus provides the following approximate percentage of the U.S. Recommended Adult Daily Allowances (U.S. RDA):

	% U.S. RDA
B_1	221.4
B_2	125
B_6	80
Vitamin C	333.3
Niacin	83.3
Pantothenic Acid	9

Minerals

One capsule of Heptuna Plus provides the following approximate percentages of U.S. Recommended Adult Daily Allowances (U.S. RDA):

	% U.S. RDA
Copper	50
Molybdenum	*
Calcium	4.25
Iodine	38.46
Manganese	*
Magnesium	0.57
Phosphorous	3.63
Potassium	*

*U.S. RDA not yet established.

The precise role of minerals in human nutritional maintenance has yet to be defined. However, several trace elements (including copper, molybdenum, calcium, iodine, manganese) have been identified as being essential for animal life.

Copper: Copper has been identified as a component of several amine oxidases. Copper depletion in experimental animals results in failure to utilize ferritin iron and is accompanied by increases in hepatic iron concentration sometimes with clear evidence of hemosiderosis. Copper-dependent enzyme systems may be intimately involved in tissue iron mobilization.

Molybdenum: Molybdenum has been identified as a component of xanthine oxidase (involved in purine oxidation and possibly in the release of iron from ferritin), aldehydeoxidase, and sulfite oxidase.

Calcium: In addition to this element's well known important roles in maintenance of bone, neurologic, and muscular tissue integrity, calcium may also play a role in maintaining the integrity of cell membrance structures.

Iodine: As the central element of thyroid activity, iodine intake may influence carbohydrate and cholesterol metabolism, functions of the central nervous system, catecholamine secretion, and skeletal growth and maturation. Its exact role in the hematopoietic process, if any, has not been determined.

Manganese: The main manifestations of manganese deficiency in laboratory animals are impaired growth, disturbed or depressed reproductive function, skeletal abnormalities, and nervous disorders. Its exact role in the hematopoietic process, if any, has not been determined.

Magnesium: Magnesium plays a fundamental role in most reactions that include phosphate transfer, and it is believed to be essential for the structural stabilization of nucleic acids. Magnesium depletion has been known to impair homeostasis of potassium and calcium. Deficiency of magnesium almost always occurs as a consequence of some underlying disease, including malabsorption syndromes.

Phosphorus: Hypophosphatemia may cause a marked decrease in erythrocytic concentrations of ATP and of 2,3 diphosphoglycerate. Acute hemolytic-type anemia may develop in severe deficiency states.

Potassium: Potassium is an essential mineral in electrolyte maintenance and in maintaining electrical excitability of cells and acid-base homeostasis. Its exact role in the hematopoietic process, if any, has not been determined.

Contraindications: Hemachromatosis and hemosiderosis are contraindications to iron therapy. Previous hypersensitivity to any of the components of Heptuna Plus contraindicates its use.

Precautions: Anemia is a manifestation of an underlying disease process. While Heptuna Plus provides components useful in the management of certain anemias, appropriate attention should be directed to an etiological diagnosis and treatment of the underlying causes of the anemia.

Resistance to the effects of exogenous intrinsic factor has been reported. Local intestinal antibodies which render exogenous intrinsic factor inactive have been noted to develop in approximately 50% of patients treated within one year of continuous oral therapy. If resistance develops, parenteral therapy or oral therapy with large doses of vitamin B_{12} may be necessary to circumvent normal active transport mechanisms and adequately treat the patient.

Although this product contains vitamin B_{12} (as Stablets®) with intrinsic factor concentrate (non-inhibitory) and desiccated liver, it is not as reliable as parenterally administered cyanocobalamin (vitamin B_{12}) in the management of pernicious anemia. Some patients with pernicious anemia may not respond to orally ingested cobalamin concentrate (vitamin B_{12}). There is no known way to predict which patients will respond or which patients may cease to respond.

Information for Patients: As Heptuna Plus contains substantial amounts of iron, patients should be advised that gastrointestinal reactions such as diarrhea or constipation may occur with usage. Patients should be cautioned against concomitant usage of Heptuna Plus and tetracycline, or its analogs, so as to avoid a chelation interaction which would reduce the amounts of antibiotic and iron or divalent ions available for gastrointestinal absorption.

Laboratory Tests: Periodic clinical and laboratory monitoring are considered essential to proper use of hematopoietics. The following laboratory tests may be useful in evaluating patients' response to therapy: peripheral blood smears, reticulocyte count, serum iron, iron binding capacity, serum B_{12}, serum folic acid, hemoglobin and hematocrit, mean corpuscular volume.

Drug Interactions: The following drug/drug interactions may occur with the use of Heptuna Plus.

Agent	Interaction
Tetracycline and derivatives	Complexation of antibiotic and iron or divalent ions (such as calcium) decrease availability of component for gastric absorption. This may be avoided by administration of Heptuna Plus at least one hour before tetracycline-type agent.
Levodopa	Doses of pyridoxine of approximately 5 mg (three capsules Heptuna Plus provide 4.8 mg B_6) or more per day may reduce the beneficial effects of levodopa in parkinsonian disease. This is thought to be due to increased transamination of levodopa. Patients receiving this combination should be carefully observed for unwanted variations in parkinson control.
Lithium	The presence of iodine in Heptuna Plus may enhance the hypothyroid and goiterogenic potential of these two components. Patients receiving lithium and Heptuna Plus should have baseline and periodic thyroid status checks.

Laboratory Interactions: Heptuna Plus contains iodine 0.05 mg (as potassium iodide) as an active component and the iodinated dye tetraiodofluorescein (FD and C#3) in the capsule shell. These agents may interfere with I^{131} or other diagnostic radioiodine neucleotide testing procedures. Other than changes induced from the therapeutic effects of the components of Heptuna Plus, no other interferences with laboratory testing procedures have been identified.

Carcinogenesis, Mutagenesis, Impairment of Fertility: The potential for Heptuna Plus to impair fertility or act as a carcinogen or a mutagen has not been studied *in vivo* or *in vitro*.

Use in Pregnancy

Category C: Animal reproductive studies have not been conducted with Heptuna Plus. It is also not known whether Heptuna Plus can cause fetal harm when administered to a pregnant woman or can affect reproductive capacity. Heptuna Plus should be given to a pregnant woman only if clearly needed.

Nursing Mothers: It is not known whether this drug is excreted in human milk. Because many drugs are excreted in human milk, caution should be exercised when Heptuna Plus is administered to a nursing woman.

Pediatric Use: Safety and effectiveness in children have not been established.

Adverse Reactions:

Ferrous Sulfate: The most frequent adverse reactions to Heptuna Plus are those associated with oral iron therapy. An incidence of gastrointestinal discomfort in 19.5% to 27% of patients receiving "iron placebo" tablets has been reported. The gastrointestinal complaints usually noted are diarrhea, constipation, nausea, epigastric pain, ructus, vomiting, and black staining of stools. Reduction in dosage or administration with meals may minimize these effects.

In extremely rare instances, skin rash suggesting allergy has been noted following the oral administration of desiccated liver preparations.

Iodine: Allergic reactions, including angioedema, rashes, lymphadenopathy, eosinophilia, arteritis, and febrile reactions have been reported with iodine usage. Also, acne, swelling of salivary glands, iodine coryza, and stomach upsets have been reported. Iodine use may precipitate hypo- or hyperthyroid activity and goiter.

B Complex Vitamins: Adverse reactions to these water-soluble vitamins are rare:

—Thiamine; Hypersensitivity reactions are rare and have been reported mostly with parenteral administration.

—Pyridoxine; Allergic reactions have been reported, but are rare.

—Cyanocobalamine/Cobalamine; Mild forms of polycythemia, and peripheral vascular thrombosis during recovery from pernicious anemia treated with B_{12} have been observed. Use of high dose oral vitamin B_{12} has been associated with the appearance of acne.

Minerals: No adverse reactions other than those specified for iodine have been reported with orally administered minerals as supplied in Heptuna Plus.

Overdosage:

Acute Toxicity: Toxicity may result from overdosage due to ingestion of ferrous sulfate. In young children 300 mg of elemental iron may be fatal. The remainder of the ingredients are essentially nontoxic (water-soluble vitamins) or present in such small amounts as to be nontoxic even with overdosage.

Symptoms: Symptoms may occur 30 to 60 minutes after ingestion. Danger may exist for 24-48 hours. Acute gastroenteritis, vomiting, diarrhea, dehydration, collapse, and coma ending in death may occur. A severe acidosis may also be present. The diarrhea may initially be watery, becoming bloody and then tarry.

Dialyzability: It is known that iron, magnesium, potassium, iodide, and phosphate are dialyzable. Dialysis may not be effective in removing vitamin B_{12} or copper. The effect of dialysis on the other components in Heptuna Plus is not certain.

Management: Management should be directed primarily at the treatment of iron toxicity. Acute toxicity may occur in young children after ingestion of 1 gram of ferrous sulfate (equivalent to 3 capsules of Heptuna Plus). In adults iron toxicity is rare and is most likely to occur only after ingestion of more than 50 grams of ferrous sulfate (equivalent to 150 capsules of Heptuna Plus). Treatment involves gastric lavage and/or use of absorbents. A 1% sodium bicarbonate lavage fluid may be useful to prevent further iron absorption. Lavage must be performed with caution after the first hour of an overdosage because of the potential for gastric necrosis and perforation. Shock and acid-base imbalances should be treated with standard methods. Serum iron levels should be monitored and deferoxamine mesylate therapy initiated if necessary. Other chelating agents should be used only if deferoxamine mesylate is not available or otherwise contraindicated, as it may form toxic complexes with iron.

Dosage and Administration: For many patients one capsule of Heptuna Plus daily will provide sufficient amounts of hematopoietic factors for therapeutic results. If the severity and etiology of the anemia so indicate, 1 capsule three times a day (approximately every six hours) may be prescribed. Therapy with Heptuna Plus may be continued until patient response indicates discontinuation of therapy.

How Supplied: Heptuna Plus capsules are available as red and white gelatin capsules, in bottles of 100.

[*Shown in Product Identification Section*]

MARAX® ℞

(ephedrine sulfate, theophylline, hydroxyzine HCl)

TABLETS AND DF SYRUP

Contents:

	Each Tablet Contains:	Each Teaspoon (5 ml.) Syrup Contains:
Ephedrine Sulfate	25 mg.	6.25 mg.
Theophylline	130 mg.	32.50 mg.
Atarax® (hydroxyzine HCl)	10 mg.	2.5 mg.
Alcohol (Ethyl Alcohol)		5% v/v.

Actions: The action of ephedrine as a vasoconstrictor is well known. It is therefore of significant benefit in symptomatic relief of the congestion occurring in bronchial asthma. As a bronchodilator, it has a slower onset but longer duration of action than does epinephrine, which, in contrast to ephedrine, is not effective upon oral administration.

The diverse actions of theophylline—bronchospasmolytic, cardiovascular, and diuretic—are well established, and make it a particularly useful drug in the treatment of bronchial asthma, both in the acute attack and in the prophylactic therapy of the disease.

Atarax (hydroxyzine HCl) modifies the central stimulatory action of ephedrine preventing excessive excitation in patients on Marax therapy.

In animal studies Atarax (hydroxyzine HCl) has demonstrated antiserotonin activity and antispasmodic potency of a nonspecific nature.

Marax-DF Syrup produces an expectorant action wherein the tenacity of the sputum is decreased and the ease of expectoration is increased.

Indications

Based on a review of this drug by the National Academy of Sciences-National Research Council and/or other information, FDA has classified the indications as follows:

"Possibly" Effective: For controlling bronchospastic disorders.

Final classification of the less than effective indication requires further investigation.

Contraindications: Because of the ephedrine, Marax is contraindicated in cardiovascular disease, hyperthyroidism, and hypertension. This drug is contraindicated in individuals who have shown hypersensitivity to the drug or its components.

Hydroxyzine, when administered to the pregnant mouse, rat, and rabbit induced fetal abnormalities in the rat at doses substantially above the human therapeutic range. Clinical data in human beings are inadequate to establish safety in early pregnancy. Until such data are available, hydroxyzine is contraindicated in early pregnancy.

Precautions: Because of the ephedrine component this drug should be used with caution in elderly males or those with known prostatic hypertrophy.

The potentiating action of hydroxyzine, although mild, must be taken into consideration when the drug is used in conjunction with central nervous system depressants; and when other central nervous system depressants are administered concomitantly with hydroxyzine their dosage should be reduced. Patients should be cautioned that hydroxyzine can increase the effect of alcohol.

Patients should be warned—because of the hydroxyzine component—of the possibility of drowsiness occurring and cautioned against

Continued on next page

Roerig—Cont.

driving a car or operating dangerous machinery while taking this drug.

Adverse Reactions: With large doses of ephedrine, excitation, tremulousness, insomnia, nervousness, palpitation, tachycardia, precordial pain, cardiac arrhythmias, vertigo, dryness of the nose and throat, headache, sweating, and warmth may occur. Because ephedrine is a sympathomimetic agent some patients may develop vesical sphincter spasm and resultant urinary hesitation, and occasionally acute urinary retention. This should be borne in mind when administering preparations containing ephedrine to elderly males or those with known prostatic hypertrophy. At the recommended dose for Marax, a side effect occasionally reported is palpitation, and this can be controlled with dosage adjustment, additional amounts of concurrently administered Atarax (hydroxyzine HCl), or discontinuation of the medication. When ephedrine is given three or more times daily patients may develop tolerance after several weeks of therapy.

Theophylline when given on an empty stomach frequently causes gastric irritation accompanied by upper abdominal discomfort, nausea, and vomiting. Administration of the medication after meals will serve to minimize this side effect. Theophylline may cause diuresis and cardiac stimulation. The amount of Atarax (hydroxyzine HCl) present in Marax has not resulted in disturbing side effects. When used alone specifically as a tranquilizer in the normal dosage range (25 to 50 mg. three or four times a day), side effects are infrequent; even at these higher doses, no serious side effects have been reported and confirmed to date. Those which do occasionally occur when Atarax (hydroxyzine HCl) is used alone are drowsiness, xerostomia and, at extremely high doses, involuntary motor activity, unsteadiness of gait, neuromuscular weakness, all of which may be controlled by reduction of the dosage or discontinuation of the medication.

With the relatively low dose of Atarax (hydroxyzine HCl) in Marax, these effects are not likely to occur. In addition, the ataractic action of Atarax (hydroxyzine HCl) may modify the cardiac stimulatory action of ephedrine, and concurrently, increasing the amount of Atarax (hydroxyzine HCl) may control or abolish this undesirable effect of ephedrine.

Dosage and Administration: The dosage of Marax should be adjusted according to the severity of complaints, and the patient's individual toleration.

Tablets: In general, an adult dose of 1 tablet, 2 to 4 times daily, should be sufficient. Some patients are controlled adequately with ½ to 1 tablet at bedtime. The time interval between doses should not be shorter than four hours. The dosage for children over 5 years of age and for adults who are sensitive to ephedrine, is one-half the usual adult dose. Clinical experience to date has been confined to ages above 5 years.

Syrup: The dose for children over 5 years of age is 1 teaspoon (5 ml.), 3 to 4 times daily. Dosage for children 2 to 5 years of age is ½ to 1 teaspoon (2.5-5 ml.), 3 to 4 times daily. Not recommended for children under 2 years of age.

How Supplied: Marax Tablets are available as scored, dye free, m-shaped tablets in bottles of 100 and 500.

Marax-DF Syrup is available in pints and gallons as a colorless syrup free of all coal tar dyes, and should be dispensed in tight, light-resistant containers (USP).

[*Shown in Product Identification Section*]

NAVANE® ℞
(thiothixene) CAPSULES
NAVANE®
(thiothixene hydrochloride) CONCENTRATE

Description: Navane (thiothixene) is a thioxanthene derivative. Specifically, it is the *cis* isomer of N,N-dimethyl-9-[3-(4-methyl-1-piperazinyl)-propylidene] thioxanthene-2-sulfonamide.

The thioxanthenes differ from the phenothiazines by the replacement of nitrogen in the central ring with a carbon-linked side chain fixed in space in a rigid structural configuration. An N,N-dimethyl sulfonamide functional group is bonded to the thioxanthene nucleus.

Actions: Navane is a psychotropic agent of the thioxanthene series. Navane possesses certain chemical and pharmacological similarities to the piperazine phenothiazines and differences from the aliphatic group of phenothiazines.

Indications: Navane is effective in the management of manifestations of psychotic disorders. Navane has not been evaluated in the management of behavioral complications in patients with mental retardation.

Contraindications: Navane is contraindicated in patients with circulatory collapse, comatose states, central nervous system depression due to any cause, and blood dyscrasias. Navane is contraindicated in individuals who have shown hypersensitivity to the drug. It is not known whether there is a cross sensitivity between the thioxanthenes and the phenothiazine derivatives, but this possibility should be considered.

Warnings:

Usage in Pregnancy—Safe use of Navane during pregnancy has not been established. Therefore, this drug should be given to pregnant patients only when, in the judgment of the physician, the expected benefits from the treatment exceed the possible risks to mother and fetus. Animal reproduction studies and clinical experience to date have not demonstrated any teratogenic effects.

In the animal reproduction studies with Navane, there was some decrease in conception rate and litter size, and an increase in resorption rate in rats and rabbits. Similar findings have been reported with other psychotropic agents. After repeated oral administration of Navane to rats (5 to 15 mg/kg/day), rabbits (3 to 50 mg/kg/day), and monkeys (1 to 3 mg/kg/day) before and during gestation, no teratogenic effects were seen.

Usage in Children—The use of Navane in children under 12 years of age is not recommended because safe conditions for its use have not been established.

As is true with many CNS drugs, Navane may impair the mental and/or physical abilities required for the performance of potentially hazardous tasks such as driving a car or operating machinery, especially during the first few days of therapy. Therefore, the patient should be cautioned accordingly.

As in the case of other CNS-acting drugs, patients receiving Navane (thiothixene) should be cautioned about the possible additive effects (which may include hypotension) with CNS depressants and with alcohol.

Precautions: An antiemetic effect was observed in animal studies with Navane; since this effect may also occur in man, it is possible that Navane may mask signs of overdosage of toxic drugs and may obscure conditions such as intestinal obstruction and brain tumor.

In consideration of the known capability of Navane and certain other psychotropic drugs to precipitate convulsions, extreme caution should be used in patients with a history of convulsive disorders or those in a state of alcohol withdrawal, since it may lower the convulsive threshold. Although Navane potentiates the actions of the barbiturates, the dosage of the anticonvulsant therapy should not be reduced when Navane is administered concurrently.

Though exhibiting rather weak anticholinergic properties, Navane should be used with caution in patients who might be exposed to extreme heat or who are receiving atropine or related drugs.

Use with caution in patients with cardiovascular disease.

Caution as well as careful adjustment of the dosages is indicated when Navane is used in conjunction with other CNS depressants.

Also, careful observation should be made for pigmentary retinopathy, and lenticular pigmentation (fine lenticular pigmentation has been noted in a small number of patients treated with Navane for prolonged periods). Blood dyscrasias (agranulocytosis, pancytopenia, thrombocytopenic purpura), and liver damage (jaundice, biliary stasis), have been reported with related drugs.

Neuroleptic drugs elevate prolactin levels; the elevation persists during chronic administration. Tissue culture experiments indicate that approximately one-third of human breast cancers are prolactin dependent *in vitro*, a factor of potential importance if the prescription of these drugs is contemplated in a patient with a previously detected breast cancer. Although disturbances such as galactorrhea, amenorrhea, gynecomastia, and impotence have been reported, the clinical significance of elevated serum prolactin levels is unknown for most patients. An increase in mammary neoplasms has been found in rodents after chronic administration of neuroleptic drugs. Neither clinical studies nor epidemiologic studies conducted to date, however, have shown an association between chronic administration of these drugs and mammary tumorigenesis; the available evidence is considered too limited to be conclusive at this time.

Adverse Reactions:

NOTE: Not all of the following adverse reactions have been reported with Navane. However, since Navane has certain chemical and pharmacologic similarities to the phenothiazines, all of the known side effects and toxicity associated with phenothiazine therapy should be borne in mind when Navane is used.

Cardiovascular effects: Tachycardia, hypotension, lightheadedness, and syncope. In the event hypotension occurs, epinephrine should not be used as a pressor agent since a paradoxical further lowering of blood pressure may result. Nonspecific EKG changes have been observed in some patients receiving Navane. These changes are usually reversible and frequently disappear on continued Navane therapy. The incidence of these changes is lower than that observed with some phenothiazines. The clinical significance of these changes is not known.

CNS effects: Drowsiness, usually mild, may occur although it usually subsides with continuation of Navane therapy. The incidence of sedation appears similar to that of the piperazine group of phenothiazines but less than that of certain aliphatic phenothiazines. Restlessness, agitation and insomnia have been noted with Navane. Seizures and paradoxical exacerbation of psychotic symptoms have occurred with Navane infrequently.

Hyperreflexia has been reported in infants delivered from mothers having received structurally related drugs.

In addition, phenothiazine derivatives have been associated with cerebral edema and cerebrospinal fluid abnormalities.

Extrapyramidal symptoms, such as pseudoparkinsonism, akathisia and dystonia have been reported. Management of these extrapyramidal symptoms depends upon the type and severity. Rapid relief of acute symptoms may require the use of an injectable antiparkinson agent. More slowly emerging symptoms may be managed by reducing the dosage of Navane and/or administering an oral antiparkinson agent.

Persistent Tardive Dyskinesia: As with all antipsychotic agents tardive dyskinesia may appear in some patients on long term therapy or may occur after drug therapy has been discontinued. The risk seems to be greater in elderly patients on high-dose therapy, especially females. The symptoms are persistent and in some patients appear to be irreversible. The syndrome is characterized by rhythmical involuntary movements of the tongue, face, mouth or jaw (e.g., protrusion of tongue, puffing of cheeks, puckering of mouth, chewing movements). Sometimes these may be accompanied by involuntary movements of extremities.

There is no known effective treatment for tardive dyskinesia; antiparkinsonism agents usually do not alleviate the symptoms of this syndrome. It is suggested that all antipsychotic agents be discontinued if these symptoms appear.

Should it be necessary to reinstitute treatment, or increase the dosage of the agent, or switch to a different antipsychotic agent, the syndrome may be masked.

It has been reported that fine vermicular movements of the tongue may be an early sign of the syndrome and if the medication is stopped at that time, the syndrome may not develop.

Hepatic effects: Elevations of serum transaminase and alkaline phosphatase, usually transient, have been infrequently observed in some patients. No clinically confirmed cases of jaundice attributable to Navane have been reported.

Hematologic effects: As is true with certain other psychotropic drugs, leukopenia and leucocytosis, which are usually transient, can occur occasionally with Navane. Other antipsychotic drugs have been associated with agranulocytosis, eosinophilia, hemolytic anemia, thrombocytopenia and pancytopenia.

Allergic reactions: Rash, pruritus, urticaria, photosensitivity and rare cases of anaphylaxis have been reported with Navane. Undue exposure to sunlight should be avoided. Although not experienced with Navane, exfoliative dermatitis and contact dermatitis (in nursing personnel), have been reported with certain phenothiazines.

Endocrine disorders: Lactation, moderate breast enlargement and amenorrhea have occurred in a small percentage of females receiving Navane (thiothixene). If persistent, this may necessitate a reduction in dosage or the discontinuation of therapy. Phenothiazines have been associated with false positive pregnancy tests, gynecomastia, hypoglycemia, hyperglycemia and glycosuria.

Autonomic effects: Dry mouth, blurred vision, nasal congestion, constipation, increased sweating, increased salivation and impotence have occurred infrequently with Navane therapy. Phenothiazines have been associated with miosis, mydriasis, and adynamic ileus.

Other adverse reactions: Hyperpyrexia, anorexia, nausea, vomiting, diarrhea, increase in appetite and weight, weakness or fatigue, polydipsia, and peripheral edema.

Although not reported with Navane, evidence indicates there is a relationship between phenothiazine therapy and the occurrence of a systemic lupus erythematosus-like syndrome.

NOTE: Sudden deaths have occasionally been reported in patients who have received certain phenothiazine derivatives. In some cases the cause of death was apparently cardiac arrest or asphyxia due to failure of the cough reflex. In others, the cause could not be determined nor could it be established that death was due to phenothiazine administration.

Dosage and Administration: Dosage of Navane should be individually adjusted depending on the chronicity and severity of the condition. In general, small doses should be used initially and gradually increased to the optimal effective level, based on patient response. Some patients have been successfully maintained on once-a-day Navane therapy.

The use of Navane in children under 12 years of age is not recommended because safe conditions for its use have not been established.

In milder conditions, an initial dose of 2 mg. three times daily. If indicated, a subsequent increase to 15 mg./day total daily dose is often effective.

In more severe conditions, an initial dose of 5 mg. twice daily.

The usual optimal dose is 20 to 30 mg. daily. If indicated, an increase to 60 mg./day total daily dose is often effective. Exceeding a total daily dose of 60 mg. rarely increases the beneficial response.

Overdosage: Manifestations include muscular twitching, drowsiness and dizziness. Symptoms of gross overdosage may include CNS depression, rigidity, weakness, torticollis, tremor, salivation, dysphagia, hypotension, disturbances of gait, or coma.

Treatment: Essentially symptomatic and supportive. Early gastric lavage is helpful. Keep patient under careful observation and maintain an open airway, since involvement of the extrapyramidal system may produce dysphagia and respiratory difficulty in severe overdosage. If hypotension occurs, the standard measures for managing circulatory shock should be used (I.V. fluids and/or vasoconstrictors).

If a vasoconstrictor is needed, levarterenol and phenylephrine are the most suitable drugs. Other pressor agents, including epinephrine, are not recommended, since phenothiazine derivatives may reverse the usual pressor action of these agents and cause further lowering of blood pressure.

If CNS depression is present, recommended stimulants include amphetamine, dextroamphetamine, or caffeine and sodium benzoate. Stimulants that may cause convulsions (e. g. picrotoxin or pentylenetetrazol) should be avoided. Extrapyramidal symptoms may be treated with antiparkinson drugs.

There are no data on the use of peritoneal or hemodialysis, but they are known to be of little value in phenothiazine intoxication.

How Supplied: Navane (thiothixene) is available as capsules containing 1 mg, 2 mg, 5 mg, and 10 mg of thiothixene in bottles of 100, 1,000 and unit-dose pack of 100 (10 × 10's).

Navane (thiothixene) is also available as capsules containing 20 mg of thiothixene in bottles of 100, 500 and unit-dose pack of 100 (10 × 10's).

Navane (thiothixene hydrochloride) Concentrate is available in 120 ml (4 oz.) bottles with an accompanying dropper calibrated at 2 mg, 3 mg, 4 mg, 5 mg, 6 mg, 8 mg, and 10 mg and in 30 ml (1 oz.) bottles with an accompanying dropper calibrated at 2 mg, 3 mg, 4 mg, and 5 mg. Each ml. contains thiothixene hydrochloride equivalent to 5 mg. of thiothixene. Contains alcohol, U.S.P. 7.0% v/v. (small loss unavoidable).

[*Shown in Product Identification Section*]

NAVANE®

(thiothixene hydrochloride)
Intramuscular
2 mg./ml. 5 mg./ml. † ℞

Description: Navane (thiothixene hydrochloride) is a thioxanthene derivative. Specifically, it is the *cis* isomer of N,N-dimethyl-9-[3-(4-methyl-1-piperazinyl)-propylidene] thioxanthene-2-sulfonamide.

The thioxanthenes differ from the phenothiazines by the replacement of nitrogen in the central ring with a carbon-linked side chain fixed in space in a rigid structural configuration. An N,N-dimethyl sulfonamide functional group is bonded to the thioxanthene nucleus.

†Navane Intramuscular contains in each ml. thiothixene HCl equivalent to 2 mg. of thiothixene, dextrose 5% w/v, benzyl alcohol 0.9% w/v, and propyl gallate 0.02% w/v.

Navane (thiothixene hydrochloride) Intramuscular For Injection, when reconstituted with 2.2 ml of Sterile Water for Injection, contains in each ml thiothixene hydrochloride equivalent to 5 mg of thiothixene, and 59.6 mg of mannitol.

Actions: Navane is a psychotropic agent of the thioxanthene series. Navane possesses certain chemical and pharmacological similarities to the piperazine phenothiazines and differences from the aliphatic group of phenothiazines. Navane's mode of action has not been clearly established.

Indications: Navane is effective in the management of manifestations of psychotic disorders. Navane has not been evaluated in the management of behavioral complications in patients with mental retardation.

Contraindications: Navane is contraindicated in patients with circulatory collapse, comatose states, central nervous system depression due to any cause, and blood dyscrasias. Navane is contraindicated in individuals who have shown hypersensitivity to the drug. It is not known whether there is a cross sensitivity between the thioxanthenes and the phenothiazine derivatives, but this possibility should be considered.

Warnings: Usage in Pregnancy—Safe use of Navane during pregnancy has not been established. Therefore, this drug should be given to pregnant patients only when, in the judgment of the physician, the expected benefits from treatment exceed the possible risks to mother and fetus. Animal reproductive studies and clinical experience to date have not demonstrated any teratogenic effects.

In the animal reproduction studies with Navane, there was some decrease in conception rate and litter size, and an increase in resorption rate in rats and rabbits, changes which have been similarly reported with other psychotropic agents. After repeated oral administration of Navane to rats (5 to 15 mg./kg./day), rabbits (3 to 50 mg./kg./day), and monkeys (1 to 3 mg./kg./day) before and during gestation, no teratogenic effects were seen. (See Precautions).

Usage in Children—The use of Navane in children under 12 years of age is not recommended because safety and efficacy in the pediatric age group have not been established.

As is true with many CNS drugs, Navane may impair the mental and/or physical abilities required for the performance of potentially hazardous tasks such as driving a car or operating machinery, especially during the first few days of therapy. Therefore, the patient should be cautioned accordingly.

As in the case of other CNS-acting drugs, patients receiving Navane should be cautioned about the possible additive effects (which may include hypotension) with CNS depressants and with alcohol.

Precautions: An antiemetic effect was observed in animal studies with Navane (thiothixene hydrochloride); since this effect may also occur in man, it is possible that Navane may mask signs of overdosage of toxic drugs and may obscure conditions such as intestinal obstruction and brain tumor.

In consideration of the known capability of Navane and certain other psychotropic drugs to precipitate convulsions, extreme caution should be used in patients with a history of convulsive disorders, or those in a state of alcohol withdrawal since it may lower the convulsive threshold. Although Navane potentiates the actions of the barbiturates, the dosage of the anticonvulsant therapy should not be reduced when Navane is administered concurrently.

Continued on next page

Roerig—Cont.

Caution as well as careful adjustment of the dosage is indicated when Navane is used in conjunction with other CNS depressants other than anticonvulsant drugs.
Though exhibiting rather weak anticholinergic properties, Navane should be used with caution in patients who are known or suspected to have glaucoma, or who might be exposed to extreme heat, or who are receiving atropine or related drugs.
Use with caution in patients with cardiovascular disease.
Also, careful observation should be made for pigmentary retinopathy, and lenticular pigmentation (fine lenticular pigmentation has been noted in a small number of patients treated with Navane for prolonged periods).
Blood dyscrasias (agranulocytosis, pancytopenia, thrombocytopenic purpura), and liver damage (jaundice, biliary stasis), have been reported with related drugs.
Undue exposure to sunlight should be avoided. Photosensitive reactions have been reported in patients on Navane.
As with all intramuscular preparations, Navane Intramuscular should be injected well within the body of a relatively large muscle. The preferred sites are the upper outer quadrant of the buttock (i.e., gluteus maximus) and the mid-lateral thigh.
The deltoid area should be used only if well developed such as in certain adults and older children, and then only with caution to avoid radial nerve injury. Intramuscular injections should not be made into the lower and mid-thirds of the upper arm. As with all intramuscular injections, aspiration is necessary to help avoid inadvertent injection into a blood vessel.
Neuroleptic drugs elevate prolactin levels; the elevation persists during chronic administration. Tissue culture experiments indicate that approximately one-third of human breast cancers are prolactin dependent *in vitro*, a factor of potential importance if the prescription of these drugs is contemplated in a patient with a previously detected breast cancer. Although disturbances such as galactorrhea, amenorrhea, gynecomastia, and impotence have been reported, the clinical significance of elevated serum prolactin levels is unknown for most patients. An increase in mammary neoplasms has been found in rodents after chronic administration of neuroleptic drugs. Neither clinical studies nor epidemiologic studies conducted to date, however, have shown an association between chronic administration of these drugs and mammary tumorigenesis; the available evidence is considered too limited to be conclusive at this time.

Adverse Reactions:

NOTE: Not all of the following adverse reactions have been reported with Navane. However, since Navane has certain chemical and pharmacologic similarities to the phenothiazines, all of the known side effects and toxicity associated with phenothiazine therapy should be borne in mind when Navane is used.
Cardiovascular effects: Tachycardia, hypotension, lightheadedness, and syncope. In the event hypotension occurs, epinephrine should not be used as a pressor agent since a paradoxical further lowering of blood pressure may result. Nonspecific EKG changes have been observed in some patients receiving Navane. These changes are usually reversible and frequently disappear on continued Navane therapy. The clinical significance of these changes is not known.
CNS effects: Drowsiness, usually mild, may occur although it usually subsides with continuation of Navane therapy. The incidence of sedation appears similar to that of the piperazine group of phenothiazines, but less than that of certain aliphatic phenothiazines. Restlessness, agitation and insomnia have been noted with Navane. Seizures and paradoxical exacerbation of psychotic symptoms have occurred with Navane infrequently.
Hyperreflexia has been reported in infants delivered from mothers having received structurally related drugs.
In addition, phenothiazine derivatives have been associated with cerebral edema and cerebrospinal fluid abnormalities.
Extrapyramidal symptoms, such as pseudoparkinsonism, akathisia, and dystonia have been reported. Management of these extrapyramidal symptoms depends upon the type and severity. Rapid relief of acute symptoms may require the use of an injectable antiparkinson agent. More slowly emerging symptoms may be managed by reducing the dosage of Navane and/or administering an oral antiparkinson agent.
Persistent Tardive Dyskinesia: As with all antipsychotic agents tardive dyskinesia may appear in some patients on long term therapy or may occur after drug therapy has been discontinued. The risk seems to be greater in elderly patients on high-dose therapy, especially females. The symptoms are persistent and in some patients appear to be irreversible. The syndrome is characterized by rhythmical involuntary movements of the tongue, face, mouth or jaw (e.g., protrusion of tongue, puffing of cheeks, puckering of mouth, chewing movements). Sometimes these may be accompanied by involuntary movements of extremities.
There is no known effective treatment for tardive dyskinesia; antiparkinsonism agents usually do not alleviate the symptoms of this syndrome. It is suggested that all antipsychotic agents be discontinued if these symptoms appear.
Should it be necessary to reinstitute treatment, or increase the dosage of the agent, or switch to a different antipsychotic agent, the syndrome may be masked.
It has been reported that fine vermicular movements of the tongue may be an early sign of the syndrome and if the medication is stopped at that time, the syndrome may not develop.
Hepatic effects: Elevations of serum transaminase and alkaline phosphatase, usually transient, have been infrequently observed in some patients. No clinically confirmed cases of jaundice attributable to Navane (thiothixene hydrochloride) have been reported.
Hematologic effects: As is true with certain other psychotropic drugs, leukopenia and leucocytosis, which are usually transient, can occur occasionally with Navane. Other antipsychotic drugs have been associated with agranulocytosis, eosinophilia, hemolytic anemia, thrombocytopenia and pancytopenia.
Allergic reactions: Rash, pruritus, urticaria, and rare cases of anaphylaxis have been reported with Navane. Undue exposure to sunlight should be avoided. Although not experienced with Navane, exfoliative dermatitis, contact dermatitis (in nursing personnel), have been reported with certain phenothiazines.
Endocrine disorders: Lactation, moderate breast enlargement and amenorrhea have occurred in a small percentage of females receiving Navane. If persistent, this may necessitate a reduction in dosage or the discontinuation of therapy. Phenothiazines have been associated with false positive pregnancy tests, gynecomastia, hypoglycemia, hyperglycemia, and glycosuria.
Autonomic effects: Dry mouth, blurred vision, nasal congestion, constipation, increased sweating, increased salivation, and impotence have occurred infrequently with Navane therapy. Phenothiazines have been associated with miosis, mydriasis, and adynamic ileus.
Other adverse reactions: Hyperpyrexia, anorexia, nausea, vomiting, diarrhea, increase in appetite and weight, weakness or fatigue, polydipsia and peripheral edema.
Although not reported with Navane, evidence indicates there is a relationship between phenothiazine therapy and the occurrence of a systemic lupus erythematosus-like syndrome.
NOTE: Sudden deaths have occasionally been reported in patients who have received certain phenothiazine derivatives. In some cases the cause of death was apparently cardiac arrest or asphyxia due to failure of the cough reflex. In others, the cause could not be determined nor could it be established that death was due to phenothiazine administration.

Dosage and Administration:

Preparation

Navane (thiothixene hydrochloride) Intramuscular Solution is ready for use as supplied.
Navane (thiothixene hydrochloride) Intramuscular For Injection must be reconstituted with 2.2 ml of Sterile Water for Injection.

For Intramuscular Use Only

Dosage of Navane should be individually adjusted depending on the chronicity and severity of the condition. In general, small doses should be used initially and gradually increased to the optimal effective level, based on patient response.
Usage in children under 12 years of age is not recommended.
Where more rapid control and treatment of acute behavior is desirable, the intramuscular form of Navane may be indicated. It is also of benefit where the very nature of the patient's symptomatology, whether acute or chronic, renders oral administration impractical or even impossible.
For treatment of acute symptomatology or in patients unable or unwilling to take oral medication, the usual dose is 4 mg. of Navane Intramuscular administered 2 to 4 times daily. Dosage may be increased or decreased depending on response. Most patients are controlled on a total daily dosage of 16 to 20 mg. The maximum recommended dosage is 30 mg./day. An oral form should supplant the injectable form as soon as possible. It may be necessary to adjust the dosage when changing from the intramuscular to oral dosage forms. Dosage recommendations for Navane Capsules and Concentrate can be found in the Navane oral package insert.
Overdosage: Manifestations include muscular twitching, drowsiness, and dizziness. Symptoms of gross overdosage may include CNS depression, rigidity, weakness, torticollis, tremor, salivation, dysphagia, hypotension, disturbances of gait, or coma.
Treatment: Essentially symptomatic and supportive. Keep patient under careful observation and maintain an open airway, since involvement of the extrapyramidal system may produce dysphagia and respiratory difficulty in severe overdosage. If hypotension occurs, the standard measures for managing circulatory shock should be used (I.V. fluids and/or vasoconstrictors).
If a vasoconstrictor is needed, levarterenol and phenylephrine are the most suitable drugs. Other pressor agents, including epinephrine, are not recommended, since phenothiazine derivatives may reverse the usual pressor elevating action of these agents and cause further lowering of blood pressure.
If CNS depression is present and specific therapy is indicated, recommended stimulants include amphetamine, dextroamphetamine, or caffeine and sodium benzoate. Picrotoxin or pentylenetetrazol should be avoided. Extrapyramidal symptoms may be treated with antiparkinson drugs.
There are no data on the use of peritoneal or hemodialysis, but they are known to be of little value in phenothiazine intoxication.
How Supplied: Navane (thiothixene hydrochloride) Intramuscular Solution is available in a 2 ml. amber glass vial in packages of 10 vials. Each ml. contains thiothixene hydrochlo-

ride equivalent to 2 mg. of thiothixene, dextrose 5% w/v, benzyl alcohol 0.9% w/v, and propyl gallate 0.02% w/v.

Navane (thiothixene hydrochloride) Intramuscular For Injection is available in amber glass vials in packages of 10 vials. When reconstituted with 2.2 ml of Sterile Water for Injection, each ml contains thiothixene hydrochloride equivalent to 5 mg of thiothixene, and 59.6 mg of mannitol. The reconstituted solution of Navane Intramuscular For Injection may be stored for 48 hours at room temperature before discarding.

SINEQUAN® ℞
(doxepin HCl)
Capsules
Oral Concentrate

Description: SINEQUAN (doxepin hydrochloride) is one of a class of psychotherapeutic agents known as dibenzoxepin tricyclic compounds. The molecular formula of the compound is $C_{19}H_{21}NO \cdot HCl$ having a molecular weight of 316. It is a white crystalline solid readily soluble in water, lower alcohols and chloroform.

Chemistry: SINEQUAN (doxepin HCl) is a dibenzoxepin derivative and is the first of a family of tricyclic psychotherapeutic agents. Specifically, it is an isomeric mixture of 1-Propanamine, 3-dibenz[*b,e*]oxepin-11(6*H*)ylidene-*N,N*-dimethyl-, hydrochloride.

Actions: The mechanism of action of SINEQUAN (doxepin HCl) is not definitely known. It is not a central nervous system stimulant nor a monoamine oxidase inhibitor. The current hypothesis is that the clinical effects are due, at least in part, to influences on the adrenergic activity at the synapses so that deactivation of norepinephrine by reuptake into the nerve terminals is prevented. Animal studies suggest that doxepin HCl does not appreciably antagonize the antihypertensive action of guanethidine. In animal studies anticholinergic, antiserotonin and antihistamine effects on smooth muscle have been demonstrated. At higher than usual clinical doses, norepinephrine response was potentiated in animals. This effect was not demonstrated in humans.

At clinical dosages up to 150 mg per day, SINEQUAN can be given to man concomitantly with guanethidine and related compounds without blocking the antihypertensive effect. At dosages above 150 mg per day blocking of the antihypertensive effect of these compounds has been reported.

There have been no reports of physical dependency or withdrawal symptoms associated with SINEQUAN therapy. This is consistent with the virtual absence of euphoria as a side effect and the lack of addiction potential characteristic of this type of chemical compound.

Indications: SINEQUAN is recommended for the treatment of:

1. Psychoneurotic patients with depression and/or anxiety.
2. Depression and/or anxiety associated with alcoholism (not to be taken concomitantly with alcohol).
3. Depression and/or anxiety associated with organic disease (the possibility of drug interaction should be considered if the patient is receiving other drugs concomitantly).
4. Psychotic depressive disorders with associated anxiety including involutional depression and manic-depressive disorders.

The target symptoms of psychoneurosis that respond particularly well to SINEQUAN include anxiety, tension, depression, somatic symptoms and concerns, sleep disturbances, guilt, lack of energy, fear, apprehension and worry.

Clinical experience has shown that SINEQUAN is safe and well-tolerated even in the elderly patient. Owing to lack of clinical experience in the pediatric population, SINEQUAN is not recommended for use in children under 12 years of age.

Contraindications: SINEQUAN is contraindicated in individuals who have shown hypersensitivity to the drug. Possibility of cross sensitivity with other dibenzoxepines should be kept in mind.

SINEQUAN is contraindicated in patients with glaucoma or a tendency to urinary retention. These disorders should be ruled out, particularly in older patients.

Warnings: The once-a-day dosage regimen of SINEQUAN in patients with intercurrent illness or patients taking other medications should be carefully adjusted. This is especially important in patients receiving other medications with anticholinergic effects.

Usage in Geriatrics

The use of SINEQUAN on a once-a-day dosage regimen in geriatric patients should be adjusted carefully based on the patient's condition.

Usage in Pregnancy

Reproduction studies have been performed in rats, rabbits, monkeys and dogs and there was no evidence of harm to the animal fetus. The relevance to humans is not known. Since there is no experience in pregnant women who have received this drug, safety in pregnancy has not been established. There are no data with respect to the secretion of the drug in human milk and its effect on the nursing infant.

Usage in Children

The use of SINEQUAN in children under 12 years of age is not recommended because safe conditions for its use have not been established.

MAO Inhibitors

Serious side effects and even death have been reported following the concomitant use of certain drugs with MAO inhibitors. Therefore, MAO inhibitors should be discontinued at least two weeks prior to the cautious initiation of therapy with SINEQUAN. The exact length of time may vary and is dependent upon the particular MAO inhibitor being used, the length of time it has been administered, and the dosage involved.

Usage with Alcohol

It should be borne in mind that alcohol ingestion may increase the danger inherent in any intentional or unintentional SINEQUAN overdosage. This is especially important in patients who may use alcohol excessively.

Precautions: Since drowsiness may occur with the use of this drug, patients should be warned of the possibility and cautioned against driving a car or operating dangerous machinery while taking the drug. Patients should also be cautioned that their response to alcohol may be potentiated.

Since suicide is an inherent risk in any depressed patient and may remain so until significant improvement has occurred, patients should be closely supervised during the early course of therapy. Prescriptions should be written for the smallest feasible amount.

Should increased symptoms of psychosis or shift to manic symptomatology occur, it may be necessary to reduce dosage or add a major tranquilizer to the dosage regimen.

Adverse Reactions:

NOTE: Some of the adverse reactions noted below have not been specifically reported with SINEQUAN use. However, due to the close pharmacological similarities among the tricyclics, the reactions should be considered when prescribing SINEQUAN (doxepin HCl).

Anticholinergic Effects: Dry mouth, blurred vision, constipation, and urinary retention have been reported. If they do not subside with continued therapy, or become severe, it may be necessary to reduce the dosage.

Central Nervous System Effects: Drowsiness is the most commonly noticed side effect. This tends to disappear as therapy is continued. Other infrequently reported CNS side effects are confusion, disorientation, hallucinations, numbness, paresthesias, ataxia, and extrapyramidal symptoms and seizures.

Cardiovascular: Cardiovascular effects including hypotension and tachycardia have been reported occasionally.

Allergic: Skin rash, edema, photosensitization, and pruritus have occasionally occurred.

Hematologic: Eosinophilia has been reported in a few patients. There have been occasional reports of bone marrow depression manifesting as agranulocytosis, leukopenia, thrombocytopenia, and purpura.

Gastrointestinal: Nausea, vomiting, indigestion, taste disturbances, diarrhea, anorexia, and aphthous stomatitis have been reported. (See anticholinergic effects.)

Endocrine: Raised or lowered libido, testicular swelling, gynecomastia in males, enlargement of breasts and galactorrhea in the female, raising or lowering of blood sugar levels have been reported with tricyclic administration.

Other: Dizziness, tinnitus, weight gain, sweating, chills, fatigue, weakness, flushing, jaundice, alopecia, and headache have been occasionally observed as adverse effects.

Dosage and Administration: For most patients with illness of mild to moderate severity, a starting daily dose of 75 mg is recommended. Dosage may subsequently be increased or decreased at appropriate intervals and according to individual response. The usual optimum dose range is 75 mg/day to 150 mg/day.

In more severely ill patients higher doses may be required with subsequent gradual increase to 300 mg/day if necessary. Additional therapeutic effect is rarely to be obtained by exceeding a dose of 300 mg/day.

In patients with very mild symptomatology or emotional symptoms accompanying organic disease, lower doses may suffice. Some of these patients have been controlled on doses as low as 25-50 mg/day.

The total daily dosage of SINEQUAN may be given on a divided or once-a-day dosage schedule. If the once-a-day schedule is employed the maximum recommended dose is 150 mg/day. This dose may be given at bedtime. **The 150 mg capsule strength is intended for maintenance therapy only and is not recommended for initiation of treatment.**

Anti-anxiety effect is apparent before the antidepressant effect. Optimal antidepressant effect may not be evident for two to three weeks.

Overdosage:

A. Signs and Symptoms
   1. Mild: Drowsiness, stupor, blurred vision, excessive dryness of mouth.
   2. Severe: Respiratory depression, hypotension, coma, convulsions, cardiac arrhythmias and tachycardias.

   Also: urinary retention (bladder atony), decreased gastrointestinal motility (paralytic ileus), hyperthermia (or hypothermia), hypertension, dilated pupils, hyperactive reflexes.

B. Management and Treatment
   1. Mild: Observation and supportive therapy is all that is usually necessary.
   2. Severe: Medical management of severe SINEQUAN overdosage consists of aggressive supportive therapy. If the patient is conscious, gastric lavage, with appropriate precautions to prevent pulmonary aspiration, should be performed even though SINEQUAN is rapidly absorbed. The use of activated charcoal has been recommended, as has been continuous gastric lavage with saline for 24 hours or more. An adequate airway should be established in comatose patients and assisted ventilation used if necessary. EKG monitoring may be required for several days, since relapse after apparent recovery has been reported. Arrhythmias

Continued on next page

Roerig—Cont.

should be treated with the appropriate antiarrhythmic agent. It has been reported that many of the cardiovascular and CNS symptoms of tricyclic antidepressant poisoning in adults may be reversed by the slow intravenous administration of 1 mg to 3 mg of physostigmine salicylate. Because physostigmine is rapidly metabolized, the dosage should be repeated as required. Convulsions may respond to standard anticonvulsant therapy, however, barbiturates may potentiate any respiratory depression. Dialysis and forced diuresis generally are not of value in the management of overdosage due to high tissue and protein binding of SINEQUAN.

Supply:
SINEQUAN is available as capsules containing doxepin HCl equivalent to: 10 mg, 75 mg, and 100 mg doxepin; bottles of 100, 1000, and unit-dose packages of 100 (10 × 10's).
25 mg and 50 mg doxepin: bottles of 100, 1000, 5000, and unit-dose packages of 100 (10 × 10's).
150 mg doxepin: bottles of 50, 500, and unit-dose packages of 100 (10 × 10's).
SINEQUAN Oral Concentrate is available in 120 ml bottles with an accompanying dropper calibrated at 5 mg, 10 mg, 15 mg, 20 mg, and 25 mg. Each ml contains doxepin HCl equivalent to 10 mg doxepin. Just prior to administration, SINEQUAN Oral Concentrate should be diluted with approximately 120 ml of water, whole or skimmed milk, or orange, grapefruit, tomato, prune or pineapple juice. SINEQUAN Oral Concentrate is not physically compatible with a number of carbonated beverages. For those patients requiring antidepressant therapy who are on methadone maintenance, SINEQUAN Oral Concentrate and methadone syrup can be mixed together with Gatorade®, lemonade, orange juice, sugar water, Tang®, or water; but not with grape juice. Preparation and storage of bulk dilutions is not recommended.

Literature Available: Yes.
[*Shown in Product Identification Section*]

SPECTROBID®
(bacampicillin HCl)
TABLETS and POWDER for ORAL SUSPENSION

Description: SPECTROBID (bacampicillin HCl) is a member of the ampicillin class of semi-synthetic penicillins derived from the basic penicillin nucleus: 6-aminopenicillanic acid. SPECTROBID, as well as ampicillin and other ampicillin analogues, is acid resistant and suitable for oral administration.
SPECTROBID is the hydrochloride salt of 1-ethoxycarbonyloxyethyl ester of ampicillin, available either as tablets or as a microencapsulated oral suspension. During the process of absorption from the gastrointestinal tract, SPECTROBID is hydrolyzed rapidly to ampicillin, a well characterized and effective antibacterial agent. Each 400 mg tablet of SPECTROBID is chemically equivalent to 280 mg of ampicillin, and 125 mg/5 ml of the oral suspension is chemically equivalent to 87.5 mg of ampicillin.
Chemically, SPECTROBID is 1′-ethoxycarbonyloxyethyl-6-(D-α aminophenylacetamide)-penicillinate hydrochloride. It has a molecular weight of 501.96.

Actions:
Clinical Pharmacology
SPECTROBID is characterized by its more complete and more rapid absorption from the GI tract than ampicillin. SPECTROBID tablets of 400 mg, 800 mg, and 1600 mg have provided ampicillin peak serum concentrations of 7.9, 12.9, and 20.1 mcg/ml. These peak levels are approximately three times the levels obtained with administration of equivalent amounts of ampicillin. The areas-under-the-serum-concentration curves obtained during the first 6 hours were 24.8 and 12.9 mcg/ml/hr., when bacampicillin HCl 800 mg and ampicillin 500 mg were administered to adults. (See Graph 1.) Graph 2 shows the serum ampicillin curves following a 28 mg/kg dose of bacampicillin HCl and a 25 mg/kg dose of ampicillin in infants and young children. The areas-under-the-serum-concentration-curves were 28.2 and 13.1 respectively.
The absorption of the SPECTROBID oral suspension was shown to be equivalent to that of the 400 mg tablet in fasting adult volunteers. A 400 mg dose of suspension gave a peak serum ampicillin concentration of 7.6 mcg/ml and the tablet gave a peak of 7.2 mcg/ml. In fasting pediatric patients a 12.5 mg/kg dose provided a peak of 8.4 mcg/ml.
After oral administration of SPECTROBID tablet or suspension, ampicillin activity in serum peaks at 0.7–0.9 hours (compared to 1.5–2.0 hours after administration of ampicillin). Serum ampicillin half-life is 1.1 hours after either SPECTROBID or ampicillin administration.
Peak tissue and body fluid ampicillin concentrations also are higher after administration of SPECTROBID. Utilizing a special skin window technique to determine ampicillin levels, therapeutic levels in the interstitial fluid were higher and more prolonged after SPECTROBID than after ampicillin administration.
SPECTROBID is stable in the presence of gastric acid. SPECTROBID oral suspension absorption is affected by food. Food does not retard absorption of SPECTROBID tablets which may be given without regard to meals. SPECTROBID is virtually completely absorbed (98%), with about 75% of a given dose being recoverable in the urine as active ampicillin within 8 hours of administration. Urinary excretion can be delayed by concurrent administration of probenecid. The active moiety of SPECTROBID (i.e., ampicillin) diffuses readily into most body tissues and fluids. In serum, ampicillin is only 20% protein-bound, compared to 60–90% for other penicillins.

Microbiology
SPECTROBID per se has no *in vitro* antibacterial activity and owes its *in vivo* bactericidal activity to the parent compound, ampicillin. The ampicillin class of penicillins (including SPECTROBID) has a broad spectrum of activity against many gram-negative and gram-positive bacteria. Like other penicillins, the ampicillin class of penicillins inhibits the synthesis of cell wall mucopeptide.
Ampicillin class antibiotics are inactivated by β-lactamases produced by certain strains of *Enterobacter, Citrobacter, Haemophilus infuenzae,* and *Escherichia coli,* and by most strains of staphylococci and indole-positive *Proteus* spp. Ampicillin class antibiotics are not active against *Pseudomonas, Klebsiella,* or *Serratia* spp.

Susceptibility Testing:
Elution Technique: For the automated method of susceptibility testing (i.e., Autobac™), gram-negative organisms should be tested with the 4.5 mcg ampicillin elution disk, while gram-positive organisms should be tested with the 0.22 mcg disk.
Diffusion Technique: For the Kirby-Bauer method of susceptibility testing, a 10 mcg ampicillin diffusion disk should be used. With this procedure, a laboratory report of "susceptible" indicates that the infecting organism is likely to respond to SPECTROBID therapy, and a report of "resistant" indicates that the infecting organism is not likely to respond to therapy. An "intermediate susceptibility" report suggests that the infecting organism would be susceptible to SPECTROBID if a high dosage is used or if the infection is confined to tissues and fluids (e.g., urine) in which high antibiotic levels are attained.
Dilution Techniques: Broth or agar dilution methods may be used to determine the minimal inhibitory concentration (MIC) value for susceptibility of bacterial isolates to SPECTROBID. Since SPECTROBID per se has no *in vitro* activity, ampicillin powder should be used in a twofold concentration series of the antibiotic prepared in either broth (in tubes) or agar (in petri plates). Tubes should be inoculated to contain 10^4 to 10^5 organisms/ml or plates "spotted" with 10^3 to 10^4 organisms.

Indications and Usage:
SPECTROBID is indicated for the treatment of the following infections when caused by ampicillin-susceptible organisms:

1. Upper and Lower Respiratory Tract Infections (including acute exacerbations of chronic bronchitis) due to streptococci (β-hemolytic streptococci, *Streptococcus pyogenes*), pneumococci (*Streptococcus pneumoniae*), nonpenicillinase-producing staphylococci and *H. influenzae;*
2. Urinary Tract Infections due to *E. coli, Proteus mirabilis,* and *Streptococcus faecalis* (enterococci);
3. Skin and Skin Structure Infections due to streptococci and susceptible staphylococci;
4. Gonorrhea (acute uncomplicated urogenital infections) due to *Neisseria gonorrhoeae.*

Bacteriological studies to determine the causative organisms and their suspectibility to SPECTROBID (i.e., ampicillin) should be performed. Therapy may be instituted prior to obtaining results of susceptibility testing. Indicated surgical procedures should be performed.

Contraindications:
The use of ampicillin class antibiotics is contraindicated in individuals with a history of an allergic reaction to any of the penicillin antibiotics.

Warnings: Serious and occasional fatal hypersensitivity (anaphylactic) reactions have been reported in patients on penicillin therapy. Although anaphylaxis is more frequent following parenteral therapy, it has occurred in patients on oral penicillins. These reactions are more apt to occur in individuals with a history of penicillin hypersensitivity and/or hypersensitivity to multiple allergens.
There have been reports of individuals with a history of penicillin hypersensitivity who have experienced severe reactions when treated with cephalosporins. Before therapy with a penicillin, careful inquiry should be made concerning previous hypersensitivity reactions to penicillins, cephalosporins, and other allergens.
IF AN ALLERGIC REACTION OCCURS, THE DRUG SHOULD BE DISCONTINUED AND THE APPROPRIATE THERAPY INSTITUTED. SERIOUS ANAPHYLACTOID REACTIONS REQUIRE IMMEDIATE EMERGENCY TREATMENT WITH EPINEPHRINE. OXYGEN, INTRAVENOUS STEROIDS, AND AIRWAY MANAGEMENT, INCLUDING INTUBATION, SHOULD ALSO BE ADMINISTERED AS INDICATED.

Precautions:
1. General: The possibility of superinfections with mycotic or bacterial pathogens should be kept in mind during therapy. If superinfections occur (usually involving *Aerobacter, Pseudomonas,* or *Candida*), the drug should be discontinued and appropriate therapy instituted.
As with any potent agent, it is advisable to check periodically for organ system dysfunction during prolonged therapy. This includes renal, hepatic, and hematopoietic systems and is particularly important in prematures, neonates, and patients with liver or renal impairments.
A high percentage of patients with mononucleosis who receive ampicillin develop a skin rash. Thus, ampicillin class antibiotics should not be administered to patients with mononucleosis.

2. Clinically Significant Drug Interactions: The concurrent administration of allopurinol and ampicillin increases substantially the incidence of rashes in patients receiving both drugs as compared to patients receiving ampicillin alone. It is not known whether this potentiation of ampicillin rashes is due to allopurinol or the hyperuricemia present in these patients. There are no data available on the incidence of rash in patients treated concurrently with SPECTROBID (bacampicillin HCl) and allopurinol. SPECTROBID should not be co-administered with Antabuse (disulfiram).

3. Drug and Laboratory Test Interactions: When testing for the presence of glucose in urine using Clinitest™, Benedict's Solution, or Fehling's Solution, high urine concentrations of ampicillin may result in false-positive reactions. Therefore, it is recommended that glucose tests based on enzymatic glucose oxidase reactions (such as Clinistix™ or Testape™) be used.

Following administration of ampicillin to pregnant women a transient decrease in plasma concentration of total conjugated estriol, estriol-glucuronide, conjugated estrone and estradiol, has been noted.

4. Pregnancy Category B: Reproduction studies have been performed in mice and rats at SPECTROBID doses of up to 750 mg/kg (more than 25 times the human dose) and have revealed no evidence of impaired fertility or harm to the fetus due to SPECTROBID.

There are, however, no adequate and well controlled studies in pregnant women. Because animal reproduction studies are not always predictive of human response, this drug should be used during pregnancy only if clearly needed.

5. Carcinogenesis, Mutagenesis, Impairment of Fertility: No carcinogenicity or mutagenicity studies were conducted. No impairment of fertility and no significant effect on general reproductive performance was observed in rats administered oral doses of up to 750 mg/kg of bacampicillin HCl per day prior to and during mating and gestation. In addition, bacampicillin HCl caused no drug-related effects on the reproductive organs of rats or dogs receiving daily oral doses of up to 800 and 650 mg/kg respectively for 6 months.

6. Labor and Delivery: Oral ampicillin class antibiotics are generally poorly absorbed during labor. Studies in guinea pigs showed that intravenous administration of ampicillin decreased the uterine tone, frequency of contractions, height of contractions, and duration of contractions. However, it is not known whether use of SPECTROBID in humans during labor or delivery has immediate or delayed adverse effects on the fetus, prolongs the duration of labor, or increases the likelihood that forceps delivery or other obstetrical intervention or resuscitation of the newborn will be necessary.

7. Nursing Mothers: Ampicillin class antibiotics are excreted in milk; therefore, caution should be exercised when ampicillin class antibiotics are administered to a nursing woman.

8. Pediatric Use: SPECTROBID tablets are indicated for children weighing 25 kg or more. The SPECTROBID oral suspension is indicated for children and infants weighing less than 25 kg or in those children not able to swallow a tablet.

Adverse Reactions: As with other penicillins, it may be expected that untoward reactions will be essentially limited to sensitivity phenomena. They are more likely to occur in individuals who have previously demonstrated hypersensitivity to penicillins and in those with a history of allergy, asthma, hay fever, or urticaria.

In well controlled clinical trials conducted in the U.S. the most frequent adverse reactions to SPECTROBID were epigastric upset (2%) and diarrhea (2%). Increased dosage may result in an increased incidence of diarrhea. In the same clinical trials the most frequent adverse effects for amoxicillin were diarrhea (4%) and nausea (2%).

The following adverse reactions have been reported for ampicillin.

Gastrointestinal: diarrhea, gastritis, stomatitis, nausea, vomiting, glossitis, black "hairy" tongue, enterocolitis, and pseudomembranous colitis.

Hypersensitivity Reactions: skin rashes, urticaria, erythema multiforme, and an occasional case of exfoliative dermatitis. These reactions may be controlled with antihistamines and, if necessary, systemic corticosteroids. Whenever such reactions occur, the drug should be discontinued, unless the opinion of the physician dictates otherwise.

Serious and occasional fatal hypersensitivity (anaphylactic) reactions can occur with oral penicillins. (See Warnings).

Liver: A moderate rise in serum glutamic oxaloacetic transaminase (SGOT) has been noted in some ampicillin treated patients, but the significance of this finding is unknown. In well controlled clinical trials no difference was noted between ampicillin and SPECTROBID with regard to the incidence of liver function test abnormalities.

Hemic and Lymphatic Systems: Anemia, thrombocytopenia, thrombocytopenic purpura, eosinophilia, leukopenia, and agranulocytosis have been reported during therapy with penicillins. These reactions are usually reversible on discontinuation of therapy and are believed to be hypersensitivity phenomena.

Dosage and Administration: SPECTROBID tablets may be given without regard to meals. SPECTROBID oral suspension should be administered to fasting patients.

UPPER RESPIRATORY TRACT INFECTIONS (including otitis media) due to streptococci, pneumococci, nonpenicillinase-producing staphylococci and *H. influenzae;*

URINARY TRACT INFECTIONS due to *E. coli, Proteus mirabilis,* and *Streptococcus faecalis;*

SKIN AND SKIN STRUCTURES INFECTIONS due to streptococci and susceptible staphylococci;

Usual Dosage

Adults: 1 × 400 mg tablet every 12 hours (for patients weighing 25 kg or more).

Children: 25 mg/kg per day in 2 equally divided doses at 12 hour intervals.

IN SEVERE INFECTIONS OR THOSE CAUSED BY LESS SUSCEPTIBLE ORGANISMS:

Usual Dosage

Adults: 2 × 400 mg tablets every 12 hours (for patients weighing 25 kg or more).

Children: 50 mg/kg per day in 2 equally divided doses at 12 hour intervals.

LOWER RESPIRATORY TRACT INFECTIONS due to streptococci, pneumococci, nonpenicillinase-producing staphylococci, and *H. influenzae:*

Usual Dosage

Adults: 2 × 400 mg tablets every 12 hours (for patients weighing 25 kg or more).

Children: 50 mg/kg per day in 2 equally divided doses at 12 hour intervals.

GONORRHEA—acute uncomplicated urogenital infections due to *N. gonorrhoeae* (males and females):

1.6 grams (4 × 400 mg tablet plus 1 gram probenecid) as a single oral dose.

No pediatric dosage has been established.

Cases of gonorrhea with a suspected lesion of syphilis should have dark field examination before receiving SPECTROBID and monthly serological tests for a minimum of four months. Larger doses may be required for stubborn or severe infections.

It should be recognized that in the treatment of chronic urinary tract infections, frequent bacteriological and clinical appraisals are necessary. Smaller doses than those recommended above should not be used. In stubborn infections, therapy may be required for several weeks. It may be necessary to continue clinical and/or bacteriological follow-up for several months after cessation of therapy. Except for gonorrhea, treatment should be continued for a minimum of 48 to 72 hours beyond the time that the patient becomes asymptomatic or evidence of bacterial eradication has been obtained.

IT IS RECOMMENDED THAT THERE BE AT LEAST 10 DAYS' TREATMENT FOR ANY INFECTION CAUSED BY HEMOLYTIC STREPTOCOCCI TO PREVENT THE OCCURRENCE OF ACUTE RHEUMATIC FEVER OR GLOMERULONEPHRITIS.

Directions for Mixing Oral Suspension:

Prepare suspension at the time of dispensing as follows:

Prior to reconstitution, tap bottle to thoroughly loosen powder. Add the required amount (see table below) of water to the contents of the bottle in approximately two equally divided portions and SHAKE WELL after each addition. Let stand at least 30 minutes and SHAKE WELL just prior to administering each dose. Each level teaspoon (5 ml) will contain 125 mg of bacampicillin HCl.

Final Volume after reconstitution	Amount of Water Required for reconstitution
70 ml	53 ml
100 ml	75 ml
140 ml	106 ml
200 ml	150 ml

Reconstituted suspension *must be stored under refrigeration and discarded after 10 days.*

GRAPH 1.
Comparison of Bacampicillin HCl 800 mg, Ampicillin 500 mg, and Amoxicillin 500 mg

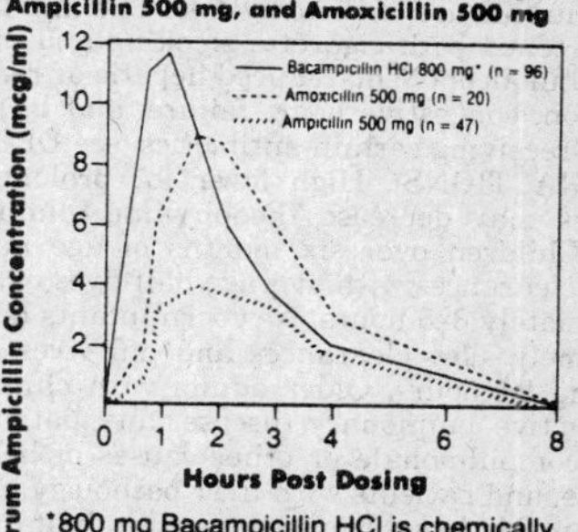

*800 mg Bacampicillin HCl is chemically equivalent to 560 mg of Ampicillin

GRAPH 2.
Crossover Comparison of Bacampicillin HCl Oral Suspension (28 mg/kg)* with Ampicillin Oral Suspension (25 mg/kg) in Fasted Infants and Children (n = 7).

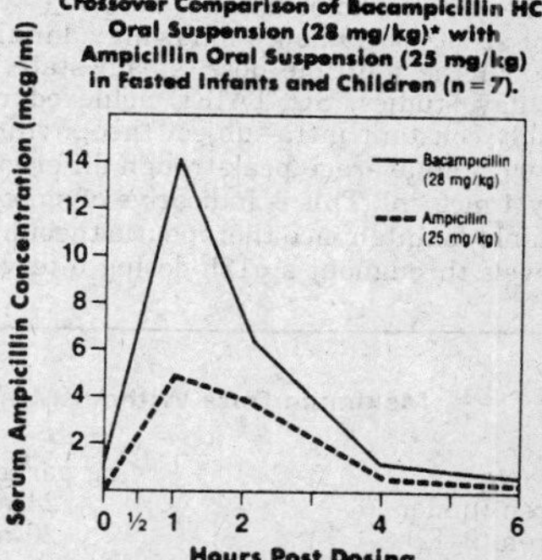

*equivalent to 19.5 mg/kg of Ampicillin

Continued on next page

Roerig—Cont.

How Supplied:
SPECTROBID (bacampicillin HCl) Tablets 400 mg (NDC 0049-0350-66): white, film-coated, oblong, unscored are available in bottles of 100.
SPECTROBID (bacampicillin HCl) Powder for Oral Suspension.
Each 5 ml of reconstituted suspension contains 125 mg of bacampicillin HCl.
Bottles containing the following volumes are available: 70 ml (NDC 0049-0357-37), 100 ml (NDC 0049-0357-44), 140 ml (NDC 0049-0357-49), 200 ml (NDC 0049-0357-91).

[*Shown in Product Identification Section*]

SUSTAIRE® ℞
theophylline (anhydrous)
SUSTAINED RELEASE TABLETS

Description: SUSTAIRE Sustained Release Tablets contain anhydrous theophylline, with no color additives. SUSTAIRE is available in two strengths: 100 mg and 300 mg; each tablet is scored for flexibility of dose. Theophylline, a xanthine compound, is a white, odorless crystalline powder, having a bitter taste.

Actions: The pharmacologic actions of theophylline are as a bronchodilator, pulmonary vasodilator, and smooth muscle relaxant since the drug directly relaxes the smooth muscle of the bronchial airways and pulmonary blood vessels. Theophylline also possesses other actions typical of the xanthine derivatives: coronary vasodilator, diuretic, cardiac stimulant, and skeletal muscle stimulant. The actions of theophylline may be mediated through inhibition of phosphodiesterase and a resultant increase in intracellular cyclic AMP which could mediate smooth muscle relaxation.
No development of tolerance appears to occur with chronic use of theophylline. The half-life is shortened with cigarette smoking and prolonged in alcoholism, reduced hepatic or renal function, congestive heart failure, and in patients receiving certain antibiotics (see DRUG INTERACTIONS). High fever for prolonged periods may decrease theophylline elimination. Children over six months of age have rapid clearances with average half-lives of approximately 3–5 hours. Newborn infants have extremely slow clearances and half-lives exceeding 24 hours. Older adults with chronic obstructive pulmonary disease, any patients with cor pulmonale or other causes of heart failure, and patients with liver pathology may have much lower clearances with half-lives that exceed 24 hours. The half-life in nonsmokers averages 7–9 hours.
In single dose studies, SUSTAIRE, administered at 8 mg/kg body weight, produced mean peak theophylline blood levels of 7.5 ± 1.9 mcg/ml at 9.2 ± 1.9 hours following administration. In the multiple dose, steady-state, 3 and 5 day studies, SUSTAIRE achieved remarkably constant intra-subject theophylline levels with an average peak-trough difference of only 4 mcg/ml. This is indicative of smooth and stable maintenance therapeutic theophylline levels throughout a q12h dosing interval.

Indications: Symptomatic relief and/or prevention of asthma and reversible bronchospasm associated with chronic bronchitis and emphysema.

Contraindications: SUSTAIRE is contraindicated in individuals who have shown hypersensitivity to any of its components or xanthine derivatives.

Warnings: Excessive theophylline doses may be associated with toxicity; serum theophylline levels should be monitored to assure maximum benefit with minimum risk. Incidence of toxicity increases at serum levels greater than 20 mcg/ml. High blood levels of theophylline resulting from conventional doses are correlated with clinical manifestations of toxicity in patients with lowered body plasma clearances, patients with liver dysfunction or chronic obstructive lung disease, and patients who are older than 55 years of age—particularly males. There are often no early signs of less serious theophylline toxicity such as nausea and restlessness, which may be the first signs of toxicity. Many patients who have higher theophylline serum levels exhibit a tachycardia. Theophylline products may worsen pre-existing arrhythmias.

Usage in Pregnancy: Safe use in pregnancy has not been established relative to possible adverse effects on fetal development, but neither have adverse effects on fetal development been established. This is, unfortunately, true for most anti-asthmatic medications. Therefore, use of theophylline in pregnant women should be balanced against the risk of uncontrolled asthma.

Precautions: SUSTAIRE TABLETS SHOULD NOT BE CHEWED OR CRUSHED.
Theophylline should not be administered concurrently with other xanthine medications. It should be used with caution in patients with severe cardiac disease, severe hypoxemia, hypertension, hyperthyroidism, acute myocardial injury, cor pulmonale, congestive heart failure, liver disease, in the elderly (particularly males), and in neonates. Great caution should be used in giving theophylline to patients in congestive heart failure since these patients show markedly prolonged theophylline blood level curves. Use theophylline cautiously in patients with history of peptic ulcer. Theophylline may occasionally act as a local irritant to the G.I. tract although gastrointestinal symptoms are more commonly central and associated with high serum concentrations above 20 mcg/ml.

Adverse Reactions: The most consistent adverse reactions are usually due to overdose and are:
Gastrointestinal: nausea, vomiting, epigastric pain, hematemesis, diarrhea.
Central Nervous System: headaches, irritability, restlessness, insomnia, reflex hyperexcitability, muscle twitching, clonic and tonic generalized convulsions.
Cardiovascular: palpitation, tachycardia, extrasystoles, flushing, hypotension, circulatory failure, life threatening ventricular arrhythmias.
Respiratory: tachypnea
Renal: albuminuria, increased excretion of renal tubular cells and red blood cells; potentiation of diuresis.
Others: hyperglycemia and inappropriate ADH syndrome.

Drug Interactions:

Drug	Effect
Theophylline with Furosemide	Increased diuresis
Theophylline with Hexamethonium	Decreased chronotropic effect
Theophylline with Reserpine	Tachycardia
Theophylline with Cyclamycin, TAO® (troleandomycin) Erythromycin or Lincomycin	Increased theophylline blood levels

Overdosage:
Management

A. If potential oral overdose is established and seizure has not occurred:
1) Induce vomiting.
2) Administer a cathartic. (This is particularly important if sustained release preparations have been taken.)
3) Administer activated charcoal.

B. Patient is having a seizure:
1) Establish an airway.
2) Administer O_2
3) Treat the seizure with intravenous diazepam: 0.1 to 0.3 mg/kg up to 10 mg.
4) Monitor vital signs. Maintain blood pressure and provide adequate hydration.

C. Post Seizure Coma:
1) Maintain airway and oxygenation.
2) If a result of oral medication, follow above recommendations to prevent absorption of drug; but intubation and lavage will have to be performed instead of inducing emesis, and the cathartic and charcoal will need to be introduced via a large bore gastric lavage tube.
3) Continue to provide full supportive care and adequate hydration while waiting for drug to be metabolized. In general, the drug is metabolized sufficiently rapidly so as to not warrant consideration of dialysis.

Dosage and Administration: Therapeutic serum levels associated with optimal likelihood for benefit and minimal risk of toxicity are considered to be between 10 and 20 mcg/ml. There is a great variation from patient to patient in dosage needed in order to achieve a therapeutic blood level due to variable rates of elimination. Because of this wide variation from patient to patient, and the relatively narrow therapeutic range, dosage must be individualized.
THE AVERAGE INITIAL CHILDREN'S (UNDER 9 YEARS OF AGE) DOSE IS ONE SUSTAIRE 100 mg TABLET q12h.
THE AVERAGE INITIAL CHILDREN'S (AGES 9–12) DOSE IS ONE HALF (150 mg) OF A SUSTAIRE 300 mg TABLET q12h.
THE AVERAGE INITIAL ADOLESCENT (AGES 12–16) DOSE IS TWO SUSTAIRE 100 mg TABLETS q12h.
THE AVERAGE INITIAL ADULT DOSE IS ONE SUSTAIRE 300 mg TABLET q12h.
If the desired response is not achieved with the above AVERAGE INITIAL DOSAGE recommendations and there are no adverse reactions, the dose may be safely increased by 2–3 mg/kg body weight per day at 3 day intervals until the following MAXIMUM DOSE WITHOUT MEASUREMENT OF SERUM CONCENTRATION or a maximum of 900 mg in any 24 hour period, whichever is less, is attained:
[See table left].
If doses higher than those contained in the above MAXIMUM DOSE WITHOUT MEAS-

Maximum Dose Without Measurement Of Serum Concentration

	mg per kg body weight*	dose per interval
Children (under 9)	24 mg per day	12 mg q12h**
Children (9–12)	20 mg per day	10 mg q12h
Adolescents (12–16)	18 mg per day	9 mg q12h
Adults	13 mg per day	6.5 mg q12h

*Use ideal body weight for obese patients.
**Some children under 9 may require 8 mg q8h.

UREMENT OF SERUM CONCENTRATION are necessary, it is recommended that serum theophylline levels be monitored. Check serum theophylline levels between 3 and 8 hours after a dose. It is important that the patient will have missed *no* doses during the previous 72 hours and that dosing intervals will have been reasonably typical with *no* added doses during that period of time. DOSAGE ADJUSTMENT BASED ON SERUM THEOPHYLLINE MEASUREMENTS WHEN THESE INSTRUCTIONS HAVE NOT BEEN FOLLOWED, MAY RESULT IN RECOMMENDATIONS THAT PRESENT RISK OF TOXICITY TO THE PATIENT.

How Supplied: SUSTAIRE 100 mg and 300 mg Sustained Release Tablets are available in bottles of 100, and Unit-dose packages of 100 (10 × 10's).

Storage Conditions: Keep tightly closed. Store at controlled room temperature 15–30° C (59–86° F).

[*Shown in Product Identification Section*]

TAO® ℞

(troleandomycin)
Capsules and Oral Suspension

Description: TAO (troleandomycin) is a synthetically derived acetylated ester of oleandomycin, an antibiotic elaborated by a species of *Streptomyces antibioticus.* It is a white crystalline compound, insoluble in water, but readily soluble and stable in the presence of gastric juice. The compound has a molecular weight of 814 and corresponds to the empirical formula $C_{41}H_{67}NO_{15}$.

Actions: TAO is an antibiotic shown to be active *in vitro* against the following gram-positive organisms:
Streptococcus pyogenes
Diplococcus pneumoniae

Susceptibility plate testing: If the Kirby-Bauer method of disc sensitivity is used, a 15 mcg. oleandomycin disc should give a zone of over 18 mm. when tested against a troleandomycin sensitive bacterial strain.

Indications:
Diplococcus pneumoniae
Pneumococcal pneumonia due to susceptible strains.
Streptococcus pyogenes
Group A beta-hemolytic streptococcal infections of the upper respiratory tract.

Injectable benzathine penicillin G is considered by the American Heart Association to be the drug of choice in the treatment and prevention of streptococcal pharyngitis and in long term prophylaxis of rheumatic fever.

Troleandomycin is generally effective in the eradication of streptococci from the nasopharynx. However, substantial data establishing the efficacy of TAO in the subsequent prevention of rheumatic fever are not available at present.

Contraindications: Troleandomycin is contraindicated in patients with known hypersensitivity to this antibiotic.

Warnings: Usage in Pregnancy: Safety for use in pregnancy has not been established.

The administration of troleandomycin has been associated with an allergic type of cholestatic hepatitis. Some patients receiving troleandomycin for more than two weeks or in repeated courses have shown jaundice accompanied by right upper quadrant pain, fever, nausea, vomiting, eosinophilia, and leukocytosis. The changes have been reversible on discontinuance of the drug. Liver function tests should be monitored in patients on such dosage, and the drug discontinued if abnormalities develop. Reports in the literature have suggested that the concurrent use of ergotamine-containing drugs and troleandomycin may induce ischemic reactions. Therefore, the concurrent use of ergotamine-containing drugs and troleandomycin should be avoided.

Studies in chronic asthmatic patients have suggested that the concurrent use of theophylline and troleandomycin may result in elevated serum concentrations of theophylline. Therefore, it is recommended that patients receiving such concurrent therapy be observed for signs of theophylline toxicity, and that therapy be appropriately modified if such signs develop.

Precautions: Troleandomycin is principally excreted by the liver.

Caution should be exercised in administering the antibiotic to patients with impaired hepatic function.

Adverse Reactions: The most frequent side effects of troleandomycin preparations are gastrointestinal, such as abdominal cramping and discomfort, and are dose related. Nausea, vomiting, and diarrhea occur infrequently with usual oral doses.

During prolonged or repeated therapy, there is a possibility of overgrowth of nonsusceptible bacteria or fungi. If such infections occur, the drug should be discontinued and appropriate therapy instituted.

Mild allergic reactions such as urticaria and other skin rashes have occurred. Serious allergic reactions, including anaphylaxis, have been reported.

Dosage and Administration: Clinical judgment based on the type of infection and its severity should determine dosage within the below listed ranges.

Adults: 250 to 500 mg. 4 times a day
Children: 125 to 250 mg. (3-5 mg./lb. or 6.6 to 11 mg./kg.) every 6 hours

When used in streptococcal infection, therapy should be continued for ten days.

How Supplied:
TAO is supplied as:
Capsules 250 mg.: Each capsule contains troleandomycin equivalent to 250 mg. of oleandomycin; bottle of 100 capsules.
Ready-Mixed Oral Suspension: Each teaspoonful (5 ml.) contains troleandomycin equivalent to 125 mg. of oleandomycin; 60 ml. bottle and pint bottle.

[*Shown in Product Identification Section*]

UROBIOTIC®-250 ℞

Each capsule contains
Oxytetracycline hydrochloride equivalent to 250 mg. oxytetracycline
Sulfamethizole ....250 mg.
Phenazopyridine hydrochloride ....50 mg.

CAPSULES

Actions: Urobiotic-250 is a product designed for use specifically in urinary tract infections. Terramycin (oxytetracycline HCl) is a widely used antibiotic with clinically proved activity against gram-positive and gram-negative bacteria, rickettsiae, spirochetes, large viruses, and certain protozoa. Terramycin is well tolerated and well absorbed after oral administration. It diffuses readily through the placenta and is present in the fetal circulation. It diffuses into the pleural fluid, and under some circumstances, into the cerebrospinal fluid. Oxytetracycline HCl appears to be concentrated in the hepatic system and is excreted in the bile. It is excreted in the urine and in the feces, in high concentrations, in a biologically active form.

Sulfamethizole is a chemotherapeutic agent active against a number of important gram-positive and gram-negative bacteria. This sulfonamide is well absorbed, has a low degree of acetylation, and is extremely soluble. Because of these features and its rapid renal excretion, sulfamethizole has a low order of toxicity and provides prompt and high concentrations of the active drug in the urinary tract.

Phenazopyridine is an orally absorbed agent which produces prompt and effective local analgesia and relief of urinary symptoms by virtue of its rapid excretion in the urinary tract. These effects are confined to the genitourinary system and are not accompanied by generalized sedation or narcosis.

Indications

Based on a review of this drug by the National Academy of Sciences-National Research Council and/or other information, FDA has classified the indications as follows:

"Lacking substantial evidence of effectiveness as a fixed combination":

Urobiotic-250 is indicated in the therapy of a number of genitourinary infections caused by susceptible organisms. These infections include the following: pyelonephritis, pyelitis, ureteritis, cystitis, prostatitis, and urethritis.

Since both Terramycin and sulfamethizole provide effective levels in blood, tissue, and urine, Urobiotic-250 provides a multiple antimicrobial approach at the site of infection. Both antibacterial components are active against the most common urinary pathogens, including *Escherichia coli, Pseudomonas aeruginosa, Aerobacter aerogenes, Streptococcus faecalis, Streptococcus hemolyticus, and Micrococcus pyogenes.* Urobiotic-250 is particularly useful in the treatment of infections caused by bacteria more sensitive to the combination than to either component alone. The combination is also of value in those cases with mixed infections, and in those instances where the causative organism is unknown pending laboratory isolation.

Final classification of the less than effective indications require further investigation. Clinical studies to substantiate the efficacy of Urobiotic-250 are ongoing. Completion of these ongoing studies will provide data for final classification of these indications.

Contraindications: This drug is contraindicated in individuals who have shown hypersensitivity to any of its components.

This drug, because of the sulfonamide component, should not be used in patients with a history of sulfonamide sensitivities, and in pregnant females at term.

Warnings: If renal impairment exists, even usual oral or parenteral doses may lead to excessive systemic accumulation of the drug and possible liver toxicity. Under such conditions, lower than usual doses are indicated and if therapy is prolonged, tetracycline serum level determinations may be advisable.

Oxytetracycline HCl, which is one of the ingredients of Urobiotic-250, may form a stable calcium complex in any bone-forming tissue with no serious harmful effects reported thus far in humans. However, use of oxytetracycline during tooth development (last trimester of pregnancy, neonatal period and early childhood) may cause discoloration of the teeth (yellow-grey-brownish). This effect occurs mostly during long term use of the drug but it also has been observed in usual short treatment courses.

Because of its sulfonamide content, this drug should be used only after critical appraisal in patients with liver damage, renal damage, urinary obstruction, or blood dyscrasias. Deaths have been reported from hypersensitivity reactions, agranulocytosis, aplastic anemia, and other blood dyscrasias associated with sulfonamide administration. When used intermittently, or for a prolonged period, blood counts and liver and kidney function tests should be performed.

Certain hypersensitive individuals may develop a photodynamic reaction precipitated by exposure to direct sunlight during the use of this drug. This reaction is usually of the photoallergic type which may also be produced by

Continued on next page

Roerig—Cont.

other tetracycline derivatives. Individuals with a history of photosensitivity reactions should be instructed to avoid exposure to direct sunlight while under treatment with this or other tetracycline drugs, and treatment should be discontinued at first evidence of skin discomfort.
NOTE: Reactions of a photoallergic nature are exceedingly rare with Terramycin (oxytetracycline HCl). Phototoxic reactions are not believed to occur with Terramycin.
Precautions: As with all antibiotic preparations, use of this drug may result in overgrowth of nonsusceptible organisms, including fungi. If superinfection occurs, the antibiotic should be discontinued and appropriate specific therapy should be instituted. This drug should be used with caution in persons having histories of significant allergies and/or asthma.
Adverse Reactions: Glossitis, stomatitis, proctitis, nausea, diarrhea, vaginitis, and dermatitis, as well as reactions of an allergic nature, may occur during oxytetracycline HCl therapy, but are rare. If adverse reactions, individual idiosyncrasy, or allergy occur, discontinue medication. Rare instances of esophagitis and esophageal ulcerations have been reported in patients receiving capsule forms of drugs in the tetracycline class. Most of these patients took medications immediately before going to bed. (See Dosage and Administration.)
With oxytetracycline therapy bulging fontanels in infants and benign intracranial hypertension in adults have been reported in individuals receiving full therapeutic dosages. These conditions disappeared rapidly when the drug was discontinued.
As in all sulfonamide therapy, the following reactions may occur: nausea, vomiting, diarrhea, hepatitis, pancreatitis, blood dyscrasias, neuropathy, drug fever, skin rash, injection of the conjunctiva and sclera, petechiae, purpura, hematuria and crystalluria. The dosage should be decreased or the drug withdrawn, depending upon the severity of the reaction.
Dosage and Administration: Urobiotic-250 is recommended in adults only. A dose of 1 capsule four times daily is suggested. In refractory cases 2 capsules four times a day may be used. Therapy should be continued for a minimum of seven days or until bacteriologic cure in acute urinary tract infections.
Administration of adequate amounts of fluid along with capsule forms of drugs in the tetracycline class is recommended to wash down the drugs and reduce the risk of esophageal irritation and ulceration. (See Adverse Reactions.)
To aid absorption of the drug, it should be given at least one hour before or two hours after eating. Aluminum hydroxide gel given with antibiotics has been shown to decrease their absorption and is contraindicated.
Supply: Urobiotic-250 capsules: bottles of 50, and unit dose packages of 100 (10 x 10's).
Literature Available: Yes.
[*Shown in Product Identification Section*]

IDENTIFICATION PROBLEM?

Consult PDR's

Product Identification Section

where you'll find over 900

products pictured actual size

and in full color.

William H. Rorer, Inc.

500 VIRGINIA DRIVE
FORT WASHINGTON, PA 19034

ANANASE® ℞

(bromelains)
Anti-inflammatory enzyme

Description: Ananase (bromelains) is a concentrate of proteolytic enzymes derived from the pineapple plant. Each yellow, enteric coated tablet (Ananase-50) contains 50,000 Rorer Units*. Each orange, enteric coated tablet (Ananase-100) contains 100,000 Rorer Units*.
Actions: Ananase as adjunctive therapy is designed to supplement and augment standard therapeutic procedures for reduction of inflammation and edema, to ease pain, speed healing and accelerate tissue repair. This is the basic purpose of proteolytic enzyme therapy in general.
While the mode of action of proteolytic enzymes has not been finally established, it seems most probable that depolymerization of fibrin and permeability modifications of venules and lymphatics underlie the action.

Indications: Based on a review of this drug by the National Academy of Sciences—National Research Council and/or other information, FDA has classified the indications as follows:
"Possibly effective" for relieving symptomatology related to episiotomy.
"Lacking substantial evidence of effectiveness" for reduction of inflammation and edema in postoperative tissue reactions and in accidental trauma.
Final classification of the less-than-effective indications requires further investigation.

Contraindications: Contraindicated in patients known to be hypersensitive to the drug or to pineapple or its products.
Warnings: USE IN PREGNANCY—Safe use of this drug in pregnancy has not been established.
Due to limited clinical experience, the use of this drug in children 12 years of age and under is not recommended.
Keep this and all drugs out of the reach of children. In case of accidental overdose, seek professional assistance or contact a poison control center immediately.
Precautions: Ananase should be used with caution in patients with abnormalities of the blood clotting mechanism, such as hemophilia, or with severe hepatic or renal disease. Patients on anticoagulant therapy should be observed carefully because of possible potentiation of the anticoagulant effect by Ananase.
Adverse Reactions: While seldom observed, sensitivity manifested by urticaria or skin rash has occurred. There has been no report of anaphylactoid reaction. One case of hypofibrinogenemia and several cases of menorrhagia and metrorrhagia possibly related to the drug have been reported. Nausea, vomiting or diarrhea have rarely been reported. Adverse reactions are usually reversible upon discontinuation of the drug.
Dosage and Administration:
Usual adult dose: Initially, 100,000 units four times daily. For maintenance, 100,000 units twice daily, or 50,000 units four times daily.

* One Rorer Unit of protease activity is defined as that amount of enzyme which will so hydrolyze a standardized casein substrate at pH 7.0 and 25°C as to cause an increase in absorbance at 280 nm. of 1×10^{-5} per minute of reaction time.

How Supplied: Ananase®-50 (bromelains) is available as yellow tablets of 50,000 Rorer units in bottles of 100 tablets (NDC 0067-0120-68) and 500 tablets (NDC 0067-0120-74).
Ananase®-100 (bromelains) is available as orange tablets of 100,000 Rorer units in bottles of 100 tablets (NDC 0067-0122-68) and 500 tablets (NDC 0067-0122-74).
[*Shown in Product Identification Section*]

ASCRIPTIN®

Aspirin, Alumina and Magnesia Tablets, Rorer
Aspirin with Maalox®

Formula: Each tablet contains:
Aspirin .... (5 grains) 325 mg
Maalox®:
Magnesium Hydroxide .... 75 mg
Dried Aluminum Hydroxide Gel ..... 75 mg
Description: Ascriptin® is an excellent analgesic, antipyretic and anti-inflammatory agent for general use, particularly where there is concern over aspirin-induced gastric distress. When large doses are used, as in arthritis and rheumatic disorders, gastric discomfort is rare.
Indications: As an analgesic for the relief of pain in such conditions as headache, neuralgia, minor injuries and dysmenorrhea. As an analgesic and antipyretic in colds and influenza. As an analgesic and anti-inflammatory agent in arthritis and other rheumatic diseases. As an inhibitor of platelet aggregation, see TIA's indications.
Usual adult dose: Two or three tablets four times daily. For children under 12, at the discretion of the physician. As an inhibitor of platelet aggregation, see TIA's dosage information.
For Recurrent TIA's in Men
Indications: For reducing the risk of recurrent transient ischemic attacks (TIA's) or stroke in men who have had transient ischemia of the brain due to fibrin platelet emboli. There is inadequate evidence that aspirin or buffered aspirin is effective in reducing TIA's in women at the recommended dosage. There is no evidence that aspirin or buffered aspirin is of benefit in the treatment of completed strokes in men or women.
Precautions: (1) Patients presenting with signs and symptoms of TIA's should have a complete medical and neurologic evaluation. Consideration should be given to other disorders which resemble TIA's.
(2) Attention should be given to risk factors: it is important to evaluate and treat, if appropriate, other diseases associated with TIA's and stroke such as hypertension and diabetes.
(3) Concurrent administration of absorbable antacids at therapeutic doses may increase the clearance of salicylates in some individuals. The concurrent administration of nonabsorbable antacids may alter the rate of absorption of aspirin, thereby resulting in a decreased acetylsalicylic acid/salicylate ratio in plasma. The clinical significance on TIA's of these decreases in available aspirin is unknown.
Dosage: 1300 mg a day, in divided doses of 650 mg twice a day or 325 mg four times a day.
Warning: Keep this and all drugs out of the reach of children. In case of accidental overdose, seek professional assistance or contact a poison control center immediately.
Supplied: Bottles of 50 tablets (NDC 0067-0135-50), 100 tablets (NDC 0067-0135-68), and 225 tablets (NDC 0067-0135-77) with child-resistant caps. Bottles of 500 tablets (NDC 0067-0135-74) without child-resistant closures (for arthritic patients). Military Stock #NSN 6505-00-135-2783. V.A. Stock #6505-00-890-1979A (bottles of 500).
[*Shown in Product Identification Section*]

ASCRIPTIN® A/D Arthritic Doses
Aspirin, Alumina and Magnesia Tablets, Rorer
Aspirin with Maalox® for increased buffering in Arthritic Doses
Aspirin, Alumina and Magnesia Tablets, Rorer

Formula: Each capsule shaped tablet contains:

Aspirin .... (5 grains) 325 mg
Maalox®:
Magnesium Hydroxide .... 150 mg
Dried Aluminum Hydroxide Gel ... 150 mg

Description: Ascriptin® A/D is a highly buffered analgesic, anti-inflammatory and antipyretic agent for use in the treatment of rheumatoid arthritis, osteoarthritis and other arthritic conditions. It is formulated with added Maalox® to provide increased neutralization of gastric acid thus improving the likelihood of GI tolerance when large antiarthritic doses of aspirin are used.

Indications: As an analgesic, anti-inflammatory and antipyretic agent in rheumatoid arthritis, osteoarthritis and other arthritic conditions.

Usual Adult Dose: Two or three tablets, four times daily, or as directed by the physician for arthritis therapy. For children under twelve, at the discretion of the physician.

Drug Interaction Precaution: Do not use if patient is taking a tetracycline antibiotic.

Warning: Keep this and all drugs out of the reach of children. In case of accidental overdose, seek professional assistance or contact a poison control center immediately.

Supplied: Available in bottles of 100 tablets (NDC 0067-0137-68), and 225 tablets (NDC 0067-0137-77) with child-resistant caps and in special bottles of 500 tablets (without child-resistant closures) for arthritic patients (NDC 0067-0137-74).

[*Shown in Product Identification Section*]

ASCRIPTIN® WITH CODEINE Ⓒ ℞
for the relief of severe pain...
with the protection of Maalox®

Description—Tablets for Oral Use:

Ascriptin® with Codeine No. 2. Each white tablet contains aspirin 325 mg; codeine phosphate 15 mg and Maalox® (magnesium hydroxide and dried aluminum hydroxide) 150 mg.

Ascriptin® with Codeine No. 3. Each white tablet contains aspirin 325 mg; codeine phosphate 30 mg and Maalox® (magnesium hydroxide and dried aluminum hydroxide) 150 mg.

Ascriptin® with Codeine is an analgesic, antipyretic, and anti-inflammatory designed to give effective relief from severe pain with minimal aspirin-induced gastric distress.

Aspirin, a salicylate, occurs as a white odorless, crystalline powder which possesses a slightly bitter taste. Aspirin is an analgesic, anti-inflammatory and antipyretic.

Codeine is an alkaloid obtained from opium (or prepared from morphine by methylation) and occurs as colorless or white crystals. Codeine effloresces slowly in dry air and is affected by light. Codeine is an analgesic and an antitussive.

In addition, Maalox® is added to the formula to help reduce gastric distress caused by aspirin. Studies show that the addition of Maalox® has no effect on the bioavailability of the two active drugs.

Clinical Pharmacology: Aspirin alleviates pain both centrally and peripherally. Orally ingested salicylates are absorbed rapidly, partly from the stomach but mostly from the small intestine. Appreciable concentrations are found in plasma in less than 30 minutes; after a single dose, a peak value is reached in about 2 hours and then gradually declines. Rate of absorption is determined by many factors, particularly the disintegration and dissolution rates if tablets are given, the pH at the mucosal surfaces, and gastric emptying time. In man, the absorption half-time for unbuffered aspirin is about 30 minutes, for buffered aspirin about 20 minutes, and for an aspirin solution only slightly less. What differences do exist probably have no therapeutic significance, since the rate-limiting factor in the onset of effects is accumulation of these drugs at their sites of action. The presence of food delays absorption of salicylates.

The biotransformation of aspirin takes place mainly in the liver and normally follows first-order kinetics. Salicylates are excreted mainly by the kidney. Codeine is a narcotic analgesic. Once absorbed, it is metabolized by the liver and excreted chiefly in the urine, largely in inactive forms. A small fraction (approximately 10%) of administered codeine is demethylated to form morphine, and both free and conjugated morphine can be found in the urine after therapeutic doses of codeine. Codeine has an exceptionally low affinity for the opioid receptor, and the analgesic effect of codeine may be due to its conversion to morphine. The half-life of codeine in plasma is 2.5 to 3 hours.

Maalox® provides neutralization of gastric acid, thus increasing the likelihood of G.I. tolerance with the aspirin component.

Indications: Ascriptin® with Codeine No. 2 and Ascriptin® with Codeine No. 3 are indicated for the relief of pain of all degrees of severity up to that which requires morphine.

Contraindications: Hypersensitivity or allergy to aspirin or codeine.

Warnings: Usage in ambulatory patients. Ascriptin® with Codeine may impair the mental and/or physical abilities required for the performance of potentially hazardous tasks such as driving a car or operating machinery. The patient using this drug should be cautioned accordingly.

Interaction with other central nervous system depressants. Patients receiving other narcotic analgesics, general anesthetics, phenothiazines, tranquilizers, sedative-hynotics or other CNS depressants (including alcohol) concomitantly with Ascriptin® with Codeine may exhibit an additive CNS depression. When such combined therapy is contemplated, the dose of one or both agents should be reduced. Do not use if patient is taking a tetracycline antibiotic.

Precautions: Usage in pregnancy. PREGNANCY CATEGORY C—Animal reproduction studies have not been conducted with **Ascriptin® with Codeine.** It is also not known whether **Ascriptin® with Codeine** can cause fetal harm when administered to pregnant women or can affect reproduction capacity. **Ascriptin® with Codeine** should be given to a pregnant woman only if clearly needed. It is not known whether this drug is excreted in human milk. Because many drugs are excreted in human milk, caution should be exercised when Ascriptin® with Codeine is administered to nursing women.

Head injury and increased intracranial pressure: The respiratory depressant effects of narcotics and their capability to elevate cerebrospinal fluid pressure may be markedly exaggerated in the presence of head injury, other intracranial lesions or a pre-existing increase in intracranial pressure. Furthermore, narcotics produce adverse reactions which may obscure the clinical course of patients with head injuries.

Acute abdominal conditions: The administration of **Ascriptin® with Codeine** or other narcotics may obscure the diagnosis or clinical course in patients with acute abdominal conditions.

History of allergy: Patients who have a history of allergies may also be hypersensitive or intolerant to aspirin. A history of reaction to other chemicals, asthma or the occurrence of nasal polyps are warning signs. Epinephrine is the drug of choice to treat a reaction should one occur.

Special risk patients: Codeine should be given with caution to certain patients such as the elderly or debilitated and those with severe impairment of hepatic or renal function, hypothyroidism, Addison's disease, and prostatic hypertrophy or urethral stricture. Long-term animal studies to determine carcinogenicity of the ingredients in **Ascriptin® with Codeine** have not been carried out.

Safety and effectiveness in children under 12 years of age, have not been established.

Adverse Reactions: The most frequently observed adverse reactions to codeine include lightheadedness, dizziness, sleepiness, nausea and vomiting. These effects seem to be more prominent in ambulatory than in nonambulatory patients, and some of these adverse reactions may be alleviated if the patient lies down. Less frequent adverse reactions include euphoria, dysphoria, constipation and pruritus.

The most frequently observed reactions to aspirin include headache, vertigo, ringing in the ears, mental confusion, drowsiness, sweating, thirst, nausea, and vomiting. Occasionally, patients experience gastric irritation and bleeding with aspirin. Some patients are unable to take salicylates without developing nausea and vomiting. Hypersensitivity may be manifested by a skin rash or even an anaphylactic reaction. Most of the side effects of aspirin occur only after repeated administration of large doses.

Drug Abuse and Dependence: Codeine can produce drug dependence of the morphine type, and therefore, has the potential for being abused. Psychic dependence, physical dependence and tolerance may develop upon repeated administration of this drug and it should be prescribed and administered with the same degree of caution appropriate to the user of other oral narcotic-containing medications. Like other narcotic-containing medications, the drug is subject to the Federal Controlled Substances Act.

Management of Overdosage: Signs and Symptoms: Serious overdose with **Ascriptin® with Codeine** is characterized by respiratory depression (a decrease in respiratory rate and/ or tidal volume. Cheyne-Stokes respiration, cyanosis), extreme somnolence progressing to stupor or coma, skeletal muscle flaccidity, cold and clammy skin, and sometimes bradycardia and hypotension. In severe overdosage, apnea, circulatory collapse, cardiac arrest and death may occur. The ingestion of very large amounts of this drug may, in addition, result in acute hepatic toxicity.

Treatment: Primary attention should be given to the reestablishment of adequate respiratory exchange through provision of a patent airway and the institution of assisted or controlled ventilation. The narcotic antagonist, naloxone, is a specific antidote against respiratory depression which may result from overdosage or unusual sensitivity to narcotics, including codeine. Therefore, an appropriate dose of naloxone (usual initial adult dose: 0.4 mg) should be administered, preferably by the intravenous route, and simultaneously with efforts at respiratory resuscitation. Since the duration of action of codeine may exceed that of the antagonist, the patient should be kept under continued surveillance and repeated doses of the antagonist should be administered as needed to maintain adequate respiration.

Continued on next page

This product information was prepared in August 1982. Information concerning these products may be obtained by addressing William H. Rorer, 500 Virginia Drive, Fort Washington, PA 19034.

Rorer—Cont.

An antagonist should not be administered in the absence of clinically significant respiratory or cardiovascular depression.
Oxygen, intravenous fluids, vasopressors and other supportive measures should be employed as indicated.
Gastric emptying may be useful in removing unabsorbed drug.
Salicylate poisoning represents an acute medical emergency. The treatment is largely symptomatic. From 10 to 30 g of aspirin has caused death in adults, but much larger amounts (130 g of aspirin, in one case) have been ingested without fatal outcome.
Initial therapy must be directed to correction of hyperthemia, dehydration and maintenance of adequate renal function. Intravenous fluids should be administered promptly, the type and amount based on interpretation of laboratory data on acid-base balance.
Measures to rid the body rapidly of salicylate should be immediately undertaken. Sodium bicarbonate administration is effective and rapid, if an alkaline urine can be produced. Forced diuresis with alkalinizing solution appears to be better than alkali alone; acetazolamide can be added to this combination if a more rapid effect is necessary and only if systemic acidosis is avoided. Potassium should be administered with the bicarbonate to prevent further depletion of intracellular potassium.
In severe intoxication, extrarenal measures such as exchange transfusion, peritoneal dialysis, hemodialysis, and hemoperfusion are the most effective measures available for the removal of salicylate. Hemodialysis in adults and older children and exchange transfusion or peritoneal dialysis in infants should be considered seriously in all salicylate-intoxicated patients whose clinical condition is deteriorating despite otherwise appropriate therapy and in those who have associated serious disease.
Dosage and Administration: Dosage should be adjusted according to the severity of the pain and the response of the patient. It may occasionally be necessary to exceed the usual dosage recommended below in cases of more severe pain or in those patients who have become tolerant to the analgesic effect of narcotics.
Ascriptin® with Codeine is given orally.
Usual Adult Dose: Ascriptin® with Codeine No. 2—two tablets every 3 to 4 hours when necessary. **Ascriptin® with Codeine No. 3**—one or two tablets every 3 to 4 hours as necessary.
Drug Interactions: The CNS depressant effect of **Ascriptin® with Codeine** may be additive with that of other CNS depressants. See WARNINGS.
Keep this and all drugs out of the reach of children. In case of accidental overdose, seek professional assistance or contact a poison control center immediately.
Ascriptin® with Codeine No. 2: (Aspirin 325 mg, Maalox® 150 mg, codeine phosphate 15 mg) is available in bottles of 100 tablets. Tablets are marked on one side with the name Rorer and the Identification Number 142; the other side displays the number 2. (NDC 0067-0142-68)
Ascriptin® with Codeine No. 3: (Aspirin 325 mg, Maalox® 150 mg, codeine phosphate 30 mg) in bottles of 100 tablets. Tablets are marked on one side with the name Rorer and the Identification Number 143; the other side displays the number 3. (NDC 0067-0143-68) DEA number required.
[*Shown in Product Identification Section*]

CAMALOX®
High-potency antacid

Description: Camalox® Suspension is a carefully balanced formulation of 200 mg. magnesium hydroxide, 225 mg. aluminum hydroxide and 250 mg. calcium carbonate per teaspoonful (5 ml). This combination of ingredients produces an antacid capability that exceeds that of other leading ethical products in terms of quantity of acid neutralized as well as the speed and duration of antacid activity as measured by laboratory tests. The formulation also minimizes the possibilities of both constipation and diarrhea. Camalox is prepared by a unique process*. This process enhances its texture and vanilla-mint flavor, making it especially palatable even for patients who must take antacids for extended periods.
Camalox® Tablets contain 200 mg. magnesium hydroxide, 225 mg. aluminum hydroxide and 250 mg. calcium carbonate per tablet and have a delicate vanilla-mint flavor. They compare favorably with Camalox Suspension in terms of potency, as well as speed and duration of antacid activity, thus, Camalox Tablets overcome the usual deficiencies of antacid tablets. As measured by the *in vitro* test for acid neutralizing capacity, Camalox Tablets exceed the antacid capabilities of the leading ethical antacid suspensions as well as tablets. In addition, the special manufacturing process* developed by Rorer contributes importantly to the flavor and to the texture of the tablets. Patients can take Camalox Tablets in full dosage day after day without tiring of the taste.
Acid Neutralizing Capacity
Camalox Suspension—36.0 mEq/2 teaspoonfuls
Camalox Tablets—36.0 mEq/2 tablets
Sodium Content
Camalox Suspension—2.5 mg/5 ml
Camalox Tablets—1.5 mg/tablet
Indications: A high potency antacid for the symptomatic relief of hyperacidity associated with the diagnosis of peptic ulcer, gastritis, peptic esophagitis, gastric hyperacidity, heartburn or hiatal hernia.
Directions for Use: Camalox Suspension—two to four teaspoonfuls, four times a day, taken one-half hour after meals and at bedtime, or as directed by a physician.
Camalox Tablets—each Camalox Tablet is equivalent to one teaspoonful of Camalox Suspension. Two to four tablets, well-chewed, one-half to one hour after meals and at bedtime, or as directed by a physician.
Patient Warnings: Do not take more than 16 teaspoonfuls or tablets in a 24-hour period or use the maximum dosage for more than two weeks or use if you have kidney disease except under the advice and supervision of a physician. Keep this and all drugs out of the reach of children. In case of accidental overdose, seek professional assistance or contact a poison control center immediately.
DRUG INTERACTION PRECAUTION: Do not use with patients taking a prescription antibiotic drug containing any form of tetracycline or phenytoin. As with all aluminum-containing antacids, Camalox may prevent the proper absorption of tetracycline or phenytoin.
How Supplied: Camalox Suspension—white liquid in convenient 12 fluid ounce (355 ml) plastic bottles (NDC 0067-0180-71).
Camalox Tablets—Bottles of 50 tablets (NDC 0067-0185-50).
Rationale: Recent studies reveal that clinical symptoms of gastroesophageal reflux correlate with lower esophageal sphincter (LES) incompetency. Although the mechanism of action is unknown, gastric alkalinization has been shown to increase LES pressure.
Camalox is an ideal antacid for the treatment of reflux esophagitis. The balanced formulation of Camalox exerts its neutralizing effect faster and longer than the leading ethical antacids providing prompt symptomatic relief.
Camalox has been shown to produce significant increases in LES pressure providing a physiological barrier against reflux.**
Because Camalox is a high potency antacid with excellent acid neutralizing capacity, fewer and smaller doses are possible.
The refreshing vanilla-mint flavor and smooth texture of Camalox have earned a high level of patient acceptance and wearability. Available in equally effective dosage forms . . . physician-preferred suspension and convenient tablets.

---

*Patent No. 3,843,778
**Higgs, R.H., Smyth, R.D., and Castell, D.O., Gastric Alkalinization—Effect on Lower-Esophageal-Sphincter Pressure and Serum Gastrin, N. Engl. J. Med. *291*:486-490, 1974.
[*Camalox Tablets shown in Product Identification Section*]

CHARDONNA®-2 ℞
brand of belladonna extract with phenobarbital

REFORMULATED WITHOUT CHARCOAL

Description: Each Chardonna-2 tablet contains: phenobarbital 15 mg (WARNING: may be habit forming) and belladonna extract 15 mg.
Actions: Chardonna-2 tablets produce antispasmodic, antisecretory and sedative effects. Belladonna acts to inhibit gastric secretion and gastrointestinal motility. The sedative action of phenobarbital allays anxiety accompanying functional gastrointestinal disorders.

Indications: Based on a review of similar drugs by the National Academy of Sciences-National Research Council and/or other information, FDA has classified the indications as follows:
"Possibly effective" as adjunctive therapy in the treatment of peptic ulcer and "possibly effective" in the treatment of irritable bowel syndrome (irritable colon, spastic colon, mucous colitis) and acute enterocolitis.
Final classification of less-than-effective indications requires further investigation.

Contraindications: Chardonna-2 is contraindicated in persons with a known intolerance to any of the ingredients, a history of porphyria or marked impairment of hepatic or renal function, respiratory disease in the presence of dyspnea or obstruction, glaucoma or obstructive uropathy.
Precautions: Use with caution in patients with increased intraocular pressure, prostatic hypertrophy or moderate hepatic or renal disease. Barbiturates are known to stimulate hepatic microsomal enzymes and alter metabolism of certain drugs. Therefore, Chardonna-2 should be used with caution in patients on anticoagulant or corticosteroid therapy. Elderly or debilitated persons may react to barbiturates with marked excitement or depression. Patients should also be warned about the combined effects of central nervous system depressant drugs and alcohol.
Adverse Reactions: Blurred vision, dry mouth, vertigo, tachycardia, urinary retention, flushing or dryness of the skin, drowsiness, lethargy, headache, skin eruptions, nausea and vomiting.
Adult Dosage: Usually given one-half hour before meals and at bedtime. One or two tablets, q.i.d.
Warning: Keep this and all drugs out of the reach of children. In case of accidental overdose, seek professional assistance or contact a poison control center immediately.
Supplied: Bottles of 100 (NDC 0067-0202-68). DEA number required.
[*Shown in Product Identification Section*]

EMETROL®

For nausea and vomiting

Description: Emetrol is an oral solution containing balanced amounts of levulose (fructose) and dextrose (glucose) and orthophosphoric acid with controlled hydrogen ion concentration. Pleasantly mint flavored.

Action: Emetrol quickly relieves nausea and vomiting by local action on the wall of the hyperactive G.I. tract. It reduces smooth-muscle contraction in direct proportion to the amount used. Unlike systemic antiemetics, Emetrol works almost immediately to control both nausea and active vomiting—and it is free from toxicity or side effects.

Indications: For nausea and vomiting.

Advantages:

1. ***Fast action***—works almost immediately by local action on contact with the hyperactive G. I. tract.
2. ***Effectiveness***—reported completely effective in epidemic vomiting—reduces smooth-muscle contractions in direct proportion to the amount used—stops both nausea and active vomiting.
3. ***Safety***—no toxicity or side effects—won't mask symptoms of organic pathology.
4. ***Convenience***—can be recommended over the phone for any member of the family, even the children—no Rx required.
5. ***Patient acceptance***—a low cost that patients appreciate—a pleasant mint flavor that both children and adults like.

Usual dose: *Epidemic and other functional vomiting (intestinal "flu", G.I. grippe, etc.); or nausea and vomiting due to psychogenic factors:* Infants and children, one or two teaspoonfuls at 15 minute intervals until vomiting ceases; adults, one or two tablespoonfuls in same manner. If first dose is rejected, resume dosage schedule in five minutes. *Regurgitation in infants:* One or two teaspoonfuls ten or fifteen minutes before each feeding; in refractory cases, two or three teaspoonfuls one-half hour before feedings. *"Morning sickness":* One or two tablespoonfuls on arising, repeated every three hours or whenever nausea threatens.

Emetrol may also be used in motion sickness and in nausea and vomiting due to drug therapy or inhalation anesthesia; in teaspoonful dosage for young children, tablespoonful dosage for older children and adults.

Important: *DO NOT DILUTE or permit oral fluids immediately before or for at least 15 minutes after dose.*

Warning: Keep this and all drugs out of the reach of children. In case of accidental overdose, seek professional assistance or contact a poison control center immediately.

Supplied: Bottles of 3 fluid ounces (89 ml) (NDC 0067-0240-58) and 1 pint (473 ml) (NDC 0067-0240-74).

FEDAHIST® GYROCAPS®, SYRUP TABLETS, EXPECTORANT

Description: **Fedahist®** is a combination of pseudoephedrine hydrochloride (1-phenyl-2 methylaminopropan-1-ol hydrochloride) and chlorpheniramine maleate (2-[p-chloro-a(2-dimethylaminoethyl) benzyl] pyridine maleate 1:1) as an oral antihistamine-decongestant.

FEDAHIST® GYROCAPS® (timed release capsules) ℞

Each white and yellow capsule contains:
Pseudoephedrine Hydrochloride ....65 mg
Chlorpheniramine Maleate ....10 mg
in a special base that provides for a prolonged, therapeutic effect.

FEDAHIST® EXPECTORANT (NONALCOHOLIC)

Each 5 ml (teaspoonful) contains:
Guaifenesin ....100 mg
Pseudoephedrine Hydrochloride ....30 mg
Chlorpheniramine Maleate ....2 mg
in pleasant-tasting, cherry-flavored syrup.

FEDAHIST® TABLETS (SCORED, DYE-FREE)

Each tablet contains:
Pseudoephedrine Hydrochloride ....60 mg
Chlorpheniramine Maleate ....4 mg

FEDAHIST® SYRUP (NONALCOHOLIC)

Each 5 ml (teaspoonful) contains:
Pseudoephedrine Hydrochloride ....30 mg
Chlorpheniramine Maleate ....2 mg
in pleasant-tasting, grape-flavored syrup.

Clinical Pharmacology: **Fedahist®** provides the antihistaminic activity of chlorpheniramine maleate with the vasoconstrictive actions of pseudoephedrine hydrochloride.

At the recommended oral dosage, pseudoephedrine has little or no pressor effects in normotensive adults, and is not known to produce drowsiness.

Chlorpheniramine is an antihistamine which acts on H_1 receptors as an antagonist. It is well absorbed and has a duration of 4 to 6 hours. (The Gyrocaps® formulation provides a longer therapeutic effect up to 12 hours.) Plasma half-life is approximately 22 hours. Degradation products of chlorpheniramine's metabolic transformation by the liver are almost completely excreted in 24 hours via the kidney. The alkylamines, of which chlorpheniramine is the prototype, are among the most potent H_1 blockers. Although not so prone as others to cause drowsiness, a significant proportion of patients do experience this effect. CNS stimulation is more common in chlorpheniramine than in other groups of H_1 blockers.

Pseudoephedrine is a sympathomimetic amine with peripheral effects similar to epinephrine and central effects similar to, but less intense than, amphetamines. Therefore, it has the potential for excitatory side effects. Pseudoephedrine at the recommended oral dosage has little or no pressor effect in normotensive adults.

Pseudoephedrine is an orally effective nasal decongestant. Patients taking pseudoephedrine orally have not been reported to experience the rebound congestion sometimes experienced with frequent repeated use of topical decongestants.

Indications and Usage: **Fedahist®** is indicated for the symptomatic relief of seasonal and perennial allergic rhinitis, and eustachian tube congestion.

Contraindications:

Use in Newborn or Premature Infants: This drug should not be used in newborn or premature infants.

Antihistamines are contraindicated in the following conditions: hypersensitivity to chlorpheniramine maleate and other antihistamines of similar chemical structure; monoamine oxidase inhibitor therapy (see Drug Interactions Section).

Fedahist® is also contraindicated in patients with hypersensitivity or idiosyncrasy to sympathomimetic amines. Sympathomimetic amines are contraindicated in patients with severe hypertension, severe coronary artery disease, and in patients on MAO inhibitor therapy. Patient idiosyncrasy to adrenergic agents may be manifested by insomnia, dizziness, weakness, tremor or arrhythmias.

Warnings: Antihistamines should be used with considerable caution in patients with: narrow angle glaucoma; stenosing peptic ulcer; pyloroduodenal obstruction; symptomatic prostatic hypertrophy; bladder neck obstruction.

Use in Children: In infants and children especially, antihistamines in **overdosage** may cause hallucinations, convulsions or death.

As in adults, antihistamines may diminish mental alertness in children. In the young child particularly, they may produce excitation.

Use with CNS Depressants: Chlorpheniramine maleate has additive effects with alcohol and other CNS depressants (hypnotics, sedatives, tranquilizers, etc.)

Use in Activities Requiring Mental Alertness: Patients should be warned about engaging in activities requiring mental alertness, such as driving a car or operating appliances, machinery, etc.

Use in the Elderly (approximately 60 years or older): Antihistamines are more likely to cause dizziness, sedation, hypotension in elderly patients.

The elderly are more likely to have adverse reactions to sympathomimetics. Overdosage of sympathomimetics in this age group may cause hallucinations, convulsions, CNS depression, and death. Therefore, safe use of a short-acting sympathomimetic should be demonstrated in the individual elderly patient before considering the use of a sustained-action formulation.

Sympathomimetic amines should be used judiciously and sparingly in patients with hypertension, diabetes mellitus, ischemic heart disease, increased intraocular pressure, hyperthyroidism, and prostatic hypertrophy. Sympathomimetics may produce central nervous system stimulation with convulsions or cardiovascular collapse with accompanying hypotension.

Do not exceed recommended dosage.

Precautions:

General: Chlorpheniramine maleate has an atropine-like action and therefore should be used with caution in patients with: a history of bronchial asthma, increased intraocular pressure, hyperthyroidism, cardiovascular disease and hypertension.

Pseudoephedrine should be used with caution in patients with diabetes, hypertension, cardiovascular disease and hyper-reactivity to ephedrine.

Drug Interactions: MAO inhibitors prolong and intensify the anticholinergic (drying) effects of antihistamines. MAO inhibitors and beta adrenergic blockers increase the effects of pseudoephedrine (sympathomimetics).

Sympathomimetics may reduce the antihypertensive effects of methyldopa, mecamylamine, reserpine and veratrum alkaloids.

Carcinogenicity: Studies show that the ingredients in **Fedahist®** have no carcinogenic effects on animals or humans.

Use in Pregnancy: The safety of the ingredients in **Fedahist®** for use during pregnancy has not been established.

Pregnancy Category C: Animal reproduction studies have not been conducted with **Fedahist®**. It is also not known whether **Fedahist®** can cause fetal harm when administered to a pregnant woman or can affect reproduction capacity.

There have been no reports that pseudoephedrine increases the risk of fetal abnormalities if administered during pregnancy. If this drug is used during pregnancy, the possibility of fetal harm appears remote. Because studies cannot rule out the possibility of harm, however, **Fedahist®** should be used during pregnancy only if clearly needed.

Nonteratogenic Effects

Nursing Mothers: Because of the potential for serious adverse reactions in nursing infants from **Fedahist®** a decision should be made whether to discontinue nursing or to discontinue the drug, taking into account the importance of the drug to the mother.

Adverse Reactions: Slight to moderate drowsiness occurs relatively infrequently with

Continued on next page

This product information was prepared in August 1982. Information concerning these products may be obtained by addressing William H. Rorer, 500 Virginia Drive, Fort Washington, PA 19034.

Rorer—Cont.

chlorpheniramine maleate. Other possible side effects common to antihistamines in general include:

General: Urticaria, drug rash, anaphylactic shock, photosensitivity, excessive perspiration, chills, dryness of mouth, nose, and throat.

Cardiovascular System: hypotension, headache, palpitations, tachycardia, extrasystoles.

Hematologic System: hemolytic anemia, thrombocytopenia, agranulocytosis.

Nervous System: sedation, dizziness, disturbed coordination, fatigue, confusion, restlessness, excitation, nervousness, tremor, irritability, insomnia, euphoria, paresthesias, blurred vision, diplopia, vertigo, tinnitus, acute labryinthitis, hysteria, neuritis, convulsions.

Gastrointestinal System: epigastric distress, anorexia, nausea, vomiting, diarrhea, constipation.

Genitourinary System: urinary frequency, difficult urination, urinary retention, early menses.

Respiratory System: thickening of bronchial secretions, tightness of chest and wheezing, nasal stuffiness.

Individuals hyper-reactive to pseudoephedrine may display reactions such as tachycardia, palpitations, headache, dizziness or nausea. Sympathomimetic drugs have been associated with certain untoward reactions including fear, anxiety, tenseness, restlessness, tremor, weakness, pallor, respiratory difficulty, dysuria, insomnia, hallucinations, convulsions, CNS depression, arrhythmias, and cardiovascular collapse with hypotension.

Overdosage: In the event of overdosage, emergency treatment should be started immediately. Manifestations of antihistamine overdosage may vary from central nervous system depression (sedation, apnea, cardiovascular collapse) to stimulation (insomnia, hallucinations, tremors or convulsions). Other signs and symptoms may be dizziness, tinnitus, ataxia, blurred vision and hypotension. Stimulation is particularly likely in children, as are atropine-like signs and symptoms (dry mouth; fixed, dilated pupils; flushing, hyperthermia and gastrointestinal symptoms).

Treatment: The patient should be induced to vomit, even if emesis has occurred spontaneously. Pharmacologic vomiting by the administration of ipecac syrup is a preferred method. However, vomiting should not be induced in patients with impaired consciousness. The action of ipecac is facilitated by physical activity and by the administration of eight to twelve fluid ounces of water. If emesis does not occur within fifteen minutes, the dose of ipecac should be repeated. Precautions against aspiration must be taken, especially in infants and children. Following emesis, any drug remaining in the stomach may be absorbed by activated charcoal administered as a slurry with water. If vomiting is unsuccessful, or contraindicated, gastric lavage should be performed. Isotonic and one-half isotonic saline are the lavage solutions of choice. Saline cathartics, such as milk of magnesia, draw water into the bowel by osmosis and, therefore, may be valuable for their action in rapid dilution of bowel content. After emergency treatment the patient should continue to be medically monitored. Treatment of the signs and symptoms of overdosage is symptomatic and supportive.

Stimulants (analeptic agents) should not be used. Vasopressors may be used to treat hypotension. Short-acting barbiturates, diazepam or paraldehyde may be administered to control seizures. Hyperpyrexia, especially in children, may require treatment with tepid water sponge baths or a hypothermic blanket. Apnea is treated with ventilatory support.

Dosage and Administration:

FEDAHIST® GYROCAPS® (Timed Release Capsules)

Dosage: Adults and children 12 years and older: one capsule twice a day. Not recommended for children under 12 years.

FEDAHIST® EXPECTORANT (NONALCOHOLIC)

Dosage: Adults and children 12 years and over: two teaspoonfuls every 6 hours not to exceed 8 teaspoonfuls in 24 hours.
Children 6 to 12 years: one teaspoonful every 6 hours not to exceed 4 teaspoonfuls in 24 hours.
Children 2 to under 6 years; one-half teaspoonful every 6 hours not to exceed 2 teaspoonfuls in 24 hours.
Do not give to children under 6 years except under the advice and supervision of a physician.

FEDAHIST® TABLETS (SCORED, DYE-FREE)

Dosage: Adults and children 12 and over: one tablet every 6 hours not to exceed 4 tablets in 24 hours.
Children 6 to under 12 years: one-half tablet every 6 hours not to exceed 2 tablets in 24 hours.
Do not give to children under 6 years except under the advice and supervision of a physician.

FEDAHIST® SYRUP (NONALCOHOLIC)

Dosage: Adults and children 12 years and over: two teaspoonfuls every 6 hours not to exceed 8 teaspoonfuls in 24 hours.
Children 6 to under 12 years: one teaspoonful every 6 hours not to exceed 4 teaspoonfuls in 24 hours.
Children 2 to under 6 years: one-half teaspoonful every 6 hours not to exceed 2 teaspoonfuls in 24 hours.
Do not give to children under 6 years except under the advice and supervision of a physician.

KEEP THIS AND ALL MEDICATION OUT OF THE REACH OF CHILDREN. In case of accidental overdose, seek professional assistance or contact a poison control center immediately.

Supplied:
FEDAHIST® GYROCAPS® ℞: Available in bottles of 100 (NDC 0067-1053-68).
FEDAHIST® TABLETS: Available in bottles of 100 (NDC 0067-0050-68).
FEDAHIST® SYRUP: Available in 4 oz bottles (NDC 0067-0052-60).
FEDAHIST® EXPECTORANT: Available in 4 oz bottles (NDC 0067-0054-60).

Fedahist® Gyrocaps®
Manufactured by
Cord Laboratories, Inc.
Broomfield, CO 80020
For
William H. Rorer, Inc.

[*Fedahist® Gyrocaps® and Tablets Shown in Product Identification Section*]

FERMALOX®
Hematinic

Formula: Each *uncoated* tablet contains: Ferrous Sulfate 200 mg; Maalox® (magnesium-aluminum hydroxide) 200 mg.

Advantages: "A less irritating, more easily tolerated medicinal iron compound (Fermalox) fills an important need in the treatment of iron-deficiency states. The demonstration of effective absorption by means of the radioactive iron tracer, plus thousands of clinical cases showing satisfactory rise of hemoglobin level, fully establishes the efficacy of this medicament. In addition, the almost complete absence of the common adverse reactions to ordinary iron medicaments enables the physician to continue use of the drug until a satisfactory therapeutic result is obtained."[1]

Indications: For use as a hematinic in iron-deficiency conditions as may occur with: rapid growth, pregnancy, blood loss, menorrhagia, post-surgical convalescence, pathologic bleeding.

Usual Adult Dose: Two tablets daily; in mild cases dosage may be reduced to one tablet daily.

Warning: Keep this and all drugs out of the reach of children. In case of accidental overdose, seek professional assistance or contact a poison control center immediately.

Supplied: Bottles of 100 tablets (NDC 0067-0260-68) with child-resistant caps.

1. *Price, A.H., Erf, L., and Bierly, J.:* **J.A.M.A. 167***:1612 (July 26), 1958.*

[*Shown in Product Identification Section*]

GEMNISYN™ OTC
(acetaminophen and aspirin)
Double Strength Analgesic For Pain

Description: Each Gemnisyn™ tablet contains aspirin 325 mg (5 gr) and acetaminophen 325 mg (5 gr) for increased assurance of analgesia in adults compared to a standard analgesic dosage unit.

Indications: For relief of pain requiring increased analgesic strength when the usual doses of mild analgesics are inadequate.

Contraindications: Sensitivity to aspirin or acetaminophen.

Adult Dosage: 1 or 2 Gemnisyn tablets every 4 to 6 hours while pain persists, not to exceed 6 tablets in any 24-hour period.

Warning: Use with caution in the presence of peptic ulcer, asthma, liver damage or with anticoagulant therapy. Not recommended for children under 12. Patient Precaution: If pain persists for more than 10 days, consult your physician.
Keep this and all drugs out of the reach of children. In case of accidental overdose, seek professional assistance or contact a poison control center immediately.

Overdosage: A massive overdosage of acetaminophen may cause hepatotoxicity. Since clinical and laboratory evidence may be delayed for up to one week, close clinical monitoring and serial hepatic enzyme determinations are recommended.

Supplied: Plastic bottle of 100 tablets.
NDC 0067-0171-68

[*Shown in Product Identification Section*]

MAALOX®
Antacid
Magnesia and Alumina Oral Suspension and Tablets, Rorer
A Balanced Formulation of Magnesium and Aluminum Hydroxides

Description: Maalox Suspension is a balanced combination of magnesium and aluminum hydroxides. . . first in order of preference for all routine purposes of antacid medication. The high neutralizing power of magnesium hydroxide and the established acid binding capacity of aluminum hydroxide support the reputation of Maalox for reliable antacid action.

MAALOX® SUSPENSION: 225 mg Aluminum Hydroxide Equivalent to Dried Gel, USP, and 200 mg Magnesium Hydroxide per 5 ml.
MAALOX® No. 1 TABLETS: (200 mg Magnesium Hydroxide, 200 mg Dried Aluminum Hydroxide Gel)
MAALOX® No. 2 TABLETS: (400 mg Magnesium Hydroxide, 400 mg Dried Aluminum Hydroxide Gel)

Acid Neutralizing Capacity
Maalox® Suspension—27 mEq/2 teaspoonfuls
Maalox No. 1 Tablets—17 mEq/2 tablets
Maalox No. 2 Tablets—18 mEq/tablet

Sodium Content
Maalox® Suspension—1.35 mg/tsp. (5 ml) or .06 mEq (5 ml)
Maalox No. 1 Tablets—0.84 mg/tablet or 0.036 mEq/tablet
Maalox No. 2 Tablets—1.84 mg/tablet or .08 mEq/tablet

Indications: As an antacid for symptomatic relief of hyperacidity associated with the diagnosis of peptic ulcer, gastritis, peptic esophagitis, gastric hyperacidity, heartburn or hiatal hernia.

Advantages: Many patients prefer Maalox whether they are taking it for occasional heartburn or routinely on an ulcer therapy regimen. Once started on Maalox, patients tend to stay on Maalox because of effectiveness, taste, low sodium and non-constipating characteristics... four important reasons for Maalox® when prolonged antacid therapy is necessary.

Directions for use:
MAALOX® SUSPENSION: Two to four teaspoonfuls, four times a day, taken twenty minutes to one hour after meals and at bedtime, or as directed by a physician.
MAALOX NO. 1 TABLETS: Two to four tablets, well chewed, twenty minutes to one hour after meals and at bedtime, or as directed by a physician.
MAALOX NO. 2 TABLETS: One or two tablets, well chewed, twenty minutes to one hour after meals and at bedtime, or as directed by a physician. May be followed with milk or water.

Patient Warnings:
Do not take more than 16 teaspoonfuls of Maalox Suspension, 16 Maalox No. 1 Tablets or 8 Maalox No. 2 Tablets in a 24-hour period or use the maximum dosage for more than 2 weeks or use if you have kidney disease, except under the supervision of a physician.

Drug Interaction Precaution: Do not use with patients taking a prescription antibiotic drug containing any form of tetracycline or phenytoin. As with all aluminum-containing antacids, Maalox® may prevent the proper absorption of the tetracycline or phenytoin. Keep this and all drugs out of the reach of children.

Supplied:
MAALOX SUSPENSION is available in bottles of 12 fluid ounces (355 ml) (NDC 0067-0330-73), plastic bottles of 5 fluid ounces (148 ml) (NDC 0067-0330-62) and 26 fluid ounces (769 ml) (NDC 0067-0330-44).
Military Stock #NSN 6505-00-680-0133; V.A. Stock #6505-00-074-0993A [bottles of 6 fluid ounces (177 ml)].
MAALOX NO. 1 TABLETS (400 mg) available in bottles of 100 tablets (NDC 0067-0335-68).
MAALOX NO. 2 TABLETS (800 mg) available in bottles of 50 (NDC 0067-0337-50) and 250 tablets (NDC 0067-0337-70). Also available in boxes of 24 (NDC 0067-0337-24) and 100 (NDC 0067-0337-67) tablets in easy-to-carry strips.
V.A. Stock #6505-00-993-3507A [boxes of 100 tablets (in cellophane strips)].

[*Maalox No. 1 Tablets and Maalox No. 2 Tablets shown in Product Identification Section*]

MAALOX® PLUS
Antacid-Antiflatulent
Alumina, Magnesia and Simethicone Oral Suspension and Tablets, Rorer

☐ **Lemon swiss creme flavor... the taste preferred by physician and patient.**
☐ **Physician-proven Maalox® formula for antacid effectiveness.**
☐ **Simethicone, at a recognized clinical dose, for antiflatulent action.**

Description: Maalox® Plus, a balanced combination of magnesium and aluminum hydroxides plus simethicone, is a non-constipating, lemon-flavored, antacid-antiflatulent.
Composition: To provide symptomatic relief of hyperacidity plus alleviation of gas symptoms, each teaspoonful/tablet contains:

Active Ingredients	Maalox Plus Per Tsp. (5 ml)	Per Tablet
Magnesium Hydroxide	200 mg	200 mg
Aluminum Hydroxide	225 mg	200 mg
Simethicone	25 mg	25 mg

To aid in establishing proper dosage schedules, the following information is provided:

	Minimum Recommended Dosage: Per 2 Tsp. (10 ml)	Per 2 Tablets
Acid neutralizing capacity	27 mEq	17 mEq
Sodium content	2.6 mg	2.0 mg
Sugar content	None	1.1 g
Lactose content	None	None

Indications: As an antacid for symptomatic relief of hyperacidity associated with the diagnosis of peptic ulcer, gastritis, peptic esophagitis, gastric hyperacidity, heartburn or hiatal hernia. As an antiflatulent to alleviate the symptoms of gas, including postoperative gas pain.
Advantages: Among antacids, Maalox Plus is uniquely palatable—an important feature which encourages patients to follow your dosage directions. Maalox Plus has the time proven, nonconstipating, low sodium Maalox formula—useful for those patients suffering from the problems associated with hyperacidity. Additionally, Maalox Plus contains simethicone to alleviate discomfort associated with entrapped gas.
Directions for Use:
MAALOX® PLUS SUSPENSION: Two to four teaspoonfuls, four times a day, taken twenty minutes to one hour after meals and at bedtime, or as directed by a physician.
MAALOX® PLUS TABLETS: Two to four tablets, well chewed, four times a day, taken twenty minutes to one hour after meals and at bedtime, or as directed by a physician.
Patient Warnings: Do not take more than 16 teaspoonfuls or 16 tablets in a 24-hour period or use the maximum dosage for more than two weeks or use if you have kidney disease except under the advice and supervision of a physician.
Drug Interaction Precaution: Do not use with patients taking a prescription antibiotic containing any form of tetracycline or phenytoin. As with all aluminum-containing antacids, Maalox Plus may prevent the proper absorption of the tetracycline or phenytoin. Keep this and all drugs out of the reach of children. In case of accidental overdose, seek professional assistance or contact a poison control center immediately.
Supplied:
MAALOX PLUS SUSPENSION is available in a plastic 12 fluid ounce (355 ml) bottle (NDC 0067-0332-71).
MAALOX PLUS TABLETS are available in bottles of 50 tablets (NDC 0067-0339-50) and boxes of 100 tablets (NDC 0067-0339-67) in handy portable strips and convenience packs of 12 tablets (NDC 0067-0339-29).

[*Maalox® Plus Tablets shown in Product Identification Section*]

MAALOX® TC
(Therapeutic Concentrate)

Descriptions and Actions: Maalox® TC is a potent, concentrated, balanced formulation of 300 mg magnesium hydroxide and 600 mg aluminum hydroxide per teaspoonful (5 ml). This formulation produces a therapeutic concentrated antacid that exceeds standard antacids in acid neutralizing capacity and acid consuming capacity.
Maalox® TC is formulated to reduce the need to alter therapy due to treatment induced changes in bowel habits. Palatability is enhanced by a pleasant-tasting peppermint flavor.

Acid Neutralizing Capacity	28.3 mEq/5 ml
Acid Consuming Capacity	49.2/ml*
Sodium Content:	
mg Na/ml	.16
mg Na/mEq ANC	.03

*(ml N/10 HCl/gm)

Indications: Maalox® TC is indicated for the prevention of stress-induced upper gastrointestinal hemorrhage. As an antacid, for the symptomatic relief of hyperacidity associated with the diagnosis of peptic ulcer and other gastrointestinal conditions where a high degree of acid neutralization is desired.
Directions for Use: PREVENTION OF STRESS-INDUCED UPPER GASTROINTESTINAL HEMORRHAGE: 1) Aspirate stomach via nasogastric tube* and record pH. 2) Instill 10 ml of Maalox® TC followed by 30 ml of water via nasogastric tube. Clamp tube. 3) Wait one hour. Aspirate stomach and record pH. 4a) If pH equals or exceeds 4.0, apply drainage or intermittent suction for one hour, then repeat the cycle. 4b) If pH is less than 4.0, instill double (20 ml) Maalox® TC followed by 30 ml of water. Clamp tube. 5) Wait one hour. If pH equals or exceeds 4.0, see number 7. If pH is still less than 4.0, instill double (40 ml) Maalox® TC followed by 30 ml of water. Clamp tube. 6) Wait one hour. If pH equals or exceeds 4.0, see number 7. If pH is still less than 4.0, instill double (80 ml)** Maalox® TC followed by 30 ml of water. 7) Drain for one hour and repeat cycle with the effective dosage of Maalox® TC.

* If nasogastric tube is not in place, administer 20 ml of Maalox® TC orally q2h.
**In a recent clinical study[1], 20 ml of Maalox® TC, q2h, was sufficient in more than 85 percent of the patients. No patient studied required more than 80 ml of Maalox® TC q2h.

IN HYPERACID STATES FOR SYMPTOMATIC RELIEF: One or two teaspoonfuls as needed between meals and at bedtime or as directed by a physician. Higher dosage regimens may be employed under the direct supervision of a physician in the treatment of active peptic ulcer disease.
Precaution: Aluminum-magnesium hydroxide containing antacids should be used with caution in patients with renal impairment.
Patient Warnings:
Warning: Do not take more than 8 teaspoonfuls in a 24-hour period, or use the maximum dosage of this product for more than two weeks or use if you have kidney disease except under the advice and supervision of a physician. Keep this and all drugs out of the reach of children. In case of accidental overdose seek professional assistance or contact a poison control center immediately.

Continued on next page

This product information was prepared in August 1982. Information concerning these products may be obtained by addressing William H. Rorer, 500 Virginia Drive, Fort Washington, PA 19034.

Rorer—Cont.

Adverse Effects: Occasional regurgutation and mild diarrhea have been reported with the dosage recommended for the prevention of stress-induced upper gastrointestinal hemorrhage.
Drug Interaction Precaution: Do not take this product if you are presently taking a prescription antibiotic drug containing any form of tetracycline or phenytoin. As with all aluminum containing antacids, Maalox® TC may prevent the proper absorption of tetracycline or phenytoin.
How Supplied: Maalox® TC is available in bottles of 12 fluid ounces (355 ml) (NDC 0067-0334-73), 6 fluid ounces (NDC 0067-0334-75), and 15 ml (NDC 0067-0334-15), and 30 ml (NDC 0067-0334-22) patient cups.

PAREPECTOLIN® Ⓒ
Antidiarrheal

Contains opium (1/4 grain) 15 mg. per fluid ounce. *(Warning: may be habit forming.)*
Formula: Each fluid ounce of creamy white suspension contains:
Paregoric (equivalent) ......3.7 ml
Pectin ......162 mg
Kaolin ......5.5 g
(Alcohol 0.69%).
Indications: For symptomatic relief of diarrhea.
Action: The kaolin adsorbs irritants and forms a protective coating on intestinal mucosa. Pectin acts to consolidate the stool. Paregoric is very useful in diarrhea because it has a soothing action and allays griping pains.
Advantages: Because Parepectolin contains paregoric (equivalent), it effectively controls both diarrhea and colicky cramps. It is a stable suspension that tastes good.
Usual Adult Dose: One or two tablespoonfuls after each loose bowel movement for no more than four doses in twelve hours.
Usual Children's Dose: One or two teaspoonfuls after each loose bowel movement for no more than four doses in twelve hours.
Pediatric Dosage:

One year	1/2 teaspoonful
Three years	1 1/2 teaspoonfuls
Six years	2 teaspoonfuls

after each loose bowel movement for no more than four doses in twelve hours.
Warning: Keep this and all drugs out of the reach of children. In case of accidental overdose, seek professional assistance or contact a poison control center immediately.
Supplied: Bottles of 4 (118 ml) (NDC 0067-0660-60) and 8 (237 ml) (NDC 0067-0660-66) fluid ounces.

PERDIEM™

Actions: Perdiem™ with its gentle action does not produce disagreeable side effects. The vegetable mucilages of Perdiem soften the stool and provide pain-free evacuation of the bowel. Perdiem is effective as an aid to elimination for the hemorrhoid or fissure patient prior to and following surgery.
Composition: Contains Natural Vegetable Derivatives. Active ingredients are 82 percent psyllium (Plantago Hydrocolloid) and 18 percent senna (Cassia Pod Concentrate).
Indication: For relief of constipation.
Patient Warning: Should not be used in the presence of undiagnosed abdominal pain. Frequent or prolonged use without the direction of a physician is not recommended. Such use may lead to laxative dependence. Should not be used in patients with a history of esophageal disorders.
Directions For Use—ADULTS: In the evening and/or before breakfast, 1–2 rounded teaspoonfuls of Perdiem granules should be placed in the mouth and swallowed with at least 8 fl. oz of cool beverage. Additional liquid would be helpful. Perdiem granules should not be chewed.
After Perdiem takes effect (usually after 24 hours, but possibly not before 36–48 hours): reduce the morning and evening doses to one rounded teaspoonful. Subsequent doses should be adjusted after adequate laxation is obtained.
In Obstinate Cases: Perdiem may be taken more frequently, up to two rounded teaspoonfuls every six hours.
For Patients Habituated To Strong Purgatives: Two rounded teaspoonfuls of Perdiem in the morning and evening may be required along with half the usual dose of the purgative being used. The purgative should be discontinued as soon as possible and the dosage of Perdiem granules reduced when and if bowel tone shows lessened laxative dependence.
For Colostomy Patients: To ensure formed stools, give one to two rounded teaspoonfuls of Perdiem in the evening.
During Pregnancy: Give one to two rounded teaspoonfuls each evening.
For Clinical Regulation: For patients confined to bed, for those of inactive habits, and in the presence of cardiovascular disease where straining must be avoided, one rounded teaspoonful of Perdiem taken once or twice daily will provide regular bowel habits.
For children: From age 7–11 years, give one rounded teaspoonful one to two times daily. From age 12 and older, give adult dosage.
Note: It is extremely important that Perdiem be taken with at least 8 fl oz of cool liquid. Psyllium containing preparations, because of their bulk-forming action, should be used with caution in patients with hiatal hernia.
Keep this and all drugs out of the reach of children. In case of accidental overdose, seek professional assistance or contact a poison control center immediately.
How Supplied: Granules; 100 gram (3.5 oz) (NDC 46213-0690-68) and 250 gram (8.8 oz) (NDC 46213-0690-70) cans.
Dist. by William H. Rorer, Inc.
[Perdiem™ Granules Shown in Product Identification Section]

SLO-BID™ 100 mg, 200 mg and 300 mg Gyrocaps® ℞
(theophylline, anhydrous)
Timed Release Capsules

Description: Slo-bid™ Gyrocaps® 300 mg, 200 mg or 100 mg anhydrous theophylline in a long-acting dye-free capsule. Theophylline is a white odorless crystalline powder, having a bitter taste, and is chemically related to theobromine and caffeine. Slo-bid™ has been specially formulated to provide therapeutic serum levels when administered *every 12 hours*, and minimizes the peaks and valleys of serum levels commonly found with shorter acting theophylline products.
Clinical Pharmacology: The pharmacologic actions of theophylline include stimulation of respiration, augmentation of cardiac inotropy and chronotropy, relaxation of smooth muscles, including those in the bronchi and blood vessels (other than cerebral vessels) and diuresis. The main use of theophylline has been in the treatment of reversible airway obstruction. Theophylline is considered a potent medication for the control of chronic asthma. No development of tolerance occurs with chronic use of theophylline. The half-life is shortened with cigarette smoking and prolonged in alcoholism, reduced hepatic or renal function, congestive heart failure, and in patients receiving antibiotics such as lincomycin, clindamycin, troleandomycin, or erythromycin. High fever for prolonged periods and certain viral illnesses may decrease theophylline elimination. Newborn infants have extremely slow clearances and theophylline half-lives exceeding 24 hours. Older adults with chronic obstructive pulmonary disease, and patients with cor pulmonale or other causes of heart failure and patients with liver pathology may have much lower clearances with half-lives that exceed 24 hours.
Indications: For relief and/or prevention of symptoms from asthma and reversible bronchospasm associated with chronic bronchitis and emphysema.
Contraindications: Slo-bid™ is contraindicated in individuals who have shown hypersensitivity to any of its components or to xanthine derivatives.
Warnings: Status asthmaticus is a medical emergency. Optimal therapy frequently requires additional medication including corticosteroids when the patient is not rapidly responsive to bronchodilators.
Since excessive theophylline doses may be associated with toxicity, periodic measurement of serum theophylline levels is recommended to assure maximal benefit without excessive risk. Incidence of toxicity increases at serum levels greater than 20 μg/ml. Although early signs of theophylline toxicity, such as nausea and restlessness, are often seen, in some cases ventricular arrhythmias or seizures may be the first signs of toxicity.
Many patients who have excessive theophylline serum levels exhibit tachycardia. Theophylline preparations may worsen pre-existing arrhythmias.
Usage in Pregnancy: Safe use in pregnancy has not been established relative to possible adverse effects on fetal development, but neither have adverse effects on fetal development been established. This is, unfortunately, true for most anti-asthmatic medications. Therefore, use of theophylline in pregnant women should be balanced against the risk of uncontrolled asthma.
Precautions: Mean half-life in smokers is shorter than non-smokers. Therefore, smokers may require larger doses of theophylline.
Theophylline should not be administered concurrently with other xanthine preparations. Use with caution in patients with severe cardiac disease, severe hypoxemia, hypertension, hyperthyroidism, acute myocardial injury, cor pulmonale, congestive heart failure, liver disease, and in the elderly (especially males) and in neonates. Great caution should be used in giving theophylline to patients with congestive heart failure. Such patients have shown markedly prolonged theophylline blood levels with theophylline persisting in serum for long periods following discontinuation of the drug.
Use theophylline cautiously in patients with a history of peptic ulcer. Theophylline may occasionally act as a local gastrointestinal irritant, although G.I. symptoms are more commonly centrally mediated and associated with high serum concentration.
Adverse Reactions: The most consistent adverse reactions are due usually to overdose, and are:
Gastrointestinal: nausea, vomiting, epigastric pain, hematemesis, diarrhea.
Central nervous system: headaches, irritability, restlessness, insomnia, reflex hyperexcitability, muscle twitching, clonic and tonic generalized convulsions.
Cardiovascular: palpitation, tachycardia, extrasystoles, flushing, hypotension, circulatory failure, ventricular arrhythmias.
Respiratory: tachypnea.
Renal: albuminuria, increased excretion of renal tubular cells and red blood cells, potentiation of diuresis.
Others: hyperglycemia and inappropriate ADH syndrome.
Drug Interactions:

Drug	Effect
Aminophylline with Lithium Carbonate	Increased excretion of Lithium Carbonate

Aminophylline with Propranolol	Antagonism of Propranolol effect
Theophylline with Cimetidine	Increased theophylline blood levels
Theophylline with Furosemide	Increased Diuresis
Theophylline with Hexamethonium	Decreased Hexamethonium-induced Chronotropic effect
Theophylline with Reserpine	Tachycardia
Theophylline with clindamycin, lincomycin, troleandomycin or erythromycin	Increased theophylline blood levels
Theophylline with Chlordiazepoxide	Chlordiazepoxide-induced fatty acid metabolism

Dosage and Administration:
Note: Due to their slower rate of absorption sustained release theophylline products are not designed for use in conditions requiring rapid theophyllinization.
Chronic Asthma: Theophyllinization is a treatment of first choice for the management of chronic asthma (to prevent symptoms and maintain patent airways). Slow clinical titration is generally preferred to assure acceptance and safety of the medication.
Initial Dose: 16 mg/kg/day or 400 mg/day (whichever is lower) in 2 divided doses at twelve hour intervals for the Gyrocaps® THE AVERAGE INITIAL CHILDREN'S (15 to 20 kg) DOSE IS ONE SLO-BID™ Gyrocaps® 100 mg CAPSULE q12h. THE AVERAGE INITIAL ADULT AND CHILDREN'S (over 25 kg) DOSE IS ONE SLO-BID™ Gyrocaps® 200 mg CAPSULE q12h.
Increased Dose: The above dosage may be increased in approximately 25% increments at 2 to 3 day intervals so long as no intolerance is observed until the maximum dose indicated below is reached.
MAXIMUM DOSE WITHOUT MEASUREMENT OF SERUM CONCENTRATION:
Not to exceed the following: (WARNING: DO NOT ATTEMPT TO MAINTAIN ANY DOSE THAT IS NOT TOLERATED.)

Age 6 months to 9 years—24 mg/kg/day
Age 9 years to 12 years—20 mg/kg/day
Age 12 years to 16 years—18 mg/kg/day
Age > 16 years—13 mg/kg/day
NOTE: Use ideal body weight for obese patients

Measurement of serum theophylline concentration during chronic therapy: If the above maximum doses are to be maintained or exceeded, serum theophylline measurement is recommended. This should be obtained at the approximate time of peak absorption during chronic therapy for the product used (3 to 5 hours for sustained release preparations). It is important that the patient will have missed *no* doses during the previous 48 hours and that dosing intervals will have been reasonably typical with no added doses during that period of time.
DOSAGE ADJUSTMENT BASED ON SERUM THEOPHYLLINE MEASUREMENTS, WHEN THESE INSTRUCTIONS HAVE NOT BEEN FOLLOWED, MAY RESULT IN RECOMMENDATIONS THAT PRESENT RISK OF TOXICITY TO THE PATIENT.
FINAL DOSAGE ADJUSTMENT: Caution should be exercised for younger children who cannot complain of minor side effects. Older adults, those with cor pulmonale, congestive heart failure, and/or liver disease may have unusually low dosage requirements, and thus may experience toxicity at the maximum dosage recommended above.
It is important that no patient be maintained on any dosage that he/she is not tolerating. In instructing patients to increase dosage according to the schedule above, they should be instructed not to take a subsequent dose if apparent side effects occur and to resume therapy at a lower dose once adverse effects have disappeared.
Overdosage:
Management
A. If potential overdose is established and seizure has not occurred:
1. Induce vomiting.
2. Administer a cathartic (this is particularly important if sustained release preparations have been taken).
3. Administer activated charcoal.
B. If patient is having seizure:
1. Establish an airway.
2. Administer oxygen.
3. Treat the seizure with intravenous diazepam, 0.1 to 0.3 mg/kg up to 10 mg.
4. Monitor vital signs, maintain blood pressure and provide adequate hydration.
C. Post-Seizure Coma:
1. Maintain airway and oxygenation.
2. Follow above recommendations to prevent absorption of drug, but intubation and lavage will have to be performed instead of inducing emesis, and the cathartic and charcoal will need to be introduced via a large bore gastric lavage tube.
3. Continue to provide full supportive care and adequate hydration while waiting for drug to be metabolized. In general, the drug is metabolized sufficiently rapidly so as to not warrant consideration of dialysis.

How Supplied: Slo-bid™ Gyrocaps® 100 mg are available in bottles of 100 (NDC 0067-0100-68), Slo-bid™ Gyrocaps® 200 mg are available in bottles of 100 (NDC 0067-0200-68) and Slo-bid™ Gyrocaps® 300 mg are available in bottles of 100 (NDC 0067-0300-68).

SLO-PHYLLIN® (theophylline, anhydrous) ℞
SYRUP, TABLETS, GYROCAPS® (timed release capsules)

Description: SLO-PHYLLIN® 80 SYRUP (theophylline, anhydrous) is a nonalcoholic, sugar free solution. Each 15 ml. contains: theophylline, anhydrous, U.S.P., 80 mg with sodium benzoate, 18 mg and methylparaben, 3 mg added as preservatives.
SLO-PHYLLIN® TABLETS (theophylline, anhydrous) are scored, dye-free tablets containing 100 mg and 200 mg of theophylline, anhydrous, U.S.P.
SLO-PHYLLIN® GYROCAPS® (theophylline, anhydrous timed release capsules) are bead filled, hard gelatin capsules containing 60 mg, 125 mg and 250 mg of theophylline, anhydrous, U.S.P. in a special base that provides for a prolonged therapeutic effect.
Theophylline, a xanthine compound, is a white, odorless, crystalline powder, having a bitter taste. It contains one molecule of hydration or is anhydrous.
Clinical Pharmacology: Theophylline directly relaxes the smooth muscle of the bronchial airways and pulmonary blood vessels, thus acting mainly as a brochodilator, pulmonary vasodilator and smooth muscle relaxant. The drug also possesses other actions typical of the xanthine derivatives: coronary vasodilator, diuretic, cardiac stimulant, cerebral stimulant, and skeletal muscle stimulant. The actions of theophylline may be mediated through inhibition of phosphodiesterase and a resultant increase in intracellular cyclic AMP which could mediate smooth muscle relaxation. At concentrations higher than attained *in vivo*, theophylline also inhibits the release of histamine by mast cells.
In vitro, theophylline has been shown to react synergistically with beta agonists that increase intracellular cyclic AMP through the stimulation of adenyl cyclase (isoproterenol), but synergism has not been demonstrated in patient studies and more data are needed to determine if theophylline and beta agonists have clinically important additive effects *in vivo*.
Apparently, no development of tolerance occurs with chronic use of theophylline.
The half-life is shortened with cigarette smoking. The half-life is prolonged in alcoholism, reduced hepatic or renal function, congestive heart failure, and in patients receiving antibiotics such as TAO (troleandomycin), erythromycin and clindamycin. High fever for prolonged periods may decrease theophylline elimination.

Theophylline Elimination Characteristics

	Theophylline Clearance Rates (mean ± S.D.)	Half-life Average (mean ± S.D.)
Children (over 6 months of age):	1.45 ± .58 ml/kg/min	3.7 ± 1.1 hours
Adult non-smokers with uncomplicated asthma	.65 ± .19 ml/kg/min	8.7 ± 2.2 hours

Newborn infants have extremely slow clearances and theophylline half-lives exceeding 24 hours which approach those seen for older children after about 3–6 months.
Older adults with chronic obstructive pulmonary disease, any patients with cor pulmonale or other causes of heart failure, and patients with liver pathology may have much lower clearances with half-lives that may exceed 24 hours.
The half-life of theophylline in smokers (1 to 2 packs/day) averaged 4 to 5 hours among various studies, much shorter than the half-life in non-smokers who averaged about 7 to 9 hours. The increase in theophylline clearance caused by smoking is probably the result of induction of drug-metabolizing enzymes that do not readily normalize after cessation of smoking. It appears that between 3 months and 2 years may be necessary for normalization of the effect of smoking on theophylline pharmacokinetics.
Indications: For relief and/or prevention of symptoms of asthma and reversible bronchospasm associated with chronic bronchitis and emphysema.
Contraindications: Individuals who have shown hypersensitivity to any of its components.
Warnings: Status asthmaticus is a medical emergency. Optimal therapy frequently requires additional medication including corticosteroids when the patient is not rapidly responsive to bronchodilators.
Excessive theophylline doses may be associated with toxicity and measurement of serum theophylline levels is recommended to assure maximal benefit without excessive risk. Incidence of toxicity increases at levels greater than 20 μg/ml. Morphine, curare, and stilbamidine should be used with caution in patients with airflow obstruction since they stimulate histamine release and can induce asthmatic attacks. They may also suppress respiration leading to respiratory failure. Alternative drugs should be chosen whenever possible.
There is an excellent correlation between high blood levels of theophylline resulting from conventional doses and associated clinical manifestations of toxicity in (1) patients with lowered body plasma clearances (due to transient cardiac decompensation), (2) patients with

Continued on next page

This product information was prepared in August 1982. Information concerning these products may be obtained by addressing William H. Rorer, 500 Virginia Drive, Fort Washington, PA 19034.

Rorer—Cont.

liver dysfunction or chronic obstructive lung disease, (3) patients who are older than 55 years of age, particularly males.

There are often no early signs of less serious theophylline toxicity such as nausea and restlessness, which may appear in up to 50 percent of patients prior to onset of convulsions. Ventricular arrhythmias or seizures may be the first signs of toxicity.

Many patients who have higher theophylline serum levels exhibit tachycardia.

Theophylline products may worsen pre-existing arrhythmias.

Usage in Pregnancy: Safe use in pregnancy has not been established relative to possible adverse effects on fetal development, but neither have adverse effects on fetal development been established. This is, unfortunately, true for most antiasthmatic medications. Therefore, use of theophylline in pregnant women should be balanced against the risk of uncontrolled asthma.

Precautions: Mean half-life in smokers is shorter than non-smokers, therefore, smokers may require larger doses of theophylline. Theophylline should not be administered concurrently with other xanthine medications. Use with caution in patients with severe cardiac disease, severe hypoxemia, hypertension, hyperthyroidism, acute myocardial injury, cor pulmonale, congestive heart failure, liver disease, and in the elderly (especially males) and in neonates. Great caution should especially be used in giving theophylline to patients in congestive heart failure. Such patients have shown markedly prolonged theophylline blood level curves with theophylline persisting in serum for long periods following discontinuation of the drug.

Use theophylline cautiously in patients with history of peptic ulcer. Theophylline may occasionally act as a local irritant to G.I. tract although gastrointestinal symptoms are more commonly central and associated with serum concentrations over 20 μg/ml.

Adverse Reactions: The most consistent adverse reactions are usually due to overdose and are:

1. Gastrointestinal: nausea, vomiting, epigastric pain, hematemesis, diarrhea.
2. Central nervous system: headaches, irritability, restlessness, insomnia, reflex hyperexcitability, muscle twitching, clonic and tonic generalized convulsions.
3. Cardiovascular: palpitation, tachycardia, extrasystoles, flushing, hypotension, circulatory failure, life threatening ventricular arrhythmias.
4. Respiratory: tachypnea.
5. Renal: albuminuria, increased excretion of renal tubular cells and red blood cells; potentiation of diuresis.
6. Others: hyperglycemia and inappropriate ADH syndrome.

Drug Interactions: Toxic synergism with ephedrine has been documented and may occur with some other sympathomimetic bronchodilators.

DRUG	EFFECT
Aminophylline with Lithium Carbonate	Increased excretion of Lithium Carbonate
Aminophylline with Propranolol	Antagonism of Propranolol effect
Theophylline with Cimetidine	Increased theophylline blood levels
Theophylline with Furosemide	Increased Diuresis of Furosemide
Theophylline with Hexamethonium	Decreased Hexamethonium-induced chronotropic effect
Theophylline with Reserpine	Reserpine-induced Tachycardia
Theophylline with Chlordiazepoxide	Chlordiazepoxide-induced fatty acid mobilization
Theophylline with Cyclamycin (TAO= troleandomycin): erythromycin, lincomycin	Increased Theophylline plasma levels

Overdosage:

Management: A. If potential oral overdose is established and seizure has not occurred:

1) Induce vomiting.
2) Administer a cathartic (this is particularly important if sustained release preparations have been taken).
3) Administer activated charcoal.

B. If patient is having a seizure:

1) Establish an airway.
2) Administer O_2.
3) Treat the seizure with intravenous diazepam, 0.1 to 0.3 mg/kg up to 10 mg.
4) Monitor vital signs, maintain blood pressure and provide adequate hydration.

C. Post-seizure Coma:

1) Maintain airway and oxygenation.
2) If a result of oral medication, follow above recommendations to prevent absorption of drug, but intubation and lavage will have to be performed instead of inducing emesis, and the cathartic and charcoal will need to be introduced via a large bore gastric lavage tube.
3) Continue to provide full supportive care and adequate hydration while waiting for drug to be metabolized. In general, the drug is metabolized sufficiently rapidly so as to not warrant consideration of dialysis.

D. Animal studies suggest that phenobarbital may decrease theophylline toxicity. There is as yet, however, insufficient data to recommend pretreatment of an overdosage with phenobarbital.

Dosage and Administration: Therapeutic serum levels associated with optimal likelihood for benefit and minimal risk of toxicity are considered to be between 10 μg/ml and 20 μg/ml. Levels above 20 μg/ml may produce toxic effects. There is great variation from patient to patient in dosage needed in order to achieve a therapeutic blood level because of variable rates of elimination. Because of this wide variation from patient to patient, and the relatively narrow therapeutic blood level range, dosage must be individualized and monitoring of theophylline serum levels is highly recommended.

Dosage should be calculated on the basis of lean (ideal) body weight where mg/kg doses are stated. Theophylline does not distribute into fatty tissue.

Giving theophylline with food may prevent the rare cases of stomach irritation; and though absorption may be slower, it is still complete. When rapidly absorbed products such as solutions and uncoated tablets with rapid dissolution are used, dosing to maintain "around the clock" blood levels generally requires administration every 6 hours to obtain the greatest efficacy for clinical use in children; dosing intervals up to 8 hours may be satisfactory for adults because of their slower elimination.

Children, and adults requiring higher than average doses, may benefit from products with slower absorption which may allow longer dosing intervals and/or less fluctuation in serum concentration over a dosing interval during chronic therapy.

Slo-Phyllin® Gyrocaps® may be administered every 8 to 12 hours depending upon the patient's age and elimination rate. Due to their rapid elimination rates, most childrn require administration of the Gyrocaps® every 8 hours, but dosing intervals of up to 12 hours may be satisfactory for adults.

Dosage for Patient Population

ACUTE SYMPTOMS OF ASTHMA REQUIRING RAPID THEOPHYLLINIZATION

Note: Due to their slower rate of absorption, sustained release theophylline products are not designed for use in conditions requiring rapid theophyllinization.

I. Not currently receiving theophylline products.

(See table below.)

Group	Oral Loading Dose (Theophylline)	Maintenance Dose for Next 12 Hours (Theophylline)	Maintenance Dose Beyond 12 Hours (Theophylline)
1. Children 6 months to 9 years	6 mg/kg	4 mg/kg q4h	4 mg/kg q6h
2. Children age 9–16 and young adult smokers	6 mg/kg	3 mg/kg q4h	3 mg/kg q6h
3. Otherwise healthy non-smoking adults	6 mg/kg	3 mg/kg q6h	3 mg/kg q8h
4. Older patients and patients with cor pulmonale	6 mg/kg	2 mg/kg q6h	2 mg/kg q8h
5. Patients with congestive heart failure, liver failure	6 mg/kg	2 mg/kg q8h	1–2 mg/kg q12h

II. Those currently receiving theophylline products: Determine, where possible, the time, amount, route of administration and form of the patient's last dose.

The loading dose for theophylline will be based on the principle that each .5 mg/kg of theophylline administered as a loading dose will result in a 1 mcg/ml increase in serum theophylline concentration. Ideally, then, the loading dose should be deferred if a serum theophylline concentration can be rapidly obtained. If this is not possible, the clinician must exercise his judgment in selecting a dose based on the potential for benefit and risk. When there is sufficient respiratory distress to warrant a small risk, 2.5 mg/kg of theophylline is likely to increase the serum concentration when administered as a loading dose in rapidly absorbed form by only about 5 μg/ml. If the patient is not already experiencing theophylline toxicity, this is unlikely to result in dangerous adverse effects.

Subsequent to the modified decision regarding loading dose in this group of patients, the subsequent maintenance dosage recommendations are the same as those described above.

Comments: To achieve optimal therapeutic theophylline dosage, it is recommended to monitor serum theophylline concentrations. However, it is not always possible or practical to obtain a serum theophylline level.

Patients should be closely monitored for signs of toxicity. The present data suggest that the above dosage recommendations will achieve therapeutic serum concentrations with minimal risk of toxicity for most patients. However, some risk of toxic serum concentrations is still present. Adverse reactions to theophylline often occur when serum theophylline levels exceed 20 μg/ml.

CHRONIC ASTHMA: Theophyllinization is a treatment of first choice for the management of chronic asthma (to prevent symptoms and maintain patent airways). Slow clinical titration is generally preferred to assure acceptance and safety of the medication.

Initial Dose: 16 mg/kg/day or 400 mg/day (whichever is lower) in 3 to 4 divided doses at 6 to 8 hour intervals for the Syrup and Tablets or 2 to 3 divided doses at 8 to 12 hour intervals for the Gyrocaps®.

Increased Dose: The above dosage may be increased in approximately 25 percent increments at 2 to 3 day intervals so long as no intolerance is observed, until the maximum indicated below is reached.

Maximum dose without measurement of serum concentration:
Not to exceed the following: (WARNING: DO NOT ATTEMPT TO MAINTAIN ANY DOSE THAT IS NOT TOLERATED.)
Age 6 months to 9 years—24 mg/kg/day
Age 9 to 12 years—20 mg/kg/day
Age 12 to 16 years—18 mg/kg/day
Age > 16 years—13 mg/kg/day or 900 mg/day (WHICHEVER IS LESS)

Note: Use ideal body weight for obese patients.

Measurement of serum theophylline concentration during chronic therapy: If the above maximum doses are to be maintained or exceeded, serum theophylline measurement is recommended. This should be obtained at the approximate time of peak absorption during chronic therapy for the product used (1 to 2 hours for liquids and plain uncoated tabets that undergo rapid dissolution, 3 to 5 hours for sustained release preparations). It is important that the patient will have missed *no* doses during the previous 48 hours and that dosing intervals will have been reasonably typical with no added doses during that period of time. DOSAGE ADJUSTMENT BASED ON SERUM THEOPHYLLINE MEASUREMENTS WHEN THESE INSTRUCTIONS HAVE NOT BEEN FOLLOWED MAY RESULT IN RECOMMENDATIONS THAT PRESENT RISK OF TOXICITY TO THE PATIENT.

Final dosage adjustment: Caution should be exercised for younger children who cannot complain of minor side effects. Older adults, those with cor pulmonale, congestive heart failure, and/or liver disease may have unusually low dosage requirements and thus may experience toxicity at the maximal dosage recommended above.

It is important that no patient be maintained on any dosage that he is not tolerating. In instructing patients to increase dosage according to the schedule above, they should be instructed not to take a subsequent dose if apparent side effects occur and to resume therapy at a lower dose once adverse effects have disappeared.

Keep this and all drugs out of the reach of children. In case of accidental overdose, seek professional assistance or contact a poison control center immediately.

How Supplied:
Slo-Phyllin® 80 Syrup (theophylline, anhydrous 80 mg/15 ml) nonalcoholic, orange color in 4 oz. (NDC 0067-0354-60), pint (NDC 0067-0354-16), and gallon (NDC 0067-0354-28) bottles, and 15 ml unit dose bottles (NDC 0067-0354-17).

Slo-Phyllin® 100 mg Tablets (theophylline, anhydrous) scored, dye-free, white, round, convex tablet, in bottles of 100 (NDC 0067-0351-68) and 1000 (NDC 0067-0351-82), unit dose strip packages (NDC 0067-0351-01).

Theophylline Elimination Characteristics

	Theophylline Clearance Rates (mean±S.D.)	Half-life Average (mean±S.D.)
Children (over 6 months of age):	1.45±.58 ml/kg/min	3.7±1.1 hours
Adult non-smokers with uncomplicated asthma:	.65±.19 ml/kg/min	8.7±2.2 hours

Slo-Phyllin® 200 mg. Tablets (theophylline, anhydrous) scored, dye-free, white, round, flat faced tablet, in bottles of 100 (NDC 0067-0352-68) and 1000 (NDC 0067-0352-82), unit dose strip packages (NDC 0067-0352-01).

Slo-Phyllin® 60 Gyrocaps® (theophylline, anhydrous timed release capsules 60 mg), white bead filled capsules, in bottles of 100 (NDC 0067-1354-68) and 1000 (NDC 0067-1354-82).

Slo-Phyllin® 125 Gyrocaps® (theophylline, anhydrous timed release capsules 125 mg), brown bead filled capsules, in bottles of 100 (NDC 0067-1355-68) and 1000 (NDC 0067-1355-82), unit dose strip packages (NDC 0067-1355-01).

Slo-Phyllin® 250 Gyrocaps® (theophylline, anhydrous timed release capsules 250 mg), purple bead filled capsules, in bottles of 100 (NDC 0067-1356-68) and 1000 (NDC 0067-1356-82), unit dose strip packages (NDC 0067-1356-01).

Recommended Dosage of SLO-PHYLLIN® Tablets or Gyrocaps® for Various Body Weights*

Weight		Dose (in mg)			
lbs.	kg	3 mg/kg	4 mg/kg	5 mg/kg	6 mg/kg
22	10	30	40	50	60
33	15	45	60	75	90
44	20	60	80	100	120
55	25	75	100	125	150
66	30	90	120	150	180
88	40	120	160	200	240
110	50	150	200	250	300
132	60	180	240	300	360
154	70	210	280	350	420
176	80	240	320	400	480
198	90	270	360	450	540
220	100	300	400	500	600

*Note: For obese patients, dosage should be calculated on the basis of lean (ideal) body weight.

Recommended Dosage of SLO-PHYLLIN® 80 Syrup for Various Body Weights

Weight		Dose (in tsp.)		
lbs.	kg	3 mg/kg	4 mg/kg	5 mg/kg
20	9	1 tsp	1⅓ tsp	1½ tsp
40	18	2 tsp	2½ tsp	3 tsp
60	27	3 tsp	4 tsp	5 tsp
79	36	4 tsp	5 tsp	6½ tsp

The therapeutic serum theophylline concentration is considered to be between 10 and 20 μg/ml. This range may best be reached by individualizing the patient's dosage while concomitantly monitoring the serum theophylline concentrations.

Slo-Phyllin® 80 Syrup U.S. Patent #3928609

[Slo-Phyllin® Tablets and Gyrocaps® Shown in Product Identification Section]

Slo-Phyllin® Gyrocaps®
Manufactured by
Cord Laboratories, Inc.
Broomfield, CO 80020
For
William H. Rorer, Inc.

SLO–PHYLLIN® GG CAPSULES, SYRUP ℞

(theophylline, anhydrous with guaifenesin)

Description: Each **Slo-Phyllin® GG** soft gelatin capsule or tablespoonful (15 ml) of liquid contains 150 mg of theophylline (anhydrous) and 90 mg of guaifenesin, as an oral bronchodilator-expectorant. Theophylline (1, 3-dimethylxanthine), a xanthine compound, is a white, odorless crystalline powder, having a bitter taste.

Guaifenesin (3-[2-methoxyphenoxy] 1,2-propanediol), a guaiacol compound, is a white to slightly yellow crystalline powder with a bitter, aromatic taste.

Clinical Pharmacology:
Theophylline: Theophylline directly relaxes the smooth muscle of the bronchial airways and pulmonary blood vessels, thus acting mainly as a bronchodilator, pulmonary vasodilator and smooth muscle relaxant. The drug also possesses other actions typical of the xanthine derivatives: coronary vasodilator, diuretic, cardiac stimulant, cerebral stimulant, and skeletal muscle stimulant. The actions of theophylline may be mediated through inhibition of phosphodiesterase and a resultant increase in intracellular cyclic AMP, which could mediate smooth muscle relaxation. At concentrations higher than attained **in vivo**, theophylline also inhibits the release of histamine by mast cells.

In vitro, theophylline has been shown to react synergistically with beta agonists that increase intracellular cyclic AMP through the stimulation of adenyl cyclase (isoproterenol), but synergism has not been demonstrated in patient studies and more data are needed to determine if theophylline and beta agonists have clinically important additive effects **in vivo**. Apparently, no development of tolerance occurs with chronic use of theophylline.

The half-life is shortened with cigarette smoking. The half-life is prolonged in alcoholism, reduced hepatic or renal function, congestive heart failure, and in patients receiving antibiotics such as TAO (troleandomycin), erthromycin and clindamycin. High fever for prolonged periods may decrease theophylline elimination.

[See table above].

Newborn infants have extremely slow clearances and theophylline half-lives exceeding 24 hours which approach those seen for older children after about 3-6 months. Older adults with chronic obstructive pulmonary disease, any patients with cor pulmonale or other causes of heart failure, and patients with liver pathology may have much lower clearances with half-lives that may exceed 24 hours.

The half-life of theophylline in smokers (1 to 2 packs/day) averaged 4 to 5 hours among various studies, much shorter than the half-life in non-smokers who averaged about 7 to 9 hours. The increase in theophylline clearance caused by smoking is probably the result of induction of drug-metabolizing enzymes that do not

Continued on next page

This product information was prepared in August 1982. Information concerning these products may be obtained by addressing William H. Rorer, 500 Virginia Drive, Fort Washington, PA 19034.

Rorer—Cont.

readily normalize after cessation of smoking. It appears that between 3 months and 2 years may be necessary for normalization of the effect of smoking on theophylline pharmacokinetics.

Guaifenesin: Guaifenesin increases respiratory tract secretions, possibly by stimulating the Goblet cells. Guaifenesin appears to be well absorbed, but its pharmacokinetics have not been thoroughly studied.

Indications and Usage: For relief and/or prevention of symptoms of asthma and reversible bronchospasm associated with chronic bronchitis and emphysema.

Contraindications: In individuals who have shown hypersensitivity to any of its components.

Warnings: Status asthmaticus is a medical emergency. Optimal therapy frequently requires additional medication including corticosteroids when the patient is not rapidly responsive to bronchodilators.
Excessive theophylline doses may be associated with toxicity. Therefore, monitoring of serum theophylline levels is recommended to assure maximal benefit without excessive risk. Incidence of toxicity increases at levels greater than 20 μg/ml. Morphine, curare, and stilbamidine should be used with caution in patients with airflow obstruction since they stimulate histamine release and can induce asthmatic attacks. They may also suppress respiration leading to respiratory failure. Alternative drugs should be chosen whenever possible.
There is an excellent correlation between high blood levels of theophylline resulting from conventional doses and associated clinical manifestations of toxicity in (1) patients with lowered body plasma clearances (due to transient cardiac decompensation), (2) patients with liver dysfunction or chronic obstructive lung disease, (3) patients who are older than 55 years of age, particularly males.
There are often no early signs of less serious theophylline toxicity such as nausea and restlessness, which may appear in up to 50 percent of patients prior to onset of convulsions. Ventricular arrhythmias or seizures may be the first signs of toxicity.
Many patients who have higher theophylline serum levels exhibit tachycardia.
Theophylline products may worsen pre-existng arrhythmias.

Precautions:
General: Theophylline.
Mean half-life in smokers is shorter than nonsmokers, therefore, smokers may require larger doses of theophylline. Theophylline should not be administered concurrently with other xanthine medications. Use with caution in patients with severe cardiac disease, severe hypoxemia, hypertension, hyperthyroidism, acute myocardial injury, cor pulmonale, congestive heart failure, liver disease, and in the elderly (especially males) and in neonates. Great caution should especially be used in giving theophylline to patients in congestive heart failure. Such patients have shown markedly prolonged theophylline blood level curves with theophylline persisting in serum for long periods following discontinuation of the drug. Use theophylline cautiously in patients with history of peptic ulcer. Theophylline may occasionally act as a local irritant to the G.I. tract although gastrointestinal symptoms are more commonly central and associated with serum concentrations over 20 μg/ml.
Drug Interactions: Toxic synergism with ephedrine has been documented and may occur with some other sympathomimetic bronchodilators.

DRUG	EFFECT
Aminophylline with lithium carbonate	Increased excretion of lithium carbonate
Aminophylline with propranolol	Antagonism of propranolol effect
Theophylline with Cimetidine	Increased theophylline blood levels
Theophylline with furosemide	Increased diuresis of furosemide
Theophylline with hexamethonium	Decreased hexamethonium-induced chronotropic effect
Theophylline with reserpine	Reserpine-induced tachycardia
Theophylline with chlordiazepoxide	Chlordiazepoxide-induced fatty acid mobilization
Theophylline with Cyclamycin (TAO= troleandomycin): erythromycin, clindamycin, lincomycin	Increased theophylline plasma levels

Drug Laboratory Test Interactions: Theophylline may increase uric acid levels and urinary catecholamines. Metabolites of guaifenesin may contribute to increased urinary 5-hydroxy-indoleacetic acid readings, when determined with nitrosonaphthol reagent.
Carcinogenicity:
Studies have shown that theophylline exhibits no carcinogenic effects on animals or humans.
Usage in Pregnancy:
Teratogenic effects:
Pregnancy Category C—Animal reproduction studies have not been conducted with **Slo-Phyllin® GG**. It is also not known whether **Slo-Phyllin® GG** can cause fetal harm when administered to a pregnant woman or can affect reproduction capacity. Therefore, it should be given to a pregnant woman only if clearly needed.
Nonteratogenic effects:
Theophylline may be excreted in the milk and cause irritability in the nursing infant. Therefore, caution should be exercised when **Slo-Phyllin® GG** is administered to a nursing mother.
Adverse Reactions: The frequency of adverse reactions is related to serum theophylline levels and is usually not a problem at levels below 20 mcg/ml. The most consistent adverse reactions are usually due to overdosage and, while all have not been reported with **Slo-Phyllin® GG**, the following reactions may be considered when theophylline is administered. Central nervous system: clonic and tonic generalized convulsions, muscle twitching, reflex hyperexcitability, headaches, insomnia, restlessness, and irritability. Cardiovascular: circulatory failure, life threatening ventricular arrhythmias, hypotension, extrasystoles, tachycardia, palpitation, and flushing. Gastrointestinal: hematemesis, vomiting, diarrhea, epigastric pain, and nausea. Renal: increased excretion of renal tubular cells and red blood cells, albuminuria, and potentiation of diuresis. Respiratory: tachypnea. Others: hyperglycemia and inappropriate ADH syndrome.
Overdosage:
Symptoms
Nervousness, agitation, headache, insomnia, vomiting, tachycardia, extrasystoles, hyperreflexia. fasciculations and clonic and tonic convulsions. Children may be particularly prone to restlessness and hyperactivity that can proceed to convulsions.

Management

A. If potential oral overdose is established and seizure has not occurred.
   1. Induce vomiting.
   2. Administer a cathartic (this is particularly important if sustained release preparations have been taken).
   3. Administer activated charcoal.
   4. Monitor vital signs, maintain blood pressure and provide adequate hydration.
B. If patient is having a seizure.
   1. Establish an airway.
   2. Administer O_2.
   3. Treat the seizure with intravenous diazepam 0.1 to 0.3 mg/kg up to 10 mg.
   4. Monitor vital signs, maintain blood pressure and provide adequate hydration.
C. Post-seizure coma.
   1. Maintain airway and oxygenation.
   2. If a result of oral medication, follow above recommendations to prevent absorption of drug, but intubation and lavage will have to be performed instead of inducing emesis and the cathartic and charcoal will need to be introduced via a large bore gastric lavage tube.
   3. Continue to provide full supportive care and adequate hydration while waiting for drug to be metabolized. In general, the drug is metabolized sufficiently rapidly enough so as to not warrant consideration of dialysis.
D. Animal studies suggest that phenobarbital may decrease theophylline toxicity. There are as yet, however, insufficient data to recommend pretreatment of an overdosage with phenobarbital.

General
The oral LD_{50} of the theophylline in mice is 350 mg/kg. The oral LD_{50} of guaifenesin in mice is 1725 mg/kg. In humans, adverse reactions often occur when serum theophylline levels exceed 20 μg/ml. Information of physiological variables which influence excretion of theophylline can be found under the heading "Clinical Pharmacology."
Dosage and Administration:
General
Therapeutic serum levels associated with optimal likelihood for benefit and minimal risk of toxicity are considered to be between 10 μg/ml and 20 μg/ml. Levels above 20 μg/ml may produce toxic effects. There is great variation from patient to patient in dosage needed in order to achieve a therapeutic blood level because of variable rates of elimination. Because of this wide variation from patient to patient and the relatively narrow therapeutic blood level range, dosage must be individualized and monitoring of serum theophylline levels is highly recommended.
Dosage should be calculated on the basis of lean (ideal) body weight where mg/kg doses are stated. Theophylline does not distribute into fatty tissue.
Giving theophylline with food may prevent the rare case of stomach irritation and, although absorption may be slower, it is still complete. When rapidly absorbed products such as solutions and soft gelatin capsules with rapid dissolution are used, dosing to maintain "around the clock" blood levels generally requires administration every 6 hours to obtain the greatest efficacy for clinical use in children; dosing intervals up to 8 hours may be satisfactory for adults because of their slower elimination. Children and adults requiring higher than average doses may benefit from products with slower absorption which may allow longer dosing intervals and/or less fluctuation in serum concentration over a dosing interval during chronic therapy.
Acute symptoms of asthma requiring rapid theophyllinization
Note: Due to their slower rate of absorption, sustaned release theophylline products are not designed for use in conditions requiring rapid theophyllinization.

Group	Oral Loading Dose (Theophylline)	Maintenance Dose for Next 12 hrs. (Theophylline)	Maintenance Dose Beyond 12 hrs. (Theophylline)
1. Children 6 months to 9 years	6 mg/kg	4 mg/kg q4hrs.	4 mg/kg q6hrs
2. Children 9–16 and young adult smokers	6 mg/kg	3 mg/kg q4hrs.	3 mg/kg q6hrs
3. Otherwise healthy non-smoking adults	6 mg/kg	3 mg/kg q6hrs	3 mg/kg q8hrs
4. Older patients and patients with cor pulmonale	6 mg/kg	2 mg/kg q6hrs	2 mg/kg q8hrs
5. Patients with congestive heart failure, liver failure	6 mg/kg	2 mg/kg q8hrs	1–2 mg/kg q12hrs

I. Not currently receiving theophylline products.
(See table above)
II. Those currently receiving theophylline products: Determine, where possible, the time, amount, route of administration and form of the patient's last dose.
The loading dose for theophylline will be based on the principle that each 5 mg/kg of theophylline administered as a loading dose will result in a 1 mcg/ml increase in serum theophylline concentration. Ideally, then, the loading dose should be deferred if a serum theophylline concentration can be rapidly obtained. If this is not possible, the clinician must exercise his judgment in selecting a dose based on the potential of benefit to risk. When there is sufficient respiratory distress to warrant a small risk, 2.5 mg/kg of theophylline is likely to increase the serum concentration when administered as a loading dose in rapidly absorbed form by only about 5 μg/ml. If the patient is not already experiencing theophylline toxicity, this is unlikely to result in dangerous adverse effects.
Once the determination is made regarding the loading dose in this group of patients, subsequent maintenance dosage recommendations are the same as those described above.
Comments: To achieve optimal therapeutic theophylline dosage, it is recommended that serum theophylline concentrations be monitored. However, it is not always possible or practical to obtain a serum theophylline level. Patients should be closely monitored for signs of toxicity. The present data suggest that the above dosage recommendations will achieve therapeutic serum concentrations with minimal risk of toxicity for most patients.
However, some risk of toxic serum concentration is still present. Adverse reactions to theophylline often occur when serum theophylline levels exceed 20 μg/ml.
Chronic Asthma: Theophyllinization is a treatment of first choice for the management of chronic asthma (to prevent symptoms and maintain patent airways). Slow clinical titration is generally preferred to assure acceptance and safety of the medication.
Initial dose: 16 mg/kg/day or 400 mg/day (whichever is lower) in 3 to 4 divided doses at 6 to 8 hours intervals for the Syrup and Capsules.
Increased dose: The above dosage may be increased in approximately 25 percent increments at 2 to 3 day intervals so long as no intolerance is observed, until the maximum indicated below is reached.
Maximum dose without measurement of serum concentration:
Not to exceed the following: **(WARNING: DO NOT ATTEMPT TO MAINTAIN ANY DOSE THAT IS NOT TOLERATED.)**
Age 6 months to 9 years ....24 mg/kg/day
Age 9 to 12 years ....20 mg/kg/day
Age 12 to 16 years ....18 mg/kg/day
Age > 16 years ....13 mg/kg/day or 900 mg/day (WHICHEVER IS LESS)
Note: Use ideal body weight for obese patients.
Measurement of serum theophylline concentration during chronic therapy:
If the above maximum doses are to be maintained or exceeded, serum theophylline measurement is recommended. This should be obtained at the approximate time of peak absorption during chronic therapy for the product used (1 to 2 hours for liquids, soft gelatin capsules, and plain uncoated tablets that undergo rapid dissolution, 3 to 5 hours for sustained release preparations). It is important that the patient will have missed **no** doses during the previous 48 hours and that dosing intervals will have been reasonably typical with no added doses during that period of time. **DOSAGE ADJUSTMENT BASED ON SERUM THEOPHYLLINE MEASUREMENTS WHEN THESE INSTRUCTIONS HAVE NOT BEEN FOLLOWED MAY RESULT IN RECOMMENDATIONS THAT PRESENT RISK OF TOXICITY TO THE PATIENT.**
Final Dosage Adjustment: Caution should be exercised for younger children who cannot complain of minor side effects. Older adults, those with cor pulmonale, congestive heart failure, and/or liver disease may have unusually low dosage requirements and thus may experience toxicity at the maximal dosage recommended above.
It is important that no patient be maintained on any dosage that he is not tolerating. In instructing patients to increase dosage according to the schedule above, they should be instructed not to take a subsequent dose if apparent side effects occur and to resume therapy at a lower dose once adverse effects have disappeared.
[See table below].
KEEP THIS AND ALL MEDICATION OUT OF THE REACH OF CHILDREN. In case of accidental overdose, seek professional assistance or contact a poison control center immediately.

Body Weight Expressed in Kilos	Lbs	Dosage of Slo-Phyllin® GG Syrup Calculated at Approximately: 3mg Per Kilo	4mg Per Kilo	5mg Per Kilo
9	20	½ tsp	¾ tsp	1 tsp
18	40	1 tsp	1½ tsp	2 tsp
27	60	1½ tsp	2 tsp	2¾ tsp
36	79	2 tsp	3 tsp	3½ tsp
45	99	2¾ tsp	3½ tsp	4½ tsp
54	118	3¼ tsp	4½ tsp	5½ tsp

Administered every six (6) hours.

Supplied:
Slo-Phyllin® GG Syrup is lemon-vanilla flavored, nonalcoholic, dye-free, and each 15 ml tablespoonful contains theophylline, anhydrous 150 mg and guaifenesin 90 mg. Available in 16 oz. bottles (NDC 0067-0357-16).
Slo-Phyllin® GG Capsules are white, liquid filled, and each soft gelatin capsule contains theophylline, anhydrous 150 mg and guaifenesin 90 mg. Available in bottles of 100 capsules (NDC 0067-2358-68).

Slo-Phyllin® GG Capsules
Manufactured by
R. P. Scherer Corporation
Detroit, MI 48226
For
William H. Rorer, Inc.

[Slo-Phyllin® GG Capsules Shown in Product Identification Section]

Ross Laboratories
COLUMBUS, OH 43216

ADVANCE®
Nutritional Beverage

Usage: As a nutritional beverage more appropriate than cow milk for healthy, growing, older babies.
Availability:
Concentrated Liquid: 13-fl-oz cans; 12 per case; No. 03313.
Ready To Feed: 32-fl-oz cans; 6 per case; No. 03301.
Preparation: Standard 16 Cal/fl oz dilution is one part Concentrated Liquid to one part water. Ready To Feed requires no dilution. For hospital use, prebottled ADVANCE is available in the Ross Hospital Formula System.
Composition: Concentrated Liquid
Ingredients: Ⓤ Water, corn syrup, nonfat milk, soy oil, soy protein isolate, corn oil, mono- and diglycerides, soy lecithin, minerals (calcium phosphate tribasic, potassium citrate, magnesium chloride, ferrous sulfate, zinc sulfate, cupric sulfate, manganese sulfate), vitamins (ascorbic acid, alpha-tocopheryl acetate, niacinamide, calcium pantothenate, vitamin A palmitate, thiamine chloride hydrochloride, pyridoxine hydrochloride, riboflavin, folic acid, vitamin D_3, cyanocobalamin) and carrageenan.

Approximate Analysis (wt/liter):	Concentrated		Standard Dilution*	
Protein	40.0	g	20.0	g
Fat	54.0	g	27.0	g
Carbohydrate	110.0	g	55.0	g
Minerals (Ash)	7.0	g	3.5	g
Calcium	1.02	g	0.51	g
Phosphorus	0.78	g	0.39	g
Sodium (maximum)	0.60	g	0.30	g
Magnesium	128	mg	64	mg
Iron	24	mg	12	mg
Zinc	12	mg	6.0	mg
Copper	1.8	mg	0.9	mg
Iodine	0.12	mg	60	mcg
Manganese	68	mcg	34	mcg
Water	843	g	920	g
Crude Fiber	0	g		
Calories per fl oz	32		16	
Calories per 100 ml	108		54	

Vitamins Per Liter (Standard Dilution*)

Vitamin A	2400	I.U.
Vitamin D	400	I.U.
Vitamin E	18	I.U.
Vitamin C	50	mg
Thiamine (Vitamin B_1)	0.75	mg
Riboflavin (Vitamin B_2)	0.90	mg

Continued on next page

Ross—Cont.

Niacin (mg equiv.)	10	
Vitamin B_6	0.60	mg
Pantothenic Acid	4.0	mg
Folic Acid	0.10	mg
Vitamin B_{12}	2.5	mcg

*Standard dilution is equal parts ADVANCE Concentrated Liquid and water.

Composition: Ready To Feed
Ingredients: Ⓤ Water, corn syrup, nonfat milk, soy oil, soy protein isolate, corn oil, mono- and diglycerides, soy lecithin, minerals (calcium phosphate tribasic, potassium citrate, magnesium chloride, ferrous sulfate, zinc sulfate, cupric sulfate, manganese sulfate), vitamins (ascorbic acid, alpha-tocopheryl acetate, niacinamide, calcium pantothenate, vitamin A palmitate, thiamine chloride hydrochloride, pyridoxine hydrochloride, riboflavin, folic acid, vitamin D_3, cyanocobalamin) and carrageenan.

Approximate Analysis (wt/liter):

Protein	20.0	g
Fat	27.0	g
Carbohydrate	55.0	g
Minerals (Ash)	3.5	g
Calcium	0.51	g
Phosphorus	0.39	g
Sodium (maximum)	0.30	g
Magnesium	64	mg
Iron	12	mg
Zinc	6.0	mg
Copper	0.9	mg
Iodine	60	mcg
Manganese	34	mcg
Water	920	g
Crude Fiber	0	g
Calories per fl oz	16	
Calories per 100 ml	54	

Vitamins Per Liter:

Vitamin A	2400	I.U.
Vitamin D	400	I.U.
Vitamin E	18	I.U.
Vitamin C	50	mg
Thiamine (Vitamin B_1)	0.75	mg
Riboflavin (Vitamin B_2)	0.90	mg
Niacin (mg equiv.)	10	
Vitamin B_6	0.60	mg
Pantothenic Acid	4.0	mg
Folic Acid	0.10	mg
Vitamin B_{12}	2.5	mcg

Vitamin/Mineral Content of Ensure (Ready To Use)

Vitamins/Minerals	Per 8 Fl Oz		Percent U.S. RDA* (Per 8 Fl Oz)
Vitamin A	625	I.U.	12.5
Vitamin D	50	I.U.	12.5
Vitamin E	7.5	I.U.	25.0
Vitamin K_1	35	mcg	**
Vitamin C	38	mg	62.5
Folic Acid	50	mcg	12.5
Thiamine (Vitamin B_1)	0.38	mg	25.0
Riboflavin (Vitamin B_2)	0.43	mg	25.0
Vitamin B_6	0.50	mg	25.0
Vitamin B_{12}	1.5	mcg	25.0
Niacin	5.0	mg	25.0
Choline	0.13	g	**
Biotin	38	mcg	12.5
Pantothenic Acid	1.25	mg	12.5
Sodium	0.20	g	**
Potassium	0.37	g	**
Chloride	0.34	g	**
Calcium	0.13	g	12.5
Phosphorus	0.13	g	12.5
Magnesium	50	mg	12.5
Iodine	19	mcg	12.5
Manganese	0.50	mg	**
Copper	0.25	mg	12.5
Zinc	3.75	mg	25.0
Iron	2.25	mg	12.5

*For adults and children 4 or more years of age.
**U.S. RDA not established.

The addition of iron to this beverage conforms to the recommendation of the Committee on Nutrition of the American Academy of Pediatrics.

ENSURE®
Liquid Nutrition

Usage: For complete, balanced nutrition. Ensure can be used as a full liquid diet, liquid supplement or tube feeding. Ensure is useful whenever the patient's medical, surgical or psychological state precludes normal food intake and/or leads to inadequate nutrition.
Ensure is appropriate for use in situations where low residue is a primary consideration, as in preoperative diets or as a preparatory diet for barium enema examination. The amount of fecal residue produced by Ensure is comparable to that produced by a chemically defined elemental diet.

Features:
Ensure is complete nutrition. Caloric density: 1.06 Calories per ml, 250 Calories per 8 fl oz, 1000 Calories per quart from a balanced distribution of protein, fat and carbohydrate (caloric distribution: protein, 14%; fat, 31.5%; carbohydrate, 54.5%). Vitamin/mineral levels in two quarts (2000 Calories) of Ensure meet or surpass 100% of the U.S. RDA for adults and children 4 or more years of age.
Ensure provides protein of high biologic value, a fat source (corn oil) easily digested, and a lactose-free formulation. Ensure has a low osmolality of 450 mOsm/kg water.

Dosage and Administration:
Ready To Use: Shake well. Do not add water for a standard 1 Calorie/ml feeding. Ensure may be stored (unopened) and fed at room temperature. Once opened, any unused Ensure should be covered, refrigerated and discarded if not used within 48 hours. Ensure is delicious when chilled.
Powder: To prepare an 8-fl-oz glassful: Put ¾ cup of cold water in a glass. Gradually stir in ½ cup Ensure Powder and mix until dissolved. Reconstituted Ensure should be used promptly or covered, refrigerated and used within 24 hours. Once can of Ensure Powder has been opened, contents should be used within 3 weeks. Opened can should be covered with overcap and stored in a cool, dry place, but not refrigerated.

- **Oral Feeding:** Ensure may be used for total nutrition, or with and between meals for added nutritional support.
- **Tube Feeding:** Follow physician's instructions. When initiating feeding, the flow rate, volume and dilution are dependent on patient condition and tolerance.

Additional fluid requirements should be met by giving water orally with or after feedings, or when flushing the feeding tube. Care should be taken to avoid contamination of this product during preparation and administration.
[See table left].

Under no circumstances should Ensure be administered parenterally.

Availability:
Ready To Use:
8-fl-oz bottles; 24 per case; Vanilla, No. 708.
8-fl-oz cans; 4 six-packs per case; Chocolate, No. 701; Black Walnut, No. 703; Coffee, No. 704;

Sample Administration Schedule For ENSURE

Continuous Drip or Pump Controlled Delivery

Day	Time	Strength	Rate (ml/hr)	Volume (ml)	Calories
1	1st 8 hours	Full	50	400	400
	2nd 8 hours	Full	75	600	600
	3rd 8 hours	Full	100	800	800
					1800 *Total Calories*
2	24 hours	Full	100–125	2400–3000	2400–3000 *Total Calories*

Intermittent Drip

Day	Time	Strength	Rate (5–10 ml/min)	Volume (ml)	Calories
1	7am–11pm	Full	100 ml q 2 hr (7am, 9am)	200	200
			150 ml q 2 hr (11am, 1pm, 3pm)	450	450
			200 ml q 2 hr (5pm, 7pm, 9pm, 11pm)	800	800
					1450 *Total Calories*
2	7am–11pm	Full	250 ml q 2 hr (8 feedings) up to	2000	2000 *Total Calories*
			400 ml q 3 hr (5 feedings)	2000	2000 *Total Calories*

Strawberry, No. 705; Eggnog, No. 710; Vanilla, No. 711.
32-fl-oz cans; 6 per case; Vanilla, No. 733.
Powder:
14-oz (400 g) cans; 6 per case; Vanilla, No. 750.
Composition: Ready To Use Vanilla (Other Ready To Use flavors and Vanilla Powder at standard dilution have similar composition and nutrient values. For specific information, see product labels.)
Ingredients: Ⓤ Water, hydrolyzed corn starch, sucrose, sodium and calcium caseinates, corn oil, soy protein isolate, potassium citrate, magnesium chloride, soy lecithin, calcium phosphate tribasic, natural and artificial flavoring, potassium chloride, sodium citrate, choline chloride, ascorbic acid, carrageenan, vitamin concentrate (alpha-tocopheryl acetate, vitamin A palmitate, phylloquinone, vitamin D_3), zinc sulfate, ferrous sulfate, niacinamide, manganous chloride, calcium pantothenate, cupric sulfate, thiamine chloride hydrochloride, pyridoxine hydrochloride, riboflavin, biotin, folic acid and cyanocobalamin.
Approximate Analysis (g/8 fl oz): Protein, 8.8; Fat, 8.8; Carbohydrate, 34.3; Ash, 1.4; Moisture, 199.5. Calories per ml, 1.06; Calories per fl oz, 31.8.
(See table on top preceding page)

ENSURE PLUS®
High Calorie Liquid Nutrition

Usage: As a high-calorie liquid food providing complete, balanced nutrition. Caloric density is 1500 Calories per liter, 50% greater than most other liquid feedings. Ensure Plus is intended for use when extra calories and correspondingly higher concentrations of protein and most other nutrients are needed to achieve a required calorie intake in a limited volume. When utilized to provide total nutrition, Ensure Plus can deliver the high-calorie intakes required by severely ill or traumatized patients who are nutritionally depleted, and who may not be able to tolerate large-volume intakes. As a dietary supplement, Ensure Plus can supply extra calories and protein for those patients unable or unwilling to consume adequate nutrition.
Ensure Plus is appropriate for use in situations where low residue is a primary consideration, as in preoperative diets or as a preparatory diet for barium enema examination. The amount of fecal residue produced by Ensure Plus is comparable to that produced by a chemically defined elemental diet.

Sample Administration Schedule For ENSURE PLUS
For patients who need 3000 Cal/day or more, or those who are fluid restricted.

Continuous Drip or Pump Controlled Delivery

Day	Time	Strength	Rate (ml/hr)	Volume (ml)	Calories
1	1st 8 hours	½	50	400	300
	2nd 8 hours	½	75	600	450
	3rd 8 hours	½	100	800	600
					1350 *Total Calories*
2	1st 8 hours	½	125	1000	750
	2nd 8 hours	Full	100–125	800–1000	1200–1500
	3rd 8 hours	Full	100–125	800–1000	1200–1500
					3150–3750 *Total Calories*
3	24 hours	Full	100–125	2400–3000	3600–4500 *Total Calories*

Intermittent Drip

Day	Time	Strength	Rate (5–10 ml/min)	Volume (ml)	Calories
1	7am–11pm	½	100 ml q 2 hr (7am, 9am)	200	150
		½	150 ml q 2 hr (11am, 1pm, 3pm)	450	338
		½	200 ml q 2 hr (5pm, 7pm, 9pm, 11pm)	800	600
					1088 *Total Calories*
2	7am–11pm	½	250 ml q 2 hr (7am, 9am, 11am)	750	563
		Full	250 ml q 2 hr (1pm, 3pm, 5pm, 7pm, 9pm, 11pm)	1500	2250
					2813 *Total Calories*
3	7am–11pm	Full	250 ml q 2 hr (8 feedings) up to	2000	3000 *Total Calories*
			400 ml q 3 hr (5 feedings)	2000	3000 *Total Calories*

Features:
Ensure Plus provides complete nutrition with low residue. Caloric density: 1.5 Calories per ml, 355 Calories per 8 fl oz, 1420 Calories per quart from a balanced distribution of protein, fat and carbohydrate (caloric distribution: protein, 14.7%; fat, 32.0%; carbohydrate, 53.3%). 2400 Cal (1.7 quarts) of Ensure Plus meet or surpass 100% of the U.S. RDA for vitamins and minerals for adults and children 4 or more years of age.
Ensure Plus provides sufficient protein (55 grams/liter) to meet the demands of severe illness. The fat source (corn oil) is easily digested, and Ensure Plus is a lactose-free feeding. Osmolality (600 mOsm/kg water) is moderate, even though caloric density is 50% greater than standard liquid feedings.
Dosage and Administration: Ensure Plus is ready to use and does not require dilution with water. Ensure Plus may be stored (unopened) and fed at room temperature. Once opened, remaining Ensure Plus should be covered, refrigerated and discarded if not used within 48 hours. Ensure Plus is delicious when chilled.

- **Oral Feeding:** Ensure Plus may be used for total nutrition, or with and between meals for added nutritional support.
- **Tube Feeding:** Follow physician's instructions. When initiating feeding, the flow rate, volume and dilution are dependent on patient condition and tolerance.

Additional fluid requirements should be met by giving water orally with or after feedings, or when flushing the feeding tube. Care should be taken to avoid contamination of this product during preparation and administration.
[See table above].

Vitamin/Mineral Content of Ensure Plus (Ready To Use)

Vitamins/Minerals	Per 8 Fl Oz		% U.S. RDA* (Per 8 Fl Oz)
Vitamin A	890	I.U.	17.8
Vitamin D	70	I.U.	17.5
Vitamin E	10.7	I.U.	35.7
Vitamin K_1	50	mcg	**
Vitamin C	38	mg	62.5
Folic Acid	75	mcg	18.8
Thiamine (Vitamin B_1)	0.63	mg	41.3
Riboflavin (Vitamin B_2)	0.65	mg	37.5
Vitamin B_6	0.75	mg	37.5
Vitamin B_{12}	2.25	mcg	37.5
Niacin	7.5	mg	37.5
Biotin	56	mcg	18.7
Choline	125	mg	**
Pantothenic Acid	2.0	mg	20
Sodium	0.27	g	**
Potassium	0.55	g	**
Chloride	0.47	g	**
Calcium	0.15	g	15
Phosphorus	0.15	g	15
Magnesium	75	mg	18.8
Manganese	0.50	mg	**
Iodine	25	mcg	16.3
Copper	0.38	mg	18.8
Iron	3.38	mg	18.8
Zinc	5.63	mg	37.5

*For adults and children 4 or more years of age.
**U.S. RDA not established.

Continued on next page

Ross—Cont.

Under no circumstances should Ensure Plus be administered parenterally.

Availability: 8-fl-oz bottles; 24 per case; Vanilla, No. 741.
8-fl-oz cans; 4 six-packs per case; Chocolate, No. 702; Vanilla, No. 707; Eggnog, No. 716; Coffee, No. 717; Strawberry, No. 718.

Composition: Ready To Use Vanilla (Other flavors have similar composition. For specific information, see product labels.)

Ingredients: ⓤ Water, hydrolyzed corn starch, sodium and calcium caseinates, corn oil, sucrose, soy protein isolate, magnesium chloride, potassium citrate, soy lecithin, calcium phosphate tribasic, natural and artificial flavoring, sodium citrate, potassium chloride, choline chloride, ascorbic acid, vitamin concentrate (alpha-tocopheryl acetate, vitamin A palmitate, phylloquinone, vitamin D_3), zinc sulfate, ferrous sulfate, carrageenan, niacinamide, calcium pantothenate, manganous chloride, cupric sulfate, thiamine chloride hydrochloride, pyridoxine hydrochloride, riboflavin, folic acid, biotin and cyanocobalamin.

Approximate Analysis (g/8 fl oz): Protein, 13.0; Fat, 12.6; Carbohydrate, 47.3; Ash, 2.2; Moisture, 182.0. Calories per ml, 1.5; Calories per fl oz, 44.4.
(See table on bottom preceding page)

FLEXIFLO® ENTERAL DELIVERY SYSTEM

A complete delivery system specially designed for enteral feeding.

FLEXIFLO® Enteral Nutrition Pump

Peristaltic pump with constant-speed motor allows accurate flow control from 50 to 200 ml/hr in 25-ml increments. The Flexiflo Pump, designed for enteral feeding, is simple to operate, quiet and reliable.

Availability: Pump; 1 pump per case; retail unit, No. 64; lease unit, No. 72.

FLEXIFLO® Enteral Pump Set

For use with the Flexiflo Pump, the set has a specially formulated insert, sight chamber, colored flow regulation tabs and a tip adapter compatible with most indwelling feeding tubes.

Availability: Pump set; 24 individually packed sets per case; No. 65.

FLEXITAINER® Enteral Nutrition Container

Ready-to-use, large-volume, one-liter container combining the best features of a bottle and a bag. . . collapsible with a rigid neck and a large opening for easy filling, and graduated measurements for both filling and delivery.

Availability: Container; 24 per case; No. 69.

FLEXIFLO® Gravity Gavage Set

Offers a means to administer a tube feeding via gravity. Attaches to either 8-oz bottles of formula or to the Flexitainer. Set is composed of a feeding cap, clear plastic sight chamber, air vent protected by bacteria-retentive filter, flow regulator (CAIR® Clamp), and tip adapter compatible with most indwelling feeding tubes.

Availability: Gavage set; 24 individually packed sets per case; No. 61.

FORTA™ PUDDING

Usage: To provide balanced nutrition in a delicious, easy-to-eat form.

Features: High caloric density—50 Cal/oz provides 250 Calories per 5-oz serving. Balanced caloric distribution—high-quality protein plus appropriate levels of fat and carbohydrates.
Low sodium content—0.22 g per serving (155 mg per 100 g)—appropriate for diets requiring moderate sodium intake. Each 5-oz serving provides at least 17% of the U.S. RDA for vitamins and minerals.
Easy-open 5-oz cans are ready to serve at room temperature or chilled. Four flavors (Vanilla, Chocolate, Butterscotch, Tapioca) provide taste and texture variety.

Availability:
Ready To Eat: 5-oz cans; 12 four-packs per case; Chocolate, No. 790; Vanilla, No. 792; Tapioca, No. 794; Butterscotch, No. 798.

Composition: Vanilla (Other flavors have similar composition. For specific information, see product packaging.)

Ingredients: Water, nonfat milk, sucrose, partially hydrogenated soybean oil, modified food starch, magnesium sulfate, sodium stearoyl-2-lactylate, sodium phosphate dibasic, artificial flavor, ascorbic acid, ferrous sulfate, choline chloride, zinc sulfate, alpha-tocopheryl acetate, niacinamide, FD&C yellow #5, manganous chloride, calcium pantothenate, cupric sulfate, vitamin D_3 concentrate, vitamin A palmitate, potassium citrate, pyridoxine hydrochloride, thiamine chloride hydrochloride, riboflavin, phylloquinone, folic acid, biotin and cyanocobalamin.

Vitamins/Minerals	Per Can (5 oz)		Percent U.S. RDA* 250 Calories
Vitamin A	833	I.U.	17
Vitamin D	67	I.U.	17
Vitamin E	5.0	I.U.	17
Vitamin C	15	mg	25
Folic Acid	67	mcg	17
Thiamine (Vitamin B_1)	0.25	mg	17
Riboflavin (Vitamin B_2)	0.28	mg	17
Vitamin B_6	0.33	mg	17
Vitamin B_{12}	1.0	mcg	17
Niacin	3.3	mg	17
Choline	25	mg	**
Biotin	50	mcg	17
Pantothenic Acid	1.66	mg	17
Sodium	0.22	g	**
Potassium	0.30	g	**
Chloride	0.21	g	**
Calcium	0.20	g	20
Phosphorus	0.20	g	20
Magnesium	67	mg	17
Iodine	60	mcg	40
Manganese	0.66	mg	**
Copper	0.33	mg	17
Zinc	3.0	mg	20
Iron	3.0	mg	17

*For adults and children 4 or more years of age.
**U.S. RDA not established.

Approximate Analysis (per 5-oz serving): Protein, 6.8 g; Fat, 9.7 g; Carbohydrate, 34.0 g; Minerals (Ash), 0.6 g; Moisture, 90.6 g. Calories per serving, 250.
(See table below)

ISOMIL®

Soy Protein Formula

Usage: As a beverage for infants, children and adults with allergy or sensitivity to cow milk. A feeding in patients with disorders where lactose should be avoided: lactase deficiency, lactose intolerance and galactosemia. A feeding following diarrhea.

Availability:
Powder: 14-oz cans; measuring scoop enclosed; 6 per case; No. 00107. 1.07-oz packets; 12 four-packet cartons per case; No. 00219.
Concentrated Liquid: 13-fl-oz cans; 24 per case; No. 02110.
Ready To Feed: (Prediluted 20 Cal/fl oz) 32-fl-oz cans; 6 per case; No. 00230.
8-fl-oz cans; 4 six-packs per case; No. 00173.
For hospital use, prebottled ISOMIL is available in the Ross Hospital Formula System.

Preparation:
Powder: Standard 20 Cal/fl oz dilution is 1 level scoop of Isomil Powder for each 2 fl oz of warm water; or, 1 packet (1.07 oz) for each 7 fl oz of warm water.
Concentrated Liquid—Standard 20 Cal/fl oz dilution is one part Concentrated Liquid to one part water.
Note: All forms of Isomil should be shaken well before feeding.

Composition: Powder

Ingredients: (Pareve, ⓤ) 25.2% corn syrup solids, 25.2% sucrose, 17.5% soy protein isolate, 13.5% corn oil, 13.5% coconut oil, minerals (1.5% calcium phosphate tribasic, 1.0% potassium citrate, 0.4% potassium chloride, 0.3% magnesium chloride, calcium carbonate, sodium chloride, ferrous sulfate, zinc sulfate, cupric sulfate, potassium iodide), vitamins (ascorbic acid, choline chloride, alpha-tocopheryl acetate, niacinamide, calcium pantothenate, vitamin A palmitate, thiamine chloride hydrochloride, riboflavin, pyridoxine hydrochloride, phylloquinone, folic acid, biotin, vitamin D_3, cyanocobalamin) and L-methionine.
[See table on top next page].

Vitamins Per Liter (Standard Dilution*):

Vitamin A	2500	I.U.
Vitamin D	400	I.U.
Vitamin E	17	I.U.
Thiamine (Vitamin B_1)	0.40	mg
Riboflavin (Vitamin B_2)	0.60	mg
Vitamin B_6	0.40	mg
Vitamin K_1	0.15	mg
Niacin (mg equiv.)	9.0	
Vitamin C	55	mg
Folic Acid	0.10	mg
Vitamin B_{12}	3.0	mcg
Pantothenic Acid	5.0	mg
Biotin	30	mcg

* Standard dilution is 1 level scoop of Isomil Powder for each 2 fl oz of warm water; or, 1 packet (1.07 oz) for each 7 fl oz of warm water.

Composition: Concentrated Liquid

Ingredients: (Pareve, ⓤ) 74% water, 7.3% corn syrup, 5.7% sucrose, 4.4% soy protein isolate, 4.0% soy oil, 2.6% coconut oil, 1.0% modified corn starch, minerals (calcium phosphate tribasic, potassium citrate, potassium chloride, magnesium chloride, sodium chloride, ferrous sulfate, zinc sulfate, cupric sulfate, manganese sulfate, potassium iodide), mono- and diglycerides, soy lecithin, vitamins (ascorbic acid, choline chloride, alpha-tocopheryl acetate, niacinamide, calcium pantothenate, vitamin A palmitate, thiamine chloride hydrochloride, riboflavin, pyridoxine hydrochloride, phylloquinone, folic acid, biotin, vitamin D_3, cyanocobalamin), L-methionine and carrageenan.

Approximate Analysis (wt/liter):	Concentrated	Standard Dilution*
Protein	40.0 g	20.0 g
Fat	72.0 g	36.0 g
Carbohydrate	136.0 g	68.0 g
Minerals (Ash)	7.5 g	3.8 g
Calcium	1.4 g	0.70 g
Phosphorus	1.0 g	0.50 g
Sodium	0.60 g	0.30 g
Potassium	1.42 g	0.71 g
Chloride	1.06 g	0.53 g
Magnesium	0.10 g	50 mg
Iron	24 mg	12 mg
Zinc	10 mg	5.0 mg
Copper	1.0 mg	0.50 mg
Iodine	0.20 mg	0.10 mg
Manganese	0.40 mg	0.20 mg
Water	805.7 g	901.6 g
Crude Fiber	0 g	
Calories per fl oz	40	20
Calories per 100 ml	136	68

Vitamins Per Liter (Standard dilution*):

Vitamin A	2500 I.U.
Vitamin D	400 I.U.
Vitamin E	20 I.U.
Vitamin C	55 mg
Thiamine (Vitamin B_1)	0.40 mg
Riboflavin (Vitamin B_2)	0.60 mg
Vitamin B_6	0.40 mg
Niacin (mg equiv.)	9.0
Folic acid	0.10 mg
Vitamin B_{12}	3.0 mcg
Pantothenic Acid	5.0 mg
Biotin	30 mcg
Vitamin K_1	0.15 mg

*Standard dilution is one part Isomil Concentrated Liquid to one part water.

Composition: Ready To Feed

Ingredients: (Pareve, ⓤ) 86.4% water, 4.0% corn syrup, 3.1% sucrose, 2.3% soy protein isolate, 2.0% soy oil, 1.4% coconut oil, minerals (calcium phosphate dibasic, calcium carbonate, potassium citrate, potassium chloride, calcium phosphate monobasic, magnesium chloride, ferrous sulfate, sodium chloride, zinc sulfate, cupric sulfate, manganese sulfate, potassium iodide), mono- and diglycerides, soy lecithin, vitamins (ascorbic acid, choline chloride, alpha-tocopheryl acetate, niacinamide, calcium pantothenate, vitamin A palmitate, thiamine chloride hydrochloride, riboflavin, pyridoxine hydrochloride, phylloquinone, folic acid, biotin, vitamin D_3, cyanocobalamin), carrageenan and L-methionine.

Approximate Analysis (wt/liter):

Protein	20.0 g
Fat	36.0 g
Carbohydrate	68.0 g
Minerals (Ash)	3.8 g
Calcium	0.70 g
Phosphorus	0.50 g
Sodium	0.30 g
Potassium	0.71 g
Chloride	0.53 g
Magnesium	50 mg
Iron	12 mg
Zinc	5.0 mg
Copper	0.50 mg
Iodine	0.10 mg
Manganese	0.20 mg
Water	901.6 g
Crude Fiber	0 g
Calories per fl oz	20
Calories per 100 ml	68

Approximate Analysis:	Powdered (wt/packet)	Standard Dilution* (wt/liter)
Protein	4.6 g	20.0 g
Fat	8.3 g	36.0 g
Carbohydrate	15.6 g	68.0 g
Minerals (Ash)	0.9 g	3.8 g
Calcium	0.16 g	0.70 g
Phosphorus	0.12 g	0.50 g
Sodium	70 mg	0.30 g
Potassium	0.16 g	0.71 g
Chloride	0.12 g	0.53 g
Magnesium	12 mg	50 mg
Iron	2.8 mg	12 mg
Zinc	1.2 mg	5.0 mg
Copper	0.12 mg	0.50 mg
Iodine	23 mcg	0.10 mg
Manganese	46 mcg	0.20 mg
Moisture	0.8 g	901.6 g
Crude Fiber	0 g	
Calories per fl oz	155	20
Calories per 100 ml		68

Vitamins Per Liter:

Vitamin A	2500 I.U.
Vitamin D	400 I.U.
Vitamin E	20 I.U.
Vitamin C	55 mg
Thiamine (Vitamin B_1)	0.40 mg
Riboflavin (Vitamin B_2)	0.60 mg
Vitamin B_6	0.40 mg
Niacin (mg equiv.)	9.0
Folic acid	0.10 mg
Vitamin B_{12}	3.0 mcg
Pantothenic Acid	5.0 mg
Biotin	30 mcg
Vitamin K_1	0.15 mg

The addition of iron to this formula conforms to the recommendation of the Committee on Nutrition of the American Academy of Pediatrics.

ISOMIL® SF

Sucrose-Free Soy Protein Formula

Usage: As a beverage for infants, children and adults with an allergy or sensitivity to cow milk and sucrose. A feeding following acute diarrhea. A feeding in patients with disorders where lactose and sucrose should be avoided.

Availability:

Concentrated Liquid: 13-fl-oz cans; 12 per case; No. 00119.

Ready To Feed: (Prediluted, 20 Cal/fl oz) 32-fl-oz cans; 6 per case; No. 00128.

For hospital use, prebottled ISOMIL SF is available in the Ross Hospital Formula System.

Preparation:

Concentrated Liquid: Standard 20 Cal/fl oz dilution is one part Isomil SF Concentrated Liquid to one part water.

Note: All forms of Isomil SF should be shaken well before feeding.

Composition: Concentrated Liquid

Ingredients: (Pareve, ⓤ) 75.7% water, 13.2% corn syrup solids, 4.2% soy protein isolate, 4.0% soy oil, 2.6% coconut oil, minerals (calcium phosphate tribasic, potassium citrate, potassium chloride, magnesium chloride, calcium carbonate, sodium chloride, ferrous sulfate, zinc sulfate, cupric sulfate, potassium iodide), mono- and diglycerides, soy lecithin, vitamins (ascorbic acid, choline chloride, alpha-tocopheryl acetate, niacinamide, calcium pantothenate, vitamin A palmitate, thiamine chloride hydrochloride, riboflavin, pyridoxine hydrochloride, phylloquinone, folic acid, biotin, vitamin D_3, cyanocobalamin) and L-methionine.

Approximate Analysis (wt/liter):	Concentrated	Standard Dilution*
Protein	40.0 g	20.0 g
Fat	72.0 g	36.0 g
Carbohydrate	136.0 g	68.0 g
Minerals (Ash)	7.5 g	3.8 g
Calcium	1.4 g	0.70g
Phosphorus	1.0 g	0.50g
Sodium	0.60g	0.30g
Potassium	1.42g	0.71g
Chloride	1.06g	0.53g
Magnesium	0.10g	50 mg
Iron	24 mg	12 mg
Zinc	10 mg	5.0 mg
Copper	1.0 mg	0.50mg
Iodine	0.20mg	0.10mg
Manganese	0.40mg	0.20mg
Water	805.7 g	901.6 g
Crude Fiber	0 g	
Calories per fl oz	40	20
Calories per 100 ml	136	68

Vitamins Per Liter (Standard dilution*):

Vitamin A	2500 I.U.
Vitamin D	400 I.U.
Vitamin E	20 I.U.
Vitamin C	55 mg
Thiamine (Vitamin B_1)	0.40 mg
Riboflavin (Vitamin B_2)	0.60 mg
Vitamin B_6	0.40 mg
Niacin (mg equiv.)	9.0
Folic acid	0.10 mg
Vitamin B_{12}	3.0 mcg
Pantothenic acid	5.0 mg
Biotin	30 mcg
Vitamin K_1	0.15 mg

* Standard dilution is one part Isomil SF Concentrated Liquid to one part water.

Composition: **Ready to Feed**

Ingredients: (Pareve, ⓤ) 87.3% water, 6.7% corn syrup solids, 2.3% soy protein isolate, 2.0% soy oil, 1.4% coconut oil, minerals (calcium phosphate dibasic, potassium citrate, calcium carbonate, potassium chloride, calcium phosphate monobasic, magnesium chloride, ferrous sulfate, sodium chloride, zinc sulfate, cupric sulfate, potassium iodide), mono- and diglycerides, soy lecithin, vitamins (ascorbic acid, choline chloride, alpha-tocopheryl acetate, niacinamide, calcium pantothenate, vitamin A palmitate, thiamine chloride hydrochloride, riboflavin, pyridoxine hydrochloride, phylloquinone, folic acid, biotin, vitamin D_3, cyanocobalamin), carrageenan and L-methionine.

Approximate Analysis (wt/liter):

Protein	20.0 g
Fat	36.0 g
Carbohydrate	68.0 g
Minerals (Ash)	3.8 g
Calcium	0.70 g
Phosphorus	0.50 g
Sodium	0.30 g
Potassium	0.71 g
Chloride	0.53 g
Magnesium	50 mg

Continued on next page

Ross—Cont.

Iron	12	mg
Zinc	5.0	mg
Copper	0.50	mg
Iodine	0.10	mg
Manganese	0.20	mg
Water	901.6	g
Crude Fiber	0	g
Calories per fl oz	20	
Calories per 100 ml	68	

Vitamins Per Liter:

Vitamin A	2500 I.U.	
Vitamin D	400 I.U.	
Vitamin E	20 I.U.	
Vitamin C	55	mg
Thiamine (Vitamin B_1)	0.40	mg
Riboflavin (Vitamin B_2)	0.60	mg
Vitamin B_6	0.40	mg
Niacin (mg equiv.)	9.0	
Folic Acid	0.10	mg
Vitamin B_{12}	3.0	mcg
Pantothenic acid	5.0	mg
Biotin	30	mcg
Vitamin K_1	0.15	mg

The addition of iron to this formula conforms to the recommendation of the Committee on Nutrition of the American Academy of Pediatrics.

OSMOLITE®
Isotonic Liquid Nutrition

Usage: As an isotonic liquid food providing complete, balanced nutrition. Osmolite has been designed for patients particularly sensitive to hyperosmotic feedings or suffering from fat maldigestion/malabsorption. Osmolite may be used as a tube feeding (nasogastric, nasoduodenal or jejunal) or as an oral feeding.

Features:

- Complete, balanced nutrition—1.06 Calories per ml, 250 Calories per 8-fl-oz feeding, 1000 Calories per quart from a balanced distribution of protein, fat, and carbohydrate (caloric distribution: protein, 14.0%; fat, 31.4%; carbohydrate, 54.6%). Vitamin/mineral levels in two quarts (2000 Calories) of Osmolite meet or exceed 100% of the U.S. RDA for adults and children 4 or more years of age.
- Isotonicity—The osmolality is 300 mOsm/kg water, equaling the osmotic pressure of plasma. Osmolite will not contribute to osmotically induced diarrhea and is indicated when feeding problems suggest a sensitivity to hyperosmotic feedings.
- Lactose-free—Osmolite will not contribute to lactose-associated diarrhea. Polycose® Glucose Polymers is the carbohydrate source, which is a readily available and easily digested source of calories.
- High biologic value protein—Osmolite provides a full complement of amino acids to meet the National Research Council's profile for high quality proteins and has a Calorie-to-nitrogen ratio of 178:1.
- Readily absorbed fats—Osmolite contains a high level of essential fatty acids, as well as medium-chain triglycerides as 15% of total calories (50% of fat calories) to facilitate rapid, effective absorption of fat calories.
- Osmolite is a low-residue feeding. The amount of fecal residue produced by Osmolite is comparable to that produced by a chemically defined, elemental diet. Therefore, Osmolite is appropriate for use in situations where low residue is a primary consideration.
- Low electrolyte levels—23.9 mEq of sodium, 25.9 mEq of potassium, and 23.8 mEq of chloride per liter permit the use of Osmolite with many electrolyte-controlled diets, yet electrolyte levels are adequate for most hospitalized patients.
- Unflavored—The mild, acceptable taste makes Osmolite particularly appropriate for use with patients experiencing altered or heightened taste perceptions (eg, individuals undergoing radiation or chemotherapy treatment). Osmolite is particularly effective orally with patients rejecting conventional, sweet-tasting feedings. The addition of Vari-Flavors® Flavor Pacs helps to combat flavor fatigue experienced by patients receiving full liquid diets and liquid supplements.
- Convenient—Osmolite is ready to use. No mixing is required. Potential for contamination during preparation is reduced.

Sample Administration Schedule for OSMOLITE
Continuous Drip or Pump Controlled Delivery

Day	Time	Strength	Rate (ml/hr)	Volume (ml)	Calories
1	1st 8 hours	Full	50	400	400
	2nd 8 hours	Full	75	600	600
	3rd 8 hours	Full	100	800	800
					1800 *Total Calories*
2	24 hours	Full	100–125	2400–3000	2400–3000 *Total Calories*

Intermittent Drip

Day	Time	Strength	Rate (5–10 ml/min)	Volume (ml)	Calories
1	7am–11pm	Full	100 ml q 2 hr (7am, 9am)	200	200
		Full	150 ml q 2 hr (11am, 1pm, 3pm)	450	450
		Full	200 ml q 2 hr (5pm, 7pm, 9pm, 11pm)	800	800
					1450 *Total Calories*
2	7am–11pm	Full	250 ml q 2 hr (8 feedings) up to	2000	2000 *Total Calories*
			400 ml q 3 hr (5 feedings)	2000	2000 *Total Calories*

Dosage and Administration: Dilution is not required. Osmolite may be stored (unopened) and fed at room temperature. Once opened, Osmolite should be covered and refrigerated. Any unused portion should be discarded if not used within 48 hours.

Oral Feeding: Osmolite may be used as a sole source of nutrition or as a supplement with and between meals for added nutritional support.

Tube Feeding: Follow physician's instructions. When initiating feeding, the flow rate, volume and dilution are dependent on patient condition and tolerance.

Additional fluid requirements should be met by giving water orally with or after feedings, or when flushing the feeding tube. Care should be taken to avoid contamination of this product during preparation and administration.

[See table below].

Under no circumstances should Osmolite be administered parenterally.

Availability:

Ready To Use:
8-fl-oz bottles; 24 per case; No. 715.
8-fl-oz cans; 4 six-packs per case; No. 709.
32-fl-oz cans; 6 per case; No. 738.

Composition:

Ingredients: Ⓤ Water, hydrolyzed corn starch, sodium and calcium caseinates, medium-chain triglycerides (fractionated coconut oil), corn oil, soy protein isolate, soy oil, potassium citrate, soy lecithin, calcium phosphate tribasic, magnesium sulfate, choline chloride, magnesium chloride, ascorbic acid, carrageenan, vitamin concentrate (alpha-tocopheryl acetate, vitamin A palmitate, phylloquinone, vitamin D_3), zinc sulfate, ferrous sulfate, niacinamide, manganous chloride, calcium pantothenate, cupric sulfate, thiamine chloride hydrochloride, pyridoxine hydrochloride, riboflavin, biotin, folic acid and cyanocobalamin.

Approximate Analysis (g/8 fl oz): Protein, 8.8; Fat, 9.1; Carbohydrate, 34.3; Ash, 1.3; Moisture, 199.1. Calories per ml, 1.06; Calories per fl oz, 31.8.

[See table on bottom next page].

PEDIAFLOR® Drops ℞
Sodium Fluoride Oral Solution, USP

Description:
One dropperful (1.0 ml) provides:
Fluoride (as sodium fluoride) .... 0.5 mg

Indications and Usage: As an aid in the prevention of dental caries in infants and children.

Contraindications: Should be used only where the fluoride content of the drinking water supply is known to be 0.7 parts per million or less.

Precautions: The recommended dosage should not be exceeded since chronic overdosage of fluoride may result in mottling of tooth enamel and osseous changes.

Overdosage: In children, acute ingestion of 10 to 20 mg of sodium fluoride may cause excessive salivation and gastrointestinal disturbances; 500 mg may be fatal. Oral and/or intravenous fluids containing calcium may be indicated.

Dosage and Administration: Daily dosage—under 2 years of age, one-half dropperful or less daily; 2 years of age, one dropperful daily; 3 years of age or older, two dropperfuls or less daily; or as directed by physician or dentist.

Availability: 50-ml bottles, calibrated dropper enclosed; Rx; **NDC** 0074-0101-50.

PEDIALYTE®
Oral Electrolyte Solution

Usage: For maintenance of water and electrolytes during mild to moderate diarrhea in infants and children; for maintenance and replacement of water and electrolytes following corrective parenteral therapy for severe diarrhea.

- Specifically formulated for home management of mild to moderate diarrhea.
- Supplies calories in the form of glucose to help avoid ketosis.
- Ready to use—no mixing or dilution necessary.
- Identical forms for either home or hospital use.

Availability: 8-fl-oz bottles; 4 six-packs per case; No. 160; **NDC** 0074-5759-24. 32-fl-oz cans; six per case; No. 236; **NDC** 0074-5759-06. For hospital use, prebottled PEDIALYTE is available in the Ross Hospital Formula System.

Dosage: For maintenance and replacement of losses in mild to moderate diarrhea of infants and young children.[1]
[See table right].

Pedialyte Dosage

WEIGHT (lb)	7	10	13	17	20	22	24	28	30	32	34	36	38	40
WEIGHT (kg)	3.18	4.54	5.90	7.71	9.07	9.98	10.89	12.70	13.61	14.51	15.42	16.33	17.24	18.14
Approximate Surface Area (square meters)	.21	.26	.30	.35	.40	.44	.47	.53	.58	.61	.64	.67	.71	.74
Pedialyte-Fl-oz/day for maintenance	10-14	13-17	15-20	17-23	20-26	22-29	23-31	26-35	29-38	30-40	32-42	33-44	35-47	37-49
Pedialyte-Fl-oz/day for maintenance and replacement	15-19	19-24	24-29	29-35	33-40	37-44	40-47	45-54	49-59	52-62	55-66	58-69	61-73	65-77

Above administration guide does not apply to infants less than 1 week of age.
For children 5 years and older: 2 quarts or more daily.

Administration of Pedialyte should begin with discontinuance of usual foods and liquids. Intake of Pedialyte should be adjusted to meet individual needs. Daily intake should be divided into frequent feedings.

Ingredients: Ⓤ Water, dextrose, potassium citrate, sodium chloride, sodium citrate, citric acid, magnesium chloride and calcium chloride.

Provides:

	Per 8 fl oz	Per Liter
Sodium (mEq)	7.1	30
Potassium (mEq)	4.7	20
Calcium (mEq)	0.9	4
Magnesium (mEq)	0.9	4
Chloride (mEq)	7.1	30
Citrate (mEq)	6.6	28
Dextrose (grams)	11.8	50
Calories	48	200

Reference:

1. Dosage recommendation extrapolated from Kaplan, SA: Fluid therapy in pediatrics, in Gellis, SS; Kagan BM: *Current Pediatric Therapy-5*. Philadelphia: WB Saunders Co, 1971, pp 718–719.

PEDIAMYCIN® ℞
erythromycin ethylsuccinate

Description: Erythromycin is produced by a strain of *Streptomyces erythraeus* and belongs to the macrolide group of antibiotics. It is basic and readily forms salts with acids. The base, the stearate salt and the esters are poorly soluble in water. Erythromycin ethylsuccinate is an ester of erythromycin suitable for oral administration. The premixed suspension, granules and drops for oral administration are intended primarily for pediatric use but can also be used in adults.

Pediamycin 400 (erythromycin ethylsuccinate oral suspension), 400 mg erythromycin activity per teaspoonful (5 ml), is a premixed suspension with an appealing cherry flavor, supplied in pint (16 fl oz) bottles and 100-ml bottles. Its form and flavor make it especially suitable for older children unwilling or unable to swallow capsules or tablets.

Pediamycin Liquid (erythromycin ethylsuccinate oral suspension), 200 mg erythromycin activity per teaspoonful (5 ml), is a premixed suspension with an appealing cherry flavor, supplied in pint (16 fl oz) bottles and 100-ml bottles. Its form and flavor make it especially suitable for infants and children, and for older children unwilling or unable to swallow capsules or tablets.

Pediamycin Suspension and *Pediamycin Drops* (erythromycin ethylsuccinate for oral suspension), 200 mg erythromycin activity per teaspoonful (5 ml), 100 mg erythromycin activity per dropperful (2.5 ml), are pleasant-tasting cherry-flavored oral suspensions, dispensed as granules of erythromycin ethylsuccinate reconstituted with water. Pediamycin granules are packaged in 60-ml, 100-ml and 150-ml (Suspension), and 50-ml (Drops) bottles. A calibrated dropper is supplied with the 50-ml bottles.

Actions:

Microbiology

Biochemical tests demonstrate that erythromycin inhibits protein synthesis of the pathogen without directly affecting nucleic acid synthesis. Antagonism has been demonstrated between clindamycin and erythromycin.

NOTE: Many strains of *Hemophilus influenzae* are resistant to erythromycin alone but are susceptible to erythromycin and sulfonamides together. Staphylococci resistant to erythromycin may emerge during a course of erythromycin therapy. Culture and susceptibility testing should be performed.

Disc Susceptibility Tests

Quantitative methods that require measurement of zone diameters give the most precise estimates of antibiotic susceptibility. One recommended procedure (21 CFR section 460.1) uses erythromycin class discs for testing susceptibility; interpretations correlate zone diameters of this disc test with MIC values for erythromycin. With this procedure, a report from the laboratory of "susceptible" indicates that the infecting organism is likely to respond to therapy. A report of "resistant" indicates that the infective organism is not likely to respond to therapy. A report of "intermediate susceptibility" suggests that the organism would be susceptible if higher doses were used.

Clinical Pharmacology: Erythromycin binds to the 50 S ribosomal subunits of susceptible bacteria and suppresses protein synthesis.

Orally administered erythromycin ethylsuccinate suspensions are readily and reliably absorbed. Comparable serum levels of erythromycin are achieved in the fasting and the nonfasting states.

Erythromycin diffuses readily into most body fluids. Only low concentrations are normally achieved in the spinal fluid, but passage of the drug across the blood-brain barrier increases in meningitis. In the presence of normal hepatic function, erythromycin is concentrated in the liver and excreted in the bile; the effect of hepatic dysfunction on excretion of erythromycin by the liver into the bile is not known. Less than 5 percent of the orally administered dose of erythromycin is excreted in active form in the urine.

Erythromycin crosses the placental barrier and is excreted in breast milk.

Indications: *Streptococcus pyogenes* (Group A beta-hemolytic streptococcus): Upper and lower respiratory tract, skin, and soft tissue infections of mild to moderate severity.

Injectable benzathine penicillin G is considered by the American Heart Association to be the drug of choice in the treatment and prevention of streptococcal pharyngitis and in long-term prophylaxis of rheumatic fever.

When oral medication is preferred for treatment of the above conditions, penicillin G or V, or erythromycin is the alternate drug of choice.

Vitamin/Mineral Content of Osmolite

Vitamins/Minerals	Per 8 Fl Oz		Percent U.S. RDA* (Per 8 Fl Oz)
Vitamin A	625	I.U.	12.5
Vitamin D	50	I.U.	12.5
Vitamin E	7.5	I.U.	25.0
Vitamin K_1	35	mcg	**
Vitamin C	38	mg	62.5
Folic Acid	50	mcg	12.5
Thiamine (Vitamin B_1)	0.38	mg	25.0
Riboflavin (Vitamin B_2)	0.43	mg	25.0
Vitamin B_6	0.50	mg	25.0
Vitamin B_{12}	1.5	mcg	25.0
Niacin	5.0	mg	25.0
Choline	0.13	g	**
Biotin	38	mcg	12.5
Pantothenic Acid	1.25	mg	12.5
Sodium	0.13	g	**
Potassium	0.24	g	**
Chloride	0.20	g	**
Calcium	0.13	g	12.5
Phosphorus	0.13	g	12.5
Magnesium	50	mg	12.5
Iodine	19	mcg	12.5
Manganese	0.50	mg	**
Copper	0.25	mg	12.5
Zinc	3.7	mg	25.0
Iron	2.2	mg	12.5

*For adults and children 4 or more years of age.
**U.S. RDA not established.

Continued on next page

Ross—Cont.

When oral medication is given, the importance of strict adherence by the patient to the prescribed dosage regimen must be stressed. A therapeutic dose should be administered for at least 10 days.

Alpha-hemolytic streptococci (viridans group): Although no controlled clinical efficacy trials have been conducted, oral erythromycin has been suggested by the American Heart Association and American Dental Association for use in a regimen for prophylaxis against bacterial endocarditis in patients hypersensitive to penicillin who have congenital heart disease, or rheumatic or other acquired valvular heart disease when they undergo dental procedures and surgical procedures of the upper respiratory tract.[1] Erythromycin is not suitable prior to genitourinary or gastrointestinal tract surgery. NOTE: When selecting antibiotics for the prevention of bacterial endocarditis the physician or dentist should read the full joint statement of the American Heart Association and the American Dental Association.[1]

Staphylococcus aureus: Acute infections of skin and soft tissue of mild to moderate severity. Resistant organisms may emerge during treatment.

Streptococcus (Diplococcus) pneumoniae: Upper respiratory tract infections (e.g., otitis media, pharyngitis) and lower respiratory tract infections (e.g., pneumonia) of mild to moderate degree.

Mycoplasma pneumoniae (Eaton agent, PPLO): For respiratory infections due to this organism.

Hemophilus influenzae: For upper respiratory tract infections of mild to moderate severity when used concomitantly with adequate doses of sulfonamides. (See sulfonamide labeling for appropriate prescribing information.) The concomitant use of the sulfonamides is necessary since not all strains of *Hemophilus influenzae* are susceptible to erythromycin at the concentrations of the antibiotic achieved with usual therapeutic doses.

Treponema pallidum: Erythromycin is an alternate choice of treatment for primary syphilis in patients allergic to the penicillins. In treatment of primary syphilis, spinal fluid examinations should be done before treatment and as part of follow-up after therapy.

Corynebacterium diphtheriae: As an adjunct to antitoxin, to prevent establishment of carriers, and to eradicate the organism in carriers.

Corynebacterium minutissimum: For the treatment of erythrasma.

Entamoeba histolytica: In the treatment of intestinal amebiasis only. Extra-enteric amebiasis requires treatment with other agents.

Listeria monocytogenes: Infections due to this organism.

Bordetella pertussis: Erythromycin is effective in eliminating the organism from the nasopharynx of infected individuals, rendering them non-infectious. Some clinical studies suggest that erythromycin may be helpful in the prophylaxis of pertussis in exposed susceptible individuals.

Legionnaires' Disease: Although no controlled clinical efficacy studies have been conducted, *in vitro* and limited preliminary clinical data suggest that erythromycin may be effective in treating Legionnaires' Disease.

Contraindications: Erythromycin is contraindicated in patients with known hypersensitivity to this antibiotic.

Precautions: Erythromycin is principally excreted by the liver. Caution should be exercised in administering the antibiotic to patients with impaired hepatic function. There have been reports of hepatic dysfunction, with or without jaundice occurring in patients receiving oral erythromycin products.

Areas of localized infection may require surgical drainage in addition to antibiotic therapy. Recent data from studies of erythromycin reveal that its use in patients who are receiving high doses of theophylline may be associated with an increase of serum theophylline levels and potential theophylline toxicity. In case of theophylline toxicity and/or elevated serum theophylline levels, the dose of theophylline should be reduced while the patient is receiving concomitant erythromycin therapy.

Usage during pregnancy and lactation: The safety of erythromycin for use during pregnancy has not been established.

Erythromycin crosses the placental barrier. Erythromycin also appears in breast milk.

Adverse Reactions: The most frequent side effects of oral erythromycin preparations are gastrointestinal, such as abdominal cramping and discomfort, and are dose related. Nausea, vomiting and diarrhea occur infrequently with usual oral doses.

During prolonged or repeated therapy, there is a possibility of overgrowth of nonsusceptible bacteria or fungi. If such infections occur, the drug should be discontinued and appropriate therapy instituted.

Allergic reactions ranging from urticaria and mild skin eruptions to anaphylaxis have occurred.

Dosage and Administration: Erythromycin ethylsuccinate suspensions may be administered without regard to meals.

Children: Age, weight and severity of the infection are important factors in determining the proper dosage. In mild to moderate infections the usual dosage of erythromycin ethylsuccinate for children is 30 to 50 mg/kg/day in equally divided doses. For more severe infections this dosage may be doubled.

Adults: 400 mg erythromycin ethylsuccinate every 6 hours is the usual dose. Dosage may be increased up to 4 g per day according to the severity of the infections.

If twice-a-day dosage is desired in either adults or children, one-half of the total daily dose may be given every 12 hours. Doses may also be given three times daily if desired by administering one-third of the total daily dose every 8 hours.

The following approximate dosage schedule is suggested for using *Pediamycin Liquid* (erythromycin ethylsuccinate oral suspension), *Pediamycin Suspension* and *Pediamycin Drops* (erythromycin ethylsuccinate for oral suspension) in the treatment of mild to moderate infections by susceptible organisms.

Body Weight	Dose	Frequency	Approximate Daily Dosage
Under 10 lb (4.5 kg)	40 mg/kg/day (20 mg/lb/day) in divided doses		
10–15 lb (4.5 to 6.8 kg)	½ dropperful (50 mg) or 1 dropperful (100 mg)	4 times/day / 2 times/day	200 mg
15–25 lb (6.8 to 11.3 kg)	1 dropperful (100 mg) ½ teaspoonful (100 mg) or 2 dropperfuls (200 mg) 1 teaspoonful (200 mg)	4 times/day / 2 times/day	400 mg
25–50 lb (11.3 to 22.7 kg)	1 teaspoonful (200 mg) or 2 teaspoonfuls (400 mg)	4 times/day / 2 times/day	800 mg
50–100 lb (22.7 to 45.4 kg)	1½ teaspoonfuls (300 mg) or 3 teaspoonfuls (600 mg)	4 times/day / 2 times/day	1200 mg
over 100 lb (45.4 kg)	2 teaspoonfuls (400 mg) or 4 teaspoonfuls (800 mg)	4 times/day / 2 times/day	1600 mg

The following approximate dosage schedule is suggested for using *Pediamycin 400* (erythromycin ethylsuccinate oral suspension) in the treatment of mild to moderate infections by susceptible organisms.

Body Weight	Dose	Frequency	Approximate Daily Dosage
25–50 lb (11.3 to 22.7 kg)	1 teaspoonful (400 mg)	2 times/day	800 mg
50–100 lb (22.7 to 45.4 kg)	1½ teaspoonfuls (600 mg)	2 times/day	1200 mg
over 100 lb (45.4 kg)	2 teaspoonfuls (800 mg)	2 times/day	1600 mg

The total daily dosage must be administered in equally divided doses.

In the treatment of streptococcal infections, a therapeutic dosage of erythromycin ethylsuccinate should be administered for at least 10 days. In continuous prophylaxis against recurrences of streptococcal infections in persons with a history of rheumatic heart disease, the usual dosage is 400 mg twice a day.

For prophylaxis against bacterial endocarditis[1] in patients with congenital heart disease, or rheumatic or other acquired valvular heart disease when undergoing dental procedures or surgical procedures of the upper respiratory tract, give 1.6 g (20 mg/kg for children) orally 1 ½ to 2 hours before the procedure, and then, 800 mg (10 mg/kg for children) orally every 6 hours for 8 doses.

For treatment of primary syphilis: Adults: 48 to 64 g given in divided doses over a period of 10 to 15 days.

For intestinal amebiasis: Adults: 400 mg four times daily for 10 to 14 days. Children: 30 to 50 mg/kg/day in divided doses for 10 to 14 days.

For use in pertussis: Although optimal dosage and duration have not been established, doses of erythromycin utilized in reported clinical studies were 40 to 50 mg/kg/day, given in divided doses for 5 to 14 days.

For treatment of Legionnaires' Disease: Although optimal doses have not been established, doses utilized in reported clinical data were those recommended above (1.6 to 4 g daily in divided doses).

How Supplied: *Pediamycin 400* (erythromycin ethylsuccinate oral suspension, USP) is supplied in 1 pint bottles (**NDC** 0074-0211-16). It provides erythromycin ethylsuccinate equivalent to 400 mg erythromycin per teaspoonful (5 ml).

Pediamycin Liquid (erythromycin ethylsuccinate oral suspension, USP) is supplied in 1 pint bottles (**NDC** 0074-0202-16). It provides erythromycin ethylsuccinate equivalent to 200 mg erythromycin per teaspoonful (5 ml).

Pediamycin Suspension (erythromycin ethylsuccinate for oral suspension, USP) is available for teaspoon dosage in 100-ml (**NDC** 0074-0206-13) and 150-ml (**NDC** 0074-0206-09) bottles, in

the form of granules to be reconstituted with 77 ml and 115 ml of water, respectively. It provides erythromycin ethylsuccinate equivalent to 200 mg erythromycin per teaspoonful (5 ml).
Pediamycin Drops (erythromycin ethylsuccinate for oral suspension, USP) is available for dropper dosage in 50-ml bottles (**NDC** 0074-0207-50), in the form of granules to be reconstituted with 38 ml of water, providing 100 mg of erythromycin activity per dropperful (2.5 ml). Dropper marked for 100 mg (dropperful), 75 mg and 50 mg (half dropperful) doses is enclosed in the carton.
Pediamycin Liquid and *Pediamycin 400* require refrigeration to preserve taste. Refrigeration by patient is not required if used within 14 days.

Reference:

1. American Heart Association. 1977. Prevention of Bacterial Endocarditis. Circulation 56:139A-143A.

PEDIAZOLE® ℞

erythromycin ethylsuccinate and sulfisoxazole acetyl for oral suspension

Description: Pediazole is a combination of erythromycin ethylsuccinate, USP and sulfisoxazole acetyl, USP. When reconstituted with water as directed on the label, the granules form a white, strawberry-banana flavor suspension which provides 200 mg erythromycin activity and the equivalent of 600 mg of sulfisoxazole per teaspoonful (5 ml).
Erythromycin is produced by a strain of *Streptomyces erythraeus* and belongs to the macrolide group of antibiotics. It is basic and readily forms salts and esters. Erythromycin ethylsuccinate is an ester of erythromycin.
Sulfisoxazole acetyl or N^1-acetyl sulfisoxazole is an ester of sulfisoxazole. Chemically, sulfisoxazole is N^1-(3,4-dimethyl-5-isoxazolyl) sulfanilamide.

Actions:

Clinical Pharmacology: Orally administered erythromycin ethylsuccinate suspension is reliably and readily absorbed and serum levels are comparable when administered to patients in either the fasting or non-fasting state. After absorption, erythromycin diffuses readily into most body fluids. In the presence of normal hepatic function, erythromycin is concentrated in the liver and excreted in the bile; the effect of hepatic dysfunction on excretion of erythromycin by the liver into the bile is not known. After oral administration, less than 5 percent of the activity of the administered dose can be recovered in the urine.
Erythromycin crosses the placental barrier but fetal plasma levels are generally low.
Sulfisoxazole acetyl is deacetylated by enzymatic hydrolysis in the gastrointestinal tract from which it is readily absorbed as sulfisoxazole. Sulfisoxazole exists in the blood primarily bound to serum proteins as well as conjugated and in the active or free form. Metabolic pathways include N^4-acetylation and oxidation with approximately 80 percent of an administered dose being excreted by the kidney within 24 hours.
Serum half-life for total erythromycin and free sulfisoxazole is about 1.5 and 6 hours, respectively.
Microbiology: Pediazole has been formulated to contain sulfisoxazole for concomitant use with erythromycin. The mode of action of erythromycin is by inhibition of protein synthesis without affecting nucleic acid synthesis. Sulfonamides, including sulfisoxazole, possess bacteriostatic activity. This bacteriostatic agent acts by means of competitively inhibiting bacterial synthesis of folic acid (pteroylglutamic acid) from para-aminobenzoic acid. Resistance to erythromycin blood levels ordinarily achieved has been demonstrated by some strains of *Hemophilus influenzae.* Pediazole is usually active against *Hemophilus influenzae in vitro,* including ampicillin-resistant strains.
Quantitative methods that require measurements of zone diameters give the most precise estimates of antibiotic susceptibility. One such standardized procedure, the ASM-2 method published by the National Committee for Clinical Laboratory Standards (NCCLS), has been recommended for use with discs to test susceptibility to erythromycin and sulfisoxazole. Interpretation involves correlation of the diameters obtained in the disc test with Minimal Inhibitory Concentrations (MIC) values for erythromycin and sulfisoxazole.
If the standardized ASM-2 procedure of disc susceptibility is used, a 15 mcg erythromycin disc should give a zone diameter of at least 18 mm when tested against an erythromycin-susceptible bacterial strain and a 250-300 mcg sulfisoxazole disc should give a zone diameter of at least 17 mm when tested against a sulfisoxazole-susceptible bacterial strain.
In vitro sulfonamide sensitivity tests are not always reliable because media containing excessive amounts of thymidine are capable of reversing the inhibitory effect of sulfonamides which may result in false resistant reports. The tests must be carefully coordinated with bacteriological and clinical responses. When the patient is already taking sulfonamides follow-up cultures should have aminobenzoic acid added to the isolation media but not to subsequent susceptibility test media.

Indication: For treatment of ACUTE OTITIS MEDIA in children that is caused by susceptible strains of *Hemophilus influenzae.*

Contraindications: Known hypersensitivity to either erythromycin or sulfonamides.
Infants less than 2 months of age.
Pregnancy at term and during the nursing period, because sulfonamides pass into the placental circulation and are excreted in human breast milk and may cause kernicterus in the infant.

Warnings: *Usage in Pregnancy* (SEE ALSO: CONTRAINDICATIONS): The safe use of erythromycin or sulfonamides in pregnancy has not been established. The teratogenic potential of most sulfonamides has not been thoroughly investigated in either animals or humans. However, a significant increase in the incidence of cleft palate and other bony abnormalities of offspring has been observed when certain sulfonamides of the short, intermediate and long-acting types were given to pregnant rats and mice at high oral doses (7 to 25 times the human therapeutic dose).
Reports of deaths have been associated with sulfonamide administration from hypersensitivity reactions, agranulocytosis, aplastic anemia and other blood dyscrasias. The presence of clinical signs such as sore throat, fever, pallor, purpura or jaundice may be early indications of serious blood disorders. Complete blood counts should be done frequently in patients receiving sulfonamides.
The frequency of renal complications is considerably lower in patients receiving the most soluble sulfonamides such as sulfisoxazole. Urinalysis with careful microscopic examination should be obtained frequently in patients receiving sulfonamides.

Precautions: Erythromycin is principally excreted by the liver. Caution should be excercised in administering the antibiotic to patients with impaired hepatic function. There have been reports of hepatic dysfunction, with or without jaundice occurring in patients receiving oral erythromycin products.
Recent data from studies of erythromycin reveal that its use in patients who are receiving high doses of theophylline may be associated with an increase of serum theophylline levels and potential theophylline toxicity. In case of theophylline toxicity and/or elevated serum theophylline levels, the dose of theophylline should be reduced while the patient is receiving concomitant erythromycin therapy.
Surgical procedures should be performed when indicated.
Sulfonamide therapy should be given with caution to patients with impaired renal or hepatic function and in those patients with a history of severe allergy or bronchial asthma. In the presence of a deficiency in the enzyme glucose-6-phosphate dehydrogenase, hemolysis may occur. This reaction is frequently dose-related. Adequate fluid intake must be maintained in order to prevent crystalluria and renal stone formation.

Adverse Reactions: The most frequent side effects of oral erythromycin preparations are gastrointestinal, such as abdominal cramping and discomfort, and are dose-related. Nausea, vomiting and diarrhea occur infrequently with usual oral doses. During prolonged or repeated therapy, there is a possibility of overgrowth of nonsusceptible bacteria or fungi. If such infections occur, the drug should be discontinued and appropriate therapy instituted. The overall incidence of these latter side effects reported for the combined administration of erythromycin and a sulfonamide is comparable to those observed in patients given erythromycin alone. Mild allergic reactions such as urticaria and other skin rashes have occurred. Serious allergic reactions, including anaphylaxis, have been reported with erythromycin.
The following untoward effects have been associated with the use of sulfonamides:
Blood Dyscrasias: Agranulocytosis, aplastic anemia, thrombocytopenia, leukopenia, hemolytic anemia, purpura, hypoprothrombinemia and methemoglobinemia.
Allergic Reactions: Erythema multiforme (Stevens-Johnson syndrome), generalized skin eruptions, epidermal necrolysis, urticaria, serum sickness, pruritus, exfoliative dermatitis, anaphylactoid reactions, periorbital edema, conjunctival and scleral injection, photosensitization, arthralgia and allergic myocarditis.
Gastrointestinal Reactions: Nausea, emesis, abdominal pains, hepatitis, diarrhea, anorexia, pancreatitis and stomatitis.
CNS Reactions: Headache, peripheral neuritis, mental depression, convulsions, ataxia, hallucinations, tinnitus, vertigo and insomnia.
Miscellaneous Reactions: Drug fever, chills and toxic nephrosis with oliguria or anuria. Periarteritis nodosa and LE phenomenon have occurred.
The sulfonamides bear certain chemical similarities to some goitrogens, diuretics (acetazolamide and the thiazides) and oral hypoglycemic agents. Goiter production, diuresis and hypoglycemia have occurred rarely in patients receiving sulfonamides. Cross-sensitivity may exist with these agents.
Rats appear to be especially susceptible to the goitrogenic effects of sulfonamides, and long-term administration has produced thyroid malignancies in the species.

Dosage and Administration: PEDIAZOLE SHOULD NOT BE ADMINISTERED TO INFANTS UNDER 2 MONTHS OF AGE BECAUSE OF CONTRAINDICATIONS OF SYSTEMIC SULFONAMIDES IN THIS AGE GROUP.
For Acute Otitis Media in Children: The dose of Pediazole can be calculated based on the erythromycin component (50 mg/kg/day) or the sulfisoxazole component (150 mg/kg/day to a maximum of 6 g/day). Pediazole should be administered in equally divided doses four times a day for 10 days. It may be administered without regard to meals.
The following approximate dosage schedule is recommended for using Pediazole:

Continued on next page

Ross—Cont.

Children: Two months of age or older

Weight	Dose—every 6 hours
Less than 8 kg (less than 18 lb)	Adjust dosage by body weight
8 kg (18 lb)	½ teaspoonful (2.5 ml)
16 kg (35 lb)	1 teaspoonful (5 ml)
24 kg (53 lb)	1½ teaspoonfuls (7.5 ml)
Over 45 kg (over 100 lb)	2 teaspoonfuls (10 ml)

How Supplied: Pediazole Suspension is available for teaspoon dosage in 100-ml (**NDC** 0074-8030-13), 150-ml (**NDC** 0074-8030-43) and 200-ml (**NDC** 0074-8030-53) bottles, in the form of granules to be reconstituted with water. The suspension provides erythromycin ethylsuccinate equivalent to 200 mg erythromycin activity and sulfisoxazole acetyl equivalent to 600 mg sulfisoxazole per teaspoonful (5 ml).

POLYCOSE®
Glucose Polymers

Usage: As a source of calories (derived solely from carbohydrate) for persons with increased caloric needs or those unable to meet their caloric needs with usual food intake. Polycose is particularly useful in supplying carbohydrate calories for protein, electrolyte and fat restricted diets. It may be used to increase the caloric density of traditional foods, liquids, and tube feedings.

Features:

* Water soluble, therefore, mixes readily with most foods and beverages to increase caloric density.
* Minimally sweet, as compared to glucose and other dietary carbohydrates, which helps improve patient acceptance.
* Absorbed as rapidly as glucose with negligible gut residue.
* Osmolality is approximately one-fifth that of pure glucose solutions of comparable caloric density. This helps reduce potential for osmotic diarrhea.
* Low in electrolytes, Polycose may be used in the dietary management of those patients whose intake of electrolytes is restricted.

Dosage and Administration: Polycose may be added to most foods and beverages, or mixed in water, with or without flavoring, in amounts determined by taste, caloric requirement and tolerance. Small, frequent feedings are more desirable than large amounts given infrequently. Polycose may be used for extended periods with diets containing all other essential nutrients, or as an oral adjunct to intravenous administration of nutrients. Polycose is not a balanced diet and should not be used as a sole source of nutrition. If indicated, solutions of Polycose may be administered via feeding tube. Refrigerate any unused dissolved Polycose Powder and opened Polycose Liquid and discard if not used after 24 hours. Concentrated solutions become more viscous when cold; thus serving at room temperature is advised. **Not for parenteral use.** UNDILUTED POLYCOSE LIQUID SHOULD NOT BE FED TO INFANTS OR COMATOSE PATIENTS WITHOUT PHYSICIAN SUPERVISION.

Availability:

Powder: 14-ounce (400 g) cans; 6 per case; No. 746.

Liquid: (43% w/w aqueous solution): 4-fl-oz bottles; 48 per case; No. 749.

Composition:

Powder: Ⓤ Glucose polymers derived from controlled hydrolysis of corn starch.

Approximate Analysis (per 100 grams):

Carbohydrate		94 g
Moisture		6 g
Minerals (Ash)	Does not exceed	0.5 g
Calcium	Does not exceed	30 mg (1.5 mEq)
Sodium	Does not exceed	110 mg (4.8 mEq)
Potassium	Does not exceed	10 mg (0.3 mEq)
Chloride	Does not exceed	223 mg (6.3 mEq)
Phosphorus	Does not exceed	5 mg

Approximate Caloric Equivalents:
1 Tablespoon (8 g) = 30 Calories; 100 g = 380 Calories; 1 av oz = 108 Calories

Composition:

Liquid: Ⓤ (43% w/w aqueous solution): Water and glucose polymers derived from controlled hydrolysis of corn starch.

Approximate Analysis (per 100 ml):

Carbohydrate		50 g
Moisture		70 g
Minerals (Ash)	Does not exceed	0.25 g
Calcium	Does not exceed	20 mg (1.0 mEq)
Sodium	Does not exceed	70 mg (3.0 mEq)
Potassium	Does not exceed	6 mg 0.15 mEq)
Chloride	Does not exceed	140 mg (3.9 mEq)
Phosphorus	Does not exceed	3 mg

Approximate Caloric Equivalents:
1 ml = 2 Calories; 1 fl oz = 60 Calories; 100 ml = 200 Calories.

PRAMET® FA ℞
Vitamin/Mineral Prescription for the Expectant and New Mother

Description: Each Pramet FA Filmtab® Film-Sealed oral tablet provides:

Vitamins	
Vitamin A (as acetate and palmitate) 1.2 mg	4000 I.U.
Vitamin D (ergocalciferol, 10 mcg)	400 I.U.
Vitamin C (ascorbic acid)	100 mg
Folic Acid	1 mg
Vitamin B_1 (thiamine mononitrate)	3 mg
Vitamin B_2 (riboflavin)	2 mg
Niacinamide	10 mg
Vitamin B_6 (pyridoxine hydrochloride)	5 mg
Vitamin B_{12} (cyanocobalamin)	3 mcg
Pantothenic Acid (as calcium pantothenate)	0.92 mg
Minerals	
Calcium (as calcium carbonate)	250 mg
Iodine (as calcium iodate)	100 mcg
Elemental Iron* (300 mg ferrous sulfate USP)	60 mg
Copper (as cupric chloride)	0.15 mg

* In controlled-release form—Gradumet®

Indications and Usage: To help prevent vitamin and mineral deficiencies during and after pregnancy and for treatment of megaloblastic anemias. One mg of folic acid has been found to be effective therapy for megaloblastic anemias of pregnancy and lactation.

Warning: Folic acid alone is improper therapy in the treatment of pernicious anemia and other megaloblastic anemias where vitamin B_{12} is deficient.

Precaution: Folic acid may mask the presence of pernicious anemia in that hematologic remission may occur while neurologic manifestations remain progressive.

Adverse Reaction: Allergic sensitization has been reported following both oral and parenteral administration of folic acid.

Overdosage: Acute overdosage of iron may cause nausea and vomiting and, in severe cases, cardiovascular collapse and death. The estimated lethal dose of orally ingested elemental iron is 300 mg per kg body weight. Serum iron and total iron-binding capacity may be used as guides for use of chelating agents such as deferoxamine.

Dosage and Administration: One tablet daily, or as directed by physician.

How Supplied: 100-tablet bottles; ℞; **NDC** 0074-0147-01.

[*Shown in Product Identification Section*]

PRAMILET® FA ℞
Prenatal Vitamin/Mineral Preparation

Description: Each Pramilet FA Filmtab® Film-Sealed oral tablet provides:

Vitamins	
Vitamin A (as acetate and palmitate) 1.2 mg	4000 I.U.
Vitamin D (ergocalciferol, 10 mcg)	400 I.U.
Vitamin C (as sodium ascorbate)	60 mg
Folic Acid	1 mg
Vitamin B_1 (thiamine mononitrate)	3 mg
Vitamin B_2 (riboflavin)	2 mg
Niacinamide	10 mg
Vitamin B_6 (pyridoxine hydrochloride)	3 mg
Vitamin B_{12} (cyanocobalamin)	3 mcg
Calcium Pantothenate	1 mg
Minerals	
Calcium (as calcium carbonate)	250 mg
Iodine (as calcium iodate)	100 mcg
Elemental Iron (as ferrous fumarate)	40 mg
Magnesium (as magnesium oxide)	10 mg
Copper (as cupric chloride)	0.15 mg
Zinc (as zinc oxide)	0.085 mg

Indications and Usage: To help prevent vitamin and mineral deficiencies during and after pregnancy and for treatment of megaloblastic anemias. One mg of folic acid has been found to be effective therapy for megaloblastic anemias of pregnancy and lactation.

Warning: Folic acid alone is improper therapy in the treatment of pernicious anemia and other megaloblastic anemias where vitamin B_{12} is deficient.

Precaution: Folic acid may mask the presence of pernicious anemia in that hematologic remission may occur while neurologic manifestations remain progressive.

Adverse Reaction: Allergic sensitization has been reported following both oral and parenteral administration of folic acid.

Overdosage: Acute overdosage of iron may cause nausea and vomiting and, in severe cases, cardiovascular collapse and death. The estimated lethal dose of orally ingested elemental iron is 300 mg per kg body weight. Serum iron and total iron-binding capacity may be used as guides for use of chelating agents such as deferoxamine.

Dosage and Administration: One tablet daily, or as directed by physician.

How Supplied: 100-tablet bottles; ℞; **NDC** 0074-0121-01.

[*Shown in Product Identification Section*]

RCF™
Ross Carbohydrate Free Soy Protein Formula Base

Usage: For use in the dietary management of persons unable to tolerate the type or amount of carbohydrate in milk or conventional infant formulas: most of these patients have intractable diarrhea and are not able to tolerate other formulas. This product has been formulated to contain no carbohydrates. Carbohydrate must be added before feeding.

Availability:

Concentrated Liquid only: 13-fl-oz cans; 12 per case; No. 108.

Preparation:

RCF is for use only under the direction of a physician. Physician's instructions must include the amount and type of carbohydrate and the amount of water to be added to RCF. Standard dilution is one part Formula Base to one part prescribed carbohydrate and water solution.

A full-strength, 20 Calories per fluid ounce, formula may be prepared with one of the following typical carbohydrates:
[See table right].

Carbohydrate Source	Amount of Carbohydrate	Water	RCF Formula Base
Table Sugar	4* level tablespoonfuls	12 fl oz	one 13-fl-oz can
Dextrose Powder (hydrous)	6* level tablespoonfuls	12 fl oz	one 13-fl-oz can
Polycose® Glucose Polymers Powder	7* level tablespoonfuls	12 fl oz	one 13-fl-oz can

* Approximately the 52 grams needed for 20 Cal/fl oz formula.

Composition: Concentrated Liquid
Ingredients: (Pareve, ⓤ) 87% water, 4.4% soy protein isolate, 4.2% soy oil, 2.8% coconut oil, minerals (calcium phosphates [mono- and tribasic], potassium citrate, potassium chloride, magnesium chloride, calcium carbonate, sodium chloride, zinc sulfate, cupric sulfate), carrageenan, mono- and diglycerides, soy lecithin, vitamins (ascorbic acid, choline chloride, alpha-tocopheryl acetate, niacinamide, calcium pantothenate, vitamin A palmitate, riboflavin, thiamine chloride hydrochloride, pyridoxine, hydrochloride, phylloquinone, biotin, folic acid, vitamin D_3, cyanocobalamin) and L-methionine.
[See table below and on next page].

Approximate Analysis (wt/liter):	Concentrated	Standard Dilution
Protein	40.0 g	20.0 g
Fat	72.0 g	36.0 g
Carbohydrate	0.1 g	*
Minerals (Ash)	7.5 g	3.8 g
Calcium	1.4 g	0.70 g
Phosphorus	1.0 g	0.50 g
Sodium	0.60 g	0.30 g
Potassium	1.42 g	0.71 g
Chloride	1.06 g	0.53 g
Magnesium	0.10 g	50 mg
Iron	3.0 mg	1.5 mg
(This product is deficient in iron; an additional 5.3 mg iron per liter should be supplied from other sources.)		
Zinc	10 mg	5.0 mg
Copper	1.0 mg	0.50 mg
Iodine	0.20 mg	0.10 mg
Manganese	0.40 mg	0.20 mg
Water	885.0 g	*
Crude Fiber	0 g	
Calories per fl oz	24	*
Calories per 100 ml	81	*

RONDEC–DM™ Syrup ℞
RONDEC–DM™ Drops ℞

Description:
Antihistamine/Decongestant/Antitussive for oral use.
Rondec-DM™ Syrup
Each teaspoonful (5 ml) contains carbinoxamine maleate, 4 mg; pseudoephedrine hydrochloride, 60 mg; dextromethorphan hydrobromide, 15 mg; less than 0.6% alcohol.
Rondec-DM™ Drops
Each dropperful (1 ml) contains carbinoxamine maleate, 2 mg; pseudoephedrine hydrochloride, 25 mg; dextromethorphan hydrobromide, 4 mg; less than 0.6% alcohol.
Carbinoxamine maleate (2-[p-Chloro-α-[2-(dimethylamino) ethoxy]benzyl]pyridine maleate) is one of the ethanolamine class of H_1 antihistamines.
Pseudoephedrine hydrochloride (Benzenemethanol,α-[1-(methylamino) ethyl]-, [S-(R*, R*)]-, hydrochloride) is the hydrochloride of pseudoephedrine, a naturally occurring dextrorotatory stereoisomer of ephedrine.
Dextromethorphan hydrobromide (Morphinan, 3-methoxy-17-methyl-, (9α, 13α, 14α)-, hydrobromide, monohydrate) is the hydrobromide of d-form racemethorphan.
Clinical Pharmacology: Antihistaminic, decongestant and antitussive actions.
Carbinoxamine maleate possesses H_1 antihistaminic activity and mild anticholinergic and sedative effects. Serum half-life for carbinoxamine is estimated to be 10 to 20 hours. Virtually no intact drug is excreted in the urine.
Pseudoephedrine hydrochloride is an oral sympathomimetic amine which acts as a decongestant to respiratory tract mucous membranes. While its vasoconstrictor action is similar to that of ephedrine, pseudoephedrine has less pressor effect in normotensive adults. Serum half-life for pseudoephedrine is 6 to 8 hours. Acidic urine is associated with faster elimination of the drug. About one half of the administered dose is excreted in the urine.
Dextromethorphan hydrobromide is a nonnarcotic antitussive with effectiveness equal to codeine. It acts in the medulla oblongata to elevate the cough threshold. Dextromethorphan does not produce analgesia or induce tolerance, and has no potential for addiction. At usual doses, it will not depress respiration or inhibit ciliary activity. Dextromethorphan is rapidly metabolized, with trace amounts of the parent compound in blood and urine. About one half of the administered dose is excreted in the urine as conjugated metabolites.
Indications and Usage: For symptomatic relief of the common cold, nasopharyngitis with postnasal drip, bronchitis and related respiratory conditions.
Contraindications: Patients with hypersensitivity or idiosyncrasy to any ingredients, patients taking monoamine oxidase (MAO) inhibitors, patients with narrow-angle glaucoma, urinary retention, peptic ulcer, severe hypertension or coronary artery disease, or patients undergoing an asthmatic attack.
Warnings:
Use in Pregnancy: Safety for use during pregnancy has not been established.
Nursing Mothers: Use with caution in nursing mothers.
Special Risk Patients: Use with caution in patients with hypertension or ischemic heart disease, and persons over 60 years.
Precautions: Before prescribing medication to suppress or modify cough, identify and provide therapy for the underlying cause of cough. Use with caution in patients with hypertension, heart disease, asthma, hyperthyroidism, increased intraocular pressure, diabetes mellitus and prostatic hypertrophy.
Information for Patients: Avoid alcohol and other CNS depressants while taking these products. Patients sensitive to antihistamines may experience moderate to severe drowsiness. Patients sensitive to sympathomimetic amines may note mild CNS stimulation. While taking these products, exercise care in driving or operating appliances, machinery, etc.
Drug Interactions: Antihistamines may enhance the effects of tricyclic antidepressants, barbiturates, alcohol, and other CNS depressants. MAO inhibitors prolong and intensify the anticholinergic effects of antihistamines. Sympathomimetic amines may reduce the antihypertensive effects of reserpine, veratrum alkaloids, methyldopa and mecamylamine. Effects of sympathomimetics are increased with MAO inhibitors and beta-adrenergic blockers. The cough suppressant action of dextromethorphan and narcotic antitussives are additive.
Pregnancy Category C.: Animal reproduction studies have not been conducted with Rondec-DM. It is also not known whether these products can cause fetal harm when administered to a pregnant woman or affect reproduction capacity. Give to pregnant women only if clearly needed.
Adverse Reactions:
Antihistamines: Sedation, dizziness, diplopia, vomiting, dry mouth, headache, nervousness, nausea, anorexia, heartburn, weakness, polyuria and dysuria and, rarely, excitability in children.
Sympathomimetic Amines: Convulsions, CNS depression, cardiac arrhythmias, respiratory difficulty, increased heart rate or blood pressure, hallucinations, tremors, nervousness, insomnia, weakness, pallor and dysuria.
Dextromethorphan: Drowsiness and GI disturbance.
Overdosage: No information is available as to specific results of an overdose of these products. The signs, symptoms and treatment described below are those of H_1 antihistamine, ephedrine and dextromethorphan overdose.
Symptoms: Should antihistamine effects predominate, central action constitutes the greatest danger. In the small child, predominant symptoms are excitation, hallucination, ataxia, incoordination, tremors, flushed face and fever. Convulsions, fixed and dilated pupils, coma, and death may occur in severe cases. In the adult, fever and flushing are uncommon; excitement leading to convulsions and postictal depression is often preceded by drowsiness and coma. Respiration is usually not seriously depressed; blood pressure is usually stable.
Should sympathomimetic symptoms predominate, central effects include restlessness, dizziness, tremor, hyperactive reflexes, talkativeness, irritability and insomnia. Cardiovascular and renal effects include difficulty in micturition, headache, flushing, palpitation, cardiac arrhythmias, hypertension with subsequent hypotension and circulatory collapse. Gastrointestinal effects include dry mouth, metallic taste, anorexia, nausea, vomiting, diarrhea and abdominal cramps.
Dextromethorphan may cause respiratory depression with a large overdose.
Treatment: *a*) Evacuate stomach as condition warrants. Activated charcoal may be useful. *b*) Maintain a nonstimulating environment. *c*) Monitor cardiovascular status. *d*) Do not give stimulants. *e*) Reduce fever with cool sponging. *f*) Treat respiratory depression with naloxone if dextromethorphan toxicity is suspected. *g*) Use sedatives or anticonvulsants to control CNS excitation and convulsions. *h*) Physostig-

Continued on next page

Ross—Cont.

mine may reverse anticholinergic symptoms. *i*) Ammonium chloride may acidify the urine to increase urinary excretion of pseudoephedrine. *j*) Further care is symptomatic and supportive.

Dosage and Administration:
Dosage:

Age	Dose*	Frequency*
Rondec-DM Syrup		
18 months–6 years	½ teaspoonful (2.5 ml)	q.i.d.
adults and children 6 years and over	1 teaspoonful (5 ml)	q.i.d.
Rondec-DM Drops for oral use only		
1–3 months	¼ dropperful (¼ ml)	q.i.d.
3–6 months	½ dropperful (½ ml)	q.i.d.
6–9 months	¾ dropperful (¾ ml)	q.i.d.
9–18 months	1 dropperful (1 ml)	q.i.d.

*In mild cases or in particularly sensitive patients, less frequent or reduced doses may be adequate.

How Supplied: Rondec-DM Syrup, grape-flavored, in 16-fl-oz (1-pint) bottles, **NDC** 0074-5640-16; and 4-fl-oz bottles, **NDC** 0074-5640-04. Dispense in USP tight, light-resistant, glass container. Avoid exposure to excessive heat.

Rondec-DM Drops, grape-flavored, in 30-ml bottles for dropper dosage. Calibrated, shatterproof dropper enclosed in each carton. Container meets safety closure requirements. **NDC** 0074-5639-30. Avoid exposure to excessive heat.

RONDEC® Drops ℞
RONDEC® Syrup ℞
RONDEC® Tablet ℞
RONDEC-TR® Tablet ℞

Description: Antihistamine/Decongestant for oral use.

For infants
RONDEC® Drops
Each dropperful (1 ml) contains carbinoxamine maleate, 2 mg; pseudoephedrine hydrochloride, 25 mg.

For young children
RONDEC® Syrup
Each teaspoonful (5 ml) contains carbinoxamine maleate, 4 mg; pseudoephedrine hydrochloride, 60 mg.

For adults and children 6 years and over
RONDEC® Tablet
Each Filmtab® tablet contains carbinoxamine maleate, 4 mg; pseudoephedrine hydrochloride, 60 mg.

For adults and children 12 years and over
RONDEX-TR® Tablet
Each timed-release Filmtab tablet contains carbinoxamine maleate, 8 mg; pseudoephedrine hydrochloride, 120 mg.

Carbinoxamine maleate (2-[p-Chloro-α-[2-(dimethylamino)ethoxy] benzyl] pyridine maleate) is one of the ethanolamine class of H_1 antihistamines.

Pseudoephedrine hydrochloride (Benzenemethanol, α-[1-(methylamino)ethyl]-, [S-(R*, R*)]-, hydrochloride) is the hydrochloride of pseudoephedrine, a naturally occurring dextrorotatory stereoisomer of ephedrine.

Clinical Pharmacology: Antihistaminic and decongestant actions.

Carbinoxamine maleate possesses H_1 antihistaminic activity and mild anticholinergic and sedative effects. Serum half-life for carbinoxamine is estimated to be 10 to 20 hours. Virtually no intact drug is excreted in the urine.

Pseudoephedrine hydrochloride is an oral sympathomimetic amine which acts as a decongestant to respiratory tract mucous membranes. While its vasoconstrictor action is similar to that of ephedrine, pseudoephedrine has less pressor effect in normotensive adults. Serum half-life for pseudoephedrine is 6 to 8 hours. Acidic urine is associated with faster elimination of the drug. About one half of the administered dose is excreted in the urine.

Indications and Usage: For symptomatic relief of seasonal and perennial allergic rhinitis and vasomotor rhinitis.

Rondec Drops, Rondec Syrup and Rondec Tablet, are immediate-release dosage forms allowing titration of dose up to four times a day. Rondec-TR Tablet utilizes a gradual-release mechanism providing approximately a 12-hour therapeutic effect, thus allowing twice-daily dosage.

Contraindications: Patients with hypersensitivity or idiosyncrasy to any ingredients, patients taking monoamine oxidase (MAO) inhibitors, patients with narrow-angle glaucoma, urinary retention, peptic ulcer, severe hypertension or coronary artery disease, or patients undergoing an asthmatic attack.

Warnings:
Use in Pregnancy: Safety for use during pregnancy has not been established.
Nursing Mothers: Use with caution in nursing mothers.
Special Risk Patients: Use with caution in patients with hypertension or ischemic heart disease, and persons over 60 years.

Precautions: Use with caution in patients with hypertension, heart disease, asthma, hyperthyroidism, increased intraocular pressure, diabetes mellitus and prostatic hypertrophy.
Information for Patients: Avoid alcohol and other CNS depressants while taking these products. Patients sensitive to antihistamines may experience moderate to severe drowsiness. Patients sensitive to sympathomimetic amines may note mild CNS stimulation. While taking these products, exercise care in driving or operating appliances, machinery, etc.
Drug Interactions: Antihistamines may enhance the effects of tricyclic antidepressants, barbiturates, alcohol, and other CNS depressants. MAO inhibitors prolong and intensify the anticholinergic effects of antihistamines. Sympathomimetic amines may reduce the antihypertensive effects of reserpine, veratrum alkaloids, methyldopa and mecamylamine. Effects of sympathomimetics are increased with MAO inhibitors and beta-adrenergic blockers.

Pregnancy Category C.: Animal reproduction studies have not been conducted with these products. It is also not known whether these products can cause fetal harm when administered to a pregnant woman or affect reproduction capacity. Give to pregnant women only if clearly needed.

Adverse Reactions: Antihistamines: Sedation, dizziness, diplopia, vomiting, dry mouth, headache, nervousness, nausea, anorexia, heartburn, weakness, polyuria and dysuria and, rarely, excitability in children.
Sympathomimetic Amines: Convulsions, CNS depression, cardiac arrhythmias, respiratory difficulty, increased heart rate or blood pressure, hallucinations, tremors, nervousness, insomnia, weakness, pallor and dysuria..

Overdosage: No information is available as to specific results of an overdose of these products. The signs, symptoms and treatment described below are those of H_1 antihistamine and ephedrine overdose.
Symptoms: Should antihistamine effects predominate, central action constitutes the greatest danger. In the small child, symptoms include excitation, hallucination, ataxia, incoordination, tremors, flushed face and fever. Convulsions, fixed and dilated pupils, coma and death may occur in severe cases. In the adult, fever and flushing are uncommon; excitement leading to convulsions and postictal depression is often preceded by drowsiness and coma. Respiration is usually not seriously depressed; blood pressure is usually stable.
Should sympathomimetic symptoms predominate, central effects include restlessness, dizziness, tremor, hyperactive reflexes, talkativeness, irritability and insomnia. Cardiovascular and renal effects include difficulty in micturition, headache, flushing, palpitation, cardiac arrhythmias, hypertension with subsequent hypotension and circulatory collapse. Gastrointestinal effects include dry mouth, metallic taste, anorexia, nausea, vomiting, diarrhea and abdominal cramps.
Treatment: *a*) Evacuate stomach as condition warrants. Activated charcoal may be useful. *b*) Maintain a nonstimulating environment. *c*) Monitor cardiovascular status. *d*) Do not give stimulants. *e*) Reduce fever with cool sponging. *f*) Support respiration. *g*) Use sedatives or anticonvulsants to control CNS excitation and convulsions. *h*) Physostigmine may reverse anticholinergic symptoms. *i*) Ammonium chloride may acidify the urine to increase excretion of pseudoephedrine. *j*) Further care is symptomatic and supportive.

Dosage and Administration:
Dosage:

Age	Dose*	Frequency*
Rondec Drops for oral use only		
1–3 months	¼ dropperful (¼ml)	q.i.d.
3–6 months	½ dropperful (½ml)	q.i.d.
6–9 months	¾ dropperful (¾ml)	q.i.d.
9–18 months	1 dropperful (1 ml)	q.i.d.
Rondec Syrup and Rondec Tablet		
18 months–6 years	½ teaspoonful (2.5 ml)	q.i.d.
adults and children 6 years and over	1 teaspoonful (5 ml) or 1 tablet	q.i.d.
Rondec-TR Tablet adults and children		
12 years and over	1 tablet	b.i.d.

*In mild cases or in particularly sensitive patients, less frequent or reduced doses may be adequate.

How Supplied: Rondec Drops, berry-flavored, in 30-ml bottles for dropper dosage, **NDC** 0074-5783-30. Calibrated shatterproof dropper enclosed in each carton. Container meets safety closure requirements. Avoid exposure to excessive heat.

Rondec Syrup, berry-flavored, in 16-fl-oz (1-pint) bottles, **NDC** 0074-5782-16; and 4-fl-oz bottles, **NDC** 0074-5782-04. Dispense in USP tight glass container. Avoid exposure to excessive heat.

Vitamins Per Liter (Standard Dilution):**

Vitamin	Amount	Unit	Vitamin	Amount	Unit
Vitamin A	2500	I.U.	Niacin (mg equiv.)	9.0	
Vitamin D	400	I.U.	Folic Acid	0.10	mg
Vitamin E	20	I.U.	Vitamin B_{12}	3.0	mcg
Vitamin C	55	mg	Pantothenic Acid	5.0	mg
Thiamine (Vitamin B_1)	0.40	mg	Biotin	30	mcg
Riboflavin (Vitamin B_2)	0.60	mg	Vitamin K_1	0.15	mg
Vitamin B_6	0.40	mg			

* Varies depending on quantity of carbohydrate and water used. If carbohydrate is not added to this product, a 1:1 dilution with water provides approximately 12 Cal/fl oz (40.5 Cal/100 ml).

** Standard dilution is one part Formula Base to one part prescribed carbohydrate and water solution.

Rondec Tablet, Filmtab tablets, in bottles of 100, **NDC** 0074-5726-13; and bottles of 500, **NDC** 0074-5726-53. Each orange-colored tablet marked with Ross "R" and the number 5726 for professional identification. Dispense in USP tight container.

[*Shown in Product Identification Section*]

Rondec-TR Tablet, Filmtab tablets, in bottles of 100, **NDC** 0074-6240-13. Each blue-colored tablet marked with Ross "R" and the number 6240 for professional identification. Dispense in USP tight container.

[*Shown in Product Identification Section*]

ROSS HOSPITAL FORMULA SYSTEM

Similac® infant formula products for hospital nursery use

SIMILAC 13, Ready To Feed, 13 Cal/fl oz
Availability:
4-fl-oz nursing bottles; 48 per case; No. 408.

SIMILAC 20, Ready To Feed, 20 Cal/fl oz
Availability:
4-fl-oz nursing bottles; 48 per case; No. 415.
8-fl-oz nursing bottles; 24 per case; No. 841.

SIMILAC 24, Ready To Feed, 24 Cal/fl oz
Availability:
4-fl-oz nursing bottles; 48 per case; No. 404.

SIMILAC 24 LBW, Ready To Feed, 24 Cal/fl oz
Availability:
4-fl-oz nursing bottles; 48 per case; No. 422.

SIMILAC 27, Ready To Feed, 27 Cal/fl oz
Availability:
4-fl-oz nursing bottles; 48 per case; No. 427.

SIMILAC WITH IRON 13, Ready To Feed, 13 Cal/fl oz
Availability:
4-fl-oz nursing bottles; 48 per case; No. 413.

SIMILAC WITH IRON 20, Ready To Feed, 20 Cal/fl oz
Availability:
4-fl-oz nursing bottles; 48 per case; No. 426.
8-fl-oz nursing bottles; 24 per case; No. 858.

SIMILAC WITH IRON 24, Ready To Feed, 24 Cal/fl oz
Availability:
4-fl-oz nursing bottles; 48 per case; No. 403.

SIMILAC WITH WHEY 20, Ready To Feed, 20 Cal/fl oz
Availability:
4-fl-oz nursing bottles; 48 per case; No. 442.
8-fl-oz nursing bottles; 24 per case; No. 822.

SIMILAC PM 60/40, Ready To Feed, 20 Cal/fl oz
Availability:
4-fl-oz nursing bottles; 48 per case; No. 424.

SIMILAC SPECIAL CARE™ 20, Ready To Feed, 20 Cal/fl oz
Availability:
4-fl-oz nursing bottles; 48 per case; No. 439.

SIMILAC SPECIAL CARE 24, Ready To Feed, 24 Cal/fl oz
Availability:
4-fl-oz nursing bottles; 48 per case; No. 433.

ISOMIL 20, Ready To Feed, 20 Cal/fl oz
Availability:
4-fl-oz nursing bottles; 48 per case; No. 406.
8-fl-oz nursing bottles; 24 per case; No. 871.

ISOMIL® SF 20, Ready To Feed, 20 Cal/fl oz
Availability:
8-fl-oz nursing bottles; 24 per case; No. 801.

PEDIALYTE, Ready To Use, **NDC** 0074-5759-57
Availability:
8-fl-oz nursing bottles; 24 per case; No. 806.

ADVANCE, Ready To Feed
Availability:
8-fl-oz nursing bottles; 24 per case; No. 804.

5% GLUCOSE WATER, Ready To Feed
Availability:
4-fl-oz nursing bottles; 48 per case; No. 405.

10% GLUCOSE WATER, Ready To Feed
Availability:
4-fl-oz nursing bottles; 48 per case; No. 410.

STERILIZED WATER, Ready To Feed
Availability:
4-fl-oz nursing bottles; 48 per case; No. 432.
8-fl-oz nursing bottles; 24 per case; No. 879.

VOLU-FEED®, Ross Volumetric Feeding System
Availability:
Volu-Feed Nursers; 100 per case; No. 080.
Volu-Feed Dispensing Caps; 250 per case; No. 081.

Redi-Nurser® System: Self-contained feeding system with a sterilized nipple attached to a 4-fl-oz nursing bottle is available in eight different varieties of infant feeding.

Component Nipple System
Availability:
Regular Nipple; 250 per case; No. 079.
Premature Nipple; 250 per case; No. 094.
Special Care Nipple; 250 per case; No. 095.

SIMILAC®
Infant Formula

Usage: When an infant formula is needed if the decision is made to discontinue breast-feeding before age 1 year, if a supplement to breast-feeding is needed, or as a routine feeding if breast-feeding is not adopted.

Availability:

Powder: 1-lb cans, measuring scoop enclosed; 12 per case; No. 00139.
1.06-oz packets; 12 four-packet cartons per case; No. 00231.

Concentrated Liquid: 13-fl-oz cans; 24 per case; No. 00264.

Ready To Feed: (Prediluted, 20 Cal/fl oz)
32-fl-oz (quart) cans; 6 per case; No. 00232.
8-fl-oz cans; 4 six-packs per case; No. 00177.
4-fl-oz nursing bottles; 6 per carry-home carton, 8 cartons per case; No. 00480.
8-fl-oz nursing bottles; 6 per carry-home carton, 4 cartons per case; No. 00880.
For hospital use, SIMILAC in disposable nursing bottles is available in the Ross Hospital Formula System.

Preparation:

Powder: Standard 20 Cal/fl oz dilution is 1 level, unpacked scoop Powder (8.74 g) for each 2 fl oz water; or, 1 packet (30.1 g) for each 7 fl oz water.

Concentrated Liquid: Standard 20 Cal/fl oz dilution is 1 part Concentrated Liquid to 1 part water.

Composition: Powder

Ingredients: ⓤ Nonfat milk, lactose, corn oil, coconut oil, vitamins (ascorbic acid, alpha-tocopheryl acetate, niacinamide, calcium pantothenate, vitamin A palmitate, thiamine chloride hydrochloride, pyridoxine hydrochloride, riboflavin, folic acid, phylloquinone, vitamin D_3, cyanocobalamin) and minerals (zinc sulfate, ferrous sulfate, cupric sulfate, manganese sulfate).

Approximate Analysis:	Powdered (wt/100 g)	Standard Dilution* (wt/liter)
Fat	27.4 g	36.1 g
Carbohydrate	54.9 g	72.3 g
Protein	11.8 g	15.5 g
Minerals (Ash)	3.1 g	4.1 g
Calcium	0.39 g	0.51 g
Phosphorus	0.30 g	0.39 g
Magnesium	31 mg	41 mg
Zinc	3.8 mg	5.0 mg
Copper	0.46 mg	0.60 mg
Iodine	76 mcg	0.10 mg
Manganese	26 mcg	34 mcg
Iron	1.1 mg	1.5 mg
(This product, like milk, is deficient in iron; an additional 5.3 mg iron per liter should be supplied from other sources.)		
Moisture	2.0 g	902.5 g
Crude Fiber	0 g	
Calories	145 per av oz	20 per fl oz

Vitamins Per Liter (Standard dilution*):

Vitamin A	2500 I.U.
Vitamin D	400 I.U.
Vitamin E	15 I.U.
Vitamin C	55 mg
Thiamine (Vitamin B_1)	0.65 mg
Riboflavin (Vitamin B_2)	1.0 mg
Niacin (mg equiv.)	7.0
Vitamin B_6	0.40 mg
Pantothenic acid	3.0 mg
Folic acid	0.10 mg
Vitamin K_1	27 mcg
Vitamin B_{12}	1.5 mcg

*Standard dilution: 1 level, unpacked scoop of Similac Powder (8.74 g) for each 2 fl oz water; or, 1 packet (30.1 g) for each 7 fl oz water.

Composition: Concentrated Liquid

Ingredients: ⓤ Water, nonfat milk, lactose, soy oil, coconut oil, mono- and diglycerides, soy lecithin, vitamins (ascorbic acid, alpha-tocopheryl acetate, niacinamide, calcium pantothenate, vitamin A palmitate, thiamine chloride hydrochloride, pyridoxine hydrochloride, riboflavin, folic acid, vitamin D_3, cyanocobalamin), carrageenan, minerals (zinc sulfate, ferrous sulfate, cupric sulfate, manganese sulfate).

Approximate Analysis (wt/liter):	Concentrated	Standard Dilution*
Fat	72.2 g	36.1 g
Carbohydrate	144.6 g	72.3 g
Protein	31.0 g	15.5 g
Minerals (Ash)	7.2 g	3.6 g
Calcium	1.0 g	0.51 g
Phosphorus	0.77 g	0.39 g
Magnesium	82 mg	41 mg
Zinc	10 mg	5.0 mg
Copper	1.2 mg	0.60 mg
Iodine	0.20 mg	0.10 mg
Manganese	68 mcg	34 mcg
Iron	3.0 mg	1.5 mg
(This product, like milk, is deficient in iron; an additional 5.3 mg iron per liter should be supplied from other sources.)		
Water	805.9 g	902.0 g
Crude Fiber	0 g	
Calories per fl oz	40	20
Calories per 100 ml	135	68

Vitamins Per Liter (Standard dilution*):

Vitamin A	2500 I.U.
Vitamin D	400 I.U.
Vitamin E	20 I.U.
Vitamin C	55 mg
Thiamine (Vitamin B_1)	0.65 mg
Riboflavin (Vitamin B_2)	1.0 mg
Niacin (mg equiv.)	7.0
Vitamin B_6	0.40 mg
Folic Acid	0.10 mg
Pantothenic acid	3.0 mg
Vitamin B_{12}	1.5 mcg

*Standard dilution is equal parts Similac Concentrated Liquid and water.

Composition: Ready To Feed

Ingredients: ⓤ Water, nonfat milk, lactose, soy oil, coconut oil, mono- and diglycerides, soy lecithin, vitamins (ascorbic acid, alpha-tocopheryl acetate, niacinamide, calcium pantothenate, vitamin A palmitate, thiamine chloride hydrochloride, pyridoxine hydrochloride, riboflavin, folic acid, vitamin D_3, cyanocobalamin), carrageenan and minerals (zinc sulfate, ferrous sulfate, cupric sulfate, manganese sulfate).

Continued on next page

Ross—Cont.

Approximate Analysis:	(wt/liter)
Fat	36.1 g
Carbohydrate	72.3 g
Protein	15.5 g
Minerals (Ash)	3.3 g
Calcium	0.51 g
Phosphorus	0.39 g
Magnesium	41 mg
Zinc	5.0 mg
Copper	0.60 mg
Iodine	0.10 mg
Manganese	34 mcg
Iron	1.5 mg
(This product, like milk, is deficient in iron; an additional 5.3 mg iron per liter should be supplied from other sources.)	
Water	902.3 g
Crude Fiber	0 g
Calories per fl oz	20
Calories per 100 ml	68

Vitamins Per Liter:	
Vitamin A	2500 I.U.
Vitamin D	400 I.U.
Vitamin E	20 I.U.
Vitamin C	55 mg
Thiamine (Vitamin B_1)	0.65 mg
Riboflavin (Vitamin B_2)	1.0 mg
Niacin (mg equiv.)	7.0
Vitamin B_6	0.40 mg
Folic Acid	0.10 mg
Pantothenic Acid	3.0 mg
Vitamin B_{12}	1.5 mcg

SIMILAC® PM 60/40
Infant Formula

Usage: For infants in the lower range of homeostatic capacity; for those who are problem feeders; those who are predisposed to hypocalcemia; and those whose renal, digestive or cardiovascular functions would benefit from lowered mineral levels.

Availability: Powder only: 1-lb cans, measuring scoop enclosed; 6 per case; No. 00850.

Preparation: Standard 20 Cal/fl oz dilution is one level, unpacked scoop (8.56 g) Powder for each 2 fl oz of water.

Higher caloric feedings are prepared by adding 8.56 g (1 level, unpacked scoopful) of Similac PM 60/40 to the following amounts of water:

For:	Water:	Yields:
24 Cal/oz	48 cc	55 cc (1.8 fl oz)
27 Cal/oz	42 cc	49 cc (1.6 fl oz)
30 Cal/oz	37 cc	44 cc (1.5 fl oz)

Ingredients: Ⓤ Demineralized whey solids, coconut oil, lactose, corn oil, calcium sodium caseinate, minerals (calcium hydroxide, potassium chloride, potassium phosphate dibasic, magnesium chloride, sodium chloride, zinc sulfate, ferrous sulfate, cupric sulfate, manganous chloride), mono- and diglycerides, soy lecithin and vitamins (ascorbic acid, alpha-tocopheryl acetate, niacinamide, calcium pantothenate, vitamin A palmitate, thiamine chloride hydrochloride, riboflavin, pyridoxine hydrochloride, phylloquinone, folic acid, vitamin D_3, cyanocobalamin).

Approximate Analysis:	Powder (wt/100 g)	Standard Dilution* (wt/liter)
Fat	26.85 g	35.4 g
Protein	11.95 g	15.7 g
Lactalbumin and lactoglobulin	60 %	
Casein	40 %	
Carbohydrate	57.50 g	75.7 g
Minerals (Ash)	1.70 g	2.2 g
Calcium	0.30 g	0.40 g
Phosphorus	0.15 g	0.20 g
Sodium	0.12 g	0.16 g
Potassium	0.44 g	0.58 g
Chloride	0.34 g	0.45 g
Magnesium	32 mg	42 mg
Zinc	3.0 mg	4.0 mg
Iron	2.0 mg	2.6 mg
(This product, like milk, is deficient in iron; an additional 4.2 mg iron per liter should be supplied from other sources.)		
Copper	0.30 mg	0.40 mg
Iodine	30 mcg	40 mcg
Manganese	26 mcg	34 mcg
Moisture	2.0 g	900.5 g
Crude Fiber	0 g	
Calories	145 per av oz	20 per fl oz
Calories per 100 ml		68

Vitamins Per Liter (Standard Dilution*):	
Vitamin A	2500 I.U.
Vitamin D	400 I.U.
Vitamin E	15 I.U.
Vitamin C	55 mg
Thiamine (Vitamin B_1)	0.65 mg
Riboflavin (Vitamin B_2)	1.0 mg
Niacin (mg equiv.)	7.3
Vitamin B_6	0.30 mg
Folic acid	50 mcg
Pantothenic Acid	3.0 mg
Vitamin K_1	27 mcg
Vitamin B_{12}	1.5 mcg

*Standard dilution is 1 level scoop of Powder for each 2 fl oz water or 131.7 g of Powder diluted to 1 liter.

Precautions: In conditions where the infant is losing abnormal quantities of one or more electrolytes, it may be necessary to supply electrolytes from sources other than the formula. With premature infants weighing less than 1500 g at birth, it may be necessary to supply an additional source of sodium, calcium and phosphorus during the period of very rapid growth.

SIMILAC® WITH IRON
Infant Formula

Usage: When an iron-containing infant formula is needed if the decision is made to discontinue breast-feeding before age 1 year, if a supplement to breast-feeding is needed, or as a routine feeding if breast-feeding is not adopted.

Availability: Powder: 1-lb cans, measuring scoop enclosed; 12 per case; No. 00360.
1.06-oz packets; 12 four-packet cartons per case; No. 00235.

Concentrated Liquid: 13-fl-oz cans; 24 cans per case; No. 00414.

Ready To Feed: (Prediluted, 20 Cal/fl oz)
32-fl-oz (quart) cans; 6 per case; No. 00241.
8-fl-oz cans; 4 six-packs per case; No. 00179.
4-fl-oz nursing bottles; 6 per carry-home carton, 8 cartons per case; No. 06201.
8-fl-oz nursing bottles; 6 per carry-home carton, 4 cartons per case; No. 06202.
For hospital use, prebottled SIMILAC WITH IRON in disposable nursing bottles is available in the Ross Hospital Formula System.

Preparation:

Powder: Standard 20 Cal/fl oz dilution is 1 level, unpacked scoop Powder (8.74 g) for each 2 fl oz of water; or, 1 packet (30.1 g) for each 7 fl oz water.

Concentrated Liquid: Standard 20 Cal/fl oz of dilution is 1 part Concentrated Liquid to 1 part water.

Composition: Powder

Ingredients: Ⓤ Nonfat milk, lactose, corn oil, coconut oil, vitamins (ascorbic acid, alpha-tocopheryl acetate, niacinamide, calcium pantothenate, vitamin A palmitate, thiamine chloride hydrochloride, pyridoxine hydrochloride, riboflavin, folic acid, phylloquinone, vitamin D_3, cyanocobalamin) and minerals (ferrous sulfate, zinc sulfate, cupric sulfate, manganese sulfate).

Approximate Analysis:	Powdered (wt/100 g)	Standard Dilution* (wt/liter)
Fat	27.4 g	36.1 g
Carbohydrate	54.9 g	72.3 g
Protein	11.8 g	15.5 g
Minerals (Ash)	3.1 g	4.1 g
Calcium	0.39 g	0.51 g
Phosphorus	0.30 g	0.39 g
Magnesium	31 mg	41 mg
Iron	9.1 mg	12 mg
Zinc	3.8 mg	5.0 mg
Copper	0.46 mg	0.60 mg
Iodine	76 mcg	0.10 mg
Manganese	26 mcg	34 mcg
Moisture	2.0 g	902.5 g
Crude Fiber	0 g	
Calories	145 per av oz	20 per fl oz

Vitamins Per Liter (Standard dilution*):	
Vitamin A	2500 I.U.
Vitamin D	400 I.U.
Vitamin E	15 I.U.
Vitamin C	55 mg
Thiamine (Vitamin B_1)	0.65 mg
Riboflavin (Vitamin B_2)	1.0 mg
Niacin (mg equiv.)	7.0
Vitamin B_6	0.40 mg
Pantothenic acid	3.0 mg
Folic acid	0.10 mg
Vitamin K_1	27 mcg
Vitamin B_{12}	1.5 mcg

*Standard dilution: 1 level, unpacked scoop of Similac With Iron Powder (8.74 g) for each 2 fl oz water; or, 1 packet (30.1 g) for each 7 fl oz water.

Composition: Concentrated Liquid

Ingredients: Ⓤ Water, nonfat milk, lactose, soy oil, coconut oil, mono- and diglycerides, soy lecithin, vitamins (ascorbic acid, alpha-tocopheryl acetate, niacinamide, calcium pantothenate, vitamin A palmitate, thiamine chloride hydrochloride, pyridoxine hydrochloride, riboflavin, folic acid, vitamin D_3, cyanocobalamin), carrageenan, minerals (ferrous sulfate, zinc sulfate, cupric sulfate, manganese sulfate).

Approximate Analysis: (wt/liter)	Concentrated	Standard Dilution*
Fat	72.2 g	36.1 g
Carbohydrate	144.6 g	72.3 g
Protein	31.0 g	15.5 g
Minerals (Ash)	7.4 g	3.7 g
Calcium	1.0 g	0.51 g
Phosphorus	0.77 g	0.39 g
Magnesium	82 mg	41 mg
Iron	24 mg	12 mg
Zinc	10 mg	5.0 mg
Copper	1.2 mg	0.60 mg
Iodine	0.20 mg	0.10 mg
Manganese	68 mcg	34 mcg
Water	805.7 g	901.9 g
Crude Fiber	0 g	
Calories per fl oz	40	20
Calories per 100 ml	135	68

Vitamins Per Liter (Standard dilution*):	
Vitamin A	2500 I.U.
Vitamin D	400 I.U.
Vitamin E	20 I.U.
Vitamin C	55 mg
Thiamine (Vitamin B_1)	0.65 mg
Riboflavin (Vitamin B_2)	1.0 mg
Niacin (mg equiv.)	7.0
Vitamin B_6	0.40 mg
Folic acid	0.10 mg

Pantothenic acid	3.0 mg
Vitamin B_{12}	1.5 mcg

*Standard dilution is equal parts Similac With Iron Concentrated Liquid and water.

Composition: Ready To Feed

Ingredients: Ⓤ Water, nonfat milk, lactose, soy oil, coconut oil, mono- and diglycerides, soy lecithin, vitamins (ascorbic acid, alpha-tocopheryl acetate, niacinamide, calcium pantothenate, vitamin A palmitate, thiamine chloride hydrochloride, pyridoxine hydrochloride, riboflavin, folic acid, vitamiin D_3, cyanocobalamin), carrageenan and minerals (ferrous sulfate, zinc sulfate, cupric sulfate, manganese sulfate).

Approximate Analysis:	(wt/liter)
Fat	36.1 g
Carbohydrate	72.3 g
Protein	15.5 g
Minerals (Ash)	3.3 g
Calcium	0.51 g
Phosphorus	0.39 g
Magnesium	41 mg
Iron	12 mg
Zinc	5.0 mg
Copper	0.60 mg
Iodine	0.10 mg
Manganese	34 mcg
Water	902.3 g
Crude Fiber	0 g
Calories per fl oz	20
Calories per 100 ml	68

Vitamins Per Liter:	
Vitamin A	2500 I.U.
Vitamin D	400 I.U.
Vitamin E	20 I.U.
Vitamin C	55 mg
Thiamine (Vitamin B_1)	0.65 mg
Riboflavin (Vitamin B_2)	1.0 mg
Niacin (mg equiv.)	7.0
Vitamin B_6	0.40 mg
Folic acid	0.10 mg
Pantothenic Acid	3.0 mg
Vitamin B_{12}	1.5 mcg

The addition of iron to this formula conforms to the recommendation of the Committee on Nutrition of the American Academy of Pediatrics.

SIMILAC® WITH WHEY

Infant Formula

Usage: When an iron-fortified, whey-predominant-protein formula is desired for feeding term infants if the decision is made to discontinue breast-feeding before age 1, if a supplement to breast-feeding is needed, or as a routine feeding if breast-feeding is not adopted.

Availability:

Powder: 1-lb cans, measuring scoop enclosed; 6 per case; No. 00372.

Concentrated Liquid: 13-fl-oz cans; 12 per case; No. 00352.

Ready To Feed: (prediluted, 20 Cal/fl oz) 32-fl-oz cans; 6 per case; No. 00312.

For hospital use, SIMILAC WITH WHEY in disposable nursing bottles is available in the Ross Hospital Formula System.

Preparation:

Powder: Standard (20 Cal/fl oz) dilution is 1 level, unpacked scoop Powder (8.74 g) for each 2 fl oz of water.

Concentrated Liquid: Standard (20 Cal/fl oz) dilution is one part Concentrated Liquid to one part water.

Composition: Powder

Ingredients: Ⓤ Nonfat milk, lactose, corn oil, coconut oil, demineralized whey solids, minerals (calcium phosphate tribasic, sodium chloride, magnesium chloride, potassium citrate, ferrous sulfate, zinc sulfate, cupric sulfate, manganese sulfate) and vitamins (ascorbic acid, alpha-tocopheryl acetate, niacinamide, calcium pantothenate, vitamin A palmitate, thiamine chloride hydrochloride, riboflavin, pyridoxine hydrochloride, folic acid, phylloquinone, vitamin D_3, biotin, cyanocobalamin).

Approximate Analysis:	Powder (wt/100 g)	Standard Dilution* (wt/liter)
Protein	11.8 g	15.5 g
(Lactoglobulin and Lactalbumin 60%, Casein 40%)		
Fat	27.4 g	36.1 g
Carbohydrate	54.9 g	72.3 g
Minerals (Ash)	2.6 g	3.4 g
Calcium	0.30 g	0.40 g
Phosphorus	0.23 g	0.30 g
Sodium	0.18 g	0.24 g
Potassium	0.57 g	0.75 g
Chloride	0.33 g	0.43 g
Magnesium	38 mg	50 mg
Iron	9.1 mg	12 mg
Zinc	3.8 mg	5.0 mg
Copper	0.46 mg	.60 mg
Iodine	76 mcg	0.10 mg
Manganese	26 mcg	34 mcg
Moisture	2.5 g	902.5 g
Crude Fiber	0 g	
Calories	145 per av oz	20 per fl oz

Vitamins Per Liter (Standard dilution*):	
Vitamin A	2500 I.U.
Vitamin D	400 I.U.
Vitamin E	15 I.U.
Vitamin C	55 mg
Thiamine (Vitamin B_1)	0.65 mg
Riboflavin (Vitamin B_2)	1.0 mg
Niacin (mg equiv.)	7.0
Vitamin B_6	0.40 mg
Pantothenic acid	3.0 mg
Folic acid	0.10 mg
Vitamin K_1	27 mcg
Biotin	11 mcg
Vitamin B_{12}	1.5 mcg

*Standard dilution: 1 level, unpacked scoop of Similac With Whey Powder (8.74 g) for each 2 fl oz water.

Composition: Concentrated Liquid

Ingredients: Ⓤ Water, nonfat milk, lactose, soy oil, coconut oil, demineralized whey solids, minerals (calcium phosphate tribasic, sodium chloride, potassium citrate, ferrous sulfate, magnesium chloride, zinc sulfate, cupric sulfate, manganese sulfate), soy lecithin, mono- and diglycerides, vitamins (ascorbic acid, alpha-tocopheryl acetate, niacinamide, calcium pantothenate, vitamin A palmitate, thiamine chloride hydrochloride, riboflavin, pyridoxine hydrochloride, folic acid, vitamin D_3, biotin, cyanocobalamin) and carrageenan.

Vitamins Per Liter (Standard dilution*):	
Vitamin A	2500 I.U.
Vitamin D	400 I.U.
Vitamin E	20 I.U.
Vitamin C	55 mg
Thiamine (Vitamin B_1)	0.65 mg
Riboflavin (Vitamin B_2)	1.0 mg
Niacin (mg equiv.)	7.0
Pantothenic acid	3.0 mg
Vitamin B_6	0.40 mg
Folic acid	0.10 mg
Biotin	11 mcg
Vitamin B_{12}	1.5 mcg

*Standard dilution is equal parts Similac With Whey Concentrated Liquid and water.

Composition: Ready To Feed

Ingredients: Ⓤ Water, nonfat milk, lactose, soy oil, coconut oil, demineralized whey solids, minerals (calcium phosphate tribasic, sodium chloride, potassium citrate, ferrous sulfate, magnesium chloride, zinc sulfate, cupric sulfate, manganese sulfate), soy lecithin, mono- and diglycerides, vitamins (ascorbic acid, alphatocopheryl acetate, niacinamide, calcium pantothenate, vitamin A palmitate, thiamine chloride hydrochloride, riboflavin, pyridoxine hydrochloride, folic acid, vitamin D_3, biotin, cyanocobalamin) and carrageenan.

Approximate Analysis (wt/liter):	
Protein	15.5 g
(Lactoglobulin and Lactalbumin 60%, Casein 40%)	
Fat	36.1 g
Carbohydrate	72.3 g
Minerals (Ash)	3.4 g
Calcium	0.40 g
Phosphorus	0.30 g
Sodium	0.24 g
Potassium	0.75 g
Chloride	0.43 g
Magnesium	50 mg
Iron	12 mg
Zinc	5.0 mg
Copper	0.60 mg
Iodine	0.10 mg
Manganese	34 mcg
Water	902.5 g
Crude Fiber	0 g
Calories per fl oz	20
Calories per 100 ml	68

Vitamins Per Liter:	
Vitamin A	2500 I.U.
Vitamin D	400 I.U.
Vitamin E	20 I.U.
Vitamin C	55 mg
Thiamine (Vitamin B_1)	0.65 mg
Riboflavin (Vitamin B_2)	1.0 mg
Niacin (mg equiv.)	7.0
Pantothenic acid	3.0 mg
Vitamin B_6	0.40 mg
Folic acid	0.10 mg
Biotin	11 mcg
Vitamin B_{12}	1.5 mcg

The addition of iron to this formula conforms to the recommendation of the Committee on Nutrition of the American Academy of Pediatrics.

VARI-FLAVORS® Flavor Pacs

Usage: To provide flavor variety for patients receiving full liquid diets and liquid supplements.

Features:

Five flavors (Pecan, Cherry, Lemon, Orange, Strawberry) offer patients variety and encourage acceptance of liquid diets and liquid supplements.

Vari-Flavors Flavor Pacs may be added to and will mix readily with Ross Medical Nutritionals—Vanilla Ensure®, Vanilla Ensure Plus®, Osmolite®, and Vital® High Nitrogen. Flavor Pacs may be stored for use in the dietary department, at nursing stations, or by patient's bedside.

Availability:

One-gram packets; 24 per dispenser carton; Pecan, No. 720; Cherry, No. 722; Lemon, No. 724; Orange, No. 726; Strawberry, No. 728; Assorted flavors, No. 730.

Instructions for Use: Tap Pac lightly to shake contents to bottom. Tear off corner of packet. Pour contents into suitable dry serving container. Add 8 ounces of one of the Ross Medical Nutritional products listed above. Allow flavor to dissolve for a few seconds. Stir until flavor is mixed and serve.

Composition: Dextrose, artificial flavoring and coloring (Strawberry, Cherry, Orange). Dextrose and artificial flavoring (Pecan). Dextrose, artificial flavoring, and FD & C Yellow #5 as coloring (Lemon).

When used as directed, Vari-Flavors contribute trace amounts of minerals and less than 1

Continued on next page

Ross—Cont.

gram of dextrose. The addition of a single Vari-Flavors Pac (1 gram) to one of the Ross Medical Nutritional products listed above increases total calories per 8-oz serving by approximately 4 Calories, and increases osmolality (mOsm/kg water) approximately as follows:

Orange 15	Pecan 20
Cherry 20	Strawberry 30
Lemon 20	

VI-DAYLIN® ADC Drops

Dietary Supplement of Vitamins A, D and C

Description: One dropperful (1 ml) provides:

Vitamins		% U.S. RDA*	% U.S. RDA**
Vitamin A	1500 I.U.	100	60
Vitamin D	400 I.U.	100	100
Vitamin C	35 mg	100	87

Ingredients: Propylene glycol, polysorbate 80, sodium ascorbate, ascorbic acid, vitamin A palmitate, methylparaben (preservative), propylparaben (preservative), and ergocalciferol in a glycerin-water vehicle with added artificial pineapple-fruit flavoring and caramel coloring. Contains only a trace (less than ½%) of alcohol.

*% U.S. Recommended Daily Allowance for infants.

**% U.S. Recommended Daily Allowance for children under 4 years of age.

Indications and Usage: Dietary supplement of vitamins A, D and C for infants and children under 4 years of age.

Dosage and Administration: One dropperful daily, or as directed by physician.

How Supplied:
50-ml bottles, calibrated dropper enclosed; OTC; **NDC** 0074-0105-04.

VI-DAYLIN® Drops

Multivitamin Supplement

Description: One dropperful (1 ml) provides:

Vitamins		% U.S. RDA*	% U.S. RDA**
Vitamin A	1500 I.U.	100	60
Vitamin D	400 I.U.	100	100
Vitamin E	5 I.U.	100	50
Vitamin C	35 mg	100	87
Thiamine (Vitamin B_1)	0.5 mg	100	71
Riboflavin (Vitamin B_2)	0.6 mg	100	75
Niacin	8 mg	100	88
Vitamin B_6	0.4 mg	100	57
Vitamin B_{12}	1.5 mcg	75	50

This product does not contain the essential vitamin folic acid.

Ingredients: Ascorbic acid, d-alpha tocopheryl acid succinate, niacinamide, benzoic acid (preservative), ferric ammonium citrate (stabilizer), vitamin A palmitate, riboflavin-5'-phosphate sodium, methylparaben (preservative), thiamine hydrochloride, pyridoxine hydrochloride, ergocalciferol, disodium edetate (stabilizer) and cyanocobalamin in a glycerin-water vehicle with added artificial flavoring. Contains only a trace (less than ½%) of alcohol.

*% U.S. Recommended Daily Allowance for infants.

**% U.S. Recommended Daily Allowance for children under 4 years of age.

Indications and Usage: Multivitamin supplement for infants and children under 4 years of age.

Dosage and Administration: One dropperful daily, or as directed by physician.

How Supplied:
50-ml bottles, calibrated dropper enclosed; OTC; **NDC** 0074-0103-04.

VI-DAYLIN®/F ADC Drops ℞

ADC Vitamins/Fluoride

Description: One dropperful (1 ml) provides:
Fluoride 0.25 mg

Vitamins		% U.S. RDA*	% U.S. RDA**
Vitamin A	1500 I.U.	100	60
Vitamin D	400 I.U.	100	100
Vitamin C	35 mg	100	87

Ingredients: Sodium ascorbate, vitamin A palmitate, ascorbic acid, ergocalciferol and sodium fluoride. Alcohol, approximately 0.4%.

*% U.S. Recommended Daily Allowance for infants.

**% U.S. Recommended Daily Allowance for children under 4 years of age.

Indications and Usage: As an aid in the prevention of dental caries in infants and children, and in the prophylaxis of vitamin A, D and C deficiencies.

Contraindications: Should be used only where the fluoride content of the drinking water supply is known to be 0.7 parts per million or less.

Precautions: The recommended dosage should not be exceeded since chronic overdosage of fluoride may result in mottling of tooth enamel and osseous changes.

Overdosage: In children, acute ingestion of 10 to 20 mg of sodium fluoride may cause excessive salivation and gastrointestinal disturbances; 500 mg may be fatal. Oral and/or intravenous fluids containing calcium may be indicated.

Dosage and Administration: One dropperful daily, or as directed by physician or dentist.

How Supplied:
50-ml bottles, calibrated dropper enclosed; Rx; **NDC** 0074-1106-50.

VI-DAYLIN®/F ADC + IRON Drops ℞

ADC Vitamins/Fluoride/Iron Supplement

Description: One dropperful (1.0 ml) provides:
Fluoride 0.25 mg

Vitamins		% U.S. RDA*	% U.S. RDA**
Vitamin A	1500 I.U.	100	60
Vitamin D	400 I.U.	100	100
Vitamin C	35 mg	100	87
Minerals			
Iron	10 mg	66	100

Ingredients: Ascorbic acid, ferrous sulfate, vitamin A palmitate, sodium fluoride and ergocalciferol.

*% U.S. Recommended Daily Allowance for infants.

**% U.S. Recommended Daily Allowance for children under 4 years of age.

Indications and Usage: As an aid in the prevention of dental caries in infants and children, and in the prophylaxis of iron and vitamin A, D and C deficiencies.

Contraindications: Should be used only where the fluoride content of the drinking water supply is known to be 0.7 parts per million or less.

Precautions: The recommended dosage should not be exceeded since chronic overdosage of fluoride may result in mottling of tooth enamel and osseous changes. In infants, oral iron-containing preparations may cause temporary darkening of the membrane covering the teeth.

Overdosage: In children, acute ingestion of 10 to 20 mg of sodium fluoride may cause excessive salivation and gastrointestinal disturbances; 500 mg may be fatal. Oral and/or intravenous fluids containing calcium may be indicated.

Acute overdosage of iron may cause nausea and vomiting and, in severe cases, cardiovascular collapse and death. The estimated lethal dose of orally ingested elemental iron is 300 mg per kg body weight. Serum iron and total iron-binding capacity may be used as guides for use of chelating agents such as deferoxamine.

Dosage and Administration: One dropperful daily, or as directed by physician or dentist.

How Supplied: 50-ml bottles, calibrated dropper enclosed; ℞; **NDC** 0074-8929-50.

VI-DAYLIN®/F Drops ℞

Multivitamins/Fluoride

Description: One dropperful (1.0 ml) provides:
Fluoride 0.25 mg

Vitamins		% U.S. RDA*	% U.S. RDA**
Vitamin A	1500 I.U.	100	60
Vitamin D	400 I.U.	100	100
Vitamin E	5 I.U.	100	50
Vitamin C	35 mg	100	87
Thiamine (Vitamin B_1)	0.5 mg	100	71
Riboflavin (Vitamin B_2)	0.6 mg	100	75
Niacin	8 mg	100	88
Vitamin B_6	0.4 mg	100	57

Ingredients: Ascorbic acid, niacinamide, d-alpha tocopheryl acid succinate, riboflavin-5'-phosphate sodium, sodium fluoride, vitamin A palmitate, thiamine hydrochloride, pyridoxine hydrochloride and ergocalciferol. No artificial sweeteners. Alcohol content less than 0.1%.

*% U.S. Recommended Daily Allowance for infants.

**% U.S. Recommended Daily Allowance for children under 4 years of age.

Indications and Usage: As an aid in the prevention of dental caries in infants and children, and in the prophylaxis of appropriate vitamin deficiencies.

Contraindications: Should be used only where the fluoride content of the drinking water supply is known to be 0.7 parts per million or less.

Precautions: The recommended dosage should not be exceeded since chronic overdosage of fluoride may result in mottling of tooth enamel and osseous changes.

Overdosage: In children, acute ingestion of 10 to 20 mg of sodium fluoride may cause excessive salivation and gastrointestinal disturbances; 500 mg may be fatal. Oral and/or intravenous fluids containing calcium may be indicated.

Dosage and Administration: One dropperful daily, or as directed by physician or dentist.

How Supplied: 50-ml bottles, calibrated dropper enclosed; Rx; **NDC** 0074-1104-50.

VI-DAYLIN®/F + IRON Chewable ℞

Multivitamins/Fluoride/Iron

Description: Each chewable tablet provides:
Fluoride (as sodium fluoride) 1 mg
[See table on top next page].

Indications and Usage: As an aid in the prevention of dental caries in children, and in the prophylaxis of iron and appropriate vitamin deficiencies.

Contraindications: Should be used only where the fluoride content of the drinking water supply is known to be 0.7 parts per million or less.

Precautions: The recommended dosage should not be exceeded since chronic overdosage of fluoride may result in mottling of tooth enamel and osseous changes.

Dosage and Administration: Children 3 years of age or older, one chewable tablet daily; age 2-3 years, ½ chewable tablet daily; or as directed by physician or dentist.

Overdosage: In children, acute ingestion of 10 to 20 mg of sodium fluoride may cause excessive salivation and gastrointestinal disturbances; 500 mg may be fatal. Oral and/or intra-

			% U.S. RDA*	% U.S. RDA**
Vitamins				
Vitamin A (as palmitate, 0.75 mg)	2500	I.U.	100	50
Vitamin D (as ergocalciferol, 10 mg)	400	I.U.	100	100
Vitamin E (as dl-alpha tocopheryl acetate)	15	I.U.	150	50
Vitamin C (as sodium ascorbate, 40 mg; ascorbic acid, 20 mg)	60	mg	150	100
Folic Acid	0.3	mg	150	75
Vitamin B_1 (as thiamine mononitrate)	1.05	mg	150	70
Vitamin B_2 (as riboflavin)	1.2	mg	150	70
Niacin (as niacinamide)	13.5	mg	150	67
Vitamin B_6 (as pyridoxine hydrochloride)	1.05	mg	150	52
Vitamin B_{12} (as cyanocobalamin)	4.5	mcg	150	75
Minerals				
Iron (as ferrous fumarate)	12	mg	120	66

*% U.S. Recommended Daily Allowance for children under 4 years of age.
**% U.S. Recommended Daily Allowance for adults and children 4 or more years of age.

venous fluids containing calcium may be indicated.

Acute overdosage of iron may cause nausea and vomiting and, in severe cases, cardiovascular collapse and death. The estimated lethal dose of orally ingested elemental iron is 300 mg per kg body weight. Serum iron and total iron-binding capacity may be used as guides for use of chelating agents such as deferoxamine.

How Supplied: 100-tablet bottles; ℞; **NDC** 0074-7621-13.

[Shown in Product Identification Section]

VI-DAYLIN®/F + IRON Drops ℞
Multivitamins/Fluoride/Iron Supplement

Description: One dropperful (1.0 ml) provides:

			% U.S. RDA*	% U.S. RDA**
Fluoride	0.25	mg		
Vitamins				
Vitamin A	1500	I.U.	100	60
Vitamin D	400	I.U.	100	100
Vitamin E	5	I.U.	100	50
Vitamin C	35	mg	100	87
Thiamine (Vitamin B_1)	0.5	mg	100	71
Riboflavin (Vitamin B_2)	0.6	mg	100	75
Niacin	8	mg	100	88
Vitamin B_6	0.4	mg	100	57
Minerals				
Iron	10	mg	66	100

Ingredients: Ascorbic acid, ferrous sulfate, niacinamide, d-alpha tocopheryl acid succinate, vitamin A palmitate, riboflavin-5′-phosphate sodium, thiamine hydrochloride, sodium fluoride, pyridoxine hydrochloride and ergocalciferol. Alcohol content less than 0.1%.

*% U.S. Recommended Daily Allowance for infants.

**% U.S. Recommended Daily Allowance for children under 4 years of age.

Indications and Usage: As an aid in the prevention of dental caries in infants and children and in the prophylaxis of iron and appropriate vitamin deficiencies.

Contraindications: Should be used only where the fluoride content of the drinking water supply is known to be 0.7 parts per million or less.

Precautions: The recommended dosage should not be exceeded since chronic overdosage of fluoride may result in mottling of tooth enamel and osseous changes. In infants, oral iron-containing preparations may cause temporary darkening of the membrane covering the teeth.

Overdosage: In children, acute ingestion of 10 to 20 mg of sodium fluoride may cause excessive salivation and gastrointestinal disturbances; 500 mg may be fatal. Oral and/or intravenous fluids containing calcium may be indicated.

Acute overdosage of iron may cause nausea and vomiting and, in severe cases, cardiovascular collapse and death. The estimated lethal dose of orally ingested elemental iron is 300 mg per kg body weight. Serum iron and total iron-binding capacity may be used as guides for use of chelating agents such as deferoxamine.

Dosage and Administration: One dropperful daily, or as directed by physician or dentist.

How Supplied: 50-ml bottles, calibrated dropper enclosed; ℞; **NDC** 0074-8928-50.

VI-DAYLIN® PLUS IRON Drops
Multivitamins/Iron Supplement

Description: One dropperful (1 ml) provides:

			% U.S. RDA*	% U.S. RDA**
Vitamins				
Vitamin A	1500	I.U.	100	60
Vitamin D	400	I.U.	100	100
Vitamin E	5	I.U.	100	50
Vitamin C	35	mg	100	87
Thiamine (Vitamin B_1)	0.5	mg	100	71
Riboflavin (Vitamin B_2)	0.6	mg	100	75
Niacin	8	mg	100	88
Vitamin B_6	0.4	mg	100	57
Vitamin B_{12}	1.5	mcg	75	50
Minerals				
Iron	10	mg	66	100

This product does not contain the essential vitamin folic acid.

Ingredients: Ascorbic acid, ferrous sulfate, d-alpha-tocopheryl acid succinate, niacinamide, sodium ascorbate, vitamin A palmitate, benzoic acid (preservative), riboflavin-5′-phosphate sodium, thiamine hydrochloride, methylparaben (preservative), pyridoxine hydrochloride, ergocalciferol and cyanocobalamin in a glycerin-water vehicle with added artificial coloring and flavoring.

*% U.S. Recommended Daily Allowance for infants.

**% U.S. Recommended Daily Allowance for children under 4 years of age.

Indications and Usage: Multivitamin supplement with iron for infants and children under 4 years of age.

Administration and Dosage: One dropperful daily, or as directed by physician.

How Supplied: 50-ml bottles, calibrated dropper enclosed; OTC; **NDC** 0074-0116-01.

VI-DAYLIN® PLUS IRON ADC Drops
Dietary Supplement of Vitamins A, D and C with Iron

Description: One dropperful (1 ml) provides:

			% U.S. RDA*	% U.S. RDA**
Vitamins				
Vitamin A	1500	I.U.	100	60
Vitamin D	400	I.U.	100	100
Vitamin C	35	mg	100	87
Minerals				
Iron	10	mg	66	100

Ingredients: Polysorbate 80, ferrous sulfate, ascorbic acid, sodium ascorbate, vitamin A palmitate, benzoic acid (preservative), ergocalciferol and methylparaben (preservative) in a glycerin-water vehicle with added artificial flavoring and coloring.

*% U.S. Recommended Daily Allowance for infants.

** % U.S. Recommended Daily Allowance for children under 4 years of age.

Indications and Usage: Dietary supplement of vitamins A, D and C with iron for infants and children under 4 years of age.

Dosage and Administration: One dropperful daily, or as directed by physician.

How Supplied: 50-ml bottles; calibrated dropper enclosed; OTC; **NDC** 0074-0117-01.

VI-DAYLIN® Chewable
Multivitamin Supplement

Description: Each chewable tablet provides:

			%U.S. RDA*	%U.S. RDA**
Vitamins				
Vitamin A	2500	I.U.	100	50
Vitamin D	400	I.U.	100	100
Vitamin E	15	I.U.	150	50
Vitamin C	60	mg	150	100
Folic Acid	0.3	mg	150	75
Thiamine (Vitamin B_1)	1.05	mg	150	70
Riboflavin (Vitamin B_2)	1.2	mg	150	70
Niacin	13.5	mg	150	67
Vitamin B_6	1.05	mg	150	52
Vitamin B_{12}	4.5	mcg	150	75

Ingredients: Sucrose and dextrins, sodium ascorbate, niacinamide, dl-alpha tocopheryl acetate, ascorbic acid, vitamin A palmitate, riboflavin, pyridoxine hydrochloride, thiamine mononitrate, ergocalciferol, folic acid and cyanocobalamin. Made with natural sweeteners, artificial flavoring and artificially colored with natural ingredients.

*% U.S. Recommended Daily Allowance for children under 4 years of age.

**% U.S. Recommended Daily Allowance for adults and children 4 or more years of age.

Indications and Usage: Multivitamin supplement for children and adults.

Dosage and Administration: One chewable tablet daily or as directed by physician.

How Supplied: 100-tablet bottles; OTC; **NDC** 0074-4519-13.

[Shown in Product Identification Section]

VI-DAYLIN®/F Chewable ℞
Multivitamins/Fluoride

Description: Each chewable tablet provides:

			%U.S. RDA*	%U.S. RDA**
Fluoride (as sodium fluoride)	1	mg		
Vitamins				
Vitamin A (as palmitate, 0.75 mg)	2500	I.U.	100	50
Vitamin D (ergocalciferol, 10 mcg)	400	I.U.	100	100
Vitamin E (dl-alpha tocopheryl acetate)	15	I.U.	150	50
Vitamin C (as sodium ascorbate, 40 mg; ascorbic acid, 20 mg)	60	mg	150	100
Folic Acid	0.3	mg	150	75
Vitamin B_1(as thiamine mononitrate)	1.05	mg	150	70
Vitamin B_2 (as riboflavin)	1.2	mg	150	70
Niacin (as niacinamide)	13.5	mg	150	67
Vitamin B_6 (as pyridoxine hydrochloride)	1.05	mg	150	52
Vitamin B_{12} (as cyanocobalamin)	4.5	mcg	150	75

*% U.S. Recommended Daily Allowance for children under 4 years of age.

**% U.S. Recommended Daily Allowance for adults and children 4 or more years of age.

Indications and Usage: As an aid in the prevention of dental caries in children and in

Continued on next page

Ross—Cont.

the prophylaxis of appropriate vitamin deficiencies.
Contraindications: Should not be used where the fluoride content of the drinking water supply is known to be greater than 0.7 parts per million.
Precautions: The recommended use and dosage of Vi-Daylin/F Chewable should not be exceeded, since chronic overdosage of fluoride may result in mottling of tooth enamel and osseous changes.
Overdosage: In children, acute ingestion of 10 to 20 mg of sodium fluoride may cause excessive salivation and gastrointestinal disturbances; 500 mg may be fatal. Oral and/or intravenous fluids containing calcium may be indicated.
Dosage and Administration: Children 3 years of age or older, 1 chewable tablet daily; age 2 to 3 years, ½ chewable tablet daily; or as directed by physician or dentist.
How Supplied: 100-tablet bottles; Rx; **NDC** 0074-7626-13.
[*Shown in Product Identification Section*]

VI-DAYLIN® + IRON Chewable
Multivitamin/Iron Supplement

Description: Each chewable tablet provides:

Vitamins			% U.S. RDA*	% U.S. RDA**
Vitamin A	2500	I.U.	100	50
Vitamin D	400	I.U.	100	100
Vitamin E	15	I.U.	150	50
Vitamin C	60	mg	150	100
Folic Acid	0.3	mg	150	75
Thiamine (Vitamin B_1)	1.05	mg	150	70
Riboflavin (Vitamin B_2)	1.2	mg	150	70
Niacin	13.5	mg	150	67
Vitamin B_6	1.05	mg	150	52
Vitamin B_{12}	4.5	mcg	150	75
Minerals				
Iron	12	mg	120	66

Ingredients: Sucrose and dextrins, mannitol, sodium ascorbate, niacinamide, ferrous fumarate, dl-alpha tocopheryl acetate, ascorbic acid, vitamin A palmitate, riboflavin, pyridoxine hydrochloride, thiamine mononitrate, ergocalciferol, folic acid and cyanocobalamin. Made with natural sweeteners, artificial flavoring and coloring.
*% U.S. Recommended Daily Allowance for children under 4 years of age.
**%U.S. Recommended Daily Allowance for adults and children 4 or more years of age.
Indications and Usage: Multivitamin supplement with iron for children and adults.
Dosage and Administration: One tablet daily, or as directed by physician.
How Supplied:
100-tablet bottles; OTC; **NDC** 0074-4520-13.
[*Shown in Product Identification Section*]

VI-DAYLIN® Liquid
Multivitamin Supplement

Description: One teaspoonful (5 ml) provides:

Vitamins			% U.S. RDA*	% U.S. RDA**
Vitamin A	2500	I.U.	100	50
Vitamin D	400	I.U.	100	100
Vitamin E	15	I.U.	150	50
Vitamin C	60	mg	150	100
Thiamine (Vitamin B_1)	1.05	mg	150	70
Riboflavin (Vitamin B_2)	1.2	mg	150	70
Niacin	13.5	mg	150	68
Vitamin B_6	1.05	mg	150	50
Vitamin B_{12}	4.5	mcg	150	75

This product does not contain the essential vitamin folic acid.
*% U.S. Recommended Daily Allowance for children under 4 years of age.
**% U.S. Recommended Daily Allowance for adults and children 4 or more years of age.
Ingredients: Glucose, sucrose, ascorbic acid, polysorbate 80, dl-alpha tocopheryl acetate, niacinamide, acacia, cysteine hydrochloride (stabilizer), benzoic acid (preservative), vitamin A palmitate, methylparaben (preservative), pyridoxine hydrochloride, riboflavin, thiamine hydrochloride, ergocalciferol and cyanocobalamin in an aqueous vehicle with added natural citrus flavoring and added color. Contains only a trace of alcohol (not more than ½%).
Indications and Usage: Multivitamin supplement for children and adults.
Dosage and Administration: One teaspoonful daily, or as directed by physician.
How Supplied:
16-fl-oz (pint) bottles; OTC; **NDC** 0074-3606-03.
8-fl-oz bottles; OTC; **NDC** 0074-3606-02.

VI-DAYLIN® PLUS IRON Liquid
Multivitamins/Iron Supplement

Description: One teaspoonful (5 ml) provides:

Vitamins			% U.S. RDA*	% U.S. RDA**
Vitamin A	2500	I.U.	100	50
Vitamin D	400	I.U.	100	100
Vitamin E	15	I.U.	150	50
Vitamin C	60	mg	150	100
Thiamine (Vitamin B_1)	1.05	mg	150	70
Riboflavin (Vitamin B_2)	1.2	mg	150	70
Niacin	13.5	mg	150	68
Vitamin B_6	1.05	mg	150	50
Vitamin B_{12}	4.5	mcg	150	75
Minerals				
Iron	10	mg	100	55

This product does not contain the essential vitamin folic acid.
*% U.S. Recommended Daily Allowance for children under 4 years of age.
**% U.S. Recommended Daily Allowance for adults and children 4 or more years of age.
Ingredients: Glucose, sucrose, ascorbic acid, ferrous gluconate, polysorbate 80, dl-alpha tocopheryl acetate, niacinamide, acacia, cysteine hydrochloride (stabilizer), benzoic acid (preservative), methylparaben (preservative), vitamin A palmitate, riboflavin-5′-phosphate sodium, pyridoxine hydrochloride, thiamine hydrochloride, propylparaben (preservative), ergocalciferol and cyanocobalamin in an aqueous vehicle with added natural citrus flavoring and added coloring. Contains only a trace of alcohol (not more than ½%).
Indications and Usage: Multivitamin supplement with iron for children and adults.
Dosage and Administration: One teaspoonful daily, or as directed by physician.
How Supplied:
16-fl-oz (pint) bottles; OTC; **NDC** 0074-6992-03.
8-fl-oz bottles; OTC; **NDC** 0074-6992-02.

VITAL® HIGH NITROGEN
Nutritionally Complete Partially Hydrolyzed Diet

Usage: As a source of total or supplemental nutrition for patients with impaired gastrointestinal function (limited digestion/absorption). Vital High Nitrogen has been designed to meet the nutritional needs of stressed patients with the following conditions:

- Inflammatory bowel disease, including Crohn's disease and ulcerative colitis
- Preoperative bowel preparation and postoperative management
- Diagnostic procedures, such as colon radiography and colonoscopy
- Alimentary tract fistulae
- Cancer, including periods of management by radiation and chemotherapy
- Hypermetabolic conditions, such as those associated with trauma, major burns, multiple fractures, and major sepsis
- Pancreatic insufficiency states
- Short bowel syndrome
- Nonspecific maldigestive and malabsorptive states

Vital High Nitrogen may be used as a tube feeding (nasogastric, nasoduodenal or jejunal) or as an oral feeding.
Features:

- Complete Nutrition—In standard dilution, Vital High Nitrogen provides 1 Calorie per ml and 300 Calories per serving (1 packet). Caloric distribution: protein, 16.7%; fat, 9.3%; carbohydrate, 74.0%. Five servings (1500 Calories) meet or exceed 100% of the U.S. RDA for vitamins and minerals for adults and children 4 or more years of age.
- High Levels of Nitrogen—Vital High Nitrogen provides 62.5 g of protein (10 g nitrogen) in 1500 Calories insuring high levels of available nitrogen for the stressed patient. Vital High Nitrogen also supplies a protein system of peptides fortified with free essential amino acids designed for maximum nitrogen absorption. The total Calorie/nitrogen ratio of 150:1 allows for effective protein sparing and utilization and meets the Calorie/nitrogen ratio recommended for nutritional support of the catabolic patient.
- Fat Source—45% of fat from medium-chain triglycerides, 55% from safflower oil. Medium-chain triglycerides for immediate fat absorption. High quantities of essential fatty acids.
- Good Taste—Vital High Nitrogen is significantly more palatable and acceptable than diets composed solely of crystalline amino acids. The mild, appealing vanilla flavor ensures better patient acceptance of an elemental feeding with no disturbing aftertaste. The addition of Vari-Flavors® Flavor Pacs helps to combat flavor fatigue experienced by patients receiving full liquid diets and liquid supplements.
- Low Osmolality—(460 mOsm/kg water) The osmolality of Vital High Nitrogen may help to avoid gastrointestinal distress and dumping syndrome commonly associated with elemental feedings.
- Low Fecal Residue—The fecal residue produced by Vital High Nitrogen is comparable to that produced by traditional elemental diets.
- Low Renal Solute Load—(Sodium 17 mEq/liter, .38 g/liter; Potassium 30 mEq/liter, 1.17 g/liter; Chloride 19 mEq/liter, .67 g/liter). The electrolyte levels are appropriate for moderately electrolyte-restricted diets, yet adequate for most hospitalized patients. Renal solute load is approximately 306 mOsm/liter at standard dilution.

Dosage and Administration:
Mixing Instructions: One packet of Vital High Nitrogen (79 g) Powder is to be mixed with 255 ml of water for standard dilution of 1 Calorie per ml. Pour 255 ml (8.5 fl oz) of cold water into a container. Empty contents of one packet into container and mix until powder dissolves. Yields approximately 300 ml. Prepare only the amount intended for a single day's serving. Refrigerate after preparation. Shake before use. Store unopened powder in a cool, dry place. UNDER NO CIRCUMSTANCES SHOULD VITAL HIGH NITROGEN BE ADMINISTERED PARENTERALLY.
Additional fluid requirements should be met by giving water orally with or after feedings, or by flushing the gavage tube.

- **Tube Feeding:** Follow physician's instructions. Flow rate, volume and dilution of feeding depend on patient's nutritional needs and tolerance for tube feedings. Care should be taken to avoid contamination of this product during preparation and administration.

[See table above].

- **Oral Feeding:** Serving Vital High Nitrogen chilled may enhance its vanilla flavor and increase palatability. Servings may provide total nutrition or supplemental nutrition with and between meals.

Availability: 2.79-oz (79 g) packets of water-soluble Powder (vanilla flavor); 24 packets per case; No. 766.

Composition:

Ingredients: Hydrolyzed corn starch, protein components (partially hydrolyzed whey and meat, and soy), sucrose, minerals (potassium phosphate dibasic, calcium phosphate tribasic, magnesium sulfate, magnesium chloride, sodium chloride, ferrous sulfate, zinc sulfate, manganous chloride, cupric sulfate), safflower oil, amino acids (L-tyrosine, L-leucine, L-valine, L-isoleucine, L-phenylalanine, L-histidine, L-methionine, L-threonine, L-tryptophan), medium-chain triglycerides (fractionated coconut oil), artificial and natural flavor, vitamins (choline chloride, ascorbic acid, alpha-tocopheryl acetate, niacinamide, calcium pantothenate, vitamin A palmitate, riboflavin, pyridoxine hydrochloride, thiamine chloride hydrochloride, folic acid, biotin, phylloquinone, vitamin D_3, cyanocobalamin), mono- and diglycerides, and soy lecithin.

Approximate Analysis: (grams)	**Per 300 Calories*** (1 packet)	**Per 1500 Calories*** (5 packets)
Protein	12.5	62.5
Fat	3.25	16.25
Carbohydrate	56.5	282.5
Minerals (Ash)	1.6	8.0
Moisture (Max)	5.2	26.0

* In standard dilution (79 g of Vital High Nitrogen Vanilla Powder mixed in 255 ml of water).

Vitamins/ Minerals	**Per 300 Calories**	**Per 1500 Calories**	**Percent U.S. RDA** 1500 Calories**
Vitamin A, (I.U.)	1000	5000	100
Vitamin D, (I.U.)	80	400	100
Vitamin E, (I.U.)	12	60	200
Vitamin C, mg	18	90	150
Folic acid, mg	0.08	0.4	100
Thiamine (Vitamin B_1), mg	0.3	1.5	100
Riboflavin (Vitamin B_2), mg	0.34	1.7	100
Vitamin B_6, mg	0.44	2.2	100
Vitamin B_{12}, mcg	1.2	6	100
Niacin, mg	4	20	100
Biotin, mg	0.06	0.3	100
Pantothenic Acid, mg	2	10	100
Vitamin K_1, mcg	56	280	***
Choline, mg	40	200	***
Calcium, mg	200	1000	100
Phosphorus, mg	200	1000	100
Sodium, mg	140	700	***
Potassium, mg	400	2000	***
Chloride, mg	270	1350	***
Magnesium, mg	80	400	100
Iodine, mcg	30	150	100
Manganese, mg	0.75	3.75	***
Copper, mg	0.4	2	100
Zinc, mg	3	15	100
Iron, mg	3.6	18	100

** For adults and children 4 or more years of age.

*** U.S. RDA not established.

Sample Administration Schedule VITAL® High Nitrogen Continuous Drip or Pump Controlled Delivery

Day	Time	Strength	Rate (ml/hr)	Volume (ml)	Calories
1	1st 8 hours	½	50	400	200
	2nd 8 hours	½	75	600	300
	3rd 8 hours	½	100	800	400
					900 *Total Calories*
2	1st 8 hours	¾	100	800	600
	2nd 8 hours	¾	100	800	600
	3rd 8 hours	¾	100	800	600
					1800 *Total Calories*
3	1st 8 hours	Full	100	800	800
	2nd 8 hours	Full	100–125	800–1000	800–1000
	3rd 8 hours	Full	100–125	800–1000	800–1000
					2400–2800 *Total Calories*

Intermittent Drip

Day	Time	Strength	Rate (5–10 ml/min)	Volume (ml)	Calories
1	7am–11pm	½	100 ml q 2 hr (7am, 9am, 11am)	300	150
		½	200 ml q 2 hr (1pm, 3pm, 5pm)	600	300
		½	300 ml q 2 hr (7pm, 9pm, 11pm)	900	450
					900 *Total Calories*
2	7am–11pm	¾	300 ml q 2 hr (7am, 9am, 11am, 1pm, 3pm, 5pm, 7pm, 9pm)	2400	1800 *Total Calories*
3	7am–11pm	Full	300 ml q 3 hr (5 feedings) up to 300 ml q 2 hr (8 feedings)	1500–2400	1500–2400 *Total Calories*

Rotex Pharmaceuticals, Inc.

P.O. BOX 19283
ORLANDO, FL. 32814

ARTHROGESIC™ TABLETS ℞

Each tablet contains: Magnesium Salicylate 600 mg., Phenyltoloxamine Citrate 30 mg. (NDC 31190-006-01).

NASALSPAN® ℞

Each capsule contains: Chlorpheniramine Maleate 8 mg., d-Pseudoephedrine Hydrochloride 120 mg. (NDC 31190-002-01).

NASALSPAN® EXPECTORANT ℞

Each teaspoonful (5 cc) contains: Pseudoephedrine HCl 30 mg., Dextromethorphan 10 mg., Guaifenesin 50 mg., Sodium Citrate 75 mg., Citric Acid 20 mg. (NDC 31190-007-01).

ROGESIC™ CAPSULES ℞

Each capsule contains: Butalbital 50 mg., Caffeine 40 mg., Acetaminophen 325 mg. (NDC 31190-088-01).

ROGESIC™ #3 TABLETS Ⓒ ℞

Each tablet contains:

Acetaminophen N.F. ....325.0 mg.
Codeine Phosphate U.S.P. ....30.0 mg.
(WARNING: May be habit forming)
Butalbital N.F. ....50.0 mg.
(WARNING: May be habit forming)
Caffeine ....40.0 mg.

ROPRES™ ℞

Each tablet contains: Trichlormethiazide 4 mg., Reserpine 0.1 mg. (NDC 31190-003-01).

ROTHAV®-150 ℞

Each tablet contains: Ethaverine Hydrochloride 150 mg. (NDC 31190-001-01).

ROVITE™

Each tablet contains: Ascorbic Acid 500 mg., Thiamine HCl (Vitamin B-1) 50 mg., Riboflavin (Vitamin B-2) 25 mg., Pyridoxine HCl (Vitamin B-6) 50 mg., Pantothenic Acid as Calcium Pantothenate 50 mg., Niacinamide 50 mg., Vitamin B-12 10 mcg., Zinc Sulfate 40 mg., Magnesium Sulfate 35 mg. (NDC 31190-005-01).

ROVITE™ TONIC ℞

Each 30 ml contains:

Thiamine Hydrochloride (B_1) .... 2.50 mg.
Riboflavin (B_2) .... 2.50 mg.
Pyridoxine Hydrochloride (B_6) .... 1.0 mg.
Vitamin B_{12} (Cyanocobalamin) .... 5.0 mcg.
Dexpanthenol .... 5.0 mg.
Niacin .... 10.0 mg.
Ferric Pyrophosphate .... 20.0 mg.
Alcohol .... 15.0 %

In a palatable special wine base. (NDC 31190-099-01)

Rowell Laboratories, Inc.
210 MAIN STREET W.
BAUDETTE, MN 56623

BALNEOL®
Perianal cleansing lotion

Composition: Contains water, mineral oil, propylene glycol, glyceryl stearate/PEG-100 stearate, PEG-40 stearate, laureth-4, PEG-4 dilaurate, lanolin oil, sodium acetate, carbomer-934, triethanolamine, methyl paraben, dioctyl sodium sulfosuccinate, fragrance, acetic acid.
Action and Uses: BALNEOL is a soothing, emollient cleanser for hygienic cleansing of irritated perianal and external vaginal areas. It helps relieve itching and other discomforts, helps stop irritation due to toilet tissue. BALNEOL gently yet thoroughly cleanses and provides a soothing, protecting film.
Administration and Dosage: For cleansing without discomfort after each bowel movement, a small amount of BALNEOL is spread on tissue or cotton and used to wipe the perianal area. Also used between bowel movements and at bedtime for additional comfort. For cleansing and soothing the external vaginal area: to be used on clean tissue or cotton as often as necessary.
Caution: In all cases of rectal bleeding, consult physician promptly. If irritation persists or increases, discontinue use and consult physician.
How Supplied: 1 oz. and 4 oz. plastic bottle.

CIN-QUIN™ ℞
(Quinidine Sulfate)

How Supplied: CIN-QUIN 100 Tablets™ (Quinidine Sulfate 100 mg.) white tablet embossed "ROWELL 4024".
CIN-QUIN 200 Tablets™ (Quinidine Sulfate 200 mg.) white tablet embossed "ROWELL 4028".
CIN-QUIN 300 Tablets™ (Quinidine Sulfate 300 mg.) white tablet embossed "ROWELL 4032".
CIN-QUIN 200 Capsules™ (Quinidine Sulfate 200 mg.) No. 2 clear capsule imprinted "ROWELL 4016" in black.
CIN-QUIN 300 Capsules™ (Quinidine Sulfate 300 mg.) No. 0 clear capsule imprinted "ROWELL 4020" in black. Supplied in bottles of 100's, 1000's and in unit-dose boxes of 100.

COLREX COMPOUND CAPSULES™ Ⓒ
COLREX COMPOUND ELIXIR™ Ⓒ

Composition: COLREX COMPOUND CAPSULES—Codeine Phosphate*, 16 mg.; Acetaminophen, 325 mg.; Phenylephrine HCl, 10 mg.; Chlorpheniramine Maleate, 2 mg.
COLREX COMPOUND ELIXIR—Codeine Phosphate*, 8 mg.; Acetaminophen, 120 mg.; Chlorpheniramine Maleate, 1 mg.; Phenylephrine HCl, 5 mg.; Alcohol 9.5% v/v. SUGAR FREE.
*WARNING: May be habit forming.
Action and Uses: COLREX COMPOUND combines antitussive, antihistaminic, decongestant, analgesic and antipyretic actions.
Indications: Adjunct for temporary relief of cough, congestion, headache and muscle soreness of common colds and upper respiratory infections. Infections should be identified and, if bacterial, given appropriate antimicrobial therapy.
Precautions: Codeine may cause constipation, and an occasional patient may display idiosyncratic response to it. Chlorpheniramine, especially with codeine, may cause drowsiness; use with caution in patients who operate machinery. Phenylephrine may cause gastric upset and, because of its sympathomimetic effect, should be used with caution in cardiovascular disease, thyrotoxicosis and diabetes.
Dosages: COLREX COMPOUND CAPSULES—Adults, 1 or 2 capsules three or four times daily. Children 6 to 12, 1 capsule three or four times daily. Not recommended for children under 6.
COLREX COMPOUND ELIXIR—Children 2 to 6, 1 teaspoonful three or four times daily. Children 6 to 12, 2 teaspoonsful three or four times daily. Adults, 2 to 4 teaspoonsful three or four times daily.
How Supplied: CAPSULES—Yellow, imprinted "ROWELL 0840".
In bottles of 100 and 1000; ELIXIR—In bottles of 60 ml., 480 ml., 1 gallon.

CORTENEMA® ℞
(Hydrocortisone Retention Enema)
Disposable Unit for Rectal Use Only

Each disposable unit (60 ml.) contains: Hydrocortisone, 100 mg. in an aqueous solution containing carboxypolymethylene, polysorbate 80, and methylparaben, 0.18% as a preservative.
Description: CORTENEMA is a convenient disposable single-dose hydrocortisone enema designed for ease of self-administration. Hydrocortisone is a naturally occurring glucocorticoid (adrenal corticosteroid), which similarly as its acetate and sodium hemisuccinate derivatives, is partially absorbed following rectal administration. Absorption studies in ulcerative colitis patients have shown up to 50% absorption of hydrocortisone administered as CORTENEMA and up to 30% of hydrocortisone acetate administered in an identical vehicle.
Actions: CORTENEMA provides the potent anti-inflammatory effect of hydrocortisone. Because this drug is absorbed from the colon, it acts both topically and systemically. Although rectal hydrocortisone, used as recommended for CORTENEMA, has a low incidence of reported adverse reactions, prolonged use presumably may cause systemic reactions associated with oral dosage forms.
Indications: CORTENEMA is indicated as adjunctive therapy in the treatment of ulcerative colitis, especially distal forms, including ulcerative proctitis, ulcerative proctosigmoiditis, and left-sided ulcerative colitis. It has proved useful also in some cases involving the transverse and ascending colons.
Contraindications: Systemic fungal infections; and ileocolostomy during the immediate or early postoperative period.
Warnings: In severe ulcerative colitis, it is hazardous to delay needed surgery while awaiting response to medical treatment.
Damage to the rectal wall can result from careless or improper insertion of an enema tip.
In patients on corticosteroid therapy subjected to unusual stress, increased dosage of rapidly acting corticosteroids before, during, and after the stressful situation is indicated.
Corticosteroids may mask some signs of infection, and new infections may appear during their use. There may be decreased resistance and inability to localize infection when corticosteroids are used.
Prolonged use of corticosteroids may produce posterior subcapsular cataracts, glaucoma with possible damage to the optic nerves, and may enhance the establishment of secondary ocular infections due to fungi or viruses.
Usage in pregnancy: Since adequate human reproduction studies have not been done with corticosteroids, the use of these drugs in pregnancy, nursing mothers or women of childbearing potential requires that the possible benefits of the drug be weighed against the potential hazards to the mother and embryo or fetus. Infants born of mothers who have received substantial doses of corticosteroids during pregnancy, should be carefully observed for signs of hypoadrenalism.
Average and large doses of hydrocortisone or cortisone can cause elevation of blood pressure, salt and water retention, and increased excretion of potassium. These effects are less likely to occur with the synthetic derivatives except when used in large doses. Dietary salt restriction and potassium supplementation may be necessary. All corticosteroids increase calcium excretion.
While on corticosteroid therapy patients should not be vaccinated against smallpox. Other immunization procedures should not be undertaken in patients who are on corticosteroids, especially on high dose, because of possible hazards of neurological complications and a lack of antibody response.
If corticosteroids are indicated in patients with latent tuberculosis or tuberculin reactivity, close observation is necessary as reactivation of the disease may occur. During prolonged corticosteroid therapy, these patients should receive chemoprophylaxis.
Precautions: CORTENEMA Hydrocortisone Retention Enema should be used with caution where there is a probability of impending perforation, abscess or other pyogenic infection; fresh intestinal anastomoses; obstruction; or extensive fistulas and sinus tracts. Use with caution in presence of active or latent peptic ulcer; diverticulitis; renal insufficiency; hypertension; osteoporosis; and myasthenia gravis.
Steroid therapy might impair prognosis in surgery by increasing the hazard of infection. If infection is suspected, appropriate antibiotic therapy must be administered, usually in larger than ordinary doses.
Drug-induced secondary adrenocortical insufficiency may occur with prolonged CORTENEMA therapy. This is minimized by gradual reduction of dosage. This type of relative insufficiency may persist for months after discontinuation of therapy; therefore, in any situation of stress occurring during that period, hormone therapy should be reinstituted. Since mineralocorticoid secretion may be impaired, salt and/or a mineralocorticoid should be administered concurrently.
There is an enhanced effect of corticosteroids on patients with hypothyroidism and in those with cirrhosis.
Corticosteroids should be used cautiously in patients with ocular herpes simplex because of possible corneal perforation.
The lowest possible dose of corticosteroid should be used to control the condition under treatment, and when reduction in dosage is possible, the reduction should be gradual.
Psychic derangement may appear when corticosteroids are used, ranging from euphoria, insomnia, mood swings, personality changes, and severe depression, to frank psychotic manifestations. Also, existing emotional instability or psychotic tendencies may be aggravated by corticosteroids.
Aspirin should be used cautiously in conjunction with corticosteroids in hypoprothrombinemia.
Growth and development of infants and children on prolonged corticosteroid therapy should be carefully observed.
Adverse Reactions: Local pain or burning, and rectal bleeding attributed to CORTENEMA have been reported rarely. Apparent exacerabtions or sensitivity reactions also occur rarely. The following adverse reactions should be kept in mind whenever corticosteroids are given by rectal administration.
Fluid and Electrolyte Disturbances: Sodium retention; fluid retention; congestive heart failure in susceptible patients; potassium loss; hypokalemic alkalosis; hypertension. Musculoskeletal: Muscle Weakness; steroid myopathy; loss of muscle mass; osteoporosis; vertebral compression fractures; aseptic necrosis of femoral and humeral heads; pathologic fracture of long bones. Gastrointestinal: Peptic ulcer with possible perforation and hemorrhage; pancreatitis; abdominal distention; ulcerative esophagitis. Dermatologic: Impaired wound healing; thin fragile skin; petechiae and ecchymoses;

facial erythema; increased sweating; may suppress reactions to skin tests. Neurological: Convulsions; increased intracranial pressure with papilledema (pseudo-tumor cerebri) usually after treatment; vertigo; headache. Endocrine: Menstrual irregularities; development of Cushingoid state; suppression of growth in children; secondary adrenocortical and pituitary unresponsiveness, particularly in times of stress, as in trauma, surgery or illness; decreased carbohydrate tolerance; manifestations of latent diabetes mellitus; increased requirements for insulin or oral hypoglycemic agents in diabetics. Ophthalmic: Posterior subcapsular cataracts; increased intraocular pressure; glaucoma; exophthalmos. Metabolic: Negative nitrogen balance due to protein catabolism.

Dosage and Administration: The use of CORTENEMA Hydrocortisone Retention Enema is predicated upon the concomitant use of modern supportive measures such as rational dietary control, sedatives, anti-diarrheal agents, antibacterial therapy, blood replacement if necessary, etc.

The usual course of therapy is one CORTENEMA nightly for 21 days, or until the patient comes into remission both clinically and proctologically. Clinical symptoms usually subside promptly within 3 to 5 days. Improvement in the appearance of the mucosa, as seen by sigmoidoscopic examination, may lag somewhat behind clinical improvement. Difficult cases may require as long as 2 or 3 months of CORTENEMA treatment. Where the course of therapy extends beyond 21 days, CORTENEMA should be discontinued gradually by reducing administration to every other night for 2 or 3 weeks.

If clinical or proctologic improvement fail to occur within 2 or 3 weeks after starting CORTENEMA, discontinue its use.

Symptomatic improvement, evidenced by decreased diarrhea and bleeding; weight gain; improved appetite; lessened fever; and decrease in leukocytosis, may be misleading and should not be used as the sole criterion in judging efficacy. Sigmoidoscopic examination and X-ray visualization are essential for adequate monitoring of ulcerative colitis. Biopsy is useful for differential diagnosis.

Patient instructions for administering CORTENEMA are enclosed in each box of seven units. We recommend that the patient lie on his left side during administration and for 30 minutes thereafter, so that the fluid will distribute throughout the left colon. Every effort should be made to retain the enema for at least an hour and, preferably, all night. This may be facilitated by prior sedation and/or antidiarrheal medication, especially early in therapy, when the urge to evacuate is great.

How Supplied: CORTENEMA Hydrocortisone 100 mg. Retention Enema is supplied as disposable single-dose bottles with lubricated rectal applicator tips, in boxes of seven × 60 ml. (NDC 0032-1904-82) and boxes of one × 60 ml. (NDC 0032-1904-73).

DERMACORT® CREAM AND LOTION ℞

(Buffered 1% Hydrocortisone)

Caution: Federal law prohibits dispensing without a prescription.

Description: DERMACORT (Hydrocortisone) 1% Cream and Lotion are topical corticosteroids. Each contains hydrocortisone 1% in a pH-adjusted Cream and Lotion containing stearyl alcohol, cetyl alcohol, isopropyl palmitate, citric acid, polyoxyethylene 40 stearate, dibasic sodium phosphate, propylene glycol, water, and sorbic acid as a preservative.

Hydrocortisone has the chemical name Pregn-4-ene-3, 20-dione, 11, 17, 21-trihydroxy-, (11β)-; empirical formula $C_{21}H_{30}O_5$; molecular weight 362.47; Chemical Abstract Service registry number 50-23-7, and has the chemical structure:

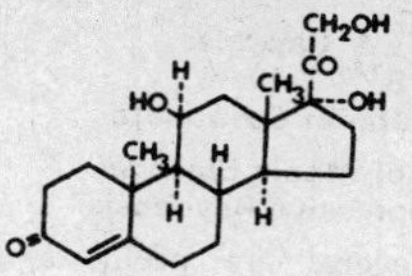

Clinical Pharmacology: Topical corticosteroids share anti-inflammatory, antipruritic and vasoconstrictive actions.

The mechanism of anti-inflammatory activity of the topical corticosteroids is unclear. Various laboratory methods, including vasoconstrictor assays, are used to compare and predict potencies and/or clinical efficacies of the topical corticosteroids. There is some evidence to suggest that a recognizable correlation exists between vasoconstrictor potency and therapeutic efficacy in man.

Pharmacokinetics: The extent of percutaneous absorption of topical corticosteroids is determined by many factors including the vehicle, the integrity of the epidermal barrier, and the use of occlusive dressings.

Topical corticosteroids can be absorbed from normal intact skin. Inflammation and/or other disease processes in the skin increase percutaneous absorption. Occlusive dressings substantially increase the percutaneous absoprtion of topical corticosteroids. Thus, occlusive dressings may be a valuable therapeutic adjunct for treatment of resistant dermatoses. (See DOSAGE AND ADMINISTRATION.)

Once absorbed through the skin, topical corticosteroids are handled through pharmacokinetic pathways similar to systemically administered corticosteroids. Corticosteroids are bound to plasma proteins in varying degrees. Corticosteroids are metabolized primarily in the liver and are then excreted by the kidneys. Some of the topical corticosteroids and their metabolites are also excreted into the bile.

Indications and Usage: Topical corticosteroids are indicated for the relief of the inflammatory and pruritic manifestations of corticosteroid-responsive dermatoses.

Contraindications: Topical corticosteroids are contraindicated in those patients with a history of hypersensitivity to any of the components of the preparation.

Precautions:

General: Systemic absorption of topical corticosteroids has produced reversible hypothalamic pituitary-adrenal (HPA) axis suppression, manifestations of Cushing's syndrome, hyperglycemia, and glucosuria in some patients.

Conditions which augment systemic absorption include the application of the more potent steroids, use over large surface areas, prolonged use, and the addition of occlusive dressings.

Therefore, patients receiving a large dose of a potent topical steroid applied to a large surface area or under an occlusive dressing should be evaluated periodically for evidence of HPA axis suppression by using the urinary-free cortisol and ACTH stimulation tests. If HPA axis suppression is noted, an attempt should be made to withdraw the drug, to reduce the frequency of application, or to substitute a less potent steroid.

Recovery of HPA axis function is generally prompt and complete upon discontinuation of the drug. Infrequently, signs and symptoms of steroid withdrawal may occur, requiring supplemental systemic corticosteroids.

Children may absorb proportionally larger amounts of topical corticosteroids and thus be more susceptible to systemic toxicity (see PRECAUTIONS—Pediatric Use).

If irritation develops, topical corticosteroids should be discontinued and appropriate therapy instituted.

In the presence of dermatological infections, the use of an appropriate antifungal or antibacterial agent should be instituted. If a favorable response does not occur promptly, the corticosteroid should be discontinued until the infection has been adequately controlled.

Information for the Patient: Patients using topical corticosteroids should receive the following information and instructions:

1. This medication is to be used as directed by the physician. It is for external use only. Avoid contact with the eyes.
2. Patients should be advised not to use this medication for any disorder other than for which it was prescribed.
3. The treated skin area should not be bandaged or otherwise covered or wrapped as to be occlusive unless directed by the physician.
4. Patients should report any signs of local adverse reactions especially under occlusive dressing.
5. Parents of pediatric patients should be advised not to use tight-fitting diapers or plastic pants on a child being treated in diaper area, as these garments may constitute occlusive dressings.

Laboratory Tests: The following tests may be helpful in evaluating the HPA axis suppresson:

Urinary-free cortisol test
ACTH stimulation test

Carcinogensis, Mutagenesis, and Impairment of Fertility: Long-term animal studies have not been performed to evaluate the carcinogenic potential or the effect on fertility of topical corticosteroids.

Studies to determine mutagenicity with prednisolone and hydrocortisone have revealed negative results.

Pregnancy Category C: Corticosteroids are generally teratogenic in laboratory animals when administered systemically at relatively low dosage levels. The more potent corticosteroids have been shown to be teratogenic after dermal application in laboratory animals. There are no adequate and well-controlled studies in pregnant women on teratogenic effects from topically applied corticosteroids. Therefore, topical corticosteroids should be used during pregnancy only if the potential benefit justifies the potential risk to the fetus. Drugs of this class should not be used extensively on pregnant patients, in large amounts, or for prolonged periods of time.

Nursing Mothers: It is not know whether topical administration of corticosteroids could result in sufficient systemic absorption to produce detectable quantities in breast milk. Systemically administered corticosteroids are secreted into breast milk in quantities not likely to have a deleterious effect on the infant. Nevertheless, caution should be exercised when topical corticosteroids are administered to a nursing woman.

Pediatric Use: *Pediatric patients may demonstrate greater susceptibility to topical corticosteroid-induced HPA axis suppression and Cushing's syndrome than mature patients because of a larger skin surface area to body weight ratio.*

Hypothalamic-pituitary-adrenal (HPA) axis suppression, Cushing's syndrome, and intracranial hypertension have been reported in children receiving topical corticosteroids. Manifestations of adrenal suppression in children include linear growth retardation, delayed weight gain, low plasma cortisol levels, and absence of response to ACTH stimulation. Manifestations of intracranial hypertension include bulging fontanelles, headaches, and bilateral papilledema.

Administration of topical corticosteroids to children should be limited to the least amount compatible with an effective therapeutic regi-

Continued on next page

Rowell—Cont.

men. Chronic corticosteroid therapy may interfere with the growth and development of children.

Adverse Reactions: The following local adverse reactions are reported infrequently with topical corticosteroids, but may occur more frequently with the use of occlusive dressings. These reactions are listed in an approximate decreasing order of occurrence:

Burning
Itching
Irritation
Dryness
Folliculitis
Hypertrichosis
Acneiform eruptions
Hypopigmentation
Perioral dermatitis
Allergic contact dermatitis
Maceration of the skin
Secondary infection
Skin atrophy
Striae
Miliaria

Overdosage: Topically applied corticosteroids can be absorbed in sufficient amounts to produce systemic effects (see PRECAUTIONS).

Dosage and Administration: Topical corticosteroids are generally applied to the affected area as a thin film from one to four times daily depending on the severity of the condition.

Occlusive dressings may be used for the management of psoriasis or recalcitrant conditions.

If an infection develops, the use of occlusive dressings should be discontinued and appropriate antimicrobial therapy instituted.

How Supplied:

DERMACORT (Hydrocortisone) Cream 1% is available in 1 lb (454 g) jars. (NDC 0032-6002-68).

DERMACORT (Hydrocortisone) Lotion 1% is available in 120 ml (4 Fl. oz.) bottles. (NDC 0032-6008-74).

Store at room temperature in tight containers. Avoid freezing.

Pl230 40M 1E DECEMBER, 1981

DEXONE™ ℞
(Dexamethasone Tablets)

How Supplied:

DEXONE 0.5™ (Dexamethasone 0.5mg) (yellow) embossed "ROWELL 3205"

DEXONE 0.75™ (Dexamethasone 0.75mg) (light green) embossed "ROWELL 3210"

DEXONE 1.5™ (Dexamethasone 1.5mg) (pink) embossed "ROWELL 3215"

DEXONE 4™ (Dexamethasone 4.0 mg) (white) embossed "ROWELL 3220"

Each supplied in bottles of 100's and in unit-dose boxes of 100.

HYDROCIL® INSTANT

Description: A concentrated hydrophilic mucilloid containing 95% psyllium. Hydrocil Instant mixes instantly, is sugar-free, low in potassium and contains less than 10 mg. of sodium per dose.

Indications: Hydrocil Instant is a natural bulk forming fiber useful in the treatment of constipation and other conditions as directed by a physician.

Directions: The usual adult dose is one packet or scoopful poured into an 8 oz. glass. Add water, fruit juices or other liquid and stir. It mixes instantly. Drink immediately. Take in the morning and night or as directed by a physician. Follow each dose with another glass of liquid.

How Supplied: In unit-dose packets of 3.7 grams that are available in boxes of 30's or 500's. Also in 250 gram jars with a measuring scoop. Each packet or scoopful, 3.7 grams, contains one usual adult dose of psyllium hydrophilic mucilloid, 3.5 grams.

LITHONATE® Capsules ℞
LITHOTABS™ Tablets ℞
Brands of Lithium Carbonate

For Control of Manic Episodes in Manic-Depressive Psychosis.

Caution: Federal law prohibits dispensing without prescription.

WARNING

Lithium toxicity is closely related to serum lithium levels, and can occur at doses close to therapeutic levels. Facilities for prompt and accurate serum lithium determinations should be available before initiating therapy.

Description:

LITHONATE: Each peach-colored capsule contains 300 mg of lithium carbonate.

LITHOTABS: Each scored, white, film-coated tablet contains 300 mg of lithium carbonate.

Lithium carbonate is a white, light, alkaline powder with molecular formula $Li_2\ CO_3$ and molecular weight 73.89. Lithium is an element of the alkali-metal group with atomic number 3, atomic weight 6.94 and an emission line at 671 nm on the flame photometer.

Indications: Lithium is indicated in the treatment of manic episodes of manic depressive illness. Maintenance therapy prevents or diminishes the intensity of subsequent episodes in those manic-depressive patients with a history of mania.

Typical symptoms of mania include pressure of speech, motor hyperactivity, reduced need for sleep, flight of ideas, grandiosity, elation, poor judgment, aggressiveness, and possibly hostility. When given to a patient experiencing a manic episode, lithium may produce a normalization of symptomatology within 1 to 3 weeks.

Warnings: Lithium should generally not be given to patients with significant renal or cardiovascular disease, severe debilitation or dehydration, or sodium depletion, and to patients receiving diuretics, since the risk of lithium toxicity is very high in such patients. If the psychiatric indication is life-threatening, and if such a patient fails to respond to other measures, lithium treatment may be undertaken with extreme caution, including daily serum lithium determinations and adjustment to the usually low doses ordinarily tolerated by these individuals. In such instances, hospitalization is a necessity.

Lithium toxicity is closely related to serum lithium levels, and can occur at doses close to therapeutic levels (see DOSAGE AND ADMINISTRATION).

Lithium therapy has been reported in some cases to be associated with morphologic changes in the kidneys. The relationship between such changes and renal function has not been established.

Outpatients and their families should be warned that the patient must discontinue lithium therapy and contact his physician if such clinical signs of lithium toxicity as diarrhea, vomiting, tremor, mild ataxia, drowsiness, or muscular weakness occur.

Lithium may prolong the effects of neuromuscular blocking agents. Therefore, neuromuscular blocking agents should be given with caution to patients receiving lithium.

Lithium may impair mental and/or physical abilities. Caution patients about activities requiring alertness (e.g., operating vehicles or machinery).

Combined use of haloperidol and lithium: An encephalopathic syndrome (characterized by weakness, lethargy, fever, tremulousness and confusion, extrapyramidal symptoms, leucocytosis, elevated serum enzymes, BUN and FBS) followed by irreversible brain damage has occurred in a few patients treated with lithium plus haloperidol. A causal relationship between these events and the concomitant administration of lithium and haloperidol has not been established; however, patients receiving such combined therapy should be monitored closely for early evidence of neurological toxicity and treatment discontinued promptly if such signs appear. The possibility of similar adverse interactions with other antipsychotic medications exists.

Usage in Pregnancy: Adverse effects on nidation in rats, embryo viability in mice, and metabolism in-vitro of rat testis and human spermatozoa have been attributed to lithium, as have teratogenicity in submammalian species and cleft palates in mice. Studies in rats, rabbits and monkeys have shown no evidence of lithium-induced teratology.

There are lithium birth registries in the United States and elsewhere; however there are at the present time insufficient data to determine the effects of lithium on human fetuses. Therefore, at this point, lithium should not be used in pregnancy, especially the first trimester, unless in the opinion of the physician, the potential benefits outweigh the possible hazards.

Usage in Nursing Mothers: Lithium is excreted in human milk. Nursing should not be undertaken during lithium therapy except in rare and unusual circumstances where, in the view of the physician, the potential benefits to the mother outweigh possible hazards to the child.

Usage in Children: Since information regarding the safety and effectiveness of lithium in children under 12 years of age is not available, its use in such patients is not recommended at this time.

Precautions: The ability to tolerate lithium is greater during the acute manic phase and decreases when manic symptoms subside (see DOSAGE AND ADMINISTRATION)

The distribution space of lithium approximates that of total body water. Lithium is primarily excreted in urine with insignificant excretion in feces. Renal excretion of lithium is proportional to its plasma concentration. The half-elimination time of lithium is approximately 24 hours. Lithium decreases sodium reabsorption by the renal tubules which could lead to sodium depletion. Therefore, it is essential for the patient to maintain a normal diet, including salt, and an adequate fluid intake (2500–3000 ml.) at least during the initial stabilization period. Decreased tolerance to lithium has been reported to ensue from protracted sweating or diarrhea and, if such occur, supplemental fluid and salt should be administered.

In addition to sweating and diarrhea, concomitant infection with elevated temperatures may also necessitate a temporary reduction or cessation of medication.

Previously existing underlying disorders do not necessarily constitute a contraindication to lithium treatment; where hypothyroidism exists, careful monitoring of thyroid function during lithium stabilization and maintenance allows for correction of changing thyroid parameters, if any, where hypothyroidism occurs during lithium stablilization and maintenance, supplemental thyroid treatment may be used.

Indomethacin (50 mg t.i.d.) has been reported to increase steady-state plasma lithium levels from 30 to 59 percent. There is also some evidence that other nonsteroidal, anti-inflammatory agents may have a similar effect. When such combinations are used, increased plasma lithium level monitoring is recommended.

Adverse Reactions: Adverse reactions are seldom encountered at serum lithium levels below 1.5 mEq./l., except in the occasional patient sensitive to lithium. Mild to moderate toxic reactions may occur at levels from 1.5 – 2.5 mEq./l., and moderate to severe reactions may be seen at levels from 2.0 – 2.5 mEq./l., depending upon individual response to the drug.

Fine hand tremor, polyuria and mild thirst may occur during initial therapy for the acute manic phase, and may persist throughout treatment. Transient and mild nausea and general discomfort may also appear during the first few days of lithium administration.

These side effects are an inconvenience rather than a disabling condition, and usually subside with continued treatment or a temporary reduction or cessation of dosage. If persistent, a cessation of dosage is indicated.

Diarrhea, vomiting, drowsiness, muscular weakness and lack of coordination may be early signs of lithium intoxication, and can occur at lithium levels below 2.0 mEq./l. At higher levels, giddiness, ataxia, blurred vision, tinnitus and a large output of dilute urine may be seen. Serum lithium levels above 3.0 mEq./l. may produce a complex clinical picture involving multiple organs and organ systems. Serum lithium levels should not be permitted to exceed 2.0 mEq./l. during the acute treatment phase.

The following toxic reactions have been reported and appear to be related to serum lithium levels, including levels within the therapeutic range.

Neuromuscular: tremor, muscle hyperirritability (fasciculations, twitching, clonic movements of whole limbs), ataxia, choreoathetotic movements, hyperactive deep tendon reflexes.

Central Nervous System: blackout spells, epileptiform seizures, slurred speech, dizziness, vertigo, incontinence of urine or feces, somnolence, psychomotor retardation, restlessness, confusion, stupor, coma.

Cardiovascular: cardiac arrhythmia, hypotension, peripheral circulatory collapse.

Gastrointestinal: anorexia, nausea, vomiting, diarrhea.

Genitourinary: albuminuria, oliguria, polyuria, glycosuria.

Dermatologic: drying and thinning of hair, anesthesia of skin, chronic folliculitis, xerosis cutis exacerbation of psoriasis.

Autonomic Nervous System: blurred vision, dry mouth.

Miscellaneous: fatigue, lethargy, tendency to sleep, dehydration, weight loss, transient scotomata.

Thyroid Abnormalities: Euthyroid goiter and/or hypothyroidism (including myxedema) accompanied by lower T_3 and T_4. I_{131}iodine uptake may be elevated. (See Precautions) Paradoxically, rare cases of hyperthyroidism have been reported.

EEG Changes: diffuse slowing, widening of frequency spectrum, potentiation and disorganization of background rhythm.

EKG Changes: reversible flattening, isoelectricity or inversion of T-waves.

Miscellaneous reactions unrelated to dosage are: transient electroencephalographic and electrocardiographic changes, leucocytosis, headache, diffuse nontoxic goiter with or without hypothyroidism, transient hyperglycemia, generalized pruritis with or without rash, cutaneous ulcers, albuminuria, worsening of organic brain syndromes, excessive weight gain, edematous swelling of ankles or wrists, and thirst or polyuria, sometimes resembling diabetes insipidus and metallic taste.

A single report has been received of the development of painful discoloration of fingers and toes and coldness of the extremities within one day of the starting of treatment of lithium. The mechanism through which these symptoms (resembling Raynaud's Syndrome) developed is not known. Recovery followed discontinuance.

Dosage and Administration:

Acute Mania: Optimal patient response can usually be established and maintained with the following dosages:

LITHONATE ....600 mg t.i.d.
LITHOTABS ....600 mg t.i.d.

Such doses will normally produce an effective serum lithium level ranging between 1.0 and 1.5 mEq./l. Dosage must be individualized according to serum levels and clinical response. Regular monitoring of the patient's clinical state and of serum lithium levels is necessary. Serum levels should be determined twice per week during the acute phase, and until the serum level and clinical condition of the patient have been stabilized.

Long-term Control: The desirable serum lithium levels are 0.6 to 1.2 mEq./l. Dosage will vary from one individual to another, but usually the following will maintain this level:

LITHONATE ....300 mg t.i.d. or q.i.d.
LITHOTABS ....300 mg t.i.d. or q.i.d.

Serum lithium levels in uncomplicated cases receiving maintenance therapy during remission should be monitored at least every two months.

Patients abnormally sensitive to lithium may exhibit toxic signs at serum levels of 1.0 to 1.5 mEq./l. Elderly patients often respond to reduced dosage, and may exhibit signs of toxicity at serum levels ordinarily tolerated by other patients.

N. B.: Blood samples for serum lithium determinations are drawn 8 – 12 hours after the previous dose when lithium concentrations are relatively stable. Total reliance must not be placed on serum levels alone. Accurate patient evaluation requires both clinical and laboratory analysis.

Overdosage: The toxic levels for lithium are close to the therapeutic levels. It is therefore important that patients and their families be cautioned to watch for early toxic symptoms and to discontinue the drug and inform the physician should they occur. Toxic symptoms are listed in detail under ADVERSE REACTIONS.

Treatment: No specific antidote for lithium poisoning is known. Early symptoms of lithium toxicity can usually be treated by reduction or cessation of dosage of the drug and resumption of the treatment at a lower dose after 24 to 48 hours. In severe cases of lithium poisoning, the first and foremost goal of treatment consists of elimination of this ion from the patient.

Treatment is essentially the same as that used in barbiturate poisoning: 1) gastric lavage. 2) correction of fluid and electrolyte imbalance and 3) regulation of kidney functioning. Urea, mannitol, and aminophylline all produce significant increases in lithium excretion. Infection prophylaxis, regular chest X-rays, and preservation of adequate respiration are essential.

How Supplied:

LITHONATE (Lithium Carbonate 300 mg) peach colored, No. 2 capsules, imprinted "ROWELL 7512" in red are supplied in bottles of 100's (unit-of-use) and 1000's, and in unit-dose boxes of 100's.

LITHOTABS (Lithium Carbonate 300 mg) scored, white, film-coated tablets embossed "ROWELL 7516" are supplied in bottles of 100's & 1000's.

ORASONE™ ℞

(Prednisone Tablets)

How Supplied:

ORASONE 1™ (Prednisone 1 mg) (pink)
ORASONE 5™ (Prednisone 5 mg) (white)
ORASONE 10™ (Prednisone 10 mg) (blue)
ORASONE 20™ (Prednisone 20 mg) (yellow)
ORASONE 50™ (Prednisone 50 mg) (white)

Each Supplied in bottles of 100's and 1000's and in unit-dose boxes of 100. Tablets are color coded and monogrammed with "ROWELL" and mg strength.

PROCTOCORT™ ℞

(Buffered 1% Hydrocortisone Cream)

Caution: Federal law prohibits dispensing without a prescription.

Description: PROCTOCORT (Hydorcortisone) 1% Cream a topical corticosteroid contains hydrocortisone 1% in a Ph-adjusted Cream containing stearyl alcohol, cetyl alcohol, isopropyl palmitate, citric acid, polyoxyethylene 40 stearate, dibasic sodium phosphate, propylene glycol, water, and sorbic acid as a preservative. Hydrocortisone has the chemical name Pregn-4-ene-3, 20-dione, 11, 17, 21-trihydroxy-, (11β)-; empirical formula $C_{21}H_{30}O_5$; molecular weight 362.47; Chemical Abstract Service registry number 50-23-7, and has the chemical structure:

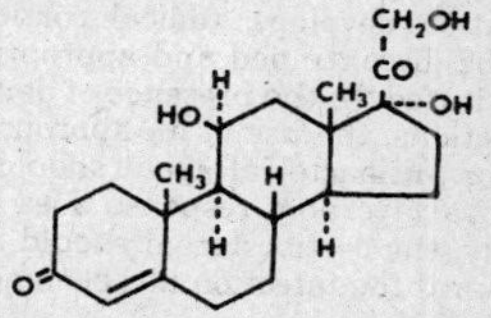

Clinical Pharmacology: Topical corticosteroids share anti-inflammatory, antipruritic and vasoconstrictive actions.

The mechanism of anti-inflammatory activity of the topical corticosteroids is unclear. Various laboratory methods, including vasoconstrictor assays, are used to compare and predict potencies and/or clinical efficacies of the topical corticosteroids. There is some evidence to suggest that a recognizable correlation exists between vasoconstrictor potency and therapeutic efficacy in man.

Pharmacokinetics: The extent of percutaneous absorption of topical corticosteroids is determined by many factors including the vehicle, the integrity of the epidermal barrier, and the use of occlusive dressings.

Topical corticosteroids can be absorbed from normal intact skin. Inflammation and/or other disease processes in the skin increase percutaneous absorption. Occlusive dressings substantially increase the percutaneous absorption of topical corticosteroids. Thus, occlusive dressings may be a valuable therapeutic adjunct for treatment of resistant dermatoses (See DOSAGE AND ADMINISTRATION)

Once absorbed through the skin, topical corticosteroids are handled through pharmacokinetic pathways similar to systemically administered corticosteroids. Corticosteroids are bound to plasma proteins in varying degrees. Corticosteroids are metabolized primarily in the liver and are then excreted by the kidneys. Some of the topical corticosteroids and their metabolities are also excreted into the bile.

Indication and Usage: Topical corticosteroids are indicated for the relief of the inflammatory and pruritic manifestations of corticosteroid-responsive dermatoses.

Contraindications: Topical corticosteroids are contraindicated in those patients with a history of hypersensitivity to any of the components of the preparation.

Precautions:

General: Systemic absorption of topical corticosteroids has produced reversible hypothalamic pituitary-adrenal (HPA) axis suppression, manifestations of Cushing's syndrome, hyperglycemia, and glucosuria in some patients. Conditions which augment systemic absorption include the application of the more potent steroids, use over large surface areas, prolonged use, and the addition of occlusive dressings.

Therefore, patients receiving a large dose of a potent topical steroid applied to a large surface area or under an occlusive dressing should be evaluated periodically for evidence of HPA axis suppression by using the urinary-free cor-

Continued on next page

Rowell—Cont.

tisol and ACTH stimulation tests. If HPA axis supression is noted, an attempt should be made to withdraw the drug, to reduce the frequency of application, or to substitute a less potent steroid.
Recovery of HPA axis function is generally prompt and complete upon discontinuation of the drug. Infrequency, signs and symptoms of steroid withdrawal may occur, requiring supplemental systemic corticosteroids.
Children may absorb proportionally larger amounts of topical corticosteroids and thus be more susceptible to systemic toxicity (see PRECAUTIONS—Pediatric Use).
If irritation develops, topical corticosteroids should be discontinued and appropriate therapy instituted. In the presence of dermatological infections, the use of an appropriate antifungal or antibacterial agent should be instituted. If a favorable response does not occur promptly, the corticosteroid should be discontinued until the infection has been adequately controlled.
Information for the Patient: Patients using topical corticosteroids should receive the following information and instructions:
1. This medication is to be used as directed by the physician. It's for external use only. Avoid contact with the eyes.
2. Patients should be advised not to use this medication for any disorder other than for which it was pescribed.
3. The treated skin area should not be bandaged or otherwise covered or wrapped as to be occlusive unless directed by the physician.
4. Patients should report any signs of local adverse reactions especially under occlusive dressing.
5. Parents of pediatric patients should be advised not to use tight-fitting diapers or plastic pants on a child being treated in diaper area, as these garments may constitute occlusive dressings.

Laboratory Tests: The following tests may be helpful in evaluating the HPA axis suppression:
Urinary-free cortisol test—ACTH stimulation test
Carcinogenesis, Mutagenesis, and Impairment of Fertility: Long-term animal studies have not been performed to evaluate the carcinogenic potential or the effect on fertility of topical corticosteroids. Studies to determine mutagenicity with prednisolone and hydrocortisone have revealed negative results.
Pregnancy Category C: Corticosteroids are generally teratogenic in laboratory animals when administered systemically at relatively low dosage levels. The more potent corticosteroids have been shown to be teratogenic after dermal application in laboratory animals. There are no adequate and well-controlled studies in pregnant women on teratogenic effects from topically applied corticosteroids. Therefore, topical corticosteroids should be used during pregnancy only if the potential benefit justifies the potential risk to the fetus. Drugs of this class should not be used extensively on pregnant patients, in large amounts, or for prolonged periods of time.
Nursing Mothers: It is not known whether topical administration of corticosteroids could result in sufficient systemic absorption to produce detectable quantities in breast milk. Systemically administered corticosteroids are secreted into breast milk in quantities not likely to have a deleterious effect on the infant. Nevertheless, caution should be exercised when topical corticosteroids are administered to a nursing woman.
Pediatric Use: *Pediatric patients may demonstrate greater susceptibility to topical corticosteroid-induced HPA axis suppression and Cushing's syndrome than mature patients because of a larger skin surface area in body weight ratio.*
Hypothalamic-pituitary-adrenal (HPA) axis suppression, Cushing's syndrome, and intracranial hypertension have been reported in children receiving topical corticosteroids. Manifestations of adrenal suppression in children include linear growth retardation, delayed weight gain, low plasma cortisol levels, and absence of response to ACTH stimulation. Manifestations of intracranial hypertension include bulging fontanelles, headaches, and bilateral papilledema.
Administration of topical corticosteroids to children should be limited to the least amount compatible with an effective therapeutic regimen. Chronic corticosteroid therapy may interfere with the growth and development of children.
Adverse Reactions: The following local adverse reactions are reported infrequently with topical corticosteroids, but may occur more frequently with the use of occlusive dressings. These reactions are listed in an approximate decreasing order of occurrence:
Burning, Itching, Irritation, Dryness, Folliculitis, Hypertrichosis, Acneiform eruptions, Hypopigmentation, Perioral dermatitis, Allergic contact dermatitis, Maceration of the skin, Secondary infection, Skin atrophy, Striae & Millaria.
Overdosage: Topically applied corticosteroids can be absorbed in sufficient amounts to produce systemic effects (see PRECAUTIONS).
Dosage and Administration: Topical corticosteroids are generally applied to the affected area as a thin film from three to four times daily depending on the severity of the condition.
Occlusive dressings may be used for the management of psoriasis or recalcitrant conditions. If an infection develops, the use of occlusive dressings should be discontinued and appropriate antimicrobial therapy instituted.
How Supplied: PROCTOCORT (Hydrocortisone) 1% Cream is supplied in 30 Gram tubes with tear-off label. A reusable measured dose applicator and 12 finger cots are included with each tube. (NDC 0032-1920-61).
Store at room temperature. Avoid freezing.
PL125 65C 16E March, 1982

PROCTODON™
(Buffered 1% Diperodon Cream)

Composition: Diperodon HCl 1% and vitamins A and D in a soft, water-miscible cream base.
Action and Uses: PROCTODON provides the local anesthetic action of diperodon HCl, the healing effects of vitamins A and D and the lubricant effect of the soft, cream base buffered to pH 5.5. The buffer re-establishes the normal acidity of the skin and counteracts the alkalinity frequently encountered in the conditions treated. As a lubricant and anesthetic, PROCTODON facilitates rectal digital examinations and alleviates the pain of postoperative bowel movements. Applied to the wound edges, PROCTODON eliminates much of the pain following repair of fistula in ano and pilonidal cyst. It is useful pre- and postoperatively in hemorrhoidectomy and after incision of thrombosed or sclerosed anorectal veins. External or internal application is useful for relief of pain or itching associated with proctitis, papillitis, cryptitis, uncomplicated hemorrhoids and pruritis ani.
Precautions: Where rectal applicator is used, exert great care to avoid injury to rectal wall. If signs of allergic reaction occur, discontinue medication. Burning or stinging may occur in an occasional patient. Irritation or allergic reactions are rarely encountered.
Administration and Dosage: Apply liberally to the affected area, two to four times daily, or in the case of postoperative wound treatment, whenever the dressing is changed. For internal use, PROCTODON may be administered with a lubricated rectal applicator (see precautions) or with a "finger cot".
How Supplied: 30 gram tubes with patient instructions, a reusable measured dose applicator and finger cots.

VIO-BEC®
(Therapeutic B Complex with C)

Composition:

Thiamine Mononitrate (B_1)	25 mg.
Riboflavin (B_2)	25 mg.
Pyridoxine HCl (B_6)	25 mg.
Calcium Pantothenate	40 mg.
Nicotinamide	100 mg.
Ascorbic Acid	500 mg.

VIO-BEC is a high-potency therapeutic source of B complex vitamins and Vitamin C. It contains only synthetic vitamins (no liver or yeast), therefore, is well tolerated and does not produce unpleasant aftertaste. It does not contain Vitamin B-12 or Folic Acid for they are known to interfere with accurate diagnosis of hematologic status. VIO-BEC is promoted to the medical profession only, for use in conditions requiring high-potency nutritional supplementation.
Action and Uses: VIO-BEC is indicated for treatment of deficiencies in vitamin B complex and vitamin C. It is recommended as a part of the therapeutic regimen in alcoholism, chronic illness, malnutrition, surgery (particularly of the G. I. tract), and other stress conditions leading to increased nutritional demands. Subclinical nutritional deficiencies characterized by anorexia, irritability, fatigability, nervousness and weakness may respond to VIO-BEC.
Dosage: One VIO-BEC capsule daily.
How Supplied: Capsules (brown, imprinted "ROWELL 1216") in bottles of 100 and 1000 and unit dose boxes of 100.

VIO-BEC FORTE™ ℞
Therapeutic B-Complex with Folic Acid, C, E, Zinc and Copper

Composition: Each film-coated tablet contains: Thiamine Mononitrate (B-1) 25 mg., Riboflavin (B-2) 25 mg., Pyridoxine Hydrochloride (B-6) 25 mg., Ascorbic Acid (C) 500 mg., Calcium Pantothenate 40 mg., Nicotinamide 100 mg., dl-alpha Tocopheryl Acetate N.F. (E) 30 I.U., Cyanocobalamin (B-12) 5 mcg., Folic Acid 0.5 mg., Zinc 25 mg. (from Zinc Sulfate), Copper 3 mg. (from Copper Sulfate).
Warnings: Folic acid alone is inappropriate in therapy of pernicious anemia and other megaloblastic anemias where vitamin B-12 is deficient and oral vitamin B-12 is therapeutically ineffective.
Precautions: Folic acid, especially in doses above 1.0 mg./day, may obscure pernicious anemia by temporary hematologic remission while neurologic involvement remains progressive.
Adverse Reactions: Allergic sensitization has been reported after administration of folic acid.
Dosage: As indicated by clinical need, usually 1 tablet daily.
How Supplied: Capsule shaped tablet (film-coated brown and imprinted "ROWELL 1218") in bottles of 100 and unit-dose boxes of 100.

Products are cross-indexed by

generic and chemical names

in the

YELLOW SECTION

Roxane Laboratories, Inc.

P.O. 16532
COLUMBUS, OH 43216

HOSPITAL UNIT DOSE

Hospital Unit Dose—Roxane, was developed to aid in improved drug distribution and administration. With Hospital Unit Dose, each single unit of medication moves from our quality controlled production lines to the patient's bedside in tamper resistant containers, labeled for positive identification, thus protecting dosage integrity to the point of administration.
The following products are currently available in Hospital Unit Dose:
Acetaminophen Elixir USP 160mg/5ml, 325mg/10.15ml, 650mg/20.3ml
Acetaminophen Suppositories 120mg, 650mg
Acetaminophen Tablets USP 325mg, 650mg
Acetaminophen 300 mg with Codeine Phosphate 30 mg tablets
Acetaminophen 300 mg with Codeine Phosphate 60 mg tablets
Aluminum Hydroxide Gel USP (Flavored) 30ml
Aluminum Hydroxide, Concentrate, 20 ml, 30 ml
Aluminum and Magnesium Hydroxides with Simethicone I 15ml, 30ml
Aluminum and Magnesium Hydroxides with Simethicone II 15ml, 30 ml
Aminophylline Tablets USP 100mg, 200mg
Amitriptyline Hydrochloride Tablets USP 10mg, 25mg, 50mg, 75mg, 100mg, 150mg
Aromatic Cascara Fluidextract USP 5ml
Ascorbic Acid Tablets USP 250mg, 500mg
Aspirin Suppositories USP 300mg, 600mg
Bisacodyl Suppositories USP 10mg
Bisacodyl Tablets USP 5mg
Bisacodyl Patient Pack
Calcium Gluconate Tablets USP
Castor Oil USP 30ml, 60ml
Castor Oil Flavored 30ml, 60ml
Chloral Hydrate Syrup USP 500mg/10ml, 1g/10ml
Chloral Hydrate Capsules USP 500mg
Chlordiazepoxide Hydrochloride Capsules USP 10mg, 25mg
Chlorpheniramine Maleate Tablets USP 4mg
Chlorpromazine Hydrochloride Tablets USP 10mg, 25mg, 50mg, 100mg, 200mg
Cocaine Hydrochloride Topical Solution 4%/4 ml, 10%/4 ml
Codeine Sulfate Tablets USP 30mg, 60mg
Dexamethasone Tablets USP 0.5 mg, 0.75mg, 1.5mg, 2mg, 4mg
Dihydrotachysterol Tablets USP 0.125mg, 0.2mg
Diluent (Flavored) for Oral Use 15 ml
Diphenhydramine Hydrochloride Elixir USP 25mg/10ml
Diphenhydramine Hydrochloride Capsules USP 50mg
Diphenoxylate Hydrochloride 2.5mg and Atropine Sulfate 0.025mg Tablets USP
Diphenoxylate Hydrochloride and Atropine Sulfate Oral Solution USP 4 ml, 10 ml
Docusate Sodium Capsules USP 50mg, 100mg, 250mg
Docusate Sodium Syrup USP 50mg/15ml, 100mg/30ml
Docusate Sodium 100mg with Casanthranol 30mg Capsules
Ferrous Sulfate Liquid 300mg/5ml
Ferrous Sulfate Tablets USP 300mg
Glycerin Oral Solution USP 180 ml
Guaifenesin Syrup USP 100mg/5ml, 200mg/10ml, 300mg/15ml
Hydrochlorothiazide Tablets USP 25mg, 50mg
Imipramine Hydrochloride Tablets USP 10mg, 25mg, 50mg
Ipecac Syrup USP 15ml, 30ml
Isoetharine Hydrochloride 0.125%, 4ml
Isoetharine Hydrochloride 0.1% 2.5ml
Isoetharine Hydrochloride 0.2% 2.5ml
Isoxsuprine Hydrochloride Tablets USP 10mg, 20mg
Kaolin-Pectin Suspension 30ml
Kaolin-Pectin Suspension Concentrated 20ml
Lithium Carbonate Capsules USP 300mg
Lithium Carbonate Tablets USP 300mg
Lithium Citrate Syrup 8 mEq per 5 ml, 16 mEq per 10 ml
Magnesia and Alumina Oral Suspension USP 30ml
Milk of Magnesia USP 15ml, 30ml
Milk of Magnesia Concentrated Flavored 10ml, 15ml, 20ml
Milk of Magnesia—Cascara Suspension Concentrated 15 ml
Milk of Magnesia—Mineral Oil Emulsion 30ml
Milk of Magnesia—Mineral Oil Emulsion (Flavored) 30ml
Mineral Oil-Light Sterile 10ml, 30ml
Mineral Oil USP 30ml
Morphine Sulfate Tablets 15mg, 30mg
Morphine Sulfate Oral Solution 10mg/5ml, 20mg/10ml
Neomycin Sulfate Tablets USP 500 mg
Niacin Tablets USP 50mg, 100mg
Oxycodone Hydrochloride Tablets 5mg
Oxycodone Hydrochloride 5mg and Acetaminophen 325mg Tablets
Oxycodone Hydrochloride 4.5mg, Oxycodone Terephthalate 0.38mg and Aspirin 325mg Tablets
Oxycodone Hydrochloride 2.25mg, Oxycodone Terephthalate 0.19mg, and Aspirin 325mg Tablets
Papaverine Hydrochloride Prolonged Release Capsules 150mg
Paregoric USP 5ml
Phenobarbital Elixir USP 20mg/5ml
Phenobarbital Tablets USP 15mg, 30mg, 60mg, 100mg
Potassium Chloride Oral Solution USP 5% (20mEq/30ml)
Potassium Chloride Oral Solution USP 10% (15mEq/11.25ml)
Potassium Chloride Oral Solution USP 10% (20mEq/15ml)
Potassium Chloride Oral Solution USP 10% (30mEq/22.5ml)
Potassium Chloride Oral Solution USP 10% (40mEq/30ml)
Potassium Chloride for Oral Solution USP 20mEq/4g
Potassium Chloride USP Powder Unflavored 20mEq/1.5g
Potassium Gluconate Elixir USP 20mEq/15ml
Potassium Iodide Liquid 500mg/15ml
Potassium Phosphates Oral Solution, 30ml
Prednisolone Tablets USP 5mg
Prednisone Tablets USP 1mg, 2.5mg, 5mg, 10mg, 20mg, 25mg, 50mg
Propantheline Bromide Tablets USP 15mg
Propoxyphene Hydrochloride Capsules USP 65 mg
Pseudoephedrine Hydrochloride Tablets USP 30mg, 60mg
Pseudoehedrine Hydrochloride Syrup USP 60mg/10ml
Pseudoephedrine Hydrochloride 60mg and Triprolidine Hydrochloride 2.5mg/10ml Syrup
Pseudoephedrine Hydrochloride 60mg and Triprolidine Hydrochloride 2.5mg Tablet
Quinidine Sulfate Tablets USP 200mg, 300mg
Quinine Sulfate Capsules USP 200mg, 325mg
Sodium Chloride Inhalation USP (Normal Saline) Sterile 0.9% 3ml, 5ml
Sodium Phosphates Oral Solution USP 30ml
Sulfisoxazole Tablets USP 500mg
Terpin Hydrate and Codeine Elixir USP 5ml
Theophylline Elixir 80mg/15ml, 160mg/30ml

As research continues, new Roxane Laboratories' products will be available in Hospital Unit Dose packages.

DIHYDROTACHYSTEROL TABLETS USP ℞

Description: Each tablet contains:
Dihydrotachysterol .. 0.125 mg, 0.2 mg; or 0.4 mg
Dihydrotachysterol is a synthetic reduction product of tachysterol, a close isomer of vitamin D. Chemically Dihydrotachysterol is *9, 10-Secoergosta-5,7,22-tri-en-3β-ol.*
Dihydrotachysterol acts as a blood calcium regulator.

Clinical Pharmacology: Dyhydrotachysterol is hydroxylated in the liver to 25-hydroxydihydrotachysterol, which is the major circulating active form of the drug. It does not undergo further hydroxylation by the kidney and therefore is the analogue of 1,25-dihydroxyvitamin D. Dihydrotachysterol is effective in the elevation of serum calcium by stimulating intestinal calcium absorption and mobilizing bone calcium in the absence of parathyroid hormone and of functioning renal tissue. Dihydrotachysterol also increases renal phosphate excretion. In contrast to parathyroid extract, Dihydrotachysterol is active when taken orally, exerts a slow but persistent effect, and may be used for long periods without increasing the dosage or causing tolerance. Dihydrotachysterol is faster-acting than pharmacologic doses of vitamin D and is less persistent after cessation of treatment, thus decreasing the risk of accumulation and of hypercalcemia.

Indications and Usage: Dihydrotachysterol is indicated for the treatment of acute, chronic, and latent forms of postoperative tetany, idiopathic tetany, and hypoparathyroidism.

Contraindications: Contraindicated in patients with hypercalcemia, abnormal sensitivity to the effects of vitamin D, and hypervitaminosis D.

Precautions:

General: The difference between therapeutic dose and intoxicating dose may be small in any patient and therefore dosage must be individualized and periodically reevaluated.
In patients with renal osteodystrophy accompanied by hyperphosphatemia, maintenance of a normal serum phosphorus level by dietary phosphate restriction and/or administration of aluminum gels as intestinal phosphate binders is essential to prevent metastatic calcification.
Because of its effect on serum calcium, Dihydrotachysterol should be administered to pregnant patients or to patients with renal stones only when, in the judgment of the physician, the potential benefits outweigh the possible hazards.

Laboratory tests: **To prevent hypercalcemia, treatment should always be controlled by regular determinations of blood calcium level, which should be maintained within the normal range.**

Drug interactions: Administration of thiazide diuretics to hypoparathyroid patients who are concurrently being treated with Dihydrotachysterol may cause hypercalcemia.

Pregnancy: Teratogenic effects — Pregnancy Category C: Animal reproduction studies have shown fetal abnormalities in several species associated with hypervitaminosis D. These are similar to the supravalvular aortic stenosis syndrome described in infants by Black in England (1963). This syndrome was characterized by supravalvular aortic stenosis, elfin facies, and mental retardation.
There are no adequate and well-controlled studies in pregnant women. Dihydrotachysterol should be used during pregnancy only if the potential benefit justifies the potential risk to the fetus.

Nursing mothers: It is not known whether this drug is excreted in human milk. Because many drugs are excreted in human milk, caution should be exercised when Dihydrotachysterol is administered to a nursing woman.

Continued on next page

Roxane—Cont.

Overdosage: The effects of Dihydrotachysterol can persist for up to one month after cessation of treatment.
Manifestations: Toxicity associated with Dihydrotachysterol is similar to that seen with large doses of vitamin D. Overdosage is manifested by symptoms of hypercalcemia, i.e., weakness, headache, anorexia, nausea, vomiting, abdominal cramps, diarrhea, constipation, vertigo, tinnitus, ataxia, hypotonia, lethargy, depression, amnesia, disorientation, hallucinations, syncope, and coma. Impairment of renal function may result in polyuria, polydipsia, and albuminuria. Widespread calcification of soft tissues, including heart, blood vessels, kidneys, and lungs, can occur. Death can result from cardiovascular or renal failure.
Treatment: Treatment of overdosage consists of withdrawal of Dihydrotachysterol, bed rest, liberal intake of fluids, a low-calcium diet, and administration of a laxative. Hypercalcemic crisis with dehydration, stupor, coma, and azotemia requires more vigorous treatment. The first step should be hydration of the patient. Intravenous saline may quickly and significantly increast urinary calcium excretion. A loop diuretic (furosemide or ethacrynic acid) may be given with the saline infusion to further increase renal calcium excretion. Other reported therapeutic measures include dialysis or the administration of citrates, sulfates, phosphates, corticosteroids, EDTA (ethylenediaminetetraacetic acids), and mithramycin via appropriate regimens.
Dosage and Administration: The dosage depends on the nature and seriousness of the disorder and should be adapted to each individual patient. Serum calcium levels should be maintained between 9 to 10 mg per 100 ml.
The following dosage schedule will serve as a guide:
Initial dose: 0.8 mg to 2.4 mg daily for several days.
Maintenance dose: 0.2 mg to 1.0 mg daily as required for normal serum calcium levels. The average maintenance dose is 0.6 mg daily. This dose may be supplemented with 10 to 15 grams of calcium lactate or gluconate by mouth daily.
How Supplied:
0.125 mg white tablets.
NDC 0054-8172-25: Unit dose, 10 tablets per strip, 10 strips per shelf pack, 10 shelf packs per shipper.
NDC 0054-4190-19: Bottles of 50 tablets.
0.2 mg pink tablets.
NDC 0054-8182-25: Unit dose, 10 tablets per strip, 10 strips per shelf pack, 10 shelf packs per shipper.
NDC 0054-4189-25: Bottles of 100 tablets.
0.4 mg white tablets.
NDC 0054-4191-19: Bottles of 50 tablets.

LITHIUM CARBONATE ℞
CAPSULES AND TABLETS USP, 300 mg

WARNING
Lithium toxicity is closely related to serum lithium levels, and can occur at doses close to therapeutic levels. Facilities for prompt and accurate serum lithium determinations should be available before initiating therapy.

Description: Each capsule or tablet for oral administration contains:
Lithium Carbonate .... 300 mg
Lithium Carbonate is a white, light alkaline powder with molecular formula Li_2CO_3 and molecular weight 73.89. Lithium is an element of the alkali-metal group with atomic number 3, atomic weight 6.94 and an emission line at 671 nm on the flame photometer. Lithium acts as an antimanic.
Clinical Pharmacology: Preclinical studies have shown that lithium alters sodium transport in nerve and muscle cells and effects a shift toward intraneuronal metabolism of catecholamines, but the specific biochemical mechanism of lithium action in mania is unknown.
Indications and Usage: Lithium carbonate is indicated in the treatment of manic episodes of Bipolar Disorder. Bipolar Disorder, Manic (DSM-III) is equivalent to Manic Depressive illness, Manic, in the older DSM-II terminology.
Lithium is also indicated as a maintenance treatment for individuals with a diagnosis of Bipolar Disorder. Maintenance therapy reduces the frequency of manic episodes and diminishes the intensity of those episodes which may occur.
Typical symptoms of mania include pressure of speech, motor hyperactivity, reduced need for sleep, flight of ideas, grandiosity, or poor judgment, aggressiveness, and possibly hostility. When given to a patient experiencing a manic episode, lithium may produce a normalization of symptomatology within 1 to 3 weeks.
Contraindications: Lithium should generally not be given to patients with significant renal or cardiovascular disease, severe debilitation or dehydration, or sodium depletion, and to patients receiving diuretics, since the risk of lithium toxicity is very high in such patients. If the psychiatric indication is life-threatening, and if such a patient fails to respond to other measures, lithium treatment may be undertaken with extreme caution, including daily serum lithium determinations and adjustment to the usualy low doses ordinarily tolerated by these individuals. In such instances, hospitlization is a necessity.
Warnings: Lithium may cause fetal harm when administered to a pregnant woman. There have been reports of lithium having adverse effects on nidation in rats, embryo viability in mice, and metabolism in-vitro of rat testis and human spermatozoa have been attributed to lithium, as have teratogenicity in submammalian species and cleft palates in mice. Studies in rats, rabbits and monkeys have shown no evidence of lithium-induced teratology. Data from lithium birth registries suggest an increase in cardiac and other anomalies, especially Ebstein's anomaly. If the patient becomes pregnant while taking lithium, she should be apprised of the potential risk to the fetus. If possible, lithium should be withdrawn for at least the first trimester unless it is determined that this would seriously endanger the mother.
Chronic lithium therapy may be associated with diminution of renal concentrating ability, occasionally presenting as nephrogenic diabetes insipidus, with polyuria and polydipsia. Such patients should be carefully managed to avoid dehydration with resulting lithium retention and toxicity. This condition is usually reversible when lithium is discontinued.
Morphologic changes with glomerular and interstitial fibrosis and nephron-atrophy have been reported in patients on chronic lithium therapy. Morphologic changes have been seen in bipolar patients never exposed to lithium. The relationship between renal functional and morphologic changes and their association with lithium therapy has not been established.
To date, lithium in therapeutic doses has not been reported to cause end-stage renal disease. When kidney function is assessed, for baseline data prior to starting lithium therapy or thereafter, routine urinalysis and other tests may be used to evaluate tubular function (e.g., urine specific gravity or osmolality following a period of water deprivation, or 24-hour urine volume) and glomerular function (e.g., serum creatinine or creatinine clearance). During lithium therapy, progressive or sudden changes in renal function, even within the normal range, indicate the need for reevaluation of treatment.
Lithium toxicity is closely related to serum lithium levels, and can occur at doses close to therapeutic levels (see DOSAGE AND ADMINISTRATION).
Precautions:
General: The ability to tolerate lithium is greater during the acute manic phase and decreases when manic symptoms subside (See DOSAGE AND ADMINISTRATION).
The distribution space of lithium approximates that of total body water. Lithium is primarily excreted in urine with insignificant excretion in feces. Renal excretion of lithium is proportional to its plasma concentration. The half-life of elimination of lithium is approximately 24 hours. Lithium decreases sodium reabsorption by the renal tubules which could lead to sodium depletion. Therefore, it is essential for the patient to maintain a normal diet, including salt, and an adequate fluid intake (2500-3000 ml) at least during the initial stabilization period. Decreased tolerance to lithium has been reported to ensue from protracted sweating or diarrhea and, if such occur, supplemental fluid and salt should be administered.
In addition to sweating and diarrhea, concomitant infection with elevated temperatures may also necessitate a temporary reduction or cessation of medication.
Previously existing underlying thyroid disorders do not necessarily constitute a contraindication to lithium treatment; where hypothyroidism exists, careful monitoring of thyroid function during lithium stabilization and maintenance allows for correction of changing thyroid parameters, if any. Where hypothyroidism occurs during lithium stabilization and maintenance, supplemental thyroid treatment may be used.
Information for the patients: Outpatients and their families should be warned that the patient must discontinue lithium therapy and contact his physician if such clinical signs of lithium toxicity as diarrhea, vomiting, tremor, mild ataxia, drowsiness, or muscular weakness occur.
Lithium may impair mental and/or physical abilities. Caution patients about activities requiring alertness (e.g., operating vehicles or machinery).
Drug interactions: Combined use of haloperidol and lithium: An encephalopathic syndrome (characterized by weakness, lethargy, fever, tremulousness and confusion, extrapyramidal symptoms, leucocytosis, elevated serum enzymes, BUN and FBS) followed by irreversible brain damage has occurred in a few patients treated with lithium plus haloperidol. A causal relationship between these events and the concomitant administration of lithium and haloperidol has not been established; however, patients receiving such combined therapy should be monitored closely for early evidence of neurological toxicity and treatment discontinued promptly if such signs appear.
The possibility of similar adverse interactions with other antipsychotic medication exists.
Lithium may prolong the effects of neuromuscular blocking agents. Therefore, neuromuscular blocking agents should be given with caution to patients receiving lithium.
Indomethacin (50 mg t.i.d.) has been reported to increase steady state plasma lithium levels from 30 to 59 percent. There is also evidence that other non-steroidal, anti-inflammatory agents may have a similar effect. When such combinations are used, increased plasma lithium level monitoring is recommended.
Pregnancy: Teratogenic effects—Pregnancy Category D, See "Warnings" section.
Nursing mothers: Lithium is excreted in human milk. Nursing should not be undertaken during lithium therapy except in rare and unusual circumstances where, in the view of the physician, the potential benefits to the mother outweigh possible hazards to the child.

Pediatric use: Since information regarding the safety and effectiveness of lithium in children under 12 years of age is not available, its use in such patients is not recommended at this time.

Adverse Reactions:

Lithium toxicity: The likelihood of toxicity increases with increasing serum lithium levels. Serum lithium levels greater than 1.5 mEq/l carry a greater risk than lower levels. However, patients sensitive to lithium may exhibit toxic signs at serum levels below 1.5 mEq/l.

Diarrhea, vomiting, drowsiness, muscular weakness and lack of coordination may be early signs of lithium toxicity, and can occur at lithium levels below 2.0 mEq/l. At higher levels, giddiness, ataxia, blurred vision, tinnitus and a large output of dilute urine may be seen. Serum lithium levels above 3.0 mEq/l may produce a complex clinical picture involving multiple organs and organ systems. Serum lithium levels should not be permitted to exceed 2.0 mEq/l during the acute treatment phase.

Fine hand tremor, polyuria and mild thirst may occur during initial therapy for the acute manic phase, and may persist throughout treatment. Transient and mild nausea and general discomfort may also appear during the first few days of lithium administration.

These side effects are an inconvenience rather than a disabling condition, and usually subside with continued treatment or a temporary reduction or cessation of dosage. If persistent, a cessation of dosage is indicated.

The following adverse reactions have been reported and do not appear to be directly related to serum lithium levels.

Neuromuscular: tremor, muscle hyperirritability (fasciculations, twitching, clonic movements of whole limbs), ataxia, choreo-athetotic movements, hyperactive deep tendon reflexes.

Central Nervous System: blackout spells, epileptiform seizures, slurred speech, dizziness, vertigo, incontinence of urine or feces, somnolence, psychomotor retardation, restlessness, confusion, stupor, coma.

Cardiovascular: cardiac arrhythmia, hypotension, peripheral circulatory collapse.

Gastrointestinal: anorexia, nausea, vomiting, diarrhea.

Genitourinary: albuminuria, oliguria, polyuria, glycosuria.

Dermatologic: drying and thinning of hair, anesthesia of skin, chronic folliculitis, xerosis cutis, alopecia and exacerbation of psoriasis.

Autonomic Nervous System: blurred vision, dry mouth.

Miscellaneous: fatigue, lethargy, tendency to sleep, dehydration, weight loss, transient scotomata.

Thyroid Abnormalities: euthyroid goiter and/or hypothyroidism (including myxedema) accompanied by lower T_3 and T_4. Iodine 131 uptake may be elevated. (See PRECAUTIONS). Paradoxically, rare cases of hyperthyroidism have been reported.

EEG Changes: diffuse slowing, widening of frequency spectrum, potentiation and disorganization of background rhythm.

EKG Changes: reversible flattening, isoelectricity or inversion of T-waves.

Miscellaneous: fatigue, lethargy, transient scotomata, dehydration, weight loss, tendency to sleep.

Miscellaneous reactions unrelated to dosage are: transient electroencephalographic and electrocardiographic changes, leucocytosis, headache, diffuse nontoxic goiter with or without hypothyroidism, transient hyperglycemia, generalized pruritis with or without rash, cutaneous ulcers, albuminuria, worsening of organic brain syndromes, excessive weight gain, edematous swelling of ankles or wrists, and thirst or polyuria, sometimes resembling diabetes insipidus, and metallic taste.

A single report has been received of the development of painful discoloration of fingers and toes and coldness of the extremities within one day of the starting of treatment of lithium. The mechanism through which these symptoms (resembling Raynaud's Syndrome) developed is not known. Recovery followed discontinuance.

Overdosage: The toxic levels for lithium are close to the therapeutic levels. It is therefore important that patients and their families be cautioned to watch for early symptoms and to discontinue the drug and inform the physician should they occur. Toxic symptoms are listed in detail under ADVERSE REACTIONS.

Treatment: No specific antidote for lithium poisoning is known. Early symptoms of lithium toxicity can usually be treated by reduction or cessation of dosage of the drug and resumption of the treatment at a lower dose after 24 to 48 hours. In severe cases of lithium poisoning, the first and foremost goal of treatment consists of elimination of this ion from the patient.

Treatment is essentially the same as that used in barbiturate poisoning: 1) gastric lavage, 2) correction of fluid and electrolyte imbalance and 3) regulation of kidney functioning. Urea, mannitol, and aminophylline all produce significant increases in lithium excretion. Hemodialysis is an effective and rapid means of removing the ion from the severely toxic patient. Infection prophylaxis, regular chest X-rays, and preservation of adequate respiration are essential.

Dosage and Administration:

Acute Mania: Optimal patient response to Lithium Carbonate usually can be established and maintained with 600 mg t.i.d. Such doses will normally produce an effective serum lithium level ranging between 1.0 and 1.5 mEq/l. Dosage must be individualized according to serum levels and clinical response. Regular monitoring of the patient's clinical state and of serum lithium levels is necessary. Serum levels should be determined twice per week during the acute phase, and until the serum level and clinical condition of the patient have been stabilized.

Long-term Control: The desirable serum lithium levels are 0.6 to 1.2 mEq/l. Dosage will vary from one individual to another, but usually 300 mg t.i.d. or q.i.d. will maintain this level. Serum lithium levels in uncomplicated cases receiving maintenance therapy during remission should be monitored at least every two months.

Patients abnormally sensitive to lithium may exhibit toxic signs at serum levels of 1.0 to 1.5 mEq/l. Elderly patients often respond to reduced dosage, and may exhibit signs of toxicity at serum levels ordinarily tolerated by other patients.

N.B.: Blood samples for serum lithium determination should be drawn immediately prior to the next dose when lithium concentrations are relatively stable (i.e., 8–12 hours after the previous dose.) Total reliance must not be placed on serum levels alone. Accurate patient evaluation requires both clinical and laboratory analysis.

How Supplied:

300 mg flesh-colored capsules.

NDC 0054-8527-25: Unit dose, 10 capsules per strip, 10 strips per shelf pack, 10 shelf packs per shipper.

NDC 0054-2527-25: Bottles of 100 capsules.

NDC 0054-2527-31: Bottles of 1000 capsules.

300 mg white, scored tablets.

NDC 0054-8528-25: Unit dose, 10 tablets per strip, 10 strips per shelf pack, 10 shelf packs per shipper.

(For Institutional Use Only).

NDC 0054-4527-25: Bottles of 100 tablets.

NDC 0054-4527-31: Bottles of 1000 tablets.

LITHIUM CITRATE SYRUP USP ℞

8 mEq of Lithium per 5 ml

SUGAR FREE

FOR ORAL ADMINISTRATION ONLY

WARNING

Lithium toxicity is closely related to serum lithium levels, and can occur at doses close to therapeutic levels. Facilities for prompt and accurate serum lithium determinations should be available before initiating therapy.

Description: Lithium Citrate Syrup is a palatable oral dosage form of lithium ion. Lithium citrate is prepared in solution from lithium hydroxide and citric acid in a ratio approximating di-lithium citrate:

Each 5 ml of Lithium Citrate Syrup contains 8 mEq of lithium ion (Li^+), equivalent to the amount of lithium in 300 mg of lithium carbonate and alcohol 0.3% v/v. Lithium is an element of the alkali-metal group with atomic number 3, atomic weight 6.94, and an emission line at 671nm on the flame photometer.

How Supplied:

Lithium Citrate Syrup, 8 mEq per 5 ml

NDC 0054-3527-63: Bottles of 500 ml.

Refer to Lithium Carbonate Capsules and Tablets heading for complete text.

METHADONE HYDROCHLORIDE ©

ORAL SOLUTION USP

(WARNING: May be habit forming)

Description: Each 5 ml of Methadone Hydrochloride Oral Solution contains:

Methadone Hydrochloride .... 5 or 10 mg

(**Warning:** May be habit forming)

Alcohol 8%

Chemically, Methadone Hydrochloride is 3-Heptanone, 6-(dimethylamino)-4,4-diphenyl-, hydrochloride.

Methadone Hydrochloride acts as a narcotic analgesic.

Clinical Pharmacology: Methadone Hydrochloride is a synthetic narcotic analgesic with multiple actions quantitatively similar to those of morphine, the most prominent of which involve the central nervous system and organs composed of smooth muscle.

When administered orally, methadone is approximately one-half as potent as when given parenterally. Oral administration results in a delay of the onset, a lowering of the peak, and an increase in the duration of analgesic effect.

Indications and Usage: Methadone Hydrochloride Oral Solution is indicated for the relief of severe chronic pain.

Contraindications: Hypersensitivity to methadone.

Warnings: Methadone Hydrochloride, a narcotic, is a Schedule II controlled substance under the Federal Controlled Substances Act.

DRUG DEPENDENCE — METHADONE CAN PRODUCE DRUG DEPENDENCE OF THE MORPHINE TYPE AND, THEREFORE, HAS THE POTENTIAL FOR BEING ABUSED. PSYCHIC DEPENDENCE, PHYSICAL DEPENDENCE, AND TOLERANCE MAY DEVELOP UPON REPEATED ADMINISTRATION OF METHADONE, AND IT SHOULD BE PRESCRIBED AND ADMINISTERED WITH THE SAME DEGREE OF CAUTION APPROPRIATE TO THE USE OF MORPHINE.

Interaction with Other Central-Nervous-System Depressants—Methadone should be used with caution and in reduced dosage in patients who are concurrently receiving other narcotic analgesics, general anesthetics, phenothiazines, other tranquilizers, sedative-hypnotics, tricyclic antidepressants, and other C.N.S. depressants (including alcohol). Respiratory depres-

Continued on next page

Roxane—Cont.

sion, hypotension, and profound sedation or coma may result.
Head Injury and Increased Intracranial Pressure—The respiratory depressant effects of methadone and its capacity to elevate cerebrospinal-fluid pressure may be markedly exaggerated in the presence of increased intracranial pressure. Furthermore, narcotics produce side effects that may obscure the clinical course of patients with head injuries. In such patients, methadone must be used with caution and only if it is deemed essential.
Asthma and Other Respiratory Conditions—Methadone should be used with caution in patients having an acute asthmatic attack, in those with chronic obstructive pulmonary disease or cor pulmonale, and in individuals with a substantially decreased respiratory reserve, preexisting respiratory depression, hypoxia, or hypercapnia. In such patients, even usual therapeutic doses of narcotics may decrease respiratory drive while simultaneously increasing airway resistance to the point of apnea.
Hypotensive Effects—The administration of methadone may result in severe hypotension in an individual whose ability to maintain his blood pressure has already been compromised by a depleted blood volume or concurrent administration of such drugs as the phenothiazines or certain anesthetics.
Use in Ambulatory Patients—Methadone may impair the mental and/or physical abilities required for the performance of potentially hazardous tasks, such as driving a car or operating machinery. The patient should be cautioned accordingly.
Methadone, like other narcotics, may produce orthostatic hypotension in ambulatory patients.
Use in Pregnancy—Safe use in pregnancy has not been established in relation to possible adverse effects on fetal development. Therefore, methadone should not be used in pregnant women unless, in the judgment of the physician, the potential benefits outweigh the possible hazards.
Methadone is not recommended for obstetric analgesia because its long duration of action increases the probability of respiratory depression in the newborn.
Use in Children—Methadone is not recommended for use as an analgesic in children, since documented clinical experience has been insufficient to establish a suitable dosage regimen for the pediatric age group.
Precautions:
Interaction with Rifampin—The concurrent administration of rifampin may possibly reduce the blood concentration of methadone. The mechanism by which rifampin may decrease blood concentrations of methadone is not fully understood, although enhanced microsomal drug-metabolized enzymes may influence drug disposition.
Acute Abdominal Conditions—The administration of methadone or other narcotics may obscure the diagnosis or clinical course in patients with acute abdominal conditions.
Interaction with Monoamine Oxidase (MAO) Inhibitors—Therapeutic doses of meperidine have precipitated severe reactions in patients concurrently receiving monoamine oxidase inhibitors or those who have received such agents within 14 days. Similar reactions thus far have not been reported with methadone; but if the use of methadone is necessary in such patients, a sensitivity test should be performed in which repeated small incremental doses are administered over the course of several hours while the patient's condition and vital signs are under careful observation.
Special-Risk Patients—Methadone should be given with caution and the initial dose should be reduced in certain patients, such as the elderly or debilitated and those with severe impairment of hepatic or renal function, hypothyroidism, Addison's disease, prostatic hypertrophy, or urethral stricture.
Adverse Reactions: THE MAJOR HAZARDS OF METHADONE, AS OF OTHER NARCOTIC ANALGESICS, ARE RESPIRATORY DEPRESSION AND, TO A LESSER DEGREE, CIRCULATORY DEPRESSION, RESPIRATORY ARREST, SHOCK, AND CARDIAC ARREST HAVE OCCURRED.
The most frequently observed adverse reactions include lightheadedness, dizziness, sedation, nausea, vomiting, and sweating. These effects seem to be more prominent in ambulatory patients and in those who are not suffering severe chronic pain. In such individuals, lower doses are advisable. Some adverse reactions may be alleviated in the ambulatory patient if he lies down.
Other adverse reactions include the following:
Central Nervous Systems—Euphoria, dysphoria, weakness, headache, insomnia, agitation, disorientation, and visual disturbances.
Gastrointestinal—Dry mouth, anorexia, constipation, and biliary tract spasm.
Cardiovascular—Flushing of the face, bradycardia, palpitation, faintness, and syncope.
Genitourinary—Urinary retention or hesitancy, antidiuretic effect, and reduced libido and/or potency.
Allergic—Pruritus, urticaria, other skin rashes, edema, and, rarely, hemorrhagic urticaria.
Administration and Dosage:
For Relief of Severe Chronic Pain—Dosage should be adjusted according to the severity of the pain and the response of the patient. Occasionally it may be necessary to exceed the usual dosage recommended in cases of exceptionally severe chronic pain or in those patients who have become tolerant to the analgesic effect of narcotics.
The usual adult dosage is 5 mg (5 ml) to 20 mg (20 ml) every six to eight hours.
Overdosage:
Symptoms—Serious overdosage of methadone is characterized by respiratory depression (a decrease in respiratory rate and/or tidal volume, Cheyne-Stokes respiration, cyanosis), extreme somnolence progressing to stupor or coma, maximally constricted pupils, skeletal-muscle flaccidity, cold and clammy skin, and sometimes, bradycardia and hypotension. In severe overdosage, particularly by the intravenous route, apnea, circulatory collapse, cardiac arrest, and death may occur.
Treatment—Primary attention should be given to the reestablishment of adequate respiratory exchange through provision of a patent airway and institution of assisted or controlled ventilation. If a nontolerant person, especially a child, takes a large dose of methadone, effective narcotic antagonists are available to counteract the potentially lethal respiratory depression. **The physician must remember, however, that methadone is a long-acting depressant (36 to 48 hours), whereas the antagonists act for much shorter periods (one to three hours).** The patient must, therefore, be monitored continuously for recurrence of respiratory depression and treated repeatedly with the narcotic antagonist as needed. If the diagnosis is correct and respiratory depression is due only to overdosage of methadone, the use of other respiratory stimulants is not indicated.
An antagonist should not be administered in the absence of clinically significant respiratory or cardiovascular depression. Intravenously administered narcotic antagonists (naloxone, nalorphine, and levallorphan) are the drugs of choice to reverse signs of intoxication. These agents should be given repeatedly until the patient's status remains satisfactory. The hazard that the narcotic agent will further depress respiration is less likely with the use of naloxone.
Oxygen, intravenous fluids, vasopressors, and other supportive measures should be employed as indicated.
How Supplied:
Methadone Hydrochloride Oral Solution
5 mg per 5 ml
NDC 0054-3555-63: Bottles of 500 ml.
10 mg per 5 ml
NDC 0054-3556-63: Bottles of 500 ml.
Caution: Federal law prohibits dispensing without prescription.

MORPHINE SULFATE ORAL SOLUTION Ⓒ
(WARNING: May be habit forming.)
MORPHINE SULFATE TABLETS Ⓒ
(WARNING: May be habit forming.)

Description:
Each 5 ml of Morphine Sulfate Oral Solution contains:
Morphine Sulfate .... 10 or 20 mg
(WARNING: May be habit forming.)
Alcohol 10%
Each tablet for oral administration contains:
Morphine Sulfate .... 15 or 30 mg
(WARNING: May be habit forming.)
Chemically, Morphine Sulfate is, Morphinan-3,6-diol, 7,8-didehydro-4,5-epoxy-17-methyl-, ($5\alpha,6\alpha$)-, sulfate (2:1) (salt), pentahydrate.
Morphine Sulfate acts as a narcotic analgesic.
Clinical Pharmacology: The major effects of morphine are on the central nervous system and the bowel. Opioids act as agonists, interacting with stereospecific and saturable binding sites or receptors in the brain and other tissues.
Morphine is about two-thirds absorbed from the gastrointestinal tract with the maximum analgesic effect occurring 60 minutes post administration.
Indications and Usage: Morphine is indicated for the relief of severe pain.
Contraindications: Hypersensitivity to morphine; respiratory insufficiency or depression; severe CNS depression; attack of bronchial asthma; heart failure secondary to chronic lung disease; cardiac arrhythmias; increased intracranial or cerebrospinal pressure; head injuries; brain tumor; acute alcoholism; delerium tremens; convulsive disorders; after biliary tract surgery; suspected surgical abdomen; surgical anastomosis; concomitantly with MAO inhibitors or within 14 days of such treatment.
Warnings: Morphine can cause tolerance, psychological and physical dependence. Withdrawal will occur on abrupt discontinuation or administration of a narcotic antagonist.
Interaction with Other Central-Nervous-System Depressants—Morphine should be used with caution and in reduced dosage in patients who are concurrently receiving other narcotic analgesics, general anesthetics, phenothiazines, other tranquilizers, sedative-hypnotics, tricyclic antidepressants, and other CNS depressants (including alcohol). Respiratory depression, hypotension, and profound sedation or coma may result.
Precautions:
General:
Head Injury and Increased Intracranial Pressure—The respiratory depressant effects of morphine and its capacity to elevate cerebrospinal-fluid pressure may be markedly exaggerated in the presence of increased intracranial pressure. Furthermore, narcotics produce side effects that may obscure the clinical course of patients with head injuries. In such patients, morphine must be used with caution and only if it is deemed essential.
Asthma and Other Respiratory Conditions—Morphine should be used with caution in patients having an acute asthmatic attack, in those with chronic obstructive pulmonary disease or cor pulmonale, and in individuals with a substantially decreased respiratory reserve, preexisting respiratory depression, hypoxia, or hypercapnia. In such patients, even usual ther-

apeutic doses of narcotics may decrease respiratory drive while simultaneously increasing airway resistance to the point of apnea.

Hypotensive Effect—The administration of morphine may result in severe hypotension in an individual whose ability to maintain his blood pressure has already been compromised by a depleted blood volume or concurrent administration of such drugs as the phenothiazines or certain anesthetics.

Special-Risk Patients—Morphine should be given with caution and the initial dose should be reduced in certain patients, such as the elderly or debilitated and those with severe impairment of hepatic or renal function, hypothyroidism, Addison's disease, prostatic hypertrophy, or urethral stricture.

Acute Abdominal Conditions—The administration of morphine or other narcotics may obscure the diagnosis or clinical course in patients with acute abdominal conditions.

Information for patients:

Use in Ambulatory Patients—Morphine may impair the mental and/or physical abilities required for the performance of potentially hazardous tasks, such as driving a car or operating machinery. The patient should be cautioned accordingly.

Morphine, like other narcotics, may produce orthostatic hypotension in ambulatory patients.

Patients should be cautioned about the combined effects of alcohol or other central nervous system depressants with morphine.

Drug interactions:

Generally, effects of morphine may be potentiated by alkalizing agents and antagonized by acidifying agents. Analgesic effect of morphine is potentiated by chlorpromazine and methocarbamol. CNS depressants such as anaesthetics, hypnotics, barbiturates, phenothiazines, chloral hydrate, glutethimide, sedatives, MAO inhibitors (including procarbazine hydrochloride), antihistamines, β-blockers (propranolol), alcohol, furazolidone and other narcotics may enhance the depressant effects of morphine.

Morphine may increase anticoagulant activity of coumarin and other anticoagulants.

Carcinogenicity/Mutagenicity:

Long-term studies to determine the carcinogenic and mutagenic potential of morphine are not available.

Pregnancy:

Teratogenic Effects—Pregnancy Category C: Animal reproduction studies have not been conducted with morphine. It is also not known whether morphine can cause fetal harm when administered to a pregnant woman or can affect reproduction capacity. Morphine should be given to a pregnant woman only if clearly needed.

Labor and Delivery:

Morphine readily crosses the placental barrier and, if administered during labor, may lead to respiratory depression in the neonate.

Nursing Mothers:

Morphine has been detected in human milk. For this reason, caution should be exercised when morphine is administered to a nursing woman.

Pediatric Usage:

Safety and effectiveness in children have not been established.

Adverse Reactions: THE MAJOR HAZARDS OF MORPHINE AS OF OTHER NARCOTIC ANALGESICS, ARE RESPIRATORY DEPRESSION AND, TO A LESSER DEGREE, CIRCULATORY DEPRESSION, RESPIRATORY ARREST, SHOCK, AND CARDIAC ARREST HAVE OCCURRED.

The most frequently observed adverse reactions include lightheadedness, dizziness, sedation, nausea, vomiting, and sweating. These effects seem to be more prominent in ambulatory patients and in those who are not suffering severe pain. In such individuals, lower doses are advisable. Some adverse reactions may be alleviated in the ambulatory patient if he lies down.

Other adverse reactions include the following:

Central Nervous System—Euphoria, dysphoria, weakness, headache, insomnia, agitation, disorientation, and visual disturbances.

Gastrointestinal—Dry mouth, anorexia, constipation, and biliary tract spasm.

Cardiovascular—Flushing of the face, bradycardia, palpitation, faintness, and syncope.

Genitourinary—Urinary retention or hesitancy, anti-diuretic effect, and reduced libido and/or potency.

Allergic—Pruritus, urticaria, other skin rashes, edema, and, rarely hemorrhagic urticaria.

Treatment of the most frequent adverse reactions:

Constipation—Ample intake of water or other liquids should be encouraged. Concommitant administration of a stool softener and a peristaltic stimulant with the narcotic analgesic can be an effective preventive measure for those patients in need of therapeutics. If elimination does not occur for two days, an enema should be administered to prevent impaction. In the event diarrhea occurs, seepage around a fecal impaction is a possible cause to consider before antidiarrheal measures are employed.

Nausea and Vomiting—Phenothiazines and antihistamines can be effective treatments for nausea of the medullary and vestibular sources respectively. However, these drugs may potentiate the side effects of the narcotic or the antinauseant.

Drowsiness (sedation)—Once pain control is achieved, undesirable sedation can be minimized by titrating the dosage to a level that just maintains a tolerable pain or pain free state.

Drug Abuse and Dependence: Morphine Sulfate, a narcotic, is a Schedule II controlled substance under the Federal Controlled Substance Act. As with other narcotics, some patients may develop a physical and psychological dependence on morphine. They may increase dosage without consulting a physician and subsequently may develop a physical dependence on the drug. In such cases, abrupt discontinuance may precipitate typical withdrawal symptoms, including convulsions. Therefore the drug should be withdrawn gradually from any patient known to be taking excessive dosages over a long period of time.

In treating the terminally ill patient the benefit of pain relief may outweigh the possibility of drug dependence. ***The chance of drug dependence is substantially reduced when the patient is placed on scheduled narcotic programs instead of a "pain to relief-of-pain" cycle typical of a PRN regimen.***

Overdosage:

Signs and Symptoms: Serious overdose with morphine is characterized by respiratory depression (a decrease in respiratory rate and/or tidal volume, Cheyne-Stokes respiration, cyanosis), extreme somnolence progressing to stupor or coma, skeletal muscle flaccidity, cold or clammy skin, and sometimes bradycardia and hypotension. In severe overdosage, apnea, circulatory collapse, cardiac arrest and death may occur.

Treatment: Primary attention should be given to the re-establishment of adequate respiratory exchange through provision of a patent airway and the institution of assisted or controlled ventilation. The narcotic antagonist naloxone is a specific antidote against respiratory depression which may result from overdosage or unusual sensitivity to narcotics, including morphine. Therefore, an appropriate dose of naloxone (usual initial adult dose: 0.4 mg) should be administered, preferably by the intravenous route and simultaneously with efforts at respiratory resuscitation. Since the duration of action of morphine may exceed that of the antagonist, the patient should be kept under continued surveillance and repeated doses of the antagonist should be administered as needed to maintain adequate respiration.

An antagonist should not be administered in the absence of clinically significant respiratory or cardiovascular depression.

Oxygen, intravenous fluids, vasopressors and other supportive measures should be employed as indicated.

Gastric emptying may be useful in removing unabsorbed drug.

Dosage and Administration: ORAL SOLUTION—Usual Adult Oral Dose: 10 to 20 mg every 4 hours or as directed by physician. TABLETS—15 to 30 mg every 4 hours or as directed by physician. Dosage is a patient dependent variable, therefore increased dosage may be required to achieve adequate analgesia.

For control of chronic, agonizing pain in patients with certain terminal diseases, this drug should be administered on a regularly scheduled basis, every 4 hours, at the lowest dosage level that will achieve adequate analgesia.

Note: Medication may suppress respiration in the elderly, the very ill, and those patients with respiratory problems, therefore lower doses may be required.

Morphine Dosage Reduction: During the first two to three days of effective pain relief, the patient may sleep for many hours. This can be misinterpreted as the effect of excessive analgesic dosing rather than the first sign of relief in a pain exhausted patient. The dose, therefore, should be maintained for at least three days before reduction, if respiratory activity and other vital signs are adequate.

Following successful relief of severe pain, periodic attempts to reduce the narcotic dose should be made. Smaller doses or complete discontinuation of the narcotic analgesic may become feasible due to a physiologic change or the improved mental state of the patient.

How Supplied:

Morphine Sulfate Oral Solution

(Unflavored).

10 mg per 5 ml.

NDC 0054-8585-04: Unit dose Patient Cup™ filled to deliver 5 ml (10 mg Morphine Sulfate), ten 5 ml Patient Cups™ per shelf pack, ten shelf packs per shipper.

NDC 0054-8586-04: Unit dose Patient Cup™ filled to deliver 10 ml (20 mg Morphine Sulfate), ten 10 ml Patient Cups™ per shelf pack, ten shelf packs per shipper.

NDC 0054-3785-63: Bottles of 500 ml.

20 mg per 5 ml.

NDC 0054-3786-63: Bottles of 500 ml.

Tablets

15 mg white scored, identified (54/733) tablets.

NDC 0054-8582-11: Unit dose, 25 tablets per card (reverse numbered), 10 cards per shipper.

NDC 0054-4582-25: Bottles of 100 tablets.

30 mg white scored, identified (54/262) tablets.

NDC 0054-8583-11: Unit dose, 25 tablets per card (reverse numbered), 10 cards per shipper.

NDC 0054-4583-25: Bottles of 100 Tablets.

DEA Order Form Required

Caution: Federal law prohibits dispensing without prescription.

OXYCODONE HYDROCHLORIDE TABLET AND ORAL SOLUTION ©

Description:

Each tablet contains:

Oxycodone Hydrochloride .... 5 mg

(WARNING: May be habit forming)

Each 5 ml Oral Solution contains:

Oxycodone Hydrochloride .... 5 mg

(WARNING: May be habit forming)

Oxycodone is 14-hydroxydihydrocodeinone, a white odorless crystalline powder which is derived from the opium alkaloid, thebaine.

Continued on next page

Roxane—Cont.

Actions: The analgesic ingredient, oxycodone, is a semisynthetic narcotic with multiple actions qualitatively similar to those of morphine; the most prominent of these involve the central nervous system and organs composed of smooth muscle. The principal actions of therapeutic value of oxycodone are analgesia and sedation.
Oxycodone is similar to codeine and methadone in that it retains at least one half of its analgesic activity when administered orally.
Indications: For the relief of moderate to moderately severe pain.
Contraindications: Hypersensitivity to oxycodone.
Warnings:
Drug Dependence: Oxycodone can produce drug dependence of the morphine type, and therefore, has the potential for being abused. Psychic dependence, physical dependence and tolerance may develop upon repeated administration of this drug, and it should be prescribed and administered with the same degree of caution appropriate to the use of other oral narcotic-containing medications. Like other narcotic-containing medications, this drug is subject to the Federal Controlled Substances Act.
Usage in ambulatory patients: Oxycodone may impair the mental and/or physical abilities required for the performance of potentially hazardous tasks such as driving a car or operating machinery. The patient using this drug should be cautioned accordingly.
Interaction with other central nervous system depressants: Patients receiving other narcotic analgesics, general anesthetics, phenothiazines, other tranquilizers, sedative-hypnotics or other CNS depressants (including alcohol) concomitantly with oxycodone hydrochloride may exhibit an additive CNS depression. When such combined therapy is contemplated, the dose of one or both agents should be reduced.
Usage in pregnancy: Safe use in pregnancy has not been established relative to possible adverse effects on fetal development. Therefore, this drug should not be used in pregnant women unless, in the judgment of the physician, the potential benefits outweigh the possible hazards.
Usage in children: This drug should not be administered to children.
Precautions:
Head injury and increased intracranial Pressure: The respiratory depressant effects of narcotics and their capacity to elevate cerebrospinal fluid pressure may be markedly exaggerated in the presence of head injury, other intracranial lesions or a pre-existing increase in intracranial pressure. Furthermore, narcotics produce adverse reactions which may obscure the clinical course of patients with head injuries.
Acute abdominal conditions: The administration of this drug or other narcotics may obscure the diagnosis or clinical course in patients with acute abdominal conditions.
Special risk patients: This drug should be given with caution to certain patients such as the elderly, or debilitated, and those with severe impairment of hepatic or renal function, hypothyroidism, Addison's disease and prostatic hypertrophy or urethral stricture.
Adverse Reactions: The most frequently observed adverse reactions include light headedness, dizziness, sedation, nausea and vomiting. These effects seem to be more prominent in ambulatory than in nonambulatory patients, and some of these adverse reactions may be alleviated if the patient lies down.
Other adverse reactions include euphoria, dysphoria, constipation, skin rash and pruritus.
Dosage and Administration: Dosage should be adjusted to the severity of the pain and the response of the patient. It may occasionally be necessary to exceed the usual dosage recommended below in cases of more severe pain or in those patients who have become tolerant to the analgesic effects of narcotics. This drug is given orally. The usual adult dose is one 5 mg tablet or 5 ml every 6 hours as needed for pain.
Drug Interactions: The CNS depressant effects of oxycodone hydrochloride may be additive with that of other CNS depressants. See WARNINGS.
Management of Overdosage:
Signs and Symptoms: Serious overdose of oxycodone hydrochloride is characterized by respiratory depression (a decrease in respiratory rate and/or tidal volume, Cheyne-Stokes respiration, cyanosis), extreme somnolence progessing to stupor or coma skeletal muscle flaccidity, cold and clammy skin, and sometimes bradycardia and hypotension. In severe overdosage, apnea, circulatory collapse, cardiac arrest and death may occur.
Treatment: Primary attention should be given to the reestablishment of adequate respiratory exchange through provision of a patent airway and the institution of assisted or controlled ventilation. The narcotic antagonist naloxone is a specific antidote against respiratory depression which may result from overdosage or unusual sensitivity to narcotics, including oxycodone. Therefore, an appropriate dose of naloxone (usual initial adult dose: 0.4 mg) should be administered, preferably by the intravenous route, simultaneously with efforts at respiratory resuscitation. Since the duration of action of oxycodone may exceed that of the antagonist, the patient should be kept under continued surveillance and repeated doses of the antagonist, should be administered as needed to maintain adequate respiration.
An antagonist should not be administered in the absence of clinically significant respiratory or cardiovascular depression.
Oxygen, intravenous fluids, vasopressors and other supportive measures should be employed as indicated.
Gastric emptying may be useful in removing unabsorbed drug.
How Supplied:
5 mg white scored tablets.
NDC 0054-8657-11: Unit dose, 25 tablets per strip (reverse numbered), 1 strip per shelf pack, 10 shelf packs per shipper.
NDC 0054-4657-25: Bottles of 100 tablets.
5 mg per 5 ml oral solution.
NDC 0054-3682-63: Bottles of 500 ml.
DEA Order Form Required
Caution: Federal law prohibits dispensing without prescription.

POTASSIUM CHLORIDE ORAL SOLUTION USP, POTASSIUM CHLORIDE POWDER USP, and POTASSIUM CHLORIDE for ORAL SOLUTION USP ℞

Description:
Potassium Chloride Oral Solution: 5, 10 or 20%:
Each 30 ml 5% solution contains potassium 20 mEq and chloride 20 mEq
Each 30 ml 10% solution contains potassium 40 mEq and chloride 40 mEq
Each 30 ml 20% solution contains potassium 80 mEq and chloride 80 mEq
The 5% and 10% solutions are cocoanut flavored, and the 20% solution is grapefruit flavored. Alcohol 5%.
Potassium Chloride Powder, 1.5 g packet (for oral solution); Potassium Chloride for Oral Solution (Cherry Flavored), 4 g packet:
Each packet contains potassium 20 mEq and chloride 20 mEq
Potassium Chloride is chemically KCl. Potassium Chloride is an electrolyte replenisher.
How Supplied:
POTASSIUM CHLORIDE ORAL SOLUTION USP, 5%
20 mEq of potassium per 30 ml
NDC 0054-8715-04: Unit dose Patient Cups™ filled to deliver 30 ml, ten 30 ml Patient Cups™ per shelf pack, ten shelf packs per shipper.
NDC 0054-3715-63: Bottles of 500 ml.
NDC 0054-3715-75: Bottles of 5 liter.
POTASSIUM CHLORIDE ORAL SOLUTION USP, 10%
15 mEq of potassium per 11.25 ml
NDC 0054-8711-04: Unit dose Patient Cups™ filled to deliver 11.25 ml, ten 11.25 ml Patient Cups™ per shelf pack, ten shelf packs per shipper.
20 mEq of potassium per 15 ml
NDC 0054-8714-04: Unit dose Patient Cups™ filled to deliver 15ml, ten 15ml patient Cups™ per shelf pack, ten shelf packs per shipper.
30 mEq of potassium per 22.5 ml
NDC 0054-8712-04: Unit dose Patient Cups™ filled to deliver 22.5 ml, ten 22.5 ml Patient Cups™ per shelf pack, ten shelf packs per shipper.
40 mEq potassium pr 30 ml
NDC 0054-8713-04: Unit dose Patient Cups™ filled to deliver 30ml, ten 30ml Patient Cups™ per shelf pack, ten shelf packs per shipper.
NDC 0054-3716-54: Bottles of 180 ml.
NDC 0054-3716-63: Bottles of 500 ml.
NDC 0054-3716-68: Bottles of 1 liter.
NDC 0054-3716-75: Bottles of 5 liter.
POTASSIUM CHLORIDE ORAL SOLUTION USP, 20%
80 mEq of potassium per 30 ml
NDC 0054-3714-54: Bottles of 180 ml.
NDC 0054-3714-63: Bottles of 500 ml.
NDC 0054-3714-68: Bottles of 1 liter.
NDC 0054-3714-75: Bottles of 5 liter.
POTASSIUM CHLORIDE POWDER USP
20 mEq of potassium per 1.5 g (unflavored)
NDC 0054-8490-13: Unit dose, 1.5 g packets, 30 packets per carton.
NDC 0054-8490-25: Unit dose, 1.5 g packets, 100 packets per carton.
POTASSIUM CHLORIDE for ORAL SOLUTION USP
20 mEq of potassium per 4 g (cherry flavored)
NDC 0054-8716-13: Unit dose, 4 g packets, 30 packets per carton.
NDC 0054-8716-25: Unit dose, 4 g packets 100 packets per carton.

PREDNISONE TABLETS USP ℞

1 mg, 2.5 mg, 5 mg, 10 mg, 20 mg, 25 mg, or 50 mg

How Supplied:
1 mg white, scored tablets.
NDC 0054-8739-25: Unit dose, 10 tablets per strip, 10 strips per shelf pack, ten shelf packs per shipper.
NDC 0054-4741-25: Bottles of 100 tablets.
NDC 0054-4741-31: Bottles of 1000 tablets.
2.5 mg white, scored tablets.
NDC 0054-8740-25: Unit dose, 10 tablets per strip, 10 strips per shelf pack, 10 shelf packs per shipper.
NDC 0054-4742-25: Bottles of 100 tablets.
NDC 0054-4742-31: Bottles of 1000 tablets.
5 mg white, scored tablets.
NDC 0054-8724-25: Unit dose, 10 tablets per strip, 10 strips per shelf pack, ten shelf packs per shipper.
NDC 0054-4728-25: Bottles of 100 tablets.
NDC 0054-4728-31: Bottles of 1000 tablets.
10 mg white, scored tablets.
NDC 0054-8725-25: Unit dose, 10 tablets per strip, 10 strips per shelf pack, 10 shelf packs per shipper.
NDC 0054-4730-25: Bottles of 100 tablets.
NDC 0054-4730-29: Bottles of 500 tablets.
20 mg white, scored tablets.
NDC 0054-8726-25: Unit dose, 10 tablets per strip, 10 strips per shelf pack, 10 shelf packs per shipper.

NDC 0054-4729-25: Bottles of 100 tablets.
NDC 0054-4729-29: Bottles of 500 tablets.
25 mg white, scored tablets.
NDC 0054-8747-25: Unit dose, 10 tablets per strip, 10 strips per shelf pack, 10 shelf packs per shipper.
NDC 0054-4747-25: Bottles of 100 tablets.
50 mg white, scored tablets.
NDC 0054-8729-25: Unit dose, 10 tablets per strip, 10 strips per shelf pack, 10 shelf packs per shipper.
NDC 0054-4733-25: Bottles of 100 tablets.

Rystan Company, Inc.
**470 MAMARONECK AVE.
WHITE PLAINS, NY 10605**

CHLORESIUM® Ointment and Solution
Water-soluble chlorophyll derivatives

(See PDR For Nonprescription Drugs)

DERIFIL® Tablets and Powder
Water-soluble chlorophyll derivatives

(See PDR For Nonprescription Drugs)

PANAFIL® Ointment ℞
PANAFIL®—White Ointment ℞

Composition: PANAFIL contains standardized papain 10%; urea, U.S.P. 10%; and water-soluble chlorophyll derivatives, 0.5% in a hydrophilic base. PANAFIL—White is identical except that the chlorophyll derivatives are omitted.
Action and Uses: For enzymatic debridement and promotion of normal healing (and deodorization, with regular PANAFIL) of surface lesions, particularly where healing is retarded by necrotic tissue, fibrinous or purulent debris, or eschar.
Administration and Dosage: Apply directly to lesion once or twice daily and cover with gauze. At each redressing, irrigate lesion with mild cleansing solution (*not* hydrogen peroxide solution which may inactivate papain) to remove any accumulation of liquefied necrotic material.
Side Effects: An occasional itching or stinging sensation is sometimes associated with the first application of proteolytic enzymes.
Precautions: Not to be used in eyes.
How Supplied: PANAFIL—1 oz. tubes, 1 lb. jars.
PANAFIL—White—1 oz. tubes.

SDA Pharmaceuticals, Inc.
**919 THIRD AVENUE
NEW YORK, NY 10022**

ANOREXIN™ OTC
**Capsules
Anorectic for simple exogenous obesity
contains:
phenylpropanolamine HCl 25 mg
caffeine 100 mg**

One-Span™ OTC
**Sustained Release Capsules
contains:
phenylpropanolamine HCl 50 mg
caffeine 200 mg**

Description: Each capsule contains phenylpropanolamine HCl, an anorexiant, and caffeine, a mild stimulant.
Indication: ANOREXIN is indicated as adjunctive therapy in a regimen of weight reduction based on caloric restriction in the management and control of simple exogenous obesity.
Caution: Do not exceed recommended dosage. Discontinue use if rapid pulse, dizziness or palpitations occur. Do not use if high blood pressure, heart, kidney, diabetes, thyroid or other disease is present, or if pregnant or lactating, nor to be used by anyone under the age of 18, except on physician's advice. Keep this and all drugs out of the reach of children. In case of accidental overdose seek professional assistance or contact a Poison Control Center immediately.
Precaution: Avoid use if taking prescription, anti-hypertensive or anti-depressive drugs containing monoamine oxidase inhibitors or other medication containing sympathomimetic amines. Avoid continuous use longer than 3 months.
Adverse Reactions: Side effects are rare when taken as directed. Nausea or nasal dryness may occasionally occur.
Dosage and Administration:
ANOREXIN™ Capsules: One capsule 30–60 minutes before each meal three times a day with one or two full glasses of water.
ANOREXIN™ One-Span™ Sustained Release Capsules: One capsule with a full glass of water once a day mid-morning (10:00 A.M.)
How Supplied:
ANOREXIN™ Capsules: Bottles of 50, packaged with 1200 calorie ANOREXIN Diet Plan.
ANOREXIN™ One-Span™ Sustained Release Capsules: Bottles of 21; packaged with 1200 calorie ANOREXIN Diet Plan.
Reference: Griboff, Solomon, I., M.D., F.A.C.P. et al., A Double-Blind Clinical Evaluation of a Phenylpropanolamine-Caffeine Combination and a Placebo in the Treatment of Exogenous Obesity, Current Therapeutic Research 17, 6:535, (1975) June.
Silverman, H.I., D.Sc., Kreger, B.E., M.D., Lewis, G.P., M.D., et. al., Lack of Side Effects from Orally Administered Phenylpropanolamine and Phenylpropanolamine with Caffeine: A Controlled Three-Phase Study, Current Therapeutic Research 28, 2:185 (1980) August.

Sandoz Pharmaceuticals
**(Division of Sandoz, Inc.)
ROUTE 10
EAST HANOVER, NJ 07936**

BELLADENAL® ℞
Tablets
BELLADENAL–S®
Tablets

The following prescribing information is based on official labeling in effect on November 1, 1982.
Composition: Each Belladenal *Tablet* and Belladenal-S Tablet contains 0.25 mg Bellafoline® (levorotatory alkaloids of belladonna, as malates), and 50 mg phenobarbital, USP. (Warning: May be habit forming.)
Properties and Therapeutics: Superior antispasmodic/anticholinergic. The natural levorotatory alkaloids of belladonna (Bellafoline) in Belladenal give the antispasmodic-anticholinergic action of belladonna with only minimal central side effects. One Belladenal or Belladenal-S Tablet has the antispasmodic-anticholinergic action of 27 minims of tincture belladonna. Both Belladenal Tablets and Belladenal-S Tablets are scored to permit dosage adjustments necessary for optimal control of symptoms.

Indications
Based on a review of this drug by the National Academy of Sciences—National Research Council and/or other information, FDA has classified the indications as follows:
"Possibly" effective: As adjunctive therapy in the treatment of peptic ulcer and in the treatment of the irritable bowel syndrome (irritable colon, spastic colon, mucous colitis) and acute enterocolitis.
Final classification of the less-than-effective indications requires further investigation.

Contraindications: Glaucoma, elevated intraocular pressure, advanced hepatic or renal disease. Hypersensitivity to any of the components.
Precautions: Due to presence of a barbiturate, may be habit forming. Caution is advised in the elderly.
Belladenal-S Tablets contain FD&C Yellow No. 5 (tartrazine) which may cause allergic-type reactions (including bronchial asthma) in certain susceptible individuals. Although the overall incidence of FD&C Yellow No. 5 (tartrazine) sensitivity in the general population is low, it is frequently seen in patients who also have aspirin hypersensitivity.
Side Effects: Urinary retention, blurred vision, dry mouth, flushing or drowsiness may occur.
Usual Dosage: Belladenal Tablets—Adults: 2 to 4 tablets per day, in divided doses of ¼ to ½ tablet. Children: ¼ to ½ tablet one to four times daily, according to age. Tablets are scored so that they can be divided easily.
Belladenal-S Tablets—Adults: One tablet in the morning and one at night.
Supplied: Belladenal Tablets (compressed, white, scored) in bottles of 100. Belladenal-S Tablets (compressed, scored tablets of tri-colored pattern: salmon pink, emerald green and white) in bottles of 100.
Company's Product Identification Mark(s): Belladenal Tablets embossed 78-28 on 1 side and scored on reverse side. Belladenal-S Tablets embossed 78-27 on 1 side and scored on reverse side.
[BED-Z12 Issued February 8, 1980]
[*Shown in Product Identification Section*]

CAFERGOT® ℞
**(ergotamine tartrate and caffeine) tablets, USP
(ergotamine tartrate and caffeine) suppositories, USP**
CAFERGOT® P-B
Tablets and Suppositories

The following prescribing information is based on official labeling in effect on November 1, 1982.
Description: Each *Cafergot Tablet* contains: 1 mg Gynergen® (ergotamine tartrate, USP) and 100 mg caffeine, USP. Each *Cafergot Suppository* contains: 2 mg Gynergen® (ergotamine tartrate, USP); 100 mg caffeine, USP; tartaric acid, NF; cocoa butter, NF.
Each *Cafergot P-B Tablet* contains: 1 mg Gynergen® (ergotamine tartrate, USP); 100 mg caffeine, USP; 0.125 mg Bellafoline® (levorotatory alkaloids of belladonna, as malates); 30 mg pentobarbital sodium, USP, (*Warning:* May be habit forming). Each *Cafergot P-B Suppository* contains: 2 mg Gynergen® (ergotamine tartrate, USP); 100 mg caffeine, USP; 0.25 mg Bellafoline® (levorotatory alkaloids of belladonna, as malates); 60 mg pentobarbital, USP. (*Warning:* May be habit forming); tartaric acid, NF; malic acid, lactose, USP; cocoa butter, NF.
Cafergot Suppositories and Cafergot P-B Suppositories are *sealed* in foil to afford protection from cocoa butter leakage. If an unavoidable period of exposure to heat softens the suppository, it should be chilled in ice-cold water to solidify it before removing the foil.
Actions: Ergotamine is an alpha adrenergic blocking agent with a direct stimulating effect on the smooth muscle of peripheral and cranial blood vessels and produces depression of central vasomotor centers. The compound also has

Continued on next page

Sandoz—Cont.

the properties of serotonin antagonism. In comparison to hydrogenated ergotamine, the adrenergic blocking actions are less pronounced and vasoconstrictive actions are greater.
Caffeine, also a cranial vasoconstrictor, is added to further enhance the vasoconstrictive effect without the necessity of increasing ergotamine dosage.
For individuals experiencing excessive nausea and vomiting during migraine attacks the further addition of the anticholinergic and antiemetic alkaloids of belladonna and pentobarbital for reduction of nervous tension has been provided.
Many migraine patients experience excessive nausea and vomiting during attacks, making it impossible for them to retain any oral medication. In such cases, therefore, the only practical means of medication is through the rectal route where medication may reach the cranial vessels directly, evading the splanchnic vasculature and the liver.
Indications:
Cafergot
Indicated as therapy to abort or prevent vascular headache, e.g., migraine, migraine variants, or so-called "histaminic cephalalgia".
Cafergot P-B
Indicated as therapy to abort or prevent vascular headache complicated by tension and gastrointestinal disturbances.
Contraindications: Peripheral vascular disease, coronary heart disease, hypertension, impaired hepatic or renal function, sepsis and pregnancy. Hypersensitivity to any of the components.
Precautions: Although signs and symptoms of ergotism rarely develop even after long term intermittent use of the orally or rectally administered drugs, care should be exercised to remain within the limits of recommended dosage.
Adverse Reactions: Vasoconstrictive complications, at times of a serious nature, may occur. These include pulselessness, weakness, muscle pains and paresthesias of the extremities and precordial distress and pain. Although these effects occur most commonly with long-term therapy at relatively high doses, they have also been reported with short-term or normal doses. Other adverse effects include transient tachycardia or bradycardia, nausea, vomiting, localized edema and itching. Drowsiness may occur with Cafergot P-B.
Dosage and Administration: Procedure: For the best results, dosage should start at the first sign of an attack. Adults: *Orally*—2 tablets at start of attack; 1 additional tablet every ½ hour, if needed for full relief (maximum 6 tablets per attack, 10 per week). *Rectally*—1 suppository at start of attack; second suppository after 1 hour, if needed for full relief (maximum 2 suppositories per attack, 5 per week).
Maximum Adult Dosage:
Orally: Total dose for any one attack should not exceed 6 tablets.
Rectally: Two suppositories is the maximum dose for an individual attack.
Total weekly dosage should not exceed 10 tablets or 5 suppositories.
In carefully selected patients, with due consideration of maximum dosage recommendations, administration of the drug at bedtime may be an appropriate short-term preventive measure.
Overdosage: The toxic effects of an acute overdosage of Cafergot are due primarily to the ergotamine component. The amount of caffeine is such that its toxic effects will be overshadowed by those of ergotamine. Symptoms include vomiting; numbness, tingling, pain and cyanosis of the extremities associated with diminished or absent peripheral pulses; hypertension or hypotension; drowsiness, stupor, coma, convulsions and shock. A case has been reported of reversible bilateral papillitis with ring scotomata in a patient who received five times the recommended daily adult dose over a period of 14 days.
Treatment consists of removal of the offending drug by induction of emesis, gastric lavage, and catharsis. Maintenance of adequate pulmonary ventilation, correction of hypotension, and control of convulsions are important considerations. Treatment of peripheral vasospasm should consist of warmth, but not heat, and protection of the ischemic limbs. Vasodilators may be used with benefit but caution must be exercised to avoid aggravating an already existent hypotension.
How Supplied: Cafergot Tablets flesh pink colored, sugar coated. Bottles of 250 and cartons of three SigPak® (dispensing unit) packages, each containing 30 tablets in individual blisters. Cafergot Suppositories (sealed in fuchsia-colored aluminum foil) in boxes of 12.
Cafergot P-B Tablets bright green, sugar coated. Bottles of 250 and cartons of three SigPak® (dispensing unit) packages, each containing 30 tablets in individual blisters. Cafergot P-B Suppositories (sealed in blue aluminum foil) in boxes of 12.
Company's Product Identification Mark(s):
Cafergot Tablets imprinted "Cafergot" on one side, triangle (S) other side.
Cafergot P-B Tablets imprinted "78-36" on 1 side, triangle (S) other side.
Cafergot Suppositories imprinted "CAFERGOT triangle (S) SANDOZ 78-33".
Cafergot P-B Suppositories imprinted "CAFERGOT P-B triangle (S) SANDOZ 78-35".
[CAF-Z18 Issued May 29, 1981]
[*Shown in Product Identification Section*]

CEDILANID® -D ℞
(deslanoside) injection, USP

The following prescribing information is based on official labeling in effect on November 1, 1982.
Description: The cardiac (or digitalis) glycosides are a closely related group of drugs having in common specific and powerful effects on the myocardium. These drugs are found in a number of plants. The term "digitalis" is used to designate the whole group. Typically, the glycosides are composed of three portions, a steroid nucleus, a lactone ring, and a sugar (hence "glycosides").
Cedilanid-D (deslanoside) is provided as ampul solution containing the cardioactive glycoside, desacetyl lanatoside C. This agent is prepared by controlled alkaline hydrolysis of lanatoside C, a glycoside obtained from digitalis lanata.
Supplied in ampuls of 2 ml. Each 2 ml contains:
deslanoside, USP .... 0.4 mg
citric acid, USP, q.s. to................. pH 6.2±0.3
sodium phosphate, USP...................... 10.6 mg
alcohol, USP .... 9.8% by vol.
glycerin, USP .... 15% by wt.
water for injection, USP, q.s. to 2 ml
Action: The digitalis glycosides have qualitatively the same therapeutic effect on the heart. They (1) increase the force of myocardial contraction, (2) increase the refractory period of the atrioventricular (A-V) node, and (3) to a lesser degree, affect the sinoatrial (S-A) node and conduction system via the parasympathetic and sympathetic nervous systems.
Cedilanid-D (deslanoside) has its onset of action in about 5 minutes after intravenous administration and reaches peak effect in 2-4 hours. Therapeutic action persists for 2 to 5 days.
Indications:

1. "Congestive heart failure," all degrees, is the primary indication. The increased cardiac output results in diuresis and general amelioration of the disturbances characteristic of right (venous congestion, edema) and left (dyspnea, orthopnea, cardiac asthma) heart failure.
   Digitalis, generally, is most effective in "low output" failure and less effective in "high output" (bronchopulmonary insufficiency, infection, hyperthyroidism) heart failure.
   Digitalis should be continued after failure is abolished unless some known precipitating factor is corrected.
2. "Atrial fibrillation"— especially when the ventricular rate is elevated. Digitalis rapidly reduces ventricular rates and eliminates the pulse deficit. Palpitation, precordial distress or weakness are relieved and any concomitant congestive failure ameliorated.
   Digitalis is continued in doses necessary to maintain the desired ventricular rate and other clinical effects.
3. "Atrial flutter" digitalis slows the heart and regular sinus rhythm may appear. Frequently the flutter is converted to atrial fibrillation with a slow ventricular rate. Stopping digitalis at this point may be followed by restoration of sinus rhythm, especially if the flutter was of the paroxysmal type. It is preferable, however, to continue digitalis if failure ensues or if atrial flutter is a frequent occurrence.
4. "Paroxysmal atrial tachycardia" digitalis may be used, especially if it is resistant to lesser measures. Depending on the urgency, a more rapid acting parenteral preparation may be preferable to initiate digitalization, although if failure has ensued or paroxysms recur frequently, digitalis is maintained by oral administration.
   Digitalis is not indicated in sinus tachycardia or premature systoles in the absence of heart failure.

"Cardiogenic shock"—the value of digitalis is not established, but the drug is often employed, especially when the condition is accompanied by pulmonary edema. Digitalis seems to adversely affect shock due to infections.
Contraindications: The presence of toxic effects (See "Overdosage") induced by any digitalis preparation is an absolute contraindication to all of the glycosides.
"Allergy," though rare, does occur. It may not extend to all preparations and another may be tried.
"Ventricular Fibrillation"
"Ventricular tachycardia," unless congestive failure supervenes after a protracted episode not itself due to digitalis.
Warnings: Many of the arrhythmias for which digitalis is advised are identical with those reflecting digitalis intoxication. If the possibility of digitalis intoxication cannot be excluded, cardiac glycosides should be temporarily withheld if permitted by the clinical situation.
The patient with congestive heart failure may complain of nausea and vomiting. These symptoms may also be indications of digitalis intoxication. A clinical determination of the cause of these symptoms must be attempted before further drug administration.
Precautions: "Potassium depletion" sensitizes the myocardium to digitalis and toxicity is apt to develop even with usual dosage. Hypokalemia also tends to reduce the positive inotropic effect of digitalis.
Potassium wastage may result from diuretic, corticosteroid, hemodialysis and other therapy. It is apt to accompany malnutrition, old age and long-standing congestive heart failure.
"Acute myocardial infarction," severe pulmonary disease, or far advanced heart failure are apt to be more sensitive to digitalis and more prone to disturbances of rhythm.
"Calcium" affects contractility and excitability of the heart in a manner similar to that of digitalis. Calcium may produce serious arrhythmias in digitalized patients.

"Myxedema"—Digitalis requirements are less because excretion rate is decreased and blood levels are significantly higher.
"Incomplete AV block," especially patients subject to Stokes Adams attacks, may develop advanced or complete heart block. Heart failure in these patients can usually be controlled by other measures and by increasing the heart rate.
"Chronic constrictive pericarditis," is apt to respond unfavorably.
"Idiopathic hypertrophic subaortic stenosis" must be managed extremely carefully. Unless cardiac failure is severe it is doubtful whether digitalis should be employed.
"Renal insufficiency" delays the excretion of digitalis and dosage must be adjusted accordingly in patients with renal disease.
NOTE: This applies also to potassium administration should it become necessary.
Electrical conversion of arrhythmias may require adjustment of digitalis dosage.
Adverse Reactions: Gynecomastia, uncommon.
Overdosage, Toxic Effects: "Gastrointestinal"—anorexia, nausea, vomiting, diarrhea—are the most common early symptoms of overdosages in the adult.
Uncontrolled heart failure may also produce such symptoms.
"Central Nervous System"—headache, weakness, apathy, visual disturbances.
"Cardiac Disturbances"—
Arrhythmias —"ventricular premature beats" is the most common.
Paroxysmal and nonparoxysmal nodal rhythms, atrioventricular (inference) dissociation and paroxysmal atrial tachycardia (PAT) with block are also common arrhythmias due to digitalis overdosage.
Conduction Disturbances—excessive slowing of the pulse is a clinical sign of digitalis overdosage. Atrioventricular block of increasing degree, may proceed to complete heart block.
NOTE: The electrocardiogram is fundamental in determining the presence and nature of these toxic disturbances. Digitalis may also induce other changes (as of the ST segment), but these provide no measure of the degree of digitalization.
TREATMENT OF TOXIC ARRHYTHMIAS: Digitalis is discontinued until after all signs of toxicity are abolished. This may be all that is necessary if toxic manifestations are not severe and appear after the time for peak effect of the drug.
Potassium salts are commonly used. Potassium chloride in divided doses totaling 4 to 6 gm. for adults provided renal function is adequate.
When correction of the arrhythmia is urgent, potassium is administered intravenously in a solution of 5 percent dextrose in water, a total of 40-100 mEq. (40 mEq. per 500 ml.) at the rate of 40 mEq. per hour unless limited by pain due to local irritation.
Additional amounts may be given if the arrhythmia is uncontrolled and the potassium well tolerated.
Electrocardiographic monitoring is indicated to avoid potassium toxicity, e.g. peaking of T waves.
CAUTION: Potassium should not be used and may be dangerous for severe or complete heart block due to digitalis and not related to any tachycardia.
Chelating agents to bind calcium may also be used to counteract the arrhythmia effect of digitalis toxicity, hypokalemia and of elevated serum calcium which may also precipitate digitalis toxicity.
Four grams (0.8 percent solution) of the disodium salt of EDTA is dissolved in 500 ml of 5 percent dextrose in water (50 mg per ml) and administered over a period of 2 hours unless the arrhythmia is controlled before the infusion is completed.
A continuous electrocardiogram should be observed so that the infusion may be promptly stopped when the desired effect is achieved.
Other counteracting agents are: Quinidine, procainamide, and beta adrenergic blocking agents.
Dosage and Administration: "Parenteral" administration should be used only when the drug cannot be taken orally, or rapid digitalization is very urgent.
Parenteral digitalization can be obtained within 12 hours by giving 8 ml (1.6 mg) *either intramuscularly* or *intravenously.* By the I.V. route the dose may be given as one injection or in portions of 4 ml each. By I.M. route, 4 ml portions are injected at each of 2 sites.
After parenteral digitalization with Cedilanid-D (deslanoside) maintenance therapy may be accomplished by starting administration of an oral preparation, within 12 hours.
How Supplied:
Ampuls, 2 ml size (2 ml contains 0.4 mg deslanoside, USP) Boxes of 20 ampuls.
Being chemically pure and of constant potency, deslanoside, USP is standardized by weight; the ampul solution of Cedilanid-D (deslanoside) contains in each 2 ml:
deslanoside, USP .... 0.4 mg
citric acid, USP q.s. to.................. pH 6.2±0.3
sodium phosphate, USP.................. 10.6 mg
alcohol, USP .... 9.8% by vol.
glycerin, USP .... 15% by wt.
water for injection, USP, q.s. to 2 ml
[CED-Z16 Issued October 10, 1980]

D.H.E. 45® Injection ℞
(dihydroergotamine mesylate) injection, USP

The following prescribing information is based on official labeling in effect on November 1, 1982.
Description: DHE-45® is hydrogenated ergotamine as the mesylate. It is a clear, colorless, stable ampul solution containing per ml:
dihydroergotamine
mesylate, USP .... 1 mg
methanesulfonic acid/sodium
hydroxide .... q.s. to pH 3.75±0.5
alcohol, USP .... 6.1% by vol.
glycerin, USP .... 15% by wt.
water for injection, USP, q.s. to.................. 1 ml
Actions: Dihydroergotamine is an alpha adrenergic blocking agent with a direct stimulating effect on the smooth muscle of peripheral and cranial blood vessels, and produces depression of central vasomotor centers. The compound also has the properties of serotonin antagonism. In comparison to ergotamine, the adrenergic blocking actions are more pronounced, the vasoconstrictive actions somewhat less pronounced, and there is reduced incidence and degree of nausea and vomiting.
Onset of action occurs in 15 to 30 minutes following intramuscular administration and persists for 3-4 hours.
Repeated dosage at 1 hour intervals up to 3 hours may be required to obtain maximal effect.
Indications: As therapy to abort or prevent vascular headache, e.g., migraine, migraine variants, or so-called "histaminic cephalalgia" when rapid control is desired or when other routes of administration are not feasible.
Contraindications: Peripheral vascular disease, coronary heart disease, hypertension, impaired hepatic or renal function, sepsis and pregnancy. Hypersensitivity.
Adverse Reactions: Numbness and tingling of fingers and toes, muscle pains in the extremities, weakness in the legs, precordial distress and pain, transient tachycardia or bradycardia, nausea, vomiting, localized edema and itching.
Dosage and Administration: *For vascular headache,* 1 ml intramuscularly at first warning sign of headache, repeated at 1 hour intervals to a total of 3 ml. Optimal results are obtained by titrating the dose for several headaches to find the minimal effective dose for each patient and this dose should then be employed at onset of subsequent attacks. Where more rapid effect is desired, the intravenous route may be employed to a maximum of 2 ml. Total weekly dosage should not exceed 6 ml.
Overdosage: Failure to observe the upper limits of repeated parenteral dosage may result in eventual onset of the peripheral toxic signs and symptoms of ergotism. Treatment includes discontinuance of the drug, warmth, vasodilators, and good nursing care to prevent tissue damage.
How Supplied: As a clear, colorless and stable solution in ampuls containing:
dihydroergotamine
mesylate, USP.................. 1 mg
methanesulfonic acid/sodium
hydroxide .... q.s. to pH 3.75±0.5
alcohol, USP .... 6.1% by vol.
glycerin, USP .... 15% by wt.
water for injection, USP, q.s. to .... 1 ml
Ampuls, 1 ml size—boxes of 20.
To assure constant potency, protect the ampuls from light and heat. In the event the ampul solution becomes discolored, it should not be used.
[D.H.E.-Z15 Issued November 3, 1980]

DIAPID® Nasal Spray ℞
(lypressin)
nasal solution, USP

The following prescribing information is based on official labeling in effect on November 1, 1982.
Description: Diapid® (lypressin) Nasal Spray contains synthetic lysine-8-vasopressin with an activity of 50 USP Posterior Pituitary (Pressor) Units per ml (0.185 mg/ml). Lysine-8-vasopressin is a polypeptide and is one of the two known naturally occurring molecular forms of mammalian posterior pituitary antidiuretic hormone. This synthetic polypeptide is present as a protein-free substance in Diapid Nasal Spray. Unlike preparations of posterior pituitary antidiuretic hormone of animal origin, Diapid is completely free of oxytocin and foreign proteins. The molecular formula of lysine-8-vasopressin is $C_{46}H_{65}N_{13}O_{12}S_2$.
Action: The principal pharmacologic action of lysine-8-vasopressin, the active ingredient of Diapid (lypressin) Nasal Spray, is similar to that of arginine-8-vasopressin, the posterior pituitary antidiuretic hormone occurring in man. Diapid Nasal Spray increases the rate of reabsorption of solute free water from the distal renal tubules, without significantly modifying the rate of glomerular filtration, producing a fall in free water clearance and an increase in urinary osmolality. The rates of solute and creatinine excretion noted with therapeutic doses of Diapid Nasal Spray suggest that sodium clearance and glomerular filtration rates are essentially unaltered by this hormone.
Diapid Nasal Spray is relatively free of oxytocic activity when used within the recommended therapeutic dose levels.
It possesses little pressor activity, the ratio of pressor to antidiuretic activity being in the range of 1:1000.
The antidiuretic effect produced by Diapid Nasal Spray begins rapidly and usually reaches a peak within 30 to 120 minutes. Its usual duration of action is 3 to 8 hours.
Indications: Diapid Nasal Spray is indicated for the control or prevention of the symptoms and complications of diabetes insipidus due to deficiency of endogenous posterior pituitary antidiuretic hormone. These symptoms and complications include polydipsia, polyuria, and dehydration. It is particularly useful in patients with diabetes insipidus who have become unresponsive to other forms of therapy or who experience various types of local and/or systemic reactions, allergic reactions, or other undesirable effects (e.g., excessive fluid retention) from preparations of posterior pituitary antidiuretic hormone of animal origin.

Continued on next page

Sandoz—Cont.

Contraindications: There are no known contraindications to the use of Diapid® (lypressin) Nasal Spray.
Warnings: The safety of this drug in pregnancy has not been established. The possibility of risk to the mother and unborn child should be weighed against potential benefits before the drug is administered to women of childbearing age.
Precautions: Cardiovascular pressor effects with Diapid Nasal Spray are minimal or absent when it is administered as a nasal spray in therapeutic doses. Nevertheless, it should be used with caution in patients for whom such effects would not be desirable because mild blood pressure elevation has been noted in unanesthetized subjects who received lypressin intravenously. Large doses intranasally may cause coronary artery constriction and caution should be observed in treating patients with coronary artery disease.
The effectiveness of Diapid (lypressin) Nasal Spray may be lessened in patients with nasal congestion, allergic rhinitis, and upper respiratory infections because these conditions may interfere with absorption of the drug by the nasal mucosa. In this event, larger doses of Diapid Nasal Spray, or adjunctive therapy, may be needed.
Patients with a known sensitivity to anti-diuretic hormone should be tested for sensitivity to Diapid.
Adverse Reactions: With clinical use of Diapid (lypressin) Nasal Spray, adverse reactions have been infrequent and mild. To date, such reactions have included rhinorrhea, nasal congestion, irritation and pruritus of the nasal passages, nasal ulceration, headache, conjunctivitis, heartburn secondary to excessive nasal administration with drippage into the pharynx, and abdominal cramps and increased bowel movements. Inadvertent inhalation of Diapid Nasal Spray has resulted in substernal tightness, coughing, and transient dyspnea. In one patient, an overdose of Diapid Nasal Spray caused marked, but transient, fluid retention. Tolerance or tachyphylaxis to Diapid Nasal Spray has not been reported to date.
Hypersensitivity manifested by a positive skin test.
Dosage and Administration: Patients should be instructed to administer 1 or 2 sprays of Diapid® (lypressin) Nasal Spray to one or both nostrils whenever frequency of urination becomes increased or significant thirst develops. (One spray provides approximately 2.0 USP Posterior Pituitary [Pressor] Units.) The usual dosage for adults and children is 1 or 2 sprays in each nostril 4 times daily. An additional dose at bedtime is often helpful to eliminate nocturia, if it is not controlled with the regular daily dosage. For patients requiring more than 2 sprays per nostril every 4 to 6 hours, it is recommended that the time interval between doses be reduced rather than increasing the number of sprays at each dose. (More than 2 or 3 sprays in each nostril usually results in wastage because the unabsorbed excess will drain posteriorly, by way of the nasopharynx, into the digestive tract where it will be inactivated.)
Diapid Nasal Spray permits individualization of dosage necessary to control the symptoms of diabetes insipidus. Patients quickly learn to regulate their dosage in accordance with their degree of polyuria and thirst, and once determined, daily requirements remain fairly stable for months or years. Although most patients require 1 or 2 sprays of Diapid (lypressin) Nasal Spray in each nostril 4 times daily, dosage has ranged from 1 spray per day at bedtime to 10 sprays in each nostril every 3-4 hours. Requirements of the larger doses may represent greater severity of disease or other phenomena, such as poor nasal absorption. A seeming requirement for large doses of lypressin may be due to the presence of mixed hypothalamic-hypophyseal and nephrogenic diabetes insipidus, the latter condition being unresponsive to administration of antidiuretic hormone.
Diapid Nasal Spray is conveniently administered, from a compact and portable, plastic squeeze bottle, by inserting the nozzle of the bottle into the nostril and squeezing once firmly to deliver each short spray.
NOTE: To assure that a uniform, well-diffused spray is delivered, the bottle of Diapid Nasal Spray should be held upright and the patient should be in a vertical position with head upright.
Supplied: Diapid Nasal Spray is supplied in a plastic bottle that contains 8 ml of solution. Each ml of solution contains lypressin (0.185 mg) equivalent to 50 USP Posterior Pituitary (Pressor) Units and the following: propylparaben, NF, methylparaben, NF, sodium phosphate, NF, citric acid, USP, sodium chloride, USP, sorbitol solution, USP, glycerin, USP, sodium acetate, USP, acetic acid, NF, chlorobutanol, NF, (0.1%-0.002%), purified water, USP.
This product has an expiration date of 36 months.

[DIA-Z11 Issued September 17, 1980]

FIOGESIC® Tablets

The following prescribing information is based on official labeling in effect on November 1, 1982.
Composition: Each Tablet contains Calurin® (calcium carbaspirin) 382 mg, equivalent to 300 mg aspirin; phenylpropanolamine hydrochloride, USP 25 mg; pheniramine maleate 12.5 mg; pyrilamine maleate, USP 12.5 mg.
Actions and Uses: For prompt, temporary relief of headache, sinus and nasal congestion, pain and fever due to sinusitis, common cold, or influenza. FIOGESIC promotes sinus and nasal decongestion and drainage with phenylpropanolamine, an orally used alpha adrenergic sympathomimetic approximately equal in potency to ephedrine but with less CNS stimulation, plus two antihistamines, pheniramine maleate and pyrilamine maleate. Calurin®, a freely soluble aspirin complex, alleviates pain and fever.
Contraindications: Sensitivity to any of the ingredients.
Caution: Not for children under 6. Individuals with high blood pressure, heart disease, diabetes, or thyroid disease should use only as directed by a physician. This preparation may cause drowsiness. Do not drive or operate machinery while taking this medication.
Side Effects: Drowsiness, blurred vision, cardiac palpitations, flushing, dizziness, nervousness, or gastrointestinal upsets may occur occasionally.
Dosage: Adults—Two tablets followed by one or two tablets every four hours, up to six per day. Children (6 to 12 years)—one-half to one tablet every four hours up to four tablets per day.
Supplied: Fiogesic Oblong Inlay-Tablets (white with yellow inlay) in bottles of 100.
Company's Product Identification Mark(s): Tablets embossed FIOGESIC on 1 side, SANDOZ other side.

[*Shown in Product Identification Section*]

FIORINAL® Ⓒ
Tablets and Capsules

The following prescribing information is based on official labeling in effect on December 15, 1982.
Description: Each Fiorinal® tablet or capsule for oral administration contains: Sandoptal® (butalbital, USP), 50 mg (Warning: May be habit forming); aspirin, USP, 325 mg; caffeine, USP, 40 mg.
Butalbital, 5-allyl-5-isobutyl-barbituric acid, a white odorless crystalline powder; is a short- to intermediate-acting barbiturate.
Actions: Pharmacologically, Fiorinal combines the analgesic properties of aspirin with the anxiolytic and muscle relaxant properties of Sandoptal.
The clinical effectiveness of Fiorinal in tension headache has been established in double-blind, placebo-controlled, multi-clinic trials. A factorial design study compared Fiorinal with each of its major components. This study demonstrated that each component contributes to the efficacy of Fiorinal in the treatment of the target symptoms of tension headache (headache pain, psychic tension, and muscle contraction in the head, neck and shoulder region). For each symptom and the symptom complex as a whole, Fiorinal was shown to have significantly superior clinical effects to either component alone.
Indications: Fiorinal is indicated for the relief of the symptom complex of tension (or muscle contraction) headache.
Contraindications: Hypersensitivity to aspirin, caffeine, or barbiturates. Patients with porphyria.
Warnings:
Drug Dependency: Prolonged use of barbiturates can produce drug dependence, characterized by psychic dependence, and less frequently, physical dependence and tolerance. The abuse liability of Fiorinal is similar to that of other barbiturate-containing drug combinations. Caution should be exercised when prescribing medication for patients with a known propensity for taking excessive quantities of drugs, which is not uncommon in patients with chronic tension headache.
Use in Ambulatory Patients: Fiorinal may impair the mental and/or physical abilities required for the performance of potentially hazardous tasks, such as driving a car or operating machinery. The patient should be cautioned accordingly. Central Nervous System depressant effects of butalbital may be additive with those of other CNS depressants. Concurrent use with other sedative-hypnotics or alcohol should be avoided. When such combined therapy is necessary, the dose of one or more agents may need to be reduced.
Use in Pregnancy: Adequate studies have not been performed in animals to determine whether this drug affects fertility in males or females, has teratogenic potential, or has other adverse effects on the fetus. While there are no well-controlled studies in pregnant women, over twenty years of marketing and clinical experience does not include any positive evidence of adverse effects on the fetus. Although there is no clearly defined risk, such experience cannot exclude the possibility of infrequent or subtle damage to the human fetus. Fiorinal should be used in pregnant women only when clearly needed.
Nursing Mothers: The effects of Fiorinal on infants of nursing mothers are not known. Salicylates and barbiturates are excreted in the breast milk of nursing mothers. The serum levels in infants are believed to be insignificant with therapeutic doses.
Precautions: Salicylates should be used with extreme caution in the presence of peptic ulcer or coagulation abnormalities.
Pediatric Use: Safety and effectiveness in children below the age of 12 have not been established.
Adverse Reactions: The most frequent adverse reactions are drowsiness and dizziness. Less frequent adverse reactions are lightheadedness and gastrointestinal disturbances including nausea, vomiting, and flatulence.
Overdosage: The toxic effects of acute overdosage of Fiorinal are attributable mainly to its barbiturate component, and, to a lesser extent, aspirin. Because toxic effects of caffeine occur in very high dosages only, the possibility of significant caffeine toxicity from Fiorinal

overdosage is unlikely. Symptoms attributable to *acute barbiturate poisoning* include drowsiness, confusion, and coma; respiratory depression; hypotension; shock. Symptoms attributable to *acute aspirin poisoning* include hyperpnea; acid-base disturbances with development of metabolic acidosis; vomiting and abdominal pain; tinnitus; hyperthermia; hypoprothrombinemia; restlessness; delirium; convulsions. *Acute caffeine poisoning* may cause insomnia, restlessness, tremor, and delirium; tachycardia and extrasystoles. *Treatment* consists primarily of management of barbiturate intoxication and the correction of the acid-base imbalance due to salicylism. Vomiting should be induced mechanically or with emetics in the conscious patient. Gastric lavage may be used if the pharyngeal and laryngeal reflexes are present and if less than four hours have elapsed since ingestion. A cuffed endotracheal tube should be inserted before gastric lavage of the unconscious patient and when necessary to provide assisted respiration. Diuresis, alkalinization of the urine, and correction of electrolyte disturbances should be accomplished through administration of intravenous fluids such as 1% sodium bicarbonate in 5% dextrose in water. Meticulous attention should be given to maintaining adequate pulmonary ventilation. Correction of hypotension may require the administration of levarterenol bitartrate or phenylephrine hydrochloride by intravenous infusion. In severe cases of intoxication, peritoneal dialysis, hemodialysis, or exchange transfusion may be lifesaving. Hypoprothrombinemia should be treated with Vitamin K, intravenously.

Dosage and Administration: One or two tablets or capsules every four hours. Total daily dose should not exceed six tablets or capsules.

How Supplied: Fiorinal Capsules: Color is dark green, with darker green band, in packages of 100 and 500. Also available in ControlPak® package, 25 capsules (continuous reverse numbered roll of sealed blisters). Fiorinal Tablets: Pale orange, compressed tablets 11 mm. diameter, 5.5 mm. thickness, in packages of 100 and 1000.

Company's Product Identification Mark(s): Tablets imprinted "FIORINAL" on one side, "SANDOZ" other side, and Capsules imprinted "FIORINAL" on one half of capsule and "SANDOZ 78-103" on other half.

[FIO-ZZ20 Issued December 15, 1982]

[Shown in Product Identification Section]

FIORINAL® with CODEINE Ⓒ
Capsules
No. 1, 2 and 3

The following prescribing information is based on official labeling in effect on November 1, 1982.

Composition: Each Fiorinal with Codeine *Capsule* contains: 50 mg Sandoptal® (butalbital, USP), (Warning: May be habit forming.) 40 mg caffeine, USP; and 325 mg aspirin, USP. In addition, Fiorinal with Codeine #1, #2, #3 also contain, respectively, codeine phosphate, USP 7.5 mg (1/8 gr.), 15 mg (1/4 gr.) and 30 mg (1/2 gr.). (Warning: May be habit forming.)

Indications: "Fiorinal with Codeine" raises the threshold of pain and discomfort and can be used in a great variety of painful conditions short of those which require morphine.

Action and Uses: Analgesic, antitussive, and antipyretic. The analgesic-sedative action of Fiorinal complements and increases the time-tested action of codeine. This enhanced analgesic-sedative effect is particularly well-suited for acute, short-range periods of pain and discomfort frequently seen in office practice. The formulation of "Fiorinal with Codeine" provides additional benefits for patients who have developed a cycle of pain, anxiety, tension which reinforces the pain experienced by the patients.

"Fiorinal with Codeine" is indicated for all types of pain associated with medical and surgical aftercare, postpartum pain, dysmenorrhea, neuritis, pleurisy, sciatica, neuralgia, sinusitis, pharyngitis, tonsillitis, otitis, febrile diseases, dental pain following extractions, headache, bursitis, arthritis, rheumatism, low back pain, dislocations, strains, sprains, fractures, etc. The analgesic, antitussive-antipyretic action of this product makes it particularly well-suited for the patient with upper respiratory infections such as acute colds, bronchitis, influenza, and pneumonia.

Contraindication: Hypersensitivity to any of the components.

Precaution: May be habit forming due to presence of codeine and barbiturate.

Side Effects: Nausea, vomiting, constipation, dizziness, skin rash, drowsiness, and miosis are possible side effects. Overdosage is primarily manifested by drowsiness.

Adult Dosage: 1 or 2 capsules, repeated if necessary up to 6 per day, or as directed by physician.

Supplied: Fiorinal with Codeine: 7.5 mg (1/8 gr) imprinted triangle (S) with F-C #1 on one half, SANDOZ 78-105 other half, color is red and yellow; 15 mg (1/4 gr) imprinted triangle (S) with F-C#2 on one half, SANDOZ 78-106 other half, color is gray and yellow; 30 mg (1/2 gr) imprinted triangle (S) with F-C#3 on one half; SANDOZ 78-107 other half, color is blue and yellow. In bottles of 100.

Fiorinal with Codeine No. 3 (1/2 gr) also in ControlPak® package, 25 capsules (continuous reverse numbered roll of sealed blisters).

Company's Product Identification Mark(s): All capsules imprinted triangle (S) with F-C #1, 2 and 3 on one half, SANDOZ plus NDC number other half.

[FWC-Z14 Issued October 1, 1982]

[Shown in Product Identification Section]

GYNERGEN® ℞
(ergotamine tartrate) tablets, USP

The following prescribing information is based on official labeling in effect on November 1, 1982.

Composition: Each Gynergen *Tablet* contains 1 mg ergotamine tartrate, USP.

Action and Uses: Long term usage has established the fact that Gynergen (ergotamine tartrate) is effective in controlling 90% of acute migraine attacks, so that it is now considered specific for the treatment of this headache syndrome. Being non-narcotic, it has the added virtue of avoiding the dangers inherent in the repeated use of narcotics in the treatment of frequently-recurring headache, such as migraine.

Indications: Vascular headache, e.g. migraine, histaminic cephalalgia (cluster headache).

Contraindications: Peripheral vascular disease, coronary heart disease, hypertension, impaired hepatic or renal function, sepsis, and pregnancy. Hypersensitivity.

Side Effects: Numbness and tingling of fingers and toes, muscle pains in the extremities, weakness in the legs, precordial distress and pain, transient tachycardia or bradycardia, nausea, vomiting, localized edema and itching.

Usual Dose: Average dose is 2 to 6 tablets per attack. Total weekly dosage should not exceed 10 tablets.

Supplied: Tablets (ivory gray, sugarcoated) in bottles of 100.

Company's Product Identification Mark(s): Tablets imprinted 78–48 on one side, SANDOZ other side.

[GYN-Z14 Issued September 30, 1980]

HYDERGINE® ℞
(ergoloid mesylates) tablets, USP (ORAL)
(ergoloid mesylates) tablets, USP (SUBLINGUAL)
(ergoloid mesylates) liquid

The following prescribing information is based on official labeling in effect on November 1, 1982.

Description:

Hydergine tablet 1 mg and **Hydergine sublingual tablet 1 mg,** each contains ergoloid mesylates USP as follows: dihydroergocornine mesylate 0.333 mg, dihydroergocristine mesylate 0.333 mg, and dihydroergocryptine (dihydro-alpha-ergocryptine and dihydro-beta-ergocryptine in the proportion of 2:1) mesylate 0.333 mg, representing a total of 1 mg.

Hydergine sublingual tablet 0.5 mg, each contains ergoloid mesylates USP as follows: dihydroergocornine mesylate 0.167 mg, dihydroergocristine mesylate 0.167 mg, and dihydroergocryptine (dihydro-alpha-ergocryptine and dihydro-beta-ergocryptine in the proportion of 2:1) mesylate 0.167 mg, representing a total of 0.5 mg.

Hydergine liquid 1mg/ml, each ml contains ergoloid mesylates USP as follows: dihydroergocornine mesylate 0.333 mg, dihydroergocristine mesylate 0.333 mg, and dihydroergocryptine (dihydro-alpha-ergocryptine and dihydro-beta-ergocryptine in the proportion of 2:1) mesylate 0.333 mg, representing a total of 1 mg; alcohol, USP, 30% by volume.

Pharmacokinetic Properties: Bioequivalence studies were performed in which Hydergine tablets were administered orally and Hydergine sublingual tablets were administered sublingually to human subjects. Hydergine tablets are rapidly but incompletely absorbed from the gastrointestinal tract. Following administration, the oral tablets resulted in slightly higher peak levels when compared to the sublingual dosage form. Hydergine substance undergoes a rapid first pass liver metabolism and less than 50% of the therapeutic moiety reaches the systemic circulation. The peak plasma levels of single, orally administered doses are achieved within one hour and by 24 hours the plasma levels are not detectable.

Actions: There is no specific evidence which clearly establishes the mechanism by which Hydergine tablets, sublingual tablets, and liquid produce mental effects, nor is there conclusive evidence that the drug particularly affects cerebral arteriosclerosis or cerebrovascular insufficiency.

Indications: A proportion of individuals over sixty who manifest signs and symptoms of an idiopathic decline in mental capacity (i.e., cognitive and interpersonal skills, mood, self-care, apparent motivation) can experience some symptomatic relief upon treatment with Hydergine preparations. The identity of the specific trait(s) or condition(s), if any, which would usefully predict a response to Hydergine therapy is not known. It appears, however, that those individuals who do respond come from groups of patients who would be considered clinically to suffer from some ill-defined process related to aging or to have some underlying dementing condition (i.e., primary progressive dementia, Alzheimer's dementia, senile onset, multi-infarct dementia).

Before prescribing Hydergine therapy, the physician should exclude the possibility that the patient's signs and symptoms arise from a potentially reversible and treatable condition. Particular care should be taken to exclude delirium and dementiform illness secondary to systemic disease, primary neurological disease, or primary disturbance of mood.

Hydergine® (ergoloid mesylates) preparations are not indicated in the treatment of acute or

Continued on next page

Sandoz—Cont.

chronic psychosis, regardless of etiology (see CONTRAINDICATIONS section).

The decision to use Hydergine therapy in the treatment of an individual with a symptomatic decline in mental capacity of unknown etiology should be continually reviewed since the presenting clinical picture may subsequently evolve sufficiently to allow a specific diagnosis and a specific alternative treatment. In addition, continued clinical evaluation is required to determine whether any initial benefit conferred by Hydergine therapy persists with time.

The efficacy of Hydergine therapy was evaluated using a special rating scale known as the SCAG (Sandoz Clinical-Assessment Geriatric). The specific items on this scale on which modest but statistically significant changes were observed at the end of twelve weeks include: mental alertness, confusion, recent memory, orientation, emotional lability, self-care, depression, anxiety/fears, cooperation, sociability, appetite, dizziness, fatigue, bothersome(-ness), and an overall impression of clinical status.

Contraindications: Hydergine tablets, sublingual tablets, and liquid are contraindicated in individuals who have previously shown hypersensitivity to the drug. Hydergine preparations are also contraindicated in patients who have psychosis, acute or chronic, regardless of etiology.

Precautions: *Practitioners are advised that because the target symptoms are of unknown etiology careful diagnosis should be attempted before prescribing Hydergine tablets, sublingual tablets, and liquid.*

Adverse Reactions: Hydergine tablets, sublingual tablets, and liquid have not been found to produce serious side effects. Some sublingual irritation, transient nausea, and gastric disturbances have been reported. Hydergine tablets, sublingual tablets, and liquid do not possess the vasoconstrictor properties of the natural ergot alkaloids.

Dosage and Administration: 1 mg three times daily.

Alleviation of symptoms is usually gradual and results may not be observed for 3–4 weeks.

How Supplied:

Hydergine tablets (for oral use):

1 mg, round, white, packages of 100 and 500.

Hydergine sublingual tablets:

1 mg, oval, white, packages of 100, & 1000.

0.5 mg, round, white, packages of 100 and 1000.

Hydergine liquid:

1 mg/ml. Bottles of 100 ml with an accompanying dropper graduated to deliver 1 mg.

Company's Product Identification Mark(s):

Hydergine oral tablets 1 mg embossed "HYDERGINE 1" on one side, triangle (S) other side.

Hydergine sublingual tablets 1 mg embossed "HYDERGINE" on one side, "78–77" other side.

Hydergine sublingual tablets 0.5 mg embossed "HYDERGINE 0.5" on one side, triangle (S) other side.

[HYG-ZZ20 Issued May 3, 1982]

[*Shown in Product Identification Section*]

MELLARIL® ℞

(thioridazine) HCl tablets, USP

(thioridazine) HCl oral solution, USP

MELLARIL-S®

(thioridazine) oral suspension, USP

The following prescribing information is based on official labeling in effect on November 1, 1982.

Description: Mellaril® (thioridazine) is 2-methylmercapto-10-[2- (N-methyl-2-piperidyl) ethyl] phenothiazine

The presence of a thiomethyl radical ($S\text{-}CH_3$) in position 2, conventionally occupied by a halogen, is unique and could account for the greater toleration obtained with recommended doses of thioridazine as well as a greater specificity of psychotherapeutic action.

Clinical Pharmacology: Mellaril (thioridazine) is effective in reducing excitement, hypermotility, abnormal initiative, affective tension and agitation through its inhibitory effect on psychomotor functions. Successful modification of such symptoms is the prerequisite for, and often the beginning of, the process of recovery in patients exhibiting mental and emotional disturbances.

Thioridazine's basic pharmacological activity is similar to that of other phenothiazines, but certain specific qualities have come to light which support the observation that the clinical spectrum of this drug shows significant differences from those of the other agents of this class. Minimal antiemetic activity and minimal extrapyramidal stimulation, notably pseudoparkinsonism, are distinctive features of this drug.

Indications: For the management of manifestations of psychotic disorders.

For the short-term treatment of moderate to marked depression with variable degrees of anxiety in adult patients and for the treatment of multiple symptoms such as agitation, anxiety, depressed mood, tension, sleep disturbances, and fears in geriatric patients.

For the treatment of severe behavioral problems in children marked by combativeness and/or explosive hyperexcitable behavior (out of proportion to immediate provocations), and in the short-term treatment of hyperactive children who show excessive motor activity with accompanying conduct disorders consisting of some or all of the following symptoms: impulsivity, difficulty sustaining attention, aggressivity, mood lability, and poor frustration tolerance.

Contraindications: In common with other phenothiazines, Mellaril (thioridazine) is contraindicated in severe central nervous system depression or comatose states from any cause. It should also be noted that hypertensive or hypotensive heart disease of extreme degree is a contraindication of phenothiazine administration.

Warnings: It has been suggested in regard to phenothiazines in general, that people who have demonstrated a hypersensitivity reaction (e.g. blood dyscrasias, jaundice) to one may be more prone to demonstrate a reaction to others. Attention should be paid to the fact that phenothiazines are capable of potentiating central nervous system depressants (e.g. anesthetics, opiates, alcohol, etc.) as well as atropine and phosphorus insecticides. Physicians should carefully consider benefit versus risk when treating less severe disorders.

Reproductive studies in animals and clinical experience to date have failed to show a teratogenic effect with Mellaril (thioridazine). However, in view of the desirability of keeping the administration of all drugs to a minimum during pregnancy, Mellaril (thioridazine) should be given only when the benefits derived from treatment exceed the possible risks to mother and fetus.

Precautions: Leukopenia and/or agranulocytosis and convulsive seizures have been reported but are infrequent. Mellaril (thioridazine) has been shown to be helpful in the treatment of behavioral disorders in epileptic patients, but anticonvulsant medication should also be maintained. Pigmentary retinopathy, which has been observed primarily in patients taking larger than recommended doses, is characterized by diminution of visual acuity, brownish coloring of vision, and impairment of night vision; examination of the fundus discloses deposits of pigment. The possibility of this complication may be reduced by remaining within the recommended limits of dosage. Where patients are participating in activities requiring complete mental alertness (e.g., driving) it is advisable to administer the phenothiazines cautiously and to increase the dosage gradually. Female patients appear to have a greater tendency to orthostatic hypotension than male patients. The administration of epinephrine should be avoided in the treatment of drug-induced hypotension in view of the fact that phenothiazines may induce a reversed epinephrine effect on occasion. Should a vasoconstrictor be required, the most suitable are levarterenol and phenylephrine.

Neuroleptic drugs elevate prolactin levels; the elevation persists during chronic administration. Tissue culture experiments indicate that approximately one-third of human breast cancers are prolactin dependent in vitro, a factor of potential importance if the prescription of these drugs is contemplated in a patient with a previously detected breast cancer. Although disturbances such as galactorrhea, amenorrhea, gynecomastia, and impotence have been reported, the clinical significance of elevated serum prolactin levels is unknown for most patients. An increase in mammary neoplasms has been found in rodents after chronic administration of neuroleptic drugs. Neither clinical studies nor epidemiologic studies conducted to date, however, have shown an association between chronic administration of these drugs and mammary tumorigenesis; the available evidence is considered too limited to be conclusive at this time.

It is recommended that a daily dose in excess of 300 mg. be reserved for use only in severe neuropsychiatric conditions.

Adverse Reactions: In the recommended dosage ranges with Mellaril (thioridazine), most side effects are mild and transient.

Central Nervous System: Drowsiness may be encountered on occasion, especially where large doses are given early in treatment. Generally, this effect tends to subside with continued therapy or a reduction in dosage. Pseudoparkinsonism and other extrapyramidal symptoms may occur but are infrequent. Nocturnal confusion, hyperactivity, lethargy, psychotic reactions, restlessness and headache have been reported but are extremely rare.

Autonomic Nervous System: Dryness of mouth, blurred vision, constipation, nausea, vomiting, diarrhea, nasal stuffiness, and pallor have been seen.

Endocrine System: Galactorrhea, breast engorgement, amenorrhea, inhibition of ejaculation, and peripheral edema have been described.

Skin: Dermatitis and skin eruptions of the urticarial type have been observed infrequently. Photosensitivity is extremely rare.

Cardiovascular System: ECG changes have been reported (see Phenothiazine Derivatives: Cardiovascular Effects).

Other: Rare cases described as parotid swelling have been reported following administration of Mellaril (thioridazine).

PHENOTHIAZINE DERIVATIVES: It should be noted that efficacy, indications and untoward effects have varied with the different phenothiazines. It has been reported that old age lowers the tolerance for phenothiazines. The most common neurological side effects in these patients are parkinsonism and akathisia. There appears to be an increased risk of agranulocytosis and leukopenia in the geriatric population. The physician should be aware that the following have occurred with one or more phenothiazines and should be considered whenever one of these drugs is used:

Autonomic Reactions: Miosis, obstipation, anorexia, paralytic ileus.

Cutaneous Reactions: Erythema, exfoliative dermatitis, contact dermatitis.

Blood Dyscrasias: Agranulocytosis, leukopenia, eosinophilia, thrombocytopenia, anemia, aplastic anemia, pancytopenia.

Allergic Reactions: Fever, laryngeal edema, angioneurotic edema, asthma.

Hepatotoxicity: Jaundice, biliary stasis.

Cardiovascular Effects: Changes in the terminal portion of the electrocardiogram, including prolongation of the Q-T interval, lowering and inversion of the T-wave and appearance of a wave tentatively identified as a bifid T or a U wave have been observed in some patients receiving the phenothiazine tranquilizers, including Mellaril (thioridazine). To date, these appear to be due to altered repolarization and not related to myocardial damage. They appear to be reversible. While there is no evidence at present that these changes are in any way precursors of any significant disturbance of cardiac rhythm, it should be noted that several sudden and unexpected deaths apparently due to cardiac arrest have occurred in patients previously showing characteristic electrocardiographic changes while taking the drug. The use of periodic electrocardiograms has been proposed but would appear to be of questionable value as a predictive device. Hypotension, rarely resulting in cardiac arrest.

Extrapyramidal Symptoms: Akathisia, agitation, motor restlessness, dystonic reactions, trismus, torticollis, opisthotonus, oculogyric crises, tremor, muscular rigidity, akinesia.

Persistent Tardive Dyskinesia: As with all antipsychotic agents, tardive dyskinesia may appear in some patients on long-term therapy or may occur after drug therapy has been discontinued. This risk seems to be greater in elderly patients on high-dose therapy, especially females. The symptoms are presistent and in some patients appear to be irreversible. The syndrome is characterized by rhythmical involuntary movements of the tongue, face, mouth or jaw (e.g., protrusion of tongue, puffing of cheeks, puckering of mouth, chewing movements). Sometimes these may be accompanied by involuntary movements of extremities.

There is no known effective treatment for tardive dyskinesia; anti-parkinsonism agents usually do not alleviate the symptoms of this syndrome. It is suggested that all antipsychotic agents be discontinued if these symptoms appear.

Should it be necessary to reinstitute treatment, or increase the dosage of the agent, or switch to a different antipsychotic agent, the syndrome may be masked.

It has been reported that fine vermicular movements of the tongue may be an early sign of the syndrome and if the medication is stopped at that time, the syndrome may not develop.

Endocrine Disturbances: Menstrual irregularities, altered libido, gynecomastia, lactation, weight gain, edema. False positive pregnancy tests have been reported.

Urinary Disturbances: Retention, incontinence.

Others: Hyperpyrexia. Behavioral effects suggestive of a paradoxical reaction have been reported. These include excitement, bizarre dreams, aggravation of psychoses, and toxic confusional states. More recently, a peculiar skin-eye syndrome has been recognized as a side effect following long-term treatment with phenothiazines. This reaction is marked by progressive pigmentation of areas of the skin or conjunctiva and/or accompanied by discoloration of the exposed sclera and cornea. Opacities of the anterior lens and cornea described as irregular or stellate in shape have also been reported. Systemic lupus erythematosus-like syndrome.

Dosage: Dosage must be individualized according to the degree of mental and emotional disturbance. In all cases, the smallest effective dosage should be determined for each patient.

ADULTS: *Psychotic manifestations:* The usual starting dose is 50 to 100 mg. three times a day, with a gradual increment to a maximum of 800 mg. daily if necessary. Once effective control of symptoms has been achieved, the dosage may be reduced gradually to determine the minimum maintenance dose. The total daily dosage ranges from 200 to 800 mg., divided into two to four doses.

For the short-term treatment of moderate to marked depression with variable degrees of anxiety in adult patients and for the treatment of multiple symptoms such as agitation, anxiety, depressed mood, tension, sleep disturbances, and fears in geriatric patients: The usual starting dose is 25 mg. three times a day. Dosage ranges from 10 mg. two to four times a day in milder cases to 50 mg. three or four times a day for more severely disturbed patients. The total daily dosage range is from 20 mg to a maximum of 200 mg.

CHILDREN: Mellaril (thioridazine) is not intended for children under 2 years of age. For children aged 2 to 12 the dosage of thioridazine hydrochloride ranges from 0.5 mg to a maximum of 3.0 mg/Kg per day. For children with moderate disorders 10 mg two or three times a day is the usual starting dose. For hospitalized, severely disturbed, or psychotic children, 25 mg two to three times daily is the usual starting dose. Dosage may be increased gradually until optimum therapeutic effect is obtained or the maximum has been reached.

Supplied:

MELLARIL (thioridazine) HCl

Tablets: 10 mg, 15 mg, 25 mg, 50 mg, 100 mg, 150 mg and 200 mg thioridazine hydrochloride, USP. Packages of 100 and 1000 tablets. Also, for wholly tax-supported institutions only, packages of 4800 (48 × 100) and 5000 tablets.

Concentrate—30 mg/ml: Each ml contains 30 mg thioridazine hydrochloride, USP, alcohol, USP, 3.0% by volume. Immediate containers: Amber glass bottles of 4 fl. oz (118 ml) as follows:

4 fl. oz bottles, in cartons of 12 bottles, with an accompanying dropper graduated to deliver 10 mg, 25 mg and 50 mg of thioridazine hydrochloride, USP. Also, for wholly tax-supported institutions only, gallon cartons of 32 x 4 oz. bottles, each with the same dropper.

Concentrate—100 mg/ml: Each ml contains 100 mg thioridazine hydrochloride, USP, alcohol, 4.2% by volume, *4 fl. oz bottles,* in cartons of 12 bottles, with an accompanying dropper graduated to deliver 100 mg, 150 mg and 200 mg of thioridazine hydrochloride.

Remarks: Store and dispense: Below 86°F; tight, amber glass bottle.

The Concentrate may be diluted with distilled water, acidified tap water, or suitable juices. Each dose should be so diluted just prior to administration—preparation and storage of bulk dilutions is not recommended.

MELLARIL-S (thioridazine)

Suspension—25 mg/5 ml: Each 5 ml contains thioridazine, USP, equivalent to 25 mg thioridazine hydrochloride, USP. Buttermint-flavored in pint bottles.

Suspension—100 mg/5 ml: Each 5 ml contains thioridazine, USP, equivalent to 100 mg thioridazine hydrochloride, USP. Buttermint-flavored in pint bottles.

Company's Product Identification Mark(s): 10 mg and 15 mg tablets branded with NDC number on one side, triangle (S) other side. All other tablet strengths branded MELLARIL on one side, triangle (S) other side.

[MEL-Z35 Issued May 5, 1982]

[*Shown in Product Identification Section*]

MESANTOIN® Tablets ℞
(mephenytoin) tablets, USP

The following prescribing information is based on official labeling in effect on November 1, 1982.

Description: Mesantoin® (mephenytoin) is 3- methyl 5,5-phenyl-ethyl-hydantoin. It may be considered to be the hydantoin homolog of the barbiturate mephobarbital.

Actions: Mephenytoin exhibits pharmacologic effects similar to both diphenylhydantoin and the barbiturates in antagonizing experimental seizures in laboratory animals. Mephenytoin produces behavioral and electroencephalographic effects in man which are similar to those produced by barbiturates.

Indications: For the control of grand mal, focal, Jacksonian, and psychomotor seizures in those patients who have been refractory to less toxic anticonvulsants.

Contraindications: Hypersensitivity to hydantoin products.

Warnings: Mephenytoin should be used only after safer anticonvulsants have been given an adequate trial and have failed.

As with all anticonvulsants, dose reduction must be gradual so as to minimize the risk of precipitating seizures.

Patients should be cautioned about possible additive effects of alcohol and other CNS depressants. Acute alcohol intoxication may increase the anticonvulsant effect due to decreased metabolic breakdown. Chronic alcohol abuse may result in decreased anticonvulsant effect due to enzyme induction.

Usage in Pregnancy: The effects of mephenytoin in human pregnancy and nursing infants are unknown.

Recent reports suggest an association between the use of anticonvulsant drugs by women with epilepsy and an elevated incidence of birth defects in children born to these women. Data are more extensive with respect to diphenylhydantoin and phenobarbital, but these are also the most commonly prescribed anticonvulsants; less systematic or anecdotal reports suggest a possible similar association with the use of all known anticonvulsant drugs.

The reports suggesting an elevated incidence of birth defects in children of drug-treated epileptic women cannot be regarded as adequate to prove a definite cause and effect relationship. There are intrinsic methodologic problems in obtaining adequate data on drug teratogenicity in humans; the possibility also exists that other factors, e.g., genetic factors or the epileptic condition itself, may be more important than drug therapy in leading to birth defects. The great majority of mothers on anticonvulsant medication deliver normal infants. It is important to note than anticonvulsant drugs should not be discontinued in patients in whom the drug is administered to prevent major seizures because of the strong possibility of precipitating status epilepticus with attendant hypoxia and threat to life. In individual cases where the severity and frequency of the seizure disorder are such that the removal of medication does not pose a serious threat to the patient, discontinuation of the drug may be considered prior to and during pregnancy, although it cannot be said with any confidence that even minor seizures do not pose some hazards to the developing embryo or fetus.

The prescribing physician will wish to weigh these considerations in treating or counseling epileptic women of child-bearing potential.

Precautions: The patient taking Mesantoin (mephenytoin) must be kept under close medical supervision at all times since serious adverse reactions may emerge.

Because the primary site of degradation is the liver, it is recommended that screening tests of liver function precede introduction of the drug. Some patients may show side reactions as the result of individual sensitivity. These reactions can be broken down into three types respectively according to severity: 1) blood dyscrasias; 2) skin and mucous membrane manifestations; and 3) central effects. The blood, skin and mucous membrane manifestations are the more important since they can be more serious in nature. Since mephenytoin has been reported to produce blood dyscrasia in certain instances, the patient must be instructed that in the event any unusual symptoms develop (e.g. sore throat, fever, mucous membrane

Continued on next page

Sandoz—Cont.

bleeding, glandular swelling, cutaneous reaction), he must discontinue the drug and report for examination immediately. It is recommended that blood examinations be made (total white cell count and differential count) during the initial phase of administration. Such tests are best made: a) before starting medication; b) after 2 weeks on a low dosage; c) again after 2 weeks when full dosage is reached; d) thereafter, monthly for a year; e) from then on, every 3 months. If the neutrophils drop to between 2500 and 1600/cu.mm., counts are made every 2 weeks. Stop medication if the count drops to 1600.

Adverse Reactions: A number of side effects and toxic reactions have been reported with Mesantoin (mephenytoin) as well as with other hydantoin compounds. Many of these appear to be dose related while others seem to be a manifestation of a hypersensitivity reaction to these drugs.

Blood Dyscrasias
Leukopenia, neutropenia, agranulocytosis, thrombocytopenia and pancytopenia have occurred. Eosinophilia, monocytosis, and leukocytosis have been described. Simple anemia, hemolytic anemia, megaloblastic anemia and aplastic anemia have occurred but are uncommon.

Skin and Mucous Membrane Manifestations
Maculopapular, morbilliform, scarlatiniform, urticarial, purpuric (associted with thrombocytopenia) and non-specific skin rashes have been reported. Exfoliative dermatitis, erythema multiforme (Stevens-Johnson Syndrome), toxic epidermal necrolysis and fatal dermatitides have been described on rare occasions. Skin pigmentation and rashes associated with a lupus erythematosus syndrome have also been reported.

Central Effects
Drowsiness is dose-related and may be reduced by a reduction in dose. Ataxia, diplopia, nystagmus, dysarthria, fatigue, irritability, choreiform movements, depression and tremor have been encountered.
Nervousness, nausea, vomiting, sleeplessness and dizziness may occur during the initial stages of therapy. Generally, these symptoms are transient, often disappearing with continued treatment.
Mental confusion and psychotic disturbances and increased seizures have been reported, but a definite causal relationship with the drug is uncertain.

Miscellaneous
Hepatitis, jaundice and nephrosis have been reported but a definite cause and effect relationship between the drug and these effects has not been established.
Alopecia, weight gain, edema, photophobia, conjunctivitis and gum hyperplasia have been encountered.
Polyarthropathy, pulmonary fibrosis, lupus erythematosus syndrome, and lymphadenopathy which simulates Hodgkin's Disease have also been observed.

Dosage and Administration: Dosage of antiepileptic therapy should be adjusted to the needs of the individual patient. Maintenance dosage is that smallest amount of antiepileptic necessary to suppress seizures completely or reduce their frequency. Optimum dosage is attained by starting with ½ or 1 tablet of Mesantoin (mephenytoin) per day during the first week and thereafter increasing the daily dose by ½ or 1 tablet at weekly intervals. No dose should be increased until it has been taken for at least one week.
The average dose of Mesantoin for adults ranges from 2 to 6 tablets (0.2 to 0.6 Gm) daily. In some instances it may be necessary to administer as much as 8 tablets or more daily in order to obtain full seizure control. Children usually require from 1 to 4 tablets (0.1 Gm to 0.4 Gm) according to nature of seizures and age.
When the physician wishes to replace the anticonvulsant now being employed with Mesantoin (mephenytoin), he should give ½ or 1 tablet of Mesantoin daily during the first week and gradually increase the daily dose at weekly intervals while gradually reducing that of the drug being discontinued. The transition can be made smoothly over a period of three to six weeks. If seizures are not completely controlled with the dose so attained, the daily dose should then be increased by a one-tablet increment at weekly intervals to the point of maximum effect. If the patient had also been receiving phenobarbital, it is well to continue it until the transition is completed, at which time gradual withdrawal of the phenobarbital may be tried.

How Supplied: Each tablet contains 100 mg mephenytoin and is scored to permit half-tablet dosage. Packages of 100 and 1,000 tablets. (Pale pink, compressed, scored).

Company's Product Identification Mark(s): Tablets embossed 78-52 and scored on one side, SANDOZ triangle S on other side.

[MES—Z13 Issued November 14, 1980]

[Shown in Product Identification Section]

METHERGINE® ℞

(methylergonovine maleate) injection, USP
(methylergonovine maleate) tablets, USP

The following prescribing information is based on official labeling in effect on November 1, 1982.

Description: Each Methergine *Tablet* contains 0.2 mg (1/320 gr.) methylergonovine maleate, USP Methergine *Injection* contains per ml: 0.2 mg (1/320 gr.) methylergonovine maleate, USP; 0.25 mg tartaric acid, NF; 3 mg sodium chloride, USP; and water for injection, USP, q.s. to 1 ml.

Actions: Methergine induces a rapid and sustained tetanic uterotonic effect which shortens the third stage of labor and reduces blood loss. The onset of action after i.v. administration is immediate; after i.m. administration, 2 to 5 minutes, and after oral administration, 5 to 10 minutes.

Indications: For routine management after delivery of the placenta; postpartum atony and hemorrhage; subinvolution. Under full obstetric supervision, it may be given in the second stage of labor following delivery of the anterior shoulder.

Contraindications: Hypertension; toxemia; pregnancy; and hypersensitivity.

Warning: This drug should not be administered i.v. routinely because of the possibility of inducing sudden hypertensive and cerebrovascular accidents. If i.v. administration is considered essential as a lifesaving measure, Methergine should be given slowly over a period of no less than 60 seconds with careful monitoring of blood pressure.

Precautions: Caution should be exercised in the presence of sepsis, obliterative vascular disease, hepatic or renal involvement.

Adverse Reactions: Nausea; vomiting; transient hypertension; dizziness; headache; tinnitus; diaphoresis and palpitation; temporary chest pain; and dyspnea.

Dosage and Administration: Intramuscularly: One ml, 0.2 mg (1/320 grain) after delivery of the anterior shoulder, after delivery of the placenta, or during the puerperium. May be repeated as required, at intervals of 2-4 hours. *Intravenously: SEE WARNING SECTION.* Dosage same as intramuscular. *Orally:* One tablet, 0.2 milligram (1/320 grain) 3 or 4 times daily in the puerperium for a maximum of 1 week.

How Supplied: Tablets in packages of 100 and 1000; Injection in 1 ml ampuls, boxes of 20 and 100.

Remarks: Methergine injection is a clear and colorless solution. In the event the ampul solution becomes discolored, it should not be used.

Company's Product Identification Mark(s): Tablets imprinted 78-54 on 1 side, SANDOZ other side.

[Met-Z14 Issued September 2, 1980]

[Shown in Product Identification Section]

PAMELOR® ℞

(nortriptyline HCl), capsules, USP
(nortriptyline HCl) oral solution, USP

The following prescribing information is based on official labeling in effect on November 1, 1982.

Description: Pamelor® (nortriptyline HCl) is 5-(3-methylaminopropylidene)-10, 11-dihydro-5H-dibenzo [a,d] cycloheptene hydrochloride. Its molecular weight is 299.8, and its empirical formula is $C_{19}H_{21}N \cdot HCl$.

Actions: The mechanism of mood elevation by tricyclic antidepressants is at present unknown. Pamelor is not a monoamine oxidase inhibitor. It inhibits the activity of such diverse agents as histamine, 5-hydroxytryptamine, and acetylcholine. It increases the pressor effect of norepinephrine but blocks the pressor response of phenethylamine. Studies suggest that Pamelor interferes with the transport, release, and storage of catecholamines. Operant conditioning techniques in rats and pigeons suggest that Pamelor has a combination of stimulant and depressant properties.

Indications: Pamelor is indicated for the relief of symptoms of depression. Endogenous depressions are more likely to be alleviated than are other depressive states.

Contraindications: The use of Pamelor or other tricyclic antidepressants concurrently with a monoamine oxidase (MAO) inhibitor is contraindicated. Hyperpyretic crises, severe convulsions, and fatalities have occurred when similar tricyclic antidepressants were used in such combinations. It is advisable to have discontinued the MAO inhibitor for at least two weeks before treatment with Pamelor is started. Patients hypersensitive to Pamelor should not be given the drug.
Cross-sensitivity between Pamelor and other dibenzazepines is a possibility.
Pamelor is contraindicated during the acute recovery period after myocardial infarction.

Warnings: Patients with cardiovascular disease should be given Pamelor only under close supervision because of the tendency of the drug to produce sinus tachycardia and to prolong the conduction time. Myocardial infarction, arrhythmia, and strokes have occurred. The antihypertensive action of guanethidine and similar agents may be blocked. Because of its anticholinergic activity, Pamelor should be used with great caution in patients who have glaucoma or a history of urinary retention. Patients with a history of seizures should be followed closely when Pamelor is administered, inasmuch as this drug is known to lower the convulsive threshold. Great care is required if Pamelor is given to hyperthyroid patients or to those receiving thyroid medication, since cardiac arrhythmias may develop.
Pamelor may impair the mental and/or physical abilities required for the performance of hazardous tasks, such as operating machinery or driving a car; therefore, the patient should be warned accordingly.
Excessive consumption of alcohol in combination with nortriptyline therapy may have a potentiating effect, which may lead to the danger of increased suicidal attempts or overdosage, especially in patients with histories of emotional disturbances or suicidal ideation.
Use in Pregnancy—Safe use of Pamelor during pregnancy and lactation has not been established; therefore, when the drug is administered to pregnant patients, nursing mothers, or

women of childbearing potential, the potential benefits must be weighed against the possible hazards. Animal reproduction studies have yielded inconclusive results.

Use in Children—This drug is not recommended for use in children, since safety and effectiveness in the pediatric age group have not been established.

Precautions: The use of Pamelor in schizophrenic patients may result in an exacerbation of the psychosis or may activate latent schizophrenic symptoms. If the drug is given to overactive or agitated patients, increased anxiety and agitation may occur. In manic-depressive patients, Pamelor may cause symptoms of the manic phase to emerge.

Administration of reserpine during therapy with a tricyclic antidepressant has been shown to produce a "stimulating" effect in some depressed patients.

Troublesome patient hostility may be aroused by the use of Pamelor. Epileptiform seizures may accompany its administration, as is true of other drugs of its class.

Close supervision and careful adjustment of the dosage are required when Pamelor is used with other anticholinergic drugs and sympathomimetic drugs.

The patient should be informed that the response to alcohol may be exaggerated.

When it is essential, the drug may be administered with electroconvulsive therapy, although the hazards may be increased. Discontinue the drug for several days, if possible, prior to elective surgery.

The possibility of a suicidal attempt by a depressed patient remains after the initiation of treatment; in this regard, it is important that the least possible quantity of drug be dispensed at any given time.

Both elevation and lowering of blood sugar levels have been reported.

Adverse Reactions: Note: Included in the following list are a few adverse reactions that have not been reported with this specific drug. However, the pharmacologic similarities among the tricyclic antidepressant drugs require that each of the reactions be considered when nortriptyline is administered.

Cardiovascular—Hypotension, hypertension, tachycardia, palpitation, myocardial infarction, arrhythmias, heart block, stroke.

Psychiatric—Confusional states (especially in the elderly) with hallucinations, disorientation, delusions; anxiety, restlessness, agitation; insomnia, panic, nightmares; hypomania; exacerbation of psychosis.

Neurologic—Numbness, tingling, paresthesias of extremities; incoordination, ataxia, tremors; peripheral neuropathy; extrapyramidal symptoms; seizures, alteration in EEG patterns; tinnitus.

Anticholinergic—Dry mouth and, rarely, associated sublingual adenitis; blurred vision, disturbance of accommodation, mydriasis; constipation, paralytic ileus; urinary retention, delayed micturition, dilation of the urinary tract.

Allergic—Skin rash, petechiae, urticaria, itching, photosensitization (avoid excessive exposure to sunlight); edema (general or of face and tongue), drug fever, cross-sensitivity with other tricyclic drugs.

Hematologic—Bone-marrow depression, including agranulocytosis; eosinophilia; purpura; thrombocytopenia.

Gastrointestinal—Nausea and vomiting, anorexia, epigastric distress, diarrhea, peculiar taste, stomatitis, abdominal cramps, black-tongue.

Endocrine—Gynecomastia in the male, breast enlargement and galactorrhea in the female; increased or decreased libido, impotence; testicular swelling; elevation or depression of blood sugar levels.

Other—Jaundice (simulating obstructive); altered liver function; weight gain or loss; perspiration; flushing; urinary frequency, nocturia; drowsiness, dizziness, weakness, fatigue; headache; parotid swelling; alopecia.

Withdrawal Symptoms—Though these are not indicative of addiction, abrupt cessation of treatment after prolonged therapy may produce nausea, headache, and malaise.

Dosage and Administration: Pamelor is not recommended for children.

Pamelor is administered orally in the form of capsules or liquid. Lower than usual dosages are recommended for elderly patients and adolescents. Lower dosages are also recommended for outpatients than for hospitalized patients who will be under close supervision. The physician should initiate dosage at a low level and increase it gradually, noting carefully the clinical response and any evidence of intolerance.

Following remission, maintenance medication may be required for a longer period of time at the lowest dose that will maintain remission.

If a patient develops minor side-effects, the dosage should be reduced. The drug should be discontinued promptly if adverse effects of a serious nature or allergic manifestations occur.

Usual Adult Dose—25 mg three or four times daily; dosage should begin at a low level and be increased as required. As an alternate regimen, the total daily dosage may be given once-a-day. When doses above 100 mg daily are administered, plasma levels of nortriptyline should be monitored and maintained in the optimum range of 50-150 ng/ml. Doses above 150 mg per day are not recommended.

Elderly and Adolescent Patients—30 to 50 mg per day, in divided doses, or the total daily dosage may be given once-a-day.

Overdosage: Toxic overdosage may result in confusion, restlessness, agitation, vomiting, hyperpyrexia, muscle rigidity, hyperactive reflexes, tachycardia, ECG evidence of impaired conduction, shock, congestive heart failure, stupor, coma, and C.N.S. stimulation with convulsions followed by respiratory depression. Deaths have occurred following overdosage with drugs of this class.

No specific antidote is known. General supportive measures are indicated, with gastric lavage. Respiratory assistance is apparently the most effective measure when indicated. The use of C.N.S. depressants may worsen the prognosis.

The administration of barbiturates for control of convulsions alleviates an increase in the cardiac work load but should be undertaken with caution to avoid potentiation of respiratory depression.

Intramuscular paraldehyde or diazepam provides anticonvulsant activity with less respiratory depression than do the barbiturates; diazepam seems to be preferred.

The use of digitalis and/or physostigmine may be considered in case of serious cardiovascular abnormalities or cardiac failure.

The value of dialysis has not been established.

How Supplied:

Solution: Pamelor (nortriptyline HCl) USP, equivalent to 10 mg base per 5 ml is supplied in 16-fluid-ounce bottles. Alcohol content 4%.

Capsules: Pamelor (nortriptyline HCl) USP, equivalent to 10 mg, 25 mg and 75 mg base, are supplied in bottles of 100. The 10 mg and 25 mg capsules are available in boxes of 100 individually labeled blisters, each containing 1 capsule. The 25 mg capsules are also available in bottles of 500.

[PAM-Z8 Issued April 15, 1982]

[*Shown in Product Identification Section*]

PARLODEL® ℞

(bromocriptine mesylate) tablets, USP
(bromocriptine mesylate) capsules

The following prescribing information is based on official labeling in effect November 1, 1982.

Description: Parlodel® (bromocriptine mesylate) is a potent dopamine receptor agonist that inhibits prolactin secretion. This activity represents a new therapeutic use for specific peptide ergot alkaloid derivatives. Each Parlodel (bromocriptine mesylate) tablet for oral administration contains 2½ mg and each capsule contains 5 mg bromocriptine (as the mesylate). Parlodel (bromocriptine mesylate) is chemically designated as (1) Ergotaman-3',-6',18-trione,2-bromo-12'-hydroxy-2'- (1-methylethyl) -5'- (2-methylpropyl)-,(5'α) monomethanesulfonate (salt); (2) 2-bromoergocryptine monomethanesulfonate (salt).*

*U.S. Pat. Nos. 3,752,814 and 3,752,888

Clinical Pharmacology: Parlodel (bromocriptine mesylate) is a dopamine receptor agonist, which activates post-synaptic dopamine receptors. The dopaminergic neurons in the tuberoinfundibular process modulate the secretion of prolactin from the anterior pituitary by secreting a prolactin inhibitory factor (thought to be dopamine); in the corpus striatum the dopaminergic neurons are involved in the control of motor function. Clinically, Parlodel (bromocriptine mesylate) has been shown to significantly reduce plasma levels of prolactin in patients with hyperprolactinemia. Pharmacologic experiments have demonstrated the efficacy and selectivity of bromocriptine in inhibiting prolactin secretion in several mammalian species under various experimental conditions. Studies have shown that bromocriptine suppresses physiological lactation in several species as well as galactorrhea in pathological hyperprolactinemic states at dose levels that do not affect other tropic hormones from the anterior pituitary. Experiments have demonstrated that bromocriptine induces long lasting stereotyped behavior in rodents and turning behavior in rats having unilateral lesions in the substantia nigra. These actions, characteristic of those produced by dopamine, are inhibited by dopamine antagonists and suggest a direct action of bromocriptine on striatal dopamine receptors.

Parlodel (bromocriptine mesylate) is a nonhormonal, nonestrogenic agent which inhibits the secretion of prolactin in humans, with little or no effect on other pituitary hormones, except in patients with acromegaly, where it lowers elevated blood levels of growth hormone.

In about 75% of cases of galactorrhea associated with amenorrhea, in the absence of demonstrable pituitary tumor, Palodel (bromocriptine mesylate) therapy suppresses the galactorrhea completely, or almost completely, and reinitiates normal ovulatory menstrual cycles.

Menses are usually reinitiated prior to complete suppression of galactorrhea; the time for this on average is 6–8 weeks. However, some patients respond within a few days.

Galactorrhea may take longer to control depending on the degree of stimulation of the mammary tissue prior to therapy. At least a 75% reduction in secretion is usually observed after 8–12 weeks. Some patients may fail to respond even after 24 weeks of therapy.

Parlodel (bromocriptine mesylate), by virtue of its ability to inhibit prolactin secretion, acts to prevent physiological lactation in women when therapy is started after delivery and continued for two to three weeks. There is no evidence that Parlodel (bromocriptine mesylate) acts on the mammary tissues to prevent lactation, as is the case with estrogen-containing preparations.

Parlodel (bromocriptine mesylate) produces its therapeutic effect in the treatment of Parkinson's disease, a clinical condition characterized by a progressive deficiency in dopamine synthesis in the substantia nigra, by directly stimulating the dopamine receptors in the corpus striatum. In contrast, levodopa exerts its therapeutic effect only after conversion to dopamine by the neurons of the substantia nigra,

Continued on next page

Sandoz—Cont.

which are known to be numerically diminished in this patient population.

Pharmacokinetics: The pharmacokinetics and metabolism of bromocriptine in human subjects were studied with the help of radioactively labeled drug. 28% of an oral dose was absorbed from the gastrointestinal tract. The blood levels following a 2½ mg dose were in the range of 2–3 ng equivalents/ml. Plasma levels were in the range of 4–6 ng equivalents/ml indicating that the red blood cells did not contain appreciable amounts of drug and /or metabolites. *In vitro* experiments showed that the drug was 90–96% bound to serum albumin.

Bromocriptine was completely metabolized prior to excretion. The major route of excretion of absorbed drug was via the bile. Only 2.5–5.5% of the dose was excreted in the urine. Almost all (84.6%) of the administered dose was excreted in the feces in 120 hours.

Indications and Usage:

Amenorrhea/Galactorrhea

Parlodel (bromocriptine mesylate), a dopamine receptor agonist, is indicated for the short-term treatment of amenorrhea/galactorrhea associated with hyperprolactinemia due to varied etiologies, excluding demonstrable pituitary tumors. It is not indicated in patients with normal prolactin levels.

Female Infertility

Parlodel (bromocriptine mesylate) tablets are indicated in the treatment of female infertility associated with hyperprolactinemia in the absence of a demonstrable pituitary tumor.

Prevention of Physiological Lactation

Parlodel (bromocriptine mesylate) tablets are indicated for the prevention of physiological lactation, (secretion, congestion, and engorgement) occurring:

1. After parturition when the mother elects not to breast feed the infant, or when breast feeding is contraindicated.
2. After stillbirth or abortion.

The physician should keep in mind that the incidence of significant painful engorgement is low and usually responsive to appropriate supportive therapy. In contrast with supportive therapy, Parlodel (bromocriptine mesylate) prevents the secretion of prolactin, thus inhibiting lactogenesis and the subsequent development of secretion, congestion and engorgement.

Once Parlodel (bromocriptine mesylate) therapy is stopped, 18% to 40% of patients experience rebound of breast secretion, congestion or engorgement, which is usually mild to moderate in severity.

Parkinson's Disease

Parlodel (bromocriptine mesylate) tablets or capsules are indicated in the treatment of the signs and symptoms of idiopathic or postencephalitic Parkinson's disease. As adjunctive treatment to levodopa (alone or with a peripheral decarboxylase inhibitor), Parlodel (bromocriptine mesylate) therapy may provide additional therapeutic benefits in those patients who are currently maintained on optimal dosages of levodopa, those who are beginning to deteriorate (develop tolerance) to levodopa therapy, and those who are experiencing "end of dose failure" on levodopa therapy. Parlodel (bromocriptine mesylate) may permit a reduction of the maintenance dose of levodopa and, thus may ameliorate the occurence and/or severity of adverse reactions associated with long-term levodopa therapy such as abnormal involuntary movements (e.g. dyskinesias) and the marked swings in motor function ("on-off" phenomenon). Continued efficacy of Parlodel (bromocriptine mesylate) during treatment of more than two years has not been established. Data are insufficient to evaluate potential benefit from treating newly diagnosed Parkinson's disease with Parlodel (bromocriptine mesylate). Studies have shown, however, significantly more adverse reactions (notably nausea, hallucinations, confusion and hypotension) in Parlodel (bromocriptine mesylate) treated patients than in levodopa/carbidopa treated patients. Patients unresponsive to levodopa are poor candidates for Parlodel (bromocriptine mesylate) therapy.

Contraindications: Sensitivity to any ergot alkaloids.

Warnings: Since hyperprolactinemia with amenorrhea/galactorrhea and infertility has been found in patients with pituitary tumors (Forbes-Albright syndrome), a complete evaluation of the sella turcica is indicated before treatment with Parlodel (bromocriptine mesylate). Although Parlodel (bromocriptine mesylate) therapy will effectively lower plasma levels of prolactin in patients with pituitary tumors, this does not obviate the necessity of radiotherapy or surgical procedures where appropriate.

If pregnancy occurs during Parlodel (bromocriptine mesylate) administration, treatment should be discontinued immediately. Careful observation of these patients throughout pregnancy is mandatory. Small prolactin-secreting adenomas not detected previously may rapidly increase in size during pregnancy. Optic nerve compression may occur and emergency pituitary surgery or other appropriate measures may be necessary.

Symptomatic hypotension can occur in patients treated with Parlodel (bromocriptine mesylate) for any indication.

In postpartum studies with Parlodel, decreases in supine systolic and diastolic pressures of greater than 20 mm and 10 mm Hg, respectively, have been observed in almost 30% of patients receiving Parlodel (bromocriptine mesylate). On occasion, the drop in supine systolic pressure was as much as 50–59 mm of Hg. Since decreases in blood pressure are frequently noted during the puerperium independent of drug therapy, it is likely that many of these decreases in blood pressure observed with Parlodel (bromocriptine mesylate) therapy were not drug induced. **However, Parlodel (bromocriptine mesylate) is known to cause hypotension in some patients; therefore, Parlodel (bromocriptine mesylate) therapy for prevention of postpartum lactation should not be initiated until the vital signs have been stabilized and no sooner than four hours after delivery.** Periodic monitoring of the blood pressure, particularly during the first few days of therapy, is advisable. Furthermore, care should be exercised when Parlodel (bromocriptine mesylate) is administered concomitantly with other medications known to lower blood pressure.

In clinical trials for the treatment of patients with amenorrhea/galactorrhea or for the prevention of postpartum lactation, dizziness (8–16%) and syncope (less than 1%) have been reported in patients receiving Parlodel. Dizziness (9%) drowsiness (8%) and faintness/fainting (8%) have also been reported in patients treated with Parlodel (bromocriptine mesylate) for Parkinson's disease. Therefore, patients receiving this drug should be cautioned with regard to engaging in activities requiring rapid and precise responses, such as driving an automobile or operating machinery.

Long-term treatment (6–36 months) with Parlodel (bromocriptine mesylate) in doses ranging from 20–100 mg/day has been associated with pulmonary infiltrates, pleural effusion and thickening of the pleura in a few patients. In most instances in which Parlodel treatment was terminated, the changes slowly reverted towards normal.

Precautions: Safety and efficacy of Parlodel (bromocriptine mesylate) have not been established in patients with renal or hepatic disease. Phenothiazines should be avoided during Parlodel (bromocriptine mesylate) therapy. Care should be exercised when administering Parlodel (bromocriptine mesylate) therapy concomitantly with other medications known to lower blood pressure.

Amenorrhea/Galactorrhea

Treatment of women suffering from amenorrhea/galactorrhea with Parlodel (bromocriptine mesylate) may result in restoration of fertility. Therefore, patients who do not desire pregnancy should be advised to use contraceptive measures, other than the oral contraceptives, during treatment with Parlodel (bromocriptine mesylate). Since pregnancy may occur prior to reinitiation of menses, as an additional precaution, a pregnancy test is recommended at least every four weeks during the amenorrheic period, and, once menses are reinitiated, every time a patient misses a menstrual period.

Parlodel (bromocriptine mesylate) therapy has been demonstrated to be effective in the short-term management of amenorrhea/galactorrhea. Data are not available on the safety or effectiveness of its use in long-term continuous dosage, or in patients given repeated courses of treatment following recurrence of amenorrhea/galactorrhea after initial treatment. Recurrence rates are reportedly very high, ranging from 70 to 80% in domestic and foreign studies.

Female Infertility

Treatment of patients with Parlodel (bromocriptine mesylate) tablets should be discontinued as soon as the diagnosis of pregnancy has been established. Patients must be monitored closely throughout pregnancy for signs and symptoms which may develop if a previously undetected prolactin-secreting tumor enlarges.

Physiological Lactation

Decreases in blood pressure are common during the puerperium and, since Parlodel therapy is known to produce hypotension in some patients, the drug should not be administered until the vital signs have been stabilized.

Parkinson's Disease

Safety during long-term use for more than two years at the doses required for parkinsonism has not been established.

As with any chronic therapy, periodic evaluation of hepatic, hematopoietic, cardiovascular, and renal function is recommended. Symptomatic hypotension can occur and therefore caution should be exercised when treating patients receiving antihypertensive drugs.

High doses of Parlodel (bromocriptine mesylate) may be associated with confusion and mental disturbances. Since parkinsonian patients may manifest mild degrees of dementia, caution should be used when treating such patients.

Parlodel (bromocriptine mesylate) administered alone or concomitantly with levodopa may cause hallucinations (visual or auditory). Hallucinations usually resolve with dosage reduction; occasionally, discontinuation of Parlodel (bromocriptine mesylate) is required. Rarely, after high doses, hallucinations have persisted for several weeks following discontinuation of Parlodel (bromocriptine mesylate).

As with levodopa, caution should be exercised when administering Parlodel (bromocriptine mesylate) to patients with a history of myocardial infarction who have a residual atrial, nodal, or ventricular arrhythmia.

Nursing Mothers

Since it prevents lactation, Parlodel (bromocriptine mesylate) should not be administered to mothers who elect to breast feed their offspring.

Pediatric Use

Safety and efficacy of Parlodel (bromocriptine mesylate) have not been established in children under the age of 15.

Use in Pregnancy

In human studies with Parlodel (bromocriptine mesylate) there have been 1276 reported pregnancies, which have yield 1109 live and 4 stillborn infants from women who took Parlodel (bromocriptine mesylate) during early pregnancy. Among the 1113 infants, 37 cases of congenital anomalies have been reported. There were 9 major malformations which included 3 limb reduction defects and 28 minor malformations which included 8 hip dislocations. The total incidence of malformations (3.3%) and the incidence of spontaneous abortions (11%) in this group of pregnancies does not exceed that generally reported for such occurrences in the population at large. There were three hydatidiform moles, two of which occurred in the same patient.

Adverse Reactions:

Amenorrhea/Galactorrhea/Female Infertility

The incidence of adverse effects is quite high (68%) but these are generally mild to moderate in degree. Therapy was discontinued in approximately 6% of patients because of adverse effects. These in decreasing order of frequency are: nausea 51%, headache 18%, dizziness 16%, fatigue 8%, abdominal cramps 7%, lightheadedness 6%, vomiting 5%, nasal congestion 5%, constipation 3% and diarrhea 3%.

A slight hypotensive effect may accompany Parlodel (bromocriptine mesylate) treatment. The occurence of adverse reactions may be lessened by temporarily reducing dosage to one-half tablet two or three times daily.

Physiological Lactation

23% of patients treated within the recommended dosage range for the prevention of physiological lactation had at least one side effect, but they were generally mild to moderate in degree. Therapy was discontinued in approximately 3% of patients. The most frequently occurring adverse reactions were: headache 10%, dizziness 8%, nausea 7%, vomiting 3%, fatigue 1.0%, syncope 0.7%, diarrhea 0.4% and cramps 0.4%. Decreases in blood pressure (≥ 20 mmHg systolic and ≥ 10 mmHG diastolic) occurred in 28% of patients at least once during the first three postpartum days; these were usually of a transient nature. Two reports of fainting in the puerperium may possibly be related to this effect.

Parkinson's Disease

In clinical trials in which bromocriptine was administered with concomitant reduction in the dose of levodopa/carbidopa, the most common newly appearing adverse reactions were: nausea, abnormal involuntary movements, hallucinations, confusion, "on-off" phenomenon, dizziness, drowsiness, faintness/fainting, vomiting, asthenia, abdominal discomfort, visual disturbance, ataxia, insomnia, depression, hypotension, shortness of breath, constipation, and vertigo.

Less common adverse reactions which may be encountered include: anorexia, anxiety, blepharospasm, dry mouth, dysphagia, edema of the feet and ankles, erythromelalgia, epileptiform seizure, fatigue, headache, lethargy, mottling of skin, nasal stuffiness, nervousness, nightmares, paresthesia, skin rash, urinary frequency, urinary incontinence, urinary retention, and rarely, signs and symptoms of ergotism such as tingling of fingers, cold feet, numbness, muscle cramps of feet and legs or exacerbation of Raynaud's syndrome.

Abnormalities in laboratory tests may include elevations in blood urea nitrogen, SGOT, SGPT, GGPT, CPK, alkaline phosphatase and uric acid, which are usually transient and not of clinical significance.

Dosage and Administration:

Amenorrhea/Galactorrhea

The therapeutic dosage of Parlodel (bromocriptine mesylate) is one 2½ mg tablet, two or three times daily, with meals. The duration of treatment should not exceed six months. It is recommended that treatment commence with one tablet daily, increasing to a therapeutic dosage within the first week, to reduce the possibility of adverse reactions.

Female Infertility

The therapeutic dosage of Parlodel (bromocriptine mesylate) is one 2½ mg tablet, two or three times daily, with meals. It is recommended that treatment commence with one tablet daily, increasing to a therapeutic dosage within the first week, to reduce the possibility of adverse reactions. In order to reduce the likelihood of prolonged exposure to Parlodel (bromocriptine mesylate) in an unsuspected pregnancy, a mechanical contraceptive should be used in conjunction with Parlodel (bromocriptine mesylate) therapy until normal ovulatory menstrual cycles have been restored. Contraception should then be discontinued. If menstruation does not occur within 3 days of the expected date, Parlodel (bromocriptine mesylate) therapy should be discontinued and a pregnancy test performed.

Prevention of Physiological Lactation

Therapy should be started only after the patient's vital signs have been stabilized and no sooner than four hours after delivery. The recommended therapeutic dosage is one 2½ mg tablet of Parlodel (bromocriptine mesylate) twice daily with meals. The usual dosage range is from one 2½ mg tablet daily to one 2½ mg tablet three times daily with meals. Parlodel (bromocriptine mesylate) therapy should be continued for 14 days; however, therapy may be given for up to 21 days if necessary.

Parkinson's Disease

The basic principle of Parlodel (bromocriptine mesylate) therapy is to initiate treatment at a low dosage and, on an individual basis, increase the daily dosage slowly until a maximum therapeutic response is achieved. The dosage of levodopa during this introductory period should be maintained, if possible. The initial dose of Parlodel (bromocriptine mesylate) is one-half of a 2½ mg tablet twice daily with meals. Assessments are advised at two week intervals during dosage titration to ensure that the lowest dosage producing an optimal therapeutic response is not exceeded. If necessary, the dosage may be increased every 14 to 28 days by 2½ mg per day with meals. Should it be advisable to reduce the dosage of levodopa because of adverse reactions, the daily dosage of Parlodel (bromocriptine mesylate), if increased, should be accomplished gradually in small (2½ mg) increments.

The safety of Parlodel (bromocriptine mesylate) has not been demonstrated in dosages exceeding 100 mg per day.

How Supplied:

Tablets, 2½ mg

Round, white, scored tablets, each containing 2½ mg bromocriptine (as the mesylate) in packages of 30. Embossed "PARLODEL 2½" on one side and scored on reverse side.

Capsules, 5 mg

Caramel and white capsules, each containing 5 mg bromocriptine (as the mesylate) in packages of 30 and 100. Imprinted "PARLODEL 5 mg" on one half and triangle (S) on other half.

[PAR-Z6 Issues May 3, 1982]

PLEXONAL® Tablets ©III

The following prescribing information is based on official labeling in effect on November 1, 1982.

Composition: Each Plexonal *Tablet* contains: 45 mg barbital sodium, 25 mg butalbital sodium (Sandoptal® sodium), Warning: May be habit forming. 15 mg phenobarbital sodium, USP, 0.16 mg dihydroergotamine mesylate, USP, 0.08 mg scopolamine hydrobromide, USP.

Properties and Therapeutics: Plexonal provides a sedative-relaxant effect for patients with symptoms such as anxiety, tension, irritability, restlessness and insomnia. A balanced action is achieved through the use of three barbiturates with differing rates of action and dissipation, potentiated by scopolamine and dihydroergotamine.

Indications: Anxiety, tension, nervousness, irritability, apprehension, restlessness, hyperexcitability, insomnia.

Contraindications: Severely depressed or comatose states. Hypersensitivity to any of the components.

Precautions: Use with caution in the presence of hepatic disease, fever, hyperthyroidism, diabetes mellitus, severe anemia. Due to presence of barbiturates, may be habit forming.

Side Effects: Drowsiness, skin rashes, gastrointestinal disturbances may occur.

Dosage: For daytime sedation—1 tablet, 2 to 4 times daily; range, 2 to 6 tablets per day. To promote sleep—2 to 4 tablets, ½ hour before bedtime.

Supplied: Triangular tablets (white, sugar-coated) in bottles of 100.

Company Product Identification Mark(s): Tablets imprinted 78—on 1 side, and—57 other side.

[PLX-Z10 Issued November 3, 1980]

[*Shown in Product Identification Section*]

RESTORIL® ©

(temazepam) capsules

The following prescribing information is based on official labeling in effect on November 1, 1982.

Description: Restoril® (temazepam) is a benzodiazepine hypnotic agent. The chemical name is 7-chloro-1,3-dihydro-3-hydroxy-1-methyl-5-phenyl-2H-1,4-benzodiazepin-2-one.

Temazepam is a white, crystalline substance, very slightly soluble in water and sparingly soluble in alcohol USP. It has a molecular weight of 300.7.

Restoril (temazepam) capsules, 15 mg and 30 mg, are for oral administration.

Clinical Pharmacology: Restoril (temazepam) improved sleep parameters in clinical studies. Residual medication effects ("hangover") were essentially absent. Early morning awakening, a particular problem in the geriatric patient, was significantly reduced.

In sleep laboratory studies, Restoril (temazepam) significantly improved sleep maintenance parameters [e.g., wake time after sleep onset, total sleep time and the number of nocturnal awakenings]. There was no significant reduction in sleep latency. REM sleep was essentially unchanged, slow wave sleep was decreased and no rebound effects occurred in these sleep stages. Transient sleep disturbance, mainly during the first night, occurred after withdrawal of the drug. In these studies, there was no evidence of tolerance when patients were given Restoril nightly for approximately one month.

A single and a multiple dose absorption, distribution, metabolism and excretion (ADME) study using ^{3}H-labeled drug, as well as a bioavailability study, were carried out in normal volunteers. Absorption was complete and detectable blood levels were achieved at 20-40 minutes; peak concentration was reached at 2-3 hours. There was minimal (approximately 8%) first pass metabolism.

The only significant metabolite present in blood was the O-conjugate. The unchanged drug was 96% bound to plasma proteins. The blood level decline of the parent drug was biphasic with the short half-life ranging from 0.4-0.6 hours and the terminal half-life from 9.5-12.4 hours (mean: 10 hours), depending on the study population and method of determination. Metabolites were formed with a half-life of 10 hours and excreted with a half-life of approximately 2 hours. Thus, formation of the major metabolite is the rate limiting step in the biodisposition of temazepam. There is no accumulation of metabolites. The area under the blood concentration/time curve was directly proportional to the dose in the 0-45 mg range.

Continued on next page

Sandoz—Cont.

Temazepam was completely metabolized prior to excretion; 80-90% of the dose appeared in the urine. The major metabolite was the O-conjugate of temazepam (90%); the O-conjugate of N-demethyl temazepam was a minor metabolite (7%). There were no active metabolites.
At a dose of 30 mg once-a-day for 8 weeks, no evidence of enzyme induction was found in man.
The steady state plasma concentration measured under therapeutic sleep laboratory conditions was 382 ± 192 ng/ml, 2.5 hours after a 30 mg dose, and 26 ng/ml at 24 hours. On a once-a-day regimen, steady state was attained on the third day.
Indications and Usage: Restoril (temazepam) is indicated for the relief of insomnia associated with the complaints of difficulty in falling asleep, frequent nocturnal awakenings, and/or early morning awakenings. In clinical trials there is a perception by patients that Restoril (temazepam) decreases sleep latency, but sleep laboratory studies have not confirmed such an effect when the drug was administered within 30 minutes of retiring.
Since insomnia is often transient and intermittent, the prolonged administration of Restoril (temazepam) is generally not necessary or recommended. Restoril (temazepam) has been employed for sleep maintenance for up to 35 consecutive nights of drug administration in sleep laboratory studies.
Since insomnia may be a symptom of several other disorders, the possibility that the complaint may be related to a condition for which there is more specific treatment should be considered.
Contraindications: Benzodiazepines may cause fetal damage when administered during pregnancy. An increased risk of congenital malformations associated with the use of diazepam and chlordiazepoxide during the first trimester of pregnancy has been suggested in several studies. Transplacental distribution has resulted in neonatal CNS depression following the ingestion of therapeutic doses of a benzodiazepine hypnotic during the last weeks of pregnancy.
Reproduction studies in animals with temazepam were performed in rats and rabbits. In a perinatal-postnatal study in rats, oral doses of 60 mg/kg/day resulted in increasing nursling mortality. Teratology studies in rats demonstrated increased fetal resorptions at doses of 30 and 120 mg/kg in one study and increased occurrence of rudimentary ribs, which are considered skeletal variants, in a second study at doses of 240 mg/kg or higher. In rabbits, occasional abnormalities such as exencephaly and fusion or asymmetry of ribs were reported without dose relationship. Although these abnormalities were not found in the concurrent control group, they have been reported to occur randomly in historical controls. At doses of 40 mg/kg or higher, there was an increased incidence of the 13th rib variant when compared to the incidence in concurrent and historical controls.
Restoril (temazepam) is contraindicated in pregnant women. If there is a likelihood of the patient becoming pregnant while receiving temazepam, she should be warned of the potential risk to the fetus. Patients should be instructed to discontinue the drug prior to becoming pregnant. The possibility that a woman of childbearing potential may be pregnant at the time of institution of therapy should be considered.
Warnings: Patients receiving Restoril (temazepam) should be cautioned about possible combined effects with alcohol and other CNS depressants.

Precautions

General

Since the risk of the development of oversedation, dizziness, confusion and/or ataxia increases, substantially with larger doses of benzodiazepines in elderly and debilitated patients, 15 mg of Restoril® (temazepam) is recommended as the initial dosage for such patients.
Restoril (temazepam) should be administered with caution in severly depressed patients or those in whom there is any evidence of latent depression; it should be recognized that suicidal tendencies may be present and protective measures may be necessary.
If Restoril (temazepam) is to be combined with other drugs having known hypnotic properties or CNS-depressant effects, consideration should be given to potential additive effects.

Information for Patients

Patients receiving Restoril (temazepam) should be cautioned about possible combined effects with alcohol and other CNS depressants. Patients should be cautioned not to operate machinery or drive a motor vehicle after ingesting the drug. Patients should also be advised that they may experience disturbed nocturnal sleep for the first or second night after discontinuing the drug.

Laboratory Tests

The usual precautions should be observed in patients with impaired renal or hepatic function. Abnormal liver function tests as well as blood dyscrasias have been reported with benzodiazepines.

Carcinogenesis, Impairment of Fertility

No carcinogenic potential was demonstrated in long-term studies in mice and rats. Fertility in male and female rats was not adversely affected by Restoril (temazepam).

Pregnancy

Pregnancy Category X. See Contraindications.

Nursing Mothers

It is not known whether this drug is excreted in human milk. Because many drugs are excreted in human milk, caution should be exercised when Restoril (temazepam) is administered to a nursing woman.

Pediatric Use

Safety and effectiveness in children below the age of 18 years have not been established.
Adverse Reactions: During clinical studies in which 795 patients received Restoril (temazepam), the drug was well tolerated. Side effects were usually mild and transient. These 795 patients included 175 subjects who received Restoril (temazepam) during daytime waking hours, sometimes in excess of recommended therapeutic dosage, in studies to evaluate dosage levels for safety and pharmacokinetic profiles.
The most common adverse reactions were drowsiness (17%), dizziness (7%), and lethargy (5%).
Other side effects include confusion, euphoria and relaxed feeling (2-3%). Less commonly reported were weakness, anorexia and diarrhea (1-2%). Rarely reported were tremor, ataxia, lack of concentration, loss of equilibrium, falling and palpitations (less than 1%). Hallucinations, horizontal nystagmus and paradoxical reactions, including excitement, stimulation and hyperactivity were rare (less than 0.5%).

Drug Abuse and Dependence

Controlled Substance

Restoril (temazepam) is a controlled substance in Schedule IV.

Abuse and Dependence

Withdrawal symptoms following abrupt discontinuation of benzodiazepines have been reported in patients receiving excessive doses over extended periods of time. These symptoms (including convulsions) are similar to those seen after barbiturate withdrawal. Although infrequently seen, milder withdrawal symptoms have also been reported following abrupt discontinuance of benzodiazepines taken continuously, generally at higher therapeutic levels, for at least several months. As with any hypnotic, caution must be exercised in administering Restoril (temazepam) to individuals known to be addiction-prone or those whose history suggests they may increase the dosage on their own initiative. It is desirable to limit repeated prescriptions without adequate medical supervision.
Overdosage: Manifestations of acute overdosage of Restoril (temazepam) can be expected to reflect the CNS effects of the drug and include somnolence, confusion and coma, with reduced or absent reflexes, respiratory depression and hypotension. If the patient is conscious, vomiting should be induced mechanically or with emetics. Gastric lavage should be employed utilizing concurrently a cuffed endotracheal tube if the patient is unconscious to prevent aspiration and pulmonary complications. Maintenance of adequate pulmonary ventilation is essential. The use of pressor agents intravenously may be necessary to combat hypotension. Fluids should be administered intravenously to encourage diuresis. The value of dialysis has not been determined. If excitation occurs, barbiturates should not be used. It should be borne in mind that multiple agents may have been ingested.
The oral LD_{50} was 1963 mg/kg in mice, 1833 mg/kg in rats and >2400 mg/kg in rabbits.
Dosage and Administration: The recommended usual adult dose is 30 mg before retiring. In some patients, 15 mg may be sufficient. As with all medications, dosage should be individualized for maximal beneficial effects. In elderly and/or debilitated patients it is recommended that therapy be initiated with 15 mg until individual responses are determined.
How Supplied: Restoril (temazepam) capsules-15 mg, maroon and pink, imprinted "RESTORIL 15 mg"; 30 mg, maroon and blue, imprinted "RESTORIL 30 mg". Packages of 100, 500 and ControlPak® packages of 25 capsules (continuous reverse-numbered roll of sealed blisters).

[RES-Z2 Issued November 1, 1981]

[*Shown in Product Identification Section*]

SANOREX® Ⓒ
(mazindol) tablets, USP

The following prescribing information is based on official labeling in effect on November 1, 1982.
Description: Sanorex (mazindol) is an imidazoiso-indole anorectic agent. It is chemically designated as 5-p-chloro-phenyl-5-hydroxy-2, 3- dihydro-5H-imidazo (2,1-a) isoindole, a tautomeric form of 2-[2'-(p-chlorobenzoyl) phenyl]-2-imidazoline.
Actions: Sanorex, (mazindol), although an isoindole, has pharmacologic activity similar in many ways to the prototype drugs used in obesity, the amphetamines. Actions include central nervous system stimulation in humans and animals, as well as such amphetamine-like effects in animals as the production of stereotyped behavior. Animal experiments also suggest certain differences from phenethylamine anorectic drugs, e.g., amphetamine, with respect to site and mechanism of action; for example, mazindol appears to exert its primary effects on the limbic system. The significance of these differences for humans is uncertain. It does not cause brain norepinephrine depletion in animals; on the other hand, it does appear to inhibit storage site uptake of norepinephrine as is suggested by its marked potentiation of the effect of exogenous norepinephrine on blood pressure in dogs (see WARNINGS) and on smooth muscle contraction *in vitro*.
Tolerance has been demonstrated with all drugs of this class in which this phenomenon has been studied.
Drugs used in obesity are commonly known as "anorectics" or "anorexigenics." It has not been established, however, that the action of

such drugs in treating obesity is exclusively one of appetite suppression. Other central nervous system actions, or metabolic effects may be involved as well.
Adult obese subjects instructed in dietary management and treated with anorectic drugs, lose more weight on the average than those treated with placebo and diet, as determined in relatively short-term clinical trials.
The average magnitude of increased weight loss of drug-treated patients over placebo-treated patients in studies of anorectics in general is ordinarily only a fraction of a pound a week. The rate of weight loss is greatest in the first weeks of therapy for both drug and placebo subjects and tends to decrease in succeeding weeks.
The amount of weight loss associated with the use of Sanorex (mazindol), as with other anorectic drugs, varies from trial to trial, and the increased weight loss appears to be related in part to variables other than the drugs prescribed, such as the interaction between physician-investigator and the patient, the population treated, and the diet prescribed. The importance of non-drug factors in such weight loss has not been elucidated.
The natural history of obesity is measured in years, whereas, most studies cited are restricted to a few weeks' duration; thus, the total impact of drug-induced weight loss over that of diet alone must be considered clinically limited.
Indication: Sanorex (mazindol) is indicated in the management of exogenous obesity as a short-term (a few weeks) adjunct in a regimen of weight reduction based on caloric restriction. The limited usefulness of agents of this class (see ACTIONS) should be measured against possible risk factors inherent in their use, such as those described below.
Contraindications: Glaucoma; hypersensitivity or idiosyncrasy to Sanorex (mazindol).
Agitated states.
Patients with a history of drug abuse.
During or within 14 days following the administration of monoamine oxidase inhibitors, (hypertensive crises may result).
Warnings: Tolerance to the effect of many anorectic drugs may develop within a few weeks; if this occurs, the recommended dose should not be exceeded in an attempt to increase the effect; rather, the drug should be discontinued.
Sanorex (mazindol) may impair the ability of the patient to engage in potentially hazardous activities such as operating machinery or driving a motor vehicle; the patient should therefore be cautioned accordingly.
Drug Interactions: Sanorex (mazindol) may decrease the hypotensive effect of guanethidine; patients should be monitored accordingly.
Sanorex (mazindol) may markedly potentiate the pressor effect of exogenous catecholamines. If it should be necessary to give a pressor amine agent (e.g., levarterenol or isoproterenol) to a patient in shock (e.g., from a myocardial infarction) who has recently been taking Sanorex® (mazindol) extreme care should be taken in monitoring blood pressure at frequent intervals and initiating pressor therapy with a low initial dose and careful titration.
Drug Dependence: Sanorex (mazindol) shares important pharmacologic properties with amphetamines. Amphetamines and related stimulant drugs have been extensively abused and can produce tolerance and severe psychologic dependence. In this regard, the manifestations of chronic overdosage or withdrawal of Sanorex (mazindol) have not been determined in humans. Abstinence effects have been observed in dogs after abrupt cessation for prolonged periods. There was some self-administration of the drug in monkeys. EEG studies and "liking" scores in human subjects yielded equivocal results. While the abuse potential of Sanorex (mazindol) has not been further defined, the possibility of dependence should be kept in mind when evaluating the desirability of including Sanorex (mazindol) as part of a weight reduction program.
Usage in Pregnancy: Sanorex (mazindol) was studied in reproduction experiments in rats and rabbits and an increase in neonatal mortality and a possible increased incidence of rib anomalies in rats were observed at relatively high doses.
Although these studies have not indicated important adverse effects, use of mazindol by women who are or may become pregnant requires that the potential benefit be weighed against the possible hazard to mother and infant.
Usage in Children: Sanorex (mazindol) is not recommended for use in children under 12 years of age.
Precautions: Insulin requirements in diabetes mellitus may be altered in association with the use of mazindol and the concomitant dietary regimen.
The least amount feasible should be prescribed or dispensed at one time in order to minimize the possibility of overdosage.
Use only with caution in hypertension with monitoring of blood pressure, since evidence is insufficient to rule out a possible adverse effect on blood pressure in some hypertensive patients. The drug is not recommended in severely hypertensive patients. The drug is not recommended for patients with symptomatic cardiovascular disease including arrhythmias.
Adverse Reactions: The most common adverse effects of Sanorex (mazindol) are dry mouth, tachycardia, constipation, nervousness and insomnia.
Cardiovascular: Palpitation, tachycardia.
Central Nervous System: Overstimulation, restlessness, dizziness, insomnia, dysphoria, tremor, headache, depression, drowsiness, weakness.
Gastrointestinal: Dryness of the mouth, unpleasant taste, diarrhea, constipation, nausea, other gastrointestinal disturbances.
Skin: Rash, excessive sweating, clamminess.
Endocrine: Impotence, changes in libido have rarely been observed with Sanorex (mazindol).
Eye: Treatment of dogs with high doses of Sanorex (mazindol) for long periods resulted in some corneal opacities, reversible on cessation of medication. No such effect has been observed in humans.
Dosage and Administration: Usual dosage is 1 mg three times daily, one hour before meals, or 2 mg once daily, one hour before lunch. The lowest effective dose should be used. To determine the lowest effective dose, therapy with Sanorex (mazindol) may be initiated at 1 mg once a day, and adjusted to the need and response of the patient. Should G.I. discomfort occur, Sanorex (mazindol) may be taken with meals.
Overdosage: There are no data as yet on acute overdosage with Sanorex (mazindol) in humans.
Manifestations of acute overdosage with amphetamines and related substances include restlessness, tremor, rapid respiration, dizziness. Fatigue and depression may follow the stimulatory phase of overdosage. Cardiovascular effects include tachycardia, hypertension and circulatory collapse. Gastrointestinal symptoms include nausea, vomiting and abdominal cramps. While similar manifestations of overdosage may be seen with Sanorex (mazindol), their exact nature has yet to be determined. The management of acute intoxication is largely symptomatic. Data are not available on the treatment of acute intoxication with Sanorex (mazindol) by hemodialysis or peritoneal dialysis, but the substance is poorly soluble except at very acid pH.
How Supplied: Sanorex (mazindol) is available in 1 mg elliptical, white tablets and in 2 mg round, white scored tablets, in packages of 100.
Company's Product Indentification Mark(s): 1 mg tablets embossed SANOREX on 1 side, 78-71 other side. 2 mg tablets scored 78-66 on 1 side, SANDOZ other side.
[SNX-Z10 Issued December 18, 1981]
[*Shown in Product Identification Section*]

SANSERT® ℞

(methysergide maleate) tablets, USP

The following prescribing information is based on official labeling in effect on November 1, 1982.

WARNING
Retroperitoneal Fibrosis, Pleuropulmonary Fibrosis and Fibrotic Thickening of Cardiac Valves May Occur in Patients Receiving Long-term Methysergide Maleate Therapy. Therefore, This Preparation Must be Reserved for Prophylaxis in Patients Whose Vascular Headaches Are Frequent and/or Severe and Uncontrollable and Who Are Under Close Medical Supervision.
(*See Also "Warnings" Section.*)

Composition: Each Sansert tablet contains 2 mg methysergide maleate, USP.
Actions: Sansert (methysergide maleate) has been shown, *in vitro* and *in vivo*, to inhibit or block the effects of serotonin, a substance which may be involved in the mechanism of vascular headaches. Serotonin has been variously described as a central neurohumoral agent or chemical mediator, as a "headache substance" acting directly or indirectly to lower pain threshold (others in this category include tyramine; polypeptides, such as bradykinin; histamine; and acetylcholine), as an intrinsic "motor hormone" of the gastrointestinal tract, and as a "hormone" involved in connective tissue reparative processes. Suggestions have been made by investigators as to the mechanism whereby methysergide produces its clinical effects, but this has not been finally established.
Indications: For the prevention or reduction of intensity and frequency of vascular headaches in the following kinds of patients:
1. Patients suffering from one or more severe vascular headaches per week.
2. Patients suffering from vascular headaches that are uncontrollable or so severe that preventive therapy is indicated regardless of the frequency of the attack.
Contraindications: Pregnancy, peripheral vascular disease, severe arteriosclerosis, severe hypertension, coronary artery disease, phlebitis or cellulitis of the lower limbs, pulmonary disease, collagen diseases or fibrotic processes, impaired liver or renal function, valvular heart disease, debilitated states and serious infections.
Warnings: With long-term, uninterrupted administration, retroperitoneal fibrosis or related conditions—pleuropulmonary fibrosis and cardiovascular disorders with murmurs or vascular bruits have been reported. Patients must be warned to report immediately the following symptoms: cold, numb, and painful hands and feet; leg cramps on walking; any type of girdle, flank, or chest pain, or any associated symptomatology. Should any of these symptoms develop, methysergide should be discontinued. Continuous administration should not exceed 6 months. There must be a drug-free interval of 3-4 weeks after each 6-month course of treatment. The dosage should be reduced gradually during the last 2-3 weeks of each treatment course to avoid "headache rebound."
The drug is not recommended for use in children.

Continued on next page

Sandoz—Cont.

Precautions: All patients receiving Sansert (methysergide maleate) should remain under constant supervision of the physician and be examined regularly for the development of fibrotic or vascular complications. (See Adverse Reactions).

The manifestations of retroperitoneal fibrosis, pleuropulmonary fibrosis, and vascular shutdown have shown a high incidence of regression once Sansert is withdrawn. These facts should be borne in mind to avoid unnecessary surgical intervention. Cardiac murmurs, which may indicate endocardial fibrosis, have shown varying degrees of regression, with complete disappearance in some and persistence in others.

Sansert has been specifically designed for the prophylaxis of vascular headache and has no place in the management of the acute attack.

Sansert tablets contain FD&C Yellow No. 5 (tartrazine) which may cause allergic-type reactions (including bronchial asthma) in certain susceptible individuals. Although the overall incidence of FD&C Yellow No. 5 (Tartrazine) sensitivity in the general population is low, it is frequently seen in patients who also have aspirin hypersensitivity.

Adverse Reactions: Within the recommended dose levels, the following side effects have been reported:

1) Fibrotic Complications

Fibrotic changes have been observed in the retroperitoneal, pleuropulmonary, cardiac, and other tissues, either singly or, very rarely, in combination.

Retroperitoneal Fibrosis: This non-specific fibrotic process is usually confined to the retroperitoneal connective tissue above the pelvic brim and may present clinically with one or more symptoms such as general malaise, fatigue, weight loss, backache, low grade fever (elevated sedimentation rate), urinary obstruction (girdle or flank pain, dysuria, polyuria, oliguria, elevated BUN), vascular insufficiency of the lower limbs (leg pain, Leriche syndrome, edema of legs, thrombophlebitis). The single most useful diagnostic procedure in suspected cases of retroperitoneal fibrosis is intravenous pyelography. Typical deviation and obstruction of one or both ureters may be observed.

Pleuropulmonary Complications: A similar nonspecific fibrotic process, limited to the pleural and immediately subjacent pulmonary tissues, usually presents clinically with dyspnea, tightness and pain in the chest, pleural friction rubs, and pleural effusion. These findings may be confirmed by chest X-ray.

Cardiac Complications: Nonrheumatic fibrotic thickenings of the aortic root and of the aortic and mitral valves usually present clinically with cardiac murmurs and dyspnea.

Other Fibrotic Complications: Several cases of fibrotic plaques simulating Peyronie's disease have been described.

2) Cardiovascular Complications

Encroachment of retroperitoneal fibrosis on the aorta, inferior vena cava and their common iliac branches may result in vascular insufficiency of the lower limbs, the presenting features of which are mentioned under retroperitoneal fibrosis.

Intrinsic vasoconstriction of large and small arteries, involving one or more vessels or merely a segment of a vessel, may occur at any stage of therapy. Depending on the vessel involved, this complication may present with chest pain, abdominal pain, or cold, numb, painful extremities with or without paresthesias and diminished or absent pulses. Progression to ischemic tissue damage has rarely been reported. Prompt withdrawal of the drug at the first signs of impaired circulation is recommended (See Warnings) to obviate such effects.

Postural hypotension and tachycardia have also been observed.

3) Gastrointestinal Symptoms

Nausea, vomiting, diarrhea, heartburn, abdominal pain. These effects tend to appear early and can frequently be obviated by gradual introduction of the medication and by administration of the drug with meals.

Constipation and elevation of gastric HCl have also been reported.

4) CNS Symptoms

Insomnia, drowsiness, mild euphoria, dizziness, ataxia, lightheadedness, hyperesthesia, unworldly feelings (described variously as "dissociation," "hallucinatory experiences," etc.). Some of these symptoms may be associated with vascular headaches, per se, and may, therefore, be unrelated to the drug.

5) Dermatological Manifestations

Facial flush, telangiectasia, and nonspecific rashes have rarely been reported. Increased hair loss may occur, but in many instances the tendency has abated despite continued therapy.

6) Edema

Peripheral edema, and more rarely, localized brawny edema may occur.

Dependent edema has responded to lowered doses, salt restriction, or diuretics.

7) Weight Gain

Weight gain may be a reason to caution patients regarding their caloric intake.

8) Hematological Manifestations

Neutropenia, eosinophilia.

9) Miscellaneous

Weakness, arthralgia, myalgia.

Dosage and Administration: Usual adult dose 4 to 8 mg daily. Tablets to be given with meals.

Note: There must be a medication-free interval of 3-4 weeks after every 6-month course of treatment (see WARNINGS).

No pediatric dosage has been established.

If, after a 3-week trial period, efficacy has not been demonstrated, longer administration of Sansert (methysergide maleate) is unlikely to be of benefit.

How Supplied: Bottles of 100 tablets, each tablet containing 2 mg of methysergide maleate, USP.

Company's Product Identification Mark(s): Imprinted 78-58 on 1 side, SANDOZ other side.

[SAN-Z17 Issued February 1, 1980]

[*Shown in Product Identification Section*]

SYNTOCINON® ℞

(oxytocin) injection, USP

The following prescribing information is based on official labeling in effect on November 1, 1982.

Description: Syntocinon (oxytocin) injection is a synthetic polypeptide consisting of eight amino acids the commercial synthesis of which was first achieved by Sandoz Laboratories.

For intravenous or intramuscular administration.

Each 1 ml of Syntocinon solution contains 10 USP or International Units of oxytocin and the following inactive ingredients:

sodium acetate, USP ....1 mg
sodium chloride, USP ....0.017 mg
chlorobutanol, NF 0.5%
alcohol, USP ....0.61% by vol.
acetic acid, NF, qs to ....pH 4 ± .3
water for injection, USP, qs to ....1 ml

The Syntocinon solution in each ampul is sterile.

Syntocinon (oxytocin) is an oxytocic agent that, when given in appropriate doses during pregnancy, is capable of elicitng graded increases in uterine motility from a moderate increase in the rate and force of spontaneous motor activity to sustained tetanic contraction.

Syntocinon (oxytocin) is an octapeptide.

Action: The pharmacologic and clinical properties of Syntocinon (oxytocin) are identical with the naturally occurring oxytocic principle of the posterior lobe of the pituitary. Syntocinon (oxytocin) injection does not contain the amino acids characteristic of vasopressin, and therefore lacks cardiovascular effects. Syntocinon (oxytocin) exerts a selective action on the smooth musculature of the uterus, particularly toward the end of pregnancy, during labor and immediately following delivery. Oxytocin stimulates rhythmic contractions of the uterus, increases the frequency of existing contractions, and raises the tone of the uterine musculature.

Indications:

> **IMPORTANT NOTICE**
> Syntocinon (oxytocin) injection is indicated for the medical rather than the elective induction of labor. Available data and information are inadequate to define the benefits to risks considerations in the use of the drug product for elective induction. Elective induction of labor is defined as the initiation of labor for convenience in an individual with a term pregnancy who is free of medical indications.

Antepartum: Syntocinon (oxytocin) is indicated for the initiation or improvement of uterine contractions, where this is desirable and considered suitable, in order to achieve early vaginal delivery for fetal or maternal reasons. It is indicated for (1) induction of labor in patients with a medical indication for the initiation of labor, such as Rh problems, maternal diabetes, pre-eclampsia at or near term, when delivery is in the best interest of mother and fetus or when membranes are prematurely ruptured and delivery is indicated; (2) stimulation or reinforcement of labor, as in selected cases of uterine inertia; (3) as adjunctive therapy in the management of incomplete or inevitable abortion. In the first trimester currettage is generally considered primary therapy. In the second trimester abortion, oxytocin infusion will often be successful in emptying the uterus. Other means of therapy, however, may be required in such cases.

Postpartum: Syntocinon (oxytocin) injection is indicated to produce uterine contractions during the third stage of labor and to control postpartum bleeding or hemorrhage.

Contraindications: Syntocinon (oxytocin) injection is contraindicated in any of the following conditions: Significant cephalopelvic disproportion; unfavorable fetal positions or presentations which are undeliverable without conversion prior to delivery, i.e., (transverse lies); in obstetrical emergencies where the benefit-to-risk ratio for either the fetus or the mother favors surgical intervention; in cases of fetal distress where delivery is not imminent; prolonged use in uterine inertia or severe toxemia; hypertonic uterine patterns; patients with hypersensitivity to the drug; induction or augmentation of labor in those cases where vaginal delivery is contraindicated, such as cord presentation or prolapse, total placenta previa, and vasa previa.

Warnings: Syntocinon (oxytocin) when given for induction or stimulation of labor, must be administered only by the intravenous route and with adequate medical supervision in a hospital.

Precautions:

1. All patients receiving intravenous oxytocin must be under continuous observation by trained personnel with a thorough knowledge of the drug and qualified to identify complications. A physician qualified to manage any complications should be immediately available.

2. When properly administered, oxytocinon should stimulate uterine contractions similar to those seen in normal labor. Overstimulation of the uterus by improper administration can be hazardous to both mother and fetus. Even with proper administration and adequate supervision, hypertonic contractions can occur in patients whose uteri are hypersensitive to oxytocin.

3. Except in unusual circumstances, oxytocin should not be administered in the following conditions: prematurity, borderline cephalopelvic disproportion, previous major surgery on the cervix or uterus including cesarean section, over-distention of the uterus, grand multiparity, or invasive cervical carcinoma. Because of the variability of the combinations of factors which may be present in the conditions listed above, the definition of "unusual circumstances" must be left to the judgment of the physician. The decision can only be made by carefully weighing the potential benefits which oxytocin can provide in a given case against rare but definite potential for the drug to produce hypertonicity or tetanic spasm.

4. Maternal deaths due to hypertensive episodes, subarchnoid hemorrhage, rupture of the uterus, and fetal deaths due to various causes have been reported associated with the use of parental oxytocic drugs for induction of labor or for augmentation in the first and second stages of labor.

5. Oxytocin has been shown to have an intrinsic antidiuretic effect, acting to increase water reabsorption from the glomerular filtrate. Consideration should, therefore, be given to the possibility of water intoxication, particularly when oxytocin is administered continuously by infusion and the patient is receiving fluids by mouth.

Adverse reactions: The following adverse reactions have been reported: Fetal bradycardia, neonatal jaundice, anaphylactic reaction, postpartum hemorrhage, cardiac arrhythmia, fatal afibrinogenemia, nausea, vomiting, premature ventricular contractions and pelvic hematoma.

Excessive dosage or hypersensitivity to the drug may result in uterine hypertonicity, spasm, tetanic contraction, or rupture of the uterus.

The possibility of increased blood loss and afibrinogenemia should be kept in mind when administering the drug.

Severe water intoxication with convulsions and coma has occurred, associated with a slow oxytocin infusion over a 24-hour period. Maternal death due to oxytocin-induced water intoxication has been reported.

Dosage and Administration: Dosage of oxytocin is determined by uterine response. The following dosage information is based upon the various regimens and indications in general use.

A. Induction or Stimulation of Labor

Intravenous infusion (drip method) is the only acceptable method of administration for the induction or stimulation of labor.

Accurate control of the rate of infusion flow is essential. An infusion pump or other such device and frequent monitoring of strength of contractions and fetal heart rate are necessary for the safe administration of oxytocin for the induction or stimulation of labor. If uterine contractions become too powerful, the infusion can be abruptly stopped, and oxytocic stimulation of the uterine musculature will soon wane.

1. An intravenous infusion of non-oxytocin containing solution should be started. Physiologic electrolyte solution should be used except under unusual circumstances.

2. To prepare the usual solution for infusion, the contents of one 1-ml ampule is combined aseptically with 1,000 ml of nonhydrating diluent. The combined solution, rotated in the infusion bottle to insure thorough mixing contains 10 mU/ml. Add the container with dilute oxytocic solution to the system through use of a constant infusion pump or other such device, to control accurately the rate of infusion.

3. The initial dose should be no more than 1–2 mU/min. The dose may be gradually increased in increments of no more than 1 to 2 mU/min. until a contraction pattern has been established, which is similar to normal labor.

4. The fetal heart rate, resting uterine tone, and the frequency, duration, and force of contractions should be monitored.

5. The oxytocin infusion should be discontinued immediately in the event of uterine hyperactivity or fetal distress. Oxygen should be administered to the mother. The mother and the fetus must be evaluated by the responsible physician.

B. Control of Postpartum Uterine Bleeding

1. *Intravenous Infusion (Drip Method):* To control postpartum bleeding, 10 to 40 units of oxytocin may be added to 1,000 ml of a nonhydrating diluent and run at a rate necessary to control uterine atony.

2. *Intramuscular Administration:* 1 ml (10 units) of oxytocin can be given after delivery of the placenta.

C. Treatment of Incomplete or Inevitable Abortion

Intravenous infusion with physiologic saline solution, 500 ml, or 5% dextrose in physiologic saline solution to which 10 units of Syntocinon® (oxytocin) have been added should be infused at a rate of 20 to 40 drops per minute.

How Supplied: Syntocinon (oxytocin) injection, ampuls, 1 ml (10 USP units) size, boxes of 20 and 100.

Store and dispense: Below 77°F; DO NOT FREEZE

[SYT-Z16 Issued July 9, 1980]

SYNTOCINON® NASAL SPRAY ℞

(oxytocin) nasal solution, USP

The following prescribing information is based on official labeling in effect on November 1, 1982.

Description: Each ml. contains 40 USP Units (International Units) Syntocinon (oxytocin) and the following: dried sodium phosphate, USP, citric acid, USP, sodium chloride, USP, glycerin, USP, sorbitol solution, USP, methylparaben, NF, propylparaben, NF, chlorobutanol, NF max. 0.05%, purified water, USP.

Oxytocin is one of the polypeptide hormones of the posterior lobe of the pituitary gland. The pharmacologic and clinical properties of Syntocinon (oxytocin) are identical with *the oxytocic and the galactokinetic* principle of the natural hormone. Syntocinon was synthesized on a commercial scale by Sandoz, and was introduced for clinical use in 1957.

Since oxytocin, a polypeptide, is subject to inactivation by the proteolytic enzymes of the alimentary tract, it is *not absorbed from the gastrointestinal tract.* Intranasal application of the spray preparation, however, is a practical and effective method of administration.

Action: Syntocinon Nasal Spray acts specifically on the myoepithelial elements surrounding the alveoli of the breast, causing them to contract and thus force milk into the larger ducts where it is more readily available to the baby.

Indication: Initial milk let-down.

Contraindications: Pregnancy; hypersensitivity.

Dosage and Administration: One spray into one or both nostrils 2 to 3 minutes before nursing or pumping of breasts.

Note: The squeeze bottle should be held in upright position when administering drug to the nose and patient should be in a sitting position rather than lying down. If preferred, the solution can be instilled in drop form by inverting the squeeze bottle and exerting very gentle pressure on its walls.

Supplied: Syntocinon (oxytocin) Nasal Spray in squeeze bottles containing 2 ml oxytocin solution or 5 ml oxytocin solution.

[SYT-ZZ10 Issued October 1, 1980]

VISKEN® ℞

(pindolol) tablets

The following prescribing information is based on official labeling in effect on November 1, 1982.

Description: Visken® (pindolol), a synthetic beta-adrenergic receptor blocking agent with intrinsic sympathomimetic activity is 4-(2-hydroxy-3-isopropylaminopropoxy)-indole.

Clinical Pharmacology: Visken (pindolol) is a non-selective beta-adrenergic antagonist (beta-blocker) which possesses intrinsic sympathomimetic activity (ISA) in therapeutic dosage ranges but does not possess quinidine-like membrane stabilizing activity.

Pharmacodynamics: In standard pharmacologic tests in man and animals, Visken (pindolol) attenuates increases in heart rate, systolic blood pressure, and cardiac output resulting from exercise and isoproterenol administration, thus confirming its beta-blocking properties. The ISA or partial agonist activity of VISKEN (pindolol) is mediated directly at the adrenergic receptor sites and may be blocked by other beta-blockers. In catecholamine depleted animal experiments, ISA is manifested as an increase in the inotropic and chronotropic activity of the myocardium. In man, ISA is manifested by a smaller reduction in the resting heart rate (4–8 beats/min) than is seen with drugs lacking ISA. There is also a smaller reduction in resting cardiac output. The clinical significance of this observation has not been evaluated and there is no evidence, or reason to believe, that exercise cardiac output is less affected by Visken (pindolol).

Visken (pindolol) has been shown in controlled, double-blind clinical studies to be an effective antihypertensive agent when used as monotherapy, or when added to therapy with thiazide-type diuretics. Divided dosages in the range of 10 mg—60 mg daily have been shown to be effective. As monotherapy, Visken (pindolol) is as effective as propranolol, α-methyldopa, hydrochlorothiazide and chlorthalidone in reducing systolic and diastolic blood pressure. The effect on blood pressure is not orthostatic, i.e. Visken (pindolol) was equally effective in reducing the supine and standing blood pressure. In open, long term studies up to four (4) years, no evidence of diminution of the blood pressure lowering response was observed.

An average 3 pound increase in body weight has been noted in patients treated with Visken (pindolol) alone, a larger increase than was observed with propranolol or placebo. The weight gain appeared unrelated to blood pressure response and was not associated with an increased risk of heart failure, although edema was more common than in control patients.

Visken (pindolol) does not have a consistent effect on plasma renin activity.

The mechanism of the antihypertensive effects of beta-blocking agents has not been established, but several mechanisms have been postulated: 1) an effect on the central nervous system resulting in a reduced sympathetic outflow to the periphery, 2) competitive antagonism of catecholamines at peripheral (especially cardiac) adrenergic receptor sites, leading to decreased cardiac output, 3) an inhibition of renin release. These mechanisms appear less likely for pindolol than other beta-blockers in view of the modest effect on resting cardiac output and renin.

Beta-blockade therapy is useful when it is necessary to suppress the effects of beta-adrenergic agonists in order to achieve therapeutic goals. However, in certain clinical situations, (e.g., cardiac failure, heart block, bronchospasm) the preservation of an adequate sympathetic tone may be necessary to maintain vital functions. Although a beta-antagonist with ISA such as Visken (pindolol) does not eliminate sympathetic tone entirely, there is no con-

Continued on next page

Sandoz—Cont.

trolled evidence that it is safer than other beta-blockers in such conditions as heart failure, heart block, or bronchospasm or is less likely to cause those conditions. In single dose studies of the effects of beta-blockers on FEV_1, Visken (pindolol) was indistinguishable from other non-cardioselective agents in its reduction of FEV_1, and its reduction in the effectiveness of an exogenous beta agonist.

Exacerbation of angina and, in some cases, myocardial infarction and ventricular dysrhythmias have been reported after abrupt discontinuation of therapy with beta-adrenergic blocking agents in patients with coronary artery disease. Abrupt withdrawal of these agents in patients without coronary artery disease has resulted in transient symptoms, including tremulousness, sweating, palpitation, headache, and malaise. Several mechanisms have been proposed to explain these phenomena, among them increased sensitivity to catecholamines because of increased numbers of beta receptors.

Pharmacokinetics and Metabolism: Visken (pindolol) is rapidly and reproducibly absorbed (greater than 95%), achieving peak plasma concentrations within one hour of drug administration. Visken (pindolol) has no significant first-pass effect. The blood concentrations are proportional in a linear manner to the administered dose in the range of 5–20 mg. Upon repeated administration to the same subject, variation is minimal. After a single dose, intersubject variation for peak plasma concentrations was about 4 fold (e.g. 45–167 ng/ml for a 20 mg dose). Upon multiple dosing, intersubject variation decreased to 2–2.5 fold. Visken (pindolol) is only 40% bound to plasma proteins and is evenly distributed between plasma and red cells. The volume of distribution in healthy subjects is about 2 L/kg.

Visken (pindolol) undergoes extensive metabolism in animals and man. In man, 35–40% is excreted unchanged in the urine and 60–65% is metabolized primarily to hydroxy-metabolites which are excreted as glucuronides and ethereal sulfates. The polar metabolites are excreted with a half-life of approximately 8 hours and thus multiple dosing therapy (q.8H) results in a less than 50% accumulation in plasma. About 6–9% of an administered intravenous dose is excreted by the bile into the feces.

The disposition of Visken (pindolol) after oral administration is monophasic with a half-life in healthy subjects or hypertensive patients with normal renal function of approximately 3–4 hours. Following t.i.d. administration (q.8H), no significant accumulation of Visken (pindolol) is observed.

In elderly hypertensive patients with normal renal function the half-life of Visken (pindolol) is more variable, averaging about 7 hours, but with values as high as 15 hours.

In hypertensive patients with renal diseases, the half-life is within the range expected for healthy subjects. However, a significant decrease (50%) in volume of distribution (V_D) is observed in uremic patients and V_D appears to be directly correlated to creatinine clearance. Therefore, renal drug clearance is significantly reduced in uremic patients, resulting in a significant decrease in urinary excretion of unchanged drug. Uremic patients with a creatinine clearance of less than 20 ml/min generally excreted less than 15% of the administered dose unchanged in the urine.

In patients with histologically diagnosed cirrhosis of the liver, the elimination of Visken (pindolol) was more variable in rate and generally significantly slower than in healthy subjects. The total body clearance of Visken (pindolol) in cirrhotic patients ranged from about 50 ml/min to 300 ml/min and was directly correlated to antipyrine clearance. The half-life ranged from 2.5 hours to greater than 30 hours. These findings strongly suggest that caution should be exercised in dosage adjustments of Visken (pindolol) in such patients.

The bioavailability of Visken (pindolol) is not significantly affected by co-administration of food, hydralazine, hydrochlorothiazide or aspirin. Visken (pindolol) has no effect on warfarin activity or the clinical effectiveness of digoxin, although small transient decreases in plasma digoxin concentrations were noted.

Indications and Usage: Visken (pindolol) is indicated in the management of hypertension. It may be used alone or concomitantly with other antihypertensive agents, particularly with a thiazide type diuretic.

Contraindications: Visken (pindolol) is contraindicated in: 1) bronchial asthma; 2) overt cardiac failure; 3) cardiogenic shock; 4) second and third degree heart block; 5) severe bradycardia; (see Warnings).

Warnings:

Cardiac Failure: Sympathetic stimulation may be a vital component supporting circulatory function in patients with congestive heart failure, and its inhibition by beta-blockade may precipitate more severe failure. Although beta-blockers should be avoided in overt congestive heart failure, if necessary, Visken (pindolol) can be used with caution in patients with a history of failure who are well-compensated, usually with digitalis and diuretics. Beta-adrenergic blocking agents do not abolish the inotropic action of digitalis on heart muscle.

In Patients Without A History of Cardiac Failure: In patients with latent cardiac insufficiency, continued depression of the myocardium with beta-blocking agents over a period of time can in some cases lead to cardiac failure. At the first sign or symptom of impending cardiac failure, patients should be fully digitalized and/or be given a diuretic, and the response observed closely. If cardiac failure continues, despite adequate digitalization and diuretic, Visken (pindolol) therapy should be withdrawn (gradually if possible).

Exacerbation of Ischemic Heart Disease Following Abrupt Withdrawal: Hypersensitivity to catecholamines has been observed in patients withdrawn from beta-blocker therapy; exacerbation of angina and, in some cases, myocardial infarction have occurred after *abrupt* discontinuation of such therapy. When discontinuing chronically administered Visken (pindolol), particularly in patients with ischemic heart disease, the dosage should be gradually reduced over a period of one to two weeks and the patient should be carefully monitored. If angina markedly worsens or acute coronary insufficiency develops, Visken (pindolol) administration should be reinstituted promptly, at least temporarily, and other measures appropriate for the management of unstable angina should be taken. Patients should be warned against interruption or discontinuation of therapy without the physician's advice. Because coronary artery disease is common and may be unrecognized, it may be prudent not to discontinue Visken (pindolol) therapy abruptly even in patients treated only for hypertension.

Nonallergic Bronchospasm (e.g., chronic bronchitis, emphysema)—Patients with Bronchospastic Diseases Should in General Not Receive Beta-Blockers: Visken (pindolol) should be administered with caution since it may block bronchodilation produced by endogenous or exogenous catecholamine stimulation of $beta_2$ receptors.

Major Surgery: Because beta blockade impairs the ability of the heart to respond to reflex stimuli and may increase the risks of general anesthesia and surgical procedures, resulting in protracted hypotension or low cardiac output, it has generally been suggested that such therapy should be withdrawn several days prior to surgery. Recognition of the increased sensitivity to catecholamines of patients recently withdrawn from beta-blocker therapy, however, has made this recommendation controversial. If possible, beta-blockers should be withdrawn well before surgery takes place. In the event of emergency surgery, the anesthesiologist should be informed that the patient is on beta-blocker therapy. The effects of Visken (pindolol) can be reversed by administration of beta-receptor agonists such as isoproterenol, dopamine, dobutamine, or levarterenol. Difficulty in restarting and maintaining the heart beat has also been reported with beta-adrenergic receptor blocking agents.

Diabetes and Hypoglycemia: Beta-adrenergic blockade may prevent the appearance of premonitory signs and symptoms (e.g., tachycardia and blood pressure changes) of acute hypoglycemia. This is especially important with labile diabetics. Beta-blockade also reduces the release of insulin in response to hyperglycemia; therefore, it may be necessary to adjust the dose of antidiabetic drugs.

Thyrotoxicosis: Beta-adrenergic blockade may mask certain clinical signs (e.g., tachycardia) of hyperthyroidism. Patients suspected of developing thyrotoxicosis should be managed carefully to avoid abrupt withdrawal of beta-blockade which might precipitate a thyroid crisis.

Precautions:

Impaired Renal or Hepatic Function: Beta-blocking agents should be used with caution in patients with impaired hepatic or renal function. Poor renal function has only minor effects on Visken (pindolol) clearance, but poor hepatic function may cause blood levels of Visken (pindolol) to increase substantially.

Information for Patients: Patients, especially those with evidence of coronary artery insufficiency, should be warned against interruption or discontinuation of Visken (pindolol) therapy without the physician's advice. Although cardiac failure rarely occurs in properly selected patients, patients being treated with beta-adrenergic blocking agents should be advised to consult the physician at the first sign or symptom of impending failure.

Drug Interactions: Catecholamine-depleting drugs (e.g., reserpine) may have an additive effect when given with beta-blocking agents. Patients receiving Visken (pindolol) plus a catecholamine depleting agent should, therefore, be closely observed for evidence of hypotension and/or marked bradycardia which may produce vertigo, syncope, or postural hypotension. Visken (pindolol) has been used with a variety of antihypertensive agents, including hydrochlorothiazide, hydralazine, and guanethidine without unexpected adverse interactions.

Carcinogenesis, Mutagenesis, Impairment of Fertility: In chronic oral toxicologic studies (one to two years) in mice, rats, and dogs, Visken (pindolol) did not produce any significant toxic effects. In two-year oral carcinogenicity studies in rats and mice in doses as high as 59 mg/kg/day and 124 mg/kg/day (50 and 100 times the maximum recommended human dose), respectively, Visken (pindolol) did not produce any neoplastic, preneoplastic, or non-neoplastic pathologic lesions. In fertility and general reproductive performance studies in rats, Visken (pindolol) caused no adverse effects at a dose of 10 mg/kg.

In the male fertility and general reproductive performance test in rats, definite toxicity characterized by mortality and decreased weight gain was observed in the group given 100 mg/kg/day. At 30 mg/kg/day, decreased mating was associated with testicular atrophy and /or decreased spermatogenesis. This response is not clearly drug related, however, as there was no dose response relationship within this experiment and no similar effect on testes of rats administered Visken (pindolol) as a dietary admixture for 104 weeks. There appeared to be an increase in prenatal mortality in males given 100 mg/kg but development of offspring was not impaired.

In females administered Visken (pindolol) prior to mating through day 21 of lactation, mating behavior was decreased at 100 mg/kg and 30 mg/kg. At these dosages there also was increased mortality of offspring. Prenatal mortality was increased at 10 mg/kg but there was not a clear dose response relationship in this experiment. There was an increased resorption rate at 100 mg/kg observed in females necropsied on the 15th day of gestation.

Pregnancy—Category B: Studies in rats and rabbits exceeding 100 times the maximum recommended human doses, revealed no embryotoxicity or teratogenicity. Since there are no adequate and well-controlled studies in pregnant women, and since animal reproduction studies are not always predictive of human response, Visken (pindolol), as with any drug, should be employed during pregnancy only if the potential benefit justifies the potential risk to the fetus.

Nursing Mothers: Since Visken (pindolol) is secreted in human milk, nursing should not be undertaken by mothers receiving the drug.

Pediatric Use: Safety and effectiveness in children have not been established.

Clinical Laboratory: Minor persistent elevations in serum transaminases (SGOT, SGPT) have been noted in 7% of patients during Visken (pindolol) administration, but progressive elevations were not observed and liver injury has not been reported in the medical literature over a ten (10) year period of marketing. Alkaline phosphatase, lactic acid dehydrogenase (LDH) and uric acid are also elevated on rare occasions. The significance of these findings is unknown.

Adverse Reactions: Most adverse reactions have been mild. The incidences listed in the following table are derived from 12 week comparative double-blind, parallel design trials in hypertensive patients given Visken (pindolol) as monotherapy, given various active control drugs as monotherapy, or given placebo. Data for Visken (pindolol) and the positive controls were pooled from several trials because no striking differences were seen in the individual studies, with one exception. The frequency of edema was noticeably higher in positive control trials (16% Visken (pindolol) vs 9% positive control) than in placebo controlled trials (6% Visken (pindolol) vs 3% placebo). The table includes adverse reactions reported in greater than 2% of Visken (pindolol) patients and other selected important reactions.

[See table above].

The following selected (potentially important) adverse reactions were seen in 2% or fewer patients and their relationship to Visken (pindolol) is uncertain. AUTONOMIC NERVOUS SYSTEM: hyperhidrosis; CARDIOVASCULAR: bradycardia, claudication, cold extremities, heart block, hypotension, syncope, tachycardia; GASTROINTESTINAL: diarrhea, vomiting; RESPIRATORY: wheezing; UROGENITAL: impotence, pollakiuria; MISCELLANEOUS: eye discomfort or burning eyes.

Potential Adverse Effects: In addition, other adverse effects not listed above have been reported with other beta-adrenergic blocking agents and should be considered potential adverse effects of Visken (pindolol).

Central Nervous System: Reversible mental depression progressing to catatonia; an acute reversible syndrome characterized by disorientation for time and place, short-term memory loss, emotional lability, slightly clouded sensorium, and decreased performance on neuropsychometrics.

Cardiovascular: Intensification of AV block. See CONTRAINDICATIONS.

Allergic: Erythematous rash; fever combined with aching and sore throat; laryngospasm; respiratory distress.

Hematologic: Agranulocytosis; thrombocytopenic and nonthrombocytopenic purpura.

Gastrointestinal: Mesenteric arterial thrombosis; ischemic colitis.

Body System/Adverse Reaction	Total (Volunteered and Elicited) Visken (pindolol) (N = 322) %	Active Controls* (N = 188) %	Placebo (N = 78) %
Central Nervous System			
Anxiety	4	<1	1
Bizarre or Many Dreams	8	3	8
Dizziness	17	23	8
Fatigue	15	19	12
Hallucinations	1	0	0
Insomnia	19	8	12
Lethargy	3	6	4
Nervousness	11	5	9
Weakness	7	5	4
Autonomic Nervous System			
Paresthesia	5	2	8
Visual Disturbances	4	3	4
Cardiovascular			
Dyspnea	9	8	9
Edema	11	9	3
Heart Failure	2	<1	0
Palpitations	2	2	0
Weight Gain	3	5	0
Musculo-Skeletal			
Chest Pain	5	3	5
Joint Pain	11	6	8
Muscle Cramps	8	2	0
Muscle Pain	12	12	9
Gastrointestinal			
Abdominal Discomfort	7	7	5
Nausea	7	4	1
Skin			
Pruritus	2	<1	0
Rash	2	3	3

*Active Controls: Patients received either propranolol, α-methyldopa or a diuretic (hydrochlorothiazide or chlorthalidone).

Miscellaneous: Reversible alopecia; Peyronie's disease.

The oculomucocutaneous syndrome associated with the beta-blocker practolol has not been reported with Visken (pindolol) during investigational use and extensive foreign experience amounting to over 4 million patient-years.

Overdosage: No specific information on emergency treatment of overdosage is available. Therefore, on the basis of the pharmacologic actions of Visken (pindolol), the following general measures should be employed as appropriate in addition to gastric lavage:

Excessive Bradycardia: administer atropine; if there is no response to vagal blockade, administer isoproterenol cautiously.

Cardiac Failure: digitalize the patient and/or administer diuretic. It has been reported that glucagon may be useful in this situation.

Hypotension: administer vasopressors, e.g., epinephrine or levarterenol, with serial monitoring of blood pressure. (There is evidence that epinephrine may be the drug of choice.)

Bronchospasm: administer a beta$_2$ stimulating agent such as isoproterenol and/or a theophylline derivative.

A case of an acute overdosage has been reported with an intake of 500 mg of Visken (pindolol) by a hypertensive patient. Blood pressure increased and heart rate was ≥80 beat/min. Recovery was uneventful. In another case 250 mg of Visken (pindolol) was taken with 150 mg diazepam and 50 mg nitrazepam, producing coma and hypotension. The patient recovered in 24 hours.

Dosage and Administration: The dosage of Visken (pindolol) should be individualized. The recommended initial dose of Visken (pindolol) is 10 mg b.i.d. alone or in combination with other antihypertensive agents. Many patients will respond to 15 mg per day (5 mg t.i.d.). The antihypertensive response usually occurs within the first week of treatment. If a satisfactory reduction in blood pressure does not occur within 2–3 weeks, the dose may be adjusted in increments of 10 mg per day at 2–3 week intervals up to a maximum of 60 mg per day.

How Supplied: White, round, scored tablets: 5 mg and 10 mg, packages of 100. 5 mg tablets embossed "VISKEN 5" on one side, and "78–111" and scored on other side (NDC 0078-0111-05). 10 mg tablets embossed "VISKEN 10" on one side, and "78–73" and scored on other side (NDC 0078-0073-05).

[VIS-Z2 Issued September 1, 1982]

Saron Pharmacal Corp.
1640 CENTRAL AVENUE
ST. PETERSBURG, FL 33712

AL-R DYE-FREE ℞
6 mg and 12 mg T.D. capsules
(chlorpheniramine maleate)

How Supplied: Bottles of 100.

BUTABELL HMB ℞

Each pink-coated tablet contains:

Butabarbital .... 15 mg
(Warning —may be habit forming)
Hyoscyamine sulfate 0.1037
Atropine sulfate 0.0194
Hyoscine hydrobromide .... 0.0065 mg

How Supplied: Bottles of 100.

CARDABID ℞

Description: Each light purple and clear T.D. capsule contains 2.5 mg nitroglycerin.

How Supplied: Bottles of 100.

CEREBID ℞

Description: Each red/clear CEREBID TD capsule contains papaverine hydrochloride, 150 mg. Each grey/clear CEREBID-200 TD

Continued on next page

Saron—Cont.

capsule contains papaverine hydrochloride, 200 mg.
How Supplied: Bottles of 100.

EMFASEEM ℞

Description: Each blue and white capsule contains:
Dyphylline (Dihydroxy-propyltheophylline)............200 mg.
Guaifenesin............100 mg.
How Supplied: Bottles of 100.

HCV CREME ℞

Contains:
Hydrocortisone Alcohol............1%
Iodochlorhydroxyquin............3%
How Supplied: 15 gram and 45 gram econo-pak tubes.

MEGA-VITA™ DYE-FREE ℞

Description: Each three, white, film-coated tablets contains:

Ascorbic Acid (Vitamin C)	500 mg.
Niacinamide	500 mg.
Pyridoxine HCl (Vitamin B6)	50 mg.
Thiamine HCl (Vitamin B1)	25 mg.
Riboflavin (Vitamin B2)	10 mg
Vitamin B12 (Cyanocobalamin)	50 mcg.
Folic Acid	150 mcg.
Vitamin E (d-Alpha Tocopheryl Acid Succinate)	200 IU
Pantothenic Acid (d-Calcium Panthothenate)	10 mg.
Vitamin A (as Palmitate)	2500 IU
Vitamin D2	333 IU
Magnesium Oxide, USP	50 mg.
Zinc Sulfate, USP	50 mg.

How Supplied: Bottles of 100.
Also available as a hematinic and as a tonic.

PULM™ 100 mg. TD, DYE-FREE ℞

Description: Each clear with white pellets capsule contains:
Theophylline (anhydrous)............100 mg.
How Supplied: Bottles of 100.

PULM™ 200 mg. TD, DYE-FREE ℞

Description: Each clear with white pellets capsule contains:
Theophylline (anhydrous)............200 mg.
How Supplied: Bottles of 100.

PULM™ 300 mg. TD, DYE-FREE ℞

Description: Each clear with white pellets capsule contains:
Theophylline (anhydrous)............300 mg.
How Supplied: Bottles of 100.

SAROFLEX™ DYE-FREE ℞

Each tan capsule contains:
Chlorzoxazone............250 mg
Acetaminophen............300 mg
How Supplied: Bottles of 100.

SAROLAX™ DYE-FREE ℞

Each brown and yellow capsule contains:
Dioctyl Sodium Sulfosuccinate............200 mg
Phenolphthalein Yellow............15 mg
Dehydrocholic Acid............20 mg
How Supplied: Bottles of 100.

Products are cross-indexed by generic and chemical names in the **YELLOW SECTION**

Savage Laboratories

a division of Byk-Gulden, Inc.
1000 MAIN ST.
POST OFFICE BOX 1000
MISSOURI CITY, TX 77459

BREXIN® Capsules and Liquid ℞

Description:
Capsules: Each maroon and yellow capsule for oral administration contains pseudoephedrine hydrochloride USP 60 mg, carbinoxamine maleate USP 4 mg, guaifenesin USP 100 mg.
Liquid: A red, pleasantly flavored, sweet tasting liquid for oral administration. Each teaspoonful (5 ml) contains: pseudoephedrine hydrochloride USP 30 mg, carbinoxamine maleate USP 2 mg, guaifenesin USP 100 mg.
This product contains ingredients of the following therapeutic classes: antihistamine, decongestant and expectorant.
Clinical Pharmacology: Carbinoxamine maleate is an ethanolamine-type antihistamine. Drugs in this group of histamine antagonists are potent and effective. Like all antihistamines, however, sedation has been observed with the use of carbinoxamine maleate, but it is generally mild.
Pseudoephedrine hydrochloride is a sympathomimetic which acts predominantly on alpha receptors and has little action on beta receptors. It therefore functions as an oral nasal decongestant with minimal CNS stimulation.
Guaifenesin is an expectorant which exerts its action by stimulation of reflexes from the stomach and acts through the nauseant effect which increases the output from the secretory glands of the respiratory tract.
Indications: Temporary relief of cough, nasal congestion and other symptoms associated with colds or seasonal or perennial allergic vasomotor rhinitis (hay fever).
Contraindications: Patients with severe hypertension, severe coronary artery disease, in patients on MAO inhibitor therapy and in nursing mothers. Also contraindicated in patients with narrow-angle glaucoma, urinary retention, peptic ulcer or in patients with a hypersensitivity to any of its ingredients.
Warnings: Considerable caution should be exercised in patients with hypertension, diabetes mellitus, ischemic heart disease, hyperthyroidism, increased intraocular pressure and prostatic hypertrophy. The elderly (60 years or older) are more likely to exhibit adverse reactions.
Antihistamines may cause excitability, especially in children. At dosages higher than the recommended dose, nervousness, dizziness or sleeplessness may occur.
Precautions:
General: Caution should be exercised in patients with high blood pressure, heart disease, diabetes or thyroid disease. The antihistamine in this product may exhibit additive effects with other CNS depressants, including alcohol.
Information for Patients: Antihistamine may cause drowsiness and ambulatory patients who operate machinery or motor vehicles should be cautioned accordingly.
Drug Interactions: MAO inhibitors and beta adrenergic blockers increase the effects of sympathomimetics. Sympathomimetics may reduce the antihypertensive effects of methyldopa, mecamylamine, reserpine and veratrum alkaloids. Concomitant use of antihistamines with alcohol and other CNS depressants may have an additive effect.
Pregnancy: The safety of use of this product in pregnancy has not been established.
Adverse Reactions: Adverse reactions include drowsiness, lassitude, nausea, giddiness, dryness of mouth, blurred vision, cardiac palpitations, flushing, increased irritability or excitement (especially in children).
Dosage and Administration: Capsules: Usual adult dose is one capsule 3 or 4 times a day.
Liquid: Adults and older children, 1 to 2 teaspoonfuls; children 6 to 12 years of age, 1 teaspoonful; children 2 to 6 years of age, ½ teaspoonful. This dose may be given every four hours.
How Supplied:
Capsules: NDC 0281-1945-53, bottle of 100.
NDC 0281-1945-56, bottle of 500.
Liquid: NDC 0281-1946-74, pint.
Store and dispense in tight containers as defined in the USP. Dispense in child resistant containers. Store between 59°–86°F.
Caution: Federal Law prohibits dispensing without prescription.
[*Shown in Product Identification Section*]

BREXIN® L.A. Capsules ℞

Description: A red and clear colored capsule containing red and blue colored beads. Each capsule for oral administration contains: chlorpheniramine maleate USP 8 mg, pseudoephedrine hydrochloride USP 120 mg, in a specially prepared base to provide prolonged action.
How Supplied: NDC 0281-1934-53, bottle of 100 capsules.
[*Shown in Product Identification Section*]

CHROMAGEN® CAPSULES ℞

Composition: Each maroon soft gelatin capsule contains ferrous fumarate USP 200 mg, ascorbic acid USP 250 mg, cyanocobalamin USP 10 mcg, desiccated stomach substance 100 mg.
Indications: For the treatment of all anemias responsive to oral iron therapy, such as hypochromic anemia associated with pregnancy, chronic or acute blood loss, dietary restriction, metabolic disease and post-surgical convalescence.
Administration and Dosage: Usual adult dose is 1 capsule daily.
Contraindications: Hemochromatosis and hemosiderosis are contraindications to iron therapy.
Side Effects: Average capsule doses in sensitive individuals or excessive dosage may cause nausea, skin rash, vomiting, diarrhea, precordial pain, or flushing of the face and extremities.
Supply:
NDC 0281-4285-53, bottle of 100.
NDC 0281-4285-56, bottle of 500.
[*Shown in Product Identification Section*]

DILOR® Tablets ℞
(dyphylline)

Composition: Each blue, scored tablet contains dyphylline (dihydroxypropyl theophylline) 200 mg; each white scored tablet contains dyphylline (dihydroxypropyl theophylline) 400 mg.
Description: Dyphylline [7-(2,3-Dihydroxypropyl) theophylline] [$C_{10}H_{14}N4\ O_4$] is a white, extremely bitter, amorphous solid, freely soluble in water and soluble to the extent of 2 gm in 100 ml alcohol.
Actions: As a xanthine derivative, dyphylline possesses the peripheral vasodilator and bronchodilator actions characteristic of theophylline. It has diuretic and myocardial stimulant effects, and is effective orally. Dyphylline may show fewer side effects than aminophylline, but its blood levels and possibly its activity are also lower.
Indications: For relief of acute bronchial asthma and for reversible bronchospasm associated with chronic bronchitis and emphysema.
Contraindications: In individuals who have shown hypersensitivity to any of its components. Dyphylline should not be administered

concurrently with other xanthine preparations.

Warnings: Status asthmaticus is a medical emergency. Excessive doses may be expected to be toxic. In children treated with dyphylline elixir, the alcoholic vehicle of the drug product poses a truly significant factor of drug dependence including all three components of tolerance, physical dependence and compulsive abuse.

Usage in Pregnancy: Safe use in pregnancy has not been established relative to possible adverse effects on fetal development. Therefore, dyphylline should not be used in pregnant women unless, in the judgment of the physician, the potential benefits outweigh the possible hazards.

Precautions: Use with caution in patients with severe cardiac disease, hypertension, hyperthyroidism, or acute myocardial injury. Particular caution in dose administration must be exercised in patients with peptic ulcers, since the condition may be exacerbated. Chronic oral administration in high doses (500 to 1,000 mg.) is usually associated with gastrointestinal irritation. Great caution should be used in giving dyphylline to patients in congestive heart failure. Such patients have shown markedly prolonged blood level curves which have persisted for long periods following discontinuation of the drug.

Adverse Reactions: Note: Included in this listing which follows are a few adverse reactions which may not have been reported with this specific drug. However, pharmacological similarities among the xanthine drugs require that each of the reactions be considered when dyphylline is administered. The most consistent adverse reactions are: 1. Gastrointestinal irritation: nausea, vomiting, and epigastric pain, generally preceded by headache, hematemesis, diarrhea. 2. Central nervous system stimulation: irritability, restlessness, insomnia, reflex hyperexcitability, muscle twitching, clonic and tonic generalized convulsions, agitation. 3. Cardiovascular: palpitation, tachycardia, extra systoles, flushing, marked hypotension, and circulatory failure. 4. Respiratory: tachypnea, respiratory arrest. 5. Renal: albuminuria, increased excretion of renal tubule and red blood cells. 6. Others: fever, dehydration.

Overdosage:

Symptoms:

In infants and small children: agitation, headache, hyperreflexia, fasciculations, and clonic and tonic convulsions.

In adults: nervousness, insomnia, nausea, vomiting, tachycardia and extra systoles.

Therapy:

Discontinue drug immediately.

No specific treatment.

Ipecac syrup for oral ingestion.

Avoid sympathomimetics.

Supportive treatment for hypotension, seizure, arrhythmias and dehydration.

Sedatives such as short acting barbiturates will help control central nervous system stimulation.

Restore the acid-base balance with lactate or bicarbonate.

Oxygen and antibiotics provide supportive treatment as indicated.

Drug Interactions: Toxic synergism with ephedrine and other sympathomimetic bronchodilator drugs may occur.

Recent controlled studies suggest that the addition of ephedrine to adequate dosage regimens of dyphylline produces no increase in effectiveness over that of dyphylline alone, but does produce an increase in toxic effects.

Dosage and Administration: When administered orally it produces less nausea than aminophylline and other alkaline theophylline compounds. Absorption orally appears to be faster on an empty stomach; preferably the drug is to be given at six hour intervals. Adults: Usual Adult Dose: 15 mg/kg every 6 hours up to 4 times a day. The dosage should be individualized by titration to the condition and response of the patient.

Pulmonary functional measurements before and after a period of treatment allow an objective assessment of whether or not therapy should be continued in patients with chronic bronchitis and emphysema.

Supply: Tablets,

200 mg– NDC 0281-1115-53, Bottle of 100.
NDC 0281-1115-57, Bottle of 1000.
NDC 0281-1115-63, Unit dose, Box of 100
NDC 0281-1115-67, Unit dose, Box of 10 × 100

400 mg– NDC 0281-1116-53, Bottle of 100.
NDC 0281-1116-57, Bottle of 1000.
NDC 0281-1116-63, Unit dose, Box of 100
NDC 0281-1116-67, Unit dose, Box of 10 × 100

Also Available: Dilor Elixir, Dyphylline 160 mg/15 ml; and Dilor Injectable, dyphylline 250 mg/ml.

[Shown in Product Identification Section]

DILOR-G® ℞

Composition: Each pink, scored tablet contains dyphylline 200 mg, guaifenesin USP 200 mg; oral liquid: each teaspoonful (5 ml) contains dyphylline 100 mg, guaifenesin USP 100 mg.

Supply: Tablets, NDC 0281-1124-53, bottle of 100.
NDC 0281-1124-57, bottle of 1000.
NDC 0281-1124-63, unit dose, 1 × 100.
Liquid, NDC 0281-1127-74, pint.
NDC 0281-1127-76, gallon.

[Shown in Product Identification Section]

DITATE®–DS ℞
(testosterone enanthate USP and estradiol valerate USP injection)

Each ml contains: testosterone enanthate USP 180 mg, estradiol valerate USP 8 mg, benzyl alcohol NF 2%. In sesame oil NF.

How Supplied: NDC 0281-5807-32, box of ten 2 ml single-dose vials.

NDC 0281-5807-43, box of ten 2 ml single-dose syringes.

HOMO-TET® ℞
(tetanus immune globulin USP)

Composition: A solution of gamma globulin 16.5%±1.5% prepared from venous blood of human subjects hyperimmunized with tetanus toxoid.

Supply: NDC 0281-7740-11, 250 unit single-dose vial.
NDC 0281-7740-12, 250 unit pre-filled disposable syringe.

IMMUGLOBIN® ℞
(immune globulin USP)

Composition: Each ml. contains Gamma Globulin 16.5%±1.5%. Standardized for measles and polio antibody content.

Supply: NDC 0281-7770-16, 10 ml vial.

MYTREX™ Cream and Ointment ℞
(nystatin neomycin gramicidin triamcinolone)

Description: Mytrex is available as a cream in an aqueous vanishing cream base and as an ointment in a polyethylene and mineral oil USP base. Each gram of the cream or ointment provides 100,000 units nystatin USP, neomycin sulfate USP equivalent to 2.5 mg neomycin base, 0.25 mg gramicidin NF, and 1 mg triamcinolone acetonide USP. The cream also contains polysorbate 60 NF, alcohol USP, aluminum hydroxide compressed gel, titanium dioxide USP, glyceryl monostearate, polyethylene glycol monostearate 400, simethicone, sorbic acid NF, propylene glycol USP, ethylenediamine USP, polyoxyethylene fatty alcohol ether, sorbitol solution USP, methyl paraben NF, propyl paraben NF, hydrochloric acid NF, white petrolatum USP, and purified water USP.

Actions: Triamcinolone acetonide is primarily effective because of its anti-inflammatory, antipruritic, and vasoconstrictive actions. Nystatin provides specific anticandidal activity and the two topical antibiotics, neomycin and gramicidin, provide antibacterial activity.

Indications

Based on a review of these drugs by the National Academy of Sciences-National Research Council and/or other information, FDA has classified the indications as follows:

Possibly effective: In
—cutaneous candidiasis
—superficial bacterial infections
—the following conditions when complicated by candidal and/or bacterial infection: atopic, eczematoid, stasis, nummular, contact, or seborrheic dermatitis; neuro-dermatitis and dermatitis venenata
—infantile eczema
—lichen simplex chronicus
—the Cream is also possibly effective in pruritus ani and pruritus vulvae

Final classification of the less-than-effective indications requires further investigation.

Contraindications: Topical steroids are contraindicated in viral diseases of the skin, such as vaccinia and varicella. The preparations are also contraindicated in fungal lesions of the skin except candidiasis, and in those patients with a history of hypersensitivity to any of their components.

The preparations are not for ophthalmic use nor should they be applied in the external auditory canal of patients with perforated eardrums. Topical steroids should not be used when circulation is markedly impaired.

Warnings: Because of the potential hazard of nephrotoxicity and ototoxicity, prolonged use or use of large amounts of these products should be avoided in the treatment of skin infections following extensive burns, trophic ulceration, and other conditions where absorption of neomycin is possible.

Usage in Pregnancy: Although topical steroids have not been reported to have an adverse effect on the fetus, the safety of topical steroid preparations during pregnancy has not been absolutely established; therefore, they should not be used extensively on pregnant patients, in large amounts, or for prolonged periods of time.

Precautions: As with any antibiotic preparation, prolonged use may result in overgrowth of nonsusceptible organisms, including fungi other than Candida. Constant observation of the patient is essential. Should superinfection due to nonsusceptible organisms occur, suitable concomitant anti-microbial therapy must be administered. If a favorable response does not occur promptly, application of Mytrex Cream and Ointment should be discontinued until the infection is adequately controlled by other anti-infective measures.

If extensive areas are treated or if the occlusive technique is used, the possibility exists of increased systemic absorption of the corticosteroid and suitable precautions should be taken. If irritation develops, the product should be discontinued and appropriate therapy instituted.

Adverse Reactions: Hypersensitivity to nystatin is extremely uncommon. Sensitivity reactions following the topical use of gramici-

Continued on next page

Savage—Cont.

din are rarely encountered. Hypersensitivity to neomycin has been reported and articles in the current medical literature indicate an increase in its prevalence.
The following local adverse reactions have been reported with topical corticosteroids either with or without occlusive dressings: burning sensations, itching, irritation, dryness, folliculitis, secondary infection, skin atrophy, striae, miliaria, hypertrichosis acneiform eruption, maceration of the skin and hypopigmentation. Contact sensitivity to a particular dressing material or adhesive may occur occasionally.
Ototoxicity and nephrotoxicity have been reported.
Dosage and Administration: Mytrex Cream—Rub into affected areas two to three times daily.
Mytrex Ointment—Apply a thin film to the affected areas two to three times daily.
Occlusive Dressing Technique:
Cream: Gently rub a small amount of the cream into the lesion until it disappears. Reapply the Cream leaving a thin coating on the lesion and cover with a pliable nonporous film. If needed, additional moisture may be provided by covering the lesion with a dampened clean cotton cloth before the plastic film is applied or by briefly soaking the affected area in water. The frequency of changing dressings is best determined on an individual basis. Reapplication is essential at each dressing change.
Ointment: Apply the Ointment leaving a thin coating on the lesion and cover with a pliable nonporous film. If needed, additional moisture may be provided by covering the lesions with a dampened clean cotton cloth before the plastic film is applied or by briefly soaking the affected area in water.
The frequency of changing dressings is best determined on an individual basis. Reapplication is essential at each dressing change.
How Supplied:
Cream: NDC 0281-3311-44, 15 gram tube.
NDC 0281-3311-45, 30 gram tube.
NDC 0281-3311-46, 60 gram tube.
NDC 0281-3311-49, 120 gram jar.
Ointment: NDC 0281-3318-44, 15 gram tube.
NDC 0281-3318-45, 30 gram tube.
NDC 0281-3318-46, 60 gram tube.
Caution: Federal law prohibits dispensing without prescription.
FOR EXTERNAL USE ONLY

SĀTRIC™ Tablets (metronidazole USP) ℞

WARNING: Metronidazole has been shown to be carcinogenic in mice and possibly carcinogenic in rats. (*See Warnings*). Unnecessary use of this drug should be avoided. Its use should be reserved for the conditions described in the Indications and Usage section below.

Description: Sātric (metronidazole) is a 1-(β-hydroxyethyl)-2-methyl-nitroimidazole. Metronidazole is classified therapeutically as an antiprotozoal (Trichomonas). It occurs as pale yellow crystals that are slightly soluble in water and alcohol. Metronidazole has the following structural formula:

CH_2CH_2OH / O_2N / N / CH_3 / N

Clinical Pharmacology: Metronidazole possesses direct Trichomonacidal and amebacidal activity against *Trichomonas vaginalis* and *Entamoeba histolytica*. Metronidazole is usually well absorbed after oral administration. The peak serum level is reached in about one hour with an average elimination half-life in healthy humans of eight hours.
Pharmacologically, metronidazole appears to be practically inert. Large doses in experimental animals affect neither the cardiovascular system nor respiration.
Metronidazole is usually well absorbed after oral administration. Some patients fail to respond to treatment, however, and in such cases, a low systemic concentration of the drug may be responsible. Whether this is due to relatively poor absorption from the gastrointestinal tract or to a rapid rate of metabolic transformation is open to question.
The major route of elimination of metronidazole and its metabolites is via the urine (60–80% of the dose), with fecal excretion accounting for 6–15% of the dose. The metabolites that appear in the urine result primarily from side-chain oxidation [1-(β-hydroxyethyl)-2-hydroxymethyl-5-nitroimidazole and 2-methyl-5-nitroimidazole-1-yl-acetic acid] and glucuronide conjugation, with unchanged metronidazole accounting for approximately 20% of the total. Renal clearance of metronidazole is approximately 10 ml/min/1.73m^2.
The urine of some patients may be reddish-brown in color due to the presence of water soluble pigments derived from the drug.
Metronidazole is the major component appearing in the plasma, with lesser quantities of the 2-hydroxymethyl metabolite also being present. Less than 20% of the circulating metronidazole is bound to plasma proteins. Both the parent compound and the metabolite possess *in vitro* trichomonacidal activity.
Metronidazole appears in cerebrospinal fluid, saliva, and breast milk in concentrations similar to those found in plasma. Bactericidal concentrations of metronidazole have also been detected in pus from hepatic abscesses. Plasma concentrations of metronidazole are proportional to the administered dose. Oral administration of 250 mg, 500 mg, or 2,000 mg produced peak plasma concentrations of 6 mcg/ml, 12 mcg/ml and 40 mcg/ml, respectively. Studies reveal no significant bioavailability differences between males and females, however, because of weight differences, the resulting plasma levels in males are generally lower.
Decreased renal function does not alter the single-dose pharmacokinetics of metronidazole. However, plasma clearance of metronidazole is decreased in patients with decreased liver function.
Microbiology: Metronidazole posseses direct trichomonacidal and amebacidal activity against *Trichomonas Vaginalis* and *Entamoeba histolytica.* The *in vitro* minimal inhibitory concentration (MIC) for most strains of these organisms is 1 mcg/ml or less. Metronidazole's mechanism of antiprotozoal action is unknown.
Indications and Usage:
Symptomatic Trichomoniasis: Sātric is indicated for the treatment of symptomatic trichomoniasis in females and males when the presence of trichomonad has been confirmed by appropriate laboratory procedures (wet smears and/or cultures).
Asymptomatic Trichomoniasis: Sātric is indicated in the treatment of asymptomatic females when the organism is associated with endocervicitis, cervicitis, or cervical erosion. Since there is evidence that presence of the trichomonad can interfere with accurate assessment of abnormal cytological smears, additional smears should be performed after eradication of the parasite.
Treatment of Asymptomatic Consorts: T. vaginalis infection is a venereal disease. Therefore, asymptomatic sexual partners of treated patients should be treated simultaneously if the organism has been found to be present in order to prevent reinfection of the partner. The decision as to whether to treat an asymptomatic male partner with a negative culture or one in whom no culture has been attempted is an individual one. In making this decision, it should be noted that there is evidence that women may become reinfected if the consort is not treated. Also, since there can be considerable difficulty in isolating the organism from the asymptomatic male carrier, negative smears and cultures cannot be relied upon in this regard. In any event, the consort should be treated with Sātric in cases of reinfection.
Amebiasis: Sātric is indicated in the treatment of acute intestinal amebiasis (amebic dysentery) and amebic liver abscess.
In amebic liver abscess, Sātric therapy does not obviate the need for aspiration or drainage of pus.
Contraindications: Sātric is contraindicated in patients with active organic disease of the central nervous system (*See Adverse Reactions.*)
Sātric is contraindicated during the first trimester of pregnancy (*See Warnings.*)
Sātric is also contraindicated in patients with a prior history of hypersensitivity to metronidazole.
Warnings:
Convulsive Seizures and *Peripheral Neuropathy:* Convulsive seizures and peripheral neuropathy, the latter characterized mainly by numbness or paresthesia of an extremity, have been reported in patients treated with metronidazole. The appearance of abnormal neurologic signs demands the prompt discontinuation of Sātric therapy. Sātric should be administered with caution to patients with central nervous system diseases.
Tumorigenicity Studies in Rodents: Metronidazole has shown evidence of tumorigenic activity in a number of studies involving chronic, oral administration in mice and rats. Most prominent among the effects in the mouse was the promotion of pulmonary tumorigenesis. This has been observed in all five reported studies in that species, including one study in which animals were dosed on an intermittent schedule (administration during every fourth week only). The published results of one of the mouse studies indicate an increase in the incidence of malignant lymphomas as well as pulmonary neoplasms associated with lifetime feeding of the drug. All these effects are statistically significant.
Two long-term toxicity studies in the rat have been completed. There was a statistically significant increase in the incidence of various neoplasms, particularly mammary tumors, among female rats administered metronidazole over that noted in the concurrent female control groups. Two lifetime tumorigenicity studies in hamsters have been performed and reported to be negative.
Precautions:
General: Patients with severe hepatic disease metabolize metronidazole slowly, with resultant accumulation of metronidazole and its metabolites in the plasma. Accordingly, for such patients, doses below those usually recommended should be administered cautiously.
Known or previously unrecognized candidiasis may present more prominent symptoms during therapy with Sātric and requires treatment with a candicidal agent.
Laboratory Tests: Sātric (metronidazole) is a nitroimidazole and should be used with care in patients with evidence of, or history of blood dyscrasia. A mild leukopenia has been observed during its administration, however, no persistent hematologic abnormalities attributable to metronidazole have been observed in clinical studies. Total and differential leukocyte counts are recommended before and after therapy for trichomoniasis and amebiasis, especially if a second course of therapy is necessary.
Drug Interactions: Metronidazole has been reported to potentiate the anticoagulant effect

of coumarin and warfarin resulting in a prolongation of prothrombin time. This possible drug interaction should be considered when Sātric is prescribed for patients on this type of anti-coagulant therapy.

Alcoholic beverages should not be consumed during Sātric therapy because abdominal cramps, nausea, vomiting, headache, and flushing may occur.

Drug/Laboratory Test Interactions: Metronidazole may interfere with certain chemical analyses for serum glutamic oxalacetic transaminase, resulting in decreased values. Values of zero may be observed.

Carcinogenesis: (*See Warnings*).

Pregnancy: Teratogenic Effects—Pregnancy Category B: Metronidazole crosses the placental barrier and enters the fetal circulation rapidly. Reproduction studies have been performed in rabbits and rats at doses up to five times the human dose and have revealed no evidence of impaired fertility or harm to the fetus due to metronidazole. There are, however, no adequate and well-controlled studies in pregnant women. Because animal reproduction studies are not always predictive of human response, and because metronidazole is a carcinogen in rodents, this drug should be used during pregnancy only if clearly needed. (*See Contraindications*).

Use of Sātric for trichomoniasis in the second and third trimesters should be restricted to those in whom local palliative treatment has been inadequate to control symptoms.

Nursing Mothers: Because of the potential for tumorigenicity shown for metronidazole in mouse and rat studies, a decision should be made whether to discontinue nursing or to discontinue the drug, taking into account the importance of the drug to the mother. Metronidazole is secreted in breast milk in concentrations similar to those found in plasma.

Pediatric Use: Safety and effectiveness in children have not been established, except for the treatment of amebiasis.

Adverse Reactions: By far the most common adverse reactions have been referable to the gastrointestinal tract, particularly nausea, sometimes accompanied by headache, anorexia and occasionally vomiting, diarrhea, epigastric distress and abdominal cramping; constipation has also been reported. A metallic, sharp, unpleasant taste is not unusual. Furry tongue, glossitis and stomatitis have occurred these may be associated with a sudden overgrowth of *Candida* which may occur during effective therapy. Proliferation of *Candida* also may occur in the vagina.

A moderate leukopenia may be observed occasionally. If this occurs, the total leukocyte count may be expected to return to normal after the course of medication is completed.

If patients receiving Sātric drink alcoholic beverages, they may experience abdominal distress, nausea, vomiting, flushing, or headache. A modification of the taste of alcoholic beverages has also been reported.

Dizziness, vertigo, incoordination, ataxia, convulsive seizures and peripheral neuropathy have been reported. Numbness or paresthesia of an extremity and fleeting joint pains sometimes resembling "serum sickness" have been experienced, as have confusion, irritability, depression, weakness, insomnia, and a mild erythematous eruption.

Urticaria, flushing, nasal congestion, dryness of the mouth (or vagina or vulva), pruritus, dysuria, cystitis and a sense of pelvic pressure have been reported.

Very rarely dyspareunia fever, polyuria, incontinence, decrease of libido, proctitis, and pyuria have occurred in patients receiving the drug.

Instances of darkened urine have been reported and this manifestation has been the subject of a special investigation. Although the pigment which is probably responsible for this phenomenon has not been positively identified, it is almost certainly a metabolite of metronidazole. It seems certain that it is of no clinical significance and may be encountered only when Sātric is administered in higher-than-recommended doses.

Flattening of the T-wave may be seen in electrocardiographic tracings.

Overdosage: Single oral doses of metronidazole, up to 15 g, have been reported in suicide attempts and accidental overdoses. Symptoms reported include nausea, vomiting and ataxia. Oral metronidazole has been studied as a radiation sensitizer in the treating of malignant tumors. Neurotoxic effects, including seizures and peripheral neuropathy, have been reported after 5 to 7 days of doses of 6 to 10.4 g every other day.

Treatment: There is no specific antidote for Sātric overdose; therefore, management of the patient should consist of symptomatic and supportive therapy.

Dosage and Administration:

Trichomoniasis: In The Female: The recommended dosage is one 250 mg tablet orally 3 times daily for 7 days.

One day therapy with 2 g of Sātric administered either as a single dose or divided doses (4 tablets twice a day) is efficacious. Cure rates may be higher for the 7 day regimen.

Selection of the appropriate treatment mode should be individualized. One day therapy often maximizes compliance, while 7 day therapy decreases the possibility of reinfection by her sexual partner(s). Certain patients may tolerate one form of therapy over the other.

Pregnant patients should not be treated during the first trimester with either regimen. If treated during the second or third trimester, the one day course of therapy should not be used, as it results in higher serum levels which reach the fetal circulation. (*See Contraindications and Precautions*).

When repeat courses of the drug are required, it is recommended that an interval of 4 to 6 weeks elapse between courses and that the presence of the trichomonad be reconfirmed by appropriate laboratory measures. Total and differential leukocyte counts should be made before and after retreatment. (*See Precautions—Laboratory Tests*).

In The Male: One 250 mg tablet 3 times daily for 7 days is recommended as a course of treatment, however, treatment may be individualized as for the female.

Amebiasis: Adults: For Acute Intestinal Amebiasis (Acute Amebic Dysentery): 750 mg orally 3 times daily for 5 to 10 days.

For Amebic Liver Abscess: 500 mg or 750 mg orally 3 times daily for 5 to 10 days.

Children: 35 to 50 mg/kg of body weight/24 hours divided into 3 doses, orally for 10 days.

How Supplied: Available in tablets containing 250 mg and 500 mg of metronidazole USP. Each tablet of 250 mg is imprinted 3681. It is a white, to off white round, convex tablet, packaged in bottles of 100 and 250 tablets.

Each tablet of 500 mg is imprinted Z3007. It is a white to off white oblong, concave tablet, packaged in bottles of 60 and 4 tablets.

NDC 0281-3681-53, bottle of 100

NDC 0281-3681-55, bottle of 250

Dispense in well closed, light resistant containers as defined in the USP.

Store below 86°F (30°C).

Manufactured by
Zenith Laboratories, Inc.
Northvale, New Jersey 07647
Distributed by
SAVAGE LABORATORIES
a division of Byk-Gulden, Inc.
Missouri City, Texas 77459

[*Shown in Product Identification Section*]

TRYMEX™ ℞

Triamcinolone Acetonide Cream U.S.P. and Ointment U.S.P.

Description: Trymex Cream U.S.P., 0.025% contains: 0.25 mg of Triamcinolone Acetonide per gram in a base containing Emulsifying Wax, Cetyl Alcohol, Isopropyl Palmitate, Sorbitol Solution, Glycerin, Lactic Acid, Benzyl Alcohol and Purified Water.

Trymex Cream U.S.P., 0.1% contains: 1 mg of Triamcinolone Acetonide per gram in a base containing Emulsifying Wax, Cetyl Alcohol, Isopropyl Palmitate, Sorbitol Solution, Glycerin, Lactic Acid, Benzyl Alcohol and Purified Water.

Trymex Cream U.S.P., 0.5% contains: 5 mg of Triamcinolone Acetonide per gram in a base containing Emulsifying Wax, Cetyl Alcohol, Isopropyl Palmitate, Sorbitol Solution, Glycerin, Lactic Acid, Benzyl Alcohol and Purified Water.

Trymex Ointment U.S.P., 0.025% contains: 0.25 mg of Triamcinolone Acetonide per gram in a base containing White Petrolatum and Mineral Oil.

Trymex Ointment U.S.P., 0.1% contains: 1 mg of Triamcinolone Acetonide per gram in a base containing white Petrolatum and Mineral Oil.

Actions: Topical steroids are primarily effective because of their anti-inflammatory, antipruritic and vasoconstrictive actions.

Indications: For relief of the inflammatory manifestations of corticosteroid-responsive dermatoses.

Contraindications: Topical steroids are contraindicated in those patients with a history of hypersensitivity to any of the components of the preparation.

Precautions: If irritation develops, the product should be discontinued and appropriate therapy instituted.

In the presence of an infection the use of an appropriate antifungal or antibacterial agent should be instituted.

If a favorable response does not occur promptly, the corticosteroid should be discontinued until the infection has been adequately controlled.

If extensive areas are treated or if the occlusive technique is used, there will be increased systemic absorption of the corticosteroid and suitable precautions should be taken, particularly in children and infants. Although topical steroids have not been reported to have an adverse effect on human pregnancy, the safety of their use in pregnant women has not absolutely been established. In laboratory animals, increases in incidence of fetal abnormalities have been associated with exposure of gestating females to topical corticosteroids in some cases at rather low dosage levels. Therefore, drugs of this class should not be used extensively on pregnant patients, in large amounts, or for prolonged periods of time.

The product is not for ophthalmic use.

Adverse Reactions: The following local adverse reactions have been reported with topical corticosteroids especially under occlusive dressings.

Burning
Itching
Irritation
Dryness
Folliculitis
Hypertrichosis
Acneiform eruptions
Hypopigmentation
Perioral dermatitis
Allergic contact dermatitis
Maceration of the skin
Secondary infection
Skin atrophy
Striae
Miliaria

Continued on next page

Savage—Cont.

Dosage and Administration: Trymex Cream U.S.P., 0.025%: Apply to the affected area two to four times daily. Rub in gently.
Trymex Cream U.S.P., 0.1% and 0.5%: Apply to the affected area two to three times daily. Rub in gently.
Trymex Ointment U.S.P., 0.025%: Apply a thin film to the affected area two to four times daily.
Trymex Ointment U.S.P., 0.1%: Apply a thin film to the affected area two to three times daily.
Occlusive Dressing Technique. Trymex Cream U.S.P., 0.025%, 0.1% and 0.5%: Gently rub a small amount of the preparation into the lesion until it disappears. Reapply the preparation leaving a thin coating on the lesion and cover with a pliable nonporous film. If needed, additional moisture may be provided by covering the lesion with a dampened clean cotton cloth before the plastic film is applied or by briefly soaking the affected area in water. The frequency of changing dressings is best determined on an individual basis. Reapplication of the preparation is essential at each dressing change.
Trymex Ointment U.S.P., 0.025% and 0.1%: Apply a thin coat of the ointment to the affected area and cover with a pliable nonporous film. If desired, the lesion may be moistened with a dampened clean cotton cloth before the plastic film is applied. The frequency of changing dressings is best determined on an individual basis. Reapplication of the preparation is essential at each dressing change.
Storage: Store the creams at room temperature; avoid freezing. Store the ointments at room temperature.
How Supplied:
Trymex Cream U.S.P., 0.025%
NDC 0281-3622-44, 15 gram tube
NDC 0281-3622-48, 80 gram tube
NDC 0281-3622-87, 1 pound jar
Trymex Cream U.S.P., 0.1%
NDC 0281-3625-44, 15 gram tube
NDC 0281-3625-48, 80 gram tube
NDC 0281-3625-87, 1 pound jar
Trymex Cream U.S.P., 0.5%
NDC 0281-3627-44, 15 gram tube
Trymex Ointment U.S.P., 0.025%
NDC 0281-3633-44, 15 gram tube
NDC 0281-3633-48, 80 gram tube
Trymex Ointment U.S.P., 0.1%
NDC 0281-3636-44, 15 gram tube
NDC 0281-3636-48, 80 gram tube
Caution: Federal law prohibits dispensing without prescription.
FOR EXTERNAL USE ONLY

TRYSUL® ℞
Triple Sulfa Vaginal Cream

Description: Active Ingredients: sulfathiazole 3.42%, sulfacetamide 2.86%, sulfabenzamide 3.70% and urea 0.64%
In a Base Containing: Glyceryl monostearate, cetyl alcohol, stearic acid, lecithin, peanut oil, diethylaminoethyl steramide, phosphoric acid, propylene glycol, ethoxylated cholesterol, methyl paraben 0.15% and propyl paraben 0.05% as preservatives, and purified water.
Indications: Trysul is indicated for the treatment of haemophilus vaginalis vaginitis. It may also be used as a deodorant for saprophytic infection following radiation therapy.
Contraindications: Sulfonamide sensitivity and kidney disease.
Warning: Keep out of reach of children.
Caution: Federal law prohibits dispensing without prescription.

Store at room temperature.
Dosage: One applicatorfull intravaginally twice daily for 4 to 6 days. The dosage may then be reduced one-half to one-quarter.
How Supplied: NDC 0281-3790-47, 78 g tube with measured dose applicator.

ZIPAN-25® and ZIPAN-50® ℞
(promethazine hydrochloride injection USP)

Composition: ZiPAN-25: Each ml contains promethazine hydrochloride USP 25 mg; ZiPAN-50: Each ml contains promethazine hydrochloride USP 50 mg.
Supply:
ZIPAN-25, NDC 0281-1410-16, 10 ml vial.
NDC 0281-1410-24, 25 × 1 ml ampules.
ZIPAN-50, NDC 0281-1411-16, 10 ml vial.
NDC 0281-1411-24, 25 × 1 ml ampules.

The R. Schattner Company
Pharmaceutical Division
4000 MASSACHUSETTS AVE., N.W.
WASHINGTON, DC 20016

ORADERM® LIP BALM
(Effective surface anesthetic and antiseptic)

Composition: A hypo-allergenic, "ALL-WEATHER™", lip balm incorporating sodium phenolate, sodium tetraborate and phenol in a specially prepared protective base containing an anionic emulsifier.
Action: ORADERM is both an anesthetic and antiseptic hypo-allergenic lip balm containing no "caines" or antibiotics. It is specifically designed to maintain lip hygiene by reducing the oral bacterial flow and to relieve local dryness, soreness and irritations. It protects against infection while bringing symptomatic relief. Lasting surface anesthesia is obtained, usually in seconds. ORADERM is an effective antimicrobial against a wide range of gram negative and gram positive bacteria and fungi for infection control. ORADERM is a soothing protectant which cools and promotes healing of the lip tissues.
Indications: ORADERM may be used in adjunctive therapy, as a topical *anesthetic* and *antiseptic* in labial manifestations of systemic disease. It is indicated for prompt temporary symptomatic relief of pain and discomfort associated with: *sunburn, windburn, cold sores* (lesions and cracking), *dryness* (from fever, mouth breathing and lip licking), *herpetic lesions* (fever blisters), *dermatitis venenata* (from lipstick), cheilitis (chronic and simplex), *perleche* (angular stomatitis), *abrasions* (lip biting, etc.)
Hypo-allergenic: In controlled university studies, ORADERM was found to be non-toxic, non-sensitizing and hypo-allergenic.
Administration: Apply liberally to the labial tissues, as often as necessary.
How Supplied: Pocket-size ⅛ oz.
NO PRESCRIPTION NECESSARY.

Products are listed alphabetically in the **PINK SECTION.**

Henry Schein, Inc.
5 HARBOR PARK DRIVE
PORT WASHINGTON, NY 11050

COMPREHENSIVE LIST OF SCHEIN GENERIC PRODUCTS

NDC 0364	PRODUCT
	Acetazolamide Tablets ℞
04-0001	250 mg, 100's
04-0002	250 mg, 1000's
	Aminophylline Tablets ℞
00-0401	1½ gr C/T, 100's
00-0402	1½ gr C/T, 1000's
00-0501	3 gr C/T, 100's
00-0502	3 gr C/T, 1000's
	Amitriptyline HCl Tablets ℞
05-7301	10 mg, 100's
05-7302	10 mg, 1000's
05-7401	25 mg, 100's
05-7402	25 mg, 1000's
05-7501	50 mg, 100's
05-7502	50 mg, 1000's
05-7601	75 mg, 100's
05-7701	100 mg, 100's
05-7801	150 mg, 100's
	Amoxicillin Trihydrate Capsules ℞
20-4001	250 mg, 100's
20-4005	250 mg, 500's
	(D.S.S.)
20-4150	500 mg, 50's
	Amoxicillin Trihydrate Powder ℞ For Oral Suspension
72-1561	125 mg, 100 ml
72-1562	125 mg, 150 ml
72-1661	250 mg, 100 ml
72-1662	250 mg, 150 ml
	Ampicillin Trihydrate Capsules ℞
20-0101	250 mg, 100's
20-0105	250 mg, 500's
20-0201	500 mg, 100's
20-0205	500 mg, 500's
	Ampicillin Trihydrate Powder For Oral Suspension ℞
20-0361	125 mg, 100 ml
20-0363	125 mg, 200 ml
20-0461	250 mg, 100 ml
20-0463	250 mg, 200 ml
	Antispasmodic Tablets ℞ (Atropine Derivatives, Hyoscyamine, Phenobarbital)
00-2002	1000's
00-2003	5000's
	Antispasmodic Elixir ℞ (Atropine Derivatives, Hyoscyamine, Phenobarbital)
70-0216	Pt
70-0299	Gal
	Apap Tablets OTC
00-2204	5 gr, 250's
00-2202	5 gr, 1000's
	Apap Extra Strength Capsules OTC
04-2601	500 mg, 100's
04-2602	500 mg, 1000's
	Apap Extra Strength Tablets OTC
05-5304	500 mg, 250's
05-5302	500 mg, 1000's
	Apap 300 mg with Codeine Tablets Ⓒ III
03-2301	15 mg, 100's
03-2401	30 mg, 100's
03-2402	30 mg, 1000's
03-2601	60 mg, 100's
03-2602	60 mg, 1000's
	Apap with Codeine Elixir Ⓒ
72-0716	Pt
	Aspirin 325 mg with Codeine Tablets Ⓒ III
05-4001	30 mg, 100's
05-4002	30 mg, 1000's
05-4101	60 mg, 100's
	Azo-Sulfisoxazole Tablets ℞
00-4102	1000's

Bromanyl Expectorant C
(Ammonium Chloride, Bromodiphenhydramine HCl, Codeine Phosphate, Diphenhydramine HCl, Potassium Guaicolsulfonate)
72-6516 Pt
72-6599 Gal

Bromphen Compound Tablets ℞
(Brompheniramine Maleate, Phenylephrine HCl, Phenylpropanolamine HCl)
05-8401 100's
05-8402 1000's

Bromphen Comp. Elixir - Sugar Free ℞
(Brompheniramine Maleate, Phenylephrine HCl, Phenylpropanolamine)
72-8116 Pt
72-8199 Gal

Bromphen Expectorant ℞
Brompheniramine Maleate, Guaifenesin, Phenylephrine HCl, Phenylpropanolamine)
72-7916 Pt
72-7999 Gal

Bromphen DC Expectorant C
(Brompheniramine Maleate, Codeine Phosphate, Guaifenesin, Phenylephrine HCl, Phenylpropanolamine)
72-8016 Pt
72-8099 Gal

Chloral Hydrate Capsules C
00-6101 7½ gr, 100's
00-6102 7½ gr, 1000's

Chlordiazepoxide HCl Capsules C
04-3601 5 mg, 100's
04-3605 5 mg, 500's
04-3602 5 mg, 1000's
04-3701 10 mg, 100's
04-3705 10 mg, 500's
04-3702 10 mg, 1000's
04-3801 25 mg, 100's
04-3805 25 mg, 500's

Chloroserpine - 250 Tablets ℞
(Chlorothiazide, Reserpine)
04-2201 100's
04-2202 1000's

Chloroserpine - 500 Tablets ℞
(Chlorothiazide, Reserpine)
04-2301 100's
04-2302 1000's

Chlorothiazide Tablets ℞
03-8901 250 mg, 100's
03-8902 250 mg, 1000's
03-9001 500 mg, 100's
03-9002 500 mg, 1000's

Chlorpromazine HCl Tablets ℞
03-8001 10 mg, 100's
03-8002 10 mg, 1000's
03-8101 25 mg, 100's
03-8102 25 mg, 1000's
03-8201 50 mg, 100's
03-8202 50 mg, 1000's
03-8301 100 mg, 100's
03-8302 100 mg, 1000's
03-8401 200 mg, 100's
03-8402 200 mg, 1000's

Chlorthalidone Tablets ℞
05-9201 25 mg, 100's
05-9202 25 mg, 1000's
05-9301 50 mg, 100's
05-9302 50 mg, 1000's

Chlorzone Forte Tablets ℞
(Acetaminophen, Chlorzoxazone)
04-6201 100's
04-6202 1000's

Clipoxide Capsules ℞
(Chlordiazepoxide HCl, Clidinium Bromide)
05-5901 100's
05-5905 500's

Cloxacillin Sodium Capsules ℞
20-6101 250 mg, 100's
20-6201 500 mg, 100's

Conjugated Estrogens Tablets - Coated ℞
00-7801 .625 mg, 100's
00-7802 .625 mg, 1000's
00-7901 1.25 mg, 100's
00-7902 1.25 mg, 1000's
00-8001 2.5 mg, 100's
00-8002 2.5 mg, 1000's

Cyclandelate Capsules ℞
05-7001 200 mg, 100's
05-7002 200 mg, 1000's
05-7101 400 mg, 100's
05-7102 400 mg, 1000's

Cyproheptadine HCl Tablets ℞
04-9901 4 mg, 100's
04-9905 4 mg, 500's

Dexamethasone Tablets - Pentagonal Shaped ℞
03-9701 .25 mg, 100's
03-9702 .25 mg, 1000's
03-9801 .50 mg, 100's
03-9802 .50 mg, 1000's
00-9801 .75 mg, 100's
00-9802 .75 mg, 1000's
03-9901 1.5 mg, 100's

Dexchlor Repeat Action Tablets ℞
(Dexchlorpheniramine Maleate)
05-8501 4 mg, 100's
05-8601 6 mg, 100's
05-8602 6 mg, 1000's

Diethylpropion HCl Tablets C
03-2901 25 mg, 100's
03-2902 25 mg, 1000's

Diethylpropion HCl Timed Tablets C
04-4001 75 mg, 100's
04-4004 75 mg, 250's

Dihydrocodeine Compound Capsules C-III
(Dihydrocodeinone Bitartrate, Aspirin, Caffeine, Promethazine)
05-8301 100's

Dioctocal Capsules - Docusate Calcium USP OTC
05-8901 240 mg, 100's

Diphenhydramine HCl Capsules ℞
01-1602 25 mg, 1000's
01-1702 50 mg, 1000's

Diphenhydramine Elixir ℞
70-2316 Pt
70-2399 Gal

Diphenhydramine Cough Syrup OTC
72-2216 Pt
72-2299 Gal

Diphenoxylate & Atropine Tablets C
04-4901 100's
04-4905 500's
04-4902 1000's

Diphenoxylate & Atropine Liquid (DPXL) C
73-3658 2 oz

Dipyridamole Tablets ℞
05-1101 25 mg, 100's
05-1102 25 mg, 1000's
05-9601 50 mg, 100's
05-9602 50 mg, 1000's
05-5201 75 mg, 100's
05-5205 75 mg, 500's

Disulfiram ℞
03-3601 250 mg, 100's
03-3750 500 mg, 50's
03-3705 500 mg, 500's

Doxycycline Hyclate Capsules ℞
20-3250 50 mg, 50's
20-3350 100 mg, 50's

Docusate Sodium Capsules (D.S.S.) OTC
01-1301 100 mg, 100's
01-1302 100 mg, 1000's
01-1401 250 mg, 100's
01-1402 250 mg, 1000's

D.S.S. Syrup-Docusate Sodium OTC
71-9216 Pt
71-9299 Gal

Docusate Sodium with Casanthranol Capsules (D.S.S.) OTC
(Casanthranol, Docusate Sodium)
01-1501 100's
01-1502 1000's

D.S.S. with Casanthrol Syrup OTC
(Docusate Sodium, Casanthrol)
71-6816 Pt
71-6899 Gal

Duo-Hist Timed Release Tablets ℞
(Dexbrompheniramine Maleate, Pseudoephedrine Sulfate)
05-4201 100's
05-4205 500's

Erythromycin Estolate Capsules ℞
05-3001 250 mg, 100's

Erythromycin Stearate Tablets ℞
20-0501 250 mg, 100's
20-0505 250 mg, 500's
20-3801 500 mg, 100's

Erythromycin Tablets E/C ℞
20-3101 250 mg, 100's
20-3105 250 mg, 500's

Erythromycin Ethylsuccinate Granules ℞
20-5761 200 mg, 100 ml

Erythromycin Ethylsuccinate Suspension ℞
20-6716 200 mg, Pt

Furosemide Tablets ℞
05-6801 20 mg, 100's
05-6802 20 mg, 1000's
05-1401 40 mg, 100's
05-1402 40 mg, 1000's

Glutethimide Tablets C-III
02-9601 100's
02-9602 1000's

H-H-R Tablets ℞
(Hydralazine, Hydrochlorothiazide, Reserpine)
03-6101 100's
03-6102 1000's

Hydralazine HCl Tablets ℞
01-4402 25 mg, 1000's
01-4502 50 mg, 1000's

Hydralazine-Thiazide Capsules ℞
06-1601 25/25, 100's
06-1701 50/50, 100's
06-1801 100/50, 100's

Hydralazine-Thiazide Tablets ℞
03-5801 100's
03-5802 1000's

Hydrochlorothiazide Tablets ℞
03-2201 25 mg, 100's
03-2202 25 mg, 1000's
03-2801 50 mg, 100's
03-2802 50 mg, 1000's
03-5301 50 mg (Y), 100's
03-5302 50 mg (Y), 1000's
04-2101 100 mg, 100's
04-2102 100 mg, 1000's

Hydro-Ergoloid Sublingual Tablets ℞
(Dihydroergocornine, Dihydroergocrystine, Dihydroergokryptine, Hydrogenated Ergot Alkaloids)
04-1501 0.5 mg, 100's
04-1502 0.5 mg, 1000's
04-4601 1.0 mg, 100's
04-4602 1.0 mg, 1000's

Hydroserpine #1 Tablets ℞
(Hydrochlorothiazide, Reserpine)
03-5401 100's
03-5402 1000's

Hydroserpine #2 Tablets ℞
(Hydrochlorothiazide, Reserpine)
03-5501 100's
03-5502 1000's

Hydroxyzine HCl Tablets ℞
04-9401 10 mg, 100's
04-9405 10 mg, 500's
04-9501 25 mg, 100's

Continued on next page

Schein—Cont.

04-9505 25 mg, 500's
04-9601 50 mg, 100's
04-9605 50 mg, 500's

Hydroxyzine HCl Syrup ℞
72-7316 Pt
72-7399 Gal

Hydroxyzine Pamoate Capsules ℞
04-8301 25 mg, 100's
04-8305 25 mg, 500's
04-8401 50 mg, 100's
04-8405 50 mg, 500's
04-8501 100 mg, 100's
04-8505 100 mg, 500's

Imipramine HCl Tablets ℞
04-4301 10 mg, 100's
04-4302 10 mg, 1000's
04-0601 25 mg, 100's
04-0602 25 mg, 1000's
04-3501 50 mg, 100's
04-3502 50 mg, 1000's

Isosorbide Dinitrate Oral Tablets ℞
03-4001 5 mg, 100's
03-4002 5 mg, 1000's
03-4101 10 mg, 100's
03-4102 10 mg, 1000's
05-0901 20 mg, 100's
05-0902 20 mg, 1000's

Isosorbide Dinitrate Sublingual Tablets ℞
03-6701 2.5 mg, 100's
03-6702 2.5 mg, 1000's
03-6801 5.0 mg, 100's
03-6802 5.0 mg, 1000's

Isosorbide Dinitrate Timed Capsules ℞
03-4201 40 mg, 100's
03-4202 40 mg, 1000's

Isosorbide Dinitrate Timed Tablets ℞
04-0101 40 mg, 100's
04-0102 40 mg, 1000's

Isoxsuprine HCl Tablets ℞
03-9301 10 mg, 100's
03-9302 10 mg, 1000's
03-9401 20 mg, 100's
03-9402 20 mg, 1000's

Meclizine HCl MLT Tablets ℞
04-1101 12.5 mg, 100's
04-1102 12.5 mg, 1000's
04-1201 25 mg, 100's
04-1202 25 mg, 1000's

Meprobamate Tablets Ⓒ
01-6001 200 mg, 100's
01-6002 200 mg, 1000's
01-6101 400 mg, 100's
01-6102 400 mg, 1000's

Mepro Compound Tablets Ⓒ
(Aspirin, Ethoheptazine Citrate, Meprobamate)
05-5701 100's
05-5705 500's

Methenamine Mandelate Tablets ℞
01-6502 0.5 mg, 1000's
01-6605 1.0 mg, 500's

Methenamine Mandelate Forte Suspension ℞
71-9416 Pt

Methocarbamol Tablets ℞
03-4601 500 mg, 100's
03-4605 500 mg, 500's
03-4701 750 mg, 100's
03-4705 750 mg, 500's

Methocarbamol w/Aspirin Tablets ℞
04-9201 100's
04-9205 500's

Methyclothiazide Tablets ℞
06-1901 2.5 mg, 100's
06-2001 5.0 mg, 100's
06-2002 5.0 mg, 1000's

Methylprednisolone Tablets ℞
04-6701 4 mg, 100's

Metronidazole Oral Tablets ℞
05-9501 250 mg, 100's
05-9504 250 mg, 250's

Nitrofurantoin Tablets ℞
03-0901 50 mg, 100's
03-0902 50 mg, 1000's
03-1001 100 mg, 100's
03-1002 100 mg, 1000's

Nitrofurantoin Capsules ℞
03-3101 50 mg, 100's
03-3105 50 mg, 500's
03-3201 100 mg, 100's
03-3205 100 mg, 500's

Nitrolin Timed Capsules ℞
(Nitroglycerin)
01-7401 2.5 mg, 100's
04-3201 6.5 mg, 100's

Nylidrin HCl Tablets ℞
03-9101 6 mg, 100's
03-9102 6 mg, 1000's
03-9201 12 mg, 100's
03-9202 12 mg, 1000's

Nystatin Oral Tablets ℞
20-5101 500,000 uts, 100's

Oxacillin Sodium Capsules ℞
20-5901 250 mg, 100's
20-6001 500 mg, 100's

Oxacillin Sodium Powder ℞
20-6461 250 mg, 100 ml

Oxytetracycline HCl Capsules ℞
20-0701 250 mg, 100's
20-0702 250 mg, 1000's

Papaverine HCl Timed Capsules ℞
01-8101 150 mg, 100's
01-8102 150 mg, 1000's

Penicillin VK Tablets ℞
20-2001 250 mg Rd, 100's
20-2002 250 mg Rd, 1000's
20-2101 250 mg Oval, 100's
20-2102 250 mg Oval, 1000's
20-2201 500 mg Rd, 100's
20-2202 500 mg Rd, 1000's
20-5801 500 mg Oval, 100's
20-5802 500 mg Oval, 1000's

Penicillin VK Powder For Oral Suspension ℞
20-2361 125 mg, 100 ml
20-2363 125 mg, 200 ml
20-2461 250 mg, 100 ml
20-2463 250 mg, 200 ml

Pentaerythritol Tetranitrate Tablets (PETN) ℞
01-8402 10 mg, 1000's
01-8502 20 mg, 1000's

Pentaerythritol Tetranitrate Timed Capsules ℞
01-8901 80 mg, 100's
01-8902 80 mg, 1000's

Pentaerythritol Tetranitrate Timed Tablets ℞
05-3101 80 mg, 100's
05-3102 80 mg, 1000's

Phenobarbital Tablets Ⓒ
02-0002 ¼ gr, 1000's
02-0302 ½ gr, 1000's
02-0602 1½ gr, 1000's

Phentermine HCl Capsules Ⓒ
05-6301 15 mg, 100's
05-6302 15 mg, 1000's
03-3501 30 mg (Y), 100's
03-3502 30 mg (Y), 1000's
05-3802 30 mg (B/C), 1000's

Phenylbutazone Tablets ℞
05-3701 100 mg, 100's
05-3702 100 mg, 1000's

Phenytoin Sodium Capsules - Prompt Action ℞
01-1902 100 mg, 1000's

Prednisolone Tablets ℞
02-1701 5 mg, 100's
02-1702 5 mg, 1000's

Prednisone Tablets ℞
02-1801 5 mg, 100's
02-1802 5 mg, 1000's
04-6101 10 mg, 100's
04-6105 10 mg, 500's
04-4201 20 mg, 100's
04-4205 20 mg, 500's
05-5601 50 mg, 100's

Primidone Tablets ℞
03-6601 250 mg, 100's
03-6602 250 mg, 1000's

Probenecid Tablets ℞
03-1401 100's
03-1402 1000's

Probenecid with Colchicine Tablets ℞
03-1501 100's
03-1502 1000's

Procainamide HCl Capsules ℞
02-1901 250 mg, 100's
02-1902 250 mg, 1000's
03-4301 375 mg, 100's
03-4302 375 mg, 1000's
03-4401 500 mg, 100's
03-4402 500 mg, 1000's

Prochlor-Iso Timed Release Capsules ℞
(Isopropamide Iodide, Prochlorperazine)
04-7401 100's
04-7405 500's

Propantheline Bromide Tablets ℞
03-0401 15 mg, 100's
03-0402 15 mg, 1000's

Propoxyphene HCl Capsules Ⓒ
03-1201 65 mg, 100's
03-1205 65 mg, 500's

Propoxyphene Compound 65 Ⓒ
03-1301 100's
03-1302 1000's

Propoxyphene & Apap Tablets 65/650 Ⓒ
03-9601 100's
03-9605 500's

Pseudoephedrine HCl Tablets
05-9801 30 mg, 100's OTC
02-2502 60 mg, 1000's ℞

Pseudoephedrine Syrup OTC
70-5416 Pt
70-5499 Gal

Quadrahist Timed Release Tablets ℞
(Chlorpheniramine, Phenylephrine, Phenylpropanolamine, Phenyltoloxamine)
05-8101 100's
05-8102 1000's

Quadrahist Pediatric Syrup ℞
(Chlorpheniramine, Phenylephrine, Phenylpropanolamine, Phenyltoloxamine)
73-3216 Pt

Quadrahist Syrup ℞
(Chlorpheniramine, Phenylephrine, Phenylpropanolamine, Phenyltoloxamine)
71-8116 Pt
71-8199 Gal

Quinidine Gluconate Tablets ℞
06-0401 324 mg, 100's
06-0404 324 mg, 250's

Quinidine Sulfate Tablets ℞
02-2901 200 mg, 100's
02-2902 200 mg, 1000's
02-8201 300 mg, 100's

Quinine Sulfate Capsules ℞
02-3001 5 gr. 100's
02-3002 5 gr. 1000's

Quinine Sulfate Tablets ℞
05-6001 260 mg, 100's

Reserpine Tablets ℞
02-3402 0.25 mg, 1000's
02-3403 0.25 mg, 5000's

Soprodol Tablets (Carisoprodol) ℞
04-7501 100's
04-7505 500's

Soprodol Compound Tablets ℞
(Carisoprodol, Phenacetin)
04-7601 100's
04-7605 500's

Spironazide Tablets ℞
(Hydrochlorothiazide, Spironolactone)

05-1301 100's
05-1302 1000's

Spironolactone Tablets ℞
05-1201 100's
05-1202 1000's

Sulfasalazine Tablets ℞
04-4401 500 mg, 100's
04-4405 500 mg, 500's

Sulfatrim Tablets ℞
(Trimethoprim, Sulfamethoxazole)
20-6801 100's

Sulfatrim D/S Tablets ℞
(Trimethoprim, Sulfamethoxazole)
20-6901 100's
20-6905 500's

Sulfisoxazole Tablets ℞
02-6502 0.5 gm, 1000's

T-E-P Tablets ℞
(Ephedrine, Theophylline, Phenobarbital)
02-6602 1000's

Tetracycline HCl Capsules ℞
20-2601 250 mg O/Y, 100's
20-2602 250 mg O/Y, 1000's
20-2701 250 mg B/Y, 100's
20-2702 250 mg B/Y, 1000's
20-2901 500 mg Bk/Y, 100's
20-2902 500 mg Bk/Y, 1000's

Theozine Tablets ℞
(Ephedrine Sulfate, Hydroxyzine HCl, Theophylline)
05-3501 100's
05-3505 500's

Theozine Syrup - Dye Free ℞
(Ephedrine Sulfate, Hydroxyzine HCl, Theophylline)
72-4616 Pt
72-4699 Gal

L-Thyroxine Tables ℞
02-7702 0.1 mg, 1000's
02-7802 0.2 mg, 1000's

Tolbutamide Tablets ℞
04-7701 0.5 gm, 100's
04-7702 0.5 gm, 1000's

Triafed Tablets ℞
(Pseudoephedrine, Triprolidine)
03-8501 100's
03-8502 1000's

Triafed Syrup ℞
(Pseudoephedrine, Triprolidine)
71-7216 Pt
71-7299 Gal

Triafed-C Expectorant Ⓒ
(Codeine Phosphate, Guaifenesin, Pseudoephedrine HCl, Triprolidine HCl)
71-7316 Pt
71-7399 Gal

Triamcinolone Tablets ℞
03-5201 4 mg, 100's
03-5205 4 mg, 500's

Trichlormethiazide Tablets ℞
03-0702 4 mg, 1000's

Trifluoperazine Tablets ℞
06-0001 1 mg, 100's
06-0101 2 mg, 100's
06-0102 2 mg, 1000's
06-0201 5 mg, 100's
06-0202 5 mg, 1000's
06-0301 10 mg, 100's

Tuss-Ade Timed Capsules ℞
(Caramiphen Edisylate, Phenylpropanolamine)
06-1405 500's

Polyvitamin-Fluoride Drops ℞
(Sodium Fluoride, Vitamins with Fluoride)
71-7057 50 ml

Polyvitamin-Fluoride Tablets ℞
(Sodium Fluoride, Vitamins with Fluoride)
10-7501 100's
10-7502 1000's

Cardec DM Drops ℞
(Carbinoxamine Maleate, Dextromethorphan Hydrobromide, Pseudoephedrine HCl)
72-7756 30 ml

Cardec DM Syrup ℞
(Carbinoxamine Maleate, Dextromethorphan Hydrobromide, Pseudoephedrine HCl)
73-1816 Pt
73-1899 Gal

Cyproheptadine HCl Syrup 125
72-7216 Pt
72-7299 Gal

Decongestant Elixir OTC
(Chlorpheniramine, Menthol, Phenylpropanolamine)
72-2316 Pt
72-2399 Gal

Decongestant Expectorant Ⓒ
(Codeine Phosphate, Guaifenesin, Phenylpropanolamine)
72-2516 Pt
72-2599 Gal

Decongestant-AT (Antitussive) Liquid Ⓒ
(Chlorpheniramine Maleate, Codeine Phosphate, Phenylpropanolamine)
72-5016 Pt
72-5099 Gal

Detussin Liquid Ⓒ-III
(Hydrocodone Bitartrate, Pseudoephedrine)
72-5716 Pt
72-5799 Gal

Detussin Expectorant Ⓒ-III
(Hydrocodone Bitartrate, Guaifenesin, Pseudoephedrine)
72-5816 Pt
72-5899 Gal

Erythromycin Ethyl Succinate Suspension ℞
20-7016 400 mg, Pt

Guiatuss Syrup OTC
(Guaifenesin)
70-2516 Pt
70-2599 Gal

Guiatuss A-C Syrup Ⓒ
(Codeine Phosphate, Guaifenesin)
70-2616 Pt
70-2699 Gal

Guiatuss D-M Syrup OTC
(Dextromethorphan, Guaifenesin)
70-2716 Pt
70-2799 Gal

Hydrocodone Syrup Ⓒ-III
72-5416 Pt
72-5499 Gal

Iophen-C Liquid Ⓒ
(Chlorpheniramine Maleate, Codeine Phosphate, Iodinated Glycerol)
73-2816 Pt

Kaolin-Pectin Mixture OTC
70-3016 Pt
70-3099 Gal

Kaolin, Pectin, Belladonna Mixture OTC
70-3116 Pt
70-3199 Gal

Kaolin-Pectin PG Mixture Ⓒ
72-6616 Pt
72-6699 Gal

Lidocaine HCl 2% Viscous Solution OTC
72-8261 100 ml

Phenobarbital Elixir Ⓒ
70-4616 Pt
70-4699 Gal

Potassium Chloride Liquid 10% Sugar Free ℞
70-4716 Pt
70-4799 Gal

Potassium Chloride Concentrate 20% ℞
71-6616 Pt
71-6699 Gal

Potassium Gluconate Elixir ℞
70-4816 Pt
70-4899 Gal

Tetracycline HCl Syrup ℞
20-3058 2 oz
20-3016 Pt

Theophylline Elixir ℞
70-6016 Pt
70-6099 Gal

Theophylline KI Elixir ℞
72-6716 Pt
72-6799 Gal

Fluocinolone Acetonide Cream 0.01% ℞
72-6272 15 gm
72-6258 60 gm

Fluocinolone Acetonide Cream 0.025% ℞
72-6372 15 gm
72-6358 60 gm

Gentamicin Cream 0.1% ℞
(Gentamicin Sulfate)
73-0572 15 gm

Gentamicin Ointment 0.1% ℞
(Gentamicin Sulfate)
73-3872 15 gm

Lindane Lotion ℞
73-2658 2 oz
73-2616 Pt

Lindane Shampoo ℞
73-2758 2 oz
73-2716 Pt

Nystatin Cream ℞
72-1072 15 mg

Nyst-olone Cream ℞
(Gramicidin, Neomycin Sulfate, Nystatin, Triamcinolone Acetonide)
72-1472 15 gm
72-1458 60 gm
72-1416 1 lb

Nyst-olone Ointment ℞
(Gramicidin, Neomycin Sulfate, Nystatin, Triamcinolone Acetonide)
72-7672 15 gm

Oxymeta-12 OTC
(Oxymetazoline HCl)
73-2072 15 ml

Pyrinal Liquid OTC
(Piperonyl Butoxide, Pyrethrins)
71-7858 2 oz

Selenium Sulfide Lotion 2½% ℞
71-6977 4 oz

Triamcinolone Acetonide Cream 0.025% ℞
72-1172 15 gm
72-1160 80 gm
72-1116 1 lb

Triamcinolone Acetonide Cream 0.1% ℞
72-1272 15 gm
72-1260 80 gm
72-1216 1 lb

Triamcinolone Acetonide Cream 0.5% ℞
72-1372 15 gm

Triple Sulfa Vaginal Cream ℞
(Sulfabenzamide, Sulfacetamide, Sulfathiazole)
72-8437 2.75 oz

Aminophylline Suppositories ℞
71-1612 250 mg 12's

Nystatin Vaginal Tablets ℞
72-0915 15's
72-0930 30's

Vaginal Sulfa Suppositories ℞
(Allantoin, Aminacrine HCl, Sulfanilamide)
73-2216 16's

Allopurinol Tablets ℞
06-3201 100 mg, 100's
06-3202 100 mg, 1000's

Continued on next page

Schein—Cont.

06-3301 300 mg, 100's
06-3305 300 mg, 500's
Aminophylline Oral Liquid ℞
73-4276 8 oz

NEW PRODUCTS ADDITIONS

Cafetrate-PB Suppositories ℞
(Caffeine, Ergotamine Tartrate)
73-4910 10's
Dicloxacillin Sodium Capsules ℞
20-7001 250 mg, 100's
20-7101 500 mg, 100's
Doxycycline Tablets ℞
20-6350 50 mg, 50's
Effervescent Potassium Tablets ℞
06-3530 25 meg, 30's
Erythromycin Ethylsuccinate Tablets ℞
20-7401 400 mg, 100's
Hydro-Ergoloid Oral Tablets ℞
06-2201 1.0 mg, 100's
06-2205 1.0 mg, 500's
Isosorbide Dinitrate Oral Tablets ℞
06-2801 30 mg 100's
06-2802 30 mg 1000's
Isosorbide Dinitrate Sublingual Tablets ℞
06-2701 10 mg 100's
06-2702 10 mg 1000's
Liothyronine Sodium Tablets ℞
06-2401 25 mcg, 100's
06-2501 50 mcg, 100's
Nitroglycerin Ointment 2% ℞
73-0658 60 gm
Phenylbutazone Capsules ℞
06-3401 100 mg, 100's
06-3402 100 mg, 1000's
Sulfinpyrazone Tablets ℞
06-2601 100 mg, 100's
Trimethobenzamide HCl Suppositories ℞
73-4710 100 mg, 10's
73-4810 200 mg, 10's
Warfarin Sodium Tablets ℞
06-3901 2.5 mg, 100's
06-4001 5.0 mg, 100's
06-4002 5.0 mg, 1000's

Schering Corporation
GALLOPING HILL ROAD
KENILWORTH, NJ 07033

Product Identification Codes

To provide quick and positive identification of Schering Products, we have imprinted the product identification number of the National Drug Code on most tablets and capsules. In some cases, identification letters also appear. For convenience, a complete list of all Schering products and their identification codes, where appropriate, follow:

Product Listing

Product **Code**

A&D™ Hand Cream* OTC
A&D™ Ointment* OTC
AFRIN®* OTC
oxymetazoline HCl
Nasal Spray 0.05%
Menthol Nasal Spray 0.05%
Nose Drops 0.05%
Pediatric Nose Drops 0.025%
AFRINOL®* OTC
pseudoephedrine sulfate
Repetabs Tablets Long-Acting Nasal Decongestant 258
AKRINOL® Cream† ℞
acrisorcin, USP
CELESTONE® ℞
betamethasone, USP
Cream†
Phosphate Injection
Soluspan® Suspension
Syrup
Tablets 0.6 mg 011/BDA
CHLOR-TRIMETON®* OTC
chlorpheniramine maleate
Allergy Syrup
Allergy Tablets 4 mg 080/TW
Long-Acting Allergy Repetabs® Tablets 8 mg 374
12 mg Allergy Repetabs Tablets 009/AAE
CHLOR-TRIMETON®* OTC
chlorpheniramine maleate/
pseudoephedrine sulfate
Decongestant Tablets 901
Long-Acting Decongestant Repetabs® Tablets
CHLOR-TRIMETON® † ℞
chlorpheniramine maleate, USP
Injection 10 mg/ml
100 mg/ml
COD LIVER OIL CONCENTRATE* OTC
Capsules
Tablets
Tablets with Vitamin C
CORICIDIN®* OTC
Cough Syrup
D® Decongestant Tablets 371
DEMILETS® Tablets
MEDILETS® Tablets
Nasal Mist
Sinus Headache Tablets (Extra Strength) Tablets 171
CORIFORTE® Capsules† 432 ℞
CORILIN® Infant Liquid† ℞
DEMAZIN®* OTC
Repetabs Tablets 133
Syrup
DERMOLATE™* OTC
hydrocortisone 0.5%
Anti-Itch Cream
Anal-Itch Ointment
Anti-Itch Spray
Scalp-Itch Lotion
DIPROSONE® ℞
betamethasone dipropionate, USP
Aerosol 0.1%
Cream 0.05%
Lotion 0.05%
Ointment 0.05%
DISMISS® Douche* OTC
DISOPHROL®* OTC
CHRONOTAB® Tablets 85-WMH/231
DISOPHROL® † Tablets WBS/866 ℞
DRIXORAL®* Sustained Action Tablets OTC
EMKO®* OTC
BECAUSE® Contraceptor®*
PRE-FIL® Vaginal Contraceptive Foam
Vaginal Contraceptive Foam
ESTINYL® Tablets ℞
estinyl estradiol, USP
0.02 mg 298/ER
0.05 mg 070/EM
0.5 mg 150/EP
ETRAFON® Tablets ℞
perphenazine, USP-amitriptyline hydrochloride, USP
Tablets (2–10) ANA/287
Tablets (2–25) ANC/598
A Tablets (4–10) ANB/119
Forte Tablets (4–25) ANE/720
FULVICIN® P/G Tablets ℞
griseofulvin ultramicrosize, USP
125 mg 228
165 mg 654
250 mg 507
330 mg 352
FULVICIN U/F® Tablets ℞
griseofulvin, (microsize), USP
250 mg AUF/948
500 mg AUG/496
GARAMYCIN® Injectables ℞
gentamicin sulfate, USP
Disposable Syringes 1.5 ml (60 mg)
Disposable Syringes 2.0 ml (80 mg)
Injectable 2 ml vial (80 mg)
Injectable 20 ml vial (800 mg)
Intrathecal 2 ml (4 mg) ampul
Pediatric Injectable 2 ml vial (20 mg)
I.V. Piggyback Injection– 60 ml (60 mg), 80 ml (80 mg)
GARAMYCIN® Topicals ℞
gentamicin sulfate, USP
Cream
Ointment
Ophthalmic Ointment
Ophthalmic Solution
GITALIGIN® Tablets† WAR/617 ℞
gitalin
GYNE-LOTRIMIN® ℞
clotrimazole, USP
Vaginal Cream 1%
Vaginal Tablets 100 mg 734
HYPERSTAT® I.V. Injection ℞
diazoxide, USP
LOTRIMIN® ℞
clotrimazole, USP
Cream 1%
Solution 1%
METICORTELONE® Acetate† ℞
prednisolone acetate, USP
Aqueous Suspension
METICORTEN® Tablets† ℞
prednisone, USP
1 mg KEM/843
5 mg ABB/172
METI-DERM® Cream† ℞
prednisolone, USP
METIMYD® ℞
prednisolone acetate, USP/
sulfacetamide sodium, USP
Ophthalmic Ointment
Ophthalmic Solution
METRETON® Ophthalmic/Otic Solution ℞
prednisolone sodium phosphate, USP
MOL-IRON®* OTC
Chronosule® Capsules
Liquid
Tablets
Tablets with Vitamin C
MY OWN®* OTC
Feminine Deodorant Spray Mist
Towelettes
NAQUA® Tablets ℞
trichlormethiazide, USP
2 mg AHG/822
4 mg AHH/547
NAQUIVAL® Tablets ℞
trichlormethiazide,
USP/reserpine, USP AHT/394
OPTIMINE® Tablets ℞
azatadine maleate, USP 282
OPTIMYD® Ophthalmic Solution† ℞
prednisolone sodium phosphate, USP/
sulfacetamide sodium, USP
ORETON® ℞
methyltestosterone, USP
Methyl Tablets 10 mg JD/311
25 mg JE/499
Methyl Buccal Tablets BE/970
ORETON® Pellets† ℞
testosterone, USP
OTOBIONE® Otic Suspension† ℞
OTOBIOTIC® Otic Solution ℞
polymyxin B sulfate, USP and
hydrocortisone, USP
PAXIPAM® Tablets Ⓒ ℞
halazepam
20 mg 251
40 mg 538
PERMITIL® ℞
fluphenazine hydrochloride, USP
CHRONOTAB® Tablets
1mg WKJ/840
Oral Concentrate
Tablets 0.25 mg WBK/122
2.5 mg WDR/442
5 mg WFF/550
10 mg WFG/316

POLARAMINE® ℞
dexchlorpheniramine maleate, USP
Expectorant†
Repetabs® Tablets 4 mg AGA/095
6 mg AGB/148
Syrup
Tablets 2 mg AGT/820

PROGLYCEM® ℞
diazoxide, USP
Capsules 50 mg PBA/205
100 mg PBB/830
Suspension

PROVENTIL® ℞
albuterol
Inhaler

PROVENTIL® ℞
albuterol sulfate
Syrup
Tablets 2 mg 252
4 mg 573

RELA® Tablets† ℞
carisoprodol **AHR/160**

SEBIZON® Lotion† ℞
sodium sulfacetamide, USP 10%

SODIUM SULAMYD® ℞
sodium sulfacetamide, USP
Ophthalmic Ointment 10%
Ophthalmic Solution 10%
Ophthalmic Solution 30% w/v

SOLGANAL® Suspension ℞
aurothioglucose, USP

SUNRIL®* Capsules OTC

THEOVENT® Long-Acting Capsules ℞
theophylline anhydrous, USP
125 mg 402
250 mg 753

TINACTIN®* OTC
tolnaftate, USP
Cream 1%
Liquid Aerosol
Powder 1%
Powder Aerosol 1%
Solution 1%

TINDAL® Tablets† BBA/968 ℞
acetophenazine maleate, USP

TREMIN® † ℞
trihexyphenidyl hydrochloride, USP
Tablets 2 mg AKH/892
5 mg AKJ/596

TRILAFON® ℞
perphenazine, USP
Concentrate
Injection
Repetabs® Tablets ADX/141
Tablets 2 mg ADH/705
4 mg ADK/940
8 mg ADJ/313
16 mg ADM/077

TRINALIN™ Long-Acting ℞
Antihistamine/Decongestant
Repetabs® Tablets 703

VALISONE® ℞
betamethasone valerate, USP
Cream 0.1%
Lotion 0.1%
Ointment 0.1%
Reduced Strength Cream 0.01%

VANCENASE® Nasal Inhaler ℞
beclomethasone dipropionate, USP

VANCERIL® Oral Inhaler ℞
beclomethasone dipropionate, USP

* For complete prescribing information see PDR for Nonprescription Drugs.
† For complete prescribing information contact the Schering Professional Services Department.

CELESTONE® ℞
brand of betamethasone, USP
Tablets
Syrup

Description: Glucocorticoids are adrenocortical steroids, both naturally occurring and synthetic, that are readily absorbed from the gastrointestinal tract. A derivative of prednisolone, CELESTONE has a 16β-methyl group that enhances the anti-inflammatory action of the molecule and reduces the sodium- and water-retaining properties of the fluorine atom bound at carbon 9.
The formula for betamethasone is $C_{22}H_{29}FO_5$ and has a molecular weight of 392.47. Chemically, it is 9-fluoro-11β, 17,21-trihydroxy-16β-methylpregna-1,4-diene-3,20-dione.
Betamethasone is a white to practically white, odorless, crystalline powder. It melts at about 240°C with some decomposition. Betamethasone is sparingly soluble in acetone, alcohol, dioxane, and methanol; very slightly soluble in chloroform and ether; and is insoluble in water.
Each CELESTONE **Tablet** contains 0.6 mg. betamethasone, USP.
CELESTONE **Syrup** contains 0.6 mg betamethasone, USP in each 5 ml and less than 1% alcohol.
Actions: Naturally occurring glucocorticoids (hydrocortisone and cortisone), which also have salt-retaining properties, are used as replacement therapy in adrenocortical deficiency states. Their synthetic analogs, such as betamethasone, are primarily used for their potent anti-inflammatory effects in disorders of many organ systems.
Glucocorticoids, such as betamethasone, cause profound and varied metabolic effects. In addition, they modify the body's immune response to diverse stimuli.
Indications:
Endocrine disorders: primary or secondary adrenocortical insufficiency (hydrocortisone or cortisone is the first choice; synthetic analogs may be used in conjunction with mineralocorticoids where applicable; in infancy mineralocorticoid supplementation is of particular importance).
congenital adrenal hyperplasia
nonsuppurative thyroiditis
hypercalcemia associated with cancer
Rheumatic disorders: as adjunctive therapy for short-term administration (to tide the patient over an acute episode or exacerbation) in:
psoriatic arthritis
rheumatoid arthritis, including juvenile rheumatoid arthritis (selected cases may require low-dose maintenance therapy)
ankylosing spondylitis
acute and subacute bursitis
acute nonspecific tenosynovitis
acute gouty arthritis
post-traumatic osteoarthritis
synovitis of osteoarthritis
epicondylitis
Collagen diseases: during an exacerbation or as maintenance therapy in selected cases of:
systemic lupus erythematosus
acute rheumatic carditis
Dermatologic diseases:
pemphigus
bullous dermatitis herpetiformis
severe erythema multiforme (Stevens-Johnson syndrome)
exfoliative dermatitis
mycosis fungoides
severe psoriasis
severe seborrheic dermatitis
Allergic states: control of severe or incapacitating allergic conditions intractable to adequate trials of conventional treatment:
seasonal or perennial allergic rhinitis
serum sickness
bronchial asthma
contact dermatitis
atopic dermatitis
drug hypersensitivity reactions
Ophthalmic diseases: severe acute and chronic allergic and inflammatory processes involving the eye and its adnexa, such as:
allergic conjunctivitis
keratitis
allergic corneal marginal ulcers
herpes zoster ophthalmicus
iritis and iridocyclitis
chorioretinitis
anterior segment inflammation
diffuse posterior uveitis and choroiditis
optic neuritis
sympathetic ophthalmia
Respiratory diseases:
symptomatic sarcoidosis
Loffler's syndrome not manageable by other means
berylliosis
fulminating or disseminated pulmonary tuberculosis when used concurrently with appropriate antituberculous chemotherapy
aspiration pneumonitis
Hematologic disorders:
idiopathic thrombocytopenic purpura in adults
secondary thrombocytopenia in adults
acquired (autoimmune) hemolytic anemia
erythroblastopenia (RBC anemia)
congenital (erythroid) hypoplastic anemia
Neoplastic diseases: for palliative management of:
leukemias and lymphomas in adults
acute leukemia of childhood
Edematous states: to induce a diuresis or remission of proteinuria in the nephrotic syndrome, without uremia, of the idiopathic type or that due to lupus erythematosus.
Gastrointestinal diseases: to tide the patient over a critical period of the disease in:
ulcerative colitis
regional enteritis
Miscellaneous: tuberculous meningitis with subarachnoid block or impending block when used concurrently with appropriate antituberculous chemotherapy; trichinosis with neurologic or myocardial involvement.
Contraindications: CELESTONE **Tablets** and **Syrup** are contraindicated in systemic fungal infections.
Warnings: In patients on corticosteroid therapy subjected to unusual stress, increased dosage of rapidly acting corticosteroids before, during, and after the stressful situation is indicated.
Corticosteroids may mask some signs of infection, and new infections may appear during their use. There may be decreased resistance and inability to localize infection when corticosteroids are used.
Prolonged use of corticosteroids may produce posterior subcapsular cataracts, glaucoma with possible damage to the optic nerves, and may enhance the establishment of secondary ocular infections due to fungi or viruses.
Average and large doses of hydrocortisone or cortisone can cause elevation of blood pressure, salt and water retention, and increased excretion of potassium. These effects are less likely to occur with the synthetic derivatives except when used in large doses. Dietary salt restrictions and potassium supplementation may be necessary. All corticosteroids increase calcium excretion.
While on corticosteroid therapy patients should not be vaccinated against smallpox. Other immunization procedures should not be undertaken in patients who are on corticosteroids, especially on high doses, because of possible hazards of neurological complications and a lack of antibody response.
The use of CELESTONE **Syrup** and **Tablets** in active tuberculosis should be restricted to those cases of fulminating or disseminated tuberculosis in which the corticosteroid is used for the management of the disease in conjunction with an appropriate antituberculous regimen.
If corticosteroids are indicated in patients with latent tuberculosis or tuberculin reactivity, close observation is necessary as reactivation of the disease may occur. During prolonged

Continued on next page

Information on Schering products appearing on these pages is effective as of September 30, 1982.

Schering—Cont.

corticosteroid therapy, these patients should receive chemoprophylaxis.

Usage in pregnancy: Since adequate human reproduction studies have not been done with corticosteroids, the use of these drugs in pregnancy, nursing mothers or women of childbearing potential requires that the possible benefits of the drug be weighed against the potential hazards to the mother and embryo or fetus. Infants born of mothers who have received substantial doses of corticosteroids during pregnancy should be carefully observed for signs of hypoadrenalism.

Precautions: Drug-induced secondary adrenocortical insufficiency may be minimized by gradual reduction of dosage. This type of relative insufficiency may persist for months after discontinuation of therapy; therefore, in any situation of stress occurring during that period, hormone therapy should be reinstituted. Since mineralocorticoid secretion may be impaired, salt and/or a mineralocorticoid should be administered concurrently.

There is an enhanced effect of corticosteroids on patients with hypothyroidism and in those with cirrhosis.

Corticosteroids should be used cautiously in patients with ocular herpes simplex because of possible corneal perforation.

The lowest possible dose of corticosteroid should be used to control the condition under treatment, and when reduction in dosage is possible, the reduction should be gradual.

Psychic derangements may appear when corticosteroids are used, ranging from euphoria, insomnia, mood swings, personality changes, and severe depression to frank psychotic manifestations. Also, existing emotional instability or psychotic tendencies may be aggravated by corticosteroids.

Aspirin should be used cautiously in conjunction with corticosteroids in hypoprothrombinemia.

Steroids should be used with caution in nonspecific ulcerative colitis, if there is a probability of impending perforation, abscess or other pyogenic infection; diverticulitis; fresh intestinal anastomoses; active or latent peptic ulcer; renal insufficiency; hypertension; osteoporosis; and myasthenia gravis.

Growth and development of infants and children on prolonged corticosteroid therapy should be carefully observed.

Adverse Reactions:

Fluid and electrolyte disturbances: sodium retention, fluid retention, congestive heart failure in susceptible patients, potassium loss, hypokalemic alkalosis, hypertension.

Musculoskeletal: muscle weakness, steroid myopathy, loss of muscle mass, osteoporosis, vertebral compression fractures, aseptic necrosis of femoral and humeral heads, pathologic fractures of long bones.

Gastrointestinal: peptic ulcer with possible perforation and hemorrhage, pancreatitis, abdominal distention, ulcerative esophagitis.

Dermatologic: impaired wound healing, thin fragile skin, petechiae and ecchymoses, facial erythema, increased sweating, may suppress reactions to skin tests.

Neurological: convulsions, increased intracranial pressure with papilledema (pseudotumor cerebri) usually after treatment, vertigo, headache.

Endocrine: menstrual irregularities; development of Cushingoid state; suppression of growth in children; secondary adrenocortical and pituitary unresponsiveness, particularly in times of stress, as in trauma, surgery or illness; decreased carbohydrate tolerance; manifestations of latent diabetes mellitus; increased requirements of insulin or oral hypoglycemic agents in diabetics.

Ophthalmic: posterior subcapsular cataracts, increased intraocular pressure, glaucoma, exophthalmos.

Metabolic: negative nitrogen balance due to protein catabolism.

Dosage and Administration: The initial dosage of CELESTONE may vary from 0.6 mg. to 7.2 mg. per day depending on the specific disease entity being treated. In situations of less severity lower doses will generally suffice, while in selected patients higher initial doses may be required. The initial dosage should be maintained or adjusted until a satisfactory response is noted. If after a reasonable period of time there is a lack of satisfactory clinical response, betamethasone should be discontinued and the patient transferred to other appropriate therapy. IT SHOULD BE EMPHASIZED THAT DOSAGE REQUIREMENTS ARE VARIABLE AND MUST BE INDIVIDUALIZED ON THE BASIS OF THE DISEASE UNDER TREATMENT AND THE RESPONSE OF THE PATIENT. After a favorable response is noted, the proper maintenance dosage should be determined by decreasing the initial drug dosage in small decrements at appropriate time intervals until the lowest dosage which will maintain an adequate clinical response is reached. It should be kept in mind that constant monitoring is needed in regard to drug dosage. Included in the situations which may make dosage adjustments necessary are changes in clinical status secondary to remissions or exacerbations in the disease process, the patient's individual drug responsiveness, and the effect of patient exposure to stressful situations not directly related to the disease entity under treatment; in this latter situation it may be necessary to increase the dosage of betamethasone for a period of time consistent with the patient's condition. If after long-term therapy the drug is to be stopped, it is recommended that it be withdrawn gradually rather than abruptly.

How Supplied: CELESTONE **Tablets**, 0.6 mg., pink, compressed, scored tablets impressed with the Schering trademark and product identification letters, BDA, or numbers, 011; bottles of 100 and 500. Also available, CELESTONE Tablet Pack (For Six Day Therapy), 0.6 mg., 21 tablets and CELESTONE **Syrup**, 0.6 mg. per 5 ml., orange-red colored liquid; 4 oz. bottle.

Store **Tablets** between 2° and 30°C (36° and 86°F). Additionally, protect the **Tablet Pack** from excessive moisture.

Protect **Syrup** from light.

Copyright © 1968, 1977, Schering Corporation. All rights reserved.

[*Shown in Product Identification Section*]

CELESTONE® Phosphate ℞
brand of betamethasone sodium phosphate, USP
Injection

Description: CELESTONE Phosphate Injection is a sterile, aqueous solution containing in each ml.: 4.0 mg. betamethasone sodium phosphate, USP equivalent to 3.0 mg. betamethasone alcohol; 10 mg. dibasic sodium phosphate; 0.1 mg. edetate disodium; 3.2 mg. sodium bisulfite; and 5.0 mg. phenol as preservative. The pH is adjusted to approximately 8.5 with sodium hydroxide.

The formula for betamethasone sodium phosphate is $C_{22}H_{28}FNa_2O_8P$ and has a molecular weight of 516.41. Chemically, it is 9-fluoro-11β,17,21- trihydroxy -16β-methylpregna-1,4-diene-3,20-dione 21-(disodium phosphate).

Betamethasone sodium phosphate is a white to practically white, odorless powder, and is hygroscopic. Betamethasone sodium phosphate is freely soluble in water and methanol and is practically insoluble in acetone and chloroform.

Actions: Naturally occurring glucocorticoids (hydrocortisone), which also have salt-retaining properties, are used as replacement therapy in adrenocortical deficiency states. Their synthetic analogs are primarily used for their potent anti-inflammatory effects in disorders of many organ systems.

Glucocorticoids cause profound and varied metabolic effects. In addition, they modify the body's immune responses to diverse stimuli.

Indications: When oral therapy is not feasible and the strength, dosage form, and route of administration of the drug reasonably lend the preparation to the treatment of the condition, the **intravenous or intramuscular use** of CELESTONE Phosphate Injection is indicated as follows:

Endocrine disorders:

Primary or secondary adrenocortical insufficiency (hydrocortisone or cortisone is the drug of choice; synthetic analogs may be used in conjunction with mineralocorticoids where applicable; in infancy, mineralocorticoid supplementation is of particular importance).

Acute adrenocortical insufficiency (hydrocortisone or cortisone is the drug of choice; mineralocorticoid supplementation may be necessary, particularly when synthetic analogs are used).

Preoperatively and in the event of serious trauma or illness, in patients with known adrenal insufficiency or when adrenocortical reserve is doubtful.

Shock unresponsive to conventional therapy if adrenocortical insufficiency exists or is suspected.

Congenital adrenal hyperplasia.

Nonsuppurative thyroiditis.

Hypercalcemia associated with cancer.

Rheumatic disorders: As adjunctive therapy for short-term administration (to tide the patient over an acute episode or exacerbation) in:

Post-traumatic osteoarthritis.

Synovitis of osteoarthritis.

Rheumatoid arthritis, including juvenile rheumatoid arthritis (selected cases may require low-dose maintenance therapy).

Acute and subacute bursitis.

Epicondylitis.

Acute nonspecific tenosynovitis.

Acute gouty arthritis.

Psoriatic arthritis.

Ankylosing spondylitis.

Collagen diseases: During an exacerbation or as maintenance therapy in selected cases of:

Systemic lupus erythematosus.

Acute rheumatic carditis.

Dermatologic diseases:

Pemphigus.

Severe erythema multiforme (Stevens-Johnson syndrome).

Exfoliative dermatitis.

Bullous dermatitis herpetiformis.

Severe seborrheic dermatitis.

Severe psoriasis.

Mycosis fungoides.

Allergic states. Control of severe or incapacitating allergic conditions intractable to adequate trials of conventional treatment in:

Bronchial asthma.

Contact dermatitis.

Atopic dermatitis.

Serum sickness.

Seasonal or perennial allergic rhinitis.

Drug hypersensitivity reactions.

Urticarial transfusion reactions.

Acute noninfectious laryngeal edema (epinephrine is the drug of first choice).

Ophthalmic diseases: Severe, acute and chronic allergic and inflammatory processes involving the eye, such as:

Herpes zoster ophthalmicus.

Iritis, iridocyclitis.

Chorioretinitis.

Diffuse posterior uveitis and choroiditis.

Optic neuritis.

Sympathetic ophthalmia.

Anterior segment inflammation.

Allergic conjunctivitis.

Allergic corneal marginal ulcers.
Keratitis.
Gastrointestinal diseases: To tide the patient over a critical period of disease in:
Ulcerative colitis—(systemic therapy).
Regional enteritis—(systemic therapy).
Respiratory diseases:
Symptomatic sarcoidosis.
Berylliosis.
Fulminating or disseminated pulmonary tuberculosis when used concurrently with appropriate antituberculous chemotherapy.
Loffler's syndrome not manageable by other means.
Aspiration pneumonitis.
Hematologic disorders:
Acquired (autoimmune) hemolytic anemia.
Idiopathic thrombocytopenic purpura in adults (I.V. only; I.M. administration is contraindicated).
Secondary thrombocytopenia in adults.
Erythroblastopenia (RBC anemia).
Congenital (erythroid) hypoplastic anemia.
Neoplastic diseases: For palliative management of:
Leukemias and lymphomas in adults.
Acute leukemia of childhood.
Edematous states. To induce diuresis or remission of proteinuria in the nephrotic syndrome, without uremia, of the idiopathic type or that due to lupus erythematosus.
Miscellaneous:
Tuberculous meningitis with subarachnoid block or impending block when used concurrently with appropriate antituberculous chemotherapy.
Trichinosis with neurologic or myocardial involvement.
When the strength and dosage form of the drug lend the preparation to the treatment of the condition, the **intra-articular or soft tissue administration** of CELESTONE Phosphate Injection is indicated as adjunctive therapy for short-term administration (to tide the patient over an acute episode or exacerbation) in:
Synovitis of osteoarthritis.
Rheumatoid arthritis.
Acute and subacute bursitis.
Acute gouty arthritis.
Epicondylitis.
Acute nonspecific tenosynovitis.
Post-traumatic osteoarthritis.
When the strength and dosage form of the drug lend the preparation to the treatment of the condition, the **intralesional administration** of CELESTONE Phosphate Injection is indicated for:
Keloids.
Localized hypertrophic, infiltrated, inflammatory lesions of: lichen planus, psoriatic plaques, granuloma annulare, and lichen simplex chronicus (neurodermatitis).
Discoid lupus erythematosus.
Necrobiosis lipoidica diabeticorum.
Alopecia areata.
CELESTONE Phosphate injection may also be useful in cystic tumors of an aponeurosis or tendon (ganglia).

Contraindications: CELESTONE Phosphate Injection is contraindicated in systemic fungal infections.

Warnings: In patients on corticosteroid therapy subjected to any unusual stress, increased dosage of rapidly acting corticosteroids before, during, and after the stressful situation is indicated.
Corticosteroids may mask some signs of infection, and new infections may appear during their use. There may be decreased resistance and inability to localize infection when corticosteroids are used.
Prolonged use of corticosteroids may produce posterior subcapsular cataracts, glaucoma with possible damage to the optic nerves, and may enhance the establishment of secondary ocular infections due to fungi or viruses.
Average and large doses of cortisone or hydrocortisone can cause elevation of blood pressure, salt and water retention, and increased excretion of potassium. These effects are less likely to occur with the synthetic derivatives except when used in large doses. Dietary salt restriction and potassium supplementation may be necessary. All corticosteroids increase calcium excretion.
While on Corticosteroid Therapy Patients Should Not Be Vaccinated Against Smallpox. Other Immunization Procedures Should Not Be Undertaken in Patients Who are on Corticosteroids, Especially in High Doses, Because of Possible Hazards of Neurological Complications and Lack of Antibody Response.
The use of CELESTONE Phosphate Injection in active tuberculosis should be restricted to those cases of fulminating or disseminated tuberculosis in which the corticosteroid is used for the management of the disease in conjunction with appropriate antituberculous regimen.
If corticosteroids are indicated in patients with latent tuberculosis or tuberculin reactivity, close observation is necessary as reactivation of the disease may occur. During prolonged corticosteroid therapy, these patients should receive chemoprophylaxis.
Because rare instances of anaphylactoid reactions have occurred in patients receiving parenteral corticosteroid therapy, appropriate precautionary measures should be taken prior to administration, especially when the patient has a history of allergy to any drug.
Usage in pregnancy: Since adequate human reproduction studies have not been done with corticosteroids, the use of these drugs in pregnancy, nursing mothers, or women of childbearing potential requires that the possible benefits of the drug be weighed against the potential hazards to the mother and embryo or fetus. Infants born to mothers who have received substantial doses of corticosteroids during pregnancy should be carefully observed for signs of hypoadrenalism.

Precautions: Drug-induced secondary adrenocortical insufficiency may be minimized by gradual reduction of dosage. This type of relative insufficiency may persist for months after discontinuation of therapy; therefore, in any situation of stress occurring during that period, hormone therapy should be reinstituted. Since mineralocorticoid secretion may be impaired, salt and/or a mineralocorticoid should be administered concurrently.
There is an enhanced effect of corticosteroids in patients with hypothyroidism and in those with cirrhosis.
Corticosteroids should be used cautiously in patients with ocular herpes simplex for fear of corneal perforation.
The lowest possible dose of corticosteroid should be used to control the condition under treatment, and when reduction in dosage is possible, the reduction must be gradual.
Psychic derangements may appear when corticosteroids are used, ranging from euphoria, insomnia, mood swings, personality changes, and severe depression to frank psychotic manifestations. Also, existing emotional instability or psychotic tendencies may be aggravated by corticosteroids.
Aspirin should be used cautiously in conjunction with corticosteroids in hypoprothrombinemia.
Steroids should be used with caution in nonspecific ulcerative colitis, if there is a probability of impending perforation, abscess or other pyogenic infection, also in diverticulitis, fresh intestinal anastomoses, active or latent peptic ulcer, renal insufficiency, hypertension, osteoporosis, and myasthenia gravis. Growth and development of infants and children on prolonged corticosteroid therapy should be carefully followed.
The following additional precautions also apply for parenteral corticosteroids. Intra-articular injection of a corticosteroid may produce systemic as well as local effects.
Appropriate examination of any joint fluid present is necessary to exclude a septic process. A marked increase in pain accompanied by local swelling, further restriction of joint motion, fever, and malaise are suggestive of septic arthritis. If this complication occurs and the diagnosis of sepsis is confirmed, appropriate antimicrobial therapy should be instituted.
Local injection of a steroid into a previously infected joint is to be avoided.
Corticosteroids should not be injected into unstable joints.
The slower rate of absorption by intramuscular administration should be recognized.

Adverse Reactions:
Fluid and electrolyte disturbances: sodium retention; fluid retention; congestive heart failure in susceptible patients; potassium loss; hypokalemic alkalosis; hypertension.
Musculoskeletal: muscle weakness; steroid myopathy; loss of muscle mass; osteoporosis; vertebral compression fractures; aseptic necrosis of femoral and humeral heads; pathologic fracture of long bones.
Gastrointestinal: peptic ulcer with possible subsequent perforation and hemorrhage; pancreatitis; abdominal distention; ulcerative esophagitis.
Dermatologic: impaired wound healing; thin fragile skin; petechiae and ecchymoses; facial erythema; increased sweating; may suppress reactions to skin tests.
Neurological: convulsions; increased intracranial pressure with papilledema (pseudotumor cerebri) usually after treatment; vertigo; headache.
Endocrine: menstrual irregularities; development of Cushingoid state; suppression of growth in children; secondary adrenocortical and pituitary unresponsiveness, particularly in times of stress, as in trauma, surgery or illness; decreased carbohydrate tolerance; manifestations of latent diabetes mellitus; increased requirements for insulin or oral hypoglycemic agents in diabetics.
Ophthalmic: posterior subcapsular cataracts; increased intraocular pressure; glaucoma; exophthalmos.
Metabolic: negative nitrogen balance due to protein catabolism.
The following *additional* adverse reactions are also related to parenteral corticosteroid therapy: rare instances of blindness associated with intralesional therapy around the face and head; hyperpigmentation or hypopigmentation; subcutaneous and cutaneous atrophy; sterile abscess; postinjection flare (following intra-articular use); charcot-like arthropathy.

Dosage and Administration: The initial dosage of parenterally administered betamethasone may vary up to 9.0 mg. per day depending on the specific disease entity being treated. In situations of less severity, lower doses will generally suffice while in selected patients higher initial doses may be required. Usually the parenteral dosage ranges are one-third to one-half the 12-hourly oral dose. However, in certain overwhelming, acute, life-threatening situations, administration in dosages exceeding the usual dosages may be justified and may be in multiples of the oral dosages.
The initial dosage should be maintained or adjusted until a satisfactory response is noted. If after a reasonable period of time there is a lack of satisfactory clinical response, CELESTONE Phosphate Injection should be discontinued and the patient transferred to other appropriate therapy. *It Should Be Emphasized that Dosage Requirements are Variable and Must Be Individualized on the Basis of*

Continued on next page

Schering—Cont.

the Disease Under Treatment and the Response of the Patient. After a favorable response is noted, the proper maintenance dosage should be determined by decreasing the initial drug dosage in small decrements at appropriate time intervals until the lowest dosage which will maintain an adequate clinical response is reached. It should be kept in mind that constant monitoring is needed in regard to drug dosage. Included in the situations which may make dosage adjustments necessary are changes in clinical status secondary to remissions or exacerbations in the disease process, the patient's individual drug responsiveness, and the effect of patient exposure to stressful situations not directly related to the disease entity under treatment; in this latter situation it may be necessary to increase dosage of CELESTONE Phosphate Injection for a period of time consistent with the patient's condition. If after long-term therapy the drug is to be stopped, it is recommended that it be withdrawn gradually rather than abruptly.

How Supplied: CELESTONE Phosphate Injection, 4.0 mg. per ml. (equivalent to 3.0 mg. per ml. betamethasone alcohol), 1 ml. ampules, box of six; 5 ml. multiple-dose vials, box of one.

Protect from freezing.

Protect from light.

Copyright © 1973, 1977, Schering Corporation. All rights reserved.

CELESTONE® SOLUSPAN® * ℞

Suspension
brand of sterile betamethasone sodium phosphate
and betamethasone acetate suspension, USP
6 mg. per ml.

Description: Each ml. of CELESTONE SOLUSPAN* Suspension contains: 3.0 mg. betamethasone as betamethasone sodium phosphate; 3.0 mg. betamethasone acetate; 7.1 mg. dibasic sodium phosphate; 3.4 mg. monobasic sodium phosphate; 0.1 mg. edetate disodium; and 0.2 mg. benzalkonium chloride. It is a sterile, aqueous suspension with a pH between 6.8 and 7.2.

The formula for betamethasone sodium phosphate is $C_{22}H_{28}FNa_2O_8P$ with a molecular weight of 516.41. Chemically it is 9-Fluoro-11β, 17,21-trihydroxy-16β-methylpregna-1,4-diene-3,20-dione 21-(disodium phosphate).

The formula for betamethasone acetate is $C_{24}H_{31}FO_6$ with a molecular weight of 434.50. Chemically it is 9-Fluoro-11β,17,21-trihydroxy-16β-methylpregna-1, 4-diene-3, 20-dione 21-acetate.

Betamethasone sodium phosphate is a white to practically white, odorless powder, and is hygroscopic. It is freely soluble in water and in methanol, but is practically insoluble in acetone and in chloroform.

Betamethasone acetate is a white to creamy white, odorless powder that sinters and resolidifies at about 165°C, and remelts at about 200°C–220°C with decomposition. It is practically insoluble in water, but freely soluble in acetone, and is soluble in alcohol and in chloroform.

*brand of rapid and repository injectable.

Actions: Naturally occurring glucocorticoids (hydrocortisone), which also have salt-retaining properties, are used as replacement therapy in adrenocortical deficiency states. Their synthetic analogs are primarily used for their potent anti-inflammatory effects in disorders of many organ systems.

Betamethasone sodium phosphate, a soluble ester, provides prompt activity, while betamethasone acetate is only slightly soluble and affords sustained activity.

Glucocorticoids cause profound and varied metabolic effects. In addition, they modify the body's immune responses to diverse stimuli.

Indications: When oral therapy is not feasible and the strength, dosage form, and route of administration of the drug reasonably lend the preparation to the treatment of the condition, CELESTONE SOLUSPAN Suspension for **intramuscular use** is indicated as follows:

Endocrine disorders: Primary or secondary adrenocortical insufficiency (hydrocortisone or cortisone is the drug of choice; synthetic analogs may be used in conjunction with mineralocorticoids where applicable; in infancy, mineralocorticoid supplementation is of particular importance).

Acute adrenocortical insufficiency (hydrocortisone or cortisone is the drug of choice; mineralocorticoid supplementation may be necessary, particularly when synthetic analogs are used).

Preoperatively and in the event of serious trauma or illness, in patients with known adrenal insufficiency or when adrenocortical reserve is doubtful. Shock unresponsive to conventional therapy if adrenocortical insufficiency exists or is suspected. Congenital adrenal hyperplasia. Nonsuppurative thyroiditis. Hypercalcemia associated with cancer.

Rheumatic disorders: As adjunctive therapy for short-term administration (to tide the patient over an acute episode or exacerbation) in: post-traumatic osteoarthritis; synovitis of osteoarthritis; rheumatoid arthritis; acute and subacute bursitis; epicondylitis; acute nonspecific tenosynovitis; acute gouty arthritis; psoriatic arthritis; ankylosing spondylitis; juvenile rheumatoid arthritis (selected cases may require low-dose maintenance therapy).

Collagen disease: During an exacerbation or as maintenance therapy in selected cases of: systemic lupus erythematosus; acute rheumatic carditis.

Dermatologic diseases: Pemphigus: severe erythema multiforme (Stevens-Johnson syndrome); exfoliative dermatitis; bullous dermatitis herpetiformis; severe seborrheic dermatitis; severe psoriasis; mycosis fungoides.

Allergic states: Control of severe or incapacitating allergic conditions intractable to adequate trials of conventional treatment in: bronchial asthma; contact dermatitis; atopic dermatitis; serum sickness; seasonal or perennial allergic rhinitis; drug hypersensitivity reactions; urticarial transfusion reactions; acute noninfectious laryngeal edema (epinephrine is the drug of first choice).

Ophthalmic diseases: Severe, acute and chronic allergic and inflammatory processes involving the eye, such as: herpes zoster ophthalmicus; iritis, iridocyclitis; chorioretinitis; diffuse posterior uveitis and choroiditis; optic neuritis; sympathetic ophthalmia; anterior segment inflammation; allergic conjunctivitis; allergic corneal marginal ulcer; keratitis.

Gastrointestinal diseases: To tide the patient over a critical period of disease in: ulcerative colitis—(systemic therapy); regional enteritis—(systemic therapy).

Respiratory diseases: Symptomatic sarcoidosis; berylliosis; fulminating or disseminated pulmonary tuberculosis, when concurrently accompanied by appropriate antituberculous chemotherapy; aspiration pneumonitis; Loffler's syndrome not manageable by other means.

Hematologic disorders: Acquired (autoimmune) hemolytic anemia. Secondary thrombocytopenia in adults. Erythroblastopenia (RBC anemia). Congenital (erythroid) hypoplastic anemia.

Neoplastic diseases: For palliative management of: leukemias and lymphomas in adults; acute leukemia of childhood.

Edematous state: To induce diuresis or remission of proteinuria in the nephrotic syndrome, without uremia, of the idiopathic type or that due to lupus erythematosus.

Miscellaneous: Tuberculous meningitis with subarachnoid block or impending block when concurrently accompanied by appropriate antituberculous chemotherapy. Trichinosis with neurologic or myocardial involvement.

When the strength and dosage form of the drug lend the preparation to the treatment of the condition, the **intra-articular or soft tissue administration** of CELESTONE SOLUSPAN Suspension is indicated as adjunctive therapy for short-term administration (to tide the patient over an acute episode or exacerbation) in: synovitis of osteoarthritis; rheumatoid arthritis; acute and subacute bursitis; acute gouty arthritis; epicondylitis; acute nonspecific tenosynovitis; post-traumatic osteoarthritis.

When the strength and dosage form of the drug lend the preparation to the treatment of the condition, the **intralesional administration** of CELESTONE SOLUSPAN Suspension is indicated for: keloids; localized hypertrophic, infiltrated, inflammatory lesions of lichen planus, psoriatic plaques, granuloma annulare, and lichen simplex chronicus (neurodermatitis); discoid lupus erythematosus; necrobiosis lipoidica diabeticorum; alopecia areata.

CELESTONE SOLUSPAN Suspension may also be useful in cystic tumors of an aponeurosis or tendon (ganglia).

Contraindications:
CELESTONE SOLUSPAN Suspension is contraindicated in systemic fungal infections.

Warnings: CELESTONE SOLUSPAN should not be administered intravenously.

In patients on corticosteroid therapy subjected to any unusual stress, increased dosage of rapidly acting corticosteroids before, during, and after the stressful situation is indicated.

Corticosteroids may mask some signs of infection, and new infections may appear during their use. There may be decreased resistance and inability to localize infection when corticosteroids are used.

Prolonged use of corticosteroids may produce posterior subcapsular cataracts, glaucoma with possible damage to the optic nerves, and may enhance the establishment of secondary ocular infections due to fungi or viruses.

CELESTONE SOLUSPAN contains two betamethasone esters one of which, betamethasone sodium phosphate, disappears rapidly from the injection site. The potential for systemic effect produced by the soluble portion of CELESTONE SOLUSPAN should therefore be taken into account by the physician when using the drug.

Average and large doses of cortisone or hydrocortisone can cause elevation of blood pressure, salt and water retention, and increased excretion of potassium. These effects are less likely to occur with the synthetic derivatives except when used in large doses. Dietary salt restriction and potassium supplementation may be necessary. All corticosteroids increase calcium excretion.

While on Corticosteroid Therapy Patients Should Not Be Vaccinated Against Smallpox. Other Immunization Procedures Should Not Be Undertaken in Patients Who Are on Corticosteroids, Especially in High Doses, Because of Possible Hazards of Neurological Complications and Lack of Antibody Response.

The use of CELESTONE SOLUSPAN Suspension in active tuberculosis should be restricted to those cases of fulminating or disseminated tuberculosis in which the corticosteroid is used for the management of the disease in conjunction with appropriate antituberculous regimen.

If corticosteroids are indicated in patients with latent tuberculosis or tuberculin reactivity, close observation is necessary as reactivation of the disease may occur. During prolonged corticosteroid therapy, these patients should receive chemoprophylaxis.

Because rare instances of anaphylactoid reactions have occurred in patients receiving parenteral corticosteroid therapy, appropriate precautionary measures should be taken prior to administration, especially when the patient has a history of allergy to any drug.

Usage in pregnancy: Since adequate human reproduction studies have not been done with corticosteroids, the use of these drugs in pregnancy, nursing mothers, or women of childbearing potential requires that the possible benefits of the drug be weighed against the potential hazards to the mother and embryo or fetus. Infants born of mothers who have received substantial doses of corticosteroids during pregnancy should be carefully observed for signs of hypoadrenalism.

Precautions: Drug-induced secondary adrenocortical insufficiency may be minimized by gradual reduction of dosage. This type of relative insufficiency may persist for months after discontinuation of therapy; therefore, in any situation of stress occurring during that period, hormone therapy should be reinstituted. Since mineralocorticoid secretion may be impaired, salt and/or a mineralocorticoid should be administered concurrently.

There is an enhanced effect of corticosteroids in patients with hypothyroidism and in those with cirrhosis.

Corticosteroids should be used cautiously in patients with ocular herpes simplex for fear of corneal perforation.

The lowest possible dose of corticosteroid should be used to control the condition under treatment, and when reduction in dosage is possible, the reduction must be gradual.

Psychic derangements may appear when corticosteroids are used, ranging from euphoria, insomnia, mood swings, personality changes, and severe depression to frank psychotic manifestations. Also, existing emotional instability or psychotic tendencies may be aggravated by corticosteroids.

Aspirin should be used cautiously in conjunction with corticosteroids in hypoprothrombinemia.

Steroids should be used with caution in nonspecific ulcerative colitis, if there is a probability of impending perforation, abscess or other pyogenic infection, also in diverticulitis, fresh intestinal anastomoses, active or latent peptic ulcer, renal insufficiency, hypertension, osteoporosis, and myasthenia gravis.

Growth and development of infants and children on prolonged corticosteroid therapy should be carefully followed.

The following additional precautions also apply for parenteral corticosteroids. **Intra-articular injection of a corticosteroid may produce systemic as well as local effects.**

Appropriate examination of any joint fluid present is necessary to exclude a septic process. A marked increase in pain accompanied by local swelling, further restriction of joint motion, fever, and malaise are suggestive of septic arthritis. If this complication occurs and the diagnosis of sepsis is confirmed, appropriate antimicrobial therapy should be instituted.

Local injection of a steroid into a previously infected joint is to be avoided.

Corticosteroids should not be injected into unstable joints.

The slower rate of absorption by intramuscular administration should be recognized.

Adverse Reactions:

Fluid and electrolyte disturbances: sodium retention; fluid retention; congestive heart failure in susceptible patients; potassium loss; hypokalemic alkalosis; hypertension.

Musculoskeletal: muscle weakness; steroid myopathy; loss of muscle mass; osteoporosis; vertebral compression fractures; aseptic necrosis of femoral and humeral heads; pathologic fracture of long bones.

Gastrointestinal: peptic ulcer with possible subsequent perforation and hemorrhage; pancreatitis; abdominal distention; ulcerative esophagitis.

Dermatologic: impaired wound healing; thin fragile skin; petechiae and ecchymoses; facial erythema; increased sweating; may suppress reactions to skin tests.

Neurological: convulsions; increased intracranial pressure with papilledema (pseudotumor cerebri) usually after treatment; vertigo; headache.

Endocrine: menstrual irregularities; development of Cushingoid state; suppression of growth in children; secondary adrenocortical and pituitary unresponsiveness, particularly in times of stress, as in trauma, surgery, or illness; decreased carbohydrate tolerance; manifestations of latent diabetes mellitus; increased requirements for insulin or oral hypoglycemic agents in diabetics.

Ophthalmic: posterior subcapsular cataracts; increased intraocular pressure; glaucoma; exophthalmos.

Metabolic: negative nitrogen balance due to protein catabolism.

The following *additional* adverse reactions are related to parenteral corticosteroid therapy: rare instances of blindness associated with intralesional therapy around the face and head; hyperpigmentation or hypopigmentation; subcutaneous and cutaneous atrophy; sterile abscess; post-injection flare (following intra-articular use); charcot-like arthropathy.

Dosage and Administration: The initial dosage of CELESTONE SOLUSPAN Suspension may vary from 0.5 to 9.0 mg. per day depending on the specific disease entity being treated. In situations of less severity, lower doses will generally suffice while in selected patients higher initial doses may be required. Usually the parenteral dosage ranges are one-third to one-half the oral dose given every 12 hours. However, in certain overwhelming, acute, life-threatening situations, administration in dosages exceeding the usual dosages may be justified and may be in multiples of the oral dosages.

The initial dosage should be maintained or adjusted until a satisfactory response is noted. If after a reasonable period of time there is a lack of satisfactory clinical response, CELESTONE SOLUSPAN Suspension should be discontinued and the patient transferred to other appropriate therapy. *It Should Be Emphasized That Dosage Requirements Are Variable and Must Be Individualized on the Basis of the Disease Under Treatment and the Response of the Patient.* After a favorable response is noted, the proper maintenance dosage should be determined by decreasing the initial drug dosage in small decrements at appropriate time intervals until the lowest dosage which will maintain an adequate clinical response is reached. It should be kept in mind that constant monitoring is needed in regard to drug dosage. Included in the situations which may make dosage adjustments necessary are changes in clinical status secondary to remissions or exacerbations in the disease process, the patient's individual drug responsiveness, and the effect of patient exposure to stressful situations not directly related to the disease entity under treatment; in this latter situation it may be necessary to increase the dosage of CELESTONE SOLUSPAN Suspension for a period of time consistent with the patient's condition. If after long-term therapy the drug is to be stopped, it is recommended that it be withdrawn gradually rather than abruptly.

If coadministration of a local anesthetic is desired, CELESTONE SOLUSPAN Suspension may be mixed with 1% or 2% lidocaine hydrochloride, using the formulations which do not contain parabens. Similar local anesthetics may also be used. Diluents containing methylparaben, propylparaben, phenol, etc., should be avoided since these compounds may cause flocculation of the steroid. The required dose of CELESTONE SOLUSPAN Suspension is first withdrawn from the vial into the syringe. The local anesthetic is then drawn in, and the syringe shaken briefly. **Do not inject local anesthetics into the vial of CELESTONE SOLUSPAN Suspension.**

Bursitis, tenosynovitis, peritendinitis. In acute subdeltoid, subacromial, olecranon, and prepatellar bursitis, one intrabursal injection of 1.0 ml. CELESTONE SOLUSPAN Suspension can relieve pain and restore full range of movement. Several intrabursal injections of corticosteroids are usually required in recurrent acute bursitis and in acute exacerbations of chronic bursitis. Partial relief of pain and some increase in mobility can be expected in both conditions after one or two injections. Chronic bursitis may be treated with reduced dosage once the acute condition is controlled. In tenosynovitis and tendinitis, three or four local injections at intervals of one to two weeks between injections are given in most cases. Injections should be made into the affected tendon sheaths rather than into the tendons themselves. In ganglions of joint capsules and tendon sheaths, injection of 0.5 ml. directly into the ganglion cysts has produced marked reduction in the size of the lesions. *Rheumatoid arthritis and osteoarthritis.* Following intra-articular administration of 0.5 to 2.0 ml. of CELESTONE SOLUSPAN Suspension, relief of pain, soreness, and stiffness may be experienced. Duration of relief varies widely in both diseases. Intra-articular Injection—CELESTONE SOLUSPAN Suspension is well tolerated in joints and periarticular tissues. There is virtually no pain on injection, and the "secondary flare" that sometimes occurs a few hours after intra-articular injection of corticosteroids has not been reported with CELESTONE SOLUSPAN Suspension. Using sterile technique, a 20- to 24-gauge needle on an empty syringe is inserted into the synovial cavity, and a few drops of synovial fluid are withdrawn to confirm that the needle is in the joint. The aspirating syringe is replaced by a syringe containing CELESTONE SOLUSPAN Suspension and injection is then made into the joint.

Recommended Doses for Intra-articular Injection

Size of joint	Location	Dose (ml.)
Very Large	Hip	1.0-2.0
Large	Knee, Ankle, Shoulder	1.0
Medium	Elbow, Wrist	0.5-1.0
Small (Metacarpophalangeal, interphalangeal) (Sternoclavicular)	Hand Chest	0.25-0.5

A portion of the administered dose of CELESTONE SOLUSPAN Suspension is absorbed systemically following intra-articular injection. In patients being treated concomitantly with oral or parenteral corticosteroids, especially those receiving large doses, the systemic absorption of the drug should be considered in determining intra-articular dosage. *Dermatologic conditions.* In intralesional treatment, 0.2 ml./sq. cm. of CELESTONE SOLUSPAN Suspension is injected intradermally (not subcutaneously) using a tuberculin syringe with a 25-gauge, ½-inch needle. Care should be taken to deposit a uniform depot of medication intradermally. A total of no more than 1.0 ml. at weekly intervals is recommended. *Disorders of the foot.* A tuberculin syringe with a 25-gauge, ¾-inch needle is suitable for most injections into the foot. The following

Continued on next page

Information on Schering products appearing on these pages is effective as of September 30, 1982.

Schering—Cont.

doses are recommended at intervals of three days to a week.

Diagnosis	CELESTONE SOLUSPAN Suspension Dose (ml.)
Bursitis	
under heloma durum or heloma molle	0.25-0.5
under calcaneal spur	0.5
over hallux rigidus or digiti quinti varus	0.5
Tenosynovitis, periostitis of cuboid	0.5
Acute gouty arthritis	0.5-1.0

How Supplied: CELESTONE SOLUSPAN Suspension, 5 ml. multiple-dose vial, box of one (NDC-0085-0566-05). Shake well before using. Store between 2° and 25°C (36° and 77°F). **Protect from light.**

Copyright © 1969, 1978, Schering Corporation. All rights reserved.

DIPROSONE®

brand of betamethasone dipropionate, USP
Cream 0.05%
Ointment 0.05%
Lotion 0.05% w/w
Topical Aerosol 0.1% w/w
(potency expressed as betamethasone)
For Dermatologic Use Only—
Not for Ophthalmic Use

Description: DIPROSONE **Cream, Ointment, Lotion,** and **Topical Aerosol** contain betamethasone dipropionate, USP, a synthetic adrenocorticosteroid, for dermatologic use. Betamethasone, an analog of prednisolone, has high corticosteroid activity and slight mineralocorticoid activity. Betamethasone dipropionate is the 17,21-dipropionate ester of betamethasone.

Chemically, betamethasone dipropionate is 9-Fluoro-11β, 17, 21-trihydroxy-16β-methylpregna-1, 4-diene-3, 20-dione 17, 21-dipropionate, with the empirical formula $C_{28}H_{37}FO_7$, a molecular weight of 504.6.

Betamethasone dipropionate is a white to creamy white, odorless crystalline powder, insoluble in water.

Each gram of DIPROSONE **Cream** 0.05% contains: 0.64 mg betamethasone dipropionate, USP (equivalent to 0.5 mg betamethasone), in a hydrophilic emollient cream consisting of purified water, mineral oil, white petrolatum, polyethylene glycol 1000 monocetyl ether, cetostearyl alcohol, monobasic sodium phosphate, and phosphoric acid; 4-chloro-*m*-cresol and propylene gylcol as preservatives.

Each gram of DIPROSONE **Ointment** 0.05% contains: 0.64 mg betamethasone dipropionate, USP (equivalent to 0.5 mg betamethasone), in an ointment base of mineral oil and white petrolatum.

Each gram of DIPROSONE **Lotion** 0.05% w/w contains: 0.64 mg betamethasone dipropionate, USP (equivalent to 0.5 mg betamethasone), in a lotion base of isopropyl alcohol (46.8%) and purified water slightly thickened with carboxy vinyl polymer; the pH is adjusted to approximately 4.7 with sodium hydroxide.

DIPROSONE **Topical Aerosol** 0.1% w/w contains: 6.4 mg betamethasone dipropionate, USP (equivalent to 5.0 mg betamethasone), in a vehicle of mineral oil and caprylic/capric triglyceride; also containing 10% isopropyl alcohol and sufficient inert hydrocarbon (propane and isobutane) propellant to make 85 grams. The aerosol spray deposits betamethasone dipropionate equivalent to approximately 0.1% betamethasone in a nonvolatile, almost invisible film. A three-second spray delivers betamethasone dipropionate equivalent to approximately 0.06 mg betamethasone.

Clinical Pharmacology: The corticosteroids are a class of compounds comprising steroid hormones secreted by the adrenal cortex and their synthetic analogs. In pharmacologic doses corticosteroids are used primarily for their anti-inflammatory and/or immunosuppressive effects.

Topical corticosteroids, such as betamethasone dipropionate, are effective in the treatment of corticosteroid-responsive dermatoses primarily because of their anti-inflammatory, antipruritic, and vasoconstrictive actions. However, while the physiologic, pharmacologic, and clinical effects of the corticosteroids are well-known, the exact mechanisms of their actions in each disease are uncertain. Betamethasone dipropionate, a corticosteroid, has been shown to have topical (dermatologic) and systemic pharmacologic and metabolic effects characteristic of this class of drugs.

Pharmacokinetics: The extent of percutaneous absorption of topical corticosteroids is determined by many factors including the vehicle, the integrity of the epidermal barrier, and the use of occlusive dressings. (See **DOSAGE AND ADMINISTRATION** section.)

Topical corticosteroids can be absorbed from normal intact skin. Inflammation and/or other disease processes in the skin increase percutaneous absorption. Occlusive dressings substantially increase the percutaneous absorption of topical corticosteroids. (See **DOSAGE AND ADMINISTRATION** section.)

Once absorbed through the skin, topical corticosteroids are handled through pharmacokinetic pathways similar to systemically administered corticosteroids. Corticosteroids are bound to plasma proteins in varying degrees. Corticosteroids are metabolized primarily in the liver and are then excreted by the kidneys. Some of the topical corticosteroids and their metabolites are also excreted into the bile.

Indications and Usage: DIPROSONE **Cream, Ointment Lotion,** and **Topical Aerosol** are indicated for relief of the inflammatory and pruritic manifestations of corticosteroid-responsive dermatoses.

Contraindications: DIPROSONE **Cream, Ointment, Lotion,** and **Topical Aerosol** are contraindicated in patients who are hypersensitive to betamethasone dipropionate, to other corticosteroids, or to any ingredient in these preparations.

Precautions: General: Systemic absorption of topical corticosteroids has produced reversible hypothalamic-pituitary-adrenal (HPA) axis suppression, manifestations of Cushing's syndrome, hyperglycemia, and glucosuria in some patients.

Conditions which augment systemic absorption include the application of the more potent steroids, use over large surface areas, prolonged use, and the addition of occlusive dressings. (See **DOSAGE AND ADMINISTRATION** section.)

Therefore, patients receiving a large dose of a potent topical steroid applied to a large surface area should be evaluated periodically for evidence of HPA axis suppression by using the urinary free cortisol and ACTH stimulation tests. If HPA axis suppression is noted, an attempt should be made to withdraw the drug, to reduce the frequency of application, or to substitute a less potent steroid.

Recovery of HPA axis function is generally prompt and complete upon discontinuation of the drug. Infrequently, signs and symptoms of steroid withdrawal may occur, requiring supplemental systemic corticosteroids.

Children may absorb proportionally larger amounts of topical corticosteroids and thus be more susceptible to systemic toxicity. (See **PRECAUTIONS-Pediatric Use.**)

If irritation develops, topical corticosteroids should be discontinued and appropriate therapy instituted.

In the presence of dermatological infections, the use of an appropriate antifungal or antibacterial agent should be instituted. If a favorable response does not occur promptly, the corticosteroid should be discontinued until the infection has been adequately controlled.

Information for Patients: Patients using topical corticosteroids should receive the following information and instructions:

1. This medication is to be used as directed by the physician. It is for external use only. Avoid contact with the eyes.
2. Patients should be advised not to use this medication for any disorder other than for which it was prescribed.
3. The treated skin area should not be bandaged or otherwise covered or wrapped as to be occlusive. (See **DOSAGE AND ADMINISTRATION** section.)
4. Patients should report any signs of local adverse reactions.
5. Parents of pediatric patients should be advised not to use tight-fitting diapers or plastic pants on a child being treated in the diaper area, as these garments may constitute occlusive dressing. (See **DOSAGE AND ADMINISTRATION** section.)
6. When using DIPROSONE **Topical Aerosol,** the patient should be advised of the following:
   - the spray should be kept away from the eyes or other mucous membranes
   - avoid freezing tissues by not spraying for more than three seconds, at a distance of not less than six inches between the nozzle and the skin
   - use only as directed; intentional misuse by deliberately concentrating and inhaling the container contents can be harmful or fatal
   - the container contents are under pressure; do not puncture the container
   - the container mixture is flammable; do not use or store the container near heat or an open flame; exposure to temperatures above 120° Fahrenheit may cause bursting; never throw container into a fire or incinerator
   - keep out of the reach of children

Laboratory Tests: The following tests may be helpful in evaluating HPA axis suppression:

Urinary free cortisol test
ACTH stimulation test

Carcinogenesis, Mutagenesis, and Impairment of Fertility: Long-term animal studies have not been performed to evaluate the carcinogenic potential or the effect on fertility of topical corticosteroids.

Studies to determine mutagenicity with prednisolone have revealed negative results.

Pregnancy Category C: Corticosteroids are generally teratogenic in laboratory animals when administered systemically at relatively low dosage levels. The more potent corticosteroids have been shown to be teratogenic after dermal application in laboratory animals. There are no adequate and well-controlled studies in pregnant women on teratogenic effects from topically applied corticosteroids. Therefore, topical corticosteroids should be used during pregnancy only if the potential benefit justifies the potential risk to the fetus. Drugs of this class should not be used extensively on pregnant patients, in large amounts, or for prolonged periods of time.

Nursing Mothers: It is not known whether topical administration of corticosteroids could result in sufficient systemic absorption to produce detectable quantities in breast milk. Systemically administered corticosteroids are secreted into breast milk in quantities not likely to have a deleterious effect on the infant. Nevertheless, caution should be exercised when topical corticosteroids are prescribed for a nursing woman.

Pediatric use: Pediatric patients may demonstrate greater susceptibility to topical corticosteroid-induced HPA axis suppression and

Cushing's syndrome than mature patients because of a larger skin surface area to body weight ratio.
Hypothalamic-pituitary-adrenal (HPA) axis suppression, Cushing's syndrome, and intracranial hypertension have been reported in children receiving topical corticosteroids. Manifestations of adrenal suppression in children include linear growth retardation, delayed weight gain, low plasma cortisol levels, and absence of response to ACTH stimulation. Manifestations of intracranial hypertension include bulging fontanelles, headaches, and bilateral papilledema.
Administration of topical corticosteroids to children should be limited to the least amount compatible with an effective therapeutic regimen. Chronic corticosteroid therapy may interfere with the growth and development of children.

Adverse Reactions: The following local adverse reactions are reported infrequently when DIPROSONE Products are used as recommended in the **DOSAGE AND ADMINISTRATION** section. These reactions are listed in an approximate decreasing order of occurrence: burning; itching; irritation; dryness; folliculitis; hypertrichosis; acneiform eruptions; hypopigmentation; perioral dermatitis; allergic contact dermatitis; maceration of the skin; secondary infection; skin atrophy; striae; miliaria.
Systemic absorption of topical corticosteroids has produced reversible hypothalamic-pituitary-adrenal (HPA) axis suppression, manifestations of Cushing's syndrome, hyperglycemia, and glucosuria in some patients.

Overdosage: Topically applied corticosteroids can be absorbed in sufficient amounts to produce systemic effects. (See **PRECAUTIONS.**)

Dosage and Administration: DIPROSONE **Cream:** Apply a thin film of DIPROSONE **Cream** 0.05% to the affected skin areas once daily. In some cases, a twice daily dosage may be necessary.
DIPROSONE **Ointment:** Apply a thin film of DIPROSONE **Ointment** to the affected skin areas once daily. In some cases, a twice daily dosage may be necessary.
DIPROSONE **Lotion:** Apply a few drops of DIPROSONE **Lotion** to the affected area and massage lightly until it disappears. Apply twice daily, in the morning and at night. For the most effective and economical use, apply nozzle very close to affected area and gently squeeze bottle.
DIPROSONE **Topical Aerosol:** Apply sparingly to the affected skin area three times a day. The container may be held upright or inverted during use. The spray should be directed onto the affected area from a distance of not less than six inches and applied for only three seconds. For the most effective and economical use, a three-second spray is sufficient to cover an area about the size of the hand.
DIPROSONE Products are not to be used with occlusive dressings.

How Supplied: DIPROSONE **Cream** 0.05% is supplied in 15-, 45-, and 110- gram tubes and 430-gram jars; boxes of one.
(NDC-0085-0853—)
DIPROSONE **Lotion** 0.05% w/w is available in 20 ml (18.7 g) and 60 ml (56.2 g) plastic squeeze bottles; boxes of one. **Protect from light. Store in carton until contents are used.**
(NDC-0085-0028—)
DIPROSONE **Ointment** 0.05% is supplied in 15- and 45- gram tubes; boxes of one.
(NDC-0085-0510—)
DIPROSONE **Topical Aerosol** 0.1% w/w is supplied as a 85-gram spray can.
(NDC-0085-0475-06)
Store all DIPROSONE preparations between 2° and 30°C (36° and 86°F).
Revised 4/82
Copyright © 1974, 1982, Schering Corporation. All rights reserved.

ESTINYL® ℞

brand of ethinyl estradiol, USP
Tablets

BOXED WARNINGS

1. ESTROGENS HAVE BEEN REPORTED TO INCREASE THE RISK RATIO OF ENDOMETRIAL CARCINOMA.
Three independent case control studies have reported an increased risk ratio of endometrial cancer in postmenopausal women exposed to exogenous estrogens for prolonged periods.[1–3] This risk ratio was independent of the other risk factors for endometrial cancer. These studies are further supported by the report that incidence rates of endometrial cancer have increased sharply since 1969 in eight different areas of the United States with population-based cancer reporting systems, an increase which may be related to the rapidly expanding use of estrogens during the last decade.[4]
The three case control studies reported that the risk ratio of endometrial cancer in estrogen users was about 4.5 to 13.9 times greater than in nonusers. The risk ratio appears to depend on both duration of treatment[1] and on estrogen dose.[3] In view of these reports, when estrogens are used for the treatment of menopausal symptoms, the lowest dose that will control symptoms should be utilized and medication should be discontinued as soon as possible. When prolonged treatment is medically indicated, the patient should be reassessed on at least a semiannual basis to determine the need for continued therapy.
Although the evidence must be considered preliminary, one study suggests that cyclic administration of low doses of estrogen may carry less risk than continuous administration[3]; it therefore appears prudent to utilize such a regimen.
Close clinical surveillance of all women taking estrogens is important. In all cases of undiagnosed persistent or recurring abnormal vaginal bleeding, adequate diagnostic measures should be undertaken to rule out malignancy.
There is no evidence at present that "natural" estrogens are more or less hazardous than "synthetic" estrogens at equiestrogenic doses.

2. ESTROGENS SHOULD NOT BE USED DURING PREGNANCY.
The use of estrogens during early pregnancy may seriously damage the offspring. It has been reported that females exposed in utero to diethylstilbestrol, a non-steroidal estrogen, may have an increased risk of developing in later life a form of vaginal or cervical cancer that is ordinarily extremely rare.[5,6] This risk has been estimated statistically as not greater than 4 per 1000 exposures.[7] In certain studies, a high percentage of such exposed women (from 30 to 90 percent) have been found to have vaginal adenosis,[8–11] epithelial changes of the vagina and cervix. Although these changes are histologically benign, it is not known whether they are precursors of malignancy. Although similar data are not available with the use of other estrogens, it cannot be presumed they would not induce similar changes.
Several reports suggest an association between intrauterine fetal exposure to female sex hormones and congenital anomalies, including congenital heart defects and limb reduction defects.[12–15] One case control study[15] estimated a 4.7 fold increased risk of limb reduction defects in infants exposed in utero to sex hormones (oral contraceptives, hormone withdrawal tests for pregnancy, or attempted treatment for threatened abortion). Some of these exposures were very short and involved only a few days of treatment. The data suggest that the risk of limb reduction defects in exposed fetuses is somewhat less than 1 per 1000.
In the past, estrogens have been used during pregnancy to treat threatened or habitual abortion. There is considerable evidence that estrogens are ineffective for these indications.
If ESTINYL is used during pregnancy, or if the patient becomes pregnant while taking this drug, she should be apprised of the potential risks to the fetus, and the advisability of pregnancy continuation.

Description: ESTINYL Tablets contain ethinyl estradiol, a potent synthetic estrogen having the chemical name, 19-Nor-17α-pregna-1,3,5(10)-trien-20-yne-3,17-diol.
ESTINYL for oral administration is available in tablets containing 0.02, 0.05, or 0.5 mg. ethinyl estradiol, USP.

Clinical Pharmacology: Ethinyl estradiol promotes growth of the endometrium and thickening, stratification and cornification of the vagina. It causes growth of the ducts of the mammary gland, but inhibits lactation. It also inhibits the anterior pituitary and causes capillary dilatation, fluid retention and protein anabolism.

Indications: ESTINYL Tablets are indicated in the treatment of: 1) Moderate to severe *vasomotor* symptoms associated with the menopause. (There is no evidence that estrogens are effective for nervous symptoms or depression which might occur during menopause, and they should not be used to treat these conditions.) 2) Female hypogonadism. 3) Prostatic carcinoma—palliative therapy of advanced disease. 4) Breast cancer (for palliation only) in appropriately selected women, such as those who are more than 5 years postmenopausal with progressing inoperable or radiation-resistant disease.
ESTINYL HAS NOT BEEN SHOWN TO BE EFFECTIVE FOR ANY PURPOSE DURING PREGNANCY AND ITS USE MAY CAUSE SEVERE HARM TO THE FETUS (SEE BOXED WARNING ABOVE).

Contraindications: Estrogens should not be used in women (or men) with any of the following conditions:
1. Known or suspected cancer of the breast except in appropriately selected patients being treated for metastatic disease.
2. Known or suspected estrogen-dependent neoplasia.
3. Known or suspected pregnancy (See Boxed Warning).
4. Undiagnosed abnormal genital bleeding.
5. Active thrombophlebitis or thromboembolic disorders.
6. A past history of thrombophlebitis, thrombosis or thromboembolic disorders associated with previous estrogen use (except when used in treatment of breast or prostatic malignancy).

Warnings: 1. *Induction of malignant neoplasms.* Long-term continuous administration of natural and synthetic estrogens in certain animal species increases the frequency of carcinomas of the breast, cervix, vagina, and liver. There is now evidence that estrogens increase the risk of carcinoma of the endometrium in humans. (See Boxed Warning.)
At the present time there is no satisfactory evidence that estrogens given to postmenopausal women increase the risk of cancer of the

Continued on next page

Information on Schering products appearing on these pages is effective as of September 30, 1982.

Schering—Cont.

breast,[16] although a recent long-term follow-up of a single physician's practice has raised this possibility.[17] Because of the animal data, there is a need for caution in prescribing estrogens for women with a strong family history of breast cancer or who have breast nodules, fibrocystic disease, or abnormal mammograms. Estrogens have been reported to be associated with carcinoma of the male breast and suspicious lesions in males receiving estrogen therapy should be investigated accordingly.

2. *Gallbladder disease.* A recent study has reported a 2- to 3-fold increase in the risk of surgically confirmed gallbladder disease in women receiving postmenopausal estrogens,[16] similar to the 2-fold increase previously noted in users of oral contraceptives.[18,22] In the case of oral contraceptives, the increased risk appeared after two years of use.[22]

3. *Effects similar to those caused by estrogen-progestagen oral contraceptives.* There are several serious adverse effects of oral contraceptives, most of which have not, up to now, been documented as consequences of postmenopausal estrogen therapy. This may reflect the comparatively low doses of estrogen used in postmenopausal women. It would be expected that the larger doses of estrogen used to treat prostatic or breast cancer are more likely to result in these adverse effects, and, in fact, it has been shown that there is an increased risk of thrombosis in men receiving estrogens for prostatic cancer.[19–22]

a. *Thromboembolic disease* It is now well established that users of oral contraceptives have an increased risk of various thromboembolic and thrombotic vascular diseases, such as thrombophlebitis, pulmonary embolism, stroke and myocardial infarction.[22–29] Cases of retinal thrombosis, mesenteric thrombosis, and optic neuritis have been reported in oral contraceptive users. There is evidence that the risk of several of these adverse reactions is related to the dose of the drug.[30,31] An increased risk of postsurgery thromboembolic complications has also been reported in users of oral contraceptives.[32,33] If feasible, estrogen should be discontinued at least 4 weeks before surgery of the type associated with an increased risk of thromboembolism, or during periods of immobilization.

While an increased rate of thromboembolic and thrombotic disease in postmenopausal users of estrogen has not been found,[16,34] this does not rule out the possibility that such an increase may be present or that subgroups of women who have underlying risk factors or who are receiving relatively large doses of estrogens may have increased risk. Therefore, estrogens should not be used in persons with active thrombophlebitis or thromboembolic disorders, and they should not be used (except in treatment of malignancy) in persons with a history of such disorders in association with estrogen use. They should be used with caution in patients with cerebral vascular or coronary artery disease and only for those in whom estrogens are clearly needed.

Large doses of estrogen (5 mg. conjugated estrogens per day), comparable to those used to treat cancer of the prostate and breast, have been shown in a large prospective clinical trial in men[35] to increase the risk of nonfatal myocardial infarction, pulmonary embolism and thrombophlebitis. When estrogen doses of this size are used, any of the thromboembolic and thrombotic adverse effects associated with oral contraceptive use should be considered a clear risk.

b. *Hepatic adenoma* Benign hepatic adenomas appear to be associated with the use of oral contraceptives.[36–38] Although benign, and rare, these may rupture and may cause death through intra-abdominal hemorrhage. Such lesions have not yet been reported in association with other estrogen or progestagen preparations but should be considered in estrogen users having abdominal pain and tenderness, abdominal mass, or hypovolemic shock. Hepatocellular carcinoma has also been reported in women taking estrogen-containing oral contraceptives.[37] The relationship of this malignancy to these drugs is not known at this time.

c. *Elevated blood pressure* Increased blood pressure is not uncommon in women using oral contraceptives. There is now a report that this may occur with use of estrogens in the menopause[39] and blood pressure should be monitored with estrogen use, especially if high doses are used.

d. *Glucose tolerance* A worsening of glucose tolerance has been observed in a significant percentage of patients on estrogen-containing oral contraceptives. For this reason, diabetic patients should be carefully observed while receiving estrogen.

4. *Hypercalcemia* Administration of estrogens may lead to severe hypercalcemia in patients with breast cancer and bone metastases. If this occurs, the drug should be stopped and appropriate measures taken to reduce the serum calcium level.

Precautions:

General Precautions

1. A complete medical and family history should be taken prior to the initiation of any estrogen therapy. The pretreatment and periodic physical examinations should include special reference to blood pressure, breasts, abdomen, and pelvic organs, and should include a Papanicolaou smear. As a general rule, estrogen should not be prescribed for longer than one year without another physical examination being performed.

2. Fluid retention—Because estrogens may cause some degree of fluid retention, conditions which might be influenced by this factor, such as epilepsy, migraine, and cardiac or renal dysfunction, require careful observation.

3. Certain patients may develop undesirable manifestations of excessive estrogenic stimulation, such as abnormal or excessive uterine bleeding, mastodynia, etc.

4. Oral contraceptives appear to be associated with an increased incidence of mental depression.[22] Although it is not clear whether this is due to the estrogenic or progestagenic component of the contraceptive, patients with a history of depression should be carefully observed.

5. Preexisting uterine leiomyomata may increase in size during estrogen use.

6. The pathologist should be advised of estrogen therapy when relevant specimens are submitted.

7. Patients with a past history of jaundice during pregnancy have an increased risk of recurrence of jaundice while receiving estrogen-containing oral contraceptive therapy. If jaundice develops in any patient receiving estrogen, the medication should be discontinued while the cause is investigated.

8. Estrogens may be poorly metabolized in patients with impaired liver function and they should be administered with caution in such patients.

9. Because estrogens influence the metabolism of calcium and phosphorus, they should be used with caution in patients with metabolic bone diseases that are associated with hypercalcemia or in patients with renal insufficiency.

10. Because of the effects of estrogens on epiphyseal closure, they should be used judiciously in young patients in whom bone growth is not complete.

11. Certain endocrine and liver function tests may be affected by estrogen-containing oral contraceptives. The following similar changes may be expected with larger doses of estrogen: Increased sulfobromophthalein retention; increased prothrombin and factors VII, VIII, IX, and X; decreased antithrombin 3; increased norepinephrine-induced platelet aggregation; increased thyroid binding globulin (TBG) leading to increased circulating total thyroid hormone, as measured by PBI, T4 by column, or T4 by radioimmunoassay. Free T3 resin uptake is decreased, reflecting the elevated TBG; free T4 concentration is unaltered; impaired glucose tolerance; decreased pregnanediol excretion; reduced response to metyrapone test; reduced serum folate concentration; increased serum triglyceride and phospholipid concentration.

12. ESTINYL Tablets, .02 mg. contain FD&C Yellow No. 5 (tartrazine) which may cause allergic-type reactions (including bronchial asthma) in certain susceptible individuals. Although the overall incidence of FD&C Yellow No. 5 (tartrazine) sensitivity in the general population is low, it is frequently seen in patients who also have aspirin hypersensitivity.

Information for the Patient: See text of Patient Package Insert.

Pregnancy Category X. See Contraindications and Boxed Warning above.

Nursing Mothers: As a general principle, the administration of any drug to nursing mothers should be done only when clearly necessary, since many drugs are excreted in human milk.

Adverse Reactions: (See Warnings regarding induction of neoplasia, adverse effects on the fetus, increased incidence of gallbladder disease, and adverse effects similar to those of oral contraceptives, including thromboembolism.) The following additional adverse reactions have been reported with estrogenic therapy, including oral contraceptives:

Genitourinary system: Breakthrough bleeding, spotting, change in menstrual flow; dysmenorrhea; premenstrual-like syndrome; amenorrhea during and after treatment; increase in size of uterine fibromyomata; vaginal candidiasis; change in cervical eversion and in degree of cervical secretion; cystitis-like syndrome.

Breasts: Tenderness, enlargement, secretion.

Gastrointestinal: Nausea, vomiting; abdominal cramps, bloating; cholestatic jaundice.

Skin: Chloasma or melasma which may persist when drug is discontinued; erythema multiforme; erythema nodosum; hemorrhagic eruption; loss of scalp hair; hirsutism.

Eyes: Steepening of corneal curvature; intolerance to contact lenses.

CNS: Headache, migraine, dizziness; mental depression; chorea.

Miscellaneous: Increase or decrease in weight; reduced carbohydrate tolerance; aggravation of porphyria; edema; changes in libido.

Acute Overdosage: Numerous reports of ingestion of large doses of estrogen-containing oral contraceptives by young children indicate that serious ill effects do not occur. Overdosage of estrogen may cause nausea, and withdrawal bleeding may occur in females.

Dosage and Administration: 1. *Given cyclically for short-term use only.*

For treatment of moderate to severe *vasomotor* symptoms associated with the menopause: The lowest dose that will control symptoms should be chosen and medication should be discontinued as promptly as possible. Administration should be cyclic (eg, 3 weeks on and 1 week off). Attempts to discontinue or taper medication should be made at 3- to 6-month intervals. The usual dosage range is one 0.02 mg. or 0.05 mg. tablet daily. In some instances, the effective dose may be as low as one 0.02 mg. tablet every other day. A useful dosage schedule for early menopause, while spontaneous menstruation continues, is 0.05 mg. once a day for twenty-one days and then a rest period for seven days. This can be continued cyclically indefinitely adding a progestational agent during the latter part of the cycle. For the initial treatment of the late menopause, the same regimen is indicated with the 0.02 mg. ESTINYL Tablet for the first few cycles, after which the 0.05 mg. dosage may be substituted. In more severe cases, such as those due to surgical and roentgenologic castration, one 0.05 mg. tablet may be administered three times daily at the start of treatment. With adequate clinical improvement, usually obtainable in a few weeks, the dosage may be reduced to one 0.05 mg. tablet daily and the patient continued thereafter on a maintenance dosage as in the average case. At the discretion of the physician, a progestational agent may be added during the latter part of a planned cycle.

2. *Given cyclically.*

Female hypogonadism: One 0.05 mg. tablet is given one to three times daily during the first two weeks of a theoretical menstrual cycle. This is followed by progesterone during the last half of the arbitrary cycle. This regimen is continued for three to six months. The patient is then allowed to go untreated for two months to determine whether or not she can maintain the cycle without hormonal therapy. If not, additional courses of therapy may be prescribed.

3. *Given chronically.*

Inoperable progressing prostatic cancer: From three 0.05 mg. to four 0.5 mg. tablets may be administered daily for palliation.

Inoperable progressing breast cancer in appropriately selected postmenopausal women (See Indications): Two 0.5 mg. tablets three times daily for palliation.

Treated patients with an intact uterus should be monitored closely for signs of endometrial cancer and appropriate diagnostic measures should be taken to rule out malignancy in the event of persistent or recurring abnormal vaginal bleeding.

How Supplied: ESTINYL Tablets 0.02 mg., beige, sugar-coated tablets branded in black with the Schering trademark and either product indentification numbers, 298, or letters, ER; bottles of 100 and 250.

ESTINYL Tablets 0.05 mg., pink, sugar-coated tablets branded in black with the Schering trademark and either product identification numbers, 070, or letters, EM; bottles of 100 and 250.

ESTINYL Tablets 0.5 mg., peach-colored, compressed, scored tablets impressed with the Schering trademark and either product identification numbers, 150, or letters, EP; bottle of 100.

Store between 2° and 30° C (36° and 86° F).

Patient package inserts are being dispensed with this product. They are available to physicians upon request. Physician references available on request.

Copyright © 1968, 1980, Schering Corporation. All rights reserved.

[*Shown in Product Identification Section*]

ETRAFON® ℞

brand of perphenazine, USP—amitriptyline hydrochloride, USP

ETRAFON 2-10 TABLETS (2-10)
ETRAFON TABLETS (2-25)
ETRAFON-A TABLETS (4-10)
ETRAFON-FORTE TABLETS (4-25)

Description: ETRAFON Tablets contain perphenazine, USP and amitriptyline hydrochloride, USP. Perphenazine is a piperazinyl phenothiazine having the chemical formula, $C_{21}H_{26}ClN_3OS$. Amitriptyline hydrochloride is a dibenzocycloheptadiene derivative having the chemical formula, $C_{20}H_{23}N.HCl$.

ETRAFON Tablets are available in multiple strengths to afford dosage flexibility for optimum management. They are available as ETRAFON 2-10 Tablets, 2 mg perphenazine and 10 mg amitriptyline hydrochloride; ETRAFON Tablets, 2 mg perphenazine and 25 mg amitriptyline hydrochloride. ETRAFON-A Tablets, 4 mg perphenazine and 10 mg amitriptyline hydrochloride; and ETRAFON-FORTE Tablets, 4 mg perphenazine and 25 mg amitriptyline hydrochloride.

Actions: ETRAFON combines the tranquilizing action of perphenazine with the antidepressant properties of amitriptyline hydrochloride. Perphenazine acts on the central nervous system and has a greater behavioral potency than other phenothiazine derivatives whose side chains do not contain a piperazine moiety. Amitriptyline hydrochloride is a tricyclic antidepressant. It is not a monoamine oxidase inhibitor, but its mechanism of action in man is not known.

Indications: ETRAFON Tablets are indicated for the treatment of patients with moderate to severe anxiety and/or agitation and depressed mood; patients with depression in whom anxiety and/or agitation are moderate or severe; patients with anxiety and depression associated with chronic physical disease; patients in whom depression and anxiety cannot be clearly differentiated.

Schizophrenic patients who have associated symptoms of depression should be considered for therapy with ETRAFON.

Many patients presenting symptoms such as agitation, anxiety, insomnia, psychomotor retardation, functional somatic complaints, a feeling of tiredness, loss of interest, and anorexia have responded to therapy with ETRAFON Tablets.

Contraindications: ETRAFON Tablets are contraindicated in comatose or greatly obtunded patients and in patients receiving large doses of central nervous system depressants (barbiturates, alcohol, narcotics, analqesics, or antihistamines); in the presence of existing blood dyscrasias, bone marrow depression, or liver damage; and in patients who have shown hypersensitivity to ETRAFON Tablets, its components, or related compounds.

ETRAFON Tablets are also contraindicated in patients with suspected or established subcortical brain damage, with or without hypothalamic damage, since a hyperthermic reaction with temperatures in excess of 104°F may occur in such patients, sometimes not until 14 to 16 hours after drug administration. Total body ice-packing is recommended for such a reaction; antipyretics may also be useful.

ETRAFON should not be given concomitantly with a monoamine oxidase inhibiting compound. Hyperpyretic crises, severe convulsions and deaths have occurred in patients receiving tricyclic antidepressant and monoamine oxidase inhibiting drugs simultaneously. In patients who have been receiving a monoamine oxidase inhibitor, it is recommended that two weeks or longer elapse before the start of treatment with ETRAFON Tablets to permit recovery from the effects of the MAO inhibitor and to avoid possible potentiation. Treatment with ETRAFON Tablets should be initiated cautiously in such patients, with gradual increase in dosage until a satisfactory response is obtained.

Amitriptyline hydrochloride is not recommended for use during the acute recovery phase following myocardial infarction.

Warnings: Patients with cardiovascular disorders should be watched closely. Tricyclic antidepressant drugs, including amitriptyline hydrochloride, particularly when given in high doses, have been reported to produce arrhythmias, sinus tachycardia, and prolongation of the conduction time. Myocardial infarction and stroke have been reported with drugs of this class.

ETRAFON should not be given concomitantly with guanethidine or similarly acting compounds, since amitriptyline, like other tricyclic antidepressants, may block the antihypertensive effect of these compounds.

If hypotension develops, epinephrine should not be administered, since its action is blocked and partially reversed by perphenozine. If a vasopressor is needed, norepinephrine may be used. Severe, acute hypotension has occurred with the use of phenothiazines and is particularly likely to occur in patients with mitral insufficiency or pheochromocytoma. Rebound hypertension may occur in pheochromocytoma patients.

Perphenazine can lower the convulsive threshold in susceptible individuals; it should be used with caution in patients with convulsive disorders. If the patient is being treated with an anticonvulsant agent, increased dosage of that agent may be required when ETRAFON Tablets are used concomitantly.

Because of the anticholinergic activity of amitriptyline hydrochloride, ETRAFON should be used with caution in patients with glaucoma, increased ocular pressure, and those in whom urinary retention is present or anticipated. In patients with angle-closure glaucoma even average doses may precipitate an attack.

Close supervision is required when amitriptyline hydrochloride is given to hyperthyroid patients or those receiving thyroid medication.

ETRAFON Tablets may impair the mental and/or physical abilities required for the performance of potentially hazardous tasks, such as driving a car or operating machinery, the patient should be warned accordingly.

Usage in Children: Since a dosage for children has not been established, ETRAFON is not recommended for use in children.

Usage in Pregnancy: Safe use of ETRAFON Tablets during pregnancy and lactation has not been established; therefore, in administering the drug to pregnant patients, nursing mothers, or women who may become pregnant, the possible benefits must be weighed against the possible hazards to mother and child.

Precautions: The possibility of suicide in depressed patients remains during treatment and until significant remission occurs. This type of patient should not have easy access to large quantities of this drug.

Perphenazine

As with all phenothiazine compounds, perphenazine should not be used indiscriminately. Caution should be observed in giving it to patients who have previously exhibited severe adverse reactions to other phenothiazines. Some of the untoward actions of perphenazine tend to appear more frequently when high doses are used. However, as with other phenothiazine compounds, patients receiving perphenazine in any dosage should be kept under close supervision.

Neuroleptic drugs elevate prolactin levels; the elevation persists during chronic administration. Tissue culture experiments indicate that approximately one-third of human breast cancers are prolactin dependent *in vitro*, a factor of potential importance if the prescription of these drugs is contemplated in a patient with a previously detected breast cancer. Although disturbances such as galactorrhea, amenorrhea, gynecomastia, and impotence have been reported, the clinical significance of elevated serum prolactin levels is unknown for most patients. An increase in mammary neoplasms has been found in rodents after chronic administration of neuroleptic drugs. Neither clinical studies nor epidemiologic studies conducted to date, however, have shown an association between chronic administration of these drugs and mammary tumorigenesis; the available evidence is considered too limited to be conclusive at this time.

The antiemetic effect of perphenazine may obscure signs of toxicity due to overdosage of other drugs, or render more difficult the diagnosis of disorders such as brain tumors or intestinal obstruction.

Adynamic ileus occasionally occurs with phenothiazine therapy and if severe, can result in

Continued on next page

Information on Schering products appearing on these pages is effective as of September 30, 1982.

Schering—Cont.

complications and death. It is of particular concern in psychiatric patients who may fail to seek treatment of the condition.
A significant, not otherwise explained, rise in body temperature may suggest individual intolerance to perphenazine, in which case ETRAFON should be discontinued.
Patients on large doses of a phenothiazine drug who are undergoing surgery should be watched carefully for possible hypotensive phenomena. Moreover, reduced amounts of anesthetics or central nervous system depressants may be necessary.
Since phenothiazines and central nervous system depressants (opiates, analgesics, antihistamines, barbiturates) can potentiate each other, less than the usual dosage of the added drug is recommended, and caution is advised, when they are administered concomitantly.
Use with caution in patients who are receiving atropine or related drugs because of additive anticholinergic effects and also in patients who will be exposed to extreme heat or organic phosphate insecticides.
The use of alcohol should be avoided, since additive effects and hypotension may occur. Patients should be cautioned that their response to alcohol may be increased while they are being treated with ETRAFON Tablets. The risk of suicide and the danger of overdose may be increased in patients who use alcohol excessively due to it potentiation of the drug's effect.
Blood counts and hepatic and renal functions should be checked periodically. The appearance of signs of blood dyscrasias requires the discontinuance of the drug and institution of appropriate therapy. If abnormalities in hepatic tests occur, phenothiazine treatment should be discontinued. Renal function in patients on long-term therapy should be monitored; if blood urea nitrogen (BUN) becomes abnormal, treatment with the drug should be discontinued.
The use of phenothiazine derivatives in patients with diminished renal function should be undertaken with caution.
Use with caution in patients suffering from respiratory impairment due to acute pulmonary infections, or in chronic respiratory disorders such as severe asthma or emphysema.
In general, phenothiazines do not produce psychic dependence. Gastritis, nausea and vomiting, dizziness, and tremulousness have been reported following abrupt cessation of high-dose therapy. Reports suggest that these symptoms can be reduced by continuing concomitant antiparkinson agents for several weeks after the phenothiazine is withdrawn.
The possibility of liver damage, corneal and lenticular deposits, and irreversible dyskinesias should be kept in mind when patients are on long-term therapy.
Because photosensitivity has been reported, undue exposure to the sun should be avoided during phenothiazine treatment.

Amitriptyline Hydrochloride

In manic-depressive psychosis, depressed patients may experience a shift toward the manic phase if they are treated with an antidepressant drug. Patients with paranoid symptomatology may have an exaggeration of such symptoms. The tranquilizing effect of ETRAFON has seemed to reduce the likelihood of this effect.
When amitriptyline hydrochloride is given with anticholinergic agents or sympathomimetic drugs, including epinephrine combined with local anesthetics, close supervision and careful adjustment of dosages are required.
Paralytic ileus may occur in patients taking tricyclic antidepressants in combination with anticholinergic-type drugs.
Concurrent use of large doses of ethchlorvynol should be used with caution, since transient delirium has been reported in patients receiving this drug in combination with amitriptyline hydrochloride.
This drug may enhance the response to alcohol and the effects of barbiturates and other CNS depressants.
Concurrent administration of amitriptyline hydrochloride and electroshock therapy may increase the hazards of therapy. Such treatment should be limited to patients for whom it is essential.
Discontinue the drug several days before elective surgery, if possible.
Both elevation and lowering of blood sugar levels have been reported.
The usefulness of amitriptyline in the treatment of depression has been amply demonstrated; however, it should be realized that abuse of amitriptyline among a narcotic-dependent population is not uncommon.

Adverse Reactions: Adverse reactions to ETRAFON Tablets are the same as those to its components, perphenazine and amitriptyline hydrochloride. There have been no reports of effects peculiar to the combination of these components in ETRAFON Tablets.

Perphenazine

Not all of the following adverse reactions have been reported with perphenazine; however, pharmacological similarities among various phenothiazine derivatives require that each be considered. With the piperazine group (of which perphenazine is an example), the extrapyramidal symptoms are more common, and others (e.g., sedative effects, jaundice, and blood dyscrasias) are less frequently seen.

CNS Effects: *Extrapyramidal reactions:* opisthotonus, trismus, torticollis, retrocollis, aching and numbness of the limbs, motor restlessness, oculogyric crisis, hyperreflexia, dystonia, including protrusion, discoloration, aching and rounding of the tongue, tonic spasm of the masticatory muscles, tight feeling in the throat, slurred speech, dysphagia, akathisia, dyskinesia, parkinsonism, and ataxia. Their incidence and severity usually increase with an increase in dosage, but there is considerable individual variation in the tendency to develop such symptoms. Extrapyramidal symptoms can usually be controlled by the concomitant use of effective antiparkinsonian drugs, such as benztropine mesylate, and/or by reduction in dosage.
Persistent tardive dyskinesia: As with all antipsychotic agents, tardive dyskinesia may appear in some patients on long-term therapy or may appear after drug therapy has been discontinued. Alhough the risk appears to be greater in elderly patients on high-dose therapy, especially females it may occur in either sex and in children. The symptoms are persistent and in some patients appear to be irreversible. The syndrome is characterized by rhythmical, involuntary movements of the tongue, face, mouth or jaw (eg, protrusion of tongue, puffing of cheeks, puckering of mouth, chewing movements). Sometimes these may be accompanied by involuntary movements of the extremities. There is no known effective treatment for tardive dyskinesia; antiparkinsonism agents usually do not alleviate the symptoms of this syndrome. It is suggested that all antipsychotic agents be discontinued if these symptoms appear. Should it be necessary to reinstitute treatment, or increase the dosage of the agent, or switch to a different antipsychotic agent, the syndrome may be masked. It has been reported that fine, vermicular movements of the tongue may be an early sign of the syndrome, and if the medication is stopped at that time the syndrome may not develop.
Other CNS effects include cerebral edema; abnormality of cerebrospinal fluid proteins; convulsive seizures, particularly in patients with EEG abnormalities or a history of such disorders; and headaches.
Drowsiness may occur, particularly during the first or second week, after which it generally disappears. If troublesome, lower the dosage. Hypnotic effects appear to be minimal, especially in patients who are permitted to remain active.
Adverse behavioral effects include paradoxical exacerbation of psychotic symptoms, catatonic-like states, paranoid reactions, lethargy, paradoxical excitement, restlessness, hyperactivity, nocturnal confusion, bizarre dreams, and insomnia. Hyperreflexia has been reported in the newborn when a phenothiazine was used during pregnancy.

Autonomic Effects: dry mouth or salivation, nausea, vomiting, diarrhea, anorexia, constipation, obstipation, fecal impaction, urinary retention, frequency or incontinence, polyuria, bladder paralysis, nasal congestion, pallor, adynamic ileus, myosis, mydiasis, blurred vision, glaucoma, perspiration, hypertension, hypotension, and a change in pulse rate occasionally may occur. Significant autonomic effects have been infrequent in patients receiving less than 24 mg perphenazine daily.

Allergic Effects: urticaria, erythema, eczema, exfoliative dermatitis, pruritus, photosensitivity, asthma, fever, anaphylactoid reactions, laryngeal edema, and angioneurotic edema; contact dermatitis in nursing personnel administering the drug; and in extremely rare instances, individual idiosyncrasy or hypersensitivity to phenothiazines has resulted in cerebral edema, circulatory collapse, and death.

Endocrine Effects: lactation, galactorrhea, moderate breast enlargement in females and gynecomastia in males on large doses, disturbances in the menstrual cycle, amenorrhea, changes in libido, inhibition of ejaculation, false positive pregnancy tests, hyperglycemia, hypoglycemia, glycosuria, syndrome of inappropriate ADH (antidiuretic hormone) secretion.

Cardiovascular Effects: Postural hypotension, tachycardia (especially with sudden marked increase in dosage), bradycardia, cardiac arrest, faintness, and dizziness. Occasionally the hypotensive effect may produce a shock-like condition. ECG changes, nonspecific, (quinidine-like effect) usually reversible, have been observed in some patients receiving phenothiazine tranquilizers.
Sudden death has occasionally been reported in patients who have received phenothiazines. In some cases the death was apparently due to cardiac arrest; in others the cause appeared to be asphyxia due to cardiac arrest; in others the cause appeared to be asphyxia due to failure of the cough reflex. In some patients, the cause could not be determined nor could it be established that the death was due to the phenothiazine.

Hematological Effects: agranulocytosis, eosinophilia, leukopenia, hemolytic anemia, thrombocytopenic purpura, and pancytopenia. Most cases of agranulocytosis have occurred between the fourth and tenth weeks of therapy. Patients should be watched closely especially during that period for the sudden appearance of sore throat or signs of infection. If white blood cell and differential cell counts show significant cellular depression, discontinue the drug and start appropriate therapy. However, a slightly lowered white count is not in itself an indication to discontinue the drug.

Other Effects: Special considerations in long-term therapy include pigmentation of the skin, occurring chiefly in the exposed areas; ocular changes consisting of deposition of fine particulate matter in the cornea and lens, progressing in more severe cases to starshaped lenticular opacities; epithelial keratopathies; and pigmentary retinopathy. Also noted: peripheral edema, reversed epinephrine effect, increase in PBI not attributable to an increase in thyroxine, parotid swelling (rare), hyperpyrexia, systemic lupus erythematosus-like syndrome, increases in appetite and weight, polyphagia, photophobia, and muscle weakness.

Liver damage (biliary stasis) may occur. Jaundice may occur, usually between the second and fourth weeks of treatment, and is regarded as a hypersensitivity reaction. Incidence is low. The clinical picture resembles infectious hepatitis but with laboratory features of obstructive jaundice. It is usually reversible; however, chronic jaundice has been reported.

Amitriptyline Hydrochloride

Although activation of latent schizophrenia has been reported with antidepressant drugs, including amitriptyline hydrochloride, it may be prevented with ETRAFON Tablets in some cases because of the antipsychotic effect of perphenazine. A few instances of epileptiform seizures have been reported in chronic schizophrenic patients during treatment with amitriptyline hydrochloride.

Note: Included in the listing which follows are a few adverse reactions which have not been reported with this specific drug. However, pharmacological similarities among the tricyclic antidepressant drugs require that each of the reactions be considered when amitriptyline hydrochloride is administered.

Allergic: Rash, pruritus, urticaria, photosensitization, edema of face and tongue.

Anticholinergic: Dry mouth, blurred vision, disturbance of accommodation, constipation, paralytic ileus, urinary retention, dilatation of urinary tract.

Cardiovascular: Hypotension, hypertension, tachycardia, palpitations, myocardial infarction, arrhythmias, heart block, stroke.

CNS and Neuromuscular: Confusional states, disturbed concentration, disorientation, delusions, hallucinations, excitement, jitteriness, anxiety, restlessness, insomnia, nightmares, numbness, tingling, and paresthesias of the extremities, peripheral neuropathy, incoordination, ataxia, tremors, seizures, alteration in EEG patterns, extrapyramidal symptoms, tinnitus.

Endocrine: Testicular swelling and gynecomastia in the male, breast enlargement and galactorrhea in the female, increased or decreased libido, elevation and lowering of blood sugar levels, syndrome of inappropriate ADH (antidiuretic hormone secretion).

Gastrointestinal: Nausea, epigastric distress, heartburn, vomiting, anorexia, stomatitis, peculiar taste, diarrhea, jaundice, parotid swelling, black tongue. Rarely hepatitis has occurred (including altered liver function and jaundice).

Hematologic: Bone marrow depression including agranulocytosis, leukopenia, eosinophilia, purpura, thrombocytopenia.

Other: Dizziness, weakness, fatigue, headache, weight gain or loss, increased perspiration, urinary frequency, mydriasis, drowsiness, alopecia.

Withdrawal Symptoms: Abrupt cessation of treatment after prolonged administration may produce nausea, headache, and malaise. These are not indicative of addiction.

Dosage and Administration:

Initial Dosage

In psychoneurotic patients whose anxiety and depression warrant combined therapy, one ETRAFON Tablet (2–25) or one ETRAFON-FORTE Tablet (4–25) three or four times a day is recommended.

In elderly patients, adolescents and other patients as indicated, one ETRAFON-A Tablet (4–10) may be administered three or four times a day as initial dosage. This dosage may be adjusted as required to produce an adequate response.

In more severely ill patients with schizophrenia, two ETRAFON-FORTE Tablets (4–25) three times a day are recommended as the initial dosage. If necessary, a fourth dose may be given at bedtime. The total daily dosage should not exceed eight tablets of any strength.

Maintenance Dosage

Depending on the condition being treated, the onset of therapeutic response may vary from a few days to a few weeks or even longer. After a satisfactory response is noted, dosage should be reduced to the smallest dose which is effective for relief of the symptoms for which ETRAFON Tablets are being administered. A useful maintenance dosage is one ETRAFON Tablet (2–25) or one ETRAFON-FORTE Tablet (4–25) two to four times a day. In some patients, maintenance dosage is required for many months. ETRAFON 2–10 Tablets (2–10) and ETRAFON-A Tablets (4–10) can be used to increase flexibility in adjusting maintenance dosage to the lowest amount consistent with relief of symptoms.

Overdosage: In the event of overdosage, emergency treatment should be started immediately. All patients suspected of having taken an overdose should be hospitalized as soon as possible.

Manifestations: Overdosage of perphenazine primarily involves the extrapyramidal mechanism and produces the same side effects described under ADVERSE REACTIONS, but to a more marked degree. It is usually evidenced by stupor or coma; children may have convulsive seizures.

High doses may cause temporary confusion, disturbed concentration, or transient visual hallucinations. Overdosage may cause drowsiness; hypothermia; tachycardia and other arrhythmic abnormalities—for example, bundle branch block; ECG evidence of impaired conduction; congestive heart failure; dilated pupils; convulsions; severe hypotension; stupor; and coma. Other symptoms may be agitation, hyperactive reflexes, muscle rigidity, vomiting, hyperpyrexia, or any of the adverse reactions listed for perphenazine or amitriptyline hydrochloride.

Overdosage with tricyclic antidepressants (TCAs), such as imipramine, doxepin, or amitriptyline may result in plasma TCA levels of 1,000 ng/ml or higher. Such levels more accurately define patients who are at risk for major medical complications of overdosage than does the amount of drug ingested based on patient history. In one study, all patients with TCA levels of this magnitude had a QRS duration of 100 msec or more on a routine ECG within the first 24 hours following overdose.

In the absence of TCA blood level determinations, a QRS of 100 msec or more suggests a greater likelihood of serious complications.

Oculomotor paresis (loss of conjugate movement in the so-called doll's eyes maneuver) as a manifestation of amitriptyline overdosage has been reported as being significant in the differential diagnosis of a patient in light coma.

Treatment: Treatment is symptomatic and supportive. There is no specific antidote. Th patient should be induced to vomit even if emesis has occurred spontaneously. Pharmacologic vomiting by the administration of ipecac syrup is a preferred method. It should be noted that ipecac has a central mode of action in addition to its local gastric irritant properties, and the central mode of action may be blocked by the antiemetic effect of ETRAFON Tablets. Vomiting should not be induced in patients with impaired consciousness. The action of ipecac is facilitated by physical activity and by the administration of 8 to 12 fluid ounces of water. If emesis does not occur within 15 minutes, the dose of ipecac should be repeated. Precautions against aspiration must be taken, especially in infants and children. Following emesis, any drug remaining in the stomach may be adsorbed by activated charcoal administered as a slurry with water. If vomiting is unsuccessful or contraindicated, gastric lavage should be performed. Isotonic and one-half isotonic saline are the lavage solutions of choice. Saline cathartics, such as milk of magnesia, draw water into the bowel by osmosis and therefore may be valuable for their action in rapid dilution of bowel content.

Standard measures (oxygen, intravenous fluids, corticosteroids) should be used to manage circulatory shock or metabolic acidosis. An open airway and adequate fluid intake should be maintained. Body temperature should be regulated. Hypothermia is expected, but severe hyperthermia may occur and must be treated vigorously. (See CONTRAINDICATIONS.)

An electrocardiogram should be taken and close monitoring of cardiac function instituted if there is any sign of abnormality. Cardiac arrhythmias may be treated with neostigmine, pyridostigmine, or propranolol. Digitalis should be considered for cardiac failure. Close monitoring of cardiac function is advisable for not less than five days.

Vasopressors such as norepinephrine may be used to treat hypotension, but epinephrine should NOT be used.

The intravenous administration of 1 to 3 mg physostigmine salicylate has been reported to reverse the symptoms of tricyclic antidepressant poisoning and therefore, should be considered in the symptomatic treatment of the central anticholinergic effects due to overdosage with ETRAFON Tablets. Because physostigmine is rapidly metabolized, it should be readministered as required, especially if life-threatening signs, such as arrhythmias, convulsions, or deep coma recur or persist.

Anticonvulsants (an inhalation anesthetic, diazepam, or paraldehyde) are recommended for control of convulsions, since perphenazine increases the central nervous system depressant action, but not the anticonvulsant action of barbiturates.

If acute parkinson-like symptoms result from perphenazine intoxication, benztropine mesylate or diphenhydramine may be administered.

Central nervous system depression may be treated with nonconvulsant doses of CNS stimulants. Avoid stimulants that may cause convulsions (e.g., picrotoxin and pentylenetetrazol).

Signs of arousal may not occur for 48 hours. Dialysis is of no value because of low plasma concentrations of the drug.

Since overdosage is often deliberate, patients may attempt suicide by other means during the recovery phase. Deaths by deliberate or accidental overdosage have occurred with this class of drugs.

How Supplied: ETRAFON 2–10 Tablets (perphenazine 2 mg. and amitriptyline hydrochloride 10 mg.): deep yellow, sugar-coated tablets branded in blue-black with the Schering trademark and either product identification letters, ANA or numbers, 287; bottles of 100 and 500 and box of 100 for unit-dose dispensing (10 strips of 10 tablets each).

ETRAFON Tablets (perphenazine 2 mg. and amitriptyline hydrochloride 25 mg.): pink, sugar-coated tablets branded in red with the Schering trademark and either product identification letters, ANC or numbers, 598; bottles of 100 and 500 and box of 100 for unit-dose dispensing (10 strips of 10 tablets each).

ETRAFON-A Tablets (perphenazine 4 mg. and amitriptyline hydrochloride 10 mg.): orange, sugar-coated tablets branded in blue-black with the Schering trademark and either product identification letters, ANB or numbers, 119; bottles of 100 and 500 and box of 100 for unit-dose dispensing (10 strips of 10 tablets each).

ETRAFON-FORTE Tablets (perphenazine 4 mg. and amitriptyline hydrochloride 25 mg.): red, sugar-coated tablets branded in blue with the Schering trademark and either product identification letters, ANE or numbers, 720;

Continued on next page

Information on Schering products appearing on these pages is effective as of September 30, 1982.

Schering—Cont.

bottles of 100 and 500 and box of 100 for unit-dose dispensing (10 strips of 10 tablets each).
Store all ETRAFON Tablets between 2° and 30°C (36° and 86°F). In addition, protect unit-dose packages from excessive moisture.
Copyright © 1969, 1980 Schering Corporation. All rights Reserved.
[*Shown in Product Identification Section*]

FULVICIN® P/G ℞
brand of griseofulvin ultramicrosize Tablets, USP

Description: FULVICIN P/G Tablets contain ultramicrosize crystals of griseofulvin, an antibiotic derived from a species of *Penicillium.* Griseofulvin crystals are partly dissolved in polyethylene glycol 6000 and partly dispersed throughout the tablet matrix.
Each FULVICIN P/G Tablet contains 125 mg or 250 mg griseofulvin ultramicrosize.
Actions: Microbiology Griseofulvin is fungistatic with *in vitro* activity against various species of *Microsporum, Epidermophyton,* and *Trichophyton.* It has no effect on bacteria or on other genera of fungi.
Human Pharmacology Following oral administration, griseofulvin is deposited in the keratin precursor cells and has a greater affinity for diseased tissue. The drug is tightly bound to the new keratin which becomes highly resistant to fungal invasions.
Controlled bioavailability studies of FULVICIN P/G have demonstrated comparable values to blood levels regarded as adequate.
The efficiency of gastrointestinal absorption of ultramicrocrystalline griseofulvin is approximately twice that of the conventional microsized griseofulvin. This factor permits the oral intake of half as much griseofulvin per tablet but there is no evidence, at this time, that this confers any significant clinical differences in regard to safety and efficacy.
Indications: FULVICIN P/G Tablets are indicated for the treatment of ringworm infections of the skin, hair, and nails, namely: tinea corporis, tinea pedis, tinea cruris, tinea barbae, tinea capitis, tinea unguium (onychomycosis) when caused by one or more of the following genera of fungi: *Trichophyton rubrum, Trichophyton tonsurans, Trichophyton mentagrophytes, Trichophyton interdigitale, Trichophyton verrucosum, Trichophyton megninii, Trichophyton gallinae, Trichophyton crateriforme, Trichophyton sulphureum, Trichophyton schoenleinii, Microsporum audouinii, Microsporum canis, Microsporum gypseum,* and *Epidermophyton floccosum.*
Note: Prior to therapy, the type of fungi responsible for the infection should be identified. The use of this drug is not justified in minor or trivial infections which will respond to topical agents alone.
Griseofulvin is not effective in the following: bacterial infections, candidiasis (moniliasis), histoplasmosis, actinomycosis, sporotrichosis, chromoblastomycosis, coccidioidomycosis, North American blastomycosis, cryptococcosis (torulosis), tinea versicolor, and nocardiosis.
Contraindications: This drug is contraindicated in patients with porphyria, hepatocellular failure, and in individuals with a history of hypersensitivity to griseofulvin.
Warnings: *Prophylactic Usage:* Safety and efficacy of griseofulvin for prophylaxis of fungal infections have not been established.
Animal Toxicology: Chronic feeding of griseofulvin, at levels ranging from 0.5–2.5% of the diet, resulted in the development of liver tumors in several strains of mice, particularly in males. Smaller particle sizes result in an enhanced effect. Lower oral dosage levels have not been tested. Subcutaneous administration of relatively small doses of griseofulvin once a week during the first three weeks of life has also been reported to induce hepatomata in mice. Although studies in other animal species have not yielded evidence of tumorigenicity, these studies were not of adequate design to form a basis for conclusions in this regard.
In subacute toxicity studies, orally administered griseofulvin produced hepatocellular necrosis in mice, but this has not been seen in other species. Disturbances in porphyrin metabolism have been reported in griseofulvin-treated laboratory animals. Griseofulvin has been reported to have a colchicine-like effect on mitosis and cocarcinogenicity with methylcholanthrene in cutaneous tumor induction in laboratory animals.
Usage in Pregnancy: The safety of this drug during pregnancy has not been established.
Animal Reproduction Studies: It has been reported in the literature that griseofulvin was found to be embryotoxic and teratogenic on oral administration to pregnant rats. Pups with abnormalities have been reported in the litters of a few bitches treated with griseofulvin. Additional animal reproduction studies are in progress.
Suppression of spermatogenesis has been reported to occur in rats, but investigation in man failed to confirm this.
Precautions: Patients on prolonged therapy with any potent medication should be under close observation. Periodic monitoring of organ system function, including renal, hepatic, and hematopoietic, should be done.
Since griseofulvin is derived from species of *Penicillium,* the possibility of cross sensitivity with penicillin exists; however, known penicillin-sensitive patients have been treated without difficulty.
Since a photosensitivity reaction is occasionally associated with griseofulvin therapy, patients should be warned to avoid exposure to intense natural or artificial sunlight. Should a photosensitivity reaction occur, lupus erythematosus may be aggravated.
Griseofulvin decreases the activity of warfarin-type anticoagulants so that patients receiving these drugs concomitantly may require dosage adjustment of the anticoagulant during and after griseofulvin therapy.
Barbiturates usually depress griseofulvin activity, and concomitant administration may require a dosage adjustment of the antifungal agent.
Adverse Reactions: When adverse reactions occur, they are most commonly of the hypersensitivity type, such as skin rashes, urticaria, and rarely, angioneurotic edema, and may necessitate withdrawal of therapy and appropriate countermeasures. Paresthesias of the hands and feet have been reported rarely after extended therapy. Other side effects reported occasionally are oral thrush, nausea, vomiting, epigastric distress, diarrhea, headache, fatigue, dizziness, insomnia, mental confusion, and impairment of performance of routine activities.
Proteinuria and leukopenia have been reported rarely. Administration of the drug should be discontinued if granulocytopenia occurs.
When rare, serious reactions occur with griseofulvin, they are usually associated with high dosages, long periods of therapy, or both.
Dosage and Administration: Accurate diagnosis of the infecting organism is essential. Identification should be made either by direct microscopic examination of a mounting of infected tissue in a solution of potassium hydroxide or by culture on an appropriate medium.
Medication must be continued until the infecting organism is completely eradicated as indicated by appropriate clinical or laboratory examination. Representative treatment periods are tinea capitis, 4 to 6 weeks; tinea corporis, 2 to 4 weeks; tinea pedis, 4 to 8 weeks; tinea unguium—depending on rate of growth—fingernails, at least 4 months; toenails, at least 6 months.
General measures in regard to hygiene should be observed to control sources of infection or reinfection. Concomitant use of appropriate topical agents is usually required particularly in treatment of tinea pedis. In some forms of athlete's foot, yeasts and bacteria may be involved as well as fungi. Griseofulvin will not eradicate the bacterial or monilial infection.
Adults: Daily administration of 250 mg (as a single dose or in divided amounts) will give a satisfactory response in most patients with tinea corporis, tinea cruris, and tinea capitis. For those fungus infections more difficult to eradicate, such as tinea pedis and tinea unguium, a divided daily dose of 500 mg is recommended.
Children: Approximately 2.5 mg per pound of body weight per day is an effective dose for most children. On this basis, the following dosage schedule is suggested: Children weighing 30 to 50 pounds—62.5 mg to 125 mg daily. Children weighing over 50 pounds—125 mg to 250 mg daily.
Children 2 years of age and younger—dosage has not been established.
Clinical experience with griseofulvin in children with tinea capitis indicates that a single daily dose is effective. Clinical relapse will occur if the medication is not continued until the infecting organism is eradicated.
How Supplied: FULVICIN P/G Tablets, 125 mg, white, compressed, scored tablets impressed with the Schering trademark and product identification numbers, 228; bottle of 100.
FULVICIN P/G Tablets, 250 mg, white, compressed, scored tablets impressed with the Schering trademark and product identification numbers, 507; bottle of 100.
Store at controlled room temperature 15°C to 30°C (59°F to 86°F).
Copyright © 1976, 1978, Schering Corporation. All rights reserved.
[*Shown in Product Identification Section*]

FULVICIN® P/G 165 and 330 ℞
brand of griseofulvin ultramicrosize, USP Tablets

Description: FULVICIN P/G Tablets contain ultramicrosize crystals of griseofulvin, an antibiotic derived from a species of *Penicillium.* Griseofulvin crystals are partly dissolved in polyethylene glycol 8000 and partly dispersed throughout the tablet matrix.
Each FULVICIN P/G Tablet contains 165 mg or 330 mg griseofulvin ultramicrosize.
Actions: Microbiology: Griseofulvin is fungistatic with *in vitro* activity against various species of *Microsporum, Epidermophyton,* and *Trichophyton.* It has no effect on bacteria or on other genera of fungi.
Human Pharmacology: Following oral administration, griseofulvin is deposited in the keratin precursor cells and has a greater affinity for diseased tissue. The drug is tightly bound to the new keratin which becomes highly resistant to fungal invasions.
The efficiency of gastrointestinal absorption of ultramicrocrystalline griseofulvin is approximately one and one-half times that of the conventional microsize griseofulvin. This factor permits the oral intake of two-thirds as much ultramicrocrystalline griseofulvin as the microsize form. However, there is currently no evidence that this lower dose confers any significant clinical differences with regard to safety and/or efficacy.
Indications: FULVICIN P/G Tablets are indicated for the treatment of ringworm infections of the skin, hair, and nails, namely: tinea corporis, tinea pedis, tinea cruris, tinea barbae, tinea capitis, tinea unguium (onychomycosis) when caused by one or more of the following genera of fungi: *Trichophyton rubrum, Trichophyton tonsurans, Trichophyton mentagrophytes, Trichophyton interdigitale, Trichophyton verrucosum, Trichophyton megninii, Tri-*

chophyton gallinae, Trichophyton crateriforme, Trichophyton sulphureum, Trichophyton schoenleinii, Microsporum audouinii, Microsporum canis, Microsporum gypseum, and *Epidermophyton floccosum.*

Note: Prior to therapy, the type of fungi responsible for the infection should be identified. The use of this drug is not justified in minor or trivial infections which will respond to topical agents alone.

Griseofulvin is not effective in the following: bacterial infections, candidiasis (moniliasis), histoplasmosis, actinomycosis, sporotrichosis, chromoblastomycosis, coccidioidomycosis, North American blastomycosis, cryptococcosis (torulosis), tinea versicolor, and nocardiosis.

Contraindications: This drug is contraindicated in patients with porphyria, hepatocellular failure, and in individuals with a history of hypersensitivity to griseofulvin.

Warnings: *Prophylactic Usage:* Safety and efficacy of griseofulvin for prophylaxis of fungal infections have not been established.

Animal Toxicology: Chronic feeding of griseofulvin, at levels ranging from 0.5–2.5% of the diet, resulted in the development of liver tumors in several strains of mice, particularly in males. Smaller particle sizes result in an enhanced effect. Lower oral dosage levels have not been tested. Subcutaneous administration of relatively small doses of griseofulvin once a week during the first three weeks of life has also been reported to induce hepatomata in mice. Thyroid tumors, mostly adenomas but some carcinomas, have been reported in male rats receiving griseofulvin at levels of 2.0%, 1.0%, and 0.2% of the diet, and in female rats receiving the two higher dose levels. Although studies in other animal species have not yielded evidence of tumorigenicity, these studies were not of adequate design to form a basis for conclusions in this regard.

In subacute toxicity studies, orally administered griseofulvin produced hepatocellular necrosis in mice, but this has not been seen in other species. Disturbances in porphyrin metabolism have been reported in griseofulvin-treated laboratory animals. Griseofulvin has been reported to have a colchicine-like effect on mitosis and cocarcinogenicity with methylcholanthrene in cutaneous tumor induction in laboratory animals.

Usage in Pregnancy: The safety of this drug during pregnancy has not been established.

Animal Reproduction Studies: It has been reported in the literature that griseofulvin was found to be embryotoxic and teratogenic on oral administration to pregnant rats. Pups with abnormalities have been reported in the litters of a few bitches treated with griseofulvin.

Suppression of spermatogenesis has been reported to occur in rats, but investigation in man failed to confirm this.

Precautions: Patients on prolonged therapy with any potent medication should be under close observation. Periodic monitoring of organ system function, including renal, hepatic, and hematopoietic, should be done.

Since griseofulvin is derived from species of *Penicillium*, the possibility of cross-sensitivity with penicillin exists; however, known penicillin-sensitive patients have been treated without difficulty.

Since a photosensitivity reaction is occasionally associated with griseofulvin therapy, patients should be warned to avoid exposure to intense natural or artificial sunlight.

Lupus erythematosus or lupus-like syndromes have been reported in patients receiving griseofulvin.

Griseofulvin decreases the activity of warfarin-type anticoagulants so that patients receiving these drugs concomitantly may require dosage adjustment of the anticoagulant during and after griseofulvin therapy.

Barbiturates usually depress griseofulvin activity, and concomitant administration may require a dosage adjustment of the antifungal agent.

The effects of alcohol may be potentiated by griseofulvin, producing such effects as tachycardia and flush.

Adverse Reactions: When adverse reactions occur, they are most commonly of the hypersensitivity type, such as skin rashes, urticaria, and rarely, angioneurotic edema, and may necessitate withdrawal of therapy and appropriate countermeasures. Paresthesias of the hands and feet have been reported rarely after extended therapy. Other side effects reported occasionally are oral thrush, nausea, vomiting, epigastric distress, diarrhea, headache, fatigue, dizziness, insomnia, mental confusion, and impairment of performance of routine activities.

Proteinuria and leukopenia have been reported rarely. Administration of the drug should be discontinued if granulocytopenia occurs.

When rare, serious reactions occur with griseofulvin, they are usually associated with high dosages, long periods of therapy, or both.

Dosage and Administration: Accurate diagnosis of the infecting organism is essential. Identification should be made either by direct microscopic examination of a mounting of infected tissue in a solution of potassium hydroxide or by culture on an appropriate medium.

Medication must be continued until the infecting organism is completely eradicated as indicated by appropriate clinical or laboratory examination. Representative treatment periods are tinea capitis, 4 to 6 weeks, tinea corporis, 2 to 4 weeks, tinea pedis, 4 to 8 weeks, tinea unguium—depending on rate of growth—fingernails, at least 4 months; toenails, at least 6 months.

General measures in regard to hygiene should be observed to control sources of infection or reinfection. Concomitant use of appropriate topical agents is usually required particularly in treatment of tinea pedis. In some forms of athlete's foot, yeasts and bacteria may be involved as well as fungi. Griseofulvin will not eradicate the bacterial or monilial infection.

Adults: Daily administration of 330 mg (as a single dose or in divided amounts) will give a satisfactory response in most patients with tinea corporis, tinea cruris, and tinea capitis. For those fungus infections more difficult to eradicate, such as tinea pedis and tinea unguium, a divided daily dosage of 660 mg is recommended.

Children: Approximately 3.3 mg per pound of body weight per day is an effective dose for most children. On this basis, the following dosage schedule is suggested: Children weighing 30 to 50 pounds—82.5 mg to 165 mg daily. Children weighing over 50 pounds—165 mg to 330 mg daily.

Children 2 years of age and younger—dosage has not been established.

Clinical experience with griseofulvin in children with tinea capitis indicates that a single daily dose is effective. Clinical relapse will occur if the medication is not continued until the infecting organism is eradicated.

How Supplied: FULVICIN P/G Tablets, 165 mg, off-white, oval, compressed, scored tablets impressed with the product name (FULVICIN P/G) and product identification numbers, 654; bottle of 100.

FULVICIN P/G Tablets, 330 mg, off-white, oval, compressed, scored tablets impressed with the product name (FULVICIN P/G) and product identification numbers, 352; bottle of 100.

Store between 2° and 30°C (36° and 86°F).

Revised 2/82

Copyright © 1982, Schering Corporation. All rights reserved.

[*Shown in Product Identification Section*]

FULVICIN-U/F®

brand of griseofulvin, USP

Tablets ℞

Description: FULVICIN-U/F Tablets contain microsize crystals of griseofulvin, an antibiotic derived from a species of *Penicillium.*

Actions: Microbiology: Griseofulvin is fungistatic with *in vitro* activity against various species of *Microsporum, Epidermophyton,* and *Trichophyton.* It has no effect on bacteria or on other genera of fungi.

Human Pharmacology: Griseofulvin absorption from the gastrointestinal tract varies considerably among individuals mainly because of insolubility of the drug in aqueous media of the upper G.I. tract. The peak serum level found in fasting adults given 0.5 g. occurs at about four hours and ranges between 0.5 to 1.5 mcg./ml. The serum level may be increased by giving the drug with a meal with a high fat content.

Griseofulvin is deposited in the keratin precursor cells and has a greater affinity for diseased tissue. The drug is tightly bound to the new keratin which becomes highly resistant to fungal invasions.

Indications: FULVICIN-U/F Tablets are indicated for the treatment of ringworm infections of the skin, hair, and nails, namely: tinea corporis, tinea pedis, tinea cruris, tinea barbae, tinea capitis, tinea unguium (onychomycosis) when caused by one or more of the following genera of fungi: *Trichophyton rubrum, Trichophyton tonsurans, Trichophyton mentagrophytes, Trichophyton interdigitale, Trichophyton verrucosum, Trichophyton megninii, Trichophyton gallinae, Trichophyton crateriforme, Trichophyton sulphureum, Trichophyton schoenleinii, Microsporum audouinii, Microsporum canis, Microsporum gypseum,* and *Epidermophyton floccosum.*

Note: Prior to therapy, the type of fungi responsible for the infection should be identified. The use of this drug is not justified in minor or trivial infections which will respond to topical agents alone.

Griseofulvin is not effective in the following: bacterial infections, candidiasis (moniliasis), histoplasmosis, actinomycosis, sporotrichosis, chromoblastomycosis, coccidioidomycosis, North American blastomycosis, cryptococcosis (torulosis), tinea versicolor, and nocardiosis.

Contraindications: This drug is contraindicated in patients with porphyria, hepatocellular failure, and in individuals with a history of hypersensitivity to griseofulvin.

Warnings: Prophylactic usage: Safety and efficacy of griseofulvin for prophylaxis of fungal infections have not been established.

Animal toxicology: Chronic feeding of griseofulvin, at levels ranging from 0.5-2.5% of the diet, resulted in the development of liver tumors in several strains of mice, particularly in males. Smaller particle sizes result in an enhanced effect. Lower oral dosage levels have not been tested. Subcutaneous administration of relatively small doses of griseofulvin, once a week, during the first three weeks of life has also been reported to induce hepatomata in mice. Thyroid tumors, mostly adenomas but some carcinomas, have been reported in male rats receiving griseofulvin at levels of 2.0%, 1.0%, and 0.2% of the diet, and in female rats receiving the two higher dose levels. Although studies in other animal species have not yielded evidence of tumorigenicity, these studies were not of adequate design to form a basis for conclusions in this regard.

In subacute toxicity studies, orally administered griseofulvin produced hepatocellular necrosis in mice, but this has not been seen in

Continued on next page

Information on Schering products appearing on these pages is effective as of September 30, 1982.

Schering—Cont.

other species. Disturbances in porphyrin metabolism have been reported in griseofulvin-treated laboratory animals. Griseofulvin has been reported to have a colchicine-like effect on mitosis and cocarcinogenicity with methylcholanthrene in cutaneous tumor induction in laboratory animals.

Usage in pregnancy: The safety of this drug during pregnancy has not been established.

Animal reproduction studies: It has been reported in the literature that griseofulvin was found to be embryotoxic and teratogenic on oral administration to pregnant rats. Pups with abnormalities have been reported in the litters of a few bitches treated with griseofulvin.

Suppression of spermatogenesis has been reported to occur in rats, but investigation in man failed to confirm this.

Precautions: Patients on prolonged therapy with any potent medication should be under close observation. Periodic monitoring of organ system functions, including renal, hepatic, and hematopoietic, should be done.

Since griseofulvin is derived from species of *Penicillium,* the possibility of cross sensitivity with penicillin exists; however, known penicillin-sensitive patients have been treated without difficulty.

Since a photosensitivity reaction is occasionally associated with griseofulvin therapy, patients should be warned to avoid exposure to intense natural or artificial sunlight.

Lupus erythematosus or lupus-like syndromes have been reported in patients receiving griseofulvin.

Griseofulvin decreases the activity of warfarin-type anticoagulants so that patients receiving these drugs concomitantly may require dosage adjustment of the anticoagulant during and after griseofulvin therapy.

Barbiturates usually depress griseofulvin activity and concomitant administration may require a dosage adjustment of the antifungal agent.

The effects of alcohol may be potentiated by griseofulvin, producing such effects as tachycardia and flush.

Adverse Reactions: When adverse reactions occur, they are most commonly of the hypersensitivity type, such as skin rashes, urticaria, and rarely, angioneurotic edema, and may necessitate withdrawal of therapy and appropriate countermeasures. Paresthesias of the hands and feet have been reported rarely after extended therapy. Other side effects reported occasionally are oral thrush, nausea, vomiting, epigastric distress, diarrhea, headache, fatigue, dizziness, insomnia, mental confusion, and impairment of performance of routine activities.

Proteinuria and leukopenia have been reported rarely. Administration of the drug should be discontinued if granulocytopenia occurs.

When rare, serious reactions occur with griseofulvin, they are usually associated with high dosages, long periods of therapy, or both.

Dosage and Administration: Accurate diagnosis of the infecting organism is essential. Identification should be made either by direct microscopic examination of a mounting of infected tissue in a solution of potassium hydroxide or by culture on an appropriate medium. Medication must be continued until the infecting organism is completely eradicated as indicated by appropriate clinical or laboratory examination. Representative treatment periods are for tinea capitis, four to six weeks; tinea corporis, two to four weeks; tinea pedis, four to eight weeks; tinea unguium, depending on the rate of growth, fingernails, at least four months; toenails, at least six months.

General measures in regard to hygiene should be observed to control sources of infection or reinfection. Concomitant use of appropriate topical agents is usually required, particularly in treatment of tinea pedis. In some forms of athlete's foot, yeasts and bacteria may be involved as well as fungi. Griseofulvin will not eradicate the bacterial or monilial infection.

Adults: Daily administration of 500 mg. (as a single dose or in divided amounts), will give a satisfactory response in most patients with tinea corporis, tinea cruris, and tinea capitis. For those fungus infections more difficult to eradicate, such as tinea pedis and tinea unguium, daily dosage of 1.0 g. is recommended.

Children: Approximately 5 mg. per pound of body weight per day is an effective dose for most children. On this basis the following dosage schedule for children is suggested:

Children weighing 30 to 50 pounds—125 mg. to 250 mg. daily.

Children weighing over 50 pounds—250 mg. to 500 mg. daily.

Clinical experience with griseofulvin in children with tinea capitis indicates that a single daily dose is effective. Clinical relapse will occur if the medication is not continued until the infecting organism is eradicated.

How Supplied: FULVCIN-U/F Tablets, 250 mg.: white, compressed, scored tablets impressed with the Schering trademark and product identification letters, AUF, or numbers, 948; bottles of 60 and 250.

FULVICIN-U/F Tablets, 500 mg.: white, compressed, scored tablets impressed with the Schering trademark and product identification letters, AUG, or numbers, 496; bottles of 60 and 250.

Store between 2° and 30° C (36° and 86° F).

Revised 8/80

Copyright © 1968, 1980, Schering Corporation. All rights reserved.

[*Shown in Product Identification Section*]

GARAMYCIN® ℞

brand of gentamicin sulfate, USP
Cream 0.1%
and
Ointment 0.1%
For Dermatologic Use

Description: Each gram of GARAMYCIN **Cream** 0.1% contains 1.7 mg. gentamicin sulfate, USP equivalent to 1.0 mg. gentamicin base, with 1.0 mg. methylparaben and 4.0 mg. butylparaben as preservatives, in a bland emulsion-type vehicle composed of stearic acid, propylene glycol monostearate, isopropyl myristate, propylene glycol, polysorbate 40, sorbitol solution and purified water.

Each gram of GARAMYCIN **Ointment** 0.1% contains 1.7 mg. gentamicin sulfate, USP equivalent to 1.0 mg. gentamicin base, with 0.5 mg. methylparaben and 0.1 mg. propylparaben as preservatives in a bland, unctuous petrolatum base.

Actions: GARAMYCIN, a wide-spectrum antibiotic, provides highly effective topical treatment in primary and secondary bacterial infections of the skin. GARAMYCIN may clear infections that have not responded to other topical antibiotic agents. In impetigo contagiosa and other primary skin infections, treatment three or four times daily with GARAMYCIN usually clears the lesions promptly. In secondary skin infections, GARAMYCIN facilitates the treatment of the underlying dermatosis by controlling the infection. Bacteria susceptible to the action of GARAMYCIN include sensitive strains of streptococci (group A beta-hemolytic, alpha-hemolytic), *Staphylococcus aureus* (coagulase positive, coagulase negative, and some penicillinase-producing strains), and the gram-negative bacteria, *Pseudomonas aeruginosa, Aerobacter aerogenes, Escherichia coli, Proteus vulgaris,* and *Klebsiella pneumoniae.*

Indications: *Primary skin infections:* Impetigo contagiosa, superficial folliculitis, ecthyma, furunculosis, sycosis barbae, and pyoderma gangrenosum. *Secondary skin infections:* Infectious eczematoid dermatitis, pustular acne, pustular psoriasis, infected seborrheic dermatitis, infected contact dermatitis (including poison ivy), infected excoriations, and bacterial superinfections of fungal or viral infections. Note: GARAMYCIN is a bactericidal agent that is not effective against viruses or fungi in skin infections. GARAMYCIN is useful in the treatment of infected skin cysts and certain other skin abscesses when preceded by incision and drainage to permit adequate contact between the antibiotic and the infecting bacteria. Good results have been obtained in the treatment of infected stasis and other skin ulcers, infected superficial burns, paronychia, infected insect bites and stings, infected lacerations and abrasions, and wounds from minor surgery. Patients sensitive to neomycin can be treated with gentamicin, although regular observation of patients sensitive to topical antibiotics is advisable when such patients are treated with any topical antibiotic. GARAMYCIN **Ointment** helps retain moisture and has been useful in infection on dry eczematous or psoriatic skin. GARAMYCIN **Cream** is recommended for wet, oozing primary infections, and greasy, secondary infections, such as pustular acne or infected seborrheic dermatitis. If a water-washable preparation is desired, GARAMYCIN **Cream** is preferable. GARAMYCIN **Ointment** and **Cream** have been used successfully in infants over one year of age as well as in adults and children.

Contraindications: This drug is contraindicated in individuals with a history of sensitivity reactions to any of its components.

Precautions: Use of topical antibiotics occasionally allows overgrowth of nonsusceptible organisms, including fungi. If this occurs, or if irritation, sensitization, or superinfection develops, treatment with gentamicin should be discontinued and appropriate therapy instituted.

Adverse Reactions: In patients with dermatoses treated with gentamicin, irritation (erythema and pruritus) that did not usually require discontinuance of treatment has been reported in a small percentage of cases. There was no evidence of irritation or sensitization, however, in any of these patients patch-tested subsequently with gentamicin on normal skin. Possible photosensitization has been reported in several patients but could not be elicited in these patients by reapplication of gentamicin followed by exposure to ultraviolet radiation.

Dosage and Administration: A small amount of GARAMYCIN **Cream** or **Ointment** should be applied gently to the lesions three or four times daily. The area treated may be covered with a gauze dressing if desired. In impetigo contagiosa, the crusts should be removed before application of GARAMYCIN to permit maximum contact between the antibiotic and the infection. Care should be exercised to avoid further contamination of the infected skin. Infected stasis ulcers have responded well to GARAMYCIN under gelatin packing.

How Supplied: GARAMYCIN **Cream** 0.1%, and GARAMYCIN **Ointment** 0.1%, 15 g. tubes.

Store between 2° and 30° C (36° and 86° F).

Revised 1/81

Copyright © 1966, 1981 Schering Corporation. All rights reserved.

GARAMYCIN® ℞

brand of gentamicin sulfate, USP
Ophthalmic Solution—Sterile
Ophthalmic Ointment—Sterile
Each ml or gram contains gentamicin sulfate, USP equivalent to 3.0 mg gentamicin

Description: Gentamicin sulfate is a water-soluble antibiotic of the aminoglycoside group active against a wide variety of pathogenic gram-negative and gram-positive bacteria.

GARAMYCIN **Ophthalmic Solution** is a sterile, aqueous solution buffered to approximately pH 7 for use in the eye. Each ml. contains gentamicin sulfate (equivalent to 3.0 mg. gentamicin), disodium phosphate, monosodium phosphate, sodium chloride, and benzalkonium chloride as a preservative.

GARAMYCIN **Ophthalmic Ointment** is a sterile ointment, each gram containing gentamicin sulfate (equivalent to 3.0 mg. gentamicin) in a bland base of white petrolatum, with methylparaben and propylparaben as preservatives.

Actions: The gram-positive bacteria against which gentamicin sulfate is active include coagulase-positive and coagulase-negative staphylococci, including certain strains that are resistant to penicillin; Group A beta-hemolytic and nonhemolytic streptococci; and *Diplococcus pneumoniae.* The gram-negative bacteria against which gentamicin sulfate is active include certain strains of *Pseudomonas aeruginosa,* indole-positive and indole-negative *Proteus* species, *Escherichia coli, Klebsiella pneumoniae* (Friedlander's bacillus), *Haemophilus influenza* and *Haemophilus aegyptius* (Koch-Weeks bacillus), *Aerobacter aerogenes, Moraxella lacunata* (diplobacillus of Morax-Axenfeld), and *Neisseria* species, including *Neisseria gonorrhoeae.* Although significant resistant organisms have not been isolated from patients treated with gentamicin at the present time, this may occur in the future as resistance has been produced with difficulty *in vitro* by repeated exposures.

Indications: GARAMYCIN **Ophthalmic Solution** and **Ointment** are indicated in the topical treatment of infections of the external eye and its adnexa caused by susceptible bacteria. Such infections embrace conjunctivitis, keratitis and keratoconjunctivitis, corneal ulcers, blepharitis and blepharoconjunctivitis, acute meibomianitis, and dacryocystitis.

Contraindications: GARAMYCIN **Ophthalmic Solution** and **Ointment** are contraindicated in patients with known hypersensitivity to any of the components.

Warnings: GARAMYCIN **Ophthalmic Solution** is not for injection. It should never be injected subconjunctivally, nor should it be directly introduced into the anterior chamber of the eye.

Precautions: Prolonged use of topical antibiotics may give rise to overgrowth of nonsusceptible organisms, such as fungi. Should this occur, or if irritation or hypersensitivity to any component of the drug develops, discontinue use of the preparation and institute appropriate therapy.

Ophthalmic ointments may retard corneal healing.

Adverse Reactions: Transient irritation has been reported with the use of GARAMYCIN **Ophthalmic Solution.**

Occasional burning or stinging may occur with the use of GARAMYCIN **Ophthalmic Ointment.**

Dosage and Administration: GARAMYCIN **Ophthalmic Solution:** instill one or two drops into the affected eye every four hours. In severe infections, dosage may be increased to as much as two drops once every hour.

GARAMYCIN **Ophthalmic Ointment:** apply a small amount to the affected eye two to three times a day.

How Supplied: GARAMYCIN **Ophthalmic Solution—Sterile,** 5 ml. plastic dropper bottle, sterile, boxes of one and six.

GARAMYCIN **Ophthalmic Ointment—Sterile,** 3.5g, boxes of one and six.

Store GARAMYCIN Ophthalmic Ointment and Solution between 2° and 30°C (36° and 86°F).

Revised 1/81

Copyright © 1969, 1981, Schering Corporation. All rights reserved.

GARAMYCIN® Injectable ℞

brand of gentamicin sulfate injection, USP 40 mg. per ml.

Each ml. contains gentamicin sulfate, USP equivalent to 40 mg. gentamicin.

For Parenteral Administration

WARNINGS

Patients treated with aminoglycosides should be under close clinical observation because of the potential toxicity associated with their use.

As with other aminoglycosides, GARAMYCIN Injectable is potentially nephrotoxic. The risk of nephrotoxicity is greater in patients with impaired renal function and in those who receive high dosage or prolonged therapy.

Neurotoxicity manifested by ototoxicity, both vestibular and auditory, can occur in patients treated with GARAMYCIN Injectable primarily in those with pre-existing renal damage and in patients with normal renal function treated with higher doses and/or for longer periods than recommended. Other manifestations of neurotoxicity may include numbness, skin tingling, muscle twitching and convulsions.

Renal and eighth cranial nerve function should be closely monitored, especially in patients with known or suspected reduced renal function at onset of therapy and also in those whose renal function is initially normal but who develop signs of renal dysfunction during therapy. Urine should be examined for decreased specific gravity, increased excretion of protein, and the presence of cells or casts. Blood urea nitrogen, serum creatinine, or creatinine clearance should be determined periodically. When feasible, it is recommended that serial audiograms be obtained in patients old enough to be tested, particularly high-risk patients. Evidence of ototoxicity (dizziness, vertigo, tinnitus, roaring in the ears or hearing loss) or nephrotoxicity requires dosage adjustment or discontinuance of the drug. As with the other aminoglycosides, on rare occasions changes in renal and eighth cranial nerve function may not become manifest until soon after completion of therapy.

Serum concentrations of aminoglycosides should be monitored when feasible to assure adequate levels and to avoid potentially toxic levels. When monitoring gentamicin peak concentrations, dosage should be adjusted so that prolonged levels above 12 mcg/ml are avoided. When monitoring gentamicin trough concentrations, dosage should be adjusted so that levels above 2 mcg/ml are avoided. Excessive peak and/or trough serum concentrations of aminoglycosides may increase the risk of renal and eighth cranial nerve toxicity. In the event of overdose or toxic reactions, hemodialysis or peritoneal dialysis will aid in removal of gentamicin from the blood.

Concurrent and/or sequential systemic or topical use of other potentially neurotoxic and/or nephrotoxic drugs, such as cisplatin, cephaloridine, kanamycin, amikacin, neomycin, polymyxin B, colistin, paromomycin, streptomycin, tobramycin, vancomycin, and viomycin, should be avoided. Other factors which may increase patient risk of toxicity are advanced age and dehydration.

The concurrent use of gentamicin with potent diuretics, such as ethacrynic acid or furosemide, should be avoided, since certain diuretics by themselves may cause ototoxicity. In addition, when administered intravenously, diuretics may enhance aminoglycoside toxicity by altering the antibiotic concentration in serum and tissue.

Description: Gentamicin sulfate, USP, a water-soluble antibiotic of the aminoglycoside group, is derived from *Micromonospora purpurea,* an actinomycete. GARAMYCIN Injectable is a sterile, aqueous solutions for parenteral administration. Each ml. contains gentamicin sulfate, USP equivalent to 40 mg. gentamicin base, 1.8 mg. methylparaben and 0.2 mg. propylparaben as preservatives, 3.2 mg. sodium bisulfite, and 0.1 mg. edetate disodium.

Clinical Pharmacology: After intramuscular administration of GARAMYCIN Injectable, peak serum concentrations usually occur between 30 and 60 minutes and serum levels are measurable for six to eight hours. When gentamicin is administered by intravenous infusion over a two-hour period, the serum concentrations are similar to those obtained by intramuscular administration.

In patients with normal renal function, peak serum concentrations of gentamicin (mcg/ml) are usually up to four times the single intramuscular dose (mg/kg); for example, a 1.0 mg/kg injection in adults may be expected to result in a peak serum concentration up to 4 mcg/ml; a 1.5 mg/kg dose may produce levels up to 6 mcg/ml. While some variation is to be expected due to a number of variables such as age, body temperature surface area and physiological differences, the individual patient given the same dose tends to have similar levels in repeated determinations. Gentamicin administered at 1.0 mg/kg every eight hours for the usual 7- to 10-day treatment period to patients with normal renal function does not accumulate in serum.

Gentamicin, like all aminoglycosides, may accumulate in the serum and tissues of patients treated with higher doses and for prolonged periods, particularly in the presence of impaired renal function. In adult patients, treatment with gentamicin dosages of 4 mg/kg/day or higher for seven to ten days may result in a slight, progressive rise in both peak and trough concentrations. In patients with impaired renal function, gentamicin is cleared from the body more slowly than in patients with normal renal function. The more severe the impairment, the slower the clearance. (Dosage must be adjusted.)

Since gentamicin is distributed in extracellular fluid, peak serum concentrations may be lower than usual in adult patients who have a large volume of this fluid. Serum concentrations of gentamicin in febrile patients may be lower than those in afebrile patients given the same dose. When body temperature returns to normal serum concentrations of the drug may rise. Febrile and anemic states may be associated with a shorter than usual serum half-life. (Dosage adjustment is usually not necessary.)

In severely burned patients, the half-life may be significantly decreased and resulting serum concentrations may be lower than anticipated from the mg/kg dose.

Protein binding studies have indicated that the degree of gentamicin binding is low; depending upon the methods used for testing, this may be between 0 and 30%.

After initial administration to patients with normal renal function, generally 70% or more of the gentamicin dose is recoverable in the urine in 24 hours, concentrations in urine above 100 mcg/ml may be achieved. Little, if any, metabolic transformation occurs; the drug is excreted principally by glomerular filtration. After several days of treatment, the

Continued on next page

Information on Schering products appearing on these pages is effective as of September 30, 1982.

Schering—Cont.

amount of gentamicin excreted in the urine approaches the daily dose administered. As with other aminoglycosides, a small amount of the gentamicin dose may be retained in the tissues, especially in the kidneys. Minute quantities of aminoglycosides have been detected in the urine weeks after drug administration was discontinued. Renal clearance of gentamicin is similar to that of endogenous creatinine.

In patients with marked impairment of renal function, there is a decrease in the concentration of aminoglycosides in urine and in their penetration into defective renal parenchyma. This decreased drug excretion, together with the potential nephrotoxicity of aminoglycosides, should be considered when treating such patients who have urinary tract infections.

Probenecid does not affect renal tubular transport of gentamicin.

The endogenous creatinine clearance rate and the serum creatinine level have a high correlation with the half-life of gentamicin in serum. Results of these tests may serve as guides for adjusting dosage in patients with renal impairment (see DOSAGE AND ADMINISTRATION).

Following parenteral administration, gentamicin can be detected in serum, lymph, tissues, sputum, and in pleural, synovial, and peritoneal fluids. Concentrations in renal cortex sometimes may be eight times higher than the usual serum levels. Concentrations in bile, in general, have been low and have suggested minimal biliary excretion. Gentamicin crosses the peritoneal as well as the placental membranes. Since aminoglycosides diffuse poorly into the subarachnoid space after parenteral administration, concentrations of gentamicin in cerebrospinal fluid are often low and dependent upon dose, rate of penetration, and degree of meningeal inflammation. There is minimal penetration of gentamicin into ocular tissues following intramuscular or intravenous administration.

Microbiology: *In vitro* tests have demonstrated that gentamicin is a bactericidal antibiotic which acts by inhibiting normal protein synthesis in susceptible microorganisms. It is active against a wide variety of pathogenic bacteria including *Escherichia coli, Proteus* species, (indole-positive and indole-negative), *Pseudomonas aeruginosa,* species of the *Klebsiella-Enterobacter-Serratia* group. *Citrobacter* species and *Staphylococcus* species (including penicillin- and methicillin-resistant strains). Gentamicin is also active *in vitro* against species of *Salmonella* and *Shigella.* The following bacteria are usually resistant to aminoglycosides; *Streptococcus pneumoniae,* most species of streptococci, particularly group D and anaerobic organisms, such as *Bacteroides* species or *Clostridium* species.

In vitro studies have shown that an aminoglycoside combined with an antibiotic that interferes with cell wall synthesis may act synergistically against some group D streptococcal strains. The combination of gentamicin and penicillin G has a synergistic bactericidal effect against virtually all strains of *Streptococcus faecalis* and its varieties *(S. faecalis* var. *liquifaciens, S. faecalis* var. *zymogenes), S. faecium* and *S. durans.* An enhanced killing effect against many of these strains has also been shown *in vitro* with combinations of gentamicin and ampicillin, carbenicillin, nafcillin, or oxacillin.

The combined effect of gentamicin and carbenicillin is synergistic for many strains of *Pseudomonas aeruginosa. In vitro* synergism against other gram-negative organisms has been shown with combinations of gentamicin and cephalosporins.

Gentamicin may be active against clinical isolates of bacteria resistant to other aminoglycosides. Bacteria resistant to one aminoglycoside may be resistant to one or more other aminoglycosides. Bacterial resistance to gentamicin is generally developed slowly.

Susceptibility Testing: If the disc method of susceptibility testing used is that described by Bauer *et al. (Am J Clin Path* 45:493, 1966; *Federal Register* 37:20525-20529, 1972), a disc containing 10 mcg. of gentamicin should give a zone of inhibition of 13mm. or more to indicate susceptibility of the infecting organism. A zone of 12mm. or less indicates that the infecting organism is likely to be resistant. In certain conditions it may be desirable to do additional susceptibility testing by the tube or agar dilution method; gentamicin substance is available for this purpose.

Indications and Usage: GARAMYCIN Injectable is indicated in the treatment of serious infections caused by susceptible strains of the following microorganisms: *Pseudomonas aeruginosa, Proteus* species (indole-positive and indole-negative). *Escherichia coli, Klebsiella-Enterobacter-Serratia* species, *Citrobacter* species and *Staphylococcus* species (coagulase-positive and coagulase-negative).

Clinical studies have shown GARAMYCIN Injectable to be effective in bacterial neonatal sepsis; bacterial septicemia; and serious bacterial infections of the central nervous system (meningitis), urinary tract, respiratory tract, gastrointestinal tract (including peritonitis), skin, bone and soft tissue (including burns).

Aminoglycosides, including gentamicin, are not indicated in uncomplicated initial episodes of urinary tract infections unless the causative organisms are susceptible to these antibiotics and are not susceptible to antibiotics having less potential for toxicity.

Specimens for bacterial culture should be obtained to isolate and identify causative organisms and to determine their susceptibility to gentamicin.

GARAMYCIN may be considered as initial therapy in suspected or confirmed gram-negative infections, and therapy may be instituted before obtaining results of susceptibility testing. The decision to continue therapy with this drug should be based on the results of susceptibility tests, the severity of the infection, and the important additional concepts contained in the "WARNINGS Box" above. If the causative organisms are resistant to gentamicin, other appropriate therapy should be instituted.

In serious infections when the causative organisms are unknown GARAMYCIN may be administered as initial therapy in conjunction with a penicillin-type or cephalosporin-type drug before obtaining results of susceptibility testing. If anaerobic organisms are suspected as etiologic agents, consideration should be given to using other suitable antimicrobial therapy in conjunction with gentamicin. Following identification of the organism and its susceptibility, appropriate antibiotic therapy should then be continued.

GARAMYCIN has been used effectively in combination with carbenicillin for the treatment of life-threatening infections caused by *Pseudomonas aeruginosa.* It has also been found effective when used in conjunction with a penicillin-type drug for the treatment of endocarditis caused by group D streptococci.

GARAMYCIN Injectable has also been shown to be effective in the treatment of serious staphylococcal infections. While not the antibiotic of first choice, GARAMYCIN Injectable may be considered when penicillins or other less potentially toxic drugs are contraindicated and bacterial susceptibility tests and clinical judgment indicate its use. It may also be considered in mixed infections caused by susceptible strains of staphylococci and gram-negative organisms.

In the neonate with suspected bacterial sepsis or staphylococcal pneumonia, a penicillin-type drug is also usually indicated as concomitant therapy with gentamicin.

Contraindications: Hypersensitivity to gentamicin is a contraindication to its use. A history of hypersensitivity or serious toxic reactions to other aminoglycosides may contraindicate use of gentamicin because of the known cross-sensitivity of patients to drugs in this class.

Warnings: (See "WARNINGS Box" above.)

Precautions: Neurotoxic and nephrotoxic antibiotics may be absorbed in significant quantities from body surfaces after local irrigation or application. The potential toxic effect of antibiotics administered in this fashion should be considered.

Increased nephrotoxicity has been reported following concomitant administration of aminoglycoside antibiotics and cephalosporins.

Neuromuscular blockade and respiratory paralysis have been reported in the cat receiving high doses (40 mg/kg) of gentamicin. The possibility of these phenomena occurring in man should be considered if aminoglycosides are administered by any route to patients receiving anesthetics, or to patients receiving neuromuscular blocking agents, such as succinylcholine, tubocurarine, or decamethonium, or in patients receiving massive transfusions of citrate-anticoagulated blood. If neuromuscular blockade occurs, calcium salts may reverse it.

Aminoglycosides should be used with caution in patients with neuromuscular disorders, such as myasthenia gravis or parkinsonism, since these drugs may aggravate muscle weakness because of their potential curare-like effects on the neuromuscular junction.

Elderly patients may have reduced renal function which may not be evident in the results of routine screening tests, such as BUN or serum creatinine. A creatinine clearance determination may be more useful. Monitoring of renal function during treatment with gentamicin, as with other aminoglycosides, is particularly important in such patients.

Cross-allergenicity among aminoglycosides has been demonstrated.

Patients should be well hydrated during treatment.

Although the *in vitro* mixing of gentamicin and carbenicillin results in a rapid and significant inactivation of gentamicin, this interaction has not been demonstrated in patients with normal renal function who received both drugs by different routes of administration. A reduction in gentamicin serum half-life has been reported in patients with severe renal impairment receiving carbenicillin concomitantly with gentamicin.

Treatment with gentamicin may result in overgrowth of nonsusceptible organisms. If this occurs, appropriate therapy is indicated.

See "WARNINGS Box" regarding concurrent use of potent diuretics and regarding concurrent and/or sequential use of other neurotoxic and/or nephrotoxic antibiotics and for other essential information.

Usage in Pregnancy—Safety for use in pregnancy has not been established.

Adverse Reactions: *Nephrotoxicity:* Adverse renal effects, as demonstrated by the presence of casts, cells, or protein in the urine or by rising BUN, NPN, serum creatinine or oliguria, have been reported. They occur more frequently in patients with a history of renal impairment and in patients treated for longer periods or with larger dosage than recommended.

Neurotoxicity: Serious adverse effects on both vestibular and auditory branches of the eighth nerve have been reported, primarily in patients with renal impairment and in patients on high doses and/or prolonged therapy. Symptoms include dizziness, vertigo, tinnitus, roaring in the ears and also hearing loss, which, as with the other aminoglycosides, may be irreversible. Hearing loss is usually manifested initially by diminution of high-tone acuity. Other factors which may increase the risk of toxicity include excessive dosage, dehydration and previous exposure to other ototoxic drugs.

Numbness, skin tingling, muscle twitching and convulsions have also been reported.

Note: The risk of toxic reactions is low in patients with normal renal function who do not receive GARAMYCIN Injectable at higher doses or for longer periods of time than recommended.

Other reported adverse reactions possibly related to gentamicin include: respiratory depression, lethargy, confusion, depression, visual disturbances, decreased appetite, weight loss, and hypotension and hypertension; rash, itching, urticaria, generalized burning, laryngeal edema, anaphylactoid reactions, fever, and headache, nausea, vomiting, increased salivation, and stomatitis; purpura, pseudotumor cerebri, acute organic brain syndrome, pulmonary fibrosis, alopecia, joint pain, transient hepatomegaly, and splenomegaly.

Laboratory abnormalities possibly related to gentamicin include: increased levels of serum transaminase (SGOT, SGPT), serum LDH and bilirubin; decreased serum calcium, magnesium, sodium and potassium; anemia, leukopenia, granulocytopenia, transient agranulocytosis, eosinophilia, increased and decreased reticulocyte counts, and thrombocytopenia.

While local tolerance of GARAMYCIN Injectable is generally excellent, there has been an occasional report of pain at the injection site. Subcutaneous atrophy or fat necrosis suggesting local irritation has been reported rarely.

Overdosage: In the event of overdose or toxic reactions, hemodialysis or peritoneal dialysis will aid in the removal of gentamicin from the blood.

Dosage and Administration: GARAMYCIN Injectable may be given intramuscularly or intravenously. The patient's pretreatment body weight should be obtained for calculation of correct dosage. The dosage of aminoglycosides in obese patients should be based on an estimate of the lean body mass. It is desirable to limit the duration of treatment with aminoglycosides to short term.

PATIENTS WITH NORMAL RENAL FUNCTION

Adults: The recommended dosage of GARAMYCIN Injectable for patients with serious infections and normal renal function is 3 mg/kg/day, administered in three equal doses every eight hours (Table I).

For patients with life-threatening infections, dosages up to 5 mg/kg/day may be administered in three or four equal doses. This dosage should be reduced to 3 mg/kg/day as soon as clinically indicated (Table I).

It is desirable to measure both peak and trough serum concentrations of gentamicin to determine the adequacy and safety of the dosage. When such measurements are feasible, they should be carried out periodically during therapy to assure adequate but not excessive drug levels. For example, the peak concentration (at 30 to 60 minutes after intramuscular injection) is expected to be in the range of 4 to 6 mcg/ml. When monitoring peak concentrations after intramuscular or intravenous administration, dosage should be adjusted so that prolonged levels above 12 mcg/ml are avoided. When monitoring trough concentrations (just prior to the next dose), dosage should be adjusted so that levels above 2 mcg/ml are avoided. Determination of the adequacy of a serum level for a particular patient must take into consideration the susceptibility of the causative organism, the severity of the infection, and the status of the patient's host-defense mechanisms.

In patients with extensive burns, altered pharmacokinetics may result in reduced serum concentrations of aminoglycosides. In such patients treated with gentamicin, measurement of serum concentrations is recommended as a basis for dosage adjustment.

TABLE I
DOSAGE SCHEDULE GUIDE FOR ADULTS WITH NORMAL RENAL FUNCTION
(Dosage at Eight-Hour Intervals)
40 mg. per ml.

Patient's Weight* kg	(lb)	Usual Dose For Serious Infections 1 mg/kg q8h (3 mg/kg/day)		Dose for Life-Threatening Infections (Reduce as Soon as Clinically Indicated) 1.7 mg/kg q8h** (5 mg/kg/day)	
		mg/dose q8h	ml/dose	mg/dose q8h	ml/dose
40	(88)	40	1.0	66	1.6
45	(99)	45	1.1	75	1.9
50	(110)	50	1.25	83	2.1
55	(121)	55	1.4	91	2.25
60	(132)	60	1.5	100	2.5
65	(143)	65	1.6	108	2.7
70	(154)	70	1.75	116	2.9
75	(165)	75	1.9	125	3.1
80	(176)	80	2.0	133	3.3
85	(187)	85	2.1	141	3.5
90	(198)	90	2.25	150	3.75
95	(209)	95	2.4	158	4.0
100	(220)	100	2.5	166	4.2

* The dosage of aminoglycosides in obese patients should be based on an estimate of the lean body mass.

** For q6h schedules, dosage should be recalculated.

Children: 6 to 7.5 mg/kg/day. (2.0 to 2.5 mg/kg administered every 8 hours.)

Infants and Neonates: 7.5 mg/kg/day. (2.5 mg/kg administered every 8 hours.)

Premature or Full-Term Neonates One Week of Age or Less: 5 mg/kg/day. (2.5 mg/kg administered every 12 hours).

For further information concerning the use of gentamicin in infants and children, see GARAMYCIN Pediatric Injectable Product Information.

The usual duration of treatment for all patients is seven to ten days. In difficult and complicated infections, a longer course of therapy may be necessary. In such cases monitoring of renal, auditory, and vestibular functions is recommended, since toxicity is more apt to occur with treatment extended for more than ten days. Dosage should be reduced if clinically indicated.

For Intravenous Administration

The intravenous administration of gentamicin may be particularly useful for treating patients with bacterial septicemia or those in shock. It may also be the preferred route of administration for some patients with congestive heart failure, hematologic disorders, severe burns, or those with reduced muscle mass. For intermittent intravenous administration in adults, a single dose of GARAMYCIN Injectable may be diluted in 50 to 200 ml. of sterile isotonic saline solution or in a sterile solution of dextrose 5% in water, in infants and children, the volume of diluent should be less. The solution may be infused over a period of one-half to two hours.

The recommended dosage for intravenous and intramuscular administration is identical.

GARAMYCIN Injectable should not be physically premixed with other drugs, but should be administered separately in accordance with the recommended route of administration and dosage schedule.

PATIENT WITH IMPAIRED RENAL FUNCTION

Dosage must be adjusted in patients with impaired renal function. Whenever possible serum concentrations of gentamicin should be monitored. One method of dosage adjustment is to increase the interval between administration of the usual doses. Since the serum creatinine concentration has a high correlation with the serum half-life of gentamicin, this laboratory test may provide guidance for adjustment of the interval between doses. The interval between doses (in hours) may be approximated by multiplying the serum creatinine level (mg/100 ml) by 8. For example, a patient weighing 60 kg. with a serum creatinine level of 2.0 mg/100 ml could be given 60 mg. (1 mg/kg) every 16 hours (2 × 8).

In patients with serious systemic infections and renal impairment, it may be desirable to administer the antibiotic more frequently but in reduced dosage. In such patients, serum concentrations of gentamicin should be measured so that adequate but not excessive levels result. A peak and trough concentration measured intermittently during therapy will provide optimal guidance for adjusting dosage. After the usual initial dose, a rough guide for determining reduced dosage at eight-hour intervals is to divide the normally recommended dose by the serum creatinine level (Table II). For example, after an initial dose of 60 mg. (1 mg/kg), a patient weighing 60 kg. with a serum creatinine level of 2.0 mg/100 ml could be given 30 mg. every eight hours (60÷2). It should be noted that the status of renal function may be changing over the course of the infectious process.

It is important to recognize that deteriorating renal function may require a greater reduction in dosage than that specified in the above guidelines for patients with stable renal impairment.

TABLE II
DOSAGE ADJUSTMENT GUIDE FOR PATIENTS WITH RENAL IMPAIRMENT
(Dosage at Eight-Hour Intervals After the Usual Initial Dose)

Serum Creatinine (mg %)	Approximate Creatinine Clearance Rate (ml/min/1.73M²)	Percent of Usual Doses Shown in Table I
≤ 1.0	> 100	100
1.1–1.3	70–100	80
1.4–1.6	55–70	65
1.7–1.9	45–55	55
2.0–2.2	40–45	50
2.3–2.5	35–40	40
2.6–3.0	30–35	35
3.1–3.5	25–30	30
3.6–4.0	20–25	25
4.1–5.1	15–20	20
5.2–6.6	10–15	15
6.7–8.0	< 10	10

In adults with renal failure undergoing hemodialysis, the amount of gentamicin removed from the blood may vary depending upon several factors including the dialysis method used. An eight-hour hemodialysis may reduce serum concentrations of gentamicin by approximately 50%. The recommended dosage at the end of each dialysis period is 1 to 1.7 mg/kg depending upon the severity of infection. In children, a dose of 2 mg/kg may be administered.

The above dosage schedules are not intended as rigid recommendations but are provided as guides to dosage when the measurement of gentamicin serum levels is not feasible.

A variety of methods are available to measure gentamicin concentrations in body fluids; these include microbiologic, enzymatic and radioimmunoassay techniques.

Continued on next page

Information on Schering products appearing on these pages is effective as of September 30, 1982.

Schering—Cont.

How Supplied: GARAMYCIN Injectable, 40 mg. per ml., for parenteral administration, is supplied in 2 ml. (80 mg.) vials, boxes of 1 and 25; 20 ml. (800 mg) vials, box of 5; and in 1.5 ml. (60 mg.) and 2 ml. (80 mg.) disposable syringes, each in boxes of 1 and 10.
Also available, GARAMYCIN Pediatric Injectable, 10 mg. per ml., for parenteral administration, supplied in 2 ml. (20 mg) vials; box of one.
GARAMYCIN Injectable is a clear, stable solution that requires no refrigeration.
Store between 2° and 30°C (36° and 86°F).

Schering Pharmaceutical Corporation (PR)
Manati, Puerto Rico 00701
An Affiliate of Schering Corporation
Kenilworth, N.J. 07033

Copyright © 1968, 1981, Schering Corporation. All rights reserved.

GARAMYCIN® PEDIATRIC ℞

Injectable
brand of gentamicin sulfate injection, USP 10 mg. per ml.
Each ml. contains gentamicin sulfate, USP equivalent to 10 mg. gentamicin.
For Parenteral Administration

WARNINGS

Patients treated with aminoglycosides should be under close clinical observation because of the potential toxicity associated with their use.
As with other aminoglycosides, GARAMYCIN Pediatric Injectable is potentially nephrotoxic. The risk of nephrotoxicity is greater in patients with impaired renal function and in those who receive high dosage or prolonged therapy. Neurotoxicity manifested by ototoxicity, both vestibular and auditory, can occur in patients treated with GARAMYCIN Pediatric Injectable, primarily in those with pre-existing renal damage and in patients with normal renal function treated with higher doses and/or for longer periods than recommended. Other manifestations of neurotoxicity may include numbness, skin tingling, muscle twitching, and convulsions.
Renal and eighth cranial nerve function should be closely monitored, especially in patients with known or suspected reduced renal function at onset of therapy and also in those whose renal function is initially normal but who develop signs of renal dysfunction during therapy. Urine should be examined for decreased specific gravity, increased excretion of protein, and the presence of cells or casts. Blood urea nitrogen, serum creatinine, or creatinine clearance should be determined periodically. When feasible, it is recommended that serial audiograms be obtained in patients old enough to be tested, particularly high-risk patients. Evidence of ototoxicity (dizziness, vertigo, tinnitus, roaring in the ears or hearing loss) or nephrotoxicity requires dosage adjustment or discontinuance of the drug. As with the other aminoglycosides, on rare occasions changes in renal and eighth cranial nerve function may not become manifest until soon after completion of therapy.
Serum concentrations of aminoglycosides should be monitored when feasible to assure adequate levels and to avoid potentially toxic levels. When monitoring gentamicin peak concentrations, dosage should be adjusted so that prolonged levels above 12 mcg/ml are avoided. Excessive peak and/or trough serum concentrations of aminoglycosides may increase the risk of renal and eighth cranial nerve toxicity. In the event of overdose or toxic reactions, hemodialysis or peritoneal dialysis will aid in the removal of gentamicin from the blood. In the newborn infant, exchange transfusions may also be considered.
Concurrent and/or sequential systemic or topical use of other potentially neurotoxic and/or nephrotoxic drugs, such as cisplatin, cephaloridine, kanamycin, amikacin, neomycin, polymyxin B, colistin, paromomycin, streptomycin, tobramycin, vancomycin, and viomycin, should be avoided. Another factor which may increase patient risk of toxicity is dehydration.
The concurrent use of gentamicin with potent diuretics, such as ethacrynic acid or furosemide, should be avoided, since certain diuretics by themselves may cause ototoxicity. In addition, when administered intravenously, diuretics may enhance aminoglycoside toxicity by altering the antibiotic concentration in serum and tissue.

Description: Gentamicin sulfate, USP, a water-soluble antibiotic of the aminoglycoside group, is derived from *Micromonospera purpurea*, an actinonmycete. GARAMYCIN Pediatric Injectable is a sterile, aqueous solution for parenteral administration. Each ml. contains gentamicin sulfate, USP equivalent to 10 mg. gentamicin base, 1.3 mg. methylparaben and 0.2 mg. propylparaben as preservatives, 3.2 mg. sodium bisulfate; and 0.1 mg. edetate disodium.

Clinical Pharmacology: After intramuscular administration of GARAMYCIN Pediatric Injectable, peak serum concentrations usually occur between 30 and 60 minutes and serum levels are measurable for 6 to 12 hours. In infants, a single dose of 2.5 mg/kg usually provides a peak serum level in the range of 3 to 5 mcg/ml. When gentamicin is administered by intravenous infusion over a two-hour period, the serum concentrations are similar to those obtained by intramuscular administration.
Age markedly affects the peak concentrations: in one report, a 1 mg/kg dose produced mean peak concentrations of 1.58, 2.03, and 2.81 mcg/ml in patients 6 months to 5 years old, 5 to 10 years old, and over 10 years old, respectively.
In infants one week to six months of age, the half-life is 3 to 3½ hours. In full-term and large premature infants less than one week old, the appropriate serum half-life of gentamicin is 5½ hours. In small premature infants, the half-life is inversely related to birth weight. In premature infants weighing less than 1500 grams, the half-life is 11½ hours; in those weighing 1500 to 2000 grams, the half-life is 8 hours; in those weighing over 2000 grams, the half-life is approximately 5 hours.
While some variation is to be expected due to a number of variables such as age, body temperature, surface area and physiologic differences, the individual patient given the same dose tends to have similar levels in repeated determinations.
Gentamicin, like all aminoglycosides, may accumulate in the serum and tissues of patients treated with higher doses and for prolonged periods, particularly in the presence of impaired or immature renal function. In patients with immature or impaired renal function, gentamicin is cleared from the body more slowly than in patients with normal renal function. The more severe the impairment, the slower the clearance. (Dosage must be adjusted.)
Since gentamicin is distributed in extracellular fluid, peak serum concentrations may be lower than usual in patients who have a large volume of this fluid. Serum concentrations of gentamicin in febrile patients may be lower than those in afebrile patients given the same dose. When body temperature returns to normal, serum concentrations of the drug may rise. Febrile and anemic states may be associated with a shorter than usual serum half-life. (Dosage adjustment is usually not necessary.) In severly burned patients, the half-life may be significantly decreased and resulting serum concentrations may be lower than anticipated from the mg/kg/dose.
Protein binding studies have indicated that the degree of gentamicin binding is low, depending upon the methods used for testing, this may be between 0 and 30%.
In neonates less than 3 days old, approximately 10% of the administered dose is excreted in 12 hours; in infants 5 to 40 days old, approximately 40% is excreted over the same period. Excretion of gentamicin correlates with postnatal age and creatinine clearance. Thus, with increasing postnatal age and concomitant increase in renal maturity, gentamicin is excreted more rapidly. Little, if any metabolic transformation occurs; the drug is excreted principally by glomerular filtration. After several days of treatment, the amount of gentamicin excreted in the urine approaches, but does not equal, the daily dose administered. As with other aminoglycosides, a small amount of the gentamicin dose may be retained in the tissues, especially in the kidneys. Minute quantities of aminoglycosides have been detected in the urine of some patients weeks after drug administration was discontinued. Renal clearance of gentamicin is similar to that of endogenous creatinine.
In patients with marked impairment of renal function, there is a decrease in the concentration of aminoglycosides in urine and in their penetration into defective renal parenchyma. This decreased drug excretion, together with the potential nephrotoxicity of aminoglycosides, should be considered when treating such patients who have urinary tract infections.
Probenecid does not affect renal tubular transport of gentamicin.
The endogenous creatinine clearance rate and the serum creatinine level have a high correlation with the half-life of gentamicin in serum. Results of these tests may serve as guides for adjusting dosage in patients with renal impairment. (see DOSAGE AND ADMINISTRATION).
Following parenteral administration, gentamicin can be detected in serum, lymph, tissues, sputum and in pleural, synovial, peritoneal fluids. Concentrations in renal cortex sometimes may be eight times higher than the usual serum levels. Concentrations in bile, in general, have been low and have suggested minimal biliary excretion. Gentamicin crosses the peritoneal as well as the placental membranes. Since aminoglycosides diffuse poorly into the subarachnoid space after parenteral administration, concentrations of gentamicin in cerebrospinal fluid are often low and dependent upon dose, rate of penetration, and degree of meningeal inflammation. There is minimal penetration of gentamicin into ocular tissues following intramuscular or intravenous administration.

Microbiology: *In vitro* tests have demonstrated that gentamicin is a bactericidal antibiotic which acts by inhibiting normal protein synthesis in susceptible microorganisms. It is active against a wide variety of pathogenic bacteria including *Escherichia coli, Proteus* species (indole-positive and indole-negative). *Pseudomonas aeruginosa,* species of *Klebsiella-Enterobacter-Serratia* group, *Citrobacter* species, and *Staphylococcus* species (including penicillin- and methicillin-resistant strains). Gentamicin is also active *in vitro* against species of *Salmonella* and *Shigella.* The following bacteria are usually resistant to aminoglycosides. *Streptococcus pneumoniae,* most species of streptococci, particularly group D and anaerobic organisms, such as *Bacteroides* species or *Clostridium* species.

In vitro studies have shown that an aminoglycoside combined with an antibiotic that interferes with cell wall synthesis may act synergistically against some group D streptococcal strains. The combination of gentamicin and penicillin G has a synergistic bacterial effect against virtually all strains of *Streptococcus faecalis* and its varieties *(S. faecalis* var. *liquifaciens, S. faecalis* var. *zymogenes), S. faecium* and *S. durans.* An enhanced killing effect against many of these strains has also been shown *in vitro* with combinations of gentamicin and ampicillin, carbenicillin, nafcillin, or oxacillin.

The combined effect of gentamicin and carbenicillin is synergistic for many strains of *Pseudomonas aeruginosa. In vitro* synergism against other gram-negative organisms has been shown with combinations of gentamicin and cephalosporins.

Gentamicin may be active against clinical isolates of bacteria resistant to other aminoglycosides. Bacteria resistant to one aminoglycoside may be resistant to one or more other aminoglycosides. Bacterial resistance to gentamicin is generally developed slowly.

Susceptibility Testing: If the disc method of susceptibility testing used is that described by Bauer *et al (Am J Clin Path* 45:493, 1966; *Federal Register* 37:20525–20529, 1972), a disc containing 10 mcg. of gentamicin should give a zone of inhibition of 13 mm. or more to indicate susceptibility of the infecting organism. A zone of 12 mm. or less indicates that the infecting organism is likely to be resistant. In certain conditions it may be desirable to do additional susceptibility testing by the tube or agar dilution method; gentamicin substance is available for this purpose.

Indications and Usage: GARAMYCIN Pediatric Injectable is indicated in the treatment of serious infections caused by susceptible strains of the following microorganisms: *Pseudomonas aeruginosa, Proteus* species (indole-positive and indole-negative), *Escherichia coli, Klebsiella-Enterobacter-Serratia* species, *Citrobacter* species, and *Staphyloccous* species (coagulase-positive and coagulase-negative).

Clinical studies have shown GARAMYCIN Pediatric Injectable to be effective in bacterial neonatal sepsis; bacterial septicemia; and serious bacterial infections of the central nervous system (meningitis), urinary tract, respiratory tract, gastrointestinal tract (including peritonitis), skin, bone and soft tissue (including burns).

Aminoglycosides, including gentamicin, are not indicated in uncomplicated initial episodes of urinary tract infections unless the causative organisms are susceptible to these antibiotics and are not susceptible to antibiotics having less potential for toxicity.

Specimens for bacterial culture should be obtained to isolate and identify causative organisms and to determine their susceptibility to gentamicin.

GARAMYCIN may be considered as initial therapy in suspected or confirmed gram-negative infections, and therapy may be instituted before obtaining results of susceptibility testing. The decision to continue therapy with this drug should be based on the results of susceptibility tests, the severity of the infection, and the important additional concepts contained in the "WARNINGS Box" above. If the causative organisms are resistant to gentamicin, other appropriate therapy should be instituted.

In serious infections when the causative organisms are unknown, GARAMYCIN may be administered as initial therapy in conjunction with a penicillin-type or cephalosporin-type drug before obtaining results of susceptibility testing. If anaerobic organisms are suspected as etiologic agents, consideration should be given to using other suitable antimicrobial therapy in conjunction with gentamicin. Following identification of the organism and its susceptibility, appropriate antibiotic therapy should then be continued.

GARAMYCIN has been used effectively in combination with carbenicillin for the treatment of life-threatening infections caused by *Pseudomonas aeruginosa.* It has also been found effective when used in conjunction with a penicillin-type drug for the treatment of endocarditis caused by group D streptococci.

GARAMYCIN Pediatric Injectable has also been shown to be effective in the treatment of serious staphylococcal infections. While not the antibiotic of first choice, GARAMYCIN Pediatric Injectable may be considered when penicillins or other less potentially toxic drugs are contraindicated and bacterial susceptibility tests and clinical judgment indicate its use. It may also be considered in mixed infections caused by susceptible strains of staphylococci and gram-negative organisms.

In the neonate with suspected bacterial sepsis or staphylococcal pneumonia, a penicillin-type drug is also usually indicated as concomitant therapy with gentamicin.

Contraindications: Hypersensitivity to gentamicin is a contraindication to its use. A history of hypersensitivity or serious toxic reactions to other aminoglycosides may contraindicate use of gentamicin because of the known cross-sensitivity of patients to drugs in this class.

Warnings: (See "WARNINGS Box" above.)

Precautions: Neurotoxic and nephrotoxic antibiotics may be absorbed in significant quantities from body surfaces after local irrigation or application. The potential toxic effect of antibiotics administered in this fashion should be considered.

Increased nephrotoxicity has been reported following concomitant administration of aminoglycoside antibiotics and cephalosporins.

Neuromuscular blockade and respiratory paralysis have been reported in the cat receiving high doses (40 mg/kg) of gentamicin. The possibility of these phenomena occurring in man should be considered if aminoglycosides are administered by any route to patients receiving anesthetics, or to patients receiving neuromuscular blocking agents, such as succinylcholine, tubocurarine, or decamethonium, or in patients receiving massive transfusions of citrate anticoagulated blood. If neuromuscular blockade occurs, calcium salts may reverse it.

Aminoglycosides should be used with caution in patients with neuromuscular disorders, such as myasthenia gravis or parkinsonism, since these drugs may aggravate muscle weakness because of their potential curare-like effects on the neuromuscular junction.

Cross-allergenicity among aminoglycosides has been demonstrated.

Patients should be well hydrated during treatment.

Although the *in vitro* mixing of gentamicin and carbenicillin results in a rapid and significant inactivation of gentamicin, this interaction has not been demonstrated in patients with normal renal function who received both drugs by different routes of administration. A reduction in gentamicin serum half-life has been reported in patients with severe renal impairment receiving carbenicillin concomitantly with gentamicin.

Treatment with gentamicin may result in overgrowth of nonsusceptible organisms. If this occurs, appropriate therapy is indicated. See "WARNINGS Box" regarding concurrent and/or sequential use of other neurotoxic and /or nephrotoxic antibiotics and for other essential information.

Usage in Pregnancy—Safety for use in pregnancy has not been established.

Adverse Reactions: *Nephrotoxicity* Adverse renal effects, as demonstrated by the presence of casts, cells or protein in the urine or by rising BUN, NPN, serum creatinine or oliguria, have been reported. They occur more frequently in patients treated for longer periods or with larger dosages than recommended.

Neurotoxicity Serious adverse effects on both vestibular and auditory branches of the eighth nerve have been reported, primarily in patients with renal impairment and in patients on high doses and/or prolonged therapy. Symptoms include dizziness, vertigo, tinnitus, roaring in the ears and also hearing loss, which, as with the other aminoglycosides, may be irreversible. Hearing loss is usually manifested initially by diminution of high-tone acuity. Other factors which may increase the risk of toxicity include excessive dosage, dehydration and previous exposure to other ototoxic drugs.

Numbness, skin tingling, muscle twitching and convulsions have also been reported.

Note: The risk of toxic reactions is low in neonates, infants and children with normal renal function who do not receive GARAMYCIN Pediatric Injectable at higher doses or for longer periods of time than recommended.

Other reported adverse reactions possibly related to gentamicin include: respiratory depression, lethargy, confusion, depression, visual disturbances, decreased appetite, weight loss and hypotension and hypertension; rash, itching, urticaria, generalized burning, laryngeal edema, anaphylactoid reactions, fever, and headache; nausea, vomiting, increased salivation, and stomatitis; purpura, pseudotumor cerebri, acute organic brain syndrome, pulmonary fibrosis, alopecia, joint pain, transient hepatomegaly, and splenomegaly.

Laboratory abnormalities possibly related to gentamicin include: increased levels of serum transaminase (SGOT, SGPT), serum LDH and bilirubin; decreased serum calcium, magnesium, sodium, and potassium; anemia, leukopenia, granulocytopenia, transient agranulocytosis, eosinophilia, increased and decreased reticulocyte counts, and thrombocytopenia.

When local tolerance of GARAMYCIN Pediatric Injectable is generally excellent, there has been an occasional report of pain at the injection site. Subcutaneous atrophy or fat necrosis suggesting local irritation has been reported rarely.

Overdosage: In the event of overdose or toxic reactions, hemodialysis or peritoneal dialysis will aid in the removal of gentamicin from the blood. In the newborn infant, exchange transfusions may also be considered.

Dosage and Administration: GARAMYCIN Pediatric Injectable may be given intramuscularly or intravenously. The patient's pretreatment body weight should be obtained for calculation of correct dosage. The dosage of aminoglycosides in obese patients should be based on an estimate of the lean body mass. It is desirable to limit the duration of treatment with aminoglycosides to short term.

PATIENTS WITH NORMAL RENAL FUNCTION

Children: 6 to 7.5 mg/kg/day. (2.0 to 2.5 mg/kg administered every 8 hours.)

Infants and Neonates: 7.5 mg/kg/day. (2.5 mg/kg administered every 8 hours.)

Premature or Full-Term Neonates One Week of Age or Less: 5 mg/kg/day. (2.5 mg/kg administered every 12 hours.)

It is desirable to measure both peak and trough serum concentrations of gentamicin to determine the adequacy and safety of the dosage. When such measurements are feasible, they should be carried out periodically during therapy to assure adequate but not excessive drug levels. For example, the peak concentration (at 30 to 60 minutes after intramuscular injection)

Continued on next page

Information on Schering products appearing on these pages is effective as of September 30, 1982.

Schering—Cont.

is expected to be in the range of 3 to 5 mcg/ml. When monitoring peak concentrations after intramuscular or intravenous administration dosage should be adjusted so that prolonged levels above 12 mcg/ml ware avoided. When monitoring trough concentrations (just prior to the next dose), dosage should be adjusted so that levels above 2 mcg/ml are avoided. Determination of the adequacy of a serum level for a particular patient must take into consideration the susceptibility of the causative organism, the severity of the infection, and the status of the patient's host-defense mechanisms.
In patients with extensive burns, altered pharmacokinetics may result in reduced serum concentrations of aminoglycosides. In such patients treated with gentamicin, measurement of serum concentrations is recommended as a basis for dosage adjustment.
The usual duration of treatment is seven to ten days. In difficult and complicated infections, a longer course of therapy may be necessary. In such cases monitoring of renal, auditory, and vestibular functions is recommended, since toxicity is more apt to occur with treatment extended for more than ten days. Dosage should be reduced if clinically indicated.

For Intravenous Administration

The intravenous administration of gentamicin may be particularly useful for treating patients with bacterial septicemia or those in shock. It may also be the preferred route of administration for some patients with congestive heart failure, hematologic disorders, severe burns, or those with reduced muscle mass.
For intermittent intravenous administration, a single dose of GARAMYCIN Pediatric Injectable may be diluted in sterile isotonic saline solution or in a sterile solution of dextrose 5% in water. The solution may be infused over a period of one-half to two hours.
The recommended dosage of intravenous and intramuscular administration is identical.
GARAMYCIN Pediatric Injectable should not be physically premixed with other drugs, but should be administered separately in accordance with the recommended route of administration and dosage schedule.

PATIENTS WITH IMPAIRED RENAL FUNCTION

Dosage must be adjusted in patients with impaired renal function. Whenever possible, serum concentrations of gentamicin should be monitored. One method of dosage adjustment is to increase the interval between administration of the usual doses. Since the serum creatinine concentration has a high correlation with the serum half-life of gentamicin, this laboratory test may provide guidance for adjustment of the interval between doses. In adults, the interval between doses (in hours) may be approximated by multiplying the serum creatinine level (mg/100 ml) by 8. For example, a patient weighing 60 kg. with a serum creatinine level of 2.0 mg/100 ml could be given 60 mg. (1 mg/kg) every 16 hours (2 × 8). These guidelines may be considered when treating infants and children with serious renal impairment.
In patients with serious systemic infections and renal impairment, it may be desirable to administer the antibiotic more frequently but in reduced dosage. In such patients, serum concentrations of gentamicin should be measured so that adequate but not excessive levels result. A peak and trough concentration measured intermittently during therapy will provide optimal guidance for adjusting dosage. After the usual initial dose, a rough guide for determining reduced dosage at eight-hour intervals is to divide the normally recommended dose by the serum creatinine level (Table 1). For example, after an initial dose of 20 mg. (2.0 mg/kg), a child weighing 10 kg with a serum creatinine level of 2.0 mg/100 ml could be given 10 mg. every eight hours (20 ÷ 2). It should be noted that the status of renal function may be changing over the course of the infectious process. It is important to recognize that deteriorating renal function may require a greater reduction in dosage than that specified in the above guidelines for patients with stable renal impairment.

TABLE 1
DOSAGE ADJUSTMENT GUIDE FOR PATIENTS WITH RENAL IMPAIRMENT
(Dosage at Eight-Hour Intervals After the Usual Initial Dose)

Serum Creatinine (mg %)	Approximate Creatinine Clearance Rate (ml/min/1.73M²)	Percent of Usual Doses Shown Above
≤ 1.0	> 100	100
1.1–1.3	70–100	80
1.4–1.6	55–70	65
1.7–1.9	45–55	55
2.0–2.2	40–45	50
2.3–2.5	35–40	40
2.6–3.0	30–35	35
3.1–3.5	25–30	30
3.6–4.0	20–25	25
4.1–5.1	15–20	20
5.2–6.6	10–15	15
6.7–8.0	< 10	10

In patients with renal failure undergoing hemodialysis, the amount of gentamicin removed from the blood may vary depending upon several factors including the dialysis method used. An eight-hour hemodialysis may reduce serum concentrations of gentamicin by approximately 50%. In children, the recommended dose at the end of each dialysis period is 2.0 to 2.5 mg/kg depending upon the severity of infection.
The above dosage schedules are not intended as rigid recommendations but are provided as guides to dosage when the measurement of gentamicin serum levels is not feasible.
A variety of methods are available to measure gentamicin concentrations in body fluids; these include microbiologic, enzymatic and radioimmunoassay techniques.
How Supplied: GARAMYCIN Pediatric Injectable, 10 mg. per ml., for parenteral administration, supplied in 2 ml. (20 mg.) vials; box of one.
Also available, GARAMYCIN Injectable, 40 mg. per ml., for parenteral administration, supplied in 2 ml. (80 mg.) vials, boxes of 1 and 25; 20 ml (800 mg) vials, box of 5; and in 1.5 ml. (60 mg.) and 2 ml. (80 mg.) disposable syringes, each in boxes of 1 and 10.
GARAMYCIN Pediatric Injectable is a clear, stable solution that requires no refrigeration.
Store between 2° and 30°C (36° and 86°F).

Schering Pharmaceutical Corporation (PR)
Manati, Puerto Rico 00701
An Affiliate of Schering Corporation
Kenilworth, N.J. 07033

Copyright © 1968, 1981, Schering Corporation. All rights reserved.

GARAMYCIN® I.V. ℞
Piggyback Injection **Sterile**
brand of gentamicin sulfate, USP
1 mg per ml
Each ml contains gentamicin sulfate, USP equivalent to 1 mg gentamicin.
For Intermittent Intravenous Infusion

Warnings: Patients treated with aminoglycosides should be under close clinical observation because of the potential toxicity associated with their use.
As with other aminoglycosides, gentamicin sulfate is potentially nephrotoxic. The risk of nephrotoxicity is greater in patients with impaired renal function and in those who receive high dosage or prolonged therapy.
Neurotoxicity manifested by ototoxicity, both vestibular and auditory, can occur in patients treated with gentamicin sulfate, primarily in those with preexisting renal damage and in patients with normal renal function treated with higher doses and/or for longer periods than recommended. Other manifestations of neurotoxicity may include numbness, skin tingling, muscle twitching and convulsions.
Renal and eighth cranial nerve function should be closely monitored, especially in patients with known or suspected reduced renal function at onset of therapy and also in those whose renal function is initially normal but who develop signs of renal dysfunction during therapy. Urine should be examined for decreased specific gravity, increased excretion of protein, and the presence of cells or casts. Blood urea nitrogen, serum creatinine, or creatinine clearance should be determined periodically. When feasible, it is recommended that serial audiograms be obtained in patients old enough to be tested, particularly high-risk patients. Evidence of ototoxicity (dizziness, vertigo, tinnitus, roaring in the ears or hearing loss) or nephrotoxicity requires dosage adjustment or discontinuance of the drug. As with the other aminoglycosides, on rare occasions changes in renal and eighth cranial nerve function may not become manifest until soon after completion of therapy.
Serum concentrations of aminoglycosides should be monitored when feasible to assure adequate levels and to avoid potentially toxic levels. When monitoring gentamicin peak concentrations, dosage should be adjusted so that prolonged levels above 12 mcg/ml are avoided. When monitoring gentamicin trough concentrations, dosage should be adjusted so that levels above 2 mcg/ml are avoided. Excessive peak and/or trough serum concentrations of aminoglycosides may increase the risk of renal and eighth cranial nerve toxicity. In the event of overdose or toxic reactions, hemodialysis or peritoneal dialysis will aid in removal of gentamicin from the blood.
Concurrent and/or sequential systemic or topical use of other potentially neurotoxic and/or nephrotoxic drugs, such as cisplatin, cephaloridine, kanamycin, amikacin, neomycin, polymyxin B, colistin, paromomycin, tobramycin, vancomycin, and viomycin, should be avoided. Other factors which may increase patient risk of toxicity are advanced age and dehydration.
The concurrent use of gentamicin with potent diuretics, such as ethacrynic acid or furosemide, should be avoided, since certain diuretics by themselves may cause ototoxicity. In addition, when administered intravenously, diuretics may enhance aminoglycoside toxicity by altering the antibiotic concentration in serum and tissue.

Description: Gentamicin sulfate, USP, a water-soluble antibiotic of the aminoglycoside group, is derived from *Micromonospora purpurea*, an actinomycete. GARAMYCIN I.V. Piggyback Injection is a sterile, aqueous solution for intravenous infusion. Each ml contains gentamicin sulfate, USP, equivalent to 1 mg gentamicin base; and 8.9 mg sodium chloride. It does not contain preservatives.
Clinical Pharmacology: When gentamicin sulfate is administered by intravenous infusion over a two-hour period, the serum concentrations are similar to those obtained by intramuscular administration. Peak serum concen-

trations following intravenous administration occur 30 to 60 minutes following cessation of infusion. Serum levels are measurable for 6 to 8 hours.
In patients with normal renal function, peak serum concentrations of gentamicin (mcg/ml) are usually up to four times the single intramuscular dose (mg/kg); for example, a 1.0 mg/kg injection in adults may be expected to result in a peak serum concentration up to 4 mcg/ml; a 1.5 mg/kg dose may produce levels up to 6 mcg/ml. While some variation is to be expected due to a number of variables such as age, body temperature, surface area, and physiologic differences, the individual patient given the same dose tends to have similar levels in repeated determinations. Gentamicin administered at 1.0 mg/kg every eight hours for the usual 7- to 10-day treatment period to patients with normal renal function does not accumulate in the serum.
Gentamicin, like all aminoglycosides, may accumulate in the serum and tissues of patients treated with higher doses and for prolonged periods, particularly in the presence of impaired renal function. In adult patients, treatment with gentamicin dosages of 4 mg/kg/day or higher for seven to ten days may result in a slight, progressive rise in both peak and trough concentrations. In patients with impaired renal function, gentamicin is cleared from the body more slowly than in patients with normal renal function. The more severe the impairment, the slower the clearance. (Dosage must be adjusted.)
Since gentamicin is distributed in extracellular fluid, peak serum concentrations may be lower than usual in adult patients who have a large volume of this fluid. Serum concentrations of gentamicin in febrile patients may be lower than those in afebrile patients given the same dose. When body temperature returns to normal, serum concentrations of the drug may rise. Febrile and anemic states may be associated with a shorter than usual serum half-life. (Dosage adjustment is usually not necessary.)
In severely burned patients, the half-life may be significantly decreased and resulting serum concentrations may be lower than anticipated from the mg/kg dose.
Protein binding studies have indiciated that the degree of gentamicin binding is low; depending upon the methods used for testing, this may be between 0 and 30%.
After initial administration to patients with normal renal function, generally 70% or more of the gentamicin dose is recoverable in the urine in 24 hours; concentrations in urine above 100 mcg/ml may be achieved. Little, if any, metabolic transformation occurs; the drug is excreted principally by glomerular filtration. After several days of treatment, the amount of gentamicin excreted in the urine approaches the daily dose administered. As with other aminoglycosides, a small amount of the gentamicin dose may be retained in the tissues, especially in the kidneys. Minute quantities of aminoglycosides have been detected in the urine weeks after drug administration was discontinued. Renal clearance of gentamicin is similar to that of endogenous creatinine.
In patients with marked impairment of renal function, there is a decrease in the concentration of aminoglycosides in urine and in their penetration into defective renal parenchyma. This decreased drug excretion, together with the potential nephrotoxicity of aminoglycosides, should be considered when treating such patients who have urinary tract infections.
Probenecid does not affect renal tubular transport of gentamicin.
The endogenous creatinine clearance rate and the serum creatinine level have a high correlation with the half-life of gentamicin in serum. Results of these tests may serve as guides for adjusting dosage in patients with renal impairment (see DOSAGE AND ADMINISTRATION).

Following parenteral administration, gentamicin can be detected in serum, lymph, tissues, sputum, and in pleural, synovial, and peritoneal fluids. Concentrations in renal cortex sometimes may be eight times higher than the usual serum levels. Concentrations in bile, in general, have been low and have suggested minimal biliary excretion. Gentamicin crosses the peritoneal as well as the placental membranes. Since aminoglycosides diffuse poorly into the subarachnoid space after parenteral administration, concentrations of gentamicin in cerebrospinal fluid are often low and dependent upon dose, rate of penetration, and degree of meningeal inflammation. There is minimal penetration of gentamicin into ocular tissues following intramuscular or intravenous administration.

Microbiology: *In vitro* tests have demonstrated that gentamicin is a bactericidal antibiotic which acts by inhibiting normal protein synthesis in susceptible microorganisms. It is active against a wide variety of pathogenic bacteria including *Escherichia coli, Proteus* species (indole-positive and indole-negative). *Pseudomonas aeruginosa*, species of the *Klebsiella-Enterobacter-Serratia* group, *Citrobacter* species and *Staphylococcus* species (including penicillin- and methicillin-resistant strains). Gentamicin is also active *in vitro* against species of *Salmonella* and *Shigella*. The following bacteria are usually resistant to aminoglycosides: *Streptococcus pneumoniae*, most species of streptococci, particularly group D and anaerobic organisms, such as *Bacteroides* species or *Clostridium* species.
In vitro studies have shown that an aminoglycoside combined with an antibiotic that interferes with cell wall synthesis may act synergistically against some group D streptococcal strains. The combination of gentamicin and penicillin G has a synergistic bactericidal effect against virtually all strains of *Streptococcus faecalis* and its varieties *(S. faecalis* var. *liquifaciens, S. Faecalis* var. *zymogenes), S. faecium* and *S. durans*. An enhanced killing effect against many of these strains has also been shown *in vitro* with combinations of gentamicin and ampicillin, carbenicillin, nafcillin, or oxacillin.
The combined effect of gentamicin and carbenicillin is synergistic for many strains of *Pseudomonas aeruginosa*. *In vitro* synergism against other gram-negative organisms has been shown with combinations of gentamicin and cephalosporins.
Gentamicin may be active against clinical isolates of bacteria resistant to other aminoglycosides.
Bacteria resistant to one aminoglycoside may be resistant to one or more other aminoglycosides. Bacterial resistance to gentamicin is generally developed slowly.

Susceptibility Testing: If the disc method of susceptibility testing used is that described by Bauer *et al.* (*Am J Clin Path* 45:493, 1966; *Federal Register* 37:20527-20529, 1972), a disc containing 10 mcg of gentamicin should give a zone of inhibition of 13mm or more to indicate susceptibility of the infecting organism. A zone of 12mm or less indicates that the infecting organism is likely to be resistant. In certain conditions it may be desirable to do additional susceptibility testing by the tube or agar dilution method; gentamicin substance is available for this purpose.

Indications and Usage: GARAMYCIN I.V. Piggyback Injection is indicated in the treatment of serious infections caused by susceptible strains of the following microorganisms: *Pseudomonas aeruginosa, Proteus* species (indole-positive and indole-negative), *Escherichia coli, Klebsiella-Enterobacter-Serratia* species, *Citrobacter* species and *Staphylococcus* species (coagulase-postive and coagulase-negative). Clinical studies have shown GARAMYCIN to be effective in bacterial neonatal sepsis; bacterial septicemia; and serious bacterial infections of the central nervous system (meningitis), urinary tract, respiratory tract, gastrointestinal tract (including peritonitis), skin, bone and soft tissue (including burns). Aminoglycosides, including gentamicin, are not indicated in uncomplicated initial episodes of urinary tract infections unless the causative organisms are susceptible to these antibiotics and are not susceptible to antibiotics having less potential for toxicity.
Specimens for bacterial culture should be obtained to isolate and identify causative organisms and to determine their susceptibility to gentamicin.
GARAMYCIN may be considered as initial therapy in suspected or confirmed gram-negative infections, and therapy may be instituted before obtaining results of susceptibility testing. The decision to continue therapy with this drug should be based on the results of susceptibility tests, the severity of the infection, and the important additional concepts contained in the "WARNINGS Box" above. If the causative organisms are resistant to gentamicin, other appropriate therapy should be instituted.
In serious infections when the causative organisms are unknown, GARAMYCIN may be administered as initial therapy in conjunction with a penicillin-type or cephalosporin-type drug before obtaining results of susceptibility testing. If anaerobic organisms are suspected as etiologic agents, consideration should be given to using other suitable antimicrobial therapy in conjunction with gentamicin. Following identification of the organism and its susceptibility, appropriate antibiotic therapy should then be continued. GARAMYCIN has been used effectively in combination with carbenicillin for the treatment of life-threatening infections caused by *Pseudomonas aeruginosa*. It has also been found effective when used in conjunction with a penicillin-type drug for the treatment of endocarditis caused by group D streptococci.
GARAMYCIN has also been shown to be effective in the treatment of serious staphylococcal infections. While not the antibiotic of first choice, GARAMYCIN may be considered when penicillins or other less potentially toxic drugs are contraindicated and bacterial susceptibility tests and clinical judgment indicate its use. It may also be considered in mixed infections caused by susceptible strains of staphylococci and gram-negative organisms.
In the neonate with suspected bacterial sepsis or staphylococcal pneumonia, a penicillin-type drug is also usually indicated as concomitant therapy with gentamicin.

Contraindications: Hypersensitivity to gentamicin is a contraindication to its use. A history of hypersensitivity or serious toxic reactions to other aminoglycosides may contraindicate use of gentamicin because of the known cross-sensitivity of patients to drugs in this class.

Warnings: (See "WARNINGS Box" above.)

Precautions: Neurotoxic and nephrotoxic antibiotics may be absorbed in significant quantities from body surfaces after local irrigation or application. The potential toxic effect of antibiotics administered in this fashion should be considered.
Increased nephrotoxicity has been reported following concomitant administration of aminoglycoside antibiotics and cephalosporins.
Neuromuscular blockade and respiratory paralysis have been reported in the cat receiving high doses (40 mg/kg) of gentamicin. The possibility of these phenomena occurring in man should be considered if aminoglycosides are

Continued on next page

Information on Schering products appearing on these pages is effective as of September 30, 1982.

Schering—Cont.

administered by any route to patients receiving anesthetics, or to patients receiving neuromuscular blocking agents, such as succinylcholine, tubocurarine, or decamethonium, or in patients receiving massive transfusions of citrate-anticoagulated blood. If neuromuscular blockade occurs, calcium salts may reverse it. Aminoglycosides should be used with caution in patients with neuromuscular disorders, such as myasthenia gravis or parkinsonism, since these drugs may aggravate muscle weakness because of their potential curare-like effects on the neuromuscular junction.
Elderly patients may have reduced renal function which may not be evident in the results of routine screening tests, such as BUN or serum creatinine. A creatinine clearance determination may be more useful. Monitoring of renal function during treatment with gentamicin, as with other aminoglycosides, is particularly important in such patients.
Cross-allergenicity among aminoglycosides has been demonstrated.
Patients should be well hydrated during treatment.
Although the *in vitro* mixing of gentamicin and carbenicillin results in a rapid and significant inactivation of gentamicin, this interaction has not been demonstrated in patients with normal renal function who received both drugs by different routes of administration. A reduction in gentamicin serum half-life has been reported in patients with severe renal impairment receiving carbenicillin concomitantly with gentamicin.
Treatment with gentamicin may result in overgrowth of nonsusceptible organisms. If this occurs, appropriate therapy is indicated. See "WARNINGS Box" regarding concurrent use of potent diuretics and regarding concurrent and/or sequential use of other neurotoxic and/or nephrotoxic antibiotics and for other essential information.
Usage in Pregnancy—Safety for use in pregnancy has not been established.
Adverse Reactions: *Nephrotoxicity* Adverse renal effects, as demonstrated by the presence of casts, cells, or protein in the urine or by rising BUN, NPN, serum creatinine or oliguria, have been reported. They occur more frequently in patients with a history of renal impairment and in patients treated for longer periods or with larger dosage than recommended.
Neurotoxicity Serious adverse effects of both vestibular and auditory branches of the eighth nerve have been reported, primarily in patients with renal impairment and in patients on high doses and/or prolonged therapy. Symptoms include dizziness, vertigo, tinnitus, roaring in the ears and also hearing loss, which, as with the other aminoglycosides, may be irreversible. Hearing loss is usually manifested initially by diminution of high-tone acuity. Other factors which may increase the risk of toxicity include excessive dosage, dehydration and previous exposure to other ototoxic drugs.
Numbness, skin tingling, muscle twitching and convulsions have also been reported.
Note: The risk of toxic reactions is low in patients with normal renal function who do not receive GARAMYCIN at higher doses or for longer periods of time than recommended.
Other reported adverse reactions possibly related to gentamicin include: respiratory depression, lethargy, confusion, depression, visual disturbances, decreased appetite, weight loss, and hypotension and hypertension; rash, itching, urticaria, generalized burning, laryngeal edema, anaphylactoid reactions, fever, and headache; nausea, vomiting, increased salivation, and stomatitis; purpura, pseudotumor cerebri, acute organic brain syndrome, pulmonary fibrosis, alopecia, joint pain, transient hepatomegaly, and splenomegaly.
Laboratory abnormalities possibly related to gentamicin include: increased levels of serum transaminase (SGOT, SGPT), serum LDH and bilirubin; decreased serum calcium, magnesium, sodium and potassium; anemia, leukopenia, granulocytopenia, transient agranulocytosis, eosinophilia, increased and decreased reticulocyte counts, and thrombocytopenia.
While local tolerance of GARAMYCIN is generally excellent, there has been an occasional report of pain at the injection site. Subcutaneous atrophy or fat necrosis suggesting local irritation has been reported rarely.
Overdosage: In the event of overdose or toxic reactions, hemodialysis or peritoneal dialysis will aid in the removal of gentamicin from the blood.
Dosage and Administration: GARAMYCIN I.V. Piggyback Injection should only be administered intravenously. This product does not contain a preservative system; the contents must be used promptly after the seal is broken. Any unused portion must be discarded. DO NOT RETAIN FOR LATER USE.

TABLE I
DOSAGE SCHEDULE GUIDE FOR ADULTS WITH NORMAL RENAL FUNCTION
(Dosage at Eight-Hour Intervals)
1 mg/ml

Patient's Weight* kg (lb)	Usual Dose for Serious Infections 1 mg/kg q8h (3 mg/kg/day)	Dose for Life-Threatening Infections (Reduce As Soon As Clinically Indicated) 1.7 mg/kg q8h** (5 mg/kg/day)
	mg/dose	mg/dose
40 (88)	40	66
45 (99)	45	75
50 (110)	50	83
55 (121)	55	91
60 (132)	60	100
65 (143)	65	108
70 (154)	70	116
75 (165)	75	125
80 (176)	80	133
85 (187)	85	141
90 (198)	90	150
95 (209)	95	158
100 (220)	100	166

* The dosage of aminoglycosides in obese patients should be based on an estimate of the lean body mass.
** For q6h schedules, dosage should be recalculated.

It is desirable to limit the duration of treatment with aminoglycosides to short-term.
The usual duration of treatment for all patients is seven to ten days. In difficult and complicated infections, a longer course of therapy may be necessary. In such cases monitoring of renal auditory, and vestibular functions is recommended, since toxicity is more apt to occur with treatment extended for more than ten days. Dosage should be reduced if clinically indicated.
The patient's pretreatment body weight should be obtained for calculation of correct dosage. The dosage of aminoglycosides in obese patients should be based on an estimate of the lean body mass.
In patients with extensive burns, altered pharmacokinetics may result in reduced serum concentrations of aminoglycosides. In such patients treated with gentamicin, measurement of serum concentrations is recommended as a basis for dosage adjustment.
It is desirable to measure both peak and trough serum concentrations of gentamicin to determine the adequacy and safety of the dosage. When such measurements are feasible, they should be carried out periodically during therapy to assure adequate but not excessive drug levels. For example, the peak concentrations (at 30 to 60 minutes following cessation of infusion) is expected to be in the range of 4 to 6 mcg/ml. When monitoring peak concentrations, dosage should be adjusted so that prolonged levels above 12 mcg/ml are avoided. When monitoring trough concentrations (just prior to the next dose), dosage should be adjusted so that levels above 2 mcg/ml are avoided. Determination of the adequacy of a serum level for a particular patient must take into consideration the susceptibility of the causative organism, the severity of the infection, and the status of the patient's host-defense mechanisms.
The intravenous administration of gentamicin may be particularly useful for treating patients with bacterial septicemia or those in shock. It may also be the preferred route of administration for some patients with congestive heart failure, hematologic disorders, severe burns, or those with reduced muscle mass. The solution may be infused over a period of one-half to two hours.
GARAMYCIN I.V. Piggyback Injection should not be physically premixed with other drugs but should be administered separately in accordance with the recommended route of administration and dosage schedule.
The dosage recommendations which follow are not intended as rigid schedules, but are provided as guides for initial therapy or when the measurement of gentamicin serum levels during therapy is not feasible.

PATIENTS WITH NORMAL RENAL FUNCTION

Adults: The recommended dosage of GARAMYCIN I.V. Piggyback Injection for patients with serious infections and normal renal function is 3 mg/kg/day, administered in three equal doses every eight hours (Table I).
For patients with life-threatening infections, dosages up to 5 mg/kg/day may be administered in three or four equal doses. This dosage should be reduced to 3 mg/kg/day as soon as clinically indicated (Table I).
[See table left].
Children: 6 to 7.5 mg/kg/day (2.0 to 2.5 mg/kg administered every 8 hours.)
Infants and Neonates: 7.5 mg/kg/day (2.5 mg/kg administered every 8 hours).
Premature or Full-Term Neonates one week of age or less: 5 mg/kg/day (2.5 mg/kg administered every 12 hours).
Note: For further information concerning the use of gentamicin in infants and children, see GARAMYCIN Pediatric Injectable Product Information.

PATIENTS WITH IMPAIRED RENAL FUNCTION

Dosage must be adjusted in patients with impaired renal function. Whenever possible serum concentrations of gentamicin should be monitored. One method of dosage adjustment is to increase the interval between administration of the usual doses. Since the serum creatinine concentration has a high correlation with the serum half-life of gentamicin, this laboratory test may provide guidance for adjustment of the interval between doses. The interval between doses (in hours) may be approximated by multiplying the serum creatinine level (mg/100 ml) by 8. For example, a patient weighing 60 kg with a serum creatinine level of 2.0 mg/100 ml could be given 60 mg (1 mg/kg every 16 hours (2 × 8).

In patients with serious systemic infections and renal impairment, it may be desirable to administer the antibiotic more frequently but in reduced dosage. In such patients, serum concentrations of gentamicin should be measured so that adequate but not excessive levels result. A peak and trough concentration measured intermittently during therapy will provide optimal guidance for adjusting dosage. After the usual initial dose, a rough guide for determining reduced dosage at eight-hour intervals is to divide the normally recommended dose by the serum creatinine level (Table II). For example, after an initial dose of 60 mg (1 mg/kg), a patient weighing 60 kg with a serum creatinine level of 2.0 mg/100 ml could be given 30 mg every eight hours (60 ÷ 2). It should be noted that the status of renal function may be changing over the course of the infectious process.

It is important to recognize that deteriorating renal function may require a greater reduction in dosage than that specified in the above guidelines for patients with stable renal impairment.

[See table above].

In adults with renal failure undergoing hemodialysis, the amount of gentamicin removed from the blood may vary depending upon several factors including the dialysis method used. An eight-hour hemodialysis may reduce serum concentrations of gentamicin by approximately 50%. The recommended dosage at the end of each dialysis period is 1 to 1.7 mg/kg depending upon the severity of infection. In children, a dose of 2 mg/kg may be administered.

A variety of methods are available to measure gentamicin concentrations in body fluids; these include microbiologic, enzymatic and radio-immunoassay techniques.

INSTRUCTIONS FOR THE ADMINISTRATION OF GARAMYCIN I.V. PIGGYBACK INJECTION (For proper apparatus setup see accompanying Instruction Sheet).

THIS PRODUCT IS IN A READY-TO-USE FORM AND IS INTENDED FOR USE ONLY AS AN I.V. PIGGYBACK.

If the prescribed dose is exactly 60 or 80 mg, use the appropriate unit; if the prescribed dose is higher or lower than that of the supplied unit, adjustments can be made in either piggyback unit. If the dose is higher that the contents of the 80 mg unit, the additional amount should be removed from a vial of GARAMYCIN Injectable (40 mg/ml) and added to the 80 mg piggyback unit. If the prescribed dose is less, decrements can be made by removing and discarding the appropriate amount from either unit. **It should be kept in mind that each ml of the piggyback unit contains 1 mg of gentamicin.**

The following are specific examples of dosage adjustment:

- to prepare a 90 mg dose, remove ¼ ml from a vial of GARAMYCIN Injectable (40 mg/ml) and add to the 80 mg piggyback unit.
- to prepare a 70 mg dose, either remove and discard 10 ml from the 80 mg piggyback unit or add the 10 ml from the 80 mg piggyback unit to the 60 mg piggyback unit.
- to prepare a 40 mg dose, remove and discard 20 ml from the 60 mg piggyback unit.

Observe all precautions for sterile technique when adding or removing contents of these units.

How Supplied: GARAMYCIN I.V. Piggyback Injection, 1 mg per ml for intravenous infusion, is supplied in 60 ml (60 mg) and 80 ml (80 mg) units; box of one.

Store between 2° and 30°C (36° and 86°F).

Also available, GARAMYCIN Injectable, 40 mg per ml, for parenteral administration, is supplied in 2 ml (80 mg) vials; boxes of 1 and 25; and 20 ml vials; box of 5; and in 1.5 ml (60 mg) and 2 ml (80 mg) disposable syringes, each in boxes of 1 and 10.

GARAMYCIN Pediatric Injectable, 10 mg per ml for parenteral administration, supplied in 2 ml (20 mg) vials; box of one.

GARAMYCIN Products are clear, stable solutions that require no refrigeration.

Schering Pharmaceutical Corporation (P.R.),
Manati, Puerto Rico 00701
An Affiliate of Schering Corporation, Kenilworth, N.J. 07033

Revised 3/81

© 1968, 1980, 1981, Schering Corporation. All rights reserved.

TABLE II
DOSAGE ADJUSTMENT GUIDE FOR PATIENTS WITH RENAL IMPAIRMENT
(Dosage at Eight-Hour Intervals After the Usual Initial Dose)

Serum Creatinine (mg %)	Approximate Creatinine Clearance Rate (ml/min/1.73M²)	Percent of Usual Doses Shown in Table I
≤1.0	>100	100
1.1-1.3	70-100	80
1.4-1.6	55-70	65
1.7-1.9	45-55	55
2.0-2.2	40-45	50
2.3-2.5	35-40	40
2.6-3.0	30-35	35
3.1-3.5	25-30	30
3.6-4.0	20-25	25
4.1-5.1	15-20	20
5.2-6.6	10-15	15
6.7-8.0	<10	10

GARAMYCIN® Intrathecal ℞
brand of gentamicin sulfate, USP
Injection 2.0 mg/ml

FOR DIRECT ADMINISTRATION INTO THE CEREBROSPINAL FLUID SPACES OF THE CENTRAL NERVOUS SYSTEM

WARNINGS

GARAMYCIN Intrathecal Injection is intended as adjunctive therapy in patients with central nervous system infections.

Since patients considered for treatment with GARAMYCIN Intrathecal Injection will usually be receiving concomitant treatment with intramuscular or intravenous gentamicin sulfate, all warnings and precautions for this or other concomitantly administered agents must be observed. Moreover, when the drug is administered by more than one route, additive effects must be considered. (See GARAMYCIN Injectable or GARAMYCIN Pediatric Injectable Product Information.) Laboratory studies in animals have shown that gentamicin sulfate, when administered directly into the central nervous system, has caused neurologic disturbances, including adverse effects on the eighth cranial nerve. The risk of direct administration of a potentially neurotoxic drug into the cerebrospinal fluid spaces of the central nervous system must be weighed against the potential benefit to be derived from this route of administration.

Description: Gentamicin sulfate, USP, a water-soluble antibiotic of the aminoglycoside group, is derived from *Micromonospora purpurea*, an actinomycete. GARAMYCIN Intrathecal Injection is a sterile, aqueous solution for direct administration into the cerebrospinal fluid spaces of the central nervous system. Each ml contains: gentamicin sulfate, USP equivalent to 2.0 mg gentamicin base; and 8.5 mg sodium chloride.

Clinical Pharmacology: Since gentamicin sulfate and other aminoglycosides diffuse poorly into the subarachnoid space after systemic administration, concentrations of these antibiotics in the lumbar or ventricular cerebrospinal fluid (CSF) are often low. Following intramuscular or intravenous administration of the usual doses, gentamicin concentrations in CSF in the absence of infection are usually less than 1 mcg/ml. In acute meningitis, slightly higher concentrations are obtained but these vary and are usually well below the peak serum concentration. CSF concentrations which are attained following intravenous or intramuscular administration of gentamicin sulfate tend to become lower as meningeal inflammation subsides. GARAMYCIN Intrathecal Injections are intended to increase the concentration of gentamicin in the CSF when used as part of the management of patients with central nervous system infections.

When GARAMYCIN Intrathecal Injection is given concomitantly with systemically administered gentamicin sulfate, the CSF levels are substantially increased depending upon the location of the injection. Peak CSF concentrations which follow intralumbar administration generally occur at 1 to 6 hours after injection. Factors which affect the concentration of gentamicin in the CSF following injection into cerebrospinal fluid spaces are the dose administered, the site of the injection (intralumbar, intraventricular), the volume in which the dose is diluted, and the presence or absence of obstruction to the CSF flow. There appears to be considerable inter-patient variation.

The half-life of gentamicin in the CSF of adults who received intralumbar injections is approximately 5.5 hours; this is somewhat longer than that in serum.

In one pharmacokinetic study in adults, a 3 to 4 mg. intralumbar injection resulted in a mean CSF concentration of 6.2 mcg/ml 24 hours after injection. The mean CSF concentration was

Continued on next page

Information on Schering products appearing on these pages is effective as of September 30, 1982.

Schering—Cont.

noted to decrease with time; during days 1 through 6 of treatment with GARAMYCIN Intrathecal Injection by the intralumbar route, the mean 24-hour concentration was 9.9 mcg/ml, while during days 7 through 13, the mean concentration was 3.7 mcg/ml.
In another study in adults, CSF levels were measured at varying intervals after intralumbar administration of gentamicin sulfate. During days 1 through 6 of treatment, a 4 mg. dose produced a mean CSF level of 2.4 mcg/ml 24 hours after injection, while during days 7 through 13, the same dose produced a mean 24-hour level of 0.5 mcg/ml.
Following intralumbar administration there may be limited upward diffusion of the drug, presumably because of the direction of the CSF flow. Intraventricular administration produces high concentrations in the ventricles and throughout the central nervous system. Adequate levels will usually result from dosing every 24 hours, but it is desirable to manage each patient's infection with serial monitoring of gentamicin serum and CSF concentrations.
Microbiology: *In vitro* tests have demonstrated that gentamicin is a bactericidal antibiotic which acts by inhibiting normal protein synthesis in susceptible microorganisms. It is active against a wide variety of pathogenic bacteria including *Escherichia coli, Proteus* species (indole-positive and indole-negative), *Pseudomonas aeruginosa,* species of the *Klebsiella-Enterobacter-Serratia* group, *Citrobacter* species, and *Staphlococcus* species (including penicillin- and methicillin-resistant strains). Gentamicin is also active *in vitro* against species of *Salmonella* and *Shigella.* The following bacteria are usually resistant to aminoglycosides: *Streptococcus pneumoniae,* most species of streptococci, particularly group D and anaerobic organisms, such as *Bacteroides* species or *Clostridium* species.
In vitro studies have shown that an aminoglycoside combined with an antibiotic that interferes with cell wall synthesis may act synergistically against some group D streptococcal strains. The combination of gentamicin sulfate and penicillin G has a synergistic bactericidal effect against virtually all strains of *Streptococcus faecalis* and its varieties *(S. faecalis* var. *liquifaciens, S. faecalis* var. *zymogenes), S. faecium* and *S. durans.* An enhanced killing effect against many of these strains has also been shown *in vitro* with combinations of gentamicin and ampicillin, carbenicillin, nafcillin, or oxacillin.
The combined effect of gentamicin and carbenicillin is synergistic for many strains of *Pseudomonas aeruginosa.*
Gentamicin may be active against clinical isolates of bacteria resistant to other aminoglycosides. However, bacteria resistant to one aminoglycoside may be resistant to one or more other aminoglycosides.
Susceptibility Testing: If the disc method of susceptibility testing used is that described by Bauer *et al* (*Am J Clin Path* **45**:493, 1966; *Federal Register* **37**:20527–20529, 1972), a disc containing 10 mcg. of gentamicin, when tested against a bacterial strain susceptible to gentamicin, should give a zone of inhibition of $\geq$ 13 mm. A zone of $\leq$ 12 mm. indicates resistance. In certain conditions it may be desirable to do additional susceptibility testing by the broth or agar dilution method; gentamicin substance is available for this purpose.
Indications and Usage: GARAMYCIN Intrathecal Injection is indicated as adjunctive therapy to systemically administered gentamicin sulfate in the treatment of serious central nervous system infections (meningitis, ventriculitis) caused by susceptible *Pseudomonas* species.
Bacteriologic tests should be performed to determine that the causative organisms are *Pseudomonas* species susceptible to gentamicin.
Contraindications: Hypersensitivity to gentamicin sulfate is a contraindication to its use. A history of hypersensitivity or serious toxic reactions to aminoglycosides may also contraindicate use of gentamicin sulfate because of the known cross-sensitivity of patients to drugs in this class.
Warnings: (See "WARNINGS Box" above and the WARNINGS listed in the Product Information for GARAMYCIN Injectable and GARAMYCIN Pediatric Injectable.)
Precautions: (See PRECAUTIONS listed in the Product Information for GARAMYCIN Injectable and GARAMYCIN Pediatric Injectable.)
In a patient with a seven-year history of multiple sclerosis who was treated with gentamicin sulfate by intralumbar injection, disseminated microscopic lesions of the brain stem were reported at autopsy. Lesions observed were: tissue rarefaction with loss and marked swelling of axis cylinders with occasional calcification, loss of oligodendroglia and astroglia, and a poor inflammatory response.
Safety and efficacy in children below the age of three months have not been established.
Adverse Reactions: Local tolerance to GARAMYCIN Intrathecal Injection has been good. Local reactions of arachnoiditis or burning at the injection site have been reported rarely.
Because the recommended dosage of GARAMYCIN Intrathecal Injection is low, the potential for systemic adverse effects is minimal. However, GARAMYCIN Intrathecal Injection is recommended as adjunctive therapy with other antibiotics, such as parenteral gentamicin sulfate, which should be administered in full therapeutic dosages. Evidence of eighth nerve dysfunction, changes in renal function, leg cramps, rash, fever, convulsions, and an increase in cerebrospinal fluid protein have been reported in patients who were treated concomitantly with GARAMYCIN Intrathecal Injection and the parenteral preparation of gentamicin.
Administration of excessive (40 to 160 mg.) doses of the parenteral formulation of gentamicin sulfate (which contains a preservative system) by the various intrathecal routes has been reported to produce neuromuscular disturbances, e.g., ataxia, paresis, and incontinence.
Dosage and Administration: GARAMYCIN Intrathecal Injection is intended for administration directly into the cerebrospinal fluid spaces of the central nervous system.
The dosage will vary depending upon factors, such as age and weight of the patient, site of injection, degree of obstruction to cerebrospinal fluid flow and the amount of cerebrospinal fluid estimated to be present. In general, the recommended dose for infants 3 months of age and older (see PRECAUTIONS) and children is 1 to 2 mg. once a day. For adults, 4 to 8 mg. may be administered once a day.
Administration of GARAMYCIN Intrathecal Injection should be continued as long as sensitive organisms are demonstrated in the cerebrospinal fluid. Since the intralumbar or intraventricular dose is administered immediately after specimens are taken for laboratory study, treatment should usually be continued for at least one day after negative results have been obtained from CSF cultures and/or stained smears.
The suggested method for administering GARAMYCIN Intrathecal Injection into the lumbar area is as follows: the desired quantity of GARAMYCIN Intrathecal Injection is drawn up carefully from the ampule into a 5- or 10-ml. sterile syringe. After the lumbar puncture is performed and a specimen of the spinal fluid is removed for laboratory tests, the syringe containing GARAMYCIN Intrathecal Injection is inserted into the hub of the spinal needle. A quantity of cerebrospinal fluid (approximately 10% of the estimated total CSF volume) is allowed to flow into the syringe and mix with the GARAMYCIN Intrathecal Injection. The resultant solution is then injected over a period of 3 to 5 minutes with the bevel of the needle directed upward.
If the cerebrospinal fluid is grossly purulent, or if it is unobtainable, GARAMYCIN Intrathecal Injection may be diluted with sterile normal saline before injection.
GARAMYCIN Intrathecal Injection may also be administered directly into the subdural space or directly into the ventricles, including administration by use of an implanted reservoir.
How Supplied: GARAMYCIN Intrathecal Injection, 2.0 mg. per ml., is supplied in 2 ml. ampules; box of 25.
Store below 30°C (86°F).
NOTE: This preparation does not contain any preservative. Once opened, contents should be used immediately and unused portions should be discarded.
Animal Pharmacology and Toxicology: In dogs, an 8-hour perfusion of the ventriculosubarachnoid system with a solution containing 40 mcg/ml (~5 mg. or ~0.3 mg/kg) gentamicin produced no seizure activity or change in vital signs during administration. No morphological changes were observed when the dogs were sacrificed at 10 and 90 days following infusion.
The effects of repeated intrathecal injections of gentamicin at 0.1 and 0.3 mg/kg were evaluated in tranquilized beagle puppies. Transient flaccid paralysis was observed on the first day when the drug was administered rapidly (i.e., in less than 5 seconds), but no adverse effects were observed thereafter when the drug was administered less rapidly (i.e., over a period of approximately 30 seconds). No drug-related changes were found on histological examination of the cerebellum, brain stem or cephalic cord. In cats, gentamicin administered intracisternally at one-hour intervals in doses of up to 50 mg/kg did not produce any abnormalities in the electroencephalogram. In another study in cats, gentamicin sulfate given daily by the intracisternal route for up to 7 days caused neurologic disturbances, including adverse effects on the eighth cranial nerve.
In rabbits intracisternal injection of gentamicin at doses 50 and 100 times the therapeutic dose produced peak CSF concentrations of 160 and 180 mcg/ml, respectively. These doses were associated with changes in the myelin sheath predominantly of the lateral columns of the upper cervical cord, and some changes in glial cells and lesions in the medulla oblongata. In addition to a high incidence of mortality, the animals demonstrated weakness, ataxia and paralysis. At doses of one and ten times the therapeutic dose (providing peak levels of 16.5 and 40 mcg/ml CSF), no morphologic changes occurred and there were no drug-related symptoms identified.

Schering Pharmaceutical Corporation (PR)
Manati, Puerto Rico 00701
An Affiliate of Schering Corporation
Kenilworth, New Jersey 07033

Copyright © 1979, 1981, Schering Corporation. All rights reserved.

GYNE-LOTRIMIN® ℞
brand of clotrimazole, USP
Vaginal Tablets, Vaginal Cream 1%

Description: GYNE-LOTRIMIN is clotrimazole [1-(*o*-Chloro-*α*, *α*-diphenylbenzyl) imidazole], a synthetic antifungal agent having the chemical formula $C_{22}H_{17}ClN_2$.
Each GYNE-LOTRIMIN Vaginal Tablet contains 100 mg clotrimazole, USP dispersed in lactose, povidone, corn starch, and magnesium stearate.

Each applicatorful of GYNE-LOTRIMIN Vaginal Cream contains approximately 50 mg clotrimazole, USP dispersed in sorbitan monostearate, polysorbate 60, cetyl esters wax, cetearyl alcohol, 2-octyldodecanol, purified water, and as preservative, benzyl alcohol (1%).

Actions: Clotrimazole is a broad-spectrum antifungal agent that inhibits the growth of pathogenic yeasts. Clotrimazole exhibits fungicidal activity *in vitro* against *Candida albicans* and other species of the genus *Candida*.

No single-step or multiple-step resistance to clotrimazole has developed during successive passages of *Candida albicans*.

Indications: GYNE-LOTRIMIN is indicated for the local treatment of patients with vulvovaginal candidiasis (moniliasis). The diagnosis should be confirmed by KOH smears and/or cultures. Other pathogens commonly associated with vulvovaginitis (*Trichomonas* and *Hemophilus vaginalis*) should be ruled out by appropriate laboratory methods.

Studies have shown that women taking oral contraceptives had a cure rate similar to those not taking oral contraceptives.

Contraindications: GYNE-LOTRIMIN Vaginal Tablets and Vaginal Cream are contraindicated in women who have shown hypersensitivity to any of the components of the preparation.

Precautions: Laboratory Tests: If there is a lack of response to GYNE-LOTRIMIN, appropriate microbiological studies should be repeated to confirm the diagnosis and rule out other pathogens before instituting another course of antimycotic therapy.

Application of ^{14}C-labeled clotrimazole has shown negligible absorption (peak of 0.03 mcg/ml of serum 24 hours after insertion of a 100 mg tablet; peak serum level of 0.01 mcg/ml 24 hours after insertion of vaginal cream containing 50 mg of active drug) from both normal and inflamed human vaginal mucosa.

Usage in Pregnancy: While GYNE-LOTRIMIN Vaginal Tablets and Cream have not been studied in the first trimester of pregnancy, use in the second and third trimesters has not been associated with ill effects. Follow-up reports now available on 71 neonates of 177 pregnant patients treated with GYNE-LOTRIMIN Vaginal Tablets reveal no adverse effects or complications attributable to GYNE-LOTRIMIN therapy.

Adverse Reactions: Eighteen (1.6%) of the 1116 patients treated with GYNE-LOTRIMIN Vaginal Tablets in double-blind studies reported complaints during therapy that were possibly drug-related. Mild burning occurred in six patients while other complaints, such as skin rash, itching, vulval irritation, lower abdominal cramps and bloating, slight cramping, slight urinary frequency, and burning or irritation in the sexual partner, occurred rarely. Three (0.5%) of the 653 patients treated with GYNE-LOTRIMIN Vaginal Cream reported complaints during therapy that were possibly drug-related. Vaginal burning occurred in one patient; erythema, irritation and burning in another; intercurrent cystitis was reported in the third.

Dosage and Administration: *Nonpregnant Patients:* Either of the following GYNE-LOTRIMIN Vaginal Tablets regimens (they are similarly effective) may be used in nonpregnant patients:

Two tablets inserted intravaginally at bedtime for three nights, or one tablet inserted intravaginally at bedtime for seven nights.

Pregnant Patients: Only one regimen is recommended for pregnant patients: One tablet inserted intravaginally at bedtime for seven nights. The three-day regimen did not prove to be effective in pregnant patients.

In the event of treatment failure, other pathogens commonly responsible for vaginitis should be ruled out before instituting another course of antimycotic therapy. There are no studies to show whether a second course of clotrimazole would be effective in patients who fail to respond to the initial course.

GYNE-LOTRIMIN Vaginal Cream has been found to be effective when used from seven to fourteen days; studies have shown that patients treated for fourteen days had a significantly higher cure rate. The recommended dose is one applicatorful of cream (approximately 5 grams) intravaginally preferably at bedtime.

How Supplied: GYNE-LOTRIMIN Vaginal Tablets, 100 mg, white, uncoated tablets impressed with the trademark (GYNE-LOTRIMIN) and/or the Schering trademark and product identification numbers, 734; carton of six tablets for three-day treatment regimen and carton of seven tablets for seven-day treatment regimen; with plastic applicator and patient instructions.

Store between 2° and 30°C (36° and 86°F).

GYNE-LOTRIMIN Vaginal Cream 1% is supplied in 45-gram tubes with a measured-dose applicator; box of one for seven-day treatment; box of two for fourteen-day treatment.

Store between 2° and 30°C (36° and 86°F).

Copyright 1976, 1982, Schering Corporation.

HYPERSTAT® I.V. ℞

brand of diazoxide, USP

Injection

FOR INTRAVENOUS USE IN HOSPITALIZED PATIENTS ONLY

Description: HYPERSTAT I.V. Injection is a rapidly acting antihypertensive agent. Each ampule (20 ml.) contains 300 mg. diazoxide USP, a nondiuretic benzothiadiazine derivative, in a clear, colorless, aqueous solution; the pH is adjusted to approximately 11.6 with sodium hydroxide. Diazoxide is 7-chloro-3-methyl-2*H*-1, 2, 4-benzothiadiazine 1, 1-dioxide.

Actions: HYPERSTAT I.V. Injection produces a prompt reduction in blood pressure by relaxing smooth muscle in the peripheral arterioles. Cardiac output is increased as blood pressure is reduced by diazoxide; coronary and cerebral blood flow are maintained. Renal blood flow is increased after an initial decrease. Diazoxide has no known direct action on the central nervous system.

Patients refractory to other antihypertensive agents usually remain responsive to diazoxide. Diazoxide is extensively bound to serum protein (>90%). The plasma half-life is 28 ± 8.3 hours; however, the duration of its antihypertensive effect is variable, generally lasting less than 12 hours. Although an antihypertensive response has been obtained with slow intravenous injection, in general, a greater antihypertensive effect is obtained with rapid intravenous administration.

Indications: HYPERSTAT I.V. Injection is indicated for the emergency reduction of blood pressure in malignant hypertension in hospitalized patients, when prompt and urgent decrease of diastolic pressure is required. Treatment with orally effective antihypertensive agents should be instituted as soon as the hypertensive emergency is controlled.

HYPERSTAT I.V. Injection is ineffective against hypertension due to pheochromocytoma.

Contraindications: HYPERSTAT I.V. Injection should not be used in the treatment of compensatory hypertension, such as that associated with aortic coarctation or arteriovenous shunt.

The drug should not be used in patients hypersensitive to diazoxide, other thiazides, or to other sulfonamide derived drugs, unless the potential benefits outweigh the possible risks.

Warnings: *Myocardial Lesions in Animals* Intravenous administration of diazoxide in dogs has been shown to induce subendocardial necrosis and necrosis of papillary muscles. These lesions, which are also produced by other vasodilator drugs (i.e., hydralazine, minoxidil) and by catecholamines, are presumed to be related to anoxia resulting from a combination of reflex tachycardia and decreased blood pressure.

Rapid decrease of blood pressure The use of diazoxide intravenously in severe hypertension has been associated with cerebral infarction, myocardial infarction, angina, and permanent blindness secondary to optic nerve infarction. One instance of optic nerve infarction was reported when control of blood pressure (i.e., diastolic pressure of 100 mmHg) was achieved over a 24-hour period. Caution must be observed when reducing severely elevated blood pressure. The desired blood pressure should be achieved over a period of days if this is compatible with the patient's status. If hypotension severe enough to require therapy occurs, it will usually respond to the administration of sympathomimetic agents, such as norepinephrine. If hypotension severe enough to require therapy occurs, it will usually respond to the administration of sympathomimetic agents, such as norepinephrine.

Hyperglycemia occurs in the majority of patients, but usually requires treatment only in patients with diabetes mellitus; it will respond to the usual management, including insulin. Therefore, blood glucose levels should be monitored, especially in patients with diabetes or in those requiring multiple injections of diazoxide. Hyperglycemia and hyperosmolar coma associated with transient cataracts developed in one infant receiving repeated daily doses of oral diazoxide. The disturbed carbohydrate metabolism was successfully treated with insulin. Cataracts have been observed in a few animals receiving repeated daily doses of intravenous or oral diazoxide.

Since diazoxide causes sodium retention, repeated injections may precipitate edema and congestive heart failure. This retention responds characteristically to diuretic agents if adequate renal function exists. It should be noted that concurrently administered thiazides may potentiate the antihypertensive, hyperglycemic, and hyperuricemic actions of diazoxide (See DRUG INTERACTIONS).

Since increased volume of extracellular fluid may be a cause of treatment failure in nonresponsive patients, it may be advisable to reduce this increased volume by means of a diuretic agent. (See DRUG INTERACTIONS.)

Although no evidence of excessive anticoagulant effects has been reported, patients, especially those who are hypoalbuminemic and receive HYPERSTAT I.V. Injection and coumarin or its derivatives, may require reduction in dosage of the anticoagulant (See DRUG INTERACTIONS).

HYPERSTAT I.V. Injection should be administered with caution to patients being treated concurrently with methyldopa or reserpine, or with drugs which act by direct peripheral vasodilatation, especially hydralazine, the nitrites and papaverine-like compounds.

Usage in Pregnancy: The safety of HYPERSTAT I.V. Injection in pregnancy has not yet been established.

Information is not available concerning the passage of HYPERSTAT in breast milk. However, it is known that diazoxide crosses the placental barrier and appears in cord blood. Like other thiazides, the drug may produce fetal or neonatal hyperbilirubinemia, thrombocytopenia, altered carbohydrate metabolism, and possibly other adverse reactions that have occurred in adults.

Continued on next page

Information on Schering products appearing on these pages is effective as of September 30, 1982.

Schering—Cont.

Usage in Children: The safety of HYPERSTAT I.V. Injection in children has not yet been established.

Precautions: HYPERSTAT (diazoxide) I.V. Injection is a potent antihypertensive agent requiring close monitoring of the patient's blood pressure at frequent intervals. Its administration may occasionally cause hypotension requiring treatment with sympathomimetic drugs. Therefore, adequate facilities to treat such untoward reactions should be available when HYPERSTAT I.V. Injection is used.

HYPERSTAT I.V. Injection should be administered only into a peripheral vein. Because the alkalinity of the solution is irritating to tissue, extravascular injection or leakage should be avoided; subcutaneous administration has produced inflammation and pain without subsequent necrosis. If leakage into subcutaneous tissue occurs, the area should be treated conservatively.

Maximal antihypertensive effects occur after rapid administration (within 30 seconds) into the vein; a slower injection may fail to reduce blood pressure or produce a very brief response.

As with any potent antihypertensive agent, HYPERSTAT I.V. Injection should be used with care in patients who have impaired cerebral or cardiac circulation, that is, patients in whom abrupt and brief reductions in blood pressure might be detrimental or those in whom concurrent tachycardia may be deleterious.

Special attention is required for patients with diabetes mellitus and those in whom retention of salt and water may present serious problems (See Warnings). Nondiabetic patients may have a transient, reversible, and clinically insignificant increase in blood glucose following HYPERSTAT I.V. Injection.

Since peritoneal dialysis or hemodialysis can reduce levels of diazoxide in the blood, patients undergoing dialysis may require more than one injection.

Adverse Reactions:

Frequent and serious adverse reactions: Sodium and water retention after repeated injections, especially important in patients with impaired cardiac reserve; hyperglycemia frequently requiring treatment in diabetic patients, especially after repeated injections.

Infrequent but serious adverse reactions: Hypotension to shock levels; myocardial ischemia, usually transient and manifested by angina, atrial and ventricular arrythmias, and marked electrocardiographic changes, but occasionally leading to myocardial infarction; cerebral ischemia, usually transient but occasionally leading to infarction and manifested by unconsciousness, convulsions, paralysis, confusion, or focal neurological deficit, such as numbness of the hands; optic nerve infarction following too rapid decrease in severely elevated blood pressure; persistent retention of nitrogenous wastes after repeated injections; hypersensitivity reactions, such as rash, leukopenia, and fever. Rarely, acute pancreatitis has been reported. Papilledema, induced by plasma volume expansion secondary to the administration of diazoxide, was reported in one patient who had received 11 injections over a 22-day period.

Other adverse reactions: Vasodilative phenomena, such as orthostatic hypotension, sweating, flushing, and generalized or localized sensations of warmth; supraventricular tachycardia and palpitation; bradycardia; various transient neurological findings secondary to alterations in regional blood flow to the brain, such as headache (sometimes throbbing), dizziness, lightheadedness, sleepiness (also reported as lethargy, somnolence or drowsiness), euphoria or "funny feeling", ringing in the ears and momentary hearing loss, and weakness of short duration; chest discomfort or nonanginal "tightness in the chest"; transient hyperglycemia in nondiabetic patients; transient retention of nitrogenous wastes; and various respiratory and gastrointestinal findings secondary to the relaxation of smooth muscle, such as dyspnea, cough and choking sensation; nausea and vomiting and/or abdominal discomfort, anorexia, alteration in taste, parotid swelling, salivation, dry mouth, lacrimation, ileus, constipation and diarrhea. Also, warmth or pain along the injected vein; cellulitus without sloughing and/or phlebitis at the site of extravasation; back pain; and increased nocturia. Apprehension or anxiety, malaise and blurred vision occurred on single occasions.

Drug Interactions: Since diazoxide is highly bound to serum protein, it may displace other substances which are also bound to protein, such as bilirubin or coumarin and its derivatives, resulting in higher blood levels of these substances. A drug interaction has also been reported for oral diazoxide and diphenylhydantoin, such that their concomitant administration may result in a loss of seizure control. These potential interactions must be considered when administering HYPERSTAT I.V. Injection. The concomitant administration of diazoxide with thiazides or other commonly used potent diuretics may potentiate the hyperglycemic, hyperuricemic, and antihypertensive effects of diazoxide. HYPERSTAT I.V. Injection should be administered with caution to patients being treated concurrently with methyldopa or reserpine, or with drugs which act by direct peripheral vasodilatation, especially hydralazine, the nitrites and papaverine-like compounds.

Overdosage: Overdosage of HYPERSTAT I.V. Injection may cause an undesirable hypotension. Usually, this can be controlled with sympathomimetic agents, such as norepinephrine; failure of the blood pressure to rise in response to such an agent suggests that the hypotension may have been caused by something other than diazoxide. Excessive hyperglycemia resulting from overdosage will respond to conventional therapy of hyperglycemia.

Diazoxide may be removed from the blood by peritoneal dialysis or hemodialysis.

Animal Pharmacology and Toxicology: In studies involving a number of species, including the rat, cat, dog, and monkey, diazoxide has been shown to exert significant antihypertensive actions through its direct effect on peripheral arterioles, which neither impairs cardiac function nor seriously diminishes perfusion of kidneys. In addition, in each species tested, including the rat, dog, and monkey, diazoxide elicits hyperglycemia, increased serum-free fatty acids and decreased plasma insulin levels by a mechanism thought to involve both suppression of insulin release and enhanced catecholamine action.

Although the data are not conclusive, reproduction and teratology studies in several species of animals indicate that diazoxide, when administered during the critical period of embryo formation, may interfere with normal fetal development, possibly through altered glucose metabolism. Parturition was occasionally prolonged in animals treated at term.

Dosage and Administration: HYPERSTAT I.V. Injection is administered undiluted and rapidly by intravenous injections of 1 to 3 mg/kg, up to a maximum of 150 mg. This dose may then be repeated at intervals of 5 to 15 minutes until a satisfactory reduction in blood pressure has been achieved.

Recent studies have shown that minibolus administration of HYPERSTAT Injection (doses of 1 to 3 mg/kg repeated at intervals of 5 to 15 minutes) is as effective as the administration of 300 mg in a single dose in reducing blood pressure while offering improved safety. Minibolus administration provides a more gradual reduction in blood pressure and thus avoids the circulatory and neurological risks associated with acute hypotension.

It should only be given into a peripheral vein. Do not administer it intramuscularly, subcutaneously, or into body cavities. Avoid extravasation of the drug into subcutaneous tissues.

The response to HYPERSTAT I.V. Injection varies from patient to patient. Generally, blood pressure decreases within five minutes, often within one to two minutes, to the lowest level achieved. The blood pressure increases relatively rapidly in the next 10 to 30 minutes, and then more slowly over the following 2 to 12 hours, nearly reaching but rarely exceeding the pretreatment level. The response to successive injections is frequently better than that to the initial injection.

Treatment of hypertensive emergencies with HYPERSTAT I.V. Injection should be limited to a few days and a regimen of oral antihypertensive medications should be instituted as soon as possible.

With the patient recumbent, the calculated dose of HYPERSTAT I.V. Injection is administered intravenously in 30 seconds or less. Slow intravenous injection may fail to reduce the blood pressure or may produce an exceedingly short response.

Repeated administration of HYPERSTAT I.V. Injection at intervals of 4 to 24 hours usually will maintain the blood pressure below pretreatment levels until a regimen of oral antihypertensive medication becomes effective. The interval between injections may be adjusted by the duration of the response to each injection. It is usually unnecessary to continue treatment with HYPERSTAT I.V. Injection for more than four to five days.

Following the use of HYPERSTAT I.V. Injection, the blood pressure should be monitored closely until it has stabilized. Thereafter, measurements taken hourly during the balance of the effect will indicate any unusual response. A further decrease in blood pressure at 30 minutes or more after injection should be investigated for causes other than the action of HYPERSTAT I.V. Injection. It is preferable that the patient remain recumbent for half an hour after injection. In ambulatory patients, the blood pressure should be measured with the patient standing before surveillance is ended.

Since repeated administration of HYPERSTAT I.V. Injection can lead to sodium and water retention, administration of a diuretic may be necessary both for maximal blood pressure reduction and to avoid congestive failure. (see DRUG INTERACTIONS.)

How Supplied: HYPERSTAT I.V. Injection is supplied in a 20 ml. ampule containing 300 mg. diazoxide in a clear, colorless aqueous solution; box of one ampule.

Protect from light and freezing.

Store between 2° and 30°C (36° and 86°F).

Revised 4/81

Copyright © 1972, 1981 Schering Corporation. All rights reserved.

LOTRIMIN® ℞

brand of clotrimazole, USP

Cream 1%

Solution 1%

For Dermatologic Use

Description: LOTRIMIN is clotrimazole [1-(o-chloro-α,α-diphenylbenzyl) imidazole], a synthetic antifungal agent having the chemical formula, $C_{22}H_{17}ClN_2$.

Each gram of LOTRIMIN Cream contains 10 mg. clotrimazole in a vanishing cream base of sorbitan monostearate, polysorbate 60, cetyl esters wax, cetearyl alcohol, 2-octyldodecanol, purified water and, as preservative, benzyl alcohol (1%).

Each ml. of LOTRIMIN Solution contains 10 mg. clotrimazole in a nonaqueous vehicle of polyethylene glycol 400.

Actions: Clotrimazole is a broad-spectrum, antifungal agent that inhibits the growth of pathogenic dermatophytes, yeasts, and *Malassezia furfur.* Clotrimazole exhibits fungicidal activity *in vitro* against isolates of *Trichophyton rubrum, Trichophyton mentagrophytes, Epidermophyton floccosum, Microsporum canis,* and *Candida albicans.*

No single-step or multiple-step resistance to clotrimazole has developed during successive passages of *Candida albicans* and *Trichophyton mentagrophytes.*

Indications: LOTRIMIN Cream and Solution are indicated for the topical treatment of the following dermal infections: tinea pedis, tinea cruris, and tinea corporis due to *Trichophyton rubrum, Trichophyton mentagrophytes, Epidermophyton floccosum,* and *Microsporum canis;* candidiasis due to *Candida albicans;* and tinea versicolor due to *Malassezia furfur.*

Contraindications: LOTRIMIN Cream and Solution are contraindicated in individuals who have shown hypersensitivity to any of its components.

Warnings: LOTRIMIN Cream and Solution are not for ophthalmic use.

Precautions: In the first trimester of pregnancy, LOTRIMIN Cream and Solution should be used only when considered essential to the welfare of the patient.

If irritation or sensitivity develops with the use of LOTRIMIN, treatment should be discontinued and appropriate therapy instituted.

Adverse Reactions: The following adverse reactions have been reported in connection with the use of this product: erythema, stinging, blistering, peeling, edema, pruritus, urticaria, and general irritation of the skin.

Dosage and Administration: Gently massage sufficient LOTRIMIN Cream or Solution into the affected and surrounding skin areas twice a day, in the morning and evening.

Clinical improvement, with relief of pruritus, usually occurs within the first week of treatment. If a patient shows no clinical improvement after four weeks of treatment with LOTRIMIN, the diagnosis should be reviewed.

How Supplied: LOTRIMIN Cream 1% is supplied in 15, 30, 45 and 90-gram tubes; boxes of one. LOTRIMIN Solution 1% is supplied in 10 ml. and 30 ml. plastic bottles; boxes of one.

Store between 2° and 30°C (36° and 86°F).

Copyright © 1975, 1981, Schering Corporation. All rights reserved.

METIMYD® ℞

brand of prednisolone acetate, USP and sulfacetamide sodium, USP

Ophthalmic Suspension–Sterile
Ophthalmic Ointment–Sterile

Description: METIMYD Ophthalmic **Suspension** is a steroid/anti-infective sterile preparation having a pH range of 7.0 to 7.4. Each ml contains: 5 mg prednisolone acetate, USP; 100 mg sulfacetamide sodium, USP; disodium hydrogen phosphate, sodium dihydrogen phosphate, tyloxapol, sodium thiosulfate, edetate disodium, and purified water; 5 mg phenylethyl alcohol and 0.25 mg benzalkonium chloride as preservatives.

METIMYD Ophthalmic **Ointment** is a steroid/anti-infective sterile preparation containing in each gram: 5 mg prednisolone acetate, USP and 100 mg sulfacetamide sodium, USP; 0.5 mg methylparaben and 0.1 mg propylparaben as preservatives, in a bland, unctuous base of mineral oil and white petrolatum.

The empirical formula for prednisolone acetate, a 1-unsaturated analog of hydrocortisone acetate, is $C_{23}H_{30}O_6$. The molecular weight is 402.49. Chemically it is 11β,17,21-trihydroxypregna-1,4-diene-3,20-dione 21-acetate.

Prednisolone acetate is a nearly odorless, white to practically white, crystalline powder. It is slightly soluble in acetone, alcohol, and chloroform, and practically insoluble in water.

Sulfacetamide sodium, $C_8H_9N_2NaO_3S \cdot H_2O$, is a sulfonamide antibacterial agent with a molecular weight of 254.24. Chemically it is *N*-[(4-aminophenyl)sulfonyl]-, acetamide, monosodium salt, monohydrate.

Sulfacetamide sodium is an odorless, white, crystalline powder. It is freely soluble in water, sparingly soluble in alcohol and practically insoluble in benzene, chloroform, and ether.

Clinical Pharmacology: Corticosteroids suppress the inflammatory response to a variety of agents and they probably delay or slow healing. Since corticoids may inhibit the body's defense mechanism against infection, a concomitant antimicrobial drug may be used when this inhibition is considered to be clinically significant in a particular case.

The anti-infective component in the combination is included to provide action against specific organisms susceptible to it. Sulfacetamide sodium inhibits the growth of susceptible strains of *Pseudomonas aeruginosa, Staphylococcus aureus* and *albus, Klebsiella pneumoniae, Escherichia coli,* and *Enterobacter aerogenes.*

When a decision is made to administer both a corticoid and an antimicrobial, the administration of such drugs in combination has the advantages of greater patient compliance and convenience and added assurance that the appropriate dosage of both drugs is administered. There is also assured compatibility of ingredients when both types of drug are in the same formulation and, particularly, that the correct volume of drug is delivered and retained.

The relative potency of corticosteroids depends on the molecular structure, concentration, and release from the vehicle.

Indications and Usage: METIMYD Ophthalmic Suspension or **Ointment** is indicated for ocular inflammation when concurrent use of an antimicrobial and a steroid is judged necessary.

Contraindications: METIMYD is contraindicated in: epithelial herpes simplex keratitis (dendritic keratitis), vaccinia, varicella, and many other viral diseases of the cornea or conjunctiva; mycobacterial infection of the eye; and fungal diseases of ocular structures. METIMYD is contraindicated in individuals with known or suspected hypersensitivity to any of the ingredients of the preparation, or to other sulfonamides, or other corticosteroids. (Hypersensitivity to the antibacterial component occurs at a higher rate than for other components.) The use of these combinations is always contraindicated after uncomplicated removal of a corneal foreign body.

Warnings: Prolonged use may result in glaucoma, with damage to the optic nerve, defects in visual acuity and fields of vision, and in posterior subcapsular cataract formation. Prolonged use may suppress the host response and thus increase the hazard of secondary ocular infections. In those diseases causing thinning of the cornea or sclera, perforations have been known to occur with the use of topical steroids. In acute purulent conditions of the eye, steroids may mask infection or enhance existing infection. If these products are used for 10 days or longer, intraocular pressure should be routinely monitored even though this may be difficult in children and uncooperative patients.

Employment of steroid medication in the treatment of herpes simplex requires great caution.

A significant percentage of staphylococcal isolates are completely resistant to sulfonamides.

Precautions: The initial prescription and renewal of the medication order beyond 20 ml of METIMYD Ophthalmic **Suspension** or beyond 8 g of the **Ointment** should be made by a physician only after examination of the patient with the aid of magnification, such as slitlamp biomicroscopy and where appropriate, fluorescein staining.

The possibility of fungal infections of the cornea should be considered after prolonged steroid dosing.

Sensitization may recur when a sulfonamide is readministered irrespective of the route of administration and cross-sensitivity among different sulfonamides may occur. (See ADVERSE REACTIONS.) Cross-allergenicity among corticosteroids has been demonstrated. If signs of hypersensitivity or other untoward reactions occur, discontinue use of the preparation.

Adverse Reactions: Adverse reactions have occurred which can be attributed to the steroid component, the anti-infective component, or the combination. Exact incidence figures are not available since no denominator of treated patients is available.

Instances of Stevens-Johnson syndrome and systemic lupus erythematosus (in one case producing a fatal outcome) have been reported following the use of ophthalmic sulfonamide containing preparations.

The reactions due to the steroid component in decreasing order of frequency are: elevation of intraocular pressure (IOP) with possible development of glaucoma, and infrequent optic nerve damage; posterior subcapsular cataract formation; and delayed wound healing.

Corticosteroid-containing preparations can also cause acute anterior uveitis or perforation of the globe. Mydriasis, loss of accommodation, and ptosis have occasionally been reported following local use of corticosteroids.

Secondary Infection: The development of secondary infection has occurred after use of combinations containing steroids and antimicrobials. Fungal infections of the cornea are particularly prone to develop coincidentally with long-term applications of the steroid. The possibility of fungal invasion must be considered in any persistent corneal ulceration where steriod treatment has been used.

Secondary bacterial ocular infection following suppression of host responses also occurs.

Dosage and Administration: METIMYD Ophthalmic Suspension: Two or three drops should be instilled into the conjunctival sac every one to two hours during the day and at bedtime until a favorable response is obtained.

METIMYD Ophthalmic Ointment: A thin film should be applied three or four times daily and once at bedtime until a favorable response is obtained.

The initial prescription of METIMYD Ophthalmic should *not* be more than 20 ml of the **Suspension** or 8 g of the **Ointment** and the prescription should not be refilled without further evaluation as outlined in the PRECAUTIONS Section.

Dosage should be adjusted according to the specific needs of the patient. METIMYD Ophthalmic **Suspension** or **Ointment** dosage may be reduced, but care should be taken not to discontinue therapy prematurely. In chronic conditions, withdrawal of treatment should be carried out by gradually decreasing the frequency of application.

How Supplied: METIMYD Ophthalmic Suspension, 5 ml dropper bottle; box of one. **Store between 2° and 30°C (36° and 86°F). Clumping may occur on long standing at high temperatures. Shake well before using. Protect from light.**

METIMYD Ophthalmic Ointment, 3.5 g applicator tube; box of one. **Store between 2° and 30°C (36° and 86°F).**

Revised 6/81

Copyright©1969, 1981, Schering Corporation. All rights reserved.

Continued on next page

Information on Schering products appearing on these pages is effective as of September 30, 1982.

Schering—Cont.

METRETON® ℞

brand of prednisolone sodium phosphate, USP (0.5% prednisolone phosphate equivalent)
Ophthalmic/Otic Solution—Sterile

Description: METRETON Ophthalmic/Otic Solution is a clear, sterile, aqueous solution. Each ml. contains 5.5 mg. prednisolone sodium phosphate, USP (equivalent to 5.0 mg. prednisolone phosphate), edetate disodium, monobasic sodium phosphate, dibasic sodium phosphate, tyloxapol, purified water, U.S.P.; sodium hydroxide to adjust pH to approximately 7.8; benzalkonium chloride and phenylethyl alcohol are added as preservatives.

Actions: METRETON Ophthalmic/Otic Solution inhibits the inflammatory response to inciting agents of a mechanical, chemical or immunological nature. No generally accepted explanation of this steroid property has been advanced.

Indications: METRETON Ophthalmic/Otic Solution is indicated for the treatment of the following conditions.

Eye: steroid-responsive inflammatory conditions of the palpebral and bulbar conjunctiva, cornea and anterior segment of the globe, such as allergic conjunctivitis, acne rosacea, superficial punctate keratitis, herpes zoster keratitis, iritis, cyclitis, selected infective conjunctivitis when the inherent hazard of steroid use is accepted to obtain an advisable diminution in edema and inflammation; corneal injury from chemical or thermal burns or penetration of foreign bodies.

Ear: steroid-responsive inflammatory conditions of the external auditory canal, such as allergic otitis externa, selected purulent and nonpurulent infective otitis externa when the hazard of steroid use is accepted to obtain an advisable diminution in edema and inflammation.

Contraindications: Hypersensitivity to a component of this medication contraindicates its use.

Eye: METRETON Ophthalmic/Otic Solution should not be used in acute superficial herpes simplex keratitis or in other viral infections of the cornea and conjunctiva, such as vaccinia and varicella. It is also contraindicated in patients with tuberculosis of the eye or in those with fungal infections of ocular structures.

Ear: METRETON Ophthalmic/Otic Solution is contraindicated if the tympanic membrane is perforated or in those patients with fungal infections of external ear structures.

Warnings: *Eye:* METRETON Ophthalmic/Otic Solution is not effective in mustard gas keratitis and in Sjogren's keratoconjunctivitis. Steroids should be used with great caution in the treatment of stromal herpes simplex; frequent slit-lamp microscopy is mandatory.

Prolonged use of this medication may result in glaucoma, damage to the optic nerve, defects in visual acuity and fields of vision, posterior subcapsular cataract formation, or may aid in the establishment of secondary ocular infections from pathogens liberated from ocular tissues. In those diseases causing thinning of the cornea or sclera, perforation has been known to occur with the use of topical steriods.

Acute, purulent, untreated infection of the eye may be masked or activity enhanced by the presence of steroid medication.

Ear: Acute, purulent, untreated infection of the ear may be masked or activity enhanced by the presence of steroid medication.

Usage in Pregnancy The safety of intensive or protracted use of topical steroids during pregnancy has not been substantiated.

Precautions: *Eye:* Since fungal infections of the cornea are particularly prone to develop coincidentally with long-term local steroid applications, fungus invasion must be considered in any persistent corneal ulceration where a steroid is in use or has been used. Intraocular pressure should be checked frequently.

Ear: If symptoms in the ear persist, the presence of a fungus infection must be considered.

Adverse Reactions: Glaucoma with optic nerve damage, visual acuity and field defects, posterior subcapsular cataract formation, secondary ocular infections from pathogens, including herpes simplex liberated from ocular tissues, perforation of the globe.

Rarely, stinging or burning may occur.

Dosage and Administration: The duration of treatment will vary with the type of lesion and may extend from a few days to several weeks, depending on therapeutic response. Relapses, more common in chronic, active lesions than in self-limited conditions, usually respond to retreatment.

Eye Instill one or two drops of METRETON Ophthalmic/Otic Solution into the conjunctival sac every hour during the day and every two hours during the night as initial therapy. When a favorable response is observed, reduce dosage to one drop every four hours. Later, further reduction in dosage to one drop three or four times daily may suffice to control symptoms.

Ear Clean the aural canal thoroughly and sponge dry. Instill the solution directly into the aural canal. A suggested initial dosage is three or four drops two or three times a day. When a favorable response is obtained, reduce dosage gradually and eventually discontinue.

If preferred, the aural canal may be packed with a gauze wick saturated with solution. Keep the wick moist with the preparation and remove from the ear after 12 to 24 hours. Treatment may be repeated as often as necessary at the discretion of the physician.

How Supplied: METRETON Ophthalmic/Otic Solution, 5-ml. plastic dropper bottle, box of one.

Store between 2° and 30°C (36° and 86°F). Protect from light.

Store in carton until contents are used.

Revised 7/80

Copyright© 1973, 1980. Schering Corporation. All rights reserved.

NAQUA® ℞

brand of trichlormethiazide, USP
Tablets

Description: NAQUA Tablets contain trichlormethiazide, USP, an antihypertensive agent and diuretic of the benzothiadiazine series having the chemical formula, $C_8H_8Cl_3N_3O_4S_2$. Each NAQUA Tablet contains 2 or 4 mg. trichlormethiazide.

Actions: The mechanism of action results in an interference with the renal tubular mechanism of electrolyte reabsorption. At maximal therapeutic dosage all thiazides are approximately equal in their diuretic potency. The mechanism whereby thiazides function in the control of hypertension is unknown.

Indications: NAQUA Tablets are indicated as adjunctive therapy in edema associated with congestive heart failure, hepatic cirrhosis, and corticosteroid and estrogen therapy.

NAQUA Tablets have also been found useful in edema due to various forms of renal dysfunction, such as: nephrotic syndrome; acute glomerulonephritis; and chronic renal failure.

NAQUA Tablets are indicated in the management of hypertension either as the sole therapeutic agent or to enhance the effectiveness of other antihypertensive drugs in the more severe forms of hypertension.

Usage in Pregnancy The routine use of diuretics in an otherwise healthy woman is inappropriate and exposes the mother and fetus to unnecessary hazard. Diuretics do not prevent development of toxemia in pregnancy, and there is no satisfactory evidence that they are useful in the treatment of developed toxemia. Edema during pregnancy may arise from pathological causes or from the physiologic and mechanical consequences of pregnancy. Thiazides are indicated in pregnancy when edema is due to pathologic causes, just as they are in the absence of pregnancy (however, see WARNINGS, below). Dependent edema in pregnancy, resulting from restriction of venous return by the expanded uterus, is properly treated through elevation of the lower extremities and use of support hose; use of diuretics to lower intravascular volume in this case is illogical and unnecessary. There is hypervolemia during normal pregnancy which is harmful to neither the fetus nor the mother (in the absence of cardiovascular disease), but which is associated with edema, including generalized edema, in the majority of pregnant women. If this edema produces discomfort, increased recumbency will often provide relief. In rare instances, this edema may cause extreme discomfort which is not relieved by rest. In these cases, a short course of diuretics may provide relief and may be appropriate.

Contraindications: NAQUA Tablets are contraindicated in patients with anuria.

Hypersensitivity to this or other sulfonamide-derived drugs is a contraindication to the use of this product.

Warnings: Thiazides should be used with caution in severe renal disease. In patients with renal disease, thiazides may precipitate azotemia. Cumulative effects of the drug may develop in patients with impaired renal function.

Thiazides should be used with caution in patients with impaired hepatic function or progressive liver disease, since minor alterations of fluid and electrolyte balance may precipitate hepatic coma.

Thiazides may add to or potentiate the action of other antihypertensive drugs. Potentiation occurs with ganglionic or peripheral adrenergic blocking drugs.

Sensitivity reactions may occur in patients with a history of allergy or bronchial asthma.

The possibility of exacerbation or activation of systemic lupus erythematosus has been reported.

Usage in Pregnancy Thiazides cross the placental barrier and appear in cord blood. The use of thiazides in pregnant women requires that the anticipated benefit be weighed against possible hazards to the fetus. These hazards include fetal or neonatal jaundice, thrombocytopenia, and possibly other adverse reactions which have occurred in the adult.

Nursing Mothers Thiazides appear in breast milk. If use of the drug is deemed essential, the patient should stop nursing.

Precautions: Periodic determination of serum electrolytes to detect possible electrolyte imbalance should be performed at appropriate intervals.

All patients receiving thiazide therapy should be observed for clinical signs of fluid or electrolyte imbalance, namely, hyponatremia, hypochloremic alkalosis, hypokalemia, hypomagnesemia, and changes in serum and urinary calcium. Serum and urine electrolyte determinations are particularly important when the patient is vomiting excessively or receiving parenteral fluids. Medications such as digitalis derivatives are sensitive to changes in serum electrolytes. Warning signs, irrespective of cause, are: dryness of mouth, thirst, weakness, lethargy, drowsiness, restlessness, muscle pains or cramps, muscular fatigue, hypotension, oliguria, tachycardia, and gastrointestinal disturbances such as nausea and vomiting.

Hypokalemia may develop with thiazides as with any other potent diuretic, especially with brisk diuresis, when severe cirrhosis is present, or during concomitant use of corticosteroids or ACTH.

Interference with adequate oral electrolyte intake will also contribute to hypokalemia.

Digitalis therapy may exaggerate metabolic effects of hypokalemia especially with reference to myocardial activity.

Any chloride deficit is generally mild and usually does not require specific treatment except under extraordinary circumstances (as in liver disease or renal disease). Dilutional hyponatremia may occur in edematous patients in hot weather; appropriate therapy is water restriction, rather than administration of salt, except in rare instances when the hyponatremia is life-threatening. In actual salt depletion, appropriate replacement is the therapy of choice.

Hyperuricemia may occur or frank gout may be precipitated in certain patients receiving thiazide therapy.

Insulin requirements in diabetic patients may be increased, decreased, or unchanged. Latent diabetes mellitus may become manifest during thiazide administration; diabetic complications such as reversible oculomotor paresis may occur.

Thiazide drugs may increase the responsiveness to tubocurarine.

The antihypertensive effects of the drug may be enhanced in the post-sympathectomy patient.

Thiazides may decrease arterial responsiveness to norepinephrine. This diminution is not sufficient to preclude effectiveness of the pressor agent for therapeutic use.

If progressive renal impairment becomes evident, as indicated by a rising nonprotein nitrogen or blood urea nitrogen, a careful reappraisal of therapy is necessary with consideration given to withholding or discontinuing diuretic therapy.

Thiazides may decrease serum PBI levels without signs of thyroid disturbance.

Adverse Reactions: *Gastrointestinal System Reactions:* anorexia; gastric irritation; nausea; vomiting; cramping; diarrhea; constipation; jaundice (intrahepatic cholestatic jaundice); pancreatitis.

Central Nervous System Reactions: dizziness; vertigo; paresthesias; headache; xanthopsia.

Hematologic Reactions: leukopenia; agranulocytosis; thrombocytopenia; aplastic anemia.

Dermatologic—Hypersensitivity Reactions: purpura; photosensitivity; rash; urticaria; necrotizing angiitis (vasculitis, cutaneous vasculitis).

Cardiovascular Reaction: Orthostatic hypotension may occur and may be aggravated by alcohol, barbiturates or narcotics.

Other: hyperglycemia; glycosuria; hyperuricemia; muscle spasm; weakness; restlessness.

Whenever adverse reactions are moderate or severe, thiazide dosage should be reduced or therapy withdrawn.

Dosage and Administration: Therapy should be individualized according to patient response. This therapy should be titrated to gain maximal therapeutic response as well as the minimal dose possible to maintain that therapeutic response.

Edematous Conditions The usual dosage of NAQUA Tablets for diuretic effect is 1 to 4 mg. daily.

Hypertension The usual dosage of NAQUA Tablets for antihypertensive effect is 2 to 4 mg. daily.

How Supplied: NAQUA Tablets, 2 mg., pink, clover-shaped, compressed tablets impressed with the letter S and product identification letters, AHG, or numbers 822; bottles of 100 and 1000.

NAQUA Tablets, 4 mg., aqua, clover-shaped, compressed tablets impressed with the letter S and product identification letters, AHH, or numbers 547; bottles of 100 and 1000.

Revised 11/79

Copyright © 1968, 1980, Schering Corporation. All rights reserved.

[*Shown in Product Identification Section*]

NAQUIVAL® ℞

brand of trichlormethiazide, USP—reserpine, USP

Tablets

> **Warning**
> This fixed combination drug is not indicated for initial therapy of hypertension. Hypertension requires therapy titrated to the individual patient. If the fixed combination represents the dosage so determined, its use may be more convenient in patient management. The treatment of hypertension is not static, but must be reevaluated as conditions in each patient warrant.

Description: Each NAQUIVAL Tablet contains 4 mg. NAQUA® (brand of trichlormethiazide, USP) and 0.1 mg. reserpine, USP. Trichlormethiazide is an antihypertensive agent and diuretic of the benzothiadiazine series having the chemical formula, $C_8H_8Cl_3N_3O_4S_2$. The antihypertensive agent, reserpine, is a rauwolfia alkaloid having the chemical formula, $C_{33}H_{40}N_2O_9$.

Actions: NAQUIVAL Tablets combine the antihypertensive and diuretic properties of trichlormethiazide with the antihypertensive actions of reserpine; maximum antihypertensive effects are achieved with minimal doses of each ingredient.

Indications: NAQUIVAL Tablets are indicated for the treatment of hypertension (see box warning).

Contraindications: NAQUIVAL Tablets are contraindicated in patients with anuria.

Hypersensitivity to this or other sulfonamide-derived drugs is a contraindication to the use of this product.

The routine use of diuretics in an otherwise healthy pregnant woman with or without mild edema is contraindicated and possibly hazardous.

The presence of an active peptic ulcer, ulcerative colitis, or severe depression contraindicates the use of reserpine.

Warnings: NAQUIVAL Tablets should be withdrawn at least three weeks prior to elective surgery or electroconvulsive therapy because of the reserpine activity.

If parenteral antihypertensive therapy is indicated for a patient receiving NAQUIVAL Tablets, the physician should be alert to the possible synergism of reserpine and trichlormethiazide with such drugs, especially those administered by rapid infusion, e.g., diazoxide.

Sympathomimetics should be used with caution in patients who are receiving reserpine, since its antihypertensive effects may be reduced.

NAQUIVAL Tablets should be used with caution in severe renal disease. In patients with renal disease, thiazides may precipitate azotemia. Cumulative effects of the drug may develop in patients with impaired renal function.

Thiazides should be used with caution in patients with impaired hepatic function or progressive liver disease, since minor alterations of fluid and electrolyte balance may precipitate hepatic coma.

Thiazides may be additive or potentiative of the action of other antihypertensive drugs. Potentiation occurs with ganglionic or peripheral adrenergic blocking drugs or vasodilators.

Sensitivity reactions may occur in patients with a history of allergy or bronchial asthma.

The possibility of exacerbation or activation of systemic lupus erythematosus has been reported.

Usage in Pregnancy Usage of thiazides in women of childbearing age requires that the potential benefits of the drug be weighed against its possible hazards to the fetus. These hazards include fetal or neonatal jaundice, thrombocytopenia, and possibly other adverse reactions which have occurred in the adult.

The safety of reserpine for use during pregnancy or lactation has not been established; therefore, it should be used in pregnant patients or in women of childbearing age only when, in the judgment of the physician, its use is deemed essential to the welfare of the patient.

Nursing Mothers Thiazides cross the placental barrier and appear in cord blood and breast milk.

Precautions: Periodic determination of serum electrolytes to detect possible electrolyte imbalance should be performed at appropriate intervals.

All patients receiving thiazide therapy should be observed for clinical signs of fluid or electrolyte imbalance, namely, hyponatremia, hypochloremic alkalosis, hypokalemia, hypomagnesemia, and changes in serum and urinary calcium. Serum and urine electrolyte determinations are particularly important when the patient is vomiting excessively or receiving parenteral fluids. Medications such as digitalis derivatives are sensitive to changes in serum electrolytes. Warning signs, irrespective of cause, are: dryness of mouth, thirst, weakness, lethargy, drowsiness, restlessness, muscle pains or cramps, muscular fatigue, hypotension, oliguria, tachycardia, and gastrointestinal disturbances such as nausea and vomiting.

Hypokalemia may develop with thiazides as with any other potent diuretic, especially with brisk diuresis, when severe cirrhosis is present, or during concomitant use of corticosteroids or ACTH.

Interference with adequate oral electrolyte intake will also contribute to hypokalemia.

Digitalis therapy may exaggerate metabolic effects of hypokalemia especially with reference to myocardial activity.

Any chloride deficit is generally mild and usually does not require specific treatment except under extraordinary circumstances (as in liver disease or renal disease). Dilutional hyponatremia may occur in edematous patients in hot weather; appropriate therapy is water restriction, rather than administration of salt, except in rare instances when the hyponatremia is life-threatening. In actual salt depletion, appropriate replacement is the therapy of choice.

Hyperuricemia may occur or frank gout may be precipitated in certain patients receiving thiazide therapy.

Insulin requirements in diabetic patients may be increased, decreased, or unchanged. Latent diabetes mellitus may become manifest during thiazide administration; diabetic complications such as reversible oculomotor paresis may occur.

Thiazide drugs may increase the responsiveness to tubocurarine.

The antihypertensive effects of the drug may be enhanced in the post-sympathectomy patient.

Thiazides may decrease arterial responsiveness to norepinephrine. This diminution is not sufficient to preclude effectiveness of the pressor agent for therapeutic use.

If progressive renal impairment becomes evident, as indicated by a rising nonprotein nitrogen or blood urea nitrogen, a careful reappraisal of therapy is necessary with consideration given to withholding or discontinuing diuretic therapy.

Thiazides may decrease serum PBI levels without signs of thyroid disturbance.

Reserpine may augment secretory and motor activity of the gastrointestinal tract, and gas-

Continued on next page

Information on Schering products appearing on these pages is effective as of September 30, 1982.

Schering—Cont.

tric hyperacidity, peptic ulceration, and mucous colitis may develop. Patients undergoing emergency surgery should be watched for precipitous falls in blood pressure; vasopressor agents such as levarterenol should be available.

Reserpine may precipitate biliary colic in patients with gallstones.

Because of the decreased sympathetic tone caused by reserpine catecholamine depletion, special care should be exercised in treating patients with a history of bronchial asthma.

NAQUIVAL Tablets contain FD&C Yellow No. 5 (tartrazine) which may cause allergic-type reactions (including bronchial asthma) in certain susceptible individuals. Although the overall incidence of FD&C Yellow No. 5 (tartrazine) sensitivity in the general population is low, it is frequently seen in patients who also have aspirin hypersensitivity.

Adverse Reactions: *Autonomic Reactions:* nasal stuffiness; dryness of the mouth; blurred vision; flushing of the face.

Gastrointestinal System Reactions: anorexia; gastric irritation; nausea; vomiting; cramping; diarrhea; constipation; jaundice (intrahepatic cholestatic jaundice); pancreatitis.

Central Nervous System Reactions: dizziness; vertigo; paresthesias; headache; xanthopsia; depression; central nervous system sensitization manifested as dull sensorium, deafness, glaucoma, uveitis, and optic atrophy.

Hematologic Reactions: leukopenia; agranulocytosis; thrombocytopenia; aplastic anemia.

Dermatologic—Hypersensitivity Reactions: purpura; photosensitivity; rash; urticaria; necrotizing angiitis (vasculitis, cutaneous vasculitis).

Cardiovascular Reactions: Ectopic cardiac rhythms, particularly when used concurrently with digitalis; orthostatic hypotension may occur and may be aggravated by alcohol, barbiturates or narcotics.

Other: hyperglycemia; glycosuria; hyperuricemia; muscle spasm; weakness; restlessness; drowsiness; weight gain; dyspnea; dyskinesia; impotence and decreased libido; conjunctival injection.

Whenever adverse reactions are moderate or severe, NAQUIVAL dosage should be reduced or therapy withdrawn.

Dosage and Administration: The dosage of NAQUIVAL should be determined by individual titration (see box warning).

Initial dosage with NAQUIVAL is frequently one tablet twice a day, with reduction to maintenance levels as therapeutic benefits become manifest. When NAQUIVAL is used with ganglionic blocking agents, careful downward adjustment of these drugs should be made to avoid precipitous blood pressure falls.

How Supplied: NAQUIVAL Tablets: peach-colored, scored, compressed tablets impressed with the Schering Trademark and product identification letters, AHT or numbers, 394; bottles of 100 and 500.

Store between 2° and 30°C (36° and 86°F).

Revised 11/79

Copyright © 1968, 1980, Schering Corporation. All rights reserved.

[*Shown in Product Identification Section*]

OPTIMINE® ℞

brand of azatadine maleate

Tablets

Description: OPTIMINE Tablets contain azatadine maleate, an antihistamine having the empirical formula, $C_{20}H_{22}N_2 \cdot 2C_4H_4O_4$, the chemical name, 6,11-Dihydro-11-(1-methyl-4-piperidylidene)-5*H*-benzo[5,6]cyclohepta [1,2-*β*] pyridine maleate (1:2).

The molecular weight of azatadine maleate is 522.54. It is a white to off-white powder and is very soluble in water and soluble in alcohol.

Each OPTIMINE Tablet contains 1 mg azatadine maleate.

Clinical Pharmacology: Azatadine maleate is an antihistamine related to cyproheptadine, with antiserotonin, anticholinergic (drying), and sedative effects.

Antihistamines competitively antagonize those pharmacological effects of histamine which are mediated through activation of histamine H_1-receptor sites on effector cells. Histamine-related allergic reactions and tissue injury are blocked or diminished in intensity. Antihistamines antagonize the vasodilator effect of endogenously released histamine, especially in small vessels, and mitigate the effect of histamine which results in increased capillary permeability and edema formation. As consequences of these actions, antihistamines antagonize the physiological manifestations of histamine release in the nose following antigen-antibody interactions, such as congestion related to vascular engorgement, mucosal edema, and profuse, watery secretion, and irritation and sneezing resulting from histamine action on afferent nerve terminals.

Phamacokinetic studies in normal volunteers dosed orally with radio-labeled azatadine maleate show that the drug is readily absorbed with peak plasma levels at about four hours after dosing. Approximately 50% of the drug is excreted in the urine within five days after administration of a single dose, and no evidence of drug accumulation was seen after daily dosing for 30 days. The elimination half-life of azatadine maleate, based on plasma radioactivity, was approximately 9 hours. Approximately 20% of the drug is excreted unchanged and extensive conjugation of the drug and its metabolites occurs. Azatadine maleate is minimally bound to plasma protein.

While the antihistamines have not been studied for passage through the blood-brain and placental barriers, the occurrence of pharmacologic effects in the central nervous system and in the newborn indicate presence of the drug.

Indications and Usage: OPTIMINE Tablets are indicated for the treatment of perennial and seasonal allergic rhinitis and chronic urticaria.

Contraindications: Antihistamines *should NOT* be used to treat lower respiratory tract symptoms, including asthma.

Antihistamines, including azatadine maleate, are also contraindicated in patients hypersensitive to this medication and to other antihistamines of similar chemical structure, and in patients receiving monoamine oxidase inhibitor therapy. (See Drug Interactions.)

Warnings: Antihistamines should be used with caution in patients with narrow angle glaucoma, stenosing peptic ulcer; pyloroduodenal obstruction; and urinary bladder obstruction due to symptomatic prostatic hypertrophy and narrowing of the bladder neck.

Use with CNS Depressants: Antihistamines have additive effects with alcohol and other CNS depressants (hypnotics, sedatives, tranquilizers, etc.).

Use in Activities Requiring Mental Alertness: Patients should be warned about engaging in activities requiring mental alertness, such as driving a car or operating certain appliances, machinery, etc., until their response to this medication has been determined.

Use in Patients approximately 60 years or older: Antihistamines are more likely to cause dizziness, sedation, and hypotension in patients over 60 years of age.

Precautions: General: Azatadine maleate has an atropine-like action and therefore should be used with caution in patients with: a history of bronchial asthma; increased intraocular pressure; hyperthyroidism; cardiovascular disease; hypertension.

Information for Patients:

1. Antihistamines may cause drowsiness.
2. Patients taking antihistamines should not engage in activities requiring mental alertness, such as driving a car or operating machinery, certain appliances, etc., until their response to this medication has been determined.
3. Alcohol or other sedative drugs may enhance the drowsiness caused by antihistamines.
4. Patients should not take this medication if they are receiving a monoamine oxidase (MAO) inhibitor, or if they are receiving oral anticoagulants.
5. This medication should not be given to children less than 12 years of age.

Drug Interactions: MAO inhibitors prolong and intensify the anticholinergic and sedative effects of antihistamines. Additive effects may occur from the concomitant use of antihistamines with tricyclic antidepressants. (See also WARNINGS.) The action of oral anticoagulants may be diminished by antihistamines.

Drug/Laboratory Test Interaction: Antihistamines should be discontinued about four days prior to skin testing procedures since these drugs may prevent or diminish otherwise positive reactions to dermal reactivity indicators.

Carcinogenesis, Mutagenesis, and Impairment of Fertility: Long-term oral dosing studies with azatadine maleate in rats and mice showed no evidence of carcinogenesis. No mutagenic effect was seen in a dominant lethal assay study in mice dosed with azatadine maleate orally and intraperitoneally. There was no impairment of fertility in rats fed azatadine maleate at doses greater than 150 times the recommended human daily dose.

Pregnancy Category B: Reproduction studies have been performed in rats and rabbits at doses up to 188 times and 38 times, respectively, the human dose and have revealed no evidence of impaired fertility or harm to the fetus due to azatadine maleate. There are, however, no adequate and well-controlled studies in pregnant women. Because animal reproduction studies are not always predictive of human response, this drug should be used during pregnancy only if clearly needed. (See **Non-Teratogenic Effects.**)

Non-Teratogenic Effects: Antihistamines should not be used in the third trimester of pregnancy because newborns and premature infants may have severe reactions, such as convulsions, to them.

Nursing Mothers: It is not known whether this drug is excreted in human milk. However, certain antihistamines are known to be excreted in human milk in low concentration. Because of the higher risk of antihistamines for infants generally and for newborns and prematures in particular, a decision should be made whether to discontinue nursing or to discontinue the drug, taking into account the importance of the drug to the mother.

Pediatric Use: Safety and effectiveness in children below the age of 12 years have not been established.

Adverse Reactions: Slight to moderate drowsiness may occur with azatadine maleate. Other possible side effects common to antihistamines in general include: (the most frequent are underlined).

General: urticaria, drug rash, anaphylactic shock, photosensitivity, excessive perspiration, chills, dryness of mouth, nose, and throat.

Cardiovascular: hypotension, headache, palpitations, tachycardia, extrasystoles.

Hematologic: hemolytic anemia, hypoplastic anemia, thrombocytopenia, agranulocytosis.

Nervous: sedation, sleepiness, dizziness, vertigo, tinnitus, acute labyrinthitis, disturbed coordination, fatigue, confusion, restlessness, excitation, nervousness, tremor, irritability, insomnia, euphoria, paresthesias, blurred vision diplopia, hysteria, neuritis, convulsions.

Gastrointestinal: epigastric distress, anorexia, nausea, vomiting, diarrhea, constipation.

Genitourinary: urinary frequency, difficult urination, urinary retention, early menses.

Respiratory: thickening of bronchial secretions, tightness of chest and wheezing, nasal stuffiness.

Drug Abuse and Dependence: There is no information to indicate that abuse or dependency occurs with azatadine maleate.

Overdosage: In the event of overdosage, emergency treatment should be started immediately.

Manifestations: Antihistamine overdosage effects may vary from central nervous system depression (sedation, apnea, diminished mental alertness, cardiovascular collapse) to stimulation (insomnia, hallucinations, tremors or convulsions) to death. Other signs and symptoms may be dizziness, tinnitus, ataxia, blurred vision, and hypotension. Stimulation is particularly likely in children, as are atropine-like signs and symptoms (dry mouth; fixed, dilated pupils; flushing; hyperthermia; and gastrointestinal symptoms).

Treatment: The patient should be induced to vomit, even if emesis has occurred spontaneously. Pharmacologic vomiting by the administration of ipecac syrup is a preferred method. However, vomiting should not be induced in patients with impaired consciousness. The action of ipecac is facilitated by physical activity and by the administration of 8 to 12 fluid ounces of water. If emesis does not occur within fifteen minutes, the dose of ipecac should be repeated. Precautions against aspiration must be taken, especially in infants and children. Following emesis, any drug remaining in the stomach may be adsorbed by activated charcoal administered as a slurry with water. If vomiting is unsuccessful or contraindicated, gastric lavage should be performed. Physiologic saline solution is the lavage solution of choice, particularly in children. In adults, tap water can be used; however, as much as possible of the amount administered should be removed before the next instillation. Saline cathartics, such as milk of magnesia, draw water into the bowel by osmosis and, therefore, may be valuable for their action in rapid dilution of bowel content. Dialysis is of little value in antihistamine poisoning. After emergency treatment, the patient should continue to be medically monitored.

Treatment of the signs and symptoms of overdosage is symptomatic and supportive. Stimulants (analeptic agents) should not be used. Vasopressors may be used to treat hypotension. Short acting barbiturates, diazepam, or paraldehyde may be administered to control seizures. Hyperpyrexia, especially in children, may require treatment with tepid water sponge baths or a hypothermic blanket. Apnea is treated with ventilatory support.

Dosage and Administration: DOSAGE SHOULD BE INDIVIDUALIZED ACCORDING TO THE NEEDS AND THE RESPONSE OF THE PATIENT.

OPTIMINE Tablets are not recommended for use in children under 12 years of age.

The usual adult dosage is 1 or 2 mg, twice a day.

How Supplied: OPTIMINE Tablets, 1 mg. white, compressed, scored tablets impressed with the Schering trademark and product identification numbers, 282; bottle of 100.

Store between 2°and 30°C (36°and 86°F).

Revised 5/81

Copyright © 1973, 1981, Schering Corporation. All rights reserved.

[*Shown in Product Identification Section*]

ORETON® Methyl ℞

brand of methyltestosterone, USP
Tablets
Buccal Tablets

Description: ORETON **Methyl** Tablets and **Buccal** Tablets contain methyltestosterone, USP, a synthetic androgen. Androgens are steroids that develop and maintain primary and secondary male sex characteristics. ORETON **Methyl** Tablets are to be taken orally. ORETON **Methyl Buccal** Tablets are NOT to be swallowed but are to be placed in the lower or upper buccal pouches.

Androgens are derivatives of cyclopentanoperhydrophenanthrene. Endogenous androgens are C-19 steroids with a side chain at C-17, and with two angular methyl groups. Testosterone is the primary endogenous androgen. In their active form, all drugs in the class have a 17-beta-hydroxy group. 17-alpha alkylation (methyltestosterone) increases the pharmacologic activity per unit weight compared to testosterone when given orally.

Methyltestosterone is the 17α-methyl derivative of testosterone, the true testicular hormone. Chemically, methyltestosterone is 17β-Hydroxy-17-methylandrost-4-en-3-one, with the empirical formula $C_{20}H_{30}O_2$, a molecular weight of 302.5.

Methyltestosterone is a white to creamy-white, odorless, slightly hygroscopic powder. It is practically insoluble in water, soluble in alcohol and other organic solvents.

ORETON **Methyl** Tablets contain either 10 mg or 25 mg of methyltestosterone, USP.

Each ORETON **Methyl Buccal** Tablet contains 10 mg methyltestosterone, USP.

Clinical Pharmacology: Endogenous androgens are responsible for the normal growth and development of the male sex organs and for maintenance of secondary sex characteristics. These effects include the growth and maturation of prostate, seminal vesicles, penis, and scrotum: the development of male hair distribution, such as beard, pubic, chest, and axillary hair; laryngeal enlargement, vocal chord thickening, alterations in body musculature, and fat distribution. Drugs in this class also cause retention of nitrogen, sodium, potassium, phosphorus, and decreased urinary excretion of calcium. Androgens have been reported to increase protein anabolism and decrease protein catabolism. Nitrogen balance is improved only when there is sufficient intake of calories and protein.

Androgens are responsible for the growth spurt of adolescence and for the eventual termination of linear growth which is brought about by fusion of the epiphyseal growth centers. In children, exogenous androgens accelerate linear growth rates, but may cause a disproportionate advancement in bone maturation. Use over long periods may result in fusion of the epiphyseal growth centers and termination of the growth process. Androgens have been reported to stimulate the production of red blood cells by enhancing the production of erythropoietic stimulating factor.

During exogenous administration of androgens, endogenous testosterone release is inhibited through feedback inhibition of pituitary luteinizing hormone (LH). With large doses of exogenous androgens, spermatogenesis may also be suppressed through feedback inhibition of pituitary follicle stimulating hormone (FSH).

There is a lack of substantial evidence that androgens are effective in fractures, surgery, convalescence, and functional uterine bleeding.

Pharmacokinetics: Testosterone given orally is metabolized by the gut and 44 percent is cleared by the liver in the first pass. Oral doses as high as 400 mg per day are needed to achieve clinically effective blood levels for full replacement therapy. The synthetic androgen (methyltestosterone) is less extensively metabolized by the liver and has a longer half-life. It is more suitable than testosterone for oral administration. Additionally, buccal administration permits the methyltestosterone to be absorbed directly into the systemic venous return so that the unmetabolized hormone is carried directly to the tissues. The buccal tablets have approximately twice the potency of the orally ingested methyltestosterone.

Testosterone in plasma is 98 percent bound to a specific testosterone-estradiol binding globulin, and about one percent is free. Generally, the amount of this sex-hormone binding globulin in the plasma will determine the distribution of testosterone between free and bound forms, and the free testosterone concentration will determine its half-life.

About 90 percent of a dose of testosterone is excreted in the urine as glucuronic and sulfuric acid conjugates of testosterone and its metabolites; about 6 percent of a dose is excreted in the feces, mostly in the unconjugated form. Inactivation of testosterone occurs primarily in the liver. Testosterone is metabolized to various 17-keto steroids through two different pathways. As reported in the literature, the half-life of testosterone varies considerably, ranging from 10 to 100 minutes.

In many tissues the activity of testosterone appears to depend on reduction to dihydrotestosterone, which binds to cytosol receptor proteins. The steroid-receptor complex is transported to the nucleus where is initiates transcription events and cellular changes related to androgen action.

Indications and Usage: ***In the male:*** ORETON **Methyl** Tablets and **Methyl Buccal** Tablets are indicated for replacement therapy in conditions associated with a deficiency or absence of endogenous testosterone:

Primary hypogonadism (congenital or acquired)—testicular failure due to cryptorchidism, bilateral torsion, orchitis, vanishing testis syndrome; or orchidectomy.

Hypogonadotropic hypogonadism (congenital or acqurie d)—idopathic gonadotropin of LHRH deficiency, or pituitary-hypothalamic injury from tumors, trauma, or radiation.

If the above conditions occur prior to puberty, androgen replacement therapy will be needed during the adolescent years for development of secondary sexual characteristics. Prolonged androgen treatment will be required to maintain sexual characteristics in these and other males who develop testosterone deficiency after puberty.

Androgens may be used to stimulate puberty in carefully selected males with clearly delayed puberty. These patients usually have a familial pattern of delayed puberty that is not secondary to a pathological disorder; puberty is expected to occur spontaneously at a relatively late date. Brief treatment with conservative doses may occasionally be justified in these patients if they do not respond to psychological support. The potential adverse effect on bone maturation should be discussed with the patient and parents prior to androgen administration. An X-ray of the hand and wrist to determine bone age should be obtained every 6 months to assess the effect of treatment on the epiphyseal centers. (See WARNINGS.)

In the female: ORETON **Methyl** Tablets and **Methyl Buccal** Tablets may be used secondarily in women with advancing inoperable metastatic (skeletal) mammary cancer who are 1 to 5 years postmenopausal. Primary goals of therapy in these women include ablation of the ovaries. Other methods of counteracting estrogen activity are adrenalectomy, hypophysec-

Continued on next page

Information on Schering products appearing on these pages is effective as of September 30, 1982.

Schering—Cont.

tomy, and/or antiestrogen therapy. This treatment has also been used in premenopausal women with breast cancer who have benefited from oophorectomy and are considered to have a hormone-responsive tumor. Judgment concerning androgen therapy should be made by an oncologist with expertise in this field.
Androgens, such as methyltestosterone, have been used for the management of postpartum breast pain and engorgement.
Contraindications: ORETON **Methyl** and **Methyl Buccal** Tablets are contraindicated for use in men with carcinomas of the breast or with known or suspected carcinomas of the prostate, and in women who are or may become pregnant.
When administered to pregnant women, androgens cause virilization of the external genitalia of the female fetus. This virilization includes clitoromegaly, abnormal vaginal development, and fusion of genital folds to form a scrotal-like structure. The degree of masculinization is related to the amount of drug given and to the age of the fetus, and is most likely to occur in the female fetus when the drugs are given in the first trimester. If the patient becomes pregnant while taking these drugs, she should be apprised of the potential hazard to the fetus.
Warnings: In patients with breast cancer, androgen therapy may cause hypercalcemia by stimulating osteolysis. In this case, the drugs should be discontinued.
Prolonged use of high doses of androgens has been associated with the development of peliosis hepatis and hepatic neoplasms including hepatocellular carcinoma. (See PRECAUTIONS:—**Carcinogenesis, Mutagenesis, Impairment of Fertility.**). Peliosis hepatis can be a life-threatening or fatal complication.
Cholestatic hepatitis and jaundice occur with 17-alpha-alkylandrogens (such as methyltestosterone) at a relatively low dose. If cholestatic hepatitis with jaundice appears or if liver function tests become abnormal, the androgen should be discontinued and the etiology should be determined. Drug-induced jaundice is reversible when the medication is discontinued.
Geriatric patients treated with androgens may be at an increased risk for the development of prostatic hypertrophy and prostatic carcinoma.
Edema with or without congestive heart failure may be a serious complication in patients with preexisting cardiac, renal, or hepatic disease. In addition to discontinuation of the drug, diuretic therapy may be required.
Gynecomastia frequently develops and occasionally persists in patients being treated for hypogonadism.
Androgen therapy should be used cautiously in healthy males with delayed puberty. The effect on bone maturation should be monitored by assessing bone age of the wrist and hand every 6 months. In children, androgen treatment may accelerate bone maturation without producing compensatory gain in linear growth. This adverse effect may result in compromised adult stature. The younger the child the greater the risk of compromising final mature height.
Precautions: General: Women should be observed for signs of virilization (deepening of the voice, hirsutism, acne, clitoromegaly and menstrual irregularities). Discontinuation of drug therapy at the time of evidence of mild virilism is necessary to prevent irreversible virilization. Such virilization is usual following androgen use at high doses. A decision may be made by the patient and the physician that some virilization will be tolerated during treatment for breast carcinoma.
Priapism or excessive sexual stimulation may develop. Males, especially the elderly, may become overstimulated. In treating males for symptoms of climacteric, avoid stimulation to the point of increasing the nervous, mental, and physical activities beyond the patient's cardiovascular capacity.
Oligospermia and reduced ejaculatory volume may occur after prolonged administration or excessive dosage.
Information for the Patients: The physician should instruct patients to report any of the following side effects of androgens:
Adult or Adolescent Males: Too frequent or persistent erections of the penis.
Women: Hoarseness, acne, changes in menstrual periods, or more hair on the face.
All Patients: Any nausea, vomiting, changes in skin color or ankle swelling.
Any male adolescent patient receiving androgens for delayed puberty should have bone development checked every six months.
Patients should be instructed in the proper taking of ORETON **Methyl Buccal** Tablets. These tablets should **NOT** be swallowed. They should be placed in the space between the gum and cheek and allowed to dissolve, so that the medication enters the body through the lining of the cheek. Avoid eating, drinking, chewing, or smoking while the buccal tablet is in place. The mouth should be rinsed with water after the tablet has dissolved completely.
Laboratory Tests: Women with disseminated breast carcinomas should have frequent determination of urine and serum calcium levels during the course of androgen therapy. (See WARNINGS.)
Because of the hepatoxicity associated with the use of 17-alpha-alkylated androgens, liver function tests should be obtained periodically.
Periodic (every 6 months) X-ray examinations of bone age should be made during treatment of prepubertal males to determine the rate of bone maturation and the effects of androgen therapy on the epiphyseal centers.
Hemoglobin and hematocrit should be checked periodically for polycythemia in patients who are receiving high doses of androgens.
Drug Interactions: Anticoagulants C-17 substituted derivatives of testosterone, such as methandrostenolone, have been reported to decrease the anticoagulant requirements of patients receiving oral anticoagulants. Patients receiving oral anticoagulant therapy require close monitoring especially when androgens are started or stopped.
Oxyphenbutazone Concurrent administration of oxyphenbutazone and androgens may result in elevated serum levels of oxyphenbutazone.
Insulin In diabetic patients the metabolic effects of androgens may decrease blood glucose and insulin requirements.
Drug/Laboratory Test Interferences: Androgens may decrease levels of thyroxine-binding globulin, resulting in decreased total T_4 serum levels and increased resin uptake of T_3 and T_4. Free thyroid hormone levels remain unchanged, however, and there is no clinical evidence of thyroid dysfunction.
Carcinogenesis, Mutagenesis, Impairment of Fertility: *Animal Data:* Testosterone has been tested by subcutaneous injection and implantation in mice and rats. The implant induced cervical-uterine tumors in mice which metastasized in some cases. There is suggestive evidence that injection of testosterone into some strains of female mice increases their susceptibility to hepatoma. Testosterone is also known to increase the number of tumors and decrease the degree of differentiation of chemically induced carcinomas of the liver in rats.
Human Data: There are rare reports of hepatocellular carcinoma in patients receiving long-term therapy with androgens in high doses. Withdrawal of the drugs did not lead to regression of the tumors in all cases.
Geriatric patients treated with androgens may be at an increased risk for the development of prostatic hypertrophy and prostatic carcinoma.
Information on mutagenesis is unknown.
Pregnancy: ***Teratogenic Effects—Pregnancy Category X:*** See CONTRAINDICATIONS.
Nursing Mothers: It is not known whether androgens are excreted in human milk. Because many drugs are excreted in human milk and because of the potential for serious adverse reactions in nursing infants from androgens, a decision should be made whether to discontinue nursing or to discontinue the drug, taking into account the importance of the drug to the mother.
Pediatric Use: Androgen therapy should be used very cautiously in children and only by specialists who are aware of the adverse effects on bone maturation. Skeletal maturation must be monitored every six months by an X-ray of the hand and wrist. (See INDICATIONS AND USAGE, and WARNINGS.)
Adverse Reactions: Endocrine and Urogenital: ***Female:*** The most common side effects of androgen therapy are amenorrhea and other menstrual irregularities, inhibition of gonadotropin secretion, and virilization, including deepening of the voice and clitoral enlargement. The latter usually is not reversible after androgens are discontinued. When administered to a pregnant woman, androgens cause virilization of external genitalia of the female fetus.
Male: Gynecomastia, and excessive frequency and duration of penile erections. Oligospermia may occur at high dosages. (See CLINICAL PHARMACOLOGY.)
Skin and appendages: Hirsutism, male pattern of baldness, and acne.
Fluid and Electrolyte Disturbances: Retention of sodium, chloride, water, potassium, calcium, and inorganic phosphates.
Gastrointestinal: Nausea, cholestatic jaundice, alterations in liver function tests, rarely hepatocellular neoplasms and peliosis hepatitis (See WARNINGS.)
Hematologic: Suppression of clotting factors, II, V, VII, and X, bleeding in patients on concomitant anticoagulant therapy, and polycythemia.
Nervous System: Increased or decreased libido, headache, anxiety, depression, and generalized paresthesiae.
Metabolic: Increased serum cholesterol.
Miscellaneous: Stomatitis with buccal preparations; rarely anaphylactoid reactions.
Overdosage: Overdose of medication may be reflected in the occurrence of the signs and symptoms associated with testosterone-anabolic drugs. Nausea and early appearance of the manifestations of edema should be looked for. However, there has been no report of acute overdosage with androgens.
Dosage and Administration: Dosage must be strictly individualized. The suggested dosage for androgens varies depending on the age, sex, and diagnosis of the individual patient. Adjustments and duration of dosage will depend upon the patient's response and the appearance of adverse reactions.
Males: In the androgen-deficient male the following guideline for replacement therapy indicates the usual initial dosages:
[See table left].
Various dosage regimens have been used to induce pubertal changes in hypogonadal males; some experts have advocated lower dos-

	Route	Dose	Frequency
ORETON **Methyl** Tablets	Oral	10–50 mg	Daily
ORETON **Methyl Buccal** Tablets	Buccal	5–25 mg*	Daily

* NOTE: ORETON **Methyl Buccal** Tablets have approximately twice the potency of the orally ingested ORETON **Methyl** Tablets.

	Route	Dose	Frequency
ORETON **Methyl** Tablets			
breast cancer	oral	50–200 mg	daily
postpartum breast pain and engorgement	oral	80 mg	daily (3 to 5 days)
ORETON **Methyl Buccal** Tablets			
breast cancer	buccal	25–100 mg*	daily
postpartum breast pain and engorgement	buccal	40 mg*	daily (3 to 5 days)

* NOTE: ORETON **Methyl Buccal** Tablets have approximately twice the potency of the orally ingested ORETON **Methyl** Tablets.

ages initially, gradually increasing the dose as puberty progresses, with or without a decrease to maintenance levels. Other experts emphasize that higher dosages are needed to induce pubertal changes and lower dosages can be used for maintenance after puberty. The chronological and skeletal ages must be taken into consideration, both in determining the initial doses and in adjusting the dose.

Dosages used in delayed puberty generally are in the lower ranges of those given above, and are for limited duration, for example, 4 to 6 months.

Females: Women with metastatic breast carcinoma must be followed closely because androgen therapy occasionally appears to accelerate the disease. Thus, many experts prefer to use the shorter acting androgen preparations rather than those with prolonged activity for treating breast carcinoma particularly during the early stages of androgen therapy.

Guideline dosages of androgens for use in the palliative treatment of women with metastatic breast cancer and for the prevention of postpartum breast pain and engorgement are:

[See table above].

Administration of Buccal Tablets: ORETON **Methyl Buccal** Tablets should NOT be swallowed, since the hormone is meant to be absorbed through the oral mucous membranes. Place the buccal tablet in the upper or lower buccal pouch between the gum and cheek; let the tablet dissolve completely. Avoid eating, drinking, chewing, or smoking while the buccal tablet is in place. Proper oral hygienic measures (e.g., rinsing mouth with water) are particularly important after the use of buccal tablets.

How Supplied: ORETON **Methyl Buccal** Tablets, 10 mg, compressed, lavender-colored, oval tablets impressed with the Schering trademark and product identification letters, BE, or numbers, 970; bottle of 100 (NDC–0085–0970–06).

Store between 2° and 30°C (36° and 86°F).

NOTE: Color of tablets may fade; potency and effectiveness are not impaired.

ORETON **Methyl** Tablets, 10 mg, compressed, white, round tablets impressed with the Schering trademark and product identification letters, JD, or numbers 311; bottle of 100 (NDC–0085–0311–06).

ORETON **Methyl** Tablets, 25 mg, compressed, peach-colored, round tablets impressed with the Schering trademark and product identification letters, JE, or numbers, 499; bottle of 100 (NDC–0085–0499–06).

Revised 9/81

Copyright © 1968, 1981, Schering Corporation. All rights reserved.

[*Shown in Product Identification Section*]

OTOBIOTIC® ℞

brand of polymyxin B sulfate, USP and hydrocortisone, USP
Sterile Otic Solution

Description: OTOBIOTIC Otic Solution is a sterile, antibacterial solution containing an anti-inflammatory agent for use in the external ear. Each ml contains polymyxin B sulfate, USP equivalent to 10,000 units polymyxin B and 5.0 mg hydrocortisone, USP in a propylene glycol, glycerin vehicle which also contains edetate disodium, sodium bisulfite, anhydrous sodium sulfite, and purified water. The pH of the solution ranges from 5.0 to 7.0.

Actions: Polymyxin B sulfate is effective against *Pseudomonas aeruginosa* and some other gram-negative organisms, including strains of *Escherichia*, that commonly cause otitis externa. The addition of hydrocortisone to the antibiotic affords an anti-inflammatory effect and relief against allergic manifestations and pruritus and reduces the possibility of hypersensitivity and tissue reaction.

Indications: OTOBIOTIC Otic Solution is indicated for the treatment of superficial bacterial infections of the external auditory canals caused by organisms susceptible to the action of the antibiotic.

Contraindications: OTOBIOTIC Otic Solution is contraindicated in those individuals who are hypersensitive to corticosteroids, polymyxin or colistin, or to any of its other components, and in infections due to herpes simplex, vaccinia, and zoster varicella viruses or to fungi.

Perforated tympanic membranes are frequently considered a contraindication to the use of external ear canal medication.

Warnings: As with other antibiotic preparations, prolonged treatment with OTOBIOTIC Otic Solution may result in overgrowth of nonsusceptible organisms and fungi.

Infections of the external auditory canals can be of mixed microbial origin and occasionally may be caused by both bacteria and fungi. If the infection is not improved after one week, bacterial and fungal cultures and susceptibility tests should be done to verify the identity of the organism and to determine whether therapy should be changed.

Patients who prefer to warm the medication before using it should be cautioned against heating the solution above body temperature in order to avoid loss of potency.

Precautions: If sensitization or irritation occurs, treatment with OTOBIOTIC Otic Solution should be discontinued promptly. Treatment with OTOBIOTIC Otic Solution should not be continued for longer than ten days.

OTOBIOTIC Otic Solution is not for ophthalmic use.

Dosage and Administration: The external auditory canal should be thoroughly cleansed and dried with a sterile cotton applicator before administration of OTOBIOTIC Otic Solution.

For adults, four drops of the solution should be instilled into the affected ear three or four times a day. For infants and children, three drops, instilled into the affected ear three or four times a day, are suggested because of the smaller capacity of the ear canal.

The patient should lie with the affected ear upward and then the drops should be instilled. This position should be maintained for five minutes to facilitate penetration of the drops into the ear canal. Repeat, if necessary, for the opposite ear.

Note: When placing the dropper in the bottle and during use, do not allow the dropper to touch affected area, fingers, or any other surface. This precaution is necessary to preserve the sterility of the solution.

How Supplied: OTOBIOTIC Otic Solution, 15 ml bottle with sterile dropper packaged separately; box of one.

Store between 2° and 8°C (36° and 46°F).

Copyright © 1981, Schering Corporation. All rights reserved.

PAXIPAM® Ⓒ

brand of halazepam
Tablets

Description: PAXIPAM Tablets contain halazepam, a benzodiazepine derivative having the chemical name, 7-chloro-1,3-dihydro-5-phenyl-1-(2,2,2-trifluoroethyl)-2*H*-1, 4-benzodiazepin-2-one. Each PAXIPAM Tablet contains 20 mg or 40 mg halazepam. The compound is a white to light cream-colored powder with a molecular weight of 352.8.

Clinical Pharmacology: Central nervous system agents of the 1,4-benzodiazepine class presumably exert their effects by binding at stereo specific receptors at several sites within the central nervous system. Their exact mechanism of action is unknown. Clinically, all benzodiazepines cause a dose-related central nervous system depressant activity varying from mild impairment of task performance to hypnosis.

Halazepam is rapidly and well-absorbed and primarily excreted in the urine. Maximum plasma concentration of halazepam is achieved between one and three hours following oral administration. Studies involving 12 normal subjects indicate the median half-life of elimination of halazepam following a 40 mg dose is approximately 14 hours. The major active plasma metabolite of halazepam is N-desmethyldiazepam. Maximum plasma concentrations of N-desmethyldiazepam usually occur within three to six hours. This metabolite has a half-life of elimination of approximately 50 to 100 hours. Less than one percent of the dose is excreted in the urine as unchanged drug. The major metabolite of halazepam in the urine is a conjugate, 3-hydroxyhalazepam. As with other benzodiazepines, enterohepatic recycling of halazepam and its metabolites may occur in uremic patients.

The degree of plasma protein binding of benzodiazepines is high. Since binding is to serum albumin, the extent of binding is dependent on the albumin concentration. In chronic alcoholics, patients with cirrhosis, and newborns, reduced binding may occur. Protein binding may be greatly reduced in patients with renal insufficiency. Since hepatic biotransformation is the predominant route for the metabolism of benzodiazepines, the disposition of these drugs may be impaired in patients with chronic liver disease. Oral dosing of rats with halazepam for a brief period induced the synthesis of hepatic microsomal drug-metabolizing enzymes. As a result, assuming similar responses in humans, the metabolism of other drugs metabolized in the liver may be increased. The transplacental transfer of halazepam has not been studied. However, other benzodiazepines readily cross the placental barrier. Following administration of halazepam to lactating women, halazepam and its major metabolite, N-desmethyldiazepam, were present in the milk.

Indications and Usage: PAXIPAM Tablets are indicated for the management of anxiety disorders or the short-term relief of the symptoms of anxiety. Anxiety or tension associated with the stress of everyday life usually does not require treatment with an anxiolytic.

The effectiveness of PAXIPAM Tablets for long-term use, that is, more than *four* months, has not been established.

The physician should periodically reassess the usefulness of the drug for the individual patient.

Continued on next page

Information on Schering products appearing on these pages is effective as of September 30, 1982.

Schering—Cont.

Contraindications: PAXIPAM Tablets are contraindicated in patients with known sensitivity to this drug or other benzodiazepines. It may be used in patients with open angle glaucoma who are receiving appropriate therapy, but is contraindicated in acute narrow angle glaucoma.

Warnings: PAXIPAM Tablets are not of value in the treatment of psychotic patients and should not be employed in lieu of appropriate treatment for psychosis. PAXIPAM Tablets are also not recommended as the primary treatment for major depressive disorders. Because of its depressant CNS effects, patients receiving PAXIPAM Tablets should be cautioned against engaging in hazardous occupations requiring complete mental alertness, such as operating machinery or driving a motor vehicle. For the same reason, patients should be cautioned about the simultaneous ingestion of alcohol and other CNS depressant drugs during treatment with PAXIPAM Tablets.

Benzodiazepines can potentially cause fetal harm when administered to pregnant women. If PAXIPAM Tablets are used during pregnancy, or if the patient becomes pregnant while taking this drug, she should be apprised of the potential hazard to the fetus. Because of experience with other members of the benzodiazepine class, PAXIPAM Tablets are assumed to be capable of causing an increased risk of congenital abnormalities when administered to a pregnant woman during the first trimester. Because use of these drugs is rarely a matter of urgency, their use during the first trimester should almost always be avoided. The possibility that a woman of childbearing potential may be pregnant at the time of institution of therapy should be considered. Patients should be advised that if they become pregnant during therapy or intend to become pregnant, they should communicate with their physicians about the desirability of discontinuing the drug.

Precautions: General: If PAXIPAM Tablets are to be combined with other psychotropic agents or anticonvulsant drugs, careful consideration should be given to the pharmacology of the agents to be employed, particularly with compounds which might potentiate the action of benzodiazepines (See Drug Interactions section).

As with other psychotropic medications, the usual precautions with respect to administration of the drug and size of the prescription are indicated for severely depressed patients or those in whom there is reason to expect concealed suicidal ideation or plans.

In elderly and debilitated patients, it is recommended that the dosage be limited to the smallest effective amount to preclude the development of ataxia or oversedation (See DOSAGE AND ADMINISTRATION section). The usual precautions in treating patients with impaired renal or hepatic function should be observed.

Information for Patients: To assure safe and effective use of benzodiazepines, the following information and instructions should be given to the patient:

1. Inform your physician about any alcohol consumption and medicine you are taking now, including drugs you buy without a prescription. Alcohol should generally not be used during treatment with benzodiazepines.
2. Inform your physician if you are planning to become pregnant, if you are pregnant, or if you become pregnant while you are taking this medication.
3. Inform your physician if you are nursing.
4. Until you experience how this medicine affects you, do not drive a car or operate potentially dangerous machinery, etc.
5. If benzodiazepines are used in large doses and/or for an extended period of time, they produce habituation, emotional and physical dependence. Therefore, do not increase the dose even if you think that the drug "does not work anymore."
6. Do not stop taking the drug abruptly without consulting your physician, since withdrawal symptoms can occur.

Laboratory Tests: Laboratory tests are not ordinarily required in otherwise healthy patients.

Drug Interactions: The benzodiazepines, including PAXIPAM Tablets, produce additive CNS depressant effects when co-administered with other psychotropic medications, anticonvulsants, antihistaminics, ethanol, and other drugs which themselves produce CNS depression.

Pharmacokinetic interactions with benzodiazepines have been reported. For example, cimetidine has been reported to reduce diazepam clearance. However, it is not known at this time whether a similar interaction occurs with PAXIPAM Tablets.

Drug/Laboratory Test Interactions: Although interactions between benzodiazepines and commonly employed clinical laboratory tests have occasionally been reported, there is no consistent pattern for a specific drug or specific test.

Carcinogenesis, Mutagenesis, Impairment of Fertility: The results of oral oncogenicity studies in rats and mice treated at doses 5 to 50 times the usual 120 mg daily human dose revealed no evidence of carcinogenicity or other significant pathology. Studies regarding mutagenesis have not been done. Reproduction studies performed in rats have revealed no evidence of impaired fertility.

Pregnancy: Teratogenic Effects: Pregnancy Category D: (See WARNINGS section).

Nonteratogenic Effects: The child born of a mother who is on benzodiazepines may be at some risk for withdrawal symptoms from the drug during the postnatal period. Also, neonatal flaccidity has been reported in children born of mothers who had been receiving benzodiazepines.

Labor and Delivery: PAXIPAM Tablets have no established use in labor or delivery.

Nursing Mothers: Halazepam and its major metabolites are excreted in the milk of lactating postpartum women. Since neonates metabolize benzodiazepines more slowly than adults, and since accumulation of the drug and its metabolites to toxic levels is possible in neonates, the drug should not be given to nursing mothers.

For example, chronic administration of the closely related benzodiazepine, diazepam, to nursing mothers has been reported to cause their infants to become lethargic and lose weight.

Pediatric Use: Safety and effectiveness in children below the age of 18 years have not been established.

Adverse Reactions: Central Nervous System: The most frequent adverse reactions to PAXIPAM Tablets were CNS disturbances. The most common of these were drowsiness, which occurred in approximately 29 per 100 patients. Other CNS disturbances occurred in approximately 9 per 100 patients (e.g., headache, apathy, psychomotor retardation, disorientation, confusion, euphoria, dysarthria, depression, syncope). Less frequent CNS disturbances were: dizziness, which occurred in approximately 8 per 100 patients; ataxia which occurred in 5 per 100 patients; fatigue, which occurred in approximately 4 per 100 patients; and visual disturbances and paradoxical reaction, which occurred in 1 per 100 patients. Sleep disturbances, changes in libido, and auditory disturbances occurred in fewer than 1 per 100 patients.

Gastrointestinal: Less frequent adverse reactions were: gastrointestinal disturbances (e.g., sense of seasickness, nausea, constipation, increased salivation, difficulty in swallowing, vomiting, gastric disorder). which occurred in approximately 9 per 100 patients; change in appetite, which occurred in approximately 1 per 100 patients; and dry mouth, which occurred in approximately 3 per 100 patients.

Hematologic: Clinically unimportant fluctuations in the white blood and differential counts were reported in less than 5% of 761 patients.

Hepatic: Small to moderate elevations of the following hepatic enzymes were reported; alkaline phosphatase in 20 (2.8%) of 705 patients; SGOT in 35 (5.4%) of 647 patients; SGPT in 3 (<1%) of 336 patients. No serious abnormalities were seen.

The following adverse reactions were reported to occur rarely in those patients treated with PAXIPAM Tablets.

Cardiovascular: Cardiovascular disturbances (e.g., tachycardia, bradycardia, hypotension) were reported to occur in approximately 2 per 100 patients.

Musculoskeletal: Muscular disturbances were reported to occur in approximately 2 per 100 patients.

Other: The following adverse reactions occurred in fewer than 1 per 100 patients: allergic manifestations, genitourinary disturbance, paresthesias, and respiratory disturbance.

Adverse Reactions not reported with the use of PAXIPAM Tablets, but reported with the use of other benzodiazepines are: jaundice, agranulocytosis, edema, slurred speech, minor menstrual irregularities, dystonia, pruritus, incontinence, urinary retention, and diplopia.

Drug Abuse and Dependence: Physical and Psychological Dependence: Withdrawal symptoms (similar in character to those noted with barbiturates and alcohol) have occurred following abrupt discontinuance of benzodiazepines. These can range from mild dysphoria and insomnia to a major syndrome which may include abdominal and muscle cramps, vomiting, sweating, tremor, and convulsions. These signs and symptoms, especially the more serious ones, are generally more common in those patients who have received excessive doses over an extended period of time. However, withdrawal symptoms have also been reported following abrupt discontinuance of benzodiazepines taken continuously, at therapeutic levels, for several months. Consequently, after extended therapy, abrupt discontinuation should generally be avoided and a gradual tapering in dosage followed.

Patients with a history of seizures or epilepsy, regardless of their concomitant anti-seizure drug therapy, should not be abruptly withdrawn from any CNS depressant agent, including PAXIPAM Tablets. Addiction-prone individuals (such as drug addicts or alcoholics) should be under careful surveillance when receiving halazepam or other psychotropic agents because of the predisposition of such patients to habituation and dependence.

Controlled Substance Class: PAXIPAM is a controlled substance under the Controlled Substance Act and has been assigned by the Drug Enforcement Administration to Schedule IV.

Overdosage: Manifestations of PAXIPAM Tablets overdosage include somnolence, confusion, impaired coordination, diminished reflexes, and coma.

No delayed reactions (e.g., organ toxicity) or clinical laboratory abnormalities have been reported.

General Treatment Of Overdose: Overdosage reports with halazepam are limited. Respiration, pulse, and blood pressure should be monitored, as in all cases of drug overdosage. General supportive measures should be employed, along with immediate gastric lavage. Intravenous fluids should be administered and an adequate airway maintained. Hypotension may be combated by the use of Levophed® (levarterenol) or Aramine® (metaraminol). Dialysis is of limited value. Animal experiments have suggested that forced diuresis or hemodialysis are probably of little value in treating overdosage. As with the management of intentional overdosing with any drug, it should be borne in mind that multiple agents may have been ingested.

Dosage and Administration: Dosage should be individualized for maximum beneficial effect. While the usual daily dosages given below will meet the needs of most patients, there will be some who require higher doses. In such cases, dosage should be increased cautiously to avoid adverse effects.

PAXIPAM Tablets are administered orally in divided doses and the dosage should be individualized according to the severity of symptoms and response of the patient. To facilitate dosing, the tablets are scored. The usual recommended dose is 20 to 40 mg three or four times a day.

The response of the patient to several days of treatment will permit the physician to adjust the dose upward or downward. The optimal dosage usually ranges from 80 to 160 mg daily. In debilitated patients or the elderly (70 years or older), the initial recommended dosage is 20 mg once or twice a day. The dose should be adjusted as needed and tolerated.

If side effects occur with the starting dose, the dose should be lowered.

How Supplied: PAXIPAM Tablets, 20 mg, orange, compressed, scored tablets impressed with the Schering trademark and product identification numbers, 251; bottles of 100 and 500 and boxes of 100 for unit-dose dispensing (10 strips of 10 tablets each).

PAXIPAM Tablets, 40 mg, white, compressed, scored tablets impressed with the Schering trademark and product identification numbers, 538; bottles of 100 and 500 and boxes of 100 for unit-dose dispensing (10 strips of 10 tablets each).

Store between 2° and 30°C (36° and 86°F). In addition, protect unit-dose packages from excessive moisture.

Animal Pharmacology and/or Animal Toxicology: In animal studies, the anti-anxiety activity of halazepam was demonstrated by its ability to induce calming effects in normally aggressive species, such as the monkey, and to alleviate suppressed behavior in animals placed in a conflict situation. Halazepam was also shown to block aggressive behavior invoked by stressful stimuli.

Halazepam has relatively little effect on autonomic function and unlike major tranquilizers such as chlorpromazine or haloperidol, it does not cause extrapyramidal side effects. As with other CNS depressants, halazepam at relatively high doses produces transient cardiovascular depressant effects, but no EKG disturbances were seen in dogs.

A battery of tests were performed in monkeys to evaluate the abuse potential of PAXIPAM. Although PAXIPAM did cause physical dependence and positive drug-seeking behavior, these effects were judged to be weaker than those caused by diazepam or chlordiazepoxide in each case. However, the abuse potential of PAXIPAM in man in comparison with that of diazepam or chlordiazepoxide remains to be established.

Revised 9/81

Copyright, © 1981, Schering Corporation. All rights reserved.

[*Shown in Product Identification Section*]

PERMITIL® ℞

brand of fluphenazine hydrochloride, USP Tablets, Oral Concentrate, CHRONOTAB® Tablets

Description: PERMITIL products are formulations of fluphenazine hydrochloride, USP a phenothiazine of the piperazine group. It is available as Tablets, 0.25, 2.5, 5, and 10 mg; Oral Concentrate, 5 mg fluphenazine hydrochloride per ml and alcohol 1%; and CHRONOTAB (brand of repeat-action tablet) Tablets, 0.5 mg fluphenazine hydrochloride in the tablet coating and 0.5 mg in the core.

Actions: Fluphenazine hydrochloride has actions at all levels of the central nervous system, as well as on other organ systems. However, the site and mechanism of action of therapeutic effect are not known.

Indications: PERMITIL **Tablets, Oral Concentrate,** and CHRONOTAB **Tablets** are indicated for the management of manifestations of psychotic disorders.

PERMITIL has not been shown effective in the management of behavioral complications in patients with mental retardation.

Contraindications: PERMITIL products are contraindicated in comatose or greatly obtunded patients and in patients receiving large doses of central nervous system depressants (barbiturates, alcohol, narcotics, analgesics, or antihistamines); in the presence of existing blood dyscrasias, bone marrow depression, or liver damage; and in patients who have shown hypersensitivity to PERMITIL products, their components, or related compounds.

PERMITIL products are also contraindicated in patients with suspected or established subcortical brain damage, with or without hypothalamic damage, since a hyperthermic reaction with temperatures in excess of 104° F may occur in such patients, sometimes not until 14 to 16 hours after drug administration. Total body ice-packing is recommended for such a reaction; antipyretics may also be useful.

Warnings: If hypotension develops epinephrine should not be administered since its action is blocked and partially reversed by fluphenazine hydrochloride. If a vasopressor is needed, norepinephrine may be used. Severe, acute hypotension has occurred with the use of phenothiazines and is particularly likely to occur in patients with mitral insufficiency or pheochromocytoma. Rebound hypertension may occur in pheochromocytoma patients.

PERMITIL products can lower the convulsive threshold in susceptible individuals; they should be used with caution in alcohol withdrawal and in patients with convulsive disorders. If the patient is being treated with an anticonvulsant agent, increased dosage of that agent may be required when PERMITIL products are used concomitantly.

PERMITIL products should be used with caution in patients with psychic depression.

Fluphenazine hydrochloride may impair the mental and/or physical abilities required for the performance of hazardous tasks such as driving a car or operating machinery; therefore, the patient should be warned accordingly.

Usage in Children Safety and effectiveness in children have not been established; therefore, PERMITIL products are not recommended for use in children.

Usage in Pregnancy Safe use of fluphenazine hydrochloride during pregnancy and lactation has not been established; therefore, in administering the drug to pregnant patients, nursing mothers, or women who may become pregnant, the possible benefits must be weighed against the possible hazards to mother and child.

Precautions: The possibility of suicide in depressed patients remains during treatment and until significant remission occurs. This type of patient should not have access to large quantities of this drug.

As with all phenothiazine compounds, fluphenazine hydrochloride should not be used indiscriminately. Caution should be observed in giving it to patients who have previously exhibited severe adverse reactions to other phenothiazines. Some of the untoward actions of fluphenazine hydrochloride tend to appear more frequently when high doses are used. However, as with other phenothiazine compounds, patients receiving PERMITIL products in any dosage should be kept under close supervision.

Neuroleptic drugs elevate prolactin levels; the elevation persists during chronic administration. Tissue culture experiments indicate that approximately one-third of human breast cancers are prolactin dependent *in vitro*, a factor of potential importance if the prescription of these drugs is contemplated in a patient with a previously detected breast cancer. Although disturbances such as galactorrhea, amenorrhea, gynecomastia, and impotence have been reported, the clinical significance of elevated serum prolactin levels is unknown for most patients. An increase in mammary neoplasms has been found in rodents after chronic administration of neuroleptic drugs. Neither clinical studies nor epidemiologic studies conducted to date, however, have shown an association between chronic administration of these drugs and mammary tumorigenesis; the available evidence is considered too limited to be conclusive at this time.

The antiemetic effect of fluphenazine hydrochloride may obscure signs of toxicity due to overdosage of other drugs, or render more difficult the diagnosis of disorders such as brain tumors or intestinal obstruction.

Adynamic ileus occasionally occurs with phenothiazine therapy and if severe can result in complications and death. It is of particular concern in psychiatric patients, who may fail to seek treatment of the condition.

A significant, not otherwise explained, rise in body temperature may suggest individual intolerance to fluphenazine hydrochloride in which case it should be discontinued.

Patients on large doses of a phenothiazine drug who are undergoing surgery should be watched carefully for possible hypotensive phenomena. Moreover, reduced amounts of anesthetics or central nervous system depressants may be necessary.

Since phenothiazines and central nervous system depressants (opiates, analgesics, antihistamines, barbiturates) can potentiate each other, less than the usual dosage of the added drug is recommended, and caution is advised, when they are administered concomitantly.

Use with caution in patients who are receiving atropine or related drugs because of additive anticholinergic effects and also in patients who will be exposed to extreme heat or phosphorus insecticides.

The use of alcohol should be avoided, since additive effects and hypotension may occur. Patients should be cautioned that their response to alcohol may be increased while they are being treated with PERMITIL products. The risk of suicide and the danger of overdose may be increased in patients who use alcohol excessively due to its potentiation of the drug's effect.

Blood counts and hepatic and renal functions should be checked periodically. The appearance of signs of blood dyscrasias requires the discontinuance of the drug and institution of appropriate therapy. If abnormalities in hepatic tests occur, phenothiazine treatment should be discontinued. Renal function in patients on long-term therapy should be monitored: if blood urea nitrogen (BUN) becomes abnormal, treatment with the drug should be discontinued.

The use of phenothiazine derivatives in patients with diminished renal function should be undertaken with caution.

Use with caution in patients suffering from respiratory impairment due to acute pulmonary infections, or in chronic respiratory disorders such as severe asthma or emphysema.

Continued on next page

Information on Schering products appearing on these pages is effective as of September 30, 1982.

Schering—Cont.

In general, phenothiazines, including fluphenazine hydrochloride, do not produce psychic dependence. Gastritis, nausea and vomiting, dizziness, and tremulousness have been reported following abrupt cessation of high-dose therapy. Reports suggest that these symptoms can be reduced by continuing concomitant antiparkinson agents for several weeks after the phenothiazine is withdrawn.
The possibility of liver damage, corneal and lenticular deposits, and irreversible dyskinesias should be kept in mind when patients are on long-term therapy.
Because photosensitivity has been reported, undue exposure to the sun should be avoided during phenothiazine treatment.
PERMITIL CHRONOTAB **Tablets** and PERMITIL **Tablets** 0.25 mg. contain FD&C Yellow No. 5 (tartrazine) which may cause allergic-type reactions (including bronchial asthma) in certain susceptible individuals. Although the overall incidence of FD&C Yellow No. 5 (tartrazine) sensitivity in the general population is low, it is frequently seen in patients who also have aspirin hypersensitivity.
Adverse Reactions: Not all of the following adverse reactions have been reported with this specific drug, however, pharmacological similarities among various phenothiazine derivatives require that each be considered. In the case of the piperazine group (of which fluphenazine hydrochloride is an example), the extrapyramidal symptoms are more common, and others (e.g., sedative effects, jaundice, and blood dyscrasias) are less frequently seen.
CNS Effects: *Extrapyramidal reactions:* opisthotonus, trismus, torticollis, retrocollis, aching and numbness of the limbs, motor restlessness, oculogyric crisis, hyperreflexia, dystonia, including protrusion, discoloration, aching and rounding of the tongue, tonic spasm of the masticatory muscles, tight feeling in the throat, slurred speech, dysphagia, akathisia, dyskinesia, parkinsonism, and ataxia. Their incidence and severity usually increase with an increase in dosage, but there is considerable individual variation in the tendency to develop such symptoms. Extrapyramidal symptoms can usually be controlled by the concomitant use of effective antiparkinsonian drugs, such as benztropine mesylate, and/or by reduction in dosage.
Persistent tardive dyskinesia: As with all antipsychotic agents, tardive dyskinesia may appear in some patients on long-term therapy or may appear after drug therapy has been discontinued. Although the risk appears to be greater in elderly patients on high-dose therapy, especially females, it may occur in either sex and in children. The symptoms are persistent and in some patients appear to be irreversible. The syndrome is characterized by rhythmical, involuntary movements of the tongue, face, mouth or jaw (e.g., protrusion of tongue, puffing of cheeks, puckering of mouth, chewing movements). Sometimes these may be accompanied by involuntary movements of the extremities. There is no known effective treatment for tardive dyskinesia; antiparkisonism agents usually do not alleviate the symptoms of this syndrome. It is suggested that all antipsychotic agents be discontinued if these symptoms appear. Should it be necessary to reinstitute treatment, or increase the dosage of the agent, or switch to a different antipsychotic agent the syndrome may be masked. It has been reported that fine, vermicular movements of the tongue may be an early sign of the syndrome, and if the medication is stopped at that time the syndrome may not develop.
Other CNS effects include cerebral edema; abnormality of cerebrospinal fluid proteins; convulsive seizures, particularly in patients with EEG abnormalities or a history of such disorders; and headaches.
Drowsiness may occur, particularly during the first or second week, after which it generally disappears. If troublesome, lower the dosage. Hypnotic effects appear to be minimal, especially in patients who are permitted to remain active.
Adverse behavioral effects include paradoxical exacerbation of psychotic symptoms, catatonic-like states, paranoid reactions, lethargy, paradoxical excitement, restlessness, hyperactivity, nocturnal confusion, bizarre dreams, and insomnia.
Hyperreflexia has been reported in the newborn when a phenothiazine was used during pregnancy.
Autonomic Effects: dry mouth or salivation, nausea, vomiting, diarrhea, anorexia, constipation, obstipation, fecal impaction, urinary retention, frequency or incontinence, bladder paralysis, polyuria, nasal congestion, pallor, adynamic ileus, myosis, mydriasis, blurred vision, glaucoma, perspiration, hypertension, hypotension, and change in pulse rate occasionally may occur. Significant autonomic effects have been infrequent in patients receiving less than 6 mg fluphenazine hydrochloride daily.
Allergic Effects: urticaria, erythema, eczema, exfoliative dermatitis, pruritus, photosensitivity, asthma, fever, anaphylactoid reactions, laryngeal edema, and angioneurotic edema; contact dermatitis in nursing personnel administering the drug; and in extremely rare instances, individual idiosyncrasy or hypersensitivity to phenothiazines has resulted in cerebral edema, cirulatory collapse, and death.
Edocrine Effects: lactation, galactorrhea, moderate breast enlargement in females and gynecomastia in males on large doses, disturbances in the menstrual cycle, amenorrhea, changes in libido, inhibition of ejaculation, syndrome of inappropriate ADH (antidiuretic hormone) secretion, false positive pregnancy tests, hyperglycemia, hypoglycemia, glycosuria.
Cardiovascular Effects: postural hypotension, tachycardia (especially with sudden marked increase in dosage), bradycardia, cardiac arrest, faintness, and dizziness. Occasionally the hypotensive effect may produce a shock-like condition. ECG changes, nonspecific, (quinidine-like effect) usually reversible, have been observed in some patients receiving phenothiazine tranquilizers.
Sudden death has occasionally been reported in patients who have received phenothiazines. In some cases the death was apparently due to cardiac arrest; in others, the cause appeared to be asphyxia due to failure of the cough reflex. In some patients, the cause could not be determined nor could it be established that the death was due to the phenothiazine.
Hematological Effects: agranulocytosis, eosinophilia, leukopenia, hemolytic anemia, thrombocytopenic purpura, and pancytopenia. Most cases of agranulocytosis have occurred between the fourth and tenth weeks of therapy. Patients should be watched closely especially during that period for the sudden appearance of sore throat or signs of infection. If white blood cell and differential cell counts show significant cellular depression, discontinue the drug and start appropriate therapy. However, a slightly lowered white count is not in itself an indiction to discontinue the drug.
Other Effects: Special considerations in long-term therapy include pigmentation of the skin, occurring chiefly in the exposed area; ocular changes consisting of deposition of fine particulate matter in the cornea and lens, progressing in more severe cases to star-shaped lenticular opacities; epithelial keratopathies; and pigmentary retinopathy. Also noted: peripheral edema, reversed epinephrine effect, increase in PBI not attributable to an increase in thyroxine, parotid swelling (rare), hyperpyrexia, systemic lupus erythematosus-like syndrome, increases in appetite and weight, polyphagia, photophobia, and muscle weakness.
Liver damage (biliary stasis) may occur. Jaundice may occur usually between the second and fourth weeks of treatment and is regarded as a hypersensitivity reaction. Incidence is low. The clinical picture resembles infectious hepatitis but with laboratory features of obstructive jaundice. It is usually reversible; however, chronic jaundice has been reported.
Dosage and Administration: In all cases the smallest effective dose should be used. Doses should be initiated at a low level and increased gradually to determine clinical response. Patients who are acutely ill may respond to lower doses than those who are chronically ill. Acutely ill patients may require a rapid increase of dosage. Elderly and debilitated patients and adolescents may respond to low dosages. Outpatients should receive smaller dosages than are given to hospitalized patients who are under close supervision.
Adults: The total daily dose ranges from 0.5 mg. to 10 mg. and is usually administered in divided doses. In general, a daily dose in excess of 3 mg. is rarely necessary. A dose in excess of 20 mg. should be used with caution.
Administration of an adequate dose should be continued for sufficiently long periods in order to obtain maximum benefits. After maximum therapeutic response is obtained, dosage may be decreased gradually to a maintenance level.
Geriatric patients: Reduced dosage is usually recommended.
PERMITIL **Oral Concentrate** is a palatable liquid preparation, suitable for administration with the following diluents: water, saline, Seven-Up, homogenized milk, carbonated orange beverage, and pineapple, apricot, prune, orange, V-8, tomato, and grapefruit juices. PERMITIL Oral Concentrate should not be mixed with beverages containing caffeine (coffee, cola) tannics (tea), or pectinates (apple juice) since physical incompatability may result.
PERMITIL CHRONOTAB **Tablets** are suggested for those conditions in which a prolonged effect from a single tablet is desired.
Overdosage: In the event of overdosage, emergency treatment should be started immediately. All patients suspected of having taken an overdose should be hospitalized as soon as possible.
Manifestations: Overdosage of fluphenazine hydrochloride primarily involves the extrapyramidal mechanism and produces the same side effects described under ADVERSE REACTIONS, but to a more marked degree. It is usually evidenced by stupor or coma; children may have convulsive seizures.
Treatment: Treatment is symptomatic and supportive. There is no specific antidote. The patient should be induced to vomit even if emesis has occurred spontaneously. Pharmacologic vomiting by the administration of ipecac syrup is a preferred method. It should be noted that ipecac has a central mode of action in addition to its local gastric irritant properties, and the central mode of action may be blocked by the antiemetic effect of PERMITIL products.
Vomiting should not be induced in patients with impaired consciousness. The action of ipecac is facilitated by physical activity and by the administration of 8 to 12 fluid ounces of water. If emesis does not occur within 15 minutes, the dose of ipecac should be repeated. Precautions against aspiration must be taken, especially in infants and children. Following emesis, any drug remaining in the stomach may be adsorbed by activated charcoal administered as a slurry with water. If vomiting is unsuccessful or contraindicated, gastric lavage should be performed. Isotonic and one-half isotonic saline are the lavage solutions of choice. Saline cathartics, such as milk of magnesia, draw water into the bowel by osmosis

and therefore may be valuable for their action in rapid dilution of bowel content.

Standard measures (oxygen, intravenous fluids, corticosteroids) should be used to manage circulatory shock or metabolic acidosis. An open airway and adequate fluid intake should be maintained. Body temperature should be regulated. Hypothermia is expected, but severe hyperthermia may occur and must be treated vigorously. (See CONTRAINDICATIONS.)

An electrocardiogram should be taken and close monitoring of cardiac function instituted if there is any sign of abnormality. Cardiac arthythmias may be treated with neostigmine, pyridostigmine, or propranolol. Digitalis should be considered for cardiac failure. Close monitoring of cardiac function is advisable for not less than the five days. Vasopressors such as norepinephrine may be used to treat hypotension, but epinephrine should NOT be used.

Anticonvulsants (an inhalation anesthetic, diazepam or paraldehyde) are recommended for control of convulsions, since fluphenazine hydrochloride increases the central nervous system depressant action, but not the anticonvulsant action, of barbiturates.

If acute parkinson-like symptoms result from fluphenazine hydrochloride intoxication, benztropine mesylate or diphenhydramine may be administered.

Central nervous system depression may be treated with non-convulsant doses of CNS stimulants. Avoid stimulants that may cause convulsions (e.g., picrotoxin and pentylenetetrazol).

Signs of arousal may not occur for 48 hours.

Dialysis is of no value because of low plasma concentrations of the drug.

Since overdosage is often deliberate, patients may attempt suicide by other means during the recovery phase. Deaths by deliberate or accidental overdosage have occurred with this class of drugs.

How Supplied: PERMITIL **Tablets,** 0.25 mg., sugar-coated, bright green tablets branded in black with the Schering trademark and product identification letters, WBK, or numbers, 122; bottle of 100.

PERMITIL **Tablets,** 2.5 mg., compressed, scored, light orange, oval tablets impressed with the Schering trademark and product identification letters, WDR, or numbers, 442; bottle of 100.

PERMITIL **Tablets,** 5 mg., compressed, scored, purple-pink, oval tablets impressed with the Schering trademark and product identification letters WFF, or numbers, 550; bottle of 100.

PERMITIL **Tablets,** 10 mg., compressed, scored, light red, oval tablets impressed with the Schering trademark and product identification letters, WFG, or numbers, 316; bottle of 1000.

PERMITIL **Oral Concentrate,** 5 mg. per ml., a straw-colored, unflavored syrup; bottle of 4 fluid ounces (118 ml), with dropper calibrated both in mg. of fluphenazine hydrochloride and in ml. of concentrate. **Protect from light and dispense only in amber bottles.**

PERMITIL CHRONOTAB **Tablets,** 1 mg., sugar-coated, yellow tablets branded in black with the Schering trademark and product identification letters, WKJ, or numbers, 840; bottles of 60 and 250.

Store PERMITIL Tablets, Oral Concentrate, and CHRONOTAB Tablets between 2° and 30°C (36° and 86°F).

Copyright © 1964, 1980, Schering Corporation. All rights reserved.

[*Shown in Product Identification Section*]

POLARAMINE® ℞

brand of dexchlorpheniramine maleate, USP
REPETABS® Tablets
Tablets
Syrup

Description: POLARAMINE products contain dexchlorpheniramine maleate, USP, an antihistamine having the formula, $C_{16}H_{19}ClN_2 \cdot C_4H_4O_4$, and a molecular weight of 390.87. Chemically, it is (+)-2-[*p*-Chloro-α-[2-(dimethylamino)ethyl] benzyl] pyridine maleate (1:1).

POLARAMINE REPETABS (brand of repeat-action tablets) Tablets (4 mg and 6 mg) contain respectively 2 or 3 mg dexchlorpheniramine maleate, USP in an outer layer for prompt effect and 2 or 3 mg in an inner core for release three to six hours after ingestion.

POLARAMINE **Tablets** contain 2 mg dexchlorpheniramine maleate, USP.

POLARAMINE **Syrup** contains 2 mg dexchlorpheniramine maleate, USP per 5 ml, in pleasant-tasting vehicle containing 6% alcohol.

Dexchlorpheniramine maleate is a white, odorless, crystalline powder which in aqueous solution has a pH of between 4 and 5. It is freely soluble in water, soluble in alcohol and in chloroform, but only slightly soluble in benzene or ether.

Clinical Pharmacology: POLARAMINE (dexchlorpheniramine maleate) is an antihistamine with anticholinergic properties. It is capable of producing a slight to moderate sedative effect. Antihistamines appear to compete with histamine for receptor sites on effector cells and are of value clinically in the prevention and relief of many allergic manifestations.

In vitro and *in vivo* assays of the antihistamine potencies of the optically active isomers of chlorpheniramine demonstrate that the predominant activity is in the dextro-isomer. The dextro-isomer is approximately two times more active than the racemic compound. Since dexchlorpheniramine is the dextro-isomer and active moiety of chlorpheniramine, it can be assumed that experience with chlorpheniramine also applies to dexchlorpheniramine.

Chlorpheniramine maleate 4 mg given to fasting human volunteers produced prompt blood levels after oral administration. Peak blood levels were approximately 7 ng/ml at an average time of 3 hours after administration. The half-life of chlorpheniramine maleate ranged from 20 to 24 hours. Following a single dose of tritium-labeled chlorpheniramine maleate to humans, the drug was found to be extensively metabolized whether given orally or by intravenous administration. The drug and metabolites were primarily excreted in the urine, with 19% of the dose appearing in 24 hours and a total of 34% in 48 hours.

Another study in volunteers has demonstrated that a REPETABS Tablet containing 12 mg chlorpheniramine maleate gives essentially identical plasma levels of drug as 12 mg of chlorpheniramine given in divided doses.

In a study in normal volunteers, a high flow rate of acidic urine resulted in a high excretion rate of chlorpheniramine maleate. Over a concentration range of 0.28 to 1.24 mcg/ml of plasma, chlorpheniramine maleate was 72 to 69% bound to plasma protein, respectively.

Indications and Usage: POLARAMINE is indicated for the treatment of perennial and seasonal allergic rhinitis; vasomotor rhinitis; allergic conjunctivitis; mild, uncomplicated allergic skin manifestations of urticaria and angioedema; amelioration of allergic reactions to blood or plasma; and dermographism. They are also indicated as therapy for anaphylactic reactions adjunctive to epinephrine and other standard measures after the acute manifestations have been controlled.

Contraindications: Hypersensitivity to dexchlorpheniramine maleate or other antihistamines of similar chemical structure contraindicates the use of POLARAMINE.

Drug products containing dexchlorpheniramine maleate should not be used in newborn or premature infants because of the possibility of severe reactions such as convulsions.

Antihistamines *should not* be used to treat lower respiratory tract symptoms. Antihistamines are also contraindicated for use in conjunction with monoamine oxidase inhibitor therapy.

Warnings: Dexchlorpheniramine, as with all antihistamines, should be used with caution in patients with narrow angle glaucoma, stenosing peptic ulcer, pyloroduodenal obstruction, symptomatic prostatic hypertrophy, and bladder neck obstruction.

Overdoses of antihistamines may cause hallucinations, convulsions, or death, especially in infants and children.

Products containing dexchlorpheniramine maleate have additive effects with alcohol and other CNS depressants (hypnotics, sedatives, tranquilizers, etc.). Patients should not engage in activities requiring mental alertness, such as driving a car or operating machinery.

Antihistamines are more likely to cause dizziness, sedation, and hypotension in elderly patients (approximately 60 years or older).

Precautions: *General:* Dexchlorpheniramine maleate has an atropine-like action and therefore products containing it should be used with caution in patients with: a history of bronchial asthma; increased intraocular pressure; hyperthyroidism; cardiovascular disease; hypertension.

Information for Patients:

1. Dexchlorpheniramine may cause slight to moderate drowsiness.
2. Patients should not engage in activities requiring mental alertness, such as driving or operating machinery.
3. Alcohol or other sedative drugs may enhance the drowsiness caused by antihistamines.
4. Patients should not take POLARAMINE in conjunction with a monoamine oxidase inhibitor or oral anticoagulant.

Drug Interactions: Dexchlorpheniramine maleate may cause severe hypotension when given in conjunction with a monoamine oxidase inhibitor.

Alcohol and other sedative drugs will potentiate the sedative effects of dexchlorpheniramine. (See WARNINGS.)

The action of oral anticoagulants may be inhibited by antihistamines.

Carcinogenesis, Mutagenesis, Impairment of Fertility: Although there have been no oncogenic or mutagenic studies on dexchlorpheniramine, a 103-week oncogenic study in rats on the racemic mixture, chlorpheniramine, did not produce an increase in the incidence of tumors in the drug-treated groups, as compared with the controls.

An Ames mutagenicity test performed on chlorpheniramine and its nitrosation product was negative. An early study in rats with chlorpheniramine maleate revealed a reduction in fertility in female rats at doses approximately 67 times the human dose. More recent studies in rabbits and rats, using more appropriate methodology and doses up to approximately 50 and 85 times the human dose, showed no reduction in fertility in the animals.

Pregnancy Category B: Reproduction studies have been performed in rabbits and rats at doses up to 50 times and 85 times the human dose, respectively, and have revealed no evidence of harm to the fetus due to chlorpheniramine maleate. (See above, "*Impairment of Fertility.*") There are, however, no adequate and

Continued on next page

Information on Schering products appearing on these pages is effective as of September 30, 1982.

Schering—Cont.

well-controlled studies in pregnant women. Because animal reproduction studies are not always predictive of human response, this drug should be used during the first two trimesters of pregnancy only if clearly needed. Dexchlorpheniramine maleate should not be used in the third trimester of pregnancy because newborn and premature infants may have severe reactions to antihistamines. (See CONTRAINDICATIONS.)

Nonteratogenic Effects: Studies of chlorpheniramine maleate done in rats revealed a decrease in the postnatal survival rate of pups of animals dosed with 33 and 67 times the human dose.

Nursing Mothers: It is not known whether this drug is excreted in human milk. Because certain other antihistamines are known to be excreted in human milk, and because dexchlorpheniramine maleate is contraindicated in newborn and premature infants, caution should be exercised when it is administered to a nursing woman.

Pediatric Use: Safety and effectiveness of the 4 and 6 mg REPETABS Tablets in children below the ages of 6 and 12 years, respectively, have not been established. Safety and effectiveness of the Tablets and Syrup in children below the age of 2 years have not been established.

Adverse Reactions: Slight to moderate drowsiness is the most frequent side effect of dexchlorpheniramine maleate. Other possible side effects of antihistamines include:

General: urticaria, drug rash, anaphylactic shock, photosensitivity, excessive perspiration, chills, dryness of mouth, nose, and throat.

Cardiovascular System: headache, palpitations, tachycardia, extrasystoles, hypotension.

Hematologic System: hemolytic anemia, hypoplastic anemia, thrombocytopenia, agranulocytosis.

Nervous System: sedation, dizziness, vertigo, tinnitus, acute labyrinthitis, disturbed coordination, fatigue, confusion, restlessness, excitation, nervousness, tremor, irritability, insomnia, euphoria, paresthesias, blurred vision, hysteria, neuritis, convulsions.

Gastrointestinal System: epigastric distress, anorexia, nausea, vomiting, diarrhea, constipation.

Genitourinary System: urinary frequency, difficult urination, urinary retention, early menses.

Respiratory System: thickening of bronchial secretions, tightness of chest, wheezing, nasal stuffiness.

Overdosage: In the event of overdosage, emergency treatment should be started immediately.

Manifestations of antihistamine overdosage may vary from central nervous system depression (sedation, apnea, diminished mental alertness, cardiovascular collapse) to stimulation (insomnia, hallucinations, tremors, or convulsions) to death. Other signs and symptoms may be dizziness, tinnitus, ataxia, blurred vision, and hypotension. Stimulation is particularly likely in children, as are atropine-like signs and symptoms (dry mouth; fixed, dilated pupils; flushing; hyperthermia; and gastrointestinal symptoms).

Treatment—The patient should be induced to vomit, even if emesis has occurred spontaneously. Pharmacologic vomiting by the administration of ipecac syrup is a preferred method. However, vomiting should not be induced in patients with impaired consciousness. The action of ipecac is facilitated by physical activity and by the administration of eight to twelve fluid ounces of water. If emesis does not occur within fifteen minutes, the dose of ipecac should be repeated. Precautions against aspiration must be taken, especially in infants and children. Following emesis, any drug remaining in the stomach may be adsorbed by activated charcoal administered as a slurry with water. If vomiting is unsuccessful or contraindicated, gastric lavage should be performed. Isotonic and one-half isotonic saline are the lavage solutions of choice. Saline cathartics, such as milk of magnesia, draw water into the bowel by osmosis and therefore may be valuable for their action in rapid dilution of bowel content. Dialysis is of little value in antihistamine poisoning. After emergency treatment, the patient should continue to be medically monitored.

Treatment of the signs and symptoms of overdosage is symptomatic and supportive. *Stimulants* (analeptic agents) should *not* be used. Vasopressors may be used to treat hypotension. Short-acting barbiturates, diazepam, or paraldehyde may be administered to control seizures. Hyperpyrexia, especially in children, may require treatment with tepid water sponge baths or a hypothermic blanket. Apnea is treated with ventilatory support.

In mice, the oral LD_{50} of dexchlorpheniramine is 258 mg/kg. In humans, the estimated lethal dose of racemic chlorpheniramine is 5 to 10 mg/kg. Thus a dose of 2.5 to 5 mg/kg of dexchlorpheniramine should be similarly regarded.

Dosage and Administration: DOSAGE SHOULD BE INDIVIDUALIZED ACCORDING TO THE NEEDS AND RESPONSE OF THE PATIENT.

Adults and children 12 years or older: one 4 or 6 mg POLARAMINE REPETABS Tablet at bedtime or every 8 to 10 hours during the day.

Children 6 to 12 years: one 4 mg REPETABS Tablet daily, taken preferably at bedtime.

POLARAMINE **Tablets**—Adults and children 12 years of age and over: one tablet every 4 to 6 hours. Children 6 through 11 years: one-half tablet every 4 to 6 hours. Children 2 through 5 years: one-quarter tablet every 4 to 6 hours.

POLARAMINE **Syrup**—Adults and children 12 years of age and over: 1 teaspoonful (2 mg) every 4 to 6 hours. Children 6 through 11 years: one-half teaspoonful (1 mg) every 4 to 6 hours. Children 2 through 5 years: one-quarter teaspoonful (½ mg) every 4 to 6 hours.

How Supplied: POLARAMINE REPETABS Tablets, 4 mg, light red, sugar-coated, oval tablets branded in blue-black with the Schering trademark and product identification letters, AGA, or numbers, 095; bottle of 100.

POLARAMINE REPETABS Tablets, 6 mg, bright red, sugar-coated, oval tablets branded in white with the Schering trademark and product identification letters, AGB, or numbers, 148; bottles of 100 and 1000.

POLARAMANE **Tablets**, 2 mg, red, compressed, oval tablets impressed with the Schering trademark and either product identification letters, AGT, or numbers, 820; bottle of 100.

POLARAMINE **Syrup**, 2 mg per 5 ml, red-orange-colored, orange-like flavored liquid; 16-fluid ounce (473 ml) bottle.

Store POLARAMINE Tablets and Syrup between 2° and 30°C (36° to 86°F).

Copyright © 1968, 1980, Schering Corporation. All rights reserved.

[*Shown in Product Identification Section*]

PROGLYCEM® ℞

brand of diazoxide, USP
Capsules
Suspension
FOR ORAL ADMINISTRATION

Description: PROGLYCEM (diazoxide; 7-chloro-3-methyl-2*H*-1, 2, 4-benzothiadiazine 1, 1-dioxide) is a benzothiadiazine derivative. PROGLYCEM **Capsules** contain either 50 or 100 mg. diazoxide, USP. The **Suspension** contains 50 mg. of diazoxide, USP in each milliliter and has a chocolate-mint flavor; alcohol content is approximately 7.25%.

Actions: Diazoxide administered orally produces a prompt dose-related increase in blood glucose level, due primarily to an inhibition of insulin release from the pancreas, and also to an extrapancreatic effect.

The hyperglycemic effect begins within an hour and generally lasts no more than eight hours in the presence of normal renal function.

PROGLYCEM decreases the excretion of sodium and water, resulting in fluid retention which may be clinically significant.

The effects on blood pressure are usually not marked with the oral preparation. This contrasts with the intravenous preparation of diazoxide (see Adverse Reactions).

Other pharmacologic actions of PROGLYCEM include increased pulse rate; increased serum uric acid levels due to decreased excretion; increased serum levels of free fatty acids; decreased chloride excretion; decreased paraaminohippuric acid (PAH) clearance with no appreciable effect on glomerular filtration rate.

The concomitant administration of a benzothiazide diuretic may intensify the hyperglycemic and hyperuricemic effects of PROGLYCEM. In the presence of hypokalemia, hyperglycemic effects are also potentiated.

PROGLYCEM-induced hyperglycemia is reversed by the administration of insulin or tolbutamide.

The inhibition of insulin release by PROGLYCEM is antagonized by alpha-adrenergic blocking agents.

PROGLYCEM is extensively bound (more than 90%) to serum proteins, and is excreted by the kidneys. The plasma half-life following i.v. administration is 28±8.3 hours. Limited data on oral administration revealed a half-life of 24 and 36 hours in two adults. In four children aged four months to six years, the plasma half-life varied from 9.5 to 24 hours on long-term oral administration. The half-life may be prolonged following overdosage, and in patients with impaired renal function.

Indications: PROGLYCEM (oral diazoxide) is useful in the management of hypoglycemia due to hyperinsulinism associated with the following conditions:

Adults: Inoperable islet cell adenoma or carcinoma, or extrapancreatic malignancy.

Infants and Children: Leucine sensitivity, islet cell hyperplasia, nesidioblastosis, extrapancreatic malignancy, islet cell adenoma, or adenomatosis. PROGLYCEM may be used preoperatively as a temporary measure, and postoperatively, if hypoglycemia persists.

PROGLYCEM should be used only after a diagnosis of hypoglycemia due to one of the above conditions has been definitely established. When other specific medical therapy or surgical management either has been unsuccessful or is not feasible, treatment with PROGLYCEM should be considered.

Contraindications: The use of PROGLYCEM for functional hypoglycemia is contraindicated. The drug should not be used in patients hypersensitive to diazoxide or to other thiazides unless the potential benefits outweigh the possible risks.

Warnings: The antidiuretic property of diazoxide may lead to significant fluid retention, which in patients with compromised cardiac reserve, may precipitate congestive heart failure. The fluid retention will respond to conventional therapy with diuretics.

It should be noted that concomitantly administered thiazides may potentiate the hyperglycemic and hyperuricemic actions of diazoxide (see Drug Interactions and Animal Pharmacology and Toxicology).

Ketoacidosis and nonketotic hyperosmolar coma have been reported in patients treated with recommended doses of PROGLYCEM usually during intercurrent illness. Prompt recognition and treatment are essential (see Overdosage), and prolonged surveillance fol-

lowing the acute episode is necessary because of the long drug half-life of approximately 30 hours. The occurrence of these serious events may be reduced by careful education of patients regarding the need for monitoring the urine for sugar and ketones and for prompt reporting of abnormal findings and unusual symptoms to the physician.

Transient cataracts occurred in association with hyperosmolar coma in an infant, and subsided on correction of the hyperosmolarity. Cataracts have been observed in several animals receiving daily doses of intravenous or oral diazoxide.

Usage in Pregnancy: Reproduction studies using the oral preparation in rats have revealed increased fetal resorptions and delayed parturition, as well as fetal skeletal anomalies; evidence of skeletal and cardiac teratogenic effects in rabbits has been noted with intravenous administration. The drug has also been demonstrated to cross the placental barrier in animals and cause degeneration of the fetal pancreatic beta cells (see Animal Pharmacology and Toxicology). Since there are no adequate data on fetal effects of this drug when given to pregnant women, safety in pregnancy has not been established. When the use of PROGLYCEM in pregnant women is considered, the indications should be limited to those specified above for adults (see Indications), and the potential benefits to the mother must be weighed against possible harmful effects to the fetus.

Precautions: **Treatment with PROGLYCEM should be initiated under close clinical supervision, with careful monitoring of blood glucose and clinical response until the patient's condition has stabilized. This usually requires several days. If not effective in two to three weeks, the drug should be discontinued.**

Prolonged treatment requires regular monitoring of the urine for sugar and ketones, especially under stress conditions, with prompt reporting of any abnormalities to the physician. Additionally, blood sugar levels should be monitored periodically by the physician to determine the need for dose adjustment.

The effects of diazoxide on the hematopoietic system and the level of serum uric acid should be kept in mind; the latter should be considered particularly in patients with hyperuricemia or a history of gout.

In some patients, higher blood levels have been observed with the liquid than with the capsule formulation of PROGLYCEM. Dosage should be adjusted as necessary in individual patients if changed from one formulation to the other.

Since the plasma half-life of diazoxide is prolonged in patients with impaired renal function, a reduced dosage should be considered. Serum electrolyte levels should also be evaluated for such patients.

The antihypertensive effect of other drugs may be enhanced by PROGLYCEM, and this should be kept in mind when administering it concomitantly with antihypertensive agents.

Because of protein binding, administration of PROGLYCEM with coumarin or its derivatives may require reduction in the dosage of the anticoagulant, although there has been no reported evidence of excessive anticoagulant effect. In addition, PROGLYCEM may possibly displace bilirubin from albumin; this should be kept in mind particularly when treating newborns with increased bilirubinemia.

Adverse Reactions:

Frequent and Serious: ***Sodium and fluid retention*** **is most common in young infants and in adults and may precipitate congestive heart failure in patients with compromised cardiac reserve. It usually responds to diuretic therapy (see Drug Interactions).**

Infrequent but Serious: Diabetic ketoacidosis and hyperosmolar nonketotic coma may develop very rapidly. Conventional therapy with insulin and restoration of fluid and electrolyte balance are usually effective if instituted promptly. Prolonged surveillance is essential in view of the long half-life of PROGLYCEM (see Overdosage).

Other frequent adverse reactions are: *Hirsutism* of the lanugo type, mainly on the forehead, back and limbs, occurs most commonly in children and women and may be cosmetically unacceptable. It subsides on discontinuation of the drug.

Hyperglycemia **or** ***glycosuria*** **may require reduction in dosage** in order to avoid progression to ketoacidosis or hyperosmolar coma.

Gastrointestinal intolerance **may include anorexia, nausea, vomiting, abdominal pain, ileus, diarrhea, transient loss of taste.** ***Tachycardia, palpitations, increased levels of serum uric acid*** **are common.**

Thrombocytopenia **with or without** ***purpura*** **may require discontinuation of the drug.** ***Neutropenia*** **is transient, is not associated with increased susceptibility to infection, and ordinarily does not require discontinuation of the drug.** ***Skin rash, headache, weakness,*** **and** ***malaise*** **may also occur.**

Other adverse reactions which have been observed are:

Cardiovascular: Hypotension occurs occasionally, which may be augmented by thiazide diuretics given concurrently. A few cases of transient hypertension, for which no explanation is apparent, have been noted. Chest pain has been reported rarely.

Hematologic: eosinophilia; decreased hemoglobin/hematocrit; excessive bleeding; decreased IgG. *Hepato-renal:* increased SGOT, alkaline phosphatase; azotemia, decreased creatinine clearance, reversible nephrotic syndrome, decreased urinary output, hematuria, albuminuria. *Neurologic:* anxiety, dizziness, insomnia, polyneuritis, paresthesia, pruritus, extrapyramidal signs. *Ophthalmologic:* transient cataracts, subconjunctival hemorrhage, ring scotoma, blurred vision, diplopia, lacrimation. *Skeletal, integumentary;* monilial dermatitis, herpes, advance in bone age; loss of scalp hair. *Systemic:* fever, lymphadenopathy. *Other:* gout, acute pancreatitis/pancreatic necrosis, galactorrhea, enlargement of lump in breast.

Drug Interactions: Since diazoxide is highly bound to serum protein, it may displace other substances which are also bound to protein, such as bilirubin or coumarin and its derivatives, resulting in higher blood levels of these substances. A drug interaction has also been reported for oral diazoxide and diphenylhydantoin, such that their concomitant administration may result in a loss of seizure control. These potential interactions must be considered when administering PROGLYCEM Capsules or Suspension. The concomitant administration of thiazides or other commonly used potent diuretics may potentiate the hyperglycemic and hyperuricemic effects of diazoxide.

Dosage and Administration: Patients should be under close clinical observation when treatment with PROGLYCEM is initiated. The clinical response and blood glucose level should be carefully monitored until the patient's condition has stabilized satisfactorily; in most instances, this may be accomplished in several days. If administration of PROGLYCEM is not effective after two or three weeks, the drug should be discontinued.

The dosage of PROGLYCEM must be individualized based on the severity of the hypoglycemic condition and the blood glucose level and clinical response of the patient. The dosage should be adjusted until the desired clinical and laboratory effects are produced with the least amount of the drug. Special care should be taken to assure accuracy of dosage in infants and young children.

Adults and children: The usual daily dosage is 3 to 8 mg/kg, divided into two or three equal doses every 8 or 12 hours. In certain instances, patients with refractory hypoglycemia may require higher dosages. Ordinarily, an appropriate starting dosage is 3 mg/kg/day, divided into three equal doses every eight hours. Thus, an average adult would receive a starting dosage of approximately 200 mg. daily.

Infants and newborns: The usual daily dosage is 8 to 15 mg/kg, divided into two or three equal doses every 8 or 12 hours. An appropriate starting dosage is 10 mg/kg/day, divided into three equal doses every eight hours.

Overdosage: An overdosage of PROGLYCEM causes marked hyperglycemia which may be associated with ketoacidosis. It will respond to prompt insulin administration and restoration of fluid and electrolyte balance. Because of the drug's long half-life (approximately 30 hours), the symptoms of overdosage require prolonged surveillance for periods up to seven days, until the blood sugar level stabilizes within the normal range. One investigator reported successful lowering of diazoxide blood levels by peritoneal dialysis in one patient and by hemodialysis in another.

How Supplied: PROGLYCEM **Capsules,** 50 mg., half opaque, orange and half clear capsules, branded in black with the Schering trademark and product identification letters, PBA, or numbers, 205; bottle of 100.

PROGLYCEM **Capsules,** 100 mg., opaque orange capsules, branded in black with the Schering trademark and product identification letters, PBB, or numbers, 830; bottle of 100.

PROGLYCEM **Suspension,** 50 mg/ml, a chocolate-mint flavored suspension; bottle of 30 ml. with dropper calibrated to deliver 10, 20, 30, 40 and 50 mg. diazoxide. Shake well before each use. Protect from light.

Animal Pharmacology and Toxicology: Oral diazoxide in the mouse, rat, rabbit, dog, pig, and monkey produces a rapid and transient rise in blood glucose levels. In dogs, increased blood glucose is accompanied by increased free fatty acids, lactate, and pyruvate in the serum. In mice, a marked decrease in liver glycogen and an increase in the blood urea nitrogen level occur.

In acute toxicity studies, the LD_{50} for oral diazoxide suspension is >5000 mg/kg in the rat, >522 mg/kg in the neonatal rat, between 1900 and 2572 mg/kg in the mouse, and 210 mg/kg in the guinea pig. Although the oral LD_{50} was not determined in the dog, a dosage of up to 500 mg/kg was well tolerated.

In subacute oral toxicity studies, diazoxide at 400 mg/kg in the rat produced growth retardation, edema, increases in liver and kidney weights, and adrenal hypertrophy. Daily dosages up to 1080 mg/kg for three months produced hyperglycemia, an increase in liver weight and an increase in mortality. In dogs given oral diazoxide at approximately 40 mg/kg/day for one month, no biologically significant gross or microscopic abnormalities were observed. Cataracts, attributed to markedly disturbed carbohydrate metabolism, have been observed in a few dogs given repeated daily doses of oral or intravenous diazoxide. The lenticular changes resembled those which occur experimentally in animals with increased blood sugar levels. In chronic toxicity studies, rats given a daily dose of 200 mg/kg diazoxide for 52 weeks had a decrease in weight gain and an increase in heart, liver, adrenal, and thyroid weights. Mortality in drug-treated and control groups was not different. Dogs treated with diazoxide at dosages of 50, 100, and 200 mg/kg/day for 82 weeks had higher blood glucose levels than controls. Mild bone marrow stimulation and increased pancreas weights were evident in the drug-treated dogs; several developed inguinal hernias, one had a testicular seminoma, and another had a

Continued on next page

Information on Schering products appearing on these pages is effective as of September 30, 1982.

Schering—Cont.

mass near the penis. Two females had inguinal mammary swellings. The etiology of these changes was not established. There was no difference in mortality between drug-treated and control groups. In a second chronic oral toxicity study, dogs given milled diazoxide at 50, 100, and 200 mg/kg/day had anorexia and severe weight loss, causing death in a few. Hematologic, biochemical, and histologic examinations did not indicate any cause of death other than inanition. After one year of treatment, there is no evidence of herniation or tissue swelling in any of the dogs.

When diazoxide was administered at high dosages concomitantly with either chlorothiazide to rats or trichlormethiazide to dogs, increased toxicity was observed. In rats, the combination was nephrotoxic; epithelial hyperplasia was observed in the collecting tubules. In dogs, a diabetic syndrome was produced which resulted in ketosis and death. Neither of the drugs given alone produced these effects.

Although the data are inconclusive, reproduction and teratology studies in several species of animals indicate that diazoxide, when administered during the critical period of embryo formation, may interfere with normal fetal development, possibly through altered glucose metabolism. Parturition was occasionally prolonged in animals treated at term. Intravenous administration of diazoxide to pregnant sheep, goats, and swine produced in the fetus an appreciable increase in blood glucose level and degeneration of the beta cells of the islets of Langerhans. The reversibility of these effects was not studied.

Copyright © 1972, 1979, Schering Corporation. All rights reserved.

[*Shown in Product Identification Section*]

PROVENTIL® Inhaler ℞
brand of albuterol
Bronchodilator Aerosol
FOR ORAL INHALATION ONLY

Description: The active component of PROVENTIL Inhaler is albuterol (α^1-[(*tert*-butylamino)methyl]-4-hydroxy-*m*-xylene-α,α'-diol), a relatively selective $beta_2$-adrenergic bronchodilator.

Albuterol is the official generic name in the United States. The international generic name for the drug is salbutamol. The molecular weight of albuterol is 239.3.

PROVENTIL Inhaler is a metered-dose aerosol unit for oral inhalation. It contains a microcrystalline suspension of albuterol in propellants (trichloromonofluoromethane and dichlorodifluoromethane) with oleic acid. Each actuation delivers from the mouthpiece 90 mcg of albuterol. Each canister provides at least 200 inhalations.

Clinical Pharmacology: The prime action of beta-adrenergic drugs is to stimulate adenyl cyclase, the enzyme which catalyzes the formation of cyclic-3′,5′-adenosine monophosphate (cyclic AMP) from adenosine triphosphate (ATP). The cyclic AMP thus formed mediates the cellular responses. By virtue of its relatively selective action on $beta_2$- adrenoceptors, albuterol relaxes smooth muscle of the bronchi, uterus, and vascular supply to skeletal muscle, but may have less cardiac stimulant effects than does isoproterenol.

Albuterol is longer acting than isoproterenol by any route of administration in most patients because it is not a substrate for the cellular uptake processes for catecholamines nor for catechol-*O*-methyl transferase.

Because of its gradual absorption from the bronchi, systemic levels of albuterol are low after inhalation of recommended doses. Studies undertaken with four subjects administered tritiated albuterol, resulted in maximum plasma concentrations occurring within two to four hours. Due to the sensitivity of the assay method, the metabolic rate and half-life of elimination of albuterol in plasma could not be determined. However, urinary excretion provided data indicating that albuterol has an elimination half-life of 3.8 hours. Approximately 72 percent of the inhaled dose is excreted within 24 hours in the urine, and consists of 28 percent of unchanged drug and 44 percent as metabolite.

Results of animal studies show that albuterol does not pass the blood-brain barrier.

The effects of rising doses of albuterol and isoproterenol aerosols were studied in volunteers and asthmatic patients. Results in normal volunteers indicated that albuterol is ½ to ¼ as active as isoproterenol in producing increases in heart rate. In asthmatic patients similar cardiovascular differentiation between the two drugs was also seen.

Indications and Usage: PROVENTIL Inhaler is indicated for the relief of bronchospasm in patients with reversible obstructive airway disease.

In controlled clinical trials the onset of improvement in pulmonary function was within 15 minutes, as determined by both maximal midexpiratory flow rate (MMEF) and FEV_1. MMEF measurements also showed that near maximum improvement in pulmonary function generally occurs within 60 to 90 minutes following 2 inhalations of albuterol and that clinically significant improvement generally continues for 3 to 4 hours in most patients. In clinical trials, some patients with asthma showed a therapeutic response (defined by maintaining FEV_1 values 15 percent or more above base line) which was still apparent at 6 hours. Continued effectiveness of albuterol was demonstrated over a 13-week period in these same trials.

Contraindications: PROVENTIL Inhaler is contraindicated in patients with a history of hypersensitivity to any of its components.

Warnings: As with other adrenergic aerosols, the potential for paradoxical bronchospasm should be kept in mind. If it occurs, the preparation should be discontinued immediately and alternative therapy instituted.

Fatalities have been reported in association with excessive use of inhaled sympathomimetic drugs. The exact cause of death is unknown, but cardiac arrest following the unexpected development of a severe acute asthmatic crisis and subsequent hypoxia is suspected.

The contents of PROVENTIL Inhaler are under pressure. Do not puncture. Do not use or store near heat or open flame. Exposure to temperatures above 120°F may cause bursting. Never throw container into fire or incinerator. Keep out of reach of children.

Precautions: Although it has less effect on the cardiovascular system than isoproterenol at recommended dosages, albuterol is a sympathomimetic amine and as such should be used with caution in patients with cardiovascular disorders, including coronary insufficiency and hypertension, in patients with hyperthyroidism or diabetes mellitus, and in patients who are unusually responsive to sympathomimetic amines.

Large doses of intravenous albuterol have been reported to aggravate preexisting diabetes and ketoacidosis. The relevance of this observation to the use of PROVENTIL Inhaler is unknown, since the aerosol dose is much lower than the doses given intravenously.

Although there have been no reports concerning the use of PROVENTIL Inhaler during labor and delivery, it has been reported that high doses of albuterol administered intravenously inhibit uterine contractions. Although this effect is extremely unlikely as a consequence of aerosol use, it should be kept in mind.

Information For Patients: The action of PROVENTIL Inhaler may last up to six hours and therefore it should not be used more frequently than recommended. Do not increase the number or frequency of doses without medical consultation. If symptoms get worse, medical consultation should be sought promptly. While taking PROVENTIL Inhaler, other inhaled medicines should not be used unless prescribed.

See illustrated Patient Instructions For Use.

Drug Interactions: Other sympathomimetic aerosol bronchodilators or epinephrine should not be used concomitantly with albuterol.

Albuterol should be administered with caution to patients being treated with monoamine oxidase inhibitors or tricyclic antidepressants, since the action of albuterol on the vascular system may be potentiated.

Beta-receptor blocking agents and albuterol inhibit the effect of each other.

Carcinogenesis, Mutagenesis, and Impairment of Fertility: In a 2 year study in the rat, albuterol sulfate caused a significant dose-related increase in the incidence of benign leiomyomata of the mesovarium at doses corresponding to 111, 555, and 2,800 times the maximum human inhalational dose. The relevance of these findings to humans is not known. An 18-month study in mice revealed no evidence of tumorigenicity. Studies with albuterol revealed no evidence of mutagenesis. Reproduction studies in rats revealed no evidence of impaired fertility.

Teratogenic Effects — Pregnancy Category C: Albuterol has been shown to be teratogenic in mice when given in doses corresponding to 14 times the human dose. There are no adequate and well-controlled studies in pregnant women. Albuterol should be used during pregnancy only if the potential benefit justifies the potential risk to the fetus. A reproduction study in CD-1 mice with albuterol (0.025, 0.25, and 2.5 mg/kg, corresponding to 1.4, 14, and 140 times the maximum human inhalational dose) showed cleft palate formation in 5 of 111 (4.5 percent) fetuses at 0.25 mg/kg and in 10 of 108 (9.3 percent) fetuses at 2.5 mg/kg. None were observed at 0.025 mg/kg. Cleft palate also occurred in 22 of 72 (30.5 percent) fetuses treated with 2.5 mg/kg isoproterenol (positive control). A reproduction study in Stride Dutch rabbits revealed cranioschisis in 7 of 19 (37 percent) fetuses at 50 mg/kg, corresponding to 2,800 times the maximum human inhalational dose.

Nursing Mothers: It is not known whether this drug is excreted in human milk. Because of the potential for tumorigenicity shown for albuterol in animal studies, a decision should be made whether to discontinue nursing or to discontinue the drug, taking into account the importance of the drug to the mother.

Pediatric Use: Safety and effectiveness in children below the age of 12 years have not been established.

Adverse Reactions: The adverse reactions of albuterol are similar in nature to those of other sympathomimetic agents, although the incidence of certain cardiovascular effects is less with albuterol. A 13-week double-blind study compared albuterol and isoproterenol aerosols in 147 asthmatic patients. The results of this study showed that the incidence of cardiovascular effects was: palpitations, less than 10 per 100 with albuterol and less than 15 per 100 with isoproterenol. The incidences of tachycardia and increased blood pressure were 10 per 100 and less than 5 per 100, respectively, with both drugs. In the same study, both drugs caused tremor or nausea in less than 15 patients per 100; dizziness or heartburn in less than 5 per 100 patients. Nervousness occurred in less than 10 per 100 patients receiving albuterol and in less than 15 per 100 patients receiving isoproterenol.

In addition, albuterol, like other sympathomimetic agents, can cause adverse reactions such as hypertension, angina, vomiting, vertigo, central stimulation, insomnia, headache, unusual taste, and drying or irritation of the oropharynx.

Overdosage: Exaggeration of the effects listed in ADVERSE REACTIONS can occur. Anginal pain and hypertension may result.

The oral LD_{50} in male and female rats and mice was greater than 2,000 mg/kg. The aerosol LD_{50} could not be determined.

Dialysis is not appropriate treatment for overdosage of PROVENTIL Inhaler. The judicious use of a cardioselective beta-receptor blocker, such as metoprolol tartrate, is suggested, bearing in mind the danger of inducing an asthmatic attack.

Dosage and Administration: The usual dosage for adults and children 12 years and older is 2 inhalations repeated every 4 to 6 hours; in some patients, 1 inhalation every 4 hours may be sufficient. More frequent administration or a larger number of inhalations is not recommended. The use of PROVENTIL Inhaler can be continued as medically indicated to control recurring bouts of bronchospasm. During this time most patients gain optimal benefit from regular use of the inhaler. Safe usage for periods extending over several years has been documented.

If a previously effective dosage regimen fails to provide the usual relief, medical advice should be sought immediately as this is often a sign of seriously worsening asthma which would require reassessment of therapy.

How Supplied: PROVENTIL Inhaler, 17.0 g canister; box of one. Each actuation delivers 90 mcg of albuterol from the mouthpiece. It is supplied with an oral adapter and patient's instructions; (NDC-0085-0614-02).

Store between 15° and 30°C (59° to 86°F). Shake well before using.

Copyright© 1981, Schering Corporation. All rights reserved.

[*Shown in Product Identification Section*]

PROVENTIL® ℞
brand of albuterol sulfate
Tablets

Description: PROVENTIL Tablets contain albuterol sulfate, a relatively selective $beta_2$-adrenergic bronchodilator. Albuterol sulfate has the chemical name α^1-[(*tert*-Butylamino) methyl]-4-hydroxy-*m*-xylene-α,α'-diol sulfate (2:1) (salt).

Albuterol sulfate has a molecular weight of 576.7 and the empirical formula $(C_{13}H_{21}NO_3)_2 \cdot H_2SO_4$. Albuterol sulfate is a white crystalline powder, soluble in water and slightly soluble in ethanol.

The international generic name for albuterol base is salbutamol.

Each PROVENTIL Tablet contains 2 or 4 mg of albuterol as 2.4 and 4.8 mg of albuterol sulfate, respectively.

Clinical Pharmacology: The prime action of beta-adrenergic drugs is to stimulate adenyl cyclase, the enzyme which catalyzes the formation of cyclic-3′,5′-adenosine monophosphate (cyclic AMP) from adenosine triphosphate (ATP). The cyclic AMP thus formed mediates the cellular responses. Based on pharmacologic studies in animals, albuterol appears to exert direct and preferential action on $beta_2$-adrenoceptors including those of the bronchial tree and uterus, and may have less cardiac stimulant effect than isoproterenol, when given in the usual recommended dose.

Albuterol is longer acting than isoproterenol in most patients by any route of administration because it is not a substrate for the cellular uptake processes for catecholamines nor for catechol-*O*-methyl transferase.

In three normal volunteers given tablets containing 6 mg tritiated albuterol sulfate, the maximum plasma concentrations of albuterol occurred within 2.5 hours. In other studies, the analysis of peak plasma samples indicated that the metabolite of albuterol represented 80% of the radioactivity present. Albuterol was shown to have a plasma half-life ranging from 2.7 to 5.0 hours when administered orally. Analysis of urine samples showed that 76% of the dose was excreted over 3 days, with the majority of the dose being excreted within the first 24 hours. Sixty percent of this radioactivity was shown to be the metabolite. Feces collected over this period contained 4% of the administered dose.

Animal studies show that albuterol does not pass the blood-brain barrier.

Indications and Usage: PROVENTIL Tablets are indicated for the relief of bronchospasm in patients with reversible obstructive airway disease.

In controlled clinical trials in patients with asthma, the onset of improvement in pulmonary function, as measured by maximal midexpiratory flow rate, MMEF, was noted within 30 minutes after a dose of PROVENTIL Tablets with peak improvement occurring between 2 to 3 hours. In controlled clinical trials in which measurements were conducted for 6 hours, significant clinical improvement in pulmonary function (defined as maintaining a 15% or more increase in FEV_1 and a 20% or more increase in MMEF over baseline values) was observed in 60% of patients at 4 hours and in 40% at 6 hours. No decrease in the effectiveness of PROVENTIL Tablets has been reported in patients who received long-term treatment with the drug in uncontrolled studies for periods up to 6 months.

Contraindications: PROVENTIL Tablets are contraindicated in patients with a history of hypersensitivity to any of its components.

Precautions: General: Although albuterol usually has minimal effects on the $beta_1$-adrenoceptors of the cardiovascular system at the recommended dosage, occasionally the usual cardiovascular and CNS stimulatory effects common to all sympathomimetic agents have been seen with patients treated with albuterol necessitating discontinuation. Therefore, albuterol should be used with caution in patients with cardiovascular disorders, including coronary insufficiency and hypertension, in patients with hyperthyroidism or diabetes mellitus, and in patients who are unusually responsive to sympathomimetic amines.

Large doses of intravenous albuterol have been reported to aggravate preexisting diabetes mellitus and ketoacidosis. The relevance of this observation to the use of PROVENTIL Tablets is unkown.

Although there have been no reports concerning the use of PROVENTIL Tablets during labor and delivery, high doses of albuterol administered intravenously are reported to inhibit uterine contractions. Although this effect is extremely unlikely as a consequence of oral use, it should be kept in mind.

Information for Patients: The action of PROVENTIL Tablets may last for six hours or longer and therefore it should not be taken more frequently than recommended. Do not increase the dose or frequency of medication without medical consultation. If symptoms get worse, medical consultation should be sought promptly.

Drug Interactions: The concomitant use of PROVENTIL Tablets and other oral sympathomimetic agents is not recommended since such combined use may lead to deleterious cardiovascular effects. This recommendation does not preclude the judicious use of an aerosol bronchodilator of the adrenergic stimulant type in patients receiving PROVENTIL Tablets. Such concomitant use, however, should be individualized and not given on a routine basis. If regular coadministration is required, then alternative therapy should be considered.

Albuterol should be administered with extreme caution to patients being treated with monoamine oxidase inhibitors or tricyclic antidepressants, since the action of albuterol on the vascular system may be potentiated.

Beta-receptor blocking agents and albuterol inhibit the effect of each other.

Carcinogenesis, Mutagenesis, and Impairment of Fertility: Albuterol sulfate, like other agents in its class, caused a significant dose-related increase in the incidence of benign leiomyomas of the mesovarium in a 2-year study in the rat, at doses corresponding to 3, 16, and 78 times the maximum human oral dose. In another study this effect was blocked by the coadministration of propranolol. The relevance of these studies to humans is not known. An 18-month study in mice and a lifetime study in hamsters revealed no evidence of tumorigenicity. Studies with albuterol revealed no evidence of mutagenesis. Reproduction studies in rats revealed no evidence of impaired fertility.

Teratogenic Effects—Pregnancy Category C: Albuterol has been shown to be teratogenic in mice when given subcutaneously in doses corresponding to 0.4 times the maximum human oral dose. There are no adequate and well-controlled studies in pregnant women. Albuterol should be used during pregnancy only if the potential benefit justifies the potential risk to the fetus. A reproduction study in CD-1 mice with albuterol showed cleft palate formation in 5 of 111 (4.5%) fetuses at 0.25 mg/kg and in 10 of 108 (9.3%) fetuses at 2.5 mg/kg, none were observed at 0.025 mg/kg. Cleft palate also occurred in 22 of 72 (30.5%) fetuses treated with 2.5 mg/kg isoproterenol (positive control). A reproduction study in Stride Dutch rabbits revealed cranioschisis in 7 of 19 (37%) fetuses at 50 mg/kg, corresponding to 78 times the maximum human oral dose.

Nursing Mothers: It is not known whether this drug is excreted in human milk. Because of the potential for tumorigenicity shown for albuterol in animal studies, a decision should be made whether to discontinue nursing or to discontinue the drug, taking into account the importance of the drug to the mother.

Pediatric Use: Safety and effectiveness in children below the age of 12 years have not been established.

Adverse Reactions: The adverse reactions to albuterol are similar in nature to those of other sympathomimetic agents. The most frequent adverse reactions to PROVENTIL Tablets were nervousness and tremor, with each occurring in approximately 20 of 100 patients. Other reported reactions were headache, 7 of 100 patients; tachycardia and palpitations, 5 of 100 patients; muscle cramps, 3 of 100 patients; insomnia, nausea, weakness, and dizziness, each occurred in 2 of 100 patients. Drowsiness, flushing, restlessness, irritability, chest discomfort, and difficulty in micturition each occurred in less than 1 of 100 patients.

In addition, albuterol, like other sympathomimetic agents, can cause adverse reactions such as hypertension, angina, vomiting, vertigo, central stimulation, unusual taste, and drying or irritation of the oropharynx.

The reactions are generally transient in nature, and it is usually not necessary to discontinue treatment with PROVENTIL Tablets. In selected cases, however, dosage may be reduced temporarily; after the reaction has subsided, dosage should be increased in small increments to the optimal dosage.

Overdosage: Manifestations of overdosage include anginal pain, hypertension and exaggeration of the effects listed in **ADVERSE REACTIONS.**

The oral LD_{50} in rats and mice was greater than 2,000 mg/kg.

Continued on next page

Information on Schering products appearing on these pages is effective as of September 30, 1982.

Schering—Cont.

Dialysis is not appropriate treatment for overdosage of PROVENTIL Tablets. The judicious use of a cardioselective beta-receptor blocker, such as metoprolol tartrate, is suggested, bearing in mind the danger of inducing an asthmatic attack.

Dosage and Administration: The following dosages of PROVENTIL Tablets are expressed in terms of albuterol base.

Usual Dose: The usual starting dosage for adults and children 12 years and over is 2 mg or 4 mg three or four times a day.

Dosage Adjustment: Doses above 4 mg, four times a day should be used only when the patient fails to respond. If a favorable response does not occur with the 4 mg initial dosage, it should be cautiously increased step wise up to a maximum of 8 mg four times a day as tolerated.

Elderly Patients and Those Sensitive to Beta-Adrenergic Stimulators: An initial dosage of 2 mg three or four times a day is recommended for elderly patients and for those with a history of unusual sensitivity to beta-adrenergic stimulators. If adequate bronchodilatation is not obtained, dosage may be increased gradually to as much as 8 mg three or four times a day.

The total daily dose should not exceed 32 mg in adults and children 12 years and over.

How Supplied: PROVENTIL Tablets, 2 mg albuterol as the sulfate, white, round, compressed tablets, impressed with the product name (PROVENTIL) and the number 2 on one side, and product identification numbers, 252, and scored on the other; bottles of 100 and 500. (NDC 0085-0252-__)

PROVENTIL Tablets, 4 mg albuterol as the sulfate, white, round, compressed tablets, impressed with the product name (PROVENTIL) and the number 4 on one side, and product identification numbers, 573, and scored on the other; bottles of 100 and 500. (NDC 0085-0573-__)

Store between 2° and 30°C (36° and 86°F).

Copyright © 1982, Schering Corporation. All rights reserved.

Revised 3/82

Sodium SULAMYD® ℞

brand of sulfacetamide sodium, USP

Ophthalmic Solution 30%—Sterile
Ophthalmic Solution 10%—Sterile
Ophthalmic Ointment 10%—Sterile

Description: Sodium SULAMYD is available in three ophthalmic forms:

Ophthalmic Solution 30% contains in each ml. of sterile aqueous solution 300 mg. sulfacetamide sodium, USP, 1.5 mg. sodium thiosulfate, with 0.5 mg. methylparaben and 0.1 mg. propylparaben added as preservatives, and sodium dihydrogen phosphate as buffer.

Ophthalmic Solution 10% contains in each ml. of sterile aqueous solution 100 mg. sulfacetamide sodium, USP, 3.1 mg. sodium thiosulfate, and 5 mg. methylcellulose, with 0.5 mg. methylparaben and 0.1 mg. propylparaben added as preservatives and sodium dihydrogen phosphate as buffer.

Ophthalmic Ointment 10% is a sterile ointment, each gram containing 100 mg. sulfacetamide sodium, USP, with 0.5 mg. methylparaben, 0.1 mg. propylparaben and 0.25 mg. benzalkonium chloride added as preservatives, and sorbitan monolaurate and water in a bland, unctuous, petrolatum base.

Actions: Sodium SULAMYD exerts a bacteriostatic effect against a wide range of gram-positive and gram-negative microorganisms by restricting, through competition with para-aminobenzoic acid, the synthesis of folic acid which bacteria require for growth.

Indications: Sodium SULAMYD is indicated for the treatment of conjunctivitis, corneal ulcer, and other superficial ocular infections due to susceptible microorganisms, and as adjunctive treatment in systemic sulfonamide therapy of trachoma.

Contraindications: Sodium SULAMYD is contraindicated in individuals with known or suspected sensitivity to sulfonamides or to any of the ingredients of the preparations.

Precautions: Sodium SULAMYD products are incompatible with silver preparations. Ophthalmic ointments may retard corneal healing. Non-susceptible organisms, including fungi, may proliferate with the use of these preparations. Sulfonamides are inactivated by the para-aminobenzoic acid present in purulent exudates.

Sensitization may recur when a sulfonamide is re-administered irrespective of the route of administration, and cross sensitivity between different sulfonamides may occur. If signs of sensitivity or other untoward reactions occur, discontinue use of the preparation.

Adverse Reactions: Sulfacetamide sodium may cause local irritation. Transient stinging or burning has been reported with the 30% solution of sulfacetamide sodium.

Although sensitivity reactions to sulfacetamide sodium are rare, an isolated incident of Stevens-Johnson syndrome was reported in a patient who had experienced a previous bullous drug reaction to an orally administered sulfonamide and a single instance of local hypersensitivity was reported which progressed to a fatal syndrome resembling systemic lupus erythematosus.

Dosage and Administration: Sodium SULAMYD Ophthalmic Solution 30%. *For conjunctivitis or corneal ulcer:* instill one drop into lower conjunctival sac every two hours or less frequently according to severity of infection. *For trachoma:* Two drops every two hours; concomitant systemic sulfonamide therapy is indicated.

Sodium SULAMYD Ophthalmic Solution 10%. One or two drops into the lower conjunctival sac every two or three hours during the day and less often at night.

Sodium SULAMYD Ophthalmic Ointment 10%. Apply a small amount four times daily and at bedtime. The ointment may be used adjunctively with either of the solution forms.

How Supplied: Sodium SULAMYD Ophthalmic Ointment 10%, 3.5 g tube, box of one. **Store away from heat.**

Sodium SULAMYD Ophthalmic Solution 30%, 15 ml. dropper bottle, box of one. **Store between 2° and 30°C (36° and 86°F).**

Sodium SULAMYD Ophthalmic Solution 10%, 5 ml. dropper bottle, box of 25; 15 ml. dropper bottle, box of one. **Store between 2° and 30°C (36° and 86°F).**

On long standing, sulfonamide solutions will darken in color and should be discarded.

Revised 6/81

Copyright © 1969, 1981, Schering Corporation. All rights reserved.

SOLGANAL® ℞

brand of sterile aurothioglucose

Suspension, USP
FOR INTRAMUSCULAR INJECTION ONLY—
NOT FOR INTRAVENOUS USE

WARNINGS

> Physicians planning to use SOLGANAL Suspension should thoroughly familiarize themselves with its toxicity and its benefits. The possibility of toxic reactions should always be explained to the patient before starting therapy. Patients should be warned to report promptly any symptom suggesting toxicity. Before **each** injection of SOLGANAL Suspension, the physician should review the results of laboratory work and see the patient to determine the presence or absence of adverse reactions, since some of these can be severe or even fatal.

Description: SOLGANAL is a sterile suspension, for **intramuscular injection only.** SOLGANAL Suspension is an antiarthritic agent which is absorbed gradually following intramuscular injection, producing a therapeutically desired prolonged effect.

Each ml contains 50 mg of aurothioglucose, USP in sterile sesame oil with 2% aluminum monostearate; 1 mg propylparaben is added as preservative. Aurothioglucose contains approximately 50% gold by weight.

The empirical formula for aurothioglucose is $C_6H_{11}AuO_5S$; the molecular weight is 392.18. Chemically it is (1-Thio-D-glucopyranosato) gold.

Aurothioglucose is a nearly odorless, yellow powder which is stable in air. An aqueous solution is unstable on long standing. Aurothioglucose is freely soluble in water but practically insoluble in acetone, in alcohol, in chloroform, and in ether.

Clinical Pharmacology: Although the mechanism of action is not well understood, gold compounds have been reported to decrease synovial inflammation and retard cartilage and bone destruction.

Gold is absorbed from injection sites, reaching peak concentration in blood in four to six hours. Following a single intramuscular injection of 50 mg SOLGANAL Suspension in each of two patients, peak serum levels were about 235 mcg/dl in one patient and 450 mcg/dl in the other. In plasma, 95% is bound to the albumin fraction. Approximately 70% of the gold is eliminated in the urine and approximately 30% in the feces. When a standard weekly treatment schedule is followed, approximately 40% of the administered dose is excreted each week, and the remainder is excreted over a longer period. The biological half-life of gold salts following a single 50 mg dose has been reported to range from 3 to 27 days. Following successive weekly doses, the half-life increases and may be 14 to 40 days after the third dose and up to 168 days after the eleventh weekly dose.

After the initial injection, the serum level of gold rises sharply and declines over the next week. Peak levels with aqueous preparations are higher and decline faster than those with oily preparations. Weekly administration produces a continuous rise in the basal value for several months, after which the serum level becomes relatively stable. After a standard weekly dose, considerable individual variation in the levels of gold has been found. A steady decline in gold levels occurs when the interval between injections is lengthened, and small amounts may be found in the serum for months after discontinuance of therapy. The incidence of toxic reactions is apparently unrelated to the plasma level of gold, but it may be related to the cumulative body content of gold.

Storage of gold in human tissues is dependent upon organ mass as well as upon the concentration of gold. Therefore, tissues having the highest gold levels (weight/weight) do not necessarily contain the greatest total amounts of gold. The major depots, in decreasing order of total gold content, are the bone marrow, liver, skin, and bone, accounting for approximately 85% of body gold. The highest concentrations of gold are found in the lymph nodes, adrenal glands, liver, kidneys, bone marrow, and spleen. Relatively small concentrations are found in articular structures.

Gold passes the blood-brain barrier in hamsters.

Transfer of gold across the human placenta at the twentieth week of pregnancy has been documented. The placenta showed numerous gold deposits and smaller amounts were detected in the fetal liver and kidneys; other tissues provided no evidence of gold deposition.

Gold is excreted into human milk in significant amounts and trace amounts can be demonstrated in the blood of nursing infants. (See PRECAUTIONS, "*Nursing Mothers*.")

Indications and Usage: (SOLGANAL Suspension is indicated for the adjunctive treatment of early active rheumatoid arthritis (both of the adult and juvenile types) not adequately controlled by other anti-inflammatory agents and conservative measures. In chronic, advanced cases of rheumatoid arthritis, gold therapy is less valuable.

Antirheumatic measures such as salicylates and other anti-inflammatory drugs (both steroidal and non-steroidal) may be continued after initiation of gold therapy. After improvement commences, these measures may be discontinued slowly as symptoms permit.

See Precautions, "*Laboratory Tests*" and **Dosage and Administration.**

Contraindications: A history of known hypersensitivity to any component of SOLGANAL Suspension contraindicates its use. Gold therapy is contraindicated in patients with uncontrolled diabetes mellitus, severe debilitation, systemic lupus erythematosus, renal disease, hepatic dysfunction, uncontrolled congestive heart failure, marked hypertension, agranulocytosis, other blood dyscrasias, or hemorrhagic diathesis; or if there is a history of infectious hepatitis. Patients who recently have had radiation, and those who have developed severe toxicity from previous exposure to gold or other heavy metals should not receive SOLGANAL Suspension.

Urticaria, eczema, and colitis are also contraindications.

Gold therapy is usually contraindicated in pregnancy. (See PRECAUTIONS, "*Usage in Pregnancy*".)

Gold salts should not be used with penicillamine (See MANAGEMENT OF ADVERSE REACTIONS) or antimalarials. The safety of coadministration with immunosuppressive agents other than corticosteroids has not been established.

Warnings: The following signs should be considered danger signals of gold toxicity, and no additional injection should be given unless further studies reveal some other cause for their presence; rapid reduction of hemoglobin, leukopenia (WBC below 4000/cu mm), eosinophilia above 5%, platelet count below 100,000/cu mm, albuminuria, hematuria, pruritus, dermatitis, stomatitis, jaundice, and petechiae.

Effects that may occur immediately following an injection, or at any time during gold therapy, include: anaphylactic shock, syncope, bradycardia, thickening of the tongue, difficulty in swallowing and breathing, and angioneurotic edema. If such effects are observed, treatment with SOLGANAL Suspension should be discontinued.

Tolerance to gold usually decreases with advancing age. Diabetes mellitus or congestive heart failure should be under control before gold therapy is instituted.

SOLGANAL Suspension should be used with extreme caution in patients with: skin rash, hypersensitivity to other medications, or a history of renal or liver disease.

Precautions: *General:* Before **each** injection, the physician should personally check the patient for adverse reactions and inquiry should be made regarding pruritus, rash, sore mouth, indigestion, and metallic taste. The patient should be observed for at least 15 minutes following each injection. (See also "*Laboratory Tests*".)

Patients with HLA-D locus histocompatibility antigens DRw2 and DRw3 may have a genetic predisposition to develop certain toxic reactions, such as proteinuria, during treatment with gold or D-penicillamine.

SOLGANAL Suspension should be used with caution in patients with compromised cardiovascular or cerebral circulation.

Information for Patients:

1. Promptly report to the physician any unusual symptoms such as pruritus (itching), rash, sore mouth, indigestion, or metallic taste.
2. Increased joint pain may occur for one or two days after an injection and usually subsides after the first few injections.
3. Exposure to sunlight or artificial ultraviolet light should be minimized.
4. Careful oral hygiene is recommended in conjunction with therapy.
5. Patients should be aware of potential hazards if they become pregnant while receiving gold therapy. (See "*Usage in Pregnancy*".)

Laboratory Tests: Before treatment is started, a complete blood count, platelet count, and urinalysis should be done to serve as reference points. Since gold therapy is usually contraindicated in pregnant patients, pregnancy should be ruled out before treatment is started. Throughout the treatment period, urinalysis should be repeated prior to each injection, and complete blood cell and platelet counts should be performed every two weeks. A platelet count is indicated any time that purpura or ecchymosis occurs.

Drug Interactions: Drug interactions have not been reported. (See **Contraindications.**)

Carcinogenesis, Mutagenesis, and Impairment of Fertility: Renal adenomas developed in rats receiving an injectable gold product similar to SOLGANAL Suspension at doses of 2 mg/kg weekly for 46 weeks, followed by 6 mg/kg daily for 47 weeks. These doses were higher and administered more frequently than the recommended human doses. The adenomas were similar histologically to those produced by chronic administration of other gold compounds and heavy metals, such as lead or nickel.

Renal tubular cell neoplasia consisting of renal adenoma and adenocarcinoma were noted in a dose-response relationship in another study in rats using daily intramuscular doses of 3 mg/kg and 6 mg/kg for up to 2 years. These doses were higher and were administered more frequently than the recommended human doses. In this same study, sarcomas at the injection site occurred in some rats but their numbers were not sufficient to demonstrate a dose-response relationship.

No report of renal adenoma or sarcoma at the injection site in man in association with the use of SOLGANAL Suspension has been received.

Gold compounds have not been studied for evaluation of mutagenesis.

Gold sodium thiomalate given subcutaneously did not adversely affect fertility or reproductive performance.

Usage in Pregnancy: Gold therapy is usually contraindicated in pregnant patients. The patient should be warned about the hazards of becoming pregnant while on gold therapy. Rheumatoid arthritis frequently improves when the patient becomes pregnant, thereby eliminating the need for gold therapy. The potential nephrotoxicity of gold should not be superimposed on the increased renal burden which normally occurs in pregnancy and hence, gold therapy should be discontinued upon recognition of pregnancy unless continued use is required in an individual case. The slow excretion of gold and its persistence in body tissues after discontinuation of treatment should be kept in mind when a woman of child-bearing potential being treated with gold plans to become pregnant.

Pregnancy Category C: Gold sodium thiomalate administered subcutaneously, a route not used clinically, has been shown to be teratogenic during the organogenic period in rats and rabbits when given in doses 140 and 175 times, respectively, the usual human dose. Hydrocephalus and microphthalmia were the malformations observed in rats when gold sodium thiomalate was administered at a dose of 25 mg/kg/day from day 6 through day 15 of gestation. In rabbits, limb defects and gastroschisis were the malformations observed when gold sodium thiomalate was administered at doses of 20 to 45 mg/kg/day from day 6 through day 18 of gestation.

Gold compounds administered orally to rabbits from days 6 through 18 of pregnancy resulted in the occurrence of abdominal defects, such as gastroschisis and umbilical hernia; anomalies of the brain, heart, lung, and skeleton; and microphthalmia.

The administration of excessive doses of gold-containing compounds during pregnancy in the above studies was toxic to the mothers and their embryos; the embryotoxic effects probably were secondary to maternal toxicity. Therefore, the significance of these findings in relation to human use is unknown.

There are no adequate and well-controlled studies with SOLGANAL Suspension in pregnant women. Extensive clinical experience with SOLGANAL Suspension has not demonstrated human teratogenicity.

Nursing Mothers: Gold has been demonstated in the milk of lactating mothers. In one patient, a total dose of 135 mg of gold thioglucose was given during the postpartum period. Samples of the maternal milk and urine, and samples of red blood cells and serum of the mother and child were evaluated by atomic absorption spectrophotometry. Trace amounts of gold appeared in the serum and red blood cells of the nursing offspring. It has been postulated that this may be the cause of unexplained rashes, nephritis, hepatitis, and hematologic aberrations in the nursing infants of mothers treated with gold. Because of the potential for serious adverse reactions in nursing infants, a decision should be made whether to discontinue nursing or to discontinue the gold therapy, taking into account the importance of the drug to the mother. The slow excretion of gold and its persistence in the mother after discontinuation of treatment should be kept in mind.

Pediatric Use: Safety and effectiveness in children below the age of six years have not been established.

Adverse Reactions: Adverse reactions to gold therapy may occur at any time during treatment or many months after therapy has been discontinued. The incidence of toxic reactions is apparently unrelated to the plasma level of gold, but it may be related to the cumulative body content of gold. Higher than conventional dosage schedules may increase the occurrence and severity of toxicity. Severe effects are most common after 300 to 500 mg have been administered.

Cutaneous Reactions: Dermatitis is the most common reaction. Pruritus should be considered a warning signal of an impending cutaneous reaction. Erythema and occasionally the more severe reactions such as papular, vesicular, and exfoliative dermatitis leading to alopecia and shedding of the nails may occur. Chrysiasis (gray-to-blue pigmentation) has been reported, especially on photoexposed areas. Gold dermatitis may be aggravated by exposure to sunlight, or an actinic rash may develop.

Mucous Membrane Reactions: Stomatitis is the second most common adverse reaction. Shallow ulcers on the buccal membranes, on the borders of the tongue and on the palate, diffuse glossitis, or gingivitis may be preceded

Continued on next page

Information on Schering products appearing on these pages is effective as of September 30, 1982.

Schering—Cont.

by the sensation of metallic taste. Careful oral hygiene is recommended. Inflammation of the upper respiratory tract, pharyngitis, gastritis, colitis, tracheitis, and vaginitis have also been reported. Conjunctivitis is rare.

Renal Reactions: Nephrotic syndrome or glomerulitis with hematuria, which is usually relatively mild, subsides completely if recognized early and treatment is discontinued. These reactions become severe and chronic if gold therapy is continued after their onset. Therefore, it is important to perform a urinalysis before each injection and to discontinue treatment promptly if proteinuria or hematuria develops.

Hematologic Reactions: Although rare, blood dyscrasias, including granulocytopenia, agranulocytosis, thrombocytopenia with or without purpura, leukopenia, eosinophilia, panmyelopathy, hemorrhagic diathesis, and hypoplastic and aplastic anemia, have been reported. These reactions may occur separately or in combination.

Nitritoid and Allergic Reactions: These reactions, which may rarely occur with SOLGANAL Suspension and which resemble anaphylactoid effects, include flushing, fainting, dizziness, sweating, malaise, weakness, nausea, and vomiting.

Miscellaneous Reactions: On rare occasions, gastrointestinal symptoms, i.e., nausea, vomiting, colic, anorexia, abdominal cramps, diarrhea, ulcerative enterocolitis, and headache have been reported.

There have been rare reports of iritis and corneal ulcers. Transient, asymptomatic gold deposits in the cornea or conjunctiva may occur. Other reported reactions include encephalitis, immunological destruction of the synovia, EEG abnormalities, intrahepatic cholestasis, hepatitis with jaundice, toxic hepatitis, acute yellow atrophy, peripheral neuritis, gold bronchitis, pulmonary injury manifested by interstitial pneumonitis or fibrosis, fever, and partial or complete hair loss.

Less common but more severe effects that may occur shortly after an injection or at any time during gold therapy include: anaphylactic shock, syncope, bradycardia, thickening of the tongue, difficulty in swallowing and breathing, and angioneurotic edema. If they are observed, treatment with SOLGANAL Suspension should be discontinued.

Arthralgia may occur for one or two days after an injection and usually subsides after the first few injections. The mechanism of the transient increase in rheumatic symptoms after injection of gold (the so-called nonvasomotor postinjection reaction) is unknown. These reactions are usually mild but occasionally may be so severe that treatment is stopped prematurely.

Management of Adverse Reactions: In the event of toxic reactions, gold therapy should be discontinued immediately.

In the presence of mild reactions, it may be sufficient to discontinue the administration of SOLGANAL Suspension for a short period and then to resume treatment with smaller doses.

Dermatitis and pruritus may respond to soothing lotions, other appropriate antipruritic treatment, or topical glucocorticoids.

If dermatitis or stomatitis becomes severe or spreads, systemic glucocorticoid treatment may be indicated. For renal, hematologic, and most other adverse reactions, glucocorticoids may be required in larger doses and for a longer time than for dermatologic reactions. Often this treatment may be required for many months because of the slow elimination of gold from the body.

If severe adverse reactions do not improve with steroid treatment in patients who receive large doses of gold, a chelating agent, such as dimercaprol (BAL), may be used. In one case, it was reported that penicillamine was beneficial in the treatment of gold-induced thrombocytopenia. Adjunctive use of an anabolic steroid with other drugs (i.e., BAL, penicillamine, and corticosteroids) may contribute to recovery of bone marrow deficiency.

In the presence of severe or idiosyncratic reactions, treatment with SOLGANAL Suspension should not be reinstituted.

Overdosage: Overdosage resulting from too rapid increases in dosing with SOLGANAL Suspension will be manifested by rapid appearance of toxic reactions, particularly those relating to renal damage, such as hematuria, proteinuria, and to hematologic effects, such as thrombocytopenia and granulocytopenia. Other toxic effects, including fever, nausea, vomiting, diarrhea, and various skin disorders such as papulovesicular lesions, urticaria, and exfoliative dermatitis, all attended with severe pruritus, may develop. Treatment consists of prompt discontinuation of the medication, and early administration of dimercaprol. Specific supportive therapy should be given for the renal and hematologic complications. (See also MANAGEMENT OF ADVERSE REACTIONS above).

Dosage and Administration: Adults—The usual dosage schedule for the intramuscular administration of SOLGANAL is as follows: first dose, 10 mg; second and third doses, 25 mg; fourth and subsequent doses, 50 mg. The interval between doses is one week. The 50 mg dose is continued at weekly intervals until 0.8 to 1.0 g SOLGANAL has been given. If the patient has improved and has exhibited no sign of toxicity, the 50 mg dose may be continued many months longer, at three- to four-week intervals. A weekly dose above 50 mg is usually unnecessary and contraindicated; the tendency in gold therapy is toward lower dosage. With this in mind, it may eventually be established that a 25 mg dose is the one of choice. If no improvement has been demonstrated after a total administration of 1.0 g of SOLGANAL Suspension, the necessity for gold therapy should be reevaluated.

Children 6 to 12 years—one-fourth of the adult dose, governed chiefly by body weight, not to exceed 25 mg per dose.

SOLGANAL Suspension should be injected **intramuscularly,** (preferably intragluteally), **never intravenously.** The patient should be lying down and should remain recumbent for approximately 10 minutes after the injection. The vial should be thoroughly shaken in order to suspend all of the active material. Heating the vial to body temperature (by immersion in warm water) will facilitate drawing the suspension into the syringe. An 18-gauge, 1½-inch needle is recommended for depositing the preparation deep into the muscular tissue. For obese patients, an 18-gauge, 2-inch needle may be used. The site usually selected for injection is the upper outer quadrant of the gluteal region.

NOTE: Shake the vial in horizontal position before the dose is withdrawn. Needle and syringe must be dry. The patient should be observed for at least 15 minutes following each injection.

How Supplied: SOLGANAL Suspension is available in 10 ml multiple-dose vials containing 5% (50 mg/ml) aurothioglucose; box of one. **Shake well before using. Store between 0° and 30°C (32° and 86°F). Protect from light. Store in carton until contents are used.**

Copyright © 1963, 1981, Schering Corporation. All rights reserved.

THEOVENT® ℞

brand of theophylline anhydrous, USP
Long-Acting Capsules

Description: THEOVENT Long-Acting Capsules are a specially formulated preparation of anhydrous theophylline which is gradually released for prolonged therapeutic effect after oral administration. The product is formulated so that most of the dose is released after leaving the stomach, thereby minimizing exposure of the gastric mucosa to the potentially irritating effects of theophylline. Each capsule contains either 125 mg or 250 mg of anhydrous theophylline, USP.

Anhydrous theophylline is 3,7-Dihydro-1,3-dimethyl-1*H*-purine-2,6-dione, anhydrous.

Anhydrous theophylline is a xanthine compound having the chemical formula, $C_7H_8N_4O_2$, with a molecular weight of 180.17. It is a white, odorless, crystalline powder which is stable in air and has a bitter taste. Theophylline is slightly soluble in water, freely soluble in solutions of alkali hydroxides and in ammonia, while only slightly soluble in alcohol, chloroform, or ether.

Clinical Pharmacology: Theophylline directly relaxes the smooth muscle of the bronchial airways and pulmonary blood vessels, thus acting mainly as a bronchodilator, pulmonary vasodilator, and smooth muscle relaxant. It produces an increase in vital capacity and counteracts the entrapment of residual air. Its bronchodilating action helps relieve wheezing, coughing, and other respiratory symptoms associated with reversible bronchospasm.

Theophylline also possesses other actions typical of the xanthine derivatives: coronary vasodilation; diuretic; and skeletal muscle, cardiac, and cerebral stimulation. Its actions may be mediated through inhibition of phosphodiesterase and a resultant increase in intracellular cyclic AMP which could mediate smooth muscle relaxation. Theophylline also inhibits the release of histamine by mast cells *in vitro* at concentrations higher than those usually attained clinically.

In vitro theophylline has been shown to react synergistically with appropriate beta agonists (e.g., isoproterenol), by increasing intracellular cyclic AMP through stimulation of adenyl cyclase, but therapeutic synergistic bronchodilation has not been demonstrated in clinical studies. More data are needed to determine if theophylline and beta agonists have clinically important therapeutic additive effects.

Tolerance (tachyphylaxis) does not appear to develop with prolonged use of theophylline.

The elimination characteristics of theophylline are as follows:

Patient Population	Theophylline Plasma Clearance Rates (mean ± S.D.)	Average Half-Life (mean ± S.D.)
Children (over 6 months of age)	1.45 ± .58 ml/kg/min	3.7 ± 1.1 hours
Adult non-smokers with uncomplicated asthma	.65 ± .19 ml/kg/min	8.7 ± 2.2 hours

The half-life is shortened by cigarette smoking and also by a low carbohydrate, high protein diet. Conversely, the half-life is prolonged by a high carbohydrate, low protein diet, and also in patients with alcoholism, reduced hepatic or renal functions, congestive heart failure, and in patients receiving certain antibiotics, such as troleandomycin, erythromycin, lincomycin, or clindamycin. High fever for prolonged periods may decrease theophylline elimination.

THEOVENT Long-Acting Capsules *are not indicated* for young children or infants. It should be noted that newborn infants have extremely slow theophylline clearances with a half-life exceeding 24 hours.

In infants 3 to 6 months old, these elimination characteristics are similar to those in older children.

Older adults with chronic obstructive pulmonary disease, patients with cor pulmonale or other causes of heart failure, and patients with liver disease may have much lower clearances with a half-life that may exceed 24 hours.

The half-life of the theophylline in smokers (of 1 to 2 packs of cigarettes per day) averaged 4 to 5 hours among various studies, much shorter than the half-life in non-smokers, which averaged about 7 to 9 hours. The increase in theophylline clearance caused by smoking is probably the result of induction of drug-metabolizing enzymes. After cessation of smoking, normalization of theophylline pharmacokinetics may not occur for 3 months to 2 years.

In a well-controlled study in normal adult males, a single dose of 500 mg THEOVENT Long-Acting Capsules, administered as 2 capsules each containing 250 mg, resulted in a mean peak serum concentration of 7.5 mcg/ml at 4.6 hours after administration. The relative bioavailability of THEOVENT Long-Acting Capsules was complete compared to that of a standard theophylline syrup.

In a multiple-dose study in which asthmatic adults received 500 mg THEOVENT Long-Acting Capsules every 12 hours, therapeutic levels of theophylline were achieved by the second day of therapy and were maintained within the optimal therapeutic range of 10 to 20 mcg/ml from the second day through the last treatment day (day 4) of the study. In chronic therapy of patients requiring higher than average doses, the gradual absorption of theophylline from THEOVENT Long-Acting Capsules, as compared with that of non-sustained release theophylline products, may minimize the fluctuation (peaks and troughs) in serum concentrations and permit longer intervals between dosing.

Studies suggest that 1-demethylation of theophylline to 3-methylxanthine is the principal biotransformation pathway of theophylline elimination. Only 10% of an administered dose of theophylline appears unchanged in the urine. Principal metabolites are 3-methylxanthine, 1,3-dimethyluric acid, and 1-methyluric acid. Animal experiments have shown that theophylline enters the cerebrospinal fluid. The degree of protein binding (55% to 63%) of theophylline at the therapeutic serum concentration has little effect on theophylline distribution. Theophylline distributes well into breast milk; the average ratio of milk to serum concentration of the drug was approximately 0.7, and milk concentrations paralleled the time course of serum concentrations.

Indications and Usage: THEOVENT Long-Acting Capsules are indicated for relief and/or prevention of reversible bronchospasm associated with asthma, chronic bronchitis, or emphysema. Use of theophylline is a treatment of first choice for the management of chronic asthma to prevent symptoms and maintain patent airways.

Contraindications: This product is contraindicated in individuals who have shown hypersensitivity to any of its components, to aminophylline, or to other xanthines, e.g., theobromine or caffeine.

Warnings: Status asthmaticus is a medical emergency. When the patient is not rapidly responsive to bronchodilators, optimal therapy requires additional medication, including corticosteroids. Severe episodes of bronchospasm may require inhalant and/or parenteral therapy or a rapidly acting theophylline preparation.

Although early signs of theophylline toxicity, such as nausea and restlessness, are often seen, in some cases more serious signs such as ventricular arrhythmias or convulsions may be the first signs of toxicity. It is important to discontinue doses which are not tolerated. In situations where therapy is to be resumed, it should be at a lower dosage after all signs of toxicity have disappeared.

Patients with higher than the recommended therapeutic theophylline serum levels are more likely to experience tachycardia than patients whose levels are within the recommended therapeutic range. Theophylline products may worsen preexisting arrhythmias. (See *Drug Interactions* under Precautions.)

Precautions: *General:* Theophylline should not be administered concurrently with other xanthine medications such as aminophylline and caffeine. Use theophylline with caution in patients with severe cardiac disease, arrhythmias, acute myocardial injury, congestive heart failure, cor pulmonale, hypertension, severe hypoxemia, hyperthyroidism, liver or renal disease, dehydration, and in the elderly (especially males over 55 years of age). In patients with a peptic ulcer or a history of peptic ulcer, their condition may be exacerbated. Theophylline may occasionally act as a local gastrointestinal irritant, especially in high doses and during chronic use, but gastrointestinal symptoms are more commonly central and associated with serum concentrations exceeding 20 mcg/ml.

Factors known to influence body clearance of theophylline are:

Increased Clearance	Decreased Clearance
Cigarette smoking	Increasing age Congestive heart failure Liver disease Pulmonary edema Concurrent infection Concomitant use of any of the following: erythromycin troleandomycin clindamycin lincomycin

In the presence of any of the above factors, it is advisable to monitor theophylline serum levels periodically. Other circumstances in which it is advisable to monitor serum levels include: unexplained poor control of asthma; occurrence of toxic symptoms; addition or removal of other drugs from the therapeutic regimen which affect the metabolism of theophylline; use of unusually high doses.

Information for Patients:

1. Contact a physician immediately if vomiting, nausea, restlessness, convulsions, or irregular heartbeat occurs.
2. Take only the dosage which has been prescribed; especially do not take a larger dose, or take the drug more frequently, or for a longer time than directed.
3. Do not take other medicines, especially those for asthma or breathing problems, except under advice and supervision of a physician.
4. Avoid drinking large amounts of caffeine-containing beverages, such as tea, coffee (except decaffeinated), cocoa, and cola drinks or eating large amounts of chocolate while taking this medicine, since these products may add to the side effects of theophylline.

Laboratory Tests: Periodic measurement of theophylline serum levels is recommended to assure maximal benefit from the drug with minimal risk of toxicity. The incidence of toxicity increases sharply at serum levels greater than 20 mcg/ml. For purposes of monitoring serum theophylline concentrations, serum should be obtained at the time of peak drug absorption (2 to 5 hours after ingestion). In the preceding 48 hours, dosage should have been reasonably typical of the prescribed regimen and no doses should have been missed or added. INCREASING DOSAGE BASED ON SERUM THEOPHYLLINE MEASUREMENTS WHEN THESE INSTRUCTIONS HAVE NOT BEEN FOLLOWED MAY INCREASE THE RISK OF TOXICITY TO THE PATIENT. Generally, the optimum therapeutic serum levels of theophylline are between 10 and 20 mcg/ml; higher levels may produce toxic effects. There are wide interpatient and intrapatient variations in the dosage needed to achieve and maintain therapeutic serum levels. Because of these wide variations and the relatively narrow range between therapeutic and toxic serum levels, dosage must be individualized, and serum level monitoring is recommended, particularly when prolonged use is planned. (See also Clinical Pharmacology and Warnings sections).

High serum levels of theophylline in association with manifestations of toxicity may result from conventional doses in clinical situations such as: lowered body plasma clearances (due to transient cardiac decompensation); liver dysfunction or chronic obstructive lung disease; age of 55 years or more, particularly in males.

Further, in the presence of any of the factors discussed under PRECAUTIONS, *General,* it is especially advisable to monitor theophylline serum levels periodically. (See also DOSAGE AND ADMINISTRATION.)

Drug Interactions: (See also PRECAUTIONS, *General.*) Toxic synergism with ephedrine has been documented and may occur with some other sympathomimetic bronchodilators. Recent controlled studies suggest that the addition of ephedrine to dosage regimens of theophylline results in an increase in toxic effects, but not in efficacy, when compared to theophylline alone. The concurrent use of theophylline and sympathomimetic drugs is of particular concern in the presence of arrhythmias. Following is a list of other drugs and the effects seen from their interaction with theophylline.

DRUG	EFFECT
lithium carbonate	increased excretion of lithium carbonate
propranolol	antagonism of propranolol
furosemide	increased diuresis
reserpine	tachycardia
troleandomycin erythromycin lincomycin, or clindamycin	increased theophylline blood levels

Drug/Laboratory Test Interactions: Theophylline may increase the results of tests for urinary catecholamines, plasma free fatty acids, serum uric acid, bilirubin, and sedimentation rate. Theophylline may decrease the results of ^{131}I uptake tests.

Carcinogenesis, Mutagenesis, Impairment of Fertility: No long-term study of theophylline has been done in animals to evaluate carcinogenic potential. Theophylline has been reported to cause chromosomal breakage in human cells in culture at concentrations approximately 35 times the maximum therapeutic serum concentrations.

Pregnancy Category C: Theophylline has been shown to be teratogenic in mice when given in doses 30 times the adult human dose. It was not teratogenic when administered to Br46-Wistar II rats prior to mating and at various stages of gestation. As with most anti-asthmatic medications, there are no adequate and well-controlled studies in pregnant women. Theophylline should be used during pregnancy only if the potential benefits justify the potential risks to the fetus. To be considered in the benefit-risk assessment are the dangers of uncontrolled asthma in pregnant women and the reported presence of theophylline in cord serum.

Nonteratogenic Effects: Theophylline levels have been found in cord serum and there have been reports of slight tachycardia and jitteriness in neonates whose mothers received theophylline up to the time of delivery.

Continued on next page

Information on Schering products appearing on these pages is effective as of September 30, 1982.

Schering—Cont.

Nursing Mothers: It has been reported that theophylline distributes readily into breast milk. One nursing infant experienced mild symptoms of irritability, fretfulness, and insomnia on the days the mother took aminophylline. Four other asthmatic mothers receiving theophylline did not observe any irritability in their nursing children. Caution should be exercised when theophylline is administered to a nursing woman.

Pediatric Use: Safety and effectiveness of THEOVENT Long-Acting Capsules in children below the age of 6 years have not been established.

Adverse Reactions: Most adverse reactions are usually due to overdose and include:

Gastrointestinal: hematemesis, nausea, epigastric pain, vomiting, diarrhea.

Central Nervous System: clonic and tonic generalized convulsions, muscle twitching, headaches, irritability, restlessness, insomnia, reflex hyperexcitability.

Cardiovascular: life-threatening ventricular arrhythmias, circulatory failure, extrasystoles, hypotension, tachycardia, palpitations, flushing.

Respiratory: tachypnea.

Renal: albuminuria, increased excretion of renal tubular cells and red blood cells; potentiation of diuresis.

Others: hyperglycemia and inappropriate anti-diuretic hormone syndrome. Methylxanthines may cause persistence of benign breast tumors.

Overdosage: ALTHOUGH EARLY EVIDENCE OF THEOPHYLLINE TOXICITY, SUCH AS NAUSEA AND RESTLESSNESS, IS OFTEN SEEN, IN SOME CASES MORE SERIOUS SIGNS, SUCH AS VENTRICULAR ARRHYTHMIAS OR CONVULSIONS, MAY BE THE FIRST MANIFESTATIONS OF TOXICITY.

Management: Emergency treatment should be started immediately.

A. If overdose is established and seizure has not occurred:
   1. Induce vomiting, even if emesis has occurred spontaneously; the administration of ipecac syrup is the preferred method. Emesis should not be induced in patients with impaired consciousness. The action of ipecac is facilitated by physical activity and the administration of 8 to 12 ounces of water. If emesis does not occur within 15 minutes, the dose of ipecac should be repeated. Precautions against aspiration must be taken, especially in infants and children. If vomiting is unsuccessful or contraindicated, gastric lavage should be performed.
   2. Administer a cathartic (this is particularly important if a sustained-release preparation has been taken).
   3. Administer activated charcoal.

B. If the patient is having a seizure:
   1. Establish an airway.
   2. Administer oxygen.
   3. Treat the seizure with intravenous diazepam 0.1 to 0.3 mg/kg up to 10 mg.
   4. Monitor vital signs, maintain blood pressure, and provide adequate hydration.

C. Post-Seizure Coma:
   1. Maintain airway and oxygenation.
   2. Follow above recommendations to prevent absorption of drug, but perform intubation and lavage instead of inducing emesis. Introduce the cathartic and charcoal via a large bore gastric lavage tube.
   3. Continue to provide full supportive care and adequate hydration while waiting for the drug to be metabolized, which generally occurs rapidly enough that dialysis is not necessary.

D. General:
   Treatment is symptomatic and supportive. *Stimulants (analeptic agents) should not be used.* If atrial arrhythmia occurs during treatment with theophylline, lidocaine should be administered with caution, since both drugs may produce accelerated atrioventricular conduction.

Intravenous fluids may be required to overcome dehydration, acid-base imbalance, and hypotension; the latter may also be treated with vasopressors. Apnea will require ventilatory support. Hyperpyrexia, especially in children, may be treated with tepid water sponge baths or a hypothermic blanket. Theophylline serum levels should be monitored until they fall below 20 mcg/ml. After emergency treatment, medical monitoring should be continued.

Theophylline is dialyzable; peritoneal and hemodialyses are effective means of removing theophylline and may be useful adjuncts in the management of overdosage. In one case of massive overdose, charcoal hemoperfusion over a 6-hour period rapidly removed theophylline from the serum with notable clinical improvement. Charcoal hemoperfusion should be considered in patients with severe theophylline intoxication as a possible means of preventing irreversible central nervous system damage.

Animal studies suggest that phenobarbital may decrease theophylline toxicity, but at present there are insufficient data to recommend it as a treatment for theophylline overdosage. Following the unsuccessful trial of the other preferable modalities of theophylline overdosage treatment mentioned above, phenobarbital should only be considered for trial in those patients who are awake.

The oral LD_{50} of theophylline is 100 mg/kg in cats and 300 to 400 mg/kg in rabbits.

Dosage and Administration: The usual initial dosage is: For adults 17 years and older—one or two 250 mg capsules every 12 hours.

For adolescents, 13 through 16 years—one 250 mg capsule every 12 hours.

For children, 9 through 12 years—one or two 125 mg capsules every 12 hours.

For children, 6 through 8 years—one 125 mg capsule every 12 hours.

Patients currently maintained on non-sustained release theophylline or aminophylline products: The total daily dose of a non-sustained release product may be replaced by administering one-half (½) of the equivalent amount of anhydrous theophylline given as THEOVENT Long-Acting Capsules, every 12 hours.

DOSAGE MUST BE ADJUSTED ACCORDING TO THE NEEDS AND RESPONSE OF THE PATIENT. In order to achieve optimal therapeutic dosage, especially if doses higher than those recommended above are required, monitoring of serum theophylline concentrations is recommended. (See PRECAUTIONS, *Laboratory Tests.*)

Dosage should be calculated on the basis of lean (ideal) body weight. Theophylline does not distribute into fatty tissue.

Giving theophylline with food may prevent stomach irritation; although absorption may be slower, it is still complete. If the desired response is not achieved with the recommended usual initial dosage and there are no adverse reactions, the dose may be increased by 2 to 3 mg/kg body weight per day at 3-day intervals, until the following MAXIMUM DOSE WITHOUT MEASUREMENT OF SERUM CONCENTRATION is attained, or until a maximum of 1000 mg is taken in any 24-hour period, whichever occurs first.

MAXIMUM DOSE WITHOUT MEASUREMENT OF SERUM CONCENTRATION

Age	Daily Dose* (mg/kg of body weight)	Dose per 12-hour Interval (mg/kg of body weight)
Adults	13	6.5
Adolescents 13–16 years	18	9
Children 9–12 years	20	10
Children 6–8 years	24	12†

* Use ideal body weight for obese patients
†Some children under 9 years may require 8 mpk q8h

How Supplied: THEOVENT Long-Acting Capsules, 125 mg, dark green and yellow capsules, branded in blue with the Schering trademark and product identification numbers, 402; bottle of 100 and 500.

THEOVENT Long-Acting Capsules, 250 mg, dark green and clear capsules, branded in blue with the Schering trademark and product identification numbers, 753; bottles of 100 and 500.

Store between 2° and 30°C (36° and 86°F).

Revised 11/80

Copyright © 1979, 1980, Schering Corporation. All rights reserved.

[*Shown in Product Identification Section*]

TRILAFON® ℞

brand of perphenazine, USP
Tablets
REPETABS® Tablets
Concentrate
Injection

Description: TRILAFON products contain perphenazine, USP (4-[3-(2-chlorophenothiazin-10-yl)propyl]-1-piperazineethanol), a piperazinyl phenothiazine having the chemical formula, $C_{21}H_{26}ClN_3OS$. It is available as **Tablets,** 2, 4, 8 and 16 mg.; REPETABS (brand of repeat-action tablets) **Tablets,** 4 mg. in an outer layer for immediate effect and 4 mg. in an inner core for release three to six hours later; **Concentrate,** 16 mg. perphenazine per 5 ml. and alcohol less than 0.1%; and **Injection,** perphenazine 5 mg., disodium citrate 24.6 mg., sodium bisulfite 2 mg., and Water for Injection, USP, per 1 ml.

Actions: Perphenazine has actions at all levels of the central nervous system, particularly the hypothalamus. However, the site and mechanism of action are not known.

Indications: Perphenazine is indicated for use in the management of the manifestations of psychotic disorders; and for the control of severe nausea and vomiting in adults.

TRILAFON has not been shown effective in the management of behavioral complications in patients with mental retardation.

Contraindications: TRILAFON products are contraindicated in comatose or greatly obtunded patients and in patients receiving large doses of central nervous system depressants (barbiturates, alcohol, narcotics, analgesics, or antihistamines); in the presence of existing blood dyscrasias, bone marrow depression, or liver damage; and in patients who have shown hypersensitivity to TRILAFON products, their components, or related compounds.

TRILAFON products are also contraindicated in patients with suspected or established subcortical brain damage, with or without hypothalamic damage, since a hyperthermic reaction with temperatures in excess of 104°F may occur in such patients, sometimes not until 14 to 16 hours after drug administration. Total body ice-packing is recommended for such a reaction; antipyretics may also be useful.

Warnings: If hypotension develops, epinephrine should not be administered since its action is blocked and partially reversed by perphenazine. If a vasopressor is needed, norepinephrine may be used. Severe, acute hypotension has occurred with the use of phenothiazines and is particularly likely to occur in patients with mitral insufficiency or pheochromocytoma. Rebound hypertension may occur in pheochromocytoma patients.

TRILAFON products can lower the convulsive threshold in susceptible individuals; they should be used with caution in alcohol withdrawal and in patients with convulsive disorders. If the patient is being treated with an anticonvulsant agent, increased dosage of that agent may be required when TRILAFON products are used concomitantly.

TRILAFON products should be used with caution in patients with psychic depression.

Perphenazine may impair the mental and/or physical abilities required for the performance of hazardous tasks such as driving a car or operating machinery; therefore, the patient should be warned accordingly.

TRILAFON products are not recommended for children under 12 years of age.

Usage in Pregnancy: Safe use of TRILAFON during pregnancy and lactation has not been established; therefore, in administering the drug to pregnant patients, nursing mothers, or women who may become pregnant, the possible benefits must be weighed against the possible hazards to mother and child.

Precautions: The possibility of suicide in depressed patients remains during treatment and until significant remission occurs. This type of patient should not have access to large quantities of this drug.

As with all phenothiazine compounds, perphenazine should not be used indiscriminately. Caution should be observed in giving it to patients who have previously exhibited severe adverse reactions to other phenothiazines. Some of the untoward actions of perphenazine tend to appear more frequently when high doses are used. However, as with other phenothiazine compounds, patients receiving TRILAFON products in any dosage should be kept under close supervision.

Neuroleptic drugs elevate prolactin levels; the elevation persists during chronic administration Tissue culture experiments indicate that approximately one-third of human breast cancers are prolactin dependent *in vitro*, a factor of potential importance if the prescription of these drugs is contemplated in a patient with a previously detected breast cancer. Although disturbances such as galactorrhea, amenorrhea, gynecomastia, and impotence have been reported the clinical significance of elevated serum prolactin levels is unknown for most patients. An increase in mammary neoplasms has been found in rodents after chronic administration of neuroleptic drugs. Neither clinical studies nor epidemiologic studies conducted to date, however, have shown an association between chronic administration of these drugs and mammary tumorigenesis, the available evidence is considered too limited to be conclusive at this time.

The antiemetic effect of perphenazine may obscure signs of toxicity due to overdosage of other drugs, or render more difficult the diagnosis of disorders such as brain tumors or intestinal obstruction.

A significant, not otherwise explained, rise in body temprature may suggest individual intolerance to perphenazine, in which case it should be discontinued.

Patients on large doses of a phenothiazine drug who are undergoing surgery should be watched carefully for possible hypotensive phenomena. Moreover, reduced amounts of anesthetics or central nervous system depressants may be necessary.

Since phenothiazines and central nervous system depressants (opiates, analgesics, antihistamines, barbiturates) can potentiate each other, less than the usual dosage of the added drug is recommended, and caution is advised, when they are administered concomitantly.

Use with caution in patients who are receiving atropine or related drugs because of additive anticholinergic effects and also in patients who will be exposed to extreme heat or phosphorus insecticides.

The use of alcohol should be avoided, since additive effects and hypotension may occur. Patients should be cautioned that their response to alcohol may be increased while they are being treated with TRILAFON products. The risk of suicide and the danger of overdose may be increased in patients who use alcohol excessively due to its potentiation of the drug's effect.

Blood counts and hepatic and renal functions should be checked periodically. The appearance of signs of blood dyscrasias requires the discontinuance of the drug and institution of appropriate therapy. If abnormalities in hepatic tests occur, phenothiazine treatment should be discontinued. Renal function in patients on long-term therapy should be monitored; if blood urea nitrogen (BUN) becomes abnormal, treatment with the drug should be discontinued.

The use of phenothiazine derivatives in patients with diminished renal function should be undertaken with caution.

Use with caution in patients suffering from respiratory impairment due to acute pulmonary infections, or in chronic respiratory disorders such as severe asthma or emphysema.

In general, phenothiazines, including perphenazine, do not produce psychic dependence. Gastritis, nausea and vomiting, dizziness, and tremulousness have been reported following abrupt cessation of high-dose therapy. Reports suggest that these symptoms can be reduced by continuing concomitant antiparkinson agents for several weeks after the phenothiazine is withdrawn.

The possiblity of liver damage, corneal and lenticular deposits, and irreversible dyskinesias should be kept in mind when patients are on long-term therapy.

Because photosensitivity has been reported, undue exposure to the sun should be avoided during phenothiazine treatment.

Adverse Reactions: Not all of the following adverse reactions have been reported with this specific drug; however, pharmacological similarities among various phenothiazine derivatives require that each be considered. In the case of the piperazine group (of which perphenazine is an example) the extrapyramidal symptoms are more common, and others (e.g., sedative effects, jaundice, and blood dyscrasias) are less frequently seen.

CNS Effects: *Extrapyramidal reactions:* opisthotonus, trismus, torticollis, retrocollis, aching and numbness of the limbs, motor restlessness, oculogyric crisis, hyperreflexia, dystonia, including protrusion, discoloration, aching and rounding of the tongue, tonic spasm of the masticatory muscles, tight feeling in the throat, slurred speech, dysphagia, akathisia, dyskinesia, parkinsonism, and ataxia. Their incidence and severity usually increase with an increase in dosage, but there is considerable individual variation in the tendency to develop such symptoms. Extrapyramidal symptoms can usually be controlled by the concomitant use of effective antiparkinsonian drugs. Such as benztropine mesylate, and/or by reduction in dosage. In some instances, however, these extrapyramidal reactions may persist after discontinuation of treatment with perphenazine.

Persistent tardive dyskinesia: As with all antipsychotic agents, tardive dyskinesia may appear in some patients on long-term therapy or may appear after drug therapy has been discontinued. Although the risk appears to be greater in elderly patients on high-dose therapy, especially females, it may occur in either sex and in children. The symptoms are persistent and in some patients appear to be irreversible. The syndrome is characterized by rhythmical, involuntary movements of the tongue, face, mouth, or jaw (e.g. protrusion of tongue, puffing of cheeks, puckering of mouth, chewing movements). Sometimes these may be accompanied by involuntary movements of the extremities. There is no known effective treatment for tardive dyskinesia; antiparkinsonism agents usually do not alleviate the symptoms of this syndrome. It is suggested that all antipsychotic agents be discontinued if these symptoms appear. Should it be necessary to reinstitute treatment, or increase the dosage of the agent, or switch to a different antipsychotic agent, the syndrome may be masked. It has been reported that fine, vermicular movements of the tongue may be an early sign of the syndrome, and if the medication is stopped at that time the syndrome may not develop.

Other CNS effects include cerebral edema; abnormality of cerebrospinal fluid proteins; convulsive seizures, particularly in patients with EEG abnormalities or a history of such disorders, and headaches.

Drowsiness may occur, particularly during the first or second week, after which it generally disappears. If troublesome, lower the dosage. Hypnotic effects appear to be minimal, especially in patients who are permitted to remain active.

Adverse behavioral effects include paradoxical exacerbation of psychotic symptoms, catatonic-like states, paranoid reactions, lethargy, paradoxical excitement, restlessness, hyperactivity, nocturnal confusion, bizarre dreams, and insomnia.

Hyperreflexia has been reported in the newborn when a phenothiazine was used during pregnancy.

Autonomic Effects: dry mouth or salivation, nausea, vomiting, diarrhea, anorexia, constipation, obstipation, fecal impaction, urinary retention, frequency or incontinence, bladder paralysis, polyuria, nasal congestion, pallor, adynamic ileus, myosis, mydriasis, blurred vision, glaucoma, perspiration, hypertension, hypotension, and change in pulse rate occasionally may occur. Significant autonomic effects have been infrequent in patients receiving less than 24 mg. perphenazine daily.

Adynamic ileus occasionally occurs with phenothiazine therapy and if severe can result in complications and death. It is of particular concern in psychiatric patients, who may fail to seek treatment of this condition.

Allergic Effects: urticaria, erythema, eczema, exfoliative dermatitis, pruritus, photosensitivity, asthma, fever, anaphylactoid reactions, laryngeal edema, and angioneurotic edema; contact dermatitis in nursing personnel administering the drug, and in extremely rare instances, individual idiosyncrasy or hypersensitivity to phenothiazines has resulted in cerebral edema, circulatory collapse, and death.

Endocrine Effects: lactation, galactorrhea, moderate breast enlargement in females and gynecomastia in males on large doses, disturbances in the menstrual cycle, amenorrhea, changes in libido, inhibition of ejaculation, syndrome of inappropriate ADH (antidiuretic hormone) secretion, false positive pregnancy tests, hyperglycemia, hypoglycemia, glycosuria.

Cardiovascular Effects: postural hypotension, tachycardia (especially with sudden marked increase in dosage), bradycardia, cardiac arrest, faintness, and dizziness. Occasionally the hypotensive effect may produce a shock-like condition. ECG changes, nonspecific, (quindine-like effect) usually reversible, have been observed in some patients receiving phenothiazine tranquilizers.

Information on Schering products appearing on these pages is effective as of September 30, 1982.

Continued on next page

Schering—Cont.

Sudden death has occasionally been reported in patients who have received phenothiazines. In some cases the death as apparently due to cardiac arrest; in others, the cause appeared to be asphyxia due to failure of the cough reflex. In some patients, the cause could not be determined nor could it be established that the death was due to the phenothiazine.

Hematological Effects: agranulocytosis, eosinophilia, leukopenia, hemolytic anemia, thrombocytopenic purpura, and pancytopenia. Most cases of agranulocytosis have occurred between the fourth and tenth weeks of therapy. Patients should be watched closely especially during that period for the sudden appearance of sore throat or signs of infection. If white blood cell and differential cell counts show significant cellular depression, discontinue the drug and start appropriate therapy. However, a slightly lowered white count is not in itself an indication to discontinue the drug.

Other Effects: Special considerations in long-term therapy include pigmentation of the skin, occurring chiefly in the exposed areas, occular changes consisting of deposition of fine particulate matter in the cornea and lens, progressing in more severe cases to star-shaped lenticular opacities; epithelial keratopathies; and pigmentary retinopathy. Also noted: peripheral edema, reversed epinephrine effect, increase in PBI not attributable to an increase in thyroxine, parotid swelling (rare), hyperpyrexia, systemic lupus erythematosus-like syndrome, increases in appetite and weight, polyphagia, photophobia, and muscle weakness.

Liver damage (biliary stasis) may occur. Jaundice may occur, usually between the second and fourth weeks of treatment and is regarded as a hypersensitivity reaction. Incidence is low. The clinical picture resembles infectious hepatitis but with laboratory features of obstructive jaundice. It is usually reversible; however, chronic jaundice has been reported.

Side effects with intramuscular TRILAFON **Injection** have been infrequent and transient. Dizziness or significant hypotension after treatment with TRILAFON **Injection** is a rare occurrence.

Dosage and Administration: Dosage must be individualized and adjusted according to the severity of the condition and the response obtained. As with all potent drugs, the best dose is the lowest dose that will produce the desired clinical effect. Since extrapyramidal symptoms increase in frequency and severity with increased dosage, it is important to employ the lowest effective dose. These symptoms have disappeared upon reduction of dosage, withdrawal of the drug or administration of an anti-parkinsonian agent.

Prolonged administration of doses exceeding 24 mg. daily should be reserved for hospitalized patients or patients under continued observation for early detection and management of adverse reactions. An antiparkinsonian agent, such as trihexyphenidyl hydrochloride or benztropine mesylate, is valuable in controlling drug-induced, extrapyramidal symptoms.

TRILAFON **Tablets** and REPETABS **Tablets**

Suggested dosages for **Tablets** and REPETABS **Tablets** for various conditions follow:

Moderately disturbed non-hospitalized psychotic patients:

Tablets 4 to 8 mg. t.i.d., or one or two REPETABS **Tablets** b.i.d., initially; reduce as soon as possible to minimum effective dosage.

Hospitalized psychotic patients: **Tablets** 8 to 16 mg. b.i.d. to q.i.d. or one to four REPETABS **Tablets** b.i.d.; avoid dosages in excess of 64 mg. daily.

Severe nausea and vomiting in adults: **Tablets** 8 to 16 mg. daily in divided doses or one REPETABS **Tablet** b.i.d.; 24 mg. occasionally may be necessary; early dosage reduction is desirable. Two REPETABS **Tablets** may be administered in acute cases.

TRILAFON **INJECTION**—Intramuscular Administration

The injection is used when rapid effect and prompt control of acute or intractable conditions is required or when oral administration is not feasible. TRILAFON **Injection**, administered by deep intramuscular injection, is well tolerated. The injection should be given with the patient seated or recumbent, and the patient should be observed for a short period after administration.

Therapeutic effect is usually evidenced in 10 minutes and is maximal in 1 to 2 hours. The average duration of effective action is 6 hours, occasionally 12 to 24 hours.

Pediatric dosage has not yet been established. Children over 12 years may receive the lowest limit of adult dosage.

The usual initial dose is 5 mg. (1 ml.). This may be repeated every 6 hours. Ordinarily, the total daily dosage should not exceed 15 mg. in ambulatory patients or 30 mg. in hospitalized patients. When required for satisfactory control of symptoms in severe conditions, in initial 10 mg. intramuscular dose may be given. Patients should be placed on oral therapy as soon as practicable. Generally, this may be achieved within 24 hours. In some instances, however, patients have been maintained on injectable therapy for several months. It has been established that TRILAFON **Injection** is more potent than TRILAFON **Tablets.** Therefore, equal or higher dosage should be used when the patient is transferred to oral therapy after receiving the injection.

Psychotic conditions: While 5 mg. of the **Injection** has a definite tranquilizing effect, it may be necessary to use 10 mg. doses to initiate therapy in severely agitated states. Most patients will be controlled and amendable to oral therapy within a maximum of 24 to 48 hours. Acute conditions (hysteria, panic reaction) often respond well to a single dose whereas in chronic conditions, several injections may be required. When transferring patients to oral therapy, it is suggested that increased dosage be employed to maintain adequate clinical control. This should be followed by gradual reduction to the minimal effective maintenance dose.

Severe nausea and vomiting in adults: To obtain rapid control of vomiting, administer 5 mg. (1 ml); in rare instances it may be necessary to increase the dosage to 10 mg., in general, higher dosage should be given only to hospitalized patients.

TRILAFON **Injection**—Intravenous Administration

The intravenous administration of TRILAFON **Injection** is seldom required. This route of administration should be used with particular caution and care and only when absolutely necessary to control severe vomiting, intractable hiccoughs, or acute conditions, such as violent retching during surgery. Its use should be limited to recumbent, hospitalized adults in doses not exceeding 5 mg. When employed in this manner, intravenous injection ordinarily should be given as a diluted solution by either fractional injection or a slow drip infusion. In the surgical patient, slow infusion of no more than 5 mg. is preferred. When administered in divided doses, TRILAFON **Injection** should be diluted to 0.5 mg/ml (1 ml mixed with 9 ml. of psysiologic saline solution), and not more than 1 mg. per injection given at not less than one-to two-minute intervals. Intravenous injection should be discontinued as soon as symptoms are controlled and should not exceed 5 mg. The possibility of hypotensive and extrapyramidal side effects should be considered and appropriate means for management kept available. Blood pressure and pulse should be monitored continuously during intravenous administration. Pharmacologic and clinical studies indicate that intravenous administration of norepinephrine should be useful in alleviating the hypotensive effect.

TRILAFON **Concentrate**

In hospitalized psychotic patients, the usual dosage range is 8 to 16 mg. b.i.d. to q.i.d., depending on the severity of symptoms and individual response. Although a number of investigators have employed higher dosage, a total daily dose of more than 64 mg. ordinarily is not required. The **Concentrate** should be diluted only with water, saline, Seven-Up, homogenized milk, carbonated orange drink and pineapple, apricot, prune, orange. V-8, tomato, and grapefruit juices. Trilafon Concentrate should not be mixed with beverages containing caffeine (coffee, cola) tannics (tea), or pectinates (apple juice) since physical incompatibility may result. Suggested dilution is approximately two fluid ounces of diluent for each 5 ml. (16 mg.) teaspoonful of TRILAFON **Concentrate.** For convenience in measuring smaller doses, a graduated dropper marked to measure 8 mg. or 4 mg. is supplied with each bottle.

Overdosage: In the event of overdosage, emergency treatment should be started immediately. All patients suspected of having taken an overdose should be hospitalized as soon as possible.

Manifestations: Overdosage of perphenazine primarily involves the extrapyramidal mechanism and produces the same side effects described under ADVERSE REACTIONS, but to a more marked degree. It is usually evidenced by stupor or coma; children may have convulsive seizures.

Treatment: Treatment is symptomatic and supportive. There is no specific antidote. The patient should be induced to vomit even if emesis has occurred spontaneously. Pharmacologic vomiting by the administration of ipecac syrup is a preferred method. It should be noted that ipecac has a central mode of action in addition to its local gastric irritant properties, and the central mode of action may be blocked by the antiemetic effect of TRILAFON products. Vomiting should not be induced in patients with impaired consciousness. The action of ipecac is facilitated by physical activity and by the administration of 8 to 12 fluid ounces of water. If emesis does not occur within 15 minutes, the dose of ipecac should be repeated. Precautions against aspiration must be taken, especially in infants and children. Following emesis, any drug remaining in the stomach may be adsorbed by activated charcoal administered as a slurry with water. If vomiting is unsuccessful or contraindicated, gastric lavage should be performed. Isotonic and one-half isotonic saline are the lavage solutions of choice. Saline cathartics, such as milk of magnesia, draw water into the bowel by osmosis and therefore may be valuable for their action in rapid dilution of bowel content.

Standard measures (oxygen, intravenous fluids, corticosteroids) should be used to manage circulatory shock or metabolic acidosis. An open airway and adequate fluid intake should be maintained. Body temperature should be regulated. Hypothermia is expected, but severe hyperthermia may occur and must be treated vigorously. (See CONTRAINDICATIONS.)

An electrocardiogram should be taken and close monitoring of cardiac function instituted if there is any sign of abnormality. Cardiac arrhythmias may be treated with neostigmine, pyridostigmine, or propranolol. Digitalis should be considered for cadiac failure. Close monitoring of cardiac function is advisable for not less than five days. Vasopressors such as norepinephrine may be used to treat hypotension, but epinephrine should NOT be used.

Anticonvulsants (an inhalation anesthetic, diazepam, or paraldehyde) are recommended for control of convulsions, since perphenazine increases the central nervous system depressant action, but not the anticonvulsant action, of barbiturates.

If acute parkinson-like symptoms result from perphenazine intoxication, benztropine mesylate or diphenydramine may be administered.

Central nervous system depression may be treated with non-convulsant doses of CNS stimulants. Avoid stimulants that may cause convulsions (e.g., picrotoxin and pentylenetetrazol).

Signs of arousal may not occur for 48 hours.

Dialysis is of no value because of low plasma concentrations of the drug.

Since overdosage is often deliberate, patients may attempt suicide by other means during the recovery phase. Deaths by deliberate or accidental overdosage have occurred with this class of drugs.

How Supplied: TRILAFON **Tablets** (2 mg.): gray, sugar-coated tablets branded in black with the Schering trademark and either product identification letters, ADH, or numbers 705; bottles of 100 and 500.

TRILAFON **Tablets** (4 mg.): gray, sugar-coated tablets branded in green with the Schering trademark and either product identification letters, ADK, or numbers, 940; bottles of 100 and 500.

TRILAFON **Tablets** (8 mg.): gray, sugar-coated tablets branded in blue with the Schering trademark and either product identification letters, ADJ, or numbers 313; bottles of 100 and 500.

TRILAFON **Tablets** (16 mg.): gray, sugar-coated tablets branded in red with the Schering trademark and either product identification letters, ADM, or numbers, 077; bottles of 100 and 500.

TRILAFON REPETABS **Tablets** (8 mg.): white, sugar-coated tablets branded in gray with the Schering trademark and either product identification letters, ADX, or numbers, 141; bottle of 100.

TRILAFON **Concentrate,** 16 mg. per 5 ml., 4 fluid ounce (118 ml.) bottle with graduated dropper. The **Concentrate** is light-sensitive and should be dispensed in amber bottles. **Protect from light. Store in carton until contents are used. Shake well.**

TRILAFON **Injection,** 5 mg. per ml., 1-ml. ampul for intramuscular or intravenous use, box of 100. Keep package closed to protect from light. Exposure may cause discoloration. Slight yellowish discoloration will not alter potency or therapeutic efficacy; if markedly discolored, ampul should be discarded. **Protect from light. Store in carton until contents are used.**

Store all TRILAFON Tablets and TRILAFON Concentrate between 2° and 30°C (36° and 86°F).

Copyright©1969, 1980, Schering Corporation. All rights reserved.

[*Shown in Product Identification Section*]

TRINALIN™ ℞

brand of azatadine maleate and pseudoephedrine sulfate, USP

Long-Acting Antihistamine/Decongestant REPETABS® Tablets

Description: TRINALIN Long-Acting Antihistamine/Decongestant REPETABS (brand of repeat-action tablets) Tablets contain 1 mg azatadine maleate in the tablet coating and 120 mg pseudoephedrine sulfate, USP, equally distributed between the tablet coating and the barrier-coated core. Following ingestion, the two active components in the coating are quickly liberated; release of the decongestant in the core is delayed for several hours.

Azatadine maleate is an antihistamine having the empirical formula, $C_{20}H_{22}N_2 \cdot 2C_4H_4O_4$, the chemical name, 6,11-Dihydro-11-(1-methyl-4-piperidylidene)-5*H*-benzo[5,6]cyclohepta[1,2-*b*]pyridine maleate (1:2).

The molecular weight of azatadine maleate is 522.54. Azatadine maleate is a white to off-white powder and is very soluble in water and soluble in alcohol.

Pseudoephedrine sulfate, a sympathomimetic amine, is a salt of pseudoephedrine, one of the naturally occurring alkaloids obtained from various species of the plant *Ephedra.* The empirical formula for pseudoephedrine sulfate is $(C_{10}H_{15}NO)_2 \cdot H_2SO_4$; the chemical name is Benzenemethanol, α-[1-(methylamino)ethyl]-, [*S*-(*R**, *R**)]-, sulfate (2:1) (salt).

The molecular weight of pseudoephedrine sulfate is 428.56. It is a white to off-white crystal or powder, very soluble in water, freely soluble in alcohol, and sparingly soluble in chloroform.

Clinical Pharmacology: Azatadine maleate is an antihistamine, related to cyproheptadine, with antiserotonin, anticholinergic (drying), and sedative effects. Antihistamines appear to compete with histamine for histamine H_1-receptor sites on effector cells. The antihistamines antagonize those pharmacological effects of histamine which are mediated through activation of H_1-receptor sites and thereby reduce the intensity of allergic reactions and tissue injury response involving histamine release. Antihistamines antagonize the vasodilator effect of endogenously released histamine, especially in small vessels, and mitigate the effect of histamine which results in increased capillary permeability and edema formation. As consequences of these actions, antihistamines antagonize the physiological manifestations of histamine release in the nose following antigen-antibody interaction, such as congestion related to vascular engorgement, mucosal edema, and profuse, watery secretion, and irritation and sneezing resulting from histamine action on afferent nerve terminals.

Pseudoephedrine sulfate (d-isoephedrine sulfate) is an orally effective nasal decongestant which appears to exert its sympathomimetic effect indirectly, predominantly through release of adrenergic mediators from post-ganglionic nerve terminals. In effective recommended oral dosage, pseudoephedrine sulfate produces minimal other sympathomimetic effects, such as pressor activity and CNS stimulation. Use of an orally administered vasoconstrictor for shrinkage of congested nasal mucosa has several advantages: a) it produces a gradual but sustained decongestant effect, causing little, if any "rebound" congestion; b) it facilitates shrinkage of swollen mucosa in upper respiratory areas that are relatively inaccessible to topically applied sprays or drops; c) it relieves nasal obstruction without the additional irritation that may result from local medication.

Pseudoephedrine passes through the blood-brain and placental barriers. While the antihistamines have not been studied systematically for passage through these barriers, the occurrence of pharmacologic effects in the central nervous system and in newborns indicate presence of the drug.

Following administration of the two drugs to normal volunteers in either a single TRINALIN REPETABS Tablet or similar doses in two conventional pseudoephedrine sulfate tablets and a conventional tablet of azatadine maleate, the blood levels of pseudoephedrine and the urinary excretion of azatadine showed that the TRINALIN REPETABS Tablets are bioequivalent to the conventional dosage forms. The apparent elimination half-life of pseudoephedrine in TRINALIN REPETABS Tablets was approximately 6½ hours. The apparent elimination of half-life of azatadine maleate (available from the outer layer of the TRINALIN REPETABS Tablets or from the conventional azatadine maleate tablet) was approximately 12 hours.

Indications and Usage: TRINALIN Long-Acting Antihistamine/Decongestant REPETABS Tablets are indicated for the relief of the symptoms of upper respiratory mucosal congestion in perennial and allergic rhinitis, and for the relief of nasal congestion and eustachian tube congestion. Analgesics, antibiotics, or both may be administered concurrently, when indicated.

Contraindications: Antihistamines should not be used to treat lower respiratory tract symptoms, including asthma.

This product is contraindicated in patients with narrow-angle glaucoma or urinary retention, and in patients receiving monoamine oxidase (MAO) inhibitor therapy or within ten days of stopping such treatment. (See Drug Interactions section.) It is also contraindicated in patients with severe hypertension, severe coronary artery disease, hyperthyroidism, and in those who have shown hypersensitivity or idiosyncrasy to its components, to adrenergic agents, or to other drugs of similar chemical structures. Manifestations of patient idiosyncrasy to adrenergic agents include: insomnia, dizziness, weakness, tremor, or arrhythmias.

Warnings: TRINALIN REPETABS Tablets should be used with considerable caution in patients with: stenosing peptic ulcer, pyloroduodenal obstruction, urinary bladder obstruction due to symptomatic prostatic hypertrophy, or narrowing of the bladder neck. It should also be administered with caution to patients with cardiovascular disease, including hypertension or ischemic heart disease; increased intraocular pressure (See CONTRAINDICATIONS); diabetes mellitus, or in patients receiving digitalis or oral anticoagulants.

Central nervous system stimulation and convulsions or cardiovascular collapse with accompanying hypotension may be produced by sympathomimetics.

Do not exceed recommended dosage.

Use in Activities Requiring Mental Alertness: Patients should be warned about engaging in activities requiring mental alertness, such as driving a car or operating appliances, machinery, etc.

Use in Patients Approximately 60 Years and Older: Antihistamines are more likely to cause dizziness, sedation, and hypotension in patients over 60 years of age. In these patients, sympathomimetics are also more likely to cause adverse reactions, such as confusion, hallucinations, convulsions, CNS depression, and death. For this reason, before considering the use of a repeat-action formulation, the safe use of a short-acting sympathomimetic in that particular patient should be demonstrated.

Precautions: General: Because of the atropine-like action of antihistamines, this product should be used with caution in patients with a history of bronchial asthma.

Information for Patients:

1. Products containing antihistamines may cause drowsiness.
2. Patients should not engage in activities requiring mental alertness, such as driving or operating machinery or appliances.
3. Alcohol or other sedative drugs may enhance the drowsiness caused by antihistamines.
4. Patients should not take TRINALIN REPETABS Tablets if they are receiving a monoamine oxidase inhibitor or within 10 days of stopping such treatment, or if they are receiving oral anticoagulants.
5. This medication should not be given to children less than 12 years of age.

Drug Interactions: MAO inhibitors prolong and intensify the effects of antihistamines. Concomitant use of antihistamines with alcohol, tricyclic antidepressants, barbiturates, or other central nervous system depressants may have an additive effect. The action of oral anti-

Continued on next page

Information on Schering products appearing on these pages is effective as of September 30, 1982.

Schering—Cont.

coagulants may be inhibited by antihistamines.
When sympathomimetic drugs are given to patients receiving monoamine oxidase inhibitors, hypertensive reactions, including hypertensive crises, may occur. The antihypertensive effects of methyldopa, mecamylamine, reserpine, and veratrum alkaloids may be reduced by sympathomimetics. Beta-adrenergic blocking agents may also interact with sympathomimetics. Increased ectopic pacemaker activity can occur when pseudoephedrine is used concomitantly with digitalis. Antacids increase the rate of absorption of pseudoephedrine, while kaolin decreases it.
Drug/Laboratory Test Interactions: The *in vitro* addition of pseudoephedrine to sera containing the cardiac isoenzyme MB of serum creatine phosphokinase progressively inhibits the activity of the enzyme. The inhibition becomes complete over six hours.
Carcinogenesis, Mutagenesis, and Impairment of Fertility: There is no animal or laboratory study of the mixture of azatadine maleate and pseudoephedrine sulfate to evaluate carcinogenesis or mutagenesis. Reproduction studies of this mixture in rats showed no evidence of impaired fertility.
Pregnancy Category C: Retarded fetal development and the presence of angulated hyoid wings were seen in the offspring of pregnant rabbits administered TRINALIN at about 12.5 times and 5 times the recommended human dosage, respectively; increased resorption was noted at about 25 times the human dosage. A decreased survival rate at day 21 was seen in rat pups born of mothers given TRINALIN during pregnancy at a dose about 12.5 times the human dosage. There are no adequate and well-controlled studies in pregnant women. TRINALIN REPETABS Tablets should be used during pregnancy only if the potential benefits to the mother justify the potential risks to the infant. (See Nonteratogenic Effects.)
Nonteratogenic Effects: Antihistamines should not be used in the third trimester of pregnancy, because newborns and premature infants may have severe reactions to them such as convulsions.
Nursing Mothers: It is not known whether these drugs are excreted in human milk. However, certain antihistamines and sympathomimetics are known to be excreted in human milk. Because of the higher risks of antihistamines for infants generally and for newborns and prematures in particular, a decision should be made whether to discontinue nursing or to discontinue the drug, taking into account the importance of the drug to the mother.
There is a report of irritability, excessive crying and disturbed sleeping patterns in a nursing infant whose mother had taken a product containing an antihistamine and pseudoephedrine.
Pediatric use: Safety and effectiveness in children below the age of 12 years have not been established.
Adverse Reactions: The following adverse reactions are associated with antihistamine and sympathomimetic drugs. (Those adverse reactions which occur most frequently with the antihistamines are underlined.)
General: Urticaria, drug rash, anaphylactic shock, photosensitivity, excessive perspiration, chills, dryness of mouth, nose, and throat.
Cardiovascular: Hypertension (see CONTRAINDICATIONS and WARNINGS), hypotension, arrhythmias and cardiovascular collapse, headache, palpitations, extrasystoles, tachycardia, angina.
Hematologic: Hemolytic anemia, hypoplastic anemia, thrombocytopenia, agranulocytosis.
Central Nervous System: Sedation, sleepiness, dizziness, vertigo, tinnitus, acute labyrinthitis, disturbed coordination, fatigue, mydriasis, confusion, restlessness, excitation, nervousness, tension, tremor, irritability, insomnia, euphoria, paresthesias, blurred vision, hysteria, neuritis, convulsions, fear, anxiety, hallucinations, CNS depression, weakness, pallor.
Gastrointestinal: Epigastric distress, anorexia, nausea, vomiting, diarrhea, constipation, abdominal cramps.
Genitourinary: Urinary frequency, urinary retention, dysuria, early menses.
Respiratory: Thickening of bronchial secretions, tightness of chest and wheezing, nasal stuffiness, respiratory difficulty.
Drug Abuse and Dependence: There is no information to indicate that abuse or dependency occurs with azatadine maleate.
Pseudoephedrine, like other central nervous system stimulants, has been abused. At high doses, subjects commonly experience an elevation of mood, a sense of increased energy and alertness, and decreased appetite. Some individuals become anxious, irritable, and loquacious. In addition to the marked euphoria, the user experiences a sense of markedly enhanced physical strength and mental capacity. With continued use, tolerance develops, the user increases the dose, and toxic signs and symptoms appear. Depression may follow rapid withdrawal.
Overdosage: In the event of overdosage, emergency treatment should be started immediately.
Manifestations of overdosage may vary from central nervous system depression (sedation, apnea, diminished mental alertness, cyanosis, coma, cardiovascular collapse) to stimulation (insomnia, hallucinations, tremors, or convulsions) to death. Other signs and symptoms may be euphoria, excitement, tachycardia, palpitations, thirst, perspiration, nausea, dizziness, tinnitus, ataxia, blurred vision, and hypertension or hypotension. Stimulation is particularly likely in children, as are atropine-like signs and symptoms (dry mouth; fixed, dilated pupils, flushing; hyperthermia; and gastrointestinal symptoms).
In large doses sympathomimetics may give rise to giddiness, headache, nausea, vomiting, sweating, thirst, tachycardia, precordial pain, palpitations, difficulty in micturition, muscular weakness and tenseness, anxiety, restlessness, and insomnia. Many patients can present a toxic psychosis with delusions and hallucinations. Some may develop cardiac arrhythmias, circulatory collapse, convulsions, coma, and respiratory failure.
The oral LD_{50} of the mixture of the two drugs in mature rats and mice was greater than 1700 mg/kg and 600 mg/kg, respectively.
Treatment—The patient should be induced to vomit, even if emesis has occurred spontaneously. Pharmacologically induced vomiting by the administration of ipecac syrup is a preferred method. However, vomiting should not be induced in patients with impaired consciousness. The action of ipecac is facilitated by physical activity and by the administration of eight to twelve fluid ounces of water. If emesis does not occur within fifteen minutes, the dose of ipecac should be repeated. Precautions against aspiration must be taken, especially in infants and children. Following emesis, any drug remaining in the stomach may be adsorbed by activated charcoal administered as a slurry with water. If vomiting is unsuccessful or contraindicated, gastric lavage should be performed. Isotonic and one-half isotonic saline are the lavage solutions of choice. Saline cathartics, such as milk of magnesia, draw water into the bowel by osmosis and therefore may be valuable for their action in rapid dilution of bowel content. Dialysis is of little value in antihistamine poisoning. After emergency treatment the patient should continue to be medically monitored.
Treatment of the signs and symptoms of overdosage is symptomatic and supportive. Stimulants (analeptic agents) should not be used. Vasopressors may be used to treat hypotension. Short-acting barbiturates, diazepam, or paraldehyde may be administered to control seizures. Hyperpyrexia, especially in children, may require treatment with tepid water sponge baths or a hypothermic blanket. Apnea is treated with ventilatory support.
Dosage and Administration: TRINALIN REPETABS Tablets ARE NOT INTENDED FOR USE IN CHILDREN UNDER 12 YEARS OF AGE. The usual adult dosage is one tablet twice a day.
How Supplied: TRINALIN REPETABS Tablets contain 1 mg azatadine maleate and 120 mg pseudoephedrine sulfate. TRINALIN REPETABS Tablets are coral-colored, sugar-coated tablets branded in black with the Schering trademark, or the product name and product identification numbers, 703; bottle of 100 (NDC-0085-0703-04).
Store between 2° and 30°C (36° and 86°F).
Copyright © 1981, Schering Corporation. All rights reserved.
Revised 11/81
[*Shown in Product Identification Section*]

VALISONE® ℞

brand of betamethasone valerate, USP
Cream 0.1%
Lotion 0.1%
Ointment 0.1%
Reduced Strength Cream 0.01%
For Dermatologic Use Only–Not for Ophthalmic Use

Description: VALISONE contains betamethasone valerate, USP (9-Fluoro-11β,17,21-trihydroxy-16β-methylpregna-1,4-diene-3,20-dione 17-valerate).
Each gram of VALISONE **Cream** 0.1% contains 1.2 mg. betamethasone valerate, (equivalent to 1.0 mg. betamethasone) in a soft, white, hydrophilic cream of water, mineral oil, petrolatum, polyethylene glycol 1000 monocetyl ether, cetearyl alcohol, monobasic sodium phosphate, and phosphoric acid; chlorocresol and propylene glycol as preservatives.
VALISONE **Lotion** 0.1% contains in each gram betamethasone valerate, equivalent to 1.0 mg. betamethasone in a vehicle consisting of isopropyl alcohol (47.5%) and water slightly thickened with carboxy vinyl polymer; the pH is adjusted to approximately 4.7 with sodium hydroxide.
Each gram of VALISONE **Ointment** 0.1% contains 1.2 mg. betamethasone valerate (equivalent to 1.0 mg. betamethasone) in an ointment base of liquid and white petrolatum, and hydrogenated lanolin.
Each gram of VALISONE **Reduced Strength Cream** 0.01% contains 0.12 mg betamethasone valerate, (equivalent to 0.1 mg betamethasone) in a hydrophilic, emollient cream consisting of purified water, mineral oil, white petrolatum, polyethylene glycol 1000 monocetyl ether, cetearyl alcohol, monobasic sodium phosphate, and phosphoric acid; chlorocresol and propylene glycol as preservatives.
Actions: VALISONE **Cream, Reduced Strength Cream, Lotion** and **Ointment** are primarily effective because of their anti-inflammatory, antipruritic, and vasoconstrictive actions.
Indications: VALISONE **Cream, Reduced Strength Cream, Lotion** and **Ointment** are indicated for the relief of the inflammatory manifestations of corticosteroid-responsive dermatoses.
Contraindications: VALISONE **Cream, Reduced Strength Cream, Lotion** and **Ointment** are contraindicated in those patients with a history of hypersensitivity to any of the components of the preparations.

Precautions: If irritation develops with the use of VALISONE **Cream, Reduced Strength Cream, Lotion** or **Ointment,** treatment should be discontinued and appropriate therapy instituted.

In the presence of an infection, the use of an appropriate antifungal or antibacterial agent should be instituted. If a favorable response does not occur promptly, the corticosteroid should be discontinued until the infection has been adequately controlled.

It should be recognized that any of the side effects reported following systemic use of corticosteroids, including adrenal suppression, may also occur following their topical use, especially in infants and children. Systemic absorption of topically applied steroids will be increased if extensive body surface areas are treated or if the occlusive technique is used. Therefore, under these circumstances, suitable precautions should be taken when long-term use is anticipated, particularly in infants and children.

Although topical steroids have not been reported to have an adverse effect on human pregnancy, the safety of their use in pregnant women has not been absolutely established. In laboratory animals, increases in incidence of fetal abnormalities have been associated with exposure of gestating females to topical corticosteroids, in some cases at rather low dosage levels. Therefore, drugs of this class should not be used on pregnant patients in large amounts or for prolonged periods of time.

VALISONE **Cream, Reduced Strength Cream, Lotion** and **Ointment** are not for ophthalmic use.

Adverse Reactions: The following local adverse reactions have been reported with topical corticosteroids, especially under occlusive dressings: burning; itching; irritation; dryness; folliculitis; hypertrichosis; acneiform eruptions; hypopigmentation; perioral dermatitis; allergic contact dermatitis; maceration of the skin; secondary infection; skin atrophy; striae; miliaria.

Dosage and Administration:

VALISONE **Cream**

Apply a thin film of VALISONE **Cream** to the affected skin areas one to three times a day. Clinical Studies of VALISONE have indicated that dosage only once or twice a day is often feasible and effective.

VALISONE **Reduced Strength Cream**

Apply a thin film of VALISONE **Reduced Strength Cream** to the affected skin areas one to three times a day. Commonly, treatment twice a day is adequate. In some cases, treatment three times a day is necessary; in others, once a day suffices.

VALISONE **Reduced Strength Cream** 0.01% has an aqueous, hydrophilic base that softens and moisturizes the skin. Although occlusive dressings are required infrequently, they may enhance therapeutic efficacy in certain refractory lesions of psoriasis and other dermatoses that are difficult to treat.

VALISONE **Lotion**

Apply a few drops of VALISONE **Lotion** to the affected area and massage lightly until it disappears. Apply twice daily, in the morning and at night. Dosage may be increased in stubborn cases. Following improvement, apply once daily.

For the most effective and economical use, apply nozzle to affected area and gently squeeze bottle.

VALISONE **Ointment**

Apply a thin film of VALISONE **Ointment** to the affected skin areas one to three times a day.

Clinical studies of VALISONE have indicated that dosage only once or twice a day is often feasible and effective.

How Supplied: VALISONE **Cream** 0.1% is supplied in 5-, 15-, and 45-gram tubes; boxes of one.

VALISONE **Reduced Strength Cream** 0.01% is supplied in 15- and 60-gram tubes; boxes of one.

VALISONE **Lotion** 0.1% (containing 1.0 mg. betamethasone as the valerate per gram of lotion) is available in 20 ml. and 60 ml. plastic squeeze bottles; boxes of one. **Protect from light. Store in carton until contents are used.**

VALISONE **Ointment** 0.1% is supplied in 5-, 15-, and 45-gram tubes; boxes of one.

Store all VALISONE products between 2° and 30°C (36° and 86°F).

Copyright © 1969, 1978, Schering Corporation. All rights reserved.

VANCENASE™ Nasal Inhaler ℞

brand of beclomethasone dipropionate, USP
For Nasal Inhalation Only

Description: Beclomethasone dipropionate, USP, the active component of VANCENASE Nasal Inhaler, is an anti-inflammatory steroid having the chemical name, 9-Chloro-11β,17,21-trihydroxy-16β-methylpregna-1, 4-diene-3, 20-dione 17,21-dipropionate.

Beclomethasone dipropionate is a white to creamy-white odorless powder with a molecular weight of 521.25. It is very slightly soluble in water; very soluble in chloroform; and freely soluble in acetone and in alcohol.

VANCENASE Nasal Inhaler is a metered-dose aerosol unit containing a microcrystalline suspension of beclomethasone dipropionate-trichloromonofluoromethane clathrate in a mixture of propellants (trichloromonofluoromethane and dichlorodifluoromethane) with oleic acid. Each canister contains beclomethasone dipropionate-trichloromonofluoromethane clathrate having a molecular proportion of beclomethasone dipropionate to trichloromonofluoromethane between 3:1 and 3:2. Each actuation delivers from the nasal adapter a quantity of clathrate equivalent to 42 mcg of beclomethasone dipropionate, USP. The contents of one canister provide at least 200 metered doses.

Clinical Pharmacology: Beclomethasone 17,21-dipropionate is a diester of beclomethasone, a synthetic corticosteroid which is chemically related to dexamethasone. Beclomethasone differs from dexamethasone only in having a chlorine at the 9-α position in place of a fluorine. Animal studies showed that beclomethasone dipropionte has potent glucocorticoid and weak mineralocorticoid activity. The mechanisms for the anti-inflammatory action of beclomethasone dipropionate are unknown. The precise mechanism of the aerosolized drug's action in the nose is also unknown. Biopsies of nasal mucosa obtained during clinical studies showed no histopathologic changes when beclomethasone dipropionate was administered intranasally.

The effects of beclomethasone dipropionate on hypothalamic-pituitary-adrenal (HPA) function have been evaluated in adult volunteers, by other routes of administration. Studies are currently being undertaken with beclomethasone dipropionate by the intranasal route, which may demonstrate that there is more or that there is less absorption by this route of administration. There was no suppression of early morning plasma cortisol concentrations when beclomethasone dipropionate was administered in a dose of 1000 mcg/day for one month as an oral aerosol or for three days by intramuscular injection. However, partial suppression of plasma cortisol concentration was observed when beclomethasone dipropionate was administered in doses of 2000 mcg/day either by oral aerosol or intramuscularly. Immediate suppression of plasma cortisol concentrations was observed after single doses of 4000 mcg of beclomethasone dipropionate. Suppression of HPA function (reduction of early morning plasma cortisol levels) has been reported in adult patients who received 1600 mcg daily doses of oral beclomethasone dipropionate for one month. In clinical studies using beclomethasone dipropionate intranasally, there was no evidence of decreased adrenal insufficiency.

Beclomethasone dipropionate is sparingly soluble. When given by nasal inhalation in the form of an aerosolized suspension, the drug is deposited primarily in the nasal passages. A portion of the drug is swallowed. Absorption occurs rapidly from all respiratory and gastrointestinal tissues. There is no evidence of tissue storage of beclomethasone dipropionate or its metabolites. *In vitro* studies, have shown that tissue other than the liver (lung slices) can rapidly metabolize beclomethasone dipropionate to beclomethasone 17-monopropionate and more slowly to free beclomethasone (which has very weak anti-inflammatory activity). However, irrespective of the route of entry, the principal route of excretion of the drug and its metabolites is the feces. In humans, 12% to 15% of an orally administered dose of beclomethasone dipropionate is excreted in the urine as both conjugated and free metabolites of the drug. The half-life of beclomethasone dipropionate in humans is approximately 15 hours. Studies have shown that the degree of binding to plasma proteins is 87%.

Indications and Usage: VANCENASE Nasal Inhaler is indicated for the relief of the symptoms of seasonal or perennial rhinitis, in those cases poorly responsive to conventional treatment.

Clinical studies have shown that improvement is usually apparent within a few days. However, symptomatic relief may not occur in some patients for as long as two weeks. Although systemic effects are minimal at recommended doses, VANCENASE should not be continued beyond three weeks in the absence of significant symptomatic improvement. VANCENASE should not be used in the presence of untreated localized infection involving the nasal mucosa.

Contraindications: Hypersensitivity to any of the ingredients of this preparation contraindicates its use.

Warnings: The replacement of a systemic corticosteroid with VANCENASE Nasal Inhaler can be accompanied by signs of adrenal insufficiency.

When transferred to VANCENASE Nasal Inhaler, careful attention must be given to patients previously treated for prolonged periods with systemic corticosteroids. This is particularly important in those patients who have associated asthma or other clinical conditions, where too rapid a decrease in systemic corticosteroids may cause a severe exacerbation of their symptoms.

Studies have shown that the combined administration of alternate day prednisone systemic treatment and orally inhaled beclomethasone increased the likelihood of HPA suppression compared to a therapeutic dose of either one alone. Therefore, VANCENASE treatment should be used with caution in patients already on alternate day prednisone regimens for any disease.

Precautions: *General:* During withdrawal from oral steroids, some patients may experience symptoms of withdrawal, e.g., joint and/or muscular pain, lassitude, and depression.

In clinical studies with beclomethasone dipropionate administered intranasally, the development of localized infections of the nose and pharynx with *Candida albicans* has occurred only rarely. When such an infection develops, it may require treatment with appropriate local therapy or discontinuance of treatment with VANCENASE Nasal Inhaler.

Continued on next page

Information on Schering products appearing on these pages is effective as of September 30, 1982.

Schering—Cont.

Beclomethasone dipropionate is absorbed into the circulation. Use of excessive doses of VANCENASE Nasal Inhaler may suppress HPA function.
VANCENASE should be used with caution, if at all, in patients with active or quiescent tuberculous infections of the respiratory tract, or in untreated fungal, bacterial, systemic viral infections, or ocular herpes simplex.
Because of the inhibitory effect of corticosteroids on wound healing, patients who have experienced recent nasal septal ulcers, nasal surgery, or trauma should not use a nasal corticosteroid until healing has occurred.
Although systemic effects have been minimal with recommended doses, this potential increases with excessive doses. Therefore, larger than recommended doses should be avoided.
Information for Patients: Patients should use VANCENASE Nasal Inhaler at regular intervals since its effectiveness depends on its regular use. The patient should take the medication as directed. It is not acutely effective and the prescribed dosage should not be increased. Instead, nasal vasoconstrictors or oral antihistamines may be needed until the effects of VANCENASE Nasal Inhaler are fully manifested. One to two weeks may pass before full relief is obtained. The patient should contact the doctor if symptoms do not improve, or if the condition worsens, or if sneezing or nasal irritation occurs. For the proper use of this unit and to attain maximum improvement, the patient should read and follow the accompanying Patient's Instructions carefully.
Carcinogenesis, Mutagenesis, Impairment of Fertility: Treatment of rats for a total of 95-weeks, 13 weeks by inhalation and 82 weeks by the oral route, resulted in no evidence of carcinogenic activity. Mutagenic studies have not been performed.
Impairment of fertility, as evidenced by inhibition of the estrus cycle in dogs, was observed following treatment by the oral route. No inhibition of the estrus cycle in dogs was seen following treatment with beclomethasone dipropionte by the inhalation route.
Pregnancy Category C: Like other corticoids, parenteral (subcutaneous) beclomethasone dipropionate has been shown to be teratogenic and embryocidal in the mouse and rabbit when given in doses approximately ten times the human dose. In these studies beclomethasone was found to produce fetal resorption, cleft palate, agnathia, microstomia, absence of tongue, delayed ossification, and agenesis of the thymus. No teratogenic or embryocidal effects have been seen in the rat when beclomethasone dipropionate was administered by inhalation at ten times the human dose or orally at 1000 times the human dose. There are no adequate and well-controlled studies in pregnant women. Beclomethasone dipropionate should be used during pregnancy only if the potential benefit justifies the potential risk to the fetus.
Nonteratogenic effects: Hypoadrenalism may occur in infants born of mothers receiving corticosteroids during pregnancy. Such infants should be carefully observed.
Nursing Mothers: It is not known whether beclomethasone dipropionate is excreted in human milk. Because other corticosteroids are excreted in human milk, caution should be exercised when VANCENASE Nasal Inhaler is administered to nursing women.
Pediatric Use: Safety and effectiveness in children below the age of 12 years have not been established.
Adverse Reactions: In general, side effects in clinical studies have been primarily associated with the nasal mucous membranes. Adverse reactions reported in controlled clinical trials and long-term open studies in patients treated with VANCENASE are described below.
Sensations of irritation and burning in the nose (11 per 100 patients) following the use of VANCENASE Nasal Inhaler have been reported. Also, occasional sneezing attacks (10 per 100 patients) have occurred immediately following the use of the intranasal inhaler.
Localized infections of the nose and pharynx with *Candida albicans* have occurred rarely. (see PRECAUTIONS)
Less than 2 per 100 patients reported transient episodes of bloody discharge from the nose.
Ulceration of the nasal mucosa has been reported rarely. Systemic corticosteroid side effects were not reported during the controlled clinical trials. If recommended doses are exceeded, however, or if individuals are particularly sensitive, symptoms of hypercorticism, i.e., Cushing's syndrome could occur.
Dosage and Administration: Adults and Children 12 years of age and over: the usual dosage is one inhalation (42 mcg) in each nostril two to four times a day (total dose 168–336 mcg/day). Patients can often be maintained on a maximum dose of one inhalation in each nostril three times a day (252 mcg/day).
In patients who respond to VANCENASE Nasal Inhaler, an improvement of the symptoms of seasonal or perennial rhinitis usually becomes apparent within one to five days after the start of VANCENASE Inhaler therapy.
The therapeutic effects of corticosteroids, unlike those of decongestants are not immediate. This should be explained to the patient in advance in order to ensure cooperation and continuation of treatment with the prescribed dosage regimen.
VANCENASE Nasal Inhaler is **not** recommended for children below 12 years of age.
In the presence of excessive nasal mucus secretion or edema of the nasal mucosa, the drug may fail to reach the site of intended action. In such cases it is advisable to use a nasal vasoconstrictor during the first two to three days of VANCENASE Nasal Inhaler therapy.
Directions for Use: Illustrated PATIENT INSTRUCTIONS for proper use accompany each package of VANCENASE Nasal Inhaler.
CONTENTS UNDER PRESSURE. Do not puncture. Do not use or store near heat or open flame. Exposure to temperatures above 120°F may cause bursting. Never throw container into fire or incinerator. Keep out of reach of children.
Overdosage: When used at excessive doses, systemic corticosteroid effects such as hypercorticism and adrenal suppression may appear. If such symptoms appear, the dosage should be decreased.
The oral LD_{50} of beclomethasone dipropionate is greater than 1 g/kg in rodents. One canister of VANCENASE Nasal Inhaler contains 8.4 mg of beclomethasone dipropionate, therefore acute overdosage is unlikely.
How Supplied: VANCENASE Nasal Inhaler, 16.8 g canister; box of one. Supplied with nasal adapter and PATIENT'S INSTRUCTIONS; (NDC 0085-0041-06).
Store between 2° and 30°C (36° and 86°F).
Revised 9/81
Copyright ©1981, Schering Corporation. All rights reserved.
[*Shown in Product Identification Section*]

VANCERIL® Inhaler ℞

brand of beclomethasone dipropionate, USP
FOR ORAL INHALATION ONLY

Description: Beclomethasone dipropionate, the active component of VANCERIL Inhaler, is an anti-inflammatory steroid having the chemical name 9-Chloro-11β,17-21-trihydroxy-16 β-methylpregna-1,4-diene-3, 20-dione 17,21-dipropionate.
VANCERIL Inhaler is a metered-dose aerosol unit containing a microcrystalline suspension of beclomethasone dipropionate-trichloromonofluoromethane clathrate in a mixture of propellants (trichloromonofluoromethane and dichlorodifluoromethane) with oleic acid. Each canister contains beclomethasone dipropionate-trichloromonofluoromethane clathrate having a molecular proportion of beclomethasone dipropionate to trichloromonofluoromethane between 3:1 and 3:2. Each actuation delivers from the mouthpiece a quantity of clathrate equivalent to 42 mcg. of beclomethasone dipropionate. The contents of one canister provide at least 200 oral inhalations.
Clinical Pharmacology: Beclomethasone 17,21-dipropionate is a diester of beclomethasone, a synthetic corticosteriod which is chemically related to prednisolone. Beclomethasone differs from prednisolone only in having a chlorine at the 9-alpha and a methyl group at the 16-beta position in place of hydrogen. Animal studies showed that beclomethasone dipropionate has potent anti-inflammatory activity. When administered systemically to mice, the anti-inflammatory activity was accompanied by other typical features of glucocorticoid action including thymic involution, liver glycogen deposition, and pituitary-adrenal suppression. However, after systemic administration to rats, the anti-inflammatory action was associated with little or no effect on other tests of glucocorticoid activity.
Beclomethasone dipropionate is sparingly soluble and is poorly mobilized from subcutaneous or intramuscular injection sites. However, systemic absorption occurs after all routes of administration. When given to animals in the form of an aerosolized suspension of the trichloromonofluoromethane clathrate, the drug is deposited in the mouth and nasal passages, the trachea and principal bronchi, and in the lung; a considerable portion of the drug is also swallowed. Absorption occurs rapidly from all respiratory and gastrointestinal tissues, as indicated by the rapid clearance of radioactively labeled drug from local tissues and appearance of tracer in the circulation. There is no evidence of tissue storage of beclomethasone dipropionate or its metabolites. Lung slices can metabolize beclomethasone dipropionate rapidly to beclomethasone 17-monopropionate and more slowly to free beclomethasone (which has very weak anti-inflammatory activity). However, irrespective of the route of administration (injection, oral, or aerosol), the principal route of excretion of the drug and its metabolites is the feces. Less than 10% of the drug and its metabolites is excreted in the urine. In humans, 12% to 15% of an orally administered dose of beclomethasone dipropionate was excreted in the urine as both conjugated and free metabolites of the drug.
The mechanisms responsible for the anti-inflammatory action of beclomethasone dipropionate are unknown. The precise mechanism of the aerosolized drug's action in the lung is also unknown.
Indications: VANCERIL Inhaler is indicated only for patients who require chronic treatment with corticosteroids for control of the symptoms of bronchial asthma. Such patients would include those already receiving systemic corticosteroids, and selected patients who are inadequately controlled on a non-steroid regimen and in whom steroid therapy has been withheld because of concern over potential adverse effects.
VANCERIL Inhaler is NOT indicated:
1. For relief of asthma which can be controlled by bronchodilators and other non-steroid medications.
2. In patients who require systemic corticosteroid treatment infrequently.
3. In the treatment of non-asthmatic bronchitis.

Contraindications: VANCERIL Inhaler is contraindicated in the primary treatment of status asthmaticus or other acute episodes of asthma where intensive measures are required.

Hypersensitivity to any of the ingredients of this preparation contraindicates its use.

Warnings:

Particular care is needed in patients who are transferred from systemically active corticosteroids to VANCERIL Inhaler because deaths due to adrenal insufficiency have occurred in asthmatic patients during and after transfer from systemic corticosteroids to aerosol beclomethasone dipropionate. After withdrawal from systemic corticosteroids, a number of months are required for recovery of hypothalamic-pituitary-adrenal (HPA) function. During this period of HPA suppression, patients may exhibit signs and symptoms of adrenal insufficiency when exposed to trauma, surgery or infections, particularly gastroenteritis. Although VANCERIL Inhaler may provide control of asthmatic symptoms during these episodes, it does NOT provide the systemic steroid which is necessary for coping with these emergencies. During periods of stress or a severe asthmatic attack, patients who have been withdrawn from systemic corticosteroids should be instructed to resume systemic steroids (in large doses) immediately and to contact their physician for further instruction. These patients should also be instructed to carry a warning card indicating that they may need supplementary systemic steroids during periods of stress or a severe asthma attack. To assess the risk of adrenal insuffficiency in emergency situations, routine tests of adrenal cortical function, including measurement of early morning resting cortisol levels, should be performed periodically in all patients. An early morning resting cortisol level may be accepted as normal only if it falls at or near the normal mean level.

Localized infections with *Candida albicans* or *Aspergillus niger* have occurred frequently in the mouth and pharynx and occasionally in the larynx. Positive cultures for oral *Candida* may be present in up to 75% of patients. Although the frequency of clinically apparent infection is considerably lower, these infections may require treatment with appropriate antifungal therapy or discontinuance of treatment with VANCERIL Inhaler.

VANCERIL Inhaler is not to be regarded as a bronchodilator and is not indicated for rapid relief of bronchospasm.

Patients should be instructed to contact their physician immediately when episodes of asthma which are not responsive to bronchodilators occur during the course of treatment with VANCERIL. During such episodes, patients may require therapy with systemic corticosteroids.

There is no evidence that control of asthma can be achieved by the administration of VANCERIL in amounts greater than the recommended doses.

Transfer of patients from systemic steroid therapy to VANCERIL Inhaler may unmask allergic conditions previously suppressed by the systemic steroid therapy, e.g., rhinitis, conjunctivitis, and eczema.

Precautions: During withdrawal from oral steroids, some patients may experience symptoms of systemically active steroid withdrawal, e.g., joint and/or muscular pain, lassitude and depression, despite maintenance or even improvement of respiratory function (See DOSAGE AND ADMINISTRATION for details).

In responsive patients, beclomethasone dipropionate may permit control of asthmatic symptoms without suppression of HPA function, as discussed below (See CLINICAL STUDIES). Since beclomethasone dipropionate is absorbed into the circulation and can be systemically active, the beneficial effects of VANCERIL Inhaler in minimizing or preventing HPA dysfunction may be expected only when recommended dosages are not exceeded.

The long-term effects of beclomethasone dipropionate in human subjects are still unknown. In particular, the local effects of the agent on developmental or immunologic processes in the mouth, pharynx, trachea, and lung are unknown. There is also no information about the possible long-term systemic effects of the agent.

The potential effects of VANCERIL on acute, recurrent, or chronic pulmonary infections, including active or quiescent tuberculosis, are not known. Similarly, the potential effects of long-term administration of the drug on lung or other tissues are unknown.

Pulmonary infiltrates with eosinophilia may occur in patients on VANCERIL Inhaler therapy. Although it is possible that in some patients this state may become manifest because of systemic steroid withdrawal when inhalational steroids are administered, a causative role for beclomethasone dipropionate and/or its vehicle cannot be ruled out.

Use in Pregnancy: Glucocorticoids are known teratogens in rodent species and beclomethasone dipropionate is no exception.

Teratology studies were done in rats, mice, and rabbits treated with subcutaneous beclomethasone dipropionate. Beclomethasone dipropionate was found to produce fetal resorptions, cleft palate, agnathia, microstomia, absence of tongue, delayed ossification and partial agenesis of the thymus. Well-controlled trials relating to fetal risk in humans are not available. Glucocorticoids are secreted in human milk. It is not known whether beclomethasone dipropionate would be secreted in human milk but it is safe to assume that it is likely. The use of beclomethasone dipropionate in pregnancy, nursing mothers, or women of childbearing potential requires that the possible benefits of the drug be weighed against the potential hazards to the mother, embryo, or fetus. Infants born of mothers who have received substantial doses of corticosteroids during pregnancy should be carefully observed for hypoadrenalism.

Adverse Reactions: Deaths due to adrenal insufficiency have occurred in asthmatic patients during and after transfer from systemic corticosteroids to aerosol beclomethasone dipropionate (See WARNINGS).

Suppression of HPA function (reduction of early morning plasma cortisol levels) have been reported in adult patients who received 1600 mcg. daily doses of VANCERIL for one month. A few patients on VANCERIL have complained of hoarseness or dry mouth. Bronchospasm and rash have been reported rarely.

Dosage and Administration: Adults: The usual dosage is two inhalations (84 mcg.) given three or four times a day. In patients with severe asthma, it is advisable to start with 12 to 16 inhalations a day and adjust the dosage downward according to the response of the patient. The maximal daily intake should not exceed 20 inhalations, 840 mcg. (0.84 mg.), in adults.

Children 6 to 12 years of age: The usual dosage is one or two inhalations (42 to 84 mcg.) given three or four times a day according to the response of the patient. The maximal daily intake should not exceed ten inhalations, 420 mcg. (0.42 mg.), in children 6 to 12 years of age. Insufficient clinical data exist with respect to the administration of VANCERIL Inhaler in children below the age of 6. Rinsing the mouth after inhalation is advised.

Patients receiving bronchodilators by inhalation should be advised to use the bronchodilator before VANCERIL Inhaler in order to enhance penetration of beclomethasone dipropionate into the bronchial tree. After use of an aerosol bronchodilator, several minutes should elapse before use of the VANCERIL Inhaler to reduce the potential toxicity from the inhaled fluorocarbon propellants in the two aerosols.

Different considerations must be given to the following groups of patients in order to obtain the full therapeutic benefit of VANCERIL Inhaler.

Patients not receiving systemic steroids: The use of VANCERIL Inhaler is straightforward in patients who are inadequately controlled with non-steroid medications but in whom systemic steroid therapy has been withheld because of concern over potential adverse reactions. In patients who respond to VANCERIL, an improvement in pulmonary function is usually apparent within one to four weeks after the start of VANCERIL Inhaler.

Patients receiving systemic steroids: In those patients dependent on systemic steroids, transfer to VANCERIL and subsequent management may be more difficult because recovery from impaired adrenal function is usually slow. Such suppression has been known to last for up to 12 months. Clinical studies, however, have demonstrated that VANCERIL may be effective in the management of these asthmatic patients and may permit replacement or significant reduction in the dosage of systemic corticosteroids.

The patient's asthma should be reasonably stable before treatment with VANCERIL Inhaler is started. Initially, the aerosol should be used concurrently with the patient's usual maintenance dose of systemic steroid. After approximately one week, gradual withdrawal of the systemic steroid is started by reducing the daily or alternate daily dose. The next reduction is made after an interval of one or two weeks, depending on the response of the patient. Generally, these decrements should not exceed 2.5 mg. of prednisone or its equivalent. A slow rate of withdrawal cannot be overemphasized. During withdrawal, some patients may experience symptoms of systemically active steroid withdrawal, e.g., joint and/or muscular pain, lassitude and depression, despite maintenance or even improvement of respiratory function. Such patients should be encouraged to continue with the Inhaler but should be watched carefully for objective signs of adrenal insufficiency, such as hypotension and weight loss. If evidence of adrenal insufficiency occurs, the systemic steroid dose should be boosted temporarily and thereafter further withdrawal should continue more slowly.

During periods of stress or a severe asthma attack, transfer patients will require supplementary treatment with systemic steroids. Exacerbations of asthma which occur during the course of treatment with VANCERIL Inhaler should be treated with a short course of systemic steroid which is gradually tapered as these symptoms subside. There is no evidence that control of asthma can be achieved by administration of VANCERIL in amounts greater than the recommended doses.

Directions for Use: Illustrated patient instructions for proper use accompany each package of VANCERIL Inhaler.

CONTENTS UNDER PRESSURE. Do not puncture. Do not use or store near heat or open flame. Exposure to temperatures above 120°F. may cause bursting. Never throw container into fire or incinerator. Keep out of reach of children.

How Supplied: VANCERIL Inhaler 16.8 g canister supplied with an oral adapter and patient's instructions; box of one. (NDC-0085-0736-04). VANCERIL Inhaler REFILL Canister with Patient's Instructions; box of one. (NDC-0085-0736-01).

Continued on next page

Information on Schering products appearing on these pages is effective as of September 30, 1982.

Schering—Cont.

Store between 2° and 30°C (36° and 86°F).

Animal Pharmacology and Toxicology: Studies in a number of animal species including rats, rabbits, and dogs have shown no unusual toxicity during acute experiments. However, the effects of beclomethasone dipropionate in producing signs of glucocorticoid excess during chronic administration by various routes were dose related.

Clinical Studies: The effects of beclomethasone dipropionate on hypothalamic-pituitary-adrenal (HPA) function have been evaluated in adult volunteers. There was no suppression of early morning plasma cortisol concentrations when beclomethasone dipropionate was administered in a dose of 1000 mcg./day for one month as an aerosol or for three days by intramuscular injection. However, partial suppression of plasma cortisol concentration was observed when beclomethasone dipropionate was administered in doses of 2000 mcg./day either intramuscularly or by aerosol. Immediate suppression of plasma cortisol concentrations was observed after single doses of 4000 mcg. of beclomethasone dipropionate.

In one study, the effects of beclomethasone dipropionate on HPA function were examined in patients with asthma. There was no change in basal early morning plasma cortisol concentrations or in the cortisol responses to tetracosactrin (ACTH 1:24) stimulation after daily administration of 400, 800 or 1200 mcg. of beclomethasone dipropionate for 28 days. After daily administration of 1600 mcg. each day for 28 days, there was a slight reduction in basal cortisol concentrations and a statistically significant ($p < .01$) reduction in plasma cortisol responses to tetracosactrin stimulation. The effects of a more prolonged period of beclomethasone dipropionate administration on HPA function have not been evaluated. However, a number of investigators have noted that when systemic corticosteroid therapy in asthmatic subjects can be replaced with recommended doses of beclomethasone dipropionate, there is gradual recovery of endogenous cortisol concentrations to the normal range. There is still no documented evidence of recovery from other adverse systemic corticosteroid-induced reactions during prolonged therapy of patients with beclomethasone dipropionate.

Clinical experience has shown that some patients with bronchial asthma who require corticosteroid therapy for control of symptoms can be partially or completely withdrawn from systemic corticosteroid if therapy with beclomethasone dipropionate aerosol is substituted. Beclomethasone dipropionate aerosol is not effective for all patients with bronchial asthma or at all stages of the disease in a given patient.

The early clinical experience has revealed several new problems which may be associated with the use of beclomethasone dipropionate by inhalation for treatment of patients with bronchial asthma:

1. There is a risk of adrenal insufficiency when patients are transferred from systemic corticosteroids to aerosol beclomethasone dipropionate. Although the aerosol may provide adequate control of asthma during the transfer period, it does not provide the systemic steroid which is needed during acute stress situations. Deaths due to adrenal insufficiency have occurred in asthmatic patients during and after transfer from systemic corticosteroids to aerosol beclomethasone dipropionate. (See WARNINGS.)
2. Transfer of patients from systemic steroid therapy to beclomethasone dipropionate aerosol may unmask allergic conditions which were previously controlled by the systemic steroid therapy, e.g., rhinitis, conjunctivitis, and eczema.
3. Localized infections with *Candida albicans* or *Aspergillus niger* have occurred frequently in the mouth and pharynx and occasionally in the larynx. It has been reported that up to 75% of the patients who receive prolonged treatment with beclomethasone dipropionate have positive oral cultures for *Candida albicans*. The incidence of clinically apparent infection is considerably lower but may require therapy with appropriate antifungal agents or discontinuation of treatment with beclomethasone dipropionate aerosol.

The long-term effects of beclomethasone dipropionate in human subjects are still unknown. In particular, the local effects of the agent on developmental or immunologic processes in the mouth, pharynx, trachea and lung are unknown. There is also no information about the possible long-term systemic effects of the agent. The possible relevance of the data in animal studies to results in human subjects cannot be evaluated.

Revised 6/81

Copyright © 1973, 1980, 1981, Schering Corporation. All rights reserved.

[*Shown in Product Identification Section*]

Information on Schering products appearing on these pages is effective as of September 30, 1982.

Schmid Products Company

Division of Schmid Laboratories, Inc.
ROUTE 46 WEST
LITTLE FALLS, NJ 07424

RAMSES® BENDEX® ℞
FLEXIBLE CUSHIONED DIAPHRAGM
(Arc-ing Spring)

Composition: Noted for its unusual rim design—a rust-resistant arc-ing spring encased in a cushion of soft rubber tubing. The BENDEX Diaphragm retains all the features of the regular RAMSES Diaphragm, *plus the hinge mechanism.* Lateral flexibility supplies the proper degree of spring tension without discomfort, permitting complete freedom of movement while maintaining anterior-posterior rigidity and a spermtight fit against the vaginal walls.

Action and Uses: Provides complete comfort and safety to the patient with structural abnormalities such as cystocele or rectocele. Use does not impair future planned pregnancy and does not alter female physiology. Recommended for use with RAMSES Contraceptive Vaginal Jelly in combined technique of conception control.

Note: See under RAMSES Contraceptive Vaginal Jelly for full disclosure.

Administration and Dosage: Easily inserted, slips readily into place without the use of an introducer, and easily removed. Insert diaphragm up to one hour before coitus, according to instructions in "Information for Patients" in package circular. Diaphragm should be left in place at least 8 hours after coitus.

Side Effects: None.

Precautions: None.

Contraindications: None.

How Supplied: RAMSES BENDEX Diaphragm: Package #603, Bendex and 1¼ oz. tube of Ramses Vaginal Jelly; package #703, Bendex and 3 oz. tube Ramses Vaginal Jelly in zipper kit. Diaphragms prescribed in sizes 65–90 mm.

RAMSES® ℞
FLEXIBLE CUSHIONED DIAPHRAGM

Composition: A coral-colored rim with a dome of pure gum rubber. Rim construction: spring coil encased in soft rubber to buffer spring pressure; flexible in all planes, thus permitting ready adjustment to muscular action of vagina.

Action and Uses: Provides dependable barrier to sperm, with complete comfort to patient. Use does not impair future planned pregnancy and does not impair female physiology. Recommended for use with RAMSES Contraceptive Vaginal Jelly in combined technique of conception control.

Note: See under RAMSES Contraceptive Vaginal Jelly for full disclosure.

Administration and Dosage: Easily inserted, placed and removed. Insert diaphragm up to one hour before coitus, according to instructions for "Information for Patients" in package circular. Diaphragm should be left in place at least 8 hours after last coitus.

Side Effects: None.

Precautions: None.

Contraindications: None.

How Supplied: RAMSES DIAPHRAGM: Package #602; diaphragm and 1¼ oz. tube RAMSES Vaginal Jelly, package #701 diaphragm, introducer, and 3 oz. tube RAMSES Vaginal Jelly in zipper kit. Diaphragms prescribed in sizes 55–90 mm.

RAMSES® Contraceptive Vaginal Jelly

Composition: Active Ingredient: Nonoxynol-9, 5%.

Action and Uses: RAMSES® Contraceptive Vaginal Jelly is effective for birth control by jelly-alone technique or with a diaphragm. It is colorless, non-staining and contains a fast acting spermicide to instantly immobilize sperm. It is safe, will not liquify at body temperature, pleasantly scented, water soluble and acceptable to both partners. Store at room temperature.

Dosage and Administration: For complete instructions, please read pamphlet.

RAMSES® Jelly-Alone Technique

One applicatorful of RAMSES® Jelly is sufficient for one intercourse and should be inserted just prior to intercourse. Remove cap from tube and replace it with applicator, gently turning applicator until it is firmly attached. Squeeze tube from the bottom forcing the jelly into the applicator until the plunger is pushed out as far as it will go and the barrel is filled. After detaching from the tube, hold the filled applicator by the barrel and insert well into the vagina. Press the plunger completely thus depositing the correct amount of contraceptive jelly in front of the cervix. Remove the applicator, holding it by the barrel while the plunger is still depressed.

One applicatorful of RAMSES® Jelly is sufficient for one act of intercourse only. An additional applicatorful is required each time intercourse is repeated.

RAMSES® Jelly With Diaphragm

For maximum protection, the combined use of a diaphragm and RAMSES® Jelly is recommended. Prior to inserting your diaphragm put about a teaspoonful of RAMSES® Jelly into the dome of the diaphragm and spread a small amount around the rim. This provides the proper lubrication for easy insertion and the jelly forms a seal and barrier to sperm. If intercourse occurs more than six hours after insertion, or if repeated intercourse takes place, an additional application of RAMSES® Jelly is necessary. Do not remove the diaphragm, just put more RAMSES® Jelly into the vagina with the applicator taking care not to dislodge the diaphragm.

It is important that the diaphragm remain in place for at least six hours after intercourse. Removal of the diaphragm before this time may increase the risk of becoming pregnant. If you wish, the diaphragm may be left in place for up to 24 hours.

Precaution: If your doctor advised against pregnancy for medical reasons you should discuss your birth control method with him so

that both you and your doctor are satisfied that the method you have selected is right for you.
Side Effects: No significant side effects reported to date. If burning or irritation of the vagina or penis is experienced discontinue use and consult your physician.
Warning: Keep out of the reach of children.

SAF–T–COIL® ℞
Intra-Uterine Contraceptive Device

U.S. Patents 3,374,788; 3,234,938; 3,590,816; and 3,630,190.

Description: Saf-T-Coil is a double coil intrauterine contraceptive device made of a plastic material, Ethylene-vinyl acetate copolymer, with barium sulfate added for radiopacity and release agents. The Saf-T-Coil is provided sterile in three sizes. Saf-T-Coil 33-S, the standard size, is 37 mm in width by 32 mm in length. Saf-T-Coil 32-S, the intermediate size, is 29 mm in width and 30 mm in length. Saf-T-Coil 25-S Nullip, the small size, is 25 mm in width by 20 mm in length. The components in the package include the Saf-T-Coil with monofilament nylon sutures. In addition, disposable plastic insertion tube with adjustable blue stop, plastic plunger, and uterine sound are included (packages containing 33-SX, 32-SX, and 25-SX Nullip do not include the uterine sound).
Mode of Action: The exact mechanism by which the inert Saf-T-Coil attains effective conception control has not been conclusively demonstrated. IUD's seem to interfere in some manner with nidation in the endometrium, probably through foreign body reaction in the uterus.
Indications: Saf-T-Coil is indicated for contraception.
Contraindications: IUD's should not be inserted when the following conditions exist:
1. Pregnancy or suspicion of pregnancy.
2. Abnormalities of the uterus resulting in distortion of the uterine cavity.
3. Acute pelvic inflammatory disease or a history of repeated pelvic inflammatory disease.
4. Post partum endometritis or infected abortion in the past 3 months.
5. Known or suspected uterine or cervical malignancy including unresolved, abnormal "Pap" smear.
6. Genital bleeding of unknown etiology.
7. Untreated acute cervicitis until infection is controlled.

Warnings:
1. Pregnancy—a. Long-term effects. Long-term effects on the off-spring when pregnancy occurs with Saf-T-Coil in place are unknown.
b. Septic abortion. Reports have indicated an increased incidence of septic abortion associated in some instances with septicemia, septic shock, and death in patients becoming pregnant with an IUD in place. Most of these reports have been associated with the midtrimester of pregnancy. In some cases, the initial symptoms have been insidious and not easily recognized. If pregnancy should occur with an IUD in place, the IUD should be removed if the string is visible or, if removal proves to be or would be difficult, termination of the pregnancy should be considered and offered the patient as an option bearing in mind that the risks associated with an elective abortion increase with gestational age.
c. Continuation of pregnancy: If the patient chooses to continue the pregnancy, she must be warned of the increased risk of spontaneous abortion and of the increased risk of sepsis, including death if the pregnancy continues with the IUD in place. The patient must be closely observed and she must be advised to report all abnormal symptoms, such as flu-like syndrome, fever, abdominal cramping, and pain, bleeding, or vaginal discharge, immediately because generalized symptoms of septicemia may be insidious.
2. Ectopic pregnancy. a. A pregnancy that occurs with an IUD in place is more likely to be ectopic than a pregnancy occurring without an IUD in place. Accordingly, patients who become pregnant while using the IUD should be carefully evaluated for the possibility of an ectopic pregnancy.
b. Special attention should be directed to patients with delayed menses, slight metrorrhagia and/or unilateral pelvic pain and to those patients who wish to terminate a pregnancy because of IUD failure to determine whether ectopic pregnancy has occurrred.
3. Pelvic infection. Pelvic infection may occur with the IUD in place and at times results in the development of tubo-ovarian abscesses or general peritonitis. Appropriate aerobic and anaerobic bacteriological studies should be done and antibiotic therapy initiated. If the infection does not show a marked clinical improvement within 24 to 48 hours, the IUD should be removed and the continuing treatment reassessed based upon the results of culture and sensitivity tests.
4. Embedment. Partial penetration or lodging of the IUD in the endometrium can result in difficult removals.
5. Perforation. Partial or total perforation of the uterine wall or cervix may occur with the use of IUD's. The possibility of perforation must be kept in mind during insertion and at the time of any subsequent examination. If perforation occurs, the IUD should be removed. Adhesions, foreign body reactions, and intestinal obstruction may result if an IUD is left in the peritoneal cavity.

Precautions:
1. Patient counseling. Prior to insertion the physician, nurse, or other trained health professional must provide the patient with the Patient Brochure. The patient should be given the opportunity to read the brochure and discuss fully any questions she may have concerning the IUD as well as other methods of contraception.
2. Patient evaluation and clinical considerations. a. A complete medical history should be obtained to determine conditions that might influence the selection of an IUD. Physical examination should include a pelvic examination, "Pap" smear, gonorrhea culture and, if indicated, appropriate tests for other forms of venereal disease.
b. The uterus should be carefully sounded prior to insertion to determine the degree of patency of the endocervical canal and the internal os, and the direction and depth of the uterine cavity. In occasional cases, severe cervical stenosis may be encountered. Do not use excessive force to overcome this resistance.
c. The uterus should sound to a depth of 6 to 8 centimeters (cm). Insertion of an IUD into a uterine cavity measuring less than 6.5 cm by sounding may increase the incidence of expulsion, bleeding and pain.
d. The possibility of insertion in the presence of an existing undetermined pregnancy is reduced if insertion is performed during or shortly following a menstrual period. The IUD should not be inserted post partum or postabortion until involution of the uterus is completed. The incidence of perforation and expulsion is greater if involution is not completed.
e. IUD's should be used with caution in those patients who have anemia or a history of menorrhagia or hypermenorrhea. Patients experiencing menorrhagia and/or metrorrhagia following IUD insertion may be at risk for the development of hypochromic microcytic anemia. Also, IUD's should be used with caution in patients receiving anticoagulants or having a coagulopathy.
f. Syncope, bradycardia, or other neurovascular episodes may occur during insertion or removal of IUD's especially in patients with a previous disposition to these conditions.
g. Patients with valvular or congenital heart disease are more prone to develop subacute bacterial endocarditis than patients who do not have valvular or congenital heart disease. Use of an IUD in these patients may represent a potential source of septic emboli.
h. Use of an IUD in those patients with acute cervicitis should be postponed until proper treatment has cleared up the infection.
i. Since an IUD may be expelled or displaced, patients should be reexamined and evaluated shortly after the first postinsertion menses, but definitely within 3 months after insertion. Thereafter, annual examination with appropriate medical and laboratory examination should be carried out.
j. The patient should be told that some bleeding and cramps may occur during the first few weeks after insertion, but if these symptoms continue or are severe she should report them to her physician. She should be instructed on how to check after each menstrual period to make certain that the thread still protrudes from the cervix, and she should be cautioned that there is no contraceptive protection if the IUD is expelled. She should be cautioned not to pull on the thread and displace the IUD. If partial expulsion occurs, removal is indicated and a new IUD may be inserted.
k. The use of medical diathermy (shortwave and microwave) in patients with metal-containing IUD's may cause heat injury to the surrounding tissue. Therefore, medical diathermy to the abdominal and sacral areas should not be used.*

Adverse Reactions: These adverse reactions are not listed in any order of frequency or severity.
Reported adverse reactions include: endometritis, spontaneous abortion, septic abortion, septicemia, perforation of the uterus and cervix, embedment, fragmentation of the IUD, pelvic infection, vaginitis, leukorrhea, cervical erosion, pregnancy, ectopic pregnancy, difficult removal, complete or partial expulsion of the IUD, intermenstrual spotting, prolongation of menstrual flow, anemia, pain and cramping, dysmenorrhea, backaches, dyspareunia, neurovascular episodes including bradycardia and syncope secondary to insertion. Perforation into the abdomen has been followed by abdominal adhesions, intestinal penetration, intestinal obstruction, and cystic masses in the pelvis.

Directions for Use:
Insertion Technique
Preparation for Insertion: For insertion of Saf-T-Coil 33-S, 32-S and 25-S Nullip use Saf-T-Sound where indicated (physician use own appropriate uterine sound for 33-SX, 32-SX and 25-SX Nullip). To facilitate insertion, have at hand sponges, an antiseptic solution and sterile speculum, tenaculum, uterine sound and scissors.
1) Cleanse vagina and cervix with an antiseptic solution.
2) Peel the transparent cover of the sterile package about ⅓ length and remove Saf-T-Sound.
3) Gently probe the cervical canal with the uterine sound to determine the depth, position and direction of the uterus and to check for any abnormality.
4) Leave the sound in position for a few moments to slightly dilate the cervix, to align the cervical canal, and to ease the way for passage of the insertion tube.
5) Remove the sound and note the depth of the uterine cavity.

Continued on next page

Schmid—Cont.

Loading the Insertion Tube

1) With the Saf-T-Coil on the package insert card, position the adjustable blue stop on the insertion tube 1.5 cm less than the depth of the uterine cavity as measured by the uterine sound. Rotate the blue stop, if necessary, to be sure its tabs are in the same plane as coils of Saf-T-Coil. Bend insertion tube (containing Saf-T-Coil) to approximate the natural curvature of the canal as determined with the uterine sound. Grasping the protruding end of the plunger, slowly pull Saf-T-Coil into insertion tube until nodule on the end of the coil contacts the distal end of the insertion tube and remains in place. NOTE: Do not hold Saf-T-Coil in the insertion tube more than 5 minutes to prevent loss of its 'memory'.
   Push plunger back into insertion tube as far as possible without advancing Saf-T-Coil.

Introducing Device into Uterus

While holding the tenaculum in one hand, gently introduce the distal end of the loaded insertion tube into the cervical os. Carefully advance it into the uterus until the blue stop is flush with the cervix, keeping the tabs of the blue stop parallel to the frontal plane of the body.

Meticulous care should be exercised at this point to avoid excessive pressure against the fundus.

Depositing the Saf-T-Coil

Hold plunger in place and retract insertion tube over the plunger. This releases Saf-T-Coil, without pressure, into proper position within the uterine cavity. (If there is any question as to its having attained its proper position, withdraw at once into the insertion tube and reinsert as described above).

Completing the Insertion

Wait a full minute, to allow Saf-T-Coil to assume its original configuration. Withdraw the insertion tube until the sutures become visible. With scissors, clip sutures leaving about 2 inches of sutures exposed. (Sutures may be shortened at a later date, if desired).

Do not leave patient unattended. Observe patient several minutes after insertion for signs of syncope, severe cramping, abnormal bleeding, or extrusion of the coil.

Clinical Studies: Different event rates have been recorded with the use of different IUD's. Inasmuch as these rates are usually derived from separate studies conducted by different investigators in several population groups, they cannot be compared with precision. Furthermore, event rates tend to be lower as clinical experience is expanded, possibly due to retention in the clinical study of those patients who accept the treatment regimen and do not discontinue due to adverse reactions or pregnancy. In clinical trials conducted by Tietze (1967), Solish and Majzlin (1968), Tietze and Lewit (1970), Hayes (1973) and Laufe, *et al* (1974) with the Saf-T-Coil, use effectiveness was determined as follows for parous and nulliparous women, as tabulated by the life table method. (Rates are expressed as events per 100 women through 12 and 24 months of use). This experience is based on 46,721 women/months of use including 4,231 women who completed 12 months of use and 1,842 women who completed 24 months of use.

[See table below].

	12 Months		24 Months	
	Parous	Nulliparous	Parous	Nulliparous
Pregnancy	2.4 (0.42-2.8)	—	3.1 (0.42-3.8)	—
Expulsion	18.3 (7.8-29.0)	—	18.8 (9.0-21.5)	—
Medical removal	15.6 (4.8-18.7)	—	23.2 (9.0-27.0)	—
Continuation rate	70.4 (55.2-88.0)	—	59.8 (57.0-81.5)	—

References:

Hayes, O.J.: *A Clinical Evaluation of the Intrauterine Device for Control of Contraception.* South. Med. J. 66:254 (1973).

Laufe, L.E., Brickner, P.B., Ryser, P.E., and Ammer, J.L.: *An Evaluation of the Use-Effectiveness of the Saf-T-Coil in Private Practice.* Contraception 9:23 (1974).

Solish, G.I. and Majzlin, G.: *The Majzlin Spring IUCD.* Presented at the Sixth Annual Meeting of the Am. Assoc. of Planned Parenthood Physicians, Apr. 16-17, 1968.

Tietze, C. and Lewit, S.: *Evaluation of Intrauterine Devices: Ninth Progress Report of the Operative Statistical Program.* Studies in Family Planning. A publication of The Population Council. No. 55, (1970).

Tietze, C.: *Report of a New IUD: The Double Coil.* Advances in Planned Parenthood, III:85 (1967).

Long Term Experience: An additional extensive study extending for five years relating actual field experience of the Florida Public Health Clinics has been reported. That study included 27,712 patients with 541,248 women months of use of the Saf-T-Coil. Event rates reported include 0.8% for pregnancy, 11.9% for expulsion, 8.0% for medical removal and continuation rate increased from 75% in 1967 to 80% in 1971. That study indicates that physicians and other medical personnel of diverse background and training are able to achieve outstanding use-effectiveness with the Saf-T-Coil when the device is properly inserted.

Reference:

Caraway, A.F., and Vaughn, B.J.: *Florida's Five Year Experience with the Double Coil IUD.* J. Reprod. Med. 10:170 (1973).

How Supplied: SAF-T-COIL is available in three sizes: 33-S (standard) for the multiparous patient; 32-S (intermediate) for the primiparous patient and the person who cannot accommodate the 33-S; and 25-S Nullip (small) for the nulliparous patient. Each package of SAF-T-COIL (33-S, 32-S, and 25-S Nullip) is enclosed with a SAF-T-SOUND in a sterile, peel package. SAF-T-SOUND is a sterile, disposable intrauterine probe that assists in more accurate placement of the SAF-T-COIL. SAF-T-COIL 33-SX, 32-SX and 25-SX Nullip are also available without the SAF-T-SOUND included in the package. Physician instructions and patient instructions are provided with each package. There are six SAF-T-COIL units per carton. SAF-T-COIL/SAF-T-SOUND units are available from Surgical Supply Dealers.

Federal law restricts this device to sale by or on the order of a physician.

*Not associated with Saf-T-Coil.

VAGISEC PLUS® SUPPOSITORIES ℞
VAGISEC® MEDICATED DOUCHE LIQUID CONCENTRATE

Description: VAGISEC PLUS SUPPOSITORIES contain a combination of trichomonacidal and bactericidal agents and provide continued medication by gradual liquefaction. Each vaginal suppository contains the following ingredients:

9-aminoacridine HCl	6.00 mg.
Polyoxyethylene nonyl phenol	5.25 mg.
Sodium edetate	0.66 mg.
Sodium dioctyl sulfosuccinate	0.07 mg.

in a polyethylene glycol base containing glycerin and citric acid.

VAGISEC MEDICATED DOUCHE LIQUID CONCENTRATE contains a combination of polyoxyethylene nonyl phenol sodium edetate, and sodium dioctyl sulfosuccinate, a complex proven to be effective trichomonacide when used as a vaginal douche (Vagisec Liquid).

Clinical Pharmacology: 9-aminoacridine is a broad-spectrum anti-infective of extensive medical acceptance for the topical treatment of bacterial infections. The combination of polyoxyethylene nonyl phenol, sodium edetate, and sodium dioctyl sulfosuccinate is a trichomonacide which when in solution and diluted disintegrates the flagellates through marked changes in surface tension.

Indications and Usage: The Vagisec Liquid/Suppository regimen is indicated for the specific treatment, in adults, of vaginitis, as evidenced by pruritus, malodorous leukorrhea, erythema of the vaginal mucosa, dyspareunia, caused by Trichomonas vaginalis and mixed vaginal infections complicated by a bacterial moiety.

The presence of trichomonads can be established by a hanging drop mount preparation of the discharge from the posterior fornix and confirmed by cultures grown on STS medium; the atypical bacterial moiety can be identified by examination of gram-stained preparations of smeared vaginal secretions.

Contraindications: Douching is not recommended during pregnancy. VAGISEC Medicated Douche and VAGISEC PLUS Suppositories are spermicidal and should not be used when the patient is trying to conceive.

Precautions: *General:* The full course of therapy must be completed to eliminate the infecting micro-organisms from the vagina. It is generally desirable to continue treatment through the menses in order to guard against potential flare-ups since the presence of blood favors the rapid growth of Trichomonas. Recurrence of vaginitis often indicates extravaginal foci or infection in cervical, vestibular and urethral glands, etc. or reinfection by the sexual partner.

Information for Patients: During treatment, patient should refrain from intercourse, or the partner should wear a prophylactic. To prevent flare-ups after completion of therapy and for continued vaginal cleanliness, the patient is advised to continue with VAGISEC Liquid as a regular douche, but no more than twice weekly unless otherwise directed by physician.

Laboratory Tests: No patient should be considered cured until cultures on STS medium and gram-stained preparations of smeared vaginal secretions, taken at monthly intervals for 3 months following treatment, show absence of trichomonads and a return to the normal vaginal bacterial flora.

Adverse Reactions: No significant adverse reactions have been reported to date for Vagisec Plus Suppositories or Vagisec Liquid. Any minor irritation is generally relieved by discontinuance of douche for 24 hours.

Overdosage: *Antidote:* Copious use of water. The dilute Vagisec solution is non-toxic.

Dosage & Administration: *Office Treatment (Adult):* For the treatment of vaginal trichomoniasis and mixed vaginal infections, best results are obtained by scrubbing the vagina with VAGISEC Liquid, diluted 1:100 by the physician in the office: 3 scrubs the first week, 2 the second. A suppository is inserted after each office scrub in the Liquid/Suppository regimen. Patient should be instructed to continue treatment at home. *Home Treatment:* The combination douche and suppositories (Liquid/Suppository regimen) is recommended for home use. The usual daily home treatment is VAGISEC Medicated Douche in the morning, followed by a VAGISEC PLUS Suppository inserted deep in the vagina, using tip of finger, and a second suppository inserted in like manner at bedtime for a period of 14 days. Treatment should be omitted the night and morning preceding an office visit. In chronic or stubborn cases, therapy may be repeated with no interval between courses. The Liquid/Suppository regimen may be continued through-

out the menstrual cycle. It is advisable to continue treatment through two menstrual periods. Patients should be reexamined 3 days after home treatment has been discontinued. The full course of therapy must be completed to eliminate the infecting micro-organisms from the vagina. No patient should be considered cured until vaginal smears or cultures, taken at monthly intervals for 3 months following treatment, show absence of trichomonads and a return to the normal vaginal flora.
How Supplied: VAGISEC PLUS® SUPPOSITORIES—box of 28 plastic-wrapped 3 gram suppositories. VAGISEC® MEDICATED DOUCHE LIQUID CONCENTRATE—4 oz. plastic bottle with instructions for dilution and douching.
Caution: Federal law prohibits dispensing VAGISEC PLUS Suppositories without prescription.

Sclavo Inc.
5 MANSARD COURT
WAYNE, NJ 07470

COMPLETE INFORMATION FOR THE BELOW LISTED PRODUCTS IS FURNISHED IN THE PACKAGING.

ANTIRABIES SERUM (equine) USP ℞
CHOLERA VACCINE, USP ℞
DIPHTHERIA ANTITOXIN (equine) USP ℞
DIPHTHERIA TOXOID, USP ℞
DIPHTHERIA AND TETANUS TOXOIDS ADSORBED, USP (For Pediatric Use) ℞
SclavoTest®-PPD ℞
Tuberculin Purified Protein Derivative (PPD)
Multiple Puncture Device
For product information, consult Diagnostic Product Information Section.
TETANUS ANTITOXIN (equine) USP ℞
TETANUS TOXOID, ADSORBED, USP ℞
TETANUS AND DIPHTHERIA TOXOIDS ADSORBED, USP (For Adult Use) ℞

Scot-Tussin Pharmacal Co., Inc.
50 CLEMENCE STREET
POST OFFICE BOX 8217
CRANSTON, RI 02920

Scot-Tussin National Drug Code

NDC 0372	Product
0001-04	SCOT-TUSSIN® Syrup
0001-16	
0001-28	
0002-04	SCOT-TUSSIN® Sugar-Free
0002-16	
0002-28	
0010-16	S-T DECONGEST™ Sugar-Free, Dye Free
0006-04	S-T EXPECTORANT™ Sugar-Free, Dye Free
0006-16	
0006-28	
0017-16	TUSSIREX™ w/CODEINE Syrup
0017-28	
0018-16	TUSSIREX™ w/CODEINE Sugar-Free
0018-28	

S-T FORTE™ Syrup
S-T FORTE™ SUGAR-FREE Ⓒ

This is the text of the latest official Package Circular dated Nov. '69.

Alcohol 5% by volume.
Caution: Federal Law prohibits dispensing without a prescription.
Composition: Each teaspoonful (5 ml) contains:
Hydrocodone Bitartrate, U.S.P. ....25 mg.
(Warning: May be habit forming.)
Phenylephrine HCl U.S.P. ....5.0 mg.
Phenylpropanolamine HCl, U.S.P. ....5.0 mg.
Pheniramine Maleate, U.S.P.............13.33 mg.
Guaifenesin, U.S.P...............................80.0 mg.
Administration and Dosage:
Average Adult Dosage: One teaspoonful 3 or 4 times a day as indicated, not to exceed 4 teasp. in any 24 hours.
Children: 6 to 12 years, half teasp. 3 or 4 times a day as indicated, not to exceed 2 teasp. in any 24 hours.
Children: 3 to 6 years, ½ teasp.; 1 to 3 years 20 drops; 6 mos. to 1 year 10 drops.
Side Effects: S-T Forte is usually well tolerated, but if drowsiness or nausea or other side effects occur, discontinue its use immediately. Keep this and all medications out of the reach of children.
Action and Uses: S-T Forte, "The 5-action cough medicine", gives 5-action symptomatic relief of stubborn coughs and nasal congestion due to colds or hay fever. It contains: HYDROCODONE BITARTRATE, U.S.P. an excellent narcotic antitussive. PHENYLEPHRINE HCl U.S.P., an orally effective vasoconstrictor for relief of nasal congestion and bronchial spasm. PHENYLPROPANOLAMINE HCl, U.S.P., a well known decongestant used to shrink engorged mucous membranes caused by hay fever and allergic rhinitis. PHENIRAMINE MALEATE, U.S.P., one of the most potent antihistamines on a weight basis. GUAIFENESIN, U.S.P., an effective expectorant in the treatment of coughs.
Precautions and Contraindications: S-T Forte contains Hydrocodone Bitartrate and may be habit forming; therefore should be used with caution and only when indicated, not for a prolonged period of time. It should be used with caution in patients sensitive to antihistamines and to sympathomimetic products, or patients suffering with arteriosclerosis, hypertension or hyperthyroidism. Patients taking S-T Forte should not drive vehicles or operate machinery.
How Supplied:
Syrup: Pints NDC 0372-0004-16; Gallons NDC 0372-0004-28.
Sugar-Free: Pints NDC 0372-0005-16; Gallons NDC 0372-0005-28.
S-T Forte is a schedule 3 controlled substance.

VITA-PLUS H™*
(Hematinic)
SUGAR-FREE Liquid

Preliminary listing only.
Complete information furnished in the packaging.
Each teaspoonful (5 ml.) contains:
1-Lysine Mono HCl .... 100 mg.
Vitamin B_1 .... 10 mg.
Vitamin B_{12} (Cobalamin Conc.) ..... 25 mcgm.
Vitamin B_6 .... 5 mg.
Iron Pyrophosphate soluble .... 100 mg.
(Equivalent to 22 mg. elemental iron)
In a palatable Sorbitol Base.
How Supplied: 4 oz. NDC 0372-0021-04
8 oz. NDC 0372-0021-08
16 oz. NDC 0372-0021-16
gallons NDC 0372-0021-28
*TM since 1956

Products are cross-indexed by generic and chemical names in the **YELLOW SECTION**

Searle Pharmaceuticals Inc.
BOX 5110
CHICAGO, IL 60680

Searle Consumer Products*
Division of Searle Pharmaceuticals Inc.
BOX 5110
CHICAGO, IL 60680

Searle & Co.†
SAN JUAN, PUERTO RICO 00936

Alphabetic Product Listing
List#, Prod. ID# (NDC§), Form, Strength

46 †Aldactazide, 1011, Tablet, 25 mg/25 mg
39 †Aldactone, 1001, Tablet, 25 mg
134 †Aldactone, 1031, Tablet, 100 mg
96 Aminophyllin Injection, 1213, Ampul IV, 250 mg/10 ml
95 Aminophyllin Injection, 1223, Ampul IV, 500 mg/20 ml
18 †Aminophyllin, 1231, Tablet, 100 mg
44 †Aminophyllin, 1251, Tablet, 200 mg
47 †Amodrine, 1291, Tablet
43 †Anavar, 1401, Tablet, 2.5 mg
40 †Banthine, 1501, Tablet, 50 mg
563 Calan, 1853, Ampul, 5 mg/2 ml.
626 Calan, 1851, Tablet, 80 mg
632 Calan, 1861, Tablet, 120 mg
511 Chlorthalidone, 531, Tablet, 25 mg
512 Chlorthalidone, 541, Tablet, 50 mg
152 Cu-7, 708, Unit
146 Cu-7/Mark 7, 708, Unit
1596 *Comfolax, 1552, Capsule, 100 mg
1966 *Comfolax-*plus*, 1572, Capsule, 100 mg/30 mg
163 †Demulen Compack, 71, Tablet, 1 mg/50 mcg
172 †Demulen Refill, 71, Tablet, 1 mg/50 mcg
181 †Demulen Triopak, 71, Tablet, 1 mg/50 mcg
156 †Demulen-28 Compack, 71 (0081), Tablet, 1 mg/50 mcg
164 †Demulen-28 Refill, 71 (0081), Tablet, 1 mg/50 mcg
139 †Demulen 1/35-21 Compack, 151, Tablet, 1 mg/35 mcg
51 †Demulen 1/35-21 Refill, 151 Tablet, 1 mg/35 mcg
80 †Demulen 1/35-28 Compack, 151 (0161), Tablet, 1 mg/35 mcg
108 †Demulen 1/35-28 Refill, 151 (0161), Tablet, 1 mg/35 mcg
251 Diulo, 501, Tablet, 2½ mg
273 Diulo, 511, Tablet, 5 mg
285 Diulo, 521, Tablet, 10 mg
34 Dramamine Injection, 1703, Ampul, 50 mg/1 ml
72 Dramamine, 1701, Tablet, 50 mg (500s, 1,000s, 2,500s)
73 Dramamine, 1736, Liquid, 12.5 mg/4 ml, 16 oz
74 Dramamine Injection, 1724, Vial, 250 mg/5 ml
112 Dramamine 1701, Unit-Dose, Tablet, 50 mg
7012 *Dramamine, 1701, Tablet, 50 mg (12s, 36s, 100s)
7303 *Dramamine, 1736, Liquid, 12.5 mg/4 ml, 3 oz
56 †Enovid, 51, Tablet, 5 mg/75 mcg
22 †Enovid Calendar-Pack, 51, Tablet, 5 mg/75 mcg
67 †Enovid, 101, Tablet, 10 mg/(9.85 mg/0.15 mg)

Continued on next page

Searle—Cont.

153 †Enovid-E 21 Compack, 131, Tablet, 2.5 mg/0.1 mg
191 †Enovid-E 21 Refill, 131, Tablet, 2.5 mg/0.1 mg
27231 *Equal, 8109, Powder, Packets
26931 *Equal, 8201, Sweet-Tabs, Pocket Pak
111 †Flagyl, 1831, Tablet, 250 mg
155 †Flagyl, 500 (1821), Tablet, 500 mg
270 Flagyl I.V., 1804, Vial (partial fill, lyoph. pwd.), 500 mg
261 Flagyl I.V. RTU, 1844, Vial, 500 mg/100 ml
661 Flagyl I.V. RTU, 1847, Plastic Container, 500 mg/100 ml
639 Furosemide, 571, Tablet USP, 20 mg
640 Furosemide, 581, Tablet USP, 40 mg
1093 *Icy Hot, 2008, Balm, 3½ oz
1097 *Icy Hot, 2008, Balm, 7 oz
2801 *Icy Hot, 2018, Rub, 1¼ oz
2803 *Icy Hot, 2018, Rub, 3 oz
81 †Lomotil, 61, Tablet, 2.5 mg/0.025 mg
94 †Lomotil Liquid, 66, 2.5 mg/0.025 mg per 5 ml
154 Mark-7 Sound, 709, Unit
5407 *Metamucil, 2209, Powder, 7 oz
5414 *Metamucil, 2209, Powder, 14 oz
5421 *Metamucil, 2209, Powder, 21 oz
54100 *Metamucil, 2209, Powder, Unit-Dose, Packets, 7 g, 100s
1716 *Metamucil Instant Mix, 2219, Packet, 16s
1730 *Metamucil Instant Mix, 2219, Packet, 30s
17100 *Metamucil Instant Mix, 2219, Unit-Dose, Packets, 100s
26516 *Metamucil Instant Mix, Orange Flavor, 2259, Packet, 16s
26530 *Metamucil Instant Mix, Orange Flavor, 2259, Packet, 30s
25407 *Metamucil Orange Flavor, 2229, Powder, 7 oz
25414 *Metamucil Orange Flavor, 2229, Powder, 14 oz
25421 *Metamucil Orange Flavor, 2229, Powder, 21 oz
6907 *Metamucil Strawberry Flavor, 2269, Powder, 7 oz
6914 *Metamucil Strawberry Flavor, 2269, Powder, 14 oz
6921 *Metamucil Strawberry Flavor, 2269, Powder, 21 oz
580 Nitrodisc, 2058, Transdermal Pad, 5 mg (8 cm^2)
581 Nitrodisc, 2068, Transdermal Pad, 10 mg (16 cm^2)
123 †Norpace, 2752, Capsule, 100 mg
906 †Norpace, 2762, Capsule, 150 mg
256 †Norpace CR, 2732, Capsule, 100 mg
278 †Norpace CR, 2742, Capsule, 150 mg
129 †Ovulen-21 Compack, 401, Tablet, 1 mg/0.1 mg
137 †Ovulen-21 Refill, 401, Tablet, 1 mg/0.1 mg
133 †Ovulen-21 Triopak, 401, Tablet, 1 mg/0.1 mg
130 †Ovulen-28 Compack, 401 (0421), Tablet, 1 mg/0.1 mg
141 †Ovulen-28 Refill, 401 (0421), Tablet, 1 mg/0.1 mg
28 †Pro-Banthīne, 601, Tablet, 15 mg
121 †Pro-Banthīne Unit-Dose, 601, Tablet, 15 mg
9 †Pro-Banthīne, 611, Tablet, 7½ mg
29 †Pro-Banthīne w/Phenobarbital, 631, Tablet, 15 mg/15 mg
132 †Pro-Banthīne w/Pheno Unit-Dose, 631, Tablet, 15 mg/15 mg
4903 *Prompt, 2249, Powder, 2½ oz
4906 *Prompt, 2249, Powder, 5 oz
4913 *Prompt, 2249, Powder, Packets, 12s
20 Tatum-T, 508, Unit

* Products of Searle Consumer Products (those not shown in this publication are included in the PDR for Nonprescription Drugs).
†Products of Searle & Co.
[Products without reference marks are Searle Pharmaceuticals Inc. products.]
§When the product ID# is not the same as the NDC#, the NDC# appears in parentheses.

Searle Pharmaceuticals Inc.

BOX 5110
CHICAGO, IL 60680

AMINOPHYLLIN INJECTION™ ℞
(aminophylline injection USP)

Description: Aminophyllin Injection is a sterile solution of theophylline in water for injection prepared with the aid of ethylenediamine. Aminophyllin Injection contains anhydrous theophylline USP 19.7 mg/ml and ethylenediamine USP 3.6 mg/ml (equivalent to aminophylline dihydrate 25 mg/ml) in water for injection.
Aminophylline is a 2:1 complex of theophylline ($C_7H_8N_4O_2$) and ethylenediamine ($C_2H_8N_2$).
Aminophylline is white or slightly yellowish granules or powder, having a slight ammoniacal odor and a bitter taste.

Clinical Pharmacology: Theophylline directly relaxes the smooth muscle of the bronchial airways and pulmonary blood vessels, thus acting mainly as a bronchodilator and smooth muscle relaxant. The drug also possesses other actions typical of the xanthine derivatives: coronary vasodilator, cardiac stimulant, diuretic, cerebral stimulant, and skeletal muscle stimulant. The actions of theophylline may be mediated through inhibition of phosphodiesterase and an increase in intracellular cyclic AMP, which can mediate smooth muscle relaxation. *In vitro*, theophylline inhibits the release of histamine by mast cells at concentrations generally higher than attained *in vivo*. *In vitro*, theophylline has been shown to react synergistically with beta agonists that increase intracellular cyclic AMP through the stimulation of adenyl cyclase (isoproterenol), but synergism has not been demonstrated in clinical studies. More data are needed to determine if theophylline and beta agonists have a clinically important additive effect *in vivo*.
The half-life of theophylline is shortened with cigarette-smoking. It is prolonged in alcoholism, reduced hepatic or renal function, and congestive heart failure, and in patients receiving cimetidine or antibiotics such as troleandomycin, erythromycin, and clindamycin. High fever for prolonged periods may reduce the rate of theophylline elimination. Apparently, no development of tolerance occurs with chronic use of theophylline.

Theophylline Elimination Characteristics

	Theophylline Clearance Rates (mean ± S.D.)	Half-life Average (mean ± S.D.)
Children (over 6 months of age):	1.45 ± 0.58 ml/kg/min	3.7 ± 1.1 hours
Adult nonsmokers with uncomplicated asthma	0.65 ± 0.19 ml/kg/min	8.7 ± 2.2 hours

Newborn infants have extremely slow theophylline clearance rates. The theophylline half-life in newborn infants may exceed 24 hours. Not until after about 3 to 6 months do these rates approach those seen in older children.
Older adults with chronic obstructive pulmonary disease, any patients with cor pulmonale or other causes of heart failure, and patients with liver pathology may have much slower clearance rates with half-lives that may exceed 24 hours.
The half-life of theophylline in smokers (1 to 2 packs/day) averaged 4 to 5 hours among various studies, much shorter than the half-life in nonsmokers which averaged about 7 to 9 hours. The increase in theophylline clearance caused by smoking is probably the result of induction of drug-metabolizing enzymes that do not readily normalize after cessation of smoking. It appears that between 3 months and 2 years may be necessary for normalization of the effect of smoking on theophylline pharmacokinetics.

Indications and Usage: Aminophyllin Injection is indicated for relief of acute bronchial asthma and for reversible bronchospasm associated with chronic bronchitis and emphysema.

Contraindications: Patients with a history of hypersensitivity to aminophylline or its components (theophylline or ethylenediamine) should not be treated with Aminophyllin Injection (aminophylline).

Warnings: Status asthmaticus is a medical emergency. Optimal therapy frequently requires additional medication including corticosteroids when the patient is not rapidly responsive to bronchodilators.
Excessive theophylline doses may be associated with toxicity. The determination of theophylline serum levels is recommended to assure maximal benefit without excessive risk. Incidence of toxicity increases at theophylline serum levels greater than 20 mcg/ml.
Morphine and curare should be used with caution in patients with airflow obstruction because they stimulate histamine release and can induce asthmatic attacks. They may also suppress respiration leading to respiratory failure. Alternative drugs should be chosen whenever possible.
There is an excellent correlation between high serum levels of theophylline resulting from conventional doses and associated clinical manifestations of toxicity in (1) patients with lowered body plasma clearances (due to transient cardiac decompensation), (2) patients with liver dysfunction or chronic obstructive lung disease, (3) patients who are older than 55 years of age, particularly males.
Less serious signs of theophylline toxicity such as nausea and restlessness may appear in up to 50% of patients. However, serious side effects such as ventricular arrhythmias and convulsions may appear as the first signs of toxicity. Many patients who have high theophylline serum levels exhibit tachycardia. Theophylline products may worsen preexisting arrhythmias.
Aminophylline injection should not be injected rapidly (no more than 25 mg/min) or through a central venous catheter. Intravenous doses given too rapidly or excessive doses given by any route of administration may be expected to be toxic, causing gastrointestinal, central nervous system, cardiovascular, and/or respiratory symptoms (see *OVERDOSAGE*). Some children may be unusually sensitive to aminophylline. Toxic synergism with ephedrine and other sympathomimetic drugs may occur.
Caution should be used when aminophylline is given to patients with impaired liver function. Serum levels in such patients may persist longer than expected.

Precautions: Mean half-life in smokers is shorter than in nonsmokers; therefore smokers may require larger doses of aminophylline. Aminophylline should not be administered concurrently with other xanthine medications.

Use with caution in patients with severe cardiac disease, severe hypoxemia, hypertension, hyperthyroidism, acute myocardial injury, cor pulmonale, congestive heart failure, or liver disease, and in the elderly (especially males) and in neonates.

In particular, great caution should be used in giving aminophylline to patients in congestive heart failure. Frequently, such patients have markedly prolonged theophylline serum levels with theophylline persisting in serum for long periods following discontinuation of the drug.

Convulsions may be seen in patients with aminophylline overdosage with serum levels of 30 to 50 mcg/ml or higher. Aminophylline may lower the seizure threshold.

Use aminophylline cautiously in patients with a history of peptic ulcer since the disease may be exacerbated. Methylxanthines are known to increase gastric acidity. Theophylline may occasionally act as a local irritant to the G.I. tract although gastrointestinal symptoms are more commonly centrally mediated and associated with serum drug concentrations over 20 mcg/ml.

DRUG INTERACTIONS. In patients receiving cimetidine or the antibiotics troleandomycin, erythromycin, lincomycin, or clindamycin concurrently with theophylline preparations, elevated serum levels of theophylline may result. Therefore, such patients should be watched carefully for signs of toxicity to theophylline and the dose of aminophylline decreased if necessary. If ephedrine or other sympathomimetic drugs are given concomitantly with aminophylline, toxic synergism may occur.

Interaction	Effect
With lithium carbonate	Increased excretion of lithium carbonate
With propranolol	Antagonism of propranolol effect
With cimetidine	Increased theophylline serum levels
With troleandomycin, erythromycin, lincomycin or clindamycin	Increased theophylline plasma levels

LABORATORY TEST INTERACTIONS: When serum levels of theophylline are measured by spectrophotometric methods, coffee, tea, cola beverages, chocolate, and acetaminophen contribute to falsely high values.

USE IN PREGNANCY: Safe use in pregnancy has not been established relative to possible adverse effects on fetal development, but neither have adverse effects on fetal development been established. This is true for most antiasthmatic medications. Use of aminophylline in pregnant women should be balanced against the risk of uncontrolled asthma.

Adverse Reactions: The most consistent adverse reactions are usually due to overdose and are:

1. Gastrointestinal: nausea, vomiting, epigastric pain, hematemesis, diarrhea.
2. Central nervous system: headaches, irritability, restlessness, insomnia, reflex hyperexcitability, muscle twitching, clonic and tonic generalized convulsions.
3. Cardiovascular: palpitation, tachycardia, extra systoles, flushing, hypotension, circulatory failure, life-threatening ventricular arrhythmias.
4. Respiratory: tachypnea.
5. Renal: albuminuria, microhematuria, potentiation of diuresis.
6. Others: hyperglycemia and inappropriate ADH (antidiuretic hormone) syndrome; rash (ethylenediamine).

Overdosage:

Management of Toxic Symptoms:

1. Discontinue drug immediately.
2. There is no known specific antidote.
3. Treatment is supportive and symptomatic.
4. Avoid administration of sympathomimetic drugs.
5. Theophylline is dialyzable; charcoal hemoperfusion should be considered in severe theophylline toxic reactions.
6. Administer intravenous fluids, oxygen, and other supportive measures to prevent hypotension, correct dehydration and acid-base imbalance.
7. For hyperthermia, use a cooling blanket or give sponge baths as necessary.
8. Maintain patent airway and use artificial respiration (mechanical ventilation) in case of respiratory depression.
9. Control convulsions with appropriate parenteral medication(s) such as short-acting barbiturates, diazepam (0.1 to 0.3 mg/kg up to 10 mg), or phenytoin.
10. Monitor theophylline serum levels until below 20 mcg/ml.

Aminophylline Dosage for Patient Population

A. Not currently receiving theophylline products.

Group	Loading Dose* (mg/kg)	Maintenance Dose for Next 12 Hours (mg/kg/hr)	Maintenance Dose Beyond 12 Hours (mg/kg/hr)
1. Children 6 months to 9 years	6 (5)†	1.2 (1.0)†	1.0 (0.8)†
2. Children age 9 to 16 and young adult smokers	6 (5)	1.0 (0.8)	0.8 (0.65)
3. Otherwise healthy nonsmoking adults	6 (5)	0.7 (0.6)	0.5 (0.4)
4. Older patients and patients with cor pulmonale	6 (5)	0.6 (0.5)	0.3 (0.24)
5. Patients with congestive heart failure, liver disease	6 (5)	0.5 (0.4)	0.1–0.2 (0.08–0.16)

* Administer slowly, no faster than 25 mg/min.
† Equivalent anhydrous theophylline indicated in parentheses.

Dosage and Administration: Therapeutic theophylline serum levels associated with optimal likelihood for benefit and minimal risk of toxicity are considered to be between 10 and 20 mcg/ml. Levels above 20 mcg/ml may produce toxic effects. There is great variation from patient to patient in dosage needed in order to achieve a therapeutic serum level because of variable rates of elimination. Because of this wide interpatient variation and the relatively narrow therapeutic serum level range, dosage must be individualized. Monitoring of theophylline serum levels is highly recommended. Continuous cardiac monitoring may offer additional safety. Patients should be closely monitored for signs of toxicity. Dosage should be temporarily discontinued and resumed later at a lower dose if any signs of theophylline toxicity are present.

Dosage should be calculated on the basis of lean (ideal) body weight where mg/kg doses are stated. Theophylline does not distribute into fatty tissue.

Due to the marked variation in theophylline metabolism in infants, this drug is not recommended for infants under 6 months of age. [See table above].

B. Currently receiving theophylline products: Determine, where possible, the time, amount, route of administration, and form of the patient's last dose.

The loading dose for theophylline is based on the principle that each 0.5 mg/kg of theophylline administered as a loading dose will result in a 1 mcg/ml increase in serum theophylline concentration. Ideally, the loading dose should be deferred if serum theophylline concentration can be rapidly obtained. If this is not possible, the clinician must exercise judgment in selecting a dose based on the potential for benefit and risk. When there is sufficient respiratory distress to warrant a small risk, 2.5 mg/kg of intravenous anhydrous theophylline (3.1 mg/kg of intravenous aminophylline) is likely to increase the serum concentration when administered as a loading dose in rapidly absorbed form by approximately 5 mcg/ml. If the patient is not already experiencing theophylline toxicity, this is unlikely to result in dangerous adverse effects.

Subsequent to the decision regarding modification of the loading dose in this group of patients, the maintenance dosage recommendations are the same as those described above.

Aminophyllin Injection in intravenous ampuls and vials of 10 ml (250 mg) or 20 ml (500 mg) can either be injected very slowly by syringe or, more conveniently, may be infused in a small quantity (usually 100 or 200 ml) of 5% dextrose injection or 0.9% sodium chloride injection. This solution is sometimes given "piggyback" through an I.V. system already in place. Do not exceed the rate of 25 mg/min. Thereafter, maintenance therapy can be administered by a large volume infusion to deliver the desired amount of drug each hour.

Aminophylline is compatible with most commonly used I.V. solutions.

Oral therapy should be substituted for intravenous aminophylline as soon as adequate improvement is achieved.

Parenteral drug products should be inspected visually for particulate matter and discoloration prior to administration, whenever solution and container permit. Use only if solution is clear, no crystals are present, and vial seal is intact.

Unused amount of solution should be discarded immediately following withdrawal of any portion of contents.

INTRAVENOUS ADMIXTURE INCOMPATIBILITY: Although there have been reports of aminophylline precipitating in acidic media, these reports do not apply to the dilute solutions found in intravenous infusions. Aminophyllin Injection (aminophylline) should not be mixed in a syringe with other drugs but should be added separately to the intravenous solution.

When an intravenous solution containing aminophylline is given "piggyback," the intravenous system already in place should be turned off while the aminophylline is infused if there is a potential problem with admixture incompatibility.

The following may be incompatible when mixed with aminophylline in intravenous fluids: anileridine HCl, ascorbic acid, chlorproma-

Continued on next page

Searle Pharm.—Cont.

zine, codeine phosphate, dimenhydrinate, epinephrine HCl, erythromycin gluceptate, hydralazine HCl, insulin, levorphanol tartrate, meperidine HCl, methadone HCl, methicillin sodium, morphine sulfate, norepinephrine bitartrate, oxytetracycline HCl, penicillin G potassium, phenobarbital sodium, phenytoin sodium, prochlorperazine maleate, promazine HCl, promethazine HCl, tetracycline HCl, vancomycin HCl, vitamin B complex with C.

How Supplied:
Ampuls: 10-ml (250 mg) or 20-ml (500 mg) ampuls, aqueous solution, USP; cartons of 25 and boxes of 100.
Vials: 10-ml (250 mg) or 20-ml (500 mg) single-dose vials, aqueous solution, USP; cartons of 25 and boxes of 100.
Store below 86°F (30°C) and protect from light and from freezing.

[*Tablets Shown in Product Identification Section*]

CALAN® ℞
(verapamil hydrochloride)
For Intravenous Injection

Description: Calan (verapamil HCl) is a slow-channel inhibitor or calcium antagonist. Each 2-ml sterile ampul (for intravenous administration) contains 5 mg verapamil HCl and 17 mg sodium chloride in water for injection. Hydrochloric acid is used for pH adjustment. The pH of the solution is between 4.1 and 6.0. Protect contents from light.
Verapamil hydrochloride is benzeneacetonitrile, α-[3- [[2-(3, 4-dimethoxyphenyl) ethyl] methylamino] propyl] -3, 4- dimethoxy-α-(1-methylethyl) hydrochloride.
Verapamil HCl is an almost white, crystalline powder, practically free of odor, with a bitter taste. It is soluble in water, chloroform, and methanol. Verapamil HCl is not chemically related to other antiarrhythmic drugs.

Clinical Pharmacology:
Mechanism of Action: Calan (verapamil HCl) inhibits the calcium ion (and possibly sodium ion) influx through slow channels into conductile and contractile myocardial cells and vascular smooth muscle cells. The antiarrhythmic effect of Calan appears to be due to its effect on the slow channel in cells of the cardiac conductile system.
Electrical activity through the SA and AV nodes depends, to a significant degree, upon calcium influx through the slow channel. By inhibiting this influx, Calan slows AV conduction and prolongs the effective refractory period within the AV node in a rate-related manner, reducing elevated ventricular rate in patients with supraventricular tachycardia due to atrial flutter and/or atrial filbrillation. By interrupting reentry at the AV node, Calan can restore normal sinus rhythm in patients with paroxysmal supraventricular tachycardias (PSVT), including Wolff-Parkinson-White (W-P-W) syndrome. Calan has no effect on conduction across accessory bypass tracts. Calan does not alter the normal atrial action potential or intraventricular conduction time but depresses amplitude, velocity of depolarization, and conduction in depressed atrial fibers.
In the isolated rabbit heart, concentrations of Calan that markedly affect SA nodal fibers or fibers in the upper and middle regions of the AV node have very little effect on fibers in the lower AV node (NH region) and no effect on atrial action potentials or His bundle fibers.
Calan does not induce bronchoconstriction or peripheral arterial spasm.
Calan has a local anesthetic action that is 1.6 times that of procaine on an equimolar basis. It is not known whether this action is important at the doses used in man.
Calan does not alter total serum calcium levels.
Hemodynamics: In animals and man, Calan (verapamil HCl) reduces afterload and myocardial contractility. In most patients, including those with organic cardiac disease, the negative inotropic action of Calan is countered by reduction of afterload, and cardiac index is usually not reduced, but in patients with moderately severe to severe cardiac dysfunction (pulmonary wedge pressure above 20 mm Hg, ejection fraction less than 20%), acute worsening of heart failure may be seen. Peak therapeutic effects occur within 3 to 5 minutes after a bolus injection. The commonly used intravenous doses of 5-10 mg Calan produce transient, usually asymptomatic, reduction in normal systemic arterial pressure, systemic vascular resistance and contractility; left ventricular filling pressure is slightly increased.
Pharmacokinetics: Intravenously administered Calan (verapamil HCl) has been shown to be rapidly metabolized in both humans and animals. Following intravenous infusion in man, verapamil is eliminated bi-exponentially, with a rapid early distribution phase (half-life, about 4 minutes) and a slower terminal elimination phase (half-life, 2-5 hours). In healthy men, orally administered Calan undergoes extensive metabolism in the liver, with 12 metabolites having been identified, most in only trace amounts. The major metabolites have been identified as various N- and O-dealkylated products of Calan. Approximately 70% of an administered dose is excreted in the urine and 16% or more in the feces within 5 days. About 3% to 4% is excreted as unchanged drug.

Indications and Usage: Calan (verapamil HCl) is indicated for the treatment of supraventricular tachyarrhythmias, including:

- Rapid conversion to sinus rhythm of paroxysmal supraventricular tachycardias, including those associated with accessory bypass tracts (Wolff-Parkinson-White [W-P-W] and Lown-Ganong-Levine [L-G-L] syndromes). When clinically advisable, appropriate vagal maneuvers (eg, Valsalva maneuver) should be attempted prior to Calan administration.
- Temporary control of rapid ventricular rate in atrial flutter or atrial fibrillation.

In controlled studies in the United States, about 60% of patients with supraventricular tachycardia converted to normal sinus rhythm within 10 minutes after intravenous verapamil HCl. Uncontrolled studies reported in the world literature describe a conversion rate of about 80%. About 70% of patients with atrial flutter and/or fibrillation with a fast ventricular rate respond with a decrease in heart rate of at least 20%. Conversion of atrial flutter or fibrillation to sinus rhythm is uncommon (about 10%) after verapamil HCl and may reflect the spontaneous conversion rate, since the conversion rate after placebo was similar. The effect of a single injection lasts for 30-60 minutes when conversion to sinus rhythm does not occur.
Because a small fraction (< 1.0%) of patients treated with verapamil HCl respond with life-threatening adverse responses (rapid ventricular rate in atrial flutter/fibrillation, marked hypotension, or extreme bradycardia/asystole—see *Warnings*), the initial use of intravenous verapamil HCl should, if possible, be in a treatment setting with monitoring and resuscitation facilities, including D.C.-cardioversion capability. As familiarity with the patient's response is gained, an office setting would be acceptable.

Contraindications:
Verapamil HCl is contraindicated in:
1. Severe hypotension or cardiogenic shock
2. Second- or third-degree AV block
3. Sick sinus syndrome (except in patients with a functioning artificial ventricular pacemaker)
4. Severe congestive heart failure (unless secondary to a supraventricular tachycardia amenable to verapamil therapy)
5. Patients receiving **intravenous** beta-adrenergic blocking drugs (eg, propranolol). **Intravenous** verapamil and **intravenous** beta-adrenergic blocking drugs should not be administered in close proximity to each other (within a few hours), since both may have a depressant effect on myocardial contractility and AV conduction.

Warnings:
CALAN SHOULD BE GIVEN AS A SLOW INTRAVENOUS INJECTION OVER AT LEAST A TWO-MINUTE PERIOD OF TIME. (See *Dosage and Administration.*)
Hypotension: Intravenous verapamil often produces a decrease in blood pressure below baseline levels that is usually transient and asymptomatic but may result in dizziness. Systolic pressure less than 90 mm Hg and/or diastolic pressure less than 60 mm Hg was seen in 5%-10% of patients in controlled U.S. trials in supraventricular tachycardia and in about 10% of the patients with atrial flutter/fibrillation. The incidence of symptomatic hypotension observed in studies conducted in the U.S. was approximately 1.5%. Three of the five symptomatic patients required pharmacologic treatment (levarterenol [norepinephrine] bitartrate IV, metaraminol bitartrate IV, or 10% calcium gluconate IV). All recovered without sequelae.
Rapid Ventricular Response in Atrial Flutter/Fibrillation: Patients with atrial flutter/fibrillation and an accessory AV pathway (eg, Wolff-Parkinson-White or Lown-Ganong-Levine syndromes) may develop increased antegrade conduction across the aberrant pathway bypassing the AV node, producing a very rapid ventricular response after receiving verapamil (or digitalis). This has been reported in 1% of the patients treated in controlled double-blind trials in the U.S. Treatment is usually D.C.-cardioversion. Cardioversion has been used safely and effectively after intravenous Calan. (See *Adverse Reactions* including suggested treatment of adverse reactions.)
Extreme Bradycardia/Asystole: Verapamil slows conduction across the AV node and rarely may produce second- or third-degree AV block, bradycardia, and, in extreme cases, asystole. This is more likely to occur in patients with a sick sinus syndrome (SA nodal disease), which is more common in older patients. Bradycardia associated with sick sinus syndrome was reported in 0.3% of the patients treated in controlled double-blind trials in the U.S. The total incidence of bradycardia (ventricular rate less than 60 beats/min) was 1.2% in these studies. Asystole in patients other than those with sick sinus syndrome is usually of short duration (few seconds or less), with spontaneous return to AV nodal or normal sinus rhythm. If this does not occur promptly, appropriate treatment should be initiated immediately. (See *Adverse Reactions* including suggested treatment of adverse reactions.)
Heart Failure: When heart failure is not severe or rate related, it should be controlled with optimum digitalization and diuretics, as appropriate, before Calan is used.
In patients with moderately severe to severe cardiac dysfunction (pulmonary wedge pressure above 20 mm Hg, ejection fraction less than 20%), acute worsening of heart failure may be seen.
Concomitant Antiarrhythmic Therapy:
Digitalis
Intravenous verapamil has been used concomitantly with digitalis preparations without the occurrence of serious adverse effects. However, since both drugs slow AV conduction, patients should be monitored for AV block or excessive bradycardia.
Quinidine—Procainamide
Intravenous verapamil has been administered to a small number of patients receiv-

ing oral quinidine and oral procainamide without the occurrence of serious adverse effects.

Beta-Adrenergic Blocking Drugs
Intravenous verapamil has been administered to patients receiving **oral** beta blockers without the development of serious adverse effects. However, since both drugs may depress myocardial contractility or AV conduction, these possibilities should be considered. On rare occasions, the concomitant administration of **intravenous** beta blockers and **intravenous** verapamil has resulted in serious adverse reactions (see *Contraindications*), especially in patients with severe cardiomyopathy, congestive heart failure, or recent myocardial infarction.

Disopyramide
Until data on possible interactions between verapamil and all forms of disopyramide phosphate are obtained, disopyramide should not be administered within 48 hours before or 24 hours after verapamil administration.

Heart Block: Calan prolongs AV conduction time. While high-degree AV block has not been observed in controlled clinical trials in the U.S., a low percentage (less than 0.5%) has been reported in the world literature. Development of second- or third-degree AV block or unifascicular, bifascicular, or trifascicular bundle branch block requires reduction in subsequent doses or discontinuation of verapamil and institution of appropriate therapy, if needed. (See *Adverse Reactions* and *Concomitant Antiarrhythmic Therapy.*)

Hepatic and Renal Failure: Significant hepatic and renal failure should not increase the effects of a single intravenous dose of Calan but may prolong its duration. Repeated injections of intravenous Calan in such patients may lead to accumulation and an excessive pharmacologic effect of the drug. There is no experience to guide use of multiple doses in such patients, and this generally should be avoided. If repeated injections are essential, blood pressure and PR interval should be closely monitored and smaller repeat doses should be utilized. Data on the clearance of verapamil by dialysis are not yet available.

Premature Ventricular Contractions: During conversion to normal sinus rhythm or marked reduction in ventricular rate, a few benign complexes of unusual appearance (sometimes resembling premature ventricular contractions) may be seen after treatment with verapamil. Similar complexes are seen during spontaneous conversion of supraventricular tachycardia, after D.C.-cardioversion and other pharmacologic therapy. These complexes appear to have no clinical significance.

Precautions:

Drug Interactions: (See *Warnings: Concomitant Antiarrhythmic Therapy.*) Intravenous verapamil has been used concomitantly with other cardioactive drugs (especially digitalis and quinidine) without evidence of serious negative drug interactions, except, in rare instances, when patients with severe cardiomyopathy, congestive heart failure, or recent myocardial infarction were given **intravenous** beta-adrenergic blocking agents or disopyramide. Drug interaction studies are ongoing. As verapamil is highly bound to plasma proteins, it should be administered with caution to patients receiving other highly protein-bound drugs.

Pregnancy: Pregnancy Category B. Reproduction studies have been performed in rats and rabbits. At doses up to 2.5 and 1.5 times the human **oral** dose, respectively, no evidence of impaired fertility or harm to the fetus due to verapamil was revealed. There are, however, no adequate and well-controlled studies in pregnant women. Because animal reproduction studies are not always predictive of human response, this drug should be used during pregnancy only if clearly needed.

Labor and Delivery: There have been few controlled studies to determine whether the use of verapamil during labor or delivery has immediate or delayed adverse effects on the fetus, or whether it prolongs the duration of labor or increases the need for forceps delivery or other obstetric intervention. Such adverse experiences have not been reported in the literature, despite a long history of use of intravenous Calan in Europe in the treatment of cardiac side effects of beta-adrenergic agonist agents used to treat premature labor.

Nursing Mothers: It is not known whether this drug is excreted in human milk. Because many drugs are excreted in human milk and because of the potential for adverse reactions in nursing infants from verapamil, nursing should be discontinued while verapamil is administered.

Pediatrics: Controlled studies with verapamil have not been conducted in pediatric patients, but uncontrolled experience with intravenous administration in more than 250 patients, about half under 12 months of age and about 25% newborn, indicates that results of treatment are similar to those in adults. The most commonly used single doses in patients up to 12 months of age have ranged from 0.1 to 0.2 mg/kg of body weight, while in patients aged 1 to 15 years, the most commonly used single doses ranged from 0.1 to 0.3 mg/kg of body weight. Most of the patients received the lower dose of 0.1 mg/kg once, but in some cases, the dose was repeated once or twice every 10 to 30 minutes.

Adverse Reactions: The following reactions were reported with intravenous verapamil use in controlled U.S. clinical trials involving 324 patients:

Cardiovascular: Symptomatic hypotension (1.5%); bradycardia (1.2%); severe tachycardia (1.0%). The worldwide experience in open clinical trials in more than 7,900 patients was similar.

Central Nervous System Effects: Dizziness (1.2%); headache (1.2%).

Gastrointestinal: Nausea (0.9%); abdominal discomfort (0.6%).

The following reactions were reported in single patients: emotional depression, rotary nystagmus, sleepiness, vertigo, muscle fatigue, or diaphoresis.

Suggested Treatment of Acute Cardiovascular Adverse Reactions*

The frequency of these adverse reactions was quite low, and experience with their treatment has been limited.

(See table below)

Overdosage: Treatment of overdosage should be supportive. Beta-adrenergic stimulation or parenteral administration of calcium solutions may increase calcium ion flux across the slow channel. These pharmacologic interventions have been effectively used in treatment of deliberate overdosage with oral verapamil. Clinically significant hypotensive reactions or high-degree AV block should be treated with vasopressor agents or cardiac pacing, respectively. Asystole should be handled by the usual measures including isoproterenol hydrochloride, other vasopressor agents, or cardiopulmonary resuscitation (see *Suggested Treatment of Acute Cardiovascular Adverse Reactions*).

Dosage and Administration: For intravenous use only. The recommended intravenous doses of Calan (verapamil HCl) are as follows:

ADULT:

Initial dose—5-10 mg (0.075–0.15 mg/kg body weight) given as an intravenous bolus over 2 minutes.

Repeat dose—10 mg (0.15 mg/kg body weight) 30 minutes after the first dose if the initial response is not adequate.

Older Patients—The dose should be administered over at least 3 minutes to minimize the risk of untoward drug effects.

PEDIATRIC:

Initial dose

0-1 year: 0.1–0.2 mg/kg body weight (usual single dose range: 0.75–2 mg) should be administered as an intravenous bolus over 2 minutes (*under continuous ECG monitoring*).

1-15 years: 0.1–0.3 mg/kg body weight (usual single dose range: 2–5 mg) should be administered as an intravenous bolus over 2 minutes. *Do not exceed 5 mg.*

Repeat dose

0-1 year: 0.1–0.2 mg/kg body weight (usual single dose range: 0.75–2 mg) 30 minutes after the first dose if the initial response is not adequate (*under continuous ECG monitoring*).

1-15 years: 0.1–0.3 mg/kg body weight (usual single dose range: 2-5 mg) 30 minutes after the first dose if the initial re-

Adverse Reaction	Proven Effective Treatment	Treatment With Good Theoretical Rationale	Supportive Treatment
1. Symptomatic hypotension requiring treatment	Norepinephrine bitartrate IV Metaraminol bitartrate IV Isoproterenol HCl IV	Dopamine HCl IV Dobutamine HCl IV	Intravenous fluids Trendelenburg position
2. Bradycardia, AV block, Asystole	Isoproterenol HCl IV Norepinephrine bitartrate IV Atropine sulfate IV Cardiac pacing	. . .	Intravenous fluids (slow drip)
3. Rapid ventricular rate (due to antegrade conduction in flutter/fibrillation with W-P-W or L-G-L syndromes)	D.C.-cardioversion (high energy may be required) Procainamide IV Lidocaine HCl IV	. . .	Intravenous fluids (slow drip)

*Actual treatment and dosage should depend on the severity of the clinical situation and the judgment and experience of the treating physician.

Continued on next page

Searle Pharm.—Cont.

sponse is not adequate. *Do not exceed 10 mg as a single dose.*

NOTE: Parenteral drug products should be inspected visually for particulate matter and discoloration prior to administration, whenever solution and container permit.

How Supplied: Calan is supplied in 2-ml, individually packaged ampuls in cartons of 10. Each milliliter contains verapamil hydrochloride 2.5 mg, and sodium chloride 8.5 mg.

Store at 59° to 86° F (15° to 30° C) and protect from light.

[*Shown in Product Identification Section*]

CALAN® Tablets ℞
(verapamil hydrochloride)

Description: Calan (verapamil HCl) is a calcium ion influx inhibitor (slow-channel blocker or calcium ion antagonist) available for oral administration in sugar-coated tablets containing 80 mg or 120 mg of verapamil hydrochloride.

Verapamil hydrochloride is benzeneacetonitrile, α -[3- [[2- (3, 4-dimethoxyphenyl) ethyl] methylamino] propyl] -3, 4- dimethoxy-α -(1-methylethyl) hydrochloride.

Verapamil HCl is an almost-white, crystalline powder, practically free of odor, with a bitter taste. It is a soluble in water, chloroform, and methanol. Verapamil HCl is not chemically related to other cardioactive drugs.

Clinical Pharmacology: Calan is a calcium ion influx inhibitor (slow-channel blocker or calcium ion antagonist) that exerts its pharmacologic effects by modulating the influx of ionic calcium across the cell membrane of the arterial smooth muscle as well as in conductile and contractile myocardial cells.

Mechanism of action: The precise mechanism of action of Calan as an antianginal agent remains to be fully determined, but includes the following two mechanisms:

1. *Relaxation and prevention of coronary artery spasm:* Calan dilates the main coronary arteries and coronary arterioles, both in normal and ischemic regions, and is a potent inhibitor of coronary artery spasm, whether spontaneous or ergonovine-induced. This property increases myocardial oxygen delivery in patients with coronary artery spasm and is responsible for the effectiveness of Calan in vasospastic (Prinzmetal's or variant) as well as unstable angina at rest. Whether this effect plays any role in classical effort angina is not clear, but studies of exercise tolerance have not shown an increase in the maximum exercise rate–pressure product, a widely accepted measure of oxygen utilization. This suggests that, in general, relief of spasm or dilation of coronary arteries is not an important factor in classical angina.
2. *Reduction of oxygen utilization:* Calan regularly reduces arterial pressure at rest and at a given level of exercise by dilating peripheral arterioles and reducing the total peripheral resistance (afterload) against which the heart works. This unloading of the heart reduces myocardial energy consumption and oxygen requirements and probably accounts for the effectiveness of Calan in chronic stable effort angina.

Electrical activity through the SA and AV nodes depends, to a significant degree, on calcium influx through the slow channel. By inhibiting this influx, Calan slows AV conduction and prolongs the effective refractory period within the AV node in a rate-related manner. It can interfere with sinus node impulse generation and induce sinus arrest in patients with sick sinus syndrome; it also can induce atrioventricular block, although this has been seen rarely in clinical use. Calan may shorten the antegrade effective refractory period of the accessory bypass tracts. Calan does not alter the normal atrial action potential or intraventricular conduction time, but depresses amplitude, velocity of depolarization, and conduction in depressed atrial fibers.

Calan (verapamil HCl) has a local anesthetic action that is 1.6 times that of procaine on an equimolar basis. It is not known whether this action is important at the doses used in man.

Calan does not alter total serum calcium levels.

Pharmacokinetics and metabolism: More than 90% of the orally administered dose of Calan is absorbed. Because of rapid biotransformation of verapamil during its first pass through the portal circulation, absolute bioavailability ranges from 20% to 35%. Peak plasma concentrations are reached between 1 and 2 hours after oral administration. Chronic oral administration of 120 mg of verapamil every 6 hours resulted in plasma levels of verapamil ranging from 125 to 400 ng/ml, with higher values reported occasionally. A close relationship exists between verapamil plasma concentration and prolongation of the PR interval. The mean elimination half-life in single-dose studies ranged from 2.8 to 7.4 hours. In these same studies, after repetitive dosing, the half-life increased to a range from 4.5 to 12.0 hours (after less than 10 consecutive doses given 6 hours apart). Half-life may increase during titration due to saturation of hepatic enzyme systems as plasma verapamil levels rise. A linear correlation seems to exist between the verapamil dose administered and verapamil plasma levels.

Verapamil is highly bound to plasma proteins. In healthy men, orally administered Calan undergoes extensive metabolism in the liver. Twelve metabolites have been identified in plasma; all except norverapamil are present in trace amounts only. Norverapamil can reach steady-state plasma concentrations approximately equal to those of verapamil itself. The major metabolites of verapamil have been identified as various N- and O-dealkylated products of verapamil. Approximately 70% of an administered dose is excreted as metabolites in the urine and 16% or more in the feces within 5 days. About 3% to 4% is excreted in the urine as unchanged drug. Approximately 90% is bound to plasma proteins. In patients with hepatic insufficiency, metabolism is delayed and elimination half-life prolonged up to 14 to 16 hours (see *Precautions*); the volume of distribution is increased and plasma clearance reduced to about 30% of normal. Verapamil clearance values suggest that patients with liver dysfunction may attain therapeutic verapamil plasma concentrations with one third of the oral daily dose required for patients with normal liver function.

Hemodynamics and myocardial metabolism: In animals and man, Calan (verapamil HCl) reduces afterload and myocardial contractility. In most patients, including those with organic cardiac disease, the negative inotropic action of Calan is countered by reduction of afterload, and cardiac index is usually not reduced. However, in patients with severe left ventricular dysfunction (eg, pulmonary wedge pressure above 20 mm Hg or ejection fraction less than 30%), or in patients taking beta-adrenergic blocking agents, or other cardiodepressant drugs, deterioration of ventricular function may occur (see *Drug interactions*).

Pulmonary function: Calan does not induce bronchoconstriction and, hence, does not impair ventilatory function.

Indications and Usage: Calan tablets are indicated for the treatment of angina pectoris, including:

1. Angina at rest, including:
   - Vasospastic (Prinzmetal's variant) angina
   - Unstable (crescendo, preinfarction) angina
2. Chronic stable angina (classic effort-associated angina)

Contraindications: Verapamil HCl is contraindicated in:

1. Severe left ventricular dysfunction (see *Warnings*)
2. Hypotension (systolic pressure less than 90 mm Hg) or cardiogenic shock
3. Sick sinus syndrome (except in patients with a functioning artificial ventricular pacemaker)
4. Second- or third-degree AV block

Warnings: Heart failure: Verapamil has a negative inotropic effect, which in most patients is compensated by its afterload reduction (decreased peripheral vascular resistance) properties without a net impairment of ventricular performance. In clinical studies involving 1,166 patients, 11 (0.9%) developed congestive heart failure or pulmonary edema. Congestive heart failure/pulmonary edema led to discontinuation or reduction of dosage of verapamil in 6 patients (0.5%). Verapamil should be avoided in patients with severe left ventricular dysfunction (eg, ejection fraction less than 30%) or moderate to severe symptoms of cardiac failure and in patients with any degree of ventricular dysfunction if they are receiving a beta-blocker (see *Drug interactions*). Patients with milder ventricular dysfunction should, if possible, be controlled with optimum doses of digitalis and/or diuretics before verapamil treatment. **(Note interactions with digoxin under *Precautions.*)**

Hypotension: Occasionally, the pharmacologic action of verapamil may produce a decrease in blood pressure below normal levels, which may result in dizziness or symptomatic hypotension. Hypotension is usually asymptomatic, orthostatic, mild, and can be controlled by a decrease in the Calan (verapamil HCl) dose. The incidence of hypotension observed in 1,166 patients enrolled in clinical trials was 2.9%.

Elevated liver enzymes: Occasional elevations of transaminase and alkaline phosphatase have been reported. Two patients had marked elevations of transaminase with recurrent elevation upon rechallenge with verapamil. Although liver biopsies were not performed, the potential for hepatocellular-type injury with verapamil appears to exist. Worldwide experience has not revealed similar cases, and the incidence of this injury is not known. Patients receiving verapamil should have liver enzyme levels monitored periodically.

Atrial flutter/fibrillation with accessory bypass tract: Patients with atrial flutter and/or fibrillation and an accessory AV pathway (eg, Wolff-Parkinson-White or Lown-Ganong-Levine syndromes) may develop increased antegrade conduction across the aberrant pathway bypassing the AV node, producing a very rapid ventricular response after receiving verapamil (or digitalis). Treatment is usually D.C.-cardioversion. Cardioversion has been used safely and effectively after oral Calan.

Atrioventricular block: The effect of verapamil on AV conduction and the SA node leads to first-degree AV block and transient bradycardia, sometimes accompanied by nodal escape rhythms, fairly commonly during the peaks of serum concentration. Higher degrees of AV block, however, were infrequently observed (0.8%). Marked first-degree block or progressive development to second- or third-degree AV block requires a reduction in dosage or, in rare instances, discontinuation of verapamil HCl and institution of appropriate therapy, depending on the clinical situation.

Patients with hypertrophic cardiomyopathy (IHSS): In 120 patients with hypertrophic cardiomyopathy (most of them refractory or intolerant to propranolol) who received therapy with verapamil at doses up to 720 mg/day, a variety of serious adverse effects was seen. Three patients died in pulmonary edema; all had a past history of severe left ventricular outflow obstruction and left ventricular dysfunction. Eight other patients had pulmonary edema and/or severe hypotension; abnormally high (greater than 20 mm Hg) pulmonary wedge pressure and a marked left ventricular outflow obstruction were present in most of these patients. Concomitant administration of quinidine preceded the severe hypotension in 3 of the 8 patients (2 of whom developed pulmonary edema). Sinus bradycardia occurred in 11% of the patients, second-degree AV block in 4%, and sinus arrest in 2%. It must be appreciated that this group of patients had a serious disease with a high mortality rate. Most adverse effects responded well to dose reduction, and only rarely did verapamil use have to be discontinued.

Precautions:

General

Use in patients with impaired hepatic function: Since verapamil is highly metabolized by the liver, it should be administered cautiously to patients with impaired hepatic function. Severe liver dysfunction prolongs the elimination half-life of verapamil to about 14 to 16 hours; hence, approximately 30% of the dose given to patients with normal liver function should be administered to these patients. Careful monitoring for abnormal prolongation of the PR interval or other signs of excessive pharmacologic effects (see *Overdosage*) should be carried out.

Use in patients with impaired renal function: About 70% of an administered dose of verapamil is excreted as metabolites in the urine. Until further data are available, verapamil should be administered cautiously to patients with impaired renal function. These patients should be carefully monitored for abnormal prolongation of the PR interval or other signs of overdosage (see *Overdosage*).

Drug interactions

Beta-blockers: Controlled studies in small numbers of patients suggest that the concomitant use of Calan (verapamil HCl) and beta-blocking agents may be beneficial in patients with chronic stable angina, but available information is not sufficient to predict with confidence the effects of concurrent treatment, especially in patients with left ventricular dysfunction or cardiac conduction abnormalities. The combination can have adverse effects on cardiac function. In one study involving 15 patients treated with high doses of propranolol (median dose, 480 mg/day; range, 160 to 1,280 mg/day) for severe angina, with preserved left ventricular function (ejection fraction greater than 35%), the hemodynamic effects of additional therapy with verapamil HCl were assessed using invasive methods. The addition of verapamil to high-dose beta-blockers induced modest negative inotropic and chronotropic effects that were not severe enough to limit short-term (48 hours) combination therapy in this study. These modest cardiodepressant effects persisted for greater than 6 but less than 30 hours after abrupt withdrawal of beta-blockers and were closely related to plasma levels of propranolol. The primary verapamil/beta-blocker interaction in this study appeared to be hemodynamic rather than electrophysiologic.

In 3 other studies involving 51 patients, verapamil did not induce negative inotropic or chronotropic effects in patients with preserved left ventricular function receiving low or moderate doses of propranolol (less than or equal to 320 mg/day). Because of the still limited experience with combination therapy, verapamil should be used alone, if possible. If combined therapy is used, close surveillance of vital signs and clinical status should be carried out and the need for concomitant treatment with propranolol reassessed periodically. Combined therapy should usually be avoided in patients with atrioventricular conduction abnormalities and those with depressed left ventricular function.

Digitalis: Chronic verapamil treatment increases serum digoxin levels by 50% to 70% during the first week of therapy, and this can result in digitalis toxicity. Maintenance digitalization doses should be reduced when verapamil is administered and the patient should be carefully monitored to avoid over- or underdigitalization. Whenever overdigitalization is suspected, the daily dose of digoxin should be reduced or temporarily discontinued. On discontinuation of Calan (verapamil HCl) use, the patient should be monitored to avoid underdigitalization.

Antihypertensive agents: Verapamil administered concomitantly with oral antihypertensive agents (eg, vasodilators, diuretics) may have an additive effect on lowering blood pressure. Patients receiving these combinations should be appropriately monitored. In patients who have recently received drugs such as methyldopa, which attenuate alpha-adrenergic response, combined therapy of verapamil and propranolol should probably be avoided (severe hypotension may occur).

Disopyramide: Until data on possible interactions between verapamil and disopyramide are obtained, disopyramide should not be administered within 48 hours before or 24 hours after verapamil administration.

Quinidine: In a small number of patients with hypertrophic cardiomyopathy (IHSS), concomitant use of verapamil and quinidine resulted in significant hypotension. Until further data are obtained, combined therapy of verapamil and quinidine in patients with hypertrophic cardiomyopathy should probably be avoided.

Nitrates: Verapamil has been given concomitantly with short- and long-acting nitrates without any undesirable drug interactions. The pharmacologic profile of both drugs and the clinical experience suggest beneficial interactions.

Carcinogenesis, mutagenesis, impairment of fertility: Adequate animal carcinogenicity studies have not been performed with verapamil. An 18-month toxicity study in rats, at a low multiple (6-fold) of the maximum recommended human dose, and not the maximum tolerated dose, did not suggest a tumorigenic potential. A 2-year carcinogenicity study will be carried out in rats.

Verapamil was not mutagenic in the Ames test in 5 test strains at 3 mg per plate with or without metabolic activation.

Studies in female rats at daily dietary doses up to 5.5 times (55 mg/kg/day) the maximum recommended human dose did not show impaired fertility. Effects on male fertility have not been determined.

Pregnancy: Pregnancy Category C. Reproduction studies have been performed in rabbits and rats at oral doses up to 1.5 (15 mg/kg/day) and 6 (60 mg/kg/day) times the human oral daily dose, respectively, and have revealed no evidence of teratogenicity. In the rat, however, this multiple of the human dose was embryocidal and retarded fetal growth and development, probably because of adverse maternal effects reflected in reduced weight gains of the dams. This oral dose has also been shown to cause hypotension in rats. There are no adequate and well-controlled studies in pregnant women. Because animal reproduction studies are not always predictive of human response, this drug should be used during pregnancy only if clearly needed.

Labor and delivery: It is not known whether the use of verapamil during labor or delivery has immediate or delayed adverse effects on the fetus, or whether it prolongs the duration of labor or increases the need for forceps delivery or other obstetric intervention. Such adverse experiences have not been reported in the literature, despite a long history of use of verapamil in Europe in the treatment of cardiac side effects of beta-adrenergic agonist agents used to treat premature labor.

Nursing mothers: It is not known whether this drug is excreted in human milk. Because many drugs are excreted in human milk and because of the potential for adverse reactions in nursing infants from verapamil, nursing should be discontinued while verapamil is administered. Studies in rats at 2.5 times the maximum recommended human dose revealed no evidence of an effect of verapamil on lactation or weaning.

Animal pharmacology and/or animal toxicology: Chronic animal toxicology studies indicate that verapamil causes lenticular and/or suture line changes at 30 mg/kg/day or greater, and frank cataracts at 62.5 mg/kg/day or greater in the beagle dog but not in the rat. These effects are thought to be species specific. Development of cataracts due to verapamil has not been reported in man.

Adverse Reactions: Serious adverse reactions are rare when Calan (verapamil HCl) therapy is initiated with upward dose titration within the recommended single and total daily dose. The following reactions to orally administered verapamil were reported from clinical studies involving 1,166 patients with angina or arrhythmia.

Adverse reactions occurred at a similar rate in controlled clinical trials and uncontrolled clinical experience.

Cardiovascular: Hypotension (2.9%), peripheral edema (1.7%), AV block: third-degree (0.8%), bradycardia: HR <50/min (1.1%), CHF or pulmonary edema (0.9%).

Central nervous system: Dizziness (3.6%), headache (1.8%), fatigue (1.1%).

Gastrointestinal: Constipation (6.3%), nausea (1.6%).

The following reactions, reported in less than 0.5% of patients, occurred under circumstances where a causal relationship is not certain, and are therefore mentioned to alert the physician to a possible relationship: confusion, paresthesia, insomnia, somnolence, equilibrium disorders, blurred vision, syncope, muscle cramps, shakiness, claudication, hair loss, macular eruptions, and spotty menstruation.

In addition, more serious adverse events were observed, not readily distinguishable from the natural history of the disease in these patients. Of the 1,166 patients evaluated, 16 (1.4%) had myocardial infarctions. Nine of these 16 patients had myocardial infarctions while being treated for unstable angina, 4 of these were receiving placebo, the remaining 5 received verapamil.

The daily dose of verapamil was reduced in 6.3% and discontinued in 5.5% of the 1,166 patients. In general, the highest incidence of adverse reactions was seen in the dose-titration periods in all the studies.

Treatment of acute cardiovascular adverse reactions: The frequency of cardiovascular adverse reactions that require therapy is rare; hence, experience with their treatment is limited. Whenever severe hypotension or complete AV block occur following oral administration of verapamil, the appropriate emergency measures should be applied immediately; eg, intravenously administered isoproterenol HCl, norepinephrine bitartrate, atropine sulfate (all in the usual doses), or calcium gluconate (10% solution). In patients with hypertrophic cardiomyopathy (IHSS), alpha-adrenergic agents (phenylephrine HCl, metaraminol bitartrate, or methoxamine HCl) should be used to maintain blood pressure and isoproterenol and norepinephrine should be avoided. If further support is necessary, dopamine HCl or dobutamine HCl may be administered. Actual treatment and dosage should depend on the severity of the clinical situation and the judgment and experience of the treating physician.

Overdosage: Treatment of overdosage should be supportive. Beta-adrenergic stimulation or parenteral administration of calcium solutions may increase calcium ion flux across the slow channel, and have been used effec-

Continued on next page

Searle Pharm.—Cont.

tively in treatment of deliberate overdosage with verapamil. Clinically significant hypotensive reactions or fixed high-degree AV block should be treated with vasopressor agents or cardiac pacing, respectively. Asystole should be handled by the usual measures, including cardiopulmonary resuscitation.

Dosage and Administration: The dose of verapamil must be individualized by titration. Calan (verapamil HCl) is available in 80-mg and 120-mg tablets. The usual initial dose is 80 mg every 6 to 8 hours. Dosage may be increased at daily (eg, patients with unstable angina) or weekly intervals until optimum clinical response is obtained. In general, maximum effects of any given dosage would be apparent during the first 24 to 48 hours of therapy, but note that between 24 and 48 hours, the half-life of verapamil increases; therefore, the maximum response may be delayed. The total daily dose ranges from 240 to 480 mg. The optimum daily dose for most patients ranges from 320 to 480 mg. The usefulness and safety of dosages exceeding 480 mg/day in angina pectoris have not been established.

How Supplied:

Calan 80-mg tablets are round, yellow, sugar coated, with Calan 80 imprinted on one side, supplied as:

NDC Number	Size
0025-1851-31	bottle of 100
0025-1851-51	bottle of 500
0025-1851-34	carton of 100 unit dose

Calan 120-mg tablets are round, white, sugar coated, with Calan 120 imprinted on one side, supplied as:

NDC Number	Size
0025-1861-31	bottle of 100
0025-1861-51	bottle of 500
0025-1861-34	carton of 100 unit dose

Store at 59° to 86°F (15° to 30°C).

Manufactured for:
Searle Pharmaceuticals Inc.

[*Shown in Product Identification Section*]

CU-7® ℞
(intrauterine copper contraceptive)

Description: The plastic component of the Cu-7 is composed of pharmaceutical grade polypropylene homopolymer with barium sulfate added to render it radiopaque. Its shape approximates the number 7. It is substantially smaller than previously available intrauterine devices; the vertical dimension measures 36 mm and the horizontal, 26 mm.

Coiled around the vertical limb is 89 mg of copper wire providing approximately 200 mm^2 of exposed copper surface area. A retrieval thread is fastened to the free end of the vertical limb of the Cu-7.

The Cu-7 is supplied with a simple tubular plastic inserter. All components are sterile.

[*The following sections apply to both Cu-7 and Tatum-T.*]

Mode of Action: Available data indicate that the contraceptive effectiveness of the Cu-7 or Tatum-T is enhanced by a minute quantity of copper released continuously from the coiled copper into the uterine cavity.

The exact mechanism by which metallic copper enhances the contraceptive effect of an IUD has not been conclusively demonstrated. Various hypotheses have been advanced, the most common being that copper placed in the uterus interferes with enzymatic or other processes that regulate blastocyst implantation.

Animal studies suggest that copper may play an additional role by reduction of sperm transport within the uterine environment.

Indication and Usage: The Cu-7 or Tatum-T is indicated for contraception.

Contraindications: The Cu-7 or Tatum-T should not be inserted when any of the following conditions exist: pregnancy or suspicion of pregnancy; abnormalities of the uterus resulting in distortion of the uterine cavity; acute pelvic inflammatory disease, a history of repeated or recent pelvic inflammatory disease, or a history of severe pelvic inflammatory disease; genital actinomycosis; postpartum endometritis or infected abortion in the past three months; known or suspected uterine or cervical disease such as hyperplasia or carcinoma including unresolved, abnormal Pap test; vaginal bleeding of unknown etiology; untreated acute cervicitis until infection is controlled; diagnosed Wilson's disease; known or suspected allergy to copper; previous ectopic pregnancy; significant anemia; and valvular heart disease, leukemia, or use of chronic corticosteroid therapy because of the increased susceptibility to infection with certain microorganisms which may possibly be introduced at the time of an IUD insertion.

Warnings:

1. *Pregnancy:* (a) *Long-term effects.* The long-term effects on the offspring of the presence of copper in the uterus when pregnancy occurs with the Cu-7 or Tatum-T are unknown.

(b) *Septic abortion.* Reports have indicated an increased incidence of septic abortion associated in some instances with septicemia, septic shock and death in patients becoming pregnant with an IUD in place. Most of these reports have been associated with the mid-trimester of pregnancy. In some cases, the initial symptoms have been insidious and not easily recognized. If pregnancy should occur with a Cu-7 or Tatum-T in situ, the Cu-7 or Tatum-T should be removed if the thread is visible or, if removal proves to be or would be difficult, interruption of the pregnancy should be considered and offered to the patient as an option, bearing in mind that the risks associated with an elective abortion increase with gestational age.

(c) *Continuation of pregnancy.* If the patient chooses to continue the pregnancy and the Cu-7 or Tatum-T remains in situ, she must be warned of the increased risk of spontaneous abortion and the increased risk of sepsis, including death. The patient must be closely observed and she must be advised to report immediately all abnormal symptoms, such as flu-like syndrome, fever, abdominal cramping and pain, bleeding, or vaginal discharge, because generalized symptoms of septicemia may be insidious.

2. *Ectopic pregnancy:* (a) A pregnancy which occurs with an IUD in situ is more likely to be ectopic than a pregnancy occurring without an IUD. Therefore, patients who become pregnant while using a Cu-7 or Tatum-T should be carefully evaluated for the possibility of an ectopic pregnancy.

(b) Special attention should be directed to patients with delayed menses, slight metrorrhagia and/or unilateral pelvic pain, and to those patients who wish to interrupt a pregnancy occurring in the presence of a Cu-7 or Tatum-T, to determine whether ectopic pregnancy has occurred.

3. *Pelvic infection:* An increased risk of pelvic inflammatory disease associated with the use of IUDs has been reported. While unconfirmed, this risk appears to be greatest for young women who are nulliparous and/or who have a multiplicity of sexual partners. Salpingitis can result in tubal damage and occlusion, thereby threatening future fertility. Therefore, it is recommended that patients be taught to look for symptoms of pelvic inflammatory disease. The decision to use an IUD in a particular case must be made by the physician and patient with the consideration of a possible deleterious effect on future fertility.

Pelvic infection may occur with a Cu-7 or Tatum-T in situ and at times result in the development of tubo-ovarian abscesses or general peritonitis. The symptoms of pelvic infection include: new development of menstrual disorders (prolonged or heavy bleeding), abnormal vaginal discharge, abdominal or pelvic pain, dyspareunia, fever. The symptoms are especially significant if they occur following the first two or three cycles after insertion. Appropriate aerobic and anaerobic bacteriologic studies should be done and antibiotic therapy initiated promptly. If the infection does not show marked clinical improvement within 24 to 48 hours, the Cu-7 or Tatum-T should be removed and the continuing treatment reassessed on the basis of the results of culture and sensitivity tests. Genital actinomycosis has been associated primarily with long-term IUD use. It has been reported with the use of copper-bearing IUDs as well. Treatment requires prompt removal of the IUD and appropriate antibiotic therapy.

4. *Embedment:* Partial penetration or lodging of the Cu-7 or Tatum-T in the endometrium or myometrium can result in a difficult removal. This may occur more frequently in smaller uteri. (See removal instructions.)

5. *Perforation:* Partial or total perforation of the uterine wall or cervix may occur with the use of the Cu-7 or Tatum-T, usually during insertions into patients sooner than two months after abortion or delivery, or in uterine cavities too small for the Cu-7 or Tatum-T. The possibility of perforation must be kept in mind during insertion and at the time of any subsequent examination. If perforation occurs, laparotomy or laparoscopy should be performed as soon as medically feasible and the Cu-7 or Tatum-T removed. Abdominal adhesions, intestinal penetration, intestinal obstruction, and local inflammatory reaction with abscess formation and erosion of adjacent viscera may result if the Cu-7 or Tatum-T is left in the peritoneal cavity.

6. *Medical diathermy:* The use of medical diathermy (short-wave and microwave) in a patient with a metal-containing IUD may cause heat injury to the surrounding tissue. Therefore, medical diathermy to the abdominal and sacral areas should not be used on patients using a Cu-7 or Tatum-T.

7. *Effects of copper:* Additional amounts of copper available to the body from the Cu-7 or Tatum-T may precipitate symptoms in women with undiagnosed Wilson's disease. The incidence of Wilson's disease is 1 in 200,000.

Precautions:

1. *Patient counseling.* Prior to the insertion the physician, nurse, or other trained health professional must provide the patient with the Patient Brochure. The patient should be given the opportunity to read the brochure and discuss fully any questions she may have concerning the Cu-7 or Tatum-T as well as other methods of contraception.

2. *Patient evaluation and clinical considerations.* (a) A complete medical history should be obtained to determine conditions that might influence the selection of an IUD. A physical examination should include a pelvic examination, Pap test, gonorrhea culture, and, if indicated, appropriate tests for other forms of genital disease including genital actinomycosis, which usually can be detected by the Pap test. The physician should determine that the patient is not pregnant.

(b) The uterus should be carefully sounded prior to the insertion to determine the degree of patency of the endocervical canal and the internal os, and the direction and depth of the uterine cavity. Exercise care to avoid perforation with the sound. DO NOT USE THE Cu-7 OR Tatum-T INSERTION INSTRUMENT AS A SOUND. In occasional cases, severe cervical stenosis may be encountered. Do not use excessive force to overcome this resistance.

(c) The uterus usually sounds to a depth of 6 to 8 cm. Insertion of a Cu-7 or Tatum-T into a uterine cavity measuring less than 6.5 cm by sounding may increase the incidence of pain, bleeding, partial or complete expulsion, perforation, and possibly pregnancy.

(d) To reduce the possibility of insertion in the presence of an existing undetermined pregnancy, the optimal time for insertion is the latter part of the menstrual flow or one or two days thereafter. The Cu-7 or Tatum-T should not be inserted post partum or post abortion until involution of the uterus is complete. The incidence of perforation and expulsion is greater if involution is not complete.

It is, however, necessary to place the Cu-7 or Tatum-T as high as possible within the uterine cavity to help avoid partial or complete expulsion that could result in pregnancy.

Since the Cu-7 or Tatum-T represents a different design in intrauterine contraception, physicians are cautioned that it is imperative for them to become thoroughly familiar with the instructions for use before attempting placement of the Cu-7 or Tatum-T.

(e) IUDs should be used with caution in those patients who have an anemia or a history of menorrhagia or hypermenorrhea. Patients experiencing menorrhagia and/or metrorrhagia following IUD insertion may be at risk for the development of hypochromic microcytic anemia. Also, IUDs should be used with caution in patients receiving anticoagulants or having a coagulopathy.

(f) Syncope, bradycardia or other neurovascular episodes may occur during insertion or removal of IUDs, especially in patients with a previous disposition to these conditions.

(g) Patients with valvular or congenital heart disease are more prone to develop subacute bacterial endocarditis than patients who do not have valvular or congenital heart disease. Use of an IUD in these patients may represent a potential source of septic emboli. See *Contraindications.*

(h) Use of an IUD in those patients with acute cervicitis should be postponed until proper treatment has cleared up the infection.

(i) Since the Cu-7 or Tatum-T may be partially or completely expelled, patients should be reexamined and evaluated shortly after the first postinsertion menses, but definitely within three months after insertion. Thereafter annual examination with appropriate medical and laboratory evluation, and a Pap test, including examination for *Actinomyces* organisms, should be carried out. The Cu-7 or Tatum-T should be replaced every three years.

(j) The patient should be told that some bleeding or cramping may occur during the first few weeks after insertion, but if these symptoms continue or are severe she should report them to her physician. She should be instructed on how to check after each menstrual period to make certain that the thread still protrudes from the cervix and cautioned that there is no contraceptive protection if the Cu-7 or Tatum-T has been expelled. She should also be cautioned not to dislodge the Cu-7 or Tatum-T by pulling on the thread. If a partial expulsion occurs, removal is indicated and a new Cu-7 or Tatum-T may be inserted. The patient should be told to return within three years for removal of the Cu-7 or Tatum-T and for replacement if desired.

(k) A copper-induced urticarial allergic skin reaction may develop in women using a copper-containing IUD. If symptoms of such an allergic response occur, the patient should be instructed to tell the consulting physician that a copper-containing device is being used.

(l) The Cu-7 or Tatum-T should be removed for the following medical reasons: menorrhagia and/or metrorrhagia producing significant anemia; uncontrolled pelvic infection; genital actinomycosis; intractable pain often aggravated by intercourse, dyspareunia; pregnancy, if the thread is visible; endometrial or cervical malignancy; uterine or cervical perforation; or any indication of partial expulsion.

(m) If the retrieval thread cannot be visualized it may have retracted into the uterus or have been broken off, or the Cu-7 or Tatum-T may have been expelled. Localization usually can be made by feeling with a probe; if not, x-ray or sonography can be used. When the physician elects to recover a Cu-7 or Tatum-T with the thread not visible, the removal instructions should be considered.

(n) If any patient with a Cu-7 or Tatum-T suddenly develops overt clinical hepatitis or abnormal liver function tests, appropriate diagnostic procedures should be initiated.

(o) It has been reported that IUDs may be less effective in insulin-dependent diabetics.

Adverse Reactions: Perforations of uterus and cervix have occurred. Perforation into the abdomen has been followed by abdominal adhesions, intestinal penetration, intestinal obstruction, local inflammatory reaction with abscess formation and erosion of adjacent viscera. Pregnancy has occurred with the Cu-7 or Tatum-T in situ and when the Cu-7 or Tatum-T has been partially or completely expelled.

The incidence of spontaneous abortion, when conception occurs with intrauterine devices in situ, appears to be increased over that in unprotected women. Insertion cramping, usually of no more than a few seconds' duration, may occur; however, some women may experience residual cramping for several hours or even days. Intermenstrual spotting or bleeding, or prolonged or increased menstrual flow may occur.

Pelvic infection including salpingitis with tubal damage or occlusion has been reported. This may result in future infertility. Complete or partial expulsion of the Cu-7 or Tatum-T may sometimes occur, particularly in those patients with uteri measuring less than 6.5 cm by sounding. Urticarial allergic skin reaction may occur. The following complaints have also been reported with IUDs although their relation to the Cu-7 or Tatum-T has not been established: amenorrhea or delayed menses, backaches, cervical erosion, cystic masses in the pelvis, vaginitis, leg pain or soreness, weight loss or gain, nervousness, dyspareunia, cystitis, endometritis, septic abortion, septicemia, leukorrhea, ectopic pregnancy, difficult removal, uterine embedment, anemia, pain, neurovascular episodes including bradycardia and syncope secondary to insertion, dysmenorrhea, and fragmentation of the IUD.

[*The following sections do not apply to Tatum-T. See* **Directions for Use, Clinical Studies, Procedure for Insertion, and Removal of the Tatum-T** *under that product's heading.*]

Directions for Use: The Cu-7 is to be placed within the uterine cavity. See the *Procedure for Insertion* that follows, which describes two insertion techniques.

The small diameter of the Cu-7 facilitates easy insertion in nulligravidous and nulliparous, as well as parous, women. The optimal time of insertion is during the latter part of the menstrual flow or one or two days thereafter. The cervical canal is relatively more patent at this time, and there is little chance that the patient may be pregnant.

Present information indicates that efficacy is retained for 36 months. There is no evidence that contraceptive efficacy decreases with time up to three years of use, but unless new data support a longer period of efficacy and safety, the Cu-7 must be removed within 36 months from the date of insertion and a new one inserted if desired. If partial expulsion occurs, removal is indicated, and a new Cu-7 may be inserted. Removal of the Cu-7 may also be indicated in the event of heavy or persistent bleeding.

The physician should become thoroughly familiar with the instructions for use before attempting insertion or removal of the Cu-7.

Clinical Studies: Different event rates have been reported with the use of different intrauterine contraceptives. Inasmuch as these rates are usually derived from separate studies conducted by different investigators in several population groups, a comparison cannot be made with precision. Even in different studies with the same contraceptive, considerably different rates are likely to be obtained because of differing characteristics of the study population. Furthermore, event rates per unit of time tend to be lower as clinical experience is expanded, possibly due to retention in the clinical study of those patients who accept the treatment regimen, not having discontinued due to adverse reactions or pregnancy, so that those remaining in the study were those less susceptible. In clinical trials of the Cu-7 conducted by Searle, use effectiveness was determined as follows for parous and nulliparous women, as tabulated by the life table method. (Rates are expressed as cumulative events per 100 women through 12, 24, and 36 months of use.)

This experience encompasses 373,948 woman-months of use, including 12 months for 11,288 women, 24 months for 7,518, and 36 months for 3,371.

Cumulative rates were:

[See table above].

	12 Months		24 Months		36 Months	
	Parous	**Nulliparous**	**Parous**	**Nulliparous**	**Parous**	**Nulliparous**
Pregnancy	1.9	1.7	3.0	2.6	3.5	3.1
Expulsion	5.6	7.8	6.7	9.0	7.2	9.4
Medical removal	10.9	13.7	18.3	20.9	24.8	28.7
Continuation	69.8	65.9	45.7	45.8	21.6	17.8

Cu-7® Insertion Instrument

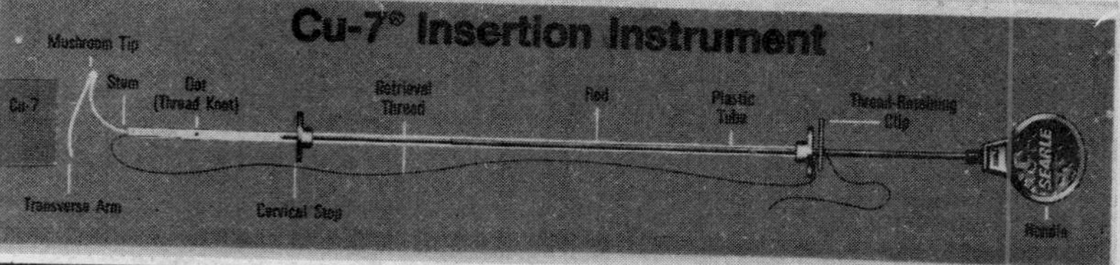

Procedure for Insertion

The Cu-7 may be inserted easily at any time during the menstrual cycle. It is *not* necessary to delay insertion until a menstrual flow is in progress; however, the possibility of existing undetermined pregnancy is lessened if insertion is made during or shortly following a menstrual period.

The cervix should be cleansed with antiseptic solution and its anterior lip grasped with a tenaculum prior to sounding the uterus and insertion of the Cu-7. Insertion of the Cu-7 into a severely anteverted or severely retroverted uterus may be difficult unless sufficient tension is applied to the tenaculum. Determination of the depth and direction of the uterine cavity should be made with a sound prior to insertion.

An aseptic technique should be employed. Sterile gloves are recommended; however, the sterile sheath covering the Cu-7 in the package

Continued on next page

Searle Pharm.—Cont.

may be used to avoid handling any part of the copper figure seven or the tube which will enter the cervical canal.

To load the Cu-7 into the tube, fold the transverse arm against the copper-clad stem and push it into the tube until only the mushroom tip protrudes. Center the dot (thread knot) on the stem of the plastic carrier with the long axis (horizontal plane) of the cervical stop.

Caution: DO NOT leave the Cu-7 folded in the tube longer than two minutes or the plastic will lose its "memory"; it will then fail to resume its original configuration within the uterus and thus invite loss of effectiveness and early expulsion.
DO NOT remove the thread-retaining clip from the insertion rod until after insertion has been made and you are ready to deposit the Cu-7 within the uterine cavity.
DO NOT force the insertion. It is generally believed that most perforations occur at the time of insertion, although the perforation may not be detected until some time later. The position of the uterus should be determined during the pre-insertion examination. Great care must be exercised during the pre-insertion sounding and subsequent insertion.
Note: If the uterine cavity measures under 6.5 cm, the incidence of pain, bleeding, partial or complete expulsion, perforation, and possibly pregnancy increases. Insertion is not recommended into a uterus which sounds under 5.5 cm.

Release Technique

Note: After sounding, the cervical stop should be set at the depth measured on the sound. *See Figure 1.* Load the Cu-7 into the tube and immediately begin the insertion. DO NOT leave the Cu-7 in the tube longer than 2 minutes.

1. Apply tension with the tenaculum and gently insert the loaded instrument through the cervical canal, *see Figure 2,* to the fundus, *see Figure 3,* at which time the cervical stop should be at the cervix. Pinch the thread-retaining clip to the tube-stop during insertion to prevent the tube from crimping. The end of the rod should be touching the end of the Cu-7 at all times. Keep the cervical stop in the horizontal plane until it reaches the cervix. DO NOT FORCE.

2. Hold the rod firmly with the cervical stop at the cervix and free the thread by pressing the thread-retaining clip from the rod. Release the Cu-7 into the uterine cavity by *withdrawing* the tube to ½ inch from the handle. (DO NOT PUSH ON THE HANDLE; perforation could result.) *See Figure 4.*

3. Hold the tube still (do not withdraw further) and gently push the rod all of the way into the tube to correctly seat the Cu-7 entirely within the uterine cavity. *See Figure 5.*

4. Withdraw the insertion instrument and cut the thread at least 2 in (5 cm) from the external os. DO NOT PULL OUT EXCESS THREAD BEFORE CUTTING. *See Figure 6.*

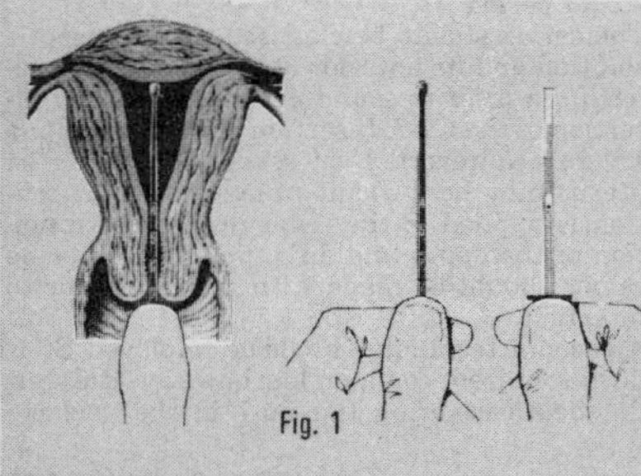
Fig. 1

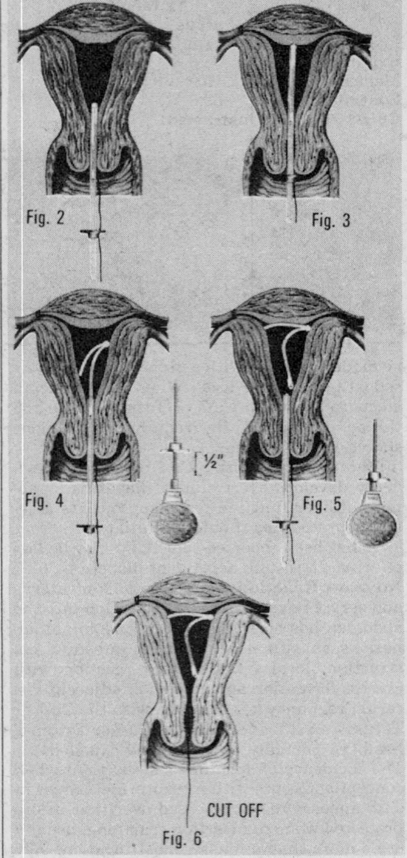

Fig. 2 Fig. 3 Fig. 4 Fig. 5 Fig. 6

Push-In Technique

Note: The cervical stop has been preset on the tube at 34 mm from the proximal end. *See Figure 1.* This will allow proper placement of the Cu-7 in a uterus which sounds to 2¾ in (7.0 cm) using *this* insertion technique only. (Since the cervical stop may have moved during shipment, this measurement should be verified.) If the uterus sounds to a depth greater than 2¾ in (7.0 cm), the cervical stop should be moved farther from the end of the tube by that many inches (centimeters). If the uterus sounds to a depth less than 2¾ in (7.0 cm), the cervical stop should be moved that much closer to the end of the tube.

1. Apply tension with the tenaculum and gently insert the loaded instrument through the cervical canal to the cervical stop, *see Figure 2.* Pinch the thread-retaining clip to the tube-stop during insertion to prevent the tube from crimping. The end of the rod should be touching the end of the Cu-7 at all times. Keep the cervical stop in the horizontal plane until it reaches the cervix. DO NOT FORCE.

2. Hold the tube firmly; remove the thread-retaining clip by pressing it off the rod and gently push the rod, *see Figure 3,* all the way into the tube to correctly seat the Cu-7 entirely within the uterine cavity. *See Figure 4.*

3. Withdraw the insertion instrument and cut the thread at least 2 in (5 cm) from the external os. DO NOT PULL OUT EXCESS THREAD BEFORE CUTTING. *See Figure 5.*

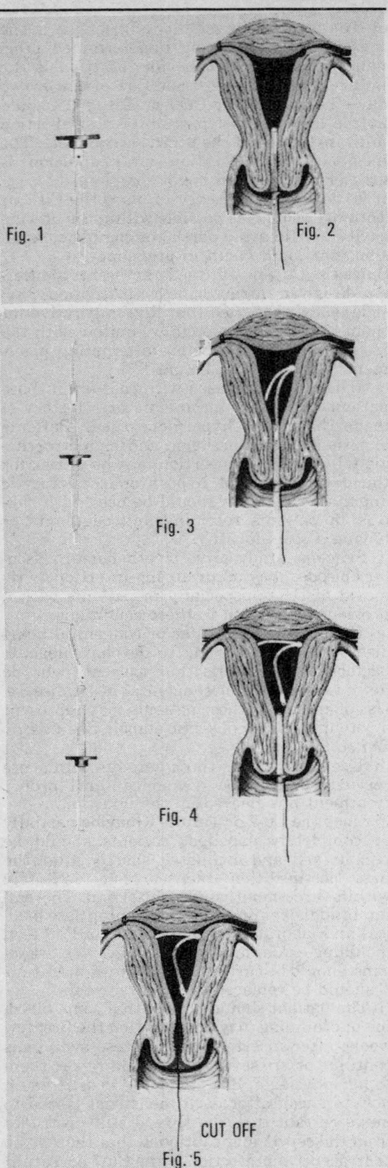

Fig. 1 Fig. 2 Fig. 3 Fig. 4 Fig. 5

Removal of the Cu-7

ROUTINE REMOVAL—THREAD VISIBLE:

1. DO NOT exert a sudden pull or jerk on the retrieval thread. Exert a firm, steady pull on the thread. A jerk may cause the thread to break.

2. A ring (sponge) forceps, with its smooth edges and minimal crushing force, is a good instrument with which to grasp the thread.

3. Other instruments may be used, but care must be exerted to avoid crushing or cutting the thread.

4. Avoid winding or angulating the thread about the jaws of the withdrawal instrument.

5. Utilize the minimum force needed to remove the Cu-7.

6. Should resistance be encountered, dislodge the Cu-7 by the aseptic use of a slim instrument (e.g., uterine dressing forceps) before making further removal attempts.

THREAD NOT VISIBLE: If the Cu-7 is in the uterus and the thread is not visible, the following procedures should be considered when you elect to recover it:

1. Aseptic use of a slim instrument (e.g., uterine dressing forceps) will frequently permit removal in the office.

2. Hysteroscopy under hospital conditions may be required.

3. D & C and also suction aspiration have been used as alternative measures.

NOTE: If intrauterine manipulative procedures are required, allow an appropriate healing period before inserting a new Cu-7.

How Supplied: Available in boxes of 10, 30, and 100 sterile units (Cu-7 with an inserter), and sufficient patient brochures and identification cards.

[*Shown in Product Identification Section*]

DIULO™ ℞
(metolazone)

Description: Each Diulo tablet contains 2½, 5, or 10 mg of metolazone, a diuretic/saluretic/antihypertensive drug. Metolazone has the molecular formula $C_{16}H_{16}ClN_3O_3S$. The chemical name of metolazone is 7-chloro-1, 2, 3, 4-tetrahydro-2-methyl-4-oxo-3-o-tolyl-6-quinazolinesulfonamide. Metolazone is only sparingly soluble in water, but more soluble in plasma, blood, alkali, and organic solvents.

Actions: Diulo (metolazone) is a diuretic/saluretic/antihypertensive drug whose action results in an interference with the renal tubular mechanism of electrolyte reabsorption. The mechanism of this action is unknown. Diulo acts primarily to inhibit sodium reabsorption at the cortical diluting site and in the proximal convoluted tubule. Sodium and chloride ions are excreted in approximately equivalent amounts. The increased delivery of sodium to the distal-tubular exchange site may result in increased potassium excretion.

Drug Interaction Studies: In animals pretreated with metolazone, the drug did not alter the characteristic effect of heparin on clotting time nor protamine antagonism; dicumarol on prothrombin time nor Vitamin K antagonism; the response of guanethidine, reserpine and hydralazine to cardiovascular parameters nor the pressor response of the subsequent dose of norepinephrine.

Metolazone and furosemide, administered concurrently have produced marked diuresis in some patients whose edema or ascites was refractory to treatment with maximum recommended doses of these or other diuretics administered alone. The mechanism of this interaction is not known.

In clinical usage, metolazone does not inhibit carbonic anhydrase. Its proximal action has been evidenced in humans by increased excretion of phosphate and magnesium ions, by markedly increased fractional excretion of sodium in patients with severely compromised glomerular filtration, and in animals by the results of micropuncture studies. Decrease in calcium ion excretion has not been noted.

At maximum therapeutic dosage Diulo is approximately equal to thiazide diuretics in its diuretic potency. However, Diulo may produce diuresis in patients with glomerular filtration rates below 20 ml/min.

When Diulo is given, diuresis and saluresis usually begin within one hour and persist for 12 to 24 hours depending on dosage. Maximum effect occurs about two hours after administration. At the higher recommended dosages, effect may be prolonged beyond 24 hours. *A single daily dose is recommended.* For most patients the duration of effect can be varied by adjusting the daily dose.

The prolonged duration of action of Diulo is attributed to protein binding and enterohepatic recycling. A small amount of Diulo is metabolized and the fraction so changed is nontoxic. The primary route of excretion is renal.

The mechanism whereby diuretics function in the control of hypertension is unknown; both renal and extra-renal actions may be involved. An antihypertensive effect may be seen as early as three to four days after Diulo has been started. Administration for three to four weeks, however, is usually required for optimum antihypertensive effect.

Indications and Usage: Diulo (metolazone) is indicated in the management of hypertension either as the sole therapeutic agent or to enhance the effectiveness of other antihypertensive drugs in the more severe forms of hypertension.

Diulo (metolazone) is indicated for the treatment of salt and water retention including

— edema accompanying congestive heart failure

— edema accompanying renal diseases, including the nephrotic syndrome, and states of diminished renal function.

Usage in Pregnancy: The routine use of diuretics in an otherwise healthy woman is inappropriate and exposes mother and fetus to unnecessary hazard. Diuretics do not prevent development of toxemia of pregnancy, and there is no satisfactory evidence that they are useful in the treatment of developed toxemia.

Edema during pregnancy may arise from pathological causes or from the physiologic and mechanical consequences of pregnancy. Diulo is indicated in pregnancy when edema is due to pathologic causes, just as it is in the absence of pregnancy (however, see *Precautions,* below). Dependent edema in pregnancy, resulting from restriction of venous return by the expanded uterus, is properly treated through elevation of the lower extremities and use of support hose; use of diuretics to lower intravascular volume in this case is illogical and unnecessary. There is hypervolemia during normal pregnancy which is harmful to neither the fetus nor the mother (in the absence of cardiovascular disease), but which is associated with edema, including generalized edema, in the majority of pregnant women. If this edema produces discomfort, increased recumbency will often provide relief. In rare instances, this edema may cause extreme discomfort which is not relieved by rest. In these cases, a short course of diuretics may provide relief and may be appropriate.

Contraindications: Anuria.

Hepatic coma or pre-coma; known allergy or hypersensitivity to metolazone.

Warnings: While not reported to date, cross-allergy theoretically may occur when metolazone is given to patients known to be allergic to sulfonamide-derived drugs, thiazides, or quinethazone.

Hypokalemia may occur, with consequent weakness, cramps, and cardiac dysrhythmias. Hypokalemia is a particular hazard in digitalized patients; dangerous or fatal arrhythmias may be precipitated.

Azotemia and hyperuricemia may be noted or precipitated during the administration of metolazone. Infrequently, gouty attacks have been reported in persons with history of gout. If azotemia and oliguria worsen during treatment of patients with severe renal disease, Diulo should be discontinued.

Until additional data have been obtained, Diulo is not recommended for patients in the pediatric age group.

Unusually large or prolonged effects on volume and electrolytes may result when metolazone and furosemide are administered concurrently. It is recommended that concurrent administration of these diuretics for treatment of resistant edema be started under hospital conditions in order to provide for adequate monitoring.

When Diulo is used with other antihypertensive drugs, particular care must be taken, especially during initial therapy. Dosage of other antihypertensive agents, especially the ganglionic blockers, should be reduced.

Diulo may be given with a potassium-sparing diuretic when indicated. In this circumstance, diuresis may be potentiated and dosages should be reduced. Potassium retention and hyperkalemia may result; the serum potassium should be determined frequently. Potassium supplementation is contraindicated when a potassium-sparing diuretic is given.

Precautions: Periodic determination of serum electrolytes to detect possible electrolyte imbalance should be performed at appropriate intervals. Blood urea nitrogen, uric acid, and glucose levels should be assessed at intervals during diuretic therapy.

All patients receiving Diulo (metolazone) therapy should be observed for clinical signs of fluid and/or electrolyte imbalance; namely, hyponatremia, hypochloremic alkalosis, and hypokalemia. Serum and urine electrolyte determinations are particularly important when the patient is vomiting excessively or receiving parenteral fluids. Medication such as digitalis may also influence serum electrolytes. Warning signs, irrespective of cause, are: dryness of mouth, thirst, weakness, lethargy, drowsiness, restlessness, muscle pains or cramps, muscular fatigue, hypotension, oliguria, tachycardia, and gastrointestinal disturbances such as nausea and vomiting.

The serum potassium should be determined at regular intervals, and potassium supplementation instituted whenever indicated. Hypokalemia will be more common in association with intensive or prolonged diuretic therapy, with concomitant steroid or ACTH therapy, and with inadequate electrolyte intake.

While not reported to date for metolazone, related diuretics have increased responsiveness to tubocurarine and decreased arterial responsiveness to norepinephrine. Accordingly, it may be advisable to discontinue Diulo three days before elective surgery.

Caution should be observed when administering Diulo to hyperuricemic or gouty patients.

Diulo exerts minimal effects on glucose metabolism; insulin requirements may be affected in diabetics, and hyperglycemia and glycosuria may occur in patients with latent diabetes.

Chloride deficit and hypochloremic alkalosis may occur. In patients with severe edema accompanying cardiac failure or renal disease, a low-salt syndrome may be produced; hot weather and a low-salt diet will contribute.

Caution should be observed when administering Diulo to patients with severely impaired renal function. As most of the drug is excreted by the renal route, cumulative effects may be seen in this circumstance.

Orthostatic hypotension may occur; this may be potentiated by alcohol, barbiturates, narcotics, or concurrent therapy with other antihypertensive drugs.

While not reported for metolazone, use of other diuretics has been associated on rare occasions with pathological changes in the parathyroid glands and with hypercalcemia. This possibility should be kept in mind with clinical use of Diulo.

Usage in Pregnancy:

Diulo crosses the placental barrier and appears in cord blood. The use of Diulo in pregnant women requires that the anticipated benefit be weighed against possible hazards to the fetus. These hazards include fetal or neonatal jaundice, thrombocytopenia, and possibly other adverse reactions which have occurred in the adult.

Nursing Mothers

Metolazone appears in breast milk. If use of the drug is deemed essential, the patient should stop nursing.

Adverse Reactions: Adverse reactions encountered during therapy with potent medications should be considered in two groups: those that represent extension of the expected pharmacologic actions of the drug, and those which are pharmacologically unexpected, idiosyncratic, specially toxic, due to allergy or hypersensitivity, or due to unexplained causes.

For Diulo (metolazone), adverse reactions constituting extensions of the expected pharmacologic actions of this potent diuretic/ saluretic/ antihypertensive drug may include:

Continued on next page

Searle Pharm.—Cont.

Gastrointestinal reactions: constipation.
Central nervous system reactions: syncope, dizziness, drowsiness.
Cardiovascular reactions: orthostatic hypotension, excessive volume depletion, hemoconcentration, venous thrombosis.
Other reactions: dryness of the mouth, symptomatic and asymptomatic hypokalemia, hyponatremia, hypochloremia; hypochloremic alkalosis, hypophosphatemia, hyperuricemia, hyperglycemia, glycosuria, increase in BUN or creatinine, fatigue, muscle cramps or spasm, weakness, restlessness sometimes resulting in insomnia.
In the second classification, adverse reactions to Diulo may include:
Gastrointestinal reactions: nausea, vomiting, anorexia, diarrhea, abdominal bloating, epigastric distress, intrahepatic cholestatic jaundice, hepatitis.
Central nervous system reactions: vertigo, headache, paresthesias.
Hematologic reactions: leukopenia, aplastic anemia.
Dermatologic-hypersensitivity reactions: urticaria and other skin rashes, purpura, necrotizing angiitis (cutaneous vasculitis).
Cardiovascular reactions: palpitation, chest pain.
Other reactions: chills, acute gouty attacks, transient blurred vision.
Adverse reactions which have occurred with other diuretics include:
pancreatitis, xanthopsia, agranulocytosis, thrombocytopenia, and photosensitivity. These reactions should be considered as possible occurrences with clinical usage of Diulo.
Whenever adverse reactions are moderate or severe, Diulo dosage should be reduced or therapy withdrawn.
Dosage and Administration: Therapy should be individualized according to patient response. Programs of therapy with Diulo (metolazone) should be titrated to gain a maximal initial therapeutic response, and to determine the minimal dose possible to maintain that therapeutic response.
Diulo is a potent drug with a prolonged, 12- to 24-hour duration of action. When an initially-desired therapeutic effect has been obtained, it is ordinarily advisable to reduce the dosage of Diulo to a lower maintenance level. The time interval required for the initial higher-dosage regimen may vary from days in edematous states to three or four weeks in the treatment of elevated blood pressure.
The daily dosage depends on the severity of each patient's condition, sodium intake, and responsiveness. Therefore, dosage adjustment is usually necessary during the course of therapy. A decision to reduce the daily dosage of Diulo from a higher induction level to a lower maintenance level should be based on the results of thorough clinical and laboratory evaluations. If antihypertensive drugs or diuretics are given concurrently with Diulo, careful dosage adjustment may be necessary.
Usual Dosage
Suitable initial dosages will usually fall in the ranges given:
Edema of cardiac failure: Diulo 5–10 mg, once daily
Edema of renal disease: Diulo 5–20 mg, once daily
Mild to moderate essential hypertension: Diulo 2½–5 mg, once daily
For patients with congestive cardiac failure who tend to experience paroxysmal nocturnal dyspnea, it is usually advisable to employ a dosage near the upper end of the range, to ensure prolongation of diuresis and saluresis for a full 24-hour period.
How Supplied: Diulo (metolazone) is supplied as tablets containing 2½, 5, and 10 mg of metolazone.
Diulo 2½ mg tablets are round, pink tablets with SEARLE debossed on one side and 501 on the other side.
Diulo 5 mg tablets are round, blue tablets with SEARLE debossed on one side and 511 on the other side.
Diulo 10 mg tablets are round, yellow tablets with SEARLE debossed on one side and 521 on the other side.
Available in bottles of 100 and 500 tablets, and cartons of 100 unit-dose individually blister-sealed tablets.
[*Shown in Product Identification Section*]

DRAMAMINE® Liquid
DRAMAMINE® Tablets
DRAMAMINE INJECTION™ ℞
(dimenhydrinate)

Description: Dimenhydrinate is the chlorotheophylline salt of the antihistaminic agent diphenhydramine. Dimenhydrinate contains not less than 53% and not more than 56% of diphenhydramine, and not less than 44% and not more than 47% of 8-chlorotheophylline, calculated on the dried basis.
Actions: While the precise mode of action of dimenhydrinate is not known, it has a depressant action on hyperstimulated labyrinthine function.
Indications: Dramamine is indicated for the prevention and treatment of the nausea, vomiting, or vertigo of motion sickness.
Warning: Caution should be used when Dramamine is given in conjunction with certain antibiotics which may cause ototoxicity, since Dramamine is capable of masking ototoxic symptoms and an irreversible state may be reached.
Precautions and Adverse Reactions: Drowsiness may be experienced by some patients, especially on high dosage, although this action frequently is not undesirable in some conditions for which the drug is used. However, because of possible drowsiness, patients taking Dramamine should be cautioned against operating automobiles or dangerous machinery. Patients should also avoid alcoholic beverages while taking medication. Dramamine should not be used in the presence of asthma, glaucoma, or enlargement of the prostate gland, except on advice of a physician. If pregnant or nursing a baby, the patient should consult a physician or pharmacist before using this product.
Dosage and Administration: *Dramamine Tablets:* To prevent motion sickness, the first dose should be taken one-half to one hour before starting your activity. Additional medication depends on travel conditions. *Adults*—Nausea or vomiting may be expected to be controlled for approximately four hours with 50 mg of Dramamine, and prevented by a similar dose every four hours. Its administration may be attended by some degree of drowsiness in some patients, and 100 mg every four hours may be given in conditions in which drowsiness is not objectionable or is even desirable. The usual adult dosage is 1 to 2 tablets every four to six hours, not to exceed 8 tablets in 24 hours. *Children 6 to 12 years:* ½ to 1 tablet every six to eight hours, not to exceed 3 tablets in 24 hours. *Children 2 to 6 years:* Up to ½ tablet every six to eight hours, not to exceed 1½ tablets in 24 hours. Children may also be given Dramamine (dimenhydrinate) cherry-flavored liquid in accordance with directions for use. Not for frequent or prolonged use except on advice of a physician. Do not exceed recommended dosage.
Dramamine Injection (dimenhydrinate) is supplied in 1-ml ampuls and in 5-ml serum-type vials, each containing 50 mg/ml of Dramamine dissolved in a solution containing 5% benzyl alcohol, 50% propylene glycol, and water q.s.
Adults: For *intramuscular administration* each milliliter (50 mg) of solution is injected as needed, but for *intravenous therapy* each milliliter (50 mg) of solution is diluted in 10 ml of Sodium Chloride Injection USP and injected over a period of two minutes.
Children: The intramuscular dosage of Dramamine Injection for children should be 1.25 mg/kg of body weight or 37.5 mg/m² of body surface, four times a day, up to 300 mg daily.
Dramamine Liquid: To prevent motion sickness, the first dose should be taken one-half to one hour before starting your activity. Additional medication depends on travel conditions. *Dosage: Adults:* 4 to 8 teaspoonfuls every four to six hours, not to exceed 32 teaspoonfuls in 24 hours. *Children 6 to 12 years:* 2 to 4 teaspoonfuls (4 ml per teaspoonful) every six to eight hours, not to exceed 12 teaspoonfuls in 24 hours. *Children 2 to 6 years:* 1 to 2 teaspoonfuls every six to eight hours, not to exceed 6 teaspoonfuls in 24 hours. *Children under 2 years:* only on advice of a physician.
Not for frequent or prolonged use except on advice of a physician. Do not exceed recommended dosage. Use of a measuring device is recommended for all liquid medication.
How Supplied: Dramamine (dimenhydrinate) is supplied in the following dosage forms and package sizes:
For parenteral use—**ampuls**, 1 ml (50 mg); cartons of 5, 25, and 100; **vials**, rubber-capped, serum type, 5 ml (250) mg); cartons of 5, 25, and 100.
For oral use—scored white **tablets** of 50 mg, USP, with SEARLE debossed on one side and 1701 on the other side; bottles of 36, 100, 500, 1,000, and 2,500, packets of 12 tablets, and cartons of 100 unit-dose individually blister-sealed tablets; **liquid**, 12.5 mg/4 ml, ethyl alcohol 5%, bottles of 3 fl oz and 16 fl oz.
[*Please note: Dramamine Tablets and Liquid are also shown in the PDR For Nonprescription Drugs.*]
[*Tablets are shown in Product Identification Section*]

FLAGYL I.V.™ ℞
(metronidazole hydrochloride)
FLAGYL I.V.™ RTU® ℞
(metronidazole)
For Intravenous Infusion Only

Warning
Metronidazole has been shown to be carcinogenic in mice and rats (see *Warnings*). Its use, therefore, should be reserved for serious anaerobic infections where, in the judgment of the physician, the benefit outweighs the possible risk.

Description: Flagyl I.V., sterile (metronidazole hydrochloride), and Flagyl I.V. RTU, sterile (metronidazole), are parenteral dosage forms of the synthetic antibacterial agents 1-(β-hydroxyethyl)-2- methyl-5- nitroimidazole hydrochloride and 1-(β-hydroxyethyl)-2-methyl-5-nitroimidazole, respectively.
Each single-dose vial of lyophilized Flagyl I.V. contains sterile, nonpyrogenic metronidazole hydrochloride, equivalent to 500 mg metronidazole, and 415 mg mannitol.
Each Flagyl I.V. RTU 100-ml single-dose glass vial or plastic container contains a sterile, nonpyrogenic, isotonic, buffered solution of 500 mg metronidazole, 47.6 mg sodium phosphate, 22.9 mg citric acid, and 790 mg sodium chloride in Water for Injection USP. Flagyl I.V. RTU has a tonicity of 310 mOsm/L and a pH of 5 to 7. Each container contains 14 mEq of sodium.
The plastic container is fabricated from a specially formulated polyvinyl chloride plastic. Water can permeate from inside the container into the overwrap in amounts insufficient to affect the solution significantly. Solutions in

contact with the plastic container can leach out certain of its chemical components in very small amounts within the expiration period, e.g., di 2-ethylhexyl phthalate (DEHP), up to 5 parts per million. However, the safety of the plastic has been confirmed in tests in animals according to USP biological tests for plastic containers as well as by tissue culture toxicity studies.

Clinical Pharmacology: Metronidazole is a synthetic antibacterial compound. Disposition of metronidazole in the body is similar for both oral and intravenous dosage forms, with an average elimination half-life in healthy humans of eight hours.

The major route of elimination of metronidazole and its metabolites is via the urine (60–80% of the dose), with fecal excretion accounting for 6–15% of the dose. The metabolites that appear in the urine result primarily from side-chain oxidation [1-(β-hydroxyethyl)-2-hydroxymethyl-5-nitroimidazole and 2-methyl-5-nitroimidazole-1-yl-acetic acid] and glucuronide conjugation, with unchanged metronidazole accounting for approximately 20% of the total. Renal clearance of metronidazole is approximately 10 ml/min/1.73m^2.

Metronidazole is the major component appearing in the plasma, with lesser quantities of the 2-hydroxymethyl metabolite also being present Less than 20% of the circulating metronidazole is bound to plasma proteins. Both the parent compound and the metabolite possess *in vitro* bactericidal activity against most strains of anaerobic bacteria.

Metronidazole appears in cerebrospinal fluid, saliva, and breast milk in concentrations similar to those found in plasma. Bactericidal concentrations of metronidazole have also been detected in pus from hepatic abscesses.

Plasma concentrations of metronidazole are proportional to the administered dose. An eight-hour intravenous infusion of 100–4,000 mg of metronidazole in normal subjects showed a linear relationship between dose and peak plasma concentration.

In patients treated with Flagyl I.V., using a dosage regimen of 15 mg/kg loading dose followed six hours later by 7.5 mg/kg every six hours, peak steady-state plasma concentrations of metronidazole averaged 25 mcg/ml with trough (minimum) concentrations averaging 18 mcg/ml.

Decreased renal function does not alter the single-dose pharmacokinetics of metronidazole. However, plasma clearance of metronidazole is decreased in patients with decreased liver function.

Microbiology: Metronidazole is active *in vitro* against most obligate anaerobes, but does not appear to possess any clinically relevant activity against facultative anaerobes or obligate aerobes. Against susceptible organisms, metronidazole is generally bactericidal at concentrations equal to or slightly higher than the minimal inhibitory concentrations. Metronidazole has been shown to have *in vitro* and clinical activity against the following organisms:

Anaerobic gram-negative bacilli, including:
- *Bacteroides* species, including the *Bacteroides fragilis* group (*B. fragilis, B. distasonis, B. ovatus, B. thetaiotaomicron, B. vulgatus*)
- *Fusobacterium* species.

Anaerobic gram-positive bacilli, including:
- *Clostridium* species and susceptible strains of *Eubacterium*

Anaerobic gram-positive cocci, including:
- *Peptococcus* species
- *Peptostreptococcus* species

Susceptibility Tests: Bacteriologic studies should be performed to determine the causative organisms and their susceptibility to metronidazole; however, the rapid routine susceptibility testing of individual isolates of anaerobic bacteria is not always practical, and therapy may be started while awaiting these results.

Quantitative methods give the most accurate estimates of susceptibility to antibacterial drugs. A standardized agar dilution method and a broth microdilution method are recommended.[1]

Control strains are recommended for standardized susceptibility testing. Each time the test is performed, one or more of the following strains should be included: *Clostridium perfringens* ATCC 13124, *Bacteroides fragilis* ATCC 25285, and *Bacteroides thetaiotaomicron* ATCC 29741. The mode metronidazole MICs for those three strains are reported to be 0.25, 0.25, and 0.5 mcg/ml, respectively.

A clinical laboratory test is considered under acceptable control if the results of the control strains are within one doubling dilution of the mode MICs reported for metronidazole.

A bacterial isolate may be considered susceptible if the MIC value for metronidazole is not more than 16 mcg/ml. An organism is considered resistant if the MIC is greater than 16 mcg/ml. A report of "resistant" from the laboratory indicates that the infecting organism is not likely to respond to therapy.

Indications and Usage: Flagyl I.V. (metronidazole hydrochloride) and Flagyl I.V. RTU (metronidazole) are indicated in the treatment of serious infections caused by susceptible anaerobic bacteria. Indicated surgical procedures should be performed in conjunction with Flagyl I.V. or Flagyl I.V. RTU therapy. In a mixed aerobic and anaerobic infection, antibiotics appropriate for the treatment of the aerobic infection should be used in addition to Flagyl I.V. or Flagyl I.V. RTU.

Flagyl I.V. and Flagyl I.V. RTU are effective in *Bacteroides fragilis* infections resistant to clindamycin, chloramphenicol, and penicillin.

INTRA-ABDOMINAL INFECTIONS, including peritonitis, intra-abdominal abscess, and liver abscess, caused by *Bacteroides* species including the *B. fragilis* group (*B. fragilis, B. distasonis, B. ovatus, B. thetaiotaomicron, B. vulgatus*), *Clostridium* species, *Eubacterium* species, *Peptococcus* species, and *Peptostreptococcus* species.

SKIN AND SKIN STRUCTURE INFECTIONS caused by *Bacteroides* species including the *B. fragilis* group, *Clostridium* species, *Peptococcus* species, *Peptostreptococcus* species, and *Fusobacterium* species.

GYNECOLOGIC INFECTIONS, including endometritis, endomyometritis, tubo-ovarian abscess, and postsurgical vaginal cuff infection, caused by *Bacteroides* species including the *B. fragilis* group, *Clostridium* species, *Peptococcus* species, and *Peptostreptococcus* species.

BACTERIAL SEPTICEMIA caused by *Bacteroides* species including the *B. fragilis* group, and *Clostridium* species.

BONE AND JOINT INFECTIONS, as adjunctive therapy, caused by *Bacteroides* species including the *B. fragilis* group.

CENTRAL NERVOUS SYSTEM (CNS) INFECTIONS, including meningitis and brain abscess, caused by *Bacteroides* species including the *B. fragilis* group.

LOWER RESPIRATORY TRACT INFECTIONS, including pneumonia, empyema, and lung abscess, caused by *Bacteroides* species including the *B. fragilis* group.

ENDOCARDITIS caused by *Bacteroides* species including the *B. fragilis* group.

Contraindications: Flagyl I.V. and Flagyl I.V. RTU are contraindicated in patients with a prior history of hypersensitivity to metronidazole or other nitroimidazole derivatives.

Warnings:

Convulsive Seizures and Peripheral Neuropathy: Convulsive seizures and peripheral neuropathy, the latter characterized mainly by numbness or paresthesia of an extremity, have been reported in patients treated with metronidazole. The appearance of abnormal neurologic signs demands the prompt evaluation of the benefit/risk ratio of the continuation of therapy.

Tumorigenicity in Rodents: Metronidazole has shown evidence of carcinogenic activity in studies involving chronic, oral administration in mice and rats, but similar studies in the hamster gave negative results. Also, metronidazole has shown mutagenic activity in a number of *in vitro* assay systems, but studies in mammals *(in vivo)* failed to demonstrate a potential for genetic damage.

Precautions:

General: Patients with severe hepatic disease metabolize metronidazole slowly, with resultant accumulation of metronidazole and its metabolites in the plasma. Accordingly, for such patients, doses below those usually recommended should be administered cautiously.

Administration of solutions containing sodium ions may result in sodium retention. Care should be taken when administering Flagyl I.V. RTU to patients receiving corticosteroids or to patients predisposed to edema.

Known or previously unrecognized candidiasis may present more prominent symptoms during therapy with Flagyl I.V. or Flagyl I.V. RTU and requires treatment with a candicidal agent.

Laboratory Tests: Metronidazole is a nitroimidazole, and Flagyl I.V. or Flagyl I.V. RTU should be used with care in patients with evidence of or history of blood dyscrasia. A mild leukopenia has been observed during its administration; however, no persistent hematologic abnormalities attributable to metronidazole have been observed in clinical studies. Total and differential leukocyte counts are recommended before and after therapy.

Drug Interactions: Metronidazole has been reported to potentiate the anticoagulant effect of warfarin and other oral coumarin anticoagulants, resulting in a prolongation of prothrombin time. This possible drug interaction should be considered when Flagyl I.V. or Flagyl I.V. RTU is prescribed for patients on this type of anticoagulant therapy.

Alcoholic beverages should not be consumed during metronidazole therapy because abdominal cramps, nausea, vomiting, headaches, and flushing may occur.

Drug/Laboratory Test Interactions: Metronidazole may interfere with certain chemical analyses for serum glutamic oxalacetic transaminase, resulting in decreased values. Values of zero may be observed.

Carcinogenesis: See *Warnings.*

Pregnancy: Metronidazole crosses the placental barrier and enters the fetal circulation rapidly. Reproduction studies have been performed in rabbits and rats at doses up to five times the human dose and have revealed no evidence of impaired fertility or harm to the fetus due to metronidazole. There are, however, no adequate and well-controlled studies in pregnant women. Because animal reproduction studies are not always predictive of human response, and because metronidazole is a carcinogen in rodents, these drugs should be used during pregnancy only if clearly needed.

Nursing Mothers: Because of the potential for tumorigenicity shown for metronidazole in mouse and rat studies, a decision should be made whether to discontinue nursing or to discontinue the drug, taking into account the importance of the drug to the mother. Metronidazole is secreted in breast milk in concentrations similar to those found in plasma.

Pediatric Use: Safety and effectiveness in children have not been established.

Adverse Reactions: The two most serious adverse reactions reported in patients treated with Flagyl I.V. have been convulsive seizures and peripheral neuropathy, the latter characterized mainly by numbness or paresthesia of an extremity. Since persistent peripheral neu-

Continued on next page

Searle Pharm.—Cont.

ropathy has been reported in some patients receiving prolonged oral administration of Flagyl® (metronidazole), patients should be observed carefully if neurologic symptoms occur and a prompt evaluation made of the benefit/risk ratio of the continuation of therapy.
The following reactions have also been reported during treatment with Flagyl I.V.:

Gastrointestinal: Nausea, vomiting, abdominal discomfort, diarrhea, and an unpleasant metallic taste.

Hematopoietic: Reversible neutropenia (leukopenia).

Dermatologic: Erythematous rash and pruritus.

Central Nervous System: Headache, dizziness, and syncope.

Local Reactions: Thrombophlebitis after intravenous infusion. This reaction can be minimized or avoided by avoiding prolonged use of indwelling intravenous catheters.

Other: Fever. Instances of a darkened urine have also been reported, and this manifestation has been the subject of a special investigation. Although the pigment which is probably responsible for this phenomenon has not been positively identified, it is almost certainly a metabolite of metronidazole and seems to have no clinical significance.

The following adverse reactions have been reported during treatment with oral Flagyl (metronidazole):

Gastrointestinal: Nausea, sometimes accompanied by headache, anorexia and occasionally vomiting; diarrhea, epigastric distress, abdominal cramping, and constipation.

Mouth: A sharp, unpleasant metallic taste is not unusual. Furry tongue, glossitis, and stomatitis have occurred; these may be associated with a sudden overgrowth of *Candida* which may occur during effective therapy.

Hematopoietic: Reversible neutropenia (leukopenia).

Cardiovascular: Flattening of the T-wave may be seen in electrocardiographic tracings.

Central Nervous System: Convulsive seizures, peripheral neuropathy, dizziness, vertigo, incoordination, ataxia, confusion, irritability, depression, weakness, and insomnia.

Hypersensitivity: Urticaria, erythematous rash, flushing, nasal congestion, dryness of mouth (or vagina or vulva), and fever.

Renal: Dysuria, cystitis, polyuria, incontinence, a sense of pelvic pressure, and darkened urine.

Other: Proliferation of *Candida* in the vagina, dyspareunia, decrease of libido, proctitis, and fleeting joint pains sometimes resembling "serum sickness." If patients receiving metronidazole drink alcoholic beverages, they may experience abdominal distress, nausea, vomiting, flushing, or headache. A modification of the taste of alcoholic beverages has also been reported.

Overdosage: Use of dosages of Flagyl I.V. (metronidazole hydrochloride) higher than those recommended has been reported. These include the use of 27 mg/kg three times a day for 20 days, and the use of 75 mg/kg as a single loading dose followed by 7.5 mg/kg maintenance doses. No adverse reactions were reported in either of the two cases.
Single oral doses of metronidazole, up to 15 g, have been reported in suicide attempts and accidental overdoses. Symptoms reported include nausea, vomiting, and ataxia.
Oral metronidazole has been studied as a radiation sensitizer in the treatment of malignant tumors. Neurotoxic effects, including seizures and peripheral neuropathy, have been reported after 5 to 7 days of doses of 6 to 10.4 g every other day.
Treatment: There is no specific antidote for overdose; therefore, management of the patient should consist of symptomatic and supportive therapy.

Dosage and Administration: The recommended dosage schedule for *adults* is:
Loading dose:
15 mg/kg infused over one hour (approximately 1 g for a 70-kg adult).
Maintenance Dose:
7.5 mg/kg infused over one hour every six hours (approximately 500 mg for a 70-kg adult). The first maintenance dose should be instituted six hours following the initiation of the loading dose.
Parenteral therapy may be changed to oral Flagyl (metronidazole) when conditions warrant, based upon the severity of the disease and the response of the patient to Flagyl I.V. or Flagyl I.V. RTU (metronidazole) treatment. The usual adult oral dosage is 7.5 mg/kg every six hours.
A maximum of 4.0 g should not be exceeded during a 24-hour period.
Patients with severe hepatic disease metabolize metronidazole slowly, with resultant accumulation of metronidazole and its metabolites in the plasma. Accordingly, for such patients, doses below those usually recommended should be administered cautiously. Close monitoring of plasma metronidazole levels[2] and toxicity is recommended.
The dose of Flagyl I.V. or Flagyl I.V. RTU should not be specifically reduced in anuric patients since accumulated metabolites may be rapidly removed by dialysis.
The usual duration of therapy is 7 to 10 days; however, infections of the bone and joint, lower respiratory tract, and endocardium may require longer treatment.
CAUTION: Flagyl I.V. (metronidazole hydrochloride) or Flagyl I.V. RTU (metronidazole) is to be administered by slow intravenous drip infusion only, either as a continuous or intermittent infusion. I.V. admixtures containing metronidazole and other drugs should be avoided. Additives should not be introduced into the Flagyl I.V. RTU solution. If used with a primary intravenous fluid system, the primary solution should be discontinued during metronidazole infusion. DO NOT USE EQUIPMENT CONTAINING ALUMINUM (EG, NEEDLES, CANNULAE) THAT WOULD COME IN CONTACT WITH THE DRUG SOLUTION.

FLAGYL I.V.
Flagyl I.V. <u>cannot</u> be given by direct intravenous injection (I.V. bolus) because of the low pH (0.5 to 2.0) of the reconstituted product. FLAGYL I.V. MUST BE FURTHER DILUTED AND NEUTRALIZED FOR I.V. INFUSION.
Flagyl I.V. is prepared for use in two steps:
NOTE: ORDER OF MIXING IS IMPORTANT
A. Reconstitution
B. Dilution in intravenous solution followed by pH neutralization with sodium bicarbonate injection into the dilution.

Reconstitution: To prepare the solution, add 4.4 ml of one of the following diluents and mix thoroughly: Sterile Water for Injection, USP; Bacteriostatic Water for Injection, USP; 0.9% Sodium Chloride Injection, USP; or Bacteriostatic 0.9% Sodium Chloride Injection, USP. The resultant approximate withdrawal volume is 5.0 ml with an approximate concentration of 100 mg/ml.
The pH of the reconstituted product will be in the range of 0.5 to 2.0. Reconstituted Flagyl I.V. is clear, and pale yellow to yellow-green in color.

Dilution in Intravenous Solutions: Properly reconstituted Flagyl I.V. may be added to a glass or plastic I.V. container not to exceed a concentration of 8 mg/ml. Any of the following intravenous solutions may be used: 0.9% Sodium Chloride Injection, USP; 5% Dextrose Injection, USP; or Lactated Ringer's Injection, USP.

NEUTRALIZATION IS REQUIRED PRIOR TO ADMINISTRATION
The final product should be mixed thoroughly and used within 24 hours.

Neutralization For Intravenous Infusion: Neutralize the intravenous solution containing Flagyl I.V. with approximately 5 mEq of sodium bicarbonate injection for each 500 mg of Flagyl I.V. used. Mix thoroughly. The pH of the neutralized intravenous solution will be approximately 6.0 to 7.0. Carbon dioxide gas will be generated with neutralization. It may be necessary to relieve gas pressure within the container.

Note: When the contents of one vial (500 mg) are diluted and neutralized to 100 ml, the resultant concentration is 5 mg/ml. Do not exceed an 8 mg/ml concentration of Flagyl I.V. in the neutralized intravenous solution, since neutralization will decrease the aqueous solubility and precipitation may occur. DO NOT REFRIGERATE NEUTRALIZED SOLUTIONS; otherwise, precipitation may occur.

Storage and Stability: Reconstituted vials of Flagyl I.V. are chemically stable for 96 hours when stored below 86°F (30°C) in room light. Use diluted and neutralized intravenous solutions containing Flagyl I.V. within 24 hours of mixing.

FLAGYL I.V. RTU
Flagyl I.V. RTU is a ready-to-use isotonic solution. **NO DILUTION OR BUFFERING IS REQUIRED.** Each container of Flagyl I.V. RTU contains 14 mEq of sodium.

Directions for use of plastic container:
CAUTION: Do not use plastic containers in series connections. Such use could result in air embolism due to residual air (approximately 15 ml) being drawn from the primary container before administration of the fluid from the secondary container is complete.
To open. Tear overwrap down side at slit and remove solution container. Check for minute leaks by squeezing inner bag firmly. If leaks are found discard solution as sterility may be impaired.
Preparation for administration.
1. Suspend container from eyelet support.
2. Remove plastic container from outlet port at bottom of container.
3. Attach administration set. Refer to complete directions accompanying set.

Parenteral drug products should be inspected visually for particulate matter and discoloration prior to administration, whenever solution and container permit. Do not use if cloudy or precipitated or if the seal is not intact.
Use sterile equipment. It is recommended that the intravenous administration apparatus be replaced at least once every 24 hours.

How Supplied:
FLAGYL I.V.
Flagyl I.V., sterile (metronidazole hydrochloride), is supplied in single-dose lyophilized vials each containing 500 mg metronidazole equivalent, individually packaged in cartons of 10 vials.
Flagyl I.V., prior to reconstitution, should be stored below 86°F (30°C) and protected from light.

FLAGYL I.V. RTU
In plastic container: Flagyl I.V. RTU, sterile (metronidazole), is supplied in 100-ml single-dose containers, each containing an isotonic, buffered solution of 500 mg metronidazole, individually packaged in boxes of 24.
In glass: Flagyl I.V. RTU, sterile (metronidazole), is supplied in 100-ml single-dose vials, each containing an isotonic, buffered solution of 500 mg metronidazole, individually packaged in cartons of 6 vials.

Flagyl I.V. RTU should be stored at controlled room temperature, 59° to 86° F (15° to 30°C), and protected from light.

1. Proposed standard: PSM-11—Proposed Reference Dilution Procedure for Antimicrobic Susceptibility Testing of Anaerobic Bacteria, National Committee for Clinical Laboratory Standards, and Sutter, et al.: Collaborative Evaluation of a Proposed Reference Dilution Method of Susceptibility Testing of Anaerobic Bacteria, Antimicrob. Agents Chemother. *16:*495–502 (Oct.) 1979; and Tally, et al: *In Vitro* Activity of Thienamycin, Antimicrob. Agents Chemother. *14:*436–438 (Sept.) 1978.

2. Ralph, E.D., and Kirby, W.M.M.: Bioassay of Metronidazole With Either Anaerobic or Aerobic Incubation, J. Infect. Dis. *132:*587–591 (Nov.) 1975; or Gulaid, et al.: Determination of Metronidazole and Its Major Metabolites in Biological Fluids by High Pressure Liquid Chromatography, Br. J. Clin. Pharmacol. *6:*430–432, 1978.

[*Shown in Product Identification Section*]

NITRODISC™ ℞
(nitroglycerin)
5 mg/24 hr; 10 mg/24 hr

Description: The Nitrodisc pad incorporates a patented Microseal Drug Delivery™ system consisting of a solid, nitroglycerin-impregnated polymer bonded to a flexible, non-sensitizing adhesive bandage. It is designed to be applied topically. Nitrodisc provides constant and controlled drug delivery over a uniform skin surface area for 24 hours.
Nitrodisc is available in two strengths which release either 5 mg or 10 mg of nitroglycerin during a 24-hour period. The 5 mg/24 hr system contains 16 mg nitroglycerin over an 8 cm^2 releasing surface. The 10 mg/24 hr system contains 32 mg nitroglycerin over a 16 cm^2 releasing surface (see *How Supplied* section).
Actions: When a Nitrodisc pad is applied to the skin, nitroglycerin is absorbed continuously through the skin into the systemic circulation. This results in active drug reaching the target organs (heart and peripheral vasculature) before being inactivated by the liver. Nitroglycerin is a smooth muscle relaxant with vascular effects manifested predominantly by venous dilation and pooling. The major beneficial effect of nitroglycerin in angina pectoris is due to a reduction in myocardial oxygen consumption secondary to vascular smooth muscle relaxation and consequent reduced cardiac preload and afterload. In addition, a direct effect of nitroglycerin on the coronary vessels is recognized as well.
In clinical studies, transdermal absorption of nitroglycerin from Nitrodisc occurred in a continuous and well-controlled manner for a minimum of 24 hours. Therapeutic plasma levels were attained within 1 hour after the application of the pad and remained in the therapeutic range for 24 hours. Plasma levels of nitroglycerin were still detectable 30 minutes after removal of the system.
The amount of nitroglycerin released (5 mg/24 hr or 10 mg/24 hr) represents the mean absorption rates through skin determined during clinical evaluations. Absorption may vary among individuals.
Indications and Usage: Nitrodisc is indicated for the prevention and treatment of angina pectoris due to coronary artery disease.
Contraindications: Nitrodisc (nitroglycerin) is contraindicated in patients known to be intolerant of organic nitrate drugs, and in patients with marked anemia, increased intraocular pressure, or increased intracranial pressure.
Warnings: In patients with acute myocardial infarction or congestive heart failure, Nitrodisc should be used under careful clinical and/or hemodynamic monitoring.
In terminating treatment of patients with angina, both the dosage and frequency of application must be gradually reduced over a period of 4 to 6 weeks to prevent potential withdrawal reactions, which are characteristic of all vasodilators in the nitrate class.
Precautions: Symptoms of hypotension, such as faintness, weakness, or dizziness, particularly orthostatic hypotension, may be due to overdosage. When these symptoms occur, the dosage should be reduced or use of the product discontinued.
Nitrodisc is not intended for immediate relief of anginal attacks. For this purpose, occasional use of sublingual preparations may be necessary.
Adverse Reactions: Transient headache is the most common side effect, especially when higher doses of the drug are used. These headaches should be treated with mild analgesics while Nitrodisc therapy is continued. When such headaches are unresponsive to treatment, the nitroglycerin dosage should be reduced or use of the product discontinued.
Adverse reactions reported less frequently include hypotension, increased heart rate, faintness, flushing, dizziness, nausea, vomiting, and dermatitis. These symptoms are attributable to the known pharmacologic effects of nitroglycerin, but may be symptoms of overdosage. When they persist, Nitrodisc (nitroglycerin) dose should be reduced or use of the product discontinued.
Dosage and Administration: A Nitrodisc pad should be applied once each day. To use the pad, follow the instructions on the package. Nitrodisc should be applied to a skin site free of hair and not subject to excessive movement. It should not be applied to the distal parts of the extremities. A suitable area should be shaved free of hair, if necessary. The application site should be changed slightly each time to avoid undue skin irritation. A new pad should be applied if the product loosens.
The optimal dosage regimen should be selected based upon the clinical response, the side effects, and the effects of therapy upon blood pressure and heart rate. It is recommended that therapy be initiated with the smaller pad, and that the larger pad be utilized when a greater response is desired. In the event that higher doses are necessary, multiple pads may be applied.
Patient Instructions for Application: These are provided with the product.
How Supplied:

Nitrodisc	5 mg/ 24 hr	10 mg/ 24 hr
Drug released per 24 hours	5 mg	10 mg
Total drug content	16 mg	32 mg
Drug releasing surface	8 cm^2	16 cm^2

Nitrodisc (nitroglycerin) pads are supplied in cartons of 30. Store at a controlled room temperature of 59°–86°F (15°–30°C). **Do not refrigerate.** Extremes of temperature and humidity should be avoided.

[*Shown in Product Identification Section*]

TATUM-T™ ℞
(intrauterine copper contraceptive)

Description: The plastic component of the Tatum-T (intrauterine copper contraceptive) is composed of polyethylene with barium sulfate added to render it radiopaque. Its shape approximates the letter T. The vertical dimension measures 36 mm and the horizontal, 32 mm.
Coiled around the vertical limb is 120 mg of copper wire providing approximately 210 mm^2 of exposed copper surface area. A polyethylene retrieval thread is fastened to the free end of the vertical limb of the Tatum-T.
The Tatum-T is supplied with a simple tubular plastic inserter. All components are sterile.

For **Mode of Action, Indications and Usage, Contraindications, Warnings, Precautions,** and **Adverse Reactions,** *see Cu-7 (intrauterine copper contraceptive) under this manufacturer.*

Directions for Use: The Tatum-T is to be placed within the uterine cavity. See the *Procedure for Insertion* for the insertion technique. The optimal time of insertion is during the latter part of the menstrual flow or one or two days thereafter. The cervical canal is relatively more patent at this time, and there is little chance that the patient may be pregnant.
Present information indicates that efficacy is retained for 36 months. There is no evidence that contraceptive efficacy decreases with time up to three years of use, but unless new data support a longer period of efficacy and safety, the Tatum-T must be removed within 36 months from the date of insertion and a new one inserted if desired. If partial expulsion occurs, removal is indicated, and a new Tatum-T may be inserted. Removal of the Tatum-T may also be indicated in the event of heavy or persistent bleeding.
The physician should become thoroughly familiar with the instructions for use before attempting insertion or removal of the Tatum-T.
Clinical Studies: Different event rates have been reported with the use of different intrauterine contraceptives. Inasmuch as these rates are usually derived from separate studies conducted by different investigators in several population groups, a comparison cannot be made with precision. Even in different studies with the same contraceptive, considerably different rates are likely to be obtained because of differing characteristics of the study population. Furthermore, event rates per unit of time tend to be lower as clinical experience is expanded, possibly due to retention in the clinical study of those patients who accept the treatment regimen, not having discontinued due to adverse reactions or pregnancy, so that those remaining in the study were those less susceptible. In clinical trials of the Tatum-T conducted in the United States and Canada, use effectiveness was determined as follows for parous and nulliparous women, as tabulated by the life-table method. (Rates are expressed as cumulative events per 100 women through 12, 24, and 36 months of use.)
This experience encompasses 236,060 woman-months of use, including 12 months for 8,232 women, 24 months for 4,247, and 36 months for 1,408.
Cumulative rates were:
[See table on next page].
Procedure for Insertion
Physicians are cautioned that it is imperative that they become thoroughly familiar with the instructions for insertion before attempting placement of the "T." The insertion technique is different in several respects from that employed with other intrauterine contraceptives currently available; particular attention should be paid to the illustrations and instructions.
The Tatum-T may be inserted easily at any time during the menstrual cycle. It is *not* necessary to delay insertion until a menstrual flow is in progress; however, the possibility of existing undetermined pregnancy is lessened if insertion is made during or shortly following a menstrual period.
The cervix should be cleansed with antiseptic solution and its anterior lip grasped with a tenaculum prior to sounding the uterus and insertion of the Tatum-T. Insertion of the Tatum-T into a severely anteverted or severely retro-

Continued on next page

Searle Pharm.—Cont.

verted uterus may be difficult unless sufficient tension is applied to the tenaculum. Determination of the depth and direction of the uterine cavity should be made with a sound prior to insertion.
An aseptic technique should be employed. Sterile gloves are recommended; however, the package itself may be used to set the cervical stop and to load the "T" into the insertion tube. A small loading device is contained within the package to facilitate this step. Exercise care to avoid contaminating the "T" or that part of the tube which will enter the cervical canal.

Caution:
DO NOT load the "T" into the tube until after the cervical stop on the tube has been set to the sounded depth nor leave it loaded longer than 2 minutes. The plastic of the Tatum-T is soft and it will lose its "memory"; it will then fail to return to its "T" configuration within the uterus and thus invite loss of effectiveness and early expulsion.
DO NOT push the "T" into the tube so that less than ¼ inch of the frame protrudes; placement may be improper; the arms may be damaged. If more than ¼ inch protrudes, the risk of perforation is increased.
DO NOT remove the thread-retaining clip from the insertion rod until after insertion has been made and you are ready to deposit the Tatum-T within the uterine cavity. The thread-retaining clip on the rod prevents the "T" and/or rod from falling to a non-sterile surface. When held against the end of the tube during the loading procedure, it helps to keep the "T" from being pushed too far into the tube and prevents premature ejection of the "T" during the insertion procedure.
DO NOT force the insertion. It is generally believed that most perforations occur at the time of insertion, although the perforation may not be detected until some time later. The position of the uterus should be determined during the pre-insertion examination. Great care must be exercised during the pre-insertion sounding and subsequent insertion.
Note: If the uterine cavity measures under 6.5 cm, the incidence of pain, bleeding, partial or complete expulsion, perforation, and possibly pregnancy, increases. Insertion is not recommended into a uterus that sounds under 6.0 cm.

1. Sterile gloves are recommended for the insertion procedure. If sterile gloves are used, the instrument may be removed from the package when setting the cervical stop and loading it into the insertion tube. If sterile gloves are not used then the package containing the "T" should be used for these procedures. (The package should be torn open just over halfway.)
2. After sounding, adjust the ¼-in-thick blue cervical stop on the tube. The edge closer to the handle must be set at the sounded depth of the uterus, *see Figure 1,* because the "T" protrudes ¼ in from the end of the tube. If the package is being used to set the cervical stop, do not put the sound inside the package since it could contaminate the "T".
3. The plastic loading device affixed to the cardboard backing near the "T" will help facilitate loading the "T" into the tube. NOTE: It is easier to load the "T" when the sides of the loading device are not squeezed together. For this reason it is best to hold the cardboard backing and not the device. Free the insertion instrument from the cardboard mount. Holding the insertion instrument midway between the cervical stop and the handle, push the insertion rod and tube so that the arms of the "T" slide into the cul-de-sac of the loading device. *See Figure 2.* The arms of the "T" are now folded against the tube. Retract the tube and rod together until the tube clears the arms of the "T". Again push the insertion instrument towards the loading device, trapping the arms of the "T" in the tube until ¼ in (~0.6 cm) of the folded "T" protrudes and the end of the rod just touches the stem of the "T". *See Figure 3.* To release the "T" from the loading device, rotate the insertion instrument 90° and slide the inserter out. If the package is being used to maintain sterility, the insertion instrument should not be completely removed from the package until the cervical stop has been aligned. Align the folded arms of the "T" with the wings of the cervical stop. After the cervical stop has been aligned, open the package the rest of the way.
4. Immediately apply gentle traction on the uterus with a tenaculum and insert the Tatum-T through the cervical canal up to the fundus. *See Figure 4.* Maintain or align the cervical stop at the cervix in a horizontal plane.
5. Press the thread-retaining clip back toward the handle to free the thread. Hold the rod firmly, but without undue pressure against the stem of the "T," and withdraw the tube to about ½ in (1.3 cm) from the handle. This frees the arms of the "T" but still keeps the stem end in the tube. *See Figure 5. Push the tube back until the cervical stop touches the cervix. See Figure 6.* This holds the "T" near the fundus while the rod is removed.
6. Hold the tube still and withdraw the insertion rod.
7. Withdraw the tube, depositing the "T" in the uterus. Cut the thread about 2 in (5 cm) from the external os. DO NOT PULL OUT EXCESS THREAD BEFORE CUTTING.

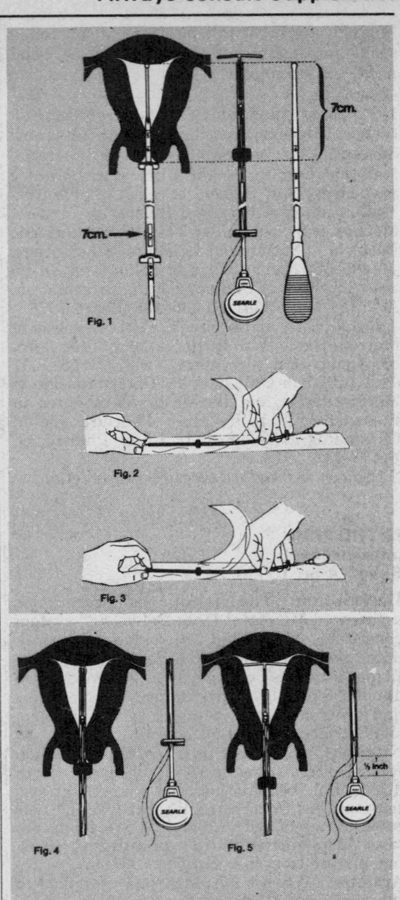

Removal of the Tatum-T

ROUTINE REMOVAL—THREAD VISIBLE:

1. DO NOT exert a sudden pull or jerk on the retrieval thread. Exert a firm, steady pull on the thread. A jerk may cause the thread to break.

2. A ring (sponge) forceps, with its smooth edges and minimal crushing force, is a good instrument with which to grasp the thread.

3. Other instruments may be used, but care must be exerted to avoid crushing or cutting the thread.

4. Avoid winding or angulating the thread about the jaws of the withdrawal instrument.

5. Utilize the minimum force needed to remove the Tatum-T.

6. Should resistance be encountered, dislodge the Tatum-T with a probe or uterine sound before making further removal attempts.

THREAD NOT VISIBLE: It the Tatum-T is in the uterus, and the thread is not visible, the following procedures should be considered when you elect to recover it:

1. Aseptic use of a slim instrument (e.g., uterine dressing forceps) will frequently permit removal in the office.

2. Hysteroscopy under hospital conditions may be required.

3. D & C and also suction aspiration have been used as alternative measures.

	12 Months		24 Months		36 Months	
	Parous	Nulliparous	Parous	Nulliparous	Parous	Nulliparous
Pregnancy	3.0	2.1	4.9	4.5	6.0	5.8
Expulsion	7.8	8.0	9.8	9.6	10.8	10.9
Medical removal	10.9	13.9	18.2	21.9	23.3	26.9
Continuation	73.4	71.4	55.0	53.9	41.9	40.1

Tatum-T Placement Instrument

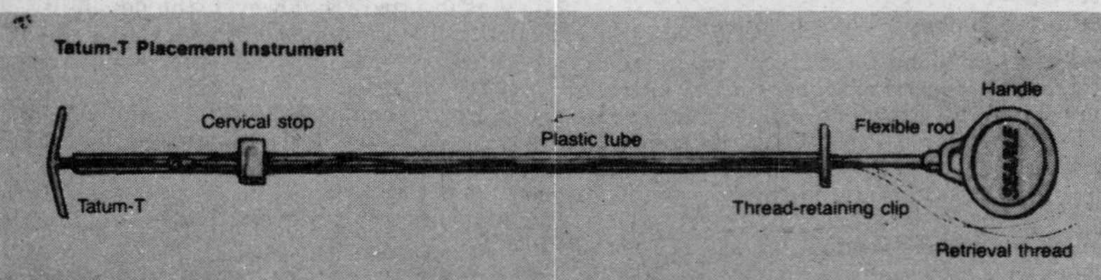

NOTE: If intrauterine manipulative procedures are required, allow an appropriate healing period before inserting a new Tatum-T.

How Supplied: Available in boxes of 10, 25, and 50 sterile units (Tatum-T with an inserter), and sufficient patient brochures and identification cards.

[*Shown in Product Identification Section*]

The preceding prescribing information for Searle Pharmaceuticals Inc. was current on November 15, 1982.

Searle Consumer Products

Division of Searle Pharmaceuticals Inc.
BOX 5110
CHICAGO, IL 60680

COMFOLAX®
(docusate sodium USP)

For a complete description of this product, please see the PDR for Nonprescription Drugs.

COMFOLAX-*plus* ®
(docusate sodium with casanthranol)

For a complete description of this product, please see the PDR for Nonprescription Drugs.

DRAMAMINE®
(dimenhydrinate)

Product information for all forms of Dramamine is now shown under Searle Pharmaceuticals Inc. in this publication, and for the forms shown below in the PDR for Nonprescription Drugs.
The OTC forms of Dramamine are available as follows:

How Supplied: *For Oral Use*—Scored, white **tablets** of 50 mg, USP, with SEARLE debossed on one side and 1701 on the other side, in packets of 12, and in bottles of 36 and 100; **liquid,** 12.5 mg/4 ml, in bottles of 3 fl oz.

METAMUCIL®
(psyllium hydrophilic mucilloid)

Description: Metamucil is a bulk laxative that provides a bland, nonirritating bulk and promotes normal elimination. It contains refined hydrophilic mucilloid, a highly efficient dietary fiber, derived from the husk of the psyllium seed *(Plantago ovata)*. An equal amount of dextrose, a carbohydrate, is added as a dispersing agent. Each dose contains about 1 mg of sodium, 31 mg of potassium, and 14 calories. Carbohydrate content is approximately 3.5 g; psyllium mucilloid content is 3.4 g.

Actions: Metamucil is uniform, instantly miscible, palatable, and nonirritative in the gastrointestinal tract.

Indications: Metamucil is indicated in the management of chronic constipation, in irritable bowel syndrome, as adjunctive therapy in constipation of duodenal ulcer and diverticular disease, in the bowel management of patients with hemorrhoids, and for constipation during pregnancy, convalescence, and senility.

Dosage and Administration: The usual adult dosage is one rounded teaspoonful (7 g) stirred into a standard 8-oz glass of cool water or other suitable liquid and taken orally one to three times a day, depending on the need and response. It may require continuing use for 2 or 3 days to provide optimal benefit. Best results are observed if each dose is followed by an additional glass of liquid.

Contraindications: Intestinal obstruction, fecal impaction.

How Supplied: Powder, containers of 7 oz, 14 oz, and 21 oz, and cartons of 100 unit-dose (7g) packets.

Is This Product OTC: Yes. See also PDR For Nonprescription Drugs.

INSTANT MIX METAMUCIL®
(psyllium hydrophilic mucilloid)

Description: Instant Mix Metamucil is provided in premeasured, single-dose packets for oral use. It contains refined hydrophilic mucilloid, a highly efficient dietary fiber, derived from the husk of the psyllium seed *(Plantago ovata)*, together with citric acid, sucrose (a carbohydrate), potassium bicarbonate, calcium carbonate, flavoring, and sodium bicarbonate. Each dose contains approximately 7 mg of sodium, 60 mg of calcium, 280 mg of potassium, and less than 4 calories. Carbohydrate content is 0.9 g; psyllium mucilloid content is 3.6 g.

Actions: Instant Mix Metamucil, effervescent and requiring no stirring, is uniform, instantly miscible, palatable, and nonirritative in the gastrointestinal tract.

Indications: Instant Mix Metamucil is indicated for its smoothage effect in the management of chronic constipation, in irritable bowel syndrome, as adjunctive therapy in constipation of duodenal ulcer and diverticular disease, in the bowel management of patients with hemorrhoids, and for constipation during pregnancy, convalescence, and senility.

Contraindications: Intestinal obstruction, fecal impaction.

Dosage and Administration: The usual adult dosage is the contents of one packet, taken one to three times daily as follows: 1. Entire contents of a packet are poured into a standard 8-oz water glass. 2. The glass is slowly filled with cool water. 3. Entire contents are drunk immediately. (An additional glass of water may be taken for best results.)

How Supplied: Cartons of 16 and 30 single-dose (6.4 g) packets, and cartons of 100 unit-dose (6.4 g) packets.

Is This Product OTC: Yes. See also PDR For Nonprescription Drugs.

Orange Flavor METAMUCIL®
Strawberry Flavor METAMUCIL®
(psyllium hydrophilic mucilloid)

Description: Metamucil is a bulk laxative that provides a bland, nonirritating bulk and promotes normal elimination. It contains refined hydrophilic mucilloid, a highly efficient dietary fiber, derived from the husk of the psyllium seed (*Plantago ovata*), with sucrose (a carbohydrate) as a dispersing agent, citric acid, flavoring, and coloring. Each dose contains about 1 mg of sodium, 31 mg of potassium, and 28 calories. Carbohydrate content is approximately 7.1 g; psyllium mucilloid content is 3.4 g.

Actions: Metamucil is uniform, instantly miscible, palatable, and nonirritative in the gastrointestinal tract.

Indications: Metamucil is indicated in the management of chronic constipation, in irritable bowel syndrome, as adjunctive therapy in constipation of duodenal ulcer and diverticular disease, in the bowel management of patients with hemorrhoids, and for constipation during pregnancy, convalescence, and senility.

Contraindications: Intestinal obstruction, fecal impaction.

Dosage and Administration: The usual adult dosage is one rounded tablespoonful (11 g) stirred into a standard 8-oz glass of cool water and taken orally one to three times a day, depending on the need and response. It may require continuing use for 2 or 3 days to provide optimal benefit. Best results are observed if each dose is followed by an additional glass of liquid.

How Supplied: Powder, containers of 7 oz, 14 oz, and 21 oz.

Is This Product OTC: Yes. See also PDR For Nonprescription Drugs.

Orange Flavor
INSTANT MIX METAMUCIL®
(psyllium hydrophilic mucilloid)

Description: Orange Flavor Instant Mix Metamucil is provided in premeasured, single-dose packets for oral use. It contains refined hydrophilic mucilloid, a highly efficient dietary fiber derived from the husk of the psyllium seed (*Plantago ovata*), together with sucrose (a carbohydrate), citric acid, potassium bicarbonate, flavoring, coloring, and sodium bicarbonate. Each dose contains approximately 6 mg of sodium, 307 mg of potassium, and 4½ calories. Carbohydrate content is about 1.1 g; psyllium mucilloid content is 3.6 g.

Actions: Instant Mix Metamucil, effervescent and requiring no stirring, is uniform, instantly miscible, palatable, and nonirritative in the gastrointestinal tract.

Indications: Instant Mix Metamucil is indicated in the management of chronic constipation, in irritable bowel syndrome, as adjunctive therapy in constipation of duodenal ulcer and diverticular disease, in the bowel management of patients with hemorrhoids, and for constipation during pregnancy, convalescence, and senility.

Contraindications: Intestinal obstruction, fecal impaction.

Dosage and Administration: The usual adult dosage is the contents of one packet, taken one to three times daily as follows: 1. Entire contents of a packet are poured into a standard 8-oz water glass. 2. The glass is slowly filled with cool water. 3. Entire contents are drunk immediately. (An additional glass of water may be taken for best results.)

How Supplied: Cartons of 16 and of 30 single-dose packets.

Is This Product OTC: Yes. See also PDR for Nonprescription Drugs.

The preceding prescribing information for Searle Consumer Products was current on November 1, 1982.

Searle & Co.

SAN JUAN, PUERTO RICO 00936

ALDACTAZIDE® ℞
(spironolactone with hydrochlorothiazide)

Warning

Spironolactone, an ingredient of Aldactazide, has been shown to be a tumorigen in chronic toxicity studies in rats (see *Warnings*). Aldactazide should be used only in those conditions described under *Indications*. Unnecessary use of this drug should be avoided.

Fixed-dose combination drugs are not indicated for initial therapy of edema or hypertension. Edema or hypertension requires therapy titrated to the individual patient. If the fixed combination represents the dosage so determined, its use may be more convenient in patient management. The treatment of hypertension and edema is not static, but must be reevaluated as conditions in each patient warrant.

Description: Each tablet of Aldactazide contains 25 mg of spironolactone (Aldactone®) and 25 mg of hydrochlorothiazide.

Spironolactone is 17-hydroxy-7α-mercapto-3-oxo-17α-pregn-4-ene-21-carboxylic acid γ-lactone acetate. Hydrochlorothiazide is 6-

Continued on next page

Searle & Co.—Cont.

chloro-3,4-dihydro-2H-1,2,4-benzothiadiazine-7-sulfonamide 1,1-dioxide.

Actions: Aldactazide is a combination of two diuretic agents with different but complementary mechanisms and sites of action, thereby providing additive diuretic and antihypertensive effects. Additionally, the spironolactone component helps to minimize the potassium loss characteristically induced by the thiazide component.

The diuretic effect of spironolactone is mediated through its action as a specific pharmacologic antagonist of aldosterone, primarily by competitive binding of receptors at the aldosterone-dependent sodium-potassium exchange site in the distal convoluted renal tubule. Hydrochlorothiazide promotes the excretion of sodium and water primarily by inhibiting their reabsorption in the cortical diluting segment of the renal tubule.

Aldactazide is effective in significantly lowering the systolic and diastolic blood pressure in many patients with essential hypertension, even when aldosterone secretion is within normal limits.

Both spironolactone and hydrochlorothiazide reduce exchangeable sodium, plasma volume, body weight and blood pressure. The diuretic and antihypertensive effects of the individual components are potentiated when spironolactone and hydrochlorothiazide are given concurrently.

Clinical Pharmacology: In the human, the bioavailability of both spironolactone and hydrochlorothiazide from orally administered Aldactazide tablets is approximately 90 percent when compared with equivalent doses of the individual components administered in an optimally-absorbed solution (spironolactone in polyethylene glycol 400).

Spironolactone is rapidly and extensively metabolized. The primary metabolite is canrenone which attains peak serum levels at two to four hours following single oral administration. Canrenone plasma concentrations decline in two distinct phases, being rapid in the first 12 hours and slower from 12 to 96 hours. The log-linear phase half-life of canrenone, following multiple doses of Aldactone (spironolactone), is between 13 and 24 hours. Both spironolactone and canrenone are more than 90-percent bound to plasma proteins. The metabolites of spironolactone are excreted primarily in urine, but also in bile.

Hydrochlorothiazide is rapidly absorbed following oral administration. Onset of action is observed within one hour and persists for 6 to 12 hours. Plasma concentrations attain peak levels at one to two hours and decline with a half-life of four to five hours. Hydrochlorothiazide undergoes only slight metabolic alteration and is excreted in urine. It is distributed throughout the extracellular space, with essentially no tissue accumulation except in the kidney.

Indications: Spironolactone, an ingredient of Aldactazide, has been shown to be a tumorigen in chronic toxicity studies in rats (see *Warnings* section). Aldactazide should be used only in those conditions described below. Unnecessary use of this drug should be avoided.

Aldactazide is indicated for:

Edematous conditions for patients with:

Congestive heart failure: For the management of edema and sodium retention when the patient is only partially responsive to, or is intolerant of, other therapeutic measures. The treatment of diuretic-induced hypokalemia in patients with congestive heart failure when other measures are considered inappropriate. The treatment of patients with congestive heart failure taking digitalis when other therapies are considered inadequate or inappropriate.

Cirrhosis of the liver accompanied by edema and/or ascites: Aldosterone levels may be exceptionally high in this condition. Aldactazide is indicated for maintenance therapy together with bed rest and the restriction of fluid and sodium.

The nephrotic syndrome: For nephrotic patients when treatment of the underlying disease, restriction of fluid and sodium intake, and the use of other diuretics do not provide an adequate response.

Essential hypertension

For patients with essential hypertension in whom other measures are considered inadequate or inappropriate. In hypertensive patients for the treatment of a diuretic-induced hypokalemia when other measures are considered inappropriate.

Usage in Pregnancy. The routine use of diuretics in an otherwise healthy woman is inappropriate and exposes mother and fetus to unnecessary hazard. Diuretics do not prevent development of toxemia of pregnancy, and there is no satisfactory evidence that they are useful in the treatment of developing toxemia.

Edema during pregnancy may arise from pathologic causes or from the physiologic and mechanical consequences of pregnancy. Aldactazide is indicated in pregnancy when edema is due to pathologic causes just as it is in the absence of pregnancy (however, see *Warnings* section). Dependent edema in pregnancy, resulting from restriction of venous return by the expanded uterus, is properly treated through elevation of the lower extremities and use of support hose; use of diuretics to lower intravascular volume in this case is unsupported and unnecessary. There is hypervolemia during normal pregnancy which is harmful to neither the fetus nor the mother (in the absence of cardiovascular disease), but which is associated with edema, including generalized edema, in the majority of pregnant women. If this edema produces discomfort, increased recumbency will often provide relief. In rare instances, this edema may cause extreme discomfort which is not relieved by rest. In these cases, a short course of diuretics may provide relief and may be appropriate.

Contraindications: Aldactazide is contraindicated in patients with anuria, acute renal insufficiency, significant impairment of renal function or hyperkalemia and in patients who are allergic to thiazide diuretics or to other sulfonamide-derived drugs. Aldactazide may also be contraindicated in acute or severe hepatic failure.

Warnings: Potassium supplementation, either in the form of medication or as a diet rich in potassium, should not ordinarily be given in association with Aldactazide therapy. Excessive potassium intake may cause hyperkalemia in patients receiving Aldactazide (see *Precautions* section). Aldactazide should not be administered concurrently with other potassium-sparing diuretics.

Sulfonamide derivatives, including thiazides, have been reported to exacerbate or activate systemic lupus erythematosus.

Spironolactone has been shown to be a tumorigen in chronic toxicity studies performed in rats, with its proliferative effects manifested on endocrine organs and the liver. In one study using 25, 75 and 250 times the usual daily human dose (2 mg/kg) there was a statistically significant dose-related increase in benign adenomas of the thyroid and testes. In female rats there was a statistically significant increase in malignant mammary tumors at the mid-dose only. In male rats there was a dose-related increase in proliferative changes in the liver. At the highest dosage level (500 mg/kg) the range of effects included hepatocytomegaly, hyperplastic nodules and hepatocellular carcinoma; the last was not statistically significant at a value of $p = 0.05$.

Precautions: Patients receiving Aldactazide therapy should be carefully evaluated for possible disturbances of fluid and electrolyte balance. Hyperkalemia may occur in patients with impaired renal function or excessive potassium intake and can cause cardiac irregularities which may be fatal. Consequently, no potassium supplement should ordinarily be given with Aldactazide. Hyperkalemia can be treated promptly by the rapid intravenous administration of glucose (20 to 50 percent) and regular insulin, using 0.25 to 0.5 units of insulin per gram of glucose. This is a temporary measure to be repeated as required. Aldactazide should be discontinued and potassium intake (including dietary potassium) restricted.

Hypokalemia may develop as a result of profound diuresis, particularly when Aldactazide is used concomitantly with loop diuretics, glucocorticoids or ACTH. Hypokalemia may exaggerate the effects of digitalis therapy. Potassium depletion may induce signs of digitalis intoxication at previously tolerated dosage levels.

Warning signs of possible fluid and electrolyte imbalance include dryness of the mouth, thirst, weakness, lethargy, drowsiness, restlessness, muscle pains or cramps, muscular fatigue, hypotension, oliguria, tachycardia and gastrointestinal symptoms.

Aldactazide therapy may cause a transient elevation of BUN. This appears to represent a concentration phenomenon rather than renal toxicity, since the BUN returns to normal after Aldactazide is discontinued. Progressive elevation of BUN is suggestive of the presence of preexisting renal impairment.

Reversible hyperchloremic metabolic acidosis, usually in association with hyperkalemia, has been reported to occur in some patients with decompensated hepatic cirrhosis, even in the presence of normal renal function.

Dilutional hyponatremia, manifested by dryness of the mouth, thirst, lethargy and drowsiness, and confirmed by a low serum sodium level, may be induced, especially when Aldactazide is administered in combination with other diuretics. A true low-salt syndrome may rarely develop with Aldactazide therapy and may be manifested by increasing mental confusion similar to that observed with hepatic coma. This syndrome is differentiated from dilutional hyponatremia in that it does not occur with obvious fluid retention. Its treatment requires that diuretic therapy be discontinued and sodium administered.

Gynecomastia may develop in association with the use of spironolactone, and physicians should be alert to its possible onset. The development of gynecomastia appears to be related to both dosage level and duration of therapy and is normally reversible when Aldactazide is discontinued. In rare instances some breast enlargement may persist.

Thiazides have been demonstrated to alter the metabolism of uric acid and carbohydrates, with possible development of hyperuricemia, gout and decreased glucose tolerance. Thiazides may temporarily exaggerate abnormalities of glucose metabolism in diabetic patients or cause abnormalities to appear in patients with latent diabetes.

Both spironolactone and hydrochlorothiazide reduce the vascular responsiveness to norepinephrine. Therefore, caution should be exercised in the management of patients subjected to regional or general anesthesia while they are being treated with Aldactazide. Thiazides may also increase the responsiveness to tubocurarine. The antihypertensive effects of hydrochlorothiazide may be enhanced in patients who have undergone sympathectomy.

Pathologic changes in the parathyroid gland with hypercalcemia and hypophosphatemia have been observed in patients on prolonged thiazide therapy. Thiazides may also decrease serum PBI levels without evidence of alteration of thyroid function.

Usage in Pregnancy. Spironolactone or its metabolites may, and hydrochlorothiazide does, cross the placental barrier. Therefore, the use of Aldactazide in pregnant women requires that the anticipated benefit be weighed against possible hazards to the fetus. These hazards include fetal or neonatal jaundice, thrombocytopenia, and possible other adverse reactions which have been reported in the adult.

Nursing Mothers. Canrenone, a metabolite of spironolactone, and hydrochlorothiazide appear in breast milk. If use of these drugs is deemed essential, an alternative method of infant feeding should be instituted.

Adverse Reactions: Gynecomastia is observed not infrequently. Other adverse reactions that have been reported in association with the use of spironolactone are: gastrointestinal symptoms including cramping and diarrhea, drowsiness, lethargy, headache, maculopapular or erythematous cutaneous eruptions, urticaria, mental confusion, drug fever, ataxia, inability to achieve or maintain erection, irregular menses or amenorrhea, postmenopausal bleeding, hirsutism and deepening of the voice. Carcinoma of the breast has been reported in patients taking spironolactone, but a cause and effect relationship has not been established.

Adverse reactions reported in association with the use of thiazides include: gastrointestinal symptoms (anorexia, nausea, vomiting, diarrhea, abdominal cramps), purpura, thrombocytopenia, leukopenia, agranulocytosis, dermatologic symptoms (cutaneous eruptions, pruritus, erythema multiforme), paresthesia, acute pancreatitis, jaundice, dizziness, vertigo, headache, xanthopsia, photosensitivity, necrotizing angiitis, aplastic anemia, orthostatic hypotension, muscle spasm, weakness and restlessness. Adverse reactions are usually reversible upon discontinuation of Aldactazide.

Dosage and Administration: Optimal dosage should be established by individual titration of the components (see Box Warning).

Edema in adults (*congestive heart failure, hepatic cirrhosis or nephrotic syndrome*). The usual maintenance dose of Aldactazide is four tablets daily administered in a single dose or in divided doses but may range from one to eight tablets daily depending on the response to the initial titration. In some instances it may be desirable to administer separate tablets of either Aldactone (spironolactone) or hydrochlorothiazide in addition to Aldactazide in order to provide optimal individual therapy.

The onset of diuresis with Aldactazide occurs promptly and, due to prolonged effect of the spironolactone component, persists for two to three days after Aldactazide is discontinued.

Edema in children. The usual daily maintenance dose of Aldactazide should be that which provides 0.75 to 1.5 mg of spironolactone per pound of body weight (1.65 to 3.3 mg/kg).

Essential hypertension. Although the dosage will vary depending on the results of titration of the individual ingredients, many patients will be found to have an optimal response to the amount of hydrochlorothiazide and spironolactone contained in two to four tablets of Aldactazide per day given in a single dose or in divided doses.

Concurrent potassium supplementation is not recommended when Aldactazide is used in the long-term management of hypertension or in the treatment of most edematous conditions, since the spironolactone content of Aldactazide is usually sufficient to minimize loss induced by the hydrochlorothiazide component.

How Supplied: Aldactazide is supplied as scored, white tablets with SEARLE and 1011 debossed on the scored side and ALDACTAZIDE on the other side, each tablet containing 25 mg of Aldactone (spironolactone) and 25 mg of hydrochlorothiazide; bottles of 100, 500, 1,000, and 2,500, and cartons of 100 unit-dose individually blister-sealed tablets.

[*Shown in Product Identification Section*]

ALDACTONE® ℞
(spironolactone)

> **Warning**
>
> Spironolactone has been shown to be a tumorigen in chronic toxicity studies in rats (see *Warnings*). Aldactone should be used only in those conditions described under *Indications*. Unnecessary use of this drug should be avoided.

Description: Aldactone oral tablets contain 25 mg or 100 mg of spironolactone, 17-hydroxy-7α - mercapto -3- oxo-17α -pregn -4- ene-21-carboxylic acid γ-lactone acetate.

Spironolactone is practically insoluble in water, soluble in alcohol, and freely soluble in benzene and in chloroform.

Actions: Aldactone (spironolactone) is a specific pharmacologic antagonist of aldosterone, acting primarily through competitive binding of receptors at the aldosterone-dependent sodium-potassium exchange site in the distal convoluted renal tubule. Aldactone causes increased amounts of sodium and water to be excreted, while potassium is retained. Aldactone acts both as a diuretic and as an antihypertensive drug by this mechanism. It may be given alone or with other diuretic agents which act more proximally in the renal tubule.

Increased levels of the mineralocorticoid, aldosterone, are present in primary and secondary hyperaldosteronism. Edematous states in which secondary aldosteronism is usually involved include congestive heart failure, hepatic cirrhosis, and the nephrotic syndrome. By competing with aldosterone for receptor sites, Aldactone provides effective therapy for the edema and ascites in those conditions. Aldactone counteracts secondary aldosteronism induced by the volume depletion and associated sodium loss caused by active diuretic therapy.

Aldactone is effective in lowering the systolic and diastolic blood pressure in patients with primary hyperaldosteronism. It is also effective in most cases of essential hypertension, despite the fact that aldosterone secretion may be within normal limits in benign essential hypertension.

Through its action in antagonizing the effect of aldosterone, Aldactone inhibits the exchange of sodium for potassium in the distal renal tubule and helps to prevent potassium loss.

Aldactone has not been demonstrated to elevate serum uric acid, to precipitate gout or to alter carbohydrate metabolism.

Clinical Pharmacology: In the human, the bioavailability of spironolactone from orally administered Aldactone tablets exceeds 90 percent when compared with an optimally absorbed solution (spironolactone in polyethylene glycol 400). Spironolactone is rapidly and extensively metabolized. The primary metabolite is canrenone which attains peak serum levels at two to four hours following single oral administration. In the dose range of 25 to 200 mg, an approximately linear relationship exists between a single dose of spironolactone and plasma levels of canrenone. Plasma concentrations of canrenone decline in two distinct phases, the first phase lasting from 3 to 12 hours, being more rapid than the second phase lasting from 12 to 96 hours. Following multiple doses, the steady state plasma elimination half-life of canrenone is longer (19.2 ± 6.57 versus 12.5 ± 3.39 hours; means $\pm$ SD) when 200 mg of spironolactone is given once a day than when 50 mg is given four times a day. Both spironolactone and canrenone are more than 90-percent bound to plasma proteins. The metabolites of spironolactone are excreted primarily in urine, but also in bile.

Indications: Aldactone (spironolactone) is indicated in the management of:

Primary hyperaldosteronism for:

Establishing the diagnosis of primary hyperaldosteronism by therapeutic trial.

Short-term preoperative treatment of patients with primary hyperaldosteronism.

Long-term maintenance therapy for patients with discrete aldosterone-producing adrenal adenomas who are judged to be poor operative risks, or who decline surgery.

Long-term maintenance therapy for patients with bilateral micro- or macronodular adrenal hyperplasia (idiopathic hyperaldosteronism).

Edematous conditions for patients with:

Congestive heart failure: For the management of edema and sodium retention when the patient is only partially responsive to, or is intolerant of, other therapeutic measures. Aldactone is also indicated for patients with congestive heart failure taking digitalis when other therapies are considered inappropriate.

Cirrhosis of the liver accompanied by edema and/or ascites: Aldosterone levels may be exceptionally high in this condition. Aldactone is indicated for maintenance therapy together with bed rest and the restriction of fluid and sodium.

The nephrotic syndrome: For nephrotic patients when treatment of the underlying disease, restriction of fluid and sodium intake, and the use of other diuretics do not provide an adequate response.

Essential hypertension

Usually in combination with other drugs, Aldactone is indicated for patients who cannot be treated adequately with other agents or for whom other agents are considered inappropriate.

Hypokalemia

For the treatment of patients with hypokalemia when other measures are considered inappropriate or inadequate. Aldactone is also indicated for the prophylaxis of hypokalemia in patients taking digitalis when other measures are considered inadequate or inappropriate.

Usage in Pregnancy. The routine use of diuretics in an otherwise healthy woman is inappropriate and exposes mother and fetus to unnecessary hazard. Diuretics do not prevent development of toxemia of pregnancy, and there is no satisfactory evidence that they are useful in the treatment of developing toxemia.

Edema during pregnancy may arise from pathologic causes or from the physiologic and mechanical consequences of pregnancy.

Aldactone is indicated in pregnancy when edema is due to pathologic causes just as it is in the absence of pregnancy (however, see *Warnings* section). Dependent edema in pregnancy, resulting from restriction of venous return by the expanded uterus, is properly treated through elevation of the lower extremities and use of support hose; use of diuretics to lower intravascular volume in this case is unsupported and unnecessary. There is hypervolemia during normal pregnancy which is harmful to neither the fetus nor the mother (in the absence of cardiovascular disease), but which is associated with edema, including generalized edema, in the majority of pregnant women. If this edema produces discomfort, increased recumbency will often provide relief. In rare instances, this edema may cause extreme discomfort which is not relieved by rest. In these cases, a short course of diuretics may provide relief and may be appropriate.

Contraindications: Aldactone is contraindicated for patients with anuria, acute renal insufficiency, significant impairment of renal function, or hyperkalemia.

Warnings: Potassium supplementation, either in the form of medication or as a diet rich in potassium, should not ordinarily be given in

Continued on next page

Searle & Co.—Cont.

association with Aldactone therapy. Excessive potassium intake may cause hyperkalemia in patients receiving Aldactone (see *Precautions* section). Aldactone should not be administered concurrently with other potassium-sparing diuretics.

Spironolactone has been shown to be a tumorigen in chronic toxicity studies performed in rats, with its proliferative effects manifested on endocrine organs and the liver. In one study using 25, 75 and 250 times the usual daily human dose (2 mg/kg) there was a statistically significant dose-related increase in benign adenomas of the thyroid and testes. In female rats there was a statistically significant increase in malignant mammary tumors at the mid-dose only. In male rats there was a dose-related increase in proliferative changes in the liver. At the highest dosage level (500 mg/kg) the range of effects include hepatocytomegaly, hyperplastic nodules and hepatocellular carcinoma; the last was not statistically significant at a value of $p = 0.05$.

Precautions: Because of the diuretic action of Aldactone (spironolactone), patients should be carefully evaluated for possible disturbances of fluid and electrolyte balance. Hyperkalemia may occur in patients with impaired renal function or excessive potassium intake and can cause cardiac irregularities which may be fatal. Consequently, no potassium supplement should ordinarily be given with Aldactone. Hyperkalemia can be treated promptly by the rapid intravenous administration of glucose (20 to 50 percent) and regular insulin, using 0.25 to 0.5 units of insulin per gram of glucose. This is a temporary measure to be repeated as required. Aldactone should be discontinued and potassium intake (including dietary potassium) restricted.

Reversible hyperchloremic metabolic acidosis, usually in association with hyperkalemia, has been reported to occur in some patients with decompensated hepatic cirrhosis, even in the presence of normal renal function.

Hyponatremia, manifested by dryness of the mouth, thirst, lethargy and drowsiness, and confirmed by a low serum sodium level, may be caused or aggravated, especially when Aldactone is administered in combination with other diuretics.

Gynecomastia may develop in association with the use of spironolactone, and physicians should be alert to its possible onset. The development of gynecomastia appears to be related to both dosage level and duration of therapy and is normally reversible when Aldactone is discontinued. In rare instances some breast enlargement may persist.

Aldactone therapy may cause a transient elevation of BUN, especially in patients with preexisting renal impairment. Aldactone may cause mild acidosis.

When used in combination with other diuretics or antihypertensive agents Aldactone potentiates their effects. Therefore, the dosage of such drugs, particularly the ganglionic blocking agents, should be reduced by at least 50 percent when Aldactone is added to the regimen.

Spironolactone reduces the vascular responsiveness to norepinephrine. Therefore, caution should be exercised in the management of patients subjected to regional or general anesthesia while they are being treated with Aldactone.

Usage in Pregnancy. Spironolactone or its metabolites may cross the placental barrier. Therefore, the use of Aldactone in pregnant women requires that the anticipated benefit be weighed against possible hazard to the fetus.

Nursing Mothers. Canrenone, a metabolite of spironolactone, appears in breast milk. If use of the drug is deemed essential, an alternative method of infant feeding should be instituted.

Adverse Reactions: Gynecomastia is observed not infrequently. Other adverse reactions that have been reported in association with Aldactone are: gastrointestinal symptoms including cramping and diarrhea, drowsiness, lethargy, headache, maculopapular or erythematous cutaneous eruptions, urticaria, mental confusion, drug fever, ataxia, inability to achieve or maintain erection, irregular menses or amenorrhea, postmenopausal bleeding, hirsutism and deepening of the voice. Carcinoma of the breast has been reported in patients taking spironolactone, but a cause and effect relationship has not been established. Adverse reactions are usually reversible upon discontinuation of the drug.

Dosage and Administration: **Primary hyperaldosteronism.** Aldactone may be employed as an initial diagnostic measure to provide presumptive evidence of primary hyperaldosteronism while patients are on normal diets.

Long test: Aldactone (spironolactone) is administered at a daily dosage of 400 mg for three to four weeks. Correction of hypokalemia and of hypertension provides presumptive evidence for the diagnosis of primary hyperaldosteronism.

Short test: Aldactone is administered at a daily dosage of 400 mg for four days. If serum potassium increases during Aldactone administration but drops when Aldactone is discontinued, a presumptive diagnosis of primary hyperaldosteronism should be considered.

After the diagnosis of hyperaldosteronism has been established by more definitive testing procedures, Aldactone may be administered in doses of 100 to 400 mg daily in preparation for surgery. For patients who are considered unsuitable for surgery, Aldactone may be employed for long-term maintenance therapy at the lowest effective dosage determined for the individual patient.

Edema in adults (*congestive heart failure, hepatic cirrhosis or nephrotic syndrome*). An initial daily dosage of 100 mg of Aldactone administered in either single or divided doses is recommended, but may range from 25 to 200 mg daily. When given as the sole agent for diuresis, Aldactone should be continued for at least five days at the initial dosage level, after which it may be adjusted to the optimal therapeutic or maintenance level administered in either single or divided daily doses. If, after five days, an adequate diuretic response to Aldactone has not occurred, a second diuretic which acts more proximally in the renal tubule may be added to the regimen. Because of the additive effect of Aldactone when administered concurrently with such diuretics, an enhanced diuresis usually begins on the first day of combined treatment; combined therapy is indicated when more rapid diuresis is desired. The dosage of Aldactone should remain unchanged when other diuretic therapy is added.

Edema in children. The initial daily dosage should provide approximately 1.5 mg of Aldactone per pound of body weight (3.3 mg/kg) administered in either single or divided doses. For small children, Aldactone tablets may be pulverized and administered as a suspension in cherry syrup, NF. When refrigerated, such a suspension is stable for one month.

Essential hypertension. For adults, an initial daily dosage of 50 to 100 mg of Aldactone administered in either single or divided doses is recommended. Aldactone may also be given with diuretics which act more proximally in the renal tubule or with other antihypertensive agents. Treatment with Aldactone should be continued for at least two weeks, since the maximum response may not occur before this time. Subsequently, dosage should be adjusted according to the response of the patient.

Hypokalemia. Aldactone in a dosage ranging from 25 mg to 100 mg daily is useful in treating a diuretic-induced hypokalemia, when oral potassium supplements or other potassium-sparing regimens are considered inappropriate.

How Supplied: Aldactone 25 mg tablets are round, white, scored tablets with SEARLE and 1001 debossed on the scored side and ALDACTONE on the other side; bottles of 100, 500, 1,000, and 2,500, and cartons of 100 unit-dose individually blister-sealed tablets.

Aldactone 100 mg tablets are round, white, scored tablets with SEARLE and 1031 debossed on the scored side and ALDACTONE 100 MG on the other side; bottles of 100, and cartons of 100 unit-dose individually blister-sealed tablets.

[*Shown in Product Identification Section*]

AMINOPHYLLIN™ Tablets ℞
(aminophylline)

Description: Each tablet contains 100 or 200 mg of aminophylline USP, calculated as the dihydrate. Aminophylline USP (anhydrous) is a soluble complex containing approximately 85% anhydrous theophylline and 15% ethylenediamine. Aminophylline is white or slightly yellowish granules or powder, having a slight ammoniacal odor and a bitter taste.

Actions: Aminophylline directly relaxes the smooth muscle of the bronchial airways and pulmonary blood vessels, thus acting mainly as a bronchodilator, pulmonary vasodilator, and smooth muscle relaxant. The drug also possesses other actions typical of the xanthine derivatives: coronary vasodilator, diuretic, cardiac stimulant, cerebral stimulant, and skeletal muscle stimulant.

Indications: Aminophyllin Tablets are indicated for the relief and/or prevention of symptoms from asthma and reversible bronchospasm associated with chronic bronchitis and emphysema.

Contraindications: Aminophylline should not be administered to patients with active peptic ulcer disease, since it may increase the volume and acidity of gastric secretions.

Patients with a history of hypersensitivity to aminophylline or theophylline should not be treated with the drug.

Aminophylline should not be administered with other xanthine preparations.

Warnings: Excessive doses may be expected to be toxic. Some children may be unusually sensitive to aminophylline. Toxic synergism with ephedrine and other sympathomimetic bronchodilator drugs may occur.

Usage in Pregnancy. Safe use in pregnancy has not been established relative to possible adverse effects on fetal development. Therefore, aminophylline should not be used in pregnant women unless, in the judgment of the physician, the potential benefits outweigh the possible hazards.

Precautions: Use with caution in patients with severe cardiac disease, hypertension, hyperthyroidism, or acute myocardial injury. Particular caution in dose administration must be exercised in patients with a history of peptic ulcer since the condition may be exacerbated. Chronic oral administration in high doses may be associated with gastrointestinal irritation.

Caution should be used in giving aminophylline to patients in congestive heart failure. Serum levels in such patients have persisted for long periods following discontinuation of the drug.

The addition of ephedrine or other sympathomimetic drugs to regimens of aminophylline increases the toxicity potential and may result in symptoms of overdosage, due to the additive pharmacological effects of these compounds.

Adverse Reactions: The most consistent adverse reactions observed with *therapeutic* amounts of aminophylline are:

1. Gastrointestinal: Nausea, vomiting, anorexia, bitter aftertaste, dyspepsia, heavy feeling in the stomach, and gastrointestinal distress.

2. Central nervous system: Dizziness, vertigo, light-headedness, headache, nervousness, insomnia, and agitation.
3. Cardiovascular: Palpitation, tachycardia, flushing, and extrasystoles.
4. Respiratory: Increase in respiratory rate.
5. Dermatologic: Urticaria.

Overdosage: The most consistent reactions observed with *toxic* overdoses of aminophylline are:

1. Gastrointestinal: Nausea, vomiting, epigastric pain, hematemesis, and diarrhea.
2. Central nervous system: In addition to those cited above, the patient may exhibit hyperreflexia, fasciculations, and clonic and tonic convulsions. These are especially prone to occur in cases of overdosage in infants and small children.
3. Cardiovascular: In addition to those outlined above, marked hypotension and circulatory failure may be manifest.
4. Respiratory: Tachypnea and respiratory arrest may occur.
5. Renal: Albuminuria and microhematuria may occur. Increased excretion of renal tubular cells has been observed.
6. General systemic effects: Syncope, collapse, fever, and dehydration.

Management of Toxic Symptoms:

1. Discontinue drug immediately.
2. There is no known specific antidote.
3. Gastric lavage.
4. Emetic medication may be of value.
5. Avoid administration of sympathomimetic drugs.
6. Intravenous fluids, oxygen, and other supportive measures to prevent hypotension and overcome dehydration.
7. Central nervous system stimulation and seizures may respond to short-acting barbiturates.
8. Monitor serum levels until below 20 mcg/ml.

Dosage and Administration: The oral dose for adults should be adjusted according to the need and response of the patient. Usually a daily dose in the range of 600 to 1600 mg, administered in 3 or 4 divided doses, will provide the desired therapeutic effect. Similarly, the dose for children should be adjusted according to the response. An oral dose of 12 mg/kg/24 hours, administered in four divided doses, will usually provide the desired therapeutic effect in children.

Therapeutic serum levels are considered to be between 10 mcg/ml and 20 mcg/ml. Levels above 20 mcg/ml may produce toxic effects. There is great variation from patient to patient in dosage needed to achieve a therapeutic serum level and in the duration of action of oral aminophylline. Because of these wide variations and the relatively narrow therapeutic serum-level range, dosage must be individualized with monitoring of theophylline serum levels, particularly when prolonged use is planned.

How Supplied: Aminophyllin Tablets are supplied as:

Round, white, scored tablets with SEARLE debossed on one side and 1231 on the other side, each tablet containing 100 mg of aminophylline; bottles of 100, 500, 1,000, and 2,500, and cartons of 100 unit-dose individually blister-sealed tablets.

Oval, white, scored tablets with SEARLE debossed on one side and 1251 on the other side, each tablet containing 200 mg of aminophylline; bottles of 100, 500, 1,000, and 2,500, and cartons of 100 unit-dose individually blister-sealed tablets.

[*Shown in Product Identification Section*]

ANAVAR® ℞
(oxandrolone)

Description: Anavar is 17β-hydroxy-17α-methyl-2-oxa-5α-androstan-3-one.

Actions: Anabolic steroids are synthetic derivatives of testosterone. Anavar is used primarily for its protein anabolic effect and its catabolism-inhibiting effect on tissue. Nitrogen balance is improved by anabolic agents, but only when the intake of calories and protein is sufficient. It has not been established whether this positive nitrogen balance indicates a primary benefit in the utilization of protein-building dietary substances.

Some clinical effects and adverse reactions reported demonstrate the androgenic properties of drugs of this class. Complete dissociation of anabolic from androgenic effects has not been achieved. The actions of anabolic steroids are therefore similar to those of male sex hormones with the possibility that serious disturbances of growth and sexual development may be caused if given to young children. They suppress the gonadotrophic functions of the pituitary and may exert a direct effect upon the testes.

Indications and Usage: Anavar is indicated as an anabolic agent to promote weight gain after weight loss following extensive surgery, chronic infections, or severe trauma, and in some patients who without definite pathophysiologic reasons fail to gain or to maintain normal weight, to offset the protein catabolism associated with prolonged administration of corticosteroids, and for the relief of the bone pain frequently accompanying osteoporosis.

Contraindications:

1. Carcinoma of the prostate or male breast.
2. Carcinoma of the breast in some women.
3. Pregnancy, because of possible masculinization of the fetus.
4. Nephrosis or the nephrotic phase of nephritis.
5. Hypercalcemia.

Warning: Anabolic steroids do not enhance athletic ability.

Precautions:

1. Hypercalcemia may develop both spontaneously and as a result of hormonal therapy in women with disseminated breast carcinoma. Anavar therapy should be discontinued if hypercalcemia develops.
2. Use cautiously in patients with cardiac, renal, or hepatic disease. Edema may occur occasionally. Concomitant administration with adrenal steroids or ACTH may increase the edema.
3. The drug should be discontinued until the etiology is determined in patients in whom amenorrhea or menstrual irregularities develop.
4. Anabolic steroids may cause an increased response to anticoagulants. It may be necessary to decrease the dosage of an anticoagulant in order to maintain the prothrombin time at the desired therapeutic level.
5. Anabolic steroids have been shown to alter the results of glucose tolerance tests. Diabetic patients hould be carefully observed, and the dosage of insulin or oral hypoglycemic agents adjusted accordingly.
6. Liver function should be checked at regular intervals in patients receiving Anavar since it contains a 17α-alkyl group.
7. Anabolic steroids should be cautiously used in patients with benign prostatic hypertrophy.
8. The serum cholesterol may increase during therapy. Therefore, caution is required in administering these agents to patients with a history of myocardial infarction or coronary artery disease. Serial determinations of serum cholesterol should be made and therapy adjusted accordingly.

Adverse Reactions: The following adverse reactions have been associated with use of anabolic steroids:

1. In *males:*
   Prepubertal
   Phallic enlargement
   Increased frequency of erections
   Postpubertal
   Inhibition of testicular function and oligospermia
   Gynecomastia
2. In *females:*
   Hirsutism, male-pattern baldness, deepening of the voice, and clitoral enlargement. (These changes are usually irreversible even after prompt discontinuance of therapy and are not prevented by concomitant use of estrogens.)
   Menstrual irregularities
   Masculinization of the fetus
3. *In both sexes*
   There have been rare reports of hepatocellular neoplasms, including carcinoma, and peliosis hepatis in association with androgenic-anabolic steroid therapy.
   Nausea, abdominal fullness, loss of appetite, vomiting, burning of the tongue
   Increased or decreased libido
   Acne (especially in females and prepubertal males)
   Inhibition of gonadotropin secretion
   Bleeding in patients on concomitant anticoagulant therapy
   Premature closure of epiphyses in children
   Jaundice associated with 17α-alkyl substitutions
4. *Alterations have occurred in the results of the following clinical laboratory tests:*
   Metyrapone test
   Glucose tolerance test
   Thyroid-function tests: a decrease in the PBI, thyroxine-binding capacity, and radioactive iodine uptake.
   Fluid and electrolytes: retention of sodium, chlorides, water, potassium, phosphates, and calcium
   Liver function tests, mainly with the oral preparations having 17α-alkyl substitutions:
   Increased:
   BSP
   SGOT
   Serum bilirubin
   Alkaline phosphatase
   Serum cholesterol
   Suppression of clotting factors II, V, VII, and X
   Decreased 17-ketosteroid excretion (with oral 17α-alkyl substitutions)

Dosage and Administration: Therapy with anabolic steroids is adjunctive to and not a replacement for conventional therapy. The duration of therapy with Anavar (oxandrolone) will depend on the response of the patient and the possible appearance of adverse reactions. Therapy should be intermittent.

Adults. The *average adult dosage* of Anavar is one 2.5-mg tablet two to four times daily. However, the response of individuals to anabolic steroids varies, and a daily dosage of as little as 2.5 mg or as much as 20 mg may be required to achieve the desired response. A course of therapy of two to four weeks is usually adequate. This may be repeated intermittently as indicated.

Children. For children the *total daily dosage* of Anavar is 0.25 mg per kilogram or 0.125 mg per pound of body weight. This may be repeated intermittently as indicated.

How Supplied: Anavar is supplied as oval, white, scored, 2.5-mg tablets with SEARLE debossed on one side and 1401 on the other side; bottles of 100.

[*Shown in Product Identification Section*]

Continued on next page

Searle & Co.—Cont.

DEMULEN® ℞
DEMULEN-28® ℞
DEMULEN 1/35™-21 ℞
DEMULEN 1/35™-28 ℞
(ethynodiol diacetate with ethinyl estradiol)

OVULEN-21® ℞
OVULEN-28® ℞
(ethynodiol diacetate with mestranol)

ENOVID-E® 21 ℞
ENOVID® 5 mg ℞
ENOVID® 10 mg ℞
(norethynodrel with mestranol)

Description:
Demulen and Demulen-28. Each white tablet contains 1 mg of ethynodiol diacetate and 50 mcg of ethinyl estradiol. Each pink tablet in the Demulen-28 package is a placebo containing no active ingredients.
Demulen 1/35™-21 and Demulen 1/35™-28. Each white tablet contains 1 mg of ethynodiol diacetate and 35 mcg of ethinyl estradiol. Each blue tablet in the Demulen 1/35™-28 package is a placebo, containing no active ingredients.
Ovulen-21 and Ovulen-28. Each white tablet contains 1 mg of ethynodiol diacetate and 0.1 mg of mestranol. Each pink tablet in the Ovulen-28 package is a placebo containing no active ingredients.
Enovid-E 21. Each tablet contains 2.5 mg of norethynodrel and 0.1 mg of mestranol.
Enovid 5 mg. Each tablet contains 5 mg of norethynodrel and 75 mcg of mestranol.
Enovid 10 mg. Each tablet contains 9.85 mg of norethynodrel and 0.15 mg of mestranol.
The chemical name for norethynodrel is 17α-ethynyl-17-hydroxy-5(10)-estren-3-one, for mestranol it is 3-methoxy-19-nor-17α-pregna-1,3,5(10)-trien-20-yn-17-ol, for ethynodiol diacetate it is 19-nor-17α-pregn-4-en-20-yne-3β,17-diol diacetate, and for ethinyl estradiol it is 19-nor-17α-pregna-1, 3, 5(10)-trien-20-yne-3,17-diol.
Therapeutic Class: Oral contraceptive (except for Enovid 10 mg). Estrogen-progestogen combination (Enovid 5 mg and 10 mg only).

Clinical Pharmacology: Combination oral contraceptives act primarily through the mechanism of gonadotropin suppression due to the estrogenic and progestational activity of their components. Although the primary mechanism of action is inhibition of ovulation, alterations in the genital tract, including changes in the cervical mucus (which reduce sperm penetration) and the endometrium (which reduce the likelihood of implantation) may also contribute to contraceptive effectiveness.
Enovid 5 mg or Enovid 10 mg, when used for the treatment of endometriosis, may be administered to induce changes in areas of endometriosis similar to those that occur during pregnancy. In many instances when Enovid 5 mg or Enovid 10 mg is taken continuously the areas of endometriosis develop a decidua-like response followed by necrosis, which may result in destruction of the abnormally located tissue and resolution of the lesions.

Indications and Usage: Demulen, Demulen 1/35™, Ovulen, Enovid-E, and Enovid 5 mg are indicated for the prevention of pregnancy in women who elect to use oral contraceptives as a method of contraception.
Enovid 5 mg and Enovid 10 mg are indicated for the treatment of endometriosis, for the treatment of hypermenorrhea, and for the production of cyclic withdrawal bleeding.
NOTE: The contraindication, warning, precaution, and adverse reaction information in this monograph also applies when Enovid 5 mg is prescribed for indications other than contraception or when Enovid 10 mg is prescribed.
Oral contraceptives are highly effective. The pregnancy rate in women using conventional combination oral contraceptives (containing 35 mcg or more of ethinyl estradiol or 50 mcg or more of mestranol) is generally reported to be less than one pregnancy per 100 woman-years of use. Slightly higher rates (somewhat more than one pregnancy per 100 woman-years of use) are reported for some combination products containing 35 mcg or less of ethinyl estradiol, and rates on the order of three pregnancies per 100 woman-years are reported for the progestogen-only oral contraceptives.
These rates are derived from separate studies conducted by different investigators in several population groups; therefore, a precise comparison cannot be made. Furthermore, pregnancy rates tend to be lower as clinical studies are continued, possibly due to selective retention in the longer studies of those patients who accept the treatment regimen and do not discontinue as a result of adverse reactions, pregnancy, or other reasons. In Table 1 ranges of pregnancy rates as reported in the literature[1] are shown for other means of contraception. The efficacy of these means of contraception, except for the IUD, depends upon the degree of adherence to the method.
In clinical trials with Ovulen, 5,938 patients completed 83,463 cycles, and a total of 8 pregnancies were reported. This represents a pregnancy rate of 0.12 per 100 woman-years.
In clinical trials with Enovid-E, 1,657 patients completed 28,400 cycles, and a total of 8 pregnancies were reported. This represents a pregnancy rate of 0.34 per 100 woman-years.
In clinical trials with Demulen, 2,256 patients completed 30,409 cycles, and a total of 30 pregnancies were reported. This represents a pregnancy rate of 1.18 per 100 woman-years.
In clinical trials with Demulen 1/35, 1,231 patients completed 14,641 cycles, and a total of 15 pregnancies were reported. This represents a pregnancy rate of 1.23 per 100 woman-years.
In clinical trials with Demulen 1/35, the incidence of delayed or breakthrough bleeding was 44% at cycle 6. Although this rate is higher than for other similar products, only 9.9% of the patients dropped out of the study due to bleeding.

Table 1
Pregnancies per 100 Woman-Years

Method	*Range*
IUD	<1 to 6
Diaphragm with spermicidal cream or gel	2 to 20
Condom	3 to 36
Spermicidal aerosol foams	2 to 29
Spermicidal gels and creams	4 to 36
Periodic abstinence (rhythm), all types	<1 to 47
1. Calendar method	14 to 47
2. Temperature method	1 to 20
3. Temperature method (intercourse only in post-ovulatory phase)	<1 to 7
4. Mucus method	1 to 25
No contraception	60 to 80

Dose-related Risk of Thromboembolism From Oral Contraceptives: Studies have shown a positive association between the dose of estrogens in oral contraceptives and the risk of thromboembolism[2,96,97] (see *Warning* No. 1). For this reason, it is prudent and in keeping with good principles of therapeutics to minimize exposure to estrogen. The oral contraceptive product prescribed for any given patient should be that product which contains the least amount of estrogen that is compatible with an acceptable pregnancy rate and patient acceptance. It is recommended that new users of oral contraceptives be started on preparations containing 50 mcg or less of estrogen.

Contraindications: Oral contraceptives should not be used in women with any of the following conditions:

1. Thrombophlebitis or thromboembolic disorders.
2. A past history of deep vein thrombophlebitis or thromboembolic disorders.
3. Cerebral vascular disease, myocardial infarction or coronary artery disease, or a past history of these conditions.
4. Known or suspected carcinoma of the breast.
5. Known or suspected estrogen-dependent neoplasia.
6. Undiagnosed abnormal genital bleeding.
7. Known or suspected pregnancy (see *Warning* No. 5).
8. Past or present, benign or malignant liver tumors among women who developed these tumors during the use of oral contraceptives or other estrogen-containing products (see *Warning* No. 4).

WARNINGS

Cigarette-smoking increases the risk of serious cardiovascular side effects from oral contraceptive use. This risk increases with age and with heavy smoking (15 or more cigarettes per day) and is quite marked in women over 35 years of age. Women who use oral contraceptives should be strongly advised not to smoke.

The use of oral contraceptives is associated with increased risk of several serious conditions including venous and arterial thromboembolism, thrombotic and hemorrhagic stroke, myocardial infarction, visual disorders, hepatic tumors, gallbladder disease, hypertension, and fetal abnormalities. Practitioners prescribing oral contraceptives should be familiar with the following information relating to these and other risks.

1. *Thromboembolic Disorders and Other Vascular Problems.* An increased risk of thromboembolic and thrombotic disease associated with the use of oral contraceptives is well established. One study in Great Britain[3] demonstrated an increased relative risk for fatal venous thromboembolism; several British[4,5,14,22,92] and U.S. [6–8,23,98–101,126] studies demonstrated an increased relative risk for nonfatal venous thromboembolism. U.S. studies[6,9,10,99,101–103] demonstrated an increased relative risk for stroke, which had not been shown in prior British studies.[3–5] In these studies it was estimated that users of oral contraceptives were 1.9 to 11 times more likely than nonusers to manifest these diseases without evident cause (Table 2). In a British study of idiopathic deep vein thrombosis and pulmonary embolism, the projected annual hospitalization rates for women aged 16–40 were 47 per 100,000 users and 5 for nonusers.[77] In one British mortality study,[3] overall excess mortality due to pulmonary embolism or stroke was on the order of 1.3 to 3.4 deaths annually per 100,000 users and increased with age.

Cerebrovascular Disorders: In a collaborative U.S. study[9,10] of cerebrovascular disorders in women with and without predisposing causes, it was estimated that the risk of hemorrhagic stroke was 2.0 times greater in users than in nonusers, and the risk of thrombotic stroke was 4.0[10] to 9.5[9] times greater in users than in nonusers (Table 2). Analysis of mortality trends in 21 countries indicates that, since oral contraceptives first became available, changes in mortality from nonrheumatic heart disease and hypertension, cerebrovascular disease, and all nonrheumatic cardiovascular disease among women aged 15 to 44 years have been associated with changes in the prevalence of oral contraceptive use in each country.[11]

Table 2. *Summary of Relative Risks of Thromboembolic Disorders and Other Vascular Prob-*

lems in Oral Contraceptive Users Compared with Nonusers.

Disorders	*Relative Risk*
Idiopathic thromboembolic disease	2 to 11 times greater
Postsurgery thromboembolic complications	4 to 7 times greater
Thrombotic stroke	4 to 9.5 times greater
Hemorrhagic stroke	2.0 to 2.3 times greater
Myocardial infarction	2 to 12 times greater

In May 1974 the Royal College of General Practitioners[12] issued an interim report of its continuing large-scale prospective study comparing a user group with a nonuser group. It stated: "A statistically significant higher rate of reporting of cerebrovascular accidents in Takers is evident, but the numbers are too small to justify an estimation of the degree of risk." A 1981 analysis of data from this study was reported[13] to show a 4-fold increased mortality from circulatory diseases, mainly from myocardial infarction and hemorrhagic stroke, in users. The excess mortality was associated with age and smoking in users.

In October 1976 an interim report was issued on the long-term follow-up study of the British Family Planning Association.[14] There was a highly significant association between oral contraceptive use and stroke, although total numbers were small in this study also. The increase in risk of venous thrombosis and pulmonary embolism among users was about 4-fold and was statistically highly significant. In later reports[15] it was noted that mortality from nonrheumatic heart disease was greater in women who had ever used oral contraceptives. In the Walnut Creek prospective study,[99,101,102] the risk of subarachnoid hemorrhage was associated with heavy smoking, age, and use of the pill.

Myocardial Infarction: An increased risk of myocardial infarction associated with the use of oral contraceptives has been reported in Great Britain,[16–19,136] confirming a previously suspected association.[3] The morbidity study[16,17] found that the greater the number of underlying risk factors for coronary artery disease (cigarette-smoking, hypertension, hypercholesterolemia, obesity, diabetes, history of preeclamptic toxemia), the higher the risk of developing myocardial infarction, regardless of whether the patient was an oral contraceptive user or not. Oral contraceptives were considered an additional risk factor.

The annual excess rate of fatal myocardial infarction in British oral contraceptive users was estimated to be approximately 3.5 cases per 100,000 women users in the 30- to 39-year age group and 20 per 100,000 women users in the 40- to 44-year age group.[19] (These estimates are based on British vital statistics, which show acute myocardial infarction death rates 2 to 3 times less than in the U.S. for women in these age groups. In an attempt to extrapolate these figures to U.S. women, it was estimated that the annual excess rates in users are 25.7 cases per 100,000 for women aged 30–39 with predisposing conditions versus 1.5 cases without; corresponding estimates for women aged 40–44 were 86.2 versus 5.1.[78]) The annual excess rate of hospitalization for nonfatal myocardial infarction in married British oral contraceptive users was estimated to be approximately 3.5 per 100,000 women users in the 30- to 39-year age group and 47 per 100,000 women users in the 40- to 44-year age group.[16]

Smoking is considered a major predisposing condition to myocardial infarction. In terms of relative risk, it has been estimated[20] that oral contraceptive users who do not smoke are about twice as likely to have a fatal myocardial infarction as nonusers who do not smoke. Oral contraceptive users who are also smokers have about a 5-fold increased risk of fatal infarction compared to users who do not smoke, but about a 10- to 12-fold increased risk compared to nonusers who do not smoke. Furthermore, the amount of smoking is also an important factor. In determining the importance of these relative risks, however, the baseline rates for various age groups, as shown in Table 3, must be given serious consideration. The importance of other predisposing conditions mentioned above in determining relative and absolute risks has not been quantified; it is likely that the same synergistic action exists, but perhaps to a lesser extent.

Similar findings relating nonfatal and fatal myocardial infarction, oral contraceptives, smoking, and age were subsequently published in the U.S.[91,99,104–108]

Table 3. *Estimated Annual Mortality Rate per 100,000 Women from Myocardial Infarction by Use of Oral Contraceptives, Smoking Habits, and Age in Years*[20]

	Myocardial infarction			
	Women aged 30–39		Women aged 40–44	
Smoking habits	Users	Non-users	Users	Non-users
All smokers ..	10.2	2.6	62.0	15.9
Heavy*	13.0	5.1	78.7	31.3
Light	4.7	0.9	28.6	5.7
Nonsmokers .	1.8	1.2	10.7	7.4
Smokers and nonsmokers	5.4	1.9	32.8	11.7

*15 or more cigarettes per day

Risk of Dose: Reports of thromboembolism following the use of oral contraceptives containing 50 mcg or more of estrogen received by drug safety committees in Great Britain, Sweden, and Denmark were compared with the distribution expected from market research estimates of sales.[2] A positive correlation was found between the dose of estrogen and the reporting of thromboembolism, including coronary thrombosis, in excess of that predicted by sales estimates. Preparations containing 100 mcg or more of estrogen were associated with a higher risk of thromboembolism than those containing 50 to 80 mcg of estrogen. The authors' analysis did suggest, however, that the quantity of estrogen may not be the sole factor involved. Any influence on the part of the progestogens was not considered, which may have been responsible for certain discrepancies in the data. No significant differences were detected between preparations containing the same dose of estrogen nor between the two estrogens ethinyl estradiol and mestranol. A subsequent study of a similar nature in Great Britain found a positive association between the dose of progestogen or estrogen and certain thromboembolic conditions,[96] which is consistent with findings of the Royal College study.[12,92,135] Swedish authorities noted decreased reporting of thromboembolic episodes when higher estrogen preparations were no longer prescribed.[97] Careful epidemiologic studies to determine the degree of thromboembolic risk associated with progestogen-only oral contraceptives have not been performed. Cases of thromboembolic disease have been reported in women using these products, and they should not be presumed to be free of excess risk.

The relative risk of oral contraceptive use one month prior to hospitalization for various types of thromboembolism was calculated in a U.S. retrospective case-control study.[8] If no account is taken of the relative estrogenic potency of different estrogens and if any possible influence of the different progestogenic components is ignored, the products employed may be divided into those containing less than 100 mcg and those containing 100 mcg or more of estrogen. For all cases combined, the larger dose category was associated with only a slightly higher relative risk; for the idiopathic subgroup, the relative risk was approximately doubled with the larger estrogen content, but the confidence limits overlapped considerably and the differences, therefore, were not statistically significant. Apparently there was less of an increased relative risk for the sub-group with predispositions to thromboembolism.[98]

The risk of thromboembolic and thrombotic disorders, both in users and in nonusers of oral contraceptives, increases with age. Oral contraceptives have been considered an independent risk factor for these events.

Estimate of Excess Mortality from Circulatory Diseases: A large prospective study[13] carried out in the U.K. provided estimates of the mortality rate per 100,000 women per year from diseases of the circulatory system for users and nonusers of oral contraceptives according to age, smoking habits, and duration of use. The overall annual excess death rate from circulatory diseases for oral contraceptive users was estimated at 23 per 100,000 for women of all ages. The rates for nonsmokers and smokers, respectively, were: ages 25–34, 2 and 10 per 100,000; ages 35–44, 15 and 48 per 100,000; and ages 45 and older, 41 and 179 per 100,000. The risk was statistically significant only in cigarette-smokers over age 34. The majority of deaths were due to subarachnoid hemorrhage or ischemic heart disease. Relative risk for women who had ever used oral contraceptives rose with increasing parity, a new observation that needs confirmation.

The available data from a variety of sources have been analyzed[21] to estimate the risk of death associated with various methods of contraception. The estimates of risk of death for each method included the combined risk of the contraceptive method (eg, thromboembolic and thrombotic disease in the case of oral contraceptives) plus the risk attributable to pregnancy or abortion in the event of method failure. This latter risk varies with the effectiveness of the contraceptive method. The findings of this analysis are shown in Figure 1.[21] The

Figure 1 Estimated annual number of deaths associated with control of fertility and no control per 100 000 nonsterile women by regimen of control and age of woman

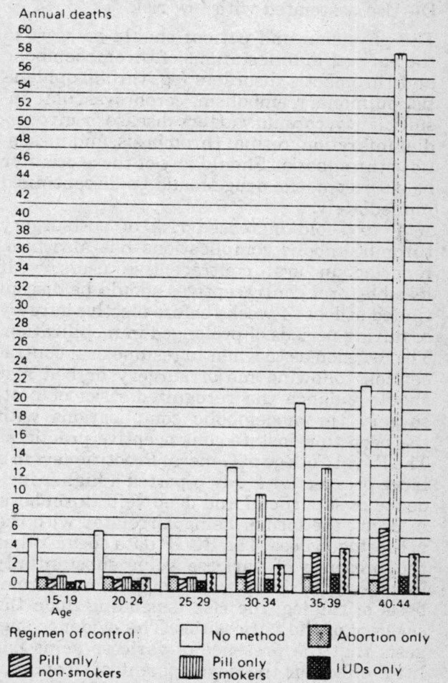

Continued on next page

Searle & Co.—Cont.

study concluded that the mortality associated with all methods of birth control is low and below that associated with childbirth, except for that associated with oral contraceptives in women over 40 who smoke. (The rates given for pill only/smokers for each age group are for smokers as a class. For "heavy" smokers [more than 15 cigarettes a day], the rates given would be about double; for "light" smokers [less than 15 cigarettes a day], about 50 percent.[20]) The mortality associated with oral contraceptive use in nonsmokers over 40 is higher than with any other method of contraception in that age group. The lowest mortality is associated with the condom or diaphragm backed up by early legal abortion.

The risk of thromboembolic and thrombotic disease associated with oral contraceptives increases with age after approximately age 30 and, for myocardial infarction, is further increased by hypertension, hypercholesterolemia, obesity, diabetes, or history of preeclamptic toxemia and especially by cigarette-smoking.[20,78,79]

Based on the data currently available, the following table gives a gross estimate of the risk of death from circulatory disorders associated with the use of oral contraceptives:

Table 4. *Smoking Habits and Other Predisposing Conditions—Risk Associated with Use of Oral Contraceptives*

Age	Below 30	30–39	40+
Heavy smokers	C	B	A
Light smokers	D	C	B
Nonsmokers (no predisposing conditions)	D	C,D	C
Nonsmokers (other predisposing conditions)	C	C,B	B,A

A—Use associated with very high risk.
B—Use associated with high risk.
C—Use associated with moderate risk.
D—Use associated with low risk.

The physician and patient should be alert to the earliest manifestations of thromboembolic and thrombotic disorders (eg, thrombophlebitis, pulmonary embolism, cerebrovascular insufficiency, coronary artery disease or myocardial infarction, retinal thrombosis, and mesenteric thrombosis). Should any of these occur or be suspected, the drug should be discontinued immediately.

A 4- to 7-fold increased risk of postsurgery thromboembolic complications has also been reported in oral contraceptive users.[22,23] If feasible, oral contraceptives should be discontinued at least 4 weeks before elective surgery or during periods of prolonged immobilization. The decision as to when to resume oral contraception following major surgery or bed rest should balance the recognized risks of postsurgery thromboembolic complications with the need to reinstate contraceptive practices.

The Royal College of General Practitioners in a large prospective study reported a higher incidence of superficial and deep vein thrombosis in users, the former being correlated with the progestogen dose. The RCGP data suggest that the presence of varicose veins substantially increases the risk of superficial venous thrombosis of the leg, the risk depending upon the severity of the varicosities. The evidence suggests that the presence of varicose veins has little effect on the development of deep vein thrombosis in the leg.[92] Other prospective studies have also reported a higher incidence of venous thrombosis in users.[14,99–101,109]

2. *Ocular Lesions.* There have been reports of neuro-ocular lesions such as optic neuritis or retinal thrombosis associated with the use of oral contraceptives. Discontinue medication if there is unexplained, gradual or sudden, partial or complete loss of vision; proptosis or diplopia; papilledema; or any evidence of retinal vascular lesions. Appropriate diagnostic and therapeutic measures should be instituted.

3. *Carcinoma.* Long-term continuous administration of either natural or synthetic estrogens in certain animal species increases the frequency of certain carcinomas, and/or nonmalignant neoplasms, such as those of the breast, uterus, cervix, vagina, ovary, liver, and pituitary. Certain synthetic progestogens, none currently contained in oral contraceptives, have been noted to increase the incidence of mammary nodules, benign and malignant, in dogs.

There is now evidence that estrogens increase the risk of carcinoma of the endometrium in humans. In several independent, retrospective case-control studies,[24–28,80,93] an increased relative risk (2.2 to 13.9 times) was reported, associating endometrial carcinoma with the prolonged use of estrogens in postmenopausal women who took estrogen replacement medication to relieve menopausal symptoms. This risk was independent of the other known risk factors for endometrial cancer and appeared to depend both on duration of treatment[24,27,28] and on estrogen dose.[26–28] These findings are supported by the observation that incidence rates of endometrial cancer have increased sharply since 1969 in 8 different areas of the U.S. with population-based cancer-reporting systems, an increase which may be related to the rapidly expanding use of estrogens during the past decade.[29] There is no evidence at present that "natural" estrogens are more or less hazardous than "synthetic" estrogens at equiestrogenic doses.

One publication[30] reported on the first 30 cases submitted by physicians to a registry of cases of adenocarcinoma of the endometrium in women under 40 on oral contraceptives. Of the adenocarcinomas found in women without predisposing risk factors for adenocarcinoma of the endometrium (eg, irregular bleeding at the time oral contraceptives were first given, polycystic ovaries), nearly all occurred in women who had used a sequential oral contraceptive. These products are no longer marketed. No statistical association has been reported suggesting an increased risk of endometrial cancer in users of conventional combination or progestogen-only oral contraceptives, although individual cases have been reported.

Several studies[7,31–35,99,121,122] have shown no increased risk of breast cancer to women taking oral contraceptives or estrogens. In one study,[36,37] however, while no overall increased risk of breast cancer was noted in women treated with oral contraceptives, a greater risk was suggested for the subgroups of oral contraceptive users with documented benign breast disease and for long-term (2–4 years) users. Another study[123] reported increased risk of breast cancer in women who had used the pill for more than 4 years before their first full-term pregnancy. One other study[38] indicated an increasing risk of breast cancer in women taking menopausal estrogens, which increased with duration of follow-up. Several other studies have also shown oral contraceptives[127–129,133] or estrogens[130] to be associated with breast cancer, particularly in connection with other risk factors[127–129] and long duration of use.[127,128,130] A reduced occurrence of benign breast tumors in users of oral contraceptives has been well documented.[7,12,14,31,36,39,40,86,99]

Some epidemiologic studies[41,81–84,99,109,120] have suggested an increased risk of cervical dysplasia, erosion, and carcinoma in long-term pill users; however, cause and effect has not been established. There have been other reports of microglandular dysplasia of the cervix in users.

In summary, there is at present no consistent evidence from human studies of an increased risk of cancer associated with oral contraceptives.[42] Close clinical surveillance of all women taking oral contraceptives is, nevertheless, essential. In all cases of undiagnosed persistent or recurrent abnormal vaginal bleeding, nonfunctional causes should be borne in mind and appropriate diagnostic measures should be taken to rule out malignancy. Women who have a strong family history of breast cancer or who have breast nodules, fibrocystic disease, recurrent cystic mastitis, abnormal mammograms, or cervical dysplasia should be monitored with particular care if they elect to use oral contraceptives.

4. *Hepatic Lesions (adenomas, hepatomas, hamartomas, regenerating nodules, focal nodular hyperplasia, hemangiomas, hepatocellular carcinoma, etc).* Benign hepatic adenomas and other hepatic lesions have been associated with the use of oral contraceptives.[43–46,85] One study[46] reported that oral contraceptive formulations with high "hormonal potency" were associated with a higher risk than lower-potency formulations, as was age over 30 years. Although benign, these hepatic lesions may rupture and may cause death through intra-abdominal hemorrhage. This has been reported in short-term as well as long-term users of oral contraceptives. Two studies related risk with duration of use of the contraceptive, the risk being much greater after 4 or more years of oral contraceptive use.[45,46] Long-term users of oral contraceptives have an estimated annual incidence of hepatocellular adenoma of 3 to 4 per 100,000.[46] While such hepatic lesions are rare, they should be considered in women presenting with abdominal pain and tenderness, abdominal mass, or shock. Patients with liver tumors have demonstrated variable clinical features, which may make preoperative diagnosis difficult. About one quarter of the cases presented because of abdominal masses; up to one half had signs and symptoms of acute intraperitoneal hemorrhage. Routine radiologic and laboratory studies may not be helpful. Liver scans may clearly show a focal defect. Hepatic arteriography or computed tomography may be useful procedures in diagnosing primary liver neoplasms.

A few cases of hepatocellular carcinoma have been reported in women taking oral contraceptives.[44] The relationship of these drugs to this type of malignancy is not known at this time. Oral contraceptives are contraindicated if there are past or present, benign or malignant liver tumors among women who developed these tumors during the use of oral contraceptives or other estrogen-containing products.

5. *Use In or Immediately Preceding Pregnancy, Birth Defects in Offspring, and Malignancy in Offspring.* The use of female sex hormones, both estrogens and progestogens, during early pregnancy may seriously damage the offspring. It has been reported that females exposed in utero to diethylstilbestrol and other nonsteroidal estrogens have an increased risk of developing in later life a form of vaginal or cervical cancer that is ordinarily extremely rare.[47,48] This risk has been estimated to be on the order of 1 in 1,000 exposures or less.[49,50] Although there is no evidence at the present time that oral contraceptives further enhance the risk of developing this type of malignancy, such patients should be monitored with particular care if they elect to use oral contraceptives instead of other methods of contraception. Furthermore, a high percentage of such exposed women (from 30 to 90%) have been found to have adenosis (epithelial changes) of the vagina and cervix.[51–55] Although these changes are histologically benign, it is not known whether this condition is a precursor of malignancy. DES-exposed daughters appear to have an increased risk of unfavorable outcome of pregnancy.[110–112] DES-exposed male children may develop abnormalities of the urogenital tract[56–58,131] and sperm.[131] Although similar data are not available for the use of other estro-

gens, it cannot be presumed that they would not induce similar changes.

Several reports suggest an association between fetal exposure to female sex hormones, including oral contraceptives, and congenital anomalies,[59–64,94,113–116] including multiple congenital anomalies described by the acronym VACTERL, for vertebral, anal, cardiac, tracheoesophageal, renal, and limb defects.[61,62,113] There appears to be a preferential expression of these defects by exposed male offspring.[63,65,115,121] In one case-control study[63] it was estimated that there was a 4.7-fold increased risk of limb-reduction defects in infants exposed in utero to sex hormones (oral contraceptives, hormonal withdrawal tests for pregnancy, or attempted treatment for threatened abortion). Some of these exposures were very short and involved only a few days of treatment. The data suggest that the risk of limb-reduction defects in exposed fetuses is somewhat less than 1 in 1,000 live births. In a large prospective study,[64] cardiovascular defects in children born to women who received female hormones, including oral contraceptives, during early pregnancy occurred at a rate of 18.2 per 1,000 births, compared to 7.8 per 1,000 for children not so exposed in utero. These results are statistically significant. The incidence of twin births may be increased for women who conceive shortly after discontinuing use of the pill.[14,63,117,118,124]

In the past, female sex hormones have been used during pregnancy in an attempt to treat threatened or habitual abortion. There is considerable evidence that estrogens are ineffective for these indications, and there is no evidence from well-controlled studies that progestogens are effective for these uses.

There is some evidence that triploidy and possibly other types of polyploidy are increased among abortuses from women who become pregnant soon after stopping oral contraceptives.[66] Embryos with these anomalies are virtually always aborted spontaneously. Whether there is an overall increase in spontaneous abortion of pregnancies conceived soon after stopping the oral contraceptives is unknown. The safety of this product in pregnancy has not been demonstrated. Pregnancy should be ruled out before initiating or continuing the contraceptive regimen. Pregnancy should always be considered if withdrawal bleeding does not occur. It is recommended that for any patient who has missed 2 consecutive periods, pregnancy should be ruled out before continuing the contraceptive regimen. If the patient has not adhered to the prescribed schedule, the possibility of pregnancy should be considered at the time of the first missed period, and further use of oral contraceptives should be withheld until pregnancy has been ruled out. If pregnancy is confirmed, the patient should be apprised of the potential risks to the fetus, and the advisability of continuation of the pregnancy should be discussed in the light of these risks.

It is recommended that women who discontinue oral contraceptives with the intent of becoming pregnant use an alternative form of contraception for a period of time before attempting to conceive. Many clinicians recommend 3 months, although no precise information is available on which to base this recommendation.

The administration of progestogen-only or progestogen-estrogen combinations to induce withdrawal bleeding should not be used as a test of pregnancy.

6. *Gallbladder Disease.* Reports of studies[7,8,12,14,33] indicate an increased risk for surgically confirmed gallbladder disease in users of oral contraceptives or estrogens. In one study,[12] an increased risk appeared after 2 years of use and doubled after 4 or 5 years of use. In one of the other studies[7] an increased risk was apparent between 6 and 12 months of use.

7. *Carbohydrate and Lipid Metabolism.* A decrease in glucose tolerance has been observed in a significant percentage of patients on oral contraceptives. For this reason, prediabetic and diabetic patients should be carefully observed while receiving oral contraceptives. An increase in triglycerides and total phospholipids has been observed in patients receiving oral contraceptives.[67] The clinical significance of this finding remains to be defined.

8. *Elevated Blood Pressure.* An increase in blood pressure has been reported in patients receiving oral contraceptives.[12,69,109] There is evidence that the degree of hypertension may correlate directly with increasing dosage of progestogen.[86] In some women, hypertension may occur within a few months of beginning oral contraceptive use. The prevalence of hypertension in users is low in the first year of use, and may be no higher than that in a comparable group of nonusers. The prevalence in users increases, however, with longer exposure and, in the fifth year of use, is 2½ to 3 times the reported prevalence in the first year. Age is also strongly correlated with the development of hypertension in oral contraceptive users.

Women with a history of elevated blood pressure (hypertension), preexisting renal disease, a history of toxemia or elevated blood pressure during pregnancy, a familial tendency to hypertension or its consequences, or a history of excessive weight gain or fluid retention during the menstrual cycle may be more likely to develop elevation of blood pressure when given oral contraceptives and, therefore, should be monitored closely.[68] Even though elevated blood pressure may remain within the "normal" range, the clinical implications of elevations should not be ignored and close surveillance is indicated, particularly for women with other risk factors for cardiovascular disease or stroke.[69] High blood pressure may or may not persist after discontinuation of the oral contraceptive.

9. *Headache.* The onset or exacerbation of migraine or development of headache of a new pattern which is recurrent, persistent, or severe, requires discontinuation of oral contraceptives and evaluation of the cause.

10. *Bleeding Irregularities.* Breakthrough bleeding, spotting, and amenorrhea are frequent reasons for discontinuance of oral contraceptives. In breakthrough bleeding, as in all cases of irregular vaginal bleeding, nonfunctional causes should be borne in mind. In patients with undiagnosed persistent or recurrent abnormal vaginal bleeding, adequate diagnostic measures are indicated to rule out pregnancy or malignancy. If a pathologic basis has been excluded, passage of time or a change to another formulation may correct the bleeding problem. A change to an oral contraceptive with a higher estrogen content, while potentially useful in minimizing menstrual irregularity, should be made only when considered necessary since this may increase the risk of thromboembolic disease.

Women with a past history of oligomenorrhea or secondary amenorrhea or young women who have not established regular cycles may have a tendency to remain anovulatory or to become amenorrheic after discontinuation of oral contraceptives. Women with these preexisting problems should be informed of these possibilities and encouraged to use other contraceptive methods. Post-use anovulation, possibly prolonged, may also occur in women without previous irregularities. A higher incidence of galactorrhea and of pituitary tumors (eg, adenomas) has been associated with amenorrhea in former users compared with nonusers.[87] One study[70] reported a 16-fold increased prevalence of pituitary prolactin-secreting tumors among patients with postpill amenorrhea when galactorrhea was present.

11. *Ectopic Pregnancy.* Contraceptive failure may result in either ectopic or intrauterine pregnancy. In failures with combination-type oral contraceptives, the ratio of ectopic to intrauterine pregnancies is no higher than in women who are not receiving oral contraceptives.

12. *Breast Feeding.* Oral contraceptives given in the postpartum period may interfere with lactation. There may be a decrease in the quantity and quality of the breast milk. Furthermore, a small fraction of the hormonal agents in oral contraceptives has been identified in the milk of mothers receiving these drugs.[71,88,89] The effects, if any, on the breast-fed child have not been determined. If feasible, the use of oral contraceptives should be deferred until the infant has been weaned.

13. *Infertility.* There is evidence of fertility impairment in women discontinuing oral contraceptives in comparison with those discontinuing other methods.[14,90,132] The impairment appears to be independent of the duration of use. While the impairment diminishes with time, there is still an appreciable difference in the results in nulliparous women 30 months after discontinuation of birth control; the difference is negligible after 42 months. For parous women the difference is no longer apparent 30 months after cessation of contraception.

Precautions:

General. 1. A complete medical and family history should be taken and a thorough physical examination should be performed prior to the initiation of oral contraceptives. The pretreatment and periodic physical examinations should include special reference to blood pressure, breasts, abdomen, and pelvic organs, including a Pap smear and relevant laboratory tests. As a general rule, oral contraceptives should not be prescribed for longer than one year without the performance of another physical examination (see *Warnings*).

2. Preexisting uterine leiomyomata may increase in size during oral contraceptive use.

3. Oral contraceptives appear to be associated with an increased incidence of mental depression. Therefore, patients with a history of depression should be carefully observed and the drug discontinued if depression recurs to a serious degree. Patients becoming significantly depressed while taking oral contraceptives should stop the medication and use an alternative method of contraception in an attempt to determine whether the symptom is drug related.

4. Oral contraceptives may cause some degree of fluid retention. They should be prescribed with caution, and only with careful monitoring, in patients with conditions which might be aggravated by fluid retention, such as convulsive disorders, migraine syndrome, asthma, or cardiac, hepatic, or renal dysfunction.

5. Patients with a past history of jaundice during pregnancy have an increased risk of recurrence of jaundice and should be carefully observed while receiving oral contraceptives. If jaundice develops in any patient receiving such drugs, the medication should be discontinued while the cause is investigated. Cholestatic jaundice has been reported after combined treatment with oral contraceptives and troleandomycin.

6. Steroid hormones may be poorly metabolized in patients with impaired liver function and should be administered with caution in such patients.

7. Oral contraceptive users may have disturbances in normal tryptophan metabolism, which may result in a relative pyridoxine deficiency. The clinical significance of this is unknown, although megaloblastic anemia has been reported.

8. Serum folate levels may be depressed by oral contraceptive therapy. Since the pregnant woman is predisposed to folate deficiency and the incidence of folate deficiency increases with lengthening gestation, it is possible that if

Continued on next page

Searle & Co.—Cont.

a woman becomes pregnant shortly after stopping oral contraceptives, she may have a greater chance of developing folate deficiency and complications attributable to this deficiency.

9. The pathologist should be advised of oral contraceptive therapy when relevant specimens are submitted.

10. Certain endocrine and liver function tests may be affected by estrogen-containing oral contraceptives. Therefore, it is recommended that any abnormal tests be repeated after the drug has been withdrawn for two months. The following alterations in laboratory results have been observed with the use of oral contraceptives:

a. Hepatic function: Increased sulfobromophthalein retention and other abnormalities in tests of liver function.
b. Coagulation tests: Increased prothrombin and coagulation factors VII, VIII, IX, and X; decreased antithrombin III; increased platelet aggregability.
c. Thyroid function: Increased thyroid-binding globulin (TBG) leading to increased circulating total thyroid hormone, as measured by protein-bound iodine (PBI) or T^4 by column or radioimmunoassay. Free T^3 resin uptake is decreased, reflecting the elevated TBG; free T^4 concentration is unaltered.
d. Decreased pregnanediol excretion.
e. Reduced response to metyrapone test.
f. Increased blood transcortin and corticosteroid levels.
g. Increased blood triglyceride and phospholipid concentrations.
h. Reduced serum folate concentration.
i. Impaired glucose tolerance.
j. Altered plasma levels of trace minerals (eg, increased ceruloplasmin).

11. The influence of prolonged oral contraceptive therapy on pituitary, ovarian, adrenal, hepatic, or uterine function, or on the immune response, has not been established.

12. Treatment with oral contraceptives may mask the onset of the climacteric. (See *Warnings* section regarding risks in this age group.)

Information for the Patient. See patient labeling printed at end.

Drug Interactions. Oral contraceptives may be rendered less effective and increased incidence of breakthrough bleeding may occur by virtue of drug interaction with rifampin, isoniazid, ampicillin, neomycin, penicillin V, tetracycline, chloramphenicol, sulfonamides, nitrofurantoin, barbiturates, phenytoin, primidone, phenylbutazone, analgesics, tranquilizers, and antimigraine preparations.[72–74,95,125] Oral contraceptives may alter the effectiveness of other types of drugs, such as oral anticoagulants, anticonvulsants, tranquilizers (eg, diazepam), tricyclic antidepressants, antihypertensive agents (eg, guanethidine), vitamins, and hypoglycemic agents.[72,119,134] (See *Precaution* No. 5.)

Carcinogenesis. See *Warnings* No. 3 and 4 for information on the carcinogenic potential of oral contraceptives.

Pregnancy. Pregnancy category X. See *Contraindication* No. 7 and *Warning* No. 5.

Nursing Mothers. See *Warning* No. 12.

Adverse Reactions: An increased risk of the following serious adverse reactions has been associated with the use of oral contraceptives (see *Warnings*).

Thrombophlebitis and thrombosis
Pulmonary embolism
Myocardial infarction and coronary thrombosis
Cerebral thrombosis
Cerebral hemorrhage
Hypertension
Gallbladder disease
Benign adenomas and other hepatic lesions, with or without intra-abdominal bleeding
Congenital anomalies

There is evidence of an association between the following conditions and the use of oral contraceptives, although confirmatory studies have not been done:

Mesenteric thrombosis
Budd-Chiari syndrome
Neuro-ocular lesions, (eg, retinal thrombosis and optic neuritis)

The following adverse reactions have been reported in patients receiving oral contraceptives and are believed to be drug related:

Nausea and vomiting
(Usually the most common adverse reactions, occurring in approximately 10% or fewer patients during the first cycle. Other reactions, as a general rule, are seen much less frequently or only occasionally.)
Gastrointestinal symptoms (eg, abdominal cramps and bloating)
Breakthrough bleeding
Spotting
Change in menstrual flow
Dysmenorrhea
Amenorrhea during and after use
Infertility after discontinuation
Edema
Chloasma or melasma, which may persist when the drug is discontinued
Breast changes: tenderness, enlargement, and secretion
Change in weight (increase or decrease)
Change in cervical erosion and secretion
Endocervical hyperplasia
Possible diminution in lactation when given immediately post partum
Cholestatic jaundice
Migraine
Increase in size of uterine leiomyomata
Rash (allergic)
Mental depression
Reduced tolerance to carbohydrates
Vaginal candidiasis
Change in corneal curvature (steepening)
Intolerance to contact lenses

The following adverse reactions or conditions have been reported in users of oral contraceptives, and the association has been neither confirmed nor refuted:

Premenstrual-like syndrome
Cataracts
Changes in libido
Chorea
Changes in appetite
Cystitis-like syndrome
Headache
Paresthesia
Nervousness
Dizziness
Auditory disturbances
Rhinitis
Fatigue
Backache
Hirsutism
Loss of scalp hair
Erythema multiforme
Erythema nodosum
Hemorrhagic eruption
Hemolytic uremic syndrome
Itching
Vaginitis
Porphyria
Impaired renal function
Anemia
Pancreatitis
Hepatitis
Colitis
Gingivitis
Dry socket
Lupus erythematosus
Rheumatoid arthritis
Pituitary tumors (eg, adenoma) with amenorrhea and/or galactorrhea after OC use
Malignant melanoma
Endometrial, cervical, and breast carcinoma (see *Warning* No. 3)

Acute Overdosage: Serious ill effects have not been reported following the acute ingestion of large doses of oral contraceptives by young children.[75,76] Overdosage may cause nausea, and withdrawal bleeding might occur in females.

Dosage and Administration:

Contraception: Demulen, Demulen-28, Demulen 1/35™-21, Demulen 1/35™-28, Ovulen-21, Ovulen-28, Enovid-E 21, and Enovid 5 mg.

To achieve maximum contraceptive effectiveness, oral contraceptives must be taken exactly as directed and at intervals of 24 hours.

IMPORTANT: The patient should be instructed to use an additional method of protection until after the first week of administration *in the initial cycle.* The possibility of ovulation and conception prior to initiation of use should be considered.

Enovid 5 mg 20-Tablet Dosage Schedule: The patient should take one tablet daily for twenty consecutive days beginning each 20-tablet course on day 5 of her menstrual cycle or eight days after taking the last pill from the previous cycle, whichever occurs first. The first day of menstruation is counted as day 1.

Demulen, Demulen-28, Demulen 1/35™-21, Demulen 1/35™-28, Ovulen-21, Ovulen-28 and Enovid-E 21 Dosage Schedules: The Demulen, Demulen 1/35™-21 Ovulen-21, and Enovid-E 21 Compack® tablet dispensers contain 21 tablets arranged in three numbered rows of 7 tablets each.

The Demulen-28, Demulen 1/35™-28, and Ovulen-28 tablet dispensers contain 21 white active tablets arranged in three numbered rows of 7 tablets each, followed by a fourth row of 7 pink (blue for Demulen 1/35™-28) placebo tablets.

Days of the week are printed above the tablets, starting with Sunday on the left.

Two dosage schedules are described, one of which may be more convenient or suitable than the other for an individual patient.

Schedule #1: Sunday Start: The patient begins taking Demulen, Demulen-28, Demulen 1/35™-21, Demulen 1/35™-28, Ovulen-21, Ovulen-28, or Enovid-E 21 from the first row of her package, one tablet daily, starting on the first Sunday after the onset of menstruation. If the patient's period begins on a Sunday she takes her first tablet that very same day. The 21st tablet or the 28th tablet, depending on whether the patient is taking the 21- or 28-tablet course, will then be taken on a Saturday.

Subsequent Cycles:

21-tablet course—The patient begins a new 21-tablet course on the eighth day, Sunday, after taking her last tablet. All subsequent cycles will also begin on Sunday, one tablet being taken each day for three weeks followed by a week of no pill-taking.

28-tablet course—The patient begins a new 28-tablet course on the next day, Sunday, and all subsequent cycles will also begin on Sunday, one tablet being taken each and every day.

With a Sunday-start schedule, a woman whose period begins on the day of or one to four days before taking the first tablet should expect a diminution of flow and fewer menstrual days. The initial cycle will likely be shortened by from one to five days. Thereafter, cycles should be about 28 days in length.

Schedule #2: Day 5 Start: The patient begins taking Demulen, Demulen 1/35™-21, Ovulen-21, or Enovid-E 21 from the first row of her package, one tablet daily, starting with the pill day which corresponds to day 5 of her menstrual cycle; the first day of menstruation is counted as day 1. After the last (Saturday) tablet in row #3 has been taken, if any remain in the first row, the patient completes her 21-tablet schedule starting with Sunday in row #1.

Subsequent Cycles: The patient begins a new 21-tablet course on the eighth day after taking her last tablet, again starting the same day of the week on which she began her first course. All subsequent cycles will also begin on that same day, one tablet being taken each day for three weeks followed by a week of no pill-taking.

Postpartum Administration. Ovulen-21 and Ovulen-28 oral contraceptives may be prescribed at the first postpartum examination regardless of whether or not the patient has experienced spontaneous menstruation. In non-nursing mothers, administration may be initiated immediately after delivery if desired or on the first Sunday after delivery. If preferred the tablets may be started on the day the patient leaves the hospital. (For nursing mothers see *Warning* No. 12.)

Hypermenorrhea; Production of Cyclic Withdrawal Bleeding: Enovid 5 mg or 10 mg only. Most patients with hypermenorrhea may be expected to respond to Enovid 5-mg or 10-mg therapy within 24 to 48 hours. Regular withdrawal bleeding may then be induced by cyclic administration. Vaginal bleeding at times other than the regular menstrual period requires that a diagnosis be established prior to beginning therapy.

For emergency control of severe bleeding in patients with hypermenorrhea give 20 to 30 mg of Enovid daily until the bleeding is controlled, then reduce the daily dose to 10 mg and continue through day 24 of the cycle. Then discontinue Enovid and withdrawal flow usually will begin approximately two to three days later.

Cyclic withdrawal bleeding may be produced after treatment in this initial cycle by giving the patient 5 to 10 mg of Enovid 5 mg or 10 mg daily from day 5 through day 24 of the next two or three cycles. A new course of Enovid therapy should be started on day 5 of her menstrual cycle or eight days after the last pill from the previous cycle, whichever occurs first. The first day of menstruation is counted as day 1.

Endometriosis: Enovid 5 mg or 10 mg only. A daily dose of Enovid should be given for six to nine months or longer on the following schedule: 5 or 10 mg should be given for two weeks beginning on day 5 of a menstrual cycle. This daily dose should be given continuously (without cyclic interruption) and increased 5 or 10 mg at two-week intervals until the patient is receiving 20 mg daily. This dose of 20 mg should be continued for six to nine months and further increased (up to 40 mg daily) if breakthrough bleeding occurs.

Therapy may be discontinued after six months if the disease is mild and the lesions are no longer palpable. If the disorder is more severe continue treatment for nine months or longer. When surgery is contemplated prior administration of Enovid may facilitate the surgical procedure. (See *Warning* No. 1 concerning discontinuation prior to elective surgery.)

Special Notes: *Spotting or Breakthrough Bleeding.* If spotting (bleeding insufficient to require a pad) or breakthrough bleeding (heavier bleeding similar to a menstrual flow) occurs when these products are used for contraception the patient should continue taking her tablets as directed. The incidence of spotting or breakthrough bleeding is minimal, most frequently occurring in the first cycle. Ordinarily spotting or breakthrough bleeding will stop within a week. Usually the patient will begin to cycle regularly within two or three courses of tablet-taking. If breakthrough bleeding occurs while the patient is taking Enovid for hypermenorrhea she should immediately increase the daily dosage by 5 or 10 mg until bleeding has been controlled for three days, after which the original dosage usually may be resumed. In the event of spotting or breakthrough bleeding organic causes should be borne in mind. (See *Warning* No. 10.)

Missed Menstrual Periods. Withdrawal flow will normally occur two or three days after the last active tablet is taken. Failure of withdrawal bleeding ordinarily does not mean that the patient is pregnant, providing the dosage schedule has been correctly followed. (See *Warning* No. 5.)

If the patient has *not* adhered to the prescribed dosage regimen, the possibility of pregnancy should be considered after the first missed period, and oral contraceptives should be withheld until pregnancy has been ruled out.

If the patient has adhered to the prescribed regimen and misses two consecutive periods, pregnancy should be ruled out before continuing the contraceptive regimen.

The first intermenstrual interval after discontinuing the tablets is usually prolonged; consequently, a patient for whom a 28-day cycle is usual might not begin to menstruate for 35 days or longer. Ovulation in such prolonged cycles will occur correspondingly later in the cycle. Post-treatment cycles after the first one, however, are usually typical for the individual woman prior to taking tablets. (See *Warnings* No. 10 and 11.)

Missed Tablets (Contraception). If a woman misses taking one active tablet the missed tablet should be taken as soon as it is remembered. In addition, the next tablet should be taken at the usual time. If two consecutive tablets are missed the dosage should be doubled for the next two days. The regular schedule should then be resumed, but an additional method of protection is recommended for the remainder of the cycle.

While there is little likelihood of ovulation if only one active tablet is missed, the possibility of spotting or breakthrough bleeding is increased and should be expected if two or more successive active tablets are missed. However, the possibility of ovulation increases with each successive day that scheduled active tablets are missed.

If one or more placebo tablets of Demulen-28, Demulen 1/35™-28, or Ovulen-28 are missed, the Demulen-28, Demulen 1/35™-28, or Ovulen-28 schedule should be resumed on the following Sunday (the eighth day after the last white tablet was taken). Omission of placebo tablets in the 28-tablet courses does not increase the possibility of conception provided that this schedule is followed.

How Supplied:

Demulen: Each white Demulen tablet is round in shape, with a debossed SEARLE on one side and 71 on the other side, and contains 1 mg of ethynodiol diacetate and 50 mcg of ethinyl estradiol.

Demulen is packaged in cartons of 6 Compack tablet dispensers of 21 tablets each; in cartons of 12 and 48 Compack refills of 21 tablets each; and in cartons of 10 Triopak™ tablet containers, each Triopak containing 1 Compack tablet dispenser and 2 refills of 21 tablets each.

Demulen-28 is packaged in cartons of 6 Compack tablet dispensers and in cartons of 12 Compack refills. Each Compack and refill contain 21 white Demulen tablets and 7 pink placebo tablets. (Placebo tablets have a debossed SEARLE on one side and a "P" on the other side.)

Demulen 1/35:

Each white Demulen 1/35 tablet is round in shape, with a debossed SEARLE on one side and 151 and design on the other side, and contains 1 mg of ethynodiol diacetate and 35 mcg of ethinyl estradiol.

Demulen 1/35™-21 is packaged in cartons of 6 Compack tablet dispensers of 21 tablets each, and in cartons of 12 and 48 Compack refills of 21 tablets each.

Demulen 1/35™-28 is packaged in cartons of 6 Compack tablet dispensers and in cartons of 12 Compack refills. Each Compack and refill contains 21 white Demulen 1/35 tablets and 7 blue placebo tablets. (Placebo tablets have a debossed SEARLE on one side and a "P" on the other side.)

Ovulen: Each white Ovulen tablet is pentagonal in shape, with a debossed SEARLE on one side and 401 on the other side, and contains 1 mg of ethynodiol diacetate and 0.1 mg of mestranol.

Ovulen-21 is packaged in cartons of 6 Compack tablet dispensers of 21 tablets each; in cartons of 12 and 48 Compack refills of 21 tablets each; and in cartons of 10 and boxes of 100 Triopak™ tablet containers, each Triopak containing 1 Compack tablet dispenser and 2 refills of 21 tablets each.

Ovulen-28 is packaged in cartons of 6 Compack tablet dispensers and in cartons of 12 Compack refills. Each Compack and refill contains 21 white Ovulen tablets and 7 pink placebo tablets. (Placebo tablets have a debossed SEARLE on one side and a "P" on the other side.)

Enovid-E: Each Enovid-E tablet is pale pink, round in shape, with a debossed SEARLE E on one side and 131 on the other side, and contains 2.5 mg of norethynodrel and 0.1 mg of mestranol.

Enovid-E 21 is packaged in cartons of 6 Compack tablet dispensers of 21 tablets each, and in cartons of 12 Compack refills of 21 tablets each.

Enovid 5 mg: Each Enovid 5 mg tablet is pink, round in shape, with a debossed SEARLE 5 on one side and 51 on the other side, and contains 5 mg of norethynodrel and 75 mcg of mestranol. Enovid 5 mg is packaged in cartons of 6 Calendar-Pack™ tablet dispensers of 20 tablets each and in bottles of 100 tablets each.

Enovid 10 mg: Each Enovid 10 mg tablet is coral colored, round in shape, with a debossed SEARLE 10 on one side and 101 on the other side, and contains 9.85 mg of norethynodrel and 0.15 mg of mestranol. Enovid 10 mg is packaged in bottles of 50 tablets each.

References:

1. Population Reports, Series H, No. 2 (May) 1974; Series I, No. 1 (June) 1974; Series B, No. 3 (May) 1979; Series H, No. 3 (Jan.) 1975; Series H, No. 4 (Jan.) 1976; Population Information Program, Geo. Washington U. Medical Center, Washington, D.C. **2.** Inman, W. H. W., et al.: Br. Med. J. *2*:203 (April 25) 1970. **3.** Inman, W. H. W., et al.: Br. Med. J. *2*:193 (April 27) 1968. **4.** Royal College of General Practitioners: J. Coll. Gen. Pract. *13*:267 (May) 1967. **5.** Vessey, M. P., et al.: Br. Med. J. *2*:651 (June 14) 1969. **6.** Sartwell, P. E., et al.: Am. J. Epidemiol. *90*:365 (Nov.) 1969. **7.** Boston Collaborative Drug Surveillance Programme: Lancet *1*:1399 (June 23) 1973. **8.** Stolley, P.D., et al.: Am. J. Epidemiol. *102*:197 (Sept.) 1975. **9.** Collaborative Group for the Study of Stroke in Young Women: N. Engl. J. Med. *288*:871 (April 26) 1973.

10. Collaborative Group for the Study of Stroke in Young Women: J.A.M.A. *231*:718 (Feb. 17) 1975. **11.** Beral, V.: Lancet *2*:1047 (Nov. 13) 1976. **12.** Royal College of General Practitioners: Oral Contraceptives and Health, New York, Pitman Publ. Corp., May 1974. **13.** Layde, P., et al.: Lancet *1*:541 (March 7) 1981. **14.** Vessey, M., et al.: J. Biosoc. Sci. *8*:373 (Oct.) 1976. **15.** Vessey, M., et al.: Lancet *2*:731 (Oct. 8) 1977; *1*:549 (March 7) 1981. **16.** Mann, J. I., et al.: Br. Med. J. *2*:241 (May 3) 1975. **17.** Mann, J. I., et al.: Br. Med. J. *3*:631 (Sept. 13) 1975. **18.** Mann, J. I., et al.: Br. Med. J. *2*:245 (May 3) 1975. **19.** Mann, J. I., et al.: Br. Med. J. *2*:445 (Aug. 21) 1976.

20. Jain, A. K.: Stud. Fam. Plann. *8*:50 (March) 1977. **21.** Tietze, C.: Fam. Plann. Perspect. *9*:74 (March-April) 1977. **22.** Vessey, M. P., et al.: Br. Med. J. *3*:123 (July 18) 1970. **23.** Greene, G. R., et al.: Am. J. Public Health *62*:680 (May) 1972. **24.** Ziel, H. K., et al.: N. Engl. J. Med.

Continued on next page

Searle & Co.—Cont.

293:1167 (Dec. 4) 1975. **25.** Smith, D. C., et al.: N. Engl. J. Med. *293*:1164 (Dec. 4) 1975. **26.** Mack, T. M., et al.: N. Engl. J. Med. *294*:1262 (June 3) 1976. **27.** Gray, L. A., et al.: Obstet. Gynecol. *49*:385 (April) 1977. **28.** McDonald, T. W., et al.: Am. J. Obstet. Gynecol. *127*:572 (March 15) 1977. **29.** Weiss, N. S., et al.: N. Engl. J. Med. *294*:1259 (June 3) 1976.
30. Silverberg, S. G., et al.: Cancer *39*:592 (Feb.) 1977. **31.** Vessey, M. P., et al.: Br. Med. J. *3*:719 (Sept. 23) 1972. **32.** Vessey, M. P., et al.: Lancet *1*:941 (April 26) 1975. **33.** Boston Collaborative Drug Surveillance Program: N. Engl. J. Med.*290*:15 (Jan. 3) 1974. **34.** Arthes, F. G., et al.: Cancer *28*:1391 (Dec.) 1971. **35.** Casagrande, J., et al.: J. Natl. Cancer Inst. *56*:839 (April) 1976. **36.** Fasal, E., et al.: J. Natl. Cancer Inst. *55*:767 (Oct.) 1975. **37.** Paffenbarger, R. S., et al.: Cancer *49*:1887 (April Suppl.) 1977. **38.** Hoover, R., et al.: N. Engl. J. Med. *295*:401 (Aug. 19) 1976. **39.** Kelsey, J. L., et al.: Am. J. Epidemiol. *107*:236 (March) 1978.
40. Ory, H., et al.: N. Engl. J. Med. *294*:419 (Feb. 19) 1976. **41.** Stern, E., et al.: Science *196*:1460 (June 24) 1977. **42.** Population Reports, Series A, No. 4 (May) 1977: Population Information Program, Geo. Washington U. Medical Center, Washington, D.C. **43.** Baum, J. K., et al.: Lancet *2*:926 (Oct. 27) 1973. **44.** Mays, E. T., et al.: J.A.M.A. *235*:730 (Feb. 16) 1976. **45.** Edmondson, H. A., et al.: N. Engl. J. Med. *294*:470 (Feb. 26) 1976. **46.** Rooks, J. B., et al.: J.A.M.A. *242*:644 (Aug. 17) 1979. **47.** Herbst, A. L., et al.: N. Engl. J. Med. *284*:878 (April 22) 1971. **48.** Greenwald, P., et al.: N. Engl. J. Med. *285*:390 (Aug. 12) 1971. **49.** Lanier, A. P., et al.: Mayo Clin. Proc. *48*:793 (Nov.) 1973.
50. Herbst, A. L., et al.: Am. J. Obstet. Gynecol. *128*:43 (May 1) 1977. **51.** Herbst, A. L., et al.: Obstet. Gynecol. *40*:287 (Sept.) 1972. **52.** Herbst, A. L., et al.: Am. J. Obstet. Gynecol. *118*:607 (March 1) 1974. **53.** Herbst, A. L., et al.: N. Engl. J. Med. *292*:334 (Feb. 13) 1975. **54.** Stafl, A., et al.: Obstet. Gynecol. *43*:118 (Jan.) 1974. **55.** Sherman, A. I., et al.: Obstet. Gynecol. *44*:531 (Oct.) 1974. **56.** Bibbo, M., et al.: J. Reprod. Med. *15*:29 (July) 1975. **57.** Gill, W., et al.: J. Reprod. Med. *16*:147 (April) 1976. **58.** Henderson, B., et al.: Pediatrics *58*:505 (Oct.) 1976. **59.** Gal, I., et al.: Nature *240*:241 (Nov. 24) 1972.
60. Levy, E. P., et al.: Lancet *1*:611 (March 17) 1973. **61.** Nora, J. J., et al.: Lancet *1*:941 (April 28) 1973. **62.** Nora, A. H., et al.: Arch. Environ. Health *30*:17 (Jan.) 1975; Adv. Plann. Parent. *12*:156, 1978. **63.** Janerich, D. T., et al.: N. Engl. J. Med. *291*:697 (Oct. 3) 1974. **64.** Heinonen, O. P., et al.: N. Engl. J. Med. *296*:67 (Jan. 13) 1977. **65.** Nora, J. J., et al.: N. Engl. J. Med. *291*:731 (Oct. 3) 1974. **66.** Carr, D. H.: Can. Med. Assoc. J. *103*:343 (Aug. 15 & 29) 1970. **67.** Wynn, V., et al.: Lancet *2*:720 (Oct. 1) 1966. **68.** Laragh, J. H.: Am. J. Obstet. Gynecol. *126*:141 (Sept.) 1976. **69.** Fisch, I. R., et al.: J.A.M.A. *237*:2499 (June 6) 1977.
70. Van Campenhout, J., et al.: Fertil. Steril. *28*:728 (July) 1977. **71.** Laumas, K. R., et al.: Am. J. Obstet. Gynecol. *98*:411 (June 1) 1967. **72.** Stockley, I.: Pharmaceut. J. *216*:140 (Feb. 14) 1976. **73.** Hempel, E., et al.: Drugs *12*:442 (Dec.) 1976. **74.** Bessot, J.-C., et al.: Nouv. Presse Med. *6*:1568 (April 30) 1977. **75.** Francis, W. G., et al.: Can. Med. Assoc. J. *92*:191 (Jan. 23) 1965. **76.** Verhulst, H. L., et al.: J. Clin. Pharmacol. *7*:9 (Jan.-Feb.) 1967. **77.** Vessey, M. P., et al.: Br. Med. J. *2*:199 (April 27) 1968. **78.** Ory, H. W.: J.A.M.A. *237*:2619 (June 13) 1977. **79.** Jain, A. K.: Am. J. Obstet. Gynecol. *126*:301 (Oct. 1) 1976.
80. Ziel, H. K., et al.: Am. J. Obstet. Gynecol. *124*:735 (April 1) 1976. **81.** Peritz, E., et al.: Am. J. Epidemiol. *106*:462 (Dec.) 1977. **82.** Ory, H. W., et al.: in Garattini, S., and Berendes, H. (eds.), Pharmacology of Steroid Contraceptive Drugs, Raven Press, N.Y., 1977. **83.** Goldacre, M. J., et al.: Br. Med. J. *1*:748 (March 25) 1978. **84.** Meisels, A., et al.: Cancer *40*:3076 (Dec.) 1977. **85.** Klatskin, G.: Gastroenterology *73*:386 (Aug.) 1977. **86.** Kay, C. R.: Lancet *1*:624 (March 19) 1977. **87.** March, C. M., et al.: Fertil. Steril. *28*:346 (March) 1977. **88.** Saxena, B. N., et al.: Contraception *16*:605 (Dec.) 1977. **89.** Nilsson, S., et al.: Contraception *17*:131 (Feb.) 1978.
90. Vessey, M. P., et al.: Br. Med. J. *1*:265 (Feb. 4) 1978. **91.** Jick, H., et al.: J.A.M.A. *239*:1403, 1407 (April 3) 1978. **92.** Kay, C. R.: J. Royal Coll. Gen. Pract. *28*:393 (July) 1978. **93.** Hoogerland, D. L., et al.: Gynecol. Oncol. *6*:451 (Oct.) 1978. **94.** Lorber, C. A., et al.: Fertil. Steril. *31*:21 (Jan.) 1979. **95.** Bacon, J. F., et al.: Br. Med. J. *280*:293 (Feb. 2) 1980. **96.** Meade, T. W., et al.: Br. Med. J. *280*:1157 (May 10) 1980. **97.** Böttiger, L. E., et al.: Lancet *1*:1097 (May 24) 1980. **98.** Maquire, M. G., et al.: Am. J. Epidemiol. *110*:188 (Aug.) 1979. **99.** Ramcharan, S., et al.: The Walnut Creek Contraceptive Drug Study, Vol. 3, U.S. Govt. Ptg. Off., 1981,; J. Reprod. Med. *25*:346 (Dec.) 1980.
100. Petitti, D. B., et al.: Am. J. Epidemiol. *108*:480 (Dec.) 1978. **101.** Petitti, D. B., et al.: J.A.M.A. *242*:1150 (Sept. 14) 1979. **102.** Petitti, D. B., et al.: Lancet *2*:234 (July 29) 1978. **103.** Jick, H., et al.: Ann. Int. Med. *88*:58 (July) 1978. **104.** Jick, H., et al.: J.A.M.A. *240*:2548 (Dec. 1) 1978. **105.** Shapiro, S., et al.: Lancet *1*:743 (April 7) 1979. **106.** Rosenberg, L., et al.: Am. J. Epidemiol. *111*:59 (Jan.) 1980. **107.** Kreuger, D. E., et al.: Am. J. Epidemiol. *111*:655 (June) 1980. **108.** Arthes, F. G., et al.: Chest *70*:574 (Nov.) 1976. **109.** Hoover, R., et al.: Am. J. Public Health *18*:335 (April) 1978.
110. Herbst, A. L., et al.: J. Reprod. Med. *24*:62 (Feb.) 1980. **111.** Barnes, A. B., et al.: N. Engl. J. Med. *302*:609 (March 13) 1980. **112:** Cousins, L., et al.: Obstet. Gynecol. *56*:70 (July) 1980.
113. Nora, J. J., et al.: J.A.M.A. *240*:837 (Sept. 1) 1978. **114.** Aarskog, D.: N. Engl. J. Med. *300*:75 (Jan. 11) 1979. **115.** Janerich, D. T., et al.: Am. J. Epidemiol. *112*:73 (July) 1980. **116.** Kasan, P. N., et al.: Br. J. Obstet. Gynaecol. *87*:545 (July) 1980. **117.** Rothman, K. J.: N. Engl. J. Med. *297*:468 (Sept. 1) 1977. **118.** Bracken, M. B.: Am. J. Obstet. Gynecol. *133*:432 (Feb. 15) 1979. **119.** De Teresa, E., et al.: Br. Med. J. *2*:1260 (Nov. 17) 1979.
120. Swan, S., et al.: Am. J. Obstet. Gynecol. *139*:52 (Jan. 1) 1981. **121.** Kay, C. R.: Br. Med. J. *282*:2089 (June 27) 1981. **122.** Vessey, M. P., et al.: Br. Med. J. *282*:2093 (June 27) 1981. **123.** Pike, M. C., et al.: Br. J. Cancer *43*:72 (Jan.) 1981. **124.** Harlap, S., et al.: Obstet. Gynecol. *55*:447 (April) 1980. **125.** Back, D. J., et al.: Drugs *21*:46 (Jan.) 1981. **126.** Porter, J. B., et al.: Obstet. Gynecol. *59*:229 (March) 1982. **127.** Lees, A.W., et al.: Int. J. Cancer *22*:700, 1978.
128. Brinton, L. A., et al.: J. Natl. Cancer Inst. (JNCl) *62*:37 (Jan.) 1979. **129.** Black, M. M.: Pathol. Res. Pract. *166*:491. 1980; Cancer *46*:2747 (Dec.) 1980.
130. Hoover, R., et al.: JNCl *67*:815 (Oct.) 1981. **131.** Gill, W. B., et al.: J. Urol. *122*:36 (July) 1979. **132.** Linn. S., et al.: J.A.M.A. *247*:629 (Feb. 5) 1982. **133.** Clavel, F., et al.: Bull. Cancer (Paris) *68*:449 (Dec.) 1981. **134.** Abernethy, D. R., et al.: N. Engl. J. Med. *306*:791 (April 1) 1982. **135.** Kay, C. R.: Am. J. Obstet. Gynecol. *142*:762 (March 15) 1982. **136.** Adam, S. A., et al.: Br. J. Obstet. Gynaecol. *88*:838 (Aug.) 1981.

Brief Summary of Patient Labeling

Cigarette-smoking increases the risk of serious adverse effects on the heart and blood vessels from oral contraceptive use. This risk increases with age and with heavy smoking (15 or more cigarettes per day) and is quite marked in women over 35 years of age. Women who use oral contraceptives should not smoke.

In the detailed leaflet, " What You Should Know About Oral Contraceptives," which you have received, the risks and benefits of oral contraceptives are discussed in much more detail. This leaflet also provides information on other forms of contraception. Please take time to read it carefully for it may have been recently revised.
If you have any questions or problems regarding this information, contact your doctor.

Oral contraceptives taken as directed are about 99% effective in preventing pregnancy. (The mini-pill, however, is somewhat less effective.) Forgetting to take your pills increases the chance of pregnancy.
Women who have or have had clotting disorders, cancer of the breast or sex organs, unexplained vaginal bleeding, stroke, heart attack, chest pains on exertion (angina pectoris), liver tumors associated with the use of the pill or with other estrogen-containing products, or who suspect they may be pregnant should not use oral contraceptives.
Most side effects of the pill are not serious. The most common side effects are nausea, vomiting, bleeding between menstrual periods, weight gain, and breast tenderness. However, proper use of oral contraceptives requires that they be taken under your doctor's continuing supervision, because they can be associated with serious side effects which may be fatal. Fortunately, these are very uncommon. The serious side effects are:

1. Blood clots in the legs, arms, lungs, brain, heart, eyes, abdomen, or elsewhere in the body.
2. Bleeding in the brain (hemorrhage) as a result of bursting of a blood vessel.
3. Disorders of vision.
4. Liver tumors, which may rupture and cause severe bleeding.
5. Birth defects if the pill is taken during pregnancy.
6. High blood pressure.
7. Gallbladder disease.

The symptoms associated with these serious side effects are discussed in the detailed leaflet given you with your supply of pills. Notify your doctor if you notice any unusual physical disturbance while taking the pill.
Breast cancer and other cancers have developed in certain animals when given the estrogens in oral contraceptives for long periods. These findings suggest that oral contraceptives may also cause cancer in humans. However, studies to date in women taking currently marketed oral contraceptives have not confirmed that oral contraceptives cause cancer in humans.
Caution: Oral contraceptives are of no value in the prevention or treatment of venereal disease.
Various drugs, such as antibiotics, may also decrease the effectiveness of oral contraceptives.

Detailed Patient Labeling: What You Should Know About Oral Contraceptives

Oral contraceptives (the pill) are the most effective way (except for sterilization) to prevent pregnancy if you follow the directions for their use and are careful not to skip doses or take them irregularly. They are also convenient and, for most women, free of serious or unpleasant side effects. Oral contraceptives must always be taken under the continuing supervision of a doctor.
It is important that any woman who considers using an oral contraceptive understands the risks involved. Although the oral contraceptives have important advantages over other methods of contraception, they have certain risks that no other method has. Only you can decide whether the advantages are worth these

risks. This leaflet will tell you about the most important risks. It will explain how you can help your doctor prescribe the pill as safely as possible by telling him/her about yourself and being alert for the earliest signs of trouble. And it will tell you how to use the pill properly, so that it will be as effective as possible. THERE IS MORE DETAILED INFORMATION AVAILABLE IN THE LEAFLET PREPARED FOR DOCTORS. Your pharmacist can show you a copy; you may need your doctor's help in understanding parts of it.

Enovid 5 mg or 10 mg can be prescribed as a treatment for endometriosis and as a treatment for hypermenorrhea and regulating periods. If you are taking Enovid 5 mg or 10 mg for one of these other conditions besides contraception the warning information in the detailed leaflet also applies, so please read this leaflet.

Caution: Oral contraceptives are of no value in the prevention or treatment of venereal disease.

Cigarette-smoking increases the risk of serious adverse effects on the heart and blood vessels from oral contraceptive use. This risk increases with age and with heavy smoking (15 or more cigarettes per day) and is quite marked in women over 35 years of age. Women who use oral contraceptives should not smoke.

Who Should Not Use Oral Contraceptives:
You should not use oral contraceptives:

A. If you have any of the following conditions:
   1. Blood clots in the legs, lungs, or elsewhere in the body.
   2. Chest pains on exertion (angina pectoris).
   3. Known or suspected cancer of the breast or sex organs, such as the womb (uterus), vagina, or cervix.
   4. Unusual vaginal bleeding that has not been diagnosed by your doctor.
   5. Known or suspected pregnancy (one or more menstrual periods missed).

B. If you have had any of the following conditions:
   1. Heart attack or stroke (clots or bleeding in the brain).
   2. Blood clots in the legs, lungs, or elsewhere in the body.
   3. Liver tumor associated with use of the pill or other estrogen-containing products.

C. If you have scanty or irregular periods or are a young woman without a regular cycle, you should use another method of contraception because, if you use the pill, you may have difficulty becoming pregnant or may fail to have menstrual periods after discontinuing the pill.

Deciding to Use Oral Contraceptives. If you do not have any of the conditions listed above and are thinking about using oral contraceptives, to help you decide, you need information about the advantages and risks of oral contraceptives and of other contraceptive methods as well. This leaflet describes the advantages and risks of oral contraceptives. Except for sterilization, the intrauterine device (IUD), and abortion, which have their own specific risks, the only risks of other methods of contraception are those due to pregnancy should the method fail. Your doctor can answer questions you may have with respect to other methods of contraception, and further questions you may have on oral contraceptives after reading this leaflet.

1. *What Oral Contraceptives Are and How They Work.*

Oral contraceptives are of two types. The most common, often simply called "the pill," is a *combination* of an estrogen and a progestogen, the two kinds of female hormones. The amount of estrogen and progestogen can vary, but the amount of estrogen is more important because both the effectiveness and some of the dangers of oral contraceptives have been related to the amount of estrogen. This combination oral contraceptive works principally by preventing release of an egg from the ovary during the cycle in which the pills are taken. When the amount of estrogen is 50 micrograms or more, and the pill is taken as directed, oral contraceptives are more than 99% effective (that is, there would be less than one pregnancy in 100 women using the pill for one year). Pills that contain 20 to 35 micrograms of estrogen vary slightly in effectiveness, ranging from 98% to more than 99% effective.

The second type of oral contraceptive, often called the mini-pill, contains only a progestogen. It works in part by preventing release of an egg from the ovary, but also by keeping sperm from reaching the egg and by making the womb (uterus) less receptive to any fertilized egg that reaches it. The mini-pill is less effective than the combination oral contraceptive, about 97% effective. In addition, the mini-pill has a tendency to cause irregular bleeding, which may be quite inconvenient, or cessation of bleeding entirely. The mini-pill is used despite its lower effectiveness in the hope that it will prove not to have some of the serious side effects of the estrogen-containing pill, but it is not yet certain that the mini-pill does in fact have fewer serious side effects. The following discussion, while based mainly on information about the combination pills, should be considered to apply as well to the mini-pill.

2. *Other Nonsurgical Ways to Prevent Pregnancy.*

As this leaflet will explain, oral contraceptives have several serious risks. Other methods of contraception have lesser risks or none at all. They are also less effective than oral contraceptives, but, used properly, may be effective enough for many women. The following table gives reported pregnancy rates (the number of women out of 100 who would become pregnant in one year) for these methods:

Pregnancies per 100 Women per Year

Method	*Range*
Intrauterine device (IUD)	less than 1 to 6
Diaphragm with spermicidal cream or jelly	2 to 20
Condom (rubber)	3 to 36
Spermicidal aerosol foams	2 to 29
Spermicidal jellies or creams	4 to 36
Periodic abstinence (rhythm), all types	less than 1 to 47
1. Calendar method	14 to 47
2. Temperature method	1 to 20
3. Temperature method (intercourse only in postovulatory phase)	less than 1 to 7
4. Mucus method	1 to 25
No contraception	60 to 80

These figures (except for the IUD) vary widely because people differ in how well they use each method. Very faithful users of the various methods obtain the best results, except for users of the periodic abstinence (rhythm) calendar method. Effective use of these methods, except for the IUD, requires somewhat more effort than simply taking a single pill every day, but it is an effort that many couples undertake successfully. Your doctor can tell you a great deal more about these methods of contraception and their effectiveness.

3. *The Dangers of Oral Contraceptives.*

a. *Circulatory Disorders (Blood Clots, Strokes, and Heart Attacks).* Blood clots occasionally form in the blood vessels of the body and, though rare, are the most common of the serious side effects of oral contraceptives. Clotting can result in a stroke (a clot in the brain), a heart attack (a clot in a blood vessel of the heart), or a pulmonary embolus (a clot that forms in the legs or abdominal region, then breaks off and travels to the lungs), or loss of a limb (a clot in a blood vessel in, or leading to, an arm or leg). Clots can also form in the blood vessels of the intestines or liver. Any of these events can be fatal (lead to death). Clots also occur rarely in the blood vessels of the eye, resulting in blindness or impairment of vision in that eye. There is some evidence that the risk of clotting may increase with higher estrogen doses. It is therefore important for your doctor to keep the dose of estrogen as low as possible, so long as the oral contraceptive used has an acceptable pregnancy rate and doesn't cause unacceptable changes in the menstrual pattern.. Higher doses of progestogen have also been suggested as increasing the risk of clotting. Furthermore, cigarette-smoking by oral contraceptive users increases the risk of serious adverse effects on the heart and blood vessels. This risk increases with age and with heavy smoking (15 or more cigarettes per day) and begins to become quite marked in women over 35 years of age. For this reason, women who use oral contraceptives should not smoke.

The risk of abnormal clotting increases with age both in users and in nonusers of oral contraceptives, but the increased risk with the oral contraceptives appears to be present at all ages.

For oral contraceptive users in general, it has been estimated that in women between the ages of 25 and 34 the risk of death due to circulatory disorders in nonsmokers is about 1 in 23,000 per year. In contrast, for nonusers of the pill the risk is about 1 in 37,000 per year. Estimates of the risk of death due to circulatory disorders can be made, depending upon the woman's age, whether or not she uses oral contraceptives, and whether or not she smokes cigarettes. In the age group 25–34 years, women who use the pill have a risk of 1 in 7,000 (for smokers) to 1 in 23,000 (for nonsmokers) per year. This may be compared to the corresponding risk in women who have not used the pill: 1 in 24,000 (for smokers) to 1 in 37,000 (for nonsmokers) per year. The risks are greater in older women; thus, in the age group 35–44 years, women who use the pill have a risk of 1 in 1,600 (for smokers) to 1 in 4,700 (for nonsmokers) per year. The corresponding risk for women who have not used the pill is 1 in 6,600 (for smokers) to 1 in 16,000 (for nonsmokers) per year.

For women aged 16 to 40 it is estimated that about 1 in 2,000 using oral contraceptives will be hospitalized each year because of abnormal clotting in the veins or lungs. Among nonusers of the same age, about 1 in 20,000 would be hospitalized each year for these disorders.

Strokes are caused by a bursting blood vessel in the brain (hemorrhage) or a loss of blood circulation to the brain due to blood clots. When they occur, paralysis of all or part of the body may result; death can result. The risk of strokes due to clots or hemorrhages in the brain has been reported to be increased in pill users when compared with nonusers.

It has been estimated that pill users are twice as likely as nonusers to have a stroke due to a bursting blood vessel in the brain. It has further been estimated that pill users are 4 to 10 times as likely as nonusers to have a stroke due to clotting in a blood vessel in or leading to the brain.

It has been reported that women using the pill may have a greater risk of heart attack than nonusers. Even without the pill the risk of having a heart attack increases with age and is also increased by additional risk factors such as high blood pressure, high blood cholesterol, obesity, diabetes, cigarette-smoking, or the occurrence during pregnancy of high blood pressure, swelling of the legs, or protein in the urine. Without any risk factors present, the

Continued on next page

Searle & Co.—Cont.

use of oral contraceptives alone may double the risk of heart attack. However, the combination of cigarette-smoking, especially heavy smoking, and oral contraceptive use greatly increases the risk of heart attack. Oral contraceptive users who smoke are about five times more likely to have a heart attack than users who do not smoke, and about ten times more likely to have a heart attack than nonusers who do not smoke. It has been estimated that users between the ages of 30 and 39 who smoke have about a 1 in 10,000 chance each year of having a fatal heart attack compared to about a 1 in 50,000 chance in users who do not smoke, and about a 1 in 100,000 chance in nonusers who do not smoke. In the age group 40 to 44, the risk is about 1 in 1,700 per year for users who smoke compared to about 1 in 10,000 for users who do not smoke, and to about 1 in 14,000 per year for nonusers who do not smoke. Heavy smoking (about 15 cigarettes or more a day) further increases the risk. If you do not smoke and have none of the other heart attack risk factors described above, you will have a smaller risk than listed. If you have several heart attack risk factors, the risk may be considerably greater than listed.
The above are average figures for Great Britain; comparable estimates for the U.S. have been higher.
Oral contraceptives should never be used at any age by women who have had a stroke, a heart attack, or chest pains on exertion (angina pectoris), or who have had blood clots in the legs, lungs, or elsewhere.
Anyone using the pill who has severe leg or chest pains, coughs up blood, has difficulty in breathing, severe headache or vomiting, dizziness or fainting, disturbances of vision or speech, weakness, numbness, or pain in an arm or leg should call her doctor immediately and stop taking the pill, and use another method of contraception.
b. *Formation of tumors.* When certain animals are given the female sex hormone estrogen (which is an ingredient in oral contraceptives) continuously for long periods, cancers may develop in organs such as the breast, cervix, vagina, liver, womb, ovary, and pituitary. These findings suggest that oral contraceptives may cause cancer in humans. However, studies to date in women taking currently marketed oral contraceptives have not confirmed that oral contraceptives cause cancer in humans, but it remains possible they will be discovered in the future to do so. Several studies have found no increase in breast cancer in users, although it has been suggested that oral contraceptives might cause an increase in breast cancer in women who already have benign (noncancerous) breast disease (for example, cysts) or in long-term (2–4 years) users.
Women with a family history of breast cancer or who have breast nodules (lumps), fibrocystic disease (breast cysts), or abnormal mammograms (x-ray pictures of the breasts), or who were exposed to the estrogen diethylstilbestrol (DES) during their mother's pregnancy, or who have abnormal Pap smears should be followed very closely by their doctors if they choose to use oral contraceptives instead of another method of contraception. Many studies have shown that women taking oral contraceptives have less risk of getting benign (noncancerous) breast disease than those who have not used oral contraceptives. There is strong evidence that estrogens (one component of combination-type oral contraceptives), when given for periods of more than one year to women after the menopause (change-of-life), increase the risk of cancer of the womb (uterus). There is also some evidence that the sequential oral contraceptive, a kind of oral contraceptive that is no longer sold, may increase the risk of cancer of the womb. There is no evidence, however, that the oral contraceptives now available increase the risk of this type of cancer, although some individual cases have been reported. Cancer of the cervix may develop more readily in long-term users of the pill, particularly if they have had preexisting abnormal Pap smears. Cervical erosion and cell abnormalities have been reported to be more frequent in pill users.
Very rarely, oral contraceptive users may have a noncancerous tumor of the liver. These tumors do not spread, but they may rupture and cause internal bleeding, which may be fatal. This has been reported in short-term as well as long-term users, although increasing duration of use increases the risk. Long-term users have an estimated annual incidence of 3 to 4 per 100,000. One study reported that oral contraceptive products with a high "hormonal potency" were associated with a higher risk than lower-potency products, as was age over 30 years. A few cases of cancer of the liver have been reported in women using oral contraceptives, but it is not yet known whether the drug caused them.
A type of skin cancer that has been linked to exposure to sunlight (malignant melanoma) has been reported to be more frequent among pill users. It was not possible to determine what the effect was of greater exposure to sunlight in users.
c. *Dangers to a developing baby if oral contraceptives are used in or immediately preceding pregnancy.* Oral contraceptives should not be taken by pregnant women because they may damage the developing baby. There is an increased risk to the baby of abnormalities of such parts of the body as the backbone, anus, heart, windpipe, esophagus, kidneys, arms, and legs. In addition, the developing female child whose mother has received DES, a synthetic estrogen, during pregnancy has a risk of getting cancer of the vagina or cervix in her teens or young adulthood. This risk is estimated to be about 1 in 1,000 exposures or less. DES-exposed daughters appear to have an increased risk of unfavorable outcome of pregnancy. Abnormalities of the urinary and sex organs and sperm have been reported in DES-exposed male babies as well. It is possible that other estrogens, such as the estrogens in oral contraceptives, could have the same effect in the baby if the mother takes them during pregnancy.
Occasionally women who are taking the pill miss periods. It has been reported to occur as frequently as several times each year in some women, depending on various factors such as age and prior history. (Your doctor is the best source of information about this.) The pill should not be used when you are pregnant or suspect you may be pregnant. Very rarely, women who are using the pill as directed become pregnant. The likelihood of becoming pregnant is higher if you occasionally miss one or two pills. Therefore, if you miss a period you should consult your physician before continuing to take the pill. If you miss a period, especially if you have not taken the pill regularly, you should use an alternative method of contraception until pregnancy has been ruled out; if you have missed more than one pill at any time, you should immediately start using an additional method of contraception and complete your pill cycle.
You should not attempt to become pregnant for at least three months after discontinuing oral contraceptives. Use another method of contraception during this period of time. The reason for this is that during this period there may be an increased risk of miscarriage and deformity to the baby, or an increased chance of having twins. Whether there is an overall increase in miscarriage in women who become pregnant soon after stopping the pill as compared with women who did not use the pill is not known, but it is possible that there may be. If, however, you do become pregnant soon after stopping oral contraceptives, and do not have a miscarriage, there is no evidence that the baby has an increased risk of being abnormal.
d. *Gallbladder disease.* Women who use oral contraceptives have a greater risk than nonusers of having gallbladder disease requiring surgery. The increased risk may first appear within one year of use and may double after 4 or 5 years of use.
e. *Other side effects of oral contraceptives.* Some women using oral contraceptives experience unpleasant side effects from the pill which are not dangerous and are not likely to damage their health. Some of these side effects are similar to symptoms women experience in early pregnancy and may be temporary. Your breasts may feel tender, be enlarged, or have a discharge; nausea and vomiting or other stomach or intestinal problems may occur; you may gain or lose weight, and your ankles may swell. A spotty darkening of the skin, particularly of the face, is possible and may persist after the drug is discontinued. An allergic or other type of rash or vaginal yeast infection might occur. You may notice unexpected vaginal bleeding, change in discharge, or changes in your menstrual period. Irregular bleeding is frequently seen when the mini-pill or the combination oral contraceptives containing less than 50 micrograms of estrogen are used. These should all be reported to your doctor.
Other side effects include worsening of migraine, asthma, convulsive disorders (such as epilepsy), and kidney, liver, or heart disease because of a tendency for water to be retained in the body when oral contraceptives are used. Other side effects are painful periods, growth of preexisting fibroid tumors of the womb; mental depression; and liver problems with jaundice (yellowing of the whites of the eyes or of the skin). Your doctor may find that levels of sugar and fatty substances in your blood are elevated; the long-term effects of these changes are not known. Some women develop high blood pressure while taking oral contraceptives, which ordinarily, but not always, returns to the original levels when the oral contraceptive is stopped. The degree of blood pressure rise may be related to the amount of progestogen in the pill. Women with a history of increased blood pressure, kidney disease, or toxemia during pregnancy (increased blood pressure, swelling of the legs, protein in the urine, or convulsions), or a family tendency to high blood pressure or its consequences (stroke, heart disease, kidney disease, blood vessel problems), or a history of excessive weight gain or swelling of the legs during their menstrual cycle, may be more likely to develop increased blood pressure when given oral contraceptives; therefore, they should have their blood pressure taken frequently. High blood pressure predisposes one to stroke, heart attacks, kidney disease, and other diseases of the blood vessels. The effect of prolonged use of oral contraceptives on several of your organs (pituitary, liver, ovaries, womb, and adrenals) or immune system is not known at this time.
Other conditions, although not proved to be caused by oral contraceptives, are occasionally reported. These include more frequent urination and some discomfort when urinating, kidney disease, nervousness, dizziness, hearing problems, inflammation of the nasal passages, loss of scalp hair, an increase in body hair, an increase or decrease in sex drive, appetite changes, gum disease, dry socket, cataracts, a need for a change in contact lens prescription or inability to use contact lenses, tiredness, backache, vaginal infections, itching, anemia, bloodcell breakdown with kidney failure, headache, symptoms similar to those you get before a period; breast, womb, and cervical cancer; inflammation of the pancreas, liver, or colon; chorea (spasmodic movements), burning or prickly sensation, and rheumatoid arthritis.

After you stop using oral contraceptives, there may be a delay before you are able to become pregnant or before you resume having menstrual periods. This is especially true of women who had irregular menstrual cycles prior to the use of oral contraceptives.

One study showed that this delay in becoming pregnant can persist to 30 months after stopping the pill, especially if you have never had children, and does not depend on how long you have used the pill. Very rarely there may be secretions from the breast associated with the absence of periods, which might be due to a noncancerous tumor of the pituitary gland requiring surgery. This may occur more frequently in former users of the pill than in nonusers. As discussed previously, you should wait at least three months after stopping the pill before you try to become pregnant. During the first three months after stopping oral contraceptives, use another form of contraception. You should consult your doctor before resuming use of oral contraceptives after childbirth, especially if you plan to nurse your baby. Drugs in oral contraceptives are known to appear in the milk, and the long-range effect on babies is not known at this time. Furthermore, oral contraceptives may cause a decrease in your milk supply as well as in the quality of the milk.

4. *Comparison of the Risks of Oral Contraceptives and Other Contraceptive Methods.*

The many studies on the risks and effectiveness of oral contraceptives and other methods of contraception have been analyzed to estimate the risk of death associated with various methods of contraception. This risk has two parts: (a) the risk of the method itself (for example, the risk that oral contraceptives might cause death due to abnormal blood clotting), and (b) the risk of death due to pregnancy or abortion in the event the method should fail. The results of this analysis are shown in the following bar graph. The height of the bars indicates the number of deaths per 100,000 women each year. There are six sets of bars, each set referring to a specific age group of women. Within each set of bars, there is a single bar for each of the different contraceptive methods.

For oral contraceptives, there are two bars —one for smokers and the other for nonsmokers. The analysis is based on present knowledge and new information could, of course, alter it. The analysis shows that the risk of death from all methods of birth control is low and below that associated with the risks of childbirth, *except for oral contraceptives in women over 40 who smoke.* The risk of death associated with pill use in nonsmokers over 40 is higher than with any other method of contraception in that age group. It shows that the lowest risk of death is associated with the condom or diaphragm (traditional contraception) backed up by early legal abortion in case of failure of the condom or diaphragm to prevent pregnancy. Also, at any age, the risk of death (due to unexpected pregnancy) from use of traditional contraception, even without a backup of abortion, is generally the same as, or less than, that from use of oral contraceptives.

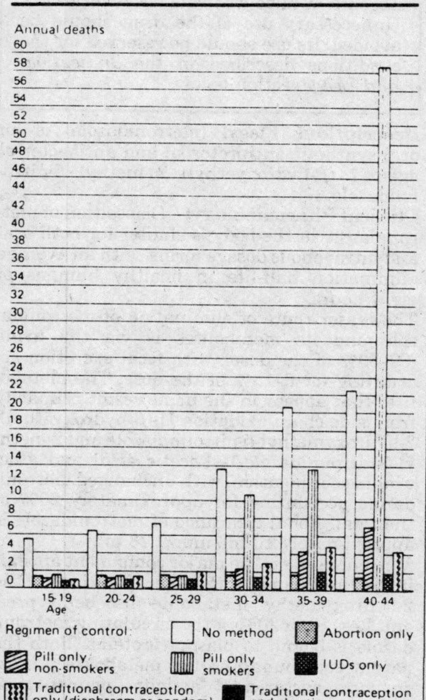
Figure 1 Estimated annual number of deaths associated with control of fertility and no control per 100 000 nonsterile women by regimen of control and age of woman

How to Use Oral Contraceptives as Safely and Effectively as Possible, Once You Have Decided to Use Them:

1. *What to Tell Your Doctor.* You can make use of the pill as safe as possible, by telling your doctor if you have any of the following:

a. Conditions that mean you should not use oral contraceptives:

If you *now* have any of the following:

1. Blood clots in the legs, lungs, or elsewhere in the body.
2. Chest pains on exertion (angina pectoris).
3. Known or suspected cancer of the breast or sex organs, such as the womb (uterus), vagina, or cervix.
4. Unusual vaginal bleeding that has not been diagnosed by your doctor.
5. Known or suspected pregnancy (one or more menstrual periods missed).

If you have *ever* had any of the following:

1. Heart attack or stroke (clots or bleeding in the brain).
2. Blood clots in the legs, lungs, or elsewhere in the body.
3. Liver tumor associated with use of the pill or other estrogen-containing products.

b. Inform your doctor of the following conditions since s/he will want to watch them closely or they might cause him/her to suggest another method of contraception:

A family history of breast cancer
Breast nodules (lumps), fibrocystic disease (breast cysts), abnormal mammograms (x-ray pictures of the breasts), or abnormal Pap smears
Diabetes
High blood pressure
High blood cholesterol
Cigarette-smoking
Migraine
Heart or kidney disease
Asthma
Problems during a prior pregnancy
Epilepsy
Mental depression
Fibroid tumors of the womb
History of jaundice (yellowing of the whites of the eyes or of the skin)
Gallbladder disease
Varicose veins
Tuberculosis
Plans for elective surgery
Previous problems with your periods (irregularities)
Use of any of the following kinds of drugs, which might interact with the pill: antibiotics (such as rifampin, ampicillin, and tetracycline), sulfa drugs, drugs for epilepsy or migraine, painkillers, tranquilizers, sedatives or sleeping pills, blood-thinning drugs, vitamins, drugs being used for the treatment of depression, high blood pressure, or high blood sugar (diabetes)

c. Once you are using oral contraceptives, you should be alert for signs of a serious adverse effect and call your doctor immediately if any of these occur:

Sharp pain in the chest, coughing up of blood, or sudden shortness of breath (indicating possible clots in the lungs).
Pain in the calf (possible clot in the leg).
Crushing chest pain or heaviness (indicating possible heart attack).
Sudden severe headache or vomiting, dizziness or fainting, disturbance of vision or speech, or weakness or numbness in an arm or leg (indicating a possible stroke).
Sudden partial or complete loss of vision (indicating a possible clot in the blood vessels of the eye).
Abnormal vaginal bleeding.
Breast discharge or lumps (you should ask your doctor to show you how to examine your own breasts).
Severe and/or persistent pain or a mass in the abdomen (indicating a possible tumor of the liver, which might have ruptured).
Severe depression.
Yellowing of the whites of the eyes or of the skin (jaundice).
Unusual swelling.
Other unusual conditions.

2. *How to Take the Pill So That It is Most Effective. Dosage Schedules.* See later sections in this leaflet concerning spotting, breakthrough bleeding, forgotten pills, and missed menstruation.

When you first begin to use the pill, you should use an additional method of protection until you have taken your first seven pills.

To remove a pill, press down on it. The pill will drop through a hole in the bottom of the Compack®.

The "20-pill" Schedule. Enovid® 5 mg may be prescribed on the 20-pill schedule. The Enovid 5 mg package is a Calendar-Pack™. Sometimes Enovid 5 mg is dispensed in a bottle.

Take a pill each day for 20 consecutive days, beginning each pill cycle on day 5 after your period starts, just as you did during the first pill cycle, or on the eighth day after having taken the last pill, whichever occurs first. Count the day you start to menstruate as day 1. Continue this 20-pill schedule, cycle after cycle, regardless of whether your flow has or has not ceased when you start or whether you happen to spot or experience unexpected (breakthrough) bleeding during a cycle.

You will probably have your periods about every 27 days.

The Two "three weeks on—one week off" Schedules. Your Demulen, Demulen 1/35™-21, Ovulen 21, or Enovid-E 21 Compack contains 21 tablets arranged in three numbered rows with the days of the week printed above them.

Day-5 Schedule. If you are to begin on day 5, count the day you start to menstruate as day 1 and determine which day to start. Start in row #1 with the pill under the day which corresponds to day 5 after your flow began. Continue to take one pill each day on consecutive days of the week.

After the last (Saturday) pill in row #3 has been taken, if any remain in the first row, complete your 21-pill schedule by taking one pill daily starting with Sunday in row #1. Then stop for one week before starting to take the pills again. Begin your next pill cycle on the same day of the week that you began the first cycle.

Sunday Schedule. Start taking the pills on the first Sunday after your period begins unless your period begins on Sunday. If your period begins on Sunday start taking the pill that very same day.

Continued on next page

Searle & Co.—Cont.

Begin in row #1 and take your pills, one each day on consecutive days, for three weeks (21 days), then stop taking them for one week (7 days) before starting to take the pills again on Sunday.
Whether you begin on "day 5" or on Sunday, continue taking your pills as directed, month after month, regardless of whether your flow has or has not ceased or whether you may have experienced spotting or unexpected (breakthrough) bleeding during your pill cycle. You will probably have your period about every 28 days.
The "Pill-a-day" Schedule. Your Demulen-28, Demulen 1/35™-28, or Ovulen-28 Compack contains 28 pills arranged in four numbered rows of seven pills each with the days of the week printed above them.
You must take your pills in order, one pill each day. Begin with the Sunday pill in row #1.
1—Start taking the pills on the first Sunday after your period begins unless your period begins on Sunday. *If your period begins on Sunday start taking the pills that very same day.*
2—Continue to take one pill each day on consecutive days of the week.
3—After the Saturday pill in row #1 has been taken begin taking pills in row #2, and so on, until the Saturday pill in row #4 has been taken.
4—Replace the Refill in your Compack at once, and begin a new pill cycle the next day, starting with the Sunday pill in row #1.
You will probably have your period about every 28 days, while you are taking the pink (blue for Demulen 1/35™-28) pills.
Continue your pill-a-day schedule, month after month, regardless of whether your flow ceases while you are taking the colored pills, or whether you experience spotting or unexpected (breakthrough) bleeding during a cycle.
Take your pill faithfully every "pill day"!
It is important that you take a pill without fail every pill day at intervals of 24 hours for two reasons. First, your ovaries may release an egg and therefore you may become pregnant if you do not take your pills regularly. Second, you may spot or start to flow between your periods. This may be inconvenient.
Take your pill at the same time every day!
You are probably wondering why the same time of day is important. By taking your pill at the same time every day it becomes a good habit, and you are much less likely to forget. You may wish to keep your pills in the medicine cabinet near your toothbrush as a reminder to take them when you brush your teeth at night. The best time to take your daily pill may be either with your evening meal or at bedtime. You may find it helpful to associate your pill-taking with something else you do every day at a particular time.
Another very important reason for you to take your pills as "regular as clockwork" is that you are protected best when you take one every 24 hours; they are made to work that way. Just remember that once every day is not the same as once every 24 hours. Here is why: Suppose you were to take your Monday pill in the morning when you get up, and then not take your Tuesday pill till the evening before you go to bed. True, you will have taken a pill each day, on Monday and on Tuesday—but the time between pill-taking will probably have been more than 36 hours, or more than 1½ days! You might spot. Chances are you would still be protected and would not get pregnant, but why risk it when it is so easy to guarantee yourself maximal protection by taking your pill faithfully every pill day and at the same time every pill day?
In summary, you should take the pills exactly as directed and at intervals of 24 hours in order to achieve maximum contraceptive effectiveness.
Spotting. This is a slight staining between your menstrual periods which may not even require a pad. Some women spot even though they take their pills exactly as directed. Many women spot although they have never taken the pills. Spotting does not mean that your ovaries are releasing an egg. Spotting may be the result of irregular pill-taking. Getting back on schedule will usually stop it.
If you should spot while taking the pills you should not be alarmed because spotting usually stops by itself within a few days. It seldom occurs after the first pill cycle. Consult your doctor if spotting persists for more than a few days or if it occurs after the second cycle.
Unexpected (Breakthrough) Bleeding. Unexpected (breakthrough) bleeding does not mean your ovaries have released an egg. It seldom occurs, but when it does happen it is most common in the first pill cycle. It is a flow much like a regular period, requiring the use of a pad or tampon.
If you experience breakthrough bleeding use a pad or tampon and continue with your schedule. Usually your periods will become regular within a few cycles. Breakthrough bleeding will seldom bother you again.
Consult your doctor if breakthrough bleeding does not stop within a week or if it occurs after the second cycle.
Forgotten Pills. There is little likelihood of your getting pregnant if only one active pill is missed; however, the possibility increases with each successive day that the scheduled active pills are missed. If you forget to take a pill one day, take two the next day—the one you forgot as soon as you remember and your regular pill at your usual time.
If you forget your pills (except the inactive colored pills in Demulen-28, Demulen 1/35-28, or Ovulen-28) on two consecutive days, do not be surprised if you spot or start to flow. You should take two pills each day for the next two days, and use an additional method of protection for the remainder of the cycle.
If you are using Demulen-28, Demulen 1/35™-28, or Ovulen-28 and forget to take one or more colored pills, begin a new cycle on the next Sunday; use a new package and start taking the white pills. Missing the colored pills does not increase your chances of getting pregnant providing the white pill schedule has been followed.
Missed Menstruation. At times there may be no menstrual period after a cycle of pills. Therefore, if you miss one menstrual period but have taken the pills *exactly as you were supposed to,* continue as usual into the next cycle. You may wish to call your doctor. If you have not taken the pills correctly and miss a menstrual period, *you may be pregnant* and should stop taking oral contraceptives until your doctor determines whether or not you are pregnant. Until you can get to your doctor, use another form of contraception. If two consecutive menstrual periods are missed, you should stop taking the pills until it is determined whether you are pregnant. If you do become pregnant while using oral contraceptives, you should discuss the risks to the developing baby with your doctor.
3. *Periodic Examinations.* Your doctor will take a complete medical and family history before prescribing oral contraceptives. At that time and about once a year thereafter, s/he will generally examine your blood pressure, breasts, abdomen, and internal female organs (including a Pap smear test for cancer of the cervix) and perform certain laboratory tests. Certain health problems or conditions in your medical or family history may require that your doctor see you more frequently while you are taking the pill.
4. *Using Enovid for Purposes Other Than Contraception.* Since dosage schedules for these uses must be individualized for each patient, please follow the directions of your doctor.
Summary: Oral contraceptives are the most effective method, except sterilization, for preventing pregnancy. Other methods, when used conscientiously, are also very effective and have fewer risks. The serious side effects of oral contraceptives are uncommon, and the pill is a very convenient method for preventing pregnancy.
Women who use oral contraceptives should not smoke.
If you have certain conditions or have had these conditions in the past, you should not use oral contraceptives because of increased risk. These conditions are listed in this leaflet. If you do not have these conditions, and decide to use the pill, please read this leaflet carefully so that you can use the pill safely and effectively. Be certain to read new revisions of this leaflet.
Based on your doctor's assessment of your medical needs, this drug has been prescribed for you. Do not give it to anyone else.
See your doctor regularly, ask any questions you may have about the use of the pill, and report any special problems that may arise.
[*These products are shown in the Product Identification Section.*]

ENOVID–E® 21 ℞
(norethynodrel with mestranol)

See Demulen under Searle & Co. for Enovid-E 21 prescribing information.
[*Shown in Product Identification Section.*]

ENOVID® 5 mg ℞
ENOVID® 10 mg ℞
(norethynodrel with mestranol)

See Demulen under Searle & Co. for Enovid 5 mg and Enovid 10 mg prescribing information.
[*Shown in Product Identification Section.*]

FLAGYL® Tablets ℞
(metronidazole)

> **Warning**
> Metronidazole has been shown to be carcinogenic in mice and rats (see *Warnings*). Unnecessary use of the drug should be avoided. Its use should be reserved for the conditions described in the *Indications and Usage* section below.

Description: Flagyl (metronidazole) is an oral synthetic antiprotozoal and antibacterial agent, 1-(β-hydroxyethyl)-2-methyl-5-nitroimidazole.
Clinical Pharmacology: Disposition of metronidazole in the body is similar for both oral and intravenous dosage forms, with an average elimination half-life in healthy humans of eight hours.
The major route of elimination of metronidazole and its metabolites is via the urine (60–80% of the dose), with fecal excretion accounting for 6–15% of the dose. The metabolites that appear in the urine result primarily from side-chain oxidation [1-(β-hydroxyethyl)-2-hydroxymethyl-5-nitroimidazole and 2-methyl-5-nitroimidazole-1-yl-acetic acid] and glucuronide conjugation, with unchanged metronidazole accounting for approximately 20% of the total. Renal clearance of metronidazole is approximately 10 ml/min/1.73 m^2.
Metronidazole is the major component appearing in the plasma, with lesser quantities of the 2-hydroxymethyl metabolite also being present. Less than 20% of the circulating metronidazole is bound to plasma proteins. Both the parent compound and the metabolite possess *in vitro* bactericidal activity against most strains of anaerobic bacteria and *in vitro* trichomonacidal activity.

Metronidazole appears in cerebrospinal fluid, saliva, and breast milk in concentrations similar to those found in plasma. Bactericidal concentrations of metronidazole have also been detected in pus from hepatic abscesses.

Following oral administration metronidazole is well absorbed, with peak plasma concentrations occurring between one and two hours after administration. Plasma concentrations of metronidazole are proportional to the administered dose. Oral administration of 250 mg, 500 mg, or 2,000 mg produced peak plasma concentrations of 6 mcg/ml, 12 mcg/ml, and 40 mcg/ml, respectively. Studies reveal no significant bioavailability differences between males and females; however, because of weight differences, the resulting plasma levels in males are generally lower.

Decreased renal function does not alter the single-dose pharmacokinetics of metronidazole. However, plasma clearance of metronidazole is decreased in patients with decreased liver function.

Microbiology: *Trichomonas vaginalis, Entamoeba histolytica.* Flagyl (metronidazole) possesses direct trichomonacidal and amebacidal activity against *T. vaginalis* and *E. histolytica.* The *in vitro* minimal inhibitory concentration (MIC) for most strains of these organisms is 1 mcg/ml or less.

Anaerobic Bacteria. Metronidazole is active *in vitro* against most obligate anaerobes, but does not appear to possess any clinically relevant activity against facultative anaerobes or obligate aerobes. Against susceptible organisms, metronidazole is generally bactericidal at concentrations equal to or slightly higher than the minimal inhibitory concentrations. Metronidazole has been shown to have *in vitro* and clinical activity against the following organisms:

Anaerobic gram-negative bacilli, including:
- *Bacteroides* species including the *Bacteroides fragilis* group (*B. fragilis, B. distasonis, B. ovatus, B. thetaiotaomicron, B. vulgatus)*
- *Fusobacterium* species

Anaerobic gram-positive bacilli, including:
- *Clostridium* species and susceptible strains of of *Eubacterium*

Anaerobic gram-positive cocci, including:
- *Peptococcus* species
- *Peptostreptococcus* species

Susceptibility Tests: Bacteriologic studies should be performed to determine the causative organisms and their susceptibility to metronidazole; however, the rapid, routine susceptibility testing of individual isolates of anaerobic bacteria is not always practical, and therapy may be started while awaiting these results.

Quantitative methods give the most precise estimates of susceptibility to antibacterial drugs. A standardized agar dilution method and a broth microdilution method are recommended.[1]

Control strains are recommended for standardized susceptibility testing. Each time the test is performed, one or more of the following strains should be included: *Clostridium perfringens* ATCC 13124, *Bacteroides fragilis* ATCC 25285, and *Bacteroides thetaiotaomicron* ATCC 29741. The mode metronidazole MICs for those three strains are reported to be 0.25, 0.25, and 0.5 mcg/ml, respectively.

A clinical laboratory is considered under acceptable control if the results of the control strains are within one doubling dilution of the mode MICs reported for metronidazole.

A bacterial isolate may be considered susceptible if the MIC value for metronidazole is not more than 16 mcg/ml. An organism is considered resistant if the MIC is greater than 16 mcg/ml. A report of "resistant" from the laboratory indicates that the infecting organism is not likely to respond to therapy.

Indications and Usage:

Symptomatic Trichomoniasis. Flagyl is indicated for the treatment of symptomatic trichomoniasis in females and males when the presence of the trichomonad has been confirmed by appropriate laboratory procedures (wet smears and/or cultures).

Asymptomatic Trichomoniasis. Flagyl is indicated in the treatment of asymptomatic females when the organism is associated with endocervicitis, cervicitis, or cervical erosion. Since there is evidence that presence of the trichomonad can interfere with accurate assessment of abnormal cytological smears, additional smears should be performed after eradication of the parasite.

Treatment of Asymptomatic Consorts. T. vaginalis infection is a venereal disease. Therefore, asymptomatic sexual partners of treated patients should be treated simultaneously if the organism has been found to be present, in order to prevent reinfection of the partner. The decision as to whether to treat an asymptomatic male partner who has a negative culture or one for whom no culture has been attempted is an individual one. In making this decision, it should be noted that there is evidence that a woman may become reinfected if her consort is not treated. Also, since there can be considerable difficulty in isolating the organism from the asymptomatic male carrier, negative smears and cultures cannot be relied upon in this regard. In any event, the consort should be treated with Flagyl in cases of reinfection.

Amebiasis. Flagyl is indicated in the treatment of acute intestinal amebiasis (amebic dysentery) and amebic liver abscess.

In amebic liver abscess, Flagyl therapy does not obviate the need for aspiration or drainage of pus.

Anaerobic Bacterial Infections. Flagyl is indicated in the treatment of serious infections caused by susceptible anaerobic bacteria. Indicated surgical procedures should be performed in conjunction with Flagyl therapy. In a mixed aerobic and anaerobic infection, antibiotics appropriate for the treatment of the aerobic infection should be used in addition to Flagyl. In the treatment of most serious anaerobic infections, Flagyl I.V.™ (metronidazole hydrochloride) or Flagyl I.V.™RTU™ (metronidazole) is usually administered initially. This may be followed by oral therapy with Flagyl (metronidazole) at the discretion of the physician.

INTRA-ABDOMINAL INFECTIONS, including peritonitis, intra-abdominal abscess, and liver abscess, caused by *Bacteroides* species including the *B. fragilis* group (*B. fragilis, B. distasonis, B. ovatus, B. thetaiotaomicron, B. vulgatus), Clostridium* species, *Eubacterium* species, *Peptococcus* species, and *Peptostreptococcus* species.

SKIN AND SKIN STRUCTURE INFECTIONS caused by *Bacteroides* species including the *B. fragilis* group, *Clostridium* species, *Peptococcus* species, *Peptostreptococcus* species, and *Fusobacterium* species.

GYNECOLOGIC INFECTIONS, including endometritis, endomyometritis, tubo-ovarian abscess, and post-surgical vaginal cuff infection, caused by *Bacteroides* species including the *B. fragilis* group, *Clostridium* species, *Peptococcus* species, and *Peptostreptococcus* species.

BACTERIAL SEPTICEMIA caused by *Bacteroides* species including the *B. fragilis* group, and *Clostridium* species.

BONE AND JOINT INFECTIONS, as adjunctive therapy, caused by *Bacteroides* species including the *B. fragilis* group.

CENTRAL NERVOUS SYSTEM (CNS) INFECTIONS, including meningitis and brain abscess, caused by *Bacteroides* species including the *B. fragilis* group.

LOWER RESPIRATORY TRACT INFECTIONS, including pneumonia, empyema, and lung abscess, caused by *Bacteroides* species including the *B. fragilis* group.

ENDOCARDITIS caused by *Bacteroides* species including the *B. fragilis* group.

Contraindications: Flagyl is contraindicated in patients with a prior history of hypersensitivity to metronidazole or other nitroimidazole derivatives.

In patients with trichomoniasis, Flagyl is contraindicated during the first trimester of pregnancy. (See *Warnings.*)

Warnings: *Convulsive Seizures and Peripheral Neuropathy:* Convulsive seizures and peripheral neuropathy, the latter characterized mainly by numbness or paresthesia of an extremity, have been reported in patients treated with metronidazole. The appearance of abnormal neurologic signs demands the prompt discontinuation of Flagyl therapy. Flagyl should be administered with caution to patients with central nervous system diseases.

Tumorigenicity in Rodents: Metronidazole has shown evidence of carcinogenic activity in a number of studies involving chronic, oral administration in mice and rats.

Prominent among the effects in the mouse was the promotion of pulmonary tumorigenesis. This has been observed in all six reported studies in that species, including one study in which the animals were dosed on an intermittent schedule (administration during every fourth week only). At very high dose levels (approx. 500 mg/kg/day) there was a statistically significant increase in the incidence of malignant liver tumors in males. Also, the published results of one of the mouse studies indicate an increase in the incidence of malignant lymphomas as well as pulmonary neoplasms associated with lifetime feeding of the drug. All these effects are statistically significant.

Several long-term, oral-dosing studies in the rat have been completed. There were statistically significant increases in the incidence of various neoplasms, particularly in mammary and hepatic tumors, among female rats administered metronidazole over those noted in the concurrent female control groups.

Two lifetime tumorigenicity studies in hamsters have been performed and reported to be negative.

Mutagenicity Studies: Although metronidazole has shown mutagenic activity in a number of *in vitro* assay systems, studies in mammals (*in vivo*) have failed to demonstrate a potential for genetic damage.

Precautions:

General: Patients with severe hepatic disease metabolize metronidazole slowly, with resultant accumulation of metronidazole and its metabolites in the plasma. Accordingly, for such patients, doses below those usually recommended should be administered cautiously.

Known or previously unrecognized candidiasis may present more prominent symptoms during therapy with Flagyl and requires treatment with a candicidal agent. Vaginitis due to organisms other than *T. vaginalis* does not respond to Flagyl.

Laboratory Tests: Flagyl (metronidazole) is a nitroimidazole and should be used with care in patients with evidence of or history of blood dyscrasia. A mild leukopenia has been observed during its administration; however, no persistent hematologic abnormalities attributable to metronidazole have been observed in clinical studies. Total and differential leukocyte counts are recommended before and after therapy for trichomoniasis and amebiasis, especially if a second course of therapy is necessary, and before and after therapy for anaerobic infection.

Drug Interactions: Metronidazole has been reported to potentiate the anticoagulant effect of warfarin and other oral coumarin anticoagulants, resulting in a prolongation of prothrombin time. This possible drug interaction should be considered when Flagyl is prescribed for patients on this type of anticoagulant therapy.

Alcoholic beverages should not be consumed during Flagyl therapy because abdominal

Continued on next page

Searle & Co.—Cont.

cramps, nausea, vomiting, headaches, and flushing may occur.

Drug/Laboratory Test Interactions: Metronidazole may interfere with certain chemical analyses for serum glutamic oxalacetic transaminase, resulting in decreased values. Values of zero may be observed.

Carcinogenesis: See *Warnings.*

Pregnancy: Metronidazole crosses the placental barrier and enters the fetal circulation rapidly. Reproduction studies have been performed in rabbits and rats at doses up to five times the human dose and have revealed no evidence of impaired fertility or harm to the fetus due to metronidazole. There are, however, no adequate and well-controlled studies in pregnant women. Because animal reproduction studies are not always predictive of human response, and because metronidazole is a carcinogen in rodents, this drug should be used during pregnancy only if clearly needed (see *Contraindications*)

Use of Flagyl for trichomoniasis in the second and third trimesters should be restricted to those in whom local palliative treatment has been inadequate to control symptoms.

Nursing Mothers: Because of the potential for tumorigenicity shown for metronidazole in mouse and rat studies, a decision should be made whether to discontinue nursing or to discontinue the drug, taking into account the importance of the drug to the mother. Metronidazole is secreted in breast milk in concentrations similar to those found in plasma.

Pediatric Use: Safety and effectiveness in children have not been established, except for the treatment of amebiasis.

Adverse Reactions: The two most serious adverse reactions reported in patients treated with Flagyl (metronidazole) have been convulsive seizures and peripheral neuropathy, the latter characterized mainly by numbness or paresthesia of an extremity. Since persistent peripheral neuropathy has been reported in some patients receiving prolonged administration of Flagyl, patients should be specifically warned about these reactions and should be told to stop the drug and report immediately to their physicians if any neurologic symptoms occur.

The most common adverse reactions reported have been referable to the gastrointestinal tract, particularly nausea, sometimes accompanied by headache, anorexia, and occasionally vomiting; diarrhea; epigastric distress; and abdominal cramping. Constipation has also been reported.

The following reactions have also been reported during treatment with Flagyl (metronidazole):

Mouth: A sharp, unpleasant metallic taste is not unusual. Furry tongue, glossitis, and stomatitis have occurred; these may be associated with a sudden overgrowth of *Candida* which may occur during effective therapy.

Hematopoietic: Reversible neutropenia (leukopenia).

Cardiovascular: Flattening of the T-wave may be seen in electrocardiographic tracings.

Central Nervous System: Convulsive seizures, peripheral neuropathy, dizziness, vertigo, incoordination, ataxia, confusion, irritability, depression, weakness, and insomnia.

Hypersensitivity: Urticaria, erythematous rash, flushing, nasal congestion, dryness of mouth (or vagina or vulva), and fever.

Renal: Dysuria, cystitis, polyuria, incontinence, and a sense of pelvic pressure. Instances of darkened urine have been reported, and this manifestation has been the subject of a special investigation. Although the pigment which is probably responsible for this phenomenon has not been positively identified, it is almost certainly a metabolite of metronidazole and seems to have no clinical significance.

Other: Proliferation of *Candida* in the vagina, dyspareunia, decrease of libido, proctitis, and fleeting joint pains sometimes resembling "serum sickness." If patients receiving Flagyl drink alcoholic beverages, they may experience abdominal distress, nausea, vomiting, flushing, or headache. A modification of the taste of alcoholic beverages has also been reported.

Overdosage: Single oral doses of metronidazole, up to 15 g, have been reported in suicide attempts and accidental overdoses. Symptoms reported include nausea, vomiting, and ataxia. Oral metronidazole has been studied as a radiation sensitizer in the treatment of malignant tumors. Neurotoxic effects, including seizures and peripheral neuropathy, have been reported after 5 to 7 days of doses of 6 to 10.4 g every other day.

Treatment: There is no specific antidote for Flagyl overdose; therefore, management of the patient should consist of symptomatic and supportive therapy.

Dosage and Administration:

Trichomoniasis:

In the Female:

One-day treatment—two grams of Flagyl, given either as a single dose or in two divided doses of one gram each given in the same day.

Seven-day course of treatment—250 mg three times daily for seven consecutive days. There is some indication from controlled comparative studies that cure rates as determined by vaginal smears, signs and symptoms, may be higher after a seven-day course of treatment than after a one-day treatment regimen.

The dosage regimen should be individualized. Single-dose treatment can assure compliance, especially if administered under supervision, in those patients who cannot be relied on to continue the seven-day regimen. A seven-day course of treatment may minimize reinfection of the female long enough to treat sexual contacts. Further, some patients may tolerate one course of therapy better than the other.

Pregnant patients should not be treated during the first trimester with either regimen. If treated during the second or third trimester, the one-day course of therapy should not be used, as it results in higher serum levels which reach the fetal circulation. (See *Contraindications* and *Precautions.*)

When repeat courses of the drug are required, it is recommended that an interval of four to six weeks elapse between courses and that the presence of the trichomonad be reconfirmed by appropriate laboratory measures. Total and differential leukocyte counts should be made before and after retreatment.

In the Male: Treament should be individualized as for the female.

Amebiasis:

Adults:

For acute intestinal amebiasis (acute amebic dysentery): 750 mg orally three times daily for 5 to 10 days.

For amebic liver abscess: 500 mg or 750 mg orally three times daily for 5 to 10 days.

Children: 35 to 50 mg/kg/24 hours, divided into three doses, orally for 10 days.

Anaerobic Bacterial Infections: In the treatment of most serious anaerobic infections, Flagyl I.V.™ (metronidazole hydrochloride) or Flagyl I.V.™RTU™ (metronidazole) is usually administered initially.

The usual adult *oral* dosage is 7.5 mg/kg every six hours (approx. 500 mg for a 70-kg adult). A maximum of 4.0 g should not be exceeded during a 24-hour period.

The usual duration of therapy is 7 to 10 days; however, infections of the bone and joint, lower respiratory tract, and endocardium may require longer treatment.

Patients with severe hepatic disease metabolize metronidazole slowly, with resultant accumulation of metronidazole and its metabolites in the plasma. Accordingly, for such patients, doses below those usually recommended should be administered cautiously. Close monitoring of plasma metronidazole levels[2] and toxicity is recommended.

The dose of Flagyl should not be specifically reduced in anuric patients since accumulated metabolites may be rapidly removed by dialysis.

How Supplied:

Flagyl 250-mg tablets are round, blue, film coated, with SEARLE and 1831 debossed on one side and FLAGYL and 250 on the other side; bottles of 100, 250, 500, 1,000, and 2,500, and cartons of 100 unit-dose individually blister-sealed tablets.

Flagyl 500-mg tablets are oblong, blue, film coated, with FLAGYL debossed on one side and 500 on the other side; bottles of 100 and 500, and cartons of 100 unit-dose individually blister-sealed tablets.

Storage and Stability: Store below 86°F (30°C) and protect from light.

1. Proposed standard: PSM-11—Proposed Reference Dilution Procedure for Antimicrobic Susceptibility Testing of Anaerobic Bacteria, National Committee for Clinical Laboratory Standards, and Sutter, et al.: Collaborative Evaluation of a Proposed Reference Dilution Method of Susceptibility Testing of Anaerobic Bacteria, Antimicrob. Agents Chemother. *16:*495–502 (Oct.) 1979; and Tally, et al.: *In Vitro* Activity of Thienamycin, Antimicrob. Agents Chemother. *14:*436–438 (Sept.) 1978.

2. Ralph, E.D., and Kirby, W.M.M.: Bioassay of Metronidazole With Either Anaerobic or Aerobic Incubation, J. Infect. Dis. *132:*587–591 (Nov.) 1975; or Gulaid, et al.: Determination of Metronidazole and Its Major Metabolites in Biological Fluids by High Pressure Liquid Chromatography, Br. J. Clin. Pharmacol. *6:*430–432, 1978.

[*Shown in Product Identification Section*]

•LOMOTIL® Liquid Ⓒ
•LOMOTIL® Tablets Ⓒ
(diphenoxylate hydrochloride with atropine sulfate)

Description: Each Lomotil tablet and each 5 ml of Lomotil liquid contains:

Diphenoxylate hydrochloride............ 2.5 mg
(Warning—May be habit forming.)
Atropine sulfate .... 0.025 mg

Diphenoxylate hydrochloride is ethyl 1-(3-cyano-3,3-diphenylpropyl)-4-phenylisonipecotate monohydrochloride.

Atropine sulfate is endo-(±)-α-(hydroxymethyl)benzeneacetic acid 8-methyl-8-azabicyclo [3.2.1]oct-3-yl ester sulfate (2:1) (salt) monohydrate.

Important Information: Lomotil is classified as a Schedule V controlled substance by federal law. Diphenoxylate hydrochloride is chemically related to the narcotic meperidine. Therefore, in case of overdosage, treatment is similar to that for meperidine or morphine intoxication, in which prolonged and careful monitoring is essential. Respiratory depression may be evidenced as late as 30 hours after ingestion and may recur in spite of an initial response to narcotic antagonists. A subtherapeutic amount of atropine sulfate is present to discourage deliberate overdosage. LOMOTIL IS *NOT* AN INNOCUOUS DRUG AND DOSAGE RECOMMENDATIONS SHOULD BE STRICTLY ADHERED TO, ESPECIALLY IN CHILDREN. KEEP THIS AND

ALL MEDICATIONS OUT OF REACH OF CHILDREN.

Clinical Pharmacology: Diphenoxylate is rapidly and extensively metabolized in man by ester hydrolysis to diphenoxylic acid (difenoxine), which is biologically active and the major circulating metabolite in the blood. After a 5-mg oral dose of carbon-14 labeled diphenoxylate hydrochloride in ethanolic solution was given to three healthy volunteers, an average of 14% of the drug plus its metabolites over a four-day period was excreted in the urine and 49% in the feces. Urinary excretion of the unmetabolized drug constituted less than 1% of the dose, and diphenoxylic acid plus its glucuronide conjugate constituted about 6% of the dose. In a sixteen-subject cross-over bioavailability study, a linear relationship in the dose range of 2.5 to 10 mg was found between the dose of diphenoxylate hydrochloride (given as Lomotil liquid) and the peak plasma concentration, the area under the plasma concentration-time curves, and the amount of diphenoxylic acid excreted in the urine. In the same study the bioavailability of the tablet compared with an equal dose of the liquid was approximately 90%. The average peak plasma concentration of diphenoxylic acid following ingestion of four 2.5-mg tablets was 163 ng/ml at about 2 hours, and the elimination half-life of diphenoxylic acid was approximately 12 to 14 hours.

In studies with male rats, diphenoxylate hydrochloride was found to inhibit the hepatic microsomal enzyme system at a dosage of 2 mg/kg/day. Therefore, diphenoxylate has the potential to prolong the biological half-lives of drugs for which the rate of elimination is dependent on the microsomal drug metabolizing enzyme system.

Indications: Lomotil is effective as adjunctive therapy in the management of diarrhea.

Contraindications: Lomotil is contraindicated in children under 2 years of age due to a decreased margin of safety in younger age groups, in patients with a known hypersensitivity to diphenoxylate hydrochloride or atropine, and in patients who have obstructive jaundice. Lomotil is also contraindicated in the treatment of diarrhea associated with pseudomembranous enterocolitis.

Warnings: Lomotil should be used with special caution in young children because of the greater variability of response in this age group. The use of Lomotil does not preclude the administration of appropriate fluid and electrolyte therapy. Dehydration, particularly in younger children, may further influence the variability of response to Lomotil and may predispose to delayed diphenoxylate intoxication. Drug-induced inhibition of peristalsis may result in fluid retention in the intestine, which may further aggravate dehydration and electrolyte imbalance. If severe dehydration or electrolyte imbalance is manifested, Lomotil should be withheld until appropriate corrective therapy has been initiated.

Antiperistaltic agents may prolong and/or worsen diarrhea associated with organisms that penetrate the intestinal mucosa (toxigenic *E. coli, Salmonella, Shigella*), and pseudomembranous enterocolitis associated with broad-spectrum antibiotics. Antiperistaltic agents should not be used in these conditions.

In some patients with acute ulcerative colitis, agents which inhibit intestinal motility or prolong intestinal transit time have been reported to induce toxic megacolon. Consequently, patients with acute ulcerative colitis should be carefully observed and Lomotil therapy should be discontinued promptly if abdominal distention occurs or if other untoward symptoms develop.

Since the chemical structure of diphenoxylate hydrochloride is similar to that of meperidine hydrochloride, the concurrent use of Lomotil with monoamine oxidase inhibitors may, in theory, precipitate hypertensive crisis.

Lomotil should be used with extreme caution in patients with advanced hepatorenal disease and in all patients with abnormal liver function since hepatic coma may be precipitated. Diphenoxylate hydrochloride may potentiate the action of barbiturates, tranquilizers and alcohol. Therefore, the patient should be closely observed when these medications are used concomitantly.

Precautions: Because a subtherapeutic dose of atropine has been added to the diphenoxylate hydrochloride to discourage deliberate overdosage, consideration should be given to the precautions relating to the use of atropine. In children, Lomotil should be used with caution since signs of atropinism may occur even with recommended doses, particularly in patients with Down's syndrome.

Drug Abuse and Dependence: In doses used for the treatment of diarrhea, whether acute or chronic, diphenoxylate has not produced addiction.

Diphenoxylate hydrochloride is devoid of morphine-like subjective effects at therapeutic doses. At high doses it exhibits codeine-like subjective effects. The dose which produces antidiarrheal action is widely separated from the dose which causes central nervous system effects. The insolubility of diphenoxylate hydrochloride in commonly available aqueous media precludes intravenous self-administration. A dose of 100-300 mg/day, which is equivalent to 40-120 tablets, administered to humans for 40 to 70 days, showed opiate withdrawal symptoms. Since addiction to diphenoxylate hydrochloride is possible at high doses, the recommended dosage should not be exceeded.

Usage in Pregnancy: The use of any drug during pregnancy, lactation, or in women of childbearing age requires that the potential benefits of the drug be weighed against any possible hazard to the mother and child.

Teratology: Experiments on the effect of Lomotil in three animal species (rabbit, rat and mouse) demonstrated no evidence of teratogenicity in 300 fetuses exposed to Lomotil during the critical phase of embryonic development. Controls treated with thalidomide demonstrated 20% fetal abnormality.

At 20 mg/kg/day, growth was retarded in female rats. Upon mating, a marked contraceptive action was recorded, and out of 27 matings, only 4 rats conceived and bore 25 normal young. Peri- and postnatal studies were normal. In rabbits the compound was devoid of embryotoxicity, of teratogenicity, and of effects on male and female fertility.

Nursing Mothers: Effects of diphenoxylate hydrochloride or atropine sulfate may be evident in the infants of nursing mothers taking Lomotil since these compounds are excreted in breast milk.

Pediatric Use: Lomotil is contraindicated in children under 2 years of age and should be used with special caution in young children due to the greater variability of response. (See *Contraindications* and *Warnings* sections.) In case of accidental ingestion by children, see *Overdosage* section for recommended treatment.

Adverse Reactions: Atropine effects, such as dryness of the skin and mucous membranes, flushing, hyperthermia, tachycardia, and urinary retention may occur, especially in children. Other adverse reactions reported with Lomotil use are:

Gastrointestinal: anorexia, nausea, vomiting, abdominal discomfort, paralytic ileus, toxic megacolon.

Allergic: pruritus, swelling of gums, giant urticaria, angioneurotic edema.

Nervous system: dizziness, drowsiness/sedation, headache, malaise/lethargy, restlessness, euphoria, depression, respiratory depression, coma, numbness of extremities.

Overdosage:

Diagnosis and Treatment: Caution patients to adhere strictly to recommended dosage schedules. The medication should be kept out of reach of children, since accidental overdosage may result in severe, even fatal, respiratory depression. In the event of overdosage (initial signs may include dryness of the skin and mucous membranes, flushing, hyperthermia, and tachycardia followed by lethargy or coma, hypotonic reflexes, nystagmus, pinpoint pupils and respiratory depression), induction of vomiting, gastric lavage, establishment of a patent airway and possibly mechanically assisted respiration are advised.

A narcotic antagonist without agonist activity (e.g., naloxone) should be used in the treatment of respiratory depression caused by Lomotil. When a narcotic antagonist is administered intravenously the onset of action is generally apparent within two minutes. It may also be administered subcutaneously or intramuscularly, providing a slightly less rapid onset of action but a more prolonged effect.

To counteract respiratory depression caused by Lomotil overdosage, the following dosage schedule for the narcotic antagonist Narcan® (naloxone hydrochloride) should be followed:

Adult Dosage: The usual initial adult dose of Narcan is 0.4 mg (1 ml) administered intravenously. If respiratory function does not adequately improve after the initial dose the same I.V. dose may be repeated at two- to three-minute intervals.

Children: The usual initial dose of Narcan for children is 0.01 mg/kg of body weight administered intravenously and repeated at two- to three-minute intervals if necessary.

Following initial improvement of respiratory function, repeat doses of Narcan may be required to counteract recurrent respiratory depression. Supplemental intramuscular doses of Narcan may be utilized to produce a longer-lasting effect.

Since the duration of action of diphenoxylate hydrochloride is longer than that of naloxone hydrochloride, improvement of respiration following administration may be followed by recurrent respiratory depression. Consequently, continuous observation is necessary until the effect of diphenoxylate hydrochloride on respiration (which effect may persist for many hours) has passed. The period of observation should extend over at least 48 hours, preferably under continuous hospital care.

It should be noted that, although signs of overdosage and respiratory depression may not be evident soon after ingestion of diphenoxylate hydrochloride, respiratory depression may occur from 12 to 30 hours later.

Dosage and Administration:

Adults: The recommended initial dosage is two Lomotil tablets four times daily or 10 ml (two regular teaspoonfuls) of Lomotil liquid four times daily (20 mg per day). Most patients will require this dosage until initial control has been achieved, after which the dosage may be reduced to meet individual requirements. Control may often be maintained with as little as 5 mg (two tablets or 10 ml of liquid) daily.

Children: Lomotil is contraindicated in children under 2 years of age. Lomotil should be used with special caution in young children due to the variable response in this age group. *In children 2 to 12 years of age use Lomotil liquid. Do not use Lomotil tablets for this age group.*

For children 2 to 12 years of age, the recommended initial dosage of Lomotil liquid is 0.3 to 0.4 mg/kg daily administered in divided doses. The following schedule will usually fulfill dosage requirements:

Continued on next page

Searle & Co.—Cont.

Age:	*Dosage:*
2 to 5 years (13 to 20 kg)	4 ml (2 mg) t.i.d.
5 to 8 years (20 to 27 kg)	4 ml (2 mg) q.i.d.
8 to 12 years (27 to 36 kg)	4 ml (2 mg) 5 times daily

Reduction of dosage may be made as soon as initial control of symptoms has been achieved. Maintenance dosage may be as low as one-fourth of the initial daily dosage. If no response occurs within 48 hours, Lomotil is unlikely to be effective.

Do not exceed recommended dosage.

How Supplied:

Tablets—white, with SEARLE debossed on one side and 61 on the other side and containing 2.5 mg of diphenoxylate hydrochloride and 0.025 mg (1/2,400 grain) of atropine sulfate; bottles of 100, 500, 1,000, and 2,500, and cartons of 100 unit-dose individually blister-sealed tablets.

Liquid—containing 2.5 mg of diphenoxylate hydrochloride and 0.025 mg (1/2,400 grain) of atropine sulfate per 5 ml; bottles of 2 oz.

A plastic dropper calibrated in increments of ½ ml (¼ mg) with a capacity of 2 ml (1 mg) accompanies each 2-oz bottle of Lomotil liquid. Only this plastic dropper should be used when measuring Lomotil liquid for administration.

[*Tablets shown in Product Identification Section*]

NORPACE® CAPSULES ℞
(disopyramide phosphate)
NORPACE® CR CAPSULES ℞
(disopyramide phosphate)
Controlled-Release

Description

Norpace (disopyramide phosphate) is an antiarrhythmic drug available for oral administration in immediate-release and controlled-release capsules containing 100 mg or 150 mg of disopyramide base, present as the phosphate. The base content of the phosphate salt is 77.6%. The chemical name of Norpace is α-[2-(diisopropylamino) ethyl]-α-phenyl-2-pyridineacetamide phosphate.

Norpace is freely soluble in water, and the free base (pKa 10.4) has an aqueous solubility of 1 mg/ml. The chloroform: water partition coefficient of the base is 3.1 at pH 7.2.

Norpace is a racemic mixture of *d*- and *l*-isomers. This drug is not chemically related to other antiarrhythmic drugs.

Norpace CR (controlled-release) capsules are designed to afford a gradual and consistent release of disopyramide. Thus, for maintenance therapy, Norpace CR provides the benefit of less frequent dosing (every 12 hours) as compared with the every-6-hour-dosage schedule of immediate-release Norpace capsules.

Clinical Pharmacology

Mechanisms of Action

Norpace (disopyramide phosphate) is a Type 1 antiarrhythmic drug (ie, similar to procainamide and quinidine). *In animal studies* Norpace decreases the rate of diastolic depolarization (phase 4) in cells with augmented automaticity, decreases the upstroke velocity (phase 0) and increases the action potential duration of normal cardiac cells, decreases the disparity in refractoriness between infarcted and adjacent normally perfused myocardium and has no effect on alpha- or beta-adrenergic receptors.

Electrophysiology

In man, Norpace at therapeutic plasma levels shortens the sinus node recovery time, lengthens the effective refractory period of the atrium and has a minimal effect on the effective refractory period of the AV node. Little effect has been shown on AV-nodal and His-Purkinje conduction times or QRS duration. However, prolongation of conduction in accessory pathways occurs.

Hemodynamics

At recommended oral doses, Norpace rarely produces significant alterations of blood pressure in patients without congestive heart failure (see *Warnings*). With intravenous Norpace, either increases in systolic/diastolic or decreases in systolic blood pressure have been reported, depending on the infusion rate and the patient population. Intravenous Norpace may cause cardiac depression with an approximate mean 10% reduction of cardiac output, which is more pronounced in patients with cardiac dysfunction.

Anticholinergic Activity

The *in vitro* anticholinergic activity of Norpace is approximately 0.06% that of atropine; however, the usual dose for Norpace is 150 mg every 6 hours and for Norpace CR 300 mg every 12 hours compared to 0.4–0.6 mg for atropine (see *Warnings* and *Adverse Reactions* for anticholinergic side effects).

Pharmacokinetics

Following oral administration of immediate-release Norpace, disopyramide phosphate is rapidly and almost completely absorbed, and peak plasma levels are usually attained within 2 hours. The usual therapeutic plasma levels of disopyramide base are 2–4 mcg/ml and at these concentrations protein binding varies from 50–65%. Because of concentration-dependent protein binding, it is difficult to predict the concentration of the free drug when total drug is measured.

The mean plasma half-life of disopyramide in healthy humans is 6.7 hours (range of 4 to 10 hours). In six patients with impaired renal function (creatinine clearance less than 40 ml/min), disopyramide half-life values were 8 to 18 hours.

In healthy men about 50% of a given dose of disopyramide is excreted in the urine as the unchanged drug, about 20% as the mono-N-dealkylated metabolite and 10% as the other metabolites. The plasma concentration of the major metabolite is approximately one tenth that of disopyramide. Altering the urinary pH in man does not affect the plasma half-life of disopyramide.

In a crossover study in healthy subjects, the bioavailability of disopyramide from Norpace CR capsules was similar to that from the immediate-release capsules. With a single 300-mg oral dose, peak disopyramide plasma concentrations of 3.23 $\pm$ 0.75 mcg/ml (mean $\pm$ SD) at 2.5 $\pm$ 2.3 hours were obtained with the immediate-release capsules (two 150-mg) and 2.22 $\pm$ 0.47 mcg/ml at 4.9 $\pm$ 1.4 hours with Norpace CR capsules (two 150-mg). The elimination half-life of disopyramide was 8.31 $\pm$ 1.83 hours with the immediate-release capsules and 11.65 $\pm$ 4.72 hours with Norpace CR capsules. The amount of disopyramide and mono-N-dealkylated metabolite excreted in the urine in 48 hours was 128 and 48 mg, respectively, with the immediate-release capsules and 112 and 33 mg, respectively, with Norpace CR capsules. The differences in the urinary excretion of either constituent were not statistically significant.

Following multiple doses, steady-state plasma levels of between 2 and 4 mcg/ml were attained following either 150 mg every-6-hour-dosing with immediate-release capsules or 300 mg every-12-hour-dosing with Norpace CR capsules.

Indications

Norpace or Norpace CR should be prescribed only after appropriate electrocardiographic assessment.

Norpace and Norpace CR are indicated for suppression and prevention of recurrence of the following cardiac arrhythmias when they occur singly or in combination:

1. Unifocal premature (ectopic) ventricular contractions.
2. Premature (ectopic) ventricular contractions of multifocal origin.
3. Paired premature ventricular contractions (couplets).
4. Episodes of ventricular tachycardia (persistent ventricular tachycardia is ordinarily treated with D.C. cardioversion).

In controlled trials of ambulatory patients, 150 mg of Norpace every 6 hours was as effective as 325 mg of quinidine every 6 hours in reducing the frequency of ventricular ectopic activity. Norpace was equally effective in digitalized and nondigitalized patients. Norpace is also equally effective in the treatment of primary cardiac arrhythmias and those which occur in association with organic heart disease including coronary artery disease.

Oral disopyramide phosphate has not been adequately studied in patients with acute myocardial infarction or in patients with persistent ventricular tachycardia or atrial arrhythmias.

Norpace CR should not be used initially if rapid establishment of disopyramide plasma levels is desired.

Type 1 antiarrhythmic drugs are usually not effective in treating arrhythmias secondary to digitalis intoxication and, therefore, Norpace or Norpace CR is not indicated for such cases.

The value of antiarrhythmic drugs in preventing sudden death in patients with serious ventricular ectopic activity has not been established.

Contraindications

Norpace and Norpace CR are contraindicated in the presence of cardiogenic shock, preexisting second- or third-degree AV block (if no pacemaker is present), or known hypersensitivity to the drug.

Warnings

Negative Inotropic Properties:
Heart Failure/Hypotension

Norpace or Norpace CR may cause or worsen congestive heart failure or produce severe hypotension as a consequence of its negative inotropic properties. Hypotension has been observed primarily in patients with primary cardiomyopathy or inadequately compensated congestive heart failure. Norpace or Norpace CR should not be used in patients with uncompensated or marginally compensated congestive heart failure or hypotension unless the congestive heart failure or hypotension is secondary to cardiac arrhythmia. Patients with a history of heart failure may be treated with Norpace or Norpace CR, but careful attention must be given to the maintenance of cardiac function, including optimal digitalization. If hypotension occurs or congestive heart failure worsens, Norpace or Norpace CR, should be discontinued and, if necessary, restarted at a lower dosage only after adequate cardiac compensation has been established.

QRS Widening

Although it is unusual, significant widening (greater than 25%) of the QRS complex may occur during Norpace or Norpace CR administration; in such cases Norpace or Norpace CR should be discontinued.

Q-T Prolongation

As with other Type 1 antiarrhythmic drugs, prolongation of the Q-T interval (corrected) and worsening of the arrhythmia, including ventricular tachycardia and ventricular fibrillation, may occur. Patients who have evidenced prolongation of the Q-T interval in response to quinidine may be at particular risk. If a Q-T prolongation of greater than 25% is observed and if ectopy continues, the patient should be monitored closely, and

consideration be given to discontinuing Norpace or Norpace CR.

Hypoglycemia

In rare instances significant lowering of blood glucose values has been reported during Norpace administration. The physician should be alert to this possibility, especially in patients with congestive heart failure, chronic malnutrition, hepatic, renal or other diseases or drugs (eg, beta adrenoceptor blockers, alcohol) which could compromise preservation of the normal glucoregulatory mechanisms in the absence of food. In these patients the blood glucose levels should be carefully followed.

Concomitant Antiarrhythmic Therapy

The concomitant use of Norpace or Norpace CR with other Type 1 antiarrhythmic agents (such as quinidine or procainamide) and/or propranolol should be reserved for patients with life-threatening arrhythmias who are demonstrably unresponsive to single-agent antiarrhythmic therapy. Such use may produce serious negative inotropic effects, or may excessively prolong conduction. This should be considered particularly in patients with any degree of cardiac decompensation or those with a prior history thereof. Patients receiving more than one antiarrhythmic drug must be carefully monitored.

Heart Block

If first-degree heart block develops in a patient receiving Norpace or Norpace CR, the dosage should be reduced. If the block persists despite reduction of dosage, continuation of the drug must depend upon weighing the benefit being obtained against the risk of higher degrees of heart block. Development of second- or third-degree AV block or unifascicular, bifascicular or trifascicular block requires discontinuation of Norpace or Norpace CR therapy, unless the ventricular rate is adequately controlled by a temporary or implanted ventricular pacemaker.

Anticholinergic Activity

Because of its anticholinergic activity, disopyramide phosphate should not be used in patients with glaucoma, myasthenia gravis or urinary retention unless adequate overriding measures are taken; these consist of the topical application of potent miotics (eg, pilocarpine) for patients with glaucoma, and catheter drainage or operative relief for patients with urinary retention. Urinary retention may occur in patients of either sex as a consequence of Norpace or Norpace CR administration, but males with benign prostatic hypertrophy are at particular risk. In patients with a family history of glaucoma, intraocular pressure should be measured before initiating Norpace or Norpace CR therapy. Disopyramide phosphate should be used with special care in patients with myasthenia gravis since its anticholinergic properties could precipitate a myasthenic crisis in such patients.

Precautions

Atrial Tachyarrhythmias

Patients with atrial flutter or fibrillation should be digitalized prior to Norpace or Norpace CR administration to ensure that drug-induced enhancement of AV conduction does not result in an increase of ventricular rate beyond physiologically acceptable limits.

Conduction Abnormalities

Care should be taken when prescribing Norpace or Norpace CR for patients with sick sinus syndrome (bradycardia-tachycardia syndrome), Wolff-Parkinson-White syndrome (WPW), or bundle branch block. The effect of disopyramide phosphate in these conditions is uncertain at present.

Cardiomyopathy

Patients with myocarditis or other cardiomyopathy may develop significant hypotension in response to the usual dosage of disopyramide phosphate, probably due to cardiodepressant mechanisms. Therefore, a loading dose of Norpace should not be given to such patients and initial dosage and subsequent dosage adjustments should be made under close supervision (see *Dosage and Administration*).

Drug Interactions

If phenytoin or other hepatic enzyme inducers are taken concurrently with Norpace or Norpace CR, lower plasma levels of disopyramide may occur. Monitoring of disopyramide plasma levels is recommended in such concurrent use to avoid ineffective therapy. Other antiarrhythmic drugs (eg, quinidine, procainamide, lidocaine, propranolol) have occasionally been used concurrently with Norpace but no specific drug interaction studies have been conducted (see *Warnings*). Excessive widening of the QRS complex and/or prolongation of the Q-T interval may occur in these situations. Norpace does not increase serum digoxin levels.

Renal Impairment

More than 50% of disopyramide is excreted in the urine unchanged. Therefore Norpace dosage should be reduced in patients with impaired renal function (see *Dosage and Administration*). The electrocardiogram should be carefully monitored for prolongation of PR interval, evidence of QRS widening or other signs of overdosage (see *Overdosage*).

Norpace CR is not recommended for patients with severe renal insufficiency (creatinine clearance 40 ml/min or less).

Hepatic Impairment

Hepatic impairment also causes an increase in the plasma half-life of disopyramide. Dosage should be reduced for patients with such impairment. The electrocardiogram should be carefully monitored for signs of overdosage (see *Overdosage*).

Patients with cardiac dysfunction have a higher potential for hepatic impairment; this should be considered when administering Norpace or Norpace CR.

Potassium Imbalance

Antiarrhythmic drugs may be ineffective in patients with hypokalemia, and their toxic effects may be enhanced in patients with hyperkalemia. Therefore, potassium abnormalities should be corrected before starting Norpace or Norpace CR therapy.

Pregnancy

Reproduction studies in rats and teratology studies performed both in rats and in rabbits have revealed minimal evidence of impaired fertility. No fetal anomalies were attributable to Norpace. Disopyramide has been found in human fetal blood. However, well-controlled studies of Norpace have not been performed in pregnant women and experience with Norpace during pregnancy is limited; therefore the possibility of damage to the fetus cannot be excluded. **Norpace has been reported to stimulate contractions of the pregnant uterus.** Norpace or Norpace CR should be used in pregnant women only when it is clearly indicated and the benefit/risk ratio has been carefully evaluated.

Labor and Delivery

It is not known whether the use of Norpace or Norpace CR during labor or delivery has immediate or delayed adverse effects on the fetus, or whether it prolongs the duration of labor or increases the need for forceps delivery or other obstetric intervention.

Nursing Mothers

Studies in rats have shown that the concentration of disopyramide and its metabolites is between one and three times greater in milk than it is in plasma. Following oral administration, disopyramide has been detected in human milk at a concentration not exceeding that in plasma. Therefore, if use of the drug is deemed essential, an alternative method of infant feeding should be instituted.

Adverse Reactions

The adverse reactions which were reported in Norpace clinical trials encompass observations in 1,500 patients, including 90 patients studied for at least 4 years. The most serious adverse reactions are hypotension and congestive heart failure. The most common adverse reactions, which are dose dependent, are associated with the anticholinergic properties of the drug. These may be transitory, but may be persistent or can be severe. Urinary retention is the most serious anticholinergic effect.

The following reactions were reported in 10–40% of patients:

Anticholinergic: dry mouth (32%), urinary hesitancy (14%), constipation (11%)

The following reactions were reported in 3–9% of patients:

Anticholinergic: blurred vision, dry nose/eyes/throat

Genitourinary: urinary frequency and urgency

Gastrointestinal: nausea, pain/bloating/gas

General: dizziness, general fatigue/muscle weakness, headache, malaise, aches/pains

The following reactions were reported in 1–3% of patients:

Anticholinergic: urinary retention

Genitourinary: impotence

Cardiovascular: hypotension with or without congestive heart failure, increased congestive heart failure (see *Warnings*), cardiac conduction disturbances (see *Warnings*), edema/weight gain, shortness of breath, syncope, chest pain

Gastrointestinal: anorexia, diarrhea, vomiting

Dermatologic: generalized rash/dermatoses, itching

Central nervous system: nervousness

Other: hypokalemia, elevated cholesterol/triglycerides

The following reactions were reported in less than 1%:

Depression, insomnia, dysuria, numbness/tingling, elevated liver enzymes, AV block, elevated BUN, elevated creatinine, decreased hemoglobin/hematocrit

Hypoglycemia has been reported in association with Norpace administration (see *Warnings*). Infrequent occurrences of reversible cholestatic jaundice, fever, and respiratory difficulty have been reported in association with disopyramide therapy as have rare instances of thrombocytopenia, reversible agranulocytosis, and gynecomastia. Rarely, acute psychosis has been reported following Norpace therapy, with prompt return to normal mental status when therapy was stopped. The physician should be aware of these possible reactions and should discontinue Norpace or Norpace CR therapy promptly if they occur.

Dosage and Administration

The dosage of Norpace or Norpace CR must be individualized for each patient on the basis of response and tolerance. The usual adult dosage of Norpace or Norpace CR is 400 to 800 mg per day given in divided doses. The recommended dosage for most adults in 600 mg/day given in divided doses (either 150 mg every 6 hours for immediate-release Norpace or 300 mg every 12 hours for Norpace CR). For patients whose body weight is less than 110 pounds (50 kg), the recommended dosage is 400 mg/day given in divided doses (either 100 mg every 6 hours for immediate-release Norpace or 200 mg every 12 hours for Norpace CR).

For patients with cardiomyopathy or possible cardiac decompensation, a loading dose, as discussed below, should not be given and initial dosage should be limited to 100 mg of immediate-release Norpace every 6 hours. Subsequent dosage adjustments should be made gradually, with close monitoring for the possi-

Continued on next page

Searle & Co.—Cont.

ble development of hypotension and/or congestive heart failure (see *Warnings*).
For patients with moderate renal insufficiency (creatinine clearance greater than 40 ml/min) or hepatic insufficiency, the recommended dosage is 400 mg/day given in divided doses (either 100 mg every 6 hours for immediate-release Norpace or 200 mg every 12 hours for Norpace CR).
For patients with severe renal insufficiency (C_{cr}40 ml/min or less), the recommended dosage of immediate-release Norpace is 100 mg at intervals shown in the table below, with or without an initial loading dose of 150 mg.

IMMEDIATE-RELEASE NORPACE DOSAGE INTERVAL FOR PATIENTS WITH RENAL INSUFFICIENCY

Creatinine clearance (ml/min)	40–30	30–15	less than 15
Approximate maintenance-dosing interval	q 8 hr	q 12 hr	q 24 hr

The above dosing schedules are for Norpace immediate-release capsules; Norpace CR is not recommended for patients with severe renal insufficiency.
For patients in whom rapid control of ventricular arrhythmia is essential, an initial loading dose of 300 mg of immediate-release Norpace (200 mg for patients whose body weight is less than 110 pounds) is recommended, followed by the appropriate maintenance dosage. Therapeutic effects are usually attained 30 minutes to 3 hours after administration of a 300-mg loading dose. If there is no response nor evidence of toxicity within 6 hours of the loading dose, 200 mg of immediate-release Norpace every 6 hours may be prescribed instead of the usual 150 mg. If there is no response to this dosage within 48 hours, either Norpace should then be discontinued or the physician should consider hospitalizing the patient for careful monitoring while subsequent immediate-release Norpace doses of 250 or 300 mg every 6 hours are given. A limited number of patients with severe refractory ventricular tachycardia have tolerated daily doses of Norpace up to 1600 mg per day (400 mg every 6 hours) resulting in disopyramide plasma levels up to 9 mcg/ml. If such treatment is warranted, it is essential that patients be hospitalized for close evaluation and continuous monitoring.
Norpace CR should not be used initially if rapid establishment of disopyramide plasma levels is desired.

Transferring to Norpace or Norpace CR
The following dosage schedule based on theoretical considerations rather than experimental data is suggested for transferring patients with normal renal function from either quinidine sulfate or procainamide therapy (Type 1 antiarrhythmic agents) to Norpace or Norpace CR therapy:
Norpace or Norpace CR should be started using the regular maintenance schedule **without a loading dose** 6–12 hours after the last dose of quinidine sulfate or 3–6 hours after the last dose of procainamide.
In patients where withdrawal of quinidine sulfate or procainamide is likely to produce life-threatening arrhythmias, the physician should consider hospitalization of the patient. When transferring a patient from immediate-release Norpace to Norpace CR, the maintenance schedule of Norpace CR may be started 6 hours after the last dose of immediate-release Norpace.

Pediatric Dosage
Controlled clinical studies have not been conducted in pediatric patients; however, the following suggested dosage table is based on published clinical experience.
Total daily dosage should be divided and equal doses administered orally every 6 hours or at intervals according to individual patient needs. Disopyramide plasma levels and therapeutic response must be monitored closely. Patients should be hospitalized during the initial treatment period, and dose titration should start at the lower end of the ranges provided below.

SUGGESTED TOTAL DAILY DOSAGE*

Age (years)	Disopyramide (mg/kg body weight/day)
Under 1	10 to 30
1 to 4	10 to 20
4 to 12	10 to 15
12 to 18	6 to 15

* Dosage is expressed in milligrams of disopyramide base. Since Norpace (disopyramide phosphate) 100-mg capsules contain 100 mg of disopyramide base, the pharmacist can readily prepare a 1-mg/ml to 10-mg/ml liquid suspension by adding the entire contents of Norpace capsules to cherry syrup, NF. The resulting suspension, when refrigerated, is stable for one month and should be thoroughly shaken before the measurement of each dose. The suspension should be dispensed in an amber glass bottle with a child-resistant closure.

Norpace CR capsules should not be used to prepare the above suspension.

Overdosage

Symptoms
Five patients who took deliberate overdoses of oral disopyramide phosphate developed an early loss of consciousness after an apneic period, followed by cardiac arrhythmias and loss of spontaneous respiration, leading to death.
Toxic plasma levels of disopyramide produce excessive widening of the QRS complex and Q-T interval, worsening of congestive heart failure, hypotension, varying kinds and degrees of conduction disturbance, bradycardia, and finally asystole. Obvious anticholinergic effects are also observed.

Treatment
Discontinue use of the drug. No specific antidote for disopyramide phosphate has been identified; treatment of overdosage should be symptomatic and may include the administration of isoproterenol, dopamine, intra-aortic balloon counterpulsation, and mechanically assisted respiration. Hemodialysis or hemoperfusion with charcoal may be employed to lower serum concentration of the drug.
The electrocardiogram should be monitored, and supportive therapy with cardiac glycosides and diuretics should be given as required.
If progressive AV block should develop, endocardial pacing should be implemented. In case of any impaired renal function, measures to increase the glomerular filtration rate may reduce the toxicity (disopyramide is excreted primarily by the kidney).
The anticholinergic effects can be reversed with neostigmine at the discretion of the physician.
Altering the urinary pH in humans does not affect the plasma half-life or the amount of disopyramide excreted in the urine.

How Supplied

Norpace (disopyramide phosphate) is supplied in hard gelatin capsules containing either 100 mg or 150 mg of disopyramide base, present as the phosphate.
Norpace 100-mg capsules are white and orange, with markings SEARLE, 2752, Norpace, and 100 MG.
Norpace 150-mg capsules are brown and orange, with markings SEARLE, 2762, Norpace, and 150 MG.
Available in bottles of 100, 500, 1,000, and 2,500 capsules, and cartons of 100 unit-dose individually blister-sealed capsules.
Norpace CR (disopyramide phosphate) Controlled-Release is supplied as specially prepared controlled-release beads in hard gelatin capsules containing either 100 mg or 150 mg of disopyramide base, present as the phosphate.
Norpace CR 100-mg capsules are white and light green, with markings SEARLE, 2732, NORPACE CR, and 100 mg. Norpace CR 150-mg capsules are brown and light green, with markings SEARLE, 2742, NORPACE CR, and 150 mg.
Available in bottles of 100 and 500 capsules, and cartons of 100 unit-dose individually blister-sealed capsules.
Certain manufacturing operations for Norpace CR have been performed by G. D. Searle & Co. LTD., Morpeth, England.
[*Shown in Product Identification Section*]

OVULEN-21® ℞
OVULEN-28® ℞
(ethynodiol diacetate with mestranol)

See Demulen under Searle & Co. for Ovulen prescribing information.
[*Shown in Product Identification Section*]

PRO-BANTHĪNE® Tablets ℞
(propantheline bromide USP)

Description: Pro-Banthīne tablets contain 15 mg or 7½ mg of propantheline bromide, (2-hydroxyethyl)diisopropylmethylammonium bromide xanthene-9-carboxylate.
Clinical Pharmacology: Pro-Banthīne inhibits gastrointestinal motility and diminishes gastric acid secretion. The drug also inhibits the action of acetylcholine at the postganglionic nerve endings of the parasympathetic nervous system.
After oral administration to man, propantheline bromide is extensively metabolized primarily by hydrolysis to the inactive materials xanthene-9-carboxylic acid and (2-hydroxyethyl)diisopropylmethylammonium bromide, approximately half of which occurs in the gastrointestinal tract prior to its absorption. After a single 15-mg oral dose of carbon-14 labeled drug given to a healthy man, 390 ng/ml peak plasma concentration of total-^{14}C material is attained at 6 hours. Unmetabolized drug represents only a small proportion of the total-^{14}C materials. The plasma half-life of the total-^{14}C material is about 9 hours, and approximately 70 percent of the dose is excreted in the urine, mostly as metabolites. The urinary excretion of the intact propantheline is about 5 percent after oral administration, and about 20 percent after intravenous administration.
Indications: Pro-Banthīne is effective as adjunctive therapy in the treatment of peptic ulcer.
Contraindications: Pro-Banthīne (propantheline bromide) is contraindicated in patients with:

1. Glaucoma, since mydriasis is to be avoided.
2. Obstructive disease of the gastrointestinal tract (pyloroduodenal stenosis, achalasia, paralytic ileus, etc).
3. Obstructive uropathy (eg, bladder-neck obstruction due to prostatic hypertrophy).
4. Intestinal atony of elderly or debilitated patients.
5. Severe ulcerative colitis or toxic megacolon complicating ulcerative colitis.
6. Unstable cardiovascular adjustment in acute hemorrhage.

7. Myasthenia gravis.

Warnings: In the presence of a high environmental temperature, heat prostration (fever and heat stroke due to decreased sweating) can occur with the use of Pro-Banthīne.

Diarrhea may be an early symptom of incomplete intestinal obstruction, especially in patients with ileostomy or colostomy. In this instance treatment with Pro-Banthīne would be inappropriate and possibly harmful.

Pro-Banthīne may produce drowsiness or blurred vision. The patient should be cautioned regarding activities requiring mental alertness, such as operating a motor vehicle or other machinery or performing hazardous work, while taking this drug.

With overdosage, a curare-like action may occur (ie, neuromuscular blockade leading to muscular weakness and possible paralysis).

Patients with severe cardiac disease should be given this medication with caution if an increase in heart rate is undesirable.

Use in Pregnancy: Reproduction studies have not been performed in animals. Information on possible adverse effects to the fetus is limited to uncontrolled data derived from marketing experience. Such experience has revealed no evidence of toxicity to mother or fetus. There are no controlled studies in animals or humans to determine whether this drug affects fertility in human males or females, has teratogenic potential, or has other adverse effects on the fetus. It should be used during pregnancy only when, in the opinion of the physician, the benefits outweigh any possible risk.

Use in Nursing Mothers: Information regarding the secretion of Pro-Banthīne (propantheline bromide) in breast milk is limited to uncontrolled data derived from marketing experience. Such experience does not suggest that significant quantities of Pro-Banthīne are secreted in breast milk.

Pediatric Use: Since there is inadequate experience with the use of Pro-Banthīne in children, safety and efficacy in children have not been established.

Precautions: Pro-Banthīne (propantheline bromide) should be used with caution in the elderly and in all patients with autonomic neuropathy, hepatic or renal disease, hyperthyroidism, coronary heart disease, congestive heart failure, cardiac tachyarrhythmias, hypertension, or hiatal hernia associated with reflux esophagitis, since anticholinergics may aggravate this condition.

In patients with ulcerative colitis, large doses of Pro-Banthīne may suppress intestinal motility to the point of producing paralytic ileus and, for this reason, may precipitate or aggravate toxic megacolon, a serious complication of the disease.

Adverse Reactions: Varying degrees of drying of salivary secretions may occur as well as decreased sweating. Ophthalmic side effects include blurred vision, mydriasis, cycloplegia, and increased ocular tension. Other reported adverse reactions include urinary hesitancy and retention, tachycardia, palpitations, loss of the sense of taste, headache, nervousness, mental confusion, drowsiness, weakness, dizziness, insomnia, nausea, vomiting, constipation, bloated feeling, impotence, suppression of lactation, and allergic reactions or drug idiosyncracies including anaphylaxis, urticaria and other dermal manifestations.

Overdosage: The symptoms of overdosage with Pro-Banthīne progress from an intensification of the usual side effects to CNS disturbances (from restlessness and excitement to psychotic behavior), circulatory changes (flushing, fall in blood pressure, circulatory failure), respiratory failure, paralysis, and coma.

Measures to be taken are (1) immediate lavage of the stomach and (2) injection of physostigmine 0.5 to 2 mg intravenously, and repeated as necessary up to a total of 5 mg. Fever may be treated symptomatically (alcohol sponging, ice packs).

Excitement of a degree which demands attention may be managed with sodium thiopental 2% solution given slowly intravenously or chloral hydrate (100–200 ml of a 2% solution) by rectal infusion. In the event of progression of the curare-like effect to paralysis of the respiratory muscles, artificial respiration should be instituted and maintained until effective respiratory action returns.

Dosage and Administration: The usual initial adult dose of Pro-Banthīne tablets is 15 mg taken 30 minutes before each meal and 30 mg at bedtime (a total of 75 mg daily). Subsequent dosage adjustment should be made according to the patient's individual response and tolerance. The administration of one 7½-mg tablet three times a day is convenient for patients with mild manifestations and for geriatric patients and for those of small stature.

Drug Interactions: Concurrent use of Pro-Banthīne (propantheline bromide) with slow-dissolving tablets of digoxin may cause increased serum digoxin levels. This interaction can be avoided by using only those digoxin tablets that rapidly dissolve by USP standards. Anticholinergics may delay absorption of other medication given concomitantly. Excessive cholinergic blockade may occur if Pro-Banthīne is given concomitantly with belladonna alkaloids or synthetic and semisynthetic anticholinergic agents (eg, antispasmodics, antiparkinsonism agents), phenothiazine, tricyclic antidepressants, quinidine, antihistamines, or procainamide.

How Supplied: *For oral use: Tablets:* Pro-Banthīne 15-mg tablets are sugar coated, peach colored, with SEARLE imprinted on one side and 601 on the other side; bottles of 100, 500 and 1,000, and cartons containing 100 unit-dose, individually blister-sealed tablets.

Pro-Banthīne 7½-mg tablets are sugar coated, white, with SEARLE imprinted on one side and 611 on the other side; bottles of 100 and 500.

[*Shown in Product Identification Section*]

PRO–BANTHĪNE® with PHENOBARBITAL Tablets ℞
(propantheline bromide with phenobarbital)

Description:

Each Pro-Banthīne with Phenobarbital tablet contains:

propantheline bromide .... 15 mg
phenobarbital .... 15 mg
(Warning: May be habit forming.)

Propantheline bromide is (2-hydroxyethyl) diisopropylmethylammonium bromide xanthene-9-carboxylate.

For *Clinical Pharmacology* see Pro-Banthīne Tablets.

Indications:

Based on a review of this drug by the National Academy of Sciences—National Research Council and/or other information, FDA has classified the indications as follows:

"Possibly" effective: as adjunctive therapy in the treatment of peptic ulcer and in the treatment of the irritable bowel syndrome (irritable colon, spastic colon, mucous colitis, acute enterocolitis, and functional gastrointestinal disorders).

Final classification of the less-than-effective indications requires further investigation.

For *Contraindications, Warnings* (except for the *Use in Pregnancy* section, which follows), *Precautions, Adverse Reactions,* and *Overdosage* see Pro-Banthīne Tablets.

Use in Pregnancy: Reproduction studies with this combination of medications have not been performed in animals. However, a study in rats concluded that the administration of phenobarbital given as a single daily subcutaneous dose of 40 mg/kg from the twelfth to the nineteenth day of pregnancy resulted in altered reproductive function in the female offspring, as evidenced by delayed onset of puberty, disorders in the estrous cycle, and infertility. An increased incidence of congenital malformations in humans has also been reported in response to phenobarbital exposure in utero. Consequently, Pro-Banthīne with Phenobarbital should be used during pregnancy only when, in the opinion of the physician, the benefits outweigh any possible risk.

Dosage and Administration: The usual adult dosage of Pro-Banthīne with Phenobarbital is one or two tablets three or four times daily.

For *Drug Interactions* see Pro-Banthīne Tablets.

How Supplied: *For Oral Use:* Tablets: Pro-Banthīne with Phenobarbital tablets containing 15 mg of propantheline bromide and 15 mg of phenobarbital are sugar coated, ivory colored, with SEARLE imprinted on one side and 631 on the other side; bottles of 100 and 500, and cartons containing 100 unit-dose, individually blister-sealed tablets.

[*Shown in Product Identification Section*]

The preceding prescribing information for Searle & Co. was current on November 15, 1982.

The Seatrace Company
POST OFFICE BOX 363
GADSDEN, AL 35902

ACUCRON TABLETS ℞
Composition:

Acetaminophen .... 300 mg.
Salicylamide .... 200 mg.
Phenyltoloxamine .... 20 mg.

DURASAL TABLETS ℞
Composition:

Magnesium Salicylate .... 600 mg.

DYLINE GG LIQUID ℞
Composition:

Diphylline .... 100 mg./teaspoonful
Guaifenesin .... 100 mg./teaspoonful

DYLINE GG TABLETS
Composition:

Diphylline .... 200 mg.
Guaifenesin .... 200 mg.

LOBAC CAPSULES ℞
Composition:

Chlorzoxazone .... 250 mg.
Acetaminophen .... 300 mg.

N D CLEAR T.D. CAPSULES ℞
Composition:

Chlorpheniramine Maleate .... 8 mg.
Pseudoephedrine Hydrochloride .... 120 mg.

VERSACAPS ℞

Description:

Each Timed Disintegrating Capsule Contains:
Brompheniramine Maleate ....4 mg
Pseudoephedrine Hydrochloride ....60 mg
Guaifenesin ....300 mg

Versacaps provides a continuous release of medication which affords effects for ten to twelve hours.

Actions and Uses: Versacaps provide simultaneous expectorant, decongestant, bronchodilator and antihistaminic effects. Combines the potent antihistiminic action of brompheniramine maleate with the rapid and sustained

Continued on next page

Seatrace—Cont.

decongestant effect of pseudoephedrine on the swollen mucosa of the respiratory tract. Guaifenesin, an ether, is capable of being partially eliminated by way of the expired air, and is therefore able to exert a local expectorant action in the respiratory passages. Guaifenesin makes expectoration freer and easier, because the respiratory tract secretions are made more fluid and thereby more easily expelled.
Indications: Versacaps are indicated for the symptomatic relief of cough in conditions such as: the common cold, acute bronchitis, allergic asthma, broncholitis, emphysema, and tracheobrochitis. Versacaps are also indicated for relief of nasal congestion, chronic rhinitis, allergic rhinitis, and post nasal drip of chronic sinusitis.
Contraindications: Severe hypertension or severe cardiac disease, sensitivity to antihistamines or sympathomimetic agents.
Warnings: Use with caution in patients suffering from hypertension, cardiac disease or hyperthyroidism.
Precautions: Although pseudoephedrine hydrochloride causes virtually no pressor effect in normotensive patients, it should be used with caution in patients with hypertension.
Adverse Reactions: The great majority of patients will have no side effects. Only certain patients, sensitive to one or another of the ingredients, may note mild stimulation or mild sedation. As with other preparations containing antihistamines, drowsiness may occur in some patients; if so, it is usually transitory, disappearing within a few days of continued therapy or upon reduction of dosage. Other side effects produced by antihistamine drugs include dizziness and dryness of the mouth. Gastrointestinal irritation has been reported.
Usual Adult Dosage: Two capsules every 12 hours; one capsule in mild cases.
Children 6–12: 1 capsule every 12 hours.
How Supplied: In bottles of 100 and 1000. Dispense in a tight, light resistant container as defined in the National Formulary.
Caution: Federal law prohibits dispensing without a prescription.
CONTAINS NO FD&C YELLOW DYE No. 5 (DYE FREE)

SERES Laboratories, Inc.
3331 INDUSTRIAL DRIVE
BOX 470
SANTA ROSA, CA 95402

CANTHARONE® ℞
(cantharidin collodion)
For External Use Only

Description: CANTHARONE®, cantharidin collodion, is a topical liquid containing 0.7% cantharidin in a film-forming vehicle containing acetone, ethocel and flexible collodion. Ether 35%, alcohol 11%. The active ingredient, cantharidin, is a vesicant. The chemical name is Hexahydro-3aα, 7aα-dimethyl-4β, 7β-epoxyisobenzofuran-1, 3-dione. $C_{10}H_{12}O_4$
Clinical Pharmacology: The vesicant action of cantharidin is the result of its primary acantholytic action. Its effectiveness against warts is presumed to result from the "exfoliation" of the tumor as a consequence of its acantholytic action. The lytic action of cantharidin does not go beyond the epidermal cells, the basal layer remains intact and there is minimal effect on the corium; as a result there is no scarring from topical application.

Indications and Usage: Cantharone® is indicated for removal of warts and molluscum contagiosum. It is designed for topical application by a physician. Painless application and the absence of instruments makes it especially useful for treating children. See Dosage and Administration section for specific directions for use.
Contraindications: Cantharone® is not recommended for treatment of mosaic warts.
Warnings: Cantharidin is a strong vesicant and Cantharone® may product blisters if it comes in contact with normal skin or mucous membrane. If spilled on skin, wipe off at once, using acetone, alcohol or tape remover. Then wash vigorously with warm soapy water and rinse well. If spilled on mucous membrane or in eyes, flush with water, remove precipitated collodion, and flush with water for an additional 15 minutes. Residual pigment changes may occur. Patients vary in their sensitivity to cantharidin and in rare cases tingling, burning or extreme tenderness may develop. In these cases the patient should remove tape and soak the area in cool water for 10 to 15 minutes, repeating as required for relief. If soreness persists, puncture blister using sterile technique, apply antiseptic and cover with a Band-Aid. It is advisable to treat only one or two lesions on the first visit, until the sensitivity of the patient is known. For external use only.
Precautions: There have been no adequate and well-controlled studies on the use of cantharidin in pregnant women or nursing mothers, therefore the use of Cantharone® during pregnancy or in nursing mothers is not recommended.
Cantharone® is flammable; keep away from heat, sparks and flame.
Adverse Reactions: The development of annular warts following Cantharone® therapy has been reported in a small percentage of patients. These lesions are superficial and, although they may alarm some patients, present little problem. Treatment consists of patient reassurance and re-treatment using either Cantharone® or other procedures. There has been one report of chemical lymphangitis following use of Cantharone® in combination with salicylic acid plaster.
Dosage and Administration: *Ordinary and periungual warts*—No cutting or prior treatment is required. (Occasionally nails must be trimmed to expose subungual warts to medication.) Apply Cantharone® directly to the lesion; cover the growth completely using an applicator stick. Allow a few seconds for a thin membrane to form and cover with a piece of non-porous plastic adhesive tape e.g. Blenderm. Instruct patient to remove tape in 24 hours and replace with a loose Band-Aid. On next visit remove necrotic tissue and re-apply Cantharone® to any growth remaining. Defer second treatment if inflammation is intense. A single application may suffice for normally keratinized skin.
Plantar warts—Pare away keratin covering the wart: avoid cutting viable tissue. Using a Q-tip or applicator stick, apply Cantharone® to both the wart and a 1–3mm margin around the wart. Allow a few minutes to dry. Secure with non-porous plastic adhesive tape. Leave in place for a week, then debride. If any viable wart tissue remains after debridement, re-apply a small amount of Cantharone® and bandage as above. Three or more such treatments may be required for large lesions. When destruction of wart is complete, the healed site will appear smooth, with normal skin lines.
Palpebral warts—Using a toothpick or fine probe, apply a small amount of Cantharone® to the surface of the wart. Avoid touching surrounding normal skin or applying inside the eye lashes. Leave lesion uncovered. Repeat in a week or ten days if any growth remains.
Molluscum contagiosum—Coat each lesion with a thin film of Cantharone®. In one week, treat any new lesions the same way and retreat any resistant lesions with Cantharone®, this time covering with a small piece of occlusive tape. The tape should be removed in 6 to 8 hours.
How Supplied: 7.5 mL bottles (NDC 50694-096-01). Close tightly immediately after use. Keep away from heat.
Revised Sept. 1982
Direct inquiries to Kathryn MacLeod, Ph.D.

CANTHARONE PLUS™ ℞
For External Use Only

Description: CANTHARONE PLUS™ is a topical liquid containing 30% salicylic acid, 5% podophyllin, 1% cantharidin in a film-forming vehicle containing 0.5% octylphenyl-polyethylene glycol, cellosolve, ethocel, collodion, castor oil and acetone.
Salicylic acid is a deratolytic. The chemical name is 2-Hydroxybenzoic acid. Podophyllin is a caustic. It is an extract of the rhizomes and roots of Podophyllum peltatum. Cantharidin is a vesicant, the chemical name is Hexahydro-3aα, 7aα-dimethyl-4β, 7β-epoxyisobenzofuran-1, 3-dione.
How Supplied: 7.5 mL bottles (NDC 50694-097-01). Close tightly immediately after use. Keep away from heat. Do not refrigerate.
Revised Sept. 1982
Direct inquiries to Kathryn MacLeod, Ph.D.

Serono Laboratories, Inc.
280 POND STREET
RANDOLPH, MA 02368

Serono Laboratories, Inc. will be pleased to answer inquiries about the following products:

ASELLACRIN® ℞
(somatropin)

FOR INTRAMUSCULAR INJECTION

Description: Asellacrin (somatropin) is a sterile, lyophilized, purified somatropic hormone extracted from the human pituitary gland.
The potency of Asellacrin (somatropin) is determined by bioassay in hypophysectomized rats and is designated in International Units (IU). Each 10 ml vial contains 10 IU of somatropin and 40 mg of mannitol. After reconstitution, each milliliter of Asellacrin (somatropin) contains 2 IU of somatropin and 8 mg of mannitol as well as other pituitary hormones as shown below:

Follitropin (FSH)	less than 0.714 IU
Lutropin (LH)	less than or equal to 17.85 IU
Corticotropin (ACTH)	less than or equal to .014 IU
Thyrotropin (TSH)	less than 0.071 IU
Prolactin (PRL)	less than or equal to 2.86 IU

The pH is adjusted between 6 and 8 with hydrochloric acid and/or sodium hydroxide.
Clinical Pharmacology:
A. Skeletal Growth
Asellacrin (somatropin) stimulates linear growth in patients with pituitary growth hormone deficiency. The measurable increase in growth (body length) after somatropin administration results from its effect on cartilaginous growth areas of the long bones. It is known that somatropin's effect is mediated by a sulfation factor, or somatomedin which permits the incorporation of sulfate into cartilage. Somatomedin is low in serum of the growth hormone deficient patients whose growth hormone deficiency is the result of hypopituitarism or hypophysectomy, whereas its presence can be demonstrated after somatropin therapy.
B. Cellular Growth
In addition to its effect on the skeleton, somatropin brings about an increase in the muscular and visceral mass. In muscle tissue the increase in mass is observed by a corresponding increase in number and dimension of muscular fiber cells.

C. Carbohydrate Metabolism
The diabetogenic effect of somatropin is well-known in clinical medicine. Acromegalic patients often suffer from diabetes mellitus while hypopituitary children experience hypoglycemia. In healthy patients, very large doses of somatropin can interfere with glucose tolerance.
A simultaneous increase in the plasma insulin level is observed upon somatropin administration.
The diabetogenic activity of somatropin is perhaps due to several concomitant factors:
a. Reduced transport of glucose into peripheral tissues
b. Increased release of glucose from the liver
c. Reduced concentration of insulin at the muscular level
d. Reduced glycolysis resulting from the block of the enzyme triose phosphate dehydrogenase, mediated by non-esterified fatty acids.

D. Protein Metabolism
Asellacrin (somatropin) is an anabolic agent that stimulates intracellular transport of amino acids and net retention of nitrogen, which can be quantitated by observing the decline in urinary nitrogen excretion and BUN. At the subcellular level, somatropin may stimulate the duplication of DNA, the synthesis of messenger ribonucleic acid (mRNA), the activation of cyclic AMP and the subsequent coupling of amino acids with their respective transfer RNA's. The increase of mRNA observed by some investigators may perhaps point to mRNA synthesis as the primary process in turn provoking protein synthesis.

E. Fat Metabolism
Somatropin stimulates intracellular lipolysis, increases the plasma concentration of free fatty acids and stimulates the oxidation of fatty acids. In the diabetic patient, somatropin has been shown to accentuate ketogensis.

F. Connective Tissue Metabolism
Somatropin stimulates the synthesis of chondroitin sulfate and collagen as well as the urinary excretion of hydroxyproline.

G. Mineral Metabolism
Somatropin induces the net retention of phosphorus and potassium and to a lesser degree sodium. Somatropin induces the increased intestinal absorption of calcium and the increased renal tubular reabsorption of phosphorus with increased serum and inorganic phosphate. Increased serum alkaline phosphatase may also be observed during somatropin therapy.

Indications and Usage: Growth failure due to a deficiency of pituitary growth hormone is the only indication for Asellacrin (somatropin) administration. The criteria for treatment are as follows:

1. Other causes for growth failure should be eliminated. Disorders of the pulmonary, cardiac, gastrointestinal and central nervous system and nutritional disorders which interfere with growth should be ruled out. There should be no evidence of a specific bone or cartilage disorder such as achondroplasia or other chondrodystrophy. The patient must not have psychosocial dwarfism. Primary hypothyroidism should be eliminated by appropriate laboratory testing. An abnormality of the X-chromosome should be ruled out by a karyotype in girls whenever indicated.
2. Patients must show significant short stature and/or a retarded growth rate. Patients with congenital growth hormone deficiency should be below the third percentile for height and growing at a rate of less than 5.0 cm/year over at least one year of continuous observation by the same physician. Height should be compared to appropriate standards for age. The most suitable are those compiled by the National Center for Health Statistics. Charts based on these standards are generally available. Patients with acquired growth hormone deficiency should also have grown less than 5.0 cm/year and should have been observed continuously by the same physician for at least 12 months.
3. Skeletal maturation should be compatible with a beneficial response to therapy. Epiphyseal maturation should be incomplete. In general, the response to therapy is diminished when the bone age is advanced beyond 13 to 14 years. While this is not a contraindication to the use of Asellacrin (somatropin), epiphyseal maturation should be below 12 to 13 years to increase the likelihood of a beneficial response.
4. The diagnosis of pituitary growth hormone deficiency should be confirmed by objective tests of growth hormone function. There must be failure to increase the serum concentration of growth hormone above 5 to 7 ng/ml in response to two standard stimuli. The stimuli which may be used are insulin-induced hypoglycemia, an intravenous infusion of arginine, oral L-DOPA, or subcutaneous or intramuscular glucagon. Suitable modifications of such procedures, such as pretreatment with estrogen or the administration of propranolol, may also be employed. Fasting serum growth hormone concentrations or the growth hormone response to exercise or sleep are not regarded as definitive tests for documentation of the diagnosis.
5. Tests of other pituitary hormone deficiency should be carried out. Additional deficiencies should be recognized and treated where appropriate.

Deficiency of thyrotropin (TSH) must be treated before definitive testing for growth hormone deficiency can be performed. Patients must have been euthyroid for 4 to 8 weeks prior to testing. They must also have been observed for at least 6 months while euthyroid to determine whether the growth rate meets the criteria for treatment. Corticotropin (ACTH) deficiency should also be appropriately treated, as should deficiency of antidiuretic hormone. If indicated, gonadotropin deficiency may be treated concomitantly with Asellacrin (somatropin) administration, but this may rapidly advance epiphyseal maturation and limit the long-term response to therapy.

Contraindications: Asellacrin (somatropin) is ineffective, and should not be used, in patients with closed epiphyses.
Asellacrin (somatropin) is contraindicated in the face of any progression of underlying intracranial lesion. Intracranial lesions must be inactive for 12 months prior to instituting therapy and Asellacrin (somatropin) should be discontinued if there is evidence of recurrent activity.

Warnings: In spite of rigorous requirements for the collection of pituitary glands used in the preparation of Asellacrin, the risk of transmitting hepatitis cannot be excluded. The risk can be considered extremely small as no cases have been reported.

Precautions: Asellacrin (somatropin) should be used only be physicians experienced in the diagnosis and management of patients with pituitary growth hormone deficiency.
Because of its diabetogenic actions, which include the induction of hyperglycemia and ketosis, Asellacrin (somatropin) should be used with caution in patients with diabetes mellitus or with a family history of diabetes mellitus. Regular urine testing for evidence of glycosuria should be carried out in all patients.
Subcutaneous administration of Asellacrin (somatropin) may lead to local lipoatrophy or lipodystrophy and may enhance the development of neutralizing antibodies. The injections must be intramuscular and the injection site should be rotated.
Bone age must be monitored annually during Asellacrin (somatropin) administration especially in patients who are pubertal and/or receiving concomitant thyroid replacement therapy. Under these circumstances, epiphyseal maturation may progress rapidly to closure.
Concomitant glucocorticoid therapy may inhibit the response of Asellacrin (somatropin) and should not exceed 10–15 mg hydrocortisone equivalent/M^2 body surface area during the administration of Asellacrin (somatropin).
Patients with growth hormone deficiency secondary to an intracranial lesion should be examined frequently for progression or recurrence of the underlying disease process.

Adverse Reactions: Antibodies to somatropin are formed in 30–40% of the patients who have received somatropin prepared by similar methods. In general, these antibodies are not neutralizing and do not interfere with the response to Asellacrin (somatropin) administration. Approximately 5% of treated patients developed neutralizing antibodies and failed to respond to somatropin. Therefore, testing for antisomatropin antibodies should be carried out in any patient with well-documented growth hormone deficiency who fails to respond to therapy.

Dosage and Administration: Reconstitute each vial with 5 ml of Bacteriostatic Water for Injection (U.S.P.) only. Each vial of reconstituted Asellacrin (somatropin) provides 2 IU somatropin per ml, 10 IU per vial.
It is recommended that Asellacrin (somatropin) be given initially as 1 ml (2 IU) intramuscularly, three times a week, with a minimum of 48 hours between injections.
If at any time during the continuous Asellacrin (somatropin) administration the growth rate does not exceed 2.5 cm (1 in) in a 6-month period the dose may be doubled for the next 6 months. This may be done with or without the presence of antibodies to Asellacrin (somatropin). If there is still no satisfactory response, Asellacrin (somatropin) should be discontinued and the patient reinvestigated.
Treatment should be discontinued when the patient has reached a satisfactory adult height, when the epiphyses have fused, or when the patient ceases to respond to Asellacrin (somatropin) administration.

Storage: Unreconstituted vials of Asellacrin (somatropin) may be stored at room temperature (15°–30°C/59°–86°F).
Reconstituted vials must be refrigerated (2°–8°C/36°–46°F) and used within one month.

How Supplied: Asellacrin (somatropin), in sterile lyophilized form, is available in 2 IU and 10 IU vials. Vials are packaged individually.

PERGONAL® ℞
(menotropins)

Description: Pergonal® (menotropins) is a purified preparation of gonadotropins extracted from the urine of postmenopausal women. Each ampule of Pergonal® contains 75 I.U. of follicle-stimulating hormone (FSH) activity and 75 I.U. of luteinizing hormone (LH) activity plus 10 mg lactose in a sterile, lyophilized form.
Pergonal® is biologically standardized for FSH and LH (ICSH) gonadotropin activities in terms of the Second International Reference Preparation for Human Menopausal Gonadotropins established in September, 1964, by the Expert Committee on Biological Standards of the World Health Organization.

Actions:
WOMEN:
Pergonal® administered for nine to twelve days produces ovarian follicular growth in women who do not have primary ovarian failure. Treatment with Pergonal® in most instances results only in follicular growth and maturation. In order to effect ovulation, hCG (human chorionic gonadotropin) must be given following the administration of Pergonal® when clinical assessment of the patient indi-

Continued on next page

Serono—Cont.

cates that sufficient follicular maturation has occurred.

MEN:

Pergonal® administered concomitantly with human chorionic gonadotropin (hCG) for at least three months induces spermatogenesis in men with primary or secondary pituitary hypofunction who have achieved adequate masculinization with prior hCG therapy.

Indications:

WOMEN:

Pergonal® and human chorionic gonadotropin (hCG) given in a sequential manner are indicated for the induction of ovulation and pregnancy in the anovulatory infertile patient, in whom the cause of anovulation is functional and is not due to primary ovarian failure.

MEN:

Pergonal® with concomitant hCG is indicated for the stimulation of spermatogenesis in men who have primary or secondary hypogonadotropic hypogonadism.

Pergonal® with concomitant hCG has proven effective in inducing spermatogenesis in men with primary hypogonadotropic hypogonadism due to a congenital factor or prepuberal hypophysectomy and in men with secondary hypogonadotropic hypogonadism due to hypophysectomy, craniopharyngioma, cerebral aneurysm or chromophobe adenoma.

Selection of Patients:

WOMEN:

1. Before treatment with Pergonal® is instituted, a thorough gynecologic and endocrinologic evaluation must be performed. This should include a hysterosalpingogram (to rule out uterine and tubal pathology) and documentation of anovulation by means of basal body temperature, serial vaginal smears, examination of cervical mucus, determination of urinary pregnanediol and endometrial biopsy.
2. Primary ovarian failure should be excluded by the determination of gonadotropin levels.
3. Careful examination should be made to rule out the presence of an early pregnancy.
4. Patients in late reproductive life have a greater predilection to endometrial carcinoma as well as a higher incidence of anovulatory disorders. Cervical dilation and curettage should always be done for diagnosis before starting Pergonal® (menotropins) therapy in such patients.
5. Evaluation of the husband's fertility potential should be included in the workup.

MEN:

Patient selection should be made based on a documented lack of pituitary function. Prior to hormonal therapy, these patients will have low testosterone levels and low or absent gonadotropin levels. Patients with primary hypogonadotropic hypogonadism will have a subnormal development of masculinization, and those with secondary hypogonadotropic hypogonadism will have decreased masculinization.

Contraindications:

WOMEN:

1. A high gonadotropin level indicating primary ovarian failure.
2. The presence of overt thyroid and adrenal dysfunction.
3. An organic intracranial lesion such as a pituitary tumor.
4. The presence of any cause of infertility other than anovulation, as stated in the indications.
5. In patients with abnormal bleeding of undetermined origin.
6. In patients with ovarian cysts or enlargement not due to polycystic ovary syndrome.
7. Pregnancy

MEN:

1. Normal gonadotropin levels indicating normal pituitary function.
2. Elevated gonadotropin levels indicating primary testicular failure.
3. Infertility disorders other than hypogonadotropic hypogonadism.

Warnings: Pergonal® is a drug that should only be used by physicians who are thoroughly familiar with infertility problems. It is a potent gonadotropic substance capable of causing mild to severe adverse reactions in women. In female patients it must be used with a great deal of care.

Precautions:

WOMEN:

1. Diagnosis Prior to Therapy
   Careful attention should be given to diagnosis in candidates for Pergonal® therapy. (See sections headed "Indications" and "Selection of Patients").
2. Overstimulation of the Ovary During Pergonal® Therapy.
   In order to minimize the hazard associated with the occasional abnormal ovarian enlargement associated with Pergonal® -hCG therapy, the lowest dose consistent with expectation of good results should be used.
   Mild to moderate uncomplicated ovarian enlargement which may be accompanied by abdominal distension and/or abdominal pain occurs in approximately 20% of those treated with Pergonal® and hCG, and generally regresses without treatment within two or three weeks.
   The hyperstimulation syndrome characterized by sudden ovarian enlargement accompanied by ascites with or without pain and/or pleural effusion occurs in approximately 0.4% of patients when the recommended dose is administered. In studies performed the overall incidence of the hyperstimulation syndrome was 1.3%.
   If hyperstimulation occurs, treatment should be stopped and the patient hospitalized. The hyperstimulation syndrome develops rapidly over a period of three to four days and generally occurs during the two week period immediately following treatment. The phenomenon of hemoconcentration associated with fluid loss in the abdominal cavity has been seen to occur and should be thoroughly assessed in the following manner: 1) fluid intake and output, 2) weight, 3) hematocrit, 4) serum and urinary electrolytes, and 5) urine specific gravity. These determinations are to be performed daily or more often if the need arises. Treatment is primarily symptomatic and would consist primarily of bed rest, fluid and electrolyte replacement and analgesics if needed. The ascitic fluid should never be removed because of the potential danger of injury to the ovary.
   Hemoperitoneum may occur from ruptured ovarian cysts. This is usually the result of pelvic examination. If this does occur, and if bleeding becomes such that surgery is required, the conservative approach with partial resection of the enlarged ovary or ovaries is generally adequate.
   Intercourse should be prohibited in those patients in whom significant ovarian enlargement occurs after ovulation because of the danger of hemoperitoneum resulting from ruptured ovarian cysts.
3. Arterial Thromboembolism
   Arterial thromboembolism following Pergonal® (menotropins) and hCG therapy has been reported in two patients, one of whom died (1).
4. Multiple Births
   Of the pregnancies following therapy with Pergonal® and hCG, 80% have resulted in single births and 20% in multiple births, most of which have been twins. Fifteen percent of the total pregnancies resulted in twins, of which 93% were viable (78 surviving infants from 43 sets of twins). Five per cent of the total pregnancies have resulted in three or more conceptuses, of which only 20% were viable (nine surviving infants from three sets of triplets, four surviving infants from four sets of quadruplets, and no surviving infants from four sets of quintuplets). The patient and her husband should be advised of the frequency and potential hazards of multiple pregnancy before starting treatment.

Adverse Reactions:

WOMEN:

1. Ovarian Enlargement
2. Hyperstimulation Syndrome
3. Hemoperitoneum
4. Arterial Thromboembolism (see "Precautions" above).
5. Sensitivity to Pergonal®
   Three patients experienced febrile reactions after the administration of Pergonal®. It is not clear whether or not these were pyrogenic responses or possibly allergic reactions.
6. Defects at Birth
   From 287 completed pregnancies following Pergonal®-hCG therapy, five incidents of birth defects have been reported. One infant had multiple congenital anomalies consisting of imperforate anus, aplasia of the sigmoid colon, third degree hypospadias, cecovesicle fistula, bifid scrotum, meningocele, bilateral internal tibial torsion, and right metatarsus adductus. Another infant was born with an imperforate anus and possible congenital heart lesions; another had a supernumerary digit; another was born with hypospadias and exstrophy of the bladder; and the fifth child had Down's syndrome. None of the investigators felt that these defects were drug-related.

MEN:

1. Gynecomastia may occur occasionally during Pergonal®-hCG therapy. This is a known effect of hCG treatment.
2. Erythrocytosis (hct 50% hgb 17.8 g%) was recorded in 1 patient.

Dosage and Administration for Intramuscular Administration

WOMEN:

1. Treatment for Induction of Ovulation
   Treatment with Pergonal® in most instances results only in follicular growth and maturation. In order to effect ovulation, hCG must be given following the administration of Pergonal® when clinical assessment of the patient indicates that sufficient follicular maturation has occurred. This is indirectly estimated by the estrogenic effect upon the target organs. These indices of estrogenic activity include:
   a) Changes in the vaginal smear
   b) Appearance and volume of the cervical mucus
   c) Spinnbarkeit, and
   d) Ferning of the cervical mucus.

If available, the urinary excretion of estrogens is a more reliable index of follicular maturation.

The clinical confirmation of ovulation, with the exception of pregnancy, is obtained by indirect indices of progesterone production. The indices most generally used are as follows:

a) a rise in basal body temperature
b) change of the cervical mucus from a "fern" pattern to a "cellular" pattern
c) vaginal cytology characteristic of the luteal phase of the menstrual cycle
d) increase in urinary pregnanediol, and
e) menstruation following the shift in basal body temperature.

Because of the subjectivity of the various tests for the determination of follicular maturation and ovulation, it cannot be over-emphasized that the physician should choose tests with which he is thoroughly familiar.

2. Dosage of Pergonal®
The dose of Pergonal® to produce maturation of the follicle must be individualized for each patient. It is recommended that the initial dose to any patient should be 75 I.U. of FSH and 75 I.U. of LH (one ampule) per day, **ADMINISTERED INTRAMUSCULARLY**, for nine to twelve days followed by hCG, 10,000 I.U., one day after the last dose of Pergonal®. The hyperstimulation syndrome has never occurred with administration of 75 I.U. of FSH and 75 I.U. of LH (one ampule) per day for up to twelve days. Administration of Pergonal® should not exceed 12 days. The patient should be treated until indices of estrogenic activity, as indicated under Item 1 above, are equivalent to or greater than those of the normal individual. If urinary estrogen determinations are available, they may be useful as a guide to therapy. If the total estrogen excretion is less than 100 mcg/24 hours or the estriol excretion is less than 50 mcg/24 hours prior to hCG administration, the hyperstimulation syndrome is less likely to occur. If the estrogen values are greater than this it is not advisable to administer hCG because the hyperstimulation syndrome is more likely to occur. If the ovaries are abnormally enlarged on the last day of Pergonal® therapy, hCG should not be administered in this course of therapy; this will reduce the chances of development of the hyperstimulation syndrome. If there is evidence of ovulation but no pregnancy, repeat this dosage regime for at least two more courses before increasing the dose of Pergonal® to 150 I.U. of FSH and 150 I.U. of LH (two ampules) per day for nine to twelve days. As before, this dose should be followed by 10,000 I.U. of hCG one day after the last dose of Pergonal®. 150 I.U. of FSH and 150 I.U. of LH (two ampules) of Pergonal® per day has proven to be the most effective dose. If evidence of ovulation is present, but pregnancy does not ensue, repeat the same dose for two more courses. Doses larger than this are not recommended.
During treatment with both Pergonal® and hCG and during a two-week post-treatment period, patients should be examined at least every other day for signs of excessive ovarian stimulation. It is recommended that Pergonal® administration be stopped if the ovaries become abnormally enlarged or abdominal pain occurs. Most of of ovarian hyperstimulation occurs after treatment has been discontinued and reaches its maximum at about seven to ten days post-ovulation. Patients should be followed for at least two week after hCG administration.
The couple should be encouraged to have intercourse daily beginning on the day prior to the administration of hCG until ovulation becomes apparent from the indices employed for the determination of progestational activity. Care should be taken to insure insemination. In the light of the foregoing indices and parameters mentioned, it should become obvious that, unless a physician is willing to devote considerable time to these patients and be familiar with and conduct the necessary laboratory studies, he should not use Pergonal® (menotropins).

3. How to Administer Pergonal®
Dissolve the contents of one ampule of Pergonal® in one to two ml. of sterile saline and **ADMINISTER INTRAMUSCULARLY** immediately. Any unused reconstituted material should be discarded.

MEN:

1. Dosage of Pergonal®
Prior to concomitant therapy with Pergonal® (hMG) and hCG, pretreatment with hCG alone (5000 IU three times a week) is required. Treatment should continue for a period sufficient to achieve serum testosterone levels within the normal range and masculinization as judged by the appearance of secondary sex characteristics. Such pretreatment may require four to six months, then the recommended dose of Pergonal® is one ampule **ADMINISTERED INTRAMUSCULARLY**, three times a week and the recommended dose of hCG is 2,000 IU twice a week. Therapy should be carried on for a minimum of four more months to insure detecting spermatozoa in the ejaculate, as it takes 74 ± 4 days in the human male for germ cells to reach the spermatozoa stage.
In one clinical series consisting of nine patients, 4 patients produced 2 million sperm per ejaculate with a dosage of Pergonal® of 25 IU every other day concomitantly with 2,000 IU hCG three times a week. When 38 IU of Pergonal® every other day was administered, 7 of the 9 subjects produced at least 2 million sperm per ejaculate, and at the higher dose of 75 I.U. of Pergonal® every other day, 8 of the 9 subjects were sperm positive at 2 million per ejaculate. In this series, Pergonal® was administered concomitantly with 2,000 IU hCG three times a week, after achievement of adequate masculinization with prior hCG therapy. The nonresponder had a history of surgical orchiopexy to repair bilateral cryptorchidism at the age of 12, and this may have complicated the response of his testes to gonadotropin replacement. The results obtained in this series are in keeping with very recent studies quantitating the production rate of FSH in the human as approximately 30 or 40 IU a day.
If the patient has not responded with evidence of increased spermatogenesis at the end of four months therapy, treatment may continue with one ampule of Pergonal® three times a week, or the dose can be increased to two ampules (150 IU FSH and 150 IU LH) three times a week, with the hCG dose unchanged.

2. How to Administer Pergonal®
Dissolve the contents of one ampule of Pergonal® in one to two ml of sterile saline and **ADMINISTER INTRAMUSCULARLY** immediately. Any unused reconstituted material should be discarded.

How Supplied: Each ampule of Pergonal® (menotropins) contains 75 I.U. of FSH and 75 I.U. of LH (ICSH). By biological assay, one I.U. of LH for the Second International Reference Preparation (2nd-IRP) for hMG is biologically equivalent to approximately ½ I.U. of human chorionic gonadotropin (hCG).

Clinical Studies:

WOMEN:

The results of the clinical experience and effectiveness of the administration of Pergonal® (menotropins) to 1,286 patients in 3,002 courses of therapy are summarized below. The values include patients who were treated with other than the recommended dosage regime. The values for the presently recommended dosage regime are essentially the same, except for the fact that the hyperstimulation syndrome has not occurred with administration of 75 I.U. of Pergonal® per day for 9 to 12 days and the incidence of the hyperstimulation syndrome with administration of 150 I.U. of Pergonal® per day for 9 to 12 days has not exceeded 0.4%.

	%
Patients ovulating	75
Patients pregnant	25
Patients aborting	25*
Multiple pregnancies	20†
Twins	15†
Three or more conceptuses	5†
Fetal abnormalities	1.7†
Hyperstimulation syndrome	1.3

* Based on total pregnancies
† Based on total deliveries

Results by diagnosis group are summarized below. (These values include patients who were treated with other than the present recommended dosage regime).
[See table above].

	% Pts. Ovul.	% Pts. Preg.	% Abort	% Multi Preg.	% Twins	% 3 or More Conceptuses	% Hyper-stim. Syndr.
Primary Amenorrhea	62	22	14	25	25	0	0
Secondary Amenorrhea	61	28	24	28	18	10	1.9
Secondary Amen. with Galactorrhea	77	42	21	41	31	10	1.2
Polycystic Ovaries	76	26	39	17	17	0	1.1
Anovulatory Cycles	77	24	15	14	9	5	2.0
Miscellaneous	83	20	36	2	2	0	0.1

MEN:

Clinical results of the treatment of men with primary or secondary hypogonadotropic hypogonadism are as follows:
In the Serono Cooperative study, with an adequate treatment period of 3 to 8 months, 60 of 70 men with primary hypogonadotropic hypogonadism and 8 of 11 men with secondary hypogonadotropic hypogonadism responded with mean increases in their sperm counts from less than 5 to 24 million spermatozoa per milliliter of ejaculate. Forty-one wives of 54 men with primary hypogonadotropic hypogonadism desiring offspring and 7 wives of men with secondary hypogonadotropic hypogonadism conceived. Patients treated with Pergonal® and hCG for less than 3 months or with Pergonal® alone did not respond to therapy.
A world-wide data search revealed that of 160 recorded pregnancies as the result of use of Pergonal® -hCG in men, there were 7 spontaneous abortions, one ectopic pregnancy and 3 congenital anomalies at birth (esophageal atresia in a female infant which was later corrected by surgery, unilateral cryptorchidism, inguinal hernia).

References:

1. Mozes, M., Bogokowsky, H., Antebi, E., et al.: Thromboembolic phenomena after ovarian stimulation with human gonadotropins, Lancet 2:1213–1215, 1965.

PROFASI HP® ℞
(chorionic gonadotropin)
FOR INJECTION, U.S.P.

Description: Human chorionic gonadotropin (HCG), a polypeptide hormone produced by the human placenta, is composed of an alpha and a beta sub-unit. The alpha sub-unit is essentially identical to the alpha sub-unit of the human pituitary gonadotropins, luteinizing hormone (LH) and follicle-stimulating hormone (FSH), as well as to the alpha sub-unit of human thyroid-stimulating hormone (TSH). The beta sub-units of these hormones differ in amino acid sequence. Chorionic Gonadotropin

Continued on next page

Serono—Cont.

is derived from the urine of pregnant women. It is standardized by a biological assay procedure.

Actions: The action of HCG is virtually identical to that of pituitary LH, although HCG appears to have a small degree of FSH activity as well. It stimulates production of gonadal steroid hormones by stimulating the Interstitial cells, (Leydig cells) of the testis to produce androgens and the corpus luteum of the ovary to produce progesterone. Andorgen stimulation in the male leads to the development of secondary sex characteristics and may stimulate testicular descent when no anatomical impediment to descent is present. This descent is usually reversible when HCG is discontinued. During the normal menstrual cycle, LH participates with FSH in the development and maturation of the normal ovarian follicle, and the mid-cycle LH surge triggers ovulation. HCG can substitute for LH in this function. During a normal pregnancy, HCG secreted by the placenta maintains the corpus luteum after LH secretion decreases, supporting continued secretion of estrogen and progesterone and preventing menstruation. HCG HAS NO KNOWN EFFECT ON FAT MOBILIZATION, APPETITE OR SENSE OF HUNGER, OR BODY FAT DISTRIBUTION.

Indications: HCG HAS NOT BEEN DEMONSTRATED TO BE EFFECTIVE ADJUNCTIVE THERAPY IN THE TREATMENT OF OBESITY. THERE IS NO SUBSTANTIAL EVIDENCE THAT IT INCREASES WEIGHT LOSS BEYOND THAT RESULTING FROM CALORIC RESTRICTION, THAT IT CAUSES A MORE ATTRACTIVE OR "NORMAL" DISTRIBUTION OF FAT, OR THAT IT DECREASES THE HUNGER AND DISCOMFORT ASSOCIATED WITH CALORIE-RESTRICTED DIETS.

1. Prepubertal cryptorchidism not due to anatomical obstruction. In general, HCG is thought to induce testicular descent in situations when descent would have occurred at puberty. HCG thus may help predict whether or not orchiopexy will be needed in the future. Although, in some cases, descent following HCG administration is permanent, in most cases, the response is temporary. Therapy is usually instituted between the ages of 4 and 9.
2. Selected cases of hypogonadotropic hypogonadism (hypogonadism secondary to a pituitary deficiency) in males.
3. Induction of ovulation in the anovulatory, infertile woman in whom the cause of anovulation is secondary and not due to primary ovarian failure, and who has been appropriately pre-treated with human menotropins.

Contraindications: Precocious puberty, prostatic carcinoma or other androgen-dependent neoplasm, prior allergic reaction to HCG.

Warnings: HCG should be used in conjunction with human menopausal gonadotropins only by physicians experienced with infertility problems who are familiar with the criteria for patient selection, contraindications, warnings, precautions, and adverse reactions described in the package insert for menotropins. The principal serious adverse reactions during this use are: (1) Ovarian hyperstimulation, a syndrome of sudden ovarian enlargement, ascites with or without pain, and/or pleural effusion, (2) Rupture of ovarian cysts with resultant hemoperitoneum, (3) Multiple births, and (4) Arterial thromboembolism. If the hyperstimulation syndrome occurs, treatment should be stopped and the patient hospitalized.

Precautions: Induction of androgen secretion by HCG may induce precocious puberty in patients treated for cryptorchidism. Therapy should be discontinued if signs of precocious puberty occur.

Since androgens may cause fluid retention, HCG should be used with caution in patients with cardiac or renal disease, epilepsy, migraine, or asthma.

Adverse Reactions: Headache, irritability, restlessness, depression, fatigue, edema, precocious puberty, gynecomastia, pain at the site of injection.

Dosage and Administration (Intramuscular Use Only): The dosage regimen employed in any particular case will depend upon the indication for use, the age and weight of the patient, and the physician's preference. The following regimens have been advocated by various authorities.

Prepubertal cryptorchidism not due to anatomical obstruction.

1. 4,000 U.S.P. Units three times weekly for three weeks.
2. 5,000 U.S.P. Units every second day for four injections.
3. 15 injections of 500 to 1,000 U.S.P. Units over a period of six weeks.
4. 500 U.S.P. Units three times weekly for four to six weeks. If this course of treatment is not successful, another is begun one month later giving 1,000 U.S.P. Units per injection.

Selected cases of hypogonadotropic hypogonadism in males.

1. 500 to 1,000 U.S.P. Units three times a week for three weeks, followed by the same dose twice a week for three weeks.
2. 4,000 U.S.P. Units three times weekly for six to nine months, following which the dosage may be reduced to 2,000 U.S.P. Units three times weekly for an additional three months.

Induction of ovulation in the anovulatory, infertile woman in whom the cause of anovulation is secondary and not due to primary ovarian failure and who has been appropriately pretreated with human menotropins (See prescribing information for menotropins for dosage and administration for that drug product). 5,000 to 10,000 U.S.P. Units one day following the last dose of menotropins. (A dosage of 10,000 U.S.P. Units is recommended in the labeling for menotropins).

IMPORTANT: USE COMPLETELY WITHIN 60 DAYS AFTER RECONSTITUTION, REFRIGERATE AFTER RECONSTITUTION.

How Supplied: The freeze-dried, stabilized active principle is supplied in the two vial package including Bacteriostatic Water for Injection as diluent. When reconstituted, each vial contains in U.S.P. Units:

VIAL SIZE:	10 ml.	10 ml.
Chorionic Gonadotropin	5,000 U.	10,000 U.
Mannitol, U.S.P.	50 mg.	100 mg.
Benzyl Alcohol, N.F.	0.9%	0.9%

with Sodium Phosphate Dibasic and Sodium Phosphate Monobasic to adjust pH.

The product is assayed in accord with the U.S.P. method and potencies refer to U.S.P. Units (International Units) defined in terms of the U.S.P. Chorionic Gonadotropin Reference Standard.

Caution: Federal law prohibits dispensing without prescription.

Directions For Reconstitution: TWO-VIAL PACKAGE: withdraw sterile air from lyophilized vial and inject into diluent vial. Remove 10 ml. from diluent and add to lyophilized vial; agitate gently until solution is complete.

Revised January 1982

SEROPHENE® ℞
(clomiphene citrate tablets, U.S.P.)

Description: Each scored white tablet contains:

Clomiphene Citrate USP 50 mg. Clomiphene citrate is designated chemically as 2-[p-(2-chloro-1,2-diphenylvinyl) phenoxy] triethylamine dihydrogen citrate and is represented structurally as:

$(C_2H_5)_2NCH_2CH_2O$–C6H4–C(C6H5) = C(Cl)–C6H5 · $C_6H_8O_7$

As shown, one molecule of citric acid is chemically bound with one molecule of the organic base, clomiphene.

Clomiphene citrate is a chemical analog of other triarylethylene compounds such as chlorotrianisene and the cholesterol inhibitor, triparanol.

Actions: Clomiphene citrate, an orally-administered, non-steroidal agent, may induce ovulation in selected anovulatory women. It is a drug of considerable pharmacologic potency. Careful evaluation and selection of the patient and close attention to the timing of the dose is mandatory prior to treatment with clomiphene citrate. Conservative selection and management of the patient contribute to successful therapy of anovulation. Clomiphene citrate induces ovulation in most selected anovulatory patients. The various criteria for ovulation include: an ovulation peak of estrogen excretion followed by a biphasic basal body temperature curve; urinary excretion of pregnanediol at post-ovulatory levels and, endometrial histologic findings characteristic of the luteal phase.

A review of eleven publications appearing between 1964 and 1978 showed that pregnancy occurred in 35% of 5154 patients with ovulatory dysfunction who received clomiphene citrate.

[See table left].

PREGNANCIES FOLLOWING CLOMIPHENE CITRATE U.S.P.[a]			(Range)
Number of Patients	=	5154	
Percent of Patients Ovulating[b]	=	75	(50-94)%
Percent of Ovulatory Cycles	=	53	(33-69)%
Percent of Patients Pregnant	=	35	(11-52)%
Percent Patients Pregnant / Percent Patients Ovulating	=	46	(22-61)%
Percent Live Births	=	86	(74-99.8)%
Percent Abortions	=	14	(0.2-26)%
Percent of Single Births	=	90	(67-100)%
Percent Surviving	=	99	(98.2-100)%
Percent of Multiple Births	=	10	(0-33)%
Percent Surviving	=	96	(82-100)%

a) includes patients receiving other than recommended dosage regimen.
b) average from studies

Clomiphene citrate therapy appears to mediate ovulation through increased output of pituitary gonadotropins. These stimulate the maturation and endocrine activity of the ovarian follicle which is followed by the development and function of the corpus luteum. Increased urinary excretion of gonadotropins and estrogen suggest involvement of the pituitary.

Studies with ^{14}C labeled clomiphene citrate have shown that is readily absorbed orally in humans, and is excreted principally in the feces. An average of 51% of the administered dose was excreted after 5 days. After intravenous administration 37% was excreted in 5 days. The appearance of ^{14}C in the feces six weeks after administration suggests that the remaining drug and/or metabolites are slowly excreted from a sequestered enterohepatic recirculation pool.

Indications: Clomiphene citrate is indicated for the treatment of ovulatory failure in patients desiring pregnancy, and whose husbands are fertile and potent. Impediments to this goal must be excluded or adequately treated before beginning therapy. Administration of clomiphene citrate is indicated only in patients with demonstrated ovulatory dysfunction and in whom the following conditions apply:

1. Normal liver function.
2. Physiologic indications of normal endogenous estrogen (as estimated from vaginal smears, endometrial biopsy, assay of urinary estrogen, or from bleeding in response to progesterone). Reduced estrogen levels, while less favorable, do not prevent successful therapy.
3. Clomiphene citrate therapy is not effective for those patients with primary pituitary or ovarian failure. It cannot substitute for appropriate therapy of other disturbances leading to ovulatory dysfunction, e.g., diseases of the thyroid or adrenals.
4. Particularly careful evaluation prior to clomiphene citrate therapy should be done in patients with abnormal uterine bleeding. It is most important that neoplastic lesions are detected.

Contraindications:

Pregnancy

Although no direct effect of clomiphene citrate therapy on the human fetus has been seen, clomiphene citrate should not be administered in cases of suspected pregnancy as such effects have been reported in animals. To prevent inadvertent clomiphene citrate administration during early pregnancy, the basal body temperature should be recorded throughout all treatment cycles, and therapy should be discontinued if pregnancy is suspected. If the basal body temperature following clomiphene citrate is biphasic and is not followed by menses, the possibility of an ovarian cyst and/or pregnancy should be excluded. Until the correct diagnosis has been determined, the next course of therapy should be delayed.

Liver Disease

Patients with liver disease or a history of liver dysfunction should not receive clomiphene citrate therapy.

Abnormal Uterine Bleeding

Clomiphene citrate is contraindicated in patients with abnormal uterine bleeding.

Warnings:

Visual Symptoms

Patiens should be warned that blurring and/or other visual symptoms may occur occasionally with clomiphene citrate therapy. These may make activities such as driving or operating machinery more hazardous than usual, particularly under conditions of variable lighting. While their significance is not yet understood (see ADVERSE REACTIONS), patients having any visual symptoms, should discontinue treatment and have a complete ophthalmologic evaluation.

Precautions:

Diagnosis Prior to Clomiphene Citrate Therapy

Careful evaluation should be given to candidates for clomiphene citrate therapy. A complete pelvic examination should be performed prior to treatment and repeated before each subsequent course. Clomiphene citrate should not be given to patients with an ovarian cyst, as further ovarian enlargement may result.
Since the incidence of endometrial carcinoma and of ovulatory disorders increases with age, endometrial biopsy should always exclude the former as causative in such patients. If abnormal uterine bleeding is present, full diagnostic measures are necessary.

Ovarian Overstimulation During Treatment with Clomiphene Citrate

To minimize the hazard associated with the occasional abnormal ovarian enlargement during clomiphene citrate therapy (see ADVERSE REACTIONS), the lowest dose producing good results should be chosen. Some patients with polycystic ovary syndrome are unusually sensitive to gonadotropin and may have an exaggerated response to usual doses of clomiphene citrate. Maximal enlargement of the ovary, whether abnormal or physiologic, does not occur until several days after discontinuation of clomiphene citrate. The patient complaining of pelvic pains after receiving clomiphene citrate should be examined carefully. If enlargement of the ovary occurs, clomiphene citrate therapy should be withheld until the ovaries have returned to pretreatment size, and the dosage or duration of the next course should be reduced. The ovarian enlargement and cyst formation following clomiphene citrate therapy regress spontaneously within a few days or weeks after discontinuing treatment. Therefore, unless a strong indication for laparotomy exists, such cystic enlargement always should be managed conservatively.

Multiple Pregnancy

In the reviewed publications, the incidence of multiple pregnancies was increased during those cycles in which clomiphene citrate was given. Among the 1803 pregnancies on which the outcome was reported, 90% were single and 10% twins. Less than 1% of the reported deliveries resulted in triplets or more.
Of these multiple pregnancies, 96-99% resulted in the births of live infants. The patient and her husband should be advised of the frequency and potential hazards of multiple pregnancy before starting treatment.

Adverse Reactions:

Symptoms

Side effects are not prominent at the recommended dosage of clomiphene citrate and infrequently interfere with treatment. Side effects tend to occur more frequently at higher doses and in the longer treatment courses used in some early studies. The more common side effects and the percent of patients experiencing them include vasomotor flushes (11%), abdominal discomfort (7.4%), abnormal uterine bleeding (0.5%), ovarian enlargement (14%), breast tenderness (2.1%), and visual symptoms (1.6%). The vasomotor symptoms resemble menopausal "hot flushes", and are not usually severe. They promptly disappear after treatment is discontinued. Abdominal discomfort may resemble ovulatory (mittelschmerz) or premenstrual phenomena, or that due to ovarian enlargement. In addition, nausea and vomiting (2.1%), nervousness and insomnia (1.9%), headache (1%), dizziness and lightheadedness (1%), increased urination (0.9%), depression and fatigue (0.8%), urticaria and allergic dermatitis (0.6%), weight gain (0.4%), and reversible hair loss (0.3%) have been reported.
When clomiphene citrate is administered at the recommended dose, abnormal ovarian enlargement (see PRECAUTIONS) is infrequent, although the usual cyclic variation in ovarian size may be exaggerated. Similarly, mid-cycle ovarian pain (mittelschmerz) may be accentuated. With prolonged or higher dosage, ovarian enlargement and cyst formation (usually luteal) may occur more often and the luteal phase of the cycle may be prolonged. Patients with polycystic ovary disease may be unusually sensitive to clomiphene therapy. Rare occurrences of massive ovarian enlargement have been reported, for example, in a patient with polycystic ovary syndrome whose clomiphene citrate therapy consisted of 100 mg daily for 14 days. Since abnormal ovarian enlargement usually regresses spontaneously, most of these patients should be treated conservatively.

The incidence of visual symptoms (see WARNINGS for further recommendations), usually described as "blurring" or spots or flashes (scintillating scotomata), correlates with increasing total dose. The symptoms disappear within a few days or weeks after clomiphene citrate is discontinued. This may be due to intensification and/or prolongation of after-images. Symptoms often appear first, or are accentuated, upon exposure to a more brightly lit environment. While measured visual acuity has not generally been affected, in one patient taking 200 mg daily, visual blurring developed on the seventh day of treatment, and progressed to severe diminution of visual acuity by the tenth day. No other abnormality was coincident, and the visual acuity was normal by the third day after treatment was stopped. Ophthalmologically definable scotomata and electroetinographic retinal function changes have also been reported.

BSP Laboratory Studies

Greater than 5% retention of sulfobromophthalein (BSP) has been reported in approximately 10 to 20% of patients in whom it was measured. Retention was usually minimal but was elevated during prolonged clomiphene citrate administration or with apparently unrelated liver disease. In some patients, preexisting BSP retention decreased even though clomiphene citrate therapy was continued. Other liver function tests were usually normal.

Other Laboratory Studies

Clomiphene citrate has not been reported to cause a significant abnormality in hematologic or renal tests, in protein bound iodine, or in serum cholesterol levels.

Birth Defects

Of 1803 births following clomiphene-citrate administration, 45 infants with birth defects were reported for a cumulative rate of 2.5%. Six cases of Down's Syndrome, one neonatal death with multiple malformations and one case each of the following were reported: extropia, club foot, tibial torsion, blocked tear duct and hemangioma. The other congenital abnormalities were not described. The investigators did not report that these were presumed to be due to therapy. The cumulative rate of congenital abnormalities does not exceed that reported in the general population.

Dosage and Administration:

General Considerations

Physicians experienced in managing gynecologic or endocrine disorders should supervise the work-up and treatment of candidate patients for clomiphene citrate therapy. Patients should be chosen for clomiphene citrate therapy only after careful diagnostic evaluation (see INDICATIONS). The plan of therapy should be outlined in advance. Impediments to achieving the goal of therapy must be excluded or adequately treated before beginning clomiphene citrate.
In determining a starting dose schedule, efficacy must be balanced against potential side effects. For example, the available data so far suggests that ovulation and pregnancy are slightly more attainable with 100 mg/day for 5 days then with 50 mg/day for 5 days. As the dosage is increased, however, ovarian overstimulation and other side effects may be expected to increase. Although the data do not yet establish a relationship between dose level and multiple births, it is reasonable that such a correlation exists on pharmacologic grounds.
For these reasons, treatment of the usual patient should initiate with a 50 mg daily dose for 5 days. The dose may be increased only in those patients who do not respond to the first course (see Recommended Dosage). Special treatment with lower dosage over shorter duration is particularly recommended if unusual sensitivity to pituitary gonadotropin is suspected, includ-

Continued on next page

Serono—Cont.

ing patients with polycystic ovary syndrome (see Precautions).

Recommended Dosage

The recommended dosage for the first course of clomiphene citrate is 50 mg (1 tablet) daily for 5 days. Therapy may be started at any time if the patient has had no recent uterine bleeding. If progestin-induced bleeding is intended or if spontaneous uterine bleeding occurs prior to therapy, the regimen of 50 mg daily for 5 days should be started on or about the fifth day of the cycle. When ovulation occurs at this dosage, there is no advantage to increasing the dose in subsequent cycles of treatment.

If ovulation does not appear to have occurred after the first course of therapy, a second course of 100 mg daily (two 50 mg tablets given as a single daily dose) for 5 days may be started. This course may begin as early as 30 days after the previous one. Increasing the dosage or duration of therapy beyond 100 mg/day for 5 days should not be undertaken.

The majority of patients who respond do so during the first course of therapy, and 3 courses constitute an adequate therapeutic trial. If ovulatory menses do not occur, the diagnosis should be re-evaluated. Treatment beyond this is not recommended in the patient who does not exhibit evidence of ovulation.

Pregnancy

Properly timed coitus is very important for good results. For regularity of cyclic ovulatory response it is also important that each course of clomiphene citrate be started on or about the first day of the cycle, once ovulation has been established. As with other therapeutic modalities, Serophene therapy follows the rule of diminishing returns, such that likelihood of conception diminishes with each succeeding course of therapy. If pregnancy has not been achieved after 3 ovulatory responses to Serophene, further treatment is not generally recommended. Before starting treatment. Patients should be advised of the possibility and potential hazards of multiple pregnancy if conception occurs following clomiphene citrate therapy.

Long-Term Cyclic Therapy—Not Recommended

Since the relative safety of long-term cyclic therapy has not yet been conclusively demonstrated, and since the majority of patients will ovulate following 3 courses, long-term cyclic therapy is not recommended.

How Supplied: Serophene is available as 50 mg scored white tablets, packaged in cartons of 30. Each carton contains 3 strips of 10 tablets, each in 1 2 × 5 arrangement.

PRODUCT INFORMATION: AVAILABLE ONLY ON PRESCRIPTION

For additional information, please contact:
Serono Laboratories, Inc.
Director of Clinical Affairs
280 Pond Street
Randolph, MA 02368
800-225-5185 (Toll free, outside MA)
617-963-8154 (Inside MA)

Products are cross-indexed

by product classifications

in the

BLUE SECTION

Smith Kline & French Laboratories

Division of SmithKline Beckman Corporation
1500 SPRING GARDEN ST.
P.O. BOX 7929
PHILADELPHIA, PA 19101

SK&F Co.

Carolina, P.R. 00630
Subsidiary of SmithKline Beckman Corporation

SK&F Lab Co.

Carolina, P.R. 00630
Subsidiary of SmithKline Beckman Corporation

Menley & James Laboratories

a SmithKline company
P.O. BOX 8082
PHILADELPHIA, PA 19101

SK&F PRODUCT CODE INDEX

Code	Product, Form and Strength
C44	'Compazine' *Spansule* capsules 10 mg.
C46	'Compazine' *Spansule* capsules 15 mg.
C47	'Compazine' *Spansule* capsules 30 mg.
C49	'Compazine' *Spansule* capsules 75 mg.
C60	'Compazine' Suppositories 2 ½ mg.
C61	'Compazine' Suppositories 5 mg.
C62	'Compazine' Suppositories 25 mg.
C66	'Compazine' Tablets 5 mg.
C67	'Compazine' Tablets 10 mg.
C69	'Compazine' Tablets 25 mg.
D14	'Cytomel' Tablets 5 mcg.
D16	'Cytomel' Tablets 25 mcg.
D17	'Cytomel' Tablets 50 mcg.
D62	'Darbid' Tablets 5 mg.
E12	'Dexedrine' *Spansule* capsules 5 mg.
E13	'Dexedrine' *Spansule* capsules 10 mg.
E14	'Dexedrine' *Spansule* capsules 15 mg.
E19	'Dexedrine' Tablets 5 mg.
E33	'Dibenzyline' Capsules 10 mg.
J09	'Eskalith' Tablets 300 mg.
J10	'Eskalith' Controlled Release Tablets 450 mg.
K77	'Hispril' *Spansule* capsules 5 mg.
120	'SK-Amitriptyline' Tablets 10 mg.
121	'SK-Amitriptyline' Tablets 25 mg.
123	'SK-Amitriptyline' Tablets 50 mg.
124	'SK-Amitriptyline' Tablets 75 mg.
131	'SK-Amitriptyline' Tablets 100 mg.
132	'SK-Amitriptyline' Tablets 150 mg.
101	'SK-Ampicillin' Capsules 250 mg.
102	'SK-Ampicillin' Capsules 500 mg.
174	'SK-APAP' Tablets 325 mg.
494	'SK-APAP' with Codeine Tablets 300 mg./15 mg.
496	'SK-APAP' with Codeine Tablets 300 mg./30 mg.
497	'SK-APAP' with Codeine Tablets 300 mg./60 mg.
133	'SK-Bamate' Tablets 200 mg.
134	'SK-Bamate' Tablets 400 mg.
176	'SK-Chloral Hydrate' Capsules 500 mg.
419	'SK-Chlorothiazide' Tablets 250 mg.
420	'SK-Chlorothiazide' Tablets 500 mg.
374	'SK-Dexamethasone' Tablets 0.5 mg.
376	'SK-Dexamethasone' Tablets 0.75 mg.
377	'SK-Dexamethasone' Tablets 1.5 mg.
303	'SK-Diphenhydramine' Capsules 25 mg.
304	'SK-Diphenhydramine' Capsules 50 mg.
423	'SK-Diphenoxylate' Tablets 2.5 mg./.025 mg.
367	'SK-Erythromycin' Tablets 250 mg.
369	'SK-Erythromycin' Tablets 500 mg.
340	'SK-Furosemide' Tablets 20 mg.
341	'SK-Furosemide' Tablets 40 mg.
363	'SK-Hydrochlorothiazide' Tablets 25 mg.
364	'SK-Hydrochlorothiazide' Tablets 50 mg.
441	'SK-Lygen' Capsules 5 mg.
442	'SK-Lygen' Capsules 10 mg.
443	'SK-Lygen' Capsules 25 mg.
111	'SK-Penicillin G' Tablets 400,000 units
112	'SK-Penicillin G' Tablets 800,000 units
116	'SK-Penicillin VK' Tablets 250 mg.
117	'SK-Penicillin VK' Tablets 500 mg.
136	'SK-Phenobarbital' Tablets 15 mg.
137	'SK-Phenobarbital' Tablets 30 mg.
321	'SK-Pramine' Tablets 10 mg.
322	'SK-Pramine' Tablets 25 mg.
323	'SK-Pramine' Tablets 50 mg.
339	'SK-Prednisone' Tablets 5 mg.
499	'SK-Probenecid' Tablets 500 mg.
310	'SK-Propantheline Bromide' Tablets 15 mg.
171	'SK-Quinidine Sulfate' Tablets 200 mg.
169	'SK-Reserpine' Tablets 0.25 mg.
463	'SK-65' Capsules 65 mg.
467	'SK-65 Compound' Capsules
474	'SK-65 APAP' Tablets
163	'SK-Soxazole' Tablets 500 mg.
126	'SK-Tetracycline' Capsules 250 mg.
127	'SK-Tetracycline' Capsules 500 mg.
409	'SK-Tolbutamide' Tablets 500 mg.
S03	*'Stelazine' Tablets 1 mg.
S04	*'Stelazine' Tablets 2 mg.
S06	*'Stelazine' Tablets 5 mg.
S07	*'Stelazine' Tablets 10 mg.
T01	'Temaril' *Spansule* capsules 5 mg.
T03	'Temaril' Tablets 2.5 mg.
T63	'Thorazine' *Spansule* capsules 30 mg.
T64	'Thorazine' *Spansule* capsules 75 mg.
T66	'Thorazine' *Spansule* capsules 150 mg.
T67	'Thorazine' *Spansule* capsules 200 mg.
T69	'Thorazine' *Spansule* capsules 300 mg.
T70	'Thorazine' Suppositories 25 mg.
T71	'Thorazine' Suppositories 100 mg.
T73	'Thorazine' Tablets 10 mg.
T74	'Thorazine' Tablets 25 mg.
T76	'Thorazine' Tablets 50 mg.
T77	'Thorazine' Tablets 100 mg.
T79	'Thorazine' Tablets 200 mg.
V90	'Urispas' Tablets 100 mg.

*A product of SK&F Co., Carolina, P.R. 00630, Subsidiary of SmithKline Beckman Corporation, Philadelphia, Pa.

ACNOMEL® CREAM

acne therapy

Marketed by Menley & James Laboratories, a SmithKline company.
(See PDR For Nonprescription Drugs)

ANCEF® ℞

(brand of sterile cefazolin sodium)
(lyophilized)

Description: Ancef (sterile cefazolin sodium, SK&F) is a semi-synthetic cephalosporin for parenteral administration. It is the sodium salt of 3-{[(5-methyl-1,3,4-thiadiazol-2-yl)thio]methyl} -8-oxo-7-[2- (1H-tetrazol-1-yl) acetamido]-5 - thia -1- azabicyclo [4.2.0] oct-2-ene-2-carboxylic acid.

The sodium content is 46 mg. per gram of cefazolin.

'Ancef' is supplied in vials equivalent to 250 mg., 500 mg. or 1 gram of cefazolin; in "Piggyback" Vials for intravenous admixture equivalent to 500 mg. or 1 gram of cefazolin; and in Pharmacy Bulk Vials equivalent to 5 grams or 10 grams of cefazolin.

Clinical Pharmacology:

Human Pharmacology: The following tables demonstrate the blood levels and duration of cefazolin following the administration of 'Ancef'.

TABLE 1
Duration of Blood Levels of Cefazolin
250 mg. I.M. Dose (Figures are μg./ml.)

	Time After Injection in Hours				
	½	1	2	4	6
CEFAZOLIN	15.5	17.0	13.0	5.1	2.5

TABLE 2
500 mg. I.M. Dose (Figures are μg./ml.)

	Time After Injection in Hours					
	½	1	2	4	6	8
CEFAZOLIN	36.2	36.8	37.9	15.5	6.3	3.0

TABLE 3
1 gram I.M. Dose (Figures are μg./ml.)

	Time After Injection in Hours						
	½	1	2	4	6	8	10
CEFAZOLIN*	60.1	63.8	54.3	29.3	13.2	7.1	< 4.1

*Average of the two studies

Clinical pharmacology studies in patients hospitalized with infections indicate that Ancef (sterile cefazolin sodium, SK&F) produces mean peak serum levels approximately equivalent to those seen in normal volunteers.

In a study (using normal volunteers) of constant intravenous infusion with dosages of 3.5 mg./kg. for 1 hour (approximately 250 mg.) and 1.5 mg./kg. the next two hours (approximately 100 mg.), 'Ancef' produced a steady serum level at the third hour of approximately 28 μg./ml. The following table shows the average serum concentration and average half life of cefazolin after I.V. injection of a single 1 gram dose of 'Ancef'.

TABLE 4
1 gram I.V. Dose (Figures are μg./ml.)

	Time After Injection, Min.			
	5	15	30	60
CEFAZOLIN	188.4	135.8	106.8	73.7

1 gram. I.V. Dose (Figures are μg./ml.)

	Time After Injection, Min.			
	120	240	Peak	Half-life in Hours
CEFAZOLIN	45.6	16.5	190.0	1.4

Controlled studies on adult normal volunteers, receiving 1 gram 4 times a day for 10 days, monitoring CBC, SGOT, SGPT, bilirubin, alkaline phosphatase, BUN, creatinine, and urinalysis, indicated no clinically significant changes attributed to 'Ancef'.

'Ancef' is excreted unchanged in the urine. In the first six hours approximately 60% of the drug is excreted in the urine and this increases to 70%–80% within 24 hours. 'Ancef' achieves peak urine concentrations of approximately 2400 μg./ml. and 4000 μg./ml. respectively following 500 mg. and 1 gram intramuscular doses.

In patients undergoing peritoneal dialysis (2 l./hr.), 'Ancef' produced mean serum levels of approximately 10 and 30 μg./ml. after 24 hours' instillation of a dialyzing solution containing 50 mg./l. and 150 mg./l., respectively. Mean peak levels were 29 μg./ml. (range 13-44 μg./ml.) with 50 mg./l. (three patients), and 72 μg./ml. (range 26-142 μg./ml.) with 150 mg./l. (six patients). Intraperitoneal administration of 'Ancef' is usually well tolerated.

Bile levels in patients without obstructive biliary disease can reach or exceed serum levels by up to five times; however, in patients with obstructive biliary disease, bile levels of 'Ancef' are considerably lower than serum levels (< 1.0 μg./ml.). In synovial fluid, the 'Ancef' level becomes comparable to that reached in serum at about four hours after drug administration. Studies of cord blood show prompt transfer of 'Ancef' across the placenta. 'Ancef' is present in very low concentrations in the milk of nursing mothers.

Microbiology: *In vitro* tests demonstrate that the bactericidal action of cephalosporins results from inhibition of cell wall synthesis. Ancef (sterile cefazolin sodium, SK&F) is active against the following organisms *in vitro* and in clinical infections:

Staphylococcus aureus (penicillin-sensitive and penicillin-resistant)
Group A beta-hemolytic streptococci and other strains of streptococci (many strains of enterococci are resistant)
Streptococcus pneumoniae (formerly *D. pneumoniae*)
Escherichia coli
Proteus mirabilis
Klebsiella species
Enterobacter aerogenes
Hemophilus influenzae

Most strains of *Enterobacter cloacae* and indole positive Proteus (*P. vulgaris, P. morgani, P. rettgeri*) are resistant. Methicillin-resistant staphylococci, serratia, pseudomonas, mima, herellea species are almost uniformly resistant to cefazolin.

Disc Susceptibility Tests

Quantitative methods that require measurement of zone diameters give the most precise estimates of antibiotic susceptibility. One such procedure* has been recommended for use with discs for testing susceptibility to cephalosporin class antibiotics. Interpretations correlate diameters of the disc test with MIC values for 'Ancef'. With this procedure, a report from the laboratory of "susceptible" indicates that the infecting organism is likely to respond to therapy. A report of "resistant" indicates that the infecting organism is not likely to respond to therapy. A report of "intermediate susceptibility" suggests that the organism would be susceptible if high dosage is used, or if the infection is confined to tissues and fluids (e.g., urine) in which high antibiotic levels are attained.

Indications and Usage: Ancef (sterile cefazolin sodium, SK&F) is indicated in the treatment of the following serious infections due to susceptible organisms:

RESPIRATORY TRACT INFECTIONS due to *Streptococcus pneumoniae* (formerly *D. pneumoniae*), *Klebsiella* species, *Hemophilus influenzae, Staphylococcus aureus* (penicillin-sensitive and penicillin-resistant), and group A beta-hemolytic streptococci.

Injectable benzathine penicillin is considered to be the drug of choice in treatment and prevention of streptococcal infections, including the prophylaxis of rheumatic fever.

'Ancef' is effective in the eradication of streptococci from the nasopharynx; however, data establishing the efficacy of 'Ancef' in the subsequent prevention of rheumatic fever are not available at present.

URINARY TRACT INFECTIONS due to *Escherichia coli, Proteus mirabilis, Klebsiella* species, and some strains of enterobacter and enterococci.

SKIN AND SKIN STRUCTURE INFECTIONS due to *Staphylococcus aureus* (penicillin-sensitive and penicillin-resistant), group A beta-hemolytic streptococci and other strains of streptococci.

BILIARY TRACT INFECTIONS due to *Escherichia coli*, various strains of streptococci, *Proteus mirabilis, Klebsiella* species and *Staphylococcus aureus*.

BONE AND JOINT INFECTIONS due to *Staphylococcus aureus*.

GENITAL INFECTIONS (i.e., prostatitis, epididymitis) due to *Escherichia coli, Proteus mirabilis, Klebsiella* species, and some strains of enterococci.

SEPTICEMIA due to *Streptococcus pneumoniae* (formerly *D. pneumoniae*), *Staphylococcus aureus* (penicillin-sensitive and penicillin-resistant), *Proteus mirabilis, Escherichia coli*, and *Klebsiella* species.

ENDOCARDITIS due to *Staphylococcus aureus* (penicillin-sensitive and penicillin-resistant) and group A beta-hemolytic streptococci.

Appropriate culture and susceptibility studies should be performed to determine susceptibility of the causative organism to 'Ancef'.

PERIOPERATIVE PROPHYLAXIS: The prophylactic administration of 'Ancef' preoperatively, intraoperatively, and postoperatively may reduce the incidence of certain postoperative infections in patients undergoing surgical procedures which are classified as contaminated or potentially contaminated (e.g., vaginal hysterectomy, and cholecystectomy in high-risk patients such as those over 70 years of age, with acute cholecystitis, obstructive jaundice, or common duct bile stones).

The perioperative use of 'Ancef' may also be effective in surgical patients in whom infection at the operative site would present a serious risk (e.g., during open-heart surgery and prosthetic arthroplasty).

The prophylactic administration of 'Ancef' should usually be discontinued within a 24-hour period after the surgical procedure. In surgery where the occurrence of infection may be particularly devastating (e.g., open-heart surgery and prosthetic arthroplasty), the prophylactic administration of 'Ancef' may be continued for 3 to 5 days following the completion of surgery.

If there are signs of infection, specimens for cultures should be obtained for the identification of the causative organism so that appropriate therapy may be instituted.

(See Dosage and Administration.)

Contraindications: ANCEF (STERILE CEFAZOLIN SODIUM, SK&F) IS CONTRAINDICATED IN PATIENTS WITH KNOWN ALLERGY TO THE CEPHALOSPORIN GROUP OF ANTIBIOTICS.

Warnings: BEFORE CEFAZOLIN THERAPY IS INSTITUTED, CAREFUL INQUIRY SHOULD BE MADE CONCERNING PREVIOUS HYPERSENSITIVITY REACTIONS TO CEPHALOSPORINS AND PENICILLIN. CEPHALOSPORIN C DERIVATIVES SHOULD BE GIVEN CAUTIOUSLY IN PENICILLIN-SENSITIVE PATIENTS.

SERIOUS ACUTE HYPERSENSITIVITY REACTIONS MAY REQUIRE EPINEPHRINE AND OTHER EMERGENCY MEASURES.

There is some clinical and laboratory evidence of partial cross-allergenicity of the penicillins and the cephalosporins. Patients have been reported to have had severe reactions (including anaphylaxis) to both drugs.

Any patient who has demonstrated some form of allergy, particularly to drugs, should receive antibiotics cautiously. No exception should be made with regard to 'Ancef'.

Precautions:

General—Prolonged use of Ancef (sterile cefazolin sodium, SK&F) may result in the overgrowth of nonsusceptible organisms. Careful clinical observation of the patient is essential.

When 'Ancef' is administered to patients with low urinary output because of impaired renal function, lower daily dosage is required (see Dosage and Administration).

Continued on next page

Smith Kline & French—Cont.

Drug Interactions—Probenecid may decrease renal tubular secretion of cephalosporins when used concurrently, resulting in increased and more prolonged cephalosporin blood levels.

Drug/Laboratory Test Interactions—A false positive reaction for glucose in the urine may occur with Benedict's solution, Fehling's solution, or with Clinitest® tablets, but not with enzyme-based tests such as Clinistix® and Tes-Tape®.

Positive direct and indirect antiglobulin (Coombs) tests have occurred; these may also occur in neonates whose mothers received cephalosporins before delivery.

Carcinogenesis/Mutagenesis — Mutagenicity studies and long-term studies in animals to determine the carcinogenic potential of 'Ancef' have not been performed.

Pregnancy—Teratogenic Effects—Pregnancy Category B. Reproduction studies have been performed in rats, mice and rabbits at doses up to 25 times the human dose and have revealed no evidence of impaired fertility or harm to the fetus due to 'Ancef'. There are, however, no adequate and well-controlled studies in pregnant women. Because animal reproduction studies are not always predictive of human response, this drug should be used during pregnancy only if clearly needed.

Labor and Delivery—When cefazolin has been administered prior to caesarean section, drug levels in cord blood have been approximately one quarter to one third of maternal drug levels. The drug appears to have no adverse effect on the fetus.

Nursing Mothers—'Ancef' is present in very low concentrations in the milk of nursing mothers. Caution should be exercised when 'Ancef' is administered to a nursing woman.

Pediatric Use—Safety and effectiveness for use in prematures and infants under one month of age have not been established. See Dosage and Administration for recommended dosage in children over one month.

Adverse Reactions: The following reactions have been reported:

Gastrointestinal: Diarrhea, oral candidiasis (oral thrush), vomiting, nausea, stomach cramps, anorexia.

Allergic: Anaphylaxis, eosinophilia, itching, drug fever, skin rash.

Hematologic: Neutropenia, leukopenia, thrombocythemia.

Hepatic and Renal: Transient rise in SGOT, SGPT, BUN and alkaline phosphatase levels has been observed without clinical evidence of renal or hepatic impairment.

Local Reactions: Rare instances of phlebitis have been reported at site of injection. Pain at the site of injection after intramuscular administration has occurred infrequently. Some induration has occurred.

Other Reactions: Genital and anal pruritus (including vulvar pruritus, genital moniliasis, and vaginitis).

Dosage and Administration: Ancef (sterile cefazolin sodium, SK&F) may be administered intramuscularly or intravenously after reconstitution.

DILUTION TABLE*

Vial Size	Diluent to Be Added	Approximate Available Volume	Approximate Average Concentration
250 mg.	2.0 ml.	2.0 ml.	125 mg./ml.
500 mg.	2.0 ml.	2.2 ml.	225 mg./ml.
1 gram	2.5 ml.	3.0 ml.	330 mg./ml.

* See labeling on "Piggyback" Vials (500 mg. and 1 gram) and Pharmacy Bulk Vials (5 and 10 grams) for their reconstitution directions.

Intramuscular Administration—Reconstitute with Sterile Water for Injection, Bacteriostatic Water for Injection or Sodium Chloride Injection, according to the dilution table above. Shake well until dissolved. 'Ancef' should be injected into a large muscle mass. Pain on injection is infrequent with 'Ancef'. Reconstituted 'Ancef' is stable for 24 hours at room temperature and for 96 hours if stored under refrigeration. However, the solution is light sensitive and should be protected from light until used.

Intravenous Administration—Ancef (sterile cefazolin sodium, SK&F) may be administered by intravenous injection or by continuous or intermittent infusion. Total daily dosages are the same as with intramuscular injection.

Intermittent intravenous infusion: 'Ancef' can be administered along with primary intravenous fluid management programs in a volume control set or in a separate, secondary I.V. bottle. Reconstituted 500 mg. or 1 gram of 'Ancef' may be diluted in 50 to 100 ml. of one of the following intravenous solutions:

- Sodium Chloride Injection
- 5% or 10% Dextrose Injection
- 5% Dextrose in Lactated Ringer's Injection
- 5% Dextrose and 0.9% Sodium Chloride Injection (also may be used with 5% Dextrose and 0.45% or 0.2% Sodium Chloride Injection)
- Lactated Ringer's Injection
- Invert Sugar 5% or 10% in Sterile Water for Injection
- Ringer's Injection
- 5% Sodium Bicarbonate in Sterile Water for Injection

'Ancef' is stable in these intravenous fluids for 24 hours at room temperature and 96 hours if stored under refrigeration (5°C).

Direct intravenous injection: Reconstituted 500 mg. or 1 gram of 'Ancef' should be diluted with Sterile Water for Injection. The Sterile Water for Injection may be added to the 'Ancef' vial to achieve a total volume of 10 ml. Inject solution slowly over 3 to 5 minutes. May be administered directly into vein or through tubing for patient receiving the above parenteral fluids.

Parenteral drug products should be inspected visually for particulate matter and discoloration prior to administration, whenever solution and container permit.

Usual Adult Dosage

Type of Infection	Dose	Frequency
Moderate to severe infections	500 mg. to 1 gram	every 6 to 8 hrs.
Mild infections caused by susceptible gram + cocci	250 mg. to 500 mg.	every 8 hours
Acute, uncomplicated urinary tract infections	1 gram	every 12 hours
Pneumococcal pneumonia	500 mg.	every 12 hours
Severe, life-threatening infections (e.g., endocarditis, septicemia)*	1 gram to 1.5 grams	every 6 hours

* In rare instances, doses of up to 12 grams of 'Ancef' per day have been used.

Dosage Adjustment for Patients with Reduced Renal Function

'Ancef' may be used in patients with reduced renal function with the following dosage adjustments: Patients with a creatinine clearance of 55 ml./min. or greater or a serum creatinine of 1.5 mg. % or less can be given full doses. Patients with creatinine clearance rates of 35 to 54 ml./min. or serum creatinine of 1.6 to 3.0 mg. % can also be given full doses but dosage should be restricted to at least 8 hour intervals. Patients with creatinine clearance rates of 11 to 34 ml./min. or serum creatinine of 3.1 to 4.5 mg. % should be given ½ the usual dose every 12 hours. Patients with creatinine clearance rates of 10 ml./min. or less or serum creatinine of 4.6 mg. % or greater should be given ½ the usual dose every 18 to 24 hours. All reduced dosage recommendations apply after an initial loading dose appropriate to the severity of the infection. Patients undergoing peritoneal dialysis: See Human Pharmacology.

Perioperative Prophylactic Use

To prevent postoperative infection in contaminated or potentially contaminated surgery, recommended doses are:

a. 1 gram I.V. or I.M. administered ½ hour to 1 hour prior to the start of surgery.
b. For lengthy operative procedures (e.g., 2 hours or more), 500 mg. to 1 gram I.V. or I.M. during surgery (administration modified depending on the duration of the operative procedure).
c. 500 mg. to 1 gram I.V. or I.M. every 6 to 8 hours for 24 hours postoperatively.

It is important that (1) the preoperative dose be given just (½ to 1 hour) prior to the start of surgery so that adequate antibiotic levels are present in the serum and tissues at the time of initial surgical incision; and (2) 'Ancef' be administered, if necessary, at appropriate intervals during surgery to provide sufficient levels of the antibiotic at the anticipated moments of greatest exposure to infective organisms.

In surgery where the occurrence of infection may be particularly devastating (e.g., open-heart surgery and prosthetic arthroplasty), the prophylactic administration of 'Ancef' may be continued for 3 to 5 days following the completion of surgery.

Pediatric Dosage

In children, a total daily dosage of 25 to 50 mg. per kg. (approximately 10 to 20 mg. per pound) of body weight, divided into three or four equal doses, is effective for most mild to moderately severe infections. Total daily dosage may be increased to 100 mg. per kg. (45 mg. per pound) of body weight for severe infections. Since safety for use in premature infants and in infants under one month has not been established, the use of 'Ancef' in these patients is not recommended.

Pediatric Dosage Guide

Weight		25 mg./kg./Day Divided into 3 Doses		25 mg./kg./Day Divided into 4 Doses	
Lbs.	Kg.	Approximate Single Dose mg./q8h	Vol. (ml.) needed with dilution of 125 mg./ml.	Approximate Single Dose mg./q6h	Vol. (ml.) needed with dilution of 125 mg./ml.
10	4.5	40 mg.	0.35 ml.	30 mg.	0.25 ml.
20	9.0	75 mg.	0.60 ml.	55 mg.	0.45 ml.
30	13.6	115 mg.	0.90 ml.	85 mg.	0.70 ml.
40	18.1	150 mg.	1.20 ml.	115 mg.	0.90 ml.
50	22.7	190 mg.	1.50 ml.	140 mg.	1.10 ml.

Weight		50 mg./kg./Day Divided into 3 Doses		50 mg./kg./Day Divided into 4 Doses	
Lbs.	Kg.	Approximate Single Dose mg./q8h	Vol. (ml.) needed with dilution of 225 mg./ml.	Approximate Single Dose mg./q6h	Vol. (ml.) needed with dilution of 225 mg./ml.
10	4.5	75 mg.	0.35 ml.	55 mg.	0.25 ml.
20	9.0	150 mg.	0.70 ml.	110 mg.	0.50 ml.
30	13.6	225 mg.	1.00 ml.	170 mg.	0.75 ml.
40	18.1	300 mg.	1.35 ml.	225 mg.	1.00 ml.
50	22.7	375 mg.	1.70 ml.	285 mg.	1.25 ml.

In children with mild to moderate renal impairment (creatinine clearance of 70 to 40 ml./min.), 60 percent of the normal daily dose given in equally divided doses every 12 hours should be sufficient. In patients with moderate impairment (creatinine clearance of 40 to 20 ml./min.), 25 percent of the normal daily dose given in equally divided doses every 12 hours should be adequate. Children with severe renal impairment (creatinine clearance of 20 to 5 ml./min.) may be given 10 percent of the normal daily dose every 24 hours. All dosage recommendations apply after an initial loading dose.

How Supplied: Ancef (sterile cefazolin sodium, SK&F)—supplied in vials equivalent to 250 mg., 500 mg or 1 gram of cefazolin; in "Piggyback" Vials for intravenous admixture equivalent to 500 mg. or 1 gram of cefazolin; and in Pharmacy Bulk Vials equivalent to 5 grams or 10 grams of cefazolin.

Military—Vial, 1 gram, 6505-01-010-0832; vial, 500 mg., 6505-01-010-0833.

---

* Bauer, A.W.; Kirby, W.M.M.; Sherris, J.C., and Turck, M.: Antibiotic Testing by a Standardized Single Disc Method, Am. J. Clin. Path. 45:493, 1966. Standardized Disc Susceptibility Test, Federal Register 39:19182-19184, 1974.

ANSPOR® ℞

(brand of cephradine)
Capsules, 250 mg. and 500 mg.
and
for Oral Suspension, 125 mg./5 ml. and 250 mg./5 ml.

Description: Anspor (cephradine, SK&F) is a semisynthetic cephalosporin antibiotic chemically designated as 7-[D-2-amino-2-(1,4-cyclohexadien-1-yl) acetamido] -3- methyl -8- oxo-5-thia -1- azabicyclo[4.2.0]-oct-2-ene-2-carboxylic acid.

Each Anspor (cephradine, SK&F) Capsule contains 250 mg. or 500 mg. of cephradine. 'Anspor' for Oral Suspension is available in bottles containing 2.5 grams or 5 grams of cephradine, which after reconstitution with 61 ml. of water, respectively, provides 125 mg. or 250 mg. of cephradine per 5 ml. teaspoonful.

Clinical Pharmacology:

Human Pharmacology: Anspor (cephradine, SK&F) is acid stable. It is rapidly absorbed after oral administration in the fasting state. Following doses of 250 mg. and 500 mg. in normal adult volunteers, average peak serum levels within one hour were approximately 9 and 16.5 mcg. per ml. respectively. The presence of food in the gastrointestinal tract delays the absorption but does not affect the total amount of cephradine absorbed. Over 90 percent of the drug is excreted unchanged in the urine within 6 hours. Peak urine concentrations are approximately 1600 mcg. per ml. following a 250 mg. dose and 3200 mcg. per ml. following a 500 mg. dose.

Microbiology: *In vitro* tests demonstrate that the cephalosporins are bactericidal because of their inhibition of cell-wall synthesis. Cephradine is active against the following organisms *in vitro* and in clinical infections:

Beta-hemolytic streptococci
Staphylococci, including coagulase-positive, coagulase-negative, and penicillinase-producing strains
Streptococcus pneumoniae (formerly *D. pneumoniae*)
Escherichia coli
Proteus mirabilis
Klebsiella sp.
Hemophilus influenzae

Note—Some strains of enterococci *(Streptococcus faecalis)* are resistant to cephradine. It is not active against most strains of *Enterobacter* sp., *Pr. morganii,* and *Pr. vulgaris.* It has no activity against *Pseudomonas* or *Herellea* species. When tested by *in vitro* methods, staphylococci exhibit cross-resistance between cephradine and methicillin-type antibiotics.

Disc Susceptibility Tests: Quantitative methods that require measurement of zone diameters give the most precise estimates of antibiotic susceptibility. One recommended procedure (21 CFR § 460.1) uses cephalosporin class discs for testing susceptibility; interpretations correlate zone diameters of this disc test with MIC values for cephradine. With this procedure, a report from the laboratory of "resistant" indicates that the infecting organism is not likely to respond to therapy. A report of "intermediate susceptibility" suggests that the organism would be susceptible if the infection is confined to the urinary tract, as high antibiotic levels can be obtained in the urine, or if high dosage is used in other types of infection.

Indications and Usage: Anspor (cephradine, SK&F) Capsules and 'Anspor' for Oral Suspension are indicated in the treatment of the following infections when caused by susceptible strains of designated microorganisms:

Infections of the respiratory tract (e.g., tonsillitis, pharyngitis, and lobar pneumonia) caused by group A beta-hemolytic streptococci and *Streptococcus pneumoniae* (formerly *D. pneumoniae*).

(Penicillin is the usual drug of choice in the treatment and prevention of streptococcal infections, including the prophylaxis of rheumatic fever. 'Anspor' is generally effective in the eradication of streptococci from the nasopharynx; substantial data establishing the efficacy of 'Anspor' in the subsequent prevention of rheumatic fever are not available at present.)

Otitis media caused by group A beta-hemolytic streptococci, *Streptococcus pneumoniae* (formerly *D. pneumoniae*), *Hemophilus influenzae* and staphylococci.

Skin and skin structure infections caused by staphylococci (penicillin-susceptible and penicillin-resistant) and beta-hemolytic streptococci.

Infections of the urinary tract, including prostatitis, caused by *Escherichia coli, Pr. mirabilis,* and *Klebsiella* sp.

Note—Culture and susceptibility tests should be initiated prior to and during therapy. Renal function studies should be performed when indicated.

Contraindications: Cephradine is contraindicated in patients with known hypersensitivity to the cephalosporin group of antibiotics.

Warnings: BEFORE CEPHRADINE THERAPY IS INSTITUTED, CAREFUL INQUIRY SHOULD BE MADE CONCERNING PREVIOUS HYPERSENSITIVITY REACTIONS TO CEPHALOSPORINS AND PENICILLIN. CEPHALOSPORIN C DERIVATIVES SHOULD BE GIVEN CAUTIOUSLY IN PENICILLIN-SENSITIVE PATIENTS.

SERIOUS ACUTE HYPERSENSITIVITY REACTIONS MAY REQUIRE EPINEPHRINE AND OTHER EMERGENCY MEASURES.

There is some clinical and laboratory evidence of partial cross-allergenicity of the penicillins and the cephalosporins. Patients have been reported to have had severe reactions (including anaphylaxis) to both drugs.

Any patient who has demonstrated some form of allergy, particularly to drugs, should receive antibiotics cautiously. No exception should be made with regard to 'Anspor'.

Pseudomembranous colitis has been reported with the use of cephalosporins (and other broad-spectrum antibiotics); therefore, it is important to consider its diagnosis in patients who develop diarrhea in association with antibiotic use.

Treatment with broad-spectrum antibiotics alters normal flora of the colon and may permit overgrowth of clostridia. Studies indicate a toxin produced by *Clostridium difficile* is one primary cause of antibiotic-associated colitis. Cholestyramine and colestipol resins have been shown to bind the toxin *in vitro.*

Mild cases of colitis may respond to drug discontinuance alone.

Moderate to severe cases should be managed with fluid, electrolyte and protein supplementation as indicated.

When the colitis is not relieved by drug discontinuance or when it is severe, oral vancomycin is the treatment of choice for antibiotic-associated pseudomembranous colitis produced by *C. difficile.* Other causes of colitis should also be considered.

Precautions:

General—Patients should be followed carefully so that any side effects or unusual manifestations of drug idiosyncrasy may be detected. If a hypersensitivity reaction occurs, the drug should be discontinued and the patient treated with the usual agents, e.g., pressor amines, antihistamines, or corticosteroids.

Administer cephradine with caution in the presence of markedly impaired renal function. In patients with known or suspected renal impairment, careful clinical observation and appropriate laboratory studies should be made prior to and during therapy as cephradine accumulates in the serum and tissues. See DOSAGE AND ADMINISTRATION section for information on treatment of patients with impaired renal function.

Prolonged use of antibiotics may promote the overgrowth of nonsusceptible organisms. Should superinfection occur during therapy, appropriate measures should be taken.

'Anspor', as with all cephalosporins, should be prescribed with caution in individuals with a history of gastrointestinal disease, particularly colitis.

Information for Patients—Cephradine may be taken without regard to meals, unless gastrointestinal irritation occurs.

Diabetic patients receiving 'Anspor' should be cautioned to check with physicians before changing diet or dosage of diabetes medication. A false positive reaction for glucose in the urine may occur with Benedict's solution, Fehling's solution, or with Clinitest® tablets, but not with enzyme-based tests such as Clinistix® and Tes-Tape®.

Laboratory Tests—In chronic urinary tract infections, frequent bacteriologic tests are necessary during drug therapy and may be necessary for several months afterwards.

Drug Interactions—Probenecid may decrease renal tubular secretion of cephalosporins when used concurrently, resulting in increased and more prolonged cephalosporin blood levels.

Drug/Laboratory Test Interactions—After treatment with cephradine, a false positive reaction for glucose in the urine may occur with Benedict's solution, Fehling's solution, or with Clinitest® tablets, but not with enzyme-based tests such as Clinistix® and Tes-Tape®.

A false positive direct Coombs test has been reported after treatment with other cephalosporins; therefore, it should be recognized that a positive Coombs test may be due to the drug.

Carcinogenesis/Mutagenesis — Mutagenicity studies and long-term studies in animals to determine the carcinogenic potential of 'Anspor' have not been performed.

Pregnancy—*Teratogenic Effects*—Pregnancy Category B. Reproduction studies have been performed in mice and rats receiving doses up to four times the maximum human dose and have revealed no evidence of impaired fertility

Continued on next page

Smith Kline & French—Cont.

or harm to the fetus due to cephradine. There are, however, no adequate and well-controlled studies in pregnant women. Because animal reproduction studies are not always predictive of human response, this drug should be used during pregnancy only if clearly needed.

Nursing Mothers—Cephradine is present in very low concentrations in the milk of nursing mothers. Caution should be exercised when cephradine is administered to a nursing woman.

Pediatric Use—Safety and effectiveness for use in infants under nine months of age have not been established. See DOSAGE AND ADMINISTRATION section for recommended dosage in children over nine months.

Adverse Reactions: As with other cephalosporins, untoward reactions are limited essentially to gastrointestinal disturbances and to hypersensitivity phenomena. The latter are more likely to occur in individuals who have previously demonstrated hypersensitivity and those with a history of allergy, asthma, hay fever, or urticaria.

The following adverse reactions have been reported following the use of cephradine:

Gastrointestinal: Diarrhea or loose stools, vomiting, glossitis, nausea, abdominal pain and heartburn.

Symptoms of pseudomembranous colitis can appear during antibiotic treatment.

Nausea and vomiting have been reported rarely.

Allergic: Anaphylaxis, mild urticaria or skin rash, pruritus, joint pains.

Hematologic: Mild, transient eosinophilia, leukopenia and neutropenia.

Liver: Transient mild rise of SGOT, SGPT, and total bilirubin has been observed with no evidence of hepatocellular damage.

Renal: Transitory rises in BUN have been observed in some patients treated with cephalosporins; their frequency increases in patients over 50 years old. In adults for whom serum creatinine determinations were performed, the rise in BUN was not accompanied by a rise in serum creatinine.

Other: Dizziness and tightness in the chest and candidal vaginitis.

Dosage and Administration: Anspor (cephradine, SK&F) may be given without regard to meals.

Adults: For skin and soft-tissue and respiratory tract infections (other than lobar pneumonia), the usual dose is 250 mg. every 6 hours or 500 mg. every 12 hours. For acute infections of the urinary tract, including prostatitis, and pneumococcal lobar pneumonia, the usual dose is 500 mg. every 6 hours or 1 gram every 12 hours. Severe or chronic infections may require larger doses.

Children: No adequate information is available on the efficacy of b.i.d. regimens in children under nine months of age. The usual dose in children over nine months of age is 25 to 50 mg./kg./day administered in equally divided doses every 6 or 12 hours. For otitis media due to *H. influenzae,* doses are from 75 to 100 mg./kg./day administered in equally divided doses every 6 or 12 hours. Doses for children should not exceed doses recommended for adults. The maximum dose should not exceed 4 grams per day.

All patients, regardless of age and weight: Larger doses (up to 1 gram, q.i.d.) may be given for severe or chronic infections.

As with antibiotic therapy generally, therapy should be continued for a minimum of 48 to 72 hours after the patient becomes asymptomatic or evidence of bacterial eradication has been obtained. In infections caused by group A beta-hemolytic streptococci, a minimum of 10 days of treatment is recommended to guard against the risk of rheumatic fever or glomerulonephritis. In the treatment of chronic urinary tract infection, frequent bacteriologic and clinical appraisal is necessary during therapy and may be necessary for several months afterwards. Persistent infections may require treatment for several weeks. Prolonged intensive therapy is recommended for prostatitis. Doses smaller than those indicated are not recommended.

Patients with Impaired Renal Function

Not on Dialysis: The following initial dosage schedule is suggested as a guideline based on creatinine clearance. Further modification in the dosage schedule may be required because of individual variations in absorption.

Creatinine Clearance	Dose	Time Interval
>20 ml./min.	500 mg.	6 hours
5–20 ml./min.	250 mg.	6 hours
<5 ml./min.	250 mg.	12 hours

On Chronic, Intermittent Hemodialysis:

250 mg. Start
250 mg. at 12 hours
250 mg. 36–48 hours (after start)

Children may require dosage modification proportional to their weight and severity of infection.

How Supplied: Anspor (cephradine, SK&F) is available as 'Anspor' Capsules in 250 mg. in bottles of 100 and in Single Unit Packages of 100 (intended for institutional use only); and in 500 mg. in bottles of 20 and 100 and in Single Unit Packages of 100 (intended for institutional use only). 'Anspor' is also available as 'Anspor' for Oral Suspension which, after reconstitution, provides 125 mg. or 250 mg. of cephradine per 5 ml. teaspoonful in a pleasant, fruit-flavored suspension in 100 ml. bottles.

Notes on Stability: 'Anspor' Capsules—Do not store above 86°F.; keep bottle tightly closed. 'Anspor' for Oral Suspension—Prior to reconstitution, do not store above 86°F. After reconstitution, suspensions retain their potency for seven days at room temperature and for 14 days if refrigerated.

Military—Capsules, 250 mg., 100's, 6505-01-009-9531.

[*Shown in Product Identification Section*]

BENZEDREX® INHALER

nasal decongestant

Marketed by Menley & James Laboratories, a SmithKline company.
(See PDR For Nonprescription Drugs)

COMBID® SPANSULE® CAPSULES ℞

Description: Each 'Combid' *Spansule* capsule contains 10 mg. of prochlorperazine, as the maleate, and isopropamide iodide equivalent to 5 mg. of isopropamide.

The prochlorperazine component is so prepared that an initial dose is released promptly and the remaining medication is released gradually over a prolonged period. The isopropamide iodide component is not in sustained release form because it can provide 10 to 12 hours of antisecretory-antispasmodic action.

Actions: A single 'Combid' *Spansule* capsule b.i.d. (every 12 hours) can provide the following actions: (1) reduction of gastric secretion, (2) inhibition of spasm and motility, (3) relief of anxiety and tension, and (4) control of nausea and vomiting.

Indications

Based on a review of this drug by the National Academy of Sciences—National Research Council and/or other information, FDA has classified the indications as follows:

Possibly effective: As adjunctive therapy in peptic ulcer and in the irritable bowel syndrome (irritable colon, spastic colon, mucous colitis, functional gastrointestinal disorders); functional diarrhea.

Final classification of the less-than-effective indications requires further investigation.

Contraindications: Known hypersensitivity to prochlorperazine maleate and/or isopropamide iodide, existing drug-induced C.N.S. depression, glaucoma, pyloric obstruction, prostatic hypertrophy, bladder neck obstruction, obstructive intestinal lesions and/or ileus, intestinal atony of the elderly or debilitated patient, unstable cardiovascular status in acute hemorrhage, severe ulcerative colitis, toxic megacolon complicating ulcerative colitis; myasthenia gravis, bone marrow depression, jaundice, hepatic disease, blood dyscrasias. Children under 12 years of age.

Because of the antiemetic action of the prochlorperazine component, 'Combid' *Spansule* capsules should not be used where nausea and vomiting are believed to be a manifestation of intestinal obstruction or brain tumor.

Warnings: Use cautiously in patients with a past history of jaundice, hepatic abnormality or blood dyscrasias. Because of possible additive effects, caution patients about concomitant use of alcohol and other C.N.S. depressants. Also, caution patients about activities requiring alertness (e.g., operating vehicles or machinery).

In patients with ulcerative colitis, large doses of isopropamide iodide may suppress intestinal motility to the point of producing paralytic ileus, and the use of this drug may precipitate or aggravate the serious complication of toxic megacolon.

In the presence of a high environmental temperature, heat prostration (fever and heat stroke due to decreased sweating) can occur. In patients with diarrhea due to incomplete intestinal obstruction (especially those with ileostomy or colostomy), treatment with isopropamide iodide would be inappropriate and possibly harmful. With overdosage, a curare-like action, due to the isopropamide iodide component, may occur.

Usage in Pregnancy: Use of any drug in pregnancy, lactation, or in women who may bear children requires that the potential benefit of the drug be weighed against its possible hazards to the mother and child. As with all anticholinergic drugs, an inhibiting effect on lactation may occur.

Nursing Mothers: There is evidence that phenothiazines are excreted in breast milk.

Precautions: Patients who have shown a sensitivity reaction to other drugs may be more liable to have such a reaction to prochlorperazine.

Since the iodine in isopropamide iodide may alter PBI test results and will suppress I^{131} uptake, it is suggested that 'Combid' *Spansule* capsules be discontinued one week prior to these tests. Also, iodine skin rash may occur rarely.

Use with caution in elderly patients and patients with autonomic neuropathy, hepatic or renal disease, hyperthyroidism, coronary heart disease, congestive heart failure, cardiac arrhythmia, hypertension and nonobstructive prostatic hypertrophy. Anticholinergic drugs may aggravate gastroesophageal reflux. Investigate any tachycardia before giving anticholinergic (atropine-like) drugs, since they may increase the heart rate.

Neuroleptic drugs elevate prolactin levels; the elevation persists during chronic administration. Tissue culture experiments indicate that approximately one-third of human breast cancers are prolactin-dependent in vitro, a factor of potential importance if the prescribing of these drugs is contemplated in a patient with a previously detected breast cancer. Although disturbances such as galactorrhea, amenorrhea, gynecomastia, and impotence have been reported, the clinical significance of elevated serum prolactin levels is unknown for most patients. An increase in mammary neoplasms has been found in rodents after chronic administration of neuroleptic drugs. Neither clinical nor epidemiologic studies conducted to date, however, have shown an association between chronic administration of these drugs and mammary tumorigenesis; the available evidence is considered too limited to be conclusive at this time.

Drugs which lower the seizure threshold, including phenothiazine derivatives, should not be used with 'Amipaque'.* 'Combid' should be discontinued at least 48 hours before myelography, should not be resumed for at least 24 hours postprocedure, and should not be used for the control of nausea and vomiting occurring either prior to myelography or postprocedure.

Long-Term Therapy: Long-term therapy with neuroleptic agents, including prochlorperazine, has been reported to result in the appearance of tardive dyskinesia in some patients. To lessen the likelihood of this adverse reaction related to cumulative drug effect, patients in whom long-term 'Combid' therapy is indicated should be evaluated periodically to determine whether the dosage could be lowered or drug therapy discontinued.

Adverse Reactions:

Isopropamide Iodide: Xerostomia (dry mouth); urinary hesitancy and retention; tachycardia; palpitations; mydriasis (dilatation of the pupils); cycloplegia; blurred vision; constipation; bloated feeling; nausea; dysphagia; fever; nasal congestion.

Other adverse reactions possible with anticholinergics include: increased ocular tension; loss of taste; headaches; nervousness; drowsiness; weakness; dizziness; insomnia; vomiting; impotence; suppression of lactation; severe allergic reaction or drug idiosyncrasies, including anaphylaxis; urticaria and other dermal manifestations; some degree of mental confusion and /or excitement, especially in elderly persons. Decreased sweating may occur. It should be noted that adrenergic innervation of the eccrine sweat glands on the palms and soles makes complete control of sweating impossible. An end point of complete anhidrosis cannot occur because large drug doses would be required, and this would produce severe side effects from parasympathetic paralysis.

Prochlorperazine or Other Phenothiazine Derivatives: Adverse reactions with different phenothiazines vary in type, frequency, and mechanism of occurrence, i.e., some are dose-related, while others involve individual patient sensitivity. Some adverse reactions may be more likely to occur, or occur with greater intensity, in patients with special medical problems, e.g., patients with mitral insufficiency or pheochromocytoma have experienced severe hypotension following recommended doses of certain phenothiazines.

Not all of the following adverse reactions have been observed with every phenothiazine derivative, but they have been reported with one or more and should be borne in mind when drugs of this class are administered.

Extrapyramidal symptoms (opisthotonos, oculogyric crisis, hyperreflexia, dystonia, akathisia, dyskinesia, pseudo-parkinsonism) have been reported. (These symptoms usually subside several hours after 'Combid' is discontinued; if troublesome to the patient, mild sedation or injectable 'Benadryl'† may be useful.) As with all antipsychotic agents, persistent or tardive dyskinesia may appear after long-term therapy—especially in elderly female patients on high doses. Symptoms are persistent and in some patients irreversible. The syndrome is characterized by rhythmical involuntary movements of the tongue, face, mouth or jaw, sometimes accompanied by involuntary movements of extremities. Fine vermicular movements of the tongue may be an early sign; if these appear, discontinuation of medication is suggested.

Other adverse reactions include drowsiness; dizziness; grand mal convulsions; altered cerebrospinal fluid proteins; cerebral edema; intensification and prolongation of the action of central nervous system depressants (opiates, analgesics, antihistamines, barbiturates, alcohol), atropine, heat, organophosphorus insecticides; autonomic reactions (dryness of mouth, nasal congestion, headache, nausea, constipation, obstipation, adynamic ileus, inhibition of ejaculation); reactivation of psychotic processes, catatonic-like states; hypotension (sometimes fatal); cardiac arrest; blood dyscrasias (pancytopenia, thrombocytopenic purpura, leukopenia, agranulocytosis, eosinophilia); liver damage (jaundice, biliary stasis); endocrine disturbances (lactation, galactorrhea, gynecomastia, priapism, menstrual irregularities, false positive pregnancy tests); skin disorders (photosensitivity, itching, erythema, urticaria, eczema up to exfoliative dermatitis); other allergic reactions (asthma, laryngeal edema, angioneurotic edema, anaphylactoid reactions); peripheral edema; reversed epinephrine effect; hyperpyrexia; a systemic lupus erythematosus-like syndrome; pigmentary retinopathy; with prolonged administration of substantial doses, skin pigmentation, epithelial keratopathy, and lenticular and corneal deposits.

EKG changes—particularly nonspecific, usually reversible Q and T wave distortions—have been observed in some patients receiving phenothiazine tranquilizers. Their relationship to myocardial damage has not been confirmed.

Although phenothiazines cause neither psychic nor physical dependence, sudden discontinuance in long-term psychiatric patients may cause temporary symptoms, e.g., nausea and vomiting, dizziness, tremulousness.

Note: There have been occasional reports of sudden death in patients receiving phenothiazines. In some cases, the cause appeared to be asphyxia due to failure of the cough reflex. In others, the cause could not be determined. There is not sufficient evidence to establish a relationship between such deaths and the administration of phenothiazines.

Dosage and Administration: *Adults and children over 12*—One 'Combid' *Spansule* capsule b.i.d. (every 12 hours). Some patients may require only one capsule every 24 hours (on arising). Only the exceptional patient will require two capsules in the morning and two at night.

Overdosage: (See also Adverse Reactions)

Symptoms of 'Combid' overdosage may be those of either isopropamide iodide or prochlorperazine overdosage.

Isopropamide Iodide: *Symptoms*—May include dryness of mouth, dysphagia, thirst, blurred vision, dilated pupils, photophobia, fever, rapid pulse and respiration, disorientation. Depression and circulatory collapse may result from severe overdosage.

Treatment—Gastric lavage, repeated several times.

Respiratory depression should be promptly treated by the use of oxygen and stimulants. If marked excitement is present, one of the short-acting barbiturates, chloral hydrate, or gas anesthesia may be used. Otherwise do not administer sedation. Hyperpyrexia may be treated with physical cooling measures. Force fluids by mouth or, if necessary, by intravenous administration.

While pilocarpine or similar drugs are sometimes recommended for the relief of dry mouth, many authorities feel that these drugs are not indicated, since they relieve the minor peripheral effect but do not influence the more serious central effects and, thus, may merely mask signs of drug activity. If photophobia occurs, the patient should be kept in a darkened room. It is not known whether isopropamide is dialyzable.

Prochlorperazine: *Symptoms*—Primarily involvement of the extrapyramidal mechanism producing some of the dystonic reactions described above.

Symptoms of central nervous system depression to the point of somnolence or coma. Agitation and restlessness may also occur. Other possible manifestations include convulsions, fever, and autonomic reactions such as hypotension, dry mouth and ileus.

Treatment—Essentially symptomatic and supportive. Early gastric lavage is helpful. Keep patient under observation and maintain an open airway, since involvement of the extrapyramidal mechanism may produce dysphagia and respiratory difficulty in severe overdosage. **Do not attempt to induce emesis because a dystonic reaction of the head or neck may develop that could result in aspiration of vomitus.** Extrapyramidal symptoms may be treated with anti-parkinsonism drugs, barbiturates, or 'Benadryl'.

If administration of a stimulant is desirable, amphetamine, dextroamphetamine, or caffeine with sodium benzoate is recommended. Stimulants that may cause convulsions (e.g., picrotoxin or pentylenetetrazol) should be avoided.

If hypotension occurs, the standard measures for managing circulatory shock should be initiated. If it is desirable to administer a vasoconstrictor, 'Levophed' and 'Neo-Synephrine'‡ are most suitable. Other pressor agents, including epinephrine, are not recommended because phenothiazine derivatives may reverse the usual elevating action of these agents and cause a further lowering of blood pressure.

Limited experience indicates that phenothiazines are *not* dialyzable.

Special note on 'Spansule' capsules—Since much of the 'Spansule' capsule medication is coated for gradual release, therapy directed at reversing the effects of the ingested drugs and at supporting the patient should be continued for as long as overdosage symptoms remain. Saline cathartics are useful for hastening evacuation of pellets that have not already released medication.

How Supplied: In bottles of 50 and 500; in Single Unit Packages of 100 (intended for institutional use only).

Military—Capsules, 500's, 6505-00-935-9817

---

*Trademark Reg. U.S. Pat. Off.: 'Amipaque' for metrizamide, Winthrop Laboratories.

†Trademark Reg. U.S. Pat. Off.: 'Benadryl' for diphenhydramine hydrochloride, Parke-Davis.

‡'Levophed' and 'Neo-Synephrine' are the trademarks (Reg. U.S. Pat. Off.) of Winthrop Laboratories for its brands of levarterenol and phenylephrine respectively.

[*Shown in Product Identification Section*]

COMPAZINE® ℞

(brand of prochlorperazine)

Description: **Tablets**—Each tablet contains 5 mg., 10 mg., or, for severe neuropsychiatric conditions, 25 mg. of prochlorperazine as the maleate.

Spansule® sustained release capsules—Each 'Spansule' capsule contains 10 mg., 15 mg., 30 mg., or, for severe neuropsychiatric conditions, 75 mg. of prochlorperazine as the maleate, so prepared that an initial dose is released promptly and the remaining medication is released gradually over a prolonged period. (In general, dosage recommendations for other oral forms of the drug may be applied to 'Spansule' capsules on the basis of the total daily dose in milligrams.)

Ampuls, 2 ml. (5 mg./ml.)—Each ml. contains, in aqueous solution, 5 mg. prochlorperazine as the edisylate, 1 mg. sodium sulfite, 1 mg. sodium bisulfite, 8 mg. sodium phosphate and 12 mg. sodium biphosphate.

Continued on next page

Smith Kline & French—Cont.

Multiple-dose Vials, 10 ml. (5 mg./ml.)—Each ml. contains, in aqueous solution, 5 mg. prochlorperazine as the edisylate, 5 mg. sodium biphosphate, 12 mg. sodium tartrate, 0.9 mg. sodium saccharin and 0.75% benzyl alcohol as preservative.

Disposable Syringes, 2 ml. (5 mg./ml.)—Each ml. contains, in aqueous solution, 5 mg. prochlorperazine as the edisylate, 5 mg. sodium biphosphate, 12 mg. sodium tartrate, 0.9 mg. sodium saccharin, and 0.75% benzyl alcohol as preservative.

Suppositories—Each suppository contains 2½ mg., 5 mg., or 25 mg. of prochlorperazine; with glycerin, glyceryl monopalmitate, glyceryl monostearate, hydrogenated cocoanut oil fatty acids and hydrogenated palm kernel oil fatty acids.

Syrup—Each 5 ml. (one teaspoonful) contains 5 mg. of prochlorperazine as the edisylate.

Indications: Management of the manifestations of psychotic disorders; management of psychoneurotic patients displaying primarily symptoms of moderate to severe anxiety and tension; and for control of severe nausea and vomiting.

'Compazine' has not been shown effective in the management of behavioral complications in patients with mental retardation.

Contraindications: In comatose or greatly depressed states due to central nervous system depressants; and in the presence of bone marrow depression.

Do not use in pediatric surgery.

Do not use in children under 2 years of age or under 20 lbs. Do not use in children for conditions for which dosage has not been established.

Warnings: The extrapyramidal symptoms which can occur secondary to 'Compazine' may be confused with the central nervous system signs of an undiagnosed primary disease responsible for the vomiting, e.g., Reye's syndrome or other encephalopathy. The use of 'Compazine' and other potential hepatotoxins should be avoided in children and adolescents whose signs and symptoms suggest Reye's syndrome.

Patients who have demonstrated a hypersensitivity reaction (e.g., blood dyscrasias, jaundice) with a phenothiazine should not be reexposed to any phenothiazine, including Compazine (prochlorperazine, SK&F), unless in the judgment of the physician the potential benefits of treatment outweigh the possible hazard.

'Compazine' may impair mental and/or physical abilities, especially during the first few days of therapy. Therefore, caution patients about activities requiring alertness (e.g., operating vehicles or machinery).

Phenothiazines may intensify or prolong the action of central nervous system depressants (e.g., alcohol, anesthetics, narcotics).

Usage in Pregnancy: Safety for the use of 'Compazine' during pregnancy has not been established. Therefore, it is recommended that the drug be given to pregnant patients only when, in the judgment of the physician, the potential benefits outweigh the possible hazards.

Nursing Mothers: There is evidence that phenothiazines are excreted in the breast milk of nursing mothers.

Precautions: The antiemetic action of 'Compazine' may mask the signs and symptoms of overdosage of other drugs and may obscure the diagnosis and treatment of other conditions such as intestinal obstruction, brain tumor and Reye's syndrome (See Warnings).

'Compazine' should be used cautiously with cancer chemotherapy drugs that cause vomiting at toxic levels because vomiting, as a sign of toxicity, may be obscured.

Because hypotension may occur, large doses and parenteral administration should be used cautiously in patients with impaired cardiovascular systems. To minimize the occurrence of hypotension after initial injection, keep patient lying down and observe for at least ½ hour. If hypotension occurs after parenteral or oral dosing, place patient in head-low position with legs raised. If a vasoconstrictor is required, 'Levophed' and 'Neo-Synephrine'* are suitable. Other pressor agents, including epinephrine, should not be used because they may cause a paradoxical further lowering of blood pressure.

Aspiration of vomitus has occurred in a few post-surgical patients who have received 'Compazine' as an antiemetic. Although no causal relationship has been established, this possibility should be borne in mind during surgical aftercare.

Deep sleep, from which patients can be aroused, and coma have been reported, usually with overdosage.

Neuroleptic drugs elevate prolactin levels; the elevation persists during chronic administration. Tissue culture experiments indicate that approximately one-third of human breast cancers are prolactin-dependent in vitro, a factor of potential importance if the prescribing of these drugs is contemplated in a patient with a previously detected breast cancer. Although disturbances such as galactorrhea, amenorrhea, gynecomastia and impotence have been reported, the clinical significance of elevated serum prolactin levels is unknown for most patients. An increase in mammary neoplasms has been found in rodents after chronic administration of neuroleptic drugs. Neither clinical nor epidemiologic studies conducted to date, however, have shown an association between chronic administration of these drugs and mammary tumorigenesis; the available evidence is considered too limited to be conclusive at this time.

As with all drugs which exert an anticholinergic effect, and/or cause mydriasis, prochlorperazine should be used with caution in patients with glaucoma.

Phenothiazines can diminish the effect of oral anticoagulants.

Phenothiazines can produce alpha-adrenergic blockade.

Concomitant administration of propranolol with phenothiazines results in increased plasma levels of both drugs.

Phenothiazines may lower the convulsive threshold; dosage adjustments of anticonvulsants may be necessary. Potentiation of anticonvulsant effects does not occur. However, it has been reported that phenothiazines may interfere with the metabolism of 'Dilantin'† and thus precipitate 'Dilantin' toxicity.

Long-Term Therapy: To lessen the likelihood of adverse reactions related to cumulative drug effect, patients with a history of long-term therapy with Compazine (prochlorperazine, SK&F) and/or other neuroleptics should be evaluated periodically to decide whether the maintenance dosage could be lowered or drug therapy discontinued.

Children with acute illnesses (e.g., chickenpox, C.N.S. infections, measles, gastroenteritis) or dehydration seem to be much more susceptible to neuromuscular reactions, particularly dystonias, than are adults. In such patients, the drug should be used only under close supervision.

Some solid oral dosage forms of 'Compazine' contain FD&C Yellow #5 (tartrazine) which may cause allergic-type reactions (including bronchial asthma) in certain susceptible individuals. Although the overall incidence of FD&C Yellow #5 (tartrazine) sensitivity in the general population is low, it is frequently seen in patients who also have aspirin sensitivity. The solid oral dosage forms of 'Compazine' which contain FD&C Yellow #5 are in the process of being reformulated to remove it. For specific information, contact Smith Kline &French Laboratories (outside Pa., call toll-free: 1-800-523-4835, ext. 4262; in Pa., call collect: 215-751-4262).

Drugs which lower the seizure threshold, including phenothiazine derivatives, should not be used with 'Amipaque'.†† As with other phenothiazine derivatives, 'Compazine' should be discontinued at least 48 hours before myelography, should not be resumed for at least 24 hours postprocedure, and should not be used for the control of nausea and vomiting occurring either prior to myelography or postprocedure.

Adverse Reactions: Drowsiness, dizziness, amenorrhea, blurred vision, skin reactions and hypotension may occur.

Cholestatic jaundice has occurred. If fever with grippe-like symptoms occurs, appropriate liver studies should be conducted. If tests indicate an abnormality, stop treatment. There have been a few observations of fatty changes in the livers of patients who have died while receiving the drug. No causal relationship has been established.

Leukopenia and agranulocytosis have occurred. Warn patients to report the sudden appearance of sore throat or other signs of infection. If white blood cell and differential counts indicate leukocyte depression, stop treatment and start antibiotic and other suitable therapy.

Neuromuscular (Extrapyramidal) Reactions

These symptoms are seen in a significant number of hospitalized mental patients. They may be characterized by motor restlessness, be of the dystonic type, or they may resemble parkinsonism.

Depending on the severity of symptoms, dosage should be reduced or discontinued. If therapy is reinstituted, it should be at a lower dosage. Should these symptoms occur in children or pregnant patients, the drug should be stopped and not reinstituted. In most cases barbiturates by suitable route of administration will suffice. (Or, injectable 'Benadryl'§ may be useful.) In more severe cases, the administration of an anti-parkinsonism agent, except levodopa, usually produces rapid reversal of symptoms. Suitable supportive measures such as maintaining a clear airway and adequate hydration should be employed.

Motor Restlessness: Symptoms may include agitation or jitteriness and sometimes insomnia. These symptoms often disappear spontaneously. At times these symptoms may be similar to the original neurotic or psychotic symptoms. Dosage should not be increased until these side effects have subsided.

If this phase becomes too troublesome, the symptoms can usually be controlled by a reduction of dosage or concomitant administration of a barbiturate.

Dystonias: Symptoms may include: spasm of the neck muscles, sometimes progressing to torticollis; extensor rigidity of back muscles, sometimes progressing to opisthotonos; carpopedal spasm, trismus, swallowing difficulty, oculogyric crisis and protrusion of the tongue. These usually subside within a few hours, and almost always within 24 to 48 hours, after the drug has been discontinued.

In mild cases, reassurance or a barbiturate is often sufficient. *In moderate cases,* barbiturates will usually bring rapid relief. *In more severe adult cases,* the administration of an anti-parkinsonism agent, except levodopa, usually produces rapid reversal of symptoms. *In children,* reassurance and barbiturates will usually control symptoms. (Or, injectable 'Benadryl' may be useful. Note: See 'Benadryl' prescribing information for appropriate *children's* dosage.) If appropriate treatment with anti-parkinsonism agents or 'Benadryl' fails to reverse the signs and symptoms, the diagnosis should be reevaluated.

Pseudo-parkinsonism: Symptoms may include: mask-like facies; drooling; tremors; pill-rolling motion; cogwheel rigidity; and shuffling gait. Reassurance and sedation are important. In most cases these symptoms are readily controlled when an anti-parkinsonism agent is administered concomitantly. Anti-parkinsonism agents should be used only when required. Generally, therapy of a few weeks to two or three months will suffice. After this time patients should be evaluated to determine their need for continued treatment. (Note: Levodopa has not been found effective in pseudo-parkinsonism.) Occasionally it is necessary to lower the dosage of 'Compazine' or to discontinue the drug.

Persistent Tardive Dyskinesia: As with all antipsychotic agents, tardive dyskinesia may appear in some patients on long-term therapy or may appear after drug therapy has been discontinued. This condition appears in all age groups. However, the risk appears to be greater in elderly patients on high-dose therapy, especially females. The symptoms are persistent and in some patients appear to be irreversible. The syndrome is characterized by rhythmical involuntary movements of the tongue, face, mouth or jaw (e.g., protrusion of tongue, puffing of cheeks, puckering of mouth, chewing movements). Sometimes these may be accompanied by involuntary movements of extremities. In rare instances, these involuntary movements of the extremities are the only manifestations of tardive dyskinesia.

There is no known effective treatment for tardive dyskinesia; anti-parkinsonism agents do not alleviate the symptoms of this syndrome. It is suggested that all antipsychotic agents be discontinued if these symptoms appear. Should it be necessary to reinstitute treatment, or increase the dosage of the agent, or switch to a different antipsychotic agent, the syndrome may be masked.

It has been reported that fine vermicular movements of the tongue may be an early sign of the syndrome and if the medication is stopped at that time the syndrome may not develop.

Contact Dermatitis: Avoid getting the Injection solution on hands or clothing because of the possibility of contact dermatitis.

Adverse Reactions Reported with Compazine (prochlorperazine, SK&F) or Other Phenothiazine Derivatives: Adverse reactions with different phenothiazines vary in type, frequency, and mechanism of occurrence, i.e., some are dose-related, while others involve individual patient sensitivity. Some adverse reactions may be more likely to occur, or occur with greater intensity, in patients with special medical problems, e.g., patients with mitral insufficiency or pheochromocytoma have experienced severe hypotension following recommended doses of certain phenothiazines.

Not all of the following adverse reactions have been observed with every phenothiazine derivative, but they have been reported with one or more and should be borne in mind when drugs of this class are administered: extrapyramidal symptoms (opisthotonos, oculogyric crisis, hyperreflexia, dystonia, akathisia, dyskinesia, parkinsonism) some of which have lasted months and even years—particularly in elderly patients with previous brain damage; grand mal and petit mal convulsions; altered cerebrospinal fluid proteins; cerebral edema; intensification and prolongation of the action of central nervous system depressants (opiates, analgesics, antihistamines, barbiturates, alcohol), atropine, heat, organophosphorus insecticides; autonomic reactions (dryness of mouth, nasal congestion, headache, nausea, constipation, obstipation, adynamic ileus, inhibition of ejaculation, priapism); reactivation of psychotic processes, catatonic-like states; hypotension (sometimes fatal); cardiac arrest; blood dyscrasias (pancytopenia, thrombocytopenic purpura, leukopenia, agranulocytosis, eosinophilia, hemolytic anemia, aplastic anemia); liver damage (jaundice, biliary stasis); endocrine disturbances (lactation, galactorrhea, gynecomastia, menstrual irregularities, false positive pregnancy tests); skin disorders (photosensitivity, itching, erythema, urticaria, eczema up to exfoliative dermatitis); other allergic reactions (asthma, laryngeal edema, angioneurotic edema, anaphylactoid reactions); peripheral edema; reversed epinephrine effect; hyperpyrexia; mild fever after large I.M. doses; increased appetite; increased weight; a systemic lupus erythematosus-like syndrome; pigmentary retinopathy; with prolonged administration of substantial doses, skin pigmentation, epithelial keratopathy, and lenticular and corneal deposits.

EKG changes—particularly nonspecific, usually reversible Q and T wave distortions—have been observed in some patients receiving phenothiazine tranquilizers. Their relationship to myocardial damage has not been confirmed.

Although phenothiazines cause neither psychic nor physical dependence, sudden discontinuance in long-term psychiatric patients may cause temporary symptoms, e.g., nausea and vomiting, dizziness, tremulousness.

Note: There have been occasional reports of sudden death in patients receiving phenothiazines. In some cases, the cause appeared to be asphyxia due to failure of the cough reflex. In others, the cause could not be determined. There is not sufficient evidence to establish a relationship between such deaths and the administration of phenothiazines.

Dosage and Administration: Note on Injection: It is recommended that Compazine (prochlorperazine, SK&F) Injection not be mixed with other agents in the syringe. This solution should be protected from light. Slight yellowish discoloration will not alter potency. If markedly discolored, solution should be discarded. When administered I.V., do not use bolus injection.

Dosage and Administration—Adults: (For children's dosage and administration, see below.) Dosage should be increased more gradually in debilitated or emaciated patients.

Elderly Patients: In general, dosages in the lower range are sufficient for most elderly patients. Since they appear to be more susceptible to hypotension and neuromuscular reactions, such patients should be observed closely. Dosage should be tailored to the individual, response carefully monitored, and dosage adjusted accordingly. Dosage should be increased more gradually in elderly patients.

1. To Control Severe Nausea and Vomiting or to Control Excessive Anxiety: Adjust dosage to the response of the individual. Begin with the lowest recommended dosage.

Oral Dosage: Usually 5 or 10 mg. 3 or 4 times daily; by 'Spansule' capsule, usually one 15 mg. capsule on arising or one 10 mg. capsule q12h.

Rectal Dosage: 25 mg. twice daily.

I.M. Dosage: Initially 5 to 10 mg. (1–2 ml.) injected *deeply* into the upper outer quadrant of the buttock. If necessary, repeat every 3 or 4 hours. Total I.M. dosage should not exceed 40 mg. per day.

Subcutaneous administration is not advisable because of local irritation.

2. Adult Surgery (for severe nausea and vomiting): Total parenteral dosage should not exceed 40 mg. per day. Hypotension is a possibility if the drug is given by I.V. injection or infusion.

I.M. Dosage: 5 to 10 mg. (1–2 ml.) 1 to 2 hours before induction of anesthesia (repeat once in 30 minutes, if necessary), or to control acute symptoms during and after surgery (repeat once if necessary).

I.V. Injection: 5 to 10 mg. (1–2 ml.) 15 to 30 minutes before induction of anesthesia, or to control acute symptoms during or after surgery. Repeat once if necessary. The rate of administration should not exceed 5 mg./ml./min. When administered I.V., do not use bolus injection.

I.V. Infusion: 20 mg. (4 ml.) per liter of isotonic solution. Add to I.V. infusion 15 to 30 minutes before induction.

3. In Adult Psychiatry: Adjust dosage to the response of the individual and according to the severity of the condition. Begin with the lowest recommended dose. Although response ordinarily is seen within a day or two, longer treatment is usually required before maximal improvement is seen.

Oral Dosage: *In relatively mild conditions,* as seen in private psychiatric practice or in outpatient clinics, dosage is 5 or 10 mg. 3 or 4 times daily.

In moderate to severe conditions, for hospitalized or adequately supervised patients, usual starting dosage is 10 mg. 3 or 4 times daily. Increase dosage gradually until symptoms are controlled or side effects become bothersome. When dosage is increased by small increments every 2 or 3 days, side effects either do not occur or are easily controlled. Some patients respond satisfactorily on 50 to 75 mg. daily.

In more severe disturbances, optimum dosage is usually 100 to 150 mg. daily.

I.M. Dosage: For immediate control of severely disturbed adults, inject an initial dose of 10 to 20 mg. (2–4 ml.) *deeply* into the upper outer quadrant of the buttock. Many patients respond shortly after the first injection. If necessary, however, repeat the initial dose every 2 to 4 hours (or, in resistant cases, every hour) to gain control of the patient. More than 3 or 4 doses are seldom necessary. After control is achieved, switch patient to an oral form of the drug at the same dosage level or higher. If, in rare cases, parenteral therapy is needed for a prolonged period, give 10 to 20 mg. (2–4 ml.) every 4 to 6 hours. Pain and irritation at the site of injection have seldom occurred.

Subcutaneous administration is not advisable because of local irritation.

Dosage and Administration—Children:

Do not use in pediatric surgery.

Children seem more prone to develop extrapyramidal reactions, even on moderate doses. Therefore, use lowest effective dosage. Tell parents not to exceed prescribed dosage, since the possibility of adverse reactions increases as dosage rises.

Occasionally the patient may react to the drug with signs of restlessness and excitement; if this occurs, do not administer additional doses. Take particular precaution in administering the drug to children with acute illnesses or dehydration (see under Dystonias).

When writing a prescription for the 2½ mg. size suppository, write "2½," not "2.5"; this will help avoid confusion with the 25 mg. adult size.

1. Severe Nausea and Vomiting in Children: Compazine (prochlorperazine, SK&F) should not be used in children under 20 pounds in weight or two years of age. It should not be used in conditions for which children's dosages have not been established. Dosage and frequency of administration should be adjusted according to the severity of the symptoms and the response of the patient. The duration of activity following intramuscular administration may last up to 12 hours. Subsequent doses may be given by the same route if necessary.

Oral or Rectal Dosage: More than one day's therapy is seldom necessary.

Weight	Usual Dosage	Not to Exceed
under 20 lbs.	not recommended	
20–29 lbs.	2½ mg. 1 or 2 times a day	7.5 mg. per day
30–39 lbs.	2½ mg. 2 or 3 times a day	10 mg. per day

Continued on next page

Smith Kline & French—Cont.

40–85 lbs.	2½ mg. 3 times a day or 5 mg. 2 times a day	15 mg. per day

I.M. Dosage: Calculate each dose on the basis of 0.06 mg. of the drug per lb. of body weight; give by deep I.M. injection. Control is usually obtained with one dose.

2. In Child Psychiatry:

Oral or Rectal Dosage: For children 2 to 12 years, starting dosage is 2½ mg. 2 or 3 times daily. Do not give more than 10 mg. the first day. Then increase dosage according to patient's response.

FOR AGES 2–5, total daily dosage usually does not exceed 20 mg.

FOR AGES 6–12, total daily dosage usually does not exceed 25 mg.

I.M. Dosage: For ages under 12, calculate each dose on the basis of 0.06 mg. of Compazine (prochlorperazine, SK&F) per lb. of body weight; give by deep I.M. injection. Control is usually obtained with one dose. After control is achieved, switch the patient to an oral form of the drug at the same dosage level or higher.

Overdosage: (See also Adverse Reactions.)

Symptoms—Primarily involvement of the extrapyramidal mechanism producing some of the dystonic reactions described above.

Symptoms of central nervous system depression to the point of somnolence or coma. Agitation and restlessness may also occur. Other possible manifestations include convulsions, EKG changes and cardiac arrhythmias, fever, and autonomic reactions such as hypotension, dry mouth and ileus.

Treatment—It is important to determine other medications taken by the patient since multiple dose therapy is common in overdosage situations. Treatment is essentially symptomatic and supportive. Early gastric lavage is helpful. Keep patient under observation and maintain an open airway, since involvement of the extrapyramidal mechanism may produce dysphagia and respiratory difficulty in severe overdosage. **Do not attempt to induce emesis because a dystonic reaction of the head or neck may develop that could result in aspiration of vomitus.** Extrapyramidal symptoms may be treated with anti-parkinsonism drugs, barbiturates, or 'Benadryl'. See prescribing information for these products. Care should be taken to avoid increasing respiratory depression.

If administration of a stimulant is desirable, amphetamine, dextroamphetamine, or caffeine with sodium benzoate is recommended.

Stimulants that may cause convulsions (e.g., picrotoxin or pentylenetetrazol) should be avoided.

If hypotension occurs, the standard measures for managing circulatory shock should be initiated. If it is desirable to administer a vasoconstrictor, 'Levophed' and 'Neo-Synephrine' are most suitable. Other pressor agents, including epinephrine, are not recommended because phenothiazine derivatives may reverse the usual elevating action of these agents and cause a further lowering of blood pressure.

Limited experience indicates that phenothiazines are *not* dialyzable.

Special note on 'Spansule' capsules—Since much of the 'Spansule' capsule medication is coated for gradual release, therapy directed at reversing the effects of the ingested drug and at supporting the patient should be continued for as long as overdosage symptoms remain. Saline cathartics are useful for hastening evacuation of pellets that have not already released medication.

How Supplied:

Tablets—5 and 10 mg., in bottles of 100 and 1000; in Single Unit Packages of 100 (intended for institutional use only). For use in severe neuropsychiatric conditions, 25 mg., in bottles of 100 and 1000.

'Spansule' capsules—10, 15 and 30 mg., in bottles of 50 and 500; in Single Unit Packages of 100 (intended for institutional use only). For use in severe neuropsychiatric conditions, 75 mg., in bottles of 50. **Ampuls**—2 ml. (5mg./ml.), in boxes of 10, 100 and 500. **Multiple-dose Vials**—10 ml. (5 mg./ml.), in boxes of 1, 20 and 100.

Disposable Syringes—2 ml. (5 mg./ml.), individually packaged in boxes of 10 and 100.

Suppositories—2½ mg. (for young children), 5 mg. (for older children) and 25 mg. (for adults), in boxes of 12. **Syrup**—5 mg./teaspoonful (5 ml.), in 4 fl. oz. bottles.

Military—Injection 2 ml., 100's, 6505-00-656-1610; Suppositories 2½ mg., 12's, 6505-00-133-5213; 25 mg., 12's, 6505-00-133-5214; Tablets 5 mg., 1000's, 6505-00-022-1328, and S.U.P. 100's 6505-00-118-2563; 10 mg., 1000's, 6505-00-022-1329.

---

*'Levophed' and 'Neo-Synephrine' are the trademarks (Reg. U.S. Pat. Off.) of Winthrop Laboratories for its brands of levarterenol and phenylephrine respectively.

†Trademark Reg. U.S. Pat. Off.: 'Dilantin' for diphenylhydantoin, Parke-Davis.

††Trademark Reg. U.S. Pat. Off.: 'Amipaque' for metrizamide, Winthrop Laboratories.

§Trademark Reg. U.S. Pat. Off.: 'Benadryl' for diphenhydramine hydrochloride, Parke-Davis.

[*Shown in Product Identification Section*]

CYTOMEL® TABLETS ℞

(brand of liothyronine sodium)
[L-triiodothyronine]

Description: 'Cytomel' contains liothyronine (L-triiodothyronine or LT_3) as the sodium salt. 25 mcg. of liothyronine is equivalent to approximately 1 grain of desiccated thyroid or thyroglobulin and 0.1 mg. of L-thyroxine.

Actions: 'Cytomel' contains liothyronine sodium, a synthetic form of a natural thyroid hormone, with all pharmacologic activities of the natural substance. Thyroid hormone acts to promote the synthesis of protein. It increases the metabolic rate of the body, presumably by, among other things, increasing oxygen consumption, altering enzymes (particularly those that affect growth), and altering the permeability of the mitochondrial membranes of cells.

Since liothyronine sodium is not firmly bound to serum protein, 'Cytomel' is readily available to body tissues. Following oral administration, about 85% of the dose is absorbed from the gastrointestinal tract. The onset of activity of liothyronine sodium is rapid, occurring within a few hours. Maximum pharmacologic response occurs within two or three days, providing early clinical response. The biological half-life is about 2½ days. The drug has a rapid cutoff of activity which permits quick dosage adjustment and facilitates control of the effects of overdosage, should they occur.

'Cytomel' can be used in patients allergic to desiccated thyroid or thyroid extract derived from pork or beef.

Indications:

1. Cytomel (liothyronine sodium, SK&F) is indicated for thyroid replacement in patients with inadequate endogenous thyroid hormone production. These include mild hypofunction, cretinism, and myxedema. Replacement therapy will be effective only in manifestations of hypothyroidism.
2. Simple (non-toxic) goiter: 'Cytomel' may be used therapeutically in an attempt to reduce the size of such a goiter.
3. For use in the T_3 suppression test to differentiate suspected *hyper*thyroidism from euthyroidism. (See special instructions under Dosage and Administration.)

Contraindication: Uncorrected adrenal insufficiency.

Warnings:

> Drugs with thyroid hormone activity, alone or together with other therapeutic agents, have been used for the treatment of obesity. In euthyroid patients, doses within the range of daily hormonal requirements are ineffective for weight reduction. Larger doses may produce serious or even life-threatening manifestations of toxicity, particularly when given in association with sympathomimetic amines such as those used for their anorectic effects.

Cytomel (liothyronine sodium, SK&F) should not be used in the presence of cardiovascular disease unless thyroid-replacement therapy is clearly indicated. In such cases, it should be used with caution and initiated at a low dosage, with due consideration for its relatively rapid onset of action. Starting dosage is 5 mcg. daily, and should be increased by no more than 5 mcg. increments at two-week intervals.

Morphologic hypogonadism and nephrosis should be ruled out before the drug is administered. If hypopituitarism is present, the adrenal deficiency must be corrected prior to starting the drug.

Myxedematous patients are very sensitive to thyroid; dosage should be started at a very low level and increased gradually.

Severe and prolonged hypothyroidism can lead to a decreased level of adrenocortical activity commensurate with the lowered metabolic state. When thyroid-replacement therapy is administered, the metabolism increases at a greater rate than adrenocortical activity. This can precipitate adrenocortical insufficiency. Therefore, in severe and prolonged hypothyroidism, supplemental adrenocortical steroids may be necessary.

In rare instances the administration of thyroid hormone may precipitate a hyperthyroid state or may aggravate existing hyperthyroidism.

Precautions: Since liothyronine sodium is not as firmly bound to serum protein as thyroxine, the PBI usually remains at levels below normal during full replacement therapy using Cytomel (liothyronine sodium, SK&F).

As with all thyroid preparations, thyroid gland function reflected by ^{131}I thyroid uptake may be depressed by 'Cytomel', particularly when dosage exceeds 75 mcg. daily. This effect disappears rapidly, and useful ^{131}I thyroid uptake values may be obtained usually within two weeks following discontinuance of the drug.

Adverse Reactions: Overdosage will produce signs and symptoms of hyperthyroidism, such as nervousness, cardiac arrhythmias, angina pectoris, and menstrual irregularities. (See Overdosage section.) Medication should be interrupted until symptoms disappear, then resumed in smaller doses. Therapy can usually be resumed after one or two days.

In rare instances, allergic skin reactions have been reported.

Dosage and Administration: Optimum dosage is usually determined by the patient's clinical response. Confirmatory tests include: Radioactive Iodine T_3 Resin Uptake, BMR, Thyro Binding Index (TBI), and the Achilles Tendon Reflex test.

Once-a-day dosage is recommended; although Cytomel (liothyronine sodium, SK&F) has a rapid cutoff, its metabolic effects persist for a few days following discontinuance.

Mild Hypothyroidism: Recommended starting dosage is 25 mcg. daily. Daily dosage then may be increased by 12.5 or 25 mcg. every one or two weeks. Usual maintenance dose is 25–75 mcg. daily. Smaller doses may be fully effective in some patients, while dosage of 100 mcg. daily may be required in others.

Myxedema: Recommended starting dosage is 5 mcg. daily. This may be increased by 5 to 10 mcg. daily every one or two weeks. When 25 mcg. daily is reached, dosage may often be increased by 12.5 or 25 mcg. every one or two weeks. Usual maintenance dose is 50 to 100 mcg. daily.

Cretinism: Since the mother provides little or no thyroid hormone to the fetus, infants with thyroid dysfunction will require replacement therapy from birth. Treatment should be initiated as early as possible to avoid permanent physical and mental changes.

Recommended starting dosage is 5 mcg. daily, with a 5 mcg. increment every three to four days until the desired response is achieved. Infants a few months old may require only 20 mcg. daily for maintenance. At 1 year, 50 mcg. daily may be required. Above 3 years, full adult dosage may be necessary.

Simple (non-toxic) goiter: Recommended starting dosage is 5 mcg. daily. This dosage may be increased by 5 to 10 mcg. daily every one or two weeks. When 25 mcg. daily is reached, dosage may be increased every week or two by 12.5 or 25 mcg. Usual maintenance dosage is 75 mcg. daily.

In the elderly or in children, therapy should be started with 5 mcg. daily and increased only by 5 mcg. increments at the recommended intervals.

When switching a patient to 'Cytomel' from thyroid, L-thyroxine or thyroglobulin, discontinue the other medication, initiate 'Cytomel' at a low dosage, and increase gradually according to the patient's response. When selecting a starting dosage, bear in mind that this drug has a rapid onset of action, and that residual effects of the other thyroid preparation may persist for the first several weeks of therapy.

Special Instructions for T_3 Suppression Test: When ^{131}I Thyroid Uptake is in the borderline-high range, administer 75-100 mcg. of Cytomel (liothyronine sodium, SK&F) daily for 7 days, then repeat ^{131}I Thyroid Uptake test. In the hyperthyroid patient, 24-hour ^{131}I Thyroid Uptake will not be affected significantly. In the euthyroid patient, 24-hour ^{131}I Thyroid Uptake will drop to less than 20%.

Overdosage: *Symptoms*—Headache, irritability, nervousness, sweating, tachycardia, increased bowel motility, and menstrual irregularities. Angina pectoris or congestive heart failure may be induced or aggravated. Shock may also develop. Massive overdosage may result in symptoms resembling thyroid storm. Chronic excessive dosage will produce the signs and symptoms of hyperthyroidism. *Treatment*—In shock, supportive measures and treatment of unrecognized adrenal insufficiency should be considered.

How Supplied: In three dosage strengths: 5 mcg. tablets in bottles of 100; 25 mcg. tablets (scored) in bottles of 100 and 1000; and 50 mcg. tablets (scored) in bottles of 100.

Military—Tablets 5 mcg., 100's, 6505-00-660-1609; 25 mcg., 1000's, 6505-00-066-4875.

[*Shown in Product Identification Section*]

DARBID® TABLETS, 5 mg. ℞
(brand of isopropamide iodide)

Description: Each tablet contains isopropamide iodide equivalent to 5 mg. of isopropamide.

Chemically, Darbid (isopropamide iodide, SK&F) is 3-carbamoyl-3, 3-diphenylpropyl) diisopropylmethyl ammonium iodide.

Actions: Darbid (isopropamide iodide, SK&F) is a synthetic anticholinergic that produces 10- to 12-hour gastric acid antisecretory effect and gastrointestinal antispasmodic response in man.

Indications

Based on a review of this drug by the National Academy of Sciences—National Research Council and/or other information, FDA has classified the indications as follows:

Effective: As adjunctive therapy in peptic ulcer.

Probably effective: In the irritable bowel syndrome (irritable colon, spastic colon, mucous colitis, acute enterocolitis, and functional gastrointestinal disorders).

Final classification of the less-than-effective indications requires further investigation.

IT SHOULD BE NOTED AT THIS POINT IN TIME THAT THERE IS A LACK OF CONCURRENCE AS TO THE VALUE OF ANTICHOLINERGICS IN THE TREATMENT OF GASTRIC ULCER. IT HAS NOT BEEN SHOWN CONCLUSIVELY WHETHER ANTICHOLINERGIC DRUGS AID IN THE HEALING OF A PEPTIC ULCER, DECREASE THE RATE OF RECURRENCES, OR PREVENT COMPLICATION.

FUNCTIONAL DISORDERS ARE OFTEN RELIEVED BY VARYING COMBINATIONS OF SEDATIVES, REASSURANCE, PHYSICIAN INTEREST, AMELIORATION OF ENVIRONMENTAL FACTORS, ETC.

To be effective, dosage must be titrated to the individual patient's needs.

Contraindications: Glaucoma; obstructive uropathy (e.g., bladder neck obstruction due to prostatic hypertrophy); obstructive disease of the gastrointestinal tract (as in achalasia, pyloroduodenal stenosis, etc.); obstructive or paralytic ileus, intestinal atony of the elderly or debilitated patient; unstable cardiovascular status in acute hemorrhage; severe ulcerative colitis; toxic megacolon complicating ulcerative colitis; myasthenia gravis.

Warnings: In the presence of a high environmental temperature, heat prostration (fever and heat stroke due to decreased sweating) can occur.

In patients with diarrhea due to incomplete intestinal obstruction (especially those with ileostomy or colostomy), treatment with Darbid (isopropamide iodide, SK&F) would be inappropriate and possibly harmful.

'Darbid' may produce drowsiness or blurred vision. In this event, the patient should be warned not to engage in activities requiring mental alertness such as operating a motor vehicle or other machinery or perform hazardous work while taking this drug.

Usage in Pregnancy: In pregnancy, lactation, and in women who may bear children, the potential benefits of the drug must be weighed against possible hazards.

Precautions: Use cautiously in elderly patients.

Since the iodine in isopropamide iodide may alter PBI test results and will suppress I^{131} uptake, it is suggested that therapy be discontinued one week prior to these tests. Also, iodine skin rash may occur rarely.

Use with caution in patients with:

Autonomic neuropathy.

Hepatic or renal disease.

Ulcerative colitis (large doses may suppress intestinal motility to the point of producing paralytic ileus, and the use of this drug may precipitate or aggravate the serious complication of toxic megacolon).

Hyperthyroidism, coronary heart disease, congestive heart failure, cardiac arrhythmia, hypertension and nonobstructing prostatic hypertrophy.

Hiatal hernia associated with reflux esophagitis (anticholinergic drugs may aggravate this condition).

It should be noted that the use of anticholinergic drugs in the treatment of gastric ulcer may produce a delay in gastric emptying time (antral stasis) and, thus, complicate therapy.

Do not rely on the use of the drug in the presence of complication of biliary tract disease.

Investigate any tachycardia before giving anticholinergic (atropine-like) drugs, since they may increase the heart rate.

With overdosage, a curare-like action may occur.

Adverse Reactions: Anticholinergics produce certain pharmacological effects which may be desirable or undesirable, depending upon the individual patient's response. The physician must delineate these.

Adverse reactions which have occurred with Darbid (isopropamide iodide, SK&F) include: xerostomia (dry mouth); urinary hesitancy and retention; blurred vision; tachycardia; palpitations; mydriasis (dilatation of the pupils); cycloplegia; constipation; bloated feeling; nausea; dysphagia; fever; and nasal congestion.

Other adverse reactions possible with anticholinergics include: increased ocular tension; loss of taste; headaches; nervousness; drowsiness; weakness; dizziness; insomnia; vomiting; impotence; suppression of lactation; severe allergic reaction or drug idiosyncrasies including anaphylaxis; urticaria and other dermal manifestations; some degree of mental confusion and/or excitement, especially in elderly persons.

Decreased sweating may occur. It should be noted that adrenergic innervation of the eccrine sweat glands on the palms and soles makes complete control of sweating impossible. An end point of complete anhidrosis cannot occur because large doses of drug would be required, and this would produce severe side effects from parasympathetic paralysis.

Dosage and Administration: Not for use in children under 12. Adults and children over 12—Usual starting dose is one 5 mg. tablet b.i.d. (every 12 hours). Patients with severe symptoms may require two 5 mg. tablets b.i.d., or more. Dosage should be individualized and titrated to the patient's need for greatest therapeutic effect.

Overdosage: Involves the cardiovascular, respiratory, gastrointestinal, central and peripheral nervous systems.

SYMPTOMS—May include dryness of mouth, dysphagia, thirst, blurred vision, dilated pupils, photophobia, fever, rapid pulse and respiration, disorientation. Depression and circulatory collapse may result from severe overdosage. TREATMENT—Gastric lavage, repeated several times.

Respiratory depression should be promptly treated by the use of oxygen and stimulants. If marked excitement is present, one of the short-acting barbiturates, chloral hydrate, or gas anesthesia may be used. Otherwise do not administer sedation. Hyperpyrexia may be treated with physical cooling measures. Force fluids by mouth or, if necessary, by intravenous administration.

While pilocarpine or similar drugs are sometimes recommended for the relief of dry mouth, many authorities feel that these drugs are not indicated, since they relieve the minor peripheral effect but do not influence the more serious central effects and, thus, may merely mask signs of drug activity. If photophobia occurs, the patient should be kept in a darkened room.

How Supplied: In bottles of 50.

[*Shown in Product Identification Section*]

DEXEDRINE® Ⓒ
(brand of dextroamphetamine sulfate)
SPANSULE® CAPSULES, TABLETS and ELIXIR

Warning:

AMPHETAMINES HAVE A HIGH POTENTIAL FOR ABUSE. THEY SHOULD

Continued on next page

Smith Kline & French—Cont.

THUS BE TRIED ONLY IN WEIGHT REDUCTION PROGRAMS FOR PATIENTS IN WHOM ALTERNATIVE THERAPY HAS BEEN INEFFECTIVE. ADMINISTRATION OF AMPHETAMINES FOR PROLONGED PERIODS OF TIME IN OBESITY MAY LEAD TO DRUG DEPENDENCE AND MUST BE AVOIDED. PARTICULAR ATTENTION SHOULD BE PAID TO THE POSSIBILITY OF SUBJECTS OBTAINING AMPHETAMINES FOR NON-THERAPEUTIC USE OR DISTRIBUTION TO OTHERS, AND THE DRUGS SHOULD BE PRESCRIBED OR DISPENSED SPARINGLY.

Description: Dexedrine (dextroamphetamine sulfate, SK&F) is the dextro isomer of the compound *d,l*-amphetamine sulfate, a sympathomimetic amine of the amphetamine group. Chemically, dextroamphetamine is *d*-alpha-methylphenethylamine, and is present in all forms of 'Dexedrine' as the neutral sulfate.

Spansule® sustained release capsules—Each 'Spansule' sustained release capsule contains dextroamphetamine sulfate, 5 mg., 10 mg., or 15 mg., so prepared that an initial dose is released promptly and the remaining medication is released gradually over a prolonged period.

Tablets—Each tablet contains dextroamphetamine sulfate, 5 mg.

Elixir—Each 5 ml. (one teaspoonful) contains dextroamphetamine sulfate, 5 mg., and alcohol, 10%.

Actions: Amphetamines are sympathomimetic amines with CNS stimulant activity. Peripheral actions include elevation of systolic and diastolic blood pressures and weak bronchodilator and respiratory stimulant action.

There is neither specific evidence which clearly establishes the mechanism whereby amphetamines produce mental and behavioral effects in children, nor conclusive evidence regarding how these effects relate to the condition of the central nervous system.

Drugs of this class used in obesity are commonly known as "anorectics" or "anorexigenics." It has not been established, however, that the action of such drugs in treating obesity is primarily one of appetite suppression. Other central nervous system actions, or metabolic effects, may be involved, for example.

Adult obese subjects instructed in dietary management and treated with "anorectic" drugs lose more weight on the average than those treated with placebo and diet, as determined in relatively short-term clinical trials.

The magnitude of increased weight loss of drug-treated patients over placebo-treated patients is only a fraction of a pound a week. The rate of weight loss is greatest in the first weeks of therapy for both drug and placebo subjects and tends to decrease in succeeding weeks. The origins of the increased weight loss due to the various possible drug effects are not established. The amount of weight loss associated with the use of an "anorectic" drug varies from trial to trial, and the increased weight loss appears to be related in part to variables other than the drug prescribed, such as the physician-investigator, the population treated, and the diet prescribed. Studies do not permit conclusions as to the relative importance of the drug and nondrug factors on weight loss.

The natural history of obesity is measured in years, whereas the studies cited are restricted to a few weeks' duration; thus, the total impact of drug-induced weight loss over that of diet alone must be considered clinically limited.

'Dexedrine' *Spansule* capsules are formulated to release the active drug substance *in vivo* in a more gradual fashion than the standard formulation, as demonstrated by blood levels. The formulation has not been shown superior in effectiveness over the same dosage of the standard, noncontrolled-release formulations given in divided doses.

Indications: Dexedrine (dextroamphetamine sulfate, SK&F) is indicated:

1. **In Narcolepsy.**
2. As an integral part of a total treatment program which typically includes other remedial measures (psychological, educational, social) for a stabilizing effect in children with a behavioral syndrome characterized by the following group of developmentally inappropriate symptoms: moderate to severe distractibility, short attention span, hyperactivity, emotional lability, and impulsivity. The diagnosis of this syndrome should not be made with finality when these symptoms are only of comparatively recent origin. Nonlocalizing (soft) neurological signs, learning disability, and abnormal EEG may or may not be present, and a diagnosis of central nervous system dysfunction may or may not be warranted.
3. **In Exogenous Obesity,** as a short-term (a few weeks) adjunct in a regimen of weight reduction based on caloric restriction, for patients refractory to alternative therapy, e.g., repeated diets, group programs, and other drugs. The limited usefulness of amphetamines (see ACTIONS) should be weighed against possible risks inherent in use of the drug, such as those described below.

Contraindications: Advanced arteriosclerosis, symptomatic cardiovascular disease, moderate to severe hypertension, hyperthyroidism, known hypersensitivity or idiosyncrasy to the sympathomimetic amines, glaucoma.

Agitated states.

Patients with a history of drug abuse.

During or within 14 days following the administration of monoamine oxidase inhibitors (hypertensive crises may result).

Warnings: When tolerance to the "anorectic" effect develops, the recommended dose should not be exceeded in an attempt to increase the effect; rather, the drug should be discontinued.

Amphetamines may impair the ability of the patient to engage in potentially hazardous activities such as operating machinery or vehicles; the patient should therefore be cautioned accordingly.

Usage in Pregnancy: Safe use in pregnancy has not been established. Reproduction studies in mammals at high multiples of the human dose have suggested both an embryotoxic and a teratogenic potential. Use of amphetamines by women who are or who may become pregnant, and especially those in the first trimester of pregnancy, requires that the potential benefit be weighed against the possible hazard to mother and infant.

Usage in Children: Amphetamines are not recommended for use as anorectic agents in children under 12 years of age, or in children under 3 years of age with the behavioral syndrome described under INDICATIONS.

Clinical experience suggests that in psychotic children, administration of amphetamines may exacerbate symptoms of behavior disturbance and thought disorder.

Amphetamines have been reported to exacerbate motor and phonic tics and Tourette's syndrome.

Data are inadequate to determine whether chronic administration of amphetamines may be associated with growth inhibition; therefore, growth should be monitored during treatment.

Precautions: Caution is to be exercised in prescribing amphetamines for patients with even mild hypertension.

Insulin requirements in diabetes mellitus may be altered in association with the use of amphetamines and the concomitant dietary regimen.

Amphetamines may decrease the hypotensive effect of guanethidine.

The least amount feasible should be prescribed or dispensed at one time in order to minimize the possibility of overdosage.

Drug treatment is not indicated in all cases of the behavioral syndrome and should be considered only in light of the complete history and evaluation of the child. The decision to prescribe amphetamines should depend on the physician's assessment of the chronicity and severity of the child's symptoms and their appropriateness for his/her age. Prescription should not depend solely on the presence of one or more of the behavioral characteristics.

When these symptoms are associated with acute stress reactions, treatment with amphetamines is usually not indicated.

Long-term effects of amphetamines in children have not been well established.

These products contain FD&C Yellow #5 (tartrazine), which may cause allergic-type reactions (including bronchial asthma) in certain susceptible individuals. Although the overall incidence of FD&C Yellow #5 (tartrazine) sensitivity in the general population is low, it is frequently seen in patients who also have aspirin hypersensitivity.

Adverse Reactions: *Cardiovascular:* Palpitation, tachycardia, elevation of blood pressure. *Central nervous system:* Overstimulation, restlessness, dizziness, insomnia, euphoria, dyskinesia, dysphoria, tremor, headache; rarely, psychotic episodes at recommended doses. *Gastrointestinal:* Dryness of the mouth, unpleasant taste, diarrhea, constipation, other gastrointestinal disturbances. Anorexia and weight loss may occur as undesirable effects when amphetamines are used for other than the anorectic effect. *Allergic:* Urticaria. *Endocrine:* Impotence, changes in libido.

Drug Abuse and Dependence: Dexedrine (dextroamphetamine sulfate, SK&F) is a Schedule II controlled substance.

Amphetamines have been extensively abused. Tolerance, extreme psychological dependence, and severe social disability have occurred. There are reports of patients who have increased the dosage to many times that recommended. Abrupt cessation following prolonged high dosage administration results in extreme fatigue and mental depression; changes are also noted on the sleep EEG.

Manifestations of chronic intoxication with amphetamines include severe dermatoses, marked insomnia, irritability, hyperactivity, and personality changes. The most severe manifestation of chronic intoxication is psychosis, often clinically indistinguishable from schizophrenia.

Dosage and Administration: Regardless of indication, amphetamines should be administered at the lowest effective dosage and dosage should be individually adjusted. Late evening doses—particularly with the 'Spansule' capsule form—should be avoided because of the resulting insomnia.

Narcolepsy: Usual dose 5 to 60 milligrams per day in divided doses, depending on the individual patient response.

Narcolepsy seldom occurs in children under 12 years of age; however, when it does, Dexedrine (dextroamphetamine sulfate, SK&F) may be used. The suggested initial dose for patients aged 6-12 is 5 mg. daily; daily dose may be raised in increments of 5 mg. at weekly intervals until optimal response is obtained. In patients 12 years of age and older, start with 10 mg. daily; daily dosage may be raised in increments of 10 mg. at weekly intervals until optimal response is obtained. If bothersome adverse reactions appear (e.g., insomnia or anorexia), dosage should be reduced. 'Spansule' capsules may be used for once-a-day dosage wherever appropriate. With tablets or elixir, give first dose on awakening; additional doses (1 or 2) at intervals of 4 to 6 hours.

Behavioral Syndrome in Children: Not recommended for children under 3 years of age.

In children from 3 to 5 years of age, start with 2.5 mg. daily, by tablet or elixir; daily dosage may be raised in increments of 2.5 mg. at weekly intervals until optimal response is obtained.

In children 6 years of age and older, start with 5 mg. once or twice daily; daily dosage may be raised in increments of 5 mg. at weekly intervals until optimal response is obtained. Only in rare cases will it be necessary to exceed a total of 40 milligrams per day.

'Spansule' capsules may be used for once-a-day dosage wherever appropriate.

With tablets or elixir, give first dose on awakening; additional doses (1 or 2) at intervals of 4 to 6 hours.

Where possible, drug administration should be interrupted occasionally to determine if there is a recurrence of behavioral symptoms sufficient to require continued therapy.

Exogenous Obesity: Usual dosage is one 10 or 15 mg. 'Spansule' capsule daily, taken in the morning, or up to 30 mg. daily by tablets or elixir, taken in divided doses of 5 to 10 mg. 30 to 60 minutes before meals. Not recommended for this use in children under 12 years of age.

Overdosage: SYMPTOMS—Manifestations of acute overdosage with amphetamines include restlessness, tremor, hyperreflexia, rapid respiration, confusion, assaultiveness, hallucinations, panic states.

Fatigue and depression usually follow the central stimulation.

Cardiovascular effects include arrhythmias, hypertension or hypotension and circulatory collapse. Gastrointestinal symptoms include nausea, vomiting, diarrhea, and abdominal cramps. Fatal poisoning is usually preceded by convulsions and coma.

TREATMENT—Management of acute amphetamine intoxication is largely symptomatic and includes gastric lavage and sedation with a barbiturate. Experience with hemodialysis or peritoneal dialysis is inadequate to permit recommendation in this regard. Acidification of the urine increases amphetamine excretion. If acute, severe hypertension complicates amphetamine overdosage, administration of intravenous phentolamine (Regitine®, CIBA) has been suggested. However, a gradual drop in blood pressure will usually result when sufficient sedation has been achieved.

Since much of the 'Spansule' capsule medication is coated for gradual release, therapy directed at reversing the effects of the ingested drug and at supporting the patient should be continued for as long as overdosage symptoms remain. Saline cathartics are useful for hastening the evacuation of pellets that have not already released medication.

How Supplied:

'Spansule' capsules—Gelatin capsules having a natural body and brown cap, filled with small light orange, medium orange and dark orange pellets; 5 mg., in bottles of 50; 10 mg. and 15 mg., in bottles of 50 and 500.

Tablets—Pastel orange, triangular-shaped, single scored, compressed tablets; 5 mg., in bottles of 100 and 1000.

Elixir—A clear, orange-colored, orange-flavored liquid, containing 5 mg./5 ml., in 16 fl. oz. (473 ml.) bottles.

Military—Tablets 5 mg., 100's, 6505-00-106-8715.

[*Shown in Product Identification Section*]

DIBENZYLINE® Capsules ℞

(brand of phenoxybenzamine hydrochloride)

Description: Each capsule contains phenoxybenzamine hydrochloride, 10 mg.

Actions: Dibenzyline (phenoxybenzamine hydrochloride, SK&F) is a long-acting, adrenergic, α-receptor blocking agent which can produce and maintain "chemical sympathectomy" by oral administration. It increases blood flow to the skin, mucosa and abdominal viscera, and lowers both supine and erect blood pressures. It has no effect on the parasympathetic system.

Indication: Pheochromocytoma, to control episodes of hypertension and sweating. If tachycardia is excessive, it may be necessary to use a beta-blocking agent concomitantly.

Contraindications: Conditions where a fall in blood pressure may be undesirable.

Warning: 'Dibenzyline'-induced *alpha*-adrenergic blockade leaves *beta*-adrenergic receptors unopposed. Compounds that stimulate both types of receptors may therefore produce an exaggerated hypotensive response and tachycardia.

Precautions: Phenoxybenzamine hydrochloride has shown *in vitro* mutagenic activity in the Ames test and in the mouse lymphoma assay; it has not shown mutagenic activity in the micronucleus test in mice. In rats and mice repeated intraperitoneal administration of phenoxybenzamine hydrochloride resulted in peritoneal sarcomas. The clinical significance of such test results is not established. Nevertheless, these results should be given consideration in determining the benefit-risk ratio as it applies to the individual patient.

Administer with caution in patients with marked cerebral or coronary arteriosclerosis or renal damage. Adrenergic blocking effect may aggravate symptoms of respiratory infections.

Dibenzyline (phenoxybenzamine hydrochloride, SK&F) should not be used in diseases involving the larger blood vessels where direct-acting vasodilators are preferred therapy.

Adverse Reactions: Nasal congestion, miosis, postural hypotension, tachycardia and inhibition of ejaculation may occur. These so-called "side effects" are actually evidence of adrenergic blockade and vary according to the degree of blockade. Furthermore, they tend to decrease as therapy is continued. Gastrointestinal irritation, drowsiness and fatigue have also been reported.

Dosage and Administration: The dosage should be adjusted to fit the needs of each patient. Small initial doses should be *slowly* increased until the desired effect is obtained or the side effects from blockade become troublesome. *After each increase, the patient should be observed on that level for at least 4 days before instituting another increase.* The dosage should be carried to a point where symptomatic relief and/or objective improvement are obtained, but not so high that the side effects from blockade become troublesome.

Initially, 10 mg. daily. After at least 4 days, the daily dosage may be increased by 10 mg., and similarly increased thereafter until optimum dosage is reached. Dosage range is usually 20–60 mg. daily. NOTE: At least 2 weeks are usually required to reach the optimal dosage level in most patients. At this time improvement in these patients will usually be observed. But it may be several more weeks before the *full* benefits of the drug become apparent.

Overdosage: *Symptoms*—These are largely the result of block of the sympathetic nervous system and of the circulating epinephrine. They may include postural hypotension resulting in dizziness or fainting; tachycardia, particularly postural; vomiting; lethargy; shock.

Treatment—When symptoms and signs of overdosage exist, discontinue the drug. Treatment of circulatory failure, if present, is a prime consideration. In cases of mild overdosage, recumbent position with legs elevated usually restores cerebral circulation. In the more severe cases, the usual measures to combat shock should be instituted. Usual pressor agents are *not* effective. Epinephrine is contraindicated because it stimulates both α and β receptors; since α receptors are blocked, the net effect of epinephrine administration is vasodilation and a further drop in blood pressure (epinephrine reversal).

The patient may have to be kept flat for 24 hours or more in the case of overdose, as the effect of the drug is prolonged. Leg bandages and an abdominal binder may shorten the period of disability.

I.V. infusion of levarterenol bitartrate* may be used to combat severe hypotensive reactions, because it stimulates α receptors primarily. Although Dibenzyline (phenoxybenzamine hydrochloride, SK&F) is an α adrenergic blocking agent, a sufficient dose of levarterenol bitartrate will overcome this effect.

How Supplied: Bottles of 100.

*Available as Levophed® Bitartrate (brand of levarterenol bitartrate) from Winthrop Laboratories.

[*Shown in Product Identification Section*]

DYAZIDE® Capsules ℞

('Dyazide' is a product of SK&F Co., Carolina, P.R. 00630, Subsidiary of SmithKline Beckman Corporation, Philadelphia, Pa.)

> **Warning:**
> This fixed combination drug is not indicated for initial therapy of edema or hypertension. Edema or hypertension requires therapy titrated to the individual patient. If the fixed combination represents the dosage so determined, its use may be more convenient in patient management. The treatment of hypertension and edema is not static, but must be reevaluated as conditions in each patient warrant.

Description: Each maroon and white 'Dyazide' capsule contains 50 mg. of Dyrenium® (brand of triamterene), a potassium-sparing agent, and 25 mg. of hydrochlorothiazide.

'Dyrenium' is 2, 4, 7-triamino-6-phenylpteridine.

Hydrochlorothiazide is 6-chloro-3, 4-dihydro-2*H*-1, 2, 4-benzothiadiazine-7-sulfonamide 1, 1-dioxide.

At 50°C., triamterene is practically insoluble in water (less than 0.1%). It is soluble in formic acid, sparingly soluble in methoxyethanol, and very slightly soluble in alcohol.

Hydrochlorothiazide is slightly soluble in water. It is soluble in dilute ammonia, dilute aqueous sodium hydroxide, and dimethylformamide. It is sparingly soluble in methanol.

Action: 'Dyazide' is a diuretic/antihypertensive drug product that combines the natriuretic, hydrochlorothiazide, and the potassium-sparing natriuretic, triamterene, each of which complements the action of the other. The hydrochlorothiazide component blocks the reabsorption of sodium and chloride ions, and thereby increases the quantity of sodium traversing the distal tubule and the volume of water excreted. A portion of the additional sodium presented to the distal tubule is exchanged there for potassium and hydrogen ions. With continued use of hydrochlorothiazide and depletion of sodium, compensatory mechanisms tend to increase this exchange and may produce excessive loss of potassium, hydrogen and chloride ions. Hydrochlorothiazide also decreases the excretion of calcium and uric acid, may increase the excretion of iodide and may reduce glomerular filtration rate. The exact mechanism of the antihypertensive effect of hydrochlorothiazide is not known.

The triamterene component of 'Dyazide' exerts its diuretic effect on the distal renal tubule to inhibit the reabsorption of sodium in exchange for potassium and hydrogen ions. Its natriuretic activity is limited by the amount of sodium reaching its site of action. Although it blocks the increase in this exchange that is

Continued on next page

Smith Kline & French—Cont.

stimulated by mineralocorticoids (chiefly aldosterone) it is not a competitive antagonist of aldosterone and its activity can be demonstrated in adrenalectomized rats and patients with Addison's disease. As a result the dose of triamterene required is not proportionally related to the level of mineralocorticoid activity, but is dictated by the response of the individual patient, and the kaliuretic effect of concomitantly administered drugs. By inhibiting the distal tubular exchange mechanism, triamterene maintains or increases the sodium excretion and reduces the excess loss of potassium, hydrogen, and chloride ions induced by hydrochlorothiazide. As with hydrochlorothiazide, triamterene may reduce glomerular filtration and renal plasma flow. Via this mechanism it may reduce uric acid excretion although it has no tubular effect on uric acid reabsorption or secretion. Triamterene does not affect calcium excretion. No predictable antihypertensive effect has been demonstrated for triamterene.

Duration of diuretic activity and effective dosage range of the hydrochlorothiazide and triamterene components of 'Dyazide' are similar. Onset of diuresis with 'Dyazide' takes place within one hour, peaks at two-three hours and tapers off during the subsequent seven to nine hours.

Indications: This combination drug finds its usefulness primarily in the treatment of edema. Any usefulness of triamterene when used with a thiazide in hypertension will derive from its potassium-sparing effect. Either its main diuretic effect or potassium-sparing effect when used with a thiazide drug should be determined by individual titration. (See box warning.)

When the fixed combination represents the dosage determined by titration, 'Dyazide' is indicated as adjunctive therapy in edema associated with congestive heart failure, hepatic cirrhosis and the nephrotic syndrome. It is also indicated in corticosteroid and estrogen induced edema and idiopathic edema.

When the potassium-sparing action of its Dyrenium (triamterene, SK&F CO.) component is warranted and the fixed combination represents the dosage determined by titration, 'Dyazide' is indicated in the management of hypertension as determined by individual dosage titration of all agents employed. (See box warning.)

Usage in Pregnancy. The routine use of diuretics in an otherwise healthy woman is inappropriate and exposes mother and fetus to unnecessary hazard. Diuretics do not prevent development of toxemia of pregnancy, and there is no satisfactory evidence that they are useful in the treatment of developed toxemia. Edema during pregnancy may arise from pathological causes or from the physiologic and mechanical consequences of pregnancy. Diuretics are indicated in pregnancy when edema is due to pathologic causes, just as they are in the absence of pregnancy (however, see Warnings, below). Dependent edema in pregnancy, resulting from restriction of venous return by the expanded uterus, is properly treated through elevation of the lower extremities and use of support hose; use of diuretics to lower intravascular volume in this case is illogical and unnecessary. There is hypervolemia during normal pregnancy which is harmful to neither the fetus nor the mother (in the absence of cardiovascular disease), but which is associated with edema, including generalized edema, in the majority of pregnant women. If this edema produces discomfort, increased recumbency will often provide relief. In rare instances, this edema may cause extreme discomfort which is not relieved by rest. In these cases, a short course of diuretics may provide relief and may be appropriate.

Contraindications: 'Dyazide' should not be given to patients receiving other potassium-sparing agents such as spironolactone or amiloride. Two deaths have been reported in patients receiving concomitant spironolactone and Dyrenium (triamterene, SK&F CO.) or 'Dyazide'. In one case dosage recommendations were exceeded; in the other serum electrolytes were not properly monitored.

'Dyazide' is contraindicated for further use in patients who exhibit anuria or progressive renal dysfunction, including increasing oliguria and increasing azotemia or in patients who develop hyperkalemia while on the drug.

'Dyazide' should not be used in patients with pre-existing elevated serum potassium, as is sometimes seen in patients with impaired renal function. Increasing hepatic dysfunction in patients on 'Dyazide' contraindicates further use of the preparation. Hypersensitivity to either drug in the preparation or to other sulfonamide-derived drugs is a contraindication.

Warnings: Patients should not be placed on dietary potassium supplements, potassium salts, or potassium-containing salt substitutes in conjunction with 'Dyazide' unless they develop hypokalemia or their dietary intake of potassium is markedly impaired. Because of the potassium conserving effect of Dyrenium (triamterene, SK&F CO.), hypokalemia is an uncommon occurrence with the use of 'Dyazide'. If the need for supplementary potassium is demonstrated by repeated low serum potassium determinations a form other than potassium tablets should be used since these have been implicated in the development of nonspecific small bowel lesions consisting of stenosis with or without ulceration.

Abnormal elevation of serum potassium, though uncommon, is potentially the most severe electrolyte disturbance with 'Dyazide' therapy. Hyperkalemia has been reported and in some cases has been associated with cardiac irregularities. Hyperkalemia is more likely to occur in patients who are severely ill, with relatively small urine volumes (less than one liter per day), or in elderly or diabetic patients with confirmed or suspected renal insufficiency. Acute transient hyperkalemia has been observed during intravenous glucose tolerance testing of diabetics dosed with the Dyrenium (triamterene, SK&F CO.) component of 'Dyazide'. Fatalities due to hyperkalemia have been reported, accordingly no potassium supplements should ordinarily be given with 'Dyazide' therapy, and periodic determinations of serum potassium should be made. If hyperkalemia develops, withdraw 'Dyazide', substitute a thiazide alone, and restrict potassium intake.

If hyperkalemia is present or suspected, an electrocardiogram should be obtained. If the ECG shows no widening of the QRS or arrhythmia in the presence of hyperkalemia, it is usually sufficient to discontinue 'Dyazide' and any potassium supplementation and substitute a thiazide alone. Sodium polystyrene sulfonate (Kayexalate®, Winthrop) may be administered to enhance the excretion of excess potassium. **The presence of a widened QRS complex or arrhythmia in association with hyperkalemia requires prompt additional therapy.** For tachyarrhythmia, infuse 44 mEq. of sodium bicarbonate or 10 ml. of 10% calcium gluconate or calcium chloride over several minutes. For asystole, bradycardia or A-V block transvenous pacing is also recommended.

The effect of calcium and sodium bicarbonate is transient and repeated administration may be required. When indicated by the clinical situation, excess K+ may be removed by dialysis or oral or rectal administration of Kayexalate®. Infusion of glucose and insulin has also been used to treat hyperkalemia.

Sensitivity reactions may occur in patients with or without a history of allergy or bronchial asthma.

The possibility of exacerbation or activation of systemic lupus erythematosus has been reported with thiazide diuretics.

Usage in Pregnancy. Thiazides cross the placental barrier and appear in cord blood. The use of thiazides in pregnant women requires that the anticipated benefit be weighed against possible hazards to the fetus. These hazards include fetal or neonatal jaundice, thrombocytopenia, and possibly other adverse reactions which have occurred in the adult.

Nursing Mothers. Thiazides appear and triamterene may appear in breast milk. If use of the drug product is deemed essential, the patient should stop nursing.

Usage in Children

Adequate information on the use of 'Dyazide' in children is not available.

Precautions: Electrolyte imbalance, often encountered in such conditions as heart failure, renal disease, or cirrhosis of the liver. may also be aggravated by diuretics, and should be considered during 'Dyazide' therapy when using high doses for prolonged periods or in patients on a salt-restricted diet. Serum determinations of electrolytes should be performed, and are particularly important if the patient is vomiting excessively or receiving fluids parenterally. Possible fluid and electrolyte imbalance may be indicated by such warning signs as: dry mouth, thirst, weakness, lethargy, drowsiness, restlessness, muscle pain or cramps, muscular fatigue, hypotension, oliguria, tachycardia, and gastrointestinal symptoms.

Because of the potassium-sparing characteristic of Dyrenium (triamterene, SK&F CO.), hypokalemia is uncommon with 'Dyazide' but may occur in some cases when the 'Dyrenium' component is unable to completely compensate for the potassium-wasting effect of the hydrochlorothiazide component or the disease. The myocardial effects of digitalis may be exaggerated in patients with hypokalemia. In these patients signs of digitalis intoxication may be produced by previously tolerated doses of digitalis.

Hypokalemia is uncommon with 'Dyazide' but should it develop, corrective measures should be taken such as potassium supplementation or increased dietary intake of potassium-rich foods. Institute such measures cautiously with frequent determinations of serum potassium levels. Discontinue corrective measures immediately if laboratory determinations reveal an abnormal elevation of serum potassium. Discontinue 'Dyazide' and substitute a thiazide diuretic alone until potassium levels return to normal.

Although any chloride deficit is generally mild and usually does not require specific treatment except under extraordinary circumstances (as in liver disease or renal disease), chloride replacement may be required in the treatment of metabolic alkalosis. Dilutional hyponatremia may occur in edematous patients in hot weather; appropriate therapy is water restriction, rather than administration of salt, except in rare instances when the hyponatremia is life threatening. In actual salt depletion, appropriate replacement is the therapy of choice.

'Dyazide' may produce an elevated blood urea nitrogen level, creatinine level, or both. This apparently is secondary to a reversible reduction of glomerular filtration rate or a depletion of intravascular fluid volume (pre-renal azotemia) rather than renal toxicity; levels return to normal when 'Dyazide' is discontinued. Elevated levels are seldom seen with every-other-day therapy. If azotemia increases, discontinue 'Dyazide'. Cumulative effects of the drug may develop in patients with impaired renal function. Periodic BUN or serum creatinine determinations should be made, especially in elderly patients and in patients with suspected or confirmed renal insufficiency.

Triamterene has been found in renal stones in association with the other usual calculus components. Therefore, 'Dyazide' should be used with caution in patients with histories of stone formation.

A possible interaction resulting in acute renal failure has been reported in a few patients on 'Dyazide' when treated with indomethacin, a nonsteroidal anti-inflammatory agent. Caution is advised in administering nonsteroidal anti-inflammatory agents with 'Dyazide'.

Thiazides should be used with caution in patients with impaired hepatic function. They can precipitate hepatic coma in patients with severe liver disease. Potassium depletion induced by the thiazide may be important in this connection. Administer 'Dyazide' cautiously and be alert for such early signs of impending coma as confusion, drowsiness and tremor; if mental confusion increases discontinue 'Dyazide' for a few days. Attention must be given to other factors that may precipitate hepatic coma, such as blood in the gastrointestinal tract or preexisting potassium depletion.

Patients should be observed regularly for the possible occurrence of blood dyscrasias, liver damage, or other idiosyncratic reactions. There have been reports of blood dyscrasias in patients receiving 'Dyrenium'. Leukopenia, thrombocytopenia, agranulocytosis, and aplastic and hemolytic anemia have been reported with the thiazides. Cirrhotics with splenomegaly may have marked variations in their blood pictures—including thrombocyte and leukocyte levels—which are not related to drug therapy. Since the 'Dyrenium' component of 'Dyazide' is a weak folic acid antagonist, it may contribute to the appearance of megaloblastosis in cases where folic acid stores are depleted. Periodic blood studies in these patients are recommended.

The antihypertensive effects of 'Dyazide' may be enhanced in the post-sympathectomy patient.

Diabetes mellitus which has been latent may become manifest during thiazide administration.

Thiazides may cause hyperglycemia and glycosuria, and alter insulin requirements in diabetes. 'Dyazide' may have similar effects; concurrent use with chlorpropamide may increase the risk of severe hyponatremia. Hyperuricemia may be observed, with possible occurrence of gout. Dyrenium (triamterene, SK&F CO.) may cause a decreasing alkali reserve with the possibility of metabolic acidosis.

Thiazides may add to or potentiate the action of other antihypertensive drugs. See Dosage and Administration for concomitant use with other antihypertensive drugs.

Thiazides have been shown to decrease arterial responsiveness to norepinephrine (an effect attributed to loss of sodium). This diminution is not sufficient to preclude effectiveness of the pressor agent for therapeutic use. Thiazides have also been shown to increase the paralyzing effect of nondepolarizing muscle relaxants such as tubocurarine (an effect attributed to potassium loss); consequently caution should be observed in patients undergoing surgery.

Thiazides may decrease serum PBI levels without signs of thyroid disturbance.

Calcium excretion is decreased by thiazides. Pathologic changes in the parathyroid glands with hypercalcemia and hypophosphatemia have been observed in a few patients on prolonged thiazide therapy. The common complications of hyperparathyroidism such as renal lithiasis, bone resorption, and peptic ulceration have not been seen. Thiazides should be discontinued before carrying out tests for parathyroid function.

'Dyrenium' and quinidine have similar fluorescence spectra; thus, 'Dyazide' will interfere with the fluorescent measurement of quinidine.

Lithium generally should not be given with diuretics because they reduce its renal clearance and increase the risk of lithium toxicity. Read circulars for lithium preparations before use of such concomitant therapy with 'Dyazide'.

Concurrent use of hydrochlorothiazide with amphotericin B or corticosteroids or corticotropin (ACTH) may intensify electrolyte imbalance, particularly hypokalemia, although the presence of triamterene minimizes the hypokalemic effects.

The effects of oral anticoagulants may be decreased when used concurrently with hydrochlorothiazide; dosage adjustments may be necessary.

Adverse Reactions: Side effects observed in association with the use of 'Dyazide' include: muscle cramps, weakness, dizziness, headache and dry mouth; anaphylaxis, rash, urticaria, photosensitivity, purpura and other dermatological conditions; nausea and vomiting, diarrhea, constipation, and other gastrointestinal disturbances (such nausea can usually be prevented by giving the drug after meals). It should be noted that symptoms of nausea and vomiting can also be indicative of electrolyte imbalance (see Precautions). Postural hypotension (may be aggravated by alcohol, barbiturates, or narcotics). Impotence has been reported in a few patients on 'Dyazide', although a causal relationship has not been established. Triamterene has been found in renal stones in association with the other usual calculus components (see Precautions).

Thiazides alone have been known to cause necrotizing vasculitis, paresthesias, icterus, pancreatitis, xanthopsia, and respiratory distress including pneumonitis and pulmonary edema, transient blurred vision, sialadenitis, and vertigo. Rare incidents of acute interstitial nephritis have been reported with the use of 'Dyazide'.

Newborn, whose mothers had received thiazides during pregnancy, in rare instances have developed thrombocytopenia or pancreatitis.

Dosage and Administration: As determined by individual titration. (See box warning.)

Adults:

The usual dose is one or two capsules twice daily after meals. Some patients may be maintained on one capsule daily or every other day. Maximum daily dose should not exceed four capsules, and at this dosage, the incidence of side effects may increase.

Since 'Dyazide' has an antihypertensive effect, hypotensive drugs used concomitantly should be added at reduced dosage—at least one half the usual dosage—particularly if it is a ganglionic or peripheral adrenergic blocking agent. Adjust dosage as indicated.

Children:

Adequate information on the use of 'Dyazide' in children is not available.

Note: Potassium supplementation used concurrently with other diuretics should be discontinued when titrating with Dyrenium (triamterene, SK&F CO.). They should not be reinstituted when the patient is placed on 'Dyazide' unless the triamterene component does not completely compensate for the potassium loss.

Overdosage: Electrolyte imbalance is the major concern (See Warnings section). Symptoms reported include: polyuria, nausea, vomiting, weakness, lassitude, fever, flushed face, and hyperactive deep tendon reflexes. If hypotension occurs, it may be treated with pressor agents such as levarterenol to maintain blood pressure. Carefully evaluate the electrolyte pattern and fluid balance. Induce immediate evacuation of the stomach through emesis or gastric lavage. There is no specific antidote.

Although triamterene is largely protein-bound (approximately 67%), there may be some benefit to dialysis in cases of overdosage.

How Supplied: 'Dyazide' is supplied in gelatin capsules having an opaque white body and maroon cap, with tapered ends, in bottles of 1000 capsules; in Single Unit Packages (unit-dose) of 100 (intended for institutional use only); in Patient-Pak™ unit-of-use bottles of 100.

[Shown in Product Identification Section]

DYRENIUM® ℞
(brand of triamterene)

('Dyrenium' is a product of SK&F Co., Carolina, P.R. 00630, Subsidiary of SmithKline Beckman Corporation, Philadelphia, Pa.)

Description: Each capsule contains triamterene, 50 mg. or 100 mg.

Dyrenium (triamterene, SK&F CO.) is 2,4,7-triamino-6-phenylpteridine.

Action: Dyrenium (triamterene, SK&F CO.) has a unique mode of action; it inhibits the reabsorption of sodium ions in exchange for potassium and hydrogen ions at that segment of the distal tubule under the control of adrenal mineralocorticoids (especially aldosterone). This activity takes place through a direct effect on the renal tubule and not by competitive aldosterone antagonism; it is not directly related to the level of aldosterone secretion.

The fraction of filtered sodium reaching this distal tubular exchange site is relatively small, and the amount which is exchanged depends on the level of mineralocorticoid activity. Thus, the degree of natriuresis and diuresis produced by inhibition of the exchange mechanism is necessarily limited. Increasing the amount of available sodium and the level of mineralocorticoid activity by the use of more proximally-acting diuretics will increase the degree of diuresis and potassium conservation.

'Dyrenium' occasionally causes increases in serum potassium which, in some instances, can result in hyperkalemia. It does not produce alkalosis because it does not cause excessive excretion of titratable acid and ammonium.

Indications: Dyrenium (triamterene, SK&F CO.) is indicated in the treatment of edema associated with congestive heart failure, cirrhosis of the liver, and the nephrotic syndrome; also in steroid-induced edema, idiopathic edema, and edema due to secondary hyperaldosteronism.

'Dyrenium' may be used alone or with other diuretics either for its added diuretic effect or its potassium-conserving potential. It also promotes increased diuresis when patients prove resistant or only partially responsive to thiazides or other diuretics because of secondary hyperaldosteronism.

Usage in Pregnancy. The routine use of diuretics in an otherwise healthy woman is inappropriate and exposes mother and fetus to unnecessary hazard. Diuretics do not prevent development of toxemia of pregnancy, and there is no satisfactory evidence that they are useful in the treatment of developed toxemia.

Edema during pregnancy may arise from pathological causes or from the physiologic and mechanical consequences of pregnancy. Diuretics are indicated in pregnancy when edema is due to pathologic causes, just as they are in the absence of pregnancy (however, see Warnings, below). Dependent edema in pregnancy, resulting from restriction of venous return by the expanded uterus, is properly treated through elevation of the lower extremities and use of support hose; use of diuretics to lower intravascular volume in this case is illogical and unnecessary. There is hypervolemia during normal pregnancy which is harmful to neither the fetus nor the mother (in the absence of cardiovascular disease), but which is associated with edema, including generalized edema, in the majority of pregnant women. If this edema produces discomfort, increased recumbency will often provide relief. In rare instances, this edema may cause extreme discomfort which is not relieved by rest. In these

Continued on next page

Smith Kline & French—Cont.

cases, a short course of diuretics may provide relief and may be appropriate.

Contraindications: Dyrenium (triamterene, SK&F CO.) should not be given to patients receiving other potassium-sparing agents such as spironolactone or amiloride. Two deaths have been reported in patients receiving concomitant spironolactone and 'Dyrenium': In one case, dosage recommendations were exceeded; in the other, serum electrolytes were not properly monitored.

Anuria. Severe or progressive kidney disease or dysfunction with the possible exception of nephrosis. Severe hepatic disease. Hypersensitivity to the drug.

'Dyrenium' should not be used in patients with preexisting elevated serum potassium, as is sometimes seen in patients with impaired renal function or azotemia, or in patients who develop hyperkalemia while on the drug. Patients should not be placed on dietary potassium supplements, potassium salts, or potassium-containing salt substitutes in conjunction with 'Dyrenium'.

Warnings: Patients should be observed regularly for the possible occurrence of blood dyscrasias, liver damage, or other idiosyncratic reactions. There have been reports of blood dyscrasias in patients receiving Dyrenium (triamterene, SK&F CO.).

Periodic BUN and serum potassium determinations should be made to check kidney function, especially in patients with suspected or confirmed renal insufficiency. It is particularly important to make serum potassium determinations in elderly or diabetic patients receiving the drug; these patients should be observed carefully for possible adverse serum potassium increases.

Usage in Pregnancy. Triamterene has been shown to cross the placental barrier and appear in the cord blood of ewes; this may occur in humans. The use of 'Dyrenium' in pregnant women requires that the anticipated benefit be weighed against possible hazards to the fetus. These possible hazards include adverse reactions which have occurred in the adult.

Nursing Mothers. Triamterene appears in cow's milk; this may occur in humans. If use of the drug is deemed essential, the patient should stop nursing.

Precautions: Dyrenium (triamterene, SK&F CO.) tends to conserve potassium rather than to promote its excretion as do many diuretics and, occasionally, can cause increases in serum potassium which, in some instances, can result in hyperkalemia. In rare instances, hyperkalemia has been associated with cardiac irregularities.

Hyperkalemia will rarely occur in patients with adequate urinary output, but it is a possibility if large doses are used for considerable periods of time.* If hyperkalemia is observed, 'Dyrenium' should be withdrawn. Because 'Dyrenium' conserves potassium, it has been theorized that in patients who have received intensive therapy or been given the drug for prolonged periods, a rebound kaliuresis could occur upon abrupt withdrawal. In such patients withdrawal of 'Dyrenium' should be gradual.

Electrolyte imbalance often encountered in such diseases as congestive heart failure, renal disease, or cirrhosis may be aggravated or caused independently by any effective diuretic agent including 'Dyrenium'. The use of full doses of a diuretic when salt intake is restricted can result in a low-salt syndrome.

'Dyrenium' can cause mild nitrogen retention which is reversible upon withdrawal of the drug and is seldom observed with intermittent (every-other-day) therapy.

Triamterene has been found in renal stones in association with other usual calculus components. Therefore, 'Dyrenium' should be used with caution in patients with histories of stone formation.

By the very nature of their illness, cirrhotics with splenomegaly sometimes have marked variations in their blood pictures. Since 'Dyrenium' is a weak folic acid antagonist, it may contribute to the appearance of megaloblastosis in cases where folic acid stores have been depleted. Therefore, periodic blood studies in these patients are recommended.

Although 'Dyrenium' has not proved to be a consistent antihypertensive agent, the physician should be aware of a possible lowering of blood pressure. Concomitant use with antihypertensive drugs may result in an additive effect.

'Dyrenium' may cause a decreasing alkali reserve with the possibility of metabolic acidosis. 'Dyrenium' and quinidine have similar fluorescence spectra; thus, 'Dyrenium' will interfere with the fluorescent measurement of quinidine.

A possible interaction resulting in acute renal failure has been reported in a few subjects when indomethacin, a nonsteroidal anti-inflammatory agent, was given with triamterene. Caution is advised in administering nonsteroidal anti-inflammatory agents with triamterene.

Lithium generally should not be given with diuretics because they reduce its renal clearance and increase the risk of lithium toxicity. Read circulars for lithium preparations before use of such concomitant therapy with 'Dyrenium'.

Adverse Reactions: There have been occasional reports of diarrhea, nausea and vomiting, and other gastrointestinal disturbances. Such nausea can usually be prevented by giving the drug after meals. It should be noted that symptoms of nausea and vomiting can also be indicative of electrolyte imbalance (see Precautions). Weakness, headache, dry mouth, anaphylaxis, photosensitivity, and rash have also been reported. Only rarely has it been necessary to discontinue therapy because of these side effects.

Triamterene has been found in renal stones in association with the other usual calculus components. Rare occurrences of acute interstitial nephritis have been reported with use of triamterene.

Note on Gout and Diabetes: In special studies, investigators found that Dyrenium (triamterene, SK&F CO.) has little or no effect on serum uric acid levels or carbohydrate metabolism. However, it has elevated uric acid, especially in persons predisposed to gouty arthritis.

Dosage and Administration: **Adult Dosage**
Dosage should be titrated to the needs of the individual patient. When used alone, the usual starting dose is 100 mg. twice daily after meals. When combined with another diuretic, the total daily dosage of each agent should usually be lowered initially, and then adjusted to the patient's needs. The total daily dosage should not exceed 300 mg.

Onset of action is 2–4 hours after ingestion. Most patients will respond to Dyrenium (triamterene, SK&F CO.) during the first day of treatment. Maximum therapeutic effect, however, may not be seen for several days. Duration of diuresis depends on several factors, especially renal function, but it generally tapers off 7–9 hours after administration.

When 'Dyrenium' is added to other diuretic therapy or when patients are switched to 'Dyrenium' from other diuretics, all potassium supplementation should be discontinued.

Overdosage: In the event of overdosage it can be theorized that electrolyte imbalance would be the major concern, with particular attention to possible hyperkalemia. Other symptoms that might be seen would be nausea and vomiting, other g.i. disturbances, and weakness. It is conceivable that some hypotension could occur. As with an overdose of any drug, immediate evacuation of the stomach should be induced through emesis and gastric lavage. Careful evaluation of the electrolyte pattern and fluid balance should be made. There is no specific antidote.

Although triamterene is largely protein-bound (approximately 67%), there may be some benefit to dialysis in cases of overdosage.

How Supplied: 50 mg. capsules, in bottles of 100, in Single Unit Packages of 100 (intended for institutional use only). 100 mg. capsules in bottles of 100 and 1000, in Single Unit Packages of 100 (intended for institutional use only).

Military—Capsules 100 mg., 100's, 6505-00-982-9143.

---

*In making laboratory checks, blood samples require careful handling to prevent hemolysis on standing with resulting false serum potassium readings.

[*Shown in Product Identification Section*]

ECOTRIN®
Duentric® Coated Aspirin

Composition: Each Ecotrin tablet contains 325 mg. (5 gr.) aspirin, specially processed with Duentric® coating to prevent disintegration in the stomach and minimize the possibility of consequent gastric irritation.

Indications: When your physician recommends regular use of aspirin, Ecotrin may be taken—particularly for temporary relief of minor aches and pains of arthritis and rheumatism. The Ecotrin tablet has a Duentric coating designed to protect against gastric upset caused by plain, uncoated aspirin. Because Ecotrin passes through the stomach before dissolving in the intestine, initial relief may take longer.

Usual Dosage: One or 2 tablets every 4 hours as necessary, with water or fruit juice. Do not exceed 12 tablets in 24 hours unless directed by a physician. Children—as recommended by physician.

Warning: If under medical care, do not use without physician's approval. If pain persists more than 10 days or redness is present, or in arthritic or rheumatic conditions affecting children under 12, consult a physician immediately. Discontinue use if dizziness, ringing in ears or impaired hearing occurs. If you experience persistent or unexplained stomach upset, consult a physician.

Keep this and all medicines out of reach of children. In case of accidental overdose contact a physician or poison control center immediately. Caution: If pregnant or nursing, consult a physician before taking this or any medicine.

EASY-OPENING CAP available on 250 tablet bottle—intended for households without young children.

How Supplied: Five grain tablets in bottles of 36, 100, 250 and 1000.

Physician Information: High aspirin dosage is recommended in arthritis and rheumatic conditions (40-80 gr. daily) and in acute rheumatic fever (up to 120 gr. daily), in divided doses. In arthritic and rheumatic conditions concomitant use of Ecotrin may permit a reduction in steroid dosage.

Marketed by Menley & James Laboratories, a SmithKline company.

Maximum Strength
ECOTRIN®
Duentric® Coated Aspirin

Composition: Each Maximum Strength Ecotrin tablet contains 500 mg. (7.69 gr.) aspirin, specially processed with Duentric® coating to prevent disintegration in the stomach and minimize the possibility of consequent gastric irritation.

Indications: When your physician recommends regular use of aspirin, Ecotrin may be taken—particularly for temporary relief of minor aches and pains of arthritis and rheumatism. The Maximum Strength Ecotrin tablet has a Duentric coating designed to protect against gastric upset caused by plain, uncoated aspirin. Because Ecotrin passes through the stomach before dissolving in the intestine, initial relief may take longer.

Usual Dosage: Two tablets every 6 hours as necessary, with water or fruit juice. Do not exceed 8 tablets in 24 hours unless directed by a physician. Children—as recommended by a physician.

Warning: If under medical care, do not use without your physician's approval. If pain persists more than 10 days or redness is present, or in arthritic or rheumatic conditions affecting children under 12, consult a physician immediately. Discontinue use if dizziness, ringing in ears or impaired hearing occurs. If you experience persistent or unexplained stomach upset, consult a physician.

Keep this and all medicines out of reach of children. In case of accidental overdose, contact a physician or poison control center immediately. Caution: If pregnant or nursing, consult a physician before taking this or any medicine. EASY-OPENING CAP available on 150 tablet bottle—intended for households without young children.

How Supplied: 500 mg. (7.69 grain) tablets, in bottles of 24, 60 and 150.

Physician Information: High aspirin dosage is recommended in arthritis and rheumatic conditions (40-80 gr. daily) and in acute rheumatic fever (up to 120 gr. daily), in divided doses. In arthritic and rheumatic conditions, concomitant use of Ecotrin may permit a reduction in steroid dosage.

Marketed by Menley & James Laboratories, a SmithKline company.

ESKALITH® ℞
(brand of lithium carbonate)
Capsules, 300 mg.
Tablets, 300 mg.

ESKALITH CR® ℞
(brand of lithium carbonate)
Controlled Release Tablets, 450 mg.

WARNING

Lithium toxicity is closely related to serum lithium levels, and can occur at doses close to therapeutic levels. Facilities for prompt and accurate serum lithium determinations should be available before initiating therapy (see DOSAGE AND ADMINISTRATION).

Description: 'Eskalith' contains lithium carbonate, a white, light alkaline powder with molecular formula Li_2CO_3 and molecular weight 73.89. Lithium is an element of the alkali-metal group with atomic number 3, atomic weight 6.94 and an emission line at 671 nm on the flame photometer.

'Eskalith CR' tablets 450 mg. are designed to release a portion of the dose initially and the remainder gradually; the release pattern of the controlled release tablets reduces the variability in lithium blood levels seen with the immediate release dosage forms.

Actions: Preclinical studies have shown that lithium alters sodium transport in nerve and muscle cells and effects a shift toward intraneuronal metabolism of catecholamines, but the specific biochemical mechanism of lithium action in mania is unknown.

Indications: Eskalith (lithium carbonate, SK&F) is indicated in the treatment of manic episodes of manic-depressive illness. Maintenance therapy prevents or diminishes the intensity of subsequent episodes in those manic-depressive patients with a history of mania.

Typical symptoms of mania include pressure of speech, motor hyperactivity, reduced need for sleep, flight of ideas, grandiosity, elation, poor judgment, aggressiveness, and possibly hostility. When given to a patient experiencing a manic episode, 'Eskalith' may produce a normalization of symptomatology within 1 to 3 weeks.

Warnings: Lithium should generally not be given to patients with significant renal or cardiovascular disease, severe debilitation or dehydration, or sodium depletion, and to patients receiving diuretics, since the risk of lithium toxicity is very high in such patients. If the psychiatric indication is life-threatening, and if such a patient fails to respond to other measures, lithium treatment may be undertaken with extreme caution, including daily serum lithium determinations and adjustment to the usually low doses ordinarily tolerated by these individuals. In such instances, hospitalization is a necessity.

Chronic lithium therapy may be associated with diminution of renal concentrating ability, occasionally presenting as nephrogenic diabetes insipidus, with polyuria and polydipsia. Such patients should be carefully managed to avoid dehydration with resulting lithium retention and toxicity. This condition is usually reversible when lithium is discontinued.

Morphologic changes with glomerular and interstitial fibrosis and nephron atrophy have been reported in patients on chronic lithium therapy. Morphologic changes have also been seen in manic-depressive patients never exposed to lithium. The relationship between renal functional and morphologic changes and their association with lithium therapy have not been established.

When kidney function is assessed, for baseline data prior to starting lithium therapy or thereafter, routine urinalysis and other tests may be used to evaluate tubular function (e.g., urine specific gravity or osmolality following a period of water deprivation, or 24-hour urine volume) and glomerular function (e.g., serum creatinine or creatinine clearance). During lithium therapy, progressive or sudden changes in renal function, even within the normal range, indicate the need for reevaluation of treatment.

An encephalopathic syndrome (characterized by weakness, lethargy, fever, tremulousness and confusion, extrapyramidal symptoms, leukocytosis, elevated serum enzymes, BUN and FBS) followed by irreversible brain damage has occurred in a few patients treated with lithium plus haloperidol. A causal relationship between these events and the concomitant administration of lithium and haloperidol has not been established; however, patients receiving such combined therapy should be monitored closely for early evidence of neurologic toxicity and treatment discontinued promptly if such signs appear. The possibility of similar adverse interactions with other antipsychotic medication exists.

Lithium toxicity is closely related to serum lithium levels, and can occur at doses close to therapeutic levels (see DOSAGE AND ADMINISTRATION).

Outpatients and their families should be warned that the patient must discontinue lithium carbonate therapy and contact his physician if such clinical signs of lithium toxicity as diarrhea, vomiting, tremor, mild ataxia, drowsiness, or muscular weakness occur.

Lithium carbonate may impair mental and/or physical abilities. Caution patients about activities requiring alertness (e.g., operating vehicles or machinery).

Lithium may prolong the effects of neuromuscular blocking agents. Therefore, neuromuscular blocking agents should be given with caution to patients receiving lithium.

Usage in Pregnancy: Adverse effects on implantation in rats, embryo viability in mice, and metabolism *in vitro* of rat testes and human spermatozoa have been attributed to lithium, as have teratogenicity in submammalian species and cleft palates in mice.

In humans, lithium carbonate may cause fetal harm when administered to a pregnant woman. Data from lithium birth registries suggest an increase in cardiac and other anomalies, especially Ebstein's anomaly. If this drug is used during pregnancy, or if a patient becomes pregnant while taking this drug, the patient should be apprised of the potential hazard to the fetus.

Usage in Nursing Mothers: Lithium is excreted in human milk. Nursing should not be undertaken during lithium therapy except in rare and unusual circumstances where, in the view of the physician, the potential benefits to the mother outweigh possible hazards to the child.

Usage in Children: Since information regarding the safety and effectiveness of lithium carbonate in children under 12 years of age is not available, its use in such patients is not recommended at this time.

Precautions: The ability to tolerate lithium is greater during the acute manic phase and decreases when manic symptoms subside (see DOSAGE AND ADMINISTRATION).

The distribution space of lithium approximates that of total body water. Lithium is primarily excreted in urine with insignificant excretion in feces. Renal excretion of lithium is proportional to its plasma concentration. The half-life of elimination of lithium is approximately 24 hours. Lithium decreases sodium reabsorption by the renal tubules which could lead to sodium depletion. Therefore, it is essential for the patient to maintain a normal diet, including salt, and an adequate fluid intake (2500–3000 ml.) at least during the initial stabilization period. Decreased tolerance to lithium has been reported to ensue from protracted sweating or diarrhea and, if such occur, supplemental fluid and salt should be administered. In addition to sweating and diarrhea, concomitant infection with elevated temperatures may also necessitate a temporary reduction or cessation of medication.

Previously existing underlying thyroid disorders do not necessarily constitute a contraindication to lithium treatment; where hypothyroidism exists, careful monitoring of thyroid function during lithium stabilization and maintenance allows for correction of changing thyroid parameters, if any; where hypothyroidism occurs during lithium stabilization and maintenance, supplemental thyroid treatment may be used.

Indomethacin has been reported to increase steady state plasma lithium levels from 30 to 59 percent. There is also some evidence that other nonsteroidal anti-inflammatory agents may have a similar effect. When such combinations are used, increased plasma lithium level monitoring is recommended.

Adverse Reactions: Adverse reactions are seldom encountered at serum lithium levels below 1.5 mEq./l., except in the occasional patient unusually sensitive to lithium. Mild to moderate toxic reactions may occur at levels from 1.5 to 2.5 mEq./l., and moderate to severe reactions may be seen at levels from 2.0 to 2.5 mEq./l., depending upon the individual response to the drug.

Fine hand tremor, polyuria, and mild thirst may occur during initial therapy for the acute manic phase, and may persist throughout treatment. Transient and mild nausea and general discomfort may also appear during the first few days of lithium administration.

These side effects are an inconvenience rather than a disabling condition, and usually subside with continued treatment or a temporary reduction or cessation of dosage. If persistent, a cessation of dosage is indicated.

Continued on next page

Smith Kline & French—Cont.

Diarrhea, vomiting, drowsiness, muscular weakness, and lack of coordination may be early signs of lithium intoxication, and can occur at lithium levels below 2.0 mEq./l. At higher levels, ataxia, giddiness, tinnitus, blurred vision, and a large output of dilute urine may be seen. Serum lithium levels above 3.0 mEq./l. may produce a complex clinical picture, involving multiple organs and organ systems. Serum lithium levels should not be permitted to exceed 2.0 mEq./l. during the acute treatment phase.

The following reactions have been reported and appear to be related to serum lithium levels, including levels within the therapeutic range: **Neuromuscular/Central Nervous System**—tremor, muscle hyperirritability (fasciculations, twitching, clonic movements of whole limbs), ataxia, choreo-athetotic movements, hyperactive deep tendon reflex, extrapyramidal symptoms, blackout spells, epileptiform seizures, slurred speech, dizziness, vertigo, incontinence of urine or feces, somnolence, psychomotor retardation, restlessness, confusion, stupor, coma, tongue movements, tics, tinnitus, hallucinations, poor memory, slowed intellectual functioning, startled response; **Cardiovascular**—cardiac arrhythmia, hypotension, peripheral circulatory collapse, bradycardia; **Gastrointestinal**—anorexia, nausea, vomiting, diarrhea, gastritis, salivary gland swelling, abdominal pain, excessive salivation, flatulence, indigestion; **Genitourinary**—albuminuria, oliguria, polyuria, glycosuria, decreased creatinine clearance; **Dermatologic**—drying and thinning of hair, alopecia, anesthesia of skin, chronic folliculitis, xerosis cutis, psoriasis or its exacerbation, itching, angioedema; **Autonomic**—blurred vision, dry mouth; **Thyroid Abnormalities**—euthyroid goiter and/or hypothyroidism (including myxedema) accompanied by lower T_3 and T_4. I^{131} uptake may be elevated. (See Precautions.) Paradoxically, rare cases of hyperthyroidism have been reported; **EEG Changes**—diffuse slowing, widening of the frequency spectrum, potentiation and disorganization of background rhythm; **EKG Changes**—reversible flattening, isoelectricity or inversion of T-waves; **Miscellaneous**—fatigue, lethargy, transient scotomata, dehydration, weight loss, tendency to sleep, transient electroencephalographic and electrocardiographic changes, leukocytosis, headache, diffuse nontoxic goiter with or without hypothyroidism, transient hyperglycemia, generalized pruritus with or without rash, cutaneous ulcers, albuminuria, worsening of organic brain syndromes, excessive weight gain, edematous swelling of ankles or wrists, thirst or polyuria, sometimes resembling diabetes insipidus, metallic taste, dysgeusia/taste distortion, salty taste, swollen lips, tightness in chest, impotence/sexual dysfunction, swollen and/or painful joints, fever, polyarthralgia, hypertoxicity, dental caries.

A few reports have been received of the development of painful discoloration of fingers and toes and coldness of the extremities within one day of the starting of treatment with lithium. The mechanism through which these symptoms (resembling Raynaud's syndrome) developed is not known. Recovery followed discontinuance.

Dosage and Administration: Immediate release capsules and tablets are usually given t.i.d. or q.i.d. Doses of controlled release tablets are usually given b.i.d. (approximately 12-hour intervals). When initiating therapy with immediate release or controlled release lithium, dosage must be individualized according to serum levels and clinical response.

When switching a patient from immediate release capsules or tablets to the 'Eskalith CR' Controlled Release Tablets, give the same total daily dose when possible. Most patients on maintenance therapy are stabilized on 900 mg. daily, e.g., 450 mg. 'Eskalith CR' b.i.d. When the previous dosage of immediate release lithium is not a multiple of 450 mg., for example, 1500 mg., initiate 'Eskalith CR' dosage at the multiple of 450 mg. nearest to, but *below*, the original daily dose, i.e., 1350 mg. When the two doses are unequal, give the larger dose in the evening. In the above example, with a total daily dosage of 1350 mg., generally 450 mg. 'Eskalith CR' should be given in the morning and 900 mg. 'Eskalith CR' in the evening. If desired, the total daily dosage of 1350 mg. can be given in three equal 450 mg. 'Eskalith CR' doses. These patients should be monitored at 1–2 week intervals, and dosage adjusted if necessary, until stable and satisfactory serum levels and clinical state are achieved.

When patients require closer titration than that available with 'Eskalith CR' doses in increments of 450 mg., immediate release capsules or tablets should be used.

Acute Mania—Optimal patient response to Eskalith (lithium carbonate, SK&F) can usually be established and maintained with 1800 mg. per day in divided doses. Such doses will normally produce the desired serum lithium level ranging between 1.0 and 1.5 mEq./l.

Dosage must be individualized according to serum levels and clinical response. Regular monitoring of the patient's clinical state and serum lithium levels is necessary. Serum levels should be determined twice per week during the acute phase, and until the serum level and clinical condition of the patient have been stabilized.

Long-Term Control—The desirable serum lithium levels are 0.6 to 1.2 mEq./l. Dosage will vary from one individual to another, but usually 900 mg. to 1200 mg. per day in divided doses will maintain this level. Serum lithium levels in uncomplicated cases receiving maintenance therapy during remission should be monitored at least every two months.

Patients abnormally sensitive to lithium may exhibit toxic signs at serum levels of 1.0 to 1.5 mEq./l. Elderly patients often respond to reduced dosage, and may exhibit signs of toxicity at serum levels ordinarily tolerated by other patients.

N.B.: Blood samples for serum lithium determinations should be drawn immediately prior to the next dose when lithium concentrations are relatively stable (i.e., 8–12 hours after the previous dose). Total reliance must not be placed on serum levels alone. Accurate patient evaluation requires both clinical and laboratory analysis.

Overdosage: The toxic levels for lithium are close to the therapeutic levels. It is therefore important that patients and their families be cautioned to watch for early toxic symptoms and to discontinue the drug and inform the physician should they occur. Toxic symptoms are listed in detail under ADVERSE REACTIONS.

Treatment

No specific antidote for lithium poisoning is known. Early symptoms of lithium toxicity can usually be treated by reduction or cessation of dosage of the drug and resumption of the treatment at a lower dose after 24 to 48 hours. In severe cases of lithium poisoning, the first and foremost goal of treatment consists of elimination of this ion from the patient. Treatment is essentially the same as that used in barbiturate poisoning: 1) gastric lavage, 2) correction of fluid and electrolyte imbalance, and 3) regulation of kidney function. Urea, mannitol, and aminophylline all produce significant increases in lithium excretion. Hemodialysis is an effective and rapid means of removing the ion from the severely toxic patient. Infection prophylaxis, regular chest X-rays, and preservation of adequate respiration are essential.

How Supplied:
ESKALITH (lithium carbonate, SK&F) Capsules available as 300 mg. yellow and gray capsules in bottles of 100 and 500.
ESKALITH (lithium carbonate, SK&F) Tablets available as 300 mg. round, gray, single scored tablets in bottles of 100.
ESKALITH CR (lithium carbonate, SK&F) Controlled Release Tablets available as 450 mg. round, buff, single scored tablets in bottles of 100.

[*Shown in Product Identification Section*]

FEOSOL® ELIXIR
Hematinic

Description: Feosol Elixir, an unusually palatable iron elixir, provides the body with ferrous sulfate—iron in its most efficient form. The standard elixir for simple iron deficiency and iron-deficiency anemia when the need for such therapy has been determined by a physician.

Each 5 ml. (1 teaspoonful) contains ferrous sulfate USP, 220 mg. (44 mg. of elemental iron); alcohol, 5%.

Usual Dosage: *Adults*—1 to 2 teaspoonfuls three times daily. *Children*—½ to 1 teaspoonful three times daily preferably between meals. *Infants*—as directed by physician. Mix with water or fruit juice to avoid temporary staining of teeth; do not mix with milk or wine-based vehicles.

Warning: The treatment of any anemic condition should be under the advice and supervision of a physician. Since oral iron products interfere with absorption of oral tetracycline antibiotics, these products should not be taken within two hours of each other. Occasional gastrointestinal discomfort (such as nausea) may be minimized by taking with meals and by beginning with one teaspoonful the first day, two the second, etc. until the recommended dosage is reached. Iron-containing medication may occasionally cause constipation or diarrhea, and liquids may cause temporary staining of the teeth (this is less likely when diluted). Keep this and all medicines out of reach of children. In case of accidental overdose, contact a physician or poison control center immediately.

How Supplied: A clear orange liquid in 12 fl. oz. bottles.

Also Available: Feosol® Tablets, Feosol® Spansule® capsules.

Marketed by Menley & James Laboratories, a SmithKline company.

FEOSOL® SPANSULE® CAPSULES
Hematinic

Description: Feosol *Spansule* capsules provide the body with ferrous sulfate—iron in its most efficient form—for simple iron deficiency and iron-deficiency anemia, when the need for such therapy has been determined by a physician.

The special *Spansule* capsule formulation—ferrous sulfate in pellets—reduces stomach upset, a common problem with iron.

Formula: Each capsule contains 167 mg. of dried ferrous sulfate USP (50 mg. of elemental iron), equivalent to 250 mg. of ferrous sulfate USP.

Usual Dosage: *Adults and Children*—One to two Feosol *Spansule* capsules daily, depending on severity of iron deficiency. Children too young to swallow the capsule can be given the contents in a spoonful of soft, cool food (applesauce, custard, etc.). *Children under 6*—Use Feosol® Elixir.

Warnings: The treatment of any anemic condition should be under the advice and supervision of a physician. Since oral iron products interfere with absorption of oral tetracycline antibiotics, these products should not be taken within two hours of each other. Keep this and all medicines out of reach of children. In case of accidental overdose, contact a physi-

cian or poison control center immediately. Iron-containing medicine may occasionally cause constipation or diarrhea.
How Supplied: Bottles of 30, 100 and 500 capsules; in Single Unit Packages of 100 capsules (intended for institutional use only).
Also available in Tablets and Elixir.
Marketed by Menley & James Laboratories, a SmithKline company.

FEOSOL® TABLETS
Hematinic

Description: Feosol Tablets provide the body with ferrous sulfate, iron in its most efficient form, for iron deficiency and iron-deficiency anemia when the need for such therapy has been determined by a physician. The distinctive triangular-shaped tablet has a special coating to prevent oxidation and improve palatability.
Formula: Each tablet contains 200 mg. of dried ferrous sulfate USP (65 mg. of elemental iron), equivalent to 325 mg. (5 grains) of ferrous sulfate USP.
Usual Dosage: *Adults*—one tablet 3 to 4 times daily, after meals and upon retiring. *Children 6 to 12 years*—one tablet three times a day after meals. *Children under 6 years and infants*—use Feosol® Elixir.
Warning: The treatment of any anemic condition should be under the advice and supervision of a physician. Since oral iron products interfere with absorption of oral tetracycline antibiotics, these products should not be taken within two hours of each other.
Occasional gastrointestinal discomfort (such as nausea) may be minimized by taking with meals and by beginning with one tablet the first day, two the second, etc. until the recommended dosage is reached. Iron-containing medication may occasionally cause constipation or diarrhea.
Keep this and all medicines out of reach of children. In case of accidental overdose, contact a physician or poison control center immediately.
How Supplied: Bottles of 100 and 1000 tablets; in Single Unit Packages of 100 tablets (intended for institutional use only).
Also available in Spansule® capsules and Elixir.
Marketed by Menley & James Laboratories, a SmithKline company.

FEOSOL PLUS®
Iron plus vitamins

Description: For use in iron deficiency and iron-deficiency anemia where additional vitamins are indicated.
Modified Formula (No prescription required):
Formula: Each Feosol Plus capsule contains:

Dried ferrous sulfate (equivalent to 325 mg. ferrous sulfate USP; 65 mg. of elemental iron)	200 mg.
Folic acid	0.2 mg.
Ascorbic acid (Vitamin C)	50 mg.
Thiamine HCl (Vitamin B_1)	2 mg.
Riboflavin (Vitamin B_2)	2 mg.
Pyridoxine HCl (Vitamin B_6)	2 mg.
Vitamin B_{12} (activity equivalent) (derived from streptomyces fermentation)	5 mcg.
Nicotinic acid (niacin)	20 mg.

Usual Dosage: *Adults and Children (over 3 yrs.)* One capsule twice daily or as directed by physician.
Warning: The treatment of any anemic condition should be under the advice and supervision of a physician.
Since oral iron products tend to interfere with absorption of oral tetracycline antibiotics, these products should not be taken within two hours of each other.
Keep this and all medicines out of reach of children. In case of accidental overdose, contact a physician or poison control center immediately. Iron-containing medication may occasionally cause constipation or diarrhea.
How Supplied: Bottles of 100 capsules.
Marketed by Menley & James Laboratories, a SmithKline company.

HISPRIL® ℞
(brand of diphenylpyraline hydrochloride)
SPANSULE® CAPSULES 5 mg.

Description: Hispril®, brand of diphenylpyraline HCl, is an antihistamine.
Each 'Spansule' capsule contains diphenylpyraline hydrochloride, 5 mg., so prepared that an initial dose is released promptly and the remaining medication is released gradually over a prolonged period.
Actions: Diphenylpyraline hydrochloride is an antihistamine with anticholinergic (drying) and sedative side effects. Antihistamines appear to compete with histamine for cell receptor sites on effector cells.
Indications: For the symptomatic treatment of perennial and seasonal allergic rhinitis; vasomotor rhinitis; allergic conjunctivitis due to inhalant allergens and foods; mild, uncomplicated allergic skin manifestations of urticaria and angioedema; amelioration of allergic reactions to blood or plasma; dermographism; and as therapy for anaphylactic reactions adjunctive to epinephrine and other standard measures after the acute manifestations have been controlled.
Contraindications:
Use in Newborn or Premature Infants—This drug should *not* be used in newborn or premature infants.
Use in Nursing Mothers—Because of the higher risk of antihistamines for infants generally and for newborns and prematures in particular, antihistamine therapy is contraindicated in nursing mothers.
Use in Lower Respiratory Disease—Antihistamines *should NOT* be used to treat lower respiratory tract symptoms including asthma.
Antihistamines are also contraindicated in the following conditions:
Hypersensitivity to diphenylpyraline hydrochloride and other antihistamines of similar chemical structure
Monoamine oxidase inhibitor therapy (See Drug Interactions section)
Warnings: Antihistamines should be used with considerable caution in patients with:
Narrow angle glaucoma
Stenosing peptic ulcer
Pyloroduodenal obstruction
Symptomatic prostatic hypertrophy
Bladder neck obstruction
Use in Children—In infants and children, especially, antihistamines in *overdosage* may cause hallucinations, convulsions, or death.
As in adults, antihistamines may diminish mental alertness in children. In the young child, particularly, they may produce excitation.
Use in Pregnancy—Experience with this drug in pregnant women is inadequate to determine whether there exists a potential for harm to the developing fetus.
Use with CNS Depressants—Diphenylpyraline hydrochloride has additive effects with alcohol and other CNS depressants (hypnotics, sedatives, tranquilizers, etc.).
Use in Activities Requiring Mental Alertness—Patients should be warned about engaging in activities requiring mental alertness as driving a car or operating appliances, machinery, etc.
Use in the Elderly (approximately 60 years or older)—Antihistamines are more likely to cause dizziness, sedation, and hypotension in the elderly than in younger patients.
Precautions: Diphenylpyraline hydrochloride has an atropine-like action and, therefore, should be used with caution in patients with:
History of bronchial asthma
Increased intraocular pressure
Hyperthyroidism
Cardiovascular disease
Hypertension
Drug Interactions—MAO inhibitors prolong and intensify the anticholinergic (drying) effects of antihistamines.
Adverse Reactions: The most frequent adverse reactions are underlined:
1. **General:** Urticaria, drug rash, anaphylactic shock, photosensitivity, excessive perspiration, chills, dryness of mouth, nose, and throat.
2. **Cardiovascular System:** Hypotension, headache, palpitations, tachycardia, extrasystoles.
3. **Hematologic System:** Hemolytic anemia, thrombocytopenia, agranulocytosis.
4. **Nervous System:** <u>Sedation, sleepiness, dizziness, disturbed coordination,</u> fatigue, confusion, restlessness, excitation, nervousness, tremor, irritability, insomnia, euphoria, paresthesias, blurred vision, diplopia, vertigo, tinnitus, acute labyrinthitis, hysteria, neuritis, convulsions.
5. **G.I. System:** <u>Epigastric distress,</u> anorexia, nausea, vomiting, diarrhea, constipation.
6. **G.U. System:** Urinary frequency, difficult urination, urinary retention, early menses.
7. **Respiratory System:** <u>Thickening of bronchial secretions,</u> tightness of chest and wheezing, nasal stuffiness.

Overdosage: Antihistamine overdosage reactions may vary from central nervous system depression to stimulation. Stimulation is particularly likely in children. Atropine-like signs and symptoms—dry mouth; fixed, dilated pupils; flushing; and gastrointestinal symptoms may also occur. Marked cerebral irritation, resulting in jerking of muscles and possible convulsions, may be followed by deep stupor.
If vomiting has not occurred spontaneously the patient should be induced to vomit. This is best done by having him drink a glass of water or milk after which he should be made to gag. Precautions against aspiration must be taken, especially in infants and children.
If vomiting is unsuccessful gastric lavage is indicated within 3 hours after ingestion and even later if large amounts of milk or cream were given beforehand. Isotonic or ½ isotonic saline is the lavage solution of choice.
Saline cathartics, as milk of magnesia, by osmosis draw water into the bowel and, therefore, are valuable for their action in rapid dilution of bowel content.
Do not treat CNS depression with analeptics which might precipitate convulsions. Use only short-acting depressants to treat convulsions.
Stimulants should *not* be used.
If a vasoconstrictor is required for hypotension, levarterenol bitartrate, USP, may be used. Other pressor agents, including epinephrine, should not be used as they may cause a paradoxical further lowering of blood pressure.
Special note on 'Spansule' capsules—Since much of the 'Spansule' capsule medication is coated for gradual release, therapy directed at reversing the effects of the ingested drug and at supporting the patient should be continued for as long as overdosage symptoms remain. Saline cathartics are useful for hastening evacuation of pellets that have not already released medication.
Dosage and Administration: DOSAGE SHOULD BE INDIVIDUALIZED ACCORDING TO THE NEEDS AND THE RESPONSE OF THE PATIENT.

Continued on next page

Smith Kline & French—Cont.

Adults—One capsule (5 mg.), q12h.
Older Children (6–12 years)—One 5 mg. capsule daily is usually sufficient. The physician should bear in mind that in children a higher incidence and a greater degree of antihistaminic side effects may be encountered. Do not use in children under 6 years.
How Supplied: Bottles of 50 capsules.
[*Shown in Product Identification Section*]

ORNACOL®
Relieves coughing and nasal congestion.

Marketed by Menley & James Laboratories, a SmithKline company.
(See PDR For Nonprescription Drugs)

ORNADE® SPANSULE® CAPSULES ℞

Description: Each 'Ornade' *Spansule* capsule contains 75 mg. of phenylpropanolamine hydrochloride and 12 mg. of chlorpheniramine maleate, so prepared that an initial dose is released promptly and the remaining medication is released gradually over a prolonged period. A single capsule dose produces blood levels comparable to those produced by administration of three 25 mg. doses of phenylpropanolamine hydrochloride and three 4 mg. doses of chlorpheniramine maleate in conventional release form given at four-hour intervals.
Actions: Phenylpropanolamine hydrochloride is a decongestant that provides vasoconstriction similar to that of ephedrine, but with less CNS stimulation.
Chlorpheniramine maleate is an antihistamine with anticholinergic (drying) and sedative side effects. Antihistamines appear to compete with histamines for H_1 cell receptor sites on effector cells.

Indications
For symptomatic relief of nasal congestion, runny nose, sneezing, itchy nose or throat, and itchy and watery eyes as may occur with the common cold or in allergic rhinitis (e.g., hay fever).
N.B.: A final determination has not been made on the effectiveness of this drug combination in accordance with efficacy requirements of the 1962 Amendments to the Food, Drug and Cosmetic Act.

Contraindications: Hypersensitivity to either ingredient; severe hypertension; coronary artery disease; stenosing peptic ulcer; pyloroduodenal or bladder neck obstruction.
'Ornade' *Spansule* capsules should NOT be used to treat lower respiratory tract conditions, including asthma.
As with any product containing a sympathomimetic, 'Ornade' *Spansule* capsules should NOT be used in patients taking MAO inhibitors.
Because of the higher risk of antihistamine side effects in infants generally, and for newborns and prematures in particular, antihistamine therapy is contraindicated in nursing mothers. This drug product should NOT be used in newborn or premature infants.
Warnings: Caution patients about activities requiring alertness (e.g., operating vehicles or machinery). Patients should also be warned about the possible additive effects of alcohol and other CNS depressants (hypnotics, sedatives, tranquilizers, etc.).
Precautions: Use with caution in patients with narrow-angle glaucoma, hypertension, cardiovascular disease, prostatic hypertrophy, hyperthyroidism, or diabetes. Patients taking this medication should be cautioned not to take simultaneously other products containing phenylpropanolamine HCl or amphetamines.
Use in Children: In infants and children, antihistamines in *overdosage* may cause hallucinations, convulsions, or death.
As in adults, antihistamines may diminish mental alertness in children. In the young child, particularly, they may produce excitation.
Use in Pregnancy: Experience with this drug in pregnant women is inadequate to determine whether there exists a potential for harm to the developing fetus. Therefore, 'Ornade' *Spansule* capsules should be used in pregnant women only when clearly needed in the judgment of the physician.
Use in the Elderly (approximately 60 years or older): The risk of dizziness, sedation, and hypotension is greater in the elderly patient.
Adverse Reactions:
General: excessive dryness of nose, throat, or mouth; headache; rash; weakness.
Cardiovascular System: angina pain; palpitations; hypertension; hypotension.
Hematologic: thrombocytopenia; leukopenia; hemolytic anemia; agranulocytosis.
Nervous System: drowsiness; nervousness or insomnia; dizziness; irritability; incoordination; tremor; convulsions; visual disturbances.
GI System: nausea; vomiting; epigastric distress; diarrhea; abdominal pain; anorexia; constipation.
GU System: difficulty in urination; dysuria.
Respiratory System: tightness of chest.
Dosage and Administration: Adults and children over 12 years of age—one capsule every 12 hours.
'Ornade' *Spansule* capsules should not be used in children under 12. For children 2 to 12 years of age, Ornade 2® Liquid for Children (a non-sustained release preparation) is available.
Overdosage: Symptoms may vary from central nervous system depression to stimulation. Also, atropine-like signs and symptoms (dry mouth; fixed, dilated pupils; flushing, etc.) as well as gastrointestinal symptoms may occur. Marked cerebral irritation resulting in jerking of muscles and possible convulsions may be followed by deep stupor and respiratory failure. Acute hypertension or cardiovascular collapse with accompanying hypotension may occur.
Treatment of Overdosage: Immediate evacuation of the stomach should be induced by emesis and gastric lavage. Since much of the 'Spansule' capsule medication is coated for gradual release, saline cathartics should be administered to hasten evacuation of pellets that have not already released medication.
Respiratory depression should be treated promptly with oxygen. Do not treat respiratory or CNS depression with analeptics that might precipitate convulsions; if convulsions or marked CNS excitement occurs, only short-acting barbiturates or chloral hydrate should be used.
Supplied: In bottles of 50 and 500 capsules, and in Single Unit Packages of 100 capsules (intended for institutional use only).
[*Shown in Product Identification Section*]

ORNADE 2® Liquid for Children

Description: Each 5 ml. teaspoonful of 'Ornade 2' Liquid for Children contains 12.5 mg. of phenylpropanolamine hydrochloride, 2 mg. of chlorpheniramine maleate, and alcohol 5%.
Actions: Phenylpropanolamine hydrochloride provides vasoconstriction similar to that of ephedrine but with less CNS stimulation. Chlorpheniramine maleate is an antihistamine (H_1-receptor antagonist) with anticholinergic (drying) and sedative side effects. Antihistamines appear to compete with histamine for H_1-receptor sites on effector cells.
Indications: For relief of runny nose, sneezing, itchy nose or throat, itchy and watery eyes or nasal congestion as may occur in the common cold or in allergic rhinitis such as hay fever.
Contraindications: Hypersensitivity to either ingredient, severe hypertension or severe coronary artery disease. 'Ornade 2' Liquid for Children should NOT be used to treat lower respiratory tract conditions such as asthma. As in any product containing a sympathomimetic, 'Ornade 2' Liquid for Children should NOT be used in patients taking MAO inhibitors.
Adverse Reactions: Drowsiness; excessive dryness of nose, throat or mouth; nervousness or insomnia may occur on rare occasions with 'Ornade 2' Liquid for Children but is usually mild and transitory. Other reported adverse reactions with the components of this formulation include: nausea, vomiting, epigastric distress, diarrhea, rash, dizziness, weakness, tightness of chest, angina pain, abdominal pain, irritability, palpitation, headache, incoordination, tremor, difficulty in urination, dysuria, thrombocytopenia, leukopenia, convulsions, hypertension, hypotension, anorexia, constipation, visual disturbances.
Dosage: Adults and children 12 and over—2 teaspoonfuls every four hours. Children 6 to 12—1 teaspoonful every four hours. For children 2 to 6 years, oral dosage is ½ teaspoon every 4 to 6 hours. Do not exceed 6 doses in 24 hours.
Note: Because 'Ornade 2' Liquid for Children may be purchased without a prescription, the following warnings and information appear on package labelling:
"**Warnings:** May cause drowsiness. Use caution in activities requiring alertness (e.g., operating vehicles or heavy machinery).
"Do not take this product if you are presently taking a prescription antihypertensive or antidepressant drug containing a monoamine oxidase inhibitor except on the advice of a physician. Individuals with asthma, glaucoma, high blood pressure, heart disease, enlarged prostate, diabetes or thyroid disease should use only under the advice and supervision of a physician.
"Avoid alcoholic beverages while taking this product. Do not exceed recommended dosage because at higher doses nervousness, dizziness, or sleeplessness may occur. May cause excitability, especially in children.
"If symptoms do not improve within 7 days or are accompanied by high fever, consult your physician before continuing use.
"Keep this and all drugs out of the reach of children. In case of accidental overdose, seek professional assistance or contact a poison control center immediately."
Overdosage: Symptoms may vary from central nervous system depression to stimulation. Also, atropine-like signs and symptoms (dry mouth; fixed, dilated pupils; flushing, etc.) as well as gastrointestinal symptoms may occur. Marked cerebral irritation resulting in jerking of muscles and possible convulsions may be followed by deep stupor and respiratory failure. Acute hypertension or cardiovascular collapse with accompanying hypotension may occur.
Treatment of Overdosage: Immediate evacuation of the stomach should be induced by emesis and gastric lavage. Respiratory depression should be treated promptly with oxygen. Do not treat respiratory or CNS depression with analeptics which might precipitate convulsions; if convulsions or marked CNS excitement occur, only short-acting barbiturates or chloral hydrate should be used.
Supplied: In 4 fl. oz. bottles with safety closure and 16 fl. oz. bottles.

ORNEX®
decongestant/analgesic

Marketed by Menley & James Laboratories, a SmithKline company.
(See PDR For Nonprescription Drugs)

PAREDRINE® 1% ℞
(brand of hydroxyamphetamine hydrobromide)
with BORIC ACID, OPHTHALMIC SOLUTION

Description: Hydroxyamphetamine hydrobromide, 1%, in distilled water. Made tear-isotonic with 2% boric acid, and preserved with thimerosal, 1:50,000.
Action: Dilates the pupil; probably by stimulating the dilator muscles of the iris.
Indication: To dilate the pupil; produces a pupillary dilatation which lasts for a few hours.
Contraindication: Narrow-angle glaucoma.
Precautions: Use with caution in patients with hypertension, hyperthyroidism and diabetes.
Adverse Reactions: With widely dilated pupils there will likely be increased intraocular pressure, photophobia and blurring of vision.
Dosage and Administration: Instil 1 or 2 drops into the conjunctival sac.
Overdosage: *Symptoms*—Dilatation of pupils. *Treatment*—Dilute pilocarpine (1%) may be administered if desired. Instil one drop at intervals. Repeat as necessary. **Accidental ingestion**—*Symptoms*—These may include marked rise in blood pressure, palpitation, cardiac arrhythmias, substernal discomfort, headache, sweating, nausea, vomiting and gastrointestinal irritation. *Treatment*—Sedation is indicated. Further treatment is symptomatic. Shock, if present, should be treated promptly. If hypertension is prominent, measures should be taken to lower blood pressure.
How Supplied: ½ fl. oz. bottles.

PARNATE® ℞
(brand of tranylcypromine sulfate)

Before prescribing, the physician should be familiar with the entire contents of this prescribing information.
Description: Each tablet contains tranylcypromine sulfate equivalent to 10 mg. of tranylcypromine.
Chemically, tranylcypromine sulfate is (±)-*trans*-2-phenylcyclopropylamine sulfate (2:1).
Action: Tranylcypromine is a non-hydrazine monoamine oxidase inhibitor with a rapid onset of activity. It increases the concentration of epinephrine, norepinephrine, and serotonin in storage sites throughout the nervous system, and in theory, this increased concentration of monoamines in the brainstem is the basis for its antidepressant activity. When tranylcypromine is withdrawn, monoamine oxidase activity is recovered in 3 to 5 days, although the drug is excreted in 24 hours.

Indications
Based on a review of this drug by the National Academy of Sciences—National Research Council and/or other information, FDA has classified the indications as follows:
Probably effective: For symptomatic relief of severe reactive or endogenous depression in hospitalized or closely supervised patients who have not responded to other antidepressant therapy.
Final classification of the less-than-effective indications requires further investigation.

Summary of Contraindications: Parnate (tranylcypromine sulfate, SK&F) should not be administered in combination with any of the following: MAO inhibitors or dibenzazepine derivatives; sympathomimetics (including amphetamines); some central nervous system depressants (including narcotics and alcohol); antihypertensive, diuretic, antihistaminic, sedative or anesthetic drugs; cheese or other foods with a high tyramine content; or excessive quantities of caffeine.
Parnate (tranylcypromine sulfate, SK&F) should not be administered to any patient beyond 60 years of age or with a confirmed or suspected cerebrovascular defect or to any patient with cardiovascular disease, hypertension or history of headache.
(For complete discussion of contraindications and warnings, see below.)
Contraindications: Parnate (tranylcypromine sulfate, SK&F) is contraindicated:
1. In patients with cerebrovascular defects or cardiovascular disorders
Parnate (tranylcypromine sulfate, SK&F) should not be administered to any patient with a confirmed or suspected cerebrovascular defect or to any patient with cardiovascular disease or hypertension. The drug should also be withheld from individuals beyond the age of 60 because of the possibility of existing cerebral sclerosis with damaged vessels.
2. In the presence of pheochromocytoma
Parnate (tranylcypromine sulfate, SK&F) should not be used in the presence of pheochromocytoma since such tumors secrete pressor substances.
3. In combination with MAO inhibitors or with dibenzazepine-related entities
Parnate (tranylcypromine sulfate, SK&F) should not be administered together or in rapid succession with other MAO inhibitors or with dibenzazepine-related entities. Hypertensive crises or severe convulsive seizures may occur in patients receiving such combinations.
In patients being transferred to 'Parnate' from another MAO inhibitor or from a dibenzazepine-related entity, allow a medication-free interval of at least a week, then initiate 'Parnate' using half the normal starting dosage for at least the first week of therapy. Similarly, at least a week should elapse between the discontinuance of 'Parnate' and the administration of another MAO inhibitor or a dibenzazepine-related entity.

Other MAO inhibitors presently known to be marketed in this country:

Generic Name	Trademark
Isocarboxazid	'Marplan' (Roche Laboratories)
Pargyline HCl	'Eutonyl' (Abbott Laboratories)
Pargyline HCl and methyclothiazide	'Eutron' (Abbott Laboratories)
Phenelzine sulfate	'Nardil' (Warner-Chilcott Laboratories)

Dibenzazepine-related entities and other tricyclic drugs presently known to be marketed in this country:

Generic Name	Trademark
Amitriptyline HCl	'Elavil' (Merck Sharp & Dohme)
	'SK-Amitriptyline' (Smith Kline &French)
Perphenazine and amitriptyline HCl	'Etrafon' (Schering)
	'Triavil' (Merck Sharp & Dohme)
Desipramine HCl	'Norpramin' (Merrell-National)
	'Pertofrane' (USV)
Imipramine HCl	'Imavate' (Robins)
	'Presamine' (USV)
	'SK-Pramine' (Smith Kline &French)
	'Tofranil' (Geigy Pharmaceuticals)
Nortriptyline HCl	'Aventyl' (Eli Lilly & Co.)
	'Pamelor' (Sandoz)
Protriptyline HCl	'Vivactil' (Merck Sharp & Dohme)
Doxepin HCl	'Adapin' (Pennwalt)
	'Sinequan' (Pfizer)
Carbamazepine	'Tegretol' (Geigy Pharmaceuticals)
Cyclobenzaprine HCl	'Flexeril' (Merck Sharp & Dohme)
Amoxapine	'Asendin' (Lederle)
Maprotiline HCl	'Ludiomil' (CIBA)
Trimipramine maleate	'Surmontil' (Ives)

4. In combination with sympathomimetics
Parnate (tranylcypromine sulfate, SK&F) should not be administered in combination with sympathomimetics, including amphetamines, and over-the-counter drugs such as cold, hay fever or weight-reducing preparations that contain vasoconstrictors.
During 'Parnate' therapy, it appears that certain patients are particularly vulnerable to the effects of sympathomimetics when the activity of certain enzymes is inhibited. Use of sympathomimetics and compounds such as methyldopa, dopamine, levodopa and tryptophane with 'Parnate' may precipitate hypertension, headache, and related symptoms.
5. In combination with cheese or other foods with a high tyramine content
Hypertensive crises have sometimes occurred during Parnate (tranylcypromine sulfate, SK&F) therapy after ingestion of foods with a high tyramine content. In general, the patient should avoid protein foods in which aging or protein breakdown is used to increase flavor. In particular, patients should be instructed not to take foods such as cheese (particularly strong or aged varieties), sour cream, Chianti wine, sherry, beer, pickled herring, liver, canned figs, raisins, bananas or avocados (particularly if overripe), chocolate, soy sauce, the pods of broad beans (fava beans), yeast extracts, or meat prepared with tenderizers.
Additional Contraindications: In general, the physician should bear in mind the possibility of a lowered margin of safety when Parnate (tranylcypromine sulfate, SK&F) is administered in combination with potent drugs.
1. 'Parnate' should not be used in combination with some central nervous system depressants such as narcotics and alcohol, or with hypotensive agents. A marked potentiating effect on these classes of drugs has been reported.
2. Anti-parkinsonism drugs should be used with caution in patients receiving 'Parnate' since severe reactions have been reported.
3. 'Parnate' should not be used in patients with a history of liver disease or in those with abnormal liver function tests.
4. Excessive use of caffeine in any form should be avoided in patients receiving 'Parnate'.
Warning to Physicians: Parnate (tranylcypromine sulfate, SK&F) is a potent agent with the capability of producing serious side effects. 'Parnate' is not recommended in those severe endogenous depressions in which electroconvulsive therapy is the treatment of choice or in those depressive reactions where other antidepressant drugs may be effective.
It should be reserved for patients who are either hospitalized or under close supervision and who have not responded satisfactorily to other antidepressant therapy.
Before prescribing, the physician should be completely familiar with the full material on dosage, side effects, and contraindications on these pages, with the principles of MAO inhibitor therapy and the side effects of this class of drugs. Also, the physician should be familiar with the symptomatology of mental depressions and alternate methods of treatment to aid in the careful selection of patients for 'Parnate' therapy. In depressed patients, the possi-

Continued on next page

Smith Kline & French—Cont.

bility of suicide should always be considered and adequate precautions taken.

Pregnancy Warning: Use of any drug in pregnancy, during lactation, or in women of childbearing age requires that the potential benefits of the drug be weighed against its possible hazards to mother and child. Animal reproductive studies show that Parnate (tranylcypromine sulfate, SK&F) passes through the placental barrier into the fetus of the rat. Also, it passes into milk of the lactating dog. The absence of a harmful action of 'Parnate' on fertility or on postnatal development by either prenatal treatment or from the milk of treated animals has not been demonstrated.

Warning to the Patient: Patients should be instructed to report promptly the occurrence of headache or other unusual symptoms.

Patients should be warned against eating the foods listed in Section 5 under Contraindications while on Parnate (tranylcypromine sulfate, SK&F) therapy. Also, they should be told not to drink alcoholic beverages.

Patients should be warned against self-medication with proprietary (over-the-counter) drugs such as cold, hay fever or weight-reducing preparations that contain pressor agents. They should be advised not to consume excessive amounts of caffeine in any form.

Warnings: Hypertensive Crises: The most important reaction associated with Parnate (tranylcypromine sulfate, SK&F) is the occurrence of hypertensive crises which have sometimes been fatal.

These crises are characterized by some or all of the following symptoms: occipital headache which may radiate frontally, palpitation, neck stiffness or soreness, nausea or vomiting, sweating (sometimes with fever and sometimes with cold, clammy skin) and photophobia. Either tachycardia or bradycardia may be present, and associated constricting chest pain and dilated pupils may occur. **Intracranial bleeding, sometimes fatal in outcome, has been reported in association with the paradoxical increase in blood pressure.**

In all patients taking 'Parnate' blood pressure should be followed closely to detect evidence of any pressor response. It is emphasized that full reliance should not be placed on blood pressure readings, but that the patient should also be observed frequently.

Therapy should be discontinued immediately upon the occurrence of palpitation or frequent headaches during 'Parnate' therapy. These signs may be prodromal of a hypertensive crisis.

Important: Recommended treatment in hypertensive crises

If a hypertensive crisis occurs, Parnate (tranylcypromine sulfate, SK&F) should be discontinued and therapy to lower blood pressure should be instituted immediately. Headache tends to abate as blood pressure is lowered. On the basis of present evidence, phentolamine (available as 'Regitine'*) is recommended. (The dosage reported for phentolamine is 5 mg. i.v.) Care should be taken to administer this drug slowly in order to avoid producing an excessive hypotensive effect. Fever should be managed by means of external cooling. Other symptomatic and supportive measures may be desirable in particular cases. Do not use parenteral reserpine.

Precautions: Hypotension—Hypotension has been observed during Parnate (tranylcypromine sulfate, SK&F) therapy. Symptoms of postural hypotension are seen most commonly but not exclusively in patients with pre-existent hypertension; blood pressure usually returns rapidly to pretreatment levels upon discontinuation of the drug. At doses above 30 mg. daily, postural hypotension is a major side effect and may result in syncope. Dosage increases should be made more gradually in patients showing a tendency toward hypotension at the beginning of therapy. Postural hypotension may be relieved by having the patient lie down until blood pressure returns to normal. Also, when 'Parnate' is combined with those phenothiazine derivatives or other compounds known to cause hypotension, the possibility of additive hypotensive effects should be considered.

Other Precautions: There have been reports of drug dependency in patients using doses of tranylcypromine significantly in excess of the therapeutic range. Some of these patients had a history of previous substance abuse. The following withdrawal symptoms have been reported: restlessness, anxiety, depression, confusion, hallucinations, headache, weakness and diarrhea.

Drugs which lower the seizure threshold, including MAO inhibitors, should not be used with 'Amipaque'. † As with other MAO inhibitors, Parnate (tranylcypromine sulfate, SK&F) should be discontinued at least 48 hours before myelography and should not be resumed for at least 24 hours postprocedure.

In depressed patients, the possibility of suicide should always be considered and adequate precautions taken. Exclusive reliance on drug therapy to prevent suicidal attempts is unwarranted, as there may be a delay in the onset of therapeutic effect or an increase in anxiety and agitation. Also, of course, some patients fail to respond to drug therapy or may respond only temporarily.

MAO inhibitors may have the capacity to suppress anginal pain that would otherwise serve as a warning of myocardial ischemia. The usual precautions should be observed in patients with impaired renal function since there is a possibility of accumulative effects in such patients.

Although excretion is rapid, inhibition of MAO may persist for a few days. It is, therefore, suggested that the drug be discontinued seven days before elective surgery to allow time for recovery of enzymatic activity before anesthetic agents are given.

Because the influence of Parnate (tranylcypromine sulfate, SK&F) on the convulsive threshold is variable in animal experiments, suitable precautions should be taken if epileptic patients are treated.

Some MAO inhibitors have contributed to hypoglycemic episodes in diabetic patients receiving insulin or oral hypoglycemic agents. Therefore, 'Parnate' should be used with caution in diabetics using these drugs.

'Parnate' may aggravate coexisting symptoms in depression, such as anxiety and agitation.

Use 'Parnate' with caution in hyperthyroid patients because of their increased sensitivity to pressor amines.

'Parnate' should be administered with caution to patients receiving disulfiram (Antabuse®‡). In a single study, rats given high intraperitoneal doses of *d* or *l* isomers of tranylcypromine sulfate plus disulfiram experienced severe toxicity including convulsions and death. Additional studies in rats given high oral doses of racemic tranylcypromine sulfate ('Parnate') and disulfiram produced no adverse interaction.

Adverse Reactions: Overstimulation which may include increased anxiety, agitation and manic symptoms is usually evidence of excessive therapeutic action. Dosage should be reduced, or a phenothiazine tranquilizer should be administered concomitantly.

Patients may experience restlessness or insomnia; may notice some weakness, drowsiness, episodes of dizziness, or dry mouth; or may report nausea, diarrhea, abdominal pain, or constipation. Most of these effects can be relieved by lowering the dosage or by giving suitable concomitant medication.

Tachycardia, significant anorexia, edema, palpitation, blurred vision, chills, and impotence have each been reported.

Headaches without blood pressure elevation have occurred.

Rare instances of hepatitis and skin rash have been reported.

Impaired water excretion compatible with the syndrome of inappropriate secretion of antidiuretic hormone (SIADH) has been reported.

Tinnitus, muscle spasm and tremors, paresthesia and urinary retention have been reported so rarely that the role of Parnate (tranylcypromine sulfate, SK&F) cannot be established.

Blood toxicity has not been reported.

Dosage and Administration: Dosage should be adjusted to the requirements of the individual patient. Improvement should be seen within 48 hours to three weeks after starting therapy.

1. Recommended starting dosage is 20 mg. per day—10 mg. in the morning and 10 mg. in the afternoon.
2. This dosage may be continued for two weeks.
3. If no signs of a response appear, dosage may be increased to 30 mg. daily—20 mg. in the morning and 10 mg. in the afternoon.
4. This dosage may be continued for a week. If no improvement occurs, continued administration is unlikely to be beneficial.
5. When a satisfactory response is obtained, dosage may usually be reduced to a maintenance level.
6. Some patients will be maintained on 20 mg. per day; many will need only 10 mg. daily.
7. Although dosages above 30 mg. daily have been used, the physician should bear in mind that the likelihood of side effects increases as dosage is raised.
8. When ECT is being administered concurrently, 10 mg. b.i.d. can usually be given during the series, then reduced to 10 mg. daily for maintenance therapy.

Dosage increases should be made in increments of 10 mg. per day and ordinarily at intervals of one to three weeks. It is important that the lowest effective dose be used.

Reduction from peak to maintenance dosage is desirable before withdrawal. If withdrawn prematurely, original symptoms will recur. Although no tendency to produce rebound depressions of greater intensity has been seen, this is a theoretical possibility.

Overdosage: *Symptoms:* The characteristic symptoms that may be caused by overdosage are usually those described in the preceding paragraphs.

However, an intensification of these symptoms and sometimes severe additional manifestations may be seen, depending on the degree of overdosage and on individual susceptibility. Some patients exhibit insomnia, restlessness and anxiety, progressing in severe cases to agitation, mental confusion and incoherence. Hypotension, dizziness, weakness and drowsiness may occur, progressing in severe cases to extreme dizziness and shock. A few patients have displayed hypertension with severe headache and other symptoms. Rare instances have been reported in which hypertension was accompanied by twitching or myoclonic fibrillation of skeletal muscles with hyperpyrexia, sometimes progressing to generalized rigidity and coma.

Treatment: Gastric lavage is helpful if performed early. Treatment should normally consist of general supportive measures, close observation of vital signs and steps to counteract specific symptoms as they occur, since MAO inhibition may persist. The management of hypertensive crises is described under Hypertensive Crises.

External cooling is recommended if hyperpyrexia occurs. Barbiturates have been reported to help relieve myoclonic reactions, but frequency of administration should be controlled carefully because Parnate (tranylcypromine sulfate, SK&F) may prolong barbiturate activity. When hypotension requires treatment, the standard measures for managing circulatory shock should be initiated. If pressor agents are used, the rate of infusion should be regulated by careful observation of the patient because an exaggerated pressor response sometimes occurs in the presence of MAO inhibition. Remember that the toxic effect of 'Parnate' may be delayed or prolonged following the last dose of the drug. Therefore, the patient should be closely observed for at least a week.

How Supplied: Tablets, containing tranylcypromine sulfate equivalent to 10 mg. of tranylcypromine, in bottles of 100 and 1000.

Clinical Studies: There have been only a small number of controlled studies (e.g., 1,2,3,4) of the effectiveness of Parnate (tranylcypromine sulfate, SK&F) in comparison to placebo or other antidepressant drugs, embracing comparatively few subjects. These and other studies disclose a remarkably high incidence, about 50 percent, of favorable placebo effect and a statistically significant but small superiority of 'Parnate' and other antidepressant drugs over placebo. No statistically significant superiority of 'Parnate' over other antidepressant drugs, including other MAO inhibitors, has been regularly demonstrated. However, clinical experience also indicates that some patients who fail to respond satisfactorily to one therapy may respond to another.

References:

1. Bartholomew, A.A.: An evaluation of tranylcypromine ('Parnate') in the treatment of depression, *M. J. Australia 1:*655 (May 5) 1962.
2. Khanna, J.L., et al.: A study of certain effects of tranylcypromine, a new antidepressant, *J. New Drugs 3:*227, 1963.
3. Spear, F.G., et al.: A comparison of subjective responses to imipramine and tranylcypromine, *Brit. J. Psychiat. 110:*53, 1964.
4. Janacek, J., et al.: Pargyline and tranylcypromine in the treatment of hospitalized depressed patients, *J. New Drugs 3:*309, 1963.

*Trade Mark Reg. U.S. Pat. Off.: 'Regitine' for phentolamine mesylate, U.S.P., CIBA.
†Trademark Reg. U.S. Pat. Off.: 'Amipaque' for metrizamide, Winthrop Laboratories.
‡Trademark of Ayerst Laboratories.

[*Shown in Product Identification Section*]

PRAGMATAR® OINTMENT

Marketed by Menley & James Laboratories, a SmithKline company.
(See PDR For Nonprescription Drugs)

SK–LINE®

SK–AMITRIPTYLINE™ ℞
(amitriptyline HCl, SK&F)
Tablets: 10 mg. (No. 120), 25 mg. (No. 121), 50 mg. (No. 123), 75 mg. (No. 124), 100 mg. (No. 131), 150 mg. (No. 132).

SK–AMPICILLIN® ℞
(ampicillin, SK&F)
Capsules: 250 mg. (No. 101), 500 mg. (No. 102).
For Oral Suspension: 125 mg./5 ml. (No. 103), 250 mg./5 ml. (No. 104), 100 mg./ml. (No. 109).

SK–AMPICILLIN-N® ℞
(sterile ampicillin sodium, SK&F)
Injection: 500 mg. (No. 106).

SK–APAP™ OTC
(acetaminophen, SK&F)
Tablets: 325 mg. (No. 174).
Elixir: 120 mg./5 ml. (contains alcohol) (No. 175).

SK–APAP™ with CODEINE Ⓒ
(acetaminophen, codeine phosphate)
Tablets: 300 mg./15 mg. (No. 494), 300 mg./30 mg. (No. 496), 300 mg./60 mg. (No. 497).

SK–BAMATE™ Ⓒ
(meprobamate, SK&F)
Tablets: 200 mg. (No. 133), 400 mg. (No. 134).

SK–CHLORAL HYDRATE™ Ⓒ
(chloral hydrate, SK&F)
Capsules: 500 mg. (No. 176).

SK–CHLOROTHIAZIDE™ ℞
(chlorothiazide, SK&F)
Tablets: 250 mg. (No. 419), 500 mg. (No. 420).

SK–DEXAMETHASONE™ ℞
(dexamethasone, SK&F)
Tablets: 0.5 mg. (No. 374), 0.75 mg. (No. 376), 1.5 mg. (No. 377).

SK–DIPHENHYDRAMINE™ ℞
(diphenhydramine hydrochloride, SK&F)
Capsules: 25 mg. (No. 303), 50 mg. (No. 304).
Elixir: 12.5 mg./5 ml. (No. 305).

SK–DIPHENOXYLATE™ Ⓒ
(diphenoxylate HCl, atropine sulfate)
Tablets: 2.5 mg./.025 mg. (No. 423).

SK–ERYTHROMYCIN™ ℞
(erythromycin stearate, SK&F)
Tablets: 250 mg. (No. 367), 500 mg. (No. 369).

SK–FUROSEMIDE™ ℞
(furosemide, SK&F)
Tablets: 20 mg. (No. 340), 40 mg. (No. 341).

SK–HYDROCHLOROTHIAZIDE™ ℞
(hydrochlorothiazide, SK&F)
Tablets: 25 mg. (No. 363), 50 mg. (No. 364).

SK–LYGEN® Ⓒ
(chlordiazepoxide hydrochloride, SK&F)
Capsules: 5 mg. (No. 441), 10 mg. (No. 442), 25 mg. (No. 443).

SK–METHOCARBAMOL™ ℞
(methocarbamol, SK&F)
Tablets: 500 mg. (No. 470), 750 mg. (No. 471).

SK–PENICILLIN G™ ℞
(penicillin G potassium, SK&F)
Tablets: 400,000 units (No. 111), 800,000 units (No. 112).
For Oral Solution: 200,000 units/5 ml. (No. 113), 400,000 units/5 ml. (No. 114).

SK–PENICILLIN VK™ ℞
(penicillin V potassium, SK&F)
Tablets: 250 mg. (No. 116), 500 mg. (No. 117).
For Oral Solution: 125 mg./5 ml. (No. 118), 250 mg./5 ml. (No. 119).

SK–PHENOBARBITAL™ Ⓒ
(phenobarbital, SK&F)
Tablets: 15 mg. (No. 136), 30 mg. (No. 137).

SK–POTASSIUM CHLORIDE™ ℞
(potassium chloride, SK&F)
Oral Solution: 40 mEq./30 ml.—10% Solution (No. 456), 80 mEq./30 ml.—20% Solution (No. 457).

SK–PRAMINE™ ℞
(imipramine hydrochloride, SK&F)
Tablets: 10 mg. (No. 321), 25 mg. (No. 322), 50 mg. (No. 323).

SK–PREDNISONE™ ℞
(prednisone, SK&F)
Tablets: 5 mg. (No. 339).

SK–PROBENECID™ ℞
(probenecid, SK&F)
Tablets: 500 mg. (No. 499).

SK–PROPANTHELINE BROMIDE™ ℞
(propantheline bromide, SK&F)
Tablets: 15 mg. (No. 310).

SK–QUINIDINE SULFATE™ ℞
(quinidine sulfate, SK&F)
Tablets: 200 mg. (No. 171).

SK–RESERPINE™ ℞
(reserpine, SK&F)
Tablets: 0.25 mg. (No. 169).

SK–65® Ⓒ
(propoxyphene hydrochloride, SK&F)
Capsules: 65 mg. (No. 463).

SK–65 APAP® Ⓒ
Each tablet: 65 mg. propoxyphene HCl, 650 mg. acetaminophen (No. 474).

SK–65® COMPOUND Ⓒ
Each capsule: 65 mg. propoxyphene HCl, 227 mg. aspirin, 162 mg. phenacetin, 32.4 mg. caffeine (No. 467).

SK–SOXAZOLE™ ℞
(sulfisoxazole, SK&F)
Tablets: 500 mg. (No. 163).

SK–TERPIN HYDRATE and CODEINE ™ Ⓒ
(brand of terpin hydrate and codeine)
Elixir: 4 fl. oz. (118 ml.) (No. 354).

SK–TETRACYCLINE™ CAPSULES ℞
(tetracycline hydrochloride, SK&F)
250 mg. (No. 126), 500 mg. (No. 127).

SK–TETRACYCLINE™ SYRUP ℞
(tetracycline oral suspension, SK&F)
125 mg./5 ml. (No. 125).

SK–TOLBUTAMIDE™ ℞
(brand of tolbutamide)
Tablets: 500 mg. (No. 409).

Continued on next page

Smith Kline & French—Cont.

STELAZINE® ℞
(brand of trifluoperazine hydrochloride)

('Stelazine' is a product of SK&F Co., Carolina, P.R. 00630, Subsidiary of SmithKline Beckman Corporation, Philadelphia, Pa.)

Description: Tablets—Each tablet contains trifluoperazine, 1 mg., 2 mg., 5 mg., or 10 mg., as the hydrochloride.

Multiple-dose Vials, 10 ml. (2 mg./ml.)—Each ml. contains, in aqueous solution, trifluoperazine, 2 mg., as the hydrochloride; sodium tartrate, 4.75 mg.; sodium biphosphate, 11.6 mg.; sodium saccharin, 0.3 mg.; benzyl alcohol, 0.75%, as preservative.

Concentrate (intended for institutional use only)—Each ml. contains trifluoperazine, 10 mg., as the hydrochloride.

N.B.: The Concentrate is for use in severe neuropsychiatric conditions when oral medication is preferred and other oral forms are considered impractical.

Indications

Based on a review of this drug by the National Academy of Sciences—National Research Council and/or other information, FDA has classified the indications as follows:

Effective: For the management of the manifestations of psychotic disorders.

Possibly effective: To control excessive anxiety, tension and agitation as seen in neuroses or associated with somatic conditions.

'Stelazine' has not been shown effective in the management of behavioral complications in patients with mental retardation.

Final classification of the less-than-effective indications requires further investigation.

Contraindications: Comatose or greatly depressed states due to central nervous system depressants, and in cases of existing blood dyscrasias, bone marrow depression and pre-existing liver damage.

Warnings: Patients who have demonstrated a hypersensitivity reaction (e.g., blood dyscrasias, jaundice) with a phenothiazine should not be re-exposed to any phenothiazine, including Stelazine (trifluoperazine HCl, SK&F), unless in the judgment of the physician the potential benefits of treatment outweigh the possible hazard.

'Stelazine' may impair mental and/or physical abilities, especially during the first few days of therapy. Therefore, caution patients about activities requiring alertness (e.g., operating vehicles or machinery).

If agents such as sedatives, narcotics, anesthetics, tranquilizers, or alcohol are used either simultaneously or successively with the drug, the possibility of an undesirable additive depressant effect should be considered.

Usage in Pregnancy: Animal reproductive studies and clinical experience to date have not demonstrated any teratogenic effect from Stelazine (trifluoperazine HCl, SK&F). However, as with any medication, it should be used in pregnant patients only when, in the judgment of the physician, it is necessary for the welfare of the patient.

Nursing Mothers: There is evidence that phenothiazines are excreted in the breast milk of nursing mothers.

Precautions: Thrombocytopenia and anemia have been reported in patients receiving the drug. Agranulocytosis and pancytopenia have also been reported—warn patients to report the sudden appearance of sore throat or other signs of infection. If white blood cell and differential counts indicate cellular depression, stop treatment and start antibiotic and other suitable therapy.

Jaundice of the cholestatic type of hepatitis or liver damage has been reported. If fever with grippe-like symptoms occurs, appropriate liver studies should be conducted. If tests indicate an abnormality, stop treatment.

One result of therapy may be an increase in mental and physical activity. For example, a few patients with angina pectoris have complained of increased pain while taking the drug. Therefore, angina patients should be observed carefully and, if an unfavorable response is noted, the drug should be withdrawn.

Because hypotension has occurred, large doses and parenteral administration should be avoided in patients with impaired cardiovascular systems. To minimize the occurrence of hypotension after initial injection, keep patient lying down and observe for at least ½ hour. If hypotension occurs from parenteral or oral dosing, place patient in head-low position with legs raised. If a vasoconstrictor is required, 'Levophed' and 'Neo-Synephrine'* are suitable. Other pressor agents, including epinephrine, should not be used as they may cause a paradoxical further lowering of blood pressure.

Since certain phenothiazines have been reported to produce retinopathy, the drug should be discontinued if ophthalmoscopic examination or visual field studies should demonstrate retinal changes.

An antiemetic action of 'Stelazine' may mask the signs and symptoms of toxicity or overdosage of other drugs and may obscure the diagnosis and treatment of other conditions such as intestinal obstruction, brain tumor and Reye's syndrome.

With prolonged administration at high dosages, the possibility of cumulative effects, with sudden onset of severe central nervous system or vasomotor symptoms, should be kept in mind.

Neuroleptic drugs elevate prolactin levels; the elevation persists during chronic administration. Tissue culture experiments indicate that approximately one-third of human breast cancers are prolactin-dependent in vitro, a factor of potential importance if the prescribing of these drugs is contemplated in a patient with a previously detected breast cancer. Although disturbances such as galactorrhea, amenorrhea, gynecomastia and impotence have been reported, the clinical significance of elevated serum prolactin levels is unknown for most patients. An increase in mammary neoplasms has been found in rodents after chronic administration of neuroleptic drugs. Neither clinical nor epidemiologic studies conducted to date, however, have shown an association between chronic administration of these drugs and mammary tumorigenesis; the available evidence is considered too limited to be conclusive at this time.

As with all drugs which exert an anticholinergic effect, and/or cause mydriasis, trifluoperazine should be used with caution in patients with glaucoma.

Phenothiazines may diminish the effect of oral anticoagulants.

Phenothiazines can produce alpha-adrenergic blockade.

Concomitant administration of propranolol with phenothiazines results in increased plasma levels of both drugs.

Phenothiazines may lower the convulsive threshold; dosage adjustments of anticonvulsants may be necessary. Potentiation of anticonvulsant effects does not occur. However, it has been reported that phenothiazines may interfere with the metabolism of 'Dilantin'† and thus precipitate 'Dilantin' toxicity.

Drugs which lower the seizure threshold, including phenothiazine derivatives, should not be used with 'Amipaque'.‡ As with other phenothiazine derivatives, 'Stelazine' should be discontinued at least 48 hours before myelography, should not be resumed for at least 24 hours postprocedure, and should not be used for the control of nausea and vomiting occurring either prior to myelography or postprocedure.

Long-Term Therapy: To lessen the likelihood of adverse reactions related to cumulative drug effect, patients with a history of long-term therapy with Stelazine (trifluoperazine HCl, SK&F) and/or other neuroleptics should be evaluated periodically to decide whether the maintenance dosage could be lowered or drug therapy discontinued.

Adverse Reactions: Drowsiness, dizziness, skin reactions, rash, dry mouth, insomnia, amenorrhea, fatigue, muscular weakness, anorexia, lactation, blurred vision and neuromuscular (extrapyramidal) reactions.

Neuromuscular (Extrapyramidal) Reactions

These symptoms are seen in a significant number of hospitalized mental patients. They may be characterized by motor restlessness, be of the dystonic type, or they may resemble parkinsonism.

Depending on the severity of symptoms, dosage should be reduced or discontinued. If therapy is reinstituted, it should be at a lower dosage. Should these symptoms occur in children or pregnant patients, the drug should be stopped and not reinstituted. In most cases barbiturates by suitable route of administration will suffice. (Or, injectable 'Benadryl'§ may be useful.) In more severe cases, the administration of an anti-parkinsonism agent, except levodopa, usually produces rapid reversal of symptoms. Suitable supportive measures such as maintaining a clear airway and adequate hydration should be employed.

Motor Restlessness: Symptoms may include agitation or jitteriness and sometimes insomnia. These symptoms often disappear spontaneously. At times these symptoms may be similar to the original neurotic or psychotic symptoms. Dosage should not be increased until these side effects have subsided.

If this phase becomes too troublesome, the symptoms can usually be controlled by a reduction of dosage or concomitant administration of a barbiturate.

Dystonias: Symptoms may include: spasm of the neck muscles, sometimes progressing to torticollis; extensor rigidity of back muscles, sometimes progressing to opisthotonos; carpopedal spasm, trismus, swallowing difficulty, oculogyric crisis and protrusion of the tongue. These usually subside within a few hours, and almost always within 24 to 48 hours, after the drug has been discontinued.

In mild cases, reassurance or a barbiturate is often sufficient. *In moderate cases,* barbiturates will usually bring rapid relief. *In more severe adult cases,* the administration of an anti-parkinsonism agent, except levodopa, usually produces rapid reversal of symptoms. Also, intravenous caffeine with sodium benzoate seems to be effective. *In children,* reassurance and barbiturates will usually control symptoms. (Or, injectable 'Benadryl' may be useful.) Note: See 'Benadryl' prescribing information for appropriate children's dosage. If appropriate treatment with anti-parkinsonism agents or 'Benadryl' fails to reverse the signs and symptoms, the diagnosis should be reevaluated.

Pseudo-parkinsonism: Symptoms may include: mask-like facies; drooling; tremors; pill-rolling motion; cogwheel rigidity; and shuffling gait. Reassurance and sedation are important. In most cases these symptoms are readily controlled when an anti-parkinsonism agent is administered concomitantly. Anti-parkinsonism agents should be used only when required. Generally, therapy of a few weeks to two or three months will suffice. After this time patients should be evaluated to determine their need for continued treatment. (Note: Levodopa has not been found effective in pseudo-parkinsonism.) Occasionally it is necessary to lower the dosage of 'Stelazine' or to discontinue the drug.

Persistent Tardive Dyskinesia: As with all antipsychotic agents, tardive dyskinesia may appear in some patients on long-term therapy or may appear after drug therapy has been discontinued. This condition appears in all age groups. However, the risk appears to be greater in elderly patients on high-dose therapy, especially females. The symptoms are persistent and in some patients appear to be irreversible. The syndrome is characterized by rhythmical involuntary movements of the tongue, face, mouth or jaw (e.g., protrusion of tongue, puffing of cheeks, puckering of mouth, chewing movements). Sometimes these may be accompanied by involuntary movements of extremities. In rare instances, these involuntary movements of the extremities are the only manifestations of tardive dyskinesia.

There is no known effective treatment for tardive dyskinesia; anti-parkinsonism agents do not alleviate the symptoms of this syndrome. It is suggested that all antipsychotic agents be discontinued if these symptoms appear. Should it be necessary to reinstitute treatment, or increase the dosage of the agent, or switch to a different antipsychotic agent, the syndrome may be masked.

It has been reported that fine vermicular movements of the tongue may be an early sign of the syndrome and if the medication is stopped at that time the syndrome may not develop.

Adverse Reactions Reported with Stelazine (trifluoperazine HCl, SK&F) or Other Phenothiazine Derivatives: Adverse effects with different phenothiazines vary in type, frequency, and mechanism of occurrence, i.e., some are dose-related, while others involve individual patient sensitivity. Some adverse effects may be more likely to occur, or occur with greater intensity, in patients with special medical problems, e.g., patients with mitral insufficiency or pheochromocytoma have experienced severe hypotension following recommended doses of certain phenothiazines.

Not all of the following adverse reactions have been observed with every phenothiazine derivative, but they have been reported with one or more and should be borne in mind when drugs of this class are administered: extrapyramidal symptoms (opisthotonos, oculogyric crisis, hyperreflexia, dystonia, akathisia, dyskinesia, parkinsonism) some of which have lasted months and even years—particularly in elderly patients with previous brain damage; grand mal and petit mal convulsions; altered cerebrospinal fluid proteins; cerebral edema; intensification and prolongation of the action of central nervous system depressants (opiates, analgesics, antihistamines, barbiturates, alcohol), atropine, heat, organophosphorus insecticides; autonomic reactions (dryness of mouth, nasal congestion, headache, nausea, constipation, obstipation, adynamic ileus, priapism, inhibition of ejaculation); reactivation of psychotic processes, catatonic-like states; hypotension (sometimes fatal); cardiac arrest; blood dyscrasias (pancytopenia, thrombocytopenic purpura, leukopenia, agranulocytosis, eosinophilia, hemolytic anemia, aplastic anemia); liver damage (jaundice, biliary stasis); endocrine disturbances (lactation, galactorrhea, gynecomastia, menstrual irregularities, false positive pregnancy tests); skin disorders (photosensitivity, itching, erythema, urticaria, eczema up to exfoliative dermatitis); other allergic reactions (asthma, laryngeal edema, angioneurotic edema, anaphylactoid reactions); peripheral edema; reversed epinephrine effect; hyperpyrexia; mild fever after large I.M. doses; increased appetite; increased weight; a systemic lupus erythematosus-like syndrome; pigmentary retinopathy; with prolonged administration of substantial doses, skin pigmentation, epithelial keratopathy, and lenticular and corneal deposits.

EKG changes—particularly nonspecific, usually reversible Q and T wave distortions—have been observed in some patients receiving phenothiazine tranquilizers. Their relationship to myocardial damage has not been confirmed. Although phenothiazines cause neither psychic nor physical dependence, sudden discontinuance in long-term psychiatric patients may cause temporary symptoms, e.g., nausea and vomiting, dizziness, tremulousness.

Note: There have been occasional reports of sudden death in patients receiving phenothiazines. In some cases, the cause appeared to be asphyxia due to failure of the cough reflex. In others, the cause could not be determined. There is not sufficient evidence to establish a relationship between such deaths and the administration of phenothiazines.

Dosage and Administration: Dosage should be adjusted to the needs of the individual. The lowest effective dosage should always be used. Dosage should be increased more gradually in debilitated or emaciated patients. When maximum response is achieved, dosage may be reduced gradually to a maintenance level. Because of the inherent long action of the drug, patients may be controlled on convenient b.i.d. administration; some patients may be maintained on once-a-day administration. When Stelazine (trifluoperazine HCl, SK&F) is administered by intramuscular injection, equivalent oral dosage may be substituted once symptoms have been controlled.

Elderly Patients: In general, dosages in the lower range are sufficient for most elderly patients. Since they appear to be more susceptible to hypotension and neuromuscular reactions, such patients should be observed closely. Dosage should be tailored to the individual, response carefully monitored, and dosage adjusted accordingly. Dosage should be increased more gradually in elderly patients.

1. Adult Dosage

Oral (for office patients and outpatients): 1 or 2 mg. twice daily. It is seldom necessary to exceed 4 mg. a day except in patients with more severe conditions and in discharged mental patients.

Oral (for hospitalized patients or those under close supervision): Usual starting dosage is 2 mg. to 5 mg. b.i.d. (Small or emaciated patients should always be started on the lower dosage.) Most patients will show optimum response on 15 mg. or 20 mg. daily, although a few may require 40 mg. a day or more. Optimum therapeutic dosage levels should be reached within two or three weeks.

When the Concentrate dosage form is to be used, it should be added to 60 ml. (2 fl. oz.) or more of diluent *just prior to administration* to insure palatability and stability. Vehicles suggested for dilution are: tomato or fruit juice, milk, simple syrup, orange syrup, carbonated beverages, coffee, tea, or water. Semisolid foods (soup, puddings, etc.) may also be used.

Intramuscular (for prompt control of severe symptoms): Usual dosage is 1 mg. to 2 mg. (½-1 ml.) by deep intramuscular injection q4-6h, p.r.n. More than 6 mg. within 24 hours is rarely necessary.

Only in very exceptional cases should intramuscular dosage exceed 10 mg. within 24 hours. Injections should not be given at intervals of less than 4 hours because of a possible cumulative effect.

Note: Stelazine (trifluoperazine HCl, SK&F) Injection has been usually well tolerated and there is little, if any, pain and irritation at the site of injection.

The Injection should be protected from light. Exposure may cause discoloration. Slight yellowish discoloration will not alter potency or efficacy. If markedly discolored, the solution should be discarded.

2. Dosage for Psychotic Children

Dosage should be adjusted to the weight of the child and severity of the symptoms. These dosages are for children, ages 6 to 12, who are hospitalized or under close supervision.

Oral: The starting dosage is 1 mg. administered once a day or b.i.d. Dosage may be increased gradually until symptoms are controlled or until side effects become troublesome.

While it is usually not necessary to exceed dosages of 15 mg. daily, some older children with severe symptoms may require higher dosages.

Intramuscular: There has been little experience with the use of Stelazine (trifluoperazine HCl, SK&F) Injection in children. However, if it is necessary to achieve rapid control of severe symptoms, 1 mg. (½ ml.) of the drug may be administered intramuscularly once or twice a day.

Overdosage (See also under Adverse Reactions.):

Symptoms—Primarily involvement of the extrapyramidal mechanism producing some of the dystonic reactions described above. Symptoms of central nervous system depression to the point of somnolence or coma. Agitation and restlessness may also occur. Other possible manifestations include convulsions, EKG changes and cardiac arrhythmias, fever, and autonomic reactions such as hypotension, dry mouth and ileus.

Treatment—It is important to determine other medications taken by the patient since multiple dose therapy is common in overdosage situations. Treatment is essentially symptomatic and supportive. Early gastric lavage is helpful. Keep patient under observation and maintain an open airway, since involvement of the extrapyramidal mechanism may produce dysphagia and respiratory difficulty in severe overdosage. **Do not attempt to induce emesis because a dystonic reaction of the head or neck may develop that could result in aspiration of vomitus.** Extrapyramidal symptoms may be treated with anti-parkinsonism drugs, barbiturates, or 'Benadryl'. See prescribing information for these products. Care should be taken to avoid increasing respiratory depression. If administration of a stimulant is desirable, amphetamine, dextroamphetamine, or caffeine with sodium benzoate is recommended. Stimulants that may cause convulsions (e.g., picrotoxin or pentylenetetrazol) should be avoided.

If hypotension occurs, the standard measures for managing circulatory shock should be initiated. If it is desirable to administer a vasoconstrictor, 'Levophed' and 'Neo-Synephrine' are most suitable. Other pressor agents, including epinephrine, are not recommended because phenothiazine derivatives may reverse the usual elevating action of these agents and cause a further lowering of blood pressure.

Limited experience indicates that phenothiazines are *not* dialyzable.

How Supplied:

Tablets, 1 mg. and 2 mg., in bottles of 100 and 1000; in Single Unit Packages of 100 (intended for institutional use only).

For psychiatric patients who are hospitalized or under close supervision:

Tablets, 5 mg. and 10 mg., in bottles of 100 and 1000; in Single Unit Packages of 100 (intended for institutional use only).

Multiple-dose Vials, 10 ml. (2 mg./ml.), in boxes of 1 and 20.

Concentrate (intended for institutional use only)—10 mg./ml., in 2 fl. oz. bottles and in cartons of 12 bottles.

Each bottle is packaged with a graduated dropper.

The Concentrate form is light-sensitive. For this reason, it should be protected from light and dispensed in amber bottles. *Refrigeration is not required.*

Note: Although there is little likelihood of contact dermatitis due to the drug, persons with

Continued on next page

Smith Kline & French—Cont.

known sensitivity to phenothiazine drugs should avoid direct contact.

Military—Tablets 1 mg., 1000's, 6505-00-022-1336, and S.U.P. 100's, 6505-00-132-0132; 2 mg., 1000's, 6505-00-022-1337; 5 mg., 1000's, 6505-00-022-1338; 10 mg., 1000's, 6505-00-180-5973, and S.U.P. 100's, 6505-00-132-0188.

*'Levophed' and 'Neo-Synephrine' are the trademarks (Reg. U.S. Pat. Off.) of Winthrop Laboratories for its brands of levarterenol and phenylephrine respectively.
†Trademark Reg. U.S. Pat. Off.: 'Dilantin' for diphenylhydantoin, Parke-Davis.
‡Trademark Reg. U.S. Pat. Off.: 'Amipaque' for metrizamide, Winthrop Laboratories.
§Trademark Reg. U.S. Pat. Off.: 'Benadryl' for diphenhydramine hydrochloride, Parke-Davis.

[*Shown in Product Identification Section*]

TAGAMET® ℞

(brand of cimetidine tablets cimetidine hydrochloride liquid and cimetidine hydrochloride injection)

('Tagamet' is a product of SK&F Lab Co., Carolina, P.R. 00630, Subsidiary of SmithKline Beckman Corporation, Philadelphia, Pa.)

Description: 'Tagamet' (brand of cimetidine) is a histamine H_2 receptor antagonist. Chemically it is *N''*-cyano-N-methyl-*N'*-[2-[[(5-methyl-1H-imidazol-4-yl) methyl] thio]-ethyl]-guanidine.

(The liquid and injection dosage forms contain cimetidine as the hydrochloride.)

Cimetidine has a bitter taste and characteristic odor.

Tablets: Each tablet contains 200 mg. or 300 mg. of cimetidine.

Liquid: Each 5 ml. teaspoonful contains, in aqueous solution, cimetidine hydrochloride equivalent to cimetidine, 300 mg.; alcohol, 2.8%.

Vials: Each 2 ml. vial contains, in aqueous solution, cimetidine hydrochloride equivalent to cimetidine, 300 mg.; phenol, 10 mg.

Multiple-dose Vials: 8 ml. (300 mg./2 ml.): Each 2 ml. contains, in aqueous solution, cimetidine hydrochloride equivalent to cimetidine, 300 mg.; phenol, 10 mg.

Clinical Pharmacology: 'Tagamet' (brand of cimetidine) competitively inhibits the action of histamine at the histamine H_2 receptors of the parietal cells and thus represents a new class of pharmacological agents, the histamine H_2-receptor antagonists.

'Tagamet' is not an anticholinergic agent. Studies have shown that 'Tagamet' inhibits both daytime and nocturnal basal gastric acid secretion. 'Tagamet' also inhibits gastric acid secretion stimulated by food, histamine, pentagastrin, caffeine and insulin.

Antisecretory Activity

1) **Acid Secretion:** *Basal:* Oral 'Tagamet' 300 mg. inhibited basal gastric acid secretion by 100% for at least two hours and by at least 90% throughout the 4 hour study in fasting duodenal ulcer patients.

The gastric pH in all subjects was increased to 5.0 or greater for at least 2¼ hours.

Nocturnal: Nighttime basal secretion in fasting duodenal ulcer patients was inhibited by a 300 mg. dose of 'Tagamet' by 100% for at least one hour and by a mean of 89% over a seven hour period. Gastric pH was increased to 5.0 or greater in most of the patients for three to four hours.

'Tagamet' 300 mg. reduced non-stimulated acid concentration by 70–100% and the non-stimulated volume of gastric secretion by 20–50%.

Food Stimulated: During the first hour after a standard experimental meal, oral 'Tagamet' 300 mg. inhibited gastric acid secretion in duodenal ulcer patients by at least 50%. During the subsequent two hours 'Tagamet' inhibited gastric acid secretion by at least 75%.

The effect of a 300 mg. breakfast dose of 'Tagamet' continued for at least four hours and there was partial suppression of the rise in gastric acid secretion following the luncheon meal in duodenal ulcer patients. This suppression of gastric acid output was enhanced and could be maintained by another 300 mg. dose of 'Tagamet' given with lunch.

In another study, 'Tagamet' 300 mg. given with the meal increased gastric pH as compared with placebo.

	Mean Gastric pH	
	'Tagamet'	Placebo
1 hour	3.5	2.6
2 hours	3.1	1.6
3 hours	3.8	1.9
4 hours	6.1	2.2

The effects of oral 'Tagamet' 300 mg. and propantheline bromide on food-stimulated gastric acid secretion were compared in 7 duodenal ulcer patients. Propantheline bromide was titrated to maximally tolerated dosages—the average dose was 45 mg. 'Tagamet' 300 mg. reduced gastric acid output by 67% vs. 27% ($p<0.05$) for propantheline bromide.

Chemically Stimulated: Oral 'Tagamet' (brand of cimetidine) significantly inhibited gastric acid secretion stimulated by betazole (an isomer of histamine), pentagastrin, caffeine and insulin as follows:

Stimulant	Stimulant Dose	'Tagamet'	% Inhibition
Betazole	1.5mg/kg (sc)	300mg (po)	85% at 2½ hours
Pentagastrin	6mcg/kg/hr (iv)	100mg/hr (iv)	60% at 1 hour
Caffeine	5mg/kg/hr (iv)	300mg (po)	100% at 1 hour
Insulin	0.03 units/kg/hr (iv)	100mg/hr (iv)	82% at 1 hour

When food and betazole were used to stimulate secretion, inhibition of hydrogen ion concentration usually ranged from 45–75% and the inhibition of volume ranged from 30–65%.

2) **Pepsin:** Oral 'Tagamet' 300 mg. reduced total pepsin output as a result of the decrease in volume of gastric juice.

3) **Intrinsic Factor:** Intrinsic factor secretion was studied with betazole as a stimulant. Oral 'Tagamet' 300 mg. inhibited the rise in intrinsic factor concentration produced by betazole, but some intrinsic factor was secreted at all times.

4) **Serum Gastrin:** A single oral dose of 'Tagamet' 300 mg. augments the normal serum gastrin increase in response to a meal. This effect is probably attributable to the action of the drug in inhibiting food-stimulated gastric acid secretion. 'Tagamet' does not increase nocturnal serum gastrin levels in fasting patients. Studies of serum gastrin levels in short-term therapy have shown a slight or no increase. Studies are continuing for evaluation of the long-term effects, if any, of 'Tagamet' on serum gastrin.

Other

Lower Esophageal Sphincter Pressure and Gastric Emptying

'Tagamet' has no effect on lower esophageal sphincter (LES) pressure or the rate of gastric emptying.

Pharmacokinetics

'Tagamet' is rapidly absorbed after oral administration and peak levels occur in 45–90 minutes. The half-life of 'Tagamet' is approximately 2 hours. Both oral and parenteral (IV or IM) administration provide comparable periods of therapeutically effective blood levels; blood concentrations remain above that required to provide 80% inhibition of basal gastric acid secretion for 4–5 hours following a dose of 300 mg.

The principal route of excretion of 'Tagamet' is the urine. Following parenteral administration, most of the drug is excreted as the parent compound; following oral administration, the drug is more extensively metabolized, the sulfoxide being the major metabolite. Following a single oral dose, 48% of the drug is recovered from the urine after 24 hours as the parent compound. Following IV or IM administration, approximately 75% of the drug is recovered from the urine after 24 hours as the parent compound.

Clinical Trials:

Duodenal Ulcer

'Tagamet' (brand of cimetidine) has been shown to be effective in the treatment of active duodenal ulcer and, at reduced dosage, in the prevention of recurrent ulcer.

Active Ulcer: In worldwide double-blind clinical studies, endoscopically evaluated duodenal ulcer healing rates with 'Tagamet' were consistently higher than those of the placebo controls. In many of the studies, these differences were statistically significant.

In a multicenter, double-blind controlled U.S. study on endoscopically diagnosed duodenal ulcers earlier healing was seen in the 'Tagamet' patients as shown below:

	'Tagamet'†	Placebo†
Inpatients		
week 1	15/43 (35%)	12/51 (24%)
week 2	24/43 (56%*)	18/49 (37%)
Outpatients		
week 1	20/87 (23%)	14/91 (15%)
week 2	12/26 (46%*)	7/27 (26%)
week 4	16/28 (57%)	13/27 (48%)
week 6	22/29 (76%)	17/27 (63%)

†All patients were permitted p.r.n. antacids for relief of pain.
*$p<0.05$

In this study, 'Tagamet'-treated patients reported a general reduction in both daytime and nocturnal pain, and they also consumed less antacid.

While short-term treatment with 'Tagamet' can result in complete healing of the duodenal ulcer, acute therapy will not prevent ulcer recurrence after 'Tagamet' has been discontinued. Some follow-up studies have reported that the rate of recurrence once therapy was discontinued was slightly higher for patients healed on 'Tagamet' than for patients healed on other forms of therapy; however, the 'Tagamet'-treated patients generally had more severe disease.

Recurrent Ulcer: Extended treatment with a reduced dose of 'Tagamet' has been shown to decrease the recurrence of duodenal ulcer. In double-blind multicenter studies, 400 mg. of 'Tagamet', taken at bedtime, resulted in a significantly lower incidence of duodenal ulcer recurrence in patients treated for up to one year.

PERCENT RECURRING IN EACH QUARTER

Double-Blind Studies Conducted in the U.S.

Quarter	'Tagamet' 400 mg. h.s.	Placebo
I	7% (3/46)	22% (11/49)
II	7% (2/28)	46% (13/28)
III	6% (1/16)	10% (1/10)
IV	– (0/4)	33% (1/3)
Total	13% (6/46)	53% (26/49)

Double-Blind Studies Conducted in Europe

Quarter	'Tagamet' 400 mg. h.s.	Placebo
I	5% (8/179)	32% (108/333)
II	10% (14/143)	24% (45/184)
III	5% (4/78)	21% (17/82)
IV	5% (2/44)	20% (10/49)
Total	16% (28/179)	54% (180/333)

Pathological Hypersecretory Conditions (such as Zollinger-Ellison Syndrome)
'Tagamet' significantly inhibited gastric acid secretion and reduced occurrence of diarrhea, anorexia and pain in patients with pathological hypersecretion associated with Zollinger-Ellison Syndrome, systemic mastocytosis and multiple endocrine adenomas. Use of 'Tagamet' was also followed by healing of intractable ulcers.

Indications:
'Tagamet' (brand of cimetidine) is indicated in:
(1) Short-term treatment of active duodenal ulcer. Since most patients heal within 6-8 weeks, there is rarely reason to use 'Tagamet' at full dosage for longer periods. Concomitant antacids should be given as needed for relief of pain. However, simultaneous administration of 'Tagamet' and antacids is not recommended, since antacids have been reported to interfere with the absorption of 'Tagamet'.
(2) Prophylactic use in duodenal ulcer patients, at reduced dosage, to prevent ulcer recurrence in patients likely to need surgical treatment, e.g., as demonstrated by a history of recurrence or complications, and in patients with concomitant illness in whom surgery would constitute a greater than usual risk. Limitation of use to this population is recommended because the consequences of very long-term use, i.e., beyond one year, of continuous 'Tagamet' therapy are not known.
(3) The treatment of pathological hypersecretory conditions (i.e., Zollinger-Ellison Syndrome, systemic mastocytosis, multiple endocrine adenomas).

Contraindications: There are no known contraindications to the use of 'Tagamet' (brand of cimetidine). However, the physician should refer to the Precautions section regarding usage in pregnant, nursing, or pediatric patients.

Precautions: 'Tagamet' (brand of cimetidine) has demonstrated a weak antiandrogenic effect. In animal studies this was manifested as reduced prostate and seminal vesicle weights. However, there was no impairment of mating performance or fertility, nor any harm to the fetus in these animals at doses 9 to 56 times the full therapeutic dose of 'Tagamet', as compared with controls. The cases of gynecomastia seen in patients treated for one month or longer may be related to this effect.
One study without a parallel control reported that the concentration of sperm in 7 males was reduced during treatment with 'Tagamet' 300 mg. q.i.d., for 9 weeks. In only one patient did the count fall below 50 million/ml. (i.e., 43 million/ml.). After the treatment period the concentrations returned to pretreatment levels.
However, a controlled, double-blind study on spermatogenesis in 30 normal males who received 'Tagamet' (300 mg. q.i.d. or 400 mg. h.s.) or placebo for six months did not demonstrate any effect of 'Tagamet' on spermatogenesis, sperm count, motility, morphology or fertilizing capacity *in vitro*. Blood levels of androgen and gonadotropin were unchanged.
In a 24-month toxicity study conducted in rats, at dose levels of 150, 378 and 950 mg./kg./day (approximately 9 to 56 times the recommended human dose), there was a small increase in the incidence of benign Leydig cell tumors in each dose group; when the combined drug-treated groups and control groups were compared, this increase reached statistical significance. In a subsequent 24-month study, there were no differences between the rats receiving 150 mg./kg./day and the untreated controls. However, a statistically significant increase in benign Leydig cell tumor incidence was seen in the rats that received 378 and 950 mg./kg./day. These tumors were common in control groups as well as treated groups and the difference became apparent only in aged rats.
Rare instances of cardiac arrhythmias and hypotension have been reported following the rapid administration of 'Tagamet' HCl (brand of cimetidine hydrochloride) Injection by intravenous bolus.
Symptomatic response to 'Tagamet' therapy does not preclude the presence of a gastric malignancy.
Use in Elderly/Severely Ill Patients: Reversible confusional states have been observed on occasion, usually in elderly and/or severely ill patients, such as those with renal insufficiency or organic brain syndrome; overdosage may have played a role in some cases. These confusional states generally cleared within 48 hours of drug withdrawal.
Drug Interactions: 'Tagamet', apparently through an effect on certain microsomal enzyme systems, has been reported to reduce the hepatic metabolism of warfarin-type anticoagulants, phenytoin, propranolol, chlordiazepoxide, diazepam, lidocaine and theophylline, thereby delaying elimination and increasing blood levels of these drugs.
Clinically significant effects have been reported with the warfarin anticoagulants; therefore, close monitoring of prothrombin time is recommended, and adjustment of the anticoagulant dose may be necessary when 'Tagamet' is administered concomitantly. Interaction with phenytoin, lidocaine and theophylline has also been reported to produce adverse clinical effects.
Dosage of the drugs mentioned above and other similarly metabolized drugs, particularly those of low therapeutic ratio or in patients with renal and/or hepatic impairment, may require adjustment when starting or stopping concomitantly administered 'Tagamet' to maintain optimum therapeutic blood levels.
Additional clinical experience may reveal other drugs affected by the concomitant administration of 'Tagamet'.
Decreased white blood cell counts, including agranulocytosis, have been reported in 'Tagamet'-treated patients who also received antimetabolites, alkylating agents or other drugs and/or treatment known to produce neutropenia.
Usage in Pregnancy: There has been no experience to date with the use of 'Tagamet' in pregnant patients. However, animal studies have demonstrated that 'Tagamet' crosses the placental barrier. Teratology studies (100–950 mg./kg./day) have shown no effects attributable to 'Tagamet' on litter parameters or early development of the young.
'Tagamet' should not be used in pregnant patients or women of childbearing potential unless, in the judgment of the physician, the anticipated benefits outweigh the potential risks.
Nursing Mothers: Cimetidine is secreted in human milk and, as a general rule, nursing should not be undertaken while a patient is on a drug.
Pediatric Use: Clinical experience in children is limited. Therefore, 'Tagamet' therapy cannot be recommended for children under 16, unless, in the judgment of the physician, anticipated benefits outweigh the potential risks. In very limited experience, doses of 20–40 mg./kg. per day have been used.

Adverse Reactions: Mild and transient diarrhea, dizziness, somnolence and rash have been reported in a small number of patients, e.g., approximately 1 in 100, during treatment with 'Tagamet' (brand of cimetidine). A few cases of headache, ranging from mild to severe, have been reported; these cleared on withdrawal of the drug.
There have been rare reports of reversible arthralgia and myalgia; exacerbation of joint symptoms in patients with preexisting arthritis has also been reported. Such symptoms have usually been alleviated by a reduction in 'Tagamet' (brand of cimetidine) dosage. A few cases of polymyositis have been reported, but no causal relationship has been established.
Mild gynecomastia has been reported in patients treated for one month or longer. In patients being treated for pathological hypersecretory states, this occurred in about 4 percent of cases while in all others the incidence was 0.3% to 1% in various studies. No evidence of induced endocrine dysfunction was found, and the condition remained unchanged or returned toward normal with continuing 'Tagamet' treatment.
Reversible impotence has been reported in patients with pathological hypersecretory disorders, e.g., Zollinger-Ellison Syndrome, receiving 'Tagamet', particularly in high doses, for at least 12 months (range 12–79 months, mean 38 months). However, in large-scale surveillance studies at regular dosage, the incidence has not exceeded that commonly reported in the general population. Furthermore, in controlled long-term studies in patients receiving a single daily bedtime dose, the incidence of reversible impotence did not differ significantly between the 'Tagamet' and placebo groups.
Decreased white blood cell counts in 'Tagamet'-treated patients (approximately 1 per 100,000 patients), including agranulocytosis (approximately 3 per million patients), have been reported, including a few reports of recurrence on rechallenge. These patients generally had serious concomitant illnesses and received drugs and/or treatment known to produce neutropenia. Thrombocytopenia (approximately 3 per million patients) and a few cases of aplastic anemia have also been reported.
Regularly observed small increases in plasma creatinine and some increases in serum transaminase have been reported. These did not progress with continued therapy and disappeared at the end of therapy.
Rare cases of fever, interstitial nephritis, hepatitis and pancreatitis, which cleared on withdrawal of the drug, have been reported.
There has been reported a single case of biopsy-proven periportal hepatic fibrosis in a patient receiving 'Tagamet'.

Dosage and Administration:
Duodenal Ulcer
Active Ulcer: The recommended adult oral dosage for duodenal ulcer is 300 mg. four times a day, with meals and at bedtime.
Concomitant antacids should be given as needed for relief of pain. However, simultaneous administration of 'Tagamet' and antacids is not recommended, since antacids have been reported to interfere with the absorption of 'Tagamet'.
While healing with 'Tagamet' often occurs during the first week or two, treatment should be continued for 4–6 weeks unless healing has been demonstrated by endoscopic examination.
Prophylaxis of Recurrent Ulcer: In those patients in whom prophylactic use is indicated, 400 mg. (two 200 mg. tablets) at bedtime is recommended. Prophylactic treatment with higher or more frequent doses does not improve effectiveness.
Pathological Hypersecretory Conditions (such as Zollinger-Ellison Syndrome)
Recommended adult oral dosage: 300 mg. four times a day with meals and at bedtime. In some patients it may be necessary to administer 'Tagamet' 300 mg. doses more frequently. Doses should be adjusted to individual patient needs, but should not usually exceed 2400 mg. per day and should continue as long as clinically indicated.
Parenteral Administration
In some hospitalized patients with pathological hypersecretory conditions or intractable ulcers, or in patients who are unable to take

Continued on next page

Smith Kline & French—Cont.

oral medication, 'Tagamet' may be administered parenterally according to the following recommendations:
Intramuscular injection: 300 mg. q 6 hours (no dilution necessary). Transient pain at the site of injection has been reported.
Intermittent intravenous infusion: 300 mg. q 6 hours. Dilute 'Tagamet' HCl Injection, 300 mg., in 100 ml. of Dextrose Injection (5%) or other compatible i.v. solution (see Stability of 'Tagamet' HCl Injection) and infuse over 15–20 minutes. In some patients it may be necessary to increase dosage. When this is necessary the increases should be made by more frequent administration of a 300 mg. dose, but should not exceed 2400 mg. per day. **Intravenous injection:** 300 mg. q 6 hours. Dilute 'Tagamet' HCl Injection, 300 mg., in Sodium Chloride Injection (0.9%) or other compatible i.v. solution (see Stability of 'Tagamet' HCl Injection) to a total volume of 20 ml. and inject over a period of not less than 2 minutes (see Precautions).

Dosage Adjustment for Patients with Impaired Renal Function

Patients with severely impaired renal function have been treated with 'Tagamet'. However, such usage has been very limited. On the basis of this experience the recommended dosage is 300 mg. q 12 hours orally or by intravenous injection. Should the patient's condition require, the frequency of dosing may be increased to q 8 hours or even further with caution. In severe renal failure accumulation may occur and the lowest frequency of dosing compatible with an adequate patient response should be used. When liver impairment is also present, further reductions in dosage may be necessary. Hemodialysis reduces the level of circulating 'Tagamet'. Ideally, the dosage schedule should be adjusted so that the timing of a scheduled dose coincides with the end of hemodialysis.

Stability of 'Tagamet' HCl Injection

'Tagamet' HCl (brand of cimetidine hydrochloride) Injection is stable for 48 hours at normal room temperature when added to or diluted with most commonly used intravenous solutions, e.g., Sodium Chloride Injection (0.9%), Dextrose Injection (5% or 10%), Lactated Ringer's Solution, 5% Sodium Bicarbonate Injection.

Overdosage: The usual measures to remove unabsorbed material from the gastrointestinal tract, clinical monitoring and supportive therapy should be employed. Studies in animals indicate that toxic doses are associated with respiratory failure and tachycardia which may be controlled by assisted respiration and the administration of a beta-blocker.

Human experience with gross overdosage is limited. However, in the few cases which have been reported, doses up to 10 grams have not been associated with any untoward effects.

How Supplied:

Pale Green Tablets: 200 mg. tablets in bottles of 100; 300 mg. tablets in bottles of 100 and Single Unit Packages of 100 (intended for institutional use only).
Liquid: 300 mg./5 ml., in 8 fl. oz. (237 ml.) amber glass bottles.
Injection: 300 mg./2 ml. in single-dose vials and in 8 ml. multiple-dose vials, in packages of 10.
Military—Tablets, 300 mg., 6505-01-050-3547

[*Shown in Product Identification Section*]

TELDRIN® MULTI-SYMPTOM ALLERGY RELIEVER CAPSULES
Allergy Capsules

Marketed by Menley & James Laboratories
a SmithKline company
(See PDR For Nonprescription Drugs)

TELDRIN®
Chlorpheniramine maleate
TIMED-RELEASE ALLERGY CAPSULES, 8 mg. and 12 mg.

Marketed by Menley & James Laboratories,
a SmithKline company.
(See PDR For Nonprescription Drugs)

TEMARIL® ℞
(brand of trimeprazine tartrate)
Tablets, Syrup and Spansule® capsules

Description: 'Temaril', available as trimeprazine tartrate, a phenothiazine derivative, is 10-[3-(dimethylamino)-2-methylpropyl]-phenothiazine tartrate.
Trimeprazine tartrate is a white to off-white odorless, crystalline powder readily soluble in water.
Tablets—Each tablet contains trimeprazine tartrate equivalent to 2.5 mg. of trimeprazine.
Syrup—Each 5 ml. (one teaspoonful) contains trimeprazine tartrate equivalent to 2.5 mg. of trimeprazine, and alcohol, 5.7%.
Spansule® sustained release capsules—Each 'Spansule' capsule contains trimeprazine tartrate equivalent to 5 mg. of trimeprazine, so prepared that an initial dose is released promptly and the remaining medication is released gradually over a prolonged period.
Actions: Temaril (trimeprazine tartrate, SK&F), a phenothiazine, possesses antipruritic and antihistaminic properties with anticholinergic (drying) and sedative side effects.
Indications: Treatment of pruritic symptoms in urticaria. Relief of pruritic symptoms in a variety of allergic and non-allergic conditions including atopic dermatitis, neurodermatitis, contact dermatitis, pityriasis rosea, poison ivy dermatitis, eczematous dermatitis, pruritus ani and vulvae, and drug rash.
Contraindications: Temaril (trimeprazine tartrate, SK&F) is contraindicated: in comatose patients; in patients who have received large amounts of central nervous system depressants (alcohol, barbiturates, narcotics, etc.); in patients with bone marrow depression; in patients who have demonstrated an idiosyncrasy or hypersensitivity to 'Temaril' or other phenothiazines; in newborn or premature children; and in nursing mothers. It should not be used in children who are acutely ill and/or dehydrated, as there is an increased susceptibility to dystonias in such patients.
Warnings: Temaril (trimeprazine tartrate, SK&F) may impair the mental and/or physical ability required for the performance of potentially hazardous tasks, such as driving a vehicle or operating machinery. Similarly, it may impair mental alertness in children. The concomitant use of alcohol or other central nervous system depressants may have an additive effect. Patients should be warned accordingly.
'Temaril' should be used with extreme caution in patients with:

- Asthmatic attack
- Narrow-angle glaucoma
- Prostatic hypertrophy
- Stenosing peptic ulcer
- Pyloroduodenal obstruction
- Bladder neck obstruction
- Patients receiving monoamine oxidase inhibitors

Usage in Pregnancy: The safe use of 'Temaril' has not been established with respect to the possible adverse effects upon fetal development. Therefore, it should not be used in women of childbearing potential. Jaundice and prolonged extrapyramidal symptoms have been reported in infants whose mothers received phenothiazines during pregnancy.
Usage in Children: 'Temaril' should be used with caution in children who have a history of sleep apnea or a family history of sudden infant death syndrome (SIDS). It should also be used with caution in young children, in whom it may cause excitation.
Overdosage may produce hallucinations, convulsions and sudden death.
Usage in Elderly Patients (60 years or older): Elderly patients are more prone to develop the following side effects from phenothiazines:

- Hypotension
- Syncope
- Toxic confusional states
- Extrapyramidal symptoms, especially parkinsonism
- Excessive sedation

Precautions: Temaril (trimeprazine tartrate, SK&F) may significantly affect the actions of other drugs. It may increase, prolong or intensify the sedative action of central nervous system depressants such as anesthetics, barbiturates or alcohol. When 'Temaril' is administered concomitantly the dose of a narcotic or barbiturate should be reduced to ¼ or ½ the usual amount. In the patient with pain, receiving treatment with narcotics, excessive amounts of 'Temaril' may lead to restlessness and motor hyperactivity. 'Temaril' can block and even reverse the usual pressor effect of epinephrine.
'Temaril' should be used cautiously in persons with acute or chronic respiratory impairment, particularly children, as it may suppress the cough reflex.
This drug should be used cautiously in persons with cardiovascular disease, impairment of liver function, or those with a history of ulcer disease.
Since 'Temaril' has a slight antiemetic action, it may obscure signs of intestinal obstruction, brain tumor, or overdosage of toxic drugs.
Phenothiazines have been shown to elevate prolactin levels; the elevation persists during chronic administration. Tissue culture experiments indicate that approximately one-third of human breast cancers are prolactin-dependent in vitro, a factor of potential importance if the prescribing of these drugs is contemplated in a patient with a previously detected breast cancer. Although disturbances such as galactorrhea, amenorrhea, gynecomastia, and impotence have been reported, the clinical significance of elevated serum prolactin levels is unknown for most patients. An increase in mammary neoplasms has been found in rodents after chronic administration of neuroleptic drugs. Neither clinical nor epidemiologic studies conducted to date, however, have shown an association between chronic administration of these drugs and mammary tumorigenesis; the available evidence is considered too limited to be conclusive at this time.
Drugs which lower the seizure threshold, including phenothiazine derivatives, should not be used with 'Amipaque'.* As with other phenothiazine derivatives, 'Temaril' should be discontinued at least 48 hours before myelography, should not be resumed for at least 24 hours postprocedure, and should not be used for the control of nausea and vomiting occurring either prior to myelography or postprocedure.
Adverse Reactions: Temaril (trimeprazine tartrate, SK&F) may produce adverse reactions attributable to both phenothiazines and antihistamines.
Note: Not all of the following adverse reactions have been reported with 'Temaril'; however, pharmacological similarities among the phenothiazine derivatives require that each be considered when 'Temaril' is administered. There have been occasional reports of sudden death in patients receiving phenothiazine derivatives chronically.
C.N.S. Effects: Drowsiness is the most common C.N.S. effect of this drug. Extrapyramidal reactions (opisthotonos, dystonia, akathisia, dyskinesia, parkinsonism) occur, particularly with high doses. (See Overdosage section for management of extrapyramidal symptoms).

Hyperreflexia has been reported in the newborn when a phenothiazine was used during pregnancy. Other reported reactions include dizziness, headache, lassitude, tinnitus, incoordination, fatigue, blurred vision, euphoria, diplopia, nervousness, insomnia, tremors and grand mal seizures, excitation, catatonic-like states, neuritis and hysteria, oculogyric crises, disturbing dreams/nightmares, pseudoschizophrenia, and intensification and prolongation of the action of C.N.S. depressants (opiates, analgesics, antihistamines, barbiturates, alcohol), atropine, heat, organophosphorus insecticides.

Cardiovascular Effects: Postural hypotension is the most common cardiovascular effect of phenothiazines. Reflex tachycardia may be seen. Bradycardia, faintness, dizziness and cardiac arrest have been reported. ECG changes, including blunting of T waves and prolongation of the Q-T interval, may be seen.

Gastrointestinal: Anorexia, nausea, vomiting, epigastric distress, diarrhea, constipation, and dry mouth may occur. Increased appetite and weight gain have also been reported.

Genitourinary: Urinary frequency and dysuria, urinary retention, early menses, induced lactation, gynecomastia, decreased libido, inhibition of ejaculation and false positive pregnancy tests have been reported.

Respiratory: Thickening of bronchial secretions, tightness of the chest, wheezing and nasal stuffiness may occur.

Allergic Reactions: These include urticaria, dermatitis, asthma, laryngeal edema, angioneurotic edema, photosensitivity, lupus erythematosus-like syndrome and anaphylactoid reactions.

Other Reported Reactions: Leukopenia, agranulocytosis, pancytopenia, hemolytic anemia, elevation of plasma cholesterol levels and thrombocytopenic purpura have been reported. Jaundice of the obstructive type has also been reported; it is usually reversible but chronic jaundice has been reported. Erythema, peripheral edema, and stomatitis have been reported. High or prolonged glucose tolerance curves, glycosuria, elevated spinal fluid proteins and reversed epinephrine effects may also occur.

Long-Term Therapy Considerations: After prolonged phenothiazine administration at high dosage, pigmentation of the skin has occurred, chiefly in the exposed areas. Ocular changes consist of the appearance of lenticular and corneal opacities, epithelial keratopathies and pigmentary retinopathy. Vision may be impaired.

Dosage and Administration:

Tablets and Syrup:

Adults: Usual dosage is 2.5 mg. q.i.d.

Children over three years: Usual dosage is 2.5 mg. h.s., or t.i.d. if needed.

Children 6 months to 3 years: Usual dosage is 1.25 mg. (1/2 teaspoonful of syrup) h.s., or t.i.d. if needed.

'Spansule' capsules:

Adults: Usual daily dosage is 1 capsule q12h.

Children over 6 years of age: 1 capsule daily. This product form is not recommended for children under 6 years of age. Use tablets or syrup for their dosage flexibility.

Because some side effects appear to be dose-related, it is important to use the lowest effective dosage.

Drug Interactions: MAO inhibitors and thiazide diuretics prolong and intensify the anticholinergic effects of 'Temaril'. Combined use of MAO inhibitors and phenothiazines may result in hypertension and extrapyramidal reactions.

Narcotics: The C.N.S. depressant and analgesic effects of narcotics are potentiated by phenothiazines.

The following drugs may result in potentiation of phenothiazine effects:

Oral contraceptives
Progesterone
Reserpine
Nylidrin hydrochloride

Management of Overdosage: Signs and symptoms of 'Temaril' overdosage range from mild depression of the central nervous system and cardiovascular system to profound hypotension, respiratory depression and unconsciousness. Stimulation may be evident, especially in children and geriatric patients. Atropine-like signs and symptoms—dry mouth, fixed, dilated pupils, flushing, etc.—as well as gastrointestinal symptoms may occur. The treatment of overdosage is essentially symptomatic and supportive. Early gastric lavage may be beneficial. **Do not administer emetics or attempt to induce vomiting because a dystonic reaction of the head or neck might result in aspiration of vomitus.** Extrapyramidal symptoms may be treated with anti-parkinsonism drugs, barbiturates, or 'Benadryl'.†

Avoid analeptics, which may cause convulsions. Severe hypotension usually responds to the administration of levarterenol or phenylephrine. EPINEPHRINE SHOULD NOT BE USED, since its use in a patient with partial adrenergic blockade may further lower the blood pressure. Additional measures include oxygen and intravenous fluids. Limited experience with dialysis indicates that it is not helpful.

Special note on 'Spansule' capsules—Since much of the 'Spansule' capsule medication is coated for gradual release, therapy directed at reversing the effects of the ingested drug and at supporting the patient should be continued for as long as overdosage symptoms remain. Saline cathartics are useful for hastening evacuation of pellets that have not already released medication.

How Supplied:

'Temaril' Tablets—2.5 mg. trimeprazine/tablet in bottles of 100 and 1000; Single Unit Packages of 100 (intended for institutional use only).

'Temaril' Syrup—2.5 mg. trimeprazine/5 ml. (teaspoonful) and alcohol 5.7%, in 4 fl. oz. bottles.

'Temaril' Spansule capsules—5 mg. trimeprazine/capsule in bottles of 50; Single Unit Packages of 100 (intended for institutional use only).

Military—Tablets 2.5 mg., 1000's, 6505-00-935-9826.

*Trademark Reg. U.S. Pat. Off.: 'Amipaque' for metrizamide, Winthrop Laboratories.

†Trademark Reg. U.S. Pat. Off.: 'Benadryl' for diphenhydramine hydrochloride, Parke-Davis.

[*Shown in Product Identification Section*]

THORAZINE® ℞

(brand of chlorpromazine)

Description: Thorazine (chlorpromazine, SK&F) is 10-(3-dimethylaminopropyl)-2-chlorphenothiazine, a dimethylamine derivative of phenothiazine. It is present in oral and injectable forms as the hydrochloride salt, and in the suppositories as the base.

Actions: The precise mechanism whereby the therapeutic effects of chlorpromazine are produced is not known. The principal pharmacological actions are psychotropic. It also exerts sedative and antiemetic activity. Chlorpromazine has actions at all levels of the central nervous system—primarily at subcortical levels—as well as on multiple organ systems. Chlorpromazine has strong antiadrenergic and weaker peripheral anticholinergic activity; ganglionic blocking action is relatively slight. It also possesses slight antihistaminic and antiserotonin activity.

Indications: For the management of manifestations of psychotic disorders.

To control nausea and vomiting.

For relief of restlessness and apprehension before surgery.

For acute intermittent porphyria.

As an adjunct in the treatment of tetanus.

To control the manifestations of the manic type of manic-depressive illness.

For relief of intractable hiccups.

For the treatment of severe behavioral problems in children marked by combativeness and/or explosive hyperexcitable behavior (out of proportion to immediate provocations), and in the short-term treatment of hyperactive children who show excessive motor activity with accompanying conduct disorders consisting of some or all of the following symptoms: impulsivity, difficulty sustaining attention, aggressivity, mood lability and poor frustration tolerance.

Based on a review of this drug by the National Academy of Sciences—National Research Council and/or other information, FDA has classified the other indication as follows:

Possibly effective: For control of excessive anxiety, tension and agitation as seen in neuroses.

Final classification of the less-than-effective indication requires further investigation.

Contraindications: Comatose states, presence of large amounts of C.N.S. depressants (alcohol, barbiturates, narcotics, etc.) and in the presence of bone marrow depression.

Warnings: The extrapyramidal symptoms which can occur secondary to 'Thorazine' may be confused with the central nervous system signs of an undiagnosed primary disease responsible for the vomiting, e.g., Reye's syndrome or other encephalopathy. The use of 'Thorazine' and other potential hepatotoxins should be avoided in children and adolescents whose signs and symptoms suggest Reye's syndrome.

Patients who have demonstrated a hypersensitivity reaction (e.g., blood dyscrasias, jaundice with a phenothiazine) should not be reexposed to any phenothiazine, including Thorazine (chlorpromazine, SK&F), unless in the judgment of the physician the potential benefits of treatment outweigh the possible hazard.

'Thorazine' may impair mental and/or physical abilities, especially during the first few days of therapy. Therefore, caution patients about activities requiring alertness (e.g., operating vehicles or machinery).

The use of alcohol with this drug should be avoided due to possible additive effects and hypotension.

'Thorazine' may counteract the antihypertensive effect of guanethidine and related compounds.

Usage in Pregnancy: Safety for the use of 'Thorazine' during pregnancy has not been established; therefore, it is recommended that the drug be given to pregnant patients only when, in the judgment of the physician, it is essential. The potential benefits should clearly outweigh possible hazards. There are reported instances of jaundice, prolonged extrapyramidal signs or hyperreflexia in newborn infants whose mothers had received 'Thorazine'.

Reproductive studies in rodents have demonstrated a potential for embryotoxicity, increased neonatal mortality and nursing transfer of the drug. Tests in the offspring of the drug-treated rodents demonstrate decreased performance. The possibility of permanent neurological damage cannot be excluded.

Nursing Mothers: There is evidence that chlorpromazine is excreted in the breast milk of nursing mothers.

Continued on next page

Smith Kline & French—Cont.

Precautions: Thorazine (chlorpromazine, SK&F) should be administered cautiously to persons with cardiovascular or liver disease. There is evidence that patients with a history of hepatic encephalopathy due to cirrhosis have increased sensitivity to the C.N.S. effects of 'Thorazine' (i.e., impaired cerebration and abnormal slowing of the EEG).

Because of its C.N.S. depressant effect, 'Thorazine' should be used with caution in patients with chronic respiratory disorders such as severe asthma, emphysema and acute respiratory infections, particularly in children.

Because 'Thorazine' can suppress the cough reflex, aspiration of vomitus is possible.

Thorazine (chlorpromazine, SK&F) prolongs and intensifies the action of C.N.S. depressants such as anesthetics, barbiturates and narcotics. When 'Thorazine' is administered concomitantly, about ¼ to ½ the usual dosage of such agents is required. When 'Thorazine' is not being administered to reduce requirements of C.N.S. depressants, it is best to stop such depressants before starting 'Thorazine' treatment. These agents may subsequently be reinstated at low doses and increased as needed.

Note: 'Thorazine' does *not* intensify the anticonvulsant action of barbiturates. Therefore, dosage of anticonvulsants, including barbiturates, should *not* be reduced if 'Thorazine' is started. Instead, start 'Thorazine' at low doses and increase as needed.

Use with caution in persons who will be exposed to extreme heat, organophosphorus insecticides, and in persons receiving atropine or related drugs.

'Thorazine' tablets have recently been reformulated to remove FD&C Yellow #5 (tartrazine). Reformulated lots can be identified by the wording "Modified Formula" on the immediate container labels.

However, until the transition process is complete, some lots of 'Thorazine' tablets containing FD&C Yellow #5 (tartrazine) will still be in stock. FD&C Yellow #5 (tartrazine) may cause allergic-type reactions (including bronchial asthma) in certain susceptible individuals. Although the overall incidence of FD&C Yellow #5 (tartrazine) sensitivity in the general population is low, it is frequently seen in patients who also have aspirin sensitivity.

For specific information, contact Smith Kline &French Laboratories (outside Pa., call toll-free: 1-800-523-4835, ext. 4262; in Pa., call collect: 215-751-4262).

Neuroleptic drugs elevate prolactin levels; the elevation persists during chronic administration. Tissue culture experiments indicate that approximately one-third of human breast cancers are prolactin-dependent in vitro, a factor of potential importance if the prescribing of these drugs is contemplated in a patient with a previously detected breast cancer. Although disturbances such as galactorrhea, amenorrhea, gynecomastia and impotence have been reported, the clinical significance of elevated serum prolactin levels is unknown for most patients. An increase in mammary neoplasms has been found in rodents after chronic administration of neuroleptic drugs. Neither clinical nor epidemiologic studies conducted to date, however, have shown an association between chronic administration of these drugs and mammary tumorigenesis; the available evidence is considered too limited to be conclusive at this time.

As with all drugs which exert an anticholinergic effect, and/or cause mydriasis, chlorpromazine should be used with caution in patients with glaucoma.

Chlorpromazine diminishes the effect of oral anticoagulants.

Phenothiazines can produce alpha-adrenergic blockade.

Chlorpromazine may lower the convulsive threshold; dosage adjustments of anticonvulsants may be necessary. Potentiation of anticonvulsant effects does not occur. However, it has been reported that chlorpromazine may interfere with the metabolism of 'Dilantin' * and thus precipitate 'Dilantin' toxicity.

Concomitant administration with propranolol results in increased plasma levels of both drugs.

Drugs which lower the seizure threshold, including phenothiazine derivatives, should not be used with 'Amipaque'.† As with other phenothiazine derivatives, 'Thorazine' should be discontinued at least 48 hours before myelography, should not be resumed for at least 24 hours postprocedure, and should not be used for the control of nausea and vomiting occurring either prior to myelography or postprocedure.

Long-Term Therapy: To lessen the likelihood of adverse reactions related to cumulative drug effect, patients with a history of long-term therapy with 'Thorazine' and/or other neuroleptics should be evaluated periodically to decide whether the maintenance dosage could be lowered or drug therapy discontinued.

Antiemetic Effect: The antiemetic action of 'Thorazine' may mask the signs and symptoms of overdosage of other drugs and may obscure the diagnosis and treatment of other conditions such as intestinal obstruction, brain tumor and Reye's syndrome (See Warnings).

'Thorazine' should be used cautiously with cancer chemotherapy drugs that cause vomiting at toxic levels because vomiting, as a sign of toxicity, may be obscured.

Abrupt Withdrawal: Like other phenothiazines, Thorazine (chlorpromazine, SK&F) is not known to cause psychic dependence and does not produce tolerance or addiction. There may be, however, following abrupt withdrawal of high-dose therapy, some symptoms resembling those of physical dependence such as gastritis, nausea and vomiting, dizziness and tremulousness. These symptoms can usually be avoided or reduced by gradual reduction of the dosage or by continuing concomitant anti-parkinsonism agents for several weeks after 'Thorazine' is withdrawn.

Adverse Reactions:

Drowsiness, usually mild to moderate, may occur, particularly during the first or second week, after which it generally disappears. If troublesome, dosage may be lowered.

Jaundice: Overall incidence has been low, regardless of indication or dosage. Most investigators conclude it is a sensitivity reaction. Most cases occur between the second and fourth weeks of therapy. The clinical picture resembles infectious hepatitis, with laboratory features of obstructive jaundice, rather than those of parenchymal damage. It is usually promptly reversible on withdrawal of the medication; however, chronic jaundice has been reported.

There is no conclusive evidence that preexisting liver disease makes patients more susceptible to jaundice. Alcoholics with cirrhosis have been successfully treated with Thorazine (chlorpromazine, SK&F) without complications. Nevertheless, the medication should be used cautiously in patients with liver disease. Patients who have experienced jaundice with a phenothiazine should not, if possible, be reexposed to 'Thorazine' or other phenothiazines.

If fever with grippe-like symptoms occurs, appropriate liver studies should be conducted. If tests indicate an abnormality, stop treatment.

Liver function tests in jaundice induced by the drug may mimic extrahepatic obstruction; withhold exploratory laparotomy until extrahepatic obstruction is confirmed.

Hematological Disorders, including agranulocytosis, eosinophilia, leukopenia, hemolytic anemia, aplastic anemia, thrombocytopenic purpura and pancytopenia, though rare, have been reported.

Agranulocytosis—Warn patients to report the sudden appearance of sore throat or other signs of infection. If white blood cell and differential counts indicate cellular depression, stop treatment and start antibiotic and other suitable therapy.

Most cases have occurred between the 4th and 10th weeks of therapy; patients should be watched closely during that period.

Moderate suppression of white blood cells is not an indication for stopping treatment unless accompanied by the symptoms described above.

Cardiovascular:

Hypotensive Effects—Postural hypotension, simple tachycardia, momentary fainting and dizziness may occur after the first injection; occasionally after subsequent injections; rarely, after the first oral dose. Usually recovery is spontaneous and symptoms disappear within ½ to 2 hours. Occasionally, these effects may be more severe and prolonged, producing a shock-like condition.

To minimize hypotension after initial injection, keep patient lying down and observe for at least ½ hour. To control hypotension, place patient in head-low position with legs raised. If a vasoconstrictor is required, 'Levophed' and 'Neo-Synephrine'‡ are the most suitable. Other pressor agents, including epinephrine, should not be used as they may cause a paradoxical further lowering of blood pressure.

EKG Changes—particularly nonspecific, usually reversible Q and T wave distortions—have been observed in some patients receiving phenothiazine tranquilizers, including Thorazine (chlorpromazine, SK&F). Their relationship to myocardial damage has not been confirmed.

Note: Sudden death, apparently due to cardiac arrest, has been reported, but there is not sufficient evidence to establish a relationship between such deaths and the administration of the drug.

C.N.S. Reactions:

Neuromuscular (Extrapyramidal) Reactions—Neuromuscular reactions include dystonias, motor restlessness, pseudo-parkinsonism and tardive dyskinesia, and appear to be dose-related. They are discussed in the following paragraphs:

Dystonias: Symptoms may include spasm of the neck muscles, sometimes progressing to acute, reversible torticollis; extensor rigidity of back muscles, sometimes progressing to opisthotonos; carpopedal spasm, trismus, swallowing difficulty, oculogyric crisis and protrusion of the tongue.

These usually subside within a few hours, and almost always within 24 to 48 hours after the drug has been discontinued.

In mild cases, reassurance or a barbiturate is often sufficient. *In moderate cases,* barbiturates will usually bring rapid relief. *In more severe adult cases,* the administration of an anti-parkinsonism agent, except levodopa, usually produces rapid reversal of symptoms. *In children,* reassurance and barbiturates will usually control symptoms. (Or, parenteral 'Benadryl'§ may be useful. See 'Benadryl' prescribing information for appropriate children's dosage.) If appropriate treatment with anti-parkinsonism agents or 'Benadryl' fails to reverse the signs and symptoms, the diagnosis should be reevaluated.

Suitable supportive measures such as maintaining a clear airway and adequate hydration should be employed when needed. If therapy is reinstituted, it should be at a lower dosage. Should these symptoms occur in children or pregnant patients, the drug should not be reinstituted.

Motor Restlessness: Symptoms may include agitation or jitteriness and sometimes insomnia. These symptoms often disappear spontaneously. At times these symptoms may be similar to the original neurotic or psychotic symptoms. Dosage should not be increased until these side effects have subsided.

If these symptoms become too troublesome, they can usually be controlled by a reduction of dosage or concomitant administration of a barbiturate.

Pseudo-parkinsonism: Symptoms may include: mask-like facies, drooling, tremors, pill-rolling motion, cogwheel rigidity and shuffling gait. In most cases these symptoms are readily controlled when an anti-parkinsonism agent is administered concomitantly. Anti-parkinsonism agents should be used only when required. Generally, therapy of a few weeks to two or three months will suffice. After this time patients should be evaluated to determine their need for continued treatment. (Note: Levodopa has not been found effective in neuroleptic-induced pseudo-parkinsonism.) Occasionally it is necessary to lower the dosage of Thorazine (chlorpromazine, SK&F) or to discontinue the drug.

Persistent Tardive Dyskinesia: As with all antipsychotic agents, tardive dyskinesia may appear in some patients on long-term therapy or may appear after drug therapy has been discontinued. This condition appears in all age groups. However, the risk appears to be greater in elderly patients on high-dose therapy, especially females. The symptoms are persistent and in some patients appear to be irreversible. The syndrome is characterized by rhythmical involuntary movements of the tongue, face, mouth or jaw (e.g., protrusion of tongue, puffing of cheeks, puckering of mouth, chewing movements). Sometimes these may be accompanied by involuntary movements of extremities. In rare instances, these involuntary movements of the extremities are the only manifestations of tardive dyskinesia.

There is no known effective treatment for tardive dyskinesia; anti-parkinsonism agents do not alleviate the symptoms of this syndrome. It is suggested that all antipsychotic agents be discontinued if these symptoms appear. Should it be necessary to reinstitute treatment, or increase the dosage of the agent, or switch to a different antipsychotic agent, the syndrome may be masked.

It has been reported that fine vermicular movements of the tongue may be an early sign of the syndrome and if the medication is stopped at that time the syndrome may not develop.

Adverse Behavioral Effects—Psychotic symptoms and catatonic-like states have been reported rarely.

Other C.N.S. Effects—Cerebral edema has been reported.

Convulsive seizures *(petit mal* and *grand mal)* have been reported, particularly in patients with EEG abnormalities or history of such disorders.

Abnormality of the cerebrospinal fluid proteins has also been reported.

Allergic Reactions of a mild urticarial type or photosensitivity are seen. Avoid undue exposure to sun. More severe reactions, including exfoliative dermatitis, have been reported occasionally.

Contact dermatitis has been reported in nursing personnel; accordingly, the use of rubber gloves when administering 'Thorazine' liquid or injectable is recommended.

Endocrine Disorders: Lactation and moderate breast engorgement may occur in females on large doses. If persistent, lower dosage or withdraw drug. False-positive pregnancy tests have been reported, but are less likely to occur when a serum test is used. Amenorrhea and gynecomastia have also been reported. Hyperglycemia, hypoglycemia and glycosuria have been reported.

Autonomic Reactions: Occasional dry mouth; nasal congestion; constipation; adynamic ileus; urinary retention; priapism; miosis and mydriasis.

Special Considerations in Long-Term Therapy: Skin pigmentation and ocular changes have occurred in some patients taking substantial doses of Thorazine (chlorpromazine, SK&F) for prolonged periods.

Skin Pigmentation—Rare instances of skin pigmentation have been observed in hospitalized mental patients, primarily females who have received the drug usually for three years or more in dosages ranging from 500 mg. to 1500 mg. daily. The pigmentary changes, restricted to exposed areas of the body, range from an almost imperceptible darkening of the skin to a slate gray color, sometimes with a violet hue. Histological examination reveals a pigment, chiefly in the dermis, which is probably a melanin-like complex. The pigmentation may fade following discontinuance of the drug.

Ocular Changes—Ocular changes have occurred more frequently than skin pigmentation and have been observed both in pigmented and nonpigmented patients receiving Thorazine (chlorpromazine, SK&F) usually for two years or more in dosages of 300 mg. daily and higher. Eye changes are characterized by deposition of fine particulate matter in the lens and cornea. In more advanced cases, star-shaped opacities have also been observed in the anterior portion of the lens. The nature of the eye deposits has not yet been determined. A small number of patients with more severe ocular changes have had some visual impairment. In addition to these corneal and lenticular changes, epithelial keratopathy and pigmentary retinopathy have been reported. Reports suggest that the eye lesions may regress after withdrawal of the drug.

Since the occurrence of eye changes seems to be related to dosage levels and/or duration of therapy, it is suggested that long-term patients on moderate to high dosage levels have periodic ocular examinations.

Etiology—The etiology of both of these reactions is not clear, but exposure to light, along with dosage/duration of therapy, appears to be the most significant factor. If either of these reactions is observed, the physician should weigh the benefits of continued therapy against the possible risks and, on the merits of the individual case, determine whether or not to continue present therapy, lower the dosage, or withdraw the drug.

Other Adverse Reactions: Mild fever may occur after large I.M. doses. Hyperpyrexia has been reported. Increases in appetite and weight sometimes occur. Peripheral edema and a systemic lupus erythematosus-like syndrome have been reported.

Note: There have been occasional reports of sudden death in patients receiving phenothiazines. In some cases, the cause appeared to be asphyxia due to failure of the cough reflex. In others, the cause could not be determined. There is not sufficient evidence to establish a relationship between such deaths and the administration of phenothiazines.

Dosage and Administration: Adjust dosage to individual and the severity of his condition, recognizing that the milligram for milligram potency relationship among all dosage forms has not been precisely established clinically. It is important to increase dosage until symptoms are controlled. Dosage should be increased more gradually in debilitated or emaciated patients. In continued therapy, gradually reduce dosage to the lowest effective maintenance level, after symptoms have been controlled for a reasonable period.

In general, dosage recommendations for other oral forms of the drug may be applied to Spansule® brand sustained release capsules on the basis of total daily dosage in milligrams.

Increase parenteral dosage only if hypotension has not occurred. Before using I.M., see Important Notes on Injection.

Elderly Patients: In general, dosages in the lower range are sufficient for most elderly patients. Since they appear to be more susceptible to hypotension and neuromuscular reactions, such patients should be observed closely. Dosage should be tailored to the individual, response carefully monitored, and dosage adjusted accordingly. Dosage should be increased more gradually in elderly patients.

General Medicine:

Adults: EXCESSIVE ANXIETY, TENSION AND AGITATION—*Oral:* 10 mg. t.i.d. or q.i.d., or 25 mg. b.i.d. or t.i.d. MORE SEVERE CASES—*Oral:* 25 mg. t.i.d. After 1 or 2 days, daily dosage may be increased by 20 to 50 mg. semiweekly, until patient becomes calm and cooperative. (Maximum improvement may not be seen for weeks or even months.) Continue optimum dosage for 2 weeks; then gradually reduce to maintenance level. Daily dosage of 200 mg. is not unusual. Some patients require higher dosages (e.g., 800 mg. daily is not uncommon in discharged mental patients).

PROMPT CONTROL OF SEVERE SYMPTOMS—*I.M.:* 25 mg. (1 ml.). If necessary, repeat in 1 hour. Subsequent doses should be oral, 25 to 50 mg. t.i.d.

NAUSEA AND VOMITING—*Oral:* 10 to 25 mg. q4-6h, p.r.n., increased, if necessary. *I.M.:* 25 mg. (1 ml.). If no hypotension occurs, give 25 to 50 mg. q3-4h, p.r.n., until vomiting stops. Then switch to oral dosage. *Rectal:* One 100 mg. suppository q6-8h, p.r.n. In some patients, half this dose will do.

INTRACTABLE HICCUPS—*Oral:* 25 to 50 mg. t.i.d. or q.i.d. If symptoms persist for 2-3 days, give 25 to 50 mg. (1-2 ml.) I.M. Should symptoms persist, use *slow* I.V. infusion with patient flat in bed: 25 to 50 mg. (1-2 ml.) in 500 to 1,000 ml. of saline. Follow blood pressure closely.

ACUTE INTERMITTENT PORPHYRIA—*Oral:* 25 to 50 mg. t.i.d. or q.i.d. Can usually be discontinued after several weeks, but maintenance therapy may be necessary for some patients. *I.M.:* 25 mg. (1 ml.) t.i.d. or q.i.d. until patient can take oral therapy.

TETANUS—*I.M.:* 25 to 50 mg. (1-2 ml.) given 3 or 4 times daily, usually in conjunction with barbiturates. Total doses and frequency of administration must be determined by the patient's response, starting with low doses and increasing gradually. *I.V.:* 25 to 50 mg. (1-2 ml.). Dilute to at least 1 mg. per ml. and administer at a rate of 1 mg. per minute.

Children: NAUSEA AND VOMITING—Thorazine (chlorpromazine, SK&F) should generally not be used in children under 6 months of age. It should not be used in conditions for which children's dosages have not been established. Dosage and frequency of administration should be adjusted according to the severity of the symptoms and response of the patient. The duration of activity following intramuscular administration may last up to 12 hours. Subsequent doses may be given by the same route if necessary. *Oral:* ¼ mg./lb. body weight q4-6h (e.g., 40 lb. child—10 mg. q4-6h). *Rectal:* ½ mg./lb. body weight q6-8h, p.r.n. (e.g., 20-30 lb. child—half of a 25 mg. suppository q6-8h). *I.M.:* ¼ mg./lb. body weight q6-8h, p.r.n. *Maximum I.M. Dosage:* Children up to 5 yrs. (or 50 lbs.), not over 40 mg./day; 5-12 yrs. (or 50-100 lbs.), not over 75 mg./day except in severe cases. (For mental and emotional disorders, see Psychiatry, below.)

TETANUS—*I.M.* or *I.V.:* ¼ mg./lb. body weight q6-8h. When given I.V., dilute to at least 1 mg./ml. and administer at rate of 1 mg. per 2 minutes. In children up to 50 lbs., do not exceed 40 mg. daily; 50 to 100 lbs., do not exceed 75 mg., except in severe cases.

Surgery:

Adults: PREOPERATIVE—*Oral:* 25 to 50 mg., 2 to 3 hours before the operation. *I.M.:* 12.5 to 25 mg. (0.5-1 ml.), 1 to 2 hours before operation.

DURING SURGERY—Administer only to control acute nausea and vomiting. *I.M.:* 12.5 mg. (0.5 ml.). Repeat in ½ hour if necessary and if no hypotension occurs. *I.V.:* 2 mg. per fractional injection, at 2-minute intervals. Do not

Continued on next page

Smith Kline & French—Cont.

exceed 25 mg. Dilute to 1 mg./ml., i.e., 1 ml. (25 mg.) mixed with 24 ml. of saline. POSTOPERATIVE—*Oral:* 10 to 25 mg. q4-6h, p.r.n. *I.M.:* 12.5 to 25 mg. (0.5-1 ml.). Repeat in 1 hour if necessary and if no hypotension occurs.

Children: Thorazine (chlorpromazine, SK&F) should generally not be used in children under 6 months of age except where potentially lifesaving. It should not be used in conditions for which specific children's dosages have not been established. PREOPERATIVE—¼ mg./lb. body weight, either *orally* 2 to 3 hours before operation, or *I.M.* 1 to 2 hours before. DURING SURGERY—*I.M.:* ⅛ mg./lb. body weight. Repeat in ½ hour if necessary and if no hypotension occurs. *I.V.:* 1 mg. per fractional injection at 2-minute intervals and not exceeding recommended I.M. dosage. Always dilute to 1 mg./ml., i.e., 1 ml. (25 mg.) mixed with 24 ml. of saline. POSTOPERATIVE—¼ mg./lb. body weight, either *orally* q4-6h, p.r.n., or *I.M.* Repeat in 1 hour if necessary and if no hypotension occurs.

Psychiatry:
Increase dosage gradually until symptoms are controlled. Maximum improvement may not be seen for weeks or even months. Continue optimum dosage for 2 weeks; then gradually reduce dosage to the lowest effective maintenance level.

Adults: OFFICE PATIENTS OR OUTPATIENTS—*Oral:* 10 mg. t.i.d. or q.i.d., or 25 mg. b.i.d. or t.i.d. MORE SEVERE CASES —*Oral:* 25 mg. t.i.d. After 1 or 2 days, daily dosage may be increased by 20-50 mg. at semiweekly intervals until patient becomes calm and cooperative. PROMPT CONTROL OF SEVERE SYMPTOMS—*I.M.:* 25 mg. (1 ml.). If necessary, repeat in 1 hour. Subsequent doses should be oral, 25-50 mg. t.i.d.
HOSPITALIZED PATIENTS: ACUTELY AGITATED, MANIC, OR DISTURBED—*I.M.:* 25 mg. (1 ml.). If necessary, give additional 25 to 50 mg. injection in 1 hour. Increase subsequent I.M. doses gradually over several days—up to 400 mg. q4-6h in exceptionally severe cases —until patient is controlled. Usually patient becomes quiet and cooperative within 24 to 48 hours and oral doses may be substituted and increased until the patient is calm. 500 mg. a day is generally sufficient. While gradual increases to 2,000 mg. a day or more may be necessary, there is usually little therapeutic gain to be achieved by exceeding 1,000 mg. a day for extended periods. In general, dosage levels should be lower in the elderly, the emaciated and the debilitated. LESS ACUTELY AGITATED PATIENTS—*Oral:* 25 mg. t.i.d. Increase gradually until effective dose is reached—usually 400 mg. daily.

Children: OFFICE PATIENTS OR OUTPATIENTS—Select route of administration according to severity of patient's condition and increase dosage gradually as required. *Oral:* ¼ mg./lb. body weight q4-6h, p.r.n. (e.g., for 40 lb. child—10 mg. q4-6h). *Rectal:* ½ mg./lb. body weight q6-8h, p.r.n. (e.g., for 20-30 lb. child —half a 25 mg. suppository q6-8h). *I.M.:* ¼ mg./lb. body weight q6-8h, p.r.n.
HOSPITALIZED PATIENTS—As with outpatients, start with low doses and increase dosage gradually. In severe behavior disorders or psychotic conditions, higher dosages (50-100 mg. daily, and in older children, 200 mg. daily or more) may be necessary. There is little evidence that behavior improvement in severely disturbed mentally retarded patients is further enhanced by doses beyond 500 mg. per day. *Maximum I.M. Dosage:* Children up to 5 years (or 50 lbs.), not over 40 mg./day; 5-12 years (or 50-100 lbs.), not over 75 mg./day except in unmanageable cases.

Important Notes on Injection: Inject slowly, deep into upper outer quadrant of buttock. Because of possible hypotensive effects, reserve parenteral administration for bedfast patients or for acute ambulatory cases, and keep patient lying down for at least ½ hour after injection. If irritation is a problem, dilute Injection with saline or 2% procaine; mixing with other agents in the syringe is not recommended. Subcutaneous injection is not advised. Avoid injecting undiluted Thorazine (chlorpromazine, SK&F) into vein. I.V. route is only for severe hiccups and surgery.
Because of the possibility of contact dermatitis, avoid getting solution on hands or clothing. Protect from light, or discoloration may occur. Slight yellowing will not alter potency. Discard if markedly discolored.

Note on Concentrate: When the Concentrate is to be used, add the desired dosage of Concentrate to 60 ml. (2 fl. oz.) or more of diluent *just prior to administration.* This will insure palatability and stability. Vehicles suggested for dilution are: tomato or fruit juice, milk, simple syrup, orange syrup, carbonated beverages, coffee, tea, or water. Semisolid foods (soups, puddings, etc.) may also be used. The Concentrate is light sensitive; it should be protected from light and dispensed in amber glass bottles. *Refrigeration is not required.*

Overdosage: (See also Adverse Reactions.)

Symptoms—Primarily symptoms of central nervous system depression to the point of somnolence or coma. Hypotension and extrapyramidal symptoms.
Other possible manifestations include agitation and restlessness, convulsions, fever, autonomic reactions such as dry mouth and ileus, EKG changes and cardiac arrhythmias.

Treatment—It is important to determine other medications taken by the patient since multiple dose therapy is common in overdosage situations. Treatment is essentially symptomatic and supportive. Early gastric lavage is helpful. Keep patient under observation and maintain an open airway, since involvement of the extrapyramidal mechanism may produce dysphagia and respiratory difficulty in severe overdosage. **Do not attempt to induce emesis because a dystonic reaction of the head or neck may develop that could result in aspiration of vomitus.** Extrapyramidal symptoms may be treated with anti-parkinsonism drugs, barbiturates, or 'Benadryl'. See prescribing information for these products. Care should be taken to avoid increasing respiratory depression.
If administration of a stimulant is desirable, amphetamine, dextroamphetamine, or caffeine with sodium benzoate is recommended. Stimulants that may cause convulsions (e.g., picrotoxin or pentylenetetrazol) should be avoided.
If hypotension occurs, the standard measures for managing circulatory shock should be initiated. If it is desirable to administer a vasoconstrictor, 'Levophed' and 'Neo-Synephrine' are most suitable. Other pressor agents, including epinephrine, are not recommended because phenothiazine derivatives may reverse the usual elevating action of these agents and cause a further lowering of blood pressure.
Limited experience indicates that phenothiazines are *not* dialyzable.
Special note on 'Spansule' capsules—Since much of the 'Spansule' capsule medication is coated for gradual release, therapy directed at reversing the effects of the ingested drug and at supporting the patient should be continued for as long as overdosage symptoms remain. Saline cathartics are useful for hastening evacuation of pellets that have not already released medication.

How Supplied: Tablets—Each tablet contains chlorpromazine hydrochloride, 10 mg., 25 mg. or 50 mg., in bottles of 100 and 1000; in Single Unit Packages of 100 (intended for institutional use only). For use in severe neuropsychiatric conditions, 100 mg. and 200 mg., in bottles of 100 and 1000; in Single Unit Packages of 100 (intended for institutional use only).

Spansule® brand of sustained release capsules—Each 'Spansule' capsule contains chlorpromazine hydrochloride, so prepared that an initial dose is released promptly and the remaining medication is released gradually over a prolonged period. Available as 30 mg., 75 mg., 150 mg. or 200 mg., in bottles of 50 and 500; in Single Unit Packages of 100 (intended for institutional use only). For use in severe neuropsychiatric conditions, 300 mg., in bottles of 50; in Single Unit Packages of 100 (intended for institutional use only).

Ampuls—1 ml. and 2 ml. (25 mg./ml.), in boxes of 10, 100 and 500. Each ml. contains, in aqueous solution, chlorpromazine hydrochloride, 25 mg.; ascorbic acid, 2 mg.; sodium bisulfite, 1 mg.; sodium sulfite, 1 mg.; sodium chloride, 6 mg.

Multiple-dose Vials—10 ml. (25 mg./ml.), in boxes of 1, 20 and 100. Each ml. contains, in aqueous solution, chlorpromazine hydrochloride, 25 mg.; ascorbic acid, 2 mg.; sodium bisulfite, 1 mg.; sodium sulfite, 1 mg.; sodium chloride, 1 mg. Contains benzyl alcohol, 2%, as a preservative.

Syrup—Each 5 ml. (one teaspoonful) contains chlorpromazine hydrochloride, 10 mg., in 4 fl. oz. bottles.

Suppositories—Each suppository contains chlorpromazine, 25 mg. or 100 mg., glycerin, glyceryl monopalmitate, glyceryl monostearate, hydrogenated cocoanut oil fatty acids, hydrogenated palm kernel oil fatty acids, in boxes of 12.

Concentrate (intended for institutional use only)—*30 mg./ml.:* Each ml. contains chlorpromazine hydrochloride, 30 mg., in 4 fl. oz. bottles, in cartons of 36 bottles, and in 1 gallon bottles. *100 mg./ml.:* Each ml. contains chlorpromazine hydrochloride, 100 mg., in 8 fl. oz. bottles, in cartons of 12.

Military—Concentrate 30 mg./ml., 4 fl. oz., 6505-00-660-1664; Injection 2 ml., 6's, 6505-00-597-5843; Tablets 25 mg., S.U.P. 100's, 6505-00-118-2529, and 1000's, 6505-00-022-1326; Tablets 50 mg., S.U.P. 100's, 6505-00-132-0371, and 1000's, 6505-00-022-1327; Tablets 100 mg., S.U.P. 100's, 6505-00-132-0372, and 1000's, 6505-00-935-9820.

---

*Trademark Reg. U.S. Pat. Off.: 'Dilantin' for diphenylhydantoin, Parke-Davis.
†Trademark Reg. U.S. Pat. Off.: 'Amipaque' for metrizamide, Winthrop Laboratories.
‡'Levophed' and 'Neo-Synephrine' are the trademarks (Reg. U.S. Pat. Off.) of Winthrop Laboratories for its brands of levarterenol and phenylephrine respectively.
§Trademark Reg. U.S. Pat. Off.: 'Benadryl' for diphenhydramine hydrochloride, Parke-Davis.

[*Shown in Product Identification Section*]

TROPH-IRON®
Vitamins B_1, B_{12} and Iron

Marketed by Menley & James Laboratories, a SmithKline company.
(See PDR For Nonprescription Drugs)

TROPHITE®
Vitamins B_1 and B_{12}

Marketed by Menley & James Laboratories, a SmithKline company.
(See PDR For Nonprescription Drugs)

Modified Formula
TUSS-ORNADE® ℞
LIQUID

Description: Each 5 ml. (1 teaspoonful) of 'Tuss-Ornade' Liquid contains caramiphen edisylate, 6.7 mg.; phenylpropanolamine hy-

drochloride, 12.5 mg.; and alcohol, 5.0%, in a preparation that contains no sugar or dyes.
(**Note:** The concentrations of the antitussive and decongestant components have been adjusted so that on the new recommended daily dosage schedule of q4h—contrasted to q6h for the original formula—the usual adult daily dose now is 40 mg. of caramiphen edisylate and 75 mg. of phenylpropanolamine HCl, compared to 20 mg. of caramiphen edisylate and 60 mg. of phenylpropanolamine HCl for the original formula. The antihistamine and anticholinergic ingredients have been removed, and the alcohol content reduced.)

Actions: The 'Tuss-Ornade' formula contains caramiphen edisylate, a synthetic, nonnarcotic cough suppressant, and phenylpropanolamine hydrochloride, a vasoconstrictor with decongestant action on nasal and upper respiratory tract mucosal membranes.

> **Indications:**
> For the symptomatic relief of coughs and nasal congestion associated with common colds.
> N.B.: A final determination has not been made on the effectiveness of this drug combination in accordance with efficacy requirements of the 1962 Amendments to the Food, Drug and Cosmetic Act.

Contraindications: Hypersensitivity to either of the components; concurrent MAO inhibitor therapy; severe hypertension; bronchial asthma; coronary artery disease.
Do not use 'Tuss-Ornade' Liquid in children under 15 pounds or in children less than six months of age.

Warnings: Caution patients about activities requiring alertness (e.g., operating vehicles or machinery). Patients should also be warned about the possible additive effects of alcohol and other CNS depressants.

Precautions: Use with caution in persons with cardiovascular disease, glaucoma, prostatic hypertrophy, thyroid disease or diabetes. Use with caution in patients in whom productive cough is desirable to clear excessive secretions from the bronchial tree. Patients taking this medication should be cautioned not to take simultaneously other products containing phenylpropanolamine HCl or amphetamines.

Usage in Pregnancy: Safe use in pregnancy has not been established. This drug should not be used in pregnancy, nursing mothers, or women of childbearing potential unless, in the judgment of the physician, the anticipated benefits outweigh the potential risks.

Adverse Reactions: Adverse effects associated with products containing a centrally acting antitussive or sympathomimetic amine may occur and include: nausea, gastrointestinal upset, diarrhea, constipation, dizziness, drowsiness, nervousness, insomnia, anorexia, weakness, tightness of chest, angina pain, irritability, palpitations, headache, incoordination, tremor, difficulty in urination, dysuria, hypertension, hypotension, visual disturbances.

Dosage and Administration: Adults and children over 12 years—2 teaspoonfuls every 4 hours; do not exceed 12 teaspoonfuls in 24 hours. Children 6 to 12 years—1 teaspoonful every 4 hours; do not exceed 6 teaspoonfuls in 24 hours. Children 2 to 6 years—½ teaspoonful every 4 hours; do not exceed 3 teaspoonfuls in 24 hours. Data are not available on which to base dosage recommendations for children under 2 years of age. **Do not use in children under 15 pounds or less than 6 months old.**

Overdosage: Symptoms—May include dryness of mouth, dysphagia, thirst, blurred vision, dilated pupils, photophobia, fever, rapid pulse and respiration, disorientation, dizziness, nausea, fainting, tachycardia, and either excitation or depression of the central nervous system.
Treatment—Immediate evacuation of the stomach should be induced by emesis and gastric lavage, repeated as necessary.
Respiratory depression should be treated promptly with oxygen and respiratory stimulants. Do not treat respiratory or CNS depression with analeptics that might precipitate convulsions. If marked excitement occurs, a short-acting barbiturate or chloral hydrate may be used.

Supplied: 'Tuss-Ornade' Liquid is supplied as a fruit flavored liquid, in 16 fl. oz. bottles.

TUSS-ORNADE® SPANSULE® CAPSULES ℞

Description: Each 'Tuss-Ornade' *Spansule* capsule contains 40 mg. of caramiphen edisylate and 75 mg. of phenylpropanolamine hydrochloride, so prepared that an initial dose is released promptly and the remaining medication is released gradually over a prolonged period.

Actions: The 'Tuss-Ornade' formula contains caramiphen edisylate, a synthetic, nonnarcotic cough suppressant, and phenylpropanolamine hydrochloride, a vasoconstrictor with decongestant action on nasal and upper respiratory tract mucosal membranes.

Pharmacokinetics: At steady-state conditions, the following peak levels are reached after the oral administration of a 'Spansule' capsule: 24 ng./ml. caramiphen in 4.6 hours; 200 ng./ml. phenylpropanolamine in 5.5 hours; the half-lives are approximately 11 and 8 hours, respectively.

> **Indications:**
> For the symptomatic relief of coughs and nasal congestion associated with common colds.
> N.B.: A final determination has not been made on the effectiveness of this drug combination in accordance with efficacy requirements of the 1962 Amendments to the Food, Drug and Cosmetic Act.

Contraindications: Hypersensitivity to either of the components; concurrent MAO inhibitor therapy; severe hypertension; bronchial asthma; coronary artery disease.
Do not use 'Tuss-Ornade' *Spansule* capsules in children under 12 years of age.

Warnings: Caution patients about activities requiring alertness (e.g., operating vehicles or machinery). Patients should also be warned about the possible additive effects of alcohol and other CNS depressants.

Precautions: Use with caution in persons with cardiovascular disease, glaucoma, prostatic hypertrophy, thyroid disease or diabetes. Use with caution in patients in whom productive cough is desirable to clear excessive secretions from the bronchial tree. Patients taking this medication should be cautioned not to take simultaneously other products containing phenylpropanolamine HCl or amphetamines.

Usage in Pregnancy: Safe use in pregnancy has not been established. This drug should not be used in pregnancy, nursing mothers, or women of childbearing potential unless, in the judgment of the physician, the anticipated benefits outweigh the potential risks.

Adverse Reactions: Adverse effects associated with products containing a centrally acting antitussive or sympathomimetic amine may occur and include: nausea, gastrointestinal upset, diarrhea, constipation, dizziness, drowsiness, nervousness, insomnia, anorexia, weakness, tightness of chest, angina pain, irritability, palpitation, headache, incoordination, tremor, difficulty in urination, dysuria, hypertension, hypotension, visual disturbances.

Dosage and Administration: 'Tuss-Ornade' *Spansule* capsules: Adults and children over 12 years of age—one 'Tuss-Ornade' *Spansule* capsule every 12 hours. **Do not use in children under 12 years of age.**

Overdosage: Symptoms—May include dryness of mouth, dysphagia, thirst, blurred vision, dilated pupils, photophobia, fever, rapid pulse and respiration, disorientation, dizziness, nausea, fainting, tachycardia, and either excitation or depression of the central nervous system.
Treatment—Immediate evacuation of the stomach should be induced by emesis and gastric lavage, repeated as necessary.
Respiratory depression should be treated promptly with oxygen and respiratory stimulants. Do not treat respiratory or CNS depression with analeptics that might precipitate convulsions. If marked excitement occurs, a short-acting barbiturate or chloral hydrate may be used.
Since much of the 'Spansule' capsule medication is coated for gradual release, saline cathartics should be administered to hasten evacuation of pellets that have not already released medication.

Supplied: 'Tuss-Ornade' *Spansule* capsules: in bottles of 50 and 500 capsules.
[*Shown in Product Identification Section*]

URISPAS® ℞
(brand of flavoxate HCl)
100 mg. tablets
Urinary tract spasmolytic

Description: Urispas (brand of flavoxate HCl) is a synthetic antispasmodic offered specifically for the relief of symptoms associated with various urologic disorders. 'Urispas' exerts its effect directly on the muscle.
Chemically, flavoxate hydrochloride is 2-piperidinoethyl 3-methyl-4-oxo-2-phenyl-4*H*-1-benzopyran-8-carboxylate hydrochloride. The empirical formula of flavoxate hydrochloride is $C_{24}H_{25}NO_4 \bullet HCl$.

Action: Flavoxate hydrochloride counteracts smooth muscle spasm of the urinary tract.

Indications: Urispas (brand of flavoxate HCl) is indicated for symptomatic relief of dysuria, urgency, nocturia, suprapubic pain, frequency and incontinence as may occur in cystitis, prostatitis, urethritis, urethrocystitis/urethrotrigonitis. 'Urispas' is not indicated for definitive treatment, but is compatible with drugs used for the treatment of urinary tract infections.

Contraindications: Urispas (brand of flavoxate HCl) is contraindicated in patients who have any of the following obstructive conditions: pyloric or duodenal obstruction, obstructive intestinal lesions or ileus, achalasia, gastrointestinal hemorrhage, and obstructive uropathies of the lower urinary tract.

Warnings: Urispas (brand of flavoxate HCl) should be given cautiously in patients with suspected glaucoma.

Usage in Pregnancy—Safety in women who are or may become pregnant has not been established. Therefore, Urispas (brand of flavoxate HCl) should not be given except when the expected benefits outweigh the possible hazards.

Usage in Children—This drug cannot be recommended for infants and children under 12 years of age because safety and efficacy have not been demonstrated in this age group.

Precautions: In the event of drowsiness and blurred vision, the patient should not operate a motor vehicle or machinery or participate in activities where alertness is required.

Adverse Reactions: Adverse reactions reported include nausea and vomiting, dry mouth, nervousness, vertigo, headache, drowsiness, blurred vision, increased ocular tension, disturbance in eye accommodation, urticaria and other dermatoses, mental confusion especially in the elderly patient, dysuria, tachycardia and palpitation, hyperpyrexia, eosino-

Continued on next page

Smith Kline & French—Cont.

philia and leukopenia (1 case which was reversible upon discontinuation of the drug).
Dosage and Administration: Adults and children over twelve years of age: one or two 100 mg. tablets three or four times a day. With improvement of symptoms, the dose may be reduced. This drug cannot be recommended for infants and children under 12 years of age because safety and efficacy have not been demonstrated in this age group.
How Supplied: 100 mg. tablets, in bottles of 100; in Single Unit Packages of 100 (intended for institutional use only).
Military—Tablets, 100 mg., 100's, 6505-00-172-3420.

[*Shown in Product Identification Section*]

VONTROL® ℞
(brand of diphenidol)

'Vontrol' may cause hallucinations, disorientation, or confusion. For this reason, its use is limited to patients who are hospitalized or under comparable, continuous, close, professional supervision. Even then, the physician should carefully weigh the benefits against the possible risks and give due consideration to alternate therapeutic measures.
Description: 'Vontrol', α, α-diphenyl-1-piperidinebutanol, is a compound not related to the antihistamines, phenothiazines, barbiturates, or other agents with antivertigo or antiemetic action.
Actions: 'Vontrol' (diphenidol, SK&F) apparently exerts a specific antivertigo effect on the vestibular apparatus to control vertigo and inhibits the chemoreceptor trigger zone to control nausea and vomiting.
Indications (See Warnings):
1) VERTIGO—'Vontrol' is indicated in peripheral (labyrinthine) vertigo and associated nausea and vomiting, as seen in such conditions as: Meniere's disease, middle- and inner-ear surgery (labyrinthitis).
2) NAUSEA AND VOMITING—'Vontrol' is indicated in the control of nausea and vomiting, as seen in such conditions as: postoperative states, malignant neoplasms and labyrinthine disturbances.

Contraindications: Known hypersensitivity to the drug is a contraindication. Anuria is a contraindication. (Since approximately 90% of the drug is excreted in the urine, renal shutdown could cause systemic accumulation.)
Warnings: 'Vontrol' (diphenidol, SK&F) may cause hallucinations, disorientation or confusion. For this reason, its use is limited to patients who are hospitalized or under comparable, continuous, close, professional supervision. Even then, the physician should carefully weigh the benefits against the possible risks and give due consideration to alternate therapeutic measures.
The incidence of auditory and visual hallucinations, disorientation and confusion appears to be less than ½% or approximately one in 350 patients. The reaction has usually occurred within three days of starting the drug in recommended dosage and has subsided spontaneously usually within three days after discontinuation of the drug. Patients on 'Vontrol' should be observed closely and in the event of such a reaction the drug should be stopped.
Usage in Pregnancy: Use of any drug in pregnancy, lactation or in women of childbearing age requires that the potential benefits of the drug be weighed against its possible hazards to the mother and child.
In animal teratogenesis and reproduction studies of 'Vontrol' (diphenidol, SK&F), there were no significant differences between drug-treated groups and untreated control groups, except as noted under animal Reproduction Studies (see "Pharmacology [animal]").
In 936 patients who received 'Vontrol' during pregnancy, the incidences of normal and abnormal birth were comparable to those reported in the literature for the average population of pregnant patients. And in no instance was there any evidence that 'Vontrol' played a part in birth abnormality (see "In Pregnancy").
'Vontrol' is not indicated for use in nausea and vomiting of pregnancy, since the therapeutic value and safety in this indication have not yet been determined.
Precautions: The antiemetic action of 'Vontrol' (diphenidol, SK&F) may mask signs of overdose of drugs (e.g., digitalis) or may obscure diagnosis of conditions such as intestinal obstruction and brain tumor.
Although there have been no reports of blood dyscrasias with 'Vontrol', patients should be observed regularly for any idiosyncratic reactions.
'Vontrol' has a weak peripheral anticholinergic effect and should be used with care in patients with glaucoma, obstructive lesions of the gastrointestinal and genitourinary tracts, such as stenosing peptic ulcer, prostatic hypertrophy, pyloric and duodenal obstruction, and organic cardiospasm.
Intravenous administration to persons with a history of sinus tachycardia may be undesirable because this procedure may initiate an episode in such patients.
Several patients were reported to have had a transient decrease in systolic and diastolic blood pressure, up to 20 mm. Hg., following parenteral use of 'Vontrol'.
'Vontrol' Tablets contain FD&C Yellow #5 (tartrazine) which may cause allergic-type reactions (including bronchial asthma) in certain susceptible individuals. Although the overall incidence of FD&C Yellow #5 (tartrazine) sensitivity in the general population is low, it is frequently seen in patients who also have aspirin hypersensitivity.
Adverse Reactions: Auditory and visual hallucinations, disorientation and confusion have been reported. Drowsiness, overstimulation, depression, sleep disturbance, dry mouth, g.i. irritation (nausea and indigestion), or blurred vision may occur.
Rarely, slight dizziness, skin rash, malaise, headache, or heartburn may occur. Mild jaundice of questionable relationship to the use of 'Vontrol' (diphenidol, SK&F) has been reported. Slight, transient lowering of blood pressure has been reported in a few patients.
(See laboratory studies under "Pharmacology [human]".)
Dosage and Administration (See Warnings)
Adults—for Vertigo or Nausea and Vomiting: The usual dose is one tablet (25 mg.) every four hours as needed. Some patients may require two tablets (50 mg.).
Children—for Nausea and Vomiting: These recommendations are for nausea and vomiting only. There has been no experience with 'Vontrol' in vertigo in children.
Unit doses in children are best calculated by body weight: usually 0.4 mg./lb.
Children's doses usually should not be given more often than every four hours. However, if symptoms persist after the first dose, administration may be repeated after one hour. Thereafter, doses may be given every four hours as needed.
The total dose in 24 hours should not exceed 2.5 mg./lb.
NOTE: The drug is not recommended for use in infants under six months or 25 pounds. The dosage for children 50 to 100 pounds is one tablet (25 mg.).
Overdosage: In the event of overdosage, the patient should be managed according to his symptoms. Treatment is essentially supportive, with maintenance of blood pressure and respiration, plus careful observation. Early gastric lavage may be indicated depending on the amount of overdose and nature of symptoms.
How Supplied: Bottles of 100—Each tablet contains 25 mg. diphenidol as the hydrochloride.
Pharmacology (animal): 'Vontrol' (diphenidol, SK&F) exerts its antiemetic effect primarily by inhibiting the chemoreceptor trigger zone, as evidenced by its activity in blocking emesis induced by apomorphine in dogs. In this regard 'Vontrol', as the hydrochloride salt, has a potency equal to the potent phenothiazine antiemetic, chlorpromazine hydrochloride. In animals 'Vontrol' has only weak parasympatholytic activity and no significant sedative, tranquilizing or antihistaminic action or effects on blood pressure, heart rate, respiration or the electrocardiogram.
Subacute and chronic toxicity studies in rats and dogs, in which large doses of 'Vontrol', as the hydrochloride salt, were administered orally and intramuscularly for periods up to one year, revealed no significant effects on hematology, liver function, kidney function or blood glucose determinations. Histological examination of the animals' tissues did not reveal any significant lesions attributable to administration of 'Vontrol'.
Reproduction Studies: Teratogenesis and reproduction studies were carried out in rats and rabbits. In rats, 'Vontrol' (diphenidol, SK&F), as the hydrochloride salt, was fed daily to male and female animals in doses of 20 mg./kg. and 40 mg./kg. (approximately three and six times the maximum recommended daily dose in adult humans) for 60 days before mating, and during mating, gestation and lactation for each of two litters. There were no significant differences between drug-treated and untreated control groups with regard to conception rate, litter size, live birth or viability in either of the two litters. There was no congenital anomaly among the offspring. In rabbits, 'Vontrol', as the hydrochloride salt, was fed in the diets in doses of 5 mg./kg. or 75 mg./kg. (approximately equal to, and 12 times as much as, the maximum recommended daily dose in adult humans) from the first day of gestation through the 26th or 27th day of gestation, when the young were delivered by Cesarean section. There were no significant differences between drug-treated and control groups with regard to number and weight of fetuses, numbers of resorption sites or viable fetuses. There was also no statistically significant difference between drug-treated and control groups with regard to the total percentage of underdeveloped fetuses. However, when data were calculated on the basis of a ratio between underdeveloped fetuses and number of pregnant does, an adverse dose-related effect was observed in the high-dose test group.
Pharmacology (human): Three double-blind controlled studies comparing 'Vontrol' (diphenidol, SK&F) to placebo were carried out: one in 32 male volunteers over a four-week period; one in 45 volunteers of whom 15 were studied for 12 weeks and 17 for 24 weeks; and one in 48 volunteers of whom 36 were studied for 12 weeks.
In the first study 'Vontrol', as the hydrochloride salt, was given orally in daily doses that were started at 75 mg. during the first week and graduated up to 200 mg. by the fourth week. In the second study, one group received 'Vontrol' orally, as the hydrochloride salt, titrated up to 500 mg. daily, then down to 200 mg. daily; another group received a maximum of 200 mg. daily. In the third study, patients received oral doses of 200 mg. to 300 mg. of 'Vontrol' daily, as the hydrochloride or pamoate salts.
The studies included these laboratory determinations: complete blood counts (including hemoglobin and hematocrit determinations), urinalyses (including microscopic examination), serum alkaline phosphatase, serum bilirubin, and bromsulphalein retention. The

studies also included records of weight and blood pressure and, in one, electrocardiograms. In two of these studies, clinical laboratory changes were seen among volunteers in both treated and control groups. The changes included: extrasystoles, white cells in the urine, increase in prothrombin time, rise in hematocrit, rise in leucocytes, rise in eosinophils, and rise or reduction in neutrophils. At no time in any study did changes in the treated group differ significantly from those in the control group.
'Vontrol', as the hydrochloride salt, was given orally to 17 children (aged five to 15). Total daily doses ranged from 90 to 240 mg. Complete blood counts and, in some patients, urinalyses were done before treatment and after approximately four days of treatment. There was no significant difference between pre- and post-treatment laboratory determinations in any child. No side effects were seen.
Excretion: Following oral administration of 'Vontrol' (diphenidol, SK&F) to dogs, as the hydrochloride or pamoate salts, and to humans, as the hydrochloride salt, peak blood concentration of the drug generally occurs in one and a half to three hours. In dogs and rats, virtually all of an oral dose of C^{14}-labeled 'Vontrol' is excreted in the urine and feces within three to four days, as determined by radioactivity counts. Approximately the same percentage of an administered dose appeared in the urine of dogs following either oral administration of the hydrochloride salt or rectal administration of the free base.
In Pregnancy: Investigators kept follow-up records on 936 patients who had received 'Vontrol' (diphenidol, SK&F) at some time during pregnancy, primarily during the first trimester.
Of the 936 women, 864 (92%) had normal births of normal infants.
Seventy-two (8%) of the women experienced some birth abnormality. Of the 72, six patients had premature but otherwise normal infants, 40 patients aborted, 10 had stillbirths, and 16 had infants with miscellaneous defects. These included hernias, congenital heart defects, hydrocephalus, internal strabismus, anencephalus, enlarged thyroid, and hypospadia. These incidences of abnormal birth are lower than those generally reported in the literature for the average population of pregnant patients. And in no instance was there any evidence that the administration of 'Vontrol' played a part in birth abnormality.
[Shown in Product Identification Section]

Springbok Pharmaceuticals, Inc.
12502 SOUTH GARDEN STREET
HOUSTON, TX 77071

E.N.T. Syrup ℞
Sugar-free decongestant

Each 5 ml. (one teaspoonful) orange-colored syrup contains:
Brompheniramine maleate .... 4 mg.
Phenylephrine hydrochloride .... 5 mg.
Phenylpropanolamine hydrochloride . 5 mg.
Alcohol .... 2.3 %
How Supplied:
Bottles of 16 fluid ounces NDC 50821-376-16
Bottles of one gallon NDC 50821-376-28

E.N.T. Tablets ℞
Adult dose decongestant

Each prolonged-action, scored tablet contains:
Phenylephrine hydrochloride ....25 mg.
Phenylpropanolamine hydrochloride ...50 mg.
Chlorpheniramine maleate ....8 mg.
How Supplied:
Bottles of 100 tablets NDC 50821-378-01
Bottles of 500 tablets NDC 50821-378-05

STOPAYNE Capsules ℞ Ⓒ
Analgesic

Each blue/white capsule imprinted STOPAYNE/819 contains:
Codeine phosphate ....30 mg.
(Warning: May be habit-forming)
Promethazine hydrochloride ....6.25 mg.
Acetaminophen ....357 mg.
How Supplied:
Bottles of 100 capsules NDC 50821-819-01
Bottles of 500 capsules NDC 50821-819-05
U/D Packs of 100 capsules NDC 50821-819-03

STOPAYNE Syrup ℞ Ⓒ
Analgesic, antipyretic

Each 5 ml. (one teaspoonful) red-colored syrup contains:
Acetaminophen ....120 mg.
Promethazine hydrochloride ....6.25 mg.
Codeine phosphate ....5 mg.
(Warning: May be habit-forming)
Alcohol 10%
How Supplied:
Bottles of 4 fluid ounces NDC 50821-820-04
Bottles of 16 fluid ounces NDC 50821-820-16

E. R. Squibb & Sons, Inc.
GENERAL OFFICES
P.O. BOX 4000
PRINCETON, NJ 08540

UNILOG®
(Tablet and Capsule Identification Code)
NUMERICAL INDEX

Unilog Number **Product**

F16 Principen with Probenecid
(Ampicillin-Probenecid Capsules)
113 Velosef '250' Capsules
(Cephradine Capsules USP) 250 mg.
114 Velosef '500' Capsules
(Cephradine Capsules USP) 500 mg.
147 Velosef Tablets
(Cephradine Tablets) 1 g.
160 Ethril '250'
(Erythromycin Stearate Tablets USP) 250 mg.
161 Ethril '500'
(Erythromycin Stearate Tablets USP) 500 mg.
164 Pentids Tablets
(Penicillin G Potassium Tablets USP) 200,000 u.
165 Pentids '400' Tablets
(Penicillin G Potassium Tablets USP) 400,000 u.
168 Pentids '800' Tablets
(Penicillin G Potassium Tablets USP) 800,000 u.
194 Vitamin C Tablets 100 mg.
196 Vitamin C Tablets 250 mg.
197 Vitamin C Tablets 500 mg.
201 Aspirin Tablets USP, 324 mg. (5 gr.)
207 Corgard (Nadolol Tablets) 40 mg.
208 Corgard (Nadolol Tablets) 120 mg.
230 Trimox '250' Capsules
(Amoxicillin Capsules USP) 250 mg.
231 Trimox '500' Capsules
(Amoxicillin Capsules USP) 500 mg.
241 Corgard (Nadolol Tablets) 80 mg.
246 Corgard (Nadolol Tablets) 160 mg.
341 Theragran-Z Tablets
355 Valadol Tablets
(Acetaminophen Tablets USP) 325 mg. (5 gr.)
429 Florinef Acetate
(Fludrocortisone Acetate Tablets USP) 0.1 mg.
431 Pronestyl Tablets
(Procainamide Hydrochloride Tablets) 250 mg.
434 Pronestyl Tablets
(Procainamide Hydrochloride Tablets) 375 mg.
438 Pronestyl Tablets
(Procainamide Hydrochloride Tablets) 500 mg.
452 Capoten (Captopril Tablets) 25 mg.
455 Oragrafin Sodium Capsules
(Ipodate Sodium Capsules USP) 500 mg.
457 Mycostatin Vaginal Tablets
(Nystatin Vaginal Tablets USP) 100,000 u.
478 Engran-HP Tablets
(Multi-Vitamin and Multi-Mineral Supplement)
482 Capoten (Captopril Tablets) 50 mg.
485 Capoten (Captopril Tablets) 100 mg.
504 Kenacort
(Triamcinolone Tablets USP) 2 mg.
512 Kenacort
(Triamcinolone Tablets USP) 4 mg.
518 Kenacort
(Triamcinolone Tablets USP) 8 mg.
535 Theragran Hematinic
(Therapeutic Formula Vitamin Tablets with Hematinics)
537 Niacin Tablets NF, 500 mg.
549 Iron and Vitamin C Tablets
573 Ora-Testryl
(Fluoxymesterone Tablets USP) 5 mg.
580 Mycostatin Oral Tablets
(Nystatin Tablets USP) 500,000 u.
598 Neomycin Sulfate Tablets USP, 500 mg.
603 Sumycin '500' Tablets
(Tetracycline Hydrochloride Tablets USP) 500 mg.
605 Naturetin-2.5
(Bendroflumethiazide Tablets USP) 2.5 mg.
606 Naturetin-5
(Bendroflumethiazide Tablets USP) 5 mg.
610 Niacin Tablets NF, 25 mg.
611 Niacin Tablets NF, 50 mg.
612 Niacin Tablets NF, 100 mg.
615 Propoxyphene Hydrochloride Capsules USP, 65 mg.
618 Naturetin-10
(Bendroflumethiazide Tablets USP) 10 mg.
619 Propoxyphene Hydrochloride and APC Capsules USP
623 Noctec Capsules
(Chloral Hydrate Capsules USP) 250 mg. (3¾ grains)
626 Noctec Capsules
(Chloral Hydrate Capsules USP) 500 mg. (7½ grains)
637 Nydrazid Tablets
(Isoniazid Tablets USP) 100 mg.
648 Veetids '500' Tablets
(Penicillin V Potassium Tablets USP) 500 mg. (800,000 u.)
649 Trigot
(Ergoloid Mesylates Tablets) 0.5 mg.
654 Trigot
(Ergoloid Mesylates Tablets) 1 mg.
655 Sumycin '250' Capsules
(Tetracycline Hydrochloride Capsules USP) 250 mg.
663 Sumycin '250' Tablets
(Tetracycline Hydrochloride Tablets USP) 250 mg.
684 Veetids '250' Tablets
(Penicillin V Potassium Tablets USP) 250 mg. (400,000 u.)
690 Teslac Tablets
(Testolactone Tablets USP) 50 mg.
692 Tolbutamide Tablets USP, 500 mg.
694 Hydrochlorothiazide Tablets USP, 50 mg.

Continued on next page

Squibb—Cont.

713 Raudixin
(Rauwolfia Serpentina Tablets USP) 50 mg.
718 Chlordiazepoxide Hydrochloride Capsules USP, 5 mg.
727 Chlordiazepoxide Hydrochloride Capsules USP, 10 mg.
736 Chlordiazepoxide Hydrochloride Capsules USP, 25 mg.
756 Pronestyl Capsules
(Procainamide Hydrochloride Capsules USP) 375 mg.
757 Pronestyl Capsules
(Procainamide Hydrochloride Capsules USP) 500 mg.
758 Pronestyl Capsules
(Procainamide Hydrochloride Capsules USP) 250 mg.
763 Sumycin '500' Capsules
(Tetracycline Hydrochloride Capsules USP) 500 mg.
769 Rauzide Tablets
(50 mg. powdered Rauwolfia serpentina with 4 mg. bendroflumethiazide)
775 Pronestyl-SR Tablets
(Procainamide Hydrochloride Tablets) 500 mg.
776 Raudixin
(Rauwolfia Serpentina Tablets USP) 100 mg.
779 Mysteclin-F Capsules
(Tetracycline - Amphotericin B Capsules) 250 mg. c̄ 50 mg.
780 Rau-Sed
(Reserpine Tablets USP) 0.25 mg.
788 Vitamin B_{12} Capsules 25 mcg.
823 Theragran Tablets
825 Theragran-M Tablets
829 Chlorothiazide Tablets USP, 500 mg.
830 Hydrea Capsules
(Hydroxyurea Capsules USP) 500 mg.
863 Prolixin Tablets
(Fluphenazine Hydrochloride Tablets USP) 1 mg.
864 Prolixin Tablets
(Fluphenazine Hydrochloride Tablets USP) 2.5 mg.
876 Trigesic Tablets
(Analgesic Compound)
877 Prolixin Tablets
(Fluphenazine Hydrochloride Tablets USP) 5 mg.
887 Terfonyl Tablets
(Trisulfapyrimidines Tablets USP) 500 mg.
889 Vitamin E Capsules 100 I.U.
915 Vitamin B_1 Tablets 50 mg.
916 Vitamin B_1 Tablets 100 mg.
917 Amitid Tablets
(Amitriptyline Hydrochloride Tablets USP) 10 mg.
918 Amitid Tablets
(Amitriptyline Hydrochloride Tablets USP) 25 mg.
921 Vesprin Tablets
(Triflupromazine Hydrochloride Tablets USP) 10 mg.
922 Vesprin Tablets
(Triflupromazine Hydrochloride Tablets USP) 25 mg.
923 Vesprin Tablets
(Triflupromazine Hydrochloride Tablets USP) 50 mg.
942 Amitid Tablets
(Amitriptyline Hydrochloride Tablets USP) 50 mg.
943 Amitid Tablets
(Amitriptyline Hydrochloride Tablets USP) 75 mg.
955 Amitid Tablets
(Amitriptyline Hydrochloride Tablets USP) 100 mg.
956 Prolixin Tablets
(Fluphenazine Hydrochloride Tablets USP) 10 mg.
971 Principen '250' Capsules
(Ampicillin Capsules USP) 250 mg.
974 Principen '500' Capsules
(Ampicillin Capsules USP) 500 mg.

CAPOTEN® TABLETS ℞
(Captopril Tablets)

Description: CAPOTEN (captopril) is the first of a new class of antihypertensive agents, a specific competitive inhibitor of angiotensin I-converting enzyme (ACE), the enzyme responsible for the conversion of angiotensin I to angiotensin II.
CAPOTEN (captopril) is designated chemically as 1-[(2S)-3-mercapto-2-methylpropionyl]-L-proline [MW 217.29].
Captopril is a white to off-white crystalline powder with a slight acid-sulfhydryl odor; it is soluble in water (approx. 50 mg./ml.), methanol, and ethanol and sparingly soluble in chloroform and ethyl acetate.
CAPOTEN (captopril tablets) is available as scored tablets for oral administration.

Clinical Pharmacology

Mechanism of Action: The mechanism of action of captopril has not yet been fully elucidated. It appears to lower blood pressure primarily through suppression of the renin-angiotensin-aldosterone system, yet it is antihypertensive even in low-renin hypertension. Renin, an enzyme synthesized by the kidneys, is released into the circulation where it acts on a plasma globulin substrate to produce angiotensin I, a relatively inactive decapeptide. Angiotensin I is then converted by angiotensin-converting enzyme (ACE) to angiotensin II, a potent endogenous vasoconstrictor substance. Angiotensin II also stimulates aldosterone secretion from the adrenal cortex, thereby contributing to sodium and fluid retention.
CAPOTEN (captopril) prevents the conversion of angiotensin I to angiotensin II by inhibition of ACE, a peptidyldipeptide carboxy hydrolase. This inhibition has been demonstrated in both healthy human subjects and in animals by showing that the elevation of blood pressure caused by exogenously administered angiotensin I was attenuated or abolished by captopril. In animal studies, captopril did not alter the pressor responses to a number of other agents, including angiotensin II and norepinephrine, indicating specificity of action.
ACE is identical to "bradykininase," and captopril may also interfere with the degradation of the vasodepressor peptide, bradykinin. However, the effectiveness of captopril in therapeutic doses appears to be unrelated to potentiation of the actions of bradykinin.
Inhibition of ACE results in decreased plasma angiotensin II and increased plasma renin activity (PRA), the latter resulting from loss of negative feedback on renin release caused by reduction in angiotensin II. The reduction of angiotensin II leads to decreased aldosterone secretion, and, as a result, to small increases in serum potassium.
The antihypertensive effects persist for a longer period of time than does demonstrable inhibition of circulating ACE. It is not known whether the ACE present in vascular endothelium is inhibited longer than the ACE in circulating blood.

Pharmacokinetics: After oral administration of therapeutic doses of CAPOTEN (captopril tablets), rapid absorption occurs with peak blood levels at about one hour. The presence of food in the gastrointestinal tract reduces absorption by about 30 to 40 percent; captopril therefore should be given one hour before meals. Based on carbon-14 labeling, average minimal absorption is approximately 75 percent. In a 24-hour period, over 95 percent of the absorbed dose is eliminated in the urine; 40 to 50 percent is unchanged drug; most of the remainder is the disulfide dimer of captopril and captopril-cysteine disulfide.
Approximately 25 to 30 percent of the circulating drug is bound to plasma proteins. The apparent elimination half-life for total radioactivity in blood is probably less than 3 hours. An accurate determination of half-life of unchanged captopril is not, at present, possible, but it is probably less than 2 hours.
In patients with normal renal function, absorption and disposition of a labeled dose are not altered after seven days of captopril administration. In patients with renal impairment, however, retention of captopril occurs (see DOSAGE AND ADMINISTRATION).

Pharmacodynamics: Administration of CAPOTEN (captopril tablets) results in a reduction of peripheral arterial resistance in hypertensive patients with either no change, or an increase, in cardiac output. There is an increase in renal blood flow following administration of CAPOTEN (captopril tablets) and glomerular filtration rate is usually unchanged. In patients with heart failure, decreased peripheral resistance, reduced pulmonary capillary wedge pressure, and increased cardiac output have been observed.
Reductions of blood pressure are often maximal 60 to 90 minutes after oral administration of an individual dose of CAPOTEN (captopril tablets). The duration of effect appears to be dose related. The reduction in blood pressure may be progressive, so to achieve maximal therapeutic effects, several weeks of therapy may be required. The blood pressure lowering effects of captopril and thiazide-type diuretics appear to be additive. In contrast, captopril and beta-blockers have a less than additive effect.
Blood pressure is lowered to about the same extent in both standing and supine positions. Orthostatic effects and tachycardia are infrequent but may occur in volume-depleted patients. Abrupt withdrawal of CAPOTEN (captopril tablets) has not been associated with a rapid increase in blood pressure.
Studies in rats and cats indicate that CAPOTEN (captopril) does not cross the blood-brain barrier to any significant extent.

Indications and Usage: Because serious adverse effects have been reported (see WARNINGS), CAPOTEN (captopril tablets) is indicated for treatment of hypertensive patients who on multidrug regimens have either failed to respond satisfactorily or developed unacceptable side effects.
Usually, multidrug regimens include combinations of a diuretic, a sympathetic nervous system-active agent (such as a beta-blocker) and a vasodilator.
CAPOTEN (captopril tablets) is effective alone, but in the population described above, it should usually be used in combination with a thiazide-type diuretic. The blood pressure lowering effects of captopril and thiazides appear to be additive.

Warnings

Proteinuria: Total urinary proteins greater than 1 g per day were seen in 1.2 percent of patients receiving captopril and the nephrotic syndrome occurred in about one-fourth of these cases. The existence of prior renal disease increased the likelihood of the development of proteinuria. About 60 percent of affected patients had evidence of prior renal disease; the remainder had no known renal dysfunction. In most cases, proteinuria subsided or cleared within six months whether or not captopril was continued, but some patients had persistent proteinuria. Parameters of renal function, such as BUN and creatinine, were seldom altered in the patients with proteinuria.
Membranous glomerulopathy was found in nearly all of the proteinuric patients receiving captopril who were biopsied, and may be drug related. This is uncertain, however, since patients were not biopsied prior to treatment and

membranous glomerulopathy may be associated with hypertension in the absence of captopril treatment.

Since most cases of proteinuria occurred by the eighth month of therapy with captopril, patients receiving captopril should have urinary protein estimates (dip-stick on first morning urine, or quantitative 24-hour urine) prior to therapy, at approximately monthly intervals for the first nine months of treatment, and periodically thereafter. When proteinuria is persistent and/or at low levels, 24-hour quantitative determinations provide greater precision. For patients who develop proteinuria exceeding 1 g/day, or proteinuria that is increasing, the benefits and risks of continuing captopril should be evaluated.

Neutropenia/Agranulocytosis: Neutropenia ($<300/mm^3$) associated with myeloid hypoplasia (that was probably drug related) was observed in about 0.3 percent of patients treated with captopril. About half of the neutropenic patients developed systemic or oral cavity infections or other features of the syndrome of agranulocytosis. Most of the neutropenic patients had severe hypertension and renal functional impairment, and about half had systemic lupus erythematosus (SLE), or another autoimmune/collagen disorder. Multiple concomitant drug therapy was common, including immunosuppressive therapy in a few cases. Daily doses of captopril in the leukopenic patients were relatively high, particularly in view of their diminished renal function.

The neutropenia appeared 3 to 12 weeks after starting captopril, and it developed relatively slowly, the white count falling to its nadir over 10 to 30 days. Neutrophils returned to normal in about two weeks (other than in two patients who died of sepsis).

Capotril should be used with caution in patients with impaired renal function, serious autoimmune disease (particularly SLE), or who are exposed to other drugs known to affect the white cells or immune response.

In patients at particular risk (as noted above), white blood cell and differential counts should be performed before starting treatment, at approximately two-week intervals for about the first three months of therapy, and periodically thereafter.

The risk of neutropenia in patients who are less seriously ill or who receive lower dosages appears to be smaller, and it is sufficient in these patients to have white blood cell counts every two weeks for the first three months of captopril therapy, and periodically thereafter. Differential counts should be performed when leukocytes are $<4000/mm^3$, or the pretreatment white count is halved.

All patients treated with captopril should be told to report any signs of infection (e.g., sore throat; fever). If infection is suspected, counts should be performed without delay.

Since discontinuation of captopril and other drugs has generally led to prompt return of the white count to normal, upon confirmation of neutropenia (neutrophil count $<1000/mm^3$) the physician should withdraw captopril and closely follow the patient's course.

Hypotension: Excessive hypotension was rarely seen in hypertensive patients but is a possible consequence of captopril use in severely salt/volume depleted persons such as those treated vigorously with diuretics, for example, patients with severe congestive heart failure (see PRECAUTIONS [Drug Interactions]).

Precautions

General: *Impaired Renal Function*—Some patients with renal disease, particularly those with severe renal artery stenosis, have developed increases in BUN and serum creatinine after reduction of blood pressure with captopril. Captopril dosage reduction and/or discontinuation of diuretic may be required. For some of these patients, it may not be possible to normalize blood pressure and maintain adequate renal perfusion (see CLINICAL PHARMACOLOGY, DOSAGE AND ADMINISTRATION, ADVERSE REACTIONS [Altered Laboratory Findings]).

Surgery/Anesthesia—In patients undergoing major surgery or during anesthesia with agents that produce hypotension, captopril will block angiotensin II formation secondary to compensatory renin release. If hypotension occurs and is considered to be due to this mechanism, it can be corrected by volume expansion.

Information for Patients: Patients should be told to report promptly any indication of infection (e.g., sore throat, fever), which may be a sign of neutropenia, or of progressive edema, which might be related to proteinuria and nephrotic syndrome.

All patients should be cautioned that excessive perspiration and dehydration may lead to an excessive fall in bloood pressure because of reduction in fluid volume. Other causes of volume depletion such as vomiting or diarrhea may also lead to a fall in blood pressure; patients should be advised to consult with the physician.

Patients should be warned against interruption or discontinuation of antihypertensive medications without the physician's advice.

Patients should be informed that CAPOTEN (captopril tablets) should be taken one hour before meals (see DOSAGE AND ADMINISTRATION).

Drug Interactions: *Hypotension—Patients on Diuretic Therapy*—Patients on diuretics and especially those in whom diuretic therapy was recently instituted, as well as those on severe dietary salt restriction or dialysis, may occasionally experience a precipitous reduction of blood pressure within the first three hours after receiving the initial dose of captopril.

The possibility of hypotensive effects can be minimized by either discontinuing the diuretic or increasing the salt intake approximately one week prior to initiation of treatment with CAPOTEN (captopril tablets). Alternatively, provide medical supervision for at least three hours after the initial dose. If hypotension occurs, the patient should be placed in a supine position and, if necessary, receive an intravenous infusion of normal saline. This transient hypotensive response is not a contraindication to further doses which can be given without difficulty once the blood pressure has increased after volume expansion.

Agents Causing Renin Release—Captopril's effect will be augmented by antihypertensive agents that cause renin release.

Agents Affecting Sympathetic Activity—The sympathetic nervous system may be especially important in supporting blood pressure in patients receiving captopril alone or with diuretics. Therefore, agents affecting sympathetic activity (e.g., ganglionic blocking agents or adrenergic neuron blocking agents) should be used with caution. Beta-adrenergic blocking drugs add some further antihypertensive effect to captopril, but the overall response is less than additive.

Agents Increasing Serum Potassium—Since captopril decreases aldosterone production, elevation of serum potassium may occur. Potassium-sparing diuretics or potassium supplements should be given only for documented hypokalemia, and then with caution, since they may lead to a significant increase of serum potassium.

If the patient has received spironolactone at any time up to several months prior to captopril therapy, the serum potassium should be determined frequently, since the effect of spironolactone perists.

Drug/Laboratory Test Interaction: Captopril may cause a false-positive urine test for acetone.

Carcinogenesis, Mutagenesis and Impairment of Fertility: Two-year studies with doses of 50 to 1350 mg./kg./day in mice and rats failed to show any evidence of carcinogenic potential. Studies in rats have revealed no impairment of fertility.

Animal Toxicology: Chronic oral toxicity studies were conducted in rats (2 years), dogs (47 weeks; 1 year), mice (2 years), and monkeys (1 year). Significant drug-related toxicity included effects on hematopoiesis, renal toxicity, erosion/ulceration of the stomach, and variation of retinal blood vessels.

Reductions in hemoglobin and/or hematocrit values were seen in mice, rats, and monkeys at doses 50 to 150 times the maximum recommended human dose (MRHD). Anemia, leukopenia, thrombocytopenia, and bone marrow suppression occurred in dogs at doses 8 to 30 times MRHD. The reductions in hemoglobin and hematocrit values in rats and mice were only significant at 1 year and returned to normal with continued dosing by the end of the study. Marked anemia was seen at all dose levels (8 to 30 times MRHD) in dogs, whereas moderate to marked leukopenia was noted only at 15 to 30 times MRHD and thrombocytopenia at 30 times MRHD. The anemia could be reversed upon discontinuation of dosing. Bone marrow suppression occurred to a varying degree, being associated only with dogs that died or were sacrificed in a moribund condition in the 1-year study. However, in the 47-week study at a dose 30 times MRHD, bone morrow suppression was found to be reversible upon continued drug administration.

Captopril caused hyperplasia of the juxtaglomerular apparatus of the kidneys at doses 7 to 200 times the MRHD in rats and mice, at 20 to 60 times MRHD in monkeys, and at 30 times the MRHD in dogs.

Gastric erosions/ulcerations were increased in incidence at 20 and 200 times MRHD in male rats and at 30 and 65 times MRHD in dogs and monkeys, respectively. Rabbits developed gastric and intestinal ulcers when given oral doses approximately 30 times MRHD for only 5 to 7 days.

In the two-year rat study, irreversible and progressive variations in the caliber of retinal vessels (focal sacculations and constrictions) occurred at all dose levels (7 to 200 times MRHD) in a dose-related fashion. The effect was first observed in the 88th week of dosing, with a progressively increased incidence thereafter, even after cessation of dosing.

Pregnancy: Category C: Captopril was embryocidal in rabbits when given in doses 2 to 70 times (on a mg./kg. basis) the maxium recommended human dose. The marked embryocidal effect in rabbits was most probably due to the particularly marked decrease in blood pressure caused by the drug in this species.

Captopril given to pregnant rats at 400 times the recommended human dose continuously during gestation and lactation caused a reduction in neonatal survival.

No teratogenic effects (malformations) have been observed after large doses of captopril in hamsters, rats, and rabbits.

There are no adequate and well-controlled studies in pregnant women. Captopril should be used during pregnancy only if the potential benefit justifies the potential risk to the fetus.

Nursing Mothers: Concentrations of captopril in human milk are approximately one percent of those in maternal blood. The effect of low levels of captopril on the nursing infant has not been determined. Caution should be exercised when captopril is administered to a nursing woman, and, in general, nursing should be interrupted.

Pediatric Use: Safety and effectiveness in children have not been established although there is limited experience with the use of captopril in children from 2 months to 15 years of age with secondary hypertension and varying

Continued on next page

Squibb—Cont.

degrees of renal insufficiency. Dosage, on a weight basis, was comparable to that used in adults. CAPOTEN (captopril tablets) should be used in children only if other measures for controlling blood pressure have not been effective.

Adverse Reactions: Reported incidences are based on clinical trials involving approximately 4000 patients.

Renal—One to two of 100 patients developed proteinuria (see WARNINGS).

Each of the following has been reported in approximately 1 to 2 of 1000 patients and are of uncertain relationship to drug use: renal insufficiency, renal failure, polyuria, oliguria, and urinary frequency.

Hematologic—Neutropenia/agranulocytosis that was probably drug related occurred in about 0.3 percent of patients treated with captopril (see WARNINGS). Two of these patients developed sepsis and died.

Dermatologic—Rash, often with pruritus, and sometimes with fever and eosinophilia, occurred in about 10 of 100 patients, usually during the first four weeks of therapy. It is usually maculopapular, and rarely urticarial. The rash is usually mild and disappears within a few days of dosage reduction, short-term treatment with an antihistaminic agent, and/or discontinuing therapy; remission may occur even if captopril is continued. Pruritus, without rash, occurs in about 2 of 100 patients. Between 7 and 10 percent of patients with skin rash have shown an eosinophilia and/or positive ANA titers. A reversible associated pemphigoid-like lesion, and photosensitivity, have also been reported.

Angioedema of the face, mucous membranes of the mouth, or of the extremities has been observed in approximately 1 of 100 patients and is reversible on discontinuance of captopril therapy. One case of laryngeal edema has been reported.

Flushing or pallor has been reported in 2 to 5 of 1000 patients.

Cardiovascular—Hypotension occurred in approximately 2 of 100 patients. See PRECAUTIONS (Drug Interactions) for discussion of hypotension on initiation of captopril therapy. Tachycardia, chest pain, and palpitations have each been observed in approximately 1 of 100 patients.

Angina pectoris, myocardial infarction, Raynaud's syndrome, and congestive heart failure have each occurred in 2 to 3 of 1000 patients.

Dysgeusia—Approximately 7 of 100 patients developed a diminution or loss of taste perception. Taste impairment is reversible and usually self-limited even with continued drug administration (2 to 3 months). Weight loss may be associated with the loss of taste.

The following have been reported in about 0.5 to 2 percent of patients but did not appear at increased frequency compared to placebo or other treatments used in controlled trials: gastric irritation, abdominal pain, nausea, vomiting, diarrhea, anorexia, constipation, aphthous ulcers, peptic ulcer, dizziness, headache, malaise, fatigue, insomnia, dry mouth, dyspnea, paresthesias.

Altered Laboratory Findings: Elevations of liver enzymes have been noted in a few patients but no causal relationship to captopril use has been established. A single case of hepatocellular injury with secondary cholestasis has been reported in association with captopril administration.

A transient elevation of BUN and serum creatinine may occur, especially in patients who are volume-depleted or who have renovascular hypertension. In instances of rapid reduction of longstanding or severely elevated blood pressure, the glomerular filtration rate may decrease transiently, also resulting in transient rises in serum creatinine and BUN.

Small increases in the serum potassium concentration frequently occur, especially in patients with renal impairment (see PRECAUTIONS).

Overdosage: Correction of hypotension would be of primary concern. Volume expansion with an intravenous infusion of normal saline is the treatment of choice for restoration of blood pressure.

Captopril may be removed from the general circulation by hemodialysis.

Dosage and Administration: CAPOTEN (captopril tablets) should be taken one hour before meals. Dosage must be individualized.

Initiation of therapy requires consideration of recent antihypertensive drug treatment, the extent of blood pressure elevation, salt restriction, and other clinical circumstances. If possible, discontinue the patient's previous antihypertensive drug regimen for one week before starting CAPOTEN (captopril tablets).

The initial dose of CAPOTEN (captopril tablets) is 25 mg. t.i.d. If satisfactory reduction of blood pressure has not been achieved after one or two weeks, the dose may be increased to 50 mg. t.i.d.

If the blood pressure has not been satisfactorily controlled after another one to two weeks, a modest dose of a thiazide-type diuretic (e.g., hydrochlorothiazide, 25 mg. daily) should be added. The diuretic dose may be increased at one- to two-week intervals until its highest usual antihypertensive dose is reached.

If further blood pressure reduction is required, the dose of CAPOTEN (captopril tablets) may be increased to 100 mg. t.i.d. and then, if necessary, to 150 mg. t.i.d. (while continuing the diuretic). The usual dose range is 25 to 150 mg. t.i.d. A maximum daily dose of 450 mg. CAPOTEN (captopril tablets) should not be exceeded.

For patients with accelerated or malignant hypertension, when temporary discontinuation of current antihypertensive therapy is not practical, or when prompt titration to more normotensive blood pressure levels is indicated, current antihypertensive medication may be stopped and CAPOTEN (captopril tablets) dosage promptly initiated at 25 mg. t.i.d., under close medical supervision. The daily dose of CAPOTEN (captopril tablets) may be increased every 24 hours until a satisfactory blood pressure response is obtained or the maximum dose of CAPOTEN (captopril tablets) is reached. In this regimen, addition of a more potent diuretic, e.g., furosemide, may also be indicated.

Beta-blockers may also be used in conjunction with CAPOTEN (captopril tablets) therapy (see PRECAUTIONS [Drug Interactions]), but the effects of the two drugs are less than additive.

Dosage Adjustment in Renal Impairment—Because CAPOTEN (captopril tablets) is excreted primarily by the kidneys, excretion rates are reduced in patients with impaired renal function. These patients will take longer to reach steady-state captopril levels and will reach higher steady-state levels for a given daily dose than patients with normal renal function. Therefore, these patients may respond to smaller or less frequent doses.

Accordingly, for patients with significant renal impairment, initial daily dosage of CAPOTEN (captopril tablets) should be reduced, and smaller increments utilized for titration, which should be quite slow (one- to two-week intervals). After the desired therapeutic effect has been achieved, the dose should be slowly back-titrated to determine the minimal effective dose. When concomitant diuretic therapy is required, a loop diuretic (e.g., furosemide), rather than a thiazide diuretic, is preferred in patients with severe renal impairment.

How Supplied: CAPOTEN (captopril tablets) is available as white tablets in potencies of 25, 50, and 100 mg. in bottles of 100, and in UNIMATIC® single-dose packs of 100 tablets. Bottles contain desiccant and charcoal. The 25 mg. tablet is a biconvex rounded square with a quadrisect bar; the 50 and 100 mg. tablets are biconvex ovals with a bisect bar. Captopril tablets may exhibit a slight sulfurous odor.

Storage: Do not store above 86° F. Keep bottles tightly closed (protect from moisture).

[*Shown in Product Identification Section*]

CARDIOGRAFIN® ℞
(Diatrizoate Meglumine Injection USP 85%)

(See Diagnostic Section)

CHOLOGRAFIN® MEGLUMINE ℞
(Iodipamide Meglumine Injection USP 52%)

(See Diagnostic Section)

CHOLOGRAFIN® MEGLUMINE FOR INFUSION ℞
(Iodipamide Meglumine Injection USP 10.3%)

(See Diagnostic Section)

CHOLOVUE® ℞
(Iodoxamate Meglumine Injection 40.3%)

(See Diagnostic Section)

CHOLOVUE® FOR INFUSION ℞
(Iodoxamate Meglumine Injection 9.9%)

(See Diagnostic Section)

CORGARD® ℞
(Nadolol Tablets)

Description: CORGARD (nadolol) is a synthetic nonselective beta-adrenergic receptor blocking agent chemically described as 2, 3-Naphthalenediol, 5-[3-[(1,1-dimethylethyl) amino]-2-hydroxypropoxy]-1,2,3,4-tetrahydro-, cis-. Nadolol is a white crystalline powder, slightly soluble in water and freely soluble in ethanol.

CORGARD (nadolol) is available as tablets for oral administration.

Clinical Pharmacology: CORGARD (nadolol) is a nonselective beta-adrenergic receptor blocking agent. Clinical pharmacology studies have demonstrated beta-blocking activity by showing (1) reduction in heart rate and cardiac output at rest and on exercise, (2) reduction of systolic and diastolic blood pressure at rest and on exercise, (3) inhibition of isoproterenol-induced tachycardia, and (4) reduction of reflex orthostatic tachycardia.

CORGARD (nadolol) specifically competes with beta-adrenergic receptor agonists for available beta receptor sites; it inhibits both the $beta_1$ receptors located chiefly in cardiac muscle and the $beta_2$ receptors located chiefly in the bronchial and vascular musculature, inhibiting the chronotropic, inotropic, and vasodilator responses to beta-adrenergic stimulation proportionately. CORGARD (nadolol) has no intrinsic sympathomimetic activity and, unlike some other beta-adrenergic blocking agents, nadolol has little direct myocardial depressant activity and does not have an anesthetic-like membrane-stabilizing action. Animal and human studies show that CORGARD (nadolol) slows the sinus rate and depresses AV conduction. In dogs, only minimal amounts of nadolol were detected in the brain relative to amounts in blood and other organs and tissues. In controlled clinical studies, CORGARD (nadolol) at doses of 40 to 320 mg./day has been shown to decrease both standing and supine blood pressure, the effect persisting for approximately 24 hours after dosing.

The mechanism of the antihypertensive effects of beta-adrenergic receptor blocking agents has not been established; however, factors that may be involved include (1) competitive antagonism of catecholamines at peripheral (non-CNS) adrenergic neuron sites (especially cardiac) leading to decreased cardiac output, (2) a central effect leading to reduced tonic-sympathetic nerve outflow to the periphery, and (3) suppression of renin secretion by blockade of the beta-adrenergic receptors responsible for renin release from the kidneys.

By blocking catecholamine-induced increases in heart rate, velocity and extent of myocardial contraction, and blood pressure, CORGARD (nadolol) generally reduces the oxygen requirements of the heart at any given level of effort, making it useful for many patients in the long-term management of angina pectoris. On the other hand, nadolol can increase oxygen requirements by increasing left ventricular fiber length and end diastolic pressure, particularly in patients with heart failure.

Although beta-adrenergic receptor blockade is useful in treatment of angina and hypertension, there are also situations in which sympathetic stimulation is vital. For example, in patients with severely damaged hearts, adequate ventricular function may depend on sympathetic drive. Beta-adrenergic blockade may worsen AV block by preventing the necessary facilitating effects of sympathetic activity on conduction. $Beta_2$-adrenergic blockade results in passive bronchial constriction by interfering with endogenous adrenergic bronchodilator activity in patients subject to bronchospasm and may also interfere with exogenous bronchodilators in such patients.

Absorption of nadolol after oral dosing is variable, averaging about 30 percent. Peak serum concentrations of nadolol usually occur in three to four hours after oral administration and the presence of food in the gastrointestinal tract does not affect the rate or extent of nadolol absorption. Approximately 30 percent of the nadolol present in serum is reversibly bound to plasma protein.

Unlike many other beta-adrenergic blocking agents, nadolol is not metabolized and is excreted unchanged, principally by the kidneys. The half-life of therapeutic doses of nadolol is about 20 to 24 hours, permitting once-daily dosage. Because nadolol is excreted predominantly in the urine, its half-life increases in renal failure (see PRECAUTIONS and DOSAGE AND ADMINISTRATION). Steady-state serum concentrations of nadolol are attained in six to nine days with once-daily dosage in persons with normal renal function. Because of variable absorption and different individual responsiveness, the proper dosage must be determined by titration.

Exacerbation of angina and, in some cases, myocardial infarction and ventricular dysrhythmias have been reported after abrupt discontinuation of therapy with beta-adrenergic blocking agents in patients with coronary artery disease. Abrupt withdrawal of these agents in patients without coronary artery disease has resulted in transient symptoms, including tremulousness, sweating, palpitation, headache, and malaise. Several mechanisms have been proposed to explain these phenomena, among them increased sensitivity to catecholamines because of increased numbers of beta receptors.

Indications and Usage:

Angina Pectoris—CORGARD (nadolol) is indicated for the long-term management of patients with angina pectoris.

Hypertension—CORGARD (nadolol) is indicated in the management of hypertension; it may be used alone or in combination with other antihypertensive agents, especially thiazide-type diuretics.

Contraindications: Nadolol is contraindicated in bronchial asthma, sinus bradycardia and greater than first degree conduction block, cardiogenic shock, and overt cardiac failure (see WARNINGS).

Warnings:

Cardiac Failure—Sympathetic stimulation may be a vital component supporting circulatory function in patients with congestive heart failure, and its inhibition by beta-blockade may precipitate more severe failure. Although beta-blockers should be avoided in overt congestive heart failure, if necessary, they can be used with caution in patients with a history of failure who are well-compensated, usually with digitalis and diuretics. Beta-adrenergic blocking agents do not abolish the inotropic action of digitalis on heart muscle.

IN PATIENTS WITHOUT A HISTORY OF HEART FAILURE, continued use of beta-blockers can, in some cases, lead to cardiac failure. Therefore, at the first sign or symptom of heart failure, the patient should be digitalized and/or treated with diuretics, and the response observed closely, or nadolol should be discontinued (gradually, if possible).

Exacerbation of Ischemic Heart Disease Following Abrupt Withdrawal—Hypersensitivity to catecholamines has been observed in patients withdrawn from beta-blocker therapy; exacerbation of angina and, in some cases, myocardial infarction have occurred after *abrupt* discontinuation of such therapy. When discontinuing chronically administered nadolol, particularly in patients with ischemic heart disease, the dosage should be gradually reduced over a period of one to two weeks and the patient should be carefully monitored. If angina markedly worsens or acute coronary insufficiency develops, nadolol administration should be reinstituted promptly, at least temporarily, and other measures appropriate for the management of unstable angina should be taken. Patients should be warned against interruption or discontinuation of therapy without the physician's advice. Because coronary artery disease is common and may be unrecognized, it may be prudent not to discontinue nadolol therapy abruptly even in patients treated only for hypertension.

Nonallergic Bronchospasm (e.g., chronic bronchitis, emphysema)—PATIENTS WITH BRONCHOSPASTIC DISEASES SHOULD IN GENERAL NOT RECEIVE BETA-BLOCKERS. Nadolol should be administered with caution since it may block bronchodilation produced by endogenous or exogenous catecholamine stimulation of $beta_2$ receptors.

Major Surgery—Because beta-blockade impairs the ability of the heart to respond to reflex stimuli and may increase the risks of general anesthesia and surgical procedures, resulting in protracted hypotension or low cardiac output, it has generally been suggested that such therapy should be withdrawn several days prior to surgery. Recognition of the increased sensitivity to catecholamines of patients recently withdrawn from beta-blocker therapy, however, has made this recommendation controversial. If possible, beta-blockers should be withdrawn well before surgery takes place. In the event of emergency surgery, the anesthesiologist should be informed that the patient is on beta-blocker therapy. The effects of nadolol can be reversed by administration of beta-receptor agonists such as isoproterenol, dopamine, dobutamine, or levarterenol. Difficulty in restarting and maintaining the heart beat has also been reported with beta-adrenergic receptor blocking agents.

Diabetes and Hypoglycemia—Beta-adrenergic blockade may prevent the appearance of premonitory signs and symptoms (e.g., tachycardia and blood pressure changes) of acute hypoglycemia. This is especially important with labile diabetics. Beta-blockade also reduces the release of insulin in response to hyperglycemia; therefore, it may be necessary to adjust the dose of antidiabetic drugs.

Thyrotoxicosis—Beta-adrenergic blockade may mask certain clinical signs (e.g., tachycardia) of hyperthyroidism. Patients suspected of developing thyrotoxicosis should be managed carefully to avoid abrupt withdrawal of beta-adrenergic blockade which might precipitate a thyroid storm.

Precautions:

Impaired Hepatic or Renal Function—Nadolol should be used with caution in patients with impaired hepatic or renal function (see DOSAGE AND ADMINISTRATION).

Information for Patients—Patients, especially those with evidence of coronary artery insufficiency, should be warned against interruption or discontinuation of nadolol therapy without the physician's advice. Although cardiac failure rarely occurs in properly selected patients, patients being treated with beta-adrenergic blocking agents should be advised to consult the physician at the first sign or symptom of impending failure.

Drug Interactions—Catecholamine-depleting drugs (e.g., reserpine) may have an additive effect when given with beta-blocking agents. Patients treated with nadolol plus a catecholamine-depleting agent should therefore be closely observed for evidence of hypotension and/or excessive bradycardia which may produce vertigo, syncope, or postural hypotension.

Carcinogenesis, Mutagenesis, Impairment of Fertility—In chronic oral toxicologic studies (one to two years) in mice, rats, and dogs, nadolol did not produce any significant toxic effects. In two-year oral carcinogenic studies in rats and mice, nadolol did not produce any neoplastic, preneoplastic, or nonneoplastic pathologic lesions. In fertility and general reproductive performance studies in rats, nadolol caused no adverse effects.

Pregnancy—Teratogenic Effects: Pregnancy Category C. In animal reproduction studies with nadolol, evidence of embryo- and fetotoxicity was found in rabbits, but not in rats or hamsters, at doses 5 to 10 times greater (on a mg./kg. basis) than the maximum indicated human dose. No teratogenic potential was observed in any of these species.

There are no adequate and well-controlled studies in pregnant women. Nadolol should be used during pregnancy only if the potential benefit justifies the potential risk to the fetus.

Nursing Mothers—It is not known whether this drug is excreted in human milk. Because many drugs are excreted in human milk, caution should be exercised when nadolol is administered to a nursing woman.

Animal studies showed that nadolol is found in the milk of lactating rats.

Pediatric Use—Safety and effectiveness in children have not been established.

Adverse Reactions: Most adverse effects have been mild and transient and have rarely required withdrawal of therapy.

Cardiovascular—Bradycardia with heart rates of less than 60 beats per minute occurs commonly, and heart rates below 40 beats per minute and/or symptomatic bradycardia were seen in about 2 of 100 patients. Symptoms of peripheral vascular insufficiency, usually of the Raynaud type, have occurred in approximately 2 of 100 patients. Cardiac failure, hypotension, and rhythm/conduction disturbances have each occurred in about 1 of 100 patients. Single instances of first degree and third degree heart block have been reported; intensification of AV block is a known effect of beta-blockers (see also CONTRAINDICATIONS, WARNINGS, and PRECAUTIONS).

Central Nervous System—Dizziness or fatigue have each been reported in approximately 2 of 100 patients; paresthesias, sedation, and change in behavior have each been reported in approximately 6 of 1000 patients.

Respiratory—Bronchospasm has been reported in approximately 1 of 1000 patients (see CONTRAINDICATIONS and WARNINGS).

Continued on next page

Squibb—Cont.

Gastrointestinal—Nausea, diarrhea, abdominal discomfort, constipation, vomiting, indigestion, anorexia, bloating, and flatulence have been reported in 1 to 5 of 1000 patients.
Miscellaneous—Each of the following has been reported in 1 to 5 of 1000 patients: rash; pruritus; headache; dry mouth, eyes, or skin; impotence or decreased libido; facial swelling; weight gain; slurred speech; cough; nasal stuffiness; sweating; tinnitus; blurred vision.
Sleep disturbances have been reported, but their relationship to drug usage is not clear.
The oculomucocutaneous syndrome associated with the beta-blocker practolol has not been reported with nadolol.
Potential Adverse Effects: In addition, other adverse effects not reported with nadolol have been reported with other beta-adrenergic blocking agents and should be considered potential adverse effects of nadolol.
Central Nervous System—Reversible mental depression progressing to catatonia; visual disturbances; hallucinations; an acute reversible syndrome characterized by disorientation for time and place, short-term memory loss, emotional lability with slightly clouded sensorium, and decreased performance on neuropsychometrics.
Gastrointestinal—Mesenteric arterial thrombosis; ischemic colitis.
Hematologic—Agranulocytosis; thrombocytopenic or nonthrombocytopenic purpura.
Allergic—Fever combined with aching and sore throat; laryngospasm; respiratory distress.
Miscellaneous—Reversible alopecia; Peyronie's disease; erythematous rash.
Overdosage: Nadolol can be removed from the general circulation by hemodialysis.
In addition to gastric lavage, the following measures should be employed, as appropriate. In determining the duration of corrective therapy, note must be taken of the long duration of the effect of nadolol.
Excessive Bradycardia—Administer atropine (0.25 to 1.0 mg.). If there is no response to vagal blockade, administer isoproterenol cautiously.
Cardiac Failure—Administer a digitalis glycoside and diuretic. It has been reported that glucagon may also be useful in this situation.
Hypotension—Administer vasopressors, e.g., epinephrine or levarterenol. (There is evidence that epinephrine may be the drug of choice.)
Bronchospasm—Administer a beta$_2$-stimulating agent and/or a theophylline derivative.
Dosage and Administration: DOSAGE MUST BE INDIVIDUALIZED. CORGARD (NADOLOL) MAY BE ADMINISTERED WITHOUT REGARD TO MEALS.
Angina Pectoris—The usual initial dose is 40 mg. CORGARD (nadolol) once daily. Dosage should be gradually increased in 40 to 80 mg. increments at 3- to 7-day intervals until optimum clinical response is obtained or there is pronounced slowing of the heart rate. The usual maintenance dose range is 80 to 240 mg. administered once daily, with most patients responding to 160 mg. or less daily.
The usefulness and safety in angina pectoris of dosage exceeding 240 mg. per day have not been established. If treatment is to be discontinued, reduce the dosage gradually over a period of one to two weeks (see WARNINGS).
Hypertension—The usual initial dose is 40 mg CORGARD (nadolol) once daily, whether it is used alone or in addition to diuretic therapy. Dosage may be gradually increased in 40 to 80 mg. increments until optimum blood pressure reduction is achieved. The usual maintenance dose is 80 to 320 mg., administered once daily. In rare instances, daily doses up to 640 mg. may be needed.
Dosage Adjustment in Renal Failure—Absorbed nadolol is excreted principally by the kidneys and, although nonrenal elimination does occur, dosage adjustments are necessary in patients with renal impairment. The following dose intervals are recommended:

Creatinine Clearance (ml/min/1.73m^2)	Dosage Interval (hours)
>50	24
31–50	24–36
10–30	24–48
<10	40–60

How Supplied: CORGARD Tablets (Nadolol Tablets) are supplied as scored tablets containing 40, 80, 120, or 160 mg. nadolol per tablet in bottles of 100 and 1000 tablets and in Unimatic® unit-dose packs of 100 tablets. The 40 mg. and 80 mg. tablets are also available in convenience packages containing 4 blister cards of 7 tablets each.
Storage: Store at room temperature; avoid excessive heat. Protect from light. Keep bottle tightly closed. Dispense in tight, light-resistant containers.
[*Shown in Product Identification Section*]

CRYSTICILLIN® 300 A.S. ℞
CRYSTICILLIN® 600 A.S. ℞
(Sterile Penicillin G Procaine Suspension USP)

Description: Crysticillin 300 A.S. and Crysticillin 600 A.S. are aqueous suspensions providing 300,000 u. per ml. and 600,000 u. per 1.2 ml. (500,000 u./ml.) penicillin G procaine, respectively. The vials providing 300,000 u. per ml. also contain 0.13% methylparaben, 0.02% propylparaben, and 0.25% phenol as preservatives; 0.5% lecithin; 0.5% povidone; 1% sodium citrate; not more than 0.01% sodium formaldehyde sulfoxylate; and 0.075% sodium carboxymethylcellulose. The vials providing 600,000 u. per 1.2 ml. also contain 0.13% methylparaben, 0.02% propylparaben, and 0.18% phenol as preservatives; 0.3% povidone; 1% sodium citrate; 0.05% sodium carboxymethylcellulose; not more than 0.03% sodium formaldehyde sulfoxylate; and 2.3% lecithin.
Clinical Pharmacology: Penicillin G is bactericidal against penicillin-susceptible microorganisms during the stage of active multiplication. It acts by inhibiting biosynthesis of cell-wall mucopeptide. It is not active against the penicillinase-producing bacteria, which include many strains of staphylococci. Penicillin G is highly active *in vitro* against staphylococci (except penicillinase-producing strains), streptococci (groups A, C, G, H, L, and M), and pneumococci. Other organisms susceptible *in vitro* to penicillin G are *Neisseria gonorrhoeae, Corynebacterium diphtheriae, Bacillus anthracis,* Clostridia, *Actinomyces bovis, Streptobacillus moniliformis, Listeria monocytogenes,* and Leptospira; *Treponema pallidum* is extremely susceptible.
Susceptibility plate testing: If the Kirby-Bauer method of disc susceptibility is used, a 10 u. penicillin disc should give a zone greater than 28 mm. when tested against a penicillin-susceptible bacterial strain.
Penicillin G procaine is an equimolar compound of procaine and penicillin G administered intramuscularly as a suspension. It dissolves slowly at the site of injection, giving a plateau type of blood level at about four hours which falls slowly during the next 15 to 20 hours.
Approximately 60 percent of penicillin G is bound to serum protein. The drug is distributed throughout the body tissues in widely varying amounts. Highest levels are found in the kidneys with lesser amounts in the liver, skin, and intestines. Penicillin G penetrates into all other tissues to a lesser degree with a very small level found in the cerebrospinal fluid. The drug is excreted rapidly by tubular excretion in patients with normal kidney function. In neonates and young infants, and in individuals with impaired kidney function, excretion is considerably delayed. Approximately 60 to 90 percent of a dose of parenteral penicillin G is excreted in the urine within 24 to 36 hours.
Indications and Usage: Crysticillin 300 A.S. and Crysticillin 600 A.S. (Sterile Penicillin G Procaine Suspension USP) are indicated in the treatment of moderately severe infections due to penicillin G-susceptible microorganisms. Therapy should be guided by bacteriological studies, including susceptibility tests, and by clinical response. Note: severe pneumonia, empyema, bacteremia, pericarditis, meningitis, peritonitis, and septic arthritis are better treated with aqueous penicillin G during the acute stage; when high, sustained serum levels are required, aqueous penicillin G, either I.M. or I.V. should be used.
The following infections will usually respond to adequate dosage:
Streptococcal infections Group A without bacteremia—Moderately severe to severe infections of the upper respiratory tract, skin and skin structures infections, scarlet fever, and erysipelas. Note: streptococci in groups A, C, G, H, L, and M are very susceptible to penicillin G. Other groups, including group D (enterococcus) are resistant. Aqueous penicillin is recommended for streptococcal infections with bacteremia.
Pneumococcal infections—Moderately severe infections of the respiratory tract.
Staphylococcal infections—penicillin G susceptible—Moderately severe infections of the skin and skin structures. Note: reports indicate an increasing number of strains of staphylococci resistant to penicillin G, emphasizing the need for culture and susceptibility studies in treating suspected staphylococcal infections. Indicated surgical procedures should be performed.
Vincent's gingivitis and pharyngitis (fusospirochetosis)—Moderately severe infections of the oropharynx. Note: necessary dental care should be accomplished in infections involving the gum tissue.
Syphilis (*T. pallidum*)—All stages; **Gonorrheal infections** (acute and chronic—without bacteremia)—With adequate recommended doses; **Treponema**—Yaws, Bejel, Pinta; **Diphtheria**—as an adjunct to antitoxin for the prevention of the carrier state; **Anthrax; Rat-bite fever** (*S. moniliformis* and *S. minus*); **Erysipeloid.**
Subacute bacterial endocarditis (group A streptococcus)—Only in extremely susceptible infections. **Prophylaxis against bacterial endocarditis**—Although no controlled clinical efficacy studies have been conducted, aqueous crystalline penicillin G for injection and penicillin G procaine suspension have been suggested by the American Heart Association and the American Dental Association for use as part of a combined parenteral-oral regimen for prophylaxis against bacterial endocarditis in patients with congenital heart disease or rheumatic or other acquired valvular heart disease when they undergo dental procedures and surgical procedures of the upper respiratory tract.[1] Since it may happen that *alpha* hemolytic streptococci relatively resistant to penicillin may be found when patients are receiving continuous oral penicillin for secondary prevention of rheumatic fever, prophylactic agents other than penicillin may be chosen for these patients and prescribed in addition to their continuous rheumatic fever prophylactic regimen. **NOTE: When selecting antibiotics for the prevention of bacterial endocarditis, the physician or dentist should read the full joint statement of the American Heart Association and the American Dental Association.[1]**
Contraindications: Contraindicated in patients with a history of hypersensitivity to procaine or any penicillin.
Warnings: Serious and occasional fatal hypersensitivity (anaphylactoid) reactions have been reported in patients on penicillin therapy. Although anaphylaxis is more frequent follow-

ing parenteral administration, it has occurred in patients on oral penicillins. These reactions are more apt to occur in individuals with a history of sensitivity to multiple allergens.

There have been well-documented reports of individuals with a history of penicillin hypersensitivity who have experienced severe hypersensitivity reactions when treated with cephalosporins. Before therapy with a penicillin, careful inquiry should be made concerning previous hypersensitivity reactions to penicillins, cephalosporins, and other allergens. If an allergic reaction occurs, the drug should be discontinued and the patient treated with the usual agents, e.g., pressor amines, antihistamines, and corticosteroids. Serious anaphylactoid reactions are not controlled by antihistamines alone, and require such emergency measures as the immediate use of epinephrine, aminophylline, oxygen, and intravenous corticosteroids.

Immediate toxic reactions to procaine may occur in some individuals, particularly when a large single dose is administered in the treatment of gonorrhea (4.8 million u.). These reactions may be manifested by mental disturbances including anxiety, confusion, agitation, depression, weakness, seizures, hallucinations, combativeness, and expressed "fear of impending death." The reactions noted in carefully controlled studies occurred in approximately one in 500 patients treated for gonorrhea. Reactions are transient, lasting from 15 to 30 minutes.

Precautions: Penicillin should be used with caution in individuals with histories of significant allergies and/or asthma.

A small percentage of patients are sensitive to procaine. If there is a history of sensitivity, make the usual test: inject intradermally 0.1 ml. of a 1 to 2% procaine hydrochloride solution. Development of an erythema, wheal, flare or eruption indicates procaine sensitivity. Sensitivity should be treated by the usual methods, and procaine penicillin preparations should not be used. Antihistamines appear beneficial in the treatment of procaine reactions.

The use of antibiotics may result in overgrowth of nonsusceptible organisms. Constant observation of the patient is essential. If new infections due to bacteria or fungi appear during therapy, the drug should be discontinued and appropriate measures taken. Whenever allergic reactions occur, penicillin should be withdrawn unless, in the opinion of the physician, the condition being treated is life-threatening and amenable only to penicillin therapy.

Care should be taken to avoid accidental intravenous administration.

In prolonged therapy with penicillin, and particularly with high dosage schedules, periodic evaluation of the renal and hematopoietic systems is recommended.

In streptococcal infections, therapy must be sufficient to eliminate the organism (10 days minimum); otherwise the sequelae of streptococcal disease may occur. Cultures should be taken following the completion of treatment to determine whether streptococci have been eradicated.

In suspected staphylococcal infections, proper laboratory studies, including susceptibility tests, should be performed.

When treating gonococcal infections in which primary or secondary syphilis may be suspected, proper diagnostic procedures, including darkfield examinations, should be done. In all cases in which concomitant syphilis is suspected, monthly serological tests should be made for at least four months. All cases of penicillin-treated syphilis should receive clinical and serological examinations every six months for at least two or three years.

Adverse Reactions: Penicillin is a substance of low toxicity, but does possess a significant index of sensitization. The hypersensitivity reactions reported are skin rashes ranging from maculopapular eruptions to exfoliative dermatitis; urticaria; and serum sickness-like reactions including chills, fever, edema, arthralgia, and prostration. Hemolytic anemia, leukopenia, thrombocytopenia, neuropathy, and nephropathy are infrequent reactions and are usually associated with high doses of parenteral penicillin. Severe and often fatal anaphylaxis has been reported; these reactions require emergency measures (see WARNINGS). As with other treatments for syphilis, the Jarisch-Herxheimer reaction has been reported.

Procaine toxicity manifestations have been reported (see WARNINGS). Procaine hypersensitivity reactions have not been reported with this drug.

Dosage and Administration:

For intramuscular use only

The product is ready for immediate injection after vigorous shaking of the vial to insure a uniform suspension.

Injection is made rapidly by the intramuscular route. The preferred site is the upper outer quadrant of the gluteal area. Injections are easier to make and there is less likelihood of needle blockage if a small bore syringe is used; use a 20-gauge needle. Avoid using a syringe with a loosely-fitting plunger as crystals may creep between the walls and cause it to "freeze". Remove the needle and plunger from the syringe soon after injection to prevent "freezing" of the remaining crystals.

The usual dosage recommendation is as follows:

Streptococcal infections (Group A)—moderately severe to severe tonsillitis, erysipelas, scarlet fever, infections of the upper respiratory tract, and skin and skin structures infections: 600,000 to 1,200,000 u. daily for a minimum of 10 days.

Pneumococcal infections (uncomplicated)—moderately severe: 600,000 to 1,200,000 u. daily.

Staphylococcal infections—moderately severe to severe: 600,000 to 1,200,000 u. daily.

Vincent's gingivitis and pharyngitis (fusospirochetosis): 600,000 to 1,200,000 u. daily.

Syphilis—*Primary, secondary and latent* with a negative spinal fluid in adults and children over 12 years of age: 600,000 u. daily for eight days—total 4,800,000 u.; *Late* (tertiary, neurosyphilis and latent syphilis with positive or no spinal fluid examination): 600,000 u. daily for 10 to 15 days—total 6 to 9 million u.; *Congenital* (under 32 kg. [70 lb.] body weight): 10,000 u./kg./day for 10 days.

Gonorrheal infections (uncomplicated): 4.8 million u. divided into at least two doses at one visit for males and females; one gram of oral probenecid is given 30 minutes before the injections. Follow-up cultures should be obtained from the original site(s) of infection 7 to 14 days after therapy. In women, it is also desirable to obtain culture test-of-cure from both the endocervical and anal canals. Note: gonorrheal endocarditis should be treated intensively with aqueous penicillin G.

Yaws, Bejel, and Pinta—treat same as syphilis in corresponding stage of disease.

Diphtheria—*adjunctive therapy with antitoxin:* 300,000 to 600,000 u. daily; **Anthrax**—cutaneous: 600,000 to 1,200,000 u. daily; **Rat-bite fever** (*S. moniliformis* and *S. minus*) and **Erysipeloid:** 600,000 to 1,200,000 u. daily.

Bacterial endocarditis (group A streptococcus) —only in extremely susceptible infections: 600,000 to 1,200,000 u. daily.

Prophylaxis against bacterial endocarditis—For prophylaxis against bacterial endocarditis[1] in patients with congenital heart disease or rheumatic or other acquired valvular heart disease when undergoing dental procedures or surgical procedures of the upper respiratory tract, use a combined parenteral-oral regimen. One million units of aqueous crystalline penicillin G (30,000 u./kg. in children) mixed with 600,000 u. of penicillin G procaine (600,000 u. for children) should be given intramuscularly one-half to one hour before the procedure. Oral penicillin V (phenoxymethyl penicillin), 500 mg. for adults or 250 mg. for children less than 60 lb., should be given every six hours for eight doses. Doses for children should not exceed recommendations for adults for a single dose or for a 24-hour period.

How Supplied: Crysticillin 300 A.S. (Sterile Penicillin G Procaine Suspension USP) is available in 10 ml. vials; Crysticillin 600 A.S. is available in 12 ml. vials.

Storage: Store below 15° C. (59° F.); avoid freezing.

Reference: 1. American Heart Association. 1977. Prevention of bacterial endocarditis. Circulation 56:139A-143A.

CYSTOGRAFIN® ℞

(Diatrizoate Meglumine Injection USP 30%)

(See Diagnostic Section)

DELATESTRYL® ℞

(Testosterone Enanthate Injection USP)

Description: Delatestryl is a sterile solution of testosterone enanthate for intramuscular use. Chemically, testosterone enanthate is androst-4-en-3-one,17-[(1-oxoheptyl)oxy]-,(17β)-.

Clinical Pharmacology: Delatestryl is intended for androgen therapy, particularly when prolonged action is desirable. Following a single intramuscular injection, the androgenic effect is sustained over a period of about four weeks. This continuous flow of hormone is thought to resemble closely the endogenous production of testosterone.

Testosterone enanthate is primarily used for its protein anabolic effect and its catabolic inhibiting effect on tissue. Nitrogen balance is improved with anabolic agents but only when there is sufficient intake of calories and protein. Whether this positive nitrogen balance is of primary benefit in the utilization of protein-building dietary substances has not been established.

Enhancement of protein anabolism is manifest by conservation of sodium, nitrogen, phosphorus, potassium, sulfur, and water in the proportions of physiologic protein tissues, and of calcium with additional phosphorus in the proportions of physiologic osseous tissues.

Certain clinical effects and adverse reactions demonstrate the androgenic properties of this class of drugs. Complete dissociation of anabolic and androgenic effects has not been achieved. The actions of anabolic steroids are therefore similar to those of male sex hormones with the possibility of causing serious disturbances of growth and sexual development if given to young children. They suppress the gonadotropic functions of the pituitary and may exert a direct effect upon the testes.

Indications and Usage: In males, Delatestryl (Testosterone Enanthate Injection USP) is indicated in the treatment of eunuchism, eunuchoidism, deficiency after castration, male climacteric-like symptoms when these are secondary to androgen deficiency, and oligospermia.

Contraindications: Androgens are contraindicated in male patients with prostatic or breast cancer, in those elderly patients in whom overstimulation is to be avoided, and in those cases of benign prostatic hypertrophy with obstructive symptoms. Androgens are also contraindicated in patients with nephrosis or the nephrotic phase of nephritis.

Precautions: If symptomatic hypercalcemia occurs, discontinue androgen therapy and institute appropriate measures.

Caution is required in administering androgens to patients with cardiac, renal, or hepatic disease. Edema may occur occasionally. Con-

Continued on next page

Squibb—Cont.

comitant administration with adrenal steroids or ACTH may add to the edema.
Anabolic steroids may increase sensitivity to anticoagulants. Dosage of the anticoagulant may have to be decreased in order to maintain the prothrombin time at the desired therapeutic level.
Anabolic steroids have been shown to alter glucose tolerance tests. Diabetics should be followed carefully and the insulin or oral hypoglycemic dosage adjusted accordingly.
Serum cholesterol may increase or decrease during therapy. Because of its hypercholesterolemic effects, caution is required when administering this drug to patients with a history of myocardial infarction or coronary artery disease. Serial determinations of serum cholesterol should be made and therapy adjusted accordingly. A cause and effect relationship between myocardial infarction and hypercholesterolemia has not been established.
Inhibition of testicular function and decrease in ejaculatory volume may occur when the drug is administered in doses greater than those used for replacement therapy in hypogonadal males.
Adverse Reactions: In males, the following postpubertal adverse reactions have occurred: inhibition of testicular function, testicular atrophy and oligospermia, impotence, chronic priapism, gynecomastia, epididymitis, and bladder irritability. In addition, the following reactions are known to occur with anabolic steroids: increased or decreased libido, flushing of the skin, acne, habituation, excitation and sleeplessness, chills, leukopenia, and bleeding in patients on concomitant anticoagulant therapy. There have been rare reports of hepatocellular neoplasms and peliosis hepatis in association with long-term androgenic-anabolic steroid therapy.
Intramuscular preparations of anabolic steroids have been associated with urticaria at the injection site, postinjection induration, and furunculosis.
Alterations may occur in the following clinical laboratory tests: metyrapone test, fasting blood sugar (FBS), and glucose tolerance test; thyroid function tests [decrease in protein-bound iodine (PBI), thyroxine-binding capacity, and radioactive iodine uptake, and an increase in T_3 uptake by the red blood cells or resin; free thyroxine levels remain normal and the altered tests usually persist for two to three weeks after stopping anabolic therapy]; electrolytes (retention of sodium, chloride, water, potassium, calcium, and inorganic phosphates); blood coagulation tests (increase in clotting factors II, V, VII, and X); and miscellaneous laboratory tests (decreased creatinine and creatine excretion lasting up to two weeks after discontinuing therapy and increased 17-ketosteroid excretion).
Dosage and Administration: When properly given, injections of Delatestryl (Testosterone Enanthate Injection USP) are well tolerated. Care should be taken to inject the preparation deeply into the gluteal muscle following the usual precautions for intramuscular administration. In general, total doses above 400 mg. per month are not required because of the prolonged action of the preparation. Injections more frequently than every two weeks are rarely indicated. NOTE: Use of a wet needle or wet syringe may cause the solution to become cloudy; however, this does not affect the potency of the material.
In male hypogonadism (i.e., eunuchism, eunuchoidism, severe deficiency after castration, male climacteric-like symptoms when secondary to androgen deficiency), the suggested dosage is 200 to 400 mg. every four weeks. Androgen therapy is regarded as replacement therapy, being effective only as long as continued.
In the treatment of oligospermia, the suggested dosage is 100 to 200 mg. every four to six weeks for the development and maintenance of testicular tubular function; for suppression and rebound stimulation, the recommended dosage is 200 mg. every week for 6 to 12 weeks.
How Supplied: Delatestryl (Testosterone Enanthate Injection USP) is available in multiple dose vials of 5 ml. and Unimatic® single-dose preassembled syringes of 1 ml. Each ml. of sterile solution provides 200 mg. testosterone enanthate in sesame oil with 0.5% chlorobutanol (chloral derivative) as a preservative. (The Unimatic single dose preassembled syringe has a 20-gauge needle and is 1½" long.)
Storage: Vials should be stored at room temperature. Warming and shaking the vial will redissolve any crystals that may have formed during storage at low temperatures. Unimatic single-dose preassembled syringes should be stored at room temperature.

DIATRIZOATE MEGLUMINE INJECTION USP 76% ℞

(See Diagnostic Section)

FUNGIZONE® ℞
(Amphotericin B)
CREAM/LOTION/OINTMENT

Description: Fungizone Cream (Amphotericin B Cream USP) contains the antifungal antibiotic Amphotericin B USP at a concentration of 3% (30 mg./gram) in a pleasantly tinted aqueous vehicle, which also contains titanium dioxide, thimerosal, propylene glycol, cetearyl alcohol (and) ceteareth-20, white petrolatum, methylparaben, propylparaben, sorbitol solution, glyceryl monostearate, polyethylene glycol monostearate, simethicone, and sorbic acid.
Fungizone Lotion (Amphotericin B Lotion USP) contains the antifungal antibiotic Amphotericin B USP at a concentration of 3% (30 mg./ml.) in a tinted aqueous lotion vehicle, which is pleasantly scented, and also contains thimerosal, titanium dioxide, guar gum, propylene glycol, cetyl alcohol, stearyl alcohol, sorbitan monopalmitate, polysorbate 20, glyceryl monostearate, polyethylene glycol monostearate, simethicone, sorbic acid, methylparaben, and propylparaben.
Fungizone Ointment (Amphotericin B Ointment USP) contains the antifungal antibiotic Amphotericin B USP at a concentration of 3% (30 mg./gram) in a tinted form of Plastibase® (Plasticized Hydrocarbon Gel), a polyethylene and mineral oil gel base with titanium dioxide.
Clinical Pharmacology: Amphotericin B is an antibiotic with antifungal activity which is produced by a strain of *Streptomyces nodosus.* It has been shown to exhibit greater *in vitro* activity than nystatin against *Candida* (Monilia) *albicans.* In clinical studies involving cutaneous and mucocutaneous candidal infections, results with topical preparations of amphotericin B were comparable to those obtained with nystatin in similar formulations.
Although amphotericin B exhibits some *in vitro* activity against the superficial dermatophytes (ringworm organisms), it has not demonstrated an effectiveness *in vivo* on topical application. Amphotericin B has no significant effect either *in vitro* or clinically against gram-positive or gram-negative bacteria, or viruses.
Indications and Usage: Fungizone (Amphotericin B) topical preparations are indicated in the treatment of cutaneous and mucocutaneous mycotic infections caused by Candida (Monilia) species.
Contraindications: The preparations are contraindicated in patients with a history of hypersensitivity to any of their components.
Precautions: Should a reaction of hypersensitivity occur the drug should be immediately withdrawn and appropriate measures taken.
Adverse Reactions: Fungizone Cream (Amphotericin B Cream USP)—No evidence of any systemic toxicity or side effects has been observed during or following the use of the Cream. The preparation is usually well tolerated by all age groups. It is not a primary irritant and apparently has only a slight sensitizing potential. It may have a "drying" effect on some skin, and local irritation characterized by erythema, pruritus, or a burning sensation sometimes occurs, particularly in intertriginous areas.
Fungizone Lotion (Amphotericin B Lotion USP)—No evidence of any systemic toxicity or side effects has been observed during or following even prolonged, intensive and extensive application of the Lotion. The preparation is extremely well tolerated by all age groups, including infants, even when therapy must be continued for many months. It is not a primary irritant and apparently has only a slight sensitizing potential. Local intolerance, which seldom occurs, has included increased pruritus with or without other subjective or objective evidence of local irritation, or exacerbation of preexisting candidal lesions. Allergic contact dermatitis is rare.
Fungizone Ointment (Amphotericin B Ointment USP)—No evidence of any systemic toxicity or side effects has been observed during or following even prolonged, intensive and extensive application of the Ointment. The preparation is usually well tolerated by all age groups. It is not a primary irritant and apparently has only a slight sensitizing potential. However, it is well to remember that any oleaginous ointment vehicle may occasionally irritate when applied to moist, intertriginous areas.
Dosage and Administration: Fungizone (Amphotericin B) Cream, Lotion, or Ointment should be applied liberally to the candidal lesions two to four times daily. Duration of therapy depends on individual patient response. Intertriginous lesions usually respond within a few days, and treatment may be completed in one to three weeks. Similarly, candidiasis of the diaper area, perleche, and glabrous skin lesions usually clear in one to two weeks. Interdigital (erosio) lesions may require two to four weeks of intensive therapy; paronychias also require relatively prolonged therapy, and those onychomycoses which respond may require several months or more of treatment. (Relapses are frequently encountered in the last three clinical conditions.)
NOTE: When rubbed into the lesion, the Cream discolors the skin minimally. The Lotion and Ointment do not stain the skin when thoroughly rubbed into the lesion although nail lesions may be stained. The patient should be informed that any discoloration of fabrics from the Cream may be removed by hand-washing the fabric with soap and warm water, that any discoloration of fabrics from the Lotion is readily removed with soap and warm water, or that any discoloration of fabrics from the Ointment may be removed by applying a standard cleaning fluid.
How Supplied: Fungizone Cream (Amphotericin B Cream USP) is supplied in tubes of 20 grams.
Fungizone Lotion (Amphotericin B Lotion USP) is supplied in 30 ml. plastic squeeze bottles (Military Depot Item, NSN 6505-00-890-1486).
Fungizone Ointment (Amphotericin B Ointment USP) is supplied in tubes of 20 grams.
Storage: Store the Cream and Lotion at room temperature; avoid freezing. Store the Ointment at room temperature.

FUNGIZONE® INTRAVENOUS ℞
(Amphotericin B for Injection USP)

> **WARNING**
> This drug should be used *primarily* for treatment of patients with progressive and potentially fatal fungal infections; it should not be used to treat the common clinically inapparent forms of fungal disease which show only positive skin or serologic tests.

Description: Fungizone Intravenous (Amphotericin B for Injection USP) is an antifungal antibiotic derived from a strain of *Streptomyces nodosus.* Crystalline amphotericin B is insoluble in water; therefore, the antibiotic is "solubilized" by the addition of sodium desoxycholate to form a mixture which provides a colloidal dispersion for parenteral administration.

Actions:

Microbiology

Amphotericin B shows a high order of *in vitro* activity against many species of fungi. *Histoplasma capsulatum, Coccidiodes immitis, Candida* species, *Blastomyces dermatitidis, Rhodotorula, Cryptococcus neoformans, Sporotrichum schenckii, Mucor mucedo,* and *Aspergillus fumigatus* are all inhibited by concentrations of amphotericin B ranging from 0.03 to 1.0 mcg./ml. *in vitro.* The antibiotic is without effect on bacteria, rickettsiae, and viruses.

Clinical Pharmacology

Amphotericin B is fungistatic or fungicidal depending on the concentration obtained in body fluids and the susceptibility of the fungus. The drug probably acts by binding to sterols in the fungus cell membrane with a resultant change in membrane permeability which allows leakage of a variety of small molecules. Mammalian cell membranes also contain sterols and it has been suggested that the damage to human cells and fungal cells may share common mechanisms.

An initial intravenous infusion of 1 to 5 mg. of amphotericin B per day, gradually increased to 0.65 mg./kg. daily, produces peak plasma concentrations of approximately 2 to 4 mcg./ml. which can persist between doses since the plasma half-life of amphotericin B is about 24 hours. (For recommended dosages, see the DOSAGE AND ADMINISTRATION section.)

It has been reported that amphotericin B is highly bound (>90%) to plasma proteins and is poorly dialyzable.

Amphotericin B is excreted very slowly by the kidneys with two to five percent of a given dose being excreted in biologically active form. After treatment is discontinued, the drug can be detected in the urine for at least seven weeks. The cumulative urinary output over a seven-day period amounts to approximately 40 percent of the amount of drug infused.

Details of tissue distribution and possible metabolic pathways are not known.

Indications: Fungizone Intravenous should be administered primarily to patients with progressive, potentially fatal infections. This potent drug should not be used to treat the common inapparent forms of fungal disease which show only positive skin or serologic tests.

Fungizone Intravenous (Amphotericin B for Injection USP) is specifically intended to treat cryptococcosis (torulosis); North American blastomycosis; the disseminated forms of moniliasis, coccidioidomycosis, and histoplasmosis; mucormycosis (phycomycosis) caused by species of the genera *Mucor, Rhizopus, Absidia, Entomophthora,* and *Basidiobolus;* sporotrichosis (*Sporothrix schenckii* [formerly *Sporotrichum schenckii*]); aspergillosis (*Aspergillus fumigatus*).

Amphotericin B may be helpful in the treatment of American mucocutaneous leishmaniasis, but is not the drug of choice in primary therapy.

Contraindications: This product is contraindicated in those patients who have shown hypersensitivity to it unless, in the opinion of the physician, the condition requiring treatment is life-threatening and amenable only to amphotericin B therapy.

Warnings: Amphotericin B is frequently the only effective treatment available for potentially fatal fungal disease. In each case, its possible life-saving benefit must be balanced against its untoward and dangerous side effects.

Usage in Pregnancy: Safety for use in pregnancy has not been established; therefore, it should be used during pregnancy only if the possible benefits to be derived outweigh the potential risks involved.

Precautions: Prolonged therapy with amphotericin B is usually necessary. Unpleasant reactions are quite common when the drug is given parenterally at therapeutic dosage levels. **Some of these reactions are potentially dangerous.** Hence, amphotericin B should be used parenterally only in hospitalized patients or those under close clinical observation by medically trained personnel and should be reserved for those patients in whom a diagnosis of the progressive, potentially fatal forms of susceptible mycotic infections has been firmly established, preferably by positive culture or histologic study.

Corticosteroids should not be administered concomitantly unless they are necessary to control drug reactions. Other nephrotoxic antibiotics and antineoplastic agents such as nitrogen mustard should not be given concomitantly except with great caution.

Laboratory facilities must be available to perform blood urea nitrogen and serum creatinine or endogenous creatinine clearance tests. These determinations should be made at least weekly during therapy. If the BUN exceeds 40 mg. per 100 ml. or the serum creatinine exceeds 3.0 mg. per 100 ml. the drug should be discontinued or the dosage markedly reduced until renal function is improved. Weekly hemograms and serum potassium determinations are also advisable. Low serum magnesium levels have also been noted during treatment with amphotericin B. Therapy should be discontinued if liver function test results (elevated bromsulphalein, alkaline phosphatase and bilirubin) are abnormal.

Whenever medication is interrupted for a period longer than seven days, therapy should be resumed by starting with the lowest dosage level, e.g., 0.25 mg./kg. of body weight, and increased gradually as outlined under DOSAGE AND ADMINISTRATION.

Adverse Reactions: While some few patients may tolerate full intravenous doses of amphotericin B without difficulty, most will exhibit some intolerance, often at less than the full therapeutic dosage. They may be made less severe by giving aspirin, antihistamines, and antiemetics. Administration of the drug on alternate days may decrease anorexia and phlebitis. Intravenous administration of small doses of adrenal corticosteroids just prior to or during the amphotericin B infusion may decrease febrile reactions. The dosage and duration of such corticosteroid therapy should be kept to a minimum. Adding a small amount of heparin to the infusion may lessen the incidence of thrombophlebitis. Extravasation may cause chemical irritation.

The adverse reactions that are most commonly observed are: fever (sometimes with shaking chills); headache; anorexia; weight loss; nausea and vomiting; malaise; dyspepsia; diarrhea; generalized pain including muscle and joint pains, cramping epigastric pain, and local venous pain at the injection site with phlebitis and thrombophlebitis; and normochromic, normocytic anemia. Abnormal renal function including hypokalemia, azotemia, hyposthenuria, renal tubular acidosis and nephrocalcinosis is also commonly observed, and usually improves upon interruption of therapy; however, some permanent impairment often occurs, especially in those patients receiving large amounts (over 5 g.) of amphotericin B. Supplemental alkali medication may decrease renal tubular acidosis complications.

The following adverse reactions occur less frequently or rarely: anuria; oliguria; cardiovascular toxicity including arrhythmias, ventricular fibrillation, cardiac arrest, hypertension, and hypotension; coagulation defects; thrombocytopenia; leukopenia; agranulocytosis; eosinophilia; leukocytosis; melena or hemorrhagic gastroenteritis; maculopapular rash; hearing loss; tinnitus; transient vertigo; blurred vision or diplopia; peripheral neuropathy; convulsions and other neurologic symptoms; pruritus (without rash); anaphylactoid reactions; acute liver failure; and flushing.

Dosage and Administration: Fungizone Intravenous (Amphotericin B for Injection USP) should be administered by *slow* intravenous infusion. Intravenous infusion should be given over a period of approximately six hours observing the usual precautions for intravenous therapy. The recommended concentration for intravenous infusion is 0.1 mg./ml. (1 mg./10 ml.).

Dosage must be adjusted to the specific requirements of each patient since tolerance to amphotericin B varies individually. Therapy is usually instituted with a daily dose of 0.25 mg./kg. of body weight and **gradually** increased as tolerance permits. There are insufficient data presently available to define total dosage requirements and duration of treatment necessary for eradication of mycoses such as phycomycosis. The optimal dose is unknown. Total daily dosage may range up to 1.0 mg./kg. of body weight or alternate day dosages ranging up to 1.5 mg./kg. Several months of therapy are usually necessary; a shorter period of therapy may produce an inadequate response and lead to relapse.

CAUTION: Under no circumstances should a total daily dosage of 1.5 mg./kg. be exceeded.

Therapy with intravenous amphotericin B for sporotrichosis has ranged up to nine months. The usual dose per injection is 20 mg.

Aspergillosis has been treated with amphotericin B intravenously for a period up to 11 months with a total dose up to 3.6 g.

Rhinocerebral phycomycosis, a fulminating disease, generally occurs in association with diabetic ketoacidosis. It is, therefore, imperative that rapid restoration of diabetic control be instituted before successful treatment with Fungizone Intravenous (Amphotericin B for Injection USP) can be accomplished. In contradistinction, pulmonary phycomycosis, which is more common in association with hematologic malignancies, is often an incidental finding at autopsy. A cumulative dose of at least 3 g. of amphotericin B is recommended. Although a total dose of 3 to 4 g. will infrequently cause lasting renal impairment, this would seem a reasonable minimum where there is clinical evidence of invasion of the deep tissues; since rhinocerebral phycomycosis usually follows a rapidly fatal course, the therapeutic approach must necessarily be more aggressive than that used in more indolent mycoses.

Preparation of Solutions: Reconstitute as follows: An initial concentrate of 5 mg. amphotericin B per ml. is first prepared by rapidly expressing 10 ml. Sterile Water for Injection USP *without a bacteriostatic agent* directly into the lyophilized cake, using a sterile needle (minimum diameter: 20 gauge) and syringe. Shake the vial immediately until the colloidal solution is clear. The infusion solution, providing 0.1 mg. amphotericin B per ml., is then obtained by further dilution (1:50) with 5% Dextrose Injection USP *of pH above 4.2.* The pH of

Continued on next page

Squibb—Cont.

each container of Dextrose Injection should be ascertained before use. Commercial Dextrose Injection usually has a pH above 4.2; however, if it is below 4.2, then 1 or 2 ml. of buffer should be added to the Dextrose Injection before it is used to dilute the concentrated solution of amphotericin B. The recommended buffer has the following composition:

Dibasic sodium phosphate (anhydrous)	1.59 g.
Monobasic sodium phosphate (anhydrous)	0.96 g.
Water for Injection USP	qs. 100.0 ml.

The buffer should be sterilized before it is added to the Dextrose Injection, either by filtration through a bacterial retentive stone, mat, or membrane, or by autoclaving for 30 minutes at 15 lb. pressure (121° C.).

CAUTION: Aseptic technique must be strictly observed in all handling, since no preservative or bacteriostatic agent is present in the antibiotic or in the materials used to prepare it for administration. **All entries into the vial or into the diluents must be made with a sterile needle. Do not reconstitute with saline solutions. The use of any diluent other than the ones recommended or the presence of a bacteriostatic agent** (e.g., benzyl alcohol) **in the diluent may cause precipitation of the antibiotic. Do not use the initial concentrate or the infusion solution if there is any evidence of precipitation or foreign matter in either one.**

An in-line membrane filter may be used for intravenous infusion of amphotericin B; **however, the mean pore diameter of the filter should not be less than 1.0 micron in order to assure passage of the antibiotic dispersion.**

How Supplied: Fungizone Intravenous is supplied in vials as a sterile lyophilized cake (which may partially reduce to powder following manufacture) providing 50 mg. amphotericin B and 41 mg. sodium desoxycholate with 20.2 mg. sodium phosphates as a buffer. At the time of manufacture, the air in the container is replaced by nitrogen.

Storage: Prior to reconstitution, Fungizone Intravenous (Amphotericin B for injection USP) should be stored in the refrigerator, protected against exposure to light. The concentrate (5 mg. amphotericin B per ml. after reconstitution with 10 ml. Sterile Water for Injection USP) may be stored in the dark, at room temperature for 24 hours, or at refrigerator temperatures for one week with minimal loss of potency and clarity. Any unused material should then be discarded. Solutions prepared for intravenous infusion (0.1 mg. or less amphotericin B per ml.) should be used promptly after preparation and should be protected from light during administration.

GASTROGRAFIN® ℞
(Diatrizoate Meglumine and Diatrizoate Sodium Solution USP)

(See Diagnostic Section)

HALCIDERM® CREAM ℞
(Halcinonide Cream 0.1%)

Description: The topical corticosteroids constitute a class of primarily synthetic steroids used as anti-inflammatory and antipruritic agents. The steroids in this class include halcinonide. Halcinonide is designated chemically as 21-Chloro-9-fluoro-11β, 16α,17-trihydroxypregn-4-ene-3,20-dione cyclic 16,17-acetal with acetone.

Each gram of 0.1% Halciderm Cream (Halcinonide Cream) contains 1 mg. halcinonide in a hydrophilic vanishing cream base consisting of propylene glycol, dimethicone 350, castor oil, cetearyl alcohol (and) ceteareth-20, propylene glycol stearate, white petrolatum, and purified water. This formulation is water-washable, greaseless, and nonstaining, with moisturizing and emollient properties.

Clinical Pharmacology: Topical corticosteroids share anti-inflammatory, antipruritic and vasoconstrictive actions.

The mechanism of anti-inflammatory activity of the topical corticosteroids is unclear. Various laboratory methods, including vasoconstrictor assays, are used to compare and predict potencies and/or clinical efficacies of the topical corticosteroids. There is some evidence to suggest that a recognizable correlation exists between vasoconstrictor potency and therapeutic efficacy in man.

Pharmacokinetics: The extent of percutaneous absorption of topical corticosteroids is determined by many factors including the vehicle, the integrity of the epidermal barrier, and the use of occlusive dressings.

Topical corticosteroids can be absorbed from normal intact skin. Inflammation and/or other disease processes in the skin increase percutaneous absorption. Occlusive dressings substantially increase the percutaneous absorption of topical corticosteroids. Thus, occlusive dressings may be a valuable therapeutic adjunct for treatment of resistant dermatoses (see DOSAGE AND ADMINISTRATION).

Once absorbed through the skin, topical corticosteroids are handled through pharmacokinetic pathways similar to systemically administered corticosteroids. Corticosteroids are bound to plasma proteins in varying degrees. Corticosteroids are metabolized primarily in the liver and are then excreted by the kidneys. Some of the topical corticosteroids and their metabolites are also excreted into the bile.

Indications and Usage: Halciderm Cream is indicated for the relief of the inflammatory and pruritic manifestations of corticosteroid-responsive dermatoses.

Contraindication: Topical corticosteroids are contraindicated in those patients with a history of hypersensitivity to any of the components of the preparations.

Precautions: General: Systemic absorption of topical corticosteroids has produced reversible hypothalamic-pituitary-adrenal (HPA) axis suppression, manifestations of Cushing's syndrome, hyperglycemia, and glucosuria in some patients.

Conditions which augment systemic absorption include the application of the more potent steroids, use over large surface areas, prolonged use, and the addition of occlusive dressings.

Therefore, patients receiving a large dose of any potent topical steroid applied to a large surface area or under an occlusive dressing should be evaluated periodically for evidence of HPA axis suppression by using the urinary free cortisol and ACTH stimulation tests, and for impairment of thermal homeostasis. If HPA axis suppression or elevation of the body temperature occurs, an attempt should be made to withdraw the drug, to reduce the frequency of application, substitute a less potent steroid, or use a sequential approach when utilizing the occlusive technique.

Recovery of HPA axis function and thermal homeostasis are generally prompt and complete upon discontinuation of the drug. Infrequently, signs and symptoms of steroid withdrawal may occur, requiring supplemental systemic corticosteroids. Occasionally, a patient may develop a sensitivity reaction to a particular occlusive dressing material or adhesive and a substitute material may be necessary.

Children may absorb proportionally larger amounts of topical corticosteroids and thus be more susceptible to systemic toxicity (see PRECAUTIONS, Pediatric Use).

If irritation develops, topical corticosteroids should be discontinued and appropriate therapy instituted.

In the presence of dermatological infections, the use of an appropriate antifungal or antibacterial agent should be instituted. If a favorable response does not occur promptly, the corticosteroid should be discontinued until the infection has been adequately controlled.

Information for the Patient: Patients using topical corticosteroids should receive the following information and instructions:

1. This medication is to be used as directed by the physician. It is for external use only. Avoid contact with the eyes.
2. Patients should be advised not to use this medication for any disorder other than for which it was prescribed.
3. The treated skin area should not be bandaged or otherwise covered or wrapped as to be occlusive unless directed by the physician.
4. Patients should report any signs of local adverse reactions especially under occlusive dressing.
5. Parents of pediatric patients should be advised not to use tight-fitting diapers or plastic pants on a child being treated in the diaper area, as these garments may constitute occlusive dressings.

Laboratory Tests: A urinary free cortisol test and ACTH stimulation test may be helpful in evaluating HPA axis suppression.

Carcinogenesis, Mutagenesis, and Impairment of Fertility: Long-term animal studies have not been performed to evaluate the carcinogenic potential or the effect on fertility of topical corticosteroids. Studies to determine mutagenicity with prednisolone and hydrocortisone showed negative results.

Pregnancy: Teratogenic Effects: Category C. Corticosteroids are generally teratogenic in laboratory animals when administered systemically at relatively low dosage levels. The more potent corticosteroids have been shown to be teratogenic after dermal application in laboratory animals. There are no adequate and well-controlled studies in pregnant women on teratogenic effects from topically applied corticosteroids. Therefore, topical corticosteroids should be used during pregnancy only if the potential benefit justifies the potential risk to the fetus. Drugs of this class should not be used extensively on pregnant patients, in large amounts, or for prolonged periods of time.

Nursing Mothers: It is not known whether topical administration of corticosteroids could result in sufficient systemic absorption to produce detectable quantities in breast milk. Systemically administered corticosteroids are secreted into breast milk in quantities **not** likely to have a deleterious effect on the infant. Nevertheless, caution should be exercised when topical corticosteroids are administered to a nursing woman.

Pediatric Use: Pediatric patients may demonstrate greater susceptibility to topical corticosteroid-induced HPA axis suppression and Cushing's syndrome than mature patients because of a larger skin surface area to body weight ratio.

HPA axis suppression, Cushing's syndrome, and intracranial hypertension have been reported in children receiving topical corticosteroids. Manifestations of adrenal suppression in children include linear growth retardation, delayed weight gain, low plasma cortisol levels, and absence of response to ACTH stimulation. Manifestations of intracranial hypertension include bulging fontanelles, headaches, and bilateral papilledema.

Administration of topical corticosteroids to children should be limited to the least amount compatible with an effective therapeutic regimen. Chronic corticosteroid therapy may interfere with the growth and development of children.

Adverse Reactions: The following local adverse reactions are reported infrequently with topical corticosteroids, but may occur more frequently with the use of occlusive dressings (reactions are listed in an approximate decreasing order of occurrence): burning, itching, irritation, dryness, folliculitis, hypertrichosis, acneiform eruptions, hypopigmentation, perioral dermatitis, allergic contact dermatitis, maceration of the skin, secondary infection, skin atrophy, striae, and miliaria.

Overdosage: Topically applied corticosteroids can be absorbed in sufficient amounts to produce systemic effects (see PRECAUTIONS, General).

Dosage and Administration: Apply Halciderm Cream (Halcinonide Cream) 0.1% to the affected area one to three times daily. Rub in gently.

Occlusive Dressing Technique: Occlusive dressings may be used for the management of psoriasis or other recalcitrant conditions. Gently rub a small amount of the cream into the lesion until it disappears. Reapply the preparation leaving a thin coating on the lesion, cover with a pliable nonporous film, and seal the edges. If needed, additional moisture may be provided by covering the lesion with a dampened clean cotton cloth before the nonporous film is applied or by briefly wetting the affected area with water immediately prior to applying the medication. The frequency of changing dressings is best determined on an individual basis. It may be convenient to apply the cream under an occlusive dressing in the evening and to remove the dressing in the morning (i.e., 12-hour occlusion). When utilizing the 12-hour occlusion regimen, additional cream should be applied, without occlusion, during the day. Reapplication is essential at each dressing change. If an infection develops, the use of occlusive dressings should be discontinued and appropriate antimicrobial therapy instituted.

How Supplied: Available in 15 g., 30 g., and 60 g. tubes.

Storage: Store at room temperature; avoid freezing and refrigeration.

HALOG® ℞
(Halcinonide)
CREAM/OINTMENT/SOLUTION

Description: The topical corticosteroids constitute a class of primarily synthetic steroids used as anti-inflammatory and antipruritic agents. The steroids in this class include halcinonide. Halcinonide is designated chemically as 21-Chloro-9-fluoro-11β,16α,17-trihydroxypregn-4-ene-3,20-dione cyclic 16,17-acetal with actone.

Each gram of 0.025% Halog Cream (Halcinonide Cream) contains 0.25 mg. halcinonide in a specially formulated cream base consisting of glyceryl monostearate NF XII, cetyl alcohol, cetyl esters wax, polysorbate 60, propylene glycol, dimethicone 350, and purified water.

Each gram of 0.1% Halog Cream (Halcinonide Cream) contains 1 mg. halcinonide in a specially formulated cream base consisting of glyceryl monostearate NF XII, cetyl alcohol, isopropyl palmitate, dimethicone 350, polysorbate 60, titanium dioxide, propylene glycol, and purified water.

Each gram of 0.025% Halog Ointment (Halcinonide Ointment) contains 0.25 mg. halcinonide in Plastibase® (Plasticized Hydrocarbon Gel), a polyethylene and mineral oil gel base with polyethylene glycol 400, polyethylene glycol 6000 distearate, polyethylene glycol 300, polyethylene glycol 1540, and butylated hydroxytoluene as a preservative. Each gram of 0.1% Halog Ointment (Halcinonide Ointment) contains 1 mg. halcinonide in Plastibase, a polyethylene and mineral oil gel base with polyethylene glycol 400, polyethylene glycol 6000 distearate, polyethylene glycol 300, polyethylene glycol 1540, and butylated hydroxytoluene as a preservative.

Each ml. of 0.1% Halog Solution (Halcinonide Solution) contains 1 mg. halcinonide with edetate disodium, polyethylene glycol 300, purified water, and butylated hydroxytoluene as a preservative.

Clinical Pharmacology: Topical corticosteroids share anti-inflammatory, antipruritic and vasoconstrictive actions.

The mechanism of anti-inflammatory activity of the topical corticosteroids is unclear. Various laboratory methods, including vasoconstrictor assays, are used to compare and predict potencies and/or clinical efficacies of the topical corticosteroids. There is some evidence to suggest that a recognizable correlation exists between vasoconstrictor potency and therapeutic efficacy in man.

Pharmacokinetics: The extent of percutaneous absorption of topical corticosteroids is determined by many factors including the vehicle, the integrity of the epidermal barrier, and the use of occlusive dressings.

Topical corticosteroids can be absorbed from normal intact skin. Inflammation and/or other disease processes in the skin increase percutaneous absorption. Occlusive dressings substantially increase the percutaneous absorption of topical corticosteroids. Thus, occlusive dressings may be a valuable therapeutic adjunct for treatment of resistant dermatoses (see DOSAGE AND ADMINISTRATION).

Once absorbed through the skin, topical corticosteroids are handled through pharmacokinetic pathways similar to systemically administered corticosteroids. Corticosteroids are bound to plasma proteins in varying degrees. Corticosteroids are metabolized primarily in the liver and are then excreted by the kidneys. Some of the topical corticosteroids and their metabolites are also excreted into the bile.

Indications and Usage: Halog (Halcinonide) preparations are indicated for the relief of the inflammatory and pruritic manifestations of corticosteroid-responsive dermatoses.

Contraindications: Topical corticosteroids are contraindicated in those patients with a history of hypersensitivity to any of the components of the preparations.

Precautions: General: Systemic absorption of topical corticosteroids has produced reversible hypothalamic-pituitary-adrenal (HPA) axis suppression, manifestations of Cushing's syndrome, hyperglycemia, and glucosuria in some patients.

Conditions which augment systemic absorption include the application of the more potent steroids, use over large surface areas, prolonged use, and the addition of occlusive dressings.

Therefore, patients receiving a large dose of any potent topical steroid applied to a large surface area or under an occlusive dressing should be evaluated periodically for evidence of HPA axis suppression by using the urinary free cortisol and ACTH stimulation tests, and for impairment of thermal homeostasis. If HPA axis suppression or elevation of the body temperature occurs, an attempt should be made to withdraw the drug, to reduce the frequency of application, substitute a less potent steroid, or use a sequential approach when utilizing the occlusive technique.

Recovery of HPA axis function and thermal homeostasis are generally prompt and complete upon discontinuation of the drug. Infrequently, signs and symptoms of steroid withdrawal may occur, requiring supplemental systemic corticosteroids. Occasionally, a patient may develop a sensitivity reaction to a particular occlusive dressing material or adhesive and a substitute material may be necessary.

Children may absorb proportionally larger amounts of topical corticosteroids and thus be more susceptible to systemic toxicity (see PRECAUTIONS, Pediatric Use).

If irritation develops, topical corticosteroids should be discontinued and appropriate therapy instituted.

In the presence of dermatological infections, the use of an appropriate antifungal or antibacterial agent should be instituted. If a favorable response does not occur promptly, the corticosteroid should be discontinued until the infection has been adequately controlled.

Information for the Patient: Patients using topical corticosteroids should receive the following information and instructions:

1. This medication is to be used as directed by the physician. It is for external use only. Avoid contact with the eyes.
2. Patients should be advised not to use this medication for any disorder other than for which it was prescribed.
3. The treated skin area should not be bandaged or otherwise covered or wrapped as to be occlusive unless directed by the physician.
4. Patients should report any signs of local adverse reactions especially under occlusive dressing.
5. Parents of pediatric patients should be advised not to use tight-fitting diapers or plastic pants on a child being treated in the diaper area, as these garments may constitute occlusive dressings.

Laboratory Tests: A urinary free cortisol test and ACTH stimulation test may be helpful in evaluating HPA axis suppression.

Carcinogenesis, Mutagenesis, and Impairment of Fertility: Long-term animal studies have not been performed to evaluate the carcinogenic potential or the effect on fertility of topical corticosteroids. Studies to determine mutagenicity with prednisolone and hydrocortisone showed negative results.

Pregnancy: Teratogenic Effects: Category C. Corticosteroids are generally teratogenic in laboratory animals when administered systemically at relatively low dosage levels. The more potent corticosteroids have been shown to be teratogenic after dermal application in laboratory animals. There are no adequate and well-controlled studies in pregnant women on teratogenic effects from topically applied corticosteroids. Therefore, topical corticosteroids should be used during pregnancy only if the potential benefit justifies the potential risk to the fetus. Drugs of this class should not be used extensively on pregnant patients, in large amounts, or for prolonged periods of time.

Nursing Mothers: It is not known whether topical administration of corticosteroids could result in sufficient systemic absorption to produce detectable quantities in breast milk. Systemically administered corticosteroids are secreted into breast milk in quantities **not** likely to have a deleterious effect on the infant. Nevertheless, caution should be exercised when topical corticosteroids are administered to a nursing woman.

Pediatric Use: Pediatric patients may demonstrate greater susceptibility to topical corticosteroid-induced HPA axis suppression and Cushing's syndrome than mature patients because of a larger skin surface area to body weight ratio.

HPA axis suppression, Cushing's syndrome, and intracranial hypertension have been reported in children receiving topical corticosteroids. Manifestations of adrenal suppression in children include linear growth retardation, delayed weight gain, low plasma cortisol levels, and absence of response to ACTH stimulation. Manifestations of intracranial hypertension include bulging fontanelles, headaches, and bilateral papilledema.

Administration of topical corticosteroids to children should be limited to the least amount compatible with an effective therapeutic regimen. Chronic corticosteroid therapy may in-

Continued on next page

Squibb—Cont.

terfere with the growth and development of children.

Adverse Reactions: The following local adverse reactions are reported infrequently with topical corticosteroids, but may occur more frequently with the use of occlusive dressings (reactions are listed in an approximate decreasing order of occurrence): burning, itching, irritation, dryness, folliculitis, hypertrichosis, acneiform eruptions, hypopigmentation, perioral dermatitis, allergic contact dermatitis, maceration of the skin, secondary infection, skin atrophy, striae, and miliaria.

Overdosage: Topically applied corticosteroids can be absorbed in sufficient amounts to produce systemic effects (see PRECAUTIONS, General).

Dosage and Administration: Halog Cream (Halcinonide Cream): Apply the 0.025% or the 0.1% Halog Cream (Halcinonide Cream) to the affected area two to three times daily. Rub in gently.

Halog Ointment (Halcinonide Ointment): Apply a thin film of the 0.025% or the 0.1% Halog Ointment (Halcinonide Ointment) to the affected area two to three times daily.

Halog Solution (Halcinonide Solution) 0.1%: Apply to the affected area two to three times daily.

Occlusive Dressing Technique: Occlusive dressings may be used for the management of psoriasis or other recalcitrant conditions.

Halog Cream (Halcinonide Cream) 0.025% and 0.1%: Gently rub a small amount of the cream into the lesion until it disappears. Reapply the preparation leaving a thin coating on the lesion, cover with a pliable nonporous film, and seal the edges. If needed, additional moisture may be provided by covering the lesion with a dampened clean cotton cloth before the nonporous film is applied or by briefly wetting the affected area with water immediately prior to applying the medication. The frequency of changing dressings is best determined on an individual basis. It may be convenient to apply the cream under an occlusive dressing in the evening and to remove the dressing in the morning (i.e., 12-hour occlusion). When utilizing the 12-hour occlusion regimen, additional cream should be applied, without occlusion, during the day. Reapplication is essential at each dressing change. If an infection develops, the use of occlusive dressings should be discontinued and appropriate antimicrobial therapy instituted.

Halog Ointment (Halcinonide Ointment) 0.025% and 0.1%: Apply a thin film of the ointment to the lesion, cover with a pliable nonporous film, and seal the edges. If needed, additional moisture may be provided by covering the lesion with a dampened clean cotton cloth before the nonporous film is applied or by briefly wetting the affected area with water immediately prior to applying the medication. The frequency of changing dressings is best determined on an individual basis. It may be convenient to apply the ointment under an occlusive dressing in the evening and to remove the dressing in the morning (i.e., 12-hour occlusion). When utilizing the 12-hour occlusion regimen, additional ointment should be applied, without occlusion, during the day. Reapplication is essential at each dressing change. If an infection develops, the use of occlusive dressings should be discontinued and appropriate antimicrobial therapy instituted.

Halog Solution (Halcinonide Solution) 0.1%: Apply the solution to the lesion, cover with a pliable nonporous film, and seal the edges. If needed, additional moisture may be provided by covering the lesion with a dampened clean cotton cloth before the nonporous film is applied or by briefly wetting the affected area with water immediately prior to applying the medication. The frequency of changing dressings is best determined on an individual basis. It may be convenient to apply the solution under an occlusive dressing in the evening and to remove the dressing in the morning (i.e., 12-hour occlusion). When utilizing the 12-hour occlusion regimen, additional solution should be applied, without occlusion, during the day. Reapplication is essential at each dressing change. If an infection develops, the use of occlusive dressings should be discontinued and appropriate antimicrobial therapy instituted.

How Supplied: 0.025% Cream—Tubes of 15 g. and 60 g.; jars of 240 g. (8 oz.). 0.1% Cream—Tubes of 15 g., 30 g., and 60 g.; jars of 240 g. (8 oz.). [0.1% Cream, 60 g.—V.A. Depot Item NSN 6505-01-007-9895A]. 0.025% Ointment—Tubes of 15 g. and 60 g. 0.1% Ointment—Tubes of 15 g., 30 g., and 60 g.; jars of 240 g. (8 oz.). 0.1% Solution—Plastic squeeze bottles of 20 ml. and 60 ml.

Storage: Store the 0.025% and 0.1% Creams at room temperature; avoid excessive heat (104°F). Store the 0.025% and 0.1% Ointments at room temperature; avoid excessive heat (104°F). Store the Solution at room temperature; avoid freezing and temperatures above 104°F.

HYDREA® ℞

(Hydroxyurea Capsules USP)

Description: Hydrea (Hydroxyurea Capsules USP) is an antineoplastic agent, available for oral use as capsules providing 500 mg. hydroxyurea. Hydroxyurea occurs as an essentially tasteless, white crystalline powder.

Actions: Mechanism of Action

The precise mechanism by which hydroxyurea produces its cytotoxic effects cannot, at present, be described. However, the reports of various studies in tissue culture in rats and man lend support to the hypothesis that hydroxyurea causes an immediate inhibition of DNA synthesis without interfering with the synthesis of ribonucleic acid or of protein. This hypothesis explains why, under certain conditions, hydroxyurea may induce teratogenic effects.

Three mechanisms of action have been postulated for the increased effectiveness of concomitant use of hydroxyurea therapy with irradiation on squamous cell (epidermoid) carcinomas of the head and neck. *In vitro* studies utilizing Chinese hamster cells suggest that hydroxyurea (1) is lethal to normally radioresistant S-stage cells, and (2) holds other cells of the cell cycle in the G1 or pre-DNA synthesis stage where they are most susceptible to the effects of irradiation. The third mechanism of action has been theorized on the basis of *in vitro* studies of HeLa cells: it appears that hydroxyurea, by inhibition of DNA synthesis, hinders the normal repair process of cells damaged but not killed by irradiation, thereby decreasing their survival rate; RNA and protein syntheses have shown no alteration.

Absorption, Metabolism, Fate and Excretion

After oral administration in man, hydroxyurea is readily absorbed from the gastrointestinal tract. The drug reaches peak serum concentrations within 2 hours; by 24 hours the concentration in the serum is essentially zero. Approximately 80 percent of an oral or intravenous dose of 7 to 30 mg./kg. may be recovered in the urine within 12 hours.

Animal Pharmacology and Toxicology

The oral LD_{50} of hydroxyurea is 7330 mg./kg. in mice and 5780 mg./kg. in rats, given as a single dose.

In subacute and chronic toxicity studies in the rat, the most consistent pathological findings were an apparent dose-related mild to moderate bone marrow hypoplasia as well as pulmonary congestion and mottling of the lungs. At the highest dosage levels (1260 mg./kg./day for 37 days then 2520 mg./kg./day for 40 days), testicular atrophy with absence of spermatogenesis occurred; in several animals, hepatic cell damage with fatty metamorphosis was noted. In the dog, mild to marked bone marrow depression was a consistent finding except at the lower dosage levels. Additionally, at the higher dose levels (140 to 420 mg. or 140 to 1260 mg./kg./week given 3 or 7 days weekly for 12 weeks), growth retardation, slightly increased blood glucose values, and hemosiderosis of the liver or spleen were found; reversible spermatogenic arrest was noted. In the monkey, bone marrow depression, lymphoid atrophy of the spleen, and degenerative changes in the epithelium of the small and large intestines were found. At the higher, often lethal, doses (400 to 800 mg./kg./day for 7 to 15 days), hemorrhage and congestion were found in the lungs, brain and urinary tract. Cardiovascular effects (changes in heart rate, blood pressure, orthostatic hypotension, EKG changes) and hematological changes (slight hemolysis, slight methemoglobinemia) were observed in some species of laboratory animals at doses exceeding clinical levels.

Indications and Usage: Significant tumor response to Hydrea (Hydroxyurea Capsules USP) has been demonstrated in melanoma, resistant chronic myelocytic leukemia, and recurrent, metastatic, or inoperable carcinoma of the ovary.

Hydrea used concomitantly with irradiation therapy is intended for use in the local control of primary squamous cell (epidermoid) carcinomas of the head and neck, excluding the lip.

Contraindications: Hydroxyurea is contraindicated in patients with marked bone marrow depression, i.e., leukopenia (less than 2500 WBC) or thrombocytopenia (less than 100,000), or severe anemia.

Warnings: Treatment with hydroxyurea should not be initiated if bone marrow function is markedly depressed (—see CONTRAINDICATIONS). Bone marrow suppression may occur, and leukopenia is generally its first and most common manifestation. Thrombocytopenia and anemia occur less often, and are seldom seen without a preceding leukopenia. However, the recovery from myelosuppression is rapid when therapy is interrupted. It should be borne in mind that bone marrow depression is more likely in patients who have previously received radiotherapy or cytotoxic cancer chemotherapeutic agents; hydroxyurea should be used cautiously in such patients.

Patients who have received irradiation therapy in the past may have an exacerbation of postirradiation erythema.

Severe anemia must be corrected with whole blood replacement before initiating therapy with hydroxyurea.

Erythrocytic abnormalities: megaloblastic erythropoiesis, which is self-limiting, is often seen early in the course of hydroxyurea therapy. The morphologic change resembles pernicious anemia, but is not related to vitamin B_{12} or folic acid deficiency. Hydroxyurea may also delay plasma iron clearance and reduce the rate of iron utilization by erythrocytes, but it does not appear to alter the red blood cell survival time.

Hydroxyurea should be used with caution in patients with marked renal dysfunction.

Elderly patients may be more sensitive to the effects of hydroxyurea, and may require a lower dose regimen.

Usage in Pregnancy—Drugs which affect DNA synthesis, such as hydroxyurea, may be potential mutagenic agents. The physician should carefully consider this possibility before administering this drug to male or female patients who may contemplate conception.

Hydrea (Hydroxyurea Capsules USP) is a known teratogenic agent in animals. Therefore, hydroxyurea should not be used in women who are or may become pregnant unless in the judgment of the physician the potential benefits outweigh the possible hazards.

Precautions: Therapy with hydroxyurea requires close supervision. The complete status of the blood, including bone marrow examination, if indicated, as well as kidney function and liver function should be determined prior to, and repeatedly during, treatment. The determination of the hemoglobin level, total leukocyte counts, and platelet counts should be performed at least once a week throughout the course of hydroxyurea therapy. If the white blood cell count decreases to less than 2500/mm^3, or the platelet count to less than 100,000/mm^3, therapy should be interrupted until the values rise significantly toward normal levels. Anemia, if it occurs, should be managed with whole blood replacement, without interrupting hydroxyurea therapy.

Adverse Reactions: Adverse reactions have been primarily bone marrow depression (leukopenia, anemia, and occasionally thrombocytopenia), and less frequently gastrointestinal symptoms (stomatitis, anorexia, nausea, vomiting, diarrhea, and constipation), and dermatological reactions such as maculopapular rash and facial erythema. Dysuria and alopecia occur very rarely. Large doses may produce moderate drowsiness. Neurological disturbances have occurred extremely rarely and were limited to headache, dizziness, disorientation, hallucinations, and convulsions. Hydroxyurea occasionally may cause temporary impairment of renal tubular function accompanied by elevations in serum uric acid, BUN, and creatinine levels. Abnormal BSP retention has been reported. Fever, chills, malaise, and elevation of hepatic enzymes have also been reported.

Adverse reactions observed with combined hydroxyurea and irradiation therapy are similar to those reported with the use of hydroxyurea alone. These effects primarily include bone marrow depression (anemia and leukopenia), and gastric irritation. Almost all patients receiving an adequate course of combined hydroxyurea and irradiation therapy will demonstrate concurrent leukopenia. Platelet depression (less than 100,000 cells/mm^3) has occurred rarely and only in the presence of marked leukopenia. Gastric distress has also been reported with irradiation alone and in combination with hydroxyurea therapy.

It should be borne in mind that therapeutic doses of irradiation alone produce the same adverse reactions as hydroxyurea; combined therapy may cause an increase in the incidence and severity of these side effects.

Although inflammation of the mucous membranes at the irradiated site (mucositis) is attributed to irradiation alone, some investigators believe that the more severe cases are due to combination therapy.

Dosage and Administration: Because of the rarity of melanoma, resistant chronic myelocytic leukemia, carcinoma of the ovary, and carcinomas of the head and neck in children, dosage regimens have not been established.

All dosage should be based on the patient's actual or ideal weight, whichever is less.

NOTE: If the patient prefers, or is unable to swallow capsules, the contents of the capsules may be emptied into a glass of water and taken immediately. Some inert material used as a vehicle in the capsule may not dissolve, and may float on the surface.

Solid Tumors

Intermittent Therapy: 80 mg./kg. administered orally as a *single* dose every *third* day

Continuous Therapy: 20 to 30 mg./kg. administered orally as a *single* dose *daily*

The intermittent dosage schedule offers the advantage of reduced toxicity since patients on this dosage regimen have rarely required complete discontinuance of therapy because of toxicity.

Concomitant Therapy with Irradiation (*Carcinoma of the head and neck*)—80 mg./kg. administered orally as a *single* dose every *third* day.

Administration of Hydrea (Hydroxyurea Capsules USP) should be begun at least seven days before initiation of irradiation and continued during radiotherapy as well as indefinitely afterwards provided that the patient may be kept under adequate observation and evidences no unusual or severe reactions.

Irradiation should be given at the maximum dose considered appropriate for the particular therapeutic situation; adjustment of irradiation dosage is not usually necessary when Hydrea is used concomitantly.

Resistant Chronic Myelocytic Leukemia

Until the intermittent therapy regimen has been evaluated, CONTINUOUS therapy (20 to 30 mg./kg. administered orally as a *single* dose *daily*) is recommended.

An adequate trial period for determining the antineoplastic effectiveness of Hydrea is six weeks of therapy. When there is regression in tumor size or arrest in tumor growth, therapy should be continued indefinitely. Therapy should be interrupted if the white blood cell count drops below 2500/mm^3, or the platelet count below 100,000/mm^3. In these cases, the counts should be rechecked after three days, and therapy resumed when the counts rise significantly toward normal values. Since the hematopoietic rebound is prompt, it is usually necessary to omit only a few doses. If prompt rebound has not occurred during combined hydroxyurea and irradiation therapy, irradiation may also be interrupted. However, the need for postponement of irradiation has been rare; radiotherapy has usually been continued using the recommended dosage and technique.

Anemia, if it occurs, should be corrected with whole blood replacement, without interrupting hydroxyurea therapy. Because hematopoiesis may be compromised by extensive irradiation or by other antineoplastic agents, it is recommended that Hydrea be administered cautiously to patients who have recently received extensive radiation therapy or chemotherapy with other cytotoxic drugs.

Pain or discomfort from inflammation of the mucous membranes at the irradiated site (mucositis) is usually controlled by measures such as topical anesthetics and orally administered analgesics. If the reaction is severe, hydroxyurea therapy may be temporarily interrupted; if it is extremely severe, irradiation dosage may, in addition, be temporarily postponed. However, it has rarely been necessary to terminate these therapies.

Severe gastric distress, such as nausea, vomiting, and anorexia resulting from combined therapy may usually be controlled by temporary interruption of Hydrea (Hydroxyurea Capsules USP) administration; rarely has the additional interruption of irradiation been necessary.

How Supplied: Bottles of 100.

Storage: Store at room temperature; avoid excessive heat; keep bottle tightly closed. Dispense in tight containers.

[*Shown in Product Identification Section*]

INSULIN, SQUIBB®/NOVO™

Squibb carries a full line of insulins sold under the name Squibb®/Novo™. These insulins are manufactured under exacting quality controls and meet all official standards for purity, stability, consistency, and sterility. The insulin in these products has undergone special purification during manufacture, resulting in a reduction of noninsulin protein material (proinsulin) in the formulations to less than 25 parts per million of insulin.* If the word "purified" is in the name of the product, the proinsulin has been reduced to less than ten parts per million.* In Actrapid®, Semitard®, Monotard®, Protaphane™ NPH, and Lentard® and Ultratard® the proinsulin content is less than or equal to one part per million.* The following is a list along with a brief description of each of the insulin preparations available.

*By weight of dry insulin.

STANDARD INSULINS

INSULIN INJECTIONS USP (REGULAR)

Sometimes also called unmodified, ordinary, or plain insulin. The neutral solution is prepared with insulin obtained from pork pancreas. Regular insulin is "unmodified," nothing has been added to change the speed or duration of its action. The product is a clear colorless solution made from zinc-insulin crystals. The onset of action of this insulin is evident in approximately 30 minutes to 1 hour from the time of administration, and its effect persists for approximately 6 to 8 hours.

How Supplied: U-40 (40 units per ml.) and U-100 (100 units per ml.) in 10 ml. vials. The identifying label symbol is R.

ISOPHANE INSULIN SUSPENSION USP
(NPH Insulin)

The neutral suspension is prepared with insulin obtained from beef pancreas; the insulin is combined with precisely adjusted amounts of protamine and zinc, with which it forms tiny crystals. These crystals make the liquid cloudy or milky when the vial is shaken. The vial must be carefully shaken or rotated before withdrawing each dose so that the contents are uniformly mixed. The onset of action of this insulin is evident in approximately 1 to 1½ hours from the time of administration, and its effect persists for approximately 24 hours.

How Supplied: U-40 (40 units per ml.) and U-100 (100 units per ml.). The identifying label symbol is N.

LENTE® Insulin
(Insulin Zinc Suspension USP)

The neutral suspension is prepared with insulin obtained from beef pancreas; the insulin is combined with zinc to form minute particles in suspension that make the liquid cloudy or milky when the vial is shaken. The vial must be carefully shaken or rotated before withdrawing each dose so that the contents are uniformly mixed. The onset of action of this insulin is evident in approximately 1 to 1½ hours from the time of administration, and its effect persists for approximately 24 hours.

How Supplied: U-40 (40 units per ml.) and U-100 (100 units per ml.). The identifying label symbol is L.

LENTE® is a licensed TM of Novo Industri A/S.

PROTAMINE ZINC INSULIN SUSPENSION USP

Protamine Zinc Insulin Suspension USP is sometimes referred to as PZI Insulin. The suspension is prepared with insulin obtained from beef pancreas; the insulin is combined with precisely adjusted amounts of protamine and zinc, with which it forms tiny crystals. These crystals make the liquid cloudy or milky when the vial is shaken. The vial must be carefully shaken or rotated before withdrawing each dose so that the contents are uniformly mixed. The onset of action of this insulin is evident in approximately 4 to 8 hours from the time of administration, and its effect persists for approximately 36 hours.

How Supplied: U-100 (100 units per ml.). The identifying label symbol is P.

Continued on next page

Squibb—Cont.

SEMILENTE® Insulin
(Prompt Insulin Zinc Suspension USP)

The suspension is prepared with insulin obtained from beef pancreas; the insulin is combined with zinc to form minute particles in suspension that make the liquid cloudy or milky when the vial is shaken. The vial must be carefully shaken or rotated before withdrawing each dose so that the contents are uniformly mixed. The onset of action of this insulin is evident in approximately 30 minutes to one hour from the time of administration and its effect persists for approximately 12 to 16 hours.
How Supplied: U-100 (100 units per ml.). The identifying label symbol is S.
SEMILENTE® is a licensed TM of Novo Industri A/S.

ULTRALENTE® Insulin
(Extended Insulin Zinc Suspension USP)

The suspension is prepared with insulin obtained from beef pancreas; the insulin is combined with zinc to form a product that has a prolonged duration of activity. This combination of zinc and insulin, in the form of minute particles in suspension, make the liquid cloudy or milky when the vial is shaken. The vial must be carefully shaken or rotated before withdrawing each dose so that the contents are uniformly mixed. The onset of action of this insulin is evident in approximately 4 to 8 hours from the time of administration, and its effect persists for more than 36 hours.
How Supplied: U-100 (100 units per ml.). The identifying label symbol is U.
ULTRALENTE® is a licensed TM of Novo Industri A/S.

PURIFIED INSULINS

PURIFIED PORK INSULIN INJECTION (REGULAR)

The neutral solution is prepared with insulin obtained from pork pancreas. Regular insulin is "unmodified;" nothing has been added to change the speed or duration of its action. The product is a clear colorless solution made from zinc-insulin crystals. The onset of action of this insulin is evident in approximately 30 minutes to 1 hour from the time of administration, and its effect persists for approximately 6 to 8 hours.
How Supplied: U-100 (100 units per ml.). The identifying label symbol is R.

ISOPHANE PURIFIED BEEF INSULIN SUSPENSION
(NPH Insulin)

The neutral suspension is prepared with insulin obtained from beef pancreas; the insulin is combined with precisely adjusted amounts of protamine and zinc, with which it forms tiny crystals. These crystals make the liquid cloudy or milky when the vial is shaken. The vial must be carefully shaken or rotated before withdrawing each dose so that the contents are uniformly mixed. The onset of action of this insulin is evident in approximately 1 to 1½ hours from the time of administration, and its effect persists for approximately 24 hours.
How Supplied: U-100 (100 units per ml.). The identifying label symbol is N.

PURIFIED BEEF INSULIN ZINC SUSPENSION
(LENTE®)

The suspension is prepared with insulin obtained from beef pancreas; the insulin is combined with zinc to form minute particles in suspension that make the liquid cloudy or milky when the vial is shaken. The vial must be carefully shaken or rotated before withdrawing each dose so that the contents are uniformly mixed. The onset of action of this insulin is evident in approximately 1 to 1½ hours from the time of administration, and its effect persists for approximately 24 hours.
How Supplied: U-100 (100 units per ml.). The identifying label symbol is L.
LENTE® is a licensed TM of Novo Industri A/S.

ACTRAPID®
Purified Pork Insulin Injection (Purified Regular)

Actrapid is a neutral solution of porcine purified insulin. It is a clear colorless solution. The effect of Actrapid® begins after approximately ½ hour, is maximal between 2½ and 5 hours, and terminates after approximately 8 hours.
How Supplied: U-100 (100 units per ml.). The identifying label symbol is A.

LENTARD®
Purified Pork and Beef Insulin Zinc Suspension (Purified Lente®)

Lentard is a neutral suspension of 30% amorphous porcine purified insulin and 70% crystalline bovine purified insulin. When agitated gently the liquid appears white and cloudy. The vial must be gently agitated so that the contents are uniformly mixed before filling the syringe. The effect of Lentard® begins after approximately 2½ hours, is maximal between 7 and 15 hours, and terminates after approximately 24 hours.
How Supplied: U-100 (100 units per ml.). The identifying label symbol is L.

MONOTARD®
Purified Pork Insulin Zinc Suspension (Purified Monospecies Lente®)

Monotard® is a neutral suspension of porcine purified insulin. 30% is present in amorphous form and 70% in crystalline form. When agitated gently the liquid appears white and cloudy. The vial must be gently agitated so that the contents are uniformly mixed before filling the syringe. The effect of Monotard® begins after approximately 2½ hours, is maximal between 7 and 15 hours, and terminates after approximately 22 hours.
How Supplied: U-100 (100 units per ml.). The identifying label symbol is M.
Lente® is a registered trademark of Novo Industri A/S.

PROTAPHANE™ NPH
Isophane Purified Pork Insulin Suspension (Purified NPH)

Protaphane™ NPH is a neutral suspension of porcine purified insulin crystals with protamine and zinc. When agitated gently, the liquid appears white and cloudy. The vial must be gently agitated so that the contents are uniformly mixed before filling the syringe. The effect of Protaphane™NPH begins after approximately 1-1½ hours, is maximal between 4 and 12 hours, and terminates after approximately 24 hours.
How Supplied: U-100 (100 units per ml.). The identifying label symbol is N.

SEMITARD®
Prompt Purified Pork Insulin Zinc Suspension (Purified Semilente®)

Semitard® is a neutral suspension of amorphous porcine purified insulin. When agitated gently the liquid appears white and cloudy. The vial must be gently agitated so that the contents are uniformly mixed before filling the syringe. The effect of Semitard® begins after approximately 1½ hours, is maximal between 5 and 10 hours and terminates after approximately 16 hours.
How Supplied: U-100 (100 units per ml.). The identifying label symbol is S.

ULTRATARD®
Extended Purified Beef Insulin Zinc Suspension (Purified Ultralente®)

Ultratard® is a neutral suspension of crystalline bovine purified insulin. When agitated gently the liquid appears white and cloudy. The vial must be gently agitated so that the contents are uniformly mixed before filling the syringe. The effect of Ultratard® begins after approximately 4 hours, is maximal between 10 and 30 hours, and terminates after approximately 36 hours.
How Supplied: U-100 (100 units per ml.). The identifying label symbol is U.

KENALOG® ℞
Triamcinolone Acetonide USP CREAM/LOTION/OINTMENT/SPRAY

Description: The topical corticosteroids constitute a class of primary synthetic steroids used as anti-inflammatory and antipruritic agents. The steroids in this class include triamcinolone acetonide. Triamcinolone acetonide is designated chemically as 9-Fluoro-11β, 16α, 17, 21,-tetrahydroxypregna-1,4-diene-3, 20-dione cyclic 16, 17-acetal with acetone.
Each gram of 0.025%, 0.1%, and 0.5% Kenalog Cream (Triamcinolone Acetonide Cream) provides 0.25 mg, 1 mg, or 5 mg. triancinolone acetonide, respectively, in a vanishing cream base containing propylene glycol, cetearyl alcohol (and) ceteareth-20, white petrolatum, sorbitol solution, glyceryl monostearate, polyethylene glycol monostearate, simethicone, sorbic acid, and purified water.
Each ml of 0.025% and 0.1% Kenalog Lotion (Triamcinolone Acetonide Lotion) provides 0.25 mg. and 1 mg. triamcinolone acetonide, respectively, in a lotion base containing propylene glycol, cetyl alcohol, stearyl alcohol, sorbitan monopalmitate, polysorbate 20, simethicone, and purified water.
Each gram of 0.025%, 0.1%, and 0.5% Kenalog Ointment (Triamcinolone Acetonide Ointment) provides 0.25 mg, 1 mg, or 5 mg. triamcinolone acetonide, respectively, in Plastibase® (Plasticized Hydrocarbon Gel), a polyethylene and mineral oil gel base.
Kenalog Spray (Triamcinolone Acetonide Topical Aerosol) is **for dermatologic use only.** A two-second application, which covers an area approximately the size of the hand, delivers an amount of triamcinolone acetonide not exceeding 0.2 mg. After spraying, the nonvolatile vehicle remaining on the skin contains approximately 0.2% triamcinolone acetonide. Each gram of spray provides 0.147 mg. triamcinolone acetonide in a vehicle of isopropyl palmitate, dehydrated alcolol (10.3%), and isobutane propellant.
Clinical Pharmacology: Topical corticosteroids share anti-inflammatory, antipruritic and vasoconstrictive actions.
The mechanism of anti-inflammatory activity of the topical corticosteroids is unclear. Various laboratory methods, including vasoconstrictor assays, are used to compare and predict potencies and/or clinical efficacies of the topical corticosteroids. There is some evidence to suggest that a recognizable correlation exists between vasoconstrictor potency and therapeutic efficacy in man.
Pharmacokinetics—The extent of percutaneous absorption of topical corticosteroids is determined by many factors including the vehicle, the integrity of the epidermal barrier, and the use of occlusive dressings.
Topical corticosteroids can be absorbed from normal intact skin. Inflammation and/or

other disease processes in the skin increase percutaneous absorption. Occlusive dressings substantially increase the percutaneous absorption of topical corticosteroids. Thus, occlusive dressings may be a valuable therapeutic adjunct for treatment of resistant dermatoses (see DOSAGE AND ADMINISTRATION).

Once absorbed through the skin, topical corticosteroids are handled through pharmacokinetic pathways similar to systemically administered corticosteroids. Corticosteroids are bound to plasma proteins in varying degrees. Corticosteroids are metabolized primarily in the liver and are then excreted by the kidneys. Some of the topical corticosteroids and their metabolites are also excreted into the bile.

Indications and Usage: Kenalog (Triamcinolone Acetonide) Creams, Lotions, Ointments, and Spray are indicated for relief of the inflammatory and pruritic manifestations of corticosteroid-responsive dermatoses.

Contraindications: Topical corticosteroids are contraindicated in those patients with a history of hypersensitivity to any of the components of the preparations.

Precautions: General—Systemic absorption of topical corticosteroids has produced reversible hypothalamic-pituitary-adrenal (HPA) axis suppression, manifestations of Cushing's syndrome, hyperglycemia, and glycosuria in some patients.

Conditions which augment systemic absorption include the application of the more potent steroids, use over large surface areas, prolonged use, and the addition of occlusive dressings.

Therefore, patients receiving a large dose of any potent topical steroid applied to a large surface area or under an occlusive dressing should be evaluated periodically for evidence of HPA axis suppression by using the urinary free cortisol and ACTH stimulation tests, and for impairment of thermal homeostasis. If HPA axis suppression or elevation of the body temperature occurs, an attempt should be made to withdraw the drug, to reduce the frequency of application, substitute a less potent steroid, or use a sequential approach when utilizing the occlusive technique.

Recovery of HPA axis function and thermal homeostasis are generally prompt and complete upon discontinuation of the drug. Infrequently, signs and symptoms of steroid withdrawal may occur, requiring supplemental systemic corticosteroids. Occasionally, a patient may develop a sensitivity reaction to a particular occlusive dressing material or adhesive and a substitute material may be necessary.

Children may absorb proportionally larger amounts of topical corticosteroids and thus be more susceptible to systemic toxicity (see PRECAUTIONS, Pediatric Use).

If irritation develops, topical corticosteroids should be discontinued and appropriate therapy instituted.

In the presence of dermatological infections, the use of an appropriate antifungal or antibacterial agent should be instituted. If a favorable response does not occur promptly, the corticosteroid should be discontinued until the infection has been adequately controlled.

Information for the Patient: Patients using topical corticosteroids should receive the following information and instructions:

1. This medication is to be used as directed by the physician. It is for external use only. Avoid contact with the eyes.
2. Patients should be advised not to use this medication for any disorder other than for which it was prescribed.
3. The treated skin area should not be bandaged or otherwise covered or wrapped as to be occlusive unless directed by the physician.
4. Patients should report any signs of local adverse reactions especially under occlusive dressing.
5. Parents of pediatric patients should be advised not to use tight-fitting diapers or plastic pants on a child being treated in the diaper area, as these garments may constitute occlusive dressings.

Laboratory Tests—A urinary free cortisol test and ACTH stimulation test may be helpful in evaluating HPA axis suppression.

Carcinogenesis, Mutagenesis, and Impairment of Fertility—Long-term animal studies have not been performed to evaluate the carcinogenic potential or the effect on fertility of topical corticosteroids.

Studies to determine mutagenicity with prednisolone and hydrocortisone showed negative results.

Pregnancy: Teratogenic Effects—Category C. Corticosteroids are generally teratogenic in laboratory animals when administered systemically at relatively low dosage levels. The more potent corticosteroids have been shown to be teratogenic after dermal application in laboratory animals. There are no adequate and well-controlled studies in pregnant women on teratogenic effects from topically applied corticosteroids. Therefore, topical corticosteroids should be used during pregnancy only if the potential benefit justifies the potential risk to the fetus. Drugs of this class should not be used extensively on pregnant patients, in large amounts, or for prolonged periods of time.

Nursing Mothers—It is not known whether topical administration of corticosteroids could result in sufficient systemic absorption to produce detectable quantities in breast milk. Systemically administered corticosteroids are secreted into breast milk in quantities **not** likely to have a deleterious effect on the infant. Nevertheless, caution should be exercised when topical corticosteroids are administered to a nursing woman.

Pediatric Use—**Pediatric patients may demonstrate greater susceptibility to topical corticosteroid-induced HPA axis suppression and Cushing's syndrome than mature patients because of a larger skin surface area to body weight ratio.**

HPA axis suppression, Cushing's syndrome, and intracranial hypertension have been reported in children receiving topical corticosteroids. Manifestations of adrenal suppression in children include linear growth retardation, delayed weight gain, low plasma cortisol levels, and absence of response to ACTH stimulation. Manifestations of intracranial hypertension include bulging fontanelles, headaches, and bilateral papilledema.

Administration of topical corticosteroids to children should be limited to the least amount compatible with an effective therapeutic regimen. Chronic corticosteroid therapy may interfere with the growth and development of children.

Adverse Reactions: The following local adverse reactions are reported infrequently with topical corticosteroids, but may occur more frequently with the use of occlusive dressings (reactions are listed in an approximate decreasing order of occurrence): burning, itching, irritation, dryness, folliculitis, hypertrichosis, acneiform eruptions, hypopigmentation, perioral dermatitis, allergic contact dermatitis, maceration of the skin, secondary infection, skin atrophy, striae, and miliaria.

Overdosage: Topically applied corticosteroids can be absorbed in sufficient amounts to produce systemic effects (see PRECAUTIONS, General).

Dosage and Administration: Kenalog Cream (Triamcinolone Acetonide Cream) 0.025%: Apply to the affected area two to four times daily. Rub in gently.

Kenalog Cream (Triamcinolone Acetonide Cream) 0.1% or 0.5%: Apply, as appropriate, to the affected area two to three times daily. Rub in gently.

Kenalog Lotion (Triamcinolone Acetonide Lotion) 0.025%: Apply to the affected area two to four times daily. Rub in gently.

Kenalog Lotion (Triamcinolone Acetonide Lotion) 0.1%): Apply to the affected area two to three times daily. Rub in gently.

Kenalog Ointment (Triamcinolone Acetonide Ointment) 0.025%: Apply a thin film to the affected area two to four times daily.

Kenalog Ointment (Triamcinolone Acetonide Ointment) 0.1% or 0.5%: Apply a thin film, as appropriate, to the affected area two to three times daily.

Kenalog Spray (Triamcinolone Acetonide Topical Aerosol): Directions for use of the spray can are provided on the label. The preparation may be applied to any area of the body, but when it is sprayed about the face, care should be taken to see that the eyes are covered, and that inhalation of the spray is avoided. Three or four applications daily are generally adequate.

Occlusive Dressing Technique—Kenalog Cream (Triamcinolone Acetonide Cream) 0.025%, 0.1%, and 0.5% and Kenalog Lotion (Triamcinolone Acetonide Lotion) 0.025% and 0.1%: Occlusive dressings may be used for the management of psoriasis or other recalcitrant conditions. Gently rub a small amount of the preparation into the lesion until it disappears. Reapply the preparation leaving a thin coating on the lesion, cover with a pliable nonporous film, and seal the edges. If needed, additional moisture may be provided by covering the lesion with a dampened clean cotton cloth before the nonporous film is applied or by briefly wetting the affected area with water immediately prior to applying the medication. The frequency of changing dressings is best determined on an individual basis. It may be convenient to apply the preparation under an occlusive dressing in the evening and to remove the dressing in the morning (i.e., 12-hour occlusion). When utilizing the 12-hour occlusion regimen, additional preparation should be applied, without occlusion, during the day. Reapplication is essential at each dressing change.

If an infection develops, the use of occlusive dressings should be discontinued and appropriate antimicrobial therapy instituted.

Kenalog Ointment (Triamcinolone Acetonide Ointment) 0.025%, 0.1% and 0.5% and Kenalog Spray (Triamcinolone Acetonide Topical Aerosol): Occlusive dressings may be used for the management of psoriasis or other recalcitrant conditions. Apply a thin coating of the preparation onto the lesion, cover with a pliable nonporous film, and seal the edges. If needed, additional moisture may be provided by covering the lesion with a dampened clean cotton cloth before the nonporous film is applied or by briefly wetting the affected area with water immediately prior to applying the medication. The frequency of changing dressings is best determined on an individual basis. It may be convenient to apply the preparation under an occlusive dressing in the evening and to remove the dressing in the morning (i.e., 12-hour occlusion). When utilizing the 12-hour occlusion regimen, additional preparation should be applied, without occlusion, during the day. Reapplication is essential at each dressing change.

If an infection develops, the use of occlusive dressings should be discontinued and appropriate antimicrobial therapy instituted.

How Supplied: The 0.025% Cream and Ointment are supplied in 15 g. and 80 g. tubes, and 240 g. (8 oz.) jars. The 0.1% Cream and Ointment are supplied in 15 g., 60 g., and 80 g. tubes and in 240 g. (8 oz.) jars. The 0.5% Cream and Ointment are supplied in 20 g. tubes and 240 g. (8 oz.) jars. The 0.1% and 0.025% Creams are also supplied in 5.25 lb. jars. The 0.025% Lotion is supplied in 60 ml. plastic

Continued on next page

Squibb—Cont.

squeeze bottles. The 0.1% Lotion is supplied in 15 ml. and 60 ml. plastic squeeze bottles. [60 ml. bottle, V.A. Depot Item NSN 6505-00-282-5118A]. The Spray is supplied in 23 g. and 63 g. aerosol cans (each can is supplied with a spray tube applicator). [63 g. cans, Military Depot Item, NSN 6505-01-066-1325].

Storage

Store the creams and lotions at room temperature; avoid freezing. Store the ointments at room temperature. Store the spray at room temperature; avoid excessive heat.

KENALOG-H® CREAM ℞
(Triamcinolone Acetonide Cream USP 0.1%)

Description: The topical corticosteroids constitute a class of primary synthetic steroids used as anti-inflammatory and antipruritic agents. The steroids in this class include triamcinolone acetonide. Triamcinolone acetonide is designated chemically as 9-Fluoro-11β, 16α, 17, 21,-tetrahydroxypregna-1,4-diene-3, 20-dione cyclic 16, 17-acetal with acetone.

Each gram of the cream provides 1 mg. triamcinolone acetonide in a specially formulated hydrophilic vanishing cream base containing propylene glycol, dimethicone 350, castor oil, cetearyl alcohol (and) ceteareth-20, propylene glycol stearate, white petrolatum, and purified water. This formulation is water-washable, greaseless, and nonstaining, with moisturizing and emollient properties.

Clinical Pharmacology: Topical corticosteroids share anti-inflammatory, antipruritic and vasoconstrictive actions.

The mechanism of anti-inflammatory activity of the topical corticosteroids is unclear. Various laboratory methods, including vasoconstrictor assays, are used to compare and predict potencies and/or clinical efficacies of the topical corticosteroids. There is some evidence to suggest that a recognizable correlation exists between vasoconstrictor potency and therapeutic efficacy in man.

Pharmacokinetics—The extent of percutaneous absorption of topical corticosteroids is determined by many factors including the vehicle, the integrity of the epidermal barrier, and the use of occlusive dressings.

Topical corticosteroids can be absorbed from normal intact skin. Inflammation and/or other disease processes in the skin increase percutaneous absorption. Occlusive dressings substantially increase the percutaneous absorption of topical corticosteroids. Thus, occlusive dressings may be a valuable therapeutic adjunct for treatment of resistant dermatoses (see DOSAGE AND ADMINISTRATION).

Once absorbed through the skin, topical corticosteroids are handled through pharmacokinetic pathways similar to systemically administered corticosteroids. Corticosteroids are bound to plasma proteins in varying degrees. Corticosteroids are metabolized primarily in the liver and are then excreted by the kidneys. Some of the topical corticosteroids and their metabolites are also excreted into the bile.

Indications: Kenalog-H Cream (Triamcinolone Acetonide Cream) 0.1% is indicated for the relief of the inflammatory and puritic manifestations of corticosteroid-responsive dermatoses.

Contraindications: Topical corticosteroids are contraindicated in those patients with a history of hypersensitivity to any of the components of the preparations.

Precautions: General—Systemic absorption of topical corticosteroids has produced reversible hypothalamic-pituitary-adrenal (HPA) axis suppression, manifestations of Cushing's syndrome, hyperglycemia, and glycosuria in some patients.

Conditions which augment systemic absorption include the application of the more potent steroids, use over large surface areas, prolonged use, and the addition of occlusive dressings.

Therefore, patients receiving a large dose of any potent topical steroid applied to a large surface area or under an occlusive dressing should be evaluated periodically for evidence of HPA axis suppression by using the urinary free cortisol and ACTH stimulation tests, and for impairment of thermal homeostasis. If HPA axis suppression or elevation of the body temperature occurs, an attempt should be made to withdraw the drug, to reduce the frequency of application, substitute a less potent steroid, or use a sequential approach when utilizing the occlusive technique.

Recovery of HPA axis function and thermal homeostasis are generally prompt and complete upon discontinuation of the drug. Infrequently, signs and symptoms of steroid withdrawal may occur, requiring supplemental systemic corticosteroids. Occasionally, a patient may develop a sensitivity reaction to a particular occlusive dressing material or adhesive and a substitute material may be necessary.

Children may absorb proportionally larger amounts of topical corticosteroids and thus be more susceptible to systemic toxicity (see PRECAUTIONS, Pediatric Use).

If irritation develops, topical corticosteroids should be discontinued and appropriate therapy instituted.

In the presence of dermatological infections, the use of an appropriate antifungal or antibacterial agent should be instituted. If a favorable response does not occur promptly, the corticosteroid should be discontinued until the infection has been adequately controlled.

Information for the Patient—Patients using topical corticosteroids should receive the following information and instructions:

1. This medication is to be used as directed by the physician. It is for external use only. Avoid contact with the eyes.
2. Patients should be advised not to use this medication for any disorder other than for which it was prescribed.
3. The treated skin area should not be bandaged or otherwise covered or wrapped as to be occlusive unless directed by the physician.
4. Patients should report any signs of local adverse reactions especially under occlusive dressing.
5. Parents of pediatric patients should be advised not to use tight-fitting diapers or plastic pants on a child being treated in the diaper area, as these garments may constitute occlusive dressings.

Laboratory Tests—A urinary free cortisol test and ACTH stimulation test may be helpful in evaluating HPA axis suppression.

Carcinogenesis, Mutagenesis, and Impairment of Fertility—Long-term animal studies have not been performed to evaluate the carcinogenic potential or the effect on fertility of topical corticosteroids.

Studies to determine mutagenicity with prednisolone and hydrocortisone showed negative results.

Pregnancy: Teratogenic Effects—Category C. Corticosteroids are generally teratogenic in laboratory animals when administered systemically at relatively low dosage levels. The more potent corticosteroids have been shown to be teratogenic after dermal application in laboratory animals. There are no adequate and well-controlled studies in pregnant women on teratogenic effects from topically applied corticosteroids. Therefore, topical corticosteroids should be used during pregnancy only if the potential benefit justifies the potential risk to the fetus. Drugs of this class should not be used extensively on pregnant patients, in large amounts, or for prolonged periods of time.

Nursing Mothers—It is not known whether topical administration of corticosteroids could result in sufficient systemic absorption to produce detectable quantities in breast milk. Systemically administered corticosteroids are secreted into breast milk in quantities **not** likely to have a deleterious effect on the infant. Nevertheless, caution should be exercised when topical corticosteroids are administered to a nursing woman.

Pediatric Use—Pediatric patients may demonstrate greater susceptibility to topical corticosteroid-induced HPA axis suppression and Cushing's syndrome than mature patients because of a larger skin surface area to body weight ratio.

HPA axis suppression, Cushing's syndrome, and intracranial hypertension have been reported in children receiving topical corticosteroids. Manifestations of adrenal suppression in children include linear growth retardation, delayed weight gain, low plasma cortisol levels, and absence of response to ACTH stimulation. Manifestations of intracranial hypertension include bulging fontanelles, headaches, and bilateral papilledema.

Administration of topical corticosteroids to children should be limited to the least amount compatible with an effective therapeutic regimen. Chronic corticosteroid therapy may interfere with the growth and development of children.

Adverse Reactions: The following local adverse reactions are reported infrequently with topical corticosteroids, but may occur more frequently with the use of occlusive dressings (reactions are listed in an approximate decreasing order of occurrence): burning, itching, irritation, dryness, folliculitis, hypertrichosis, acneiform eruptions, hypopigmentation, perioral dermatitis, allergic contact dermatitis, maceration of the skin, secondary infection, skin atrophy, striae, and miliaria.

Overdosage: Topically applied corticosteroids can be absorbed in sufficient amounts to produce systemic effects (see PRECAUTIONS, General).

Dosage and Administration: Apply Kenalog-H Cream (Triamcinolone Acetonide Cream) 0.1% to the affected area two to three times daily. Rub in gently.

Occlusive Dressing Technique

Occlusive dressings may be used for the management of psoriasis or other recalcitrant conditions. Gently rub a small amount of the cream into the lesion until it disappears. Reapply the preparation leaving a thin coating on the lesion, cover with a pliable nonporous film, and seal the edges. If needed, additional moisture may be provided by covering the lesion with a dampened clean cotton cloth before the nonporous film is applied or by briefly wetting the affected area with water immediately prior to applying the medication. The frequency of changing dressings is best determined on an individual basis. It may be convenient to apply the cream under an occlusive dressing in the evening and to remove the dressing in the morning (i.e., 12-hour occlusion). When utilizing the 12-hour occlusion regimen, additional preparation should be applied, without occlusion, during the day. Reapplication is essential at each dressing change.

If an infection develops, the use of occlusive dressings should be discontinued and appropriate antimicrobial therapy instituted.

How Supplied: Kenalog-H Cream (Triamcinolone Acetonide Cream) 0.1% is supplied in 15 g. and 60 g. tubes.

Storage: Store at room temperature; avoid freezing.

KENALOG®-40 INJECTION ℞
(Sterile Triamcinolone Acetonide Suspension USP)

NOT FOR INTRAVENOUS OR INTRADERMAL USE

Description: Kenalog-40 Injection provides a synthetic corticosteroid with marked anti-inflammatory action. Each ml. of the sterile, aqueous suspension provides 40 mg. of triamcinolone acetonide, with sodium chloride for isotonicity, 0.9% (w/v) benzyl alcohol as a preservative, 0.75% sodium carboxymethylcellulose, and 0.04% polysorbate 80. Sodium hydroxide or hydrochloric acid may be present to adjust pH to 5.0 to 7.5. At the time of manufacture, the air in the container is replaced by nitrogen.

Actions: Naturally occurring glucocorticoids (hydrocortisone), which also have salt-retaining properties, are used as replacement therapy in adrenocortical deficiency states. Their synthetic analogs are primarily used for their potent anti-inflammatory effects in disorders of many organ systems.

Glucocorticoids cause profound and varied metabolic effects. In addition, they modify the body's immune responses to diverse stimuli.

Kenalog-40 Injection has an extended duration of effect which may be permanent, or sustained over a period of several weeks. Studies indicate that following a single intramuscular dose of 60 to 100 mg. of triamcinolone acetonide, adrenal suppression occurs within 24 to 48 hours and then gradually returns to normal, usually in 30 to 40 days. This finding correlates closely with the extended duration of therapeutic action achieved with the drug.

Indications:

Intramuscular

Where oral therapy is not feasible or is temporarily undesirable in the judgment of the physician, Kenalog-40 Injection (Sterile Triamcinolone Acetonide Suspension USP) is indicated for intramuscular use as follows:

1. *Endocrine disorders*—Primary or secondary adrenocortical insufficiency (hydrocortisone or cortisone is the drug of choice; synthetic analogs may be used in conjunction with mineralocorticoids where applicable; in infancy, mineralocorticoid supplementation is of particular importance).
Acute adrenocortical insufficiency (hydrocortisone or cortisone is the drug of choice; mineralocorticoid supplementation may be necessary, particularly when synthetic analogs are used).
Preoperatively and in the event of serious trauma or illness, in patients with known adrenal insufficiency or when adrenocortical reserve is doubtful.
Shock unresponsive to conventional therapy if adrenocortical insufficiency exists or is suspected.
Congenital adrenal hyperplasia. Nonsuppurative thyroiditis.
2. *Rheumatic disorders*—As adjunctive therapy for short-term administration (to tide the patient over an acute episode or exacerbation) in: posttraumatic osteoarthritis; synovitis of osteoarthritis; rheumatoid arthritis; acute and subacute bursitis; epicondylitis; acute nonspecific tenosynovitis; acute gouty arthritis; psoriatic arthritis; ankylosing spondylitis; juvenile rheumatoid arthritis.
3. *Collagen diseases*—During an exacerbation or as maintenance therapy in selected cases of: systemic lupus erythematosus; acute rheumatic carditis.
4. *Dermatologic diseases*—Pemphigus; severe erythema multiforme (Stevens-Johnson syndrome); exfoliative dermatitis; bullous dermatitis herpetiformis; severe seborrheic dermatitis; severe psoriasis.
5. *Allergic states*—Control of severe or incapacitating allergic conditions intractable to adequate trials of conventional treatment in: bronchial asthma; contact dermatitis; atopic dermatitis; serum sickness; seasonal or perennial allergic rhinitis; drug hypersensitivity reactions; urticarial transfusion reactions; acute noninfectious laryngeal edema (epinephrine is the drug of first choice).
6. *Ophthalmic diseases*—Severe acute and chronic allergic and inflammatory processes involving the eye, such as: herpes zoster ophthalmicus; iritis; irridocyclitis; chorioretinitis; diffuse posterior uveitis and choroiditis; optic neuritis; sympathetic ophthalmia; anterior segment inflammation.
7. *Gastrointestinal diseases*—To tide the patient over a critical period of disease in: ulcerative colitis (systemic therapy); regional enteritis (systemic therapy).
8. *Respiratory diseases*—Symptomatic sarcoidosis; berylliosis; fulminating or disseminated pulmonary tuberculosis when concurrently accompanied by appropriate antituberculous chemotherapy; aspiration pneumonitis.
9. *Hematologic disorders*—Acquired (autoimmune) hemolytic anemia.
10. *Neoplastic diseases*—For palliative management of: leukemias and lymphomas in adults; acute leukemia of childhood.
11. *Edematous state*—To induce diuresis or remission of proteinuria in the nephrotic syndrome, without uremia, of the idiopathic type or that due to lupus erythematosus.
12. *Miscellaneous*—Tuberculous meningitis with subarachnoid block or impending block when concurrently accompanied by appropriate antituberculous chemotherapy.

Intra-Articular

Kenalog-40 Injection (Sterile Triamcinolone Acetonide Suspension USP) is indicated for intra-articular or intrabursal administration, and for injections into tendon sheaths, as adjunctive therapy for short-term administration (to tide the patient over an acute episode or exacerbation) in: synovitis of osteoarthritis; rheumatoid arthritis; acute and subacute bursitis; acute gouty arthritis; epicondylitis; acute nonspecific tenosynovitis; posttraumatic osteoarthritis.

Contraindications: Corticosteroids are contraindicated in patients with systemic fungal infections. Intramuscular corticosteroid preparations are contraindicated for idiopathic thrombocytopenic purpura.

Warnings: Because it is a suspension, the preparation should **not** be administered intravenously. Strict aseptic technique is mandatory. This preparation is not recommended for children under six years of age.

When patients who are receiving corticosteroid therapy are subjected to unusual stress, increased dosage of rapidly acting corticosteroids is indicated before, during, and after the stressful situation.

Corticosteroids may mask some signs of infection, and new infections may appear during their use. There may be decreased resistance and inability to localize infection when corticosteroids are used. If an infection occurs during corticosteroid therapy, it should be promptly controlled by suitable antimicrobial therapy (see PRECAUTIONS).

Prolonged use of corticosteroids may produce posterior subcapsular cataracts, glaucoma with possible damage to the optic nerves, and may enhance the establishment of secondary ocular infections due to fungi or viruses.

Average and large doses of hydrocortisone or cortisone can cause elevation of blood pressure, salt and water retention, and increased excretion of potassium. These effects are less likely to occur with the synthetic derivatives except when they are used in large doses; dietary salt restriction and potassium supplementation may be necessary (see PRECAUTIONS). All corticosteroids increase calcium excretion.

Patients should not be vaccinated against smallpox while on corticosteroid therapy. Other immunization procedures should not be undertaken in patients who are on corticosteroids, especially on high dose, because of possible hazards of neurological complications and a lack of antibody response.

The use of triamcinolone acetonide in patients with active tuberculosis should be restricted to those cases of fulminating or disseminated tuberculosis in which the corticosteroid is used for the management of the disease in conjunction with an appropriate antituberculous regimen. If corticosteroids are indicated in patients with latent tuberculosis or tuberculin reactivity, close observation is necessary since reactivation of the disease may occur. During prolonged corticosteroid therapy, these patients should receive chemoprophylaxis.

Because rare instances of anaphylactoid reactions have occurred in patients receiving parenteral corticosteroid therapy, appropriate precautionary measures should be taken prior to administration, especially when the patient has a history of allergy to any drug.

Unless a **deep** intramuscular injection is given, local atrophy is likely to occur. (For recommendations on injection techniques, see DOSAGE AND ADMINISTRATION.) Due to the significantly higher incidence of local atrophy when the material is injected into the deltoid area, this injection site should be avoided in favor of the gluteal area. Only very unusual circumstances would warrant injection into the deltoid area.

Usage in Pregnancy: Since adequate human reproduction studies have not been done with corticosteroids, the use of these drugs in pregnancy, nursing mothers, or women of child-bearing potential requires that the possible benefits of the drug be weighed against the potential hazards to the mother and the embryo, fetus, or nursing infant. Infants born of mothers who have received substantial doses of corticosteroids during pregnancy should be carefully observed for signs of hypoadrenalism.

Precautions: Drug-induced secondary adrenocortical insufficiency may be minimized by a gradual reduction of dosage. This type of relative insufficiency may persist for months after discontinuation of therapy; therefore, in any situation of stress (such as trauma, surgery, or severe illness) occurring during that period, hormone therapy should be reinstituted. Since mineralocorticoid secretion may be impaired, salt and/or a mineralocorticoid should be administered concurrently.

There is an enhanced corticosteroid effect in patients with hypothyroidism and in those with cirrhosis.

Corticosteroids should be used cautiously in patients with ocular herpes simplex because of possible corneal perforation.

The lowest possible dose of corticosteroid should be used to control the condition being treated. A gradual reduction in dosage should be made when possible.

Psychic derangements may appear when corticosteroids are used. These may range from euphoria, insomnia, mood swings, personality changes and severe depression to frank psychotic manifestations. Existing emotional instability or psychotic tendencies may also be aggravated by corticosteroids.

Aspirin should be used cautiously in conjunction with corticosteroids in patients with hypoprothrombinemia.

Corticosteroids should be used with caution in patients with nonspecific ulcerative colitis if there is a probability of impending perforation, abscess, or other pyogenic infection. Corticosteroids should also be used cautiously in patients with diverticulitis, fresh intestinal anastomoses, active or latent peptic ulcer, renal insufficiency, hypertension, osteoporosis, acute glomerulonephritis, vaccinia, varicella, exanthema, Cushing's syndrome, antibiotic resistant infections, diabetes mellitus, congestive heart failure, chronic nephritis, thromboembolitic tendencies, thrombophlebitis, convulsive disorders, metastatic carcinoma, and myasthenia gravis.

Growth and development of infants and children on prolonged corticosteroid therapy should be carefully observed.

Although therapy with Kenalog-40 Injection (Sterile Triamcinolone Acetonide Suspension USP) will ameliorate symptoms, it is in no

Continued on next page

Squibb—Cont.

sense a cure and the hormone has no effect on the cause of the inflammation. Therefore, this method of treatment does not obviate the need for the conventional measures usually employed.

Intra-articular injection of a corticosteroid may produce systemic as well as local effects. The inadvertent injection of the suspension into the soft tissues surrounding a joint is not harmful, but may lead to the occurrence of systemic effects, and is the most common cause of failure to achieve the desired local results.

Following intra-articular steroid therapy, patients should be specifically warned to avoid overuse of joints in which symptomatic benefit has been obtained. Negligence in this matter may permit an increase in joint deterioration that will more than offset the beneficial effects of the steroid. To detect deterioration, follow-up x-ray examination is suggested in selected cases.

Overdistention of the joint capsule and deposition of steroid along the needle track should be avoided in intra-articular injection since this may lead to subcutaneous atrophy.

Corticosteroids should not be injected into unstable joints. Repeated intra-articular injection may in some cases result in instability of the joint. In selected cases, particularly when repeated injections are given, x-ray follow-up is suggested.

An increase in joint discomfort has seldom occurred. A marked increase in pain accompanied by local swelling, further restriction of joint motion, fever, and malaise are suggestive of a septic arthritis. If these complications should appear, and the diagnosis of septic arthritis is confirmed, administration of triamcinolone acetonide should be stopped, and antimicrobial therapy should be instituted immediately and continued for 7 to 10 days after all evidence of infection has disappeared. Appropriate examination of any joint fluid present is necessary to exclude a septic process.

Local injection of a steroid into a previously infected joint is to be avoided.

Kenalog-40 Injection (Sterile Triamcinolone Acetonide Suspension USP) should be administered only with full knowledge of characteristic activity of, and varied responses to, adrenocortical hormones. Like other potent corticosteroids, triamcinolone acetonide should be used under close clinical supervision. Triamcinolone acetonide can cause elevation of blood pressure, salt and water retention, and increased potassium and calcium excretion necessitating dietary salt restriction and potassium supplementation. Edema may occur in the presence of renal disease with a fixed or decreased glomerular filtration rate.

During prolonged therapy, **a liberal protein intake is essential** for counteracting the tendency to gradual weight loss sometimes associated with negative nitrogen balance, wasting and weakness of skeletal muscles.

When local or systemic microbial infections are present, therapy with triamcinolone acetonide is not recommended, but may be employed with caution and only in conjunction with appropriate antibiotic or chemotherapeutic medication. Triamcinolone acetonide may mask signs of infection and enhance dissemination of the infecting organism. Hence, all patients receiving triamcinolone acetonide should be watched for evidence of intercurrent infection. Should infection occur, vigorous, appropriate anti-infective therapy should be initiated. If possible, abrupt cessation of steroids should be avoided because of the danger of superimposing adrenocortical insufficiency on the infectious process.

Menstrual irregularities may occur, and this possibility should be mentioned to female patients past menarche.

In peptic ulcer, recurrence may be asymptomatic until perforation or hemorrhage occurs. Long-term adrenocorticoid therapy may evoke hyperacidity or peptic ulcer; therefore, as a prophylactic measure, an ulcer regimen and the administration of an antacid are highly recommended. X-rays should be taken in peptic ulcer patients complaining of gastric distress, or when therapy is prolonged. Whether or not changes are observed, an ulcer regimen is recommended.

As with other corticosteroids, the possibility of other severe reactions should be considered. If such reactions should occur, appropriate corrective measures should be instituted and use of the drug discontinued.

Continued supervision of the patient after termination of triamcinolone acetonide therapy is essential, since there may be a sudden reappearance of severe manifestations of the disease for which the patient was treated.

Adverse Reactions: Following Administration by Any Route — Patients should be watched closely for the following adverse reactions which may be associated with any corticosteroid therapy:

Fluid and electrolyte disturbances — sodium retention, fluid retention, congestive heart failure in susceptible patients, potassium loss, cardiac arrhythmias or ECG changes due to potassium deficiency, hypokalemic alkalosis, and hypertension.

Musculoskeletal — muscle weakness, fatigue, steroid myopathy, loss of muscle mass, osteoporosis, vertebral compression fractures, delayed healing of fractures, aseptic necrosis of femoral and humeral heads, pathologic fractures of long bones, and spontaneous fractures.

Gastrointestinal — peptic ulcer with possible subsequent perforation and hemorrhage, pancreatitis, abdominal distention, and ulcerative esophagitis.

Dermatologic — impaired wound healing, thin fragile skin, petechiae and ecchymoses, facial erythema, increased sweating, purpura, striae, hirsutism, acneiform eruptions, lupus erythematosus-like lesions and suppressed reactions to skin tests.

Neurological — convulsions, increased intracranial pressure with papilledema (pseudotumor cerebri) usually after treatment, vertigo, headache, neuritis or paresthesias, and aggravation of preexisting psychiatric conditions.

Endocrine — menstrual irregularities; development of the cushingoid state; suppression of growth in children; secondary adrenocortical and pituitary unresponsiveness, particularly in times of stress (e.g., trauma, surgery, or illness); decreased carbohydrate tolerance; manifestations of latent diabetes mellitus and increased requirements for insulin or oral hypoglycemic agents in diabetics.

Ophthalmic — posterior subcapsular cataracts, increased intraocular pressure, glaucoma, and exophthalmos.

Metabolic — hyperglycemia, glycosuria, and negative nitrogen balance due to protein catabolism.

Others — necrotizing angiitis, thrombophlebitis, thromboembolism, aggravation or masking of infections, insomnia, syncopal episodes, and anaphylactoid reactions.

Following Intramuscular Administration — Severe pain has been reported in a few cases. Sterile abscess formation, subcutaneous and cutaneous atrophy, hyperpigmentation and hypopigmentation and charcot-like arthropathy have also occurred.

Following Intra-Articular Administration — Undesirable reactions have included postinjection flare, transient pain, occasional irritation at the injection site, sterile abscess formation, hyperpigmentation and hypopigmentation, charcot-like arthropathy and occasional brief increase in joint discomfort.

Dosage and Administration:

General

The initial dose of Kenalog-40 Injection (Sterile Triamcinolone Acetonide Suspension USP) may vary from 2.5 to 60 mg. per day depending on the specific disease entity being treated (see **Dosage** section below). In situations of less severity, lower doses will generally suffice while in selected patients higher initial doses may be required. Usually the parenteral dosage ranges are one-third to one-half the oral dose given every 12 hours. However, in certain overwhelming, acute, life-threatening situations, administration of dosages exceeding the usual dosages may be justified and may be in multiples of the oral dosages.

The initial dosage should be maintained or adjusted until a satisfactory response is noted. If after a reasonable period of time there is a lack of satisfactory clinical response, Kenalog-40 Injection should be discontinued and the patient transferred to other appropriate therapy. **IT SHOULD BE EMPHASIZED THAT DOSAGE REQUIREMENTS ARE VARIABLE AND MUST BE INDIVIDUALIZED ON THE BASIS OF THE DISEASE UNDER TREATMENT AND THE RESPONSE OF THE PATIENT.** After a favorable response is noted, the proper maintenance dosage should be determined by decreasing the initial drug dosage in small increments at appropriate time intervals until the lowest dosage which will maintain an adequate clinical response is reached. It should be kept in mind that constant monitoring is needed in regard to drug dosage. Included in the situations which may make dosage adjustments necessary are changes in clinical status secondary to remissions or exacerbations in the disease process, the patient's individual drug responsiveness, and the effect of patient exposure to stressful situations not directly related to the disease entity under treatment; in this latter situation it may be necessary to increase the dosage of Kenalog-40 Injection for a period of time consistent with the patient's condition. If after long-term therapy the drug is to be stopped, it is recommended that it be withdrawn gradually rather than abruptly.

Dosage

Systemic: Although Kenalog-40 Injection (Sterile Triamcinolone Acetonide Suspension USP) may be administered intramuscularly for initial therapy, most physicians prefer to adjust the dose orally until adequate control is attained. Intramuscular administration provides a sustained or depot action which can be used to supplement or replace initial oral therapy. With intramuscular therapy, greater supervision of the amount of steroid used is made possible in the patient who is inconsistent in following an oral dosage schedule. In maintenance therapy, the patient-to-patient response is not uniform and, therefore, the dose must be individualized for optimal control.

For **adults and children over 12 years of age,** the suggested initial dose is 60 mg., **injected deeply into the gluteal muscle.** Subcutaneous fat atrophy may occur if care is not taken to inject the preparation intramuscularly. Dosage is usually adjusted within the range of 40 to 80 mg., depending upon patient response and duration of relief. However, some patients may be well controlled on dosages as low as 20 mg. or less. Patients with hay fever or pollen asthma who are not responding to pollen administration and other conventional therapy may obtain a remission of symptoms lasting throughout the pollen season after one injection of 40 to 100 mg.

For **children from 6 to 12 years of age,** the suggested initial dose is 40 mg., although dosage depends more on the severity of symptoms than on age or weight. There is insufficient clinical experience with Kenalog-40 Injection to recommend its use in children under six years of age.

Local: For intra-articular or intrabursal administration and for injection into tendon sheaths, the initial dose of Kenalog-40 Injection (Sterile Triamcinolone Acetonide Suspension USP) may vary from 2.5 to 5 mg. for smaller joints and from 5 to 15 mg. for larger joints depending on the specific disease entity being treated. (A more dilute form of Sterile Triamcinolone Acetonide Suspension USP is available—see ALSO AVAILABLE.) For adults, doses up to 10 mg. for smaller areas and up to 40 mg. for larger areas have usually been sufficient to alleviate symptoms. Single injections into several joints for multiple locus involvement, up to a total of 80 mg., have been given without undue reactions. A single local injection of triamcinolone acetonide is frequently sufficient, but several injections may be needed for adequate relief of symptoms. The lower dosages in the initial dosage range of triamcinolone acetonide may produce the desired effect when the corticosteroid is administered to provide a localized concentration. The site of the injection and the volume of the injection should be carefully considered when triamcinolone acetonide is administered for this purpose.

Administration

General: Shake the vial before use to insure a uniform suspension. After withdrawal, inject without delay to prevent settling in the syringe. Careful technique should be employed to avoid the possibility of entering a blood vessel or introducing infection.

Routine laboratory studies, such as urinalysis, two-hour postprandial blood sugar, determination of blood pressure and body weight and a chest x-ray should be made at regular intervals during prolonged therapy. Upper GI x-rays are desirable in patients with an ulcer history or significant dyspepsia.

Systemic: For systemic therapy, injection should be made **deeply into the gluteal muscle** to insure intramuscular delivery (see WARNINGS). For adults, a minimum needle length of 1 ½ inches is recommended. In obese patients, a longer needle may be required. Use alternate sites for subsequent injections.

Local: For treatment of joints, the usual intra-articular injection technique, as described in standard textbooks, should be followed. If an excessive amount of synovial fluid is present in the joint, some, but not all, should be aspirated to aid in the relief of pain and to prevent undue dilution of the corticosteroid.

With intra-articular or intrabursal administration, and with injection of the drug into tendon sheaths, the use of a local anesthetic may often be desirable. When a local anesthetic is used, its package insert should be read with care and all the precautions connected with its use should be observed. It should be injected into the surrounding soft tissues prior to the injection of the corticosteroid. A small amount of the anesthetic solution may be instilled into the joint.

In treating acute nonspecific tenosynovitis, care should be taken to insure that the injection of the corticosteroid is made into the tendon sheath rather than the tendon substance. Epicondylitis (tennis elbow) may be treated by infiltrating the preparation into the area of greatest tenderness.

How Supplied: In vials of 1, 5, and 10 ml. [5 ml. vial—Military Depot Item, NSN 6505-00-885-6216 and V.A. Depot Item, NSN6505-00-885-6216A].

Also Available: Kenalog-10 Injection (Sterile Triamcinolone Acetonide Suspension USP) providing 10 mg. triamcinolone acetonide per ml., with sodium chloride for isotonicity, 0.9% (w/v) benzyl alcohol as a preservative, 0.75% sodium carboxymethylcellulose, and 0.04% polysorbate 80. See package insert for full information.

Storage: Store at room temperature; avoid freezing. Protect from light.

KENALOG® -10 INJECTION ℞

(Sterile Triamcinolone Acetonide Suspension USP)

For Intra-articular, Intrabursal or Intradermal Use

NOT FOR INTRAVENOUS OR INTRAMUSCULAR USE

Description: Kenalog-10 Injection (Sterile Triamcinolone Acetonide Suspension USP) provides triamcinolone acetonide, a synthetic corticosteroid with marked anti-inflammatory action, in a sterile aqueous suspension suitable for intradermal, intra-articular, and intrabursal injection and for injection into tendon sheaths. This preparation is NOT suitable for intravenous or intramuscular use. Each ml. of the sterile aqueous suspension provides 10 mg. triamcinolone acetonide, with sodium chloride for isotonicity, 0.9% (w/v) benzyl alcohol as a preservative, 0.75% carboxymethylcellulose sodium, and 0.04% polysorbate 80; sodium hydroxide or hydrochloric acid may have been added to adjust pH between 5.0 and 7.5. At the time of manufacture, the air in the container is replaced by nitrogen.

The chemical name for triamcinolone acetonide is 9-fluoro-11β, 16α, 17, 21-tetrahydroxypregna-1,4-diene-3,20-dione cyclic 16, 17-acetal with acetone.

Clinical Pharmacology: Naturally occurring glucocorticoids (hydrocortisone), which also have salt-retaining properties, are used as replacement therapy in adrenocortical deficiency states. Their synthetic analogs are primarily used for their potent anti-inflammatory effects in disorders of many organ systems.

Glucocorticoids cause profound and varied metabolic effects. In addition, they modify the body's immune responses to diverse stimuli.

Indications and Usage:

Intra-Articular:

Kenalog-10 Injection (Sterile Triamcinolone Acetonide Suspension USP) is indicated for intra-articular or intrabursal administration, and for injections into tendon sheaths, as adjunctive therapy for short-term administration (to tide the patient over an acute episode or exacerbation) in: synovitis of osteoarthritis, rheumatoid arthritis, acute and subacute bursitis, acute gouty arthritis, epicondylitis, acute nonspecific tenosynovitis, and post-traumatic osteoarthritis.

Intradermal:

Intralesional administration of Kenalog-10 Injection is indicated for the treatment of keloids, discoid lupus erythematosus, necrobiosis lipoidica diabeticorum, alopecia areata, and localized hypertrophic, infiltrated, inflammatory lesions of: lichen planus, psoriatic plaques, granuloma annulare, and lichen simplex chronicus (neurodermatitis). Kenalog-10 Injection also may be useful in cystic tumors of an aponeurosis or tendon (ganglia).

Contraindications: Corticosteroids are contraindicated in patients with systemic fungal infections.

Warnings: Because it is a suspension, the preparation should *not* be administered intravenously. Strict aseptic technique is mandatory.

When patients who are receiving corticosteroid therapy are subjected to unusual stress, increased dosage of rapidly acting corticosteroids is indicated before, during, and after the stressful situation. Kenalog-10 Injection (Sterile Triamcinolone Acetonide Suspension USP), as a long-acting preparation, is *not* suitable for use in acute stress situations.

Corticosteroids may mask some signs of infection, and new infections may appear during their use. There may be decreased resistance and inability to localize infection when corticosteroids are used. If an infection occurs during corticosteroid therapy, it should be promptly controlled by suitable antimicrobial therapy (see PRECAUTIONS).

Prolonged use of corticosteroids may produce posterior subcapsular cataracts, glaucoma with possible damage to the optic nerves, and may enhance the establishment of secondary ocular infections due to fungi or viruses.

Average and large doses of hydrocortisone or cortisone can cause elevation of blood pressure, salt and water retention, and increased excretion of potassium. These effects are less likely to occur with the synthetic derivatives except when they are used in large doses; dietary salt restriction and potassium supplementation may be necessary (see PRECAUTIONS). All corticosteroids increase calcium excretion.

Patients should not be vaccinated against smallpox while on corticosteroid therapy. Other immunization procedures should not be undertaken in patients who are on corticosteroids, especially on high dose, because of possible hazards of neurological complications and a lack of antibody response.

The use of triamcinolone acetonide in patients with active tuberculosis should be restricted to those cases of fulminating or disseminated tuberculosis in which the corticosteroid is used for the management of the disease in conjunction with an appropriate antituberculous regimen. If corticosteroids are indicated in patients with latent tuberculosis or tuberculin reactivity, close observation is necessary since reactivation of the disease may occur. During prolonged corticosteroid therapy these patients should receive chemoprophylaxis.

Because rare instances of anaphylactoid reactions have occurred in patients receiving parenteral corticosteroid therapy, appropriate precautionary measures should be taken prior to administration, especially when the patient has a history of allergy to any drug.

Safety of use of Kenalog-10 Injection (Sterile Triamcinolone Acetonide Suspension USP) by intraturbinal, subconjunctival, subtenons, and retrobulbar injection has not been established.

Usage in Pregnancy — Since adequate human reproduction studies have not been done with corticosteroids, the use of these drugs in pregnancy, nursing mothers, or women of childbearing potential requires that the possible benefits of the drug be weighed against the potential hazards to the mother and the embryo, fetus, or nursing infant. Infants born of mothers who have received substantial doses of corticosteroids during pregnancy should be carefully observed for signs of hypoadrenalism.

Precautions: Drug-induced secondary adrenocortical insufficiency may be minimized by a gradual reduction of dosage. This type of relative insufficiency may persist for months after discontinuation of therapy; therefore, in any situation of stress (such as trauma, surgery, or severe illness) occurring during that period, hormone therapy should be reinstituted. Since mineralocorticoid secretion may be impaired, salt and/or a mineralocorticoid should be administered concurrently.

There is enhanced corticosteroid effect in patients with hypothyroidism and in those with cirrhosis.

Corticosteroids should be used cautiously in patients with ocular herpes simplex because of possible corneal perforation.

The lowest possible dose of corticosteroid should be used to control the condition being treated. A gradual reduction in dosage should be made when possible.

Psychic derangements may appear when corticosteroids are used. These may range from euphoria, insomnia, mood swings, personality changes, and severe depression, to frank psychotic manifestations. Existing emotional instability or psychotic tendencies may also be aggravated by corticosteroids.

Continued on next page

Squibb—Cont.

Aspirin should be used cautiously in conjunction with corticosteroids in patients with hypoprothrombinemia.
Corticosteroids should be used with caution in patients with nonspecific ulcerative colitis if there is a probability of impending perforation, abscess, or other pyogenic infection. Corticosteroids should also be used cautiously in patients with diverticulitis, fresh intestinal anastomoses, active or latent peptic ulcer, renal insufficiency, hypertension, osteoporosis, and myasthenia gravis.
Growth and development of infants and children on prolonged corticosteroid therapy should be carefully observed.
Although therapy with Kenalog-10 Injection (Sterile Triamcinolone Acetonide Suspension USP) may ameliorate symptoms, it is in no sense a cure and the hormone has no effect on the cause of the inflammation. Therefore, this method of treatment does not obviate the need for the conventional measures usually employed.
Intra-articular injection of a corticosteroid may produce systemic as well as local effects. The inadvertent injection of the suspension into the soft tissues surrounding a joint is not harmful, but is the most common cause of failure to achieve the desired local results.
Following intra-articular steroid therapy, patients should be specifically warned to avoid overuse of joints in which symptomatic benefit has been obtained. Negligence in this matter may permit an increase in joint deterioration that will more than offset the beneficial effects of the steroid. To detect deterioration follow-up x-ray examination is suggested in selected cases.
Overdistention of the joint capsule and deposition of steroid along the needle track should be avoided in intra-articular injection since this may lead to subcutaneous atrophy.
Corticosteroids should not be injected into unstable joints. Repeated intra-articular injection may in some cases result in instability of the joint. In selected cases, particularly when repeated injections are given, x-ray follow-up is suggested.
An increase in joint discomfort has seldom occurred. A marked increase in pain accompanied by local swelling, further restriction of joint motion, fever, and malaise are suggestive of a septic arthritis. If these complications should appear, and the diagnosis of septic arthritis is confirmed, administration of triamcinolone acetonide should be stopped, and antimicrobial therapy should be instituted immediately and continued for 7 to 10 days after all evidence of infection has disappeared. Appropriate examination of any joint fluid present is necessary to exclude a septic process.
Local injection of a steroid into a previously infected joint is to be avoided.
Kenalog-10 Injection (Sterile Triamcinolone Acetonide Suspension USP) should be administered only with full knowledge of characteristic activity of, and varied responses to, adrenocortical hormones. Like other potent corticosteroids, triamcinolone acetonide should be used under close clinical supervision. Triamcinolone acetonide can cause elevation of blood pressure, salt and water retention, and increased potassium and calcium excretion necessitating dietary salt restriction and potassium supplementation. Edema may occur in the presence of renal disease with a fixed or decreased glomerular filtration rate.
During prolonged therapy, *a liberal protein intake is essential* for counteracting the tendency to gradual weight loss sometimes associated with negative nitrogen balance, wasting and weakness of skeletal muscles.
When local or systemic microbial infections are present, therapy with triamcinolone acetonide is not recommended, but may be employed with caution and only in conjunction with appropriate antibiotic or chemotherapeutic medication. Triamcinolone acetonide may mask signs of infection and enhance dissemination of the infecting organism. Hence, all patients receiving triamcinolone acetonide should be watched for evidence of intercurrent infection. Should infection occur, vigorous, appropriate anti-infective therapy should be initiated. If possible, abrupt cessation of steroids should be avoided because of the danger of superimposing adrenocortical insufficiency on the infectious process.
Menstrual irregularities may occur, and this possibility should be mentioned to female patients past menarche.
In peptic ulcer, recurrence may be asymptomatic until perforation or hemorrhage occurs. X-rays should be taken in peptic ulcer patients complaining of gastric distress, or when therapy is prolonged. Whether or not changes are observed, an ulcer regimen is recommended.
As with other corticosteroids, the possibility of other severe reactions should be considered. If such reactions should occur, appropriate corrective measures should be instituted and use of the drug discontinued.
Continued supervision of the patient after termination of triamcinolone acetonide therapy is essential, since there may be a sudden reappearance of severe manifestations of the disease for which the patient was treated.

Adverse Reactions: Undesirable reactions following intra-articular administration of the preparation have included postinjection flare, transient pain, occasional local irritation at the injection site, sterile abscesses, hyper- and hypopigmentation, charcot-like arthropathy, and occasional brief increase in joint discomfort; following intradermal administration, rare instances of blindness associated with intralesional therapy around the face and head, transient local discomfort, sterile abscesses, hyper- and hypopigmentation, and subcutaneous and cutaneous atrophy (which usually disappears, unless the basic disease process is itself atrophic) have occurred.
Since systemic absorption may occasionally occur with intra-articular or other local administration, patients should be watched closely for the following adverse reactions which may be associated with any corticosteroid therapy:
Fluid and electrolyte disturbances—sodium retention, fluid retention, congestive heart failure in susceptible patients, potassium loss, cardiac arrythmias or ECG changes due to potassium deficiency, hypokalemic alkalosis, and hypertension.
Musculoskeletal—muscle weakness, fatigue, steroid myopathy, loss of muscle mass, osteoporosis, vertebral compression fractures, delayed healing of fractures, aseptic necrosis of femoral and humeral heads, pathologic fractures of long bones, and spontaneous fractures.
Gastrointenstinal—peptic ulcer with possible subsequent perforation and hemorrhage, pancreatitis, abdominal distention, and ulcerative esophagitis.
Dermatologic—impaired wound healing, thin fragile skin, petechiae and ecchymoses, facial erythema, increased sweating, purpura, striae, hirsutism, acneiform eruptions, lupus erythematosus-like lesions and suppressed reactions to skin tests.
Neurological—convulsions, increased intracranial pressure with papilledema (pseudotumor cerebri) usually after treatment, vertigo, headache, neuritis or paresthesias, and aggravation of pre-existing psychiatric conditions.
Endocrine—menstrual irregularities; development of the cushingoid state; suppression of growth in children; secondary adrenocortical and pituitary unresponsiveness, particularly in times of stress (e.g., trauma, surgery, or illness); decreased carbohydrate tolerance; manifestations of latent diabetes mellitus; and increased requirements for insulin or oral hypoglycemic agents in diabetics.
Ophthalmic—posterior subcapsular cataracts, increased intraocular pressure, glaucoma, and exophthalmos.
Metabolic—hyperglycemia, glycosuria, and negative nitrogen balance due to protein catabolism.
Others—necrotizing angiitis, thrombophlebitis, thromboembolism, aggravation or masking of infections, insomnia, syncopal episodes, and anaphylactoid reactions.

Dosage and Administration:
Dosage: The initial dose of Kenalog-10 Injection (Sterile Triamcinolone Acetonide Suspension USP) for intra-articular or intrabursal administration and for injection into tendon sheaths may vary from 2.5 mg. to 5 mg. for smaller joints and from 5 to 15 mg. for larger joints depending on the specific disease entity being treated. Single injections into several joints for multiple locus involvement, up to a total of 20 mg. or more, have been given without incident. For intradermal administration, the initial dose of triamcinolone acetonide will vary depending upon the specific disease entity being treated but should be limited to 1.0 mg. (0.1 ml.) per injection site, since larger volumes are more likely to produce cutaneous atrophy. Multiple sites (separated by one centimeter or more) may be so injected, keeping in mind that the greater the *total* volume employed the more corticosteroid becomes available for possible systemic absorption and subsequent corticosteroid effects. Such injections may be repeated, if necessary, at weekly or less frequent intervals.
The lower dosages in the initial dosage range of triamcinolone acetonide may produce the desired effect when the corticosteroid is administered to provide a localized concentration. The site of the injection and the volume of the injection should be carefully considered when triamcinolone acetonide is administered for this purpose. The inital dosage should be maintained or adjusted until a satisfactory response is noted. If after a reasonable period of time there is a lack of satisfactory clinical response, Kenalog-10 Injection should be discontinued and the patient transferred to other appropriate therapy. IT SHOULD BE EMPHASIZED THAT DOSAGE REQUIREMENTS ARE VARIABLE AND MUST BE INDIVIDUALIZED ON THE BASIS OF THE DISEASE UNDER TREATMENT AND THE RESPONSE OF THE PATIENT. After a favorable response is noted, the proper maintenance dosage should be determined by decreasing the initial drug dosage in small increments at appropriate time intervals until the lowest dosage which will maintain an adequate clinical response is reached. It should be kept in mind that constant monitoring is needed in regard to drug dosage. Included in the situations which may make dosage adjustments necessary are changes in clinical status secondary to remissions or exacerbations in the disease process, the patient's individual drug responsiveness, and the effect of patient exposure to stressful situations not directly related to the disease entity under treatment; in this latter situation it may be necessary to increase the dosage of Kenalog-10 Injection (Sterile Triamcinolone Acetonide Suspension USP) for a period of time consistent with the patient's condition. If the drug is to be stopped after long-term therapy, it is recommended that it be withdrawn gradually rather than abruptly.
Administration: Shake the vial before use to insure a uniform suspension. After withdrawal, inject without delay to prevent settling in the syringe. Careful technique should be employed to avoid the possibility of entering a blood vessel or introducing infection.
Routine laboratory studies, such as urinalysis, two-hour post-prandial blood sugar, determination of blood pressure and body weight, and a chest x-ray should be made at regular inter-

vals during prolonged therapy. Upper GI x-rays are desirable in patients with an ulcer history or significant dyspepsia.

For treatment of joints, the usual intra-articular injection technique, as described in standard textbooks, should be followed. If an excessive amount of synovial fluid is present in the joint, some, but not all, should be aspirated to aid in the relief of pain and to prevent undue dilution of the steroid.

With intra-articular or intrabursal administration, and with injection of Kenalog-10 Injection into tendon sheaths, the use of a local anesthetic may often be desirable. When a local anesthetic is used, its package insert should be read with care and all the precautions connected with its use should be observed. It should be injected into the surrounding soft tissue prior to the injection of the corticosteroid. A small amount of the anesthetic solution may be instilled into the joint.

In treating acute nonspecific tenosynovitis, care should be taken to insure that the injection of Kenalog-10 Injection is made into the tendon sheath rather than the tendon substance. Epicondylitis (tennis elbow) may be treated by infiltrating the preparation into the area of greatest tenderness.

For treatment of dermal lesions, Kenalog-10 Injection is injected directly into the lesion, i.e., intradermally or sometimes subcutaneously. For accuracy of dosage measurement and ease of administration, it is preferable to employ a tuberculin syringe and a small bore needle (23 to 25 gauge). Ethyl chloride spray may be used to alleviate the discomfort of the injection.

How Supplied: Kenalog-10 Injection (Sterile Triamcinolone Acetonide Suspension USP) is supplied in 5 ml. multiple-dose vials providing 10 mg. triamcinolone acetonide per ml. [Military Depot Item, NSN 6505-00-065-6772].

Storage: Store at room temperature; avoid freezing; protect from light.

KENALOG® IN ORABASE® ℞
(Triamcinolone Acetonide Dental Paste USP)

Description: Each gram of Kenalog in Orabase provides 1 mg. (0.1%) triamcinolone acetonide in emollient dental paste containing gelatin, pectin, and carboxymethylcellulose sodium in Plastibase® (Plasticized Hydrocarbon Gel), a polyethylene and mineral oil gel base.

Actions: Triamcinolone acetonide is a synthetic corticosteroid which possesses anti-inflammatory, antipruritic, and antiallergic action. The emollient dental paste acts as an adhesive vehicle for applying the active medication to the oral tissues. The vehicle provides a protective covering which may serve to temporarily reduce the pain associated with oral irritation.

Indications: Kenalog in Orabase (Triamcinolone Acetonide Dental Paste USP) is indicated for adjunctive treatment and for the temporary relief of symptoms associated with oral inflammatory lesions and ulcerative lesions resulting from trauma.

Contraindications: This preparation is contraindicated in patients with a history of hypersensitivity to any of its components.

Because it contains a corticosteroid, the preparation is contraindicated in the presence of fungal, viral, or bacterial infections of the mouth or throat.

Warning: Usage in Pregnancy—Safe use of this preparation during pregnancy has not been established with respect to possible adverse reactions upon fetal development; therefore, it should not be used in women of childbearing potential and particularly during early pregnancy unless, in the judgment of the physician or dentist, the potential benefits outweigh the possible hazards.

Precautions: Patients with tuberculosis, peptic ulcer or diabetes mellitus should not be treated with any corticosteroid preparation without the advice of the patient's physician. It should be borne in mind that the normal defensive responses of the oral tissues are depressed in patients receiving topical corticosteroid therapy. Virulent strains of oral microorganisms may multiply without producing the usual warning symptoms of oral infections. The small amount of steroid released when the preparation is used as recommended makes systemic effects very unlikely; however, they are a possibility when topical corticosteroid preparations are used over a long period of time.

If local irritation or sensitization should develop, the preparation should be discontinued and appropriate therapy instituted.

If significant regeneration or repair of oral tissues has not occurred in seven days, additional investigation into the etiology of the oral lesion is advised.

Adverse Reactions: Prolonged administration may elicit the adverse reactions known to occur with systemic steroid preparations; for example, adrenal suppression, alteration of glucose metabolism, protein catabolism, peptic ulcer activations, and others. These are usually reversible and disappear when the hormone is discontinued.

Dosage and Administration: Press a small dab (about one-quarter of an inch) to the lesion until a thin film develops. A larger quantity may be required for coverage of some lesions. For optimal results use only enough to coat the lesion with a thin film. Do not rub in. Attempting to spread this preparation may result in a granular, gritty sensation and cause it to crumble. After application, however, a smooth, slippery film develops.

The preparation should be applied at bedtime to permit steroid contact with the lesion throughout the night. Depending on the severity of symptoms, it may be necessary to apply the preparation two or three times a day, preferably after meals. If significant repair or regeneration has not occurred in seven days, further investigation is advisable.

How Supplied: 5 gram tubes (Military Depot Item, NSN 6505-00-926-8913).

Storage: Store at room temperature; keep tube tightly closed.

KINEVAC® ℞
(Sincalide for Injection)

(See Diagnostic Section)

MEDOTOPES® ℞
(Radiopharmaceuticals)

(See Diagnostic Section)

MYCOLOG® ℞
(Nystatin—Neomycin Sulfate—Gramicidin—Triamcinolone Acetonide) CREAM AND OINTMENT

Description: Mycolog (Nystatin—Neomycin Sulfate—Gramicidin—Triamcinolone Acetonide) is available as a cream in an aqueous vanishing cream base and as an ointment in Plastibase® (Plasticized Hydrocarbon Gel), a polyethylene and mineral oil gel base. Each gram of the cream or ointment provides 100,000 units nystatin, neomycin sulfate equivalent to 2.5 mg. neomycin base, 0.25 mg. gramicidin and 1 mg. triamcinolone acetonide (0.1%). The cream also contains polysorbate 60, alcohol, aluminum hydroxide concentrated wet gel, titanium dioxide, glyceryl monostearate, polyethylene glycol monostearate, simethicone, sorbic acid, propylene glycol, ethylenediamine hydrochloride, white petrolatum, cetearyl alcohol (and) ceteareth-20, methylparaben, propylparaben, and sorbitol solution.

Actions: Triamcinolone acetonide is primarily effective because of its anti-inflammatory, antipruritic, and vasoconstrictive actions. Nystatin provides specific anticandidal activity and the two topical antibiotics, neomycin and gramicidin, provide antibacterial activity.

Indications

Based on a review of these drugs by the National Academy of Sciences—National Research Council and/or other information, FDA has classified the indications as follows:

Possibly effective: In
- cutaneous candidiasis
- superficial bacterial infections
- the following conditions when complicated by candidal and/or bacterial infection: atopic, eczematoid, stasis, nummular, contact, or seborrheic dermatitis; neurodermatitis and dermatitis venenata
- infantile eczema
- lichen simplex chronicus
- the Cream is also possibly effective in pruritus ani and pruritus vulvae

Final classification of the less-than-effective indications requires further investigation.

Contraindications: Topical steroids are contraindicated in viral diseases of the skin, such as vaccinia and varicella. The preparations are also contraindicated in fungal lesions of the skin except candidiasis, and in those patients with a history of hypersensitivity to any of their components.

The preparations are not for ophthalmic use nor should they be applied in the external auditory canal of patients with perforated eardrums.

Topical steroids should not be used when circulation is markedly impaired.

Warnings: Because of the potential hazard of nephrotoxicity and ototoxicity, prolonged use or use of large amounts of these products should be avoided in the treatment of skin infections following extensive burns, trophic ulceration, and other conditions where absorption of neomycin is possible.

Usage in Pregnancy: Although topical steroids have not been reported to have an adverse effect on the fetus, the safety of topical steroid preparations during pregnancy has not been absolutely established; therefore, they should not be used extensively on pregnant patients, in large amounts, or for prolonged periods of time.

Precautions: As with any antibiotic preparation, prolonged use may result in overgrowth of nonsusceptible organisms, including fungi other than *Candida*. Constant observation of the patient is essential. Should superinfection due to nonsusceptible organisms occur, suitable concomitant antimicrobial therapy must be administered. If a favorable response does not occur promptly, application of Mycolog (Nystatin—Neomycin Sulfate—Gramicidin—Triamcinolone Acetonide) Cream or Ointment should be discontinued until the infection is adequately controlled by other anti-infective measures.

If extensive areas are treated or if the occlusive technique is used, the possibility exists of increased systemic absorption of the corticosteroid and suitable precautions should be taken. If irritation develops, the product should be discontinued and appropriate therapy instituted.

Adverse Reactions: Hypersensitivity to nystatin is extremely uncommon. Sensitivity reactions following the topical use of gramicidin are rarely encountered. Hypersensitivity to neomycin has been reported and articles in the current medical literature indicate an increase in its prevalence.

The following local adverse reactions have been reported with topical corticosteroids ei-

Continued on next page

Squibb—Cont.

ther with or without occlusive dressings: burning sensations, itching, irritation, dryness, folliculitis, secondary infection, skin atrophy, striae, miliaria, hypertrichosis, acneform eruptions, maceration of the skin and hypopigmentation. Contact sensitivity to a particular dressing material or adhesive may occur occasionally.
Ototoxicity and nephrotoxicity have been reported.
Dosage and Administration: *Mycolog Cream* (Nystatin—Neomycin Sulfate—Gramicidin—Triamcinolone Acetonide Cream) —Rub the cream into affected areas two to three times daily.
Mycolog Ointment (Nystatin—Neomycin Sulfate—Gramicidin—Triamcinolone Acetonide Ointment)—Apply a thin film of the ointment to the affected areas two to three times daily.
Occlusive Dressing Technique—Cream: Gently rub a small amount of the cream into the lesion until it disappears. Reapply the cream leaving a thin coating on the lesion and cover with a pliable nonporous film. If needed, additional moisture may be provided by covering the lesion with a dampened clean cotton cloth before the plastic film is applied or by briefly soaking the affected area in water.
The frequency of changing dressings is best determined on an individual basis. Reapplication is essential at each dressing change.
Ointment: Apply the ointment leaving a thin coating on the lesion and cover with a pliable nonporous film. If needed, additional moisture may be provided by covering the lesion with a dampened clean cotton cloth before the plastic film is applied or by briefly soaking the affected area in water.
The frequency of changing dressings is best determined on an individual basis. Reapplication is essential at each dressing change.
How Supplied: Both preparations are available in tubes of 15, 30, and 60 g. They are also available in jars of 120 g. for hospital or institutional use only. [Cream in 15 g. tubes—V.A. Depot Item, NSN6505-00-961-5504A; Cream in 120 g. jars—V.A. Depot Item, NSN6505-00-772-0245A; Ointment in 15 g. tubes—Military Depot Item, NSN 6505-01-040-5957; V.A. Depot Item, NSN6505-00-772-0244A.]
Storage: Store the cream at room temperature; avoid freezing. Store the ointment at room temperature.

MYCOSTATIN® CREAM ℞
(Nystatin Cream)
MYCOSTATIN OINTMENT ℞
(Nystatin Ointment USP)
MYCOSTATIN TOPICAL POWDER ℞
(Nystatin Topical Powder)

Description: Mycostatin Cream (Nystatin Cream) contains the antifungal antibiotic Nystatin USP at a concentration of 100,000 units per gram in an aqueous, perfumed vanishing cream base containing aluminum hydroxide concentrated wet gel, titanium dioxide, propylene glycol, cetearyl alcohol (and) ceteareth-20, white petrolatum, sorbitol solution, glyceryl monostearate, polyethylene glycol monostearate, sorbic acid and simethicone.
Mycostatin Ointment (Nystatin Ointment USP) provides 100,000 units Nystatin USP per gram in Plastibase® (Plasticized Hydrocarbon Gel), a polyethylene and mineral oil gel base.
Mycostatin Topical Powder (Nystatin Topical Powder) provides, in each gram, 100,000 units Nystatin USP dispersed in Talc USP.
Clinical Pharmacology: Nystatin is an antifungal antibiotic which is both fungistatic and fungicidal *in vitro* against a wide variety of yeasts and yeast-like fungi. It probably acts by binding to sterols in the cell membrane of the fungus with a resultant change in membrane permeability allowing leakage of intracellular components. Nystatin is a polyene antibiotic of undetermined structural formula that is obtained from *Streptomyces noursei*, and is the first well tolerated antifungal antibiotic of dependable efficacy for the treatment of cutaneous, oral and intestinal infections caused by *Candida* (Monilia) *albicans* and other Candida species. It exhibits no appreciable activity against bacteria.
Nystatin provides specific therapy for all localized forms of candidiasis. Symptomatic relief is rapid, often occurring within 24 to 72 hours after the initiation of treatment. Cure is effected both clinically and mycologically in most cases of localized candidiasis.
Indications and Usage: Mycostatin topical preparations are indicated in the treatment of cutaneous or mucocutaneous mycotic infections caused by *Candida* (Monilia) *albicans* and other Candida species.
Contraindications: Mycostatin topical preparations are contraindicated in patients with a history of hypersensitivity to any of their components.
Precautions: Should a reaction of hypersensitivity occur the drug should be immediately withdrawn and appropriate measures taken.
Adverse Reactions: Nystatin is virtually nontoxic and nonsensitizing and is well tolerated by all age groups including debilitated infants, even on prolonged administration. If irritation on topical application should occur, discontinue medication.
Dosage and Administration: The cream and the ointment should be applied liberally to affected areas twice daily or as indicated until healing is complete. The powder should be applied to candidal lesions two or three times daily until lesions have healed. For fungal infection of the feet caused by Candida species, the powder should be dusted freely on the feet as well as in shoes and socks. The cream is usually preferred to the ointment in candidiasis involving intertriginous areas; very moist lesions, however, are best treated with the topical dusting powder.
The preparations do not stain skin or mucous membranes and they provide a simple, convenient means of treatment.
How Supplied: Mycostatin Cream (Nystatin Cream) is supplied in tubes of 15 g. and 30 g. Mycostatin Ointment (Nystatin Ointment USP) is supplied in tubes of 15 g. and 30 g. Mycostatin Topical Powder (Nystatin Topical Powder) is supplied in plastic squeeze bottles of 15 g. (½ oz.) [Military Depot Item, NSN 6505-00-890-1218].
Storage: Store the cream at room temperature; avoid freezing. Store the ointment at room temperature. Store the topical powder at room temperature; avoid excessive heat; keep bottle tightly closed.

MYCOSTATIN® ORAL SUSPENSION ℞
(Nystatin Oral Suspension USP)

Description: Nystatin is an antifungal antibiotic which is both fungistatic and fungicidal *in vitro* against a wide variety of yeasts and yeast-like fungi. It is a polyene antibiotic of undetermined structural formula that is obtained from *Streptomyces noursei*. Mycostatin Oral Suspension is provided for oral administration containing 100,000 units nystatin per ml. in a vehicle containing 50% sucrose; not more than 1% alcohol by volume.
Clinical Pharmacology: Nystatin probably acts by binding to sterols in the cell membrane of the fungus with a resultant change in membrane permeability allowing leakage of intracellular components. It exhibits no appreciable activity against bacteria or trichomonads.
Following oral administration, nystatin is sparingly absorbed with no detectable blood levels when given in the recommended doses. Most of the orally administered nystatin is passed unchanged in the stool.
Indications and Usage: Mycostatin Oral Suspension is indicated for the treatment of candidiasis in the oral cavity.
Contraindication: The preparation is contraindicated in patients with a history of hypersensitivity to any of its components.
Precautions:
Usage in Pregnancy—No adverse effects or complications have been attributed to nystatin in infants born to women treated with nystatin.
Adverse Reactions: Nystatin is virtually nontoxic and nonsensitizing and is well tolerated by all age groups including debilitated infants, even on prolonged administration. Large oral doses have occasionally produced diarrhea, gastrointestinal distress, nausea, and vomiting.
Dosage and Administration: INFANTS—2 ml. (200,000 units nystatin) four times daily (1 ml. in each side of mouth).
NOTE: Limited clinical studies in premature and low birth weight infants indicate that 1 ml. four times daily is effective.
CHILDREN AND ADULTS—4-6 ml. (400,000 to 600,000 units nystatin) four times daily (one-half of dose in each side of mouth). The preparation should be retained in the mouth as long as possible before swallowing.
Continue treatment for at least 48 hours after perioral symptoms have disappeared and cultures returned to normal.
How Supplied: Mycostatin Oral Suspension (Nystatin Oral Suspension USP) is available as a pleasant-tasting, ready-to-use suspension containing 100,000 units nystatin per ml. in 60 ml. bottles (each supplied with a calibrated dropper) and UNIMATIC® bottles containing a single 5 ml. dose.
Storage: Store at room temperature; avoid freezing.

MYCOSTATIN® ORAL TABLETS ℞
(Nystatin Tablets USP)

Description: Nystatin is an antifungal antibiotic which is both fungistatic and fungicidal *in vitro* against a wide variety of yeasts and yeast-like fungi. It is a polyene antibiotic of undetermined structural formula that is obtained from *Streptomyces noursei*. Mycostatin Oral Tablets are provided for oral administration as coated tablets containing 500,000 units nystatin.
Clinical Pharmacology: Nystatin probably acts by binding to sterols in the cell membrane of the fungus with a resultant change in membrane permeability allowing leakage of intracellular components. It exhibits no appreciable activity against bacteria or trichomonads.
Following oral administration, nystatin is sparingly absorbed with no detectable blood levels when given in the recommended doses. Most of the orally administered nystatin is passed unchanged in the stool.
Indications and Usage: Mycostatin Oral Tablets (Nystatin Tablets USP) are intended for the treatment of intestinal candidiasis.
Contraindications: Mycostatin Oral Tablets are contraindicated in patients with a history of hypersensitivity to any of their components.
Precautions: Usage in Pregnancy—No adverse effects or complications have been attributed to nystatin in infants born to women treated with nystatin.
Adverse Reactions: Nystatin is virtually nontoxic and nonsensitizing and is well tolerated by all age groups including debilitated infants, even on prolonged administration. Large oral doses have occasionally produced diarrhea, gastrointestinal distress, nausea and vomiting.
Dosage and Administration: The usual therapeutic dosage is one to two tablets (500,000 to 1,000,000 units nystatin) three

times daily. Treatment should generally be continued for at least 48 hours after clinical cure to prevent relapse.

How Supplied: Mycostatin Oral Tablets (Nystatin Tablets USP) are available for oral administration as FILMLOK® tablets providing 500,000 units nystatin per tablet in bottles of 100 and UNIMATIC® cartons of 100. (Filmlok is a Squibb trademark for veneer-coated tablets.) [Bottles of 100, Military Depot Item, NSN6505-00-118-1949.]

Storage: Store at room temperature; avoid excessive heat. Dispense in tight, light-resistant containers.

[*Shown in Product Identification Section*]

MYCOSTATIN® VAGINAL TABLETS ℞
(Nystatin Vaginal Tablets USP)

Description: Nystatin is an antimycotic polyene antibiotic obtained from *Streptomyces noursei.*

Mycostatin Vaginal Tablets (Nystatin Vaginal Tablets USP) are available as diamond-shaped compressed tablets for intravaginal administration, providing 100,000 units of nystatin dispersed in lactose with ethyl cellulose, stearic acid, and starch.

Clinical Pharmacology: Nystatin is both fungistatic and fungicidal *in vitro* against a wide variety of yeats and yeast-like fungi. Nystatin acts by binding to sterols in the cell membrane of sensitive fungi with a resultant change in membrane permeability allowing leakage of intracellular components. Nystatin exhibits no appreciable activity against bacteria, protozoa, trichomonads, or viruses.

Nystatin is not absorbed from intact skin or mucous membranes.

Indications and Usage: Mycostatin Vaginal Tablets (Nystatin Vaginal Tablets USP) are effective for the local treatment of vulvovaginal candidiasis (moniliasis). The diagnosis should be confirmed, prior to therapy, by KOH smears and/or cultures. Other pathogens commonly associated with vulvovaginitis (Trichomonas and *Haemophilus vaginalis*) do not respond to nystatin and should be ruled out by appropriate laboratory methods.

Contraindications: This preparation is contraindicated in patients with a history of hypersensitivity to any of its components.

Precautions: General: Discontinue treatment if sensitization or irritation is reported during use.

Information for Patients: The patient should be informed of symptoms of sensitization or irritation and told to report them promptly.

The patient should be warned against interruption or discontinuation of medication even during menstruation and even though symptomatic relief may occur within a few days.

The patient should be advised that adjunctive measures such as therapeutic douches are unnecessary and sometimes inadvisable, but cleansing douches may be used by nonpregnant women, if desired, for esthetic purposes.

Laboratory Tests: If there is a lack of response to Mycostatin Vaginal Tablets (Nystatin Vaginal Tablets USP), appropriate microbiological studies should be repeated to confirm the diagnosis and rule out other pathogens, before instituting another course of antimycotic therapy (see INDICATIONS AND USAGE).

Carcinogenesis, Mutagenesis, Impairment of Fertility: Long-term studies in animals have not been performed to evaluate carcinogenic potential, mutagenesis, or whether this medication affects fertility in females.

Pregnancy: Teratogenic Effects: Category A. There have been no reports that use of nystatin vaginal tablets by pregnant women increases the risk of fetal abnormalities or affects later growth, development, and functional maturation of the child. Nevertheless, because the possibility of harm cannot be ruled out, nystatin vaginal tablets should be used during pregnancy only if the physician considers it essential to the welfare of the patient. Animal reproduction studies have not been conducted with nystatin vaginal tablets.

Pediatric Use: Safety and effectiveness in children have not been established.

Adverse Reactions: Nystatin is virtually nontoxic and nonsensitizing and is well tolerated by all age groups, even on prolonged administration. Rarely, irritation or sensitization may occur (see PRECAUTIONS).

Dosage and Administration: The usual dosage is one tablet (100,000 units nystatin) daily for two weeks. The tablets should be deposited high in the vagina by means of the applicator. "Instructions for the Patient" are enclosed in each package.

How Supplied: Mycostatin Vaginal Tablets (Nystatin Vaginal Tablets USP) are available in packages of 15 and 30 individually foil wrapped tablets with applicator and in UNIMATIC® cartons of 50 unit-dose packs per carton—each celloprotected unit-dose pack contains one individually foil wrapped tablet, one applicator, and one "Instructions for the Patient" leaflet.

Storage: Store in refrigerator below 15° C (59° F).

[*Shown in Product Identification Section*]

MYSTECLIN-F® CAPSULES ℞
(Tetracycline—Amphotericin B Capsules)

MYSTECLIN-F® SYRUP ℞
(Tetracycline—Amphotericin B Syrup)

> Recently, a panel of the National Academy of Sciences—National Research Council has stated that in its informed judgment Mysteclin-F is ineffective as a fixed combination. Further, it stated, "The Panel is not aware of evidence of proved efficacy of this combination in the prevention of disease due to monilial organisms, although suppression of growth of monilia may be accomplished. It should be noted that the apparent reduction of organisms in the feces may be an artifact due to residual antibiotic activity and thus may not reflect the true state in the patient. It is preferable, in the Panel's opinion, to prescribe antifungal drugs when clinically indicated, rather than to use them indiscriminately as 'prophylaxis' against an uncommon clinical entity seen during therapy with tetracyclines and other antibiotics."

Mysteclin-F Capsules (Tetracycline—Amphotericin B Capsules) are available in the equivalent of 250 mg. tetracycline hydrochloride with 50 mg. amphotericin B, buffered with potassium metaphosphate.

Mysteclin-F Syrup (Tetracycline—Amphotericin B Syrup) is a fruit-flavored syrup containing, in each 5 ml. teaspoonful, tetracycline equivalent to 125 mg. tetracycline hydrochloride, buffered with potassium metaphosphate, and 25 mg. amphotericin B.

Clinical Pharmacology: Mysteclin-F (Tetracycline—Amphotericin B) Capsules and Syrup have been designed to provide simultaneous antimicrobial therapy and anticandidal prophylaxis, a concept first developed by Squibb.

The preparations, which contain the broad spectrum antibiotic tetracycline, well known for its pronounced antimicrobial effect against a wide range of pathogenic organisms, produce exceptionally high initial tetracycline blood levels as well as excellent diffusion to tissues and body fluids.

Furthermore, these preparations also contain **prophylactic** amounts of the antifungal antibiotic, amphotericin B. This antibiotic, first isolated and described by the Squibb Institute for Medical Research, is substantially more active *in vitro* against *Candida* strains than nystatin, and has been widely used by the intravenous route in the treatment of many deep-seated mycotic infections.

Given orally, amphotericin B is extremely well tolerated and is virtually nontoxic in prophylactic doses. Although poorly absorbed from the gut, amphotericin B has a high degree of activity against *Candida* species in the intestinal tract and prevents the overgrowth of these organisms commonly associated with broad spectrum antibiotic therapy (amphotericin B has no antibacterial activity). By suppressing overgrowth of *Candida* in the gastrointestinal tract, thereby minimizing a possible reservoir of this organism, Mysteclin-F (Tetracycline—Amphotericin B) provides added protection for the patient against troublesome, or even serious, candidal superinfections, e.g., intestinal (diarrheal), anogenital, vulvovaginal, mucocutaneous candidiasis.

Note: Microorganisms that have become insensitive to one tetracycline invariably exhibit cross-resistance to other tetracyclines. In addition, gram-negative bacilli made tetracycline resistant may also show cross-resistance to chloramphenicol.

Indications and Usage: Candidal overgrowth occurs in a large number of patients taking broad spectrum antibiotics. Although it is impossible to predict exactly which patient will develop candidal complications and which will not, certain types of patients are known to be particularly susceptible to candidiasis. Among these are elderly or debilitated patients; patients on high or prolonged antibiotic dosage; diabetics; infants; patients on corticoid therapy; patients who have developed candidiasis on previous broad spectrum therapy; women, particularly during pregnancy. Because the danger of candidal complications is greatest in these patients, they are potential candidates for therapy with Mysteclin-F.

Mysteclin-F (Tetracycline—Amphotericin B) Capsules and Syrup are indicated for the many common infections, including those of the respiratory, gastrointestinal and genitourinary systems, which are amenable to tetracycline therapy. Infections caused by gram-positive and gram-negative bacteria, spirochetes, viruses of the lymphogranuloma-psittacosis-trachoma group, rickettsiae and *Endamoeba histolytica* can be expected to respond. Because of the wide range of antimicrobial activity, the preparations are particularly useful in the treatment of mixed infections due to susceptible organisms.

Mysteclin-F (Tetracycline—Amphotericin B) Capsules and Syrup are also a useful part of the armamentarium in the management of chronic cases of acne vulgaris which, in the judgment of the clinician, require long-term treatment. The cystic and pustular forms of this condition respond most satisfactorily to tetracycline therapy; the papular form may also show improvement in some individuals. Because long-term maintenance therapy with tetracycline is involved, the presence of amphotericin B in the product is a particular advantage, helping to guard against the risk of candidal overgrowth.

Note: A number of strains of staphylococci and streptococci have shown resistance to tetracyclines. A few strains of pneumococci, *E. coli* and shigellae also have been reported as resistant. Indicated laboratory studies, including sensitivity tests, should be performed.

Contraindications: These products should not be used in persons with a history of hypersensitivity to any of their components.

Warnings: THE USE OF DRUGS OF THE TETRACYCLINE CLASS DURING TOOTH DEVELOPMENT (LAST HALF OF PREGNANCY, INFANCY, AND CHILDHOOD TO AGE OF EIGHT YEARS) MAY CAUSE PER-

Continued on next page

Squibb—Cont.

MANENT DISCOLORATION OF THE TEETH (YELLOW-GRAY-BROWN). This reaction is more common during long-term use of the drugs but has been observed following repeated short-term courses. Enamel hypoplasia has also been reported. TETRACYCLINE DRUGS, THEREFORE, SHOULD NOT BE USED IN THIS AGE GROUP UNLESS OTHER DRUGS ARE NOT LIKELY TO BE EFFECTIVE OR ARE CONTRAINDICATED.
If renal impairment exists, even usual oral or parenteral doses may lead to excessive systemic accumulation of the drug and possible liver toxicity. Under such conditions, lower-than-usual doses are indicated and if therapy is prolonged, tetracycline serum level determinations may be advisable.
Certain hypersensitive individuals may develop a photodynamic reaction precipitated by exposure to direct sunlight during the use of this drug. This reaction is usually of the photoallergic type which may also be produced by other tetracycline derivatives. Individuals with a history of photosensitivity reactions should be instructed to avoid exposure to direct sunlight while under treatment with this or other tetracycline drugs and treatment should be discontinued at first evidence of skin discomfort.
NOTE: Photosensitization reactions have occurred most frequently with demethylchlortetracycline, less with chlortetracycline and very rarely with oxytetracycline and tetracycline.
Precautions: As with any antibiotic preparation, prolonged use may result in overgrowth of nonsusceptible organisms. Constant observation of the patient is essential. Should superinfection occur, the preparation should be discontinued and/or appropriate therapy instituted. *Note:* Superinfection of the bowel by staphylococci may be life threatening.
Tetracycline may form a stable calcium complex in any bone forming tissue with no serious harmful effects reported thus far in humans. However, use of tetracycline during tooth development (i.e., latter half of gestation, neonatal period and early childhood) may cause discoloration of the teeth (i.e., yellow-gray-brownish). This effect occurs mostly during long-term use of the drug but it has also been observed in usual short treatment courses.
During long-term therapy, periodic assessment of organ system function, including renal, hepatic, and hematopoietic systems, should be made.
Increased intracranial pressure with bulging fontanels has been observed in infants taking therapeutic doses of tetracycline. Occurrence has been rare and all signs and symptoms have disappeared rapidly upon cessation of treatment.
Since sensitivity reactions are more likely to occur in persons with a history of allergy, asthma, hay fever, or urticaria, the preparation should be used with caution in such individuals. Cross-sensitization among the various tetracyclines is extremely common.
In the treatment of gonorrhea, patients with a suspected lesion of syphilis should have darkfield examinations before receiving tetracycline and monthly serologic tests for a minimum of three months.
The use of tetracycline in staphylococcal infections does not preclude the need for indicated surgical procedures.
Adverse Reactions: Oral administration of amphotericin B is usually well tolerated.
The following adverse reactions have been reported with tetracycline preparations:
Gastrointestinal irritation (anorexia, epigastric distress, nausea, vomiting) as well as bulky loose stools, and diarrhea may occur. Glossitis, stomatitis, enterocolitis, proctitis, and pruritus ani may occur in some patients. Black hairy tongue, sore throat, dysphagia, and hoarseness have also been reported. However, tetracycline is generally well tolerated, undesirable gastrointestinal side effects occurring significantly less frequently than with the two analogues, oxytetracycline and chlortetracycline.
Tetracyclines may also cause maculopapular and erythematous skin rashes. A rare case of exfoliative dermatitis has been reported. Photosensitivity, manifested by an exaggerated sunburn reaction has been observed in some individuals (see *Warnings*). Onycholysis and discoloration of the nails have been reported rarely.
Rise in BUN has been reported and is apparently dose related. Urinary loss of nitrogen has been observed in some patients receiving tetracyclines and may result in negative nitrogen balance. Increased excretion of sodium has also been reported. The development of peptic ulcers and bleeding has been observed in uremic patients receiving tetracyclines.
Hypersensitivity reactions may include urticaria, serum sickness-like reactions (fever, rash, arthralgia), angioneurotic edema, and anaphylactoid shock. If allergic reactions occur, or if an individual idiosyncrasy appears, tetracycline therapy should be discontinued.
Increased intracranial pressure with bulging fontanels has been reported in infants following full therapeutic doses of tetracycline. This symptom disappears rapidly when administration of tetracycline is discontinued (see *Precautions*).
The use of tetracycline during the mineralization phase of tooth development (latter half of gestation, neonatal period, and early childhood) may cause discoloration of the teeth (yellow-gray-brownish) which may sometimes be accompanied by enamel hypoplasia (see *Warnings*).
Anemia, thrombocytopenic purpura, neutropenia, and eosinophilia have been reported. Tetracyclines may delay blood coagulation.
Hepatic cholestasis has been reported rarely, and is usually associated with high dosage levels of tetracycline.
Dosage and Administration: Dosage should be based on the tetracycline content.
Adults: For the many common infections amenable to tetracycline therapy, adults should receive a minimum of 250 mg. four times daily. Higher dosages, such as 500 mg. four times daily, may be required for severe infections or for those infections which do not respond to the smaller dose. **For children above eight years of age:** In general, the pediatric dosage should supply 10 to 20 mg. tetracycline per pound of body weight each day, in divided doses, depending on the type and severity of the infection.
Representative pediatric dosages of Mysteclin-F Syrup (Tetracycline—Amphotericin B Syrup) are as follows: 20 lbs.: ½ teaspoonful q.i.d.; 40 lbs.: 1 teaspoonful q.i.d.; 60 lbs: 1½ teaspoonfuls q.i.d.; 80 lbs.: 2 teaspoonfuls q.i.d.
Oral forms of tetracycline should be given one hour before or two hours following meals. Pediatric dosage forms (oral) should not be given with milk formulas or other calcium containing food, and should be given at least one hour prior to feeding.
Treatment of most common infections should continue for 24 to 48 hours after symptoms and fever subside. However, if the capsules or syrup are used in the treatment of streptococcal infections due to susceptible organisms, therapy should be continued for a full 10 days to guard against the risk of rheumatic fever or glomerulonephritis. Higher dosage and even more prolonged therapy is necessary for subacute bacterial endocarditis and may be required in certain staphylococcal infections.
In chronic cases of acne vulgaris which, in the judgment of the clinician, require long-term treatment, the recommended initial dosage of the capsules or syrup is 1 gram daily in divided doses. When improvement is noted, usually within one week, dosage should be gradually reduced to maintenance levels ranging from 125 to 500 mg. daily. In some patients it may be possible to maintain adequate remission of lesions with alternate-day or intermittent therapy. Tetracycline therapy of acne vulgaris should augment the other standard measures known to be of value.
How Supplied: *Mysteclin-F Capsules (Tetracycline—Amphotericin B Capsules) are available in bottles of 16 and 100 and Unimatic® unit-dose cartons of 100.
Mysteclin-F Syrup (Tetracycline—Amphotericin B Syrup) is available in bottles of 60 ml. and 240 ml. (8 oz.)
Storage: Store the capsules at room temperature; avoid excessive heat; keep tightly closed. Dispense in tight containers. Store the syrup below 30°C. (86°F.); protect from light; keep tightly closed. Dispense in tight light-resistant containers.
*[Shown in Product Identification Section]

NATURETIN®-2.5 ℞
NATURETIN®-5 ℞
NATURETIN®-10 ℞
(Bendroflumethiazide Tablets USP)

Description: Naturetin is a benzothiadiazine derivative containing a benzyl and a trifluoromethyl group. It is a potent oral diuretic and antihypertensive agent available as compressed tablets providing 2.5, 5, or 10 mg. bendroflumethiazide. The tablets contain FD&C Yellow No. 5 (tartrazine).
Clinical Pharmacology: Thiazides affect the renal tubular mechanism of electrolyte reabsorption. At maximal therapeutic dosage all thiazides are approximately equal in their diuretic potency.
Thiazides increase excretion of sodium and chloride in approximately equivalent amounts. Natriuresis causes a secondary loss of potassium and bicarbonate.
The mechanism of the antihypertensive effect of thiazides is unknown. Thiazides do not affect normal blood pressure.
Onset of action of thiazides occurs in two hours and the peak effect at about four hours. Duration of action persists for approximately six to 12 hours. Thiazides are eliminated rapidly by the kidney.
Indications and Usage: Naturetin is indicated as adjunctive therapy in edema associated with congestive heart failure, hepatic cirrhosis, and corticosteroid and estrogen therapy.
Naturetin has also been found useful in edema due to various forms of renal dysfunction such as: nephrotic syndrome, acute glomerulonephritis, and chronic renal failure.
Naturetin (Bendroflumethiazide Tablets USP) tablets are indicated in the management of hypertension either as the sole therapeutic agent or to enhance the effectiveness of other antihypertensive drugs in the more severe forms of hypertension.
Usage in Pregnancy—The routine use of diuretics in an otherwise healthy woman is inappropriate and exposes mother and fetus to unnecessary hazard. Diuretics do not prevent development of toxemia of pregnancy, and there is no satisfactory evidence that they are useful in the treatment of developed toxemia. Edema during pregnancy may arise from pathological causes or from the physiologic and mechanical consequences of pregnancy. Thiazides are indicated in pregnancy when edema is due to pathologic causes, just as they are in the absence of pregnancy (however, see WARNINGS below). Dependent edema in pregnancy, resulting from restriction of venous return by the expanded uterus, is properly treated through elevation of the lower extremities and use of support hose; use of diuretics to lower intravascular volume in this case is illogical and unnecessary. There is hypervolemia during normal pregnancy which is

harmful to neither the fetus nor the mother (in the absence of cardiovascular disease), but which is associated with edema, including generalized edema, in the majority of pregnant women. If this edema produces discomfort, increased recumbency will often provide relief. In rare instances, this edema may cause extreme discomfort which is not relieved by rest. In these cases, a short course of diuretics may provide relief and may be appropriate.

Contraindications: Bendroflumethiazide is contraindicated in anuria.

It is also contraindicated in patients who have previously demonstrated hypersensitivity to it or other sulfonamide-derived drugs.

Warnings: Thiazides should be used with caution in severe renal disease. In patients with renal disease, thiazides may precipitate azotemia. Cumulative effects of the drug may develop in patients with impaired renal function.

Thiazides should be used with caution in patients with impaired hepatic function or progressive liver disease, since minor alterations of fluid and electrolyte balance may precipitate hepatic coma.

Thiazides may be additive or may potentiate the action of other antihypertensive drugs. Potentiation occurs with ganglionic or peripheral adrenergic blocking drugs.

Sensitivity reactions may occur in patients with a history of allergy or bronchial asthma. The possibility of exacerbation or activation of systemic lupus erythematosus has been reported.

Lithium generally should not be given with diuretics; diuretic agents reduce the renal clearance of lithium and add a high risk of lithium toxicity. Refer to the package insert for lithium preparations before use of such concomitant therapy.

Usage in Pregnancy—Thiazides cross the placental barrier and appear in cord blood. The use of thiazides in pregnant women requires that the anticipated benefit be weighed against possible hazards to the fetus. These hazards include fetal or neonatal jaundice, thrombocytopenia, and possibly other adverse reactions which have occurred in the adult.

Nursing Mothers—Thiazides appear in breast milk. If use of the drug is deemed essential, the patient should stop nursing.

Precautions: Periodic determination of serum electrolytes to detect possible electrolyte imbalance should be performed at appropriate intervals.

All patients receiving thiazide therapy should be observed for clinical signs of fluid or electrolyte imbalance; namely, hyponatremia, hypochloremic alkalosis, and hypokalemia. Serum and urine electrolyte determinations are particularly important when the patient is vomiting excessively or receiving parenteral fluids. Warning signs or symptoms of fluid and electrolyte imbalance include: dryness of the mouth, thirst, weakness, lethargy, drowsiness, restlessness, muscle pains or cramps, muscular fatigue, hypotension, oliguria, tachycardia, and gastrointestinal disturbances such as nausea and vomiting.

Hypokalemia may develop, especially with brisk diuresis, when severe cirrhosis is present, or during concomitant use of corticosteroids, ACTH, or after prolonged thiazide therapy. Interference with adequate oral electrolyte intake will also contribute to hypokalemia. Hypokalemia can sensitize or exaggerate the response of the heart to the toxic effects of digitalis (e.g., increased ventricular irritability). Concurrent administration of a potassium-sparing diuretic or potassium supplements may be indicated in these patients.

Any chloride deficit is generally mild and usually does not require specific treatment except under extraordinary circumstances (as in liver disease or renal disease). Dilutional hyponatremia may occur in edematous patients in hot weather; appropriate therapy is water restriction, rather than administration of salt, except in rare instances when the hyponatremia is life threatening. In actual salt depletion, appropriate replacement is the therapy of choice. Hyperuricemia may occur or frank gout may be precipitated in certain patients receiving thiazide therapy.

Insulin requirements in diabetic patients may be increased, decreased, or unchanged. Latent diabetes mellitus may become manifest during thiazide administration.

Thiazide drugs may increase the responsiveness to tubocurarine.

The antihypertensive effects of the drug may be enhanced in the postsympathectomy patient.

Thiazides may decrease arterial responsiveness to norepinephrine. This diminution is not sufficient to preclude effectiveness of the pressor agent for therapeutic use. If emergency surgery is indicated, preanesthetic and anesthetic agents should be administered in reduced dosage.

If progressive renal impairment becomes evident, as indicated by a rising nonprotein nitrogen or blood urea nitrogen, a careful reappraisal of therapy is necessary with consideration given to withholding or discontinuing diuretic therapy.

Thiazides may decrease serum PBI levels without signs of thyroid disturbance.

Calcium excretion is decreased by thiazides. Pathological changes in the parathyroid gland with hypercalcemia and hypophosphatemia have been observed in a few patients on prolonged thiazide therapy. The common complications of hyperparathyroidism such as renal lithiasis, bone resorption, and peptic ulceration have not been seen. Thiazides should be discontinued before carrying out tests for parathyroid function.

This product contains FD&C Yellow No. 5 (tartrazine) which may cause allergic-type reactions (including bronchial asthma) in certain susceptible individuals. Although the overall incidence of FD&C Yellow No. 5 (tartrazine) sensitivity in the general population is low, it is frequently seen in patients who also have aspirin hypersensitivity.

Adverse Reactions: 1. *Gastrointestinal system*—anorexia; gastric irritation; nausea; vomiting; cramping; diarrhea; constipation; jaundice (intrahepatic cholestatic jaundice); pancreatitis; sialadenitis.

2. *Central nervous system*—dizziness; vertigo; paresthesia; headache; xanthopsia.

3. *Hematologic-leukopenia;* agranulocytosis; aplastic anemia; hemolytic anemia.

4. *Cardiovascular*—orthostatic hypotension (may be aggravated by alcohol, barbiturates, or narcotics)

5. *Hypersensitivity*—purpura; photosensitivity; rash; urticaria; necrotizing angiitis (vasculitis, cutaneous vasculitis); fever; respiratory distress including pneumonitis; anaphylactic reactions.

6. *Other*—hyperglycemia; glycosuria; hyperuricemia; muscle spasm; weakness; restlessness; transient blurred vision.

Whenever adverse reactions are moderate or severe, thiazide dosage should be reduced or therapy withdrawn.

Dosage and Administration: Therapy should be individualized according to patient response and titrated to obtain maximal therapeutic response as well as the lowest dose possible to maintain that therapeutic response and minimize side effects.

Diuretic: The usual dose is 5 mg. once daily, preferably given in the morning. To initiate therapy, doses up to 20 mg. may be given once daily or divided into two doses. A single daily dose of 2.5 to 5 mg. should suffice for maintenance.

Alternatively, intermittent therapy may be advantageous in many patients. By administering the preparation every other day or on a three to five day per week schedule, electrolyte imbalance is less likely to occur; however, the possibility still exists.

In general, the lowest dosage that achieves the therapeutic response should be employed.

Antihypertensive: The suggested initial dosage is 5 to 20 mg. daily. Maintenance dosage may range from 2.5 to 15 mg. per day depending on the individual response of the patient. When the diuretic is used with other antihypertensive agents, lower maintenance doses for each drug are usually sufficient.

How Supplied: 2.5 mg. in bottles of 100; 5 mg. (scored) in bottles of 100 and 1000; 10 mg. (scored) in bottles of 100.

Storage: Store at room temperature; avoid excessive heat. Dispense in tight containers.

[*Shown in Product Identification Section*]

NOCTEC® CAPSULES ℞ ©
(Chloral Hydrate Capsules USP)
NOCTEC® SYRUP ℞ ©
(Chloral Hydrate Syrup USP)

Description: Noctec capsules and syrup contain chloral hydrate, an effective sedative and hypnotic agent for oral administration. Chemically, chloral hydrate is 1,1-Ethanediol,2,2,2-trichloro-Chloral hydrate [MW 165.40]; its graphic formula is $CCl_3CH(OH)_2$.

Chloral hydrate occurs as colorless or white, volatile, hygroscopic crystals very soluble in water and in olive oil and freely soluble in alcohol. It has an aromatic, pungent odor and a slightly bitter, caustic taste.

Clinical Pharmacology: The mechanism of action by which the central nervous system is affected is not known. Chloral hydrate is readily absorbed from the gastrointestinal tract following oral administration; however, significant amounts of chloral hydrate have not been detected in the blood after oral administration. It is generally believed that the central depressant effects are due to the principal pharmacologically active metabolite trichloroethanol, which has a plasma half-life of 8 to 10 hours. A portion of the drug is oxidized to trichloroacetic acid (TCA) in the liver and kidneys; TCA is excreted in the urine and bile along with trichloroethanol in free or conjugated form.

Hypnotic dosage produces mild cerebral depression and quiet, deep sleep with little or no "hangover"; blood pressure and respiration are depressed only slightly more than in normal sleep and reflexes are not significantly depressed, so the patient can be awakened and completely aroused. Chloral hydrate's effect on rapid eye movement (REM) sleep is uncertain. Chloral hydrate has been detected in cerebrospinal fluid and human milk, and it crosses the placental barrier.

Indications and Usage: Noctec (Chloral Hydrate) is indicated for nocturnal sedation in all types of patients and especially for the ill, the young, and the elderly patient.

In candidates for surgery, it is a satisfactory preoperative sedative that allays anxiety and induces sleep without depressing respiration or cough reflex. In postoperative care and control of pain, it is a valuable adjunct to opiates and analgesics.

Contraindications: Chloral hydrate is contraindicated in patients with marked hepatic or renal impairment and in patients with severe cardiac disease. Oral dosage forms of chloral hydrate are contraindicated in the presence of gastritis. Chloral hydrate is also contraindicated in patients who have previously exhibited an idiosyncrasy or hypersensitivity to the drug.

Warnings: Chloral hydrate may be habit-forming. Long-term use of larger than the usual therapeutic doses may result in psychic and physical dependence; therefore, caution must be exercised when administering the

Continued on next page

Squibb—Cont.

drug to patients susceptible to drug abuse. Sudden withdrawal may result in delirium.

Chloral hydrate may increase the rate of metabolism of concomitantly administered coumarin or coumarin-related anticoagulants, thus reducing their effectiveness. Upon withdrawal of chloral hydrate, the rate of metabolism of the anticoagulant drug may decrease with a concomitant rise in plasma levels and with the possibility of a gradual increase of anticoagulant effects (i.e., development of bleeding tendency and hemorrhage). Patients on oral anticoagulant therapy who are also taking chloral hydrate should have close observation of prothrombin times.

Precautions:

General—Chloral hydrate has been reported to precipitate attacks of acute intermittent porphyria and should be used with caution in susceptible patients.

Continued use of therapeutic doses of chloral hydrate has been shown to be without deleterious effect on the heart. Large doses of chloral hydrate, however, should not be used in patients with *severe* cardiac disease (see CONTRAINDICATIONS).

Information for Patients—Chloral hydrate may cause gastrointestinal upset. The capsules should be taken with a full glass of water or fruit juice; capsules should be taken whole, and not chewed. The syrup should be diluted in half a glass of water or fruit juice.

Chloral hydrate may cause drowsiness; therefore, patients should be instructed to use caution when driving, operating dangerous machinery, or performing any hazardous task.

Patients should avoid alcohol and other CNS depressants. They should also be informed that chloral hydrate may be habit-forming.

Noctec (Chloral Hydrate) and all drugs should be kept out of the reach of children.

Patients should be warned against sudden discontinuation of chloral hydrate except under the advice of the physician; they should also be informed of symptoms that would suggest potential adverse effects.

Drug Interactions—Chloral hydrate may cause hypoprothrombinemic effects in patients taking oral anticoagulants (see WARNINGS).

Administration of chloral hydrate followed by intravenous furosemide may result in sweating, hot flashes, and variable blood pressure including hypertension due to a hypermetabolic state caused by displacement of thyroid hormone from its bound state.

Caution is recommended in combining chloral hydrate with other CNS depressants such as alcohol, barbiturates, and tranquilizers. Administration of chloral hydrate should be delayed in patients who have ingested significant amounts of alcohol in the preceding 12 to 24 hours. CNS depressants are additive in effect and the dosage should be reduced when such combinations are given concurrently.

Drug/Laboratory Test Interactions—Chloral hydrate may interfere with copper sulfate tests for glycosuria (suspected glycosuria should be confirmed by a glucose oxidase test when the patient is receiving chloral hydrate), fluorometric tests for urine catecholamines (it is recommended that the medication not be administered for 48 hours preceding the test), or urinary 17-hydroxycorticosteroid determinations (when using the Reddy, Jenkins, and Thorn procedure).

Carcinogenesis, Mutagenesis, Impairment of Fertility—Long-term studies in animals have not been performed.

Pregnancy Category C—Animal reproduction studies have not been conducted with chloral hydrate. Chloral hydrate crosses the placental barrier and chronic use during pregnancy may cause withdrawal symptoms in the neonate. It is not known whether chloral hydrate can affect reproduction capacity. Chloral hydrate should be given to a pregnant woman only if clearly needed.

Nursing Mothers—Chloral hydrate is excreted in human milk; use by nursing mothers may cause sedation in the infant.

Adverse Reactions:

Central Nervous System—Occasionally a patient becomes somnambulistic and he may be disoriented and incoherent and show paranoid behavior. Rarely, excitement, tolerance, addiction, delirium, drowsiness, staggering gait, ataxia, lightheadedness, vertigo, dizziness, nightmares, malaise, mental confusion, and hallucinations have been reported.

Hematological—Leukopenia and eosinophilia have occasionally occurred.

Dermatological—Allergic skin rashes including hives, erythema, eczematoid dermatitis, urticaria, and scarlatiniform exanthems have occasionally been reported.

Gastrointestinal—Some patients experience gastric irritation and occasionally nausea and vomiting, flatulence, diarrhea, and unpleasant taste occur.

Miscellaneous—Rarely, headache, hangover, idiosyncratic syndrome, and ketonuria have been reported.

Drug Abuse and Dependence:

Controlled Substance—Drug Enforcement Administration Schedule Ⓒ.

Abuse—Chloral hydrate may be habit-forming. Patients known to be addiction-prone and patients who actively solicit hypnotics in increasing doses are potential addicts. Many patients take higher doses of hypnotics than they admit, and slurring of speech, incoordination, tremulousness, and nystagmus should arouse suspicion. Drowsiness, lethargy, and hangover are frequently observed from excessive drug intake.

Dependence—Prolonged use of larger than usual therapeutic doses may result in psychic and physical dependence. Tolerance and psychologic dependence may develop by the second week of continued administration.

Chloral hydrate addicts may take huge doses of the drug, i.e., up to 12 g. nightly has been reported. This abuse is similar to alcohol addiction and sudden withdrawal may result in central nervous excitation, with tremor, anxiety, hallucination, or even delirium which may be fatal. In patients suffering from chronic chloral hydrate intoxication, gastritis is common and skin eruptions may develop. Parenchymatous renal injury may also occur.

Withdrawal should be undertaken in a hospital and supportive treatment similar to that used during barbiturate withdrawal is recommended.

Overdosage: The signs and symptoms of chloral hydrate overdosage resemble those of barbiturate overdosage and especially affect the CNS and cardiovascular system. They may include: hypothermia; pinpoint pupils; blood pressure falls; comatose state; slow or rapid and shallow breathing. Gastric irritation may result in vomiting and even gastric necrosis. If the patient survives, icterus due to hepatic damage and albuminuria from renal irritation may appear.

The toxic oral dose of chloral hydrate for adults is approximately 10 g.; however, death has been reported from a dose of 4 g. and some patients have survived after taking as much as 30 g.

Accidental overdosage should be treated with gastric lavage or by inducing vomiting to empty the stomach. Supportive measures may be used. Hemodialysis is reported to be effective in promoting the clearance of trichloroethanol.

Dosage and Administration: The capsules should be taken with a full glass of liquid. The syrup may be administered in a half glass of water, fruit juice, or ginger ale.

ADULTS: The usual *hypnotic* dose is 500 mg. to 1 g., taken 15 to 30 minutes before bedtime or ½ hour before surgery. The usual *sedative* dose is 250 mg. three times daily after meals. Generally, single doses or daily dosage should not exceed 2 g.

CHILDREN: The usual daily *hypnotic* dosage is 50 mg./kg. of body weight, with a maximum of 1 g. per single dose. Daily dosage may be given in divided doses, if indicated. The *sedative* dosage is half of the hypnotic dosage.

How Supplied: *Noctec Capsules (Chloral Hydrate Capsules USP) are available in potencies of 250 mg. (3¾ grains) in bottles of 100 capsules and 500 mg. (7½ grains) in bottles of 100 and Unimatic® cartons of 25 and 100 capsules.

Noctec (Chloral Hydrate) is also available as an aromatic, flavored syrup supplying 500 mg. (7½ grains) per 5 ml. teaspoonful in 473 ml. (pint) bottles, 3.8 liter (gallon) bottles, and Unimatic unit-dose bottles in cartons of 4 x 25 bottles (5 ml. each bottle).

Storage: Store Noctec (Chloral Hydrate) capsules and syrup at room temperature; avoid excessive heat. Dispense only in glass containers. Dispense the syrup in tight, light-resistant containers.

*[*Shown in Product Identification Section*]

ORAGRAFIN® CALCIUM GRANULES ℞
(Ipodate Calcium for Oral Suspension USP)

ORAGRAFIN® SODIUM CAPSULES ℞
(Ipodate Sodium Capsules USP)

(See Diagnostic Section)

O–V STATIN® ℞
(oral/vaginal therapy pack)

O-V STATIN (oral/vaginal therapy pack) is designed specifically to provide a convenient therapy pack for use in the treatment of coexisting intestinal candidiasis and vulvovaginal candidiasis.

Mycostatin® Oral Tablets
(Nystatin Tablets USP)
Mycostatin® Vaginal Tablets
(Nystatin Vaginal Tablets USP)

Description: Nystatin is an antifungal antibiotic which is both fungistatic and fungicidal *in vitro* against a wide variety of yeasts and yeast-like fungi. It is a polyene antibiotic of undetermined structural formula that is obtained from *Streptomyces noursei.*

MYCOSTATIN ORAL TABLETS (Nystatin Tablets USP) are provided for oral administration as coated tablets containing 500,000 units nystatin.

MYCOSTATIN VAGINAL TABLETS (Nystatin Vaginal Tablets USP) are provided as diamond-shaped, individually foil wrapped, compressed tablets containing 100,000 units nystatin dispersed in lactose with ethyl cellulose, stearic acid and starch.

Clinical Pharmacology: Nystatin probably acts by binding to sterols in the cell membrane of the fungus with a resultant change in membrane permeability allowing leakage of intracellular components. It exhibits no appreciable activity against bacteria or trichomonads.

Following oral administration, nystatin is sparingly absorbed with no detectable blood levels when given in the recommended doses. Most of the orally administered nystatin is passed unchanged in the stool.

Indications and Usage: O-V STATIN oral/vaginal therapy pack [Mycostatin Oral Tablets (Nystatin Tablets USP) and Mycostatin Vaginal Tablets (Nystatin Vaginal Tablets USP)] is indicated for use in the treatment of coexisting intestinal candidiasis and vulvovaginal candidiasis.

MYCOSTATIN VAGINAL TABLETS (Nystatin Vaginal Tablets USP) are effective for the local treatment of vulvovaginal candidiasis (moniliasis). The diagnosis should be confirmed, prior to therapy, by KOH smears and/or cultures. Other pathogens commonly associated with vulvovaginitis (Trichomonas and

Hemophilus vaginalis) do not respond to nystatin and should be ruled out by appropriate laboratory methods.

Contraindications: Both preparations are contraindicated in patients with a history of hypersensitivity to any of their components.

Precautions: General—Discontinue treatment if sensitization or irritation is reported during intravaginal use.

Laboratory Tests—If there is a lack of response to MYCOSTATIN VAGINAL TABLETS (Nystatin Vaginal Tablets USP), appropriate microbiological studies should be repeated to confirm the diagnosis and rule out other pathogens before instituting another course of antimycotic therapy.

Usage in Pregnancy: No adverse effects or complications have been attributed to nystatin in infants born to women treated with nystatin oral or vaginal tablets.

Adverse Reactions: Nystatin is virtually nontoxic and nonsensitizing and is well tolerated by all age groups, even on prolonged administration. Large oral doses have occasionally produced diarrhea, gastrointestinal distress, nausea and vomiting. Rarely, irritation or sensitization on intravaginal use may occur (see PRECAUTIONS).

Dosage and Administration: MYCOSTATIN ORAL TABLETS—The usual therapeutic dosage is one to two tablets (500,000 to 1,000,000 units nystatin) three times daily. Treatment should generally be continued for at least 48 hours after clinical cure to prevent relapse.

MYCOSTATIN VAGINAL TABLETS—The usual dosage is one tablet (100,000 units nystatin) daily for two weeks. The tablets should be deposited high in the vagina by means of the applicator. "Instructions for the Patient" are enclosed in each package.

Even though symptomatic relief may occur within a few days, treatment should be continued for the full course.

It is important that therapy be continued during menstruation. Adjunctive measures such as therapeutic douches are unnecessary and sometimes inadvisable. Cleansing douches may be used by nonpregnant women, if desired, for esthetic purposes.

How Supplied: O-V STATIN oral/vaginal therapy pack—containing one bottle of 42 MYCOSTATIN ORAL TABLETS (Nystatin Tablets USP, 500,000 units nystatin each) and 14 individually foil wrapped MYCOSTATIN VAGINAL TABLETS (Nystatin Vaginal Tablets USP, 100,000 units nystatin each) with one plastic applicator and one "Instructions for the Patient" leaflet.

Storage: Store in refrigerator below 15° C (59° F).

PENICILLIN G POTASSIUM FOR INJECTION USP ℞

Description: Penicillin G Potassium for Injection USP is crystalline penicillin G potassium as a sterile powder. The preparation contains approximately 27 mg. citrate buffer (composed of sodium citrate and not more than 0.94 mg. citric acid) with approximately 1.7 mEq. potassium and 0.3 mEq. sodium per million units of penicillin.

Clinical Pharmacology: Penicillin G is bactericidal against penicillin-susceptible microorganisms during the stage of active multiplication. It acts by inhibiting biosynthesis of cell-wall mucopeptide. It is not active against the penicillinase-producing bacteria, which include many strains of staphylococci. Penicillin G is highly active *in vitro* against staphylococci (except penicillinase-producing strains), streptococci (groups A, C, G, H, L, and M) and pneumococci. Other organisms sensitive *in vitro* to penicillin G are *Neisseria gonorrhoeae, Corynebacterium diphtheriae, Bacillus anthracis,* Clostridia, *Actinomyces bovis, Streptobacillus moniliformis, Listeria monocytogenes* and Leptospira; *Treponema pallidum* is extremely susceptible. Some species of gram-negative bacilli are susceptible to moderate to high concentrations of penicillin G obtained with intravenous administration. These include most strains of *Escherichia coli;* all strains of *Proteus mirabilis,* Salmonella, and Shigella; and some strains of *Enterobacter aerogenes* (formerly *Aerobacter aerogenes*) and *Alcaligenes faecalis.*

Susceptibility plate testing: If the Kirby-Bauer method of disc susceptibility is used, a 10 u. penicillin disc should give a zone greater than 28 mm. when tested against a penicillin-susceptible bacterial strain.

Aqueous penicillin G is rapidly absorbed following both intramuscular and subcutaneous injection. Approximately 60 percent of the total dose of 300,000 u. is excreted in the urine within this five-hour period. Therefore, high and frequent doses are required to maintain the elevated serum levels desirable in treating certain severe infections in individuals with normal kidney function. In neonates and young infants, and in individuals with impaired kidney function, excretion is considerably delayed.

Indications and Usage: Penicillin G Potassium for Injection USP is indicated in the treatment of severe infections caused by penicillin G-susceptible microorganisms when rapid and high penicillinemia is required. Therapy should be guided by bacteriological studies, including susceptibility tests, and by clinical response.

The following infections will usually respond to adequate dosage:

Streptococcal infections. Note: streptococci in groups A, C, G, H, L, and M are very susceptible to penicillin G. Some group D organisms are susceptible to the high serum levels obtained with aqueous penicillin G. Aqueous penicillin G potassium is the penicillin dosage form of choice for bacteremia, empyema, severe pneumonia, pericarditis, endocarditis, meningitis and other severe infections caused by susceptible strains of the gram-positive species listed above.

Pneumococcal infections; Staphylococcal infections—penicillin G-susceptible; **Anthrax; Actinomycosis; Clostridial infections** (including tetanus); **Diphtheria** (to prevent the carrier state); **Erysipeloid endocarditis** (Erysipelothrix insidiosa); **Vincent's gingivitis and pharyngitis** (fusospirochetosis)—Severe infections of the oropharynx (Note: necessary dental care should be accomplished in infections involving gum tissue.), and **lower respiratory tract and genital area infections** due to *F. fusiformisans* spirochetes; **Gram-negative bacillary infections** (bacteremias)—*(E. coli, E. aerogenes, A. faecalis,* Salmonella, Shigella and *P. mirabilis);* **Listeria infections** *(L. monocytogenes);* **Meningitis and endocarditis; Pasteurella infections** *(P. multocida): Bacteremia* and *meningitis;* **Ratbite fever** *(S. minus* or *S. moniliformis);* **Gonorrheal endocarditis and arthritis** *(N. gonorrhoeae);* **Syphilis** *(T. pallidum)* including congenital syphilis; **Meningococcic meningitis.**

Prevention of bacterial endocarditis—Although no controlled clinical efficacy studies have been conducted, aqueous crystalline penicillin G for injection and penicillin G procaine suspension have been suggested by the American Heart Association and the American Dental Association for use as part of a combined parenteral-oral regimen for prophylaxis against bacterial endocarditis in patients with congenital heart disease or rheumatic or other acquired valvular heart disease when they undergo dental procedures and surgical procedures of the upper respiratory tract.[1] Since it may happen that *alpha* hemolytic streptococci relatively resistant to penicillin may be found when patients are receiving continuous oral penicillin for secondary prevention of rheumatic fever, prophylactic agents other than penicillin may be chosen for these patients and prescribed in addition to their continuous rheumatic fever prophylactic regimen. **NOTE: When selecting antibiotics for the prevention of bacterial endocarditis the physician or dentist should read the full joint statement of the American Heart Association and the American Dental Association.[1]**

Contraindications: Contraindicated in patients with a history of hypersensitivity to any penicillin.

Warnings: Serious and occasional fatal hypersensitivity (anaphylactoid) reactions have been reported in patients on penicillin therapy. Although anaphylaxis is more frequent following parenteral administration, it has occurred in patients on oral penicillins. These reactions are more apt to occur in individuals with a history of sensitivity to multiple allergens.

There have been well-documented reports of individuals with a history of penicillin hypersensitivity who have experienced severe hypersensitivity reactions when treated with cephalosporins. Before therapy with a penicillin, careful inquiry should be made concerning previous hypersensitivity reactions to penicillins, cephalosporins, and other allergens. If an allergic reaction occurs, the drug should be discontinued and the patient treated with the usual agents, e.g., pressor amines, antihistamines, and corticosteroids. Serious anaphylactoid reactions are not controlled by antihistamines alone, and require such emergency measures as the immediate use of epinephrine, aminophylline, oxygen, and intravenous corticosteroids.

Precautions: Penicillin should be used with caution in individuals with histories of significant allergies and/or asthma.

In prolonged therapy with penicillin and particularly with high dosage schedules, periodic evaluation of the renal and hematopoietic systems is recommended.

In streptococcal infections, therapy must be sufficient to eliminate the organism (ten days minimum); otherwise the sequelae of streptococcal disease may occur. Cultures should be taken following the completion of treatment to determine whether streptococci have been eradicated.

In high doses (above 10 million u.), intravenous aqueous penicillin G potassium should be administered slowly because of the adverse effects of electrolyte imbalance from the potassium content of the penicillin. The patient's renal, cardiac and vascular status should be evaluated and if impairment of function is suspected or known to exist, a reduction in the total dosage should be considered. Frequent evaluation of electrolyte balance, and renal and hematopoietic function is recommended during therapy when high doses of intravenous aqueous penicillin G potassium are used.

Prolonged use of antibiotics may promote overgrowth of nonsusceptible organisms, including fungi. Should superinfection occur, appropriate measures should be taken. Indwelling intravenous catheters encourage superinfections and should be avoided whenever possible.

Therapy of susceptible infections should be accompanied by any indicated surgical procedures. In suspected staphylococcal infections, proper laboratory studies, including susceptibility tests, should be performed.

When treating gonococcal infections in which primary or secondary syphilis may be suspected, proper diagnostic procedures, including darkfield examinations, should be done. In all cases in which concomitant syphilis is suspected, monthly serological tests should be made for at least four months. All cases of penicillin-treated syphilis should receive clinical and serological examinations every six months for at least two or three years.

Continued on next page

Squibb—Cont.

Adverse Reactions: Penicillin is a substance of low toxicity but does possess a significant index of sensitization.
The hypersensitivity reactions reported are skin rashes ranging from maculopapular eruptions to exfoliative dermatitis; urticaria; and serum sickness-like reactions including chills, fever, edema, arthralgia and prostration. Severe and occasionally fatal anaphylaxis has occurred (see WARNINGS).
Hemolytic anemia, leukopenia, thrombocytopenia, neuropathy, and nephropathy are rarely observed adverse reactions and are usually associated with high intravenous dosage. Urticaria, other skin rashes, and serum sickness-like reactions may be controlled by antihistamines and, if necessary, corticosteroids. Whenever such reactions occur, penicillin should be discontinued unless, in the opinion of the physician, the condition being treated is life-threatening and amenable only to penicillin therapy. Patients given continuous intravenous therapy with penicillin G potassium in high dosage (10 million to 100 million u. daily) may suffer severe or even fatal potassium poisoning, particularly if renal insufficiency is present. Hyperreflexia, convulsions and coma may be indicative of this syndrome.
The Jarisch-Herxheimer reaction has been reported in patients treated for syphilis.
Dosage and Administration: Penicillin G Potassium for Injection USP may be given intramuscularly or by continuous intravenous drip.
The 10,000,000 and 20,000,000 u. preparations of Penicillin G Potassium for Injection USP should be administered by intravenous infusion only.
The usual dose recommendation is as follows:
Severe infections due to susceptible strains of streptococci, pneumococci, and staphylococci; bacteremia, pneumonia, endocarditis, pericarditis, empyema, meningitis and other severe infections: a minimum of 5 million u. daily.
Anthrax: a minimum of 5 million u./day in divided doses until cure is effected; **Actinomycosis:** 1 to 6 million u./day for cervicofacial cases; 10 to 20 million u./day for thoracic and abdominal disease; **Clostridial infections** (as adjunctive therapy to antitoxin): 20 million u./day; **Diphtheria**—adjunctive therapy to antitoxin for prevention of the carrier state: 300,000 to 400,000 u./day in divided doses for 10 to 12 days; **Erysipeloid:** *Endocarditis:* 2 to 20 million u./day for four to six weeks; **Fusospirochetal infections** (fusospirochetosis)—severe infections of the oropharynx, lower respiratory tract and genital area: 5 to 10 million u./day; **Gram-negative bacillary infections** *(E. coli, E. aerogenes, A. faecalis,* Salmonella, Shigella, and *P. mirabilis); Bacteremia:* 20 to 80 million u./ day; **Listeria infections** *(L. monocytogenes): Neonates:* 500,000 to 1 million u./day; *Adults with meningitis:* 15 to 20 million u./day for two weeks; *Adults with endocarditis:* 15 to 20 million u./ day for four weeks; **Pasteurella infections** *(P. multocida): Bacteremia* and *meningitis:* 4 to 6 million u./day for two weeks; **Rat-bite fever** *(S. minus* or *S. moniliformis):* 12 to 15 million u./day for three to four weeks.
Gonorrheal endocarditis and arthritis: a minimum of 5 million u. daily.
Syphilis—aqueous penicillin G potassium may be used in the treatment of acquired and congenital syphilis but, because of the necessity of frequent dosage, hospitalization is recommended. Dosage and duration of therapy is determined by the age of the patient and the stage of the disease.
Meningococcic meningitis: 1 to 2 million u. I.M. every two hours or continuous I.V. drip of 20 to 30 million u./day.
Prevention of bacterial endocarditis—For prophylaxis against bacterial endocarditis[1] in patients with congenital heart disease or rheumatic or other acquired valvular heart disease when undergoing dental procedures or surgical procedures of the upper respiratory tract, use a combined parenteral-oral regimen. One million units of aqueous crystalline penicillin G (30,000 u./kg. in children) mixed with 600,000 u. penicillin G procaine (600,000 u. for children) should be given intramuscularly one-half to one hour before the procedure. Oral penicillin V (phenoxymethyl penicillin), 500 mg. for adults or 250 mg. for children less than 60 lb., should be given every six hours for eight doses. Doses for children should not exceed recommendations for adults for a single dose or for a 24-hour period.
Preparation of Solutions: Solutions of penicillin should be prepared as follows: Loosen powder. Hold vial horizontally and rotate it while *slowly* directing the stream of diluent against the wall of the vial. Shake vial vigorously after all the diluent has been added. Depending on the route of administration, use Sterile Water for Injection USP, isotonic Sodium Chloride Injection USP, or Dextrose Injection USP.
NOTE: Penicillins are rapidly inactivated in the presence of carbohydrate solutions at alkaline pH.
RECONSTITUTION: 1,000,000 u. vial—add 9.6 ml., 4.6 ml., or 3.6 ml. diluent to provide 100,000 u., 200,000 u., or 250,000 u. per ml., respectively: 5,000,000 u. vial—add 23 ml., 18 ml., 8 ml., or 3 ml. diluent to provide 200,000 u., 250,000 u., 500,000 u., or 1,000,000 u. per ml., respectively. *For I.V. infusion only:* 10,000,000 u. vial—add 15.5 ml. or 5.4 ml. diluent to provide 500,000 u. or 1,000,000 u. per ml., respectively: 20,000,000 u. vial—add 31.6 ml. diluent to provide 500,000 u. per ml.
How Supplied: Penicillin G Potassium for Injection USP is available in vials providing 1, 5, 10, and 20 million units of crystalline penicillin G potassium.
Storage: The dry powder is relatively stable and may be stored at room temperature without significant loss of potency. Sterile solutions may be kept in the refrigerator one week without significant loss of potency. Solutions prepared for intravenous infusion are stable at room temperature for at least 24 hours.
Reference: 1. American Heart Association. 1977. Prevention of bacterial endocarditis. Circulation 56:139A-143A.

PENICILLIN G SODIUM FOR INJECTION USP ℞

Description: Penicillin G Sodium for Injection USP is crystalline penicillin G sodium as a sterile powder. The preparation contains 28 mg. citrate buffer (composed of sodium citrate, and not more than 0.92 mg. citric acid) and approximately 2.0 mEq. sodium per million units of penicillin.
Clinical Pharmacology: Penicillin G is bactericidal against penicillin-susceptible microorganisms during the stage of active multiplication. It acts by inhibiting biosynthesis of cell-wall mucopeptide. It is not active against the penicillinase-producing bacteria, which include many strains of staphylococci. Penicillin G is highly active *in vitro* against staphylococci (except penicillinase-producing strains), streptococci (groups A, C, G, H, L, and M) and pneumococci. Other organisms susceptible *in vitro* to penicillin G are *Neisseria gonorrhoeae, Corynebacterium diphtheriae, Bacillus anthracis,* Clostridia, *Actinomyces bovis, Streptobacillus moniliformis, Listeria monocytogenes* and Leptospira; *Treponema pallidum* is extremely susceptible. Some species of gram-negative bacilli are susceptible to moderate to high concentrations of penicillin G obtained with intravenous administration. These include most strains of *Escherichia coli;* all strains of *Proteus mirabilis,* Salmonella and Shigella; and some strains of *Enterobacter aerogenes* (formerly *Aerobacter aerogenes*) and *Alcaligenes faecalis.*
Susceptibility plate testing: If the Kirby-Bauer method of disc susceptibility is used, a 10 u. penicillin disc should give a zone greater than 28 mm. when tested against a penicillin-susceptible bacterial strain.
Aqueous penicillin G is rapidly absorbed following both intramuscular and subcutaneous injection. Approximately 60 percent of the total dose of 300,000 u. is excreted in the urine within this five-hour period. Therefore, high and frequent doses are required to maintain the elevated serum levels desirable in treating certain severe infections in individuals with normal kidney function. In neonates and young infants and in individuals with impaired kidney function, excretion is considerably delayed.
Indications and Usage: Penicillin G Sodium for Injection USP is indicated in the treatment of severe infections caused by penicillin G-susceptible microorganisms when rapid and high penicillinemia is required. Therapy should be guided by bacteriological studies, including susceptibility tests, and by clinical response.
The following infections will usually respond to adequate dosage:
Streptococcal infections. Note: streptococci in groups A, C, G, H, L, and M are very susceptible to penicillin G. Some group D organisms are susceptible to the high serum levels obtained with aqueous penicillin G. Aqueous penicillin G sodium is the penicillin dosage form of choice for bacteremia, empyema, severe pneumonia, pericarditis, endocarditis, meningitis and other severe infections caused by susceptible strains of the gram-positive species listed above.
Pneumococcal infections; Staphylococcal infections—penicillin G-susceptible; **Anthrax; Actinomycosis; Clostridial infections** (including tetanus); **Diphtheria** (to prevent the carrier state); **Erysipeloid endocarditis** *(Erysipelothrix insidiosa);* **Vincent's gingivitis and pharyngitis** (fusospirochetosis)—Severe infections of the oropharynx (Note: necessary dental care should be accomplished in infections involving gum tissue.) and **lower respiratory tract and genital area infections** due to *F. fusiformisans* spirochetes; **Gram-negative bacillary infections** (bacteremias)—*(E. coli, E. aerogenes, A. faecalis,* Salmonella, Shigella and *P. mirabilis);* **Listeria infections** *(L. monocytogenes);* **Meningitis and endocarditis; Pasteurella infections** *(P. multocida):* Bacteremia and meningitis; **Rat-bite fever** *(S. minus* or *S. moniliformis);* **Gonorrheal endocarditis and arthritis** *(N. gonorrhoeae);* **Syphilis** *(T. pallidum)* including congenital syphilis; **Meningococcic meningitis.**
Prevention of bacterial endocarditis—Although no controlled clinical efficacy studies have been conducted, aqueous crystalline penicillin G for injection and penicillin G procaine suspension have been suggested by the American Heart Association and the American Dental Association for use as part of a combined parenteral-oral regimen for prophylaxis against bacterial endocarditis in patients with congenital heart disease or rheumatic or other acquired valvular heart disease when they undergo dental procedures and surgical procedures of the upper respiratory tract.[1] Since it may happen that *alpha* hemolytic streptococci relatively resistant to penicillin may be found when patients are receiving continuous oral penicillin for secondary prevention of rheumatic fever, prophylactic agents other than penicillin may be chosen for these patients and prescribed in addition to their continuous rheumatic fever prophylactic regimen. **NOTE: When selecting antibiotics for the prevention of bacterial endocarditis the physician or dentist should read the full joint statement of the American Heart Association and the American Dental Association.[1]**
Contraindications: Contraindicated in patients with a history of hypersensitivity to any penicillin.

Warnings: Serious and occasional fatal hypersensitivity (anaphylactoid) reactions have been reported in patients on penicillin therapy. Although anaphylaxis is more frequent following parenteral administration, it has occurred in patients on oral penicillins. These reactions are more apt to occur in individuals with a history of sensitivity to multiple allergens.

There have been well-documented reports of individuals with a history of penicillin hypersensitivity who have experienced severe hypersensitivity reactions when treated with cephalosporins. Before therapy with a penicillin, careful inquiry should be made concerning previous hypersensitivity reactions to penicillins, cephalosporins, and other allergens. If an allergic reaction occurs, the drug should be discontinued and the patient treated with the usual agents, e.g., pressor amines, antihistamines, and corticosteroids. Serious anaphylactoid reactions are not controlled by antihistamines alone, and require such emergency measures as the immediate use of epinephrine, aminophylline, oxygen, and intravenous corticosteroids.

Precautions: Penicillin should be used with caution in individuals with histories of significant allergies and/or asthma.

In prolonged therapy with penicillin and particularly with high dosage schedules, periodic evaluation of the renal and hematopoietic systems is recommended.

In streptococcal infections, therapy must be sufficient to eliminate the organism (10 days minimum); otherwise the sequelae of streptococcal disease may occur. Cultures should be taken following the completion of treatment to determine whether streptococci have been eradicated.

In high doses (above 10 million u.), intravenous aqueous penicillin G sodium should be administered slowly because of the adverse effects of electrolyte imbalance from the sodium content of the penicillin. The patient's renal, cardiac and vascular status should be evaluated and if impairment of function is suspected or known to exist, a reduction in the total dosage should be considered. Frequent evaluation of electrolyte balance, and renal and hematopoietic function is recommended during therapy when high doses of intravenous aqueous penicillin G sodium are used.

Prolonged use of antibiotics may promote overgrowth of nonsusceptible organisms, including fungi. Should superinfection occur, appropriate measures should be taken. Indwelling intravenous catheters encourage superinfections and should be avoided whenever possible.

Therapy of susceptible infections should be accompanied by any indicated surgical procedures. In suspected staphylococcal infections, proper laboratory studies, including susceptibility tests, should be performed.

When treating gonococcal infections in which primary or secondary syphilis may be suspected, proper diagnostic procedures, including darkfield examinations, should be done. In all cases in which concomitant syphilis is suspected, monthly serological tests should be made for at least four months. All cases of penicillin-treated syphilis should receive clinical and serological examinations every six months for at least two or three years.

Adverse Reactions: Penicillin is a substance of low toxicity but does possess a significant index of sensitization.

The hypersensitivity reactions reported are skin rashes ranging from maculopapular eruptions to exfoliative dermatitis; urticaria; and serum sickness-like reactions including chills, fever, edema, arthralgia and prostration. Severe and occasionally fatal anaphylaxis has occurred (see WARNINGS).

Hemolytic anemia, leukopenia, thrombocytopenia, neuropathy, and nephropathy are rarely observed adverse reactions and are usually associated with high intravenous dosage. Urticaria, other skin rashes, and serum sickness-like reactions may be controlled by antihistamines and, if necessary, corticosteroids. Whenever such reactions occur, penicillin should be discontinued unless, in the opinion of the physician, the condition being treated is life-threatening and amenable only to penicillin therapy. High dosage of penicillin G sodium may result in congestive heart failure due to high sodium intake.

The Jarisch-Herxheimer reaction has been reported in patients treated for syphilis.

Dosage and Administration: Penicillin G Sodium for Injection USP may be given intramuscularly or by continuous intravenous drip. The usual dosage recommendation is as follows:

Severe infections due to susceptible strains of streptococci, pneumococci, and staphylococci; bacteremia, pneumonia, endocarditis, pericarditis, empyema, meningitis and other severe infections: a minimum of 5 million u. daily.

Anthrax: a minimum of 5 million u./day in divided doses until cure is effected; **Actinomycosis:** 1 to 6 million u./day for cervicofacial cases; 10 to 20 million u./day for thoracic and abdominal disease; **Clostridial infections** (as adjunctive therapy to antitoxin): 20 million u./day; **Diphtheria**—adjunctive therapy to antitoxin for prevention of the carrier state: 300,000 to 400,000 u./day in divided doses for 10 to 12 days; **Erysipeloid:** *Endocarditis:* 2 to 20 million u./day for four to six weeks: **Fusospirochetal infections** (fusospirochetosis)—severe infections of the oropharynx, lower respiratory tract and genital area: 5 to 10 million u./day; **Gram-negative bacillary infections** *(E. coli, E. aerogenes, A. faecalis,* Salmonella, Shigella and *P. mirabilis); Bacteremia:* 20 to 80 million u./day; **Listeria infections** *(L. monocytogenes): Neonates:* 500,000 to 1 million u./day; *Adults with meningitis:* 15 to 20 million u./day for two weeks; *Adults with endocarditis:* 15 to 20 million u./ day for four weeks; **Pasteurella infections** *(P. multocida): Bacteremia* and *meningitis:* 4 to 6 million u./day for two weeks; **Rat-bite fever** *(S. minus* or *S. moniliformis):* 12 to 15 million u./day for three to four weeks.

Gonorrheal endocarditis and arthritis: a minimum of 5 million u. daily.

Syphilis—aqueous penicillin G sodium may be used in the treatment of acquired and congenital syphilis but, because of the necessity of frequent dosage, hospitalization is recommended. Dosage and duration of therapy is determined by the age of the patient and the stage of the disease.

Meningococcic meningitis: 1 to 2 million u. I.M. every two hours or continuous I.V. drip of 20 to 30 million u./day.

Prevention of bacterial endocarditis—For prophylaxis against bacterial endocarditis[1] in patients with congenital heart disease or rheumatic or other acquired valvular heart disease when undergoing dental procedures or surgical procedures of the upper respiratory tract, use a combined parenteral-oral regimen. One million units of aqueous crystalline penicillin G (30,000 u./kg. in children) mixed with 600,000 u. penicillin G procaine (600,000 u. for children) should be given intramuscularly one-half to one hour before the procedure. Oral penicillin V (phenoxymethyl penicillin), 500 mg. for adults or 250 mg. for children less than 60 lb., should be given every six hours for eight doses. Doses for children should not exceed recommendations for adults for a single dose or for a 24-hour period.

Preparation of Solutions: Solutions of penicillin should be prepared as follows: Loosen powder. Hold vial horizontally and rotate it while *slowly* directing the stream of diluent against the wall of the vial. Shake vial vigorously after all the diluent has been added. Depending on the route of administration, use Sterile Water for Injection USP, isotonic Sodium Chloride Injection USP, or Dextrose Injection USP. NOTE: Penicillins are rapidly inactivated in the presence of carbohydrate solutions at alkaline pH.

Reconstitute with 23 ml., 18 ml., 8 ml., or 3 ml. diluent to provide concentrations of 200,000 u., 250,000 u., 500,000 u., or 1,000,000 u. per ml., respectively.

How Supplied: In vials providing 5 million units of crystalline penicillin G sodium.

Storage: The dry powder is relatively stable and may be stored at room temperature without significant loss of potency. Sterile solutions may be kept in the refrigerator one week without significant loss of potency. Solutions prepared for intravenous infusion are stable at room temperature for at least 24 hours.

Reference: 1. American Heart Association. 1977. Prevention of bacterial endocarditis. Circulation 56:139A-143A.

PENTIDS® TABLETS ℞
PENTIDS® '400' TABLETS ℞
PENTIDS® '800' TABLETS ℞
(Penicillin G Potassium Tablets USP)
PENTIDS® FOR SYRUP ℞
PENTIDS® '400' FOR SYRUP ℞
(Penicillin G Potassium for Oral Solution USP)

Description: Pentids Tablets, Pentids '400' Tablets and Pentids '800' Tablets (Penicillin G Potassium Tablets USP) are scored, compressed uncoated tablets of crystalline penicillin G potassium. Pentids '800' Tablets contain FD&C Yellow No. 5 (tartrazine).

Pentids for Syrup and Pentids '400' for Syrup (Penicillin G Potassium for Oral Solution USP) provide penicillin G potassium in flavored powder forms for preparation as syrups when liquid oral penicillin therapy is indicated, especially for infants and children. Pentids for Syrup and Pentids '400' for Syrup contain FD&C Yellow No. 5 (tartrazine).

Clinical Pharmacology: Penicillin G is bactericidal against penicillin-susceptible microorganisms during the stage of active multiplication. It acts by inhibiting biosynthesis of cell-wall mucopeptide. It is not active against the penicillinase-producing bacteria, which include many strains of staphylococci.

Penicillin G is highly active *in vitro* against staphylococci (except penicillinase-producing strains), streptococci (groups A, C, G, H, L, and M) and pneumococci. Other organisms susceptible *in vitro* to penicillin G are *Neisseria gonorrhoeae, Corynebacterium diphtheriae, Bacillus anthracis,* Clostridia, *Actinomyces bovis, Streptobacillus moniliformis, Listeria monocytogenes,* and Leptospira; *Treponema pallidum* is extremely susceptible. Some species of gram-negative bacilli are susceptible to moderate to high concentrations of penicillin G obtained with intravenous administration. These include most strains of *Escherichia coli,* all strains of *Proteus mirabilis,* Salmonella and Shigella and some strains of *Enterobacter aerogenes* (formerly *Aerobacter aerogenes*) and *Alcaligenes faecalis.*

Oral preparations of penicillin G are only slightly affected by normal gastric acidity (pH 2.0 to 3.5); however, a pH below 2.0 may partially or totally inactivate penicillin G. Oral penicillin G is absorbed in the upper small intestine, chiefly the duodenum; however, serum level and urinary excretion data indicate that only approximately 30 percent of the dose is absorbed. For this reason four to five times the dose of oral penicillin G must be given to obtain a blood level comparable to that obtained with parenteral penicillin G. Since gastric acidity, stomach emptying time, and other factors affecting absorption may vary considerably, serum levels may be appreciably reduced to nontherapeutic levels in certain individuals.

Approximately 60 percent of penicillin G is bound to serum protein. The drug is distributed throughout the body tissues in widely varying amounts. Highest levels are found in

Continued on next page

Squibb—Cont.

the kidneys with lesser amounts in the liver, skin, and intestines. Penicillin G penetrates into all other tissues to a lesser degree with very limited amounts found in the cerebrospinal fluid. The drug is excreted rapidly by tubular excretion in patients with normal kidney function. In neonates and young infants, and in individuals with impaired kidney function, excretion is considerably delayed. Normally, approximately 20 percent of a dose of oral penicillin G is excreted in the urine.

Indications and Usage: Pentids (Penicillin G Potassium) are indicated in the treatment of mild to moderately severe infections due to penicillin G-susceptible microorganisms. Therapy should be guided by bacteriological studies, including susceptibility tests, and by clinical response. Note: severe pneumonia, empyema, bacteremia, pericarditis, meningitis, and septic arthritis should not be treated with oral penicillin G during the acute stage.

Oral penicillin G is not recommended for short-term prevention of bacterial endocarditis in patients with valvular heart disease undergoing dental or surgical procedures.

Indicated surgical procedures should be performed.

The following infections will usually respond to adequate dosage:

Streptococcal infections Group A without bacteremia—Mild to moderate infections of the upper respiratory tract, skin and skin structures infections, scarlet fever, and mild erysipelas. Note: streptococci in groups A, C, G, H, L, and M are very susceptible to penicillin G. Other groups, including group D (enterococcus) are resistant.

Pneumococcal infections—Mild to moderately severe infections of the respiratory tract.

Staphylococcal infections — penicillin G-susceptible—Mild infections of the skin and skin structures. Note: reports indicate an increasing number of strains of staphylococci resistant to penicillin G, emphasizing the need for culture and susceptibility studies in treating suspected staphylococcal infections.

Vincent's gingivitis and pharyngitis (fusospirochetosis)—Mild to moderately severe infections of the oropharynx usually respond to oral penicillin G. Note: necessary dental care should be accomplished in infections involving gum tissue.

Medical conditions in which oral penicillin G therapy is indicated as prophylaxis: (A) *For the prevention of recurrence following rheumatic fever and/or chorea.* Prophylaxis with oral penicillin G on a continuing basis is effective in preventing recurrence of these conditions.

(B) *Prevention of bacteremia following tooth extraction.*

Contraindications: Contraindicated in patients with a history of hypersensitivity to any penicillin.

Warnings: Serious and occasional fatal hypersensitivity (anaphylactoid) reactions have been reported in patients on penicillin therapy. Although anaphylaxis is more frequent following parenteral administration, it has occurred in patients on oral penicillins. These reactions are more apt to occur in individuals with a history of sensitivity to multiple allergens.

There have been well-documented reports of individuals with a history of penicillin hypersensitivity who have experienced severe hypersensitivity reactions when treated with cephalosporins. Before therapy with a penicillin, careful inquiry should be made concerning previous hypersensitivity reactions to penicillins, cephalosporins, and other allergens. If an allergic reaction occurs, the drug should be discontinued and the patient treated with the usual agents, e.g., pressor amines, antihistamines, and corticosteroids. Serious anaphylactoid reactions are not controlled by antihistamines alone, and require such emergency measures as the immediate use of epinephrine, aminophylline, oxygen, and intravenous corticosteroids.

Precautions: Penicillin should be used with caution in individuals with histories of significant allergies and/or asthma.

The oral route of administration should not be relied upon in patients with severe illness, or with nausea, vomiting, gastric dilatation, cardiospasm or intestinal hypermotility.

Occasional patients will not absorb therapeutic amounts of orally administered penicillin.

In streptococcal infections, therapy must be sufficient to eliminate the organism (10 days minimum); otherwise the sequelae of streptococcal disease may occur. Cultures should be taken following completion of treatment to determine whether streptococci have been eradicated.

Prolonged use of antibiotics may promote the overgrowth of nonsusceptible organisms, including fungi. Should superinfection occur, appropriate measures should be taken.

In prolonged therapy with penicillin, and particularly with high dosage schedules, periodic evaluation of the renal and hematopoietic systems is recommended.

Pentids '800' Tablets (Penicillin G Potassium Tablets USP), Pentids for Syrup (Penicillin G Potassium for Oral Solution USP), and Pentids '400' for Syrup contain FD&C Yellow No. 5 (tartrazine) which may cause allergic-type reactions (including bronchial asthma) in certain susceptible individuals. Although the overall incidence of FD&C Yellow No. 5 (tartrazine) sensitivity in the general population is low, it is frequently seen in patients who also have aspirin hypersensitivity.

Adverse Reactions: Although the incidence of reactions to oral penicillins has been reported with much less frequency than following parenteral therapy, it should be remembered that all degrees of hypersensitivity, including fatal anaphylaxis, have been reported with oral penicillin.

The most common reactions to oral penicillin are nausea, vomiting, epigastric distress, diarrhea, and black hairy tongue. The hypersensitivity reactions reported are skin rashes ranging from maculopapular to exfoliative dermatitis; urticaria; serum sickness-like reactions including chills, fever, edema, arthralgia, and prostration; laryngeal edema; and anaphylaxis. Fever and eosinophilia may frequently be the only reactions observed. Hemolytic anemia, leukopenia, thrombocytopenia, neuropathy, and nephropathy are infrequent reactions usually associated with high doses of parenteral penicillin. Urticaria, other skin rashes, and serum sickness-like reactions may be controlled by antihistamines and, if necessary, corticosteroids. Whenever such reactions occur, penicillin should be discontinued unless, in the opinion of the physician, the condition being treated is life-threatening and amenable only to penicillin therapy. Serious anaphylactoid reactions require emergency measures (see WARNINGS).

An occasional patient may complain of sore mouth or tongue, as with any oral penicillin preparation.

Dosage and Administration: The dosage of penicillin G should be determined according to the susceptibility of the causative microorganisms and the severity of infection, and adjusted to the clinical response of the patient.

Therapy for children under 12 years of age is calculated on the basis of body weight. For infants and small children the suggested dose is 15 to 56 mg. (25,000 to 90,000 u.) per kg./day in three to six divided doses.

For maximum absorption of penicillin, dosage should be given on an empty stomach. Thus, a dose of 200,000 units should be administered one-half hour before or at least two hours after meals. The blood concentration with a dose of 400,000 units is sufficiently high to inhibit susceptible bacteria when the antibiotic is given without regard to meals but, as can be expected, the resultant concentration will be higher when it is given before meals.

The usual dosage recommendation for adults and children 12 years and over is as follows:

Streptococcal infections—mild to moderately severe—of the upper respiratory tract and including otitis media, scarlet fever and mild erysipelas: 125 mg. (200,000 u.) t.i.d. or q.i.d. for 10 days for mild infections; 250 mg. (400,000 u.) t.i.d. for 10 days for moderately severe infections; alternatively, 500 mg. (800,000 u.) may be given b.i.d.

Pneumococcal infections—mild to moderately severe—of the respiratory tract, including otitis media: 250 mg. (400,000 u.) q.i.d. until the patient has been afebrile for at least two days.

Staphylococcal infections—mild infections of skin and skin structures (culture and susceptibility tests should be performed): 125 to 250 mg. (200,000 to 400,000 u.) t.i.d. or q.i.d. until infection is cured.

Vincent's gingivitis and pharyngitis (fusospirochetosis)—mild to moderately severe infections of the oropharynx: 250 mg. (400,000 u.) t.i.d. or q.i.d.

For the prevention of recurrence following rheumatic fever and/or chorea: 125 mg. (200,000 u.) twice daily on a continuing basis.

How Supplied: *Pentids, *Pentids '400' and *Pentids '800' Tablets (Penicillin G Potassium Tablets USP) are available for oral administration as scored, uncoated tablets which provide 125 mg. (200,000 units), 250 mg. (400,000 units) and 500 mg. (800,000 units) crystalline penicillin G potassium, respectively, equivalent to 120 mg., 240 mg. and 480 mg. of penicillin G sodium reference standard; the tablets are buffered with calcium carbonate. Pentids Tablets, in bottles of 100; Pentids '400' Tablets in bottles of 16 and 100 and Unimatic® cartons of 100; and Pentids '800' Tablets in bottles of 30 and 100.

Pentids for Syrup and Pentids '400' for Syrup (Penicillin G Potassium for Oral Solution USP) are available for oral administration as powders that, when prepared as directed, provide fruit-flavored syrups respectively containing 125 mg. (200,000 units) and 250 mg. (400,000 units) of penicillin G potassium (equivalent to 120 mg. and 240 mg. penicillin G sodium reference standard) per 5 ml. teaspoonful; both preparations are buffered with sodium phosphates. Pentids for Syrup and Pentids '400' for Syrup in 100 ml. and 200 ml. bottles.

Storage: Penicillin G Potassium Tablets USP—Store at room temperature; avoid excessive heat; keep bottle tightly closed. Dispense in tight containers.

Penicillin G Potassium for Oral Solution USP—Store at room temperature prior to preparation of syrup; store syrup in refrigerator; keep bottle tightly closed; discard unused portion after 14 days. Shake well before using.

*[*Shown in Product Identification Section*]

PRINCIPEN® '250' CAPSULES ℞
PRINCIPEN® '500' CAPSULES ℞
(Ampicillin Capsules USP)
PRINCIPEN® '125' FOR ORAL SUSPENSION ℞
PRINCIPEN® '250' FOR ORAL SUSPENSION ℞
(Ampicillin for Oral Suspension USP)

Description: Principen (Ampicillin Trihydrate), a semisynthetic penicillin derived from the basic penicillin nucleus, 6- aminopenicillanic acid, is available for oral administration as Principen '250' Capsules and Principen '500' Capsules (Ampicillin Capsules USP) which provide ampicillin trihydrate equivalent to 250 mg. and 500 mg. ampicillin, respectively. It is also available as Principen '125' for Oral Suspension and Principen '250' for Oral Suspension (Ampicillin for Oral Suspension USP) which provide, after mixing, ampicillin trihydrate equivalent to 125 mg. and 250 mg. ampicillin, respectively, per 5 ml. teaspoonful.

Actions: Human Pharmacology: Ampicillin is bactericidal at low concentrations and is clinically effective not only against the gram-positive organisms usually susceptible to penicillin G but also against a variety of gram-negative organisms. It is stable in the presence of gastric acid and is well absorbed from the gastrointestinal tract. It diffuses readily into most body tissues and fluids; however, penetration into the cerebrospinal fluid and brain occurs only with meningeal inflammation. Ampicillin is excreted largely unchanged in the urine; its excretion can be delayed by concurrent administration of probenecid which inhibits the renal tubular secretion of ampicillin. In blood serum, ampicillin is the least bound of all the penicillins; an average of about 20 percent of the drug is bound to the plasma proteins as compared to 60 to 90 percent for the other penicillins. The administration of a 500 mg. dose of ampicillin trihydrate capsules results in an average peak blood serum level of approximately 3.0 mcg./ml.; the average peak serum level for the same dose of ampicillin trihydrate for oral suspension is approximately 3.4 mcg./ml.

Microbiology: The following microorganisms show *in vitro* sensitivity to ampicillin:

GRAM-POSITIVE—strains of alpha- and beta-hemolytic streptococci, *Diplococcus pneumoniae,* those strains of staphylococci which do not produce penicillinase, *Clostridium* sp., *Bacillus anthracis, Corynebacterium xerose,* and most strains of enterococci.

GRAM-NEGATIVE—*Hemophilus influenzae; Neisseria gonorrhoeae* and *N. meningitidis; Proteus mirabilis;* and many strains of Salmonella (including *S. typhosa),* Shigella, and *Escherichia coli.*

NOTE: Ampicillin is inactivated by penicillinase and therefore is ineffective against penicillinase-producing organisms including certain strains of staphylococci, *Pseudomonas aeruginosa, P. vulgaris, Klebsiella pneumoniae, Aerobacter aerogenes,* and some strains of *E. coli.* Ampicillin is not active against Rickettsia, Mycoplasma, and "large viruses" (Miyagawanella).

TESTING FOR SUSCEPTIBILITY: The invading organism should be cultured and its sensitivity demonstrated as a guide to therapy. If the Kirby-Bauer method of disc sensitivity is used, a 10 mcg. ampicillin disc should be used to determine the relative *in vitro* susceptibility.

Indications: Principen Capsules (Ampicillin Capsules USP) and Principen for Oral Suspension (Ampicillin for Oral Suspension USP) are primarily indicated for the treatment of genitourinary, respiratory, and gastrointestinal tract infections caused by susceptible strains of gram-negative bacteria (including Shigella, *S. typhosa* and other Salmonella, *E. coli, H. influenzae, N. gonorrhoeae* and *N. meningitidis,* and *P. mirabilis).* Ampicillin may also be indicated in certain infections due to susceptible gram-positive bacteria: penicillin G-sensitive staphylococci, streptococci, pneumococci, and enterococci.

Bacteriology studies to determine the causative organisms and their sensitivity to ampicillin should be performed. Therapy may be instituted prior to the results of sensitivity testing.

Contraindications: A history of a previous hypersensitivity reaction to any of the penicillins is a contraindication. Ampicillin is also contraindicated in infections caused by penicillinase-producing organisms.

Warnings: Serious and occasional fatal hypersensitivity (anaphylactoid) reactions have been reported in patients on penicillin therapy. Although anaphylaxis is more frequent following parenteral administration, it has occurred in patients on oral penicillins. These reactions are more apt to occur in individuals with a history of sensitivity to multiple allergens.

There have been well-documented reports of individuals with a history of penicillin hypersensitivity who have experienced severe hypersensitivity reactions when treated with cephalosporins. Before therapy with a penicillin, careful inquiry should be made concerning previous hypersensitivity reactions to penicillins, cephalosporins, and other allergens. If an allergic reaction occurs, the drug should be discontinued and the patient treated with the usual agents, e.g., pressor amines, antihistamines, and corticosteroids. **Serious anaphylactoid reactions require immediate emergency treatment with epinephrine. Oxygen, intravenous steroids and airway management, including intubation, should also be administered as indicated.**

Usage in Pregnancy: The safety of this drug for use in pregnancy has not been established.

Precautions: Prolonged use of antibiotics may promote the overgrowth of nonsusceptible organisms, including fungi. Should superinfection occur, appropriate measures should be taken.

Cases of gonococcal infection with a suspected lesion of syphilis should have darkfield examinations ruling out syphilis before receiving ampicillin. Patients who do not have suspected lesions of syphilis and are treated with ampicillin should have a follow-up serologic test for syphilis each month for four months to detect syphilis that may have been masked by treatment for gonorrhea. Patients with gonorrhea who also have syphilis should be given additional appropriate parenteral penicillin treatment.

Treatment with ampicillin does not preclude the need for surgical procedures, particularly in staphylococcal infections.

In prolonged therapy, and particularly with high dosage schedules, periodic evaluation of the renal, hepatic, and hematopoietic systems is recommended.

Adverse Reactions: As with other penicillins, it may be expected that untoward reactions will be essentially limited to sensitivity phenomena. They are more likely to occur in individuals who have previously demonstrated hypersensitivity to penicillin and in those with a history of allergy, asthma, hay fever, or urticaria.

The following adverse reactions have been reported as associated with the use of ampicillin:

Gastrointestinal: glossitis, stomatitis, nausea, vomiting, enterocolitis, pseudomembranous colitis, and diarrhea. These reactions are usually associated with oral dosage forms of the drug.

Hypersensitivity Reactions: an erythematous, mildly pruritic, maculopapular skin rash has been reported fairly frequently. The rash, which usually does not develop within the first week of therapy, may cover the entire body including the soles, palms, and oral mucosa. The eruption usually disappears in 3 to 7 days. Other hypersensitivity reactions that have been reported are: skin rash, pruritus, urticaria, erythema multiforme, and an occasional case of exfoliative dermatitis. Anaphylaxis is the most serious reaction experienced and has usually been associated with the parenteral dosage form of the drug.

NOTE: Urticaria, other skin rashes, and serum sickness-like reactions may be controlled by antihistamines, and, if necessary, systemic corticosteroids. Whenever such reactions occur, ampicillin should be discontinued unless, in the opinion of the physician, the condition being treated is life-threatening and amenable only to ampicillin therapy. Serious anaphylactoid reactions require emergency measures (see WARNINGS).

Liver: moderate elevation in serum glutamic oxaloacetic transaminase (SGOT) has been noted, but the significance of this finding is unknown.

Hemic and Lymphatic Systems: anemia, thrombocytopenia, thrombocytopenic purpura, eosinophilia, leukopenia, and agranulocytosis have been reported during therapy with penicillins. These reactions are usually reversible on discontinuation of therapy and are believed to be hypersensitivity phenomena.

Other adverse reactions that have been reported with the use of ampicillin are laryngeal stridor and high fever. An occasional patient may complain of sore mouth or tongue as with any oral penicillin preparation.

Dosage and Administration: *Adults, and children weighing over 20 kg.:* **For genitourinary or gastrointestinal tract infections other than gonorrhea in men and women,** the usual dose is 500 mg. q.i.d. in equally spaced doses; severe or chronic infections may require larger doses. For the treatment of gonorrhea in both men and women, a single oral dose of 3.5 grams of ampicillin administered simultaneously with 1.0 gram of probenecid is recommended. Physicians are cautioned to use no less than the above recommended dosage for the treatment of gonorrhea. Follow-up cultures should be obtained from the original site(s) of infection 7 to 14 days after therapy. In women, it is also desirable to obtain culture test-of-cure from both the endocervical and anal canals. Prolonged intensive therapy is needed for complications such as prostatitis and epididymitis. For **respiratory tract infections,** the usual dose is 250 mg. q.i.d. in equally spaced doses.

Children weighing 20 kg. or less: For **genitourinary or gastrointestinal tract infections,** the usual dose is 100 mg./kg./day total, q.i.d. in equally divided and spaced doses. For **respiratory infections,** the usual dose is 50 mg./kg./day total, in equally divided and spaced doses 3 to 4 times daily.

All patients, irrespective of age and weight: Larger doses may be required for severe or chronic infections. Although ampicillin is resistant to degradation by gastric acid, like all antibiotics given orally it should be administered at least two hours after or one-half hour before meals for maximal absorption. Except for the single dose regimen for gonorrhea referred to above, therapy should be continued for a minimum of 48 to 72 hours after the patient becomes asymptomatic or evidence of bacterial eradication has been obtained. In infections caused by hemolytic strains of streptococci, a minimum of 10 days' treatment is recommended to guard against the risk of rheumatic fever or glomerulonephritis. In the treatment of chronic urinary or gastrointestinal infections, frequent bacteriologic and clinical appraisal is necessary during therapy and may be necessary for several months afterwards. Stubborn infections may require treatment for several weeks. Smaller doses than those indicated above should not be used. Doses for children should not exceed doses recommended for adults.

How Supplied: Principen is available for oral administration as *Principen '250' Capsules and *Principen '500' Capsules (Ampicillin Capsules USP) which provide ampicillin trihydrate equivalent to 250 mg. and 500 mg. ampicillin, respectively; the 250 mg. potency in bottles of 100 and 500 and Unimatic® Unit-Dose Packs of 100 and 500; the 500 mg. potency in bottles of 16, 100, and 500 and Unimatic Unit-Dose Packs of 100 and 500. It is also available for oral administration as Principen '125' for Oral Suspension and Principen '250' for Oral Suspension (Ampicillin for Oral Suspension USP) which provide, after mixing, pleasantly flavored suspensions containing ampicillin trihydrate equivalent to 125 mg. and 250 mg. ampicillin, respectively, per 5 ml. teaspoonful; both potencies in 80, 100, 150, and 200 ml. bottles, and in Unimatic® cartons of 4 × 25 bottles (5 ml. each bottle).

Continued on next page

Squibb—Cont.

Storage: Principen Capsules—Store at room temperature; avoid excessive heat; keep bottle tightly closed. Dispense in tight containers.
Principen for Oral Suspension—Store at room temperature prior to preparation of suspension; after preparation of suspension, store at room temperature and discard unused portion after 7 days or store in refrigerator and discard unused portion after 14 days; keep bottle tightly closed. Shake well before using.
*[*Shown in Product Identification Section*]

PRINCIPEN® with PROBENECID ℞
(Ampicillin—Probenecid Capsules)

Description: Ampicillin trihydrate is a semisynthetic penicillin derived from the basic penicillin nucleus, 6-aminopenicillanic acid. Probenecid is a uricosuric and renal tubular blocking agent. Principen with Probenecid is provided in single-dose bottles containing nine capsules; each capsule contains ampicillin trihydrate equivalent to 389 mg. ampicillin and 111 mg. probenecid (9 capsules contain ampicillin trihydrate equivalent to 3.5 g. ampicillin and 1 g. probenecid).
Actions: Ampicillin is stable in the presence of gastric acid and is well absorbed from the gastrointestinal tract. It diffuses readily into most body tissues and fluids; however, penetration into the cerebrospinal fluid and brain occurs only with meningeal inflammation. Ampicillin is excreted largely unchanged in the urine; its excretion is delayed by concurrent administration of probenecid which inhibits the renal tubular secretion of ampicillin. In blood serum, ampicillin is the least bound of all the penicillins; an average of about 20 percent of the drug is bound to the plasma proteins as compared to 60 to 90 percent for the other penicillins. Probenecid inhibits the tubular reabsorption of urate, thus increasing the urinary excretion of uric acid and decreasing serum uric acid levels. It also inhibits the tubular secretion of penicillin and usually increases penicillin plasma levels by any route the antibiotic is given. A two-fold to four-fold elevation has been demonstrated for various penicillins.
Ampicillin is inactivated by penicillinase and therefore is ineffective against penicillinase-producing organisms.
Indications: Principen with Probenecid (Ampicillin—Probenecid Capsules) is indicated for the treatment of uncomplicated infection (urethral, endocervical, or rectal) caused by *Neisseria gonorrhoeae* in men and women.
Urethritis and the presence of gram-negative diplococci in urethral smears is strong presumptive evidence of gonorrhea. Culture or fluorescent antibody studies will confirm the diagnosis.
Susceptibility studies should be performed with recurrent infections or when resistant strains are encountered. Therapy may be instituted prior to obtaining results of susceptibility testing.
Contraindications: A history of a previous hypersensitivity reaction to any of the penicillins or to probenecid is a contraindication.
Probenecid is not recommended in persons with known blood dyscrasias or uric acid kidney stones or during an acute attack of gout. It is not recommended in conjunction with ampicillin in the presence of known renal impairment.
Warnings: Serious and occasional fatal hypersensitivity (anaphylactoid) reactions have been reported in patients on penicillin therapy. Although anaphylaxis is more frequent following parenteral administration, it has occurred in patients on oral penicillins. These reactions are more apt to occur in individuals with a history of sensitivity to multiple allergens.
There have been well-documented reports of individuals with a history of penicillin hypersensitivity who have experienced severe hypersensitivity reactions when treated with cephalosporins. Before therapy with a penicillin, careful inquiry should be made concerning previous hypersensitivity reactions to penicillins, cephalosporins, and other allergens. If an allergic reaction occurs, the patient should be treated with the usual agents, e.g., pressor amines, antihistamines, and corticosteroids.
Serious anaphylactoid reactions require immediate emergency treatment with epinephrine. Oxygen, intravenous steroids, and airway management, including intubation, should also be administered as indicated.
Usage in Pregnancy: The safety of these drugs for use in pregnancy has not been established.
Precautions: Cases of gonococcal infection with a suspected lesion of syphilis should have darkfield examinations ruling out syphilis before receiving ampicillin. Patients who do not have suspected lesions of syphilis and are treated with ampicillin should have a follow-up serologic test for syphilis each month for four months to detect syphilis that may have been masked by treatment for gonorrhea. Patients with gonorrhea who also have syphilis should be given additional appropriate parenteral penicillin treatment.
Adverse Reactions: Ampicillin—As with other penicillins, it may be expected that untoward reactions will be essentially limited to sensitivity phenomena. They are more likely to occur in individuals who have previously demonstrated hypersensitivity to penicillin and in those with a history of allergy, asthma, hay fever, or urticaria.
The following adverse reactions have been reported as associated with the use of ampicillin:
Gastrointestinal: glossitis, stomatitis, nausea, vomiting, enterocolitis, pseudomembranous colitis, and diarrhea. These reactions are usually associated with oral dosage forms of the drug.
Hypersensitivity Reactions: An erythematous, mildly pruritic, maculopapular skin rash has been reported fairly frequently. The rash, which usually does not develop within the first week of therapy, may cover the entire body including the soles, palms, and oral mucosa. The eruption usually disappears in three to seven days. Other hypersensitivity reactions that have been reported are: skin rash, pruritus, urticaria, erythema multiforme, and an occasional case of exfoliative dermatitis. Anaphylaxis is the most serious reaction experienced and has usually been associated with the parenteral dosage form of the drug.
NOTE: Urticaria, other skin rashes, and serum sickness-like reactions may be controlled by antihistamines, and, if necessary, systemic corticosteroids. Serious anaphylactoid reactions require emergency measures (see WARNINGS).
Liver: Moderate elevation in serum glutamic oxaloacetic transaminase (SGOT) has been noted, but the significance of this finding is unknown.
Hemic and Lymphatic Systems: Anemia, thrombocytopenia, thrombocytopenic purpura, eosinophilia, leukopenia, and agranulocytosis have been reported during therapy with penicillins. These reactions are usually reversible on discontinuation of therapy and are believed to be hypersensitivity phenomena.
Probenecid—The following are the principal adverse reactions which have been reported as associated with the use of probenecid, generally with more prolonged or repeated administration: hypersensitivity reactions (including anaphylaxis), nephrotic syndrome, hepatic necrosis, aplastic anemia; also other anemias, including hemolytic anemia related to genetic deficiency of glucose-6-phosphate dehydrogenase.
Dosage and Administration: For the treatment of gonorrhea in both men and women—3.5 g. ampicillin and 1 g. probenecid (9 capsules) is administered as a single dose.
Physicians are cautioned to use no less than the above recommended dosage.
Follow-up cultures should be obtained from the original site(s) of infection 7 to 14 days after therapy. In women, it is also desirable to obtain culture test-of-cure from both the endocervical and anal canals.
How Supplied: Principen with Probenecid (Ampicillin—Probenecid Capsules) is provided in single-dose bottles containing nine capsules; each capsule contains ampicillin trihydrate equivalent to 389 mg. ampicillin and 111 mg. probenecid (9 capsules contain ampicillin trihydrate equivalent to 3.5 g. ampicillin and 1 g. probenecid).
Storage: Store at room temperature; avoid excessive heat.

PROLIXIN® INJECTION ℞
(Fluphenazine Hydrochloride Injection USP)
PROLIXIN® TABLETS ℞
(Fluphenazine Hydrochloride Tablets USP)
PROLIXIN® ELIXIR ℞
(Fluphenazine Hydrochloride Elixir USP)

Description: Prolixin is a trifluoromethyl phenothiazine derivative.
Prolixin Injection (Fluphenazine Hydrochloride Injection USP) is available in multiple-dose vials providing 2.5 mg. fluphenazine hydrochloride per ml. **FOR INTRAMUSCULAR USE ONLY.** The preparation also includes sodium chloride for isotonicity, sodium hydroxide or hydrochloric acid to adjust the pH to 4.8 to 5.2, and 0.1% methylparaben and 0.01% propylparaben as preservatives. At the time of manufacture, the air in the vials is replaced by nitrogen.
Prolixin Tablets (Fluphenazine Hydrochloride Tablets USP) are available for oral administration as tablets providing 1, 2.5, 5, and 10 mg. fluphenazine hydrochloride. Prolixin 2.5, 5, and 10 mg. tablets contain FD&C Yellow No. 5 (tartrazine).
Prolixin Elixir (Fluphenazine Hydrochloride Elixir USP) is available as an elixir for oral administration which provides 0.5 mg. fluphenazine hydrochloride per ml. (2.5 mg. per 5 ml. teaspoonful) and contains 14% alcohol by volume.
Clinical Pharmacology: Prolixin has activity at all levels of the central nervous system as well as on multiple organ systems. The mechanism whereby its therapeutic action is exerted is unknown.
Indications and Usage: Prolixin (Fluphenazine Hydrochloride) Injection, Tablets, and Elixir are indicated in the management of manifestations of psychotic disorders.
Fluphenazine hydrochloride has not been shown effective in the management of behavorial complications in patients with mental retardation.
Contraindications: Phenothiazines are contraindicated in patients with suspected or established subcortical brain damage, in patients receiving large doses of hypnotics, and in comatose or severely depressed states. The presence of blood dyscrasia or liver damage precludes the use of fluphenazine hydrochloride. Prolixin (Fluphenazine Hydrochloride) is contraindicated in patients who have shown hypersensitivity to fluphenazine; cross-sensitivity to phenothiazine derivatives may occur.
Warnings: The use of this drug may impair the mental and physical abilities required for driving a car or operating heavy machinery.
Potentiation of the effects of alcohol may occur with the use of this drug.
Since there is no adequate experience in children who have received this drug, safety and efficacy in children have not been established.
Usage in Pregnancy: The safety for the use of this drug during pregnancy has not been estab-

lished; therefore, the possible hazards should be weighed against the potential benefits when administering this drug to pregnant patients.

Precautions: Because of the possibility of cross-sensitivity, fluphenazine hydrochloride should be used cautiously in patients who have developed cholestatic jaundice, dermatoses or other allergic reactions to phenothiazine derivatives.

Prolixin Tablets (Fluphenazine Hydrochloride Tablets USP) 2.5, 5, and 10 mg. contain FD&C Yellow No. 5 (tartrazine) which may cause allergic-type reactions (including bronchial asthma) in certain susceptible individuals. Although the overall incidence of FD&C Yellow No. 5 (tartrazine) sensitivity in the general population is low, it is frequently seen in patients who also have aspirin hypersensitivity.

Psychotic patients on large doses of a phenothiazine drug who are undergoing surgery should be watched carefully for possible hypotensive phenomena. Moreover, it should be remembered that reduced amounts of anesthetics or central nervous system depressants may be necessary.

The effects of atropine may be potentiated in some patients receiving fluphenazine because of added anticholinergic effects.

Fluphenazine hydrochloride should be used cautiously in patients exposed to extreme heat or phosphorus insecticides; in patients with a history of convulsive disorders since grand mal convulsions have been known to occur; and in patients with special medical disorders such as mitral insufficiency or other cardiovascular diseases and pheochromocytoma.

The possibility of liver damage, pigmentary retinopathy, lenticular and corneal deposits, and development of irreversible dyskinesia should be remembered when patients are on prolonged therapy.

Neuroleptic drugs elevate prolactin levels; the elevation persists during chronic administration. Tissue culture experiments indicate that approximately one-third of human breast cancers are prolactin dependent *in vitro,* a factor of potential importance if the prescription of these drugs is contemplated in a patient with a previously detected breast cancer. Although disturbances such as galactorrhea, amenorrhea, gynecomastia, and impotence have been reported, the clinical significance of elevated serum prolactin levels is unknown for most patients. An increase in mammary neoplasms has been found in rodents after chronic administration of neuroleptic drugs. Neither clinical studies nor epidemiologic studies conducted to date, however, have shown an association between chronic administration of these drugs and mammary tumorigenesis; the available evidence is considered too limited to be conclusive at this time.

Abrupt Withdrawal: In general, phenothiazines do not produce psychic dependence; however, gastritis, nausea and vomiting, dizziness, and tremulousness have been reported following abrupt cessation of high dose therapy. Reports suggest that these symptoms can be reduced if concomitant antiparkinsonian agents are continued for several weeks after the phenothiazine is withdrawn.

Facilities should be available for periodic checking of hepatic function, renal function and the blood picture. Renal function of patients on long-term therapy should be monitored; if BUN (blood urea nitrogen) becomes abnormal, treatment should be discontinued.

As with any phenothiazine, the physician should be alert to the possible development of "silent pneumonias" in patients under treatment with fluphenazine hydrochloride.

Adverse Reactions: *Central Nervous System*—The side effects most frequently reported with phenothiazine compounds are extrapyramidal symptoms including pseudoparkinsonism, dystonia, dyskinesia, akathisia, oculogyric crises, opisthotonos, and hyperreflexia. Most often these extrapyramidal symptoms are reversible; however, they may be persistent (see below). With any given phenothiazine derivative, the incidence and severity of such reactions depend more on individual patient sensitivity than on other factors, but dosage level and patient age are also determinants.

Extrapyramidal reactions may be alarming, and the patient should be forewarned and reassured. These reactions can usually be controlled by administration of antiparkinsonian drugs, such as Benztropine Mesylate or intravenous Caffeine and Sodium Benzoate Injection, and by subsequent reduction in dosage.

Persistent Tardive Dyskinesia: As with all antipsychotic agents, tardive dyskinesia may appear in some patients on long-term therapy or may occur after drug therapy has been discontinued. The risk seems to be greater in elderly patients on high-dose therapy, especially females. The symptoms are persistent and in some patients appear to be irreversible. The syndrome is characterized by rhythmical involuntary movements of the tongue, face, mouth, or jaw (e.g., protrusion of tongue, puffing of cheeks, puckering of mouth, chewing movements). Sometimes these may be accompanied by involuntary movements of the extremities. There is no known effective treatment for tardive dyskinesia; antiparkinsonism agents usually do not alleviate the symptoms of this syndrome. It is suggested that all antipsychotic agents be discontinued if these symptoms appear. Should it be necessary to reinstitute treatment, or increase the dosage of the agent, or switch to a different antipsychotic agent, the syndrome may be masked. It has been reported that fine vermicular movements of the tongue may be an early sign of the syndrome and if the medication is stopped at that time, the syndrome may not develop.

Drowsiness or lethargy, if they occur, may necessitate a reduction in dosage; the induction of a catatonic-like state has been known to occur with dosages of fluphenazine far in excess of the recommended amounts. As with other phenothiazine compounds, reactivation or aggravation of psychotic processes may be encountered.

Phenothiazine derivatives have been known to cause, in some patients, restlessness, excitement, or bizarre dreams.

Autonomic Nervous System—Hypertension and fluctuation in blood pressure have been reported with fluphenazine hydrochloride.

Hypotension has rarely presented a problem with fluphenazine. However, patients with pheochromocytoma, cerebral vascular or renal insufficiency, or a severe cardiac reserve deficiency such as mitral insufficiency appear to be particularly prone to hypotensive reactions with phenothiazine compounds and should therefore be observed closely when the drug is administered. If severe hypotension should occur, supportive measures including the use of intravenous vasopressor drugs should be instituted immediately. Levarterenol Bitartrate Injection is the most suitable drug for this purpose; *epinephrine should not be used* since phenothiazine derivatives have been found to reverse its action, resulting in a further lowering of blood pressure.

Autonomic reactions including nausea and loss of appetite, salivation, polyuria, perspiration, dry mouth, headache, and constipation may occur. Autonomic effects can usually be controlled by reducing or temporarily discontinuing dosage.

In some patients, phenothiazine derivatives have caused blurred vision, glaucoma, bladder paralysis, fecal impaction, paralytic ileus, tachycardia, or nasal congestion.

Metabolic and Endocrine—Weight change, peripheral edema, abnormal lactation, gynecomastia, menstrual irregularities, false results on pregnancy tests, impotency in men and increased libido in women have all been known to occur in some patients on phenothiazine therapy.

Allergic Reactions—Skin disorders such as itching, erythema, urticaria, seborrhea, photosensitivity, eczema and even exfoliative dermatitis have been reported with phenothiazine derivatives. The possibility of anaphylactoid reactions occurring in some patients should be borne in mind.

Hematologic—Routine blood counts are advisable during therapy since blood dyscrasias including leukopenia, agranulocytosis, thrombocytopenic or nonthrombocytopenic purpura, eosinophilia, and pancytopenia have been observed with phenothiazine derivatives. Furthermore, if any soreness of the mouth, gums, or throat, or any symptoms of upper respiratory infection occur and confirmatory leukocyte count indicates cellular depression, therapy should be discontinued and other appropriate measures instituted immediately.

Hepatic—Liver damage as manifested by cholestatic jaundice may be encountered, particularly during the first months of therapy; treatment should be discontinued if this occurs. An increase in cephalin flocculation, sometimes accompanied by alterations in other liver function tests, have been reported in patients receiving fluphenazine hydrochloride who have had no clinical evidence of liver damage.

Others—Sudden, unexpected and unexplained deaths have been reported in hospitalized psychotic patients receiving phenothiazines. Previous brain damage or seizures may be predisposing factors; high doses should be avoided in known seizure patients. Several patients have shown sudden flare-ups of psychotic behavior patterns shortly before death. Autopsy findings have usually revealed acute fulminating pneumonia or pneumonitis, aspiration of gastric contents, or intramyocardial lesions.

Although this is not a general feature of fluphenazine, potentiation of central nervous system depressants (opiates, analgesics, antihistamines, barbiturates, alcohol) may occur.

The following adverse reactions have also occurred with phenothiazine derivatives: systemic lupus erythematosus-like syndrome, hypotension severe enough to cause fatal cardiac arrest, altered electrocardiographic and electroencephalographic tracings, altered cerebrospinal fluid proteins, cerebral edema, asthma, laryngeal edema and angioneurotic edema; with long-term use—skin pigmentation, and lenticular and corneal opacities.

Dosage and Administration: *Prolixin Injection (Fluphenazine Hydrochloride Injection USP)*—The average well-tolerated parenteral starting dose for adult psychotic patients is 1.25 mg. (0.5 ml.) intramuscularly. Depending on the severity and duration of symptoms, initial total daily parenteral dosage may range from 2.5 to 10.0 mg. and should be divided and given at 6- to 8-hour intervals.

The smallest amount that will produce the desired results must be carefully determined for each individual since optimal dosage levels of this potent drug vary from patient to patient. In general, the parenteral dose for fluphenazine has been found to be approximately $\frac{1}{3}$ to $\frac{1}{2}$ the oral dose. Treatment may be instituted with a *low initial dosage,* which may be increased, if necessary, until the desired clinical effects are achieved. Dosages exceeding 10.0 mg. intramuscularly daily should be used with caution.

When symptoms are controlled, oral maintenance therapy can generally be instituted, often with single daily doses. Continued treatment, by the oral route if possible, is needed to achieve maximum therapeutic benefits; further adjustments in dosage may be necessary during the course of therapy to meet the patient's requirements.

Prolixin (Fluphenazine Hydrochloride) Tablets and Elixir—Depending on severity and duration of symptoms, total daily oral dosage for

Continued on next page

Squibb—Cont.

adult psychotic patients may range initially from 2.5 to 10.0 mg. and should be divided and given at 6- to 8-hour intervals.
The smallest amount that will produce the desired results must be carefully determined for each individual since optimal dosage levels of this potent drug vary from patient to patient. In general, the oral dose has been found to be approximately two to three times the parenteral dose of fluphenazine. Treatment is best instituted with a *low initial dosage,* which may be increased, if necessary, until the desired clinical effects are achieved. Therapeutic effect is often achieved with doses under 20 mg. daily. Patients remaining severely disturbed or inadequately controlled may require upward titration of dosage. Daily doses up to 40 mg. may be necessary; controlled clinical studies have not been performed to demonstrate safety of prolonged administration of such doses.
When symptoms are controlled, dosage can generally be reduced gradually to daily oral maintenance doses of 1.0 or 5.0 mg., often given as a single daily dose. Continued treatment is needed to achieve maximum therapeutic benefits; further adjustments in dosage may be necessary during the course of therapy to meet the patient's requirements.
For psychotic patients who have been stabilized on a fixed daily dosage of Prolixin (Fluphenazine Hydrochloride) Tablets or Elixir, conversion of therapy from oral fluphenazine hydrochloride dosage forms to the long-acting injectable Prolixin Decanoate® may be indicated [see package insert for Prolixin Decanoate (Fluphenazine Decanoate Injection) for conversion information].
For *geriatric* patients, the suggested starting dose is 1.0 to 2.5 mg. orally daily, adjusted according to the response of the patient.
Prolixin Injection (Fluphenazine Hydrochloride Injection USP) is useful when psychotic patients are unable or unwilling to take oral therapy.
How Supplied: Prolixin Injection (Fluphenazine Hydrochloride Injection USP) is available as a sterile, aqueous solution providing 2.5 mg. fluphenazine hydrochloride per ml. in multiple-dose vials of 10 ml.
*Prolixin Tablets (Fluphenazine Hydrochloride Tablets USP) are available for oral administration as sugar-coated tablets providing 1, 2.5, 5, and 10 mg. fluphenazine hydrochloride. — 1 mg. (pink) and 10 mg. (coral) in bottles of 50 and 500; 2.5 mg. (yellow) and 5 mg. (green) in bottles of 50 and 500 and Unimatic® Unit-Dose Packs of 100 [2.5 mg in bottles of 500—V.A. Depot Item, NSN6505-00-764-4322A; 5 mg. in bottles of 500—V.A. Depot Item, NSN6505-00-951-4750A.]
Prolixin Elixir (Fluphenazine Hydrochloride Elixir USP) is available as an elixir for oral administration which provides 0.5 mg. fluphenazine hydrochloride per ml. (2.5 mg. per 5 ml. teaspoonful)—(orange-flavored and colored) in bottles of 473 ml. (1 pint) and in 60 ml. dropper assembly bottles with dropper calibrated at 0.5 ml. (0.25 mg.), 1 ml. (0.5 mg.), 1.5 ml. (0.75 mg.), and 2 ml. (1 mg.). [1 pint bottles—V.A. Depot Item, NSN6505-00-764-5042A.]
Storage: Prolixin Injection should be protected from exposure to light. Parenteral solutions may vary in color from essentially colorless to light amber. If a solution has become any darker than light amber or is discolored in any other way, it should not be used. Store at room temperature; avoid freezing.
Store the tablets and elixir at room temperature; protect from light; keep tightly closed. Tablets: avoid excessive heat. Elixir: avoid freezing.
*[*Shown in Product Identification Section*]

PROLIXIN DECANOATE® ℞
(Fluphenazine Decanoate Injection)

Description: Prolixin Decanoate is the decanoate ester of a trifluoromethyl phenothiazine derivative. It is a highly potent behavior modifier with a markedly extended duration of effect. Prolixin Decanoate is available for intramuscular or subcutaneous administration, providing 25 mg. fluphenazine decanoate per ml. in a sesame oil vehicle with 1.2% (w/v) benzyl alcohol as a preservative. At the time of manufacture, the air in the vials is replaced by nitrogen.
Clinical Pharmacology: The basic effects of fluphenazine decanoate appear to be no different from those of fluphenazine hydrochloride, with the exception of duration of action. The esterification of fluphenazine markedly prolongs the drug's duration of effect without unduly attenuating its beneficial action.
Prolixin Decanoate has activity at all levels of the central nervous system as well as on multiple organ systems. The mechanism whereby its therapeutic action is exerted is unknown.
Fluphenazine differs from other phenothiazine derivatives in several respects: it is more potent on a milligram basis, it has less potentiating effect on central nervous system depressants and anesthetics than do some of the phenothiazines and appears to be less sedating, and it is less likely than some of the older phenothiazines to produce hypotension (nevertheless, appropriate cautions should be observed—see sections on PRECAUTIONS and ADVERSE REACTIONS).
Indications and Usage: Prolixin Decanoate is a long-acting parenteral antipsychotic drug intended for use in the management of patients requiring prolonged parenteral neuroleptic therapy (e.g., chronic schizophrenics). Fluphenazine decanoate has not been shown effective in the management of behavioral complications in patients with mental retardation.
Contraindications: Phenothiazines are contraindicated in patients with suspected or established subcortical brain damage.
Phenothiazine compounds should not be used in patients receiving large doses of hypnotics. Prolixin Decanoate is contraindicated in comatose or severely depressed states.
The presence of blood dyscrasia or liver damage precludes the use of fluphenazine decanoate.
Fluphenazine decanoate is not intended for use in children under 12 years of age.
Prolixin Decanoate (Fluphenazine Decanoate Injection) is contraindicated in patients who have shown hypersensitivity to fluphenazine; cross-sensitivity to phenothiazine derivatives may occur.
Warnings: The use of this drug may impair the mental and physical abilities required for driving a car or operating heavy machinery.
Physicians should be alert to the possibility that severe adverse reactions may occur which require immediate medical attention.
Potentiation of the effects of alcohol may occur with the use of this drug.
Since there is no adequate experience in children who have received this drug, safety and efficacy in children have not been established.
Usage in Pregnancy—The safety for the use of this drug during pregnancy has not been established; therefore, the possible hazards should be weighed against the potential benefits when administering this drug to pregnant patients.
Precautions: Because of the possibility of cross-sensitivity, fluphenazine decanoate should be used cautiously in patients who have developed cholestatic jaundice, dermatoses, or other allergic reactions to phenothiazine derivatives.
Psychotic patients on large doses of a phenothiazine drug who are undergoing surgery should be watched carefully for possible hypotensive phenomena. Moreover, it should be remembered that reduced amounts of anesthetics or central nervous system depressants may be necessary.
The effects of atropine may be potentiated in some patients receiving fluphenazine because of added anticholinergic effects.
Fluphenazine decanoate should be used cautiously in patients exposed to extreme heat or phosphorus insecticides.
The preparation should be used with caution in patients with a history of convulsive disorders since grand mal convulsions have been known to occur.
Use with caution in patients with special medical disorders such as mitral insufficiency or other cardiovascular diseases and pheochromocytoma.
The possibility of liver damage, pigmentary retinopathy, lenticular and corneal deposits, and development of irreversible dyskinesia should be remembered when patients are on prolonged therapy.
Outside state hospitals or other psychiatric institutions, fluphenazine decanoate should be administered under the direction of a physician experienced in the clinical use of psychotropic drugs, particularly phenothiazine derivatives. Furthermore, facilities should be available for periodic checking of hepatic function, renal function, and the blood picture. Renal function of patients on long-term therapy should be monitored; if BUN (blood urea nitrogen) becomes abnormal, treatment should be discontinued.
As with any phenothiazine, the physician should be alert to the possible development of "silent pneumonias" in patients under treatment with fluphenazine decanoate.
Neuroleptic drugs elevate prolactin levels; the elevation persists during chronic administration. Tissue culture experiments indicate that approximately one-third of human breast cancers are prolactin dependent *in vitro,* a factor of potential importance if the prescription of these drugs is contemplated in a patient with a previously detected breast cancer. Although disturbances such as galactorrhea, amenorrhea, gynecomastia, and impotence have been reported, the clinical significance of elevated serum prolactin levels is unknown for most patients. An increase in mammary neoplasms has been found in rodents after chronic administration of neuroleptic drugs. Neither clinical studies nor epidemiologic studies conducted to date, however, have shown an association between chronic administration of these drugs and mammary tumorigenesis; the available evidence is considered too limited to be conclusive at this time.
Adverse Reactions: *Central Nervous System*—The side effects most frequently reported with phenothiazine compounds are extrapyramidal symptoms including pseudoparkinsonism, dystonia, dyskinesia, akathisia, oculogyric crises, opisthotonos, and hyperreflexia. Muscle rigidity sometimes accompanied by hyperthermia has been reported following use of fluphenazine decanoate. Most often these extrapyramidal symptoms are reversible; however, they may be persistent (see below). The frequency of such reactions is related in part to chemical structure: one can expect a higher incidence with fluphenazine decanoate than with less potent piperazine derivatives or with straight-chain phenothiazines such as chlorpromazine. With any given phenothiazine derivative, the incidence and severity of such reactions depend more on individual patient sensitivity than on other factors, but dosage level and patient age are also determinants.
Extrapyramidal reactions may be alarming, and the patient should be forewarned and reassured. These reactions can usually be controlled by administration of antiparkinsonian drugs, such as Benztropine Mesylate or intravenous Caffeine and Sodium Benzoate Injection, and by subsequent reduction in dosage.

Persistent Tardive Dyskinesia: As with all antipsychotic agents, tardive dyskinesia may appear in some patients on long-term therapy or may occur after drug therapy has been discontinued. The risk seems to be greater in elderly patients on high-dose therapy, especially females. The symptoms are persistent and in some patients appear to be irreversible. The syndrome is characterized by rhythmical involuntary movements of the tongue, face, mouth or jaw (e.g., protrusion of tongue, puffing of cheeks, puckering of mouth, chewing movements). Sometimes these may be accompanied by involuntary movements of the extremities. There is no known effective treatment for tardive dyskinesia; antiparkinsonism agents usually do not alleviate the symptoms of this syndrome. It is suggested that all antipsychotic agents be discontinued if these symptoms appear. Should it be necessary to reinstitute treatment, or increase the dosage of the agent, or switch to a different antipsychotic agent, the syndrome may be masked. It has been reported that fine vermicular movements of the tongue may be an early sign of the syndrome and if the medication is stopped at that time, the syndrome may not develop.

Drowsiness or lethargy, if they occur, may necessitate a reduction in dosage; the induction of a catatonic-like state has been known to occur with dosages of fluphenazine far in excess of the recommended amounts. As with other phenothiazine compounds, reactivation or aggravation of psychotic processes may be encountered.

Phenothiazine derivatives have been known to cause, in some patients, restlessness, excitement, or bizarre dreams.

Autonomic Nervous System—Hypertension and fluctuations in blood pressure have been reported with fluphenazine.

Hypotension has rarely presented a problem with fluphenazine. However, patients with pheochromocytoma, cerebral vascular or renal insufficiency, or a severe cardiac reserve deficiency such as mitral insufficiency appear to be particularly prone to hypotensive reactions with phenothiazine compounds, and should therefore be observed closely when the drug is administered. If severe hypotension should occur, supportive measures including the use of intravenous vasopressor drugs should be instituted immediately. Levarterenol Bitartrate Injection is the most suitable drug for this purpose; *epinephrine should not be used* since phenothiazine derivatives have been found to reverse its action, resulting in a further lowering of blood pressure.

Autonomic reactions including nausea and loss of appetite, salivation, polyuria, perspiration, dry mouth, headache, and constipation may occur. Autonomic effects can usually be controlled by reducing or temporarily discontinuing dosage.

In some patients, phenothiazine derivatives have caused blurred vision, glaucoma, bladder paralysis, fecal impaction, paralytic ileus, tachycardia, or nasal congestion.

Metabolic and Endocrine—Weight change, peripheral edema, abnormal lactation, gynecomastia, menstrual irregularities, false results on pregnancy tests, impotency in men and increased libido in women have all been known to occur in some patients on phenothiazine therapy.

Allergic Reactions—Skin disorders such as itching, erythema, urticaria, seborrhea, photosensitivity, eczema and even exfoliative dermatitis have been reported with phenothiazine derivatives. The possibility of anaphylactoid reactions occurring in some patients should be borne in mind.

Hematologic—Routine blood counts are advisable during therapy since blood dyscrasias including leukopenia, agranulocytosis, thrombocytopenic or nonthrombocytopenic purpura, eosinophilia, and pancytopenia have been observed with phenothiazine derivatives. Furthermore, if any soreness of the mouth, gums, or throat, or any symptoms of upper respiratory infection occur and confirmatory leukocyte count indicates cellular depression, therapy should be discontinued and other appropriate measures instituted immediately.

Hepatic—Liver damage as manifested by cholestatic jaundice may be encountered, particularly during the first months of therapy; treatment should be discontinued if this occurs. An increase in cephalin flocculation, sometimes accompanied by alterations in other liver function tests, has been reported in patients receiving the enanthate ester of fluphenazine (a closely related compound) who have had no clinical evidence of liver damage.

Others—Sudden, unexpected and unexplained deaths have been reported in hospitalized psychotic patients receiving phenothiazines. Previous brain damage or seizures may be predisposing factors; high doses should be avoided in known seizure patients. Several patients have shown sudden flare-ups of psychotic behavior patterns shortly before death. Autopsy findings have usually revealed acute fulminating pneumonia or pneumonitis, aspiration of gastric contents, or intramyocardial lesions.

Although this is not a general feature of fluphenazine, potentiation of central nervous system depressants (opiates, analgesics, antihistamines, barbiturates, alcohol) may occur.

The following adverse reactions have also occurred with phenothiazine derivatives: systemic lupus erythematosus-like syndrome, hypotension severe enough to cause fatal cardiac arrest, altered electrocardiographic and electroencephalographic tracings, altered cerebrospinal fluid proteins, cerebral edema, asthma, laryngeal edema, and angioneurotic edema; with long-term use—skin pigmentation and lenticular and corneal opacities.

Injections of fluphenazine decanoate are extremely well tolerated, local tissue reactions occurring only rarely.

Dosage and Administration: Prolixin Decanoate (Fluphenazine Decanoate Injection) may be given intramuscularly or subcutaneously. A dry syringe and needle of at least 21 gauge should be used. Use of a wet needle or syringe may cause the solution to become cloudy.

To begin therapy with Prolixin Decanoate the following regimens are suggested:

For *most patients,* a dose of 12.5 to 25 mg. (0.5 to 1 ml.) may be given to initiate therapy. The onset of action generally appears between 24 and 72 hours after injection and the effects of the drug on psychotic symptoms becomes significant within 48 to 96 hours. Subsequent injections and the dosage interval are determined in accordance with the patient's response. When administered as maintenance therapy, a single injection may be effective in controlling schizophrenic symptoms up to four weeks or longer. The response to a single dose has been found to last as long as six weeks in a few patients on maintenance therapy.

It may be advisable that patients who have no history of taking phenothiazines should be treated initially with a shorter-acting form of fluphenazine (see HOW SUPPLIED section for the availability of the shorter-acting fluphenazine hydrochloride dosage forms) before administering the decanoate to determine the patient's response to fluphenazine and to establish appropriate dosage. For psychotic patients who have been stabilized on a fixed daily dosage of Prolixin® Tablets (Fluphenazine Hydrochloride Tablets USP) or Prolixin® Elixir (Fluphenazine Hydrochloride Elixir USP), conversion of therapy from these short-acting oral forms to the long-acting injectable Prolixin Decanoate may be indicated.

Appropriate dosage of Prolixin Decanoate should be individualized for each patient and responses carefully monitored. No precise formula can be given to convert to use of Prolixin Decanoate; however, a controlled multicentered study*, in patients receiving oral doses from 5 to 60 mg. fluphenazine hydrochloride daily, showed that 20 mg. fluphenazine hydrochloride daily was equivalent to 25 mg. (1 ml.) Prolixin Decanoate every three weeks. This represents an approximate conversion ratio of 0.5 ml. (12.5 mg.) of decanoate every three weeks for every 10 mg. of fluphenazine hydrochloride daily.

Once conversion to Prolixin Decanoate is made, careful clinical monitoring of the patient and appropriate dosage adjustment should be made at the time of each injection.

Severely agitated patients may be treated with a rapid-acting phenothiazine compound such as Prolixin Injection (Fluphenazine Hydrochloride Injection USP—see package insert accompanying that product for complete information). When acute symptoms have subsided, 25 mg. (1 ml.) of Prolixin Decanoate may be administered; subsequent dosage is adjusted as necessary.

"Poor risk" patients (those with known hypersensitivity to phenothiazines or with disorders that predispose to undue reactions): Therapy may be initiated cautiously with oral or parenteral fluphenazine hydrochloride (see package inserts accompanying these products for complete information). When the pharmacologic effects and an appropriate dosage are apparent, an equivalent dose of Prolixin Decanoate may be administered. Subsequent dosage adjustments are made in accordance with the response of the patient.

The optimal amount of the drug and the frequency of administration must be determined for each patient, since dosage requirements have been found to vary with clinical circumstances as well as with individual response to the drug.

Dosage should not exceed 100 mg. If doses greater than 50 mg. are deemed necessary, the next dose and succeeding doses should be increased cautiously in increments of 12.5 mg.

How Supplied: Prolixin Decanoate (Fluphenazine Decanoate Injection) is available in 1 ml. Unimatic® single dose preassembled syringes, 1 ml. cartridge-needle units, and 5 ml. vials, providing 25 mg. fluphenazine decanoate per ml. [5 ml. vial—V.A. Depot Item, NSN 6505-00-264-7759A; preassembled syringe—V.A. Depot Item, NSN 6505-00-282-3788A.] Prolixin (fluphenazine) is also available for oral administration as Prolixin Tablets (Fluphenazine Hydrochloride Tablets USP) providing 1, 2.5, 5, and 10 mg. fluphenazine hydrochloride per tablet, and Prolixin Elixir (Fluphenazine Hydrochloride Elixir USP) providing 0.5 mg. fluphenazine hydrochloride per ml. (2.5 mg. per 5 ml. teaspoonful).

Storage: Store at room temperature; avoid freezing and excessive heat. Protect from light.

*The Initiation of Long-Term Pharmacotherapy in Schizophrenia: Dosage and Side Effect Comparisons Between Oral and Depot Fluphenazine; N.R. Schooler; Pharmakopsych. 9:159-169, 1976.

PRONESTYL® CAPSULES ℞
(Procainamide Hydrochloride Capsules USP)

PRONESTYL® TABLETS ℞
(Procainamide Hydrochloride Tablets)

> The prolonged administration of procainamide often leads to the development of a positive anti-nuclear antibody (ANA) test with or without symptoms of lupus erythematosus-like syndrome. If a positive ANA titer develops, the benefit/risk ratio related to continued procainamide therapy should be assessed. This may necessi-

Continued on next page

Squibb—Cont.

tate consideration of alternative antiarrhythmic therapy.

Description: Pronestyl is the amide analogue of procaine hydrochloride. It is available for oral administration as capsules and FILMLOK® tablets in potencies of 250 mg., 375 mg., and 500 mg. Pronestyl tablets contain FD&C Yellow No. 5 (tartrazine). (FILMLOK is a Squibb trademark for veneer-coated tablets.)

Actions: Procainamide depresses the excitability of cardiac muscle to electrical stimulation and slows conduction in the atrium, the bundle of His, and the ventricle. The refractory period of the atrium is considerably more prolonged than that of the ventricle. Contractility of the heart is usually not affected, nor is cardiac output decreased to any extent unless myocardial damage exists. In the absence of any arrhythmia, the heart rate may occasionally be accelerated by conventional doses, suggesting that the drug possesses anticholinergic properties. Larger doses can induce atrioventricular block and ventricular extrasystoles which may proceed to ventricular fibrillation. These effects on the myocardium are reflected in the electrocardiogram; a widening of the QRS complex occurs most consistently; less regularly, the P-R and Q-T intervals are prolonged, and the QRS and T waves show some decrease in voltage.

The action of procainamide begins almost immediately after intramuscular or intravenous administration. Plasma levels after intramuscular injection are at their peak in 15 to 60 minutes. Following oral administration, plasma levels of the drug are comparable to those obtained parenterally, and are maximal within an hour; therapeutic levels are usually attained in half that time.

Therapeutic plasma levels have been reported to be 3 to 10 mcg./ml., with those for the majority of patients in the range of 4 to 8 mcg./ml. Procainamide is less readily hydrolyzed than procaine, and plasma levels decline slowly—about 10% to 20% per hour. The drug is excreted primarily in the urine, about 10% as free and conjugated p-aminobenzoic acid and about 60% in the unchanged form. The fate of the remainder is unknown.

Indications: Pronestyl (Procainamide Hydrochloride) Capsules and Tablets are indicated in the treatment of premature ventricular contractions and ventricular tachycardia, atrial fibrillation, and paroxysmal atrial tachycardia.

Contraindications: It has been suggested that procainamide be contraindicated in patients with myasthenia gravis. Hypersensitivity to the drug is an absolute contraindication; in this connection, cross sensitivity to procaine and related drugs must be borne in mind. Procainamide should not be administered to patients with complete atrioventricular heart block. Procainamide is also contraindicated in cases of second degree and third degree A-V block unless an electrical pacemaker is operative.

Precautions: During administration of the drug, evidence of untoward myocardial responses should be carefully watched for in all patients. In the presence of an abnormal myocardium, procainamide may at times produce untoward responses. In atrial fibrillation or flutter, the ventricular rate may increase suddenly as the atrial rate is slowed. Adequate digitalization reduces but does not abolish this danger. If myocardial damage exists, ventricular tachysystole is particularly hazardous. Correction of atrial fibrillation, with resultant forceful contractions of the atrium, may cause a dislodgment of mural thrombi and produce an embolic episode. However, it has been suggested that in a patient who is already discharging emboli, procainamide is more likely to stop than to aggravate the process.

Attempts to adjust the heart rate in a patient who has developed ventricular tachycardia during an occlusive coronary episode should be carried out with extreme caution. Caution is also required in marked disturbances of atrioventricular conduction such as second degree and third degree A-V block, bundle branch block, or severe digitalis intoxication, where the use of procainamide may result in additional depression of conduction and ventricular asystole or fibrillation.

Since patients with severe organic heart disease and ventricular tachycardia may also have complete heart block which is difficult to diagnose under these circumstances, this complication should always be kept in mind when treating ventricular arrhythmias with procainamide. If the ventricular rate is significantly slowed by procainamide without attainment of regular atrioventricular conduction, the drug should be stopped and the patient reevaluated as asystole may result under these circumstances.

In patients receiving normal dosage, but who have both liver and kidney disease, symptoms of overdosage (principally ventricular tachycardia and severe hypotension) may occur due to drug accumulation.

Instances of a syndrome resembling lupus erythematosus have been reported in connection with oral maintenance procainamide therapy. The mechanism of this syndrome is uncertain. Polyarthralgia, arthritis, and pleuritic pain are common symptoms; to a lesser extent fever, myalgia, skin lesions, pleural effusion and pericarditis may occur. Rare cases of thrombocytopenia or Coombs positive hemolytic anemia have been reported which may be related to this syndrome. Patients receiving procainamide for extended periods of time or in whom symptoms suggestive of a lupus-like reaction appear should have anti-nuclear antibody titers measured at regular intervals. If there is a rising titer (anti-nuclear antibody) or clinical symptoms of LE appear, the benefit/risk ratio related to continued procainamide therapy should be assessed (see boxed Warning). The LE syndrome may be reversible upon discontinuance of the drug. If discontinuation of the drug does not cause remission of the symptoms, steroid therapy may be effective. If the syndrome develops in a patient with recurrent life-threatening arrhythmias not controllable by other antiarrhythmic agents, steroid suppressive therapy may be used concomitantly with procainamide.

Pronestyl Tablets (Procainamide Hydrochloride Tablets) contain FD&C Yellow No. 5 (tartrazine) which may cause allergic-type reactions (including bronchial asthma) in certain susceptible individuals. Although the overall incidence of FD&C Yellow No. 5 (tartrazine) sensitivity in the general population is low, it is frequently seen in patients who also have aspirin hypersensitivity.

Adverse Reactions: Hypotension following oral administration is rare. Serious disturbances of cardiac rhythm such as ventricular asystole or fibrillation are more common with intravenous administration.

Large oral doses of procainamide may sometimes produce anorexia, nausea, urticaria, and/or pruritus.

A syndrome resembling lupus erythematosus has been reported in patients on oral maintenance therapy (see PRECAUTIONS). Reactions consisting of fever and chills have also been reported, including a case with fever and chills plus nausea, vomiting, abdominal pain, acute hepatomegaly, and a rise in serum glutamic oxaloacetic transaminase following single doses of the drug. Bitter taste, diarrhea, weakness, mental depression, giddiness, and psychosis with hallucinations have been reported. The possibility of such untoward effects should be borne in mind.

Hypersensitivity reactions such as angioneurotic edema and maculopapular rash have also occurred.

Agranulocytosis has occasionally followed the repeated use of the drug, and deaths have occurred. Therefore, routine blood counts are advisable during maintenance procainamide therapy. The patients should be instructed to report any soreness of the mouth, throat, or gums, unexplained fever or any symptoms of upper respiratory tract infection. If any of these should occur, and leukocyte counts indicate cellular depression, procainamide therapy should be discontinued and appropriate treatment should be instituted immediately.

Dosage and Administration: Oral administration is preferred for treatment of arrhythmias which do not require immediate suppression, or to continue treatment after control of serious arrhythmias with Pronestyl Injection (Procainamide Hydrochloride Injection USP) or other antiarrhythmic therapy.

Intravenous therapy for the treatment of serious arrhythmias including those following myocardial infarctions should be limited to use in hospitals where monitoring facilities are available (see package insert accompanying Pronestyl Injection [Procainamide Hydrochloride Injection USP] for complete information).

If oral procainamide therapy is continued for appreciable periods, electrocardiograms should be made occasionally to determine the need for the drug.

Oral dose: For ventricular tachycardia, an initial dose of 1 gram orally followed thereafter by a *total daily dose* of 50 mg./kg. of body weight given at 3 hour intervals. The suggested oral dosage for premature ventricular contractions is 50 mg./kg. of body weight daily given in divided doses at 3 hour intervals.

To provide 50 mg./kg./day: give patients weighing less than 120 lbs. 250 mg. q. 3 hours; give patients between 120 and 200 lbs. 375 mg. q. 3 hours; and give patients over 200 lbs. 500 mg. q. 3 hours. This dosage schedule is for use as a guide for treating the average patient but all patients must be considered on an individual basis.

In atrial fibrillation and paroxysmal atrial tachycardia, an initial dose of 1.25 g. may be followed in one hour by 0.75 g. if there have been no electrocardiographic changes. A dose of 0.5 to 1 g. may then be given every 2 hours until arrhythmia is interrupted or the limit of tolerance is reached. Suggested maintenance dosage is 0.5 to 1 g. every 4 to 6 hours.

How Supplied: Pronestyl Capsules (Procainamide Hydrochloride Capsules USP) providing 250 mg. and 500 mg. are available in bottles of 100 and 1000, and UNIMATIC® unit-dose cartons of 100. The capsules which provide 375 mg. are available in bottles of 100 and UNIMATIC unit-dose cartons of 100 [375 mg. capsules in bottles of 100, Military Depot Item, NSN 6505-01-015-1846]. Pronestyl Tablets (Procainamide Hydrochloride Tablets) providing 250 mg., 375 mg., and 500 mg. are available in bottles of 100 and Unimatic unit-dose cartons of 100; the 250 mg. and 500 mg. tablets are also available in bottles of 1000.

Storage: Store the capsules and tablets at room temperature; avoid excessive heat.

[*Shown in Product Identification Section*]

PRONESTYL® INJECTION ℞

(Procainamide Hydrochloride Injection USP)

Description: Procainamide hydrochloride is the amide analogue of procaine hydrochloride. It is available for parenteral use as a sterile, aqueous solution providing 100 mg. or 500 mg. per ml. The 100 mg./ml. potency contains 0.9% (w/v) benzyl alcohol and 0.09% sodium bisulfite as preservatives; pH adjusted to 4.0–6.0 with hydrochloric acid or sodium hydroxide; the 500 mg./ml. potency contains 0.1% methylparaben and not more than 0.2% sodium bisulfite as preservatives; pH adjusted with hydrochloric acid or sodium hydroxide. At the time of manufacture, the air in the containers is replaced by nitrogen.

Actions: Procainamide depresses the excitability of cardiac muscle to electrical stimulation and slows conduction in the atrium, the bundle of His, and the ventricle. The refractory period of the atrium is considerably more prolonged than that of the ventricle. Contractility of the heart is usually not affected, nor is cardiac output decreased to any extent unless myocardial damage exists. In the absence of any arrhythmia, the heart rate may occasionally be accelerated by conventional doses, suggesting that the drug possesses anticholinergic properties. Larger doses can induce atrioventricular block and ventricular extrasystoles which may proceed to ventricular fibrillation. These effects on the myocardium are reflected in the electrocardiogram; a widening of the QRS complex occurs most consistently; less regularly, the P-R and Q-T intervals are prolonged, and the QRS and T waves show some decrease in voltage.

The action of procainamide begins almost immediately after intramuscular or intravenous administration. Plasma levels after intramuscular injection are at their peak in 15 to 60 minutes. Following oral administration, plasma levels of the drug are comparable to those obtained parenterally, and are maximal within an hour; therapeutic levels are usually attained in half that time.

Therapeutic plasma levels have been reported to be 3 to 10 mcg./ml., with those for the majority of patients in the range of 4 to 8 mcg./ml. Procainamide is less readily hydrolyzed than procaine, and plasma levels decline slowly—about 10% to 20% per hour. The drug is excreted primarily in the urine, about 10% as free and conjugated p-aminobenzoic acid and about 60% in the unchanged form. The fate of the remainder is unknown.

Indications: Pronestyl Injection (Procainamide Hydrochloride Injection USP) is indicated in the treatment of ventricular extrasystoles and tachycardia, atrial fibrillation, paroxysmal atrial tachycardia, and cardiac arrhythmias associated with anesthesia and surgery.

Contraindications: It has been suggested that procainamide be contraindicated in patients with myasthenia gravis. Hypersensitivity to the drug is an absolute contraindication; in this connection, cross sensitivity to procaine and related drugs must be borne in mind. Procainamide should not be administered to patients with complete atrioventricular heart block. Procainamide is also contraindicated in cases of high-degree A-V block unless an electrical pacemaker is operative.

Precautions: During administration of the drug, evidence of untoward myocardial responses should be carefully watched for in all patients. In the presence of an abnormal myocardium, procainamide may at times produce untoward responses. In atrial fibrillation or flutter, the ventricular rate may increase suddenly as the atrial rate is slowed. Adequate digitalization reduces, but does not abolish this danger. If myocardial damage exists, ventricular tachysystole is particularly hazardous. Correction of atrial fibrillation, with resultant forceful contractions of the atrium, may cause a dislodgment of mural thrombi and produce an embolic episode. However, it has been suggested that in a patient who is already discharging emboli, procainamide is more likely to stop than to aggravate the process.

Attempts to adjust the heart rate in a patient who has developed ventricular tachycardia during an occlusive coronary episode should be carried out with extreme caution. Caution is also required in marked disturbances of atrioventricular conduction such as A-V block, bundle branch block, or severe digitalis intoxication, where the use of procainamide may result in additional depression of conduction and ventricular asystole or fibrillation.

Parenteral administration should be monitored electrocardiographically whenever practicable. If electrocardiograms give evidence of impending heart block, parenteral administration should be discontinued at once. Since patients with severe organic heart disease and ventricular tachycardia may also have complete heart block which is difficult to diagnose under these circumstances, this complication should always be kept in mind when treating ventricular arrhythmias with procainamide (especially parenterally). If the ventricular rate is significantly slowed by procainamide without attainment of regular atrioventricular conduction, the drug should be stopped and the patient re-evaluated as asystole may result under these circumstances.

In patients receiving normal dosage, but who have both liver and kidney disease, symptoms of overdosage (principally ventricular tachycardia and severe hypotension) may occur due to drug accumulation.

Instances of a syndrome resembling lupus erythematosus have been reported in connection with oral maintenance procainamide therapy. The mechanism of this syndrome is uncertain. Polyarthralgia, arthritis, and pleuritic pain are common symptoms; to a lesser extent fever, myalgia, skin lesions, pleural effusion and pericarditis may occur. Rare cases of thrombocytopenia or Coombs positive hemolytic anemia have been reported which may be related to this syndrome. Patients receiving procainamide for extended periods of time or in whom symptoms suggestive of a lupus-like reaction appear should have anti-nuclear antibody titers measured at regular intervals. The drug should be discontinued if there is a rising titer (anti-nuclear antibody) or clinical symptoms of LE appear. The LE syndrome may be reversible upon discontinuance of the drug. If discontinuation of the drug does not cause remission of the symptoms, steroid therapy may be effective. If the syndrome develops in a patient with recurrent life-threatening arrhythmias not controllable by other antiarrhythmic agents, steroid suppressive therapy may be used concomitantly with procainamide.

Adverse Reactions: Because procainamide is a peripheral vasodilator, intravenous administration may produce transient but at times severe lowering of blood pressure, particularly in conscious patients. Intramuscular injection is less likely to be accompanied by serious falls in blood pressure. Serious disturbances of cardiac rhythm such as ventricular asystole or fibrillation are also more common with intravenous administration. Precautionary measures to be followed during intravenous injection are given in the section on "DOSAGE AND ADMINISTRATION".

A syndrome resembling lupus erythematosus has been reported in patients on oral maintenance therapy (see PRECAUTIONS). Reactions consisting of fever and chills have also been reported, including a case with fever and chills plus nausea, vomiting, abdominal pain, acute hepatomegaly, and a rise in serum glutamic oxaloacetic transaminase following single doses of the drug. Bitter taste, diarrhea, weakness, mental depression, giddiness, and psychosis with hallucinations have been reported. The possibility of such untoward effects should be borne in mind.

Hypersensitivity reactions such as angioneurotic edema and maculopapular rash have also occurred.

Agranulocytosis has occasionally followed the repeated use of the drug, and deaths have occurred. Therefore, routine blood counts are advisable during maintenance procainamide therapy. The patients should be instructed to report any soreness of the mouth, throat, or gums, unexplained fever or any symptoms of upper respiratory tract infection. If any of these should occur, and leukocyte counts indicate cellular depression, procainamide therapy should be discontinued and appropriate treatment should be instituted immediately.

Dosage and Administration: Oral administration is preferred for treatment of arrhythmias which do not require immediate suppression, or to continue treatment after control of serious arrhythmias with Pronestyl Injection (Procainamide Hydrochloride Injection USP) or other antiarrhythmic therapy.

Intravenous therapy for the treatment of serious arrhythmias including those following myocardial infarction should be limited to use in hospitals where monitoring facilities are available.

Both the 100 mg./ml. and 500 mg./ml. concentrations of Pronestyl Injection (Procainamide Hydrochloride Injection USP) should be diluted prior to intravenous use to facilitate control of dosage rate.

Intramuscular dose: Intramuscular administration may be preferable to the oral route in patients with vomiting, in those who are to receive nothing *per os* before surgery, or in those in whom there is reason to believe absorption may be unreliable. A dose of 0.5 to 1 g. may be given intramuscularly, repeated every four to eight hours until oral therapy is possible.

Intravenous dose: CAUTION—Intravenous use of procainamide hydrochloride may be accompanied by a hypotensive response, sometimes marked, if the dose is excessive or administration too rapid. Therefore, to initiate therapy, the intravenous dose should be diluted in 5% Dextrose Injection USP prior to administration to facilitate control of dosage rate; the dose should be administered at a rate not greater than 25 to 50 mg. per minute by either direct intravenous administration or infusion. Slow administration allows for some initial tissue distribution.

Direct Intravenous Administration—To reduce the possibility of a hypotensive response, 100 mg. doses may be administered every five minutes by direct slow intravenous injection, at a rate not exceeding 50 mg. in any one minute, until the arrhythmia is suppressed or the maximum dosage of 1 g. has been administered. Blood pressure must be taken and the electrocardiogram read before each dose. Some effects may be seen after the first 100 or 200 mg., and it is unusual to require more than 500 to 600 mg. to achieve satisfactory antiarrhythmic effects.

To maintain therapeutic levels, an infusion may then be started at a rate of 2 to 6 mg. procainamide per minute (see Table entitled "DILUTIONS AND RATES FOR INTRAVENOUS INFUSIONS") depending on the patient's body weight, circulatory condition and renal function.

Intravenous Infusion—An alternative method of achieving and then maintaining a therapeutic plasma concentration is to infuse 500 to 600 mg. of procainamide at a constant rate over a period of 25 to 30 minutes and then changing to another infusion for maintenance at a rate of 2 to 6 mg./min. (see Table entitled "DILUTIONS AND RATES FOR INTRAVENOUS INFUSIONS"). (See table next page)

Intravenous therapy should be terminated as soon as the patient's basic cardiac rhythm appears to be stabilized and, if indicated, the patient should be placed on oral antiarrhythmic maintenance therapy. A period of about three to four hours (one half-life) should elapse after the last intravenous dose of procainamide before administering the first oral dose of procainamide.

Intravenous administration should be monitored electrocardiographically. Excessive widening of the QRS complex or prolongation of the P-R interval suggests the occurrence of myocardial toxicity. Patients should be kept in

Continued on next page

Squibb—Cont.

a supine position and blood pressure should be measured almost continuously during administration. If the fall in blood pressure exceeds 15 mm Hg, administration should be temporarily discontinued. Phenylephrine Hydrochloride Injection USP or Levarterenol Bitartrate Injection USP should be available to counteract severe hypotensive responses.
Surgical Use: For cardiac arrhythmias associated with anesthesia and surgery, the suggested parenteral dose is 0.1 to 0.5 g., preferably given intramuscularly.
How Supplied: Pronestyl Injection (Procainamide Hydrochloride Injection USP) is available as sterile, aqueous solutions in 10 ml. vials providing 100 mg. procainamide hydrochloride per ml. or 2 ml. vials providing 500 mg. procainamide hydrochloride per ml.
The solutions, which are colorless initially, may develop a slightly yellow color in time. This does not indicate a change which would prevent its use, but a solution any darker than light amber or discolored in any other way should not be used.
Pronestyl is also available for oral administration as Pronestyl Tablets (Procainamide Hydrochloride Tablets) and Pronestyl Capsules (Procainamide Hydrochloride Capsules USP) providing 250 mg., 375 mg., and 500 mg. procainamide hydrochloride (see package inserts accompanying the products for complete information).
Storage: Store Pronestyl Injection between 50° and 80° F.

PRONESTYL-SR® TABLETS ℞
(Procainamide Hydrochloride Tablets)

> The prolonged administration of procainamide often leads to the development of a positive antinuclear antibody (ANA) test with or without symptoms of lupus erythematosus-like syndrome. If a positive ANA titer develops, the benefit/risk ratio related to continued procainamide therapy should be assessed. This may necessitate consideration of alternative antiarrhythmic therapy.

Description: Procainamide hydrochloride is the amide analogue of procaine hydrochloride. Chemically, procainamide hydrochloride is p-Amino-N-[2-(diethylamino)ethyl] benzamide monohydrochloride.
Pronestyl-SR Tablets (Procainamide Hydrochloride Tablets), containing 500 mg. procainamide hydrochloride, are for oral administration. The tablet matrix is specially designed for the prolonged release of the drug in the gastrointestinal tract.
Clinical Pharmacology: Procainamide depresses the excitability of cardiac muscle to electrical stimulation and slows conduction in the atrium, the bundle of His, and the ventricle. The refractory period of the atrium is considerably more prolonged than that of the ventricle. Contractility of the heart is usually not affected, nor is cardiac output decreased to any extent unless myocardial damage exists. In the absence of any arrhythmia, the heart rate may occasionally be accelerated by conventional doses, suggesting that the drug possesses anticholinergic properties. Larger doses can induce atrioventricular block and ventricular extrasystoles which may proceed to ventricular fibrillation. These effects on the myocardium are reflected in the electrocardiogram; a widening of the QRS complex occurs most consistently; less regularly, the P-R and Q-T intervals are prolonged, and the QRS and T waves show some decrease in voltage.
Following oral administration q6h, the tablets achieve a mean steady state of procainamide (as well as procainamide plus N-acetylprocainamide) serum concentrations approximately equivalent to those from a comparable dose of Pronestyl® Capsules (Procainamide Hydrochloride Capsules USP) q3h. Pronestyl-SR Tablets (Procainamide Hydrochloride Tablets) have a half-life which is significantly longer than that of the capsules.
The specially-formulated tablet coating and core of Pronestyl-SR (Procainamide Hydrochloride Tablets) was designed to provide the biopharmaceutic characteristics of a sustained and relatively constant rate of release and absorption throughout the entire small intestine. Therapeutic plasma levels have been reported to be 3 to 10 mcg./ml., with those for the majority of patients in the range of 4 to 8 mcg./ml. Procainamide is less readily hydrolyzed than procaine, and plasma levels decline slowly—about 10 to 20 percent per hour for standard dosage forms of procainamide. The drug is excreted primarily in the urine, with an average of about 60 percent being excreted unchanged; about 10 percent is excreted as free and conjugated p-aminobenzoic acid. The fate of the remainder is unknown.
Indications and Usage: Pronestyl-SR (Procainamide Hydrochloride Tablets) are indicated in the treatment of premature ventricular contractions and ventricular tachycardia, atrial fibrillation, and paroxysmal atrial tachycardia.
Contraindications: It has been suggested that procainamide be contraindicated in patients with myasthenia gravis. Hypersensitivity to the drug is an absolute contraindication; in this connection, cross sensitivity to procaine and related drugs must be borne in mind. Procainamide should not be administered to patients with complete atrioventricular heart block. Procainamide is also contraindicated in cases of second degree and third degree A-V block unless an electrical pacemaker is operative.
Precautions: During administration of the drug, evidence of untoward myocardial responses should be carefully watched for in all patients. In the presence of an abnormal myocardium, procainamide may at times produce untoward responses. In atrial fibrillation or flutter, the ventricular rate may increase suddenly as the atrial rate is slowed. Adequate digitalization reduces, but does not abolish this danger. If myocardial damage exists, ventricular tachysystole is particularly hazardous. Correction of atrial fibrillation, with resultant forceful contractions of the atrium, may cause a dislodgment of mural thrombi and produce an embolic episode. However, it has been suggested that in a patient who is already discharging emboli, procainamide is more likely to stop than to aggravate the process.
Attempts to adjust the heart rate in a patient who has developed ventricular tachycardia during an occlusive coronary episode should be carried out with extreme caution. Caution is also required in marked disturbances of atrioventricular conduction such as second degree and third degree A-V block, bundle branch block, or severe digitalis intoxication, where the use of procainamide may result in additional depression of conduction and ventricular asystole or fibrillation.
Since patients with severe heart disease and ventricular tachycardia may also have complete heart block which is difficult to diagnose under these circumstances, this complication should always be kept in mind when treating ventricular arrhythmias with procainamide. If the ventricular rate is significantly slowed by procainamide without attainment of regular atrioventricular conduction, the drug should be stopped and the patient reevaluated as asystole may result under these circumstances.
In patients receiving normal dosage, but who have both liver and kidney disease, symptoms of overdosage (principally ventricular tachycardia and severe hypotension) may occur due to drug accumulation.
Instances of a syndrome resembling lupus erythematosus have been reported in connection with oral maintenance procainamide therapy. The mechanism of this syndrome is uncertain. Polyarthralgia, arthritis, and pleuritic pain are common symptoms; to a lesser extent fever, myalgia, skin lesions, pleural effusion and pericarditis may occur. Rare cases of thrombocytopenia or Coombs positive hemolytic anemia have been reported which may be related to this syndrome. Patients receiving procainamide for extended periods of time or in whom symptoms suggestive of lupus-like reaction appear should have anti-nuclear antibody titers measured at regular intervals. If there is a rising titer (anti-nuclear antibody) or clinical symptoms of LE appear, the drug should be discontinued. The LE syndrome may be reversible upon discontinuance of the drug. If discontinuation of the drug does not cause remission of the symptoms, steroid therapy may be effective. If the syndrome develops in a patient with recurrent life-threatening arrhythmias not controllable by other antiarrhythmic agents, steroid suppressive therapy may be used concomitantly with procainamide.
Adverse Reactions: Hypotension following oral administration is rare. Serious disturbances of cardiac rhythm such as ventricular asystole or fibrillation are more common with intravenous administration.
Large oral doses of procainamide may sometimes produce anorexia, nausea, urticaria, and/or pruritus.
A syndrome resembling lupus erythematosus has been reported in patients on oral maintenance therapy (see PRECAUTIONS). Reactions consisting of fever and chills have also been reported, including a case with fever and chills plus nausea, vomiting, abdominal pain, acute hepatomegaly, and a rise in serum glu-

DILUTIONS AND RATES FOR INTRAVENOUS INFUSIONS*
PRONESTYL INJECTION (Procainamide Hydrochloride Injection USP)

Approximate Final Concentration	Infusion Bottle Size (ml.)	ml. of Pronestyl (100 mg./ml.) to be added	ml. of Pronestyl (500 mg./ml.) to be added	Infusion Rate
0.2% (2 mg./ml.)	500	10	2	1–3 ml./min.
	250	5	1	
0.4% (4 mg./ml.)	500	20	4	0.5–1.5 ml./min.
	250	10	2	

* CAUTION: The flow rate of all intravenous infusion solutions must be closely monitored. These dilutions are calculated to deliver 2 to 6 mg. per minute at the infusion rates listed.

tamic oxaloacetic transaminase following single doses of the drug. Bitter taste, diarrhea, weakness, mental depression, giddiness, and psychosis with hallucinations have been reported. The possibility of such untoward effects should be borne in mind.
Hypersensitivity reactions such as angioneurotic edema and maculopapular rash have also occurred.
Agranulocytosis has occasionally followed the repeated use of the drug, and deaths have occurred. Therefore, routine blood counts are advisable during maintenance procainamide therapy. The patients should be instructed to report any soreness of the mouth, throat, or gums, unexplained fever or any symptoms of upper respiratory tract infection. If any of these should occur, and leukocyte counts indicate cellular depression, procainamide therapy should be discontinued and appropriate treatment should be instituted immediately.

Dosage and Administration:

Initial Therapy:

Pronestyl-SR Tablets (Procainamide Hydrochloride Tablets) are a sustained-release dosage form not intended for initial therapy. For initial therapy by oral administration, conventional oral formulations of Pronestyl (procainamide hydrochloride) are recommended (see HOW SUPPLIED).
The duration of action of procainamide hydrochloride supplied in this sustained release dosage form allows dosing at intervals of every six hours, a schedule which may encourage patient compliance.
For control of arrhythmias requiring immediate suppression, Pronestyl Injection (Procainamide Hydrochloride Injection USP)—see HOW SUPPLIED) or other antiarrhythmic therapy is recommended; following interruption of the arrhythmia, or when the limit of tolerance is reached, Pronestyl-SR is indicated for maintenance.

Maintenance Therapy:

Dosage:

Ventricular Tachycardia and Premature Ventricular Contractions—The suggested maintenance dosage of Pronestyl-SR (Procainamide Hydrochloride Tablets) is 50 mg./kg. of body weight daily given in divided doses at six hour intervals.

To provide approximately 50 mg. per kg. per day: Give patients weighing less than 120 lbs. (less than 55 kg.) 500 mg. q6h; give patients between 120 and 200 lbs. (55 to 91 kg.) 500 mg. or 1 g. q6h; and give patients over 200 lbs. (more than 91 kg.) 1 g. q6h. This dosage schedule is for use as a guide for treating the average patient; however, each patient must be considered on an individual basis.

Atrial Fibrillation and Paroxysmal Atrial Tachycardia—The suggested maintenance dosage for Pronestyl-SR is 1 g. every six hours.

Administration:

Patients should be advised not to break or chew the tablet, as this would interfere with designed dissolution characteristics.

How Supplied: Pronestyl-SR Tablets (Procainamide Hydrochloride Tablets) are available as FILMLOK® tablets containing 500 mg. procainamide hydrochloride; these tablets are unscored, biconvex, greenish-yellow elongated ovals and are available in bottles of 100 and Unimatic® cartons of 100. (FILMLOK is a Squibb trademark for veneer-coated tablets.)

Also Available: For initial therapy, available oral dosage forms include Pronestyl Capsules (Procainamide Hydrochloride Capsules USP) and conventionally-formulated capsule-shaped FILMLOK Pronestyl Tablets (Procainamide Hydrochloride Tablets); tablets and capsules are available in potencies of 250 mg., 375 mg., and 500 mg. procainamide hydrochloride. Consult the common package insert provided with these formulations for complete information.
Pronestyl is also available for parenteral use as Pronestyl Injection (Procainamide Hydrochloride Injection USP) as sterile aqueous solutions in 10 ml. vials providing 100 mg. procainamide hydrochloride per ml. or 2 ml. vials providing 500 mg. procainamide hydrochloride per ml. Consult the package insert provided with this product for complete information.

Storage: Store Pronestyl-SR Tablets (Procainamide Hydrochloride Tablets) at room temperature; avoid excessive heat.

[Shown in Product Identification Section]

RAUDIXIN® ℞

(Rauwolfia Serpentina Tablets USP)
Whole Root—Biologically Standardized

Description: Raudixin contains Powdered Rauwolfia Serpentina USP, a hypotensive agent prepared from the powdered whole root of *Rauwolfia serpentina* Benth. The powdered rauwolfia serpentina in Raudixin contains not less than 0.15 percent and not more than 0.2 percent of reserpine-rescinnamine group alkaloids, calculated as reserpine. This product contains FD&C Yellow No. 5 (tartrazine).

Clinical Pharmacology: Rauwolfia serpentina probably produces its antihypertensive effects through depletion of tissue stores of catecholamines (epinephrine and norepinephrine) from peripheral sites. By contrast, its sedative and tranquilizing properties are thought to be related to depletion of 5-hydroxytryptamine from the brain.
Rauwolfia serpentina is characterized by slow onset of action and sustained effect. Both its cardiovascular and central nervous system effects may persist following withdrawal of the drug.

Indications and Usage: Raudixin (Rauwolfia Serpentina Tablets USP) is indicated in the treatment of mild essential hypertension. It is also useful as adjunctive therapy with other antihypertensive agents in the more severe forms of hypertension.
Raudixin is also indicated for the relief of symptoms in agitated psychotic states (e.g., schizophrenia), primarily in those individuals unable to tolerate phenothiazine derivatives or those who also require antihypertensive medication.

Contraindications: The preparation is contraindicated in patients who have previously demonstrated hypersensitivity to rauwolfia. In this regard, it should be remembered that a past history of bronchial asthma or allergy may increase the possibility of drug sensitivity reactions. It is also contraindicated in patients with mental depression (especially with suicidal tendencies), active peptic ulcer, ulcerative colitis, and in patients receiving electroconvulsive therapy.

Warnings: Extreme caution should be exercised in treating patients with a history of mental depression. Discontinue the drug at the first sign of despondency, early morning insomnia, loss of appetite, impotence, or self-deprecation. Drug-induced depression may persist for several months after drug withdrawal and may be severe enough to result in suicide.

Usage in Pregnancy: Usage of rauwolfia preparations in women of childbearing age requires that the potential benefits of the drug be weighed against its possible hazards to the fetus. The hazards of using rauwolfia preparations include increased respiratory secretions, nasal congestion, cyanosis and anorexia in infants born to rauwolfia alkaloid-treated mothers.

Nursing Mothers: Rauwolfia preparations cross the placental barrier and appear in cord blood and breast milk.

Precautions: Because rauwolfia preparations increase gastrointestinal motility and secretion, this drug should be used cautiously in patients with a history of peptic ulcer, ulcerative colitis, or gallstones where biliary colic may be precipitated. Patients on high dosage should be observed carefully at regular intervals to detect possible reactivation of peptic ulcer.
Caution should be exercised when treating hypertensive patients with renal insufficiency since they adjust poorly to lowered blood pressure levels.
Use rauwolfia serpentina cautiously with digitalis and quinidine since cardiac arrhythmias have occurred with rauwolfia preparations.
Preoperative withdrawal of rauwolfia serpentina does not insure that circulatory instability will not occur. It is important that the anesthesiologist be aware of the patient's drug intake and consider this in the overall management since hypotension has occurred in patients receiving rauwolfia preparations. Anticholinergic and/or adrenergic drugs (metaraminol, norepinephrine) have been employed to treat adverse vagocirculatory effects.
This product contains FD&C Yellow No. 5 (tartrazine) which may cause allergic-type reactions (including bronchial asthma) in certain susceptible individuals. Although the overall incidence of FD&C Yellow No. 5 (tartrazine) sensitivity in the general population is low, it is frequently seen in patients who also have aspirin hypersensitivity.

Adverse Reactions: *Gastrointestinal System*—hypersecretion, nausea, vomiting, anorexia, and diarrhea. *Central Nervous System*—drowsiness, depression, nervousness, paradoxical anxiety, nightmares, rare Parkinsonian syndrome, C.N.S. sensitization manifested by dull sensorium, deafness, glaucoma, uveitis, and optic atrophy. *Cardiovascular*—angina-like symptoms, arrhythmias, particularly when used concurrently with digitalis or quinidine, and bradycardia. *Other*—nasal congestion, pruritus, rash, dryness of mouth, dizziness, headache, dyspnea, purpura, impotence or decreased libido, dysuria, muscular aches, conjunctival injection, weight gain, and extrapyramidal tract symptoms.
These reactions are usually reversible and disappear when the drug is discontinued.
Water retention with edema in patients with hypertensive vascular disease may occur rarely, but the condition generally clears with cessation of therapy, or with the administration of a diuretic agent.

Dosage and Administration: For adults, the average oral dose is 200 to 400 mg. daily, given in divided doses in the morning and evening. Higher doses should be used cautiously because serious mental depression and other side effects may be considerably increased. (Orally, 200 to 300 mg. of powdered whole root is equivalent to 0.5 mg. of reserpine.) Maintenance doses may vary from 50 to 300 mg. per day given as a single dose or as two divided doses. Concomitant use of rauwolfia serpentina and ganglionic blocking agents, guanethidine, veratrum, hydralazine, methyldopa, chlorthalidone, or thiazides necessitates careful titration of dosage with each agent.
Dosage for adolescents, children and the aged should be proportionately less than the usual adult dosage.

How Supplied: Raudixin (Rauwolfia Serpentina Tablets USP) is available for oral use as 50 and 100 mg. coated tablets, in bottles of 100 and 1000.

Storage: Store at room temperature; avoid excessive heat; keep bottle tightly closed.

[Shown in Product Identification Section]

RAUZIDE® ℞

(Powdered Rauwolfia Serpentina [50 mg.] with Bendroflumethiazide [4 mg.])

Description: Rauzide is Powdered Rauwolfia Serpentina with Bendroflumethiazide. The Powdered Rauwolfia Serpentina in Rauzide contains not less than 0.15 percent and not more than 0.2 percent of reserpine-rescinnamine group alkaloids, calculated as reserpine.

Continued on next page

Squibb—Cont.

The preparation has been designed specifically to combine the antihypertensive effects of both rauwolfia and bendroflumethiazide for the treatment of hypertension, and may be useful in those patients not adequately benefited by either component alone. This product contains FD&C Yellow No. 5 (tartrazine).

Actions: The mechanism of action of bendroflumethiazide results in an interference with the renal tubular mechanism of electrolyte reabsorption. At maximal therapeutic dosage all thiazides are approximately equal in their diuretic potency. The mechanism whereby thiazides function in the control of hypertension is unknown.

Rauwolfia serpentina probably produces its antihypertensive effects through depletion of tissue stores of catecholamines (epinephrine and norepinephrine) from peripheral sites. By contrast, its sedative and tranquilizing properties are thought to be related to depletion of 5-hydroxytryptamine from the brain.

Rauwolfia serpentina is characterized by slow onset of action and sustained effect. Both its cardiovascular and central nervous system effects may persist following withdrawal of the drug.

Either of the components of Rauzide, when administered alone, may produce a reduction of blood pressure in hypertension. When the two agents are administered simultaneously, the action of the one appears to supplement that of the other so that a hypotensive effect may be produced which is greater than that produced by either agent alone. Thus, hypertension which does not adequately respond to either drug alone may frequently respond to the combination of both drugs.

Indications: Rauzide is indicated for hypertension (see box under WARNINGS).

Contraindications: The preparation is contraindicated in patients who have previously demonstrated hypersensitivity to thiazides or other sulfonamide-derived drugs, or rauwolfia. In this regard, it should be remembered that a past history of bronchial asthma or allergy may increase the possibility of drug sensitivity reactions.

Bendroflumethiazide is contraindicated in anuria.

The routine use of diuretics in otherwise healthy pregnant women with or without mild edema is contraindicated and possibly hazardous.

Rauwolfia serpentina is contraindicated in patients with mental depression (especially with suicidal tendencies), active peptic ulcer, ulcerative colitis, and in patients receiving electroconvulsive therapy.

Warnings:

> This fixed combination drug is not indicated for initial therapy of hypertension. Hypertension requires therapy titrated to the individual patient. If the fixed combination represents the dosage so determined, its use may be more convenient in patient management. The treatment of hypertension is not static, but must be reevaluated as conditions in each patient warrant.

Bendroflumethiazide should be used with caution in severe renal disease. In patients with renal disease, thiazides may precipitate azotemia. Cumulative effects of the drug may develop in patients with impaired renal function.

Thiazides should be used with caution in patients with impaired hepatic function or progressive liver disease, since minor alterations of fluid and electrolyte balance may precipitate hepatic coma.

Thiazides may be additive or may potentiate the action of other antihypertensive drugs. Potentiation occurs with ganglionic or peripheral adrenergic blocking drugs.

Sensitivity reactions may occur in patients with a history of allergy or bronchial asthma.

The possibility of exacerbation or activation of systemic lupus erythematosus has been reported.

When using rauwolfia serpentina, extreme caution should be exercised in treating patients with a history of mental depression. Discontinue the drug at the first sign of despondency, early morning insomnia, loss of appetite, impotence, or self-deprecation. Drug-induced depression may persist for several months after drug withdrawal and may be severe enough to result in suicide.

Usage in Pregnancy—Usage of thiazides and rauwolfia preparations in women of childbearing age requires that the potential benefits of the drug be weighed against its possible hazards to the fetus. The hazards of using thiazides include fetal or neonatal jaundice, thrombocytopenia and possibly other adverse reactions which have occurred in the adult. The hazards of using rauwolfia preparations include increased respiratory secretions, nasal congestion, cyanosis and anorexia in infants born to rauwolfia alkaloid-treated mothers.

Nursing mothers—Thiazides and rauwolfia preparations cross the placental barrier and appear in cord blood and breast milk.

Precautions: This product contains FD&C Yellow No. 5 (tartrazine) which may cause allergic-type reactions (including bronchial asthma) in certain susceptible individuals. Although the overall incidence of FD&C Yellow No. 5 (tartrazine) sensitivity in the general population is low, it is frequently seen in patients who also have aspirin hypersensitivity.

Bendroflumethiazide—Periodic determination of serum electrolytes to detect possible electrolyte imbalance should be performed at appropriate intervals.

All patients receiving thiazide therapy should be observed for clinical signs of fluid or electrolyte imbalance; namely, hyponatremia, hypochloremic alkalosis, and hypokalemia. Serum and urine electrolyte determinations are particularly important when the patient is vomiting excessively or receiving parenteral fluids. Medication such as digitalis may also influence serum electrolytes. Warning signs, irrespective of cause, are: dryness of the mouth, thirst, weakness, lethargy, drowsiness, restlessness, muscle pains or cramps, muscular fatigue, hypotension, oliguria, tachycardia, and gastrointestinal disturbances such as nausea and vomiting.

Hypokalemia may develop with thiazides as with any other potent diuretic, especially with brisk diuresis, when severe cirrhosis is present, or during concomitant use of corticosteroids or ACTH.

Interference with adequate oral electrolyte intake will also contribute to hypokalemia. Digitalis therapy may exaggerate metabolic effects of hypokalemia especially with reference to myocardial activity.

Any chloride deficit is generally mild and usually does not require specific treatment except under extraordinary circumstances (as in liver disease or renal disease). Dilutional hyponatremia may occur in edematous patients in hot weather; appropriate therapy is water restriction, rather than administration of salt except in rare instances when the hyponatremia is life threatening. In actual salt depletion appropriate replacement is the therapy of choice.

Hyperuricemia may occur or frank gout may be precipitated in certain patients receiving thiazide therapy.

Insulin requirements in diabetic patients may be increased, decreased, or unchanged. Latent diabetes mellitus may become manifest during thiazide administration.

Thiazide drugs may increase the responsiveness to tubocurarine.

The antihypertensive effects of the drug may be enhanced in the post-sympathectomy patient.

Thiazides may decrease arterial responsiveness to norepinephrine. This diminution is not sufficient to preclude effectiveness of the pressor agent for therapeutic use. If emergency surgery is indicated, preanesthetic and anesthetic agents should be administered in reduced dosage.

If progressive renal impairment becomes evident, as indicated by a rising nonprotein nitrogen or blood urea nitrogen, a careful reappraisal of therapy is necessary with consideration given to withholding or discontinuing diuretic therapy.

Thiazides may decrease serum PBI levels without signs of thyroid disturbance.

Rauwolfia serpentina—Because rauwolfia preparations increase gastrointestinal motility and secretion, this drug should be used cautiously in patients with a history of peptic ulcer, ulcerative colitis, or gallstones where biliary colic may be precipitated. Patients on high dosage should be observed carefully at regular intervals to detect possible reactivation of peptic ulcer.

Caution should be exercised when treating hypertensive patients with renal insufficiency since they adjust poorly to lowered blood pressure levels.

Use Rauwolfia serpentina cautiously with digitalis and quinidine since cardiac arrhythmias have occurred with rauwolfia preparations.

Preoperative withdrawal of rauwolfia serpentina does not insure that circulatory instability will not occur. It is important that the anesthesiologist be aware of the patient's drug intake and consider this in the overall management since hypotension has occurred in patients receiving rauwolfia preparations. Anticholinergic and/or adrenergic drugs (metaraminol, norepinephrine) have been employed to treat adverse vagocirculatory effects.

Adverse Reactions: Bendroflumethiazide: *Gastrointestinal System*—anorexia, gastric irritation, nausea, vomiting, cramping, diarrhea, constipation, jaundice (intrahepatic cholestatic jaundice), and pancreatitis. *Central Nervous System*—dizziness, vertigo, paresthesias, headache, and xanthopsia. *Hematologic*—leukopenia, agranulocytosis, thrombocytopenia, and aplastic anemia. *Dermatologic-Hypersensitivity*—purpura, photosensitivity, rash, urticaria, and necrotizing angiitis (vasculitis, cutaneous vasculitis). *Cardiovascular*—Orthostatic hypotension may occur and may be aggravated by alcohol, barbiturates or narcotics. *Other*—hyperglycemia, glycosuria, occasional metabolic acidosis in diabetic patients, hyperuricemia, allergic glomerulonephritis, muscle spasm, weakness, and restlessness.

Whenever adverse reactions are moderate or severe, thiazide dosage should be reduced or therapy withdrawn.

Rauwolfia serpentina: *Gastrointestinal System*—hypersecretion, nausea, vomiting, anorexia, and diarrhea. *Central Nervous System*—drowsiness, depression, nervousness, paradoxical anxiety, nightmares, rare Parkinsonian syndrome, C.N.S. sensitization manifested by dull sensorium, deafness, glaucoma, uveitis, and optic atrophy. *Cardiovascular*—angina-like symptoms, arrhythmias, particularly when used concurrently with digitalis or quinidine, and bradycardia. *Other*—nasal congestion, pruritus, rash, dryness of mouth, dizziness, headache, dyspnea, purpura, impotence or decreased libido, dysuria, muscular aches, conjunctival injection, weight gain, and extrapyramidal tract symptoms.

These reactions are usually reversible and disappear when the drug is discontinued.

Dosage and Administration: As determined by individual titration (see box under WARNINGS). Usual dosage may range from 1 to 4 tablets daily.

How Supplied: Rauzide is available as tablets providing 50 mg. powdered rauwolfia serpentina and 4 mg. bendroflumethiazide. Bottles of 100 and 1000.
Storage: Store at room temperature; avoid excessive heat; keep bottle tightly closed.
[*Shown in Product Identification Section*]

RENOGRAFIN® -60 ℞
(Diatrizoate Meglumine and Diatrizoate Sodium Injection USP)

(See Diagnostic Section)

RENOGRAFIN® -76 ℞
(Diatrizoate Meglumine and Diatrizoate Sodium Injection USP)

(See Diagnostic Section)

RENO-M-30® ℞
(Diatrizoate Meglumine Injection USP 30%)

(See Diagnostic Section)

RENO-M-60® ℞
(Diatrizoate Meglumine Injection USP 60%)

(See Diagnostic Section)

RENO-M-DIP® ℞
(Diatrizoate Meglumine Injection USP 30%) For Intravenous Drip Infusion

(See Diagnostic Section)

RENOVIST® ℞
(Diatrizoate Meglumine and Diatrizoate Sodium Injection USP)

(See Diagnostic Section)

RENOVIST® II ℞
(Diatrizoate Meglumine and Diatrizoate Sodium Injection USP)

(See Diagnostic Section)

RENOVUE®-65 ℞
(Iodamide Meglumine Injection)

(See Diagnostic Section)

RENOVUE®-DIP ℞
(Iodamide Meglumine Injection 24%)

(See Diagnostic Section)

RUBRAMIN PC® ℞
(Cyanocobalamin Injection USP)

Description: Rubramin PC (Vitamin B_{12}) is a clear, sterile, aqueous solution with a characteristic red color. The cobalt content of the 100 mcg./ml. and 1000 mcg./ml. Rubramin PC is 4 mcg./ml. and 40 mcg./ml., respectively. The preparation contains 1% (w/v) benzyl alcohol as a preservative and sodium chloride for isotonicity; the pH has been adjusted with sodium hydroxide or hydrochloric acid.
Clinical Pharmacology: Vitamin B_{12} is essential to growth, cell reproduction, hematopoiesis, nucleoprotein and myelin synthesis. Within 48 hours after injection of 100 to 1000 mcg. of vitamin B_{12}, 50 to 98 percent of the injected dose may appear in the urine. The major portion is excreted within the first eight hours.
Indications and Usage: Rubramin PC is indicated for vitamin B_{12} deficiency due to malabsorption which may be associated with the following conditions: Addisonian (pernicious) anemia; gastrointestinal pathology, dysfunction, or surgery; fish tapeworm infestation; gluten enteropathy; sprue; thyrotoxicosis; malignancy of the pancreas or bowel; concomitant folic acid deficiency; or hepatic or renal disease.
Rubramin PC (Cyanocobalamin Injection USP) is also suitable for use as the flushing dose in the Schilling (vitamin B_{12} absorption) Test for pernicious anemia.
Contraindications: This preparation is contraindicated in patients who are sensitive to cobalt or vitamin B_{12}.
Warnings: The preparation should be protected from sunlight.
If a vitamin B_{12} deficiency is allowed to progress for more than three months, permanent degenerative spinal cord lesions may occur; such lesions have been observed when folic acid is used as the sole hematopoietic agent.
Patients who have early Leber's disease (hereditary optic nerve atrophy) have been found to suffer severe and swift optic atrophy when treated with vitamin B_{12}.
Hypokalemia and sudden death may occur when severe megaloblastic anemia is treated intensively. Lack of therapeutic response may be due to infection, uremia, concomitant treatment with chloramphenicol or misdiagnosis.
The preparation should not be administered intravenously.
Precautions: Before administering vitamin B_{12}, an intradermal test dose is recommended for patients known to be sensitive to cobalamines.
Most antibiotics, methotrexate, and pyrimethamine invalidate folic acid and vitamin B_{12} diagnostic microbiological blood assays.
Colchicine, para-aminosalicylic acid or excessive alcohol intake longer than two weeks may produce malabsorption of vitamin B_{12}. Doses of vitamin B_{12} exceeding 10 mcg. daily may produce a hematologic response in patients who have a folate deficiency. Indiscriminate administration of vitamin B_{12} may mask the true diagnosis of pernicious anemia. A dietary deficiency of only vitamin B_{12} is rare. Multiple vitamin deficiency is expected in any dietary deficiency.
Adverse Reactions: Mild transient diarrhea, polycythemia vera, peripheral vascular thrombosis, itching, transitory exanthema, feeling of swelling of entire body, pulmonary edema and congestive heart failure early in treatment, anaphylactic shock and death.
Dosage and Administration:
A. General Rules
In patients with Addisonian (pernicious) anemia, parenteral therapy with vitamin B_{12} is the recommended method of treatment and will be required for the remainder of the patient's life. Oral therapy is not dependable. Serum potassium must be watched closely the first 48 hours; and potassium should be replaced if necessary. Reticulocyte plasma count, vitamin B_{12} and folic acid levels must be obtained prior to treatment and between the fifth and seventh day of therapy.
In patients with other types of vitamin B_{12} deficiency due to malabsorption, the malabsorption should be corrected. In all patients a well balanced dietary intake should be prescribed and poor dietary habits should be corrected.
B. Dosage:
Thirty micrograms daily for 5 to 10 days followed by 100 mcg. monthly injected intramuscularly or deep subcutaneously. Folic acid should be administered concomitantly early in the treatment unless folic acid levels are adequate.
C. Schilling Test:
The flushing dose is 1000 mcg. injected intramuscularly.
How Supplied: Rubramin PC (Cyanocobalamin Injection USP) is available in 10 ml. multiple-dose vials providing 100 mcg. cyanocobalamin per ml. and in 1 ml. and 10 ml. multiple-dose vials providing 1000 mcg. cyanocobalamin per ml. Both potencies are also available in 1 ml. UNIMATIC® single-dose preassembled syringes.
Storage: Store at room temperature; avoid freezing. Protect from light.

SINOGRAFIN® ℞
(Diatrizoate Meglumine and Iodipamide Meglumine Injection)

(See Diagnostic Section)

STOMAHESIVE®
(Peristomal Covering)

Stomahesive is a covering which can be applied to the skin around the stoma of an ostomate or the skin around a fistula to protect against contact of skin with exudates. It may also be applied to pressure points of the immobile patient to help preserve skin integrity and help prevent ulceration. It is available as wafers containing gelatin, pectin, sodium carboxymethylcellulose, and polyisobutylene.
Stomahesive is for use with colostomies, ileostomies, and ileal bladders. When applied as directed, it helps protect against drainage with an effective skintight adhesion that permits an ostomy appliance to remain intact for up to seven days.
How Supplied: Boxes of 5 4″ x 4″ wafers and boxes of 3 8″ x 8″ wafers. Both packages contain application instructions and cutting guides.

STOMAHESIVE® Protective Powder

Stomahesive Protective Powder is sodium carboxymethylcellulose, pectin, gelatin—the special skin saving ingredients in Stomahesive Peristomal Covering—in powder form. Stomahesive Protective Powder can be used as a protective barrier against drainage around stomas and fistulas. This product is designed to assist with stoma management problems. It aids in healing process by blocking seepage; it fills in gaps and crevices to form a flat surface. When used with a skin barrier such as Stomahesive Peristomal Covering, a light spray of the protective powder provides an extra layer of protection.
Precaution: For external use only.
How Supplied: 1 oz. plastic squeeze bottles.

STOMAHESIVE® Sterile Wafer
(Protective Skin Barrier)

Stomahesive Sterile Wafer is a sterile covering which can be applied to the skin around the stoma of an ostomate or the skin around an abdominal fistula or a draining surgical wound to protect against contact of the skin with exudates. Stomahesive Sterile Wafer may be used immediately following surgery and reapplied as long as a sterile dressing is indicated. It is also useful in the adjunctive management of decubitus ulcers. The product is available as sterile wafers containing gelatin, pectin, carboxymethylcellulose sodium, and polyisobutylene.
Stomahesive Sterile Wafer is for postoperative use with colostomies, ileostomies, or urostomies. When applied as directed, it helps protect the skin against drainage with an effective skintight adhesion that permits an ostomy appliance to remain intact for up to seven days.
How Supplied: Boxes of five wafers, each wafer 4″ by 4″ square.

STOMAHESIVE® WAFER WITH SUR-FIT® APPLIANCE SYSTEM

The Stomahesive Wafer with Sur-Fit Appliance System is a two-piece system which consists of a 4″ × 4″ Stomahesive Wafer with Sur-Fit Flange and a Sur-Fit Pouch with matching size Sur-Fit Flange.
The round, plastic Sur-Fit Flange is welded to the surface of a Stomahesive Wafer and to a Sur-Fit Pouch. The flanges of the pouch and wafer snap together and fit precisely to insure a leak-free seal between the pouch and wafer to

Continued on next page

Squibb—Cont.

help prevent skin irritation from drainage around the stoma.
When applied as directed, the Stomahesive Wafer helps protect against drainage with an effective skintight adhesion around the stoma.
The Sur-Fit Pouch can be removed whenever necessary without disturbing the Stomahesive Wafer with Flange for up to five to seven full days.
The Sur-Fit Appliance System provides a secure, comfortable, easy-to-use appliance system for all types of colostomies, ileostomies, and urostomies.
How Supplied: Stomahesive Wafer with Sur-Fit Flange—boxes of five 4" × 4" wafers with flange openings of 1¼", 1½", 1¾", 2¼", and 2¾".
Sur-Fit Pouches—Drainable Pouch, 12" opaque; Drainable Pouch, 10" opaque; Drainable Pouch, 12" transparent; Closed-End Pouch, opaque; Urostomy Pouch, transparent, standard; Urostomy Pouch, transparent, small. All pouches are available with flange openings of 1¼", 1½", 1¾", 2¼", and 2¾" except the Closed-End Pouch which is not available in the 1¼" flange size and the Urostomy Pouch which is not available in the 2¾" flange size.
Also available—Belts suitable for use with the Sur-Fit Appliance System, adjustable up to approximately 50".

SUMYCIN® '250' TABLETS ℞
SUMYCIN® '500' TABLETS ℞
(Tetracycline Hydrochloride Tablets USP)
SUMYCIN® '250' CAPSULES ℞
SUMYCIN® '500' CAPSULES ℞
(Tetracycline Hydrochloride Capsules USP)
SUMYCIN® SYRUP ℞
(Tetracycline Oral Suspension USP)

Description: Sumycin '250' and Sumycin '500' Tablets (Tetracycline Hydrochloride Tablets USP) are available for oral administration as FILMLOK® tablets providing 250 mg. and 500 mg. tetracycline hydrochloride, respectively. (FILMLOK is a Squibb trademark for veneer-coated tablets.)
Sumycin '250' and Sumycin '500' Capsules (Tetracycline Hydrochloride Capsules USP) contain 250 mg. and 500 mg. crystalline tetracycline hydrochloride, respectively.
Sumycin Syrup (Tetracycline Oral Suspension USP) is a suspension containing, in each 5 ml. teaspoonful, tetracycline equivalent to 125 mg. tetracycline hydrochloride.
Clinical Pharmacology: The tetracyclines are primarily bacteriostatic antibiotics and are thought to exert their antimicrobial effect by the inhibition of protein synthesis. Tetracyclines are active against a wide range of gram-negative and gram-positive organisms.
The drugs in the tetracycline class have closely similar antimicrobial spectra. Microorganisms that have become insensitive to one tetracycline invariably exhibit cross-resistance to other tetracyclines. In addition, gram-negative bacilli made tetracycline-resistant may also show cross-resistance to chloramphenicol. Microorganisms may be considered susceptible if the MIC (minimum inhibitory concentration) is not more than 4 mcg./ml. and intermediate if the MIC is 4 to 12.5 mcg./ml.
Susceptibility plate testing: A tetracycline disc may be used to determine microbial susceptibility to drugs in the tetracycline class. If the Kirby-Bauer method of disc sensitivity is used, a 30 mcg. tetracycline disc should give a zone of at least 19 mm. when tested against a tetracycline-susceptible bacterial strain.
Tetracyclines are readily absorbed and are bound to plasma proteins in varying degree. They are concentrated by the liver in the bile and excreted in the urine and feces at high concentrations and in a biologically active form.
Indications and Usage: Tetracycline is indicated in infections caused by the following microorganisms.
Rickettsiae: Rocky mountain spotted fever, typhus fever and the typhus group, Q fever, rickettsialpox, tick fevers, *Mycoplasma pneumoniae* (PPLO, Eaton agent), agents of psittacosis and ornithosis, agents of *Lymphogranuloma venereum* and *Granuloma inguinale*, and the spirochetal agent of relapsing fever *(B. recurrentis)*.
The following gram-negative organisms: *H. ducreyi* (chancroid), *Pasteurella pestis* and *Past. tularensis, Bartonella bacilliformis,* Bacteroides, *Vibrio comma* and *V. fetus,* and Brucella organisms (in conjunction with streptomycin).
Because many strains of the following groups of microorganisms have been shown to be resistant to tetracyclines, culture and susceptibility testing are recommended.
The following gram-negative organisms, when bacteriologic testing indicates appropriate susceptibility to the drug: *E. coli, Enterobacter aerogenes* (formerly *A. aerogenes*), Shigella, *Mima, Herellea, H. influenzae* (respiratory infections), and Klebsiella infections (respiratory and urinary).
The following gram-positive organisms when bacteriologic testing indicates appropriate susceptibility to the drug:
1) Streptococcus species: Up to 44 percent of strains of *Streptococcus pyogenes* and 74 percent of *Streptococcus faecalis* have been found to be resistant to tetracycline drugs. Therefore, tetracyclines should not be used for streptococcal disease unless the organism has been demonstrated to be sensitive.
(For upper respiratory infections due to group A beta-hemolytic streptococci, penicillin is the usual drug of choice including prophylaxis of rheumatic fever.)
2) *D. pneumoniae.*
3) *Staphylococcus aureus* (skin and soft tissue infections). Tetracyclines are not the drugs of choice in the treatment of any type of staphylococcal infections.
When penicillin is contraindicated, tetracyclines are alternative drugs in the treatment of infections due to: *N. gonorrhoeae, T. pallidum* and *T. pertenue* (syphilis and yaws), *Listeria monocytogenes,* Clostridia, *B. anthracis, Fusobacterium fusiforme* (Vincent's infection), and *Actinomyces.*
In acute intestinal amebiasis, the tetracyclines may be a useful adjunct to amebicides.
In severe acne the tetracyclines may be useful adjunctive therapy.
Tetracyclines are indicated in the treatment of trachoma, although the infectious agent is not always eliminated, as judged by immunofluorescence.
Inclusion conjunctivitis may be treated with oral tetracyclines or with a combination of oral and topical agents.
Contraindications: This drug is contraindicated in persons who have shown hypersensitivity to any of the tetracyclines.
Warnings: THE USE OF DRUGS OF THE TETRACYCLINE CLASS DURING TOOTH DEVELOPMENT (LAST HALF OF PREGNANCY, INFANCY AND CHILDHOOD TO AGE OF EIGHT YEARS) MAY CAUSE PERMANENT DISCOLORATION OF THE TEETH (YELLOW-GRAY-BROWN). This reaction is more common during long-term use of the drugs but has been observed following repeated short-term courses. Enamel hypoplasia has also been reported. TETRACYCLINE DRUGS, THEREFORE, SHOULD NOT BE USED IN THIS AGE GROUP UNLESS OTHER DRUGS ARE NOT LIKELY TO BE EFFECTIVE OR ARE CONTRAINDICATED.
If renal impairment exists, even usual oral or parenteral doses may lead to excessive systemic accumulation of the drug and possible liver toxicity. Under such conditions, lower than usual doses are indicated and, if therapy is prolonged, serum level determinations of the drug may be advisable. The antianabolic action of tetracycline may cause an increase in BUN. While this is not a problem in those with normal renal function, in patients with significantly impaired function, higher serum levels of tetracycline may lead to azotemia, hyperphosphatemia, and acidosis.
Photosensitivity, manifested by an exaggerated sunburn reaction, has been observed in some individuals taking tetracyclines. Patients apt to be exposed to direct sunlight or ultraviolet light should be advised that this reaction can occur with tetracycline drugs, and treatment should be discontinued at the first evidence of skin erythema. NOTE: Photosensitization reactions have occurred most frequently with demeclocycline, less with chlortetracycline, and very rarely with oxytetracycline and tetracycline.
Usage in Pregnancy: (See WARNINGS about use during tooth development.)
Results of animal studies indicate that tetracyclines cross the placenta, are found in fetal tissues and can have toxic effects on the developing fetus (often related to retardation of skeletal development). Evidence of embryotoxicity has also been noted in animals treated early in pregnancy.
Usage in Newborns, Infants, and Children: (See WARNINGS about use during tooth development.)
Tetracyclines form a stable calcium complex in any bone-forming tissue. A decrease in the fibula growth rate has been observed in prematures given oral tetracycline in doses of 25 mg./kg. every six hours. This reaction was shown to be reversible when the drug was discontinued.
Tetracyclines are present in the milk of lactating women who are taking a drug in this class.
Precautions: As with other antibiotics, use of this drug may result in overgrowth of nonsusceptible organisms, including fungi. If superinfection occurs, the antibiotic should be discontinued and appropriate therapy instituted. Note: Superinfection of the bowel by staphylococci may be life-threatening.
In venereal diseases when coexistent syphilis is suspected, patients should have darkfield examinations before treatment is started and the blood serology should be repeated monthly for at least four months.
Because the tetracyclines have been shown to depress plasma prothrombin activity, patients who are on anticoagulant therapy may require downward adjustment of their anticoagulant dosage.
During long-term therapy, periodic laboratory evaluation of organ systems, including hematopoietic, renal and hepatic studies should be performed.
All infections due to group A beta-hemolytic streptococci should be treated for at least 10 days.
Since bacteriostatic drugs may interfere with the bactericidal action of penicillin, it is advisable to avoid giving tetracycline in conjunction with penicillin.
Since sensitivity reactions are more likely to occur in persons with a history of allergy, asthma, hay fever, or urticaria, the preparation should be used with caution in such individuals.
Adverse Reactions: Gastrointestinal: anorexia, epigastric distress, nausea, vomiting, diarrhea, bulky loose stools, stomatitis, sore throat, glossitis, black hairy tongue, dysphagia, hoarseness, enterocolitis, and inflammatory lesions (with candidal overgrowth) in the anogenital region, including proctitis and pruritus ani. These reactions have been caused by both the oral and parenteral administration of tetracyclines but are less frequent after parenteral use.
Skin: maculopapular and erythematous rashes. Exfoliative dermatitis has been reported but is uncommon. Onycholysis and discoloration of the nails have been reported

rarely. Photosensitivity has occurred (see WARNINGS).
Renal toxicity: rise in BUN has been reported and is apparently dose-related (see WARNINGS).
Hepatic cholestasis has been reported rarely, and is usually associated with high dosage levels of tetracycline.
Hypersensitivity reactions: urticaria, angioneurotic edema, anaphylaxis, anaphylactoid purpura, pericarditis, exacerbation of systemic lupus erythematosus, and serum sickness-like reactions, as fever, rash, and arthralgia.
When given over prolonged periods, tetracyclines have been reported to produce brown-black microscopic discoloration of thyroid glands. No abnormalities of thyroid function studies are known to occur.
Bulging fontanels have been reported in young infants following full therapeutic dosage. This sign disappeared rapidly when the drug was discontinued.
Blood: anemia, hemolytic anemia, thrombocytopenia, thrombocytopenic purpura, neutropenia and eosinophilia have been reported.
Dizziness and headache have been reported.
Dosage and Administration: Adults: Usual daily dose is 1 to 2 g.; for mild to moderate infections: 500 mg. b.i.d. or 250 mg. q.i.d.; higher dosages such as 500 mg. q.i.d. may be required for severe infections.
For children above eight years of age: Usual daily dose is 10 to 20 mg./lb. (25 to 50 mg./kg.) body weight divided in four equal doses.
Representative pediatric dosages for the syrup on a q.i.d. basis are as follows: 20 lbs.—½ teaspoonful; 40 lbs.—1 teaspoonful; 60 lbs.—1½ teaspoonfuls; and 80 lbs.—2 teaspoonfuls.
Therapy should be continued for at least 24 to 48 hours after symptoms and fever have subsided.
The treatment of brucellosis, 500 mg. tetracycline four times daily for three weeks should be accompanied by streptomycin, 1 g. intramuscularly twice daily the first week and once daily the second week.
For treatment of gonorrhea, the recommended dose is 1.5 g. initially, then 0.5 g. every six hours until a total of 9 g. have been given.
For treatment of syphilis, a total of 30 to 40 g. in equally divided doses over a period of 10 to 15 days should be given. Close followup, including laboratory tests, is recommended.
In cases of severe acne which, in the judgment of the clinician, require long-term treatment, the recommended initial dosage is 1 g. daily in divided doses. When improvement is noted, usually within one week, dosage should be gradually reduced to maintenance levels ranging from 125 mg. to 500 mg. daily. In some patients it may be possible to maintain adequate remission of lesions with alternate-day or intermittent therapy. Tetracycline therapy of acne should augment the other standard measures known to be of value.
In patients with renal impairment (see WARNINGS) total dosage should be decreased by reduction of recommended individual doses and/or by extending time intervals between doses.
In the treatment of streptococcal infections, a therapeutic dose of tetracycline should be administered for at least 10 days.
Concomitant therapy: Antacids containing aluminum, calcium, or magnesium impair absorption and should not be given to patients taking oral tetracycline.
Foods and some dairy products also interfere with absorption. Oral forms of tetracycline should be given one hour before or two hours after meals. Pediatric oral dosage forms should not be given with milk formulas and should be given at least one hour prior to feeding.
How Supplied: *Sumycin '250' Tablets (Tetracycline Hydrochloride Tablets USP) are available for oral administration as tablets containing 250 mg. tetracycline hydrochloride in bottles of 100 and 1000. *Sumycin '500' Tablets are available for oral administration as tablets containing 500 mg. tetracycline hydrochloride in bottles of 100 and 500. *Sumycin '250' Capsules (Tetracycline Hydrochloride Capsules USP) are available for oral administration as capsules containing 250 mg. tetracycline hydrochloride in bottles of 100 and 1000 and in Unimatic® Unit-Dose Packs of 100. *Sumycin '500' Capsules are available for oral administration as capsules containing 500 mg. tetracycline hydrochloride in bottles of 100 and 500 and in Unimatic Unit-Dose Packs of 100.
Sumycin Syrup (Tetracycline Oral Suspension USP) is available as a fruit-flavored suspension containing, in each 5 ml. teaspoonful, tetracycline equivalent to 125 mg. tetracycline hydrochloride buffered with potassium metaphosphate in bottles of 60 ml. and 473 ml. (1 pint).
Storage: Store the tablets and capsules at room temperature; avoid excessive heat. Store the syrup below 30° C (86° F); avoid freezing; protect from light; keep bottle tightly closed.
*[*Shown in Product Identification Section*]

TESLAC® TABLETS ℞
(Testolactone Tablets USP)

Description: Teslac (Testolactone) contains testolactone, which is chemically designated as D-Homo-17a-oxaandrosta-1, 4-diene-3, 17-dione (1-dehydrotestololactone, or Δ^1-testololactone). Testolactone is a white, odorless, crystalline solid, soluble in ethanol and slightly soluble in water.
Teslac Tablets are available for oral administration as tablets containing 50 mg. and 250 mg. testolactone.
Clinical Pharmacology: The precise mechanism by which testolactone produces its clinical antineoplastic effects is unknown at present.
Although the chemical configuration of testolactone is similar to that of certain androgenic hormones, it is devoid of androgenic activity in the doses commonly employed.
Teslac was found to be effective in approximately 15% of patients with advanced or disseminated mammary cancer evaluated according to the following criteria: 1) those with a measurable decrease in size of all demonstrable tumor masses; 2) those in whom more than 50% of non-osseous lesions decreased in size although all bone lesions remained static; and 3) those in whom more than 50% of total lesions improved while the remainder were static.
Indications and Usage: Teslac Tablets (Testolactone Tablets USP) are recommended as adjunctive therapy in the palliative treatment of advanced or disseminated breast cancer in postmenopausal women when hormonal therapy is indicated. It may also be used in women who were diagnosed as having had disseminated breast carcinoma when premenopausal, in whom ovarian function has been subsequently terminated.
Contraindications: Testolactone is contraindicated in the treatment of breast cancer in men.
Warnings: Usage in Pregnancy: Since safe use of testolactone has not been established with respect to adverse effects upon fetal development, and since this preparation is intended for use only in postmenopausal women, testolactone should not be used during pregnancy.
Precautions: Plasma calcium levels should be routinely determined in any patient receiving therapy for mammary cancer, particularly during periods of active remission of bony metastases. If hypercalcemia occurs, appropriate measures should be instituted.
Adverse Reactions: Certain signs and symptoms have been reported in association with the use of this drug but, in these instances, it is often impossible to determine the relationship of the underlying disease and drug administration to the reported reaction. Such reactions include maculopapular erythema, increase in blood pressure, paresthesia, aches and edema of the extremities, glossitis, anorexia, and nausea and vomiting. Alopecia alone and with associated nail growth disturbance have been reported rarely; these side effects subsided without interruption of treatment.
Dosage and Administration: The recommended oral dose is 250 mg. q.i.d.
In order to evaluate the response, therapy with testolactone should be continued for a minimum of three months unless there is active progression of the disease.
How Supplied: Teslac Tablets are available for oral administration as tablets containing 50 mg. or 250 mg. testolactone in bottles of 100.
Storage: Store Teslac Tablets (Testolactone Tablets USP) at room temperature; avoid excessive heat. Keep bottle tightly closed.

THERAGRAN HEMATINIC® ℞
(Therapeutic Formula Vitamin Tablets with Hematinics)

Description: Theragran Hematinic is a therapeutic iron-containing multivitamin with minerals tablet for oral administration. The tablets contain FD&C Yellow No. 5 (tartrazine).
Graphic formulas and physical/chemical information for the vitamins may be found in the US Pharmacopeia XX. Theragran Hematinic Tablets supply:

Vitamin A Acetate	(8,333 IU) 2.5 mg
Vitamin D (Ergocalciferol)	(133 IU) 3.3 mcg
Thiamine Mononitrate	3.3 mg
Riboflavin	3.3 mg
Pyridoxine Hydrochloride	3.3 mg
Niacinamide	33.3 mg
Calcium Pantothenate	11.7 mg
Vitamin E (dl-α-Tocopheryl Acetate)	(5 IU) 5 mg
Copper (as Sulfate)	0.67 mg
Magnesium (as Carbonate)	41.7 mg
Iron, elemental (as Ferrous Fumarate)	66.7 mg
Vitamin B_{12} (as Cyanocobalamin)	50 mcg
Folic Acid	0.33 mg
Vitamin C (as Sodium Ascorbate)	100 mg

Clinical Pharmacology: Vitamins and dietary minerals are fundamentally involved in vital metabolic processes, where they usually serve as oxidizing and reducing agents and as factors in various enzyme systems. These essential micronutrients are so closely interrelated that the lack of any one may affect the body requirements of others.
Metabolic Functions of Inorganic Ions—*Iron* plays an important role in oxygen and electron transport. Iron may be functional (in hemoglobin, myoglobin, heme enzymes, and cofactor and transport iron) or stored as ferritin and hemosiderin in the liver, spleen, bone marrow, and reticuloendothelial system. The hemoglobin (0.34 percent iron) content of blood is about 14 to 17 g. per 100 ml. in adult males; in adult females it ranges between 12 and 14 g. Following ingestion, ferrous iron forms low molecular chelates with amino acids, ascorbic acid, and sugars which may be solubilized and absorbed before they reach the distal small intestine. Iron is probably absorbed passively into the mucosal layer of the small intestine, then transferred actively to transferrin where it is incorporated into red blood cells in bone marrow or into all body cells. Transferrin iron may also be stored in bone marrow, liver and spleen. Iron is removed from the body in the urine, bile, sweat, feces, and via desquamation of cells.
Copper: an essential enzyme cofactor in the utilization of iron in hemoglobin synthesis.
Magnesium: an enzyme activator—certain peptidases and phosphatases require magne-

Continued on next page

Squibb—Cont.

sium for maximal activity as do virtually all reactions involving adenosine triphosphate.

Metabolic Functions of the Vitamins—*Fat Soluble Vitamins*—These tend to be stored in the body; their precise mode of action is largely unknown.

Vitamin A: essential to the production and regeneration of the visual purple of the retina; maintenance of the integrity of epithelial tissue; lysosome stability.

Vitamin D: functions in bone metabolism by regulating the intestinal absorption of calcium and phosphorus.

Vitamin E: intracellular antioxidant, important to the stability of biologic membranes.

Water Soluble Vitamins—except for vitamin B_{12}, these micronutrients are not stored in the body.

B Complex Vitamins (thiamine, riboflavin, pyridoxine, niacinamide, pantothenic acid, vitamin B_{12}, folic acid): these function, either alone or as structural components of more complex molecules, in catalytic systems where they usually function as coenzymes in carbohydrate, protein, or amino acid metabolism, synthesis of DNA and other molecules, maturation of RBCs, nerve cell function, or oxidation-reduction reactions.

Vitamin C: a coenzyme, essential to osteoid tissue; collagen formation; vascular function; tissue respiration and wound healing; facilitates absorption of iron.

Indications and Usage: Theragran Hematinic Tablets are indicated in the treatment of many of the common iron-deficiency anemias, particularly those associated with nutritional deficiency states or when nutritional requirements are high, and tropical and nontropical sprue. These iron-deficiency states include anemias associated with dietary inadequacy, convalescence, those frequently encountered in late childhood, early adolescence and old age, menorrhagia, and the anemias of women from menarche to menopause including macrocytic or microcytic anemia of pregnancy.

Iron deficiency may result in fatigue, palpitation, smooth and sore tongue, angular stomatitis, dysphagia, gastritis, enteropathy, and koilonychia, as well as anemia. In young children, depressed growth and impaired mental performance occur.

Contraindications: Hemochromatosis and hemosiderosis are contraindications to iron therapy.

Warnings: Folic acid alone is improper therapy in the treatment of pernicious anemia and other megaloblastic anemias where vitamin B_{12} is deficient.

Precautions:

General—The use of niacin-containing preparations in patients with gastritis, peptic ulcer, or asthma should be undertaken carefully.

Since iron-deficiency anemia may be a manifestation of a basic systemic disturbance such as recurrent blood loss, the underlying cause of the anemia should be determined and corrected if possible.

The ingredients in Theragran Hematinic are not sufficient nor are they intended for the treatment of pernicious anemia. Folic acid in doses above 0.1 mg. daily may obscure pernicious anemia in that hematologic remission can occur while neurological manifestations remain progressive; therefore, the possibility of pernicious anemia should be excluded before treatment with this preparation. Parenteral use of vitamin B_{12} is recommended to assure essential medical supervision of the patient (see WARNINGS).

This product contains FD&C Yellow No. 5 (tartrazine) which may cause allergic-type reactions (including bronchial asthma) in certain susceptible individuals. Although the overall incidence of FD&C Yellow No. 5 (tartrazine) sensitivity in the general population is low, it is frequently seen in patients who also have aspirin hypersensitivity.

Information for the Patient—Keep Theragran Hematinic and all other medication out of the reach of children.

Patients should be informed of symptoms of intolerance to components of this preparation; if any of these symptoms appear the patient should be advised to discontinue dosing, and to notify the physician.

Recommended dosage should not be exceeded unless directed by the physician.

Laboratory Tests—Periodic hematologic studies should be performed.

Drug Interactions—Since oral iron products interfere with absorption of oral tetracyclines, these products should not be taken within two hours of each other.

Mineral oil and bile-acid sequestrants such as cholestyramine and colestipol hydrochloride in long-term therapy have been shown to decrease the absorption of fat-soluble vitamins.

Pyridoxine hydrochloride may act as an antagonist to levodopa.

Hydralazine hydrochloride, penicillamine, isoniazid, and cycloserine may antagonize pyridoxine hydrochloride.

Phenytoin, methotrexate, and pyrimethamine may interfere with folic acid absorption.

Colestipol hydrochloride may decrease the bioavailability of niacin.

Vitamin C may decrease the hypoprothrombinemic effect of oral anticoagulants; prothrombin levels should be monitored.

Neomycin and colchicine may impair cyanocobalamin absorption.

Carcinogenesis, Mutagenesis, Impairment of Fertility—Long-term studies in animals have not been performed.

Pregnancy Category C—Animal reproduction studies have not been conducted with therapeutic formula vitamin tablets with hematinics. Controlled clinical studies have not been performed to determine if therapeutic formula vitamin tablets with hematinics can cause fetal harm when administered to a pregnant woman or can affect reproduction capacity. Theragran Hematinic should be given to a pregnant woman only if clearly needed.

Nursing Mothers—It is not known whether components of this product are excreted in human milk. Because many substances are excreted in human milk, caution should be exercised when Theragran Hematinic is administered to a nursing woman.

Pediatric Use—Safety and effectiveness in children have not been established.

Adverse Reactions: Allergic reactions, skin rashes, and gastrointestinal disturbances, such as nausea, vomiting, diarrhea, or constipation may occur.

A generalized flushing and a feeling of warmth has been reported following niacinamide therapy.

Allergic sensitization has been reported following both oral and parenteral administration of folic acid.

Dosage and Administration: The usual adult dose is one Theragran Hematinic Tablet three times daily. When prescribed in late childhood and early adolescence, dosage reduction according to the size and weight of the child should be considered by the physician. Dosage may be adjusted according to the response of the patient. Since ferrous fumarate is not likely to cause gastric upsets, dosage need not be given at mealtime.

How Supplied: Theragran Hematinic is supplied in bottles of 90 tablets.

Storage: Store at room temperature; avoid excessive heat.

[*Shown in Product Identification Section*]

THERAGRAN® LIQUID
(High Potency Vitamin Supplement)

Each 5 ml. teaspoonful contains:

			Percent US RDA*
Vitamin A	(3 mg)	10,000 IU	200
Vitamin D	(10 mcg)	400 IU	100
Vitamin C		200 mg	333
Thiamine		10 mg	667
Riboflavin		10 mg	588
Niacin		100 mg	500
Vitamin B_6		4.1 mg	205
Vitamin B_{12}		5 mcg	83
Pantothenic Acid		21.4 mg	214

*US Recommended Daily Allowance

Usage: For 12 year olds and older—1 teaspoonful daily.

How Supplied: In bottles of 4 fl. oz.

Storage: Store at room temperature; avoid excessive heat.

THERAGRAN® TABLETS
(High Potency Vitamin Supplement)

Each tablet contains:

			Percent US RDA*
Vitamin A	(3 mg)	10,000 IU	200
Vitamin D	(10 mcg)	400 IU	100
Vitamin E	(15 mg)	15 IU	50
Vitamin C		200 mg	333
Thiamine		10.3 mg	687
Riboflavin		10 mg	588
Niacin		100 mg	500
Vitamin B_6		4.1 mg	205
Vitamin B_{12}		5 mcg	83
Pantothenic Acid		18.4 mg	184

*US Recommended Daily Allowance

Usage: For 12 year olds and older—1 tablet daily.

How Supplied: Bottles of 1000; Packs of 30, 60, 100, and 180; and Unimatic® cartons of 100.

Storage: Store at room temperature; avoid excessive heat.

[*Shown in Product identification Section*]

THERAGRAN-M® TABLETS
(High Potency Vitamin Supplement with Minerals)

Each tablet contains:

			Percent US RDA*
Vitamins			
Vitamin A	(3 mg)	10,000 IU	200
Vitamin D	(10 mcg)	400 IU	100
Vitamin E	(15 mg)	15 IU	50
Vitamin C		200 mg	333
Thiamine		10.3 mg	687
Riboflavin		10 mg	588
Niacin		100 mg	500
Vitamin B_6		4.1 mg	205
Vitamin B_{12}		5 mcg	83
Pantothenic Acid		18.4 mg	184
Minerals			
Iodine		150 mcg	100
Iron		12 mg	67
Magnesium		65 mg	16
Copper		2 mg	100
Zinc		1.5 mg	10
Manganese		1 mg	**

*US Recommended Daily Allowance
**US RDA not established

Usage: For 12 year olds and older —1 tablet daily.

How Supplied: Bottles of 1000; Packs of 30, 60, 100, and 180; and Unimatic® cartons of 100.

Storage: Store at room temperture; avoid excessive heat.

[*Shown in Product Identification Section*]

THERAGRAN-Z® TABLETS
(High Potency Vitamin-Mineral Supplement with Zinc)

Each tablet contains:

		Percent US RDA*
Vitamins		
Vitamin A	(3 mg) 10,000 IU	200
Vitamin D	(10 mcg) 400 IU	100
Vitamin E	(15 mg) 15 IU	50
Vitamin C	200 mg	333
Thiamine	10.3 mg	687
Riboflavin	10 mg	588
Niacin	100 mg	500
Vitamin B_6	4.1 mg	205
Vitamin B_{12}	5 mcg	83
Pantothenic Acid	18.4 mg	184
Minerals		
Iodine	150 mcg	100
Iron	12 mg	67
Copper	2 mg	100
Zinc	22.5 mg	150
Manganese	1 mg	**

*US Recommended Daily Allowance
**US RDA not established

Usage: For 12 year olds and older — 1 tablet daily.

How Supplied: Bottles of 30 and 60.

Storage: Store at room temperature; avoid excessive heat.

[*Shown in Product Identification Section*]

TRIMOX® '250' CAPSULES ℞
TRIMOX® '500' CAPSULES ℞
(Amoxicillin Capsules USP)
TRIMOX® '125' FOR ORAL SUSPENSION ℞
TRIMOX® '250' FOR ORAL SUSPENSION ℞
(Amoxicillin for Oral Suspension USP)

Description: Trimox (amoxicillin) is a semi-synthetic antibiotic, an analog of ampicillin, with a broad spectrum of bactericidal activity against many gram-positive and gram-negative microorganisms. Chemically it is D-(-)-alpha-amino-p-hydroxybenzyl penicillin trihydrate.

Clinical Pharmacology: Amoxicillin is stable in the presence of gastric acid and may be given without regard to meals. It is rapidly absorbed after oral administration. It diffuses readily into most body tissues and fluids, with the exception of brain and spinal fluid, except when meninges are inflamed. The half-life of amoxicillin is 61.3 minutes. Most of the amoxicillin is excreted unchanged in the urine; its excretion can be delayed by concurrent administration of probenecid. Amoxicillin is not highly protein-bound. In blood serum, amoxicillin is approximately 20 percent protein-bound as compared to 60 percent for penicillin G.

Orally administered doses of 250 mg. and 500 mg. amoxicillin capsules result in average peak blood levels one to two hours after administration in the range of 3.5 mcg./ml. to 5.0 mcg./ml. and 5.5 mcg./ml. to 7.5 mcg./ml., respectively.

Orally administered doses of amoxicillin suspension 125 mg./5 ml. and 250 mg./5 ml. result in average peak blood levels one to two hours after administration in the range of 1.5 mcg./ml. to 3.0 mcg./ml. and 3.5 mcg./ml. to 5.0 mcg./ml., respectively.

Detectable serum levels are observed up to 8 hours after an orally administered dose of amoxicillin. Following a 1 g. dose and utilizing a special skin window technique to determine levels of the antibiotic, it was noted that therapeutic levels were found in the interstitial fluid. Approximately 60 percent of an orally administered dose of amoxicillin is excreted in the urine within six to eight hours.

Microbiology: Trimox (amoxicillin) is similar to ampicillin in its bactericidal action against susceptible organisms during the stage of active multiplication. It acts through the inhibition of biosynthesis of cell wall mucopeptides. *In vitro* studies have demonstrated the susceptibility of most strains of the following gram-positive bacteria: alpha- and beta-hemolytic streptococci, *Streptococcus pneumoniae* (formerly *Diplococcus pneumoniae*), nonpenicillinase-producing staphylococci, and *Streptococcus faecalis*. It is active *in vitro* against many strains of *Hemophilus influenzae, Neisseria gonorrhoeae, Escherichia coli* and *Proteus mirabilis*. Because it does not resist destruction by penicillinase, it is *not* effective against penicillinase-producing bacteria, particularly resistant staphylococci. All strains of Pseudomonas and most strains of Klebsiella and Enterobacter are resistant.

Disc Susceptibility Tests: Quantitative methods that require measurement of the diameters of zones of inhibition of microbial growth give the most precise estimates of antibiotic susceptibility. One recommended procedure (21 CFR Sec. 460.1) uses discs for testing susceptibility to ampicillin-class antibiotics. Interpretations correlate diameters of the disc test with MIC values for amoxicillin. With this procedure, a report from the laboratory of "susceptible" indicates that the infecting organism is likely to respond to therapy. A report of "resistant" indicates that the infecting organism is not likely to respond to therapy. A report of "intermediate susceptibility" suggests that the organism would be susceptible if high dosage is used, or if the infection is confined to tissues and fluids (e.g., urine) in which high antibiotic levels are attained.

Indications and Usage: Trimox (amoxicillin) is indicated in the treatment of infections due to susceptible strains of the following:

Gram-negative organisms — *H. influenzae, E. coli, P. mirabilis* and *N. gonorrhoeae*.

Gram-positive organisms — Streptococci (including *Streptococcus faecalis*), *S. pneumoniae* and nonpenicillinase-producing staphylococci.

Therapy may be instituted prior to obtaining results from bacteriological and susceptibility studies to determine the causative organisms and their susceptibility to amoxicillin.

Indicated surgical procedures should be performed.

Contraindications: The use of this drug is contraindicated in individuals with a history of an allergic reaction to any of the penicillins.

Warnings: Serious and occasionally fatal hypersensitivity (anaphylactoid) reactions have been reported in patients on penicillin therapy. Although anaphylaxis is more frequent following parenteral therapy, it has occurred in patients on oral penicillins. These reactions are more likely to occur in individuals with a history of sensitivity to multiple allergens. There have been reports of individuals with a history of penicillin hypersensitivity who have experienced severe reactions when treated with a cephalosporin. Before therapy with any penicillin, careful inquiry should be made concerning previous hypersensitivity reactions to penicillins, cephalosporins, or other allergens. If an allergic reaction occurs, appropriate therapy should be instituted and discontinuance of amoxicillin therapy considered. **Serious anaphylactoid reactions require immediate emergency treatment with epinephrine. Oxygen, intravenous steroids, and airway management, including intubation, should also be administered as indicated.**

Precautions: As with any potent drug, periodic assessment of renal, hepatic and hematopoietic function should be made during prolonged therapy.

The possibility of superinfections with mycotic or bacterial pathogens should be kept in mind during therapy. If superinfections occur (usually involving Enterobacter, Pseudomonas or Candida), amoxicillin should be discontinued and/or appropriate therapy instituted.

Usage in Pregnancy: Safety for use in pregnancy has not been established.

Adverse Reactions: As with other penicillins, it may be expected that untoward reactions will be essentially limited to sensitivity phenomena. They are more likely to occur in individuals who have previously demonstrated hypersensitivity to penicillins and in those with a history of allergy, asthma, hay fever or urticaria. The following adverse reactions have been reported as associated with the use of the penicillins:

Gastrointestinal: Glossitis, stomatitis, black "hairy" tongue, nausea, vomiting and diarrhea.

Hypersensitivity Reactions: Erythematous maculopapular rashes, urticaria, and a few cases of exfoliative dermatitis and erythema multiforme have been reported. Anaphylaxis is the most serious reaction experienced and has usually been associated with parenteral dosage forms (See WARNINGS).

NOTE: Urticaria, other skin rashes and serum sickness-like reactions may be controlled with antihistamines and, if necessary, systemic corticosteroids. Whenever such reactions occur, amoxicillin should be discontinued unless, in the opinion of the physician, the condition being treated is life-threatening and amenable only to amoxicillin therapy.

Liver: A moderate rise in serum glutamic oxaloacetic transaminase (SGOT) has been noted, but the significance of this finding is unknown.

Hemic and Lymphatic Systems: Anemia, thrombocytopenia, thrombocytopenic purpura, eosinophilia, leukopenia and agranulocytosis have been reported during therapy with the penicillins. These reactions are usually reversible on discontinuation of therapy and are believed to be hypersensitivity phenomena.

Dosage and Administration: **Infections of the ear, nose and throat** due to streptococci, pneumococci, nonpenicillinase-producing staphylococci and *H. influenzae*; **Infections of the genitourinary tract** due to *E. coli, P. mirabilis* and *S. faecalis*; **Infections of the skin and soft tissues** due to streptococci, susceptible staphylococci and *E. coli:*

USUAL DOSAGE:
Adults: 250 mg. every 8 hours
Children: 20 mg./kg./day in divided doses every 8 hours
Children weighing 20 kg. or more should be dosed according to the adult recommendations.

In severe infections or those caused by less susceptible organisms:
500 mg. every 8 hours for adults and 40 mg./kg./day in divided doses every 8 hours for children may be needed.

Infections of the lower respiratory tract due to streptococci, pneumococci, nonpenicillinase-producing staphylococci and *H. influenzae:*

USUAL DOSAGE:
Adults: 500 mg. every 8 hours
Children: 40 mg./kg./day in divided doses every 8 hours
Children weighing 20 kg. or more should be dosed according to the adult recommendations.

Gonorrhea, acute uncomplicated ano-genital and urethral infections due to *N. gonorrhoeae* (males and females):
3 grams as a single oral dose

Cases of gonorrhea with a suspected lesion of syphilis should have darkfield examinations before receiving amoxicillin, and monthly serological tests for a minimum of four months.

General: Larger doses may be required for stubborn or severe infections.

The children's dosage is intended for individuals whose weight will not cause a dosage to be calculated greater than that recommended for adults.

Continued on next page

Squibb—Cont.

It should be recognized that in the treatment of chronic urinary tract infections frequent bacteriological and clinical appraisals are necessary. Smaller doses than those recommended above should not be used. Even higher doses may be needed at times. In stubborn infections, therapy may be required for several weeks. It may be necessary to continue clinical and/or bacteriological follow-up for several months after cessation of therapy. Except for gonorrhea, treatment should be continued for a minimum of 48 to 72 hours beyond the time that the patient becomes asymptomatic or evidence of bacterial eradication has been obtained. It is recommended that there be at least 10 days' treatment for any infection caused by hemolytic streptococci to prevent the occurrence of acute rheumatic fever or glomerulonephritis.

Preparation and Storage of Oral Suspensions: Prepare the suspension at the time of dispensing. Follow the directions for constitution on the label of the package. Discard any unused suspension after 14 days. The suspension may be kept at room temperature; refrigeration is not required. **Shake well before using.**

How Supplied: Trimox (amoxicillin) is available for oral administration as *Trimox '250' Capsules and *Trimox '500' Capsules (Amoxicillin Capsules USP) which provide amoxicillin trihydrate equivalent to 250 mg. and 500 mg. amoxicillin, respectively. The 250 mg. capsules are available in bottles of 100 and 500 and in Unimatic® cartons of 100. The 500 mg. capsules are available in bottles of 50 and 500 and in Unimatic cartons of 100. Trimox is also available as Trimox '125' for Oral Suspension and Trimox '250' for Oral Suspension (Amoxicillin for Oral Suspension USP) which provide, after preparation, pleasantly flavored suspensions containing amoxicillin trihydrate equivalent to 125 mg. and 250 mg. amoxicillin, respectively, per 5 ml. teaspoonful. Available in bottles of 80, 100, and 150 ml. and Unimatic® cartons of 4 × 25 single-dose bottles, 5 ml. per bottle.

Storage: Store Trimox Capsules (Amoxicillin Capsules USP) and Trimox for Oral Suspension (Amoxicillin for Oral Suspension USP) at room temperature. Dispense the capsules in tight containers.

*[*Shown in Product Identification Section*]

VEETIDS® '250' TABLETS ℞
VEETIDS® '500' TABLETS ℞
(Penicillin V Potassium Tablets USP)
VEETIDS® '125' FOR ORAL SOLUTION ℞
VEETIDS® '250' FOR ORAL SOLUTION ℞
(Penicillin V Potassium for Oral Solution USP)

Description: Veetids (Penicillin V Potassium) is the potassium salt of semisynthetically-produced penicillin V. Veetids '125' for Oral Solution contains FD&C Yellow No. 5 (tartrazine).

Clinical Pharmacology: Penicillin V is bactericidal against penicillin-susceptible microorganisms during the stage of active multiplication. It acts by inhibiting biosynthesis of cell-wall mucopeptide. It is not active against the penicillinase-producing bacteria, which include many strains of staphylococci. Penicillin V is highly active *in vitro* against staphylococci (except penicillinase-producing strains), streptococci (groups A, C, G, H, L, and M) and pneumococci. Other organisms susceptible *in vitro* to penicillin V are *Corynebacterium diphtheriae, Bacillus anthracis,* Clostridia, *Actinomyces bovis, Streptobacillus moniliformis, Listeria monocytogenes,* Leptospira and *Neisseria gonorrhoeae; Treponema pallidum* is extremely susceptible.

Penicillin V is more resistant to inactivation by gastric acid than penicillin G; however, it has the same bacterial spectrum as penicillin G. It may be given with meals; however, blood levels are slightly higher when the drug is given on an empty stomach. Average blood levels are two to five times higher than the levels following the same dose of oral penicillin G and also show much less individual variation.

Once absorbed, penicillin V is about 75 percent bound to serum protein. Highest levels are found in the kidneys, with lesser amounts in the liver, skin, and intestines. Penicillin V penetrates into all other tissues to a lesser degree with a very small level found in the cerebrospinal fluid. The drug is excreted rapidly by tubular excretion in patients with normal kidney function. In neonates and young infants, and in individuals with impaired kidney function, excretion is considerably delayed.

Indications and Usage: Veetids (Penicillin V Potassium) are indicated in the treatment of mild to moderately severe infections due to penicillin-susceptible microorganisms. Therapy should be guided by bacteriological studies, including susceptibility tests, and by clinical response. Note: severe pneumonia, empyema, bacteremia, pericarditis, meningitis, and septic arthritis should not be treated with penicillin V during the acute stage.

Indicated surgical procedures should be performed.

The following infections will usually respond to adequate oral dosage:

Streptococcal infections Group A without bacteremia—Mild to moderate infections of the upper respiratory tract (including otitis media), scarlet fever, and mild erysipelas. Note: streptococci in groups A, C, G, H, L, and M are very susceptible to penicillin. Other groups including group D (enterococcus) are resistant.

Pneumococcal infections—Mild to moderately severe infections of the respiratory tract, including otitis media.

Staphylococcal infections — penicillin-susceptible—Mild infections of the skin and skin structures. Note: reports indicate an increasing number of strains of staphylococci resistant to penicillin, emphasizing the need for culture and susceptibility studies in treating suspected staphylococcal infections.

Vincent's gingivitis and pharyngitis (fusospirochetosis)—Mild to moderately severe infections of the oropharynx usually respond to oral penicillin. Note: necessary dental care should be accomplished in infections involving gum tissue.

Medical conditions in which oral penicillin therapy is indicated as prophylaxis: *For the prevention of recurrence following rheumatic fever and/or chorea.* Prophylaxis with oral penicillin on a continuing basis is effective in preventing recurrence of these conditions. *To prevent bacterial endocarditis.* Although no controlled clinical efficacy studies have been conducted penicillin V has been suggested by the American Heart Association and the American Dental Association for use as part of a parenteral-oral regimen and as an alternative oral regimen for prophylaxis against bacterial endocarditis in patients with congenital heart disease or rheumatic or other acquired valvular heart disease when they undergo dental procedures and surgical procedures of the respiratory tract.[1] Since it may happen that *alpha* hemolytic streptococci relatively resistant to penicillin may be found when patients are receiving continuous oral penicillin for secondary prevention of rheumatic fever, prophylactic agents other than penicillin may be chosen for these patients and prescribed in addition to their continuous rheumatic fever prophylactic regimen. Oral penicillin should not be used as adjunctive prophylaxis for genitourinary instrumentation or surgery, lower intestinal tract surgery, sigmoidoscopy, and childbirth.

NOTE: When selecting antibiotics for the prevention of bacterial endocarditis the physician or dentist should read the full joint statement of the American Heart Association and the American Dental Association.[1]

Contraindications: Contraindicated in patients with a history of hypersensitivity to any penicillin.

Warnings: Serious and occasional fatal hypersensitivity (anaphylactoid) reactions have been reported in patients on penicillin therapy. Although anaphylaxis is more frequent following parenteral administration, it has occurred in patients on oral penicillins. These reactions are more apt to occur in individuals with a history of sensitivity to multiple allergens.

There have been well-documented reports of individuals with a history of penicillin hypersensitivity who have experienced severe hypersensitivity reactions when treated with cephalosporins. Before therapy with a penicillin, careful inquiry should be made concerning previous hypersensitivity reactions to penicillins, cephalosporins, and other allergens. If an allergic reaction occurs, the drug should be discontinued and the patient treated with the usual agents, e.g., pressor amines, antihistamines, and corticosteroids. Serious anaphylactoid reactions are not controlled by antihistamines alone, and require such emergency measures as the immediate use of epinephrine, aminophylline, oxygen, and intravenous corticosteroids.

Concomitant use of oral neomycin therapy should be avoided since malabsorption of penicillin V potassium has been reported.

Precautions: Penicillin should be used with caution in individuals with histories of significant allergies and/or asthma.

The oral route of administration should not be relied upon in patients with severe illness, or with nausea, vomiting, gastric dilatation, cardiospasm or intestinal hypermotility.

Occasional patients will not absorb therapeutic amounts of orally administered penicillin.

In streptococcal infections, therapy must be sufficient to eliminate the organism (10 days minimum); otherwise the sequelae of streptococcal disease may occur. Cultures should be taken following completion of treatment to determine whether streptococci have been eradicated.

Prolonged use of antibiotics may promote the overgrowth of nonsusceptible organisms, including fungi. Should superinfection occur, appropriate measures should be taken.

In prolonged therapy with penicillin, and particularly with high dosage schedules, periodic evaluation of the renal and hematopoietic systems is recommended.

Veetids '125' for Oral Solution (Penicillin V Potassium Oral Solution USP) contains FD&C Yellow No. 5 (tartrazine) which may cause allergic-type reactions (including bronchial asthma) in certain susceptible individuals. Although the overall incidence of FD&C Yellow No. 5 (tartrazine) sensitivity in the general population is low, it is frequently seen in patients who also have aspirin hypersensitivity.

Adverse Reactions: Although the incidence of reactions to oral penicillins has been reported with much less frequency than following parenteral therapy, it should be remembered that all degrees of hypersensitivity, including fatal anaphylaxis, have been reported with oral penicillin.

The most common reactions to oral penicillin are nausea, vomiting, epigastric distress, diarrhea, and black hairy tongue. The hypersensitivity reactions reported are skin rashes ranging from maculopapular to exfoliative dermatitis; urticaria; serum sickness-like reactions including chills, fever, edema, arthralgia, and prostration; laryngeal edema; and anaphylaxis. Fever and eosinophilia may frequently be the only reactions observed. Hemolytic anemia, leukopenia, thrombocytopenia, neuropathy, and nephropathy are infrequent reactions usually associated with high doses of parenteral penicillin. Urticaria, other skin rashes, and serum sickness-like reactions may be controlled by antihistamines and, if necessary, corticosteroids. Whenever such reactions occur, penicillin should be discontinued unless, in the opinion of the physician, the condition being treated is life-threatening and amenable only to penicillin therapy. Serious anaphylactoid reactions require emergency measures (see WARNINGS).

An occasional patient may complain of sore mouth or tongue, as with any oral penicillin preparation.

Dosage and Administration: The dosage of Veetids (Penicillin V Potassium) should be determined according to the susceptibility of the causative microorganism and the severity of the infection, and adjusted to the clinical response of the patient.

For Therapeutic Use

Dosage for *children under 12 years* of age is calculated on the basis of body weight. For *infants and small children* the suggested dose is 15 to 56 mg. (25,000 to 90,000 u.) per kg./day in three to six divided doses.

The usual dosage recommendations for *adults and children 12 years and over* are as follows:

Streptococcal infections—mild to moderately severe—of the upper respiratory tract and including otitis media, scarlet fever and mild erysipelas: 125 mg. (200,000 u.) t.i.d. or q.i.d. for 10 days for mild infections; 250 mg. (400,000 u.) t.i.d. for 10 days for moderately severe infections; for mild to moderately severe streptococcal pharyngitis: 500 mg. (800,000 u.) b.i.d. may be used as an alternative regimen.

Pneumococcal infections—mild to moderately severe—of the respiratory tract, including otitis media: 250 to 500 mg. (400,000 to 800,000 u.) q.i.d. until the patient has been afebrile for at least two days.

Staphylococcal infections—mild infections of skin and skin structures (culture and susceptibility tests should be performed): 250 mg. (400,000 u.) t.i.d. or q.i.d., or 500 mg. (800,000 u.) t.i.d.

Vincent's gingivitis and pharyngitis (fusospirochetosis)—mild to moderately severe infections of the oropharynx: 250 mg. (400,000 u.) t.i.d. or q.i.d., or 500 mg. t.i.d.

For Prophylactic Use

For the prevention of recurrence following rheumatic fever and/or chorea: *Adults*—125 mg. (200,000 u.) b.i.d. on a continuing basis. Dosage for *children under 12 years* of age is calculated on the basis of body weight. For *infants and small children* the suggested dose is 15 to 56 mg. (25,000 to 90,000 u.) per kg./day in three to six divided doses.

To prevent bacterial endocarditis. For prophylaxis against bacterial endocarditis[1] in patients with congenital heart disease or rheumatic or other acquired valvular heart disease when undergoing dental procedures or surgical procedures of the upper respiratory tract, one of two regimens may be selected:

(1) For the oral regimen, give 2 g. of penicillin V (1 g. for children under 60 lb.) one-half to one hour before the procedure, and then 500 mg. (250 mg. for children under 60 lb.) every six hours for eight doses; or

(2) For the combined parenteral-oral regimen give 1,000,000 u. of aqueous crystalline penicillin G (30,000 u./kg. in children) intramuscularly mixed with 600,000 u. procaine penicillin G (600,000 u. for children) one-half to one hour before the procedure, and then oral penicillin V, 500 mg. for adults or 250 mg. for children less than 60 lb., every six hours for eight doses. Doses for children should not exceed recommendations for adults for a single dose or for a 24-hour period.

How Supplied: *Veetids '250' Tablets and *Veetids '500' Tablets (Penicillin V Potassium Tablets USP) are available for oral administration as FILMLOK® tablets providing penicillin V potassium equivalent to 250 mg. (400,000 units) and 500 mg. (800,000 units), respectively, of penicillin V. (Filmlok is a Squibb trademark for veneer-coated tablets.) Bottles of 100 and 1000, and Unimatic® cartons of 100.

Veetids '125' for Oral Solution and Veetids '250' for Oral Solution (Penicillin V Potassium for Oral Solution USP) are available as powders that, when constituted as directed, provide pleasantly flavored solutions containing penicillin V potassium equivalent to 125 mg. (200,000 units) and 250 mg. (400,000 units), respectively, of penicillin V per 5 ml. teaspoonful. Bottles of 100 ml. and 200 ml.

Storage: Store Veetids Tablets at room temperature; avoid excessive heat. Dispense in tight containers. Store Veetids for Oral Solution in dry form at room temperature; after preparation of the solution, store in refrigerator and discard unused portion after 14 days. Shake well before using. Keep tightly closed.

Reference: 1. American Heart Association. 1977. Prevention of bacterial endocarditis. Circulation 56:139A-143A.

*[*Shown in Product Identification Section*]

VELOSEF® '250' CAPSULES ℞
VELOSEF® '500' CAPSULES ℞
(Cephradine Capsules USP)
VELOSEF® TABLETS 1 GRAM ℞
(Cephradine Tablets)
VELOSEF® '125' FOR ORAL SUSPENSION ℞
VELOSEF® '250' FOR ORAL SUSPENSION ℞
(Cephradine for Oral Suspension USP)

Description: Velosef (Cephradine, Squibb) is a semisynthetic cephalosporin antibiotic; oral dosage forms include capsules containing 250 mg. and 500 mg. cephradine, tablets containing 1 g. cephradine, and cephradine for oral suspension containing, after constitution, 125 mg. and 250 mg. per 5 ml. dose. Cephradine is chemically designated as (6R,7R)-7-[(R)-2-amino-2-(1,4-cyclohexadien-1-yl) acetamido]-3-methyl-8-oxo-5-thia-1-azabicylo [4.2.0] oct-2-ene-2-carboxylic acid.

Clinical Pharmacology: Velosef (Cephradine, Squibb) is acid stable. It is rapidly absorbed after oral administration in the fasting state. Following single doses of 250 mg., 500 mg., and 1 g. in normal adult volunteers, average peak serum concentrations within one hour were approximately 9 mcg./ml., 16.5 mcg./ml., and 24.2 mcg./ml., respectively.

In vitro studies by an ultracentrifugation technique show that at therapeutic serum antibiotic concentrations, cephradine is minimally bound (8 to 17 percent) to normal serum protein. Cephradine does not pass across the blood-brain barrier to any appreciable extent. The presence of food in the gastrointestinal tract delays absorption but does not affect the total amount of cephradine absorbed. Over 90 percent of the drug is excreted unchanged in the urine within six hours. Peak urine concentrations are approximately 1600 mcg./ml., 3200 mcg./ml., and 4000 mcg./ml. following single doses of 250 mg., 500 mg., and 1 g., respectively.

Microbiology—*In vitro* tests demonstrate that the cephalosporins are bactericidal because of their inhibition of cell-wall synthesis. Cephradine is active against the following organisms *in vitro:*

- Group A beta-hemolytic streptococci
- Staphylococci, including coagulase-positive, coagulase-negative, and penicillinase-producing strains
- *Streptococcus pneumoniae* (formerly *Diplococcus pneumoniae*)
- *Escherichia coli*
- *Proteus mirabilis*
- *Klebsiella* species
- *Hemophilus influenzae*

Cephradine is not active against most strains of *Enterobacter* species, *P. morganii,* and *P. vulgaris.* It has no activity against *Pseudomonas* or *Herellea* species. When tested by *in vitro* methods, staphylococci exhibit cross-resistance between cephradine and methicillin-type antibiotics.

Note—Most strains of enterococci (*Streptococcus faecalis*) are resistant to cephradine.

Disc Susceptibility Tests—Quantitative methods that require measurement of zone diameters give the most precise estimates of antibiotic susceptibility. One recommended procedure (21 CFR Sec. 460.1) uses cephalosporin class discs for testing susceptibility; interpretations correlate zone diameters of this disc test with MIC values for cephradine. With this procedure, a report from the laboratory of "resistant" indicates that the infecting organism is not likely to respond to therapy. A report of "intermediate susceptibility" suggests that the organism would be susceptible if the infection is confined to the urinary tract, as high antibiotic levels can be obtained in the urine, or if high dosage is used in other types of infection.

Indications and Usage: Velosef Capsules (Cephradine Capsules USP), Velosef Tablets (Cephradine Tablets), and Velosef for Oral Suspension (Cephradine for Oral Suspension USP) are indicated in the treatment of the following infections when caused by susceptible strains of the designated microorganisms:

RESPIRATORY TRACT INFECTIONS (e.g., tonsillitis, pharyngitis, and lobar pneumonia) caused by group A beta-hemolytic streptococci and *S. pneumoniae* (formerly *D. pneumoniae*).

[Penicillin is the usual drug of choice in the treatment and prevention of streptococcal infections, including the prophylaxis of rheumatic fever. Velosef is generally effective in the eradication of streptococci from the nasopharynx; substantial data establishing the efficacy of Velosef (Cephradine, Squibb) in the subsequent prevention of rheumatic fever are not available at present.]

OTITIS MEDIA caused by group A beta-hemolytic streptococci, *S. pneumoniae* (formerly *D. pneumoniae*), *H. influenzae,* and staphylococci.

SKIN AND SKIN STRUCTURES INFECTIONS caused by staphylococci (penicillin-susceptible and penicillin-resistant) and beta-hemolytic streptococci.

URINARY TRACT INFECTIONS, including prostatitis, caused by *E. coli, P. mirabilis, Klebsiella* species, and enterococci (*S. faecalis*). The high concentrations of cephradine achievable in the urinary tract will be effective against many strains of enterococci for which disc susceptibility studies indicate relative resistance. It is to be noted that among beta-lactam antibiotics, ampicillin is the drug of choice for enterococcal urinary tract (*S. faecalis*) infection.

Note—Culture and susceptibility tests should be initiated prior to and during therapy.

Following clinical improvement achieved with parenteral therapy, oral cephradine may be utilized for continuation of treatment of persistent or severe conditions where prolonged therapy is indicated.

Contraindications: Cephradine is contraindicated in patients with known hypersensitivity to the cephalosporin group of antibiotics.

Warnings: *In penicillin-sensitive patients, cephalosporin derivatives should be used with great caution. There is clinical and laboratory evidence of partial cross-allergenicity of the penicillins and the cephalosporins, and there are instances of patients who have had reactions to both drug classes (including anaphylaxis after parenteral use).*

Any patient who has demonstrated some form of allergy, particularly to drugs, should receive antibiotics, including cephradine, cautiously and then only when absolutely necessary.

Continued on next page

Squibb—Cont.

Pseudomembranous colitis has been reported with the use of cephalosporins (and other broad spectrum antibiotics); therefore, it is important to consider its diagnosis in patients who develop diarrhea in association with antibiotic use. Treatment with broad spectrum antibiotics alters normal flora of the colon and may permit overgrowth of clostridia. Studies indicate a toxin produced by *Clostridium difficile* is one primary cause of antibiotic-associated colitis. Cholestyramine and colestipol resins have been shown to bind the toxin *in vitro.* Mild cases of colitis may respond to drug discontinuance alone. Moderate to severe cases should be managed with fluid, electrolyte and protein supplementation as indicated. When the colitis is not relieved by drug discontinuance or when it is severe, oral vancomycin is the treatment of choice for antibiotic-associated pseudomembranous colitis produced by *C. difficile.* Other causes of colitis should also be considered.

Precautions: General—Patients should be followed carefully so that any side effects or unusual manifestations of drug idiosyncrasy may be detected. If a hypersensitivity reaction occurs, the drug should be discontinued and the patient treated with the usual agents, e.g., pressor amines, antihistamines, or corticosteroids.

Administer cephradine with caution in the presence of markedly impaired renal function. In patients with known or suspected renal impairment, careful clinical observation and appropriate laboratory studies should be made prior to and during therapy as cephradine accumulates in the serum and tissues. See DOSAGE AND ADMINISTRATION section for information on treatment of patients with impaired renal function.

Cephradine should be prescribed with caution in individuals with a history of gastrointestinal disease, particularly colitis.

Prolonged use of antibiotics may promote the overgrowth of nonsusceptible organisms. Should superinfection occur during therapy, appropriate measures should be taken.

Indicated surgical procedures should be performed in conjunction with antibiotic therapy.

Information for Patients: Caution diabetic patients that false results may occur with urine glucose tests (see PRECAUTIONS, Drug/Laboratory Test Interactions).

Advise the patient to comply with the full course of therapy even if he begins to feel better and to take a missed dose as soon as possible. Inform the patient that this medication may be taken with food or milk since gastrointestinal upset may be a factor in compliance with the dosage regimen. The patient should report current use of any medicines and should be cautioned not to take other medications unless the physician knows and approves of their use (see PRECAUTIONS, Drug Interactions).

Laboratory Tests: In patients with known or suspected renal impairment, it is advisable to monitor renal function (see DOSAGE AND ADMINISTRATION).

Drug Interactions: When administered concurrently, the following drugs may interact with cephalosporins:

Other antibacterial agents—Bacteriostats may interfere with the bactericidal action of cephalosporins in acute infection; other agents, e.g., aminoglycosides, colistin, polymyxins, vancomycin, may increase the possibility of nephrotoxicity.

Diuretics (potent "loop diuretics," e.g., furosemide and ethacrynic acid)—Enhanced possibility for renal toxicity.

Probenecid—Increased and prolonged blood levels of cephalosporins, resulting in increased risk of nephrotoxicity.

Drug/Laboratory Test Interactions: After treatment with cephradine, a false-positive reaction for glucose in the urine may occur with Benedict's solution, Fehling's solution, or with Clinitest® tablets, but not with enzyme-based tests such as Clinistix® and Tes-Tape®. False-positive Coombs test results may occur in newborns whose mothers received a cephalosporin prior to delivery.

Cephalosporins have been reported to cause false-positive reactions in tests for urinary proteins which use sulfosalicylic acid, false elevations of urinary 17-ketosteroid values, and prolonged prothrombin times.

Carcinogenesis, Mutagenesis: Long-term studies in animals have not been performed to evaluate carcinogenic potential or mutagenesis.

Pregnancy: Teratogenic Effects/Impairment of Fertility—Category B: Reproduction studies have been peformed in mice and rats at doses up to four times the maximum indicated human dose and have revealed no evidence of impaired fertility or harm to the fetus due to cephradine. There are, however, no adequate and well-controlled studies in pregnant women. Because animal reproduction studies are not always predictive of human response, this drug should be used during pregnancy only if clearly needed.

Nursing Mothers: Since cephradine is excreted in breast milk during lactation, caution should be exercised when cephradine is administered to a nursing woman.

Pediatric Use: See DOSAGE AND ADMINISTRATION. Adequate information is unavailable on the efficacy of b.i.d. regimens in children under nine months of age.

Adverse Reactions: As with other cephalosporins, untoward reactions are limited essentially to gastrointestinal disturbances and, on occasion, to hypersensitivity phenomena. The latter are more likely to occur in individuals who have previously demonstrated hypersensitivity and those with a history of allergy, asthma, hay fever, or urticaria.

The following adverse reactions have been reported following the use of cephradine:

Gastrointestinal: Symptoms of pseudomembranous colitis can appear during treatment. Nausea and vomiting have been reported rarely.

Skin and Hypersensitivity Reactions: Mild urticaria or skin rash, pruritus, and joint pains were reported by very few patients.

Blood: Mild, transient eosinophilia, leukopenia, and neutropenia have been reported.

Liver: Transient mild rise of SGOT, SGPT, and total bilirubin have been observed with no evidence of hepatocellular damage.

Renal: Transitory rises in BUN have been observed in some patients treated with cephalosporins; their frequency increases in patients over 50 years old. In adults for whom serum creatinine determinations were performed, the rise in BUN was not accompanied by a rise in serum creatinine.

Other adverse reactions have included dizziness and tightness in the chest and candidal vaginitis.

Dosage and Administration: Velosef (Cephradine, Squibb) may be given without regard to meals.

Adults: *For respiratory tract infections (other than lobar pneumonia) and skin and skin structures infections,* the usual dose is 250 mg. every 6 hours or 500 mg. every 12 hours.

For lobar pneumonia, the usual dose is 500 mg. every 6 hours or 1 g. every 12 hours.

For uncomplicated urinary tract infections, the usual dose is 500 mg. every 12 hours. In more serious urinary tract infections, including prostatitis, 500 mg. every 6 hours or 1 g. every 12 hours may be administered.

Larger doses (up to 1 g. every 6 hours) may be given for severe or chronic infections.

Children: No adequate information is available on the efficacy of b.i.d. regimens in children under nine months of age. The usual dose in children over nine months of age is 25 to 50 mg./kg./day administered in equally divided doses every 6 or 12 hours. For otitis media due to *H. influenzae,* doses are from 75 to 100 mg./kg./day administered in equally divided doses every 6 or 12 hours, but should not exceed 4 g. per day. Dosage for children should not exceed dosage recommended for adults.

All patients, regardless of age and weight: Larger doses (up to 1 gram q.i.d.) may be given for severe or chronic infections.

As with antibiotic therapy in general, treatment should be continued for a minimum of 48 to 72 hours after the patient becomes asymptomatic or evidence of bacterial eradication has been obtained. In infections caused by group A beta-hemolytic streptococci, a minimum of 10 days of treatment is recommended to guard against the risk of rheumatic fever or glomerulonephritis. In the treatment of chronic urinary tract infection, frequent bacteriologic and clinical appraisal is necessary during therapy and may be necessary for several months afterwards. Persistent infections may require treatment for several weeks. Prolonged intensive therapy is recommended for prostatitis. Doses smaller than those indicated are not recommended.

Patients With Impaired Renal Function

A modified dosage schedule in patients with decreased renal function is necessary. Each patient should be considered individually; the following reduced dosage schedule is recommended as a guideline, based on the creatinine clearance (ml./min./1.73 m^2). In adults, the initial loading dose is 750 mg. of Velosef (Cephradine, Squibb) and the maintenance dose is 500 mg. at the time intervals listed below:

Creatinine Clearance	Time Interval
> 20 ml./min.	6–12 hours
15–19 ml./min.	12–24 hours
10–14 ml./min.	24–40 hours
5–9 ml./min.	40–50 hours
< 5 ml./min.	50–70 hours

Further modification of the dosage schedule may be necessary in children.

How Supplied: Velosef is available as *Velosef '250' Capsules and *Velosef '500' Capsules (Cephradine Capsules USP) providing 250 mg. and 500 mg. cephradine per capsule, respectively, and as *Velosef Tablets (Cephradine Tablets) providing 1 g. cephradine per tablet. The Capsules are available in bottles of 24 and 100 and Unimatic® cartons of 100. The Tablets are available in bottles of 24.

Velosef is also available as Velosef '125' for Oral Suspension and Velosef '250' for Oral Suspension (Cephradine for Oral Suspension USP) which, after constitution, provide 125 mg. and 250 mg. cephradine, respectively, per 5 ml. teaspoonful in a pleasant fruit-flavored suspension. Bottles of 100 ml. and 200 ml.

Storage: Velosef Capsules—Do not store above 86°F.; keep bottle tightly closed. Velosef Tablets—Do not store above 86°F.; keep bottle tightly closed. Dispense in tight containers. Velosef for Oral Suspension— Prior to constitution, store at room temperature; avoid excessive heat. After constitution, the suspension may be stored at room temperature or in refrigerator; when the suspension is stored at room temperature, discard unused portion after 7 days; when the suspension is stored in the refrigerator, discard unused portion after 14 days.

*[*Shown in Product Identification Section*]

VELOSEF® for INFUSION ℞

(Sterile Cephradine USP)
Sodium-Free

Description: Velosef (Cephradine, Squibb) is a semisynthetic cephalosporin antibiotic. Cephradine is designated chemically as

(6R,7R)-7- [(R)-2-amino-2-(1, 4-cyclochexadien-1-yl) acetamido]-3-methyl-8-oxo-5-thia-1- azabicyclo [4.2.0] oct-2-ene-2- carboxylic acid.

Velosef for Infusion is sterile cephradine, a white powder for constitution and intravenous administration by drip infusion; it is available in infusion bottles containing 2 g. cephradine. At the time of manufacture, the air in the container is replaced by nitrogen.

Clinical Pharmacology: Pharmacokinetic studies with Velosef for Injection (Cephradine for Injection USP) (containing sodium carbonate) and Velosef for Infusion (Sterile Cephradine USP) (sodium-free) performed by drip infusion demonstrate bioequivalence for these formulations. The mean steady-state concentration of cephradine maintained in the sera of nine normal adult volunteers during infusion of either solution was approximately 3 mcg. per ml. for each mg. of cephradine infused per hour per kg. of body weight. Serum half-life, serum clearance, and apparent volume of distribution were equivalent following intravenous infusion of either preparation.

Figure 1 depicts mean serum concentrations after administration of Velosef for Infusion (Sterile Cephradine USP) to nine normal adult volunteers at the average rate of 380 mg. cephradine per hour (5.3 mg./kg./hr.) over a four-hour period; the mean cephradine level rises rapidly and approaches a mean steady-state concentration of 17 mcg./ml. in approximately 1.5 hours. After the infusion is discontinued, the cephradine concentration decreases exponentially, declining to 1.5 mcg./ml. at 6.5 hours.

Figure 1

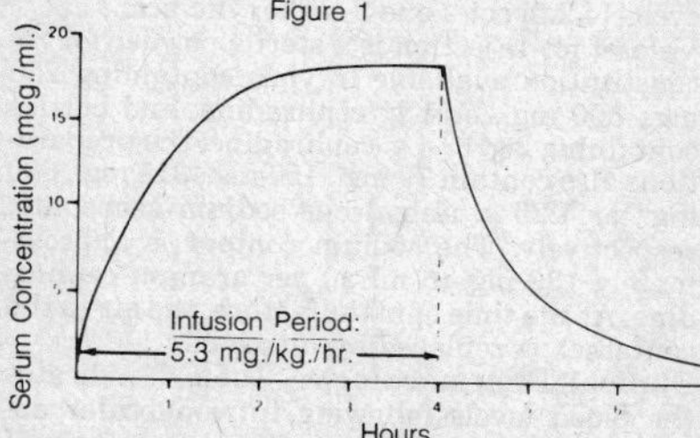

Cephradine is excreted unchanged in the urine. Between 1.5 and 4 hours after the start of the infusion depicted in Figure 1, cephradine is excreted in urine at a mean rate of 312 mg./hr.; a high concentration of cephradine in the urine exists during this period with a mean concentration of 885 mcg./ml. Studies with Velosef for Injection (Cephradine for Injection USP) demonstrate that probenecid slows tubular excretion of cephradine and increases serum concentration.

In vitro studies by an ultracentrifugation technique show that at therapeutic serum antibiotic concentrations, cephradine is minimally bound (8 to 17 percent) to normal human serum protein. Cephradine does not pass across the blood-brain barrier to any appreciable extent.

Assays of bone obtained at surgery have shown that cephradine penetrates bone tissue.

Microbiology: In vitro tests demonstrate that the cephalosporins are bactericidal because of their inhibition of cell-wall synthesis. Cephradine is active against the following organisms *in vitro:* group A beta-hemolytic streptococci; staphylococci, including coagulase-positive, coagulase-negative, and penicillinase-producing strains; *Escherichia coli; Streptococcus pneumoniae* (formerly *Diplococcus pneumoniae*); *Proteus mirabilis; Klebsiella* species; and *Hemophilus influenzae.*

It is not active against most strains of *Enterobacter* species, *Proteus morganii,* and *Proteus vulgaris.* It has no activity against *Pseudomonas* or *Herellea* species. When tested by *in vitro* methods, staphylococci exhibit cross-resistance between cephradine and methicillin-type antibiotics.

NOTE—Most strains of enterococci (*Streptococcus faecalis*) are resistant to cephradine.

Disc Susceptibility Tests: Quantitative methods that require measurement of zone diameters give the most precise estimates of antibiotic susceptibility. One recommended procedure (21 CFR Sec. 460.1) uses cephalosporin class discs for testing susceptibility; interpretations correlate zone diameters of this disc test with MIC values for cephradine. With this procedure, a report from the laboratory of "resistant" indicates that the infecting organism is not likely to respond to therapy. A report of "intermediate susceptibility" suggests that the organism would be susceptible if the infection is confined to the urinary tract, as high antibiotic levels can be obtained in the urine, or if high dosage is used in other types of infection.

Indications and Usage: Velosef for Infusion (Sterile Cephradine USP) is indicated in the treatment of the following serious infections when caused by susceptible strains of the designated microorganisms:

RESPIRATORY TRACT INFECTIONS due to *Streptococcus pneumoniae* (formerly *Diplococcus pneumoniae*), *Klebsiella* species, *H. influenzae, Staphylococcus aureus* (penicillin-susceptible and penicillin-resistant), and group A beta-hemolytic streptococci.

[Penicillin is the usual drug of choice in the treatment and prevention of streptococcal infections, including the prophylaxis of rheumatic fever. Velosef (Cephradine, Squibb) is generally effective in the eradication of streptococci from the nasopharynx; substantial data establishing the efficacy of Velosef in the subsequent prevention of rheumatic fever are not available at present.]

URINARY TRACT INFECTIONS due to *E. coli, P. mirabilis,* and *Klebsiella* species.

SKIN AND SKIN STRUCTURES INFECTIONS due to *S. aureus* (penicillin-susceptible and penicillin-resistant) and group A beta-hemolytic streptococci.

BONE INFECTIONS due to *S. aureus* (penicillin-susceptible and penicillin-resistant).

SEPTICEMIA due to *Streptococcus pneumoniae* (formerly *Diplococcus pneumoniae*), *S. aureus* (penicillin-susceptible and penicillin-resistant), *P. mirabilis,* and *E. coli.*

NOTE—Culture and susceptibility tests should be initiated prior to and during therapy.

Contraindications: Cephradine is contraindicated in patients with known hypersensitivity to the cephalosporin group of antibiotics.

Warnings: *In penicillin-sensitive patients, cephalosporin derivatives should be used with great caution. There is clinical and laboratory evidence of partial cross-allergenicity of the penicillins and the cephalosporins, and there are instances of patients who have had reactions to both drug classes (including anaphylaxis after parenteral use).*

Any patient who has demonstrated some form of allergy, particularly to drugs, should receive antibiotics, including cephradine, cautiously and then only when absolutely necessary. Serious anaphylactoid reactions require immediate emergency treatment with epinephrine. Oxygen, intravenous steroids, and airway management, including intubation, should also be administered as indicated.

Pseudomembranous colitis has been reported with the use of cephalosporins (and other broad spectrum antibiotics); therefore, it is important to consider its diagnosis in patients who develop diarrhea in association with antibiotic use. Treatment with broad spectrum antibiotics alters normal flora of the colon and may permit overgrowth of clostridia. Studies indicate a toxin produced by *Clostridium difficile* is one primary cause of antibiotic-associated colitis. Cholestyramine and colestipol resins have been shown to bind the toxin *in vitro.* Mild cases of colitis may respond to drug discontinuance alone. Moderate to severe cases should be managed with fluid, electrolyte and protein supplementation as indicated. When the colitis is not relieved by drug discontinuance or when it is severe, oral vancomycin is the treatment of choice for antibiotic-associated pseudomembranous colitis produced by *C. difficile.* Other causes of colitis should also be considered.

Precautions: General—Prolonged use of antibiotics may promote the overgrowth of nonsusceptible organisms. Should superinfection occur during therapy, appropriate measures should be taken.

When cephradine is administered to patients with markedly impaired renal function, lower daily dosage is required. (See DOSAGE AND ADMINISTRATION.) In patients with known or suspected renal impairment, careful clinical observation and appropriate laboratory studies should be conducted because cephradine in the usual recommended dosage will accumulate in the serum and tissues.

Cephradine should be prescribed with caution in individuals with a history of gastrointestinal disease, particularly colitis.

Patients should be followed carefully so that any side effects or unusual manifestations of drug idiosyncrasy may be detected. If a hypersensitivity reaction occurs, the drug should be discontinued and the patient treated with the usual agents, e.g., pressor amines, antihistamines, or corticosteroids.

To reduce the risk of phlebitis from intravenous infusion, the injection site should be changed at appropriate intervals during long-term therapy.

Information for Patients: Caution diabetic patients that false test results may occur with urine glucose tests (see PRECAUTIONS, Drug/Laboratory Test Interactions). The patient should report current use of any medicines and should be cautioned not to take other medications unless the physician knows and approves of their use (see PRECAUTIONS, Drug Interactions).

Laboratory Tests: In patients with known or suspected renal impairment, it is advisable to monitor renal function (see DOSAGE AND ADMINISTRATION).

Drug Interactions: When administered concurrently, the following drugs may interact with cephalosporins:

Other antibacterial agents—Bacteriostats may interfere with the bactericidal action of cephalosporins in acute infection; other agents, e.g., aminoglycosides, colistin, polymyxins, vancomycin, may increase the possibility of nephrotoxicity.

Diuretics (potent "loop diuretics," e.g., furosemide and ethacrynic acid)—Enhanced possibility for renal toxicity.

Probenecid—Increased and prolonged blood levels of cephalosporins, resulting in increased risk of nephrotoxicity.

Drug/Laboratory Test Interactions: After treatment with cephradine, a false-positive reaction for glucose in the urine may occur with Benedict's solution, Fehling's solution, or with Clinitest® tablets, but not with enzyme-based tests such as Clinistix® and Tes-Tape®. False-positive Coombs test results may occur in newborns whose mothers received a cephalosporin prior to delivery.

Cephalosporins have been reported to cause false-positive reactions in tests for urinary proteins which use sulfosalicylic acid, false elevations of urinary 17-ketosteroid values, and prolonged prothrombin times.

Carcinogenesis, Mutagenesis: Long-term studies in animals have not been performed to evaluate carcinogenic potential or mutagenesis.

Pregnancy: Teratogenic Effect/Impairment of Fertility: Category B: Reproduction studies have been performed in mice and rats at doses up to four times the maximum indicated human dose and have revealed no evidence of

Continued on next page

Squibb—Cont.

impaired fertility or harm to the fetus due to cephradine. There are, however, no adequate and well-controlled studies in pregnant women. Because animal reproduction studies are not always predictive of human response, this drug should be used during pregancy only if clearly needed.

Nursing Mothers: Since cephradine is excreted in breast milk during lactation, caution should be exercised when cephradine is administered to a nursing woman.

Pediatric Use: See DOSAGE AND ADMINISTRATION. Cephradine has been effectively used in infants, but all laboratory parameters have not been extensively studied in infants one month to one year of age; therefore, in the treatment of children in this age group, the benefits of the drug to the risk involved must be considered.

Since safety for use in premature infants and in infants under one month of age has not been established, the use of cephradine by injection or infusion should be based on careful consideration of the benefits of the drug against the risk involved.

Adverse Reactions: As with other cephalosporins, untoward reactions are limited essentially to gastrointestinal disturbances and, on occasion, to hypersensitivity phenomena. The latter are more likely to occur in individuals who have previously demonstrated hypersensitivity and those with a history of allergy, asthma, hay fever, or urticaria.

The following adverse reactions have been reported following the use of cephradine:

Gastrointestinal: Symptoms of pseudomembranous colitis can appear during antibiotic treatment. Nausea and vomiting have been reported rarely.

Skin and Hypersensitivity Reactions: Mild urticaria or skin rash, edema, erythema, pruritus, joint pains, and drug fever.

Blood: Mild, transient eosinophilia, leukopenia, and neutropenia.

Liver: Instances of elevated SGOT and SGPT of approximately 10 percent and 2 percent of patients, respectively, have been observed; also, a few cases of elevated total bilirubin, alkaline phosphatase and LDH have been observed. In most patients, values tended to return to normal after the end of therapy.

Renal: Mild elevations in BUN have been observed in some patients treated with cephalosporins; their frequency increases in patients over 50 years old and in children under three. In adults for whom serum creatinine determinations were performed, the rise in BUN was not accompanied by a rise in serum creatinine.

Other adverse reactions are headache, dizziness, dyspnea, paresthesia, candidal overgrowth, candidal vaginitis, isolated instances of hepatomegaly, and thrombophlebitis at the site of injection.

Dosage and Administration: Velosef for Infusion (Sterile Cephradine USP) may be administered by continuous or intermittent intravenous infusion. The infusion bottle is designed to be suspended from an I.V. stand and may also be used in any administration procedure where sequential administration of infusion solutions is intended.

Adults: The usual daily dosage of Velosef for Infusion is 2 to 4 g. of cephradine given in equally divided doses four times a day (e.g., 500 mg. to 1 g. q.i.d.). In bone infections the usual dosage is 1 g. q.i.d. A daily dose of 2 g. is adequate in uncomplicated pneumonia, skin and skin structures infections, and most urinary tract infections. In severe infections, the dosage may be increased.

The maximum daily dose should not exceed 8 g. per day.

Infants and Children: The usual dosage range of Velosef for Infusion is 50 to 100 mg./kg./day (approximately 23 to 45 mg./lb./day) in equally divided doses four times a day and should be determined by age, weight of the patient, and severity of the infection being treated.

All laboratory parameters have not been extensively studied in infants under one year of age; therefore, in the treatment of children in this age group, the benefits of the drug to the risk involved must be considered. In newborn infants, accumulation of other cephalosporin-class antibiotics (with resultant prolongation of drug half-life) has been reported.

The maximum daily pediatric dose should not exceed doses recommended for adults.

PEDIATRIC DOSAGE GUIDE

Weight lbs	Weight kg	50 mg/kg/day Approx. dose mg qid	100 mg/kg/day Approx. dose mg qid
10	4.5	56 mg	112 mg
20	9.1	114 mg	227 mg
30	13.6	170 mg	340 mg
40	18.2	227 mg	455 mg
50	22.7	284 mg	567 mg

As with antibiotic therapy generally: therapy should be continued for a minimum of 48 to 72 hours after the patient becomes asymptomatic or evidence of bacterial eradication has been obtained; in infections caused by group A beta-hemolytic streptococci, a minimum of 10 days of treatment is recommended to guard against the risk of rheumatic fever or glomerulonephritis; in the treatment of chronic urinary tract infection, frequent bacteriologic and clinical appraisal is necessary during therapy and may be necessary for several months afterwards; persistent infections may require treatment for several weeks; doses smaller than those indicated above should not be used.

Parenteral therapy may be followed by oral Velosef (Cephradine, Squibb) either as capsules or as an oral suspension.

Velosef for Infusion (Sterile Cephradine USP) should be administered only by intravenous infusion.

Renal Impairment Dosage: A modified dosage schedule in patients with decreased renal function is necessary. Each patient should be considered individually; the following reduced dosage schedule is recommended as a guideline, based on the creatinine clearance (ml./min./1.73m^2).

In adults, the initial loading dose is 750 mg. of Velosef and the maintenance dose is 500 mg. at the time intervals listed below:

Creatinine Clearance	Time Interval
>20 ml./min.	6 - 12 hours
15 - 19 ml./min.	12 - 24 hours
10 - 14 ml./min.	24 - 40 hours
5 - 9 ml./min.	40 - 50 hours
< 5 ml./min.	50 - 70 hours

Further modification of the dosage schedule may be necessary in children.

Constitution and Storage: The choice of I.V. solution and the volume to be employed are dictated by fluid and electrolyte management. Suitable I.V. solutions are: 5% Dextrose Injection USP, Lactated Ringer's Injection USP, 10% Dextrose Injection USP, Dextrose and Sodium Chloride Injection USP (5% : 0.9% or 5% : 0.45%), 10% Invert Sugar in Water for Injection, Normosol®-R, Ionosol® B with Dextrose 5%, Sodium Chloride Injection USP, or Sodium Lactate Injection USP (M/6 sodium lactate). **Do not use Sterile Water for Injection.** Aseptically add 150 ml. or 200 ml. of the I.V. solution to the infusion bottle for approximate concentrations of 13.3 mg./ml. or 10 mg./ml., respectively. *Note: Complete solution of the preparation requires a minimum of 150 ml. of diluent. Shake well until dissolved.*

Infusion solutions prepared as directed above retain potency for 48 hours at room temperature, or one week under refrigeration (5° C.). Unused solutions must be discarded after these time periods. Constituted solutions may vary in color from nearly colorless to light yellow.

Parenteral drug products should be inspected visually for particulate matter and discoloration prior to administration, whenever solution and container permit.

Store Velosef for Infusion (Sterile Cephradine USP) at room temperature in dry form; avoid excessive heat. Protect the dry form and constituted solutions from concentrated light or direct sunlight.

Extemporaneous mixtures with other antibiotics or drugs are not recommended.

How Supplied: Velosef for Infusion (Sterile Cephradine USP) is available in intravenous infusion bottles (200 ml. size) containing 2 g. cephradine.

VELOSEF® for INJECTION ℞
(Cephradine for Injection USP)

Description: Velosef (Cephradine, Squibb) is a semisynthetic cephalosporin antibiotic. Cephradine is designated chemically as (6R, 7R)-7-[(R)-2-amino-2-(1, 4-cyclohexadien-1-yl) acetamido]-3-methyl-8-oxo-5- thia-1-azabicyclo- [4.2.0] oct-2-ene-2-carboxylic acid.

Velosef for Injection is a sterile powder for reconstitution available in vials containing 250 mg., 500 mg., or 1 g. cephradine; and bottles containing 2 g. or 4 g. cephradine; the preparations also contain 79 mg., 157 mg., 315 mg., 630 mg., or 1.26 g. anhydrous sodium carbonate, respectively. The sodium content is approximately 136 mg. (6 mEq.) per gram of cephradine. At the time of manufacture, the air in the container is replaced by nitrogen.

Clinical Pharmacology: Table I indicates the blood levels following intramuscular administration of a 500 mg. or 1 g. dose to normal adults.

[See table on next page].

Figure I depicts representative mean serum concentrations after administration of a 500 mg. and 1 g. I.M. dose, and a 500 mg. oral dose of cephradine. Areas beneath the curves for the 500 mg. oral and I.M. dose are equivalent.

Figure I
VELOSEF FOR INJECTION
(Cephradine for Injection USP)

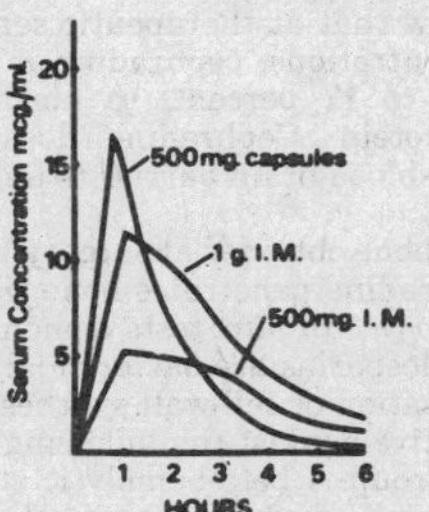

A single intravenous dose of 1 g. cephradine resulted in serum levels of approximately 86 mcg./ml. at 5 minutes, 50 mcg./ml. at 15 minutes, 26 mcg./ml. at 30 minutes, and 12 mcg./ml. at 60 minutes; these levels declined to 1 mcg./ml. at four hours.

In vitro studies by an ultracentrifugation technique show that, at therapeutic serum antibiotic concentrations, cephradine is minimally bound (8 to 17 percent) to normal human serum protein. Cephradine does not pass

across the blood-brain barrier to any appreciable extent.
Velosef (Cephradine, Squibb) is excreted unchanged in the urine. The kidneys excrete 57 to 80 percent of an intramuscular dose in the first six hours; this results in a high urine concentration, e.g., a mean urine concentration of 313 mcg./ml. within a six hour period following a 500 mg. I.M. dose. Probenecid slows tubular excretion and increases serum concentration. Assays of bone and cardiac tissue (atrial appendage) obtained at surgery have shown that cephradine penetrates these tissues.

Microbiology—In vitro tests demonstrate that the cephalosporins are bactericidal because of their inhibition of cell-wall synthesis. Cephradine is active against the following organisms *in vitro:* group A beta-hemolytic streptococci; staphylococci, including coagulase-positive, coagulase-negative, and penicillinase-producing strains; *Escherichia coli; Streptococcus pneumoniae* (formerly *Diplococcus pneumoniae); Proteus mirabilis; Klebsiella* species; and *Hemophilus influenzae.*

It is not active against most strains of Enterobacter species, *Proteus morganii,* and *Proteus vulgaris.* It has no activity against *Pseudomonas* or *Herellea* species. When tested by *in vitro* methods, staphylococci exhibit cross-resistance between cephradine and methicillin-type antibiotics.

NOTE—Most strains of enterococci (*Streptococcus faecalis*) are resistant to cephradine.

Disc Susceptibility Tests—Quantitative methods that require measurement of zone diameters give the most precise estimates of antibiotic susceptibility. One recommended procedure (21 CFR § 460.1) uses cephalosporin class discs for testing susceptibility; interpretations correlate zone diameters of this disc test with MIC values for cephradine. With this procedure, a report from the laboratory of "resistant" indicates that the infecting organism is not likely to respond to therapy. A report of "intermediate susceptibility" suggests that the organism would be susceptible if the infection is confined to the urinary tract, as high antibiotic levels can be obtained in the urine, or if high dosage is used in other types of infection.

Indications and Usage:Treatment—Velosef for Injection (Cephradine for Injection USP) is indicated in the treatment of the following serious infections when caused by susceptible strains of the designated microorganisms:

RESPIRATORY TRACT INFECTIONS due to *Streptococcus pneumoniae* (formerly *Diplococcus pneumoniae*), *Klebsiella* species, *H. influenzae, Staphylococcus aureus* (penicillin-susceptible and penicillin-resistant), and group A beta-hemolytic streptococci.

[Penicillin is the usual drug of choice in the treatment and prevention of streptococcal infections, including the prophylaxis of rheumatic fever. Velosef is generally effective in the eradication of streptococci from the nasopharynx; substantial data establishing the efficacy of Velosef in the subsequent prevention of rheumatic fever are not available at present.]

URINARY TRACT INFECTIONS due to *E. coli, P. mirabilis,* and *Klebsiella* species.

SKIN AND SKIN STRUCTURES INFECTIONS due to *S. aureus* (penicillin-susceptible and penicillin-resistant) and group A beta-hemolytic streptococci.

BONE INFECTIONS due to *S. aureus* (penicillin-susceptible and penicillin-resistant).

SEPTICEMIA due to *Streptococcus pneumoniae* (formerly *Diplococcus pneumoniae*), *S. aureus* (penicillin-susceptible and penicillin-resistant), *P. mirabilis,* and *E. coli.*

NOTE—Culture and susceptibility tests should be initiated prior to and during therapy.

Prevention: When compared to placebo in randomized controlled studies in patients undergoing vaginal hysterectomy and cesarean section, the prophylactic use of VELOSEF (cephradine) resulted in a significant reduction in the number of postoperative infections.

TABLE I
VELOSEF FOR INJECTION
(Cephradine for Injection USP)

	MEAN TIME TO PEAK SERUM LEVELS Minutes		MEAN PEAK SERUM CONCENTRATION mcg./ml.		MEAN SERUM CONCENTRATION AT 1 HR. - mcg./ml.	
	500 mg. I.M.	1 g. I.M.	500 mg. I.M.	1 g. I.M.	500 mg. I.M.	1 g. I.M.
MALES	49 (41–59)*	52 (45–61)	6.3 (5.5–7.2)	13.6 (12.2–15.1)	6.2 (5.5–6.9)	12.4 (11.0–14.0)
FEMALES	98 (87–111)	128 (103–157)	5.8 (5.1–6.6)	9.9 (8.7–11.2)	4.3 (3.5–5.2)	6.0 (4.4–8.1)

*Figures in parentheses are 95% confidence limits.

The prophylactic administration of VELOSEF perioperatively (preoperatively, intraoperatively, and postoperatively) may reduce the incidence of certain postoperative infections in patients undergoing surgical procedures (e.g., vaginal hysterectomy) that are classified as contaminated or potentially contaminated.

In patients undergoing cesarean section, intraoperative (after clamping the umbilical cord) and postoperative use of VELOSEF may reduce the incidence of certain postoperative infections.

Effective perioperative use depends on the time of administration. VELOSEF (Cephradine, Squibb) usually should be given 30 to 90 minutes before surgery, which is sufficient time to achieve effective tissue levels. Prophylactic administration should usually be stopped within 24 hours since continuing administration of any antibiotic increases the possibility of adverse reactions but, in the majority of surgical procedures, does not reduce the incidence of subsequent infection.

If there are signs of infection, specimens for culture should be obtained for identification of the causative organism so that appropriate therapy may be instituted.

Contraindications: Cephradine is contraindicated in patients with known hypersensitivity to the cephalosporin group of antibiotics.

Warnings: *In penicillin-sensitive patients, cephalosporin derivatives should be used with great caution. There is clinical and laboratory evidence of partial cross-allergenicity of the penicillins and the cephalosporins, and there are instances of patients who have had reactions to both drug classes (including fatal anaphylaxis after parenteral use).*

Any patient who has demonstrated some form of allergy, particularly to drugs, should receive antibiotics, including cephradine, cautiously and then only when absolutely necessary. Serious anaphylactoid reactions require immediate emergency treatment with epinephrine. Oxygen, intravenous steroids, and airway management, including intubation, should also be administered as indicated.

Pseudomembranous colitis has been reported with the use of cephalosporins (and other broad spectrum antibiotics); therefore, it is important to consider its diagnosis in patients who develop diarrhea in association with antibiotic use. Treatment with broad spectrum antibiotics alters normal flora of the colon and may permit overgrowth of clostridia. Studies indicate a toxin produced by *Clostridium difficile* is one primary cause of antibiotic-associated colitis. Cholestryamine and colestipol resins have been shown to bind the toxin *in vitro.* Mild cases of colitis may respond to drug discontinuance alone. Moderate to severe cases should be managed with fluid, electrolyte and protein supplementation as indicated. When the colitis is not relieved by drug discontinuance or when it is severe, oral vancomycin is the treatment of choice for antibiotic-associated pseudomembranous colitis produced by *C. difficile.* Other causes of colitis should also be considered.

Precautions: General—Prolonged use of antibiotics may promote the overgrowth of nonsusceptible organisms. Should superinfection occur during therapy, appropriate measures should be taken.

When cephradine is administered to patients with markedly impaired renal function lower daily dosage is required. (See DOSAGE AND ADMINISTRATION.) In patients with known or suspected renal impairment, careful clinical observation and appropriate laboratory studies should be conducted because cephradine in the usual recommended dosage will accumulate in the serum and tissues.

Cephradine should be prescribed with caution in individuals with a history of gastrointestinal disease, particularly colitis.

Patients should be followed carefully so that any side effects or unusual manifestations of drug idiosyncrasy may be detected. If a hypersensitivity reaction occurs, the drug should be discontinued and the patient treated with the usual agents, e.g., pressor amines, antihistamines, or corticosteroids.

Velosef for Injection (Cephradine for Injection USP) is physically compatible with most commonly used intravenous fluids and electrolyte solutions (such as 5% Dextrose Injection or Sodium Chloride Injection or M/6 sodium lactate); however, it is *not* compatible with Lactated Ringer's Injection because of the incompatibility between calcium ions and the sodium carbonate present in Velosef for Injection.

Information for Patients: Caution diabetic patients that false test results may occur with urine glucose tests (see PRECAUTIONS, Drug/Laboratory Test Interactions). The patient should report current use of any medicines and should be cautioned not to take other medications unless the physician knows and approves of their use (see PRECAUTIONS, Drug Interactions).

Laboratory Tests: In patients with known or suspected renal impairment, it is advisable to monitor renal function (see DOSAGE AND ADMINISTRATION).

Drug Interactions: When administered concurrently, the following drugs may interact with cephalosporins:

Other antibacterial agents—Bacteriostats may interfere with the bactericidal action of cephalosporins in acute infection; other agents, e.g., aminoglycosides, colistin, polymyxins, vancomycin, may increase the possibility of nephrotoxicity.

Diuretics (potent "loop diuretics," e.g., furosemide and ethacrynic acid)—Enhanced possibility for renal toxicity.

Probenecid—Increased and prolonged blood levels of cephalosporins, resulting in increased risk of nephrotoxicity.

Continued on next page

Squibb—Cont.

Drug/Laboratory Test Interactions: After treatment with cephradine, a false-positive reaction for glucose in the urine may occur with Benedict's solution, Fehling's solution, or with Clinitest® tablets, but not with enzyme-based tests such as Clinistix® and Tes-Tape®. False-positive Coombs test results may occur in newborns whose mothers received a cephalosporin prior to delivery.
Cephalosporins have been reported to cause false-positive reactions in tests for urinary proteins which use sulfosalicylic acid, false elevations of urinary 17-ketosteroid values, and prolonged prothrombin times.
Carcinogenesis, Mutagenesis: Long-term studies in animals have not been performed to evaluate carcinogenic potential or mutagenesis.
Pregnancy: Teratogenic Effects/Impairment of Fertility—Category B: Reproduction studies have been performed in mice and rats at doses up to four times the maximum indicated human dose and have revealed no evidence of impaired fertility or harm to the fetus due to cephradine. There are, however, no adequate and well-controlled studies in pregnant women. Because animal reproduction studies are not always predictive of human response, this drug should be used during pregnancy only if clearly needed.
Nursing Mothers: Since cephradine is excreted in breast milk during lactation, caution should be exercised when cephradine is administered to a nursing woman.
Pediatric Use: See DOSAGE AND ADMINISTRATION. Cephradine has been effectively used in infants, but all laboratory parameters have not been extensively studied in infants one month to one year of age; therefore, in the treatment of children in this age group, the benefits of the drug to the risk involved must be considered.
Since safety for use in premature infants and in infants under one month of age has not been established, the use of cephradine by injection or infusion should be based on careful consideration of the benefits of the drug against the risk involved.
Adverse Reactions: As with other cephalosporins, untoward reactions are limited essentially to gastrointestinal disturbances and, on occasion, to hypersensitivity phenomena. The latter are more likely to occur in individuals who have previously demonstrated hypersensitivity and those with a history of allergy, asthma, hay fever, or urticaria.
The following adverse reactions have been reported following the use of cephradine:
Gastrointestinal: Symptoms of pseudomembranous colitis can appear during antibiotic treatment. Nausea and vomiting have been reported rarely.
Skin and Hypersensitivity Reactions: Mild urticaria or skin rash, edema, erythema, pruritus, joint pains and drug fever.
Blood: Mild, transient eosinophilia, leukopenia and neutropenia.
Liver: Instances of elevated SGOT and SGPT of approximately 10 percent and 2 percent of patients, respectively, have been observed; also, a few cases of elevated total bilirubin, alkaline phosphatase and LDH have been observed. In most patients, values tended to return to normal after the end of therapy.
Renal: Mild elevations in BUN have been observed in some patients treated with cephalosporins; their frequency increases in patients over 50 years old and in children under three. In adults for whom serum creatinine determinations were performed, the rise in BUN was not accompanied by a rise in serum creatinine.
Other adverse reactions are headache, dizziness, dyspnea, paresthesia, candidal overgrowth, candidal vaginitis, isolated instances of hepatomegaly, and thrombophlebitis at the site of injection.
Pain on intramuscular injection has been experienced by some patients. Since sterile abscesses have been reported following accidental subcutaneous injection, the preparation should be administered by deep intramuscular injection.
Dosage and Administration: Adults—
Treatment: The usual daily dosage of Velosef for Injection (Cephradine for Injection USP) is 2 to 4 g. of cephradine given in equally divided doses four times a day intramuscularly or intravenously (e.g., 500 mg. to 1 g. q.i.d.). In bone infections the usual dosage is 1 g. q.i.d. administered intravenously. A dosage of 500 mg. q.i.d. is adequate in uncomplicated pneumonia, skin and skin structures and most urinary tract infections. In severe infections, the total daily dose may be increased by using a q. 4 h. dosage regimen or by increasing the dose given q.i.d.; the maximum dose should not exceed 8 g. per day.
Prevention: To prevent postoperative infection in contaminated or potentially contaminated surgery, recommended doses are as follows:
a. 1 g IV or IM administered 30 to 90 minutes prior to start of surgery.
b. 1 g every 4 to 6 hours after the first dose for one or two doses, or for up to 24 hours postoperatively.
Cesarean Section Patients: The first dose of 1 g is administered intravenously as soon as the umbilical cord is clamped. The second and third doses should be given as 1 g intravenously or intramuscularly at 6 and 12 hours after the first dose.
Infants and Children—The usual dosage range of Velosef is 50 to 100 mg./ kg./day (approximately 23 to 45 mg./lb./day) in equally divided doses four times a day and should be regulated by age, weight of the patient and severity of the infection being treated.
All laboratory parameters have not been extensively studied in infants under one year of age; therefore, in the treatment of children in this age group, the benefits of the drug to the risk involved must be considered. In newborn infants, accumulation of other cephalosporin-class antibiotics (with resultant prolongation of drug half-life) has been reported.
The maximum daily pediatric dose should not exceed doses recommended for adults. [See table entitled "Pediatric Dosage Guide" below.]
As with antibiotic therapy generally: therapy should be continued for a minimum of 48 to 72 hours after the patient becomes asymptomatic or evidence of bacterial eradication has been obtained; in infections caused by group A beta-hemolytic streptococci, a minimum of 10 days of treatment is recommended to guard against the risk of rheumatic fever or glomerulonephritis; in the treatment of chronic urinary tract infection, frequent bacteriologic and clinical appraisal is necessary during therapy and may be necessary for several months afterwards; persistent infections may require treatment for several weeks; doses smaller than those indicated above should not be used.
Parenteral therapy may be followed by oral Velosef either as capsules or as an oral suspension.
Velosef for injection (Cephradine for Injection USP) may be given intravenously or by deep intramuscular injection. To minimize pain and induration, intramuscular injections should be made into a large muscle mass, such as the gluteus or lateral aspect of the thigh.
Renal Impaired Dosage—A modified dosage schedule in patients with decreased renal function is necessary. Each patient should be considered individually; the following reduced dosage schedule is recommended as a guideline, based on the creatinine clearance (ml./min./1.73m^2).
In adults, the initial loading dose is 750 mg. of Velosef and the maintenance dose is 500 mg. at the time intervals listed below.

Creatinine Clearance	Time Interval
> 20 ml./min.	6–12 hours
15–19 ml./min.	12–24 hours
10–14 ml./min.	24–40 hours
5–9 ml./min.	40–50 hours
< 5 ml./min.	50–70 hours

Further modification of the dosage schedule may be necessary in children.
Reconstitution and Storage:
Parenteral drug products should be inspected visually for particulate matter and discoloration prior to administration, whenever solution and container permit.
For I.M. Use.—Aseptically add Sterile Water for Injection or Bacteriostatic Water for Injection (containing 0.9% [w/v] benzyl alcohol, or 0.12% methylparaben and 0.014% propylparaben) according to the following table [i.e., the table entitled "I.M. Dilution Table" next page]. Intramuscular solutions should be used within two hours at room temperature; if stored in the refrigerator at 5° C., solutions retain full potency for 24 hours. Reconstituted solutions may vary in color from light straw to yellow; however, this does not affect the potency.
For I.V. Use—Velosef (Cephradine for Injection USP) may also be administered by direct intravenous injection or by continuous or intermittent infusion. A 3 mcg./ml. serum concentration can be maintained for each mg. of cephradine per kg. body weight per hour of infusion.
For Direct I.V. Administration: Suitable diluents are Sterile Water for Injection, 5% Dextrose Injection, or Sodium Chloride Injection.
Do not use Lactated Ringer's Injection.
Aseptically add 5 ml. of diluent to the 250 mg. or 500 mg. vials, 10 ml. of diluent to the 1 g. vial, or 20 ml. of diluent to the 2 g. bottle; withdraw entire contents. The solution may be slowly injected directly into a vein over a three to five minute period or may be given as a supplementary injection through the injection site on the administration set when the infusion solution is compatible with cephradine. These Velosef (Cephradine, Squibb) solutions

VELOSEF FOR INJECTION
(Cephradine for Injection USP)

PEDIATRIC DOSAGE GUIDE

Weight		50 mg./kg./day		100 mg./kg./day	
lbs.	kg.	Approx. single dose mg. q. 6 h.	Volume needed @ 208 mg./ml. dilution	Approx. single dose mg. q. 6 h.	Volume needed @ 227 mg./ml.
10	4.5	56 mg.	0.27 ml.	112 mg.	0.5 ml.
20	9.1	114 mg.	0.55 ml.	227 mg.	1 ml.
30	13.6	170 mg.	0.82 ml.	340 mg.	1.5 ml.
40	18.2	227 mg.	1.1 ml.	455 mg.	2 ml.
50	22.7	284 mg.	1.4 ml.	567 mg.	2.5 ml.

should be used within two hours when held at room temperature; if stored at 5° C., the solutions retain full potency for 24 hours.

For Continuous or Intermittent I.V. Infusion: Suitable intravenous infusion solutions for Velosef are 5% or 10% Dextrose Injection; Sodium Chloride Injection; Sodium Lactate Injection (M/6 sodium lactate); Dextrose and Sodium Chloride Injection (5% : 0.9%) or (5% : 0.45%); 10% Invert Sugar in Water for Injection; Normosol®-R, and Ionosol® B with Dextrose 5%. Sterile Water for Injection may be used as an I.V. infusion solution for Velosef at a concentration of 30 to 50 mg./ml. (30 mg./ml. is approximately isotonic). **Do not use Lactated Ringer's Injection.**

a) To prepare a Velosef solution for transfer into an I.V. infusion bottle, aseptically add 10 ml., 20 ml., or 40 ml. of Sterile Water for Injection or a suitable infusion solution, respectively, to the 1 g. vial, or 2 g. or 4 g. bottles. Promptly withdraw the entire contents of the resulting solution and aseptically transfer to an I.V. infusion bottle. Intravenous infusion solutions containing Velosef at a concentration of five percent (50 mg./ml.) or less retain potency as noted under (b) below. The choice of I.V. infusion solution and the volume to be employed are dictated by fluid and electrolyte management.

b) Velosef may be infused directly from the 2 g. or 4 g. I.V. bottle. Reconstitute the 2 g. bottle with 40 ml. and the 4 g. bottle with 80 ml. of a suitable intravenous infusion solution; attach an I.V. administration set directly to the Velosef I.V. infusion bottle. The 2 g. and 4 g. I.V. bottles are designed to be suspended from an I.V. stand.

Intravenous infusion solutions containing Velosef retain full potency for 10 hours at room temperature or 48 hours at 5° C.; infusion solutions of Velosef in Sterile Water for Injection that are frozen immediately after reconstitution in the original container are stable for as long as six weeks when stored at −20° C.

For prolonged infusions, replace the infusion every 10 hours with a freshly prepared solution.

Extemporaneous mixtures of Velosef for Injection (Cephradine for Injection USP) with other antibiotics are not recommmended.

Protect solutions of Velosef from concentrated light or direct sunlight. Velosef for Injection may be stored at room temperature prior to reconstitution; avoid excessive heat; protect from light.

How Supplied: Velosef for Injection (Cephradine for Injection USP) is available for intramuscular or intravenous use in vials containing 250 mg., 500 mg., or 1 g. cephradine; and for intravenous use in 100 ml. infusion bottles containing 2 g. or 4 g. cephradine.

VELOSEF FOR INJECTION
(Cephradine for Injection USP)

I.M. DILUTION TABLE

Vial Size	Volume of Diluent	Approximate Available Volume	Approximate Available Concentration
250 mg.	1.2 ml.	1.2 ml.	208 mg./ml.
500 mg.	2.0 ml.	2.2 ml.	227 mg./ml.
1 g.	4.0 ml.	4.5 ml.	222 mg./ml.

VESPRIN® INJECTION ℞
(Triflupromazine Hydrochloride Injection USP)
VESPRIN® TABLETS ℞
(Triflupromazine Hydrochloride Tablets USP)
VESPRIN® HIGH-POTENCY SUSPENSION ℞
(Triflupromazine Oral Suspension USP)

Description: Vesprin is a phenothiazine derivative. It is available for parenteral use in multiple dose vials providing 10 or 20 mg. triflupromazine hydrochloride per ml., with 1.5% (w/v) benzyl alcohol as a preservative and sodium chloride for isotonicity. The pH has been adjusted to 4.5-5.2 with sodium hydroxide or hydrochloric acid. At the time of manufacture, the air in the vials is replaced by nitrogen.

Vesprin is also available for oral use as tablets providing 10, 25, and 50 mg. triflupromazine hydrochloride and as a suspension providing triflupromazine equivalent to 50 mg. triflupromazine hydrochloride per 5 ml. teaspoonful (10 mg. per ml.). Vesprin Tablets, 25 mg. and 50 mg., contain FD&C Yellow No. 5 (tartrazine).

Clinical Pharmacology: Experimental and clinical studies suggest that the phenothiazine derivatives act on the hypothalamus. These drugs are believed to depress various components of the mesodiencephalic activating system, which is involved in the control of basal metabolism and body temperature, wakefulness, vasomotor tone, emesis, and hormonal balance. In addition, the drugs exert a peripheral autonomic effect in varying degrees. However, the site and mode of action of phenothiazine derivatives including triflupromazine have not been completely elucidated.

Indications and Usage: Oral: Vesprin (Triflupromazine) is effective for oral use in the management of the manifestations of psychotic disorders (excluding psychotic depressive reactions) and for the control of severe nausea and vomiting.

Parenteral: Vesprin Injection (Triflupromazine Hydrochloride Injection USP) is effective in the management of the manifestations of psychotic disorders (excluding psychotic depressive reactions) and for the control of severe nausea and vomiting.

Triflupromazine has not been shown effective in the management of behavioral complications in patients with mental retardation.

Contraindications: Phenothiazines are contraindicated in patients with suspected or established subcortical brain damage, with or without hypothalamic damage, since a hyperthermic reaction with temperatures in excess of 104° F. may occur in such patients, sometimes not until 14 to 16 hours after drug administration. Total body ice-packing is recommended for such a reaction; antipyretics may also be useful.

Phenothiazine compounds should not be used in patients receiving large doses of hypnotics. As with other phenothiazine compounds, triflupromazine is contraindicated in comatose or severely depressed states.

The presence of blood dyscrasia or liver damage precludes the use of triflupromazine.

Warnings: The extrapyramidal symptoms which can occur secondary to administration of triflupromazine may be confused with the central nervous system signs of an undiagnosed primary disease responsible for the vomiting, e.g., Reye Syndrome or other encephalopathy. The use of triflupromazine and other potential hepatotoxins should be avoided in children and adolescents whose signs and symptoms suggest Reye Syndrome.

The use of this drug may impair the mental and physical abilities required for driving a car or operating heavy machinery.

Potentiation of the effects of alcohol may occur with the use of this drug.

Usage in Pregnancy—The safety for the use of this drug during pregnancy has not been established; therefore, the possible hazards should be weighed against the potential benefits when administering this drug to pregnant patients.

Precautions: Antiemetic Effect: The antiemetic action of triflupromazine may mask the signs and symptoms of overdosage of other drugs and may obscure the diagnosis and treatment of other conditions such as intestinal obstruction, brain tumor, and Reye Syndrome (see WARNINGS).

Because of the possibility of cross-sensitivity, this drug should be used cautiously in patients who have developed cholestatic jaundice, dermatoses, or other allergic reactions to phenothiazine derivatives.

Psychotic patients on large doses of a phenothiazine drug who are undergoing surgery should be watched carefully for possible hypotensive phenomena. Moreover, it should be remembered that reduced amounts of anesthetics or central nervous system depressants may be necessary. It is generally not recommended that triflupromazine be used prior to spinal anesthesia.

Although this is not a general feature of triflupromazine, potentiation of central nervous system depressants (opiates, analgesics, antihistamines, barbiturates, alcohol) may occur. The effects of atropine may be potentiated in some patients receiving triflupromazine.

Phenothiazines should be used with caution in patients with a history of convulsive disorders, since grand mal convulsions have been known to occur.

Patients with special medical disorders such as mitral insufficiency or pheochromocytoma and patients who have exhibited idiosyncrasy to other centrally-acting drugs may experience severe reactions to phenothiazine compounds.

The parenteral administration of triflupromazine may sometimes cause postural hypotension; to preclude its occurrence, patients should be kept under close clinical supervision, in a recumbent position if necessary.

Facilities should be available for periodic checking of hepatic function, renal function and the blood picture. Renal function of patients on long-term therapy should be monitored; if BUN (blood urea nitrogen) becomes abnormal, treatment should be discontinued.

As with any phenothiazine, the physician should be alert to the possible development of "silent pneumonias" in patients under treatment with triflupromazine.

Neuroleptic drugs elevate prolactin levels; the elevation persists during chronic administration. Tissue culture experiments indicate that approximately one-third of human breast cancers are prolactin dependent *in vitro*, a factor of potential importance if the prescription of these drugs is contemplated in a patient with a previously detected breast cancer. Although disturbances such as galactorrhea, amenorrhea, gynecomastia, and impotence have been reported, the clinical significance of elevated serum prolactin levels is unknown for most patients. An increase in mammary neoplasms has been found in rodents after chronic administration of neuroleptic drugs. Neither clinical studies nor epidemiologic studies conducted to date, however, have shown an association between chronic administration of these drugs and mammary tumorigenesis; the available evidence is considered too limited to be conclusive at this time.

Vesprin Tablets (Triflupromazine Hydrochloride Tablets USP), 25 mg. and 50 mg., contain FD&C Yellow No. 5 (tartrazine) which may cause allergic-type reactions (including bronchial asthma) in certain susceptible individu-

Continued on next page

Squibb—Cont.

als. Although the overall incidence of FD&C Yellow No. 5 (tartrazine) sensitivity in the general population is low, it is frequently seen in patients who also have aspirin hypersensitivity.

Adverse Reactions: *Central Nervous System*—The side effects most frequently reported with phenothiazine compounds are extrapyramidal symptoms including pseudoparkinsonism, dystonia, dyskinesia, akathisia, oculogyric crises, opisthotonos, and hyperreflexia. Most often these extrapyramidal symptoms are reversible; however, they may be persistent (see below). With any given phenothiazine derivative, the incidence and severity of such reactions depend more on individual patient sensitivity than on other factors, but dosage level and patient age are also determinants.

Extrapyramidal reactions may be alarming, and the patient should be forewarned and reassured. These reactions can usually be controlled by administration of antiparkinsonian drugs such as Benztropine Mesylate and by subsequent reduction in dosage.

Persistent Tardive Dyskinesia—As with all antipsychotic agents, tardive dyskinesia may appear in some patients on long-term therapy or may occur after drug therapy has been discontinued. The risk seems to be greater in elderly patients on high-dose therapy, especially females. The symptoms are persistent and in some patients appear to be irreversible. The syndrome is characterized by rhythmical involuntary movements of the tongue, face, mouth, or jaw (e.g., protrusion of tongue, puffing of cheeks, puckering of mouth, chewing movements). Sometimes these may be accompanied by involuntary movements of the extremities. There is no known effective treatment for tardive dyskinesia; antiparkinsonism agents usually do not alleviate the symptoms of this syndrome. It is suggested that all antipsychotic agents be discontinued if these symptoms appear. Should it be necessary to reinstitute treatment, or increase the dosage of the agent, or switch to a different antipsychotic agent, the syndrome may be masked. It has been reported that fine vermicular movements of the tongue may be an early sign of the syndrome and if the medication is stopped at that time, the syndrome may not develop.

Drowsiness or lethargy, if they occur, may necessitate a reduction in dosage; the induction of a catatonic-like state has been known to occur with dosages far in excess of the recommended amounts. As with other phenothiazine compounds, reactivation or aggravation of psychotic processes may be encountered.

Phenothiazine derivatives have been known to cause, in some patients, restlessness, excitement, or bizarre dreams.

Autonomic Nervous System—Hypertension and fluctuation in blood pressure have been reported with triflupromazine.

Patients with pheochromocytoma, cerebral vascular or renal insufficiency appear to be particularly prone to hypotensive reactions with phenothiazine compounds and should therefore be observed closely when the drug is administered. If severe hypotension should occur, supportive measures including the use of intravenous vasopressor drugs should be instituted immediately. Levarterenol Bitartrate Injection and Phenylephrine Hydrochloride Injection are suitable drugs for this purpose. *Epinephrine should not be used* since phenothiazine derivatives have been found to reverse its action, resulting in a further lowering of blood pressure.

Autonomic reactions including nausea and loss of appetite, salivation, polyuria, perspiration, dry mouth, headache, and constipation may occur. Autonomic effects can usually be controlled by reducing or temporarily discontinuing dosage.

In some patients, phenothiazine derivatives have caused blurred vision, glaucoma, bladder paralysis, fecal impaction, paralytic ileus, tachycardia, or nasal congestion.

Metabolic and Endocrine—Weight change, peripheral edema, abnormal lactation, gynecomastia, menstrual irregularities, false results on pregnancy tests, impotency in men, and increased libido in women have all been known to occur in some patients on phenothiazine therapy.

Allergic Reactions—Skin disorders such as itching, erythema, urticaria, seborrhea, photosensitivity, eczema, and even exfoliative dermatitis have been reported with phenothiazine derivatives. The possibility of anaphylactoid reactions occuring in some patients should be borne in mind.

Hematologic—Routine blood counts are advisable during therapy since blood dyscrasias including leukopenia, agranulocytosis, thrombocytopenic or nonthrombocytopenic purpura, eosinophilia, and pancytopenia have been observed with phenothiazine derivatives. Furthermore, if any soreness of the mouth, gums, or throat, or any symptoms of upper respiratory infection occur and confirmatory leukocyte count indicates cellular depression, therapy should be discontinued and other appropriate measures instituted immediately.

Hepatic—Liver damage as manifested by cholestatic jaundice or biliary stasis have been observed with phenothiazine derivatives, particularly during the first months of therapy; treatment should be discontinued if this occurs. An increase in cephalin flocculation, sometimes accompanied by alterations in other liver function tests has been reported in patients receiving phenothiazines who have had no clinical evidence of liver damage.

Others—Sudden, unexpected, and unexplained deaths have been reported in hospitalized psychotic patients receiving phenothiazines. Previous brain damage or seizures may be predisposing factors; high doses should be avoided in known seizure patients. Several patients have shown sudden flare-ups of psychotic behavior patterns shortly before death. Autopsy findings have usually revealed acute fulminating pneumonia or pneumonitis, aspiration of gastric contents, or intramyocardial lesions.

The following adverse reactions have also occurred with phenothiazine derivatives: systemic lupus erythematosus-like syndrome, hypotension severe enough to cause fatal cardiac arrest, altered electrocardiographic and electroencephalographic tracings, altered cerebrospinal fluid proteins, cerebral edema, potentiation of heat and of phosphorus insecticides, asthma, laryngeal edema, angioneurotic edema, and pigmentary retinopathy; with long-term use—skin pigmentation, and lenticular and corneal opacities.

Dosage and Administration: Psychotic Disorders—*Institutionalized Adult Patients:* Optimum dosage levels must be determined individually in each patient. The recommended initial dose for oral therapy is 100 mg. up to a maximum total daily dose of 150 mg. After treatment is instituted, the daily dosage should be adjusted until the desired clinical effect is obtained. Continued treatment is necessary to achieve maximum therapeutic benefits. In some patients, optimum clinical improvement may occur only after prolonged treatment. When symptoms are controlled, dosage can generally be reduced gradually to maintenance levels.

The recommended intramuscular dose is 60 mg. up to a maximum total daily dose of 150 mg.

Noninstitutionalized Adult Patients: Use the same regimen as outlined for institutionalized patients.

For patients on *maintenance therapy* following institutional care, the recommended oral dose is 30 mg. up to a maximum total daily dose of 150 mg.

Children: As in adult therapy, optimum dosage levels must be determined individually for each patient. The recommended oral dosage schedule is 2 mg./kg. (1 mg./lb.) up to a maximum total daily dose of 150 mg. in divided doses. For maintenance therapy, dosage should be increased or decreased to meet individual requirements.

When intramuscular use is indicated in children, the recommended range is 0.2 to 0.25 mg./kg. ($\frac{1}{10}$ to $\frac{1}{8}$ mg./lb.) up to a maximum total daily dose of 10 mg. The drug should not be administered to children under $2\frac{1}{2}$ years of age.

Nausea and Vomiting—For adults, the recommended dosage range for prophylaxis as well as for treatment is 1 mg. up to a maximum total daily dose of 3 mg. intravenously or 5 to 15 mg. as a single dose which may be repeated every four hours up to a maximum total daily dose of 60 mg. intramuscularly. The recommended dosage range for oral prophylaxis is 20 mg. up to a maximum total daily dose of 30 mg. For elderly or debilitated patients, the recommended intramuscular dosage is 2.5 mg. up to a maximum total daily dose of 15 mg.

Triflupromazine should generally not be used in children under $2\frac{1}{2}$ years of age. It should not be used in conditions for which children's dosages have not been established. Dosage and frequency of administration should be adjusted according to the severity of the symptoms and response of the patient. The duration of activity following intramuscular administration may last up to 12 hours. Subsequent doses may be given by the same route if necessary.

For children, the recommended dosage is 0.2 mg./kg. ($\frac{1}{10}$ mg./lb.) up to a maximum total daily dose of 10 mg. divided into three doses orally or a range of 0.2 to 0.25 mg./kg. ($\frac{1}{10}$ to $\frac{1}{8}$ mg./lb.) up to a maximum total daily dose of 10 mg. intramuscularly. Intravenous administration is not recommended for children.

How Supplied: Vesprin Injection (Triflupromazine Hydrochloride Injection USP) is available in multiple dose vials of 1 ml. providing 20 mg. per ml., and in multiple dose vials of 10 ml. providing 10 mg. per ml.

Vesprin Tablets (Triflupromazine Hydrochloride Tablets USP) are available in potencies of 10 mg., 25 mg. and 50 mg. The 10 mg. tablets are available in bottles of 50 and 500; the 25 mg. and 50 mg. tablets are available in bottles of 50.

Vesprin High-Potency Suspension (Triflupromazine Oral Suspension USP) is available as a flavored suspension providing triflupromazine equivalent to 50 mg. triflupromazine hydrochloride per 5 ml. teaspoonful (10 mg. per ml.) in bottles of 120 ml.

Storage: Store the injection, tablets and oral suspension at room temperature; protect from light. Injection: avoid freezing. Parenteral solutions may vary in color from essentially colorless to light amber. If a solution has become any darker than light amber or is discolored in any other way it should not be used. Tablets: keep tightly closed; avoid excessive heat. Oral suspension: keep tightly closed; avoid excessive heat and freezing.

For information on Squibb products, write to: Squibb Professional Services Department, Lawrenceville-Princeton Road, Princeton, N.J. 08540.

Products are cross-indexed by generic and chemical names in the

YELLOW SECTION

Standard Process Laboratories, Inc.

2023 WEST WISCONSIN AVENUE
MILWAUKEE, WI 53201

CHLOROPHYLL COMPLEX PERLES

Composition: Crude, natural chlorophyll extracted from Alfalfa and Tillandsia is a steroid rich source of fat soluble natural Vitamin K (6 Perles supply 3.3 mg. of Vitamin K). Vitamin K is indicated to be essential to the normal function of the liver and the formation of prothrombin, one of the normal constituents of the blood.
Action and Uses: Prothrombin is one of the several clotting agents in the blood. (Ref. #1) On the other hand, *water soluble* extracts of chlorophyll, being chemically altered from their natural form, contain no vitamins. Doses of synthetic Vitamin K have produced hemolytic anemia in rats and the toxicity of *synthetic* Vitamin K is attributed to increased breakdown of the red blood cells, (Ref. #2) whereas it is interesting to note, that administering *natural, fat soluble* Vitamin K, causes a prompt response by the body with the formation of prothrombin. The blood returns to its normal composition. (Ref. #3)
Administration: Three to six perles per day or as directed.
How Supplied: CHLOROPHYLL COMPLEX PERLES in bottles of 60 and 350.
Also Available: CHLOROPHYLL, FAT SOLUBLE OINTMENT in 1½-oz. tube.
References: (1) and (3) *Yearbook of Agriculture,* 1959, (U.S. Government Publication) pages 137-138. (2) *Recommended Dietary Allowances,* (Seventh Edition-1968), National Research Council Publication No. 1694, page 30.

ZYPAN TABLETS

An Enzymatic Digestive Supplement for Common Indigestion

Description: Each ZYPAN TABLET contains 1.0 gr. Pancreatin, plus 0.5 gr. of other Pancreas extracts, 1.5 gr. Pepsin (1:3000), 2.75 gr. Betaine Hydrochloride and 0.15 gr. Ammonium Chloride.
ZYPAN is a source of digestive enzymes as derived from fresh, frozen beef pancreas (as pancreatin), with betaine hydrochloride as a source of hydrochloric acid, and ammonium chloride as an acidifying agent. Pancreatin is a source of multiple digestive enzymes, notably as follows: (1) Trypsin, which breaks down *protein* into amino acids, (2) Diastase, which converts *starch* to an absorbable form, and (3) Lipase, which assists in the digestion of *fats.*
Indications: When intestinal fermentative processes result in such conditions as flatulence, bloating, and fullness after meals; a lack of digestive enzymes may be present. A long-term inability to absorb foods, because of incomplete digestion, may affect the general health. Deficient protein digestion should be a primary concern, and mere increase of protein in the diet may not correct a deficiency as efficiently as when aided by the proteolytic enzymes.
Administration: One to two tablets with each meal, or as directed.
How Supplied: Bottles of 90 tablets.

Products are cross-indexed by

generic and chemical names

in the

YELLOW SECTION

Star Pharmaceuticals, Inc.

16499 N.E. 19TH AVE.
N. MIAMI BEACH, FL 33160

MICROSUL® 0.5 Gm. & 1.0 Gm. ℞

NDC 0076-0104-03 & 04
& NDC 0076-0202-03 & 04

Each tablet contains: Sulfamethizole 0.5 Gm. & 1.0 Gm.

MICROSUL–A® ℞

NDC 0076-0105-03 & 04

Each tablet contains: Sulfamethizole 0.5 Gm. with Phenazopyridine HCl 50 mg.

NITREX® 50 mg. & 100 mg. ℞

NDC 0076-0401-03 & 04
& NDC 0076-0402-03 & 04

Each tablet contains: Nitrofurantoin USP 50 mg. & 100 mg.

PROSED® ℞

NDC 0076-0107-03 & 04

Each tablet contains: Methenamine 40.8 mg., Methylene blue 5.4 mg., Phenyl Salicylate 18.1 mg., Atropine sulfate 0.03 mg., Hyocyamine 0.03 mg., Benzoic acid 4.5 mg.

STAR–OTIC® OTC

Antibacterial–Antifungal Otic Solution
NDC 0076-0300-03

(See PDR For Nonprescription Drugs)

URO–KP–NEUTRAL® OTC

NDC 0076-0109-03 & 04

Each 4 peach capsule-shaped tablets contain:
Phosphorous ....1000 mg.
Potassium ....197.6 mg.
Sodium ....1002 mg.
Derived from Disodium Phosphate Anhydrous, Dipotassium Phosphate Anhydrous, and Sodium Monobasic Anhydrous.
How Supplied: Bottles of 100.

UROLENE BLUE® ℞

NDC 0076-0501-03 & 04

Each tablet contains: Methylene blue USP 65 mg.
How Supplied: Bottles of 100 and 1000.

VESICHOLINE® ℞

NDC 0076-0701-03 & 04

Each tablet contains: Bethanechol chloride NF 25 mg. FOR ORAL USE.

VIRILON® ℞

NDC 0076-0301-03 & 04

Each capsule contains: Methyltestosterone USP 10 mg. in controlled release pellets.
How Supplied: Bottles of 100 and 1000.

Important Notice

Before prescribing or administering any product described in PHYSICIANS' DESK REFERENCE always consult the PDR Supplement for possible new or revised information.

Steri-Med Inc.

POST OFFICE BOX 459
LINDENHURST, NY 11757

NDC 0188-	PRODUCT	
1120	Cortisone Acetate Tablets, 25 mg.	℞
9826	Dimenhydrinate Tablets, 50 mg.	
	Diphenydramine HCl	℞
8009	25 mg.	
8010	50 mg.	
8015	Hydrochlorothiazide Tablets, 50 mg.	℞
1330	Hydrocortisone Tablets, 20 mg.	℞
	Levodopa Capsules	℞
8280	250 mg.	
8281	500 mg.	
	Meprobamate Tablets	℞
1410	200 mg.	
1400	400 mg.	
	Nitrofurantoin Tablets	℞
1450	50 mg.	
1460	100 mg.	
1580	Prednisolone Tablets, 5 mg.	℞
	Prednisone Tablets	℞
1570	5 mg.	
8159	20 mg.	
1650	Quinidine Sulfate Tablets, 200 mg.	℞
	Reserpine Tablets	℞
1740	0.1 mg.	
1744	0.25 mg.	
	Sodium Sulfacetamide Ophthalmic Solution	℞
9386	10%	
9387	30%	
	Tetracycline HCl Capsules	℞
1805	250 mg.	
1806	500 mg.	

Stiefel Laboratories, Inc.

2801 PONCE DE LEON BLVD.
CORAL GABLES, FL 33134

DUOFILM® ℞

Description: Duofilm is a topical preparation containing 16.7% Salicyclic Acid, U.S.P., and 16.7% Lactic Acid, U.S.P., as the active ingredients in a base of Flexible Collodion, U.S.P.
Duofilm's pharmacologic activity is generally attributed to the keratolytic action of Salicylic Acid and Lactic Acid.
Clinical Pharmacology: The exact mode of action of Salicyclic Acid and Lactic Acid in the treatment of warts is not known. Their activity appears to be associated with keratolytic action which results in mechanical removal of epidermal cells infected with wart viruses.
Indications and Usage: Duofilm is indicated in the treatment of common warts. See Dosage and Administration section for information on frequency and duration of use.
Contraindications: Duofilm should not be used by diabetics or patients with impaired blood circulation. Do not use on moles, birthmarks, or unusual warts with hair growing from them.
Precautions: Duofilm is for external use only. Do not permit Duofilm to contact eyes or mucosal membranes. If spilled in eyes or on mucosal membranes, flush with water, remove precipitated collodion, and flush with water for an additional 15 minutes.
Duofilm should not be allowed to contact normal skin surrounding wart. Treatment should be discontinued if excessive irritation occurs. Duofilm is highly flammable and should be kept away from fire or flame. Keep bottle tightly capped when not in use. Store at controlled room temperature.

Continued on next page

Stiefel—Cont.

Adverse Reactions: A localized irritant reaction will occur if Duofilm is applied to the normal skin surrounding the wart. The irritation will normally be controlled by temporarily discontinuing use of Duofilm, and by applying the medication only to the wart site when treatment is resumed.
Dosage and Administration: Prior to the application of Duofilm, soak affected area in hot water for at least five minutes. Dry thoroughly with a clean towel.
Apply two to four drops of Duofilm directly to wart once a day using the plastic applicator. Each drop should be permitted to dry before the next is added. Duofilm should be applied with care to avoid contact with normal skin surrounding wart. Treated area should be covered by lightly applied Band-Aid.®
Clinically visible improvement will normally occur during the first two to four weeks of therapy. Maximum resolution may be expected after six to twelve weeks of drug use.
How Supplied: Duofilm is supplied in a ½ oz. bottle with plastic applicator, NDC 0145-6788-05.
See Precautions section for special handling and storage conditions.

SCABENE™ LOTION ℞
Lindane USP 1%

Description: Active ingredient: lindane USP 1%. **Inert ingredients:** 99% in a non-greasy, pleasantly scented base, containing purified water, stearic acid, glyceryl stearate laureth-23, carrageenan, triethanolamine, cetyl alcohol, aminomethyl propanol, fragrance, butylparaben, and methylparaben.
Actions: SCABENE LOTION is an ectoparasiticide for Sarcoptes scabiei (scabies), Pediculus capitis (head lice), Phthirus pubis (crab lice), and their ova.
Indications: SCABENE LOTION is indicated for the treatment of Sarcoptes scabiei (scabies), as well as infestations with Pediculus capitis (head lice), Phthirus pubis (crab lice), and their ova.
Contraindications: SCABENE LOTION is contraindicated in individuals with known hypersensitivity to the product or to any of its components.
Warning: SCABENE LOTION SHOULD BE USED WITH CAUTION ESPECIALLY ON INFANTS, CHILDREN AND IN PREGNANCY. LINDANE PENETRATES HUMAN SKIN AND HAS THE POTENTIAL FOR CNS TOXICITY. STUDIES INDICATE THAT POTENTIAL TOXIC EFFECTS OF TOPICALLY APPLIED LINDANE ARE GREATER IN THE YOUNG. Seizures have been reported after the use of lindane but a cause and effect relationship has not been established.
Simultaneous application of lotions, ointments or oils may enhance the percutaneous absorption of lindane.
Warning: Do not contaminate water by disposing of waste—DISCARD BOTTLE WHEN EMPTY—DO NOT REUSE.
Precautions: If accidental ingestion occurs, prompt institution of gastric lavage will rid the body of large amounts of the toxicant. However, since oils favor absorption, saline cathartics for intestinal evacuation should be given rather than oil laxatives. If central nervous system manifestations occur, they can be antagonized by the administration of pentobarbital or phenobarbital.
If accidental contact with the eyes occurs, flush with water. If irritation or sensitization occurs, discontinue use and consult a physician.
Adverse Reactions: Eczematous eruptions due to irritation from this product have been reported.
Administration:

CAUTION: USE ONLY AS DIRECTED. DO NOT EXCEED RECOMMENDED DOSAGE.
NOTE: PLEASE READ CAREFULLY.

Directions For Use:
Shake well before using.
Pediculosis capitis (head lice)—Apply a quantity sufficient to cover only the affected and adjacent hairy areas.
The lotion should be rubbed into scalp and hair and left in place for 12 hours followed by thorough washing.
Retreatment is usually not necessary. Demonstrable living lice after 7 days is evidence that retreatment is necessary.
Pediculosis pubis (crab lice)—Apply a sufficient quantity only to cover thinly the hair and skin of the pubic area, and if infested, the thighs, trunk, and axillary regions. The material should be rubbed into the skin and hair and left in place for 12 hours followed by a thorough washing.
Retreatment is usually not necessary. Demonstrable living lice after 7 days indicates that retreatment is necessary. Sexual contacts should be treated simultaneously.
Scabies (Sarcoptes scabiei)—The lotion should be applied to dry skin in a thin layer and rubbed in thoroughly. If crusted lesions are present, a warm bath preceding the medication is helpful. If a warm bath is used, allow the skin to dry and cool before applying the lotion. Usually one ounce is sufficient for an adult. A total body application should be made from the neck down. Scabies rarely affects the head of children or adults but may occur in infants. The lotion should be left on for 8–12 hours and should then be removed by thorough washing.
ONE APPLICATION IS USUALLY CURATIVE.
Many patients exhibit persistent pruritus after treatment; this is rarely a sign of treatment failure and is not an indication for retreatment unless living mites can be demonstrated.
Caution: Federal law prohibits dispensing without prescription.
How Supplied:
Scabene Lotion 2 ounce (59 ml.) bottle NDC 0145-7064-02
Scabene Lotion 16 ounce (472 ml.) bottle NDC 0145-7064-07

Stuart Pharmaceuticals
Div. of ICI Americas Inc.
WILMINGTON, DE 19897

ALternaGEL®
Liquid
High-Potency Aluminum Hydroxide Antacid

Composition: ALternaGEL is available as a white, pleasant-tasting, high-potency aluminum hydroxide liquid antacid.
Each 5 ml. teaspoonful contains 600 mg. aluminum hydroxide (equivalent to dried gel, USP) providing 16 milliequivalents (mEq) of acid-neutralizing capacity (ANC), and less than 2 mg. (.087 mEq) of sodium per teaspoonful.
Action and Uses: ALternaGEL is indicated for the symptomatic relief of hyperacidity associated with peptic ulcer, gastritis, peptic esophagitis, gastric hyperacidity, hiatal hernia, and heartburn.
ALternaGEL will be of special value to those patients for whom magnesium-containing antacids are undesirable, such as patients with renal insufficiency, patients requiring control of attendant G.I. complications resulting from steroid or other drug therapy, and patients experiencing the laxation which may result from magnesium or combination antacid regimens.
Dosage and Administration: One or two teaspoonfuls, as needed, between meals and at bedtime, or as directed by a physician. May be followed by a sip of water if desired.
Warnings: As with all medications, ALternaGEL should be kept out of the reach of children.
ALternaGEL may cause constipation.
Except under the advice and supervision of a physician, more than 18 teaspoonfuls should not be taken in a 24-hour period, or the maximum recommended dosage taken for more than two weeks.
Drug Interaction Precaution: ALternaGEL should not be taken concurrently with an antibiotic containing any form of tetracycline.
How Supplied: ALternaGEL is available in bottles of 12 fluid ounces and 5 fluid ounces. NDC 0038-0860.
[*Shown in Product Identification Section*]

BUCLADIN®-S SOFTAB® Tablets ℞
(buclizine hydrochloride)

Description: Buclizine hydrochloride is 1-(p-tert-Butylbenzyl) -4- (p-chloro- α -phenylbenzyl) piperazine dihydrochloride. Each tablet contains 50 mg. buclizine hydrochloride.
Actions and Uses: BUCLADIN-S (buclizine hydrochloride) acts centrally to suppress nausea and vomiting.
Indications: BUCLADIN-S is effective in the management of nausea, vomiting, and dizziness associated with motion sickness.
Contraindications: Buclizine hydrochloride, when administered to the pregnant rat, induced fetal abnormalities at doses above the human therapeutic range. Clinical data are not adequate to establish nonteratogenicity in early pregnancy. Until such data are available, buclizine hydrochloride is contraindicated for use in early pregnancy. Buclizine hydrochloride is contraindicated in individuals who have shown a previous hypersensitivity to it.
Warnings: Since drowsiness may occur with use of this drug, patients should be warned of this possibility and cautioned against engaging in activities requiring mental alertness, such as driving a car, or operating heavy machinery or appliances. Safe and effective dosage in children has not been established.
Precaution: This product contains FD&C Yellow #5 (tartrazine) which may cause allergic-type reactions (including bronchial asthma) in certain susceptible individuals. Although the overall incidence of FD&C Yellow #5 (tartrazine) sensitivity in the general population is low, it is frequently seen in patients who also have aspirin hypersensitivity.
Adverse Reactions: Occasionally drowsiness, dryness of mouth, headache, and jitteriness are encountered.
Dosage and Administration: BUCLADIN-S (buclizine hydrochloride) SOFTAB Tablets can be taken without swallowing water. Place the SOFTAB tablet in the mouth and allow it to dissolve, or the tablet may be chewed or swallowed whole.
Adults: One tablet usually serves to alleviate nausea. In severe cases, three tablets a day may be taken. The usual maintenance dosage is one tablet twice daily. In the prevention of motion sickness, one tablet taken at least ½ hour before beginning travel usually suffices. For extended travel, a second tablet may be taken after 4 to 6 hours.
How Supplied: Bottles of 100 scored, yellow, SOFTAB Tablets, identified front "STUART", reverse "864". NDC 0038-0864.
[*Shown in Product Identification Section*]

CARI-TAB® SOFTAB® Tablets ℞
(fluoride with multivitamins)

Composition: Each tablet contains: Fluoride (as 1.1 mg. sodium fluoride), 0.5 mg.; Vitamin A (as palmitate), 2,000 USP units; Vitamin D (ergocalciferol), 200 USP units; Vitamin C (as ascorbic acid, and sodium ascorbate), 75 mg.

Indications: As an aid in promoting the development of caries-resistant teeth and in preventing deficiencies of vitamins A, D, and C. Controlled studies show that fluoride must be provided in adequate amounts to infants and children by daily dietary supplementation, if natural sources are deficient, through at least the first fifteen years to achieve maximal anticariogenic effect.

CARI-TAB SOFTAB provides a pleasant tasting, raspberry flavored, convenient form for administering an optimal amount of fluoride and those vitamins which are essential to the formation of normal bones and teeth.

Dosage and Administration: It is necessary to know the fluoride content of drinking water in order to adjust the dosage of this product correctly. Where the drinking water is substantially free of fluoride (i.e. less than 3 parts per million) the following dosage schedule is recommended:

Infants, birth to two years of age: one-half tablet daily. For infant use, tablet should be crushed and mixed with food or formula.

Children, two to three years of age: one tablet daily. Tablets may be chewed or allowed to dissolve in the mouth.

Children, three to sixteen years of age: two tablets daily after a meal. Tablets may be chewed or allowed to dissolve in the mouth.

Important Note: It is recommended that the daily fluoride intake from dietary supplements such as CARI-TAB be adjusted according to the amount of fluoride contained in drinking water. In communities with less than 0.3 ppm of fluoride in the water supply, the recommended dosage is 0.25 mg. of fluoride daily between birth and two years of age, 0.5 mg. between two and three years of age, and 1.0 mg. between three and sixteen years of age. Where the water supply contains between 0.3 and 0.7 ppm of fluoride the recommendation is for no supplemental fluoride between birth and two years of age, 0.25 mg. between two and three years of age, and 0.5 mg. of fluoride between three and sixteen years of age. If the water supply contains greater than 0.7 ppm of fluoride then no supplemental fluoride is needed. When prescribing CARI-TAB the physician should make sure the child is not receiving significant amounts of fluoride from other medications.

Caution: Dental fluorosis (mottling) may result from exceeding the recommended dose. In hypersensitive individuals, fluorides occasionally cause skin eruptions such as atopic dermatitis, eczema, or urticaria. Gastric distress, headache, and weakness have also been reported. These hypersensitive reactions usually disappear promptly after discontinuation of the fluoride.

Warnings: As in the case of all medications, keep out of reach of children.

How Supplied: Bottles of 100 pink colored, scored SOFTAB tablets, identified front "STUART", reverse "680". NDC 0038-0680.

DIALOSE™ Capsules
Stool Softener

Composition: Each capsule contains docusate potassium, 100 mg.

Action and Uses: DIALOSE is indicated for treating constipation due to hardness, or lack of moisture in the intestinal contents. DIALOSE is an effective stool softener, whose gentle action will help to restore normal bowel function gradually, without griping or acute discomfort.

Dosage and Administration:

Adults: Initially, one capsule three times a day.

Children, 6 years and over: One capsule at bedtime, or as directed by physician.

Children, under 6 years: As directed by physician.

It is helpful to increase the daily intake of fluids by taking a glass of water with each dose.

When adequate laxation is obtained, the dose may be adjusted to meet individual needs.

How Supplied: Bottles of 36, 100, and 500 pink capsules, identified "STUART 470". Also available in 100 capsule unit dose boxes (10 strips of 10 capsules each).

NDC 0038-0470.

[*Shown in Product Identification Section*]

DIALOSE™ PLUS Capsules
Stool Softener
***plus* Peristaltic Activator**

Composition: Each capsule contains: docusate potassium, 100 mg. and casanthranol, 30 mg.

Action and Uses: DIALOSE PLUS is indicated for the treatment of constipation generally associated with any of the following: hardness, or lack of moisture in the intestinal contents, or decreased intestinal motility.

DIALOSE PLUS combines the advantages of the stool softener, docusate potassium, with the peristaltic activating effect of casanthranol.

Warning: As with any laxative, DIALOSE PLUS should not be used when abdominal pain, nausea, or vomiting are present. Frequent or prolonged use may result in dependence on laxatives.

Dosage and Administration:

Adults: Initially, one capsule two times a day.

Children: As directed by physician.

When adequate laxation is obtained the dose may be adjusted to meet individual needs.

It is helpful to increase the daily intake of fluids by taking a glass of water with each dose.

How Supplied: Bottles of 36, 100, and 500 yellow capsules, identified "STUART 475". Also available in 100 capsule unit dose boxes (10 strips of 10 capsules each).

NDC 0038-0475.

[*Shown in Product Identification Section*]

EFFERSYLLIUM® Instant Mix
Bulk Laxative

Composition: Each rounded teaspoonful, or individual packet (7 g.) contains psyllium hydrocolloid, 3 g.

Actions and Uses: EFFERSYLLIUM produces a soft, lubricating bulk which promotes natural elimination.

EFFERSYLLIUM is not a one-dose, fast-acting purgative or cathartic. Administration for several days may be needed to establish regularity.

Effersyllium contains less than 2.5 mg. sodium per rounded teaspoonful.

Indications: EFFERSYLLIUM is indicated to restore normal bowel habits in chronic constipation, to promote normal elimination in irritable bowel syndrome, and to ease passage of stools in presence of anorectal disorders.

Dosage and Administration:

Adults: One rounded teaspoonful, or one packet, in a glass of water one to three times a day, or as directed by physician.

Children, 6 years and over: One level teaspoonful, or one-half packet (3.5 g.) in one-half glass of water at bedtime, or as directed by physician. *Children, under 6 years:* As directed by physician.

Note: To avoid caking, always use a dry spoon to remove EFFERSYLLIUM from its container. Dosage should be placed in a dry glass. Add water, stir and drink immediately. REPLACE CAP TIGHTLY. KEEP IN A DRY PLACE.

Warning: As with all medications, keep out of the reach of children.

How Supplied: Bottles of 9 oz. and 16 oz. of tan, granular powder. Convenient pouch package 7 g. per packet in boxes of 12 or 24.

NDC 0038-0440.

FERANCEE®
Chewable Tablets

Composition: Each tablet contains: iron (from 200 mg. ferrous fumarate), 67 mg. and Vitamin C (as ascorbic acid, 49 mg. and sodium ascorbate, 114 mg.), 150 mg. Contains FD&C Yellow #5 (tartrazine) as a color additive.

Action and Uses: A pleasant tasting hematinic for iron-deficiency anemias, FERANCEE is particularly useful when chronic blood loss, onset of menses, or pregnancy create additional demands for iron supplementation. Because ferrous fumarate is unusually well-tolerated, FERANCEE can be administered between meals when iron absorption is maximal. The peach-cherry flavored chewable tablets dissolve quickly in the mouth and may be either chewed or swallowed.

Dosage and Administration:

Adults: Two tablets daily, or as directed by physician.

Children over 6 years of age: One tablet daily, or as directed by physician.

Children under 6 years of age: As directed by physician.

How Supplied: Bottles of 100 brown and yellow, two-layer tablets identified "STUART 650" on brown layer. A childproof cap is standard on each bottle as a safeguard against accidental ingestion by children.

NDC 0038-0650.

[*Shown in Product Identification Section*]

FERANCEE®-HP Tablets

Composition: Each tablet contains: iron (from 330 mg. ferrous fumarate), 110 mg.; Vitamin C (as ascorbic acid, 350 mg. and sodium ascorbate, 281 mg.), 600 mg.

Action and Uses: FERANCEE-HP is a high potency formulation of iron and vitamin C and is intended for use as either:

(1) intensive therapy for the acute and/or severe iron deficiency anemia where a high intake of elemental iron is required, or

(2) a maintenance hematinic for those patients needing a daily iron supplement to maintain normal hemoglobin levels.

The use of well-tolerated ferrous fumarate provides high levels of elemental iron with a low incidence of gastric distress. The inclusion of 600 mg. of Vitamin C per tablet serves to maintain more of the iron in the absorbable ferrous state.

Precautions: Because FERANCEE-HP contains 110 mg. of elemental iron per tablet, it is recommended that its use be limited to adults, i.e. over age 12 years. As with all medication, FERANCEE-HP should be kept out of the reach of children.

Dosage and Administration:

For acute and/or severe iron deficiency anemia, two or three tablets per day taken one tablet per dose after meals. (Each tablet provides 110 mg. elemental iron).

For maintenance of normal hemoglobin levels in most patients with a history of recurring iron deficiency anemia, one tablet per day taken after a meal should be sufficient.

How Supplied: FERANCEE-HP is supplied in bottles of 60 red, film coated, oval shaped tablets.

NDC 0038-0863.

Note: A childproof safety cap is standard on each bottle of 60 tablets as a safeguard against accidental ingestion by children.

[*Shown in Product Identification Section*]

HIBICLENS® Antiseptic Antimicrobial
Skin Cleanser
(chlorhexidine gluconate)

Description: HIBICLENS is an antiseptic antimicrobial skin cleanser possessing bactericidal activities. HIBICLENS contains 4%

Continued on next page

Stuart—Cont.

chlorhexidine gluconate, a chemically unique hexamethylenebis biguanide, in a mild, sudsing base adjusted to pH 5.0–6.5 for optimal activity and stability as well as compatability with the normal pH of the skin.

Action: HIBICLENS is bactericidal on contact. It has antiseptic activity and a persistent antimicrobial effect against a wide range of microorganisms, including gram-positive bacteria, and gram-negative bacteria such as *Pseudomonas aeruginosa*. The effectiveness of HIBICLENS is not signficantly reduced by the presence of organic matter, such as pus or blood.[1]

In a study[2] simulating surgical use, the immediate bactericidal effect of HIBICLENS after a single six-minute scrub resulted in a 99.9% reduction in resident bacterial flora, with a reduction of 99.98% after the eleventh scrub. Reductions on surgically gloved hands were maintained over the six-hour test period.

HIBICLENS displays persistent antimicrobial action. In one study[2], 93% of a radiolabeled formulation of HIBICLENS remained present on uncovered skin after five hours.

Hibiclens prevents skin infection thereby reducing the risk of cross-infection.

Indications: HIBICLENS is indicated for use as a surgical scrub, as a health-care personnel handwash, for preoperative showering and bathing, as a patient preoperative skin preparation, and as a skin wound cleanser and general skin cleanser.

Safety: The extensive use of chlorhexidine gluconate for over 20 years outside the United States has produced no evidence of absorption of the compound through intact skin. The potential for producing skin reactions is extremely low. HIBICLENS can be used many times a day without causing irritation, dryness, or discomfort. When used for cleaning superficial wounds, HIBICLENS will neither cause additional tissue injury nor delay healing.

Precautions: HIBICLENS is for topical use only. The sudsing formulation may be irritating to the eyes. If HIBICLENS should get into the eyes, rinse out promptly and thoroughly with water.

Keep out of ears. Chlorhexidine gluconate, like various other antimicrobial agents, has been reported to cause deafness when instilled in the middle ear. In the presence of a perforated eardrum particular care should be taken to prevent exposure of inner ear tissues to HIBICLENS.

HIBICLENS should not be used by persons with sensitivity to any of its components. Adverse reactions, including dermatitis and photosensitivity, are rare, but if they do occur, discontinue use. Keep this and all other drugs out of the reach of children. Avoid excessive heat (104°F).

Directions for Use:

Skin wound and general skin cleansing

Thoroughly rinse area to be cleansed with water. Apply sufficient HIBICLENS and wash gently. Rinse again thoroughly.

Patient preoperative skin preparation

Apply HIBICLENS liberally to surgical site and swab for at least two minutes. Dry with a sterile towel. Repeat procedure for an additional two minutes and dry with a sterile towel.

Health-care personnel use

SURGICAL HAND SCRUB

Wet hands and forearms with water. Scrub for 3 minutes with about 5 ml. of HIBICLENS and a wet brush, paying particular attention to the nails, cuticles, and interdigital spaces. A separate nail cleaner may be used. Rinse thoroughly. Wash for an additional 3 minutes with 5 ml. of HIBICLENS and rinse under running water. Dry thoroughly.

HAND WASH

Wet hands with water. Dispense about 5 ml. of HIBICLENS into cupped hands and wash in a vigorous manner for 15 seconds. Rinse and dry thoroughly.

How Supplied: In 15 ml. packettes and plastic disposable bottles: for general handwashing locations, 4 oz. and 8 oz. with dispenser caps, and 16 oz. filled globes; for surgical scrub areas, 32 oz. and 1 gal. The 32 oz. bottle is designed for a special foot-operated wall dispenser. A hand-operated wall dispenser is available for the 16 oz. globe. Hand pumps are available for 16 oz., 32 oz., and 1 gal. sizes. NDC 0038-0575.

References:

1. Lowbury, EJL, and Lilly, HA: The effect of blood on disinfection of surgeons' hands, Brit. J. Surg. 61:19–21 (Jan.) 1974.
2. Peterson AF, Rosenberg A, Alatary SD: Comparative evaluation of surgical scrub preparations, Surg. Gynecol. Obstet. 146:63–65 (Jan.) 1978.

[*Shown in Product Identification Section*]

HIBISTAT®
(chlorhexidine gluconate)
Germicidal Hand Rinse

Description: HIBISTAT is a germicidal hand rinse effective against a wide range of microorganisms. HIBISTAT is a clear, colorless liquid containing 0.5% w/w chlorhexidine gluconate in 70% isopropyl alcohol with emollients.

Actions and Uses: HIBISTAT is indicated for health-care personnel use as a germicidal hand rinse. HIBISTAT is for hand hygiene on physically clean hands. It is used in those situations where hands are physically clean, but in need of degerming, when routine handwashing is not convenient or desirable. HIBISTAT provides rapid germicidal action and has a persistent effect.

HIBISTAT should be used in-between patients and procedures where there are no sinks available or continued return to the sink area is inconvenient or time-consuming. HIBISTAT can be used as an alternative to detergent-based products when hands are physically clean. Also, HIBISTAT is an effective germicidal hand rinse following a soap and water handwash.

Cautions: Keep out of eyes and ears. If HIBISTAT should get into eyes or ears, rinse out promptly and thoroughly with water. Chlorhexidine gluconate has been reported to cause deafness when instilled in the middle ear through perforated ear drums. Irritation or other adverse reactions, such as dermatitis or photosensitivity are rare, but if they do occur, discontinue use. Keep this and all other drugs out of the reach of children.

Avoid excessive heat (104°F).

Directions for Use: Dispense about 5 ml. of HIBISTAT into cupped hands and rub vigorously until dry (about 15 seconds), paying particular attention to nails and interdigital spaces. HIBISTAT dries rapidly in use. No water or toweling are necessary.

How Supplied: In plastic disposable bottles of 4 oz. and 8 oz. with flip-top cap.
NDC 0038-0585.

[*Shown in Product Identification Section*]

HIBITANE® Tincture (Tinted)
HIBITANE® Tincture (Non-Tinted)
(chlorhexidine gluconate)
Patient Skin Preparation Prior to Surgery or Skin Puncture/Venipuncture

Description: HIBITANE TINCTURE is an antimicrobial skin preparation for use (1) before surgery to cleanse the operative site, and (2) before skin puncture/venipuncture. HIBITANE TINCTURE contains 0.5% chlorhexidine gluconate in 70% isopropyl alcohol. It possesses both a rapid and persistent antimicrobial effect against a wide range of microorganisms. HIBITANE TINCTURE (Tinted) contains a skin colorant for demarcation of the skin. HIBITANE TINCTURE (Non-Tinted) is slightly colored but will not stain the skin. Both products are nondetergent and ready to use without dilution.

Actions and Uses: HIBITANE Tincture offers wide-range bactericidal activity for the preparation of the skin at the surgical site and prior to skin puncture or vessel puncture. It provides rapid action on contact and maintains persistent antimicrobial effect, not being significantly affected by pus or blood.

Cautions: Keep out of eyes and ears. If HIBITANE Tincture should get into eyes or ears, rinse immediately and thoroughly with water. Chlorhexidine gluconate has been reported to cause deafness when instilled in the middle ear through perforated ear drums. Irritation or other adverse reactions such as dermatitis or photosensitivity are rare, but if they do occur, discontinue use. HIBITANE Tincture may be irritating if used on mucosal tissue. Keep this and all other drugs out of the reach of children. Avoid excessive heat (104°F).

Directions for Use:

Prior to Surgery: Apply HIBITANE Tincture liberally to the surgical site and swab for approximately 2 minutes. Allow to air dry.

Prior to Skin Puncture/Venipuncture: Swab the site with a gauze pad or cotton ball saturated with HIBITANE Tincture. Allow to air dry.

How Supplied: HIBITANE Tincture (Tinted) is supplied in plastic disposable bottles of 4 oz. NDC 0038-0580.

HIBITANE Tincture (Non-Tinted) is supplied in plastic disposable bottles of 4 oz. and 1 gal. pour package bottles. NDC 0038-0583.

[*Shown in Product Identification Section*]

KASOF® Capsules
High Strength Stool Softener

Composition: Each KASOF capsule contains docusate potassium, 240 mg.

Action and Uses: KASOF provides a highly efficient wetting action to restore moisture to the bowel, thus softening the stool to prevent straining. KASOF is especially valuable for the severely constipated, as well as patients with anorectal disorders, such as hemorrhoids and anal fissures. KASOF is ideal for patients with any condition that can be complicated by straining at stool, for example, cardiac patients. The action of KASOF does not interfere with normal peristalsis and generally does not cause griping or extreme sensation of urgency. KASOF is sodium-free, containing a unique potassium formulation, without the problems associated with sodium intake. The simple, one-a-day dosage helps assure patient compliance in maintaining normal bowel function.

Dosage and Administration: Adults: 1 KASOF capsule daily for several days, or until bowel movements are normal and gentle. It is helpful to increase the daily intake of fluids by drinking a glass of water with each dose.

How Supplied: KASOF is available in bottles of 30 and 60 brown, gelatin capsules, identified "Stuart 380".
NDC 0038-0380.

[*Shown in Product Identification Section*]

KINESED® Tablets ℞
(belladonna alkaloids and phenobarbital)

Description: KINESED is a balanced formulation providing the effective spasmolytic and anticholinergic action of the belladonna alkaloids and the sustained sedative effect of phenobarbital.

Composition: Each chewable, fruit-flavored, scored, oval tablet contains:

Phenobarbital.......................................16 mg.
(Warning: May be habit forming)
Hyoscyamine Sulfate..........................0.1 mg.

Atropine Sulfate ....0.02 mg.
Scopolamine Hydrobromide ....0.007 mg.

Action: The belladonna alkaloids (atropine sulfate, hyoscyamine sulfate, scopolamine hydrobromide) depress the activity of the postganglionic fibers of smooth muscle and secretory glands. Within recommended doses, effects on the central nervous system should be absent or minimal.

Phenobarbital is included to provide a mild sedative effect. The smooth, even sedative action of phenobarbital is well suited for the control of anxiety, tension, or other emotional overlay often associated with many functional disorders.

Indications:
Based on a review of this drug by the National Academy of Sciences—National Research Council, and/or other information, FDA has classified the indications as follows:
Possibly effective as adjunctive therapy in the treatment of peptic ulcer and in the treatment of the irritable bowel syndrome (irritable colon, spastic colon, mucous colitis) and acute enterocolitis.

Contraindications: Contraindicated in patients hypersensitive to belladonna alkaloids or barbiturates, and in patients with glaucoma or advanced hepatic or renal disease.

Precautions: As with any parasympatholytic agent, administer with caution to patients with incipient glaucoma, bladder neck obstruction, or urinary bladder atony. Prolonged use of barbiturates may result in habituation.

Side Effects: Atropine-like side reactions such as blurred vision, oral dryness, and difficult urination, may occur at high doses, but are only rarely noted at recommended dosages.

Dosage and Administration:
Adults: One or two tablets, three or four times daily; chewed, or swallowed with liquids.
Children, 2 to 12 Years: One-half to one tablet, three or four times daily; chewed, or swallowed with liquids.

How Supplied:
Bottles of 100 and 500 scored, oval, fruit-flavored, orange, chewable tablets, identified front "STUART," reverse "220." NDC 0038-0220.

[*Shown in Product Identification Section*]

MULVIDREN®-F SOFTAB® Tablets ℞
(fluoride with multivitamins)

Composition: Each tablet contains: fluoride (as 2.2 mg. sodium fluoride), 1 mg.; Vitamin A (as palmitate), 4,000 USP units; Vitamin D (ergocalciferol), 400 USP units; Vitamin C (as ascorbic acid, and sodium ascorbate), 75 mg.; thiamine mononitrate, 2 mg.; riboflavin, 2 mg.; Vitamin B_6 (as pyridoxine hydrochloride), 1.2 mg.; Vitamin B_{12} (cyanocobalamin), 3 mcg.; niacinamide, 10 mg.; calcium pantothenate, 3 mg.

Action and Uses: As an aid in promoting the development of caries-resistant teeth, MULVIDREN-F provides a source of daily fluoride supplementation in addition to full nutritional amounts of vitamins. Controlled studies show that a definite decrease in the incidence of dental caries is obtained in children receiving an optimal nutritional supply of fluoride. These studies indicate that in order to achieve maximal anticariogenic effect, fluoride must be provided throughout the stages of tooth formation and calcification. Thus, fluoride should be provided in adequate amounts to the child from birth through the first fifteen years of life. Fluoride should be made available continuously throughout this period by daily dietary supplementation if natural sources are deficient. MULVIDREN-F SOFTAB is a well-accepted and convenient form of administering fluoride for both topical and systemic effects.

Dosage and Administration: It is necessary to know the fluoride content of drinking water in order to adjust the dosage of this product correctly. Where the drinking water is substantially free of fluoride (i.e. less than 3 parts per million) the following dosage schedule is recommended:
Children, three to sixteen years of age: One tablet daily after a meal. Tablets may be chewed or allowed to dissolve in the mouth.
Children, two to three years of age: One-half tablet daily. Tablets may be chewed or crushed and mixed with food.

Important Note: It is recommended that the daily fluoride intake from dietary supplements such as MULVIDREN-F be adjusted according to the amount of fluoride contained in the drinking water. In communities with less than 0.3 ppm of fluoride in the water supply, the recommended dosage is 0.25 mg. of fluoride daily between birth and two years of age, 0.5 mg. between two and three years of age, and 1.0 mg. between 3 and 16 years of age. Where the water supply contains between 0.3 and 0.7 ppm of fluoride the recommendation is for no supplemental fluoride between birth and two years of age, 0.25 mg. between two and three years of age, and 0.5 mg. of fluoride between three and sixteen years of age. If the water supply contains greater than 0.7 ppm of fluoride then no supplemental fluoride is needed. When prescribing MULVIDREN-F, the physician should make sure the child is not receiving significant amounts of fluoride from other medications.

Precautions: Dental fluorosis (mottling) may result from exceeding the recommended dose. In hypersensitive individuals, fluorides occasionally cause skin eruptions such as atopic dermatitis, eczema or urticaria. Gastric distress, headache and weakness have also been reported. These hypersensitivity reactions usually disappear promptly after discontinuation of the fluoride. In rare cases, a delay in the eruption of teeth has been reported.

Warnings: As in the case of all medications, keep out of the reach of children.

How Supplied: On prescription only, in bottles of 100 orange colored, scored SOFTAB tablets, identified front "Stuart", reverse "710". A childproof safety cap is standard on each 100 tablet bottle as a safeguard against accidental ingestion by children. NDC 0038-710.

[*Shown in Product Identification Section*]

MYLANTA®
Liquid and Tablets
Antacid/Antiflatulent

Composition: Each chewable tablet or each 5 ml. (one teaspoonful) of liquid contains:
Aluminum hydroxide
(Dried Gel, USP in tablet and equiv.
to Dried Gel, USP in liquid) ....200 mg.
Magnesium hydroxide ....200 mg.
Simethicone ....20 mg.

Sodium Content: Typical values are 0.68 mg. (0.03 mEq) sodium per 5 ml. teaspoonful of liquid; 0.77 mg. (0.03 mEq) per tablet.

Acid Neutralizing Capacity: Each teaspoonful of MYLANTA liquid will neutralize 12.7 mEq of acid. Each MYLANTA tablet will neutralize 11.5 mEq.

Actions and Uses: MYLANTA, a well-balanced combination of two antacids and simethicone, provides consistently dependable relief of symptoms associated with gastric hyperacidity, and mucus-entrapped air or "gas". These indications include:
Common heartburn (pyrosis)
Hiatal hernia
Peptic esophagitis
Gastritis
Peptic ulcer
The soft, easy-to-chew tablets and exceptionally pleasant tasting liquid encourage patients' acceptance, thereby minimizing the skipping of prescribed doses. MYLANTA is appropriate whenever there is a need for effective relief of temporary gastric hyperacidity and mucus-entrapped gas.

Dosage and Administration: One or two teaspoonfuls of liquid or one or two tablets, well-chewed, every two to four hours between meals and at bedtime, or as directed by physician.

Warning: Magnesium hydroxide and other magnesium salts, in the presence of renal insufficiency, may cause central nervous system depression and other symptoms of hypermagnesemia.

Drug Interaction Precaution: Do not use this product for any patient receiving a prescription antibiotic containing any form of tetracycline.

How Supplied: MYLANTA is available as a white, pleasant tasting liquid suspension, and as a two-layer yellow and white chewable tablet, identified on yellow layer "STUART 620". Liquid supplied in bottles of 5 oz. and 12 oz. Tablets supplied in boxes of individually wrapped 40's and 100's, economy size bottles of 180, and consumer convenience packs of 48. Also available for hospital use in liquid unit doses of 1 oz., and bottles of 5 oz.
NDC 0038-0610 (liquid). NDC 0038-0620 (tablets).

[*Shown in Product Identification Section*]

MYLANTA®-II
Liquid and Tablets
High Potency Antacid/Antiflatulent

Composition: Each chewable tablet or each 5 ml. (one teaspoonful) of liquid contains:
Aluminum hydroxide
(Dried Gel, USP in tablet and equiv.
to Dried Gel, USP in liquid) 400 mg.
Magnesium hydroxide 400 mg.
Simethicone 30 mg.

Sodium Content: Typical values are 1.14 mg. (0.05 mEq) sodium per 5 ml. teaspoonful of liquid; 1.3 mg. (0.06 mEq) per tablet.

Acid Neutralizing Capacity: Each teaspoonful of MYLANTA-II liquid will neutralize 25.4 mEq of acid. Each MYLANTA-II tablet will neutralize 23.0 mEq.

Actions and Uses: MYLANTA-II is a high-potency antacid with an antiflatulent. The soft, easy-to-chew tablets and exceptionally pleasant tasting liquid encourage patient acceptance, thereby minimizing the skipping of prescribed doses. MYLANTA-II provides consistently dependable relief of the symptoms of peptic ulcer and other problems related to acid hypersecretion. The high potency of MYLANTA-II is achieved through its concentration of noncalcium antacid ingredients. Thus MYLANTA-II can produce both rapid and long lasting neutralization without the acid rebound associated with calcium carbonate. The balanced formula of aluminum and magnesium hydroxides minimizes undesirable bowel effects. Simethicone is effective for the relief of concomitant distress caused by mucus-entrapped gas and swallowed air.

Dosage and Administration: One or two teaspoonfuls of liquid, or one or two tablets, well-chewed, between meals and at bedtime, or as directed by physician.
Because patients with peptic ulcer vary greatly in both acid output and gastric emptying time, the amount and schedule of dosages should be varied accordingly.

Warning: Magnesium hydroxide and other magnesium salts, in the presence of renal insufficiency, may cause central nervous system depression and other symptoms of hypermagnesemia.

Drug Interaction Precaution: Do not use this product for any patient receiving a prescription antibiotic containing any form of tetracycline.

Continued on next page

Stuart—Cont.

How Supplied: MYLANTA-II is available as a white, pleasant tasting liquid suspension, and a two-layer green and white chewable tablet, identified on green layer "STUART 851". Liquid supplied in 12 oz. bottles. Tablets supplied in boxes of 60 individually wrapped chewable tablets. Also available for hospital use in liquid unit doses of 1 oz., and bottles of 5 oz. NDC 0038-0852 (liquid). NDC 0038-0851 (tablets).

[*Shown in Product Identification Section*]

MYLICON® Tablets and Drops
Antiflatulent

Composition: Each tablet or 0.6 ml. of drops contains simethicone, 40 mg.

Action and Uses: For relief of the painful symptoms of excess gas in the digestive tract. MYLICON is a valuable adjunct in the treatment of many conditions in which the retention of gas may be a problem, such as: postoperative gaseous distention, air swallowing, functional dyspepsia, peptic ulcer, spastic or irritable colon, diverticulitis.

The defoaming action of MYLICON relieves flatulence by dispersing and preventing the formation of mucus-surrounded gas pockets in the gastrointestinal tract. MYLICON acts in the stomach and intestines to change the surface tension of gas bubbles enabling them to coalesce; thus the gas is freed and is eliminated more easily by belching or passing flatus.

Dosage and Administration:

Tablets—One or two tablets four times daily after meals and at bedtime. May also be taken as needed or as directed by a physician. TABLETS SHOULD BE CHEWED THOROUGHLY.

Drops—0.6 ml. four times daily after meals and at bedtime. May also be taken as needed or as directed by a physician. Shake well before using.

How Supplied: Bottles of 100 and 500 white, scored, chewable tablets, identified front "STUART", reverse "450," and dropper bottles of 30 ml. (1 fl. oz.) pink, pleasant tasting liquid. Also available in 100 tablet unit dose boxes (10 strips of 10 tablets each).

NDC 0038-0450 (tablets).

NDC 0038-0630 (drops).

[*Shown in Product Identification Section*]

MYLICON®-80 Tablets
High-Capacity Antiflatulent

Composition: Each tablet contains simethicone, 80 mg.

Action and Uses: For relief of the painful symptoms of excess gas in the digestive tract. MYLICON-80 is a high capacity antiflatulent for adjunctive treatment of many conditions in which the retention of gas may be a problem, such as the following: air swallowing, functional dyspepsia, postoperative gaseous distention, peptic ulcer, spastic or irritable colon, diverticulitis.

MYLICON-80 has a defoaming action that relieves flatulence by dispersing and preventing the formation of mucus-surrounded gas pockets in the gastrointestinal tract. MYLICON-80 acts in the stomach and intestines to change the surface tension of gas bubbles enabling them to coalesce; thus, the gas is freed and is eliminated more easily by belching or passing flatus.

Dosage and Administration: One tablet four times daily after meals and at bedtime. May also be taken as needed or as directed by a physician. TABLETS SHOULD BE CHEWED THOROUGHLY.

How Supplied: Economical bottles of 100 and convenience packages of individually wrapped 12 and 48 pink, scored, chewable tablets identified "STUART 858". Also available in 100 tablet unit dose boxes (10 strips of 10 tablets each). NDC 0038-0858.

[*Shown in Product Identification Section*]

NOLVADEX® 10 mg. Tablets ℞
(tamoxifen citrate)

Description: NOLVADEX (tamoxifen citrate) tablets for oral administration contain 15.2 mg. of tamoxifen citrate, which is equivalent to 10 mg. of tamoxifen. It is a nonsteroidal antiestrogen.

Chemically, NOLVADEX is the trans-isomer of a triphenylethylene derivative. The chemical name is (Z)-2-[4-(1,2-diphenyl-1-butenyl) phenoxy] - N, N - dimethylethanamine 2- hydroxy-1, 2, 3-propanetricarboxylate(1:1).

NOLVADEX is intended only for oral administration; the tablets should be protected from heat and light.

Clinical Pharmacology: NOLVADEX is a nonsteroidal agent which has demonstrated potent antiestrogenic properties in animal test systems. The antiestrogenic effects may be related to its ability to compete with estrogen for binding sites in target tissues such as breast. Tamoxifen inhibits the induction of rat mammary carcinoma induced by dimethylbenzanthracene (DMBA), and causes the regression of already established DMBA-induced tumors. In this rat model, tamoxifen appears to exert its antitumor effects by binding to estrogen receptors.

In cytosols derived from human breast adenocarcinomas, tamoxifen competes with estradiol for estrogen receptor protein.

Preliminary pharmacokinetics in women using radio-labeled tamoxifen has shown that most of the radioactivity is slowly excreted in the feces, with only small amounts appearing in urine. The drug is excreted mainly as conjugates, with unchanged drug and hydroxylated metabolites accounting for 30% of the total.

Blood levels of total radioactivity following single oral doses of approximately 0.3 mg./kg. reached peak values of 0.06–0.14 μg/ml. at 4–7 hours after dosing, with only 20–30% of the drug present as tamoxifen. There was an initial half-life of 7–14 hours with secondary peaks four or more days later. The prolongation of blood levels and fecal excretion is believed to be due to enterohepatic circulation.

Indications and Usage: NOLVADEX has proven useful in the palliative treatment of advanced breast cancer in postmenopausal women. Available evidence indicates that patients who have had a recent negative estrogen receptor assay are unlikely to respond to NOLVADEX.

Contraindications: There are no known contraindications to the use of NOLVADEX.

Warnings: NOLVADEX may have oncogenic activity in animals; the possibility of this potential in humans should be considered. NOLVADEX affects reproductive function in rats at dose levels somewhat higher than the human dose. Safe use in pregnancy has not been established.

Ocular changes have been reported in a few patients treated for periods greater than one year with NOLVADEX at doses at least four times the highest recommended daily dose of 40 mg. The ocular changes consist of retinopathy and, in some patients, there are also corneal changes and a decrease in visual acuity. Ophthalmologic examinations of selected patients receiving long-term therapy with NOLVADEX at recommended doses have not detected any ocular pathology attributable to the drug.

As with other additive hormonal therapy (estrogens and androgens), hypercalcemia has been reported in some breast cancer patients with bone metastases within a few weeks of starting treatment with NOLVADEX. If hypercalcemia does occur, appropriate measures should be taken and, if severe, NOLVADEX should be discontinued.

Precautions: NOLVADEX should be used cautiously in patients with existing leukopenia or thrombocytopenia. Observations of leukopenia and thrombocytopenia occasionally have been made, but it is uncertain if these effects are due to NOLVADEX therapy. Transient decreases in platelet counts, usually to 50,000–100,000/ cu. mm., infrequently lower, have been occasionally reported in patients taking NOLVADEX for breast cancer. No hemorrhagic tendency has been recorded and the platelet counts returned to normal levels even though treatment with NOLVADEX continued. Periodic complete blood counts, including platelet counts, may be appropriate.

Usage in Pregnancy: NOLVADEX should not be used during pregnancy.

Adverse Reactions: The most frequent adverse reactions to NOLVADEX are hot flashes, nausea, and vomiting. These may occur in up to one-fourth of patients, but are rarely severe enough to require discontinuation of treatment.

Less frequently reported adverse reactions are vaginal bleeding, vaginal discharge, menstrual irregularities, and skin rash. Usually these have not been of sufficient severity to require dosage reduction or discontinuation of treatment.

Increased bone and tumor pain, and also local disease flare have occurred, which are sometimes associated with a good tumor response. Patients with increased bone pain may require additional analgesics. Patients with soft tissue disease may have sudden increases in the size of preexisting lesions, sometimes associated with marked erythema within and surrounding the lesions, and/or the development of new lesions. When they occur, the bone pain or disease flare are seen shortly after starting NOLVADEX and generally subside rapidly.

Other adverse reactions which are seen infrequently are hypercalcemia, peripheral edema, distaste for food, pruritus vulvae, depression, dizziness, light-headedness, and headache.

If adverse reactions are severe, it is sometimes possible to control them by a simple reduction of dosage without loss of control of the disease.

Overdosage: Acute overdosage in humans has not been reported. Signs observed at the highest doses following studies to determine LD_{50} in animals were respiratory difficulties and convulsions. No specific treatment for overdosage is known; treatment must be symptomatic.

Dosage and Administration: One or two 10 mg. tablets twice a day (morning and evening).

How Supplied: NOLVADEX tablets are white, round, biconvex tablets, identified "Stuart 600," containing tamoxifen as the citrate in an amount equivalent to 10 mg. of tamoxifen. The tablets are available in bottles of 60 and 250 tablets. The tablets should be protected from heat and light. NDC0038-0600.

[*Shown in Product Identification Section*]

OREXIN® SOFTAB® Tablets

Composition: Each tablet contains: thiamine mononitrate, 10 mg.; Vitamin B_6 (as pyridoxine hydrochloride), 5 mg.; and Vitamin B_{12} (cyanocobalamin), 25 mcg.

Action and Uses: OREXIN is a high-potency vitamin supplement providing thiamine mononitrate and Vitamins B_6 and B_{12}.

OREXIN SOFTAB tablets are specially formulated to dissolve quickly in the mouth. They may be chewed or swallowed. Dissolve tablet in a teaspoonful of water or fruit juice if liquid is preferred.

Dosage and Administration: One tablet daily, or as directed by physician.

How Supplied: Bottles of 100 pale pink SOFTAB tablets, identified "STUART".

NDC 0038-0280.

PROBEC®-T Tablets

Composition: Each tablet contains: Vitamin C (as ascorbic acid, 67 mg. and sodium ascorbate, 600 mg.), 600 mg.; thiamine mononitrate, 15 mg.; riboflavin, 10 mg.; Vitamin B_6 (as pyridoxine hydrochloride), 5 mg.; Vitamin B_{12} (cyanocobalamin), 5 mcg.; niacinamide, 100 mg.; calcium pantothenate, 20 mg. Contains FD&C yellow #5 (tartrazine) as a color additive.
Action and Uses: PROBEC-T is a high-potency B complex supplement with 600 mg. of Vitamin C in easy to swallow odorless tablets.
Dosage and Administration: One tablet a day with a meal, or as directed by physician.
How Supplied: Bottles of 60, salmon colored, capsule-shaped tablets.
NDC 0038-0840.

[*Shown in Product Identification Section*]

SORBITRATE® Tablets ℞
(isosorbide dinitrate)

Description: Chemistry: SORBITRATE (isosorbide dinitrate) is an organic nitrate that is designated chemically as 1,4:3,6-dianhydrosorbitol-2,5-dinitrate.
The potency of the available dosage forms is maintained under normal storage conditions. [See table right].
Mode of Action: The mechanism of action of SORBITRATE in the relief of angina pectoris is unknown at this time, although the basic pharmacologic action is to relax smooth muscle.
Since therapy at the present time is essentially empirical, clinical improvement is generally measured by a decrease in the severity of the symptoms of angina pectoris and the need for medication. Specifically, SORBITRATE reduces in number and severity the incidence of angina pectoris attacks, with concomitant reduction in nitroglycerin intake.
In the evaluation of isosorbide dinitrate in angina pectoris, clinical improvement has been customarily measured subjectively. Individual patterns of angina pectoris differ widely as does the symptomatic response to antianginal agents. In conjunction with the total management of patients with angina pectoris, isosorbide dinitrate has been generally accepted as safe and widely regarded as useful.

SORBITRATE® (isosorbide dinitrate)

FORMS	STRENGTHS	DESCRIPTION	PACKAGING
CHEWABLE Tablets	5 mg.	Green, round, scored tablets identified front "STUART", reverse "810"	Bottles of 100 and 500; and Unit Dose packages of 100. NDC 0038-0810.
	10 mg.	Yellow, round, scored tablets identified front "STUART", reverse "815 "	Bottles of 100 and Unit Dose packages of 100. NDC 0038-0815.
ORAL (Swallow) Tablets	5 mg.	Green, oval-shaped tablets identified front "STUART", reverse "770"	Bottles of 100 and 500; and Unit Dose packages of 100. NDC0038-0770.
	10 mg.	Yellow, oval-shaped tablets identified front "STUART", reverse "780"	Bottles of 100 and 500; and Unit Dose packages of 100. NDC0038-0780.
	20 mg.	Blue, oval-shaped tablets identified front "STUART", reverse "820"	Bottles of 100 and Unit Dose packages of 100. NDC 0038-0820.
SA (Swallow) Tablets (Sustained Action)	40 mg.	Yellow, round tablets identified front "STUART", reverse "880"	Bottles of 100 and Unit Dose packages of 100. NDC0038-0880.
SUBLINGUAL Tablets	2.5 mg	Round, white tablets identified "S" on one side	Bottles of 100 and 500; and Unit Dose packages of 100. NDC 0038-0853.
	5 mg.	Round, pink tablets identified "S" on one side	Bottles of 100 and 500;and Unit Dose packages of 100. NDC 0038-0760.

Indications:
Based on a review of this drug by The National Academy of Sciences—National Research Council and/or other information, FDA has classified the indications as follows:
Probably effective: Sublingual and chewable dosage forms of SORBITRATE are indicated for the treatment of acute anginal attacks and for prophylaxis in situations likely to provoke such attacks.
Possibly effective: Oral dosage forms of SORBITRATE are indicated for the relief of angina pectoris (pain of coronary artery disease). They are not intended to abort the acute anginal episode, but they are widely regarded as useful in the prophylactic treatment of angina pectoris.
Final classification of the less-than-effective indications requires further investigation.

Contraindications: A history of sensitivity to the drug.
Warnings: Data supporting the use of nitrates during the early days of the acute phase of myocardial infarction (the period during which clinical and laboratory findings are unstable) are insufficient to establish safety.
Precautions: Tolerance to this drug and cross tolerance to other nitrites and nitrates may occur. SORBITRATE SA (Sustained Action) 40 mg. tablets contain FD&C Yellow #5 (tartrazine) which may cause allergic-type reactions (including bronchial asthma) in certain susceptible individuals. Although the overall incidence of FD&C Yellow #5 (tartrazine) sensitivity in the general population is low, it is frequently seen in patients who also have aspirin hypersensitivity.
Adverse Reactions: Headache is the most common adverse reaction and may be severe and persistent. Lowering the dose and the use of analgesics will help control the headaches which usually diminish or disappear as therapy is continued. Cutaneous vasodilation with flushing may occur. Transient episodes of dizziness and weakness, as well as other signs of cerebral ischemia associated with postural hypotension, may occasionally develop. This drug can act as a physiological antagonist to norepinephrine, acetylcholine, histamine, and many other agents. An occasional individual exhibits marked sensitivity to the hypotensive effects of nitrates and severe responses (nausea, vomiting, weakness, restlessness, pallor, perspiration, and collapse) can occur even with the usual therapeutic dose. Alcohol may enhance this effect. Drug rash and/or exfoliative dermatitis may occasionally occur.
Dosage and Administration:
Route: Chewable, sublingual, sustained action, and oral tablets.
Initiating Therapy: In starting patients on SORBITRATE (isosorbide dinitrate) it is necessary to adjust the dosage until the smallest effective dose is determined. This is of particular importance in employing chewable tablets. Occasionally, severe hypotensive responses may occur with this dosage form, even with doses as low as 5 mg.
Individual Dose: 2.5 to 10 mg. is the range commonly used, although oral doses up to 30 mg. have frequently been employed. The oral and chewable tablets are scored for more accurate dosage adjustment when necessary. The usual dose for sustained action tablets is one 40 mg. tablet.
Dosage Schedule: Smallest effective dose necessary for the prevention and treatment of pain of an anginal attack. CHEWABLE SORBITRATE and SORBITRATE Sublingual may be taken P.R.N. for prompt relief of anginal pain, or at 4 to 6 hour intervals. SORBITRATE Oral may be taken 3 to 4 times daily. SORBITRATE SA sustained action oral tablets may be taken at 12 hour intervals. Although the onset of effect and the duration of effect of coronary nitrates may be quite variable, following are the generally reported ranges of these values for SORBITRATE.
Onset of Effect:
Chewable and Sublingual: 2 to 5 minutes
Oral and Sustained Action: 15 to 30 minutes
Duration of Effect:
Chewable and Sublingual: 1 to 2 hours
Oral: Estimated to be 4 to 6 hours
Sustained Action: Estimated to be up to 12 hours at a continuous controlled rate
It is recommended that the oral dosage be taken on an empty stomach. If vascular headache cannot be effectively controlled by ordinary measures, dosages may be taken with meals to minimize this side effect.
How Supplied: See table listing all forms and strengths of SORBITRATE at beginning of product information.

[*Shown in Product Identification Section*]

THE STUART FORMULA® Tablets

Composition: Each tablet contains:
Vitamins: Vitamin A (as palmitate), 5000 I.U.; Vitamin D (ergocalciferol), 400 I.U.; Vitamin E (as dl-alpha tocopheryl acetate), 15 I.U.; Vitamin C (as ascorbic acid), 60 mg.; folic acid, 0.4 mg.; thiamine (as thiamine mononitrate), 1.5 mg.; riboflavin, 1.7 mg.; niacin (as niacinamide), 20 mg.; Vitamin B_6 (as pyridoxine hy-

Continued on next page

Stuart—Cont.

drochloride), 2 mg.; Vitamin B_{12} (cyanocobalamin), 6 mcg.
Minerals: calcium 160 mg.; phosphorus, 125 mg.; iodine, 150 mcg.; iron (from 54 mg. ferrous fumarate) 18 mg.; magnesium, 100 mg.
Actions and Uses: The STUART FORMULA tablet provides a well-balanced multivitamin/multimineral formula intended for use as a daily dietary supplement for adults and children over age four.
Dosage and Administration: One tablet daily or as directed by a physician.
How Supplied: Bottles of 100, 250 and 500 white round tablets. Childproof safety caps are standard on the 100 and 250 tablet bottles as a safeguard against accidental ingestion by children.
NDC 0038-0866.
[*Shown in Product Identification Section*]

STUART PRENATAL® Tablets

Composition: Each tablet contains:

Vitamins:	% U.S. RDA*	
A (as acetate)	100%	8,000 I.U.
D (ergocalciferol)	100%	400 I.U.
E (as dl-alpha tocopheryl acetate)	100%	30 I.U.
C (ascorbic acid)	100%	60 mg.
Folic Acid	100%	0.8 mg.
Thiamine (as thiamine mononitrate)	100%	1.7 mg.
Riboflavin	100%	2 mg.
Niacin (as niacinamide)	100%	20 mg.
B_6 (as pyridoxine hydrochloride)	160%	4 mg.
B_{12} (cyanocobalamin)	100%	8 mcg.
Minerals:		
Calcium (from 679 mg. calcium sulfate anhydrous)	15%	200 mg.
Iodine (from potassium iodide)	100%	150 mcg.
Iron (from 182 mg. ferrous fumarate)	333%	60 mg.
Magnesium (from magnesium oxide)	22%	100 mg.

* Recommended Daily Allowance

Action and Uses: STUART PRENATAL is a multivitamin/multimineral supplement for pregnant and lactating women. It provides vitamins equal to 100% or more of the U.S. RDA for pregnant and lactating women, plus essential minerals, including 60 mg. of elemental iron as well-tolerated ferrous fumarate, and 200 mg. of elemental calcium (non-alkalizing and phosphorus-free). Stuart Prenatal also contains .8 mg. folic acid.
Dosage and Administration: During and after pregnancy, one tablet daily after a meal, or as directed by a physician.
How Supplied: Bottles of 100 and 500 pink capsule-shaped tablets. A childproof safety cap is standard on 100 tablet bottles as a safeguard against accidental ingestion by children.
NDC 0038-0270.
(*Shown in Product Identification Section*)

STUART PRENATAL® with Folic Acid Tablets ℞

Composition: Each tablet contains:
Vitamins: Vitamin A (as acetate), 6,000 USP units; Vitamin D (ergocalciferol), 400 USP Units; Vitamin C (ascorbic acid), 100 mg.; thiamine mononitrate, 3 mg.; riboflavin, 3 mg.; Vitamin B_6 (as pyridoxine hydrochloride), 10 mg.; Vitamin B_{12} (cyanocobalamin), 5 mcg.; niacinamide, 20 mg.; calcium pantothenate, 5.44 mg.; folic acid, 0.3 mg.
Minerals: iron (from 197 mg. ferrous fumarate), 65 mg.; calcium (from 1.2 g. calcium sulfate anhydrous), 350 mg.
Action and Uses: STUART PRENATAL with FOLIC ACID is indicated in pregnancy and during lactation to provide vitamin and mineral nutritional supplementation. Each tablet provides 350 mg. phosphorus-free calcium, and 65 mg. elemental iron. STUART PRENATAL with FOLIC ACID is high in pyridoxine hydrochloride and Vitamin C. Folic acid is added to aid in the prevention of megaloblastic anemia.
Precaution: Folic acid may partially correct the hematological damage due to Vitamin B_{12} deficiency of pernicious anemia, while the associated neurological damage progresses. This product contains FD&C Yellow #5 (tartrazine) which may cause allergic-type reactions (including bronchial asthma) in certain susceptible individuals. Although the overall incidence of FD&C Yellow #5 (tartrazine) sensitivity in the general population is low, it is frequently seen in patients who also have aspirin hypersensitivity.
Dosage and Administration: One tablet daily, to be taken after a meal, or as directed by physician.
How Supplied: Bottles of 100 light blue colored capsule-shaped tablets identified "Stuart 800". A childproof safety cap is standard on each 100 tablet bottle as a safeguard against accidental ingestion by children.
NDC 0038-0800.
[*Shown in Product Identification Section*]

STUARTINIC® Tablets

Composition: Each tablet contains: iron (from 300 mg. ferrous fumarate), 100 mg.; Vitamin C (as ascorbic acid, 300 mg. and sodium ascorbate, 225 mg.), 500 mg.; Vitamin B_{12} (cyanocobalamin), 25 mcg.; thiamine mononitrate, 6 mg.; riboflavin, 6 mg.; Vitamin B_6 (as pyridoxine hydrochloride), 1 mg.; niacinamide, 20 mg.; calcium pantothenate, 10 mg. Contains FD&C yellow #5 (tartrazine) as a color additive.
Action and Uses: STUARTINIC is a complete hematinic for patients with history of iron deficiency anemia who also lack adequate amounts of B-complex vitamins due to poor diet.
The use of well-tolerated ferrous fumarate in STUARTINIC provides a high level of elemental iron with a low incidence of gastric distress. The inclusion of 500 mg. of Vitamin C per tablet serves to maintain more of the iron in the absorbable ferrous state. The B-complex vitamins improve nutrition where B-complex deficient diets contribute to the anemia.
Precautions: Because STUARTINIC contains 100 mg. of elemental iron per tablet, use should be confined to adults, i.e. over age 12 years. As with all medications, STUARTINIC should be kept out of the reach of children.
Dosage and Administration: One tablet daily taken after a meal to maintain normal hemoglobin levels in most patients with chronic iron deficiency anemia resulting from inadequate diet. Higher doses of STUARTINIC can be taken as directed by the physician.
How Supplied: STUARTINIC is supplied in bottles of 60 and 500 yellow, film coated, oval shaped tablets. NDC 0038-0862.
Note: A childproof safety cap is standard on each bottle of 60 tablets. The physician should prescribe or recommend the bottle of 60 tablets, where appropriate, to provide that additional safeguard against accidental ingestion by children.
[*Shown in Product Identification Section*]

STUARTNATAL® 1+1 Tablets ℞

Composition: Each tablet contains:

Vitamins:	% U.S. RDA*	
A (as acetate)	100%	8,000 I.U.
D (ergocalciferol)	100%	400 I.U.
E (as dl-alpha tocopheryl acetate)	100%	30 I.U.
C (ascorbic acid)	150%	90 mg.
Folic Acid	125%	1 mg.
Thiamine (as thiamine mononitrate)	150%	2.55 mg.
Riboflavin	150%	3 mg.
Niacin (as niacinamide)	100%	20 mg.
B_6 (as pyridoxine hydrochloride)	400%	10 mg.
B_{12} (cyanocobalamin)	150%	12 mcg.
Minerals:		
Calcium (from 679 mg. calcium sulfate anhydrous)	15%	200 mg.
Iodine (from potassium iodide)	100%	150 mcg.
Iron (from 197 mg. ferrous fumarate)	361%	65 mg.
Magnesium (from magnesium oxide)	22%	100 mg.

*Recommended Daily Allowance

Action and Uses: STUARTNATAL 1+1 is indicated to provide more potent vitamin and mineral supplementation throughout pregnancy and during the postnatal period—for both the lactating and non-lactating mother. Each tablet provides vitamins equal to 100% or more of U.S. RDA for pregnant and lactating women plus essential minerals, including 1 full grain of elemental iron and 200 mg. of elemental calcium (non-alkalizing and phosphorus-free). STUARTNATAL 1+1 also offers 1 mg. folic acid to aid in the prevention of megaloblastic anemia.
Precaution: Folic acid may partially correct the hematological damage due to Vitamin B_{12} deficiency of pernicious anemia, while the associated neurological damage progresses.
Dosage and Administration: During and after pregnancy, one tablet daily after a meal, or as directed by a physician.
How Supplied: Bottles of 100 and 500 light yellow capsule-shaped tablets identified "Stuart 850". A childproof safety cap is standard on 100 tablet bottles as a safeguard against accidental ingestion by children.
NDC 0038-0850.
(*Shown in Product Identification Section*)

TENORMIN® (atenolol) ℞

Description: TENORMIN (atenolol), a synthetic, $beta_1$-selective (cardioselective) adrenoreceptor blocking agent, may be chemically described as benzeneacetamide, 4-[2'-hydroxy-3'-[(1-methylethyl) amino] propoxy]-.
TENORMIN is available as 50 mg. and 100 mg. tablets for oral administration.
Clinical Pharmacology: TENORMIN is a $beta_1$-selective (cardioselective) beta-adrenergic receptor blocking agent without membrane-stabilizing or intrinsic sympathomimetic (partial agonist) activities. This preferential effect is not absolute, however and, at higher doses, TENORMIN inhibits $beta_2$ adrenoreceptors, chiefly located in the bronchial and vascular musculature.
Pharmacokinetics and Metabolism: In man, absorption of an oral dose is rapid and consistent but incomplete. Approximately 50% of an oral dose is absorbed from the gastrointestinal tract, the remainder being excreted unchanged in the feces. Peak blood levels are reached between 2 and 4 hours after ingestion. Unlike propranolol or metoprolol, but like nadolol, TENORMIN undergoes little or no metabolism by the liver and the absorbed portion is eliminated primarily by renal excretion. TENORMIN also differs from propranolol in that only a small amount (6%–16%) is bound to proteins in the plasma. This kinetic profile results in relatively consistent plasma drug levels with about a fourfold interpatient variation.
The elimination half-life of TENORMIN is approximately 6 to 7 hours and there is no alteration of the kinetic profile of the drug by chronic administration. Following doses of 50

mg or 100 mg, both beta-blocking and antihypertensive effects persist for at least 24 hours. When renal function is impaired, elimination of TENORMIN is closely related to the glomerular filtration rate; but, significant accumulation does not occur until the creatinine clearance falls below 35 ml./min./1.73 m^2 (see DOSAGE AND ADMINISTRATION).

Pharmacodynamics.: In standard animal or human pharmacological tests, beta-adrenoreceptor blocking activity of TENORMIN has been demonstrated by: (1) reduction in resting and exercise heart rate and cardiac output, (2) reduction of systolic and diastolic blood pressure at rest and on exercise, (3) inhibition of isoproterenol-induced tachycardia, and (4) reduction in reflex orthostatic tachycardia.

A significant beta-blocking effect of TENORMIN, as measured by reduction of exercise tachycardia, is apparent within 1 hour following oral administration of a single dose. This effect is maximal at about 2 to 4 hours, and persists for at least 24 hours. The effect at 24 hours is dose-related and also bears a linear relationship to the logarithm of plasma TENORMIN concentration. However, as has been shown for all beta-blocking agents, the antihypertensive effect does not appear to be related to plasma level.

In normal subjects, the $beta_1$ selectivity of TENORMIN has been shown by its reduced ability to reverse the $beta_2$-mediated vasodilating effect of isoproterenol as compared to equivalent beta-blocking doses of propranolol. In asthmatic patients, a dose of TENORMIN producing a greater effect on resting heart rate than propranolol resulted in much less increase in airway resistance. In a placebo-controlled comparison of approximately equipotent oral doses of several beta blockers, TENORMIN produced a significantly smaller decrease of FEV_1 than nonselective beta blockers such as propranolol and, unlike those agents, did not inhibit bronchodilation in response to isoproterenol.

Consistent with its negative chronotropic effect due to beta blockade of the SA node, TENORMIN increases sinus cycle length and sinus node recovery time. Conduction in the AV node is also prolonged. TENORMIN is devoid of membrane-stabilizing activity, and increasing the dose well beyond that producing beta blockade does not further depress myocardial contractility. Several studies have demonstrated a moderate (approximately 10%) increase in stroke volume at rest and during exercise.

In controlled clinical trials TENORMIN given as a single daily dose was an effective antihypertensive agent providing 24-hour reduction of blood pressure. TENORMIN has been studied in combination with thiazide-type diuretics and the blood pressure effects of the combination are approximately additive. TENORMIN is also compatible with methyldopa, hydralazine, and prazosin, the combination resulting in a larger fall in blood pressure than with the single agents. The dose range of TENORMIN is narrow and increasing the dose beyond 100 mg. once daily is not associated with increased antihypertensive effect. The mechanisms of the antihypertensive effects of beta-blocking agents have not been established. Several possible mechanisms have been proposed and include: (1) competitive antagonism of catecholamines at peripheral (especially cardiac) adrenergic neuron sites, leading to decreased cardiac output, (2) a central effect leading to reduced sympathetic outflow to the periphery, and (3) suppression of renin activity. The results from long-term studies have not shown any diminution of the antihypertensive efficacy of TENORMIN with prolonged use.

Indications and Usage: TENORMIN is indicated in the management of hypertension. It may be used alone or concomitantly with other antihypertensive agents, particularly with a thiazide-type diuretic.

	Volunteered (U.S. Studies)		Total: Volunteered and Elicited (Foreign + U.S. Studies)	
	Atenolol (n = 164 %	Placebo (n = 206) %	Atenolol (n = 399) %	Placebo (n = 407) %
CARDIOVASCULAR				
Bradycardia	3	0	3	0
Cold Extremities	0	0.5	12	5
Postural Hypotension	2	1	4	5
Leg Pain	0	0.5	3	1
CENTRAL NERVOUS SYSTEM/NEUROMUSCULAR				
Dizziness	4	1	13	6
Vertigo	2	0.5	2	0.2
Light Headed	1	0	3	0.7
Tiredness	0.6	0.5	26	13
Fatigue	3	1	6	5
Lethargy	1	0	3	0.7
Drowsiness	0.6	0	2	0.5
Depression	0.6	0.5	12	9
Dreaming	0	0	3	1
GASTROINTESTINAL				
Diarrhea	2	0	3	2
Nausea	4	1	3	1
RESPIRATORY (see WARNINGS)				
Wheeziness	0	0	3	3
Dyspnea	0.6	1	6	4

Contraindications: TENORMIN is contraindicated in sinus bradycardia, heart block greater than first degree, cardiogenic shock, and overt cardiac failure (see WARNINGS).

Warnings: Cardiac Failure: Sympathetic stimulation is necessary in supporting circulatory function in congestive heart failure, and beta blockade carries the potential hazard of further depressing myocardial contractility and precipitating more severe failure. In hypertensive patients who have congestive heart failure controlled by digitalis and diuretics, TENORMIN should be administered cautiously. Both digitalis and atenolol slow AV conduction.

In Patients Without a History of Cardiac Failure: Continued depression of the myocardium with beta-blocking agents over a period of time can, in some cases, lead to cardiac failure. At the first sign or symptom of impending cardiac failure, patients should be fully digitalized and/or be given a diuretic and the response observed closely. If cardiac failure continues, despite adequate digitalization and diuresis, TENORMIN should be withdrawn.

Ischemic Heart Disease: Following abrupt cessation of therapy with certain beta-blocking agents in patients with coronary artery disease, exacerbations of angina pectoris and, in some cases, myocardial infarction have been reported. Therefore, such patients should be cautioned against interruption of therapy without the physician's advice. Even in the absence of overt angina pectoris, when discontinuation of TENORMIN is planned, the patient should be carefully observed and should be advised to limit physical activity to a minimum. TENORMIN should be reinstated if withdrawal symptoms occur.

Bronchospastic Diseases: PATIENTS WITH BRONCHOSPASTIC DISEASE SHOULD IN GENERAL NOT RECEIVE BETA BLOCKERS. Because of its relative $beta_1$ selectivity, however, TENORMIN may be used with caution in patients with bronchospastic disease who do not respond to, or cannot tolerate, other antihypertensive treatment. Since $beta_1$selectivity is not absolute, the lowest possible dose of TENORMIN should be used with therapy initiated at 50 mg. and a $beta_2$-stimulating agent (bronchodilator) should be made available. If dosage must be increased, dividing the dose should be considered in order to achieve lower peak blood levels.

Anesthesia and Major Surgery: As with all beta-receptor blocking drugs it may be decided to withdraw TENORMIN before surgery. In this case, 48 hours should be allowed to elapse between the last dose and anesthesia. If treatment is continued, care should be taken when using anesthetic agents which depress the myocardium such as ether, cyclopropane, and trichloroethylene.

TENORMIN, like other beta blockers, is a competitive inhibitor of beta-receptor agonists and its effects on the heart can be reversed by administration of such agents (eg, dobutamine or isoproterenol with caution, see section on OVERDOSAGE). Manifestations of excessive vagal tone (eg, profound bradycardia, hypotension) may be corrected with atropine (1–2 mg. IV).

Diabetes and Hypoglycemia: TENORMIN should be used with caution in diabetic patients if a beta-blocking agent is required. Beta blockers may mask tachycardia occurring with hypoglycemia, but other manifestations such as dizziness and sweating may not be significantly affected. TENORMIN does not potentiate insulin-induced hypoglycemia and, unlike nonselective beta blockers, does not delay recovery of blood glucose to normal levels.

Thyrotoxicosis: Beta-adrenergic blockade may mask certain clinical signs (eg, tachycardia) of hyperthyroidism. Abrupt withdrawal of beta blockade might precipitate a thyroid storm; therefore, patients suspected of developing thyrotoxicosis from whom TENORMIN is to be withdrawn should be monitored closely.

Precautions: Impaired Renal Function: The drug should be used with caution in patients with impaired renal function (see DOSAGE AND ADMINISTRATION).

Drug Interactions: Catecholamine-depleting drugs (eg, reserpine) may have an additive effect when given with beta-blocking agents. Patients treated with TENORMIN plus a catecholamine depletor should therefore be closely observed for evidence of hypotension and or marked bradycardia which may produce vertigo, syncope, or postural hypotension.

Should it be decided to discontinue therapy in patients receiving beta blockers and clonidine concurrently, the beta blocker should be discontinued several days before the gradual withdrawal of clonidine.

Carcinogenesis, Mutagenesis, Impairment of Fertility: Two long-term (maximum dosing duration of 18 or 24 months) rat studies and one long-term (maximum dosing duration of 18 months) mouse study, each employing dose levels as high as 300 mg./kg./day or 150 times the maximum recommended human dose, did not indicate a carcinogenic potential in rodents. Results of various mutagenicity studies support this finding.

Continued on next page

Stuart—Cont.

Fertility of male or female rats (evaluated at dose levels as high as 200 mg./kg./day or 100 times the maximum recommended human dose) was unaffected by atenolol administration.

Animal Toxicology: Chronic studies performed in animals have revealed the occurrence of vacuolation of epithelial cells of Brunner's glands in the duodenum of both male and female dogs at all tested dose levels of atenolol (starting at 15 mg./kg./day or 7.5 times the maximum recommended human dose) and increased incidence of atrial degeneration of hearts of male rats at 300 mg. but not 150 mg. atenolol/kg./day (150 and 75 times the maximum recommended human dose, respectively).

Usage in Pregnancy: Pregnancy Category C. Atenolol has been shown to produce a dose-related increase in embryo/fetal resorptions in rats at doses equal to or greater than 50 mg./kg. or 25 or more times the maximum recommended human dose. Although similar effects were not seen in rabbits, the compound was not evaluated in rabbits at doses above 25 mg./kg. or 12.5 times the maximum recommended human dose. There are no adequate and well-controlled studies in pregnant women. TENORMIN should be used during pregnancy only if the potential benefit justifies the potential risk to the fetus.

Nursing Mothers: It is not established to what extent this drug is excreted in human milk. Since most drugs are excreted in human milk, nursing should not be undertaken by mothers receiving TENORMIN.

Pediatric Use: Safety and effectiveness in children have not been established.

Adverse Reactions: Most adverse effects have been mild and transient.

The frequency estimates in the following table derive from controlled studies in which adverse reactions were either volunteered by the patient (U.S. studies) or elicited, eg, by checklist (foreign studies). The reported frequency of elicited adverse effects was higher for both TENORMIN and placebo-treated patients than when these reactions were volunteered. Where frequency of adverse effects for TENORMIN and placebo is similar, causal relationship to TENORMIN is uncertain.

(See table on preceding page)

MISCELLANEOUS: There have been reports of skin rashes and/or dry eyes associated with the use of beta-adrenergic blocking drugs. The reported incidence is small, and in most cases, the symptoms have cleared when treatment was withdrawn. Discontinuance of the drug should be considered if any such reaction is not otherwise explicable. Patients should be closely monitored following cessation of therapy.

Potential Adverse Effects: In addition, a variety of adverse effects have been reported with other beta-adrenergic blocking agents and may be considered potential adverse effects of TENORMIN.

HEMATOLOGIC: Agranulocytosis, nonthrombocytopenic purpura, thrombocytopenic purpura.

ALLERGIC: Fever, combined with aching and sore throat, laryngospasm, respiratory distress.

CENTRAL NERVOUS SYSTEM: Reversible mental depression progressing to catatonia, visual disturbances, hallucinations, an acute reversible syndrome characterized by disorientation of time and place, short-term memory loss, emotional lability with slightly clouded sensorium, and decreased performance on neuropsychometrics.

GASTROINTESTINAL: Mesenteric arterial thrombosis, ischemic colitis.

Creatinine Clearance (ml./min./1.73 m^2)	Atenolol Elimination Half-life (hrs.)	Maximum Dosage
15–35	16–27	50 mg. daily
<15	>27	50 mg. every other day

OTHER: Reversible alopecia, Peyronie's disease, erythematous rash, Raynaud's phenomenon.

MISCELLANEOUS: The oculomucocutaneous syndrome associated with the beta blocker practolol has not been reported with TENORMIN during investigational use and foreign marketing experience. Furthermore, a number of patients who had previously demonstrated established practolol reactions were transferred to TENORMIN with subsequent resolution or quiescence of the reaction.

Overdosage: To date, there is no known case of acute overdosage, and no specific information on emergency treatment of overdosage is available. The most common effects expected with overdosage of a beta-adrenergic blocking agent are bradycardia, congestive heart failure, hypotension, bronchospasm, and hypoglycemia.

In the case of overdosage, treatment with TENORMIN should be stopped and the patient carefully observed. TENORMIN can be removed from the general circulation by hemodialysis. In addition to gastric lavage, the following therapeutic measures are suggested if warranted:

BRADYCARDIA: Atropine or another anticholinergic drug.

HEART BLOCK (SECOND OR THIRD DEGREE): Isoproterenol or transvenous cardiac pacemaker.

CONGESTIVE HEART FAILURE: Conventional therapy.

HYPOTENSION (DEPENDING ON ASSOCIATED FACTORS): Epinephrine rather than isoproterenol or norepinephrine may be useful in addition to atropine and digitalis.

BRONCHOSPASM: Aminophylline, isoproterenol, or atropine.

HYPOGLYCEMIA: Intravenous glucose.

Dosage and Administration: The initial dose of TENORMIN is 50 mg. given as one tablet a day either alone or added to diuretic therapy. The full effect of this dose will usually be seen within 1 to 2 weeks. If an optimal response is not achieved, the dosage should be increased to TENORMIN 100 mg. given as one tablet a day. Increasing the dosage beyond 100 mg. a day is unlikely to produce any further benefit.

TENORMIN may be used alone or concomitantly with other antihypertensive agents including thiazide-type diuretics, hydralazine, prazosin, and alpha-methyldopa.

Since TENORMIN is excreted via the kidneys, dosage should be adjusted in cases of severe impairment of renal function. No significant accumulation of TENORMIN occurs until creatinine clearance falls below 35 ml./min./1.73 m^2 (normal range is 100–150 ml./min./1.73 m^2); therefore, the following maximum dosages are recommended for patients with renal impairment:

[See table above].

Patients on hemodialysis should be given 50 mg. after each dialysis; this should be done under hospital supervision as marked falls in blood pressure can occur.

How Supplied: Tablets of 50 mg. atenolol (round, flat, uncoated, white tablets identified front "Stuart", reverse "105") are supplied in monthly calendar paks of 28 tablets, bottles of 100 tablets, and unit-dose packages of 100 tablets. NDC 0038-0105.

Tablets of 100 mg. atenolol (round, flat, uncoated, white tablets identified front "Stuart", reverse "101") are supplied in bottles of 100 tablets and unit-dose packages of 100 tablets. NDC 0038-0101.

Protect from heat, light, and moisture. Store unit-dose and calendar paks at controlled room temperature.

[Shown in Product Identification Section]

Sween Corporation
SWEEN BUILDING
P.O. BOX 980
LAKE CRYSTAL, MN 56055

FORDUSTIN'®
Body Powder

Description: A non-caking natural cornstarch based body powder with Sodium Bicarbonate, Silica, Methylbenzethonium Chloride and Fragrance. National Drug Code (NDC) 11701-005.

Indications and Usage: Lubrication of skin subject to excoriation from friction. Helps absorb perspiration to aid in the protection of the skin from perspiration irritation.

Contraindications: Hypersensitivity to any components of the preparation.

Precautions and Adverse Reactions: Transmission electron microscopy and electron diffraction examinations of Fordustin' powder found the product free of any form of fibrous material (asbestiform minerals included) or inorganic materials. For External Use Only. Avoid contact with eyes. Fordustin' is not considered a primary eye or skin irritant under normal use conditions and is not toxic by oral ingestion.

Dosage and Administration: Apply liberally to areas subject to friction and perspiration irritations.

How Supplied: 3 oz. and 8 oz. containers.

GENTLE RAIN™
Shampoo and Skin Cleanser

Description: A shampoo and skin cleanser consisting of Water, Sodium Lauryl Sulfate, Ammonium Lauryl Sulfate, Cocamidopropyl Betaine, Lauramide DEA, Glycol Stearate, Hydrolyzed Animal Protein, Quaternium-33, Ethyl Hexanediol, Citric Acid, Fragrance, Quaternium-15, Tetrasodium EDTA and FD&C Yellow #5.

Indications and Usage: Gentle Rain is a luxurious, non-alkaline formulation designed to condition hair as it cleans, plus cleanse sensitive skin gently and thoroughly. The pH has been carefully adjusted for compatibility with the normal range of hair and skin. The low pH, along with the benefits of the special protein and built-in conditioning ingredients, leave hair extremely manageable and easy to care for. Used as a skin cleanser, this same combination leaves the skin soft and supple. This formulation is safe for color treated hair and gentle enough for daily use.

Contraindications: Hypersensitivity to any components of the preparation.

Precautions and Adverse Reactions: For External Use Only. May cause eye irritation. In case of eye contact, flush eyes with water. Gentle Rain is not toxic by oral ingestion and is not considered a primary skin irritant under normal use conditions.

Dosage and Administration:

Shampooing: Wet hair. Lather, rinse thoroughly and repeat.

Bathing: Apply liberally to a warm washcloth and gently wash skin. Rinse thoroughly and pat dry.

How Supplied: 4 fl.oz. and 16 fl.oz. bottles with flip-top caps, in addition to larger bulk sizes.

MEDICATED SOFT TOUCH™
Antimicrobial Lotion Skin Cleanser

Description: Medicated Soft Touch is an antimicrobial lotion skin cleanser which contains Chloroxylenol (PCMX), a well known antimicrobial agent, in a mild, densely sudsing, soap-free base, adjusted to pH 5.0–5.5 for optimal activity and maintenance of the "acid-balanced" range for healthy skin.
Indications and Usage: Medicated Soft Touch is recommended for repeated daily use as a health care personnel handwash. It decreases bacteria on the skin, reducing the risk and/or chance of cross-infection.
Contraindications: Hypersensitivity to any components of the preparation.
Precautions and Adverse Reactions: For external use only. Avoid contact with eyes. If accidental contact occurs, immediately flush eyes with water for 15 minutes and consult a physician. Keep this and all drugs out of the reach of children. Store at room temperature. Medicated Soft Touch is not toxic by oral ingestion and is not considered a primary skin irritant under normal use conditions.
Dosage and Administration: Wet skin with warm water. Spread a small amount on hands and forearms. Scrub well and rinse thoroughly with warm water after washing.
How Supplied: 16 fl. oz. and 32 fl. oz. bottles with flip-top caps, in addition to larger bulk sizes.

MICRO-GUARD™
Antimicrobial Skin Cream

Description: Micro-Guard Skin Cream contains the antimicrobial agent Chloroxylenol (PCMX) in a water washable, vanishing cream base. National Drug Code (NDC) 11701-012.
Indications and Usage: Micro-Guard is a soothing antiseptic and antifungal cream. Micro-Guard's antifungal action is effective treatment for conditions such as Athlete's Foot, Jock Itch and Ringworm, while its antiseptic activity helps prevent skin infection. Micro-Guard can be used for adjunctive topical treatment of superficial skin infections when oral antibiotic agents are concurrently being administered.
Contraindications: Micro-Guard is contraindicated in individuals who have shown hypersensitivity to any of its components.
Warnings: Micro-Guard is not for ophthalmic, otic or vaginal use.
Precautions: For external use only. Do not use near eyes. If accidental contact occurs, flush eyes immediately with water for 15 minutes and consult a physician. Keep this and all drugs out of the reach of children. If irritation occurs or if there is no improvement within two weeks, discontinue use and consult a physician.
Adverse Reactions: Micro-Guard is not considered a primary skin irritant or sensitizer, but occasional erythema, stinging and eczematous reactions have occurred following its use. If irritation or sensitivity develops with the use of Micro-Guard, treatment should be discontinued and appropriate therapy instituted.
Dosage and Administration: Gently and thoroughly cleanse affected area and pat dry. Apply a thin layer of Micro-Guard over involved area. Repeat application 2 to 3 times daily or as directed by physician.
How Supplied: 2 oz. jars.

PERI–CARE®
Water Resistant Ointment for Perineal Protection

Description: A soft petrolatum ointment with Natural Vitamins A&D, Casein, BHT, Methylbenzethonium Chloride, Chloroxylenol, Propylparaben and D & C Green #6. National Drug Code 11701-010.
Indications and Usage: Used in the perineal area, Peri-Care provides a protective barrier against urine, feces, and post operative drainage.
Contraindications: Hypersensitivity to any components of the preparation.
Precautions and Adverse Reactions: For External Use Only. Avoid contact with eyes. Peri-Care ointment is not toxic by oral ingestion and is not considered a primary eye or skin irritant under normal use conditions.
Dosage and Administration: Cleanse and rinse soiled perineal area thoroughly. Pat or air dry. Apply Peri-Care ointment liberally to perineal area to be protected. Repeat cleansing procedure promptly whenever discharge occurs and re-apply Peri-Care.
How Supplied: Unit dose packets, 2 oz. tubes, 2-oz. and 8-oz. jars.

PERI-WASH®
Perineal Area Cleanser

Description: A skin cleanser. A feces and urine emulsifier consisting of Water, TEA-Lauryl Sulfate, Amphoteric-2, Sodium Lauryl Sulfate, Propylene Glycol, Buffered with Hydrochloric Acid, PEG-75 Lanolin Oil, Vinylpyrrolidone/Styrene Copolymer, Quaternium-15, Methylbenzethonium Chloride, PEG-90M and FD&C Yellow #5. Normal skin pH. National Drug Code 11701-014.
Indications and Usage: Peri-Wash is used for daily care of the perineal area. It is indicated for cleansing of perineal areas afflicted with dermatitis and ammonia dermatitis associated with diarrhea. Through the process of emulsification, Peri-Wash makes the removal of fecal matter from the skin easier, thereby reducing the irritation and formation of denuded skin around the anus. Peri-Wash reduces or eliminates the ammonia odors from urine or feces. Peri-Wash cleanses peristomal skin. Used in ostomy appliances and urine collecting bags, it controls offensive odors. Additional uses for odor control: Cleaning bed pans, urinals, wheel chairs, soiled linens and garments, and hands.
Contraindications: Hypersensitivity to any components of the preparation.
Precautions and Adverse Reactions: For External Use Only. Peri-Wash is not toxic by oral ingestion and is not considered a primary skin irritant under normal use conditions. Peri-Wash is an eye irritant (Sodium Lauryl Sulfate) and should be rinsed thoroughly from eyes if accidental contact occurs.
Dosage and Administration: Apply liberally to perineal area. Wash and rinse thoroughly with clean warm water in the normal manner.
How Supplied: 4 fl. oz. and 8 fl. oz. bottles with spray fitment, in addition to larger bulk sizes.

PURI-CLENS™
(formerly Wound Depurant)
Wound Deodorizer and Cleanser

Description: Puri-Clens contains a safe and effective non-irritating antimicrobial ingredient, Methylbenzethonium Chloride, in a water washable, soothing base. National Drug Code (NDC) 11701-008.
Indications and Usage: Puri-Clens deodorizes wounds and aids in the removal of foreign materials and exudates. Will not delay wound healing.
Contraindications: Hypersensitivity to any components of the preparation.
Precautions and Adverse Reactions: For external use only. Do not use on animal bites or puncture wounds. Do not use for more than ten days without consulting physician. Keep this and all drugs out of the reach of children. Puri-Clens is not toxic by oral ingestion and is not considered a primary eye or skin irritant under normal use conditions.
Dosage and Administration: Apply Puri-Clens liberally to a sterile 4″ × 4″ pad. Gently and throughly cleanse wound and surrounding area. To aid in removing foreign material and exudates, dab wound carefully with clean 4″ × 4″ pad saturated with Puri-Clens. May be rinsed with sterile saline, water or hydrogen peroxide solution.
Deodorization: Apply Puri-Clens directly to wound and cover with a sterile absorbent pad. Do not use solution with occlusive dressing. Repeat one to three times daily as necessary to control odors.
How Supplied: 8 fl. oz bottles with flip top caps.

SURGI-KLEEN™
Skin cleanser and shampoo

Description: A skin cleanser consisting of Water, Sodium Lauryl Sulfate, TEA-Lauryl Sulfate, Amphoteric-2, Propylene Glycol, Buffered with Hydrochloric Acid, PEG-75 Lanolin Oil, Vinylpyrrolidone/Styrene Copolymer, Quaternium-15, Frangrance, Methylbenzethonium Chloride, PEG-90M, FD&C Yellow #5 and D&C Red #19. Normal skin pH. National Drug Code 11701-003
Indications and Usage: Surgi-Kleen, a gentle and effective liquid skin cleanser and shampoo replaces the need for all bar soap and shampoos. One container for both tasks! Containing a special refined lanolin, Surgi-Kleen helps retain a soft and supple skin. This easy-to-use, low sudsing liquid rinses free, leaving no residue or film on the skin or hair. The convenient flip-top helps reduce the incidence of cross contamination. Problem head and body odors are controlled when using this one versatile cleanser.
Contraindications: Hypersensitivity to any components of the preparation.
Precautions and Adverse Reactions: For External Use Only. Surgi-Kleen is not toxic by oral ingestion and is not considered a primary skin irritant under normal use conditions. Surgi-Kleen is an eye irritant (Sodium Lauryl Sulfate) and should be rinsed thoroughly from eyes if accidental contact occurs.
Dosage and Administration: Surgi-Kleen may be used full strength or diluted one part to three parts of water.
For Regular Bathing: Apply diluted product to moistened wash cloth and gently wash skin, rinse thoroughly and pat dry.
For Shampooing: Apply diluted or undiluted to moistened hair. Massage hair and scalp until lather develops. Then rinse thoroughly and lather again. A very small quantity of Surgi-Kleen will develop a thick, rich lather when hair is clean.
How Supplied: 8 fl. oz. and 16 fl. oz. bottles with flip-top caps, in addition to larger bulk sizes.

SWEEN CREAM®
Protective Cream

Description: A vanishing cream consisting of Water, Lanolin Oil, Cetyl Alcohol, Propylene Glycol, Natural Vitamins A & D, Sodium Lauryl Sulfate, Beeswax, BHT, Methylbenzethonium Chloride, Quaternium-15, and Fragrance. National Drug Code 11701-002.
Indications and Usage: Sween Cream is used for long-term care of incontinent, geriatric, ostomy, and para/quadraplegic skin. Apply as needed to red, sore, irritated skin such as urine scald, diaper rash, diarrheal breakdowns, rectal itch, psoriasis, minor burns, chaffing and itching. Also apply to folds of skin subject to perspiration irritation, to dry or cracked skin and to pressure sore areas. For

Continued on next page

Sween—Cont.

ostomy patients, apply a small amount around stoma area before attaching appliance to protect skin, relieve itching, and improve tape adhesion.
Contraindications: Hypersensitivity to any components of the preparation.
Precautions and Adverse Reactions: For External Use Only. Avoid contact with eyes. Sween Cream is not toxic by oral ingestion and is not considered a primary eye or skin irritant under normal use conditions.
Dosage and Administration: Apply liberally as required.
How Supplied: Unit dose packets, 2 oz. tubes, 2-oz. and 9-oz. jars.

WHIRL-SOL®
Skin Conditioner

Description: Mineral Oil, Propylene Glycol Dipelargonate, Lanolin Oil, PEG-8 Dioleate, Fragrance, D&C Green #6. National Drug Code 11701-001.
Indications and Usage: Whirl-Sol is a completely water dispersible oil easily absorbed by the skin to aid in the relief of dry, pruritic conditions. Whirl-Sol helps soothe and restore skin to a more elastic and pliable condition. It is an effective aid in treating skin problems such as soap dermatitis, pruritus senilis and hiemalis, chronic atopic dermatitis, asteatosis, xerosis, ichthyosis, psoriasis, etc. Whirl-Sol promotes a normal healthy skin with natural-like oils.
Contraindications: Hypersensitivity to any components of the preparation.
Precautions and Adverse Reactions: For External Use Only. Avoid contact with eyes. Whirl-Sol is not toxic by oral ingestion and is not considered a primary eye or skin irritant under normal use conditions. Guard against slipping in tub or shower.
Dosage and Administration: Whirl-Sol is always used with water. It is added, 6 to 10 sprays to whirlpool bathing systems, regular bath tubs, or wash basins. Apply to washcloth for use in the shower.
How Supplied: 8 fl. oz. and 16 fl. oz. bottles in addition to larger bulk sizes.

XTRACARE® II
Moisturizing Body Lotion

Description: A thick-bodied, high moisturizing cream consisting of Water, Cetyl Alcohol, Propylene Glycol, Lanolin Oil, Beeswax, Sodium Lauryl Sulfate, Quaternium-15, Fragrance and Methylbenzethonium Chloride. National Drug Code 11701-004.
Indications and Usage: Xtracare II is an unusually rich moisturizer which serves as an exceptional massage vehicle for the entire body. Its creamy consistency applies easily and uniformly to soothe and moisturize skin. The special emollient and humectant properties provide long lasting retardation of skin moisture evaporation. This leaves the skin feeling smooth, cool and comfortable without greasiness and tackiness or interference of normal skin respiration. Apply as needed for back rubs, dry skin problems and physical therapy. Especially suited for foot and lower leg care. Liberal application recommended before applying plaster casts.
Contraindications: Hypersensitivity to any components of the preparation.
Precautions and Adverse Reactions: For External Use Only. Avoid contact with eyes. Xtracare II in not toxic by oral ingestion and is not considered a primary eye or skin irritant under normal use conditions.
Dosage and Administration: Apply liberally as often as needed for dry skin management. Use as a massage lubricant for back rubs and for therapeutic muscle massage.
How Supplied: 4 fl. oz. and 8 fl. oz. bottles with dispenser caps, in addition to larger bulk sizes.

Syntex (F.P.) Inc.
HUMACAO, PUERTO RICO 00661

Syntex Laboratories, Inc
STANFORD INDUSTRIAL PARK
PALO ALTO, CA 94304

Syntex Puerto Rico, Inc.
HUMACAO, PUERTO RICO 00661

ANADROL®-50 ℞
(oxymetholone)
50 mg. Tablets

A product of Syntex Laboratories, Inc.

Description: Anadrol-50 contains 50 mg. of the steroid, oxymetholone, which has the chemical name 17 β-hydroxy-2-(hydroxymethylene)-17-methyl-5α-androstan-3-one.
Action: Anadrol-50 is a potent anabolic and androgenic drug. It enhances the production and urinary excretion of erythropoietin in patients with anemias due to bone marrow failure and often stimulates erythropoiesis in anemias due to deficient red cell production.
Indications: Anadrol-50 is indicated in the treatment of anemias caused by deficient red cell production. Acquired aplastic anemia, congenital aplastic anemia, myelofibrosis and the hypoplastic anemias due to the administration of myelotoxic drugs often respond. Anadrol-50 should not replace other supportive measures such as transfusion, correction of iron, folic acid, vitamin B_{12} or pyridoxine deficiency, antibacterial therapy and the appropriate use of corticosteroids.
Contraindications: Since anabolic agents are generally contraindicated in the following situations, before instituting therapy, the clinician must weigh the risk involved against the patients' needs.

1. Carcinoma of the prostate or breast in male patients.
2. Pregnancy—primarily because of masculinization of the fetus.
3. Infancy. Since evidence of beneficial effect in prematures and newborns is lacking, and consequences of the use of anabolic steroids in these patients are unknown, their use is not recommended.
4. Nephrosis or the nephrotic phase of nephritis.
5. Hypersensitivity.
6. Hepatic dysfunction.

Warnings: Anabolic steroids do not enhance athletic ability.
Precautions:
1. *Hepatotoxicity*
Hepatotoxic effects, including jaundice, are common with the prescribed dosage. Clinical jaundice may be painless, with or without pruritus. It may also be associated with acute hepatic enlargement and right-upper quadrant pain, which has been mistaken for acute (surgical) obstruction of the bile duct. Drug-induced jaundice is usually reversible when the medication is discontinued. Continued therapy has been associated with hepatic coma and death. Because of the hepatotoxicity associated with Anadrol-50 (oxymetholone) administration, periodic liver function tests are recommended. Hepatocellular carcinoma and peliosis hepatis,[1] a rare condition of ill-defined etiology consisting of blood-filled cysts in the liver, have been observed in patients with congenital and acquired aplastic anemia treated with oxymetholone and other androgens for prolonged periods. In some cases withdrawal of the drug has been associated with regression of the hepatic lesions.
2. *Virilization*
In the female virilization may occur. Amenorrhea usually occurs in the adult female, even in the presence of thrombocytopenia. Concomitant administration of large doses of progestational agents to control menorrhagia is not recommended.
3. *Iron deficiency*
The development of iron deficiency anemia, manifested by a low serum iron and decreased percent saturation of transferrin, has been observed in some patients treated with Anadrol-50 (oxymetholone). Periodic determination of the serum iron and iron binding capacity is recommended. If iron deficiency is detected, it should be appropriately treated with supplementary iron.
4. Leukemia has been observed in patients with aplastic anemia treated with oxymetholone. The role, if any, of oxymetholone is unclear because malignant transformation has been seen in blood dyscrasias and leukemia has been reported in patients with aplastic anemia who have not been treated with oxymetholone.
5. Caution is required in administering these agents to patients with cardiac, renal, or hepatic disease. Edema, with or without congestive heart failure, may occur occasionally. Concomitant administration with adrenal steroids or ACTH may add to the edema. This is generally controllable with appropriate diuretic and/or digitalis therapy.
6. Hypercalcemia may develop both spontaneously and as a result of hormonal therapy in women with disseminated breast carcinoma. If it develops while on this agent, the drug should be stopped.
7. Anabolic steroids may increase sensitivity to anticoagulants. Dosage of the anticoagulant may have to be decreased in order to maintain the prothrombin time at the desired therapeutic level.
8. Anabolic steroids have been shown to alter glucose tolerance tests. Diabetics should be followed carefully and the insulin or oral hypoglycemic dosage adjusted accordingly.
9. Anabolic steroids should be used with caution in patients with benign prostatic hypertrophy.
10. Serum cholesterol may increase or decrease during therapy. Therefore, caution is required in administering these agents to patients with a history of myocardial infarction or coronary artery disease. Serial determinations of serum cholesterol should be made and therapy adjusted accordingly.

Adverse Reactions:
1. *Hepatotoxicity* is the most serious adverse reaction associated with anabolic steroid therapy. Reversible increase in BSP retention occurs early and appears to be directly related to the dose. Increase in serum bilirubin, with or without an increase in the serum alkaline phosphatase and transaminases (SGOT and SGPT) indicate a higher degree of excretory dysfunction. Clinical jaundice, which is reversible when the drug is discontinued, may occur. The histologic picture is one of intrahepatic cholestasis with little or no cellular damage. Continued therapy may be associated with hepatic coma and death.
2. Virilization is the most common undesirable effect associated with anabolic steroid therapy. Acne occurs frequently in all age groups.
Prepuberal male: The first signs of virilization in the prepuberal male are phallic enlargement and an increase in frequency of erection. Hirsutism and increased skin pigmentation may also occur.
Postpuberal male: Inhibition of testicular function with oligospermia: decrease in seminal volume, alteration in libido, and impotence may occur with prolonged or intensive anabolic therapy. Gynecomastia, and testicular atrophy may occur. Chronic priapism, male-pat-

tern of hair loss, epididymitis and bladder irritability have been reported. In females, hirsutism, hoarseness or deepening of the voice, clitoral enlargement, alteration of libido, and menstrual irregularities and male-pattern baldness may occur. The voice change and clitoral enlargement are usually irreversible even after prompt discontinuance of therapy. The use of estrogens in combination with androgens will not prevent virilization in females.

3. Other adverse reactions associated with anabolic/androgenic therapy include: muscle cramps, nausea, excitation and sleeplessness, chills, bleeding in patients on concomitant anticoagulant therapy, premature closure of epiphyses in children, vomiting and diarrhea.

4. Alterations in these clinical laboratory tests:

a. The metyrapone test
b. The FBS and glucose tolerance test
c. The thyroid function tests: a decrease in the PBI, in thyroxine-binding capacity and radioactive iodine uptake and an increase in T^3 uptake by the rbc's or resin may occur. Free thyroxine is normal. Altered tests usually persist for 2-3 weeks after stopping anabolic therapy.
d. The electrolytes: retention of sodium, chlorides, water, potassium, phosphates and calcium.
e. Increased or decreased serum cholesterol.
f. Suppression of clotting factors II, V, VII, and X.
g. Increased creatine and creatinine excretion lasting up to two weeks after discontinuing therapy.
h. Decreased 17-ketosteroid excretion.

5. There have been rare reports of hepato cellular neoplasms and peliosis hepatis in association with long-term androgenic-anabolic steroid therapy.

Dosage and Administration: The recommended daily dose in children and adults, 1-5 mg./kg. body weight per day. The usual effective dose is 1-2 mg./kg./day but higher doses may be required and the dose should be individualized. Response is not often immediate and a minimum trial of three to six months should be given. Following remission, some patients may be maintained without the drug; others may be maintained on an established lower daily dosage. A continued maintenance dose is usually necessary in patients with congenital aplastic anemia.

Availability: Anadrol-50 (oxymetholone) is available in bottles of 100 white scored tablets imprinted with the code "2902" and "Syntex".

[1]Zak, F. G., Peliosis Hepatis. Am. J. Path. 26:1-15, (Jan.) 1950.

[*Shown in Product Identification Section*]

ANAPROX® ℞
(naproxen sodium)
275 mg Tablets

Manufactured for Syntex Laboratories, Inc. by Syntex Puerto Rico, Inc.

Description: ANAPROX filmcoated tablets for oral administration each contain 275 mg of naproxen sodium, which is equivalent to 250 mg naproxen with 25 mg (about 1mEq) sodium. It is a member of the arylacetic acid group of nonsteroidal anti-inflammatory drugs.

The chemical name of naproxen sodium is 2-naphthaleneacetic acid, 6-methoxy-α-methyl-, sodium salt, (−). Naproxen sodium is a white to creamy white, crystalline solid, freely soluble in water.

Clinical Pharmacology: ANAPROX, the sodium salt of naproxen, has been developed as an analgesic because it is more rapidly absorbed. Naproxen is a nonsteroidal anti-inflammatory drug with analgesic and antipyretic properties. Naproxen anion inhibits prostaglandin synthesis but beyond this its mode of action is unknown.

Naproxen sodium is rapidly and completely absorbed from the gastrointestinal tract. After administration of naproxen sodium, peak plasma levels of naproxen anion are attained at 1-2 hours with steady-state conditions normally achieved after 4-5 doses. The mean biological half-life of the anion in humans is approximately 13 hours, and at therapeutic levels it is greater than 99% albumin bound. Approximately 95% of the dose is excreted in the urine, primarily as naproxen, 6-0-desmethyl naproxen or their conjugates. The rate of excretion has been found to coincide closely with the rate of drug disappearance from the plasma. The drug does not induce metabolizing enzymes.

The drug was studied in patients with mild to moderate pain, and pain relief was obtained within 1 hour. It is not a narcotic and is not a CNS-acting drug. Controlled double-blind studies have demonstrated the analgesic properties of the drug in, for example, post-operative, post-partum, orthopedic and uterine contraction pain and dysmenorrhea. In dysmenorrheic patients, the drug reduces the level of prostaglandins in the uterus, which correlates with a reduction in the frequency and severity of uterine contractions. Analgesic action has been shown by such measures as reduction of pain intensity scores, increase in pain relief scores, decrease in numbers of patients requiring additional analgesic medication, and delay in time for required remedication. The analgesic effect has been found to last for up to 7 hours.

The drug was studied in patients with rheumatoid arthritis, osteoarthritis, juvenile arthritis, ankylosing spondylitis and acute gout. It is not a corticosteroid. Improvement in patients treated for rheumatoid arthritis has been demonstrated by a reduction in joint swelling, a reduction in pain, a reduction in duration of morning stiffness, a reduction in disease activity as assessed by both the investigator and patient, and by increased mobility as demonstrated by a reduction in walking time.

In patients with osteoarthritis, the therapeutic action of the drug has been shown by a reduction in joint pain or tenderness, an increase in range of motion in knee joints, increased mobility as demonstrated by a reduction in walking time, and improvement in capacity to perform activities of daily living impaired by the disease.

In clinical studies in patients with rheumatoid arthritis, osteoarthritis and juvenile arthritis, the drug has been shown to be comparable to aspirin and indomethacin in controlling the aforementioned measures of disease activity, but the frequency and severity of the milder gastrointestinal adverse effects (nausea, dyspepsia, heartburn) and nervous system adverse effects (tinnitus, dizziness, lightheadedness) were less than in both the aspirin- and indomethacin-treated patients. It is not known whether the drug causes less peptic ulceration than aspirin.

In patients with ankylosing spondylitis, the drug has been shown to decrease night pain, morning stiffness and pain at rest. In double-blind studies the drug was shown to be as effective as aspirin, but with fewer side effects.

In patients with acute gout, a favorable response to the drug was shown by significant clearing of inflammatory changes (e.g., decrease in swelling, heat) within 24-48 hours, as well as by relief of pain and tenderness.

The drug may be used safely in combination with gold salts and/or corticosteroids; however, in controlled clinical trials, when added to the regimen of patients receiving corticosteroids it did not appear to cause greater improvement over that seen with corticosteroids alone. Whether the drug could be used in conjunction with partially effective doses of corticosteroid for a "steroid-sparing" effect has not been adequately studied. When added to the regimen of patients receiving gold salts, the drug did result in greater improvement. Its use in combination with salicylates is not recommended because data are inadequate to demonstrate that the drug produces greater improvement over that achieved with aspirin alone. Further, there is some evidence that aspirin increases the rate of excretion of the drug.

Generally, improvement due to the drug has not been found to be dependent on age, sex, severity or duration of disease.

In ^{51}Cr blood loss and gastroscopy studies with normal volunteers, daily administration of 1100 mg of ANAPROX (naproxen sodium) has been demonstrated to cause statistically significantly less gastric bleeding and erosion than 3250 mg of aspirin.

Indications and Usage: ANAPROX® (naproxen sodium) is indicated in the relief of mild to moderate pain and for the treatment of primary dysmenorrhea.

It is also indicated for the treatment of the signs and symptoms of mild to moderately severe, acute or chronic, musculoskeletal and soft tissue inflammation.

Pediatric dosage forms have not been established for ANAPROX.

Contraindications: Naproxen sodium is contraindicated in patients who have shown hypersensitivity to it. Because the potential exists for cross-sensitivity reactions, it should not be given to patients in whom aspirin or other non-steroidal anti-inflammatory drugs induce the syndrome of asthma, rhinitis, or urticaria.

Warnings: Gastrointestinal bleeding, sometimes severe, and occasionally fatal, has been reported in patients receiving the drug. Among 960 patients treated for rheumatoid arthritis or osteoarthritis during the course of clinical trials in the United States (260 treated for more than two years), 16 cases of peptic ulceration were reported. More than half were on concomitant corticosteroid and/or salicylate therapy and about a third had a prior history of peptic ulcer. Gastrointestinal bleeding, including nine potentially serious cases, was also reported in this population. These were not always preceded by premonitory gastrointestinal symptoms. Although most of the patients with serious bleeding were receiving concomitant therapy and had a history of peptic ulcer disease, it should be kept in mind that the drug also has the potential for causing gastrointestinal bleeding on its own. Therefore, it should be administered to patients with active gastric and duodenal ulcers only under close supervision.

Precautions:
General:
***ANAPROX®* (NAPROXEN SODIUM) SHOULD NOT BE USED CONCOMITANTLY WITH THE RELATED DRUG *NAPROSYN®* (NAPROXEN) SINCE THEY BOTH CIRCULATE IN PLASMA AS THE NAPROXEN ANION.**

In chronic studies in laboratory animals, the drug has caused nephritis. Glomerular nephritis, interstitial nephritis and nephrotic syndrome have been reported in humans. This drug should therefore be used with great caution in patients with significantly impaired renal function and the monitoring of serum creatinine and/or creatinine clearance is advised in these patients.

As with other nonsteroidal anti-inflammatory drugs borderline elevations of one or more liver tests may occur in up to 15% of patients. These abnormalities may progress, may remain essentially unchanged, or may be transient with continued therapy. The SGPT (AST) test is probably the most sensitive indicator of liver dysfunction. Meaningful (3 times the upper limit of normal) elevations of SGPT or SGOT (AST) occurred in controlled clinical trials in less than 1% of patients. A patient

Continued on next page

Syntex—Cont.

with symptoms and/or signs suggesting liver dysfunction, or in whom an abnormal liver test has occurred, should be evaluated for evidence of the development of more severe hepatic reactions while on therapy with this drug. Severe hepatic reactions, including jaundice and cases of fatal hepatitis, have been reported with this drug as with other nonsteroidal anti-inflammatory drugs. Although such reactions are rare, if abnormal liver tests persist or worsen, if clinical signs and symptoms consistent with liver disease develop, or if systemic manifestations occur (e.g. eosinophilia, rash, etc.), this drug should be discontinued.

If steroid dosage is reduced or eliminated during therapy, the steroid dosage should be reduced slowly and the patients must be observed closely for any evidence of adverse effects, including adrenal insufficiency and exacerbation of symptoms of arthritis.

Patients with initial hemoglobin values of 10 grams or less who are to receive long-term therapy should have hemoglobin values determined frequently.

Peripheral edema has been observed in some patients. Since each naproxen sodium tablet contains approximately 25 mg (about 1 mEq) of sodium, this should be considered in patients whose overall intake of sodium must be markedly restricted. For these reasons, the drug should be used with caution in patients with fluid retention, hypertension or heart failure.

The antipyretic and anti-inflammatory activities of the drug may reduce fever and inflammation, thus diminishing their utility as diagnostic signs in detecting complications of presumed non-infectious, non-inflammatory painful conditions. Because of adverse eye findings in animal studies with drugs of this class it is recommended that ophthalmic studies be carried out within a reasonable period of time after starting therapy and at periodic intervals thereafter if the drug is to be used for an extended period of time.

Information for Patients:

Caution should be exercised by patients whose activities require alertness if they experience drowsiness, dizziness, vertigo or depression during therapy with the drug.

Drug Interactions:

In vitro studies have shown that naproxen anion, because of its affinity for protein, may displace from their binding sites other drugs which are also albumin-bound. Theoretically, the naproxen anion itself could likewise be displaced. Short-term controlled studies failed to show that taking the drug significantly affects prothrombin times when administered to individuals on coumarin-type anticoagulants. Caution is advised nonetheless, since interactions have been seen with other nonsteroidal agents of this class. Similarly, patients receiving the drug and a hydantoin, sulfonamide or sulfonylurea should be observed for signs of toxicity to these drugs.

Probenecid given concurrently increases naproxen anion plasma levels and extends its plasma half-life significantly.

Drug/Laboratory Test Interactions:

The drug may decrease platelet aggregation and prolong bleeding time. This effect should be kept in mind when bleeding times are determined.

The administration of the drug may result in increased urinary values for 17-ketogenic steroids because of an interaction between the drug and/or its metabolites with m-dinitrobenzene used in this assay. Although 17-hydroxy-corticosteroid measurements (Porter-Silber test) do not appear to be artifactually altered, it is suggested that therapy with the drug be temporarily discontinued 72 hours before adrenal function tests are performed.

The drug may interfere with some urinary assays of 5-hydroxy indoleacetic acid (5HIAA).

Carcinogenesis:

A two-year study was performed in rats to evaluate the carcinogenic potential of the drug. No evidence of carcinogenicity was found.

Pregnancy:

Teratogenic Effects: Pregnancy Category B. Reproduction studies have been performed in rats, rabbits and mice at doses up to six times the human dose and have revealed no evidence of impaired fertility or harm to the fetus due to the drug. There are, however, no adequate and well-controlled studies in pregnant women. Because animal reproduction studies are not always predictive of human response, the drug should not be used during pregnancy unless clearly needed. Because of the known effect of drugs of this class on the human fetal cardiovascular system (closure of ductus arteriosus), use during late pregnancy should be avoided.

Non-teratogenic Effects: As with other drugs known to inhibit prostaglandin synthesis, an increased incidence of dystocia and delayed parturition occurred in rats.

Nursing Mothers:

The naproxen anion has been found in the milk of lactating women at a concentration of approximately 1% of that found in the plasma. Because of the possible adverse effects of prostaglandin-inhibiting drugs on neonates, use in nursing mothers should be avoided.

Pediatric Use:

Pediatric dosage forms have not been established for ANAPROX® (naproxen sodium).

Adverse Reactions: Adverse reactions reported in controlled clinical trials in 960 patients treated for rheumatoid arthritis or osteoarthritis are listed below. In general, these reactions were reported 2 to 10 times more frequently than they were in studies in the 962 patients treated for mild to moderate pain or for dysmenorrhea.

Incidence greater than 1%

Gastrointestinal: The most frequent complaints reported related to the gastrointestinal tract. They were: constipation*, heartburn*, abdominal pain*, nausea*, dyspepsia, diarrhea, stomatitis. **Central Nervous System:** Headache*, dizziness*, drowsiness*, lightheadedness, vertigo. **Dermatologic:** Itching (pruritus)*, skin eruptions*, ecchymoses*, sweating, purpura. **Special Senses:** Tinnitus*, hearing disturbances, visual disturbances. **Cardiovascular:** Edema*, dyspnea*, palpitations. **General:** Thirst.

* Incidence of reported reaction between 3% and 9%. Those reactions occurring in less than 3% of the patients are unmarked.

Incidence less than 1%

Probable Causal Relationship:

The following adverse reactions were reported less frequently than 1% during controlled clinical trials and through voluntary reports since marketing. The probability of a causal relationship exists between the drug and these adverse reactions: congestive heart failure, renal disease, glomerular nephritis, interstitial nephritis, nephrotic syndrome, abnormal liver function tests, hematuria, jaundice, thrombocytopenia, leukopenia, granulocytopenia, gastrointestinal bleeding, peptic ulceration with bleeding and/or perforation, hematemesis, melena, vomiting, eosinophilia, pyrexia (chills and fever), skin rashes, menstrual disorders, myalgia and muscle weakness, alopecia, inability to concentrate, depression, malaise, dream abnormalities.

Causal Relationship Unknown:

Other reactions have been reported in circumstances in which a causal relationship could not be established. However, in these rarely reported events, the possibility cannot be excluded. Therefore these observations are being listed to serve as alerting information to the physicians: angioneurotic edema, agranulocytosis, aplastic anemia, hemolytic anemia, hypoglycemia, hyperglycemia, urticaria.

Overdosage: Significant overdosage may be characterized by drowsiness, heartburn, indigestion, nausea or vomiting. Because naproxen sodium may be rapidly absorbed, high and early blood levels should be anticipated. No evidence of toxicity or late sequelae have been reported 5 to 15 months after ingestion for three to seven days of doses equivalent to up to 3,300 mg of naproxen sodium. One patient ingested a single dose equivalent to 27.5 g of naproxen sodium and experienced mild nausea and indigestion. It is not known what dose of the drug would be life threatening. The oral LD_{50} of the drug is 543 mg/kg in rats, 1234 mg/kg in mice, 4110 mg/kg in hamsters and greater than 1000 mg/kg in dogs.

Should a patient ingest a large number of tablets, accidentally or purposefully, the stomach may be emptied and usual supportive measures employed. Animal studies suggest that the prompt administration of 5 grams of activated charcoal would tend to reduce markedly the absorption of the drug. It is not known if the drug is dialyzable.

Dosage and Administration:

For Mild to Moderate Pain and Primary Dysmenorrhea:

The recommended starting dose is two 275 mg tablets, followed by one 275 mg tablet every 6 to 8 hours, as required. The total daily dose should not exceed 5 tablets (1,375 mg).

For Mild to Moderately Severe, Acute or Chronic, Musculoskeletal and Soft Tissue Inflammation:

The recommended starting dose in adults is one 275 mg tablet twice daily (morning and evening) or one 275 mg tablet in the morning and two 275 mg tablets in the evening. During long-term administration, the dose may be adjusted up or down depending on the clinical response of the patient. A lower daily dose may suffice for long-term administration. Daily doses higher than 1100 mg in these indications have not been studied. The morning and evening doses do not have to be equal in size and the administration of the drug more frequently than twice daily is not necessary. Symptomatic improvement in arthritis usually begins within two weeks. However, if improvement is not seen within this period, a trial for an additional two weeks should be considered.

For Acute Gout:

The recommended starting dose is three 275 mg tablets, followed by one 275 mg tablet every eight hours until the attack has subsided.

How Supplied: ANAPROX® (naproxen sodium) is available in filmcoated tablets of 275 mg (light blue), in bottles of 100 tablets (NDC 18393-274-42) and 500 tablets (NDC 18393-274-62) or in cartons of 100 individually blister packed tablets (NDC 18393-274-53). Store at room temperature in well-closed containers.

[*Shown in Product Identification Section*]

BREVICON® ℞
(norethindrone with ethinyl estradiol)
Tablets

NORINYL® 1 + 35 Tablets ℞
(norethindrone with ethinyl estradiol)

NORINYL® 1 + 50 Tablets ℞
(norethindrone with mestranol)

NORINYL® 1 + 80 Tablets ℞
(norethindrone with mestranol)

NORINYL® 2 mg. Tablets ℞
(norethindrone with mestranol)

NOR–Q.D.® ℞
(norethindrone)
Tablets 0.35 mg.
Oral Contraceptives

Products of Syntex (F.P.) Inc.

Description: **BREVICON 21-DAY** Tablets provide an oral contraceptive regimen consisting of 21 blue tablets containing norethindrone 0.5 mg. with ethinyl estradiol 0.035 mg.
BREVICON 28-DAY Tablets provide a continuous oral contraceptive regimen consisting of 21 blue tablets containing norethindrone 0.5 mg. with ethinyl estradiol 0.035 mg. and 7 orange tablets containing inert ingredients.
NORINYL 1 + 35 21-DAY Tablets provide an oral contraceptive regimen consisting of 21 green tablets containing norethindrone 1 mg. with ethinyl estradiol 0.035 mg.
NORINYL 1 + 35 28-DAY Tablets provide a continuous oral contraceptive regimen consisting of 21 green tablets containing norethindrone 1 mg. with ethinyl estradiol 0.035 mg. and 7 orange tablets containing inert ingredients.
NORINYL 1 + 50 21-DAY Tablets provide an oral contraceptive regimen consisting of 21 white tablets containing norethindrone 1 mg. with mestranol 0.05 mg.
NORINYL 1 + 50 28-DAY Tablets provide a continuous oral contraceptive regimen consisting of 21 white tablets containing norethindrone 1 mg. with mestranol 0.05 mg. and 7 orange tablets containing inert ingredients.
NORINYL 1 + 80 21-DAY Tablets provide an oral contraceptive regimen consisting of 21 yellow tablets containing norethindrone 1 mg. with mestranol 0.08 mg.
NORINYL 1 + 80 28-DAY Tablets provide a continuous oral contraceptive regimen consisting of 21 yellow tablets containing norethindrone 1 mg. with mestranol 0.08 mg. and 7 orange tablets containing inert ingredients.
NORINYL 2 mg. Tablets provide an oral contraceptive regimen consisting of 20 white tablets containing norethindrone 2 mg. and mestranol 0.1 mg.
NOR-Q.D. (norethindrone) Tablets provide a continuous oral contraceptive regimen of one yellow norethindrone 0.35 mg. tablet daily.
Norethindrone is a potent progestational agent with the chemical name 17-hydroxy-19-nor-17α-pregn-4-en-20-yn-3-one. Ethinyl estradiol is an estrogen with the chemical name 19-nor-17α-pregna-1, 3, 5(10) -trien-20-yne-3, 17-diol. Mestranol is an estrogen with the chemical name 3-methoxy-19-nor-17α-pregna-1, 3, 5(10) -trien-20-yn-17-ol.
Clinical Pharmacology: Combination oral contraceptives act primarily through the mechanism of gonadotrophin suppression due to the estrogenic and progestational activity of the ingredients. Although the primary mechanism of action is inhibition of ovulation, alterations in the genital tract including changes in the cervical mucus (which increase the difficulty of sperm penetration) and the endometrium (which reduce the likelihood of implantation) may also contribute to contraceptive effectiveness.
The primary mechanism through which NOR-Q.D. prevents conception is not known, but progestogen-only contraceptives are known to alter the cervical mucus, exert a progestational effect on the endometrium, interfering with implantation, and, in some patients, suppress ovulation.
Indications and Usage: Oral contraceptives are indicated for the prevention of pregnancy in women who elect to use oral contraceptives as a method of contraception. NORINYL 2 mg. is also indicated in the treatment of hypermenorrhea.
Oral contraceptives are highly effective. The pregnancy rate in women using conventional combination oral contraceptives (containing 35 mcg. or more of ethinyl estradiol or 50 mcg. or more of mestranol) is generally reported as less than one pregnancy per 100 woman-years of use. Slightly higher rates (somewhat more than 1 pregnancy per 100 woman-years of use) are reported for some combination products containing 35 mcg. or less of ethinyl estradiol, and rates on the order of 3 pregnancies per 100 woman-years are reported for the progestogen-only oral contraceptives.
These rates are derived from separate studies conducted by different investigators in several population groups and cannot be compared precisely. Furthermore, pregnancy rates tend to be lower as clinical studies are continued, possibly due to selective retention in the longer studies of those patients who accept the treatment regimen and do not discontinue as a result of adverse reactions, pregnancy, or other reasons.
In clinical trials with BREVICON, 1,168 patients completed 16,345 cycles and a total of 3 pregnancies was reported. This represents a pregnancy rate of 0.22 per 100 woman-years. In clinical trials with NORINYL 1 + 35, 940 patients completed 14,366 cycles and a total of 2 pregnancies was reported. This represents a pregnancy rate of 0.17 per 100 woman-years. The dropout rate for medical reasons, as observed in the clinical trials conducted with BREVICON and NORINYL 1 + 35, appears to be somewhat higher than observed with higher dose combination products. The dropout rate due to menstrual disorders and irregularities was also somewhat higher, dropouts being equally split between menstrual disorders and irregularities and other medical reasons attributable to the drug.
In clinical trials with NORINYL 1 + 50 21-DAY, 3,852 patients completed 45,937 cycles and a total of 10 pregnancies was reported. This represents a pregnancy rate of 0.26 per 100 woman-years. In clinical trials with NORINYL 1 + 50 28-DAY, 1,590 patients completed 7,330 cycles and a total of 3 pregnancies was reported. This represents a pregnancy rate of 0.5 per 100 woman-years. In clinical trials with NORINYL 1 + 80 21- and 28-DAY, 3,464 patients completed 34,068 cycles and a total of 5 pregnancies was reported. This represents a pregnancy rate of 0.18 per 100 woman-years. In clinical trials with NORINYL 2 mg. 6,097 patients completed 121,233 cycles and a total of 13 pregnancies was reported. This represents a pregnancy rate of 0.13 per 100 woman-years. In clinical trials with NOR-Q.D. (norethindrone) 2,963 patients completed 25,901 cycles of therapy and a total of 55 pregnancies was reported. This represents an average pregnancy rate of 2.54 per 100 woman-years. A higher pregnancy rate of 3.72 was recorded in "fresh" patients (those who had never taken oral contraceptives prior to starting NOR-Q.D. therapy) to a large extent because of incorrect tablet intake. This compares to the lower pregnancy rate of 1.95 recorded in "changeover" patients (those switched from other oral contraceptives). This difference was found to be statistically significant. Furthermore, an even greater statistically significant difference in pregnancy rates between these two groups was found during the first six months of NOR-Q.D. therapy. Therefore, it is especially important for "fresh" patients to strictly adhere to the regimen.
Table 1 gives ranges of pregnancy rates reported in the literature[1] for other means of contraception. The efficacy of these means of contraception (except the IUD) depends upon the degree of adherence to the method.
TABLE 1. *Pregnancies per 100 Woman-Years*
IUD, less than 1–6;
Diaphragm with spermicidal products (creams or jellies), 2–20;
Condom, 3–36;
Aerosol foams, 2–29;
Jellies and creams, 4–36;
Periodic abstinence (rhythm) all types, less than 1–47;
—Calendar method, 14–47;
—Temperature method, 1–20;
—Temperature method—intercourse only in post-ovulatory phase, less than 1–7;
—Mucus method, 1–25;
No contraception, 60–80.
Dose-Related Risk of Thromboembolism From Oral Contraceptives. Studies have shown a positive association between the dose of estrogens in oral contraceptives and the risk of thromboembolism[2,3,81,82]. For this reason, it is prudent and in keeping with good principles of therapeutics to minimize exposure to estrogen. The oral contraceptive product prescribed for any given patient should be that product which contains the least amount of estrogen that is compatible with an acceptable pregnancy rate and patient acceptance. It is recommended that new acceptors of oral contraceptives should be started on preparations containing 0.05 mg or less of estrogen.
Contraindications:
1. Known or suspected pregnancy (see Warning No. 5).
2. Undiagnosed abnormal genital bleeding.
3. Oral contraceptives should not be used by women who have or have had any of the following conditions:
   a. Thrombophlebitis or thromboembolic disorders.
   b. Cerebral vascular or coronary artery disease, including myocardial infarction.
   c. Known or suspected carcinoma of the breast.
   d. Known or suspected estrogen dependent neoplasia.
   e. Benign or malignant liver tumor which developed during the use of oral contraceptives or other estrogen containing products.
4. Diplopia or any ocular lesion arising from ophthalmic vascular disease (see Warning No. 2).
5. During the period a mother is breast feeding (see Warning No. 13).
6. Classical migraine.
7. Active liver disease.
8. History of cholestatic jaundice.

Warnings:

Cigarette smoking increases the risk of serious cardiovascular side effects from oral contraceptive use. This risk increases with age and with heavy smoking (15 or more cigarettes per day) and is quite marked in women over 35 years of age. Women who use oral contraceptives should be strongly advised not to smoke.

The use of oral contraceptives is associated with increased risk of several serious conditions including thromboembolism, stroke, myocardial infarction, liver tumor, gall bladder disease, visual disturbances, fetal abnormalities, and hypertension. Practitioners prescribing oral contracep-

Continued on next page

Syntex—Cont.

tives should be familiar with the following information relating to these risks.

1. *Thromboembolic Disorders and Other Vascular Problems:* An increased risk of thromboembolic and thrombotic disease associated with the use of oral contraceptives is well established. One British study[4] demonstrated an increased relative risk for fatal venous thromboembolism, several British[5,6,11,20,72] and three American[3,7,8,21] studies demonstrated an increased relative risk for non-fatal venous thromboembolism. These studies estimate that users of oral contraceptives are 4 to 11 times more likely than nonusers to develop these diseases without evident cause (Table 2). An analysis of deaths in one British study[73] reported an excess death rate of 40% in oral contraceptive users, most of which resulted from cardiovascular disease. A somewhat similar British study[74] showed a lower death rate in oral contraceptive users than controls; here an increase in cardiovascular deaths was seen although the findings were not statistically significant. A U.S. prospective study[75] failed to disclose increased mortality rates from cardiovascular disorders. However, a selected subset of this study, analyzed as a retrospective, case-control study[76] showed significant increases in venous thromboembolism.

Cerebrovascular Disorders. Two American studies[7,9,10] demonstrated an increased relative risk for stroke, which had not been shown in prior British studies[4–6]. In a collaborative American study[9,10] of cerebrovascular disorders in women with and without predisposing causes, it was estimated that the relative risk of hemorrhagic stroke was 2.0 times greater in users than nonusers and the relative risk of thrombotic stroke was 4 to 9.5 times greater in users than in nonusers (Table 2). A British long-term, follow-up study[11] reported in 1976 a highly significant association between oral contraceptive use and stroke. Another British long-term, follow-up study[12] had suggested such an association in 1974, but the number of cases was too small to estimate the risk. Subarachnoid hemorrhage has been shown to be increased by oral contraceptive use in British[73] and American studies[75,77]. Smoking alone increases the incidence of these accidents and smoking and pill use appear to work together to produce a combined risk greater than either alone.

Myocardial Infarction. An increased relative risk of myocardial infarction associated with the use of oral contraceptives has been reported[13–15], confirming a previously suspected association[4]. One study[14,15] conducted in the United Kingdom found, as expected, that the greater the number of underlying risk factors for coronary artery disease (cigarette smoking, hypertension, hypercholesterolemia, obesity, diabetes, history of preeclamptic toxemia) the higher the risk of developing myocardial infarction, regardless of whether the patient was an oral contraceptive user or not. Oral contraceptives, however, were found to be an additional risk factor.

In terms of relative risk, it has been estimated[16,17] that oral contraceptive users who do not smoke (smoking is considered a major predisposing condition to myocardial infarction) are about twice as likely to have a fatal myocardial infarction as nonusers who do not smoke. Oral contraceptive users who are also smokers have about a 5-fold increased risk of fatal infarction compared to users who do not smoke, and about a 10- to 12-fold increased risk compared to nonusers who do not smoke. Furthermore, the number of cigarettes smoked is also an important factor. In determining the importance of these relative risks, however, the baseline rates for various age groups, as shown in Table 3, must be given serious consideration. (The estimates in Table 3 are based on British vital statistics which show acute myocardial infarction death rate 2- to 3-times less than in the U.S. for women in these age groups; consequently, actual U.S. death rates could be higher than those in Table 3[17].) The importance of other predisposing conditions mentioned above in determining relative and absolute risks has not been quantified; other synergistic actions may exist.

TABLE 2. *Summary of relative risk of thromboembolic disorders and other vascular problems in oral contraceptive users compared to nonusers*

	Relative risk, times greater
Idiopathic thromboembolic disease	4–11
Post surgery thromboembolic complications	4–6
Thrombotic stroke	4–9.5
Hemorrhagic stroke	2
Myocardial infarction	2–12
Subarachnoid hemorrhage	6–22

TABLE 3. *Estimated[16] annual mortality rate per 100,000 women from myocardial infarction by use of oral contraceptives, smoking habits, and age (in years)*

	Myocardial infarction			
	Women aged 30–39		Women aged 40–44	
Smoking habits	Users	Non-users	Users	Non-users
All smokers	10.2	2.6	62.0	15.9
Heavy*	13.0	5.1	78.7	31.3
Light	4.7	0.9	28.6	5.7
Nonsmokers	1.8	1.2	10.7	7.4
Smokers and nonsmokers	5.4	1.9	32.8	11.7

*Heavy smoker: 15 or more cigarettes per day.

Risk of Dose. In an analysis of data derived from several national adverse reaction reporting systems[2], British investigators concluded that the risk of thromboembolism including coronary thrombosis is directly related to the dose of estrogen used in oral contraceptives. Preparations containing 0.1 mg or more of estrogen were associated with a higher risk of thromboembolism than those containing 0.05–0.08 mg of estrogen. Their analysis did suggest, however, that the quantity of estrogen may not be the sole factor involved. This finding has been supported by a study in the United States[3]. A subsequent study in Great Britain[81] found a positive association between dose of progestogen or estrogen and certain thromboembolic conditions. Swedish authorities[82] noted decreased reporting of thromboembolic episodes when higher estrogen preparations were no longer prescribed. Careful epidemiological studies to determine the degree of thromboembolic risk associated with progestogen-only oral contraceptives have not been performed. Cases of thromboembolic disease have been reported in women using these products, and they should not be presumed to be free of excess risk.

Estimate of Excess Mortality from Circulatory Diseases. A large British prospective study[12,18] estimated[18] the mortality rate per 100,000 women per year from diseases of the circulatory system for users and nonusers of oral contraceptives according to age, smoking habits, and duration of use. The overall excess death rate annually from circulatory diseases for oral contraceptive users was estimated to be 20 per 100,000 (ages 15–34—5/100,000; ages 35–44—33/100,000; ages 45–49—140/100,000). The risk is concentrated in older women, in those with a long duration of use, and in cigarette smokers, and may persist after discontinuation of oral contraceptive use. It was not possible, however, to examine the interrelationships of age, smoking, and duration of use, nor to compare the effects of continuous vs. intermittent use. Although the study showed a 10-fold increase in death due to circulatory diseases in users for 5 or more years, all of these deaths occurred in women 35 or older. An update of this study[73] provided the following rates: ages 15-34—1/6700 for non-smokers and 1/2000 for smokers; ages 45 and over—1/2500 for non-smokers and 1/500 for smokers.

Risk appeared to increase with parity, but not with duration of use. Until larger numbers of women under 35 with continuous use for 5 or more years are available, it is not possible to assess the magnitude of the relative risk for this younger age group.

The available data from a variety of sources have been analyzed[19] to estimate the risk of death associated with various methods of contraception. The estimates of risk of death for each method include the combined risk of the contraceptive method (e.g., thromboembolic and thrombotic disease in the case of oral contraceptives) plus the risk attributable to pregnancy or abortion in the event of method failure. This latter risk varies with the effectiveness of the contraceptive method.

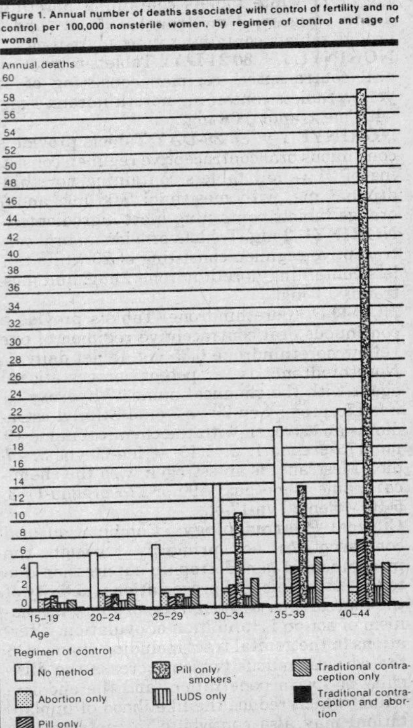

Figure 1. Annual number of deaths associated with control of fertility and no control per 100,000 nonsterile women, by regimen of control and age of woman

The findings of this analysis are shown in Figure 1 below[19]. The study concluded that the mortality associated with all methods of birth control is low and below that of childbirth, with the exception of oral contraceptives in women over 40 who smoke. (The rates given for pill only/smokers for each age group are for smokers as a class. For "heavy" smokers (more than 15 cigarettes a day), the rates given would be about double; for "light" smokers (less than 15 cigarettes a day), about 50 percent.) The lowest mortality is associated with the condom or diaphragm backed up by early abortion. The study also concluded that oral contraceptive users who smoke, especially those over the age of 30, have a greater mortality risk than oral contraceptive users who do not smoke.

The risk of thromboembolic and thrombotic disease associated with oral contraceptives increases with age after approximately age 30 and, for myocardial infarction, is further increased by hypertension, hyperlipidemias, obesity, diabetes, or history of preeclamptic toxemia and especially by cigarette smoking[16,17].

Based on the data currently available, the following chart gives a gross estimate of the risk of death from circulatory disorders associated with the use of oral contraceptives:

Smoking Habits and Other Predisposing Conditions—Risk Associated with Use of Oral Contraceptives

Age	Below 30	30–39	40+
Heavy smokers	C	B	A
Light smokers	D	C	B
Nonsmokers (no predisposing conditions)	D	C, D	C
Nonsmokers (other predisposing conditions)	C	C, B	B, A

A—Use associated with very high risk.
B—Use associated with high risk.
C—Use associated with moderate risk.
D—Use associated with low risk.

The physician and the patient should be alert to the earliest manifestations of thromboembolic and thrombotic disorders (e.g., thrombophlebitis, pulmonary embolism, cerebrovascular insufficiency, coronary occlusion, retinal thrombosis, and mesenteric thrombosis). Should any of these occur or be suspected, the drug should be discontinued immediately.

A four- to six-fold increased risk of post-surgery thromboembolic complications has been reported in oral contraceptive users[20,21]. If feasible, oral contraceptives should be discontinued at least 4 weeks before surgery of a type associated with an increased risk of thromboembolism or prolonged immobilization. The decision as to when to resume oral contraception following major surgery or bedrest should balance the recognized risks of post-surgery thromboembolic complications with the need to reinstate contraceptive practices.

Data[72] also suggest that the presence of varicose veins substantially increases the risk of superficial venous thrombosis of the leg, the risk depending on the severity of the varicosities.

2. *Ocular Lesions:* There have been reports of neuro-ocular lesions such as optic neuritis or retinal thrombosis associated with the use of oral contraceptives. Discontinue oral contraceptive medication if there is unexplained, sudden or gradual, partial or complete loss of vision; onset of proptosis or diplopia; papilledema; or retinal vascular lesions; and institute appropriate diagnostic and therapeutic measures.
3. *Carcinoma:* Long-term continuous administration of either natural or synthetic estrogen in certain animal species increases the frequency of certain tumors, benign or malignant, such as those of the breast, cervix, vagina, uterus, ovary, pituitary and liver. Certain synthetic progestogens, none currently contained in oral contraceptives, have been noted to increase the incidence of mammary nodules, benign and malignant, in dogs.

   Several retrospective case-control studies[22–27] have reported an increased relative risk (3.1 to 13.9 times) associating endometrial carcinoma with the prolonged use of estrogens in postmenopausal women who took estrogen replacement medication to relieve menopausal symptoms. One publication[28] reported on the first 30 cases submitted by physicians to a registry of cases of adenocarcinoma of the endometrium in women under 40 on oral contraceptives. Of the adenocarcinomas found in women without predisposing risk factors for adenocarcinoma of the endometrium (e.g., irregular bleeding at the time oral contraceptives were first given, polycystic ovaries) nearly all occurred in women who had used a sequential oral contraceptive. These products are no longer marketed. No statistical association has been reported suggesting an increased risk of endometrial cancer in users of conventional combination or progestogen-only oral contraceptives, although individual cases have been reported.

   Several studies[8,29–33] have shown no increased risk of breast cancer to women taking oral contraceptives or estrogens. In one study[34,35], however, while no overall increased risk of breast cancer was noted in women treated with oral contraceptives, a greater risk was suggested for the subgroups of oral contraceptive users with documented benign breast disease and for long-term (2–4 years) users. In one study, it was found that a history of breast cancer among grandmothers or aunts was significantly more frequent among breast cancer patients who had used an oral contraceptive continuously for one or more years than among non-users with breast cancer[83]. One other study[36] indicated an increasing risk of breast cancer in women taking menopausal estrogens, which increased with duration of follow-up. A reduced occurrence of benign breast tumors in users of oral contraceptives has been well documented[8,11,12,29,34,37,38]. In contrast, one author[79] suggests that extended (over 6 years) use of oral contraceptives prior to the first full term pregnancy was associated with a significant relative risk of breast cancer.

   One study[75] reported malignant melanoma more frequently in oral contraceptive users than in controls and suggests an increased incidence of urinary tract cancers and thyroid cancers.

   In a prospective study[39] of women with cervical dysplasia, there was an increase in severity and of conversion to cancer *in situ* in oral contraceptive users compared with nonusers. This became statistically significant after 3 to 4 years of use. Nonreversal of dysplasia within the first 6 months of pill use was suggested to be predictive of progression after prolonged exposure. One study[75] disclosed an increased risk of cancer of the cervix (largely carcinoma-*in-situ*) in oral contraceptive users under 40, particularly those who had used these drugs for over four years. There have been other reports of microglandular hyperplasia of the cervix in users of oral contraceptives.

   In summary, there is at present no confirmed evidence from human studies of an increased risk of cancer associated with oral contraceptives. Close clinical surveillance of all women taking oral contraceptives is, nevertheless, essential. In all cases of undiagnosed persistent or recurrent abnormal vaginal bleeding, appropriate diagnostic measures should be taken to rule out malignancy. Women with a strong family history of breast cancer or who have breast nodules, fibrocystic disease or abnormal mammograms should be monitored with particular care if they elect to use oral contraceptives instead of other methods of contraception.
4. *Liver Tumors:* Sudden severe abdominal pain or shock may be due to rupture and hemorrhage of a liver tumor. There have been reports associating benign or malignant liver tumors with oral contraceptive use[40–44]. This has been reported in short-term as well as long-term users of oral contraceptives. One study[44] reported that use of oral contraceptives with high hormonal potency and age over 30 years may further increase a woman's risk of hepatocellular adenoma. Two studies[41,44] relate risk with duration of use, the risk being much greater after 4 or more years of use. Long-term users of oral contraceptives have an estimated annual incidence of hepatocellular adenoma of 3-4 per 100,000.[44] Although it is an uncommon lesion, it should be considered in women presenting with an "acute abdomen". The tumor may cause serious or fatal hemorrhage. Patients with liver tumors have demonstrated variable clinical features which may make preoperative diagnosis difficult. Some cases presented because of right upper quadrant masses, while most had signs and symptoms of acute intraperitoneal hemorrhage. Routine radiological and laboratory studies may not be helpful. Liver scans may clearly show a focal defect. Hepatic arteriography may be a useful procedure in diagnosing primary liver neoplasm.
5. *Use in or Immediately Preceding Pregnancy, Birth Defects in Offspring, and Malignancy in Female Offspring:* The use of female sex hormones—both estrogenic and progestational agents—during early pregnancy may seriously damage the offspring. It has been shown that females exposed *in utero* to diethylstilbestrol, a nonsteroidal estrogen, have an increased risk of developing in later life a form of vaginal or cervical cancer that is ordinarily extremely rare[45,46]. This risk has been estimated to be of the order of 1 in 1,000 exposures or less[47,48]. Although there is no evidence at the present time that oral contraceptives further enhance the risk of developing this type of malignancy, such patients should be monitored with particular care if they elect to use oral contraceptives instead of other methods of contraception.

   Furthermore, a high percentage of women exposed to diethylstilbestrol (from 30 to 90%) have been found to have epithelial changes of the vagina and cervix[49–53]. Although these changes are histologically benign, it is not known whether this condition is a precursor of vaginal malignancy. Male children so exposed may develop abnormalities of the urogenital tract[54–56]. Although similar data are not available with the use of other estrogens, it cannot be presumed that they would not induce similar changes.

Continued on next page

Syntex—Cont.

An increased risk of congenital anomalies, including heart defects and limb defects, has been reported following use of sex hormones, including oral contraceptives, in pregnancy[57–61]. In one case-control study[60] it was estimated that there was a 4.7-fold increased relative risk of limb-reduction defects in infants exposed *in utero* to sex hormones (oral contraceptives, hormonal withdrawal tests for pregnancy or attempted treatment for threatened abortion). Some of these exposures were very short and involved only a few days of treatment. The data suggest that the risk of limb-reduction defects in exposed fetuses is somewhat less than 1 in 1,000 live births. In a large prospective study[61], cardiovascular defects in children born to women who received female hormones, including oral contraceptives, during early pregnancy occurred at a rate of 18.2 per 1,000 births, compared to 7.8 per 1,000 for children not so exposed *in utero*. These results are statistically significant. A Welsh study[80] identified a statistically significant excess of neural tube defects among offspring of prior users (within 3 months) of oral contraceptives than among controls. The incidence of twin births may be increased for women who conceive shortly after discontinuing use of the pill[11,60,84,85,86].

In the past, female sex hormones have been used during pregnancy in an attempt to treat threatened or habitual abortion. There is considerable evidence that estrogens are ineffective for these indications, and there is no evidence from well controlled studies that progestogens are effective for these uses.

There is some evidence that triploidy and possibly other types of polyploidy are increased among abortuses from women who become pregnant soon after ceasing oral contraceptives.[62]. Embryos with these anomalies are virtually always aborted spontaneously. Whether there is an overall increase in spontaneous abortion of pregnancies conceived soon after stopping oral contraceptives is unknown.

If the patient has not adhered to the prescribed schedule, the possibility of pregnancy should be considered at the time of the first missed period (or after 45 days from the last menstrual period if progestogen-only contraceptives are used) and further use of oral contraceptives should be withheld until pregnancy has been ruled out. It is recommended that for any patient who has missed two consecutive periods, pregnancy should be ruled out before continuing the contraceptive regimen. If pregnancy is confirmed, the patient should be apprised of the potential risks to the fetus and the advisability of continuation of the pregnancy should be discussed in the light of these risks.

It is also recommended that women who discontinue oral contraceptives with the intent of becoming pregnant use an alternate form of contraception for a period of time before attempting to conceive. Many clinicians recommend 3 months; this recommendation is supported by a study suggesting an increased frequency of neural tube defects in women impregnated during the first three months after cessation of pill use[80].

The administration of progestogen-only or progestogen-estrogen combinations to induce withdrawal bleeding should not be used as a test of pregnancy.

6. *Gall Bladder Disease:* Studies[3,8,11,12,31] report an increased risk of gall bladder disease in users of oral contraceptives or estrogens. In one study[12], an increased risk appeared after 2 years of use and doubled after 4 or 5 years of use. In another study[8], an increased risk was apparent between 6 and 12 months of use.
7. *Carbohydrate and Lipid Metabolic Effects:* A decrease in glucose tolerance has been observed in a significant percentage of patients on oral contraceptives. For this reason, prediabetic and diabetic patients should be carefully observed while receiving oral contraceptives.

   An increase in triglycerides and total phospholipids has been observed in patients receiving oral contraceptives[63]. The clinical significance of this finding is unknown.
8. *Elevated Blood Pressure:* An increase in blood pressure has been reported[12,64] with oral contraceptive use. In some women, hypertension may occur within a few months of beginning oral contraceptive use. In the first year of use, the prevalence of women with hypertension is low in users and may be no higher than that of a comparable group of nonusers. The prevalence in users increases, however, with longer exposure, and in the fifth year of use is two and a half to three times the reported prevalence in the first year. Age is also strongly correlated with the development of hypertension in oral contraceptive users. Women with a history of elevated blood pressure (hypertension), preexisting renal disease, a history of toxemia or elevated blood pressure during pregnancy, a familial tendency to hypertension or its consequences, or a history of excessive weight gain or fluid retention during the menstrual cycle may be more likely to develop elevation of blood pressure when given oral contraceptives and, therefore, should be monitored closely[65]. Even though elevated blood pressure may remain within the "normal" range, the clinical implications of elevations should not be ignored and close surveillance is indicated, particularly for women with other risk factors for cardiovascular disease or stroke[64]. High blood pressure may or may not persist after discontinuation of the oral contraceptive.
9. *Headache:* The onset or exacerbation of migraine or development of headache of a new pattern which is recurrent, persistent, or severe, requires discontinuation of oral contraceptives and evaluation of the cause.
10. *Bleeding Irregularities:* Breakthrough bleeding, spotting, and missed menses are frequent reasons for patients discontinuing oral contraceptives. In breakthrough bleeding, as in all cases of irregular bleeding from the vagina, nonfunctional causes should be borne in mind. In undiagnosed persistent or recurrent abnormal bleeding from the vagina, adequate diagnostic measures are indicated to rule out pregnancy or malignancy. If pathology has been excluded, time or a change to another formulation may solve the problem. Changing to an oral contraceptive with a higher estrogen content, while potentially useful in minimizing menstrual irregularity, should be done only if necessary since this may increase the risk of thromboembolic disease.

    Women with a past history of oligomenorrhea or secondary amenorrhea or young women without regular cycles may have a tendency to remain anovulatory or to become amenorrheic after discontinuation of oral contraceptives. Women with these preexisting problems should be advised of this possibility and encouraged to use other contraceptive methods.

    Post-use anovulation, possibly prolonged, may also occur in women without previous irregularities. A higher incidence of galactorrhea and of pituitary tumors (e.g., adenomas) has been associated with amenorrhea in former users compared with nonusers[66,67]. One study[67] reported a 16-fold increased prevalence of pituitary prolactin-secreting tumors among patients with postpill amenorrhea when galactorrhea was present.
11. *Infertility:* There is evidence of impairment of fertility in women discontinuing oral contraceptives in comparison with those discontinuing other methods of contraception. The impairment appears to be independent of the duration of use of the preparations. While the impairment diminishes with time, there is still an appreciable difference in the results in nulliparous women for the oral contraceptive and nonoral contraceptive groups 30 months after discontinuation of birth control. For parous women the difference is no longer apparent 30 months after cessation of contraception[11].
12. *Ectopic Pregnancy:* Ectopic as well as intrauterine pregnancy may occur in contraceptive failures. However, in progestogen-only oral contraceptive failures, the ratio of ectopic to intrauterine pregnancies is higher than in women who are not receiving oral contraceptives, since the drugs are more effective in preventing intrauterine than ectopic pregnancies.
13. *Breast Feeding:* Oral contraceptives given in the postpartum period may interfere with lactation. There may be a decrease in the quantity and quality of the breast milk. Furthermore, a small fraction of the hormonal agents in oral contraceptives has been identified in the milk of mothers receiving these drugs[68]. The effects, if any, on the breast fed child have not been determined. If feasible, the use of oral contraceptives should be deferred until the infant has been weaned.

Precautions:

General

1. A complete medical and family history should be taken prior to the initiation of oral contraceptives. The pretreatment and periodic physical examinations should include special reference to blood pressure, breasts, abdomen and pelvic organs, including Papanicolaou smear and relevant laboratory tests. As a general rule, oral contraceptives should not be prescribed for longer than 1 year without another physical examination being performed.
2. Under the influence of estrogen-progestogen preparations, preexisting uterine leiomyomata may increase in size.
3. Patients with a history of psychic depression should be carefully observed and the drug discontinued if depression recurs to a serious degree. Patients becoming significantly depressed while taking oral contraceptives should stop the medication and use an alternate method of contraception in an attempt to determine whether the symptom is drug related.
4. Oral contraceptives may cause some degree of fluid retention. They should be prescribed with caution, and only with careful monitoring, in patients with conditions which might be aggravated by fluid retention, such as convulsive disorders, migraine syndrome, asthma or cardiac, hepatic or renal insufficiency.
5. Patients with a past history of jaundice during pregnancy have an increased risk of recurrence of jaundice while receiving oral contraceptive therapy. If jaundice develops in any patient receiving such drugs, the medication should be discontinued.

6. Steroid hormones may be poorly metabolized in patients with impaired liver function and should be administered with caution in such patients.
7. Oral contraceptive users may have disturbances in normal tryptophan metabolism which may result in a relative pyridoxine deficiency. The clinical significance of this is unknown.
8. Serum folate levels may be depressed by oral contraceptive therapy. Since the pregnant woman is predisposed to the development of folate deficiency and the incidence of folate deficiency increases with increasing gestation, it is possible that if a woman becomes pregnant shortly after stopping oral contraceptives, she may have a greater chance of developing folate deficiency and complications attributed to this deficiency.
9. The pathologist should be advised of oral contraceptive therapy when relevant specimens are submitted.
10. Certain endocrine and liver function tests and blood components may be affected by estrogen-containing oral contraceptives. For example:
    a. Increased sulfobromophthalein retention.
    b. Increased prothrombin and factors VII, VIII, IX, and X; decreased antithrombin 3; increased norepinephrine-induced platelet aggregability.
    c. Increased thyroid binding globulin (TBG) leading to increased circulating total thyroid hormone, as measured by protein-bound iodine (PBI), T4 by column, or T4 by radioimmunoassay. Free T3 resin uptake is decreased, reflecting the elevated TBG, free T4 concentration is unaltered.
    d. Decreased pregnanediol excretion.
    e. Reduced response to metyrapone test.
    f. Increased phospholipids and triglycerides.
    g. Temporarily decreased glucose tolerance.
11. Contact lens wearers who develop visual changes or changes in lens tolerance should be assessed by an ophthalmologist and temporary or permanent cessation of wear considered.

DRUG INTERACTIONS

Oral contraceptives may be rendered less effective by virtue of drug interaction with rifampin, isoniazid, ampicillin, tetracycline, neomycin, penicillin V, chloramphenicol, sulfonamides, nitrofurantoin, barbiturates, phenytoin, primidone, analgesics, tranquilizers and antimigraine preparations[69–71,78]. Oral contraceptives may alter the effectiveness of other types of drugs, such as oral anticoagulants, anticonvulsants, tricyclic antidepressants, antihypertensive agents (e.g., guanethidine), vitamins and hypoglycemic agents[69].

INFORMATION FOR THE PATIENT

See detailed patient labeling below.

CARCINOGENESIS

See Warnings section for information on the carcinogenic potential of oral contraceptives.

PREGNANCY

Pregnancy category X. See Contraindications and Warnings.

NURSING MOTHERS

See Contraindications and Warnings.

Adverse Reactions: An increased risk of the following serious adverse reactions has been associated with the use of oral contraceptives (see Warnings):

- Thrombophlebitis, thrombosis
- Pulmonary embolism
- Coronary thrombosis
- Cerebral thrombosis
- Mesenteric thrombosis
- Liver tumors
- Cerebral hemorrhage
- Hypertension
- Gall bladder disease
- Congenital anomalies
- Neuro-ocular lesions, e.g., retinal thrombosis and optic neuritis

The following adverse reactions have been reported in patients receiving oral contraceptives and are believed to be drug related:

- Bleeding irregularities
  - Breakthrough bleeding
  - Spotting
  - Missed menses during treatment
  - Amenorrhea after treatment
- Gastrointestinal symptoms
  - Nausea
  - Vomiting
  - Bloating
  - Abdominal cramps
- Dysmenorrhea
- Infertility after discontinuance of treatment
- Edema
- Chloasma or melasma which may persist after drug is discontinued
- Breast changes: tenderness, enlargement, and secretion
- Intolerance to contact lenses
- Change in corneal curvature (steepening)
- Change in weight (increase or decrease)
- Change in cervical erosion and cervical secretion
- Possible diminution in lactation when given immediately postpartum
- Cholestatic jaundice
- Migraine
- Increase in size of uterine leiomyomata
- Rash (allergic)
- Mental depression
- Reduced tolerance to carbohydrates
- Vaginal candidiasis
- Prolaction-secreting pituitary tumors

The following adverse reactions have been reported in users of oral contraceptives, and the association has been neither confirmed nor refuted:

- Premenstrual-like syndrome
- Cataracts
- Changes in libido
- Chorea
- Changes in appetite
- Cystitis-like syndrome
- Headache
- Nervousness
- Dizziness
- Hirsutism
- Loss of hair
- Erythema multiforme
- Erythema nodosum
- Hemorrhagic eruption
- Vaginitis
- Porphyria
- Impaired renal function

Acute Overdose: Serious ill effects have not been reported following acute ingestion of large doses of oral contraceptives by young children. Overdosage may cause nausea. Withdrawal bleeding may occur in females.

Dosage and Administration: To achieve maximum contraceptive effectiveness, oral contraceptives must be taken exactly as directed and at intervals not exceeding 24 hours.

21-Day Regimen Dosage Schedule: The dosage for the initial cycle of therapy is one tablet taken each evening at bedtime from DAY 5 through DAY 25 of the menstrual cycle, counting the first day of menstrual flow as DAY 1. No tablets are taken for 7 days, then, whether bleeding has stopped or not, a new course is started of one tablet a day for 21 days. This institutes a three weeks on, one week off dosage regimen.

28-Day Regimen Dosage Schedule: The dosage for the initial cycle of therapy is one tablet taken daily beginning with DAY 5 of the menstrual cycle, counting the first day of menstrual flow as DAY 1. Tablets are taken without interruption as follows: Beginning with Tablet 1, take one tablet each evening at bedtime for 21 days, through Tablet 21. Then take orange Tablets 22 through 28, one each evening at bedtime, for 7 days. After all 28 tablets have been taken, whether bleeding has stopped or not, repeat the same dosage schedule beginning on the following day.

NORINYL 2 mg. Tablets: To prevent conception, one tablet is taken each evening at bedtime for 20 days beginning on DAY 5 of the menstrual cycle, counting the first day of menstrual flow as DAY 1. In the vast majority of women on this schedule menses occur within two to three days following the termination of each 20-day course, but tend to be scantier than normal menses. In those cases where withdrawal bleeding may be delayed until 4, 5 or 6 days after the 20-day course of therapy, the patient should start the next course of medication on the 7th day following completion of the previous 20-day course. For the treatment of hypermenorrhea, one tablet is taken each evening at bedtime from day 5 through day 24 of each menstrual cycle. Following three months of treatment of hypermenorrhea, medication may be discontinued to determine the need for further therapy.

20, 21, 28-Day Schedules: Even if spotting or breakthrough bleeding should occur, continue the medication according to the schedule. Should spotting or breakthrough bleeding persist, your physician should be notified.

Use of oral contraceptives in the event of a missed menstrual period:

1. If the patient has not adhered to the prescribed dosage regimen, the possibility of pregnancy should be considered after the first missed period and oral contraceptives should be withheld until pregnancy has been ruled out.
2. If the patient has adhered to the prescribed regimen and misses two consecutive periods, pregnancy should be ruled out before continuing the contraceptive regimen.

NOR-Q.D.® (norethindrone) is administered as a continuous daily dosage regimen starting on the first day of menstruation, i.e., one tablet each day, every day of the year. Tablets should be taken at the same time each day and continued daily, without interruption, whether bleeding occurs or not. This is especially important for patients new to progestogen alone oral contraception. The patient should be advised that if prolonged bleeding occurs, she should consult her physician. In the non-nursing mother, NOR-Q.D. may be prescribed in the post-partum period either immediately or at the first post-partum examination whether or not menstruation has resumed.

The risk of pregnancy increases with each tablet missed. If the patient misses one tablet, she should be instructed to take it as soon as she remembers and also to take her next tablet at the regular time which means she will be taking two tablets on that day. If she misses two tablets in a row, she should take one of the missed tablets as soon as she remembers, discard the other missed tablet, and take her regular tablet for that day at the proper time. Furthermore, she should use an additional method of contraception in addition to taking NOR-Q.D. until menses has appeared or pregnancy has been excluded. If more than two tablets in a row have been missed, NOR-Q.D. should be discontinued immediately and an additional method of contraception should be used until menses has appeared or pregnancy has been excluded. Whether or not the patient has adhered to the prescribed schedule, if she does not have a period within 45 days of her last period, she should stop taking NOR-Q.D. and depend upon a method of nonhormonal contraception until pregnancy has been ruled out.

How Supplied:

BREVICON® 21-DAY Tablets (21 blue norethindrone 0.5 mg. with ethinyl estradiol 0.035 mg. tablets) are available in MEMORETTE®

Continued on next page

Syntex—Cont.

Tablet Dispensers, each containing 21 tablets. Also supplied are 21-tablet refills. BREVICON® 28-DAY Tablets (21 blue norethindrone 0.5 mg. with ethinyl estradiol 0.035 mg. tablets followed by 7 orange inert tablets) are available in MEMORETTE Tablet Dispensers, each containing 28 tablets. Also supplied are 28-tablet refills.
NORINYL 1 + 35 21-DAY Tablets (21 green norethindrone 1 mg. with ethinyl estradiol 0.035 mg. tablets) are available in MEMORETTE Tablet Dispensers, each containing 21 tablets. Also supplied are 21-tablet refills.
NORINYL 1 + 35 28-DAY Tablets (21 green norethindrone 1 mg. with ethinyl estradiol 0.035 mg. tablets followed by 7 orange inert tablets) are available in MEMORETTE Tablet Dispensers, each containing 28 tablets. Also supplied are 28-tablet refills.
NORINYL® 1 + 50 21-DAY Tablets (21 white norethindrone 1 mg. with mestranol 0.05 mg. tablets) and NORINYL® 1 + 80 21-DAY Tablets (21 yellow norethindrone 1 mg. with mestranol 0.08 mg. tablets) are available in MEMORETTE® Tablet Dispensers, each containing 21 tablets. Also supplied are 21-tablet refills. NORINYL 1 + 50 28-DAY Tablets (21 white norethindrone 1 mg. with mestranol 0.05 mg. tablets followed by 7 orange inert tablets) and NORINYL 1 + 80 28-DAY Tablets (21 yellow norethindrone 1 mg. with mestranol 0.08 mg. tablets followed by 7 orange inert tablets) are available in MEMORETTE Tablet Dispensers, each containing 28 tablets. Also supplied are 28-tablet refills.
NORINYL® 2 mg. Tablets (20 white norethindrone 2 mg. with mestranol 0.1 mg. tablets) are available in MEMORETTE® Tablet Dispensers, each containing 20 tablets. Also supplied are 20-tablet refills.
NOR-Q.D.® (norethindrone) (as yellow-colored unscored tablets) is available in 42-tablet dispensers.

References:

[1] Population Reports, Series H, Number 2, May 1974; Series I, Number 1, June 1974: Series B, Number 2, January 1975; Series H, Number 3, January 1975; Series H, Number 4, January 1976 (published by the Population Information Program, The George Washington University Medical Center, 2001 S St. NW, Washington, D. C.).
[2] Inman, W., et al.: *Brit Med J* 2:203–209, 1970.
[3] Stolley, P., et al.: *Am J Epidemiol* 102:197–208, 1975.
[4] Inman, W., et al.: *Brit Med J* 2:193–199, 1968.
[5] Royal College of General Practitioners: *J Coll Gen Pract* 13:267–279, 1967.
[6] Vessey, M., et al.: *Brit Med J* 2:651–657, 1969.
[7] Sartwell, P., et al.: *Am J Epidemiol* 90:365–380, 1969.
[8] Boston Collaborative Drug Surveillance Program: *Lancet* 1:1399–1404, 1973.
[9] Collaborative Group for the Study of Stroke in Young Women: *N Engl J Med* 288:871–878, 1973.
[10] Collaborative Group for the Study of Stroke in Young Women: *JAMA* 231:718–722, 1975.
[11] Vessey, M., et al.: *J Biosoc Sci* 8:373–427, (Oct.) 1976.
[12] Royal College of General Practitioners: Oral Contraceptives and Health, London, Pitman, 1974.
[13] Mann, J., et al.: *Brit Med J* 2:245–248, 1975.
[14] Mann, J., et al.: *Brit Med J* 2:445–447, 1976.
[15] Mann, J., et al.: *Brit Med J* 2:241–245, 1975.
[16] Jain, A.: *Studies in Family Planning* 8:50–54, 1977.
[17] Ory, H.: *JAMA* 237:2619–2622, (June 13) 1977.
[18] Beral, V.: *Lancet* 2:727–731, 1977.
[19] Tietze, C.: *Family Planning Perspectives* 9:74–76, 1977.
[20] Vessey, M., et al.: *Brit Med J* 3:123–126, 1970.
[21] Greene, G., et al.: *Am J Pub Health* 62:680–685, 1972.
[22] Ziel, H., et al.: *N Engl J Med* 293:1167–1170, 1975.
[23] Gordon, J., et al.: *N Engl J Med* 297:570–571, (Sept. 15) 1977.
[24] Smith, D., et al.: *N Engl J Med* 293:1164–1167, 1975.
[25] Mack, T., et al.: *N Engl J Med* 294:1262–1267, 1976.
[26] Gray, L., et al.: *Obstet Gyncecol* 49:385–389, (April) 1977.
[27] McDonald, T., et al.: *Am J Obstet Gynecol* 127:572–580, (Mar. 20) 1977.
[28] Silverberg, S., et al.: *Cancer* 39:592–598, (Feb.) 1977).
[29] Vessey, M., et al.: *Brit Med J* 3:719–724, 1972.
[30] Vessey, M., et al.: *Lancet* 1:941–943, 1975.
[31] Boston Collaborative Drug Surveillance Program: *N Engl J Med* 290:15–19, 1974.
[32] Arthes, F., et al.: *Cancer* 28:1391–1394, 1971.
[33] Casagrande, J., et al.: *J Natl Cancer Inst* 56:839–841, (April) 1976).
[34] Fasal, E., et al.: *J Natl Cancer Inst* 55:767–773, 1975.
[35] Paffenbarger, R., et al.: *Cancer* 49:1887–1891, (April Suppl.) 1977.
[36] Hoover, R., et al.: *N Engl J Med* 295:401–405, (Aug. 19) 1976.
[37] Kelsey, J., et al.: *Internat J Epidemiol* 3:333–340, 1974.
[38] Ory, H., et al.: *N Engl J Med* 294:419–422, 1976.
[39] Stern, E., et al.: *Science* 196:1460–1462, (June 24) 1977.
[40] Mays, E., et al.: *JAMA* 235:730–732, 1976.
[41] Edmondson, H., et al.: *N Engl J Med* 294:470–472, 1976.
[42] Murphy, G.: *Am Col of Surg Bull,* (April) 1977.
[43] Klatskin, G.: *Gastroent* 73:386–394, (Aug.) 1977.
[44] Rooks, et al: *JAMA* 242:644, 1979.
[45] Herbst, A., et al.: *N Engl J Med* 284:878–881, 1971.
[46] Greenwald, P., et al.: *N Engl J Med* 285:390–392, 1971.
[47] Lanier, A., et al.: *Mayo Clin Pro* 48:793–799, 1973.
[48] Herbst, A., et al.: *Am J Obstet Gynecol* 128:43–50, 1977.
[49] Herbst, A., et al.: *Obstet Gyncecol* 40:287–298, 1972.
[50] Herbst, A., et al.: *Am J Obstet Gyncecol* 118:607–615, 1974.
[51] Herbst, A., et al.: *N Engl J Med* 292:334–339, 1975.
[52] Stafl, A., et al.: *Obstet Gynecol* 43:118–128, 1974.
[53] Sherman, A., et al.: *Obstet Gynecol* 44:531–545, 1974.
[54] Bibbo, M., et al.: *Jour of Repro Med* 15:29–32, 1975.
[55] Gill, W., et al.: *Jour of Repro Med* 16:147–153, 1976.
[56] Henderson, B., et al.: *Pediatrics* 58:505–507, 1976.
[57] Gal, I., et al.: *Nature* 216:83, 1967.
[58] Levy, E., et al.: *Lancet* 1:611, 1973.
[59] Nora, J., et al.: *Lancet* 1:941–942, 1973.
[60] Janerich, D., et al.: *N Engl J Med* 291:697–700, 1974.
[61] Heinonen, O., et al.: *N Engl J Med* 296:67–70, 1977.
[62] Carr, D.: *Canad Med Assoc J* 103:343–348, 1970.
[63] Wynn, V., et al.: *Lancet* 2:720–723, 1966.
[64] Fisch, I., et al.: *JAMA* 237:2499–2503, (June 6) 1977.
[65] Laragh, J.: *Am J Obstet Gynecol* 126:141–147, (Sept.) 1976.
[66] March, C., et al.: *Fertil and Steril* 28:346, (Mar.) 1977.
[67] Van Campenhout, J., et al.: *Fertil and Steril* 28:728–732, (July) 1977.
[68] Laumas, K., et al.: *Am J Obstet Gynecol* 98:411–413, 1967.
[69] Stockley, I.: *Pharm J* 216:140–143, (Feb. 14) 1976.
[70] Hempel, E., et al.: *Drugs* 12:442–448, (Dec.) 1976.
[71] Bessot, J.-C., et al.: *Nouv Press Med* 6:1568, (Apr. 30) 1977.
[72] Royal College of General Practitioners: *J Coll Gen Pract* 28:393–399, 1978.
[73] Layde, P. M., et al.: *Lancet* 1:541–546, 1981.
[74] Vessey, M. P., et al.: *Lancet* 1:549–550, 1981.
[75] Ramcharan, S., et al.: *The Walnut Creek Contraceptive Drug Study,* Volume III, NIH Publication 81–564, 1981.
[76] Petitti, D. B., et al.: *Am J Epidemiol* 108:480–485, 1978.
[77] Petitti, D. B., et al.: *Lancet* 2:234, 1978.
[78] Abernethy, D. R., et al.: *N Engl J Med* 306:791, 1982.
[79] Pike, M. C., et al.: *Brit J Cancer* 43:72, 1981.
[80] Kasan, P. N., et al.: *Brit J Obstet Gynecol* 87:545, 1980.
[81] Meade, T. W., et al.: *Brit Med J* 280:1157, 1980.
[82] Bottiger, L. E., et al.: *Lancet* 1:1097, 1980.
[83] Black, M. M., et al.: *Cancer* 46:2747, 1980.
[84] Rothman, E. J.: *N Engl J Med* 297:468, 1977.
[85] Bracken, M. B.: *Am J Obstet Gynecol* 133:432, 1979.
[86] Harlap, S., et al.: *Obstet Gynecol* 55:447, 1980.

Detailed Patient Labeling: Oral contraceptives ("the pill") are the most effective way (except for sterilization) to prevent pregnancy. They are also convenient and, for most women, free of serious or unpleasant side effects. Oral contraceptives must always be taken under the continuous supervision of a physician.

It is important that any woman who considers using an oral contraceptive understand the risks involved. Although the oral contraceptives have important advantages over the other methods of contraception, they have certain risks that no other method has. Only you can decide whether the advantages are worth these risks. This leaflet will tell you about the most important risks. It will explain how you can help your doctor prescribe the pill as safely as possible by telling him/her about yourself and being alert for the earliest signs of trouble. And it will tell you how to use the pill properly, so that it will be as effective as possible. There is more detailed information available in the leaflet prepared for doctors. If you need further help, ask your physician or pharmacist.

Who Should Not Use Oral Contraceptives:

A. If you have any of the following conditions you should not use the pill:
   1. Unusual vaginal bleeding that has not yet been diagnosed.
   2. Known or suspected pregnancy.
   3. Double vision or diseases related to blood vessel of the eye.
   4. Classical migraine.
   5. Active liver disease.

B. If you have or have had any of the following conditions you should not use the pill:
   1. Heart attack or stroke.
   2. Clots in the legs, lungs, brain, heart or elsewhere.
   3. Chest pain (angina pectoris).
   4. Known or suspected cancer of the breast or sex organs.
   5. Liver tumor associated with the use of the pill or other estrogen containing products.
   6. Jaundice resulting from liver abnormality.

C. Cigarette smoking increases the risk of serious adverse effects on the heart and blood vessels from oral contraceptive use.

This risk increases with age and with heavy smoking (15 or more cigarettes per day) and is quite marked in women over 35 years of age. Women who use oral contraceptives should not smoke.

D. If you have scanty or irregular periods or are a young woman without a regular cycle, you should use another method of contraception because, if you use the pill, you may have difficulty becoming pregnant or may fail to have menstrual periods after discontinuing the pill.

E. You should not use the pill during the period you are breast feeding a child.

What You Should Know About Oral Contraceptives: This leaflet describes the advantages and risks of oral contraceptives. Except for sterilization, the IUD and abortion, which have their own exclusive risks, the only risks of other methods of contraception are those due to pregnancy should the method fail or not be used conscientiously. Your doctor can answer questions you may have with respect to methods of contraception.

1. What Oral Contraceptives Are and How They Work. Oral contraceptives are of two types. The most common, often simply called "the pill", is a combination of an estrogen and a progestogen, the two kinds of female hormones. The amount of estrogen and progestogen can vary, but the amount of estrogen is most important because both the effectiveness and some of the dangers of oral contraceptives are related to the amount of estrogen. This kind of oral contraceptive works principally by preventing release of an egg from the ovary. When the amount of estrogen is 0.05 milligrams or more, and the pill is taken as directed, oral contraceptives are more than 99% effective (i.e., there would be less than one pregnancy if 100 women used the pill for 1 year). Pills that contain 0.02 to 0.035 milligrams of estrogen vary slightly in effectiveness, ranging from 98% to more than 99% effective.

The second type of oral contraceptive, often called the "mini-pill", contains only a progestogen. It works in part by preventing release of an egg from the ovary but also by keeping sperm from reaching the egg and by making the uterus (womb) less receptive to any fertilized egg that reaches it. The mini-pill is less effective than the combination oral contraceptive, about 97% effective. In addition, the progestogen-only pill has a tendency to cause irregular bleeding which may be quite inconvenient, or cessation of bleeding entirely. The progestogen-only pill is used despite its lower effectiveness in the hope that it will prove not to have some of the serious side effects of the estrogen-containing pill (see below) but it is not yet certain that the mini-pill does in fact have fewer serious side effects. The discussion below, while based mainly on information about the combination pills, should be considered to apply as well to the mini-pill.

2. Other Nonsurgical Ways to Prevent Pregnancy. As this leaflet will explain, oral contraceptives have several serious risks. Some other methods of contraception have lesser risks. They are usually less effective than oral contraceptives, but, used properly, may be effective enough for many women. The following table gives reported pregnancy rates (the number of women out of 100 who would become pregnant in 1 year) for these methods:

Pregnancies per 100 Women per Year
Intrauterine device (IUD), less than 1–6;
Diaphragm with spermicidal products (creams or jellies), 2–20;
Condom (rubber), 3–36;
Aerosol foams, 2–29;
Jellies and creams, 4–36;
Periodic abstinence (rhythm), all types, less than 1–47;
—Calendar method, 14–47;
—Temperature method, 1–20;
—Temperature method—intercourse only in post-ovulatory phase, less than 1–7;
—Mucus method, 1–25;
No contraception, 60–80.

The figures (except for the IUD) vary widely because people differ in how well they use each method. Very faithful users of the various methods, with the exception of the calendar method of periodic abstinence (rhythm), may achieve lower pregnancy rates than those given above, which are the average results for large groups of women. Except for the IUD, effective use of these methods requires somewhat more effort than simply taking a single pill every evening, but it is an effort that many couples undertake successfully. Your doctor can tell you a great deal more about these methods of contraception.

3. The Dangers of Oral Contraceptives

a. *Circulatory disorders (abnormal blood clots, strokes, and heart attacks).* Blood clots (in various blood vessels of the body) are the most common of the serious side effects of oral contraceptives. A clot can result in a stroke (if the clot is in the brain), a heart attack (if the clot is in a blood vessel of the heart), a pulmonary embolus (a clot which forms in the legs or pelvis, then breaks off and travels to the lungs), or loss of a limb (a clot in a blood vessel in or leading to an arm or leg). Any of these can cause death or disability. Clots also occur rarely in the blood vessels of the eye, resulting in blindness or impairment of vision in that eye. There is evidence that the risk of clotting increases with higher estrogen doses. It is therefore important to keep the dose of estrogen as low as possible, so long as the oral contraceptive used has an acceptable pregnancy rate and doesn't cause unacceptable changes in the menstrual pattern. The risk of abnormal clotting increases with age in both users and nonusers of oral contraceptives, but the increased risk from the contraceptive appears to be present at all ages.

In addition to blood-clotting disorders, it has been estimated that women taking oral contraceptives are twice as likely as nonusers to have a stroke due to rupture of a blood vessel in the brain.

Furthermore, cigarette smoking by oral contraceptive users increases the risk of serious adverse effects on the heart and blood vessels. This risk increases with age and with heavy smoking (15 or more cigarettes per day) and becomes quite marked in women over 35 years of age. For this reason, women who use oral contraceptives should not smoke.

For oral contraceptive users in general, it has been estimated that in women between the ages of 15 and 34 the risk of death due to a circulatory disorder is about 1 in 12,000 per year, whereas for nonusers the rate is about 1 in 50,000 per year. In the age group 35 to 44, the risk is estimated to be about 1 in 2,500 per year for oral contraceptive users and about 1 in 10,000 per year for nonusers. The risk is concentrated in older women, in those with a long duration of use, and in cigarette smokers. The effects on the circulatory system may persist after oral contraceptives are discontinued.

Even without the pill the risk of having a heart attack increases with age and is also increased by such heart attack risk factors as high blood pressure, high cholesterol, obesity, diabetes, and cigarette smoking. Without any risk factors present, the use of oral contraceptives alone may double the risk of heart attack. However, the combination of cigarette smoking, especially heavy smoking, and oral contraceptive use greatly increases the risk of heart attack. Oral contraceptive users who smoke are about 5 times more likely to have a heart attack than users who do not smoke and about 10 times more likely to have a heart attack than nonusers who do not smoke. It has been estimated that users between the ages of 30 and 39 who smoke have about a 1 in 10,000 chance each year of having a fatal heart attack compared to about a 1 in 50,000 chance in users who do not smoke, and about a 1 in 100,000 chance in nonusers who do not smoke.

In the age group 40 to 44, the risk is about 1 in 1,700 per year for users who smoke compared to about 1 in 10,000 for users who do not smoke and to about 1 in 14,000 per year for nonusers who do not smoke. These are average figures for Great Britain; comparable estimates for the U.S. may be higher. Heavy smoking (about 15 cigarettes or more a day) further increases the risk. If you do not smoke and have none of the other heart attack risk factors described above, you will have a smaller risk than listed. If you have several heart attack risk factors, the risk may be considerably greater than listed.

b. *Formation of tumors.* Studies have found that when certain animals are given the female sex hormone estrogen, which is an ingredient of oral contraceptives, continuously for long periods, cancers may develop in the breast, cervix, vagina, uterus, ovary, pituitary and liver.

These findings suggest that oral contraceptives may cause cancer in humans. However, studies to date in women taking currently marketed oral contraceptives have not confirmed that oral contraceptives cause cancer in humans. Several studies have found no increase in breast cancer in users, although one study suggested oral contraceptives might cause an increase in breast cancer in women who already have benign breast disease (e.g., cysts).

Women with a strong family history of breast cancer or who have breast nodules, fibrocystic disease, or abnormal mammograms or who were exposed to DES (diethylstilbestrol), an estrogen, during their mother's pregnancy must be followed very closely by their doctors if they choose to use oral contraceptives instead of another method of contraception. Many studies have shown that women taking oral contraceptives have less risk of getting benign breast disease than those who have not used oral contraceptives. Strong evidence has emerged that estrogens (one component of oral contraceptives) when given alone (unaccompanied by progestogen) for periods of more than one year to women after the menopause, increase the risk of cancer of the uterus (womb). There is also some evidence that a kind of oral contraceptive which is no longer marketed, the sequential oral contraceptive, may increase the risk of cancer of the uterus. There remains no evidence, however, that the oral contraceptives now available (containing estrogen and progestogen in combination or progestogen alone) increase the risk of this cancer. Cancer of the cervix may develop more readily in long-term (3–4 years) users of the pill who had preexisting abnormal Pap smears. One study reported malignant melanoma (skin cancer), urinary tract cancers, and thyroid cancers more frequently in pill users than in non-users. Benign or malignant liver tumors have been associated with short-term as well as long-term oral contraceptive use. The benign (non-malignant) tumors do not spread, but they may rupture and produce internal bleeding, which may cause death.

c. *Dangers to a developing child if oral contraceptives are used in or immediately preceding pregnancy.* Oral contraceptives should not be taken by pregnant women because they may damage the developing child. An increased risk of birth defects, including heart defects and limb defects, has been associated with the use of sex hormones, including oral contraceptives, in pregnancy. In addition, the developing female child whose mother has received DES (diethylstilbestrol), an estrogen, during pregnancy has a risk of getting cancer of the vagina

Continued on next page

Syntex—Cont.

or cervix in her teens or young adulthood. This risk is estimated to be about 1 in 1,000 exposures or less. Abnormalities of the urinary and sex organs have been reported in male offspring so exposed. It is possible that other estrogens, such as the estrogens in oral contraceptives, could have the same effect in the child if the mother takes them during pregnancy.

If you stop taking oral contraceptives to become pregnant, your doctor may recommend that you use another method of contraception for a short while. The reason for this is that there is evidence from studies in women who have had "miscarriages" soon after stopping the pill, that the lost fetuses are more likely to be abnormal. Whether there is an overall increase in "miscarriage" in women who become pregnant soon after stopping the pill as compared with women who do not use the pill is not known, but it is possible that there may be. If, however, you do become pregnant soon after stopping oral contraceptives, and do not have a miscarriage, there is no evidence that the baby has an increased risk of being abnormal.

d. *Gallbladder disease.* Women who use oral contraceptives have a greater risk than nonusers of having gallbladder disease requiring surgery. The increased risk may first appear within 1 year of use and may double after 4 to 5 years of use.

e. *Other side effects of oral contraceptives.* Some women using oral contraceptives experience unpleasant side effects that are not dangerous and are not likely to damage their health. Some of these may be temporary. Your breasts may feel tender, nausea and vomiting may occur, you may gain or lose weight, and your ankles may swell. A spotty darkening of the skin, particularly of the face, is possible and may persist. Many of these effects are seen more frequently with combination oral contraceptives containing 0.05 milligrams or more of estrogen. You may notice unexpected vaginal bleeding or changes in your menstrual period. Irregular bleeding is frequently seen when using the mini-pill or combination oral contraceptives containing less than 0.05 milligrams of estrogen.

More serious side effects include worsening of migraine, asthma, epilepsy, and kidney or heart disease because of a tendency for water to be retained in the body when oral contraceptives are used. Other side effects are growth of preexisting fibroid tumors of the uterus; mental depression; and liver problems with jaundice (yellowing of the skin). Your doctor may find that levels of sugar and fatty substances in your blood are elevated; the long-term effects of these changes are not known. Some women develop high blood pressure while taking oral contraceptives, which may persist after discontinuation. High blood pressure may lead to serious disease of the kidney and circulatory system. Your physician may wish to check your blood pressure more frequently if you have a history of toxemia of pregnancy, kidney disease or increased blood pressure.

Other reactions have been reported occasionally. These include more frequent urination and some discomfort when urinating, kidney disease, nervousness, dizziness, an increase in or loss of hair, an increase or decrease in sex drive, appetite changes, cataracts, and a need for a change in contact lens prescription or inability to use contact lenses.

After you stop using oral contraceptives, your ability to menstruate or become pregnant may be impaired. This impairment may be greater if you have never been pregnant.

As discussed previously, you should wait a few months after stopping the pill before you try to become pregnant. An increased incidence of twin births has been reported in women who have conceived soon after stopping the pill. During these few months, use another form of contraception. You should consult your physician before resuming use of oral contraceptives after childbirth, especially if you plan to nurse your baby. Drugs in oral contraceptives are known to appear in the milk, and the long-range effect on infants is not known. Furthermore, oral contraceptives may cause a decrease in your milk supply as well as in the quality of the milk.

4. Comparison of the Risks of Oral Contraceptives and Other Contraceptive Methods. The many studies on the risks and effectiveness of oral contraceptives and other methods of contraception have been analyzed to estimate the risk of death associated with various methods of contraception. This risk has two parts: (a) the risk associated with the method itself (e.g., the risk that an oral contraceptive user will die due to abnormal clotting), and (b) the risk associated with failure of the method (death due to pregnancy or abortion). The results of this analysis are shown in the bar graph below. The height of the bars is the estimated number of deaths per 100,000 women each year. There are six sets of bars, each set referring to a specific age group of women. Within each set of bars, there are two bars for oral contraceptive users, one referring to users who smoke and one referring to users who do not smoke, and five bars for other contraceptive methods including one bar representing no method of contraception. ("Traditional contraception" means diaphragm or condom.)

This analysis is based on present knowledge and new information could, of course, alter it. The analysis shows that the risk of death from all methods of birth control is low compared to the risks of childbirth, *except for oral contraceptives in women over 40 who smoke.* It shows that the lowest risk of death is associated with the condom or diaphragm (traditional contraception) backed up by early abortion in case of failure of the condom or diaphragm to prevent pregnancy. Also, at any age the risk of death (due to unexpected pregnancy) from use of traditional contraception even without a backup

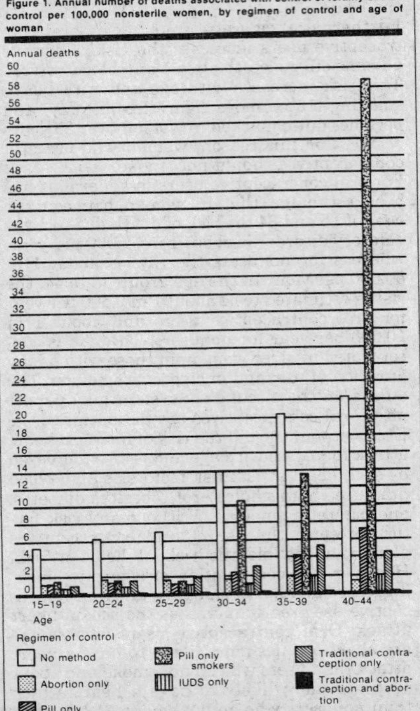

Figure 1. Annual number of deaths associated with control of fertility and no control per 100,000 nonsterile women, by regimen of control and age of woman

of abortion is generally the same as, or less than, that from use of oral contraceptives.

Careful Use of Oral Contraceptives:

1. Tell Your Doctor About Any Of The Following:

a. Present or past conditions that mean you should not use oral contraceptives:

Clots in the legs, lungs or elsewhere
A stroke, heart attack, or chest pain (angina pectoris)
Known or suspected cancer of the breast or sex organs
Irregular or scanty menstrual periods before starting to take the pill
Liver tumor associated with the use of the pill or other estrogen containing products.

b. Present conditions that mean you should not use oral contraceptives:

Unusual vaginal bleeding that has not yet been diagnosed.
Known or suspected pregnancy.

c. Conditions that your doctor will want to watch closely or which might cause him to suggest another method of contraception:

A family history of breast cancer
Breast nodules, fibrocystic disease of the breast, or an abnormal mammogram
Diabetes
High blood pressure
High cholesterol
Cigarette smoking
Migraine headaches
Heart or kidney disease
Epilepsy
Mental depression
Fibroid tumors of the uterus
Gallbladder disease
Asthma
Problems during a prior pregnancy
Plans for elective surgery
History of jaundice or other liver disease

d. Use of any of the following kinds of drugs, which might interact with the pill: antibiotics, sulfa drugs, drugs for epilepsy or migraine, pain killers, tranquilizers, sedatives or sleeping pills, blood thinning drugs, vitamins, drugs being used for the treatment of depression, high blood pressure, or high blood sugar (diabetes).

e. Once you are using oral contraceptives, you should be alert for signs of a serious adverse effect and call your doctor if they occur:

Sharp pain in the chest, coughing blood, or sudden shortness of breath (indicating possible clots in the lungs)
Pain in the calf (possible clot in the leg)
Crushing chest pain or heaviness (indicating possible heart attack)
Sudden severe headache or vomiting, dizziness or fainting, disturbance of vision or speech, or weakness or numbness in an arm or leg (indicating a possible stroke)
Sudden partial or complete loss of vision (indicating a possible clot in the eye)
Breast lumps (you should ask your doctor to show you how to examine your own breasts)
Severe pain or mass in the abdomen (indicating a possible tumor of the liver)
Severe depression
Yellowing of the skin (jaundice)
Unusual swelling.

2. How to Take the Pill So That It is Most Effective

Reduced effectiveness and an increased incidence of breakthrough bleeding have been associated with the use of oral contraceptives with antibiotics such as rifampicin, ampicillin, and tetracycline or with certain other drugs, such as barbiturates, phenylbutazone or phenytoin sodium. You should use an additional means of contraception during any cycle in which any of these drugs are taken.

Your physician has prescribed one of the following dosage schedules. Please follow the instructions appropriate for your schedule.

20-Day Schedule: Counting the onset of flow as day 1, take the first pill on day 5 of the menstrual cycle whether or not the flow has stopped. Take another pill the same time each day, preferably at bedtime, for 20 days. Then wait for 7 days, during which time a menstrual period usually occurs, and begin taking 1 pill every day on the 8th day after you took your last pill, whether or not the menstrual flow has stopped. This cycle is repeated 20 days on pills and 7 days off pills until time for the physician's examination and pill refill. If you are taking NORINYL® 2 mg Tablets for the control of excessive bleeding (hypermenorrhea), your physician may instruct you to stop taking the pills after 3 cycles to determine the need for further treatment. The information contained in this leaflet regarding who should not use the pill, the dangers of the pill and safe use of the pill applies to the use of the pill for hypermenorrhea, as well as for contraception.

21-Day Schedule: Counting the onset of flow as day 1, take the first pill on day 5 of the menstrual cycle whether or not the flow has stopped. Take another pill the same time each day, preferably at bedtime, for 21 days. Then wait for 7 days, during which time a menstrual period usually occurs, and begin taking 1 pill every day on the 8th day after you took your last pill, whether or not the menstrual flow has stopped. This cycle is repeated 21 days on pills and 7 days off pills until time for the physician's examination and pill refill.

28-Day Schedule: Counting the onset of flow as day 1, take the first pill on day 5 of the menstrual cycle whether or not the flow has stopped. Take another pill the same time each day, preferably at bedtime, for 21 days. Then take pills 22 through 28 (which are a different color) and expect a menstrual period during this week. Pills 22 through 28 contain no active drug and are included simply for your convenience—to eliminate the need for counting days. After all 28 pills have been taken, whether bleeding has stopped or not, take the first pill of the next cycle without any interruption. With the 28-day package, pills are taken every day of the year with no gap between cycles.

Important Additional Instructions for the 20-Day, 21-Day and 28-Day Schedules

The prescribed dosage schedule must be followed exactly. The chance of becoming pregnant increases with each pill missed. If you miss one pill, you should take it as soon as you remember and also take your next pill at the regular time, which means you will be taking two pills on that day. If you miss two pills in a row, you should take one of the missed pills as soon as you remember, discard the other missed pill, and take your regular pill for that day at the proper time. Furthermore, you should use an additional method of contraception in addition to taking your pills for the remainder of the cycle. If more than 2 pills in a row have been missed, discontinue taking your pills immediately and use an additional method of contraception until you have a period or your doctor determines that you are not pregnant. Missing pills numbered 22–28 (orange pills) in the 28-day schedule does not increase your chances of becoming pregnant.

At times there may be no menstrual period after a cycle of pills. Therefore, if you miss one menstrual period but have taken the pills *exactly as you were supposed to,* continue as usual into the next cycle. If you have not taken the pills correctly, and have missed a menstrual period, *you may be pregnant* and should stop taking oral contraceptives until your doctor determines whether or not you are pregnant. Until you can get to your doctor, use another form of contraception. If two consecutive menstrual periods are missed, you should stop taking pills until it is determined whether you are pregnant. If you do become pregnant while using oral contraceptives, you should discuss the risks to the developing child with your doctor.

Even if spotting or breakthrough bleeding should occur, continue the medication according to the schedule. Should spotting or breakthrough bleeding persist you should notify your physician.

NOR-Q.D.® (norethindrone) Tablets 0.35 mg. Schedule: Take the first pill on the first day of the menstrual flow, and take another pill each day, every day of the year. The pill should be taken at the same time of day, preferably at bedtime, and *continued daily, without interruption, whether bleeding occurs or not.* If prolonged bleeding occurs, you should consult your physician.

The chance of becoming pregnant increases with each pill missed. If you miss one pill, you should take it as soon as you remember and also take your next pill at the regular time, which means you will be taking two pills on that day. If you miss two pills in a row you should take one of the missed pills as soon as you remember, discard the other missed pill, and take your regular pill for that day at the proper time. Furthermore, you should use an additional method of contraception in addition to taking NOR-Q.D.® until you have a period or your doctor determines you are not pregnant. If more than 2 pills in a row have been missed, NOR-Q.D. should be discontinued immediately and an additional method of contraception should be used until you have a period or your doctor determines that you are not pregnant.

Whether or not you have missed a pill, if you have not had a period within 45 days of your last period, *you may be pregnant.* You should stop taking NOR-Q.D. until your doctor determines whether or not you are pregnant. Until you can get to your doctor, use another form of contraception. If you do become pregnant while using NOR-Q.D., you should discuss the risks to the developing child with your doctor.

3. Periodic Examination

Your doctor will take a complete medical and family history before prescribing oral contraceptives. At that time and about once a year thereafter, he will generally examine your blood pressure, breasts, abdomen, and pelvic organs (including a Papanicolaou smear).

Summary: Oral contraceptives are the most effective method, except sterilization, for preventing pregnancy. Other methods, when used conscientiously, are also very effective and have fewer risks. The serious risks of oral contraceptives are uncommon and the "pill" is a very convenient method of preventing pregnancy.

If you have certain conditions or have had these conditions in the past, you should not use oral contraceptives because the risk is too great. These conditions are listed in this leaflet. If you do not have these conditions, and decide to use the "pill", please read this leaflet carefully so that you can use the "pill" most safely and effectively.

Based on his or her assessment of your medical needs, your doctor has prescribed this drug for you. Do not give the drug to anyone else.

[*Shown in Product Identification Section*]

CARMOL® 10 OTC
10% urea lotion
for total body
dry skin care.

A product of Syntex Laboratories, Inc.

(See PDR For Nonprescription Drugs)

CARMOL® 20 OTC
20% Urea Cream
Extra strength for
rough, dry skin

A product of Syntex Laboratories, Inc.

(See PDR For Nonprescription Drugs)

CARMOL® HC ℞
(hydrocortisone acetate)
Cream 1%

A product of Syntex Laboratories, Inc.

Description: CARMOL HC contains micronized hydrocortisone acetate, USP, 10 mg./g., in a water-washable vanishing cream containing urea (10%), purified water, stearic acid, isopropyl myristate, PPG-26 oleate, isopropyl palmitate, propylene glycol, trolamine, cetyl alcohol, carbomer 940, sodium bisulfite, sodium laureth sulfate, edetate disodium, xanthan gum; scented with hypoallergenic perfume. CARMOL HC is non-lipid, non-occlusive and hypoallergenic; it contains no mineral oil, petrolatum, lanolin or parabens.

Actions: Topical steroids are primarily effective because of their anti-inflammatory, antipruritic and vasoconstrictive actions.

Indications: For relief of the inflammatory manifestations of corticosteroid-responsive dermatoses.

Contraindications: Topical steroids are contraindicated in those patients with a history of hypersensitivity to any of the components of the preparation.

Precautions: If irritation develops, the product should be discontinued and appropriate therapy instituted.

In the presence of an infection, the use of an appropriate antifungal or antibacterial agent should be instituted. If a favorable response does not occur promptly, the corticosteroid should be discontinued until the infection has been adequately controlled.

If extensive areas are treated or if the occlusive technique is used there will be increased systemic absorption of the corticosteroid and suitable precautions should be taken, particularly in children and infants.

Although topical steroids have not been reported to have an adverse effect on human pregnancy, the safety of their use in pregnant women has not absolutely been established. In laboratory animals, increases in incidences of fetal abnormalities have been associated with exposure of gestating females to topical corticosteroids, in some cases at rather low dosage levels. Therefore, drugs of this class should not be used extensively on pregnant patients, in large amounts, or for prolonged periods of time.

CARMOL® HC Cream is not for ophthalmic use.

Adverse Reactions: The following local adverse reactions have been reported with topical corticosteroids, especially under occlusive dressings: burning, itching, irritation, dryness, folliculitis, hypertrichosis, acneform eruptions, hypopigmentation, perioral dermatitis, allergic contact dermatitis, maceration of the skin, secondary infection, skin atrophy, striae, miliaria.

Dosage and Administration: Apply to affected areas 3 or 4 times daily.

How Supplied: CARMOL HC (hydrocortisone acetate) Cream, 1%, is supplied in 1 oz. tubes and 4 oz. jars. Protect from excessive heat.

Continued on next page

Syntex—Cont.

EVEX® ℞
(Esterified Estrogens)
TABLETS

A product of Syntex Laboratories, Inc.

1. ESTROGENS HAVE BEEN REPORTED TO INCREASE THE RISK OF ENDOMETRIAL CARCINOMA.
Three independent case control studies have shown an increased risk of endometrial cancer in post-menopausal women exposed to exogenous estrogens for prolonged periods.[1–3] This risk was independent of the other known risk factors for endometrial cancer. These studies are further supported by the finding that incidence rates of endometrial cancer have increased sharply since 1969 in eight different areas of the United States with population-based cancer reporting systems, an increase which may be related to the rapidly expanding use of estrogens during the last decade.[4]
The three case control studies reported that the risk of endometrial cancer in estrogen users was about 4.5 to 13.9 times greater than in nonusers. The risk appears to depend on both duration of treatment[1] and on estrogen dose.[3] In view of these findings, when estrogens are used for the treatment of menopausal symptoms, the lowest dose that will control symptoms should be utilized and medication should be discontinued as soon as possible. When prolonged treatment is medically indicated, the patient should be reassessed on at least a semiannual basis to determine the need for continued therapy. Although the evidence must be considered preliminary, one study suggests that cyclic administration of low doses of estrogen may carry less risk than continuous administration;[3] it therefore appears prudent to utilize such a regimen.
Close clinical surveillance of all women taking estrogens is important. In all cases of undiagnosed persistent or recurring abnormal vaginal bleeding, adequate diagnostic measures should be undertaken to rule out malignancy.
There is no evidence at present that "natural" estrogens are more or less hazardous than "synthetic" estrogens at equiestrogenic doses.
2. ESTROGENS SHOULD NOT BE USED DURING PREGNANCY.
The use of female sex hormones, both estrogens and progestogens, during early pregnancy may seriously damage the offspring. It has been shown that females exposed *in utero* to diethylstibestrol, a nonsteroidal estrogen, have an increased risk of developing in later life a form of vaginal or cervical cancer that is ordinarily extremely rare.[5,6] This risk has been estimated as not greater than 4 per 1000 exposures.[7] Furthermore, a high percentage of such exposed women (from 30 to 90 percent) have been found to have vaginal adenosis, epithelial changes of the vagina and cervix.[8–12] Although these changes are histologically benign, it is not known whether they are precursors of malignancy. Although similar data are not available with the use of other estrogens, it cannot be presumed they would not induce similar changes.
Several reports suggest an association between intrauterine exposure to female sex hormones and congenital anomalies, including congenital heart defects and limb reduction defects.[13–16] One case control study[16] estimated a 4.7 fold increased risk of limb reduction defects in infants exposed *in utero* to sex hormones (oral contraceptives, hormone withdrawal tests for pregnancy, or attempted treatment for threatened abortion). Some of these exposures were very short and involved only a few days of treatment. The data suggest that the risk of limb reduction defects in exposed fetuses is somewhat less than 1 per 1000.
In the past, female sex hormones have been used during pregnancy in an attempt to treat threatened or habitual abortion. There is considerable evidence that estrogens are ineffective for these indications, and there is no evidence from well controlled studies that progestogens are effective for these uses.
If EVEX is used during pregnancy, or if the patient becomes pregnant while taking this drug, she should be apprised of the potential risks to the fetus, and the advisability of pregnancy continuation.

Description: EVEX (esterified estrogens) tablets for oral administration contain either 0.625 mg. or 1.25 mg. of purified, esterified, orally active, water soluble estrogens expressed as sodium estrone sulfate.
Clinical Pharmacology: Estrogens promote growth of the endometrium; promote thickening, stratification, and cornification of the vagina; cause growth of mammary gland ducts; and inhibit the anterior pituitary gland. The ability of estrogens to promote the development of both primary and secondary sex characteristics is of benefit in female hypogonadism, where estrogens provide a substitute for deficient ovarian function.
Indications: EVEX tablets are indicated in the treatment of:

1. Moderate to severe *vasomotor* symptoms associated with the menopause. (There is no evidence that estrogens are effective for nervous symptoms or depression which might occur during menopause, and they should not be used to treat these conditions.)
2. Atrophic vaginitis.
3. Kraurosis vulvae.
4. Female hypogonadism.
5. Female castration.
6. Primary ovarian failure.
7. Breast cancer (for palliation only) in appropriately selected women and men with metastatic disease.
8. Prostatic carcinoma—palliative therapy of advanced disease.

EVEX HAS NOT BEEN SHOWN TO BE EFFECTIVE FOR ANY PURPOSE DURING PREGNANCY AND ITS USE MAY CAUSE SEVERE HARM TO THE FETUS (SEE BOXED WARNING).
Contraindications: Estrogens should not be used in women (or men) with any of the following conditions:

1. Known or suspected cancer of the breast except in appropriately selected patients being treated for metastatic disease.
2. Known or suspected estrogen-dependent neoplasia.
3 EVEX can cause fetal damage when administered to pregnant women. EVEX is contraindicated in women who are or may become pregnant. If this drug is used during pregnancy, or if the patient becomes pregnant while taking this drug, the patient should be apprised of the potential risks to the fetus, and the possibility of termination of the pregnancy should be discussed in the light of those risks. (See boxed warning).
4. Undiagnosed abnormal genital bleeding.
5. Active thrombophlebitis or thromboembolic disorders.
6. A past history of thrombophlebitis or thromboembolic disorders associated with previous estrogen use (except when used in treatment of breast or prostatic malignancy).

Warnings:

1. *Induction of malignant neoplasms.* Long term continuous administration of natural and synthetic estrogens in certain animal species increases the frequency of carcinomas of the breast, cervix, vagina, and liver. There is now evidence that estrogens increase the risk of carcinoma of the endometrium in humans. (See boxed warning.) At the present time there is no satisfactory evidence that estrogens given to postmenopausal women increase the risk of cancer of the breast,[18] although a recent long-term followup of a single physician's practice has raised this possibility.[18a] Because of the animal data there is a need for caution in prescribing estrogens for women with a strong family history of breast cancer or who have breast nodules, fibrocystic disease, or abnormal mammograms.
2. *Gall bladder disease.* A recent study has reported a 2 to 3-fold increase in the risk of surgically confirmed gall bladder disease in women receiving postmenopausal estrogens,[18] similar to the 2-fold increase previously noted in users of oral contraceptives.[19,24] In the case of oral contraceptives, the increased risk appeared after two years of use.[24]
3. *Effects similar to those caused by estrogen-progestogen oral contraceptives.* There are several serious adverse effects of oral contraceptives, most of which have not, up to now, been documented as consequences of postmenopausal estrogen therapy. This may reflect the comparatively low doses of estrogen used in postmenopausal women. It would be expected that the larger doses of estrogen used to treat prostatic or breast cancer or postpartum breast engorgement are more likely to result in these adverse effects, and, in fact, it has been shown that there is an increased risk of thrombosis in men receiving estrogens for prostatic cancer and women for postpartum breast engorgement.[20—23]

a. *Thromboembolic disease.* It is now well established that users of oral contraceptives have an increased risk of various thromboembolic and thrombotic vascular diseases, such as thrombophlebitis, pulmonary embolism, stroke, and myocardial infarction.[24–31] Cases of retinal thrombosis, mesenteric thrombosis and optic neuritis have been reported in oral contraceptive users. There is evidence that the risk of several of these adverse reactions is related to the dose of the drug.[32,33] An increased risk of post-surgery thromboembolic complications has also been reported in users of oral contraceptives.[34,35] If feasible, estrogen should be discontinued at least 4 weeks before surgery of the type associated with an increased risk of thromboembolism, or during periods of prolonged immobilization.
While an increased rate of thromboembolic and thrombotic disease in postmenopausal users of estrogens has not been found[18,36] this does not rule out the possibility that such an increase may be present or that subgroups of women who have underlying risk factors or who are receiving relatively large doses of estrogen may have increased risk. Therefore estrogens should not be used in persons with active thrombophlebitis or thromboembolic disorders, and they should not be used (except in treatment of malignancy) in persons with a history of such disorders in association with estrogen use. They should be used with caution in patients with cerebral vascular or coronary artery disease and only for those women in whom estrogens are clearly needed.

Large doses of estrogen (5 mg. esterified estrogens per day), comparable to those used to treat cancer of the prostate and breast, have been shown in a large prospective clinical trial in men[37] to increase the risk of nonfatal myocardial infarction, pulmonary embolism and thrombophlebitis. When estrogen doses of this size are used, any of the thromboembolic and thrombotic adverse effects associated with oral contraceptive use should be considered a clear risk.

b. *Hepatic adenoma.* Benign hepatic adenomas appear to be associated with the use of oral contraceptives.[38–40] Although benign, and rare, these may rupture and may cause death through intraabdominal hemorrhage. Such lesions have not yet been reported in association with other estrogen or progestogen preparations but should be considered in estrogen users having abdominal pain and tenderness, abdominal mass, or hypovolemic shock. Hepatocellular carcinoma has also been reported in women taking estrogen-containing oral contraceptives.[39] The relationship of this malignancy to these drugs is not known at this time.

c. *Elevated blood pressure.* Increased blood pressure is not uncommon in women using oral contraceptives. There is now a report that this may occur with use of estrogens in the menopause[41] and blood pressure should be monitored with estrogen use, especially if high doses are used.

d. *Glucose tolerance.* A worsening of glucose tolerance has been observed in a significant percentage of patients on estrogen-containing oral contraceptives. For this reason, diabetic patients should be carefully observed while receiving estrogen.

4. *Hypercalcemia.* Administration of estrogens may lead to severe hypercalcemia in patients with breast cancer and bone metastases. If this occurs, the drug should be stopped and appropriate measures taken to reduce the serum calcium level.

Precautions:

A. General Precautions.

1. A complete medical and family history should be taken prior to the initiation of any estrogen therapy. The pretreatment and periodic physical examinations should include special reference to blood pressure, breasts, abdomen, and pelvic organs, and should include a Papanicolaou smear. As a general rule, estrogen should not be prescribed for longer than one year without another physical examination being performed.
2. Fluid retention—Because estrogens may cause some degree of fluid retention, conditions which might be influenced by this factor such as epilepsy, migraine, and cardiac or renal dysfunction, require careful observation.
3. Certain patients may develop undesirable manifestations of excessive estrogenic stimulation, such as abnormal or excessive uterine bleeding, mastodynia, etc.
4. Oral contraceptives appear to be associated with an increased incidence of mental depression.[24] Although it is not clear whether this is due to the estrogenic or progestogenic component of the contraceptive, patients with a history of depression should be carefully observed.
5. Preexisting uterine leiomyomata may increase in size during estrogen use.
6. The pathologist should be advised of estrogen therapy when relevant specimens are submitted.
7. Patients with a past history of jaundice during pregnancy have an increased risk of recurrence of jaundice while receiving estrogen-containing oral contraceptive therapy. If jaundice develops in any patient receiving estrogen, the medication should be discontinued while the cause is investigated.
8. Estrogens may be poorly metabolized in patients with impaired liver function and they should be administered with caution in such patients.
9. Because estrogens influence the metabolism of calcium and phosphorus, they should be used with caution in patients with metabolic bone diseases that are associated with hypercalcemia or in patients with renal insufficiency.
10. Because of the effects of estrogens on epiphyseal closure, they should be used judiciously in young patients in whom bone growth is not complete.
11. Certain endocrine and liver function tests may be affected by estrogen-containing oral contraceptives. The following similar changes may be expected with larger doses of estrogen:
    a. Increased sulfobromophthalein retention.
    b. Increased prothombin and factors VII, VIII, IX, and X; decreased antithrombin 3; increased norepinephrine-induced platelet aggregability.
    c. Increased thyroid binding globulin (TBG) leading to increased circulating total thyroid hormone, as measured by PBI, T4 by column or T4 by radioimmunoassay. Free T3 resin uptake is decreased, reflecting the elevated TBG; free T4 concentration is unaltered.
    d. Impaired glucose tolerance.
    e. Decreased pregnanediol excretion.
    f. Reduced response to metyrapone test.
    g. Reduced serum folate concentration.
    h. Increased serum triglyceride and phospholipid concentration.

B. Pregnancy Category X

See Contraindications and boxed warning.

C. Nursing Mothers

As a general principle, the administration of any drug to nursing mothers should be done only when clearly necessary since many drugs are excreted in human milk.

Adverse Reactions: (See Warnings regarding induction of neoplasia, adverse effects on the fetus, increased incidence of gall bladder disease, and adverse effects similar to those of oral contraceptives, including thromboembolism.) The following additional adverse reactions have been reported with estrogenic therapy, including oral contraceptives:

1. Genitourinary system

Breakthrough bleeding
Spotting
Change in menstrual flow
Dysmenorrhea
Premenstrual-like syndrome
Amenorrhea during and after treatment
Increase in size of uterine fibromyomata
Vaginal candidiasis
Change in cervical eversion and in degree of cervical secretion
Cystitis-like syndrome

2. Breasts

Tenderness, enlargement, secretion

3. Gastrointestinal

Nausea, vomiting
Abdominal cramps, bloating
Cholestatic jaundice

4. Skin

Chloasma or melasma which may persist when drug is discontinued
Erythema multiforme
Erythema nodosum
Hemorrhagic eruption
Loss of scalp hair
Hirsutism

5. Eyes

Steepening of corneal curvature
Intolerance to contact lenses

6. CNS

Headache, migraine, dizziness
Mental depression
Chorea

7. Miscellaneous

Increase or decrease in weight
Reduced carbohydrate tolerance
Aggravation of porphyria
Edema
Changes in libido

Acute Overdosage: Numerous reports of ingestion of large doses of estrogen-containing oral contraceptives by young children indicate that serious ill effects do not occur. Overdosage of estrogen may cause nausea, and withdrawal bleeding may occur in females.

Dosage and Administration:

1. Given cyclically for short term use only:

For treatment of moderate to severe *vasomotor* symptoms, atrophic vaginitis, or kraurosis vulvae associated with the menopause.

The lowest dose that will control symptoms should be chosen and medication should be discontinued as promptly as possible.

Administration should be cyclic (e.g., 3 weeks on and 1 week off).

Attempts to discontinue or taper medication should be made at 3 to 6 month intervals.

The usual dosage ranges are as follows:

Severe vasomotor symptoms: 0.625 mg. to 1.25 mg. daily, depending on severity of symptoms. Dosage may be increased to 2.5 mg. or 3.75 mg. daily if necessary to control symptoms. Dosage should be individualized and titrated according to response.

Atrophic vaginitis and kraurosis vulvae: 1.25 mg. to 3.75 mg. daily for kraurosis vulvae and 0.3 mg. to 1.25 mg. daily for atrophic vaginitis, depending on tissue response. Careful diagnostic evaluation of vulvar lesions is indicated before therapy is instituted.

2. Given cyclically:

Female hypogonadism, female castration, and primary ovarian failure: EVEX is administered for 21 days in a dosage of 2.5 mg. to 7.5 mg. daily. If bleeding occurs before this regimen is concluded, therapy should be discontinued. This same regimen should be resumed following 7 days of no medication, thereby instituting a 3 weeks on, 1 week off dosage regimen.

3. Given chronically:

Inoperable progressing prostatic cancer: For temporary relief of local discomfort, 1.25 mg. to 2.5 mg. daily. Effectiveness can be judged by symptomatic response to therapy and by phosphatase determinations.

Inoperable progressing breast cancer in appropriately selected men and postmenopausal women (see Indications): A dose of up to 10 mg. three times daily over a period of at least three months has been used. Side effects are common in such large doses. Dose adjustment to therapeutic response is important. Treated patients with an intact uterus should be monitored closely for signs of endometrial cancer and appropriate diagnostic measures should be taken to rule out malignancy in the event of persistent or recurring abnormal vaginal bleeding.

References:

[1] Ziel, H. K. and W. D. Finkel, "Increased Risk of Endometrial Carcinoma Among Users of Conjugated Estrogens," *New England Journal of Medicine,* 293:1167-1170, 1975.

[2] Smith, D. C., R. Prentice, D. J. Thompson, and W. L. Hermann, "Association of Exogenous Estrogen and Endometrial Carcinoma," *New England Journal of Medicine,* 293:1164-1167, 1975.

[3] Mack, T. M., M. C. Pike, B. E. Henderson, R. I. Pfeffer, V. R. Gerkins, M. Arthur, and S. E. Brown, "Estrogens and Endometrial Cancer in a Retirement Community," *New England Journal of Medicine,* 294:1262-1267, 1976.

Continued on next page

Syntex—Cont.

[4] Weiss, N. S., D. R. Szekely, and D. F. Austin, "Increasing Incidence of Endometrial Cancer in the United States," *New England Journal of Medicine,* 294:1259-1262, 1976.
[5] Herbst, A. L., H. Ulfelder, and D. C. Poskanzer, "Adenocarcinoma of Vagina," *New England Journal of Medicine,* 284:878-881, 1971.
[6] Greenwald, P., J. Barlow, P. Nasca, and W. Burnett, "Vaginal Cancer after Maternal Treatment with Synthetic Estrogens," *New England Journal of Medicine,* 285:390-392, 1971.
[7] Lanier, A., K. Noller, D. Decker, L. Elveback, and L. Kurland, "Cancer and Stilbestrol. A Follow-up of 1719 Persons Exposed to Estrogens *In Utero* and Born 1943-1959," *Mayo Clinic Proceedings,* 48:793-799, 1973.
[8] Herbst, A., R. Kurman, and R. Scully, "Vaginal and Cervical Abnormalities After Exposure to Stilbestrol *In Utero*," *Obstetrics and Gynecology,* 40:287-298, 1972.
[9] Herbst, A., S. Robboy, G. Macdonald, and R. Scully, "The Effects of Local Progesterone on Stilbestrol-Associated Vaginal Adenosis," *American Journal of Obstetrics and Gynecology,* 118:607-615, 1974.
[10] Herbst, A., D. Poskanzer, S. Robboy, L. Friedlander, and R. Scully, "Prenatal Exposure to Stilbestrol, A Prospective Comparison of Exposed Female Offspring with Unexposed Controls," *New England Journal of Medicine,* 292:334-339, 1975.
[11] Stafi, A., R. Mattingly, D. Foley, and W. Fetherston, "Clinical Diagnosis of Vaginal Adenosis," *Obstetrics and Gynecology,* 43: 118-128, 1974.
[12] Sherman, A. I., M. Goldrath, A. Berlin, V. Vakhariya, F. Banooni, W. Michaels, P. Goodman, S. Brown, "Cervical-Vaginal Adenosis After *In Utero* Exposure to Synthetic Estrogens," *Obstetrics and Gynecology,* 44:531-545, 1974.
[13] Gal, I., B. Kirman, and J. Stern, "Hormone Pregnancy Tests and Congenital Malformation," *Nature* 216:83, 1967.
[14] Levy, E. P., A. Cohen, and F. C. Fraser, "Hormone Treatment During Pregnancy and Congenital Heart Defects," *Lancet,* 1:611, 1973.
[15] Nora, J. and A. Nora, "Birth Defects and Oral Contraceptives," *Lancet,* 1:941-942, 1973.
[16] Janerich, D. T., J. M. Piper, and D. M. Glebatis, "Oral Contraceptives and Congenital Limb-Reduction Defects," *New England Journal of Medicine,* 291:697-700, 1974.
[17] "Estrogens for Oral or Parenteral Use," *Federal Register,* 40:8212, 1975.
[18] Boston Collaborative Drug Surveillance Program "Surgically Confirmed Gall Bladder Disease, Venous Thromboembolism and Breast Tumors in Relation to Post-Menopausal Estrogen Therapy." *New England Journal of Medicine,* 290:15-19, 1974.
[18a] Hoover, R., L. A. Gray, Sr., P. Cole, and B. MacMahon, "Menopausal Estrogens and Breast Cancer," *New England Journal of Medicine,* 295:401-405, 1976.
[19] Boston Collaborative Drug Surveillance Program, "Oral Contraceptives and Venous Thromboembolic Disease, Surgically Confirmed Gall Bladder Disease, and Breast Tumors," *Lancet* 1:1399-1404, 1973.
[20] Daniel, D. G., H. Campbell, and A. C. Turnbull, "Puerperal Thromboembolism and Suppression of Lactation," *Lancet,* 2: 287-289, 1967.
[21] The Veterans Administration Cooperative Urological Research Group, "Carcinoma of the Prostate: Treatment Comparisons," *Journal of Urology,* 98:516-522, 1967.
[22] Bailer, J. C., "Thromboembolism and Oestrogen Therapy," *Lancet,* 2:560, 1967.
[23] Blackard, C., R. Doe, G. Mellinger, and D. Byar, "Incidence of Cardiovascular Disease and Death in Patients Receiving Diethylstilbestrol for Carcinoma of the Prostate," *Cancer,* 26:249-256, 1970.
[24] Royal College of General Practitioners, "Oral Contraception and Thromboembolic Disease," *Journal of the Royal College of General Practitioners,* 13:267-279, 1967.
[25] Inman, W. H. W., and M. P. Vessey, "Investigation of Deaths from Pulmonary, Coronary, and Cerebral Thrombosis and Embolism in Women of Child-Bearing Age," *British Medical Journal,* 2:193-199, 1968.
[26] Vessey, M. P. and R. Doll, "Investigation of Relation Between Use of Oral Contraceptives and Thromboembolic Disease. A Further Report," *British Medical Journal,* 2:651-657, 1969.
[27] Sartwell, P. E., A. T. Masi, F. G. Arthes, G. R. Greene, and H. E. Smith, "Thromboembolism and Oral Contraceptives: An Epidemiological Case Control Study," *American Journal of Epidemiology,* 90:365-380, 1969.
[28] Collaborative Group for the Study of Stroke in Young Women, "Oral Contraception and Increased Risk of Cerebral Ischemia or Thrombosis," *New England Journal of Medicine,* 288:871-878, 1973.
[29] Collaborative Group for the Study of Stroke in Young Women, "Oral Contraceptives and Stroke in Young Women: Associated Risk Factors", *Journal of the American Medical Association,* 231:718-723, 1975.
[30] Mann, J. I. and W. H. W. Inman, "Oral Contraceptives and Death fom Myocardial Infarction," *British Medical Journal,* 2:245-248, 1975.
[31] Mann, J. I., M. P. Vessey, M. Thorogood, and R. Doll, "Myocardial Infarction in Young Women with Special Reference to Oral Contraceptive Practice," *British Medical Journal,* 2:241-245, 1975.
[32] Inman, W. H. W., V. P. Vessey, B. Westerholm, and A. Engelund, "Thromboembolic Disease and the Steroidal Content of Oral Contraceptives," *British Medical Journal,* 2:203-209, 1970.
[33] Stolley, P. D., J. A. Tonascia, M. S. Tockman, P. E. Sartwell, A. H. Rutledge, and M. P. Jacobs, "Thrombosis with Low-Estrogen Oral Contraceptives," *American Journal of Epidemiology,* 102:197-208, 1975.
[34] Vessey, M. P., R. Doll, A. S. Fairbairn, and G. Glober, "Post-Operative Thromboembolism and the Use of the Oral Contraceptives," *British Medical Journal,* 3:123-126, 1970.
[35] Greene, G. R. and P. E. Sartwell, "Oral Contraceptive Use in Patients with Thromboembolism Following Surgery, Trauma or Infection," *American Journal of Public Health,* 62:680-685, 1972.
[36] Rosenberg, L., M. B. Armstrong, and H. Jick, "Myocardial Infarction and Estrogen Therapy in Postmenopausal Women," *New England Journal of Medicine,* 294:1256-1259, 1976.
[37] Coronary Drug Project Research Group, "The Coronary Drug Project: Initial Findings Leading to Modifications of Its Research Protocol, *Journal of the American Medical Association,* 214:1303-1313, 1970.
[38] Baum, J., F. Holtz, J. J. Bookstein, and E. W. Klein, "Possible Association between Benign Hepatomas and Oral Contraceptives," *Lancet,* 2:926-928, 1973.
[39] Mays, E. T., W. M. Christopherson, M. M. Mahr, and H. C. Williams, "Hepatic Changes in Young Women Ingesting Contraceptive Steroids, Hepatic Hemorrhage and Primary Hepatic Tumors," *Journal of the American Medical Association,*" 235:730-782, 1976.
[40] Edmondson, H. A., B. Henderson, and B. Benton, "Liver Cell Adenomas Associated with the Use of Oral Contraceptives," *New England Journal of Medicine,* 294:470-472, 1976.
[41] Pfeiffer, R. I. and S. Van Den Noort, "Estrogen Use and Stroke Risk in Postmenopausal Women," *American Journal of Epidemiology,* 103:445-456, 1976.

How Supplied: EVEX (esterified estrogens) is supplied as film-coated tablets in two potencies in bottles of 100 tablets: 0.625 mg. (orange) and 1.25 mg. (pink).

Patient Labeling

What You Should Know About Estrogens: Estrogens are female hormones produced by the ovaries. The ovaries make several different kinds of estrogens. In addition, scientists have been able to make a variety of synthetic estrogens. As far as we know, all these estrogens have similar properties and therefore much the same usefulness, side effects, and risks. This leaflet is intended to help you understand what estrogens are used for, the risks involved in their use, and how to use them as safely as possible.

This leaflet includes the most important information about estrogens, but not all the information. If you want to know more, you can ask your doctor or pharmacist to let you read the package insert prepared for the doctor.

Uses of Estrogen: Estrogens are prescribed by doctors for a number of purposes, including:

1. To provide estrogen during a period of adjustment when a woman's ovaries no longer produce it, in order to prevent certain uncomfortable symptoms of estrogen deficiency. (All women normally stop producing estrogens, generally between the ages of 45 and 55; this is called the menopause.)
2. To prevent symptoms of estrogen deficiency when a woman's ovaries have been removed surgically before the natural menopause.
3. To treat certain cancers in women and men.
4. To prevent painful swelling of the breasts after pregnancy in women who choose not to nurse their babies, although the usefulness of this treatment is limited and EVEX is not indicated for this use.

THERE IS NO PROPER USE OF ESTROGENS IN A PREGNANT WOMAN.

Estrogens in the Menopause: In the natural course of their lives all women eventually experience a decrease in estrogen production. This usually occurs between ages 45 and 55 but may occur earlier or later. Sometimes the ovaries may need to be removed before natural menopause by an operation, producing a "surgical menopause."

When the amount of estrogen in the blood begins to decrease, many women may develop typical symptoms: feelings of warmth in the face, neck, and chest or sudden intense episodes of heat and sweating throughout the body (called "hot flashes" or "hot flushes"). These symptoms are sometimes very uncomfortable. A few women eventually develop changes in the vagina (called "atrophic vaginitis") which cause discomfort, especially during and after intercourse.

Estrogens can be prescribed to treat these symptoms of the menopause. It is estimated that considerably more than half of all women undergoing the menopause have only mild symptoms or no symptoms at all and therefore do not need estrogens. Other women may need estrogens for a few months, while their bodies adjust to lower estrogen levels. Sometimes the need will be for periods longer than six months. In an attempt to avoid over-stimulation of the uterus (womb), estrogens are usually given cyclically during each month of use, that is, three weeks of pills followed by one week without pills.

Sometimes women experience nervous symptoms or depression during menopause. There is no evidence that estrogens are effective for such symptoms and they should not be used to

treat them, although other treatment may be needed.
You may have heard that taking estrogens for long periods (years) after the menopause will keep your skin soft and supple and keep you feeling young. There is no evidence that this is so, however, and such long-term treatment carries important risks.

The Dangers of Estrogens:

1. *Cancer of the uterus.* When estrogens are used, there is an increased risk of endometrial cancer (cancer of the uterus), particularly with prolonged use. Women taking estrogens have roughly 5 to 10 times as great a chance of getting this cancer as women who take no estrogens. To put this another way, while a postmenopausal woman not taking estrogens has one chance in a 1,000 each year of getting cancer of the uterus, a woman taking estrogens has 5 to 10 chances in 1,000 each year. For this reason *it is important to take estrogens only when you really need them.*
The risk of this cancer is greater the longer estrogens are used and also seems to be greater when larger doses are taken. For this reason *it is important to take the lowest dose of estrogen that will control symptoms and to take it only as long as it is needed.* If estrogens are needed for longer periods of time, your doctor will want to reevaluate your need for estrogens at least every six months.
Women using estrogens should report any irregular vaginal bleeding to their doctors; such bleeding may be of no importance, but it can be an early warning of cancer of the uterus. If you have undiagnosed vaginal bleeding, you should not use estrogens until a diagnosis is made and you are certain there is no cancer of the uterus.
If you have had your uterus completely removed (total hysterectomy), there is no danger of developing cancer of the uterus.
2. *Other possible cancers.* Estrogens can cause development of other tumors in animals, such as tumors of the breast, cervix, vagina, or liver, when given for a long time. At present there is no good evidence that women using estrogen in the menopause have an increased risk of such tumors, but there is no way yet to be sure they do not; and one study raises the possibility that use of estrogens in the menopause may increase the risk of breast cancer many years later. This is a further reason to use estrogens only when clearly needed. While you are taking estrogens, it is important that you go to your doctor at least once a year for a physical examination. Also, if members of your family have had breast cancer or if you have breast nodules or abnormal mammograms (breast x-rays), your doctor may wish to carry out more frequent examinations of your breasts.
3. *Abnormal Blood Clotting.* Oral contraceptives, which contain estrogens, increase the risk of blood clotting in various parts of the body. Use of estrogens alone in the menopause is not known to cause such blood clotting, but this has not been fully studied. Estrogens in large doses in the male have been shown to increase the risk of abnormal blood clotting. Abnormal blood clotting can result in a stroke (if the clot is in the brain), a heart attack (clot in a blood vessel of the heart), or a pulmonary embolus (a clot which forms in the legs or pelvis, then breaks off and travels to the lungs). Any of these can be fatal or can lead to serious disability.
If you have had clotting in the legs or lungs, or have had a stroke or heart attack, or if you have angina pectoris, estrogens should be used with great caution and only if clearly needed. Estrogens should not be used at all if you have had any of these conditions while you were using estrogens or birth control pills previously (unless they are being used to treat cancer of the breast or prostate).
Larger doses of estrogens have been shown to increase the risk of abnormal blood clotting; therefore the dosage should be kept as low as possible.
4. *Gall bladder disease.* Women who use estrogens after the menopause are more likely to develop gall bladder disease needing surgery than women who do not use estrogens. Birth control pills have a similar effect.

Special Warning About Pregnancy: You should not use estrogens if you are pregnant. If this should occur, there is a greater than usual chance that the developing child will be born with a birth defect, although the possibility remains fairly small. A female child may have an increased risk of developing cancer of the vagina or cervix later in life (in the teens or twenties). Every possible effort should be made to avoid exposure to estrogens during pregnancy. If exposure occurs, see your doctor.

Other Effects of Estrogens: In addition to the serious known risks described above, estrogens have the following side effects and potential risks:

1. *Nausea and vomiting.* The most common side effect of estrogen therapy is nausea. Vomiting is less common.
2. *Effects on breasts.* Estrogens may cause breast tenderness or enlargement and may cause the breasts to secrete a liquid. These effects are not dangerous.
3. *Effects on the uterus.* Estrogens may cause benign fibroid tumors of the uterus to get larger.
Some women will have menstrual bleeding when estrogens are stopped. But if the bleeding occurs on days you are still taking estrogens you should report this to your doctor.
4. *Effects on liver.* Women taking oral contraceptives, which contain estrogens, on rare occasions develop a tumor of the liver which can rupture and bleed into the abdomen. You should report any swelling or unusual pain or tenderness in the abdomen to your doctor immediately.
Women with a past history of jaundice (yellowing of the skin and white parts of the eyes) may get jaundice again during estrogen use. If this occurs, stop taking estrogens and see your doctor.
5. *Other effects.* Estrogens may cause excess fluid to be retained in the body. This may make some conditions worse, such as epilepsy, migraine, heart disease, or kidney disease.

Summary: Estrogens have important uses, but they have serious risks as well. You must decide, with your doctor, whether the risks are acceptable to you in view of the benefits of treatment. Except where your doctor has prescribed estrogens for use in special cases of cancer of the breast or prostate, you should not use estrogens if you have cancer of the breast or uterus, are pregnant, have undiagnosed abnormal vaginal bleeding, clotting in the legs or lungs, or have had a stroke, heart attack or angina, or clotting in the legs or lungs in the past while you were taking estrogens.
You can use estrogens as safely as possible by understanding that your doctor will require regular physical examinations while you are taking them and will try to discontinue the drug as soon as possible and use the smallest dose possible. Be alert for signs of trouble including:

1. Abnormal bleeding from the vagina.
2. Pains in the calves or chest or sudden shortness of breath, or coughing blood (indicating possible clots in the legs, heart, or lungs).
3. Severe headache, dizziness, faintness, or changes in vision (indicating possible developing clots in the brain or eye).
4. Breast lumps (you should ask your doctor how to examine your own breasts).
5. Jaundice (yellowing of the skin).
6. Mental depression.

Based on his or her assessment of your medical needs, your doctor has prescribed this drug for you. Do not give this drug to anyone else.

KATO® (potassium chloride for oral solution) 20 mEq. (1.5 g. KCl) ℞

Manufactured for Syntex Laboratories, Inc. by Syntex Puerto Rico, Inc.

Description: KATO (potassium chloride for oral solution) is a pleasantly flavored spray-dried tomato powder containing 20 mEq potassium (equivalent to 1.5 g KCl) per 6 grams of powder (one dose), and natural and artificial flavors, spices and colors with benzoic acid and potassium benzoate added as preservatives. KATO is a potassium replacement product. Each daily dose (2 packets) contains approximately 0.5 mEq sodium.

Clinical Pharmacology: As the principal intracellular cation of most body tissues, potassium is instrumental in physiological processes such as maintenance of intracellular tonicity, contractility of cardiac, skeletal, and smooth muscles, maintenance of renal function, and transmission of nervous impulses.
Potassium depletion may occur when potassium intake is insufficient to compensate for potassium loss from the G.I. tract or via renal excretion. Such loss may slowly develop during prolonged oral diuretic therapy, in hyperaldosteronism, diabetic ketoacidosis, severe diarrhea, or where potassium intake is inadequate in patients receiving prolonged parenteral nutrition.
The potassium deficit is usually accompanied by chloride depletion and is manifested by hypokalemia and a hypochloremic metabolic alkalosis. Clinical symptoms and signs include weakness, fatigue, disturbances of cardiac rhythmicity (primarily ectopic beats), EKG changes (prominent U waves) and, in severe cases, flaccid paralysis and/or impaired urinary concentration.
Potassium chloride is therefore regarded as the appropriate potassium salt for use in correcting potassium depletion states associated with metabolic alkalosis.

Indications and Usage: KATO is indicated for the treatment or prevention of potassium deficit, particularly when accompanied by hypochloremic alkalosis in conjunction with thiazide diuretic therapy, in digitalis intoxication, or as a result of long-term corticosteroid therapy, low dietary intake of potassium, or excessive vomiting or diarrhea.

Contraindications: Potassium is contraindicated in patients with: severe renal impairment involving oliguria, anuria or azotemia; untreated Addison's disease; familial periodic paralysis; acute dehydration; heat cramps; and hyperkalemia from any cause.

Warnings: Potassium intoxication may result from overdosage or from the usual therapeutic dose in patients for whom the drug is contraindicated. Hyperkalemia, when detected, must be treated immediately because lethal levels can be reached in a few hours. (See Overdosage for treatment of hyperkalemia).

Precautions:

General: Patients receiving potassium supplementation should be monitored with periodic checks of plasma potassium levels.
A high plasma concentration of potassium ion may cause death through cardiac depression, arrhythmias or arrest. Therefore, the drug should be used with caution in patients with cardiac disease.
The drug should not be used in patients with low urinary output or renal decompensation because of the heightened likelihood of overdosage.
In rare circumstances (e.g. patients with renal tubular acidosis) potassium depletion may be associated with a hyperchloremic metabolic acidosis. In such patients, potassium depletion is appropriately corrected using potassium salts other than the chloride.

Continued on next page

Syntex—Cont.

As with other concentrated potassium supplements, KATO must be reconstituted with the proper amount of water (2 oz. for 1 packet) to avoid the possibility of gastrointestinal irritation.

Drug Interactions: Concomitant administration of potassium chloride and a potassium-sparing diuretic (e.g. aldosterone antagonists or triamterene) can lead to severe hyperkalemia.

Adverse Reactions: Adverse reactions are related to the gastrointestinal system. Vomiting, diarrhea, nausea and abdominal discomfort may occur.

Overdosage: The symptoms and signs of potassium intoxication include paresthesias of the extremities, flaccid paralysis, listlessness, mental confusion, weakness and heaviness of the legs, fall in blood pressure, cardiac arrhythmias and heart block. Hyperkalemia may be associated with the following electrocardiographic abnormalities: disappearance of the P wave, widening and slurring of the QRS complex, changes of the S-T segment and tall peaked T waves.

The drug is dialyzable.

Treatment of hyperkalemia includes: 1. Elimination of potassium-containing foods and medicaments. 2. Dextrose solution 10% or 25% containing 10 units of crystalline insulin per 20 g dextrose, given i.v. with a dose of 300 cc to 500 cc in an hour. 3. Adsorption and exchange of potassium using sodium or ammonium cycle cation exchange resin, orally or as retention enema. 4. Hemodialysis or peritonial dialysis.

Warning: Digitalis toxicity can be precipitated by lowering the plasma potassium concentration too rapidly in digitalized patients.

Dosage and Administration: The usual adult dose is 1 packet of KATO (20 mEq potassium) mixed with 2 ounces of cold water twice daily. If possible it should stand for 15 minutes to allow the tomato powder to absorb moisture. The preparation should be taken with meals, if convenient. If not, drink ½ glass of water immediately after taking the medication. Larger doses may be required, but should be administered under close supervision because of the possibility of potassium intoxication.

The appropriate dosage of potassium for pediatric use may be calculated from the adult dosage according to relative total body weight.

How Supplied: KATO is available in cartons of 30 (NDC 18393-488-30) and 120 (NDC 18393-488-40) 6-gram unit dose packets (20 mEq potassium each). Store away from heat.

LIDEX® ℞
(fluocinonide)
CREAM 0.05%
OINTMENT 0.05%

LIDEX®–E ℞
(fluocinonide)
CREAM 0.05%

TOPSYN® ℞
(fluocinonide)
GEL 0.05%

Products of Syntex Laboratories, Inc.

Description: LIDEX preparations contain the active compound fluocinonide; TOPSYN gel also contains the active compound fluocinonide. Fluocinonide, which is the 21-acetate ester of fluocinolone acetonide, has the chemical formula 6α, 9-difluoro-11β, 16α, 17, 21-tetrahydroxypregna-1, 4-diene-3, 20-dione, cyclic 16, 17-acetal with acetone 21-acetate.

LIDEX cream contains fluocinonide 0.5 mg./g. in FAPG® cream, a specially formulated cream base consisting of stearyl alcohol, polyethylene glycol 8000, propylene glycol, 1,2,6-hexanetriol and citric acid. This white cream vehicle is greaseless, non-staining, anhydrous and completely water miscible. The base provides emollient and hydrophilic properties.

LIDEX ointment contains fluocinonide 0.5 mg./g. in a specially formulated ointment base consisting of Amerchol CAB (mixture of sterols and higher alcohols), white petrolatum, propylene carbonate and propylene glycol. It provides the occlusive and emollient effects desirable in an ointment.

In these formulations, the active ingredient is totally in solution.

LIDEX-E cream contains fluocinonide 0.5 mg./g. in a water-washable aqueous emollient base of stearyl alcohol, cetyl alcohol, mineral oil, propylene glycol, sorbitan monostearate, polysorbate 60, citric acid and purified water.

TOPSYN gel contains fluocinonide 0.5 mg./g. in a specially formulated gel base consisting of propylene glycol, propyl gallate, edetate disodium, and Carbopol 940 (carboxypolymethylene) with NaOH and/or HCl added to adjust the pH. This clear, colorless, thixotropic vehicle is greaseless, non-staining and completely water miscible. In this formulation, the active ingredient is totally in solution.

Actions: LIDEX preparations and TOPSYN gel are primarily effective because of their anti-inflammatory, antipruritic and vasoconstrictor actions.

Indications: For relief of the inflammatory manifestations of corticosteroid-responsive dermatoses.

Contraindications: Topical steroids are contraindicated in those patients with a history of hypersensitivity to any of the components of the preparation.

Precautions: If irritation develops, the cream should be discontinued and appropriate therapy instituted.

In the presence of an infection, the use of an appropriate antifungal or antibacterial agent should be instituted. If a favorable response does not occur promptly, the corticosteroid cream should be discontinued until the infection has been adequately controlled.

If extensive areas are treated or if occlusive technique is used, there will be increased systemic absorption of the corticosteroid and suitable precautions should be taken, particularly in children and infants.

Although topical steroids have not been reported to have an adverse effect on human pregnancy, the safety of their use in pregnant women has not absolutely been established. In laboratory animals, increases in incidences of fetal abnormalities have been associated with exposure of gestating females to topical corticosteroids, in some cases at rather low dosage levels. Therefore, drugs of this class should not be used extensively on pregnant patients, in large amounts or for prolonged periods of time.

LIDEX preparations and TOPSYN gel are not for ophthalmic use.

Adverse Reactions: The following local adverse reactions have been reported with topical corticosteroids: burning, itching, irritation, dryness, folliculitis, hypertrichosis, acneform eruptions, hypopigmentation, perioral dermatitis, allergic contact dermatitis, maceration of the skin, secondary infection, skin atrophy, striae, miliaria.

Dosage and Administration: A small amount should be gently massaged into the affected area two to four times daily for the LIDEX preparations and three or four times daily for TOPSYN gel, as needed.

How Supplied:

LIDEX (fluocinonide)
- Cream 0.05%—15g., 30g., 60g. and 120g. tubes.
- Ointment 0.05%—15g., 30g., 60g. and 120g. tubes.

LIDEX-E
- Cream 0.05%—15g., 30g., 60g. and 120g. tubes.

TOPSYN
- Gel 0.05%—15g., 30g., 60g. and 120g. tubes.

NAPROSYN® ℞
(naproxen)
Tablets

Manufactured for Syntex Laboratories, Inc. by Syntex Puerto Rico, Inc.

Description: NAPROSYN® (naproxen) tablets for oral administration each contain 250 mg, 375 mg or 500 mg of naproxen. NAPROSYN is a member of the arylacetic acid group of nonsteroidal anti-inflammatory drugs. The chemical name for naproxen is 2-naphthaleneacetic acid, 6-methoxy-α-methyl-,(+).

Naproxen is an odorless, white to off-white crystalline substance. It is lipid soluble, practically insoluble in water at low pH and freely soluble in water at high pH.

Clinical Pharmacology: NAPROSYN (naproxen) is a nonsteroidal anti-inflammatory drug with analgesic and antipyretic properties. Naproxen sodium, the sodium salt of naproxen, has been developed as an analgesic because it is more rapidly absorbed. The naproxen anion inhibits prostaglandin synthesis but beyond this its mode of action is unknown.

Naproxen is rapidly and completely absorbed from the gastrointestinal tract. After administration of naproxen, peak plasma levels of naproxen anion are attained in 2 to 4 hours, with steady-state conditions normally achieved after 4–5 doses. The mean biological half-life of the anion in humans is approximately 13 hours, and at therapeutic levels it is greater than 99% albumin bound. Approximately 95% of the dose is excreted in the urine, primarily as naproxen, 6-0-desmethyl naproxen or their conjugates. The rate of excretion has been found to coincide closely with the rate of drug disappearance from the plasma. The drug does not induce metabolizing enzymes.

The drug was studied in patients with rheumatoid arthritis, osteoarthritis, juvenile arthritis, ankylosing spondylitis and acute gout. It is not a corticosteroid. Improvement in patients treated for rheumatoid arthritis has been demonstrated by a reduction in joint swelling, a reduction in pain, a reduction in duration of morning stiffness, a reduction in disease activity as assessed by both the investigator and patient, and by increased mobility as demonstrated by a reduction in walking time.

In patients with osteoarthritis, the therapeutic action of the drug has been shown by a reduction in joint pain or tenderness, an increase in range of motion in knee joints, increased mobility as demonstrated by a reduction in walking time, and improvement in capacity to perform activities of daily living impaired by the disease.

In clinical studies in patients with rheumatoid arthritis, osteoarthritis, and juvenile arthritis, the drug has been shown to be comparable to aspirin and indomethacin in controlling the aforementioned measures of disease activity, but the frequency and severity of the milder gastrointestinal adverse effects (nausea, dyspepsia, heartburn) and nervous system adverse effects (tinnitus, dizziness, lightheadedness) were less than in both the aspirin- and indomethacin-treated patients. It is not known whether the drug causes less peptic ulceration than aspirin.

In patients with ankylosing spondylitis, the drug has been shown to decrease night pain, morning stiffness and pain at rest. In double-blind studies the drug was shown to be as effective as aspirin, but with fewer side effects.

In patients with acute gout, a favorable response to the drug was shown by significant clearing of inflammatory changes (e.g., decrease in swelling, heat) within 24–48 hours, as well as by relief of pain and tenderness.

The drug may be used safely in combination with gold salts and/or corticosteroids; however, in controlled clinical trials, when added to the regimen of patients receiving corticosteroids it did not appear to cause greater improvement over that seen with corticosteroids alone. Whether the drug could be used in conjunction with partially effective doses of corticosteroid for a "steroid-sparing" effect has not been adequately studied. When added to the regimen of patients receiving gold salts the drug did result in greater improvement. Its use in combination with salicylates is not recommended because data are inadequate to demonstrate that the drug produces greater improvement over that achieved with aspirin alone. Further, there is some evidence that aspirin increases the rate of excretion of the drug.

Generally, improvement due to the drug has not been found to be dependent on age, sex, severity or duration of disease.

The drug was studied in patients with mild to moderate pain, and pain relief was obtained within 1 hour. It is not a narcotic and is not a CNS-acting drug. Controlled double-blind studies have demonstrated the analgesic properties of the drug in, for example, post-operative, post-partum, orthopedic and uterine contraction pain and dysmenorrhea. In dysmenorrheic patients, the drug reduces the level of prostaglandins in the uterus, which correlates with a reduction in the frequency and severity of uterine contractions. Analgesic action has been shown by such measures as a reduction of pain intensity scores, increase in pain relief scores, decrease in numbers of patients requiring additional analgesic medication, and delay in time for required remedication. The analgesic effect has been found to last for up to 7 hours.

In ^{51}Cr blood loss and gastroscopy studies with normal volunteers, daily administration of 1000 mg of the drug has been demonstrated to cause statistically significantly less gastric bleeding and erosion than 3250 mg of aspirin.

Indications and Usage: NAPROSYN (naproxen) is indicated for the treatment of the signs and symptoms of mild to moderately severe, acute or chronic, musculoskeletal and soft tissue inflammation.

It is also indicated in the relief of mild to moderate pain and for the treatment of primary dysmenorrhea.

Contraindications: Naproxen is contraindicated in patients who have shown hypersensitivity to it. Because the potential exists for cross-sensitivity reactions, the drug should not be given to patients in whom aspirin or other non-steroidal anti-inflammatory drugs induce the syndrome of asthma, rhinitis, or urticaria.

Warnings: Gastrointestinal bleeding, sometimes severe, and occasionally fatal, has been reported in patients receiving the drug. Among 960 patients treated for rheumatoid arthritis or osteoarthritis during the course of clinical trials in the United States (260 treated for more than two years), 16 cases of peptic ulceration were reported. More than half were on concomitant corticosteroid and/or salicylate therapy and about a third had a prior history of peptic ulcer. Gastrointestinal bleeding, including nine potentially serious cases, was also reported in this population. These were not always preceded by premonitory gastrointestinal symptoms. Although most of the patients with serious bleeding were receiving concomitant therapy and had a history of peptic ulcer disease, it should be kept in mind that the drug also has the potential for causing gastrointestinal bleeding on its own. Therefore, it should be administered to patients with active gastric and duodenal ulcers only under close supervision.

Precautions:

General:

***NAPROSYN*® (NAPROXEN) SHOULD NOT BE USED CONCOMITANTLY WITH THE RELATED DRUG *ANAPROX*® (NAPROXEN SODIUM) SINCE THEY BOTH CIRCULATE IN PLASMA AS THE NAPROXEN ANION.**

In chronic studies in laboratory animals, the drug has caused nephritis. Glomerular nephritis, interstitial nephritis and nephrotic syndrome have been reported in humans. Naproxen should therefore be used with great caution in patients with significantly impaired renal function and the monitoring of serum creatinine and/or creatinine clearance is advised in these patients.

As with other nonsteroidal anti-inflammatory drugs borderline elevations of one or more liver tests may occur in up to 15% of patients. These abnormalities may progress, may remain essentially unchanged, or may be transient with continued therapy. The SGPT (AST) test is probably the most sensitive indicator of liver dysfunction. Meaningful (3 times the upper limit of normal) elevations of SGPT or SGOT (AST) occurred in controlled trials in less than 1% of patients. A patient with symptoms and/or signs suggesting liver dysfunction, or in whom an abnormal liver test has occurred, should be evaluated for evidence of the development of more severe hepatic reaction while on therapy with this drug. Severe hepatic reactions, including jaundice and cases of fatal hepatitis, have been reported with this drug as with other nonsteroidal anti-inflammatory drugs. Although such reactions are rare, if abnormal liver tests persist or worsen, if clinical signs and symptoms consistent with liver disease develop, or if systemic manifestations occur (e.g. eosinophilia, rash, etc.), this drug should be discontinued.

If steroid dosage is reduced or eliminated during therapy, the steroid dosage should be reduced slowly and the patients must be observed closely for any evidence of adverse effects, including adrenal insufficiency and exacerbation of symptoms of arthritis.

Patients with initial hemoglobin values of 10 grams or less who are to receive long-term therapy should have hemoglobin values determined frequently.

Peripheral edema has been observed in some patients. For this reason, the drug should be used with caution in patients with fluid retention, hypertension or heart failure.

The antipyretic and anti-inflammatory activities of the drug may reduce fever and inflammation, thus diminishing their utility as diagnostic signs in detecting complications of presumed non-infectious, non-inflammatory painful conditions.

Because of adverse eye findings in animal studies with drugs of this class it is recommended that ophthalmic studies be carried out within a reasonable period of time after starting therapy and at periodic intervals thereafter if the drug is to be used for an extended period of time.

Information for Patients:

Caution should be exercised by patients whose activities require alertness if they experience drowsiness, dizziness, vertigo or depression during therapy with the drug.

Drug Interactions:

In vitro studies have shown that naproxen anion, because of its affinity for protein, may displace from their binding sites other drugs which are also albumin-bound. Theoretically, the naproxen anion itself could likewise be displaced. Short-term controlled studies failed to show that taking the drug significantly affects prothrombin times when administered to individuals on coumarin-type anticoagulants. Caution is advised nonetheless, since interactions have been seen with other non-steroidal agents of this class. Similarly, patients receiving the drug and a hydantoin, sulfonamide or sulfonylurea should be observed for signs of toxicity to these drugs.

Probenecid given concurrently increases naproxen anion plasma levels and extends its plasma half-life significantly.

Drug/Laboratory Test Interactions:

The drug may decrease platelet aggregation and prolong bleeding time. This effect should be kept in mind when bleeding times are determined.

The administration of the drug may result in increased urinary values for 17-ketogenic steroids because of an interaction between the drug and/or its metabolites with m-dinitrobenzene used in this assay. Although 17-hydroxy-corticosteroid measurements (Porter-Silber test) do not appear to be artifactually altered, it is suggested that therapy with the drug be temporarily discontinued 72 hours before adrenal function tests are performed.

The drug may interfere with some urinary assays of 5-hydroxy indoleacetic acid (5HIAA).

Carcinogenesis:

A two-year study was performed in rats to evaluate the carcinogenic potential of the drug. No evidence of carcinogenicity was found.

Pregnancy:

Teratogenic Effects: Pregnancy Category B. Reproduction studies have been performed in rats, rabbits and mice at doses up to six times the human dose and have revealed no evidence of impaired fertility or harm to the fetus due to the drug. There are, however, no adequate and well-controlled studies in pregnant women. Because animal reproduction studies are not always predictive of human response, the drug should not be used during pregnancy unless clearly needed. Because of the known effect of drugs of this class on the human fetal cardiovascular system (closure of ductus arteriosus), use during late pregnancy should be avoided.

Non-teratogenic Effects: As with other drugs known to inhibit prostaglandin synthesis, an increased incidence of dystocia and delayed parturition occurred in rats.

Nursing Mothers:

The naproxen anion has been found in the milk of lactating women at a concentration of approximately 1% of that found in the plasma. Because of the possible adverse effects of prostaglandin-inhibiting drugs on neonates, use in nursing mothers should be avoided.

Adverse Reactions: Adverse reactions reported in controlled clinical trials in 960 patients treated for rheumatoid arthritis or osteoarthritis are listed below. In general, these reactions were reported 2 to 10 times more frequently than they were in studies in the 962 patients treated for mild to moderate pain or for dysmenorrhea.

Incidence greater than 1%

Gastrointestinal: The most frequent complaints reported related to the gastrointestinal tract. They were: constipation*, heartburn*, abdominal pain*, nausea*, dyspepsia, diarrhea, stomatitis. **Central Nervous System:** Headache*, dizziness*, drowsiness*, lightheadedness, vertigo. **Dermatologic:** Itching (pruritus)*, skin eruptions*, ecchymoses*, sweating, purpura. **Special Senses:** Tinnitus*, hearing disturbances, visual disturbances. **Cardiovascular:** Edema*, dyspnea*, palpitations. **General:** Thirst.

* Incidence of reported reactions between 3% and 9%. Those reactions occurring in less than 3% of the patients are unmarked.

Incidence less than 1%

Probable Causal Relationship:

The following adverse reactions were reported less frequently than 1% during controlled clinical trials and through voluntary reports since marketing. The probability of a causal relationship exists between the drug and these adverse reactions: congestive heart failure, renal disease, glomerular nephritis, interstitial nephritis, nephrotic syndrome, abnormal liver function tests, hematuria, jaundice, thrombocytopenia, leukopenia, granulocytopenia, gastrointestinal bleeding, peptic ulceration with bleeding and/or perforation, hematemesis,

Continued on next page

Syntex—Cont.

melena, vomiting, eosinophilia, pyrexia (chills and fever), skin rashes, menstrual disorders, myalgia and muscle weakness, alopecia, inability to concentrate, depression, malaise, dream abnormalities.

Causal Relationship Unknown:
Other reactions have been reported in circumstances in which a causal relationship could not be established. However, in these rarely reported events, the possibility cannot be excluded. Therefore these observations are being listed to serve as alerting information to the physicians: angioneurotic edema, agranulocytosis, aplastic anemia, hemolytic anemia, hypoglycemia, hyperglycemia, urticaria.

Overdosage: Significant overdosage may be characterized by drowsiness, heartburn, indigestion, nausea or vomiting. No evidence of toxicity or late sequelae have been reported 5 to 15 months after ingestion for three to seven days of doses up to 3,000 mg of naproxen. One patient ingested a single dose of 25 g of naproxen and experienced mild nausea and indigestion. It is not known what dose of the drug would be life threatening. The oral LD_{50} of the drug is 543 mg/kg in rats, 1234 mg/kg in mice, 4110 mg/kg in hamsters and greater than 1000 mg/kg in dogs.
Should a patient ingest a large number of tablets, accidentally or purposefully, the stomach may be emptied and usual supportive measures employed. Animal studies suggest that the prompt administration of 5 grams of activated charcoal would tend to reduce markedly the absorption of the drug. It is not known if the drug is dialyzable.

Dosage and Administration:
For Mild to Moderately Severe, Acute or Chronic, Musculoskeletal and Soft Tissue Inflammation:
The recommended starting dose in adults is one 250 mg tablet or one 375 mg tablet twice daily (morning and evening). During long-term administration, the dose may be adjusted up or down depending on the clinical response of the patient. A lower daily dose may suffice for long-term administration. Daily doses higher than 1000 mg in these indications have not been studied. The morning and evening doses do not have to be equal in size and the administration of the drug more frequently than twice daily is not necessary. Symptomatic improvement in arthritis usually begins within two weeks. However, if improvement is not seen within this period, a trial for an additional two weeks should be considered.
For Acute Gout:
The recommended starting dose is 750 mg, followed by 250 mg every eight hours until the attack has subsided.
For Juvenile Arthritis:
The recommended total daily dose is approximately 10 mg/kg given in two divided doses. The scored 250 mg tablet may be used to approximate this dose.
For Mild to Moderate Pain and Primary Dysmenorrhea:
The recommended starting dose is 500 mg, followed by 250 mg every 6 to 8 hours, as required. The total daily dose should not exceed 1,250 mg.

How Supplied: NAPROSYN (naproxen) is available in scored tablets of 250 mg (yellow) in bottles of 100 tablets (NDC 18393-272-42) and 500 tablets (NDC 18393-272-62) or in cartons of 100 individually blister packed tablets (NDC 18393-272-53) and in 375 mg (peach) tablets in bottles of 100 tablets (NDC 18393-273-42) and 500 tablets (NDC 18393-273-62) or in cartons of 100 individually blister packed tablets (NDC 18393-273-53). The 500 mg (yellow) tablets are available in bottles of 100 tablets (NDC 18393-277-42). Store at room temperature in well-closed containers; dispense in light-resistant containers.
[*Shown in Product Identification Section*]

NASALIDE® ℞
(flunisolide)
Nasal Solution
0.025%
For Nasal Use Only

A product of Syntex Laboratories, Inc.

Description: NASALIDE® (flunisolide) nasal solution is intended for administration as a spray to the nasal mucosa. Flunisolide, the active component of NASALIDE nasal solution, is an anti-inflammatory steroid with the chemical name: 6α-fluoro-11β, 16α, 17,21-tetrahydroxypregna-1,4-diene-3,20-dione cyclic 16,17-acetal with acetone (USAN).
Flunisolide is a white to creamy white crystalline powder with a molecular weight of 434.49. It is soluble in acetone, sparingly soluble in chloroform, slightly soluble in methanol, and practically insoluble in water. It has a melting point of about 245°C.
Each 25 ml spray bottle contains flunisolide 6.25 mg (0.25 mg/ml) in a solution of propylene glycol, polyethylene glycol 3350 and purified water buffered with citric acid/sodium citrate, with benzalkonium chloride added as a preservative, and NaOH and/or HCl added to adjust the pH to approximately 5.8. It contains no fluorocarbons.
After priming the delivery system for NASALIDE, each actuation of the unit delivers a metered droplet spray containing approximately 25 mcg of flunisolide. The size of the droplets produced by the unit is in excess of 8 microns to facilitate deposition on the nasal mucosa. The contents of one nasal spray bottle deliver at least 200 sprays.

Clinical Pharmacology: NASALIDE® (flunisolide) has demonstrated potent glucocorticoid and weak mineralocorticoid activity in classical animal test systems. As a glucocorticoid it is several hundred times more potent that the cortisol standard. Clinical studies with flunisolide have shown therapeutic activity on nasal mucous membranes with minimal evidence of systemic activity at the recommended doses.
Following administration of flunisolide to man, approximately half of the administered dose is recovered in the urine and half in the stool; 65–70% of the dose recovered in urine is the primary metabolite, which has undergone loss of the 6α fluorine and addition of a 6β hydroxy group. Flunisolide is well absorbed but is rapidly converted by the liver to the much less active primary metabolite and to glucuronate and/or sulfate conjugates. Because of first-pass liver metabolism, only 20% of the flunisolide reaches the systemic circulation when it is given orally whereas 50% of the flunisolide administered intranasally reaches the systemic circulation unmetabolized. The plasma half-life of flunisolide is 1–2 hours.
The effects of flunisolide on hypothalamic-pituitary-adrenal (HPA) axis function have been studied in adult volunteers. NASALIDE was administered intranasally as a spray in total doses over 7 times the recommended dose (2200 mcg, equivalent to 88 sprays/day) in 2 subjects for 4 days, about 3 times the recommended dose (800 mcg, equivalent to 32 sprays/day) in 4 subjects for 4 days, and over twice the recommended dose (700 mcg, equivalent to 28 sprays/day) in 6 subjects for 10 days. Early morning plasma cortisol concentrations and 24-hour urinary 17-ketogenic steroids were measured daily. There was evidence of decreased endogenous cortisol production at all three doses.
In controlled studies, NASALIDE was found to be effective in reducing symptoms of stuffy nose, runny nose and sneezing in most patients. These controlled clinical studies have been conducted in 488 adult patients at doses ranging from 8 to 16 sprays (200–400 mcg) per day and 127 children at doses ranging from 6 to 8 sprays (150–200 mcg) per day for periods as long as 3 months. In 170 patients who had cortisol levels evaluated at baseline and after 3 months or more of flunisolide treatment, there was no unequivocal flunisolide-related depression of plasma cortisol levels.
The mechanisms responsible for the anti-inflammatory action of corticosteroids and for the activity for the aerosolized drug on the nasal mucosa are unknown.

Indications: NASALIDE® (flunisolide) is indicated for the relief of the symptoms of seasonal or perennial rhinitis when effectiveness of or tolerance to conventional treatment is unsatisfactory.
Clinical studies have shown that improvement is usually apparent within a few days after starting NASALIDE. However, symptomatic relief may not occur in some patients for as long as two weeks. Although systemic effects are minimal at recommended doses, NASALIDE should not be continued beyond 3 weeks in the absence of significant symptomatic improvement.
NASALIDE should not be used in the presence of untreated localized infection involving nasal mucosa.

Contraindications: Hypersensitivity to any of the ingredients.

Warnings: The replacement of a systemic corticosteroid with a topical corticoid can be accompanied by signs of adrenal insufficiency, and in addition some patients may experience symptoms of withdrawal, e.g., joint and/or muscular pain, lassitude and depression. Patients previously treated for prolonged periods with systemic corticosteroids and transferred to NASALIDE® (flunisolide) should be carefully monitored to avoid acute adrenal insufficiency in response to stress.
When transferred to NASALIDE, careful attention must be given to patients previously treated for prolonged periods with systemic corticosteroids. This is particularly important in those patients who have associated asthma or other clinical conditions, where too rapid a decrease in systemic corticosteroids may cause a severe exacerbation of their symptoms.
The use of NASALIDE with alternate-day prednisone systemic treatment could increase the likelihood of HPA suppression compared to a therapeutic dose of either one alone. Therefore, NASALIDE treatment should be used with caution in patients already on alternate-day prednisone regimens for any disease.

Precautions:
General: In clinical studies with flunisolide administered intranasally, the development of localized infections of the nose and pharynx with *Candida albicans* has occurred only rarely. When such an infection develops it may require treatment with appropriate local therapy or discontinuance of treatment with NASALIDE® (flunisolide).
Flunisolide is absorbed into the circulation. Use of excessive doses of NASALIDE may suppress hypothalamic-pituitary-adrenal function.
Flunisolide should be used with caution, if at all, in patients with active or quiescent tuberculosis infections of the respiratory tract or in untreated fungal, bacterial or systemic viral infections or ocular herpes simplex.
Because of the inhibitory effect of corticosteroids on wound healing, in patients who have experienced recent nasal septal ulcers, recurrent epistaxis, nasal surgery or trauma, a nasal corticosteroid should be used with caution until healing has occurred.
Although systemic effects have been minimal with recommended doses, this potential increases with excessive dosages. Therefore, larger than recommended doses should be avoided.

Information for Patients: Patients should use NASALIDE at regular intervals since its effectiveness depends on its regular use. The patient should take the medication as directed. It is not acutely effective and the prescribed dosage should not be increased. Instead, nasal vasoconstrictors or oral antihistamines may be needed until the effects of NASALIDE are fully manifested. One to two weeks may pass before full relief is obtained. The patient should contact the physician if symptoms do not improve, or if the condition worsens, or if sneezing or nasal irritation occurs.

For the proper use of this unit and to attain maximum improvement, the patient should read and follow the accompanying Patient Instructions carefully.

Carcinogenesis: A 22-month study was conducted in Swiss derived mice to evaluate the carcinogenic potential of the drug. While no evidence of carcinogenicity was found, there was a slight increase in the incidence of pulmonary adenomas which was well within the range of spontaneous adenomas previously reported in the literature for untreated or control Swiss derived mice. An additional study is being conducted in a species with a lower incidence of spontaneous pulmonary tumors.

Impairment of fertility: Female rats receiving high doses of flunisolide (200 mcg/kg/day) showed some evidence of impaired fertility. Reproductive performance in the low (8 mcg/kg/day) and mid-dose (40 mcg/kg/day) groups was comparable to controls.

Pregnancy: Teratogenic effects: Pregnancy Category C. As with other corticosteroids, flunisolide has been shown to be teratogenic in rabbits and rats at doses of 40 and 200 mcg/kg/day respectively. It was also fetotoxic in these animal reproductive studies. There are no adequate and well-controlled studies in pregnant women. Flunisolide should be used during pregnancy only if the potential benefit justifies the potential risk to the fetus.

Nursing Mothers: It is not known whether this drug is excreted in human milk. Because other corticosteroids are excreted in human milk, caution should be exercised when flunisolide is administered to nursing women.

Adverse Reactions: Adverse reactions reported in controlled clinical trials and long-term open studies in 595 patients treated with NASALIDE are described below. Of these patients, 409 were treated for 3 months or longer, 323 for 6 months or longer, 259 for 1 year or longer, and 91 for 2 years or longer.

In general, side effects elicited in the clinical studies have been primarily associated with the nasal mucous membranes. The most frequent complaints were those of mild transient nasal burning and stinging, which were reported in approximately 45% of the patients treated with NASALIDE in placebo-controlled and long-term studies. These complaints do not usually interfere with treatment; in only 3% of patients was it necessary to decrease dosage or stop treatment because of these symptoms. Approximately the same incidence of mild transient nasal burning and stinging was reported in patients on placebo as was reported in patients treated with NASALIDE in controlled studies, implying that these complaints may be related to the vehicle or the delivery system. The incidence of complaints of nasal burning and stinging decreased with increasing duration of treatment.

Other side effects reported at a frequency of 5% or less were: nasal congestion, sneezing, epistaxis and/or bloody mucus, nasal irritation, watery eyes, sore throat, nausea and/or vomiting, headaches and loss of sense of smell and taste. In rare instances, nasal septal perforations were observed during the studies but a causal relationship with NASALIDE was not established.

Systemic corticosteroid side effects were not reported during the controlled clinical trials. If recommended doses are exceeded, or if individuals are particularly sensitive, symptoms of hypercorticism, i.e., Cushing's syndrome, could occur.

Overdosage: I.V. flunisolide in animals at doses up to 4 mg/kg showed no effect. One spray bottle contains 6.25 mg of NASALIDE; therefore acute overdosage is unlikely.

Dosage and Administration: The therapeutic effects of corticosteroids, unlike those of decongestants, are not immediate. This should be explained to the patient in advance in order to ensure cooperation and continuation of treatment with the prescribed dosage regimen. Full therapeutic benefit requires regular use, and is usually evident within a few days. However, a longer period of therapy may be required for some patients to achieve maximum benefit (up to 3 weeks). If no improvement is evident by that time, NASALIDE® (flunisolide) should not be continued.

Patients with blocked nasal passages should be encouraged to use a decongestant just before NASALIDE administration to ensure adequate penetration of the spray. Patients should also be advised to clear their nasal passages of secretions prior to use.

Adults: The recommended starting dose of NASALIDE is 2 sprays (50 mcg) in each nostril 2 times a day (total dose 200 mcg/day). If needed, this dose may be increased to 2 sprays in each nostril 3 times a day (total dose 300 mcg/day).

Children 6 to 14 years: The recommended starting dose of NASALIDE is one spray (25 mcg) in each nostril 3 times a day or two sprays (50 mcg) in each nostril 2 times a day (total dose 150-200 mcg/day). NASALIDE is not recommended for use in children less than 6 years of age as safety and efficacy studies, including possible adverse effects on growth, have not been conducted.

Maximum total daily doses should not exceed 8 sprays in each nostril for adults (total dose 400 mcg/day) and 4 sprays in each nostril for children under 14 years of age (total dose 200 mcg/day). Since there is no evidence that exceeding the maximum recommended dosage is more effective and increased systemic absorption would occur, higher doses should be avoided.

After the desired clinical effect is obtained, the maintenance dose should be reduced to the smallest amount necessary to control the symptoms. Approximately 15% of patients with perennial rhinitis may be maintained on as little as 1 spray in each nostril per day.

How Supplied: Each 25 ml NASALIDE® (flunisolide) nasal solution spray bottle (NDC 0033-2906-45) contains 6.25 mg (0.25 mg/ml) of flunisolide and is supplied with a pump unit, nasal adapter with dust cover and a patient leaflet of instructions.

NEO-SYNALAR® CREAM ℞

[neomycin sulfate 0.5% (0.35% neomycin base), fluocinolone acetonide 0.025%]

A product of Syntex Laboratories, Inc.

Description: NEO-SYNALAR cream contains fluocinolone acetonide, which has the chemical formula 6α, 9α-difluoro-16α-hydroxyprednisolone-16, 17-acetonide. The cream contains neomycin sulfate 5 mg./g. (3.5 mg./g. neomycin base) and fluocinolone acetonide 0.25 mg./g. in a water-washable aqueous base of stearic acid, propylene glycol, sorbitan monostearate and monooleate, polysorbate 60 and purified water with methylparaben and propylparaben as preservatives.

Actions: Topical steroids are primarily effective because of their anti-inflammatory, antipruritic and vasoconstrictive actions.

Indications:
Based on a review of this drug by the National Academy of Sciences—National Research Council and/or other information, FDA has classified the indications as follows:
"Possibly" effective:
For topical use in the adjunctive management of acute or chronic dermatoses where the dermatoses are initially infected or develop infection during treatment, when such infections are caused by organisms susceptible to neomycin.
These include: atopic dermatitis, neurodermatitis, contact dermatitis, seborrheic dermatitis, eczematous dermatitis, pruritus ani, lichen simplex chronicus, postanal surgical infections, nummular eczema, stasis dermatitis, intertrigo, exfoliative dermatitis and intertriginous psoriasis.
Final classification of the less-than-effective indications requires further investigation.

Contraindications: Topical steroids are contraindicated in those patients with a history of hypersensitivity to any of the components of the preparation.

Warnings: If local infection should continue or become severe, or in the presence of systemic infection, appropriate systemic antibacterial therapy, based on susceptibility testing, should be considered.

Because of the potential hazard of nephrotoxicity and ototoxicity, prolonged use or use of large amounts of this product should be avoided in the treatment of skin infections following extensive burns, trophic ulceration, and other conditions where absorption of neomycin is possible.

There are articles in the current medical literature that indicate an increase in the prevalence of persons sensitive to neomycin.

Precautions: If irritation develops, the cream should be discontinued and appropriate therapy instituted.

As with all antibiotics, prolonged use may result in over-growth of nonsusceptible organisms. If superinfection occurs, appropriate measures should be taken.

If extensive areas are treated there will be increased systemic absorption of the corticosteroid and suitable precautions should be taken, particularly in children and infants.

It is recommended that NEO-SYNALAR® cream not be used under occlusive dressing.

Although topical steroids have not been reported to have an adverse effect on human pregnancy, the safety of their use in pregnant women has not absolutely been established. In laboratory animals, increases in incidences of fetal abnormalities have been associated with exposure of gestating females to topical corticosteroids, in some cases at rather low dosage levels. Therefore, drugs of this class should not be used extensively on pregnant patients, in large amounts or for prolonged periods of time.

NEO-SYNALAR cream is not for ophthalmic use.

Adverse Reactions: The following local adverse reactions have been reported with topical corticosteroids: burning, itching, irritation, dryness, folliculitis, hypertrichosis, acneform eruptions, hypopigmentation, perioral dermatitis, allergic contact dermatitis, maceration of the skin, secondary infection, skin atrophy, striae, miliaria.

The following adverse reactions have been reported with the topical use of neomycin: ototoxicity and nephrotoxicity.

Dosage and Administration: A small amount should be applied lightly to the affected skin area two or three times daily, as

Continued on next page

Syntex—Cont.

needed, and rubbed in gently and thoroughly until it disappears. Since NEO-SYNALAR® cream is a water-washable vanishing cream, it is easily applied and leaves no traces.
How Supplied: NEO-SYNALAR cream—15, 30 and 60 g. tubes. Store at room temperature. Avoid freezing.

NORINYL® 1+35 Tablets ℞
(norethindrone with ethinyl estradiol)
NORINYL® 1+50 Tablets ℞
(norethindrone with mestranol)
NORINYL® 1+80 Tablets ℞
(norethindrone with mestranol)
NORINYL® 2 mg. Tablets
(norethindrone with mestranol)

Refer to entry under BREVICON® (norethindrone with ethinyl estradiol) Tablets.

NOR-Q.D.® ℞
(norethindrone)
0.35 mg. Tablets

Refer to entry under BREVICON® (norethindrone with ethinyl estradiol) Tablets.

SYNACORT™ ℞
(hydrocortisone)
CREAM 1%
CREAM 2.5%

Description: SYNACORT contains hydrocortisone, U.S.P., 10 mg./g. or 25 mg./g. in a cream containing propylene glycol, stearyl alcohol, mineral oil, cetyl alcohol, sorbitan monostearate, polysorbate 60, citric acid and purified water.
Actions: SYNACORT (hydrocortisone) creams are primarily effective because of their anti-inflammatory, antipruritic and vasoconstrictor action.
Indications: SYNACORT creams are indicated for relief of the inflammatory manifestations of corticosteroid-responsive dermatoses.
Contraindications: Topical steroids are contraindicated in those patients with a history of hypersensitivity to any of the components of the preparation.
Precautions: If irritation develops, the cream should be discontinued and appropriate therapy instituted.
In the presence of an infection, the use of an appropriate antifungal or antibacterial agent should be instituted. If a favorable response does not occur promptly, the corticosteroid cream should be discontinued until the infection has been adequately controlled.
If extensive areas are treated or if occlusive technique is used, there will be increased systemic absorption of the corticosteroid and suitable precautions should be taken, particularly in children and infants.
Although topical steroids have not been reported to have an adverse effect on human pregnancy, the safety of their use in pregnant women has not absolutely been established. In laboratory animals, increases in incidences of fetal abnormalities have been associated with exposure of gestating females to topical corticosteroids, in some cases at rather low dosage levels. Therefore, drugs of this class should not be used extensively on pregnant patients, in large amounts or for prolonged periods of time. SYNACORT creams are not for ophthalmic use.
Adverse Reactions: The following local adverse reactions have been reported with topical corticosteroids: burning, itching, irritation, dryness, folliculitis, hypertrichosis, acneform eruptions, hypopigmentation, perioral dermatitis, allergic contact dermatitis, maceration of the skin, secondary infection, skin atrophy, striae, miliaria.
Dosage and Administration: A small amount should be gently massaged into the affected area two to four times daily.
How Supplied:
SYNACORT™ (hydrocortisone) cream 1% —15 g. (NDC 0033-2519-13), 30 g. (NDC 0033-2519-14), and 60 g. tubes (NDC 0033-2519-17).
SYNACORT™ (hydrocortisone) cream 2.5% —30 g. tube (NDC 0033-2520-14).
Store at room temperature. Avoid excessive heat (above 104°F).

SYNALAR® ℞
(fluocinolone acetonide)
CREAM 0.025%
CREAM 0.01%
OINTMENT 0.025%
TOPICAL SOLUTION 0.01%

SYNALAR-HP® ℞
(fluocinolone acetonide)
CREAM 0.2%

Products of Syntex Laboratories, Inc.

Description: SYNALAR (fluocinolone acetonide) and SYNALAR-HP (fluocinolone acetonide) have the chemical name 6α, 9α-difluoro-16α-hydroxyprednisolone-16, 17-acetonide.
SYNALAR cream contains fluocinolone acetonide 0.25 mg./g. or 0.1 mg./g. in a water-washable aqueous base of stearic acid, propylene glycol, sorbitan monostearate and monooleate, polysorbate 60, purified water and citric acid with methylparaben and propylparaben as preservatives.
SYNALAR ointment contains fluocinolone acetonide 0.25 mg./g. in a white petrolatum U.S.P. vehicle.
SYNALAR topical solution contains fluocinolone acetonide 0.1 mg./ml. in a water-washable base of propylene glycol with citric acid.
SYNALAR-HP cream contains fluocinolone acetonide 2 mg./g. in a water-washable aqueous base of stearyl alcohol, cetyl alcohol, mineral oil, propylene glycol, sorbitan monostearate, polysorbate 60, purified water and citric acid with methylparaben and propylparaben as perservatives.
Action: Topical steroids are primarily effective because of their anti-inflammatory, antipruritic and vasoconstrictive actions.
Indications: For relief of the inflammatory manifestations of corticosteroid-responsive dermatoses.
Contraindications: Topical steroids are contraindicated in those patients with a history of hypersensitivity to any of the components of the preparation.
SYNALAR-HP® (fluocinolone acetonide) cream 0.2% should not be used on infants up to two years of age.
Precautions: If irritation develops, the product should be discontinued and appropriate therapy instituted.
In the presence of an infection, the use of an appropriate antifungal or antibacterial agent should be instituted. If a favorable response does not occur promptly, the corticosteroid should be discontinued until the infection has been adequately controlled.
If extensive areas are treated or if occlusive technique is used, there will be increased systemic absorption of the corticosteroid and suitable precautions should be taken, particularly in children and infants.
Although topical steroids have not been reported to have an adverse effect on human pregnancy, the safety of their use in pregnant women has not absolutely been established. In laboratory animals, increases in incidences of fetal abnormalities have been associated with exposure of gestating females to topical corticosteroids, in some cases at rather low dosage levels. Therefore, drugs of this class should not be used extensively on pregnant patients, in large amounts or for prolonged periods of time. SYNALAR and SYNALAR-HP products are not for ophthalmic use.
SYNALAR-HP cream should not be used for prolonged periods and the quantity per day should not exceed 2 g. of formulated material.
Adverse Reactions: The following local adverse reactions have been reported with topical corticosteroids: burning, itching, irritation, dryness, folliculitis, hypertrichosis, acneform eruptions, hypopigmentation, perioral dermatitis, allergic contact dermatitis, maceration of the skin, secondary infection, skin atrophy, striae, miliaria.
Dosage and Administration:
Open Therapy
Apply three or four times daily as follows: A sparing amount, sufficient to cover the affected area, should be spread evenly over the surface and rubbed in gently until it disappears. In hairy sites, the hair should be parted to allow direct contact with the lesion.
Occlusive Dressing Technique
Apply directly to the affected area, leaving a visible thin coat on the surface. Cover completely with a pliable non-porous film. Changes of dressing may be done once or twice daily as determined on an individual basis by the physician.
Some plastic films may be flammable and due care should be exercised in their use. Similarly, caution should be employed when such films are used on children or left in their proximity, to avoid the possibility of accidental suffocation.
How Supplied:
SYNALAR (fluocinolone acetonide)
Cream 0.025%—15, 30 and 60 g. tubes and 120 and 425 g. jars.
Cream 0.01%—15, 45 and 60 g. tubes and 120 and 425 g. jars.
Ointment 0.025%—15, 30, 60 and 120 g. tubes and 425 g. jars.
Topical Solution 0.01%—20 cc. and 60 cc. plastic squeeze bottles.
SYNALAR-HP® (fluocinolone acetonide)
Cream 0.2%—12 g. tubes.

SYNEMOL® ℞
(fluocinolone acetonide)
CREAM 0.025%

A product of Syntex Laboratories, Inc.

Description: SYNEMOL (fluocinolone acetonide) has the chemical name 6α,9α-difluoro-16α-hydroxyprednisolone-16, 17-acetonide. The cream contains fluocinolone acetonide 0.25 mg./g. in a water-washable aqueous emollient base of stearyl alcohol, cetyl alcohol, mineral oil, propylene glycol, sorbitan monostearate, polysorbate 60, purified water, and citric acid.
Actions: SYNEMOL (fluocinolone acetonide) cream is primarily effective because of its anti-inflammatory, antipruritic and vasoconstrictor action.
Indications: For relief of the inflammatory manifestations of corticosteroid-responsive dermatoses.
Contraindications: Topical steroids are contraindicated in those patients with a history of hypersensitivity to any of the components of the preparation.
Precautions: If irritation develops, the cream should be discontinued and appropriate therapy instituted.
In the presence of an infection, the use of an appropriate antifungal or antibacterial agent should be instituted. If a favorable response does not occur promptly, the corticosteroid cream should be discontinued until the infection has been adequately controlled.
If extensive areas are treated or if occlusive technique is used, there will be increased systemic absorption of the corticosteroid and suitable precautions should be taken, particularly in children and infants.
Although topical steroids have not been reported to have an adverse effect on human pregnancy, the safety of their use in pregnant

women has not absolutely been established. In laboratory animals, increases in incidences of fetal abnormalities have been associated with exposure of gestating females to topical corticosteroids, in some cases at rather low dosage levels. Therefore, drugs of this class should not be used extensively on pregnant patients, in large amounts or for prolonged periods of time. SYNEMOL® (fluocinolone acetonide) cream is not for ophthalmic use.

Adverse Reactions: The following local adverse reactions have been reported with topical corticosteroids: burning, itching, irritation, dryness, folliculitis, hypertrichosis, acneform eruptions, hypopigmentation, perioral dermatitis, allergic contact dermatitis, maceration of the skin, secondary infection, skin atrophy, striae, miliaria.

Dosage and Administration:

Open Therapy

SYNEMOL® (fluocinolone acetonide) cream should be applied three or four times daily as follows: a sparing amount, sufficient to cover the affected area, should be spread evenly over the surface and rubbed in gently until it disappears. In hairy sites, the hair should be parted to allow direct contact with the lesion.

Occlusive Dressing Technique

Apply SYNEMOL cream directly to the affected area, leaving a visible thin coat on the surface. Cover completely with a pliable nonporous film. Changes of dressing may be done once or twice daily as determined on an individual basis by the physician.

Some plastic films may be flammable and due care should be exercised in their use. Similarly, caution should be employed when such films are used on children or left in their proximity, to avoid the possibility of accidental suffocation.

How Supplied: Synemol® (fluocinolone acetonide) Cream 0.025%—15, 30, 60 and 120 g. tubes.

TOPIC® — OTC

Benzyl alcohol gel
Relieves itching

A product of Syntex Laboratories, Inc.

(See PDR For Nonprescription Drugs)

Thompson Medical Company, Inc.

919 THIRD AVENUE
NEW YORK, NY 10022

MAXIMUM STRENGTH APPEDRINE® — OTC

Anorectic for Weight Control

Each tablet contains:

phenylpropanolamine HCl	25 mg
caffeine	100 mg

Each three tablets contain:

Vitamin A	5000 IU
Vitamin D	400 IU
Vitamin E	30 IU
Vitamin C (Ascorbic Acid)	60 mg
Folic Acid	0.4 mg
Vitamin B_1 (Thiamine HCl)	1.5 mg
Vitamin B_2 (Riboflavin)	1.7 mg
Niacinamide	20 mg
Vitamin B_6 (Pyridoxine HCl)	2 mg
Vitamin B_{12} (Cyanocobalamin)	6 mcg
d-Calcium Pantothenate	10 mg

Description: Each tablet contains phenylpropanolamine HCl, an anorexiant and caffeine, a mild stimulant and one third of the recommended daily adult requirement of major vitamins.

Indications: Maximum Strength APPEDRINE is indicated as adjunctive therapy in the management of simple exogenous obesity in a regimen of weight reduction and control based on caloric restriction.

Caution: Do not exceed recommended dosage. Discontinue use if rapid pulse, dizziness or palpitations occur. Do not use if high blood pressure, heart, diabetes, kidney, thyroid or other disease is present or if pregnant, nursing or by anyone under the age of 18 except on the advice of a physician. Keep this and all drugs out of the reach of children. In case of accidental overdose, seek professional assistance or contact a Poison Control Center immediately.

Precaution: Avoid use if taking prescription, anti-hypertensive and anti-depressive drugs containing monoamine oxidase inhibitors or other medication containing sympathomimetic amines. Avoid continuous use longer than 3 months.

Adverse Reactions: Side effects are rare when taken as directed. Nausea or nasal dryness may occasionally occur.

Dosage and Administration: Adults: One tablet 30–60 minutes before each meal three times a day with one or two full glasses of water.

How Supplied: Maximum Strength APPEDRINE® packages of 30 and 60 tablets packaged with 1200 Calorie Extra Strength Appedrine Diet Plan.

Reference: Griboff, Solomon, I., M.D., F.A.C.P. et al., A Double-Blind Clinical Evaluation of a Phenylpropanolamine-Caffeine Combination and a Placebo in the Treatment of Exogenous Obesity, Current Therapeutic Research 17, 6:535, (1975) June.

Silverman, H.I., D.Sc., Kreger, B.E., M.D., Lewis, G.P., M.D., et. al., Lack of Side Effects from Orally Administered Phenylpropanolamine and Phenylpropanolamine with Caffeine: A Controlled Three-Phase Study, Current Therapeutic Research 28, 2:185 (1980) August.

ASPERCREME® — OTC

Description: 10% Triethanolamine Salicylate in a pleasantly scented lotion and cream.

Actions: External analgesic with rapid penetration and absorption.

Indications: An effective salicylate analgesic for temporary relief from minor pains of arthritis, rheumatism and muscular aches. Moderately effective in relieving the sensation of burning and tingling, frequently occurring in the hands and feet of elderly patients.

Contraindications: Do not use in patients manifesting idiosyncrasy to salicylates.

Warning: Use only as directed. If pain persists for more than ten days or in arthritic or rheumatic conditions affecting children under twelve years of age, consult a physician immediately. Keep out of reach of children.

Precautions: For external use only. Occasionally where this product has been used extensively, moderate peeling of the skin may occur. This is a normal reaction to salicylates on the skin, and should not warrant discontinuance of the use of the product.

Dosage and Administration: Apply to painful areas with gentle massage until absorbed into skin, three or four times daily, especially before retiring. Relief lasts for hours.

How Supplied: Lotion; 6 oz plastic bottle. Cream; 1.25 oz, 3 oz, and 5 oz plastic tube.

References: Golden, Emanuel L., M.D., A Double-Blind Comparison of Orally Ingested Aspirin and a Topically Applied Salicylate Cream in the Relief of Rheumatic Pain, Current Therapeutic Research, 24, 5:524, (1978) Sept.

Rabinowitz, Joseph L., Ph.D., Feldman, Ella S., M.D., et. al., Comparative Tissue Absorption of Oral ^{14}C—Aspirin and Topical Triethanolamine, ^{14}C—Salicylate in Human and Canine Knee Joints, J Clin Pharmacol. 1982; 22:42–48.

CONTROL Capsules — OTC

Prolonged action anorectic for weight control containing
phenylpropanolamine HCl 75 mg

Description: Phenylpropanolamine HCl is a sympathomimetic, related to ephedrine but with less CNS stimulation. Useful as an anorexiant.

Indication: CONTROL is indicated as adjunctive therapy in a regimen of weight reduction based on caloric restriction in the management and control of simple exogenous obesity.

Caution: For Adults use only.

Do not exceed recommended dose. If nervousness, dizziness, sleeplessness, rapid pulse, palpitations or other symptoms occur discontinue medication and consult your physician. If you have, or are being treated for high blood pressure, heart, diabetes, thyroid or other disease, or while pregnant, or nursing or under the age of 18 do not take this drug except under the advice of a physician. Keep this and all drugs out of the reach of children. In case of accidental overdose seek professional assistance or contact a Poison Control Center immediately.

Precaution: Avoid use if taking prescription, anti-hypertensive and anti-depressive drugs containing monoamine oxidase inhibitors or other medication containing sympathomimetic amines. Avoid continuous use for longer than 3 months.

Adverse Reactions: Side effects are rare when taken as directed. Nausea or nasal dryness may occasionally occur.

Dosage and Administration: One capsule with a full glass of water once a day at midmorning (10:00 A.M.).

How Supplied: CONTROL Capsules—Packages of 14, 28 and 56 capsules, packaged with 1200 Calorie CONTROL Diet Plan.

Reference: Griboff, Solomon, I., M.D., F.A.C.P. et al., A Double-Blind Clinical Evaluation of a Phenylpropanolamine-Caffeine Combination and a Placebo in the Treatment of Exogenous Obesity, Current Therapeutic Research 17, 6:535, (1975) June.

Silverman, H.I., D.Sc., Kreger, B.E., M.D., Lewis, G.P., M.D., et. al., Lack of Side Effects from Orally Administered Phenylpropanolamine and Phenylpropanolamine with Caffeine: A Controlled Three-Phase Study, Current Therapeutic Research 28, 2:185 (1980) August.

DEXATRIM® Capsules — OTC

Prolonged action anorectic for weight control contains

phenylpropanolamine HCl	**50 mg**
caffeine	**200 mg**

DEXATRIM® Extra Strength Capsules — OTC

phenylpropanolamine	**75 mg**
caffeine	**200 mg**

Caffeine-Free DEXATRIM® Extra Strength Capsules — OTC

phenylpropanolamine	**75 mg**

DEXATRIM® Extra Strength Plus Vitamins — OTC

Phenylpropanolamine	**75 mg**
plus multi-vitamins	

Description: Phenylpropanolamine hydrochloride is a sympathomimetic, related to ephedrine but with less CNS stimulation. Useful as an anorexiant. Caffeine is a mild stimulant.

Indication: DEXATRIM, Extra Strength DEXATRIM Capsules, Caffeine-Free DEXATRIM Extra Strength and DEXATRIM Extra Strength Plus Vitamins are indicated as adjunctive therapy in a regimen of weight reduction based on caloric restriction in the management and control of simple exogenous obesity.

Continued on next page

Thompson—Cont.

Studies comparing DEXATRIM to prescription anorexiants have shown DEXATRIM to be equally effective in helping to suppress appetite and in resultant weight loss. DEXATRIM, however, unlike prescription products, has been shown to induce little to no untoward CNS effects. When DEXATRIM was compared to mazindol in a six-week, double-blind study employing 67 outpatients, similar weight losses were reported for all subjects. DEXATRIM patients reported no significant adverse effects, while 18% of the mazindol patients reported side effects which included nervousness, nausea and insomnia.*

In a six week double-blind parallel study comparing phenylpropanolamine HCl to diethylpropion similar weight losses occurred in 62 clinically obese patients. Ninety-six percent of the patients receiving phenylpropanolamine HCl and 87% of the patients receiving diethylpropion lost weight.*

Caution: Do not exceed recommended dosage. Discontinue use if rapid pulse, dizziness or palpitations occur. Do not use if high blood pressure, heart, diabetes, kidney, thyroid or other disease is present, or if pregnant, nursing or by anyone under the age of 18 except on the advice of a physician. Keep this and all drugs out of the reach of children. In case of accidental overdose seek professional assistance or contact a Poison Control Center immediately.

Precaution: Avoid use if taking prescription, anti-hypertensive and anti-depressive drugs containing monoamine oxidase inhibitors or other medication containing sympathomimetic amines. Avoid continuous use for longer than 3 months.

Adverse Reactions: Side effects are rare when taken as directed. Nausea or nasal dryness may occasionally occur.

Dosage and Administration:

DEXATRIM® Capsules: One capsule with a full glass of water mid-morning (10:00 AM)

Extra Strength DEXATRIM® Capsules: One capsule with a full glass of water mid-morning (10:00 AM)

How Supplied:

DEXATRIM® Capsules: Packages of 28 or 56 with 1200 calorie DEXATRIM Diet Plan.

Extra Strength DEXATRIM® Capsules: Packages of 10, 20, and 40 with 1200 calorie DEXATRIM Diet Plan.

Caffeine-Free DEXATRIM® Extra Strength: Packages of 10, 20, and 40 capsules with 1200 calorie DEXATRIM Diet Plan.

DEXATRIM Extra Strength Plus Vitamins: Packages of 16 and 32 capsules with 1200 calorie DEXATRIM Diet Plan.

* Report on file, Professional Services, Thompson Medical Company, Inc. 919 Third Avenue, New York, New York 10022.

Reference: Griboff, Solomon, I., M.D., F.A.C.P. et. al., A Double-Blind Clinical Evaluation of a Phenylpropanolamine-Caffeine Combination and a Placebo in the Treatment of Exogenous Obesity, Current Therapeutic Research 17, 6:535, (1975) June.

Silverman, H.I., D.Sc., Kreger, B.E., M.D., Lewis, G.P., M.D., et. al., Lack of Side Effects from Orally Administered Phenylpropanolamine and Phenylpropanolamine with Caffeine: A Controlled Three-Phase Study, Current Therapeutic Research 28, 2:185 (1980) August.

Maximum Strength PROLAMINE™ Capsules — OTC
Continous Action Anorectic for Weight Control

Each capsule contains:

phenylpropanolamine HCl	37½ mg
caffeine	140 mg

Description: Each capsule contains phenylpropanolamine hydrochloride an anorexiant and caffeine, a mild stimulant.

Indication: Maximum Strength PROLAMINE is indicated as adjunctive therapy in the regimen of weight reduction based on caloric restriction in the management and control of simple exogenous obesity.

In a six week double-blind study of 70 obese patients comparing phenylpropanolamine HCl to a placebo, 35% of the subjects taking phenylpropanolamine HCl experienced a weight loss of 8 pounds or more. Only 9% of the subjects taking placebo lost that amount of weight. Results were statistically significant at the 0.05 probability level.[1]

Caution: Do not exceed recommended dosage. Discontinue use if rapid pulse, dizziness, or palpitations occur. Do not take if you have high blood pressure, heart disease, diabetes, kidney, thyroid, or other disease or if pregnant or lactating. Keep this and all drugs out of the reach of children. In case of accidental overdose seek professional assistance or contact a Poison Control Center immediately.

Precaution: Avoid use if taking prescription, anti-hypertensive and anti-depressive drugs containing monoamine oxidase inhibitors or other medication containing sympathomimetic amines. Avoid continuous use for longer than 3 months.

Adverse Reactions: Side effects are rare when taken as directed. Nausea and nasal dryness may occasionally occur.

Dosage and Administration: One capsule at 10 A.M. and 1 capsule at 4 P.M.

How Supplied: Maximum Strength PROLAMINE™ Capsules: Packages of 20 and 50 packaged with 1200 Calorie PROLAMINE Diet Plan.

1. Report on file, Professional Services, Thompson Medical Company, Inc. 919 Third Avenue, New York, New York 10022

Reference: Griboff, Solomon, I., M.D., F.A.C.P. et. al., A Double-Blind Clinical Evaluation of a Phenylpropanolamine-Caffeine Combination and a Placebo in the Treatment of Exogenous Obesity, Current Therapeutic Research 17, 6:535, (1975) June.

Silverman, H.I., D.Sc., Kreger, B.E., M.D., Lewis, G.P., M.D., et. al., Lack of Side Effects from Orally Administered Phenylpropanolamine and Phenylpropanolamine with Caffeine: A Controlled Three-Phase Study, Current Therapeutic Research 28, 2:185 (1980) August.

Travenol Laboratories, Inc.
Parenteral Products
ONE BAXTER PARKWAY
DEERFIELD, ILLINOIS 60015

5.5% and 8.5% TRAVASOL® (Amino Acid) Injections with Electrolytes and without Electrolytes — ℞

Description: TRAVASOL (Amino Acid) Injections are sterile, nonpyrogenic hypertonic solutions of essential and non-essential L-amino acids provided with or without electrolytes for intravenous administration.

Each 100 ml of TRAVASOL (Amino Acid) Injections with Electrolytes and without Electrolytes contain:

	5.5%	8.5%
L-Amino Acids	5.5 g	8.5 g
Total Nitrogen	924 mg	1.42 g
Approximate pH	6.0	6.0
Essential Amino Acids	**5.5%**	**8.5%**
L-Leucine	340 mg	526 mg
L-Phenylalanine	340 mg	526 mg
L-Methionine	318 mg	492 mg
L-Lysine (added as the hydrochloride salt)	318 mg	492 mg
L-Isoleucine	263 mg	406 mg
L-Valine	252 mg	390 mg
L-Histidine	241 mg	372 mg
L-Threonine	230 mg	356 mg
L-Tryptophan	99 mg	152 mg
Non-essential Amino Acids	**5.5%**	**8.5%**
L-Alanine	1.14 g	1.76 g
Aminoacetic Acid	1.14 g	1.76 g
L-Arginine	570 mg	880 mg
L-Proline	230 mg	356 mg
L-Tyrosine	22 mg	34 mg

In addition to the above, TRAVASOL (Amino Acid) Injections with Electrolytes contain in each 100 ml:

Electrolytes	**5.5%**	**8.5%**
Sodium Acetate, Hydrous, USP	431 mg	594 mg
Dibasic Potassium Phosphate	522 mg	522 mg
Sodium Chloride, USP	224 mg	154 mg
Magnesium Chloride, USP	102 mg	102 mg

TRAVASOL (Amino Acid) Injections with Electrolytes contain the following milliequivalents:

Electrolyte	**5.5%**	**8.5%**
Sodium	70 mEq/l	70 mEq/l
Potassium	60 mEq/l	60 mEq/l
Magnesium	10 mEq/l	10 mEq/l
Acetate*	100 mEq/l	135 mEq/l
Chloride	70 mEq/l	70 mEq/l
Phosphate (as $HPO_4^{=}$)	60 mEq/l (30mM)	60 mEq/l (30 mM)

*Acetate is added as sodium acetate and as acetic acid used for pH adjustment.

TRAVASOL (Amino Acid) Injections without Electrolytes contain the following anion profiles in mEq/l:

Anion	**5.5%**	**8.5%**
Acetate (1)	48 mEq/l	73 mEq/l
Chloride (2)	22 mEq/l	34 mEq/l

(1) derived from pH adjustment with acetic acid

(2) contributed by the L-Lysine Hydrochloride

Approximately 3 mEq/l Sodium Bisulfite, USP is added as stabilizer to all TRAVASOL (Amino Acid) Injections.

Actions: TRAVASOL (Amino Acid) Injections administered via central vein provide biologically utilizable source material for protein synthesis when used with concentrated calorie sources (such as hypertonic dextrose or fat emulsion), electrolytes, vitamins and minerals. Administered peripherally after appropriate dilution or with minimal calorie supplementation (such as 5% dextrose), it enhances the conservation of body protein.

Indications: TRAVASOL (Amino Acid) Injections are indicated as an adjunct in the offsetting of nitrogen loss or in the treatment of negative nitrogen balance in patients where: (1) the alimentary tract, by the oral, gastrostomy or jejunostomy route, cannot or should not be used, (2) gastrointestinal absorption of protein is impaired, or (3) metabolic requirements for protein are substantially increased, as with extensive burns.

Central Vein Administration: Central vein infusion should be considered when amino acid solutions are to be admixed with hypertonic dextrose to promote protein synthesis such as for hypercatabolic or depleted patients or those requiring long term parenteral nutrition.

Peripheral Vein Administration: For patients in whom the central vein route is not indicated, amino acid solutions mixed with low dextrose concentrations may be infused by peripheral vein when supplemented with fat emulsion.

Protein Sparing: Dilute amino acid solutions for **peripheral administration** may be used in patients who exemplify no clinically significant protein malnutrition. The purpose of the solution is to replace protein losses which occur in relation to an intercurrent phenomenon which is known or suspected to be productive of a protein loss condition for a short or moderate period of time. Protein sparing can be achieved by peripheral infusion of amino acid solutions with or without dextrose.

Contraindications:

1. Patients with renal failure—anuria [for TRAVASOL (Amino Acid) Injection with Electrolytes only]
2. Patients with severe liver disease—hepatic coma
3. Hypersensitivity to one or more amino acids.

Warnings:

1. Proper administration of TRAVASOL (Amino Acid) Injections requires a knowledge of fluid and electrolyte balance and nutrition as well as clinical expertise in recognition and treatment of the complications which may occur. FREQUENT CLINICAL EVALUATION AND LABORATORY DETERMINATIONS ARE NECESSARY FOR PROPER MONITORING DURING ADMINISTRATION. Studies should include blood sugar, serum proteins, kidney and liver function tests, electrolytes, hemogram, carbon dioxide combining power or content, serum osmolarities, blood cultures and blood ammonia levels.
2. Administration of amino acid solutions to a patient with hepatic insufficiency may result in serum amino acid imbalances, hyperammonemia, stupor and coma.
   Hyperammonemia is of SPECIAL SIGNIFICANCE IN INFANTS. This reaction appears to be related to a deficiency of the urea cycle amino acids of genetic or product origin. It is essential that blood ammonia be measured frequently in infants.
   Conservative doses of TRAVASOL (Amino Acid) Injection should be given to patients with known or suspected hepatic dysfunction. Should symptoms of hyperammonemia develop, administration should be discontinued and the patient's clinical status reevaluated.
3. Administration of amino acid solutions in the presence of impaired renal function presents special issues associated with retention of electrolytes.
4. The safety of the use of amino acid solutions in pregnant women has not been demonstrated.
5. Do not administer unless solution is clear. This solution should not be administered simultaneously with blood through the same infusion set because of the possibility of pseudoagglutination.

Precautions:

1. It is essential to provide adequate calories concurrently if parenterally administered amino acids are to be retained by the body and utilized for protein synthesis. Concentrated dextrose solutions are an effective source of such calories.
2. With the administration of TRAVASOL (Amino Acid) Injection in combination with highly concentrated dextrose solutions, hyperglycemia, glycosuria, and hyperosmolar syndrome may result. Blood and urine glucose should be monitored on a routine basis in patients receiving this therapy.
3. Sudden cessation in administration of a concentrated dextrose solution may result in insulin reaction due to continued endogenous insulin production. Parenteral nutrition mixtures should be withdrawn slowly.
4. TRAVASOL (Amino Acid) Injection with Electrolytes contains sufficient electrolytes to provide for most parenteral nutritional needs with the possible exception of potassium where supplementation may be required. However, replacement of exceptional electrolyte loss due to nasogastric suction, fistula drainage, or unusual tissue exudation may be necessary. Particular attention should be given to monitoring serum potassium levels.
   Electrolytes may be added to the TRAVASOL (Amino Acid) Injections without Electrolytes as dictated by the patient's electrolyte profile.
5. Commonly reported complications of parenteral nutrition, hyperammonemia and hyperchloremic metabolic acidosis, were not observed during clinical studies with TRAVASOL (Amino Acid) Injection. While the potassium, phosphate, metabolizable acetate anion, and amino acid profiles in TRAVASOL (Amino Acid) Injections with Electrolytes were designed to minimize or prevent occurrences of these imbalances, the physician should be aware of appropriate counter-measures if they become necessary.
6. Strongly hypertonic nutrient solutions should be administered through an indwelling intravenous catheter with the tip located in the superior vena cava.
7. Care should be taken to avoid circulatory overload, particularly in patients with cardiac insufficiency.
8. During protein sparing therapy in the absence of supporting carbohydrate metabolism, an accumulation of ketone bodies in the blood often occurs. Correction of ketonemia usually can be accomplished by administering some carbohydrates.
9. Protein sparing therapy is useful for periods up to 10-12 days. Patients requiring nutritional support thereafter should be placed on oral or parenteral regimens that employ adequate non-protein calorie components.

Special Precautions: Administration of amino acid solutions and other nutrients via central or peripheral venous catheter may be associated with complications which can be prevented or minimized by careful attention to all aspects of the procedure. This includes attention to solution preparation, administration, and patient monitoring. IT IS ESSENTIAL THAT A CAREFULLY PREPARED PROTOCOL, BASED ON CURRENT MEDICAL PRACTICES, BE FOLLOWED, PREFERABLY BY AN EXPERIENCED TEAM.

Although a detailed discussion of the complications is beyond the scope of this insert, the following summary lists those based on current literature:

1. **Technical:** The placement of a central venous catheter should be regarded as a surgical procedure. The physician should be fully acquainted with various techniques of catheter insertion as well as recognition and treatment of complications. For details of techniques and placement sites consult the medical literature. X-ray is the best means of verifying catheter placement. Complications known to occur from the placement of central venous catheters are pneumothorax, hemothorax, hydrothorax, artery puncture and transection, injury to the brachial plexus, malposition of the catheter, formation of arterio-venous fistula, phlebitis, thrombosis, cardiac arrhythmia and catheter embolus.
2. **Septic:** The constant risk of sepsis is present during administration of parenteral nutrition solution. Since contaminated solutions and infusion catheters are potential sources of infection, it is imperative that the preparation of the solution and the placement and care of catheters be accomplished under controlled aseptic conditions. If fever develops, the solution, its delivery system and the site of the indwelling catheter should be changed.
   Solutions ideally should be prepared in the hospital pharmacy under a laminar flow hood. The key factor in their preparation is careful aseptic technique to avoid inadvertent touch contamination during mixing of solutions and addition of other nutrients.
   Solutions should be used promptly after mixing. Any storage should be under refrigeration and limited to a brief period of time, preferably less than 24 hours.
3. **Metabolic:** The following metabolic complications have been reported: metabolic acidosis, hypophosphatemia, alkalosis, hyperglycemia and glycosuria, osmotic diuresis and dehydration, rebound hypoglycemia, elevated liver enzymes, hypo and hypervitaminosis, electrolyte imbalances, and hyperammonemia. Frequent clinical evaluation and laboratory determinations are necessary, especially during the first few days of therapy, to prevent or minimize these complications.

Adverse Reactions: See Warnings and Special precautions

Dosage and Administration: The total daily dose of these solutions depends on the patient's metabolic requirement and clinical response. The determination of nitrogen balance and accurate daily body weights, corrected for fluid balance, are probably the best means of assessing individual nitrogen requirements.

Recommended Dietary Allowances* of protein range from approximately 0.8 g/kg of body weight for adults to 2.2 g/kg for infants. It must be recognized, however, that protein as well as caloric requirements in traumatized or malnourished patients may be substantially increased. Daily amino acid doses of approximately 1.0 to 1.5 g/kg of body weight for adults and 2 to 3 g/kg of body weight for infants with adequate calories and generally sufficient to satisfy protein needs and promote positive nitrogen balance.

For the initial treatment of trauma or protein calorie malnutrition, higher doses of protein with corresponding quantities of carbohydrate will be necessary to promote adequate patient response to therapy. The severity of the illness being treated is the primary consideration in determining proper dose level. Such higher doses, especially in infants, must be accompanied by more frequent laboratory evaluation.

For protein sparing in well-nourished patients not receiving significant additional calories, amino acid dosages of 1.0 to 1.7 g/kg/day reduce nitrogen losses and spare body protein. If daily increases in BUN in the range of 10-15 mg% for more than three days should occur, then protein sparing therapy should be discontinued and a regimen with full non-protein calorie substrates should be adopted.

Care should be exercised to insure the maintenance of proper levels of serum potassium. Quantities of 60-180 mEq of potassium per day have been used with adequate clinical effect. It may be necessary to enhance the already present quantity of this electrolyte in TRAVASOL (Amino Acid) Injections with Electrolytes, depending primarily on the amount of carbohydrate administered to and metabolized by the patient. All serum electrolytes should be monitored frequently, especially phosphate, magnesium, and chloride.

Patients receiving TRAVASOL (Amino Acid) Injections without Electrolytes should be monitored (carefully) and their electrolyte requirements individualized.

Central Vein Administration: Hypertonic mixtures of amino acids and dextrose may be administered safely by continuous infusion through a central vein catheter with the tip located in the vena cava. Typically 500 ml of TRAVASOL (Amino Acid) Injection mixed with 500 ml of 50% Dextrose Injection, electrolytes (if indicated) and vitamins is administered over an 8 hour period. (If the rate of administration should fall behind schedule, no attempt to "catch up" to planned intake should be made.) In addition to meeting nitrogen needs, the administration rate is governed, especially during the first few days of therapy, by the patient's tolerance to dextrose. Daily

Continued on next page

Travenol—Cont.

intake of amino acids and dextrose should be increased gradually to the maximum required dose as indicated by frequent determinations of urine and blood sugar levels.

In many patients, provision of adequate calories in the form of hypertonic dextrose may require the administration of exogenous insulin to prevent hyperglycemia and glycosuria.

Parenteral nutrition may be started with infusates containing lower concentrations of dextrose; dextrose content may be gradually increased to estimated caloric needs as the patient's glucose tolerance increases.

Sudden cessation in administration of a concentrated dextrose solution may result in insulin reaction due to continued endogenous insulin production. Such solutions should be withdrawn slowly.

Peripheral Vein Administration: For patients requiring parenteral nutrition in whom the central vein route is not indicated, TRAVASOL (Amino Acid) Injection can be mixed with low concentration dextrose solutions and administered by peripheral vein with fat emulsions.

For example, to prepare a solution of 2.75% TRAVASOL (Amino Acid) Injection in 5% dextrose, aseptically transfer 500 ml of 5.5% TRAVASOL (Amino Acid) Injection with Electrolytes and 500 ml of 10% dextrose to a liter intravenous container. Each liter of the resultant solution provides 28.9 g of protein equivalent and 170 carbohydrate calories with an osmolarity of approximately 680 mOs/l.

Parenteral fat emulsion provides approximately 1.1 calories per ml and may be administered along with amino acid-dextrose solutions through a Y-type administration set to supplement caloric intake. Fat, however, should not be the sole caloric intake since studies have indicated that glucose is more nitrogen sparing in the stressed patient.

Protein Sparing: For well-nourished patients who require short-term parenteral support, TRAVASOL (Amino Acid) Injection can be administered peripherally with or without carbohydrate calories. Such infusates can be prepared by dilution of TRAVASOL (Amino Acid) Injection with Sterile Water for Injection or 5% dextrose solutions to prepare isotonic or slightly hypertonic solutions which may be administered by peripheral vein. For example, a 2.75% TRAVASOL (Amino Acid) Injection solution can be prepared by the aseptic transfer of 500 ml of 5.5% TRAVASOL (Amino Acid) Injection with Electrolytes to a half-filled intravenous liter container of Sterile Water for Injection. The resultant solution contains 2.75% amino acids, and provides 28.9 g of protein equivalent with an osmolarity of approximately 425 mOs/l.

Route: Peripheral or central vein.

Storage: It is recommended that all intravenous administration apparatus be replaced at least every 24 hours.

L-Amino Acid Solutions should be protected from light until immediately prior to use.

Protect from excessive heat (about 40°C) and freezing.

How Supplied: TRAVASOL (Amino Acid) Injection with Electrolytes and without Electrolytes are available in 5.5% and 8.5% concentrations and are supplied in 500 ml containers.

* Food and Nutrition Board National Academy of Sciences—National Research Council (Revised 1974).

8-19-20-226
April 1978

10% TRAVASOL® (Amino Acid) Injection without Electrolytes ℞

Description: 10% TRAVASOL (Amino Acid) Injection without Electrolytes is a sterile, nonpyrogenic, hypertonic solution of essential and nonessential L-amino acids provided without electrolytes.

Each 100 ml of 10% TRAVASOL (Amino Acid) Injection without Electrolytes contains:

L-Amino Acids	10.0 g
Total Nitrogen	1.65 g
Approximate pH	6.0
Essential Amino Acids	
L-leucine	730 mg
L-Isoleucine	600 mg
L-Lysine (added as the hydrochloride salt)	580 mg
L-Valine	580 mg
L-Phenylalanine	560 mg
L-Histidine	480 mg
L-Theronine	420 mg
L-Methionine	400 mg
L-Tryptophan	180 mg
Nonessential Amino Acids	
L-Alanine	2.07 g
L-Arginine	1.15 g
Aminoacetic Acid	1.03 g
L-Proline	680 mg
L-Serine	500 mg
L-Tyrosine	40 mg

10% TRAVASOL (Amino Acid) Injection without Electrolytes contains the following anions:

Anion	
Acetate (1)	87 mEq/l
Chloride (2)	40 mEq/l

(1) derived from pH adjustment with acetic acid

(2) contributed by the L-Lysine Hydrochloride

Approximately 3 mEq/l Sodium Bisulfite is added as stabilizer.

10% TRAVASOL (Amino Acid) Injection without Electrolytes contains approximately 1000 mOs/l.

Clinical Pharmacology: 10% TRAVASOL (Amino Acid) Injection without Electrolytes administered via central vein provides biologically utilizable souce material for protein synthesis when used with concentrated calorie sources (such as hypertonic dextrose or fat emulsion), electrolytes, vitamins and minerals. Administered peripherally after appropriate dilution or with minimal calorie supplementation (such as 5% dextrose), it enhances the conservation of body protein.

Indications and Usage: 10% TRAVASOL (Amino Acid) Injection without Electrolytes is indicated as an adjunct in the offsetting of nitrogen loss or in the treatment of negative nitrogen balance in patients where: (1) the alimentary tract, by the oral, gastrostomy or jejunostomy route, cannot or should not be used. (2) gastrointestinal absorption of protein is impaired, or (3) metabolic requirements for protein are substantially increased as with extensive burns.

Central Vein Administration: Central vein infusion should be considered when amino acid solutions are to be admixed with hypertonic dextrose to promote protein synthesis such as for hypercatabolic or depleted patients or those requiring long-term parenteral nutrition.

Peripheral Vein Administration: For patients in whom the central vein route is not indicated, amino acid solutions mixed with low dextrose concentrations may be infused by peripheral vein when supplemented with fat emulsion.

Protein Sparing: Dilute amino acid solutions for peripheral administration may be used in patients who exemplify no clinically significant protein malnutrition. The purpose of the solution is to replace protein losses which occur in relation to an intercurrent phenomenon which is known or suspected to be productive of a protein loss condition for a short or moderate period of time. Protein sparing can be achieved by peripheral infusion of amino acid solutions with or without dextrose.

Contraindications:

1. Hypersensitivity to one or more amino acids.
2. Severe liver disease or hepatic coma.

Warnings:

1. Proper administration of 10% TRAVASOL (Amino Acid) Injection without Electrolytes requires a knowledge of fluid and electrolyte balance and nutrition as well as clinical expertise in recognition and treatment of the complications which may occur.
   FREQUENT CLINICAL EVALUATION AND LABORATORY DETERMINATIONS ARE NECESSARY FOR PROPER MONITORING DURING ADMINISTRATION. Studies should include blood sugar, serum proteins, kidney and liver function tests, electrolytes, hemogram, carbon dioxide combining power or content, serum osmolarities, blood cultures and blood ammonia levels.
2. Administration of amino acid solutions to a patient with hepatic insufficiency may result in serum amino acid imbalances, hyperammonemia, stupor and coma.
   Hyperammonemia is of SPECIAL SIGNIFICANCE IN INFANTS. This reaction appears to be related to a deficiency of the urea cycle amino acids of genetic or product origin. It is essential that blood ammonia be measured frequently in infants.
   Conservative doses of 10% TRAVASOL (Amino Acid) Injection without Electrolytes should be given to patients with known or suspected hepatic dysfunction. Should symptoms of hyperammonemia develop, administration should be discontinued and the patient's clinical status reevaluated.
3. Administration of amino acid solutions in the presence of impaired renal function presents spcial issues associated with retention of electrolytes.
4. The safety of the use of amino acid solutions in pregnant women has not been demonstrated.
5. Do not administer unless solution is clear. This solution should not be administered simultaneously with blood through the same infusion set because of the possibility of pseudoagglutination.

Precautions:

1. It is essential adequate calories concurrently if parenterally administered amino acids are to be retained by the body and utilized for protein synthesis. Concentrated dextrose solutions are an effective source of such calories.
2. With the administration of 10% TRAVASOL (Amino Acid) injection without Electrolytes in combination with highly concentrated dextrose solutions, hyperglycemia, glycosuria, and hyperosmolar syndrome may result. Blood and urine glucose should be monitored on a routine basis in patients receiving this therapy.
3. Sudden cessation in administration of a concentrated dextrose solution may result in insulin reaction due to continued endogenous insulin production. Parenteral nutrition mixtures should be withdrawn slowly.
4. Electrolytes may be added to the 10% TRAVASOL (Amino Acid) Injection without Electrolytes as dictated by the patient's electrolyte profile.
5. The metabolizable acetate anion and amino acid profile in 10% TRAVASOL (Amino Acid) injection without Electrolytes were designed to minimize or prevent occurrences of hyperammonemia and hyperchloremic metabolic acidosis. However, the physician should be aware of appropriate countermeasures if they become necessary.
6. Strongly hypertonic nutrient solutions should be administered through an indwelling intravenous catheter with the tip located in the superior vena cava.
7. Care should be taken to avoid circulatory overload, particularly in patients with cardiac insufficiency.
8. During protein sparing therapy in the absence of supporting carbohydrate metabolism, an accumulation of ketone bodies in the blood often occurs. Correction of ketonemia

usually can be accomplished by administering some carbohydrates.

9. Protein sparing therapy is useful for periods up to 10–12 days. Patients requiring nutritional support thereafter should be placed on oral or parenteral regimens that employ adequate nonprotein calorie components.

Special Precautions: Administration of amino acid solutions and other nutrients via central or peripheral venous catheter may be associated with complications which can be prevented or minimized by careful attention to all aspects of the procedure. This includes attention to solution preparation, administration, and patient monitoring. IT IS ESSENTIAL THAT A CAREFULLY PREPARED PROTOCOL, BASED ON CURRENT MEDICAL PRACTICES, BE FOLLOWED, PREFERABLY BY AN EXPERIENCED TEAM.

Although a detailed discussion of the complications is beyond the scope of this insert, the following summary lists those based on current literature.

1. **Technical:** The placement of a central venous catheter should be regarded as a surgical procedure. The physician should be fully acquainted with various techniques of catheter insertion as well as recognition and treatment of complications. For details of techniques and placement sites consult the medical literature, X-ray is the best means of verifying catheter placement. Complications known to occur from the placement of central venous catheters are pneumothorax, hemothorax, hydrothorax, artery puncture and transection, injury to the brachial plexus, malposition of the catheter, formation of arteriovenous fistula, phlebitis, thrombosis, cardiac arrhythmia and catheter embolus.
2. **Septic:** The constant risk of sepsis is present during administration of parenteral nutrition solution. Since contaminated solutions and infusion catheters are potential sources of infection, it is imperative that the preparation of the solution and the placement and care of catheters be accomplished under controlled aseptic conditions. If fever develops, the solution, its delivery system and the site of the indwelling catheter should be changed.
   Solutions ideally should be prepared in the hospital pharmacy under a laminar flow hood. The key factor in their preparation is careful aseptic technique to avoid inadvertent touch contamination during mixing of solutions and addition of other nutrients.
   Solutions should be used promptly after mixing. Any storage should be under refrigeration and limited to a brief period of time, preferably less than 24 hours.
3. **Metabolic:** The following metabolic complications have been reported: metabolic acidosis, hypophosphatemia, alkalosis, hyperglycemia and glycosuria, osmotic diuresis and dehydraton, rebound hypoglycemia, elevated liver enzymes, hypo- and hypervitaminosis, electrolyte imbalances, and hyperammonemia. Frequent clinical evaluation and laboratory determinations are necessary, especially during the first few days of therapy, to prevent or minimize these complications.

Adverse Reactions: See Warnings and Special Precautions.

Dosage and Administration: The total daily dose of these solutions depends on the patients's metabolic requirement and clinical response. The determination of nitrogen balance and accurate daily body weights, corrected for fluid balance, are probably the best means of assessing individual nitrogen requirements.

Recommended Dietary Allowances* of protein range from approximately 0.8 g/kg of body weight for adults to 2.2 g/kg for infants. It must be recognized, however, that protein as well as caloric requirements in traumatized or malnourished patients may be increased substantially. Daily amino acid doses of approximately 1.0 to 1.5 g/kg of body weight for adults and 2 to 3 g/kg of body weight for infants with adequate calories are generally sufficient to satisfy protein needs and promote positive nitrogen balance.

For the initial treatment of trauma or protein calorie malnutrition, higher doses of protein with corresponding quantities of carbohydrate will be necessary to promote adequate patient response to therapy. The severity of the illness being treated is the primary consideration in determining proper dose level. Such higher doses, especially in infants, must be accompanied by more frequent laboratory evaluation.

For protein sparing in well-nourished patients not receiving significant additional calories, amino acid dosages of 1.0 to 1.7 g/kg/day reduce nitrogen losses and spare body protein. If daily increases in BUN in the range of 10–15 mg % for more than three days should occur, then protein sparing therapy should be discontinued and a regimen with full nonprotein calorie substrates should be adopted.

Care should be exercised to insure the maintenance of proper levels of serum potassium. Quantities of 60–180mEq of potassium per day have been used with adequate clinical effect. It may be necessary to add quantities of this electrolyte to 10% TRAVASOL (Amino Acid) Injections without Electrolytes, depending primarily on the amount of carbohydrate administered to and metabolized by the patient. All serum electrolytes should be monitored frequently and electrolyte requirements individualized.

10% TRAVASOL (Amino Acid) Injection without Electrolytes provides a concentrated source of amino acids to meet the protein requirements of patients who are fluid restricted (e.g., renal failure). Typically 250 ml of 10% TRAVASOL (Amino Acid) Injection without Electrolytes mixed with 500 ml of 70% Dextrose Injection is administered over a 12-hour period. Acceptable total daily administration volumes are dependent upon the fluid balance requirements of the patient. Extreme care should be given to prevent fluctuations of blood osmolarity and serum electrolyte concentrations. Frequent and careful monitoring is mandatory when fluid-restricted patients are receiving intravenous nutrition.

Central Vein Administration: Hypertonic mixtures of amino acids and dextrose may be administered safely by continuous infusion through a central vein catheter with the tip located in the vena cava. In addition to meeting nitrogen needs, the administration rate is governed, especially during the first few days of therapy, by the patient's tolerance to dextrose. Daily intake of amino acids and dextrose should be increased gradually to the maximum required dose as indicated by frequent determinations of urine and blood sugar levels.

In many patients, provisions of adequate calories in the form of hypertonic dextrose may require the administration of exogenous insulin to prevent hyperglycemia and glycosuria.

Parenteral nutrition may be started with infusates containing lower concentrations of dextrose, dextrose content may be gradually increased to estimated caloric needs as the patient's glucose tolerance increases.

Sudden cessation in administration of concentrated dextrose solution may result in insulin reaction due to continued endogenous insulin production. Such solutions should be withdrawn slowly.

Peripheral Vein Administration: For patients requiring parenteral nutrition in whom the central vein route is not indicated, 10% TRAVASOL (Amino Acid) Injection without Electrolytes can be mixed with low concentration dextrose solutions and administered by peripheral vein in conjunction with or without fat emulsions.

Parenteral fat emulsion provides approximately 1.1 calories per ml and may be administered along with amino acid-dextrose solutions through a Y-type administration set to supplement caloric intake. Fats, however, should not be the sole caloric intake since studies have indicated that glucose is more nitrogen sparing in the stressed patient.

Protein Sparing: For well-nourished patients who require short-term parenteral support, 10% TRAVASOL (Amino Acid) Injection without Electrolytes can be administered peripherally with or without carbohydrate calories. Infusates may also be prepared by dilution of 10% TRAVASOL (Amino Acid) Injection without Electrolytes with Sterile Water for Injection or 5% Dextrose Injection solutions to prepare isotonic or slightly hypertonic solutions which may be administered by peripheral vein. Depending upon the clinical condition of the patient, approximately 3 liters of solution may be administered per 24-hour period. When used postoperatively, the therapy should begin with 1000 ml on the first postoperative day. Thereafter, the dose may be increased to 3000 ml per day.

Route: Peripheral or central vein.

NOTE: It is recommended that all intravenous administration apparatus be replaced at least every 24 hours. Protect from light until immediately prior to use. Do not store above 40°C (104°F). Protect from freezing.

How Supplied: 10% TRAVASOL (Amino Acid) Injection without Electrolytes is available in 250 ml, 500 ml and 1000 ml containers.

*Food and Nutrition Board National Academy of Sciences—National Research Council (Revised 1974).

8-19-20-209AA

© Copyright 1979, 1980, 1981 Travenol Laboratories, Inc. All rights reserved.

Trimen Laboratories, Inc.

Pharmaceutical Division
80 TWENTY-SIXTH STREET
PITTSBURGH, PA 15222

AMAPHEN® CAPSULES ℞

(Non-Narcotic Analgesic)

Each Capsule contains:

50 mg .... Butalbital
(WARNING: May be habit forming)
40 mg .... Caffeine
325 mg .... Acetaminophen.

How Supplied: Bottles of 100's; opaque white and opaque pink capsule, imprinted "TRIMEN".

AMAPHEN® with CODEINE #3 Ⓒ

Analgesic

Each Amaphen with Codeine Capsule contains: 50 mg butalbital, U.S.P. (Warning: May be habit forming; 325 mg acetaminophen, U.S.P., and 40 mg caffeine, U.S.P.

In addition, Amaphen with Codeine also contains 30 mg of codeine phosphate, U.S.P. (Warning: May be habit forming).

How Supplied: Bottles of 100's, pink and maroon capsules, imprinted TRIMEN.

BELLERMINE–O.D™ CAPSULES ℞

Belladonna Ergotamine

Each long-acting capsule contains:

Phenobarbital .... 40.0 mg.
(Warning: May be habit forming)
Ergotamine tartrate .... 0.6 mg.
Belladonna alkaloids .... 0.2 mg.

How Supplied: Bottles of 100's, chocolate and clear with white beads, imprinted "TRIMEN".

Continued on next page

Trimen—Cont.

DYREXAN™-OD ©
Brand of Phendimetrazine Tartrate
Slow-Release Capsules 105 mg

How Supplied: Bottles of 100's, clear yellow and opaque brown 105 mg capsules imprinted with TRIMEN.

HYDREX® TABLETS ℞
(Benzthiazide 50 mg.)
Diuretic-Antihypertensive

How Supplied: Bottles of 100's, white, scored tablet embossed with logo.

KORIGESIC® TABLETS ℞
Analgesic Decongestant

Each Tablet contains: 4 mg. Chlorpheniramine Maleate, 14 mg. Phenylpropanolamine Hydrochloride, 5 mg. Phenylephrine Hydrochloride, 150 mg. Salicylamide, 200 mg. Acetaminophen, 30 mg. Caffeine.
How Supplied: Bottles of 100's, two-layer, scored blue and white tablet, embossed with logo.

NATACOMP-FA® TABLETS ℞
Multivitamin, Multimineral supplement for pregnant or lactating women

How Supplied: Bottles of 100's and 500's pink, oval, film coated tablet.

SORATE® ℞
Isosorbide Dinitrate

How Supplied:
Sorate®-5 Chewable as 5 mg orange, round, scored, chewable tablet, embossed with logo.
Sorate®-10 Chewable as 10 mg. white, round, scored, orange flavored chewable tablets, embossed with logo.
Sorate®-2.5 Sublingual as 2.5 mg lavender tablet.
Sorate®-5 Sublingual as 5 mg light green oval shaped tablet.
Sorate®-40 Capsules as 40 mg long-acting, opaque purple and clear with white beads imprinted TRIMEN.

VIOPAN-T™ TABLETS
High Potency Vitamin Mineral Formula

How Supplied: Red, film coated tablet, embossed with TRIMEN.

Tyson and Associates, Inc.
19725 SHERMAN WAY
SUITE 270
CANOGA PARK, CA 91306

AMINOPLEX™ ℞

Description: Free form amino acid supplement for adults and children 4 or more years of age. Capsules containing 740 mg of 19 free form amino acids without fillers, binders, preservatives or sugars. The composition of Aminoplex™ is: L-Lysine HCl, L-Tryptophan, L-Arginine Base, L-Isoleucine, L-Leucine, L-Alanine, L-Threonine, L-Histidine Base, L-Cystine, L-Methionine, L-Glutamine, L-Tyrosine, L-Aspartic Acid, L-Valine, L-Glutamic Acid, L-Phenylalanine, L-Glycine, L-Serine, L-Cysteine HCl.
Indications: Effective as adjunctive therapy in partially reversing negative nitrogen balance with conditions characterized by interference or malabsorption of dietary protein. Also been shown effective in heavy metal detoxification, and psychiatry.
Contraindication: Aminoplex™ is contraindicated in conditions of severe liver disease or symptoms of impending hepatic coma. Blood ammonia levels should be closely monitored in those patients with liver disease as Aminoplex™ contains 13 milligrams of nitrogen per capsule. Caution should also be used with patients with acidosis and renal impairment.
Adverse Reactions: In some sensitive patients Aminoplex™ may elicit nausea, bladder irritation, vasodilaton, or drowsiness. If hypersensitivity or other adverse reactions are encountered dosage should be reduced.
Dosage and Oral Administration: It should be noted that free form amino acids alone cannot supply sufficient calories to maintain homeostasis; therefore, it is essential to supply other dietary sources of calories. It is also important to supply the necessary vitamins and minerals which facilitate amino acid absorption and utilization.
Initially it is recommended 3 capsules T.I.D. or as recommended by the physician.
How Supplied:
740mg capsule: Bottles of 500, 250, and 100 capsules.
All individual amino acids are available upon request.
Literature Available: Product information and additional specific information are available upon request.

U. S. Chemical Marketing Group, Inc.
203 RIO CIRCLE
DECATUR, GA 30030

HEMOCYTE Injection ℞
Hematinic-Vitamin

Description: Each 2 ml. contains: Peptonized Iron 50 mg., Folic Acid 2 mg. (as Sodium Salt), Liver Injection (activity equivalent to 2 mcg. of cyanocobalamin), Cyanocobalamin 50 mcg., Benzyl Alcohol 1.5%, Phenol 0.5%.
How Supplied: 10 mg. multiple dose vial NDC 0184-0179-10.

HEMOCYTE Tablets OTC
(ferrous fumarate 324 mg.)

How Supplied:
Bottles of 100 NDC 0184-0307-60.

HEMOCYTE PLUS™ Tabules ℞
Iron-Vitamin-Mineral Complex

Description: Each tabule contains:
Ferrous Fumarate
(anhydrous) .... 324 mg.
[Equivalent to about 106 mg. of Elemental Iron]
Sodium Ascorbate (Vit. C) .... 200 mg.
Vit. B-1—Thiamine
Mononitrate .... 10 mg.
Vit. B-2—Riboflavin .... 6 mg.
Vit. B-6—Pyridoxine HCl .... 5 mg.
Vit. B-12—Cyanocobalamin
Concentrate .... 15mcg.
Folic Acid .... 1 mg.
Niacinamide .... 30 mg.
Calcium Pantothenate .... 10 mg.
Zinc Sulfate .... 80 mg.
Magnesium Sulfate .... 70 mg.
Manganese Sulfate .... 4 mg.
Copper Sulfate .... 2 mg.
How Supplied: Bottles of 100 NDC 0184-0308-60.

HEMOCYTE-F TABLETS ℞

Description: Each tablet contains:
Ferrous Fumarate ....324 mg.
Folic Acid ....1 mg.
How Supplied: Bottles of 100 NDC 0184-0306-60.

MAGSAL™ TABLETS ℞

Description: Each tablet contains:
Magnesium Salicylate .... 600 mg.
Phenyltoloxamine Citrate .... 25 mg.
How Supplied: Bottles of 100
NDC 0184-0321-60

ISOVEX® Capsules ℞
(ethaverine hydrochloride 100 mg.)

How Supplied:
Bottles of 100 NDC 0184-0204-60.
Bottles of 1000 NDC 0184-0204-80.

MEDIGESIC PLUS® Capsules ℞
Analgesic-Sedative

Description: Each capsule contains:
Butalbital* .... 50 mg
Warning: May be habit forming
Acetaminophen .... 325 mg
Caffeine .... 40 mg
*Derivative of Barbituric Acid
How Supplied:
Bottles of 100 NDC 0184-0212-60.

MEDIPLEX
Vitamin/Mineral Complex

Description: Each tabule contains:
Vitamin E—
dl-alpha Tocopherol Acetate ....60 I.U.
Vitamin C—Ascorbic Acid ....300 mg.
Vitamin B[12]—Cyanocobalmin
Concentrate ....25 mcg.
Vitamin B[1]—Thiamine ....25 mg.
Niacinamide ....100 mg.
Vitamin B[6]—Pyridoxine ....10 mg.
Vitamin B[2]—Riboflavin ....10 mg.
Calcium Pantothenate ....25 mg.
Zinc Sulfate ....80 mg.
Magnesium Sulfate ....70 mg.
Manganese Sulfate ....4 mg.
Copper Sulfate ....2 mg.
How Supplied: Bottles of 100 Tabules.
NDC 0184-0142-60

MEDIZINC Scored Tablets ℞
(zinc sulfate 220 mg.)

How Supplied: Bottles of 100 NDC 0184-0310-60.

NOREL PLUS Capsules ℞
Antihistamine-Analgesic-Decongestant

Description: Each capsule contains: Acetaminophen 325 mg., Phenyltoloxamine Dihydrogen Citrate 25 mg., Phenylpropanolamine HCl. 25 mg. and Chlorpheniramine Maleate 4 mg.
How Supplied: Bottles of 100 NDC 0184-0128-60.

U. S. Products, Inc.
16636 N.W. 54TH AVENUE
MIAMI LAKES, FL 33014

AMEBAQUIN ℞
Iodoquinol Tablets, USP
formerly Diiodohydroxyquin

Description: Iodoquinol U.S.P. (5, 7 diiodo-8-quinolinol) is a light yellowish-tan powder relatively insoluble in water and sparingly soluble in alcohol. It contains 63.9% Iodine. It is supplied as compressed tablets.
Actions: Iodoquinol possesses amebicidal activity against Entamoeba histolytica. It is especially destructive to amebae in the intestinal tract, is relatively non-toxic and produces virtually no intestinal irritation.
Absorption, distribution, fate and excretion studies on Iodoquinol are incomplete. Most of an oral dose of the drug is unabsorbed from the gastrointestinal tract. Increased blood iodine levels following ingestion of Iodoquinol, how-

ever, indicate that some systemic absorption does occur. Iodoquinol appears to be absorbed to a lesser extent with less consistency from one subject to another than is iodochlorhydroxyquin. The distribution and fate in man of absorbed Iodoquinol are unknown. Very limited studies in experimental animals suggest that a portion of the drug is distributed to tissues and that free iodine appears in the urine.
Indications: Iodoquinol is indicated for the treatment of asymptomatic intestinal amebiasis and in conjunction with other agents for treatment of mild to severe intestinal disease and hepatic abscess.
Contraindications: Known hypersensitivity to iodine and 8-hydroxyquinolines. Contraindicated in patients with hepatic damage.
Warnings: Optic neuritis, optic atrophy and peripheral neuropathy have been reported following prolonged high dosage therapy with halogenated 8-hydroxyquinolines. Long-term use of this drug, therefore, should be avoided.
Usage in Pregnancy: Safety for use in pregnancy or during lactation has not been established.
Precautions: Iodoquinol should be used with caution in patients with thyroid diseases.
Protein-bound serum iodine levels may be increased during treatment with diiodohydroxyquin and, therefore, interfere with certain thyroid function tests. These effects may persist for as long as six months after discontinuation of therapy.
Discontinue the drug if hypersensitivity reactions occur.
Adverse Reactions:
Skin: various forms of skin eruptions (acneiform papular and pustular; bullae; vegetating or tuberous iododerma), urticaria and pruritus.
Gastrointestinal: nausea, vomiting, abdominal cramps, diarrhea and pruritus ani.
Fever, chills, headache, vertigo, and enlargement of thyroid have been reported.
Optic neuritis, optic atrophy and peripheral neuropathy have been reported in association with prolonged high-dosage 8-hydroxyquinoline therapy.
Dosage and Administration: Usual Dose for Adults: 650 mg. three times a day for twenty days in asymptomatic amebiasis and when used in combination with other drugs.
Children: For twenty days, 40 mg. per Kg. of body weight daily, divided into 3 doses; the maximum dose during 24 hours is 1.95 grams.
How Supplied:
NDC 51626-103-10 Bottles of 100

CHARCOAL-ANTIDOSE™ Suspension
Activated Charcoal, U.S.P. Liquid
Ready to Use - Unit of Dosage

Indications: Emergency treatment for poisoning.
Recommended by National Poison Center Network.
Contraindications: If Patient is unconscious, do not force liquids. There are no known contraindications or side effects to activated charcoal.
Warnings: BEFORE USING, CALL POISON CENTER, EMERGENCY ROOM or PHYSICIAN IMMEDIATELY for advice.
Caution: Do not make victim vomit when acid, alkalis and petroleum products have been swallowed. Charcoal-Antidose may be of limited value for these cases. Never give Charcoal-Antidose simultaneously with syrup of ipecac as it will adsorb the ipecac and prevent emesis. Give Charcoal-Antidose after vomiting.
Actions: Charcoal-Antidose adsorbs or neutralizes poisons and is effective for virtually all chemicals (except cyanide) whether they are organic, inorganic, or large or small molecule compounds. pH is not a major factor in adsorption.
Dosage and Administration: After vomiting has occurred, shake well, and have victim drink entire contents.
How Supplied: Single dose, in oversized jars. 40 gm activated charcoal in 200 ml suspension. Manufactured under Patent No. 3917821.
NDC 51626-109-40 40 Gm Jars

CHARCOAL-ANTI-DOTE Powder
Activated Charcoal, U.S.P.

Indications: Emergency treatment for poisoning.
Approved by National Poison Center Network.
Contraindications: If Patient is unconscious, do not force liquids. There are no known contraindications or side effects to activated charcoal.
Warnings: BEFORE USING, CALL POISON CENTER, EMERGENCY ROOM or PHYSICIAN IMMEDIATELY for advice.
Caution: Do not make victim vomit when acid, alkalis and petroleum products have been swallowed. Charcoal-Anti-Dote may be of limited value for these cases. Never give Charcoal-Anti-Dote simultaneously with syrup of ipecac as it will adsorb the ipecac and prevent emesis. Give Charcoal-Anti-Dote after vomiting.
Actions: Charcoal-Anti-Dote adsorbs or neutralizes poisons and is effective for virtually all chemicals (except cyanide) whether they are organic, inorganic, or large or small molecule compounds. pH is not a major factor in adsorption.
Dosage and Administration: After vomiting has occurred, add warm water to the shoulder of the Charcoal-Anti-Dote bottle, shake well, and have victim drink entire contents.
How Supplied: Single dose, in oversized bottles. To be reconstituted with water.
NDC 51626-101-15 15 Gm Bottles
NDC 51626-102-30 30 Gm Bottles

USV Laboratories, Division
USV Pharmaceutical Corp.
TUCKAHOE, NY 10707

USV Laboratories Inc.
MANATI, P.R. 00701

USV (P.R.) Development Corp.
MANATI, P.R. 00701

AQUASOL® A DROPS — OTC

Composition: Oil-soluble vitamin A water solubilized with polysorbate 20 for faster, better absorption and utilization. Drops provide 5,000 IU vitamin A per 0.1 ml.
Actions: There is evidence that aqueous vitamin A produces a more rapid increase in the blood concentration and higher blood levels than the oily form of the vitamin.
Administration and Dosage: As a dietary supplement 0.1 ml (3 drops) for adults and children 4 or more years of age provides 100% of the U.S. RDA; 2 drops for children under 4, 133%.
How Supplied: *Drops:* 5,000 IU per 0.1 ml, bottles of 30 ml, with dropper.

AQUASOL A® — ℞
water-miscible vitamin A
50,000 USP Units (15 mg)
vitamin A per capsule
25,000 USP Units (7.5 mg)
vitamin A per capsule

Description: AQUASOL A (water-miscible vitamin A) Capsules provide 50,000 USP Units (15 mg) or 25,000 USP Units (7.5 mg) of vitamin A per capsule as retinol in the form of vitamin A alcohol, a light yellow to amber oil. One USP Unit is equivalent to one international unit (IU) and to 0.3 mcg of retinol or 0.6 mcg of beta-carotene. One molecule of beta-carotene yields two molecules of retinol, which is known as provitamin A.
Vitamin A, one of the fat-soluble vitamins, includes vitamin A itself as well as its precursors, alpha, beta, and gamma-carotene and cryptoxanthin. Of the precursors, beta-carotene predominates in nature and is the most active; on splitting, it forms two molecules of vitamin A, whereas the other precursors form only one molecule of vitamin A.

```
 CH3 CH3
   \ /
    C           CH3                 CH3
   / \           |                   |
H2C   C—CH=CH—C=CH—CH=CH—C=CHCH2OH
 |    ||
H2C   C—CH3
   \ /
    C
    H2
```

Ordinarily fat-soluble, the vitamin A in this product has been water solubilized by special processing* to enable better absorption and utilization particularly in conditions in which absorption or utilization of fats and fat-soluble substances is impaired.
Clinical Pharmacology: Retinol combines with opsin, the rod pigment in the retina, to form rhodopsin, which is necessary for visual adaptation to darkness.
Vitamin A prevents retardation of growth and preserves the integrity of the epithelial cells. Vitamin A deficiency is characterized by nyctalopia, keratomalacia, keratinization and drying of the skin, lowered resistance to infection, retardation of growth, thickening of bone, diminished production of cortical steroids, and fetal malformations. Vitamin A absorption requires bile salts, pancreatic lipase, and dietary fat. The vitamin is stored (primarily as the palmitate) in the Kupffer cells of the liver. The minimum daily requirement is approximately 20 units of vitamin A or 40 units of beta-carotene per kg of body weight. The daily Recommended Dietary Allowances (RDA) established by the National Academy of Sciences for selected categories of population are as follows: children 4-10 years of age, 2,500-3,000 units; adult males, 5,000 units; adult females, 4,000 units; pregnant women, 5,000 units; lactating women, 6,000 units.
The fat-soluble vitamins (A, D, E, and K) are absorbed by complex processes that parallel the absorption of fat. Thus, any condition that causes malabsorption of fat (e.g., celiac disease, tropical sprue, regional enteritis) may result in deficiency of one or all of these vitamins. Fat-soluble vitamins affect permeability or transport in various cell membranes and act as oxidation-reduction agents, coenzymes, or enzyme inhibitors. They are stored principally in the liver and excreted in the feces. Because these vitamins are metabolized very slowly, overdosage may produce toxic effects. Dietary fat is necessary for effective absorption of carotene, and protein is required for absorption of retinols. Protein and, possibly, zinc may be required to mobilize vitamin A reserves in the liver.
Vitamin A is more rapidly absorbed than carotene. Absorption of vitamin A from an aqueous vehicle is appreciably greater than when the drug is given in an oily solution.
Carotene is converted to vitamin A in the intestinal wall and in the liver. Vitamin A itself is found only in animal sources; it occurs in high concentrations in the liver of the cod, halibut, tuna, and shark. It is also prepared synthetically. Carotene is found only in plants.
Indications and Usage: AQUASOL A (water-miscible vitamin A) Capsules are effective

*Oil-soluble vitamin A water solubilized with polysorbate 80.

Continued on next page

USV—Cont.

for the treatment of vitamin A deficiency. Unlike fat-soluble vitamin A products, AQUASOL A Capsules are not contraindicated in the malabsorption syndrome, because of the water-solubilizing process.

Contraindications: Hypervitaminosis A. Sensitivity to any of the ingredients of this preparation.

Warnings: Avoid overdosage. Keep out of the reach of children.

Use in Pregnancy: Safety of amounts exceeding 5,000 units of vitamin A daily during pregnancy has not been established at this time. Therefore, for the protection of the fetus, the use of vitamin A in excess of the recommended dietary allowance should be avoided during normal pregnancy. Animal reproduction studies have shown fetal abnormalities associated with overdosage in several species. Malformations of the central nervous system, eye, palate, and genitourinary tract have been recorded.

Precautions: General: Protect from light. Vitamin A ingestion from fortified foods, dietary supplements, self-administered drugs and prescription drug sources should be evaluated. Prolonged daily dose administration over 25,000 units vitamin A should be under close supervision. Blood level assays are not a direct measure of liver storage. Liver storage should be adequate before discontinuing therapy. Single vitamin A deficiency is rare. Multiple vitamin deficiency is expected in any dietary deficiency.

Drug Interactions: Women receiving oral contraceptives have shown a significant increase in plasma vitamin A levels.

Pregnancy Category C: See Warnings section.

Nursing Mothers: The U.S. Recommended Dietary Allowance of vitamin A (6,000 units) is recommended for nursing mothers. Human milk supplies sufficient vitamin A for infants unless the maternal diet is grossly inadequate.

Adverse Reactions: See Overdosage section.

Overdosage: The following amounts have been found to be toxic orally. Toxicity manifestations depend on the age, dosage units, and duration of administration.

Acute toxicity—single dose (25,000 units/kg body weight)

Infant: 350,000 units

Adult: Over 2 million units

Chronic toxicity (4,000 units/kg body weight for 6 to 15 months)

Infants 3 to 6 months old: 18,500 units (water dispersed) per day for one to three months

Adult: 1 million units daily for three days, or 50,000 units daily for longer than 18 months, or 500,000 units daily for two months

Hypervitaminosis A Syndrome:

1. *General manifestations:* Fatigue, malaise, lethargy, abdominal discomfort, anorexia, and vomiting.
2. *Specific manifestations:*
   a. Skeletal: slow growth, hard tender cortical thickening over the radius and tibia, migratory arthralgia, and premature closure of the epiphysis:
   b. Central Nervous System: irritability, headache, and increased intracranial pressure as manifested by bulging fontanels, papilledema, and exophthalmos.
   c. Dermatologic: fissures of the lips, drying and cracking of the skin, alopecia, scaling, massive desquamation, and increased pigmentation.
   d. Systemic: hypomenorrhea, hepatosplenomegaly, jaundice, leukopenia, vitamin A plasma level over 1,200 units.

The treatment of hypervitaminosis A consists of immediate withdrawal of the vitamin along with symptomatic and supportive treatment.

Dosage and Administration: For adults and children over eight years of age:

1. Severe deficiency with xerophthalmia: 500,000 units daily for three days, followed by 50,000 units daily for two weeks.
2. Severe deficiency: 100,000 units daily for three days followed by 50,000 units daily for two weeks.
3. Follow-up therapy: 10,000 to 20,000 units daily for two months.

Poor dietary habits should be corrected and an abundant and well-balanced dietary intake should be prescribed.

How Supplied: AQUASOL A Capsules (water-miscible vitamin A) 50,000 USP Units vitamin A, bottles of 100 (NDC 0075-0104-00) and 500 (NDC 0075-0104-05); 25,000 USP Units vitamin A, bottles of 100 (NDC 0075-0103-00). These products are dark red, soft gelatin capsules. The 50,000 unit capsules are imprinted with the number 104, the 25,000 unit capsules with the number 103.

[*Shown in Product Identification Section*]

AQUASOL® E — OTC
(Aqueous Vitamin E Supplements, Oral)

Composition: Two potencies, 100 IU and 400 IU vitamin E per capsule; water-solubilized for more rapid and more complete absorption than oily vitamin E. Drops, 50 IU vitamin E per ml in aqueous solution.

How Supplied: 100 IU Capsules, bottles of 100; 400 IU capsules, bottles of 30. Drops, 12 ml and 30 ml.

[*Shown in Product Identification Section*]

ARLIDIN® — ℞
(nylidrin HCl)
Vasodilator/Vasorelaxant

Arlidin is a product of USV Laboratories Inc., Manati, P.R. 00701.

Description: Tablets of 6 and 12 mg nylidrin HCl.

Actions: Arlidin acts predominantly by beta-receptor stimulation. Beta stimulation with Arlidin has been demonstrated in a variety of isolated tissues from rabbits, guinea pigs and dogs. It has been shown to dilate arterioles in skeletal muscle and to increase cardiac output in the anesthetized dog and cat and in unanesthetized man.

Indications: Based on a review of this drug by the National Academy of Sciences—National Research Council and/or other information, FDA has classified the indications as follows:

"Possibly" effective whenever an increase in blood supply is desirable in vasospastic disorders such as:

Peripheral vascular disease: arteriosclerosis obliterans, thromboangiitis obliterans, diabetic vascular disease, night leg cramps, Raynaud's phenomenon and disease, ischemic ulcer, frostbite, acrocyanosis, acroparesthesia, thrombophlebitis, cold feet, legs and hands.

Circulatory disturbances of the inner ear: primary cochlear cell ischemia, cochlear stria vascular ischemia, macular or ampullar ischemia and other disturbances due to labyrinthine artery spasm or obstruction.

Final classification of the less-than-effective indications requires further investigation.

Contraindications: Acute myocardial infarction, paroxysmal tachycardia, progressive angina pectoris and thyrotoxicosis.

Warnings: In patients with cardiac disease such as tachyarrhythmias and uncompensated congestive heart failure, the benefit/risk ratio should be weighed prior to therapy and reconsidered at intervals during treatment.

Adverse Reactions: Trembling, nervousness, weakness, dizziness (not associated with labyrinthine artery insufficiency), palpitations, nausea and vomiting may occur. Postural hypotension, while not reported, may also occur.

Dosage: Orally, 3 to 12 mg three or four times a day.

How Supplied: ARLIDIN (nylidrin HCl)—White, scored tablets, 6 mg and 12 mg. Bottles of 100 and 1000. Unit-dose blister packs, boxes of 100 (10 x 10 strips).

NSN 6505-00-685-5435A, V.A. Depots (6 mg., 1000s).

[*Shown in Product Identification Section*]

AZOLID® — ℞
phenylbutazone

100 mg tablets, capsules

Important Note: AZOLID (phenylbutazone) cannot be considered a simple analgesic and should never be administered casually. Each patient should be carefully evaluated before treatment is started and should remain constantly under the close supervision of the physician. The following precautions should be observed:

1. Therapy should not be initiated until a careful, detailed history and complete hemogram and urinalysis, etc., of the patient have been made. These examinations should be made at regular, frequent intervals throughout the duration of this drug therapy.

2. Patients should be carefully selected, avoiding those in whom it is contraindicated as well as those who will respond to ordinary therapeutic measures, or those who cannot be observed at frequent intervals.

3. Patients taking AZOLID should be warned not to exceed the recommended dosage because this may lead to toxic effects. Patients should report to the physician immediately any sign of:

a. fever, sore throat, lesions in the mouth (symptoms of blood dyscrasia);
b. dyspepsia, epigastric pain, symptoms of anemia, unusual bleeding, unusual bruising, black or tarry stools, or other evidence of intestinal ulceration;
c. skin reactions;
d. significant weight gain or edema.

4. A TRIAL PERIOD OF ONE WEEK IS CONSIDERED ADEQUATE TO DETERMINE THE THERAPEUTIC EFFECT OF THE DRUG. IN THE ABSENCE OF A FAVORABLE RESPONSE, THERAPY SHOULD BE DISCONTINUED.

In patients 60 years of age and over, AZOLID should be restricted to a short-term period of no more than seven days.

5. BEFORE PRESCRIBING AZOLID FOR AN INDIVIDUAL PATIENT, READ THOROUGHLY THE INFORMATION CONTAINED UNDER EACH HEADING THAT FOLLOWS:

Description: Chemically, AZOLID is 4-butyl-1,2-diphenyl-3,5-pyrazolidinedione. It is closely related chemically to the pyrazoles.

It is very slightly soluble in water; freely soluble in acetone and in ether; soluble in alcohol.

Clinical Pharmacology: AZOLID is closely related pharmacologically, including toxic effects, to the pyrazole compounds, aminopyrine and antipyrine. It is entirely unrelated to the steroid hormones.

It has analgesic, antipyretic and anti-inflammatory actions as well as mild uricosuric properties resulting in symptomatic relief only. THE DISEASE PROCESS ITSELF IS UNALTERED BY THE DRUG.

The exact mechanism of the anti-inflammatory effects of phenylbutazone has not been elucidated, but clinical pharmacology studies have shown that phenylbutazone inhibits certain factors believed to be involved in the inflammatory process. These processes are (1) prostaglandin synthesis; (2) leucocyte migra-

tion; (3) release and/or activity of lysosomal enzymes.
Phenylbutazone is rapidly absorbed after oral administration. Tests conducted in 18 healthy adult male volunteers indicated that a peak plasma concentration of 43.3 (±3.1) mg/liter was attained within 2.5 (±1.4) hours after the ingestion of three 100-mg tablets. In these same volunteers, the apparent elimination half-life was 84 (±23) hours. About 98% of the drug is bound to human serum albumin.
Twenty-one days after oral administration of ^{14}C-labeled drug, 61% was recovered from the urine and 27% from the feces. However, only about 1% of total urinary radioactivity represents unchanged drug. The sum of nonconjugated urinary metabolites (oxyphenbutazone, γ-hydroxyphenylbutazone, p, γ-dihydroxyphenylbutazone), and phenylbutazone itself amounted to only about 10%. About 40% of the total urinary radioactivity was excreted as the C(4)-glucuronide of phenylbutazone and an additional 12% was identified as the C(4)-glucuronide of γ-hydroxyphenylbutazone.
The major metabolite of phenylbutazone in human plasma is oxyphenbutazone; steady-state plasma levels are about 50% of those of phenylbutazone. Less than 2% of the dose of phenylbutazone appears in the urine as oxyphenbutazone.

Indications: The indications for AZOLID (phenylbutazone) are as follows:
Acute gouty arthritis
Acute rheumatoid arthritis
Active ankylosing spondylitis
Short-term treatment of acute attacks of degenerative joint disease of the hips and knees not responsive to other treatment
Painful shoulder (peritendinitis, capsulitis, bursitis, and acute arthritis of that joint).

Contraindications:
AGE: Phenylbutazone is contraindicated in children 14 years of age or younger because controlled clinical trials in patients of this age group have not been conducted.
OTHER MEDICAL CONDITIONS: Phenylbutazone is contraindicated in patients with incipient cardiac failure, blood dyscrasias, pancreatitis, parotitis, stomatitis, polymyalgia rheumatica, temporal arteritis, senility, drug allergy, and in the presence of severe renal, cardiac and hepatic disease, and in patients with a history of peptic ulcer disease, or symptoms of gastrointestinal inflammation or active ulceration because serious adverse reactions or aggravation of existing medical problems can occur.
CONCOMITANT MEDICATIONS: Phenylbutazone should not be used in combination with other drugs that accentuate or share a potential for similar toxicity.
It is also inadvisable to administer phenylbutazone in combination with other potent drugs because of the possibility of increased toxic reactions from phenylbutazone and other agents. (See also PRECAUTIONS: Drug Interactions.)
Phenylbutazone is contraindicated in patients with a history or suggestion of prior toxicity, sensitivity, or idiosyncrasy to phenylbutazone or oxyphenbutazone.

Warnings: Based upon reports of clinical experience with phenylbutazone and related compounds, the following warnings should be considered by the physician prior to prescribing the drug:
GASTROINTESTINAL: Upper G.I. diagnostic tests should be performed in patients with persistent or severe dyspepsia. Peptic ulceration, reactivation of latent peptic ulcer, perforation and gastrointestinal bleeding, sometimes severe, have been reported.
As with other nonsteroidal anti-inflammatory drugs, borderline elevations of one or more liver tests may occur in up to 15% of patients. These abnormalities may progress, may remain essentially unchanged, or may be transient with continued therapy. The SGPT (ALT) test is probably the most sensitive indicator of liver dysfunction. Meaningful (three times the upper limit of normal) elevations of SGPT or SGOT (AST) occurred in controlled clinical trials in less than 1% of patients. A patient with symptoms and/or signs suggesting liver dysfunction, or in whom an abnormal liver test has occurred, should be evaluated for evidence of the development of more severe hepatic reaction while on therapy with phenylbutazone. Severe hepatic reactions, including jaundice and cases of fatal hepatitis, have been reported with phenylbutazone as with other nonsteroidal anti-inflammatory drugs. Although such reactions are rare, if abnormal liver tests persist or worsen, if clinical signs and symptoms consistent with liver disease develop, or if systemic manifestations occur (e.g. eosinophilia, rash, etc.), phenylbutazone should be discontinued.
HEMATOLOGIC: Frequent and regular hematologic evaluations should be performed on patients receiving the drug for periods over one week. Any significant change in the total white count, relative decrease in granulocytes, appearance of immature forms or fall in hematocrit should be a signal for immediate cessation of therapy and a complete hematologic investigation. Serious, sometimes fatal blood dyscrasias, including aplastic anemia have been reported to occur. Hematologic toxicity may occur suddenly or many days or weeks after cessation of treatment as manifested by the appearance of anemia, leukopenia, thrombocytopenia or clinically significant hemorrhagic diathesis. There have been published reports associating phenylbutazone with leukemia. However, the circumstances involved in these reports are such that a cause and effect relationship to the drug has not been established.

Precautions:
GENERAL: Because of potential serious adverse reactions to phenylbutazone, the following precautions should be observed in the use of the drug:
1. A careful diagnostic physical examination and history should be performed on all patients at regular intervals while the patient is receiving the drug.
2. Phenylbutazone is not recommended for chronic use in the elderly.
3. Hematologic evaluation should be performed at frequent and regular intervals and additional laboratory examinations performed as indicated.
4. Patients should be instructed to report immediately the occurrence of high fever, severe sore throat, stomatitis, salivary gland enlargement, tarry stools, unusual bleeding or bruising, sudden weight gain, or edema.
5. The drug reduces iodine uptake by the thyroid and may interfere with laboratory tests of thyroid function. (See ADVERSE REACTIONS: Endocrine-Metabolic.)
6. The patient should be cautioned regarding participation in activities requiring alertness and coordination and that the concomitant ingestion of alcohol with phenylbutazone may further impair psychomotor skills.
DRUG INTERACTIONS: Phenylbutazone is highly bound to serum proteins. If its affinity for protein binding is higher than other concurrently administered drugs, the actions and toxicity of the other drug may be increased.
Phenylbutazone accentuates the prothrombin depression produced by coumarin-type anticoagulants. When administered alone, it does not affect prothrombin activity. The pharmacologic action of insulin, and anti-diabetic and sulfonamide drugs may be potentiated by the simultaneous administration of phenylbutazone.
Concomitant administration of phenylbutazone and phenytoin may result in increased serum levels of phenytoin which could lead to increased phenytoin toxicity.
PREGNANCY CATEGORY C: Reproductive studies in animals, although inconclusive, exhibited evidence of possible embryotoxicity. It is, therefore, recommended that this drug should be used with caution during pregnancy. The benefits should be weighed against the potential risk to the fetus.
NURSING MOTHERS: Caution is also advised in prescribing phenylbutazone in nursing mothers because the drug may appear in cord blood and breast milk.
PEDIATRIC USE: Phenylbutazone is contraindicated in children 14 years of age or younger because controlled clinical trials in patients of this age group have not been conducted.

Adverse Reactions: Based upon reports of clinical experience with phenylbutazone and related compounds, the following adverse reactions have been reported.
TABLE 1: (1)* = Incidence greater than 1%; (2) = Incidence less than 1%.

Gastrointestinal
(1) Nausea*; dyspepsia/including indigestion and heartburn*; abdominal discomfort/distress*.
(2) Vomiting; abdominal distention with flatulence; constipation; diarrhea; esophagitis; gastritis; salivary gland enlargement; stomatitis, sometimes with ulceration; ulceration and perforation of the intestinal tract, including acute and reactivated peptic ulcer with perforation, hemorrhage and hematemesis; anemia due to gastrointestinal bleeding which may be occult; hepatitis, both fatal and nonfatal, sometimes associated with evidence of cholestasis.

Hematological
(1) None.
(2) Anemia; leukopenia; thrombocytopenia with associated purpura, petechiae and hemorrhage; pancytopenia; aplastic anemia; bone marrow depression; agranulocytosis and agranulocytic anginal syndrome; hemolytic anemia.

Hypersensitivity
(1) None.
(2) Urticaria; anaphylactic shock; arthralgia, drug fever; hypersensitivity angiitis (polyarteritis) and vasculitis; Lyell's syndrome; serum sickness; Stevens-Johnson syndrome; activation of systemic lupus erythematosus; aggravation of temporal arteritis in patients with polymyalgia rheumatica.

Dermatologic
(1) Rash*.
(2) Pruritis; erythema nodosum; erythema multiforme; non-thrombocytopenic purpura.

Cardiovascular, Fluid, and Electrolyte
(1) Edema/water retention*.
(2) Sodium and chloride retention; fluid retention and plasma dilution; cardiac decompensation (congestive heart failure) with edema and dyspnea; metabolic acidosis; respiratory alkalosis; hypertension; pericarditis; interstitial myocarditis with muscle necrosis and perivascular granulomata.

Renal
(1) None.
(2) Hematuria; proteinuria; ureteral obstruction with uric acid crystals; anuria; glomerulonephritis; acute tubular necrosis; cortial necrosis; renal stones; nephrotic syndrome; impaired renal function and renal failure associated with azotemia.

Central Nervous System
(1) None
(2) Headache; drowsiness; agitation; confusional states and lethargy; tremors; numbness; weakness.

Endocrine-Metabolic
(1) None.
(2) Hyperglycemia.

Special Senses
(1) Ocular: none; otic: none.
(2) Ocular: none; otic: hearing loss; tinnitus.
Adverse reactions have also been listed in a Group (3)—Causal Relationship Unknown. The reactions in this group have been reported

Continued on next page

USV—Cont.

but occurred under circumstances where a causal relationship could not be established. In some patients the reported reactions may have been unrelated to the administration of phenylbutazone. However, in these reported events, the possibility cannot be excluded. Therefore these observations are being listed to serve as alerting information to physicians. Before prescribing this drug for an individual patient, the physician should be familiar with the following:

TABLE 2: (3)=Causal Relationship Unknown —incidence less than 1%.

Hematological

Leukemia. (There have been reports associating phenylbutazone with leukemia. However, the circumstances involved in these reports are such that a cause-and-effect relationship to the drug has not been clearly established.)

Endocrine-Metabolic

Thyroid hyperplasia; goiters associated with hyperthyroidism and hypothyroidism; pancreatitis.

Special Senses

Blurred vision; optic neuritis; toxic amblyopia; scotomata; retinal detachment; retinal hemorrhage; oculomotor palsy.

Overdosage: SIGNS AND SYMPTOMS: Include any of the following: nausea, vomiting, epigastric pain, excessive perspiration, euphoria, psychosis, headaches, giddiness, vertigo, hyperventilation, insomnia, tinnitus, difficulty in hearing, edema (sodium retention), hypertension, cyanosis, respiratory depression, agitation, hallucinations, stupor, convulsions, coma, hematuria, and oliguria. Hepatomegaly, jaundice, and ulceration of the buccal or gastrointestinal mucosa have been reported as late manifestations of massive overdosage.

Reported laboratory abnormalities following overdosage include: respiratory or metabolic acidosis, impaired hepatic or renal function, and abnormalities of formed blood elements.

TREATMENT: In the alert patient, empty the stomach promptly by induced emesis followed by lavage. In the obtunded patient, secure the airway with a cuffed endotracheal tube before beginning lavage (do not induce emesis). Maintain adequate respiratory exchange; do not use respiratory stimulants. Treat shock with appropriate supportive measures. Control seizures with intravenous diazepam or short-acting barbiturates. Dialysis may be helpful if renal function is impaired.

Dosage and Administration: AZOLID (phenylbutazone) should be used at the smallest effective dosage to afford rapid relief of severe symptoms. It is contraindicated in children under 14 years of age and in senile patients.

If a favorable symptomatic response to treatment is not obtained after one week, the drug should be discontinued. When a favorable therapeutic response has been obtained, the dosage should be reduced and then discontinued as soon as possible.

In elderly patients (60 years and over) every effort must be made to discontinue therapy on, or as soon as possible after the seventh day, because of the exceedingly high risk of severe fatal toxic reactions in this age group.

To minimize gastric upset, the drug should be taken with milk or with meals.

In selecting the appropriate dosage in any specific case, consideration should be given to the patient's age, weight, general health, and any other factors that may influence his response to the drug.

Rheumatoid Arthritis, Ankylosing Spondylitis, Acute Attacks of Degenerative Joint Disease, and Painful Shoulder:

Initial Dosage: The daily dose in adult patients is 300 to 600 mg in three or four divided doses. Maximum therapeutic response is usually obtained at a total daily dose of 400 mg. A trial period of one week of therapy is considered adequate to determine the therapeutic effect of the drug. In the absence of a favorable response, therapy should be discontinued.

Maintenance Dosage: When improvement is obtained, dosage should be promptly decreased to the minimum effective level necessary to maintain relief, not exceeding 400 mg daily because of the possibility of cumulative toxicity. A satisfactory clinical response may be obtained with daily doses as low as 100 to 200 mg daily.

Acute Gouty Arthritis:

Satisfactory results are obtained after an initial dose of 400 mg followed by 100 mg every four hours. The articular inflammation usually subsides within four days and treatment should not be continued longer than one week.

How Supplied: AZOLID tablets, 100 mg (yellow, coated), and capsules, 100 mg (yellow and white), bottles of 100 (tablets: NDC 0075-0060-00; capsules: NDC 0075-0112-00) and 1000 (tablets: NDC 0075-0060-99; capsules: NDC 0075-0112-99).

[*Shown in Product Identification Section*]

Bi-K™ ℞

potassium supplement

Description: Each 15 ml (one tablespoonful) supplies 20 mEq of potassium ions as a combination of potassium gluconate and potassium citrate in a sorbitol and saccharin solution.

Indications: For use as oral potassium therapy in the prevention or treatment of hypokalemia which may occur as a result of diuretic or corticosteroid administration. It may be used in the treatment of cardiac arrhythmias due to digitalis intoxication.

Contraindications: Severe renal impairment with oliguria or azotemia, untreated Addison's disease, adynamia episodica hereditaria, acute dehydration, heat cramps and hyperkalemia from any cause. This product should not be used in patients receiving aldosterone antagonists or triamterene.

Warnings: Bi-K (potassium gluconate and potassium citrate) is a palatable form of oral potassium replacement. It appears that little if any potassium gluconate-citrate penetrates as far as the jejunum or ileum where enteric coated potassium chloride lesions have been noted. Excessive, undiluted doses of Bi-K may cause a saline laxative effect.

To minimize gastrointestinal irritation, it is recommended that Bi-K be taken with meals or diluted with water or fruit juice. A tablespoonful (15 ml) in 8 ounces of water is approximately isotonic. More than a single tablespoonful should not be taken without prior dilution.

Precautions: Potassium is a major intracellular cation which plays a significant role in body physiology. The serum level of potassium is normally 3.8–5.0 mEq/liter. While the serum or plasma level is a poor indicator of total body stores, a plasma or serum level below 3.5 mEq/liter is considered to be indicative of hypokalemia.

The most common cause of hypokalemia is excessive loss of potassium in the urine. However, hypokalemia can also occur with vomiting, gastric drainage and diarrhea.

Usually a potassium deficiency can be corrected by oral administration of potassium supplements. With normal kidney function it is difficult to produce potassium intoxication by oral administration. However, potassium supplements must be administered with caution since, usually, the exact amount of the deficiency is not accurately known. Checks on the patient's clinical status and periodic E.K.G. and/or serum potassium levels should be made. High serum potassium levels may cause death by cardiac depression, arrhythmias or arrest.

In patients with hypokalemia who also have alkalosis and a chloride deficiency, (hypokalemia hypochloremic alkalosis) there will be a requirement for chloride ions. Bi-K is not recommended for use in these patients.

Adverse Reactions: Symptoms of potassium intoxication include paresthesias of the extremities, flaccid paralysis, listlessness, mental confusion, weakness and heaviness of the legs, fall in blood pressure, cardiac arrhythmias and heart block. Hyperkalemia may exhibit the following electrocardiographic abnormalities: disappearance of the P wave, widening and slurring of the QRS complex, changes of the ST segment and tall peaked T waves.

Bi-K taken on an empty stomach in undiluted doses larger than 30 ml (two tablespoons) can produce gastric irritation with nausea, vomiting, diarrhea and abdominal discomfort.

Overdosage: The administration of oral potassium supplements to persons with normal kidney function rarely causes serious hyperkalemia. However, if the renal excretory function is impaired, potentially fatal hyperkalemia can result. It is important to note that hyperkalemia is usually asymptomatic and may be manifested only by an increased serum potassium concentration with E.K.G. changes.

Treatment measures include:

1. Elimination of potassium containing drugs or foods.
2. Intravenous administration of 300 to 500 ml/hr of a 10% dextrose solution containing 10–20 units of crystalline insulin per 1000 milliliters.
3. Correction of acidosis.
4. Use of exchange resins or peritoneal dialysis.

In treating hyperkalemia, it should be noted that patients stabilized on digitalis can develop digitalis toxicity when the serum potassium concentration is changed too rapidly.

Dosage and Administration: The usual dosage is one tablespoonful (15 ml) in 6–8 fluid ounces of water or fruit juice, two to four times a day. This will supply 40 to 80 mEq of potassium ions. The usual preventive dose of potassium is 20 mEq per day while therapeutic doses range from 30 mEq to 100 mEq per day. Because of the potential for gastrointestinal irritation, undiluted large single doses (30 ml or more) of Bi-K are to be avoided.

Deviations from this schedule may be indicated, since no average total daily dose can be defined, but must be governed by close observation for clinical effects.

How Supplied: 1 pint (16 fl. oz.).

CERESPAN® ℞

(papaverine HCl)

in sustained-release micro-dialysis cells

Composition: Each capsule provides 150 mg papaverine hydrochloride in micro-dialysis cells, uniquely processed for sustained release of medication to provide prolonged therapeutic effect.

Actions and Uses: The main actions of papaverine are exerted on cardiac and various smooth muscles. It relaxes the smooth musculature of the larger blood vessels, especially coronary, systemic peripheral, cerebral and pulmonary arteries. This relaxation may be prominent if spasm exists. The muscle cell is not paralyzed by papaverine, and still responds to drugs and other stimuli causing contraction. The antispasmodic effect is a direct one, and unrelated to muscle innervation. Papaverine is practically devoid of effects on the central nervous system.

Perhaps by its direct vasodilating action on cerebral blood vessels, papaverine increases cerebral blood flow and decreases cerebral vascular resistance in normal subjects; oxygen consumption is unaltered. These effects may explain the benefit reported from the drug in cerebral vascular encephalopathy.

Like quinidine, papaverine acts directly on heart muscle to depress conduction and prolong the refractory period. These direct actions provide the basis for its clinical trial in abrogating atrial and ventricular premature systoles and ominous ventricular arrhythmias.

The coronary vasodilator action could be an additional factor of therapeutic value when such rhythms are secondary to insufficiency or occlusion of the coronary arteries.

In patients with acute coronary thrombosis, the occurrence of ventricular rhythms is serious and requires measures designed to decrease myocardial irritability. Papaverine may have advantages over quinidine, used for a similar purpose, in that it may be given in an emergency by the intravenous route, does not depress myocardial contraction or cause cinchonism, and produces coronary vasodilation.

Indications: For the relief of cerebral and peripheral ischemia associated with arterial spasm and myocardial ischemia complicated by arrhythmias.

Precautions: Use with caution in patients with glaucoma. Hepatic hypersensitivity has been reported with gastrointestinal symptoms, jaundice, eosinophilia and altered liver function tests. Discontinue drug if these occur.

Side Effects: Although occurring rarely, the reported side effects of papaverine include nausea, abdominal distress, anorexia, constipation or diarrhea, skin rash, malaise, drowsiness, vertigo, sweating, and headache.

Administration and Dosage: One capsule every 12 hours. In difficult cases administration may be increased to one capsule every 8 hours, or two capsules every 12 hours.

How Supplied: Bottles of 100 and 1000.

[*Shown in Product Identification Section*]

For dilution in intravenous infusions only

CHROMETRACE™ ℞

Chromic Chloride Injection USP

4 mcg/ml

Chromic Chloride in Sodium Chloride Solution

Description: Chrometrace, Chromic Chloride Injection USP (4 mcg chromium/ml), is a sterile, nonpyrogenic solution intended for use as an additive to intravenous solutions for total parenteral nutrition (TPN). Each ml of solution provides:

chromic chloride ....12.18 mcg
sodium ....3.34 mg
chloride ....5.29 mg
(not including ions for pH adjustment)

The pH is approximately 2.0, adjusted with hydrochloric acid and may be adjusted with sodium hydroxide. The solution is adjusted to isotonicity with sodium chloride. The osmolarity is approximately 0.300 mOsm/ml. The solution contains no bacteriostat, antimicrobial agent, or added buffer.

Chromic chloride is chemically designated $CrCl_3$, a cystalline compound soluble in water. Sodium chloride USP is chemically designated NaCl, a white, crystalline compound freely soluble in water.

Clinical Pharmacology: Trivalent chromium is part of glucose tolerance factor, an essential activator of insulin-mediated reactions. Chromium helps to maintain normal glucose metabolism and peripheral nerve function.

Providing chromium during TPN helps prevent deficiency symptoms including impaired glucose tolerance, ataxia, peripheral neuropathy, and a confusional state similar to mild/moderate hepatic encephalopathy.

Serum chromium is bound to transferrin (siderophilin) in the beta-globulin fraction. Typical blood levels for chromium range from 1 to 5 mcg/liter, but blood levels are not considered a meaningful index of tissue stores. Administration of chromium supplements to chromium-deficient patients can result in normalization of the glucose tolerance curve from the diabetic-like curve typical of chromium deficiency. This response is viewed as a more meaningful indicator of chromium nutriture then serum chromium levels.

Excretion of chromium is via the kidneys, ranging from 3 to 50 mcg/day. Biliary excretion via the small intestine may be an ancillary route, but it is believed that only small amounts of chromium are excreted in this manner.

Indications and Usage: Chrometrace is indicated for use as a supplement to intravenous solutions given for total parenteral nutrition (TPN). Administration helps to maintain chromium serum levels and to prevent depletion of endogenous stores and subsequent deficiency symptoms.

Contraindications: Direct intramuscular or intravenous injection of Chrometrace is contraindicated, as the acidic pH of the solution (2.0) may cause considerable tissue irritation.

Warnings: None known.

Precautions: Do not use unless solution is clear and the seal is intact.

Chrometrace, Chromic Chloride Injection USP, should be used only in conjunction with a pharmacy-directed admixture program using aseptic technique in a laminar flow environment. The solution contains no preservatives; discard unused portion within 24 hours after opening.

In assessing the contribution of chromium supplements to maintenance of glucose homeostasis, consideration should be given to the possibility that the patient may be diabetic.

Pregnancy Category C. Animal reproduction studies have not been conducted with chromic chloride. It is also not known whether chromic chloride can cause fetal harm when administered to a pregnant woman or can affect reproductive capacity. Chromic chloride should be given to a pregnant woman only if clearly indicated.

Adverse Reactions: None known.

Drug Abuse and Dependence: None known.

Overdosage: Trivalent chromium administered intravenously to TPN patients has been shown to be nontoxic when given at dosage levels of up to 250 mcg/day for two consecutive weeks.

Reported toxic reactions to chromium include nausea, vomiting, ulcers of the gastrointestinal tract, renal and hepatic damage, convulsions, and coma. The acute LD_{50} for intravenous trivalent chromium in rats was reported as 10 to 18 mg/kg.

Dosage and Administration: Chrometrace contains 4 mcg chromium/ml and is administered intravenously only after dilution.

Adult: For the adult receiving TPN, the suggested additive dosage is 10 to 15 mcg chromium/day. The metabolically stable adult with intestinal fluid loss may require 20 mcg chromium/day, with frequent monitoring of blood levels as a guideline for subsequent administration.

Pediatric: For pediatric patients, the suggested additive dosage is 0.14 to 0.20 mcg/kg/day.

Parenteral drug products should be inspected visually for particulate matter and discoloration prior to administration, whenever solution and container permit. See Precautions section.

How Supplied:

Chrometrace 10-ml vials (NDC-0075-0830-22), boxes of 25.

[*Shown in Product Identification Section*]

For dilution in intravenous infusions only

COPPERTRACE™ ℞

Cupric Chloride Injection USP

0.4 mg/ml

Cupric Chloride in Sodium Chloride Solution

Description: Coppertrace, Cupric Chloride Injection USP (0.4 mg copper/ml), is a sterile nonpyrogenic solution intended for use as an additive to intravenous solutions for total parenteral nutrition (TPN). Each ml of solution provides:

cupric chloride ....0.85 mg
sodium ....3.19 mg
chloride ....5.36 mg
(not including ions for pH adjustment).

The pH is approximately 2.0, adjusted with hydrochloric acid, and may be adjusted with sodium hydroxide. The solution is adjusted to isotonicity with sodium chloride. The osmolarity is approximately 0.300 mOsm/ml. The solution contains no bacteriostat, antimicrobial agent, or added buffer.

Cupric chloride is chemically designated $CuCl_2$, a crystalline compound freely soluble in water. Sodium chloride USP is chemically designated NaCl, a white crystalline compound freely soluble in water.

Clinical Pharmacology: Copper is an essential nutrient that serves as a cofactor for serum ceruloplasmin, an oxidase necessary for proper formation of the iron carrier protein, transferrin. Copper also helps maintain normal rates of red and white blood cell formation.

Providing copper during TPN helps prevent development of the following deficiency symptoms: Leukopenia, neutropenia, anemia, depressed ceruloplasmin levels, impaired transferrin formation, and secondary iron deficiency.

Normal serum copper values range from 80 to 163 mcg/dl (mean, approximately 110 mcg/dl). The serum copper level at which deficiency symptoms appear is not precisely defined. The daily turnover of copper through ceruloplasmin is approximately 0.5 mg. Excretion of copper is through the bile (80%), directly through the intestinal wall (16%), and in urine (4%).

Indications and Usage: Coppertrace is indicated for use as a supplement to intravenous solutions given for total parenteral nutrition (TPN). Administration helps to maintain copper serum levels and to prevent depletion of endogenous stores and subsequent deficiency symptoms.

Contraindications: Direct intramuscular or intravenous injection of Coppertrace is contraindicated, as the acidic pH of the solution (2.0) may cause considerable tissue irritation.

Warnings: **Copper is eliminated via the bile. In patients with severe liver dysfunction and/or biliary tract obstruction, decreasing or omitting copper supplements entirely may be necessary.**

Precautions: Do not use unless the solution is clear and the seal is intact.

Coppertrace should be used only in conjunction with a pharmacy-directed admixture program using aseptic technique in a laminar flow environment. The solution contains no preservatives; discard unused portion within 24 hours after opening.

Twice monthly serum assays for copper and/or ceruloplasmin are suggested for monitoring copper concentrations in long-term TPN patients. As ceruloplasmin is a cuproenzyme, ceruloplasmin assays may be depressed secondary to copper deficiency.

Pregnancy Catergory C. Animal reproduction studies have not been conducted with cupric chloride. It is also not known whether cupric chloride can cause fetal harm when administered to a pregnant woman or can affect reproductive capacity. Cupric chloride should be given to a pregnant woman only if clearly indicated.

Adverse Reactions: None known.

Drug Abuse and Dependence: None known.

Overdosage: Copper toxicity can produce prostration, behavior change, diarrhea, progressive marasmus, hypotonia, photophobia and peripheral edema. Such symptoms have been reported with a serum copper level of 286

Continued on next page

USV—Cont.

mcg/dl. D-penicillamine has been reported effective as an antidote.

Dosage and Administration: Coppertrace, Cupric Chloride Injection USP, contains 0.4 mg copper/ml and is administered intravenously only after dilution.

Adult: For the adult receiving TPN, the suggested additive dosage is 0.5 to 1.5 mg copper/day.

Pediatric: For pediatric patients, the suggested additive dosage is 20 mcg copper/kg/day.

Parenteral drug products should be inspected visually for particulate matter and discoloration prior to administration, whenever solution and container permit. See Precautions section.

How Supplied: Coppertrace 10-ml vials (NDC 0075-0831-22), boxes of 25.

[*Shown in Product Identification Section*]

DEMI-REGROTON® ℞
Oral antihypertensive

See under Regroton®.

DORIDEN® Ⓒ
glutethimide USP

0.5 g tablets
0.25 g tablets

Description: DORIDEN (glutethimide), an oral hypnotic, is a piperidinedione derivative that occurs as a white, crystalline powder and is practically insoluble in water, soluble in alcohol. Its chemical name is 2-ethyl-2-phenylglutarimide with the following structural formula:

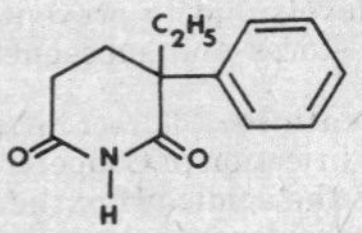

C_2H_5

Clinical Pharmacology: Doriden is erratically absorbed from the gastrointestinal tract. Following single oral doses of 500 mg, wide variations in absorption of the drug were observed, and the peak plasma concentration occurred from one to six hours after administration. The average plasma half-life is 10–12 hours. Glutethimide is a racemate; both isomers are hydroxylated; the d-isomer on the piperidinedione ring and the l-isomer on the phenyl substituent. Both hydroxylates are conjugated with glucuronic acid; the glucuronides pass into the enterohepatic circulation, and thence are excreted in the urine. Less than 2% of a usual dose is excreted in the urine unchanged. About 50% of the drug is bound to plasma proteins.

Glutethimide exhibits pronounced anticholinergic activity, which is manifested by mydriasis, inhibition of salivary secretions, and decreased intestinal motility.

Indications and Usage: Glutethimide has been shown to be effective as a hypnotic for three to seven days. It is not indicated for chronic administration. Should insomnia persist, a drug-free interval of one or more weeks should elapse before retreatment is considered. Attempts should be made to find alternative nondrug therapy in chronic insomnia.

Contraindications: Glutethimide is contraindicated in patients with known hypersensitivity to the drug. It is also contraindicated in patients with porphyria.

Warnings: The concomitant use of alcohol or other CNS depressants may produce additive CNS depressant effects.

Precautions:

Information for Patients: The patient should be warned about the possible additive effects when glutethimide is taken concomitantly with other central nervous system depressants such as alcohol.

The patient on Doriden must be warned against driving a car or operating dangerous machinery while on the drug, since glutethimide may impair the ability to perform hazardous activities requiring mental alertness or physical coordination.

Drug Interactions: Glutethimide induces hepatic microsomal enzymes resulting in increased metabolism of coumarin anticoagulants and decreased anticoagulant response.

Carcinogenesis: No carcinogenicity studies in animals have been performed.

Pregnancy/Teratogenic Effects: *Pregnancy Category C.* Animal reproduction studies have not been conducted with glutethimide. It is also not known *whether glutethimide can cause fetal harm when administered to a pregnant woman or can affect reproduction capacity. Glutethimide should be given to a pregnant woman only if clearly needed.*

Nursing Mothers: Because of the potential for serious adverse reactions in nursing infants from glutethimide, a decision should be made whether to discontinue nursing or to discontinue the drug, taking into account the importance of the drug to the mother.

Pediatric Use: Glutethimide is not recommended for use in children, because its safety and effectiveness in the pediatric age group have not been established by clinical trials.

Adverse Reactions: In clinical studies in more than 796 patients 8.6% exhibited skin rash, 2.7% reported nausea, 1.1% hangover, and 1% reported drowsiness. The following reactions occurred in less than 1% of the patient population: vertigo, headache, depression, dizziness, ataxia, confusion, edema, indigestion, lightheadedness, nocturnal diaphoresis, vomiting, dry mouth, euphoria, impaired memory, slurred speech, and tinnitus. Paradoxical excitation, blurred vision, acute hypersensitivity, porphyria, and blood dyscrasia such as thrombocytopenic purpura, aplastic anemia, and leukopenia are rare.

In cases in which a generalized skin rash occurs, the medication should be withdrawn. This rash usually clears spontaneously within a few days after drug withdrawal.

Drug Abuse and Dependence:

Controlled Substance: This drug is controlled in Schedule III.

Dependence: Both physical and psychological dependence have occurred; therefore patients should be carefully evaluated before prescribing Doriden (glutethimide). Ordinarily, an amount adequate for one week is sufficient. The patient should be reevaluated before re-prescribing, after an interval of one or more weeks. Withdrawal symptoms include nausea, abdominal discomfort, tremors, convulsions, and delirium. Newborn infants of mothers dependent on glutethimide may also exhibit withdrawal symptoms. In the presence of dependence dosage should be reduced gradually.

Overdosage:

Acute Overdosage: The single acute lethal dose of glutethimide in humans ranges from 10 g to 20 g. Although the majority of fatalities have resulted from single doses in this range, patients have died from single doses as low as 5 g and have recovered from single doses as high as 35 g. A single oral dose of 5 g usually produces severe intoxication. A plasma level of 3 mg/100 ml is indicative of severe poisoning, but the level may be higher if the patient is tolerant to the drug. However, the level may also be lower because of sequestration of the drug in body fat depots and in the gastrointestinal tract. A lower level does not preclude the possibility of severe poisoning; therefore, the extent of intoxication may not be accurately reflected by single glutethimide plasma level determinations. Serial determinations are mandatory for proper patient evaluation.

Ingestion of acutely excessive dosage of glutethimide can give rise to a life-threatening situation. The effects of glutethimide are exaggerated by concomitant ingestion of other hypnotics or sedatives such as alcohol, barbiturates, etc., and suicidal effects commonly involve multiple drugs of the sedative-hypnotic-tranquilizer types.

Signs and Symptoms: The principal signs and symptoms caused by glutethimide intoxication vary in severity in ratio to the ingested dosage, in general, and are indistinguishable from those caused by barbiturate intoxication. The degree of CNS depression often fluctuates, possibly due to irregular absorption of the drug and/or accumulation of an active toxic metabolite, 4-hydroxy-2-ethyl-2-phenyl-glutarimide (4-HG). They are: CNS depression, including coma *(profound and prolonged in severe intoxication);* hypothermia, which may be followed by fever even without apparent infection; depressed or lost deep tendon reflexes; depression or absence of corneal and pupillary reflexes; dilation of pupils; depressed or absent response to painful stimuli; inadequate ventilation (even with relatively normal respiratory rate), sometimes with cyanosis; sudden apnea, especially with manipulation such as gastric lavage or endotracheal intubation; diminished or absent peristalsis. Severe hypotension unresponsive to volume expansion, tonic muscular spasms, twitching and convulsions may occur.

Treatment: As with all forms of acute intoxication, the sooner adequate treatment is instituted, the better the prognosis. Early and vigorous cardiopulmonary supportive measures should be employed and should include:

1) Maintenance of a patent airway with assisted ventilation if necessary.
2) Monitoring of vital signs and level of consciousness.
3) Continuous electrocardiogram to detect arrhythmias.
4) Maintenance of blood pressure with plasma volume expanders and, if absolutely essential, pressor drugs.

Blood for glutethimide levels and other chemical determinations should be obtained as well as arterial blood for blood gas determinations. Vomiting should be induced if the patient is fully conscious. Gastric lavage should be done in all cases regardless of elapsed time since drug ingestion, with due caution to prevent aspiration of gastric contents or respiratory arrest during manipulation, including prior insertion of a cuffed endotracheal tube or employment of tracheostomy. Lavage with a 1:1 mixture of castor oil and water is capable of removing larger amounts of glutethimide from the stomach than with aqueous lavage. Fifty ml. of castor oil should be left in the stomach as a cathartic.

Intestinal lavage is used to remove unabsorbed Doriden (glutethimide) from the intestines (100–250 ml of 20–40% sorbitol or mannitol). If emesis or gastric lavage cannot be effected in the fully conscious patient, delay absorption of Doriden by giving one pint of water, milk or fruit juice; flour or cornstarch suspension, or activated charcoal in water. Follow up as soon as possible with production of emesis or gastric lavage.

Adequate respiratory gas exchange must be maintained and may require tracheostomy and mechanical assistance. If coma is prolonged, urine output must be monitored and maintained while preventing overhydration which might contribute to pulmonary or cerebral edema.

In *Severe Intoxication,* in addition to intensive supportive measures and symptomatic care, consideration should be given to dialysis or hemoperfusion in the following circumstances: Grade III or Grade IV coma, but the level of coma per se is not a mandatory indication for the procedure. Hemodialysis may also be required when renal shutdown or impaired renal function are manifest and in life-threatening overdose situations complicated by (a) pulmonary edema, (b) heart failure, (c) circulatory collapse, (d) significant liver disease, (e) major metabolic disturbance, (f) uremia. While aqueous hemodialysis is less effective for glutethimide than for readily water-soluble compounds that are not bound by proteins or sequestered in body fat depots, glutethimide blood levels may decline more rapidly with hemodialysis and the duration of coma may be shortened; efficacy of the procedure, however, is largely controversial. As long as significant amounts of glutethimide remain in fat depots or as an unabsorbed bolus in the intestinal tract, the fall in serum level accelerated by hemodialysis may be followed by increased absorption into the bloodstream on termination of dialysis and may require further dialysis.

Recent clinical data indicate that use of pure food-grade soybean oil as the dialysate enhances removal of glutethimide and some other lipidsoluble substances by means of hemodialysis. Peritoneal dialysis, while able to remove some glutethimide, apparently is of minimal value.

Hemoperfusion appears to be a promising technique for eliminating glutethimide from the body. Charcoal hemoperfusion utilizing acrylic hydrogel microencapsulation of activated charcoal has been reported to be simpler and more effective than hemodialysis. Similarly, a microcapsule artificial kidney has been developed utilizing activated charcoal granules encapsulated with cellulose nitrate and albumin. *Resin* hemoperfusion utilizing a column containing Amberberlite XAD-2 has demonstrated exceptionally high clearance capabilities in glutethimide intoxication and has been reported to be clinically superior to hemodialysis in patients with profound life-threatening coma and potentially lethal blood concentrations of intoxicant drugs.

Drug extraction techniques should be continued for at least two hours after the patient regains consciousness. Glutethimide is highly lipid soluble and therefore, rapidly accumulated in lipoid tissue. As the drug is removed from the bloodstream by any technique, it is gradually released from fat storage depots back into the bloodstream. Even after substantial quantities of the drug have been extracted, this blood-level rebound can cause coma to persist or recur.

As in the case of any prolonged coma, appropriate antibiotic therapy is indicated if pulmonary or other infection intervenes.

Chronic Overdosage: Signs and symptoms of chronic glutethimide intoxication (and for all drugs producing barbiturate-alcohol type of dependence in chronic overdosage) include impairment of memory and ability to concentrate, impaired gait, ataxia, tremors, hyporeflexia, and slurring of speech. Abrupt discontinuance of glutethimide after prolonged overdosage will in most cases cause withdrawal reactions ranging from nervousness and anxiety to grand mal seizures, and may include abdominal cramping, chills, numbness of extremities and dysphagia.

Treatment: Chronic glutethimide intoxication may be treated by gradual, stepwise reduction of dosage over a period of days or weeks. Watch patient carefully. If withdrawal reactions occur, they can be controlled by readministration of glutethimide, or substitution of pentobarbital, and subsequent gradual withdrawal.

Dosage and Administration: For use as a hypnotic, dosage should be individualized. The usual adult dosage is 0.25 to 0.5 g at bedtime. For elderly or debilitated patients, the initial daily dosage should not exceed 0.5 g at bedtime, in order to avoid oversedation.

How Supplied: DORIDEN (glutethimide). Tablets, 0.5 g (white, scored); bottles of 100 (NDC 0105-0354-00), 500 (NDC 0105-0354-05), 1000 (NDC 0105-0354-99) and Strip Dispensers of 100 (NDC 0105-0354-61). Tablets, 0.25 g (white, scored); bottles of 100 (NDC 0105-0353-00).

[*Shown in Product Identification Section*]

HISTASPAN-D® ℞

in sustained-release micro-dialysis cells

Composition: Each Histaspan-D capsule provides 8 mg chlorpheniramine maleate, 20 mg phenylephrine hydrochloride, and 2.5 mg methscopolamine nitrate in sustained-release micro-dialysis cells, uniquely processed for sustained release of medication to provide prolonged therapeutic effect.

Action: Histaspan-D combines the highly effective and widely used antihistamine, chlorpheniramine maleate, with a decongestant, phenylephrine hydrochloride, and a drying agent, methscopolamine nitrate, for relief of rhinorrhea, sneezing, lacrimation, nasal congestion, and other respiratory symptoms accompanying the common cold, sinusitis, hay fever and similar allergic conditions. Prolonged therapeutic effect is obtained by sustained release of medication through the micro-dialysis process.

Indications: One capsule q. 12 h. usually provides relief of rhinorrhea, sneezing, lacrimation, itching of eyes and nose, and nasal congestion accompanying upper respiratory infections such as the common cold and sinusitis; and hay fever and similar allergic conditions.

Contraindications: Hypersensitivity to any component of the drug, glaucoma, paralytic ileus, pyloric obstruction and prostatic hypertrophy.

Precautions: Use with caution in diabetes mellitus, hyperthyroidism, hypertension, cardiovascular disease, debilitated patients with chronic lung disease, in the aged and in children under age 12. Since blurred vision, drowsiness and dizziness may occur, patients should be cautioned about driving or operating machinery.

Adverse Reactions: May include drowsiness, dizziness, blurred vision, and excessive dryness of the nose, throat and mouth. Other possible adverse reactions to individual components, infrequently seen, include photophobia, tachycardia, gastrointestinal symptoms, increased irritability or excitement, flushing, incoordination, headache, nervousness, weakness and urinary disturbances.

Administration and Dosage: Adults and children over age 12, one capsule in the morning and one at night (q. 12 h.).

How Supplied: Bottles of 100 and 1000.

[*Shown in Product Identification Section*]

HISTASPAN®-PLUS ℞

in sustained-release micro-dialysis cells

Composition: Each Histaspan-Plus capsule provides 8 mg chlorpheniramine maleate and 20 mg phenylephrine hydrochloride in sustained-release micro-dialysis cells, uniquely processed for sustained release of medication to provide prolonged therapeutic effect.

Actions and Uses: Antihistaminic and decongestant for relief of nasal congestion and other respiratory symptoms accompanying the common cold, sinusitis, hay fever and similar allergic conditions.

Contraindication: Hypersensitivity to any component of the drug.

Precautions: Use with caution in diabetes mellitus, hyperthyroidism, hypertension and cardiovascular disease. Since blurred vision, drowsiness or dizziness may occur, patients should be cautioned about driving or operating machinery.

Adverse Reactions: May include drowsiness, dizziness, blurred vision, dry mouth, disturbed coordination, G.I. disturbance, tachycardia, headache, nervousness, weakness and urinary disturbances.

Dosage: Adults and children over age 12, one capsule every 12 hours.

How Supplied: Bottles of 100.

[*Shown in Product Identification Section*]

HYGROTON® ℞

(chlorthalidone USP)

Oral antihypertensive-diuretic

Hygroton is a product of USV Laboratories Inc., Manati, P.R. 00701.

Composition: Each tablet provides 25 mg, 50 mg or 100 mg chlorthalidone.

Description: Hygroton is a monosulfamyl diuretic which differs chemically from thiazide diuretics in that a double-ring system is incorporated in its structure.

Actions: Hygroton is an oral diuretic with prolonged action (48-72 hours) and low toxicity. The diuretic effect of the drug occurs within two hours of an oral dose and continues for up to 72 hours. It produces copious diuresis with greatly increased excretion of sodium and chloride. At maximal therapeutic dosage, chlorthalidone is approximately equal in its diuretic effect to comparable maximal therapeutic doses of benzothiadiazine diuretics. The site of action appears to be the cortical diluting segment of the ascending limb of Henle's loop of the nephron.

Indications: Diuretics such as Hygroton are indicated in the management of hypertension either as the sole therapeutic agent or to enhance the effect of other antihypertensive drugs in the more severe forms of hypertension.

Hygroton is indicated as adjunctive therapy in edema associated with congestive heart failure, hepatic cirrhosis, and corticosteroid and estrogen therapy.

Hygroton has also been found useful in edema due to various forms of renal dysfunction such as nephrotic syndrome, acute glomerulonephritis, and chronic renal failure.

Usage in Pregnancy: The routine use of diuretics in an otherwise healthy woman is inappropriate and exposes mother and fetus to unnecessary hazard. Diuretics do not prevent development of toxemia of pregnancy, and there is no satisfactory evidence that they are useful in the treatment of developed toxemia. Edema during pregnancy may arise from pathological causes or from the physiologic and mechanical consequences of pregnancy. Chlorthalidone is indicated in pregnancy when edema is due to pathologic causes, just as it is in the absence of pregnancy (however, see Warnings, below). Dependent edema in pregnancy, resulting from restriction of venous return by the expanded uterus, is properly treated through elevation of the lower extremities and use of support hose; use of diuretics to lower intravascular volume in this case is illogical and unnecessary. There is hypervolemia during normal pregnancy which is harmful to neither the fetus nor the mother (in the absence of cardiovascular disease), but which is associated with edema, including generalized edema, in the majority of pregnant women. If this edema produces discomfort, increased recumbency will often provide relief. In rare instances, this edema may cause extreme discomfort which is not relieved by rest. In these cases, a short course of diuretics may provide relief and may be appropriate.

Contraindications: Anuria.

Hypersensitivity to chlorthalidone or other sulfonamide-derived drugs.

Warnings: Should be used with caution in severe renal disease. In patients with renal disease, chlorthalidone or related drugs may precipitate azotemia. Cumulative effects of the

Continued on next page

USV—Cont.

drug may develop in patients with impaired renal function.
Chlorthalidone should be used with caution in patients with impaired hepatic function or progressive liver disease, since minor alterations of fluid and electrolyte balance may precipitate hepatic coma.
Chlorthalidone may add to or potentiate the action of other antihypertensive drugs. Potentiation occurs with ganglionic or peripheral adrenergic blocking drugs.
Sensitivity reactions may occur in patients with a history of allergy or bronchial asthma.
The possibility of exacerbation or activation of systemic lupus erythematosus has been reported with thiazide diuretics, which are structurally related to chlorthalidone. However, systemic lupus erythematosus has not been reported following chlorthalidone administration.
USAGE IN PREGNANCY: Reproduction studies in various animal species at multiples of the human dose showed no significant level of teratogenicity; no fetal or congenital abnormalities were observed. Animal data should not be extrapolated for clinical application.
Thiazides cross the placental barrier and appear in cord blood. The use of chlorthalidone and related drugs in pregnant women requires that the anticipated benefits of the drug be weighed against possible hazards to the fetus. These hazards include fetal or neonatal jaundice, thrombocytopenia, and possibly other adverse reactions which have occurred in the adult.
NURSING MOTHERS: Thiazides cross the placental barrier and appear in breast milk. If use of the drug is deemed essential, the patient should stop nursing.
Precautions: Periodic determination of serum electrolytes to detect possible electrolyte imbalance should be performed at appropriate intervals.
All patients receiving chlorthalidone should be observed for clinical signs of fluid or electrolyte imbalance; namely, hyponatremia, hypochloremic alkalosis, and hypokalemia. Serum and urine electrolyte determinations are particularly important when the patient is vomiting excessively or receiving parenteral fluids. Medication such as digitalis may also influence serum electrolytes. Warning signs, irrespective of cause, are: Dryness of mouth, thirst, weakness, lethargy, drowsiness, restlessness, muscle pains or cramps, muscular fatigue, hypotension, oliguria, tachycardia, and gastrointestinal disturbances such as nausea and vomiting.
Hypokalemia may develop with chlorthalidone as with any other potent diuretic, especially with brisk diuresis, when severe cirrhosis is present, or during concomitant use of corticosteroids or ACTH.
Interference with adequate oral electrolyte intake will also contribute to hypokalemia. Digitalis therapy may exaggerate metabolic effects of hypokalemia especially with reference to myocardial activity.
Any chloride deficit is generally mild and usually does not require specific treatment except under extraordinary circumstances (as in liver disease or renal disease). Dilutional hyponatremia may occur in edematous patients in hot weather; appropriate therapy is water restriction, rather than administration of salt except in rare instances when the hyponatremia is life threatening. In actual salt depletion, appropriate replacement is the therapy of choice.
Hyperuricemia may occur or frank gout may be precipitated in certain patients receiving chlorthalidone.
Insulin requirements in diabetic patients may be increased, decreased, or unchanged. Latent diabetes mellitus may become manifest during chlorthalidone administration.
Chlorthalidone and related drugs may increase the responsiveness to tubocurarine.
The antihypertensive effects of the drug may be enhanced in the postsympathectomy patient.
Chlorthalidone and related drugs may decrease arterial responsiveness to norepinephrine. This diminution is not sufficient to preclude effectiveness of the pressor agent for therapeutic use.
If progressive renal impairment becomes evident, as indicated by a rising nonprotein nitrogen or blood urea nitrogen, a careful reappraisal of therapy is necessary with consideration given to withholding or discontinuing diuretic therapy.
Chlorthalidone and related drugs may decrease serum PBI levels without signs of thyroid disturbance.
Adverse Reactions: *Gastrointestinal System Reactions:* anorexia, gastric irritation, nausea, vomiting, cramping, diarrhea, constipation, jaundice (intrahepatic cholestatic jaundice), pancreatitis; *Central Nervous System Reactions:* dizziness, vertigo, paresthesias, headache, xanthopsia; *Hematologic Reactions:* leukopenia, agranulocytosis, thrombocytopenia, aplastic anemia; *Dermatologic—Hypersensitivity Reactions:* purpura, photosensitivity, rash, urticaria, necrotizing angiitis (vasculitis) (cutaneous vasculitis), Lyell's syndrome (toxic epidermal necrolysis); *Cardiovascular Reaction:* Orthostatic hypotension may occur and may be aggravated by alcohol, barbiturates or narcotics. *Other Adverse Reactions:* hyperglycemia, glycosuria, hyperuricemia, muscle spasm, weakness, restlessness, impotence.
Whenever adverse reactions are moderate or severe, chlorthalidone dosage should be reduced or therapy withdrawn.
Dosage and Administration: Therapy should be initiated with the lowest possible dose. This dose should be titrated according to individual patient response to gain maximal therapeutic benefit while maintaining the minimal dosage possible. A single dose given in the morning with food is recommended; divided doses are unnecessary.
Hypertension. *Initiation:* Therapy, in most patients should be initiated with a single daily dose of 25 mg. If the response is insufficient after single suitable trial, the dosage may be increased to a single daily dose of 50 mg. If additional control is required, the dosage of HYGROTON may be increased to 100 mg once daily or a second antihypertensive drug (step-2 therapy) may be added. Dosage above 100 mg daily usually does not increase effectiveness. Increases in serum uric acid and decreases in serum potassium are dose-related over the 25–100 mg day range.
Maintenance: Maintenance doses may be lower than initial doses and should be adjusted according to individual patient response. Effectiveness is well sustained during continued use.
Edema. *Initiation:* Adults, initially 50 to 100 mg daily, or 100 mg on alternate days. Some patients may require 150 to 200 mg at these intervals, or up to 200 mg daily. Dosages above this level, however, do not usually produce a greater response.
Maintenance: Maintenance doses may often be lower than initial doses and should be adjusted according to the individual patient. Effectiveness is well sustained during continued use.
Overdosage: Symptoms of overdosage include nausea, weakness, dizziness and disturbances of electrolyte balance. There is no specific antidote, but gastric lavage is recommended, followed by supportive treatment. Where necessary, this may include intravenous dextrose-saline with potassium, administered with caution.
How Supplied: HYGROTON (chlorthalidone). White, single-scored tablets of 100 mg and aqua tablets of 50 mg in bottles of 100, 1000 and 5000; unit-dose blister packs, boxes of 100 (10 × 10 strips). Also, 25 mg peach-color tablets in bottles of 100 and 1000; unit-dose blister packs, boxes of 100 (10 × 10 strips). NSN 6505-00-074-9914A (100 mg, 100s), NSN 6505-00-065-4246A (100 mg, 1000s), V.A. Depots; NSN 6505-00-074-9914 (100 mg, 100s), Military Depots.
Animal Pharmacology: Biochemical studies in animals have suggested reasons for the prolonged effect of chlorthalidone. Absorption from the gastrointestinal tract is slow due to its low solubility. After passage to the liver, some of the drug enters the general circulation, while some is excreted in the bile, to be reabsorbed later. In the general circulation, it is distributed widely to the tissues, but is taken up in highest concentrations by the kidneys, where amounts have been found 72 hours after ingestion, long after it has disappeared from other tissues. The drug is excreted unchanged in the urine.

[*Shown in Product Identification Section*]

M.V.I.® ℞
Multi-Vitamin Infusion

Composition: Each 10 ml ampul† or 5 ml Concentrate vial†† provides:

ascorbic acid (C)	500 mg
vitamin A*	10,000 IU
vitamin D* (ergocalciferol)	1,000 IU
thiamine HCl (B_1)	50 mg
riboflavin (B_2)**	10 mg
pyridoxine HCl (B_6)	15 mg
niacinamide	100 mg
dexpanthenol	25 mg
vitamin E* (dl-alpha tocopheryl acetate)	5 IU

†with polysorbate 20 1%, sodium hydroxide for pH adjustment, butylated hydroxytoluene 0.003%, butylated hydroxyanisole 0.0008%; and gentisic acid ethanolamide 2.4% as preservative.
††with propylene glycol 30% and gentisic acid ethanolamide 2% as stabilizers and preservatives, sodium hydroxide for pH adjustment, polysorbate 20 1.7%, butylated hydroxytoluene 0.006%, butylated hydroxyanisole 0.0015%.
*Oil-soluble vitamins A, D and E water solubilized with polysorbate 20.
**In Concentrate as riboflavin-5-phosphate.
ORIGINAL "AQUEOUS" MULTIVITAMIN FORMULA FOR INTRAVENOUS INFUSION:
M.V.I. (Multi-Vitamin Infusion) makes available a combination of important oil-soluble and water-soluble vitamins in an aqueous solution, formulated specially for incorporation in intravenous infusions. Through special processing techniques developed in the research laboratories of USV Pharmaceutical Corporation, the liposoluble vitamins A, D and E have been solubilized in an aqueous medium, permitting intravenous administration of these vitamins.
Indications: *In Emergency Feedings*
Surgery, extensive burns, fractures and other trauma, severe infectious diseases, comatose states, etc. may provoke a "stress" situation with profound alterations in the body's metabolic demands and consequent tissue depletion of nutrients. As a result, wound healing may be impaired, enzyme activity disturbed, hematopoietic tissues affected; hypoproteinemia and edema may appear; convalescence is thus prolonged.
In such patients M.V.I. (administered in intravenous fluids under proper dilution) contributes optimum vitamin intake toward maintaining the body's normal resistance and repair processes.
Directions for Use: M.V.I. is ready for immediate use when added to intravenous infusion fluids.

For intravenous feeding, one daily dose of 10 ml of M.V.I. or 5 ml of M.V.I. Concentrate added directly to not less than 500 ml, preferably 1,000 ml, of intravenous dextrose, saline or similar infusion solutions ... plasma, protein hydrolysates, etc.
Precaution: Allergic reaction has been known to occur following intravenous administration of solutions containing thiamine.
Caution: Not to be given as a direct undiluted intravenous injection as it may give rise to dizziness, faintness, etc.
Therapeutic Note: Intravenous use should be discontinued as early as practical in favor of an oral vitamin preparation, if needed.
How Supplied: M.V.I.—10 ml ampuls, boxes of 25 and 100. NSN 6505-00-455-9955/NSN 6505-00-424-9808A. M.V.I. CONCENTRATE —5 ml vials, boxes of 25. NSN 6505-00-212-6156A. Available in 100s only.
[*Shown in Product Identification Section*]

For dilution in intravenous infusions only

M.V.I.®-12 ℞

Multi-Vitamin Infusion

Description: This is a sterile product consisting of two vials, labeled Vial 1 and Vial 2.
Each 5 ml Vial 1† provides:

ascorbic acid (C)	100 mg
vitamin A†† (retinol)	3,300 IU
vitamin D†† (ergocalciferol)	200 IU
thiamine (B_1)*	3.0 mg
riboflavin (B_2)**	3.6 mg
pyridoxine HCl (B_6)	4.0 mg
niacinamide	40.0 mg
pantothenic acid***	15.0 mg
vitamin E†† (dl-alpha tocopheryl acetate)	10 IU

† with propylene glycol 30% and gentisic acid ethanolamide 2% as stabilizers and preservatives, sodium hydroxide for pH adjustment, polysorbate 80 1.6%, polysorbate 20 0.028%, butylated hydroxytoluene 0.002%, butylated hydroxyanisole 0.0005%.
†† Oil-soluble vitamins A, D and E water solubilized with polysorbate 80.
*as the hydrochloride.
**as riboflavin-5-phosphate.
***as dexpanthenol.
Each 5 ml Vial 2 provides:

biotin	60 mcg
folic acid	400 mcg
vitamin B_{12}	5 mcg

with propylene glycol 30%; and citric acid, sodium citrate, and sodium hydroxide for pH adjustment.

"Aqueous" multivitamin formula for intravenous infusion:
M.V.I.-12 (Multi-Vitamin Infusion) makes available a combination of important oil-soluble and water-soluble vitamins in an aqueous solution, formulated specially for incorporation into intravenous infusions. Through special processing techniques developed in the research laboratories of USV Pharmaceutical Corporation, the liposoluble vitamins A, D and E have been solubilized in an aqueous medium, permitting intravenous administration of these vitamins.
Indications and Usage: This formulation is indicated as daily multivitamin maintenance dosage for adults and children aged 11 and above receiving parenteral nutrition.
It is also indicated in other situations where administration by the intravenous route is required. Such situations include surgery, extensive burns, fractures and other trauma, severe infectious diseases, and comatose states, which may provoke a "stress" situation with profound alterations in the body's metabolic demands and consequent tissue depletion of nutrients.
The physician should not await the development of clinical signs of vitamin deficiency before initiating vitamin therapy. The use of a multivitamin product obviates the need to speculate on the status of individual vitamin nutriture.
M.V.I.-12 (administered in intravenous fluids under proper dilution) contributes intake of these necessary vitamins toward maintaining the body's normal resistance and repair processes.
Patients with multiple vitamin deficiencies or with markedly increased requirements may be given multiples of the daily dosage for two or more days as indicated by the clinical status.
M.V.I.-12 does not contain vitamin K, which may have to be administered separately.
Contraindications: Known hypersensitivity to any of the vitamins in this product or a pre-existing hypervitaminosis.
Precautions:
Drug Interactions:
M.V.I.-12 is not physically compatible with KEFLIN (sodium cephalothin), ANCEF, KEFZOL (sodium cefazolin), or moderately alkaline solutions, e.g., sodium bicarbonate solution. Some of the vitamins in M.V.I.-12 may react with vitamin K bisulfite. Direct addition of M.V.I.-12 to intravenous fat emulsions is not recommended.
Adverse Reactions: Allergic reaction has been known to occur following intravenous administration of thiamine. This risk, however, is negligible if the thiamine is administered with other vitamins of the B group.
Dosage and Administration: M.V.I.-12 (Multi-Vitamin Infusion) is ready for immediate use in adults and children aged 11 and above when added to intravenous infusion fluids.
M.V.I.-12 should not be given as a direct, undiluted intravenous injection as it may give rise to dizziness, faintness, and possible tissue irritation.
For intravenous feeding, one daily dose of M.V.I.-12 (5 ml of Vial 1 plus 5 ml of Vial 2) added directly to not less than 500 ml, preferably 1,000 ml, of intravenous dextrose, saline or similar infusion solutions.
Parenteral drug products should be inspected visually for particulate matter and discoloration prior to administration, whenever solution and container permit.
After M.V.I.-12 is diluted in an intravenous infusion, the resulting solution should be refrigerated unless it is to be administered immediately, and in any event should be administered within 48 hours. Some of the vitamins in this product, particularly vitamins A and D, and riboflavin, are light sensitive, and exposure to light should be minimized.
KEEP IN REFRIGERATOR
How Supplied: M.V.I.-12 (5 ml Vial 1 and 5 ml Vial 2) boxes of 25 and cartons of 100.
[*Shown in Product Identification Section*]

For dilution in intravenous infusions only

MANGATRACE™ ℞

Manganese Chloride Injection USP

0.1 mg/ml

Manganese Chloride in Sodium Chloride Solution

Description: Mangatrace, Manganese Chloride Injection USP (0.1 mg manganese/ml), is a sterile nonpyrogenic solution intended for use as an additive to intravenous solutions for total parenteral nutrition (TPN). Each ml of solution provides:

manganese chloride	0.23 mg
sodium	3.34 mg
chloride	5.29 mg

(not including ions for pH adjustment).
The pH is approximately 2.0, adjusted with hydrochloric acid, and may be adjusted with sodium hydroxide. The solution is adjusted to isotonicity with sodium chloride. The osmolarity is approximately 0.300 mOsm/ml. The solution contains no bacteriostat, antimicrobial agent, or added buffer.
Manganese chloride is chemically designated $MnCl_2$, a deliquescent, crystalline compound soluble in water. Sodium chloride USP is chemically designated NaCl, a white crystalline compound freely soluble in water.
Clinical Pharmacology: Manganese is an essential nutrient that serves as an activator for enzymes such as polysaccharide polymerase, liver arginase, cholinesterase, and pyruvate carboxylase.
Providing manganese during TPN helps prevent development of deficiency symptoms such as nausea and vomiting, weight loss, dermatitis, and changes in growth and color of hair.
Under conditions of minimal intake, 20 mcg manganese/day is retained. Manganese is bound to a specific transport protein, transmanganin, a beta-l-globulin. Manganese is widely distributed but concentrates in the mitochondria-rich tissues such as brain, kidney, pancreas, and liver. Assays for manganese in whole blood result in concentrations ranging from 6 to 12 mcg/manganese/liter.
Excretion of manganese occurs mainly through the bile, but in the event of obstruction, ancillary excretion routes include pancreatic juice, or return into the lumen of the duodenum, jejunum, or ileum. Urinary excretion of manganese is negligible.
Indications and Usage: Mangatrace is indicated for use as a supplement to intravenous solutions given for total parenteral nutrition (TPN). Administration helps to maintain manganese serum levels and to prevent depletion of endogenous stores and subsequent deficiency symptoms.
Contraindications: Direct intramuscular or intravenous injection of Mangatrace is contraindicated, as the acidic pH of the solution (2.0) may cause considerable tissue irritation.
Warnings: **Manganese is eliminated via the bile. In patients with severe liver dysfunction and/or biliary tract obstruction, decreasing or omitting manganese supplements entirely may be necessary.**
Precautions: Do not use unless the solution is clear and the seal is intact.
Mangatrace should be used only in conjunction with a pharmacy-directed admixture program using aseptic technique in a laminar flow environment. The solution contains no preservatives; discard unused portion within 24 hours after opening.
Pregnancy Category C. Animal reproduction studies have not been conducted with manganese chloride. It is also not known whether manganese chloride can cause fetal harm when administered to a pregnant woman or can affect reproductive capacity. Manganese chloride should be given to a pregnant woman only if clearly indicated.
Adverse Reactions: None known.
Drug Abuse and Dependence: None known.
Overdosage: Manganese toxicity in TPN patients has not been reported.
Dosage and Administration: Mangatrace, Manganese Chloride Injection, contains 0.1 mg manganese/ml and is administered intravenously only after dilution.
Adult: For the adult receiving TPN, the suggested additive dosage for manganese is 0.15 to 0.8 mg/day.
Pediatric: For pediatric patients, a dosage of 2 to 10 mcg manganese/kg/day is recommended.
Periodic monitoring of manganese plasma levels is suggested as a guideline for subsequent administration.
Parenteral products should be inspected visually for particulate matter and discoloration prior to administration, whenever solution and container permit. See Precautions sections.
How Supplied: Mangatrace 10-ml vials (NDC 0075-0832-22), boxes of 25.
[*Shown in Product Identification Section*]

Continued on next page

USV—Cont.

NITROSPAN® ℞
(nitroglycerin)
in sustained-release capsules

Composition: Each capsule provides 2.5 mg or 6.5 mg nitroglycerin in a sustained-release vehicle processed to release medication gradually and continuously for prolonged therapeutic effect.

Actions: The mechanism of action of nitroglycerin in the relief of angina pectoris is not as yet known. However, its main pharmacologic action is to relax smooth muscle, principally in the smaller blood vessels, thus dilating arterioles and capillaries, especially in the coronary circulation. In therapeutic doses, nitroglycerin is thought to increase the blood supply to the myocardium which may in turn relieve myocardial ischemia, the possible functional basis for the pain of angina pectoris.

In Nitrospan the micro-dialysis cells permit smooth, continuous release of nitroglycerin, requiring only the presence of fluid in the gastrointestinal tract.

Indications: Based on a review of this drug by the National Academy of Sciences—National Research Council and/or other information, FDA has classified the indication as follows:
"Possibly" effective: For the management, prophylaxis, or treatment of anginal attacks.
Final classification of the less-than-effective indication requires further investigation.

Contraindications: Acute or recent myocardial infarction, severe anemia, closed-angle glaucoma, postural hypotension, increased intracranial pressure and idiosyncrasy to the drug.

Warnings: Nitrospan Capsules must be swallowed. FOR ORAL, NOT SUBLINGUAL USE. This form of the drug is not intended for immediate relief of anginal attacks.

Precautions: Intraocular pressure may be increased; therefore, caution is required in administering to patients with glaucoma. Tolerance to this drug and cross-tolerance to other organic nitrites and nitrates may occur. If blurring of vision, dryness of mouth or lack of benefit occurs, the drug should be discontinued.

Adverse Reactions: Severe and persistent headaches, cutaneous flushing, dizziness and weakness. Occasionally, drug rash or exfoliative dermatitis, and nausea and vomiting may occur; these responses may disappear with a decrease in dosage. Adverse effects are enhanced by ingestion of alcohol, which appears to increase absorption from the gastrointestinal tract.

Dosage and Administration: Administer the smallest effective dose 2 or 3 times daily at 8- to 12-hour intervals, unless clinical response suggests a different regimen. Discontinue if not effective.

How Supplied: Capsules: 2.5 mg (light green and clear), bottles of 100; 6.5 mg (dark green and clear), bottles of 60.
NSN 6505-00-998-5871A (2.5 mg), V.A. Depots.
[*Shown in Product Identification Section*]

OXALID® ℞
oxyphenbutazone

100 mg tablets

Important Note: OXALID (oxyphenbutazone) cannot be considered a simple analgesic and should never be administered casually. Each patient should be carefully evaluated before treatment is started and should remain constantly under the close supervision of the physician. The following cautions should be observed:

1. Therapy should not be initiated until a careful detailed history and complete physical and laboratory examination, including a complete hemogram and urinalysis, etc., of the patient have been made. These examinations should be made at regular, frequent intervals throughout the duration of this drug therapy.
2. Patients should be carefully selected, avoiding those in whom it is contraindicated as well as those who will respond to ordinary therapeutic measures, or those who cannot be observed at frequent intervals.
3. Patients taking this drug should be warned not to exceed the recommended dosage, since this may lead to toxic effects, and should discontinue the drug and report to the physician immediately any sign of:
a. Fever, sore throat, lesions in the mouth (symptoms of blood dyscrasia).
b. Dyspepsia, epigastric pain, symptoms of anemia, unusual bleeding, unusual bruising, black or tarry stools or other evidence of intestinal ulceration.
c. Skin rashes.
d. Significant weight gain or edema.
4. A trial period of one week of therapy is considered adequate to determine the therapeutic effect of the drug. In the absence of a favorable response, therapy should be discontinued.
In the elderly (sixty years and over) the drug should be restricted to short-term treatment periods only—if possible, *one week* maximum.
5. BEFORE PRESCRIBING OXALID FOR AN INDIVIDUAL PATIENT, READ THOROUGHLY THE INFORMATION CONTAINED UNDER EACH HEADING WHICH FOLLOWS:

Description and Actions: OXALID should not be considered as a simple analgesic that can be prescribed for indiscriminate use.

OXALID is closely related chemically and pharmacologically, including toxic effects, to the well-known pyrazolines (pyrazole compounds) amidopyrine and antipyrine.

Chemically, OXALID is 4-butyl-l-(*p*-hydroxyphenyl) 2-phenyl-3, 5-pyrazolidinedione monohydrate, the parahydroxy analog of phenylbutazone.

It has anti-inflammatory and antipyretic action as well as analgesic and mild uricosuric properties resulting in symptomatic relief only. THE DISEASE PROCESS ITSELF IS UNALTERED BY THIS DRUG.

Clinical Pharmacology: In man, oxyphenbutazone is completely absorbed after oral administration of OXALID. After ingestion of three 100-mg tablets, peak plasma concentration of oxyphenbutazone has been measured at 34.9 (± 5.3) mg/l within six hours. After therapeutic doses, about 98 percent of the drug is bound to human serum albumin. Elimination is mainly by biotransformation in the liver, and the plasma halflife has been measured as 72 (± 15 hours). Urinary excretion consists mostly of metabolites.

Indications: The indications for OXALID are:
Acute Gouty Arthritis
Active Rheumatoid Arthritis
Active Ankylosing Spondylitis
Short-term treatment of acute attacks of degenerative joint disease of the hips and knees not responsive to other treatment.
Painful Shoulder (peritendinitis, capsulitis, bursitis, and acute arthritis of that joint)

Contraindications:
1. *Age:* OXALID is contraindicated in children 14 years of age or younger since controlled clinical trials in patients of this age group have not been conducted.
2. *Other Medical Conditions:* OXALID is contraindicated in patients with incipient cardiac failure, blood dyscrasias, pancreatitis, parotitis, stomatitis, polymyalgia rheumatica, temporal arteritis, senility, drug allergy, and in the presence of severe renal, cardiac and hepatic disease, and in patients with a history of peptic ulcer disease, or symptoms of gastrointestinal inflammation or active ulceration because serious adverse reactions or aggravation of existing medical problems can occur.
3. *Concomitant Medications:* OXALID (oxyphenbutazone) should not be used in combination with other drugs which accentuate or share a potential for similar toxicity.
It is also inadvisable to administer OXALID in combination with other potent drugs because of the possibility of increased toxic reactions from OXALID and other agents. (See also *Drug Interactions.*)
OXALID is contraindicated in patients with a history or suggestion of prior toxicity, sensitivity, or idiosyncrasy to phenylbutazone or oxyphenbutazone.

Warnings: Based on reports of clinical experience with oxyphenbutazone and related compounds, the following warnings should be considered by the physician prior to prescribing the drug:
1. *Gastrointestinal:* Upper G.I. diagnostic tests should be performed in patients with persistent or severe dyspepsia. Peptic ulceration, reactivation of latent peptic ulcer, perforation and gastrointestinal bleeding, sometimes severe, have been reported.
As with other nonsteroidal anti-inflammatory drugs, borderline elevations of one or more liver tests may occur in up to 15% of patients. These abnormalities may progress, may remain essentially unchanged, or may be transient with continued therapy. The SGPT (ALT) test is probably the most sensitive indicator of liver dysfunction. Meaningful (three times the upper limit of normal) elevations of SGPT or SGOT (AST) occurred in controlled clinical trials in less than 1% of patients. A patient with symptoms and/or signs suggesting liver dysfunction, or in whom an abnormal liver test has occurred, should be evaluated for evidence of the development of more severe hepatic reaction while on therapy with OXALID. Severe hepatic reactions, including jaundice and cases of fatal hepatitis, have been reported with OXALID as with other nonsteroidal anti-inflammatory drugs. Although such reactions are rare, if abnormal liver tests persist or worsen, if clinical signs and symptoms consistent with liver disease develop, or if systemic manifestations occur (e.g. eosinophilia, rash, etc.), OXALID should be discontinued.
2. *Hematologic: Frequent and regular hematologic evaluations should be performed on patients receiving the drug for periods over one week.* Any significant change in the total white count, relative decrease in granulocytes, appearance of immature forms, or fall in hematocrit should be a signal for immediate cessation of therapy and a complete hematologic investigation. Serious, sometimes fatal blood dyscrasias, including aplastic anemia have been reported to occur. Hematologic toxicity may occur suddenly or many days or weeks after cessation of treatment as manifest by the appearance of anemia, leukopenia, thrombocytopenia or clinically significant hemorrhagic diathesis. There have been published reports associating oxyphenbutazone with leukemia. However, the circumstances involved in these reports are such that a cause-and-effect relationship to the drug has not been clearly established.
3. *Pregnancy:* Reproductive studies in animals, although inconclusive, exhibited evidence of possible embryotoxicity. It is, therefore, recommended that this drug should be used with caution during pregnancy. The benefits should be weighed against the potential risk to the fetus.
4. *Nursing Mothers:* Caution is also advised in prescribing OXALID in nursing mothers since the drug may appear in cord blood and breast milk.
5. Patients reporting visual disturbances while receiving the drug should discontinue treatment and have an ophthalmologic examination because ophthalmologic adverse reac-

tions have been reported (see **Adverse Reactions:** *Special Senses*).
6. In the aging (forty years and over), there appears to be an increase in the possibility of adverse reactions. OXALID should be used with commensurately greater care in the elderly and should be avoided altogether in the senile patient.
7. Like other drugs with prostaglandin synthetase inhibition activity, OXALID (oxyphenbutazone) may precipitate acute episodes of asthmatic attacks in patients with asthma.
8. OXALID increases sodium retention. Evidence of fluid retention in patients in whom there is danger of cardiac decompensation is an indication to discontinue the drug.

Precautions: Because of potential serious adverse reactions to OXALID, the following precautions should be observed in the use of the drug:
1. A careful diagnostic physical examination and history should be performed on all patients at regular intervals and while the patient is receiving the drug.
2. OXALID is not recommended for chronic use in the elderly.
3. Hematologic evaluation should be performed at frequent and regular intervals and additional laboratory examinations performed as indicated.
4. Patients should be instructed to report immediately the occurrence of high fever, severe sore throat, stomatitis, salivary gland enlargement, tarry stools, unusual bleeding or bruising, sudden weight gain, or edema.
5. The drug reduces iodine uptake by the thyroid and may interfere with laboratory tests of thyroid function (see **Adverse Reactions:** *Endocrine-Metabolic*).
6. The patient should be cautioned regarding participation in activities requiring alertness and coordination, and that the concomitant ingestion of alcohol with OXALID may further impair psychomotor skills.

Drug Interactions: OXALID is highly bound to serum proteins. If its affinity for protein binding is higher than other concurrently administered drugs, the actions and toxicity of the other drug may be increased.
OXALID accentuates the prothrombin depression produced by coumarin-type anticoagulants. When administered alone, it does not affect prothrombin activity.
The pharmacologic action of insulin, anti-diabetic, and sulfonamide drugs may be potentiated by the simultaneous administration of OXALID.
Concomitant administration of oxyphenbutazone and phenytoin may result in increased serum levels of phenytoin which could lead to increased phenytoin toxicity.

Adverse Reactions: Based upon reports of clinical experience with oxyphenbutazone and related compounds, the following adverse reactions have been reported.
The adverse reactions listed in the following table have been arranged into three groups: (1) incidence greater than 1%, (2) incidence less than 1% and (3) causal relationship unknown. The incidence for group (1) was obtained from fifty-seven (57) clinical trials reported in the literature (3713 patients). The incidence for group (2) was based on reports in clinical trials, in the literature, and on voluntary reports. The reactions in group (3) have been reported but occurred under circumstances where a causal relationship could not be established. In some patients the reported reactions may have been unrelated to the administration of the drug. However, in these reported events, the possibility cannot be excluded. Therefore these observations are being listed to serve as alerting information to physicians. Before prescribing this drug for an individual patient, the physician should be familiar with the following:

GASTROINTESTINAL (see **Warnings**)
1. Incidence greater than 1%
gastrointestinal upset
2. Incidence less than 1%
nausea
dyspepsia/including indigestion and heartburn
abdominal and epigastric distress
vomiting
abdominal distention with flatulence
constipation
diarrhea
esophagitis
gastritis
salivary gland enlargement
stomatitis, sometimes with ulceration
ulceration and perforation of the intestinal tract including acute and reactivated peptic ulcer with perforation, hemorrhage and hematemesis
anemia due to gastrointestinal bleeding which may be occult
hepatitis, both fatal and nonfatal, sometimes associated with evidence of cholestasis

HEMATOLOGICAL (see **Warnings**)
1. Incidence greater than 1%
None
2. Incidence less than 1%
anemia
leukopenia
thrombocytopenia with associated purpura, petechiae, and hemorrhage
pancytopenia
aplastic anemia
bone marrow depression
agranulocytosis and agranulocytic anginal syndrome
hemolytic anemia

HYPERSENSITIVITY
1. Incidence greater than 1%
None
2. Incidence less than 1%
urticaria
anaphylactic shock
arthralgia, drug fever
hypersensitivity angiitis (polyarteritis) and vasculitis
Lyell's syndrome
serum sickness
Stevens-Johnson syndrome
activation of systemic lupus erythematosus
aggravation of temporal arteritis in patients with polymyalgia rheumatica

DERMATOLOGIC
1. Incidence greater than 1%
None
2. Incidence less than 1%
pruritus
erythema nodosum
erythema multiforme
nonthrombocytopenic purpura

CARDIOVASCULAR, FLUID AND ELECTROLYTE
1. Incidence greater than 1%
None
2. Incidence less than 1%
sodium and chloride retention
fluid retention and plasma dilution
cardiac decompensation (congestive heart failure) with edema and dyspnea
metabolic acidosis
respiratory alkalosis
hypertension
pericarditis
interstitial myocarditis with muscle necrosis and perivascular granulomata

RENAL
1. Incidence greater than 1%
None
2. Incidence less than 1%
hematuria
proteinuria
ureteral obstruction with uric acid crystals
anuria
glomerulonephritis
acute tubular necrosis
cortical necrosis
renal stones
nephrotic syndrome
impaired renal function and renal failure associated with azotemia

CENTRAL NERVOUS SYSTEM
1. Incidence greater than 1%
None
2. Incidence less than 1%
headache
drowsiness
agitation
confusional states and lethargy
tremors
numbness
weakness

ENDOCRINE-METABOLIC (see **Precautions**)
1. Incidence greater than 1%
None
2. Incidence less than 1%
None

SPECIAL SENSES (see **Warnings**)
1. Incidence greater than 1%
Ocular: none
Otic: none
2. Incidence less than 1%
Ocular: none
Otic: hearing loss, tinnitus

(3) Causal relationship unknown—Incidence less than 1%: *Hematological* (see **Warnings**)—Leukemia (There have been reports associating oxyphenbutazone with leukemia. However, the circumstances involved in these reports are such that a cause-and-effect relationship to the drug has not been clearly established.) *Endocrine-Metabolic* (see **Precautions**)—Thyroid hyperplasia; goiters associated with hyperthyroidism and hypothyroidism; pancreatitis; hyperglycemia. *Special Senses* (see **Warnings**)—Blurred vision; optic neuritis; toxic amblyopia; scotomata; retinal detachment; retinal hemorrhage; oculomotor palsy.

Overdosage:
Signs and Symptoms: Include any of the following: nausea, vomiting, epigastric pain, excessive perspiration, euphoria, psychosis, headaches, giddiness, vertigo, hyperventilation, insomnia, tinnitus, difficulty in hearing, edema (sodium retention), hypertension, cyanosis, respiratory depression, agitation, hallucinations, stupor, convulsions, coma, hematuria, and oliguria. Hepatomegaly, jaundice, and ulceration of the buccal or gastrointestinal mucosa have been reported as late manifestations of massive overdosage.
Reported laboratory abnormalities following overdosage include: respiratory or metabolic acidosis, impaired hepatic or renal function, and abnormalities of formed blood elements.
Treatment: In the alert patient, empty the stomach promptly by induced emesis followed by lavage. In the obtunded patient, secure the airway with a cuffed endotracheal tube before beginning lavage (do not induce emesis). Maintain adequate respiratory exchange, do not use respiratory stimulants. Treat shock with appropriate supportive measures. Control seizures with intravenous diazepam or short-acting barbiturates. Dialysis may be helpful if renal function is impaired.

Dosage and Administration: OXALID (oxyphenbutazone) should be used at the smallest effective dosage to afford rapid relief of severe symptoms. It is contraindicated in children under 14 years of age and in senile patients.
If a favorable symptomatic response to treatment is not obtained after one week, the drug should be discontinued. When a favorable therapeutic response has been obtained, the dosage should be reduced and then discontinued as soon as possible.
In elderly patients (sixty years and over) every effort must be made to discontinue therapy on, or as soon as possible after the seventh day, because of the exceedingly high risk of severe fatal toxic reactions in this age group.
To minimize gastric upset, the drug should be taken with milk or with meals.

Continued on next page

USV—Cont.

In selecting the appropriate dosage in any specific case, consideration should be given to the patient's age, weight, general health, and any other factors that may influence his response to the drug.

Rheumatoid Arthritis, Ankylosing Spondylitis, Acute Attacks of Degenerative Joint Disease, and Painful Shoulder. Initial Dosage: The initial daily dose in adult patients is 300 to 600 mg as 3 to 4 divided doses. Maximum therapeutic response is usually obtained at a total daily dose of 400 mg. A trial period of one week of therapy is considered adequate to determine the therapeutic effect of the drug. In the absence of a favorable response, therapy should be discontinued.

Maintenance Dosage: When improvement is obtained, dosage should be promptly decreased to the minimum effective level necessary to maintain relief, not exceeding 400 mg daily because of the possibility of cumulative toxicity. A satisfactory clinical response may be obtained with daily doses as low as 100 to 200 mg daily.

Acute Gouty Arthritis: Satisfactory results are obtained after an initial dose of 400 mg followed by 100 mg every 4 hours. The articular inflammation usually subsides within 4 days and treatment should not be continued longer than one week.

How Supplied: 100 mg Tablets (white, round, sugar coated), bottles of 100 and 1000.

[*Shown in Product Identification Section*]

PANTHODERM® OTC
Lotion and Cream

Composition: Panthoderm Lotion and Panthoderm Cream contain dexpanthenol 2% in a water-miscible cream base.

Indications: Panthoderm relieves itching and may aid healing of skin lesions by stimulating epithelization and granulation in mild eczemas and dermatoses; itching skin, minor wounds, insect bites, poison ivy and poison oak, minor skin irritations. Also, in infants and children—diaper rash, chafing, mild skin irritations.

Administration: Apply directly to affected areas once or twice daily, or more often as needed.

How Supplied: *Lotion:* Bottles of 4 fl. oz. *Cream:* 1 oz. tube, 2 oz. and 1 lb. jars.

PERTOFRANE® ℞
(desipramine hydrochloride USP)

Pertofrane is a product of USV Laboratories Inc., Manati, P.R. 00701.

Composition: Each capsule provides 25 mg or 50 mg desipramine hydrochloride.

Description: PERTOFRANE is a metabolite of imipramine hydrochloride. It is a dibenzazepine derivative, representing the desmethyl analog of imipramine hydrochloride. Chemically, it is 10,11-dihydro-5-[3-(methylamino) propyl]-5H-dibenz [b,f] azepine Monohydrochloride, and differs from the parent substance by having only one methyl group on the side chain nitrogen.

Desipramine hydrochloride is a white, crystalline substance with a molecular weight of 302.8. It is soluble to the extent of about 10% w/v in water, and melts within a range of 5° between 208-218°C.

Actions: PERTOFRANE has been found in some studies to have a more rapid onset of action than imipramine; antidepressant efficacy is similar though potency on a weight basis may be less. The earliest manifestations consist mainly of an increase in psychomotor activity. Full treatment benefit is seldon attained before the end of the second week.

PERTOFRANE is not a monoamine oxidase inhibitor and does not act primarily as a central nervous system stimulant. Like all tricyclic antidepressants, PERTOFRANE blocks the reuptake of norepinephrine by adrenergic nerve terminals. Demethylated analogs such as desipramine are more potent in increasing norepinephrine turnover rate than the methylated compounds. However, the exact mechanism of action of tricyclics in depression is still unknown.

A mechanism of action proposed for antidepressant drugs, the biogenic amine theory, postulates that some, if not all, depression is associated with a deficiency or depletion of catecholamines and that some antidepressant drugs increase the amount of amine available at the synaptic receptor.

Desipramine is metabolized in the liver and approximately 70% is excreted in the urine.

Indications: PERTOFRANE is indicated for the relief of mental depression (see Note before How Supplied section for additional information on depressive symptomatologies often responsive to this drug).

Contraindications: The use of PERTOFRANE concomitantly or within two weeks of the administration of MAO inhibitors, is contraindicated. Hyperpyretic crises or severe convulsive seizures may occur in patients receiving such combinations. The potentiation of adverse reactions can be serious, or even fatal. When it is desired to substitute PERTOFRANE in patients receiving a monoamine oxidase inhibitor, as long an interval should elapse as the clinical situation allows, with a minimum of 14 days. Initial dosage should be low and increases should be gradual and cautiously prescribed.

The drug is contraindicated following recent myocardial infarction.

Patients with a known hypersensitivity to tricyclic antidepressants should not be given PERTOFRANE.

Warnings: As with other potent antidepressants, an activation of the psychosis may occasionally be observed in schizophrenic patients. Due to the drug's atropine-like effects and sympathomimetic potentiation, PERTOFRANE should be used only with the greatest care in patients with narrow-angle glaucoma and with urethral or ureteral spasm.

Likewise, only when patient need outweighs the risk of serious adverse reactions should the drug be used in the presence of any of the following conditions: severe coronary heart disease with EKG abnormalities, progressive heart failure, angina pectoris, paroxysmal tachycardia and active seizure disorder (this agent has been shown to lower the seizure threshold).

In some instances, desipramine and the parent compound, imipramine, have been shown to block the pharmacologic action of the antihypertensive, guanethidine, and related adrenergic neuron-blocking agents.

Hypertensive episodes have been observed during surgery in patients on desipramine hydrochloride therapy.

The concurrent use of other central nervous system drugs or alcohol may potentiate the adverse effects of desipramine hydrochloride. Since many such drugs may be used during surgery, it is recommended that desipramine hydrochloride be discontinued for as long as the clinical situation will allow prior to elective surgery.

In patients who may use alcohol excessively, it should be borne in mind that the potentiation may increase the danger inherent in any suicide attempt or overdosage.

Patients should be cautioned about the possibility of impaired ability to operate a motor vehicle or other dangerous machinery.

Usage in Pregnancy: Although teratogenic studies in mice, rats and rabbits have revealed no adverse effects, safe use of this drug in women who are or may become pregnant has not been definitely established. Therefore, PERTOFRANE (desipramine hydrochloride USP) should be withheld from these women unless the clinical situation warrants the potential risk.

In view of the lack of experience in children, the drug is not recommended for use in patients under twelve years of age.

Elderly and adolescent patients can usually be managed on lower dosage than that recommended for other patients and may not tolerate higher doses as well because of an increased incidence of adverse reactions.

Precautions: It should be kept in mind that the possibility of suicide in seriously depressed patients is inherent in the illness and may persist until remission occurs. These patients require careful supervision and protective measures during therapy.

Anxiety and increased agitation have been reported, particularly where depression is not the primary disorder. A shift to hypomanic or manic excitement may occur during therapy. Such reactions may necessitate discontinuation of the drug.

Although the anticholinergic activity of the drug is weak, in susceptible patients and in those receiving anticholinergic drugs (including antiparkinsonism agents), atropine-like effects may be more pronounced (e.g. paralytic ileus).

Caution should be observed in prescribing the drug in hyperthyroid patients and in those receiving thyroid medications. Transient cardiac arrhythmias have occurred in rare instances.

In all patients undergoing extended courses of therapy, periodic blood and liver studies for signs of toxicity should supplement careful clinical observations.

Adverse Reactions: PERTOFRANE is well tolerated by most patients and severe complications or adverse reactions are infrequent. Those most often reported cause little discomfort and seldom require discontinuation of the drug.

Nervous System: Dizziness, drowsiness, insomnia, headache and disturbed visual accommodation have been reported with the drug. In addition, tremor, unsteadiness, tinnitus and paresthesias have been reported. Occasionally, mild extrapyramidal activity, falling, and neuromuscular incoordination have been seen. A confusional state (with such symptoms as hallucinations and disorientation) may be produced, particularly in older patients and at higher dosage, and may require discontinuation of the drug. Changes in EEG patterns have been observed. Epileptiform seizures may occur. A reduction in dosage may help control some of these adverse reactions.

Gastrointestinal Tract: Anorexia, dryness of the mouth, nausea, epigastric distress, constipation and diarrhea have been reported in patients receiving PERTOFRANE. (desipramine hydrochloride USP)

Skin: Skin rashes (including photosensitization), perspiration and flushing sensations have been reported during therapy.

Liver: Transient jaundice, apparently of an obstructive nature, and liver damage have been observed in rare cases. Elevation in transaminase and changes in alkaline phosphatase have occurred and should indicate repeated liver-function profiles. If progressive elevation occurs, the drug should be discontinued.

Blood Elements: Bone-marrow depression, agranulocytosis, thrombocytopenia and purpura have been reported. If these occur, the drug should be discontinued. Transient eosinophilia has been observed in some instances.

Cardiovascular System: Orthostatic hypotension and tachycardia have been observed but seldom require discontinuation of treatment. Patients who require concomitant vasodilating therapy should be carefully supervised, particularly during the initial phases.

Genitourinary System: Urinary frequency or retention and impotence have been reported.

Endocrine System: Occasional hormonal effects, including gynecomastia, galactorrhea and breast enlargement have been reported with PERTOFRANE (desipramine hydrochloride USP). In addition, decreased libido and estrogenic effect have been noted. The exact relationship of these adverse effects to the administration of the drug has not been established.

Sensitivity: Urticaria and rare instances of drug fever and cross-sensitivity with imipramine have been observed.

Dosage and Administration: All Patients Except Geriatric and Adolescent: The usual dosage range is from 75 to 150 mg/day in divided doses or as a single daily dose. Titration to a maintenance dose should be based on clinical response and tolerance by starting in the low dose range and increasing dosage when required. When necessary, dosage may be increased, after initiation of therapy, up to 200 mg daily in divided doses. Continued therapy at the optimal dosage level should be maintained during the active phase of the depression.

It is recommended that a lower maintenance dosage be continued for at least two months after a satisfactory response has been achieved. This, too, may be given on a once-daily schedule for convenience and compliance.

In cases of relapse due to premature withdrawal of the drug, a prompt response may be obtained by immediate resumption of treatment.

Geriatric and Adolescent Patients: Elderly and adolescent patients can usually be managed on lower dosage and may not tolerate higher doses as well as other patients. Therapy in these age groups may be initiated with 25 to 50 mg daily. Dosage may be increased according to response and tolerance to a maximum of 100 mg daily. It is recommended that a lower maintenance dosage be continued for at least two months after a satisfactory response has been achieved. Therapy may be given in divided doses or as a single daily dose.

Overdosage:

Signs and Symptoms: These may vary in severity depending on several factors, including the amount absorbed, age, interval between ingestion and start of treatment, etc. In infants and young children, especially, acute overdosage in any amount must be considered serious and potentially fatal.

CNS abnormalities may include drowsiness, stupor, coma, ataxia, restlessness, agitation, hyperactive reflexes, muscle rigidity, athetoid and choreiform movements, and convulsions.

Cardiac abnormalities may include arrhythmia, tachycardia, ECG evidence of impaired conduction, and signs of congestive failure.

Respiratory depression, cyanosis, hypotension, shock, vomiting, hyperpyrexia, mydriasis, and diaphoresis may also be present.

Treatment: Because CNS involvement, respiratory depression and cardiac arrhythmia can occur suddenly, hospitalization and close observation are necessary, even when the amount ingested is thought to be small or the initial degree of intoxication appears slight or moderate. All patients with ECG abnormalities should have continuous cardiac monitoring for at least 72 hours and be closely observed until well after cardiac status has returned to normal; relapses may occur after apparent recovery.

The *slow* intravenous administration of physostigmine salicylate has been reported to reverse most of the cardiovascular and CNS effects of overdosage with tricyclic antidepressants. In adults, 1 to 3 mg has been reported to be effective. In children, start with 0.5 mg and repeat at 5 minute intervals to determine the minimum effective dose; do not exceed 2 mg. Because of the short duration of action of physostigmine, repeat the effective dose at 30 to 50 minute intervals, as necessary. Avoid rapid injection to reduce the possibility of physostigmine-induced convulsions.

In the alert patient, empty the stomach promptly by induced emesis followed by lavage. In the obtunded patient, secure the airway with a cuffed endotracheal tube before beginning lavage (do not induce emesis). Continue lavage for 24 hours or longer, depending on the apparent severity of intoxication. Use normal or half-normal saline to avoid water intoxication, especially in children. Instillation of activated charcoal slurry may help reduce absorption of desipramine.

Minimize external stimulation to reduce the tendency to convulsions. If anticonvulsants are necessary, diazepam, short-acting barbiturates, paraldehyde or methocarbamol may be useful. Do not use barbiturates if MAO inhibitors have been taken recently.

Maintain adequate respiratory exchange. Do not use respiratory stimulants.

Shock should be treated with supportive measures, such as intravenous fluids, oxygen and corticosteroids. Digitalis may increase conduction abnormalities and further irritate an already sensitized myocardium. If congestive heart failure necessitates rapid digitalization, particular care must be exercised.

Hyperpyrexia should be controlled by whatever external means are available, including ice packs and cooling sponge baths, if necessary.

Hemodialysis, peritoneal dialysis, exchange transfusions and forced diuresis have been generally reported as ineffective because of the rapid fixation of desipramine in tissues. Blood desipramine levels may not correlate with the degree of intoxication, and are unreliable indicators in the clinical management of the patient.

Note: Depressions which are most responsive to PERTOFRANE (desipramine hydrochloride USP) may be described in terms of "target symptoms." These include:

Despondency, sadness and depressed mood
Fatigue
Lack of interest and emotional response
Helplessness, hopelessness, pessimism and despair
Feelings of incapacity and inferiority
Psychomotor retardation and inhibition
Delusions of guilt and unworthiness
Psychosomatic complaints
Insomnia
Anorexia and weight loss
Depression-related anxiety and agitation
Suicidal drive

It should be borne in mind that these "target symptoms" of depression assume their proper significance only after careful history, physical and mental evaluations and other investigative procedures have confirmed a diagnosis of one of the several types of depression.

How Supplied: 25 mg Capsules (pink), bottles of 100 and 1000 (NSN 6505-00-913-0382A—V.A. Depots); 50 mg Capsules (maroon and pink), bottles of 100 and 1000.

[*Shown in Product Identification Section*]

REGROTON® ℞
DEMI-REGROTON® ℞
Oral antihypertensives

Regroton and Demi-Regroton are products of USV Laboratories Inc., Manati, P.R. 00701.

Composition: Each REGROTON tablet provides 50 mg chlorthalidone USP and 0.25 mg reserpine USP. Each DEMI-REGROTON tablet provides 25 mg chlorthalidone USP and 0.125 mg reserpine USP.

Description: REGROTON and DEMI-REGROTON are drug combinations of two well-known antihypertensive agents, chlorthalidone and reserpine.

Chemistry: A monosulfamyl diuretic, chlorthalidone differs from thiazide diuretics in that a double-ring system is incorporated in its structure. Chemically, it is 2-Chloro-5-(1-hydroxy-3-oxo-1-isoindolinyl) benzenesulfonamide.

Reserpine is a pure crystalline alkaloid from the root of Rauwolfia serpentina.

Actions: The pharmacologic effects are those of the constituent drugs. Chlorthalidone produces a saluretic effect in humans, beginning within two hours after an oral dose and continuing for as long as 72 hours. Copious diuresis is produced, with greatly increased excretion of sodium and chloride.

Reserpine, because it reduces arterial blood pressure and exerts a sedative effect, is particularly useful in the therapy of hypertension with related emotional disturbance. Reserpine is characterized by slow onset of action and sustained effect. Both its cardiovascular and central nervous system effects may persist following withdrawal of the drug. (See Precautions.)

Both chlorthalidone and reserpine have prolonged action, and the combination is thus able to exert a smooth and concerted effect over a long period. The two drugs appear to enhance each other, and this gives the combination a high degree of effectiveness. When considered necessary the combination may be prescribed together with other antihypertensive agents, which may then be given in lower dosage with lessened chance of side reactions.

Indication: Treatment of hypertension. (See box warning.)

Contraindications: Mental depression, demonstrated hypersensitivity, and most cases of severe renal or hepatic diseases are the only contraindications.

Warnings:

> These fixed combination drugs are not indicated for initial therapy of hypertension. Hypertension requires therapy titrated to the individual patient. If the fixed combination represents the dosage so determined, its use may be more convenient in patient management. The treatment of hypertension is not static, but must be reevaluated as conditions in each patient warrant.

These drugs should be used with caution in severe renal disease, since products containing chlorthalidone or similar drugs may precipitate azotemia. Cumulative effects of the drug may develop in patients with impaired renal function.

They should be used with caution in patients with impaired hepatic function or progressive liver disease, since minor alterations of fluid and electrolyte balance may precipitate hepatic coma.

REGROTON or DEMI-REGROTON may add to or potentiate the action of other antihypertensive drugs. Potentiation occurs with ganglionic or peripheral adrenergic blocking drugs.

Sensitivity reactions may occur in patients with a history of allergy or bronchial asthma.

Discontinue the drug in patients in whom mental depression develops while on the drug (the possibility of suicide should be kept in mind). In patients who have had depression, the drug should not be started. Electroshock therapy should not be given to patients taking reserpine, since severe and even fatal reactions have occurred. The drug should be stopped at least seven days before giving electroshock therapy.

In susceptible patients, peptic ulcer may be precipitated or activated, in which case the drug should be discontinued.

Usage in Pregnancy: Reproduction studies with chlorthalidone in various animal species at multiples of the human dose showed no significant level of teratogenicity; no fetal or congenital abnormalities were observed. Animal

Continued on next page

USV—Cont.

data should not be extrapolated for clinical application.
Thiazides cross the placental barrier and appear in cord blood. The use of chlorthalidone and related drugs in pregnant women requires that the anticipated benefits of the drug be weighed against possible hazards to the fetus. These hazards include fetal or neonatal jaundice, thrombocytopenia, and possibly other adverse reactions which have occurred in the adult.
REGROTON or DEMI-REGROTON should be used with care in nursing mothers since thiazides and reserpine cross the placental barrier and appear in cord blood and breast milk. Increased respiratory secretions, nasal congestion, cyanosis and anorexia may occur in infants born to reserpine-treated mothers. If use of the drug is deemed essential, the patient should stop nursing.
Precautions: Antihypertensive therapy with chlorthalidone/reserpine combinations should always be initiated cautiously in postsympathectomy patients and in those receiving ganglionic blocking agents, other potent antihypertensive drugs, or curare. At least a one-half reduction in the usual dosage of such agents may be advisable. Careful and continuous supervision of patients on such multiple-drug regimens is necessary.
Since some patients receiving Rauwolfia preparations have experienced hypotension when undergoing surgery, it may be advisable to discontinue chlorthalidone/reserpine combination drugs therapy about two weeks prior to elective surgical procedures. Emergency surgery may be carried out by using, if necessary, anticholinergic or adrenergic drugs to prevent vagocirculatory responses; other supportive measures may be used as indicated.
Because of the possibility of progression of renal damage, periodic kidney function tests are indicated. In case of a rising BUN, the drug should be stopped.
The drug should be discontinued in cases of aggravated liver dysfunction (hepatic coma may be precipitated).
Periodic determination of serum electrolytes to detect possible electrolyte imbalance should be performed at appropriate intervals.
All patients receiving chlorthalidone should be observed for clinical signs of fluid or electrolyte imbalance; namely, hyponatremia, hypochloremic alkalosis, and hypokalemia. Serum and urine electrolyte determinations are particularly important when the patient is vomiting excessively or receiving parenteral fluids. Medication such as digitalis may also influence serum electrolytes. Warning signs, irrespective of cause, are: Dryness of mouth, thirst, weakness, lethargy, drowsiness, restlessness, muscle pains or cramps, muscular fatigue, hypotension, oliguria, tachycardia, and gastrointestinal disturbances such as nausea and vomiting.
Hypokalemia may develop with chlorthalidone as with any other potent diuretic, especially with brisk diuresis, when severe cirrhosis is present, or during concomitant use of corticosteroids or ACTH.
Interference with adequate oral electrolyte intake will also contribute to hypokalemia. Digitalis therapy may exaggerate metabolic effects of hypokalemia especially with reference to myocardial activity.
Any chloride deficit is generally mild and usually does not require specific treatment except under extraordinary circumstances (as in liver disease or renal disease). Dilutional hyponatremia may occur in edematous patients in hot weather; appropriate therapy is water restriction, rather than administration of salt except in rare instances when the hyponatremia is life threatening. In actual salt depletion, appropriate replacement is the therapy of choice.
Hyperuricemia may occur or frank gout may be precipitated in certain patients receiving chlorthalidone.
Insulin requirements in diabetic patients may be increased, decreased, or unchanged. Latent diabetes mellitus may become manifest during chlorthalidone administration.
Chlorthalidone and related drugs may decrease arterial responsiveness to norepinephrine. This diminution is not sufficient to preclude effectiveness of the pressor agent for therapeutic use.
Chlorthalidone and related drugs may decrease serum PBI levels without signs of thyroid disturbance.
Because reserpine increases gastrointestinal motility and secretion, REGROTON or DEMI-REGROTON should be used cautiously in patients with ulcerative colitis or gallstones, where biliary colic may be precipitated. In susceptible patients, bronchial asthma may occur.
Adverse Reactions: Clinical trials indicate that the combination of chlorthalidone with reserpine is generally well tolerated. The adverse reactions most frequently seen include anorexia, gastric irritation, nausea, vomiting, diarrhea, constipation, nasal congestion, muscle cramps, dizziness, weakness, headache, drowsiness, and mental depression. Skin rashes, urticaria, and a case of ecchymosis have been reported. (Other dermatologic manifestations may occur—see below.)
A decreased glucose tolerance evidenced by hyperglycemia and glycosuria may develop inconsistently. This condition—usually reversible on discontinuation of therapy—responds to control with antidiabetic treatment. Diabetics and those predisposed should be checked regularly.
Hyperuricemia may be observed on occasion and acute attacks of gout have been precipitated. In cases where prolonged and significant elevation of blood uric acid concentration is considered potentially deleterious, concomitant use of a uricosuric agent is effective in reversing hyperuricemia without loss of diuretic and/or antihypertensive activity.
In addition to the reactions listed above, certain adverse reactions attributable to the drugs' components are shown below. Since REGROTON and DEMI-REGROTON combine chlorthalidone and reserpine in relatively small doses, such reactions may be less than when those drugs are used in full dosage.
Chlorthalidone: Idiosyncratic drug reactions such as aplastic anemia, purpura, thrombocytopenia, leukopenia, agranulocytosis, necrotizing angiitis and Lyell's syndrome (toxic epidermal necrolysis) have occurred, but are rare.
The remote possibility of pancreatitis should be considered when epigastric pain or unexplained gastrointestinal symptoms develop after prolonged administration.
Other reported reactions include restlessness, transient myopia, impotence or dysuria, and orthostatic hypotension, which may be potentiated when chlorthalidone is combined with alcohol, barbiturates or narcotics. Since jaundice, xanthopsia, paresthesia, and photosensitization have been documented in related compounds, the possibility of these reactions should be kept in mind.
Reserpine: The sedative effect of reserpine may lead to drowsiness or lassitude in some patients. Frequently, this effect disappears with continued administration. Nasal stuffiness sometimes occurs. Gastrointestinal reactions include increased gastric secretions, loose stools, or increased bowel frequency.
Symptoms of mental depression may occur in a small percentage of patients, although the recommended dosage of REGROTON contains substantially less reserpine than that usually implicated in such reactions. The same is true of other rare side effects recorded for reserpine, which include bradycardia and ectopic cardiac rhythms (especially when used with digitalis), pruritus, eruptions and/or flushing of skin, angina pectoris, headache, dizziness, paradoxical anxiety, nightmare, dull sensorium, muscular aches, a reversible paralysis agitans-like syndrome, blurred vision, conjunctival injection, uveitis, optic atrophy and glaucoma, increased susceptibility to colds, dyspnea, weight gain, decreased libido or impotence, dryness of the mouth, deafness, and anorexia.
Dosage and Administration:
Selection of drug and dosage should be determined by individual titration. (See box warning.) According to the requirement, the recommended dose of either REGROTON or DEMI-REGROTON is usually *one tablet once a day.* Some patients may require two tablets once a day. Divided doses are unnecessary, and a single dose given in the morning with food is recommended.
Maintenance: Maintenance dosage must be individually adjusted. Mild cases may be adequately controlled with one DEMI-REGROTON tablet daily. Optimal lowering of elevated blood pressure may require two weeks or more in some cases because of the slow onset of action of reserpine.
Combination With Other Drugs: In more severe cases, if the response to a chlorthalidone/reserpine combination alone is inadequate, potent antihypertensives may be added gradually in dosages at least 50% lower than those usually employed. Such patients should be supervised carefully and continuously. As soon as desired blood pressure levels have been attained, the lowest effective maintenance dosage should be followed.
Overdosage: Adverse reactions resulting from accidental acute overdosage may include nausea, weakness, dizziness, syncope, and disturbances of electrolyte balance. There is no specific antidote. However, the following is recommended: gastric lavage followed by supportive treatment, including intravenous dextrose-saline with potassium chloride if necessary, to be given with the usual caution. If marked hypotension results from overdosage, it can be treated with vasopressor drugs.
How Supplied: REGROTON is available as pink, round, single-scored tablets, in bottles of 100 and 1000; DEMI-REGROTON as white, round tablets, bottles of 100 and 1000.
Animal Pharmacology: In animal biochemical studies, chlorthalidone is absorbed slowly from the gastrointestinal tract, due to low solubility. After passage to the liver, some of the drug enters the general circulation, while some is excreted in the bile, to be reabsorbed later. In the general circulation, the drug is distributed widely to the tissues, but is taken up in the highest concentrations in the kidneys, where amounts have been found 72 hours after ingestion, long after it has disappeared from other tissues. The drug is excreted unchanged in the urine. The high renal concentration of chlorthalidone may be causally associated with the prolonged saluretic effect of the drug. Chlorthalidone appears to inhibit sodium and chloride reabsorption in the cortical diluting segment of ascending limb of Henle's loop. The reduction of plasma volume following diuresis is a probable mechanism in the initial antihypertensive action of the drug.
Reserpine probably produces its sedative and hypotensive effects through a depletion in tissue stores of catecholamines. The antihypertensive action of reserpine is probably due to loss of epinephrine and norepinephrine from peripheral sites. By contrast, its sedative and tranquilizing properties are thought to be related to depletion of 5-hydroxytryptamine from the brain.

[*Shown in Product Identification Section*]

TRACE ELEMENTS, See under:
Chrometrace™ (Chromic Chloride Injection USP)
Coppertrace™ (Cupric Chloride Injection USP)
Mangatrace™ (Manganese Chloride Injection USP)
Zinctrace™ (Zinc Chloride Injection USP)

For dilution in intravenous infusions only
ZINCTRACE™ ℞
Zinc Chloride Injection USP

1 mg/ml

Zinc Chloride in Sodium Chloride Solution

Description: Zinctrace, Zinc Chloride Injection USP (1 mg zinc/ml), is a sterile, nonpyrogenic solution intended for use as an additive to intravenous solutions for total parenteral nutrition (TPN).
Each ml of solution provides:
zinc chloride ....2.09 mg
sodium ....3.07 mg
chloride ....5.82 mg
(not including ions for pH adjustment).
The pH is approximately 2.0, adjusted with hydrochloric acid, and may be adjusted with sodium hydroxide. The solution is adjusted to isotonicity with sodium chloride. The osmolarity is approximately 0.300 mOsm/ml. The solution contains no bacteriostat, antimicrobial agent, or added buffer.
Zinc chloride USP is chemically designated $ZnCl_2$, a white crystalline compound freely soluble in water. Sodium chloride USP is chemically designated NaCl, a white crystalline compound freely soluble in water.
Clinical Pharmacology: Zinc is an essential nutritional requirement that serves as a cofactor for more than 70 different enzymes including carbonic anhydrase, alkaline phosphatase, lactic dehydrogenase, and both RNA and DNA polymerase. Zinc facilitates wound healing, helps maintain normal growth rates, normal skin hydration, and the senses of taste and smell.
Zinc resides in muscle, bone, skin, kidney, liver, pancreas, retina, prostate, and particularly in the red and white blood cells. Zinc binds to plasma albumin, Cl_2-macroglobulin, and some plasma amino acids including histidine, cysteine, threonine, glycine, and asparagine. Ingested zinc is excreted mainly in the stool (approximately 90%), and to a lesser extent in the urine and in perspiration.
Providing zinc during TPN helps prevent development of deficiency symptoms such as: Parakeratosis, hypogeusia, anorexia, dysosmia, geophagia, hypogonadism, growth retardation and hepatosplenomegaly.
The initial manifestations of hypozincemia in TPN are diarrhea, apathy, and depression. At plasma levels below 20 mcg zinc/dl, dermatitis followed by alopecia has been reported for TPN patients. Normal zinc plasma levels are 100 ± 12 mcg/dl.
Indications and Usage: Zinctrace is indicated for use as a supplement to intravenous solutions given for TPN. Administration helps to maintain zinc serum levels and to prevent depletion of endogenous stores and subsequent deficiency symptoms.
Contraindications: Direct intramuscular or intravenous injection of Zinctrace, is contraindicated as the acidic pH of the solution (2.0) may cause considerable tissue irritation.
Warnings: None known.
Precautions: Do not use unless the solution is clear and the seal is intact.
Zinctrace should be used only in conjunction with a pharmacy-directed admixture program using aseptic technique in a laminar flow environment. The solution contains no preservatives; discard unused portion within 24 hours after opening.
Zinctrace should not be given undiluted by direct injection into a peripheral vein because of the likelihood of infusion phlebitis and the potential for increased excretory loss of zinc from a bolus injection. Administration of zinc in the absence of copper may cause a decrease in serum copper levels. Periodic determinations of serum copper as well as zinc are suggested as a guideline for subsequent zinc administration.
Pregnancy Category C. Animal reproduction studies have not been conducted with zinc chloride. It is also not known whether zinc chloride can cause fetal harm when administered to a pregnant woman or can affect reproductive capacity. Zinc chloride should be given to a pregnant woman only if clearly needed.
Adverse Reactions: None known.
Drug Abuse and Dependence: None known.
Overdosage: Single intravenous doses of 1 to 2 mg zinc/kg body weight have been given to adult leukemic patients without toxic manifestations. However, acute toxicity was reported in an adult when 10 mg zinc was infused over a period of one hour on each of four consecutive days. Profuse sweating, decreased level of consciousness, blurred vision, tachycardia (140/min.), and marked hypothermia (94.2°F) on the fourth day were accompanied by a serum zinc concentration of 207 mcg/dl. Symptoms abated within three hours.
Hyperamylasemia may be a sign of impending zinc overdosage; patients receiving an inadvertent overdose (25 mg zinc/liter of TPN solution, equivalent to 50 to 70 mg zinc/day) developed hyperamylasemia (557 to 1850 Klein units; normal; 130 to 310).
Death resulted from an overdose in which 1683 mg zinc was delivered intravenously over the course of 60 hours to a 72-year-old patient. Symptoms of zinc toxicity included hypotension (80/40 mm Hg), pulmonary edema, diarrhea, vomiting, jaundice, and oliguria, with a serum zinc level of 4184 mcg/dl.
Calcium supplements may confer a protective effect against zinc toxicity.
Dosage and Administration: Zinctrace, Zinc Chloride Injection USP, contains 1 mg zinc/ml and is administered intravenously only after dilution.
Adult: For the metabolically stable adult receiving TPN, the suggested intravenous dosage is 2.5 to 4 mg zinc/day. An additional 2 mg zinc/day is suggested for acute catabolic states. For the stable adult with fluid loss from the small bowel, an additional 12.2 mg zinc/liter of small bowel fluid lost, or an additional 17.1 mg zinc/kg of stool or ileostomy output is recommended. Frequent monitoring of zinc blood levels is suggested for patients receiving more than the usual maintenance dosage level of zinc.
Pediatric: For full-term infants and children up to 5 years of age, 100 mcg zinc/kg/day is recommended. For premature infants (birth weight less than 1500 grams) up to 3 kg in body weight, 300 mcg zinc/kg/day is suggested.
Parenteral drug products should be inspected visually for particulate matter and discoloration prior to administration, whenever solution and container permit. See Precautions section.
How Supplied: Zinctrace 10-ml vials (NDC 0075-0833-22), boxes of 25.
[*Shown in Product Identification Section*]

Products are

listed alphabetically

in the

PINK SECTION.

Ulmer Pharmacal Company
(Div. of Physicians and Hospitals Supply Company)
2440 FERNBROOK LANE
MINNEAPOLIS, MN 55441

LOBANA® BATH OIL
(See PDR For Nonprescription Drugs)

LOBANA® BODY LOTION
(See PDR For Nonprescription Drugs)

LOBANA® BODY POWDER
(See PDR For Nonprescription Drugs)

LOBANA® BODY SHAMPOO
(See PDR For Nonprescription Drugs)

LOBANA® CONDITIONING SHAMPOO
(See PDR For Nonprescription Drugs)

LOBANA® DERM-ADE CREAM
(See PDR For Nonprescription Drugs)

LOBANA® LIQUID HAND SOAP
(See PDR For Nonprescription Drugs)

LOBANA® PERI-GARD
(See PDR For Nonprescription Drugs)

LOBANA® PERINEAL CLEANSE
(See PDR For Nonprescription Drugs)

VLEMINCKX' Solution
(Topical Acne Treatment and Scabicide)
(See PDR For Nonprescription Drugs)

The Upjohn Company
KALAMAZOO, MI 49001

The Upjohn Manufacturing Company*
BARCELONETA, PUERTO RICO 00617

The Upjohn Manufacturing Company M†
BARCELONETA, PUERTO RICO 00617

UPJOHN PRODUCT IDENTIFICATION CODE
Most capsules and tablets manufactured by The Upjohn Company, The Upjohn Manufacturing Company and The Upjohn Manufacturing Company M are imprinted with one or a combination of the following: (1) That portion of the National Drug Code (NDC) number which indicates product and strength (2) Product trademark (3) "Upjohn" or "U" (4) Dosage strength.
A complete list of oral solid dosage forms with their assigned NDC numbers is provided below.

Code #	Product	Strength
11	**FEMINONE®** Tablets (ethinyl estradiol tablets, USP)	0.05 mg
12	**CORTEF®** Tablets (hydrocortisone tablets, USP) Tablets, USP	5 mg

Continued on next page

Upjohn—Cont.

14 **HALOTESTIN**® Tablets 2 mg
(fluoxymesterone tablets, USP)
See Product Identification Section

15 **CORTISONE ACETATE** 5 mg
Tablets, USP

18 **DIDREX**™ Tablets ⒸIII 25 mg
(benzphetamine hydrochloride)
See Product Identification Section

19 **HALOTESTIN**® Tablets 5 mg
(fluoxymesterone tablets, USP)
See Product Identification Section

22 **MEDROL**® Tablets 8 mg
(methylprednisolone tablets, USP)
See Product Identification Section

23 **CORTISONE ACETATE** 10 mg
Tablets, USP

24 **DIDREX**™ Tablets 50 mg
(benzphetamine hydrochloride)
See Product Identification Section

25 **DELTA-CORTEF**® Tablets 5 mg
(prednisolone tablets, USP)

29 **XANAX**® **Tablets** 0.25 mg
(alprazolam)
See Product Identification Section

31 **CORTEF**® Tablets 10 mg
(hydrocortisone tablets, USP)

32 **DELTASONE**® Tablets 2.5 mg.
(prednisone tablets, USP)
See Product Identification Section

34 **CORTISONE ACETATE** 25 mg
Tablets, USP

36 **HALOTESTIN**® Tablets 10 mg
(fluoxymesterone tablets, USP)
See Product Identification Section

38 **HALODRIN**® Tablets
(fluoxymesterone and ethinyl estradiol)

44 **CORTEF**® Tablets 20 mg
(hydrocortisone tablets, USP)

45 **DELTASONE**® Tablets 5 mg
(prednisone tablets, USP)
See Product Identification Section

49 **MEDROL**® Tablets 2 mg
(methylprednisolone tablets, USP)
See Product Identification Section

50 **PROVERA**® Tablets 10 mg
(medroxyprogesterone acetate
Tablets, USP)
See Product Identification Section

53 **ALPHADROL**® Tablets 1.5 mg
(fluprednisolone)

55 **XANAX**® Tablets 0.5 mg
(alprazolam)
See Product Identification Section

56 **MEDROL**® Tablets 4 mg
(methylprednisolone tablets, USP)
See Product Identification Section

61 **PAMINE**® Tablets 2.5 mg
(methscopolamine bromide
tablets, USP)

62 **CALDEROL**® Capsules 20 mcg
(calcifediol)
See Product Identification Section

64 **PROVERA**® Tablets 2.5 mg
(medroxyprogesterone acetate
tablets, USP)
See Product Identification Section

65 **RESERPOID**® Tablets 0.25 mg
(reserpine tablets, USP)

70 **TOLINASE**® Tablets 100 mg
(tolazamide tablets, USP)
See Product Identification Section

73 **MEDROL**® Tablets 16 mg
(methylprednisolone tablets, USP)
See Product Identification Section

74 **CALDEROL**® Capsules 50 mcg
(calcifediol)

77 **ORTHOXINE**® Tablets 100 mg
(methoxyphenamine hydrochloride)

81 **ADEFLOR CHEWABLE**® 0.5 mg
Tablets
Fluoride and vitamins
See Product Identification Section

90 **XANAX**® Tablets 1 mg
(alprazolam)
See Product Identification Section

92 **ADEFLOR CHEWABLE**® 1 mg
Tablets
Fluoride and vitamins
See Product Identification Section

100 **ORINASE**® Tablets 0.5 Gm
(tolbutamide tablets, USP)
See Product Identification Section

101 **ALBAMYCIN**® Capsules 250 mg
(novobiocin sodium)

103 **E-MYCIN**® Tablets 250 mg
(erythromycin enteric-coated tablets)
See Product Identification Section

106 **DIOSTATE D**® Tablets
Vitamin, calcium and phosphorus
supplement

109 **CEBEFORTIS**® Tablets
Vitamins B and C

111 **SIGTAB**® Tablets
High potency vitamin supplement

114 **TOLINASE**® Tablets 250 mg
(tolazamide tablets, USP)
See Product Identification Section

115 **ADEFLOR M**® Tablets
Vitamins and minerals with fluoride

119 **UPJOHN VITAMIN C** 250 mg
Tablets

121 **LONITEN**® Tablets 2.5 mg
(minoxidil)
See Product Identification Section

122 **CEBENASE**® Tablets

137 **LONITEN**® Tablets 10 mg
(minoxidil)
See Product Identification Section

149 **UNICAP T**® Tablets
Vitamins with minerals

155 **MEDROL**® Tablets 24 mg
(methylprednisolone tablets, USP)
See Product Identification Section

165 **DELTASONE**® Tablets 20 mg
(prednisone tablets, USP)
See Product Identification Section

176 **MEDROL**® Tablets 32 mg
(methylprednisolone tablets, USP)
See Product Identification Section

193 **DELTASONE**® Tablets 10 mg
(prednisone tablets, USP)
See Product Identification Section

195 **PANMYCIN**® Tablets 250 mg
(tetracycline hydrochloride
tablets, USP)
See Product Identification Section

198 **UNICAP CHEWABLE**® Tablets
Multivitamin

225 ***CLEOCIN HCl**™ Capsules 150 mg
(clindamycin HCl capsules, USP)
See Product Identification Section

243 **ALKETS**® Tablets

251 **CALCIUM GLUCONATE** 975 mg
Tablets, USP

272 **CALCIUM LACTATE** 650 mg
Tablets, USP

284 **UNICAP M**® Tablets
Vitamins with minerals

285 **UNICAP PLUS IRON**® Tablets

310 **PANMYCIN**® Tablets 500 mg
(tetracycline hydrochloride
tablets, USP)

331 ***CLEOCIN HCl**™ Capsules 75 mg
(clindamycin HCl capsules, USP)
See Product Identification Section

336 **LINCOCIN**® Pediatric 250 mg
Capsules
(lincomycin hydrochloride capsules,
USP)

348 **UNICAP SENIOR**® Tablets
Vitamins with minerals

363 **ZYMACAP**® Capsules
Multivitamins

366 **UPJOHN VITAMIN E** 200 I.U.
Capsules

388 **DELTASONE**® Tablets 50 mg
(prednisone tablets, USP)
See Product Identification Section

412 **MAOLATE**® Tablets 400 mg
(chlorphenesin carbamate)
See Product Identification Section

477 **TOLINASE**® Tablets 500 mg
(tolazamide tablets, USP)
See Product Identification Section

500 **LINCOCIN**® Capsules 500 mg
(lincomycin hydrochloride capsules,
USP)

521 **MYCIFRADIN**® Tablets 0.5 Gm
(neomycin sulfate tablets, USP)

586 **UTICILLIN VK**® Tablets 250 mg
(penicillin V potassium tablets, USP)

664 **P-A-C**® Compound Tablets, Green
(aspirin, phenacetin and caffeine
tablets)

671 **UTICILLIN VK**® Tablets 500 mg
(penicillin V potassium tablets, USP)

677 **P-A-C**® Compound Tablets, Pink
(aspirin, phenacetin and caffeine
tablets)

686 **P-A-C**® with Codeine Ⓒ ¼ gr. (15 mg)
Tablets

692 **P-A-C**® Compound Tablets, White
(aspirin, phenacetin and caffeine
tablets)

701 **ORINASE**® Tablets 250 mg
(tolbutamide tablets, USP)
See Product Identification Section

716 **P-A-C**® with Codeine Ⓒ ½ gr. (30 mg)
Tablets

730 **PHENOLAX**® Wafers
(phenolphthalein)

733 **†MOTRIN**® **Tablets** **300 mg**
(ibuprofen)
See Product Identification Section

742 **†MOTRIN**® Tablets 600 mg
(ibuprofen)
See Product Identification Section

750 **†MOTRIN**® Tablets 400 mg
(ibuprofen)
See Product Identification Section

782 **PANMYCIN**® Capsules 250 mg
(tetracycline hydrochloride capsules,
USP)

831 **PYRROXATE**® with Codeine Ⓒ ¼ gr
Capsules

873 **SUPER D**® **Perles**
(oleovitamins A and D capsules, N.F.)

949 **URACIL MUSTARD** Capsules 1 mg

3176 **E-MYCIN**® Tablets 333 mg
(erythromycin)
See Product Identification Section

3212 **PYRROXATE**® Capsules

* Product of The Upjohn Manufacturing Company

† Product of The Upjohn Manufacturing Company M [Products without reference marks are products of The Upjohn Company]

Cleocin Pediatric is a registered trademark of The Upjohn Manufacturing Company

Cleocin HCl, Cleocin Phosphate, and *Cleocin T* are trademarks of The Upjohn Manufacturing Company

Motrin is a registered trademark of The Upjohn Manufacturing Company M

SPECIAL INFORMATION

Warning: Benzyl alcohol has been reported to be associated with a fatal "Gasping Syndrome" in premature infants. The following UPJOHN products contain benzyl alcohol:

BERUBIGEN® Sterile Solution
CLEOCIN PHOSPHATE™ Sterile Solution
CORTEF® Sterile Suspension IM
DEPO®**-Testosterone** Sterile Solution
Heparin Sodium Injection, USP, Sterile Solution
LINCOCIN® Sterile Solution
Sodium Chloride Injection (Bacteriostatic), USP, Sterile Solution
SOLU-CORTEF® Sterile Powder
SOLU-MEDROL® Sterile Powder
Water for Injection (Bacteriostatic), USP, Sterile Solution

Also, benzyl alcohol is contained in the diluent for the following products:

CYTOSAR-U® Sterile Powder
SOLU-MEDROL® Sterile Powder
TROBICIN® Sterile Powder

ADEFLOR CHEWABLE® Tablets ℞

Composition: Each 0.5 mg or 1 mg tablet contains:

Fluoride (as sodium fluoride)	0.5 mg or 1 mg
Vitamin A	4000 Int. Units
Vitamin D	400 Int. Units
Ascorbic Acid (as sodium ascorbate)	75 mg
Thiamine Mononitrate	2 mg
Riboflavin	2 mg
Niacinamide	18 mg
Pyridoxine Hydrochloride	1 mg
Calcium Pantothenate	5 mg
Cyanocobalamin	2 mcg

The palatable cherry-flavored *Adeflor Chewable* Tablets 0.5 mg or raspberry-flavored 1 mg tablets may be chewed, dissolved in the mouth or swallowed whole.

How Supplied:

0.5 mg	Bottles of 100	*NDC 0009-0081-01*
	Bottles of 500	*NDC 0009-0081-02*
1 mg	Bottles of 100	*NDC 0009-0092-01*
	Bottles of 500	*NDC 0009-0092-02*

[*Shown in Product Identification Section*]

ADEFLOR® Drops ℞

Composition: Each 0.6 ml contains:

Fluoride (as sodium fluoride)	0.5 mg
Vitamin A	2000 Int. Units
Vitamin D	400 Int. Units
Ascorbic Acid (C)	50 mg
Pyridoxine Hydrochloride (B_6)	1 mg

How Supplied: Aqueous solution in calibrated dropper bottles.

30 ml *NDC 0009-0211-01*
50 ml *NDC 0009-0211-02*

BACIGUENT® Antibiotic Ointment

(See PDR For Nonprescription Drugs)

CALDEROL® Capsules ℞
(calcifediol)

Description: *Calderol* Capsules contain calcifediol which is the colorless, crystalline monohydrate of 25-hydroxycholecalciferol prepared by chemical synthesis and is identical to the natural vitamin metabolite. Calcifediol has a calculated molecular weight of 418.67 and is soluble in organic solvents but relatively insoluble in water. Chemically, calcifediol is (5Z,7E)-9,10 - secocholesta - 5,7,10(19) - triene - 3β,25 - diol monohydrate.

The other names frequently used for 25-hydroxycholecalciferol are 25-hydroxyvitamin D_3, 25-HCC, 25-OHCC, and 25-OHD$_3$.

Calderol Capsules (calcifediol) for oral administration are available in two strengths: a white capsule containing 20 mcg calcifediol and an orange capsule containing 50 mcg calcifediol.

Clinical Pharmacology: The natural supply of vitamin D in man mainly depends on the ultraviolet rays of the sun for conversion of 7-dehydrocholesterol to vitamin D_3 (cholecalciferol). It is now known that vitamin D_3 must first be converted to 25-OHD$_3$ (25-hydroxycholecalciferol) by a vitamin D_3-25-hydroxylase enzyme (25-OHase) present in the liver. 25-Hydroxycholecalciferol is the major transport form of vitamin D_3 and can be readily monitored in the serum. It is further converted to 1,25-dihydroxycholecalciferol (1,25-$(OH)_2D_3$) and 24,25-dihydroxycholecalciferol (24,25-$(OH)_2D_3$) in the kidney. 1,25-$(OH)_2D_3$ stimulates resorption of calcium from bone and increases intestinal calcium absorption. The physiologic role of 24,25-$(OH)_2D_3$ has not been clearly established. The metabolic activity of calcifediol in clinical use appears to be related not only to its conversion to other metabolites but also due to its intrinsic activity.

When administered orally, calcifediol is rapidly absorbed from the intestine, with peak 25-OHD$_3$ concentrations in the serum reported after about 4 hours. 25-Hydroxycholecalciferol is known to be transported in blood, bound to a specific plasma protein. The terminal half-life of orally administered calcifediol in the serum is about 16 days.

Indications and Usage: *Calderol* Capsules (calcifediol) are indicated in the treatment and management of metabolic bone disease or hypocalcemia associated with chronic renal failure in patients undergoing renal dialysis.

In studies to date it has been shown to increase serum calcium levels, to decrease alkaline phosphatase and parathyroid hormone levels in some patients, to decrease subperiosteal bone resorption in some patients, and to decrease histological signs of hyperparathyroid bone disease and mineralization defects in some patients.

Contraindications: *Calderol* Capsules (calcifediol) should not be given to patients with hypercalcemia or evidence of vitamin D toxicity.

Warnings: Since calcifediol is a metabolite of vitamin D, vitamin D and its derivatives should be withheld during treatment.

Aluminum carbonate or hydroxide gels should be used to control serum phosphorus levels in patients undergoing dialysis.

Overdosage of any form of vitamin D is dangerous (see also **OVERDOSAGE**). Progressive hypercalcemia may be so severe as to require emergency attention. Chronic hypercalcemia can lead to generalized vascular calcification, nephrocalcinosis, and other soft-tissue calcification. The serum calcium times phosphorus (Ca × P) product should not be allowed to exceed 70. Radiographic and/or slit lamp evaluation of suspect anatomical regions may be useful in the early detection of this condition.

Precautions:

i) *General:* Excessive dosage of *Calderol* Capsules (calcifediol) induces hypercalcemia and in some instances hypercalciuria; therefore, early in treatment during dosage adjustment, serum calcium should be determined frequently (at least weekly). Should hypercalcemia develop, the drug should be discontinued immediately. After achieving normocalcemia, the drug may be readministered at a lower dosage. *Calderol* should be given cautiously to patients receiving digitalis, because hypercalcemia in such patients may precipitate cardiac arrhythmias.

ii) *Information for the Patient:* The patient and his or her parents or spouse should be informed about compliance with dosage instructions, adherence to instructions about diet, calcium supplementation, phosphate binder usage, and avoidance of non approved prescription drugs. Patients should also be informed about the symptoms of hypercalcemia (see **Adverse Reactions**).

iii) *Essential Laboratory Tests:* Serum calcium, phosphorus and alkaline phosphatase and 24-hour urinary calcium and phosphorus should be determined periodically. During the initial phase of the medication, serum calcium should be determined more frequently (at least weekly).

iv) *Drug Interactions:* Cholestyramine has been reported to reduce absorption of fat-soluble vitamins; as such, it may impair intestinal absorption of calcifediol. The administration of anticonvulsants has been shown to affect the calcifediol requirements in some patients.

v) *Carcinogenesis, Mutagenesis, Impairment of Fertility:* Long-term studies in animals have not been completed to evaluate the carcinogenic potential of *Calderol.* No significant effects of calcifediol on fertility and/or general reproductive performances were reported.

vi) *Use in Pregnancy:* Teratogenic effects: Pregnancy Category C: Calcifediol has been shown to be teratogenic in rabbits when given in doses of 6 to 12 times the human dose. There are no adequate and well-controlled studies in pregnant women. *Calderol* should be used during pregnancy only if the potential benefit justifies potential risk to the fetus.

When calcifediol was given orally to bred rabbits on the 6th through the 18th day of gestation, gross visceral and skeletal examination of pups indicated that the compound was teratogenic at doses of 25 and 50 mcg/kg/day. A dose of 5 mcg/kg/day was not teratogenic. In a similar study in rats, calcifediol was not teratogenic at doses up to and including 60 mcg/kg/day.

vii) *Nursing Mothers:* It is not known whether this drug is excreted in human milk. Because many drugs are excreted in human milk, caution should be exercised when *Calderol* is administered to a nursing woman.

viii) *Pediatric Use:* The safety and effectiveness of *Calderol* in children have not been established.

Adverse Reactions: Since calcifediol is an active metabolite of vitamin D, adverse effects are, in general, similar to those encountered with excessive vitamin D intake. The early and late signs and symptoms of vitamin D intoxication associated with hypercalcemia include:

a. *Early:* Weakness, headache, somnolence, nausea, vomiting, dry mouth, constipation, muscle pain, bone pain, and metallic taste.
b. *Late:* Polyuria, polydipsia, anorexia, irritability, weight loss, nocturia, conjunctivitis (calcific), pancreatitis, photophobia, rhinorrhea, pruritus, hyperthermia, decreased libido, elevated BUN, albuminuria, hypercholesterolemia, elevated SGOT and SGPT, ectopic calcification, hypertension, cardiac arrhythmias, and rarely, overt psychosis.

Overdosage: Administration of *Calderol* Capsules (calcifediol) to patients in excess of their daily requirements can cause hypercalcemia, hypercalciuria, and hyperphosphatemia. High intake of calcium and phosphate concomitant with *Calderol* may lead to similar abnormalities.

Treatment of Hypercalcemia and Overdosages: General treatment of hypercalcemia (greater than 1 mg/dl above the upper limit of the normal range) consists of discontinuation of therapy with *Calderol.* Serum calcium measurements should be performed regularly until normocalcemia ensues. Hypercalcemia usually resolves in two to four weeks. When serum calcium levels have returned to within normal limits, therapy with *Calderol* may be reinstituted at a dosage lower than prior therapy. Serum calcium levels should be obtained at least weekly after all dosage changes and subsequent dosage titration. Persistent or markedly elevated calcium levels in dialysis patients may be corrected by dialysis against a calcium-free dialysate.

Treatment of Accidental Overdosage: The treatment of acute accidental overdosage of *Calderol* should consist of general supportive measures. If drug ingestion is discovered within a relatively short time, induction of emesis or gastric lavage may be of benefit in preventing further absorption. If the drug has passed through the stomach, the administration of mineral oil may promote fecal elimination. Serial serum calcium determination, rate of urinary calcium excretion, and an assessment of electrocardiographic abnormalities due to hypercalcemia should be obtained. Such monitoring is critical in patients receiving digitalis. Discontinuation of supplemental calcium and a low calcium diet are also indicated in accidental overdosage. Because the conversion of calcifediol to 1,25-$(OH)_2D_3$ is tightly regulated by the body's needs, further measures are probably unnecessary. Should persistent and marked hypercalcemia occur, however, there are a variety of therapeutic measures that may be considered, depending on the patient's underlying condition.

Continued on next page

Upjohn—Cont.

These include the use of drugs such as phosphates and corticosteroids as well as measures to induce an appropriate forced diuresis. The use of peritoneal dialysis against a calcium-free dialysate may also be considered.

Dosage and Administration: The optimal daily dose of *Calderol* Capsules (calcifediol) must be carefully determined for each patient. The recommended initial dosage of *Calderol* is based on the assumption that each patient is receiving an adequate daily intake of calcium from dietary sources or from the addition of calcium supplements. The RDA for calcium in adults is 1000 mg. To insure that each patient receives an adequate daily intake of calcium, the physician should either prescribe a calcium supplement or instruct the patients in proper dietary measures.

Chronic Renal Failure—Dialysis Patients: The recommended initial dose of *Calderol* (calcifediol) is 300 to 350 mcg of calcifediol weekly, administered on a daily or alternate-day schedule. If a satisfactory response in the biochemical parameters and clinical manifestations of the disease state is not observed, dosage may be increased at four-week intervals. During this titration period serum calcium levels should be obtained at least weekly, and if hypercalcemia is noted, the drug should be discontinued until normocalcemia ensues.

Some patients with normal serum calcium levels may respond to doses of 20 mcg of calcifediol every other day. Most patients respond to doses between 50 and 100 mcg daily or between 100 and 200 mcg on alternate days.

How Supplied: *Calderol* Capsules (calcifediol) are available in the following strengths and package sizes:

Strength	Package Size	NDC Number
20 mcg	Bottles of 60	0009-0062-01
(white, soft elastic capsules)		
50 mcg	Bottles of 60	0009-0074-01
(orange, soft elastic capsules)		

Code 811 357 001

[*Shown in Product Identification Section*]

CHERACOL D® Cough Syrup

(See PDR For Nonprescription Drugs)

CHERACOL PLUS™ Cough Syrup

(See PDR For Nonprescription Drugs)

CITROCARBONATE® Antacid

(See PDR For Nonprescription Drugs)

CLEOCIN HCl ™ Capsules ℞

(clindamycin HCl capsules, USP)

150 mg (100's):
NSN 6505-00-159-4892 (M & VA)

WARNING

Clindamycin therapy has been associated with severe colitis which may end fatally. Therefore, it should be reserved for serious infections where less toxic antimicrobial agents are inappropriate, as described in the Indications section. It should not be used in patients with nonbacterial infections, such as most upper respiratory tract infections. Studies indicate a toxin(s) produced by *Clostridia* is one primary cause of antibiotic associated colitis. Cholestyramine and colestipol resins have been shown to bind the toxin *in vitro*. See WARNINGS section. The colitis is usually characterized by severe, persistent diarrhea and severe abdominal cramps and may be associated with the passage of blood and mucus. Endoscopic examination may reveal pseudomembranous colitis.

When significant diarrhea occurs, the drug should be discontinued or, if necessary, continued only with close observation of the patient. Large bowel endoscopy has been recommended.

Antiperistaltic agents such as opiates and diphenoxylate with atropine (Lomotil) may prolong and/or worsen the condition. Vancomycin has been found to be effective in the treatment of antibiotic associated pseudomembranous colitis produced by *Clostridium difficile*. The usual adult dosage is 500 milligrams to 2 grams of vancomycin orally per day in three to four divided doses administered for 7 to 10 days. Cholestyramine or colestipol resins bind vancomycin *in vitro*. If both a resin and vancomycin are to be administered concurrently, it may be advisable to separate the time of administration of each drug.

Diarrhea, colitis, and pseudomembranous colitis have been observed to begin up to several weeks following cessation of therapy with clindamycin.

Description: *Cleocin HCl* Capsules contain clindamycin hydrochloride, equivalent to 75 mg or 150 mg of clindamycin. *Cleocin HCl* is the hydrated hydrochloride salt of clindamycin. Clindamycin is a semi-synthetic antibiotic produced by a 7(S)-chloro-substitution of the 7(R)-hydroxyl group of the parent compound lincomycin.

Actions:

Microbiology: Clindamycin has been shown to have *in vitro* activity against isolates of the following organisms:

Aerobic gram-positive cocci, including:
- *Staphylococcus aureus*
- *Staphylococcus epidermidis* (penicillinase and nonpenicillinase producing strains). When tested by *in vitro* methods some staphylococcal strains originally resistant to erythromycin rapidly develop resistance to clindamycin.
- Streptococci (except *S. faecalis*)
- Pneumococci

Anaerobic gram-negative bacilli, including:
- Bacteroides species (including *Bacteroides fragilis* group and *Bacteroides melaninogenicus* group)
- Fusobacterium species

Anaerobic gram-positive nonsporeforming bacilli, including;
- Propionibacterium
- Eubacterium
- Actinomyces species

Anaerobic and microaerophilic gram-positive cocci, including:
- Peptococcus species
- Peptostreptococcus species
- Microaerophilic streptococci

Clostridia: Clostridia are more resistant than most anaerobes to clindamycin. Most *Clostridium perfringens* are susceptible, but other species, eg, *Clostridium sporogenes* and *Clostridium tertium*, are frequently resistant to clindamycin. Susceptibility testing should be done.

Cross resistance has been demonstrated between clindamycin and lincomycin.

Antagonism has been demonstrated between clindamycin and erythromycin.

Human Pharmacology. Serum level studies with a 150 mg oral dose of clindamycin hydrochloride in 24 normal adult volunteers showed that clindamycin was rapidly absorbed after oral administration. An average peak serum level of 2.50 mcg/ml was reached in 45 minutes; serum levels averaged 1.51 mcg/ml at 3 hours and 0.70 mcg/ml at 6 hours. Absorption of an oral dose is virtually complete (90%), and the concomitant administration of food does not appreciably modify the serum concentrations; serum levels have been uniform and predictable from person to person and dose to dose. Serum level studies following multiple doses of *Cleocin HCl* Capsules (clindamycin hydrochloride) for up to 14 days show no evidence of accumulation or altered metabolism of drug.

Serum half-life of clindamycin is increased slightly in patients with markedly reduced renal function. Hemodialysis and peritoneal dialysis are not effective in removing clindamycin from the serum.

Concentrations of clindamycin in the serum increased linearly with increased dose. Serum levels exceed the MIC (minimum inhibitory concentration) for most indicated organisms for at least six hours following administration of the usually recommended doses. Clindamycin is widely distributed in body fluids and tissues (including bones). The average biological half-life is 2.4 hours. Approximately 10% of the bio-activity is excreted in the urine and 3.6% in the feces; the remainder is excreted as bio-inactive metabolites.

Doses of up to 2 grams of clindamycin per day for 14 days have been well tolerated by healthy volunteers, except that the incidence of gastrointestinal side effects is greater with the higher doses.

No significant levels of clindamycin are attained in the cerebrospinal fluid, even in the presence of inflamed meninges.

Indications: Clindamycin is indicated in the treatment of serious infections caused by susceptible anaerobic bacteria.

Clindamycin is also indicated in the treatment of serious infections due to susceptible strains of streptococci, pneumococci, and staphylococci. Its use should be reserved for penicillin-allergic patients or other patients for whom, in the judgment of the physician, a penicillin is inappropriate. Because of the risk of colitis, as described in the WARNING box, before selecting clindamycin the physician should consider the nature of the infection and the suitability of less toxic alternatives (eg, erythromycin).

Anaerobes: Serious respiratory tract infections such as empyema, anaerobic pneumonitis and lung abscess; serious skin and soft tissue infections; septicemia; intra-abdominal infections such as peritonitis and intra-abdominal abscess (typically resulting from anaerobic organisms resident in the normal gastrointestinal tract); infections of the female pelvis and genital tract such as endometritis, nongonococcal tubo-ovarian abscess, pelvic cellulitis and postsurgical vaginal cuff infection.

Streptococci: Serious respiratory tract infections; serious skin and soft tissue infections.

Staphylococci: Serious respiratory tract infections; serious skin and soft tissue infections.

Pneumococci: Serious respiratory tract infections.

Bacteriologic studies should be performed to determine the causative organisms and their susceptibility to clindamycin.

In Vitro Susceptibility Testing: A standardized disk testing procedure* is recommended for determining susceptibility of aerobic bacteria to clindamycin. A description is contained in the *Cleocin®* Susceptibility Disk (clindamycin) insert. Using this method, the laboratory can designate isolates as resistant, intermediate, or susceptible. Tube or agar dilution methods may be used for both anaerobic and aerobic bacteria. When the directions in the *Cleocin* Susceptibility Powder insert are followed, an MIC of 1.6 mcg/ml may be considered susceptible; MICs of 1.6 to 4.8 mcg/ml may be considered intermediate and MICs greater than 4.8 mcg/ml may be considered resistant.

Cleocin Susceptibility Disks 2 mcg. See package insert for use.

Cleocin Susceptibility Powder 20 mg. See package insert for use.

For anaerobic bacteria the minimal inhibitory concentration (MIC) of clindamycin can be determined by agar dilution and broth dilution (including microdilution) techniques. If MICs are not determined routinely, the disk broth method is recommended for routine use. THE

KIRBY-BAUER DISK DIFFUSION METHOD AND ITS INTERPRETIVE STANDARDS ARE NOT RECOMMENDED FOR ANAEROBES.

*Bauer, A.W., Kirby, W.M.M., Sherris, J.C., Turck, M.; Antibiotic susceptibility testing by a standardized single disc method, *Am. J. Clin. Path.* 45:493-496, 1966. Standardized Disc Susceptibility Test, *Federal Register* 37:20527-29, 1972.

Contraindications: *Cleocin HCl* Capsules (clindamycin hydrochloride) are contraindicated in individuals with a history of hypersensitivity to preparations containing clindamycin or lincomycin.

Warnings:
See WARNING box. Studies indicate a toxin(s) produced by *Clostridia* is one primary cause of antibiotic associated colitis.[1–5] Cholestyramine and colestipol resins have been shown to bind the toxin *in vitro.* Mild cases of colitis may respond to drug discontinuance alone. Moderate to severe cases should be managed with fluid, electrolyte and protein supplementation as indicated. Vancomycin has been found to be effective in the treatment of antibiotic associated pseudomembranous colitis produced by *Clostridium difficile.* The usual adult dosage is 500 milligrams to 2 grams of vancomycin orally per day in three to four divided doses administered for 7 to 10 days. Cholestyramine or colestipol resins bind vancomycin *in vitro.* If both a resin and vancomycin are to be administered concurrently, it may be advisable to separate the time of administration of each drug. Systemic corticoids and corticoid retention enemas may help relieve the colitis. Other causes of colitis should also be considered.

A careful inquiry should be made concerning previous sensitivities to drugs and other allergens.

Usage in Pregnancy - Safety for use in pregnancy has not been established.

Usage in Newborns and Infants: When *Cleocin HCl* Capsules (clindamycin hydrochloride) are administered to newborns and infants, appropriate monitoring of organ system functions is desirable.

Nursing Mothers—Clindamycin has been reported to appear in breast milk in ranges of 0.7 to 3.8 mcg/ml.

Usage in Meningitis: Since clindamycin does not diffuse adequately into the cerebrospinal fluid, the drug should not be used in the treatment of meningitis.

Antagonism has been demonstrated between clindamycin and erythromycin *in vitro.* Because of possible clinical significance, these two drugs should not be administered concurrently.

1. Bartlett JG, et al: Antibiotic associated Pseudomembranous Colitis Due to Toxin-producing *Clostridia. N Engl J Med* 298(10):531-534, 1978.
2. George RH, et al: Identification of *Clostridium difficile* as a cause of Pseudomembranous Colitis. *Br Med J* 6114:669-671, 1978.
3. Larson HE, Price AB: Pseudomembranous Colitis Presence of Clostridial Toxin, *Lancet* 8052/3:1312-1314, 1977.
4. Rifkin GD, Fekety FR, Silva J: Antibiotic-induced Colitis Implication of a Toxin Neutralized by *Clostridium sordellii* Antitoxin. *Lancet* 8048:1103-1106, 1977.
5. Bailey WR, Scott EG: Diagnostic Microbiology. The CV Mosby Company, St. Louis, 1978.

Precautions: Review of experience to date suggests that a subgroup of older patients with associated severe illness may tolerate diarrhea less well. When clindamycin is indicated in these patients, they should be carefully monitored for change in bowel frequency.

Cleocin HCl Capsules (clindamycin hydrochloride) should be prescribed with caution in individuals with a history of gastrointestinal disease, particularly colitis.

Cleocin HCl should be prescribed with caution in atopic individuals.

During prolonged therapy, periodic liver and kidney function tests and blood counts should be performed.

Indicated surgical procedures should be performed in conjunction with antibiotic therapy.

The use of *Cleocin HCl* occasionally results in overgrowth of nonsusceptible organisms—particularly yeasts. Should superinfections occur, appropriate measures should be taken as indicated by the clinical situation.

Patients with very severe renal disease and/or very severe hepatic disease accompanied by severe metabolic aberrations should be dosed with caution, and serum clindamycin levels monitored during high-dose therapy.

Clindamycin has been shown to have neuromuscular blocking properties that may enhance the action of other neuromuscular blocking agents. Therefore, it should be used with caution in patients receiving such agents.

This product contains FD&C Yellow No. 5 (tartrazine) which may cause allergic-type reactions (including bronchial asthma) in certain susceptible individuals. Although the overall incidence of FD&C Yellow No. 5 (tartrazine) sensitivity in the general population is low, it is frequently seen in patients who also have aspirin hypersensitivity.

Adverse Reactions: The following reactions have been reported with the use of clindamycin.

Gastrointestinal: Abdominal pain, esophagitis, nausea, vomiting and diarrhea. (See **Warning** Box)

Hypersensitivity Reactions: Maculopapular rash and urticaria have been observed during drug therapy. Generalized mild to moderate morbilliform-like skin rashes are the most frequently reported of all adverse reactions. Rare instances of erythema multiforme, some resembling Stevens-Johnson syndrome, have been associated with clindamycin. A few cases of anaphylactoid reactions have been reported. If a hypersensitivity reaction occurs, the drug should be discontinued. The usual agents (epinephrine, corticosteroids, antihistamines) should be available for emergency treatment of serious reactions.

Liver: Jaundice and abnormalities in liver function tests have been observed during clindamycin therapy.

Hematopoietic: Transient neutropenia (leukopenia) and eosinophilia have been reported. Reports of agranulocytosis and thrombocytopenia have been made. No direct etiologic relationship to concurrent clindamycin therapy could be made in any of the foregoing.

Musculoskeletal: Rare instances of polyarthritis have been reported.

Dosage and Administration:
If significant diarrhea occurs during therapy, this antibiotic should be discontinued. (See **Warning** box).

Adults: *Serious infections*—150 to 300 mg every 6 hours. *More severe infections*—300 to 450 mg every 6 hours.

Children: *Serious infections*—8 to 16 mg/kg/day (4 to 8 mg/lb/day) divided into three or four equal doses. *More severe infections*—16 to 20 mg/kg/day (8 to 10 mg/lb/day) divided into three or four equal doses.

To avoid the possibility of esophageal irritation, *Cleocin HCl* Capsules (clindamycin hydrochloride) should be taken with a full glass of water.

In the treatment of anaerobic infections, *Cleocin Phosphate*™ Sterile Solution (clindamycin phosphate injection) should be used initially. This may be followed by oral therapy with *Cleocin HCl* Capsules or *Cleocin Pediatric*® Flavored Granules (clindamycin palmitate HCl) at the discretion of the physician.

In cases of β-hemolytic streptococcal infections, treatment should continue for at least 10 days.

How Supplied: *Cleocin HCl* Capsules (clindamycin hydrochloride) are available as:

75 mg Capsules. Each capsule contains clindamycin hydrochloride equivalent to 75 mg clindamycin.

Bottles of 100 *NDC 0009-0331-02*

150 mg Capsules. Each capsule contains clindamycin hydrochloride equivalent to 150 mg clindamycin.

Bottles of 16 *NDC 0009-0225-01*
Bottles of 100 *NDC 0009-0225-02*
Unit Dose Package (100) *NDC 0009-0225-03*

Toxicology: Animal toxicity studies showed the following:

LD_{50} I.P. Administration—Mouse ....361 mg/kg
LD_{50} I.V. Administration—Mouse ....245 mg/kg
LD_{50} Oral Administration—Rat ....2,618 mg/kg

One year oral toxicity studies in Spartan Sprague-Dawley rats and Beagle dogs at levels of 30, 100 and 300 mg/kg/day (3 grams/day per dog) have shown *Cleocin HCl* to be well tolerated. No appreciable difference in pathological findings has been obtained in *Cleocin HCl* treated groups of animals from comparable control groups. Rats receiving *Cleocin HCl* Capsules (clindamycin hydrochloride) at 600 mg/kg/day for six months tolerated the drug well; however, dogs dosed at this level vomited, would not eat, and lost weight.

Code 810 570 005

[*Shown in Product Identification Section*]

*Product of The Upjohn Manufacturing Company

Cleocin HCl and *Cleocin Phosphate* are trademarks of The Upjohn Manufacturing Company.
Cleocin and *Cleocin Pediatric* are registered trademarks of The Upjohn Manufacturing Company.

CLEOCIN PEDIATRIC® ℞ *

Flavored Granules
(clindamycin palmitate HCl for oral solution, USP)
Not for Injection

WARNING

Clindamycin therapy has been associated with severe colitis which may end fatally. Therefore, it should be reserved for serious infections where less toxic antimicrobial agents are inappropriate, as described in the Indications Section. It should not be used in patients with nonbacterial infections, such as most upper respiratory tract infections. Studies indicate a toxin(s) produced by *Clostridia* is one primary cause of antibiotic associated colitis. Cholestyramine and colestipol resins have been shown to bind the toxin *in vitro.* See WARNINGS section. The colitis is usually characterized by severe, persistent diarrhea and severe abdominal cramps and may be associated with the passage of blood and mucus. Endoscopic examination may reveal pseudomembranous colitis.

When significant diarrhea occurs, the drug should be discontinued or, if necessary, continued only with close observation of the patient. Large bowel endoscopy has been recommended.

Antiperistaltic agents such as opiates and diphenoxylate with atropine (Lomotil) may prolong and/or worsen the condition. Vancomycin has been found to be effective in the treatment of antibiotic associated pseudomembranous colitis produced by *Clostridium difficile.* The usual adult dosage is 500 milligrams to 2 grams of vancomycin orally per day in three to four di-

Continued on next page

Upjohn—Cont.

vided doses administered for 7 to 10 days. Cholestyramine or colestipol resins bind vancomycin *in vitro*. If both a resin and vancomycin are to be administered concurrently, it may be advisable to separate the time of administration of each drug. Diarrhea, colitis, and pseudomembranous colitis have been observed to begin up to several weeks following cessation of therapy with clindamycin.

Description: *Cleocin Pediatric* Flavored Granules contain clindamycin palmitate hydrochloride for reconstitution. Each 5 ml contains the equivalent of 75 mg clindamycin. Clindamycin palmitate hydrochloride is a water soluble hydrochloride salt of the ester of clindamycin and palmitic acid. Clindamycin is a semi-synthetic antibiotic produced by a 7(S)-chloro-substitution of the 7(R)-hydroxyl group of the parent compound lincomycin.

Actions:

Microbiology: Although clindamycin palmitate HCl is inactive *in vitro*, rapid *in vivo* hydrolysis converts this compound to the antibacterially active clindamycin.

Clindamycin has been shown to have *in vitro* activity against isolates of the following organisms:

Aerobic gram positive cocci, including:

Staphylococcus aureus
Staphylococcus epidermidis
(penicillinase and non-penicillinase producing strains). When tested by *in vitro* methods some staphylococcal strains originally resistant to erythromycin rapidly develop resistance to clindamycin.
Streptococci (except *S. faecalis*)
Pneumococci

Anaerobic gram negative bacilli, including:

Bacteroides species (including *Bacteroides fragilis* group and *Bacteroides melaninogenicus* group)
Fusobacterium species

Anaerobic gram positive nonsporeforming bacilli, including:

Propionibacterium
Eubacterium
Actinomyces species

Anaerobic and microaerophilic gram positive cocci, including:

Peptococcus species
Peptostreptococcus species
Microaerophilic streptococci

Clostridia: Clostridia are more resistant than most anaerobes to clindamycin. Most *Clostridium perfringens* are susceptible, but other species, eg, *Clostridium sporogenes* and *Clostridium tertium* are frequently resistant to clindamycin. Susceptibility testing should be done.

Cross resistance has been demonstrated between clindamycin and lincomycin.

Antagonism has been demonstrated between clindamycin and erythromycin.

Human Pharmacology: Blood level studies comparing clindamycin palmitate HCl with clindamycin hydrochloride show that both products reach their peak active serum levels at the same time, indicating a rapid hydrolysis of the palmitate to the clindamycin.

Clindamycin is widely distributed in body fluids and tissues (including bones). Approximately 10% of the biological activity is excreted in the urine. The average biological half-life after doses of *Cleocin Pediatric* is approximately two hours in children.

Serum half-life of clindamycin is increased slightly in patients with markedly reduced renal function. Hemodialysis and peritoneal dialysis do not appreciably affect the half-life of clindamycin in the serum.

Serum level studies with clindamycin palmitate HCl in normal children weighing 50-100 lbs given 2, 3 or 4 mg/kg every 6 hours (8, 12 or 16 mg/kg/day) demonstrated mean peak clindamycin serum levels of 1.24, 2.25 and 2.44 mcg/ml respectively, one hour after the first dose. By the fifth dose, the 6-hour serum concentration had reached equilibrium. Peak serum concentrations after this time would be about 2.46, 2.98 and 3.79 mcg/ml with doses of 8, 12, 16 mg/kg/day, respectively. Serum levels have been uniform and predictable from person to person and dose to dose. Multiple-dose studies in newborns and infants up to 6 months of age show that the drug does not accumulate in the serum and is excreted rapidly. Serum levels exceed the MICs for most indicated organisms for at least six hours following administration of the usually recommended doses of *Cleocin Pediatric* in adults and children.

No significant levels of clindamycin are attained in the cerebrospinal fluid, even in the presence of inflamed meninges.

Indications: *Cleocin Pediatric* Flavored Granules (clindamycin palmitate HCl) is indicated in the treatment of serious infections caused by susceptible anaerobic bacteria.

Clindamycin is also indicated in the treatment of serious infections due to susceptible strains of streptococci, pneumococci, and staphylococci. Its use should be reserved for penicillin-allergic patients or other patients for whom, in the judgment of the physician, a penicillin is inappropriate. Because of the risk of colitis, as described in the WARNING box, before selecting clindamycin the physician should consider the nature of the infection and the suitability of less toxic alternatives (eg, erythromycin).

Anaerobes: Serious respiratory tract infections such as empyema, anaerobic pneumonitis and lung abscess; serious skin and soft tissue infections; septicemia; intra-abdominal infections such as peritonitis and intra-abdominal abscess (typically resulting from anaerobic organisms resident in the normal gastrointestinal tract); infections of the female pelvis and genital tract such as endometritis, nongonococcal tubo-ovarian abscess, pelvic cellulitis and postsurgical vaginal cuff infection.

Streptococci: Serious respiratory tract infections; serious skin and soft tissue infections.

Staphylococci: Serious respiratory tract infections; serious skin and soft tissue infections.

Pneumococci: Serious respiratory tract infections.

Bacteriologic studies should be performed to determine the causative organisms and their susceptibility to clindamycin.

In Vitro Susceptibility Testing: A standardized disk testing procedure* is recommended for determining susceptibility of aerobic bacteria to clindamycin. A description is contained in the *Cleocin*® Susceptibility Disk (clindamycin) insert. Using this method, the laboratory can designate isolates as resistant, intermediate, or susceptible. Tube or agar dilution methods may be used for both anaerobic and aerobic bacteria. When the directions in the *Cleocin* Susceptibility Powder insert are followed, an MIC (minimal inhibitory concentration) of 1.6 mcg/ml may be considered susceptible; MICs of 1.6 to 4.8 mcg/ml may be considered intermediate and MICs greater than 4.8 mcg/ml may be considered resistant.

Cleocin Susceptibility Disks 2 mcg. See package insert for use.

Cleocin Susceptibility Powder 20 mg. See package insert for use.

For anaerobic bacteria the minimal inhibitory concentration (MIC) of clindamycin can be determined by agar dilution and broth dilution (including microdilution) techniques. If MICs are not determined routinely, the disk broth method is recommended for routine use. THE KIRBY-BAUER DISK DIFFUSION METHOD AND ITS INTERPRETIVE STANDARDS ARE NOT RECOMMENDED FOR ANAEROBES.

*Bauer, AW, Kirby, WMM, Sherris, JC, Turck, M.: Antibiotic susceptibility testing by a standardized single disc method, *Am J Clin Path*, **45**:493-496, 1966. Standardized Disc Susceptibility Test, *Federal Register* **37**:20527-29, 1972.

Contraindications: This drug is contraindicated in individuals with a history of hypersensitivity to preparations containing clindamycin or lincomycin.

Warnings:

See WARNING box. Studies indicate a toxin(s) produced by *Clostridia* is one primary cause of antibiotic associated colitis.[1–5] Cholestyramine and colestipol resins have been shown to bind the toxin *in vitro*. Mild cases of colitis may respond to drug discontinuance alone. Moderate to severe cases should be managed promptly with fluid, electrolyte and protein supplementation as indicated. Vancomycin has been found to be effective in the treatment of antibiotic associated pseudomembranous colitis produced by *Clostridium difficile*. The usual adult dosage is 500 milligrams to 2 grams of vancomycin orally per day in three to four divided doses administered for 7 to 10 days. Cholestyramine or colestipol resins bind vancomycin *in vitro*. If both a resin and vancomycin are to be administered concurrently, it may be advisable to separate the time of administration of each drug. Systemic corticoids and corticoid retention enemas may help relieve the colitis. Other causes of colitis should also be considered.

A careful inquiry should be made concerning previous sensitivities to drugs and other allergens.

Usage in Pregnancy—Safety for use in pregnancy has not been established.

Usage in Newborns and Infants: When *Cleocin Pediatric* Flavored Granules (clindamycin palmitate HCl) are administered to newborns and infants, appropriate monitoring of organ system functions is desirable.

Nursing Mothers—Clindamycin has been reported to appear in breast milk in ranges of 0.7 to 3.8 mcg/ml.

Usage in Meningitis: Since clindamycin does not diffuse adequately into the cerebrospinal fluid, the drug should not be used in the treatment of meningitis.

Antagonism has been demonstrated between clindamycin and erythromycin *in vitro*. Because of possible clinical significance, these two drugs should not be administered concurrently.

1. Bartlett JG, et al: Antibiotic associated Pseudomembranous Colitis Due to Toxin-producing *Clostridia*. *N Engl J Med* 298(10):531-534, 1978.
2. George RH, et al: Identification of *Clostridium difficile* as a cause of Pseudomembranous Colitis. *Br Med J* 6114:669-671, 1978.
3. Larson HE, Price AB: Pseudomembranous Colitis Presence of Clostridial Toxin. *Lancet* 8052/3:1312-1314, 1977.
4. Rifkin GD, Fekety FR, Silva J: Antibiotic-induced Colitis Implication of a Toxin Neutralized by *Clostridium sordellii* Antitoxin. *Lancet* 8048:1103-1106, 1977.
5. Bailey WR, Scott EG: Diagnostic Microbiology. The CV Mosby Company, St. Louis, 1978.

Precautions: Review of experience to date suggests that a subgroup of older patients with associated severe illness may tolerate diarrhea less well. When clindamycin is indicated in these patients, they should be carefully monitored for change in bowel frequency.

Cleocin Pediatric Flavored Granules (clindamycin palmitate HCl) should be prescribed with caution in individuals with a history of gastrointestinal disease, particularly colitis.

Cleocin Pediatric should be prescribed with caution in atopic individuals.

During prolonged therapy periodic liver and kidney function tests and blood counts should be performed.

Indicated surgical procedures should be performed in conjunction with antibiotic therapy.
The use of *Cleocin Pediatric* may result in overgrowth of nonsusceptible organisms—particularly yeasts. Should superinfections occur, appropriate measures should be taken as indicated by the clinical situation.
Patients with very severe renal disease and/or very severe hepatic disease accompanied by severe metabolic aberrations should be dosed with caution, and serum clindamycin levels monitored during high-dose therapy.
Clindamycin has been shown to have neuromuscular blocking properties that may enhance the action of other neuromuscular blocking agents. Therefore, it should be used with caution in patients receiving such agents.

Adverse Reactions: The following reactions have been reported with the use of clindamycin.

Gastrointestinal: Abdominal pain, nausea, vomiting and diarrhea. (See **Warning** box)

Hypersensitivity Reactions: Maculopapular rash and urticaria have been observed during drug therapy. Generalized mild to moderate morbilliform-like skin rashes are the most frequently reported of all adverse reactions. Rare instances of erythema multiforme, some resembling Stevens-Johnson syndrome, have been associated with clindamycin. A few cases of anaphylactoid reactions have been reported. If a hypersensitivity reaction occurs, the drug should be discontinued. The usual agents (epinephrine, corticosteroids, antihistamines) should be available for emergency treatment of serious reactions.

Liver: Jaundice and abnormalities in liver function tests have been observed during clindamycin therapy.

Hematopoietic: Transient neutropenia (leukopenia) and eosinophilia have been reported. Reports of agranulocytosis and thrombocytopenia have been made. No direct etiologic relationship to concurrent clindamycin therapy could be made in any of the foregoing.

Musculoskeletal: Rare instances of polyarthritis have been reported.

Dosage and Administration: If significant diarrhea occurs during therapy, this antibiotic should be discontinued. (See **Warning** box.)
Concomitant administration of food does not adversely affect the absorption of clindamycin palmitate HCl.
Serious infections: 8-12 mg/kg/day (4-6 mg/lb/day) divided into 3 or 4 equal doses.
Severe infections: 13-16 mg/kg/day (6.5-8 mg/lb/day) divided into 3 or 4 equal doses.
More severe infections: 17-25 mg/kg/day (8.5-12.5 mg/lb/day) divided into 3 or 4 equal doses.
In children weighing 10 kg or less, ½ teaspoon (37.5 mg) three times a day should be considered the minimum recommended dose.
In the treatment of anaerobic infections, *Cleocin Phosphate*™ Sterile Solution (clindamycin phosphate) should be used initially. This may be followed by oral therapy with *Cleocin Pediatric* or *Cleocin HCl*™ Capsules (clindamycin HCl) at the discretion of the physician.
NOTE: In cases of β-hemolytic streptococcal infections, treatment should be continued for at least 10 days.

Reconstitution instructions:
When reconstituted with water as follows, each 5 ml (teaspoon) of solution contains clindamycin palmitate HCl equivalent to 75 mg clindamycin.
Reconstitute bottles of 100 ml with **75 ml** of water. Add a large portion of the water and shake vigorously; add the remainder of the water and shake until the solution is uniform.

Storage conditions:
Store unreconstituted product at controlled room temperature 15°-30°C (59°-86°F).
Do **NOT** refrigerate the reconstituted solution; when chilled, the solution may thicken and be difficult to pour. The solution is stable for 2 weeks at room temperature.

How Supplied: *Cleocin Pediatric* Flavored Granules (clindamycin palmitate HCl for oral solution) is available as follows:
100 ml bottles *NDC 0009-0760-04*
When reconstituted as directed, each bottle yields a solution containing 75 mg of clindamycin per 5 ml.
Code 810 568 005
*Product of The Upjohn Manufacturing Company
Cleocin Pediatric and *Cleocin* are registered trademarks of The Upjohn Manufacturing Company.
Cleocin Phosphate and *Cleocin HCl* are trademarks of The Upjohn Manufacturing Company.

CLEOCIN PHOSPHATE™ ℞ *

Sterile Solution
(clindamycin phosphate injection, USP)
For Intramuscular and Intravenous Use

2 ml ampoule:
NSN 6505-00-138-8474 (M&VA)
4 ml ampoule:
NSN 6505-00-139-1318 (M&VA)

WARNING

Clindamycin therapy has been associated with severe colitis which may end fatally. Therefore, it should be reserved for serious infections where less toxic antimicrobial agents are inappropriate, as described in the Indications Section. It should not be used in patients with nonbacterial infections, such as most upper respiratory tract infections. Studies indicate a toxin(s) produced by *Clostridia* is one primary cause of antibiotic associated colitis. Cholestyramine and colestipol resins have been shown to bind the toxin *in vitro.* See WARNINGS section. The colitis is usually characterized by severe, persistent diarrhea and severe abdominal cramps and may be associated with the passage of blood and mucus. Endoscopic examination may reveal pseudomembranous colitis.
When significant diarrhea occurs, the drug should be discontinued or, if necessary, continued only with close observation of the patient. Large bowel endoscopy has been recommended.
Antiperistaltic agents such as opiates and diphenoxylate with atropine (Lomotil) may prolong and/or worsen the condition. Vancomycin has been found to be effective in the treatment of antibiotic associated pseudomembranous colitis produced by *Clostridium difficile.* The usual adult dosage is 500 milligrams to 2 grams of vancomycin orally per day in three to four divided doses administered for 7 to 10 days. Cholestyramine or colestipol resins bind vancomycin *in vitro.* If both a resin and vancomycin are to be administered concurrently, it may be advisable to separate the time of administration of each drug.
Diarrhea, colitis, and pseudomembranous colitis have been observed to begin up to several weeks following cessation of therapy with clindamycin.

Description: *Cleocin Phosphate* Sterile Solution contains clindamycin phosphate, a water soluble ester of clindamycin and phosphoric acid. Each ml contains the equivalent of 150 mg clindamycin, 0.5 mg disodium edetate and 9.45 mg benzyl alcohol added as preservative in each ml. Clindamycin is a semi synthetic antibiotic produced by a 7(S)-chloro-substitution of the 7(R)-hydroxyl group of the parent compound lincomycin.

Actions:

Microbiology: Although clindamycin phosphate is inactive *in vitro,* rapid *in vivo* hydrolysis converts this compound to the antibacterially active clindamycin.
Clindamycin has been shown to have *in vitro* activity against isolates of the following organisms:

Aerobic gram positive cocci, including:
Staphylococcus aureus
Staphylococcus epidermidis
(penicillinase and nonpenicillinase producing strains). When tested by *in vitro* methods some staphylococcal strains originally resistant to erythromycin rapidly develop resistance to clindamycin.
Streptococci (except *S. faecalis*)
Pneumococci

Anaerobic gram negative bacilli, including:
Bacteroides species (including *Bacteroides fragilis* group and *Bacteroides melaninogenicus* group)
Fusobacterium species

Anaerobic gram positive nonsporeforming bacilli, including:
Propionibacterium
Eubacterium
Actinomyces species

Anaerobic and microaerophilic gram positive cocci, including:
Peptococcus species
Peptostreptococcus species
Microaerophilic streptococci
Clostridia: Clostridia are more resistant than most anaerobes to clindamycin. Most *Clostridium perfringens* are susceptible, but other species, eg, *Clostridium sporogenes* and *Clostridium Tertium* are frequently resistant to clindamycin. Susceptibility testing should be done.
Cross resistance has been demonstrated between clindamycin and lincomycin.
Antagonism has been demonstrated between clindamycin and erythromycin.

Human Pharmacology:
Biologically inactive clindamycin phosphate is rapidly converted to active clindamycin.
By the end of short-term intravenous infusion, peak serum levels of active clindamycin are reached. Biologically inactive clindamycin phosphate disappears rapidly from the serum; the average disappearance half-life is 6 minutes; however, the serum disappearance half-life of active clindamycin is about 3 hours in adults and 2 ½ hours in children.
After intramuscular injection of clindamycin phosphate, peak levels of active clindamycin are reached within 3 hours in adults and 1 hour in children. Serum level curves may be constructed from IV peak serum levels as given in Table 1 by application of disappearance half-lives listed above.
Serum levels of clindamycin can be maintained above the *in vitro* minimum inhibitory concentrations for most indicated organisms by administration of clindamycin phosphate every 8-12 hours in adults and every 6-8 hours in children, or by continuous intravenous infusion. An equilibrium state is reached by the third dose.
The disappearance half-life of clindamycin is increased slightly in patients with markedly reduced renal or hepatic function. Hemodialysis and peritoneal dialysis are not effective in removing clindamycin from the serum. Dosage schedules need not be modified in the presence of mild or moderate renal or hepatic disease.
No significant levels of clindamycin are attained in the cerebrospinal fluid, even in the presence of inflamed meninges.
Serum assays for active clindamycin require an inhibitor to prevent *in vitro* hydrolysis of clindamycin phosphate.
[See table on next page].

Indications: *Cleocin Phosphate* Sterile Solution (clindamycin phosphate) is indicated in the treatment of serious infections caused by susceptible anaerobic bacteria.
Cleocin Phosphate is also indicated in the treatment of serious infections due to suscepti-

Continued on next page

Upjohn—Cont.

ble strains of streptococci, pneumococci, and staphylococci. Its use should be reserved for penicillin-allergic patients or other patients for whom, in the judgment of the physician, a penicillin is inappropriate. Because of the risk of colitis, as described in the WARNING box, before selecting clindamycin the physician should consider the nature of the infection and the suitability of less toxic alternatives (e.g., erythromycin).

Anaerobes: Serious respiratory tract infections such as empyema, anaerobic pneumonitis and lung abscess; serious skin and soft tissue infections; septicemia; intra-abdominal infections such as peritonitis and intra-abdominal abscess (typically resulting from anaerobic organisms resident in the normal gastrointestinal tract); infections of the female pelvis and genital tract such as endometritis, nongonococcal tubo-ovarian abscess, pelvic cellulitis and postsurgical vaginal cuff infection.

Streptococci: Serious respiratory tract infections; serious skin and soft tissue infections; septicemia.

Staphylococci: Serious respiratory tract infections; serious skin and soft tissue infections; septicemia; acute hematogenous osteomyelitis.

Pneumococci: Serious respiratory tract infections.

Adjunctive Therapy: In the surgical treatment of chronic bone and joint infections due to susceptible organisms.

Indicated surgical procedures should be performed in conjunction with antibiotic therapy.

Bacteriologic studies should be performed to determine the causative organisms and their susceptibility to clindamycin.

In Vitro Susceptibility Testing: A standardized disk testing procedure*** is recommended for determining susceptibility of aerobic bacteria to clindamycin. A description is contained in the *Cleocin®* Susceptibility Disk (clindamycin) insert. Using this method, the laboratory can designate isolates as resistant, intermediate, or susceptible. Tube or agar dilution methods may be used for both anaerobic and aerobic bacteria. When the directions in the *Cleocin* Susceptibility Powder insert are followed, an MIC (minimal inhibitory concentration) of 1.6 mcg/ml may be considered susceptible; MICs of 1.6 to 4.8 mcg/ml may be considered intermediate and MICs greater than 4.8 mcg/ml may be considered resistant.

Cleocin Susceptibility Disks 2 mcg. See package insert for use.

Cleocin Susceptibility Powder 20 mg. See package insert for use.

For anaerobic bacteria the minimal inhibitory concentration (MIC) of clindamycin can be determined by agar dilution and broth dilution (including microdilution) techniques. If MICs are not determined routinely, the disk broth method is recommended for routine use. The KIRBY-BAUER DISK DIFFUSION METHOD AND ITS INTERPRETIVE STANDARDS ARE NOT RECOMMENDED FOR ANAEROBES.

***Bauer, AW, Kirby, WMM, Sherris, JC, Turck, M: Antibiotic susceptibility testing by a standardized single disc method, *Am J Clin Path*, **45**:493-496, 1966. Standardized Disc Susceptibility Test, *Federal Register* **37**:20527-29, 1972.

Contraindications: This drug is contraindicated in individuals with a history of hypersensitivity to preparations containing clindamycin or lincomycin.

Warnings:

See WARNING box. Studies indicate a toxin(s) produced by *Clostridia* is one primary cause of antibiotic associated colitis.[1–5] Cholestyramine and colestipol resins have been shown to bind the toxin *in vitro*. Mild cases of colitis may respond to drug discontinuance alone. Moderate to severe cases should be managed promptly with fluid, electrolyte and protein supplementation as indicated. Vancomycin has been found to be effective in the treatment of antibiotic associated pseudomembranous colitis produced by *Clostridium difficile*. The usual adult dosage is 500 milligrams to 2 grams of vancomycin orally per day in three to four divided doses administered for 7 to 10 days. Cholestyramine or colestipol resins bind vancomycin *in vitro*. If both a resin and vancomycin are to be administered concurrently, it may be advisable to separate the time of administration of each drug. Systemic corticoids and corticoid retention enemas may help relieve the colitis. Other causes of colitis should also be considered.

A careful inquiry should be made concerning previous sensitivities to drugs and other allergens.

Usage in Pregnancy—Safety for use in pregnancy has not been established.

Usage in Newborns and infants: When *Cleocin Phosphate* Sterile Solution (clindamycin phosphate) is administered to newborns and infants, appropriate monitoring of organ system functions is desirable.

Nursing Mothers—Clindamycin has been reported to appear in breast milk in ranges of 0.7 to 3.8 mcg/ml.

Usage in Meningitis: Since clindamycin does not diffuse adequately into the cerebrospinal fluid, the drug should not be used in the treatment of meningitis.

Antagonism has been demonstrated between clindamycin and erythromycin *in vitro*. Because of possible clinical significance, these two drugs should not be administered concurrently.

SERIOUS ANAPHYLACTOID REACTIONS REQUIRE IMMEDIATE EMERGENCY TREATMENT WITH EPINEPHRINE. OXYGEN AND INTRAVENOUS CORTICOSTEROIDS SHOULD ALSO BE ADMINISTERED AS INDICATED.

1. Bartlett JG, et al: Antibiotic associated Pseudomembranous Colitis Due to Toxin-producing *Clostridia*. *N Engl J Med* 298(10):531-534, 1978.
2. George RH, et al: Identification of *Clostridium difficile* as a cause of Pseudomembranous Colitis. *Br Med J* 6114:669-671, 1978.
3. Larson HE, Price AB: Pseudomembranous Colitis Presence of Clostridial Toxin. *Lancet* 8052/3:1312-1314, 1977.
4. Rifkin GD, Fekety FR, Silva J: Antibiotic-induced Colitis Implication of a Toxin Neutralized by *Clostridium sordellii* Antitoxin. *Lancet* 8048:1103-1106, 1977.
5. Bailey WR, Scott EG: Diagnostic Microbiology. The CV Mosby Company, St. Louis, 1978.

Precautions: Review of experience to date suggests that a subgroup of older patients with associated severe illness may tolerate diarrhea less well. When clindamycin is indicated in these patients, they should be carefully monitored for change in bowel frequency.

Cleocin Phosphate Sterile Solution (clindamycin phosphate) should be prescribed with caution in individuals with a history of gastrointestinal disease, particularly colitis.

Cleocin Phosphate should be prescribed with caution in atopic individuals.

During prolonged therapy periodic liver and kidney function tests and blood counts should be performed.

Indicated surgical procedures should be performed in conjunction with antibiotic therapy.

The use of *Cleocin Phosphate* may result in overgrowth of nonsusceptible organisms—particularly yeasts. Should superinfections occur, appropriate measures should be taken as indicated by the clinical situation.

Cleocin Phosphate should not be injected intravenously undiluted as a bolus, but should be infused over at least 10-60 minutes as directed in the **Dosage and Administration** Section.

Patients with very severe renal disease and/or very severe hepatic disease accompanied by severe metabolic aberrations should be dosed with caution, and serum clindamycin levels monitored during high-dose therapy.

Clindamycin has been shown to have neuromuscular blocking properties that may enhance the action of other neuromuscular blocking agents. Therefore, it should be used with caution in patients receiving such agents.

Adverse Reactions: The following reactions have been reported with the use of clindamycin.

Gastrointestinal: Abdominal pain, nausea, vomiting and diarrhea (See **Warning** box).

Hypersensitivity Reactions: Maculopapular rash and urticaria have been observed during drug therapy. Generalized mild to moderate morbilliform-like skin rashes are the most frequently reported of all adverse reactions. Rare instances of erythema multiforme, some resembling Stevens-Johnson syndrome, have been associated with clindamycin. A few cases of anaphylactoid reactions have been reported. If a hypersensitivity reaction occurs, the drug should be discontinued. The usual agents (epinephrine, corticosteroids, antihistamines) should be available for emergency treatment of serious reactions.

Liver: Jaundice and abnormalities in liver function tests have been observed during clindamycin therapy.

Hematopoietic: Transient neutropenia (leukopenia) and eosinophilia have been reported. Reports of agranulocytosis and thrombocytopenia have been made. No direct etiologic relationship to concurrent clindamycin therapy could be made in any of the foregoing.

Local Reactions: Pain, induration and sterile abscess have been reported after intramuscular injection and thrombophlebitis after intravenous infusion. Reactions can be minimized or avoided by giving deep intramuscular injec-

Table 1. Average Peak Serum Concentrations After Dosing with Clindamycin Phosphate

Dosage Regimen	Clindamycin mcg/ml	Clindamycin Phosphate mcg/ml
Healthy Adult Males (Post equilibrium)		
300 mg IV in 10 min, q8h	7	15
600 mg IV in 20 min, q8h	10	23
900 mg IV in 30 min, q12h	11	29
1200 mg IV in 45 min, q12h	14	49
300 mg IM q8h	6	3
600 mg IM q12h**	9	3
Children (first dose)**		
5-7 mg/kg IV in 1 hr	10	
3-5 mg/kg IM	4	
5-7 mg/kg IM	8	

**Data in this group from patients being treated for infection

tions and avoiding prolonged use of indwelling intravenous catheters.
Musculoskeletal: Rare instances of polyarthritis have been reported.
Cardiovascular: Rare instances of cardiopulmonary arrest and hypotension have been reported following too rapid intravenous administration. (See Dosage and Administration Section)

Dosage and Administration:
If significant diarrhea occurs during therapy, this antibiotic should be discontinued. (See **Warning** box).

Adults
Parenteral (IM or IV Administration):
Serious infections due to aerobic gram-positive cocci and the more sensitive anaerobes (NOT generally including *Bacteroides fragilis, Peptococcus* species and *Clostridium* species other than *Clostridium perfringens*):
600–1200 mg/day in 2, 3 or 4 equal doses
More severe infections, particularly those due to proven or suspected *Bacteroides fragilis, Peptococcus* species, or *Clostridium* species other than *Clostridium perfringens:*
1200–2700 mg/day in 2, 3 or 4 equal doses
For more serious infections, these doses may have to be increased. In life threatening situations due to aerobes or anaerobes, these doses may be increased. Doses of as much as 4800 mg daily have been given intravenously to adults. See **Dilution and Infusion Rates** section below.
Alternatively, drug may be administered in the form of a single rapid infusion of the first dose followed by continuous IV infusion as follows:
[See table above].

Children (over 1 month of age)
Parenteral (IM or IV Administration):
Serious infections:
15–25 mg/kg/day in 3 or 4 equal doses
More severe infections:
25–40 mg/kg/day in 3 or 4 equal doses
As an alternative to dosing on a body weight basis, children may be dosed on the basis of square meters body surface: 350 mg/m^2/day for serious infections and 450 mg/m^2/day for more severe infections.
In severe infections it is recommended that children be given no less than 300 mg/day regardless of body weight.
Parenteral therapy may be changed to oral clindamycin (Pediatric or HCl) when the condition warrants and at the discretion of the physician.
In cases of β-hemolytic streptococcal infections, treatment should be continued for at least 10 days.

Dilution and Infusion Rates
Single IM injections of greater than 600 mg are not recommended. **Clindamycin phosphate must be diluted prior to IV administration to a dilution of 300 mg in 50 ml or more of diluent and infused at a rate of not more than 30 mg per minute as indicated below.** Infusion rates are as follows:

Dose	*Diluent*	*Time*
300 mg	50 ml	10 min
600 mg	100 ml	20 min
900 mg	150 ml	30 min
1200 mg	200 ml	45 min

Administration of more than 1200 mg in a single 1-hour infusion is not recommended.

Dilution and Compatibility
Physical and biological compatibility studies monitored for 24 hours at room temperature have demonstrated no inactivation or incompatibility with the use of *Cleocin Phosphate* Sterile Solution (clindamycin phosphate) in IV solutions containing NaCl, glucose, calcium or potassium and solutions containing vitamin B complex in concentrations usually used clinically. No incompatibility has been demonstrated with the antibiotics cephalothin, kanamycin, gentamicin, penicillin or carbenicillin.
The following drugs are physically incompatible with *Cleocin Phosphate:* ampicillin, phenytoin sodium, barbiturates, aminophylline, calcium gluconate, and magnesium sulfate.

To maintain serum clindamycin levels	Rapid infusion rate	Maintenance infusion rate
Above 4 mcg/ml	10 mg/min for 30 min	0.75 mg/min
Above 5 mcg/ml	15 mg/min for 30 min	1.00 mg/min
Above 6 mcg/ml	20 mg/min for 30 min	1.25 mg/min

How Supplied: Each ml of *Cleocin Phosphate* Sterile Solution contains clindamycin phosphate equivalent to 150 mg clindamycin; 0.5 mg disodium edetate; 9.45 mg benzyl alcohol added as preservative. When necessary, pH is adjusted with sodium hydroxide and/or hydrochloric acid.
The following sizes are available:

2 ml ampoule (300 mg)
25-pack *NDC 0009-0870-17*
100-pack *NDC 0009-0870-03*
4 ml ampoule (600 mg)
25-pack *NDC 0009-0775-16*
100-pack *NDC 0009-0775-03*
Code 810 020 108
[*Shown in Product Identification Section*]
*Product of The Upjohn Manufacturing Company
Cleocin Phosphate is a trademark of The Upjohn Manufacturing Company.
Cleocin is a registered trademark of The Upjohn Manufacturing Company.

CLEOCIN T™ Topical Solution ℞
(clindamycin phosphate topical solution, USP)
For External Use •
60 ml bottle
NSN 6505-01-116-5655 (M & VA)

Description: *Cleocin T* Topical Solution contains clindamycin phosphate, USP, at a concentration equivalent to 10 mg clindamycin per milliliter in an isopropyl alcohol and water solution.
Clindamycin phosphate is a water soluble ester of the semi-synthetic antibiotic produced by a 7(S)-chloro-substitution of the 7(R)-hydroxy group of the parent antibiotic lincomycin.
The solution contains isopropyl alcohol 50% v/v, propylene glycol, and water.
Clinical Pharmacology: Although clindamycin phosphate is inactive *in vitro*, rapid *in vivo* hydrolysis converts this compound to the antibacterially active clindamycin.
Clindamycin has been shown to have *in vivo* activity against isolates of *Propionibacterium acnes.* This may account for its usefulness in acne.
Cross resistance has been demonstrated between clindamycin and lincomycin.
Antagonism has been demonstrated between clindamycin and erythromycin.
Studies of penetration into human skin with radiolabelled clindamycin have shown that approximately 10% of the dose is absorbed as indicated by concentration in the stratum corneum. Microbiological assay of urine has shown varying concentrations of clindamycin.
Clindamycin activity has been demonstrated in comedonal extracts from acne patients. The mean concentration of antibiotic activity in comedonal extracts was 1.4 mcg/ml. Clindamycin *in vitro* inhibits all *Propionibacterium acnes* cultures tested (MICs 0.4 mcg/ml). Free fatty acids on the skin surface have been decreased from approximately 14% to 2% following application of clindamycin.
Indications: *Cleocin T* Topical Solution (clindamycin phosphate) is indicated in the treatment of acne vulgaris. In view of the potential for diarrhea, bloody diarrhea and pseudomembranous colitis, the physician should consider whether other agents are more appropriate. (See Contraindications, Warnings and Adverse Reactions).
Contraindications: *Cleocin T* Topical Solution (clindamycin phosphate) is contraindicated in individuals with a history of hypersensitivity to preparations containing clindamycin or lincomycin, a history of regional enteritis or ulcerative colitis, or a history of antibiotic-associated colitis.
Warnings: Orally and parenterally administered clindamycin has been associated with severe colitis which may end fatally. Use of the topical formulation results in absorption of the antibiotic from the skin surface. Diarrhea, bloody diarrhea, and colitis (including pseudomembranous colitis) have been reported with the use of topical and systemic clindamycin. Symptoms can occur after a few days, weeks or months following initiation of clindamycin therapy. They have also been observed to begin up to several weeks after cessation of therapy with clindamycin. Studies indicate a toxin(s) produced by *Clostridium difficile* is one primary cause of antibiotic-associated colitis. The colitis is usually characterized by severe persistent diarrhea and severe abdominal cramps and may be associated with the passage of blood and mucus. Endoscopic examination may reveal pseudomembranous colitis. When significant diarrhea occurs, the drug should be discontinued. Large bowel endoscopy should be considered in cases of severe diarrhea.
Antiperistaltic agents such as opiates and diphenoxylate with atropine (Lomotil) may prolong and/or worsen the condition. Vancomycin has been found to be effective in the treatment of antibiotic-associated pseudomembranous colitis produced by *Clostridium difficile.* The usual adult dosage is 500 mg to 2 grams of vancomycin orally per day in three to four divided doses administered for 7 to 10 days.
Mild cases of colitis may respond to discontinuance of clindamycin. Moderate to severe cases should be managed promptly with fluid, electrolyte, and protein supplementation as indicated. Cholestyramine and colestipol resins have been shown to bind the toxin *in vitro.* If both a resin and vancomycin are to be administered concurrently, it may be advisable to separate the time of administration of each drug. Systemic corticoids and corticoid retention enemas may help relieve the colitis. Other causes of colitis should also be considered. A careful inquiry should be made concerning previous sensitivities to drugs and other allergens.
Precautions: *Cleocin T* Topical Solution (clindamycin phosphate) contains an alcohol base which will cause burning and irritation of the eye. In the event of accidental contact with sensitive surfaces (eye, abraded skin, mucous membranes), bathe with copious amounts of cool tap water. The solution has an unpleasant taste and caution should be exercised when applying medication around the mouth.
Cleocin T Topical Solution should be prescribed with caution in atopic individuals.

Pregnancy Category B
Reproduction studies have been performed in rats and mice using subcutaneous and oral doses of clindamycin ranging from 100 to 600 mg/kg/day and have revealed no evidence of impaired fertility or harm to the fetus due to clindamycin. There are, however, no adequate and well-controlled studies in pregnant women. Because animal reproduction studies are not always predictive of human response, this drug should be used during pregnancy only if clearly needed.

Nursing Mothers
It is not known whether clindamycin is excreted in human milk following use of

Continued on next page

Upjohn—Cont.

Cleocin T Topical Solution. However, orally and parenterally administered clindamycin has been reported to appear in breast milk. As a general rule, nursing should not be undertaken while a patient is on a drug since many drugs are excreted in human milk.

Adverse Reactions: Gastrointestinal reactions are the most frequently reported adverse reactions.

Clindamycin has been associated with severe colitis which may end fatally (See WARNINGS).

Cases of diarrhea, bloody diarrhea and colitis (including pseudomembranous colitis) have been reported as adverse reactions in patients treated with topical formulations of clindamycin.

Other effects which have been reported in association with the use of topical formulations of clindamycin include:

- Abdominal pain
- Contact dermatitis
- Dryness
- Fatigue
- Gram-negative folliculitis
- Headache
- Irritation
- Oily skin
- Sensitization
- Sore throat
- Stinging of the eye
- Urinary frequency

Dosage and Administration: Apply a thin film of *Cleocin T* Topical Solution (clindamycin phosphate) twice daily to affected area.

How Supplied: *Cleocin T* Topical Solution (clindamycin phosphate) is available as follows:

30 ml applicator bottle (10 mg/ml)
NDC 0009-3116-01

60 ml applicator bottle (10 mg/ml)
NDC 0009-3116-02

The applicator is designed so that the solution may be applied directly to the involved skin.

Code 811 373 107

[*Shown in Product Identification Section*]

*Product of The Upjohn Manufacturing Company

Cleocin T is a trademark of The Upjohn Manufacturing Company.

COLESTID® Granules ℞
(colestipol hydrochloride)

Description: *Colestid* Granules consist of colestipol hydrochloride, which is a hyperlipidemia agent for oral use. *Colestid* (colestipol hydrochloride), is an insoluble, high molecular weight basic anion-exchange copolymer of diethylenetriamine and 1-chloro-2,3-epoxypropane, with approximately 1 out of 5 amine nitrogens protonated (chloride form). It is a light yellow resin which is hygroscopic and swells when placed in water or aqueous fluids. *Colestid* is tasteless and odorless.

Clinical Pharmacology: Cholesterol is the major, and probably the sole precursor of bile acids. During normal digestion, bile acids are secreted via the bile from the liver and gall bladder into the intestines. Bile acids emulsify the fat and lipid materials present in food, thus facilitating absorption. A major portion of the bile acids secreted is reabsorbed from the intestines and returned via the portal circulation to the liver, thus completing the enterohepatic cycle. Only very small amounts of bile acids are found in normal serum.

Colestid Granules (colestipol hydrochloride) bind bile acids in the intestine forming a complex that is excreted in the feces. This nonsystemic action results in a partial removal of the bile acids from the enterohepatic circulation, preventing their reabsorption. Since colestipol hydrochloride is an anion exchange resin, the chloride anions of the resin can be replaced by other anions, usually those with a greater affinity for the resin than chloride ion.

Colestipol hydrochloride is hydrophilic, but it is virtually water insoluble (99.75%) and it is not hydrolyzed by digestive enzymes. The high molecular weight polymer in *Colestid* apparently is not absorbed. Less than 0.05% of ^{14}C-labeled colestipol hydrochloride is excreted in the urine.

The increased fecal loss of bile acids due to *Colestid* administration leads to an increased oxidation of cholesterol to bile acids, a decrease in beta lipoprotein or low density lipoprotein serum levels, and a decrease in serum cholesterol levels. Although *Colestid* produces an increase in the hepatic synthesis of cholesterol in man, serum cholesterol levels fall.

There is evidence to show that this fall in cholesterol is secondary to an increased rate of cholesterol rich lipoproteins (beta or low density lipoproteins) from the plasma. Serum triglyceride levels may increase or remain unchanged in colestipol treated patients.

The decline in serum cholesterol levels with treatment with *Colestid* is usually evident by one month. When *Colestid* is discontinued, serum cholesterol levels usually return to baseline levels within one month. Cholesterol may rise even with continued use of *Colestid,* and serum levels should be determined periodically to confirm that a favorable initial response is maintained.

Colestiol is more effective than clofibrate in lowering total serum cholesterol and low density lipoprotein cholesterol in Frederickson type IIa hyperlipoproteinemia (pure hypercholesterolemia without hypertriglyceridemia) without affecting high density lipoprotein cholesterol.

In patients with heterozygous familial hypercholesterolemia who have not obtained an optimal response to colestipol hydrochloride alone in maximal doses, the combination of colestipol hydrochloride and nicotinic acid has been shown to provide effective further lowering of serum cholesterol, triglyceride, and LDL cholesterol values. Simultaneously, HDL cholesterol values increased significantly. In many such patients it is possible to normalize serum lipid values.[1–3]

Indications and Usage: Since no drug is innocuous, strict attention should be paid to the indications and contraindications, particularly when selecting drugs for chronic long-term use.

Colestid Granules (colestipol hydrochloride) are indicated as adjunctive therapy to diet for the reduction of elevated serum cholesterol in patients with primary hypercholesterolemia (elevated low density lipoproteins). *Colestid* has been shown to have no effect on or to increase triglyceride levels.

It has not been established whether the drug-induced lowering of serum colesterol or triglyceride levels has a beneficial effect, no effect, or a detrimental effect on the morbidity or mortality due to atherosclerosis including coronary heart disease. Investigations now in progress may yield an answer to this question.

Contraindications: *Colestid* Granules (colestipol hydrochloride) are contraindicated in those individuals who have shown hypersensitivity to any of its components.

Warnings: TO AVOID ACCIDENTAL INHALATION OR ESOPHAGEAL DISTRESS, *COLESTID* GRANULES (colestipol hydrochloride) SHOULD NOT BE TAKEN IN ITS DRY FORM. ALWAYS MIX COLESTID WITH WATER OR OTHER FLUIDS BEFORE INGESTING.

Precautions: Before instituting therapy with *Colestid* Granules (colestipol hydrochloride), a vigorous attempt should be made to control serum cholesterol by an appropriate dietary regimen and weight reduction; any underlying disorder that may contribute to the hypercholesterolemia should be treated.

Because it sequesters bile acids, *Colestid* may interfere with normal fat absorption and thus may prevent absorption of fat soluble vitamins such as A, D, and K. If *Colestid* resin is to be given for long periods of time, supplemental vitamin A and D should be considered.

Chronic use of *Colestid* may be associated with an increased bleeding tendency due to hypoprothrombinemia from vitamin K deficiency. This will usually respond promptly to parenteral vitamin K_1 and recurrences can be prevented by oral administration of vitamin K_1.

Serum cholesterol and triglyceride levels should be measured periodically to detect significant changes. *Colestid* may raise the serum triglycerides in long term use and, in some patients, the cholesterol levels return to baseline or rise above baseline.

Colestid may produce or severely worsen preexisting constipation. The dosage should be decreased in these patients since impaction may occur. Particular effort should be made to avoid constipation in patients with symptomatic coronary artery disease. Constipation associated with *Colestid* may aggravate hemorrhoids.

While there have been no reports of hypothyroidism induced in individuals with normal thyroid function, the theoretical possibility exists, particularly in patients with limited thyroid reserve.

Use in Pregnancy

The use of *Colestid* in pregnancy or lactation or by women of childbearing age requires that the potential benefits of drug therapy be weighed against the possible hazards to the mother and child. The safe use of *Colestid* resin by pregnant women has not been established.

Use in Children

Safety and effectiveness in children have not been established.

Drug Interactions: Since colestipol hydrochloride is an anion exchange resin, it may have a strong affinity for anions other than the bile acids. Therefore, colestipol hydrochloride resin may delay or reduce the absorption of concomitant oral medication. The interval between the administration of *Colestid* and any other medication should be as long as possible. Patients should take other drugs at least one hour before or four hours after *Colestid* to avoid impeding their absorption.

In vitro studies have indicated that *Colestid* binds a number of drugs. Studies in humans show that the absorption of chlorothiazide as reflected in urinary excretion is markedly decreased even when administered one hour before *Colestid.* The absorption of tetracycline and of penicillin G was significantly decreased when either one was given at the same time as *Colestid;* these drugs were not tested to determine the effect of administration one hour before *Colestid.*

No depressant effect on blood levels in humans was noted when *Colestid* was administered with any of the following drugs: aspirin, clindamycin, clofibrate, methyldopa, tolbutamide or warfarin. Particular caution should be observed with digitalis preparations since there are conflicting results for the effect of *Colestid* on the availability of digoxin and digitoxin. The potential for binding of these drugs if given concomitantly is present. Discontinuing *Colestid* could pose a hazard to health if a potentially toxic drug that is significantly bound to the resin has been titrated to a maintenance level while the patient was taking *Colestid.*

Adverse Reactions:

1. *Gastrointestinal*

The most common adverse reactions are confined to the gastrointestinal tract. Constipation, reported by about one patient in 10, is the major single complaint and at times is severe and occasionally accompanied by fecal impaction. Hemorrhoids may be aggravated. Most instances of constipation are mild, transient, and controlled with standard treatment. Some patients require decreased dosage or discontinuation of therapy.

Less frequent gastrointestinal complaints occurring in about one in 30 to one in 100 patients, are abdominal discomfort (abdominal pain and distention), belching, flatulence, nausea, vomiting, and diarrhea. Peptic ulceration, gastrointestinal irritation and bleeding, cholecystitis, and cholelithiasis have been reported by fewer than one in 500 patients and are not necessarily drug related.

2. *Hypersensitivity*
Urticaria and dermatitis were noted in fewer than one in 1,000 patients. Asthma and wheezing were not reported in the *Colestid* studies but have been noted during treatment with other cholesterol-lowering agents.
3. *Musculoskeletal*
Muscle and joint pains, and arthritis have had a reported incidence of less than one in 1,000 patients.
4. *Neurologic*
Headache and dizziness were noted in about one in 300 patients; anxiety, vertigo, and drowsiness were reported in fewer than one in 1,000.
5. *Miscellaneous*
Anorexia, fatigue, weakness, and shortness of breath have been seen in 1–3 patients in 1,000. Transient and modest elevations of serum glutamic oxaloacetic transaminase and of alkaline phosphatase were observed in one or more occasions in various patients treated with *Colestid* Granules (colestipol hydrochloride). Some patients have shown an increase in serum phosphorus and chloride with a decrease in sodium and potassium.

Overdose: Overdosage of *Colestid* Granules (colestipol hydrochloride) has not been reported. Should overdosage occur, however, the chief potential harm would be obstruction of the gastrointestinal tract. The location of such potential obstruction, the degree of obstruction and the presence or absence of normal gut motility would determine treatment.

Dosage and Administration: For adults, *Colestid* Granules (colestipol hydrochloride) are recommended in doses of 15–30 grams/day taken in divided doses two to four times daily. To avoid accidental inhalation or esophageal distress, *Colestid* should not be taken in its dry form. *Colestid* should always be mixed with water or other fluids before ingesting. Patients should take other drugs at least one hour before or four hours after *Colestid* to minimize possible interference with their absorption. (See DRUG INTERACTIONS).

Before *Colestid* Administration

1. Define the type of hyperlipoproteinemia.
2. Institute a trial of diet and weight reduction.
3. Establish baseline serum cholesterol and triglyceride levels.

During *Colestid* Administration

1. The patient should be carefully monitored clinically, including serum cholesterol and triglyceride levels.
2. Failure of cholesterol to fall or significant rise in triglyceride level should be considered as indications to discontinue medication.

Mixing and Administration Guide

Colestid Granules (colestipol hydrochloride) should always be taken mixed in a liquid such as orange or tomato juice, water, milk, or carbonated beverage. It may also be taken in soups or with cereals or pulpy fruits. *Colestid should never be taken in its dry form.*

With beverages

1. Add the prescribed amount of *Colestid* to a glassful (three ounces or more) of water, milk, flavored drink, or a favorite juice (orange, tomato, pineapple, or other fruit juice).
2. Stir the mixture until the medication is completely mixed. (*Colestid* will not dissolve in the liquid.) *Colestid* may also be mixed with carbonated beverages, slowly stirred in a large glass.

Rinse the glass with a small amount of additional beverage to make sure all the medication is taken.

With cereals, soups, and fruits

Colestid may be taken mixed with milk in hot or regular breakfast cereals, or even mixed in soups that have a high fluid content (tomato or chicken noodle soup). It may also be added to fruits that are pulpy such as crushed pineapple, pears, peaches, or fruit cocktail.

How Supplied: *Colestid* Granules (colestipol hydrochloride) are available as follows:
Box of 30–5 gram packets *NDC 0009-0260-01*
500 gram bottle *NDC 0009-0260-02*
Each packet or each level scoop supplies 5 grams of *Colestid*.
Store at controlled room temperature 15°-30°C (59°-86°F).

References:

1. Kane JP, Malloy MJ, Tun P et al: Normalization of low-density-lipoprotein levels in heterozygous familial hypercholesterolemia with a combined drug regimen. *N. Engl J Med* 304:251–258, 1981.
2. Illingworth DR, Phillipson BE, JH Rapp et al: Colestipol plus nicotinic acid in treatment of heterozygous familial hypercholesterolemia. *Lancet* 1:296–298, 1981.
3. Kuo PT, Kostis JB, Moreyra AE et al: Familial type II hyperlipoproteinemia with coronary heart disease: Effect of diet-colestipol-nicotinic acid treatment. *Chest* 79:286–291, 1981.

Code 810 307 001

[*Shown in Product Identification Section*]

CORTAID® Cream
(See PDR For Nonprescription Drugs)

CORTAID® Lotion
(See PDR For Nonprescription Drugs)

CORTAID® Ointment
(See PDR For Nonprescription Drugs)

CORTAID® Spray
(See PDR For Nonprescription Drugs)

CORTEF® Feminine Itch Cream
(See PDR For Nonprescription Drugs)

CORTEF® Rectal Itch Ointment
(See PDR For Nonprescription Drugs)

CYTOSAR-U® Sterile Powder ℞
(sterile cytarabine, USP)

For intravenous and subcutaneous use only

WARNING

Only physicians experienced in cancer chemotherapy should use *Cytosar-U* Sterile Powder.

For induction therapy patients should be treated in a facility with laboratory and supportive resources sufficient to monitor drug tolerance and protect and maintain a patient compromised by drug toxicity. The main toxic effect of *Cytosar-U* is bone marrow suppression with leukopenia, thrombocytopenia and anemia. Less serious toxicity includes nausea, vomiting, diarrhea and abdominal pain, oral ulceration, and hepatic dysfunction.

The physician must judge possible benefit to the patient against known toxic effects of this drug in considering the advisability of therapy with *Cytosar-U*. Before making this judgment or beginning treatment, the physician should be familiar with the following text.

Description: *Cytosar-U* Sterile Powder contains cytarabine (1-β-D-arabinofuranosylcytosine; β-cytosine arabinoside). Cytarabine is a synthetic nucleoside which differs from the normal nucleosides cytidine and deoxycytidine in that the sugar moiety is arabinose rather than ribose or deoxyribose.

Cytosar-U is an antineoplastic agent for parenteral administration. It is available as a sterile freeze-dried preparation in two sizes:

100 mg vials—when prepared as directed, each ml contains:
20 mg cytarabine (Supplied with 5 ml ampoule of Bacteriostatic Water for Injection with Benzyl Alcohol 0.945% w/v added as preservative).

500 mg vials—when prepared as directed, each ml contains:
50 mg cytarabine (Supplied with 10 ml ampoule of Bacteriostatic Water for Injection with Benzyl Alcohol 0.945% w/v added as preservative).

When necessary, the pH of *Cytosar-U* was adjusted with hydrochloric acid and/or sodium hydroxide.

Pharmacology:

Cell Culture Studies

Cytarabine is cytotoxic to a wide variety of proliferating mammalian cells in culture. It exhibits cell phase specificity, primarily killing cells undergoing DNA synthesis (S-phase) and under certain conditions blocking the progression of cells from the G_1 phase to the S-phase. Although the mechanism of action is not completely understood, it appears that cytarabine acts through the inhibition of DNA polymerase. A limited, but significant, incorporation of cytarabine into both DNA and RNA has also been reported. Extensive chromosomal damage, including chromatoid breaks, have been produced by cytarabine and malignant transformation of rodent cells in culture has been reported. Deoxycytidine prevents or delays (but does not reverse) the cytotoxic activity.

Cell culture studies have shown an antiviral effect.[1] However, efficacy against herpes zoster or smallpox could not be demonstrated in controlled clinical trials.[2–4]

Cellular Resistance and Sensitivity

Cytarabine is metabolized by deoxycytidine kinase and other nucleotide kinases to the nucleotide triphosphate, an effective inhibitor of DNA polymerase; it is inactivated by a pyrimidine nucleoside deaminase which converts it to the nontoxic uracil derivative. It appears that the balance of kinase and deaminase levels may be an important factor in determining sensitivity or resistance of the cell to cytarabine.

Animal Studies

In experimental studies with mouse tumors, cytarabine was most effective in those tumors with a high growth fraction. The effect was dependent on the treatment schedule; optimal effects were achieved when the schedule (multiple closely spaced doses or constant infusion) ensured contact of the drug with the tumor cells when the maximum number of cells were in the susceptible S-phase. The best results were obtained when courses of therapy were separated by intervals sufficient to permit adequate host recovery.

Human Pharmacology

Cytarabine is rapidly metabolized and is not effective orally; less than 20 percent of the orally administered dose is absorbed from the gastrointestinal tract.

Following rapid intravenous injection of *Cytosar-U* Sterile Powder with tritium, the disappearance from plasma is biphasic. There is an initial distributive phase with a half-life of about 10 minutes, followed by a second elimi-

Continued on next page

Upjohn—Cont.

nation phase with a half-life of about 1 to 3 hours. After the distributive phase, over 80 percent of plasma radioactivity can be accounted for by the inactive metabolite 1-β-D-arabino- furanosyluracil (ara-U). Within 24 hours about 80 percent of the administered radioactivity can be recovered in the urine, approximately 90 percent of which is excreted as ara-U.
Relatively constant plasma levels can be achieved by continuous intravenous infusion.
After subcutaneous or intramuscular administration of *Cytosar-U* labeled with tritium, peak-plasma levels of radioactivity are achieved about 20 to 60 minutes after injection and are considerably lower than those after intravenous administration.
Cerebrospinal fluid levels of cytarabine are low in comparison to plasma levels after single intravenous injection. However, in one patient in whom cerebrospinal levels were examined after 2 hours of constant intravenous infusion, levels approached 40 percent of the steady state plasma level. With intrathecal administration, levels of cytarabine in the cerebrospinal fluid declined with a first order half-life of about 2 hours. Because cerebrospinal fluid levels of deaminase are low, little conversion to ara-U was observed.

Immunosuppressive Action

Cytosar-U Sterile Powder (cytarabine) is capable of obliterating immune responses in man during administration with little or no accompanying toxicity.[5,6] Suppression of antibody responses to E-coli-VI antigen and tetanus toxoid have been demonstrated. This suppression was obtained during both primary and secondary antibody responses.
Cytosar-U also suppressed the development of cell-mediated immune responses such as delayed hypersensitivity skin reaction to dinitrochlorobenzene. However, it had no effect on already established delayed hypersensitivity reactions.
Following 5-day courses of intensive therapy with *Cytosar-U* the immune response was suppressed, as indicated by the following parameters: macrophage ingress into skin windows; circulating antibody response following primary antigenic stimulation; lymphocyte blastogenesis with phytohemagglutinin. A few days after termination of therapy there was a rapid return to normal.[7]

Indications and Usage: *Cytosar-U* Sterile Powder (cytarabine) is indicated primarily for induction and maintenance of remission in acute myelocytic leukemia of both adults and children. It has also been found useful in the treatment of other leukemias, such as acute lymphocytic leukemia, chronic myelocytic leukemia (blast phase) and erythroleukemia. *Cytosar-U* may be used alone or in combination with other antineoplastic agents; the best results are often obtained with combination therapy.
Cytosar-U has been used experimentally in a variety of neoplastic diseases. In general, few patients with solid tumors have benefited.
Remissions induced by *Cytosar-U* not followed by maintenance treatment have been brief. Maintenance therapy has extended these and provided useful and comfortable remissions with relatively little toxicity.

Acute Myelocytic Leukemia

The following tables outline the results of treatment with *Cytosar-U* alone and in combination with other chemotherapeutic agents, in the treatment of acute myelocytic leukemia in adults and children.
The treatment regimens outlined in the tables should not be compared for efficacy. These were independent studies with a number of variables involved, such as patient population, duration of disease, and previous treatment. [See Table I and II on next page].
The responsiveness and course of childhood acute myelocytic leukemia (AML) appears to be different from that in adults.[21–23] Numerous studies show response rates to be higher in children than in adults with similar treatment schedules. Experience indicates that at least with induction and initial drug responsiveness, childhood AML appears to be more similar to childhood acute lymphocytic leukemia (ALL) than to its adult variant.

Acute Lymphocytic Leukemia

Cytosar-U has been used in the treatment of acute lymphocytic leukemia in both adults and children. When *Cytosar-U* was used with other antineoplastic agents as part of a total therapy program, results were equal to or better than reported with such programs which did not include *Cytosar-U*.[24,25] Used singly, or in combination with other agents, *Cytosar-U* has also been effective in treating patients who had relapsed on other therapy. Table III summarizes the results obtained in previously treated patients. Since these are independent studies with such variables as patient population, duration of disease and previous treatment, results shown should not be used for comparing the efficacy of the outlined treatment programs. (See Table III on page 2040)

Intrathecal Use in Meningeal Leukemia

Cytosar-U has been used intrathecally in acute leukemia in doses ranging from 5 mg/m^2 to 75 mg/m^2 of body surface area. The frequency of administration varied from once a day for 4 days to once every 4 days. The most frequently used dose was 30 mg/m^2 every 4 days until cerebrospinal fluid findings were normal, followed by one additional treatment.[34–38] The dosage schedule is usually governed by the type and severity of central nervous system manifestations and the response to previous therapy.
Prophylactic therapy following the successful treatment of the acute meningeal episode may be useful. The physician should familiarize himself with the current literature before instituting such a program.
Cytosar-U given intrathecally may cause systemic toxicity and careful monitoring of the hemopoietic system is indicated. Modification of other anti-leukemia therapy may be necessary. Major toxicity is rare. The most frequently reported reactions after intrathecal administration were nausea, vomiting and fever; these reactions are mild and self-limiting. Paraplegia has been reported in at least three instances.[39] Necrotizing leukoencephalopathy occurred in 5 children; these patients had also been treated with intrathecal methotrexate and hydrocortisone, as well as by central nervous system radiation.[40] Isolated neurotoxicity has been reported.[41] Blindness occurred in two patients in remission whose treatment had consisted of combination systemic chemotherapy, prophylactic central nervous system radiation and intrathecal *Cytosar-U*.[42]
Focal leukemic involvement of the central nervous system may not respond to intrathecal *Cytosar-U* and may better be treated with radiotherapy.
Although severe reactions attributable to the diluent are uncommon, many investigators prefer to use a special diluent for intrathecal use which is physiologically similar to the spinal fluid (Elliott's B Solution).[43]

Contraindications: *Cytosar-U* Sterile Powder (cytarabine) is contraindicated in those patients who are hypersensitive to the drug.

Warnings: *Cytosar-U* Sterile Powder (cytarabine) is a potent bone marrow suppressant. Therapy should be started cautiously in patients with pre-existing drug-induced bone marrow suppression. Patients receiving this drug must be under close medical supervision and, during induction therapy, should have leukocyte and platelet counts performed daily. Bone marrow examinations should be performed frequently after blasts have disappeared from the peripheral blood. Facilities should be available for management of complications, possibly fatal, of bone marrow suppression (infection resulting from granulocytopenia and other impaired body defenses, and hemorrhage secondary to thrombocytopenia).
One case of anaphylaxis that resulted in acute cardiopulmonary arrest and required resuscitation has been reported. This occurred immediately after the intravenous administration of *Cytosar-U*.
Severe and at times fatal CNS, GI and pulmonary toxicity (different from that seen with conventional therapy regimens of *Cytosar-U*) has been reported following some experimental *Cytosar-U* dose schedules.[44–47] These reactions include reversible corneal toxicity; cerebral and cerebellar dysfunction, usually reversible; severe gastrointestinal ulceration, including pneumatosis cystoides intestinalis leading to peritonitis; sepsis and liver abscess; and pulmonary edema.
Benzyl alcohol is contained in the diluent for this product. Benzyl alcohol has been reported to be associated with a fatal "Gasping Syndrome" in premature infants.

Use in Pregnancy

Pregnancy Category C. *Cytosar-U* is known to be teratogenic in some animal species. Use of the drug in women who are or who may become pregnant should be undertaken only after due consideration of potential benefit and potential hazard to both mother and child.
A review of the literature has shown 32 reported cases where *Cytosar-U* was given during pregnancy, either alone or in combination with other cytotoxic agents.
Eighteen normal infants were delivered. Four of these had first trimester exposure. Five infants were premature or of low birth weight. Twelve of the 18 normal infants were followed up at ages ranging from six weeks to seven years, and showed no abnormalties. One apparently normal infant died at 90 days of gastroenteritis.
Two cases of congenital abnormalities have been reported, one with upper and lower distal limb defects,[48] and the other with extremity and ear deformities.[49] Both of these cases had first trimester exposure.
There were seven infants with various problems in the neonatal period, including pancytopenia; transient depression of WBC, hematocrit or platelets; electrolyte abnormalities; transient eosinophilia; and one case of increased IgM levels and hyperpyrexia possibly due to sepsis. Six of the seven infants were also premature. The child with pancytopenia died at 21 days of sepsis.
Therapeutic abortions were done in five cases. Four fetuses were grossly normal, but one had an enlarged spleen and another showed Trisomy C chromosome abnormality in the chorionic tissue.
Because of the potential for abnormalities with cytotoxic therapy, particularly during the first trimester, a patient who is or who may become pregnant while on *Cytosar-U* should be apprised of the potential risk to the fetus and the advisability of pregnancy continuation. There is a definite, but considerably reduced risk if therapy is initiated during the second or third trimester. Although normal infants have been delivered to patients treated in all three trimesters of pregnancy, follow-up of such infants would be advisable.

Precautions: Patients receiving *Cytosar-U* Sterile Powder (cytarabine) must be monitored closely. Frequent platelet and leukocyte counts and bone marrow examinations are mandatory. Consider suspending or modifying therapy when drug-induced marrow depression has resulted in a platelet count under 50,000 or a polymorphonuclear granulocyte count under 1000 per cu. mm. Counts of formed elements in

TABLE I
ACUTE MYELOCYTIC LEUKEMIA
REMISSION INDUCTION
ADULTS

Drug-Dosage Schedule*		No. Patients Evaluated	Complete Remissions	Investigator
(CYTOSAR-U) SINGLE-DRUG THERAPY				
	(infusion)			
	10 mg/m² 12 hrs/day	12	2 (17%)	Ellison[8] (1968)
	30 mg/m² 12 hrs/day	41	10 (24%)	
	10 mg/m² 24 hrs/day	9	2 (22%)	
	30 mg/m² 24 hrs/day	36	2 (6%)	
	(infusion) 200 mg/m² 24 hrs/5 days	36	9 (25%)	Bodey[9] (1969)
	10 mg/m² IV injection initially, then infusions of 30 mg/m²/12 hrs or 60 mg/m²/day for 4 days	49	21 (43%)	Goodell[10] (1970)
	(infusion therapy)			Southwest Oncology Group[11] (1974)
	800 mg/m²/2 days	53	12 (23%)	
	1000 mg/m²/5 days	60	24 (40%)	
	100 mg/m²/day 1 hr infusion	49	7 (14%)	Carey[12] (1975)
	5–12.5 mg/kg/12 hour infusion following IV synchronizing dose**	5	5 (100%)	Lampkin[13] (1976)
COMBINED THERAPY				
Cytosar-U-thioguanine		36	15 (42%)	Gee[14] (1969)
Cytosar-U-thioguanine		64	28 (44%)	Grann[15] (1974)
Cytosar-U-cyclophosphamide-prednisone-vincristine		66	32 (48%)	Bodey[16] (1974)
Cytosar-U-thioguanine		88	49 (56%)	Clarkson[17] (1975)
Cytosar-U-cyclophosphamide-vincristine		50	23 (46%)	Curtis[18] (1975)

*Unless otherwise stated all doses given until drug effect—modifications then based on hematologic response. See references
**Highly experimental-requires ability to study mitotic indices

TABLE II
ACUTE MYELOCYTIC LEUKEMIA
REMISSION INDUCTION
CHILDREN (21 and under)

Drug Therapy	No. Patients Evaluated	Complete Remissions	Investigator
Cytosar-U (5–12.5 mg/kg following IV synchronizing dose**)	16	12 (75%)	Lampkin[13] (1976)
Cytosar-U-cyclophosphamide-vincristine	60	27 (45%)	Sonley[19] (1971)
Cytosar-U-thioguanine-doxorubicin	11	8 (72%)	Hagbin[20] (1975)
Cytosar-U-thioguanine	47	20 (43%)	Pizzo[21] (1976)
Cytosar-U-cyclophosphamide	12	7 (58%)	

**Highly experimental-requires ability to study mitotic indices

the peripheral blood may continue to fall after the drug is stopped and reach lowest values after drug-free intervals of 12 to 24 days. When indicated, restart therapy when definite signs of marrow recovery appear (on successive bone marrow studies). Patients whose drug is withheld until "normal" peripheral blood values are attained may escape from control.

When large intravenous doses are given quickly, patients are frequently nauseated and may vomit for several hours postinjection. This problem tends to be less severe when the drug is infused.

The human liver apparently detoxifies a substantial fraction of an administered dose. Use the drug with caution and at reduced dose in patients whose liver function is poor.

Periodic checks of bone marrow, liver and kidney functions should be performed in patients receiving *Cytosar-U.*

Like other cytotoxic drugs, *Cytosar-U* may induce hyperuricemia secondary to rapid lysis of neoplastic cells. The clinician should monitor the patient's blood uric acid level and be prepared to use such supportive and pharmacologic measures as might be necessary to control this problem.

Adverse Reactions:

Expected Reactions

Because cytarabine is a bone marrow suppressant, anemia, leukopenia, thrombocytopenia, megaloblastosis and reduced reticulocytes can be expected as a result of its administration. The severity of these reactions are dose and schedule dependent.[50] Cellular changes in the morphology of bone marrow and peripheral smears can be expected.[51]

Following 5-day constant infusions or acute injections of 50 mg/m² to 600 mg/m², white cell depression follows a biphasic course. Regardless of initial count, dosage level, or schedule, there is an initial fall starting the first 24 hours with a nadir at days 7–9. This is followed by a brief rise which peaks around the twelfth day. A second and deeper fall reaches nadir at

Continued on next page

Upjohn—Cont.

days 15–24. Then there is rapid rise to above baseline in the next 10 days. Platelet depression is noticeable at 5 days with a peak depression occurring between days 12–15. Thereupon, a rapid rise to above baseline occurs in the next 10 days.[52]

The Cytarabine (Ara-C) Syndrome

A cytarabine syndrome has been described by Castleberry.[53] It is characterized by fever, myalgia, bone pain, occasionally chest pain, maculopapular rash, conjunctivitis and malaise. It usually occurs 6-12 hours following drug administration. Corticosteroids have been shown to be beneficial in treating or preventing this syndrome. If the symptoms of the syndrome are deemed treatable, corticosteroids should be contemplated as well as continuation of therapy with *Cytosar-U* Sterile Powder (cytarabine).

Most Frequent Adverse Reactions

- anorexia
- nausea
- vomiting
- diarrhea
- oral and anal inflammation or ulceration
- hepatic dysfunction
- fever
- rash
- thrombophlebitis
- bleeding (all sites)

Nausea and vomiting are most frequent following rapid intravenous injection.

Less Frequent Adverse Reactions

- sepsis
- pneumonia
- cellulitis at injection site
- skin ulceration
- urinary retention
- renal dysfunction
- neuritis or neural toxicity
- sore throat
- esophageal ulceration
- esophagitis
- chest pain
- abdominal pain
- freckling
- jaundice
- conjunctivitis (may occur with rash)
- dizziness
- alopecia
- anaphylaxis (See WARNINGS)

Experimental Doses

Severe and at times fatal CNS, GI and pulmonary toxicity (different from that seen with conventional therapy regimens of *Cytosar-U*) has been reported following some experimental *Cytosar-U* dose schedules.[44–47] These reactions include reversible corneal toxicity, cerebral and cerebellar dysfunction, usually reversible; severe gastrointestinal ulceration, including pneumatosis cystoides intestinalis leading to peritonitis; sepsis and liver abscess; and pulmonary edema.

Dosage and Administration: *Cytosar-U* Sterile Powder (cytarabine) is not active orally. The schedule and method of administration varies with the program of therapy to be used. *Cytosar-U* Sterile Powder may be given by intravenous infusion or injection or subcutaneously. Thrombophlebitis has occurred at the site of drug injection or infusion in some patients, and rarely patients have noted pain and inflammation at subcutaneous injection sites. In most instances, however, the drug has been well tolerated.

Patients can tolerate higher total doses when they receive the drug by rapid intravenous injection as compared with slow infusion. This phenomenon is related to the drug's rapid inactivation and brief exposure of susceptible normal and neoplastic cells to significant levels after rapid injection. Normal and neoplastic cells seem to respond in somewhat parallel fashion to these different modes of administration and no clear-cut clinical advantage has been demonstrated for either.

Clinical experience accumulated to date suggests that success with *Cytosar-U* is dependent more on adeptness in modifying day-to-day dosage to obtain maximum leukemic cell kill with tolerable toxicity than on the basic treatment schedule chosen at the outset of therapy. Toxicity necessitating dosage alteration almost always occurs.

In many chemotherapeutic programs, *Cytosar-U* is used in combination with other cytotoxic drugs. The addition of these cytotoxic drugs has necessitated changes and dose alterations. The dosage schedules for combination therapy outlined below have been reported in the literature (see references).

Dosage Schedules:

Acute myelocytic leukemia—induction remission, adults

Cytosar-U Sterile Powder (cytarabine)—200 mg/m^2 daily by continuous infusion for 5 days (120 hours)—total dose 1000 mg/m^2. This course is repeated approximately every 2 weeks. Modifications must be made and based on hematologic response.

Combined Chemotherapy

Before instituting a program of combined chemotherapy, the physician should be familiar with adverse reactions, precautions, contraindications, and warnings applicable to all the drugs involved in the program.

***Cytosar-U* and thioguanine** [14,15,17]

Cytosar U: 3.0 mg/kg every 12 hours by IV injection

Thioguanine: 2.5 mg/kg every 12 hours (orally)

Both drugs are given until bone marrow becomes hypoplastic. This usually takes from 1 week to 10 days. Following a 10 to 20 day rest period the cycle is started again.

***Cytosar-U*, cyclophosphamide, vincristine, prednisone**[16]

Cytosar-U: 100 mg/m^2/day for 5 days (rapid IV injection in divided doses-every 8 hours).

Cyclophosphamide: 100 mg/m^2/day for 5 days (rapid IV injection in divided doses-every 8 hours).

Vincristine: 2 mg by rapid IV injection, day 1 only.

Prednisone: 25 mg four times daily for 5 days.

Courses of therapy are initiated at 2-week intervals, the second course being given without regard to peripheral blood cell counts and appearance of bone marrow. When there is rapid recovery of blast cells in the peripheral blood, further courses can be reinstituted at less than the 2-week intervals. Therapy should be delayed when the bone marrow is hypocellular or if severe infection or hemorrhage develop. The dosage schedule is continued until the patient is in complete remission or until progressive disease is apparent after a minimum of five courses.

Dosage for subsequent courses is determined by the patient's response and the condition of the bone marrow.

Acute myelocytic leukemia-maintenance, adults

Maintenance programs are modifications of induction programs and, in general, use similar schedules of drug therapy as were used during induction. Most programs have a greater time spacing between courses of therapy during remission maintenance.

Acute myelocytic leukemia-induction and maintenance in children

Numerous studies have shown that childhood AML responds better than adult AML given similar regimens. Where the adult dosage is stated in terms of body weight or surface area, the children's dosage may be calculated on the same basis. When specified amounts of a drug are indicated for the adult dosage, these should be adjusted for children on the basis of such factors as age, body weight or body surface area.

Acute lymphocytic leukemia

In general, dosage schedules are similar to those used in acute myelocytic leukemia with some modifications. For dosage recommenda-

TABLE III
ACUTE LYMPHATIC LEUKEMIA
REMISSION INDUCTION
PREVIOUSLY TREATED PATIENTS

ADULTS AND CHILDREN

Drug Therapy	No. of Patients Evaluated	Complete Remissions	Response	Investigator
Cytosar-U 3–5 mg/kg/day (IV injection)	43	2 (5%)	15 (35%)	Howard[26] (1968)
Cytosar-U-asparaginase	9	8 (89%)	8 (89%)	McElwain[27] (1969)
Cytosar-U-cyclophosphamide	11	7 (64%)	9 (82%)	Bodey[28] (1970)
Cytosar-U-prednisone	83		(49%)	Nesbit[29] (1970)
Cytosar-U 150–200 mg/m^2/5 days (infusion)	34	1 (3%)	4 (12%)	Wang[30] (1970)
Cytosar-U 25 mg/kg/twice weekly (infusion)	74	24 (32%)	29 (39%)	Traggis[31] (1971)
Cytosar-U-asparaginase	22	13 (59%)	15 (68%)	Ortega[32] (1972)
Cytosar-U-thioguanine	19	9 (47%)	9 (47%)	Bryan[33] (1974)

tions see referenced literature in Table III under INDICATIONS AND USAGE.

Dosage Modification—The dosage of *Cytosar-U* must be modified or suspended when signs of serious hematologic depression appear. In general, consider discontinuing the drug if the patient has less than 50,000 platelets or 1000 polymorphonuclear granulocytes per cu mm in his peripheral blood. These guidelines may be modified depending on signs of toxicity in other systems and on the rapidity of fall in formed blood elements. Restart the drug when there are signs of marrow recovery and the above platelet and granulocyte levels have been attained. Withholding therapy until the patient's blood values are normal may result in escape of the patient's disease from control by the drug.

How Supplied: Store unreconstituted product at controlled room temperature: 15°-30°C (59°-86°F). *Cytosar-U* Sterile Powder (cytarabine) is available as a freeze-dried preparation in multidose vials of two sizes:

100 mg* vial—Must be reconstituted with 5 ml of Bacteriostatic Water for Injection with Benzyl Alcohol 0.945% w/v added as preservative, the resulting solution contains 20 mg of cytarabine per ml.

500 mg* vial—Must be reconstituted with 10 ml of Bacteriostatic Water for Injection with Benzyl Alcohol 0.945% w/v added as preservative, the resulting solution contains 50 mg of cytarabine per ml.

*When necessary, the pH was adjusted with hydrochloric acid and/or sodium hydroxide.

In this form the drug is suitable for intravenous or subcutaneous administration. The pH of the reconstituted solution is about 5. THESE SOLUTIONS MAY BE STORED AT CONTROLLED ROOM TEMPERATURE 15°-30°C (59°-86°F) FOR 48 HOURS. DISCARD ANY SOLUTION IN WHICH A SLIGHT HAZE DEVELOPS.

Chemical Stability in Infusion Solutions

Chemical stability studies were performed by ultraviolet assay on *Cytosar-U* infusion solutions. These studies showed that when the reconstituted *Cytosar-U* Sterile Powder (cytarabine) was added to Water for Injection, 5% Dextrose in Water or Sodium Chloride Injection, 94 to 96 percent of the cytarabine was present after 192 hours storage at room temperature.

References:

1. Zaky DA, Betts RF, Douglas RG, et al: Varicella-Zoster Virus and Subcutaneous Cytarabine: Correlation of In Vitro Sensitivities to Blood Levels, Antimicrob Agents Chemother *7*:229–232, 1975
2. Davis CM, VanDarsarl JV, Coltman CA Jr: Failure of Cytarabine in Varicella-Zoster Infections, JAMA *224*:122–123, 1973
3. Betts RF, Zaky DA, Douglas RG, et al: Ineffectiveness of Subcutaneous Cytosine Arabinoside in Localized Herpes Zoster, Ann Intern Med *82*:778–783, 1975
4. Dennis DT, Doberstyn EB, Awoke S, et al: Failure of Cytosine Arabinoside in Treating Smallpox; A Double-blind Study, Lancet *2*:377–379, 1974
5. Gray GD: ARA-C and Derivatives as Examples of Immunosuppressive Nucleoside Analogs, Ann NY Acad Sci *255*:372–379, 1975
6. Mitchell MS, Wade ME, DeConti RC, et al: Immunosuppressive Effects of Cytosine Arabinoside and Methotrexate in Man, Ann Intern Med *70*:535–547, 1969
7. Frei E, Ho DHW, Bodey GP, et al: Pharmacologic and Cytokinetic Studies of Arabinosyl Cytosine. In *Unifying Concepts of Leukemia*, Bibl. Hematol. No. 39. Karger, Basel 1973, pp 1085–1097
8. Ellison RR, Holland JF, Weil M, et al: Arabinosyl Cytosine: A Useful Agent in the Treatment of Acute Leukemia in Adults, Blood *32*:507–523, 1968
9. Bodey GP, Freireich EJ, Monto RW, et al: Cytosine Arabinoside (NSC-63878) Therapy for Acute Leukemia in Adults, Cancer Chemother Rep *53*:59–66, 1969
10. Goodell B, Leventhal B, Henderson E: Cytosine Arabinoside in Acute Granulocytic Leukemia, Clin Pharmacol Ther *12*:599–606, 1970
11. Southwest Oncology Group: Cytarabine for Acute Leukemia in Adults, Arch Intern Med *133*:251–259, 1974
12. Carey RW, Ribas-Mundo M, Ellison RR, et al: Comparative Study of Cytosine Arabinoside Therapy Alone and Combined with Thioguanine, Mercaptopurine or Daunorubicin in Acute Myelocytic Leukemia, Cancer *36*:1560–1566, 1975
13. Lampkin BC, McWilliam NB, Mauer AM, et al: Manipulation of the Mitotic Cycle in the Treatment of Acute Myelogenous Leukaemia, Brit J Haematol *32*:29–40, 1976
14. Gee TS, Yu KP, Clarkson BD: Treatment of Adult Acute Leukemia with Arabinosylcytosine and Thioguanine, Cancer *23*:1019–1032, 1969
15. Grann V, Erichson R, Flannery J, et al: The Therapy of Acute Granulocytic Leukemia in Patients More Than Fifty Years Old, Ann Int Med *80*:15–20, 1974
16. Bodey GP, Coltman CA, Freireich EJ, et al: Chemotherapy of Acute Leukemia; Comparison of Cytarabine Alone and in Combination with Vincristine, Prednisone, and Cyclophosphamide, Arch Intern Med *133*:260–266, 1974
17. Clarkson BD, Dowling MD, Gee TS, et al: Treatment of Acute Leukemia in Adults, Cancer *36*:775–795, 1975
18. Curtis JE, Cowan DH, Bergsagel DE, et al: Acute Leukemia in Adults: Assessment of Remission Induction with Combination Chemotherapy by Clinical and Cell-Culture Criteria, Canad Med Assoc J *113*:289–294, 1975
19. Sonley MJ, Nesbit M, Thatcher LG, et al: Cytosine Arabinoside, Cyclophosphamide and Vincristine in Children with Acute Myelogenous Leukemia, Proc Am Assoc Cancer Res *12*:87, 1971
20. Haghbin M: Acute Non-lymphoblastic Leukemia; Clinical and Morphological Characterization, Mod Prob Pediatr *16*:39–58, 1975
21. Pizzo PA, Henderson ES, Leventhal BG: Acute Myelogenous Leukemia in Children: A Preliminary Report of Combination Chemotherapy, J Pediatr *88*:125–130, 1976
22. Report of the Medical Research Council's Working Party on Leukaemia in Adults: Treatment of Acute Myeloid Leukaemia with Daunorubicin, Cytosine Arabinoside, Mercaptopurine, L-Asparaginase, Prednisone and Thioguanine: Results of Treatment with Five Multiple-Drug Schedules, Brit J Haematol *27*:373–389, 1974
23. Ansari BM, Thompson EN, Whittaker JA: A Comparative Study of Acute Myeloblastic Leukaemia in Children and Adults, Brit J Haematol *31*:269–277, 1975
24. Gee TS, Haghbin M, Dowling MD Jr, et al: Acute Lymphoblastic Leukemia in Adults and Children; Differences in Response with Similar Therapeutic Regimens, Cancer *37*:1256–1264, 1976
25. Spiers ASD, Roberts PD, Marsh GW, et al: Acute Lymphoblastic Leukaemia: Cyclical Chemotherapy with three Combinations of Four Drugs (COAP-POMP-CART Regimen). Brit Med J *4*:614–617, 1975
26. Howard JP, Albo V, Newton WA Jr: Cytosine Arabinoside: Results of a Cooperative Study in Acute Childhood Leukemia, Cancer *21*:341–345, 1968
27. McElwain TJ, Hardisty RM: Remission Induction with Cytosine Arabinoside and L-Asparaginase in Acute Lymphoblastic Leukaemia, Brit Med J *4*:596–598, 1969
28. Bodey GP, Rodriguez, V, Hart J, et al: Therapy of Acute Leukemia with the Combination of Cytosine Arabinoside (NSC-63878) and Cyclophosphamide (NSC-26271), Cancer Chemother Rep *54*:255–262, 1970
29. Nesbit ME Jr, Hammond D: Cytosine Arabinoside (ARAC) and Prednisone Therapy of Previously Treated Acute Lymphoblastic and Undifferentiated Leukemia (ALL/AUL) of Childhood, Proc Am Assoc Cancer Res *11*:59, 1970
30. Wang JJ, Selawry OS, Vietti TJ, et al: Prolonged Infusion of Arabinosyl Cytosine in Childhood Leukemia, Cancer *25*:1–6, 1970
31. Traggis DG, Dohlwitz A, Das L, et al: Cytosine Arabinoside in Acute Leukemia of Childhood, Cancer *28*:815–818, 1971
32. Ortega JA, Finklestein JZ, Ertell, et al: Effective Combination Treatment of Advanced Acute Lymphocytic Leukemia with Cytosine Arabinoside (NSC-63878) and L-Asparaginase (NSC-109229), Cancer Chemother Rep *56*:363–368, 1972
33. Bryan JH, Henderson ES, Leventhal BG: Cytosine Arabinoside and 6- Thioguanine in Refractory Acute Lymphocytic Leukemia, Cancer *33*:539–544, 1974
34. Proceedings of the Chemotherapy Conference on ARA-C: Development and Application (Cytosine Arabinoside Hydrochloride—NSC 63878), Oct. 10, 1969
35. Lay HN, Colebatch JH, Ekert H: Experiences with Cytosine Arabinoside in Childhood Leukaemia and Lymphoma, Med J Aust *2*:187–192, 1971
36. Halikowski B, Cyklis R, Armata J, et al: Cytosine Arabinoside Administered Intrathecally in Cerebromeningeal Leukemia, Acta Paediat Scand *59*:164–168, 1970
37. Wang JJ, Pratt CB: Intrathecal Arabinosyl Cytosine in Meningeal Leukemia, Cancer *25*:531–534, 1970
38. Band PR, Holland JF, Bernard J, et al: Treatment of Central Nervous System Leukemia with Intrathecal Cytosine Arabinoside, Cancer *32*:744–748, 1973
39. Saiki JH, Thompson S, Smith F, et al: Paraplegia Following Intrathecal Chemotherapy, Cancer *29*:370–374, 1972
40. Rubinstein LJ, Herman MM, Long TF, et al: Disseminated Necrotizing Leukoencephalopathy: A Complication of Treated Central System Leukemia and Lymphoma, Cancer *35*:291–305, 1975
41. Marmont Am, Damasio EE: Neurotoxicity of Intrathecal Chemotherapy for Leukaemia, Brit Med J *4*:47, 1973
42. Margileth DA, Poplack DG, Pizzo PA, et al: Blindness During Remission in Two Patients with Acute Lymphoblastic Leukemia, Cancer *39*:58–61, 1977
43. Duttera MJ, Gallelli JF, Kleinman LM, et al: Intrathecal Methotrexate, Lancet *1*:540, 1972
44. Hopen G, Mondino BJ, Johnson BL, et al: Corneal Toxicity with Systemic Cytarabine, *Am J Ophthalmol* 91:500–504, 1981
45. Lazarus HM, Herzig RH, Herzig GP, et al; Central Nervous System Toxicity of High-Dose Systemic Cytosine Arabinoside, *Cancer* 48:2577–2582, 1981.
46. Slavin RE, Dias MA, Soral R: Cytosine Arabinoside Induced Gastrointestinal Toxic Alterations in Sequential Chemo-

Continued on next page

Upjohn—Cont.

therapeutic Protocols—A Clinical Pathologic Study of 33 Patients, *Cancer* 42:1747–1759, 1978.

47. Haupt HM, Hutchins GM, Moore GW; Ara-C Lung: Noncardiogenic Pulmonary Edema Complicating Cytosine Arabinoside Therapy of Leukemia, *Am J Med* 70:256–261, 1981.
48. Shafer AI: Teratogenic Effects of Antileukemic Chemotherapy. *Arch Intern Med* 141:514–515, 1981.
49. Wagner VM, et al: Congenital Abnormalities in Baby Born to Cytarabine Treated Mother, *Lancet* 2:98–99, 1980.
50. Frei E III, Bickers JN, Hewlett JS, et al: Dose Schedule and Antitumor Studies of Arabinosyl Cytosine (NSC 63878), Cancer Res *29*:1325–1332, 1969
51. Bell WR, Whang JJ, Carbone PP, et al: Cytogenetic and Morphologic Abnormalities in Human Bone Marrow Cells during Cytosine Arabinoside Therapy, J. Hematol *27*:771–781, 1966
52. Burke PJ, Serpick AA, Carbone PP, et al: A Clinical Evaluation of Dose and Schedule of Administration of Cytosine Arabinoside (NSC 63878), Cancer Res *28*:274–279, 1968
53. Castleberry RP, Crist WM, Holbrook T, et al: The Cytosine Arabinoside (Ara-C) Syndrome, *Med Pediatr Oncol* 9:257–264, 1981.

Animal Toxicology: Toxicity of cytarabine in experimental animals, as well as activity, is markedly influenced by the schedule of administration. For example, in mice the LD_{10} for single intraperitoneal administration is greater than 6000 mg/m^2. However, when administered in 8 doses, each separated by 3 hours, the LD_{10} is less than 750 mg/m^2 total dose. Similarly, although a total dose of 1920 mg/m^2 administered as 12 injections at 6-hour intervals was lethal to beagle dogs (severe bone marrow hypoplasia with evidence of liver and kidney damage), dogs receiving the same total dose administered as 8 injections (again at 6-hour intervals) over a 48-hour period survived with minimal signs of toxicity. The most consistent observation in surviving dogs was elevated transaminase levels. In all experimental species the primary limiting toxic effect is marrow suppression with leukopenia. In addition, cytarabine causes abnormal cerebellar development in the neonatal hamster and is teratogenic to the rat fetus.

Code 810 126 003

DELTA-CORTEF® Tablets ℞

(prednisolone tablets, U.S.P.)

How Supplied: 5 mg scored tablets.

Bottles of 100 *NDC 0009-0025-01*
Bottles of 500 *NDC 0009-0025-02*

DELTASONE® Tablets ℞

(prednisone tablets, USP)

How Supplied: Scored tablets in the following strength and sizes:

2.5 mg	Bottles of 100	*NDC 0009-0032-01*
5 mg	Bottles of 100	*NDC 0009-0045-01*
	Bottles of 500	*NDC 0009-0045-02*
	Dosepak™ Unit of use (21)	*NDC 0009-0045-04*
	Unit Dose Package (100)	*NDC 0009-0045-05*
10 mg	Bottles of 100	*NDC 0009-0193-01*
	Bottles of 500	*NDC 0009-0193-02*
	Unit Dose Packages (100)	*NDC 0009-0193-03*
20 mg	Bottles of 100	*NDC 0009-0165-01*
	Bottles of 500	*NDC 0009-0165-02*
	Unit dose Packages (100)	*NDC 0009-0165-03*
50 mg	Bottles of 100	*NDC 0009-0388-01*
	Unit dose Packages (100)	*NDC 0009-0388-02*

Code 810 342 000

[*Shown in Product Identification Section*]

DEPO-MEDROL® ℞

Sterile Aqueous Suspension
(sterile methylprednisolone acetate suspension, USP)
Not for Intravenous Use

40 mg/ml (1 ml vial):
NSN 6505-00-952-0267 (M)
40 mg/ml (5 ml vial):
NSN 6505-00-890-1186A (M & VA)

Description: *Depo-Medrol* Sterile Aqueous Suspension contains methylprednisolone acetate which is the 6-methyl derivative of prednisolone. Methylprednisolone acetate is a white or practically white, odorless, crystalline powder which melts at about 215° with some decomposition. It is soluble in dioxane, sparingly soluble in acetone, in alcohol, in chloroform, and in methanol, and slightly soluble in ether. It is practically insoluble in water.

The chemical name for methylprednisolone acetate is pregna-1, 4-diene-3, 20-dione, 21-(acetyloxy)-11, 17-dihydroxy-6-methyl-,(6α, 11β)- and the molecular weight is 416.51.

Depo-Medrol Sterile Aqueous Suspension (methylprednisolone acetate) is an anti-inflammatory glucocorticoid in a sterile aqueous suspension for intramuscular, intra-articular, soft tissue or intralesional injection. It is available in three strengths: 20 mg/ml; 40 mg/ml; 80 mg/ml.

[See table below].

Actions: Naturally occurring glucocorticoids (hydrocortisone), which also have salt retaining properties, are used in replacement therapy in adrenocortical deficiency states. Their synthetic analogs are used primarily for their potent anti-inflammatory effects in disorders of many organ systems.

Glucocorticoids cause profound and varied metabolic effects. In addition, they modify the body's immune response to diverse stimuli.

Indications

A. FOR INTRAMUSCULAR ADMINISTRATION

When oral therapy is not feasible and the strength, dosage form, and route of administration of the drug reasonably lend the preparation to the treatment of the condition, the intramuscular use of *Depo-Medrol* Sterile Aqueous Suspension (methylprednisolone acetate) is indicated as follows:

1. **Endocrine Disorders**
   Primary or secondary adrenocortical insufficiency (hydrocortisone or cortisone is the drug of choice; synthetic analogs may be used in conjunction with mineralocorticoids where applicable; in infancy, mineralocorticoid supplementation is of particular importance)
   Acute adrenocortical insufficiency (hydrocortisone or cortisone is the drug of choice; mineralocorticoid supplementation may be necessary, particularly when synthetic analogs are used)
   Preoperatively and in the event of serious trauma or illness, in patients with known adrenal insufficiency or when adrenocortical reserve is doubtful
   Congenital adrenal hyperplasia
   Hypercalcemia associated with cancer
   Nonsuppurative thyroiditis
2. **Rheumatic Disorders**
   As adjunctive therapy for short-term administration (to tide the patient over an acute episode or exacerbation) in:
   Post-traumatic osteoarthritis
   Synovitis of osteoarthritis
   Rheumatoid arthritis, including juvenile rheumatoid arthritis (selected cases may require low-dose maintenance therapy)
   Acute and subacute bursitis
   Epicondylitis
   Acute nonspecific tenosynovitis
   Acute gouty arthritis
   Psoriatic arthritis
   Ankylosing spondylitis
3. **Collagen Diseases**
   During an exacerbation or as maintenance therapy in selected cases of:
   Systemic lupus erythematosus
   Systemic dermatomyositis (polymyositis)
   Acute rheumatic carditis
4. **Dermatologic Diseases**
   Pemphigus
   Severe erythema multiforme (Stevens-Johnson syndrome)
   Exfoliative dermatitis
   Bullous dermatitis herpetiformis
   Severe seborrheic dermatitis
   Severe psoriasis
   Mycosis fungoides
5. **Allergic States**
   Control of severe or incapacitating allergic conditions intractable to adequate trials of conventional treatment in:
   Bronchial asthma
   Contact dermatitis
   Atopic dermatitis
   Serum sickness
   Seasonal or perennial allergic rhinitis
   Drug hypersensitivity reactions
   Urticarial transfusion reactions
   Acute noninfectious laryngeal edema (epinephrine is the drug of first choice)
6. **Ophthalmic Diseases**
   Severe acute and chronic allergic and inflammatory processes involving the eye, such as:
   Herpes zoster ophthalmicus
   Iritis, iridocyclitis
   Chorioretinitis
   Diffuse posterior uveitis and choroiditis
   Optic neuritis
   Sympathetic ophthalmia
   Anterior segment inflammation
   Allergic conjunctivitis
   Allergic corneal marginal ulcers
   Keratitis
7. **Gastrointestinal Diseases**
   To tide the patient over a critical period of the disease in:
   Ulcerative colitis (systemic therapy)
   Regional enteritis (systemic therapy)
8. **Respiratory Diseases**
   Symptomatic sarcoidosis
   Berylliosis
   Fulminating or disseminated pulmonary tuberculosis when used concurrently with appropriate antituberculous chemotherapy
   Loeffler's syndrome not manageable by other means

Each ml of these preparations contains:	20 mg	40 mg	80 mg
Methylprednisolone Acetate	20 mg	40 mg	80 mg
Also			
Polyethylene Glycol 3350	29.6 mg	29 mg	28 mg
Sodium Chloride	8.9 mg	8.7 mg	8.5 mg
Myristyl-gamma-picolinium Chloride added as preservative	0.198 mg	0.195 mg	0.189 mg

When necessary, pH was adjusted with sodium hydroxide and/or hydrochloric acid. The pH of the finished product remains within the USP specified range; ie, 3.5 to 7.0.

Aspiration pneumonitis

9. **Hematologic Disorders**
   Acquired (autoimmune) hemolytic anemia
   Secondary thrombocytopenia in adults
   Erythroblastopenia (RBC anemia)
   Congenital (erythroid) hypoplastic anemia
10. **Neoplastic Diseases**
   For palliative management of:
   Leukemias and lymphomas in adults
   Acute leukemia of childhood
11. **Edematous States**
   To induce diuresis or remission of proteinuria in the nephrotic syndrome, without uremia, of the idiopathic type or that due to lupus erythematosus
12 **Nervous System**
   Acute exacerbations of multiple sclerosis
13. **Miscellaneous**
   Tuberculous meningitis with subarachnoid block or impending block when used concurrently with appropriate antituberculous chemotherapy
   Trichinosis with neurologic or myocardial involvement

B. FOR INTRA-ARTICULAR OR SOFT TISSUE ADMINISTRATION

Depo-Medrol is indicated as adjunctive therapy for short-term administration (to tide the patient over an acute episode or exacerbation) in:
Synovitis of osteoarthritis
Rheumatoid arthritis
Acute and subacute bursitis
Acute gouty arthritis
Epicondylitis
Acute nonspecific tenosynovitis
Post-traumatic osteoarthritis

C. FOR INTRALESIONAL ADMINISTRATION

Depo-Medrol is indicated for intralesional use in the following conditions:
Keloids
Localized hypertrophic, infiltrated inflammatory lesions of:
   lichen planus, psoriatic plaques, granuloma annulare, and lichen simplex chronicus (neurodermatitis)
Discoid lupus erythematosus
Necrobiosis lipodica diabeticorum
Alopecia areata

Depo-Medrol also may be useful in cystic tumors of an aponeurosis or tendon (ganglia).

Contraindications: Systemic fungal infections.

Warnings:

Multidose Use

Although initially sterile, any multidose use of vials may lead to contamination unless strict aseptic technique is observed. The preservative in *Depo-Medrol* Sterile Aqueous Suspension (methylprednisolone acetate) will prevent growth of most pathogenic organisms, but certain ones (eg *Serratia marcescens*) may remain viable. Particular care, such as use of disposable sterile syringes and needles, should be observed if intrasynovial use is intended.

While crystals of adrenal steroids in the dermis suppress inflammatory reactions, their presence may cause disintegration of the cellular elements and physiochemical changes in the ground substance of the connective tissue. The resultant infrequently occurring dermal and/or subdermal changes may form depressions in the skin at the injection site. The degree to which this reaction occurs will vary with the amount of adrenal steroid injected. Regeneration is usually complete within a few months or after all crystals of the adrenal steroid have been absorbed.

In order to minimize the incidence of dermal and subdermal atrophy, care must be exercised not to exceed recommended doses in injections. Multiple small injections into the area of the lesion should be made whenever possible. The technique of intra-articular and intramuscular injection should include precautions against injection or leakage into the dermis. Injection into the deltoid muscle should be avoided because of a high incidence of subcutaneous atrophy.

Depo-Medrol is Not Recommended For Intrathecal Administration.

In patients on corticosteroid therapy subjected to any unusual stress, increased dosage of rapidly acting corticosteroids before, during, and after the stressful situation is indicated.

Corticosteroids may mask some signs of infection, and new infections may appear during their use. There may be decreased resistance and inability to localize infection when corticosteroids are used. Do not use intra-articularly, intrabursally or for intratendinous administration for *local* effect in the presence of acute infection.

Prolonged use of corticosteroids may produce posterior subcapsular cataracts, glaucoma with possible damage to the optic nerves, and may enhance the establishment of secondary ocular infections due to fungi or viruses.

Usage in pregnancy. Since adequate human reproduction studies have not been done with corticosteroids, the use of these drugs in pregnancy, nursing mothers, or women of childbearing potential requires that the possible benefits of the drug be weighed against the potential hazards to the mother and embryo or fetus. Infants born of mothers who have received substantial doses of corticosteroids during pregnancy should be carefully observed for signs of hypoadrenalism.

Average and large doses of cortisone or hydrocortisone can cause elevation of blood pressure, salt and water retention, and increased excretion of potassium. These effects are less likely to occur with the synthetic derivatives except when used in large doses. Dietary salt restriction and potassium supplementation may be necessary. All corticosteroids increase calcium excretion.

While on corticosteroid therapy patients should not be vaccinated against smallpox. Other immunization procedures should not be undertaken in patients who are on corticosteroids, especially in high doses, because of possible hazards of neurological complications and lack of antibody response.

The use of *Depo-Medrol* in active tuberculosis should be restricted to those cases of fulminating or disseminated tuberculosis in which the corticosteroid is used for the management of the disease in conjunction with appropriate antituberculous regimen.

If corticosteroids are indicated in patients with latent tuberculosis or tuberculin reactivity, close observation is necessary as reactivation of the disease may occur. During prolonged corticosteroid therapy, these patients should receive chemoprophylaxis.

Because rare instances of anaphylactoid reactions have occurred in patients receiving parenteral corticosteroid therapy, appropriate precautionary measures should be taken prior to administration especially when the patient has a history of allergy to any drug.

Precautions: Drug-induced secondary adrenocortical insufficiency may be minimized by gradual reduction of dosage. This type of relative insufficiency may persist for months after discontinuation of therapy; therefore, in any situation of stress occurring during that period, hormone therapy should be reinstituted. Since mineralocorticoid secretion may be impaired, salt and/or a mineralocorticoid should be administered concurrently.

When multidose vials are used, special care to prevent contamination of the contents is essential (See WARNINGS).

There is an enhanced effect of corticosteroids in patients with hypothyroidism and in those with cirrhosis.

Corticosteroids should be used cautiously in patients with ocular herpes simplex for fear of corneal perforation.

The lowest possible dose of corticosteroid should be used to control the condition under treatment, and when reduction in dosage is possible, the reduction must be gradual.

Psychic derangements may appear when corticosteroids are used, ranging from euphoria, insomnia, mood swings, personality changes, and severe depression to frank psychotic manifestations. Also, existing emotional instability or psychotic tendencies may be aggravated by corticosteroids.

Aspirin should be used cautiously in conjunction with corticosteroids in hypoprothrombinemia.

Steroids should be used with caution in nonspecific ulcerative colitis, if there is a probability of impending perforation, abscess or other pyogenic infection. Caution must also be used in diverticulitis, fresh intestinal anastomoses, active or latent peptic ulcer, renal insufficiency, hypertension, osteoporosis, and myasthenia gravis, when steroids are used as direct or adjunctive therapy.

Growth and development of infants and children on prolonged corticosteroid therapy should be carefully followed.

The following additional precautions apply for parenteral corticosteroids. Intra-articular injection of a corticosteroid may produce systemic as well as local effects.

Appropriate examination of any joint fluid present is necessary to exclude a septic process.

A marked increase in pain accompanied by local swelling, further restriction of joint motion, fever, and malaise are suggestive of septic arthritis. If this complication occurs and the diagnosis of sepsis is confirmed, appropriate antimicrobial therapy should be instituted.

Local injection of a steroid into a previously infected joint is to be avoided.

Corticosteroids should not be injected into unstable joints.

The slower rate of absorption by intramuscular administration should be recognized.

Although controlled clinical trials have shown corticosteroids to be effective in speeding the resolution of acute exacerbations of multiple sclerosis, they do not show that corticosteroids affect the ultimate outcome or natural history of the disease. The studies do show that relatively high doses of corticosteroids are necessary to demonstrate a significant effect. (See **Dosage And Administration**).

Since complications of treatment with glucocorticoids are dependent on the size of the dose and the duration of treatment, a risk/benefit decision must be made in each individual case as to dose and duration of treatment and as to whether daily or intermittent therapy should be used.

Adverse Reactions:

Fluid and electrolyte disturbances:
   Sodium retention
   Fluid retention
   Congestive heart failure in susceptible patients
   Potassium loss
   Hypokalemic alkalosis
   Hypertension

Musculoskeletal:
   Muscle weakness
   Steroid myopathy
   Loss of muscle mass
   Osteoporosis
   Vertebral compression fractures
   Aseptic necrosis of femoral and humeral heads
   Pathologic fracture of long bones

Gastrointestinal:
   Peptic ulcer with possible subsequent perforation and hemorrhage
   Pancreatitis
   Abdominal distention
   Ulcerative esophagitis

Dermatologic:
   Impaired wound healing
   Thin fragile skin

Continued on next page

Upjohn—Cont.

Petechiae and ecchymoses
Facial erythema
Increased sweating
May suppress reactions to skin tests

Neurological:
Convulsions
Increased intracranial pressure with papilledema (pseudotumor cerebri) usually after treatment
Vertigo
Headache

Endocrine:
Menstrual irregularities
Development of Cushingoid state
Suppression of growth in children
Secondary adrenocortical and pituitary unresponsiveness, particularly in times of stress, as in trauma, surgery or illness
Decreased carbohydrate tolerance
Manifestations of latent diabetes mellitus
Increased requirements for insulin or oral hypoglycemic agents in diabetes

Ophthalmic:
Posterior subcapsular cataracts
Increased intraocular pressure
Glaucoma
Exophthalmos

Metabolic:
Negative nitrogen balance due to protein catabolism

The following *additional* adverse reactions are related to parenteral corticosteroid therapy:
Rare instances of blindness associated with intralesional therapy around the face and head
Anaphylactic reaction
Allergic or hypersensitivity reactions
Utricaria
Hyperpigmentation or hypopigmentation
Subcutaneous and cutaneous atrophy
Injection site infections following non-sterile administration (see WARNINGS)
Postinjection flare, following intra-articular use
Charcot-like arthropathy
Arachnoiditis has been reported following intrathecal administration

Dosage And Administration: Because of possible physical incompatibilities, *Depo-Medrol* Sterile Aqueous Suspension (methylprednisolone acetate) should not be diluted or mixed with other solutions.

A. Administration for Local Effect

Therapy with *Depo-Medrol* does not obviate the need for the conventional measures usually employed. Although this method of treatment will ameliorate symptoms, it is in no sense a cure and the hormone has no effect on the cause of the inflammation.

1. Rheumatoid and Osteoarthritis. The dose for intra-articular administration depends upon the size of the joint and varies with the severity of the condition in the individual patient. In chronic cases, injections may be repeated at intervals ranging from one to five or more weeks depending upon the degree of relief obtained from the initial injection. The doses in the following table are given as a general guide:

Size of Joint	*Examples*	*Range of Dosage*
Large	Knees Ankles Shoulders	20 to 80 mg
Medium	Elbows Wrists	10 to 40 mg
Small	Metacarpophalangeal Interphalangeal Sternoclavicular Acromioclavicular	4 to 10 mg

Procedure: It is recommended that the anatomy of the joint involved be reviewed before attempting intra-articular injection. In order to obtain the full anti-inflammatory effect it is important that the injection be made into the synovial space. Employing the same sterile technique as for a lumbar puncture, a sterile 20 to 24 gauge needle (on a dry syringe) is quickly inserted into the synovial cavity. Procaine infiltration is elective. The aspiration of only a few drops of joint fluid proves the joint space has been entered by the needle. *The injection site for each joint is determined by that location where the synovial cavity is most superficial and most free of large vessels and nerves.* With the needle in place, the aspirating syringe is removed and replaced by a second syringe containing the desired amount of *Depo-Medrol* Sterile Aqueous Suspension. The plunger is then pulled outward slightly to aspirate synovial fluid and to make sure the needle is still in the synovial space. After injection, the joint is moved gently a few times to aid mixing of the synovial fluid and the suspension. The site is covered with a small sterile dressing.

Suitable sites for intra-articular injection are the knee, ankle, wrist, elbow, shoulder, phalangeal, and hip joints. Since difficulty is not infrequently encountered in entering the hip joint, precautions should be taken to avoid any large blood vessels in the area. Joints not suitable for injection are those that are anatomically inaccessible such as the spinal joints and those like the sacroiliac joints that are devoid of synovial space. Treatment failures are most frequently the result of failure to enter the joint space. Little or no benefit follows injection into surrounding tissue. If failures occur when injections into the synovial spaces are certain, as determined by aspiration of fluid, repeated injections are usually futile. Local therapy does not alter the underlying disease process, and whenever possible comprehensive therapy including physiotherapy and orthopedic correction should be employed.

Following intra-articular steroid therapy, care should be taken to avoid overuse of joints in which symptomatic benefit has been obtained. Negligence in this matter may permit an increase in joint deterioration that will more than offset the beneficial effects of the steroid. Unstable joints should not be injected. Repeated intra-articular injection may in some cases result in instability of the joint. X-ray follow-up is suggested in selected cases to detect deterioration.

If a local anesthetic is used prior to injection of *Depo-Medrol,* the anesthetic package insert should be read carefully and all the precautions observed.

2. Bursitis. The area around the injection site is prepared in a sterile way and a wheal at the site made with 1 percent procaine hydrochloride solution. A 20 to 24 gauge needle attached to a dry syringe is inserted into the bursa and the fluid aspirated. The needle is left in place and the aspirating syringe changed for a small syringe containing the desired dose. After injection, the needle is withdrawn and a small dressing applied.

3. Miscellaneous: Ganglion, Tendinitis, Epicondylitis. In the treatment of conditions such as tendinitis or tenosynovitis, care should be taken, following application of a suitable antiseptic to the overlying skin, to inject the suspension into the tendon sheath rather than into the substance of the tendon. The tendon may be readily palpated when placed on a stretch. When treating conditions such as epicondylitis, the area of greatest tenderness should be outlined carefully and the suspension infiltrated into the area. For ganglia of the tendon sheaths, the suspension is injected directly into the cyst. In many cases, a single injection causes a marked decrease in the size of the cystic tumor and may effect disappearance. The usual sterile precautions should be observed, of course, with each injection.

The dose in the treatment of the various conditions of the tendinous or bursal structures listed above varies with the condition being treated and ranges from 4 to 30 mg. In recurrent or chronic conditions, repeated injections may be necessary.

4. Injections for Local Effect in Dermatologic Conditions. Following cleansing with an appropriate antiseptic such as 70% alcohol, 20 to 60 mg of the suspension is injected into the lesion. It may be necessary to distribute doses ranging from 20 to 40 mg by repeated local injections in the case of large lesions. Care should be taken to avoid injection of sufficient material to cause blanching since this may be followed by a small slough. One to four injections are usually employed, the intervals between injections varying with the type of lesion being treated and the duration of improvement produced by the initial injection.

When multidose vials are used, special care to prevent contamination of the contents is essential (See WARNINGS).

B. Administration for Systemic Effect

The intramuscular dosage will vary with the condition being treated. When employed as a temporary substitute for oral therapy, a single injection during each 24-hour period of a dose of the suspension equal to the total daily oral dose of *Medrol* ® Tablets (methylprednisolone) is usually sufficient. When a prolonged effect is desired, the weekly dose may be calculated by multiplying the daily oral dose by 7 and given as a single intramuscular injection.

Dosage must be individualized according to the severity of the disease and response of the patient. For infants and children, the recommended dosage will have to be reduced, but dosage should be governed by the severity of the condition rather than by strict adherence to the ratio indicated by age or body weight.

Hormone therapy is an adjunct to, and not a replacement for, conventional therapy. Dosage must be decreased or discontinued gradually when the drug has been administered for more than a few days. The severity, prognosis and expected duration of the disease and the reaction of the patient to medication are primary factors in determining dosage. If a period of spontaneous remission occurs in a chronic condition, treatment should be discontinued. Routine laboratory studies, such as urinalysis, two-hour postprandial blood sugar, determination of blood pressure and body weight, and a chest X-ray should be made at regular intervals during prolonged therapy. Upper GI X-rays are desirable in patients with an ulcer history or significant dyspepsia.

In patients with the **adrenogenital syndrome,** a single intramuscular injection of 40 mg every two weeks may be adequate. For maintenance of patients with **rheumatoid arthritis,** the weekly intramuscular dose will vary from 40 to 120 mg. The usual dosage for patients with **dermatologic lesions** benefited by systemic corticoid therapy is 40 to 120 mg of methylprednisolone acetate administered intramuscularly at weekly intervals for one to four weeks. In acute severe dermatitis due to poison ivy, relief may result within 8 to 12 hours following intramuscular administration of a single dose of 80 to 120 mg. In chronic contact dermatitis repeated injections at 5 to 10 day intervals may be necessary. In seborrheic dermatitis, a weekly dose of 80 mg may be adequate to control the condition.

Following intramuscular administration of 80 to 120 mg to asthmatic patients, relief may result within 6 to 48 hours and persist for several days to two weeks. Similarly in patients with allergic rhinitis (hay fever) an intramuscular dose of 80 to 120 mg may be followed by

relief of coryzal symptoms within six hours persisting for several days to three weeks.
If signs of stress are associated with the condition being treated, the dosage of the suspension should be increased. If a rapid hormonal effect of maximum intensity is required, the intravenous administration of highly soluble methylprednisolone sodium succinate is indicated.

Multiple Sclerosis

In treatment of acute exacerbations of multiple sclerosis daily doses of 200 mg of prednisolone for a week followed by 80 mg every other day for 1 month have been shown to be effective (4 mg of methylprednisolone is equivalent to 5 mg of prednisolone).

How Supplied: *Depo-Medrol* Sterile Aqueous Suspension (methylprednisolone acetate) is available in the following strengths and sizes:

20 mg/ml	5 ml vial	*NDC 0009-0274-01*
40 mg/ml	1 ml vial	*NDC 0009-0280-01*
	5 ml vial	*NDC 0009-0280-02*
	10 ml vial	*NDC 0009-0280-03*
80 mg/ml	1 ml vial	*NDC 0009-0306-01*
	1 ml *U-Ject®* Disposable Syringe	*NDC 0009-0306-04*
	5 ml vial	*NDC 0009-0306-02*

Store at controlled room temperature 15°–30° C (59°–86° F)
Code 810 341 004

[*Shown in Product Identification Section*]

DEPO-PROVERA® Sterile Aqueous Suspension ℞
(sterile medroxyprogesterone acetate suspension, USP)
400 mg/ml
2.5 ml vial
NSN 6505-01-059-9006 (VA)
10 ml vial
NSN 6505-01-059-9005 (VA)

WARNING

THE USE OF PROGESTATIONAL AGENTS DURING THE FIRST FOUR MONTHS OF PREGNANCY IS NOT RECOMMENDED

Progestational agents have been used beginning with the first trimester of pregnancy in an attempt to prevent habitual abortion or treat threatened abortion. There is no adequate evidence that such use is effective and there is evidence of potential harm to the fetus when such drugs are given during the first four months of pregnancy. Furthermore, in the vast majority of women, the cause of abortion is a defective ovum, which progestational agents could not be expected to influence. In addition, the use of progestational agents, with their uterine-relaxant properties, in patients with fertilized defective ova may cause a delay in spontaneous abortion. Therefore, the use of such drugs during the first four months of pregnancy is not recommended.

Several reports suggest an association between intrauterine exposure to female sex hormones and congenital anomalies, including congenital heart defects and limb reduction defects[1–5]. One study[4] estimated a 4.7-fold increased risk of limb reduction defects in infants exposed in utero to sex hormones (oral contraceptives, hormone withdrawal tests for pregnancy, or attempted treatment for threatened abortion). Some of these exposures were very short and involved only a few days of treatment. The data suggest that the risk of limb reduction defects in exposed fetuses is somewhat less than 1 in 1000.

If the patient is exposed to *Depo-Provera* Sterile Aqueous Suspension (medroxyprogesterone acetate) during the first four months of pregnancy or if she becomes pregnant while taking this drug, she should be apprised of the potential risks to the fetus.

Description: Medroxyprogesterone acetate is a derivative of progesterone and is active by the parenteral and oral routes of administration. It is a white to off-white, odorless crystalline powder, stable in air, melting between 200 and 210° C. It is freely soluble in chloroform, soluble in acetone and dioxane, sparingly soluble in alcohol and methanol, slightly soluble in ether and insoluble in water.

The chemical name for medroxyprogesterone acetate is Pregn-4-ene-3,20-dione, 17-(acetyloxy)-6-methyl-, (6α)-.

Depo-Provera Sterile Aqueous Suspension (medroxyprogesterone acetate) for intramuscular injection is available in 2 strengths, 100 mg/ml and 400 mg/ml medroxyprogesterone acetate.

Each ml of the **100 mg/ml** suspension contains:

Medroxyprogesterone Acetate	100 mg
Also	
Polyethylene Glycol 3350	27.6 mg
Polysorbate 80	1.84 mg
Sodium Chloride	8.3 mg
Methylparaben	1.75 mg
Propylparaben	0.194 mg

added as preservatives

Each ml of the **400 mg/ml** suspension contains:

Medroxyprogesterone Acetate	400 mg
Polyethylene Glycol 3350	20.3 mg
Sodium Sulfate Anhydrous	11 mg
Myristyl-gamma-picolinium Chloride	1.69 mg

added as preservative

When necessary, pH was adjusted with sodium hydroxide and/or hydrochloric acid.

Actions: *Depo-Provera* Sterile Aqueous Suspension (medroxyprogesterone acetate) administered parenterally in the recommended doses to women with adequate endogenous estrogen transforms proliferative endometrium into secretory endometrium.

Depo-Provera inhibits (in the usual dose range) the secretion of pituitary gonadotropin which, in turn, prevents follicular maturation and ovulation.

Because of its prolonged action and the resulting difficulty in predicting the time of withdrawal bleeding following injection, *Depo-Provera* is not recommended in secondary amenorrhea or dysfunctional uterine bleeding. In these conditions oral therapy is recommended.

Indications: Adjunctive therapy and palliative treatment of inoperable, recurrent, and metastatic endometrial carcinoma or renal carcinoma.

Contraindications:

1. Thrombophlebitis, thromboembolic disorders, cerebral apoplexy or patients with a past history of these conditions.
2. Carcinoma of the breast.
3. Undiagnosed vaginal bleeding.
4. Missed abortion.
5. As a diagnostic test for pregnancy.
6. Known sensitivity to *Depo-Provera* Sterile Aqueous Suspension (medroxyprogesterone acetate).

Warnings:

1. The physician should be alert to the earliest manifestations of thrombotic disorders (thrombophlebitis, cerebrovascular disorders, pulmonary embolism, and retinal thrombosis). Should any of these occur or be suspected, the drug should be discontinued immediately.
2. Long term toxicology studies in the monkey, dog and rat disclose:
   1) Beagle dogs receiving 75 mg/kg and 3 mg/kg every 90 days developed mammary nodules, as did some of the control animals. The nodules appearing in the control animals were intermittent in nature, whereas the nodules in the drug treated animals were larger, more numerous, persistent, and there were two high dose animals that developed breast malignancies.
   2) Two of the monkeys receiving 150 mg/kg every 90 days developed undifferentiated carcinoma of the uterus. No uterine malignancies were found in monkeys receiving 30 mg/kg, 3 mg/kg, or placebo every 90 days. Transient mammary nodules were found during the study in the control, 3 mg/kg and 30 mg/kg groups, but not in the 150 mg/kg group. At sacrifice, the only nodules extant were in three of the monkeys in the 30 mg/kg group. Upon histopathologic examination these nodules have been determined to be hyperplastic.
   3) No uterine or breast abnormalities were revealed in the rat.

   The relevance of any of these findings with respect to humans has not been established.
3. The use of *Depo-Provera* Sterile Aqueous Suspension (medroxyprogesterone acetate) for contraception is investigational since there are unresolved questions relating to its safety for this indication. Therefore, this is not an approved indication.
4. Discontinue medication pending examination if there is sudden partial or complete loss of vision, or if there is a sudden onset of proptosis, diplopia or migraine. If examination reveals papilledema or retinal vascular lesions, medication should be withdrawn.
5. Usage in pregnancy (See WARNING Box).
6. Retrospective studies of morbidity and mortality in Great Britain and studies of morbidity in the United States have shown a statistically significant association between thrombophlebitis, pulmonary embolism, and cerebral thrombosis and embolism and the use of oral contraceptives.[6–9] The estimate of the relative risk of thromboembolism in the study by Vessey and Doll[8] was about sevenfold, while Sartwell and associates[9] in the United States found a relative risk of 4.4, meaning that the users are several times as likely to undergo thromboembolic disease without evident cause as non-users. The American study also indicated that the risk did not persist after discontinuation of administration, and that it was not enhanced by long continued administration. The American study was not designed to evaluate a difference between products.
7. Following repeated injections, amenorrhea and infertility may persist for periods up to 18 months and occasionally longer.
8. The physician should be alert to the earliest manifestations of impaired liver function.

Precautions:

1. The pretreatment physical examination should include special reference to breast and pelvic organs, as well as Papanicolaou smear.
2. Because progestogens may cause some degree of fluid retention, conditions which might be influenced by this factor, such as epilepsy, migraine, asthma, cardiac or renal dysfunction, require careful observation.
3. In cases of breakthrough bleeding, as in all cases of irregular bleeding per vaginum, nonfunctional causes should be borne in mind. In cases of undiagnosed vaginal bleeding, adequate diagnostic measures are indicated.
4. Patients who have a history of psychic depression should be carefully observed and the drug discontinued if the depression recurs to a serious degree.

Continued on next page

Upjohn—Cont.

5. Any possible influence of prolonged progestin therapy on pituitary, ovarian, adrenal, hepatic or uterine functions awaits further study.
6. A decrease in glucose tolerance has been observed in a small percentage of patients on estrogen-progestin combination drugs. The mechanism of this decrease is obscure. For this reason, diabetic patients should be carefully observed while receiving progestin therapy.
7. The age of the patient constitutes no absolute limiting factor although treatment with progestins may mask the onset of the climacteric.
8. The pathologist should be advised of progestin therapy when relevant specimens are submitted.
9. Because of the occasional occurrence of thrombotic disorders, (thrombophlebitis, pulmonary embolism, retinal thrombosis, and cerebrovascular disorders) in patients taking estrogen-progestin combinations and since the mechanism is obscure, the physician should be alert to the earliest manifestation of these disorders.

Information for the Patient
See Patient Information at the end of the insert.

The patient insert should be given to all premenopausal women, except those in whom childbearing is impossible.

Adverse Reactions: (See WARNING Box for possible adverse effects on the fetus).
In a few instances there have been undesirable sequelae at the site of injection, such as residual lump, change in color of skin or sterile abscess.
The following adverse reactions have been associated with the use of *Depo-Provera* Sterile Aqueous Suspension (medroxyprogesterone acetate).
Breast—In a few instances, breast tenderness or galactorrhea have occurred.
Psychic—An occasional patient has experienced nervousness, insomnia, somnolence, fatigue or dizziness.
Thromboembolic Phenomena—Thromboembolic phenomena including thrombophlebitis and pulmonary embolism have been reported.
Skin and Mucous Membranes—Sensitivity reactions ranging from pruritus, urticaria, angioneurotic edema to generalized rash and anaphylaxis have occasionally been reported. Acne, alopecia, or hirsutism have been reported in a few cases.
Gastrointestinal—Rarely, nausea has been reported. Jaundice, including neonatal jaundice, has been noted in a few instances.
Miscellaneous—Rare cases of headache and hyperpyrexia have been reported.
The following adverse reactions have been observed in women taking progestins including *Depo-Provera:*
breakthrough bleeding
spotting
change in menstrual flow
amenorrhea
edema
change in weight
(increase or decrease)
changes in cervical erosion and
cervical secretions
cholestatic jaundice
rash (allergic) with and
without pruritus
melasma or chloasma
mental depression
A statistically significant association has been demonstrated between use of estrogen-progestin combination drugs and the following serious adverse reactions: thrombophlebitis; pulmonary embolism and cerebral thrombosis and embolism. For this reason patients on progestin therapy should be carefully observed.
Although available evidence is suggestive of an association, such a relationship has been neither confirmed nor refuted for the following serious adverse reactions: neuro-ocular lesions, eg, retinal thrombosis and optic neuritis.
The following adverse reactions have been observed in patients receiving estrogen-progestin combination drugs:
rise in blood pressure in susceptible individuals
premenstrual-like syndrome
changes in libido
changes in appetite
cystitis-like syndrome
headache
nervousness
dizziness
fatigue
backache
hirsutism
loss of scalp hair
erythema multiforme
erythema nodosum
hemorrhagic eruption
itching
In view of these observations, patients on progestin therapy should be carefully observed.
The following laboratory results may be altered by the use of estrogen-progestin combination drugs:
Increased sulfobromophthalein retention and other hepatic function tests.
Coagulation tests: increase in prothrombin factors VII, VIII, IX and X.
Metyrapone test.
Pregnanediol determination.
Thyroid function: increase in PBI, and butanol extractable protein bound iodine and decrease in T^3 uptake values.

Dosage and Administration: **The suspension is intended for intramuscular administration only.**
Endometrial or renal carcinoma—doses of 400 mg to 1000 mg of *Depo-Provera* Sterile Aqueous Suspension (medroxyprogesterone acetate) per week are recommended initially. If improvement is noted within a few weeks or months and the disease appears stabilized, it may be possible to maintain improvement with as little as 400 mg per month. Medroxyprogesterone acetate is not recommended as primary therapy, but as adjunctive and palliative treatment in advanced inoperable cases including those with recurrent or metastatic disease.

How Supplied: *Depo-Provera* Sterile Aqueous Suspension (medroxyprogesterone acetate) is available in 2 strengths:

100 mg/ml:	
5 ml vials	NDC 0009-0248-02
400 mg/ml:	
1 ml unit dose	
U-ject® Disposable Syringe	NDC 0009-0626-03
2.5 ml vial	NDC 0009-0626-01
10 ml vial	NDC 0009-0626-02

References:

1. Gal I, Kirman B, Stern J: Hormonal pregnancy tests and congenital malformation. Nature *216*:83, 1967.
2. Levy EP, Cohen A, Fraser FC: Hormone treatment during pregnancy and congenital heart defects. Lancet *1*:611, 1973.
3. Nora JJ, Nora AH: Birth defects and oral contraceptives. Lancet *1*:941–942, 1973.
4. Janerich DT, Piper JM, Glebatis DM: Oral contraceptives and congenital limb-reduction defects. N Engl J Med *291*:697–700, 1974.
5. Heinonen OP, Slone D, Monson RR, et al: Cardiovascular birth defects and antenatal exposure to female sex hormones. N Engl J Med *296*:67–70, 1977.
6. Royal College of General Practitioners: Oral contraception and thromboembolic disease. J Coll Gen Pract *13*:267–279, 1967.
7. Inman WHW, Vessey MP: Investigation of deaths from pulmonary, coronary, and cerebral thrombosis and embolism in women of child-bearing age. Br Med J *2*:193–199, 1968.
8. Vessey MP, Doll R: Investigation of relation between use of oral contraceptives and thromboembolic disease. A further report. Br Med J *2*:651–657, 1969.
9. Sartwell PE, Masi AT, Arthes FG, et al: Thromboembolism and oral contraceptives: An epidemiological case-control study. Am J Epidemiol *90*:365–380, 1969.

The text of the patient insert for progesterone and progesterone-like drugs is set forth below.

Patient Information: *Depo-Provera* Sterile Aqueous Suspension contains a progesterone (medroxyprogesterone acetate). The information below is that which the U.S. Food and Drug Administration requires be provided for all patients taking progesterones. The information below relates only to the risk to the unborn child associated with use of progesterone during pregnancy. For further information on the use, side effects and other risks associated with this product, ask your doctor.

WARNING FOR WOMEN
There is an increased risk of birth defects in children whose mothers take this drug during the first four months of pregnancy.
Medroxyprogesterone acetate is similar to the progesterone hormones naturally produced by the body. Progesterone and progesterone-like drugs are used to treat menstrual disorders, to test if the body is producing certain hormones, and to treat some forms of cancer in women. They have been used as a test for pregnancy but such use is no longer considered safe because of possible damage to a developing baby. Also, more rapid methods for testing for pregnancy are now available.
These drugs have also been used to prevent miscarriage in the first few months of pregnancy. No adequate evidence is available to show that they are effective for this purpose. Furthermore, most cases of early miscarriage are due to causes which could not be helped by these drugs.
There is an increased risk of birth defects, such as heart or limb defects, if progesterone and progesterone-like drugs are taken during the first four months of pregnancy.
The exact risk of taking this drug early in pregnancy and having a baby with a birth defect is not known. However, one study found that babies born to women who had taken sex hormones (such as progesterone-like drugs) during the first three months of pregnancy were 4 to 5 times more likely to have abnormalities of the arms or legs than if their mothers had not taken such drugs. Some of these women had taken these drugs for only a few days. The chance that an infant whose mother had taken this drug will have this type of defect is about 1 in 1,000.
If you take *Depo-Provera* Sterile Aqueous Suspension and later find you were pregnant when you took it, be sure to discuss this with your doctor as soon as possible.
Code 810 597 002

DEPO®-TESTOSTERONE ℞

Sterile Solution
(testosterone cypionate injection, USP)
For Intramuscular Use Only

How Supplied: *Depo*-Testosterone Sterile Solution is available in the following packages:
50 mg per ml. Each ml contains 50 mg testosterone cypionate, also 5.4 mg chlorobutanol anhydrous (chloral deriv.), in 874 mg cottonseed oil.

10 ml vial *NDC 0009-0303-01*

100 mg per ml. Each ml contains 100 mg testosterone cypionate, also 0.1 ml benzyl benzoate, 9.45 mg benzyl alcohol in 736 mg cottonseed oil.

1 ml vial *NDC 0009-0347-01*
10 ml vial *NDC 0009-0347-02*

200 mg per ml. Each ml contains 200 mg testosterone cypionate, also 0.2 ml benzyl benzoate, 9.45 mg benzyl alcohol, in 560 mg cottonseed oil.

1 ml vial *NDC 0009-0417-01*
10 ml vial *NDC 0009-0417-02*

DIDREX™ Tablets Ⓒ ℞
(benzphetamine hydrochloride)

Description: Benzphetamine hydrochloride is d-N-benzyl-N, α-dimethylphenethylamine hydrochloride, a white crystalline powder readily soluble in water, 95% ethanol and chloroform.

Actions: *Didrex* Tablets (benzphetamine hydrochloride) are a sympathomimetic amine with pharmacologic activity similar to the prototype drugs of this class used in obesity, the amphetamines. Actions include central nervous system stimulation and elevation of blood pressure. Tachyphylaxis and tolerance have been demonstrated with all drugs of this class in which these phenomena have been looked for.

Drugs of this class used in obesity are commonly known as "anorectics" or "anorexigenics." It has not been established, however, that the action of such drugs in treating obesity is primarily one of appetite suppression. Other central nervous system actions, or metabolic effects, may be involved, for example.

Adult obese subjects instructed in dietary management and treated with "anorectic" drugs, lose more weight on the average than those treated with placebo and diet, as determined in relatively short term clinical trials.

The magnitude of increased weight loss of drug treated patients over placebo treated patients is only a fraction of a pound a week. The rate of weight loss is greatest in the first weeks of therapy for both drug and placebo subjects and tends to decrease in succeeding weeks. The possible origins of the increased weight loss due to the various drug effects are not established. The amount of weight loss associated with the use of an "anorectic" drug varies from trial to trial, and the increased weight loss appears to be related in part to variables other than the drug prescribed, such as the physician-investigator, the population treated, and the diet prescribed. Studies do not permit conclusions as to the relative importance of the drug and nondrug factors on weight loss.

The natural history of obesity is measured in years, whereas the studies cited are restricted to a few weeks duration; thus, the total impact of drug induced weight loss over that of diet alone must be considered clinically limited.

Indications: *Didrex* Tablets (benzphetamine hydrochloride) are indicated in the management of exogenous obesity as a short term adjunct (a few weeks) in a regimen of weight reduction based on caloric restriction. The limited usefulness of agents of this class (see **Actions**) should be measured against possible risk factors inherent in their use such as those described above.

Contraindications: *Didrex* Tablets (benzphetamine hydrochloride) are contraindicated in patients with advanced arteriosclerosis, symptomatic cardiovascular disease, moderate to severe hypertension, hyperthyroidism, known hypersensitivity or idiosyncrasy to sympathomimetic amines, and agitated states, and in patients with a history of drug abuse.

Hypertensive crises have resulted when sympathomimetic amines have been used concomitantly or within 14 days following use of monamine oxidase inhibitors. *Didrex* should not be used concomitantly with other CNS stimulants.

Warnings:

Drug Dependence: *Didrex* Tablets (benzphetamine hydrochloride) are related chemically and pharmacologically to the amphetamines. Amphetamines and related stimulant drugs have been extensively abused, and the possibility of abuse of *Didrex* should be kept in mind when evaluating the desirability of including a drug as part of a weight reduction program. Abuse of amphetamines and related drugs may be associated with intense psychological dependence and severe social dysfunction. There are reports of patients who have increased the dosage to many times that recommended. Abrupt cessation following prolonged high dosage administration results in extreme fatigue and mental depression; changes are also noted on the sleep EEG. Manifestations of chronic intoxication with anorectic drugs include severe dermatoses, marked insomnia, irritability, hyperactivity, and personality changes. The most severe manifestation of chronic intoxication is psychosis, often clinically indistinguishable from schizophrenia.

Usage in Pregnancy—Safe use in pregnancy has not been established. Reproductive studies in mammals at high multiples of the human dose on some anorectic drugs have suggested both an embryotoxic and a teratogenic potential for this type of drug. Therefore, use of *Didrex* by women who are or who may become pregnant, and especially those in the first trimester of pregnancy, requires that the potential benefit be weighed against the possible hazard to mother and infant.

Usage in Children—Use of benzphetamine hydrochloride is not recommended in children under 12 years of age.

Precautions: Insulin requirements in diabetes mellitus may be altered in association with use of anorexigenic drugs and the concomitant dietary restrictions.

Psychological disturbances have been reported in patients who receive an anorectic agent together with a restrictive dietary regimen.

Didrex Tablets, 25 mg, contain FD&C Yellow No. 5 (tartrazine) which may cause allergic-type reactions (including bronchial asthma) in certain susceptible individuals. Although the overall incidence of FD&C Yellow No. 5 (tartrazine) sensitivity in the general population is low, it is frequently seen in patients who also have aspirin hypersensitivity.

Adverse Reactions: The following have been associated with the use of benzphetamine hydrochloride:

Overstimulation, restlessness, dizziness, insomnia, gastrointestinal disturbances, nausea, diarrhea, palpitation, tachycardia, elevation of blood pressure, tremor, sweating, headache, dryness of the mouth or unpleasant taste, urticaria and other allergic reactions involving the skin, changes in libido; rarely, psychotic episodes at recommended dosage; depression following withdrawal of drug.

Dosage and Administration: Dosage should be individualized according to the response of the patient. The suggested dosage ranges from 25 to 50 mg one to three times daily. Treatment should begin with 25 to 50 mg once daily with subsequent increase in individual dose or frequency according to response. A single daily dose is preferably given in mid-morning or mid-afternoon, according to the patient's eating habits. In an occasional patient it may be desirable to avoid late afternoon administration. Use of benzphetamine hydrochloride is not recommended in children under 12 years of age.

Treatment of Overdosage: (See **Warnings**)
Information concerning the effects of overdosage with *Didrex* Tablets (benzphetamine hydrochloride) is extremely limited. The following is based on experience with other anorexiants.

Management of acute amphetamine intoxication is largely symptomatic and includes sedation with a barbiturate. If hypertension is marked the use of a nitrite or rapidly acting alpha receptor blocking agent should be considered. Experience with hemodialysis or peritoneal dialysis is inadequate to permit recommendations in this regard.

How Supplied: *Didrex* Tablets (benzphetamine hydrochloride) are available in 2 strengths:

25 mg
Bottles of 100 *NDC 0009-0018-01*

50 mg
Bottles of 100 *NDC 0009-0024-01*
Bottles of 500 *NDC 0009-0024-02*
Code 810 735 201

[Shown in Product Identification Section]

E-MYCIN® Tablets ℞
(erythromycin base enteric-coated tablets)
Each tablet contains erythromycin as the base

250 mg (40's) Unit of Use
NSN 6505-01-113-4758 (M)
250 mg (100's)
NSN 6505-00-604-1223 (M)

Description: Erythromycin is produced by a strain of *Streptomyces erythraeus* and belongs to the macrolide group of antibiotics. It is basic and readily forms salts with acids. The base is a white to off-white crystals or powder slightly soluble in water, soluble in alcohol, in chloroform, and in ether. *E-Mycin* Tablets (erythromycin) are specially coated to protect the contents from the inactivating effects of gastric acidity and to permit efficient absorption of the antibiotic in the small intestine.

Actions: The mode of action of erythromycin is inhibition of protein synthesis without affecting nucleic acid synthesis. Resistance to erythromycin of some strains of *Haemophilus influenzae* and staphylococci has been demonstrated. Culture and susceptibility testing should be done. If the Kirby-Bauer method of disk susceptibility is used, a 15 mcg erythromycin disk should give a zone diameter of at least 18 mm when tested against an erythromycin susceptible organism.

Bioavailability data are available from The Upjohn Company.

E-Mycin Tablets (erythromycin base enteric-coated tablets) are well absorbed and may be given without regard to meals.

After absorption, erythromycin diffuses readily into most body fluids. In the absence of meningeal inflammation, low concentrations are normally achieved in the spinal fluid but passage of the drug across the blood-brain barrier increases in meningitis. In the presence of normal hepatic function, erythromycin is concentrated in the liver and excreted in the bile; the effect of hepatic dysfunction on excretion of erythromycin by the liver into the bile is not known. After oral administration, less than 5 percent of the activity of the administered dose can be recovered in the urine.

Erythromycin crosses the placental barrier but fetal plasma levels are low.

Indications:

Streptococcus pyogenes (Group A beta hemolytic streptococcus): For upper and lower respiratory tract, skin, and soft tissue infections of mild to moderate severity.

Injectable benzathine penicillin G is considered by the American Heart Association to be the drug of choice in the treatment and prevention of streptococcal pharyngitis and in long-term prophylaxis of rheumatic fever.

When oral medication is preferred for treatment of the above conditions, penicillin G, V, or erythromycin are alternate drugs of choice.

When oral medication is given, the importance of strict adherence by the patient to the prescribed dosage regimen must be stressed. A therapeutic dose should be administered for at least 10 days.

Alpha-hemolytic streptococci (viridans group): Although no controlled clinical efficacy trials have been conducted, oral erythromycin has been suggested by the American Heart Association and American Dental Association for use in a regimen for prophylaxis against bacterial

Continued on next page

Upjohn—Cont.

endocarditis in patients hypersensitive to penicillin who have congenital or rheumatic or other acquired valvular heart disease when they undergo dental procedures and surgical procedures of the upper respiratory tract.[1] Erythromycin is not suitable prior to genitourinary or gastrointestinal tract surgery.

Note: When selecting antibiotics for the prevention of bacterial endocarditis the physician or dentist should read the full joint statement of the American Heart Association and the American Dental Association.[1]

Staphylococcus aureus: For acute infections of skin and soft tissue of mild to moderate severity. Resistant organisms may emerge during treatment.

Streptococcus pneumoniae (Diplococcus pneumoniae): For upper respiratory tract infections (eg, otitis media, pharyngitis) and lower respiratory tract infections (eg, pneumonia) of mild to moderate degree.

Mycoplasma pneumoniae (Eaton agent, PPLO): For respiratory infections due to this organism.

Hemophilus influenzae: For upper respiratory tract infections of mild to moderate severity when used concomitantly with adequate doses of sulfonamides. Not all strains of this organism are susceptible at the erythromycin concentrations ordinarily achieved (see appropriate sulfonamide labeling for prescribing information).

Treponema pallidum: Erythromycin is an alternate choice of treatment for primary syphilis in patients allergic to the penicillins. In treatment of primary syphilis, spinal fluid examinations should be done before treatment and as part of follow-up after therapy.

Corynebacterium diphtheriae and **C. minutissimum:** As an adjunct to antitoxin, to prevent establishment of carriers, and to eradicate the organism in carriers.

In the treatment of erythrasma.

Entamoeba histolytica: In the treatment of intestinal amebiasis only. Extraenteric amebiasis requires treatment with other agents.

Listeria monocytogenes: Infections due to this organism.

Neisseria gonorrhoeae: Erythromycin lactobionate for injection in conjunction with erythromycin base orally, as an alternative drug in treatment of acute pelvic inflammatory disease caused by *N. gonorrhoeae* in female patients with a history of sensitivity to penicillin. Before treatment of gonorrhea, patients who are suspected of also having syphilis should have a microscopic examination for *T. pallidum* (by immunofluorescence or darkfield) before receiving erythromycin, and monthly serologic tests for a minimum of 4 months.

Bordetella pertussis: Erythromycin is effective in eliminating the organism from the nasopharynx of infected individuals, rendering them noninfectious. Some clinical studies suggest that erythromycin may be helpful in the prophylaxis of pertussis in exposed susceptible individuals.

Legionnaires Disease: Although no controlled clinical efficacy studies have been conducted, *in vitro* and limited preliminary clinical data suggest that erythromycin can be effective in treating Legionnaires Disease.

Contraindications: Erythromycin is contraindicated in patients with known hypersensitivity to this antibiotic.

Warning: Usage in pregnancy: Safety for use in pregnancy has not been established.

Precautions: Erythromycin is principally excreted by the liver. Caution should be exercised in administering the antibiotic to patients with impaired hepatic function.

There have been reports of hepatic dysfunction, with or without jaundice, occurring in patients receiving oral erythromycin products. Recent data from studies of erythromycin reveal that its use in patients who are receiving high doses of theophylline may be associated with an increase of serum theophylline levels and potential theophylline toxicity. In cases of theophylline toxicity and/or elevated serum theophylline levels, the dose of theophylline should be reduced while the patient is receiving concomitant erythromycin therapy.

Surgical procedures should be performed when indicated.

Adverse Reactions: The most frequent side effects of erythromycin preparations are gastrointestinal, such as abdominal cramping and discomfort, and are dose related. Nausea, vomiting, and diarrhea occur infrequently with usual oral doses.

During prolonged or repeated therapy, there is a possibility of overgrowth of nonsusceptible bacteria or fungi. If such infections occur, the drug should be discontinued and appropriate therapy instituted.

Mild allergic reactions such as urticaria and other skin rashes have occurred. Serious allergic reactions, including anaphylaxis, have been reported.

Dosage and Administration: *E-Mycin* Tablets (erythromycin base enteric-coated tablets) are well absorbed and may be given without regard to meals.

Adults: The usual dose is 250 mg four times daily or 333 mg every 8 hours.

If twice a day dosage is desired, the recommended dose is 500 mg every 12 hours.

Dosage may be increased up to 4 or more grams per day according to the severity of the infection. Twice-a-day dosing is not recommended when doses larger than 1 gram daily are administered.

Children: Age, weight, and severity of the infection are important factors in determining the proper dosage. 30 to 50 mg/kg/day, in divided doses, is the usual dose. For more severe infections, this dose may be doubled.

In the treatment of streptococcal infections, a therapeutic dosage of erythromycin should be administered for at least 10 days. In continuous **prophylaxis** of streptococcal infections in persons with a history of rheumatic heart disease, the dose is 250 mg twice a day.

For prophylaxis against bacterial endocarditis[1] in patients with rheumatic, congenital, or other acquired valvular heart disease when undergoing dental procedures or surgical procedures of the upper respiratory tract, give 1.0 gram (20 mg/kg for children) orally 1 ½–2 hours before the procedure and then 500 mg (10 mg/kg for children) orally every 6 hours for 8 doses.

For treatment of primary syphilis: 30 to 40 grams given in divided doses over a period of 10 to 15 days.

For treatment of acute pelvic inflammatory disease caused by *N. gonorrhoeae:* After initial treatment with erythromycin lactobionate for injection (500 mg every 6 hours for 3 days), the oral dosage recommendation is 250 mg every 6 hours for 7 days or 333 mg every 8 hours for 7 days.

For dysenteric amebiasis: 250 mg four times daily or 333 mg every 8 hours for 10 to 14 days, for adults; 30 to 50 mg/kg/day in divided doses for 10 to 14 days, for children.

For use in pertussis: Although optimal dosage and duration have not been established, doses of erythromycin utilized in reported clinical studies were 40 to 50 mg/kg/day, given in divided doses for 5 to 14 days.

For treatment of Legionnaires Disease: Although optimal doses have not been established, doses utilized in reported clinical data were those recommended above (1 to 4 grams erythromycin base daily in divided doses).

Treatment of Overdosage: Allergic reactions associated with acute overdosage should be handled in the usual manner—that is, by the administration of adrenalin, corticosteroids, and antihistamines as indicated and the prompt elimination of unabsorbed drug, in addition to all needed supportive measures.

How Supplied: *E-Mycin* Tablets (erythromycin base enteric-coated tablets) are available in the following packages:

250 mg Tablets

Bottles of 100	*NDC 0009-0103-02*
Bottles of 500	*NDC 0009-0103-15*
Unit dose packages (100)	*NDC 0009-0103-03*
Bottles of 40, unit of use	*NDC 0009-0103-39*

333 mg Tablets

Bottles of 100	*NDC 0009-3176-01*

[1] American Heart Association 1977. Prevention of bacterial endocarditis. Circulation *56*:139A–143A.

Code 810 386 107

[Shown in Product Identification Section]

E-MYCIN E® Liquid
(erythromycin ethylsuccinate oral suspension)

Each 5 ml (one teaspoon) of *E-Mycin E* Liquid contains erythromycin ethylsuccinate equivalent to erythromycin 200 mg or 400 mg in a pleasant tasting oral suspension suitable for oral administration.

How Supplied: *E-Mycin E* Liquid (erythromycin ethylsuccinate oral suspension) is supplied in the following sizes and strengths:

200 mg/5 ml

500 ml bottle	NDC 0009-0939-01

400 mg/5 ml

500 ml bottle	NDC 0009-0940-01

[Shown in Product Identification Section]

FLORONE® Cream **0.05%** ℞
(diflorasone diacetate)

Each gram of *Florone* Cream (diflorasone diacetate) contains 0.5 mg diflorasone diacetate in a cream base.

How Supplied: *Florone* Cream 0.05% (diflorasone diacetate), is available in 15, 30 and 60 gram tubes.

15 gram tube	NDC 0009-0199-07
30 gram tube	NDC 0009-0199-03
60 gram tube	NDC 0009-0199-05

FLORONE® Ointment, **0.05%** ℞
(diflorasone diacetate)

Each gram of *Florone* Ointment (diflorasone diacetate) contains 0.5 mg diflorasone diacetate in an ointment base:

How Supplied: *Florone* Ointment (diflorasone diacetate) 0.05% is supplied in 15, 30 and 60 gram tubes.

15 gram tube	NDC 0009-0917-01
30 gram tube	NDC 0009-0917-02
60 gram tube	NDC 0009-0917-03

GELFOAM® Sterile Sponge
(absorbable gelatin sponge, USP)

Size 12-7 mm:
NSN 6510-00-080-2053 (M)
Size 100:
NSN 6510-00-080-2054 (M)
Dental Packs, Size 4:
NSN 6510-00-064-4858 (M)

Description: *Gelfoam* Sterile Sponge is a sterile, pliable, surgical sponge prepared from specially treated, purified gelatin solution and capable of absorbing and holding within its meshes many times its weight of whole blood.

Actions: When implanted in tissues, *Gelfoam* absorbable gelatin sponge is absorbed completely in from 4 to 6 weeks without inducing excessive scar tissue formation. When applied to bleeding areas of skin or nasal, rectal, or vaginal mucosa, it completely liquefies within 2 to 5 days.

Indications:

Hemostasis: *Gelfoam* Sterile Sponge, absorbable gelatin sponge, dry or saturated with sodium chloride, is indicated in surgical procedures as an adjunct to hemostasis when control of bleeding by ligature or conventional procedures is ineffective or impractical.

Directions For Use: Pieces of *Gelfoam* Sterile Sponge, absorbable gelatin sponge, cut to the desired size, may be applied dry or saturated with sodium chloride injection. When applied dry, the pieces of *Gelfoam* should be compressed before application to the bleeding surface and then should be held in place with moderate pressure for 10 to 15 seconds. When used with saline, the pieces of *Gelfoam* should be immersed in the solution, then withdrawn, squeezed between the gloved fingers to remove the air bubbles present in the meshes, replaced in the solution, and left there until needed. The *Gelfoam* should immediately swell to its original size and shape when dropped into the solution the second time; if it does not swell, it should be removed and kneaded vigorously until all air is expelled and it does expand to its original shape when dropped into the solution. The piece of *Gelfoam* is then left wet or blotted to dampness on gauze and applied to the bleeding point. It should be held in place for 10 to 15 seconds with a pledget of cotton or small gauze sponge. Removal of the pledget of cotton or gauze is made easier by wetting it with a few drops of water to prevent pulling up the *Gelfoam,* which now encloses a firm clot. If desired, suction may be applied over the pledget of cotton or gauze to draw blood into the *Gelfoam* where it promptly clots; however, while suction hastens clotting, it is not essential, since the *Gelfoam* will draw up blood by capillary attraction and cause clotting satisfactorily. Usually the first application of *Gelfoam* will control bleeding, but if not, additional applications should be made, using fresh pieces of *Gelfoam* prepared as previously described.

When bleeding is controlled, the pieces of *Gelfoam* should be left in place; otherwise bleeding may start again. Since *Gelfoam* causes but little more cellular infiltration than the blood clot, the wound may be closed over it. When applied to bleeding skin or mucosa, *Gelfoam* will stay in place until it liquefies.

Contraindications: *Gelfoam* absorbable gelatin sponge should not be used in the closure of skin incisions as it may interfere with the healing of skin edges.

Warnings: This product should not be resterilized by heat, since heating may change its absorption time. Ethylene oxide is not recommended for resterilization since it may be trapped in the interstices of the foam. Although not reported for *Gelfoam* absorbable gelatin sponge, the gas is toxic to tissue, and may cause burns or irritation in trace amounts.

Precautions: The use of *Gelfoam* Sterile Sponge, absorbable gelatin sponge, is not recommended in the presence of frank infection. If signs of infection or abscess develop in an area where *Gelfoam* has been placed, reoperation may be necessary to remove the infected material and allow drainage.

Gelfoam should not be employed for controlling postpartum bleeding or menorrhagia.

By absorbing fluid, *Gelfoam* may expand and impinge on neighboring structures. Therefore, when placed into cavities or closed tissue spaces, minimal preliminary compression is advised and care should be exercised to avoid overpacking.

Adverse Reactions: *Gelfoam* Sterile Sponge, absorbable gelatin sponge, may form a nidus of infection and abscess formation. Giant cell granuloma in the brain has been reported at the site of *Gelfoam* implantation, as well as compression of the brain and spinal cord as a result of sterile accumulation of fluid. Excessive fibrosis and prolonged fixation of the tendon have been reported when *Gelfoam* was used about a tendon juncture in the repair of severed tendons.

Storage and Handling: *Gelfoam* absorbable gelatin sponge should be stored under normal conditions. Once the package is opened, the contents are subject to contamination. It is recommended that *Gelfoam* be used as soon as the package is opened and the unused contents discarded.

How Supplied: *Gelfoam* Sterile Sponge (absorbable gelatin sponge) is available in the following sizes:

Size 12—3 mm 20 mm × 60 mm (12 sq cm) × 3 mm [3/4 in × 2 3/8 in (1 3/4 sq in) × 1/8 in] *in boxes of 4 sponges in individual envelopes.*
NDC 0009-0301-01

Size 12—7 mm 20 mm × 60 mm (12 sq cm) × 7 mm [3/4 in × 2 3/8 in (1 3/4 sq in) × 1/4 in] *in boxes of 12 sponges in individual envelopes, and in jars of 4 sponges.*
Box NDC 0009-0315-03
Jar NDC 0009-0315-02

Size 50, 80 mm × 62.5 mm (50 sq cm) × 10 mm [3 1/8 in × 2 1/2 in (7 7/8 sq in) × 3/8 in] *in boxes of 4 sponges in individual envelopes.*
NDC 0009-0323-01

Size 100, 80 mm × 125 mm (100 sq cm) × 10 mm [3 1/8 in × 5 in (15 5/8 sq in) × 3/8 in] *in boxes of 6 sponges in individual envelopes.*
NDC 0009-0342-01

Size 200, 80 mm × 250 mm (200 sq cm) × 10 mm [3 1/8 in × 10 in (31 1/4 sq in) × 3/8 in] *in boxes of 6 sponges in individual envelopes.*
NDC 0009-0349-01

Size 2 cm (approximately 40 cm × 2 cm) [15 3/4 in × 3/4 in] *packaged in individual jars.*
NDC 0009-0364-01

Size 6 cm (approximately 40 cm × 6 cm) [15 3/4 in × 2 3/8 in] *packaged in cartons of six sponges in individual envelopes.*
NDC 0009-0371-01

Code 812 250 000

Also available:

***Gelfoam* Sterile Compressed Sponge (absorbable gelatin sponge, USP) Size 100.** For application in dry state. Sponges measure 80 mm × 125 mm and are available in boxes of 6 sponges in individual envelopes.
NDC 0009-0353-01

***Gelfoam* Sterile Dental Packs (absorbable gelatin sponge, USP), Size 2 or 4.** Each measures 10 × 20 × 7 mm or 20 × 20 × 7 mm, respectively, packaged in jars of 15 packs.
Size 2 NDC 0009-0379-01
Size 4 NDC 0009-0396-01

***Gelfoam* Sterile Prostatectomy Cones, (absorbable gelatin sponge, USP), Size 13 cm or 18 cm** (for use with Foley bag catheter). Each cone diameter measures 13 cm or 18 cm, respectively. Packaged in boxes of 6 cones in individual envelopes.
Size 13 cm NDC 0009-0449-01
Size 18 cm NDC 0009-0457-01

GELFOAM® Sterile Powder
(absorbable gelatin powder)

How Supplied: *Gelfoam* Sterile Powder (absorbable gelatin powder) is supplied in jars containing 1 gram.
NDC 0009-0433-01

HALCION® Tablets ©
(triazolam)

Description: *Halcion* Tablets contain triazolam, a triazolobenzodiazepine hypnotic agent and are available in 0.25 mg and 0.5 mg strengths for oral administration. Chemically, triazolam is 8-chloro-6-(o-chlorophenyl)-1-methyl-4H-s-triazolo-[4,3-a][1,4] benzodiazepine.

It is a white crystalline powder, soluble in alcohol and poorly soluble in water. It has a molecular weight of 343.21.

Clinical Pharmacology: Triazolam is a hypnotic with a short mean plasma half-life of 2.3 hours, and a range of 1.7–3.0 hours. Following oral administration, triazolam is readily absorbed. The mean peak concentration occurred at 1.3 hours following a single dose of triazolam ^{14}C. The nature of the relationship between dose and bioavilability of triazolam has not yet been established.

Triazolam and its metabolites, principally as conjugated glucuronides which are presumably inactive, are excreted primarily in the urine. Only small amounts of unmetabolized triazolam appear in the urine. The two primary metabolites accounted for 79.9% of urinary excretion. Urinary excretion appeared to be biphasic in its time course.

Halcion Tablets (triazolam) 0.5 mg, in two separate studies, did not affect the prothrombin times or plasma warfarin levels in male volunteers administered sodium warfarin orally.

Extremely high concentrations of triazolam do not displace bilirubin bound to human serum albumin *in vitro.*

Triazolam ^{14}C was administered orally to pregnant mice. Drug-related material appeared uniformly distributed in the fetus with ^{14}C concentrations approximately the same as in the brain of the mother.

In sleep laboratory studies, *Halcion* Tablets significantly decreased sleep latency, increased the duration of sleep and decreased the number of nocturnal awakenings. After two weeks of consecutive nightly administration, the effect of *Halcion* on total wake time is decreased, and the values recorded in the last third of the night approach baseline levels. On the first night after drug discontinuance (first post-drug night), total time asleep, percentage of time spent sleeping, and rapidity of falling asleep frequently were significantly less than on baseline (pre-drug) nights. This effect is often called "rebound" insomnia.

The type and duration of hypnotic effects and the profile of unwanted effects during administration of benzodiazepine drugs may be influenced by the biologic half-life of administered drug and any active metabolites formed. When half-lives are long, drug or metabolites may accumulate during periods of nightly administration and be associated with impairments of congnitive and motor performance during waking hours; the possibility of interaction with other psychoactive drugs or alcohol will be enhanced. In contrast, if half-lives are short, drug and metabclites will be cleared before the next dose is ingested, and carry-over effects related to excessive sedation or CNS depression should be minimal or absent. However, during nightly use for an extended period, pharmacodynamic tolerance or adaptation to some effects of benzodiazepine hypnotics may develop. If the drug has a short half-life of elimination, it is possible that a relative deficiency of the drug or its active metabolites (i.e., in relationship to the receptor site) may occur at some point in the interval between each night's use. This sequence of events may account for two clinical findings reported to occur after several weeks of nightly use of rapidly eliminated benzodiazepine hypnotics: 1) increased wakefulness during the last third of the night, and 2) the appearance of increased signs of day-time anxiety reported by one author in a selected group of patients.

Indications and Usage: *Halcion* Tablets contain triazolam which is a hypnotic agent useful in the short-term management of insomnia characterized by difficulty in falling asleep, frequent nocturnal awakenings, and/or early morning awakenings.

In polysomnographic studies in man of 1 to 42 days duration, triazolam decreased sleep latency, increased duration of sleep, and decreased the number of nocturnal awakenings.

Continued on next page

Upjohn—Cont.

It is recommended that *Halcion* not be prescribed in quantities exceeding a one-month supply.

Contraindications: *Halcion* Tablets (triazolam) are contraindicated in patients with known hypersensitivity to this drug or other benzodiazepines.

Benzodiazepines may cause fetal damage when administered during pregnancy. An increased risk of congenital malformations associated with the use of diazepam and chlordiazepoxide during the first trimester of pregnancy has been suggested in several studies. Transplacental distribution has resulted in neonatal CNS depression following the ingestion of therapeutic doses of a benzodiazepine hypnotic during the last weeks of pregnancy.

Halcion is contraindicated in pregnant women. If there is a likelihood of the patient becoming pregnant while receiving *Halcion* she should be warned of the potential risk to the fetus. Patients should be instructed to discontinue the drug prior to becoming pregnant. The possibility that a woman of childbearing potential may be pregnant at the time of institution of therapy should be considered.

Warnings: Overdosage may occur at four times the maximum recommended therapeutic dose (see DOSAGE AND ADMINISTRATION section). Patients should be cautioned *not* to exceed prescribed dosage.

Becuase of its depressant CNS effects, patients receiving triazolam should be cautioned against engaging in hazardous occupations requiring complete mental alertness such as operating machinery or driving a motor vehicle. For the same reason, patients should be cautioned about the simultaneous ingestion of alcohol and other CNS depressant drugs during treatment with *Halcion* Tablets (triazolam).

As with some but not all benzodiazepines, anterograde amnesia of varying severity and paradoxical reactions have been reported following therapeutic doses of *Halcion*.

Precautions:

General: In elderly and/or debilitated patients, it is recommended that treatment with *Halcion* Tablets (triazolam) be initiated at 0.125 mg to decrease the possibility of development of oversedation, dizziness, or impaired coordination. (See Dosage & Administration Section).

Caution should be exercised if *Halcion* is prescribed to patients with signs or symptoms of depression which could be intensified by hypnotic drugs. Suicidal tendencies may be present in such patients and protective measures may be required. Intentional overdosage is more common in these patients, and the least amount of drug that is feasible should be available to the patient at any one time.

The usual precautions should be observed in patients with impaired renal or hepatic function and chronic pulmonary insufficiency.

Information for Patients: To assure safe and effective use of *Halcion* Tablets (triazolam), the following information and instructions should be given to patients:

1. Inform your physician about any alcohol consumption and medicine you are taking now, including drugs you may buy without a prescription. Alcohol should generally not be used during treatment with hypnotics.
2. Inform your physician if you are planning to become pregnant, if you are pregnant, or if you become pregnant while you are taking this medicine.
3. Inform your physician if you are nursing.
4. Until you experience how this medication affects you, do not drive a car or operate potentially dangerous machinery, etc.
5. Do *not* increase prescribed dosage.
6. Patients should also be advised that they may experience an increase in sleep complaints (rebound insomnia) on the first night or two after discontinuing the drug.

Laboratory Tests: Laboratory tests are not ordinarily required in otherwise healthy patients.

Drug Interactions: The benzodiazepines, including triazolam, produce additive CNS depressant effects when co-administered with other psychotropic medications, anticonvulsants, anti-histaminics, ethanol, and other drugs which themselves produce CNS depression.

Pharmacokinetic interactions of benzodiazepines with other drugs have been reported. For example, cimetidine has been reported to reduce diazepam clearance. However, it is not known at this time whether a similar interaction occurs with *Halcion*.

Carcinogenesis, Mutagenesis, Impairment of Fertility: No evidence of carcinogenic potential was observed in mice during a 24-month study with *Halcion* in doses up to 4000 times the human dose.

Pregnancy:

1. Teratogenic Effects: Pregnancy Category X. See CONTRAINDICATIONS.
2. Non-Teratogenic Effects: It is to be considered that the child born of a mother who is on benzodiazepines may be at some risk for withdrawal symptoms from the drug, during the postnatal period. Also, neonatal flaccidity has been reported in an infant born of a mother who had been receiving benzodiazepines.

Nursing Mothers: Human studies have not been performed; however, studies in rats have indicated that *Halcion* and its metabolites are secreted in milk. Therfore, administration of *Halcion* to nursing mothers is not recommended.

Pediatric Use: Safety and efficacy of *Halcion* in children below the age of 18 have not been established.

Adverse Reactions: During placebo-controlled clinical studies in which 1003 patients received *Halcion* Tablets (triazolam), the most troublesome side effects were extensions of the pharmacologic activity of *Halcion*, e.g. drowsiness, dizziness, or lightheadedness.

The figures cited below are statistically adjusted estimates of untoward clinical event incidence among subjects who participated in the relatively short duration (i.e., 1 to 42 days) placebo-controlled clinical trials of *Halcion*. The figures cannot be used to predict precisely the incidence of untoward events in the course of usual medical practice where patient characteristics, and other factors often differ from those which obtained in the clinical trials. These figures cannot be compared with those obtained from other clinical studies involving related drug products and placebo as each group of drug trials are conducted under a different set of conditions.

Comparison of the cited figures, however, can provide the prescriber with some basis for estimating the relative contributions of drug and non-drug factors to the untoward event incidence rate in the population studied. Even this use must be approached cautiously, as a drug may relieve a symptom in one patient while inducing it in others. [For example, an anticholinergic, anxiolytic drug may relieve dry mouth (a sign of anxiety) in some subjects but induce it (an untoward event) in others.]

	Halcion	Placebo
Number of Patients	1003	997
% of Patients Reporting:		
Central Nervous System		
Drowsiness	14.0	6.4
Headache	9.7	8.4
Dizziness	7.8	3.1
Nervousness	5.2	4.5
Lightheadedness	4.9	0.9
Coordination Disorders/Ataxia	4.6	0.8
Gastrointestinal		
Nausea/Vomiting	4.6	3.7

In addition to the relatively common (i.e., 1% or greater) untoward events enumerated above, the following adverse events have been reported less frequently (i.e., 0.9–0.5%): euphoria, tachycardia, tiredness, confusional states/memory impairment, cramps/pain, depression, visual disturbances.

Rare (i.e., less than 0.5%) adverse reactions included constipation, taste alterations, diarrhea, dry mouth, dermatitis/allergy, dreaming/nightmares, insomnia, paresthesia, tinnitus, dysesthesia, weakness, congestion, death from hepatic failure in a patient also receiving diuretic drugs.

In addition to these untoward events, the following adverse events have been reported in association with the use of benzodiazepines: dystonia, irritability, anorexia, fatigue, sedation, slurred speech, jaundice, pruritus, dysarthria, changes in libido, menstrual irregularities, incontinence and urinary retention.

As with all benzodiazepines, paradoxical reactions such as stimulation, agitation, increased muscle spasticity, sleep disturbances, hallucinations and other adverse behavioral effects may occur in rare instances and in a random fashion. Should these occur, use of the drug should be discontinued.

Laboratory analyses were performed on all patients participating in the *Halcion* clinical program. The following incidences of abnormalities were observed in patients receiving *Halcion* and the corresponding placebo group. None of these changes were considered to be of physiological significance.

[See table left].

	Halcion		Placebo	
Number of patients	380		361	
% of Patients Reporting:	Low	High	Low	High
Hematology				
Hematocrit	*	*	*	*
Hemoglobin	*	*	*	*
Total WBC Count	1.7	2.1	*	1.3
Neutrophil Count	1.5	1.5	3.3	1.0
Lymphocyte Count	2.3	4.0	3.1	3.8
Monocyte Count	3.6	*	4.4	1.5
Eosinophil Count	10.2	3.2	9.8	3.4
Basophil Count	1.7	2.1	*	1.8
Urinalysis				
Albumin	—	1.1	—	*
Sugar	—	*	—	*
RBC/HPF	—	2.9	—	2.9
WBC/HPF	—	11.7	—	7.9
Blood Chemistry				
Creatinine	2.4	1.9	3.6	1.5
Bilirubin	*	1.5	1.0	*
SGOT	*	5.3	*	4.5
Alkaline Phosphatase	*	2.2	*	2.6

*Less than 1%

When treatment with *Halcion* is protracted, periodic blood counts, urinalysis and blood chemistry analyses are advisable.

Minor changes in EEG patterns, usually low-voltage fast activity have been observed in patients during therapy with *Halcion* and are of no known significance.

Drug Abuse and Dependence

Controlled Substance: *Halcion* Tablets (triazolam) are a Controlled Substance in Schedule IV.

Abuse and Dependence: Withdrawal symptoms similar in character to those noted with barbiturates and alcohol have occurred following abrupt discontinuance of benzodiazepine drugs. These can range from mild dysphoria to a major syndrome which may include abdominal and muscle cramps, vomiting, sweating, tremor, and convulsions.

Patients with a history of seizures should not be abruptly withdrawn from any CNS depressant agent, including *Halcion*. Addiction-prone individuals, such as drug addicts and alcoholics, should be under careful surveillance when receiving triazolam because of the predisposition of such patients to habituation and dependence. As with all hypnotics, repeat prescriptions should be limited to those who are under medical supervision.

Overdosage: Because of the potency of triazolam, overdosage may occur at 2 mg. four times the maximum recommended therapeutic dose (0.5 mg).

Manifestations of overdosage with *Halcion* Tablets (triazolam) include somnolence, confusion, impaired coordination, slurred speech, and ultimately, coma. As in all cases of drug overdosage, respiration, pulse, and blood pressure should be monitored and supported by general measures when necessary. Immediate gastric lavage should be performed. An adequate airway should be maintained. Intravenous fluids may be administered.

Experiments in animals have indicated that cardiopulmonary collapse can occur with massive intravenous doses of *Halcion* (over 100 mg/kg, more than 10,000 times the maximum daily human dose). This could be reversed with positive mechanical respiration and the intravenous infusion of levarterenol or metaraminol. Hemodialysis and forced diuresis are probably of little value. As with the management of intentional overdosage with any drug, the physician should bear in mind that multiple agents may have been ingested by the patient. The oral LD_{50} in mice is greater than 1000 mg/kg and in rats is greater than 5000 mg/kg.

Dosage and Administration: It is important to individualize the dosage of *Halcion* Tablets (triazolam) for maximum beneficial effect and to help avoid significant adverse effects. The recommended dosage range for adults is 0.25 to 0.5 mg before retiring. In geriatric and/or debilitated patients, the dosage range is 0.125 to 0.25 mg. Therapy should be initiated at 0.125 mg (half of a 0.25 mg scored tablet) until individual response is determined.

How Supplied: *Halcion* Tablets (triazolam) scored, are available in the following strengths and package sizes:

0.25 mg (powder blue):

Bottles of 100	NDC 0009-0017-01
Unit Dose Pkg (100)	NDC 0009-0017-08
Unit Dose Pkg (100)	NDC 0009-0017-17

0.5 mg (white)

Bottles of 100	NDC 0009-0027-01
Unit Dose Pkg (100)	NDC 0009-0027-08
Unit Dose Pkg (100)	NDC 0009-0027-18

Store at controlled room temperature 15°–30°C (59°–86°F).

Code 812 110 000

HALOTESTIN® Tablets ℞
(fluoxymesterone tablets, USP)

10 mg-100s
NSN 6505-01-053-8669A (VA)

Description: *Halotestin* Tablets contain fluoxymesterone which is a white or practically white odorless, crystalline powder, melting at about 240° C. with some decomposition. It is practically insoluble in water, sparingly soluble in alcohol and slightly soluble in chloroform.

Actions: In the eunuch and eunuchoid male, androgens act to stimulate and maintain the secondary sexual characteristics associated with the adult male. Androgens influence closure of the epiphyseal lines.

In males and some females, administration of androgens reduces urinary excretion of nitrogen, sodium, potassium, chloride, phosphorus and water.

Indications:

In the male

The primary indication in the male is replacement therapy in conditions associated with a deficiency or absence of endogenous testicular hormone. Androgen therapy prevents the development of atrophic changes in the accessory male sex organs following castration; as long as replacement therapy is continued, these organs can be maintained in a relatively normal state.

1. Eunuchoidism and eunuchism.
2. Climacteric symptoms when these are secondary to androgen deficiency.
3. Those symptoms of panhypopituitarism related to hypogonadism. Appropriate adrenocortical and thyroid hormone replacement therapy are still necessary, however, and are actually of primary importance.
4. Impotence due to androgen deficiency.
5. Delayed puberty, provided it has been definitely established as such, and it is not just a familial trait.

In the female

1. Prevention of postpartum breast pain and engorgement. There is no satisfactory evidence that this drug prevents or suppresses lactation.
2. Palliation of androgen-responsive, advancing, inoperable mammary cancer, in women who are more than 1 year, but less than 5 years postmenopausal, or who have been proven to have a hormone-dependent tumor as shown by previous beneficial response to castration.

Contraindications:

Carcinoma of the male breast
Carcinoma known or suspected of the prostate
Cardiac, hepatic or renal decompensation
Hypercalcemia
Liver function impairment
Prepubertal males
Pregnancy
Patients easily stimulated

Warnings:

Hypercalcemia may occur in immobilized patients and in patients with breast cancer. In patients with cancer this may indicate progression of bony metastasis. If this occurs the drug should be discontinued.

Watch female patients closely for signs of virilization. Some effects such as voice changes may not be reversible even when the drug is stopped.

Discontinue the drug if cholestatic hepatitis with jaundice appears or liver tests become abnormal.

Precautions: Patients with cardiac, renal or hepatic derangement may retain sodium and water thus forming edema. Priapism or excessive sexual stimulation may develop. Males, especially the elderly, may become overly stimulated. Oligospermia and reduced ejaculatory volume may occur after prolonged administration or excessive dosage. Hypersensitivity and gynecomastia may occur. When any of these affects appear the androgen should be stopped and if restarted, a lower dosage should be utilized.

Halotestin Tablets (fluoxymesterone) may increase sensitivity to oral anticoagulants. Dosage of the anticoagulant may require reduction in order to maintain a satisfactory therapeutic hypoprothrombinemia.

The PBI may decrease during androgen therapy without clinical significance.

This product contains FD&C Yellow No. 5 (tartrazine) which may cause allergic-type reactions (including bronchial asthma) in certain susceptible individuals. Although the overall incidence of FD&C Yellow No. 5 (tartrazine) sensitivity in the general population is low, it is frequently seen in patients who also have aspirin hypersensitivity.

Adverse Reactions:

Acne
Decreased ejaculatory volume
Gynecomastia
Edema
Hypersensitivity, including skin manifestations and anaphylactoid reactions
Priapism
Hypercalcemia (especially in immobile patients and those with metastatic breast carcinoma)
Virilization in females
Cholestatic jaundice

There have been rare reports of hepatocellular neoplasms and peliosis hepatis in association with long-term androgenic-anabolic steroid therapy.

Dosage and Administration: The dosage will vary depending upon the individual, the condition being treated, its severity, and prior androgenic therapy. The total daily oral dose may be administered singly or in divided (three or four) doses.

Male Hypogonadism—For complete replacement in eunuchs and eunuchoid patients, a daily dose of 2 to 10 mg will suffice in the majority of patients. It is usually preferable to begin treatment with full therapeutic doses which are later adjusted to individual requirements. Priapism is indicative of excessive dosage and is an indication for temporary withdrawal of the drug.

Impotence due to Testicular Deficiency; Male Climacteric—In impotency due to testicular insufficiency, this preparation may be administered in doses ranging from 2 to 10 mg daily. A similar dose may be employed in males with the climacteric syndrome.

Inoperable Carcinoma of the Breast in the Female—The recommended total daily dose for palliative therapy in advanced inoperable carcinoma of the breast is 15 to 30 mg. Because of its short action, fluoxymesterone should be administered to patients in divided, rather than single, daily doses to ensure more stable blood levels. In general, it appears necessary to continue therapy for at least one month for a satisfactory subjective response, and for 2 to 3 months for an objective response.

Postpartum Breast Engorgement—To lessen the degree and duration of painful breast engorgement, a dose of 2.5 mg may be administered when active labor has started. Thereafter, a daily dose of 5 to 10 mg, preferably in divided doses, may be given for 4 to 5 days.

How Supplied: *Halotestin* Tablets (fluoxymesterone) are available in the following strengths and sizes:

2 mg	Bottles of 100	*NDC 0009-0014-01*
5 mg	Bottles of 100	*NDC 0009-0019-06*
10 mg	Bottles of 30	*NDC 0009-0036-03*
	Bottles of 100	*NDC 0009-0036-04*

Code 810 804 000

[*Shown in Product Identification Section*]

Continued on next page

Upjohn—Cont.

HEPARIN SODIUM INJECTION, USP ℞

Sterile Solution

Description: Heparin Sodium Injection, USP, a mixture of substances having the property of prolonging the clotting time of blood, is usually obtained from the lungs of intestinal mucosa of domestic mammals used for food by man. The potency is determined by biological assay using a USP reference standard based upon units of heparin activity per milligram. The preparations of Heparin Sodium Injection are standardized aqueous solutions of the physiological anticoagulant obtained from beef lung. Slight variations in the color of heparin sodium solutions do not affect the therapeutic efficiency. Each ml of the 1,000 and 5,000 USP Units per ml preparations contains: heparin sodium 1,000 or 5,000 USP Units: 9 mg sodium chloride; 9.45 mg benzyl alcohol added as preservative. Each ml of the 10,000 USP Units per ml preparations contains: heparin sodium 10,000 USP Units; 9.45 mg benzyl alcohol added as preservative.

Actions: Heparin inhibits the clotting of blood and the formation of fibrin clots both *in vitro* and *in vivo*. In combination with a co-factor, it inactivates thrombin thus preventing the conversion of fibrinogen to fibrin. Heparin also prevents the formation of a stable fibrin clot by inhibiting the activation of the fibrin stabilizing factor.

Heparin sodium inhibits reactions which lead to clotting but does not alter the normal components of the blood. Although clotting time is prolonged by therapeutic doses, bleeding time is usually unaffected. Heparin sodium does not have fibrinolytic activity; therefore, it will not lyse existing clots.

Indications: Heparin Sodium Injection is indicated for anticoagulant therapy in prophylaxis and treatment of venous thrombosis and its extension; in low-dose regimen for prevention of postoperative deep venous thrombosis and pulmonary embolism in patients undergoing major abdominothoracic surgery who are at risk of developing thromboembolic disease (see DOSAGE AND ADMINISTRATION); for prophylaxis and treatment of pulmonary embolism; in atrial fibrillation with embolization; for diagnosis and treatment of acute and chronic consumptive coagulopathies (disseminated intravascular coagulation); for prevention of clotting in arterial and cardiac surgery; and for the prevention of cerebral thrombosis in evolving stroke.

Heparin Sodium Injection is indicated as an adjunct in treatment of coronary occlusion with acute myocardial infarction, and in prophylaxis and treatment of peripheral arterial embolism.

Heparin sodium may also be employed as an anticoagulant in blood transfusions, extracorporeal circulation, dialysis procedures, and in blood samples for laboratory purposes.

Contraindications:

Hypersensitivity to heparin.

Inability to perform suitable blood coagulation tests, e.g., the whole blood clotting time, partial thromboplastin time, etc., at required intervals.

Uncontrollable bleeding.

Warnings

> Heparin sodium should be used with extreme caution in disease states where there is increased danger of hemorrhage.

Heparin Sodium Injection, USP when used in therapeutic dosage should be regulated by frequent blood coagulation tests. If these are unduly prolonged or if hemorrhage occurs, heparin sodium should be promptly discontinued. See OVERDOSAGE section.

Some of the conditions in which increased danger of hemorrhage exists are:

Cardiovascular—subacute bacterial endocarditis, arterial sclerosis; increased capillary permeability; during and immediately following (a) spinal tap or spinal anesthesia, (b) major surgery, especially involving the brain, spinal cord, or eye.

Hematologic—conditions associated with increased bleeding tendencies such as hemophilia, some purpuras, and thrombocytopenia.

Gastrointestinal—inaccessible ulcerative lesions; continuous tube drainage of stomach or small intestine.

Heparin sodium may prolong the one-stage prothrombin time. Accordingly, when heparin sodium is given with dicumarol or warfarin sodium, a period of at least 5 hours after the last intravenous dose and 24 hours after the last subcutaneous (intrafat) dose of heparin sodium should elapse before blood is drawn, if a valid prothrombin time is to be obtained.

Drugs (such as acetylsalicylic acid, dextran, phenylbutazone, ibuprofen, indomethacin, dipyridamole and hydroxychloroquine) which interefere with platelet aggregation reactions (the main hemostatic defense of heparinized patients) may induce bleeding and should be used with caution in patients on heparin therapy.

While there is experimental evidence that heparin may antagonize the action of ACTH, insulin or corticoids, this effect has not been clearly defined.

There is also evidence in animal experiments that heparin may modify or inhibit allergic reactions. However, the application of these findings to human patients has not been fully defined.

Larger doses of heparin may be necessary in the febrile state.

The use of digitalis, tetracyclines, nicotine, or antihistamines may partially counteract the anticoagulant action of heparin. An increased resistance to heparin is frequenly encountered in cases of thrombosis, thrombophlebitis, infections with thrombosing tendency, myocardial infarction, cancer, and in the postoperative patient.

Elevation of the serum transaminases without elevation in bilirubin or alkaline phosphatase may occur in patients on heparin therapy and has been observed in normal volunteers who have received heparin. Caution should be exercised in interpreting this finding as indicative of hepatic or myocardial damage.

Because of the possibility of acute thrombocytopenia occurring when heparin is administered, platelet counts should be monitored before and during heparin therapy. If significant thrombocytopenia occurs, heparin should be immediately terminated, and oral anticoagulation substituted, if necessary. If new evidence of thrombosis appears during heparin therapy, especially in the arterial system, it should be borne in mind that it may be a paradoxical result of the therapy itself, possibly as a result of platelet aggregation. Heparin should be discontinued and oral anticoagulation employed, especially if there is associated thrombocytopenia, as noted above.

Benzyl alcohol is contained in the diluent for this product. Benzyl alcohol has been reported to be associated with a fatal "Gasping Syndrome" in premature infants.

Usage in Pregnancy

Heparin Sodium Injection should be used with caution during pregnancy, especially during the last trimester and in the immediate postpartum period.

There is no adequate information as to whether heparin may affect human fertility or have a teratogenic potential or other adverse effects to the fetus.

Heparin does not cross the placental barrier; it is not excreted in human milk.

Precautions: Because Heparin Sodium Injection is derived from animal tissue, it should be used with caution in patients with a history of allergy. Before a therapeutic dose is given to such a patient, a trial dose of 1,000 units may be advisable.

Heparin sodium should also be used with caution in the presence of mild hepatic or renal disease, hypertension, during menstruation, or in patients with indwelling catheters. A higher incidence of bleeding may be seen in women over 60 years of age.

Caution should be used when administering ACD-converted blood (i.e. blood collected in heparin sodium and later converted to ACD blood), since the anticoagulant activity of its heparin sodium content persists without loss for 22 days. ACD-converted blood may alter the coagulation system of the recipient, especially if it is given in multiple transfusions.

Adverse Reactions: Hemorrhage is the chief complication that may result from heparin therapy. An overly prolonged clotting time or minor bleeding during therapy can usually be controlled by withdrawing the drug. See OVERDOSAGE section.

The occurrence of significant gastrointestinal or urinary tract bleeding during anticoagulant therapy may indicate the presence of an underlying occult lesion.

Adrenal hemorrhage with resultant acute adrenal insufficiency has occurred during anticoagulant therapy. Therefore such treatment should be discontinued in patients who develop signs and symptoms compatible with acute adrenal hemorrhage and insufficiency. Plasma cortisol levels should be measured immediately, and vigorous therapy with intravenous corticosteroids should be instituted promptly. Initiation of therapy should not depend upon laboratory confirmation of the diagnosis, since any delay in an acute situation may result in the patient's death.

Intramuscular injection of heparin sodium frequently causes local irritation, mild pain, hematoma or ulceration, and for these reasons should be avoided. These effects are less frequently seen following deep subcutaneous (intrafat) administration. Histamine-like reactions have also been observed at the site of injection.

Hypersensitivity reactions have been reported with chills, fever, and urticaria as the most usual manifestations. Asthma, rhinitis, lacrimation, headache, nausea and vomiting, and anaphylactoid reactions have also been reported. Vasospastic reactions may develop independent of the origin of heparin, 6 to 10 days after the initiation of therapy and last for 4 to 6 hours. The affected limb is painful, ischemic and cyanosed. An artery to this limb may have been recently catheterized. After repeat injections, the reaction may gradually increase, to include generalized vasospasm, with cyanosis, tachypnea, feeling of oppression, and headache. Protamine sulfate treatment has no marked therapeutic effect. Itching and burning, especially on the plantar side of the feet, is possibly based on a similar allergic vasospastic reaction. Chest pain, elevated blood pressure, arthralgias, and/or headache have also been reported in the absence of definite peripheral vasospasm. Anaphylactic shock has been reported rarely following the intravenous administration of heparin sodium.

Elevations of serum transminases without elevation in bilirubin or alkaline phosphatase occur in a high percentage of patients receiving heparin, by either subcutaneous or intravenous route. This was also observed in normal volunteers who received heparin. Whether this represents toxicity or nonspecific stimulation of the enzymes is not known.

Necrosis of the skin has been reported at the site of subcutaneous injection of heparin, occasionally requiring skin grafting.

During clinical studies, acute reversible thrombocytopenia was reported at frequencies varying from 0 to 31%. This occurred 2 to 20 days (average 5 to 9) following the onset of therapy. In some cases this has been associated with immunologically demonstrable factors in the patients' serum resulting in *in vitro* platelet aggregation when heparin and platelets are added. In isolated cases, localized or disseminated thromboses have occurred which may have been related to *in vivo* platelet aggregation. Osteoporosis and suppression of renal function following long-term high-dose administration, suppression of aldosterone synthesis, delayed transient alopecia, priapism, and rebound hyperlipemia following discontinuation of heparin sodium have also been reported.

Dosage and Administration: Heparin sodium is not effective by oral administration and should be given by deep subcutaneous (intrafat, i.e. above iliac crest or into the abdominal fat layer) injection, by intermittent intravenous injection, or intravenous infusion. The intramuscular route of administration should be avoided because of the frequent occurrence of hematoma at the injection site.

The dosage of heparin sodium should be adjusted according to the patient's coagulation test results, which, during the first day of treatment, should be determined just prior to each injection. (There is usually no need to monitor the effect of low-dose heparin in patients with normal coagulation parameters.) Dosage is considered adequate when the whole blood clotting time is elevated approximately 2.5 to 3 times the control value.

When heparin sodium is administered by continuous intravenous infusion, coagulation tests should be performed approximately every four hours during the early stages of therapy. When it is administered intermittently by intravenous, or deep subcutaneous (intrafat) injection, coagulation tests should be performed before each injection during the early stages of treatment and daily thereafter.

When an oral anticoagulant such as warfarin sodium or similar type is administered with heparin sodium, coagulation tests and prothrombin activity should be determined at the start of therapy. For immediate anticoagulant effect, administer heparin sodium in the usual therapeutic dosage. When the results of the initial prothrombin determination are known, administer the first dose of an oral anticoagulant in the usual initial amount. Thereafter, perform a coagulation test and determine the prothrombin activity at appropriate intervals. A period of at least five hours after the last intravenous dose and 24 hours after the last subcutaneous (intrafat) dose of heparin sodium should elapse before blood is drawn if a valid prothrombin time is to be obtained. When the oral anticoagulant shows full effect and prothrombin activity is in the desired therapeutic range, heparin sodium may be discontinued and therapy continued with the oral anticoagulant.

Therapeutic anticoagulant effect with full-dose heparin: Although dosage must be adjusted for the individual patient according to the results of suitable laboratory tests, the following dosage schedules may be used as guidelines:

[See table above].

Method of Administration	Frequency	Recommended Dose [based on 150 lb (68 kg) patient]
Deep Subcutaneous (Intrafat) Injection	Initial Dose	5,000 units by I.V. injection followed by 10,000–20,000 units of a concentrated solution, subcutaneously
	Every 8 hours	8,000–10,000 units of a concentrated solution
	(or) Every 12 hours	15,000–20,000 units of a concentrated solution
Intermittent Intravenous Injection	Initial Dose	10,000 units, either undiluted or in 50–100 ml isotonic sodium chloride injection
	Every 4 to 6 hours	5,000–10,000 units, either undiluted or in 50–100 ml isotonic sodium chloride injection
Intravenous Infusion	Initial Dose	5,000 units by I.V. injection
	Continuous	20,000–40,000 units in 1,000 ml of isotonic sodium chloride solution for infusion/day

1. **By deep subcutaneous (intrafat) injection.** After an initial I.V. injection of 5,000 units, inject 10,000 to 20,000 units of a concentrated heparin sodium solution subcutaneously, followed by 8,000 to 10,000 units of a concentrated solution subcutaneously every 8 hours, or 15,000 to 20,000 units of a concentrated solution every 12 hours. A different site should be used for each injection to prevent the development of a massive hematoma.
2. **By intermittent intravenous injection.** 10,000 units initially, then 5,000 to 10,000 units every 4 to 6 hours. These amounts may be given either undiluted or diluted with 50 to 100 milliliters of isotonic sodium chloride injection.
3. **By continuous intravenous infusion.** After an initial I.V. injection of 5,000 units of heparin sodium, add 20,000 to 40,000 units to 1,000 milliliters of isotonic sodium chloride solution for infusion. For most patients, the rate of flow should be adjusted to deliver approximately 20,000 to 40,000 units in 24 hours.

Surgery of the Heart and Blood Vessels: Patients undergoing total body perfusion for open heart surgery should receive an initial dose of not less than 150 units of heparin sodium per kilogram of body weight. Frequently a dose of 300 units of heparin sodium per kilogram of body weight is used for procedures estimated to last less than 60 minutes; or 400 units/kg for those estimated to last longer than 60 minutes.

Low-dose prophylaxis of postoperative thromboembolism: A number of well-controlled clinical trials have demonstrated that low-dose heparin prophylaxis, given just prior to and after surgery, will reduce the incidence of postoperative deep vein thrombosis in the legs, as measured by the I-125 fibrinogen technique and venography, and of clinical pulmonary embolism. The most widely used dosage has been 5,000 units 2 hours before surgery and 5,000 units every 8 to 12 hours thereafter for 7 days or until the patient is fully ambulatory, whichever is longer. The heparin is given by deep subcutaneous injection in the arm or abdomen with a fine needle (25–26 gauge) to minimize tissue trauma. A concentrated solution of heparin sodium is recommended. Such prophylaxis should be reserved for patients over 40 undergoing major surgery. Patients with bleeding disorders, those having neurosurgery, spinal anesthesia, eye surgery, or potentially sanguineous operations should be excluded, as well as patients receiving oral anticoagulants or platelet-active drugs (see WARNINGS). The value of such prophylaxis in hip surgery has not been established. The possibility of increased bleeding during surgery or postoperatively should be borne in mind. If such bleeding occurs, discontinuance of heparin and neutralization with protamine sulfate is advisable. If clinical evidence of thromboembolism develops despite low-dose prophylaxis, full therapeutic doses of anticoagulants should be given unless contraindicated. All patients should be screened prior to heparinization to rule out bleeding disorders, and minitoring should be performed with appropriate coagulation tests just prior to surgery. Coagulation test values should be normal or only slightly elevated. There is usually no need for daily minitoring of the effect of low-dose heparin in patients with normal coagulation parameters.

Extracorporeal Dialysis Use: Follow equipment manufacturer's operating directions carefully.

Blood Transfusion: Addition of 400 to 600 USP Units per 100 ml of whole blood. Usually 7,500 USP heparin sodium units are added to 100 ml of Sterile Sodium Chloride Injection and mixed (or 75,000 USP Units per 1,000 ml of Sodium Chloride Injection) and from this sterile solution, 6 ml to 8 ml are added per 100 ml of whole blood. Leukocyte counts should be performed on heparinized blood within two hours after addition of the heparin. Heparinized blood should not be used for isoagglutinin, complement or erythrocyte fragility tests.

Laboratory Samples: Addition of 70 to 150 units of heparin sodium per 10 to 20 ml sample of whole blood are usually employed to prevent coagulation of the same. See comments above under "Blood Transfusion."

Overdosage: Protamine sulfate (1% solution) by slow infusion will neutralize heparin. No more than 50 mg should be given in any 10 minute period. Decreasing amounts of protamine are required as time from last heparin injection increases. Thirty minutes after a dose of heparin approximately 0.5 mg of protamine is sufficient to neutralize each mg of heparin. Single doses of protamine should not exceed 50 mg. Blood or plasma transfusions may be necessary; these dilute but do not neutralize heparin.

The *in vitro* relationship between protamine sulfate and heparin sodium may be expressed as follows:

heparin derived from beef lung
1 mg of protamine sulfate will neutralize approximately 90 USP Units of heparin sodium of beef lung origin.

heparin derived from porcine intestinal mucosa
1 mg of protamine sulfate will neutralize approximately 115 USP Units of heparin sodium of intestinal mucosa origin.

How Supplied: Heparin Sodium Injection, USP derived **from beef lung** is available in the following packages:

Continued on next page

Upjohn—Cont.

1,000 USP Units per ml
10 ml vial *NDC 0009-0268-01*
30 ml vial *NDC 0009-0268-02*
5,000 USP Units per ml
1 ml vial *NDC 0009-0291-02*
10 ml vial *NDC 0009-0291-01*
10,000 USP Units per ml
1 ml vial *NDC 0009-0317-01*
4 ml vial *NDC 0009-0317-02*
Code 810 670 008

KAOPECTATE® Anti-Diarrhea Medicine
(See PDR For Nonprescription Drugs)

KAOPECTATE CONCENTRATE®
Anti-Diarrhea Medicine
(See PDR For Nonprescription Drugs)

LINCOCIN® Capsules, Sterile Solution ℞
(lincomycin hydrochloride, USP)

WARNING
Lincomycin therapy has been associated with severe colitis which may end fatally. Therefore, it should be reserved for serious infections where less toxic antimicrobial agents are inappropriate, as described in the Indications Section. It should not be used in patients with nonbacterial infections, such as most upper respiratory tract infections. Studies indicate a toxin(s) produced by *Clostridia* is one primary cause of antibiotic associated colitis. The colitis is usually characterized by severe, persistent diarrhea and severe abdominal cramps and may be associated with the passage of blood and mucus. Endoscopic examination may reveal pseudomembranous colitis.
When significant diarrhea occurs, the drug should be discontinued or, if necessary, continued only with close observation of the patient. Large bowel endoscopy has been recommended.
Antiperistaltic agents such as opiates and diphenoxylate with atropine (Lomotil) may prolong and/or worsen the condition. Vancomycin has been found to be effective in the treatment of antibiotic associated pseudomembranous colitis produced by *Clostridium difficile.* The usual adult dose is 500 milligrams to 2 grams of vancomycin orally per day in three to four divided doses administered for 7 to 10 days. Cholestyramine or colestipol resins bind vancomycin *in vitro.* If both a resin and vancomycin are to be administered concurrently, it may be advisable to separate the time of administration of each drug.
Diarrhea, colitis, and pseudomembranous colitis have been observed to begin up to several weeks following cessation of therapy with lincomycin.

Description: *Lincocin* preparations contain lincomycin hydrochloride which is the monohydrated salt of lincomycin, a substance produced by the growth of a member of the *lincolnensis* group of *Streptomyces lincolnensis* (Fam. *Streptomycetaceae*). It is a white, or practically white, crystalline powder and is odorless or has a faint odor. Its solutions are acid and are dextrorotatory. Lincomycin hydrochloride is freely soluble in water; soluble in dimethylformamide and very slightly soluble in acetone.
Clinical Pharmacology: Microbiology—Lincomycin has been shown to be effective against most of the common gram-positive pathogens. Depending on the sensitivity of the organism and concentration of the antibiotic, it may be either bactericidal or bacteriostatic. Cross resistance has not been demonstrated with penicillin, chloramphenicol, ampicillin, cephalosporins or the tetracyclines. Despite chemical differences, lincomycin exhibits antibacterial activity similar but not identical to the macrolide antibiotics (e.g. erythromycin). Some cross resistance (with erythromycin) including a phenomenon known as dissociated cross resistance or macrolide effect has been reported. Microorganisms have not developed resistance to *Lincocin* rapidly when tested by *in vitro* or *in vivo* methods. Staphylococci develop resistance to *Lincocin* in a slow, step-wise manner based on *in vitro,* serial subculture experiments. This pattern of resistance development is unlike that shown for streptomycin.
Studies indicate that lincomycin does not share antigenicity with penicillin compounds.
Biological Studies—*In vitro* studies indicate that the spectrum of activity includes *Staphylococcus aureus, Staphylococcus albus, β-hemolytic Streptococcus, Streptococcus viridans, Diplococcus pneumoniae, Clostridium tetani, Clostridium perfringens, Corynebacterium diphtheriae and Corynebacterium acnes.*
NOTE: The drug is not active against most strains of *Streptococcus faecalis,* nor against *Neisseria gonorrhoeae, Neisseria meningitidis, Hemophilus influenzae,* or other gram-negative organisms or yeasts.
Human Pharmacology—Lincomycin is absorbed rapidly after a 500 mg oral dose, reaching peak levels in 2 to 4 hours. Levels are maintained above the MIC (minimum inhibitory concentration) for most gram-positive organisms for 6 to 8 hours. Urinary recovery of drug in a 24-hour period ranges from 1.0 to 31 percent (mean: 4.0) after a single oral dose of 500 mg of lincomycin. Tissue level studies indicate that bile is an important route of excretion. Significant levels have been demonstrated in the majority of body tissues. Although the drug is not present in significant amounts in the spinal fluid of normal volunteers, it has been demonstrated in the spinal fluid of one patient with pneumococcal meningitis.
Intramuscular administration of a single dose of 600 mg produces a peak serum level at 30 minutes with detectable levels persisting for 24 hours. Urinary excretion after this dose ranges from 1.8 to 24.8 percent (mean: 17.3).
The intravenous infusion over a 2-hour interval of 600 mg of lincomycin hydrochloride in 500 ml of 5 percent glucose in distilled water yields therapeutic levels for 14 hours. Urinary excretion ranges from 4.9 to 30.3 percent (mean: 13.8).
The biological half-life, after oral, intramuscular or intravenous administration is 5.4 ± 1.0 hours.
Hemodialysis and peritoneal dialysis do not effectively remove lincomycin from the blood.
Indications and Usage: *Lincocin* preparations (lincomycin) are indicated in the treatment of serious infections due to susceptible strains of streptococci, pneumococci, and staphylococci. Its use should be reserved for penicillin-allergic patients or other patients for whom, in the judgment of the physician, a penicillin is inappropriate. Because of the risk of colitis, as described in the WARNING box, before selecting lincomycin the physician should consider the nature of the infection and the suitability of less toxic alternatives (e.g., erythromycin).
Lincomycin has been demonstrated to be effective in the treatment of staphylococcal infections resistant to other antibiotics and susceptible to lincomycin. Staphylococcal strains resistant to *Lincocin* have been recovered; culture and susceptibility studies should be done in conjunction with therapy with *Lincocin.* In the case of macrolides, partial but not complete cross resistance may occur (see **Microbiology**).
The drug may be administered concomitantly with other antimicrobial agents when indicated.
Contraindications: This drug is contraindicated in patients previously found to be hypersensitive to lincomycin or clindamycin. It is not indicated in the treatment of minor bacterial infections or viral infections.
WARNINGS:
See WARNING box. Studies indicate a toxin(s) produced by *Clostridia* is one primary cause of antibiotic associated colitis.[1–5] Mild cases of colitis may respond to drug discontinuance alone. Moderate to severe cases should be managed promptly with fluid, electrolyte and protein supplementation as indicated. Vancomycin has been found to be effective in the treatment of antibiotic associated pseudomembranous colitis produced by *Clostridium difficile.* The usual adult dosage is 500 milligrams to 2 grams of vancomycin orally per day in three to four divided doses administered for 7 to 10 days. Cholestyramine or colestipol resins bind vancomycin *in vitro.* If both a resin and vancomycin are to be administered concurrently, it may be advisable to separate the time of administration of each drug. Systemic corticoids and corticoid retention enemas may help relieve the colitis. Other causes of colitis should also be considered.
A careful inquiry should be made concerning previous sensitivities to drugs and other allergens.
Usage in Pregnancy—Safety for use in pregnancy has not been established.
Usage in Newborn—Until further clinical experience is obtained, *Lincocin* preparations (lincomycin) are not indicated in the newborn.
Nursing Mothers—*Lincocin* has been reported to appear in breast milk in ranges of 0.5 to 2.4 mcg/ml.

1. Bailey, WR, Scott, EG, *Diagnostic Microbiology* CV Mosby Company, St. Louis, 1978.
2. Bartlett, JG, et al, "Clindamycin-associated Colitis due to a Toxin-producing Species of *Clostridium* in Hamsters" *J. Inf. Dis.* **136**(5): 701–705, (November) 1977.
3. Larson, HE, Price, AB, "Pseudomembranous Colitis: Presence of Clostridial Toxin," *Lancet,* 1312–1314 (December) 24 and 31, 1977.
4. Lusk, RH, et al, "Clindamycin-Induced Enterocolitis in Hamsters", *J. Inf. Dis.* **137**(4): 464–474 (April) 1978.
5. "Antibiotic-associated Colitis: A Progress Report", *British Med. J.* **1**:669–671 (March 18) 1978.

Precautions: Review of experience to date suggests that a subgroup of older patients with associated severe illness may tolerate diarrhea less well. When *Lincocin* preparations (lincomycin) are indicated in these patients, they should be carefully monitored for change in bowel frequency.
Lincocin should be prescribed with caution in individuals with a history of gastrointestinal disease, particularly colitis.
Lincocin, like any drug, should be used with caution in patients with a history of asthma or significant allergies.
The use of antibiotics occasionally results in overgrowth of nonsusceptible organisms—particularly yeasts. Should superinfections occur, appropriate measures should be taken. When patients with pre-existing monilial infections require therapy with *Lincocin,* concomitant antimonilial treatment should be given.
During prolonged therapy with *Lincocin,* periodic liver function studies and blood counts should be performed.
Since adequate data are not yet available in patients with pre-existing liver disease, its use in such patients is not recommended at this time unless special clinical circumstances so indicate.
Lincomycin has been shown to have neuromuscular blocking properties that may enhance the action of other neuromuscular blocking agents. Therefore, it should be used with caution in patients receiving such agents.

Indicated surgical procedures should be performed in conjunction with antibiotic therapy.

Adverse Reactions:

Gastrointestinal—Glossitis, stomatitis, nausea, vomiting. Persistent diarrhea, enterocolitis and pruritus ani. (See **Warning** box)

Hematopoietic: Neutropenia, leukopenia, agranulocytosis and thrombocytopenic purpura have been reported. There have been rare reports of aplastic anemia and pancytopenia in which *Lincocin* preparations (lincomycin hydrochloride) could not be ruled out as the causative agent.

Hypersensitivity Reactions—Hypersensitivity reactions such as angioneurotic edema, serum sickness and anaphylaxis have been reported, some of these in patients known to be sensitive to penicillin. Rare instances of erythema multiforme, some resembling Stevens-Johnson syndrome, have been associated with *Lincocin*. If an allergic reaction should occur, the drug should be discontinued and the usual agents (epinephrine, corticosteroids, antihistamines) should be available for emergency treatment.

Skin and Mucous Membranes—Skin rashes, urticaria and vaginitis and rare instances of exfoliative and vesiculobullous dermatitis have been reported.

Liver—Although no direct relationship of *Lincocin* to liver dysfunction has been established, jaundice and abnormal liver function tests (particularly elevations of serum transaminase) have been observed in a few instances.

Cardiovascular—After too rapid intravenous administration, rare instances of cardiopulmonary arrest and hypotension have been reported. (See **Dosage and Administration**).

Special Senses—Tinnitus and vertigo have been reported occasionally.

Local Reactions—Patients have demonstrated excellent local tolerance to intramuscularly administered *Lincocin*. Reports of pain following injection have been infrequent. Intravenous administration of *Lincocin* in 250 to 500 ml of 5 percent glucose in distilled water or normal saline produced no local irritation or phlebitis.

Dosage and Administration:

If significant diarrhea occurs during therapy, this antibiotic should be discontinued. (See **Warning** box).

***Oral*—Adults:** *Serious infections*—500 mg 3 times per day (500 mg approximately every 8 hours). *More severe infections*—500 mg or more 4 times per day (500 mg or more approximately every 6 hours). **Children over 1 month of age:** *Serious infections*—30 mg/kg/day (15 mg/lb/day) divided into 3 or 4 equal doses. *More severe infections*—60 mg/kg/day (30 mg/lb/day) divided into 3 or 4 equal doses.

With β-hemolytic streptococcal infections, treatment should continue for at least 10 days to diminish the likelihood of subsequent rheumatic fever or glomerulonephritis.

NOTE: For optimal absorption it is recommended that nothing be given by mouth except water for a period of one to two hours before and after oral administration of *Lincocin* preparations (lincomycin hydrochloride).

***Intramuscular*—Adults:** *Serious infections*—600 mg (2 ml) intramuscularly every 24 hours. *More severe infections*—600 mg (2 ml) intramuscularly every 12 hours or more often.

Children over 1 month of age: *Serious infections*—one intramuscular injection of 10 mg/kg (5 mg/lb) every 24 hours. *More severe infections*—one intramuscular injection of 10 mg/kg (5 mg/lb) every 12 hours or more often.

***Intravenous*—Adults:** The intravenous dose will be determined by the severity of the infection. For serious infections doses of 600 mg (2 ml of *Lincocin* Sterile Solution) to 1 gram are given every 8-12 hours. For more severe infections these doses may have to be increased. In life-threatening situations daily intravenous doses of as much as 8 grams have been given.

Intranvenous doses are given on the basis of 1 gram of lincomycin diluted in not less than 100 ml of appropriate solution (see PHYSICAL COMPATIBILITIES) and infused over a period of not less than one hour.

Dose	Vol. Diluent	Time
600 mg	100 ml	1 hr
1 gram	100 ml	1 hr
2 grams	200 ml	2 hr
3 grams	300 ml	3 hr
4 grams	400 ml	4 hr

These doses may be repeated as often as required to the limit of the maximum recommended daily dose of 8 grams of lincomycin.

Children over 1 month of age: 10-20 mg/kg/day (5-10 mg/lb/day) depending on the severity of the infection may be infused in divided doses as described above for adults.

NOTE: Severe cardiopulmonary reactions have occurred when this drug has been given at greater than the recommended concentration and rate.

Subconjunctival Injection—0.25 ml (75 mg) injected subconjunctivally will result in ocular fluid levels of antibiotic (lasting for at least 5 hours) with MIC's sufficient for most susceptible pathogens.

Patients with diminished renal function: *When therapy with Linocin is required in individuals with severe impairment of renal function, an appropriate dose is 25 to 30% of that recommended for patients with normally functioning kidneys.*

How Supplied:

Lincocin preparations (lincomycin) are available as:

250 mg Pediatric Capsules: Each capsule contains lincomycin hydrochloride equivalent to lincomycin 250 mg.

Bottles of 24 *NDC 0009-0336-01*

500 mg Capsules: Each capsule contains lincomycin hydrochloride equivalent to lincomycin 500 mg.

Bottles of 24 *NDC 0009-0500-01*
Bottles of 100 *NDC 0009-0500-02*

Sterile Solution: Each ml contains lincomycin hydrochloride equivalent to lincomycin 300 mg; also Benzyl Alcohol, 9.45 mg added as preservative—available in single dose 2 ml syringes, in 2 ml and 10 ml vials.

2 ml *U-Ject®* *NDC 0009-0600-01*
Disposable Syringe
2 ml vial *NDC 0009-0555-01*
10 ml vial *NDC 0009-0555-02*

Animal Pharmacology: *In vivo* experimental animal studies demonstrated the effectiveness of *Lincocin* preparations (lincomycin) in protecting animals infected with *Streptococcus viridans, β-hemolytic Streptococcus, Staphylococcus aureus, Diplococcus pneumoniae* and *Leptospira pomona*. It was ineffective in *Klebsiella, Pasteurella, Pseudomonas, Salmonella* and *Shigella* infections.

Clinical Studies: Experience with 345 obstetrical patients receiving this drug revealed no ill effects related to pregnancy.

Physical Compatibilities:

Physically compatible for 24 hours at room temperature unless otherwise indicated.

Infusion Solutions
Dextrose in Water, 5% and 10%
Dextrose in Saline, 5% and 10%
Ringer's Solution
Sodium Lactate 1/6 Molar
Travert 10%—Electrolyte No. 1
Dextran in Saline 6% w/v

Vitamins in Infusion Solutions
B-Complex
B-Complex with Ascorbic Acid

Antibiotics in Infusion Solutions
Penicillin G Sodium (Satisfactory for 4 hours)
Cephalothin
Tetracycline HCl
Cephaloridine
Colistimethate (Satisfactory for 4 hours)
Ampicillin
Methicillin
Chloramphenicol
Polymyxin B Sulfate

Physically Incompatible With:
Novobiocin
Kanamycin

IT SHOULD BE EMPHASIZED THAT THE COMPATIBLE AND INCOMPATIBLE DETERMINATIONS ARE PHYSICAL OBSERVATIONS ONLY, NOT CHEMICAL DETERMINATIONS. ADEQUATE CLINICAL EVALUATION OF THE SAFETY AND EFFICACY OF THESE COMBINATIONS HAS NOT BEEN PERFORMED.

Physical Compatibilities [See table above].
Code 810 174 004

LONITEN® Tablets ℞
(minoxidil)

10 mg, 100's
NSN 6505-01-088-8120(VA)

2.5 mg, 100's
NSN 6505-01-088-8121(VA)

Warnings: *Loniten* Tablets contain the powerful antihypertensive agent, minoxidil, which may produce serious adverse effects. It can cause pericardial effusion, occasionally progressing to tamponade, and angina pectoris may be exacerbated. *Loniten* should be reserved for hypertensive patients who do not respond adequately to maximum therapeutic doses of a diuretic and two other antihypertensive agents.

In experimental animals, minoxidil caused several kinds of myocardial lesions as well as other adverse cardiac effects (see Cardiac Lesions in Animals).

Loniten must be administered under close supervision, usually concomitantly with therapeutic doses of a beta-adrenergic blocking agent to prevent tachycardia and increased myocardial workload. It must also usually be given with a diuretic, frequently one acting in the ascending limb of the loop of Henle, to present serious fluid accumulation. Patients with malignant hypertension and those already receiving guanethidine (see Warnings) should be hospitalized when *Loniten* is first administered so that they can be monitored to avoid too rapid, or large orthostatic, decreases in blood pressure.

Description: *Loniten* Tablets contain minoxidil, an antihypertensive peripheral vasodilator. The chemical name for minoxidil is 2, 4-diamino-6-piperidinopyrimidine-3-oxide (mw = 209.25). It occurs as a white or off-white, odorless, crystalline solid that is soluble in water to the extent of approximately 2 mg/ml; is readily soluble in propylene glycol or ethanol; and is almost insoluble in acetone, chloroform or ethyl acetate.

Clinical Pharmacology:

1. General Pharmacologic Properties

Minoxidil is an orally effective direct acting peripheral vasodilator that reduces elevated systolic and diastolic blood pressure by decreasing peripheral vascular resistance. Microcirculatory blood flow in animals is enhanced or maintained in all systemic vascular beds. In man, forearm and renal vascular resistance

Continued on next page

Upjohn—Cont.

decline; forearm blood flow increases while renal blood flow and glomerular filtration rate are preserved.

Because it causes peripheral vasodilation, minoxidil elicits a number of predictable reactions. Reduction of peripheral arteriolar resistance and the associated fall in blood pressure trigger sympathetic, vagal inhibitory, and renal homeostatic mechanisms, including an increase in renin secretion, that lead to increased cardiac rate and output and salt and water retention. These adverse effects can usually be minimized by concomitant administration of a diuretic and a beta-adrenergic blocking agent or other sympathetic nervous system suppressant.

Minoxidil does not interfere with vasomotor reflexes and therefore does not produce orthostatic hypotension. The drug does not enter the central nervous system in experimental animals in significant amounts, and it does not affect CNS function in man.

2. Effects on Blood Pressure and Target Organs

The extent and time-course of blood pressure reduction by minoxidil do not correspond closely to its concentration in plasma. After an effective single oral dose, blood pressure usually starts to decline within one-half hour, reaches a minimum between 2 and 3 hours and recovers at an arithmetically linear rate of about 30%/day. The total duration of effect is approximately 75 hours. When minoxidil is administered chronically, once or twice a day, the time required to achieve maximum effect on blood pressure with a given daily dose is inversely related to the size of the dose. Thus, maximum effect is achieved on 10 mg/day within 7 days, on 20 mg/day within 5 days, and on 40 mg/day within 3 days.

The blood pressure response to minoxidil is linearly related to the logarithm of the dose administered. The slope of this log-linear dose-response relationship is proportional to the extent of hypertension and approaches zero at a supine diastolic blood pressure of approximately 85 mmHg.

When used in severely hypertensive patients resistant to other therapy, frequently with an accompanying diuretic and beta-blocker, *Loniten* usually decreased the blood pressure and reversed encephalopathy and retinopathy."

3. Absorption and Metabolism

Minoxidil is at least 90% absorbed from the GI tract in experimental animals and man. Plasma levels of the parent drug reach maximum within the first hour and decline rapidly thereafter. The average plasma half-life in man is 4.2 hours. Approximtely 90% of the administered drug is metabolized, predominantly by conjugation with glucuronic acid at the N-oxide position in the pyrimidine ring, but also by conversion to more polar products. Known metabolites exert much less pharmacologic effect than minoxidil itself; all are excreted principally in the urine. Minoxidil does not bind to plasma proteins, and its renal clearance corresponds to the glomerular filtration rate. In the absence of functional renal tissue, minoxidil and its metabolites can be removed by hemodialysis.

4. Cardiac Lesions in Animals

Minoxidil produced two types of cardiac lesions in non-primate species:

(a) Dog atrial lesion—
Daily oral doses of 0.5 mg/kg for several days to 1 month or longer produced a grossly visible hemorrhagic lesion of the right atrium of the dog. This lesion has not been seen in other species. Microscopic examination showed replacement of myocardial cells by proliferating fibroblasts and angioblasts; phagocytosis; and hemosiderin accumulation in macrophages.

(b) Papillary muscle lesion—
Short term treatment (about 3 days) in several species (dog, rat, minipig) produced necrosis of the papillary muscles, and, in some cases subendocardial areas of the left ventricle, lesions similar to those produced by other peripheral dilators and by beta-adrenergic receptor agonists such as isoproterenol and epinephrine. These are thought to result from myocardial ischemia resulting from reflex sympathetic or vagal withdrawal-induced tachycardia in combination with hypotension. These lesions were reduced in incidence and severity by beta-adrenergic receptor blockade.

(c) *Hemorrhagic lesions* were seen in many parts of the heart, mainly in the epicardium, endocardium, and walls of small coronary arteries and arterioles, after acute minoxidil treatment in dogs, and left atrial hemorrhagic lesions were seen in minipigs.

In addition to these lesions, longer term studies in rats, dogs, and monkeys showed cardiac hypertrophy and (in rats) cardiac dilation. In monkeys, hydrochlorothiazide partly reversed the increased heart weight, suggesting it may be related to fluid overload. In a one-year dog study, serosanguinous pericardial fluid was seen.

Autopsies of 79 patients who died from various causes and who had received minoxidil did not reveal right atrial or other hemorrhagic pathology of the kind seen in dogs. Instances of necrotic areas in the papillary muscles were seen, but these occurred in the presence of known pre-existing ischemic heart disease and did not appear different from, or more common than, lesions seen in patients never exposed to minoxidil. Studies to date cannot rule out the possibility that minoxidil can be associated with cardiac damage in humans.

Indications and Usage: Because of the potential for serious adverse effects, *Loniten* Tablets (minoxidil) are indicated only in the treatment of hypertension that is symptomatic or associated with target organ damage and is not manageable with maximum therapeutic doses of a diuretic plus two other antihypertensive drugs. At the present time use in milder degrees of hypertension is not recommended because the benefit-risk relationship in such patients has not been defined.

Loniten reduced supine diastolic blood pressure by 20 mm Hg or to 90 mm Hg or less in approximately 75% of patients, most of whom had hypertension that could not be controlled by other drugs.

Contraindications: *Loniten* Tablets (minoxidil) are contraindicated in pheochromocytoma, because it may stimulate secretion of catecholamines from the tumor through its antihypertensive action.

Warnings:

1. Salt and Water Retention; Congestive Heart Failure—concomitant use of an adequate diuretic is required—

Loniten Tablets (minoxidil) must usually be administered concomitantly with a diuretic adequate to prevent fluid retention and possible congestive heart failure; a high ceiling (loop) diuretic is *almost always* required. Body weight should be monitored closely. If *Loniten* is used without a diuretic, retention of several hundred milli-equivalents of salt and corresponding volumes of water can occur within a few days, leading to increased plasma and interstitial fluid volume and local or generalized edema. Diuretic treatment alone, or in combination with restricted salt intake, will usually minimize fluid retention, although reversible edema did develop in approximately 10% of nondialysis patients so treated. Ascites has also been reported. Diuretic effectiveness was limited mostly by disease-related impaired renal function. The condition of patients with preexisting congestive heart failure occasionally deteriorated in association with fluid retention although because of the fall in blood pressure (reduction of afterload), more than twice as many improved than worsened. Rarely, refractory fluid retention may require discontinuation of *Loniten*. Provided that the patient is under close medical supervision, it may be possible to resolve refractory salt retention by discontinuing *Loniten* for 1 or 2 days and then resuming treatment in conjunction with vigorous diuretic therapy.

2. Concomitant Treatment to Prevent Trachycardia is Usually Required—*Loniten* increases the heart rate. Angina may worsen or appear for the first time during *Loniten* treatment, probably because of the increased oxygen demands associated with increased heart rate and cardiac output. The increase in rate and the occurrence of angina generally can be prevented by the concomitant administration of a beta-adrenergic blocking drug or other sympathetic nervous system suppressant. The ability of beta-adrenergic blocking agents to minimize papillary muscle lesions in animals is further reason to utilize such an agent concomitantly. Round-the-clock effectiveness of the sympathetic suppressant should be ensured."

3. Pericardial Effusion and Tamponade—Pericardial effusion, occasionally with tamponade, has been observed in about 3% of treated patients not on dialysis, especially those with inadequate or compromised renal function. Although in many cases, the pericardial effusion was associated with a connective tissue disease, the uremic syndrome, congestive heart failure, or marked fluid retention, there have been instances in which these potential causes of effusion were not present. Patients should be observed closely for any suggestion of a pericardial disorder, and echocardiographic studies should be carried out if suspicion arises. More vigorous diuretic therapy, dialysis, pericardiocentesis, or surgery may be required. If the effusion persists, withdrawal of *Loniten* should be considered in light of other means of controlling the hypertension and the patient's clinical status.

4. *Interaction with Guanethidine:*
Although minoxidil does not itself cause orthostatic hypotension, its administration to patients already receiving guanethidine can result in profound orthostatic effects. If at all possible, guanethidine should be discontinued well before minoxidil is begun. Where this is not possible, minoxidil therapy should be started in the hospital and the patient should remain institutionalized until severe orthostatic effects are no longer present or the patient has learned to avoid activities that provoke them.

5. *Hazard of Rapid Control of Blood Pressure:*
In patients with very severe blood pressure elevation, too rapid control of blood pressure, especially with intravenous agents, can precipitate syncope, cerebrovascular accidents, myocardial infarction and ischema of special sense organs with resulting decrease or loss of vision or hearing. Patients with compromised circulation or cryoglobulinemia may also suffer ischemic episodes of the affected organs. Although such events have not been unequivocally associated with minoxidil use, total experience is limited at present.

Any patient with malignant hypertension should have initial treatment with minoxidil carried out in a hospital setting, both to assure that blood pressure is falling and to assure that it is not falling more rapidly than intended.

Precautions:

1. General—(a) **Monitor fluid and electrolyte balance and body weight** (see **Warnings:** Salt and Water Retention).

(b) **Observe patients for signs and symptoms of pericardial effusion** (see **Warnings:** Pericardial Effusion and Tamponade).

(c) **Use after myocardial infarction**—*Loniten* has not been used in patients who have had a myocardial infarction within the preceding month. It is possible that a reduction of arterial pressure with *Loniten* might further limit blood flow to the myocardium, although this might be compensated by decreased oxygen demand because of lower blood pressure.

(d) **Hypersensitivity**—Possible hypersensitivity to *Loniten*, manifested as a skin rash, has been seen in less than 1% of patients; whether the drug should be discontinued when this occurs depends on treatment alternatives.

(e) **Renal failure or dialysis patients** may require smaller doses of *Loniten* and should have close medical supervision to prevent exacerbation of renal failure or precipitation of cardiac failure.

2. **Patient Information**—The patient should be made fully aware of the importance of continuing all of his antihypertensive medications and of the nature of symptoms that would suggest fluid overload. A patient brochure has been prepared and is included with each *Loniten* package. The text of this brochure is reprinted below.

3. **Carcinogenesis, Mutagenesis and Impairment of Fertility**—Twenty-two month carcinogenicity studies in rats at doses 15 times the human dose did not provide evidence of tumorigenicity. The drug was not mutagenic in the Salmonella (Ames) test.

Rats receiving up to five times the human dose of minoxidil had a reduction in conception rate, possibly related to drug treatment. There was no evidence of increased fetal resorptions in rats but they did occur in rabbits.

4. **Use in Pregnancy-Teratogenic Effects**—Pregnancy Category C. Minoxidil has been shown to reduce the conception rate in rats and to show evidence of increased fetal absorption in rabbits when administered at five times the human dose. There was no evidence of teratogenic effects in rats and rabbits. There are no adequate and well controlled studies in pregnant women. *Loniten* should be used during pregnancy only if the potential benefit justifies the potential risk to the fetus.

5. **Nursing Mothers**—It is not known whether this drug is secreted in human milk. As a general rule, nursing should not be undertaken while a patient is on *Loniten*.

6. **Use in Pediatrics**—Total use in children has been limited to date, particularly in infants. The recommendations under Dosage and Administration can be considered only a rough guide at present and careful titration is essential.

Adverse Reactions:

1. **Salt and Water Retention** (see **Warnings:** Concomitant Use of Adequate Diuretic is Required)—Temporary edema developed in 7% of patients who were not edematous at the start of therapy.

2. **Pericardial Effusion** and **Tamponade** (see **Warnings**).

3. **Dermatologic - Hypertrichosis**—Elongation, thickening, and enhanced pigmentation of fine body hair are seen in about 80% of patients taking *Loniten* Tablets (minoxidil). This develops within 3 to 6 weeks after starting therapy. It is usually first noticed on the temples, between the eyebrows, between the hairline and the eyebrows, or in the side-burn area of the upper lateral cheek, later extending to the back, arms, legs, and scalp. Upon discontinuation of *Loniten*, new hair growth stops, but 1 to 6 months may be required for restoration to pretreatment appearance. No endocrine abnormalities have been found to explain the abnormal hair growth; thus, it is hypertrichosis without virilism. Hair growth is especially disturbing to children and women and such patients should be thoroughly informed about this effect before therapy with *Loniten* is begun.

Allergic—Rashes have been reported, including rare reports of bullous eruptions, and Stevens-Johnson Syndrome.

4. **Hematologic**—Thrombocytopenia and leukopenia (WBC < 3000/mm^3) have rarely been reported.

5. **Gastrointestinal**—Nausea and/or vomiting has been reported. In clinical trials the incidence of nausea and vomiting associated with the underlying disease has shown a decrease from pretrial levels.

6. **Miscellaneous**—Breast tenderness—This developed in less than 1% of patients.

7. **Altered Laboratory Findings**—(a) ECG changes—changes in direction and magnitude of the ECG T-waves occur in approximately 60% of patients treated with *Loniten*. In rare instances a large negative amplitude of the T-wave may encroach upon the S-T segment, but the S-T segment is not independently altered. These changes usually disappear with continuance of treatment and revert to the pretreatment state if *Loniten* is discontinued. No symptoms have been associated with these changes, nor have there been alterations in blood cell counts or in plasma enzyme concentrations that would suggest myocardial damage. Long-term treatment of patients manifesting such changes has provided no evidence of deteriorating cardiac function. At present the changes appear to be nonspecific and without identifiable clinical significance. (b) Effects of hemodilution—hematocrit, hemoglobin and erythrocyte count usually fall about 7% initially and then recover to pretreatment levels. (c) Other—Alkaline phosphatase increased varyingly without other evidence of liver or bone abnormality. Serum creatinine increased an average of 6% and BUN slightly more, but later declined to pretreatment levels.

Overdosage: There have been only a few instances of deliberate or accidental overdosage with *Loniten* Tablets (minoxidil). One patient recovered after taking 50 mg of *Loniten* Tablets together with 500 mg of a barbiturate. When exaggerated hypotension is encountered, it is most likely to occur in association with residual sympathetic nervous system blockade from previous therapy (guanethidine-like effects or alpha-adrenergic blockage), which prevents the usual compensatory maintenance of blood pressure. Intravenous administration of normal saline will help to maintain blood pressure and facilitate urine formation in these patients. Sympathomimetic drugs such as norepinephrine or epinephrine should be avoided because of their excessive cardiac stimulating action. Phenylephrine, angiotensin II, vasopressin, and dopamine all reverse hypotension due to *Loniten*, but should only be used if underperfusion of a vital organ is evident.

Dosage and Administration:

Patients over 12 years of age: The recommended initial dosage of *Loniten* Tablets (minoxidil) is 5 mg given as a single daily dose. Daily dosage can be increased to 10, 20 and then to 40 mg in single or divided doses if required for optimum blood pressure control. The effective dosage range is usually 10 to 40 mg per day. The maximum recommended dosage is 100 mg per day.

Patients under 12 years of age: The initial dosage is 0.2 mg/kg minoxidil as a single daily dose. The dosage may be increased in 50 to 100% increments until optimum blood pressure control is achieved. The effective dosage range is usually 0.25 to 1.0 mg/kg/day. The maximum recommended dosage is 50 mg daily. (see **6. Use in Pediatrics** under **Precautions**).

Dose frequency: The magnitude of within-day fluctuation of arterial pressure during therapy with *Loniten* is directly proportional to the extent of pressure reduction. If supine diastolic pressure has been reduced less than 30 mmHg, the drug need be administered only once a day; if supine diastolic pressure has been reduced more than 30 mmHg, the daily dosage should be divided into two equal parts.

Frequency of dosage adjustment: Dosage must be titrated carefully according to individual response. Intervals between dosage adjustments normally should be at least 3 days since the full response to a given dose is not obtained for at least that amount of time. **Where a more rapid management of hypertension is required, dose adjustments can be made every 6 hours if the patient is carefully monitored.**

Concomitant therapy: Diuretic and beta-blocker or other sympathetic nervous system supressant.

Diuretics: *Loniten* must be used in conjunction with a diuretic in patients relying on renal function for maintaining salt and water balance. Diuretics have been used at the following dosages when starting therapy with *Loniten:* hydrochlorothiazide (50 mg, b.i.d.) or other thiazides at equieffective dosage; chlorthalidone (50 to 100 mg, once daily); furosemide (40 mg, b.i.d.)

If excessive salt and water retention results in a weight gain of more than 5 pounds, diuretic therapy should be changed to furosemide; if the patient is already taking furosemide, dosage should be increased in accordance with the patient's requirements.

Beta-blocker or other sympathetic nervous system suppressants: When therapy with *Loniten* is begun, the dosage of a beta-adrenergic receptor blocking drug should be the equivalent of 80 to 160 mg of propranolol per day in divided doses.

If beta-blockers are contraindicated, methyldopa (250 to 750 mg, b.i.d.) may be used instead. Methyldopa must be given for at least 24 hours before starting therapy with *Loniten* because of the delay in the onset of methyldopa's action. Limited clinical experience indicates that clonidine may also be used to prevent tachycardia induced by *Loniten;* the usual dosage is 0.1 to 0.2 mg twice daily.

Sympathetic nervous system suppressants may not completely prevent an increase in heart rate due to *Loniten* but usually do prevent tachycardia. Typically, patients receiving a beta-blocker prior to initiation of therapy with *Loniten* have a bradycardia and can be expected to have an increase in heart rate toward normal when *Loniten* is added. When treatment with *Loniten* and beta-blocker or other sympathetic nervous system suppressant are begun simultaneously, their opposing cardiac effects usually nullify each other, leading to little change in heart rate.

How Supplied: *Loniten* Tablets (minoxidil) are available as round, scored, white tablets. Dosage strengths are imprinted on one convex surface. The following strengths and container sizes are available:

Strength	Container and Size	NDC Number
2.5 mg	Bottles of 100, Unit of Use	0009-0121-01
10 mg	Bottles of 100, Unit of Use	0009-0137-01

Store at controlled room temperature 15°–30°C (59°–86°F).

Patient Information: *Loniten* Tablets contain minoxidil, a powerful medicine for the treatment of high blood pressure. *Loniten* is used for the treatment of severe hypertension that is difficult to control. It must usually be taken with other medicines.

Be absolutely sure to take all of your medicines for high blood pressure according to your doctor's instructions. Do not stop taking *Loniten* unless your doctor tells you to. Do not give any of your medicine to other people.

It is important that you look for the warning signals of certain undesired effects of *Loniten*. Call your doctor if they occur. Your doctor will need to see you regularly while you are taking *Loniten*. Be sure to keep all your appointments or to arrange for new ones if you must miss one.

Do not hesitate to call your doctor if any discomforts or problems occur.

The information here is intended to help you take *Loniten* properly. It does not tell you all

Continued on next page

Upjohn—Cont.

there is to know about *Loniten.* There is a more technical leaflet that you may request from the pharmacist; you may need your doctor's help in understanding parts of that leaflet.

What is *Loniten?*

Loniten Tablets contain minoxidil which is a powerful drug for lowering the blood pressure. It works by relaxing and enlarging certain small blood vessels so that blood flows through them more easily.

Why lower blood pressure?

Your doctor has prescribed *Loniten* to lower your blood pressure and protect vital parts of your body. Uncontrolled blood pressure can cause stroke, heart failure, blindness, kidney failure, and heart attacks.

Most people with high blood pressure need to take medicines to treat it for their whole lives.

Who should take *Loniten?*

There are many people with high blood pressure, but most of them do not need *Loniten.* *Loniten* is used ONLY when your doctor decides that:

1. your high blood pressure is severe;
2. your high blood pressure is causing symptoms or damage to vital organs; and
3. other medicines did not work well enough or had very disturbing side effects.

Loniten should be taken only when a doctor prescribes it. Never give any of your *Loniten* Tablets, or any other high blood pressure medicine, to a friend or relative.

Pregnancy: In some cases doctors may prescribe *Loniten* for women who are pregnant or who are planning to have children. However, its safe use in pregnancy has not been established. Laboratory animals had a reduced ability to become pregnant and a reduced survival of offspring while taking *Loniten.* If you are pregnant or are planning to become pregnant, be sure to tell your doctor.

How to take *Loniten.*

Usually, your doctor will prescribe two other medicines along with *Loniten.* These will help lower blood pressure and will help prevent undesired effects of *Loniten.*

Often, when a medicine like *Loniten* lowers blood pressure, your body tries to return the blood pressure to the original, higher level. It does this by holding on to water and salt (so there will be more fluid to pump) and by making your heart beat faster.

To prevent this, your doctor will usually prescribe a water tablet to remove the extra salt and water from your body (a diuretic dye-u-RET-tic) and another medicine to slow your heart beat.

You must follow your doctor's instructions exactly, taking all the prescribed medicines, in the right amounts, each day. These medicines will help keep your blood pressure down.

The water tablet and heart beat medicine will help prevent the undesired effects of *Loniten.* *Loniten* Tablets come in two strengths (2 ½ milligrams and 10 milligrams) that are marked on each tablet. Pay close attention to the tablet markings to be sure you are taking the correct strength. Your doctor may prescribe half a tablet; the tablets are scored (partly cut on one side) so that you can easily break them.

When you first start taking *Loniten,* your doctor may need to see you often in order to adjust your dosage. Take all your medicine according to the schedule prescribed by your doctor. **Do not skip any doses. If you should forget a dose of *Loniten,* wait until it is time for your next dose, then continue with your regular schedule. Remember: do not stop taking *Loniten,* or any of your other high blood pressure medicines, without checking with your doctor.** Make sure that any doctor treating or examining you knows that you are taking high blood pressure medicines, including *Loniten.*

Warning Signals: Even if you take all your medicines correctly, *Loniten* may cause undesired effects. Some of these are serious and you should be on the lookout for them. **If any of the following warning signals occur, you must call your doctor immediately:**

1. *Increase in heart rate*—You should measure your heart rate by counting your pulse rate **while you are resting.** If you have an increase of 20 beats or more a minute over your normal pulse, contact your doctor immediately. If you do not know how to take your pulse rate, ask your doctor. Also ask your doctor how often to check your pulse.
2. *Rapid weight gain of more than 5 pounds*—You should weigh yourself daily. If you quickly gain five or more pounds, or if there is any swelling or puffiness in the face, hands, ankles, or stomach area, this could be a sign that you are retaining body fluids. Your doctor may have to change your drugs or change the dose of your drugs. You may also need to reduce the amount of salt you eat. A smaller weight gain (2 to 3 pounds) often occurs when treatment is started. You may lose this extra weight with continued treatment.
3. *Increased difficulty in breathing,* especially when lying down. This too may be due to an increase of body fluids. It can also happen because your high blood pressure is getting worse. In either case, you might require treatment with other medicines.
4. *New or worsening of pain in the chest, arm, or shoulder or signs of severe indigestion*—These could be signs of serious heart problems.
5. *Dizziness, lighteadedness or fainting*—These can be signs of high blood pressure or they may be side effects from one of the medicines. Your doctor may need to change or adjust the dosage of the medicines you are taking.

Other Undesired Effects: *Loniten* can cause other undesired effects such as nausea and/or vomiting that are annoying but not dangerous. Do not stop taking the drug because of these other undesired effects without talking to your doctor.

Hair growth: About 8 out of every 10 patients who have taken *Loniten* noticed that fine **body hair grew darker or longer** on certain parts of the body. This happened about three to six weeks after beginning treatment. The hair may first be noticed on the forehead and temples, between the eyebrows, or on the upper part of the cheeks. Later, hair may grow on the back, arms, legs, or scalp. Although hair growth may not be noticeable to some patients, it often is bothersome in women and children. **Unwanted hair can be controlled with a hair remover or by shaving.** The extra hair is not permanent, it disappears within 1 to 6 months of stopping *Loniten.* Nevertheless, **you should not stop taking *Loniten* without first talking to your doctor.**

A few patients have developed a rash or breast tenderness while taking *Loniten* Tablets (minoxidil), but this is unusual.

Code 810 384 105

[*Shown in Product Identification Section*]

MAOLATE® Tablets ℞
(chlorphenesin carbamate)

500's
NSN 6505-00-998-7143A (M & VA)

How Supplied: Scored tablets containing 400 mg chlorphenesin carbamate are available in the following packages.

Bottles of 50	*NDC 0009-0412-01*
Bottles of 500	*NDC 0009-0412-02*
Unit dose package (100)	*NDC 0009-0412-03*

[*Shown in Product Identification Section*]

MEDROL® Acetate Topical ℞
(methylprednisolone acetate)
For External Use Only

How Supplied: In two concentrations-2.5 mg (0.25%) or 10 mg (1.0%) methylprednisolone acetate per gram.

0.25%	7.5 gram tubes	*NDC 0009-0483-01*
	30 gram tubes	*NDC 0009-0483-02*
	1½ oz tubes	*NDC 0009-0483-03*
1%	7.5 gram tubes	*NDC 0009-0505-01*
	30 gram tubes	*NDC 0009-0505-02*

MEDROL® Tablets ℞
(methylprednisolone tablets, USP)

4 mg (500's):
NSN 6505-00-050-3068A (VA)
16 mg (50's):
NSN 6505-00-764-4358A (VA)

Description: *Medrol* Tablets contain methylprednisolone which is a glucocorticord. Glucocorticoids are adrenocortical steroids, both naturally occurring and synthetic, which are readily absorbed from the gastrointestinal tract. Methylprednisolone occurs as a white to practically white, odorless, crystalline powder. It is sparingly soluble in alcohol, in dioxane, and in methanol, slightly soluble in acetone, and in chloroform, and very slightly soluble in ether. It is practically insoluble in water.

The chemical name for methylprednisolone is pregna-1, 4-diene-3, 20-dione,11, 17, 21-trihydroxy-6-methyl-,(6α, 11β)- and the molecular weight is 374.48.

Medrol Tablets (methylprednisolone) are available as scored tablets in the following strengths: 2 mg, 4 mg, 8 mg, 16 mg, 24 mg, 32 mg.

Actions: Naturally occurring glucocorticoids (hydrocortisone and cortisone), which also have salt-retaining properties, are used as replacement therapy in adrenocortical deficiency states. Their synthetic analogs are primarily used for their potent anti-inflammatory effects in disorders of many organ systems. Glucocorticoids cause profound and varied metabolic effects. In addition, they modify the body's immune responses to diverse stimuli.

Indications: *Medrol* Tablets (methylprednisolone) are indicated in the following conditions:

1. **Endocrine Disorders**
   - Primary or secondary adrenocortical insufficiency (hydrocortisone or cortisone is the first choice; synthetic analogs may be used in conjunction with mineralocorticoids where applicable; in infancy mineralocorticoid supplementation is of particular importance).
   - Congenital adrenal hyperplasia
   - Nonsuppurative thyroiditis
   - Hypercalcemia associated with cancer
2. **Rheumatic Disorders**
   - As adjunctive therapy for short-term administration (to tide the patient over an acute episode or exacerbation) in:
   - Psoriatic arthritis
   - Rheumatoid arthritis, including juvenile rheumatoid arthritis (selected cases may require low-dose maintenance therapy)
   - Ankylosing spondylitis
   - Acute and subacute bursitis
   - Acute nonspecific tenosynovitis
   - Acute gouty arthritis
   - Post-traumatic osteoarthritis
   - Synovitis of osteoarthritis
   - Epicondylitis
3. **Collagen Diseases**
   - During an exacerbation or as maintenance therapy in selected cases of:
   - Systemic lupus erythematosus
   - Acute rheumatic carditis
   - Systemic dermatomyositis (polymyositis)

4. **Dermatologic Diseases**
   Pemphigus
   Bullous dermatitis herpetiformis
   Severe erythema multiforme (Stevens-Johnson syndrome)
   Exfoliative dermatitis
   Mycosis fungoides
   Severe psoriasis
   Severe seborrheic dermatitis
5. **Allergic States**
   Control of severe or incapacitating allergic conditions intractable to adequate trials of conventional treatment:
   Seasonal or perennial allergic rhinitis
   Serum sickness
   Bronchial asthma
   Drug hypersensitivity reactions
   Contact dermatitis
   Atopic dermatitis
6. **Ophthalmic Diseases**
   Severe acute and chronic allergic and inflammatory processes involving the eye and its adnexa such as:
   Allergic corneal marginal ulcers
   Herpes zoster ophthalmicus
   Anterior segment inflammation
   Diffuse posterior uveitis and choroiditis
   Sympathetic ophthalmia
   Allergic conjunctivitis
   Keratitis
   Chorioretinitis
   Optic neuritis
   Iritis and iridocyclitis
7. **Respiratory Diseases**
   Symptomatic sarcoidosis
   Loeffler's syndrome not manageable by other means
   Berylliosis
   Fulminating or disseminated pulmonary tuberculosis when used concurrently with appropriate antituberculous chemotherapy
   Aspiration pneumonitis
8. **Hematologic Disorders**
   Idiopathic thrombocytopenic purpura in adults
   Secondary thrombocytopenia in adults
   Acquired (autoimmune) hemolytic anemia
   Erythroblastopenia (RBC anemia)
   Congenital (erythroid) hypoplastic anemia
9. **Neoplastic Diseases**
   For palliative management of:
   Leukemias and lymphomas in adults
   Acute leukemia of childhood
10. **Edematous States**
   To induce a diuresis or remission of proteinuria in the nephrotic syndrome, without uremia, of the idiopathic type or that due to lupus erythematosus.
11. **Gastrointestinal diseases**
   To tide the patient over a critical period of the disease in:
   Ulcerative colitis
   Regional enteritis
12. **Nervous System**
   Acute exacerbations of multiple sclerosis
13. **Miscellaneous**
   Tuberculous meningitis with subarachnoid block or impending block when used concurrently with appropriate antituberculous chemotherapy.
   Trichinosis with neurologic or myocardial involvement

Contraindications: Systemic fungal infections.

Warnings: In patients on corticosteroid therapy subjected to unusual stress, increased dosage of rapidly acting corticosteroids before, during, and after the stressful situation is indicated.

Corticosteroids may mask some signs of infection and new infections may appear during their use. There may be decreased resistance and inability to localize infection when corticosteroids are used.

Prolonged use of corticosteroids may produce posterior subcapsular cataracts, glaucoma with possible damage to the optic nerves, and may enhance the establishment of secondary ocular infections due to fungi or viruses.

Usage in pregnancy: Since adequate human reproduction studies have not been done with corticosteroids, the use of these drugs in pregnancy, nursing mothers or women of childbearing potential requires that the possible benefits of the drug be weighed against the potential hazards to the mother and embryo or fetus. Infants born of mothers who have received substantial doses of corticosteroids during pregnancy should be carefully observed for signs of hypoadrenalism.

Average and large doses of hydrocortisone or cortisone can cause elevation of blood pressure, salt and water retention, and increased excretion of potassium. These effects are less likely to occur with the synthetic derivatives except when used in large doses. Dietary salt restriction and potassium supplementation may be necessary. All corticosteroids increase calcium excretion.

While on corticosteroid therapy patients should not be vaccinated against smallpox. Other immunization procedures should not be undertaken in patients who are on corticosteroids, especially on high dose, because of possible hazards of neurological complications and a lack of antibody response.

The use of *Medrol* Tablets (methylprednisolone) in active tuberculosis should be restricted to those cases of fulminating or disseminated tuberculosis in which the corticosteroid is used for the management of the disease in conjunction with an appropriate antituberculous regimen.

If corticosteroids are indicated in patients with latent tuberculosis or tuberculin reactivity, close observation is necessary as reactivation of the disease may occur. During prolonged corticosteroid therapy, these patients should receive chemoprophylaxis.

Precautions: Drug-induced secondary adrenocortical insufficiency may be minimized by gradual reduction of dosage. This type of relative insufficiency may persist for months after discontinuation of therapy; therefore, in any situation of stress occurring during that period, hormone therapy should be reinstituted. Since mineralocorticoid secretion may be impaired, salt and/or a mineralocorticoid should be administered concurrently.

There is an enhanced effect of corticosteroids on patients with hypothyroidism and in those with cirrhosis.

Corticosteroids should be used cautiously in patients with ocular herpes simplex because of possible corneal perforation.

The lowest possible dose of corticosteroid should be used to control the condition under treatment, and when reduction in dosage is possible, the reduction should be gradual.

Psychic derangements may appear when corticosteroids are used, ranging from euphoria, insomnia, mood swings, personality changes and severe depression, to frank psychotic manifestations. Also, existing emotional instability or psychotic tendencies may be aggravated by corticosteroids.

Aspirin should be used cautiously in conjunction with corticosteroids in hypoprothrombinemia.

Steroids should be used with caution in nonspecific ulcerative colitis, if there is a probability of impending perforation, abscess or other pyogenic infection; diverticulitis; fresh intestinal anastomoses; active or latent peptic ulcer; renal insufficiency; hypertension; osteoporosis; and myasthenia gravis.

Growth and development of infants and children on prolonged corticosteroid therapy should be carefully observed.

Although controlled clinical trials have shown corticosteroids to be effective in speeding the resolution of acute exacerbations of multiple sclerosis, they do not show that corticosteroids affect the ultimate outcome or natural history of the disease. The studies do show that relatively high doses of corticosteroids are necessary to demonstrate a significant effect. (See **Dosage and Administration**)

Since complications of treatment with glucocorticoids are dependent on the size of the dose and the duration of treatment, a risk/benefit decision must be made in each individual case as to dose and duration of treatment and as to whether daily or intermittent therapy should be used.

The 24 mg tablet contains FD&C Yellow No. 5 (tartrazine) which may cause allergic-type reactions (including bronchial asthma) in certain susceptible individuals. Although the overall incidence of FD&C Yellow No. 5 (tartrazine) sensitivity in the general population is low, it is frequently seen in patients who also have aspirin hypersensitivity.

Adverse Reactions:

Fluid and Electrolyte Disturbances
- Sodium retention
- Fluid retention
- Congestive heart failure in susceptible patients
- Potassium loss
- Hypokalemic alkalosis
- Hypertension

Musculoskeletal
- Muscle weakness
- Steroid myopathy
- Loss of muscle mass
- Osteoporosis
- Vertebral compression fractures
- Aseptic necrosis of femoral and humeral heads
- Pathologic fracture of long bones

Gastrointestinal
- Peptic ulcer with possible perforation and hemorrhage
- Pancreatitis
- Abdominal distention
- Ulcerative esophagitis

Dermatologic
- Impaired wound healing
- Thin fragile skin
- Petechiae and ecchymoses
- Facial erythema
- Increased sweating
- May suppress reactions to skin tests

Neurological
- Increased intracranial pressure with papilledema (pseudo-tumor cerebri) usually after treatment
- Convulsions
- Vertigo
- Headache

Endocrine
- Development of Cushingoid state
- Suppression of growth in children
- Secondary adrenocortical and pituitary unresponsiveness, particularly in times of stress, as in trauma, surgery or illness.
- Menstrual irregularities
- Decreased carbohydrate tolerance
- Manifestations of latent diabetes mellitus
- Increased requirements for insulin or oral hypoglycemic agents in diabetics

Ophthalmic
- Posterior subcapsular cataracts
- Increased intraocular pressure
- Glaucoma
- Exophthalmos

Metabolic
- Negative nitrogen balance due to protein catabolism

The following additional reactions are related to oral therapy: Urticaria and other allergic, anaphylactic or hypersensitivity reactions.

Dosage and Administration:

The initial dosage of *Medrol* Tablets (methylprednisolone) may vary from 4 mg to 48 mg per

Continued on next page

Upjohn—Cont.

day depending on the specific disease entity being treated. In situations of less severity lower doses will generally suffice while in selected patients higher initial doses may be required. The initial dosage should be maintained or adjusted until a satisfactory response is noted. If after a reasonable period of time there is a lack of satisfactory clinical response, *Medrol* should be discontinued and the patient transferred to other appropriate therapy. **IT SHOULD BE EMPHASIZED THAT DOSAGE REQUIREMENTS ARE VARIABLE AND MUST BE INDIVIDUALIZED ON THE BASIS OF THE DISEASE UNDER TREATMENT AND THE RESPONSE OF THE PATIENT.** After a favorable response is noted, the proper maintenance dosage should be determined by decreasing the initial drug dosage in small decrements at appropriate time intervals until the lowest dosage which will maintain an adequate clinical response is reached. It should be kept in mind that constant monitoring is needed in regard to drug dosage. Included in the situations which may make dosage adjustments necessary are changes in clinical status secondary to remissions or exacerbations in the disease process, the patient's individual drug responsiveness, and the effect of patient exposure to stressful situations not directly related to the disease entity under treatment; in this latter situation it may be necessary to increase the dosage of *Medrol* for a period of time consistent with the patient's condition. If after long-term therapy the drug is to be stopped, it is recommended that it be withdrawn gradually rather than abruptly.

Multiple Sclerosis

In treatment of acute exacerbations of multiple sclerosis daily doses of 200 mg of prednisolone for a week followed by 80 mg every other day for 1 month have been shown to be effective (4 mg of methylprednisolone is equivalent to 5 mg of prednisolone).

ADT® Alternate Day Therapy

Alternate day therapy is a corticosteroid dosing regimen in which twice the usual daily dose of corticoid is administered every other morning. The purpose of this mode of therapy is to provide the patient requiring long-term pharmacologic dose treatment with the beneficial effects of corticoids while minimizing certain undesirable effects, including pituitary-adrenal suppression, the Cushingoid state, corticoid withdrawal symptoms, and growth suppression in children.

The rationale for this treatment schedule is based on two major premises: (a) the anti-inflammatory or therapeutic effect of corticoids persists longer than their physical presence and metabolic effects and (b) administration of the corticosteroid every other morning allows for re-establishment of more nearly normal hypothalamic-pituitary-adrenal (HPA) activity on the off-steroid day.

A brief review of the HPA physiology may be helpful in understanding this rationale. Acting primarily through the hypothalamus a fall in free cortisol stimulates the pituitary gland to produce increasing amounts of corticotropin (ACTH) while a rise in free cortisol inhibits ACTH secretion. Normally the HPA system is characterized by diurnal (circadian) rhythm. Serum levels of ACTH rise from a low point about 10 pm to a peak level about 6 am. Increasing levels of ACTH stimulate adrenal cortical activity resulting in a rise in plasma cortisol with maximal levels occurring between 2 am and 8 am. This rise in cortisol dampens ACTH production and in turn adrenal cortical activity. There is a gradual fall in plasma corticoids during the day with lowest levels occurring about midnight.

The diurnal rhythm of the HPA axis is lost in Cushing's disease, a syndrome of adrenal cortical hyperfunction characterized by obesity with centripetal fat distribution, thinning of the skin with easy bruisability, muscle wasting with weakness, hypertension, latent diabetes, osteoporosis, electrolyte imbalance, etc. The same clinical findings of hyperadrenocorticism may be noted during long-term pharmacologic dose corticoid therapy administered in conventional daily divided doses. It would appear, then, that a disturbance in the diurnal cycle with maintenance of elevated corticoid values during the night may play a significant role in the development of undesirable corticoid effects. Escape from these constantly elevated plasma levels for even short periods of time may be instrumental in protecting against undesirable pharmacologic effects.

During conventional pharmacologic dose corticosteroid therapy, ACTH production is inhibited with subsequent suppression of cortisol production by the adrenal cortex. Recovery time for normal HPA activity is variable depending upon the dose and duration of treatment. During this time the patient is vulnerable to any stressful situation. Although it has been shown that there is considerably less adrenal suppression following a single morning dose of prednisolone (10 mg) as opposed to a quarter of that dose administered every 6 hours, there is evidence that some suppressive effect on adrenal activity may be carried over into the following day when pharmacologic doses are used. Further, it has been shown that a single dose of certain corticosteroids will produce adrenal cortical suppression for two or more days. Other corticoids, including methylprednisolone, hydrocortisone, prednisone, and prednisolone, are considered to be short acting (producing adrenal cortical suppression for 1¼ to 1½ days following a single dose) and thus are recommended for alternate day therapy.

The following should be kept in mind when considering alternate day therapy:

1) Basic principles and indications for corticosteroid therapy should apply. The benefits of *ADT* should not encourage the indiscriminate use of steroids.

2) *ADT* is a therapeutic technique primarily designed for patients in whom long-term pharmacologic corticoid therapy is anticipated.

3) In less severe disease processes in which corticoid therapy is indicated, it may be possible to initiate treatment with *ADT*. More severe disease states usually will require daily divided high dose therapy for initial control of the disease process. The initial suppressive dose level should be continued until satisfactory clinical response is obtained, usually four to ten days in the case of many allergic and collagen diseases. It is important to keep the period of initial suppressive dose as brief as possible particularly when subsequent use of alternate day therapy is intended.

Once control has been established, two courses are available: (a) change to *ADT* and then gradually reduce the amount of corticoid given every other day *or* (b) following control of the disease process reduce the daily dose of corticoid to the lowest effective level as rapidly as possible and then change over to an alternate day schedule. Theoretically, course (a) may be preferable.

4) Because of the advantages of *ADT*, it may be desirable to try patients on this form of therapy who have been on daily corticoids for long periods of time (eg, patients with rheumatoid arthritis). Since these patients may already have a suppressed HPA axis, establishing them on *ADT* may be difficult and not always successful. However, it is recommended that regular attempts be made to change them over. It may be helpful to triple or even quadruple the daily maintenance dose and administer this every other day rather than just doubling the daily dose if difficulty is encountered. Once the patient is again controlled, an attempt should be made to reduce this dose to a minimum.

5) As indicated above, certain corticosteroids, because of their prolonged suppressive effect on adrenal activity, are not recommended for alternate day therapy (eg, dexamethasone and betamethasone).

6) The maximal activity of the adrenal cortex is between 2 am and 8 am, and it is minimal between 4 pm and midnight. Exogenous corticosteroids suppress adrenocortical activity the least, when given at the time of maximal activity (am).

7) In using *ADT* it is important, as in all therapeutic situations, to individualize and tailor the therapy to each patient. Complete control of symptoms will not be possible in all patients. An explanation of the benefits of *ADT* will help the patient to understand and tolerate the possible flare-up in symptoms which may occur in the latter part of the off-steroid day. Other symptomatic therapy may be added or increased at this time if needed.

8) In the event of an acute flare-up of the disease process, it may be necessary to return to a full suppressive daily divided corticoid dose for control. Once control is again established alternate day therapy may be reinstituted.

9) Although many of the undesirable features of corticosteroid therapy can be minimized by *ADT*, as in any therapeutic situation, the physician must carefully weigh the benefit-risk ratio for each patient in whom corticoid therapy is being considered.

How Supplied:

Medrol Tablets (methylprednisolone) are available in the following strengths and sizes:

2 mg	Bottles of 100	*NDC 0009-0049-02*
4 mg	Bottles of 30	*NDC 0009-0056-01*
	Bottles of 100	*NDC 0009-0056-02*
	Bottles of 500	*NDC 0009-0056-03*
	Unit Dose Package (100)	*NDC 0009-0056-05*
	Dosepak™ Unit of use (21 tablets)	*NDC 0009-0056-04*
8 mg	Bottles of 25	*NDC 0009-0022-01*
16 mg	Bottles of 50	*NDC 0009-0073-01*
	ADT Pak® (14 tablets)	*NDC 0009-0073-02*
24 mg	Bottles of 25	*NDC 0009-0155-01*
32 mg	Bottles of 25	*NDC 0009-0176-01*

Code 810 487 105

[*Shown in Product Identification Section*]

MOTRIN® Tablets ℞ †
(ibuprofen tablets, USP)
400 mg, Unit Dose, 100's
NSN 6505-01-041-6911A (VA)
600 mg, Unit of Use, 90's
NSN 6505-01-135-9655 (VA)
600 mg, 500's
NSN 6505-01-098-0247A (VA)

Description: *Motrin* Tablets contain the active ingredient ibuprofen, which is (±)-2-(*p*-isobutylphenyl) propionic acid. Ibuprofen is a white powder with a melting point of 74–77°C and is very slightly soluble in water (<1 mg/ml) and readily soluble in organic solvents such as ethanol and acetone.

Motrin is a nonsteroidal anti-inflammatory agent. It is available in 300, 400 and 600 mg tablets for oral administration.

Clinical Pharmacology: *Motrin* Tablets contain ibuprofen which possesses analgesic and antipyretic activities. Its mode of action, like that of other nonsteroidal anti-inflammatory agents, is not completely understood, but may be related to prostaglandin synthetase inhibition. *Motrin* does not alter the course of the underlying disease.

In patients treated with *Motrin* for rheumatoid arthritis and osteoarthritis, the anti-inflammatory action of *Motrin* has been shown by reduction in joint swelling, reduction in pain, reduction in duration of morning stiffness, reduction in disease activity as assessed by both the investigator and patient; and by improved functional capacity as demonstrated by an increase in grip strength, a delay in the time to onset of fatigue, and a decrease in time to walk 50 feet.

In clinical studies in patients with rheumatoid arthritis and osteoarthritis, *Motrin* has been shown to be comparable to aspirin in controlling the aforementioned signs and symptoms of disease activity and to be associated with a statistically significant reduction in the milder gastrointestinal side effects (see ADVERSE REACTIONS). *Motrin* may be well tolerated in some patients who have had gastrointestinal side effects with aspirin, but these patients when treated with *Motrin* should be carefully followed for signs and symptoms of gastrointestinal ulceration and bleeding. Although it is not definitely known whether *Motrin* causes less peptic ulceration than aspirin, in one study involving 885 patients with rheumatoid arthritis treated for up to one year, there were no reports of gastric ulceration with *Motrin* whereas frank ulceration was reported in 13 patients in the aspirin group (statistically significant $p < .001$).

In clinical studies in patients with rheumatoid arthritis, *Motrin* has been shown to be comparable to indomethacin in controlling the aforementioned signs and symptoms of disease activity and to be associated with a statistically significant reduction of the milder gastrointestinal (see ADVERSE REACTIONS) and CNS side effects.

Motrin may be used in combination with gold salts and/or corticosteroids. When *Motrin* and placebo were compared in gold-treated rheumatoid arthritis patients, *Motrin* was consistently more effective in relieving symptoms than was placebo. However, it cannot be inferred that *Motrin* potentiates the effect of gold on the underlying disease. Whether or not *Motrin* can be used in conjunction with partially effective doses of corticosteroid for a "steroid-sparing" effect, and result in greater improvement, has not been adequately studied.

Controlled studies have demonstrated that *Motrin* is a more effective analgesic than propoxyphene for the relief of episiotomy pain, pain following dental extraction procedures, and for the relief of the symptoms of primary dysmenorrhea.

In patients with primary dysmenorrhea, *Motrin* has been shown to reduce elevated levels of prostaglandin activity in the menstrual fluid and to reduce resting and active intrauterine pressure, as well as the frequency of uterine contractions. The probable mechanism of action is to inhibit prostaglandin synthesis rather than simply to provide analgesia.

The ibuprofen in *Motrin* is rapidly absorbed when administered orally. Peak serum ibuprofen levels are generally attained one to two hours after administration. With single doses ranging from 200 mg to 800 mg, a linear dose-response relationship exists between amount of drug administered and the integrated area under the serum drug concentration vs time curve. Above 800 mg, however, the area under the curve increases less than proportional to increases in dose. There is no evidence of drug accumulation or enzyme induction.

The administration of *Motrin* Tablets either under fasting conditions or immediately before meals yields quite similar serum ibuprofen concentration-time profiles. When *Motrin* is administered immediately after a meal, there is a reduction in the rate of absorption but no appreciable decrease in the extent of absorption. The bioavailability of *Motrin* is minimally altered by the presence of food. A bioavailability study has shown that there was no interference with the absorption of *Motrin* when given in conjunction with an antacid containing both aluminum hydroxide and magnesium hydroxide.

Ibuprofen is rapidly metabolized and eliminated in the urine. The excretion of ibuprofen is virtually complete 24 hours after the last dose. The serum half-life is 1.8 to 2.0 hours. Studies have shown that following ingestion of the drug, 45% to 79% of the dose was recovered in the urine within 24 hours as metabolite A (25%), (+)-2-[p-(2hydroxymethylpropyl)-phenyl] propionic acid and metabolite B (37%), (+)-2-[p-(2carboxypropyl)-phenyl] propionic acid; the percentages of free and conjugated ibuprofen were approximately 1% and 14%, respectively.

Indications and Usage: *Motrin* Tablets (ibuprofen) are indicated for relief of the signs and symptoms of rheumatoid arthritis and osteoarthritis.

Motrin is indicated for relief of mild to moderate pain.

Motrin is also indicated for the treatment of primary dysmenorrhea.

Since there have been no controlled clinical trials to demonstrate whether or not there is any beneficial effect or harmful interaction with the use of *Motrin* in conjunction with aspirin, the combination cannot be recommended (see **Drug Interactions**).

Controlled clinical trials to establish the safety and effectiveness of *Motrin* in children have not been conducted.

Contraindications: *Motrin* Tablets (ibuprofen) should not be used in patients who have previously exhibited hypersensitivity to it, or in individuals with the syndrome of nasal polyps, angioedema and bronchospastic reactivity to aspirin or other nonsteroidal anti-inflammatory agents (see WARNINGS). Anaphylactoid reactions have occurred in such patients.

Warnings: Peptic ulceration and gastrointestinal bleeding, sometimes severe, have been reported in patients receiving *Motrin* Tablets (ibuprofen). Peptic ulceration, perforation, or severe gastrointestinal bleeding can have a fatal outcome, and although a few such reports have been received with *Motrin*, a cause and effect relationship has not been established.

Motrin should be given under close supervision to patients with a history of upper gastrointestinal tract disease, and only after consulting the ADVERSE REACTIONS section.

In patients with active peptic ulcer and active rheumatoid arthritis, attempts should be made to treat the arthritis with nonulcerogenic drugs, such as gold. If *Motrin* must be given, the patient should be under close supervision for signs of ulcer perforation or gastrointestinal bleeding.

As with other nonsteroidal anti-inflammatory agents, chronic studies in rats and monkeys have shown histologic evidence of mild renal toxicity as demonstrated by papillary edema and papillary necrosis in some animals. Renal papillary necrosis has been rarely reported in humans in association with *Motrin* treatment.

Precautions: Blurred and/or diminished vision, scotomata, and/or changes in color vision have been reported. If a patient develops such complaints while receiving *Motrin* Tablets (ibuprofen), the drug should be discontinued and the patient should have an ophthalmologic examination which includes central visual fields and color vision testing.

Fluid retention and edema have been reported in association with *Motrin*; therefore, the drug should be used with caution in patients with a history of cardiac decompensation or hypertension.

Since ibuprofen is eliminated primarily by the kidneys, patients with significantly impaired renal function should be closely monitored and a reduction in dosage should be anticipated to avoid drug accumulation. Prospective studies on the safety of *Motrin* in patients with chronic renal failure have not been conducted.

Motrin, like other nonsteroidal anti-inflammatory agents, can inhibit platelet aggregation but the effect is quantitatively less and of shorter duration than that seen with aspirin. *Motrin* has been shown to prolong bleeding time (but within the normal range) in normal subjects. Because this prolonged bleeding effect may be exaggerated in patients with underlying hemostatic defects, *Motrin* should be used with caution in persons with intrinsic coagulation defects and those on anticoagulant therapy.

Patients on *Motrin* should report to their physicians signs or symptoms of gastrointestinal ulceration or bleeding, blurred vision or other eye symptoms, skin rash, weight gain, or edema.

In order to avoid exacerbation of disease or adrenal insufficiency, patients who have been on prolonged corticosteroid therapy should have their therapy tapered slowly rather than discontinued abruptly when *Motrin* is added to the treatment program.

The antipyretic and anti-inflammatory activity of ibuprofen may reduce fever and inflammation, thus diminishing their utility as diagnostic signs in detecting complications of presumed noninfectious noninflammatory painful conditions.

As with other nonsteroidal anti-inflammatory drugs, borderline elevations of one or more liver tests may occur in up to 15% of patients. These abnormalities may progress, may remain essentially unchanged, or may be transient with continued therapy. The SGPT (ALT) test is probably the most sensitive indicator of liver dysfunction. Meaningful (3 times the upper limit of normal) elevations of SGPT or SGOT (AST) occurred in controlled clinical trials in less than 1% of patients. A patient with symptoms and/or signs suggesting liver dysfunction, or in whom an abnormal liver test has occurred, should be evaluated for evidence of the development of more severe hepatic reaction while on therapy with *Motrin*. Severe hepatic reactions, including jaundice and cases of fatal hepatitis, have been reported with ibuprofen as with other nonsteroidal anti-inflammatory drugs. Although such reactions are rare, if abnormal liver tests persist or worsen, if clinical signs and symptoms consistent with liver disease develop, or if systemic manifestations occur (e.g., eosinophilia, rash, etc.), *Motrin* should be discontinued.

Drug Interactions

Coumarin-type anticoagulants. Several short-term controlled studies failed to show that *Motrin* significantly affected prothrombin times or a variety of other clotting factors when administered to individuals on coumarin-type anticoagulants. However, because bleeding has been reported when *Motrin* and other nonsteroidal anti-inflammatory agents have been administered to patients on coumarin-type anticoagulants, the physician should be cautious when administering *Motrin* to patients on anticoagulants.

Aspirin. Animal studies show that aspirin given with nonsteroidal anti-inflammatory agents, including *Motrin*, yields a net decrease in anti-inflammatory activity with lowered blood levels of the non-aspirin drug. Single dose bioavailability studies in normal volunteers have failed to show an effect of aspirin on *Motrin* blood levels. Correlative clinical studies have not been done.

Pregnancy

Reproductive studies conducted in rats and rabbits at doses somewhat less than the maximal clinical dose did not demonstrate evidence of developmental abnormalities. However, animal reproduction studies are not always predictive of human response. As there are no adequate and well-controlled studies in pregnant women, this drug should be used during pregnancy only if clearly needed. Because of the known effects of nonsteroidal anti-inflammatory drugs on the fetal cardiovascular system (closure of ductus arteriosus), use during late pregnancy should be avoided. As with

Continued on next page

Upjohn—Cont.

other drugs known to inhibit prostaglandin synthesis, an increased incidence of dystocia and delayed parturition occurred in rats. Administration of *Motrin* is not recommended during pregnancy.

Nursing Mothers

In limited studies, an assay capable of detecting 1 mcg/ml did not demonstrate ibuprofen in the milk of lactating mothers. However, because of the limited nature of the studies, and the possible adverse effects of prostaglandin-inhibiting drugs on neonates, *Motrin* is not recommended for use in nursing mothers.

Adverse Reactions: The most frequent type of adverse reaction occurring with *Motrin* Tablets (ibuprofen) is gastrointestinal. In controlled clinical trials the percentage of patients reporting one or more gastrointestinal complaints ranged from 4% to 16%.

In controlled studies when *Motrin* was compared to aspirin and indomethacin in equally effective doses, the overall incidence of gastrointestinal complaints was about half that seen in either the aspirin- or indomethacin-treated patients.

Adverse reactions observed during controlled clinical trials at an incidence greater than 1% are listed in the following table. Those reactions listed in Column 1 encompass observations in approximately 3,000 patients. More than 500 of these patients were treated for periods of at least 54 weeks.

Still other reactions occurring less frequently than 1 in 100 were reported in controlled clinical trials and from marketing experience. These reactions have been divided into two categories: Column 2 of the following table lists reactions with therapy with *Motrin* where the probability of a causal relationship exists: for the reactions in Column 3, a causal relationship with *Motrin* has not been established.

[See table below].

Overdosage: Approximately 1½ hours after the reported ingestion of from 7 to 10 *Motrin* Tablets (ibuprofen) (400 mg), a 19-month old child weighing 12 kg was seen in the hospital emergency room, apneic and cyanotic, responding only to painful stimuli. This type of stimulus, however, was sufficient to induce respiration. Oxygen and parenteral fluids were given; a greenish-yellow fluid was aspirated from the stomach with no evidence to indicate the presence of *Motrin*. Two hours after ingestion the child's condition seemed stable; she still responded only to painful stimuli and continued to have periods of apnea lasting from 5 to 10 seconds. She was admitted to intensive care and sodium bicarbonate was administered as well as infusions of dextrose and normal saline. By four hours post-ingestion she could be aroused easily, sit by herself and respond to spoken commands. Blood level of ibuprofen was 102.9 μg/ml approximately 8½ hours after accidental ingestion. At 12 hours she appeared to be completely recovered.

In two other reported cases where children (each weighing approximately 10 kg) had taken six tablets for an estimated acute intake of approximately 120 mg/kg, there were no signs of acute intoxication or late sequelae. Blood level in one child 90 minutes after ingestion was 700 μg/ml—about 10 times the peak levels seen in absorption-excretion studies.

A 19-year old male who had taken 8,000 mg of *Motrin* Tablets over a period of a few hours complained of dizziness, and nystagmus was noted. After hospitalization, parenteral hydration and three days' bed rest, he recovered with no reported sequelae.

In cases of acute overdosage, the stomach should be emptied by vomiting or lavage, though little drug will likely be recovered if more than an hour has elapsed since ingestion. Because the drug is acidic and is excreted in the urine, it is theoretically beneficial to administer alkali and induce diuresis.

Dosage and Administration:

Do not exceed 2,400 mg total daily dose. If gastrointestinal complaints occur, administer *Motrin* Tablets (ibuprofen) with meals or milk.

Incidence Greater than 1% (but less than 3%) Probable Causal Relationship	Precise Incidence Unknown (but less than 1%) Probable Causal Relationship**	Precise Incidence Unknown (but less than 1%) Causal Relationship Unknown**
GASTROINTESTINAL Nausea*, epigastric pain*, heartburn*, diarrhea, abdominal distress, nausea and vomiting, indigestion, constipation, abdominal cramps or pain, fullness of GI tract (bloating and flatulence)	Gastric or duodenal ulcer with bleeding and/or perforation, gastrointestinal hemorrhage, melena, gastritis, hepatitis, jaundice, abnormal liver function tests	Pancreatitis
CENTRAL NERVOUS SYSTEM Dizziness*, headache, nervousness	Depression, insomnia, confusion, emotional lability, somnolence, aseptic meningitis with fever and coma	Paresthesias, hallucinations, dream abnormalities, pseudotumor cerebri
DERMATOLOGIC Rash* (including maculopapular type), pruritis	Vesiculobullous eruptions, urticaria, erythema multiforme, Stevens-Johnson syndrome, alopecia	Toxic epidermal necrolysis, photoallergic skin reactions
SPECIAL SENSES Tinnitus	Hearing loss, amblyopia (blurred and/or diminished vision, scotomata and/or changes in color vision) (see PRECAUTIONS)	Conjunctivitis, diplopia, optic neuritis, cataracts
HEMATOLOGIC	Neutropenia, agranulocytosis, aplastic anemia, hemolytic anemia (sometimes Coombs positive), thrombocytopenia with or without purpura, eosinophilia, decreases in hemoglobin and hematocrit	Bleeding episodes (eg epistaxis, menorrhagia)
METABOLIC/ENDOCRINE Decreased appetite		Gynecomastia, hypoglycemic reaction, acidosis
CARDIOVASCULAR Edema, fluid retention (generally responds promptly to drug discontinuation; see PRECAUTIONS)	Congestive heart failure in patients with marginal cardiac function, elevated blood pressure, palpitations	Arrhythmias (sinus tachycardia, sinus bradycardia)
ALLERGIC	Syndrome of abdominal pain, fever, chills, nausea and vomiting; anaphylaxis; bronchospasm (see CONTRAINDICATIONS)	Serum sickness, lupus erythematosus syndrome, Henoch-Schönlein vasculitis, angioedema
RENAL	Acute renal failure in patients with pre-existing significantly impaired renal function, decreased creatinine clearance, polyuria, azotemia, cystitis, hematuria	Renal papillary necrosis
MISCELLANEOUS	Dry eyes and mouth, gingival ulcer, rhinitis	

* Reactions occurring in 3% to 9% of patients treated with *Motrin*. (Those reactions occurring in less than 3% of the patients are unmarked).

** Reactions are classified under "*Probable Causal Relationship (PCR)*" if there has been one positive rechallenge or if three or more cases occur which might be causally related. Reactions are classified under "*Causal Relationship Unknown*" if seven or more events have been reported but the criteria for PCR have not been met.

Rheumatoid arthritis and osteoarthritis, including flare-ups of chronic disease:
Suggested Dosage: 300 mg, 400 mg, or 600 mg t.i.d. or q.i.d. The dose of *Motrin* Tablets (ibuprofen) should be tailored to each patient, and may be lowered or raised depending on the severity of symptoms either at time of initiating drug therapy or as the patient responds or fails to respond.
In general, patients with rheumatoid arthritis seem to require higher doses of *Motrin* than do patients with osteoarthritis.
The smallest dose of *Motrin* that yields acceptable control should be employed.
In chronic conditions, a therapeutic response to therapy with *Motrin* is sometimes seen in a few days to a week but most often is observed by two weeks. After a satisfactory response has been achieved, the patient's dose should be reviewed and adjusted as required.
Mild to moderate pain:
400 mg every 4 to 6 hours as necessary for relief of pain.
In controlled analgesic clinical trials, doses of *Motrin* greater than 400 mg were no more effective than the 400 mg dose.
Dysmenorrhea:
For the treatment of dysmenorrhea, beginning with the earliest onset of such pain, *Motrin* should be given in a dose of 400 mg every 4 hours as necessary for the relief of pain.
How Supplied:
Motrin Tablets (ibuprofen) are supplied as follows:
***Motrin* Tablets, 300 mg** (white)

Unit of Use Bottles of 60	NDC 0009-0733-01
Bottles of 500	NDC 0009-0733-02

***Motrin* Tablets, 400 mg** (orange)

Bottles of 500	NDC 0009-0750-02
Unit-dose package of 100	NDC 0009-0750-06
Unit of Use bottles of 100	NDC 0009-0750-25

***Motrin* Tablets, 600 mg** (peach)

Unit of Use Bottles of 60	NDC 0009-0742-01
Unit-dose package of 100	NDC 0009-0742-05
Bottles of 500	NDC 0009-0742-02
Unit of Use bottles of 100	NDC 0009-0742-03

Code 810 015 009
† Product of The Upjohn Manufacturing Company M.
Motrin is a registered trademark of The Upjohn Manufacturing Company M.
[*Shown in Product Identification Section*]

MYCIGUENT® Antibiotic Ointment
(See PDR For Nonprescription Drugs)

MYCITRACIN® Antibiotic Ointment
(See PDR For Nonprescription Drugs)

ORINASE® Tablets ℞
(tolbutamide tablets, USP)

Description: *Orinase* Tablets contain tolbutamide which is 1-butyl-3-(*p*-tolylsulfonyl) urea, which is a pure white crystalline compound practically insoluble in water but forming water soluble salts with alkalies. It has a molecular weight of 270.35; its molecular formula is $C_{12}H_{18}N_2O_3S$.
This is an oral antidiabetes agent which effectively restores blood sugar to normal ranges in selected diabetic patients. *Orinase* Tablets (tolbutamide) diminishes glycosuria and alleviates such symptoms as pruritus, polyuria, polydipsia, polyphagia. While most commonly used as the sole therapeutic agent in the management of mild to moderately severe adult-type diabetes, it has also been found of value as an adjuvant to insulin therapy in the stabilization of certain cases of labile diabetes. Such combination therapy not infrequently results in significant reduction of insulin requirement, greater freedom from threat of hypoglycemic reaction, and marked subjective improvement.
Mode of Action: Numerous studies have provided convincing evidence that the major, if not sole, mode of action of tolbutamide is that of stimulation of synthesis and release of endogenous insulin.
One factor relative to mechanism is conclusively established—that is, *Orinase Tablets (tolbutamide) will not lower blood sugar in the human subject who has no pancreatic beta cells.* Whether this agent has any significant effect after total pancreatectomy when insulin is being injected is still a moot question. If *Orinase* does exert an insulin sparing effect (and available data on this point are controversial), the mechanism of the action remains to be elucidated. It has been demonstrated that tolbutamide does not alter the rate at which labeled iodo-insulin disappears from the blood.
The Blood Sugar Lowering Effect: The blood sugar lowering effect is independent of the pituitary, adrenocortical, and neural mechanisms that exert a regulatory effect on carbohydrate metabolism. *Orinase* Tablets (tolbutamide) do not inhibit the hyperglycemic response induced by epinephrine or glucagon, and have no effect on the renal threshold for glucose excretion.
The administration of 3 grams of *Orinase* Tablets to either nondiabetics or tolbutamide-responsive diabetics will, in both instances, occasion a gradual lowering of blood sugar. Increasing the dose to 6 grams does not usually cause a response which is significantly different from that produced by a 3 gram dose. Nondiabetics show a very slight fall in blood sugar with the lowest level being reached four to five hours after dose administration. On the other hand, tolbutamide-responsive diabetics show a marked reduction of blood sugar to euglycemic levels. In these patients some decrease in blood sugar is discernible after the first hour and the nadir is seen 5 hours or more following administration. This difference between responsive diabetic and nondiabetic types of response has been emphasized in studies which employed specially prepared solutions of tolbutamide sodium. A summary of the results of these studies follows.
In nondiabetic human subjects—After the oral administration of a 3 gram dose of tolbutamide solution, healthy fasting adults usually exhibit a 30% or greater reduction in blood sugar within one hour, following which the blood sugar gradually returns to the fasting level over a period of 6 to 12 hours. With a 6 gram oral dose, the maximal fall in blood sugar is usually not significantly different from that produced by an oral dose of 3 grams. The hypoglycemic response after an oral dose of 50 mg per Kg of body weight is essentially the same as is induced by the intravenous injection of 0.1 unit of insulin per Kg of body weight.
In diabetic patients—Unlike the nondiabetic subject whose hypoglycemic response is maximal within the first hour after taking tolbutamide solution, the tolbutamide-responsive diabetic patient shows a gradually progressive blood sugar lowering effect, the maximal response being reached between 5 to 8 hours after ingestion of a single 3 gram dose; the blood sugar then rises gradually and by the 24th hour has usually returned to the pretest level. While the time of occurrence of the maximal reduction in blood sugar differs in the nondiabetic subject and the tolbutamide-responsive diabetic patient, the magnitude of the reduction, when expressed in terms of percent of the pretest blood sugar, tends to be similar. For example: in one study comparing the blood sugar lowering effect of *Orinase* (single oral dose of 50 mg per Kg of body weight) in 50 healthy adult subjects and 133 tolbutamide-responsive diabetic patients, the maximal decrease in blood sugar averaged 45.9 ± 1.8% for the normal group and 46.3 ± 1.5% for the diabetic group; the respective average mean decreases in blood sugar over the 5 hour observation period were 31.7 ± 1.4% for the normal subjects and 31.8 ± 1.2% for the diabetic patients.
Significance of the Molecular Structure: Tolbutamide is a sulfonamide but *not a sulfanilamide* derivative. While closely related to the so-called "sulfa" drugs, it differs in one important aspect. All "sulfa" drugs commonly used for treating infections have an amino group (either free or substituted) attached to the benzene ring at the *para* position. In tolbutamide, however, the amino group is replaced by a methyl group. This fundamental change in the molecular structure results in the following important characteristics of *Orinase* Tablets (tolbutamide).

1. It is devoid of chemotherapeutic effect; it *has no antibacterial activity.*
2. It cannot be measured in body fluids by the method of Bratton and Marshall.
3. It cannot be acetylated; the principal metabolite excreted in the urine is 1-butyl-3-*p*-carboxyphenylsulfonylurea.

Absorption, Degradation, and Excretion: When administered orally, *Orinase* Tablets (tolbutamide) are readily absorbed from the gastrointestinal tract. As it has no *p*-amino group, it cannot be acetylated, which is one of the common modes of metabolic degradation for the antibacterial sulfonamides. However, the presence of the *p*-methyl group renders tolbutamide susceptible to oxidation and this appears to be the principal manner of its metabolic degradation in man. The *p*-methyl group is oxidized to form a carboxyl group, converting tolbutamide into the totally inactive metabolite 1-butyl-3-*p*-carboxyphenylsulfonylurea, which can be recovered in the urine within 24 hours in amounts accounting for up to 75% of the administered dose.
Characteristics of the Metabolite:
Activity—The tolbutamide metabolite has no detectable pharmacologic effects. It has been administered orally in doses up to 6 grams and intravenously in doses up to 3 grams to normal and diabetic subjects and found devoid of hypoglycemic or other action. (When given intravenously, 71% of the 3 gram dose was excreted in the urine.)
Solubility—The tolbutamide metabolite is highly soluble over the critical acid range of urinary pH values, and its solubility increases with increase in pH. The measured solubility at pH 5 is 280 mg per 100 ml, increasing to 2000 mg per 100 ml at pH 5.5; at pH 6, by extrapolation, the solubility becomes 30,000 mg per 100 ml. Because of the marked solubility of the tolbutamide metabolite, crystalluria does not occur.
"Pseudo-albuminuria"—On very rare occasions, urine containing the tolbutamide metabolite may give a false-positive reaction for albumin by the usual test (acidification after boiling) since this procedure causes the metabolite to precipitate as flocculent particles. This problem may be circumvented by the use of bromphenol strips.
Information for modification of the sulfosalicylic acid and Esbach's tests will be supplied on request.
Indications: The principal clinical indication for *Orinase* Tablets (tolbutamide) is diabetes mellitus of the stable type without acute complications such as acidosis or ketosis. This form of diabetes has been variously described as relatively mild adult, maturity-onset, or nonketotic type.
In certain patients with labile diabetes, its use as a supplement to insulin therapy may effect stabilization of the diabetic condition and reduce insulin requirement.
Tolbutamide has been demonstrated to be exceptionally well tolerated. Certain patients removed from chlorpropamide therapy because of intolerance to usual therapeutic doses have subsequently been managed successfully on *Orinase.*

Continued on next page

Upjohn—Cont.

Selection of Patients: The basic requirement for therapy with *Orinase* Tablets (tolbutamide) is that the diabetes be adult or maturity-onset in character. The patient most likely to be responsive is one in whom the disease is relatively mild and stable and has developed sometime after the age of 30 years.

At present there is no reliable index whereby one may determine in advance the responsiveness of patients who qualify as candidates. History of an episode of diabetic coma does not necessarily disqualify a patient as a suitable candidate, but history of repeated episodes of acidosis or coma would serve as a contraindication. The only reliable method of determining responsiveness is therapeutic trial with *Orinase* for a period of at least 7 days. If the patient is already on insulin, it should be slowly withdrawn as response to *Orinase* is observed. If, during this trial period, there is absence of ketonuria plus a satisfactory reduction in blood sugar and glycosuria, the patient is responsive. The patient is considered nonresponsive if any of the following appear: ketonuria, increasing glycosuria, unsatisfactory lowering or persistent elevation of the blood sugar, or failure to obtain and hold clinical improvement.

Use in Early, Mild Diabetes: There is now considerable evidence, obtained from studies in animals and in patients with mild tolbutamide-responsive diabetes, that improvement in pancreatic beta cell function with consequent improvement in glucose tolerance occurs with prolonged administration of *Orinase* Tablets (tolbutamide). Therapy in the early, asymptomatic diabetic has produced normalization or improvement in glucose tolerance which has persisted up to 52 months. This improvement may occur after a few months of therapy, but in some instances improvement has taken place only after 10 to 14 months of continuous *Orinase* administration. Accordingly, in patients with mild, asymptomatic diabetes in whom glucose tolerance remains abnormal despite dietary therapy, it has been recommended that tolbutamide be administered in usual dosage over prolonged periods of time. Progress should be followed in these patients with glucose tolerance determinations at intervals of three to six months.

Although the long term effect of this therapy in the development of the complications of diabetes is unknown, as with other forms of antidiabetes therapy, it can reasonably be expected that improvement in the glucose tolerance or its restoration to normal may have a salutary effect on the course of the disease.

Contraindications: *Orinase* Tablets (tolbutamide) alone are not effective in juvenile or growth-onset diabetes nor in diabetes of the unstable, brittle type. Therefore, treatment of such cases requires the use of insulin, although *Orinase* may be used adjunctively when indicated.

Orinase should not be used in diabetes complicated by acidosis, ketosis, or coma; and in the presence of other acute complications such as fever, severe trauma, or infections, diabetics may require appropriate doses of insulin to insure continued control.

Orinase should not be used in patients with severe renal insufficiency.

Pregnancy Warning: The *safety* and the usefulness of *Orinase* Tablets (tolbutamide) during pregnancy have not been established at this time, either from the standpoint of the mother or the fetus. In animal studies, tolbutamide has been shown to have feticidal and teratogenic effects at doses of 1000 to 2500 mg per kg of body weight per day [Tuckmann-Duplessis, H., and Mercier-Parot, L., J. Ann. Diab. de l'Hotel Dieu (Paris) **3**:141-149, 1962; DeMeyer, R., 4e Congrèss de la Fédération Internationále du Diabète, Geneva 401-403, July 10-14, 1961; and Smithberg, M., Univ. of Minn. Med. Bull. **33**: 62-72, 1961]. It is not known at the present time whether or not this finding is applicable to human subjects. Clinical studies thus far are quite limited and experimental. Therefore, the use of *Orinase* is not recommended for the management of diabetes when complicated by *pregnancy.*

These facts should be borne in mind whenever the advisability of administering *Orinase* to women of the childbearing age is considered.

Precautions:

1. Those diagnostic and therapeutic measures which are necessary to insure optimal control of the diabetic state with insulin are equally necessary for control with tolbutamide.
2. The patient on *Orinase* Tablets (tolbutamide) must receive full and complete instructions about the nature of his disease, what he must do to prevent and detect complications, and how to control his condition.
3. He must understand that he cannot neglect his dietary restrictions, develop a careless attitude, or disregard instructions relative to body weight, exercise, personal hygiene, and avoidance of infection.
4. The patient must know how to recognize and counteract impending hypoglycemia.
5. The patient must know how and when to test for glycosuria and ketonuria.
6. During the trial period when insulin is being withdrawn, care should be taken to avoid ketosis, acidosis, and coma.
7. Caution should be observed in administering the thiazide-type diuretics to diabetic patients on therapy with *Orinase* because the thiazides have been reported to aggravate the diabetic state and to result in increased tolbutamide requirement, temporary loss of control, or even secondary failure. Response to tolbutamide is diminished in patients receiving therapy with *beta* blocking agents.
8. Very close observation and careful adjustment of dosage is mandatory in patients with impaired hepatic and/or renal function and in debilitated, malnourished or semistarved patients. In such patients severe hypoglycemia may occur and may require corrective therapy over a period of several days.
9. Tolbutamide is not an oral insulin nor a substitute for insulin. It has no blood sugar lowering effect in the absence of the pancreatic beta cells and must not be used as sole therapeutic agent in the juvenile type of diabetes.
10. Tolbutamide is of no value in diabetes complicated by acidosis and coma—here insulin is indispensable.
11. Care must be exercised in the presence of severe trauma, infection, or surgical procedures. In these circumstances it may be necessary, temporarily, to return the patient to insulin or to use insulin in addition to *Orinase.*
12. During the initial test period the patient should communicate with the physician daily, and for the first month report at least once weekly for physical examination and definitive evaluation of efficacy of diabetic control. After the first month, the patient should be examined at monthly intervals or as indicated.
13. The patient should be instructed to report immediately to his physician if he does not feel as well as usual.
14. For the protection of both patient and physician, uncooperative individuals should be considered unsuitable for treatment with this agent. Pharmacists should refill prescriptions only on the specific instruction of the physician.
15. As some diabetics are not suitable candidates for management with *Orinase,* it is essential that physicians familiarize themselves with the indications, limits of application, and the criteria for selection of patients for this therapy.
16. Patients must be under continuous medical supervision. Therapy with *Orinase* does not obviate the necessity for maintaining standard dietary regulation.

Adverse Reactions: Severe hypoglycemia, though uncommon, may occur in patients receiving *Orinase* Tablets (tolbutamide) and may mimic acute neurological disorders such as cerebral thrombosis. Certain factors, such as hepatic and renal disease, malnutrition, debility, advanced age, alcohol ingestion, and adrenal and pituitary insufficiency may predispose to hypoglycemia. Also, certain drugs may prolong or enhance the action of tolbutamide and thereby increase the risk of hypoglycemia. These include insulin, sulfonamides, oxyphenbutazone, salicylates, probenecid, monamine oxidase inhibitors, phenylbutazone, bishydroxycoumarin and phenyramidol.

Tolbutamide is mildly goitrogenic in animals in high doses, and in humans it has been reported to cause a reduction of RAI uptake after long term administration, without producing clinical hypothyroidism or thyroid enlargement.

Photosensitivity reactions and disulfiram-like reactions after ingestion of alcohol have been reported in patients taking tolbutamide.

Other untoward reactions are usually not of a serious nature and consist principally of gastrointestinal disturbances, headache, and variable allergic skin manifestations. The gastrointestinal disturbances (nausea, epigastric fullness, heartburn) and headache appear to be related to the size of the dose, and they frequently disappear when dosage is reduced to maintenance levels or the total daily dose is administered in divided portions after meals. The allergic skin manifestations (pruritus, erythema, and urticarial, morbilliform, or maculopapular eruptions) are transient reactions, which frequently disappear with continued drug administration. However, if the skin reactions persist, *Orinase* Tablets (tolbutamide) should be discontinued.

While early reports concerning the effect of sulfonylureas on body weight were inconsistent, recent reports have indicated that long-term use of *Orinase* per se has no appreciable effect in this respect.

Orinase appears to be remarkably free from gross clinical toxicity on the basis of experience accumulated during many years of clinical use. Crystalluria or other untoward effects on renal function have not been observed. Long term studies of hepatic function in human subjects and experience in over 1,000,000 diabetics have shown the incidence of tolbutamide-induced liver dysfunction to be remarkably low. Jaundice in association with the administration of tolbutamide has been rare and has cleared up readily upon discontinuance of the drug. Carcinoma of the pancreas or other extrahepatic biliary obstruction should be ruled out in instances of persistent jaundice.

Leukopenia, agranulocytosis, thrombocytopenia, hemolytic anemia, aplastic anemia, pancytopenia, hepatic porphyria and porphyria cutanea tarda have been reported.

Dosage and Administration: ***Institution of therapy and method of administration***—As with insulin therapy, there is no fixed dosage regimen for management of diabetes with *Orinase* Tablets (tolbutamide). There is no set dosage for beginning therapy in a candidate whether or not he is receiving insulin.

The average starting dose is 1 to 2 grams daily. This may be increased or decreased, depending on individual patient response. The ideal dose is the smallest amount which will maintain optimum control. This will vary considerably among patients and may be as little as 0.25

gram, particularly in elderly patients, or as much as 3 grams.
Generally, patients who do not respond to 2 grams will not respond to a higher dose; but, as with insulin therapy, dosage changes may be necessary during the course of management of a given case, and temporary increases over the 2 gram level may be required on occasion to maintain control. Maintenance dosage over 2 grams daily is seldom required.
The total daily dose may be taken either in the morning or in divided doses through the day. While either schedule is usually effective, the divided dose system is preferred by some clinicians from the standpoint of digestive tolerance (see **Adverse Reactions**). Occasionally, patients who initially respond are later found to have unsatisfactory control. This may be attributable to dietary indiscretion, emotional stress, secondary failure, or other factors. Often, temporary small increases in dosage restore control. A small percentage of patients may exhibit idiopathic loss of responsiveness after an extended period of good control. Such cases have been termed *secondary failures.*
Patients not receiving insulin—When *Orinase* is indicated, therapy is initiated as described above.
Patients receiving insulin—Patients requiring 20 units or less of insulin daily may be placed directly on *Orinase* and insulin abruptly discontinued. Patients whose insulin requirement is between 20 and 40 units daily may be started on therapy with *Orinase* with a concurrent 30 to 50% reduction in insulin dose, with further daily reduction of the insulin as response to tolbutamide is observed. In patients requiring more than 40 units of insulin daily, therapy with *Orinase* may be initiated in conjunction with a 20% reduction in insulin dose the first day, with further careful reduction of insulin as response is observed. During the withdrawal period the patient should test his urine for sugar and ketone bodies as frequently as three times daily and report the results to his physician daily. Occasionally, conversion to *Orinase* in the hospital may be advisable in candidates who required more than 40 units of insulin daily. If, during the trial period, ketosis or unsatisfactory blood or urine sugar control results, the patient should be returned to his former insulin therapy.
During the conversion period mild symptoms of hypoglycemia may occur on rare occasions. In these instances symptoms are readily corrected by administration of carbohydrate, and recurrences of hypoglycemic symptoms are avoided by more rapid withdrawal of insulin. Patients who develop ketosis, unsatisfactory lowering or persistent elevation of the blood sugar, or complications other than hypoglycemia within 24 hours after complete withdrawal of insulin should be withdrawn from tolbutamide and their former insulin therapy reinstituted. *The patient should be instructed as to the necessity of reporting to his physician immediately if any feeling of illness develops.*
Combination Therapy with Insulin: Although not universally accepted, use of *Orinase* Tablets (tolbutamide) as a supplement to insulin therapy in insulin-dependent diabetic patients with maturity-onset or growth-onset types of diabetes has been reported to decrease insulin requirements, provide easier regulation and stabilization of the diabetes, and afford an increased feeling of well being. Long term studies on this combined therapy show that the daily insulin requirement may be reduced from 10 to 70% in certain stable patients and from 10 to 50% in certain labile patients.
In insulin-resistant patients, use of the combination may be warranted in an effort to reduce the insulin requirement.
Acute Complications: During the course of intercurrent complications (e.g., ketoacidosis, severe trauma, major surgical procedures, infections, severe diarrhea, or nausea and vomiting) *supportive therapy with insulin may be necessary.* Depending upon the severity of the diabetes, the nature of the complication, and the availability of laboratory facilities, tolbutamide therapy may be continued or withdrawn while insulin is being used. Insulin is indispensable in the management of many acute complications, and all diabetics should be carefully instructed in its use.
How Supplied: *Orinase* Tablets (tolbutamide) are available in the following strengths and package sizes:
250 mg (scored, round, white)
Unit-of-Use bottles of 100 *NDC 0009-0701-01*
0.5 gram
Unit-of-Use bottles of 50 *NDC 0009-0100-01*
Unit-of-Use bottles of 100 *NDC 0009-0100-11*
Bottles of 200 *NDC 0009-0100-02*
Bottles of 500 *NDC 0009-0100-03*
Bottles of 1000 *NDC 0009-0100-05*
Unit Dose Package (100) *NDC 0009-0100-06*
Code 811 646 000
[*Shown in Product Identification Section*]

PAMINE® Tablets ℞
(methscopolamine bromide tablets, USP)

How Supplied: Each tablet contains 2.5 mg methscopolamine bromide.
Bottles of 100 *NDC 0009-0061-01*
Bottles of 500 *NDC 0009-0061-02*

PANMYCIN® Capsules ℞
(tetracycline hydrochloride capsules, USP)

How Supplied: Each capsule contains 250 mg tetracycline hydrochloride.
Bottles of 100 *NDC 0009-0782-01*
Bottles of 1000 *NDC 0009-0782-03*

PANMYCIN® Tablets ℞
(tetracycline hydrochloride tablets, USP)

How Supplied: Each tablet contains 500 mg tetracycline hydrochloride.
500 mg Bottles of 100 *NDC 0009-0310-01*

PROSTIN VR PEDIATRIC® ℞
Sterile Solution
(alprostadil)
500 micrograms per ml

WARNING
Apnea is experienced by about 10 to 12% of neonates with congenital heart defects treated with *Prostin VR Pediatric* Sterile Solution (alprostadil). Apnea is most often seen in neonates weighing less than 2 kg at birth and usually appears during the first hour of drug infusion. Therefore, respiratory status should be monitored throughout treatment, and *Prostin VR Pediatric* should be used where ventilatory assistance is immediately available.

Description: *Prostin VR Pediatric* Sterile Solution for intravascular infusion contains 500 micrograms alprostadil, more commonly known as prostaglandin E_1, in 1.0 ml dehydrated alcohol.
The chemical name for alprostadil is (11α, 13E, 15S)-11,15 dihydroxy-9-oxoprost-13-en-1-oic acid, and the molecular weight is 354.49.
Alprostadil is a white to off-white crystalline powder with a melting point between 110° and 116°C. Its solubility at 35°C is 8000 micrograms per 100 ml double distilled water.
Clinical Pharmacology: Alprostadil (prostaglandin E_1) is one of a family of naturally occurring acidic lipids with various pharmacologic effects. Vasodilation, inhibition of platelet aggregation, and stimulation of intestinal and uterine smooth muscle are among the most notable of these effects. Intravenous doses of 1 to 10 micrograms of alprostadil per kilogram of body weight lower the blood pressure in mammals by decreasing peripheral resistance. Reflex increases in cardiac output and rate accompany the reduction in blood pressure.
Smooth muscle of the ductus arteriosus is especially sensitive to alprostadil, and strips of lamp ductus markedly relax in the presence of the drug. In addition, administration of alprostadil reopened the closing ductus of newborn rats, rabbits, and lambs. These observations led to the investigation of alprostadil in infants who had congenital defects which restricted the pulmonary or systemic blood flow and who depended on a patent ductus arteriosus for adequate blood oxygenation and lower body perfusion.
In infants with restricted pulmonary blood flow, about 50% responded to alprostadil infusion with at least a 10 torr increase in blood pO_2 (mean increase about 14 torr and mean increase in oxygen saturation about 23%). In general, patients who responded best had low pretreatment blood pO_2 and were 4 days or less.
In infants with restricted systemic blood flow, alprostadil often increased pH in those having acidosis, increased systemic blood pressure, and decreased the ratio of pulmonary artery pressure to aortic pressure.
Alprostadil must be infused continuously because it is very rapidly metabolized. As much as 80% of the circulating alprostadil may be metabolized in one pass through the lungs, primarily by β- and ω-oxidation. The metabolites are excreted primarily by the kidney, and excretion is essentially complete within 24 hours after administration. No unchanged alprostadil has been found in the urine, and there is no evidence of tissue retention of alprostadil or its metabolites.
Indications and Usage: *Prostin VR Pediatric* Sterile Solution (alprostadil) is indicated for palliative, not definitive, therapy to temporarily maintain the patency of the ductus arteriosus until corrective or palliative surgery can be performed in neonates who have congenital heart defects and who depend upon the patent ductus for survival. Such congenital heart defects include pulmonary atresia, pulmonary stenosis, tricuspid atresia, tetralogy of Fallot, interruption of the aortic arch, coarctation of the aorta, or transposition of the great vessels with or without other defects.
In infants with restricted pulmonary blood flow, the increase in blood oxygenation is inversely proportional to pretreatment pO_2 values; that is, patients with low pO_2 values respond best, and patients with pO_2 values of 40 torr or more usually have little response.
Prostin VR Pediatric should be administered only by trained personnel in facilities that provide pediatric intensive care.
Contraindications: None.
Warnings: See WARNING box.
Note: *Prostin VR Pediatric* Sterile Solution (alprostadil) must be diluted before it is administered. See dilution instructions in DOSAGE AND ADMINISTRATION section.
Precautions:
General Precautions
Cortical proliferation of the long bones, first observed in dogs, has also been observed in infants during long-term infusions of alprostadil. The cortical proliferation in infants regressed after withdrawal of the drug.
Prostin VR Pediatric Sterile Solution (alprostadil) should be infused for the shortest time and at the lowest dose that will produce the desired effects. The risks of long-term infusion of *Prostin VR Pediatric* should be weighed against the possible benefits that critically ill infants may derive from its administration.
Because alprostadil inhibits platelet aggregation, use *Prostin VR Pediatric* cautiously in neonates with bleeding tendencies.

Continued on next page

Upjohn—Cont.

Prostin VR Pediatric should not be used in neonates with respiratory distress syndrome. A differential diagnosis should be made between respiratory distress syndrome (hyaline membrane disease) and cyanotic heart disease (restricted pulmonary blood flow). If full diagnostic facilities are not immediately available, cyanosis (pO_2 less than 40 torr) and restricted pulmonary blood flow apparent on an X-ray are appropriate indicators of congenital heart defects.

Necessary Monitoring: In all neonates, arterial pressure should be monitored intermittently by umbilical artery catheter, auscultation, or with a Doppler transducer. *Should arterial pressure fall significantly, decrease the rate of infusion immediately.*

In infants with restricted pulmonary blood flow, measure efficacy of *Prostin VR Pediatric* by monitoring improvement in blood oxygenation. In infants with restricted systemic blood flow, measure efficacy by monitoring improvement of systemic blood pressure and blood pH.

Drug Interactions: No drug interactions have been reported between *Prostin VR Pediatric* and the therapy standard in neonates with restricted pulmonary or systemic blood flow. Standard therapy includes antibiotics, such as penicillin and gentamicin; vasopressors, such as dopamine and isoproterenol; cardiac glycosides; and diuretics, such as furosemide.

Carcinogenesis, Mutagenesis, and Impairment of Fertility: Long-term carcinogenicity studies and fertility studies have not been done. The Ames and Alkaline Elution assays reveal no potential for mutagenesis.

Adverse Reactions:

Central Nervous System: *Apnea has been reported in about 12% of the neonates treated.* (See WARNING box.) Other common adverse reactions reported have been fever in about 14% of the patients treated and seizures in about 4%. The following reactions have been reported in less than 1% of the patients: cerebral bleeding, hyperextension of the neck, hyperirritability, hypothermia, jitteriness, lethargy, and stiffness.

Cardiovascular System: The most common adverse reactions reported have been flushing in about 10% of patients (more common after intraarterial dosing), bradycardia in about 7%, hypotension in about 4%, tachycardia in about 3%, cardiac arrest in about 1%, and edema in about 1%. The following reactions have been reported in less than 1% of the patients: congestive heart failure, hyperemia, second degree heart block, shock, spasm of the right ventricle infundibulum, supraventricular tachycardia, and ventricular fibrillation.

Respiratory System: The following reactions have been reported in less than 1% of the patients: bradypnea, bronchial wheezing, hypercapnia, respiratory depression, respiratory distress, and tachypnea.

Gastrointestinal System: The most common adverse reaction reported has been diarrhea in about 2% of the patients. The following reactions have been reported in less than 1% of the patients; gastric regurgitation, and hyperbilirubinemia.

Hematologic System: The most common hematologic event reported has been disseminated intravascular coagulation in about 1% of the patients. The following events have been reported in less than 1% of the patients: anemia, bleeding, and thrombocytopenia.

Excretory System: Anuria and hematuria have been reported in less than 1% of the patients.

Skeletal System: Cortical proliferation of the long bones has been reported. See PRECAUTIONS.

Miscellaneous: Sepsis has been reported in about 2% of the patients. Peritonitis has been reported in less than 1% of the patients. Hypokalemia has been reported in about 1%, and hypoglycemia and hyperkalemia have been reported in less than 1% of the patients.

Overdosage: Apnea, bradycardia, pyrexia, hypotension, and flushing may be signs of drug overdosage. If apnea or bradycardia occurs, discontinue the infusion, and provide appropriate medical treatment. Caution should be used in restarting the infusion. If pyrexia or hypotension occurs, reduce the infusion rate until these symptoms subside. Flushing is usually a result of incorrect intraarterial catheter placement, and the catheter should be repositioned.

Dosage and Administration: The preferred route of administration for *Prostin VR Pediatric* Sterile Solution (alprostadil) is continuous intravenous infusion into a large vein. Alternatively, *Prostin VR Pediatric* may be administered through an umbilical artery catheter placed at the ductal opening. Increases in blood pO_2 (torr) have been the same in neonates who received the drug by either route of administration.

Begin infusion with 0.1 micrograms alprostadil per kilogram of body weight per minute. After a therapeutic response is achieved (increased pO_2 in infants with restricted pulmonary blood flow or increased systemic blood pressure and blood pH in infants with restricted systemic blood flow), reduce the infusion rate to provide the lowest possible dosage that maintains the response. This may be accomplished by reducing the dosage from 0.1 to 0.05 to 0.025 to 0.01 micrograms per kilogram of body weight per minute. If response to 0.1 micrograms per kilogram of body weight per minute is inadequate, dosage can be increased up to 0.4 micrograms per kilogram of body weight per minute although, in general, higher infusion rates do not produce greater effects.

Dilution instructions: To prepare infusion solutions, dilute 1 ml of *Prostin VR Pediatric* Sterile Solution with Sodium Chloride Injection USP or Dextrose Injection USP. Dilute to volumes appropriate for the pump delivery system available. Prepare fresh infusion solutions every 24 hours. *Discard any solution more than 24 hours old.*

Sample Dilutions and Infusion Rates to Provide a Dosage of 0.1 Micrograms per Kilogram of Body Weight per Minute

Add 1 ampoule (500 micrograms) alprostadil to:	Approximate concentration of resulting solution (micrograms/ml)	Infusion rate (ml/min per kg of body weight)
250 ml	2	0.05
100 ml	5	0.02
50 ml	10	0.01
25 ml	20	0.005

Example: To provide 0.1 micrograms/kilogram of body weight per minute to an infant weighing 2.8 kilograms using a solution of 1 ampoule *Prostin VR Pediatric* in 100 ml of saline or dextrose: INFUSION RATE = 0.02 ml/min per kg × 2.8 kg = 0.056 ml/min or 3.36 ml/hr.

How Supplied: *Prostin VR Pediatric* Sterile Solution (alprostadil) is available in packages of 5—1 ml ampoules (NDC 0009-3169-01). Each ml contains 500 micrograms alprostadil in dehydrated alcohol.

Store *Prostin VR Pediatric* Sterile Solution in a refrigerator at 2°-8°C (36°-46°F).

Code 811 987 000

PROTAMINE SULFATE FOR INJECTION, USP ℞

Sterile Powder

50 mg, 250 mg

Description: Protamines are simple proteins of low molecular weight, rich in arginine and strongly basic. They occur in the sperm of salmon, and certain other species of fish.

Protamine Sulfate for Injection is available as a sterile freeze-dried preparation in two sizes: vials containing **50** mg of protamine sulfate and 45 mg of sodium chloride and vials containing **250** mg of protamine sulfate and 225 mg of sodium chloride. When reconstituted as directed, the solution contains 10 mg of protamine sulfate per ml.

When necessary pH was adjusted with sodium hydroxide and/or hydrochloric acid to conform to the USP specified range of 6.5 to 7.5.

Actions: The strongly basic nature of protamines accounts for their antiheparin effect. Protamine combines with the strongly acidic heparin to form a stable salt with the loss of anticoagulant activity. Protamine itself has an anticoagulant effect.

Indications: Antidote to heparin overdosage.

Warnings: Hyperheparinemia or bleeding has been reported in experimental animals and in some patients from 30 minutes to 18 hours after cardiac surgery (under cardiopulmonary bypass). The bleeding occurred in spite of complete neutralization of heparin with protamine sulfate after surgery. Therefore, the patient should be kept under close observation after cardiac surgery. If indicated by coagulation studies, eg, the heparin titration test with protamine and the determination of plasma thrombin time, additional doses of protamine sulfate should be given.

When protamine sulfate is administered, it should be given slowly (in 1 to 3 minutes), intravenously, in doses not exceeding 50 mg in any 10-minute period; facilities to treat shock should be available.

Reproduction studies have not been performed in animals. There is no adequate information on whether this drug may affect fertility in human males or females or have a teratogenic potential or other adverse effect on the fetus.

Precautions: Because of the anticoagulant effect of protamine, it is unwise to give more than 100 mg over a short period unless there is certain knowledge of a larger requirement.

Protamine sulfate can be inactivated by blood, and when it is used to neutralize large doses of heparin, a heparin "rebound" may be encountered. This complication is treated by additional protamine injections as needed.

Hypersensitivity reactions have been reported in patients with a history of allergy to fish. However, no definitive relationship has been established between allergic reactions to protamine sulfate and fish allergy.

Adverse Reactions: Intravenous injections of protamine may cause a sudden fall in blood pressure, bradycardia, dyspnea, or transitory flushing and a feeling of warmth. Anaphylaxis resulting in respiratory embarrassment has been reported with protamine (see PRECAUTIONS). Because fatal reactions, often resembling anaphylaxis, have been reported after administration of protamine sulfate, the drug should be given only when resuscitation techniques and treatment of anaphylactoid shock are readily available.

Dosage and Administration: Protamine sulfate is for intravenous administration only. It should be given intravenously **very slowly**—no more than 50 mg in any 10-minute period. Each mg of protamine sulfate neutralizes approximately 90 USP Units of heparin of beef lung origin or 115 USP Units of heparin derived from intestinal mucosa. After the intravenous administration of heparin, the quantity of protamine required decreases rapidly with the time elapsed after heparin injection.

Thirty minutes after a dose of heparin, the dose of protamine required for neutralization will be approximately half that required immediately after the heparin injection. Blood or plasma transfusions may also be necessary; these dilute but do not neutralize heparin. The dosage of protamine sulfate should be guided by blood coagulation studies (See Warnings).

Preparation of Solution—To prepare solution, aseptically add 5 ml of Bacteriostatic Water for Injection with Benzyl Alcohol to the vial of Protamine Sulfate for Injection **50** mg or 25 ml of the same diluent to the vial of Sterile Protamine for Injection **250** mg. Shake vial vigorously to effect complete solution. Each ml of the prepared solution will contain 10 mg of protamine sulfate. Protamine sulfate should not be mixed with other drugs without knowledge of compatibility, since protamine sulfate has been shown to be incompatible with certain antibiotics, including several of the cephalosporins and penicillins. Solutions of protamine sulfate may be kept for 24 hours if stored in a refrigerator. However, the usual precautions to maintain sterility of prepared solutions should be observed.

Storage Conditions: Store unreconstituted product at controlled room temperature 15°–30° C (59°–86° F). The reconstituted solution should be stored in a refrigerator and used within 24 hours.

How Supplied: Protamine Sulfate for Injection Sterile Powder is available in a dry stable form in rubber-capped vials, each vial containing either **50** mg protamine sulfate and 45 mg sodium chloride or **250** mg protamine sulfate and 225 mg sodium chloride. Sodium hydroxide and/or hydrochloric acid were added when necessary to adjust the pH.

Caution: The **250** mg package provides a total dose five times that in the **50** mg size and is intended only for single dose use. It is designed only for antiheparin treatment in certain instances where large doses of heparin have been given during surgery and large doses of protamine sulfate are required for neutralization after the surgical procedure.

50 mg NDC 0009-0811-03
250 mg NDC 0009-0852-01
Code 811 589 001

PROVERA® Tablets ℞
(medroxyprogesterone acetate tablets, USP)
10 mg
10s (unit of use)
NSN 6505-01-071-5605 (VA)
100s (bottle)
NSN 6505-00-890-1355 (M)

WARNING:

THE USE OF PROGESTATIONAL AGENTS DURING THE FIRST FOUR MONTHS OF PREGNANCY IS NOT RECOMMENDED

Progestational agents have been used beginning with the first trimester of pregnancy in an attempt to prevent habitual abortion or treat threatened abortion. There is no adequate evidence that such use is effective and there is evidence of potential harm to the fetus when such drugs are given during the first four months of pregnancy. Furthermore, in the vast majority of women, the cause of abortion is a defective ovum, which progestational agents could not be expected to influence. In addition, the use of progestational agents with their uterine-relaxant properties, in patients with fertilized defective ova may cause a delay in spontaneous abortion. Therefore, the use of such drugs during the first four months of pregnancy is not recommended.

Several reports suggest an association between intrauterine exposure to female sex hormones and congenital anomalies, including congenital heart defects and limb reduction defects[1–5]. One study[4] estimated a 4.7-fold increased risk of limb reduction defects in infants exposed in utero to sex hormones (oral contraceptives, hormone withdrawal tests for pregnancy, or attempted treatment for threatened abortion). Some of these exposures were very short and involved only a few days of treatment. The data suggest that the risk of limb reduction defects in exposed fetuses is somewhat less than 1 in 1,000.

If the patient is exposed to *Provera* Tablets (medroxyprogesterone acetate) during the first four months of pregnancy or if she becomes pregnant while taking this drug, she should be apprised of the potential risks to the fetus.

Description: *Provera* Tablets contain medroxyprogesterone acetate, which is a derivative of progesterone. It is a white to off-white, odorless crystalline powder, stable in air, melting between 200 and 210° C. It is freely soluble in chloroform, soluble in acetone and in dioxane, sparingly soluble in alcohol and in methanol, slightly soluble in ether, and insoluble in water.

The chemical name for medroxyprogesterone acetate is Pregn-4-ene-3,20-dione, 17-(acetyloxy)-6-methyl-, (6α)-.

Provera Tablets are available in two strengths, each tablet containing either 2.5 or 10 mg medroxyprogesterone acetate.

Actions: Medroxyprogesterone acetate, administered orally or parenterally in the recommended doses to women with adequate endogenous estrogen, transforms proliferative into secretory endometrium. Androgenic and anabolic effects have been noted, but the drug is apparently devoid of significant estrogenic activity. While parenterally administered medroxyprogesterone acetate inhibits gonadotropin production, which in turn prevents follicular maturation and ovulation, available data indicate that this does not occur when the usually recommended oral dosage is given as single daily doses.

Indications: Secondary amenorrhea; abnormal uterine bleeding due to hormonal imbalance in the absence of organic pathology, such as fibroids or uterine cancer.

Contraindications:

1. Thrombophlebitis, thromboembolic disorders, cerebral apoplexy or patients with a past history of these conditions.
2. Liver dysfunction or disease.
3. Known or suspected malignancy of breast or genital organs.
4. Undiagnosed vaginal bleeding.
5. Missed abortion.
6. As a diagnostic test for pregnancy.
7. Known sensitivity to *Provera* (medroxyprogesterone acetate).

Warnings:

1. The physician should be alert to the earliest manifestations of thrombotic disorders (thrombophlebitis, cerebrovascular disorders, pulmonary embolism, and retinal thrombosis). Should any of these occur or be suspected, the drug should be discontinued immediately.
2. Beagle dogs treated with medroxyprogesterone acetate developed mammary nodules some of which were malignant. Although nodules occasionally appeared in control animals, they were intermittent in nature, whereas the nodules in the drug-treated animals were larger, more numerous, persistent, and there were some breast malignancies with metastases. Their significance with respect to humans has not been established.
3. Discontinue medication pending examination if there is sudden partial or complete loss of vision, or if there is a sudden onset of proptosis, diplopia or migraine. If examination reveals papilledema or retinal vascular lesions, medication should be withdrawn.
4. Detectable amounts of progestin have been identified in the milk of mothers receiving the drug. The effect of this on the nursing infant has not been determined.
5. Usage in pregnancy is not recommended (See WARNING Box).
6. Retrospective studies of morbidity and mortality in Great Britain and studies of morbidity in the United States have shown a statistically significant association between thrombophlebitis, pulmonary embolism, and cerebral thrombosis and embolism and the use of oral contraceptives.[6–9] The estimate of the relative risk of thromboembolism in the study by Vessey and Doll[8] was about sevenfold, while Sartwell and associates[9] in the United States found a relative risk of 4.4, meaning that the users are several times as likely to undergo thromboembolic disease without evident cause as nonusers. The American study also indicated that the risk did not persist after discontinuation of administration, and that it was not enhanced by long continued administration. The American study was not designed to evaluate a difference between products.

Precautions:

1. The pretreatment physical examination should include special reference to breast and pelvic organs, as well as Papanicolaou smear.
2. Because progestogens may cause some degree of fluid retention, conditions which might be influenced by this factor, such as epilepsy, migraine, asthma, cardiac or renal dysfunction, require careful observation.
3. In cases of breakthrough bleeding, as in all cases of irregular bleeding per vaginum, nonfunctional causes should be borne in mind. In cases of undiagnosed vaginal bleeding, adequate diagnostic measures are indicated.
4. Patients who have a history of psychic depression should be carefully observed and the drug discontinued if the depression recurs to a serious degree.
5. Any possible influence of prolonged progestin therapy on pituitary, ovarian, adrenal, hepatic or uterine functions awaits further study.
6. A decrease in glucose tolerance has been observed in a small percentage of patients on estrogen-progestin combination drugs. The mechanism of this decrease is obscure. For this reason, diabetic patients should be carefully observed while receiving progestin therapy.
7. The age of the patient constitutes no absolute limiting factor although treatment with progestins may mask the onset of the climacteric.
8. The pathologist should be advised of progestin therapy when relevant specimens are submitted.
9. Because of the occasional occurrence of thrombotic disorders, (thrombophlebitis, pulmonary embolism, retinal thrombosis, and cerebrovascular disorders) in patients taking estrogen-progestin combinations and since the mechanism is obscure, the physician should be alert to the earliest manifestations of these disorders.

Information for the Patient

See Patient Information at the end of insert.

Adverse Reactions:

Pregnancy—(See WARNING Box for possible adverse effects on the fetus)

Breast—Breast tenderness or galactorrhea has been reported rarely.

Skin—Sensitivity reactions consisting of urticaria, pruritus, edema and generalized rash have occurred in an occasional patient. Acne, alopecia and hirsutism have been reported in a few cases.

Continued on next page

Upjohn—Cont.

Thromboembolic Phenomena—Thromboembolic phenomena including thrombophlebitis and pulmonary embolism have been reported.
The following adverse reactions have been observed in women taking progestins including *Provera* Tablets (medroxyprogesterone acetate):

breakthrough bleeding
spotting
change in menstrual flow
amenorrhea
edema
change in weight
(increase or decrease)
changes in cervical erosion
and cervical secretions
cholestatic jaundice
rash (allergic) with and
without pruritus
mental depression

A statistically significant association has been demonstrated between use of estrogen-progestin combination drugs and the following serious adverse reactions: thrombophlebitis; pulmonary embolism and cerebral thrombosis and embolism. For this reason patients on progestin therapy should be carefully observed.
Although available evidence is suggestive of an association, such a relationship has been neither confirmed nor refuted for the following serious adverse reactions:

neuro-ocular lesions, eg, retinal thrombosis
and optic neuritis.

The following adverse reactions have been observed in patients receiving estrogen-progestin combination drugs:

rise in blood pressure in susceptible individuals
premenstrual-like syndrome
changes in libido
changes in appetite
cystitis-like syndrome
headache
nervousness
dizziness
fatigue
backache
hirsutism
loss of scalp hair
erythema multiforme
erythema nodosum
hemorrhagic eruption
itching

In view of these observations, patients on progestin therapy should be carefully observed.
The following laboratory results may be altered by the use of estrogen-progestin combination drugs:
Increased sulfobromophthalein retention and other hepatic function tests.
Coagulation tests: increase in prothrombin factors VII, VIII, IX and X.
Metyrapone test.
Pregnanediol determination.
Thyroid function: increase in PBI, and butanol extractable protein bound iodine and decrease in T^3 uptake values.

Dosage and Administration:
Secondary Amenorrhea—*Provera* Tablets (medroxyprogesterone acetate) may be given in dosages of 5 to 10 mg daily for from 5 to 10 days. A dose for inducing an optimum secretory transformation of an endometrium that has been adequately primed with either endogenous or exogenous estrogen is 10 mg of *Provera* daily for 10 days. In cases of secondary amenorrhea, therapy may be started at any time. Progestin withdrawal bleeding usually occurs within three to seven days after discontinuing therapy with *Provera.*
Abnormal Uterine Bleeding Due to Hormonal Imbalance in the Absence of Organic Pathology—Beginning on the calculated 16th or 21st day of the menstrual cycle, 5 to 10 mg of *Provera* Tablets may be given daily for from 5 to 10 days. To produce an optimum secretory transformation of an endometrium that has been adequately primed with either endogenous or exogenous estrogen, 10 mg of *Provera* Tablets daily for 10 days beginning on the 16th day of the cycle is suggested. Progestin withdrawal bleeding usually occurs within three to seven days after discontinuing *Provera* therapy. Patients with a past history of recurrent episodes of abnormal uterine bleeding may benefit from planned menstrual cycling with *Provera.*

How Supplied: *Provera* Tablets (medroxyprogesterone acetate) are available in two strengths:

2.5 mg	—bottles of 25.	NDC 0009-0064-01
10 mg	—bottles of 25.	NDC 0009-0050-01
	bottles of 100.	NDC 0009-0050-02
Dosepak™	Unit-of-Use of 10	NDC 0009-0050-08

References:

1. Gal I, Kirman B, Stern J: Hormonal pregnancy tests and congenital malformation. Nature *216*:83, 1967.
2. Levy EP, Cohen A, Fraser FC: Hormone treatment during pregnancy and congenital heart defects. Lancet *1*:611, 1973.
3. Nora JJ, Nora AH: Birth defects and oral contraceptives. Lancet *1*:941–942, 1973.
4. Janerich DT, Piper JM, Glebatis DM: Oral contraceptives and congenital limb-reduction defects. N Engl J Med *291*:697–700, 1974.
5. Heinonen OP, Slone D, Monson RR, et al: Cardiovascular birth defects and antenatal exposure to female sex hormones. N Engl J Med *296*:67–70, 1977.
6. Royal College of General Practitioners: Oral contraception and thromboembolic disease. J Coll Gen Pract *13*:267–279, 1967.
7. Inman WHW, Vessey MP: Investigation of deaths from pulmonary, coronary, and cerebral thrombosis and embolism in women of child-bearing age. Br Med J *2*:193–199, 1968.
8. Vessey MP, Doll R: Investigation of relation between use of oral contraceptives and thromboembolic disease. A further report. Br Med J *2*:651–657, 1969.
9. Sartwell PE, Masi AT, Arthes FG, et al: Thromboembolism and oral contraceptives: An epidemiological case-control study. Am J Epidemiol *90*:365–380, 1969.

The text of the patient insert for progesterone and progesterone-like drugs is set forth below.
Patient Information: *Provera* Tablets contain a progesterone (medroxyprogesterone acetate). The information below is that which the U.S. Food and Drug Administration requires be provided for all patients taking progesterones. The information below relates only to the risk to the unborn child associated with use of progesterone during pregnancy. For further information on the use, side effects and other risks associated with this product, ask your doctor.

WARNING FOR WOMEN
There is an increased risk of birth defects in children whose mothers take this drug during the first four months of pregnancy.
Medroxyprogesterone acetate is similar to the progesterone hormones naturally produced by the body. Progesterone and progesterone-like drugs are used to treat menstrual disorders, to test if the body is producing certain hormones, and to treat some forms of cancer in women. They have been used as a test for pregnancy but such use is no longer considered safe because of possible damage to a developing baby. Also, more rapid methods for testing for pregnancy are now available.
These drugs have also been used to prevent miscarriage in the first few months of pregnancy. No adequate evidence is available to show that they are effective for this purpose. Furthermore, most cases of early miscarriage are due to causes which could not be helped by these drugs.
There is an increased risk of birth defects, such as heart or limb defects if progesterone and progesterone-like drugs are taken during the first four months of pregnancy. The exact risk of taking this drug early in pregnancy and having a baby with a birth defect is not known. However, one study found that babies born to women who had taken sex hormones (such as progesterone-like drugs) during the first three months of pregnancy were 4 to 5 times more likely to have abnormalities of the arms or legs than if their mothers had not taken such drugs. Some of these women had taken these drugs for only a few days. The chance that an infant whose mother had taken this drug will have this type of defect is about 1 in 1,000.
If you take *Provera* Tablets and later find you were pregnant when you took it, be sure to discuss this with your doctor as soon as possible.
Code NPA
[*Shown in Product Identification Section*]

PYRROXATE® Capsules
(See PDR For Nonprescription Drugs)

SIGTAB® Tablets

Composition: Each tablet contains:

Vitamin A	5000 IU
Vitamin D	400 IU
Vitamin E	15 IU
Vitamin C	333 mg
Folic Acid	0.4 mg
Thiamine	10.3 mg
Riboflavin	10 mg
Niacin	100 mg
Vitamin B_6	6 mg
Vitamin B_{12}	18 mcg
Pantothenic Acid	20 mg

How Supplied: Coated compressed tablets in the following sizes:

Bottles of 30	*NDC 0009-0461-01*
Bottles of 90	*NDC 0009-0461-02*
Bottles of 500	*NDC 0009-0461-03*

SOLU-B® Sterile Powder ℞
Sterile Injectable B Vitamins

Composition: Each 2 ml (when mixed) contains:

Thiamine Hydrochloride	10 mg
Riboflavin	10 mg
Pyridoxine Hydrochloride	5 mg
Calcium Pantothenate	50 mg
Niacinamide	250 mg
Also	
Methylparaben	2.56 mg
Propylparaben	0.294 mg

added as preservatives
How Supplied: Available in a 2 ml *Mix-O-Vial*® Two-Compartment Vial (5 pack)
NDC 0009-0863-02

SOLU-B® with Ascorbic Acid ℞
Sterile Powder
Sterile Injectable B and C Vitamins
***Mix-O-Vial* with Transfer Needle**
NSN 6505-00-122-3851A (VA)

Composition: Each 5 ml (when mixed) contains:

Thiamine Hydrochloride	10 mg
Riboflavin (as riboflavin and 5′-phosphate sodium)	10 mg
Niacinamide	250 mg
Pyridoxine Hydrochloride	5 mg
Sodium Pantothenate	50 mg
Ascorbic Acid	500 mg
also	
Methylparaben	6.53 mg
Propylparaben	0.752 mg

added as preservatives
When necessary, pH was adjusted with hydrochloric acid and/or sodium hydroxide.
How Supplied: Available in a 5 ml *Mix-O Vial*® Two-Compartment Vial with transfer needle.
NDC 0009-0606-01

SOLU–CORTEF® Sterile Powder ℞
(hydrocortisone sodium succinate for injection, USP)
For Intravenous or Intramuscular Administration

100 mg *Mix-O-Vial®*:
NSN 6505-00-753-9609A (M & VA)
250 mg *Mix-O-Vial*:
NSN 6505-00-951-5533A (M & VA)
500 mg *Mix-O-Vial*:
NSN 6505-00-116-5055A (VA)
1000 mg *Mix-O-Vial*:
NSN 6505-00-238-5222A (VA)

Description: *Solu-Cortef* Sterile Powder contains hydrocortisone sodium succinate as the active ingredient. Hydrocortisone sodium succinate is a white or nearly white, odorless, hygroscopic amorphous solid. It is very soluble in water and in alcohol, very slightly soluble in acetone and insoluble in chloroform. The chemical name is pregn-4-ene-3,20-dione,21-(3-carboxy-1-oxopropoxy)-11,17-dihydroxy-, monosodium salt, (11β)-and its molecular weight is 484.52.

Hydrocortisone sodium succinate is an anti-inflammatory adrenocortical steroid. This highly water-soluble sodium succinate ester of hydrocortisone permits the immediate intravenous administration of high doses of hydrocortisone in a small volume of diluent and is particularly useful where high blood levels of hydrocortisone are required rapidly.

Solu-Cortef Sterile Powder (hydrocortisone sodium succinate) is available in several packages for intravenous or intramuscular administration.

100 mg Plain—Vials containing hydrocortisone sodium succinate equivalent to 100 mg hydrocortisone, also 0.8 mg sodium biphosphate anhydrous, 8.73 mg dried sodium phosphate.

[See table above].

	100 mg *Mix-O-Vial* Each 2 ml contains: (when mixed)	250 mg *Mix-O-Vial* Each 2 ml contains: (when mixed)	500 mg *Mix-O-Vial* Each 4 ml contains: (when mixed)	1000 mg *Mix-O-Vial* Each 8 ml contains: (when mixed)
Hydrocortisone sodium succinate	equiv. to 100 mg hydrocortisone	equiv. to 250 mg hydrocortisone	equiv. to 500 mg hydrocortisone	equiv. to 1000 mg hydrocortisone
Sodium biphosphate anhydrous	0.8 mg	2 mg	4 mg	8 mg
Dried sodium phosphate	8.76 mg	21.8 mg	44 mg	88 mg
Benzyl alcohol added as preservative	18.1 mg	16.4 mg	33.4 mg	66.9 mg

When necessary, the pH of each formula was adjusted with sodium hydroxide so that the pH of the reconstituted solution is within the USP specified range of 7 to 8.

Actions: Hydrocortisone sodium succinate has the same metabolic and anti-inflammatory actions as hydrocortisone. When given parenterally and in equimolar quantities, the two compounds are equivalent in biologic activity. Following the intravenous injection of hydrocortisone sodium succinate, demonstrable effects are evident within one hour and persist for a variable period. Excretion of the administered dose is nearly complete within 12 hours. Thus, if constantly high blood levels are required, injections should be made every 4 to 6 hours. This preparation is also rapidly absorbed when administered intramuscularly and is excreted in a pattern similar to that observed after intravenous injection.

Indications: When oral therapy is not feasible, and the strength, dosage form and route of administration of the drug reasonably lend the preparation to the treatment of the condition, *Solu-Cortef* Sterile Powder (hydrocortisone sodium succinate) is indicated for intravenous or intramuscular use in the following conditions:

1. **Endocrine Disorders**
   Primary or secondary adrenocortical insufficiency (hydrocortisone or cortisone is the drug of choice; synthetic analogs may be used in conjunction with mineralocorticoids where applicable; in infancy, mineralocorticord supplementation is of particular importance)
   Acute adrenocortical insufficiency (hydrocortisone or cortisone is the drug of choice; mineralocorticoid supplementation may be necessary, particularly when synthetic analogs are used)
   Preoperatively and in the event of serious trauma or illness, in patients with known adrenal insufficiency or when adrenocortical reserve is doubtful
   Shock unresponsive to conventional therapy if adrenocortical insufficiency exists or is suspected
   Congenital adrenal hyperplasia
   Hypercalcemia associated with cancer
   Nonsuppurative thyroiditis
2. **Rheumatic Disorders**
   As adjunctive therapy for short-term administration (to tide the patient over an acute episode or exacerbation) in:
   Post-traumatic osteoarthritis
   Synovitis of osteoarthritis
   Rheumatoid arthritis, including juvenile rheumatoid arthritis (selected cases may require low-dose maintenance therapy)
   Acute and subacute bursitis
   Epicondylitis
   Acute nonspecific tenosynovitis
   Acute gouty arthritis
   Psoriatic arthritis
   Ankylosing spondylitis
3. **Collagen Diseases**
   During an exacerbation or as maintenance therapy in selected cases of:
   Systemic lupus erythematosus
   Systemic dermatomyositis (polymyositis)
   Acute rheumatic carditis
4. **Dermatologic Diseases**
   Pemphigus
   Severe erythema multiforme (Stevens-Johnson syndrome)
   Exfoliative dermatitis
   Bullous dermatitis herpetiformis
   Severe seborrheic dermatitis
   Severe psoriasis
   Mycosis fungoides
5. **Allergic States**
   Control of severe or incapacitating allergic conditions intractable to adequate trials of conventional treatment in:
   Bronchial asthma
   Contact dermatitis
   Atopic dermatitis
   Serum sickness
   Seasonal or perennial allergic rhinitis
   Drug hypersensitivity reactions
   Urticarial transfusion reactions
   Acute noninfectious laryngeal edema (epinephrine is the drug of first choice)
6. **Ophthalmic Diseases**
   Severe acute and chronic allergic and inflammatory processes involving the eye, such as:
   Herpes zoster ophthalmicus
   Iritis, iridocyclitis
   Chorioretinitis
   Diffuse posterior uveitis and choroiditis
   Optic neuritis
   Sympathetic ophthalmia
   Anterior segment inflammation
   Allergic conjunctivitis
   Allergic corneal marginal ulcers
   Keratitis
7. **Gastrointestinal Diseases**
   To tide the patient over a critical period of the disease in:
   Ulcerative colitis (systemic therapy)
   Regional enteritis (systemic therapy)
8. **Respiratory Diseases**
   Symptomatic sarcoidosis
   Berylliosis
   Fulminating or disseminated pulmonary tuberculosis when used concurrently with appropriate antituberculous chemotherapy
   Loeffler's syndrome not manageable by other means
   Aspiration pneumonitis
9. **Hematologic Disorders**
   Acquired (autoimmune) hemolytic anemia
   Idiopathic thrombocytopenic purpura in adults (IV only; IM administration is contraindicated)
   Secondary thrombocytopenia in adults
   Erythroblastopenia (RBC anemia)
   Congenital (erythroid) hypoplastic anemia
10. **Neoplastic Diseases**
    For palliative mangement of:
    Leukemias and lymphomas in adults
    Acute leukemia of childhood
11. **Edematous States**
    To induce diuresis or remission of proteinuria in the nephrotic syndrome, without uremia, of the idiopathic type or that due to lupus erythematosus
12. **Nervous System**
    Acute exacerbations of multiple sclerosis
13. **Miscellaneous**
    Tuberculous meningitis with subarachnoid block or impending block when used concurrently with appropriate antituberculous chemotherapy
    Trichinosis with neurologic or myocardial involvement

Contraindications: Systemic fungal infections.

Warnings: In patients on corticosteroid therapy subjected to unusual stress, increased dosage of rapidly acting corticosteroids before, during, and after the stressful situation is indicated.

Corticosteroids may mask some signs of infection, and new infections may appear during their use. There may be decreased resistance and inability to localize infection when corticosteroids are used.

Prolonged use of corticosteroids may produce posterior subcapsular cataracts, glaucoma with possible damage to the optic nerves, and may enhance the establishment of secondary ocular infections due to fungi or viruses.

Usage in pregnancy. Since adequate human reproduction studies have not been done with corticosteroids, the use of these drugs in pregnancy, nursing mothers, or women of childbearing potential requires that the possible benefits of the drug be weighed against the potential hazards to the mother and embryo or

Continued on next page

Upjohn—Cont.

fetus. Infants born of mothers who have received substantial doses of corticosteroids during pregnancy should be carefully observed for signs of hypoadrenalism.

Average and large doses of hydrocortisone can cause elevation of blood pressure, salt and water retention, and increased excretion of potassium. These effects are less likely to occur with the synthetic derivatives except when used in large doses. Dietary salt restriction and potassium supplementation may be necessary. All corticosteroids increase calcium excretion.

While on corticosteroid therapy patients should not be vaccinated against smallpox. Other immunization procedures should not be undertaken in patients who are on corticosteroids, especially on high dose, because of possible hazards of neurological complications and a lack of antibody response.

The use of *Solu-Cortef* Sterile Powder (hydrocortisone sodium succinate) in active tuberculosis should be restricted to those cases of fulminating or disseminated tuberculosis in which the corticosteroid is used for the management of the disease in conjunction with appropriate antituberculous regimen.

If corticosteroids are indicated in patients with latent tuberculosis or tuberculin reactivity, close observation is necessary as reactivation of the disease may occur. During prolonged corticosteroid therapy, these patients should receive chemoprophylaxis.

Because rare instances of anaphylactoid reactions (eg, bronchospasm) have occurred in patients receiving parenteral corticosteroid therapy, appropriate precautionary measures should be taken prior to administration, especially when the patient has a history of allergy to any drug.

The *Solu-Cortef* Sterile Powder 100 mg, 250 mg, 500 mg and 1000 mg *Mix-O-Vial* two-compartment vials contain benzyl alcohol. Benzyl alcohol has been reported to be associated with a fatal "Gasping Syndrome" in premature infants.

Precautions: Drug-induced secondary adrenocortical insufficiency may be minimized by gradual reduction of dosage. This type of relative insufficiency may persist for months after discontinuation of therapy; therefore, in any situation of stress occurring during that period, hormone therapy should be reinstituted. Since mineralocorticoid secretion may be impaired, salt and/or a mineralocorticoid should be administered concurrently.

There is an enhanced effect of corticosteroids in patients with hypothyroidism and in those with cirrhosis.

Corticosteroids should be used cautiously in patients with ocular herpes simplex for fear of corneal perforation.

The lowest possible dose of corticosteroid should be used to control the condition under treatment, and when reduction in dosage is possible, the reduction must be gradual.

Psychic derangements may appear when corticosteroids are used, ranging from euphoria, insomnia, mood swings, personality changes, and severe depression to frank psychotic manifestations. Also, existing emotional instability or psychotic tendencies may be aggravated by corticosteroids.

Aspirin should be used cautiously in conjunction with corticosteroids in hypoprothrombinemia.

Steroids should be used with caution in nonspecific ulcerative colitis, if there is a probability of impending perforation, abscess or other pyogenic infection, also in diverticulitis, fresh intestinal anastomoses, active or latent peptic ulcer, renal insufficiency, hypertension, osteoporosis, and myasthenia gravis.

Growth and development of infants and children on prolonged corticosteroid therapy should be carefully followed.

Although controlled clinical trials have shown corticosteroids to be effective in speeding the resolution of acute exacerbations of multiple sclerosis, they do not show that corticosteroids affect the ultimate outcome or natural history of the disease. The studies do show that relatively high doses of corticosteroids are necessary to demonstrate a significant effect. (See **Administration and Dosage**).

Since complications of treatment with glucocorticoides are dependent on the size of the dose and the duration of treatment, a risk/benefit decision must be made in each individual case as to dose and duration of treatment and as to whether daily or intermittent therapy should be used.

Adverse Reactions:

Fluid and Electrolyte Disturbances

- Sodium retention
- Fluid retention
- Congestive heart failure in susceptible patients
- Potassium loss
- Hypokalemic alkalosis
- Hypertension

Musculoskeletal

- Muscle weakness
- Steroid myopathy
- Loss of muscle mass
- Osteoporosis
- Vertebral compression fractures
- Aseptic necrosis of femoral and humeral heads
- Pathologic fracture of long bones

Gastrointestinal

- Peptic ulcer with possible perforation and hemorrhage
- Pancreatitis
- Abdominal distention
- Ulcerative esophagitis

Dermatologic

- Impaired wound healing
- Thin fragile skin
- Petechiae and ecchymoses
- Facial erythema
- Increased sweating
- May suppress reactions to skin tests

Neurological

- Convulsions
- Increased intracranial pressure with papilledema (pseudotumor cerebri) usually after treatment
- Vertigo
- Headache

Endocrine

- Menstrual irregularities
- Development of Cushingoid state
- Suppression of growth in children
- Secondary adrenocortical and pituitary unresponsiveness, particularly in times of stress, as in trauma, surgery, or illness
- Decreased carbohydrate tolerance
- Manifestations of latent diabetes mellitus
- Increased requirements for insulin or oral hypoglycemic agents in diabetics

Ophthalmic

- Posterior subcapsular cataracts
- Increased intraocular pressure
- Glaucoma
- Exophthalmos

Metabolic

- Negative nitrogen balance due to protein catabolism

The following additional reactions are related to parenteral corticosteroid therapy:

- Allergic, anaphylactic or other hypersensitivity reactions
- Hyperpigmentation or hypopigmentation
- Subcutaneous and cutaneous atrophy
- Sterile abscess

Administration and Dosage: This preparation may be administered by intravenous injection, by intravenous infusion, or by intramuscular injection, the preferred method for initial emergency use being intravenous injection. Following the initial emergency period, consideration should be given to employing a longer acting injectable preparation or an oral preparation.

Therapy is initiated by administering *Solu-Cortef* Sterile Powder (hydrocortisone sodium succinate) intravenously over a period of 30 seconds (eg, 100 mg) to 10 minutes (eg, 500 mg or more). In general, high dose corticosteroid therapy should be continued only until the patient's condition has stabilized—usually not beyond 48 to 72 hours. Although adverse effects associated with high dose, short-term corticoid therapy are uncommon, peptic ulceration may occur. Prophylactic anatacid therapy may be indicated.

When high dose hydrocortisone therapy must be continued beyond 48–72 hours, hypernatremia may occur. Under such circumstances it may be desirable to replace *Solu-Cortef* with a corticoid such as methylprednisolone sodium succinate which causes little or no sodium retention.

The initial dose of *Solu-Cortef* Sterile Powder is 100 mg to 500 mg, depending on the severity of the condition. This dose may be repeated at intervals of 2, 4 or 6 hours as indicated by the patient's response and clinical condition. While the dose may be reduced for infants and children, it is governed more by the severity of the condition and response of the patient than by age or body weight but should not be less than 25 mg daily.

Patients subjected to severe stress following corticosteroid therapy should be observed closely for signs and symptoms of adrenocortical insufficiency.

Corticoid therapy is an adjunct to, and not a replacement for, conventional therapy.

Preparation of Solutions

100 mg Plain—For intravenous or intramuscular injection, prepare solution by aseptically adding **not more than 2 ml** of Bacteriostatic Water for Injection or Bacteriostatic Sodium Chloride Injection to the contents of one vial. **For intravenous infusion,** first prepare solution by adding **not more than 2 ml** of Bacteriostatic Water for Injection to the vial; this solution may then be added to 100 to 1000 ml (but not less than 100 ml) of the following: 5% dextrose in water (or isotonic saline solution or 5% dextrose in isotonic saline solution if patient is not on sodium restriction).

Directions for using *Mix-O-Vial* Two-Compartment Vial

1. Remove protective cap, give the plunger-stopper a quarter-turn and press to force diluent into the lower compartment.
2. Gently agitate to effect solution.
3. Sterilize top of plunger-stopper with a suitable germicide.
4. Insert needle **squarely through center** of plunger-stopper until tip is just visible. Invert vial and withdraw dose.

Further dilution is not necessary for intravenous or intramuscular injection. For intravenous infusion, first prepare solution as just described. The **100 mg** solution may then be added to 100 to 1000 ml of 5% dextrose in water (or isotonic saline solution or 5% dextrose in isotonic saline solution if patient is not on sodium restriction). The **250 mg** solution may be added to 250 to 1000 ml, the **500 mg** solution may be added to 500 to 1000 ml and the **1000 mg** solution to 1000 ml of the same diluents. In cases where administration of a small volume of fluid is desirable, 100 mg to 3000 mg of *Solu-Cortef* Sterile Powder may be added to 50 ml of the above diluents. The resulting solutions are stable for at least 4 hours and may be administered either directly or by IV piggyback.

When reconstituted as directed, pH's of the solutions range from 7 to 8 and the tonicities are: 100 mg *Mix-O-Vial,* .36 osmolar; 250 mg *Mix-O-Vial,* 500 mg *Mix-O-Vial,* and the 1000 mg *Mix-O-Vial,* .57 osmolar. (Isotonic saline =.28 osmolar.)

How Supplied: *Solu-Cortef* Sterile Powder (hydrocortisone sodium succinate) is available in the following packages:
100 mg Plain—NDC 0009-0825-01
100 mg *Mix-O-Vial*—NDC 0009-0900-01
250 mg *Mix-O-Vial*—NDC 0009-0909-01
500 mg *Mix-O-Vial*—NDC 0009-0912-01
1000 mg *Mix-O-Vial*—NDC 0009-0920-01
Storage Conditions: Store unreconstituted product at controlled room temperature 15°–30°C (59°–86°F).
Store solution at controlled room temperature 15°–30°C (59°–86°F) and protect from light. Use solution only if it is clear. Unused solution should be discarded after 3 days.
Code 810 379 006

SOLU-MEDROL® Sterile Powder ℞
(methylprednisolone sodium succinate for injection, USP)
For Intravenous or Intramuscular Administration
40 mg (1 ml *Mix-O-Vial®* Two-Compartment Vial):
NSN 6505-00-768-3598A (M & VA)
125 mg (2 ml *Mix-O-Vial*):
NSN 6505-00-943-4380A (M & VA)
500 mg:
NSN 6505-00-432-1124A (VA)
1000 mg:
NSN 6505-00-104-8069A (VA)

Description: *Solu-Medrol* Sterile Powder contains methylprednisolone sodium succinate as the active ingredient. Methylprednisolone sodium succinate, USP, occurs as a white, or nearly white, odorless hygroscopic, amorphous solid. It is very soluble in water and in alcohol; it is insoluble in chloroform and is very slightly soluble in acetone.
Methylprednisolone sodium succinate is so extremely soluble in water that it may be administered in a small volume of diluent and is especially well suited for intravenous use in situations in which high blood levels of methylprednisolone are required rapidly. *Solu-Medrol* is available as **40 mg *Mix-O-Vial®*** Two-Compartment Vial—Each ml (when mixed) contains methylprednisolone sodium succinate equiv. to 40 mg methylprednisolone; also 1.6 mg sodium biphosphate anhydrous; 17.46 mg dried sodium phosphate; 25 mg lactose hydrous; 8.8 mg benzyl alcohol added as preservative. **125 mg *Mix-O-Vial*** Two-Compartment Vial—Each 2 ml (when mixed) contains methylprednisolone sodium succinate equiv. to 125 mg methylprednisolone; also 1.6 mg sodium biphosphate anhydrous; 17.4 mg dried sodium phosphate; 17.6 mg benzyl alcohol added as preservative. **500 mg Vial**—Each 8 ml (when mixed as directed) contains methylprednisolone sodium succinate equiv. to 500 mg methylprednisolone; also 6.4 mg sodium biphosphate anhydrous; 69.6 mg dried sodium phosphate; and 70.2 mg benzyl alcohol added as preservative. **1000 mg Vial**—Each 16 ml (when mixed as directed) contains methylprednisolone sodium succinate equiv. to 1000 mg methylprednisolone; also 12.8 mg sodium biphosphate anhydrous; 139.2 mg dried sodium phosphate; and 141 mg benzyl alcohol added as preservative. When necessary the pH of the 125 mg, 500 mg and 1000 mg formulas was adjusted with sodium hydroxide.
IMPORTANT—Only the accompanying diluent is to be used when dissolving the *Solu-Medrol* in vials.
Use within 48 hours after mixing
When reconstituted as directed, pH's of the solutions range from 7–8 and the tonicities are, for the 40 mg per ml solution, .50 osmolar; for the 125 mg per 2 ml, 500 mg per 8 ml and 1000 mg per 16 ml solutions, .40 osmolar. (Isotonic saline = .28 osmolar).
Actions: Methylprednisolone is a potent anti-inflammatory steroid synthesized in the Research Laboratories of The Upjohn Company. It has a greater anti-inflammatory potency than prednisolone and even less tendency than prednisolone to induce sodium and water retention.
Methylprednisolone sodium succinate has the same metabolic and anti-inflammatory actions as methylprednisolone. When given parenterally and in equimolar quantities, the two compounds are equivalent in biologic activity. The relative potency of *Solu-Medrol* Sterile Powder (methylprednisolone sodium succinate) and hydrocortisone sodium succinate, as indicated by depression of eosinophil count, following intravenous administration, is at least four to one. This is in good agreement with the relative oral potency of methylprednisolone and hydrocortisone.
Indications: When oral therapy is not feasible, and the strength, dosage form and route of administration of the drug reasonably lend the preparation to the treatment of the condition, *Solu-Medrol* Sterile Powder (methylprednisolone sodium succinate) is indicated for intravenous or intramuscular use in the following conditions:

1. Endocrine Disorders
Primary or secondary adrenocortical insufficiency (hydrocortisone or cortisone is the drug of choice; synthetic analogs may be used in conjunction with mineralocorticoids where applicable; in infancy, mineralocorticoid supplementation is of particular importance)
Acute adrenocortical insufficiency (hydrocortisone or cortisone is the drug of choice; mineralocorticoid supplementation may be necessary, particularly when synthetic analogs are used)
Preoperatively and in the event of serious trauma or illness, in patients with known adrenal insufficiency or when adrenocortical reserve is doubtful
Shock unresponsive to conventional therapy if adrenocortical insufficiency exists or is suspected
Congenital adrenal hyperplasia
Hypercalcemia associated with cancer
Nonsuppurative thyroiditis

2. Rheumatic Disorders
As adjunctive therapy for short-term administration (to tide the patient over an acute episode or exacerbation) in:
Post-traumatic osteoarthritis
Synovitis of osteoarthritis
Rheumatoid arthritis, including juvenile rheumatoid arthritis (selected cases may require low-dose maintenance therapy)
Acute and subacute bursitis
Epicondylitis
Acute nonspecific tenosynovitis
Acute gouty arthritis
Psoriatic arthritis
Ankylosing spondylitis

3. Collagen Diseases
During an exacerbation or as maintenance therapy in selected cases of:
Systemic lupus erythematosus
Systemic dermatomyositis (polymyositis)
Acute rheumatic carditis

4. Dermatologic Diseases
Pemphigus
Severe erythema multiforme (Stevens-Johnson syndrome)
Exfoliative dermatitis
Bullous dermatitis herpetiformis
Severe seborrheic dermatitis
Severe psoriasis
Mycosis fungoides

5. Allergic States
Control of severe or incapacitating allergic conditions intractable to adequate trials of conventional treatment in:
Bronchial asthma
Contact dermatitis
Atopic dermatitis
Serum sickness
Seasonal or perennial allergic rhinitis
Drug hypersensitivity reactions
Urticarial transfusion reactions
Acute noninfectious laryngeal edema (epinephrine is the drug of first choice)

6. Ophthalmic Diseases
Severe acute and chronic allergic and inflammatory processes involving the eye, such as:
Herpes zoster ophthalmicus
Iritis, iridocyclitis
Chorioretinitis
Diffuse posterior uveitis and choroiditis
Optic neuritis
Sympathetic ophthalmia
Anterior segment inflammation
Allergic conjunctivitis
Allergic corneal marginal ulcers
Keratitis

7. Gastrointestinal Diseases
To tide the patient over a critical period of the disease in:
Ulcerative colitis (systemic therapy)
Regional enteritis (systemic therapy)

8. Respiratory Diseases
Symptomatic sarcoidosis
Berylliosis
Fulminating or disseminated pulmonary tuberculosis when used concurrently with appropriate antituberculous chemotherapy
Loeffler's syndrome not manageable by other means
Aspiration pneumonitis

9. Hematologic Disorders
Acquired (autoimmune) hemolytic anemia
Idiopathic thrombocytopenic purpura in adults (IV only; IM administration is contraindicated)
Secondary thrombocytopenia in adults
Erythroblastopenia (RBC anemia)
Congenital (erythroid) hypoplastic anemia

10. Neoplastic Diseases
For palliative management of:
Leukemias and lymphomas in adults
Acute leukemia of childhood

11. Edematous States
To induce diuresis or remission of proteinuria in the nephrotic syndrome, without uremia, of the idiopathic type or that due to lupus erythematosus

12. Nervous System
Acute exacerbations of multiple sclerosis

13. Miscellaneous
Tuberculous meningitis with subarachnoid block or impending block when used concurrently with appropriate antituberculous chemotherapy
Trichinosis with neurologic or myocardial involvement

Contraindications: Systemic fungal infections.
Warnings: In patients on corticosteroid therapy subjected to any unusual stress, increased dosage of rapidly acting corticosteroids before, during, and after the stressful situation is indicated.
Corticosteroids may mask some signs of infection, and new infections may appear during their use. There may be decreased resistance and inability to localize infection when corticosteroids are used.
Prolonged use of corticosteroids may produce posterior subcapsular cataracts, glaucoma with possible damage to the optic nerves, and may enhance the establishment of secondary ocular infections due to fungi or viruses.
Usage in pregnancy. Since adequate human reproduction studies have not been done with corticosteroids, the use of these drugs in pregnancy, nursing mothers, or women of childbearing potential requires that the possible benefits of the drug be weighed against the potential hazards to the mother and embryo or fetus. Infants born of mothers who have received substantial doses of corticosteroids dur-

Continued on next page

Upjohn—Cont.

ing pregnancy should be carefully observed for signs of hypoadrenalism.
Average and large doses of cortisone or hydrocortisone can cause elevation of blood pressure, salt and water retention, and increased excretion of potassium. These effects are less likely to occur with the synthetic derivatives except when used in large doses. Dietary salt restriction and potassium supplementation may be necessary. All corticosteroids increase calcium excretion.
While on corticosteroid therapy patients should not be vaccinated against smallpox. Other immunization procedures should not be undertaken in patients who are on corticosteroids, especially on high dose, because of possible hazards of neurological complications and a lack of antibody response.
The use of *Solu-Medrol* Sterile Powder (methylprednisolone sodium succinate) in active tuberculosis should be restricted to those cases of fulminating or disseminated tuberculosis in which the corticosteroid is used for the management of the disease in conjunction with appropriate antituberculous regimen.
If corticosteroids are indicated in patients with latent tuberculosis or tuberculin reactivity, close observation is necessary as reactivation of the disease may occur. During prolonged corticosteroid therapy, these patients should receive chemoprophylaxis.
Because rare instances of anaphylactic (eg, bronchospasm) reactions have occurred in patients receiving parenteral corticosteroid therapy, appropriate precautionary measures should be taken prior to administration, especially when the patient has a history of allergy to any drug.
There are reports of cardiac arrhythmias and/or circulatory collapse and/or cardiac arrest following the rapid administration of large IV doses of *Solu-Medrol* (greater than 0.5 gram administered over a period of less than 10 minutes).
Precautions: Drug-induced secondary adrenocortical insufficiency may be minimized by gradual reduction of dosage. This type of relative insufficiency may persist for months after discontinuation of therapy; therefore, in any situation of stress occurring during that period, hormone therapy should be reinstituted. Since mineralocorticoid secretion may be impaired, salt and/or a mineralocorticoid should be administered concurrently.
There is an enhanced effect of corticosteroids on patients with hypothyroidism and in those with cirrhosis.
Corticosteroids should be used cautiously in patients with ocular herpes simplex because of possible corneal perforation.
The lowest possible dose of corticosteroid should be used to control the condition under treatment, and when reduction in dosage is possible, the reduction should be gradual.
Psychic derangements may appear when corticosteroids are used, ranging from euphoria, insomnia, mood swings, personality changes and severe depression, to frank psychotic manifestations. Also, existing emotional instability or psychotic tendencies may be aggravated by corticosteroids.
Aspirin should be used cautiously in conjunction with corticosteroids in hypoprothrombinemia.
Steroids should be used with caution in nonspecific ulcerative colitis, if there is a probability of impending perforation, abscess or other pyogenic infection; diverticulitis; fresh intestinal anastomoses; active or latent peptic ulcer; renal insufficiency; hypertension; osteoporosis; and myasthenia gravis.
Growth and development of infants and children on prolonged corticosteroid therapy should be carefully observed.
Although controlled clinical trials have shown corticosteroids to be effective in speeding the resolution of acute exacerbations of multiple sclerosis, they do not show that corticosteroids affect the ultimate outcome or natural history of the disease. The studies do show that relatively high doses of corticosteroids are necessary to demonstrate a significant effect. (See DOSAGE AND ADMINISTRATION).
Since complications of treatment with glucocorticoids are dependent on the size of the dose and the duration of treatment, a risk/benefit decision must be made in each individual case as to dose and duration of treatment and as to whether daily or intermittent therapy should be used.

Adverse Reactions:

Fluid and Electrolyte Disturbances
Sodium retention
Fluid retention
Congestive heart failure in susceptible patients
Potassium loss
Hypokalemic alkalosis
Hypertension

Musculoskeletal
Muscle weakness
Steroid myopathy
Loss of muscle mass
Severe arthralgia
Vertebral compression fractures
Aseptic necrosis of femoral and humeral heads
Pathologic fracture of long bones
Osteoporosis

Gastrointestinal
Peptic ulcer with possible perforation and hemorrhage
Pancreatitis
Abdominal distention
Ulcerative esophagitis

Dermatologic
Impaired wound healing
Thin fragile skin
Petechiae and ecchymoses
Facial erythema
Increased sweating
May suppress reactions to skin tests

Neurological
Increased intracranial pressure with papilledema (pseudo-tumor cerebri) usually after treatment
Convulsions
Vertigo
Headache

Endocrine
Development of Cushingoid state
Suppression of growth in children
Secondary adrenocortical and pituitary unresponsiveness, particularly in times of stress, as in trauma, surgery or illness
Menstrual irregularities
Decreased carbohydrate tolerance
Manifestations of latent diabetes mellitus
Increased requirements for insulin or oral hypoglycemic agents in diabetics

Ophthalmic
Posterior subcapsular cataracts
Increased intraocular pressure
Glaucoma
Exophthalmos

Metabolic
Negative nitrogen balance due to protein catabolism

The following *additional* adverse reactions are related to parenteral corticosteroid therapy:
Hyperpigmentation or hypopigmentation
Subcutaneous and cutaneous atrophy
Sterile abscess
Anaphylactic reaction with or without circulatory collapse, cardiac arrest, bronchospasm
Urticaria
Nausea and vomiting
Cardiac arrhythmias; hypotension or hypertension

Dosage and Administration: When high dose therapy is desired, the recommended dose of *Solu-Medrol* Sterile Powder (methylprednisolone sodium succinate) is 30 mg/kg administered intravenously over a 10–20 minute period. This dose may be repeated every 4 to 6 hours for 48 hours.
Therapy is initiated by administering *Solu-Medrol* intravenously over a period of one to several minutes. In general, high dose corticosteroid therapy should be continued only until the patient's condition has stabilized; usually not beyond 48 to 72 hours.
Although adverse effects associated with high dose short-term corticoid therapy are uncommon, peptic ulceration may occur. Prophylactic antacid therapy may be indicated.
In other indications initial dosage will vary from 10 to 40 mg of methylprednisolone depending on the clinical problem being treated. The larger doses may be required for short-term management of severe, acute conditions. The initial dose usually should be given intravenously over a period of one to several minutes. Subsequent doses may be given intravenously or intramuscularly at intervals dictated by the patient's response and clinical condition. Corticoid therapy is an adjunct to, and not replacement for conventional therapy.
Dosage may be reduced for infants and children but should be governed more by the severity of the condition and response of the patient than by age or size. It should not be less than 0.5 mg per kg every 24 hours.
Dosage must be decreased or discontinued gradually when the drug has been administered for more than a few days. If a period of spontaneous remission occurs in a chronic condition, treatment should be discontinued. Routine laboratory studies, such as urinalysis, two-hour postprandial blood sugar, determination of blood pressure and body weight, and a chest X-ray should be made at regular intervals during prolonged therapy. Upper GI X-rays are desirable in patients with an ulcer history or significant dyspepsia.
Solu-Medrol may be administered by intravenous or intramuscular injection or by intravenous infusion, the preferred method for initial emergency use being intravenous injection. To administer by intravenous (or intramuscular) injection, prepare solution as directed. The desired dose may be administered intravenously over a period of approximately 60 seconds. Subsequent doses may be withdrawn and administered similarly. If desired, the medication may be administered in diluted solutions by adding Water for Injection or other suitable diluent (see below) to the *Mix-O-Vial* and withdrawing the indicated dose.
To prepare solutions for intravenous infusion, first prepare the solution for injection as directed. This solution may then be added to indicated amounts of 5% dextrose in water, isotonic saline solution or 5% dextrose in isotonic saline solution.

Multiple Sclerosis
In treatment of acute exacerbations of multiple sclerosis, daily doses of 200 mg of prednisolone for a week followed by 80 mg every other day for 1 month have been shown to be effective (4 mg of methylprednisolone is equivalent to 5 mg of prednisolone).

Directions for Using the *Mix-O-Vial* Two-Compartment Vial

1. Remove protective cap, give the plunger-stopper a quarter turn and press to force diluent into the lower compartment.
2. Gently agitate to effect solution. Use solution within 48 hours.
3. Sterilize top of plunger-stopper with a suitable germicide.
4. Insert needle **squarely through center** of plunger-stopper until tip is just visible. Invert vial and withdraw dose.

Storage Conditions: Store unreconstituted product at controlled room temperature 15°–30°C (59°–86°F).
Store solution at controlled room temperature 15°–30°C (59°–86°F).

Use solution within 48 hours after mixing.

How Supplied: *Solu-Medrol* Sterile Powder (methylprednisolone sodium succinate) is available in the following packages:

40 mg *Mix-O-Vial* Two-Compartment Vial
NDC 0009-0113-01
40 mg *Mix-O-Vial* (25-Pack)
NDC 0009-0113-11
125 mg *Mix-O-Vial* Two-Compartment Vial
NDC 0009-0190-01
125 mg *Mix-O-Vial* (25-Pack)
NDC 0009-0190-08
500 mg Vial with Diluent
NDC 0009-0887-01
1000 mg Vial with Diluent
NDC 0009-0911-01
1000 mg Vial with Diluent and IV administration kit
NDC 0009-0911-05

Code 810 431 006

[*Shown in Product Identification Section*]

TOLINASE® Tablets ℞
(tolazamide tablets, USP)

250 mg (30s)
NSN 6505-01-061-6992 (VA)
250 mg (100s):
NSN 6505-00-159-4990A (VA)
250 mg (1000s):
NSN 6505-00-105-5842A (M & VA)

Tolinase Tablets contain tolazamide, an orally effective hypoglycemic agent which has been shown to be effective and safe in over 3,000 diabetic patients in a period of more than four years of clinical trials. It is effective in the mild to moderately severe maturity-onset type of diabetes. It represents the culmination of a seven year search by The Upjohn Company involving over 4,000 compounds to find an oral agent as safe as *Orinase* ® Tablets (tolbutamide) which might help fill the therapeutic gap created by sulfonylurea failures. Clinical trials have indicated that *Tolinase* is **effective in approximately one-third of failures to tolbutamide, chlorpropamide or phenformin.** It should be recognized, however, that this "salvage" rate may not be sustained and that some of these patients will also eventually fail on *Tolinase*. *Tolinase* in **once-a-day therapy** has proven to be as effective in providing satisfactory diabetic control as in multiple daily doses. **Patients must be under continuous medical supervision, particularly during the first six weeks of treatment. They should check their urines daily for sugar and acetone and should see their doctors at least once a week. *Tolinase* is not an oral insulin or an insulin substitute. It is not recommended for the juvenile diabetic or the diabetic under stress of infection, surgery, severe trauma, or in ketoacidosis or coma. It is not recommended for use in the pregnant diabetic patient. Since the primary mechanism of action is the release of endogenous insulin, occasionally hypoglycemic reactions have occurred (verified hypoglycemic reactions were reported in 0.4%). This usually results from the administration of too large a dose for the patient's immediate needs. It is imperative that the physician familiarize himself with the indications and limitations of therapy, as well as the criteria for the proper selection of patients.**

Chemistry: Tolazamide was synthesized by chemists at The Upjohn Company. The chemical name is 1-(hexahydro-1H-azepin-1-yl)-3-(*p*-tolylsulfonyl) urea.

The molecular weight is 311.40. It is a white or creamy white powder with a melting point of 165° to 173° C. The minimum solubility at 37.5° C. in aqueous buffers is 0.09 grams per liter at pH 4.5; the solubility increases logarithmically at higher and lower pH values; for example, the solubility is 1.13 grams per liter at pH 2.0 and 1.97 grams per liter at pH 7.0. Its solubility is between 4 and 5 grams per liter in 95% ethanol.

The solubility of *Tolinase* at pH 6.0 (mean urinary pH) is 27.8 mg per 100 ml. Besides the absence of crystalluria in the extensive clinical trials, the fact that small daily doses are used and that 93% of the pooled urinary extracts of man (following oral ingestion of *Tolinase*) are metabolites which are more soluble than *Tolinase* gives assurance that crystalluria should not occur.

Animal Studies: *Tolinase* Tablets (tolazamide) are five to nine and one-half times more potent than *Orinase* Tablets (tolbutamide) in glucose-primed, fasted, intact rats and four times as potent as *Orinase* in glucose-primed, fasted, adrenalectomized rats. As is true with other sulfonylurea compounds, *Tolinase* has no hypoglycemic effect in alloxanized diabetic or eviscerate rats.

Animal Toxicology: Acute toxicity is extremely low, as the mouse LD_{50} is 2200 mg per kg intraperitoneally, and the rat LD_{50} is greater than 5 grams per kg orally. One month and six month studies in dogs at doses from 12.5 to 50 mg per kg showed no significant toxicity, nor did one month and one year studies in Sprague-Dawley rats at doses from 25 to 100 mg per kg, although these rats did demonstrate marked beta cell islet hyperplasia with some resultant degeneration and fibrosis of the islet cells. Doses up to 400 mg/kg daily in the rabbit for periods of one year showed no similar changes. Doses of 100 mg/kg daily for periods up to two years in the Wistar rat produced only minimal changes in the pancreatic islets. Drug treatment of pregnant rats produced no reproductive aberrations or drug related fetal anomalies at a daily dose of 14 mg per kg. At the elevated dose of 100 mg per kg, there was a reduction in number of pups born and an increased perinatal mortality.

Absorption, Metabolism and Excretion: Isotopic techniques show that *Tolinase* Tablets (tolazamide) are well absorbed with little subject-to-subject variation. Due to slower absorption of tolazamide compared with tolbutamide or chlorpropamide, peak blood drug levels occur at four to eight hours following the oral administration of therapeutic doses. An average of 85% of the radioactivity of an oral dose appears in the urine.

Utilizing both chemical and isotopic methods, the average biological half-life is 7.0 hours. The drug does not continue to cumulate in the blood after the first four to six doses are administered. A steady or equilibrium state is reached during which the peak and nadir values do not change from day to day after the fourth to sixth dose.

Actions: As with other sulfonylureas, the primary mechanism of action appears to be stimulation of the beta cells of the pancreas with increased endogenous insulin secretion. Utilizing the immunoassay technique of Yalow and Berson, dog studies have shown *Tolinase* Tablets (tolazamide) to produce increased pancreatic venous insulin levels. Further, these levels are maintained longer than with equal doses of *Orinase* Tablets (tolbutamide) or chlorpropamide. When normal, nondiabetic, fasting volunteers are given single doses of *Tolinase* orally, the peak hypoglycemic effect occurs in one hour. Following an oral dose of 500 mg of *Tolinase* Tablets, a statistically significant hypoglycemic effect was demonstrated in nondiabetic subjects 20 hours following administration. With fasting diabetic patients, the peak hypoglycemic effect occurs at four to six hours. The duration of maximal hypoglycemic effect in fed diabetic patients is about ten hours, with the onset occurring at four to six hours and with the blood sugar levels beginning to rise at fourteen to sixteen hours.

Single-dose potency of *Tolinase* in the normal subject has been shown to be 6.7 times that of tolbutamide on a milligram basis. Clinical experience in diabetic patients has demonstrated *Tolinase* to be approximately five times more potent than tolbutamide.

Tolazamide does not appear to have an antidiuretic effect and a mild diuresis has been observed.

Indications:

1. The primary indication for *Tolinase* Tablets (tolazamide) is the stable or maturity-onset type of mild or moderately severe diabetes mellitus.
2. Approximately one-third of diabetic patients purported to be primary or secondary failures with other sulfonylurea agents or with phenformin have been reported to respond satisfactorily to therapy with *Tolinase*.
3. Some patients who have developed significant side effects or intolerance to other sulfonylurea drugs or phenformin may subsequently be successfully maintained on *Tolinase*.

Contraindications:

1. *Tolinase* Tablets (tolazamide) are not indicated in diabetic patients who have infections, severe trauma or who are undergoing surgery, who have ketosis, acidosis or coma or give a history of repeated bouts of ketoacidosis or coma.
2. It is not indicated in the therapy of juvenile or labile (brittle) diabetes.
3. Since *Tolinase* has not been studied extensively in patients with concurrent liver, renal or endocrine disease, its use is not recommended in these conditions and is contraindicated in subjects with uremia. Nevertheless, no instance of jaundice, renal or endocrine disease attributable solely to therapy with *Tolinase* has occurred.
4. In view of the question of the safety of any new drug in pregnancy, and in view of the fact that the safety and usefulness of *Tolinase* during pregnancy has not been evaluated at this time, *Tolinase* is not recommended for the treatment of the pregnant diabetic patient. Serious consideration should be giyen to the possible hazards of its use in women of child-bearing age who might become pregnant.

Precautions:

1. The diagnostic and therapeutic measures which are necessary to insure optimal control of the diabetic state with insulin or other sulfonylureas are equally necessary for control with *Tolinase* Tablets (tolazamide). No false positive tests for urinary albumin have been reported, as has been occasionally noted with other sulfonylureas.
2. The patient must receive full and complete instructions about the nature of his disease, what he must do to prevent and detect complications and how to control his condition.
3. He must understand that he cannot neglect his dietary restrictions, develop a careless attitude or disregard instructions relative to body weight, exercise, personal hygiene and avoidance of infection.
4. The patient must know how to recognize and counteract impending hypoglycemia.
5. The patient must know how and when to test for glycosuria and ketonuria.
6. During the trial period, when insulin is being withdrawn, care should be taken to avoid ketosis, acidosis and coma.
7. When *Tolinase* is administered as sole therapy to patients who have previously required combination therapy (phenformin plus sulfonylureas), careful observation of the patient is mandatory, particularly during the transitional phase.
8. Caution should be observed in administering the thiazide-type diuretics to diabetic patients on therapy with *Tolinase* because the thiazides have been reported to aggra-

Continued on next page

Upjohn—Cont.

vate diabetes mellitus and to result in increased sulfonylurea requirements.

9. Very close observation and careful adjustment of dosage is mandatory in patients who are debilitated, malnourished, semi-starved or simply not eating properly. In such patients severe hypoglycemic reactions may occur and may require corrective therapy.
10. Severe hypoglycemia, though uncommon, may occur in patients receiving *Tolinase* and may mimic acute neurological disorders such as cerebral thrombosis. Certain conditions, such as hepatic and renal disease, malnutrition, debility, advanced age, alcoholism, and adrenal and pituitary insufficiency may predispose to hypoglycemia. Also, certain drugs may prolong or enhance the action of *Tolinase* and thereby increase the risk of hypoglycemia. These include insulin, phenformin, sulfonamides, oxyphenbutazone, phenylbutazone, salicylates, probenecid and monamine oxidase inhibitors.

Adverse Reactions: *Tolinase* Tablets (tolazamide) have been generally well tolerated. In 1,784 diabetic patients specially evaluated for incidence of side effects during the clinical studies, 2.1% were discontinued from therapy because of side effects.

The following adverse reactions have been reported in connection with the use of this agent either during the clinical studies or subsequent thereto.

Gastrointestinal—Nausea and vomiting have been reported occasionally. In the clinical studies gastrointestinal symptoms related to *Tolinase* Tablets (tolazamide) were noted in 1.0% of the patients, with nausea, vomiting and gas each noted in less than 1% of the patients studied.

Hematopoietic—Rare cases of leukopenia, thrombocytopenia, agranulocytosis, and anemia have been reported.

Hypoglycemia—Hypoglycemia has been reported occasionally. Hypoglycemia is actually a physiological extension of the primary action of the drug and generally represents the result of the administration of a dose larger than that needed by the subject. Reduction in dose generally will result in alleviation of most of the mild to moderately severe hypoglycemic symptoms. Undernourished or underweight or geriatric patients, or those failing to eat properly are particularly susceptible to hypoglycemia and should be treated cautiously. It is not recommended that patients with chronic liver or kidney disease receive therapy with *Tolinase* as they may well metabolize or excrete *Tolinase* poorly and be more susceptible to hypoglycemic reactions.

Liver—Hepatic toxicity as manifested by alterations in liver function tests (bilirubin, cholesterol, SGOT, SGPT, etc.) and by cholestatic jaundice has occasionally been associated with therapy with *Tolinase.* Transient elevations in alkaline phosphatase determinations are not uncommon after initiation of sulfonylurea therapy. However, these are not necessarily drug related, inasmuch as fluctuating abnormalities of hepatic function are frequently observed in patients with diabetes mellitus.

Skin and Mucous Membranes—Hematologic and allergic reactions as manifested by urticaria and rash have been reported occasionally.

Miscellaneous—Miscellaneous symptoms of weakness, fatigue, dizziness, vertigo, malaise and headache were reported infrequently, but the relationship to therapy with *Tolinase* is difficult to assess.

Photosensitivity reactions and disulfiram-like reactions after ingestion of alcohol have been reported occasionally in patients taking tolazamide.

Selection of Patients: Generally, the basic requirement for therapy with *Tolinase* is that the diabetes be of the maturity-onset (adult) type. The patient has usually developed his diabetes after the age of 30 years. He may be a newly diagnosed diabetic or one taking less than 40 units a day of insulin. He may be one who has developed intolerance or significant side effects to phenformin, chlorpropamide or tolbutamide.

Tolinase is effective in some patients with a history of ketoacidosis or coma. Such patients must be observed very closely, however, particularly during the early transitional period.

In approximately one-third of cases reported as being primary or secondary failures to chlorpropamide, tolbutamide, or phenformin, *Tolinase* has provided satisfactory control as sole therapy in these subjects. It should be recognized, however, that this "salvage" rate may not be sustained and that some of these patients will also eventually fail on *Tolinase.*

The only reliable method of determining responsiveness to *Tolinase* is therapeutic trial, with the patient being evaluated at weekly intervals and the dose regulated according to the patient's response.

Dosage:

The newly diagnosed diabetic subject

No initial loading or priming dose is necessary. The mild to moderately severe, newly diagnosed, adult-onset diabetic should be started on from 100 mg to 250 mg of *Tolinase* Tablets (tolazamide) once a day (given with breakfast).

If the patient is malnourished, underweight, elderly, or not eating properly, the initial therapy should be 100 mg once a day.

The following is a suggested initial dose schedule for a newly diagnosed diabetic subject:

If the fasting blood sugar value is less than 200 mg% (True), start with 100 mg per day of *Tolinase* as a single daily dose.

If the fasting blood sugar is greater than 200 mg% (True), start with 250 mg per day of *Tolinase* as a single dose.

Depending upon the results of the patient's urinary glucose test at home, the weekly blood sugar determinations, and the evaluations by the physician, the dose is then either raised or lowered accordingly at weekly intervals by amounts of one tablet (100 mg or 250 mg) per day. If more than 500 mg per day is required, the dose should be divided and given twice daily. Doses larger than 1,000 mg daily doubtfully will result in improved control.

In underweight, undernourished, or geriatric patients, when increments in dosage are required, these should be on the order of ½ tablet (50 mg or 125 mg) daily at weekly intervals to help avoid hypoglycemic reactions.

Patients Receiving Other Oral Hypoglycemic Agents

When transferring patients from other oral hypoglycemic agents to *Tolinase* Tablets (tolazamide), no transitional period and no initial or priming dose is necessary. The following dose equivalents are recommended:

Tolbutamide: If receiving 1 gram per day or less, begin *Tolinase* Tablets at 100 mg per day as a single dose. If receiving more than 1 gram per day, initiate 250 mg per day as a single dose.

Chlorpropamide: 250 mg of chlorpropamide may be considered equivalent to 250 mg of *Tolinase* Tablets. The patient should be observed carefully for hypoglycemia during the transition period from chlorpropamide to *Tolinase* (1-2 weeks) due to the prolonged retention of chlorpropamide in the body and subsequent overlapping drug effect.

Acetohexamide: 100 mg of *Tolinase* Tablets may be considered equivalent to 250 mg of acetohexamide.

Phenformin: 100 mg of phenformin may be considered equivalent to 250 mg of *Tolinase* Tablets

If necessary, the dose should be adjusted (increased or decreased) weekly with increments of one tablet daily (either 100 mg or 250 mg) depending upon the patient's response. If more than 500 mg a day is required, the dose should be divided and given more often than once a day.

In underweight, undernourished, or geriatric patients, when increments in dosage are required, these should be on the order of ½ tablet (50 mg or 125 mg) daily at weekly intervals to help avoid hypoglycemic reactions.

Patients Receiving Insulin

Many maturity-onset, mild to moderate diabetic patients who have been treated only with insulin may respond satisfactorily to therapy with *Tolinase* Tablets (tolazamide).

The following schedule is recommended as based on previous insulin dosage:

Insulin dosage less than 20 units: Place directly on *Tolinase* Tablets 100 mg as a single daily dose.

Insulin dosage less than 40 units but more than 20 units: Place directly on *Tolinase* Tablets 250 mg as a single daily dose.

Insulin dosage greater than 40 units: Reduce insulin dosage 50% and start *Tolinase* Tablets 250 mg daily.

Tolinase dosage should then be adjusted on a weekly basis (or more often in the group previously requiring more than 40 units of insulin).

It is important during insulin withdrawal that the patient test his urine for glucose and acetone at least three times daily and report the results to his physician.

The appearance of significant acetonuria would make discontinuation of *Tolinase* and the return to insulin therapy mandatory.

In the event that the patient cannot be transferred completely to therapy with *Tolinase*, *Tolinase* Tablets (tolazamide) should be discontinued and the subject maintained on insulin therapy only.

When doses larger than 500 mg daily are required, a divided dosage regimen is recommended. Doses larger than 1,000 mg daily doubtfully will provide any improvement in diabetic control.

How Supplied: *Tolinase* Tablets (tolazamide) are available in the following strengths and package sizes:

100 mg (scored, round, white)
Unit-of-Use bottles of 100 *NDC 0009-0070-02*

250 mg (scored, round, white)
Unit-of-Use bottles of 100 *NDC 0009-0114-05*
Bottles of 200 *NDC 0009-0114-04*
Bottles of 1000 *NDC 0009-0114-02*
Unit Dose Packages (100) *NDC 0009-0114-06*

500 mg (scored, round, white)
Unit-of-Use bottles of 30 *NDC 0009-0477-04*
Unit-of-Use bottles of 100 *NDC 0009-0477-06*

Code 811 417 102

[*Shown in Product Identification Section*]

TROBICIN® Sterile Powder ℞
(sterile spectinomycin hydrochloride, USP)
For Intramuscular Injection

2 Gm vial
NSN 6505-00-079-7611 (M)
4 Gm vial
NSN 6505-00-079-7643 (M)

Description: *Trobicin* Sterile Powder contains spectinomycin hydrochloride which is an aminocyclitol antibiotic produced by a species of soil microorganism designated as *Streptomyces spectabilis.* Sterile spectinomycin hydrochloride is the pentahydrated dihydrochloride salt of spectinomycin.

Spectinomycin hydrochloride is isolated as a white crystalline dihydrochloride pentahydrate, molecular weight 495, and is stable in the dry state for 36 months.

Actions: Spectinomycin hydrochloride is an inhibitor of protein synthesis in the bacterial cell; the site of action is the 30S ribosomal subunit.

In vitro studies have shown spectinomycin hydrochloride to be active against most strains of *Neisseria gonorrhoeae* (minimum inhibitory concentration < 7.5 to 20 mcg/ml).

Definitive *in vitro* studies have shown no cross-resistance of *N. gonorrhoeae* between streptinomycin hydrochloride and penicillin.

The antibiotic is not significantly bound to plasma protein.

Indications: *Trobicin* Sterile Powder (spectinomycin hydrochloride) is indicated in the treatment of acute gonorrheal urethritis and proctitis in the male and acute gonorrheal cervicitis and proctitis in the female when due to susceptible strains of *Neisseria gonorrhoeae.* Men and women with known recent exposure to gonorrhea should be treated as those known to have gonorrhea.

The *in vitro* susceptibility of *Neisseria gonorrhoeae* to spectinomycin hydrochloride can be tested by agar dilution methods. *Trobicin* Susceptibility Powder is available for this purpose, and its package insert should be consulted for details.

Contraindications: The use of *Trobicin* Sterile Powder (spectinomycin hydrochloride) is contraindicated in patients previously found hypersensitive to it.

Warnings: Spectinomycin hydrochloride is not effective in the treatment of syphilis. Antibiotics used in high doses for short periods of time to treat gonorrhea may mask or delay the symptoms of incubating syphilis. Since the treatment of syphilis demands prolonged therapy with any effective antibiotic, patients being treated for gonorrhea should be closely observed clinically. All patients with gonorrhea should have a serologic test for syphilis at the time of diagnosis. Patients treated with spectinomycin hydrochloride should have a follow-up serologic test for syphilis after three months.

Usage in pregnancy: Safety for use in pregnancy has not been established.

Usage in infants and children: Safety for use in infants and children has not been established.

Precautions: The usual precautions should be observed with atopic individuals.

The clinical effectiveness of *Trobicin* Sterile Powder (spectinomycin hydrochloride) should be monitored to detect evidence of development of resistance by *Neisseria gonorrhoeae.*

Adverse Reactions: The following reactions were observed during the single dose clinical trials: soreness at the injection site, urticaria, dizziness, nausea, chills, fever and insomnia.

During multiple dose subchronic tolerance studies in normal human volunteers, the following were noted: a decrease in hemoglobin, hematocrit and creatinine clearance; elevation of alkaline phosphatase, BUN and SGPT. In single and multiple dose studies in normal volunteers, a reduction in urine output was noted. Extensive renal function studies demonstrated no consistent changes indicative of renal toxicity.

Although no clearly defined case of anaphylaxis has been reported with *Trobicin* Sterile Powder, the possibility of such reactions should be considered particularly when using antibiotics.

Dosage and Administration:

Preparation of Drug for Intramuscular Injection

Trobicin Sterile Powder, 2 gram (spectinomycin hydrochloride): reconstitute with 3.2 ml of the accompanying diluent.*

Trobicin Sterile Powder 4 gram: reconstitute with 6.2 ml of the accompanying diluent.*

*Bacteriostatic Water for Injection with Benzyl Alcohol 0.945% w/v.

Shake vials vigorously immediately after adding diluent and before withdrawing dose. It is recommended that disposable syringes and needles be used to avoid contamination with penicillin residue, especially when treating patients known to be highly sensitive to penicillin. **Use of 20 gauge needle is recommended.**

Dosage

Intramuscular injections should be made deep into the upper outer quadrant of the gluteal muscle.

Adults (Men and Women)—Inject 5 ml intramuscularly for a 2 gram dose. This is also the recommended dose for patients being treated after failure of previous antibiotic therapy.

In geographic areas where antibiotic resistance is known to be prevalent, initial treatment with 4 grams (10 ml) intramuscularly is preferred. The 10 ml injection may be divided between two gluteal injection sites.

Storage Conditions: Store unreconstituted product at controlled room temperature 15°–30°C (59°–86°F). Store prepared suspension at controlled room temperature 15°–30°C (59°–86°F) and use within 24 hours.

How Supplied: *Trobicin* Sterile Powder (spectinomycin hydrochloride) is available as:

***Trobicin* Sterile Powder, 2 gram vial—with one ampoule of Bacteriostatic Water for Injection with Benzyl Alcohol 0.945% w/v added as preservative.** When reconstituted with 3.2 ml of the accompanying diluent, each vial yields a sufficient quantity for withdrawal of 5 ml of a suspension containing 400 mg spectinomycin per ml (as the hydrochloride). 5 ml provides 2 grams spectinomycin. For intramuscular use only.

NDC 0009-0566-01

***Trobicin* Sterile Powder 4 gram vial—with one ampoule of Bacteriostatic Water for Injection with Benzyl Alcohol 0.945% w/v added as preservative.** When reconstituted with 6.2 ml of the accompanying diluent, each vial yields a sufficient quantity for withdrawal of 10 ml of a suspension containing spectinomycin hydrochloride equivalent to 400 mg spectinomycin per ml. 10 ml provides 4 grams spectinomycin. For intramuscular use only.

NDC 0009-0592-01

***Trobicin* Susceptibility Powder**—100 mg. See package insert for *in vitro* testing procedure.

Human Pharmacology: *Trobicin* Sterile Powder (spectinomycin hydrochloride) is rapidly absorbed after intramuscular injection. A single, two gram injection produces peak serum concentrations averaging about 100 mcg/ml at one hour; a single, four gram injection produces peak serum concentrations averaging 160 mcg/ml at two hours. Average serum concentrations of 15 mcg/ml for the two gram dose and 31 mcg/ml for the four gram dose were present eight hours after dosing.

Code 810 130 003

UNICAP® Capsules/Tablets

(See PDR For Nonprescription Drugs)

UNICAP CHEWABLE® Tablets

(See PDR For Nonprescription Drugs)

UNICAP M® Tablets

(See PDR For Nonprescription Drugs)

UNICAP PLUS IRON® Tablets

(See PDR For Nonprescription Drugs)

UNICAP SENIOR® Tablets

(See PDR For Nonprescription Drugs)

UNICAP T® Tablets

(See PDR For Nonprescription Drugs)

XANAX® Tablets Ⓒ
(alprazolam)

Description: *Xanax* Tablets contain alprazolam which is a triazolo analog of the 1,4 benzodiazepine class of central nervous system-active compounds.

The chemical name of alprazolam is 8-Chloro-1-methyl-6-phenyl-4H-s-triazolo[4,3-α][1,4]benzodiazepine.

Alprazolam is a white crystalline powder, soluble in methanol or ethanol but with no appreciable solublity in water at physiological pH.

Each *Xanax* tablet, for oral administration, contains, 0.25, 0.5 or 1.0 mg of alprazolam.

Clinical Pharmacology: CNS agents of the 1,4 benzodiazepine class presumably exert their effects by binding at stereo specific receptors at several sites within the central nervous system. Their exact mechanism of action is unknown. Clinically, all benzodiazepines cause a dose-related central nervous system depressant activity varying from mild impairment of task performance to hypnosis.

Following oral administration, alprazolam is readily absorbed. Peak concentrations in the plasma occur in one to two hours following administration. Plasma levels are proportionate to the dose given; over the dose range of 0.5 to 3.0 mg, peak levels of 8.0 to 37 ng/ml were observed. The mean elimination half-life of alprazolam is 12–15 hours. The predominant metabolites are α-hydroxy-alprazolam and a benzophenone derived from alprazolam. The biological activity of α-hydroxy-alprazolam is approximately one-half that of alprazolam. The benzophenone metabolite is essentially inactive. Plasma levels of these metabolites are extremely low, thus precluding precise pharmacokinetic description. However, their half-lives appear to be of the same order of magnitude as alprazolam. Alprazolam and its metabolites are excreted primarily in the urine.

The ability of *Xanax* Tablets (alprazolam) to induce human hepatic enzyme systems has not yet been determined. However, this is not a property of benzodiazepines in general. Further, *Xanax* did not affect the prothrombin or plasma warfarin levels in male volunteers administered sodium warfarin orally.

In vitro, alprazolam is bound (80 percent) to human serum protein.

Changes in the absorption, distribution, metabolism and excretion of benzodiazepines have been reported in a variety of disease states including alcoholism, impaired hepatic function and impaired renal function. Changes have also been demonstrated in geriatric patients. It has not yet been determined if similar changes occur in the pharmacokinetics of alprazolam.

Because of its similarity to other benzodiazepines, it is assumed that alprazolam undergoes transplacental passage and is excreted in human milk.

Indications and Usage: *Xanax* Tablets (alprazolam) are indicated for the management of anxiety disorders or the short-term relief of the symptoms of anxiety. Anxiety or tension associated with the stress of everyday life usually does not require treatment with an anxiolytic. Anxiety associated with depression is also responsive to *Xanax.*

The effectiveness of *Xanax* for long-term use, that is, more than four months, has not been established by systematic clinical trials. The physician should periodically reassess the usefulness of the drug for the individual patient.

Contraindications: *Xanax* Tablets (alprazolam) are contraindicated in patients with known sensitivity to this drug or other benzodiazepines. It may be used in patients with open angle glaucoma who are receiving appropriate therapy, but is contraindicated in acute narrow angle glaucoma.

Continued on next page

Upjohn—Cont.

Warnings: *Xanax* Tablets (alprazolam) are not of value in the treatment of psychotic patients and should not be employed in lieu of appropriate treatment for psychosis. Because of its depressant CNS effects, patients receiving *Xanax* should be cautioned against engaging in hazardous occupations requiring complete mental alertness such as operating machinery or driving a motor vehicle. For the same reason, patients should be cautioned about the simultaneous ingestion of alcohol and other CNS depressant drugs during treatment with *Xanax*.

Benzodiazepines can potentially cause fetal harm when administered to pregnant women. If *Xanax* is used during pregnancy, or if the patient becomes pregnant while taking this drug, the patient should be appraised of the potential hazard to the fetus. Because of experience with other members of the benzodiazepine class, *Xanax* is assumed to be capable of causing an increased risk of congenital abnormalities when administered to a pregnant woman during the first trimester. Because use of these drugs is rarely a matter of urgency, their use during the first trimester should almost always be avoided. The possibility that a woman of childbearing potential may be pregnant at the time of institution of therapy should be considered. Patients should be advised that if they become pregnant during therapy or intend to become pregnant they should communicate with their physicians about the desirability of discontinuing the drug.

Precautions

General: If *Xanax* Tablets (alprazolam) are to be combined with other psychotropic agents or anticonvulsant drugs, careful consideration should be given to the pharmacology of the agents to be employed—particularly with compounds which might potentiate the action of benzodiazepines (See Drug Interaction Section).

As with other psychotropic medications, the usual precautions with respect to administration of the drug and size of the prescription are indicated for severely depressed patients or those in whom there is reason to expect concealed suicidal ideation or plans.

In elderly and debilitated patients, it is recommended that the dosage be limited to the smallest effective amount to preclude the development of ataxia or oversedation (See Dosage and Administration Section). The usual precautions in treating patients with impaired renal or hepatic function should be observed.

Information for Patients: To assure safe and effective use of benzodiazepines, the following information and instructions should be given to patients:

1) Inform your physician about any alcohol consumption and medicine you are taking now, including drugs you may buy without a prescription. Alcohol should generally not be used during treatment with benzodiazepines.

2) Inform your physician if you are planning to become pregnant, if you are pregnant, or if you become pregnant while you are taking this medication.

3) Inform your physician if you are nursing.

4) Until you experience how this medication affects you, do not drive a car or operate potentially dangerous machinery, etc.

5) If benzodiazepines are used in large doses and/or for extended periods of time, they may produce habituation and emotional and physical dependence. Therefore, do not increase the dose even if you think the drug "does not work anymore."

6) Do not stop taking the drug abruptly without consulting your physician, since withdrawal symptoms can occur.

Laboratory Tests: Laboratory tests are not ordinarily required in otherwise healthy patients.

Drug interactions: The benzodiazepines, including *Xanax*, produce additive CNS depressant effects when co-administered with other psychotropic medications, anticonvulsants, anti-histaminics, ethanol and other drugs which themselves produce CNS depression.

Pharmacokinetic interactions with benzodiazepines have been reported. For example, cimetidine has been reported to reduce diazepam clearance. However, it is not known at this time whether a similar interaction occurs with *Xanax*.

Drug/Laboratory Test Interactions: Although interactions between benzodiazepines and commonly employed clinical laboratory tests have occasionally been reported, there is no consistent pattern for a specific drug or specific test.

Carcinogenesis, Mutagenesis, Impairment of Fertility: No evidence of carcinogenic potential was observed in rats during a 24-month study with alprazolam in doses up to 375 times the human dose.

Alprazolam was not mutagenic in the rat micronucleus test at doses up to 1250 times the human dose.

Alprazolam produced no impairment of fertility in rats at doses up to 62.5 times the human dose.

Pregnancy: Teratogenic Effects: Pregnancy Category D: (See Warnings Section)

Nonteratogenic Effects: It is to be considered that the child born of a mother who is on benzodiazepines may be at some risk for withdrawal symptoms from the drug during the postnatal period. Also, neonatal flaccidity has been reported in children born of a mother who has been receiving benzodiazepines.

Labor and Delivery: *Xanax* has no established use in labor or delivery.

Nursing Mothers: Benzodiazepines are known to be excreted in human milk. It is to be assumed that alprazolam is as well. Chronic administration of diazepam to nursing mothers has been reported to cause their infants to become lethargic and lose weight. As a general rule, nursing should not be undertaken by mothers who must use *Xanax*.

Pediatric Use: Safety and effectiveness in children below the age of 18 have not been established.

Adverse Reactions: Side effects to *Xanax* Tablets (alprazolam), if they occur are generally observed at the beginning of therapy and usually disappear upon continued medication. In the usual patient, the most frequent side effects are likely to be an extension of the pharmacological activity of *Xanax*, e.g. drowsiness or lightheadedness.

The figures cited below are statistically adjusted estimates of untoward clinical event incidence among subjects who participated in the relatively short duration (i.e., four weeks) placebo-controlled clinical trials of *Xanax*. The figures cannot be used to predict precisely the incidence of untoward events in the course of usual medical practice where patient characteristics, and other factors often differ from those which obtained in the clinical trials. These figures cannot be compared with those obtained from other clinical studies involving related drug products and placebo as each group of drug trials are conducted under a different set of conditions.

Comparison of the cited figures, however, can provide the prescriber with some basis for estimating the relative contributions of drug and non-drug factors to the untoward event incidence rate in the population studied. Even this use must be approached cautiously, as a drug may relieve a symptom in one patient while inducing it in others. [For example, an anxiolytic drug may relieve dry mouth (a symptom of anxiety) in some subjects but induces (an untoward event) in others.]

Additionally, the cited figures can provide the prescriber with an indication as to the frequency with which physician intervention (e.g. increased surveillance, decreased dosage or discontinuation of drug therapy) may be necessary because of the untoward clinical event.

[See table on next page].

In addition to the relatively common (i.e., greater than 1%) untoward events enumerated above, the following adverse events have been reported in association with the use of anxiolytic benzodiazepines: dystonia, irritability, concentration difficulties, anorexia, loss of coordination, fatigue, sedation, slurred speech, jaundice, musculoskeletal weakness, pruritus, diplopia, dysarthria, changes in libido, menstrual irregularities, incontinence and urinary retention.

As with all benzodiazepines, paradoxical reactions such as stimulation, agitation, increased muscle spasticity, sleep disturbances, hallucinations and other adverse behavioral effects may occur in rare instances and in a random fashion. Should these occur, use of the drug should be discontinued.

Laboratory analyses were performed on all patients participating in the *Xanax* clinical program. The following incidences of abnormalities were observed in patients receiving *Xanax* and the corresponding placebo group. None of these changes were considered to be of physiological significance.

	Xanax		Placebo	
	Low	High	Low	High
Hematology				
Hematocrit	*	*	*	*
Hemoglobin	*	*	*	*
Total WBC Count	1.4	2.3	1.0	2.0
Neutrophil Count	2.3	3.0	4.2	1.7
Lymphocyte Count	5.5	7.4	5.4	9.5
Monocyte Count	5.3	2.8	6.4	*
Eosinophil Count	3.2	9.5	3.3	7.2
Basophil Count	*	*	*	*
Urinalysis				
Albumin	—	*	—	*
Sugar	—	*	—	*
RBC/HPF	—	3.4	—	5.0
WBC/HPF	—	25.7	—	25.9
Blood Chemistry				
Creatinine	2.2	1.9	3.5	1.0
Bilirubin	*	1.6	*	*
SGOT	*	3.2	1.0	1.8
Alkaline Phosphatase	*	1.7	*	1.8

* Less than 1%

When *Xanax* treatment is protracted, periodic blood counts, urinalysis and blood chemistry analyses are advisable.

Minor changes in EEG patterns, usually low-voltage fast activity have been observed in patients during therapy with *Xanax* and are of no known significance.

Drug Abuse and Dependence

Physical and Psychological Dependence: Withdrawal symptoms (similar in character to those noted with barbiturates and alcohol) have occurred following abrupt discontinuance of benzodiazepines. (These can range from mild dysphoria and insomnia to a major syndrome which may include abdominal and muscle cramps, vomiting, sweating, tremor and convulsions). These signs and symptoms, especially the more serious ones, are generally more common in those patients who have received excessive doses over an extended period of time. However, withdrawal symptoms have also been reported following abrupt discontinuance of benzodiazepines taken continuously, at therapeutic levels, for several months. Consequently, after extended therapy abrupt discontinuation should generally be avoided and a gradual tapering in dosage followed.

	Treatment Emergent Symptom Incidence *Xanax*	Treatment Emergent Symptom Incidence Placebo	Incidence of Intervention Because of Symptoms *Xanax*
Number of Patients	**565**	**505**	**565**
% of Patients Reporting:			
Central Nervous System			
Drowsiness	41.0	21.6	15.1
Light-headedness	20.8	19.3	1.2
Depression	13.9	18.1	2.4
Headache	12.9	19.6	1.1
Confusion	9.9	10.0	0.9
Insomnia	8.9	18.4	1.3
Nervousness	4.1	10.3	1.1
Syncope	3.1	4.0	*
Dizziness	1.8	0.8	2.5
Akathisia	1.6	1.2	*
Tiredness/ Sleepiness	*	*	1.8
Gastrointestinal			
Dry Mouth	14.7	13.3	0.7
Constipation	10.4	11.4	0.9
Diarrhea	10.1	10.3	1.2
Nausea/ Vomiting	9.6	12.8	1.7
Increased Salivation	4.2	2.4	*
Cardiovascular			
Tachycardia/ Palpitations	7.7	15.6	0.4
Hypotension	4.7	2.2	*
Sensory			
Blurred Vision	6.2	6.2	0.4
Musculoskeletal			
Rigidity	4.2	5.3	*
Tremor	4.0	8.8	0.4
Cutaneous			
Dermatitis/ Allergy	3.8	3.1	0.6
Other			
Nasal Congestion	7.3	9.3	*
Weight Gain	2.7	2.7	*
Weight Loss	2.3	3.0	*

* None reported

Patients with a history of seizures or epilepsy, regardless of their concomitant anti-seizure drug therapy, should not be abruptly withdrawn from any CNS depressant agent, including *Xanax* Tablets (alprazolam). Addiction-prone individuals (such as drug addicts or alcoholics) should be under careful surveillance when receiving alprazolam or other psychotropic agents because of the predisposition of such patients to habituation and dependence.

Controlled Substance Class: *Xanax* is a controlled substance under the Controlled Substance Act by the Drug Enforcement Administration and has been assigned to Schedule IV.

Overdosage: Manifestations of *Xanax* Tablets (alprazolam) overdosage include somnolence, confusion, impaired coordination, diminished reflexes and coma.

No delayed reactions (e.g. organ toxicity) or clinical laboratory abnormalities have been reported.

The acute oral LD_{50} in rats is 331–2171 mg/kg. Other experiments in animals have indicated that cardiopulmonary collapse can occur following massive intravenous doses of alprazolam (over 195 mg/kg; 2000 times the maximum usual daily human dose). Animals could be resuscitated with positive mechanical ventilation and the intravenous infusion of levarterenol.

Animal experiments have suggested that forced diuresis or hemodialysis are probably of little value in treating overdosage.

General Treatment of Overdose: Overdosage reports with *Xanax* are limited. Respiration, pulse, and blood pressure should be monitored, as in all cases of drug overdosage. General supportive measures should be employed, along with immediate gastric lavage. Intravenous fluids should be administered and an adequate airway maintained. Hypotension may be combated by the use of Levophed (levarterenol) or Aramine (metaraminol). Dialysis is of limited value. As with the management of intentional overdosing with any drug, it should be borne in mind that multiple agents may have been ingested.

Dosage and Administration: Dosage should be individualized for maximum beneficial effect. While the usual daily dosages given below will meet the needs of most patients, there will be some who require higher doses. In such cases, dosage should be increased cautiously to avoid adverse effects.

Daily Dosage Schedule: The usual starting dose is 0.25 to 0.5 mg, given three times daily. This may be titrated according to the needs of the patient to a maximum total daily dose of 4 mg, given in divided doses.

In the elderly, or in the presence of debilitating disease, the usual starting dose is 0.25 mg, given two or three times daily. This may be gradually increased if needed and tolerated.

If side effects occur with the starting dose, the dose should be lowered.

How Supplied:

Xanax Tablets (alprazolam), ovoid-shaped and scored, are available as follows:

0.25 mg (white)
Bottles of 100 **NDC** 0009-0029-01
Unit-Dose Pkg (100) **NDC** 0009-0029-09

0.5 mg (peach)
Bottles of 100 **NDC** 0009-0055-01
Unit-Dose Pkg (100) **NDC** 0009-0055-02

1 mg (lavender)
Bottles of 100 **NDC** 0009-0090-01
Unit-Dose Pkg (100) **NDC** 0009-0090-02

Store at controlled room temperature 15°–30°C (59°–86°F).

Caution: Federal law prohibits dispensing without prescription.

Animal Studies: When rats were treated with alprazolam at 3, 10, and 30 mg/kg/day (37.5 to 375 times the maximum recommended human dose) orally for 2 years, a tendency for a dose related increase in the number of cataracts was observed in females and a tendency for a dose related increase in corneal vascularization was observed in males. These lesions did not appear until after 11 months of treatment.

Clinical Studies: *Xanax* Tablets (alprazolam) were compared to placebo in double blind clinical trials in patients with a diagnosis of anxiety or anxiety with associated depressive symptomatology. *Xanax* was significantly better than placebo at each of the evaluation periods of these four week studies as judged by the psychometric instruments: Physician's Global Impressions, Hamilton Anxiety Rating Scale Target Symptoms, Patient's Global Impressions and Self-Rating Symptom Scale.

Code 811 557 000

[*Shown in Product Identification Section*]

IDENTIFICATION PROBLEM?

Consult PDR's

Product Identification Section

where you'll find over 900

products pictured actual size

and in full color.

Upsher-Smith Laboratories, Inc.

14905 23RD AVE., NORTH
MINNEAPOLIS, MN 55441

ACETAMINOPHEN UNISERTS® OTC

Rectal Suppositories

Description: Acetaminophen Uniserts suppositories are supplied in 120 mg. (pediatric), 325 mg. and 650 mg. strengths. Acetaminophen Uniserts are foil strip-wrapped and unit dose labeled.

Indications: For the temporary relief of fever, minor aches, pains and headaches.

Dosage: Adults—One 650 mg. suppository every 4 to 6 hours. No more than a total of 6 suppositories in any 24-hour period.

Children (over 6)—One 325 mg. suppository every 4 to 6 hours. No more than a total of 8 suppositories in any 24-hour period.

Children (3 to 6)—One 120 mg. (pediatric) suppositories every 4 to 6 hours. No more than a total of 6 suppositories in any 24-hour period.

Children (under 3)—Consult a physician.

Warning: Severe or recurrent pain or high or continued fever may be indicative of serious illness. Under these conditions, consult a physician. Do not use consistently for more than 2 days except on the advice of a physician.

How Supplied: 120 mg., 325 mg., boxes of 12 and 50. 650 mg., boxes of 12, 50 and 500.

Continued on next page

Upsher-Smith—Cont.

HISTATAPP® ELIXIR ℞

Composition: Each 5cc contains: Brompheniramine Maleate, 4 mg.; Phenylephrine HCl, 5 mg.; Phenylpropanolamine HCl, 5 mg.
How Supplied: Grape flavored elixir in 4 fl. oz., pints and gallons.

HISTATAPP® T.D. TABLETS ℞

Composition: Each timed disintegration tablet contains: Brompheniramine Maleate, 12 mg.; Phenylephrine HCl, 15 mg.; Phenylpropanolamine HCl, 15 mg.
How Supplied: Light blue tablets in bottles of 100 and 500; unit dose boxes of 100.

KLOR-10%™ ℞
(potassium chloride oral solution, USP 10%)

How Supplied: 4 fl. oz., pints and gallons.

KLOR-CON® 20% ℞
(potassium chloride oral solution, USP 20%)

How Supplied: 4 fl. oz., pints and gallons.

KLOR-CON® Powder ℞
(Potassium Chloride for Oral Solution, U.S.P.) 20 mEq. (1.5g) per packet

Description: Each packet contains 1.5g potassium chloride providing potassium 20 mEq and chloride 20 mEq. Fruit-flavored with artificial color and sweetener (saccharin) added.
Indications: Treatment of potassium deficiency which may occur with long-term diuretic therapy, corticosteroid therapy, digitalis intoxication, low dietary intake of potassium or loss of potassium due to vomiting and diarrhea.
Contraindications: Renal impairment, untreated Addison's disease, dehydration, heat cramps and hyperkalemia. Potassium chloride should not be employed in patients receiving potassium-sparing agents such as aldosterone antagonists and triamterene.
Precautions: Potassium chloride must be administered with caution since the degree of potassium deficiency and the corresponding daily dosage is often not accurately known. Excessive or even therapeutic dosages may result in potassium intoxication. The patient should be checked frequently and periodic ECG and/or plasma potassium levels made. High plasma concentrations of potassium ion may cause cardiac depression, arrhythmias or arrest. Use with caution in the presence of cardiac disease. Patients should be cautioned to adhere to dilution instructions.
Adverse Reactions: Vomiting, diarrhea, nausea and abdominal discomfort may occur. Symptoms and signs of potassium intoxication include mental confusion, listlessness, paresthesias of the extremities, flaccid paralysis, weakness of the legs, fall in blood pressure, cardiac arrhythmias and heart block. Hyperkalemia, when detected, must be treated promptly.
Dosage and Administration: The usual adult dose is 20 to 80 mEq of potassium per day (1 packet 1 to 4 times daily after meals.) The contents of 1 packet should be dissolved in at least 4 oz cold water or fruit juice. This preparation, like other potassium supplements, must be properly diluted to avoid the possibility of gastrointestinal irritation.
How Supplied: KLOR-CON Powder 20 mEq (1.5g) (Potassium Chloride). In cartons of 30 and 100 packets.

KLOR CON®/25 Powder ℞
(Potassium Chloride for Oral Solution, U.S.P.) 25 mEq. per packet

How Supplied: Cartons of 30 and 250 packets.

SSKI® ℞
(potassium iodide oral solution, U.S.P.)

Composition: Each 0.3ml. contains potassium iodide 300 mg.
Action and Uses: An expectorant in the symptomatic treatment of chronic pulmonary diseases where tenacious mucus complicates the problem, including bronchial asthma, bronchitis and pulmonary emphysema.
Contraindications: Contraindicated in patients with hyperthyroidism or known sensitivity to iodides.
Adverse Reactions: May include gastrointestinal upset, metallic taste, minor skin eruptions, nausea, vomiting and epigastric pain. If these symptoms develop, discontinue use.
Precautions: Caution is recommended in patients during pregnancy. In some patients prolonged use of iodides can lead to hypothyroidism.
Administration and Dosage: Adults, 0.3ml. or 0.6ml. diluted in one glassful of water 3 or 4 times daily.
How Supplied: In bottles of 1 oz. (calibrated dropper, marked to deliver 0.3ml. and 0.6ml.) and 8 oz.

TROFAN®
L-Tryptophan Tablets, 0.5 Gm.

Composition: Each white, capsule shaped tablet contains L-Tryptophan, 0.5 Gm. Trofan tablets are dye-free.
How Supplied: Trofan tablets 0.5 Gm. in bottles of 30 and 100.

The Vale Chemical Co., Inc.
**1201 LIBERTY ST.
ALLENTOWN, PA 18102**

GLYCOTUSS
(Guaifenesin)

(See PDR For Nonprescription Drugs)

Verex Laboratories, Inc.
**5241 SOUTH QUEBEC STREET
ENGLEWOOD, CO 80111**

HELP™ Tablets OTC
(Constant Ordered Release Phenylpropanolamine HCl)

Description: Each tablet contains 75 mg of phenylpropanolamine, uniquely formulated to control the release of the drug after ingestion. Phenylpropanolamine is a stimulant, related to ephedrine, but has less stimulant effect on the nervous system than amphetamine like diet capsules. Constant release rate means that the tablet will release the drug slowly, at a constant rate as it dissolves in the gastrointestinal tract.
Indications and Usage: This product is indicated as a temporary diet aid for those people who wish to lose weight. The tablet is designed to be used once daily, in the morning, along with a program of dietary management and caloric restrictions. HELP has no value in causing weight reduction other than controlling appetite. Taken alone without a proper program of dietary restriction, HELP will not cause weight loss.
Warning: Use in Pregnancy: This drug should not be used during pregnancy or by mothers who are breast feeding their baby.
Precautions: This product is intended for use only by adults. Do not exceed the recommended dose of one tablet daily.
If nervousness, dizziness, sleeplessness, rapid pulse or other symptoms of stimulation occur, stop taking the drug and notify your family doctor. People with high blood pressure, heart disease, or thyroid disorders should not take this medication except under the supervision of their physician. You should not use HELP if you are taking medication for high blood pressure. Some drugs used to treat mental depression will react in an unfavorable manner with HELP. Therefore if you are being treated with medication for depression, you should talk with your doctor before starting a diet program with this drug.
Side Effects: Side effects may occur with this product which are generally a result of the stimulant effects of the drug. Reported side effects are nausea, dry nose, shaking of the hands and general irritability.
Drug Overdose: In case of accidental or intentional drug overdose, call your doctor, or contact a poison control center immediately.
Adult Dosage: One HELP tablet daily in the morning with a full glass of water or fruit juice. It is recommended that a person not take this medication longer than 60 days or as a continuous form of diet control. This product should not be used by children under 12 years of age.
How Supplied: HELP™, 75 mg. orange capsule shaped tablets embossed with the word HELP. Available in boxes of 30. (NDC 51296-003-03)

VERIN™ 650 mg. TABLETS
Aspirin (Constant Release Rate Aspirin)

Description: Each tablet contains 650 mg (10 grs) of aspirin, specially formulated to control the release rate of aspirin after ingestion. Constant release rate, means, that the tablet will release the aspirin slowly, at a constant rate, into the blood stream as it dissolves in the gastrointestinal tract.
Indications and Usage: VERIN is indicated for the treatment of osteoarthritis, rheumatoid arthritis, bursitis, tendinitis and menstrual cramps when used under the supervision of a physician. VERIN may be used by the patient for the temporary relief of pain associated with arthritis, tendinitis, bursitis or menstrual cramps. However, this drug should not be used longer than 10 days, unless the product is being used as directed by a physician. Because VERIN works slowly over a period of time, it is not recommended as a treatment for headache, muscle pains or feverish conditions.
Contraindications: This drug should not be taken by persons known to be allergic to salicylates or individuals with advanced kidney disease.
Warnings: Use in Pregnancy: VERIN, or other aspirin containing products should not be used by a woman when pregnant, except as directed by her physician.
Precautions: Many non-prescription items contain aspirin, salicylates or other aspirin like products. Precaution should be used when taking VERIN with any other non prescription drug. If you are taking VERIN, make sure you tell your doctor. People who have a recent history of gastritis or peptic ulcer should use this drug with caution. This product should not be used if you have a bleeding tendency or are taking anticoagulant drugs.
Side Effects:
Blood
Aspirin may interfere with blood clotting. Patients with a history of blood coagulation problems or individuals receiving anticoagulant drugs should avoid VERIN. Aspirin used chronically may cause an iron deficiency anemia.

Stomach
Aspirin may irritate peptic ulcers and cause heartburn. In some people, aspirin can cause a large amount of bleeding due to erosions and ulcers in the stomach and small intestine. VERIN is released slowly, and the greatest amount of active drug is released in the small intestine over a period of time, subsequently there are less gastrointestinal side effects with this form of constant release rate aspirin. For this reason, individuals who have had gastrointestinal related side effects with other aspirin preparations may tolerate VERIN.
Allergic
Allergic reactions have been noted with aspirin products. People with known sensitivity to aspirin or salicylate type drugs should not take VERIN.
Ears-Hearing
Aspirin when given in high doses may produce ringing or a buzzing noise in the ears.
Drug Interactions
Aspirin may interfere with some anticoagulant or antidiabetic drugs. Drugs to lower uric acid in patients with gout are blocked by the simultaneous use of aspirin. Some anti-arthritic drugs may produce irritation of the stomach, this effect is aggravated by aspirin. Alcohol and aspirin do not mix! Together, alcohol and aspirin may cause irritation, erosion and/or gastrointestinal bleeding.
Drug Overdose: In case of an accidental or intentional drug overdosage, call your doctor, or contact a poison control center immediately.
Dosage and Administration:
In order to achieve a constant release rate, VERIN tablets should be swallowed whole. Breaking the tablets will alter the release profile of the drug.
Adult Dosage: For mild to moderate pain associated with rheumatoid arthritis, osteoarthritis, tendinitis, bursitis as well as menstrual cramps, the initial dose of VERIN is 1300 mg (two 650 mg tablets) taken twice a day, in the morning and evening. Because VERIN releases the drug into the blood stream over 12–14 hours, the tablets need only be taken twice a day. Dosage may be increased or decreased depending upon the severity of the pain. However, you should not take more than 6 tablets in any 24 hour period. Do not continue the drug for more than 10 days unless your doctor has advised you to do so.
Dosage for Children: This drug is not intended for use in children below the age of 12 years, except at the specific direction of a physician
How Supplied: VERIN™, 650 mg white capsule shaped tablets embossed with the word VERIN. Available in bottles of 100. (NDC 51296-001-01)

Vicks Toiletry Products Division

RICHARDSON-VICKS INC.
TEN WESTPORT ROAD
WILTON, CT 06897

CLEARASIL® Super Strength Acne Treatment Cream (10% Benzoyl Peroxide) Vanishing and Tinted

(See PDR For Nonprescription Drugs)

CLEARASIL® 5% Benzoyl Peroxide Lotion Acne Treatment

(See PDR For Nonprescription Drugs)

CLEARASIL® Pore Deep Cleanser (Salicylic Acid 0.5%)

(See PDR For Nonprescription Drugs)

DENQUEL® Sensitive Teeth Toothpaste Desensitizing Dentifrice

(See PDR For Nonprescription Drugs)

TOPEX® 10% Benzoyl Peroxide Lotion Buffered* Acne Medication

***With special emollients to help prevent the overdrying effects of benzoyl peroxide**

(See PDR For Nonprescription Drugs)

Vicks Health Care Division

RICHARDSON-VICKS INC.
TEN WESTPORT ROAD
WILTON, CT 06897

DAYCARE® LIQUID DAYCARE® CAPSULES

Multi-Symptom Colds Medicine

Active Ingredients: LIQUID—per fluid ounce (2 tbs.) or CAPSULE—per **two** capsules, contains Acetaminophen 650mg., Dextromethorphan HBr 20mg., Phenylpropanolamine HCl 25mg. DAYCARE LIQUID also contains Alcohol 10%.
Indications: For temporary relief of major colds symptoms as follows:
Nasal congestion, coughing, aches and pains, fever, and cough irritated throat of a cold or flu without drowsy side effects.
Actions: VICKS DAYCARE is a decongestant, antitussive, analgesic and antipyretic. It helps clear stuffy nose, congested sinus openings. Calms, quiets coughing. Eases headache pain and the ache-all-over feeling. Reduces fever due to colds and flu. It relieves these symptoms without drowsiness. DAYCARE LIQUID is also a demulcent, it sooths a cough irritated throat.
Warning: Do not administer to children under 6 years of age unless directed by a physician. Persistent cough may indicate the presence of a serious condition. Persons with a high fever or persistent cough or with high blood pressure, diabetes, heart or thyroid disease should not use this preparation unless directed by a physician. Do not use more than ten days unless directed by a physician.
Do not exceed recommended dosage unless directed by a physician. As with all medication, keep out of reach of children.
Symptoms and Treatment of Overdosage: These symptoms are based upon medical judgement, not on actual experience, since no significant incidence of overdose has been brought to our attention in clinical or consumer experience. Ingestion of very large amounts may cause dizziness, drowsiness, nausea, diarrhea, insomnia, nervousness, anxiety, tremors, tachycardia, extrasystoles, headache, sweating, confusion and delerium. Treatment is symptomatic, with bedrest and observation.
Dosage:
ADULTS one fluid ounce (2 tbs.) LIQUID, or 2 CAPSULES.
CHILDREN (6 to 12 years) One-half ounce (1 tbs.) LIQUID, or 1 CAPSULE every 4 hours. Maximum 4 doses per day.
How Supplied: Available in: **LIQUID** with child resistant cap—6 and 10 fl. oz. bottles; **CAPSULES** in child resistant packages—8 (trial size), 20, 36 and 60.

FORMULA 44® COUGH CONTROL DISCS

Active Ingredients per disc: Dextromethorphan equivalent to Dextromethorphan Hydrobromide 5 mg., Benzocaine 1.25 mg., Special Vicks Medication (menthol, anethole, peppermint oil) 0.35% in a dark brown sugar base.
Indications: Provides temporary relief from coughs and relieves throat irritation caused by colds, flu, bronchitis.
Actions: VICKS FORMULA 44 COUGH CONTROL DISCS are antitussive, local anesthetic and demulcent cough drops. They calm, quiet coughs and help coat and soothe irritated throats.
Warning: Do not exceed recommended dosage. Do not administer to children under 4 unless directed by physician. Persistent cough may indicate presence of a serious condition. Persons with high fever or persistent cough should not use this preparation unless directed by physician. As with all medication, keep out of reach of children.
Symptoms and Treatment of Overdosage: These symptoms are based upon medical judgement, not on actual experience, since no significant incidence of overdose has been brought to our attention in clinical or consumer experience. Though unlikely, ingestion of large amounts may cause dizziness, drowsiness, nausea, vomiting, diarrhea, central excitement and a possibility of cyanosis in young children. Treatment is symptomatic, with bedrest and observation.
Dosage:
ADULTS (12 years and over) 2 discs. Dissolve in mouth. Two additional discs every three hours as needed.
CHILDREN (4 to 12 years) 1 disc. Dissolve in mouth. One additional disc every three hours as needed.
How Supplied: Available as individual foil wrapped portable packets in boxes of 24.

FORMULA 44® COUGH MIXTURE

Active Ingredients per 2 tsp. (10 ml.): Dextromethorphan Hydrobromide 15 mg., Doxylamine Succinate 7.5 mg., Sodium Citrate 500 mg. in a pleasant tasting, dark brown syrup base. Also contains Alcohol 10%.
Indications: For the temporary relief of coughs due to colds, flu, bronchitis.
Actions: VICKS FORMULA 44 COUGH MIXTURE is an antitussive, antihistamine, demulcent and expectorant. Calms and quiets coughs. Reduces sneezing and sniffling. Coats, soothes irritated throat.
Warning: Do not exceed recommended dosage unless directed by a physician. Do not administer to children under 6 years of age unless directed by a physician. Persistent cough may indicate the presence of a serious condition. Persons with a high fever or persistent cough should not use the product unless directed by a physician. FORMULA 44 may cause drowsiness. Do not drive or operate machinery while taking the product. If relief does not occur within three days, discontinue use and consult a physician. As with all medication, keep out of reach of children.
Symptoms and Treatment of Overdosage: These symptoms are based on medical judgement and not on clinical experience, since no significant incidence of overdose has been brought to our attention in clinical or consumer experience. Presenting symptom is drowsiness. Nausea, vomiting, dizziness, ataxia, mydriasis and headache may ensue with ingestion of excessive amounts. Treatment is symptomatic, with bedrest and observation.
Dosage:
Adults: 12 years and over—2 teaspoonfuls
Children: 6 to 12 years: 1 teaspoonful
Repeat every 4 hours as needed.
No more than 6 doses per day.
How Supplied: Available in 3 fl. oz., 6 fl. oz. and 8 fl. oz. bottles.

FORMULA 44D® DECONGESTANT COUGH MIXTURE

Active Ingredients per 2 tsp. (10 ml): Dextromethorphan Hydrobromide 20 mg., Phenylpropanolamine Hydrochloride 25 mg., Guaifenesin 100 mg. in a red, cherry-flavored, cooling syrup. Also contains Alcohol 10%.

Continued on next page

Vicks Health Care—Cont.

Indications: Relieves coughs, decongests nasal passages and loosens upper chest congestion due to colds, flu, bronchitis.
Actions: VICKS FORMULA 44D is an antitussive, nasal decongestant, expectorant and demulcent. It calms, quiets coughs; relieves nasal congestion; loosens phlegm, mucus; and coats, soothes an irritated throat.
Warning: Do not exceed recommended dosage unless directed by physician. Do not administer to children under 2 years of age unless directed by physician. Persistent cough may indicate the presence of a serious condition. Persons with a high fever or persistent cough or with high blood pressure, diabetes, heart or thyroid disease should not use this preparation unless directed by physician. As with all medication, keep out of reach of children.
Symptoms and Treatment of Overdosage: These symptoms are based upon medical judgement, not on actual experience, since no signifcant incidence of overdose has been brought to our attention in clinical or consumer experience. Ingestion of large amounts may cause drowsiness, dizziness, nausea, vomiting, diarrhea, central excitement, restlessness, anxiety, sweating, tremor, extrasystoles, confusion and delerium. Treatment is symptomatic, with bedrest and observation.
Dosage:
ADULTS (12 years and over): 2 teaspoonfuls
CHILDREN (6–12 years): 1 teaspoonful
(2–6 years): ½ teaspoonful
No more than 6 doses per day. Repeat every 4 hours as needed.
How Supplied: Available in 3 fl. oz., 6 fl. oz. and 8 fl. oz. bottles.

HEADWAY® CAPSULES HEADWAY® TABLETS
For colds, sinus, allergy.

Active Ingredients per two capsules or tablets: Acetaminophen 650mg., Phenylpropanolamine HCl 37.5mg., Chlorpheniramine Maleate 4mg.
Indications: Relieves nasal congestion, runny nose, sneezing, itchy watery eyes, aches and pains caused by a cold, sinus or allergy problem.
Actions: HEADWAY is a nasal decongestant, antihistamine, analgesic and antipyretic. It provides hours of effective relief from symptoms of head colds, sinus and nasal allergies.
Warning: This preparation may cause excitability, especially in children. This medication may cause drowsiness. Avoid alcoholic beverages, driving a motor vehicle, and operating heavy machinery while taking this medication. Do not give to children under 6 years of age or exceed the recommended dosage unless directed by a physician. Persons having asthma, glaucoma, high blood pressure, heart disease, diabetes, thyroid disease, high fever, or difficulty in urination due to enlargement of the prostate gland should not use this product except under the advice and supervision of a physician. Do not use for more than 10 days unless directed by physician. In case of accidental overdose, seek professional assistance or contact a Poison Control Center immediately.
Symptoms and Treatment of Overdosage: These symptoms are based upon medical judgement, not on actual experience, since no significant incidence of overdose has been brought to our attention in clinical or consumer experience. Large overdoses may cause nausea, vomiting, drowsiness, dizziness, ataxia, mydriasis, insomnia, nervousness, tachycardia and headache. Treatment is symptomatic, with bedrest and observation.
Dosage:
ADULTS—2 capsules or tablets
CHILDREN (6-12 years) 1 capsule or tablet
Dose every 4 hours, not to exceed 4 doses per day.
How Supplied: Child-proof sealed packets. Available in 16, 36 and 48 sizes for Capsules and 20, 40 and 60 sizes for tablets.

NYQUIL®
Nighttime Colds Medicine in oral liquid form.

Active Ingredients per fluid oz. (2 tbs.): Acetaminophen 600 mg., Doxylamine Succinate 7.5 mg., Ephedrine Sulfate 8.0 mg., and Dextromethorphan Hydrobromide 15.0 mg. Also contains Alcohol 25%.
Indications: For the temporary relief of major colds symptoms, as follows: stuffy nose, sniffles and sneezing, aches and pains, and coughing.
Actions: Decongestant, antihistaminic, antitussive, analgesic. Helps decongest nasal passages and sinus openings, relieves sniffles and sneezing, eases aches and pains, reduces fever, soothes headache, minor sore throat pain, and quiets coughing due to a cold. By relieving these symptoms, also helps patient get to sleep to get the rest he needs.
Warning: This preparation may cause drowsiness. Do not drive or operate machinery while taking this medication. Do not give to children under ten, unless directed by physician. If relief does not occur within three days, discontinue use and consult physician. Reduce dosage if nervousness, restlessness or sleeplessness occurs. Do not use if high blood pressure, heart disease, diabetes or thyroid disease is present unless directed by physician.
Persistent cough may indicate a serious condition. Persons with a high fever or persistent cough should not use this preparation unless directed by a physician. Do not exceed recommended dosage. As with all medication, keep out of reach of children.
Symptoms and Treatment of Overdosage: These symptoms are based on medical judgement and not on actual clinical experience, since no significant incidence of overdose has been brought to our attention in clinical or consumer experience. Presenting symptom of overdosage is drowsiness. Large overdoses may cause emesis, ataxia, nausea, vomiting, restlessness, vertigo, dysuria, palpitations, tinnitus, diaphoresis, insomnia. Treatment is symptomatic, with bedrest and observation.
Dosage and Dosage Form: A green, anise-flavored oral liquid (syrup). A plastic measuring cup with 1 and 2 tablespoonful gradations is supplied.
ADULTS (12 and over): One fluid ounce (2 tablespoonfuls) at bedtime.
CHILDREN 10 to 12: One half ounce (1 tablespoonful) at bedtime.
If confined to bed or at home, a total of 4 doses may be taken per day, each 4 hours apart.
How Supplied: Available in 6 fl. oz. and 10 fl. oz. bottles.

SINEX™
Decongestant Nasal Spray

Active Ingredients: Phenylephrine Hydrochloride 0.5%, Cetylpyridinium Chloride 0.04%, Special Vicks Blend of Aromatics (menthol, eucalyptol, camphor, methyl salicylate). Also contains Thimerosal 0.001% as a preservative.
Indications: To provide temporary relief of nasal and sinus congestion of head colds and hay fever.
Actions: VICKS SINEX is a decongestant nasal spray. The product shrinks swollen membranes to restore freer breathing; gives fast relief of nasal stuffiness and congested sinus openings; allows congested sinuses to drain; and instantly cools irritated nasal passages.
Warning: Do not exceed recommended dosage. Follow directions for use carefully. For children under 6 years, consult your physician. If condition persists consult physician. As with all medication, keep out of reach of children.
Symptoms and Treatment of Ingestion: These symptoms are based upon medical judgement, not on actual experience, since no significant incidence of overdose or ingestion has been brought to our attention in clinical or consumer experience. Though unlikely, ingestion of very large amounts may cause restlessness, anxiety, ventricular arrhythmias, nausea and gastrointestinal upset. Treatment is symptomatic, with bedrest and observation.
Directions For Use: Keep head and dispenser upright. May be used every 3 hours as needed.
ADULTS: Spray quickly, firmly 2 times up each nostril, sniffing the spray upward.
CHILDREN 6 to 12 years: Spray 1 time up each nostril.
How Supplied: Available in ½ fl. oz. and 1 fl. oz. plastic spray bottles.

SINEX™ LONG-ACTING
Decongestant Nasal Spray

Active Ingredient: Oxymetazoline Hydrochloride 0.05% in an aqueous solution containing mentholated vapors. Also contains thimerosal 0.001% as a preservative.
Indications: For temporary relief of nasal congestion due to the common cold, hay fever or other upper respiratory allergies or nasal congestion associated with sinusitis.
Actions: Oxymetazoline constricts the arterioles of the nasal passages-resulting in a nasal decongestant effect which lasts up to twelve hours, restoring freer breathing through the nose. SINEX LONG-ACTING helps decongest sinus openings and sinus passages thus promoting sinus drainage.
Warning: Do not exceed recommended dosage because symptoms may occur such as burning, stinging, sneezing or increase of nasal discharge. Do not use the product for more than three days. If symptoms persist, consult a physician. The use of this dispenser by more than one person may spread infection. In case of accidental ingestion, seek professional assistance or contact a Poison Control Center immediately. As with all medication, keep out of reach of children.
Symptoms and Treatment of Oral Ingestion: These symptoms are based upon medical judgement, not on actual experience, since no significant incidence of overdose or ingestion has been brought to our attention in clinical or consumer experience. Depending upon the amount of oral ingestion, somnolence, sedation, or deep coma may occur. With excessive ingestion, profound CNS depression may be accompanied by hypertension, bradycardia, and decreased cardiac output, which may be followed by rebound hypotension and cardiovascular collapse. Prompt gastric evacuation and intensive supportive care is indicated following marked overdosage.
Dosage and Administration: With head upright, spray 2 or 3 times in each nostril twice daily (morning and evening) or as directed by a physician. Squeeze quickly, firmly, and sniff deeply. Not recommended for children under 6 years of age.
How Supplied: Available in ½ fl. oz. and 1 fl. oz. plastic spray bottles.

TEMPO®
Antacid with Antigas Action

Description: Each soft drop contains Calcium Carbonate 414 mg., Aluminum Hydroxide 133 mg., Magnesium Hydroxide 81 mg., Simethicone 20 mg.

—Acid consuming capacity: 14 mEq per drop
—Sodium content: 2.5 mg (0.11 mEq) per drop

Indications: Dissolves quickly as you chew to afford rapid relief from symptoms of acid indigestion; heartburn, sour eructations, belching, and associated gas symptoms.

Actions: TEMPO® is an antacid and antiflatulent in a pleasant tasting, spearmint flavored, soft drop, which dissolves quickly as it is chewed, providing rapid action. It has no chalky or gritty taste.

Directions for Use: Chew one TEMPO® antacid every two or three hours as symptoms occur or as directed by a physician.

Warning: Do not take more than 12 units in a 24-hour period or use the maximum dosage for more than two weeks except under the advice and supervision of a physician. Keep this and all drugs out of reach of children.

Drug Interaction Precaution: All aluminum-containing antacids, including TEMPO®, may prevent proper absorption of tetracycline. Do not take this product if you are presently taking any form of tetracycline.

How Supplied: Foil wrapped in cartons of 10, 30 or 60 drops. Each drop is individually wrapped and enclosed in a foil-lined pouch containing 5 drops.

VAPOSTEAM®
Liquid Medication for Hot Steam Vaporizers.

Active Ingredients: Polyoxyethylene Dodecanol 1.8%, Aromatics (eucalyptus oil, camphor, menthol) 12.4%, Tincture of Benzoin 5%, in a liquid vehicle. Also contains Alcohol 55%.

Indications: For the symptomatic relief of colds, coughs, chest congestion.

Actions: VAPOSTEAM increases the action of steam to help relieve colds symptoms in the following ways: relieves coughs of colds, even croupy coughs, eases stuffy nasal congestion, loosens phlegmy chest congestion, and moistens dry, irritated breathing passages.

Warning: VAPOSTEAM is for hot steam medication only. Do not ingest.

Persistent coughing may indicate the presence of a serious condition. If symptoms persist, discontinue use and consult physician. Persons with high fever or persistent cough should not use this preparation except as directed by a physician. Keep away from open flame or extreme heat. As with all medication, keep out of reach of children.

Symptoms and Treatment of Ingestion: Based on the medical literature and clinical judgement, ingestion of large amounts may cause nausea, vomiting, epigastric pain, discomfort and weakness, coma and death. Treatment should consist of cautious gastric lavage, barbiturates for convulsions, Metrazol for coma and supportive therapy as indicated.

Dosage and Administration: In a hot steam vaporizer: Use one tablespoonful of VAPOSTEAM with each quart of water added to the vaporizer. In an open bowl: Simply add VAPOSTEAM to any ordinary bowl of hot water—2 teaspoonfuls for each pint of water—and breathe in the medicated vapors.

How Supplied: Available in 4 fl. oz. and 6 fl. oz. bottles.

VATRONOL®
Nose Drops

Active Ingredients: Ephedrine Sulfate 0.5%, Special Vicks Aromatic Blend (menthol, eucalyptol, camphor, methyl salicylate) 0.06% in an aqueous base. Also contains Thimerosal 0.001% as a preservative.

Indications: Relieves nasal congestion caused by head colds and hay fever.

Actions: VICKS VATRONOL is a decongestant nose drop. It helps restore freer breathing by relieving nasal stuffiness and congested sinus openings. VATRONOL also cools irritated nasal passages.

Warning: Do not exceed recommended dosage. Overdosage may cause nervousness, restlessness, or sleeplessness. Do not use for more than 4 consecutive days or administer to children under 6, unless directed by a physician. As with all medication, keep out of reach of children.

Symptoms and Treatment of Ingestion: These symptoms are based upon medical judgement, not on actual experience, since no significant incidence of overdose or ingestion has been brought to our attention in clinical or consumer experience. Ingestion of very large quantities may cause restlessness, anxiety, sweating, tremor, rapid pulse, extrasystoles, confusion, delirium, nausea and gastrointestinal upset. Treatment is symptomatic, with bedrest and observation.

Dosage:
ADULTS: Fill dropper to upper mark.
CHILDREN (6–12 years): Fill dropper to lower mark.

Apply up one nostril, repeat in other nostril. Repeat every 4 hours as needed.

How Supplied: Available in ½ fl. oz. and 1 fl. oz. dropper bottles.

VICKS® COUGH SILENCERS
Cough Drops

Active Ingredients per lozenge: Dextromethorphan (expressed as Dextromethorphan Hydrobromide) 2.5 mg., Benzocaine 1 mg., Special Vicks Medication (menthol, anethole, peppermint oil) 0.35% in a cooling green, sugar base.

Indications: Provides all-day relief from coughs of colds, excessive smoking, dry or irritated throats when used as directed.

Actions: VICKS COUGH SILENCERS are antitussive, local anesthetic and demulcent throat lozenges.

Warning: Do not administer to children under 4 years of age unless directed by a physician. Severe or persistent cough, sore throat, or sore throat accompanied by fever, headache, nausea and vomiting may be serious. Consult physician promptly. Persons with a high fever or persistent cough should not use this preparation unless directed by a physician. As with all medication, keep out of reach of children.

Symptoms and Treatment of Overdosage: These symptoms are based upon medical judgement, not on actual experience, since no significant incidence of overdose has been brought to our attention in clinical or consumer experience. Though unlikely, ingestion of large quantities may cause dizziness, drowsiness, nausea, vomiting, gastrointestinal upset, diarrhea, central excitement, and a possibility of cyanosis in young children. Treatment is symptomatic, with bedrest and observation.

Dosage: Age 12 and over, 2 drops, dissolve in mouth one at a time, then 1 or 2 each hour as needed. Ages 4 to 12, 1 drop, dissolve in mouth then 1 drop each hour as needed. Do not exceed recommended dosage.

How Supplied: Available in boxes of 15's.

VICKS® COUGH SYRUP
Expectorant, Antitussive Cough Syrup

Active Ingredients per 3 tsp. (15 ml.): Dextromethorphan Hydrobromide 10.5 mg., Guaifenesin 75 mg., Sodium Citrate 600 mg. in a red, cherry-flavored, syrup base. Also contains Alcohol 5%.

Indications: Provides temporary relief of coughs due to colds, helps loosen phlegm and rid passageways of bothersome mucus, and soothes a cough-irritated throat.

Actions: VICKS COUGH SYRUP is an antitussive, expectorant and demulcent. It calms, quiets coughs of colds, flu and bronchitis; loosens phlegm, promotes drainage of bronchial tubes; and coats and soothes a cough irritated throat.

Warning: Do not exceed recommended dosage. Do not administer to children under 2 years of age unless directed by a physician. Persistent cough may indicate the presence of a serious condition. Persons with a high fever or persistent cough should not use this preparation unless directed by a physician. As with all medication, keep out of reach of children.

Symptoms and Treatment of Overdosage: These symptoms are based upon medical judgement, not on actual experience, since no significant incidence of overdose has been brought to our attention in clinical or consumer experience. Ingestion of large amounts may cause drowsiness, dizziness, nausea, vomiting, diarrhea, central excitement and alkalosis. Treatment is gastric lavage and symptomatic treatment with bedrest and observation.

Dosage:
ADULTS (12 years and over): 3 teaspoonfuls
CHILDREN (6–12 years): 2 teaspoonfuls
(2–6 years): 1 teaspoonful

Repeat every 4 hours as needed.

How Supplied: Available in 3 fl. oz. and 6 fl. oz. bottles.

VICKS® INHALER
with decongestant action

Active Ingredients per inhaler: l-Desoxyephedrine 50 mg., Special Vicks Medication (menthol, camphor, methyl salicylate, bornyl acetate) 150 mg.

Indications: Provides temporary relief of nasal congestion of colds and hay fever. Decongests sinus openings.

Actions: VICKS INHALER is an intranasal inhaled decongestant. It shrinks swollen membranes and provides fast relief from a stuffy nose.

Warning: As with all medication, keep out of reach of children.

Symptoms and Treatment of Ingestion: These symptoms are based upon medical judgement, not on actual experience, since no significant incidence of overdose or ingestion has been brought to our attention in clinical or consumer experience. Though VICKS INHALER is unlikely to be ingested, consumption of large quantities of its active ingredients may cause dizziness, nervousness, headache, tachycardia, nausea and vomiting. Treatment is symptomatic, with bedrest and observation.

Directions For Use: Inhale medicated vapors through each nostril while blocking off other nostril. Use as often as needed.

VICKS INHALER is medically effective for 3 months after first use.

How Supplied: Available as a cylindrical plastic nasal inhaler (net wt. 0.007 oz.).

VICKS® THROAT LOZENGES

Active Ingredients per lozenge: Benzocaine 5 mg., Cetylpyridinium Chloride 1.66 mg., Special Vicks Medication (menthol, camphor, eucalyptus oil) in a red cooling sugar base.

Indications: For fast-acting temporary relief of minor sore throat pain, cough of colds.

Actions: VICKS THROAT LOZENGES are local anesthetic and demulcent cough drops. They temporarily soothe minor sore throat irritations—ease pain—and relieve irritation and dryness of mouth and throat.

Warning: Do not exceed recommended dosage. Severe or persistent cough, sore throat, or sore throat accompanied by high fever, headache, nausea, and vomiting may be serious. Consult physician promptly. Do not use more than 2 days or administer to children under 3 years of age unless directed by physician. As with all medication, keep out of reach of children.

Symptoms and Treatment of Overdosage: These symptoms are based upon

Continued on next page

Vicks Health Care—Cont.

medical judgement, not on actual experience, since no significant incidence of overdose has been brought to our attention in clinical or consumer experience. Though unlikely, ingestion of large amounts may cause nausea, vomiting, gastrointestinal upset, central excitement, and a possiblity of cyanosis in young children. Treatment is symptomatic, with bedrest and observation.

Dosage: ADULTS AND CHILDREN 3 years and over: allow one lozenge to dissolve slowly in mouth. Repeat hourly as needed.

How Supplied: Box of 12's.

VICKS® VAPORUB®

Decongestant Vaporizing Ointment

For use as a rub or in steam.

Active Ingredients: Special Vicks Medication (menthol, spirits of turpentine, eucalyptus oil, camphor, cedar leaf oil, myristica oil, thymol) 14% in a petrolatum base.

Indications: For the symptomatic relief of nasal congestion (up to 8 hours), bronchial mucous congestion, coughs, laryngitis and huskiness, muscular tightness and muscular aches and pains due to colds. Also for chapped hands.

Actions: The inhaled vapors of VICKS VAPORUB have a decongestant, and antitussive effect. Applied externally, the medication acts as a local analgesic. The ointment is soothing to chapped hands and skin.

Warning: For external application and use in steam only. Do not swallow or place in nostrils. If fever is present or cough or other symptoms persist, see your doctor. In case of illness in very young children, it is wise to consult your physician. To avoid possibility of fire, never expose VAPORUB to flame or place VAPORUB in any container in which you are heating water. Do not direct steam from vaporizer toward face. As with all medication, keep out of reach of children.

Symptoms and Treatment of Ingestion: These symptoms are based upon medical judgement, not on actual experience, since no significant incidence of overdose or ingestion has been brought to our attention in clinical or consumer experience. Ingestion of large quantities may cause nausea, vomitimg, abdominal discomfort, diarrhea. Theoretically, very large quantities could cause weakness, vertigo, convulsions and drowsiness. If the extent of accidental ingestion is not known, treatment should consist of cautious gastric lavage. Otherwise, supportive and symptomatic treatment as necessary. If indicated, saline cathartics, demulcents and barbiturates for convulsions. Do not induce emesis.

Dosage:

AS A RUB: For relief of head and chest cold symptoms and coughs due to colds. Rub on throat, chest and back. Cover with a dry warm cloth if desired. Repeat as needed, especially at bedtime for continous breathing relief.

For relief of muscle tightness, apply hot, moist towel to affected area. Remove towel, then massage well with VAPORUB. Cover with a dry, warm cloth if desired.

For chapped hands and skin, apply liberally as a dressing.

IN STEAM: Fill medicine cup of vaporizer with VICKS VAPORUB and follow directions of vaporizer manufacturer. VAPORUB may also be used in a steam bowl. Fill a bowl ¾ full with steaming water and add 2 teaspoonfuls of VAPORUB (after removing from heat). Then inhale steaming vapors. Add extra steaming water as steam decreases.

How Supplied: Available in 1.5 oz., 3.0 oz. and 6.0 oz. plastic jars.

Viobin Corporation

A subsidiary of A. H. Robins Co.
MONTICELLO, IL 61856

VIOKASE® ℞

(pancreatin)

Description: VIOKASE is a pancreatic enzyme concentrate of porcine origin containing standardized lipase, protease and amylase plus other pancreatic enzymes. VIOKASE is available in tablets and powder dosage form for oral administration.

The enzyme potencies of the tablets and powder are:

	Each Tablet	Each 0.75 g powder (⅓ teaspoonful)
Lipase, USP Units	6,500	15,000
Protease, USP Units	32,000	75,000
Amylase, USP	48,000	112,500

Under conditions of the USP test method (in vitro) VIOKASE has the following total digestive capacity:

	Each Tablet	Each 0.75 powder
Dietary Fat, grams	23	53
Dietary Protein, grams	32	75
Dietary Starch, grams	48	112

VIOKASE Tablets are not enteric coated.

Indication: VIOKASE is indicated as a digestive aid in cystic fibrosis and in exocrine pancreatic insufficiency usually due to chronic pancreatitis, pancreatectomy or obstruction in the pancreas caused by malignant growth.

Contraindications: There are no known contraindications for VIOKASE Tablets or Powder.

Warnings: Use with caution in patients sensitive to pork protein.

VIOKASE should not be held in the mouth as the proteolytic action may cause irritation of the mucosa.

Precautions: Avoid inhalation of the powder when administering VIOKASE. Individuals previously sensitized to trypsin, pancreatin or pancrelipase may have allergic manifestations.

Long-term studies in animals have not been performed to evaluate carcinogenic potential.

Pregnancy Category C. Animal reproduction studies have not been conducted with VIOKASE. It is also not known whether VIOKASE can cause fetal harm when administered to a pregnant woman or can affect reproduction capacity. VIOKASE should be given to a pregnant woman only if clearly needed.

It is not known whether this drug is excreted in human milk. Because many drugs are excreted in human milk, caution should be exercised when VIOKASE is administered to a nursing mother.

Adverse Reactions: The dust or finely powdered pancreatic enzyme concentrate is irritating to the nasal mucosa and the respiratory tract. It has been documented in the literature that inhalation of the air-borne powder can precipitate an asthma attack. The literature also contains several references to asthma due to inhalation in patients sensitized to pancreatic enzyme concentrates.

Overdosage of pancreatic enzyme concentrate may cause diarrhea or other transient intestinal upset.

Dosage and Administration:

Powder: Dosage for patients with cystic fibrosis: ⅓ teaspoonful (0.75 grams) with meals.

Tablets: Dosage for patients with cystic fibrosis or chronic pancreatitis—1 to 3 tablets with meals.

As a digestive aid in patients with pancreatectomy or gastrectomy—1 to 2 tablets taken at 2-hour intervals, or as directed by physician.

How Supplied:

TABLETS—bottles of 100 (NDC 0668-0013-01) and 500 tablets (NDC 0668-0013-05).

POWDER—bottles of 4 oz. (113.5 grams) (NDC 0668-0012-04) and 8 oz. (227 grams) (NDC 0668-0012-08).

Literature Available: Complete literature available upon request including information on BEEF PANCREAS POWDER for those exceptional patients allergic to pork.

Vitaline Formulas

P.O. BOX 6757
INCLINE VILLAGE, NV 89450

ENVIRO-STRESS™ with ZINC and SELENIUM

High Potency
Stress Formula with Vitamins and Minerals

Each slow release ENVIRO-STRESS tablet provides:

600 mg	Vitamin C
132 mg	Zinc Sulfate, buffered (equal to 30 mg zinc)
100 mg	Magnesium (equal to 60 mg magnesium)
25 mcg	Selenium (organically bound)
50 mg	Vitamin B1 (thiamine mononitrate)
50 mg	Vitamin B2 (riboflavin)
50 mg	Vitamin B6 (pyridoxine HCL)
25 mcg	Vitamin B12
100 mg	Niacinamide
50 mg	Pantothenic Acid
400 mcg	Folic Acid
5 mg	Para-Amino Benzoic Acid
30 I.U.	Vitamin E

ENVIRO-STRESS Tablets contain no sugar, yeast, wheat, corn, soya, salicylates, phenol, preservatives or artificial coloring agents.

Recommended Intake: Adults, 1 tablet daily or as directed by the physician.

How Supplied: Bottles of 60 and 1000 tablets.

Literature Available: Complete literature available upon request by physician.

PANCREATIN 2400 mg. N.F.

(High Lipase)

Description: Vitaline's Pancreatin 2400 mg. N.F. is an **uncoated** compressed tablet, specially buffered to prevent the destruction of unknown amounts of pancreatin by gastric pepsin. No agents have been added to the tablet formulation to mask possible undesirable attributes of odor or taste imparted by the enzymes of pancreatin. Each tablet contains no less than:

Lipase	12,000 N.F. Units
Amylase	60,000 N.F. Units
Protease	60,000 N.F. Units

Indications and Usage: Pancreatin 2400 mg. N.F. is indicated for patients with exocrine pancreatic enzyme deficiency as in:

- *chronic pancreatitis
- *pancreatectomy or gastrectomy
- *cystic fibrosis

Precautions: Use with caution in patients known to be allergic to pork protein.

Vitaline's Pancreatin 2400 mg. N.F. tablets contain no sugar, corn, wheat, soya, yeast, phenol, salicylates, preservatives or artificial coloring agents.

Dosage and Administration: Usual dosage: One or two tablets during each meal and one tablet with snacks. Occasionally a third tablet with meals may be required depending upon individual requirements for control of steatorrhea.

How Supplied: Uncoated tablets in bottles of 100, 500 and 1000 tablets.

Literature Available: Complete literature available upon request by physician.

SELENIUM 200 MCG

Description: Each tablet contains: Selenium 200 mcg (organically bound in kelp)

Advantages of Kelp Bound Selenium Source

- Free of yeast protein allergens
- High bioavailability
- Uniformly distributed selenium
- Non toxic—not extractable
- Organic selenium—selenium is contained in a colloidal polymannuronate complex
- High trace element content

Action and Uses: A convenient source of selenium for patients deficient in this essential element.

Administration and Dosage: As a dietary supplement, adults—1 tablet daily, or as directed by physician.

Side Effects: None reported.

How Supplied: Bottles of 100 and 1000.

Literature and Samples: On request by physician.

TOTAL FORMULA®

(High Potency Multivitamin/Multimineral Supplement with micro-trace elements: Chromium, Selenium and Molybdenum)

Description: Total Formula's Tablet-With-in-A-Tablet Process (vitamin core, mineral layer, calcium layer, and chlorophyll coat) protects potency and assures digestibility.

Each tablet provides:

		Percent U.S. RDA*
Vitamins:		
A (Water Soluble)	10,000 I.U.	200
D-3	400 I.U.	100
E (d alpha tocopherol succinate [water soluble])	30 I.U.	100
K (water soluble)	70 mcg	**
C (ascorbic acid)	100 mg	166
B-1 (thiamine mononitrate)	15 mg	1000
B-2 (riboflavin)	15 mg	882
B-3 (niacinamide)	40 mg	400
B-6 (pyridoxine HCL)	25 mg	1250
B-12	25 mcg	416
Folic Acid	400 mcg	100
Pantothenic Acid	25 mg	416
Biotin	300 mcg	100
Choline Bitartrate	10 mcg	**
Hesperidin Complex	10 mg	***
Citrus Bioflavinoids	10 mg	***
Inositol	10 mg	***
Rutin	10 mg	***
Para Amino Benzoic Acid	8 mg	***
Minerals:		
Calcium	100 mg	10
Magnesium	100 mg	25
Iron	20 mg	111
Manganese	6 mg	**
Iodine	100 mcg	66
Copper	2 mg	100
Potassium	25 mg	**
Zinc	30 mg	200
Phosphorus	52 mg	5
Chromium (GTF factor)	500 mcg	**
Molybdenum	100 mcg	**
Selenium	10 mcg	**

Chlorophyll coloring in coating. *Sea vegetation as binder and filler.*

*RDA—recommended daily allowance.

**Need in human nutrition established, RDA not determined. ***Need in human nutrition not determined.

Total Formula contains no yeast, soya, corn, wheat, phenol, sugar, preservatives, or artificial coloring agents.

Usage: 12-year olds and older one tablet daily or as directed by physician.

How Supplied: Bottles of 100 and 1000.

Literature and Samples: On request.

Walker, Corp & Co., Inc.

EASTHAMPTON PL. & N. COLLINGWOOD AVE. SYRACUSE, NY 13206

EVAC–U–GEN®

Description: Evac-U-Gen® is available as purple scored tablets, each containing 97.2 mg. of yellow phenolphthalein.

Action and Uses: For temporary relief of occasional constipation and to help restore a normal pattern of evacuation. A mild, non-griping, stimulant laxative in chewable, anise-flavored form, Evac-U-Gen provides softening of the feces through selective action on the intramural nerve plexus of intestinal smooth muscle, and increases the propulsive peristaltic activity of the colon.

Indications: Because of its gentle action and non-toxic nature, Evac-U-Gen is a particularly suitable laxative in pregnancy, in the presence of hemorrhoids, for children and the elderly. It is especially useful when straining at the stool is a hazard, as in hernia, cardiac or hypertensive patients.

Contraindications: Contraindicated in patients with a history of sensitivity to phenolphthalein. Evac-U-Gen should not be used when abdominal pain, nausea, vomiting, or other symptoms of appendicitis are present.

Side Effects: If skin rash appears, use of Evac-U-Gen or other preparations containing phenolphthalein should be discontinued. May cause coloration of feces or urine if they are sufficiently alkaline.

Warning: Frequent or prolonged use may result in dependence on laxatives.

Administration and Dosage: **Adults:** chew one or two tablets night or morning. **Children:** 3 to 10 years, chew ½ tablet daily. Intensity of action is proportional to dosage, but individually effective doses vary. Evac-U-Gen is usually active 6 to 8 hours after administration, but residual action may last 3 to 4 days.

How Supplied: Evac-U-Gen is available in bottles of 35, 100, 500, 1000, 2000 and 6000 tablets.

Walker Pharmacal Company

4200 LACLEDE AVENUE ST. LOUIS, MO 63108

SUCCUS CINERARIA MARITIMA ℞

(Senecio Cineraria Compound Solution) Sterile—Ophthalmic

Description: Succus Cineraria Maritima is an aqueous and glycerin solution of the total extractives of the fresh Senecio Cineraria USPH 7th (Senecio Compositae) with extract of Hamamilis Vulgaris (Witch Hazel) and boric acid USP. The Alkaloids included in the total extract include Senecine and Senecionine. Total nonvolatiles is approximately 20%. The pH is adjusted to 4.1 pH; osmotic pressure is 5.5 osmols.

Actions and Uses: Succus Cineraria Maritima applied locally to the eyes acts as a safe lymphagogue, increasing circulation in the intraocular tissues, also stimulating collateral circulation and normal metabolism, functions so necessary from the standpoint of the physiology of the eye. Clinical observation indicates the definite value of local applications of Succus Cineraria Maritima in checking, or even aborting existing opacities. The benefits attained are obviously more satisfactory when treatment is instituted in the early stage of Cataract. In cases of well advanced opacity, and where pathological changes caused by the deterioration of the Metabolic functions have occurred, as is characteristic in senility, less favorable results can be expected.

The use of Succus Cineraria Maritima, however, is justified in certain cases well past the incipient stage, particularly when an operation is not contemplated or is contraindicated. It gives comfort to the patient to know that something potentially beneficial is being done. Clinical studies of advanced stages of cataract treated with Succus Cineraria Maritima indicated that in 22.5% of these cases beneficial results were obtained. In many of the cases which did not show improvement the process of the opacity was retarded or checked. In certain cases Succus Cineraria Maritima only gives temporary relief or serves to postpone the surgical removal.

Indications: Succus Cineraria Maritima is indicated in the treatment of various cases of optic opacity caused by cataract.

Contraindications: A history of a previous hypersensitivity reaction to any of the Senecio Alkaloids or the Hamamilis Vulgaris is a contraindication.

Warning: The possibility of sensitivity reactions should be considered in patients with a history of Allergy. If excessive irritation occurs it may be advisable to dilute the dosage, or discontinue treatment. (pH of 4.1 may cause minor irritation). For topical ophthalmic use only. If excessive irritation should develop, patient should consult the prescribing physician.

Caution: Federal Law prohibits dispensing without prescription.

Caution: Not intended for use in Glaucoma.

Dosage and Administration: Succus Cineraria Maritima should be instilled in the affected eye, two drops morning and evening, or as directed by physician. Do not touch dropper tip to any surface, since this may contaminate the solution.

Supplied: In sterile ¼ oz. dropper vial (7 cc). NDC 619-4021-38.

Wallace Laboratories

P.O. BOX 1 CRANBURY, NJ 08512

AQUATENSEN® ℞

(methyclothiazide, USP 5 mg) Tablets

Description: AQUATENSEN (methyclothiazide) is a member of the benzothiadiazine (thiazide) family of drugs. It is an analogue of hydrochlorothiazide.

Clinically, AQUATENSEN is an oral diuretic-antihypertensive agent.

Actions: The diuretic and saluretic effects of AQUATENSEN result from a drug-induced inhibition of the renal tubular reabsorption of electrolytes. The excretion of sodium and chloride is greatly enhanced. Potassium excretion is also enhanced to a variable degree, as it is with the other thiazides. Although urinary excretion of bicarbonate is increased slightly, there is usually no significant change in urinary pH. Methyclothiazide has a per mg natriuretic activity approximately 100 times that of the prototype thiazide, chlorothiazide. At maximal therapeutic dosages, all thiazides are approximately equal in their diuretic/natriuretic effects.

There is significant natriuresis and diuresis within two hours after administration of a single dose of methyclothiazide. These effects reach a peak in about six hours and persist for 24 hours following oral administration of a single dose.

Like other benzothiadiazines, AQUATENSEN also has antihypertensive properties, and may be

Continued on next page

Wallace—Cont.

used for this purpose either alone or to enhance the antihypertensive action of other drugs. The mechanism by which the benzothiadiazines, including methyclothiazide, produce a reduction of elevated blood pressure is not known. However, sodium depletion appears to be involved.

AQUATENSEN is readily absorbed from the gastrointestinal tract and is excreted unchanged by the kidneys.

Indications: AQUATENSEN is indicated in the management of hypertension either as the sole therapeutic agent or to enhance the effect of other antihypertensive drugs in the more severe forms of hypertension.

AQUATENSEN is indicated as adjunctive therapy in edema associated with congestive heart failure, hepatic cirrhosis, and corticosteroid and estrogen therapy.

AQUATENSEN has also been found useful in edema due to various forms of renal dysfunction such as the nephrotic syndrome, acute glomerulonephritis and chronic renal failure.

Usage in Pregnancy. The routine use of diuretics in an otherwise healthy woman is inappropriate and exposes mother and fetus to unnecessary hazard. Diuretics do not prevent development of toxemia of pregnancy, and there is no satisfactory evidence that they are useful in the treatment of developed toxemia.

Edema during pregnancy may arise from pathological causes or from the physiological and mechanical consequences of pregnancy. Thiazides are indicated in pregnancy when edema is due to pathologic causes, just as they are in the absence of pregnancy (however, see Warnings, below). Dependent edema in pregnancy, resulting from restriction of venous return by the expanded uterus, is properly treated through elevation of the lower extremities and use of support hose; use of diuretics to lower intravascular volume in this case is illogical and unnecessary. There is hypervolemia during normal pregnancy which is harmful to neither the fetus nor the mother (in the absence of cardiovascular disease), but which is associated with edema, including generalized edema, in the majority of pregnant women. If this edema produces discomfort, increased recumbency will often provide relief. In rare instances, this edema may cause extreme discomfort which is not relieved by rest. In these cases, a short course of diuretics may provide relief and may be appropriate.

Contraindications: Renal decompensation. Hypersensitivity to this or other sulfonamide derived drugs.

Warnings: Methyclothiazide shares with other thiazides the propensity to deplete potassium reserves to an unpredictable degree.

Thiazides should be used with caution in patients with renal disease or significant impairment of renal function, since azotemia may be precipitated and cumulative drug effects may occur.

Thiazides should be used with caution in patients with impaired hepatic function or progressive liver disease, since minor alterations of fluid and electrolyte balance may precipitate hepatic coma.

Thiazides may be additive or potentiative of the action of other antihypertensive drugs. Potentiation occurs with ganglionic or peripheral adrenergic blocking drugs.

Sensitivity reactions may occur in patients with a history of allergy or bronchial asthma.

The possibility of exacerbation or activation of systemic lupus erythematosus has been reported.

Usage in Pregnancy. Thiazides cross the placental barrier and appear in cord blood. The use of thiazides in pregnant women requires that the anticipated benefit be weighed against possible hazards to the fetus. These hazards include fetal or neonatal jaundice, thrombocytopenia, and possibly other adverse reactions, that have occurred in the adult.

Nursing Mothers. Thiazides appear in breast milk. If use of the drug is deemed essential, the patient should stop nursing.

Precautions: Periodic determination of serum electrolytes should be performed at appropriate intervals for the purpose of detecting possible electrolyte imbalances such as hyponatremia, hypochloremic alkalosis, and hypokalemia. Serum and urine electrolyte determinations are particularly important when a patient is vomiting excessively or receiving parenteral fluids. All patients should be observed for other clinical signs of electrolyte imbalances such as dryness of mouth, thirst, weakness, lethargy, drowsiness, restlessness, muscle pains or cramps, muscular fatigue, hypotension, oliguria, tachycardia, and gastrointestinal disturbances such as nausea and vomiting.

Hypokalemia may develop with thiazides as with any other potent diuretic, especially when brisk diuresis occurs, severe cirrhosis is present, or when corticosteroids or ACTH are given concomitantly. Interference with the adequate oral intake of electrolytes will also contribute to the possible development of hypokalemia. Potassium depletion, even of a mild degree, resulting from thiazide use, may sensitize a patient to the effects of cardiac glycosides such as digitalis.

Any chloride deficit is generally mild and usually does not require specific treatment except under extraordinary circumstances (as in liver disease or renal disease). Dilutional hyponatremia may occur in edematous patients in hot weather; appropriate therapy is water restriction, rather than administration of salt except in rare instances when the hyponatremia is life threatening.

In actual salt depletion, appropriate replacement is the therapy of choice.

Hyperuricemia may occur or frank gout may be precipitated in certain patients receiving thiazide therapy.

Insulin requirements in diabetic patients may be increased, decreased, or unchanged. Latent diabetes mellitus may become manifest during thiazide administration.

Thiazide drugs may increase the responsiveness to tubocurarine.

The antihypertensive effects of the drug may be enhanced in the postsympathectomy patient.

Thiazides may decrease arterial responsiveness to nonrepinephrine. This diminution is not sufficient to preclude effectiveness of the pressor agent for therapeutic use.

If progressive renal impairment becomes evident as indicated by a rising nonprotein nitrogen or blood urea nitrogen, a careful reappraisal of therapy is necessary with consideration given to withholding or discontinuing diuretic therapy.

Thiazides may decrease serum PBI levels without signs of thyroid disturbance.

Thiazides have been reported, on rare occasions, to have elevated serum calcium to hypercalcemic levels. The serum calcium levels have returned to normal when the medication has been stopped. This phenomenon may be related to the ability of the thiazide diuretics to lower the amount of calcium excreted in the urine.

Adverse Reactions: *Gastrointestinal system reactions:* Anorexia, gastric irritation, nausea, vomiting, cramping, diarrhea, constipation, jaundice (intrahepatic cholestatic jaundice), pancreatitis.

Central nervous system reactions: Dizziness, vertigo, paresthesia, headache, xanthopsia.

Hematologic reactions: Leukopenia, agranulocytosis, thrombocytopenia, aplastic anemia.

Dermatologic-hypersensitivity reactions: Purpura, photosensitivity, rash, urticaria, necrotizing angiitis (vasculitis) (cutaneous vasculitis).

Cardiovascular reactions: Orthostatic hypotension may occur and may be aggravated by alcohol, barbiturates, or narcotics.

Other: Hyperglycemia, glycosuria, hypercalcemia, hyperuricemia, muscle spasm, weakness, restlessness.

There have been isolated reports that certain nonedematous individuals developed severe fluid and electrolyte derangements after only brief exposure to normal doses of thiazide and non-thiazide diuretics. The condition is usually manifested as severe dilutional hyponatremia, hypokalemia, and hypochloremia. It has been reported to be due to inappropriately increased ADH secretion and appears to be idiosyncratic. Potassium replacement is apparently the most important therapy in the treatment of this syndrome along with removal of the offending drug.

Whenever adverse reactions are severe, treatment should be discontinued.

Dosage and Administration:

AQUATENSEN (methyclothiazide) is administered orally. The usual adult dose ranges from 2.5 to 10 mg once daily.

Therapy should be individualized according to patient response. This therapy should be titrated to gain maximal therapeutic response as well as the minimal dose possible to maintain that therapeutic response.

To maintain an edema-free state or as an adjunct in the management of hypertension, 2.5 to 5.0 mg once daily is often adequate.

Maximum effective single dose is 10 mg; larger single doses do not accomplish greater diuresis, and are not recommended.

In the treatment of hypertension, methyclothiazide may be either employed alone or concurrently with other antihypertensive drugs. Combined therapy may provide adequate control of hypertension with lower dosage of the component drugs and fewer or less severe side effects.

For treatment of moderately severe or severe hypertension, supplemental use of other more potent antihypertensive agents may be indicated.

When other antihypertensive agents are to be added to the regimen, this should be accomplished gradually. Ganglionic blocking agents should be given at only half the usual dose since their effect is potentiated by pretreatment with AQUATENSEN.

Overdosage: Symptoms of overdosage include electrolyte imbalance and signs of potassium deficiency such as confusion, dizziness, muscular weakness, and gastrointestinal disturbances. General supportive measures including replacement of fluids and electrolytes may be indicated in treatment of overdosage.

How Supplied: AQUATENSEN (methyclothiazide) is supplied as a 5 mg, pink monogrammed, grooved, rectangular-shaped tablet.

NDC 0037-0153-92, bottle of 100.

NDC 0037-0153-96, bottle of 500.

Rev. 7/79

[*Shown in Product Identification Section*]

BUTISOL SODIUM® ℞ ©

(butabarbital sodium)
Tablets and Elixir
Sedative/Hypnotic

Description: BUTISOL SODIUM (butabarbital sodium) is a nonselective central nervous system depressant which is orally administered as a sedative hypnotic. Butabarbital sodium occurs as a white, bitter powder which is freely soluble in water and alcohol, but practically insoluble in benzene and ether.

The structural formula for butabarbital sodium is:

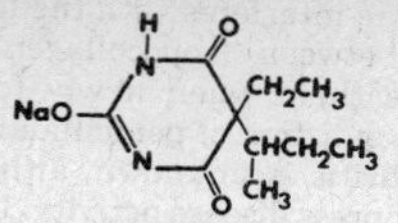

Sodium-5-*sec*-butyl-5-ethylbarbiturate

Clinical Pharmacology: Barbiturates, including BUTISOL SODIUM (butabarbital sodium), are capable of producing all levels of CNS mood alteration from excitation to mild sedation, to hypnosis, and deep coma. Overdosage can produce death. Barbiturates depress the sensory cortex, decrease motor activity, alter cerebellar function, and produce respiratory depression. With hypnotic doses, respiratory depression produced by barbiturates is similar to that which occurs during physiologic sleep with slight decrease in blood pressure and heart rate.

Pharmacokinetics: Barbiturates are weak acids that are absorbed and rapidly distributed to all tissues and fluids with high concentrations in the brain, liver, and kidneys. Barbiturates are bound to plasma and tissue proteins. The rate of absorption is increased if it is ingested as a dilute solution or taken on an empty stomach.

Barbiturates are metabolized primarily by the hepatic microsomal enzyme system, and most metabolic products are excreted in the urine. The excretion of unchanged butabarbital in the urine is negligible. BUTISOL SODIUM is classified as an intermediate acting barbiturate. The average plasma half-life for butabarbital is 100 hours in the adult.

Although variable from patient to patient, butabarbital has an onset of action of about ¾ to 1 hour, and a duration of action of about 6 to 8 hours.

Indications and Usage: BUTISOL SODIUM (butabarbital sodium) is indicated for use as a sedative or hypnotic.

Since barbiturates appear to lose their effectiveness for sleep induction and sleep maintenance after 2 weeks, use of BUTISOL SODIUM in treating insomnia should be limited to this time.

Contraindications: Barbiturates are contraindicated in patients with known barbiturate sensitivity. Barbiturates are also contraindicated in patients with a history of manifest or latent porphyria.

Warnings: Barbiturates may be habit forming (see DRUG ABUSE AND DEPENDENCE).

Acute or chronic pain: Caution should be exercised when barbiturates are administered to patients with acute or chronic pain, because paradoxical excitement could be induced, or important symptoms could be masked. However, the use of barbiturates as sedatives in the postoperative surgical period and as adjuncts to cancer chemotherapy is well established.

Use in pregnancy: Barbiturates may cause fetal damage when administered to pregnant women. Retrospective, case-controlled studies have suggested a connection between the maternal-consumption of barbiturates and a higher than expected incidence of fetal abnormalities. If this drug is used during pregnancy, or if the patient becomes pregnant while taking this drug, the patient should be apprised of the potential hazard to the fetus.

Precautions:

General: Barbiturates should be administered with caution, if at all, to patients who are mentally depressed, have suicidal tendencies, or a history of drug abuse.

Elderly or debilitated patients may react to barbiturates with marked excitement, depression, and confusion. In some persons, barbiturates repeatedly produce excitement rather than depression.

In patients with hepatic damage, barbiturates should be administered with caution and initially in reduced doses. Barbiturates should not be administered to patients showing the premonitory signs of hepatic coma.

FD&C Yellow No. 5 (tartrazine) may cause allergic-type reactions (including bronchial asthma) in certain susceptible individuals. Although the overall incidence of FD&C Yellow No. 5 (tartrazine) sensitivity in the general population is low, it is frequently seen in patients who also have aspirin hypersensitivity.

Information for the Patient: Practitioners should give the following information and instructions to patients receiving barbiturates.

The use of barbiturates carries with it an associated risk of psychological and/or physical dependence. The patient should be warned against increasing the dose of the drug without consulting a physician.

Barbiturates may impair mental and/or physical abilities required for the performance of potentially hazardous tasks, such as driving or operating machinery.

Alcohol should not be consumed while taking barbiturates. Concurrent use of the barbiturates with other CNS depressants, including other sedatives or hypnotics, alcohol, narcotics, tranquilizers, and antihistamines, may result in additional CNS depressant effects.

Laboratory Tests: Prolonged therapy with barbiturates should be accompanied by periodic laboratory evaluation of organ systems, including hematopoietic, renal, and hepatic systems (see PRECAUTIONS-General and ADVERSE REACTIONS).

Drug Interactions: Anticoagulants, doxycycline and steroidal hormones: Barbiturates can induce hepatic microsomal enzymes resulting in increased metabolism and decreased therapeutic response to these drugs. Patients stabilized on these drugs may require dosage adjustments if barbiturates are added to or withdrawn from their dosage regimen.

Phenytoin, sodium valproate, valproic acid: Because the effect of barbiturates on the metabolism of phenytoin is not predictable, phenytoin and barbiturate blood levels should be monitored if these drugs are given concurrently. Because sodium valproate and valproic acid appear to decrease barbiturate metabolism, barbiturate blood levels should be monitored and appropriate dosage adjustments made as indicated.

Central nervous system depressants: The concomitant use of alcohol or other CNS depressants may produce additive CNS depressant effects (see Information for the Patient).

Monoamine oxidase inhibitors (MAOI): MAOI prolong the effects of barbiturates, probably because metabolism of the barbiturate is inhibited.

Carcinogenesis, Mutagenesis, Impairment of Fertility: No long-term studies in animals have been performed with butabarbital sodium to determine carcinogenic and mutagenic potential, or effects on fertility.

Pregnancy: Teratogenic effects: Pregnancy Category D (See WARNINGS).

Nonteratogenic effects: Infants suffering from long-term barbiturate exposure **in utero** may have an acute withdrawal syndrome of seizures and hyperirritability from birth to a delayed onset of up to 14 days (see DRUG ABUSE AND DEPENDENCE).

Labor and delivery: Hypnotic doses of barbiturates do not appear to significantly impair uterine activity during labor. Administration of sedative-hypnotic barbiturates to the mother during labor may result in respiratory depression in the newborn. Premature infants are particularly susceptible to the depressant effects of barbiturates. If barbiturates are used during labor and delivery, resuscitation equipment should be available.

Nursing mothers: Caution should be exercised when a barbiturate is administered to a nursing woman since small amounts of some barbiturates are excreted in the milk.

Adverse Reactions: The following adverse reactions have been observed with the use of barbiturates in hospitalized patients. Because such patients may be less aware of certain of the milder adverse effects of barbiturates, the incidence of these reactions may be somewhat higher in fully ambulatory patients.

More than 1 in 100 patients: The most common adverse reaction, somnolence, is estimated to occur at a rate of 1 to 3 patients per 100.

Less than 1 in 100 patients: The most common adverse reactions estimated to occur at a rate of less than 1 in 100 patients listed below, grouped by organ system, and by decreasing order of occurrence are:

Central nervous system/psychiatric: Agitation, confusion, hyperkinesia, ataxia, CNS depression, nightmares, nervousness, psychiatric disturbance, hallucinations, insomnia, anxiety, dizziness, thinking abnormality.

Respiratory: Hypoventilation, apnea.

Cardiovascular: Bradycardia, hypotension, syncope.

Gastrointestinal: Nausea, vomiting, constipation.

Other reported reactions: Headache, hypersensitivity reactions (angioedema, skin rashes, exfoliative dermatitis), fever, liver damage.

Drug Abuse and Dependence: BUTISOL SODIUM (butabarbital sodium) is a Schedule III controlled drug.

Barbiturates may be habit-forming. Tolerance, psychological dependence, and physical dependence may occur especially following prolonged use of high doses of barbiturates. The average daily dose for the barbiturate addict is usually about 1.5 grams. As tolerance to barbiturates develops, the amount needed to maintain the same level of intoxication increases; tolerance to a fatal dosage, however, does not increase more than two-fold. As this occurs, the margin between an intoxicating dosage and fatal dosage becomes smaller.

Symptoms of barbiturate dependence are similar to those of chronic alcoholism. If an individual appears to be intoxicated with alcohol to a degree that is radically disproportionate to the amount of alcohol in his or her blood, the use of barbiturates should be suspected. The lethal dose of a barbiturate is far less if alcohol is also ingested.

The symptoms of barbiturate withdrawal can be severe and may cause death. Minor withdrawal symptoms may appear 8 to 12 hours after the last dose of a barbiturate. These symptoms usually appear in the following order: anxiety, muscle twitching, tremor of hands and fingers, progressive weakness, dizziness, distortion in visual perception, nausea, vomiting, insomnia, and orthostatic hypotension. Major withdrawal symptoms (convulsions and delirium) may occur within 16 hours and last up to 5 days after abrupt cessation of these drugs. Intensity of withdrawal symptoms gradually declines over a period of approximately 15 days.

Treatment of barbiturate dependence consists of cautious and gradual withdrawal of the drug. Barbiturate-dependent patients can be withdrawn by using a number of different withdrawal regimens. In all cases, withdrawal takes an extended period of time. One method involves initiating treatment at the patient's regular dosage level, in 3 to 4 divided doses, and decreasing the daily dose by 10 percent if tolerated by the patient.

Infants physically dependent on barbiturates may be given phenobarbital 3 to 10 mg/kg/day. After withdrawal symptoms (hyperactivity, disturbed sleep, tremors, hyperreflexia) are relieved; the dosage of phenobarbital should be gradually decreased and completely withdrawn over a 2-week period.

Overdosage: The toxic dose of barbiturates varies considerably. In general, an oral dose of 1 gram of most barbiturates produces serious

Continued on next page

Wallace—Cont.

poisoning in an adult. Death commonly occurs after 2 to 10 grams of ingested barbiturate. Symptoms of acute intoxication with barbiturates include unsteady gait, slurred speech, and sustained nystagmus. Mental signs of chronic intoxication include confusion, poor judgment, irritability, insomnia, and somatic complaints. Barbiturate intoxication may be confused with alcoholism, bromide intoxication, and with various neurological disorders.

Acute overdosage with barbiturates is manifested by CNS and respiratory depression which may progress to Cheyne-Stokes respiration, areflexia, constriction of the pupils to a slight degree (though in severe poisoning they may show paralytic dilation), oliguria, tachycardia, hypotension, lowered body temperature, and coma. Typical shock syndrome (apnea, circulatory collapse, respiratory arrest, and death) may occur.

In extreme overdose, all electrical activity in the brain may cease, in which case a "flat" EEG normally equated with clinical death cannot be accepted. This effect is fully reversible unless hypoxic damage occurs. Consideration should be given to the possibility of barbiturate intoxication even in situations that appear to involve trauma.

Complications such as pneumonia, pulmonary edema, cardiac arrhythmias, congestive heart failure, and renal failure may occur. Uremia may increase CNS sensitivity to barbiturates if renal function is impaired. Differential diagnosis should include hypoglycemia, head trauma, cerebrovascular accidents, convulsive states, and diabetic coma.

Treatment of overdosage is mainly supportive and consists of the following:

1. Maintenance of an adequate airway, with assisted respiration and oxygen administration as necessary.
2. Monitoring of vital signs and fluid balance.
3. If the patient is conscious and has not lost the gag reflex, emesis may be induced with ipecac. Care should be taken to prevent pulmonary aspiration of vomitus. After completion of vomiting, 30 grams activated charcoal in a glass of water may be administered.
4. If emesis is contraindicated, gastric lavage may be performed with a cuffed endotracheal tube in place with the patient in the face down position. Activated charcoal may be left in the emptied stomach and a saline cathartic administered.
5. Fluid therapy and other standard treatment for shock, if needed.
6. If renal function is normal, forced diuresis may aid in the elimination of the barbiturate.
7. Although not recommended as a routine procedure, hemodialysis may be used in severe barbiturate intoxications or if the patient is anuric or in shock.
8. Appropriate nursing care, including rolling patients from side-to-side every 30 minutes, to prevent hypostatic pneumonia, decubiti, aspiration, and other complications of patients with altered states of consciousness.
9. Antibiotics should be given if pneumonia is expected.

Dosage and Administration:

Usual Adult Dosage

Daytime sedative: 15 to 30 mg 3 or 4 times daily.

Bedtime hypnotic: 50 to 100 mg.

Preoperative sedative: 50 to 100 mg 60 to 90 minutes before surgery.

Usual Pediatric Dosage

Pediatric preoperative: 2 to 6 mg/kg maximum 100 mg.

Special Patient Population

Dosage should be reduced in the elderly or debilitated because these patients may be more sensitive to barbiturates. Dosage should be reduced for patients with impaired renal function or hepatic disease (see PRECAUTIONS).

How Supplied: BUTISOL SODIUM® (butabarbital sodium) 15 mg Tablets (colored lavender, imprinted "BUTISOL SODIUM" and 37/112 scored)—NDC 0037-0112-60 bottles of 100 and NDC 0037-0112-80 bottles of 1000. BUTISOL SODIUM® (butabarbital sodium) 30 mg* Tablets (colored green, imprinted "BUTISOL SODIUM" and 37/113 scored)—NDC 0037-0113-60 bottles of 100 and NDC 0037-0113-80 bottles of 1000. BUTISOL SODIUM® (butabarbital sodium) 50 mg* Tablets (colored orange, imprinted "BUTISOL SODIUM" and 37/114 scored)—NDC 0037-0114-60 bottles of 100. BUTISOL SODIUM® (butabarbital sodium) 100 mg Tablets (colored pink, imprinted "BUTISOL SODIUM" and 37/115 scored)—NDC 0037-0115-60 bottles of 100.

Dispense tablets in well-closed container.

BUTISOL SODIUM® (butabarbital sodium) elixir 30 mg/5 ml*, alcohol 7% (colored green)—NDC 0037-0110-16, bottles of pints and NDC 0037-0110-28 bottles of gallons.

Dispense elixir in tight container.

*Contains FD&C Yellow No. 5 (see PRECAUTIONS).

Distributed by WALLACE LABORATORIES
Division of
CARTER-WALLACE, INC.
Cranbury, New Jersey 08512

Tablets manufactured by McNeil Pharmaceutical Co., Dorado, P.R. 00646

Elixir manufactured by McNeil Pharmaceutical
McNeilab, Inc.
Springhouse, PA.
19477

Rev. 4/82

[*Shown in Product Identification Section*]

DEPEN® Titratabs™ ℞
(Penicillamine, Wallace)

> Physicians planning to use penicillamine should thoroughly familiarize themselves with its toxicity, special dosage considerations, and therapeutic benefits. Penicillamine should never be used casually. Each patient should remain constantly under the close supervision of the physician. Patients should be warned to report promptly any symptoms suggesting toxicity.

Description: Penicillamine is 3-mercapto-D-valine. It is a white or practically white, crystalline powder, freely soluble in water, slightly soluble in alcohol, and insoluble in ether, acetone, benzene, and carbon tetrachloride. Although its configuration is D, it is levorotatory as usually measured:

$$[\alpha]^{25}_{D} = -63^\circ \pm 5^\circ \ (C = 1, 1N \text{ NaOH}).$$

The empirical formula is $C_5H_{11}NO_2S$, giving it a molecular weight of 149.21.

It reacts readily with formaldehyde or acetone to form a thiazolidine-carboxylic acid.

Clinical Pharmacology: Penicillamine is a chelating agent recommended for the removal of excess copper in patients with Wilson's disease. From *in vitro* studies which indicate that one atom of copper combines with two molecules of penicillamine, it would appear that one gram of penicillamine should be followed by the excretion of about 200 milligrams of copper; however, the actual amount excreted is about one percent of this.

Penicillamine also reduces excess cystine excretion in cystinuria. This is done, at least in part, by disulfide interchange between penicillamine and cystine, resulting in formation of penicillamine-cysteine disulfide, a substance that is much more soluble than cystine and is excreted readily.

Penicillamine interferes with the formation of crosslinks between tropocollagen molecules and cleaves them when newly formed. The mechanism of action of penicillamine in rheumatoid arthritis is unknown, although it appears to suppress disease activity. Unlike cytotoxic immunosuppressants, penicillamine markedly lowers IgM rheumatoid factor but produces no significant depression in absolute levels of serum immunoglobulins. Also unlike cytotoxic immunosuppressants, which act on both, penicillamine *in vitro* depresses T-cell activity but not B-cell activity. *In vitro*, penicillamine dissociates macroglobulins (rheumatoid factor) although the relationship of the activity to its effect in rheumatoid arthritis is not known.

In rheumatoid arthritis, the onset of therapeutic response to DEPEN (Penicillamine, Wallace) may not be seen for two or three months. In those patients who respond, however, the first evidence of suppression of symptoms such as pain, tenderness, and swelling usually is apparent within three months. The optimum duration of therapy has not been determined. If remissions occur, they may last from months to years but usually require continued treatment (see DOSAGE AND ADMINISTRATION). In patients with rheumatoid arthritis, it is important that DEPEN be given on an empty stomach, at least one hour before meals and at least one hour apart from any other drug, food or milk. This permits maximum absorption and reduces the likelihood of metal binding.

Methodology for determining the bioavailability of penicillamine is not available; however, penicillamine is known to be a very soluble substance.

Indications: DEPEN is indicated in the treatment of Wilson's disease, cystinuria, and in patients with severe, active rheumatoid arthritis who have failed to respond to an adequate trial of conventional therapy. Available evidence suggests that DEPEN is not of value in ankylosing spondylitis.

Wilson's Disease—Wilson's disease (hepatolenticular degeneration) results from the interaction of an inherited defect and an abnormality in copper metabolism. The metabolic defect, which is the consequence of the autosomal inheritance of one abnormal gene from each parent, manifests itself in a greater positive copper balance than normal. As a result, copper is deposited in several organs and appears eventually to produce pathologic effects most prominently seen in the brain, where degeneration is widespread; in the liver, where fatty infiltration, inflammation, and hepatocellular damage progress to postnecrotic cirrhosis; in the kidney, where tubular and glomerular dysfunction results; and in the eye, where characteristic corneal copper deposits are known as Kayser-Fleischer rings.

Two types of patients require treatment for Wilson's disease: (1) the symptomatic, and (2) the asymptomatic in whom it can be assumed the disease will develop in the future if the patient is not treated.

Diagnosis, suspected on the basis of family or individual history, physical examination, or a low serum concentration of ceruloplasmin*, is confirmed by the demonstration of Kayser-Fleischer rings or, particularly in the asymptomatic patient, by the quantitative demonstration in a liver biopsy specimen of a concentration of copper in excess of 250 mcg/g dry weight.

---

*For quantitative test for serum ceruloplasmin see: Morell, A. G.; Windsor, J.; Sternlieb, I.; Scheinberg, I. H.: Measurement of the concentration of ceruloplasmin in serum by determination of its oxidase activity, in "Laboratory Diagnosis of Liver Disease," F. W. Sunderman; F. W Sunderman, Jr. (eds.), St. Louis, Warren H. Green, Inc., 1968, pp. 193-195.

Treatment has two objectives:
(1) to minimize dietary intake and absorption of copper.
(2) to promote excretion of copper deposited in tissues.

The first objective is attained by a daily diet that contains no more than one or two milligrams of copper. Such a diet should exclude, most importantly, chocolate, nuts, shellfish, mushrooms, liver, molasses, broccoli, and cereals enriched with copper, and be composed to as great an extent as possible of foods with a low copper content. Distilled or demineralized water should be used if the patient's drinking water contains more than 0.1 mg of copper per liter. For the second objective, a copper chelating agent is used. Penicillamine is the only one of these agents that is orally effective.

In symptomatic patients, this treatment usually produces marked neurologic improvement, fading of Kayser-Fleischer rings, and gradual amelioration of hepatic dysfunction and psychic disturbances.

Clinical experience to date suggests that life is prolonged with the above regimen.

Noticeable improvement may not occur for one to three months. Occasionally, neurologic symptoms become worse during initiation of therapy with DEPEN. Despite this, the drug should not be discontinued permanently, although temporary interruption may result in clinical improvement of the neurological symptoms but it carries an increased risk of developing a sensitivity reaction upon resumption of therapy (See WARNINGS).

Treatment of asymptomatic patients has been carried out for over ten years. Symptoms and signs of the disease appear to be prevented indefinitely if daily treatment with DEPEN can be continued.

Cystinuria —Cystinuria is characterized by excessive urinary excretion of the dibasic amino acids, arginine, lysine, ornithine, and cystine, and the mixed disulfide of cysteine and homocysteine. The metabolic defect that leads to cystinuria is inherited as an autosomal, recessive trait. Metabolism of the affected amino acids is influenced by at least two abnormal factors: (1) defective gastrointestinal absorption and (2) renal tubular dysfunction.

Arginine, lysine, ornithine, and cysteine are soluble substances, readily excreted. There is no apparent pathology connected with their excretion in excessive quantities.

Cystine, however, is so slightly soluble at the usual range of urinary pH that it is not excreted readily, and so crystallizes and forms stones in the urinary tract. Stone formation is the only known pathology in cystinuria.

Normal daily output of cystine is 40 to 80 mg. In cystinuria, output is greatly increased and may exceed 1 g/day. At 500 to 600 mg/day, stone formation is almost certain. When it is more than 300 mg/day, treatment is indicated.

Conventional treatment is directed at keeping urinary cystine diluted enough to prevent stone formation, keeping the urine alkaline enough to dissolve as much cystine as possible, and minimizing cystine production by a diet low in methionine (the major dietary precursor of cystine). Patients must drink enough fluid to keep urine specific gravity below 1.010, take enough alkali to keep urinary pH at 7.5 to 8, and maintain a diet low in methionine. This diet is not recommended in growing children and probably is contraindicated in pregnancy because of its low protein content (see **Precautions**).

When these measures are inadequate to control recurrent stone formation, DEPEN may be used as additional therapy. When patients refuse to adhere to conventional treatment, DEPEN may be a useful substitute. It is capable of keeping cystine excretion to near normal values, thereby hindering stone formation and the serious consequences of pyelonephritis and impaired renal function that develop in some patients.

Bartter and colleagues depict the process by which penicillamine interacts with cystine to form penicillamine-cysteine mixed disulfide as:

$$\text{CSSC} + \text{PS}' \rightleftharpoons \text{CS}' + \text{CSSP}$$
$$\text{PSSP} + \text{CS}' \rightleftharpoons \text{PS}' + \text{CSSP}$$
$$\text{CSSC} + \text{PSSP} \rightleftharpoons 2\ \text{CSSP}$$

CSSC = cystine
CS′ = deprotonated cysteine
PSSP = penicillamine
PS′ = deprotonated penicillamine sulfhydryl
CSSP = penicillamine-cysteine mixed disulfide

In this process, it is assumed that the deprotonated form of penicillamine, PS′, is the active factor in bringing about the disulfide interchange.

Rheumatoid Arthritis —Because DEPEN can cause severe adverse reactions, its use in rheumatoid arthritis should be restricted to patients who have severe, active disease and who have failed to respond to an adequate trial of conventional therapy. Even then, benefit-to-risk ratio should be carefully considered. Other measures, such as rest, physiotherapy, salicylates and corticosteroids should be used, when indicated, in conjunction with DEPEN (see **Precautions**).

Contraindications—Penicillamine should not be administered to patients with rheumatoid arthritis who are pregnant (See **Precautions**).

Patients with a history of penicillamine-related aplastic anemia or agranulocytosis should not be restarted on penicillamine (see **Warnings** and **Adverse Reactions**).

Because of its potential for causing renal damage, penicillamine should not be administered to rheumatoid arthritis patients with a history or other evidence of renal insufficiency.

Warnings: The use of penicillamine has been associated with fatalities due to certain diseases, such as aplastic anemia, agranulocytosis, thrombocytopenia, Goodpasture's syndrome, and myasthenia gravis. Because of the potential for serious hematological and renal adverse reactions, routine urinalysis, white and differential blood cell count, hemoglobin determination, and direct platelet count must be done every two weeks for the first six months of penicillamine therapy and monthly thereafter. Patients should be instructed to report promptly signs and symptoms of granulocytopenia and/or thrombocytopenia such as fever, sore throat, chills, bruising or bleeding and the above laboratory studies should be promptly repeated.

Leukopenia and thrombocytopenia have been reported to occur in up to 5% of patients during penicillamine therapy. Leukopenia is of the granulocytic series and may or may not be associated with an increase in eosinophils. A confirmed reduction in WBC below 3500 mandates discontinuance of penicillamine therapy. Thrombocytopenia may be on an idiosyncratic basis with decreased or absent megakaryocytes in the marrow, when it is part of an aplastic anemia. In other cases the thrombocytopenia is presumably on an immune basis since the number of megakaryocytes in the marrow has been reported to be normal or sometimes increased. The development of a platelet count below 100,000, even in the absence of clinical bleeding, requires at least temporary cessation of penicillamine therapy. A progressive fall in either platelet count or WBC in three successive determinations, even though values are still within the normal range, likewise requires at least temporary cessation.

Proteinuria and/or hematuria may develop during therapy and may be warning signs of membranous glomerulopathy which can progress to a nephrotic syndrome. Close observation of these patients is essential. In some patients the proteinuria disappears with continued therapy; in others penicillamine must be discontinued. When a patient develops proteinuria or hematuria the physician must ascertain whether it is a sign of drug-induced glomerulopathy or is unrelated to penicillamine.

Rheumatoid arthritis patients who develop moderate degrees of proteinuria may be continued cautiously on penicillamine therapy, provided that quantitative 24-hour urinary protein determinations are obtained at intervals of one to two weeks. Penicillamine dosage should not be increased under these circumstances. Proteinuria which exceeds 1 g/24 hours, or proteinuria which is progressively increasing requires either discontinuance of the drug or a reduction in the dosage. In some patients, proteinuria has been reported to clear following reduction in dosage.

In rheumatoid arthritis patients, penicillamine should be discontinued if unexplained gross hematuria or presistent microscopic hematuria develops.

In patients with Wilson's disease or cystinuria the risks of continued penicillamine therapy in patients manifesting potentially serious urinary abnormalities must be weighed against the expected therapeutic benefits.

When penicillamine is used in cystinuria, an annual x-ray for renal stones is advised. Cystine stones form rapidly, sometimes in six months.

Up to one year or more may be required for any urinary abnormalities to disappear after penicillamine has been discontinued.

Because of rare reports of intrahepatic cholestasis and toxic hepatitis, liver function tests are recommended every six months during therapy.

Goodpasture's syndrome has occurred rarely. The development of abnormal urinary findings associated with hemoptysis and pulmonary infiltrates on x-ray requires immediate cessation of penicillamine.

Myasthenic syndrome sometimes progressing to myasthenia gravis has been reported. In the majority of cases, symptoms of myasthenia have receded after withdrawal of penicillamine.

Pemphigoid-type reactions characterized by bullous lesions clinically indistinguishable from pemphigus have occurred and have required discontinuation of penicillamine and treatment with corticosteroids.

Once instituted for Wilson's disease or cystinuria, treatment with penicillamine should, as a rule, be continued on a daily basis. Interruptions for even a few days have been followed by sensitivity reactions after reinstitution of therapy.

Precautions: Some patients may experience drug fever, a marked febrile response to penicillamine, usually in the second or third week following initiation of therapy. Drug fever may sometimes be accompanied by a macular cutaneous eruption.

In the case of drug fever in patients with Wilson's disease or cystinuria, because no alternative treatment is available, penicillamine should be temporarily discontinued until the reaction subsides. Then penicillamine should be reinstituted with a small dose that is gradually increased until the desired dosage is attained. Systemic steroid therapy may be necessary, and is usually helpful, in such patients in whom toxic reactions develop a second or third time. In the case of drug fever in rheumatoid arthritis patients, because other treatments are available, penicillamine should be discontinued and another therapeutic alternative tried, since experience indicates that the febrile reaction will recur in a very high percentage of patients upon readministration of penicillamine.

The skin and mucous membranes should be observed for allergic reactions. Early and late

Continued on next page

Wallace—Cont.

rashes have occurred. Early rash occurs during the first few months of treatment and is more common. It is usually a generalized pruritic, erythematous, maculopapular or morbilliform rash and resembles the allergic rash seen with other drugs. Early rash usually disappears within days after stopping penicillamine and seldom recurs when the drug is restarted at a lower dosage. Pruritus and early rash may often be controlled by the concomitant administration of antihistamines. Less commonly, a late rash may be seen, usually after six months or more of treatment, and requires discontinuation of penicillamine. It is usually on the trunk, is accompanied by intense pruritus, and is usually unresponsive to topical corticosteroid therapy. Late rash may take weeks to disappear after penicillamine is stopped and usually recurs if the drug is restarted.
The appearance of drug eruption accompanied by fever, arthralgia, lymphadenopathy or other allergic manifestations usually requires discontinuation of penicillamine.
Certain patients will develop a positive antinuclear antibody (ANA) test and some of these may show a lupus erythematosus-like syndrome similar to drug-induced lupus associated with other drugs. The lupus erythematosus-like syndrome is not associated with hypocomplementemia and may be present without nephropathy. The development of a positive ANA test does not mandate discontinuance of the drug; however, the physician should be alerted to the possibility that a lupus erythematosus-like syndrome may develop in the future.
Some patients may develop oral ulcerations which in some cases have the appearance of aphthous stomatitis. The stomatitis usually recurs on rechallenge but often clears on a lower dosage. Although rare, cheilosis, glossitis and gingivostomatitis have also been reported. These oral lesions are frequently dose-related and may preclude further increase in penicillamine dosage or require discontinuation of the drug.
Hypogeusia (a blunting or diminution in taste perception) has occurred in some patients. This may last two to three months or more and may develop into a total loss of taste; however, it is usually self-limited, despite continued penicillamine treatment. Such taste impairment is rare in patients with Wilson's disease.
Penicillamine should not be used in patients who are receiving concurrent gold therapy, antimalarial or cytotoxic drugs, oxyphenbutazone or phenylbutazone because these drugs are also associated with similar serious hematologic and/or renal adverse reactions. Patients who have had gold salt therapy discontinued due to a major toxic reaction may be at greater risk of serious side effects with penicillamine, but not necessarily of the same type.
Patients who are allergic to penicillin may theoretically have cross-sensitivity to penicillamine. The possibility of reactions from contamination of penicillamine by trace amounts of penicillin has been precluded now that penicillamine is being produced synthetically rather than as a degradation product of penicillin.
Because of their dietary restrictions, patients with Wilson's disease and cystinuria should be given 25 mg/day of pyridoxine during therapy, since penicillamine increases the requirement for this vitamin. Patients also may receive benefit from a multivitamin preparation, although there is no evidence that deficiency of any vitamin other than pyridoxine is associated with penicillamine. In Wilson's disease, multivitamin preparations must be copper-free.
Rheumatoid arthritis patients whose nutrition is impaired should also be given a daily supplement of pyridoxine. Mineral supplements should not be given, since they may block the response to penicillamine.
Iron deficiency may develop, especially in children and in menstruating women. In Wilson's disease, this may be a result of adding the effects of the low copper diet, which is probably also low in iron, and the penicillamine to the effects of blood loss or growth. In cystinuria, a low methionine diet may contribute to iron deficiency, since it is necessarily low in protein. If necessary, iron may be given in short courses, but a period of two hours should elapse between administration of penicillamine and iron, since orally administered iron has been shown to reduce the effects of penicillamine.
Penicillamine causes an increase in the amount of soluble collagen. In the rat this results in inhibition of normal healing and also a decrease in tensile strength of intact skin. In man this may be the cause of increased skin friability at sites especially subject to pressure or trauma, such as shoulders, elbows, knees, toes, and buttocks. Extravasations of blood may occur and may appear as purpuric areas, with external bleeding if the skin is broken, or as vesicles containing dark blood. Neither type is progressive. There is no apparent association with bleeding elsewhere in the body and no associated coagulation defect has been found. Therapy with penicillamine may be continued in the presence of these lesions. They may disappear if dosage is reduced. Other reported effects probably due to the action of penicillamine on collagen are excessive wrinkling of the skin and development of small, white papules at venipuncture and surgical sites.
The effects of penicillamine on collagen and elastin make it advisable to consider a reduction in dosage to 250 mg/day when surgery is contemplated. Reinstitution of full therapy should be delayed until wound healing is complete.
Caution patients to report immediately any abrupt onset of pulmonary symptoms, such as exertional dyspnea, wheezing, or cough and have appropriate pulmonary function studies done to rule out obstructive bronchiolitis.
Carcinogenesis—Long-term animal carcinogenicity studies have not been done with penicillamine. There is a report that 5 to 10 autoimmune disease-prone NZB Hybrid mice developed lymphocytic leukemia after 6 months' intraperitoneal treatment with a dose of 400 mg/kg penicillamine 5 days per week.
Usage in Pregnancy—Penicillamine has been shown to be teratogenic in rats when given in doses several times higher than the highest dose recommended for human use. Skeletal defects, cleft palates and fetal toxicity (resorptions) have been reported.
Wilson's disease—There are no controlled studies in pregnant women with Wilson's disease, but experience does not include any positive evidence of adverse effects to the fetus. Reported experience* shows that continued treatment with penicillamine throughout pregnancy protects the mother against relapse of the Wilson's disease, and that discontinuation of penicillamine has deleterious effects on the mother. It indicates that the drug does not increase the risk of fetal abnormalities, but it does not exclude the possibility of infrequent or subtle damage to the fetus.

*Scheinberg, I. H., Sternlieb, I.: *N Engl J Med 293:* 1300–1302, Dec. 18, 1975.

If penicillamine is administered during pregnancy to patients with Wilson's disease, it is recommended that the daily dosage be limited to 1 g. If Caesarean section is planned, the daily dosage should be limited to 250 mg during the last six weeks of pregnancy and postoperatively until wound healing is complete.
Cystinuria—If possible, penicillamine should not be given during pregnancy to women with cystinuria. There is a report of a woman with cystinuria treated with 2 g/day of penicillamine during pregnancy who gave birth to a child with a generalized connective tissue defect that may have been caused by penicillamine. If stones continue to form in these patients, the benefits of therapy to the mother must be evaluated against the risk to the fetus.
Rheumatoid Arthritis—Penicillamine should not be administered to rheumatoid arthritis patients who are pregnant (see CONTRAINDICATIONS) and should be discontinued promptly in patients in whom pregnancy is suspected or diagnosed. Penicillamine should be used in women of childbearing potential only when the expected benefits outweigh possible hazards. Women of childbearing potential should be informed of the possible hazards of penicillamine to the developing fetus and should be advised to report promptly any missed menstrual periods or other indications of possible pregnancy.
There is a report that a woman with rheumatoid arthritis treated with less than 1 g/day of penicillamine during pregnancy gave birth (Caesarean delivery) to an infant with growth retardation, flattened face with broad nasal bridge, low set ears, short neck with loose skin folds, and unusually lax body skin.
Usage in Children—The efficacy of DEPEN in juvenile rheumatoid arthritis has not been established.
Adverse Reactions: Penicillamine is a drug with a high incidence of untoward reactions, some of which are potentially fatal. Therefore, it is mandatory that patients receiving penicillamine therapy remain under close medical supervision throughout the period of drug administration (see **Warnings** and **Precautions**).
Reported incidences (%) for the most commonly occurring adverse reactions in rheumatoid arthritis patients are noted, based on 17 representative clinical trials reported in the literature (1270 patients).
Allergic—Generalized pruritus, early and late rashes (5%), pemphigoid-type reactions and drug eruptions which may be accompanied by fever, arthralgia or lymphadenopathy have occurred (see **Warnings** and **Precautions**). Some patients may show a lupus erythematosus-like syndrome similar to drug induced lupus produced by other pharmacological agents (see **Precautions**).
Urticaria and exfoliative dermatitis have occurred. Thyroiditis has been reported but is extremely rare. Some patients may develop a migratory polyarthralgia, often with objective synovitis (see **Dosage** and **Administration**).
Gastrointestinal—Anorexia, epigastric pain, nausea, vomiting or occasional diarrhea may occur (17%). Isolated cases of reactivated peptic ulcer have occurred, as have hepatic dysfunction, cholestatic jaundice and pancreatitis. There have been a few reports of increased serum alkaline phosphatase, lactic dehydrogenase, and positive cephalin flocculation and thymol turbidity tests.
Some patients may report a blunting, diminution or total loss of taste perception (12%) or may develop oral ulcerations. Although rare, cheilosis, glossitis and gingivostomatitis have been reported (see **Precautions**).
Gastrointestinal side effects are usually reversible following cessation of therapy.
Hematological—Penicillamine can cause bone marrow depression (see **Warnings**). Leukopenia (2%) and thrombocytopenia (4%) have occurred. Fatalities have been reported as a result of thrombocytopenia, agranulocytosis and aplastic anemia. Thrombotic thrombocytopenic purpura, hemolytic anemia, red cell aplasia, monocytosis, leukocytosis, eosinophilia and thrombocytosis have also been reported.
Renal—Patients on penicillamine therapy may develop proteinuria (6%) and/or hematuria which, in some, may progress to the development of the nephrotic syndrome as a result of an immune complex membranous glomerulopathy (see **Warnings.**)

Central Nervous System—Tinnitus has been reported. Reversible optic neuritis has been reported with the administration of penicillamine and may be related to pyridoxine deficiency.

Other—Adverse reactions that have been reported rarely include thrombophlebitis; hyperpyrexia (see **Precautions**); falling hair or alopecia; myasthenia gravis (see **Warnings**); polymyositis; dermatomyositis; mammary hyperplasia; elastosis perforans serpiginosa; toxic epidermal necrolysis; anetoderma (cutaneous macular atrophy); Goodpasture's syndrome, a severe and ultimately fatal glomerulonephritis associated with intra-alveolar hemorrhage (see **Warnings**); and fatal renal vasculitis. Allergic alveolitis and obliterative bronchiolitis have been reported in patients with severe rheumatoid arthritis, some of whom were receiving penicillamine (see **Precautions**).

Increased skin friability, excessive wrinkling of skin, and development of small, white papules at venipuncture and surgical sites have been reported (See **Precautions**).

The chelating action of the drug may cause increased excretion of other heavy metals such as zinc, mercury and lead.

Dosage and Administration:

Wilson's Disease—DEPEN tablets should be given on an empty stomach, four times a day; one-half to one hour before meals and at bedtime—at least two hours after the evening meal.

Optimal dosage can be determined only by measurement of urinary copper excretion. The urine must be collected in copper-free glassware, and should be quantitatively analyzed for copper before and soon after initiation of therapy with DEPEN. Continued therapy should be monitored by doing a 24-hour urinary copper analysis every three months or so for the duration of therapy. Since a low copper diet should keep copper absorption down to less than one milligram a day, the patient probably will be in negative copper balance if 0.5 to one milligram of copper is present in a 24-hour collection of urine. To achieve this, the suggested initial dosage of DEPEN in the treatment of Wilson's disease is 1 g/day for children or adults. This may be increased, as indicated by the urinary copper analyses, but it is seldom necessary to exceed a dosage of 2 g/day.

In patients who cannot tolerate as much as 1 g/day initially, initiating dosage with 250 mg/day, and increasing gradually to the requisite amount, gives closer control of the effects of the drug and may help to reduce the incidence of adverse reactions.

Cystinuria—It is recommended that DEPEN be used along with conventional therapy. By reducing urinary cystine, it decreases crystalluria and stone formation. In some instances, it has been reported to decrease the size of, and even to dissolve, stones already formed.

The usual dosage of DEPEN in the treatment of cystinuria is 2 g/day for adults; with a range of 1 to 4 g/day. For children, dosage can be based on 30 mg/kg/day. The total daily amount should be divided into four doses. If four equal doses are not feasible, give the larger portion at bedtime. If adverse reactions necessitate a reduction in dosage, it is important to retain the bedtime dose.

Initiating dosage with 250 mg/day, and increasing gradually to the requisite amount, gives closer control of the effects of the drug and may help to reduce the incidence of adverse reactions.

In addition to taking DEPEN, patients should drink copiously. It is especially important to drink about a pint of fluid at bedtime and another pint once during the night when urine is more concentrated and more acid than during the day. The greater the fluid intake, the lower the required dosage of DEPEN.

Dosage must be individualized to an amount that limits cystine excretion to 100-200 mg/day in those with no history of stones, and below 100 mg/day in those who have had stone formation and/or pain. Thus, in determining dosage, the inherent tubular defect, the patient's size, age, and rate of growth, and his diet and water intake all must be taken into consideration.

The standard nitroprusside cyanide test has been reported useful as a qualitative measure of the effective dose*: Add 2 ml of freshly prepared 5 percent sodium cyanide to 5 ml of a 24-hour aliquot of protein-free urine and let stand ten minutes. Add 5 drops of freshly prepared 5 percent sodium nitroprusside and mix. Cystine will turn the mixture magenta. If the result is negative, it can be assumed that cystine excretion is less than 100 mg/g creatinine.

---

*Lotz, M., Potts, J. T. and Bartter, F. C.: *Brit Med J 2*:521, Aug. 28, 1965 (in Medical Memoranda).

Although penicillamine is rarely excreted unchanged, it also will turn the mixture magenta. If there is any question as to which substance is causing the reaction, a ferric chloride test can be done to eliminate doubt: Add 3 percent ferric chloride dropwise to the urine. Penicillamine will turn the urine an immediate and quickly fading blue. Cystine will not produce any change in appearance.

Rheumatoid Arthritis—The principal rule of treatment of DEPEN in rheumatoid arthritis is patience. The onset of therapeutic response is typically delayed. Two or three months may be required before the first evidence of a clinical response is noted (see **Clinical Pharmacology**).

When treatment with DEPEN has been interrupted because of adverse reactions or other reasons, the drug should be reintroduced cautiously by starting with a lower dosage and increasing slowly.

Initial Therapy

The currently recommended dosage regimen in rheumatoid arthritis begins with a single daily dose of 125 mg or 250 mg which is thereafter increased at one to three month intervals, by 125 mg or 250 mg/day, as patient response and tolerance indicate. If a satisfactory remission of symptoms is achieved, the dose associated with the remission should be continued (see Maintenance Therapy). If there is no improvement and there are no signs of potentially serious toxicity after two to three months of treatment with doses of 500–750 mg/day, increases of 250 mg/day at two to three month intervals may be continued until a satisfactory remission occurs (see Maintenance Therapy) or signs of toxicity develop (see **Warnings** and **Precautions**). If there is no discernible improvement after three to four months of treatment with 1000 to 1500 mg penicillamine/day, it may be assumed the patient will not respond and DEPEN should be discontinued.

It is important that DEPEN be given on an empty stomach at least one hour before meals and at least one hour apart from any other drug, food or milk (see **Clinical Pharmacology**).

Maintenance Therapy

The maintenance dosage of DEPEN must be individualized, and may require adjustment during the course of treatment. Many patients respond satisfactorily to a dosage within the 500–750 mg/day range. Some need less.

Changes in maintenance dosage levels may not be reflected clinically or in the erythrocyte sedimentation rate for two to three months after each dosage adjustment.

Some patients will subsequently require an increase in the maintenace dosage to achieve maximal disease suppression. In those patients who do respond, but who evidence incomplete suppression of their disease after the first six to nine months of treatment, the daily dosage of DEPEN may be increased by 125 mg or 250 mg/day at three-month intervals. It is unusual in current practice to employ a dosage in excess of 1 g/day, but up to 1.5 g/day has sometimes been required.

Management of Exacerbations

During the course of treatment some patients may experience an exacerbation of disease activity following an initial good response. These may be self-limited and can subside within twelve weeks. They are usually controlled by the addition of nonsteroidal anti-inflammatory drugs, and only if the patient has demonstrated a true "escape" phenomenon (as evidenced by failure of the flare to subside within this time period) should an increase in the maintenance dose ordinarily be considered.

In the rheumatoid patient, migratory polyarthralgia due to penicillamine is extremely difficult to differentiate from an exacerbation of the rheumatoid arthritis. Discontinuance or a substantial reduction in the dosage of DEPEN for up to several weeks will usually determine which of these processes is responsible for the arthralgia.

Duration of Therapy

The optimum duration of DEPEN therapy in rheumatoid arthritis has not been determined. If the patient has been in remission for six months or more, a gradual, stepwise dosage reduction in decrements of 125 mg or 250 mg/day at approximately three month intervals may be attempted.

Concomitant Drug Therapy

DEPEN should not be used in patients who are receiving gold therapy, antimalarial or cytotoxic drugs, oxyphenbutazone or phenylbutazone (see **Precautions**). Other measures, such as salicylates, other nonsteroidal anti-inflammatory drugs or systemic corticosteroids may be continued when DEPEN is initiated. After improvement commences, analgesic and anti-inflammatory drugs may be slowly discontinued as symptoms permit. Steroid withdrawal must be done gradually, and many months of DEPEN treatment may be required before steroids can be completely eliminated.

Dosage Frequency

Based on clinical experience, dosages up to 500 mg/day can be given as a single daily dose. Dosages in excess of 500 mg/day should be administered in divided doses.

How Supplied: DEPEN® Titratabs™ (penicillamine, Wallace) 250 mg scored, white tablets available in bottles of 100 (NDC 0037-4401-01).

Manufactured under license from
HOMBURG (Degussa), West Germany

Rev. 4/80

[*Shown in Product Identification Section*]

DEPROL® ℞ Ⓒ

(meprobamate 400 mg + benactyzine hydrochloride 1 mg)

Description: 'Deprol' is available as light pink, scored tablets, each containing meprobamate, U.S.P., 400 mg and benactyzine hydrochloride 1 mg.

Actions: 'Deprol' (meprobamate + benactyzine hydrochloride) combines the tranquilizing action of meprobamate with the antidepressant action of benactyzine hydrochloride.

Benactyzine hydrochloride

Benactyzine hydrochloride is a mild antidepressant and anticholinergic agent which in animals has been shown to reduce the autonomic response to emotion-provoking stress.

Meprobamate

Meprobamate is a carbamate derivative which has been shown in animal studies to have effects at multiple sites in the central nervous system, including the thalamus and limbic system.

Indications: Based on a review of this drug by the National Academy of Sciences—National Research Council and/or

Continued on next page

Wallace—Cont.

other information, FDA has classified the indication as follows:
"Possibly" effective: in the management of depression, both acute (reactive) and chronic. It is particularly useful in the less severe depressions and where the depression is accompanied by anxiety, insomnia, agitation, or rumination. It is also useful for management of depression and associated anxiety accompanying or related to organic illnesses.
Final classification of this indication requires further investigation.

Contraindications:
Benactyzine hydrochloride
Glaucoma and allergic or idiosyncratic reactions to benactyzine hydrochloride or related compounds.
Meprobamate
Acute intermittent porphyria as well as allergic or idiosyncratic reactions to meprobamate or related compounds such as carisoprodol, mebutamate, tybamate, or carbromal.
Warnings: The following information on meprobamate pertains to 'Deprol' (meprobamate + benactyzine hydrochloride):
Meprobamate
Drug Dependence—Physical dependence, psychological dependence, and abuse have occurred. When chronic intoxication from prolonged use occurs, it usually involves ingestion of greater than recommended doses and is manifested by ataxia, slurred speech, and vertigo. Therefore, careful supervision of dose and amounts prescribed is advised, as well as avoidance of prolonged administration, especially for alcoholics and other patients with a known propensity for taking excessive quantities of drugs.
Sudden withdrawal of the drug after prolonged and excessive use may precipitate recurrence of pre-existing symptoms, such as anxiety, anorexia, or insomnia, or withdrawal reactions, such as vomiting, ataxia, tremors, muscle twitching, confusional states, hallucinosis, and, rarely, convulsive seizures. Such seizures are more likely to occur in persons with central nervous system damage or preexistent or latent convulsive disorders. Onset of withdrawal symptoms occurs usually within 12 to 48 hours after discontinuation of meprobamate; symptoms usually cease within the next 12 to 48 hours.
When excessive dosage has continued for weeks or months, dosage should be reduced gradually over a period of one or two weeks rather than abruptly stopped. Alternatively, a short-acting barbiturate may be substituted, then gradually withdrawn.
Potentially Hazardous Tasks—Patients should be warned that this drug may impair the mental and/or physical abilities required for the performance of potentially hazardous tasks such as driving a motor vehicle or operating machinery.
Additive Effects—Since the effects of meprobamate and alcohol or meprobamate and other CNS depressants or psychotropic drugs may be additive, appropriate caution should be exercised with patients who take more than one of these agents simultaneously.

Usage in Pregnancy and Lactation
An increased risk of congenital malformations associated with the use of minor tranquilizers (meprobamate, chlordiazepoxide, and diazepam) during the first trimester of pregnancy has been suggested in several studies. Because use of these drugs is rarely a matter of urgency, their use during this period should almost always be avoided. The possibility that a woman of childbearing potential may be pregnant at the time of institution of therapy should be considered. Patients should be advised that if they become pregnant during therapy or intend to become pregnant they should communicate with their physicians about the desirability of discontinuing the drug.
Meprobamate passes the placental barrier. It is present both in umbilical cord blood at or near maternal plasma levels and in breast milk of lactating mothers at concentrations two to four times that of maternal plasma. When use of meprobamate is contemplated in breast-feeding patients, the drug's higher concentrations in breast milk as compared to maternal plasma levels should be considered.

Usage in Children—This combination is not intended for use in children.
Precautions: This product contains FD&C Yellow No. 5 (tartrazine) which may cause allergic-type reactions (including bronchial asthma) in certain susceptible individuals. Although the overall incidence of FD&C Yellow No. 5 (tartrazine) sensitivity in the general population is low, it is frequently seen in patients who also have aspirin hypersensitivity.
Meprobamate
The lowest effective dose should be administered, particularly to elderly and/or debilitated patients, in order to preclude oversedation.
The possibility of suicide attempts should be considered and the least amount of drug feasible should be dispensed at any one time.
Meprobamate is metabolized in the liver and excreted by the kidney; to avoid its excess accumulation, caution should be exercised in administration to patients with compromised liver or kidney function.
Meprobamate occasionally may precipitate seizures in epileptic patients.
Adverse Reactions: Side effects have included nausea, dryness of mouth, and other gastrointestinal symptoms; syncope; and one case each of severe nervousness and loss of power of concentration.
The following side effects, which have occurred after administration of its components alone, have either occurred or might occur when the combination is taken.
Benactyzine hydrochloride
Benactyzine hydrochloride alone, particularly in high dosage, may produce dizziness, thought-blocking, a sense of depersonalization, aggravation of anxiety, or disturbance of sleep patterns, and a subjective feeling of muscle relaxation. There may also be anticholinergic effects such as blurred vision, dryness of mouth, or failure of visual accommodation. Other reported side effects have included gastric distress, allergic response, ataxia, and euphoria.
Meprobamate
Central Nervous System—Drowsiness, ataxia, dizziness, slurred speech, headache, vertigo, weakness, paresthesias, impairment of visual accommodation, euphoria, overstimulation, paradoxical excitement, fast EEG activity.
Gastrointestinal — Nausea, vomiting, diarrhea.
Cardiovascular — Palpitations, tachycardia, various forms of arrhythmia, transient ECG changes, syncope; also, hypotensive crises (including one fatal case).
Allergic or Idiosyncratic—Allergic or idiosyncratic reactions are usually seen within the period of the first to fourth dose in patients having had no previous contact with the drug. Milder reactions are characterized by an itchy, urticarial, or erythematous maculopapular rash which may be generalized or confined to the groin. Other reactions have included leukopenia, acute nonthrombocytopenic purpura, petechiae, ecchymoses, eosinophilia, peripheral edema, adenopathy, fever, fixed drug eruption with cross reaction to carisoprodol, and cross sensitivity between meprobamate/-mebutamate and meprobamate/carbromal.
More severe hypersensitivity reactions, rarely reported, include hyperpyrexia, chills, angioneurotic edema, bronchospasm, oliguria, and anuria. Also, anaphylaxis, erythema multiforme, exfoliative dermatitis, stomatitis, proctitis, Stevens-Johnson syndrome, and bullous dermatitis, including one fatal case of the latter following administration of meprobamate in combination with prednisolone.
In case of allergic or idiosyncratic reactions to meprobamate, discontinue the drug and initiate appropriate symptomatic therapy, which may include epinephrine, antihistamines, and in severe cases corticosteroids. In evaluating possible allergic reactions, also consider allergy to excipients (information on excipients is available to physicians on request).
Hematologic (See also **Allergic or Idiosyncratic.**)—Agranulocytosis and aplastic anemia have been reported, although no causal relationship has been established. These cases rarely were fatal. Rare cases of thrombocytopenic purpura have been reported.
Other—Exacerbation of porphyric symptoms.
Dosage and Administration: The usual adult starting dosage of 'Deprol' (meprobamate +benactyzine hydrochloride) is one tablet three or four times daily, which may be increased gradually to six tablets daily and gradually reduced to maintenance levels upon establishment of relief. Doses above six tablets daily are not recommended, even though higher doses have been used by some clinicians to control depression, and in chronic psychotic patients.
Overdosage: Overdosage of 'Deprol' (meprobamate +benactyzine hydrochloride) has not differed substantially from meprobamate overdosage:
Meprobamate
Suicidal attempts with meprobamate have resulted in drowsiness, lethargy, stupor, ataxia, coma, shock, vasomotor and respiratory collapse. Some suicidal attempts have been fatal.
The following data on meprobamate tablets have been reported in the literature and from other sources. These data are not expected to correlate with each case (considering factors such as individual susceptibility and length of time from ingestion to treatment), but represent the *usual ranges* reported.
Acute simple overdose (meprobamate alone): Death has been reported with ingestion of as little as 12 gm meprobamate and survival with as much as 40 gm.
Blood Levels:
0.5—2.0 mg% represents the usual blood level range of meprobamate after therapeutic doses. The level may occasionally be as high as 3.0 mg%.
3 —10 mg% usually corresponds to findings of mild to moderate symptoms of overdosage, such as stupor or light coma.
10 —20 mg% usually corresponds to deeper coma, requiring more intensive treatment. Some fatalities occur.
At levels greater than 20 mg%, more fatalities than survivals can be expected.
Acute combined overdose (meprobamate with alcohol or other CNS depressants or psychotropic drugs): Since effects can be additive, a history of ingestion of a low dose of meprobamate plus any of these compounds (or of a relatively low blood or tissue level) cannot be used as a prognostic indicator.
In cases where excessive doses have been taken, sleep ensues rapidly and blood pressure, pulse, and respiratory rates are reduced to basal levels. Any drug remaining in the stomach should be removed and symptomatic therapy given. Should respiration or blood pressure become compromised, respiratory assistance, central nervous system stimulants, and pressor agents should be administered cautiously as indicated. Meprobamate is metabolized in the liver and excreted by the kidney. Diuresis, osmotic (mannitol) diuresis, peritoneal dialysis, and hemodialysis have been used success-

fully. Careful monitoring of urinary output is necessary and caution should be taken to avoid overhydration. Relapse and death, after initial recovery, have been attributed to incomplete gastric emptying and delayed absorption. Meprobamate can be measured in biological fluids by two methods: colorimetric (Hoffman, A.J. and Ludwig, B.J.: *J Amer Pharm Assn* **48**: 740, 1959) and gas chromatographic (Douglas, J.F. et al: *Anal Chem* **39**: 956, 1967).

How Supplied: Bottles of 100 (NDC 0037-3001-01). Bottles of 500 (NDC 0037-3001-03). Unit Dose: 500 (NDC 0037-3001-05). Unit Dose: 1000 (NDC 0037-3001-04). Rev. 7/79

[*Shown in Product Identification Section*]

DIUTENSEN® TABLETS ℞

The following text is complete prescribing information based on official labeling in effect August 1, 1981. Description: **Diutensen®** is a round, white-blue mottled tablet. Each tablet contains:

Cryptenamine ....2 mg.†
(as tannate salts)
Methyclothiazide ....2.5 mg.
†Equivalent to 260 Carotid Sinus Reflex Units.

Actions: Cryptenamine is an alkaloidal fraction obtained from *Veratrum viride* by a nonaqueous extraction procedure. The antihypertensive response to cryptenamine is widely documented. The principal mechanism of action of the drug in reducing the blood pressure involves widespread arteriolar dilatation mediated centrally, without peripheral adrenergic or ganglionic blockade. The major cardiovascular effects are reflex in nature and are mainly due to stimulation of afferent pressor receptors predominantly in the heart and carotid sinus area. These receptors initiate an increase in impulses which are interpreted by areas in the brain stem as denoting a pressure higher than that actually present. As a result, the mechanism concerned with blood pressure homeostasis is activated, sympathetic tone is decreased, vagal tone is increased, and the blood pressure is therefore reduced. Both systolic and diastolic pressures are decreased and the heart is slowed. Atropine abolishes the bradycrotic effect but only partially reverses the hypotensive effect.

Methyclothiazide is a synthetic saluretic-antihypertensive agent. It is a potent analogue of hydrochlorothiazide, being about 20 times as active by weight, as the latter compound. The renal mechanism involved in the diuretic action of methyclothiazide is indistinguishable from that elicited by chlorothiazide or hydrochlorothiazide, but the duration of action of methyclothiazide is longer than that of either of these compounds. The principle mechanism of action of methyclothiazide is the production of diuresis by inhibition of renal tubular reabsorption of electrolytes, resulting in a marked increase in the urinary excretion of sodium, chloride, and water, and moderate increase in the excretion of potassium and bicarbonate.

Indications: Based on a review of this drug by the national Academy of Sciences—National Research Council and/or other information, FDA has classified the indications as follows:
Lacking substantial evidence of effectiveness as a fixed combination for use in basic hypertensive therapy and for essential hypertension of all grades of severity. (See box warning.)
Final classification of less-than-effective indications requires further investigation.

Contraindications: DIUTENSEN is contraindicated for patients with known idiosyncrasy to *Veratrum viride* or thiazide compounds and for those who have recently experienced either coronary artery occlusion or cerebral thrombosis. Treatment with thiazide diuretics (including methyclothiazide) is also contraindicated for patients with severe renal or hepatic disease.

Warning: THIS FIXED COMBINATION DRUG IS NOT INDICATED FOR INITIAL THERAPY OF HYPERTENSION. HYPERTENSION REQUIRES THERAPY TITRATED TO THE INDIVIDUAL PATIENT. IF THE FIXED COMBINATION REPRESENTS THE DOSAGE SO DETERMINED, ITS USE MAY BE MORE CONVENIENT IN PATIENT MANAGEMENT. THE TREATMENT OF HYPERTENSION IS NOT STATIC, BUT MUST BE RE-EVALUATED AS CONDITIONS IN EACH PATIENT WARRANT.

Warnings: There have been several reports, published and unpublished, concerning nonspecific small-bowel lesions consisting of stenosis with or without ulceration, associated with the administration of enteric-coated thiazides with potassium salts. These lesions may occur with enteric-coated potassium tablets alone or when they are used with nonenteric-coated thiazides, or certain other oral diuretics. These small-bowel lesions have caused obstruction, hemorrhage, and perforation. Surgery was frequently required and deaths have occurred. Available information tends to implicate enteric-coated potassium salts although lesions of this type also occur spontaneously. Therefore, coated potassium-containing formulations should be administered only when indicated, and should be discontinued immediately if abdominal pain, distention, nausea, vomiting, or gastrointestinal bleeding ocur. Coated potassium tablets should be used only when adequate dietary supplementation is not practical.

Use in Pregnancy: USE OF ANY DRUG IN PREGNANCY, LACTATION, OR IN WOMEN OF CHILDBEARING AGE REQUIRES THAT THE POTENTIAL BENEFITS OF THE DRUG SHOULD BE WEIGHED AGAINST THE POSSIBLE HAZARDS TO THE MOTHER AND CHILD. DIUTENSEN SHOULD BE USED WITH CARE IN PREGNANT AND NURSING MOTHERS SINCE THIAZIDES CROSS THE PLACENTAL BARRIER AND APPEAR IN CORD BLOOD AND BREAST MILK. THIAZIDES MAY RESULT IN FETAL OR NEONATAL JAUNDICE, THROMBOCYTOPENIA, AND POSSIBLY OTHER ADVERSE REACTIONS WHICH HAVE OCCURRED IN THE ADULT.

Thiazides potentiate the action of other antihypertensive drugs. Therefore the dosage of these agents, especially the ganglion blockers, must be reduced by at least 50 percent as soon as thiazides are added to the regimen.

Exacerbation or activation of systemic lupus erythematosus has been reported with sulfonamide derived drugs, including thiazides.

Precautions: Cryptenamine is a potent hypotensive and occasionally bradycrotic drug. Overdosage may produce nausea and vomiting, excessive hypotension and prostration and, rarely, bronchoconstriction. If necessary, atropine sulfate (0.5 to 1.0 mg.) may be administered to reverse the bradycrotic effect. In the event of excessive fall in blood pressure, administer vasopressor drugs, such as ephedrine sulfate (30 to 50 mg.) or phenylephrine hydrochloride (5 mg.) subcutaneously. If left untended, the reaction will gradually disappear within 60 to 90 minutes.

Particular caution is warranted when treating patients with angina pectoris, coronary thrombosis, or cerebrovascular disease. Caution should also be exercised when treating hypertensive patients with chronic renal disease, since they adjust poorly to lowered blood pressure.

Special caution is warranted when treating patients with histories of bronchial asthma who may respond adversely to the cholinergic effect of cryptenamine.

The bradycrotic effect of veratrum alkaloids is additive to, but not synergistic with, that produced by morphine and related drugs.

Methyclothiazide is a potent saluretic drug. After initiation of therapy, the patient should be seen regularly to determine his individual response to therapy. Ordinarily, a total daily dose of 10 mg. (4 DIUTENSEN tablets daily), or less, is not accompanied by significant untoward reactions. However, certain patients may be unusually responsive to the saluretic effect of methyclothiazide and they may experience disturbances in electrolyte balance with subsequent development of hypokalemia. Serum electrolytes should be checked periodically during treatment, particularly in patients receiving relatively large doses of the drug. Patients who are receiving simultaneous treatment either with DIUTENSEN and digitalis or DIUTENSEN and potassium-depleting corticosteriods and those with impending hepatic coma should be carefully watched for signs and symptoms of disturbances in serum electrolyte balance. In the event evidence of electrolyte imbalance with hypokalemia is seen, it may be necessary to give supplemental potassium therapy in the form of fruit juices or direct potassium supplements of one gram, two to four times daily. In severe cases not responding to supplemental potassium therapy, it may be necessary to withdraw the drug.

Hypochloremic alkalosis occurs infrequently with methyclothiazide. Nevertheless, it is a possibility and if this condition develops, it may be treated by the addition of ammonium chloride to the dosage schedule. However, ammonium chloride should not be administered concurrently with a thiazide compound to patients with liver disease because each may cause an elevation in serum ammonia and precipitate onset of coma.

Some elevation of the blood urea nitrogen has been noted occasionally in patients receiving methyclothiazide. This reaction occurs more frequently in patients with decreased renal function. If serum nitrogen (BUN, NPN, creatinine) increases progressively, thiazide therapy should be discontinued.

As with other thiazide diuretics, hyperglycemia has been noted during treatment with methyclothiazide. If a significant elevation in blood sugar is noted, the drug should be withdrawn.

As with thiazides in general, serum uric acid has been observed to rise in a few patients treated with methyclothiazide, with overt symptoms of gout appearing in some of these. Symptoms of gout are readily controlled by treatment with colchicine.

Because some patients receiving veratrum alkaloids have experienced marked hypotension when undergoing surgical procedures, it may be advisable to discontinue treatment with DIUTENSEN for a period of approximately two weeks prior to elective surgery. Thiazide drugs may increase the responsiveness of patients to tubocurarine. Thiazides may decrease arterial responsiveness to norepinephrine and therefore should be withdrawn 48 hours before elective surgery. If emergency surgery is indicated, pre-anesthetic and anesthetic agents should be administered in reduced dosage. Emergency surgery may be carried out with the use, if necessary, of anticholinergic or adrenergic drugs to prevent vagal circulatory responses and of other supportive measures, as indicated.

Thiazides may decrease serum protein bound iodine levels without signs of thyroid disturbance.

The antihypertensive effects of these drugs may be enhanced in the post-sympathectomy patient.

Continued on next page

Wallace—Cont.

The concurrent use of DIUTENSEN with digitalis may increase the possibility of digitalis intoxication (due chiefly to the saluretic effects of methyclothiazide and perhaps to the vagotonic effects of cryptenamine). If there is evidence of myocardial irritability (extrasystoles, bigeminy, or AV block), dosage of DIUTENSEN should be reduced or discontinued.

Adverse Reactions: THIAZIDES: Varied reactions have been noted in patients treated with thiazides as follows: *Gastrointestinal:* anorexia, gastric irritation, nausea, vomiting, cramping, diarrhea, constipation, jaundice (intra-hepatic cholestatic) and pancreatitis. *Central nervous system:* vertigo, paresthesia, headache and xanthopsia. *Dermatologic-hypersensitivity:* skin rash, photosensitivity, urticaria and cutaneous vasculitis. *Hematologic:* purpura, thrombocytopenia, leukopenia, agranulocytosis and aplastic anemia.

In addition, orthostatic hypotension (aggravated when thiazides were administered in combination with either alcohol, barbiturates or narcotics), hyperglycemia, glycosuria, muscle cramps, dizziness, weakness, and restlessness have been reported.

CRYPTENAMINE: Patients treated with cryptenamine have experienced a variety of reactions as follows: excessive hypotension; prostration; anorexia; nausea and vomiting; epigastric and substernal burning, which may be mistaken for angina pectoris; unpleasant taste; salivation; sweating; hiccough; blurring of vision; mental confusion; cardiac arrhythmias; bradycardia; and, with excessive doses, bronchiolar constriction and respiratory depression.

When adverse reactions occur during treatment with DIUTENSEN, they are usually reversible and disappear when treatment is discontinued.

Dosage and Administration: As determined by individual titration (see box warning). The usual adult dosage of DIUTENSEN is 1 to 4 tablets a day depending on the individual patient response.

How Supplied:

NDC 0037-0272-92, bottle of 100
NDC 0037-0272-96, bottle of 500

Rev. 7/79

DIUTENSEN®-R TABLETS ℞

> **Warning:** THIS FIXED COMBINATION DRUG IS NOT INDICATED FOR INITIAL THERAPY OF HYPERTENSION. HYPERTENSION REQUIRES THERAPY TITRATED TO THE INDIVIDUAL PATIENT. IF THE FIXED COMBINATION REPRESENTS THE DOSAGE SO DETERMINED, ITS USE MAY BE MORE CONVENIENT IN PATIENT MANAGEMENT. THE TREATMENT OF HYPERTENSION IS NOT STATIC, BUT MUST BE RE-EVALUATED AS CONDITIONS IN EACH PATIENT WARRANT.

Description: **Diutensen®-R** is a two-component system of active ingredients containing 2.5 mg. methyclothiazide and 0.1 mg. reserpine per tablet. DIUTENSEN-R thus provides for easier titration of hypertensive patients than does a three-component system. DIUTENSEN-R tablets are round, white, pink-mottled tablets.

NOTE: DIUTENSEN-R previously contained cryptenamine tannate as a third antihypertensive agent.

Actions: *Methyclothiazide*—The predominant effects of methyclothiazide are diuresis, natriuresis, and chloruresis. The mechanism of action results in an interference with the renal tubular mechanism of electrolyte reabsorption. There is significant natriuresis and diuresis within two hours after administration of a single dose of methyclothiazide. These effects reach a peak in about six hours and persist for 24 hours following oral administration of a single dose.

In nonedematous patients the "peak" (maximum effective) natriuretic single dose of methyclothiazide is 10 mg., whereas the peak kaliuretic dose is 5 mg. Thus, doubling a daily dose of 5 mg. results in an increase of sodium output without significantly increasing potassium excretion.

Like other benzothiadiazines, methyclothiazide also has antihypertensive properties. It also may be used to enhance the antihypertensive action of other drugs. The mechanism by which benzothiadiazines, including methyclothiazide, produce a reduction of elevated blood pressure has not been definitely established. Sodium depletion, however, appears to be of primary importance.

Methyclothiazide is readily absorbed from the gastrointestinal tract and is excreted unchanged by the kidneys.

Reserpine—Reserpine is a pure crystalline alkaloid from the root of *Rauwolfia serpentina*. The drug has mild antihypertensive and bradycrotic effects in addition to sedative and tranquilizing properties.

Reserpine probably produces its antihypertensive effects through depletion of tissue stores of catecholamines (epinephrine and norepinephrine) from peripheral sites. By contrast, its sedative and tranquilizing properties are thought to be due to a depletion of 5-hydroxytryptamine from the brain.

Reserpine is characterized by slow onset of action and sustained effect. Both its cardiovascular and central nervous system effects may persist following withdrawal of the drug.

Indications: Hypertension (see box warning).

Contraindications: *Methyclothiazide*—This compound should not be used in anuric patients or those who exhibit a hypersensitivity to this or other sulfonamide derived drugs.

Reserpine—Reserpine is contraindicated in patients with known hypersensitivity, mental depression especially with suicidal tendencies, active peptic ulcer, and ulcerative colitis. It is also contraindicated in patients receiving electroconvulsive therapy.

Warnings: *Methyclothiazide* — Thiazides should be used with caution in severe renal disease. In patients with renal disease, thiazides may precipitate azotemia. Cumulative effects of the drug may develop in patients with impaired renal function.

Thiazides should be used with caution in patients with impaired hepatic function or progressive liver disease, since minor alterations of fluid and electrolyte balance may precipitate hepatic coma.

Thiazides may be additive or potentiate the action of other antihypertensive drugs. Potentiation occurs with ganglionic or peripheral adrenergic blocking drugs.

Sensitivity reactions may occur in patients with a history of allergy or bronchial asthma. The possibility of exacerbation or activation of systemic lupus erythematosus has been reported.

Reserpine—Extreme caution should be exercised in treating patients with a history of mental depression. Discontinue the drug at the first sign of despondency, early morning insomnia, loss of appetite, impotence, or self-deprecation. Drug-induced depression may persist for several months after drug withdrawal and may be severe enough to result in suicide.

Electroshock therapy should not be given to patients under treatment with reserpine since severe and even fatal reactions to such therapy have been reported in patients receiving reserpine. Reserpine should be discontinued for two weeks before electroshock therapy is given.

Use in Pregnancy: USE OF ANY DRUG IN PREGNANCY, LACTATION, OR IN WOMEN OF CHILDBEARING AGE REQUIRES THAT THE POTENTIAL BENEFITS OF THE DRUG SHOULD BE WEIGHED AGAINST THE POSSIBLE HAZARDS TO THE MOTHER AND CHILD. DIUTENSEN-R SHOULD BE USED WITH CARE IN PREGNANT AND NURSING MOTHERS SINCE METHYCLOTHIAZIDE AND RESERPINE CROSS THE PLACENTAL BARRIER AND APPEAR IN CORD BLOOD AND BREAST MILK.

THE SAFETY OF RESERPINE FOR USE DURING PREGNANCY OR LACTATION HAS NOT BEEN ESTABLISHED. INCREASED RESPIRATORY SECRETIONS, NASAL CONGESTION, CYANOSIS, AND ANOREXIA MAY OCCUR IN INFANTS BORN TO RESERPINE-TREATED MOTHERS.

THIAZIDES MAY RESULT IN FETAL OR NEONATAL JAUNDICE, THROMBOCYTOPENIA, AND POSSIBLE OTHER ADVERSE REACTIONS WHICH HAVE OCCURRED IN THE ADULT.

Precautions: *Methyclothiazide* — Periodic determination of serum electrolytes to detect possible electrolyte imbalance should be performed at appropriate intervals.

All patients receiving thiazide therapy should be observed for clinical signs of fluid or electrolyte imbalance; namely, hyponatremia, hypochloremic alkalosis, and hypokalemia. Serum and urine electrolyte determinations are particularly important when the patient is vomiting excessively or receiving parenteral fluids. Medication such as digitalis may also influence serum electrolytes. Warning signs, irrespective of cause, are: Dryness of mouth, thirst, weakness, lethargy, drowsiness, restlessness, muscle pains or cramps, muscular fatigue, hypotension, oliguria, tachycardia, and gastrointestinal disturbances such as nausea and vomiting.

Hypokalemia may develop with thiazides as with any other potent diuretic, especially with brisk diuresis, when severe cirrhosis is present, or during concomitant use of corticosteroids or ACTH.

Interference with adequate oral electrolyte intake will also contribute to hypokalemia. Digitalis therapy may exaggerate metabolic effects of hypokalemia especially with reference to myocardial activity.

Any chloride deficit is generally mild and usually does not require specific treatment except under extraordinary circumstances (as in liver disease or renal disease). Dilutional hyponatremia may occur in edematous patients in hot weather; appropriate therapy is water restriction, rather than administration of salt except in rare instances when the hyponatremia is life threatening. In actual salt depletion, appropriate replacement is the therapy of choice.

Hyperuricemia may occur or frank gout may be precipitated in certain patients receiving thiazide therapy.

Insulin requirements in diabetic patients may be increased, decreased, or unchanged. Latent diabetes mellitus may become manifest during thiazide administration.

Thiazide drugs may increase the responsiveness of tubocurarine.

The antihypertensive effects of the drug may be enhanced in the postsympathectomy patient.

Thiazides may decrease arterial responsiveness to norepinephrine. This diminution is not sufficient to preclude effectiveness of the pressor agent for therapeutic use.

If progressive renal impairment becomes evident, as indicated by a rising non-protein nitrogen or blood urea nitrogen, a careful reappraisal of therapy is necessary with consideration given to withholding or discontinuing diuretic therapy.

Thiazides may decrease serum PBI levels without signs of thyroid disturbance.

Reserpine—Because reserpine preparations increase gastrointestinal motility and secretion, this drug should be used cautiously in patients with a history of peptic ulcer, ulcerative colitis, or gallstones, where biliary colic may be precipitated.

Caution should be exercised when treating hypertensive patients with renal insufficiency since they adjust poorly to lowered blood pressure levels.

Use reserpine cautiously with digitalis and quinidine since cardiac arrhythmias have occurred with the concurrent use of rauwolfia preparations.

Preoperative withdrawal of reserpine does not assure that circulatory instability will not occur. It is important that the anesthesiologist be aware of the patient's drug intake and consider this in the overall management, since hypotension has occurred in patients receiving rauwolfia preparations. Anticholinergic and/or adrenergic drugs (metaraminol, norepinephrine) have been employed to treat adverse vagocirculatory effects.

Adverse Reactions: *Methyclothiazide:* The following adverse reactions have been associated with the use of thiazide diuretics.

Gastrointestinal: Anorexia, gastric irritation, nausea, vomiting, cramping, diarrhea, constipation, jaundice (intrahepatic cholestatic jaundice), pancreatitis.

Central nervous system: Dizziness, vertigo, parasthesia, headache, xanthopsia.

Dermatologic-Hypersensitivity: Purpura, photosensitivity, rash, urticaria, necrotizing angiitis (vasculitis) (cutaneous vasculitis).

Hematologic: Leukopenia, agranulocytosis, thrombocytopenia, aplastic anemia.

Cardiovascular: Orthostatic hypotension may occur and may be aggravated by alcohol, barbiturates or narcotics.

Miscellaneous: Hyperglycemia, glycosuria, hyperuricemia, muscle spasm, weakness, restlessness.

Reserpine—Reserpine preparations have caused gastrointestinal reactions including hypersecretion, nausea and vomiting, anorexia, and diarrhea; cardiovascular reactions including angina-like symptoms, arrhythmias particularly when used concurrently with digitalis or quinidine, and bradycardia; and central nervous system reactions including drowsiness, depression, nervousness, paradoxical anxiety, nightmares, rare parkinsonian syndrome, C.N.S. sensitization manifested by dull sensorium, deafness, glaucoma, uveitis, and optic atrophy. Nasal congestion is a frequent complaint, and pruritus, rash, dryness of mouth, dizziness, headache, dyspnea, purpura, impotence or decreased libido, dysuria, muscular aches, conjunctival injection, and weight gain have been reported. Extrapyramidal tract symptoms have also occurred. These reactions are usually reversible and disappear when the drug is discontinued.

Whenever DIUTENSEN-R therapy results in adverse reactions which are moderate or severe, dosage should be reduced or therapy withdrawn.

Dosage and Administration: As determined by individual titration (see box warning). The usual adult dosage of DIUTENSEN-R is 1 to 4 tablets a day depending on the individual patient response.

How Supplied:

NDC 0037-0274-92, bottle of 100
NDC 0037-0274-96, bottle of 500

Rev. 7/79

[*Shown in Product Identification Section*]

LUFYLLIN® Injection (dyphylline) ℞
LUFYLLIN® Elixir (dyphylline) ℞
LUFYLLIN® Tablets (dyphylline) ℞
LUFYLLIN®-400 Tablets (dyphylline) ℞

Description: Dyphylline is 7-(2,3-dihydroxypropyl) theophylline ($C_{10}H_{14}N_4O_4$), a pharmacologically active molecular modification of theophylline. This neutral theophylline derivative, stable in gastric juice, is a white, extremely bitter, amorphous solid, freely soluble in water and soluble to the extent of 2 g in 100 ml alcohol. Dyphylline contains the equivalent of approximately 70% anhydrous theophylline (on a molecular weight basis).

LUFYLLIN® Injection—Clear, colorless sterile solution. Each ml contains 250 mg dyphylline (pH adjusted with sodium hydroxide and/or hydrochloric acid).

LUFYLLIN® Elixir—is a clear red liquid. Each 15 ml (1 tablespoonful) contains 100 mg dyphylline (alcohol 20%).

LUFYLLIN® Tablets—each white, rectangular, monogrammed tablet contains 200 mg dyphylline.

LUFYLLIN®-400 Tablets—each white, capsule-shaped, monogrammed tablet contains 400 mg dyphylline.

Actions: As a xanthine derivative, dyphylline possesses the peripheral vasodilator and bronchodilator actions characteristic of theophylline. It has diuretic and myocardial stimulant effects, and is effective orally and by intramuscular injection. Dyphylline may show fewer side effects than aminophylline, but its blood levels and possibly its activity are also lower. When administered orally, it produces less nausea than aminophylline and other alkaline theophylline compounds. The injectable preparation is for intramuscular use only, and is indicated for treatment of an acute asthma attack.

Indications: For relief of acute bronchial asthma and for reversible bronchospasm associated with chronic bronchitis and emphysema.

Contraindications: In individuals who have shown hypersensitivity to any of its components. Dyphylline should not be administered concurrently with other xanthine preparations.

Warnings: Status asthmaticus is a medical emergency. Excessive doses may be expected to be toxic.

Usage in Pregnancy: Safe use in pregnancy has not been established relative to possible adverse effects on fetal development. Therefore, dyphylline should not be used in pregnant women unless, in the judgment of the physician, the potential benefits outweigh the possible hazards.

Precautions: Use with caution in patients with severe cardiac disease, hypertension, hyperthyroidism, or acute myocardial injury. Particular caution in dose administration must be exercised in patients with peptic ulcers, since the condition may be exacerbated.

Tablets only—chronic oral administration in high doses (500 to 1,000 mg) is usually associated with gastrointestinal irritation.

Great caution should be used in giving dyphylline to patients in congestive heart failure. Such patients have shown markedly prolonged blood level curves which have persisted for long periods following discontinuation of the drug.

Adverse Reactions: Note: Included in this listing which follows are a few adverse reactions which may not have been reported with this specific drug. However, pharmacological similarities among the xanthine drugs require that each of the reactions be considered when dyphylline is administered.

The most consistent adverse reactions associated with xanthine products are:

1. **Gastrointestinal:** irritation, nausea, vomiting and epigastric pain, generally preceded by headache, hematemesis, diarrhea.
2. **Central nervous system:** stimulation, irritability, restlessness, insomnia, reflex hyperexcitability, muscle twitching, clonic and tonic generalized convulsions, agitation.
3. **Cardiovascular:** palpitation, tachycardia, extra systoles, flushing, marked hypotension, and circulatory failure.
4. **Respiratory:** tachypnea, respiratory arrest.
5. **Renal:** albuminuria, increased excretion of renal tubule and red blood cells (hematuria).
6. **Others:** fever, dehydration.

Overdosage:

Symptoms: In infants and small children: agitation, headache, hyperreflexia, fasiculations, and clonic and tonic convulsions.

In adults: nervousness, insomnia, nausea, vomiting, tachycardia, and extra systoles.

Therapy: Discontinue drug immediately.
No specific treatment.
Ipecac syrup for oral ingestion.
Avoid sympathomimetics.
Supporting treatment for hypotension, seizure, arrhythmias and dehydration.
Sedatives such as short-acting barbiturates will help control central nervous system stimulation.
Restore the acid-base balance with lactate or bicarbonate.
Oxygen and antibiotics provide supportive treatment as indicated.

Drug Interactions: Toxic synergism with ephedrine and other sympathomimetic bronchodilator drugs may occur.

Recent controlled studies suggest that the addition of ephedrine to adequate dosage regimens of dyphylline produces no increase in effectiveness over that of dyphylline alone, but does produce an increase in toxic effects.

Dosage and Administration: The injectable product is for intramuscular use only and is to be injected very slowly. When administered orally, Lufylline (dyphylline) produces less nausea than aminophylline and other alkaline theophylline compounds. Absorption appears to be faster on an empty stomach. Preferably the drug is to be given at six-hour intervals.

Lufyllin Injection—Adults: Usual Dose: 1–2 ml (250–500 mg) may be injected intramuscularly, very slowly; and may be repeated if necessary.

Lufyllin Elixir—Adults: 30 ml (two tablespoonfuls) four times a day. Larger doses are generally required for the control of acute bronchial asthma. In acute asthma attack, 75 ml (5 tablespoonfuls) may be given.

Lufyllin and Lufyllin-400 Tablets—Adults: Usual Dose: 15 mg/kg every 6 hours, up to four times a day. The dosage should be individualized by titration to the condition and response of the patient.

"Therapeutic blood levels are considered to be between 10 mcg/ml and 20 mcg/ml. Levels above 20 mcg/ml may produce toxic effects. There is great variation from patient to patient in dosage needed in order to achieve a therapeutic blood level. Also, the duration of action of oral theophylline preparations varies widely from one patient to another. Because of this wide variation from patient to patient and the relatively narrow therapeutic blood level range, dosage must be individualized with monitoring of theophylline blood levels, particularly when prolonged or repeated use is planned."

Pulmonary function measurements before and after a period of treatment allow an objective assessment of whether or not therapy should be continued in patients with chronic bronchitis and emphysema.

Continued on next page

Wallace—Cont.

How Supplied:
Lufyllin Injection:
NDC 0037-0537-01, box of 25 × 2 ml ampuls.
[*Shown in Product Identification Section*]
Lufyllin Elixir:
NDC 0037-0515-68, pint bottle
NDC 0037-0515-69, gallon bottle
Lufyllin Tablets:
NDC 0037-0521-92, bottle of 100
NDC 0037-0521-97, bottle of 1000
NDC 0037-0521-85, box of 100 unit-dose individually film-sealed tablets.
[*Shown in Product Identification Section*]
Lufyllin-400 Tablets:
NDC 0037-0731-92, bottle of 100
NDC 0037-0731-97, bottle of 1000
NDC 0037-0731-85, box of 100 unit-dose individually film-sealed tablets.
[*Shown in Product Identification Section*]
Storage: Lufyllin Injection—Store below 40°C (104°F), preferably between 15° and 30°C (59° to 80°F). Excessive cold may cause formation of a precipitate. DO NOT USE if precipitate is present.
Caution: Federal (U.S.A.) law prohibits dispensing without prescription.

Lufyllin Injection is:
Distributed by
WALLACE LABORATORIES
Division of
CARTER-WALLACE, INC.
Cranbury, New Jersey 08512
Manufactured by:
Taylor Pharmacal Co.
Decatur, Illinois 62526
Lufyllin Tablets and Elixir are:
Manufactured by
WALLACE LABORATORIES
Division of
CARTER-WALLACE, INC.
Cranbury, New Jersey 08512

LUFYLLIN®–GG Tablets and Elixir ℞

Description: LUFYLLIN®-GG Tablets: Round, light yellow monogrammed tablets, scored on one side. Each tablet contains:

Dyphylline	200 mg
Guaifenesin	200 mg

LUFYLLIN®-GG Elixir: Clear yellow-orange liquid with a mild wine-like odor and taste.
Each 30 ml (two tablespoonfuls) contains:

Dyphylline	200 mg
Guaifenesin	200 mg
Alcohol	17%

Actions: LUFYLLIN (Dyphylline) is 7-(2,3-dihydroxypropyl) theophylline. It exhibits all the pharmacological effects of theophylline, including bronchodilation, vasodilation, myocardial stimulation and mild diuresis.
LUFYLLIN is completely soluble over the physiological pH range. Therapeutic dosages are readily tolerated with little or no gastric distress. LUFYLLIN effectively increases pulmonary function as determined by spirometric measurement. It is tolerated in adequate dosage levels over long periods of time without diminution of effectiveness. LUFYLLIN is neutral and stable.
LUFYLLIN-GG combines the expectorant action of guaifenesin with the bronchodilating properties of dyphylline to relieve acute bronchial asthma and reversible bronchospasm and its associated dyspnea, nonproductive cough and tracheobronchial irritation.
Indications: For relief of acute bronchial asthma and for reversible bronchospasm associated with chronic bronchitis and emphysema.
Precautions: Exercise caution with use in the presence of severe cardiac disease, renal or hepatic malfunction, glaucoma, hyperthyroidism, peptic ulcer, and concomitant use of other xanthine-containing formulations or other CNS stimulating drugs.
Adverse Reactions: May cause nausea, headache, cardiac palpitation and CNS stimulation. Postprandial administration may help to avoid gastric discomfort.
Dosage and Administration: These dosage recommendations are meant to offer a range in which one can anticipate a therapeutic response, recognizing that in the therapy of reversible bronchospasm there is considerable patient-to-patient variation; and, therefore, adjustments will probably be necessary based on the severity of symptoms and individual patient response.
Adults:
LUFYLLIN-GG Tablets and Elixir: One tablet or 30 ml (2 tablespoonfuls) four times a day. Larger doses are generally required for the control of acute bronchial asthma.
Children:
Dosages for children have not been established. Therefore, these agents are not recommended for children under six. Older children should be started on low doses which are gradually increased to the lowest effective dosage, not to exceed 5 mg/lb/day of dyphylline. Caution should be exercised in administration to children.
How Supplied:
LUFYLLIN-GG Tablets:
NDC 0037-0541-92, bottle of 100
NDC 0037-0541-97, bottle of 1000
NDC 0037-0541-85, box of 100 unit-dose individually film-sealed tablets.
[*Shown in Product Identification Section*]
LUFYLLIN-GG Elixir:
NDC 0037-0545-68, pint bottle
NDC 0037-0545-69, gallon bottle
Rev. 7/79

MALTSUPEX® OTC
(malt soup extract)
Powder, Liquid, Tablets

Composition: 'Maltsupex' is a nondiastatic extract from barley malt, which is available in powder, liquid, and tablet form. 'Maltsupex' has a gentle laxative action and promotes soft, easily passed stools. Each **Tablet** contains 750 mg of 'Maltsupex' and approximately 0.15 to 0.25 mEq of potassium. Each tablespoonful (0.5 fl oz) of **Liquid** and each heaping tablespoonful of **Powder** contains approximately 16 grams of Malt Soup Extract and 3.1 to 5.5 mEq of potassium.
Indications: 'Maltsupex' is indicated for the dietary management and treatment of functional constipation in infants and children. It is also useful in treating constipation in adults, including those with laxative dependence.
Warnings: Do not use when abdominal pain, nausea or vomiting are present. If constipation persists, consult a physician. Keep this and all medications out of the reach of children.
'Maltsupex' Powder and Liquid only—Do not use these products except under the advice and supervision of a physician if you have kidney disease.
Caution: If pregnant or nursing a baby, consult your physician or pharmacist before using this product.
Precautions: In patients with diabetes, allow for carbohydrate content of approximately 14 grams per tablespoonful of **Liquid** (56 calories), 13 grams per tablespoonful of **Powder** (52 calories), and 0.6 grams per Tablet (3 calories).
Tablets only: This product contains FD&C Yellow No. 5 (tartrazine) which may cause allergic-type reactions (including bronchial asthma) in certain susceptible individuals. Although the overall incidence of FD&C Yellow No. 5 (tartrazine) sensitivity in the general population is low, it is frequently seen in patients who also have aspirin hypersensitivity.
Dosage and Administration: General—The recommended daily dosage of 'Maltsupex' may vary from 6 to 32 grams for infants (2 years or less) and 12 to 64 grams for children and adults, accompanied by adequate fluid intake with each dose. Use the smallest dose that is effective and lower dosage as improvement occurs. Use heaping measures of the **Powder**. 'Maltsupex' **Liquid** mixes more easily if stirred first in one or two ounces of warm water.
Powder and Liquid (Usual Dosage)—
Adults: 2 tablespoonfuls (32 g) twice daily for 3 or 4 days, or until relief is noted, then 1 to 2 tablespoonfuls at bedtime for maintenance, as needed. Drink a full glass (8 oz) of liquid with each dose.
Children: 1 or 2 tablespoonfuls in 8 ounces of liquid once or twice daily (with cereal, milk or preferred beverage). **Bottle-Fed Infants (over 1 month):** ½ to 2 tablespoonfuls in the day's total formula, or 1 to 2 teaspoonfuls in a single feeding to correct constipation. To prevent constipation (as when switching to whole milk) add 1 to 2 teaspoonfuls to the day's formula or 1 teaspoonful to every second feeding. **Breast-Fed Infants (over one month):** 1 to 2 teaspoonfuls in 2 to 4 ounces of water or fruit juice once or twice daily.
Tablets—**Adults:** Start with 4 tablets (3 g) four times daily (with meals and bedtime) and adjust dosage according to response. Drink a full glass (8 oz) of liquid with each dose.
How Supplied: 'Maltsupex' is supplied in 8 ounce (NDC 0037-9101-12) and 16 ounce (NDC 0037-9101-08) jars of 'Maltsupex' Powder; 8 fluid ounce (NDC 0037-9001-12) and 1 pint (NDC 0037-9001-08) bottles of 'Maltsupex' Liquid; and in bottles of 100 'Maltsupex' Tablets (NDC 0037-9201-01).
'Maltsupex' **Powder** and **Liquid** are Distributed by
WALLACE LABORATORIES
Division of
CARTER-WALLACE, INC.
Cranbury, New Jersey 08512
'Maltsupex' **Tablets** are Manufactured by
WALLACE LABORATORIES
Division of
CARTER-WALLACE, INC.
Cranbury, New Jersey 08512
Rev. 5/82

MEPROSPAN® ℞ ©
(meprobamate, sustained-release capsules)

Description: Meprobamate is a white powder with a characteristic odor and a bitter taste. It is slightly soluble in water, freely soluble in acetone and alcohol, and sparingly soluble in ether.
Actions: Meprobamate is a carbamate derivative which has been shown in animal studies to have effects at multiple sites in the central nervous system, including the thalamus and limbic system.
Indications: 'Meprospan' (meprobamate) is indicated for the management of anxiety disorders or for the short-term relief of the symptoms of anxiety. Anxiety or tension associated with the stress of everyday life usually do not require treatment with an anxiolytic.
The effectiveness of 'Meprospan' in long-term use, that is, more than 4 months, has not been assessed by systematic clinical studies. The physician should periodically reassess the usefulness of the drug for the individual patient.
Contraindications: Acute intermittent porphyria as well as allergic or idiosyncratic reactions to meprobamate or related compounds such as carisoprodol, mebutamate, tybamate, or carbromal.
Warnings
Drug Dependence
Physical dependence, psychological dependence, and abuse have occurred. When chronic intoxication from prolonged use occurs, it usually involves ingestion of greater than recommended doses and is manifested by ataxia, slurred speech, and vertigo. Therefore, careful supervision of dose and amounts prescribed is advised, as well as avoidance of prolonged administration, especially for alcoholics and

other patients with a known propensity for taking excessive quantities of drugs.

Sudden withdrawal of the drug after prolonged and excessive use may precipitate recurrence of pre-existing symptoms, such as anxiety, anorexia, or insomnia, or withdrawal reactions, such as vomiting, ataxia, tremors, muscle twitching, confusional states, hallucinosis, and, rarely, convulsive seizures. Such seizures are more likely to occur in persons with central nervous system damage or pre-existent or latent convulsive disorders. Onset of withdrawal symptoms occurs usually within 12 to 48 hours after discontinuation of meprobamate; symptoms usually cease within the next 12 to 48 hours.

When excessive dosage has continued for weeks or months, dosage should be reduced gradually over a period of one or two weeks rather than abruptly stopped. Alternatively, a short-acting barbiturate may be substituted, then gradually withdrawn.

Potentially Hazardous Tasks

Patients should be warned that this drug may impair the mental and/or physical abilities required for the performance of potentially hazardous tasks such as driving a motor vehicle or operating machinery.

Additive Effects

Since the effects of meprobamate and alcohol or meprobamate and other CNS depressants or psychotropic drugs may be additive, appropriate caution should be exercised with patients who take more than one of these agents simultaneously.

USAGE IN PREGNANCY AND LACTATION

An increased risk of congenital malformations associated with the use of minor tranquilizers (meprobamate, chlordiazepoxide, and diazepam) during the first trimester of pregnancy has been suggested in several studies. Because use of these drugs is rarely a matter of urgency, their use during this period should almost always be avoided. The possibility that a woman of childbearing potential may be pregnant at the time of institution of therapy should be considered.

Patients should be advised that if they become pregnant during therapy or intend to become pregnant they should communicate with their physicians about the desirability of discontinuing the drug.

Meprobamate passes the placental barrier. It is present both in umbilical cord blood at or near maternal plasma levels and in breast milk of lactating mothers at concentrations two or four times that of maternal plasma. When use of meprobamate is contemplated in breast-feeding patients, the drug's higher concentration in breast milk as compared to maternal plasma levels should be considered.

Usage in Children

Meprobamate should not be administered to children under age six, since there is a lack of documented evidence for safety and effectiveness in this age group.

Precautions: The lowest effective dose should be administered, particularly to elderly and/or debilitated patients, in order to preclude oversedation.

The possibility of suicide attempts should be considered and the least amount of drug feasible should be dispensed at any one time.

Meprobamate is metabolized in the liver and excreted by the kidney; to avoid its excess accumulation, caution should be exercised in administration to patients with compromised liver or kidney function.

Meprobamate occasionally may precipitate seizures in epileptic patients.

Adverse Reactions

Central Nervous System

Drowsiness, ataxia, dizziness, slurred speech, headache, vertigo, weakness, paresthesias, impairment of visual accommodation, euphoria, overstimulation, paradoxical excitement, fast EEG activity.

Gastrointestinal

Nausea, vomiting, diarrhea.

Cardiovascular

Palpitations, tachycardia, various forms of arrhythmia, transient ECG changes, syncope; also, hypotensive crises (including one fatal case).

Allergic or Idiosyncratic

Allergic or idiosyncratic reactions are usually seen within the period of the first to fourth dose in patients having had no previous contact with the drug. Milder reactions are characterized by an itchy, urticarial, or erythematous maculopapular rash which may be generalized or confined to the groin. Other reactions have included leukopenia, acute nonthrombocytopenic purpura, petechiae, ecchymoses, eosinophilia, peripheral edema, adenopathy, fever, fixed drug eruption with cross reaction to carisoprodol, and cross sensitivity between meprobamate/mebutamate and meprobamate/carbromal.

More severe hypersensitivity reactions, rarely reported, include hyperpyrexia, chills, angioneurotic edema, bronchospasm, oliguria, and anuria. Also, anaphylaxis, erythema multiforme, exfoliative dermatitis, stomatitis, proctitis, Stevens-Johnson syndrome, and bullous dermatitis, including one fatal case of the latter following administration of meprobamate in combination with prednisolone.

In case of allergic or idiosyncratic reactions to meprobamate, discontinue the drug and initiate appropriate symptomatic therapy, which may include epinephrine, antihistamines, and in severe cases corticosteroids. In evaluating possible allergic reactions, also consider allergy to excipients (information on excipients is available to physicians on request).

Hematologic

(See also **Allergic or Idiosyncratic.**) Agranulocytosis and aplastic anemia have been reported, although no causal relationship has been established. These cases rarely were fatal. Rare cases of thrombocytopenic purpura have been reported.

Other

Exacerbation of porphyric symptoms.

Dosage and Administration: The usual adult dosage of 'Meprospan' (meprobamate, sustained-release capsules) is one to two 400 mg capsules in the morning and again at bedtime; doses above 2400 mg daily are not recommended. The usual dosage for children ages six to twelve is one 200 mg capsule in the morning and again at bedtime. Meprobamate is not recommended for children under age six.

Overdosage: Suicidal attempts with meprobamate have resulted in drowsiness, lethargy, stupor, ataxia, coma, shock, vasomotor and respiratory collapse. Some suicidal attempts have been fatal.

Overdosage experience with 'Meprospan' (meprobamate, sustained-release capsules) is limited. However, the following data on meprobamate tablets have been reported in the literature and from other sources. These data are not expected to correlate with each case (considering factors such as individual susceptibility and length of time from ingestion to treatment), but represent the *usual ranges* reported.

Acute simple overdose (meprobamate alone): Death has been reported with ingestion of as little as 12 gm meprobamate and survival with as much as 40 gm.

Blood Levels:

0.5 —2.0 mg% represents the usual blood level range of meprobamate after therapeutic doses. The level may occasionally be as high as 3.0 mg%.

3 —10 mg% usually corresonds to findings of mild to moderate symptoms of overdosage, such as stupor or light coma.

10 —20 mg% usually corresponds to deeper coma, requiring more intensive treatment. Some fatalities occur.

At levels greater than 20 mg%, more fatalities than survivals can be expected.

Acute combined overdose (meprobamate with alcohol or other CNS depressants or psychotropic drugs): Since effects can be additive, a history of ingestion of a low dose of meprobamate plus any of these compounds (or of a relatively low blood or tissue level) cannot be used as a prognostic indicator.

In cases where excessive doses have been taken, sleep ensues rapidly and blood pressure, pulse, and respiratory rates are reduced to basal levels. Any drug remaining in the stomach should be removed and symptomatic therapy given. Should respiration or blood pressure become compromised, respiratory assistance, central nervous system stimulants, and pressor agents should be administered cautiously as indicated. Meprobamate is metabolized in the liver and excreted by the kidney. Diuresis, osmotic (mannitol) diuresis, peritoneal dialysis, and hemodialysis have been used successfully. Careful monitoring of urinary output is necessary and caution should be taken to avoid overhydration. Relapse and death, after initial recovery, have been attributed to incomplete gastric emptying and delayed absorption. Meprobamate can be measured in biological fluids by two methods: colorimetric (Hoffman, A.J. and Ludwig, B.J.: *J Amer Pharm Assn 48:* 740, 1959) and gas chromatographic (Douglas, J.F. et al: *Anal Chem 39:* 956, 1967).

How Supplied: 'Meprospan' 400: Each sustained-release, blue-topped capsule contains meprobamate, U.S.P., 400 mg in bottles of 100 (NDC 0037-1301-01).

'Meprospan' 200: Each sustained-release, yellow-topped capsule contains meprobamate, U.S.P., 200 mg in bottles of 100 (NDC 0037-1401-01).

Distributed by
WALLACE LABORATORIES
Division of
CARTER-WALLACE, INC.
Cranbury, New Jersey 08512
Manufactured by KV Pharmacal, St. Louis, Mo. 63144

Rev. 10/80

MILPATH® ℞

(meprobamate + tridihexethyl chloride)

Description: 'Milpath' is available in two formulations:

'Milpath'-400 Yellow, scored tablets, each containing:

meprobamate, U.S.P. .... 400 mg
tridihexethyl chloride .... 25 mg

'Milpath'-200 Yellow, coated tablets, each containing:

meprobamate, U.S.P. .... 200 mg
tridihexethyl chloride .... 25 mg

Actions: 'Milpath' combines meprobamate, a tranquilizing agent, with tridihexethyl chloride, an anticholinergic agent.

Tridihexethyl chloride

Tridihexethyl chloride possesses antimuscarinic actions. Gastrointestinal actions include reduction in both gastric secretion and gastrointestinal motility.

Meprobamate

Meprobamate is a carbamate derivative which has been shown in animal studies to have effects at multiple sites in the central nervous system, including the thalamus and limbic system.

Indications: Based on a review of this drug by the National Academy of Sciences—National Research Council and/or other information, FDA has classified the indication as follows:

"Possibly" effective: as adjunctive therapy in the treatment of peptic ulcer and in the treatment of the irritable bowel syndrome

Continued on next page

Wallace—Cont.

(irritable colon, spastic colon, mucous colitis) and acute enterocolitis.
Final classification of this indication requires further investigation.

Contraindications:
Tridihexethyl chloride
Allergic or idiosyncratic reactions to tridihexethyl chloride or related compounds; urinary bladder-neck obstructions, such as prostatic obstructions due to hypertrophy; pyloric obstructions because of reduction of motility and tonus; organic cardiospasm (megaesophagus); glaucoma. It may also be contraindicated in stenosing gastric or duodenal ulcers with significant gastric retention.
Meprobamate
Acute intermittent porphyria as well as allergic or idiosyncratic reactions to meprobamate or related compounds such as carisoprodol, mebutamate, tybamate, or carbromal.
Warnings:
Meprobamate
Drug Dependence—Physical dependence, psychological dependence, and abuse have occurred. When chronic intoxication from prolonged use occurs, it usually involves ingestion of greater than recommended doses and is manifested by ataxia, slurred speech, and vertigo. Therefore, careful supervision of dose and amounts prescribed is advised, as well as avoidance of prolonged administration, especially for alcoholics and other patients with a known propensity for taking excessive quantities of drugs. Sudden withdrawal of the drug after prolonged and excessive use may precipitate recurrence of pre-existing symptoms, such as anxiety, anorexia, or insomnia, or withdrawal reactions, such as vomiting, ataxia, tremors, muscle twitching, confusional states, hallucinosis, and, rarely, convulsive seizures. Such seizures are more likely to occur in persons with central nervous system damage or preexistent or latent convulsive disorders. Onset of withdrawal symptoms occurs usually within 12 to 48 hours after discontinuation of meprobamate; symptoms usually cease within the next 12 to 48 hours.
When excessive dosage has continued for weeks or months, dosage should be reduced gradually over a period of one or two weeks rather than abruptly stopped. Alternatively, a short-acting barbiturate may be substituted, then gradually withdrawn.
Potentially Hazardous Tasks—Patients should be warned that this drug may impair the mental and/or physical abilities required for the performance of potentially hazardous tasks such as driving a motor vehicle or operating machinery.
Additive Effects—Since the effects of meprobamate and alcohol or meprobamate and other CNS depressants or psychotropic drugs may be additive, appropriate caution should be exercised with patients who take more than one of these agents simultaneously.

Usage in Pregnancy and Lactation
An increased risk of congenital malformations associated with the use of minor tranquilizers (meprobamate, chlordiazepoxide, and diazepam) during the first trimester of pregnancy has been suggested in several studies. Because use of these drugs is rarely a matter of urgency, their use during this period should almost always be avoided. The possibility that a woman of childbearing potential may be pregnant at the time of institution of therapy should be considered. Patients should be advised that if they become pregnant during therapy or intend to become pregnant they should communicate with their physicians about the desirability of discontinuing the drug.
Meprobamate passes the placental barrier. It is present both in umbilical cord blood at or near maternal plasma levels and in breast milk of lactating mothers at concentrations two to four times that of maternal plasma. When use of meprobamate is contemplated in breast-feeding patients, the drug's higher concentrations in breast milk as compared to maternal plasma levels should be considered.

Precautions:
Tridihexethyl chloride
Use cautiously in elderly male patients because of the possibility of prostatic hypertrophy.
Meprobamate
The lowest effective dose should be administered, particularly to elderly and/or debilitated patients, in order to preclude oversedation.
The possibility of suicide attempts should be considered and the least amount of drug feasible should be dispensed at any one time.
Meprobamate is metabolized in the liver and excreted by the kidney; to avoid its excess accumulation, caution should be exercised in administration to patients with compromised liver or kidney function.
Meprobamate occasionally may precipitate seizures in epileptic patients.
Adverse Reactions: While few of the following reactions have been reported with 'Milpath' (meprobamate + tridihexethyl chloride) administration, it is possible that side effects which have occurred with the constituents alone might also occur when the combination is taken.
Tridihexethyl chloride
At recommended dosage severe effects are rare; those reported are the occurrences typically related to administration of anticholinergic drugs. Dry mouth is fairly frequent at oral doses of 100 mg. Constipation or a "bloated" feeling sometimes occurs. Other possible anticholinergic side effects include tachycardia, bradycardia, dilation of pupils, increased ocular tension, weakness, nausea, vomiting, headache, drowsiness, urinary hesitancy or retention, and dizziness.
Meprobamate
Central Nervous System—Drowsiness, ataxia, dizziness, slurred speech, headache, vertigo, weakness, paresthesias, impairment of visual accommodation, euphoria, overstimulation, paradoxical excitement, fast EEG activity.
Gastrointestinal — Nausea, vomiting, diarrhea.
Cardiovascular — Palpitations, tachycardia, various forms of arrhythmia, transient ECG changes, syncope; also, hypotensive crises (including one fatal case).
Allergic or Idiosyncratic—Allergic or idiosyncratic reactions are usually seen within the period of the first to fourth dose in patients having had no previous contact with the drug. Milder reactions are characterized by an itchy, urticarial, or erythematous maculopapular rash which may be generalized or confined to the groin. Other reactions have included leukopenia, acute nonthrombocytopenic purpura, petechiae, ecchymoses, eosinophilia, peripheral edema, adenopathy, fever, fixed drug eruption with cross reaction to carisoprodol, and cross sensitivity between meprobamate/-mebutamate and meprobamate/carbromal.
More severe hypersensitivity reactions, rarely reported, include hyperpyrexia, chills, angioneurotic edema, bronchospasm, oliguria, and anuria. Also, anaphylaxis, erythema multiforme, exfoliative dermatitis, stomatitis, proctitis, Stevens-Johnson syndrome, and bullous dermatitis, including one fatal case of the latter following administration of meprobamate in combination with prednisolone.
In case of allergic or idiosyncratic reactions to meprobamate, discontinue the drug and initiate appropriate symptomatic therapy, which may include epinephrine, antihistamines, and in severe cases corticosteroids. In evaluating possible allergic reactions, also consider allergy to excipients (information on excipients is available to physicians on request).
Hematologic (See also **Allergic or Idiosyncratic.**)—Agranulocytosis and aplastic anemia have been reported, although no causal relationship has been established. These cases rarely were fatal. Rare cases of thrombocytopenic purpura have been reported.
Other—Exacerbation of porphyric symptoms.
Dosage and Administration: The usual adult dosage of 'Milpath'-400 (meprobamate 400 mg + tridihexethyl chloride 25 mg) is one tablet three times a day at mealtimes, and two tablets at bedtime. If a greater anticholinergic effect is desired, the usual adult dosage is two 'Milpath'-200 (meprobamate 200 mg + tridihexethyl chloride 25 mg) tablets three times a day at mealtimes, and two tablets at bedtime. Doses of meprobamate above 2400 mg daily are not recommended.
Not for use in children under age 12.
Overdosage: Although no cases of overdosage have been reported with 'Milpath' (meprobamate + tridihexethyl chloride), following is information on the separate components.
Tridihexethyl chloride
Acute overdosage of anticholinergic agents can produce dry mouth, difficulty swallowing, marked thirst; blurred vision, photophobia; flushed, hot, dry skin; rash; hyperthermia; palpitations, tachycardia with weak pulse, elevated blood pressure; urinary urgency with difficulty in micturition; abdominal distention; restlessness, confusion, delirium and other signs suggestive of an acute organic psychosis. Treatment should include removal of remaining drug from stomach after administration of Universal Antidote, and supportive and symptomatic therapy as indicated.
Meprobamate
Suicidal attempts with meprobamate have resulted in drowsiness, lethargy, stupor, ataxia, coma, shock, vasomotor and respiratory collapse. Some suicidal attempts have been fatal.
The following data on meprobamate tablets have been reported in the literature and from other sources. These data are not expected to correlate with each case (considering factors such as individual susceptibility and length of time from ingestion to treatment), but represent the *usual ranges* reported.
Acute simple overdose (meprobamate alone): Death has been reported with ingestion of as little as 12 gm meprobamate and survival with as much as 40 gm.
Blood Levels:
0.5 — 2.0 mg% represents the usual blood level range of meprobamate after therapeutic doses. The level may occasionally be as high as 3.0 mg%.
3 —10 mg% usually corresponds to findings of mild to moderate symptoms of overdosage, such as stupor or light coma.
10 —20 mg% usually corresponds to deeper coma, requiring more intensive treatment. Some fatalities occur.
At levels greater than 20 mg%, more fatalities than survivals can be expected.
Acute combined overdose (meprobamate with alcohol or other CNS depressants or psychotropic drugs): Since effects can be additive, a history of ingestion of a low dose of meprobamate plus any of these compounds (or of a relatively low blood or tissue level) cannot be used as a prognostic indicator.
In cases where excessive doses have been taken, sleep ensues rapidly and blood pressure, pulse, and respiratory rates are reduced to basal levels. Any drug remaining in the stomach should be removed and symptomatic therapy given. Should respiration or blood pressure become compromised, respiratory assistance, central nervous system stimulants, and pressor agents should be administered cautiously

as indicated. Meprobamate is metabolized in the liver and excreted by the kidney. Diuresis, osmotic (mannitol) diuresis, peritoneal dialysis, and hemodialysis have been used successfully. Careful monitoring of urinary output is necessary and caution should be taken to avoid overhydration. Relapse and death, after initial recovery, have been attributed to incomplete gastric emptying and delayed absorption. Meprobamate can be measured in biological fluids by two methods: colorimetric (Hoffman, A.J. and Ludwig, B.J.: *J Amer Pharm Assn* **48:** 740, 1959) and gas chromatographic (Douglas, J.F. et al: *Anal Chem* **39:** 956, 1967).

How supplied: 'Milpath'-400 Bottles of 100 (NDC 0037-5001-01) and 500 (NDC 0037-5001-03) 'Milpath'-200 Bottles of 100. (NDC 0037-5101-01) Rev. 1/79

[*Shown in Product Identification Section*]

MILTOWN® Tablets ℞ Ⓒ
(meprobamate)
MILTOWN® 600 Tablets ℞ Ⓒ
(meprobamate 600 mg)

Description: Meprobamate is a white powder with a characteristic odor and a bitter taste. It is slightly soluble in water, freely soluble in acetone and alcohol, and sparingly soluble in ether.

Actions: Meprobamate is a carbamate derivative which has been shown in animal studies to have effects at multiple sites in the central nervous system, including the thalamus and limbic system.

Indications: 'Miltown' (meprobamate) is indicated for the management of anxiety disorders or for the short-term relief of the symptoms of anxiety. Anxiety or tension associated with the stress of everyday life usually do not require treatment with an anxiolytic.

The effectiveness of 'Miltown' in long-term use, that is, more than 4 months, has not been assessed by systematic clinical studies. The physician should periodically reassess the usefulness of the drug for the individual patient.

Contraindications: Acute intermittent porphyria as well as allergic or idiosyncratic reactions to meprobamate or related compounds such as carisoprodol, mebutamate, tybamate, or carbromal.

Warnings:

Drug Dependence

Physical dependence, psychological dependence, and abuse have occurred. When chronic intoxication from prolonged use occurs, it usually involves ingestion of greater than recommended doses and is manifested by ataxia, slurred speech, and vertigo. Therefore, careful supervision of dose and amounts prescribed is advised, as well as avoidance of prolonged administration, especially for alcoholics and other patients with a known propensity for taking excessive quantities of drugs.

Sudden withdrawal of the drug after prolonged and excessive use may precipitate recurrence of pre-existing symptoms, such as anxiety, anorexia, or insomnia, or withdrawal reactions, such as vomiting, ataxia, tremors, muscle twitching, confusional states, hallucinosis, and, rarely, convulsive seizures. Such seizures are more likely to occur in persons with central nervous system damage or pre-existent or latent convulsive disorders. Onset of withdrawal symptoms occurs usually within 12 to 48 hours after discontinuation of meprobamate; symptoms usually cease within the next 12 to 48 hours.

When excessive dosage has continued for weeks or months, dosage should be reduced gradually over a period of one or two weeks rather than abruptly stopped. Alternatively, a short-acting barbiturate may be substituted, then gradually withdrawn.

Potentially Hazardous Tasks

Patients should be warned that this drug may impair the mental and/or physical abilities required for the performance of potentially hazardous tasks such as driving a motor vehicle or operating machinery.

Additive Effects

Since the effects of meprobamate and alcohol or meprobamate and other CNS depressants or psychotropic drugs may be additive, appropriate caution should be exercised with patients who take more than one of these agents simultaneously.

Usage in Pregnancy and Lactation

An increased risk of congenital malformations associated with the use of minor tranquilizers (meprobamate, chlordiazepoxide, and diazepam) during the first trimester of pregnancy has been suggested in several studies. Because use of these drugs is rarely a matter of urgency, their use during this period should almost always be avoided. The possibility that a woman of childbearing potential may be pregnant at the time of institution of therapy should be considered. Patients should be advised that if they become pregnant during therapy or intend to become pregnant they should communicate with their physicians about the desirability of discontinuing the drug.

Meprobamate passes the placental barrier. It is present both in umbilical cord blood at or near maternal plasma levels and in breast milk of lactating mothers at concentrations two to four times that of maternal plasma. When use of meprobamate is contemplated in breast-feeding patients, the drug's higher concentration in breast milk as compared to maternal plasma levels should be considered.

Usage in Children

'Miltown' (meprobamate)—Meprobamate should not be administered to children under age six, since there is a lack of documented evidence for safety and effectiveness in this age group.

'Miltown' 600 (meprobamate 600 mg)—This dosage form is not intended for use in children.

Precautions: The lowest effective dose should be administered, particularly to elderly and/or debilitated patients, in order to preclude oversedation.

The possibility of suicide attempts should be considered and the least amount of drug feasible should be dispensed at any one time.

Meprobamate is metabolized in the liver and excreted by the kidney; to avoid its excess accumulation, caution should be exercised in administration to patients with compromised liver or kidney function.

Meprobamate occasionally may precipitate seizures in epileptic patients.

Adverse Reactions:

Central Nervous System

Drowsiness, ataxia, dizziness, slurred speech, headache, vertigo, weakness, paresthesias, impairment of visual accommodation, euphoria, overstimulation, paradoxical excitement, fast EEG activity.

Gastrointestinal

Nausea, vomiting, diarrhea.

Cardiovascular

Palpitations, tachycardia, various forms of arrhythmia, transient ECG changes, syncope; also, hypotensive crises (including one fatal case).

Allergic or Idiosyncratic

Allergic or idiosyncratic reactions are usually seen within the period of the first to fourth dose in patients having had no previous contact with the drug. Milder reactions are characterized by an itchy, urticarial, or erythematous maculopapular rash which may be generalized or confined to the groin. Other reactions have included leukopenia, acute nonthrombocytopenic purpura, petechiae, ecchymoses, eosinophilia, peripheral edema, adenopathy, fever, fixed drug eruption with cross reaction to carisoprodol, and cross sensitivity between meprobamate/mebutamate and meprobamate/carbromal.

More severe hypersensitivity reactions, rarely reported, include hyperpyrexia, chills, angioneurotic edema, bronchospasm, oliguria, and anuria. Also, anaphylaxis, erythema multiforme, exfoliative dermatitis, stomatitis, proctitis, Stevens-Johnson syndrome, and bullous dermatitis, including one fatal case of the latter following administration of meprobamate in combination with prednisolone.

In case of allergic or idiosyncratic reactions to meprobamate, discontinue the drug and initiate appropriate symptomatic therapy, which may include epinephrine, antihistamines, and in severe cases corticosteroids. In evaluating possible allergic reactions, also consider allergy to excipients (information on excipients is available to physicians on request).

Hematologic

(See also **Allergic or Idiosyncratic.**) Agranulocytosis and aplastic anemia have been reported, although no causal relationship has been established. These cases rarely were fatal. Rare cases of thrombocytopenic purpura have been reported.

Other

Exacerbation of porphyric symptoms.

Dosage and Administration:

Doses of meprobamate above 2400 mg daily are not recommended.

'Miltown' (meprobamate)—**Adults:** the usual dosage is 1200 to 1600 mg daily, in three or four divided doses. **Children:** the usual dosage for children ages six to twelve is 100 to 200 mg two or three times daily. Meprobamate is not recommended for children under six.

'Miltown' 600 (meprobamate 600 mg)—**Adults:** the recommended dosage is one tablet twice a day. **Children:** not intended for use in children.

Overdosage: Suicidal attempts with meprobamate have resulted in drowsiness, lethargy, stupor, ataxia, coma, shock, vasomotor and respiratory collapse. Some suicidal attempts have been fatal.

The following data on meprobamate tablets have been reported in the literature and from other sources. These data are not expected to correlate with each case (considering factors such as individual susceptibility and length of time from ingestion to treatment), but represent the **usual ranges** reported.

Acute simple overdose (meprobamate alone): Death has been reported with ingestion of as little as 12 gm meprobamate and survival with as much as 40 gm.

Blood levels:

0.5 - 2.0 mg% represents the usual blood level range of meprobamate after therapeutic doses. The level may occasionally be as high as 3.0 mg%.

3 - 10 mg% usually corresponds to findings of mild to moderate symptoms of overdosage, such as stupor or light coma.

10 - 20 mg% usually corresponds to deeper coma, requiring more intensive treatment. Some fatalities occur.

At levels greater than 20 mg%, more fatalities than survivals can be expected.

Acute combined overdose (meprobamate with alcohol or other CNS depressants or psychotropic drugs): Since effects can be additive, a history of ingestion of a low dose of meprobamate plus any of these compounds (or of a relatively low blood or tissue level) cannot be used as a prognostic indicator.

In cases where excessive doses have been taken, sleep ensues rapidly and blood pressure, pulse, and respiratory rates are reduced to basal levels. Any drug remaining in the stomach should be removed and symptomatic therapy given. Should respiration or blood pressure become compromised, respiratory assistance, central nervous system stimulants, and pressor agents should be administered cautiously as indicated. Meprobamate is metabolized in

Continued on next page

Wallace—Cont.

the liver and excreted by the kidney. Diuresis, osmotic (mannitol) diuresis, peritoneal dialysis, and hemodialysis have been used successfully. Careful monitoring of urinary output is necessary and caution should be taken to avoid overhydration. Relapse and death, after initial recovery, have been attributed to incomplete gastric emptying and delayed absorption. Meprobamate can be measured in biological fluids by two methods: colorimetric (Hoffman, A.J. and Ludwig, B.J.: *J Amer Pharm Assn 48:* 740, 1959) and gas chromatographic (Douglas, J.F. et al: *Anal Chem 39:* 956, 1967).

How Supplied: 'Miltown' (meprobamate, U.S.P.) is available as 400 mg white, scored tablets in bottles of:

100 (NDC 0037-1001-01)
500 (NDC 0037-1001-03)
1000 (NDC 0037-1001-02)

and 200 mg white, sugar-coated tablets in bottles of 100 (NDC 0037-1101-01).

'Miltown' 600 is available as white, capsule-shaped tablets, each containing 600 mg meprobamate, U.S.P., in bottles of 100 (NDC 0037-1601-01).

WALLACE LABORATORIES
Division of CARTER-WALLACE, INC.
Cranbury, New Jersey 08512

Rev. 10/80

[*Shown in Product Identification Section*]

ORGANIDIN® ℞
(iodinated glycerol)
Solution, Tablets, Elixir

Description: Organidin® (iodinated glycerol), a mucolytic-expectorant, is an isomeric mixture formed by the interaction of iodine and glycerol, whose active ingredient is thought to be iodopropylidene glycerol but whose structural and chemical formulas have not been precisely established. Iodinated glycerol is a viscous, amber liquid stable in acid media, including gastric juice, which contains virtually no inorganic iodide and no free iodine. Organidin is available for oral administration as: **Solution**—5%, containing 50 mg Organidin (25 mg organically bound iodine) per ml; **Tablets**—each containing 30 mg Organidin (15 mg organically bound iodine); and **Elixir**—1.2%, containing 60 mg Organidin (30 mg organically bound iodine) per 5 ml (teaspoonful); and alcohol, 21.75% by volume.

Clinical Pharmacology: Organidin increases the output of thin respiratory tract fluid and helps liquefy tenacious mucus in the bronchial tree. Iodines are readily absorbed from the gastrointestinal tract and concentrated primarily in the secretions of the respiratory tract, but their mechanism of action as mucolytic-expectorants is not clear.

Indications and Usage: Organidin is indicated for adjunctive treatment as a mucolytic-expectorant in respiratory tract conditions such as bronchitis, bronchial asthma, pulmonary emphysema, cystic fibrosis, chronic sinusitis, or after surgery to help prevent atelectasis.

Contraindications: History of marked sensitivity to inorganic iodides; hypersensitivity to any of the ingredients or related compounds; pregnancy; newborns; and nursing mothers.

The human fetal thyroid begins to concentrate iodine in the 12th to 14th week of gestation and the use of inorganic iodides in pregnant women during this period and thereafter has rarely been reported to induce fetal goiter (with or without hypothyroidism) with the potential for airway obstruction. If the patient becomes pregnant while taking Organidin, the drug should be discontinued and the patient should be apprised of the potential risk to the fetus.

Warnings: Discontinue use if rash or other evidence of hypersensitivity appears. Use with caution or avoid use in patients with history or evidence of thyroid disease.

Precautions: General—Iodides have been reported to cause a flare-up of adolescent acne. Children with cystic fibrosis appear to have an exaggerated susceptibility to the goitrogenic effect of iodides.

Dermatitis and other reversible manifestations of iodism have been reported with chronic use of inorganic iodides. Although these have not been reported to be a problem clinically with Organidin, they should be kept in mind in patients receiving these preparations for prolonged periods.

Drug Interactions—Iodides may potentiate the hypothyroid effect of lithium and other antithyroid drugs.

Carcinogenesis, Mutagenesis, Impairment of Fertility—No long-term animal studies have been performed with Organidin.

Pregnancy—Teratogenic Effects: Pregnancy Category X (see CONTRAINDICATIONS).

Nursing Mothers—Organidin should not be administered to a nursing woman.

Adverse Reactions: Reports of gastrointestinal irritation, rash, hypersensitivity, thyroid gland enlargement, and acute parotitis have been rare.

Overdosage: Acute overdosage experience with Organidin has been rare and there have been no reports of any serious problems.

Dosage and Administration: Adults—Solution: 20 drops (60 mg) 4 times a day, with liquid. **Tablets:** 2 tablets 4 times a day, with liquid. **Elixir:** 1 teaspoonful 4 times a day.

Children—Up to one-half the adult dosage, based on the child's weight. (One drop **Solution** equals approximately 3 mg of Organidin).

How Supplied: Organidin is available as—

Solution: 5%—clear amber liquid, in 30 ml dropper bottles (NDC 0037-4211-10).

Tablets: 30 mg—round, scored, rose-colored tablets, in bottles of 100 (NDC 0037-4224-40).

[*Shown in Product Identification Section*]

Elixir: 1.2%—clear amber liquid, in bottles of one pint (NDC 0037-4213-30) and one gallon (NDC 0037-4213-40).

Storage: Store at room temperature; avoid excessive heat. Keep bottle tightly closed.

Organidin Solution and Elixir
are Distributed by
WALLACE LABORATORIES
Division of CARTER-WALLACE, INC.
Cranbury, New Jersey 08512
Manufactured by
Denver Chemical
(Puerto Rico), Inc.
Humacao, Puerto Rico 00661
Organidin Tables are
Manufactured by
WALLACE LABORATORIES
Division of CARTER-WALLACE, INC.
Cranbury, New Jersey 08512

Rev. 7/80

RONDOMYCIN® ℞
(methacycline HCl)

Description: 'Rondomycin' (methacycline HCl) is a broad-spectrum antibiotic synthetically derived from oxytetracycline. Chemical dehydration at the 6-position yields a structural homologue which is a light-yellow crystalline powder with a chemical designation of 6-methylene-5-oxytetracycline.

Actions: The tetracyclines are primarily bacteriostatic and are thought to exert their antimicrobial effect by the inhibition of protein synthesis. Tetracyclines are active against a wide range of gram-negative and gram-positive organisms.

The drugs in the tetracycline class have closely similar antimicrobial spectra, and cross-resistance among them is common. Micro-organisms may be considered susceptible if the MIC (minimum inhibitory concentration) is not more than 4.0 mcg/ml and intermediate if the MIC is 4.0 to 12.5 mcg/ml.

Susceptibility plate testing: A tetracycline disc may be used to determine microbial susceptibility to drugs in the tetracycline class. If the kirby-Bauer method of disc susceptibility testing is used, a 30 mcg tetracycline disc should give a zone of at least 19 mm when tested against a tetracycline-susceptible bacterial strain.

Tetracyclines are readily absorbed and are bound to plasma proteins in varying degree. They are concentrated by the liver in the bile and excreted in the urine and feces at high concentrations and in a biologically active form.

Indications: 'Rondomycin' (methacycline HCl) is indicated in infections caused by the following micro-organisms:

Rickettsiae (Rocky Mountain spotted fever, typhus fever and the typhus group, Q fever, rickettsialpox and tick fevers),
Mycoplasma pneumoniae (PPLO, Eaton Agent),
Agents of psittacosis and ornithosis,
Agents of lymphogranuloma venereum and granuloma inguinale,
The spirochetal agent of relapsing fever *(Borrelia recurrentis).*

The following gram-negative micro-organisms:

Haemophilus ducreyi (chancroid),
Pasteurella pestis and *Pasteurella tularensis,*
Bartonella bacilliformis,
Bacteroides species,
Vibrio comma and *Vibrio fetus,*

Brucella species (in conjunction with streptomycin).

Because many strains of the following groups of micro-organisms have been shown to be resistant to tetracyclines, culture and susceptibility testing are recommended.

'Rondomycin' (methacycline HCl) is indicated for treatment of infections caused by the following gram-negative micro-organisms, when bacteriologic testing indicates appropriate susceptibility to the drug:

Escherichia coli,
Enterobacter aerogenes (formerly *Aerobacter aerogenes),*
Shigella species,
Mima species and *Herellea* species,
Haemophilus influenzae (respiratory infections),
Klebsiella species (respiratory and urinary infections).

'Rondomycin' (methacycline HCl) is indicated for treatment of infections caused by the following gram-positive micro-organisms when bacteriologic testing indicates appropriate susceptibility to the drug:

Streptococcus species: Up to 44 percent of strains of *streptococcus pyogenes* and 74 percent of *streptococcus faecalis* have been found to be resistant to tetracycline drugs. Therefore, tetracyclines should not be used for streptococcal disease unless the organism has been demonstrated to be sensitive.

For upper respiratory infections due to group A beta-hemolytic streptococci, penicillin is the usual drug of choice, including prophylaxis of rheumatic fever.

Diplococcus pneumoniae,
Staphylococcus aureus, skin and soft tissue infections. Tetracyclines are not the drugs of choice in the treatment of any type of staphylococcal infections.

When penicillin is contraindicated, tetracyclines are alternative drugs in the treatment of infections due to:

Neisseria gonorrhoeae,
Treponema pallidum and *Treponema pertenue* (syphilis and yaws),
Listeria monocytogenes,
Clostridium species,
Bacillus anthracis,
Fusobacterium fusiforme (Vincent's infection),

Actinomyces species.
In acute intestinal amebiasis, the tetracyclines may be a useful adjunct to amebicides.
In severe acne, the tetracyclines may be useful adjunctive therapy.
Tetracyclines are indicated in the treatment of trachoma, although the infectious agent is not always eliminated, as judged by immunofluorescence.
Inclusion conjunctivitis may be treated with oral tetracyclines or with a combination of oral and topical agents.
Contraindications: This drug is contraindicated in persons who have shown hypersensitivity to any of the tetracyclines.
Warnings: THE USE OF DRUGS OF THE TETRACYCLINE CLASS DURING TOOTH DEVELOPMENT (LAST HALF OF PREGNANCY, INFANCY, AND CHILDHOOD TO THE AGE OF 8 YEARS) MAY CAUSE PERMANENT DISCOLORATION OF THE TEETH (YELLOW-GRAY-BROWN). This adverse reaction is more common during long-term use of the drugs but has been observed following repeated short-term courses. Enamel hypoplasia has also been reported. TETRACYCLINE DRUGS, THEREFORE, SHOULD NOT BE USED IN THIS AGE GROUP UNLESS OTHER DRUGS ARE NOT LIKELY TO BE EFFECTIVE OR ARE CONTRAINDICATED.
If renal impairment exists, even usual oral or parenteral doses may lead to excessive systemic accumulation of the drug and possible liver toxicity. Under such conditions, lower than usual total doses are indicated, and, if therapy is prolonged, serum level determinations of the drug may be advisable.
Photosensitivity manifested by an exaggerated sunburn reaction has been observed in some individuals taking tetracyclines. Patients apt to be exposed to direct sunlight or ultraviolet light should be advised that this reaction can occur with tetracycline drugs, and treatment should be discontinued at the first evidence of skin erythema.
The anti-anabolic action of the tetracyclines may cause an increase in BUN. While this is not a problem in those with normal renal function, in patients with significantly impaired function, higher serum levels of tetracyclines may lead to azotemia, hyperphosphatemia, and acidosis.
Usage in pregnancy. (See above "Warnings" about use during tooth development.)
Results of animal studies indicate that tetracyclines cross the placenta, are found in fetal tissues and can have toxic effects on the developing fetus (often related to retardation of skeletal development). Evidence of embryotoxicity has also been noted in animals treated early in pregnancy.
Usage in newborns, infants, and children. (See above "Warnings" about use during tooth development.)
All tetracyclines form a stable calcium complex in any bone-forming tissue. A decrease in the fibula growth rate has been observed in prematures given oral tetracycline in doses of 25 mg/kg every 6 hours. This reaction was shown to be reversible when the drug was discontinued.
Tetracyclines are present in the milk of lactating women who are taking a drug in this class.
Precautions: As with other antibiotic preparations, use of this drug may result in overgrowth of nonsusceptible organisms, including fungi. If superinfection occurs, the antibiotic should be discontinued and appropriate therapy instituted.
In venereal diseases when coexistent syphilis is suspected, darkfield examination should be done before treatment is started and the blood serology repeated monthly for at least 4 months.
Because tetracyclines have been shown to depress plasma prothrombin activity, patients who are on anticoagulant therapy may require downward adjustment of their anticoagulant dosage.
In long-term therapy, periodic laboratory evaluation of organ systems, including hematopoietic, renal and hepatic studies should be performed.
All infections due to Group A beta-hemolytic streptococci should be treated for at least 10 days.
Since bacteriostatic drugs may interfere with the bactericidal action of penicillin, it is advisable to avoid giving tetracycline in conjunction with penicillin.
Adverse Reactions:
Gastrointestinal: Anorexia, nausea, vomiting, diarrhea, glossitis, dysphagia, enterocolitis, and inflammatory lesions (with monilial overgrowth) in the anogenital region. These reactions have been caused by both the oral and parenteral administration of tetracyclines.
Skin: Maculopapular and erythematous rashes. Exfoliative dermatitis has been reported but is uncommon. Photosensitivity is discussed above. (See "Warnings".)
Renal toxicity: Rise in BUN has been reported and is apparently dose related. (See "Warnings".)
Hypersensitivity reactions: Urticaria, angioneurotic edema, anaphylaxis, anaphylactoid purpura, pericarditis and exacerbation of systemic lupus erythematosus.
Bulging fontanels in infants and benign intracranial hypertension in adults have been reported in individuals receiving full therapeutic dosages. These conditions disappeared rapidly when the drug was discontinued.
Blood: Hemolytic anemia, thrombocytopenia, neutropenia and eosinophilia have been reported.
When given over prolonged periods, tetracyclines have been reported to produce brown-black microscopic discoloration of thyroid glands. No abnormalities of thyroid function studies are known to occur.
Dosage and Administration: The usual adult dosage of 'Rondomycin' (methacycline HCl) is 600 mg daily. This may be given in four divided doses of 150 mg each or two divided doses of 300 mg each. An initial dose of 300 mg followed by 150 mg every six hours or 300 mg every 12 hours may be used in the management of more severe infections.
In uncomplicated gonorrhea, when penicillin is contraindicated, 'Rondomycin' (methacycline HCl) may be used for treating both males and females in the following clinical dosage schedule: 900 mg initially, followed by 300 mg q.i.d. for a total of 5.4 grams.
For treatment of syphilis, when penicillin is contraindicated, a total of 18 to 24 grams of 'Rondomycin' (methacycline HCl) in equally divided doses over a period of 10–15 days should be given. Close follow-up, including laboratory tests, is recommended.
In Eaton Agent pneumonia, the usual adult dosage is 900 mg daily for 6 days.
The recommended dosage schedule for children above eight years of age is 3 to 6 mg/lb of body weight per day divided into two or four equally spaced doses.
Therapy should be continued for at least 24–48 hours after symptoms and fever have subsided. It should be noted, however, that antibacterial serum levels may usually be present from 24 to 36 hours following the discontinuation of 'Rondomycin' (methacycline HCl).
Concomitant therapy: Antacids containing aluminum, calcium, or magnesium impair absorption and should no be given to patients taking oral tetracyclines.
Food and some dairy products also interfere with absorption. Oral forms of tetracycline should be given 1 hour before or 2 hours after meals. Pediatric oral dosage forms should not be given with milk formulas and should be given at least 1 hour prior to feeding.
In patients with renal impairment (see "Warnings"): Total dosage should be decreased by reduction of recommended individual doses and/or by extending time intervals between doses.
In the treatment of streptococcal infections, a therapeutic dose of tetracycline should be administered for at least 10 days.
How Supplied: 'Rondomycin'-300 is available as blue and white capsules, each containing 300 mg methacycline HCl equivalent to 280 mg methacycline base, supplied in bottles of 50 (NDC 0037-4101-06).
'Rondomycin'-150 is available as blue and white capsules, each containing 150 mg methacycline HCl equivalent to 140 mg methacycline base, supplied in bottles of 100 (NDC 0037-4001-01). Rev. 6/81

WALLACE LABORATORIES
Division of
CARTER-WALLACE, INC.
Cranbury, New Jersey 08512
[*Shown in Product Identification Section*]

RYNA™
(Liquid)
RYNA-C® Ⓒ
(Liquid)
RYNA-CX® Ⓒ
(Liquid)

Description:
Each 5 ml (one teaspoonful) of **RYNA Liquid** contains:
Chlorpheniramine maleate ....2 mg
Pseudoephedrine hydrochloride ....30 mg
in a clear, slightly yellow colored, lemon-vanilla flavored demulcent base containing no sugar, dyes, or alcohol.
Each 5 ml (one teaspoonful) of **RYNA-C Liquid** contains, in addition:
Codeine phosphate ....10 mg
(WARNING: May be habit-forming)
in a clear, colorless to slightly yellow, cinnamon-flavored, demulcent base containing no sugar, dyes, or alcohol.
Each 5 ml (one teaspoonful) of **RYNA-CX Liquid** contains:
Codeine phosphate ....10 mg
(WARNING: May be habit-forming)
Pseudoephedrine hydrochloride ....30 mg
Guaifenesin ....100 mg
in a clear, colorless, cherry-vanilla-menthol flavored demulcent base containing no sugar, dyes, or alcohol.
Actions:
Chlorpheniramine maleate in RYNA and RYNA-C is an antihistamine that antagonizes the effects of histamine.
Codeine Phosphate in RYNA-C and RYNA-CX is a centrally-acting antitussive that relieves cough.
Pseudoephedrine hydrochloride in RYNA, RYNA-C and RYNA-CX is a sympathomimetic nasal decongestant that acts to shrink swollen mucosa of the respiratory tract.
Guaifenesin in RYNA-CX is an expectorant that increases mucus flow to help prevent dryness and relieve irritated respiratory tract membranes.
Indications:
RYNA is indicated for the temporary relief of the concurrent symptoms of nasal congestion, sneezing, itchy and watery eyes, and running nose as occurs with the common cold or allergic rhinitis.
RYNA-C is indicated for the above when cough is also a concurrent symptom.
RYNA-CX is indicated for the temporary relief of the concurrent symptoms of dry, nonproductive cough and nasal congestion.
Directions: Adults: 2 teaspoonfuls every 6 hours.
Children 6-under 12 years: 1 teaspoonful every 6 hours.

Continued on next page

Wallace—Cont.

Children 2-under 6 years: ½ teaspoonful every 6 hours (see WARNINGS).

Do not exceed 4 doses in 24 hours.

Warnings: Do not give these products to children taking other medications. Do not give RYNA or RYNA-C to children under 6 years, nor RYNA-CX to children under 2 years except under the advice and supervision of a physician. Do not exceed recommended dosage unless directed by a physician because nervousness, dizziness, or sleeplessness may occur at higher doses. If symptoms do not improve within 3 days or are accompanied by high fever, discontinue use and consult a physician.

For RYNA-C and RYNA-CX only: Codeine may cause or aggravate constipation. A persistent cough may be a sign of a serious condition. Do not take these products except under the advice and supervision of a physician if you have any of the following symptoms or conditions: cough that persists more than 3 days or tends to recur; chronic cough, such as occurs with smoking, asthma, or emphysema; cough accompanied by excessive secretions, high fever, rash, or persistent headache; chronic pulmonary disease or shortness of breath; high blood pressure; thyroid disease or diabetes.

For RYNA and RYNA-C only: Do not take these products except under the advice and supervision of a physician if you have asthma, glaucoma, or difficulty in urination due to enlargement of the prostate. Both products contain an antihistamines which may cause excitability, especially in children, or drowsiness or which may impair mental alertness. Combined with alcohol, sedatives, or other depressants may have an additive effect. Do not drive motor vehicles, operate machinery, or drink alcoholic beverages while taking these products.

KEEP THIS AND ALL DRUGS OUT OF THE REACH OF CHILDREN. IN CASE OF ACCIDENTAL OVERDOSE, SEEK PROFESSIONAL ASSISTANCE OR CONTACT A POISON CONTROL CENTER IMMEDIATELY.

Caution: If pregnant or nursing a baby, consult your physician or pharmacist before using these products.

Drug Interaction Precaution: Do not take these products if you are presently taking a prescription antihypertensive or antidepressant drug containing a monoamine oxidase inhibitor, except under the advice and supervision of a physician.

How Supplied:
RYNA: bottles of 4 fl oz (NDC 0037-0638-66) and one pint (NDC 0037-0638-68).
RYNA-C: bottles of 4 fl oz (NDC 0037-0522-66) and one pint (NDC 0037-0522-68).
RYNA-CX: bottles of 4 fl oz (NDC 0037-0801-66) and one pint (NDC 0037-0801-68).

WALLACE LABORATORIES
Division of
CARTER-WALLACE, Inc.
Cranbury, New Jersey 08512

Rev. 6/82

RYNATAN® ℞
Tablets
Pediatric Suspension

Description: Rynatan® is an antihistaminic/decongestant combination available for oral administration as **Tablets** and as **Pediatric Suspension.** Each tablet contains:

Phenylephrine Tannate ....25 mg
Chlorpheniramine Tannate ....8 mg
Pyrilamine Tannate ....25 mg

Each 5 ml (teaspoonful) of the Pediatric Suspension contains:

Phenylephrine Tannate ....5 mg
Chlorpheniramine Tannate ....2 mg
Pyrilamine Tannate ....12.5 mg

Clinical Pharmacology: Rynatan combines the sympathomimetic decongestant effect of phenylephrine with the antihistaminic actions of chlorpheniramine and pyrilamine.

Indications and Usage: Rynatan is indicated for symptomatic relief of the coryza and nasal congestion associated with the common cold, sinusitis, allergic rhinitis and other upper respiratory tract conditions. Appropriate therapy should be provided for the primary disease.

Contraindications: Rynatan is contraindicated for newborns, nursing mothers and patients sensitive to any of the ingredients or related compounds.

Warnings: Use with caution in patients with hypertension, cardiovascular disease, hyperthyroidism, diabetes, narrow angle glaucoma or prostatic hypertrophy. Use with caution or avoid use in patients taking monoamine oxidase (MAO) inhibitors. This product contains antihistamines which may cause drowsiness and may have additive central nervous system (CNS) effects with alcohol or other CNS depressants (e.g., hypnotics, sedatives, tranquilizers).

Precautions: General: Antihistamines are more likely to cause dizziness, sedation and hypotension in elderly patients. Antihistamines may cause excitation, particularly in children, but their combination with sympathomimetics may cause either mild stimulation or mild sedation.

Information for Patients: Caution patients against drinking alcoholic beverages or engaging in potentially hazardous activities requiring alertness, such as driving a car or operating machinery, while using this product.

Drug Interactions: MAO inhibitors may prolong and intensify the anticholinergic effects of antihistamines and the overall effects of sympathomimetic agents.

Carcinogenesis, Mutagenesis, Impairment of Fertility: No long-term animal studies have been performed with Rynatan.

Pregnancy: Teratogenic Effects: Pregnancy Category C. Animal reproduction studies have not been conducted with Rynatan. It is also not known whether Rynatan can cause fetal harm when administered to a pregnant woman or can affect reproduction capacity. Rynatan should be given to a pregnant woman only if clearly needed.

Nursing Mothers: Rynatan should not be administered to a nursing woman.

Adverse Reactions: Adverse effects associated with Rynatan at recommended doses have been minimal. The most common have been drowsiness, sedation, dryness of mucous membranes, and gastrointestinal effects. Serious side effects with oral antihistimines or sympathomimetics have been rare.

Overdosage: Signs & Symptoms—may vary from CNS depression to stimulation (restlessness to convulsions). Antihistamine overdosage in young children may lead to convulsions and death. Atropine-like signs and symptoms may be prominent.

Treatment—Induce vomiting if it has not occurred spontaneously. Precautions must be taken against aspiration especially in infants, children and comatose patients. If gastric lavage is indicated, isotonic or half-isotonic saline solution is preferred. Stimulants should not be used. If hypotension is a problem, vasopressor agents may be considered.

Dosage and Administration: Administer the recommended dose every 12 hours.

Rynatan Tablets: Adults—1 or 2 tablets.

Rynatan Pediatric Suspension: Children over six years of age—5 to 10 ml (1 to 2 teaspoonfuls); **Children two to six years of age**—2.5 to 5 ml (½ to 1 teaspoonful); **Children under two years of age**—Titrate dose individually.

How Supplied: Rynatan® Tablets: buff, capsule-shaped, compressed tablets in bottles of 100 (NDC 0037-0713-92) and bottles of 500 (NDC 0037-0713-96)

[*Shown in Product Identification Section*]

Rynatan® Pediatric Suspension: dark-pink with strawberry-currant flavor, in pint bottles (NDC-0037-0715-68)

Storage: Rynatan Tablets—Store at room temperature; avoid excessive heat—(above 40°C/104°F).

Rynatan Pediatric Suspension—Store at controlled room temperature—between 15°C-30°C (59°F-86°F); protect from freezing.

Rev. 2/80

RYNATUSS® ℞
Tablets
Pediatric Suspension

Description: Rynatuss® is an antitussive/antihistaminic/decongestant/bronchodilator combination available for oral administration as **Tablets** and as **Pediatric Suspension.** Each tablet contains:

Carbetapentane Tannate ....60 mg
Chlorpheniramine Tannate ....5 mg
Ephedrine Tannate ....10 mg
Phenylephrine Tannate ....10 mg

Each 5 ml (teaspoonful) of the Pediatric Suspension contains:

Carbetapentane Tannate ....30 mg
Chlorpheniramine Tannate ....4 mg
Ephedrine Tannate ....5 mg
Phenylephrine Tannate ....5 mg

Clinical Pharmacology: Rynatuss combines the antitussive action of carbetapentane, the sympathomimetic decongestant effect of phenylephrine, the antihistaminic action of chlorpheniramine, and the bronchodilator action of ephedrine.

Indications and Usage: Rynatuss is indicated for the symptomatic relief of cough associated with respiratory tract conditions such as the common cold, bronchial asthma, acute and chronic bronchitis. Appropriate therapy should be provided for the primary disease.

Contraindications: Rynatuss is contraindicated for newborns, nursing mothers and patients who are sensitive to any of the ingredients or related compounds.

Warnings: Use with caution in patients with hypertension, cardiovascular disease, hyperthyroidism, diabetes, narrow angle glaucoma or prostatic hypertrophy. Use with caution or avoid use in patients taking monoamine oxidase (MAO) Inhibitors.

This product contains antihistamines which may cause drowsiness and may have additive central nervous system (CNS) effects with alcohol or other CNS depressants (e.g., hypnotics, sedatives, tranquilizers).

Precautions:

For Rynatuss Pediatric Suspension only: This product contains FD&C Yellow No. 5 (tartrazine) which may cause allergic-type reactions (including bronchial asthma) in certain susceptible individuals. Although the overall incidence of FD&C Yellow No. 5 (tartrazine) sensitivity in the general population is low, it is frequently seen in patients who also have aspirin hypersensitivity.

General: Antihistamines are more likely to cause dizziness, sedation and hypotension in elderly patients. Antihistamines may cause excitation, particularly in children, but their combination with sympathomimetics may cause either mild stimulation or mild sedation.

Information for Patients: Caution patients against drinking alcoholic beverages or engaging in potentially hazardous activities requiring alertness, such as driving a car or operating machinery, while using this product.

Drug Interactions: MAO inhibitors may prolong and intensify the anticholinergic effects of antihistamines and the overall effects of sympathomimetic agents.

Carcinogenesis, Mutagenesis, Impairment of Fertility: No long-term animal studies have been performed with Rynatuss.

Pregnancy: Teratogenic Effects: Pregnancy Category C. Animal reproduction studies have not been conducted with Rynatuss. It is also not known whether Rynatuss can cause fetal harm when administered to a pregnant woman or can affect reproduction capacity. Rynatuss should be given to a pregnant woman only if clearly needed.

Nursing Mothers: Rynatuss should not be administered to a nursing woman.

Adverse Reactions: Adverse effects associated with Rynatuss at recommended doses have been minimal. The most common have been drowsiness, sedation, dryness of mucous membranes, and gastrointestinal effects. Serious side effects with oral antihistamines or sympathomimetics have been rare.

Overdosage: Signs and Symptoms—may vary from CNS depression to stimulation (restlessness to convulsions). Antihistamine overdosage in young children may lead to convulsions and death. Atropine-like signs and symptoms may be prominent.

Treatment—Induce vomiting if it has not occurred spontaneously. Precautions must be taken against aspiration especially in infants, children and comatose patients. If gastric lavage is indicated, isotonic or half-isotonic saline solution is preferred. Stimulants should not be used. If hypotension is a problem, vasopressor agents may be considered.

Dosage and Administration: Administer the recommended dose every 12 hours.

Rynatuss Tablets: Adults—1 to 2 tablets.

Rynatuss Pediatric Suspension: Children over six years of age—5 to 10 ml (1 to 2 teaspoonfuls); **Children two to six years of age**—2.5 to 5 ml (½ to 1 teaspoonful); **Children under two years of age**—Titrate dose individually.

How Supplied:

Rynatuss® Tablets: lavender-rose, capsule-shaped, compressed tablets in bottles of 100 (NDC 0037-0717-92).

[*Shown in Product Identification Section*]

Rynatuss® Pediatric Suspension: pink with strawberry-currant flavor, in bottles of 8 fl oz (NDC 0037-0718-67) and one pint (NDC 0037-0718-68).

Storage: Rynatuss Tablets—Store at room temperature; avoid excessive heat—above 40°C (104°F).

Rynatuss Pediatric Suspension—Store at controlled room temperature—between 15°C-30°C (59°F-86°F); protect from freezing.

Rev. 2/80

SOMA® ℞
(carisoprodol)

Description: 'Soma' (carisoprodol) is available as 350 mg white tablets. Carisoprodol is N-isopropyl -2- methyl -2- propyl-1,3-propanediol dicarbamate.

Actions: Carisoprodol produces muscle relaxation in animals by blocking interneuronal activity in the descending reticular formation and spinal cord. The onset of action is rapid and effects last four to six hours.

Indications: Carisoprodol is indicated as an adjunct to rest, physical therapy, and other measures for the relief of discomfort associated with acute, painful musculoskeletal conditions. The mode of action of this drug has not been clearly identified, but may be related to its sedative properties. Carisoprodol does not directly relax tense skeletal muscles in man.

Contraindications: Acute intermittent porphyria as well as allergic or idiosyncratic reactions to carisoprodol or related compounds such as meprobamate, mebutamate, or tybamate.

Warnings:

Idiosyncratic Reactions—On very rare occasions, the first dose of carisoprodol has been followed by idiosyncratic symptoms appearing within minutes or hours. Symptoms reported include: extreme weakness, transient quadriplegia, dizziness, ataxia, temporary loss of vision, diplopia, mydriasis, dysarthria, agitation, euphoria, confusion, and disorientation. Symptoms usually subside over the course of the next several hours. Supportive and symptomatic therapy, including hospitalization, may be necessary.

Usage in Pregnancy and Lactation—Safe usage of this drug in pregnancy or lactation has not been established. Therefore, use of this drug in pregnancy, in nursing mothers, or in women of childbearing potential requires that the potential benefits of the drug be weighed against the potential hazards to mother and child. Carisoprodol is present in breast milk of lactating mothers at concentrations two to four times that of maternal plasma. This factor should be taken into account when use of the drug is contemplated in breast-feeding patients.

Usage in Children—Because of limited clinical experience, 'Soma' is not recommended for use in patients under 12 years of age.

Potentially Hazardous Tasks—Patients should be warned that this drug may impair the mental and/or physical abilities required for the performance of potentially hazardous tasks such as driving a motor vehicle or operating machinery.

Additive Effects—Since the effects of carisoprodol and alcohol or carisoprodol and other CNS depressants or psychotropic drugs may be additive, appropriate caution should be exercised with patients who take more than one of these agents simultaneously.

Drug Dependence—In dogs, no withdrawal symptoms occurred after abrupt cessation of carisoprodol from dosages as high as 1 gm/kg/day. In a study in man, abrupt cessation of 100 mg/kg/day (about five times the recommended daily adult dosage) was followed in some subjects by mild withdrawal symptoms such as abdominal cramps, insomnia, chilliness, headache, and nausea. Delirium and convulsions did not occur. In clinical use, psychological dependence and abuse have been rare, and there have been no reports of significant abstinence signs. Nevertheless, the drug should be used with caution in addiction-prone individuals.

Precautions: Carisoprodol is metabolized in the liver and excreted by the kidney; to avoid its excess accumulation, caution should be exercised in administration to patients with compromised liver or kidney function.

Adverse Reactions: Central Nervous System—Drowsiness and other CNS effects may require dosage reduction. Also observed: dizziness, vertigo, ataxia, tremor, agitation, irritability, headache, depressive reactions, syncope, and insomnia. (See also Idiosyncratic Reactions under "Warnings".)

Allergic or Idiosyncratic—Allergic or idiosyncratic reactions occasionally develop. They are usually seen within the period of the first to fourth dose in patients having had no previous contact with the drug. Skin rash, erythema multiforme, pruritus, eosinophilia, and fixed drug eruption with cross reaction to meprobamate have been reported with carisoprodol. Severe reactions have been manifested by asthmatic episodes, fever, weakness, dizziness, angioneurotic edema, smarting eyes, hypotension, and anaphylactoid shock. (See also Idiosyncratic Reactions under "Warnings".)

In case of allergic or idiosyncratic reactions to carisoprodol, discontinue the drug and initiate appropriate symptomatic therapy, which may include epinephrine, antihistamines, and in severe cases corticosteroids. In evaluating possible allergic reactions, also consider allergy to excipients (information on excipients is available to physicians on request).

Cardiovascular—Tachycardia, postural hypotension, and facial flushing.

Gastrointestinal — Nausea, vomiting, hiccup, and epigastric distress.

Hematologic — Leukopenia, in which other drugs or viral infection may have been responsible, and pancytopenia, attributed to phenylbutazone, have been reported. No serious blood dyscrasias have been attributed to carisoprodol.

Dosage and Administration: The usual adult dosage of 'Soma' (carisoprodol) is one 350 mg tablet, three times daily and at bedtime. Usage in patients under age 12 is not recommended.

Overdosage: Overdosage of carisoprodol has produced stupor, coma, shock, respiratory depression, and, very rarely, death. The effects of an overdosage of carisoprodol and alcohol or other CNS depressants or psychotropic agents can be additive even when one of the drugs has been taken in the usual recommended dosage. Any drug remaining in the stomach should be removed and symptomatic therapy given. Should respiration or blood pressure become compromised, respiratory assistance, central nervous system stimulants, and pressor agents should be administered cautiously as indicated. Carisoprodol is metabolized in the liver and excreted by the kidney. Although carisoprodol overdosage experience is limited, the following types of treatment have been used successfully with the related drug meprobamate: diuresis, osmotic (mannitol) diuresis, peritoneal dialysis, and hemodialysis (carisoprodol is dialyzable). Careful monitoring of urinary output is necessary and caution should be taken to avoid overhydration. Observe for possible relapse due to incomplete gastric emptying and delayed absorption. Carisoprodol can be measured in biological fluids by gas chromatography (Douglas, J.F. et al: *J Pharm Sci 58:* 145, 1969).

How Supplied: 'Soma' 350: Bottles of 100 (NDC 0037-2001-01) and 500 (NDC 0037-2001-03).

Rev. 8/74

[*Shown in Product Identification Section*]

SOMA® COMPOUND ℞
(carisoprodol 200 mg + phenacetin 160 mg + caffeine 32 mg)

Description: 'Soma' Compound is available as orange, scored tablets, each containing carisoprodol 200 mg, phenacetin 160 mg, and caffeine 32 mg.

Actions:

Carisoprodol

Carisoprodol produces muscle relaxation in animals by blocking interneuronal activity in the descending reticular formation and spinal cord. The onset of action is rapid and effects last four to six hours.

Phenacetin

The exact nature of the pain-relieving action of phenacetin is not understood. The main site of activity is thought to be the central nervous system.

Caffeine

Caffeine acts as a stimulant of all parts of the central nervous system, affecting first the cortex and then the medulla. Large amounts will stimulate the spinal cord.

Indications: As an adjunct to rest, physical therapy, and other measures for the relief of discomfort associated with acute, painful musculoskeletal conditions. The mode of action of carisoprodol has not been clearly identified, but may be related to its sedative properties. Carisoprodol does not directly relax tense skeletal muscles in man.

Contraindications: Acute intermittent porphyria as well as allergic or idiosyncratic reactions to phenacetin, caffeine, or carisoprodol and related compounds such as meprobamate, mebutamate, or tybamate.

Warnings:

THIS PRODUCT CONTAINS PHENACETIN. PHENACETIN, IF TAKEN IN LARGE DOSES FOR LONG PERIODS IN COMBINATION WITH OTHER ANALGESICS, IS ASSOCIATED WITH SE-

Continued on next page

Wallace—Cont.

VERE KIDNEY DISEASE AND WITH CANCER OF THE KIDNEY.

Kidney disease, often irreversible, has been noted with doses of phenacetin of 1 gm or more per day taken for 1-3 years and with total doses of 2 kg or more. It is not known whether prolonged ingestion of doses of phenacetin lower than 1 gm per day might also result in kidney disease.

Idiosyncratic Reactions
On very rare occasions, the first dose of carisoprodol has been followed by idiosyncratic symptoms appearing within minutes or hours. Symptoms reported include: extreme weakness, transient quadriplegia, dizziness, ataxia, temporary loss of vision, diplopia, mydriasis, dysarthria, agitation, euphoria, confusion, and disorientation. Symptoms usually subside over the course of the next several hours. Supportive and symptomatic therapy, including hospitalization, may be necessary.

Usage in Pregnancy and Lactation
Safe usage of this drug in pregnancy or lactation has not been established. Therefore, use of this drug in pregnancy, in nursing mothers, or in women of childbearing potential requires that the potential benefits of the drug be weighed against the potential hazards to mother and child. Carisoprodol is present in breast milk of lactating mothers at concentrations two to four times that of maternal plasma. This factor should be taken into account when use of the drug is contemplated in breast-feeding patients.

Usage in Children Under Age Five
Usage of this drug in children under age five is not recommended.

Potentially Hazardous Tasks
Patients should be warned that this drug may impair the mental and/or physical abilities required for the performance of potentially hazardous tasks such as driving a motor vehicle or operating machinery.

Additive Effects
Since the effects of carisoprodol and alcohol or carisoprodol and other CNS depressants or psychotropic drugs may be additive, appropriate caution should be exercised with patients who take more than one of these agents simultaneously.

Drug Dependence

Phenacetin
Restlessness and excitement may occur when phenacetin has been abruptly discontinued.

Caffeine
Psychological dependence has been reported.

Carisoprodol
In dogs, no withdrawal symptoms occurred after abrupt cessation of carisoprodol from dosages as high as 1 gm/kg/day. In a study in man, abrupt cessation of 100 mg/kg/day (about five times the recommended daily adult dosage) was followed in some subjects by mild withdrawal symptoms such as abdominal cramps, insomnia, chilliness, headache, and nausea. Delirium and convulsions did not occur. In clinical use, psychological dependence and abuse have been rare, and there have been no reports of significant abstinence signs. Nevertheless, the drug should be used with caution in addiction-prone individuals.

Precautions:

Phenacetin
In cases of long-term therapy, phenacetin should be administered with caution to patients with anemia or cardiac, pulmonary, renal, or hepatic disease.

Caffeine
Caffeine should not be given to persons extremely sensitive to its CNS-stimulating action.

Carisoprodol
Carisoprodol is metabolized in the liver and excreted by the kidney; to avoid its excess accumulation, caution should be exercised in administration to patients with compromised liver or kidney function.

Adverse Reactions: Drowsiness, lightheadedness, dizziness, itching, nervousness, palpitations, overdose, and idiosyncratic reactions have been reported. Side effects which have occurred after administration of the constituents alone might also occur when the combination is taken.

Phenacetin
Side effects are extremely rare with short-term use of recommended doses. Usage in large amounts or for long periods may result in gastrointestinal disturbances, anemia, methemoglobinemia, and renal damage. (See **Overdosage** section.)

Caffeine
Average doses of caffeine may rarely cause nausea, nervousness, insomnia, and diuresis. Side effects are almost always the result of overdosage. (See **Overdosage** section.)

Carisoprodol
Central Nervous System—Drowsiness and other CNS effects may require dosage reduction. Also observed: dizziness, vertigo, ataxia, tremor, agitation, irritability, headache, depressive reactions, syncope, and insomnia. (See also Idiosyncratic Reactions under **Warnings.**)
Allergic or Idiosyncratic—Allergic or idiosyncratic reactions occasionally develop. They are usually seen within the period of the first to fourth dose in patients having had no previous contact with the drug. Skin rash, erythema multiforme, pruritus, eosinophilia, and fixed drug eruption with cross reaction to meprobamate have been reported with carisoprodol. Severe reactions have been manifested by asthmatic episodes, fever, weakness, dizziness, angioneurotic edema, smarting eyes, hypotension, and anaphylactoid shock. (See also Idiosyncratic Reactions under **Warnings.**)
In case of allergic or idiosyncratic reactions to carisoprodol, discontinue the drug and initiate appropriate symptomatic therapy, which may include epinephrine, antihistamines, and in severe cases corticosteroids. In evaluating possible allergic reactions, also consider allergy to excipients (information on excipients is available to physicians on request).
Cardiovascular—Tachycardia, postural hypotension, and facial flushing.
Gastrointestinal — Nausea, vomiting, hiccup, and epigastric distress.
Hematologic — Leukopenia, in which other drugs or viral infection may have been responsible, and pancytopenia, attributed to phenylbutazone, have been reported. No serious blood dyscrasias have been attributed to carisoprodol.

Dosage and Administration: The usual adult dosage of 'Soma' Compound (carisoprodol +phenacetin +caffeine) is one or two tablets, three times daily and at bedtime. Usage in children under age five is not recommended.

Overdosage: Diagnosis and treatment are according to component signs and symptoms. Note that symptoms and signs which could develop with one component used alone would be modified in varying degrees by the presence of the other components in the combination.

Phenacetin
Acute overdosage of phenacetin can produce dyspnea, cyanosis (due to methemoglobinemia and sulfhemoglobinemia), hemolytic anemia, skin reactions with or without fever, anorexia, hypothermia, insomnia, and in severe cases: stupor, coma, vascular collapse, and death. Remove any remaining drug from stomach and institute appropriate symptomatic therapy as indicated.
For methemoglobinemia the recommended treatment is a 1% aqueous solution of methylene blue, 1 to 2 mg/kg body weight, injected intravenously over a period of several minutes. This may be repeated at hourly intervals if cyanosis has not disappeared, but the total dose should not exceed 7 mg/kg.

Caffeine
Excessive dosage of caffeine can produce restlessness, nervousness, tolerance, delirium, tinnitus, tremors, scintillating scotomata, diuresis, tachycardia, and cardiac arrhythmias. It is possible that stimulatory signs would be offset by the CNS-depressant overdosage effects of the carisoprodol present in the combination.

Carisoprodol
Overdosage of carisoprodol has produced stupor, coma, shock, respiratory depression, and, very rarely, death. The effects of an overdosage of carisoprodol and alcohol or other CNS depressants or psychotropic agents can be additive, even when one of the drugs has been taken in the usual recommended dosage. Any drug remaining in the stomach should be removed and symptomatic therapy given. Should respiration or blood pressure become compromised, respiratory assistance, central nervous system stimulants, and pressor agents should be administered cautiously as indicated. Carisoprodol is metabolized in the liver and excreted by the kidney. Although carisoprodol overdosage experience is limited, the following types of treatment have been used successfully with the related drug meprobamate: diuresis, osmotic (mannitol) diuresis, peritoneal dialysis, and hemodialysis (carisoprodol is dialyzable). Careful monitoring of urinary output is necessary and caution should be taken to avoid overhydration. Observe for possible relapse due to incomplete gastric emptying and delayed absorption. Carisoprodol can be measured in biological fluids by gas chromatography (Douglas, J.F. et al: *J Pharm Sci* **58**: 145, 1969).

How Supplied: Bottles of 100 (NDC 0037-2101-01) and 500 (NDC 0037-2101-03).

Rev. 5/79

[*Shown in Product Identification Section*]

SOMA® COMPOUND with CODEINE ©R

(carisoprodol 200 mg + phenacetin 160 mg + caffeine 32 mg + codeine phosphate 16 mg)

WARNING: May be habit-forming.

Description: 'Soma' Compound with Codeine is available as white, capsule-shaped tablets, each containing carisoprodol 200 mg, phenacetin 160 mg, caffeine 32 mg, and codeine phosphate 16 mg.

Actions:

Carisoprodol
Carisoprodol produces muscle relaxation in animals by blocking interneuronal activity in the descending reticular formation and spinal cord. The onset of action is rapid and effects last four to six hours.

Phenacetin
The exact nature of the pain-relieving action of phenacetin is not understood. The main site of activity is thought to be the central nervous system.

Caffeine
Caffeine acts as a stimulant of all parts of the central nervous system, affecting first the cortex and then the medulla. Large amounts will stimulate the spinal cord.

Codeine Phosphate
Codeine phosphate is a narcotic-analgesic whose actions are qualitatively similar to morphine, but whose potency is substantially less.

Indications: As an adjunct to rest, physical therapy, and other measures for the relief of discomfort associated with acute, painful musculoskeletal conditions when the additional action of codeine is desired. The mode of action of carisoprodol has not been clearly identified, but may be related to its sedative properties. Carisoprodol does not directly relax tense skeletal muscles in man.

Contraindications: Acute intermittent porphyria as well as allergic or idiosyncratic reactions to phenacetin, caffeine, codeine, or carisoprodol and related compounds such as meprobamate, mebutamate, or tybamate.

Warnings:

THIS PRODUCT CONTAINS PHENACETIN. PHENACETIN, IF TAKEN IN LARGE DOSES FOR LONG PERIODS IN COMBINATION WITH OTHER ANALGESICS, IS ASSOCIATED WITH SEVERE KIDNEY DISEASE AND WITH CANCER OF THE KIDNEY.

Kidney disease, often irreversible, has been noted with doses of phenacetin of 1 gm or more per day taken for 1-3 years and with total doses of 2 kg or more. It is not known whether prolonged ingestion of doses of phenacetin lower than 1 gm per day might also result in kidney disease.

Idiosyncratic Reactions
On very rare occasions, the first dose of carisoprodol has been followed by idiosyncratic symptoms appearing within minutes or hours. Symptoms reported include: extreme weakness, transient quadriplegia, dizziness, ataxia, temporary loss of vision, diplopia, mydriasis, dysarthria, agitation, euphoria, confusion, and disorientation. Symptoms usually subside over the course of the next several hours. Supportive and symptomatic therapy, including hospitalization, may be necessary.

Usage in Pregnancy and Lactation
Safe usage of this drug in pregnancy or lactation has not been established. Therefore, use of this drug in pregnancy, in nursing mothers, or in women of childbearing potential requires that the potential benefits of the drug be weighed against the potential hazards to mother and child. Carisoprodol is present in breast milk of lactating mothers at concentrations two to four times that of maternal plasma. This factor should be taken into account when use of the drug is contemplated in breast-feeding patients.

Usage in Children Under Age Five
Usage of this drug in children under age five is not recommended.

Potentially Hazardous Tasks
Patients should be warned that this drug may impair the mental and/or physical abilities required for the performance of potentially hazardous tasks such as driving a motor vehicle or operating machinery.

Additive Effects
Since the effects of carisoprodol and alcohol or carisoprodol and other CNS depressants or psychotropic drugs may be additive, appropriate caution should be exercised with patients who take more than one of these agents simultaneously.

Drug Dependence
Phenacetin
Restlessness and excitement may occur when phenacetin has been abruptly discontinued.
Caffeine
Psychological dependence has been reported.
Carisoprodol
In dogs, no withdrawal symptoms occurred after abrupt cessation of carisoprodol from dosages as high as 1 gm/kg/day. In a study in man, abrupt cessation of 100 mg/kg/day (about five times the recommended daily adult dosage) was followed in some subjects by mild withdrawal symptoms such as abdominal cramps, insomnia, chilliness, headache, and nausea. Delirium and convulsions did not occur. In clinical use, psychological dependence and abuse have been rare, and there have been no reports of significant abstinence signs. Nevertheless, the drug should be used with caution in addiction-prone individuals.
Codeine Phosphate
Codeine phosphate should be used with caution since it may result in drug dependence of the morphine type.

Precautions:
Phenacetin
In cases of long-term therapy, phenacetin should be administered with caution to patients with anemia or cardiac, pulmonary, renal or hepatic disease.
Caffeine
Caffeine should not be given to persons extremely sensitive to its CNS-stimulating action.
Carisoprodol
Carisoprodol is metabolized in the liver and excreted by the kidney; to avoid its excess accumulation, caution should be exercised in administration to patients with compromised liver or kidney function.

Adverse Reactions: These have consisted primarily of drowsiness, dizziness, and gastric complaints. Side effects which have occurred after administration of the constituents alone might also occur when the combination is taken.
Phenacetin
Side effects are extremely rare with short-term use of recommended doses. Usage in large amounts or for long periods may result in gastrointestinal disturbances, anemia, methemoglobinemia, and renal damage. (See **Overdosage** section.)
Caffeine
Average doses of caffeine may rarely cause nausea, nervousness, insomnia, and diuresis. Side effects are almost always the result of overdosage. (See **Overdosage** section.)
Codeine Phosphate
Possible side effects associated with the administration of codeine phosphate are nausea, vomiting, constipation, miosis, sedation, and dizziness.
Carisoprodol
Central Nervous System—Drowsiness and other CNS effects may require dosage reduction. Also observed: dizziness, vertigo, ataxia, tremor, agitation, irritability, headache, depressive reactions, syncope, and insomnia. (See also Idiosyncratic Reactions under **Warnings.**)
Allergic or Idiosyncratic—Allergic or idiosyncratic reactions occasionally develop. They are usually seen within the period of the first to fourth dose in patients having had no previous contact with the drug. Skin rash, erythema multiforme, pruritus, eosinophilia, and fixed drug eruption with cross reaction to meprobamate have been reported with carisoprodol. Severe reactions have been manifested by asthmatic episodes, fever, weakness, dizziness, angioneurotic edema, smarting eyes, hypotension, and anaphylactoid shock. (See also Idiosyncratic Reactions under **Warnings.**)
In case of allergic or idiosyncratic reactions to carisoprodol, discontinue the drug and initiate appropriate symptomatic therapy, which may include epinephrine, antihistamines, and in severe cases corticosteroids. In evaluating possible allergic reactions, also consider allergy to excipients (information on excipients is available to physicians on request).
Cardiovascular—Tachycardia, postural hypotension, and facial flushing.
Gastrointestinal — Nausea, vomiting, hiccup, and epigastric distress.
Hematologic — Leukopenia, in which other drugs or viral infection may have been responsible, and pancytopenia, attributed to phenylbutazone, have been reported. No serious blood dyscrasias have been attributed to carisoprodol.

Dosage and Administration: The usual adult dosage of 'Soma' Compound with Codeine (carisoprodol + phenacetin + caffeine + codeine) is one or two tablets, three times daily and at bedtime. Usage in children under age five is not recommended.

Overdosage: Diagnosis and treatment are according to component signs and symptoms. Note that symptoms and signs which could develop with one component used alone would be modified in varying degrees by the presence of the other components in the combination.
Phenacetin
Acute overdosage of phenacetin can produce dyspnea, cyanosis (due to methemoglobinemia and sulfhemoglobinemia), hemolytic anemia, skin reactions with or without fever, anorexia, hypothermia, insomnia, and in severe cases: stupor, coma, vascular collapse, and death. Remove any remaining drug from stomach and institute appropriate symptomatic therapy as indicated.
For methemoglobinemia the recommended treatment is a 1% aqueous solution of methylene blue, 1 to 2 mg/kg body weight, injected intravenously over a period of several minutes. This may be repeated at hourly intervals if cyanosis has not disappeared, but the total dose should not exceed 7 mg/kg.
Caffeine
Excessive dosage of caffeine can produce restlessness, nervousness, tolerance, delirium, tinnitus, tremors, scintillating scotomata, diuresis, tachycardia, and cardiac arrhythmias. It is possible that stimulatory signs would be offset by the CNS-depressant overdosage effect of the carisoprodol present in the combination.
Codeine Phosphate
Overdosage of codeine may produce coma, pinpoint pupils, depressed respiration, and shock. Treat symptomatically, using respiratory assistance as needed, narcotic antagonists such as nalorphine and levallorphan, and pressor agents if indicated for shock.
Carisoprodol
Overdosage of carisoprodol has produced stupor, coma, shock, respiratory depression, and, very rarely, death. Overdosage of carisoprodol plus alcohol or other CNS depressants or psychotropic drugs can be additive. Any drug remaining in the stomach should be removed and symptomatic therapy given. Should respiration or blood pressure become compromised, respiratory assistance, central nervous system stimulants, and pressor agents should be administered cautiously as indicated. Carisoprodol is metabolized in the liver and excreted by the kidney. Although carisoprodol overdosage experience is limited, the following types of treatment have been used successfully with the related drug meprobamate: diuresis, osmotic (mannitol) diuresis, peritoneal dialysis, and hemodialysis (carisoprodol is dialyzable). Careful monitoring of urinary output is necessary and caution should be taken to avoid overhydration. Observe for possible relapse due to incomplete gastric emptying and delayed absorption. Carisoprodol can be measured in biological fluids by gas chromatography (Douglas, J.F. et al: *J Pharm Sci* **58**: 145, 1969).

How Supplied: Bottles of 100 (NDC 0037-2401-01) Rev. 5/79

[*Shown in Product Identification Section*]

THEO-ORGANIDIN™ ℞
Elixir

Description: Theo-Organidin is a bronchodilator/mucolytic-expectorant combination available for oral administration as an **Elixir.** Each 15 ml (tablespoonful) contains theophylline (anhydrous), 120 mg; Organidin® (iodinated glycerol), 30 mg (15 mg organically bound iodine); and alcohol, 15% by volume.

Clinical Pharmacology: Theo-Organidin combines the bronchodilator effects of theophylline, a xanthine derivative, and the mucolytic-expectorant action of Organidin. Therapeutic blood levels of theophylline are reached in approximately 15 minutes and peak blood levels in one hour.

Indications and Usage: Theo-Organidin is indicated for symptomatic treatment in bronchial asthma and other bronchospastic conditions such as bronchitis, bronchiolitis, and pulmonary emphysema; for the relief of wheezing

Continued on next page

Wallace—Cont.

and respiratory distress due to reversible bronchospasm and tenacious mucous secretions; and for daily maintenance therapy of patients with bronchial asthma and other chronic bronchospastic pulmonary disorders.

Contraindications: History of marked sensitivity to inorganic iodides; hypersensitivity to any of the ingredients or related compounds; pregnancy; newborns; and nursing mothers. The human fetal thyroid begins to concentrate iodine in the 12th to 14th week of gestation and the use of inorganic iodides in pregnant women during this period and thereafter has rarely been reported to induce fetal goiter (with or without hypothyroidism) with the potential for airway obstruction. If the patient becomes pregnant while taking Theo-Organidin, the drug should be discontinued and the patient should be apprised of the potential risk to the fetus.

Warnings: Discontinue use if rash or other evidence of hypersensitivity appears. Use with caution or avoid use in patients with history or evidence of thyroid disease. Do not exceed recommended dosage. Do not administer more often than every 6 hours or within 12 hours after rectal administration of any preparation containing theophylline or aminophylline. Use with caution or avoid use with other xanthine derivatives or CNS stimulants.

Precautions:

General—Children have been know to exhibit marked sensitivity to the CNS stimulant action of the xanthines. Toxic synergism (i.e., CNS stimulation) may occur with other sympathomimetic bronchodilator agents, particularly in children. Iodides have been reported to cause a flare-up of adolescent acne. Children with cystic fibrosis appear to have an exaggerated susceptibility to the goitrogenic effects of iodides.

Dermatitis and other reversible manifestations of iodism have been reported with chronic use of inorganic iodides. Although these have not been reported to be a problem clinically with Organidin formulations, they should be kept in mind in patients receiving these preparations for prolonged periods.

Drug Interactions—Iodides may potentiate the hypothyroid effect of lithium and other antithyroid drugs.

Carcinogenesis, Mutagenesis, Impairment of Fertility—No long-term animal studies have been performed with Theo-Organidin.

Pregnancy—Teratogenic Effects: Pregnancy Category X (see CONTRAINDICATIONS).

Nursing Mothers—Theo-Organidin should not be administered to a nursing woman.

Adverse Reactions: Side effects sometimes seen with individual ingredients may occur and may be modified as a result of their combination. **Theophylline**—Gastric irritation, nausea, and vomiting may occur; these can be minimized by taking Theo-Organidin after meals. Palpitations and mild central nervous system stimulation (e.g., restlessness, sleeplessness) have been reported, particularly in children. **Organidin**—Reports of gastrointestinal irritation, rash, hypersensitivity, thyroid enlargement, and acute parotitis have been rare.

Overdosage: There have been no reports of any serious problems from overdosage with Theo-Organidin. However, overdosage with theophylline has been reported and the following may be expected if overdosage with Theo-Organidin should occur:

Signs and Symptoms—Toxic overdosage with theophylline may produce severe gastrointestinal adverse effects including nausea, vomiting, epigastric pain, hematemesis and diarrhea; CNS effects including insomnia, headache, irritability, restlessness, severe agitation and convulsions; cardiovascular effects including hypotension, circulatory failure, and life-threatening arrhythmias; renal effects including diuresis and hypokalemia; and respiratory arrest. Serious toxicity leading to seizures and death can occur with serum concentrations of 40 mcg/ml or more.

Treatment—There is no specific antidote for theophylline toxicity. Discontinue drug immediately. Avoid sympathomimetic agents. Emetics and gastric lavage may be of value. Provide general supportive measures to prevent hypotension, overcome hydration, and maintain adequate ventilation. Hemodialysis with the use of resin or charcoal hemoperfusion may be helpful in reducing theophylline serum levels.

Dosage and Administration: Do not exceed recommended dosage. Acute attacks of asthma can usually be terminated fairly rapidly with the recommended dosage of Theo-Organidin; but in severe attacks, or when initiating treatment, the dose may be increased by 1/2 for up to 24 hours. The need for intravenous aminophylline and/or other regimens should also be considered in the management of severe episodes.

Usual Adult Dosage: For maintenance therapy: 1–2 tablespoonfuls 3 times a day (every 6–8 hours).

For the acute asthmatic attack: 3 tablespoonfuls initially, then reduce to maintenance dosage.

Children: 1 teaspoonful per 20 lbs. (9 kg) body weight, 2–3 times daily. Children over 99 lbs (45 kg) may require adult dosage.

How Supplied: Theo-Organidin Elixir—clear amber liquid, in bottles of one pint (NDC 0037-4611-10) and one gallon (NDC 0037-4611-20).

Storage: Store at room temperature; avoid excessive heat; protect from freezing. Keep bottle tightly closed.

Distributed by
WALLACE LABORATORIES
Division of CARTER-WALLACE, INC.
Cranbury, New Jersey 08512
Manufactured by
Denver Chemical (Puerto Rico), Inc.
Humacao, Puerto Rico 00661
Rev. 2/80

TUSSI-ORGANIDIN™ Ⓒ ℞
TUSSI-ORGANIDIN™ DM
Elixir

Description: Tussi-Organidin and **Tussi-Organidin DM** are antitussive/mucolytic-expectorant/antihistaminic combinations available for oral administration as the **Elixir. Tussi-Organidin** - Each 5 ml (teaspoonful) contains: Organidin® (iodinated glycerol), 30 mg (15 mg organically bound iodine); codeine phosphate (**Warning:** May be habit-forming), 10 mg; chlorpheniramine maleate, 2 mg; and alcohol, 15% by volume.

Tussi-Organidin DM—Each 5 ml (teaspoonful) contains: Organidin (iodinated glycerol), 30 mg (15 mg organically bound iodine); dextromethorphan hydrobromide, 10 mg; chlorpheniramine maleate, 2 mg; and alcohol, 15% by volume.

Clinical Pharmacology: Tussi-Organidin combines the antitussive action of codeine with the mucolytic-expectorant action of Organidin and the antihistiminic action of chlorpheniramine.

Tussi-Organidin DM combines the non-narcotic antitussive action of dextromethorphan with the mucolytic-expectorant action of Organidin and the antihistiminic action of chlorpheniramine.

Indications and Usage: Tussi-Organidin and Tussi-Organidin DM are indicated for the symptomatic relief of irritating, nonproductive cough associated with respiratory tract conditions such as chronic bronchitis, bronchial asthma, tracheobronchitis, and the common cold; also for the symptomatic relief of cough accompanying other respiratory tract conditions such as laryngitis, pharyngitis, croup, pertussis and emphysema. Appropriate therapy should be provided for the primary disease.

Contraindications: History of marked sensitivity to inorganic iodides; hypersensitivity to any of the ingredients or related compounds; pregnancy; newborns; and nursing mothers. The human fetal thyroid begins to concentrate iodine in the 12th to 14th week of gestation and the use of inorganic iodides in pregnant women during this period and thereafter has rarely been reported to induce fetal goiter (with or without hypothyroidism) with the potential for airway obstruction. If the patient becomes pregnant while taking any of these products, the drug should be discontinued and the patient should be apprised of the potential risk to the fetus.

Warnings: These products contain an antihistamine which may cause drowsiness and may have additive central nervous system (CNS) effects with alcohol or other CNS depressants (e.g., hypnotics, sedatives, tranquilizers). Discontinue use if rash or other evidence of hypersensitivity appears. Use with caution or avoid use in patients with history or evidence of thyroid disease.

Precautions: General—Antihistamines may produce excitation, particularly in children. Iodides have been reported to cause a flare-up of adolescent acne. Children with cystic fibrosis appear to have an exaggerated susceptibility to the goitrogenic effects of iodides. Dermatitis and other reversible manifestations of iodism have been reported with chronic use of inorganic iodides. Although these have not been a problem clinically with Organidin formulations, they should be kept in mind in patients receiving these preparations for prolonged periods.

Information for Patients—Caution patients against drinking alcoholic beverages or engaging in potentially hazardous activities requiring alertness, such as driving a car or operating machinery, while using these products.

Drug Interactions—Iodides may potentiate the hypothyroid effect of lithium and other antithyroid drugs. MAO inhibitors may prolong the anticholinergic effects of antihistamines.

Carcinogenesis, Mutagenesis, Impairment of Fertility—No long-term animal studies have been performed with Tussi-Organidin or Tussi-Organidin DM.

Pregnancy—Teratogenic effects: Pregnancy Category X (see CONTRAINDICATIONS).

Nursing Mothers—Tussi-Organidin or Tussi-Organidin DM should not be administered to a nursing woman.

Adverse Reactions: Side effects with Tussi-Organidin and Tussi-Organidin DM have been rare, including those which may occur with the individual ingredients and which may be modified as a result of their combination.

Organidin—Rare side effects include gastrointestinal irritation, rash, hypersensitivity, thyroid gland enlargement, and acute parotitis.

Codeine—(Tussi-Organidin only): Nausea, vomiting, constipation, drowsiness, dizziness, and miosis have been reported.

Dextromethorphan — (Tussi-Organidin DM only): Rarely produces drowsiness or gastrointestinal disturbances.

Chlorpheniramine—The most common side effects of antihistamines have been drowsiness, sedation, dryness of the mucous membranes, and gastrointestinal effects. Less commonly reported have been dizziness, headache, heartburn, dysuria, polyuria, visual disturbances, and excitation (particularly in children). Serious adverse effects are rare.

Drug Abuse and Dependence (Tussi-Organidin only):

Controlled Substance—Schedule V.

Dependence—Codeine may be habit-forming.

Overdosage: There have been no reports of any serious problems from overdosage with Tussi-Organidin or Tussi-Organidin DM.

Dosage and Administration:
Adults: 1 to 2 teaspoonfuls every 4 hours.
Children: 1/2 to 1 teaspoonful every 4 hours.
How Supplied: Tussi-Organidin Elixir—clear red liquid, in bottles of one pint (NDC 0037-4811-10) and one gallon (NDC 0037-4811-20).
Tussi-Organidin DM Elixir—clear yellow liquid, in bottles of one pint (NDC 0037-4711-10) and one gallon (NDC 0037-4711-20).
Storage: Store at room temperature; avoid excessive heat. Keep bottle tightly closed.

Distributed by
WALLACE LABORATORIES
Division of
CARTER-WALLACE, INC.
Cranbury, New Jersey 08512
Manufactured by Denver Chemical (Puerto Rico) Inc.
Humacao, Puerto Rico 00661

Rev. 5/82

VōSoL® Otic Solution ℞
(acetic acid-nonaqueous 2%)

VōSoL® HC Otic Solution ℞
(hydrocortisone 1%, acetic acid–nonaqueous 2%)

Description: VōSoL is a nonaqueous solution of acetic acid (2%), in a propylene glycol vehicle containing propylene glycol diacetate (3%), benzethonium chloride (0.02%), and sodium acetate (0.015%). VōSoL HC also contains hydrocortisone (1%) and citric acid (0.2%).
Action: VōSoL is antibacterial, antifungal, hydrophilic, has an acid pH and a low surface tension.
VōSoL HC is, in addition, anti-inflammatory and antipruritic.

Indications: (VōSoL only)
Based on a review of this drug by the National Academy of Sciences—National Research Council and/or other information, FDA has classified the indications as follows:
Effective: For the treatment of superficial infections of the external auditory canal caused by organisms susceptible to the action of the antimicrobial.
"Possibly" effective: For prophylaxis of otitis externa in swimmers and susceptible subjects.
Final classification of the less-than-effective indication requires further investigation.

Indications: (VōSoL HC only) For the treatment of superficial infections of the external auditory canal caused by organisms susceptible to the action of the antimicrobial, complicated by inflammation.
Contraindications: These products are contraindicated in those individuals who have shown hypersensitivity to any of their components; perforated tympanic membranes are frequently considered a contraindication to the use of external ear canal medication. VōSoL HC is contraindicated in vaccinia and varicella.
Precautions: VōSoL HC only: As safety of topical steroids during pregnancy has not been confirmed, they should not be used for an extended period during pregnancy. Systemic side effects may occur with extensive use of steroids.
Vōsol and Vōsol HC: If sensitization or irritation occurs, medication should be discontinued promptly.
Dosage and Administration: Carefully remove all cerumen and debris to allow VōSoL (or VōSoL HC) to contact infected surfaces immediately. To promote continuous contact, insert a VōSoL (or VōSoL HC) saturated cotton wick in the ear with instructions to the patient to keep wick moist for the next 24 hours by occasionally adding a few drops on the wick. Remove wick after first 24 hours and continue to instill 5 drops of VōSoL (or VōSoL HC) three or four times daily thereafter.
During treatment, to prevent infection of the other ear, use VōSoL in unaffected ear 3 times daily. To help prevent otitis externa in swimmers and susceptible subjects, instill two drops of VōSoL each morning and evening.
How Supplied: VōSoL Otic Solution, in 15 ml (NDC 0037-3611-10) and 30 ml (NDC 0037-3611-30) measured-drop, safety-tip plastic bottles. VōSoL HC Otic Solution, in 10 ml measured-drop, safety-tip plastic bottle (NDC 0037-3811-12).

Distributed by
WALLACE LABORATORIES
Division of CARTER-WALLACE, INC.
Cranbury, New Jersey 08512
Manufactured by
Denver Chemical (Puerto Rico), Inc.
Humacao, Puerto Rico 00661

Rev. 8/78

[Shown in Product Identification Section]

Warner/Chilcott

Warner/Chilcott products are now marketed by Parke-Davis, Division of Warner-Lambert Company.
Please see the Parke-Davis product monographs.

Warren-Teed Laboratories

Warren-Teed products are now marketed by Adria Laboratories Inc.
Please see the Adria product monographs.

Webcon Pharmaceuticals

Division of
ALCON (Puerto Rico) INC.
P.O. BOX 1629
FORT WORTH, TX 76101

SUPPRETTES®, Webcon's identifying trademark for suppository medication in the NEOCERA® BASE, a unique blend of water-soluble Carbowaxes* that release drugs by hydrophilic action.
*TM Union Carbide.

ANESTACON® ℞
(2% lidocaine hydrochloride)

Description: A sterile anesthetic for endourethral use. Each ml contains: Active: Lidocaine Hydrochloride 20 mg (2%). Vehicle: Hydroxypropyl Methylcellulose 10 mg (1%). Preservative: Benzalkonium Chloride 0.1 mg (0.01%). Inactive: Sodium Chloride, Hydrochloric Acid and/or Sodium Hydroxide (to adjust pH), Purified Water.
Clinical Pharmacology: Lidocaine HCl acts on surface mucous membranes of the urethra to produce local anesthesia by altering the permeability of the nerve cell membrane to sodium and potassium ions, resulting in an increased threshold for electrical excitability and a decreased conduction of impulses whereby depolarization and ion exchanges are inhibited. The anesthetic effect usually begins within two to five minutes and lasts for at least 30 minutes.
Lidocaine is metabolized mainly in the liver and excreted via the kidneys. Approximately 90% of lidocaine administered is excreted in the form of various metabolites, while less than 10% is excreted unchanged.
Indications and Usage: For prevention and control of pain in procedures involving the male and female urethra and for topical treatment of painful urethritis.
Contraindications: Contraindicated in patients with a known sensitivity (allergy) to lidocaine or other drugs of a similar chemical nature.
Warnings: RESUSCITATIVE EQUIPMENT AND DRUGS SHOULD BE IMMEDIATELY AVAILABLE WHEN ANY LOCAL ANESTHETIC IS USED. Lidocaine should be used with extreme caution on traumatized mucosa or in a region of sepsis.
NOTE: After initial use, the remaining contents of the container should be discarded.
Precautions: The smallest volume that will produce effective anesthesia is recommended, and caution should be exercised to avoid overdosage. The safety and effectiveness are dependent on proper dosage, correct technique, adequate precautions, and readiness for emergencies. The debilitated, elderly, acutely ill, and children should be given reduced doses commensurate with their age and physical condition. Use cautiously in persons with known drug sensitivities or allergies.
PREGNANCY CATEGORY C: Animal reproduction studies have not been conducted with Anestacon®. It is also not known whether Anestacon can cause fetal harm when administered to a pregnant woman or can affect reproduction capacity. Anestacon should be administered to a pregnant woman only if clearly needed.
NURSING MOTHERS: It is not known whether this drug is excreted in human milk. Because many drugs are excreted in human milk, caution should be exercised when Anestacon is administered to a nursing mother.
Adverse Reactions: Adverse reactions result from high plasma levels due to excessive dosage, rapid absorption, or inadvertent intravascular injection. Hypersensitivity, idiosyncrasy, or diminished tolerance may also be the cause of reactions. Reactions due to overdosage (high plasma levels) are systemic and involve the central nervous system and the cardiovascular system.
Reactions involving the central nervous system are characterized by excitation and/or depression. Nervousness, dizziness, blurred vision or tremors may occur, followed by convulsions, unconsciousness, drowsiness, and possible respiratory arrest. Excitement may be transient or absent, and the first manifestations may be drowsiness, merging into unconsciousness and respiratory arrest.
Reactions involving the cardiovascular system include depression of the myocardium, hypotension, bradycardia, and even cardiac arrest.
Treatment of a patient with toxic manifestations consists of maintaining an airway, and supporting ventilation using oxygen and assisted or controlled respiration as required. Supportive treatment of the cardiovascular system consists of using vasopressors, preferably those that stimulate the myocardium (e.g. ephedrine, metaraminol, etc.) and intravenous fluids. Convulsions may be controlled by the intravenous administration in small increments of an ultra-short-acting barbiturate (i.e. thiopental, thiamylal) or a short-acting muscle relaxant (succinylcholine), together with oxygen. Muscle relaxants and intravenous barbiturates should only be used by those familiar with their use.
Allergic reactions are characterized by cutaneous lesions of delayed onset, urticaria, edema, or other manifestations of allergy. The detection of sensitivity by skin testing is of doubtful value.
Dosage and Administration: Dosage varies and depends upon the area to be anesthetized,

Continued on next page

Webcon—Cont.

vascularity of the tissues, individual tolerance, and the technique of anesthesia. The least volume of the drug needed to provide effective anesthesia should be administered. For specific techniques and procedures refer to standard texts. THE USUAL DOSE SHOULD NOT EXCEED 600 mg IN ANY TWELVE HOUR PERIOD.
15 ML SINGLE-DOSE CONTAINER: ADULT MALES: Immediately before use, remove the label and cap and firmly insert the sterile tip into the urethral orifice. Slowly instill 5 ml to 15 ml by exerting pressure on opposite sides of the container - the full dose should be administered in a single action without removing the tip. While waiting two to five minutes for induction of anesthesia, the urethra should be occluded with a penile clamp or by manual compression. ADULT FEMALES: The sterile tip may be used to insert about 1 ml.
240 ml CONTAINER: Note: This is for use for only one patient.
ADULT MALES: Instill slowly into the urethra 5 ml to 15 ml and allow two to five minutes for induction of anesthesia. The medication is retained in the urethra by means of a penile clamp or by manual compression of the distal urethra. ADULT FEMALES: Apply liberal amount of medication on a cotton swab and insert into urethra for two to five minutes, or a dropper may be employed to insert about 1 ml.
How Supplied: In 15 ml (NDC 0991-0300-10) and 240 ml (NDC 0991-0300-20) single-dose disposable containers.

B & O SUPPRETTES® Ⓒ ℞
No. 15A and No. 16A
(belladonna and opium rectal suppositories)

Description: Each B & O Supprette® contains (in water-soluble Neocera® Base for rectal administration):
B & O No. 15A: powdered opium* USP 30 mg (½ gr) and powdered belladonna extract USP XX 16.2 mg (equivalent to 0.203 mg or 0.0031 gr alkaloid of belladonna).
B & O No. 16A: powdered opium* USP 60 mg (1 gr) and powdered belladonna extract USP XX 16.2 mg (equivalent to 0.203 mg or 0.0031 gr alkaloid of belladonna).
Neocera® Base is a blend of polyethylene glycol and Polysorbate 60. This drug falls into the pharmacological/therapeutic class of narcotic analgesic/antispasmodic agents.
The pharmacologically active principles present in the belladonna extract component of B & O Supprettes are Atropine and Scopolamine.
Opium contains more than a score of alkaloids, the principal ones being morphine (10%), narcotine (6%), papaverine (1%) and codeine (.5%). The major pharmacologically active principle of the powdered opium component of B & O Supprettes, however, is morphine.
Clinical Pharmacology: Through its parasympatholytic action, atropine relaxes smooth muscle resulting from parasympathetic stimulation. It is the dl isomer of l-hyoscyamine and therefore exhibits the same clinical effects. It is, however, approximately one-half as active peripherally as l-hyoscyamine, the latter being the major active plant principle. The dl isomer atropine is formed during the process of isolation of the belladonna extract.[1]
Morphine, the major active principle of powdered opium, is responsible for the action of powdered opium although the other alkaloids present also contribute to it. The sedative and analgesic action of morphine, the effect desired by inclusion in B & O Supprettes of powdered opium, are thought to be due to its depressant effect on the cerebral cortex, hypothalamus and medullary centers. In large doses the opiates and their analogs also inhibit synaptic conduction in the spinothalamic tracts, depress the function of the reticular formation, the lemniscus and the thalamic relays, and inhibit spinal synaptic reflexes; but these inhibitor actions are not elicited with therapeutic doses of the drug. Moderate doses of powder opium do not alter the electroencephalogram. The action of morphine consists mainly of a descending depression of the central nervous system. It exerts its analgesic action by increasing the pain threshold or the magnitude of stimulus required to evoke pain and by dulling the sensibility or reaction to pain. In addition to its action in abolishing pain, morphine induces a sense of well being (euphoria) facilitating certain mental processes while retarding others. Upon absorption of morphine, oxidative dealkylation to produce nor-compounds appears to be the first step in the reaction sequence which imparts analgesia. Morphine is conjugated in the liver to form the 3-glucuronide which passes into the bile and is reabsorbed and excreted in the urine.
The atropine effect of the belladonna extract serves to eliminate morphine induced smooth muscle spasm without affecting the sedative analgesic action of powdered opium.[2]
Indications and Usage: B & O Supprettes are used for the relief of moderate to severe pain associated with ureteral spasm not responsive to non-narcotic analgesics and to space intervals between injections of opiates.
Contraindications: Do not use B & O Supprettes in patients suffering from glaucoma, severe hepatic or renal disease, bronchial asthma, narcotic idiosyncrasies, respiratory depression, convulsive disorders, acute alcoholism, delirium tremens and premature labor.
***Warnings:** True addiction may result from opium usage. These preparations are not recommended for use in children.
Precautions: Administer with caution to persons with a known idiosyncrasy to atropine or atropine-like compounds; to persons known to be sensitive to or addicted to morphine or morphine-like drugs; to persons with cardiac disease, incipient glaucoma or prostatic hypertrophy. Caution should be used in the administration of this drug to old and debilitated patients and patients with increased intracranial pressure, toxic psychosis and myxedema.
Pregnancy Category C. Animal studies have not been conducted with B & O Supprettes 15A and 16A. It is also not known whether B & O Supprettes 15A and 16A can affect reproduction capacity. The active principles of B & O Supprettes, atropine and morphine, are known to enter the fetal circulation. B & O Supprettes 15A and 16A therefore should be used by a pregnant woman with caution and only when clearly indicated.
Nursing Mothers: It is not known whether this drug is excreted in human milk. Because many drugs are excreted in human milk, caution should be exercised when B & O Supprettes are administered to a nursing woman.
Adverse Reactions: Belladonna may cause drowsiness, dry mouth, urinary retention, photophobia, rapid pulse, dizziness and blurred vision. Opium usage may result in constipation, nausea, vomiting. Pruritis and urticaria may occasionally occur.
Drug Abuse and Dependence: Because of their content of opium, B & O Supprettes 15A and 16A are considered as Schedule II drugs by the Drug Enforcement Agency. No data exists on chronic abuse effects or dependence characteristics of B & O Supprettes 15A and 16A.
Overdosage: As with morphine and related narcotics, overdosage is characterized by respiratory depression, pinpoint pupils and coma. Respiratory depression may be reversed by intravenous administration of naloxone hydrochloride or levallorphan tartrate. In addition, supportive measures such as oxygenation, intravenous fluids and vasopressors should be used as indicated.
Dosage and Administration: Adults: One B & O No. 15A or No. 16A Supprette rectally once or twice daily, or as recommended by the physician. Moisten finger and Supprette with water before inserting. Not recommended for use in children.
How Supplied: In strip packaged units of 12 (scored for ½ dosage). DEA order required (Schedule II).
B & O No. 15A NDC 0991-5015-75.
B & O No. 16A NDC 0991-5016-75.
References:
1. Grollman, A., and Grollman, E. F., Pharmacology and Therapeutics, 7th Edition, Lea and Febiger, Philadelphia, 1970, pp. 338 to 346.
2. Ibid., pp. 96 to 107.

CYSTOSPAZ® ℞
(Hyoscyamine Tablets USP XX)
CYSTOSPAZ-M® ℞
(Hyoscyamine Sulfate)

Description: CYSTOSPAZ® is a pale blue uncoated compressed tablet for oral administration. It contains the parasympatholytic agent hyoscyamine as the free base. Each tablet contains hyoscyamine 0.15 mg.
CYSTOSPAZ-M® is a light blue timed-release capsule containing hyoscyamine sulfate 0.375 mg.
Clinical Pharmacology: Through its parasympatholytic action, hyoscyamine relaxes smooth muscle spasm resulting from parasympathetic stimulation. It is the l-isomer of atropine and therefore exhibits the same clinical effects as atropine. It is, however, approximately twice as active peripherally as atropine, since the latter is the racemic (dl) form of hyoscyamine and d-hyoscyamine possesses only a very weak anticholinergic action. Since only one-half the atropine dose is required for l-hyoscyamine it has only one-half the unwanted central effects of atropine.[1]
Indications and Usage: In the management of disorders of the lower urinary tract associated with hypermotility. Although specific therapy is often required to remove the underlying cause of spasm, Cystospaz and Cystospaz-M are offered as antispasmodic agent dosage forms which may be combined with other forms of therapy where indicated.
Contraindications: Glaucoma, urinary bladder neck or pyloric obstruction, duodenal obstruction and cardiospasm. Hypersensitivity to any of the ingredients.
Precautions: Administer with caution to persons with known idiosyncrasy to atropine-like compounds and to patients suffering cardiac disease.
Pregnancy Category C. Animal Reproduction studies have not been conducted with Cystospaz or Cystospaz-M. It is also not known whether Cystospaz or Cystospaz-M can cause fetal harm when administered to a pregnant woman or can affect reproduction capacity. Cystospaz and Cystospaz-M should be taken by a pregnant woman only if clearly needed.
Nursing Mothers: It is not known whether this drug is excreted in human milk. Because many drugs are excreted in human milk, caution should be exercised when Cystospaz is administered to a nursing woman.
Adverse Reactions: Though rarely a problem, the side effects encountered with this class of antispasmodic-antisecretory agents (drowsiness, dryness of mouth, photophobia, constipation, urinary retention) may also be seen with this drug. If rapid pulse, dizziness or blurring of vision occurs, discontinue use immediately. Acute urinary retention may be precipitated in prostatic hypertrophy. **Note:** Slight dryness of mouth is an indication that parasympathetic blockage is effective. The patient should be warned that this may occur.
Drug Abuse and Dependence: A dependence on the use of Cystospaz or Cystospaz-M has not been reported and due to the na-

ture of its ingredients abuse of Cystospaz or Cystospaz-M is not expected.

Overdosage: Symptoms of overdosage include severe dryness of mouth and throat, dryness of skin, difficulty or inability to swallow, difficult speech, dilated pupils until iris almost disappears, restlessness and garrulity indicating an irritability of the brain, marked tremors, convulsions, respiratory failure, death.[2] In adults, symptoms of overdosage may be in the range of ingestion of 0.6 to 1 mg with doses exceeding 1–2 mg eliciting more profound toxicity.

Dosage and Administration:

Adults: Cystospaz — One or two tablets four times daily or fewer if needed. Cystospaz-M—One capsule every twelve hours.

Older Children: Reduce dosage in proportion to age and weight.

How Supplied: Cystospaz — Bottles of 100 light blue tablets NDC 0991-2225-10. Cystospaz-M—Bottles of 100 light blue timed-release capsules NDC 0991-2260-10.

References:

1. Grollman, A. and Grollman, E. F.: *Pharmacology and Therapeutics*, 7th Edition, p. 346.
2. Ibid., p. 347.

URISED® ℞

Description: URISED® is a combination of antiseptics (Methenamine, Methylene Blue, Phenyl Salicylate, Benzoic Acid) and parasympatholytics (Atropine Sulfate, Hyoscyamine) in tablet form for oral administration.

Each tablet contains: Methenamine 40.8 mg, Phenyl Salicylate 18.1 mg, Methylene Blue 5.4 mg, Benzoic Acid 4.5 mg, Atropine Sulfate 0.03 mg and Hyoscyamine 0.03 mg.

Clinical Pharmacology: Methenamine itself does not have antiseptic, irritant, or toxic properties in the urine. Methenamine, in an acid urine (pH 5.5 or below) hydrolyzes into formaldehyde within the urinary tract providing mild antiseptic activity. When given as directed and the daily urine volume is 1000 to 1500 ml, a daily urinary concentration of 3–10 mcg/ml of free formaldehyde may be expected in the urine.[1] This is approximately three times the minimal inhibitory dose of formaldehyde which must be available for most urinary tract pathogens. Methenamine is readily absorbed from the gastrointestinal tract and is rapidly excreted almost entirely in the urine.[2] Methylene Blue and Benzoic Acid are mild but effective antiseptics which contribute to the antiseptic properties of Methenamine, and Phenyl Salicylate is a mild analgesic and antipyretic. All of these compounds are readily absorbed from the gastrointestinal tract and excreted in the urine. Through parasympatholytic action, atropine and hyoscyamine relax smooth muscle spasm resulting from parasympathetic stimulation.

Indications and Usage: URISED is indicated for the relief of discomfort of the lower urinary tract caused by hypermotility resulting from inflammation or diagnostic procedures and in the treatment of cystitis, urethritis, and trigonitis when caused by organisms which maintain or produce an acid urine and are susceptible to formaldehyde.

Contraindications: Glaucoma, urinary bladder neck obstruction, pyloric or duodenal obstruction, or cardiospasm. Hypersensitivity to any of the ingredients.

Precautions: Administer with caution to persons with known idiosyncrasy to atropine-like compounds and to patients suffering from cardiac disease. Bacteriological studies of the urine may be helpful in following the patient response. Methylene Blue interferes with the analysis for some urinary components such as free formaldehyde. Drugs and/or foods which produce an alkaline urine should be restricted. Patient should be advised that the urine may become blue to blue-green and the feces may be discolored as a result of excretion of Methylene Blue. Methenamine preparations should not be given to patients taking sulfonamides since insoluble precipitates may form with formaldehyde in the urine. No known longterm animal studies have been performed to evaluate carcinogenic potential.

Pregnancy Category C. Animal reproduction studies have not been conducted with URISED TABLETS. It is also not known whether URISED TABLETS can cause fetal harm when administered to a pregnant woman or can affect reproduction capacity. URISED TABLETS should be given to a pregnant woman only if clearly needed.

Nursing Mothers: It is not known whether this drug is excreted in human milk. Because many drugs are excreted in human milk, caution should be exercised when URISED TABLETS are administered to a nursing woman.

Adverse Reactions: If pronounced dryness of the mouth, flushing, or difficulty in initiating micturition occurs, decrease dosage. If rapid pulse, dizziness or blurring of vision occurs, discontinue use immediately. Acute urinary retention may be precipitated in prostatic hypertrophy.

Drug Abuse and Dependence: A dependence on the use of URISED has not been reported and due to the nature of its ingredients, abuse of URISED is not expected.

Overdosage: By exceeding the recommended dosage of URISED, symptomology related to the overdose of its individual active ingredients may be expected as follows:

Methenamine: If large amounts of the drug (8 gm daily) are used over extended periods, bladder and gastrointestinal irritation, painful and frequent micturition, albuminuria and gross hematuria may be expected.

Methylene Blue: Symptoms of Methylene Blue overdosage associated with the overdosage of URISED are not expected to be discernible from those associated with the other active ingredients in URISED.

Phenyl Salicylate: Symptoms of Phenyl Salicylate overdosage include burning pain in throat and mouth, white necrotic lesions in the mouth, abdominal pain, vomiting, bloody diarrhea, pallor, sweating, weakness, headache, dizziness and tinnitus. The symptoms, however, are not expected to be discernible from those associated with the other active ingredients in URISED.

Atropine Sulfate, Hyoscyamine: Symptoms associated with an overdosage of URISED will most probably be manifested in the symptoms related to overdosage of the alkaloids Atropine Sulfate and Hyoscyamine. Such symptoms as dryness of mucous membranes; dilatation of pupils; hot, dry, flushed skin; hyperpyrexia; tachycardia; palpitations; elevated blood pressure; coma; circulatory collapse and death from respiratory failure can occur due to overdosage of these alkaloids.

Dosage and Administration: Adults: Two tablets four times daily. **Children (12 years and older):** Reduce dosage in proportion to age and weight.

How Supplied: Bottles of 100 (NDC 0991-2183-10), 500 (NDC 0991-2183-20) and 1000 (NDC 0991-2183-30) tablets.

References:

1. Goodman, L. S. and Gilman, G., *The Pharmacological Basis of Therapeutics*, Fifth Edition, 1006 (1975).
2. *AMA Drug Evaluation*, Third Edition, 790 (1977).

WANS® Ⓒ III

(pyrilamine maleate and pentobarbital sodium)
ANTI-NAUSEA SUPPRETTES

Description: WANS® is a combination of an antihistamine (Pyrilamine Maleate) and a sedative (Pentobarbital Sodium) in suppository form for rectal administration. Each WANS® SUPPRETTE® contains (in water-soluble Neocera® Base):

WANS® Children (blue): pyrilamine maleate 25 mg and pentobarbital sodium* 30 mg; scored for ½ dosage.

WANS® No. 1 (pink): pyrilamine maleate 50 mg and pentobarbital sodium* 50 mg; scored for ½ dosage.

WANS® No. 2 (yellow): pyrilamine maleate 50 mg and pentobarbital sodium* 100 mg; scored for ½ dosage.

***Warning: May be habit forming.**

The Neocera Base is a blend of Polyethylene Glycol 400, 1540 and 6000, Polysorbate 60 and color additives including FD&C Yellow No. 5 (Tartrazine) in WANS No. 2.

Clinical Pharmacology: Pyrilamine maleate is an antihistamine of the ethylenediamine family, which exhibits recognized antiemetic activity. Pyrilamine maleate may exhibit a noticeable stimulating effect on the central nervous system (CNS) and, on occasion, a weak CNS-depressant effect.

Pentobarbital sodium is an effective, short-acting barbiturate which acts as a general CNS-depressant. Pentobarbital sodium suppresses the vomiting center itself, and at the same time, provides sedation.

Indications and Usage: WANS® is indicated in the symptomatic treatment of nausea and vomiting. The suppository dosage form is a particularly useful method of drug administration in patients with nausea and vomiting who are unable to retain oral medication.

Contraindications: Acute intermittent porphyria, known hypersensitivity to barbiturates or antihistamines, known barbiturate addiction, in senility, severe hepatic impairment, and in the presence of uncontrolled pain, acute head injury associated with vomiting or other signs of CNS injury. Not for use in infants under 6 months of age since they are more sensitive to the central nervous system stimulating effects of pyrilamine maleate than adults. Pyrilamine maleate may cause convulsions in infants, particularly in excessive dosage.

Warnings:

Caution should be exercised when administering WANS® to children for the treatment of vomiting. Antiemetics are not recommended for treatment of uncomplicated vomiting in children and their use should be limited to prolonged vomiting of known etiology. There are three principal reasons for caution:

1. There have been some recent reports of toxic encephalopathy, characterized by a depressed level of consciousness, marked irritability and ataxia in infants and children following administration of higher-than-recommended doses of pyrilamine maleate and pentobarbital sodium combination products such as WANS®. **The recommended dosage should therefore not be exceeded.**
2. There has been some suspicion that centrally acting antiemetics may contribute, in combination with viral illnesses (a possible cause of vomiting in children), to development of Reye's syndrome, a potentially fatal acute childhood encephalopathy with visceral fatty degeneration, especially involving the liver. Although there is no confirmation of this suspicion, caution is nevertheless recommended.
3. It should also be noted that salicylates and acetaminophen are hepatotoxic at large doses. Although it is not known that at usual doses they would represent a hazard in patients with the underlying hepatic disorder of Reye's syndrome, these drugs should be avoided in

Continued on next page

Webcon—Cont.

children whose signs and symptoms could represent Reye's syndrome, unless alternative methods of controlling fever are not successful.

Barbiturates may be habit forming. Administration in the presence of pre-existing psychological disturbances may result in confusion, delirium, and accentuation of symptoms. Idiosyncratic reactions may occur and include lassitude, vertigo, nausea, vomiting, and diarrhea. Acquired sensitivity to barbiturates may result in allergic reactions including urticaria, dermatitis, and rarely, exfoliative dermatitis and degenerative changes in the liver and kidney.
Pentobarbital sodium may cause fetal harm when administered to a pregnant woman. Pentobarbital sodium can cross the placental barrier and may depress the fetal central nervous system so that respiration is not adequately established at birth. If this drug is used during pregnancy, or if the patient becomes pregnant while taking this drug, the patient should be apprised of the potential hazard to the fetus.
Precautions: General: WANS® should be administered with caution to patients with a history of drug dependence or suicidal tendencies. Caution should be exercised when the drug is used concurrently with other sedative, hypnotic, or narcotic agents. This drug should be given with caution to patients with known acute or chronic hepatic disease, fever, hyperthyroidism, diabetes mellitus, severe anemia, and congestive heart failure.
WANS® No. 2 contains FD&C Yellow No. 5 (tartrazine) which may cause allergic-type reactions (including bronchial asthma) in certain susceptible individuals. Although the overall incidence of sensitivity to FD&C Yellow No. 5 (tartrazine) in the general population is low, it is frequently seen in patients who also have aspirin hypersensitivity.
Information for Patients: Do not take alcoholic beverages or other CNS depressants while taking this product. This product may cause drowsiness. Do not drive, operate machinery, or otherwise engage in activities where impairment of alertness and coordination could result in accidents or injury.
Drug Interactions: Alcohol and other CNS depressants taken in conjunction with this product produce an additive depressant effect on the central nervous system. Patients taking other CNS depressants concomitantly with this product should be observed more frequently, especially during the initiation of therapy. Also, barbiturates and antihistamines must be used with caution in patients receiving monoamine oxidase inhibitors since these drugs may potentiate the depressant effect of the barbiturate or augment the anticholinergic effect of the antihistamine.
Carcinogenesis, Mutagenesis, Impairment of Fertility: Long-term studies in animals to evaluate the carcinogenic potential of this drug have not been performed. There is no evidence in the published literature that the ingredients of this product are carcinogenic, mutagenic, or impair fertility.
Pregnancy:
Teratogenic Effects: Pregnancy Category D. See "Warnings" section.
Non-Teratogenic Effects: Dependence of the mother on pentobarbital sodium may result in withdrawal symptoms (e.g., hyperirritability, vomiting, shrill cry) in the baby after delivery.
Nursing Mothers: Antihistamines may inhibit lactation and may be excreted in breast milk. Since the risk of adverse reactions is higher in infants, use of antihistamines is not recommended in nursing mothers. Barbiturates may also be excreted in breast milk. The effects of barbiturates in the nursing infant may include sedation and induction of hepatic metabolizing enzymes. Therefore, because of the potential for serious adverse reactions in nursing infants from the use of this product, a decision should be made whether to discontinue nursing or to discontinue the drug, taking into account the importance of the drug to the mother.
Pediatric Use: See "Contraindications" and "Warnings" sections for information regarding the use of this product in infants and children.
Adverse Reactions: Antihistamine side effects include drowsiness, potentiation of the sedative effect of barbiturates, fatigue, vertigo, incoordination, tremor, muscle weakness, dryness of the nose, mouth and throat, tinnitus, pupillary dilation and blurred vision, urinary retention, impotence, epigastric and intestinal pain, anorexia, nausea, vomiting, diarrhea, excitation, euphoria, insomnia, nervousness, palpitation, tachycardia, hypotension, hypersensitivity reactions such as allergic dermatitis, and rarely, blood dyscrasias.
Side effects associated with barbiturates include drowsiness, lethargy, sedation, paradoxic restlessness or excitement in susceptible persons, respiratory depression, coma, and delirium.
Drug Abuse and Dependence:
Controlled Substance: WANS® is a Schedule III controlled drug.
Dependence: As with other CNS-depressants, the use of pentobarbital sodium may induce a psychological dependence in some patients. Prolonged, uninterrupted use of barbiturates, even in therapeutic doses, may result in physical and psychological dependence. The symptoms of chronic intoxication are similar to those of alcohol intoxication (e.g., disorientation, ataxia, euphoria). In such cases, abrupt discontinuance may precipitate typical withdrawal symptoms, including convulsions. Therefore, the drug should be withdrawn gradually.
Abuse: Those persons who develop a psychological dependence on pentobarbital sodium may increase the dosage without consulting a physician and may subsequently develop a physical dependence on the drug.
Overdosage: Antihistamine overdosage, particularly in children, may result in hallucination, excitement, ataxia, incoordination, athetosis, convulsions and death. Mechanical ventilation and supportive care are important, and drugs likely to potentiate the effects of the antihistamine should not be given.
Overdosage of pentobarbital sodium is manifested by drowsiness, lethargy, sedation, paradoxic restlessness or excitement in susceptible persons, respiratory depression, delirium, hypothermia, latent fever, sluggishness or absence of reflexes, coma, gradual appearance of circulatory collapse, pulmonary edema and death. Supportive care is of primary importance in the treatment of barbiturate overdosage.

1. Maintain and assist respiration as indicated.
2. Support circulation with vasopressors and intravenous fluids as required.
3. Aspirate stomach contents, taking care to avoid pulmonary aspiration.
4. Use osmotic diuretic and measure intake and output of fluids.

In severe overdosage, hemodialysis may be lifesaving, especially if a vigorous diuresis cannot be maintained.
Dosage and Administration:
Children: For children 2 to 12 years of age (over 15 kg bodyweight) the usual dose is one WANS® Children, rectally, every 6 to 8 hours as required. Do not exceed three doses in 24 hours. Children 6 months to 2 years of age (less than 15 kg bodyweight) should use not more than ½ the above dosage. **Do not use in infants below the age of 6 months.** In determining the optimum dosage in infants and children, consideration should be given in each case to the age and weight of the patient, the etiology and severity of the condition being treated and the clinical response. **The above recommended dosages should not be exceeded (see "Warnings").**
Adults: Rectally, one WANS® No. 1 to inhibit mild nausea and/or vomiting or one WANS® No. 2 to control pernicious vomiting. Repeat doses for adults should be 4 to 6 hours apart; do not exceed four doses in 24 hours. The optimum dosage must be determined in each case by the clinical response. Moisten finger and SUPPRETTE® with water before inserting.
How Supplied: In foil strip packaged units of 12 (scored for ½ dosage).
WANS® CHILDREN (blue): NDC 0991-1000-75
WANS® No. 1 (pink): NDC 0991-1001-75
WANS® No. 2 (yellow): NDC 0991-1002-75
Storage: Store at room temperature. Do not refrigerate.

The Wesley Pharmacal Company, Inc.
9984 GANTRY ROAD
PHILADELPHIA, PA 19115

P.D.P. LIQUID PROTEIN
Protein Supplement
15 gm. per 30 cc - 60 Calories per 30 cc

P.D.P. PROTEIN CAPSULES
1 gm. per Capsule

P.D.P. is hydrolyzed protein (pre-digested) in which the protein has been broken down into amino acids and is utilized 100% by the body. No fats or carbohydrates are contained.
How Supplied: 1 Quart Bottles, 100 Capsules.

P.D.P. PROTEIN POWDER
Cream of Chicken Soup
Cream of Vegetable Soup
Soy Base

How Supplied: 1 lb. Containers.

URACID ℞
(dl Methionine)

Description: Each capsule contains:
dl-Methionine..0.2 gm.
Action and Uses: Management of diaper rash in infants, and the control of odor in incontinent adults. An ammonia-free urine is affected by the acid producing effect of dl-methionine on pH of urine.
Contraindications: Do not use in patients with a history of liver disease because the toxemia of the disease may be exaggerated by large doses of methionine.
Precautions: Prolonged excessive doses of methionine may result in a below-normal weight gain. Adequate protein intake should be assured during long periods of methionine therapy.
Administration and Dosages: Diaper rash in infants, empty contents of one capsule into evening formula, preferably while still warm; or it may be added to orange juice. Odor control in adults: One capsule three times daily with meals.
How Supplied:
100 bottles. NDC 0917-0240-01
1000 bottles. NDC 0917-0240-10
Literature Available: Yes.

Products are cross-indexed by generic and chemical names in the **YELLOW SECTION**

Westwood Pharmaceuticals Inc.
468 DEWITT ST.
BUFFALO, NY 14213

ALPHA KERI®
Therapeutic Bath Oil

Composition: Contains mineral oil, lanolin oil, Hydroloc™ brand of Westwood's PEG-4 dilaurate, fragrance, benzophenone-3, D&C green 6.

Action and Uses: ALPHA KERI is a water-dispersible, antipruritic oil for the care of dry skin. ALPHA KERI effectively deposits a thin, uniform, emulsified film of oil over the skin. This film helps relieve itching, lubricates and softens the skin. ALPHA KERI BATH OIL is an all-over skin moisturizer. Only Alpha Keri contains Hydroloc™ — the unique emulsifier that provides a more uniform distribution of the therapeutic oils to moisturize dry skin. ALPHA KERI is valuable as an aid in the treatment of dry, pruritic skin and mild skin irritations such as chronic atopic dermatitis; pruritus senilis and hiemalis; contact dermatitis; "bath-itch"; xerosis or asteatosis; ichthyosis; soap dermatitis; psoriasis.

Administration and Dosage: ALPHA KERI *should always be used with water, either added to water or rubbed on to wet skin.* Because of its inherent cleansing properties it is not necessary to use soap when ALPHA KERI is being used.

For exact dosage, label directions should be followed.

BATH: Added as directed to bathtub of water. For optimum relief: 10 to 20 minute soak.

SHOWER: Small amount is poured into wet washcloth and rubbed on to wet skin. Rinse. Pat dry.

SPONGE BATH: Added as directed to a basin of warm water then rubbed over entire body with washcloth.

SITZ BATH: Added as directed to tub water. Soak should last for 10 to 20 minutes.

INFANT BATH: Added as directed to basin or bathinette of water.

SKIN CLEANSING OTHER THAN BATH OR SHOWER: A small amount is rubbed on to wet skin. Rinse. Pat dry.

Precaution: The patient should be warned to guard against slipping in tub or shower.

How Supplied: 4 fl. oz. (NDC 0072-3600-04), 8 fl. oz. (NDC 0072-3600-08; NSN 6505-00-890-2027) and 16 fl. oz. (NDC 0072-3600-16) plastic bottles. Also available for patients who prefer to shower—ALPHA KERI SPRAY—5 oz. (NDC 0072-3600-05) aerosol container.

ALPHA KERI® SOAP
Non-detergent Soap

Composition: Sodium tallowate, sodium cocoate, water, mineral oil, fragrance, PEG-75, glycerin, titanium dioxide, lanolin oil, sodium chloride, BHT, EDTA, D&C Green 5, D&C Yellow 10.

Action and Uses: ALPHA KERI SOAP, rich in emollient oils, thoroughly cleanses as it soothes and softens the skin.

Indications: Adjunctive use in dry skin care.

Administration and Dosage: To be used as any other soap.

How Supplied: 4 oz. (NDC 0072-3500-04) bar.

BALNETAR®
Water-dispersible Emollient Tar

Composition: Contains WESTWOOD® TAR (equivalent to 2.5% Coal Tar USP).

Action and Uses: For temporary relief of itching and scaling due to psoriasis, eczema, and other tar-responsive dermatoses. Tar ingredient is chemically and biologically standardized to insure uniform therapeutic activity. BALNETAR exerts keratoplastic, antieczematous, antipruritic, and emollient actions. It deposits microfine particles of tar over the skin in a lubricant-moisturizing film that helps soften and remove scales and crusts, making the skin smoother and more supple. BALNETAR is an important adjunct in a wide range of dermatoses, including: atopic dermatitis; chronic eczematoid dermatitis; seborrheic dermatitis.

Contraindications: Not indicated when acute inflammation is present.

Administration and Dosage: BALNETAR *should always be used with water... either added to water or rubbed onto wet skin.* For exact dosage label directions are to be followed.

IN THE TUB—Add as directed to a bathtub of water. Soap is not used. The patient soaks for 10 to 20 minutes and then pats dry.

FOR DIRECT APPLICATION—A small amount is rubbed onto the wet skin. Excess is wiped off with tissue to help prevent staining of clothes or linens.

FOR SCALP APPLICATION —A small amount is rubbed onto the wet scalp with fingertips.

Caution: If irritation persists, discontinue use. May temporarily discolor blond, bleached or tinted hair. In rare cases BALNETAR may cause allergic sensitization attributable to coal tar.

Precaution: After use of BALNETAR, patient should avoid exposure to direct sunlight unless sunlight is being used therapeutically in a supervised, modified Goeckerman regimen. Contact with the eyes should be avoided. Patient should be cautioned against slipping when BALNETAR is used in bathtub. Also advise patient that use in a plastic or fiberglass tub may cause staining of the tub.

How Supplied: 8 fl. oz. (NDC 0072-4200-08; NSN 6505-00-928-5890) plastic shatterproof bottle.

CAPITROL® ℞
(chloroxine 2%)
Cream Shampoo

Description: CAPITROL shampoo provides 2% chloroxine (each gram contains 20 mg. chloroxine) suspended in a shampoo base containing: sodium octoxynol-3 sulfonate, PEG-6 lauramide, dextrin, stearyl alcohol/ceteareth-20, sodium lauryl sulfoacetate, dioctyl sodium sulfosuccinate, magnesium aluminum silicate, PEG-14M, EDTA, citric acid, water, color, fragrance and 1% benzyl alcohol. The pH of the shampoo is 7.0.

The chemical name of chloroxine is 5, 7-dichloro-8-hydroxyquinoline.

Actions: Chloroxine is a synthetic antibacterial compound. It has a structural similarity to a number of substituted 8-hydroxyquinolines that have been in therapeutic use for some years.

Indications: CAPITROL is indicated in the treatment of dandruff and mild to moderately severe seborrheic dermatitis of the scalp.

Contraindications: CAPITROL (chloroxine) may produce allergic contact sensitization reactions in patients who are sensitive to hydroxyquinolines or EDTA. This shampoo should not be used on acutely inflamed (exudative) lesions of the scalp.

Precautions: Patients should be advised to exercise care not to allow CAPITROL to enter the eyes. For external use only.

Adverse Reactions: Irritation and burning of the scalp and adjacent areas have been reported. Allergic type skin eruptions may occur in patients who are sensitive to any component of the shampoo. As with any medicated shampoo, chemical conjunctivitis may result if CAPITROL enters the eyes. Discoloration of light-colored hair (e.g. blond, gray or bleached) may follow use of this preparation. Dryness of the scalp and increased itching have been reported.

Dosage and Administration: CAPITROL (chloroxine) should be massaged thoroughly onto the wet scalp, avoiding contact with the eyes. Lather should remain on the scalp for approximately three minutes, then rinsed. The application should be repeated and the scalp rinsed thoroughly. Two treatments per week are usually sufficient.

Caution: Keep this and all drugs out of the reach of children.

How Supplied: 85 g. (NDC 0072-6800-02) plastic tube.

DESQUAM-X 5% GEL ℞
DESQUAM-X 10% GEL ℞
Benzoyl Peroxide

Description: DESQUAM-X 5 and DESQUAM-X 10 brand topical anti-acne gels contain benzoyl peroxide (5 and 10%) in a water-base vehicle of carbomer 940, diisopropanolamine, disodium edetate and laureth-4.

Clinical Pharmacology: The effectiveness of benzoyl peroxide in the treatment of acne vulgaris is primarily attributable to its antibacterial activity, especially with respect to *Propionibacterium acnes,* the predominant organism in sebaceous follicles and comedones.[1,2] The antibacterial activity of this compound is presumably due to the release of active or free-radical oxygen capable of oxidizing bacterial proteins.[3] In acne patients treated topically with benzoyl peroxide, resolution of the acne usually coincides with reduction in the levels of *P. acnes* and free fatty acids (FFA). Mild desquamation is another observed action of topically applied benzoyl peroxide and may also play a role in the drug's effectiveness in acne.[3] Studies also indicate that topical benzoyl peroxide may exert a sebostatic effect with a resultant reduction of skin surface lipids.[4,5] Benzoyl peroxide has been shown to be absorbed by the skin, where it is metabolized to benzoic acid and then excreted as benzoate in the urine.[6]

Laureth-4 is a non-toxic surfactant which exerts its action through cleansing and mild desquamation. The result of these actions is a drying and degreasing of the skin.[7]

Indications and Usage: DESQUAM-X (5 or 10) GEL is indicated for the topical treatment of mild to moderate acne vulgaris and as an adjunct in therapeutic regimens including antibiotics, retinoic acid products and sulfur/salicylic acid-containing preparations. DESQUAM-X GEL has been shown effective in the treatment of the following acne lesion types: papules, pustules, open and closed comedones. Clinical studies have demonstrated therapeutic response after two to three weeks. DESQUAM-X GEL may also be used as adjunctive treatment for nodulocystic acne (acne conglobata), although its effectiveness for this condition has not been proven.

Contraindications: This product should not be used in patients known to be hypersensitive to benzoyl peroxide or any of the other listed ingredients.

Precautions: **General:** Avoid contact with eyes and other mucous membranes. For external use only. In patients known to be sensitive to the following substances, there is a possibility of cross-sensitization: benzoic acid derivatives (including certain topical anesthetics) and cinnamon.

Information for Patients: This product may bleach colored fabric or hair. Concurrent use with PABA-containing sunscreens may result in transient discoloration of the skin.

Carcinogenesis, Mutagenesis, Impairment of Fertility: Based upon considerable evidence, benzyol peroxide is not considered to be a carcinogen. However, in one study, using mice known to be highly susceptible to cancer, there

Continued on next page

Westwood—Cont.

was evidence for benzoyl peroxide as a tumor promoter. Benzoyl peroxide has been found to be inactive as a mutagen in the *Ames Salmonella* and other assays, including the mouse dominant lethal assay. This assay is frequently used to assess the effect of substances on spermatogenesis.

Pregnancy (Category C): Animal reproduction studies have not been conducted with benzoyl peroxide (DESQUAM-X GEL). It is also not known whether benzoyl peroxide (DESQUAM-X GEL) can cause fetal harm when administered to a pregnant woman or can affect reproductive capacity. Benzoyl peroxide (DESQUAM-X GEL) should be given to a pregnant woman only if clearly needed.

Nursing Mothers: It is not known whether this drug is excreted in human milk. Caution should be exercised when benzoyl peroxide is administered to a nursing woman.

Pediatric Use: Safety and effectiveness in children below the age of 12 have not been established.

Adverse Reactions: Adverse reactions which may be encountered with topical benzoyl peroxide include excessive drying (manifested by marked peeling, erythema and possibly edema), and allergic contact sensitization. Excessive dryness appears to occur in approximately 2 patients in 50. Pertinent literature seems to indicate that allergic sensitization to benzoyl peroxide may occur in 10 to 25 patients in 1,000.[8,9,10] There is one reference that reports an occurrence of sensitization in 5 of 100 patients.[11]

Overdosage: In the event that excessive scaling, erythema or edema occur, the use of this preparation should be discontinued. If the reaction is judged to be due to excessive use and not allergenicity, after symptoms and signs subside, a reduced dosage schedule may be cautiously tried. To hasten resolution of the adverse effects, emollients, cool compresses and/or topical corticosteroid preparations may be used.

Dosage and Administration: DESQUAM-X GEL should be gently rubbed into all affected areas once or twice daily. Suitable cleansing of the affected area should precede application. In fair-skinned individuals or under excessively drying conditions, it is suggested that therapy be initiated with one application daily. The degree of drying or peeling may be controlled by modification of dose frequency or drug concentration. The use of DESQUAM-X GEL may be continued as long as deemed necessary.

How Supplied:

DESQUAM-X 5 GEL

1.5 oz. (42.5 g) (NDC 0072-6621-01; NSN 6505-01-036-8629) plastic tube.

3 oz. (85 g) (NDC 0072-6621-03) plastic tube.

DESQUAM-X 10 GEL

1.5 oz. (42.5 g) (NDC 0072-6721-01; NSN 6505-01-036-8628) plastic tube.

3 oz. (85 g) (NDC 0072-6721-03) plastic tube.

Store at controlled room temperature (59°-86° F).

References:

1. Kligman AM, Leyden JJ, Stewart R: New uses for benzoyl peroxide: A broad-spectrum antimicrobial agent. *Int J Derm* 16: 413–417, 1977.
2. Leyden JJ, Stewart R, Kligman AM: Updated *in vivo* methods for evaluating topical antimicrobial agents on human skin. *J Invest Dermatol* 72: 165–170, 1979.
3. Fulton JE, Farzad-Bakshandeh A, Bradley S: Studies on the mechanism of action of topical benzoyl peroxide and vitamin-A acid in acne vulgaris. *J Cut Path* 1: 171–200, 1974.
4. Fanta D, Jurecka W: Autoradiographic investigation on benzoyl peroxide treated skin. *Acta Dermatovener* 58: 361–362, 1978.
5. Fanta D, Muller MM: Effect of benzoyl peroxide on skin surface lipids. *Dermatologica* 158: 55–59, 1979.
6. Nacht S, Yeung D, Beasley J, Anjo M, Maibach HI: Benzoyl peroxide: *in vitro* and *in vivo* skin penetration and metabolic disposition. Presented to Soc for Invest Derm, June 9–14, 1979, Amsterdam.
7. Blau S, Kanof N: Polyoxyethylene lauryl ether, its use in a new keratolytic acne lotion. *Arch Dermatol* 82: 158–159, 1960.
8. Eaglstein WH: Allergic contact dermatitis to benzoyl peroxide. *Arch Dermatol* 97: 527, 1968.
9. Pace WE: A benzoyl peroxide-sulfur cream for acne vulgaris. *Canad Med Assoc J* 93: 252–253, 1965.
10. Vasarinsh P: Benzoyl peroxide-sulfur lotions in acne vulgaris—a controlled study. *Cutis* 5(1): 65–69, 1969.
11. Fanta D: Clinical and experimental studies with benzoyl peroxide in the treatment of acne. *Hautzart* 29: 481–486, 1978.
12. Slaga TJ: Skin tumor-promoting activity of benzoyl peroxide, a widely used free radical-generating compound. *Sci* 213: 1023–1024. 1981.

DESQUAM-X® WASH ℞

4% Benzoyl Peroxide

Description: DESQUAM-X WASH therapeutic acne cleanser contains benzoyl peroxide (4%) in a lathering water base of sodium octoxynol-3 sulfonate, dioctyl sodium sulfosuccinate, sodium lauryl sulfoacetate, magnesium aluminum silicate, methylcellulose and EDTA.

Clinical Pharmacology: The effectiveness of benzoyl peroxide in the treatment of acne vulgaris is primarily attributable to its antibacterial activity, especially with respect to *Propionibacterium acnes,* the predominant organism in sebaceous follicles and comedones.[1,2] The antibacterial activity of this compound is presumably due to the release of active or free-radical oxygen capable of oxidizing bacterial proteins.[3] In acne patients treated topically with benzoyl peroxide, resolution of the acne usually coincides with reduction in the levels of *P. acnes* and free fatty acids (FFA). The cleansing action of the DESQUAM-X WASH detergent base also aids in the removal of excess sebum from the skin surface. Mild desquamation is another observed action of topically applied benzoyl peroxide and may also play a role in the drug's effectiveness in acne.[3] Studies also indicate that topical benzoyl peroxide may exert a sebostatic effect with a resultant reduction of skin surface lipids.[4,5] Benzoyl peroxide has been shown to be absorbed by the skin, where it is metabolized to benzoic acid and then excreted as benzoate in the urine.[6]

Indications and Usage: DESQUAM-X WASH is indicated for the topical treatment of mild to moderate acne. In more severe cases, it may be used as an adjunct in therapeutic regimens including benzoyl peroxide gels, antibiotics, retinoic acid products and sulfur/salicylic acid-containing preparations. The improvement of the treated condition is dependent on the degree and type of acne, the frequency of use of DESQUAM-X WASH and the nature of other therapies employed.

Contraindications: This product should not be used in patients known to be sensitive to benzoyl peroxide or any of the other listed ingredients.

Precautions: General: Avoid contact with eyes and other mucous membranes. For external use only. In patients known to be sensitive to the following substances, there is a possibility of cross-sensitization: benzoic acid derivatives (including certain topical anesthetics) and cinnamon.

Information for Patients: This product may bleach colored fabric or hair. Concurrent use with PABA-containing sunscreens may result in transient discoloration of the skin.

Carcinogenesis, Mutagenesis, Impairment of Fertility: No data are available concerning potential carcinogenic, teratogenic or reproductive effects of benzoyl peroxide. DESQUAM-X WASH has been shown to lack mutagenic potential in the Ames Salmonella test.

Pregnancy (Category C): Animal reproduction studies have not been conducted with benzoyl peroxide (DESQUAM-X WASH). It is also not known whether benzoyl peroxide (DESQUAM-X WASH) can cause fetal harm when administered to a pregnant woman or can affect reproductive capacity. Benzoyl peroxide (DESQUAM-X WASH) should be given to a pregnant woman only if clearly needed.

Nursing Mothers: It is not known whether this drug is excreted in human milk. Caution should be exercised when benzoyl peroxide is administered to a nursing woman.

Pediatric Use: Safety and effectiveness in children below the age of 12 have not been established.

Adverse Reactions: Adverse reactions which may be encountered with topical benzoyl peroxide include excessive drying (manifested by marked peeling, erythema and possible edema), and allergic contact sensitization. Excessive dryness would appear to occur in approximately 2 patients in 50.

Pertinent literature would seem to indicate that allergic sensitization to benzoyl peroxide may occur in 10 to 25 patients in 1,000.[7,8,9] There is one reference that reports an occurrence of sensitization in 5 of 100 patients.[10]

Overdosage: In the event that excessive scaling, erythema or edema occur, the use of this preparation should be discontinued. If the reaction is judged to be due to excessive use and not allergenicity, after symptoms and signs subside, a reduced dosage schedule may be cautiously tried.

To hasten resolution of the adverse effects, emollients, cool compresses and/or topical corticosteroid preparations may be used.

Dosage and Administration: Shake well before use. Wash with DESQUAM-X WASH once or twice daily, avoiding contact with eyes or other mucous membranes. Wet skin areas to be treated prior to administration; apply DESQUAM-X WASH, work to a full lather, rinse thoroughly and pat dry. Drying and peeling may be modified by adjusting the dosage schedule.

How Supplied: 5 oz. (141.8 g) (NDC 0072-6900-05; NSN 6505-01-113-2627) plastic bottle. Store below 77° F. Protect from freezing.

References:

1. Kligman AM, Leyden JJ, Stewart R: New uses for benzoyl peroxide: A broad spectrum antimicrobial agent. *Int J Derm* 16: 413–417, 1977.
2. Leyden JJ, Stewart R, Kligman AM: Updated *in vivo* methods for evaluating topical antimicrobial agents on human skin. *J Invest Dermatol* 72: 165–170, 1979.
3. Fulton JE, Farzad-Bakshandeh A, Bradley S: Studies on the mechanism of action of topical benzoyl peroxide and vitamin-A acid in acne vulgaris. *J Cut Path* 1: 191–200, 1974.
4. Fanta D, Jurecka W: Autoradiographic investigation on benzoyl peroxide treated skin. *Acta Dermatovener* 58: 361–362, 1978.
5. Fanta D, Muller MM: Effect of benzoyl peroxide on skin surface lipids. *Dermatologica* 158: 55–59, 1979.
6. Nacht S, Yeung D, Beasley J, Anjo M, Maibach HI: Benzoyl peroxide *in vitro* and *in vivo* skin penetration and metabolic disposition. Presented to Soc for Invest Derm, June 9–14, 1979, Amsterdam.
7. Eaglstein WH: Allergic contact dermatitis to benzoyl peroxide. *Arch Dermatol* 97: 527, 1968.

8. Pace WE: A benzoyl peroxide-sulfur cream for acne vulgaris. *Canad Med Assoc J* 93: 252–253, 1965.
9. Vasarinsh P: Benzoyl peroxide-sulfur lotions in acne vulgaris—a controlled study. *Cutis* 5(1): 65–69, 1969.
10. Fanta D: Clinical and experimental studies with benzoyl peroxide in the treatment of acne. *Hautzart* 29: 481–486, 1978.

DESQUAM-X® 10 WASH ℞

(10% benzoyl peroxide)

Caution: Federal law prohibits dispensing without prescription.

Description: DESQUAM-X WASH (10%) is a topical therapeutic anti-acne cleanser containing benzoyl peroxide (10%) in a lathering water base of sodium octoxynol-3 sulfonate, dioctyl sodium sulfosuccinate, magnesium aluminum silicate, methylcellulose and EDTA.

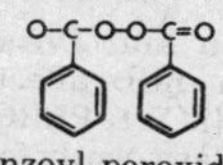

benzoyl peroxide

Clinical Pharmacology: The effectiveness of benzoyl peroxide in the treatment of acne vulgaris is primarily attributable to its antibacterial activity, especially with respect to *Propionibacterium acnes,* the predominant organism in sebaceous follicles and comedones.[1,2] The antibacterial activity of this compound is presumably due to the release of active or free-radical oxygen capable of oxidizing bacterial proteins.[3] In acne patients treated topically with benzoyl peroxide, resolution of the acne usually coincides with reduction in the levels of *P. acnes* and free fatty acids (FFA). Mild desquamation is another observed action of topically applied benzoyl peroxide and may also play a role in the drug's effectiveness in acne.[3] Studies also indicate that topical benzoyl peroxide may exert a sebostatic effect with a resultant reduction of skin surface lipids.[4,5] Benzoyl peroxide has been shown to be absorbed in the skin, where it is metabolized to benzoic acid and then excreted as benzoate in the urine.[6]

Indications and Usage: DESQUAM-X WASH (10%) is indicated for the topical treatment of mild to moderate acne. In more severe cases, it may be used as an adjunct in therapeutic regimens including benzoyl peroxide gels, antibiotics, retinoic acid products and sulfur/salicylic acid-containing preparations. The improvement of the treated condition is dependent on the degree and type of acne, the frequency of use of DESQUAM-X WASH and the nature of other therapies employed.

Contraindications: This product should not be used in patients known to be sensitive to benzoyl peroxide or any other of the listed ingredients.

Precautions: *General:* Avoid contact with eyes and other mucous membranes. For external use only. In patients known to be sensitive to the following substances, there is a possibility of cross-sensitization: benzoic acid derivatives (including certain topical anesthetics) and cinnamon.

Information for Patients: This product may bleach colored fabric or hair. Concurrent use with PABA-containing sunscreens may result in transient discoloration of the skin.

Carcinogenesis, Mutagenesis, Impairment of Fertility: Based upon considerable evidence, benzoyl peroxide is not considered to be a carcinogen. However, in one study, using mice known to be highly susceptible to cancer, there was evidence for benzoyl peroxide as a tumor promoter. Benzoyl peroxide has been found to be inactive as a mutagen in the *Ames Salmonella* and other assays, including the mouse dominant lethal assay. This assay is frequently used to assess the effect of substances on spermatogenesis.

Pregnancy (Category C): Animal reproduction studies have not been conducted with benzoyl peroxide (DESQUAM-X WASH). It is also not known whether benzoyl peroxide can cause fetal harm when administered to a pregnant woman or can affect reproductive capacity. Benzoyl peroxide should be given to a pregnant woman only if clearly needed.

Nursing Mothers: It is not known whether this drug is excreted in human milk. Caution should be exercised when benzoyl peroxide is administered to a nursing woman.

Pediatric Use: Safety and effectiveness in children below the age of 12 have not been established.

Adverse Reactions: Adverse reactions which may be encountered with topical benzoyl peroxide include excessive drying (manifested by marked peeling, erythema and possible edema), and allergic contact sensitization. Excessive dryness would appear to occur in approximately 2 patients in 50.

Pertinent literature would seem to indicate that allergic sensitization to benzoyl peroxide may occur in 10 to 25 patients in 1,000.[7,8,9] There is one reference that reports an occurrence of sensitization in 5 of 100 patients.[10]

Overdosage: In the event that excessive scaling, erythema or edema occur, the use of this preparation should be discontinued. If the reaction is judged to be due to excessive use and not allergenicity, after symptoms and signs subside, a reduced dosage schedule may be cautiously tried.

To hasten resolution of the adverse effects, emollients, cool compresses and/or topical corticosteroid preparations may be used.

Dosage and Administration: Shake well before use. Wash affected areas once or twice daily, avoiding contact with eyes or mucous membranes. Wet skin areas to be treated prior to administration; apply DESQUAM-X WASH (10%), work to a full lather, rinse thoroughly and pat dry. The amount of drying or peeling may be controlled by modification of dose frequency or drug concentration.

How Supplied: Desquam-X Wash (10%): 5 oz. plastic bottle, NDC 0072-7000-05.

Store at controlled room temperature (59°-86°F; 15°-30°C).

References:

1. Kligman AM, Leyden JJ, Stewart R: New uses for benzoyl peroxide: A broad-spectrum antimicrobial agent. *Int J Derm* 16: 413–417, 1977.
2. Leyden JJ, Stewart R, Kligman AM: Updated *in vivo* methods for evaluating topical antimicrobial agents on human skin. *J Invest Dermatol* 72:165–170, 1979.
3. Fulton JE, Farzad-Bakshandeh A, Bradley S: Studies on the mechanism of action of topical benzoyl peroxide and vitamin-A acid in acne vulgaris. *J Cut Path* 1:191–200, 1974.
4. Fanta D, Jurecka W: Autoradiographic investigation on benzoyl peroxide treated skin. *Acta Dermatovener* 58: 361–362, 1978.
5. Fanta D, Muller MM: Effect of benzoyl peroxide on skin surface lipids. *Dermatologica* 158:55–59, 1979.
6. Nacht S, Yeung D, Beasley J, Anjo M, Maibach HI: Benzoyl peroxide *in vitro* and *in vivo* skin penetration and metabolic disposition. Presented to Soc for Invest Derm, June 9-14, 1979. Amsterdam.
7. Eaglstein WH: Allergic contact dermatitis to benzoyl peroxide. *Arch Dermatol* 97:527, 1968.
8. Pace WE: A benzoyl peroxide-sulfur cream for acne vulgaris. *Canad Med Assoc J* 93:252–253, 1965.
9. Vasarinsh P: Benzoyl peroxide-sulfur lotions in acne vulgaris—a controlled study. *Cutis* 5(1):65–69, 1969.
10. Fanta D: Clinical and experimental studies with benzoyl peroxide in the treatment of acne. *Hautzart* 29:481–486, 1978.

ESTAR®

Therapeutic Tar Gel

Composition: Westwood® Tar (biologically equivalent to 5% Coal Tar USP) in a hydroalcoholic gel (13.8% alcohol).

Actions and Uses: A therapeutic aid in the treatment of eczema, psoriasis, and other tar-responsive dermatoses such as atopic dermatitis, lichen simplex chronicus, and nummular eczema. ESTAR exerts keratoplastic, antieczematous, and antipruritic actions. It is equivalent in its photodynamic activity to 5% crude coal tar in either hydrophilic ointment or petrolatum. ESTAR provides the characteristic benefits of tar therapy in a form that is readily accepted by patients and nursing staff, due to its negligible tar odor and staining potential, and the superior cosmetic qualities of its gel base. ESTAR is suitable for use in a modified Goeckerman regimen, either in the hospital or on an outpatient basis; it also can be used in follow-up treatment to help maintain remissions. Substantivity to the skin can be demonstrated by examination with a Wood's light, which shows residual microfine particles of tar on the skin several days after application.

Contraindications: ESTAR should not be applied to acutely inflamed skin or used by individuals who are known to be sensitive to coal tar.

Administration and Dosage:

Psoriasis: ESTAR can be applied at bedtime in the following manner: the patient should massage ESTAR into affected areas, allowing the gel to remain for five minutes, and then remove excess by patting with tissues. This procedure minimizes staining of skin and clothing, leaving behind an almost invisible layer of the active tar. If any staining of fabric should occur, it can be removed easily by standard laundry procedures.

The same technique of application may be used the following morning. If dryness occurs, an emollient may be applied one hour after ESTAR.

Because of ESTAR's superior substantivity and cosmetic qualities, patients who might otherwise be hospitalized for tar/UV therapy can now be treated as outpatients. The patient can easily apply ESTAR at bedtime and the following morning, then report for UV treatment that day. Laboratory tests and clinical experience to date suggest that it may be advisable to carefully regulate the length of UV exposure.

Chronic atopic dermatitis, lichen simplex chronicus, nummular eczema, and seborrheic dermatitis: One or two applications per day, as described above, are suggested. If dryness occurs, an emollient may be applied one hour after ESTAR and between applications as needed.

Caution: PROTECT TREATED AREAS FROM DIRECT SUNLIGHT, FOR AT LEAST 24 HOURS AFTER APPLICATION, UNLESS DIRECTED BY A PHYSICIAN. AVOID USE ON INFECTED, HIGHLY INFLAMED OR BROKEN SKIN. DO NOT APPLY TO GENITAL AREA. If used on the scalp, temporary discoloration of blond, bleached, or tinted hair may occur. If undue irritation develops or increases, the usage schedule should be changed or ESTAR discontinued. Contact with the eyes should be avoided. In case of contact, flush eyes with water.

Slight staining of clothing may occur. Standard laundry procedures will usually remove stains. For external use only.

How Supplied: 3 oz. (NDC 0072-7603-03; NSN 6505-01-056-2916) plastic tube.

Continued on next page

Westwood—Cont.

EURAX® CREAM/EURAX LOTION ℞
Crotamiton USP

Antipruritic/Scabicide

Description: EURAX provides 10% crotamiton, N-ethyl-o-crotonotoluidide, in a vanishing-cream or emollient-lotion base containing: glyceryl monostearate, anhydrous lanolin, PEG 6-32, glycerin, polysorbate 80, water, methyl and propylparabens, fragrance, and oxyquinoline sulfate. In addition, the cream contains mineral oil and white wax; the lotion, light mineral oil and carboxymethylcellulose sodium.
Actions: EURAX has scabicidal and antipruritic actions. The mechanisms of these actions are not known.
Indications: For eradication of scabies (*Sarcoptes scabiei*) and for symptomatic treatment of pruritic skin.
Contraindications: EURAX should not be administered to patients who are allergic to it or who manifest a primary irritation response.
Warnings and Precautions: EURAX should not be applied to acutely inflamed skin, raw, weeping surfaces, or in the eyes or mouth. Its use should be deferred until acute inflammation has subsided. If severe irritation or sensitization develops, treatment with this product should be discontinued and appropriate therapy instituted.
Adverse Reactions: Allergic sensitivity or primary irritation may occur in some patients.
Dosage and Administration: *In Scabies:* Thoroughly massage into the skin of the whole body from the chin down, paying particular attention to all folds and creases. A second application is advisable 24 hours later. Clothing and bed linen should be changed the next morning. A cleansing bath should be taken 48 hours after the last application.
In Pruritus: Massage gently into affected areas until medication is completely absorbed. Repeat as needed.
How Supplied:
Cream: 60 g (NDC 0072-2100-60; NSN 6505-00-116-0200) collapsible aluminum tubes.
Lotion: 60 g (NDC 0072-2200-60) and 454 g (NDC 0072-2200-16) amber glass bottles.

FOSTEX® MEDICATED CLEANSING BAR
Acne Skin Cleanser

Composition: Contains 2% sulfur, 2% salicylic acid, plus a combination of soapless cleansers and wetting agents.
Action and Uses: FOSTEX MEDICATED CLEANSING BAR is a surface-active, penetrating anti-seborrheic cleanser for therapeutic washing of the skin in the local treatment of acne and other skin conditions characterized by excessive oiliness. Degreases, dries and mildly desquamates.
Administration and Dosage: Use FOSTEX MEDICATED CLEANSING BAR instead of soap. Wash entire affected area 2 or 3 times daily, or as physician directs. Rinse well. The desired degree of dryness and peeling may be obtained by regulating frequency of use.
Caution: Avoid contact with eyes. In case of contact, flush with water. If undue skin irritation develops or increases, discontinue use and consult physician. For external use only.
How Supplied: 3¾ oz. (NDC 0072-3000-01; NSN 6505-00-116-1315) bar.

FOSTEX® MEDICATED CLEANSING CREAM
Acne Skin Cleanser and Dandruff Shampoo

Composition: Contains 2% sulfur, 2% salicylic acid, plus a combination of soapless cleansers and wetting agents.
Action and Uses: A penetrating antiseborrheic cleanser for the local treatment of acne, dandruff and other seborrheic skin conditions, characterized by excessive oiliness. Degreases, dries and mildly desquamates.
Administration and Dosage: AS A WASH: Wet skin; wash entire affected area with FOSTEX MEDICATED CLEANSING CREAM instead of soap. Rinse thoroughly. Use 2 or 3 times daily or as physician directs. The desired degree of dryness and peeling may be obtained by regulating frequency of use.
AS A SHAMPOO: Use liberal amount on wet scalp and hair. Shampoo thoroughly, rinse, and repeat shampoo. Rinse thoroughly. No other shampoos are required. To help keep scalp free from excessive oiliness or scaling, use FOSTEX MEDICATED CLEANSING CREAM as often as necessary or as physician directs.
Caution: Avoid contact with eyes. In case of contact, flush with water. If undue skin irritation develops or increases, discontinue use and consult physician. For external use only.
How Supplied: FOSTEX CREAM in 4 oz. (NDC 0072-3200-01; NSN 6505-01-030-9067) tube.

FOSTEX® 5% BENZOYL PEROXIDE GEL
Antibacterial Acne Gel

Composition: Contains 5% benzoyl peroxide.
Action and Uses: FOSTEX 5% BENZOYL PEROXIDE GEL is a penetrating, disappearing gel which helps kill bacteria that can cause acne. Helps prevent new pimples before they appear. Drying action promotes gentle peeling to help clear acne skin.
Indications: A topical aid for the control of acne vulgaria.
Administration and Dosage: After washing, rub FOSTEX 5% BPO into affected areas twice daily. In fair-skinned individuals or in excessively dry climates start with only one application daily. The desired degree of dryness and peeling may be obtained by regulating frequency of use.
Caution: Avoid contact with eyes, lips and mucous membranes. In case of contact, flush with water. Persons with very sensitive skin or a known allergy to benzoyl peroxide should not use this medication. If itching, redness, burning or swelling occurs, discontinue use. For external use only. May bleach dyed fabrics. Keep this and all drugs out of the reach of children. Store at controlled room temperature (59°-86°F).
How Supplied: 1.5 oz (NDC 0072-3300-02) plastic tube.

FOSTEX 10% BENZOYL PEROXIDE CLEANSING BAR
Antibacterial Acne Cleanser

Composition: 10% Benzoyl peroxide.
Action and Uses: FOSTEX 10% BENZOYL PEROXIDE CLEANSING BAR helps kill bacteria that can cause acne. Helps prevent new pimples before they appear. Drying action promotes gentle peeling to help clear your skin.
Indications: A topical aid for the control of acne vulgaris.
Administration and Dosage: Use FOSTEX 10% BENZOYL PEROXIDE CLEANSING BAR instead of soap. For best results, wash entire affected area gently with fingertips for 1 to 2 minutes, 2 to 3 times daily, or as physician directs. Rinse well. The desired degree of dryness and peeling may be obtained by regulating frequency of use.
Caution: Avoid contact with eyes, lips and mucous membranes. In case of contact, flush with water. Persons with very sensitive skin or a known allergy to benzoyl peroxide should not use this medication. If itching, redness, burning or swelling occurs, discontinue use. If symptoms persist, consult a physician. For external use only. May bleach hair and dyed fabrics. Store at controlled room temperature (59°-86°F).
How Supplied: 3 ¾ oz. (NDC 0072-2900-03) bar.

FOSTEX 10% BENZOYL PEROXIDE WASH
Antibacterial Acne Wash

Composition: 10% Benzoyl peroxide.
Action and Uses: FOSTEX 10% BENZOYL PEROXIDE WASH helps kill bacteria that can cause acne. Helps prevent new pimples before they appear. Drying action promotes gentle peeling to help clear acne skin.
Indications: A topical aid for the control of acne vulgaris.
Administration and Dosage: Shake well. Wet skin; wash entire affected are with FOSTEX 10% BENZOYL PEROXIDE WASH instead of soap. Wash gently for 1 to 2 minutes, 2 to 3 times daily, or as physician directs. The desired degree of dryness and peeling may be obtained by regulating frequency of use.
Caution: Avoid contact with eyes, lips and mucous membranes. In case of contact, flush with water. Persons with very sensitive skin or a known allergy to benzoyl peroxide should not use this medication. If itching, redness, burning or swelling occurs, discontinue use. If symptoms persist, consult a physician. May bleach dyed fabrics. Store at controlled room temperature (59°-86°F).
How Supplied: 5 oz. (NDC 0072-3100-05) plastic bottles.

FOSTRIL®
Drying Lotion for Acne

Composition: Contains 2% sulfur, in a greaseless base with laureth-4.
Action and Uses: Promotes drying and peeling of the skin in the treatment of acne. Daily use of FOSTRIL should result in a desirable degree of dryness and peeling in about 7 days. FOSTRIL removes excess oil and follicular obstruction, helping to remove comedones. It also helps prevent epithelial closure of pores and formation of new lesions.
Administration and Dosage: A thin film is applied to affected areas once or twice daily, or as directed.
Caution: If undue skin irritation develops or increases, adjust usage schedule or discontinue use. Anti-inflammatory measures may be used if necessary. For external use only. Contact with eyes should be avoided. In case of contact, flush eyes thoroughly with water.
How Supplied: 1 oz. (NDC 0072-3800-01; NSN 6505-00-116-1159) tube.

HALOTEX® CREAM/SOLUTION ℞
(Haloprogin)
Antifungal Agent

Description: Haloprogin is 3-iodo-2-propynyl 2,4,5-trichlorophenyl ether.
HALOTEX cream provides 1% haloprogin in a water-dispersible, semi-solid cream base. Each gram contains 10 mg. haloprogin solubilized in polyethylene glycol 400, polyethylene glycol 4000, diethyl sebacate and polyvinylpyrrolidone.
HALOTEX solution provides 1% (10 mg. per ml.) haloprogin in a homogenous vehicle of diethyl sebacate and 75% alcohol.
Action: HALOTEX is a synthetic antifungal agent for the treatment of superficial fungal infections of the skin.
Indications: HALOTEX cream and solution are indicated for the topical treatment of tinea pedis, tinea cruris, tinea corporis and tinea

manuum due to infection with Trichophyton rubrum, Trichophyton tonsurans, Trichophyton mentagrophytes, Microsporum canis, and Epidermophyton floccosum. It is also useful in the topical treatment of tinea versicolor due to Malassezia furfur.

Contraindications: HALOTEX preparations are contraindicated in those individuals who have shown hypersensitivity to any of the components.

Warning: USAGE IN PREGNANCY - Safety for use in pregnancy has not been established.

Precautions: In case of sensitization or irritation due to HALOTEX cream or solution or any of the ingredients, treatment with these preparations should be discontinued and appropriate therapy instituted. If a patient shows no improvement after four weeks of treatment with HALOTEX cream or solution, the diagnosis should be redetermined. In mixed infections where bacteria or nonsusceptible fungi are present, supplementary systemic anti-infective therapy may be indicated.

For external use only: KEEP OUT OF EYES.

Adverse Reactions: Reactions reported include: (1) local irritation, burning sensation, vesicle formation, and (2) increased maceration, pruritus or exacerbation of pre-existing lesions.

Dosage and Administration: HALOTEX cream and solution should be applied liberally to the affected area twice daily for two to three weeks. Interdigital lesions may require up to four weeks of therapy.

How Supplied:

CREAM

15 g (NDC 0072-7130-15) and 30 g (NDC 0072-7130-02; NSN 6505-00-118-2318) collapsible aluminum tubes.

SOLUTION

10 ml (NDC 0072-7200-10; NSN 6505-00-118-2211) and 30 ml (NDC 0072-7200-30; NSN 6505-00-118-2308) polyethylene bottles with controlled drop tip.

KERALYT® GEL ℞

Salicylic Acid

Description: KERALYT is a gel for topical administration containing 6% salicylic acid in a vehicle composed of propylene glycol, alcohol (19.4%), hydroxypropylcellulose and water. Salicylic acid is the 2-hydroxy derivative of benzoic acid.

Clinical Pharmacology: Salicylic acid has been shown to produce desquamation of the horny layer of skin while not effecting qualitative or quantitative changes in the structure of the viable epidermis.[1,2] The mechanism of action has been attributed to a dissolution of intracellular cement substance.[3] In a study of the percutaneous absorption of salicylic acid from KERALYT GEL in four patients with extensive active psoriasis, Taylor and Halprin[4] showed that the peak serum salicylate levels never exceeded 5 mg/100 ml even though more than 60% of the applied salicylic acid was absorbed. Systemic toxic reactions are usually associated with much higher serum levels (30 to 40 mg/100 ml). Peak serum levels occurred within 5 hours of the topical application under occlusion. The sites were occluded for 10 hours over the entire body surface below the neck. Since salicylates are distributed in the extracellular space, patients with a contracted extracellular space due to dehydration or diuretics have higher salicylate levels than those with a normal extracellular space.[5] (See PRECAUTIONS.)

The major metabolites identified in the urine after topical administration are salicyluric acid (52%), salicylate glucuronides (42%) and free salicylic acid (6%).[4] The urinary metabolites after percutaneous absorption differ from those after oral salicylate administration; those derived from percutaneous absorption contain more salicylate glucuronides and less salicyluric and salicylic acid. Almost 95% of a single dose of salicylate is excreted within 24 hours of its entrance into the extracellular space.[5]

Fifty to eighty percent of salicylate is protein bound to albumin. Salicylates compete with the binding of several drugs and can modify the action of these drugs; by similar competitive mechanisms other drugs can influence the serum levels of salicylate.[5] (See PRECAUTIONS.)

Indications and Usage: For Dermatologic Use: KERALYT GEL is a topical aid in the removal of excessive keratin in hyperkeratotic skin disorders, including verrucae, and the various ichthyoses (vulgaris, sex-linked and lamellar), keratosis palmaris and plantaris, keratosis pilaris, pityriasis rubra pilaris, psoriasis (including body, scalp, palms and soles).

For Podiatric Use: KERALYT GEL is a topical aid in the removal of excessive keratin on dorsal and plantar hyperkeratotic lesions. KERALYT has been reported to be useful adjunctive therapy for verrucae plantares.

Contraindications: KERALYT GEL should not be used in any patient known to be sensitive to salicylic acid or any other listed ingredients. KERALYT should not be used in children under 2 years of age.

Warnings: Prolonged use over large areas, especially in children and those patients with significant renal or hepatic impairment, could result in salicylism. Concomitant use of other drugs which may contribute to elevated serum salicylate levels should be avoided where the potential for toxicity is present. In children under 12 years of age and those patients with renal or hepatic impairment, the area to be treated should be limited and the patient monitored closely for signs of salicylate toxicity: nausea, vomiting, dizziness, loss of hearing, tinnitus, lethargy, hyperpnea, diarrhea, psychic disturbances.

In the event of salicylic acid toxicity, the use of KERALYT GEL should be discontinued. Fluids should be administered to promote urinary excretion. Treatment with sodium bicarbonate (oral or intravenous) should be instituted as appropriate.

Precautions: For external use only. Avoid contact with eyes and other mucous membranes.

Drug Interactions: (The following interactions are from a published review[5] and include reports concerning both oral and topical salicylate administration. The relationship of these interactions to the use of KERALYT GEL is not known.)

I. Due to the competition of salicylate with other drugs for binding to serum albumin the following drug interactions may occur:

DRUG	DESCRIPTION OF INTERACTION
Tolbutamide	Hypoglycemia potentiated.
Methotrexate	Decreases tubular reabsorption; clinical toxicity from methotrexate can result.

II. Drugs changing salicylate levels by altering renal tubular reabsorption:

DRUG	DESCRIPTION
Corticosteroids	Decreases plasma salicylate level; tapering doses of steroids may promote salicylism
Ammonium Sulfate	Increases plasma salicylate level.

III. Drugs with Complicated Interactions with Salicylates

DRUG	DESCRIPTION
Heparin	Salicylate decreases platelet adhesiveness and interferes with hemostasis in heparin-treated patients.
Pyrazinamide	Inhibits pyrazinamide-induced hyperuricemia.
Uricosuric Agents	Effect of probenemide, sulfinpyrazone and phenylbutazone inhibited.

The following alterations of laboratory tests have been reported during salicylate therapy.[5]

LABORATORY TESTS	EFFECT OF SALICYLATES
Thyroid Function	Decreased PBI; increased T_3 uptake.
Urinary Sugar	False negative with glucose oxidase; false positive with Clinitest with high-dose salicylate therapy (2-5g q.d.).
5-Hydroxyindole acetic acid	False negative with fluorometric test.
Acetone, ketone bodies	False positive $FeCl_3$ in Gerhardt reaction; red color persists with boiling.
17-OH corticosteroids	False reduced values with >4.8g q.d. salicylate.
Vanilmandelic acid	False reduced values.
Uric acid	May increase or decrease depending on dose.
Prothrombin	Decreased levels; slightly increased prothrombin time.

Pregnancy (Category C): Salicylic acid has been shown to be teratogenic in rats and monkeys. It is difficult to extrapolate from oral doses of acetylsalicylic acid used in these studies to topical administration as the oral dose to monkeys may represent 6 times the maximal daily human dose of salicylic acid (as supplied in one tube, 28 g, of Keralyt) when applied topically over a large body surface. There are no adequate and well-controlled studies in pregnant women. KERALYT GEL should be used during pregnancy only if the potential benefit justifies the potential risk to the fetus.

Nursing Mothers: Because of the potential for serious adverse reactions in nursing infants from the mother's use of KERALYT GEL, a decision should be made whether to discontinue nursing or to discontinue the drug, taking into account the importance of the drug to the mother.

Carcinogenesis, Mutagenesis, Impairment of Fertility: No data are available concerning potential carcinogenic or reproductive effects of KERALYT GEL. It has been shown to lack mutagenic potential in the Ames Salmonella test.

Adverse Reactions: Excessive erythema and scaling conceivably could result from use on open skin lesions.

Overdosage: See **Warnings.**

Dosage and Administraton: The preferable method of use is to apply KERALYT GEL thoroughly to the affected area and occlude the area at night. Preferably, the skin should be hydrated for at least five minutes prior to application. The medication is washed off in the morning and if excessive drying and/or irritation is observed a bland cream or lotion may be applied. Once clearing is apparent, the occasional use of KERALYT GEL will usually maintain the remission. In those areas where occlusion is difficult or impossible, application may be made more frequently; hydration by wet packs or baths prior to application apparently enhances the effect. Unless hands are being treated, hands should be rinsed thoroughly after application.

How Supplied: 1 oz. (28.4g) (NDC 0072-6500-01; NSN 6505-01-546-7319) plastic tube.

References:

1. Davies M, Marks R: Studies on the effect of salicylic acid on normal skin. *Br J Dermatol* 95: 187–192, 1976.

Continued on next page

Westwood—Cont.

2. Marks R, Davies M, Cattel A: An explanation for the keratolytic effect of salicylic acid. *J Invest Dermatol* 64: 283, 1975.
3. Huber C, Christophers E: "Keratolytic" effect of salicyic acid. *Arch Derm Res* 257: 293–297, 1977.
4. Taylor JR, Halprin KM: Percutaneous absorption of salicylic acid. *Arch Dermatol* 111: 740–743, 1975.
5. Goldsmith LA: Salicylic acid. *Int J Dermatol* 18: 32–36, 1979.
6. Wilson JG, Ritter EJ, Scott WJ, Fradlein R: Comparative distribution and embryotoxicity of acetylsalicylic acid in pregnant rats and rhesus monkeys. *Tox Appl Pharmacol* 41: 67–78, 1977.

KERI® CREME
Concentrated Moisturizer—Nongreasy Emollient

Composition: Contains water, mineral oil, talc, sorbitol, ceresin, lanolin alcohol/mineral oil, magnesium stearate, glyceryl oleate/propylene glycol, isopropyl myristate, methylparaben, propylparaben, fragrance, quaternium-15.
Actions and Uses: KERI CREME is a concentrated moisturizer and nongreasy emollient for problem dry skin—hands, face, elbows, feet, legs. KERI CREME helps retain moisture that makes skin feel soft, smooth, supple. Helps resist the drying effects of soaps, detergents and chemicals.
Administration and Dosage: A small amount is rubbed into dry skin areas as needed.
How Supplied: 2.25 oz. (NDC 0072-5800-01) tube.

KERI® FACIAL SOAP
Non-detergent Facial Soap

Composition: KERI LOTION® concentrate in a gentle, non-detergent soap containing: sodium tallowate, sodium cocoate, water, mineral oil, octyl hydroxystearate, fragrance, glycerin, titanium dioxide, PEG-75, lanolin oil, sodium dioctyl sulfosuccinate, PEG-4 dilaurate, propylparaben, PEG-40 stearate, glyceryl monostrearate, PEG-100 stearate, sodium chloride, BHT, EDTA.
Action and Uses: KERI FACIAL SOAP helps keep skin soft while thoroughly cleansing.
Administration and Dosage: To be used as facial soap.
How Supplied: 3.25 oz. (NDC 0072-4900-03) bar.

KERI® LOTION
Skin Lubricant—Moisturizer

Composition: Contains mineral oil, water, propylene glycol, glyceryl stearate/ PEG-100 stearate, PEG-40 stearate, PEG-4 dilaurate, laureth-4, lanolin oil, methylparaben, propylparaben, fragrance, carbomer-934, triethanolamine, dioctyl sodium sulfosuccinate, quaternium-15. Freshly-scented: FD&C blue 1, D&C yellow 10.
Action and Uses: KERI LOTION lubricates and helps hydrate the skin, making it soft and smooth. It relieves itching, helps maintain a normal moisture balance and supplements the protective action of skin lipids. Indicated for generalized dryness and itching; detergent hands; chapped or chafed skin; sunburn; "winter-itch"; aging, dry skin; diaper rash; heat rash.
Administration and Dosage: Apply as often as needed. Use particularly after bathing and exposure to sun, water, soaps and detergents.
How Supplied: 6½ oz. (NDC 0072-4600-56; NSN 6505-01-009-2897), 13 oz. (NDC 0072-4600-63) and 20 oz. (NDC 0072-4600-70) plastic bottles. Also available as KERI LOTION FRESHLY SCENTED—6½ oz. (NDC 0072-4500-56), 13 oz. (NDC 0072-4500-63), and 20 oz. (NDC 0072-4500-70) plastic bottles.

LOWILA® CAKE
Soap-free Skin Cleanser

Composition: Contains dextrin, sodium α olefin (C_{14}-C_{16}) sulfonate, water, boric acid, urea, sorbitol, mineral oil, PEG-14 M, lactic acid, dioctyl sodium sulfosuccinate, cellulose gum, fragrance.
Action and Uses: LOWILA CAKE is indicated when soap should not be used, for cleansing skin that is sensitive or irritated, or in dermatitic and eczematous conditions. Used for general bathing, infant bathing, routine washing of hands and face and shampooing. The pH of LOWILA CAKE helps protect the skin's normal acid mantle and create an environment favorable to therapy and healing.
Administration and Dosage: LOWILA CAKE is used in place of soap. Lathers well in both hard and soft water.
How Supplied: 3¾ oz. (NDC 0072-2304-01) bar.

PERNOX®
Medicated Lathering Scrub Cleanser for Acne

Composition: Contains 2% Sulfur, 1.5% salicylic acid, plus a combination of soapless cleansers and wetting agents and abradant polyethylene granules.
Actions and Uses: A lathering scrub cleanser for acne, oily skin. PERNOX provides microfine, uniform-size scrub particles with a rounded surface area to enable patients to achieve effective and gentle desquamation as they wash their skin. PERNOX helps loosen and remove comedones, dries, peels and degreases acne skin. It lathers abundantly and leaves the skin feeling smooth.
Contraindications: Not indicated when acute inflammation is present or in nodular or cystic acne.
Administration and Dosage: After wetting the skin, PERNOX is applied with the fingertips and massaged onto the skin for about one-half to one minute. The skin is then thoroughly rinsed. May be used instead of soap one to two times daily, or as directed.
Caution: If undue skin irritation develops or increases, adjust usage schedule or discontinue use. If necessary, anti-inflammatory measures may be used after discontinuance. For external use only. Contact with eyes should be avoided. In case of contact, flush eyes thoroughly with water.
How Supplied: 2 oz. (NDC 0072-5200-02; NSN 6505-01-035-1719), and 4 oz. (NDC 0072-5200-04) tubes; lemon scented: 2 oz. (NDC 0072-5300-02), and 4 oz. (NDC 0072-5300-04) tubes.

PERNOX® LOTION
Lathering Scrub Cleanser for Acne

Composition: Contains 2% Sulfur, 1.5% salicylic acid, plus a combination of soapless cleansers and wetting agents and abradant polyethylene granules.
Actions and Uses: PERNOX LOTION is a therapeutic scrub cleanser in lotion form that is to be used routinely instead of soap. It gently desquamates or peels acne or oily skin. PERNOX LOTION also removes excessive oil from the skin surface and will produce mild drying of the affected skin areas when used regularly. It helps skin feel fresher and smoother with each wash.
Contraindications: Not indicated when acute inflammation is present or in nodular or cystic acne.
Administration and Dosage: To be shaken well before using. PERNOX may be used instead of soap one or two times daily or as directed. The skin should be wet first and PERNOX applied with the fingertips. The lather should be massaged into skin for one-half to one minute. The patient then rinses thoroughly and pats dry.
Caution: If undue skin irritation develops or increases, adjust usage schedule or discontinue use. For external use only. Contact with eyes should be avoided. In case of contact, flush eyes with water.
How Supplied: 5 oz. (NDC 0072-7900-05) plastic bottle.

PERNOX® SHAMPOO
For Oily Hair

Composition: A blend of biodegradable cleansers and hair conditioners, containing: sodium laureth sulfate, water, lauramide DEA, quaternium 22, PEG-75 lanolin/hydrolyzed animal protein, sodium chloride, fragrance, lactic acid, sorbic acid, disodium EDTA, FD&C yellow 6, FD&C blue 1.
Actions and Uses: A gentle but thorough shampoo especially formulated to cleanse, control and condition oily hair. Especially suitable for adjunctive use with acne patients. PERNOX SHAMPOO works into a rich, pleasant lather, leaves the hair lustrous and manageable. Its special conditioners help prevent tangles and fly away hair. Gentle enough to be used every day. It contains a refreshing natural scent.
Administration and Dosage: A liberal amount is massaged into wet hair and scalp. A good lather is worked up, massaging thoroughly. This is followed by a rinse and repeat application. A final rinse is used. No other shampoos or hair conditioners are necessary. May be used as needed.
Caution: For external use only. Contact with the eyes should be avoided. In case of contact, flush eyes with water.
How Supplied: 8 fl. oz. (NDC 0072-5500-08) shatterproof plastic bottle.

PRESUN® 4 CREAMY SUNSCREEN
Moderate Sunscreen Protection

Composition: Contains Octyl dimethyl PABA.
Action and Uses: PRESUN 4 CREAMY, a water-resistant, non-staining moisturizing formula, provides 4 times an individual's natural protection. Liberal and regular use may help reduce the chance of premature aging of the skin and skin cancer from overexposure to the sun. PRESUN 4 CREAMY provides moderate protection, permits limited tanning while reducing the chance of sunburn. PRESUN 4 CREAMY maintains its degree of sunburn protection even after 40 minutes in the water.
Administration and Dosage: Shake well. Gently smooth liberal amount evenly onto **dry skin** before sun exposure. Do not rub in. Reapply to dry skin after prolonged swimming or excessive perspiration, or after towel drying. Repeated applications during prolonged sun exposure are recommended.
If used, cosmetics or emollients may be applied after PRESUN.
Warnings: For external use only. Do not use if sensitive to p-aminobenzoic acid (PABA), or related compounds (such as benzocaine, sulfonamides, aniline dyes, or PABA esters). Discontinue use if irritation or rash appears. Avoid contact with eyes. In case of contact, flush eyes with water. Keep out of the reach of children.
How Supplied: 4 oz. (NDC 0072-5904-04) plastic bottle.

PRESUN® 8; LOTION, CREAMY AND GEL
Maximal Sunscreen Protection

Composition: LOTION: Contains aminobenzoic acid (PABA), 55% (w/w) SD alcohol 40. CREAMY LOTION: Contains octyl dimethyl PABA,

oxybenzone. GEL: Contains aminobenzoic acid (PABA), 55% SD alcohol 40.
Action and Uses: PRESUN 8 provides 8 times an individual's natural protection. Liberal and regular use may reduce the chance of premature aging of the skin and skin cancer from overexposure to the sun. PRESUN 8 permits limited tanning and reduces the chance of sunburn. It gives maximum protection in the erythemogenic range, screening out the burning rays of the sun. CREAMY: A water-resistant, non-staining moisturizing formula which maintains its degree of sunburn protection even after 40 minutes in the water.
Warnings: For external use only. Do not use if sensitive to p-aminobenzoic acid (PABA), or related compounds (such as benzocaine, sulfanomides, aniline dyes, or PABA esters). Discontinue use if irritation or rash appears. Avoid contact with eyes. In case of contact, flush eyes with water. Keep out of the reach of children. LOTION: Avoid flame. Avoid contact with fabric or other materials as staining may result.
Administration and Dosage: Apply liberally and evenly to **dry skin,** let dry before dressing. CREAMY: Do not rub in. Reapply after swimming or excessive perspiration, or after towel drying. Repeated applications during prolonged sun exposure are recommended. If used, cosmetics or emollients may be applied after PRESUN.
How Supplied: Lotion: 4 fl. oz. (NDC 0072-5400-04; NSN 6505-01-037-8636) and 7 fl. oz. (NDC 0072-5400-07) plastic bottles. Creamy Lotion: 4 oz. (NDC 0072-8404-04) plastic bottle. Gel: 3 oz. (NDC 0072-7700-03) plastic tube.

PRESUN® 15 SUNSCREEN LOTION
Ultra Sunscreen Protection

Composition: Aminobenzoic acid (PABA), octyl dimethyl PABA, oxybenzone, 58% SD alcohol 40.
Actions and Uses: PRESUN 15, a clear PABA formula, provides 15 times an individual's natural protection. Liberal and regular use may reduce the chance of premature aging of the skin and skin cancer from overexposure to the sun. PRESUN 15 provides the highest degree of sunburn protection.
Administration and Dosage: Shake well. Apply liberally and evenly to **dry skin** before exposure; let dry before dressing. Reapply to dry skin after swimming or excessive perspiration, or after towel drying. Repeated applications during prolonged exposure ae recommended. If used, cosmetics or emollients may be applied after PRESUN.
Warnings: For external use only. Do not use if sensitive to p-aminobenzoic acid (PABA), or related compounds (such as benzocaine, sulfonamides, aniline dyes or PABA esters). Discontinue use if irritation or rash appars. Transient facial stinging may occur in hot, humid weather. Avoid contact with eyes. In case of contact, flush eyes with water. Avoid flame. Avoid contact with fabric or other materials as staining may result. Keep out of the reach of children.
How Supplied: 4 oz. (NDC 0072-8800-04) plastic bottle.

PRESUN®15 CREAMY SUNSCREEN
Ultra Sunscreen Protection

Composition: Octyl dimethyl PABA, oxybenzone.
Action and Uses: PRESUN 15 CREAMY, a water-resistant, non-staining moisturizing formula, provides 15 times an individual's natural protection. Liberal and regular use may help reduce the chance of premature aging of the skin and skin cancer from overexposure to the sun. PRESUN 15 CREAMY permits limited tanning while reducing the chance of sunburn. PRESUN 15 CREAMY maintains its degree of protection even after 40 minutes in the water.
Administration and Dosage: Shake well. Gently smooth liberal amount evenly onto **dry skin** before sun exposure. Do not rub in. Reapply to dry skin after prolonged swimming or excessive perspiration, or after towel drying. Repeated applications during prolonged sun exposure are recommended.
Warnings: For external use only. Do not use if sensitive to p-aminobenzoic acid (PABA), or related compounds (such as benzocaine, sulfonamides, aniline dyes, or PABA esters). Discontinue use if irritation or rash appears. Avoid contact with eyes. In case of contact, flush eyes with water. Keep out of the reach of children.
How Supplied: 4 oz. (NDC 0072-8904-04) plastic bottle.

SEBUCARE®
Antiseborrheic Scalp Lotion

Contains: 1.8% Salicylic acid, 61% alcohol, water, PPG-40 butyl ether, laureth-4, dihydroabietyl alcohol, fragrance.
Action and Uses: An aid in the treatment of dandruff, seborrhea capitis and other scaling conditions of the scalp. SEBUCARE helps control scaling, oiliness and itching. The unique base helps soften brittle hair and grooms the hair, thus eliminating the need for hair dressing which often impedes antiseborrheic treatment. SEBUCARE should be used every day in conjunction with therapeutic shampoos such as SEBULEX® or FOSTEX® CREAM.
Administration and Dosage: SEBUCARE is applied directly to scalp and massaged thoroughly with fingertips. Comb or brush as usual. Grooms as it medicates. Use once or twice daily or as directed..
Precaution: Volatile—Flame should be avoided. Contact with eyes should be avoided. In case of contact, flush eyes thoroughly with water. For external use only.
How Supplied: 4 fl. oz. (NDC 0072-4800-04) plastic bottle.

SEBULEX® and SEBULEX® CREAM
Antiseborrheic Treatment Shampoo

Composition: Contains 2% sulfur and 2% salicylic acid in SEBULYTIC® brand of surface-active cleansers and wetting agents.
Action and Uses: A penetrating therapeutic shampoo for the temporary relief of itchy scalp and the scaling of dandruff, SEBULEX helps relieve itching, remove dandruff, excess oil. It penetrates and softens the crusty, matted layers of scales adhering to the scalp, and leaves the hair soft and manageable.
Administration and Dosage: SEBULEX liquid should be shaken before being used. SEBULEX or SEBULEX CREAM is massaged into wet scalp. Lather should be allowed to remain on scalp for about 5 minutes and then rinsed. Application is repeated, followed by a thorough rinse. Initially, SEBULEX or SEBULEX CREAM can be used daily, or every other day, or as directed, depending on the condition. Once symptoms are under control, one or two treatments a week usually will maintain control of itching, oiliness and scaling.
Caution: If undue skin irritation develops or increases, discontinue use. For external use only. Contact with eyes should be avoided. In case of contact, flush eyes thoroughly with water.
How Supplied: SEBULEX in 4 oz. (NDC 0072-2700-04) and 8 oz. (NDC 0072-2700-08) plastic bottles. SEBULEX CREAM in 4 oz. (NDC 0072-2800-04) plastic tube.

SEBULEX® CONDITIONING SHAMPOO WITH PROTEIN
Antiseborrheic Treatment and Conditioning Shampoo

Composition: Contains 2% sulfur, 2% salicylic acid, water, sodium octoxynol-3 sulfonate, sodium lauryl sulfate, lauramide DEA, acetamide MEA, amphoteric-2, hydrolyzed animal protein, magnesium aluminum silicate, propylene glycol, methylcellulose, PEG-14 M, fragrance, disodium EDTA, dioctyl sodium sulfosuccinate, FD & C blue 1, D & C yellow 10.
Action and Uses: SEBULEX CONDITIONING SHAMPOO provides effective temporary control of the scaling and itching of dandruff and seborrheic dermatitis, while adding protein to the hair shaft to increase its manageability.
Administration and Dosage: SEBULEX CONDITIONING SHAMPOO should be shaken well before use. Shampoo five minutes. For optimum dandruff control and conditioning leave lather on scalp for the full five minutes. Rinse. Repeat. Use two to three times weekly to maintain control, although daily use may be continued. Consult physician for severe or unresponsive scalp conditions.
Caution: If undue skin irritation develops or increases, use should be discontinued. Contact with eyes should be avoided. In cases of contact, eyes should be flushed thoroughly with water.
How Supplied: 4 oz. (NDC 0072-2600-04) and 8 oz. (NDC 0072-2600-08) plastic bottles.

SEBUTONE® and SEBUTONE® CREAM
Antiseborrheic Tar Shampoo

Composition: WESTWOOD® TAR (equivalent to 0.5% Coal Tar USP), 2% sulfur and 2% salicylic acid in SEBULYTIC® brand of surface-active cleansers and wetting agents.
Action and Uses: A surface-active, penetrating therapeutic shampoo for the temporary relief of itchy scalp and the scaling of stubborn dandruff and psoriasis. Provides prompt and prolonged relief of itching, helps control oiliness and rid the scalp of scales and crust. Tar ingredient is chemically and biologically standardized to produce uniform therapeutic activity. Wood's light demonstrates residual microfine particles of tar on the scalp several days after a course of SEBUTONE shampoo. In addition to its antipruritic and antiseborrheic actions, SEBUTONE also helps offset excessive scalp dryness with a special moisturizing emollient.
Administration and Dosage: SEBUTONE liquid should be shaken before being used. A liberal amount of SEBUTONE or SEBUTONE CREAM is massaged into the wet scalp for 5 minutes and the scalp is then rinsed. Application is repeated, followed by a thorough rinse. Use as often as necessary to keep the scalp free from itching and scaling or as directed. No other shampoo or soap washings are required.
Caution: If undue skin irritation develops or increases, discontinue use. In rare instances, temporary discoloration of white, blond, bleached or tinted hair may occur. Contact with the eyes is to be avoided. In case of contact flush eyes with water.
How Supplied: SEBUTONE in 4 oz. (NDC 0072-5000-04) and 8 oz. (NDC 0072-5000-08) plastic bottles.
SEBUTONE CREAM in 4 oz. (NDC 0072-5100-01) tubes.

STATICIN® (ERYTHROMYCIN) 1.5% TOPICAL SOLUTION ℞

Description: STATICIN (erythromycin) 1.5% Topical Solution contains 15 mg/ml erythromycin base in a clear solution vehicle of 55% alcohol, propylene glycol, laureth-4 and fragrance.

Continued on next page

Westwood—Cont.

Actions: Although the mechanism by which STATICIN acts in reducing inflammatory lesions of acne vulgaris is unknown, it is presumably due to its antibiotic action.
Indications: STATICIN is indicated for the topical control of acne vulgaris.
Contraindications: STATICIN is contraindicated in persons who have shown hypersensitivity to erythromycin or any of the other listed ingredients.
Warning: The safe use of STATICIN during pregnancy or lactation has not been established.
Precautions: STATICIN is recommended for external use only and should be kept away from the eyes, nose, mouth and other mucous membranes. Concomitant topical acne therapy should be used with caution because a cumulative irritancy effect may occur, especially with the use of peeling, desquamating or abrasive agents.
The use of antibiotic agents may be associated with the overgrowth of antibiotic-resistant organisms. If this occurs, administration of this drug should be discontinued and appropriate measures taken.
Adverse Reactions: Adverse conditions experienced included erythema, desquamation, tenderness, dryness, pruritus and oiliness. Of a total of 193 patients exposed to the drug during clinical effectiveness trials, 155 experienced some type of adverse effect, with approximately half of the patients treated experiencing local drying of the treated areas. There was one case of a generalized urticarial reaction, possibly related to the drug, which required the use of systemic steroid therapy.
Dosage and Administration: STATICIN should be applied each morning and evening to areas usually affected by acne. These areas first should be washed, rinsed well, and patted dry. STATICIN should be applied with the fingertips and the hands washed after application. If applicator is used, apply STATICIN to the affected areas with a dabbing motion.
How Supplied: 60 ml (NDC 0072-8000-60) plastic bottle with optional applicator.
Store at controlled room temperature or lower.
U.S. Pat. 4,000,263.

TACARYL Tablets and Syrup (Methdilazine HCl) ℞
TACARYL Chewable Tablets (Methdilazine) ℞

Description: TACARYL, available as methdilazine or methdilazine HCl, a phenothiazine derivative, is 10- (1-methyl-3-pyrrolidinyl) methyl phenothiazine.
Actions: TACARYL and TACARYL HCl are phenothiazine derivatives, possessing antipruritic and antihistaminic properties with anticholinergic (drying) and sedative side effects.
Indication: TACARYL and TACARYL HCl are indicated for the symptomatic relief of pruritic symptoms in urticaria.
Contraindications: TACARYL is contraindicated in comatose states, in patients who have received large amounts of central nervous system depressants (alcohol, barbiturates, narcotics, etc.). It is contraindicated in patients who have bone marrow depression, jaundice, or in those who have demonstrated an idiosyncrasy or hypersensitivity to TACARYL or other phenothiazines. This drug is contraindicated in newborn or premature infants. Further, it should not be used in children acutely ill and dehydrated, as there may be an increased susceptibility to dystonias. Because of the higher risk of drugs of this type for infants generally and prematures in particular, TACARYL is contraindicated in nursing mothers.
Warnings: TACARYL may impair the mental and/or physical ability required for the performance of potentially hazardous tasks, such as driving a vehicle or operating machinery. Similarly, it may impair mental alertness in children. The concomitant use of alcohol or other central nervous system depressants may have an additive effect. Patients should be warned accordingly. TACARYL should be used with extreme caution in patients with: asthmatic attack, narrow-angle glaucoma, prostatic hypertrophy, stenosing peptic ulcer, pyloroduodenal obstruction, bladder neck obstruction, as well as in patients receiving monoamine oxidase inhibitors.
Usage in Pregnancy: The safe use of TACARYL has not been established with respect to the possible adverse effects upon fetal development. Therefore, it is recommended that this medication be given to pregnant patients, or women of child-bearing potential, only when in the judgment of the physician the potential benefits outweigh the possible hazards. There are reports of jaundice and prolonged extrapyramidal symptoms in infants whose mothers received phenothiazines during pregnancy.
Use in Children: TACARYL should be used with caution, as administration in the young child may result in excitation. Overdosage may produce hallucinations, convulsions, and sudden death.
Use in the Elderly (60 Years or Older): The elderly are more prone to develop the following side effects from phenothiazines: hypotension; syncope; toxic confusional states; excessive sedation; extrapyramidal signs, especially parkinsonism; akathisia; persistent dyskinesia.
Precautions: TACARYL may significantly affect the actions of other drugs. It may increase, prolong or intensify the sedative action of central nervous system depressants such as anesthetics, barbiturates or alcohol. The dose of a narcotic or barbiturate may be reduced to ¼ or ½ the usual amount when TACARYL is administered concomitantly. Excessive amounts of TACARYL, relative to a narcotic, may lead to restlessness and motor hyperactivity in the patient with pain.
Phenothiazines may block and even reverse some of the actions of epinephrine.
TACARYL should be used cautiously in persons with acute or chronic respiratory impairment, particularly children. The cough reflex can be suppressed.
TACARYL should be used cautiously in persons with cardiovascular disease, impairment of liver function or those with a history of ulcer disease.
Adverse Reactions: This drug may produce adverse reactions common to both phenothiazines and antihistamines.
Note: Not all of the following adverse reactions have been reported with this specific drug; however, pharmacological similarities among the phenothiazine derivatives require that each be considered when TACARYL is administered. There have been occasional reports of sudden death in patients receiving phenothiazine derivatives chronically.
CNS: Drowsiness is the most prominent CNS effect of this drug. Extrapyramidal reactions occur, particularly with high doses. Hyperreflexia has been reported in the newborn when a phenothiazine was used during pregnancy. Other reported reactions include dizziness, lassitude, tinnitus, incoordination, fatigue, blurred vision, euphoria, diplopia, nervousness, insomnia, tremors and grand mal seizures; excitation, catatonic-like states, neuritis and hysteria.
Cardiovascular: Postural hypotension is the most common cardiovascular effect of the phenothiazines. Reflex tachycardia may be seen. Bradycardia, faintness, dizziness and cardiac arrest have been reported. ECG changes, including blunting of T waves and prolongation of the Q-T interval, may be seen.
Gastrointestinal: Anorexia, nausea, vomiting, epigastric distress, constipation and dry mouth may occur. Diarrhea has also been reported as well as increased appetite and weight gain.
Genitourinary: Urinary frequency and dysuria, urinary retention, early menses, induced lactation, gynecomastia, decreased libido, inhibition of ejaculation and false pregnancy tests have been reported.
Respiratory: Thickening of bronchial secretions, tightness of the chest, wheezing and nasal stuffiness may occur.
Allergic Reactions: These include urticaria, dermatitis, asthma, laryngeal edema, photosensitivity, lupus erythematosus-like syndrome and anaphylactoid reactions.
Other Reported Reactions: Leukopenia, agranulocytosis, elevation of plasma cholesterol levels, thrombocytopenic purpura and jaundice of the obstructive type have been reported. The jaundice is usually reversible, but chronic jaundice has been reported. High or prolonged glucose tolerance curves, glycosuria, elevated spinal fluid proteins may also occur.
Long-Term Therapy Considerations: After prolonged administration at high dosage, pigmentation of the skin has occurred, chiefly in the exposed areas. Ocular changes consist of the appearance of lenticular and corneal opacities, epithelial keratopathies and pigmentary retinopathy. Vision may be impaired.
Dosage and Administration:
TACARYL® Hydrochloride Tablets (methdilazine HCl)
Adults: 1 tablet (8 mg.) 2 to 4 times daily.
Children over 3 years: ½ tablet (4 mg.) 2 to 4 times daily.
TACARYL® Hydrochloride Syrup (methdilazine HCl)
Adults: 2 teaspoons (8 mg.) 2 to 4 times daily.
Children over 3 years: 1 teaspoon (4 mg.) 2 to 4 times daily.
TACARYL® Chewable Tablets (methdilazine)
Adults: 2 tablets (7.2 mg.) 2 to 4 times daily.
Children over 3 years: 1 tablet (3.6 mg.) 2 to 4 times daily.
This product form should be chewed and swallowed promptly.
The above doses should be considered maximal daily doses and every effort should be made to minimize side-effects and adverse reactions, through the use of the minimal effective dosage.
Drug Interactions: MAO inhibitors and thiazide diuretics prolong and intensify the anticholinergic effects of the phenothiazines. Combined use of MAO inhibitors and phenothiazines may result in hypotension and extrapyramidal reactions.
Narcotics: The CNS depressant and analgesic effects of narcotics are potentiated by phenothiazines.
The following drugs result in potentiation of phenothiazine effect: oral contraceptives, progesterone, reserpine, nylidrin hydrochloride.
Management of Overdosage: Signs and symptoms of overdosage range from mild depression of the central nervous system and cardiovascular system, to profound hypotension, respiratory depression and unconsciousness. Stimulation may be evident, especially in children and geriatric patients. Atropine-like signs and symptoms—dry mouth; fixed, dilated pupils; flushing; etc.—as well as gastrointestinal symptoms may occur. The treatment of overdosage is essentially symptomatic and supportive. Early gastric lavage may be beneficial. Centrally acting emetics are of little use. Avoid analeptics, which may cause convulsions. Severe hypotension usually responds to the administration of levarterenol or phenylephrine. EPINEPHRINE SHOULD NOT BE USED, since its use in the patient with partial adrenergic blockade may further lower the blood pressure. Additional measures include oxygen and intravenous fluids. Limited experience with dialysis indicates that it is not helpful.

How Supplied:
TACARYL® Hydrochloride (methdilazine HCl) Tablets 8 mg. each, scored, peach colored tablet (w logo):

NDC 0072-7400-01 Bottles of 100 (with child-resistant closures)

TACARYL® Hydrochloride (methdilazine HCl) Syrup 4 mg./5 ml:

NDC 0072-7500-01 Bottles of 16 fl. oz. (1 pint) (with child-resistant closures)

TACARYL® (methdilazine) Chewable Tablets 3.6 mg. each (equivalent to 4 mg. methdilazine HCl), pink, unscored tablet (w logo):

NDC 0072-7300-01 Bottles of 100 (with child-resistant closures)

TRANSACT®
Transparent Medicated Acne Gel

Composition: Contains 2% Sulfur and 37% alcohol in a greaseless gel base with laureth-4.
Action and Uses: TRANSACT is a transparent, nonstaining and greaseless gel, which leaves a fresh, clean fragrance on the skin. It dries, peels and degreases the skin of acne patients. Its effect is controlled by frequency of application and climatic conditions.
Administration and Dosage: After washing acne skin thoroughly, a thin film is applied to affected areas once daily or as directed. A brief tingling sensation may be expected upon application. Patient should anticipate beneficial drying and peeling in 5 to 7 days. Since TRANSACT is a highly active drying agent it should be used sparingly when initiating therapy, particularly for patients with sensitive skin. 1. Patients with tender skin may best be started on one application every other day. 2. Most other patients can be started on one daily application. 3. When patients develop tolerance, applications may be increased to two and then three times daily to maintain an adequate therapeutic effect. 4. TRANSACT is also for use on the shoulders and back. In dry or cold climates skin is more reactive to TRANSACT and frequency of use should be reduced. During warm, humid months, frequency of use may be increased.
Caution: If undue skin irritation develops, usage schedule should be adjusted or TRANSACT discontinued. For external use only. Avoid contact with eyes. In case of contact, flush eyes with water.
How Supplied: 1 oz. (NDC 0072-5600-01) plastic tube.

WESTCORT® CREAM
(Hydrocortisone Valerate) 0.2%

Caution: Federal law prohibits dispensing without a prescription.
Description: WESTCORT CREAM is a topical formulation containing hydrocortisone valerate, a non-fluorinated steroid. It has the chemical name Pregn-4-ene-3, 20-dione, 11, 21-dihydroxy-17-[(1-oxopentyl) oxy]-, (11β)-; the empirical formula is: $C_{26}H_{38}O_6$; the molecular weight is 446.58, and the CAS registry number is: 57524-89-7. The structural formula is:

Each gram of WESTCORT CREAM contains 2.0 mg hydrocortisone valearate in a hydrophilic base composed of white petrolatum, stearyl alcohol, propylene glycol, amphoteric-9, carbomer 940, sodium phosphate, sodium lauryl sulfate, sorbic acid and water.

Clinical Pharmacology: Topical corticosteroids share anti-inflammatory, anti-pruritic and vasoconstrictive actions.
The mechanism of anti-inflammatory activity of the topical corticosteroids is unclear.[1] Various laboratory methods, including vasoconstrictor assays, are used to compare and predict potencies and/or clinical efficacies of the topical corticosteroids.[2] There is some evidence to suggest that a recognizable correlation exists between vasoconstrictor potency and therapeutic efficacy in man.[3]
Pharmacokinetics: The extent of percutaneous absorption of topical corticosteroids is determined by many factors including the vehicle, the integrity of the epidermal barrier, and the use of occlusive dressins.[4,5,6]
Topical corticosteroids can be absorbed from normal intact skin.[5,6,7] Inflammation and/or other disease processes in the skin increase percutaneous absorption.[8] Occlusive dressings substantially increase the percutaneous absorption of topical corticosteroids.[4,7] Thus, occlusive dressings may be a valuable therapeutic adjunct for treatment of resistant dermatoses (see DOSAGE AND ADMINISTRATION).
Once absorbed through the skin, topical corticosteroids are handled through pharmacokinetic pathways similar to systemically administered corticosteroids. Corticosteroids are bound to plasma proteins in varying degrees. Corticosteroids are metabolized primarily in the liver and are then excreted by the kidneys. Some of the topical corticosteroids and their metabolites are also excreted into the bile.
Indications and Usage: WESTCORT CREAM is indicated for the relief of the inflammatory and pruritic manifestations of the corticosteroid-responsive dermatoses.
Contraindications: Topical corticosteroids are contraindicated in those patients with a history of hypersensitivity to any of the components of the preparation.
Precautions: *General:* Systemic absorption of topical corticosteroids has produced reversible hypothalamic-pituitary-adrenal (HPA) axis suppression, manifestations of Cushing's syndrome, hyperglycemia, and glucosuria in some patients.[9]
Conditions which augment systemic absorption include the application of the more potent steroids, use over large surface areas, prolonged use, and the addition of occlusive dressings.[10]
Therefore, patients receiving a large dose of a potent topical steroid applied to a large surface area or under an occlusive dressing should be evaluated periodically for evidence of HPA axis suppression by using the urinary free cortisol and ACTH stimulation tests. If HPA axis suppression is noted, an attempt should be made to withdraw the drug, to reduce the frequency of application, or to substitute a less potent steroid.
Recovery of HPA axis function is generally prompt and complete upon discontinuation of the drug.[10] Infrequently, signs and symptoms of steroid withdrawal may occur, requiring supplemental systemic corticosteroids.[11,12]
Children may absorb proportionally larger amounts of topical corticosteroids and thus be more susceptible to systemic toxicity[13,14] (see PRECAUTIONS—Pediatric Use).
If irritation develops, topical corticosteroids should be discontinued and appropriate therapy instituted.
In the presence of dermatological infections, the use of an appropriate antifungal or antibacterial agent should be instituted. If a favorable response does not occur promptly, the corticosteroids should be discontinued until the infection has been adequately controlled.
Information for the Patient: Patients using topical corticosteroids should receive the following information and instructions:

1. This medication is to be used as directed by the physician. It is for external use only. Avoid contact with the eyes.
2. Patients should be advised not to use this medication for any disorder other than for which it was prescribed.
3. The treated skin area should not be bandaged or otherwise covered or wrapped as to be occlusive unless directed by the physician.
4. Patients should report any signs of local adverse reactions especially under occlusive dressing.
5. Parents of pediatric patients should be advised not to use tight-fitting diapers or plastic pants on a child being treated in the diaper area, as these garments may constitute occlusive dressing.

Laboratory Tests: The following tests may be helpful in evaluating the HPA axis suppression:

Urinary free cortisol test
ACTH stimulation test

Carcinogenesis, Mutagenesis, and Impairment of Fertility: Long-term animal studies have not been performed to evaluate the carcinogenic potential or the effect on fertility of topical corticosteroids.
Studies to determine mutagenicity with prednisolone and hydrocortisone have revealed negative results.[15,16]
Pregnancy Category C: Corticosteroids are generally teratogenic in laboratory animals when administered systemically at relatively low dosage levels. The more potent corticosteroids have been shown to be teratogenic after dermal application in laboratory animals. There are no adequate and well-controlld studies in pregnant women on teratogenic effects from topically applied corticosteroids. Therefore, topical corticosteroids should be used during pregnancy only if the potential benefit justifies the potential risk to the fetus. Drugs of this class should not be used extensively on pregnant patients, in large amounts, or for prolonged periods of time.
Nursing Mothers: It is not known whether topical administration of corticosteroids could result in sufficient systemic absorption to produce detectable quantities in breast milk. Systemically administered corticosteroids are secreted into breast milk in quantities *not* likely to have a deleterious effect on the infant.[17,18] Nevertheless, caution should be exercised when topical corticosteroids are administered to a nursing woman.
Pediatric Use: Pediatric patients may demonstrate greater susceptibility to topical corticosteroid-induced HPA axis suppression and Cushing's syndrome than mature patients because of a larger skin surface area to body weight ratio.
Hypothalamic-pituitary-adrenal (HPA) axis suppression, Cushing's syndrome, and intracranial hypertension have been reported in children receiving topical corticosteroids. Manifestations of adrenal suppression in children include linear growth retardation, delayed weight gain, low plasma cortisol levels, and absence of response to ACTH stimulation. Manifestations of intracranial hypertension include bulging fontanelles, headaches, and bilateral papilledema.
Administration of topical corticosteroids to children should be limited to the least amount compatible with an effective therapeutic regimen. Chronic corticosteroid therapy may interfere with the growth and development of children.
Adverse Reactions: The following local adverse reactions are reported infrequently with topical corticosteroids, but may occur more frequently with the use of occlusive dressings. These reactions are listed in an approximate decreasing order of occurrence: burning; itching; irritation; dryness; folliculitis; hypertrichosis; acneiform eruptions; hypopigmentation; perioral dermatitis; allergic contact dermati-

Continued on next page

Westwood—Cont.

tis; maceration of the skin; secondary infection; skin atrophy; striae; miliaria.

Overdosage: Topically applied corticosteroids can be absorbed in sufficient amounts to produce systemic effects (see PRECAUTIONS).

Dosage and Administration: WESTCORT CREAM should be applied to the affected area as a thin film two or three times daily depending on the severity of the condition.

Occlusive dressings may be used for the management of psoriasis or recalcitrant conditions. If an infection develops, the use of occlusive dressings should be discontinued and appropriate antimicrobial therapy instituted.

How Supplied: WESTCORT CREAM, 0.2% is supplied in the following tube sizes:

15 g NDC 0072-8100-15; NSN 6505-01-093-9901

45 g NDC 0072-8100-45; NSN 6505-01-083-9901

60 g NDC 0072-8100-60

120 g NDC 0072-8100-12.

Store below 78°F (26°C).

References:

1. Maibach HI, Stoughton RB: *Med Clin N Am* 57: 1253–64, 1973.
2. Engel JC, et al: *Arch Dermatol* 109: 863–5, 1974.
3. Barry BW: *Dermatologica* 152 (Supplement 1): 47–65, 1976.
4. McKenzie AW, Stoughton RB: *Arch Dermatol* 86: 608–10, 1962.
5. Feldmann RJ, Maibach HI: *J Invest Dermatol* 52: 89–94, 1969.
6. Feldmann RJ, Maibach HI: *J Invest Dermatol* 48: 181–3, 1967.
7. Feldmann RJ, Maibach HI: *Arch Dermatol* 91: 661–6, 1965.
8. Schaefer H, Zesch A, Stuttgen G: *Arch Dermatol Res* 258: 241–9, 1977.
9. Hendhkse JCM, Moolenaar AJ: *Dermatologica* 144: 179–86, 1972.
10. Monro DD: *Br J Dermatol* 94 (Supplement 12): 67–76, 1976.
11. Nathan AW, Rose GL: *Lancet* 1: 207, 1979.
12. May P, et al: *Arch Intern Med* 136: 612–3, 1976.
13. Johns AM, Bower BD: *Br Med J* 1: 347–8, 1970.
14. Feiwel M, James VHT, Barnett ES: *Lancet* 1: 485–7, 1969.
15. Seino Y, et al: *Cancer Res* 38: 2148–56, 1978.
16. Hemmerly J, Demeree M: *Cancer Res* 15 (Supplement 3): 69–75, 1955.
17. McKenzie SA, Selley JA, Agnew JE: *Arch Dis Child* 50: 894–6, 1975.
18. Katz FH, Duncan BR: *N Eng J Med* 293: 1154, 1975.

Wharton Laboratories, Inc.

37-02 FORTY-EIGHTH AVE.
LONG ISLAND CITY, NY 11101

NITRONG® OINTMENT ℞
(Nitroglycerin 2%)

Description: NITRONG® Ointment contains 2% nitroglycerin in a special absorptive lanolin-white petrolatum base. It acts as a prompt vasodilator effective in the relief and prevention of anginal attacks; especially suitable for application at night.

Action: When the ointment is spread on the skin, the active ingredient (nitroglycerin) is continuously absorbed through the skin into the circulation, thus exerting prolonged vasodilator effect. Nitroglycerin ointment is effective in the control of angina pectoris, regardless of the site of application.

Nitroglycerin ointment exhibits a consistently prolonged beneficial effect. After application of nitroglycerin ointment, the effect of the drug can be noted promptly. Exercise capacity is increased significantly. More importantly, exercise capacity continues to show increases in patients studied three hours after treatment. When nitroglycerin ointment is applied, a marked and consistent beneficial effect is observed on the exercise electrocardiogram and on exercise capacity, which persists essentially undiminished three to four hours after application.

Nitroglycerin ointment applied to the chest can be utilized as a slow-release preparation which is especially useful in the treatment of angina decubitus. An application of ointment at bedtime may give the patient a night's sleep without a nocturnal attack.

Indications: Prevention and treatment of angina pectoris attacks especially at night.

Precautions: A headache is a definite sign of overdosage and, therefore, dosage should be reduced. As with sublingual nitroglycerin, transient headaches may occur. In terminating treatment, dosage and frequency of application must be gradually reduced over a period of 4 to 6 weeks to prevent sudden withdrawal reactions, which are characteristic of all vasodilators in the nitrate class.

Contraindications: NITRONG ointment is contraindicated in patients known to be intolerant to the organic nitrates. May be contraindicated in patients with marked anemia, increased intraocular pressure or increased intracranial pressure.

Adverse Reactions: Occasionally elderly patients may have no untoward symptoms while recumbent but may develop postural hypotension with faintness upon suddenly arising.

Dosage and Administration: When applying the ointment, place the specially designed Dose Determining Applicator supplied with the package printed side down, and squeeze the necessary amount of ointment from the tube onto the Dose Determining Applicator, then place the Dose Determining Applicator, ointment side down, on the desired skin area, spreading it in a thin, uniform layer. Cover with plastic wrap which can be held in place with adhesive or transparent tape. The Dose Determining Applicator allows the patient to measure the amount of ointment, which can then be spread onto the skin. At the same time, the ointment is prevented from being absorbed through the fingers while applied to the skin.

Angina Pectoris: NITRONG ointment may be applied every eight (8) hours if necessary, but one application at bedtime frequently suffices for the entire night. It may also be used throughout the day, but it is particularly useful in patients who suffer from the fear of nocturnal attacks of angina pectoris.

The usual dose is 1 to 2 inches, (25 to 50 mm) containing 15 mg to 30 mg nitroglycerin as squeezed from the tube, applied every eight (8) hours, although some patients require as much as 4 or 5 inches (100 to 125 mm), and/or applications every four (4) hours. The ointment measured on the Dose Determining Applicator is spread in a thin uniform layer over the chest, abdomen or anterior thighs, without massaging or rubbing it in. The optimal dosage is determined by starting with an application of as little as 1 inch (25 mm) and increasing the dose ½ inch (12.5 mm) at a time until headache occurs, then dropping back to the largest dose which does not cause a headache. The dose should be titrated to the need of the patient in the prevention and treatment of angina pectoris. This ointment is effective in the control of angina pectoris regardless of the skin site of application. Therefore, any convenient skin area may be used, but, psychologically, many patients prefer the chest because anginal pain originates in this area.

Keep the tube tightly closed and store at room temperature (59° to 86°F).

In terminating treatment of anginal patients, both the dosage and frequency of application must be gradually reduced over a period of 4 to 6 weeks to prevent sudden withdrawal reactions, which are characteristic of all vasodilators in the nitroglycerin class.

Caution: Federal law prohibits dispensing without prescription.

How Supplied:

30 gram tube (NDC 0195-280-50)
60 gram tube (NDC 0195-280-51)
Unit Dose (1" Equivalent) (NDC 0195-280-77)

NITRONG® Tablets ℞
2.6 mg, 6.5 mg and 9 mg
(nitroglycerin, oral, controlled-release)

Description: Each NITRONG 2.6 mg. tablet for oral administration contains 2.6 mg. nitroglycerin in controlled-release form with light green granules, identified by the U.S. Ethicals trademark.

Each NITRONG 6.5 mg. tablet for oral administration contains 6.5 mg. nitroglycerin in controlled-release form with light orange granules, identified by the U.S. Ethicals trademark.

Each NITRONG 9.0 mg tablet for oral administration contains 9.0 mg nitroglycerin in controlled-release form with blue granules, identified by the U.S. Ethicals trademark.

How Supplied: NITRONG 2.6 mg. and 6.5 mg. are available in bottles of 100 tablets. NITRONG 9.0 mg. is available in bottles of 60 tablets. The tablets are scored and have a mottled appearance.

Willen Drug Company

18 NORTH HIGH STREET
BALTIMORE, MD 21202

BICITRA®—Sugar-Free ℞
(Brand of Sodium Citrate & Citric Acid Oral Solution USP)

Description: BICITRA is a stable and pleasant tasting oral systemic alkalizer containing Sodium Citrate and Citric Acid in a sugar-free base. BICITRA is the USP formula for SHOHL'S Solution.

Composition: BICITRA contains in each teaspoonful (5 ml): Sodium Citrate Dihydrate 500 mg (0.34 Molar) and Citric Acid Monohydrate 334 mg (0.32 Molar). Each ml contains 1 mEq. Sodium ion and is equivalent to 1 mEq. Bicarbonate (HCO_3).

Actions: Sodium Citrate is absorbed and metabolized to sodium bicarbonate, thus acting as a systemic alkalizer. The effects are essentially those of chlorides before absorption and those of bicarbonates subsequently. Oxidation is virtually complete so that less than 5% of Sodium Citrate is execreted in the urine unchanged.

Indications and Advantages: Bicitra is an effective alkalinizing agent and a non-particulate neutralizing buffer. It is useful in those conditions where long term maintenance of an alkaline urine is desirable, and is of value in the alleviation of chronic metabolic acidosis such as results from chronic renal insufficiency or the syndrome of renal tubular acidosis, especially when the administration of potassium salts is undesirable or contraindicated. BICITRA is also useful for buffering and neutralizing gastric hydrochloric acid quickly and effectively.

BICITRA is concentrated and when administered after meals and before bedtime, allows one to maintain an alkaline urinary pH around the clock, usually without the necessity of a 2 A.M. dose. BICITRA alkalinizes the urine without producing a systemic alkalosis in the recommended dosage. BICITRA is highly palatable, pleasant tasting and tolerable, even when administered for long periods, and offers these advantages over SHOHL'S Solution.

while supplying the equivalent sodium content. BICITRA is sugar-free.

Contraindications: Patients on sodium-restricted diet or with severe renal impairment. In certain situations, Potassium Citrate, as contained in Syrup POLYCITRA-K may be preferable.

Precautions: Should be used with caution by patients with low urinary output unless under the supervision of a physician. Patients should be directed to dilute adequately with water and preferably, to take each dose after meals to avoid saline laxative effect. Sodium salts should be used cautiously in patients with cardiac failure, hypertension, impaired renal function, peripheral and pulmonary edema and toxemia of pregnancy. Periodic examinations and determinations of serum electrolytes, particularly serum bicarbonate level, should be carried out in those patients with renal disease in order to avoid these complications.

Adverse Reactions: BICITRA is generally well tolerated without any unpleasant side effects when given in recommended doses to patients with normal renal function and urinary output. However, as with any alkalinizing agent, caution must be used in certain patients with abnormal renal mechanisms to avoid development of alkalosis, especially in the presence of hypocalcemia.

Dosage and Administration: BICITRA should be taken diluted in water followed by additional water, if desired. Palatability is enhanced if chilled before taking. ADULTS: 10 to 30 ml diluted in 1 to 3 ounces of water after meals and at bedtime, or as directed by physician. CHILDREN: 5 to 15 ml diluted in 1 to 3 ounces of water after meals and at bedtime, or as directed by physician. As a Neutralizing Buffer: 15 ml diluted with 15 ml water, taken as a single dose, or as directed by physician. Occasional patients will require more or less to achieve the desired alkalizing effect.

Overdosage: Sodium salts may cause diarrhea, nausea and vomiting, hypernoea, and convulsions.

How Supplied: 16 fl.oz. (473 ml)(NDC 11414-207-01), 1 gallon (3785 ml)(NDC 11414-207-08) and 4 fl.oz. (120 ml) hospital size (NDC 11414-207-04).

Literature Available: Yes.

NEUTRA-PHOS® Powder & Capsules
NEUTRA-PHOS®-K Powder & Capsules
Oral Phosphorus Dietary Supplement

NEUTRA-PHOS and NEUTRA-PHOS-K supply the physiologically important element—PHOSPHORUS—as inorganic orthophosphate, in a well tolerated oral compound. Each contains a chemically balanced combination of readily soluble inorganic phosphates, affording a very high source of elemental Phosphorus. Both products supply equal concentration of elemental Phosphorus.

Composition: NEUTRA-PHOS is a stable powder combination of monobasic and dibasic Sodium and Potassium Phosphates. NEUTRA-PHOS-K is a stable sodium-free powder combination of monobasic and dibasic Potassium Phosphates intended for oral use in low sodium diets. Both products form an oral solution by reconstitution with water and are neutral (pH 7.3), isotonic, pleasant tasting sources of Phosphorus. There is less than 1 calorie per average dose.

Indications: NEUTRA-PHOS and NEUTRA-PHOS-K are recommended as oral Phosphorus supplements, particularly if the diet is low in mineral intake or if needs are increased.

Advantages: NEUTRA-PHOS and NEUTRA-PHOS-K, reconstituted to an oral liquid, provide rapid absorption and utilization from the alimentary tract. This is very advantageous compared to the use of coated or uncoated tablet dosage forms. (The patient ingests a liquid rather than a slowly dissolving tablet which may cause localized irritation or inflamation in sensitive individuals.) Both products are highly concentrated and thus economically provide inorganic Phosphate. They are especially useful for long term maintenance requirements. NEUTRA-PHOS also supplies Sodium and Potassium in equimolar proportions—a decided advantage over products which supply a high amount of sodium and a low amount of potassium per dose. NEUTRA-PHOS-K supplies only Potassium and is recommended when a low sodium diet is indicated.

Electrolytes Supplied: 2-½ fluid ounces (75 ml) of the reconstituted solution or contents of 1 capsule* supplies:

Electrolyte	NEUTRA-PHOS mg.	NEUTRA-PHOS mEq
Phosphorus	250	14.25
Phosphate (PO_4)	765	—
Sodium	164	7.125
Potassium	278	7.125

Electrolyte	NEUTRA-PHOS-K mg.	NEUTRA-PHOS-K mEq
Phosphorus	250	14.25
Phosphate (PO_4)	765	—
Sodium	none	none
Potassium	556	14.25

(*reconstituted in water as per label directions. Refer to Unit Dose Capsules description.)

Average Directions for Adults and Children: 4 or more years of age: 2-½ fl. oz. (75 ml) of the oral solution, or contents of 1 capsule, equivalent to 250 mg Phosphorus, taken 4 times a day. (See Unit Dose Capsules description).

Pediatric Dose: Infants and children under 4 years of age: 2 fl. oz. (60 ml) of the oral solution, equivalent to 200 mg of Phosphorus, taken 4 times a day.

Usual Dose Range: 2-½ fl. oz. to 20 fl. oz. (75 ml to 600 ml) of the oral solution, or contents of 1 to 8 capsules (equivalent from 250 mg to 2 grams of Phosphorus) taken daily in divided doses, after meals and at bedtime. 2-½ fl. oz. (75 ml) or 1 capsule, 4 times a day supplies 1 gm. Phosphorus. 5 fl. oz. (150 ml) or 2 capsules, 3 times a day supplies 1.5 gm. Phosphorus. 5 fl. oz. (150 ml) or 2 capsules, 4 times a day supplies 2 gm. Phosphorus. (See Unit Dose Capsules description).

Precautions and Side Effects: Reconstitute powder and contents of capsules as directed before taking. Occasionally some individuals may experience a mild laxative effect for the first day or two when beginning to use NEUTRA-PHOS. If this persists to an unpleasant degree, reduce the daily intake until this effect subsides or, if necessary, discontinue its use.

How Supplied: Both products are supplied as powder concentrates, to be reconstituted with water by the patient, and are available in multiple dose or unit dose sizes.

Multiple Dose Powder Concentrate: For patient convenience, these powder concentrates are packaged in a size sufficient to make 1 gallon (3.785 Liters) and are intended for use while at home. This economical dosage form is prepared by the patient who is instructed to dissolve the entire contents of 1 bottle in sufficient water to make 1 gallon of solution. This solution is not to be diluted, but can be chilled if desired, to increase palatability. 2-½ fl. oz. (75 ml) of this solution supplies 250 mg Phosphorus (refer to electrolyte chart).

Unit Dose Capsules: These products are also supplied in pre-measured unit-dose capsules which are intended for use if the above multiple dose form precludes transportation of liquid. The contents of 1 capsule makes 2-½ fl. oz. (75 ml) of an oral suspension equal to the oral solution prepared above. To use, empty the contents of 1 capsule into ⅓ glass water (approx. 2-½ fl. oz.) and stir well before taking. Each capsule supplies 250 mg Phosphorus (refer to electrolyte chart).

NEUTRA-PHOS Powder Concentrate—2-¼ oz. (64 gm) bottle. Reconstitutes to 1 gallon Stock No. 201-01.

NEUTRA-PHOS Unit Dose Capsules—1.25 gm powder concentrate per capsule, 48 capsules per bottle Stock No. 202-01.

NEUTRA-PHOS-K Powder Concentrate—2-½ oz. (71 gm) bottle. Reconstitutes to 1 gallon Stock No. 203-01.

NEUTRA-PHOS-K Unit Dose Capsules—1.45 gm powder concentrate per capsule, 48 capsules per bottle Stock No. 204-01.

Is this product O.T.C.: Yes.

Literature Available: Yes.

POLYCITRA® Syrup ℞
POLYCITRA®-LC-Sugar-Free
(Brand of Tricitrates Oral Solution U.S.P.)

Description: Syrup POLYCITRA and POLYCITRA-LC are stable and pleasant-tasting oral systemic alkalizers containing Potassium Citrate, Sodium Citrate and Citric Acid. Syrup POLYCITRA is a sugar-base preparation. POLYCITRA-LC is a sugar-free solution, to be used by patients who desire a low-carbohydrate diet. Both products are non-alcoholic and contain identical amounts of active ingredients.

Composition: Syrup POLYCITRA and POLYCITRA-LC contains in each teaspoonful (5 ml): Potassium Citrate Monohydrate 550 mg (0.34 Molar), Sodium Citrate Dihydrate 500 mg (0.34 Molar), and Citric Acid Monohydrate 334 mg (0.32 Molar). Each ml contains 1 mEq. Potassium ion and 1 mEq. Sodium ion and is equivalent to 2 mEq. Bicarbonate (HCO_3).

Actions: Potassium Citrate and Sodium Citrate are absorbed and metabolized to potassium bicarbonate and sodium bicarbonate, thus acting as systemic alkalizers. The effects are essentially those of chlorides before absorption and those of bicarbonates subsequently. Oxidation is virtually complete so that less than 5% of the citrates are excreted in the urine unchanged.

Indications and Advantages: Syrup POLYCITRA and POLYCITRA-LC are effective alkalinizing agents useful in those conditions where long term maintenance of an alkaline urine is desirable, such as in patients with uric acid and cystine calculi of the urinary tract. In addition, they are valuable adjuvants when administered with uricosuric agents in gout therapy, since urates tend to crystallize out of an acid urine. They are also effective in correcting the acidosis of certain renal tubular disorders. Syrup POLYCITRA and POLYCITRA-LC are highly concentrated, and when administered after meals and before bedtime, allows one to maintain an alkaline urinary pH around the clock, usually without the necessity of a 2 AM dose. Syrup POLYCITRA and POLYCITRA-LC alkalinize the urine without producing a systemic alkalosis in recommended dosage. They are highly palatable, pleasant tasting and tolerable, even when administered for long periods. Syrup POLYCITRA and POLYCITRA-LC are useful as non-particulate neutralizing buffers, acting quickly and effectively on gastric hydrochloric acid.

Contraindications: Severe renal impairment with oliguria or azotemia, untreated Addison's disease or severe myocardial damage. In certain situations, when patients are on a sodium-restricted diet, the use of Potassium Citrate, as contained in Syrup POLYCITRA-K, may be preferable; or when patients are on a potassium-restricted diet, the use of Sodium Citrate, as contained in BICITRA, may be preferable.

Precautions and Warnings: Should be used with caution by patients with low urinary out-

Continued on next page

Willen—Cont.

put unless under the supervision of a physician. Patients should be directed to dilute adequately with water and preferably, to take each dose after meals, to minimize the possibility of gastrointestinal injury associated with oral ingestion of potassium salt preparations and to avoid saline laxative effect. Sodium salts should be used cautiously in patients with cardiac failure, hypertension, peripheral and pulmonary edema and toxemia of pregnancy. Concurrent administration of potassium-containing medication, potassium-sparing diuretics, or cardiac glycosides may lead to toxicity. Periodic examination and determinations of serum electrolytes, particularly serum bicarbonate level, should be carried out in those patients with renal disease in order to avoid these complications.

Adverse Reactions: Syrup POLYCITRA and POLYCITRA-LC are generally well tolerated without any unpleasant side effects when given in recommended doses to patients with normal renal function and urinary output. However, as with any alkalinizing agent, caution must be used in certain patients with abnormal renal mechanisms to avoid development of hyperkalemia or alkalosis, especially in the presence of hypocalcemia. Potassium intoxication causes listlessness, weakness, mental confusion and tingling of extremities.

Dosage and Administration: Syrup POLYCITRA and POLYCITRA-LC should be taken diluted in water, followed by additional water if desired. Palatability is enhanced if chilled before taking.

Usual Dosage: Adults: 15 to 30 ml diluted in water, four times a day after meals and at bedtime, or as directed by physician. Children: 5 to 15 ml diluted in water, four times a day after meals and at bedtime or as directed by physician.

Usual Dosage Range: 10 to 15 ml diluted with water, taken four times a day, will usually maintain a urine pH of 6.5–7.4. 15 to 20 ml diluted with water, taken four times a day, will usually maintain a urine pH of 7.0–7.6 throughout most of the 24 hours without unpleasant side effects.

As a Neutralizing Buffer: 15 ml diluted with 15 ml water, taken as a single dose, or as directed by physician.

Overdosage: Overdosage with sodium salts may cause diarrhea, nausea and vomiting, hypernoea, and convulsions. Overdosage with potassium salts may cause hyperkalemia and alkalosis, especially in the presence of renal disease.

How Supplied: Syrup POLYCITRA—16 fl oz (473 ml) (NDC 11414-205-01) and 4 fl oz (120 ml) hospital size (NDC 11414-205-04).
POLYCITRA-LC—16 fl oz (473 ml) (NDC 11414-208-01) and 4 fl oz (120 ml) hospital size (NDC 11414-208-04)

Literature Available: Yes.

POLYCITRA®-K Syrup ℞

(Potassium Citrate and Citric Acid Oral Solution U.S.P.)

How Supplied: Each teaspoonful (5 ml) contains Potassium Citrate Monohydrate 1100 mg (0.68 Molar) and Citric Acid Monohydrate 334 mg (0.32 Molar). Each ml contains 2 mEq. Potassium and is equivalent to 2 mEq Bicarbonate (HCO_3). 16 fl. oz. (473 ml) NDC 11414-206-01) and 4 fl. oz. (120 ml) hospital size (NDC 11414-206-04).

T. E. Williams Pharmaceuticals, Inc.

POST OFFICE BOX 1860
EDMOND, OK 73034

T-DRY CAPSULES ℞

Description: Each timed release capsule contains:
Chlorpheniramine Maleate ....12 mg.
Phenylpropanolamine Hydrochloride ..50 mg.
Phenylephrine Hydrochloride ....25 mg.
in a specially prepared base to provide prolonged action.
This product contains ingredients of the following therapeutic classes: antihistamine and decongestant.

Clinical Pharmacology: Chlorpheniramine maleate is an alkylamine type antihistamine. This group of antihistamines are among the most active histamine antagonists and are generaly effective in relatively low doses. The drugs are not so prone to produce drowsiness and are among the most suitable agents for day time use; but again, a significant proportion of patients do experience this effect. Phenylpropanolamine hydrochloride and phenylephrine hydrochloride are sympathomimetics which act predominantly on alpha receptors and have little action on beta receptors. They, therefore, function as oral nasal decongestants with minimal CNS stimulation.

Indications: For the temporary relief of symptoms of the common cold, allergic rhinitis (hay fever) and sinusitis.

Contraindications: Hypersensitivity to any of the ingredients. Also contraindicated in patients with severe hypertension, severe coronary artery disease, patients on MAO inhibitor therapy, patients with narrow-angle glaucoma, urinary retention, peptic ulcer and during an asthmatic attack.
Should not be used in children under 12 years, or in nursing mothers.

Warnings: Considerable caution should be exercised in patients with hypertension, diabetes mellitus, ischemic heart disease, hyperthyroidism, increased intraocular pressure and prostatic hypertrophy. The elderly (60 years or older) are more likely to exhibit adverse reactions.
Antihistamines may cause excitability, especially in children. At dosages higher than the recommended dose, nervousness, dizziness or sleeplessness may occur.

Precautions

General: Caution should be exercised in patients with high blood pressure, heart disease, diabetes or thyroid disease. The antihistamine in this product may exhibit additive effects with other CNS depressants, including alcohol.

Information for Patients: Antihistamines may cause drowsiness and ambulatory patients who operate machinery or motor vehicles should be cautioned accordingly.

Drug Interactions: MAO inhibitors and beta adrenergic blockers increase the effects of sympathomimetics. Sympathomimetics may reduce the antihypertensive effects of methyldopa, mecamylamine, reserpine and veratrum alkaloids. Concomitant use of antihistamines with alcohol and other CNS depressants may have an additive effect.

Pregnancy: The safety of use of this product in pregnancy has not been established.

Adverse Reactions: Adverse reactions include drowsiness, lassitude, nausea, giddiness, dryness of mouth, blurred vision, cardiac palpitations, flushing, increased irritability or excitement (especially in children).

Dosage and Administration: Adults and children over 12 years of age—1 capsule orally every 12 hours.

How Supplied: Bottles of 100 capsules—NDC 51189-011-01

DISPENSE IN TIGHT CONTAINERS AS DEFINED IN U.S.P.

STORE BETWEEN 59°–86°F.

DISPENSE IN CHILD-RESISTANT CONTAINERS.

Manufactured by:
CENTRAL PHARMACEUTICALS, INC.
Seymour, Indiana 47274
Distributed by:
T. E. WILLIAMS PHARMACEUTICALS, INC.
Edmond, Oklahoma 73034
Issued January 1982 8201011

T-DRY JR. CAPSULES ℞

Description: Each timed release capsule contains:
Chlorpheniramine Maleate ....6 mg.
Phenylpropanolamine Hydrochloride ..25 mg.
Phenylephrine Hydrochloride ....12.5 mg.
in a specially prepared base to provide prolonged action.
This product contains ingredients of the following therapeutic classes: antihistamine and decongestant.

Clinical Pharmacology: Chlorpheniramine maleate is an alkylamine type antihistamine. This group of antihistamines are among the most active histamine antagonists and are generally effective in relatively low doses. The drugs are not so prone to produce drowsiness and are among the most suitable agents for day time use; but again, a significant proportion of patients do experience this effect. Phenylpropanolamine hydrochloride and phenylephrine hydrochloride are sympathomimetics which act predominantly on alpha receptors and have little action on beta receptors. They, therefore, function as oral nasal decongestants with minimal CNS stimulation.

Indications: For the temporary relief of symptoms of the common cold, allergic rhinitis (hay fever) and sinusitis.

Contraindications: Hypersensitivity to any of the ingredients. Also contraindicated in patients with severe hypertension, severe coronary artery disease, patients on MAO inhibitor therapy, patients with narrow-angle glaucoma, urinary retention, peptic ulcer and during an asthmatic attack.
Should not be used in nursing mothers.

Warnings: Considerable caution should be exercised in patients with hypertension, diabetes mellitus, ischemic heart disease, hyperthyroidism, increased intraocular pressure and prostatic hypertrophy. The elderly (60 years or older) are more likely to exhibit adverse reactions.
Antihistamines may cause excitability, especially in children. At dosages higher than the recommended dose, nervousness, dizziness or sleeplessness may occur.

Precautions

General: Caution should be exercised in patients with high blood pressure, heart disease, diabetes or thyroid disease. The antihistamine in this product may exhibit additive effects with other CNS depressants, including alcohol.

Information for Patients: Antihistamines may cause drowsiness and ambulatory patients who operate machinery or motor vehicles should be cautioned accordingly.

Drug Interactions: MAO inhibitors and beta adrenergic blockers increase the effects of sympathomimetics. Sympathomimetics may reduce the antihypertensive effects of methyldopa, mecamylamine, reserpine and veratrum alkaloids. Concomitant use of antihistamines with alcohol and other CNS depressants may have an additive effect.

Pregnancy: The safety of use of this product in pregnancy has not been established.

Adverse Reactions: Adverse reactions include drowsiness, lassitude, nausea, giddiness, dryness of mouth, blurred vision, cardiac palpitations, flushing, increased irritability or excitement (expecially in children).

Dosage and Administration: Adults and children over 12 years of age - 2 capsules orally every 12 hours.

Children, 6 to 12 years of age - 1 capsule orally every 12 hours.
Not recommended for younger children.
How Supplied: Bottles of 100 capsules—NDC 51189-019-01

DISPENSE IN TIGHT CONTAINERS AS DEFINED IN USP/NF.
STORE BETWEEN 15°–30° C (59°–86° F)
DISPENSE IN CHILD-RESISTANT CONTAINERS

Manufactured by:
CENTRAL PHARMACEUTICALS, INC.
Seymour, Indiana 47274
Distributed by:
T. E. WILLIAMS PHARMACEUTICALS, INC.
Edmond, Oklahoma 73034
Issued April 1982 8204019

T-GESIC CAPSULES ℗ ℞

Description: Each scarlet and black capsule contains:
Acetaminophen ....325 mg.
Hydrocodone Bitartrate ....5 mg.
(WARNING: May be habit forming)
Butalbital NF ....50 mg.
(WARNING: May be habit forming)
Caffeine ....40 mg.
T-GESIC capsule is narcotic-analgesic for oral administration.
Acetaminophen: N-(4-Hydroxyphenyl) acetamide, $C_8H_9NO_2$, is a non-salicylate, analgesic and antipyretic which occurs as a white, odorless crystalline powder possessing a slightly bitter taste.
Hydrocodone: Is dihydrocodeinone, $C_{18}H_{21}NO_3$, a hydrogenated ketone of codeine, available as the bitartrate salt $C_{18}H_{21}NO_3 \cdot C_4H_6O_6 \cdot 2\frac{1}{2}H_2O$. It possesses the analgesic and antitussive activity of codeine.
Butalbital: 5-allyl-5-isobutylbarbituric acid, $C_{11}H_{16}N_2O_3$, a white crystalline powder, has a slightly bitter taste. Depending upon the dose it is hypnotic and sedative.
Caffeine: 3, 7-Dihydro-1,3,7-trimethyl-1H-purine-2,6-dione, $C_8H_{10}N_4O_2$, white powder; odorless and has a bitter taste. It is a mild CNS stimulant, to aid in staying awake and to restore mental alertness in fatigued patients.
Clinical Pharmacology: T-GESIC is analgesic, antitussive and antipyretic. The analgesic-sedative action of acetaminophen and butalbital increases the analgesic action of the hydrocodone bitartrate. This enhanced analgesic-sedative effect is particularly well-suited for acute, short-ranged periods of pain and discomfort frequently seen in office practice. T-GESIC provides additional benefits for patients who have developed a cycle of pain, anxiety, and tension which reinforces the pain experienced by the patients. T-GESIC is indicated for all types of pain associated with medical and surgical aftercare, postpartum pain, dysmenorrhea, neuritis, pleurisy, sciatica, neuralgia, sinusitus, pharyngitis, tonsillitis, otitis, febrile diseases, dental pain following extractions, headache, bursitis, arthritis, rheumatism, low back pain, dislocations, strains, sprains, fractures, etc. The antitussive, antipyretic action of T-GESIC makes it particularly useful for the patient with upper respiratory infections such as acute cold, bronchitis, influenza and pneumonia.
Indications and Usage: For the relief of moderate to moderately severe pain.
Contraindications: Hypersensitivity to any of the components.
Intracranial lesion associated with increased intracranial pressure. Status asthmaticus. Liver disease.
Warnings:
Respiratory Depression: At high doses or in sensitive patients, hydrocodone may produce dose-related respiratory depression by acting directly on brain stem respiratory centers. Hydrocodone also effects centers that control respiratory rhythm, and may produce irregular and periodic breathing.
Head Injury and Increased Intracranial Pressure: The respiratory depressant effects of narcotics and their capacity to elevate cerebrospinal fluid pressure may be markedly exagerated in the presence of head injury, other intracranial lesions or a preexisting increase in intracranial pressure. Furthermore, narcotics produce adverse reactions which may obscure the clinical course of patients with head injuries.
Acute Abdominal Conditions: The administration of narcotics may obscure the diagnosis or clinical course of patients with acute abdominal conditions.
Precautions:
Special Risk Patients: As with any narcotic analgesic agent, T-GESIC should be used with caution in elderly or debilitated patients and those with severe impairment of hepatic or renal function, hypothyroidism, Addison's disease, prostatic hypertrophy or urethral stricture. The usual precautions should be observed and the possibility of respiratory depression should be kept in mind.
Usage in Ambulatory Patients: T-GESIC, like all narcotics, may impair the mental and/or physical abilities required for the performance of potentially hazardous tasks, such as driving a car or operating machinery. The patient should be cautioned accordingly. Central Nervous System depressant effects of butalbital may be additive with those of other CNS depressants. Concurrent use with other sedative-hypnotics or alcohol should be avoided. When such combined therapy is necessary, the dose of one or more agents may need to be reduced.
Cough Reflex: Hydrocodone suppresses the cough reflex; as with all narcotics, caution should be exercised when T-GESIC is used postoperatively and in patients with pulmonary disease.
Drug Interactions: Patients receiving other narcotic analgesics, general anesthetics, phenothiazines, other tranquilizers, sedative-hypnotics or other CNS depressants (including alcohol) concomitantly with T-GESIC may exhibit an additive CNS depression. When such combined therapy is contemplated, the dose of one or both agents should be reduced.
Usage in Pregnancy: Pregnancy Category C. Hydrocodone has been shown to be teratogenic in hamsters when given in doses 700 times the human dose. There are no adequate and well-controlled studies in pregnant women. T-GESIC should be used during pregnancy only if the potential benefit justifies the potential risk to the fetus.
Nonteratogenic Effects: Babies born to mothers who have been taking opioids regularly prior to delivery will be physically dependent. The withdrawal signs include irritability and excessive crying, tremors, hyperactive reflexes, increased respiratory rate, increased stools, sneezing, yawning, vomiting and fever. The intensity of the syndrome does not always correlate with the duration of maternal opioid use or dose. There is no consensus on the best method of managing withdrawal. Chlorpromazine 0.7 to 1.0 mg/kg q6h, phenobarbital 2 mg/kg q6h, and paregoric 2 to 4 drops/kg q4h, have been used to treat withdrawal symptoms in infants. The duration of therapy is 4 to 28 days, with the dosage decreased as tolerated.
Labor and Delivery: As with all narcotics, administration of T-GESIC to the mother shortly before delivery may result in some degree of respiratory depression in the newborn, especially if higher doses are used.
Nursing Mothers: It is not known whether this drug is excreted in human milk. Because many drugs are excreted in human milk and because of the potential for serious adverse reactions in nursing infants from T-GESIC, a decision should be made whether to discontinue nursing or to discontinue the drug, taking into account the importance of the drug to the mother.
Pediatric Use: Safety and effectiveness in children have not been established.
Adverse Reactions:
Central Nervous System: Sedation, drowsiness, mental clouding, lethargy, impairment of mental and physical performance, anxiety, fear, dysphoria, dizziness, psychic dependence, mood changes.
Gastrointestinal System: Nausea and vomiting may occur; they are more frequent in ambulatory then in recumbent patients. The antiemetic phenothiazines are useful in suppressing these effects; however, some phenothiazine derivatives seem to be antianalgesic and to increase the amount of narcotic required to produce pain relief, while other phenothiazines reduce the amount of narcotic required to produce a given level of analgesia. Prolonged administration of T-GESIC may produce constipation.
Genitourinary System: Ureteral spasm, spasm of vesical sphincters and urinary retention have been reported.
Respiratory Depression: T-GESIC may produce dose-related respiratory depression by acting directly on brain stem respiratory centers. Hydrocodone also affects centers that control respiratory rhythm, and may produce irregular and periodic breathing. If significant respiratory depression occurs, it may be antagonized by the use naloxone hydrochloride, 0.005 mg/kg intravenously. Apply other supportive measures when indicated.
Drug Abuse and Dependence: T-GESIC is a Schedule CIII narcotic. Psychic dependence, physical dependence, and tolerance may develop upon repeated administration of narcotics; therefore, T-GESIC should be prescribed and administered with caution. However, psychic dependence is unlikely to develop when T-GESIC is used for a short time for the treatment of pain. Physical dependence, the condition in which continued administration of the drug is required to prevent the appearance of a withdrawal syndrome, assumes clinically significant proportions only after several weeks of continued narcotic use, although some mild degree of physical dependence may develop after a few days of narcotic therapy. Tolerance, in which increasingly large doses are required in order to produce the same degree of analgesia, is manifested initially by a shortened duration of analgesic effect, and subsequently by decreases in the intensity of analgesia. The rate of development of tolerance varies among patients.
Overdosage: The toxic effects of acute overdosage are attributable mainly to hydrocodone and butalbital present in T-GESIC.
Signs and Symptoms: Serious overdosage with T-GESIC is characterized by respiratory depression (a decrease in respiratory rate and /or tidal volume, Cheyne-Stokes respiration, cyanosis), extreme somnolence progressing to stupor or coma, skeletal muscle flaccidity, cold and clammy skin, and sometimes bradycardia and hypotension. In severe overdosage, apnea circulatory collapse, cardiac arrest and death may occur.
Symptoms attributable to acute barbiturate poisoning include drowsiness, confusion and coma; respiratory depression; hypotension; shock. The ingestion of very large amounts of this drug may also result in acute hepatic toxicity. Clinical and laboratory evidence of hepatotoxicity may be delayed for up to one week. Close clinical monitoring and serial hepatic enzyme determinations are therefore recommended.
Because toxic effects of caffeine occur in very high dosages only, the possibility of significant caffeine toxicity from this drug overdose is unlikely.

Continued on next page

Williams—Cont.

Treatment: Gastric lavage or induced emesis may be useful in removing unabsorbed drug from conscious patients.
Primary attention should be given to the reestablishment of adequate respiratory exchange through provision of a patent airway and the institution of assisted or controlled ventilation. The narcotic antagonist naloxone hydrochloride is a specific antidote against respiratory depression which may result from overdosage or unusual sensitivity to narcotics, including hydrocodone. Therefore, 0.005 mg/kg of naloxone hydrochloride should be administered, preferably by the intravenous route, simultaneously with ventilatory assistance. Since the duration of action of hydrocodone may exceed that of the antagonist, the patient should be kept under continued surveillance; repeated doses of the antagonist may be required to maintain adequate respiration. An antagonist should not be administered in the absence of clinically significant respiratory or cardiovascular depression. Oxygen, intravenous fluids, vasopressors and other supportive measures should be employed as indicated.
Correction of hypotension may require the administration of levarterenol bitartrate or phenylephrine hydrochloride by intravenous infusion. Specific antidotal therapy may be indicated in severe acetaminophen overdoses characterized by ingestion of 10 to 15 grams of acetaminophen. Although not an approved indication for the drug, there are reports in the literature that an oral loading dose of acetylcysteine, 140 mg/kg diluted in cola, grapefruit juice or water to a final volume three times that of acetylcysteine alone, followed by 70 mg/kg every 4 hours for 68 hours, has been found successful. If severe vomiting precludes the oral route, the 20% acetylcysteine solution can be diluted to 5% isotonic solution and administered intravenously at the same dosage for at least 15 minutes. Charcoal and cathartics should not be given if oral specific antidose therapy is elected, as they may interfere with the absorption of antidotes. Transfusion may be required for acute hemolytic anemia in severe poisoning. Fluid and electrolyte balance must be maintained and vital signs checked every 4 hours.
Acetaminophen in massive overdosage may cause hepatotoxicity. Clinical and laboratory evidence of hepatotoxicity may be delayed for up to one week. Close clinical monitoring and serial hepatic enzyme determination are therefore recommended.
Dosage and Administration: T-GESIC is given orally. The usual adult dose is 1 capsule every 6 hours. In case of more severe pain, 1 capsule every 4 hours or 2 capsules every 8 hours. Not to exceed 8 capsules in 24 hours.
How Supplied: Capsules with scarlet red cap and black body. Imprinted: T.E.W. on the cap and T-GESIC on the body. Packaged in bottles of 100, NDC-51189-015-01, and in bottles of 1000, NDC-51189-015-02.
Storage: Store at room temperature.
Revised November 1981

T-MOIST TABLETS ℞

Description: Each scored, long-acting tablet contains:
Pseudoephedrine Hydrochloride ....120 mg
Guaifenesin ....500 mg
in a special base to provide a prolonged effect.
Actions: Pseudoephedrine Hydrochloride is an effective vasoconstrictor that decongests swollen mucous membranes of the respiratory tract. The expectorant Guaifenesin enhances the flow of respiratory tract fluid, promotes ciliary action and facilitates removal of viscous, inspissated mucus. As a result, sinus, bronchial and Eustachian tube drainage is improved, and dry, nonproductive coughs become more productive and less frequent.
Indications: T-Moist is indicated in respiratory conditions such as sinusitis, pharyngitis, bronchitis and asthma, when these conditions are complicated by tenacious mucus and/or mucous plugs and congestion. T-Moist is also indicated as adjunctive therapy in serious Otitis Media and may be of value in avoiding secondary middle ear complications of nasopharyngeal congestion accompanying rhinitis.
Contraindications: T-Moist is contraindicated in individuals with known hypersensitivity to sympathomimetics, severe hypertension or in patients receiving MAO inhibitors.
Usage in Pregnancy: Since the safety of T-Moist for use in pregnancy has not been established, potential benefits should be weighed against possible adverse effects. This product should not be used by nursing mothers.
Precautions: DO NOT CRUSH OR CHEW T-MOIST TABLETS BEFORE INGESTION TO PRESERVE THE LONG-ACTING EFFECT. As with other sympathomimetics drugs, T-Moist should be used with caution in the presence of hypertension, hyperthyroidism, diabetes, heart disease, peripheral vascular disease, glaucoma and prostatic hypertrophy.
Adverse Reactions: Possible adverse reactions include nervousness, insomnia, restlessness or headache. These reactions seldom, if ever require discontinuation of therapy. Urinary retention may occur in patients with prostatic hypertrophy.
Overdosage: Since the effects of T-Moist may last up to 12 hours, treatment of overdosage directed towards supporting the patient and reversing the effects of the drug should be continued for at least that length of time.
Saline Cathartics may be useful in hastening the evacuation of unreleased medication.
Dosage: Adults and children over 12: 1 tablet twice daily (every 12 hours).
Not recommended for children under 12 years of age. Tablets may be broken in half for ease of administration without affecting release of medication but not crushed or chewed.
How Supplied: Bottles of 100 (NDC-51189-018-01)
Manufactured by: Mikart, Inc. Atlanta, Georgia 30318
Distributed by: T. E. Williams Pharmaceuticals, Inc. Edmond, Oklahoma 73083
Revised 07/82

Winthrop Laboratories
90 PARK AVENUE
NEW YORK, NY 10016

AMIPAQUE® ℞
brand of metrizamide

(See Diagnostic Section.)

ARALEN® Hydrochloride ℞
brand of chloroquine hydrochloride injection, USP

For Malaria and Extraintestinal Amebiasis

WARNING: PHYSICIANS SHOULD COMPLETELY FAMILIARIZE THEMSELVES WITH THE COMPLETE CONTENTS OF THIS LEAFLET BEFORE PRESCRIBING ARALEN.

Description: Parenteral solution, each ml containing 50 mg of the dihydrochloride salt equivalent to 40 mg of chloroquine base. ARALEN hydrochloride, a 4-aminoquinoline compound, is chemically 7-(chloro-4-[[4-diethylamino)-1-methylbutyl] amino] quinoline dihydrochloride (1:2), a white, crystalline substance, freely soluble in water.
Actions: The compound is a highly active antimalarial and amebicidal agent.
ARALEN hydrochloride has been found to be highly active against the erythrocytic forms of *Plasmodium vivax* and *malariae* and most strains of *Plasmodium falciparum* (but not the gametocytes of *P. falciparum).* The precise mechanism of action of the drug is not known.
ARALEN hydrochloride does not prevent relapses in patients with vivax or malariae malaria because it is not effective against exoerythrocytic forms of the parasite, nor will it prevent vivax or malariae infection when administered as a prophylactic. It is highly effective as a suppressive agent in patients with vivax or malariae malaria, in terminating acute attacks, and significantly lengthening the interval between treatment and relapse. In patients with falciparum malaria it abolishes the acute attack and effects complete cure of the infection, unless due to a resistant strain of *P. falciparum.*
Indications: ARALEN hydrochloride is indicated for the treatment of extraintestinal amebiasis and for treatment of acute attacks of malaria due to *P. vivax, P. malariae, P. ovale,* and susceptible strains of *P. falciparum* when oral therapy is not feasible.
Contraindications: Use of this drug is contraindicated in the presence of retinal or visual field changes either attributable to 4-aminoquinoline compounds or to any other etiology, and in patients with known hypersensitivity to 4-aminoquinoline compounds. However, in the treatment of acute attacks of malaria caused by susceptible strains of plasmodia, the physician may elect to use this drug after carefully weighing the possible benefits and risks to the patient.
Warnings: *Children and infants are extremely susceptible to adverse effects from an overdose of parenteral ARALEN and sudden deaths have been recorded after such administration. In no instance should the single dose of parenteral ARALEN administered to infants or children exceed 5 mg base per kg.*
In recent years it has been found that certain strains of *P. falciparum* have become resistant to 4-aminoquinoline compounds (including chloroquine and hydroxychloroquine) as shown by the fact that normally adequate doses have failed to prevent or cure clinical malaria or parasitemia. Treatment with quinine or other specific forms of therapy is therefore advised for patients infected with a resistant strain of parasites.
Use of ARALEN should be avoided in patients with psoriasis, for it may precipitate a severe attack of psoriasis. Some authors consider the use of 4-aminoquinoline compounds contraindicated in patients with porphyria since the condition may be exacerbated.
Irreversible retinal damage has been observed in some patients who had received long-term or high-dosage 4-aminoquinoline therapy. Retinopathy has been reported to be dose related. If there is any indication (past or present) of abnormality in the visual acuity, visual field, or retinal macular areas (such as pigmentary changes, loss of foveal reflex), or any visual symptoms (such as light flashes and streaks) which are not fully explainable by difficulties of accommodation or corneal opacities, the drug should be discontinued immediately and the patient closely observed for possible progression. Retinal changes (and visual disturbances) may progress even after cessation of therapy.
Usage in Pregnancy. Usage of this drug during pregnancy should be avoided except in the suppression or treatment of malaria when in the judgment of the physician the benefit outweighs the possible hazard. It should be noted that radioactively tagged chloroquine administered intravenously to pregnant pigmented CBA mice passed rapidly across the placenta,

accumulated selectively in the melanin structures of the fetal eyes and was retained in the ocular tissues for five months after the drug had been eliminated from the rest of the body.[1]

Precautions: Since the drug is known to concentrate in the liver, it should be used with caution in patients with hepatic disease or alcoholism or in conjunction with known hepatotoxic drugs.

The drug should be administered with caution to patients having G-6-PD (glucose-6-phosphate dehydrogenase) deficiency.

Adverse Reactions: Respiratory depression, cardiovascular collapse, shock, convulsions, and death have been reported with overdoses of ARALEN hydrochloride, brand of chloroquine hydrochloride injection, especially in infants and children.

Any of the adverse reactions associated with short-term oral administration of chloroquine phosphate must be considered a possibility with chloroquine hydrochloride. Cardiovascular effects, such as hypotension and electrocardiographic changes (particularly inversion or depression of the T-wave, widening of the QRS complex), have rarely been noted in patients receiving usual antimalarial doses of the drug. Mild and transient headache, pruritus, psychic stimulation, visual disturbances (blurring of vision and difficulty of focusing or accommodation), pleomorphic skin eruptions, and gastrointestinal complaints (anorexia, nausea, vomiting, diarrhea, abdominal cramps) have been observed.

Instances of convulsive seizures associated with oral chloroquine therapy in patients with extraintestinal amebiasis have been reported.

A few cases of a nerve type of deafness have been reported after prolonged therapy, usually in high doses. Tinnitus and reduced hearing have been reported, in a patient with preexistent auditory damage, after administration of only 500 mg once a week for a few months.

Since neuromyopathy, blood dyscrasias, lichen planus-like eruptions, and skin and mucosal pigmentary changes have been noted during prolonged oral therapy, their occurrence with this dosage form is possible.

Patients with retinal changes may be asymptomatic, especially in early cases, or may complain of nyctalopia and scotomatous vision with field defects of paracentral, pericentral ring types, and typically temporal scotomas, e.g., difficulty in reading with words tending to disappear, seeing only half an object, misty vision, and fog before the eyes. Rarely scotomatous vision may occur without observable retinal changes.

Dosage and Administration: *Malaria—*

Adult Dose. An initial dose of 4 or 5 ml (160 to 200 mg chloroquine base) may be injected intramuscularly and repeated in 6 hours if necessary. The total parenteral dosage in the first 24 hours should not exceed 800 mg chloroquine base. Treatment by mouth should be started as soon as practicable and continued until a course of approximately 1.5 g of base in 3 days is completed.

Pediatric Dose. Infants and children are extremely susceptible to overdosage of parenteral ARALEN. Severe reactions and deaths have occurred. In the pediatric age range, parenteral ARALEN dosage should be calculated in proportion to the adult dose based upon body weight. The recommended single dose in infants and children is 5 mg base per kg. This dose may be repeated in 6 hours; however, the total dose in any 24 hour period should not exceed 10 mg base per kg of body weight. Parenteral administration should be terminated and oral therapy instituted as soon as possible.

Extraintestinal Amebiasis—In adult patients not able to tolerate oral therapy, from 4 to 5 ml (160 to 200 mg chloroquine base) may be injected daily for 10 to 12 days. Oral administration should be substituted or resumed as soon as possible.

Overdosage: Inadvertent toxic doses may produce respiratory depression or shock with hypotension. Respiratory depression is treated by artificial respiration and administration of oxygen. In shock with hypotension, a potent vasopressor, such as NEO-SYNEPHRINE® hydrochloride, brand of phenylephrine hydrochloride, USP, should be given intramuscularly in doses of 2 to 5 mg.

How Supplied: Ampuls of 5 ml, boxes of 5.

Reference: 1. Ullberg, S., Lindquist, N. G., and Sjostrand, S. E.: Accumulation of chorio-retinotoxic drugs in the foetal eye, *Nature* *227*:1257, Sept. 19, 1970.

ARALEN® Phosphate ℞

brand of chloroquine phosphate tablets, USP

For Malaria and Extraintestinal Amebiasis

WARNING: PHYSICIANS SHOULD COMPLETELY FAMILIARIZE THEMSELVES WITH THE COMPLETE CONTENTS OF THIS LEAFLET BEFORE PRESCRIBING ARALEN.

Description: ARALEN phosphate, a 4-aminoquinoline compound, is chemically 7-chloro-4-[[4- (diethylamino) -1-methylbutyl]amino]-quinoline phosphate (1:2), a white, crystalline substance, freely soluble in water.

Actions: ARALEN phosphate has been found to be highly active against the erythrocytic forms of *Plasmodium vivax* and *malariae* and most strains of *Plasmodium falciparum* (but not the gametocytes of *P. falciparum*). The precise mechanism of action of the drug is not known.

ARALEN phosphate does not prevent relapses in patients with vivax or malariae malaria because it is not effective against exo-erythrocytic forms of the parasite, nor will it prevent vivax or malariae infection when administered as a prophylactic. It is highly effective as a suppressive agent in patients with vivax or malariae malaria, in terminating acute attacks, and significantly lengthening the interval between treatment and relapse. In patients with falciparum malaria it abolishes the acute attack and effects complete cure of the infection, unless due to a resistant strain of *P. falciparum*.

In vitro studies with trophozoites of *Entamoeba histolytica* have demonstrated that ARALEN phosphate also possesses amebicidal activity comparable to that of emetine.

Indications: ARALEN phosphate is indicated for the suppressive treatment and for acute attacks of malaria due to *P. vivax, P. malariae, P. ovale,* and susceptible strains of *P. falciparum.* The drug is also indicated for treatment of extraintestinal amebiasis.

Contraindications: Use of this drug is contraindicated in the presence of retinal or visual field changes either attributable to 4- aminoquinoline compounds or to any other etiology, and in patients with known hypersensitivity to 4-aminoquinoline compounds. However, in the treatment of acute attacks of malaria caused by susceptible strains of plasmodia, the physician may elect to use this drug after carefully weighing the possible benefits and risks to the patient.

Warnings: In recent years it has been found that certain strains of *P. falciparum* have become resistant to 4-aminoquinoline compounds (including chloroquine and hydroxychloroquine) as shown by the fact that normally adequate doses have failed to prevent or cure clinical malaria or parasitemia. Treatment with quinine or other specific forms of therapy is therefore advised for patients infected with a resistant strain of parasites.

Irreversible retinal damage has been observed in some patients who had received long-term or high-dosage 4-aminoquinoline therapy. Retinopathy has been reported to be dose related. When prolonged therapy with any antimalarial compound is contemplated, initial (base line) and periodic ophthalmologic examinations (including visual acuity, expert slit-lamp, funduscopic, and visual field tests) should be performed.

If there is any indication (past or present) of abnormality in the visual acuity, visual field, or retinal macular areas (such as pigmentary changes, loss of foveal reflex), or any visual symptoms (such as light flashes and streaks) which are not fully explainable by difficulties of accommodation or corneal opacities, the drug should be discontinued immediately and the patient closely observed for possible progression. Retinal changes (and visual disturbances) may progress even after cessation of therapy.

All patients on long-term therapy with this preparation should be questioned and examined periodically, including testing knee and ankle reflexes, to detect any evidence of muscular weakness. If weakness occurs, discontinue the drug.

A number of fatalities have been reported following the accidental ingestion of chloroquine, sometimes in relatively small doses (0.75 or 1 g chloroquine phosphate in one 3-year-old child). Patients should be strongly warned to keep this drug out of the reach of children because they are especially sensitive to the 4- aminoquinoline compounds.

Use of ARALEN phosphate, brand of chloroquine phosphate tablets, in patients with psoriasis may precipitate a severe attack of psoriasis. When used in patients with porphyria the condition may be exacerbated. The drug should not be used in these conditions unless in the judgment of the physician the benefit to the patient outweighs the possible hazard.

Usage in Pregnancy. Usage of this drug during pregnancy should be avoided except in the suppression or treatment of malaria when in the judgment of the physician the benefit outweighs the possible hazard. It should be noted that radioactively tagged chloroquine administered intravenously to pregnant pigmented CBA mice passed rapidly across the placenta, accumulated selectively in the melanin structures of the fetal eyes and was retained in the ocular tissues for five months after the drug had been eliminated from the rest of the body.[1]

Precautions: Since the drug is known to concentrate in the liver, it should be used with caution in patients with hepatic disease or alcoholism or in conjunction with known hepatotoxic drugs.

Complete blood cell counts should be made periodically if patients are given prolonged therapy. If any severe blood disorder appears which is not attributable to the disease under treatment, discontinuance of the drug should be considered. The drug should be administered with caution to patients having G-6-PD (glucose-6-phosphate dehydrogenase) deficiency.

Adverse Reactions: Following the administration of ARALEN phosphate in doses adequate for the treatment of an acute malarial attack or extraintestinal amebiasis, mild and transient headache, pruritus, gastrointestinal complaints (anorexia, nausea, vomiting, diar-

Continued on next page

This product information was effective as of November 19, 1982. On these and other products of Winthrop Laboratories, detailed information may be obtained on a current basis by direct inquiry to the Professional Services Department, 90 Park Avenue, New York, NY 10016 (212) 907-2525.

Winthrop—Cont.

rhea, abdominal cramps), psychic stimulation, and rarely psychotic episodes or convulsions have been observed. Cardiovascular effects, such as hypotension and electrocardiographic changes (particularly inversion or depression of the T-wave, widening of the QRS complex), have rarely been noted in patients receiving usual antimalarial doses of the drug. A few cases of a nerve type of deafness have been reported after prolonged therapy, usually in high doses. Tinnitus and reduced hearing have been reported, in a patient with preexistent auditory damage, after administration of only 500 mg once a week for a few months. Neuromyopathy, blood dyscrasias, lichen planus-like eruptions, and skin and mucosal pigmentary changes have also been noted during prolonged therapy.

When employed for the indications (malaria and extraintestinal amebiasis) and in the dosages recommended in this leaflet, visual disturbances, consisting of blurring of vision or difficulty in focusing or accommodation, occasionally may be noted; they are reversible and disappear on discontinuation of therapy. Other types of visual disturbances and ocular complications have been reported during the use of chloroquine for long-term therapy usually in daily doses exceeding 250 mg of chloroquine phosphate. These consisted of (1) reversible corneal changes (transient edema or opaque deposits in the epithelium) which may be asymptomatic or cause visual halos, focusing difficulties, or blurred vision and (2) generally irreversible, sometimes progressive, or, rarely delayed, retinal changes, such as narrowing of the arterioles, macular lesions (loss of foveal reflex, areas of edema, atrophy, and abnormal pigmentation), pallor of the optic disc, optic atrophy, and patchy retinal pigmentation.

Patients with retinal changes may be asymptomatic, especially in early cases, or may complain of nyctalopia and scotomatous vision with field defects of paracentral, pericentral ring types, and typically temporal scotomas, e.g., difficulty in reading with words tending to disappear, seeing only half an object, misty vision, and fog before the eyes. Rarely scotomatous vision may occur without observable retinal changes.

Dosage and Administration: The dosage of chloroquine phosphate is often expressed or calculated as the base. Each 500 mg tablet of ARALEN phosphate, brand of chloroquine phosphate tablets, is equivalent to 300 mg base. In infants and children the dosage is preferably calculated on the body weight.

Malaria: Suppression — **In adults,** 500 mg (= 300 mg base) on exactly the same day of each week. **In infants and children** the weekly suppressive dosage is 5 mg, calculated as base, per kg of body weight, but should not exceed the adult dose regardless of weight.

If circumstances permit, suppressive therapy should begin two weeks prior to exposure. However, failing this in adults, an initial double (loading) dose of 1 g (= 600 mg base), or in children 10 mg base/kg may be taken in two divided doses, six hours apart. The suppressive therapy should be continued for eight weeks after leaving the endemic area.

Treatment of the acute attack—**In adults,** an initial dose of 1 g (= 600 mg base) followed by an additional 500 mg (= 300 mg base) after six to eight hours and a single dose of 500 mg (= 300 mg base) on each of two consecutive days. This represents a total dose of 2.5 g chloroquine phosphate or 1.5 g base in three days.

The dosage for adults may also be calculated on the basis of body weight; this method is preferred for infants and children. A total dose representing 25 mg of base per kg of body weight is administered in three days, as follows:

First dose: 10 mg base per kg (but not exceeding a single dose of 600 mg base).

Second dose: 5 mg base per kg (but not exceeding a single dose of 300 mg base) 6 hours after first dose.

Third dose: 5 mg base per kg 18 hours after second dose.

Fourth dose: 5 mg base per kg 24 hours after third dose.

For radical cure of *vivax* and *malariae* malaria concomitant therapy with an 8- aminoquinoline compound is necessary.

Extraintestinal Amebiasis: Adults, 1 g (600 mg base) daily for two days, followed by 500 mg (300 mg base) daily for at least two to three weeks. Treatment is usually combined with an effective intestinal amebicide.

Overdosage: Chloroquine is very rapidly and completely absorbed after ingestion, and in accidental overdosage, or rarely with lower doses in hypersensitive patients, toxic symptoms may occur within thirty minutes. These consist of headache, drowsiness, visual disturbances, cardiovascular collapse, and convulsions followed by sudden and early respiratory and cardiac arrest. The electrocardiogram may reveal atrial standstill, nodal rhythm, prolonged intraventricular conduction time, and progressive bradycardia leading to ventricular fibrillation and/or arrest. Treatment is symptomatic and must be prompt with immediate evacuation of the stomach by emesis (at home, before transportation to the hospital) or gastric lavage until the stomach is completely emptied. If finely powdered, activated charcoal is introduced by stomach tube, after lavage, and within 30 minutes after ingestion of the antimalarial, it may inhibit further intestinal absorption of the drug. To be effective, the dose of activated charcoal should be at least five times the estimated dose of chloroquine ingested.

Convulsions, if present, should be controlled before attempting gastric lavage. If due to cerebral stimulation, cautious administration of an ultrashort-acting barbiturate may be tried but, if due to anoxia, it should be corrected by oxygen administration, artificial respiration or, in shock with hypotension, by vasopressor therapy. Because of the importance of supporting respiration, tracheal intubation or tracheostomy, followed by gastric lavage, may also be necessary. Peritoneal dialysis and exchange transfusions have also been suggested to reduce the level of the drug in the blood.

A patient who survives the acute phase and is asymptomatic should be closely observed for at least six hours. Fluids may be forced, and sufficient ammonium chloride (8 g daily in divided doses for adults) may be administered for a few days to acidify the urine to help promote urinary excretion in cases of both overdosage or sensitivity.

How Supplied: Tablets of 500 mg (= 300 mg base), bottles of 25.

Reference: 1. Ullberg, S., Lindquist, N. G., and Sjostrand, S. E.: Accumulation of chorio-retinotoxic drugs in the foetal eye, *Nature 227:* 1257, Sept. 19, 1970.

[*Shown in Product Identification Section*]

ARALEN® Phosphate ℞
brand of chloroquine phosphate, USP
with
PRIMAQUINE Phosphate, USP

For Malaria Prophylaxis Only

WARNING: PHYSICIANS SHOULD COMPLETELY FAMILIARIZE THEMSELVES WITH THE COMPLETE CONTENTS OF THIS LEAFLET BEFORE PRESCRIBING ARALEN PHOSPHATE WITH PRIMAQUINE PHOSPHATE.

Description: Each tablet contains ARALEN phosphate, brand of chloroquine phosphate, USP, 500 mg (equivalent to 300 mg base) and primaquine phosphate 79 mg (equivalent to 45 mg base).

Actions: ARALEN is a 4-aminoquinoline compound which is highly active against the erythrocytic forms of *Plasmodium vivax* and most strains of *Plasmodium falciparum* (but not the gametocytes of *P. falciparum).*

Primaquine is an 8-aminoquinoline compound which eliminates tissue (exo-erythrocytic) infection. Thereby, it prevents the development of the blood (erythrocytic) forms of the parasite which are responsible for relapses in vivax malaria. Primaquine phosphate is active against gametocytes of *P. falciparum.*

ARALEN phosphate with primaquine phosphate demonstrates antimalarial activity against all stages of human-malaria parasites, except for certain strains of *P. falciparum* resistant to chloroquine.

Indication: ARALEN phosphate with primaquine phosphate is intended solely for use in the prophylaxis of malaria, regardless of species, in all areas where this disease is endemic.

Contraindications: The drug is contraindicated in acutely ill patients suffering from systemic disease manifested by tendency to granulocytopenia, such as rheumatoid arthritis and lupus erythematosus. The drug is also contraindicated in those patients receiving concurrently other potentially hemolytic drugs or depressants of myeloid elements of the bone marrow.

Primaquine should not be administered to patients who have received quinacrine recently, as toxicity is increased.

Warnings: Children are especially sensitive to 4-aminoquinoline compounds. A number of fatalities have been reported following the accidental ingestion of chloroquine, sometimes in relatively small doses (0.75 or 1 g in one 3- year-old child). Patients should be strongly warned to keep these drugs out of the reach of children. Hemolytic reactions (moderate to severe) may occur after even a weekly dose of this preparation in glucose-6-phosphate dehydrogenase (G-6-PD) deficient Caucasians (particularly, in Sardinians and in individuals with a family or personal history of favism).

Usage in Pregnancy. Safe usage of this preparation in pregnancy has not been established. Therefore, use of it during pregnancy should be avoided except when in the judgment of the physician the benefit outweighs the possible hazard. It should be noted that radioactively tagged chloroquine administered intravenously to pregnant pigmented CBA mice passed rapidly across the placenta, accumulated selectively in the melanin structures of the fetal eyes and was retained in the ocular tissues for five months after the drug had been eliminated from the rest of the body.[1]

Precautions: ARALEN phosphate, brand of chloroquine phosphate, with primaquine phosphate is intended for malaria prophylaxis only; it should not be used for the treatment of clinical malaria. The recommended dosage (one tablet weekly, on the same day each week) should not be exceeded. The drug should not be taken more often than once every seven days to minimize danger of toxicity.

If the combination is prescribed for (1) an individual who has shown a previous idiosyncrasy to either chloroquine or primaquine (as manifested by dermatitis, hemolytic anemia, methemoglobinemia, or leukopenia), (2) an individual with a family or personal history of favism, or (3) an individual with erythrocytic glucose-6-phosphate dehydrogenase (G-6-PD) deficiency or nicotinamide adenine dinucleotide (NADH) methemoglobin reductase deficiency, the person should be observed closely for tolerance. The drug should be discontinued immediately if marked darkening of the urine, sudden decrease in hemoglobin concentration or leukocyte count, or severe skin reaction occurs.

In areas with endemic falciparum malaria due to strains that are resistant to the 4-aminoquinolines (chloroquine, amodiaquine, hydroxychloroquine), chemoprophylaxis with this combination alone may not be effective.

Adverse Reactions: *Gastrointestinal reactions:* anorexia, nausea, vomiting, epigastric distress, and abdominal cramps. *Hematologic reactions:* leukopenia, hemolytic anemia in glucose-6-phosphate dehydrogenase (G-6-PD) deficient individuals, methemoglobinemia in nicotinamide adenine dinucleotide (NADH) methemoglobin reductase deficient individuals.

Cardiovascular effects, such as hypotension and electrocardiographic changes (particularly inversion or depression of the T-wave, widening of the QRS complex), have rarely been noted in patients receiving usual antimalarial doses of the drug.

Visual disturbances, consisting of blurring of vision or difficulty in focusing or accommodation, have occasionally been noted when chloroquine has been employed for malaria. These symptoms are reversible and disappear on discontinuation of therapy. Other types of visual disturbances (reversible corneal changes) and ocular complications including retinal changes (narrowing of the arterioles, macular lesions, pallor of the optic disc, optic atrophy, and patchy retinal pigmentation) have been reported during the use of chloroquine for long-term therapy usually in daily doses exceeding 250 mg of chloroquine phosphate. These changes have not been reported with the use of ARALEN phosphate, brand of chloroquine phosphate, with primaquine phosphate for malaria prophylaxis.

Auditory disturbances: tinnitus and reduced hearing have been reported, in a patient with preexistent auditory damage, after administration of only 500 mg of ARALEN phosphate, brand of chloroquine phosphate, once a week for a few months.

Dosage and Administration:

Adults—Starting at least one day before entering the malarious area, one tablet weekly, taken on the same day each week. This schedule (one tablet weekly) should be continued for eight weeks after leaving the endemic area.

Children—The following dosage, based on body weight, is suggested.

Weight (lb)	ARALEN base (mg)	Primaquine base (mg)	Dose* (ml)
10-15	20	3	2.5
16-25	40	6	5.0
26-35	60	9	7.5
36-45	80	12	10.0
46-55	100	15	12.5
56-100	150	22.5	½ tab.
100+	300	45	1 tab.

*Dose based on liquid containing approximately 40 mg of chloroquine base and 6 mg of primaquine base per 5 ml (1 teaspoon) prepared from ARALEN phosphate, brand of chloroquine phosphate, with primaquine phosphate tablets. Chocolate syrup could be used to prepare a suspension (one tablet crushed and suspended in 40 ml of liquid). Shake well before use.

Overdosage: Symptoms of overdosage are due to the two drug components.

Chloroquine is very rapidly and completely absorbed after ingestion, and in accidental overdosage, or rarely with lower doses in hypersensitive patients, toxic symptoms may occur within thirty minutes. These consist of headache, drowsiness, visual disturbances, cardiovascular collapse, and convulsions followed by sudden and early respiratory and cardiac arrest. The electrocardiogram may reveal atrial standstill, nodal rhythm, prolonged intraventricular conduction time, and progressive bradycardia leading to ventricular fibrillation and/or arrest.

Symptoms of overdosage of primaquine are similar to those seen after overdosage of pamaquine. They include abdominal cramps, vomiting, burning epigastric distress, central nervous system and cardiovascular disturbances, cyanosis, methemoglobinemia, moderate leukocytosis or leukopenia, and anemia. The most striking symptoms are granulocytopenia and acute hemolytic anemia in sensitive persons. Acute hemolysis occurs, but patients recover completely if the dosage is discontinued.

Treatment is symptomatic and must be prompt with immediate evacuation of the stomach by emesis (at home, before transportation to the hospital) or gastric lavage until the stomach is completely emptied. Finely powdered, activated charcoal in a dose not less than five times the estimated dose of chloroquine ingested, if introduced by the stomach tube after lavage within thirty minutes after ingestion of the antimalarial, may inhibit further intestinal absorption of the drug.

Convulsions, if present, should be controlled before attempting gastric lavage. If due to cerebral stimulation, cautious administration of an ultrashort-acting barbiturate may be tried but, if due to anoxia, it should be corrected by oxygen administration, artificial respiration or, in shock with hypotension, by vasopressor therapy. Because of the importance of supporting respiration, tracheal intubation or tracheostomy, followed by gastric lavage, may also be necessary. Exchange transfusions have also been suggested to reduce the level of the drug in the blood.

The patient should be kept in bed and warm. If methemoglobinemia and cyanosis occur, oxygen may be administered and use of methylene blue may be considered. If collapse and hypotension or shock occur, vasopressors may be used. The patient should be observed for the possible development of leukopenia or hemolytic anemia.

A patient who survives the acute stage and is asymptomatic should be closely observed for at least six hours. Fluids may be forced, and sufficient ammonium chloride (8 g daily in divided doses for adults) may be administered for a few days to acidify the urine to help promote urinary excretion in cases of both overdosage or sensitivity.

How Supplied: Tablets, bottles of 100.

Clinical Studies: On the basis of carefully controlled preliminary clinical trials, Alving and his associates[2] found that the weekly administration of 300 mg chloroquine base and 45 mg primaquine base (administered as the phosphate salts) proved highly effective as a prophylactic against severe *P. vivax* infections with the Chesson strain and did not produce clinical hemolysis even among primaquine-sensitive American Negro adult volunteers. A weekly dose of primaquine phosphate equivalent to 45 mg primaquine base cured 90 per cent of infections.

The studies of these workers indicate that the toxicity of primaquine phosphate, as regards the production of hemolysis, is markedly diminished when administered in weekly doses. When administered with standard suppressive doses of chloroquine phosphate, its therapeutic effectiveness in the radical cure of Chesson vivax malaria is increased. Thus, a weekly dose equivalent to 60 mg of primaquine base is less toxic than 15 mg base administered daily; and a dose equivalent to 45 mg base administered weekly was found to be practically without demonstrable toxicity. A dose equivalent to 45 mg base weekly for 8 weeks was more effective in the radical cure of infections than 15 mg base daily for 14 days.

Wittmer[3] conducted a double-blind study in 24 Caucasian male adults who received ARALEN phosphate, brand of chloroquine phosphate, with primaquine phosphate once each week (Friday) for 15 weeks to determine its safety and suitability for use in Armed Forces flying personnel. The author concluded that there appear to be no contraindications to the long-term use of the combination in flying personnel since there was no effect on vision, time of useful consciousness, or psychomotor performance. No deleterious synergistic effect of the two drugs was demonstrated. Charles[4] investigated the effects of 5 weekly doses of primaquine phosphate (1 to 1.5 mg base per kg body weight) in combination with a 4-aminoquinoline antimalarial agent on the parasitemia and blood picture of 100 Ghanaian children from 2½ to 8 years old. Although the enzyme-deficiency trait (glucose-6-phosphate dehydrogenase deficiency) for primaquine sensitivity occurred in approximately 25 per cent of the group, no general evidence of hemolysis was observed. Eight of the treated subjects were positive for the glucose-6-phosphate dehydrogenase deficiency test but maintained their pretreatment hemoglobin values.

However, Ziai and his associates[5] noted that serious hematologic reactions can occur in persons with a glucose-6-phosphate dehydrogenase (G-6-PD) deficiency with the small weekly doses of chloroquine-primaquine used for malaria suppressive therapy. This has been reported primarily in patients with a family history and/or personal history of favism.

Methemoglobinemia has been discovered in individuals with nicotinamide adenine dinucleotide methemoglobin reductase deficiency.[6]

The susceptibility of primaquine-sensitive children to hemolysis by primaquine phosphate is considered to be of the same order of magnitude as that of adults on an equal drug/body weight basis.

References:

1. Ullberg, S., Lindquist, N. G., and Sjostrand, S. E.: Accumulation of chorio-retinotoxic drugs in the foetal eye, *Nature 227*:1257, Sept. 19, 1970.
2. Alving, A. S. *et al.:* Mitigation of the haemolytic effect of primaquine and enhancement of its action against exo-erythrocytic forms of the Chesson strain of *Plasmodium vivax* by intermittent regimens of drug administration, *Bull. WHO 22:*621, 1960.
3. Wittmer, J. F.: Aeromedical aspects of malaria prophylaxis with chloroquine-primaquine, *Aerospace Med. 34:*944, Oct. 1963.
4. Charles, L. J.: Observations on the haemolytic effect of primaquine in 100 Ghanaian children, *Ann. Trop. Med. 54:*460, Dec. 1960.
5. Ziai, M. *et al.:* Malaria prophylaxis and treatment in G-6-PD deficiency, *Clin. Pediat. 6:*242, April 1967.
6. Cohen, R. *et al.:* Methemoglobinemia provoked by malarial chemoprophylaxis in Vietnam, *New Eng. J. Med. 279:*1127-1131, Nov. 21, 1968.

BILOPAQUE® SODIUM ℞

brand of tyropanoate sodium, USP

(See Diagnostic Section.)

BRONKAID® Mist **OTC**

(See PDR For Nonprescription Drugs)

BRONKAID® Mist Suspension **OTC**

(See PDR For Nonprescription Drugs)

Continued on next page

This product information was effective as of November 19, 1982. On these and other products of Winthrop Laboratories, detailed information may be obtained on a current basis by direct inquiry to the Professional Services Department, 90 Park Avenue, New York, NY 10016 (212) 907-2525.

Winthrop—Cont.

BRONKAID® Tablets OTC

(See PDR For Nonprescription Drugs)

CAMPHO-PHENIQUE® OTC
Liquid and Gel

(See PDR For Nonprescription Drugs)

DANOCRINE® ℞
brand of danazol capsules, USP

Description: DANOCRINE, brand of danazol, is a synthetic androgen derived from ethisterone. Chemically, danazol is 17α-pregna-2,4-dien-20-yno[2,3-*d*]-isoxazol-17-ol.

Clinical Pharmacology: DANOCRINE suppresses the pituitary-ovarian axis by inhibiting the output of gonadotropins from the pituitary gland. The only other demonstrable hormonal effect is weak androgenic activity which is dose related. Studies have established that the drug is neither estrogenic nor progestational. DANOCRINE depresses the output of both follicle-stimulating hormone (FSH) and luteinizing hormone (LH).

Recent evidence suggests a direct inhibitory effect at gonadal sites and a binding of DANOCRINE to receptors of gonadal steroids at target organs.

Bioavailability studies indicate that blood levels do not increase proportionally with increases in the administered dose. When the dose of DANOCRINE is doubled the increase in plasma levels is only about 35% to 40%.

In the treatment of endometriosis, DANOCRINE alters the normal and ectopic endometrial tissue so that it becomes inactive and atrophic. Complete resolution of endometrial lesions occurs in the majority of cases.

Changes in vaginal cytology and cervical mucus reflect the suppressive effect of DANOCRINE on the pituitary-ovarian axis.

In the treatment of fibrocystic breast disease, DANOCRINE usually produces partial to complete disappearance of nodularity and complete relief of pain and tenderness. Changes in the menstrual pattern may occur.

Generally the pituitary-suppressive action of DANOCRINE is reversible. Ovulation and cyclic bleeding usually return within 60 to 90 days when DANOCRINE therapy is discontinued.

In the treatment of hereditary angioedema, DANOCRINE at effective doses prevents attacks of the disease characterized by episodic edema of the abdominal viscera, extremities, face, and airway which may be disabling and, if the airway is involved, fatal. In addition, DANOCRINE corrects partially or completely the primary biochemical abnormality of hereditary angioedema by increasing the levels of the deficient C1 esterase inhibitor (C1EI). As a result of this action the serum levels of the C4 component of the complement system are also increased.

Indications and Usage: *Endometriosis.* DANOCRINE is indicated for the treatment of endometriosis amenable to hormonal management.

Fibrocystic Breast Disease. Most cases of symptomatic fibrocystic breast disease may be treated by simple measures (eg, padded brassieres and analgesics).

In infrequent patients, symptoms of pain and tenderness may be severe enough to warrant treatment by suppression of ovarian function. DANOCRINE is usually effective in decreasing nodularity, pain, and tenderness. It should be stressed to the patient that this treatment is not innocuous in that it involves considerable alterations of hormone levels and that recurrence of symptoms is very common after cessation of therapy.

Hereditary Angioedema. DANOCRINE is indicated for the prevention of attacks of angioedema of all types (cutaneous, abdominal, laryngeal) in males and females.

Contraindications: DANOCRINE should not be administered to patients with:

1. Undiagnosed abnormal genital bleeding.
2. Markedly impaired hepatic, renal, or cardiac function.
3. Pregnancy.
4. Breast feeding.

Warnings: Safe use of the drug in pregnancy has not been established clinically. Therefore, a nonhormonal method of contraception should be recommended. If a patient becomes pregnant during treatment, administration of the drug should be discontinued. Continuing treatment may result in an androgenic effect on the fetus, which to date has been limited to clitoral hypertrophy and labial fusion of the external genitalia in the female fetus. If the patient becomes pregnant while taking DANOCRINE, she should be apprised of the potential risk to the fetus.

Before initiating therapy of fibrocystic breast disease with DANOCRINE, carcinoma of the breast should be excluded. However, nodularity, pain, tenderness due to fibrocystic breast disease may prevent recognition of underlying carcinoma before treatment is begun. Therefore, if any nodule persists or enlarges during treatment, carcinoma should be considered and ruled out.

Long-term experience with danazol is limited. Long-term therapy with other steroids alkylated at the 17 position has been associated with serious toxicity (cholestatic jaundice, peliosis hepatis). The physician therefore should be alert to the possibility that similar toxicity may develop after long-term therapy with danazol. Attempts should be made to determine the lowest dose that will provide adequate protection. If the drug was begun at a time of exacerbation of angioneurotic edema due to trauma, stress or other cause, periodic attempts to decrease or withdraw therapy should be considered.

Patients should be watched closely for signs of virilization. Some androgenic effects may not be reversible even when drug administration is stopped.

Precautions: Because DANOCRINE may cause some degree of fluid retention, conditions that might be influenced by this factor, such as epilepsy, migraine, or cardiac or renal dysfunction, require careful observation.

Since hepatic dysfunction has been reported in patients treated with DANOCRINE, periodic liver function tests should be performed (see ADVERSE REACTIONS section).

Check semen for volume, viscosity, sperm count and motility every 3–4 months, especially in adolescents.

Adverse Reactions: The following androgenic effects have occurred in patients receiving DANOCRINE: acne, edema, mild hirsutism, decrease in breast size, deepening of the voice, oiliness of the skin or hair, weight gain, and rarely, clitoral hypertrophy, or testicular atrophy.

Also hypoestrogenic manifestations such as flushing, sweating, vaginitis including itching, dryness, burning and vaginal bleeding, nervousness, and emotional lability have been reported.

Hepatic dysfunction, as evidenced by elevated serum enzymes and/or jaundice, has been reported in patients receiving a daily dosage of DANOCRINE of 400 mg or more. It is recommended that patients receiving DANOCRINE, brand of danazol capsules, be monitored for hepatic dysfunction by laboratory tests and clinical observation. Prolongation of prothrombin time in patients stabilized on warfarin has also been reported.

Although the following reactions have also been reported, a causal relationship to the administration of DANOCRINE has neither been confirmed nor refuted: *allergic:* skin rashes and rarely, nasal congestion; *CNS effects:* dizziness, headache, sleep disorders, fatigue, tremor, and rarely, paresthesia in extremities, visual disturbances, anxiety, depression, changes in appetite, and chills; *gastrointestinal:* gastroenteritis, and rarely, nausea, vomiting, constipation; *musculoskeletal:* muscle cramps or spasms, joint lock-up, joint swelling, and pain in back, neck, or legs; *genitourinary:* rarely, hematuria; *other:* abnormal glucose tolerance test and increased insulin requirements in diabetic patients, loss of hair, changes in libido, elevation in blood pressure, and rarely, pelvic pain.

Dosage and Administration: *Endometriosis.* In moderate to severe disease, or in patients infertile due to endometriosis, a starting dose of 800 mg given in two divided doses is recommended. Amenorrhea and a rapid response to painful symptoms is best achieved at this dosage level. Gradual downward titration to a dose sufficient to maintain amenorrhea may be considered depending upon patient response. For mild cases, an initial daily dose of 200 to 400 mg given in two divided doses is recommended and may be adjusted depending on patient response. **Therapy should begin during menstruation. Otherwise, appropriate tests should be performed to ensure that the patient is not pregnant while on DANOCRINE therapy. (See WARNINGS.) It is essential that therapy continue uninterrupted for 3 to 6 months but may be extended to 9 months if necessary.** After termination of therapy, if symptoms recur, treatment can be reinstituted.

Fibrocystic Breast Disease. The total daily dosage of DANOCRINE for fibrocystic breast disease ranges from 100 mg to 400 mg given in two divided doses depending upon patient response. **Therapy should begin during menstruation. Otherwise, appropriate tests should be performed to ensure that the patient is not pregnant while on DANOCRINE therapy.** A nonhormonal method of contraception is recommended when DANOCRINE is administered at this dose, since ovulation may not be suppressed.

In most instances, breast pain and tenderness are significantly relieved by the first month and eliminated in 2 to 3 months. Usually elimination of nodularity requires 4 to 6 months of uninterrupted therapy. Regular menstrual patterns, irregular menstrual patterns, and amenorrhea each occur in approximately one-third of patients treated with 100 mg of DANOCRINE, brand of danazol capsules. Irregular menstrual patterns and amenorrhea are observed more frequently with higher doses. Clinical studies have demonstrated that 50% of patients may show evidence of recurrence of symptoms within one year. In this event, treatment may be reinstated.

Hereditary Angioedema. The dosage requirements for continuous treatment of hereditary angioedema with DANOCRINE should be individualized on the basis of the clinical response of the patient. It is recommended that the patient be started on 200 mg, two or three times a day. After a favorable initial response is obtained in terms of prevention of episodes of edematous attacks, the proper continuing dosage should be determined by decreasing the dosage by 50% or less at intervals of one to three months or longer if frequency of attacks prior to treatment dictates. If an attack occurs the daily dosage may be increased by up to 200 mg. During the dose adjusting phase, close monitoring of the patient's response is indicated, particularly if the patient has a history of airway involvement.

How Supplied: Capsules of 200 mg (orange), bottles of 100 (NDC 0024-0305-06).

Capsules of 100 mg (yellow), bottles of 100 (NDC 0024-0304-06).

Capsules of 50 mg (orange and white), bottles of 100 (NDC 0024-0303-06).

Distributed by Winthrop Laboratories
Division of Sterling Drug Inc.
New York, NY 10016
Manufactured by
Sterling Pharmaceuticals Inc.
Barceloneta, Puerto Rico 00617
[*Shown in Product Identification Section*]

DEMEROL® Hydrochloride Ⓒ
brand of meperidine hydrochloride, USP ℞

Description: Meperidine hydrochloride is ethyl 1-methyl-4-phenylisonipecotate hydrochloride, a white crystalline substance with a melting point of 186 to 189 C. It is readily soluble in water and has a neutral reaction and a slightly bitter taste. The solution is not decomposed by a short period of boiling.

The syrup is a pleasant-tasting, nonalcoholic, banana-flavored solution containing 50 mg of DEMEROL hydrochloride, brand of meperidine hydrochloride, per 5 ml teaspoon (25 drops contain 13 mg of DEMEROL hydrochloride). The tablets contain 50 or 100 mg of the analgesic.

DEMEROL hydrochloride, brand of meperidine hydrochloride, 5 per cent solution has a specific gravity of 1.0086 at 20 C and 10 per cent solution, a specific gravity of 1.0165 at 20 C.

Clinical Pharmacology: Meperidine hydrochloride is a narcotic analgesic with multiple actions qualitatively similar to those of morphine; the most prominent of these involve the central nervous system and organs composed of smooth muscle. The principal actions of therapeutic value are analgesia and sedation. There is some evidence which suggests that meperidine may produce less smooth muscle spasm, constipation, and depression of the cough reflex than equianalgesic doses of morphine. Meperidine, in 60 to 80 mg parenteral doses, is approximately equivalent in analgesic effect to 10 mg of morphine. The onset of action is slightly more rapid than with morphine, and the duration of action is slightly shorter. Meperidine is significantly less effective by the oral than by the parenteral route, but the exact ratio of oral to parenteral effectiveness is unknown.

Indications and Usage:

For the relief of moderate to severe pain (parenteral and oral forms)

For preoperative medication (parenteral form only)

For support of anesthesia (parenteral form only)

For obstetrical analgesia (parenteral form only)

Contraindications:

Hypersensitivity to meperidine.

Meperidine is contraindicated in patients who are receiving monoamine oxidase (MAO) inhibitors or those who have recently received such agents. Therapeutic doses of meperidine have occasionally precipitated unpredictable, severe, and occasionally fatal reactions in patients who have received such agents within 14 days. The mechanism of these reactions is unclear, but may be related to a preexisting hyperphenylalaninemia. Some have been characterized by coma, severe respiratory depression, cyanosis, and hypotension, and have resembled the syndrome of acute narcotic overdose. In other reactions the predominant manifestations have been hyperexcitability, convulsions, tachycardia, hyperpyrexia, and hypertension. Although it is not known that other narcotics are free of the risk of such reactions, virtually all of the reported reactions have occurred with meperidine. If a narcotic is needed in such patients, a sensitivity test should be performed in which repeated, small, incremental doses of morphine are administered over the course of several hours while the patient's condition and vital signs are under careful observation. (Intravenous hydrocortisone or prednisolone have been used to treat severe reactions, with the addition of intravenous chlorpromazine in those cases exhibiting hypertension and hyperpyrexia. The usefulness and safety of narcotic antagonists in the treatment of these reactions is unknown.)

Solutions of DEMEROL and barbiturates are chemically incompatible.

Warnings: *Drug Dependence.* Meperidine can produce drug dependence of the morphine type and therefore has the potential for being abused. Psychic dependence, physical dependence, and tolerance may develop upon repeated administration of meperidine, and it should be prescribed and administered with the same degree of caution appropriate to the use of morphine. Like other narcotics, meperidine is subject to the provisions of the Federal narcotic laws.

Interaction with Other Central Nervous System Depressants. Meperidine should be used with great caution and in reduced dosage in patients who are concurrently receiving other narcotic analgesics, general anesthetics, phenothiazines, other tranquilizers (see Dosage and Administration), sedative-hypnotics (including barbiturates), tricyclic antidepressants, and other CNS depressants (including alcohol). Respiratory depression, hypotension, and profound sedation or coma may result.

Head Injury and Increased Intracranial Pressure. The respiratory depressant effects of meperidine and its capacity to elevate cerebrospinal fluid pressure may be markedly exaggerated in the presence of head injury, other intracranial lesions, or a preexisting increase in intracranial pressure. Furthermore, narcotics produce adverse reactions which may obscure the clinical course of patients with head injuries. In such patients, meperidine must be used with extreme caution and only if its use is deemed essential.

Intravenous Use. If necessary, meperidine may be given intravenously, but the injection should be given very slowly, preferably in the form of a diluted solution. Rapid intravenous injection of narcotic analgesics, including meperidine, increases the incidence of adverse reactions; severe respiratory depression, apnea, hypotension, peripheral circulatory collapse, and cardiac arrest have occurred. Meperidine should not be administered intravenously unless a narcotic antagonist and the facilities for assisted or controlled respiration are immediately available. When meperidine is given parenterally, especially intravenously, the patient should be lying down.

Asthma and Other Respiratory Conditions. Meperidine should be used with extreme caution in patients having an acute asthmatic attack, patients with chronic obstructive pulmonary disease or cor pulmonale, patients having a substantially decreased respiratory reserve, and patients with preexisting respiratory depression, hypoxia, or hypercapnia. In such patients, even usual therapeutic doses of narcotics may decrease respiratory drive while simultaneously increasing airway resistance to the point of apnea.

Hypotensive Effect. The administration of meperidine may result in severe hypotension in the postoperative patient or any individual whose ability to maintain blood pressure has been compromised by a depleted blood volume or the administration of drugs such as the phenothiazines or certain anesthetics.

Usage in Ambulatory Patients. Meperidine may impair the mental and/or physical abilities required for the performance of potentially hazardous tasks such as driving a car or operating machinery. The patient should be cautioned accordingly.

Meperidine, like other narcotics, may produce orthostatic hypotension in ambulatory patients.

Usage in Pregnancy and Lactation. Meperidine should not be used in pregnant women prior to the labor period, unless in the judgment of the physician the potential benefits outweigh the possible hazards, because safe use in pregnancy prior to labor has not been established relative to possible adverse effects on fetal development.

When used as an obstetrical analgesic, meperidine crosses the placental barrier and can produce depression of respiration and psychophysiologic functions in the newborn. Resuscitation may be required (see section on **OVERDOSAGE**).

Meperidine appears in the milk of nursing mothers receiving the drug.

Precautions: *Supraventricular Tachycardias.* Meperidine should be used with caution in patients with atrial flutter and other supraventricular tachycardias because of a possible vagolytic action which may produce a significant increase in the ventricular response rate.

Convulsions. Meperidine may aggravate preexisting convulsions in patients with convulsive disorders. If dosage is escalated substantially above recommended levels because of tolerance development, convulsions may occur in individuals without a history of convulsive disorders.

Acute Abdominal Conditions. The administration of meperidine or other narcotics may obscure the diagnosis or clinical course in patients with acute abdominal conditions.

Special Risk Patients. Meperidine should be given with caution and the initial dose should be reduced in certain patients such as the elderly or debilitated, and those with severe impairment of hepatic or renal function, hypothyroidism, Addison's disease, and prostatic hypertrophy or urethral stricture.

Adverse Reactions: The major hazards of meperidine, as with other narcotic analgesics, are respiratory depression and, to a lesser degree, circulatory depression; respiratory arrest, shock, and cardiac arrest have occurred.

The most frequently observed adverse reactions include lightheadedness, dizziness, sedation, nausea, vomiting, and sweating. These effects seem to be more prominent in ambulatory patients and in those who are not experiencing severe pain. In such individuals, lower doses are advisable. Some adverse reactions in ambulatory patients may be alleviated if the patient lies down.

Other adverse reactions include:

Nervous System. Euphoria, dysphoria, weakness, headache, agitation, tremor, uncoordinated muscle movements, transient hallucinations and disorientation, visual disturbances. Inadvertent injection about a nerve trunk may result in sensory-motor paralysis which is usually, though not always, transitory.

Gastrointestinal. Dry mouth, constipation, biliary tract spasm.

Cardiovascular. Flushing of the face, tachycardia, bradycardia, palpitation, hypotension (see Warnings), syncope, phlebitis following intravenous injection.

Genitourinary. Urinary retention.

Allergic. Pruritus, urticaria, other skin rashes, wheal and flare over the vein with intravenous injection.

Other. Pain at injection site; local tissue irritation and induration following subcutaneous injection, particularly when repeated; antidiuretic effect.

Continued on next page

This product information was effective as of November 19, 1982. On these and other products of Winthrop Laboratories, detailed information may be obtained on a current basis by direct inquiry to the Professional Services Department, 90 Park Avenue, New York, NY 10016 (212) 907-2525.

Winthrop—Cont.

Dosage and Administration:
For Relief of Pain
Dosage should be adjusted according to the severity of the pain and the response of the patient. While subcutaneous administration is suitable for occasional use, intramuscular administration is preferred when repeated doses are required. If intravenous administration is required, dosage should be decreased and the injection made very slowly, preferably utilizing a diluted solution. Meperidine is less effective orally than on parenteral administration. The dose of DEMEROL should be proportionately reduced (usually by 25 to 50 per cent) when administered concomitantly with phenothiazines and many other tranquilizers since they potentiate the action of DEMEROL, brand of meperidine.
Adults. The usual dosage is 50 to 150 mg intramuscularly, subcutaneously, or orally, every 3 or 4 hours as necessary.
Children. The usual dosage is 0.5 to 0.8 mg/lb intramuscularly, subcutaneously, or orally up to the adult dose, every 3 or 4 hours as necessary.
Each dose of the syrup should be taken in one-half glass of water, since if taken undiluted, it may exert a slight topical anesthetic effect on mucous membranes.
For Preoperative Medication
Adults. The usual dosage is 50 to 100 mg intramuscularly or subcutaneously, 30 to 90 minutes before the beginning of anesthesia.
Children. The usual dosage is 0.5 to 1 mg/lb intramuscularly or subcutaneously up to the adult dose, 30 to 90 minutes before the beginning of anesthesia.
For Support of Anesthesia
Repeated slow intravenous injections of fractional doses (eg, 10 mg/ml) or continuous intravenous infusion of a more dilute solution (eg, 1 mg/ml) should be used. The dose should be titrated to the needs of the patient and will depend on the premedication and type of anesthesia being employed, the characteristics of the particular patient, and the nature and duration of the operative procedure.
For Obstetrical Analgesia
The usual dosage is 50 to 100 mg intramuscularly or subcutaneously when pain becomes regular, and may be repeated at 1- to 3-hour intervals.
Overdosage: *Symptoms.* Serious overdosage with meperidine is characterized by respiratory depression (a decrease in respiratory rate and/or tidal volume, Cheyne-Stokes respiration, cyanosis), extreme somnolence progressing to stupor or coma, skeletal muscle flaccidity, cold and clammy skin, and sometimes bradycardia and hypotension. In severe overdosage, particularly by the intravenous route, apnea, circulatory collapse, cardiac arrest, and death may occur.
Treatment. Primary attention should be given to the reestablishment of adequate respiratory exchange through provision of a patent airway and institution of assisted or controlled ventilation. The narcotic antagonist, naloxone hydrochloride, is a specific antidote against respiratory depression which may result from overdosage or unusual sensitivity to narcotics, including meperidine. Therefore, an appropriate dose of this antagonist should be administered, preferably by the intravenous route, simultaneously with efforts at respiratory resuscitation.
An antagonist should not be administered in the absence of clinically significant respiratory or cardiovascular depression.
Oxygen, intravenous fluids, vasopressors, and other supportive measures should be employed as indicated.
In cases of overdosage with DEMEROL, brand of meperidine, tablets, the stomach should be evacuated by emesis or gastric lavage.
NOTE: In an individual physically dependent on narcotics, the administration of the usual dose of a narcotic antagonist will precipitate an acute withdrawal syndrome. The severity of this syndrome will depend on the degree of physical dependence and the dose of antagonist administered. The use of narcotic antagonists in such individuals should be avoided if possible. If a narcotic antagonist must be used to treat serious respiratory depression in the physically dependent patient, the antagonist should be administered with extreme care and only one-fifth to one-tenth the usual initial dose administered.
How Supplied:
For Parenteral Use
Detecto-Seal® — *Carpuject®* **Sterile Cartridge-Needle Units**—*2.5 per cent* (25 mg per 1 ml) **NDC 0024-0324-02**, *5 per cent* (50 mg per 1 ml) **NDC 0024-0325-02**, *7.5 per cent* (75 mg per 1 ml) **NDC 0024-0326-02**; and *10 per cent* (100 mg per 1 ml) **NDC 0024-0328-02** all in boxes of 10.
Each cartridge is only partially-filled based upon product volume to permit mixture with other sterile materials in accordance with the best judgment of the physician.
Uni-Amp®—5 per cent solution; ampuls of 0.5 ml (25 mg) **NDC 0024-0361-04**, 1 ml (50 mg) **NDC 0024-0362-04**, 1½ ml (75 mg) **NDC 0024-0363-04**, and 2 ml (100 mg) **NDC 0024-0364-04** all in boxes of 25; and 10 per cent solution, ampuls of 1 ml (100 mg) **NDC 0024-0365-04** in boxes of 25.
Uni-Nest™—5 per cent solution; ampuls of 0.5 ml (25 mg) **NDC 0024-0371-04**, 1 ml (50 mg) **NDC 0024-0372-04**, 1½ ml (75 mg) **NDC 0024-0373-04**, and 2 ml (100 mg) **NDC 0024-0374-04** all in boxes of 25; and *10 per cent solution,* ampuls of 1 ml (100 mg) **NDC 0024-0375-04** in boxes of 25.
Vials—5 per cent multiple-dose vials of 30 ml **NDC 0024-0329-01**, and *10 per cent* multiple-dose vials of 20 ml **NDC 0024-0311-01** all in boxes of 1.
Note: The pH of DEMEROL solutions is adjusted between 3.5 and 6.0 with sodium hydroxide or hydrochloric acid. Multiple-dose vials contain metacresol 0.1 per cent as preservative. No preservatives are added to the ampuls.
For Oral Use
Tablets of 50 mg, bottles of 100 **(NDC 0024-0335-04)** and 500 **(NDC 0024-0335-06)**; 100 mg. bottles of 100 **(NDC 0024-0337-04)** and 500 **(NDC 0024-0337-06)**.
Syrup, nonalcoholic, banana-flavored 50 mg per 5 ml teaspoon, bottles of 16 fl oz **(NDC 0024-0332-06)**.
[*Shown in Product Identification Section*]

HALEY'S M-O® OTC

(See PDR For Nonprescription Drugs)

HYPAQUE® SODIUM ℞
brand of diatrizoate sodium, USP
ORAL POWDER
HYPAQUE SODIUM ORAL SOLUTION
brand of diatrizoate sodium solution, USP

(See Diagnostic Section.)

HYPAQUE® SODIUM 20% ℞
brand of diatrizoate sodium injection, USP
Sterile Aqueous Solution

(See Diagnostic Section.)

HYPAQUE® SODIUM 25% ℞
brand of diatrizoate sodium injection, USP

(See Diagnostic Section.)

HYPAQUE-CYSTO® ℞
brand of diatrizoate meglumine injection, USP
Sterile Aqueous Solution

(See Diagnostic Section.)

HYPAQUE® MEGLUMINE 30% ℞
brand of diatrizoate meglumine injection, USP
Sterile Aqueous Solution

(See Diagnostic Section.)

HYPAQUE® SODIUM 50% ℞
brand of diatrizoate sodium injection, USP
Sterile Aqueous Injection

(See Diagnostic Section.)

HYPAQUE® MEGLUMINE 60% ℞
brand of diatrizoate meglumine injection, USP
Sterile Aqueous Injection

(See Diagnostic Section.)

HYPAQUE®-M, 75% ℞
brand of diatrizoate meglumine and diatrizoate sodium injection, USP
Sterile Aqueous Injection

(See Diagnostic Section.)

HYPAQUE®-76 ℞
brand of diatrizoate meglumine and diatrizoate sodium injection, USP
Sterile Aqueous Injection

(See Diagnostic Section.)

HYPAQUE®-M, 90% ℞
brand of diatrizoate meglumine and diatrizoate sodium injection, USP
Sterile Aqueous Injection

(See Diagnostic Section.)

LOTUSATE® Caplets® Ⓒ ℞
brand of talbutal tablets, USP

Each caplet contains 120 mg of 5-Allyl-5-*sec*-butylbarbituric acid.
How Supplied: CAPLETS of 120 mg (purple)—bottles of 100 (NDC 0024-1153-04)
For complete prescribing information contact Winthrop Laboratories Professional Services Department.

NegGram® Caplets® ℞
brand of nalidixic acid tablets, USP
NegGram® Suspension ℞
brand of nalidixic acid oral suspension, USP

Description: Nalidixic acid, an oral antibacterial agent, is 1-ethyl-1,4-dihydro-7-methyl-4-oxo-1,8-naphthyridine-3-carboxylic acid. It is a pale yellow, crystalline substance and a very weak organic acid.
Clinical Pharmacology: NegGram has marked antibacterial activity against gram-negative bacteria including *Proteus mirabilis, P. morganii, P. vulgaris,* and *P. rettgeri; Escherichia coli;* Enterobacter (Aerobacter), and Klebsiella. Pseudomonas strains are generally resistant to the drug. NegGram is bactericidal and is effective over the entire urinary pH range. Conventional chromosomal resistance to NegGram taken in full dosage has been reported to emerge in approximately 2 to 14 per cent of patients during treatment; however, bacterial resistance to NegGram has not been shown to be transferable via R factor.
Indications and Usage: NegGram is indicated for the treatment of urinary tract infections caused by susceptible gram-negative microorganisms, including the majority of Proteus strains, Klebsiella, Enterobacter (Aerobacter), and *E. coli.* Disc susceptibility testing with the 30 μg disc should be performed prior to administration of the drug, and during treatment if clinical response warrants.

Contraindications: NegGram is contraindicated in patients with known hypersensitivity to nalidixic acid and in patients with a history of convulsive disorders.

Warnings: CNS effects including brief convulsions, increased intracranial pressure, and toxic psychosis have been reported rarely. These have occurred in infants and children or in geriatric patients, usually from overdosage or in patients with predisposing factors, and have been completely and rapidly reversible upon discontinuation of the drug. If these reactions occur, NegGram should be discontinued and appropriate therapeutic measures instituted; only if rapid disappearance of CNS symptoms does not occur within 48 hours should diagnostic procedures involving risk to the patient be undertaken. (See Adverse Reactions and Overdosage.)

Precautions: Blood counts and renal and liver function tests should be performed periodically if treatment is continued for more than two weeks. NegGram should be used with caution in patients with liver disease, epilepsy, or severe cerebral arteriosclerosis. While caution should be used in patients with severe renal failure, therapeutic concentrations of NegGram in the urine, without increased toxicity due to drug accumulation in the blood, have been observed in patients on full dosage with creatinine clearances as low as 2 to 8 ml/minute.

Patients should be cautioned to avoid undue exposure to direct sunlight while receiving NegGram. Therapy should be discontinued if photosensitivity occurs.

If bacterial resistance to NegGram emerges during treatment, it usually does so within 48 hours, permitting rapid change to another antimicrobial. Therefore, if the clinical response is unsatisfactory or if relapse occurs, cultures and sensitivity tests should be repeated. Underdosage with NegGram during initial treatment (with less than 4 g per day for adults) may predispose to emergence of bacterial resistance. (See Dosage and Administration.)

Cross resistance between NegGram and other antimicrobials has been observed only with oxolinic acid.

Nalidixic acid may enhance the effects of oral anticoagulants, warfarin or bishydroxycoumarin, by displacing significant amounts from serum albumin binding sites.

When Benedict's or Fehling's solutions or Clinitest® Reagent Tablets are used to test the urine of patients taking NegGram, a false-positive reaction for glucose may be obtained, due to the liberation of glucuronic acid from the metabolites excreted. However, a colorimetric test for glucose based on an enzyme reaction (eg, with Clinistix® Reagent Strips or Tes-Tape®) does not give a false-positive reaction to the liberated glucuronic acid.

Incorrect values may be obtained for urinary 17-keto and ketogenic steroids in patients receiving NegGram, brand of nalidixic acid, because of an interaction between the drug and the *m*-dinitrobenzene used in the usual assay method. In such cases, the Porter-Silber test for 17-hydroxycorticoids may be used.

Usage in Prepubertal Children. Recent toxicological studies have shown that nalidixic acid and related drugs can produce erosions of the cartilage in weight-bearing joints and other signs of arthropathy in immature animals of most species tested. No such joint lesions have been reported in man to date. Nevertheless, until the significance of this finding is clarified, care should be exercised when prescribing this product for prepubertal children.

Usage in Pregnancy. Safe use of NegGram during the first trimester of pregnancy has not been established. However, the drug has been used during the last two trimesters without producing apparent ill effects in mother or child.

Adverse Reactions: Reactions reported after oral administration of NegGram include *CNS effects:* drowsiness, weakness, headache, and dizziness and vertigo. Reversible subjective visual disturbances without objective findings have occurred infrequently (generally with each dose during the first few days of treatment). These reactions include overbrightness of lights, change in color perception, difficulty in focusing, decrease in visual acuity, and double vision. They usually disappeared promptly when dosage was reduced or therapy was discontinued. Toxic psychosis or brief convulsions have been reported rarely, usually following excessive doses. In general, the convulsions have occurred in patients with predisposing factors such as epilepsy or cerebral arteriosclerosis. In infants and children receiving therapeutic doses of NegGram, increased intracranial pressure with bulging anterior fontanel, papilledema, and headache has occasionally been observed. A few cases of 6th cranial nerve palsy have been reported. Although the mechanisms of these reactions are unknown, the signs and symptoms usually disappeared rapidly with no sequelae when treatment was discontinued. *Gastrointestinal:* abdominal pain, nausea, vomiting, and diarrhea. *Allergic:* rash, pruritus, urticaria, angioedema, eosinophilia, arthralgia with joint stiffness and swelling, and rarely, anaphylactoid reaction. Photosensitivity reactions consisting of erythema and bullae on exposed skin surfaces usually resolve completely in 2 weeks to 2 months after NegGram is discontinued; however, bullae may continue to appear with successive exposures to sunlight or with mild skin trauma for up to 3 months after discontinuation of drug. (See Precautions.) *Other:* rarely, cholestasis, paresthesia, metabolic acidosis, thrombocytopenia, leukopenia, or hemolytic anemia, sometimes associated with glucose-6-phosphate dehydrogenase deficiency.

Dosage and Administration: *Adults.* The recommended dosage for initial therapy in adults is 1 g administered four times daily for one or two weeks (total daily dose, 4 g). For prolonged therapy, the total daily dose may be reduced to 2 g after the initial treatment period. Underdosage during initial treatment may predispose to emergence of bacterial resistance.

Children. Until further experience is gained, NegGram should not be administered to infants younger than three months. Dosage in children 12 years of age and under should be calculated on the basis of body weight. The recommended total daily dosage for initial therapy is 25 mg/lb/day (55 mg/kg/day), administered in four equally divided doses. For prolonged therapy, the total daily dose may be reduced to 15 mg/lb/day (33 mg/kg/day). NegGram Suspension or NegGram CAPLETS of 250 mg may be used. One 250 mg tablet is equivalent to one teaspoon (5 ml) of the Suspension.

Overdosage: *Manifestations:* Toxic psychosis, convulsions, increased intracranial pressure, or metabolic acidosis may occur in patients taking more than the recommended dosage. Vomiting, nausea, and lethargy may also occur following overdosage.

Treatment: Reactions are short-lived (two to three hours) because the drug is rapidly excreted. If overdosage is noted early, gastric lavage is indicated. If absorption has occurred, increased fluid administration is advisable and supportive measures such as oxygen and means of artificial respiration should be available. Although anticonvulsant therapy has not been used in the few instances of overdosage reported, it may be indicated in a severe case.

How Supplied:

Suspension (250 mg/5 ml tsp), raspberry flavored, bottles of 1 pint (NDC 0024-1318-06)

CAPLETS of 1 g, scored, bottles of 100 (NDC 0024-1323-04)

Unit Dose Pack of 100 (NDC 0024-1323-14)–10 strips of ten—1 g CAPLETS each

CAPLETS of 500 mg, scored, bottles of 56 (NDC 0024-1322-03), 500 (NDC 0024-1322-06), and 1000 (NDC 0024-1322-08)

Unit Dose Pack of 100 (NDC 0024-1322-14)–10 strips of ten-500 mg CAPLETS each

CAPLETS of 250 mg, scored, bottles of 56 (NDC 0024-1321-03)

Pharmacology: Following oral administration, NegGram, brand of nalidixic acid, is rapidly absorbed from the gastrointestinal tract, partially metabolized in the liver, and rapidly excreted through the kidneys. Unchanged nalidixic acid appears in the urine along with an active metabolite, hydroxynalidixic acid, which has antibacterial activity similar to that of nalidixic acid. Other metabolites include glucuronic acid conjugates of nalidixic acid and hydroxynalidixic acid, and the dicarboxylic acid derivative. The hydroxy metabolite represents 30 per cent of the biologically active drug in the blood and 85 per cent in the urine. Peak serum levels of active drug average approximately 20 to 40 μg per ml (90 per cent protein bound), one to two hours after administration of a 1 g dose to a fasting normal individual, with a half-life of about 90 minutes. Peak urine levels of active drug average approximately 150 to 200 μg per ml, three to four hours after administration, with a half-life of about six hours. Approximately four per cent of NegGram is excreted in the feces. Traces of nalidixic acid were found in blood and urine of an infant whose mother had received the drug during the last trimester of pregnancy.

Animal Pharmacology: NegGram (nalidixic acid) and related drugs have been shown to cause arthropathy in juvenile animals of most species tested. (See PRECAUTIONS.)

Hydroxynalidixic acid, the principal metabolite of NegGram did not produce any oculotoxic effects at any dosage level in seven species of animals including three primate species. However, oral administration of this metabolite in high doses has been shown to have oculotoxic potential, namely in dogs and cats where it produced retinal degeneration upon prolonged administration leading, in some cases, to blindness.

In experiments with NegGram itself, little if any such activity could be elicited in either dogs or cats. Sensitivity to CNS side effects in these species limited the doses of NegGram that could be used; this factor, together with a low conversion rate to the hydroxy metabolite in these species, may explain the absence of these effects.

[*Shown in Product Identification Section*]

NEO-SYNEPHRINE® OTC
oxymetazoline hydrochloride 0.05%
12 HOUR

(See PDR For Nonprescription Drugs)

Long Acting NEO-SYNEPHRINE® II OTC
xylometazoline hydrochloride

(See PDR For Nonprescription Drugs)

Continued on next page

This product information was effective as of November 19, 1982. On these and other products of Winthrop Laboratories, detailed information may be obtained on a current basis by direct inquiry to the Professional Services Department, 90 Park Avenue, New York, NY 10016 (212) 907-2525.

Winthrop—Cont.

NEO-SYNEPHRINE® Hydrochloride ℞
brand of phenylephrine hydrochloride injection, USP
1% INJECTION

Well-Tolerated Vasoconstrictor and Pressor

> **WARNING:** PHYSICIANS SHOULD COMPLETELY FAMILIARIZE THEMSELVES WITH THE COMPLETE CONTENTS OF THIS LEAFLET BEFORE PRESCRIBING NEO-SYNEPHRINE.

Description: NEO-SYNEPHRINE hydrochloride, brand of phenylephrine hydrochloride injection, is a vasoconstrictor and pressor drug chemically related to epinephrine and ephedrine.

NEO-SYNEPHRINE hydrochloride is a synthetic sympathomimetic agent in sterile form for parenteral injection. Chemically, phenylephrine hydrochloride is (−)-*m*-Hydroxy-α-[(methylamino) methyl] benzyl alcohol hydrochloride.

Clinical Pharmacology: NEO-SYNEPHRINE hydrochloride produces vasoconstriction that lasts longer than that of epinephrine and ephedrine. Responses are more sustained than those to epinephrine, lasting 20 minutes after intravenous and as long as 50 minutes after subcutaneous injection. Its action on the heart contrasts sharply with that of epinephrine and ephedrine, in that it slows the heart rate and increases the stroke output, producing no disturbance in the rhythm of the pulse.

Phenylephrine is a powerful postsynaptic alpha-receptor stimulant with little effect on the beta receptors of the heart. In therapeutic doses, it produces little if any stimulation of either the spinal cord or cerebrum. A singular advantage of this drug is the fact that repeated injections produce comparable effects.

The predominant actions of phenylephrine are on the cardiovascular system. Parenteral administration causes a rise in systolic and diastolic pressures in man and other species. Accompanying the pressor response to phenylephrine is a marked reflex bradycardia that can be blocked by atropine; after atropine, large doses of the drug increase the heart rate only slightly. In man, cardiac output is slightly decreased and peripheral resistance is considerably increased. Circulation time is slightly prolonged, and venous pressure is slightly increased; venous constriction is not marked. Most vascular beds are constricted; renal splanchnic, cutaneous, and limb blood flows are reduced but coronary blood flow is increased. Pulmonary vessels are constricted, and pulmonary arterial pressure is raised.

The drug is a powerful vasoconstrictor, with properties very similar to those of norepinephrine but almost completely lacking the chronotropic and inotropic actions on the heart. Cardiac irregularities are seen only very rarely even with large doses.

Indications and Usage: NEO-SYNEPHRINE is intended for the maintenance of an adequate level of blood pressure during spinal and inhalation anesthesia and for the treatment of vascular failure in shock, shocklike states, and drug-induced hypotension, or hypersensitivity. It is also employed to overcome paroxysmal supraventricular tachycardia, to prolong spinal anesthesia, and as a vasoconstrictor in regional analgesia.

Contraindications: NEO-SYNEPHRINE hydrochloride should not be used in patients with severe hypertension, ventricular tachycardia, or in patients who are hypersensitive to it.

Warnings: If used in conjunction with oxytocic drugs, the pressor effect of sympathomimetic pressor amines is potentiated (see Drug Interaction). The obstetrician should be warned that some oxytocic drugs may cause severe persistent hypertension and that even a rupture of a cerebral blood vessel may occur during the postpartum period.

Precautions: NEO-SYNEPHRINE hydrochloride should be employed only with extreme caution in elderly patients or in patients with hyperthyroidism, bradycardia, partial heart block, myocardial disease, or severe arteriosclerosis.

Drug Interactions—Vasopressors, particularly metaraminol, may cause serious cardiac arrhythmias during halothane anesthesia and therefore should be used only with great caution or not at all.

MAO Inhibitors—The pressor effect of sympathomimetic pressor amines is markedly potentiated in patients receiving a monoamine oxidase (MAO) inhibitor. Therefore, when initiating pressor therapy in these patients, the initial dose should be small and used with due caution. The pressor response of adrenergic agents may also be potentiated by tricyclic antidepressants.

Carcinogenesis, Mutagenesis, Impairment of Fertility—No long-term animal studies have been done to evaluate the potential of NEO-SYNEPHRINE in these areas.

Pregnancy Category C—Animal reproduction studies have not been conducted with NEO-SYNEPHRINE. It is also not known whether NEO-SYNEPHRINE can cause fetal harm when administered to a pregnant woman or can affect reproduction capacity. NEO-SYNEPHRINE should be given to a pregnant woman only if clearly needed.

Labor and Delivery—If vasopressor drugs are either used to correct hypotension or added to the local anesthetic solution, the obstetrician should be cautioned that some oxytocic drugs may cause severe persistent hypertension and that even a rupture of a cerebral blood vessel may occur during the postpartum period (see WARNINGS).

Nursing Mother—It is not known whether this drug is excreted in human milk. Because many are excreted in human milk, caution should be exercised when NEO-SYNEPHRINE hydrochloride, brand of phenylephrine hydrochloride injection, is administered to a nursing woman.

Pediatric Use—To combat hypotension during spinal anesthesia in children, a dose of 0.5 to 1 mg per 25 pounds of body weight, administered subcutaneously or intramuscularly, is recommended.

Adverse Reactions: Headache, reflex bradycardia, excitability, restlessness, and rarely arrhythmias.

Overdosage: Overdosage may induce ventricular extrasystoles and short paroxysms of ventricular tachycardia, a sensation of fullness in the head and tingling of the extremities. Should an excessive elevation of blood pressure occur, it may be immediately relieved by an α-adrenergic blocking agent, eg, phentolamine. The oral LD_{50} in the rat is 350 mg/kg, in the mouse 120 mg/kg.

Dosage and Administration:
NEO-SYNEPHRINE is generally injected subcutaneously, intramuscularly, slowly intravenously, or in dilute solution as a continuous intravenous infusion. In patients with paroxysmal supraventricular tachycardia and, if indicated, in case of emergency, NEO-SYNEPHRINE is administered directly intravenously. The dose should be adjusted according to the pressor response.

Dosage Calculations

Dose Required	*Use* **NEO-SYNEPHRINE 1%**
10 mg	1 ml
5 mg	0.5 ml
1 mg	0.1 ml

For convenience in intermittent intravenous administration, dilute 1 ml NEO-SYNEPHRINE 1% with 9 ml Sterile Water for Injection, USP, to yield 0.1% NEO-SYNEPHRINE.

Dose Required	*Use Diluted* **NEO-SYNEPHRINE** *(0.1%)*
0.1 mg	0.1 ml
0.2 mg	0.2 ml
0.5 mg	0.5 ml

Mild or Moderate Hypotension

Subcutaneously or Intramuscularly: Usual dose, from 2 to 5 mg. Range, from 1 to 10 mg. Initial dose should not exceed 5 mg.

Intravenously: Usual dose, 0.2 mg. Range, from 0.1 to 0.5 mg. Initial dose should not exceed 0.5 mg.

Injections should not be repeated more often than every 10 to 15 minutes. A 5 mg intramuscular dose should raise blood pressure for one to two hours. A 0.5 mg intravenous dose should elevate the pressure for about 15 minutes.

Severe Hypotension and Shock—Including Drug-Related Hypotension

Blood volume depletion should always be corrected as fully as possible before any vasopressor is administered. When, as an emergency measure, intraaortic pressures must be maintained to prevent cerebral or coronary artery ischemia, NEO-SYNEPHRINE hydrochloride, brand of phenylephrine hydrochloride injection, can be administered before and concurrently with blood volume replacement.

Hypotension and occasionally severe shock may result from overdosage or idiosyncrasy following the administration of certain drugs, especially adrenergic and ganglionic blocking agents, rauwolfia and veratrum alkaloids, and phenothiazine tranquilizers. Patients who receive a phenothiazine derivative as preoperative medication are especially susceptible to these reactions. As an adjunct in the management of such episodes, NEO-SYNEPHRINE hydrochloride is a suitable agent for restoring blood pressure.

Higher initial and maintenance doses of NEO-SYNEPHRINE are required in patients with persistent or untreated severe hypotension or shock. Hypotension produced by powerful peripheral adrenergic blocking agents, chlorpromazine, or pheochromocytomectomy may also require more intensive therapy.

Continuous Infusion—Add 10 mg of the drug (1 ml of 1 percent solution) to 500 ml of Dextrose Injection, USP, or Sodium Chloride Injection, USP (providing a 1:50,000 solution). To raise the blood pressure rapidly, start the infusion at about 100 to 180 drops per minute. When the blood pressure is stabilized (at a low normal level for the individual), a maintenance rate of 40 to 60 drops per minute usually suffices. If a prompt initial pressor response is not obtained, additional increments of NEO-SYNEPHRINE (10 mg or more) are added to the infusion bottle. The rate of flow is then adjusted until the desired blood pressure level is obtained. (In some cases, a more potent vasopressor, such as norepinephrine bitartrate, may be required.) Hypertension should be avoided. The blood pressure should be checked frequently. Headache and/ or bradycardia may indicate hypertension. Arrhythmias are rare.

Spinal Anesthesia—Hypotension

Routine parenteral use of NEO-SYNEPHRINE has been recommended for the prophylaxis and treatment of hypotension during spinal anesthesia. It is best administered subcutaneously or intramuscularly three or four minutes before injection of the spinal anesthetic. The total requirement for high anesthetic levels is usually 3 mg, and for lower levels, 2 mg. For hypotensive emergencies during spinal anesthesia, NEO-SYNEPHRINE may be injected intravenously, using an initial dose of 0.2 mg. Any subsequent dose should not exceed the previous dose by more than 0.1 to 0.2 mg and no more than 0.5 mg should be administered in a single dose. To combat hypotension during spinal anesthesia in children, a dose of 0.5 to 1 mg per 25 pounds of body weight, administered subcutaneously or intramuscularly, is recommended.

Prolongation of Spinal Anesthesia

The addition of 2 to 5 mg of NEO-SYNEPHRINE hydrochloride to the anesthetic solution increases the duration of motor block by as much as approximately 50 per cent without any increase in the incidence of complications such as nausea, vomiting, or blood pressure disturbances.

Vasoconstrictor for Regional Analgesia

Concentrations about ten times those employed when epinephrine is used as a vasoconstrictor are recommended. The optimum strength is 1:20,000 (made by adding 1 mg of NEO-SYNEPHRINE hydrochloride to every 20 ml of local anesthetic solution). Some pressor responses can be expected when 2 mg or more are injected.

Paroxysmal Supraventricular Tachycardia

Rapid intravenous injection (within 20 to 30 seconds) is recommended; the initial dose should not exceed 0.5 mg, and subsequent doses, which are determined by the initial blood pressure response, should not exceed the preceding dose by more than 0.1 to 0.2 mg, and should never exceed 1 mg.

How Supplied:

Solution 1 percent

Ampuls—Each 1 ml contains 10 mg of NEO-SYNEPHRINE hydrochloride, 3.5 mg of sodium chloride, 4 mg of sodium citrate, 1 mg of citric acid monohydrate, and not more than 2 mg of sodium bisulfite. The pH is adjusted between 3.0 and 5.5 with sodium citrate or citric acid.

Uni-Nest™ ampuls of 1 ml, boxes of 25 (NDC 0024-1342-04).

The air in all ampuls has been displaced by nitrogen gas.

NEO–SYNEPHRINE® Hydrochloride ℞

brand of phenylephrine hydrochloride ophthalmic solution, USP

Vasoconstrictor and Mydriatic

SOLUTIONS 2.5% AND 10%

VISCOUS SOLUTION 10%

For Use in Ophthalmology

WARNING: PHYSICIANS SHOULD COMPLETELY FAMILIARIZE THEMSELVES WITH THE COMPLETE CONTENTS OF THIS LEAFLET BEFORE PRESCRIBING NEO-SYNEPHRINE.

Description: NEO-SYNEPHRINE hydrochloride, brand of phenylephrine hydrochloride ophthalmic solution, is a sterile solution used as a vasoconstrictor and mydriatic for use in ophthalmology.

NEO-SYNEPHRINE hydrochloride is a synthetic sympathomimetic compound structurally similar to epinephrine and ephedrine.

Phenylephrine hydrochloride is (–)-*m*-Hydroxy- α- [(methylamino)methyl] benzyl alcohol hydrochloride.

Clinical Pharmacology:

NEO-SYNEPHRINE possesses predominantly α-adrenergic effects. In the eye, phenylephrine acts locally as a potent vasoconstrictor and mydriatic, by constricting ophthalmic blood vessels and the radial muscle of the iris.

The ophthalmologic usefulness of NEO-SYNEPHRINE hydrochloride is due to its rapid effect and moderately prolonged action, as well as to the fact that it produces no compensatory vasodilatation.

The action of different concentrations of ophthalmic solutions of NEO-SYNEPHRINE hydrochloride is shown in the following table:

Strength of solution (%)	Mydriasis: Maximal (minutes)	Mydriasis: Recovery time (hours)	Paralysis of accommodation
2.5	15-60	3	trace
10	10-60	6	slight

Although rare, systemic absorption of sufficient quantities of phenylephrine may lead to systemic α-adrenergic effects, such as rise in blood pressure which may be accompanied by a reflex atropine-sensitive bradycardia.

Indications and Usage: NEO-SYNEPHRINE hydrochloride is recommended for use as a decongestant and vasoconstrictor and for pupil dilatation in uveitis (posterior synechiae), wide angle glaucoma, surgery, refraction, ophthalmoscopic examination, and diagnostic procedures.

Contraindications: Ophthalmic solutions of NEO-SYNEPHRINE hydrochloride are contraindicated in persons with narrow angle glaucoma (and in those individuals who are hypersensitive to NEO-SYNEPHRINE). NEO-SYNEPHRINE hydrochloride 10 per cent ophthalmic solutions are contraindicated in infants and in patients with aneurysms.

Warnings: There have been rare reports associating the use of NEO-SYNEPHRINE 10 percent ophthalmic solutions with the development of serious cardiovascular reactions, including ventricular arrhythmias and myocardial infarctions. These episodes, some ending fatally, have usually occurred in elderly patients with preexisting cardiovascular diseases.

Precautions: Exceeding recommended dosages or applying NEO-SYNEPHRINE hydrochloride ophthalmic solutions to the instrumented, traumatized, diseased or post surgical eye or adnexa, or to patients with suppressed lacrimation, as during anesthesia, may result in the absorption of sufficient quantities of phenylephrine to produce a systemic vasopressor response.

A significant elevation in blood pressure is rare but has been reported following conjunctival instillation of recommended doses of NEO-SYNEPHRINE 10 percent ophthalmic solutions. Caution, therefore, should be exercised in administering the 10 percent solutions to children of low body weight, the elderly, and patients with insulin-dependent diabetes, hypertension, hyperthyroidism, generalized arteriosclerosis, or cardiovascular disease. The posttreatment blood pressure of these patients, and any patients who develop symptoms, should be carefully monitored.

Ordinarily, any mydriatic, including NEO-SYNEPHRINE hydrochloride, brand of phenylephrine hydrochloride ophthalmic solution, is contraindicated in patients with glaucoma, since it may occasionally raise intraocular pressure. However, when temporary dilatation of the pupil may free adhesions or when vasoconstriction of intrinsic vessels may lower intraocular tension, these advantages may temporarily outweigh the danger from coincident dilatation of the pupil.

Rebound miosis has been reported in older persons one day after receiving NEO-SYNEPHRINE hydrochloride ophthalmic solutions, and reinstillation of the drug produced a reduction in mydriasis. This may be of clinical importance in dilating the pupils of older subjects prior to retinal detachment or cataract surgery.

Due to a strong action of the drug on the dilator muscle, older individuals may also develop transient pigment floaters in the aqueous humor 30 to 45 minutes following the administration of NEO-SYNEPHRINE hydrochloride ophthalmic solutions. The appearance may be similar to anterior uveitis or to a microscopic hyphema.

To prevent pain, a drop of suitable topical anesthetic may be applied before using the 10 percent ophthalmic solution.

Drug Interaction: As with all other adrenergic drugs, when NEO-SYNEPHRINE 10 percent ophthalmic solutions or 2.5 percent ophthalmic solution is administered simultaneously with, or up to 21 days after, administration of monoamine oxidase (MAO) inhibitors, careful supervision and adjustment of dosages are required since exaggerated adrenergic effects may occur. The pressor response of adrenergic agents may also be potentiated by tricyclic antidepressants, propranolol, reserpine, guanethidine, methyldopa, and atropine-like drugs.

Carcinogenesis, Mutagenesis, Impairment of Fertility: No long-term animal studies have been done to evaluate the potential of NEO-SYNEPHRINE in these areas.

Pregnancy Category C: Animal reproduction studies have not been conducted with NEO-SYNEPHRINE. It is also not known whether NEO-SYNEPHRINE can cause fetal harm when administered to a pregnant woman or can affect reproduction capacity. NEO-SYNEPHRINE should be given to a pregnant woman only if clearly needed.

Nursing Mothers: It is not known whether this drug is excreted in milk; many are. Caution should be exercised when NEO-SYNEPHRINE hydrochloride ophthalmic solution is administered to a nursing woman.

Pediatric Use: NEO-SYNEPHRINE hydrochloride 10 percent ophthalmic solutions are contraindicated in infants. (See CONTRAINDICATIONS.) For use in older children see DOSAGE AND ADMINISTRATION.

Exceeding recommended dosages or applying NEO-SYNEPHRINE hydrochloride ophthalmic solutions to the instrumented, traumatized, diseased or postsurgical eye or adnexa, or to patients with suppressed lacrimation, as during anesthesia, may result in the absorption of sufficient quantities of phenylephrine to produce a systemic vasopressor response.

The hypertensive effects of phenylephrine may be treated with an alpha-adrenergic blocking agent such as phentolamine mesylate, 5 mg to 10 mg intravenously, repeated as necessary.

The oral LD_{50} of phenylephrine in the rat: 350 mg/kg, in the mouse: 120 mg/kg.

Dosage and Administration: Prolonged exposure to air or strong light may cause oxidation and discoloration. Do not use if solution is brown or contains a precipitate.

Vasoconstriction and Pupil Dilatation

NEO-SYNEPHRINE hydrochloride 10 percent ophthalmic solutions is especially useful when rapid and powerful dilatation of the pupil and reduction of congestion in the capillary bed are desired. A drop of a suitable topical anesthetic may be applied, followed in a few minutes by 1 drop of the NEO-SYNEPHRINE hydrochloride 10 percent ophthalmic solution on the upper limbus. The anesthetic prevents stinging and consequent dilution of the solution by lacrimation. It may occasionally be necessary to repeat the

Continued on next page

This product information was effective as of November 19, 1982. On these and other products of Winthrop Laboratories, detailed information may be obtained on a current basis by direct inquiry to the Professional Services Department, 90 Park Avenue, New York, NY 10016 (212) 907-2525.

Winthrop—Cont.

instillation after one hour, again preceded by the use of the topical anesthetic.

Uveitis: Posterior Synechiae

NEO-SYNEPHRINE hydrochloride 10 percent ophthalmic solutions may be used in patients with uveitis when synechiae are present or may develop. The formation of synechiae may be prevented by the use of the 10 percent ophthalmic solutions and atropine to produce wide dilatation of the pupil. It should be emphasized, however, that the vasoconstrictor effect of NEO-SYNEPHRINE hydrochloride may be antagonistic to the increase of local blood flow in uveal infection.

To free recently formed posterior synechiae, 1 drop of the 10 percent ophthalmic solutions may be applied to the upper surface of the cornea. On the following day, treatment may be continued if necessary. In the interim, hot compresses should be applied for five or ten minutes three times a day, with 1 drop of a 1 or 2 percent solution of atropine sulfate before and after each series of compresses.

Glaucoma

In certain patients with glaucoma, temporary reduction of intraocular tension may be attained by producing vasoconstriction of the intraocular vessels; this may be accomplished by placing 1 drop of the 10 percent ophthalmic solutions on the upper surface of the cornea. This treatment may be repeated as often as necessary.

NEO-SYNEPHRINE hydrochloride, brand of phenylephrine hydrochloride ophthalmic solution, may be used with miotics in patients with wide angle glaucoma. It reduces the difficulties experienced by the patient because of the small field produced by miosis, and still it permits and often supports the effect of the miotic in lowering the intraocular pressure. Hence, there may be marked improvement in visual acuity after using NEO-SYNEPHRINE hydrochloride in conjunction with miotic drugs.

Surgery

When a short-acting mydriatic is needed for wide dilatation of the pupil before intraocular surgery, the 10 percent ophthalmic solutions or 2.5 percent ophthalmic solution may be applied topically from 30 to 60 minutes before the operation.

Refraction

Prior to determination of refractive errors, NEO-SYNEPHRINE hydrochloride 2.5 percent ophthalmic solution may be used effectively with homatropine hydrobromide, atropine sulfate, or a combination of homatropine and cocaine hydrochloride.

For *adults*, a drop of the preferred cycloplegic is placed in each eye, followed in five minutes by 1 drop of NEO-SYNEPHRINE hydrochloride 2.5 percent ophthalmic solution and in ten minutes by another drop of the cycloplegic. In 50 to 60 minutes, the eyes are ready for refraction.

For *children*, a drop of atropine sulfate 1 percent is placed in each eye, followed in 10 to 15 minutes by 1 drop of NEO-SYNEPHRINE hydrochloride 2.5 percent ophthalmic solution and in five to ten minutes by a second drop of atropine sulfate 1 percent. In one to two hours, the eyes are ready for refraction.

For a "one application method," NEO-SYNEPHRINE hydrochloride 2.5 percent ophthalmic solution may be combined with a cycloplegic to elicit synergistic action. The additive effect varies depending on the patient. Therefore, when using a "one application method," it may be desirable to increase the concentration of the cycloplegic.

Ophthalmoscopic Examination

One drop of NEO-SYNEPHRINE hydrochloride 2.5 percent ophthalmic solution is placed in each eye. Sufficient mydriasis to permit examination is produced in 15 to 30 minutes. Dilatation lasts from one to three hours.

Diagnostic Procedures

Provocative Test for Angle Block in Patients with Glaucoma: The 2.5 percent ophthalmic solution may be used as a provocative test when latent increased intraocular pressure is suspected. Tension is measured before application of NEO-SYNEPHRINE hydrochloride and again after dilatation. A 3 to 5 mm of mercury rise in pressure suggests the presence of angle block in patients with glaucoma; however, failure to obtain such a rise does not preclude the presence of glaucoma from other causes.

Shadow Test (Retinoscopy): When dilatation of the pupil without cycloplegic action is desired for the shadow test, the 2.5 percent ophthalmic solution may be used alone.

Blanching Test: One or 2 drops of the 2.5 percent ophthalmic solution should be applied to the injected eye. After five minutes, examine for perilimbal blanching. If blanching occurs, the congestion is superficial and probably does not indicate iritis.

How Supplied: *In MONO-DROP® (plastic dropper) bottle:*

Low surface tension solutions

2.5 percent ophthalmic solution — NEO-SYNEPHRINE hydrochloride, brand of phenylephrine hydrochloride ophthalmic solution, 2.5 percent in a sterile, isotonic, buffered, low surface tension vehicle with sodium phosphate, sodium biphosphate, boric acid, and, as antiseptic preservative, benzalkonium chloride, NF, 1:7500. The pH is adjusted with phosphoric acid or sodium hydroxide.
Bottles of 15 ml (NDC 0024-1358-01)

10 percent ophthalmic solution — NEO-SYNEPHRINE hydrochloride 10 percent in a sterile, buffered, low surface tension vehicle with sodium phosphate, sodium biphosphate, and, as antiseptic preservative, benzalkonium chloride 1:10,000. The pH is adjusted with phosphoric acid or sodium hydroxide.
Bottles of 5 ml (NDC 0024-1359-01)

Viscous solution

10 percent ophthalmic solution — NEO-SYNEPHRINE hydrochloride 10 percent in a sterile, buffered, viscous vehicle with sodium phosphate, sodium biphosphate, methylcellulose, and, as antiseptic preservative, benzalkonium chloride 1:10,000. The pH is adjusted with phosphoric acid or sodium hydroxide.
Bottles of 5 ml (NDC 0024-1362-01)

NEO-SYNEPHRINE® — OTC
phenylephrine hydrochloride

(See PDR For Nonprescription Drugs)

NEO-SYNEPHRINOL™ — OTC
pseudoephedrine hydrochloride 120 mg DAY RELIEF™ Capsules

(See PDR For Nonprescription Drugs)

NTZ® SOLUTION — OTC

(See PDR For Nonprescription Drugs)

pHisoDerm® — OTC

(See PDR For Nonprescription Drugs)

pHisoHex® — ℞
brand of hexachlorophene detergent cleanser

sudsing antibacterial soapless skin cleanser

Description: pHisoHex is an antibacterial sudsing emulsion. It contains a colloidal dispersion of hexachlorophene 3% (w/w) in a stable emulsion consisting of entsufon sodium, petrolatum, lanolin cholesterols, methylcellulose, polyethylene glycol, polyethylene glycol monostearate, lauryl myristyl diethanolamide, sodium benzoate, and water. pH is adjusted with hydrochloric acid. Entsufon sodium is a synthetic detergent.

Clinical Pharmacology: pHisoHex is a bacteriostatic cleansing agent. It cleanses the skin thoroughly and has bacteriostatic action against staphylococci and other gram-positive bacteria. Cumulative antibacterial action develops with repeated use. This antibacterial residue is resistant to removal by many solvents, soaps, and detergents for several days. pHisoHex has the same slight acidity as normal skin (pH value 5.0 to 6.0).

Indications and Usage: pHisoHex is indicated for use as a surgical scrub and a bacteriostatic skin cleanser. It may also be used to control an outbreak of gram-positive infection where other infection control procedures have been unsuccessful. Use only as long as necessary for infection control.

Contraindications: pHisoHex should not be used on burned or denuded skin.

It should not be used as an occlusive dressing, wet pack, or lotion.

It should not be used routinely for prophylactic total body bathing.

It should not be used as a vaginal pack or tampon, or on any mucous membranes.

pHisoHex should not be used on persons with sensitivity to any of its components. It should not be used on persons who have demonstrated primary light sensitivity to halogenated phenol derivatives because of the possibility of cross-sensitivity to hexachlorophene.

Warnings: RINSE THOROUGHLY AFTER USE, especially from sensitive areas such as the scrotum and perineum.

Rapid absorption of hexachlorophene may occur with resultant toxic blood levels when preparations containing hexachlorophene are applied to skin lesions such as ichthyosis congenita, the dermatitis of Letterer-Siwe's syndrome, or other generalized dermatological conditions. Application to burns has also produced neurotoxicity and death.

PHISOHEX SHOULD BE DISCONTINUED PROMPTLY IF SIGNS OR SYMPTOMS OF CEREBRAL IRRITABILITY OCCUR.

Infants, especially premature infants or those with dermatoses, are particularly susceptible to hexachlorophene absorption. Systemic toxicity may be manifested by signs of stimulation (irritation) of the central nervous system, sometimes with convulsions.

Infants have developed dermatitis, irritability, generalized clonic muscular contractions and decerebrate rigidity following application of a 6 percent hexachlorophene powder. Examination of brainstems of those infants revealed vacuolization like that which can be produced in newborn experimental animals following repeated topical application of 3 percent hexachlorophene. Moreover, a study of histologic sections of premature infants who died of unrelated causes has shown a positive correlation between hexachlorophene baths and lesions in white matter of brains.

pHisoHex is intended for *external use only.* If swallowed, pHisoHex is harmful, especially to infants and children. **pHisoHex, brand of hexachlorophene detergent cleanser, should not be poured into measuring cups, medicine bottles, or similar containers since it may be mistaken for baby formula or other medications.**

Precaution: pHisoHex suds that get into the eyes accidentally during washing should be rinsed out promptly and thoroughly with water.

Adverse Reactions: Adverse reactions to pHisoHex may include dermatitis and photosensitivity. Sensitivity to hexachlorophene is rare; however, persons who have developed photoallergy to similar compounds also may become sensitive to hexachlorophene.

In persons with highly sensitive skin, the use of pHisoHex may at times produce a reaction characterized by redness and/or mild scaling or dryness, especially when it is combined with such mechanical factors as excessive rubbing or exposure to heat or cold.

Directions for Use:

Surgical Hand Scrub—

1. Wet hands and forearms with water. Apply approximately 5 ml of pHisoHex over the hands and rub into a copious lather by adding small amounts of water. Spread suds over hands and forearms and scrub well with a wet brush for 3 minutes. Pay particular attention to the nails and interdigital spaces. A separate nail cleaner may be used. *Rinse thoroughly* under running water.
2. Apply 5 ml of pHisoHex to hands again and scrub as above for another 3 minutes. *Rinse thoroughly* with running water and dry.
3. For repeat surgical scrubs during the day, scrub thoroughly with the same amount of pHisoHex for 3 minutes only. *Rinse thoroughly* with water and dry.

Bacteriostatic Cleansing—

Wet hands with water. Dispense approximately 5 ml of pHisoHex into the palm, work up a lather with water and apply to area to be cleansed.

Rinse thoroughly after each washing.

INFANT CARE: pHisoHex should not be used routinely for bathing infants. See **WARNINGS.**

PREMATURE INFANTS: See **WARNINGS.**

Use of baby skin products containing alcohol may decrease the antibacterial action of pHisoHex, brand of hexachlorophene detergent cleanser.

Treatment of Accidental Ingestion: The accidental ingestion of pHisoHex in amounts from 1 to 4 oz has caused anorexia, vomiting, abdominal cramps, diarrhea, dehydration, convulsions, hypotension and shock, and in several reported instances, fatalities.

If patients are seen early, the stomach should be evacuated by emesis or gastric lavage. Olive oil or vegetable oil (60 ml or 2 fl oz) may then be given to delay absorption of hexachlorophene, followed by a saline cathartic to hasten removal. Treatment is symptomatic and supportive; intravenous fluids (5 per cent dextrose in physiologic saline solution) may be given for dehydration. Any other electrolyte derangement should be corrected. If marked hypotension occurs, vasopressor therapy is indicated. Use of opiates may be considered if gastrointestinal symptoms (cramping, diarrhea) are severe. Scheduled medical or surgical procedures should be postponed until the patient's condition has been evaluated and stabilized.

How Supplied: pHisoHex is available in plastic squeeze bottles of 5 ounces (NDC 0024-1535-02) and 1 pint (NDC 0024-1535-06); in plastic bottles of 1 gallon (NDC 0024-1536-08) and ¼ oz (8 ml) unit packets, boxes of 50 (NDC 0024-1535-05).

The following, specially constructed, refillable dispensers made with metals and plastics compatible with pHisoHex can also be supplied: 16 oz hand operated wall dispensers; 30 oz pedal operated wall dispensers; 30 oz pedal operated wall dispenser with stand; portable stand with two 30 oz pedal operated dispensers.

Prolonged direct exposure of pHisoHex to strong light may cause brownish surface discoloration but does not affect its antibacterial or detergent properties. Shaking will disperse the color. If pHisoHex is spilled or splashed on porous surfaces, rinse off to avoid discoloration. pHisoHex should not be dispensed from, or stored in, containers with ordinary metal parts. A special type of stainless steel must be used or undesirable discoloration of the product or oxidation of metal may occur. Specially designed dispensers for hospital or office use may be obtained through your local dealer.

Directions for Cleaning Dispensers: Before initial installation and use, run an antiseptic, such as an aqueous solution of benzalkonium chloride, NF, 1:500 to 1:750, or alcohol, through the working parts; rinse with sterile water. At weekly intervals thereafter, remove dispenser and pour off remainder of pHisoHex emulsion. Rinse empty dispenser with water. Run water through the working parts by operating the dispenser. Sanitize as described above. Rinse thoroughly with sterile water.

PLAQUENIL® Sulfate ℞

brand of hydroxychloroquine sulfate tablets, USP

WARNING

PHYSICIANS SHOULD COMPLETELY FAMILIARIZE THEMSELVES WITH THE COMPLETE CONTENTS OF THIS LEAFLET BEFORE PRESCRIBING HYDROXYCHLOROQUINE.

Description: The compound is a colorless crystalline solid, soluble in water to at least 20 per cent; chemically the drug is 2-[[4-[(7-chloro-4-quinolyl)amino] pentyl] ethylamino] ethanol sulfate (1:1).

Actions: The drug possesses antimalarial actions and also exerts a beneficial effect in lupus erythematosus (chronic discoid or systemic) and acute or chronic rheumatoid arthritis. The precise mechanism of action is not known.

Indications: PLAQUENIL is indicated for the suppressive treatment and treatment of acute attacks of malaria due to *Plasmodium vivax, P. malariae, P. ovale,* and susceptible strains of *P. falciparum.* It is also indicated for the treatment of discoid and systemic lupus erythematosus, and rheumatoid arthritis.

Contraindications: Use of this drug is contraindicated (1) in the presence of retinal or visual field changes attributable to any 4-aminoquinoline compound, (2) in patients with known hypersensitivity to 4-aminoquinoline compounds and (3) for long-term therapy in children.

Warnings, General: PLAQUENIL is not effective against chloroquine-resistant strains of *P. falciparum.*

Children are especially sensitive to the 4-aminoquinoline compounds. A number of fatalities have been reported following the accidental ingestion of chloroquine, sometimes in relatively small doses (0.75 or 1 g in one 3-year-old child). Patients should be strongly warned to keep these drugs out of the reach of children.

Use of PLAQUENIL in patients with psoriasis may precipitate a severe attack of psoriasis. When used in patients with porphyria the condition may be exacerbated. The preparation should not be used in these conditions unless in the judgment of the physician the benefit to the patient outweighs the possible hazard.

Usage in Pregnancy—Usage of this drug during pregnancy should be avoided except in the suppression or treatment of malaria when in the judgment of the physician the benefit outweighs the possible hazard. It should be noted that radioactively-tagged chloroquine administered intravenously to pregnant, pigmented CBA mice passed rapidly across the placenta. It accumulated selectively in the melanin structures of the fetal eyes and was retained in the ocular tissues for five months after the drug had been eliminated from the rest of the body.[1]

Precautions, General: Antimalarial compounds should be used with caution in patients with hepatic disease or alcoholism or in conjunction with known hepatotoxic drugs.

Periodic blood cell counts should be made if patients are given prolonged therapy. If any severe blood disorder appears which is not attributable to the disease under treatment, discontinuation of the drug should be considered. The drug should be administered with caution in patients having G-6-PD (glucose-6-phosphate dehydrogenase) deficiency.

Overdosage: The 4-aminoquinoline compounds are very rapidly and completely absorbed after ingestion, and in accidental overdosage, or rarely with lower doses in hypersensitive patients, toxic symptoms may occur within 30 minutes. These consist of headache, drowsiness, visual disturbances, cardiovascular collapse, and convulsions, followed by sudden and early respiratory and cardiac arrest. The electrocardiogram may reveal atrial standstill, nodal rhythm, prolonged intraventricular conduction time, and progressive bradycardia leading to ventricular fibrillation and/or arrest. Treatment is symptomatic and must be prompt with immediate evacuation of the stomach by emesis (at home, before transportation to the hospital) or gastric lavage until the stomach is completely emptied. If finely powdered, activated charcoal is introduced by the stomach tube, after lavage, and within 30 minutes after ingestion of the tablets, it may inhibit further intestinal absorption of the drug. To be effective, the dose of activated charcoal should be at least five times the estimated dose of hydroxychloroquine ingested. Convulsions, if present, should be controlled before attempting gastric lavage. If due to cerebral stimulation, cautious administration of an ultrashort-acting barbiturate may be tried but, if due to anoxia, it should be corrected by oxygen administration, artificial respiration or, in shock with hypotension, by vasopressor therapy. Because of the importance of supporting respiration, tracheal intubation or tracheostomy, followed by gastric lavage, may also be necessary. Exchange transfusions have been used to reduce the level of 4-aminoquinoline drug in the blood.

A patient who survives the acute phase and is asymptomatic should be closely observed for at least six hours. Fluids may be forced, and sufficient ammonium chloride (8 g daily in divided doses for adults) may be administered for a few days to acidify the urine to help promote urinary excretion in cases of both overdosage and sensitivity.

MALARIA

Actions: Like chloroquine phosphate, USP, PLAQUENIL sulfate is highly active against the erythrocytic forms of *P. vivax* and *malariae* and most strains of *P. falciparum* (but not the gametocytes of *P. falciparum*).

PLAQUENIL sulfate does not prevent relapses in patients with *vivax* or *malariae* malaria because it is not effective against exo-erythrocytic forms of the parasite, nor will it prevent *vivax* or *malariae* infection when administered as a prophylactic. It is highly effective as a suppressive agent in patients with *vivax* or *malariae* malaria, in terminating acute attacks, and significantly lengthening the interval between treatment and relapse. In patients with *falciparum* malaria, it abolishes the acute attack and effects complete cure of the infection, unless due to a resistant strain of *P. falciparum.*

Indications: PLAQUENIL sulfate, brand of hydroxychloroquine sulfate tablets, is indicated for the treatment of acute attacks and suppression of malaria.

Warning: In recent years, it has been found that certain strains of *P. falciparum* have become resistant to 4-aminoquinoline compounds (including hydroxychloroquine) as shown by the fact that normally adequate doses have

Continued on next page

This product information was effective as of November 19, 1982. On these and other products of Winthrop Laboratories, detailed information may be obtained on a current basis by direct inquiry to the Professional Services Department, 90 Park Avenue, New York, NY 10016 (212) 907-2525.

Winthrop—Cont.

failed to prevent or cure clinical malaria or parasitemia. Treatment with quinine or other specific forms of therapy is therefore advised for patients infected with a resistant strain of parasites.

Adverse Reactions: Following the administration in doses adequate for the treatment of an acute malarial attack, mild and transient headache, dizziness, and gastrointestinal complaints (diarrhea, anorexia, nausea, abdominal cramps and, on rare occasions, vomiting) may occur.

Dosage and Administration: One tablet of 200 mg of hydroxychloroquine sulfate is equivalent to 155 mg base.

Malaria: Suppression—*In adults,* 400 mg (=310 mg base) on exactly the same day of each week. *In infants and children,* the weekly suppressive dosage is 5 mg, calculated as base, per kg of body weight, but should not exceed the adult dose regardless of weight.

If circumstances permit, suppressive therapy should begin two weeks prior to exposure. However, failing this, in adults an initial double (loading) dose of 800 mg (= 620 mg base), or in children 10 mg base/kg may be taken in two divided doses, six hours apart. The suppressive therapy should be continued for eight weeks after leaving the endemic area.

Treatment of the acute attack—*In adults,* an initial dose of 800 mg (= 620 mg base) followed by 400 mg (= 310 mg base) in six to eight hours and 400 mg (310 mg base) on each of two consecutive days (total 2 g hydroxychloroquine sulfate or 1.55 g base). An alternative method, employing a single dose of 800 mg (= 620 mg base), has also proved effective.

The dosage for adults may also be calculated on the basis of body weight; this method is preferred for infants and children. A total dose representing 25 mg of base per kg of body weight is administered in three days, as follows:

First dose: 10 mg base per kg (but not exceeding a single dose of 620 mg base).

Second dose: 5 mg base per kg (but not exceeding a single dose of 310 mg base) 6 hours after first dose.

Third dose: 5 mg base per kg 18 hours after second dose.

Fourth dose: 5 mg base per kg 24 hours after third dose.

For radical cure of *vivax* and *malariae* malaria concomitant therapy with an 8-aminoquinoline compound is necessary.

LUPUS ERYTHEMATOSUS AND RHEUMATOID ARTHRITIS

Indications: PLAQUENIL is useful in patients with the following disorders who have not responded satisfactorily to drugs with less potential for serious side effects: lupus erythematosus (chronic discoid and systemic) and acute or chronic rheumatoid arthritis.

Warnings: PHYSICIANS SHOULD COMPLETELY FAMILIARIZE THEMSELVES WITH THE COMPLETE CONTENTS OF THIS LEAFLET BEFORE PRESCRIBING PLAQUENIL.

Irreversible retinal damage has been observed in some patients who had received long-term or high-dosage 4-aminoquinoline therapy for discoid and systemic lupus erythematosus, or rheumatoid arthritis. Retinopathy has been reported to be dose related.

When prolonged therapy with any antimalarial compound is contemplated, initial (base line) and periodic (every three months) ophthalmologic examinations (including visual acuity, expert slit-lamp, funduscopic, and visual field tests) should be performed.

If there is any indication of abnormality in the visual acuity, visual field, or retinal macular areas (such as pigmentary changes, loss of foveal reflex), or any visual symptoms (such as light flashes and streaks) which are not fully explainable by difficulties of accommodation or corneal opacities, the drug should be discontinued immediately and the patient closely observed for possible progression. Retinal changes (and visual disturbances) may progress even after cessation of therapy.

All patients on long-term therapy with this preparation should be questioned and examined periodically, including the testing of knee and ankle reflexes, to detect any evidence of muscular weakness. If weakness occurs, discontinue the drug.

In the treatment of rheumatoid arthritis, if objective improvement (such as reduced joint swelling, increased mobility) does not occur within six months, the drug should be discontinued. Safe use of the drug in the treatment of juvenile arthritis has not been established.

Precautions: Dermatologic reactions to PLAQUENIL sulfate, brand of hydroxychloroquine sulfate tablets, may occur and, therefore, proper care should be exercised when it is administered to any patient receiving a drug with a significant tendency to produce dermatitis.

The methods recommended for early diagnosis of "chloroquine retinopathy" consist of (1) funduscopic examination of the macula for fine pigmentary disturbances or loss of the foveal reflex and (2) examination of the central visual field with a small red test object for pericentral or paracentral scotoma or determination of retinal thresholds to red. Any unexplained visual symptoms, such as light flashes or streaks should also be regarded with suspicion as possible manifestations of retinopathy.[2-6]

If serious toxic symptoms occur from overdosage or sensitivity, it has been suggested that ammonium chloride (8 g daily in divided doses for adults) be administered orally three or four days a week for several months after therapy has been stopped, as acidification of the urine increases renal excretion of the 4- aminoquinoline compounds by 20 to 90 per cent. However, caution must be exercised in patients with impaired renal function and/or metabolic acidosis.

Adverse Reactions: Not all of the following reactions have been observed with every 4-aminoquinoline compound during long-term therapy, but they have been reported with one or more and should be borne in mind when drugs of this class are administered. Adverse effects with different compounds vary in type and frequency.

CNS Reactions: irritability, nervousness, emotional changes, nightmares, psychosis, headache, dizziness, vertigo, tinnitus, nystagmus, nerve deafness, convulsions, ataxia.

Neuromuscular Reactions: extraocular muscle palsies, skeletal muscle weakness, absent or hypoactive deep tendon reflexes.

Ocular Reactions:

A. *Ciliary body:* disturbance of accommodation with symptoms of blurred vision. This reaction is dose related and reversible with cessation of therapy.

B. *Cornea:* transient edema, punctate to lineal opacities, decreased corneal sensitivity. The corneal changes, with or without accompanying symptoms (blurred vision, halos around lights, photophobia), are fairly common, but reversible. Corneal deposits may appear as early as three weeks following initiation of therapy.

The incidence of corneal changes and visual side effects appears to be considerably lower with hydroxychloroquine than with chloroquine.

C. *Retina:*

Macula: Edema, atrophy, abnormal pigmentation (mild pigment stippling to a "bull's-eye" appearance), loss of foveal reflex, increased macular recovery time following exposure to a bright light (photo-stress test), elevated retinal threshold to red light in macular, paramacular and peripheral retinal areas.

Other fundus changes include optic disc pallor and atrophy, attenuation of retinal arterioles, fine granular pigmentary disturbances in the peripheral retina and prominent choroidal patterns in advanced stage.

D. *Visual field defects:* pericentral or paracentral scotoma, central scotoma with decreased visual acuity, rarely field constriction.

The most common visual symptoms attributed to the retinopathy are: reading and seeing difficulties (words, letters, or parts of objects missing), photophobia, blurred distance vision, missing or blacked out areas in the central or peripheral visual field, light flashes and streaks.

Retinopathy appears to be dose related and has occurred within several months (rarely) to several years of daily therapy; a small number of cases have been reported several years after antimalarial drug therapy was discontinued. It has not been noted during prolonged use of weekly doses of the 4-aminoquinoline compounds for suppression of malaria.

Patients with retinal changes may have visual symptoms or may be asymptomatic (with or without visual field changes). Rarely scotomatous vision or field defects may occur without obvious retinal change.

Retinopathy may progress even after the drug is discontinued. In a number of patients, early retinopathy (macular pigmentation sometimes with central field defects) diminished or regressed completely after therapy was discontinued. Paracentral scotoma to red targets (sometimes called "premaculopathy") is indicative of early retinal dysfunction which is usually reversible with cessation of therapy.

A small number of cases of retinal changes have been reported as occurring in patients who received only hydroxychloroquine. These usually consisted of alteration in retinal pigmentation which was detected on periodic ophthalmologic examination; visual field defects were also present in some instances. A case of delayed retinopathy has been reported with loss of vision starting one year after administration of hydroxychloroquine had been discontinued.

Dermatologic Reactions: Bleaching of hair, alopecia, pruritus, skin and mucosal pigmentation, skin eruptions (urticarial, morbilliform, lichenoid, maculopapular, purpuric, erythema annulare centrifugum and exfoliative dermatitis).

Hematologic Reactions: Various blood dyscrasias such as aplastic anemia, agranulocytosis, leukopenia, thrombocytopenia (hemolysis in individuals with glucose-6- phosphate dehydrogenase (G-6-PD) deficiency).

Gastrointestinal Reactions: Anorexia, nausea, vomiting, diarrhea, and abdominal cramps.

Miscellaneous Reactions: Weight loss, lassitude, exacerbation or precipitation of porphyria and nonlight-sensitive psoriasis.

Dosage and Administration: One tablet of hydroxychloroquine sulfate, 200 mg, is equivalent to 155 mg base.

Lupus erythematosus—Initially, the average *adult* dose is 400 mg (=310 mg base) once or twice daily. This may be continued for several weeks or months, depending on the response of the patient. For prolonged maintenance therapy, a smaller dose, from 200 to 400 mg (=155 to 310 mg base) daily will frequently suffice. The incidence of retinopathy has been reported to be higher when this maintenance dose is exceeded.

Rheumatoid arthritis—The compound is cumulative in action and will require several weeks to exert its beneficial therapeutic effects, whereas minor side effects may occur relatively early. Several months of therapy may be required before maximum effects can be obtained. If objective improvement (such as reduced joint swelling, increased mobility) does not occur within six months, the drug should be discontinued. Safe use of the drug in the treatment of juvenile rheumatoid arthritis has not been established.

Initial dosage—In **adults,** from 400 to 600 mg (=310 to 465 mg base) daily, each dose to be taken with a meal or a glass of milk. In a small percentage of patients, troublesome side effects may require temporary reduction of the initial dosage. Later (usually from five to ten days), the dose may gradually be increased to the optimum response level, often without return of side effects.

Maintenance dosage—When a good response is obtained (usually in four to twelve weeks), the dosage is reduced by 50 per cent and continued at a usual maintenance level of 200 to 400 mg (=155 to 310 mg base) daily, each dose to be taken with a meal or a glass of milk. The incidence of retinopathy has been reported to be higher when this maintenance dose is exceeded.

Should a relapse occur after medication is withdrawn, therapy may be resumed or continued on an intermittent schedule if there are no ocular contraindications.

Corticosteroids and salicylates may be used in conjunction with this compound, and they can generally be decreased gradually in dosage or eliminated after the drug has been used for several weeks. When gradual reduction of steroid dosage is indicated, it may be done by reducing every four to five days the dose of cortisone by no more than from 5 to 15 mg; of hydrocortisone from 5 to 10 mg; of prednisolone and prednisone from 1 to 2.5 mg; of methylprednisolone and triamcinolone from 1 to 2 mg; and of dexamethasone from 0.25 to 0.5 mg.

How Supplied: Tablets of 200 mg (equivalent to 155 mg of base), bottles of 100.

References:

1. Ullberg, S., Lindquist, N.G., and Sjostrand, S. E.: Accumulation of chorio-retinotoxic drugs in the foetal eye, *Nature 227:*1257, Sept. 19, 1970.
2. Carr, R. E., Gouras, P., and Gunkel, R. D.: Chloroquine retinopathy. Early detection by retinal threshold test, *Arch. Ophthal. 75:*171, Feb. 1966.
3. Bernstein, H. N.: Chloroquine ocular toxicity, *Survey Ophthal. 12:*415, October 1967.
4. Percival, S. P. B. and Meanock, I.: Chloroquine: Ophthalmological safety and clinical assessment in rheumatoid arthritis, *Brit. Med. J. 3:*579, September 1968.
5. Carr, R. E., Henkind, P., Rothfield, Naomi, and Siegel, I. M.: Ocular toxicity of antimalarial drugs, *Amer. J. Ophthal. 66:*738, October 1968.
6. Young, P., White, G., and Fry, J.: Measurement of red light perception as a practical means of detecting retinal toxicity to antimalarials before it is irreversible. Paper presented at Interim Meeting of American Rheumatism Association, Atlanta, Georgia, Dec. 5-8, 1968; abstr. *Arthritis Rheum. 11:*850, December 1968.

[*Shown in Product Identification Section*]

SULFAMYLON® Cream ℞
brand of mafenide acetate cream, USP

Topical Antibacterial Agent for Adjunctive Therapy in Second- and Third-Degree Burns

Description: SULFAMYLON Cream is a soft, white, nonstaining, water-miscible cream containing the antibacterial agent, mafenide acetate (α-amino-*p*-toluenesulfonamide monoacetate).

SULFAMYLON Cream spreads easily, and can be washed off readily with water. It has a slight acetic odor. Each gram of SULFAMYLON Cream contains mafenide acetate equivalent to 85 mg of the base. The cream vehicle consists of cetyl alcohol, stearyl alcohol, cetyl esters wax, polyoxyl 40 stearate, polyoxyl 8 stearate, glycerin, and water, with methylparaben, propylparaben, sodium bisulfite, and edetate disodium as preservatives.

Actions: SULFAMYLON Cream, applied topically, produces a marked reduction in the bacterial population present in the avascular tissues of second- and third-degree burns. Reduction in bacterial growth after application of SULFAMYLON Cream has also been reported to permit spontaneous healing of deep partial-thickness burns, and thus prevent conversion of burn wounds from partial thickness to full thickness. It should be noted, however, that delayed eschar separation has occurred in some cases.

Absorption and Metabolism. Applied topically, SULFAMYLON Cream diffuses through devascularized areas, is absorbed, and rapidly converted to a metabolite (*p*-carboxybenzenesulfonamide) which is cleared through the kidneys. SULFAMYLON is active in the presence of pus and serum, and its activity is not altered by changes in the acidity of the environment.

Antibacterial Activity. SULFAMYLON exerts bacteriostatic action against many gram-negative and gram-positive organisms, including *Pseudomonas aeruginosa* and certain strains of anaerobes.

Indication: SULFAMYLON Cream is a topical antibacterial agent indicated for adjunctive therapy of patients with second- and third-degree burns.

Warnings: SULFAMYLON Cream should be administered with caution to patients with history of hypersensitivity to mafenide. It is not known whether there is cross sensitivity to other sulfonamides.

Fungal colonization in and below the eschar may occur concomitantly with reduction of bacterial growth in the burn wound. However, fungal dissemination through the infected burn wound is rare.

Usage in Pregnancy. Safe use of SULFAMYLON Cream during pregnancy has not been established. Therefore, the preparation is not recommended for the treatment of women of childbearing potential, *unless* the burned area covers more than 20 per cent of the total body surface, or the need for the therapeutic benefit of SULFAMYLON Cream is, in the physician's judgment, greater than the possible risk to the fetus.

Precautions: SULFAMYLON and its metabolite, *p*-carboxybenzenesulfonamide, inhibit carbonic anhydrase, which may result in metabolic acidosis, usually compensated by hyperventilation. In the presence of impaired renal function, high blood levels of SULFAMYLON and its metabolite may exaggerate the carbonic anhydrase inhibition. Therefore, close monitoring of acid-base balance is necessary, particularly in patients with extensive second-degree or partial thickness burns and in those with pulmonary or renal dysfunction. Some burn patients treated with SULFAMYLON Cream have also been reported to manifest an unexplained syndrome of marked hyperventilation with resulting respiratory alkalosis (slightly alkaline blood pH, low arterial pCO_2, and decreased total CO_2); change in arterial pO_2 is variable. The etiology and significance of these findings are unknown.

Mafenide acetate cream should be used with caution in burn patients with acute renal failure.

Adverse Reactions: It is frequently difficult to distinguish between an adverse reaction to SULFAMYLON Cream and the effect of a severe burn. The most frequently reported reaction was pain or a burning sensation. Allergic manifestations included rash, itching, facial edema, swelling, hives, blisters, erythema, and eosinophilia. Other reactions, which have rarely occurred, are tachypnea or hyperventilation, acidosis, increase in serum chloride, decrease in arterial pCO_2, excoriation of new skin, and bleeding of skin. A single case of bone marrow depression and a single case of an acute attack of porphyria have been reported following SULFAMYLON Cream therapy. Fatal hemolytic anemia with disseminated intravascular coagulation, presumably related to a glucose-6-phosphate dehydrogenase deficiency, has been reported following SULFAMYLON Cream therapy. Accidental ingestion of SULFAMYLON Cream has been reported to cause diarrhea.

Administration: Prompt institution of appropriate measures for controlling shock and pain is of prime importance. The burn wounds are then cleansed and debrided, and SULFAMYLON Cream, brand of mafenide acetate cream, is applied with a sterile gloved hand. Satisfactory results can be achieved with application of the cream once or twice daily, to a thickness of approximately 1/16 inch; thicker application is not recommended. The burned areas should be covered with SULFAMYLON Cream at all times. Therefore, whenever necessary, the cream should be reapplied to any areas from which it has been removed (eg, by patient activity). The routine of administration can be accomplished in minimal time, since dressings usually are not required. If individual patient demands make them necessary, however, only a thin layer of dressing should be used.

When feasible, the patient should be bathed daily, to aid in debridement. A whirlpool bath is particularly helpful, but the patient may be bathed in bed or in a shower.

The duration of therapy with SULFAMYLON Cream depends on each patient's requirements. Treatment is usually continued until healing is progressing well or until the burn site is ready for grafting. *SULFAMYLON Cream should not be withdrawn from the therapeutic regimen while there is the possibility of infection.* However, if allergic manifestations occur during treatment with SULFAMYLON Cream, discontinuation of treatment should be considered.

If acidosis occurs and becomes difficult to control, particularly in patients with pulmonary dysfunction, discontinuing SULFAMYLON Cream therapy for 24 to 48 hours while continuing fluid therapy may aid in restoring acid-base balance.

How Supplied:

Cans of 14.5 ounces (411 g)—NDC 0024-1884-09
Collapsible tubes of 4 ounces (113.4 g)
NDC 0024-1884-02
Collapsible tubes of 2 ounces (56.7 g)
NDC 0024-1884-01

TALACEN® Ⓒ ℞
Pentazocaine hydrochloride, USP, equivalent to 25 mg base and acetaminophen, USP, 650 mg.

Description: TALACEN is a combination of pentazocine hydrochloride, USP, equivalent to 25 mg base and acetaminophen, USP, 650 mg. Pentazocine is a member of the benzazocine series (also known as the benzomorphan series). Chemically, pentazocine is 1,2,3,4,5,6-hexahydro-6,11-dimethyl-3-(3-methyl-2-butenyl)-2,6-methano-3-benzazocin-8-ol, a white, crystalline substance soluble in acidic aqueous solutions.

Chemically, acetaminophen is Acetamide, *N*-(4-hydroxy-phenyl).

Continued on next page

This product information was effective as of November 19, 1982. On these and other products of Winthrop Laboratories, detailed information may be obtained on a current basis by direct inquiry to the Professional Services Department, 90 Park Avenue, New York, NY 10016 (212) 907-2525.

Winthrop—Cont.

Pentazocine is an analgesic and acetaminophen is an analgesic and antipyretic.
TALACEN is a pale blue, scored caplet for oral administration.

Clinical Pharmacology: TALACEN is an analgesic possessing antipyretic actions.
Pentazocine is an analgesic with agonist/antagonist action which when administered orally is approximately equivalent on a mg for mg basis in analgesic effect to codeine.
Acetaminophen is an analgesic and antipyretic.
Onset of significant analgesia with pentazocine usually occurs between 15 and 30 minutes after oral administration, and duration of action is usually three hours or longer. Onset and duration of action and the degree of pain relief are related both to dose and the severity of pretreatment pain. Pentazocine weakly antagonizes the analgesic effects of morphine, meperidine, and phenazocine; in addition, it produces incomplete reversal of cardiovascular, respiratory, and behavioral depression induced by morphine and meperidine. Pentazocine has about 1/50 the antagonistic activity of nalorphine. It also has sedative activity.
Pentazocine is well absorbed from the gastrointestinal tract. Plasma levels closely correspond to the onset, duration, and intensity of analgesia. The mean peak concentration in 24 normal volunteers was 1.7 hours (range 0.5 to 4.0 hours) after oral administration and the mean plasma elimination half-life was 3.6 hours (range 1.5 to 10 hours).
The action of pentazocine is terminated for the most part by biotransformation in the liver with some free pentazocine excreted in the urine. The products of the oxidation of the terminal methyl groups and glucuronide conjugates are excreted by the kidney. Elimination of approximately 60% of the total dose occurs within 24 hours. Pentazocine passes the placental barrier.
Onset of significant analgesic and antipyretic activity of acetaminophen when administered orally occurs within 30 minutes and is maximal at approximately 2½ hours. The pharmacological mode of action of acetaminophen is unknown at this time.
Acetaminophen is rapidly and almost completely absorbed from the gastrointestinal tract. In 24 normal volunteers the mean peak plasma concentration was 1 hour (range 0.25 to 3 hours) after oral administration and the mean plasma elimination half-life was 2.8 hours (range 2 to 4 hours).
The effect of pentazocine on acetaminophen plasma protein binding or vice versa has not been established. For acetaminophen there is little or no plasma protein binding at normal therapeutic doses. When toxic doses of acetaminophen are ingested and drug plasma levels exceed 90 mcg/ml, plasma binding may vary from 8% to 43%.
Acetaminophen is conjugated in the liver with glucuronic acid and to a lesser extent with sulfuric acid. Approximately 80% of acetaminophen is excreted in the urine after conjugation and about 3% is excreted unchanged. The drug is also conjugated to a lesser extent with cysteine and additionally metabolized by hydroxylation.
If TALACEN is taken every 4 hours over an extended period of time, accumulation of pentazocine and to a lesser extent, acetaminophen, may occur.

Indications and Usage: TALACEN is indicated for the relief of mild to moderate pain.

Contraindications: TALACEN should not be administered to patients who are hypersensitive to either pentazocine or acetaminophen.

Warnings: *Head Injury and Increased Intracranial Pressure.* As in the case of other potent analgesics, the potential of pentazocine for elevating cerebrospinal fluid pressure may be attributed to CO_2 retention due to the respiratory depressant effects of the drug. These effects may be markedly exaggerated in the presence of head injury, other intracranial lesions, or a preexisting increase in intracranial pressure. Furthermore, pentazocine can produce effects which may obscure the clinical course of patients with head injuries. In such patients, TALACEN must be used with extreme caution and only if its use is deemed essential.
Acute CNS Manifestations. Patients receiving pentazocine in doses of 50 mg or more have experienced, in rare instances, hallucinations (usually visual), disorientation, and confusion which have cleared spontaneously within a period of hours. The mechanism of this reaction is not known. Such patients should be very closely observed and vital signs checked. If the drug is reinstituted, it should be done with caution since the acute CNS manifestations may recur.
There have been instances of psychological and physical dependence on parenteral pentazocine in patients with a history of drug abuse, and rarely, in patients without such a history. (See DRUG ABUSE AND DEPENDENCE.)
Due to the potential for increased CNS depressant effects, alcohol should be used with caution in patients who are currently receiving pentazocine.
Pentazocine may precipitate opioid abstinence symptoms in patients receiving courses of opiates for pain relief.

Precautions: *In prescribing TALACEN for chronic use, the physician should take precautions to avoid increases in dose by the patient.*
Myocardial Infarction. As with all drugs, TALACEN should be used with caution in patients with myocardial infarction who have nausea or vomiting.
Certain Respiratory Conditions. Although respiratory depression has rarely been reported after oral administration of pentazocine, the drug should be administered with caution to patients with respiratory depression from any cause, severely limited respiratory reserve, severe bronchial asthma and other obstructive respiratory conditions, or cyanosis.
Impaired Renal or Hepatic Function. Decreased metabolism of the drug by the liver in extensive liver disease may predispose to accentuation of side effects. Although laboratory tests have not indicated that pentazocine causes or increases renal or hepatic impairment, the drug should be administered with caution to patients with such impairment.
Since acetaminophen is metabolized by the liver, the question of the safety of its use in the presence of liver disease should be considered.
Biliary Surgery. As with all strong analgesics, TALACEN should be used with caution in patients about to undergo surgery of the biliary tract since pentazocine may cause spasm of the sphincter of Oddi.
CNS Effect. Caution should be used when TALACEN is administered to patients prone to seizures; seizures have occurred in a few such patients in association with the use of pentazocine although no cause and effect relationship has been established.
Information for Patients: Since sedation, dizziness, and occasional euphoria have been noted, ambulatory patients should be warned not to operate machinery, drive cars, or unnecssarily expose themselves to hazards. Pentazocine may cause physical and psychological dependence when taken alone and may have additive CNS depressant properties when taken in combination with alcohol or other CNS depressants.
Drug Interactions. Pentazocine is a mild narcotic antagonist. Some patients previously given narcotics, including methadone for the daily treatment of narcotic dependence, have experienced withdrawal symptoms after receiving pentazocine.
Carcinogenesis, Mutagenesis, Impairment of Fertility. Carcinogenesis, mutagenesis, and impairment of fertility studies have not been done with this combination product.
Pentazocine, when administered orally or parenterally, had no adverse affect on either the reproductive capabilities or the course of pregnancy in rabbits and rats. Embryotoxic effects on the fetuses were not shown.
The daily administration of 4 mg/kg to 20 mg/kg pentazocine subcutaneously to female rats during a 14 day pre-mating period and until the 13th day of pregnancy did not have any adverse effects on the fertility rate.
There is no evidence in long-term animal studies to demonstrate that pentazocine is carcinogenic.
Pregnancy Category C. Animal reproduction studies have not been conducted with TALACEN. It is also not known whether TALACEN can cause fetal harm when administered to pregnant women or can effect reproduction capacity. TALACEN should be given to pregnant women only if clearly needed. However, animal reproduction studies with pentazocine have not demonstrated teratogenic embryotoxic effects.
Nonteratogenic Effects. There has been no experience in this regard with the combination pentazocine and acetaminophen. However, there have been rare reports of possible abstinence syndromes in newborns after prolonged use of pentazocine during pregnancy.
Labor and Delivery. Patients receiving pentazocine during labor have experienced no adverse effects other than those that occur with commonly used analgesics. TALACEN should be used with caution in women delivering premature infants. The effect of TALACEN on the mother and fetus, the duration of labor or delivery, the possibility that forceps delivery or other intervention or resuscitation of the newborn may be necessary, or the effect of TALACEN, on the later growth, development, and functional maturation of the child are unknown at the present time.
Nursing Mothers. It is not known whether this drug is excreted in human milk. Because many drugs are excreted in human milk, caution should be exercised when TALACEN is administered to a nursing woman.
Pediatric Use. Safety and effectiveness in children below the age of 12 have not been established.

Adverse Reactions: Clinical experience with TALACEN has been insufficient to define all possible adverse reactions with this combination. However, reactions reported after oral administration of pentazocine hydrochloride in 50 mg dosage include *gastrointestinal:* nausea, vomiting, infrequently constipation; and rarely abdominal distress, anorexia, diarrhea. *CNS effects:* dizziness, lightheadedness, sedation, euphoria, headache; infrequently weakness, disturbed dreams, insomnia, syncope, visual blurring and focusing difficulty, hallucinations (see *Acute CNS Manifestations* under WARNINGS); and rarely tremor, irritability, excitement, tinnitus. *Autonomic:* sweating; infrequently flushing; and rarely chills. *Allergic:* infrequently rash; and rarely urticaria, edema of the face. *Cardiovascular:* infrequently decrease in blood pressure, tachycardia. *Hematologic:* rarely depression of white blood cells (especially granulocytes), which is usually reversible, moderate transient eosinophilia. *Other:* rarely respiratory depression, urinary retention, paresthesia, toxic epidermal necrolysis.
Numerous clinical studies have shown that acetaminophen, when taken in recommended doses, is relatively free of adverse effects in most age groups, even in the presence of a variety of disease states.
A few cases of hypersensitivity to acetaminophen have been reported, as manifested by skin rashes, thrombocytopenic purpura, rarely hemolytic anemia and agranulocytosis. Occa-

sional individuals respond to ordinary doses with nausea and vomiting or diarrhea.

Drug Abuse and Dependence: *Controlled Substance.* TALACEN is a Schedule IV controlled substance.

Abuse and Dependence. There have been some reports of dependence and of withdrawal symptoms with orally administered pentazocine. There have been recorded instances of psychological and physical dependence in patients using parenteral pentazocine. Abrupt discontinuance following the extended use of parenteral pentazocine has resulted in withdrawal symptoms. Patients with a history of drug dependence should be under close supervision while receiving TALACEN. There have been rare reports of possible abstinence syndromes in newborns after prolonged use of pentazocine during pregnancy.

Some tolerance to the analgesic and subjective effects of pentazocine develops with frequent and repeated use.

Drug addicts who are given closely spaced doses of pentazocine (eg, 60 mg to 90 mg every 4 hours) develop physical dependence which is demonstrated by abrupt withdrawal or by administration of naloxone. The withdrawal symptoms exhibited after chronic doses of more than 500 mg of pentazocine per day have similar characteristics, but to a lesser degree, of opioid withdrawal and may be associated with drug seeking behavior.

Overdosage: *Manifestations.* Clinical experience with TALACEN has been insufficient to define the signs of overdosage with this product. It may be assumed that signs and symptoms of TALACEN overdose would be a combination of those observed with pentazocine overdose and acetaminophen overdose.

For pentazocine alone in single doses above 60 mg there have been reports of the occurrence of nalorphine-like psychotomimetic effects such as anxiety, nightmares, strange thoughts, and hallucinations. Marked respiratory depression associated with increased blood pressure and tachycardia have also resulted from excessive doses as have dizziness, nausea, vomiting, lethargy, and paresthesias. The respiratory depression is antagonized by naloxone (see *Treatment*).

In acute acetaminophen overdosage, dose-dependent, potentially fatal hepatic necrosis is the most serious adverse effect. Renal tubular necrosis, hypoglycemic coma, and thrombocytopenia may also occur.

In adults, a single dose of 10 g to 15 g (200 mg/kg to 250 mg/kg) of acetaminophen may cause hepatotoxicity. A dose of 25 g or more is potentially fatal. The potential seriousness of the intoxication may not be evident during the first two days of acute acetaminophen poisoning. During the first 24 hours, nausea, vomiting, anorexia, and abdominal pain occur. These may persist for a week or more. Liver injury may become evident the second day, initial signs being elevation of serum transaminase and lactic dehydrogenase activity, increased serum bilirubin concentration, and prolongation of prothrombin time. Serum albumin concentration and alkaline phosphatase activity may remain normal. The hepatotoxicity may lead to encephalopathy, coma, and death. Transient azotemia is evident in a majority of patients and acute renal failure occurs in some.

There have been reports of glycosuria and impaired glucose tolerance, but hypoglycemia may also occur. Metabolic acidosis and metabolic alkalosis have been reported. Cerebral edema and nonspecific myocardial depression have also been noted. Biopsy reveals centrolobular necrosis with sparing of the periportal area. The hepatic lesions are reversible over a period of weeks or months in nonfatal cases.

The severity of the liver injury can be determined by measurement of the plasma half-time of acetaminophen during the first day of acute poisoning. If the half-time exceeds 4 hours, hepatic necrosis is likely and if the half-time is greater than 12 hours, hepatic coma will probably occur. Only minimal liver damage has developed when the serum concentration was below 120 μg/ml at 12 hours after ingestion of the drug. If serum bilirubin concentration is greater than 4 mg/100 ml during the first 5 days, encephalopathy may occur. [See table above].

TALACEN LD_{50} VALUE

Drug	7-Day Oral LD_{50} Values, mg/kg (95% CL)	Equivalent mg/kg doses of: pentazocine (base)	acetaminophen
In Mice			
TALACEN 25–650 mg caplet granulation*	3570 (2440–5310)	75.68 (51.73–112.57)	1964 (1342–2920)
acetaminophen alone	Representative oral LD_{50} values at 7 days range from 850 (590–1200) to 2110 (1520–3310) mg/kg.		
In Rats			
TALACEN 25–650 mg caplet granulation*	10,700 (Estimate)	227	5885
acetaminophen alone	Representative oral LD_{50} values at 7 days range from 4260 (3760–4820) to 7940 (est.) mg/kg.		

* Diluents and excipients included

Rabbits tolerated the TALACEN 25–650 mg caplet granulation at single oral doses of up to 1,000 mg/kg (ie, 21.20 mg, as base, of pentazocine HCl plus 550.85 mg acetaminophen). The results of subacute (4- to 6-week) oral toxicity studies in the rat did not show any enhancement of toxicity with the TALACEN 25–650 mg caplet granulation as compared with acetaminophen alone.

Treatment. Oxygen, intravenous fluids, vasopressors, and other supportive measures should be employed as indicated. Assisted or controlled ventilation should also be considered. For respiratory depression due to overdosage or unusual sensitivity to TALACEN, parenteral naloxone (Narcan®, available through Endo Laboratories) is a specific and effective antagonist.

The toxic effects of acetaminophen may be prevented or minimized by antidotal therapy with N-acetylcysteine. In order to obtain the best possible results, N-acetylcysteine should be administered within approximately 16 hours of ingestion of the overdose.

The use of N-acetylcysteine as an antidote is currently restricted to investigational use. For information and directions for use, contact the Rocky Mountain Poison Center (800-525-6115).

Vigorous supportive therapy is required in severe intoxication. Procedures to limit the continuing absorption of the drug must be readily performed since the hepatic injury is dose dependent and occurs early in the course of intoxication. Induction of vomiting or gastric lavage, followed by oral administration of activated charcoal should be done in all cases. If hemodialysis can be initiated within the first 12 hours, it is advocated for patients with a plasma acetaminophen concentration exceeding 120 μg/ml at 4 hours after ingestion of the drug.

Dosage and Administration: *Adults.* The usual adult dose is 1 tablet every 4 hours as needed for pain relief, up to a maximum of 6 tablets per day.

The usual duration of therapy is dependent upon the condition being treated but in any case should be reviewed regularly by the physician. The effect of meals on the rate and extent of bioavailability of both pentazocine and acetaminophen has not been documented.

How Supplied: Caplets®, pale blue, scored, each containing pentazocine hydrochloride equivalent to 25 mg base and acetaminophen 650 mg.

Bottles of 100 (NDC 0024-1937-04).

Distributed by
Winthrop Laboratories
Division of Sterling Drug Inc
New York, NY 10016
Manufactured by
Sterling Pharmaceuticals Inc
Barceloneta, Puerto Rico 00617

[*Shown in Product Identification Section*]

TALWIN® Injection Ⓒ ℞
brand of pentazocine lactate injection, USP

Analgesic for Parenteral Use

Description: TALWIN injection, brand of pentazocine lactate injection, is a member of the benzazocine series (also known as the benzomorphan series). Chemically, pentazocine lactate is 1, 2, 3, 4, 5, 6-hexahydro - 6, 11 - dimethyl- 3-(3-methyl-2-butenyl) -2,6-methano-3-benzazocin-8-ol lactate, a white, crystalline substance soluble in acidic aqueous solutions.

Actions: TALWIN is a potent analgesic and 30 mg is usually as effective an analgesic as morphine 10 mg or meperidine 75 to 100 mg; however, a few studies suggest the TALWIN to morphine ratio may range from 20 to 40 mg TALWIN to 10 mg morphine. The duration of analgesia may sometimes be less than that of morphine. Analgesia usually occurs within 15 to 20 minutes after intramuscular or subcutaneous injection and within 2 to 3 minutes after intravenous injection. TALWIN weakly antagonizes the analgesic effects of morphine, meperidine, and phenazocine; in addition, it produces incomplete reversal of cardiovascular, respiratory, and behavioral depression induced by morphine and meperidine. TALWIN has about 1/50 the antagonistic activity of nalorphine. It also has sedative activity.

Indications: For the relief of moderate to severe pain. TALWIN may also be used for preoperative or preanesthetic medication and as a supplement to surgical anesthesia.

Continued on next page

This product information was effective as of November 19, 1982. On these and other products of Winthrop Laboratories, detailed information may be obtained on a current basis by direct inquiry to the Professional Services Department, 90 Park Avenue, New York, NY 10016 (212) 907-2525.

Winthrop—Cont.

Contraindication: TALWIN should not be administered to patients who are hypersensitive to it.

Warnings: Drug Dependence. *Special care should be exercised in prescribing pentazocine for emotionally unstable patients and for those with a history of drug misuse. Such patients should be closely supervised when greater than 4 or 5 days of therapy is contemplated. There have been instances of psychological and physical dependence on TALWIN in patients with such a history and, rarely, in patients without such a history. Extended use of parenteral TALWIN may lead to physical or psychological dependence in some patients. When TALWIN is abruptly discontinued, withdrawal symptoms such as abdominal cramps, elevated temperature, rhinorrhea, restlessness, anxiety, and lacrimation may occur. However, even when these have occurred, discontinuance has been accomplished with minimal difficulty. In the rare patient in whom more than minor difficulty has been encountered, reinstitution of parenteral TALWIN with gradual withdrawal has ameliorated the patient's symptoms. Substituting methadone or other narcotics for TALWIN in the treatment of the pentazocine abstinence syndrome should be avoided. There have been rare reports of possible abstinence syndromes in newborns after prolonged use of TALWIN during pregnancy.*

In prescribing parenteral TALWIN for chronic use, particularly if the drug is to be self-administered, the physician should take precautions to avoid increases in dose and frequency of injection by the patient.

Just as with all medication, the oral form of TALWIN is preferable for chronic administration.

Tissue Damage at Injection Sites. Severe sclerosis of the skin, subcutaneous tissues, and underlying muscle have occurred at the injection sites of patients who have received multiple doses of pentazocine lactate. Constant rotation of injection sites is, therefore, essential. In addition, animal studies have demonstrated that TALWIN is tolerated less well subcutaneously than intramuscularly. (See DOSAGE AND ADMINISTRATION.)

Head Injury and Increased Intracranial Pressure. As in the case of other potent analgesics, the potential of TALWIN injection for elevating cerebrospinal fluid pressure may be attributed to CO_2 retention due to the respiratory depressant effects of the drug. These effects may be markedly exaggerated in the presence of head injury, other intracranial lesions, or a preexisting increase in intracranial pressure. Furthermore, TALWIN can produce effects which may obscure the clinical course of patients with head injuries. In such patients, TALWIN must be used with extreme caution and only if its use is deemed essential.

Usage in Pregnancy. Safe use of TALWIN during pregnancy (other than labor) has not been established. Animal reproduction studies have not demonstrated teratogenic or embryotoxic effects. However, TALWIN should be administered to pregnant patients (other than labor) only when, in the judgment of the physician, the potential benefits outweigh the possible hazards. Patients receiving TALWIN during labor have experienced no adverse effects other than those that occur with commonly used analgesics. TALWIN should be used with caution in women delivering premature infants.

Acute CNS Manifestations. Patients receiving therapeutic doses of TALWIN have experienced, in rare instances, hallucinations (usually visual), disorientation, and confusion which have cleared spontaneously within a period of hours. The mechanism of this reaction is not known. Such patients should be very closely observed and vital signs checked. If the drug is reinstituted, it should be done with caution since the acute CNS manifestations may recur.

Due to the potential for increased CNS depressant effects, alcohol should be used with caution in patients who are currently receiving pentazocine.

Usage in Children. Because clinical experience in children under twelve years of age is limited, the use of TALWIN in this age group is not recommended.

Ambulatory Patients. Since sedation, dizziness, and occasional euphoria have been noted, ambulatory patients should be warned not to operate machinery, drive cars, or unnecessarily expose themselves to hazards.

Myocardial Infarction. Caution should be exercised in the intravenous use of pentazocine for patients with acute myocardial infarction accompanied by hypertension or left ventricular failure. Data suggest that intravenous administration of pentazocine increases systemic and pulmonary arterial pressure and systemic vascular resistance in patients with acute myocardial infarction.

Precautions: Certain Respiratory Conditions. The possibility that TALWIN may cause respiratory depression should be considered in treatment of patients with bronchial asthma. TALWIN injection, brand of pentazocine lactate injection, should be administered only with caution and in low dosage to patients with respiratory depression (eg, from other medication, uremia, or severe infection), severely limited respiratory reserve, obstructive respiratory conditions, or cyanosis.

Impaired Renal or Hepatic Function. Although laboratory tests have not indicated that TALWIN causes or increases renal or hepatic impairment, the drug should be administered with caution to patients with such impairment. Extensive liver disease appears to predispose to greater side effects (eg, marked apprehension, anxiety, dizziness, sleepiness) from the usual clinical dose, and may be the result of decreased metabolism of the drug by the liver.

Biliary Surgery. As with all strong analgesics, TALWIN should be used with caution in patients about to undergo surgery of the biliary tract since it may cause spasm of the sphincter of Oddi.

Patients Receiving Narcotics. TALWIN is a mild narcotic antagonist. Some patients previously given narcotics, including methadone for the daily treatment of narcotic dependence, have experienced withdrawal symptoms after receiving TALWIN.

CNS Effect. Caution should be used when TALWIN is administered to patients prone to seizures; seizures have occurred in a few such patients in association with the use of TALWIN although no cause and effect relationship has been established.

Adverse Reactions: The most commonly occurring reactions are: nausea, dizziness or lightheadedness, vomiting, euphoria.

Dermatologic Reactions: Soft tissue induration, nodules, and cutaneous depression can occur at injection sites. Ulceration (sloughing) and severe sclerosis of the skin and subcutaneous tissues (and, rarely, underlying muscle) have been reported after multiple doses.

Infrequently occurring reactions are—*respiratory:* respiratory depression, dyspnea, transient apnea in a small number of newborn infants whose mothers received TALWIN during labor; *cardiovascular:* circulatory depression, shock, hypertension; *CNS effects:* sedation, alteration of mood (nervousness, apprehension, depression, floating feeling), dreams; *gastrointestinal:* constipation, dry mouth; *dermatologic including local:* diaphoresis, sting on injection, flushed skin including plethora, dermatitis including pruritus; *other:* urinary retention, headache, paresthesia, alterations in rate or strength of uterine contractions during labor.

Rarely reported reactions include—*neuromuscular and psychiatric:* muscle tremor, insomnia, disorientation, hallucinations; *gastrointestinal:* taste alteration, diarrhea and cramps; *ophthalmic:* blurred vision, nystagmus, diplopia, miosis; *hematologic:* depression of white blood cells (especially granulocytes), which is usually reversible, moderate transient eosinophilia; *other:* tachycardia, weakness or faintness, chills, allergic reactions including edema of the face, toxic epidermal necrolysis.

See **Acute CNS Manifestations** and **Drug Dependence** under **WARNINGS.**

Dosage and Administration: Adults, Excluding Patients in Labor. The recommended single parenteral dose is 30 mg by intramuscular, subcutaneous, or intravenous route. This may be repeated every 3 to 4 hours. Doses in excess of 30 mg intravenously or 60 mg intramuscularly or subcutaneously are not recommended. Total daily dosage should not exceed 360 mg. The subcutaneous route of administration should be used only when necessary because of possible severe tissue damage at injection sites (see WARNINGS). When frequent injections are needed, the drug should be administered intramuscularly. In addition, constant rotation of injection sites (eg, the upper outer quadrants of the buttocks, mid-lateral aspects of the thighs, and the deltoid areas) is essential.

Patients in Labor. A single, intramuscular 30 mg dose has been most commonly administered. An intravenous 20 mg dose has given adequate pain relief to some patients in labor when contractions become regular, and this dose may be given two or three times at two-to three-hour intervals, as needed.

Children Under 12 Years of Age. Since clinical experience in children under twelve years of age is limited, the use of TALWIN in this age group is not recommended.

CAUTION. TALWIN should not be mixed in the same syringe with soluble barbiturates because precipitation will occur.

Overdosage: Manifestations: Clinical experience with TALWIN overdosage has been insufficient to define the signs of this condition.

Treatment: Oxygen, intravenous fluids, vasopressors, and other supportive measures should be employed as indicated. Assisted or controlled ventilation should also be considered. For respiratory depression due to overdosage or unusual sensitivity to TALWIN, parenteral naloxone (Narcan®, available through Endo Laboratories) is a specific and effective antagonist.

How Supplied: *Uni-Amp®—Individual unit dose ampuls of 1 ml (30 mg)* **NDC 0024-1924-04,** *1½ ml (45 mg)* **NDC 0024-1925-04,** *and 2 ml (60 mg)* **NDC 0024-1926-04** in boxes of 25. *Uni-Nest™ ampuls of 1 ml (30 mg)* **NDC 0024-1924-14,** *1½ ml (45 mg)* **NDC 0024-1925-14,** *and 2 ml (60 mg)* **NDC 0024-1926-14** in boxes of 25.

Each 1 ml contains pentazocine lactate equivalent to 30 mg base and 2.8 mg sodium chloride, in water for injection.

Carpuject® **Sterile Cartridge-Needle Units,** *1 ml (30 mg)* **NDC 0024-1917-02,** *1½ ml (45 mg)* **NDC 0024-1918-02,** *and 2 ml (60 mg)* **NDC 0024-1919-02, all in 2 ml cartridge,** boxes of 10. Each 1 ml contains pentazocine lactate equivalent to 30 mg base, 1 mg acetone sodium bisulfite, and 2.2 mg sodium chloride, in water for injection.

Multiple-dose vials of 10 ml **NDC 0024-1916-01,** boxes of 1. Each 1 ml contains pentazocine lactate equivalent to 30 mg base, 2 mg acetone sodium bisulfite, 1.5 mg sodium chloride, and 1 mg methylparaben as preservative, in water for injection.

The pH of TALWIN solutions is adjusted between 4 and 5 with lactic acid or sodium hydroxide. The air in the ampuls and vials has been displaced by nitrogen gas.

TALWIN® 50 Ⓒ ℞

brand of pentazocine hydrochloride tablets, USP

Analgesic for Oral Use

Description: TALWIN 50, brand of pentazocine hydrochloride tablets, is a member of the benzazocine series (also known as the benzomorphan series). Chemically, pentazocine hydrochloride is 1,2,3,4,5,6 - hexahydro - 6, 11-dimethyl-3- (3-methyl-2-butenyl)-2, 6-methano-3-benzazocin-8-ol hydrochloride, a white, crystalline substance soluble in acidic aqueous solutions.

Clinical Pharmacology: TALWIN 50 is a potent analgesic which when administered orally in a 50 mg dose appears equivalent in analgesic effect to 60 mg (1 gr) of codeine. Onset of significant analgesia usually occurs between 15 and 30 minutes after oral administration, and duration of action is usually three hours or longer. Onset and duration of action and the degree of pain relief are related both to dose and the severity of pretreatment pain. TALWIN 50 weakly antagonizes the analgesic effects of morphine, meperidine, and phenazocine; in addition, it produces incomplete reversal of cardiovascular, respiratory, and behavioral depression induced by morphine and meperidine. TALWIN 50 has about 1/50 the antagonistic activity of nalorphine. It also has sedative activity.

Indications and Usage: For the relief of moderate to severe pain

Contraindication: TALWIN 50 should not be administered to patients who are hypersensitive to it.

Warnings: *Drug Dependence. There have been instances of psychological and physical dependence on parenteral pentazocine in patients with a history of drug abuse and, rarely, in patients without such a history. Abrupt discontinuance following the extended use of parenteral pentazocine has resulted in withdrawal symptoms. There have been a few reports of dependence and of withdrawal symptoms with orally administered TALWIN 50. Patients with a history of drug dependence should be under close supervision while receiving TALWIN 50 orally. There have been rare reports of possible abstinence syndromes in newborns after prolonged use of TALWIN 50 during pregnancy.*

In prescribing TALWIN 50 for chronic use, the physician should take precautions to avoid increases in dose by the patient and to prevent the use of the drug in anticipation of pain rather than for the relief of pain.

Head Injury and Increased Intracranial Pressure. As in the case of other potent analgesics, the potential of TALWIN 50 for elevating cerebrospinal fluid pressure may be attributed to CO_2 retention due to the respiratory depressant effects of the drug. These effects may be markedly exaggerated in the presence of head injury, other intracranial lesions, or a preexisting increase in intracranial pressure. Furthermore, TALWIN 50 can produce effects which may obscure the clinical course of patients with head injuries. In such patients, TALWIN 50 must be used with extreme caution and only if its use is deemed essential.

Usage in Pregnancy. Safe use of TALWIN 50 during pregnancy (other than labor) has not been established. Animal reproduction studies have not demonstrated teratogenic or embryotoxic effects. However, TALWIN 50 should be administered to pregnant patients (other than labor) only when, in the judgment of the physician, the potential benefits outweigh the possible hazards. Patients receiving TALWIN 50 during labor have experienced no adverse effects other than those that occur with commonly used analgesics. TALWIN 50 should be used with caution in women delivering premature infants.

Acute CNS Manifestations. Patients receiving therapeutic doses of TALWIN 50 have experienced, in rare instances, hallucinations (usually visual), disorientation, and confusion which have cleared spontaneously within a period of hours. The mechanism of this reaction is not known. Such patients should be very closely observed and vital signs checked. If the drug is reinstituted, it should be done with caution since the acute CNS manifestations may recur.

Due to the potential for increased CNS depressant effects, alcohol should be used with caution in patients who are currently receiving pentazocine.

Usage in Children. Because clinical experience in children under 12 years of age is limited, administration of TALWIN 50 in this age group is not recommended.

Ambulatory Patients. Since sedation, dizziness, and occasional euphoria have been noted, ambulatory patients should be warned not to operate machinery, drive cars, or unnecessarily expose themselves to hazards.

Precautions: *Certain Respiratory Conditions.* Although respiratory depression has rarely been reported after oral administration of TALWIN 50, the drug should be administered with caution to patients with respiratory depression from any cause, severely limited respiratory reserve, severe bronchial asthma and other obstructive respiratory conditions, or cyanosis.

Impaired Renal or Hepatic Function. Decreased metabolism of the drug by the liver in extensive liver disease may predispose to accentuation of side effects. Although laboratory tests have not indicated that TALWIN 50 causes or increases renal or hepatic impairment, the drug should be administered with caution to patients with such impairment.

Myocardial Infarction. As with all drugs, TALWIN 50 should be used with caution in patients with myocardial infarction who have nausea or vomiting.

Biliary Surgery. As with all strong analgesics, TALWIN 50 should be used with caution in patients about to undergo surgery of the biliary tract since it may cause spasm of the sphincter of Oddi.

Patients Receiving Narcotics. TALWIN 50 is a mild narcotic antagonist. Some patients previously given narcotics, including methadone for the daily treatment of narcotic dependence, have experienced withdrawal symptoms after receiving TALWIN 50.

CNS Effect. Caution should be used when TALWIN 50 is administered to patients prone to seizures; seizures have occurred in a few such patients in association with the use of TALWIN 50 although no cause and effect relationship has been established.

Adverse Reactions: Reactions reported after oral administration of TALWIN 50 include *gastrointestinal:* nausea, vomiting; infrequently constipation; and rarely abdominal distress, anorexia, diarrhea. *CNS effects:* dizziness, lightheadedness, sedation, euphoria, headache; infrequently weakness, disturbed dreams, insomnia, syncope, visual blurring and focusing difficulty, hallucinations (see *Acute CNS Manifestations* under **WARNINGS);** and rarely tremor, irritability, excitement, tinnitus. *Autonomic:* sweating; infrequently flushing; and rarely chills. *Allergic:* infrequently rash; and rarely urticaria, edema of the face. *Cardiovascular:* infrequently decrease in blood pressure, tachycardia. *Hematologic:* rarely depression of white blood cells (especially granulocytes), which is usually reversible, moderate transient eosinophilia. *Other:* rarely respiratory depression, urinary retention, paresthesia, toxic epidermal necrolysis.

Dosage and Administration: *Adults.* The usual initial adult dose is 1 tablet (50 mg) every three or four hours. This may be increased to 2 tablets (100 mg) when needed. Total daily dosage should not exceed 600 mg.

When antiinflammatory or antipyretic effects are desired in addition to analgesia, aspirin can be administered concomitantly with TALWIN 50, brand of pentazocine hydrochloride tablets.

Children Under 12 Years of Age. Since clinical experience in children under 12 years of age is limited, administration of TALWIN 50 in this age group is not recommended.

Duration of Therapy. Patients with chronic pain who receive TALWIN 50 orally for prolonged periods have only rarely been reported to experience withdrawal symptoms when administration was abruptly discontinued (see WARNINGS). Tolerance to the analgesic effect has also been reported only rarely. Significant abnormalities of liver and kidney function tests have not been reported, even after prolonged administration of TALWIN 50.

Overdosage: *Manifestations:* Clinical experience with TALWIN 50 overdosage has been insufficient to define the signs of this condition.

Treatment: Oxygen, intravenous fluids, vasopressors, and other supportive measures should be employed as indicated. Assisted or controlled ventilation should also be considered. For respiratory depression due to overdosage or unusual sensitivity to TALWIN 50, parenteral naloxone (Narcan®, available through Endo Laboratories) is a specific and effective antagonist.

How Supplied: Tablets, peach color, scored, each equivalent to 50 mg base.

Bottles of 100 (NDC 0024-1921-04)

Unit Dose Pack of 100, 20 strips of 5 tablets each (NDC 0024-1921-14)

Distributed by
Winthrop Laboratories
Division of Sterling Drug Inc.
New York, NY 10016
Manufactured by
Winthrop Laboratories Inc. Barceloneta,
Puerto Rico 00617

[*Shown in Product Identification Section*]

TALWIN® Compound Ⓒ ℞

brand of pentazocine hydrochloride and aspirin tablets, USP

Description: TALWIN Compound is a combination of pentazocaine hydrochloride equivalent to 12.5 mg base and aspirin 325 mg. Pentazocine is a member of the benzazocine series (also known as the benzomorphan series). Chemically, pentazocine is 1, 2, 3, 4, 5, 6 - hexahydro - 6, 11-dimethyl-3-(3-methyl-2-butenyl)-2, 6-methano-3-benzazocin-8-ol, a white, crystalline substance soluble in acidic aqueous solutions.

Clinical Pharmacology: Pentazocine is a potent analgesic which when administered orally is approximately equivalent, on a mg for mg basis, in analgesic effect to codeine. Two Caplets® of TALWIN Compound when administered orally have the additive analgesic effect equivalent to 25 mg of TALWIN plus 650 mg of aspirin. TALWIN Compound provides the analgesic effects of pentazocine and the analgesic, antiinflammatory, and antipyretic actions of aspirin.

Onset of significant analgesia usually occurs between 15 and 30 minutes after oral administration, and duration of action is usually three hours or longer. Onset and duration of action and the degree of pain relief are related both to dose and the severity of pretreatment pain. Pentazocine weakly antagonizes the analgesic effects of morphine, meperidine, and phenazocine; in addition, it produces incomplete rever-

Continued on next page

This product information was effective as of November 19, 1982. On these and other products of Winthrop Laboratories, detailed information may be obtained on a current basis by direct inquiry to the Professional Services Department, 90 Park Avenue, New York, NY 10016 (212) 907-2525.

Winthrop—Cont.

sal of cardiovascular, respiratory, and behavioral depression induced by morphine and meperidine. Pentazocine has about $\frac{1}{50}$ the antagonistic activity of nalorphine. It also has sedative activity.

Indication and Usage: For the relief of moderate pain

Contraindications: TALWIN Compound should not be administered to patients who are hypersensitive to either pentazocine or salicylates, or in any situation where aspirin is contraindicated.

Warnings: *Drug Dependence. There have been instances of psychological and physical dependence on parenteral pentazocine in patients with a history of drug abuse, and rarely, in patients without such a history. Abrupt discontinuance following the extended use of parenteral pentazocine has resulted in withdrawal symptoms. There have been a few reports of dependence and of withdrawal symptoms with orally administered pentazocine. Patients with a history of drug dependence should be under close supervision while receiving TALWIN Compound orally. There have been rare reports of possible abstinence syndromes in newborns after prolonged use of pentazocine during pregnancy. In prescribing TALWIN Compound for chronic use, the physician should take precautions to avoid increases in dose by the patient and to prevent the use of the drug in anticipation of pain rather than for the relief of pain.*

Head Injury and Increased Intracranial Pressure. The respiratory depressant effects of pentazocine and its potential for elevating cerebrospinal fluid pressure may be markedly exaggerated in the presence of head injury, other intracranial lesions, or a preexisting increase in intracranial pressure. Furthermore, pentazocine can produce effects which may obscure the clinical course of patients with head injuries. In such patients, TALWIN Compound must be used with extreme caution and only if its use is deemed essential.

Usage in Pregnancy. Safe use of pentazocine during pregnancy (other than labor) has not been established. Animal reproduction studies have not demonstrated teratogenic or embryotoxic effects. However, TALWIN Compound should be administered to pregnant patients (other than labor) only when, in the judgment of the physician, the potential benefits outweigh the possible hazards. Patients receiving pentazocine during labor have experienced no adverse effects other than those that occur with commonly used analgesics. TALWIN Compound should be used with caution in women delivering premature infants.

Acute CNS Manifestations. Patients receiving therapeutic doses of pentazocine have experienced, in rare instances, hallucinations (usually visual), disorientation, and confusion which have cleared spontaneously within a period of hours. The mechanism of this reaction is not known. Such patients should be very closely observed and vital signs checked. If the drug is reinstituted it should be done with caution since the acute CNS manifestations may recur.

Due to the potential for increased CNS depressant effects, alcohol should be used with caution in patients who are currently receiving pentazocine.

Usage in Children. Because clinical experience in children under 12 years of age is limited, administration of TALWIN Compound in this age group is not recommended.

Ambulatory Patients. Since sedation, dizziness, and occasional euphoria have been noted, ambulatory patients should be warned not to operate machinery, drive cars, or unnecessarily expose themselves to hazards.

Other. Because of its aspirin content, TALWIN Compound should be used with caution in the presence of peptic ulcer, in conjunction with anticoagulant therapy, or in any situation where the effects of aspirin may be deleterious.

Precautions: *Certain Respiratory Conditions.* Although respiratory depression has rarely been reported after oral administration of pentazocine, TALWIN Compound should be administered with caution to patients with respiratory depression from any cause, severely limited respiratory reserve, severe bronchial asthma and other obstructive respiratory conditions, or cyanosis.

Impaired Renal or Hepatic Function. Decreased metabolism of the drug by the liver in extensive liver disease may predispose to accentuation of side effects. Although laboratory tests have not indicated that pentazocine causes or increases renal or hepatic impairment, TALWIN Compound should be administered with caution to patients with such impairment.

Myocardial Infarction. As with all drugs, TALWIN Compound should be used with caution in patients with myocardial infarction who have nausea or vomiting.

Biliary Surgery. As with all strong analgesics, TALWIN Compound should be used with caution in patients about to undergo surgery of the biliary tract since it may cause spasm of the sphincter of Oddi.

Patients Receiving Narcotics. Pentazocine is a mild narcotic antagonist. Some patients previously given narcotics, including methadone for the daily treatment of narcotic dependence, have experienced withdrawal symptoms after receiving pentazocine.

CNS Effect. Caution should be used when pentazocine is administered to patients prone to seizures. Seizures have occurred in a few such patients in association with the use of pentazocine although no cause and effect relationship has been established.

Adverse Reactions: Reactions reported after oral administration of pentazocine or TALWIN Compound include *gastrointestinal:* nausea, vomiting; infrequently constipation; and rarely abdominal distress, anorexia, diarrhea. *CNS Effects:* dizziness, lightheadedness, sedation, euphoria, headache; infrequently weakness, disturbed dreams, insomnia, syncope, visual blurring and focusing difficulty, depression, hallucinations (see *Acute CNS Manifestations* under **WARNINGS**); and rarely confusion, tremor, irritability, excitement, tinnitus. *Autonomic:* sweating; infrequently flushing; and rarely chills. *Allergic:* infrequently rash; and rarely urticaria, edema of the face. *Cardiovascular:* infrequently decrease in blood pressure, tachycardia. *Hematologic:* rarely depression of white blood cells (especially granulocytes), which is usually reversible, moderate transient eosinophilia. *Other:* rarely respiratory depression, urinary retention, paresthesia, toxic epidermal necrolysis.

Dosage and Administration: *Adults.* The usual adult dose is 2 CAPLETS three or four times a day.

Children Under 12 Years of Age. Since clinical experience in children under 12 years of age is limited, administration of TALWIN Compound in this age group is not recommended.

Duration of Therapy. Patients with chronic pain who receive pentazocine orally for prolonged periods have only rarely been reported to experience withdrawal symptoms when administration was abruptly discontinued (see WARNINGS). Tolerance to the analgesic effect of pentazocine has also been reported only rarely. Significant abnormalities of liver and kidney function tests have not been reported, even after prolonged administration of pentazocine.

Overdosage: *Manifestations:* Clinical experience with pentazocine overdosage has been insufficient to define the signs of this condition. Signs of salicylate overdosage include headache, dizziness, confusion, tinnitus, diaphoresis, thirst, nausea, vomiting, diarrhea, tachycardia, tachypnea, Kussmaul breathing, convulsions, and coma. Death is usually from respiratory failure.

Treatment: Treatment for overdosage of TALWIN Compound should include treatment for salicylate poisoning as outlined in standard references.

Oxygen, intravenous fluids, vasopressors, and other supportive measures should be employed as indicated. Assisted or controlled ventilation should also be considered. For respiratory depression due to overdosage or unusual sensitivity to pentazocine, parenteral naloxone (Narcan®, available through Endo Laboratories) is a specific and effective antagonist.

How Supplied: CAPLETS, white, each containing pentazocine hydrochloride equivalent to 12.5 mg base and aspirin 325 mg. Bottles of 100 (NDC 0024-1927-04).

Distributed by Winthrop Laboratories Division of Sterling Drug Inc., New York, NY 10016, Manufactured by Winthrop Laboratories Inc., Barceloneta, Puerto Rico 00617

TELEPAQUE® ℞

brand of iopanoic acid tablets, USP

(See Diagnostic Section.)

WinGel® OTC

(See PDR For Nonprescription Drugs)

WINSTROL® ℞

brand of stanozolol tablets, USP

ANABOLIC STEROID

Description: WINSTROL, brand of stanozolol tablets, is 17-methyl-2′*H*-5α-androst -2- eno [3, 2- c] pyrazol -17β-ol.It is a heterocyclic steroid.

Clinical Pharmacology: Anabolic steroids are synthetic derivatives of testosterone. WINSTROL is primarily used for its protein anabolic effect and its catabolic inhibiting effect on tissue. Nitrogen balance is improved with anabolic agents but only when there is sufficient intake of calories and protein. Whether this positive nitrogen balance is of primary benefit in the utilization of protein-building dietary substances has not been established.

Increases in hemoglobin levels have occurred in some patients with aplastic anemia receiving anabolic steroids.

Certain clinical effects and adverse reactions demonstrate the androgenic properties of this class of drugs. Complete dissociation of anabolic and androgenic effects has not been achieved. The actions of anabolic steroids are therefore similar to those of male sex hormones with the possibility of causing serious disturbances of growth and sexual development if given to young children. They suppress the gonadotropic functions of the pituitary and may exert a direct effect upon the testes.

Indications and Usage: WINSTROL has been effective in increasing hemoglobin levels in some patients with aplastic (congenital and idiopathic) anemia. WINSTROL should be used only after diagnosis has been established.

Based on a review of WINSTROL by the National Academy of Sciences—National Research Council and/or other information, FDA has classified the other indications as follows:

"Probably" effective: as adjunctive but not primary therapy in senile and postmenopausal osteoporosis. Equal or greater consideration should be given to diet, calcium balance, physiotherapy, and good general health-promoting measures. Anabolic steroids are without value as primary therapy. In pituitary dwarfism anabolic agents may be used with care until growth hormone is more available.

Final classification of less-than-effective indications requires further investigation.

Contraindications: The use of WINSTROL is contraindicated in the following:

1. Carcinoma of the prostate or breast in male patients.
2. Carcinoma of the breast in some females.
3. Pregnancy (because of masculinization of the fetus).
4. Nephrosis or the nephrotic phase of nephritis.

Warning: Anabolic steroids do not enhance athletic ability.

Precautions: Hypercalcemia may develop, both spontaneously and as a result of hormonal therapy, in women with disseminated breast carcinoma. If it develops during anabolic steroid therapy, the drug should be stopped.

Caution is required in administering anabolic steroids to patients with cardiac, renal, or hepatic disease. Edema may occur occasionally. Concomitant administration with adrenal steroids or ACTH may add to the edema.

If amenorrhea or menstrual irregularities develop during treatment with an anabolic steroid, the drug should be discontinued until the cause is determined.

Anabolic steroids may increase sensitivity to anticoagulants; therefore, dosage of an anticoagulant may have to be decreased in order to maintain the prothrombin time at the desired therapeutic level.

Anabolic steroids have been shown to alter glucose tolerance tests. Diabetics should be carefully observed and the insulin or oral hypoglycemic dosage adjusted accordingly.

Since WINSTROL, brand of stanozolol tablets, contains a 17-alkyl group, liver function should be checked at regular intervals in patients receiving this drug.

Anabolic steroids should be used with caution in patients with benign prostatic hypertrophy.

Serum cholesterol levels may increase or decrease during therapy with anabolic steroids. Therefore, caution is required in administering these agents to patients with a history of myocardial infarction or coronary artery disease. Serial determinations of serum cholesterol levels should be made and therapy adjusted accordingly.

Anabolic agents may accelerate epiphyseal maturation more rapidly than linear growth in children, and the effect may continue for 6 months after the drug has been stopped. Therefore, therapy should be monitored by x-ray studies at 3 to 6 month intervals and the drug discontinued well before the bone age reaches the norm for chronological age, in order to avoid the risk of compromising the adult height.

Adverse Reactions: Reactions to oral anabolic steroids include nausea and vomiting; diarrhea; increased or decreased libido; acne (especially in females and prepubertal males); habituation; excitation and insomnia; chills; bleeding in patients on concomitant anticoagulant therapy; premature closure of epiphyses in children; and jaundice with, rarely, hepatic necrosis and death.

There have been rare reports of hepatocellular neoplasms and peliosis hepatis in association with long-term androgenic-anabolic steroid therapy.

Phallic enlargement and increased frequency of erections have occurred in prepubertal males. Inhibition of testicular function, testicular atrophy and oligospermia, impotence, chronic priapism, gynecomastia, and epididymitis and bladder irritability have occurred in postpubertal males.

In females, hirsutism, male pattern baldness, deepening of the voice, and clitoral enlargement have occurred. These changes are usually irreversible even after prompt discontinuance of therapy, and are not prevented by concomitant use of estrogens. Menstrual irregularities have also occurred.

Therapy with anabolic steroids has caused alterations in these clinical laboratory tests: the metyrapone test; the fasting blood sugar and glucose tolerance test; thyroid function tests [decrease in protein-bound iodine (PBI), thyroxine-binding capacity, and radioactive iodine (RAI) uptake, and increase in T_3 uptake by the red blood cells or resin. Free thyroxine is normal. The altered tests usually persist for 2 to 3 weeks after anabolic therapy has been stopped.]; liver function tests [increased Bromsulphalein (BSP) retention, increased or decreased serum cholesterol, increased serum glutamic oxaloacetic transaminase (SGOT), increased serum bilirubin, and increased alkaline phosphatase]; serum electrolytes [retention of sodium, chloride, potassium, phosphate, calcium, and water]; blood clotting tests [suppression of clotting factors II, V, VII, and X]; increased creatine and creatinine excretion lasting up to two weeks after discontinuance of therapy; and decreased 17-ketosteroid excretion.

Dosage and Administration: The suggested initial dosage for adults is 1 tablet (2 mg) three times daily just before or with meals. Although considerably smaller doses have produced a response in some patients, consistently better results have been obtained with a daily dose of 6 mg. Higher doses have been employed in patients with bone marrow damage and patients on corticosteroid therapy.

The dosage for children should be adjusted according to age. The following routine is suggested: ½ tablet twice daily for children under 6 years and up to 1 tablet three times daily for children from 6 to 12. (See Precautions.)

For young women who appear particularly susceptible to the androgenic effects of the drug, 1 tablet twice daily appears adequate for long-term administration. If this amount does not produce the desired results, the dosage may be raised to 1 tablet three times daily.

WINSTROL, brand of stanozolol tablets, should not be given to pregnant women. (See Contraindications.)

To obtain the maximal therapeutic effect, a well-balanced diet should accompany the administration of WINSTROL.

Duration of therapy will depend on the response of the condition and the appearance of adverse reactions. Therapy should be intermittent.

Duration of therapy with WINSTROL has, in most cases, varied from several weeks to one year.

How Supplied: Tablets of 2 mg, scored, bottles of 100 (NDC 0024-2253-04)

Distributed by Winthrop Laboratories
Division of Sterling Drug Inc.
New York, NY 10016
Manufactured by
Sterling Pharmaceuticals Inc.
Barceloneta, Puerto Rico 00617

[*Shown in Product Identification Section*]

ZEPHIRAN® CHLORIDE OTC
brand of benzalkonium chloride

ANTISEPTIC

AQUEOUS SOLUTION 1:750
TINTED TINCTURE 1:750
SPRAY—TINTED TINCTURE 1:750

Description: ZEPHIRAN Chloride, brand of benzalkonium chloride, NF, a mixture of alkylbenzyldimethylammonium chlorides, is a cationic quaternary ammonium surface-acting agent. It is very soluble in water, alcohol, and acetone. Aqueous solutions of ZEPHIRAN Chloride are neutral to slightly alkaline, generally colorless, and nonstaining. They have a bitter taste, aromatic odor, and foam when shaken. ZEPHIRAN Chloride Tinted Tincture 1:750 contains alcohol 50 per cent and acetone 10 per cent by volume. ZEPHIRAN Chloride Spray—Tinted Tincture 1:750 contains alcohol 92 per cent. The Tinted Tincture and Spray also contain an orange-red coloring agent.

Clinical Pharmacology: ZEPHIRAN Chloride solutions are rapidly acting antiinfective agents with a moderately long duration of action. They are active against bacteria and some viruses, fungi, and protozoa. Bacterial spores are considered to be resistant. Solutions are bacteriostatic or bactericidal according to their concentration. The exact mechanism of bactericidal action is unknown but is thought to be due to enzyme inactivation. Activity generally increases with increasing temperature and pH. Gram-positive bacteria are more susceptible than gram-negative bacteria (TABLE 1).

TABLE 1
Highest Dilution of ZEPHIRAN Chloride Aqueous Solution Destroying the Organism in 10 but not in 5 Minutes

Organisms	20 C
Streptococcus pyogenes	1:75,000
Staphylococcus aureus	1:52,500
Salmonella typhosa	1:37,500
Escherichia coli	1:10,500

Pseudomonas is the most resistant gram-negative genus. Using the AOAC Use-Dilution Confirmation Method, no growth was obtained when *Staphylococcus aureus, Salmonella choleraesuis,* and *Pseudomonas aeruginosa* (strain PRD-10) were exposed for ten minutes at 20 C to ZEPHIRAN Chloride Aqueous Solution 1:750 and Tinted Tincture 1:750.

ZEPHIRAN Chloride Aqueous Solution 1:750 has been shown to retain its bactericidal activity following autoclaving for 30 minutes at 15 lb pressure, freezing, and then thawing.

The tubercle bacillus may be resistant to aqueous ZEPHIRAN Chloride solutions but is susceptible to the 1:750 tincture (AOAC Method, 10 minutes at 20 C).

ZEPHIRAN Chloride solutions also demonstrate deodorant, wetting, detergent, keratolytic, and emulsifying activity.

Indications and Usage: ZEPHIRAN Chloride aqueous solutions in appropriate dilutions (see Recommended Dilutions) are indicated for the antisepsis of skin, mucous membranes, and wounds. They are used for preoperative preparation of the skin, surgeons' hand and arm soaks, treatment of wounds, preservation of ophthalmic solutions, irrigations of the eye, body cavities, bladder, urethra, and vaginal douching.

ZEPHIRAN Chloride Tinted Tincture 1:750 and Spray are indicated for preoperative preparation of the skin and for treatment of minor skin wounds and abrasions.

Contraindication: The use of ZEPHIRAN Chloride solutions in occlusive dressings, casts, and anal or vaginal packs is inadvisable, as they may produce irritation or chemical burns.

Warnings: Sterile Water for Injection, USP, should be used as diluent in preparing diluted aqueous solutions intended for use on deep wounds or for irrigation of body cavities. Otherwise, freshly distilled water should be used. Tap water, containing metallic ions and organic matter, may reduce antibacterial potency. Resin deionized water should not be used since it may contain pathogenic bacteria.

Continued on next page

This product information was effective as of November 19, 1982. On these and other products of Winthrop Laboratories, detailed information may be obtained on a current basis by direct inquiry to the Professional Services Department, 90 Park Avenue, New York, NY 10016 (212) 907-2525.

Winthrop—Cont.

TABLE 2
Correct Use of ZEPHIRAN Chloride

ZEPHIRAN Chloride solutions must be prepared, stored, and used correctly to achieve and maintain their antiseptic action. Serious inactivation and contamination of ZEPHIRAN Chloride solutions may occur with misuse.

CORRECT DILUENTS	INCOMPATIBILITIES	PREFERRED FORM
Sterile Water for Injection is recommended for irrigation of body cavities. *Sterile distilled water* is recommended for irrigating traumatized tissue and in the eye. *Freshly distilled water* is recommended for skin antisepsis. *Resin deionized water* should not be used because the deionizing resins can carry pathogens (especially gram-negative bacteria); they also inactivate quaternary ammonium compounds. *Stored water* is not recommended since it may contain many organisms. *Saline* should not be used since it may decrease the antibacterial potency of ZEPHIRAN Chloride solutions.	Anionic detergents and soaps should be thoroughly rinsed from the skin or other areas prior to use of ZEPHIRAN Chloride solutions because they reduce the antibacterial activity of the solutions. Serum and protein material also decrease the activity of ZEPHIRAN Chloride solutions. Corks should not be used to stopper bottles containing ZEPHIRAN Chloride solutions. Fibers of fabrics when stored in ZEPHIRAN Chloride solutions adsorb ZEPHIRAN from the surrounding liquid. Examples are: Cotton, Gauze sponges Wool, Rayon Rubber materials Applicators or sponges, intended for a skin prep, should be stored separately and dipped in ZEPHIRAN Chloride solutions immediately before use. Under certain circumstances the following commonly encountered substances are incompatible with ZEPHIRAN Chloride solutions: Iodine, Aluminum Silver nitrate, Caramel Fluorescein, Kaolin Nitrates, Pine oil Peroxide, Zinc sulfate Lanolin, Zinc oxide Potassium permanganate, Yellow oxide of mercury	ZEPHIRAN Chloride Tinted Tincture 1:750 is recommended for preoperative skin preparation because it contains alcohol and acetone which enhance its cleansing action and promote rapid drying. ZEPHIRAN Chloride Tinted Tincture 1:750, containing acetone, is recommended when it is desirable to outline the operative site. (Aqueous solutions of ZEPHIRAN Chloride used in skin preparation have a tendency to "run off" the skin.) Caution: Because of the flammable organic solvents in ZEPHIRAN Chloride Tinted Tincture 1:750 and Spray, these products should be kept away from open flame or cautery.

Organic, inorganic, and synthetic materials and surfaces may adsorb sufficient quantities of ZEPHIRAN Chloride to significantly reduce its antibacterial potency in solutions. This has resulted in serious contamination of solutions of ZEPHIRAN Chloride with viable pathogenic bacteria. Solutions should not be stored in bottles stoppered with cork closures, but rather in those equipped with appropriate screw-caps. Cotton, wool, rayon, and other materials should not be stored in ZEPHIRAN Chloride solutions. Gauze sponges and fiber pledgets used to apply solutions of ZEPHIRAN Chloride to the skin should be sterilized and stored in separate containers. Only immediately prior to application should they be immersed in ZEPHIRAN Chloride solutions.

Since ZEPHIRAN Chloride solutions are inactivated by soaps and anionic detergents, thorough rinsing is necessary if these agents are employed prior to their use.

Antiseptics such as ZEPHIRAN Chloride solutions must not be relied upon to achieve complete sterilization, because they do not destroy bacterial spores and certain viruses, including the etiologic agent of infectious hepatitis, and may not destroy *Mycobacterium tuberculosis* and other rare bacterial strains.

ZEPHIRAN Chloride Tinted Tincture 1:750 and Spray contain flammable organic solvents and should not be used near an open flame or cautery.

If solutions stronger than 1:3000 enter the eyes, irrigate immediately and repeatedly with water. Prompt medical attention should then be obtained. Concentrations greater than 1:5000 should not be used on mucous membranes, with the exception of the vaginal mucosa (see Recommended Dilutions).

Precautions: In preoperative antisepsis of the skin, ZEPHIRAN Chloride solutions should not be permitted to remain in prolonged contact with the patient's skin. Avoid pooling of the solution on the operating table.

ZEPHIRAN Chloride solutions that are used on inflamed or irritated tissues must be more dilute than those used on normal tissues (see Recommended Dilutions). ZEPHIRAN Chloride Tinted Tincture 1:750 and Spray, which contain irritating organic solvents, should be kept away from the eyes or other mucous membranes.

Adverse Reactions: ZEPHIRAN Chloride solutions in normally used concentrations have low systemic and local toxicity and are generally well tolerated, although a rare individual may exhibit hypersensitivity.

Directions for Use:

General: For most surgical applications, the recommended concentration of ZEPHIRAN Chloride Aqueous Solution or ZEPHIRAN Chloride Tinted Tincture is 1:750 (0.13 per cent). Liberal use of the solution is recommended to compensate for any adsorption of ZEPHIRAN Chloride by cotton or other materials.

To use ZEPHIRAN Chloride Spray—Tinted Tincture 1:750, remove protective cap, hold in an UPRIGHT position several inches away from the surgical field or injured area (to prevent chilling), and apply by spraying freely.

Preoperative preparation of skin: ZEPHIRAN Chloride solutions 1:750 are recommended as an antiseptic for use on unbroken skin in the preoperative preparation of the surgical field. Detergents and soaps should be thoroughly rinsed from the skin before applying ZEPHIRAN Chloride solutions. The detergent action of ZEPHIRAN Chloride solutions, particularly when used alternately with alcohol, leaves the skin smooth and clean. When ZEPHIRAN Chloride solutions are applied by friction (using several changes of sponges), dirt, skin fats, desquamating epithelium, and superficial bacteria are effectively removed, thus exposing the underlying skin to the antiseptic activity of the solutions.

The following procedure has been found satisfactory for preparation of the surgical field. On the day prior to surgery, the operative site is shaved and then scrubbed thoroughly with ZEPHIRAN Chloride Aqueous Solution 1:750. Immediately before surgery, ZEPHIRAN Chloride Tinted Tincture 1:750 or Spray is applied to the site in the usual manner (see Precautions). If the red tinted solution turns yellow during the preparation of patient's skin for surgery, it usually indicates the presence of soap (alkali) residue which is incompatible with ZEPHIRAN solutions. Therefore, rinse thoroughly and reapply the antiseptic. Because ZEPHIRAN Chloride Tinted Tincture 1:750 contains alcohol and acetone, its cleansing action on the skin is particularly effective and it dries more rapidly than the aqueous solution. The Tinted Tincture is recommended when it is desirable to outline the operative site.

Recommended Dilutions: For specific directions, see TABLES 2 and 3.

Surgery

Preoperative preparation of skin: Aqueous solution 1:750 and Tinted Tincture 1:750 or Spray

Surgeons' hand and arm soaks: Aqueous solution 1:750
Treatment of minor wounds and lacerations: Tinted Tincture 1:750 or Spray
Irrigation of deep infected wounds: Aqueous solution 1:3000 to 1:20,000
Denuded skin and mucous membranes: Aqueous solution 1:5000 to 1:10,000

Obstetrics and Gynecology

Preoperative preparation of skin: Aqueous solution 1:750 and Tinted Tincture 1:750 or Spray
Vaginal douche and irrigation: Aqueous solution 1:2000 to 1:5000
Postepisiotomy care: Aqueous solution 1:5000 to 1:10,000
Breast and nipple hygiene: Aqueous solution 1:1000 to 1:2000

Urology

Bladder and urethral irrigation: Aqueous solution 1:5000 to 1:20,000
Bladder retention lavage: Aqueous solution 1:20,000 to 1:40,000

Dermatology

Oozing and open infections: Aqueous solution 1:2000 to 1:5000
Wet dressings by irrigation or open dressing (Use in occlusive dressings is inadvisable.): Aqueous solution 1:5000 or less

Ophthalmology

Eye irrigation: Aqueous solution 1:5000 to 1:10,000
Preservation of ophthalmic solutions: Aqueous solution 1:5000 to 1:7500
[See Table 2 on preceding page].

TABLE 3
Dilutions of ZEPHIRAN Chloride Aqueous Solution 1:750

Final Dilution	ZEPHIRAN Chloride Aqueous Solution 1:750 (parts)	Distilled Water (parts)
1:1000	3	1
1:2000	3	5
1:2500	3	7
1:3000	3	9
1:4000	3	13
1:5000	3	17
1:10,000	3	37
1:20,000	3	77
1:40,000	3	157

Accidental Ingestion: If ZEPHIRAN Chloride solution, particularly a concentrated solution, is ingested, marked local irritation of the gastrointestinal tract, manifested by nausea and vomiting, may occur. Signs of systemic toxicity include restlessness, apprehension, weakness, confusion, dyspnea, cyanosis, collapse, convulsions, and coma. Death occurs as a result of paralysis of the respiratory muscles. *Treatment:* Immediate administration of several glasses of a mild soap solution, milk, or egg whites beaten in water is recommended. This may be followed by gastric lavage with a mild soap solution. Alcohol should be avoided as it promotes absorption.

To support respiration, the airway should be clear and oxygen should be administered, employing artificial respiration if necessary. If convulsions occur, a short-acting barbiturate may be given parenterally with caution.

How Supplied:

ZEPHIRAN Chloride Aqueous Solution 1:750
Bottles of 8 fl oz (NDC 0024-2521-04) and 1 gallon (NDC 0024-2521-08)
ZEPHIRAN Chloride Tinted Tincture 1:750 (*flammable*)
Bottles of 1 gallon (NDC 0024-2523-08)
ZEPHIRAN Chloride Spray—Tinted Tincture 1:750 (*flammable*)
Bottles of
1 fl oz (NDC 0024-2527-01) and
6 fl oz (NDC 0024-2527-03)

Wyeth Laboratories

Division of American Home Products Corporation
P.O. BOX 8299
PHILADELPHIA, PA 19101

Product Identification Codes

The process of imprinting all oral solid dosage forms manufactured by Wyeth with their respective National Drug Code (NDC) numbers is at present incomplete. In the future that portion of the number indicating product and strength will appear on each tablet and capsule, together with the name Wyeth.

The following is a numerical list of NDC code numbers with their corresponding product names.

Numerical Listing

Product Ident. Code	Product
1	Equanil® (meprobamate) Tablet 400 mg. Ⓒ
2	Equanil® (meprobamate) Tablet 200 mg. Ⓒ
5	Equagesic® (meprobamate and ethoheptazine citrate with aspirin) Tablet Ⓒ
6	Serax® (oxazepam) Capsule 15 mg. Ⓒ
7	Equagesic®-M (meprobamate with aspirin) Tablet Ⓒ
13	Amphojel® (dried aluminum hydroxide gel) Tablet 0.6 Gm. (10 gr.)
16	Purodigin® (crystalline digitoxin) Tablet 0.1 mg.
19	Phenergan® (promethazine HCl) Tablet 12.5 mg.
22	Aludrox® (alumina and magnesia) Tablet
27	Phenergan® (promethazine HCl) Tablet 25 mg.
28	Sparine® (promazine HCl) Tablet 50 mg.
29	Sparine® (promazine HCl) Tablet 25 mg.
30	Zactirin® (ethoheptazine citrate with aspirin) Tablet
33	Equanil® (meprobamate) Tablet Wyseals® 400 mg. Ⓒ
35	Equanitrate® 10 (meprobamate and pentaerythritol tetranitrate) Tablet
39	Equanitrate® 20 (meprobamate and pentaerythritol tetranitrate) Tablet
44	Equanil® (meprobamate) Capsule 400 mg. Ⓒ
49	Zactirin® Compound-100 (ethoheptazine citrate with aspirin, phenacetin and caffeine) Tablet
51	Serax® (oxazepam) Capsule 10 mg. Ⓒ
52	Serax® (oxazepam) Capsule 30 mg. Ⓒ
53	Omnipen® (ampicillin) Capsule 250 mg.
56	Ovral® (each tablet contains 0.5 mg. norgestrel with 0.05 mg. ethinyl estradiol) Tablet, white
57	Unipen® [(nafcillin sodium) as the monohydrate] Capsule 250 mg.
58	Pen•Vee® K (penicillin V potassium) Tablet 125 mg.
59	Pen•Vee® K (penicillin V potassium) Tablet 250 mg.
62	Ovrette® (norgestrel) Tablet
64	Ativan® (lorazepam) Tablet 1 mg. Ⓒ
65	Ativan® (lorazepam) Tablet 2 mg. Ⓒ
71	Mazanor® (mazindol) Tablet 1 mg. Ⓒ
73	Wytensin® (guanabenz acetate) Tablet 4 mg.
74	Wytensin® (guanabenz acetate) Tablet 8 mg.
75	Nordette® (each tablet contains 0.15 mg. levonorgestrel with 0.03 mg. ethinyl estradiol) Tablet
78	Lo/Ovral® (each tablet contains 0.3 mg. norgestrel with 0.03 mg. ethinyl estradiol) Tablet, white
81	Ativan® (lorazepam) Tablet 0.5 mg. Ⓒ
85	Wygesic® (each tablet contains 65 mg. propoxyphene HCl, U.S.P., and 650 mg. acetaminophen, U.S.P.) Tablet Ⓒ
114	Purodigin® (crystalline digitoxin) Tablet 0.2 mg.
119	Amphojel® (dried aluminum hydroxide gel) Tablet 0.3 Gm. (5 gr.)
127	Purodigin® (crystalline digitoxin) Tablet 0.15 mg.
165	Bicillin® (penicillin G benzathine) Tablet 200,000 units
200	Sparine® (promazine HCl) Tablet 100 mg.
202	Sparine® (promazine HCl) Tablet 10 mg.
225	Zactane® (ethoheptazine citrate) Tablet 75 mg.
227	Phenergan® (promethazine HCl) Tablet 50 mg.
252	Proketazine® (carphenazine maleate) Tablet 25 mg.
253	Proketazine® (carphenazine maleate) Tablet 50 mg.
255	Penicillin G Potassium Tablet 200,000 units (125 mg)
256	Penicillin G Potassium Tablet 250,000 units (156 mg)
261	Mepergan® Fortis (meperidine HCl and promethazine HCl) Capsule Ⓒ
266	Secobarbital Sodium Capsule 100 mg Ⓒ
267	Phenobarbital Tablet 15 mg. Ⓒ
268	Phenobarbital Tablet 30 mg. Ⓒ
269	Phenobarbital Tablet 100 mg. Ⓒ
272	Penicillin G Potassium Tablet 400,000 units (250 mg)
285	Pentobarbital Sodium Capsule 100 mg. Ⓒ
308	Meperidine HCl Tablet 50 mg. Ⓒ
309	Omnipen® (ampicillin) Capsule 500 mg.
313	Aspirin Tablet 300 mg. (5 gr.)
317	Serax® (oxazepam) Tablet 15 mg. Ⓒ
320	Phenobarbital Tablet 60 mg. Ⓒ
322	Chloral Hydrate Capsule 500 mg. Ⓒ
325	Codeine Sulfate Tablet 15 mg. Ⓒ
326	Codeine Sulfate Tablet 30 mg. Ⓒ
327	Codeine Sulfate Tablet 60 mg. Ⓒ
360	Pathocil® (dicloxacillin sodium monohydrate) Capsule 250 mg.
389	Tetracycline HCl Capsule 250 mg.
390	Pen•Vee® K (penicillin V potassium) Tablet 500 mg.
433	Phenergan® Compound (promethazine HCl and pseudoephedrine HCl with aspirin) Tablet
434	Phenergan®-D (promethazine HCl with pseudoephedrine HCl) Tablet
443	Polymagma® Plain Tablet (each tablet contains Claysorb® [activated attapulgite] 500 mg., pectin 45 mg., hydrated alumina powder 50 mg.)
445	Ovral®-28 pink inert tablet
464	Unipen® [(nafcillin sodium) as the monohydrate] 500 mg. Tablet
471	Tetracycline HCl Capsule 500 mg.
472	Basaljel® (dried basic aluminum carbonate gel) Capsule
473	Basaljel® (dried basic aluminum carbonate gel) Swallow Tablet
486	Nordette®-28, Lo/Ovral®-28 pink inert tablet
559	Wymox® (amoxicillin) 250 mg. Capsule
560	Wymox® (amoxicillin) 500 mg. Capsule
576	Wyamycin®S (erythromycin stearate) Tablet 250 mg.
578	Wyamycin®S (erythromycin stearate) Tablet 500 mg.
614	Cyclapen®-W (cyclacillin) Tablet 250 mg.

Continued on next page

Wyeth—Cont.

615 Cyclapen®-W (cyclacillin) Tablet 500 mg.
2511 Ovral®-28 Pilpak® (21 white tablets each containing 0.5 mg. norgestrel with 0.05 mg. ethinyl estradiol and 7 pink inert tablets)
2514 Lo/Ovral®-28 Pilpak® (21 white tablets each containing 0.3 mg. norgestrel with 0.03 mg. ethinyl estradiol and 7 pink inert tablets)
2533 Nordette®-28 Pilpak® (21 light-orange tablets each containing 0.15 mg. levonorgestrel with 0.03 mg ethinyl estradiol and 7 pink inert tablets)

ALUDROX® OTC
(alumina and magnesia)
ORAL SUSPENSION • TABLETS

Composition: Nonconstipating, noncathartic, effective and palatable antacid containing, in each 5 ml. teaspoonful of suspension, 307 mg. of aluminum hydroxide as a gel, and 103 mg. of magnesium hydroxide. Each tablet contains 233 mg. aluminum hydroxide as a dried gel and 83 mg. magnesium hydroxide. Sodium content is 0.07 mEq per tablet and 0.05 mEq per 5 ml suspension.
Indications: For the symptomatic relief of hyperacidity associated with the diagnosis of peptic ulcer, gastritis, peptic esophagitis, gastric hyperacidity, and hiatal hernia.
Dosage and Administration: Two tablets or 2 teaspoonfuls (10 ml.) of suspension every four hours, or as required. Suspension may be followed by a sip of water if desired. Tablets are designed to be chewed with or without water. Two ALUDROX tablets have the capacity to neutralize 23 mEq of acid; 10 ml. of ALUDROX suspension have the capacity to neutralize 28 mEq of acid.
Drug Interaction Precautions: This product must not be taken if the patient is presently taking a prescription antibiotic drug containing any form of tetracycline.
How Supplied: *Oral Suspension*, bottles of 12 fluidounces.
Tablets, boxes of 100; each tablet is sealed in cellophane so that a day's supply can be conveniently carried.

AMPHOJEL® OTC
(aluminum hydroxide gel)
SUSPENSION • TABLETS

Composition: *Suspension*—Each 5 ml. teaspoonful contains 320 mg. of aluminum hydroxide as a gel, and not more than 0.3 mEq of sodium. *Tablets* contain a dried gel. The 0.3 Gm. (5 grain) strength is equivalent to about 1 teaspoonful of the suspension and the 0.6 Gm. (10 grain) strength is equivalent to about 2 teaspoonfuls.
Indications: For the symptomatic relief of hyperacidity associated with the diagnosis of peptic ulcer, gastritis, peptic esophagitis, gastric hyperacidity, and hiatal hernia.
Dosage: *Suspension*—two teaspoonfuls followed by a sip of water if desired, five or six times daily, between meals and at bedtime. 2 teaspoonfuls have the capacity to neutralize 13 mEq of acid. *Tablets*—Two tablets of the 0.3 Gm. strength, or one tablet of the 0.6 Gm. strength, five or six times daily between meals and at bedtime. 2 tablets have the capacity to neutralize 18 mEq of acid.
Precaution: May cause constipation.
Drug Interaction Precautions: This product must not be taken if the patient is presently taking a prescription antibiotic drug containing any form of tetracycline.
How Supplied: *Suspension*—Peppermint flavored; without flavor—bottles of 12 fluidounces. *Tablets*—a convenient auxiliary dosage form—0.3 Gm. (5 gr.), bottles of 100; 0.6 Gm. (10 gr.), boxes of 100.

ATIVAN® Ⓒ ℞
(lorazepam)

Description: Ativan (lorazepam), an antianxiety agent, has the chemical formula, 7-chloro-5-(o-chlorophenyl)-1, 3-dihydro-3-hydroxy-2H-1,4-benzodiazepin-2-one.
It is a nearly white powder almost insoluble in water. Each Ativan (lorazepam) tablet, to be taken orally, contains 0.5 mg, 1 mg or 2 mg of lorazepam.
Clinical Pharmacology: Studies in healthy volunteers show that in single high doses Ativan (lorazepam) has a tranquilizing action on the central nervous system with no appreciable effect on the respiratory or cardiovascular systems.
Ativan (lorazepam) is readily absorbed with an absolute bioavailability of 90 percent. Peak concentrations in plasma occur approximately 2 hours following administration. The peak plasma level of lorazepam from a 2 mg dose is approximately 20 ng/ml.
The mean half-life of unconjugated lorazepam in human plasma is about 12 hours and for its major metabolite, lorazepam glucuronide, about 18 hours. At clinically relevant concentrations, lorazepam is approximately 85% bound to plasma proteins. Ativan (lorazepam) is rapidly conjugated at its 3-hydroxy group into lorazepam glucuronide which is then excreted in the urine. Lorazepam glucuronide has no demonstrable CNS activity in animals. The plasma levels of lorazepam are proportional to the dose given. There is no evidence of accumulation of lorazepam on administration up to six months.
Studies comparing young and elderly subjects have shown that the pharmacokinetics of lorazepam remain unaltered with advancing age.
Indications and Usage: Ativan (lorazepam) is indicated for the management of anxiety disorders or for the short-term relief of the symptoms of anxiety or anxiety associated with depressive symptoms. Anxiety or tension associated with the stress of everyday life usually does not require treatment with an anxiolytic.
The effectiveness of Ativan (lorazepam) in long-term use, that is, more than 4 months, has not been assessed by systematic clinical studies. The physician should periodically reassess the usefulness of the drug for the individual patient.
Contraindications: Ativan (lorazepam) is contraindicated in patients with known sensitivity to the benzodiazepines or with acute narrow-angle glaucoma.
Warnings: Ativan (lorazepam) is not recommended for use in patients with a primary depressive disorder or psychosis. As with all patients on CNS-acting drugs, patients receiving lorazepam should be warned not to operate dangerous machinery or motor vehicles and that their tolerance for alcohol and other CNS depressants will be diminished.
PHYSICAL AND PSYCHOLOGICAL DEPENDENCE: Withdrawal symptoms similar in character to those noted with barbiturates and alcohol have occurred following abrupt discontinuance of benzodiazepine drugs. These symptoms include convulsions, tremor, abdominal and muscle cramps, vomiting and sweating. Addiction-prone individuals, such as drug addicts and alcoholics, should be under careful surveillance when receiving benzodiazepines because of the predisposition of such patients to habituation and dependence.
Withdrawal symptoms have also been reported following abrupt discontinuance of benzodiazepines taken continuously at therapeutic levels for several months.
Precautions: In patients with depression accompanying anxiety, a possibility for suicide should be borne in mind.
For elderly or debilitated patients, the initial daily dosage should not exceed 2 mg in order to avoid oversedation.
Ativan® (lorazepam) dosage should be terminated gradually, since abrupt withdrawal of any anti-anxiety agent may result in symptoms similar to those for which patients are being treated: anxiety, agitation, irritability, tension, insomnia, and occasional convulsions. The usual precautions for treating patients with impaired renal or hepatic function should be observed.
In patients where gastrointestinal or cardiovascular disorders coexist with anxiety, it should be noted that lorazepam has not been shown to be of significant benefit in treating the gastrointestinal or cardiovascular component.
Esophageal dilation occurred in rats treated with lorazepam for more than one year at 6 mg/kg/day. The no-effect dose was 1.25 mg/kg/day (approximately 6 times the maximum human therapeutic dose of 10 mg per day). The effect was reversible only when the treatment was withdrawn within two months of first observation of the phenomenon. The clinical significance of this is unknown. However, use of lorazepam for prolonged periods and in geriatric patients requires caution, and there should be frequent monitoring for symptoms of upper G.I. disease.
Safety and effectiveness of Ativan (lorazepam) in children of less than 12 years have not been established.
ESSENTIAL LABORATORY TESTS: Some patients on Ativan (lorazepam) have developed leukopenia, and some have had elevations of LDH. As with other benzodiazepines, periodic blood counts and liver-function tests are recommended for patients on long-term therapy.
CLINICALLY SIGNIFICANT DRUG INTERACTIONS: The benzodiazepines, including Ativan (lorazepam), produce CNS depressant effects when administered with such medications as barbiturates or alcohol.
CARCINOGENESIS AND MUTAGENESIS: No evidence of carcinogenic potential emerged in rats during an 18-month study with Ativan (lorazepam). No studies regarding mutagenesis have been performed.
PREGNANCY: Reproductive studies in animals were performed in mice, rats, and two strains of rabbits. Occasional anomalies (reduction of tarsals, tibia, metatarsals, malrotated limbs, gastroschisis, malformed skull, and microphthalmia) were seen in drug-treated rabbits without relationship to dosage. Although all of these anomalies were not present in the concurrent control group, they have been reported to occur randomly in historical controls. At doses of 40 mg/kg and higher, there was evidence of fetal resorption and increased fetal loss in rabbits which was not seen at lower doses.
The clinical significance of the above findings is not known. However, an increased risk of congenital malformations associated with the use of minor tranquilizers (chlordiazepoxide, diazepam, and meprobamate) during the first trimester of pregnancy has been suggested in several studies. Because the use of these drugs is rarely a matter of urgency, the use of lorazepam during this period should almost always be avoided. The possibility that a woman of childbearing potential may be pregnant at the time of institution of therapy should be considered. Patients should be advised that if they become pregnant, they should communicate with their physician about the desirability of discontinuing the drug.
In humans, blood levels obtained from umbilical cord blood indicate placental transfer of lorazepam and lorazepam glucuronide.

NURSING MOTHERS: It is not known whether oral lorazepam is excreted in human milk like the other benzodiazepine tranquilizers. As a general rule, nursing should not be undertaken while a patient is on a drug, since many drugs are excreted in human milk.

Adverse Reactions: Adverse reactions, if they occur, are usually observed at the beginning of therapy and generally disappear on continued medication or upon decreasing the dose. In a sample of about 3,500 anxious patients, the most frequent adverse reaction to Ativan® (lorazepam) is sedation (15.9%), followed by dizziness (6.9%), weakness (4.2%), and unsteadiness (3.4%). Less frequent adverse reactions are disorientation, depression, nausea, change in appetite, headache, sleep disturbance, agitation, dermatological symptoms, eye function disturbance, together with various gastrointestinal symptoms and autonomic manifestations. The incidence of sedation and unsteadiness increased with age.

Small decreases in blood pressure have been noted but are not clinically significant, probably being related to the relief of anxiety produced by Ativan (lorazepam).

Overdosage: In the management of overdosage with any drug, it should be borne in mind that multiple agents may have been taken.

Manifestations of Ativan (lorazepam) overdosage include somnolence, confusion, and coma. Induced vomiting and/or gastric lavage should be undertaken, followed by general supportive care, monitoring of vital signs, and close observation of the patient. Hypotension, though unlikely, usually may be controlled with Levarterenol Bitartrate Injection, USP. The usefulness of dialysis has not been determined.

Dosage and Administration: Ativan® (lorazepam) is administered orally. For optimal results, dose, frequency of administration, and duration of therapy should be individualized according to patient response. To facilitate this, 0.5 mg, 1 mg and 2 mg tablets are available.

The usual range is 2 to 6 mg/day given in divided doses, the largest dose being taken before bedtime, but the daily dosage may vary from 1 to 10 mg/day.

For anxiety, most patients require an initial dose of 2 to 3 mg/day given b.i.d. or t.i.d.

For insomnia due to anxiety or transient situational stress, a single daily dose of 2 to 4 mg may be given, usually at bedtime.

For elderly or debilitated patients, an initial dosage of 1 to 2 mg/day in divided doses is recommended, to be adjusted as needed and tolerated.

The dosage of Ativan (lorazepam) should be increased gradually when needed to help avoid adverse effects. When higher dosage is indicated, the evening dose should be increased before the daytime doses.

How Supplied: Ativan® (lorazepam) Tablets, Wyeth®, are available in the following dosage strengths in bottles of 100 and 500 tablets, and in Redipak® Strip Pack, boxes of 25:

0.5 mg, NDC 0008-0081, white, five-sided tablet with a raised "A" on one side and "WYETH" and "81" on reverse side.

1 mg, NDC 0008-0064, white, five-sided tablet with a raised "A" on one side and "WYETH" and "64" on scored reverse side.

2 mg, NDC 0008-0065, white, oval tablet with "WYETH" on one side and "65" on scored reverse side.

Store at controlled room temperature.
Keep bottles tightly closed.
Dispense in tight container.

[*Shown in Product Identification Section*]

ATIVAN® Ⓒ ℞
(lorazepam)
Injection

Description: Ativan (lorazepam) Injection, a benzodiazepine with anti-anxiety and sedative effects, is intended for intramuscular or intravenous route of administration. It has the chemical formula: 7-chloro-5-(o-chlorophenyl)-1,3-dihydro-3-hydroxy- 2 *H*-1, 4-benzodiazepin-2-one. The molecular weight is 321.2 and the C.A.S. No. is [846-49-1].

Lorazepam is a nearly white powder almost insoluble in water. Each ml of sterile injection contains either 2.0 or 4.0 mg of lorazepam, 0.18 ml polyethylene glycol 400 in propylene glycol with 2.0% benzyl alcohol as preservative.

Clinical Pharmacology: Intravenous or intramuscular administration of the recommended dose of 2–4 mg of Ativan (lorazepam) Injection to adult patients is followed by dose related effects of sedation (sleepiness or drowsiness), relief of pre-operative anxiety and lack of recall of events related to the day of surgery in the majority of patients. The clinical sedation (sleepiness or drowsiness), thus noted is such that the majority of patients are able to respond to simple instructions whether they give the appearance of being awake or asleep. The lack of recall is relative rather than absolute, as determined under conditions of careful patient questioning and testing using props designed to enhance recall. The majority of patients under these reinforced conditions had difficulty recalling peri-operative events, or recognizing props from before surgery. The lack of recall and recognition was optimum within 2 hours following intramuscular administration and 15–20 minutes after intravenous injection.

The intended effects of the recommended adult dose of lorazepam injection usually last 6–8 hours. In rare instances and where patients received greater than the recommended dose, excessive sleepiness and prolonged lack of recall were noted. As with other benzodiazepines, unsteadiness, enhanced sensitivity to CNS depressant effects of ethyl alcohol and other drugs were noted in isolated and rare cases for greater than 24 hours.

Studies in healthy adult volunteers reveal that intravenous lorazepam in doses up to 3.5 mg/70 kg does not alter sensitivity to the respiratory stimulating effect of carbon dioxide and does not enhance the respiratory depressant effects of doses of meperidine up to 100 mg/70 kg (also determined by carbon dioxide challenge) as long as patients remain sufficiently awake to undergo testing. Upper airway obstruction has been observed in rare instances where the patient received greater than the recommended dose, and was excessively sleepy and difficult to arouse. (See WARNINGS and ADVERSE REACTIONS).

Clinically employed doses of lorazepam injectable do not greatly affect the circulatory system in the supine position or employing a 70 degree tilt test. Doses of 8–10 mg of intravenous lorazepam (2 to 2½ times the maximum recommended dosage) will produce loss of lid reflexes within 15 minutes.

Studies in six (6) healthy young adults who received lorazepam injection and no other drugs revealed that visual tracking (the ability to keep a moving line centered) was impaired for a mean of eight (8) hours following administration of 4 mg of intramuscular lorazepam and four (4) hours following administration of 2 mg intramuscularly with considerable subject variation. Similar findings were noted with pentobarbital 150 and 75 mg. Although this study showed that both lorazepam and pentobarbital interfered with eye-hand coordination, the data are insufficient to predict when it would be safe to operate a motor vehicle or engage in a hazardous occupation or sport.

PHARMACOKINETICS

Injectable Ativan (lorazepam) is readily absorbed when given intramuscularly. Peak plasma concentrations occur approximately 60–90 minutes following administration and appear to be dose related, e.g. a 2.0 mg dose provides a level of approximately 20 ng/ml and a 4.0 mg dose aproximately 40 ng/ml in plasma. The mean half-life of lorazepam is about 16 hours when given intravenously or intramuscularly. Ativan (lorazepam) is rapidly conjugated at the 3-hydroxyl group into its major metabolite, lorazepam glucuronide, which is then excreted in the urine. Lorazepam glucuronide has no demonstrable CNS activity in animals. When 5 mg of intravenous lorazepam was administered to volunteers once a day for four consecutive days, a steady state of free lorazepam was achieved by the second day (approximately 52 ng/ml of plasma three hours after the first dose and approximately 62 ng/ml three hours after each subsequent dose, one day apart). At clinically relevant concentrations, lorazepam is bound 85% to plasma proteins.

Indications and Usage: Ativan (lorazepam) Injection is indicated in adult patients for preanesthetic medication, producing sedation (sleepiness or drowsiness), relief of anxiety, and a decreased ability to recall events related to the day of surgery. It is most useful in those patients who are anxious about their surgical procedure and who would prefer to have diminished recall of the events of the day of surgery. (see Information for Patients)

Contraindications: Ativan (lorazepam) Injection is contraindicated in patients with a known sensitivity to benzodiazepines or its vehicle (polyethylene glycol, propylene glycol, and benzyl alcohol) and in patients with acute narrow angle glaucoma. The use of Ativan (lorazepam) Injection intra-arterially is contraindicated because, as with other injectable benzodiazepines, inadvertent intra-arterial injection may produce arteriospasm resulting in gangrene which may require amputation. (see Warnings)

Warnings: PRIOR TO INTRAVENOUS USE, ATIVAN INJECTION SHOULD BE DILUTED WITH AN EQUAL AMOUNT OF COMPATIBLE DILUENT (SEE DOSAGE AND ADMINISTRATION). INTRAVENOUS INJECTION SHOULD BE MADE SLOWLY AND WITH REPEATED ASPIRATION. CARE SHOULD BE TAKEN TO DETERMINE THAT ANY INJECTION WILL NOT BE INTRA-ARTERIAL AND THAT PERIVASCULAR EXTRAVASATION WILL NOT TAKE PLACE.

PARTIAL AIRWAY OBSTRUCTION MAY OCCUR IN HEAVILY SEDATED PATIENTS. INTRAVENOUS LORAZEPAM, WHEN GIVEN ALONE IN GREATER THAN THE RECOMMENDED DOSE, OR AT THE RECOMMENDED DOSE AND ACCOMPANIED BY OTHER DRUGS USED DURING THE ADMINISTRATION OF ANESTHESIA, MAY PRODUCE HEAVY SEDATION, THEREFORE EQUIPMENT NECESSARY TO MAINTAIN A PATENT AIRWAY AND TO SUPPORT RESPIRATION/VENTILATION SHOULD BE AVAILABLE.

There is no evidence to support the use of lorazepam injection in coma, shock or acute alcohol intoxication at this time. Since the liver is the most likely site of conjugation of lorazepam and since excretion of conjugated lorazepam (glucuronide), is a renal function, this drug is not recommended for use in patients with hepatic and/or renal *failure.* This does not preclude use of the drug in patients with mild to moderate hepatic or renal disease. When injectable lorazepam is selected for use in patients with mild to moderate hepatic or renal disease, the lowest effective dose should be considered since drug effect may be prolonged. Experience with other benzodiazepines and limited experience with parenteral lorazepam has demonstrated that tolerance to alcoholic beverages, and other central nervous system depressants is diminished when used concomitantly.

As is true of similar CNS-acting drugs, patients receiving injectable lorazepam should not op-

Continued on next page

Wyeth—Cont.

erate machinery or engage in hazardous occupations or drive a motor vehicle for a period of 24–48 hours. Impairment of performance may persist for greater intervals because of extremes of age, concomitant use of other drugs, stress of surgery or the general condition of the patient.

Clinical trials have shown that patients over the age of 50 years may have a more profound and prolonged sedation with intravenous lorazepam. Ordinarily an initial dose of 2 mg may be adequate, unless a greater degree of lack of recall is desired.

As with all central nervous system depressant drugs, care should be exercised in patients given injectable lorazepam that premature ambulation may result in injury from falling.

There is no added beneficial effect to the addition of scopolamine to injectable lorazepam and their combined effect may result in an increased incidence of sedation, hallucination and irrational behavior.

PREGNANCY

ATIVAN® (LORAZEPAM) MAY CAUSE FETAL DAMAGE WHEN ADMINISTERED TO PREGNANT WOMEN. An increased risk of congenital malformations associated with the use of minor tranquilizers (chlordiazepoxide, diazepam and meprobamate) during the first trimester of pregnancy has been suggested in several studies. In humans, blood levels obtained from umbilical cord blood indicate placental transfer of lorazepam and lorazepam glucuronide.

Ativan Injection should not be used during pregnancy. There are insufficient data regarding obstetrical safety of parenteral lorazepam, including use in cesarean section. Such use, therefore, is not recommended.

Reproductive studies in animals were performed in mice, rats, and two strains of rabbits. Occasional anomalies (reduction of tarsals, tibia, metatarsals, malrotated limbs, gastroschisis, malformed skull and microphthalmia) were seen in drug-treated rabbits without relationship to dosage.

Although all of these anomalies were not present in the concurrent control group, they have been reported to occur randomly in historical controls. At doses of 40 mg/kg orally or 4 mg/kg intravenously and higher, there was evidence of fetal resorption and increased fetal loss in rabbits which was not seen at lower doses.

ENDOSCOPIC PROCEDURES

There are insufficient data to support the use of Ativan (lorazepam) Injection for outpatient endoscopic procedures. Inpatient endoscopic procedures require adequate recovery room observations.

Pharyngeal reflexes are not impaired when Ativan Injection is used for per-oral endoscopic procedures, therefore adequate topical or regional anesthesia is recommended to minimize reflex activity associated with such procedures.

Precautions:

GENERAL

The additive central nervous system effects of other drugs such as phenothiazines, narcotic analgesics, barbiturates, anti-depressants, scopolamine and monoamine oxidase inhibitors should be borne in mind when these other drugs are used concomitantly with or during the period of recovery from Ativan (lorazepam) Injection. (See CLINICAL PHARMACOLOGY and WARNINGS).

Extreme care must be used in administering Ativan Injection to elderly patients, very ill patients, and to patients with limited pulmonary reserve, because of the possibility that underventilation and/or hypoxic cardiac arrest may occur. Resuscitative equipment for ventilatory support should be readily available. (See WARNINGS and DOSAGE and ADMINISTRATION).

When lorazepam injection is used IV as the premedicant prior to regional or local anesthesia, the possibility of excessive sleepiness or drowsiness may interfere with patient cooperation to determine levels of anesthesia. This is most likely to occur when greater than 0.05 mg/kg is given and when narcotic analgesics are used concomitantly with the recommended dose. (See ADVERSE REACTIONS).

INFORMATION FOR PATIENTS

As appropriate, the patient should be informed of the pharmacological effects of the drug such as sedation, relief of anxiety and lack of recall and the duration of these effects (about 8 hours) so that they may adequately perceive the risks as well as the benefits to be derived from its use.

Patients who receive Ativan Injection as a premedicant should be cautioned that driving an automobile or operating hazardous machinery, or engaging in a hazardous sport should be delayed for 24–48 hours following the injection. Sedatives, tranquilizers, and narcotic analgesics may produce a more prolonged and profound effect when administered along with injectable Ativan. This effect may take the form of excessive sleepiness or drowsiness, and on rare occasions, interfere with recall and recognition of events of the day of surgery and the day after.

Getting out of bed unassisted may result in falling and injury if undertaken within 8 hours of receiving lorazepam injection. Alcoholic beverages should not be consumed for at least 24–48 hours after receiving lorazepam injectable due to the additive effects on central nervous system depression seen with benzodiazepines in general. Elderly patients should be told that Ativan (lorazepam) Injection may make them very sleepy for a period longer than six (6) to eight (8) hours following surgery.

LABORATORY TESTS

In clinical trials no laboratory test abnormalities were identified with either single or multiple doses of Ativan (lorazepam) Injection. These tests included: CBC, urinalysis, SGOT, SGPT, bilirubin, alkaline phosphatase, LDH, cholesterol, uric acid, BUN, glucose, calcium, phosphorus and total proteins.

DRUG INTERACTIONS

Ativan (lorazepam) Injection, like other injectable benzodiazepines, produces depression of the central nervous system when administered with ethyl alcohol, phenothiazines, barbiturates, MAO inhibitors and other antidepressants. When scopolamine is used concomitantly with injectable lorazepam an increased incidence of sedation, hallucinations and irrational behavior has been observed.

DRUG/LABORATORY TEST INTERACTIONS

No laboratory test abnormalities were identified when lorazepam was given alone or concomitantly with another drug, such as narcotic analgesics, inhalation anesthetics, scopolamine, atropine, and a variety of tranquilizing agents.

CARCINOGENESIS, MUTAGENESIS, IMPAIRMENT OF FERTILITY

No evidence of carcinogenic potential emerged in rats and mice during an 18-month study with oral lorazepam. No studies regarding mutagenesis have been performed. Pre-implantation study in rats was performed with oral lorazepam at a 20 mg/kg dose and showed no impairment of fertility.

PREGNANCY

Pregnancy Category D. See WARNINGS section.

LABOR AND DELIVERY

There are insufficient data to support the use of Ativan® (lorazepam) injection during labor and delivery, including cesarean section, therefore its use in this situation is not recommended.

NURSING MOTHERS

Injectable lorazepam should not be administered to nursing mothers, because like other benzodiazepines, the possibility exists that lorazepam may be excreted in human milk and sedate the infant.

PEDIATRIC USE

There are insufficient data to support efficacy or make dosage recommendations for injectable lorazepam in patients less than 18 years of age, therefore, such use is not recommended.

Adverse Reactions:

CENTRAL NERVOUS SYSTEM

The most frequent adverse effects seen with injectable lorazepam are an extension of the central nervous system depressant effects of the drug. The incidence varied from one study to another, depending on the dosage, route of administration, use of other central nervous system depressants, and the investigator's opinion concerning the degree and duration of desired sedation. Excessive sleepiness and drowsiness were the main side effects. This interfered with patient cooperation in approximately 6% (25/446) of patients undergoing regional anesthesia in that they were unable to assess levels of anesthesia in regional blocks or with caudal anesthesia. Patients over 50 years of age had a higher incidence of excessive sleepiness or drowsiness when compared with those under 50 (21/106 vs 24/245) when lorazepam was given intravenously. (see DOSAGE and ADMINISTRATION). On rare occasion (3/1580) the patient was unable to give personal identification in the operating room on arrival, and one patient fell when attempting premature ambulation in the post-operative period.

Symptoms such as restlessness, confusion, depression, crying, sobbing, and delirium occurred in about 1.3% (20/1580). One patient injured himself by picking at his post-operative incision.

Hallucinations were present in about 1% (14/1580) of patients, and were visual and self-limiting.

An occasional patient complained of dizziness, diplopia and/or blurred vision. Depressed hearing was infrequently reported during the peak effect period.

An occasional patient had a prolonged recovery room stay, either because of excessive sleepiness or because of some form of inappropriate behavior. The latter was seen most commonly when scopolamine was given concomitantly as a premedicant.

Limited information derived from patients who were discharged the day after receiving injectable lorazepam showed one patient complained of some unsteadiness of gait and a reduced ability to perform complex mental functions. Enhanced sensitivity to alcoholic beverages has been reported more than 24 hours after receiving injectable lorazepam, similar to experience with other benzodiazepines.

LOCAL EFFECTS

Intramuscular injection of lorazepam has resulted in pain at the injection site, a sensation of burning, or observed redness in the same area in a very variable incidence from one study to another. The overall incidence of pain and burning was about 17% (146/859) in the immediate post-injection period, and about 1.4% (12/859) at the 24-hour observation time. Reactions at the injection site (redness) occurred in approximately 2% (17/859) in the immediate post-injection period, and were present 24 hours later in about 0.8% (7/859).

Intravenous administration of lorazepam resulted in painful responses in 13/771 patients or approximately 1.6% in the immediate post-injection period and 24 hours later 4/771 patients or about 0.5% still complained of pain. Redness did not occur immediately following intravenous injection, but was noted in 19/771 patients at the 24-hour observation period. This incidence is similar to that observed with an intravenous infusion before lorazepam is given.

CARDIOVASCULAR SYSTEM

Hypertension (0.1%) and hypotension (0.1%) have occasionally been observed after patients have received injectable lorazepam.

RESPIRATORY SYSTEM

Five patients (5/446) who underwent regional anesthesia were observed to have partial airway obstruction. This was believed due to excessive sleepiness at the time of the procedure, and resulted in temporary underventilation. Immediate attention to the airway, employing the usual countermeasures, will usually suffice to manage this condition (see also CLINICAL PHARMACOLOGY, WARNINGS and PRECAUTIONS).

OTHER ADVERSE EXPERIENCES

Skin rash, nausea, and vomiting have occasionally been noted in patients who have received injectable lorazepam combined with other drugs during anesthesia and surgery.

Drug Abuse and Dependence: As with other benzodiazepines, Ativan (lorazepam) Injection has a low potential for abuse and may lead to limited dependence. Although there are no clinical data available for injectable lorazepam in this respect, physicians should be aware that repeated doses over a prolonged period of time may result in limited physical and psychological dependence.

Overdosage: Overdosage of benzodiazepines is usually manifested by varying degrees of central nervous system depression ranging from drowsiness to coma. In mild cases symptoms include drowsiness, mental confusion and lethargy. In more serious examples, symptoms may include ataxia, hypotonia, hypotension, hypnosis, stages one (1) to three (3) coma, and very rarely death.

Treatment of overdose is mainly supportive until the drug is eliminated from the body. Vital signs and fluid balance should be carefully monitored. An adequate airway should be maintained and assisted respiration used as needed. With normally functioning kidneys, forced diuresis with intravenous fluids and electrolytes may accelerate elimination of benzodiazepines from the body. In addition, osmotic diuretics such as mannitol may be effective as adjunctive measures. In more critical situations, renal dialysis and exchange blood transfusions may be indicated. Published reports indicate that intravenous infusion of 0.5 to 4 mg of physostigmine at the rate of 1 mg/minute may reverse symptoms and signs suggestive of central anticholinergic overdose (confusion, memory disturbance, visual disturbances, hallucinations, delirium); however, hazards associated with the use of physostigmine (i.e. induction of seizures) should be weighed against its possible clinical benefit.

Dosage and Administration:

INTRAMUSCULAR INJECTION

For the designated indications as a premedicant, the usual recommended dose of lorazepam for intramuscular injection is 0.05 mg/kg up to a maximum of 4 mg. As with all premedicant drugs, the dose should be individualized. (See also CLINICAL PHARMACOLOGY, WARNINGS, PRECAUTIONS, and ADVERSE REACTIONS).

Doses of other central nervous system depressant drugs should be ordinarily reduced (See PRECAUTIONS). *For optimum effect, measured as lack of recall, intramuscular lorazepam should be administered at least 2 hours before the anticipated operative procedure.* Narcotic analgesics should be administered at their usual pre-operative time. There are insufficient data to support efficacy to make dosage recommendations for intramuscular lorazepam in patients less than 18 years of age, therefore such use is not recommended.

INTRAVENOUS INJECTION

For the primary purpose of sedation and relief of anxiety, the usual recommended initial dose of lorazepam for intravenous injection is 2 mg total, or 0.02 mg/lb (0.044 mg/kg) whichever is smaller. This dose will suffice for sedating most adult patients, and should not ordinarily be exceeded in patients over 50 years of age. In those patients in whom a greater likelihood of lack of recall for perioperative events would be beneficial, larger doses as high as 0.05 mg/kg up to a total of 4 mg may be administered. (See CLINICAL PHARMACOLOGY, WARNINGS, PRECAUTIONS, and ADVERSE REACTIONS). Doses of other injectable central nervous system depressant drugs should ordinarily be reduced. (See PRECAUTIONS). *For optimum effect, measured as lack of recall, intravenous lorazepam should be administered 15–20 minutes before the anticipated operative procedure.*

EQUIPMENT NECESSARY TO MAINTAIN A PATENT AIRWAY SHOULD BE IMMEDIATELY AVAILABLE PRIOR TO INTRAVENOUS ADMINISTRATION OF LORAZEPAM (See WARNINGS).

There are insufficient data to support efficacy or make dosage recommendations for intravenous lorazepam in patients less than 18 years of age, therefore, such use is not recommended.

ADMINISTRATION

When given intramuscularly, Ativan® Injection, undiluted, should be injected deep in the muscle mass.

Injectable Ativan (lorazepam) can be used with atropine sulfate, narcotic analgesics, other parenterally used analgesics, commonly used anesthetics, and muscle relaxants.

Immediately prior to intravenous use, Ativan (lorazepam) Injection must be diluted with an equal volume of compatible solution. When properly diluted the drug may be injected directly into a vein or into the tubing of an existing intravenous infusion. The rate of injection should not exceed 2.0 mg per minute.

Parenteral drug products should be inspected visually for particulate matter and discoloration prior to administration whenever solution and container permit. Do not use if solution is discolored or contains a precipitate.

Ativan (lorazepam) Injection is compatible for dilution purposes with the following solutions:
Sterile Water for Injection, USP
Sodium Chloride Injection, USP
5% Dextrose Injection, USP

How Supplied: Ativan® (lorazepam) Injection, Wyeth®, is available in the following dosage strengths in multiple-dose vials and in TUBEX® Sterile Cartridge-Needle Units, packaged in boxes of 10 TUBEX:

2 mg per ml, NDC 0008-0581; 10 ml vial and 1 ml fill in 2 ml TUBEX.

4 mg per ml, NDC 0008-0570; 10 ml vial and 1 ml fill in 2 ml TUBEX.

For IM or IV injection.
Protect from light.
Keep in a refrigerator.

Directions for Dilution for IV Use: To dilute, adhere to the following procedure:

For TUBEX—

1. Extrude the entire amount of air in the half-filled TUBEX.
2. Slowly aspirate the desired volume of diluent.
3. Pull back slightly on the plunger to provide additional mixing space.
4. Immediately mix contents thoroughly by gently inverting TUBEX repeatedly until a homogenous solution results. Do not shake vigorously, as this will result in air entrapment.

For Vial—

Aspirate the desired amount of Ativan Injection into the syringe. Then proceed as described under TUBEX.

BASALJEL® — OTC

(basic aluminum carbonate gel)
SUSPENSION •CAPSULES •SWALLOW TABLETS

Composition: Suspension—each 5 ml teaspoonful contains basic aluminum carbonate gel equivalent to 400 mg aluminum hydroxide. Extra Strength Suspension—each 5 ml teaspoonful contains basic aluminum carbonate gel equivalent to 1000 mg aluminum hydroxide. Capsule contains dried basic aluminum carbonate gel equivalent to 608 mg of dried aluminum hydroxide gel or 500 mg aluminum hydroxide. Tablet contains dried basic aluminum carbonate gel equivalent to 608 mg of dried aluminum hydroxide gel or 500 mg aluminum hydroxide.

Indications: For the symptomatic relief of hyperacidity associated with the diagnosis of peptic ulcer, gastritis, peptic esophagitis, gastric hyperacidity and hiatal hernia.

Warnings: No more than 24 tablets/capsules/teaspoonfuls of BASALJEL, and no more than 12 teaspoonfuls of BASALJEL Extra Strength Suspension should be taken in a 24-hour period. Dosage should be carefully supervised since continued overdosage, in conjunction with restriction of dietary phosphorous and calcium, may produce a persistently lowered serum phosphate and a mildly elevated alkaline phosphatase. A usually transient hypercalciuria of mild degree may be associated with the early weeks of therapy.

Dosage and Administration: Suspension—two teaspoonfuls (10 ml) in water or fruit juice taken as often as every two hours up to twelve times daily. Two teaspoonfuls have the capacity to neutralize 28 mEq of acid. Extra Strength Suspension—one teaspoonful (5 ml) as often as every two hours up to twelve times daily. One teaspoonful is equivalent to two capsules or tablets and has the capacity to neutralize 22 mEq of acid. Capsules—two capsules as often as every two hours up to twelve times daily. Two capsules have the capacity to neutralize 26 mEq of acid. Swallow Tablets—two tablets as often as every two hours up to twelve times daily. Two tablets have the capacity to neutralize 28 mEq of acid. The sodium content of each dosage form is as follows: 0.1 mEq/5 ml for the suspension, 1.0 mEq/5 ml for the extra strength suspension, 0.12 mEq per capsule, and 0.09 mEq per tablet.

Precautions: May cause constipation. Adequate fluid intake should be maintained in addition to the specific medical or surgical management indicated by the patient's condition.

Drug Interaction Precautions: Alumina-containing antacids should not be used concomitantly with any form of tetracycline therapy.

How Supplied: Suspension—bottles of 12 fluidounces.
Extra Strength Suspension—bottles of 12 fluidounces.
Capsules—bottles of 100 and 500.
Swallow Tablets (scored)—bottles of 100.

BICILLIN® C-R — ℞

(penicillin G benzathine and penicillin G procaine suspension)
INJECTION

FOR DEEP INTRAMUSCULAR INJECTION ONLY

Description: Multiple-dose vials of 300,000 units per ml contain in each ml 150,000 units penicillin G benzathine and 150,000 units penicillin G procaine in a stabilized aqueous suspension with sodium citrate buffer, approximately 6 mg lecithin, 3 mg povidone, 1 mg carboxymethylcellulose, 0.5 mg sorbitan monopalmitate, 0.5 mg polyoxyethylene sorbitan mono-

Continued on next page

Wyeth—Cont.

palmitate, 1.2 mg methylparaben and 0.14 mg propylparaben.
Each TUBEX® cartridge (1 ml size) contains 600,000 units of penicillin comprising: 300,000 units penicillin G benzathine and 300,000 units penicillin G procaine in a stabilized aqueous suspension with sodium citrate buffer; and as w/v, approximately 0.5% lecithin, 0.55% carboxymethylcellulose, 0.55% povidone, 0.1% methylparaben, and 0.01% propylparaben.
Each TUBEX cartridge (2 ml size) contains 1,200,000 units of penicillin comprising: 600,000 units penicillin G benzathine and 600,000 units penicillin G procaine in a stabilized aqueous suspension with sodium citrate buffer; and as w/v, approximately 0.5% lecithin, 0.55% carboxymethylcellulose, 0.55% povidone, 0.1% methylparaben, and 0.01% propylparaben.
Each disposable syringe (2 ml size) contains 1,200,000 units of penicillin comprising: 600,000 units penicillin G benzathine and 600,000 units penicillin G procaine in a stabilized aqueous suspension with sodium citrate buffer; and as w/v, approximately 0.5% lecithin, 0.55% carboxymethylcellulose, 0.55% povidone, 0.1% methylparaben, and 0.01% propylparaben.
Each disposable syringe (4 ml size) contains 2,400,000 units of penicillin comprising: 1,200,000 units penicillin G benzathine and 1,200,000 units penicillin G procaine in a stabilized aqueous suspension with sodium citrate buffer, and as w/v, approximately 0.5% lecithin, 0.55% carboxymethylcellulose, 0.55% povidone, 0.1% methylparaben, and 0.01% propylparaben.
Bicillin C-R suspension in the multiple-dose vial, TUBEX, and disposable syringe formulations is viscous and opaque. Read "Contraindications," "Warnings," "Precautions," and "Dosage and Administration" sections prior to use.

Actions and Pharmacology: Penicillin G exerts a bactericidal action against penicillin-sensitive microorganisms during the stage of active multiplication. It acts through the inhibition of biosynthesis of cell-wall mucopeptide. It is not active against the penicillinase-producing bacteria, which include many strains of staphylococci. Penicillin G exerts high *in vitro* activity against staphylococci (except penicillinase-producing strains) streptococci (Groups A, C, G, H, L, and M), and pneumococci. Other organisms sensitive to penicillin G are *Neisseria gonorrhoeae, Corynebacterium diphtheriae, Bacillus anthracis*, Clostridia, *Actinomyces bovis, Streptobacillus moniliformis, Listeria monocytogenes*, and Leptospira. *Treponema pallidum* is extremely sensitive to the bactericidal action for penicillin G.
Sensitivity plate testing: If the Kirby-Bauer method of disc sensitivity is used, a 10-unit penicillin disc should give a zone greater than 28 mm when tested against a penicillin-sensitive bacterial strain.
Intramuscular penicillin G benzathine is absorbed very slowly into the bloodstream from the intramuscular site and converted by hydrolysis to penicillin G. This combination of hydrolysis and slow absorption results in blood serum levels much lower but much more prolonged than other parenteral penicillins.
Penicillin G procaine is an equimolecular compound of procaine and penicillin G, administered intramuscularly as a suspension. It dissolves slowly at the site of injection, giving a plateau type of blood level at about 4 hours which falls slowly over a period of the next 15-20 hours.
Approximately 60% of penicillin G is bound to serum protein. The drug is distributed throughout the body tissues in widely varying amounts. Highest levels are found in the kidneys with lesser amounts in the liver, skin, and intestines. Penicillin G penetrates into all other tissues and the spinal fluid to a lesser degree. With normal kidney function the drug is excreted rapidly by tubular excretion. In neonates and young infants and in individuals with impaired kidney function, excretion is considerably delayed.

Indications: This drug is indicated in the treatment of moderately severe infections due to penicillin-G-susceptible microorganisms that are susceptible to serum levels common to this particular dosage form. Therapy should be guided by bacteriological studies (including susceptibility testing) and by clinical response.
NOTE: When high, sustained serum levels are required, penicillin G sodium or potassium, either IM or IV, should be used. This drug should *not* be used in the treatment of venereal diseases, including syphilis, gonorrhea, yaws, bejel, and pinta.
The following infections will usually respond to adequate dosages of this drug:
Streptococcal infections Group A (without bacteremia). Moderately severe to severe infections of the upper respiratory tract, skin and soft-tissue infections, scarlet fever, and erysipelas.
NOTE: Streptococci in Groups A, C, G, H, L, and M are very sensitive to penicillin G. Other groups, including Group D (enterococci), are resistant. Penicillin G sodium or potassium is recommended for streptococcal infections with bacteremia.
Pneumococcal infections. Moderately severe pneumonia and otitis media.
NOTE: Severe pneumonia, empyema, bacteremia, pericarditis, meningitis, peritonitis, and arthritis of pneumococcal etiology are better treated with penicillin G sodium or potassium during the acute stage.

Contraindications: A previous hypersensitivity reaction to any penicillin or to procaine is a contraindication.
Do not inject into or near an artery or nerve.

Warnings: Serious and occasionally fatal hypersensitivity (anaphylactoid) reactions have been reported in patients on penicillin therapy. Although anaphylaxis is more frequent following parenteral therapy, it has occurred in patients on oral penicillins. These reactions are more apt to occur in individuals with a history of sensitivity to multiple allergens.
There have been well-documented reports of individuals with a history of penicillin hypersensitivity reactions who have experienced severe hypersensitivity reactions when treated with a cephalosporin. Before therapy with a penicillin, careful inquiry should be made concerning previous hypersensitivity reactions to penicillins, cephalosporins, and other allergens. If an allergic reaction occurs, the drug should be discontinued and the patient treated with the usual agents, e.g., pressor amines, antihistamines, and corticosteroids.
Inadvertent intravascular administration, including inadvertent direct intraarterial injection or injection immediately adjacent to arteries, of Bicillin C-R and other penicillin preparations has resulted in severe neurovascular damage, including transverse myelitis with permanent paralysis, gangrene requiring amputation of digits and more proximal portions of extremities, and necrosis and sloughing at and surrounding the injection site. Such severe effects have been reported following injections into the buttock, thigh, and deltoid areas. Other serious complications of suspected intravascular administration which have been reported include immediate pallor, mottling or cyanosis of the extremity both distal and proximal to the injection site followed by bleb formation; severe edema requiring anterior and/or posterior compartment fasciotomy in the lower extremity. The above-described severe effects and complications have most often occurred in infants and small children. Prompt consultation with an appropriate specialist is indicated if any evidence of compromise of the blood supply occurs at, proximal to, or distal to the site of injection.[1-9] See "Contraindications," "Precautions," and "Dosage and Administration."
Quadriceps femoris fibrosis and atrophy have been reported following repeated intramuscular injections of penicillin preparations into the anterolateral thigh.
Injection into or near a nerve may result in permanent neurological damage.

Precautions: Penicillin should be used with caution in individuals with histories of significant allergies and/or asthma.
Care should be taken to avoid intravenous or intraarterial administration, or injection into or near major peripheral nerves or blood vessels, since such injections may produce neurovascular damage. See "Contraindications," "Warnings," and "Dosage and Administration."
In streptococcal infections, therapy must be sufficient to eliminate the organism; otherwise the sequelae of streptococcal disease may occur. Cultures should be taken following completion of treatment to determine whether streptococci have been eradicated.
A small percentage of patients are sensitive to procaine. If there is a history of sensitivity make the usual test: Inject intradermally 0.1 ml of a 1 to 2 percent procaine solution. Development of an erythema, wheal, flare, or eruption indicates procaine sensitivity. Sensitivity should be treated by the usual methods, including barbiturates, and procaine penicillin preparations should not be used. Antihistaminics appear beneficial in treatment of procaine reactions.
The use of antibiotics may result in overgrowth of nonsusceptible organisms. Constant observation of the patient is essential. If new infections due to bacteria or fungi appear during therapy, the drug should be discontinued and appropriate measures taken.
Whenever allergic reactions occur, penicillin should be withdrawn unless, in the opinion of the physician, the condition being treated is life-threatening and amenable only to penicillin therapy.
In prolonged therapy with penicillin, and particularly with high-dosage schedules, periodic evaluation of the renal and hematopoietic systems is recommended.

Adverse Reactions: Penicillin is a substance of low toxicity but does possess a significant index of sensitization. The following hypersensitivity reactions associated with use of penicillin have been reported: Skin rashes, ranging from maculopapular eruptions to exfoliative dermatitis; urticaria; serum-sickness-like reactions, including chills, fever, edema, arthralgia, and prostration. Severe and often fatal anaphylaxis has been reported (see "Warnings").

Dosage and Administration: Shake multiple-dose vial vigorously before withdrawing the desired dose.
Shake TUBEX cartridge and disposable syringe vigorously before injecting contents.
Administer by DEEP, INTRAMUSCULAR INJECTION in the upper, outer quadrant of the buttock. In infants and small children, the midlateral aspect of the thigh may be preferable. When doses are repeated, vary the injection site.
When using the multiple-dose vial:
After selection of the proper site and insertion of the needle into the selected muscle, aspirate by pulling back on the plunger. While maintaining negative pressure for 2–3 seconds, carefully observe the neck of the syringe immediately proximal to the needle hub for appearance of blood or any discoloration. Blood or "typical blood color" may *not* be seen if a blood vessel has been entered—only a mixture of blood and Bicillin C-R. The appearance of any discoloration is reason to withdraw the needle

and discard the syringe. If it is elected to inject at another site, a new syringe and needle should be used. If no blood or discoloration appears, inject the contents of the syringe slowly. Discontinue delivery of the dose if the subject complains of severe immediate pain at the injection site or if in infants and young children symptoms or signs occur suggesting onset of severe pain.

When using the TUBEX cartridge:

The Wyeth Tubex® cartridge for this product incorporates several features that are designed to facilitate the visualization of blood on aspiration if a blood vessel is inadvertently entered.

The design of this cartridge is such that blood which enters its needle will be quickly visualized as a red or dark-colored "spot." This "spot" will appear on the barrel of the glass cartridge immediately proximal to the blue hub. Prior to injection, in order to determine where this "spot" can be seen, the operator should first insert and secure the cartridge in the Tubex syringe in the usual fashion. The needle cover should then be removed and the cartridge and syringe held in one hand with the needle pointing away from the operator. If the 2 ml metal syringe is used the glass cartridge should then be rotated by turning the plunger of the syringe clockwise until the flat bevel at the tip of the needle is pointing upward and is horizontal when viewed directly from above. An imaginary straight line then drawn from the middle of the flat bevel to the back edge of the blue hub where it joins the glass will point to the area on the glass cartridge where the "spot" can be visualized. If the 1 ml metal syringe is used it will not be possible to continue to rotate the glass cartridge clockwise once it is properly engaged and fully threaded; it can, however, then be rotated counterclockwise as far as necessary to properly orient the bevel of the needle and locate the observation area. (In this same area in some cartridges a dark spot may sometimes be visualized prior to injection. This is the proximal end of the needle and does not represent a foreign body in, or other abnormality of, the suspension.)

Thus, before the needle is inserted into the selected muscle, it is important for the operator to orient the flat bevel of the needle so that any blood which might enter after its insertion and during aspiration can be visualized in the area of the cartridge where it will appear and not be obscured by the metal syringe or other obstructions.

After selection of the proper site and insertion of the needle into the selected muscle, aspirate by pulling back on the plunger. While maintaining negative pressure for 2-3 seconds, carefully observe the barrel of the cartridge in the area previously identified (see above) for the appearance of a red or dark-colored "spot."

Blood or "typical blood color" may *not* be seen if a blood vessel has been entered—only a mixture of blood and Bicillin C-R. The appearance of *any* discoloration is reason to withdraw the needle and discard the glass Tubex cartridge. If it is elected to inject at another site, a new cartridge should be used. If no blood or discoloration appears, inject the contents of the cartridge slowly. Discontinue delivery of the dose if the subject complains of severe immediate pain at the injection site or if, especially in infants and young children, symptoms or signs occur suggesting onset of severe pain.

Some TUBEX cartridges may contain a small air bubble which may be disregarded since it does not affect administration of the product.

Because of the high concentration of suspended material in this product, the needle may be blocked if the injection is not made at a slow, steady rate.

When using the disposable syringe:

The Wyeth disposable syringe for this product incorporates several new features that are designed to facilitate its use.

A single small indentation, or "dot", has been punched into the metal ring that surrounds the neck of the syringe near the base of the needle. It is important that this "dot" be placed in a position so that it can be easily visualized by the operator following the intramuscular insertion of the syringe needle.

After selection of the proper site and insertion of the needle into the selected muscle, aspirate by pulling back on the plunger. While maintaining negative pressure for 2-3 seconds, carefully observe the barrel of the syringe immediately proximal to the location of the "dot" for appearance of blood or any discoloration. Blood or "typical blood color" may *not* be seen if a blood vessel has been entered—only a mixture of blood and Bicillin C-R. The appearance of any discoloration is reason to withdraw the needle and discard the syringe. If it is elected to inject at another site, a new syringe should be used. If no blood or discoloration appears, inject the contents of the syringe slowly. Discontinue delivery of the dose if the subject complains of severe immediate pain at the injection site or if in infants and young children symptoms or signs occur suggesting onset of severe pain.

Streptococcal infections Group A—Infections of the upper-respiratory tract, skin and soft-tissue infections, scarlet fever, and erysipelas.

The following doses are recommended:

Adults and children over 60 lbs. in weight: 2,400,000 units. Children from 30–60 lbs.: 900,000 units to 1,200,000 units. Infants and children under 30 lbs.: 600,000 units.

NOTE: Treatment with the recommended dosage is usually given at a single session using multiple IM sites when indicated. An alternative dosage schedule may be used, giving one-half (½) the total dose on day 1 and one-half (½) on day 3. This will also insure the penicillinemia required over a 10-day period; however, this alternative schedule should be used only when the physician can be assured of the patient's cooperation.

Pneumococcal infections (except pneumococcal meningitis): 600,000 units in children and 1,200,000 units in adults, repeated every 2 or 3 days until the temperature is normal for 48 hours. Other forms of penicillin may be necessary for severe cases.

How Supplied: *300,000 units per ml*—multiple-dose vials of 10 ml. *600,000 units per ml*—1 ml Tubex® Sterile Cartridge-Needle Units, packages of 10 and 50; 2 ml Tubex Sterile Cartridge-Needle Units (1,200,000 units per Tubex), packages of 10 and 50; 2 ml single-dose (1,200,000 units) disposable syringes, packages of 10; 4 ml single-dose (2,400,000 units) disposable syringes, packages of 10.

References:

1. SHAW, E.: Transverse myelitis from injection of penicillin, *Am. J. Dis. Child., 111*:548, 1966.
2. KNOWLES, J.: Accidental intra-arterial injection of penicillin. *Am. J. Dis. Child., 111*:552, 1966.
3. DARBY, C., et al: Ischemia following an intragluteal injection of benzathine-procaine penicillin G mixture in a one-year-old boy. *Clin. Pediatrics, 12*:485, 1973.
4. BROWN, L. & NELSON, A.: Postinfectious intravascular thrombosis with gangrene. *Arch. Surg., 94*:652, 1967.
5. BORENSTINE, J.: Transverse myelitis and penicillin (Correspondence). *Am. J. Dis. Child., 112*:166, 1966.
6. ATKINSON, J.: Transverse myelopathy secondary to penicillin injection. *J. Pediatrics, 75*:867, 1969.
7. TALBERT, J. et al: Gangrene of the foot following intramuscular injection in the lateral thigh: A case report with recommendations for prevention. *J. Pediatrics, 70*:110, 1967.
8. FISHER, T.: Medicolegal affairs. *Canad. Med. Assoc. J., 112*:395, 1975.
9. SCHANZER, H. et al: Accidental intra-arterial injection of penicillin G. *JAMA, 242*:1289, 1979.

BICILLIN® C-R 900/300 ℞
(penicillin G benzathine and penicillin G procaine suspension) INJECTION

FOR DEEP INTRAMUSCULAR INJECTION ONLY

Description: Each TUBEX® cartridge (2 ml size) contains 1,200,000 units of penicillin comprising: 900,000 units penicillin G benzathine and 300,000 units penicillin G procaine in a stabilized aqueous suspension with sodium citrate buffer; and as w/v, approximately 0.5% lecithin, 0.55% carboxymethylcellulose, 0.55% povidone, 0.1% methylparaben, and 0.01% propylparaben.

Bicillin C-R 900/300 suspension in the TUBEX formulation is viscous and opaque. Read "Contraindications," "Warnings," "Precautions," and "Dosage and Administration" sections prior to use.

Actions and Pharmacology: Penicillin G exerts a bactericidal action against penicillin-sensitive microorganisms during the stage of active multiplication. It acts through the inhibition of biosynthesis of cell-wall mucopeptide. It is not active against the penicillinase-producing bacteria, which include many strains of staphylococci. Penicillin G exerts high *in vitro* activity against staphylococci (except penicillinase-producing strains), streptococci (groups A, C, G, H, L, and M), and pneumococci.

Other organisms sensitive to penicillin G are *Neisseria gonorrhoeae, Corynebacterium diphtheriae, Bacillus anthracis,* Clostridia, *Actinomyces bovis, Streptobacillus moniliformis, Listeria monocytogenes,* and Leptospira. *Treponema pallidum* is extremely sensitive to the bactericidal action of penicillin G.

Sensitivity plate testing: If the Kirby-Bauer method of disc sensitivity is used, a 10-unit penicillin disc should give a zone greater than 28 mm when tested against a penicillin-sensitive bacterial strain.

Intramuscular penicillin G benzathine is absorbed very slowly into the bloodstream from the intramuscular site and converted by hydrolysis to penicillin G. This combination of hydrolysis and slow absorption results in blood serum levels much lower but much more prolonged than other parenteral penicillins.

Penicillin G procaine is an equimolecular compound of procaine and penicillin G, administered intramuscularly as a suspension. It dissolves slowly at the site of injection, giving a plateau type of blood level at about 4 hours which falls slowly over a period of the next 15–20 hours.

Approximately 60% of penicillin G is bound to serum protein. The drug is distributed throughout the body tissues in widely varying amounts. Highest levels are found in the kidneys with lesser amounts in the liver, skin, and intestines. Penicillin G penetrates into all other tissues and the spinal fluid to a lesser degree. With normal kidney function the drug is excreted rapidly by tubular excretion. In neonates and young infants and in individuals with impaired kidney function, excretion is considerably delayed.

Indications: This drug is indicated for use in children of all ages in the treatment of moderately severe infections due to penicillin-G-susceptible microorganisms that are susceptible to serum levels common to this particular dosage form. Therapy should be guided by bacteriological studies (including susceptibility testing) and by clinical response.

NOTE: When high, sustained serum levels are required, penicillin G sodium or potassium, either IM or IV, should be used. This drug

Continued on next page

Wyeth—Cont.

should *not* be used in the treatment of venereal diseases, including syphilis, gonorrhea, yaws, bejel, and pinta.
The following infections will usually respond to adequate dosages of this drug:
Streptococcal infections Group A (without bacteremia). Moderately severe to severe infections of the upper respiratory tract, skin and soft-tissue infections, scarlet fever, and erysipelas.
NOTE: Streptococci in groups A, C, G, H, L, and M are very sensitive to penicillin G. Other groups, including group D (enterococci), are resistant. Penicillin G sodium or potassium is recommended for streptococcal infections with bacteremia.
Pneumococcal infections. Moderately severe pneumonia and otitis media.
NOTE: Severe pneumonia, empyema, bacteremia, pericarditis, meningitis, peritonitis, and arthritis of pneumococcal etiology are better treated with penicillin G sodium or potassium during the acute stage.
Contraindications: A previous hypersensitivity reaction to any penicillin or to procaine is a contraindication.
Do not inject into or near an artery or nerve.
Warnings: Serious and occasionally fatal hypersensitivity (anaphylactoid) reactions have been reported in patients on penicillin therapy. Although anaphylaxis is more frequent following parenteral therapy, it has occurred in patients on oral penicillins. These reactions are more apt to occur in individuals with a history of sensitivity to multiple allergens.
There have been well-documented reports of individuals with a history of penicillin hypersensitivity reactions who have experienced severe hypersensitivity reactions when treated with a cephalosporin. Before therapy with a penicillin, careful inquiry should be made concerning previous hypersensitivity reactions to penicillins, cephalosporins, and other allergens. If an allergic reaction occurs, the drug should be discontinued and the patient treated with the usual agents, e.g., pressor amines, antihistamines, and corticosteroids.
Inadvertent intravascular administration, including inadvertent direct intraarterial injection or injection immediately adjacent to arteries, of Bicillin C-R 900/300 and other penicillin preparations has resulted in severe neurovascular damage, including transverse myelitis with permanent paralysis, gangrene requiring amputation of digits and more proximal portions of extremities, and necrosis and sloughing at and surrounding the injection site. Such severe effects have been reported following injections into the buttock, thigh, and deltoid areas. Other serious complications of suspected intravascular administration which have been reported include immediate pallor, mottling or cyanosis of the extremity both distal and proximal to the injection site followed by bleb formation; severe edema requiring anterior and/or posterior compartment fasciotomy in the lower extremity. The above-described severe effects and complications have most often occurred in infants and small children. Prompt consultation with an appropriate specialist is indicated if any evidence of compromise of the blood supply occurs at, proximal to, or distal to the site of injection.[1–9] See "Contraindications," "Precautions," and "Dosage and Administration."
Quadriceps, femoris fibrosis and atrophy have been reported following repeated intramuscular injections of penicillin preparations into the anterolateral thigh.
Injection into or near a nerve may result in permanent neurological damage.
Precautions: Penicillin should be used with caution in individuals with histories of significant allergies and/or asthma.
Care should be taken to avoid intravenous or intraarterial administration, or injection into or near major peripheral nerves or blood vessels, since such injections may produce neurovascular damage. See "Contraindications," "Warnings," and "Dosage and Administration."
In streptococcal infections, therapy must be sufficient to eliminate the organism; otherwise the sequelae of streptococcal disease may occur. Cultures should be taken following completion of treatment to determine whether streptococci have been eradicated.
A small percentage of patients are sensitive to procaine. If there is a history of sensitivity make the usual test: Inject intradermally 0.1 ml of a 1 to 2 percent procaine solution. Development of an erythema, wheal, flare, or eruption indicates procaine sensitivity. Sensitivity should be treated by the usual methods, including barbiturates, and procaine penicillin preparations should not be used. Antihistaminics appear beneficial in treatment of procaine reactions.
The use of antibiotics may result in overgrowth of nonsusceptible organisms. Constant observation of the patient is essential. If new infections due to bacteria or fungi appear during therapy, the drug should be discontinued and appropriate measures taken.
Whenever allergic reactions occur, penicillin should be withdrawn unless, in the opinion of the physician, the condition being treated is life-threatening and amenable only to penicillin therapy.
In prolonged therapy with penicillin, and particularly with high-dosage schedules, periodic evaluation of the renal and hematopoietic systems is recommended.
Adverse Reactions: Penicillin is a substance of low toxicity but does possess a significant index of sensitization. The following hypersensitivity reactions associated with use of penicillin have been reported: skin rashes, ranging from maculopapular eruptions to exfoliative dermatitis; urticaria; serum-sickness-like reactions, including chills, fever, edema, arthralgia, and prostration. Severe and often fatal anaphylaxis has been reported (see "Warnings").
Dosage and Administration: Shake TUBEX cartridge vigorously before injecting contents.
Administer by DEEP, INTRAMUSCULAR INJECTION in the upper, outer quadrant of the buttock. In infants and small children, the midlateral aspect of the thigh may be preferable. When doses are repeated, vary the injection site.
The Wyeth Tubex® cartridge for this product incorporates several features that are designed to facilitate the visualization of blood on aspiration if a blood vessel is inadvertently entered.
The design of this cartridge is such that blood which enters its needle will be quickly visualized as a red or dark-colored "spot." This "spot" will appear on the barrel of the glass cartridge immediately proximal to the blue hub. Prior to injection, in order to determine where this "spot" can be seen, the operator should first insert and secure the cartridge in the Tubex syringe in the usual fashion. The needle cover should then be removed and the cartridge and syringe held in one hand with the needle pointing away from the operator. If the 2 ml metal syringe is used the glass cartridge should then be rotated by turning the plunger of the syringe clockwise until the flat bevel at the tip of the needle is pointing upward and is horizontal when viewed directly from above. An imaginary straight line then drawn from the middle of the flat bevel to the back edge of the blue hub where it joins the glass will point to the area on the glass cartridge where the "spot" can be visualized. If the 1 ml metal syringe is used it will not be possible to continue to rotate the glass cartridge clockwise once it is properly engaged and fully threaded; it can, however, then be rotated counterclockwise as far as necessary to properly orient the bevel of the needle and locate the observation area. (In this same area in some cartridges a dark spot may sometimes be visualized prior to injection. This is the proximal end of the needle and does not represent a foreign body in, or other abnormality of, the suspension.)
Thus, before the needle is inserted into the selected muscle, it is important for the operator to orient the flat bevel of the needle so that any blood which might enter after its insertion and during aspiration can be visualized in the area of the cartridge where it will appear and not be obscured by the metal syringe or other obstructions.
After selection of the proper site and insertion of the needle into the selected muscle, aspirate by pulling back on the plunger. While maintaining negative pressure for 2–3 seconds, carefully observe the barrel of the cartridge in the area previously identified (see above) for the appearance of a red or dark-colored "spot."
Blood or "typical blood color" may *not* be seen if a blood vessel has been entered—only a mixture of blood and Bicillin C-R 900/300. The appearance of *any* discoloration is reason to withdraw the needle and discard the glass Tubex cartridge. If it is elected to inject at another site, a new cartridge should be used. If no blood or discoloration appears, inject the contents of the cartridge slowly. Discontinue delivery of the dose if the subject complains of severe immediate pain at the injection site or if, especially in infants and young children, symptoms or signs occur suggesting onset of severe pain.
Some TUBEX cartridges may contain a small air bubble which may be disregarded since it does not affect administration of the product.
Because of the high concentration of suspended material in this product, the needle may be blocked if the injection is not made at a slow, steady rate.
Streptococcal infections Group A—Infections of the upper respiratory tract, skin and soft-tissue infections, scarlet fever, and erysipelas.
A single injection of Bicillin C-R 900/300 is usually sufficient for the treatment of Group A streptococcal infections in children of all ages.
Pneumococcal infections (except pneumococcal meningitis): One TUBEX Bicillin C-R 900/300 repeated at 2- or 3-day intervals until the temperature is normal for 48 hours. Other forms of penicillin may be necessary for severe cases.
How Supplied: Bicillin® C-R 900/300 is supplied in 2 ml TUBEX® (Sterile Cartridge-Needle Unit) in packages of 10.

References:
1. SHAW, E.: Transverse myelitis from injection of penicillin. *Am. J. Dis. Child., 111:*548, 1966.
2. KNOWLES, J.: Accidental intra-arterial injection of penicillin. *Am. J. Dis. Child., 111:*552, 1966.
3. DARBY, C., et al: Ischemia following an intragluteal injection of benzathine-procaine penicillin G mixture in a one-year-old boy. *Clin. Pediatrics, 12:*485, 1973.
4. BROWN, L. & NELSON, A.: Postinfectious intravascular thrombosis with gangrene. *Arch. Surg., 94:*652, 1967.
5. BORENSTINE, J.: Transverse myelitis and penicillin (Correspondence). *Am. J. Dis. Child., 112:*166, 1966.
6. ATKINSON, J.: Transverse myelopathy secondary to penicillin injection. *J. Pediatrics, 75:*867, 1969.
7. TALBERT, J. et al: Gangrene of the foot following intramuscular injection in the lateral thigh: A case report with recommendations for prevention. *J. Pediatrics, 70:*110, 1967.

8. FISHER, T.: Medicolegal affairs. *Canad. Med. Assoc. J., 112:*395, 1975.
9. SCHANZER, H. et al: Accidental intra-arterial injection of penicillin G. *JAMA, 242:*1289, 1979.

BICILLIN® L-A ℞
(sterile penicillin G benzathine suspension)
INJECTION
FOR DEEP INTRAMUSCULAR INJECTION ONLY

Description: Each Tubex® Sterile Cartridge-Needle Unit or disposable syringe contains penicillin G benzathine in aqueous suspension with sodium citrate buffer; and as w/v, approximately 0.5% lecithin, 0.6% carboxymethylcellulose, 0.6% povidone, 0.1% methylparaben and, 0.01% propylparaben.
Each multiple-dose vial contains in each milliliter 300,000 units penicillin G benzathine with sodium citrate buffer and approx. 6 mg lecithin, 3 mg povidone, 1 mg carboxymethylcellulose, 0.5 mg sorbitan monopalmitate, 0.5 mg polyoxyethylene sorbitan monopalmitate, 1.2 mg methylparaben, and 0.14 mg propylparaben.
Bicillin L-A suspension in the multiple-dose vial, TUBEX, and disposable syringe formulations is viscous and opaque. Read "Contraindications," "Warnings," "Precautions," and "Dosage and Administration" sections prior to use.
Actions and Pharmacology: Penicillin G exerts a bactericidal action against penicillin-sensitive microorganisms during the stage of active multiplication. It acts through the inhibition of biosynthesis of cell-wall mucopeptide. It is not active against the penicillinase-producing bacteria, which include many strains of staphylococci. Penicillin G exerts high *in vitro* activity against staphylococci (except penicillinase-producing strains), streptococci (Groups A, C, G, H, L, and M), and pneumococci. Other organisms sensitive to penicillin G are: *Neisseria gonorrhoeae, Corynebacterium diphtheriae, Bacillus anthracis,* Clostridia, *Actinomyces bovis, Streptobacillus moniliformis, Listeria monocytogenes,* and Leptospira. *Treponema pallidum* is extremely sensitive to the bactericidal action of penicillin G.
Intramuscular penicillin G benzathine is absorbed very slowly into the bloodstream from the intramuscular site and converted by hydrolysis to penicillin G. This combination of hydrolysis and slow absorption results in blood serum levels much lower but much more prolonged than other parenteral penicillins.
Approximately 60% of penicillin G is bound to serum protein. The drug is distributed throughout the body tissues in widely varying amounts. Highest levels are found in the kidneys with lesser amounts in the liver, skin, and intestines. Penicillin G penetrates into all other tissues and the spinal fluid to a lesser degree. With normal kidney function the drug is excreted rapidly by tubular excretion. In neonates and young infants and in individuals with impaired kidney function, excretion is considerably delayed.
Indications: Intramuscular penicillin G benzathine is indicated in the treatment of infections due to penicillin-G-sensitive microorganisms that are susceptible to the low and very prolonged serum levels common to this particular dosage form. Therapy should be guided by bacteriological studies (including sensitivity tests) and by clinical response.
The following infections will usually respond to adequate dosage of intramuscular penicillin G benzathine:
Streptococcal infections (Group A—without bacteremia). Mild-to-moderate infections of the upper respiratory tract (e.g., pharyngitis).
Venereal infections—Syphilis, yaws, bejel, and pinta.
Medical Conditions in Which Penicillin G Benzathine Therapy Is Indicated as Prophylaxis:
Rheumatic fever and/or chorea—Prophylaxis with penicillin G benzathine has proven effective in preventing recurrence of these conditions. It has been used as follow-up prophylactic therapy for rheumatic heart disease and acute glomerulonephritis.
Contraindications: A history of a previous hypersensitivity reaction to any of the penicillins is a contraindication.
Do not inject into or near an artery or nerve.
Warnings: Serious and occasionally fatal hypersensitivity (anaphylactoid) reactions have been reported in patients on penicillin therapy. Although anaphylaxis is more frequent following parenteral therapy, it has occurred in patients on oral penicillins. These reactions are more apt to occur in individuals with a history of sensitivity to multiple allergens.
There have been well-documented reports of individuals with a history of penicillin hypersensitivity reactions who have experienced severe hypersensitivity reactions when treated with a cephalosporin. Before therapy with a penicillin, careful inquiry should be made concerning previous hypersensitivity reactions to penicillins, cephalosporins, and other allergens. If an allergic reaction occurs, the drug should be discontinued and the patient treated with the usual agents, e.g., pressor amines, antihistamines, and corticosteroids.
Inadvertent intravascular administration, including inadvertent direct intraarterial injection or injection immediately adjacent to arteries, of Bicillin L-A and other penicillin preparations has resulted in severe neurovascular damage, including transverse myelitis with permanent paralysis, gangrene requiring amputation of digits and more proximal portions of extremities, and necrosis and sloughing at and surrounding the injection site. Such severe effects have been reported following injections into the buttock, thigh, and deltoid areas. Other serious complications of suspected intravascular administration which have been reported include immediate pallor, mottling or cyanosis of the extremity both distal and proximal to the injection site followed by bleb formation; severe edema requiring anterior and /or posterior compartment fasciotomy in the lower extremity. The above-described severe effects and complications have most often occurred in infants and small children. Prompt consultation with an appropriate specialist is indicated if any evidence of compromise of the blood supply occurs at, proximal to, or distal to the site of injection.[1–9] See "Contraindications," "Precautions," and "Dosage and Administration."
Quadriceps femoris fibrosis and atrophy have been reported following repeated intramuscular injections of penicillin preparations into the anterolateral thigh.
Injection into or near a nerve may result in permanent neurological damage.
Precautions: Penicillin should be used with caution in individuals with histories of significant allergies and/or asthma.
Care should be taken to avoid intravenous or intraarterial administration, or injection into or near major peripheral nerves or blood vessels, since such injection may produce neurovascular damage. See "Contraindications," "Warnings," and "Dosage and Administration."
In streptococcal infections, therapy must be sufficient to eliminate the organism; otherwise, the sequelae of streptococcal disease may occur. Cultures should be taken following completion of treatment to determine whether streptococci have been eradicated.
Prolonged use of antibiotics may promote the overgrowth of nonsusceptible organisms, including fungi. Should superinfection occur, appropriate measures should be taken.
Adverse Reactions: The hypersensitivity reactions reported are skin eruptions (maculopapular to exfoliative dermatitis), urticaria and other serum-sicknesslike reactions, laryngeal edema, and anaphylaxis. Fever and eosinophilia may frequently be the only reaction observed. Hemolytic anemia, leukopenia, thrombocytopenia, neuropathy, and nephropathy are infrequent reactions and usually associated with high doses of parenteral penicillin. As with other treatments for syphilis, the Jarisch-Herxheimer reaction has been reported.
Dosage and Administration: Shake multiple-dose vial vigorously before withdrawing the desired dose.
Shake TUBEX cartridge and disposable syringe vigorously before injecting contents.
Administer by DEEP, INTRAMUSCULAR INJECTION in the upper, outer quadrant of the buttock. In infants and small children, the midlateral aspect of the thigh may be preferable. When doses are repeated, vary the injection site.
When using the multiple-dose vial:
After selection of the proper site and insertion of the needle into the selected muscle, aspirate by pulling back on the plunger. While maintaining negative pressure for 2–3 seconds, carefully observe the neck of the syringe immediately proximal to the needle hub for appearance of blood or any discoloration. Blood or "typical blood color" may *not* be seen if a blood vessel has been entered—only a mixture of blood and Bicillin L-A. The appearance of any discoloration is reason to withdraw the needle and discard the syringe. If it is elected to inject at another site, a new syringe and needle should be used. If no blood or discoloration appears, inject the contents of the syringe slowly. Discontinue delivery of the dose if the subject complains of severe immediate pain at the injection site or if in infants and young children symptoms or signs occur suggesting onset of severe pain.
When using the TUBEX cartridge:
The Wyeth Tubex® cartridge for this product incorporates several features that are designed to facilitate the visualization of blood on aspiration if a blood vessel is inadvertently entered.
The design of this cartridge is such that blood which enters its needle will be quickly visualized as a red or dark-colored "spot." This "spot" will appear on the barrel of the glass cartridge immediately proximal to the blue hub. Prior to injection, in order to determine where this "spot" can be seen, the operator should first insert and secure the cartridge in the Tubex syringe in the usual fashion. The needle cover should then be removed and the cartridge and syringe held in one hand with the needle pointing away from the operator. If the 2 ml metal syringe is used the glass cartridge should then be rotated by turning the plunger of the syringe clockwise until the flat bevel at the tip of the needle is pointing upward and is horizontal when viewed directly from above. An imaginary straight line then drawn from the middle of the flat bevel to the back edge of the blue hub where it joins the glass will point to the area on the glass cartridge where the "spot" can be visualized. If the 1 ml metal syringe is used it will not be possible to continue to rotate the glass cartridge clockwise once it is properly engaged and fully threaded; it can, however, then be rotated counterclockwise as far as necessary to properly orient the bevel of the needle and locate the observation area. (In this same area in some cartridges a dark spot may sometimes be visualized prior to injection. This is the proximal end of the needle and does not represent a foreign body in, or other abnormality of, the suspension.)
Thus, before the needle is inserted into the selected muscle, it is important for the operator to orient the flat bevel of the needle so that any blood which might enter after its insertion and during aspiration can be visualized in the area

Continued on next page

Wyeth—Cont.

of the cartridge where it will appear and not be obscured by the metal syringe or other obstructions.

After selection of the proper site and insertion of the needle into the selected muscle, aspirate by pulling back on the plunger. While maintaining negative pressure for 2–3 seconds, carefully observe the barrel of the cartridge in the area previously identified (see above) for the appearance of a red or dark-colored "spot."

Blood or "typical blood color" may *not* be seen if a blood vessel has been entered—only a mixture of blood and *Bicillin L-A.* The appearance of *any* discoloration is reason to withdraw the needle and discard the glass Tubex cartridge. If it is elected to inject at another site, a new cartridge should be used. If no blood or discoloration appears, inject the contents of the cartridge slowly. Discontinue delivery of the dose if the subject complains of severe immediate pain at the injection site or if, especially in infants and young children, symptoms or signs occur suggesting onset of severe pain.

Some TUBEX cartridges may contain a small air bubble which may be disregarded since it does not affect administration of the product.

Because of the high concentration of suspended material in this product, the needle may be blocked if the injection is not made at a slow, steady rate.

When using the disposable syringe:

The Wyeth disposable syringe for this product incorporates several new features that are designed to facilitate its use.

A single small indentation, or "dot", has been punched into the metal ring that surrounds the neck of the syringe near the base of the needle. It is important that this "dot" be placed in a position so that it can be easily visualized by the operator following the intramuscular insertion of the syringe needle.

After selection of the proper site and insertion of the needle into the selected muscle, aspirate by pulling back on the plunger. While maintaining negative pressure for 2–3 seconds, carefully observe the barrel of the syringe immediately proximal to the location of the "dot" for appearance of blood or any discoloration. Blood or "typical blood color" may *not* be seen if a blood vessel has been entered—only a mixture of blood and Bicillin L-A. The appearance of any discoloration is reason to withdraw the needle and discard the syringe. If it is elected to inject at another site, a new syringe should be used. If no blood or discoloration appears, inject the contents of the syringe slowly. Discontinue delivery of the dose if the subject complains of severe immediate pain at the injection site or if in infants and young children symptoms or signs occur suggesting onset of severe pain.

Some disposable syringes may contain a small air bubble which may be disregarded since it does not affect administration of the product.

Because of the high concentration of suspended material in this product, the needle may be blocked if the injection is not made at a slow, steady rate.

Streptococcal (Group A) upper respiratory infections (for example, pharyngitis).

A single injection of 1,200,000 units for adults.

A single injection of 900,000 units for older children.

A single injection of 300,000 to 600,000 units for infants and for children under 60 pounds.

Venereal infections—

Syphilis—Primary, secondary, and latent—2.4 million units (1 dose). Late (tertiary and neurosyphilis)—2.4 million units at 7-day intervals for three doses.

Congenital—under 2 years of age: 50,000 units/kg/body weight; ages 2–12 years: adjust dosage based on adult dosage schedule.

Yaws Bejel, and Pinta—1.2 million units (1 injection).

Prophylaxis—for rheumatic fever and glomerulonephritis.

Following an acute attack, penicillin G benzathine (parenteral) may be given in doses of 1,200,000 units once a month or 600,000 units every 2 weeks.

How Supplied: BICILLIN® L-A (sterile penicillin G benzathine suspension) Injection: *300,000 units per ml*—vials of 10 ml; *600,000 units per 1 ml* TUBEX® sterile cartridge-needle unit, packages of 10; *900,000 units per* TUBEX—1.5 ml fill in 2 ml size, packages of 10; *1,200,000 units per 2 ml* disposable syringe or TUBEX, packages of 10; *2,400,000 units per 4 ml* disposable syringe, packages of 10.

References:

1. SHAW, E.: Transverse myelitis from injection of penicillin. *Am. J. Dis. Child., 111:*548, 1966.
2. KNOWLES, J.: Accidental intra-arterial injection of penicillin. *Am. J. Dis. Child., 111:*552, 1966.
3. DARBY, C., et al: Ischemia following an intragluteal injection of benzathine-procaine penicillin G mixture in a one-year-old boy. *Clin. Pediatrics, 12:*485, 1973.
4. BROWN, L. & NELSON, A.: Postinfectious intravascular thrombosis with gangrene. *Arch. Surg., 94:*652, 1967.
5. BORENSTINE, J.: Transverse myelitis and penicillin (Correspondence). *Am. J. Dis. Child., 112:*166, 1966.
6. ATKINSON, J.: Transverse myelopathy secondary to penicillin injection. *J. Pediatrics, 75:*867, 1969.
7. TALBERT, J. et al: Gangrene of the foot following intramuscular injection in the lateral thigh: A case report with recommendations for prevention. *J. Pediatrics, 70:*110, 1967.
8. FISHER, T.: Medicolegal affairs. *Canad. Med. Assoc. J., 112:*395, 1975.
9. SCHANZER, H. et al: Accidental intra-arterial injection of penicillin G. *JAMA, 242:*1289, 1979.

BIOLOGICALS

For prescribing information on products listed —and for which full prescribing information is not provided—write to Professional Service, Wyeth Laboratories, Box 8299, Philadelphia, PA, 19101, or contact your local Wyeth representative.

ANTIVENIN (CROTALIDAE) POLYVALENT ℞
(equine origin)

Important: Pit viper bites may cause severe tissue damage or fatal envenomation, or both. The physician responsible for treatment of an envenomated patient should be familiar with the contents of this brochure and the pertinent medical literature concerning current concepts of first-aid and general supportive therapy as presented in the references listed at the end of this pamphlet.

Composition: Antivenin (Crotalidae) Polyvalent, Wyeth, is a refined and concentrated preparation of serum globulins obtained by fractionating blood from healthy horses immunized with the following venoms: *Crotalus adamanteus* (eastern diamond rattlesnake), *C. atrox* (western diamond rattlesnake), C. *durissus terrificus* (tropical rattlesnake, Cascabel), and Bothrops atrox ("Fer-de-lance"). Phenol, 0.25%, and thimerosal, 0.005%, are added as preservatives. The product is standardized by its ability to neutralize the lethal action of standard venoms by intravenous injection in mice.[1] Dried from the frozen state, the lyophilized serum has a moisture content of less than 1% and is soluble on addition of the diluent contained in each package (Bacteriostatic Water for Injection, USP, with preservative: 0.001% phenylmercuric nitrate).

Antivenin (Crotalidae) Polyvalent, Wyeth (hereinafter referred to as Antivenin) contains protective substances capable of neutralizing the toxic effects of venoms of crotalids (pit vipers) native to North, Central, and South America, including rattlesnakes *(Crotalus, Sistrurus);* copperhead and cottonmouth moccasins *(Agkistrodon),* including *A. halys* of Korea and Japan; the Fer-de-lance and other species of *Bothrops;* the tropical rattler (*Crotalus durissus* and similar species); the Cantil *(A. bilineatus);* and bushmaster *(Lachesis mutus)* of South and Central America.

Indication: Antivenin is indicated only for the treatment of envenomation caused by bites of those crotalids (pit vipers) specified in the immediately preceding paragraph.

Pit Viper Bites and Envenomation: The symptoms, signs, and severity of snake-venom poisoning resulting from pit viper bites depend on many factors, including, but not limited to, the following variables: species, age, and size of the biting snake; the number and location of bite(s); the depth of venom deposit by the snake's fangs; the condition of the snake's fangs and venom glands; the length of time the snake "hangs on"; the age, general health, and size of the victim; the type and efficacy of any first-aid treatment rendered in an attempt to remove venom and how soon such treatment was applied. In any venomous snake bite, the actual amount of venom introduced into the victim is always an unknown. Even the type of clothing or leg-footwear through which the snake's fangs pass may affect the amount of venom delivered by the bite. Although most North American pit vipers tend to bite and introduce venom superficially, their fangs may get hung-up in the subcutaneous tissues during the biting act and can penetrate deeper tissues during the attempt to release the bitten part. In some bites the fangs may penetrate into muscle. In such cases, the usual local superficial manifestations of envenomation may not appear early in the course of poisoning. In bites by some species, systemic evidence of envenomation may be present in the absence of significant local manifestations. It may be difficult to determine the severity of envenomation during the first several hours after a pit viper bite and estimates of severity may need to be revised as poisoning progresses. It must be remembered, too, that not all pit viper bites result in envenomation. In approximately 20% of rattlesnake bites, the snake may not inject any venom. The local and systemic symptoms and signs of envenomation include the following:

LOCAL:

Fang puncture(s).

Swelling—edema is usually seen around the site of bite within five minutes. It may progress rapidly and involve the entire extremity within an hour. More than 95% of all snakebites are inflicted on extremities.[2] Generally, however, edema spreads more slowly, usually over a period of 8 or more hours. Swelling is usually most severe following envenomation by the eastern diamondback; less severe after bites by the western diamondback, prairie, timber, red, Pacific, Mojave, and blacktailed rattlers, the sidewinder and cottonmouth moccasins; least severe after bites by copperheads, massasaugas, and pygmy rattlers.

Ecchymosis and discoloration of the skin —often appear in the area of the bite within a few hours. Vesicules may form within a few hours and are usually present at 24 hours. Hemorrhagic blebs and petechiae are common. Necrosis may develop, necessitating amputation of an extremity or a portion thereof.

Pain—frequently a complaint of the victim beginning shortly after the bite by most pit vipers. Pain may be absent after bites by Mojave rattlers.

SYSTEMIC:
Weakness; faintness; nausea; sweating; numbness or tingling around the mouth, tongue, scalp, fingers, toes, site of bite; muscle fasciculations; hypotension; prolongation of bleeding and clotting times; hemoconcentration, early followed by a decrease in erythrocytes; thrombocytopenia; hematuria; proteinuria; vomiting, including hematemesis; melena; hemoptysis; epistaxis. In fatal poisoning, a frequent cause of death is associated with destruction of erythrocytes and changes in capillary permeability, especially of the pulmonary vascular system, leading to pulmonary edema; hemoconcentration usually occurs early, probably as a result of plasma loss secondary to vascular permeability; the hemoglobin may fall, and bleeding may occur throughout the body as early as 6 hours after the bite. Renal involvement is not uncommon. Mojave rattler venom may cause neuromuscular changes leading to respiratory failure.

An estimate of the severity of envenomation should be made as soon as possible and before any Antivenin is administered. The amount (volume) of the first dose of Antivenin is determined on this estimate of severity. Every symptom, sign, laboratory-test result, and any other pertinent information should be considered in estimating severity—local manifestations; systemic manifestations, including abnormal laboratory findings; species and size of the biting snake, if known; number and location of bites(s); size and health of the patient; type of first-aid treatment rendered; and interval between bite and arrival for treatment. Russell et al,[3] and Wingert and Wainschel[4] grade severity as follows:

No envenomation—no local or systemic manifestations.

Minimal envenomation—local swelling and other local changes; no systemic manifestations; normal laboratory findings.

Moderate envenomation—swelling progressing beyond the site of bite and one or more systemic manifestations; abnormal laboratory findings, for example, a fall in hematocrit or platelets.

Severe envenomation—marked local response, severe systemic manifestations and significant alteration in laboratory findings.

Parrish and Hayes,[5] McCollough and Gennaro,[6] and Watt and Gennaro[7] have used a Grade 0 (no envenomation) through Grade IV (very severe) classification of severity which was developed for the most part in treatment of envenomation by the eastern diamondback and timber rattlers. This classification is more dependent on local manifestations, or the absence thereof, as the venoms of these species seem to be more consistent in inducing local tissue damage.

Any suspected envenomation should be treated as a medical emergency, and until careful observation provides clear evidence that envenomation has not occurred or is minimal, the following procedures are recommended:

Monitor vital signs at frequent intervals: Blood pressure, pulse, respiration.

Draw sufficient blood as soon as possible for baseline laboratory studies, including type and cross-match, CBC, hematocrit, platelet count, prothrombin time, clot retraction, bleeding and coagulation times, BUN, electrolytes, bilirubin. Some of these studies may need to be repeated at daily intervals, or less, depending on the severity of envenomation and the response to treatment. During the first 4 or 5 days of severe envenomations, hemoglobin, hematocrit, and platelet counts should be carried out several times a day.

Obtain urine samples at frequent intervals for analysis, with special attention to microscopic examination for presence of erythrocytes.

Chart fluid intake and urine output.

Measure and record the circumference of the bitten extremity just proximal to the bite and at one or more additional points each several inches closer to the trunk. Repeat measurements every 15-30 minutes to obtain information about progression of edema.

Have available and ready for immediate use: Oxygen, resuscitation equipment including airway, tourniquet, epinephrine, injectable antihistaminic agents, and corticosteroids.

Start an intravenous infusion in one or two extremities: one line to be used for supportive therapy, if needed, such as whole blood, plasma, packed red cells, specific clotting factors, platelet transfusion, plasma expanders; the other line to be used for administration of Antivenin and electrolytes.

Carry out and interpret a skin test for horse-serum sensitivity. (See Precautions section below.)

Dosage and Administration: Before administration, read Precautions and Systemic Reactions sections below. Since the possibility of a severe immediate reaction (anaphylaxis) exists whenever a horse-serum-containing product is administered, appropriate therapeutic agents, including a tourniquet, airway, oxygen, epinephrine, an injectable pressor amine, and corticosteroid, must be available and ready for immediate use. Constant attendance and observation of the patient for untoward reactions are mandatory when Antivenin is administered. Should any systemic reaction occur, administration should be discontinued immediately and appropriate treatment initiated.

The intravenous route of administration is preferred, and probably should always be used for moderate or severe envenomation. Intravenous administration is mandatory if venom-induced shock is present. To be most effective, Antivenin should be administered within 4 hours of the bite; it is less effective when given after 8 hours and may be of questionable value after 12 hours. However, it is recommended that Antivenin therapy be given in severe poisonings, even if 24 hours have elapsed since the time of the bite. It should be kept in mind that maximum blood levels of Antivenin may not be obtained for 8 or more hours after intramuscular administration.

For intravenous-drip use, prepare a 1:1 to 1:10 dilution of reconstituted Antivenin in Sodium Chloride Injection, USP, or 5% Dextrose Injection, USP. To avoid foaming, mix by gently swirling rather than shaking. Allow the initial 5 to 10 ml to infuse over a 3- to 5-minute period, with careful observation of the patient for evidence of untoward reaction. If no symptoms or signs of an immediate systemic reaction appear, continue the infusion with delivery at the maximum safe rate for intravenous fluid administration. The dilution of Antivenin to be used, the type of electrolyte solution used for dilution, and the rate of intravenous delivery of the diluted Antivenin must take into consideration the age, weight, and cardiac status of the patient; the severity of envenomation; the total amount and type of parenteral fluids it is anticipated will be given or are needed; and the interval between bite and initiation of specific therapy.

It is important to give as soon as possible the entire initial dose of Antivenin as based on the best estimate of the severity of envenomation at the time treatment is begun. The following initial doses are recommended:[3,4,8]

no envenomation—none

minimal envenomation—20-40 ml (contents of 2-4 vials)

moderate envenomation—50-90 ml (contents of 5-9 vials)

severe envenomation—100-150 ml or more (contents of 10-15 or more vials)

These recommended initial-dosage volumes are in general accord with those of others.[5-7,9]

The need for additional Antivenin must be based on the clinical response to the initial dose and continuing assessment of the severity of poisoning. If swelling continues to progress or if systemic symptoms or signs of envenomation increase in severity or if new manifestations appear, for example, fall in hematocrit or hypotension, administer an additional 10-50 ml (contents of 1-5 vials) intravenously.

Envenomation by large snakes in children or small adults requires larger doses of Antivenin. The amount administered to a child is not based on weight.

If Antivenin is given intramuscularly, it should be given into a large muscle mass, preferably the gluteal area, with care to avoid nerve trunks. Antivenin should never be injected into a finger or toe.

The effectiveness of corticosteroids in treatment of envenomation per se or venom shock is not resolved. Russell[3] and others[9,10] believe corticosteroids may mask the seriousness of hypovolemia in moderate or severe poisoning and have little, if any, effect on the local-tissue response to rattler venoms. Corticosteroids should not be given simultaneously with Antivenin on a routine basis or during the acute stage of envenomation; however, their use may be necessary to treat immediate allergic reactions to Antivenin, and corticosteroids are the agents of choice for treating serious delayed reactions to Antivenin.

Snakes' mouths do not harbor Clostridial organisms. However, appropriate tetanus prophylaxis is indicated, since tetanus spores may be carried into the fang puncture wounds by dirt present on skin at time of bite or by nonsterile first-aid procedures.

A broad-spectrum antibiotic in adequate dosage is indicated if local tissue damage is evident.

Shock following envenomation is treated like shock resulting from hypovolemia from any cause, including administration of whole blood, plasma, albumin, or other plasma expanders, as indicated.

Aspirin or codeine is usually adequate for relieving pain. Sedation with phenobarbital or mild tranquilizers may be used if indicated, but not in the presence of respiratory failure.

The bitten extremity should not be packed in ice, and so-called "cryotherapy" is contraindicated.

Technic for Reconstituting the Dried Antivenin: Pry off the small metal disc in the cap over the diaphragms of the vials of Antivenin and diluent. Swab the exposed surface of the rubber diaphragms of both vials with an appropriate germicide. With a sterile 10 ml syringe and needle, withdraw the diluent (Bacteriostatic Water for Injection, USP, containing phenylmercuric nitrate 1:100,000) from the vial of diluent and inject it into the vial of antivenin. Gentle agitation will hasten complete dissolution of the lyophilized Antivenin.

Precautions: Before administration of any product prepared from horse serum, appropriate measures must be taken in an effort to detect the presence of dangerous sensitivity: (1) A careful review of the patient's history, including any report of (a) asthma, hay fever, urticaria, or other allergic manifestations; (b) allergic reactions upon exposure to horses; and (c) prior injections of horse serum. (2) A suitable test for detection of sensitivity. A skin test should be performed in every patient prior to administration, regardless of clinical history.

Skin test—Inject intracutaneously 0.02 to 0.03 ml of a 1:10 dilution of Normal Horse Serum or Antivenin. A control test on the opposite extremity, using Sodium Chloride Injection, USP, facilitates interpretation. Use of larger amounts for the skin-test dose increases the likelihood of false-positive reactions, and in the exquisitely sensitive patient, increases the risk of a systemic reaction from the skin-test dose. A 1:100 or greater dilution should be used for preliminary skin testing if the history suggests sensitivity. A positive reaction to a skin test occurs within five to thirty minutes and is

Continued on next page

Wyeth—Cont.

manifested by a wheal with or without pseudopodia and surrounding erythema. In general, the shorter the interval between injection and the beginning of the skin reaction, the greater the sensitivity.

If the history is negative for allergy and the result of a skin test is negative, proceed with administration of Antivenin as outlined above. If the history is positive and a skin test is strongly positive, administration may be dangerous, especially if the positive sensitivity test is accompanied by systemic allergic manifestations. In such instances, the risk of administering Antivenin must be weighed against the risk of withholding it, keeping in mind that severe envenomation can be fatal. (See last paragraph of this section.)

A negative allergic history and absence of reaction to a properly applied skin test do not rule out the possibility of an immediate reaction. Also, a negative skin test has no bearing on whether or not delayed serum reactions (serum sickness) will occur after administration of the full dose.

If the history is negative, and the skin test is mildly or questionably positive, administer as follows to reduce the risk of a severe immediate systemic reaction: (a) Prepare, in separate sterile vials or syringes, 1:100 and 1:10 dilutions of Antivenin. (b) Allow at least 15 minutes between injections and proceed with the next dose if no reaction follows the previous dose. (c) Inject subcutaneously, using a tuberculin-type syringe, 0.1, 0.2, and 0.5 ml of the 1:100 dilution at 15-minute intervals; repeat with the 1:10 dilution, and finally undiluted Antivenin. (d) If a systemic reaction occurs after any injection, place a tourniquet proximal to the site of injections and administer an appropriate dose of epinephrine, 1:1000, proximal to the tourniquet or into another extremity. Wait at least 30 minutes before injecting another dose. The amount of the next dose should be the same as the last that did not evoke a reaction. (e) If no reaction occurs after 0.5 ml of undiluted Antivenin has been administered, switch to the intramuscular route and continue doubling the dose at 15-minute intervals until the entire dose has been injected intramuscularly or proceed to the intravenous route as described above under Dosage and Administration.

Obviously, if the just-described schedule is used, 3 to 5 or more hours would be required to administer the initial dose suggested for a moderate or severe envenomation, and time is an important factor in neutralization of venom in a critically ill patient. Wingert and Wainschel[4] have described a procedure based on the experience of their group which they have used in some severely envenomated patients who have positive sensitivity tests: 50 to 100 mg of diphenhydramine hydrochloride is given intravenously, followed by slow intravenous infusion of diluted Antivenin for 15 to 20 minutes while carefully observing the patient for symptoms and signs of anaphylaxis; if anaphylaxis does not occur, Antivenin is continued maintaining close observation of the patient. Patients who require Antivenin but develop signs of impending anaphylaxis in spite of this or the procedure described earlier present a difficult problem, and consultation should be sought.

Systemic Reactions: A. The immediate reaction (shock, anaphylaxis) usually occurs within 30 minutes. Symptoms and signs may develop before the needle is withdrawn and may include apprehension, flushing, itching, urticaria; edema of the face, tongue, and throat; cough, dyspnea, cyanosis, vomiting, and collapse.

B. Serum sickness usually occurs 5 to 24 days after administration. The incubation period may be less than 5 days, especially in those who have received horse-serum-containing preparations in the past. The usual symptoms and signs are malaise, fever, urticaria, lymphadenopathy, edema, arthralgia, nausea, and vomiting. Occasionally, neurological manifestations develop, such as meningismus or peripheral neuritis. Peripheral neuritis usually involves the shoulders and arms. Pain and muscle weakness are frequently present, and permanent atrophy may develop.

References:

1. GINGRICH, W. & HOHENADEL, J.: Standardization of polyvalent antivenin. "Venoms", edited by E. Buckley and N. Porges. Publication No. 44, Amer. Assoc. for the Advancement of Science, Washington, D.C., 1956, Pages 337–80.
2. PARRISH, H.: Incidence of treated snakebite in the United States. Pub. Hlth. Rep. *81*:269, 1966.
3. RUSSELL, F., et al.: Snake venom poisoning in the United States. Experiences with 550 cases. JAMA *233*:341, 1975. RUSSELL, F.: Venomous Bites and stings: Poisonous snakes. In The Merck Manual of Diagnosis and Therapy, pp. 1982–1987, 13th Ed., 1977.
4. WINGERT, W. and WAINSCHEL, J.: Diagnosis and management of envenomation by poisonous snakes. South. Med. J. *68*:1015, 1975.
5. PARRISH, H. & HAYES, R.: Hospital management of pit viper venenations. Clinical Toxicol. *3*:501, 1970.
6. McCOLLOUGH, N. & GENNARO, J.: Diagnosis, symptoms, treatment and sequelae of envenomation by *Crotalus adamanteus* and Genus *Agkistrodon*. J. Florida Med. Assoc. *55*:327, 1968.
7. WATT, C. & GENNARO, J.: Pit viper bites in South Georgia and North Florida. Tr. South. Surg. Assoc. *77*:378, 1966.
8. MINTON, S.: Venom Diseases: Snakebite. In Textbook of Medicine, P. Beeson and W. McDermott (Eds.), pp. 88–92; Saunders, Philadelphia, 1975.
9. VAN MIEROP, L.: Snakebite symposium. J. Florida Med. Assoc. *63*:101, 1976.
10. ARNOLD, R.: Treatment of snakebite. JAMA *236*:1843, 1976.
11. Poisonous Snakes of the World. U.S. Government Printing Office, Washington, D.C., NAVMED, 1965.

How Supplied: Each combination package contains one vacuum vial to yield 10 ml of serum—to be used immediately after reconstitution—(with preservatives: phenol 0.25% and thimerosal [mercury derivative] 0.005%). One vial containing 10 ml of Bacteriostatic Water for Injection, USP (with preservative: phenylmercuric nitrate 0.001%). One 1 ml vial of normal horse serum (diluted 1:10) as sensitivity testing material with preservatives: thimerosal (mercury derivative) 0.005% and phenol 0.35%. Not returnable.

ANTIVENIN (Micrurus fulvius) (equine origin) ℞

Composition: Each combination package contains one vial of lyophilized Antivenin (Micrurus fulvius) with 0.25% phenol and 0.005% thimerosal (mercury derivative) as preservatives (before lyophilization); one vial of diluent containing 10 ml. of Bacteriostatic Water for Injection, U.S.P., with phenylmercuric nitrate (1:100,000) as preservative.

How Supplied: Combination packages as described (not returnable).

CHOLERA VACCINE, U.S.P. ℞

Description: Each ml. contains 8 units each serotype antigen (Ogawa and Inaba). The preservative is 0.5% phenol.

How Supplied: Vials of 1.5 ml. and 20 ml.

DIPHTHERIA AND TETANUS TOXOIDS ADSORBED (PEDIATRIC) ℞
aluminum phosphate adsorbed, ULTRAFINED®

Description: Antigens adsorbed on aluminum phosphate. Preservative is 0.01% thimerosal (mercury derivative).

How Supplied: Vials of 5 ml.; and 0.5-ml. TUBEX® Sterile Cartridge-Needle Units, packages of 10.

DIPHTHERIA AND TETANUS TOXOIDS AND PERTUSSIS VACCINE ADSORBED ℞
aluminum phosphate adsorbed ULTRAFINED®
Triple Antigen

Description: Triple Antigen Adsorbed (Diphtheria and Tetanus Toxoids and Pertussis Vaccine Adsorbed), Wyeth, is a combination of diphtheria toxoid adsorbed, tetanus toxoid adsorbed, and pertussis vaccine. The diphtheria toxoid is prepared by cultivating a suitable strain of *Corynebacterium diphtheriae* on a modified Mueller's casein hydrolysate medium (J. Immunology *37*:103, 1939). The tetanus toxoid is prepared by growing a suitable strain of *Clostridium tetani* on a protein-free semisynthetic medium (Appl. Microbiol. *10*:146, 1962). Formaldehyde is used as the toxoiding (detoxifying) agent for both diphtheria and tetanus toxins. The final product contains no more than 0.02 percent free formaldehyde. The pertussis vaccine component is prepared by growing suitable strains of Phase I B. pertussis on a modified Cohen and Wheeler medium: casein hydrolysate medium with yeast dialyzate (Wadsworth:Standard Methods, 3rd. Ed., p. 200, Williams and Wilkins Co., 1947) supplemented with 5% agar and 4% charcoal. The preservative in the final product is 0.01% thimerosal (mercury derivative).

The aluminum content of the final product does not exceed 0.85 mg per 0.5 ml dose. During processing, hydrochloric acid and sodium hydroxide are used to adjust the pH. Sodium chloride is added to the final product to control isotonicity.

The total primary immunizing dose (1.5 ml) contains 12 protective units of pertussis vaccine.

Indication: Triple Antigen, Aluminum Phosphate Adsorbed, Wyeth, is indicated for active immunization of infants and children through 6 years of age against diphtheria, tetanus, and pertussis.[1]

Contraindications: A febrile acute respiratory infection or other active infection is reason for deferring administration.

Occurrence of any of the following signs, symptoms, or conditions following administration is a contraindication to further use of this product and/or pertussis vaccine as the single antigen: fever over 103° F (39° C); convulsion(s) with or without accompanying fever; alterations of consciousness; focal neurologic signs; screaming episodes (also called screaming fits); shock; collapse; thrombocytopenic purpura.[2]

The presence of an evolving or changing neurologic disorder is a contraindication to use.

Immunosuppressive therapy, including irradiation, corticosteroids, antimetabolites, alkylating agents, and cytotoxic agents may result in aberrant responses to active immunization procedures.

Administration should be deferred in individuals receiving such therapy.

Precautions: This product should be used for the age group between two months and the seventh birthday.

When an infant or child is returned for the next dose in the series, the parent should be questioned concerning occurrence of any symptoms and/or signs of a severe adverse reaction after the previous dose (See Contraindications; Side Effects and Adverse Reactions). If such are reported, further doses of Triple Antigen are contraindicated and active immunization against diphtheria and tetanus should be completed with Diphtheria and Tetanus Toxoids Adsorbed **(Pediatric).**

If the vial is used, rather than the TUBEX® Sterile Cartridge-Needle Unit, a separate syringe and needle which have been adequately cleaned and sterilized should be used for each patient to prevent transmission of hepatitis B virus and other infectious agents from one person to another.

Before the injection of any biological, the physician should take all precautions known for prevention of allergic or any other side reactions. This should include: A review of the patient's history regarding possible sensitivity; the ready availability of epinephrine 1:1000 and other appropriate agents used for control of immediate allergic reactions; and a knowledge of the recent literature pertaining to use of the biological concerned, including the nature of side effects and adverse reactions that may follow its use.

Side Effects and Adverse Reactions: Local reactions, manifested by erythema and induration with or without tenderness, are common after administration of Triple Antigen Adsorbed.[3] Such local reactions are usually self-limited and require no therapy. A nodule may be palpable at the injection site for a few weeks. Abscess formation at the site of injection has been reported.

Mild-to-moderate temperature elevations, accompanied by malaise occurring within several hours of administration and persisting for one to two days, occur frequently.[3]

The below-listed serious, and occasionally fatal, adverse reactions have been reported following administration of pertussis-vaccine-containing preparations. The incidence of these reactions is unknown, but they seem to be exceedingly rare. Should such reactions occur, further immunization against pertussis is contraindicated.[2] See also Contraindications and Precautions.

1. Severe temperature elevations—105° F or higher.
2. Collapse with rapid recovery.
3. Collapse followed by prolonged prostration and a shock-like state.
4. Screaming episodes characterized by a prolonged period of peculiar crying during which the infant cannot be comforted.
5. Isolated convulsion(s) with or without fever.
6. Frank encephalopathy with changes in the level of consciousness, focal neurological signs, and convulsions with or without permanent neurological and/or mental deficit.[4–9]
7. Thrombocytopenic purpura.

The occurrence of sudden-infant-death syndrome (SIDS) has been reported following administration of DTP.[10,11] The significance of these reports is unclear. It should be kept in mind that the three primary immunizing doses of DTP are usually administered to infants between the age of 2 and 6 months and that approximately 85 percent of SIDS cases occur in the period 1 through 6 months of age, with the peak incidence at age 2 to 4 months.[12,13]

Dosage and Administration: The basic immunizing course for infants and children through 6 years of age consists of three (primary) doses of 0.5 ml each at 4- to 8-week intervals, followed by a fourth (reinforcing) dose of 0.5 ml approximately one year after the third primary dose. The fourth (reinforcing) dose is an integral part of the basic immunizing course; basic immunization cannot be considered completed until the reinforcing dose has been given.

Interruption of the recommended schedule with a delay between doses does not interfere with the final immunity achieved; nor does it necessitate starting the series over again, regardless of the length of time elapsed between doses.[2] All doses should be injected intramuscularly, preferably into the midlateral muscles of the thigh or deltoid, with care to avoid major peripheral nerve trunks. The same muscle site should not be injected more than once during the course of basic immunization. It is recommended that active immunization against diphtheria, tetanus, and pertussis be started at 2 months of age.[1,2]

A routine recall (booster) dose of 0.5 ml is indicated at age 4–6 years, preferably prior to entrance into kindergarten or elementary school. If a child less than 6 years of age who has received fewer than 4 properly spaced doses of a DTP preparation is exposed to diphtheria or pertussis or suffers a wound which might possibly be contaminated with Cl. tetani spores or bacilli, it may be advisable to administer a 0.5 ml dose of this product (or the appropriate single active immunizing antigen) AND: 1. an adequate dose of the appropriate passive immunizing agent (at a different site with a different syringe); 2. an adequate course of the prophylactic therapy with an appropriate antibiotic, depending, among other factors, on the number of doses of DTP received in the past and the interval since the last dose, the duration and intimacy of exposure, and the interval between exposure and initiation of specific prophylactic measures.

For basic or recall (booster) immunization against tetanus and diphtheria of individuals over 6 years of age, the use of Tetanus and Diphtheria Toxoids Adsorbed, Aluminum Phosphate Adsorbed **(For Adult Use)** is recommended.

How Supplied: Diphtheria and Tetanus Toxoids and Pertussis Vaccine Adsorbed, Aluminum Phosphate Adsorbed, Ultrafined®, Triple Antigen, is available in vials of 7.5 ml and 0.5 ml TUBEX® Sterile Cartridge-Needle Units in packages of 10 TUBEX.

Technic for Injection: Before injection, the skin over the site to be injected should be cleansed and prepared with a suitable germicide. After insertion of the needle, aspirate to help avoid inadvertent injection into a blood vessel. Expel the antigen slowly and terminate the dose with a small bubble of air (0.1 to 0.2 ml). Do not inject intracutaneously or into superficial subcutaneous structures.

Directions for Use of Vials

Shake the vial vigorously before withdrawing each dose.

Before injection, the rubber diaphragm of the vial should be cleansed and prepared with a suitable germicide. Injections from the vial must be administered promptly to prevent settling of the material in the syringe. Flush the syringe after injection to prevent the remaining material from drying within the syringe.

References:

1. Recommendation of the Public Health Service Advisory Committee on Immunization Practices. Morbidity and Mortality Weekly Report 26 (No. 49): 401, 1977.
2. Report of the Committee on Infectious Diseases, American Academy of Pediatrics (Red Book), 1977.
3. BARKIN, R., PICHICHERO, M.: Diphtheria-pertussis-tetanus vaccine: Reactogenicity of commercial products. Pediatrics *63:*256, 1979.
4. TOOMEY, J. A.: Reactions to pertussis vaccine. J. Am. Med. Assoc. *139:*448, 1949.
5. BYERS, B. K., MOLL, F. C.: Encephalopathies following prophylactic pertussis vaccine. Pediatrics *1:*437, 1948.
6. BERG, J.: Neurological complications of pertussis immunization. Brit. Med. J. *2:*24, 1958.
7. STROM, J.: Further experience of reactions, especially of a cerebral nature, in conjunction with triple vaccination: A study based on vaccinations in Sweden. 1959–65. Brit. Med. J. *4:*320, 1967.
8. STEWART, G.: Vaccination against whooping cough. Efficacy versus risks. Lancet *1:*234, 1977.
9. KULENKAMPFF, M. et al.: Neurological complications of pertussis inoculation. Arch. Dis. Child. *49:*46, 1974.
10. Morbidity and Mortality Weekly Report: DTP vaccination and sudden infant deaths—Tennessee. *28* (No. 11):131, 1979.
11. Morbidity and Mortality Weekly Report: Follow-up on DTP vaccination and sudden infant deaths—Tennessee. *28* (No. 12):134, 1979.
12. STANDFAST, S., et al.: The epidemiology of sudden infant death in upstate New York. JAMA *241:*1127, 1979.
13. KRAUS, J., BORHANI, N.: Post-neonatal sudden unexplained death in California: A cohort study. Am. J. Epidemiol. *95:*497, 1972.

Smallpox Vaccine
Dried
Calf Lymph Type
DRYVAX® ℞
dried smallpox vaccine

Composition: During processing, not more than 100 units of polymyxin B sulfate, 200 micrograms of dihydrostreptomycin sulfate, 200 micrograms of chlortetracycline HCl and 100 micrograms of neomycin sulfate per ml are added, and trace amounts of these antibiotics may be present in the final product. Reconstituted vaccine contains 50% glycerin, 0.25% phenol and 0.005% brilliant green in Sterile Water for Injection, USP.

How Supplied: Combination package of 1 vial of Dried Smallpox Vaccine, 1 container of Diluent (0.15 ml, sufficient for 25 vaccinations), and 25 sterile bifurcated needles.

IMMUNE SERUM GLOBULIN ℞
(human), U.S.P.

Description: Immune Serum Globulin (human), U.S.P. is a sterile concentrated solution containing 16.5% (±1.5%) immunoglobulin stabilized with 0.3M glycine and containing 1:10,000 thimerosal (mercury derivative) as preservative.

How Supplied: Vials of 10 ml; and 2 ml Tubex® Sterile Cartridge-Needle Units, packages of 1.

INFLUENZA VIRUS VACCINE, SUBVIRION TYPE ℞

The formulation of influenza virus vaccine for use during each season is established by the Bureau of Biologics, Food and Drug Administration, Public Health Service. For current information about formulation, dosage and recommended use, consult product direction circular which can be obtained by writing Professional Service, Wyeth Laboratories, P.O. Box 8299, Philadelphia, PA, 19101, or through your local Wyeth representative.

RABIES VACCINE ℞
(Human Diploid-Cell Strain)
Subvirion Antigen

(*See* WYVAC® [Rabies Vaccine])

SMALLPOX VACCINE, DRIED
calf lymph type

(*See* DRYVAX® [dried smallpox vaccine])

TETANUS AND DIPHTHERIA TOXOIDS ADSORBED ℞
(for adult use)
aluminum phosphate adsorbed
ULTRAFINED®

Description: A combination of refined tetanus and diphtheria toxoids for adult use, in

Continued on next page

Wyeth—Cont.

which the fully potent antigens are adsorbed on aluminum phosphate. The preservative is 0.01% thimerosal (mercury derivative). Each dose contains no more than 2 Lf of purified diphtheria toxoid.

How Supplied: Vials of 5 ml.; and 0.5-ml. TUBEX® Sterile Cartridge-Needle Units, packages of 10.

TETANUS IMMUNE GLOBULIN ℞
(human)

Description: Tetanus Immune Globulin (Human) is a sterile 10- to 18-percent solution of human immunoglobulin prepared by the cold ethanol fractionation method from persons who have been hyperimmunized with tetanus toxoid. The final product contains 0.3 molar glycine as a stabilizer and 0.01 percent thimerosal (mercury derivative) as preservative. This product was prepared from blood that was nonreactive when tested for hepatitis B surface antigen (HBsAg).

How Supplied: 1 ml TUBEX® Sterile Cartridge-Needle Unit, packages of 10.

TETANUS TOXOID ADSORBED ℞
aluminum phosphate adsorbed, ULTRAFINED®

Description: A refined toxoid, in which the antigen is adsorbed on aluminum phosphate. The preservative is 0.01% thimerosal (mercury derivative).

How Supplied: Vials of 5 ml.; and 0.5-ml. TUBEX ® Sterile Cartridge-Needle Units, packages of 10.

TETANUS TOXOID, fluid ℞
purified, ULTRAFINED®

Description: A refined tetanus toxoid. The preservative is 0.01% thimerosal (mercury derivative).

How Supplied: Vials of 7.5 ml.; and 0.5-ml. TUBEX® Sterile Cartridge-Needle Units, packages of 10.

TYPHOID VACCINE, U.S.P. ℞

Description: Each ml. contains not more than 1000 million Salmonella typhosa (Ty-2 strain) organisms, killed and suspended in buffered sodium chloride injection. The preservative is 0.5% phenol. Contains 8 units per ml.

How Supplied: Vials of 5 ml., 10 ml., and 20 ml.

Rabies Vaccine
(Human Diploid-Cell Strain)
Subvirion Antigen
WYVAC® ℞

Description: Rabies Vaccine, Wyeth (WYVAC), is a sterile, stable, cell-culture rabies virus vaccine for human use by intramuscular injection. It is prepared with the Pasteur-derived Pitman-Moore virus strain adapted from material grown in rabbit brain—as used in the production of Semple-type vaccine—to cultivation in the Human Diploid-Cell Strain (HDCS), WI-38.[1] Seed stocks and vaccine lots have been prepared with cell-free virus harvests from infected cultures after 63 or more consecutive HDCS passages. The virus is propagated in these cells, in a chemically defined nutrient medium with normal serum albumin (human) with the following antibiotics added: neomycin sulfate, amphotericin B, and gentamicin sulfate.

The virus harvest is freed of undesirable materials and debris by membrane filtration and then concentrated to a standard antigen content by aseptic ultrafiltration. The virus particles in the concentrate are disrupted into smaller antigenic units by the addition of tri(n)butylphosphate (0.1%) and Polysorbate 80, USP (0.1%); and inactivation is completed by further treatment with beta propiolactone (0.025%). The vaccine is preserved with thimerosal (mercury derivative), added to the ultra-filtrate to a final concentration of 0.01% (1:10,000). The vaccine is stabilized by lyophilization. Each 1 ml dose of vaccine, which is colorless to faintly pink after reconstitution because of a phenol red indicator, contains approximately 2.5% normal human serum albumin and not more than 50 mcg neomycin, 2.5 mcg amphotericin, 50 mcg gentamicin, 0.01% tri(n)butylphosphate (as determined by assay), 0.1% Polysorbate 80, USP, and 0.01% thimerosal (mercury derivative).

The potency of the vaccine is equal to or greater than 2.5 International Units (IU) of rabies antigen per dose, which is established by tests in parallel with the Standard Rabies Vaccine in the NIH mouse potency test as required by the Bureau of Biologics, Food and Drug Administration.

Clinical Pharmacology: The administration of the inactivated rabies vaccine stimulates rapid production of specific antibodies.

In *preexposure trials* involving more than 2,000 volunteers, after three injections of vaccine over a four-week period, at least 99% of recipients developed antibodies. Geometric mean titers for various groups 35 days after the start of immunization were approximately ten IU, with only a few vaccinees falling below one IU [a level of 0.5 IU or a titer of equal or greater than 1:16 by the Rapid Fluorescent Focus Inhibition Test (RFFIT) is considered to be an adequate response to immunization].

In ongoing *postexposure* clinical trials utilizing a five- or six-dose regimen in conjunction with Rabies Immune Globulin, Human RIG(H), over 500 adults and children have been successfully treated. Treatment groups consisting of subjects allergic to Duck Embryo Vaccine (DEV), nonresponders to DEV, and subjects receiving primary postexposure therapy have been successfully immunized in 100% of cases. No cases of human rabies have occurred in these patients who have had varying degrees of exposure to confirmed or suspected rabid animals.[2,3,4,5]

A group of ten children, ranging in age from 2–16 years, has also been successfully treated on the same regimen.[6] All developed significant rabies antibody titers within 14 days, with a geometric mean titer (GMT) of 3.7 IU/ml at 14 days, 8.7 IU/ml at 28 days, and 20.1 IU/ml at 42 days after beginning treatment, as determined by the RFFIT.

As a result of exposure to two cases of human rabies, seventy individuals with histories of contact up to two months prior to receiving vaccine all developed protective responses. The GMTs ranged from 0.9 IU at 14 days to 14.6 IU at 42 days after a five-dose regimen, and RIG(H).

Data on persistence of antibody demonstrated that in 546 subjects who received preexposure inoculations, sera obtained at 9–12 months after primary immunization with a three-dose regimen demonstrated antibody levels of 0.5 to 8.4 IU/ml in nearly 93% of vaccinees. Single booster doses of 1.0 ml given to several different groups, immunized previously with 3 or 4 doses of WYVAC or a routine course of DEV, induced four-fold increases in titer in 99% of vaccinees. The GMT was 4.7 IU/ml by RFFIT 14–35 days after receipt of the booster dose. A small group of these individuals tested one year later still had a range of titers of 1.0–2.0 IU/ml.[7]

Indications and Usage[3]:

1. RATIONALE OF TREATMENT

In the United States and Canada, the following factors should be considered before specific antirabies treatment is indicated:

A. *Species of Biting Animal*

Carnivorous animals (especially skunks, foxes, coyotes, raccoons, dogs, bobcats, and cats) and bats are more likely than other animals to be infected with rabies. Rats, mice, squirrels, hamsters, guinea pigs, gerbils, chipmunks, and other rodents, or rabbits and hares are rarely found to be infected with rabies and have not been known to cause human rabies in the United States. Their bites almost never call for antirabies prophylaxis. Therefore, before initiating antirabies prophylaxis, the local or state health department should be consulted.

B. *Circumstances of Biting Incident*

An UNPROVOKED attack is more likely than a provoked attack to indicate that the animal is rabid. Bites inflicted on a person attempting to feed or handle an apparently healthy animal should generally be regarded as PROVOKED.

C. *Type of Exposure*

Rabies is commonly transmitted by inoculation with infectious saliva. The likelihood that rabies infection will result from exposure to a rabid animal varies with the nature and extent of the exposure. Two categories of exposure should be considered:

Bite: Any penetration of the skin by teeth.

Nonbite: Scratches, abrasions, open wounds or mucous membranes contaminated with saliva or other potentially infectious material, such as the brain from a rabid animal. In addition, there have been two instances of airborne rabies acquired in the laboratory and two probable airborne rabies cases acquired in one bat-infested cave (Frio Cave, Texas).

Casual contact with a rabid animal, such as petting the animal (without a bite or nonbite exposure as described above), does not constitute an exposure and is not an indication for prophylaxis.

The only documented cases of rabies due to human-to-human transmission occurred in patients who received corneal transplants from persons who died of rabies undiagnosed at the time of death.

Each exposure to possible rabies infection must be individually evaluated.

Local or state public health officials should be consulted if questions arise about the need for rabies prophylaxis.

II. PRE- AND POSTEXPOSURE TREATMENT OF RABIES

A. *Preexposure*

1. Adults—Immunization is indicated for physicians, veterinarians, laboratory workers, animal handlers, and other personnel working in hospitals, clinics, and diagnostic and research laboratories who are concerned with the treatment of rabid patients or animals or with the handling of rabies virus or potentially contaminated material. Immunization is also indicated for persons who may be exposed to rabid animals while living in or visiting regions where animal rabies occurs. Included in this category of risk are hunters, forest rangers, taxidermists, stock breeders, and slaughterhouse workers.

2. Children—Immunization is recommended for children living in or visiting countries where exposure to rabid animals is a constant threat. Worldwide statistics indicate that children are more at risk than adults.

B. *Postexposure*

1. Local Treatment of Wounds—Immediate and thorough local treatment of all bite wounds and scratches is perhaps the most effective preventive measure. The wound should be thoroughly cleansed immediately with soap and water.

Tetanus prophylaxis and measures to control bacterial infection should be given as indicated.

2. Specific Treatment—Postexposure antirabies treatment should always include both passive [preferably Rabies Immune Globulin of human origin—RIG(H)] and active (Rabies Vaccine) immunization, with one exception:

persons who have been previously immunized with rabies vaccine and have a documented adequate rabies antibody titer should receive only vaccine. Antirabies serum of horse origin (ARS) should only be used where human immune globulin is unavailable. The combination of globulin and vaccine is recommended for both bite exposures and nonbite exposures (as described under "Rationale of Treatment") and regardless of the interval between exposure and treatment. The sooner treatment is begun after exposure, the better.

POSTEXPOSURE RABIES TREATMENT GUIDE

The following recommendations are only a guide. They should be applied in conjunction with knowledge of the animal species involved, circumstances of the bite or other exposure, vaccination status of the animal, and presence of rabies in the region. Local and state public health officials should be consulted if questions arise about the need for rabies prophylaxis. [See table right].

Animal Species	Condition of Animal at Time of Attack	Treatment of Exposed Person (1). All bites and wounds should immediately be thoroughly cleansed with soap and water (see preceding text).
Domestic: Dog & Cat	Healthy and available for 10 days of observation	None, unless animal develops rabies (2).
	Rabid or suspected rabid	Rabies Immune Globulin (3) AND Rabies Vaccine (4).
	Unknown (escaped)	Consultation with public health officials. If treatment is indicated, give Rabies Immune Globulin (3) AND Rabies Vaccine (4).
Wild: Skunk, bat, fox, coyote, raccoon, bobcat, and other carnivores	Regard as rabid unless proven negative by laboratory test (5)	Rabies Immune Globulin (3) AND Rabies Vaccine (4).
Other: Livestock, rodents, rabbits, and hares	Consider Individually—provoked bites of squirrels, hamsters, guinea pigs, gerbils, chipmunks, rats, mice and other rodents or rabbits and hares almost never call for antirabies prophylaxis. Local or state public health officials should be consulted about questions that arise about the need for rabies prophylaxis.	

(1) If antirabies treatment is indicated, both Rabies Immune Globulin and Rabies Vaccine should be given as soon as possible, *regardless* of the interval from exposure.
(2) Begin treatment with Rabies Immune Globulin and Rabies Vaccine at first sign of rabies in biting domestic animals during the usual holding period of 10 days. The symptomatic animal should be killed immediately and tested.
(3) If Rabies Immune Globulin is not available, use antirabies serum of equine origin. Do not use more than the recommended dosage.
(4) Discontinue vaccine if fluorescent antibody tests of animal are negative.
(5) The animal should be killed and tested as soon as possible. Holding for observation is not recommended.

Contraindications: For postexposure treatment there are no known specific contraindications for the use of this vaccine. In cases of preexposure immunization, there are no known specific contraindications other than situations such as developing febrile illness.

Warnings: In both preexposure and postexposure immunization, the full 1.0 ml dose should be given intramuscularly. There are no data to establish the efficacy of using either reduced volumes of vaccine or of that injected intradermally.

Local or mild systemic adverse reactions to the vaccine are infrequent; they do not contraindicate continuing immunization and may be treated symptomatically. Neurological events reported following receipt of HDCS rabies vaccine include two cases of acute polyradiculoneuropathy (Guillain-Barré Syndrome)[8], a transient neuroparalytic illness that completely resolved within 12 weeks[9], and a focal subacute CNS disorder. While these have been temporally associated with vaccine administration, no causal relationship has been established. Should a neurological complication develop, advice and assistance on managing the patient as well as making a decision about discontinuing vaccine treatment is available from state health departments or the Center for Disease Control (CDC). Any serious reactions should be immediately reported to the state health department or the Viral Disease Division, Bureau of Epidemiology, CDC, Atlanta, Georgia (telephone 404-329-3727 during working hours or 404-329-3644 at other times).

Precautions:

GENERAL

Allergic reactions to WYVAC have not been reported; however, the possibility of this occurrence exists. Caution should be used in administering the vaccine to persons with a history of allergic disorders.

While the concentration of antibiotics in each dose of vaccine is extremely small, persons with known hypersensitivity to any of these agents could manifest an allergic reaction. While the risk is small, it should be weighed in light of the potential risk of contracting rabies. Epinephrine injection (1:1000) must be immediately available should an acute anaphylactic reaction occur due to any component of the vaccine.

DRUG INTERACTIONS

Corticosteroids and immunosuppressive agents may interfere with the development of active immunity and predispose the patient to developing rabies. They should not be administered during postexposure therapy unless essential for the treatment of other serious conditions. If rabies postexposure therapy is administered to persons receiving steroids or immunosuppressive therapy, it is especially important that serum be tested for rabies antibody to ensure that an adequate response has developed.

USAGE IN PREGNANCY—PREGNANCY CATEGORY C

Animal reproductive studies have not been conducted with WYVAC. It is also not known whether WYVAC can cause fetal harm when administered to a pregnant woman or can affect reproduction capacity. Pregnancy is not a contraindication to rabies postexposure therapy. Based on limited data, there have been no fetal abnormalities associated with rabies vaccination. If there is substantial risk of rabies exposure, preexposure treatment may also be indicated during pregnancy.

Adverse Reactions: Once initiated, rabies prophylaxis should not be interrupted or discontinued because of local, or mild systemic, adverse reactions to rabies vaccine. Usually such reactions can be successfully managed with antiinflammatory and antipyretic agents (aspirin, for example).

Local reactions to the injected vaccine, such as pain, erythema, and swelling or itching at the injection site, have been observed to be fewer and less severe than those seen with DEV and vaccine of brain-tissue origin. These reactions may occur after each injection and may persist for one to three days. Varying degrees of local erythema and induration have been observed. In a series of 1,100 subjects receiving three doses at 0, 7, and 21 or 28 days, the incidence of any local reaction was approximately 18%, subjects usually reporting soreness at the injection site.[10] In another series in patients receiving one to five doses after exposure to confirmed or suspected rabid animals, the incidence of minor local discomfort, redness, or induration was 15%.[11] However, other series report an incidence of local reactions of 10–28%.

Systemic reactions to the vaccine, such as mild nausea, headache, abdominal pain, muscle aches, dizziness, and malaise, have been encountered and are short-lived, ranging in these recorded series from 5–20% of vaccine recipients. No increase with successive doses has been noted. Rash, edema, itching, and shortness of breath are rare but have occurred.

Constitutional reactions and symptoms may arise in patients faced with a life-threatening situation and may not be caused by the vaccine. However, the development of fever, malaise, fatigue, nausea, and arthralgia merits careful observation.

The occurrence of neuroparalytic reactions, such as transverse myelitis, encephalomyelitis, Guillain-Barré Syndrome, and other cranial or peripheral neuropathies with resultant permanent neurological sequelae and/or death, have been reported in recipients of inactivated rabies vaccines of nervous-tissue and duck embryo origin. The possibility of the occurrence of such neuroparalytic or other major neurologic reactions following the use of inactivated rabies vaccines of human-diploid-cell origin should be kept in mind. Also see "Warnings" section.

Serious systemic, anaphylactic, or neuroparalytic reactions, occurring during the administration of rabies vaccines, pose a serious dilemma for the attending physician. A patient's risk of developing rabies must be carefully considered before deciding to discontinue vaccination or to choose an alternate vaccine. Moreover, the use of corticosteroids to treat life-threatening neuroparalytic reactions carries the risk of inhibiting the development of active immunity to rabies. It is especially important in these cases that the serum of the patient be tested for rabies antibodies. Advice and assistance on the management of serious adverse reactions in persons receiving rabies vaccines may be sought from the state health department or the CDC.

Dosage and Administration[3]:

DIRECTIONS FOR USE

Using a sterile syringe, inject 1.0 ml of Sterile Water for Injection, USP, into the vial of vaccine. Shake vial gently until vaccine is completely dissolved. The reconstituted vaccine should be used immediately.

Continued on next page

Wyeth—Cont.

Withdraw entire dose and inject intramuscularly, preferably into the deltoid muscle or upper, outer quadrant of the buttock. In infants and small children, the midlateral aspect of the thigh may be preferable. Care should be taken to avoid injection into or near blood vessels and nerves. After aspiration, if blood or any suspicious discoloration appears in the syringe, do not inject but instead, discard its contents and repeat procedure using fresh vaccine with new needle and syringe at a different site.

A. PREEXPOSURE IMMUNIZATION

The relatively low frequency of reactions to WYVAC makes it practical to offer preexposure immunization to persons in high-risk groups: veterinarians, animal handlers, certain laboratory workers, and persons—especially children—living in or visiting countries where rabies is a constant threat. Persons whose vocational or avocational pursuit brings them into contact with potentially rabid dogs, cats, foxes, skunks, bats, or other species at risk of having rabies should also be considered for preexposure prophylaxis.

Preexposure prophylaxis is given for several reasons. First, it may provide protection to persons with inapparent exposures to rabies. Second, it protects persons whose postexposure therapy might be expected to be delayed. Finally, although it does not eliminate the need for additional therapy after a rabies exposure, it simplifies that therapy by eliminating the need for globulin and decreasing the number of doses of vaccine needed. The last advantage is of particular importance for persons at high risk of being exposed in countries where the available rabies immunizing products may carry a high risk of adverse reactions.

Three 1-ml injections of WYVAC should be given intramuscularly (for example, in the deltoid area), 1 on each of days 0, 7, and 21 or 28.

Booster doses of vaccine: Persons with continuing risk of exposure should receive a booster dose (1 ml) every 2 years or have their serum tested for rabies antibody every 2 years and, if the titer is inadequate, have a booster dose. Persons who work with live rabies virus in research laboratories or vaccine production facilities and are at risk of inapparent exposure should have the rabies antibody titer of their serum determined every 6 months; booster doses of vaccine should be given, as needed, to maintain an adequate titer. Other laboratory workers, such as those doing rabies diagnostic tests, should have boosters every 2 years or have their serum tested for rabies antibody every 2 years and, if the titer is inadequate, have a booster dose.

B. POSTEXPOSURE IMMUNIZATION

Postexposure antirabies immunization should always include both passively administered antibody [preferably RIG(H)] and vaccine with 1 exception: persons who have been previously immunized with rabies vaccine and have a documented adequate rabies antibody titer should receive only vaccine. The combination of globulin and vaccine is recommended for both bite exposures and nonbite exposures (as described under "Rationale of Treatment") and regardless of the interval between exposure and treatment. RIG(H) is administered only once, at the beginning of postexposure therapy, as described below. The sooner treatment is begun after exposure, the better. However, there have been instances in which the decision to begin treatment was indicated as late as 6 months and longer after the exposure.

In 1977 the World Health Organization (WHO) established a recommendation for 6 intramuscular doses of HDCV based on studies in Germany and Iran of a regimen of RIG(H) or ARS and 6 doses of HDCV. Used in this way the vaccine was found to be effective in protecting 76 persons bitten by proven rabid animals and induced an excellent antibody response in all recipients. Since 1977, studies conducted by the CDC in the United States have shown that a regimen of 1 dose of RIG(H) and 5 doses of WYVAC induced an excellent antibody response in all recipients. Of 77 persons bitten by proven rabid animals and so treated, none developed rabies.

Five 1-ml doses of WYVAC should be given intramuscularly (for example, in the deltoid regions). Other routes of administration, such as the intradermal route, have not been tested for postexposure prophylaxis and should not be used. The first dose should be given as soon as possible after the exposure and be administered in conjunction with RIG(H); an additional dose should be given on each of days 3, 7, 14, and 28 after the first dose. (WHO currently recommends a sixth dose 90 days after the first dose.)

Postexposure therapy of previously immunized persons: When an immunized person with previously demonstrated rabies antibody is exposed to rabies, that person should receive 2 doses (1 ml each) of WYVAC, 1 immediately and 1 three days later. Passive immunization should not be given in these cases. If the immune status of a previously immunized person is not known, full primary postexposure antirabies treatment [RIG(H) plus 5 doses of WYVAC] may be necessary. In such cases, if antibody can be demonstrated in a serum sample collected before vaccine is given, treatment can be discontinued after at least 2 doses of WYVAC.

SEROLOGIC TESTING

The Immunization Practices Advisory Committee (ACIP) does not recommend routine serologic testing of persons who receive the recommended preexposure or postexposure treatment regimens of HDCV. Furthermore, the ACIP believes that routine serologic testing is no longer necessary following booster doses of HDCV for persons given the recommended primary HDCV vaccination with Duck Embryo Vaccine (DEV) or other rabies vaccines. Serologic testing is still recommended for persons vaccinated with DEV or those whose immune responses might be diminished by drug therapy or for other reasons.[12] If the need arises to determine the antibody status of a patient, the CDC or state health department should be contacted.

How Supplied: Rabies Vaccine (HDCS WI-38) Subvirion Antigen, WYVAC®, is supplied as a single-dose vial of lyophilized vaccine with one ampule of diluent (Sterile Water for Injection).

Storage: DO NOT FREEZE. Keep between 2°C and 8°C (35°F and 46°F).

References:

1. WIKTOR TJ, FERNANDES MV, KOPROWSKI H: Cultivation of Rabies Virus in Human Diploid Cell Strain WI-38. J Immunol *93*:353, 1964.

2. Human Diploid Cell Strain Rabies Vaccine. Center for Disease Control. Morbidity and Mortality Weekly Rep *27*:333–339, 1978.

3. Recommendations of the Public Health Service Advisory Committee on Immunization Practices—Rabies, Center for Disease Control. Morbidity and Mortality Weekly Rep *29*:265–280, 1980.

4. ANDERSON LJ, SIKES RK, LANGKOP CW, MANN JW, SMITH JS, WINKLER WG, DEITCH MW: Post-Exposure Trial with 5 Doses of HDCS Rabies Vaccine. J Inf Dis *142*:133–138, 1980.

5. ANDERSON LJ, WINKLER WG, HAFKIN B, KEENLYSIDE RA, D'ANGELO LJ, DEITCH MW: Clinical Experience with a Human Diploid Cell Rabies Vaccine. JAMA *244*:781–784, 1980.

6. SIEBER O, ROSANOFF E, DEITCH M, GOLDEN F, TENNICAN P: Post-exposure Rabies Treatment with Wyeth Rabies Human Diploid Cell Vaccine. Proceedings of 19th Interscience Conf. on Antimicrobial Agents & Chemotherapy, October 1979.

7. ROSANOFF E, DEITCH M, PLOTKIN S, WIKTOR T, SWANGO L: Clinical Trial of Human Diploid Cell Strain (HDCS) Rabies Vaccine. Proceedings of 19th Interscience Conf. on Antimicrobial Agents & Chemotherapy, October 1979.

8. BOE E, NYLAND H: Guillain-Barré Syndrome after Vaccination with Human Diploid Cell Rabies Vaccine. Scand J Infect Dis *12*:231–232, 1980.

9. BERNARD, KW (Personal Communication).

10. TINT H, ROSANOFF EI: Clinical Responses to Tri-(n)-butyl phosphate Disrupted Wyvac (WI-38) Rabies Vaccine. Symposium on Standardization of Cell Substrates for the Production of Virus Vaccines. Geneva 1976. Developments in Biological Standardization *37*:287–289, 1977.

11. Data on file, Wyeth Laboratories, Philadelphia, Pa.

12. Recommendations of the Immunization Practices Advisory Committee (ACIP). Morbidity and Mortality Weekly Rep *30*:535, 1981.

COLLYRIUM OTC
with ephedrine
SOOTHING EYE DROPS

Description: A neutral solution of boric acid and borax, containing 0.4% antipyrine, 0.1% ephedrine and not more than 0.002% thimerosal (mercury derivative).

Indications: Soothes, cleanses and refreshes tired or irritated eyes; eyes smarting from wind, sun glare, smog and minor irritants; eyes irritated by prolonged reading or television viewing or by allergies such as hay fever.

Dosage and Administration: Two or three drops in each eye as required.

Warning: If irritation persists or increases, patients are advised to discontinue use and consult physician. Dropper tip should not be allowed to touch any surface since this may contaminate solution. Do not use in conjunction with a wetting solution for contact lens or other eye lotions containing polyvinyl alcohol. Container should be kept tightly closed and stored at room temperature, approx. 77°F (25°C).

How Supplied: Bottles of ½ fl. oz. with built-in eye dropper.

COLLYRIUM OTC
a neutral borate
solution with antipyrine
SOOTHING EYE LOTION

Description: Containing 0.4% antipyrine, boric acid, borax and not more than 0.002% thimerosal (mercury derivative).

Indications: Soothes, cleanses and refreshes tired or irritated eyes resulting from long use, as in reading or close work or due to exposure to sun, strong light, irritation from dust, wind, etc.

Dosage and Administration: Patients are advised to rinse cup with clean water immediately before and after each use, and avoid contamination of rim and interior surface of cup. The half-filled cup should be pressed tightly to the eye to prevent the escape of the liquid, and the head tilted well backward. Eyelids should be opened wide and eyeball rotated to insure thorough bathing with the lotion.

Warning: If irritation persists or increases, patients are advised to discontinue use and consult physician. Do not use in conjunction with a wetting solution for contact lens or other eye lotions containing polyvinyl alcohol. Container should be kept tightly closed and kept at room temperature, approx. 77°F.

How Supplied: Bottles of 6 fl. oz. with eyecup.

CYCLAPEN®-W ℞
(cyclacillin)
Tablets and Oral Suspension

Description: Cyclapen-W (cyclacillin, Wyeth) is a semisynthetic penicillin of the ampicillin class chemically designated as a 6-(1-aminocyclohexanecarboxamido) penicillanic acid. It differs from ampicillin in having an aminocyclohexanecarboxamido substitution on the penicillin nucleus in place of the aminophenylacetamido substitution contained in ampicillin. It is available for oral administration as 250 mg and 500 mg Tablets and for Oral Suspension, bottles providing 125 mg or 250 mg Cyclapen-W per 5 ml teaspoonful when reconstituted. Cyclacillin is a white, crystalline, anhydrous powder sparingly soluble in water.

Actions: HUMAN PHARMACOLOGY
Cyclacillin is acid stable and is rapidly and well absorbed from the gastrointestinal tract and rapidly excreted in the urine after oral administration in the fasting state (Graphs I and II). Peak serum concentration is attained within 40–60 minutes after oral administration in the fasting state. Following oral doses of 250 mg and 500 mg in normal adult human subjects, the average peak serum levels (C max) were approximately 6–7 mcg/ml and 11–12 mcg/ml respectively. Measurable serum levels were present up to 4 hours.
Mean serum concentrations over time are shown in the graphs below:

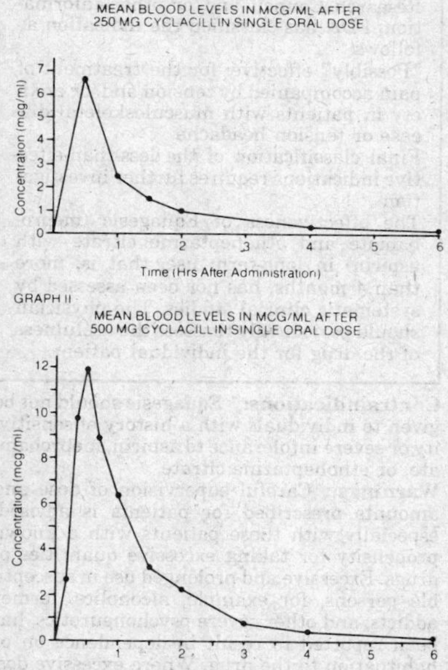

In blood, cyclacillin is one of the least-bound penicillins; an average of about 20% of the drug is bound to plasma proteins.
The biological half-life of the drug in normal adult subjects is about 30–40 minutes with renal clearance accounting for approximately 80 percent. Within 6 hours following administration, 65–70 percent of the cyclacillin dose is excreted unchanged in the urine. Additionally, approximately 15–17 percent of the dose is excreted in the urine in the form of the principal metabolite, 6-(1-aminocyclohexanecarboxamido) penicilloic acid.

Patients with Renal Failure
Cyclacillin may be safely administered to patients with reduced renal function. Normal adult subjects achieve a renal clearance of approximately 450–500 ml/min for cyclacillin. In patients with renal insufficiency (creatinine clearance less than 30 ml/min but greater than 6 ml/min), the mean renal clearance for cyclacillin was about 70 ml/min and the total body clearance was 184 ml/min, resulting in a mean biological half-life of 3.5 hours (210 min). In such patients this renal clearance accounts for approximately 38 percent of the total body clearance. In patients receiving hemodialysis the total body clearance was about 90 ml/min, resulting in a biological half-life of 8 hours (480 minutes). Due to this prolonged serum half-life of cyclacillin, patients with various degrees of renal impairment may require a change in dosage level. (See DOSAGE AND ADMINISTRATION.)

MICROBIOLOGY
Cyclacillin is an orally active, bactericidal semisynthetic penicillin for oral administration. *In vitro* studies have shown that cyclacillin is usually active against the following bacteria:

Group A beta-hemolytic streptococci
Streptococcus pneumoniae (formerly *D. pneumoniae*)
Staphylococci, non-penicillinase producers
Hemophilus influenzae
Escherichia coli
Proteus mirabilis

All strains of *Pseudomonas* and most strains of *Klebsiella* and *Enterobacter* are resistant; some strains of *Escherichia coli* and *Hemophilus influenzae* may be resistant.

DISC SUSCEPTIBILITY TESTS
Quantitative methods that require measurement of zone diameters give the most precise estimates of antibiotic susceptibility. The recommended procedure is the standardized single-disc (Kirby-Bauer) method[1,2] for testing susceptibility to ampicillin-class antibiotics of which cyclacillin is a member. The interpretation involves correlation of the diameters obtained in the disc test with minimal inhibitory concentration (MIC) values for cyclacillin obtained by the ICS method.[3]
Reports from the laboratory giving results of the standardized single-disc susceptibility test using a 10 mcg ampicillin disc[1] should be interpreted according to the following criteria:

1. Group A beta-hemolytic streptococci, *Streptococcus pneumoniae,* and staphylococci, non-penicillinase producers.
Susceptible organisms produce zones of 29 mm or greater, indicating that the tested organism is likely to respond to therapy. Organisms of intermediate susceptibility produce zones of 21–28 mm. Organisms are considered resistant if the zones are 20 mm or less, indicating that other therapy should be selected.
2. *Hemophilus influenzae* tested on chocolate agar.
Susceptible organisms produce zones of 20 mm or greater, indicating that the tested organism is likely to respond to therapy. Resistant organisms produce zones of 19 mm or less, indicating that other therapy should be selected.
3. *Escherichia coli* and *Proteus mirabilis.*
(The following information applies only to urinary-tract infections caused by these gram-negative organisms.)
If the standardized single-disc method of susceptibility testing is used, a disc containing 10 mcg of ampicillin should give a zone diameter of at least 14 mm when tested against a cyclacillin-susceptible strain of *Escherichia coli,* or *Proteus mirabilis,* a zone of 12–13 mm for a strain of intermediate susceptibility and a zone of 11 mm or less for a cyclacillin-resistant strain. Strains may be considered susceptible if the minimal inhibitory concentration (MIC) in Mueller-Hinton broth is not more than 125 mcg of cyclacillin per ml. Strains may be considered resistant if the MIC in Mueller-Hinton broth is greater than 250 mcg of cyclacillin per ml. The MIC value of ampicillin and cyclacillin can be affected by the method of assay and components and pH of the assay medium.

Indications: *Cyclapen®-W (cyclacillin) has less in vitro activity than other drugs in the ampicillin class of antibiotics, and its use should be confined to the indications listed below.*
Cyclapen-W is indicated for the treatment of the following infections:

RESPIRATORY TRACT
Tonsillitis and pharyngitis caused by Group A beta-hemolytic streptococci.
Bronchitis and pneumonia caused by *S. pneumoniae (formerly D. pneumoniae).*
Otitis Media caused by *S. pneumoniae* (formerly *D. pneumoniae), H. influenzae,* and Group A beta-hemolytic streptococci.
Acute exacerbation of chronic bronchitis caused by *H. influenzae.**
*Though clinical improvement has been shown, bacteriologic cures cannot be expected in all patients with chronic respiratory disease due to *H. influenzae.*

SKIN AND SKIN STRUCTURES (integumentary) infections caused by Group A beta-hemolytic streptococci and staphylococci, non-penicillinase producers.
URINARY-TRACT INFECTIONS caused by *E. coli* and *P. mirabilis.* (This drug should not be used in any infections caused by *E. coli* and *P. mirabilis* other than urinary-tract infections.)
NOTE: Cultures and susceptibility tests should be performed initially and during treatment to monitor the effectiveness of therapy and the susceptibility of bacteria. Therapy may be instituted prior to the results of sensitivity testing.

Contraindications: The use of this drug is contraindicated in individuals with a history of an allergic reaction to penicillins.

Warnings: CYCLACILLIN SHOULD ONLY BE PRESCRIBED FOR THE INDICATIONS LISTED IN THIS INSERT.
CYCLACILLIN HAS LESS *IN VITRO* ACTIVITY THAN OTHER DRUGS OF THE AMPICILLIN-CLASS ANTIBIOTICS. HOWEVER, CLINICAL TRIALS HAVE DEMONSTRATED THAT IT IS EFFICACIOUS FOR THE RECOMMENDED INDICATIONS.
SERIOUS AND OCCASIONAL FATAL HYPERSENSITIVITY (ANAPHYLACTOID) REACTIONS HAVE BEEN REPORTED IN PATIENTS RECEIVING PENICILLIN. ALTHOUGH ANAPHYLAXIS IS MORE FREQUENT FOLLOWING PARENTERAL ADMINISTRATION, IT HAS OCCURRED IN PATIENTS ON ORAL PENICILLINS. THESE REACTIONS ARE MORE APT TO OCCUR IN INDIVIDUALS WITH A HISTORY OF SENSITIVITY TO MULTIPLE ALLERGENS. THERE ARE REPORTS OF PATIENTS WITH A HISTORY OF PENICILLIN HYPERSENSITIVITY REACTIONS WHO EXPERIENCED SEVERE HYPERSENSITIVITY REACTIONS WHEN TREATED WITH A CEPHALOSPORIN. BEFORE THERAPY WITH A PENICILLIN, CAREFUL INQUIRY SHOULD BE MADE ABOUT PREVIOUS HYPERSENSITIVITY REACTIONS TO PENICILLINS, CEPHALOSPORINS, AND OTHER ALLERGENS. IF AN ALLERGIC REACTION OCCURS, THE DRUG SHOULD BE DISCONTINUED AND APPROPRIATE THERAPY SHOULD BE INITIATED. SERIOUS ANAPHYLACTOID REACTIONS REQUIRE IMMEDIATE EMERGENCY TREATMENT WITH EPINEPHRINE. OXYGEN, INTRAVENOUS STEROIDS, AIRWAY MANAGEMENT, INCLUDING INTUBATION, SHOULD ALSO BE ADMINISTERED AS INDICATED.

Precautions: Prolonged use of antibiotics may promote the overgrowth of nonsusceptible organisms. If superinfection occurs during therapy, appropriate measures should be taken.
PREGNANCY: Pregnancy Category B. Reproduction studies have been performed in mice

Continued on next page

Wyeth—Cont.

and rats at doses up to ten times the human dose and have revealed no evidence of impaired fertility or harm to the fetus due to cyclacillin. There are, however, no adequate and well-controlled studies in pregnant women. Because animal reproduction studies are not always predictive of human response, this drug should be used during pregnancy only if clearly needed.

NURSING MOTHERS: It is not known whether this drug is excreted in human milk. Because many drugs are excreted in human milk, caution should be exercised when cyclacillin is administered to a nursing woman.

Adverse Reactions: The oral administration of cyclacillin is generally well-tolerated.

As with other penicillins, untoward reactions of the sensitivity phenomena are likely to occur, particularly in individuals who have previously demonstrated hypersensitivity to penicillins or in those with a history of allergy, asthma, hay fever, or urticaria.

The following adverse reactions have been reported with the use of cyclacillin: diarrhea (in approximately 1 out of 20 patients treated), nausea and vomiting (in approximately 1 in 50), and skin rash (in approximately 1 in 60). Isolated instances of headache, dizziness, abdominal pain, vaginitis, and urticaria have been reported. (See WARNINGS)

Other less-frequent adverse reactions which may occur and that have been reported during therapy with other penicillins are: anemia, thrombocytopenia, thrombocytopenic purpura, leukopenia, neutropenia, and eosinophilia. These reactions are usually reversible on discontinuation of therapy.

As with other semisynthetic penicillins, SGOT elevations have been reported.

Dosage and Administration:

[See table below].

Patients with Renal Failure

Based on a dosage of 500 mg q.i.d., the following adjustment in dosage interval is recommended:

Patients with a creatinine clearance of > 50 ml/min need no dosage interval adjustment.

Patients with a creatinine clearance of 30–50 ml/min should receive full doses every 12 hours.

Patients with a creatinine clearance of between 15–30 ml/min should receive full doses every 18 hours.

Patients with a creatinine clearance of between 10–15 ml/min should receive full doses every 24 hours.

In patients with a creatinine clearance of ≤ 10 ml/min or serum creatinine values of ≥ 10 mg%, serum cyclacillin levels are recommended to determine both subsequent dosage and frequency.

How Supplied: Cyclapen®-W (cyclacillin) tablets are available in the following strengths:

250 mg, NDC 0008-0614, yellow capsule-shaped scored tablet embossed with "WYETH" and "614", supplied in bottles of 100 tablets.

500 mg, NDC 0008-0615, yellow capsule-shaped scored tablet embossed with "WYETH" and "615", supplied in bottles of 100 tablets.

Keep bottles tightly closed.

Dispense in tight containers.

Cyclapen-W (cyclacillin) for oral suspension is available in the following strengths:

125 mg per 5 ml, NDC 0008-0599, white to pinkish-white powder supplied in bottles to make 100, 150, and 200 ml of suspension.

250 mg per 5 ml, NDC 0008-0600, white to pinkish-white powder supplied in bottles to make 100, 150, and 200 ml of suspension.

After reconstituting, as directed on the package label, store under refrigeration.

Discard any unused portion after 14 days.

References:

1. BAUER, A.W., KIRBY, W.M.M., SHERRIS, J.C. and TURCK, M.; Antibiotic Testing by a Standardized Single Disc Method, Am. J. Clin. Pathol. *45*:493, 1966. Standardized Disc Susceptibility Test, FEDERAL REGISTER *37*:20527-29, 1972

2. National Committee for Clinical Laboratory Standards; Approved Standard-2; Performance Standards for Antimicrobial Disc Susceptibility Tests, 1976

3. ERICSON, H. M., and SHERRIS, J.C.; Antibiotic Sensitivity Testing Report of an International Collaborative Study, ACTA, Pathol. Microbiol. Scand., Section B:217, 1971

[*Shown in Product Identification Section*]

INFECTION*	ADULTS	CHILDREN Dosage should not result in a dose higher than that for adults.
Respiratory Tract		
Tonsillitis & Pharyngitis**	250 mg q.i.d. in equally spaced doses	body weight < 20 kg (44 lbs) 125 mg t.i.d. in equally spaced doses body weight > 20 kg (44 lbs) 250 mg t.i.d. in equally spaced doses
Bronchitis and Pneumonia		
Mild or Moderate Infections	250 mg q.i.d. in equally spaced doses	50 mg/kg/day q.i.d. in equally spaced doses
Chronic Infections	500 mg q.i.d. in equally spaced doses	100 mg/kg/day q.i.d. in equally spaced doses
Otitis Media	250 mg to 500 mg q.i.d. in equally spaced doses depending on severity	50 to 100 mg/kg/day t.i.d. in equally spaced doses depending on severity
Skin & Skin Structures	250 mg to 500 mg q.i.d. in equally spaced doses depending on severity	50 to 100 mg/kg/day in equally spaced doses depending on severity
Urinary Tract	500 mg q.i.d. in equally spaced doses	100 mg/kg/day in equally spaced doses

*As with antibiotic therapy generally, treatment should be continued for a minimum of 48 to 72 hours after the patient becomes asymptomatic or until evidence of bacterial eradication has been obtained.

**In infections caused by Group A beta-hemolytic streptococci, a minimum of 10 days of treatment is recommended to guard against the risk of rheumatic fever or glomerulonephritis.

In the treatment of chronic urinary-tract infection, frequent bacteriologic and clinical appraisal is necessary during therapy and may be required for several months afterwards.

Persistent infection may require treatment for several weeks.

Cyclacillin is not indicated in children under 2 months of age.

EQUAGESIC® Ⓒ ℞

(meprobamate and ethoheptazine citrate with aspirin)

Description: Each tablet contains 150 mg meprobamate, 75 mg ethoheptazine citrate, and 250 mg aspirin.

Indications:

Based on a review of this drug by the National Academy of Sciences—National Research Council and/or other information, FDA has classified the indication as follows:

"Possibly" effective: for the treatment of pain accompanied by tension and/or anxiety in patients with musculoskeletal disease or tension headache.

Final classification of the less-than-effective indications requires further investigation.

The effectiveness of Equagesic (meprobamate and ethoheptazine citrate with aspirin) in long-term use, that is, more than 4 months, has not been assessed by systematic clinical studies. The physician should periodically reassess the usefulness of the drug for the individual patient.

Contraindications: Equagesic should not be given to individuals with a history of sensitivity or severe intolerance to aspirin, meprobamate, or ethoheptazine citrate.

Warnings: Careful supervision of dose and amounts prescribed for patients is advised, especially with those patients with a known propensity for taking excessive quantities of drugs. Excessive and prolonged use in susceptible persons, for example, alcoholics, former addicts, and other severe psychoneurotics, has been reported to result in dependence on or habituation to the drug. Where excessive dosage has continued for weeks or months, dosage should be reduced gradually rather than abruptly stopped, since withdrawal of a "crutch" may precipitate withdrawal reaction of greater proportions than that for which the drug was originally prescribed. Abrupt discontinuance of doses in excess of the recommended dose has resulted in some cases in the occurrence of epileptiform seizures.

Special care should be taken to warn patients taking meprobamate that their tolerance to alcohol may be lowered with resultant slowing of reaction time and impairment of judgment and coordination.

USAGE IN PREGNANCY AND LACTATION

An increased risk of congenital malformations associated with the use of minor tranquilizers (meprobamate, chlordiazepoxide, and diazepam) during the first trimester of pregnancy has been suggested in several studies. Because use of these drugs is rarely a matter of

urgency, their use during this period should almost always be avoided. The possibility that a woman of childbearing potential may be pregnant at the time of institution of therapy should be considered. Patients should be advised that if they become pregnant during therapy or intend to become pregnant they should communicate with their physicians about the desirability of discontinuing the drug.

Meprobamate passes the placental barrier. It is present both in umbilical-cord blood at or near maternal plasma levels and in breast milk of lactating mothers at concentrations two to four times that of maternal plasma. When use of meprobamate is contemplated in breast-feeding patients, the drug's higher concentrations in breast milk as compared to maternal plasma levels should be considered.

Preparations containing aspirin should be kept out of the reach of children. Equagesic is not recommended for patients 12 years of age and under.

Precautions: Should drowsiness, ataxia, or visual disturbance occur, the dose should be reduced. If the symptoms continue, the patient should not operate a motor vehicle or any dangerous machinery.

Suicidal attempts with meprobamate have resulted in coma, shock, vasomotor and respiratory collapse, and anuria. Very few suicidal attempts were fatal, although some patients ingested very large amounts of the drug (20 to 40 gram). These doses are much greater than those recommended. The drug should be given cautiously, and in small amounts, to patients who have suicidal tendencies. In cases where excessive doses have been taken, sleep ensues rapidly and blood pressure, pulse, and respiratory rates are reduced to basal levels. Hyperventilation has been reported occasionally. Any drug remaining in the stomach should be removed and symptomatic treatment given. Should respiration become very shallow and slow, central-nervous-system stimulants, such as caffeine, metrazol, or amphetamine, may be cautiously administered. If severe hypotension develops, pressor amines should be used parenterally to restore blood pressure to normal levels.

Adverse Reactions: A small percentage of patients may experience nausea with or without vomiting and epigastric distress. Dizziness occurs but rarely when meprobamate and ethoheptazine citrate with aspirin is administered in the recommended dosage. The meprobamate may cause drowsiness but, as a rule, this disappears as the therapy is continued. Should drowsiness persist and be associated with ataxia, this symptom can usually be controlled by decreasing the dose, but occasionally it may be desirable to administer central stimulants such as amphetamine or mephentermine sulfate concomitantly to control drowsiness.

A clearly related side effect to the administration of meprobamate is the rare occurrence of allergic or idiosyncratic reactions. This response develops, as a rule, in patients who have had only 1–4 doses of meprobamate and have not had a previous contact with the drug. Previous history of allergy may or may not be related to the incidence of reactions.

Mild reactions are characterized by an itchy urticarial or erythematous, maculopapular rash which may be generalized or confined to the groin. Acute nonthrombocytopenic purpura with cutaneous petechiae, ecchymoses, peripheral edema, and fever have also been reported.

The more severe cases, observed only very rarely, may also have other allergic responses, including fever, fainting spells, angioneurotic edema, bronchial spasms, hypotensive crises (1 fatal case), anaphylaxis, stomatitis and proctitis (1 case), and hyperthermia. Treatment should be symptomatic, such as the administration of epinephrine, antihistamine, and possibly hydrocortisone. Meprobamate should be stopped, and reinstitution of therapy should not be attempted.

Rare cases have been reported where patients receiving meprobamate suffered from aplastic anemia (1 fatal case), thrombocytopenic purpura, agranulocytosis, and hemolytic anemia. In nearly every instance reported, other toxic agents known to have caused these conditions have been associated with the administration of meprobamate. A few cases of leukopenia during the continuous administration of meprobamate are reported; most of these returned to normal without discontinuation of the drug. Impairment of accommodation and visual acuity have been reported in rare instances.

Dosage and Administration: The usual dosage of Equagesic® (meprobamate and ethoheptazine citrate with aspirin) is one to two tablets 3 or 4 times daily as needed for the relief of pain and accompanying tension or anxiety.

Equagesic is not recommended for patients 12 years of age and under.

Overdose: Two instances of accidental or intentional significant overdosage with ethoheptazine citrate combined with aspirin have been reported. These were accompanied by symptoms of central-nervous-system depression, including drowsiness and a feeling of lightheadedness, with uneventful recovery. However, on the basis of pharmacological data, it may be anticipated that CNS stimulation could occur. Other anticipated symptoms would include nausea and vomiting. Appropriate therapy of the signs and symptoms as they appear is the only recommendation possible at this time. Overdosage with ethoheptazine combined with aspirin would probably produce the usual symptoms and signs of salicylate intoxication. Observation and treatment should include induced vomiting or gastric lavage, specific parenteral electrolyte therapy for ketoacidosis and dehydration, watching for evidence of hemorrhagic manifestations due to hypoprothrombinemia which, if it occurs, usually requires whole-blood transfusions.

How Supplied: Bottles of 50 scored tablets, and REDIPAK® (strip pack), Wyeth, boxes of 25 and 100.

[*Shown in Product Identification Section*]

EQUAGESIC®-M ℂ ℞

(meprobamate with aspirin)

Description: Each tablet of Equagesic-M contains 200 mg meprobamate and 325 mg aspirin.

Actions: Meprobamate is a carbamate derivative which has been shown (in animal and/or human studies) to have effects at multiple sites in the central nervous system, including the thalamus and limbic system.

Aspirin, acetylsalicylic acid, is a nonnarcotic analgesic with antipyretic and anti-inflammatory properties.

Indications: As an adjunct in the short-term treatment of pain accompanied by tension and/or anxiety in patients with musculoskeletal disease. Clinical trials have demonstrated that in these situations relief of pain is somewhat greater than with aspirin alone.

The effectiveness of Equagesic-M in long-term use, that is, more than 4 months, has not been assessed by systematic clinical studies. The physician should periodically reassess the usefulness of the drug for the individual patient.

Contraindications:

ASPIRIN:

Allergic or idiosyncratic reactions to aspirin or related compounds.

MEPROBAMATE:

Acute intermittent porphyria and allergic or idiosyncratic reactions to meprobamate or related compounds, such as carisoprodol, mebutamate, or carbromal.

Warnings:

ASPIRIN:

Salicylates should be used with extreme caution in patients with peptic ulcer, asthma, coagulation abnormalities, hypoprothrombinemia, vitamin K deficiency, or in those on anticoagulant therapy.

In rare instances, the use of aspirin in persons allergic to salicylates may result in life-threatening allergic episodes.

MEPROBAMATE:

DRUG DEPENDENCE: Physical dependence, psychological dependence, and abuse have occurred. Chronic intoxication from prolonged ingestion of, usually, greater-than-recommended doses is manifested by ataxia, slurred speech and vertigo. Therefore, careful supervision of dose and amounts prescribed is advised, as well as avoidance of prolonged administration, especially for alcoholics and other patients with a known propensity for taking excessive quantities of drugs.

Sudden withdrawal of the drug after prolonged and excessive use may precipitate recurrence of preexisting symptoms such as anxiety, anorexia, or insomnia, or withdrawal reactions such as vomiting, ataxia, tremors, muscle twitching, confusional states, hallucinosis, and, rarely, convulsive seizures. Such seizures are more likely to occur in persons with central-nervous-system damage or preexistent or latent convulsive disorders. Onset of withdrawal symptoms occurs usually within 12 to 48 hours after discontinuation of meprobamate; symptoms usually cease within the next 12- to 48-hour period.

When excessive dosage has continued for weeks or months, dosage should be reduced gradually over a period of 1 to 2 weeks rather than abruptly stopped. Alternatively, a short-acting barbiturate may be substituted, then gradually withdrawn.

POTENTIALLY HAZARDOUS TASKS: Patients should be warned that meprobamate may impair the mental or physical abilities required for performance of potentially hazardous tasks, such as driving or operating machinery.

ADDITIVE EFFECTS: Since CNS-suppressant effects of meprobamate and alcohol or meprobamate and other psychotropic drugs may be additive, appropriate caution should be exercised with patients who take more than one of these agents simultaneously.

USAGE IN PREGNANCY AND LACTATION

An increased risk of congenital malformations associated with the use of minor tranquilizers (meprobamate, chlordiazepoxide, and diazepam) during the first trimester of pregnancy has been suggested in several studies. Because use of these drugs is rarely a matter of urgency, their use during this period should almost always be avoided. The possibility that a woman of childbearing potential may be pregnant at the time of institution of therapy should be considered. Patients should be advised that if they become pregnant during therapy or intend to become pregnant they should communicate with their physicians about the desirability of discontinuing the drug.

Meprobamate passes the placental barrier. It is present both in umbilical-cord blood at or near maternal plasma levels and in breast milk of lactating mothers at concentrations two to four times that of maternal plasma. When use of meprobamate is contemplated in breast-feeding patients, the drug's higher concentrations in breast milk as compared to maternal plasma levels should be considered.

USAGE IN CHILDREN: Preparations containing aspirin should be kept out of the reach of children. Equagesic-M (meprobamate with

Continued on next page

Wyeth—Cont.

aspirin) is not recommended for patients 12 years of age and under.

Precautions:

ASPIRIN:

Salicylates antagonize the uricosuric activity of probenecid and sulfinpyrazone. Salicylates are reported to enhance the hypoglycemic effect of the sulfonylurea antidiabetic drugs.

MEPROBAMATE:

The lowest effective dose should be administered, particularly to elderly and/or debilitated patients, in order to preclude oversedation.

Meprobamate is metabolized in the liver and excreted by the kidney; to avoid its excess accumulation, caution should be exercised in the administration to patients with compromised liver or kidney function.

Meprobamate occasionally may precipitate seizures in epileptic patients.

The drug should be prescribed cautiously and in small quantities to patients with suicidal tendencies.

Adverse Reactions:

ASPIRIN:

Aspirin may cause epigastric discomfort, nausea, and vomiting. Hypersensitivity reactions, including urticaria, angioneurotic edema, purpura, asthma, and anaphylaxis, may rarely occur.

Patients receiving large doses of salicylates may develop tinnitus.

MEPROBAMATE:

CENTRAL NERVOUS SYSTEM: Drowsiness, ataxia, dizziness, slurred speech, headache, vertigo, weakness, paresthesias, impairment of visual accommodation, euphoria, overstimulation, paradoxical excitement, fast EEG activity.

GASTROINTESTINAL: Nausea, vomiting, diarrhea.

CARDIOVASCULAR: Palpitation, tachycardia, various forms of arrhythmia, transient ECG changes, syncope, hypotensive crisis.

ALLERGIC OR IDIOSYNCRATIC: Milder reactions are characterized by an itchy, urticarial, or erythematous maculopapular rash which may be generalized or confined to the groin.

Other reactions have included leukopenia, acute nonthrombocytopenic purpura, petechiae, ecchymoses, eosinophilia, peripheral edema, adenopathy, fever, fixed drug eruption with cross-reaction to carisoprodol, and cross-sensitivity between meprobamate/mebutamate and meprobamate/carbromal.

More severe hypersensitivity reactions, rarely reported, include hyperpyrexia, chills, angioneurotic edema, bronchospasm, oliguria, and anuria. Also, anaphylaxis, exfoliative dermatitis, stomatitis and proctitis, Stevens-Johnson syndrome and bullous dermatitis have occurred.

HEMATOLOGIC (SEE ALSO "ALLERGIC OR IDIOSYNCRATIC"): Agranulocytosis, aplastic anemia have been reported, although no causal relationship has been established, and thrombocytopenic purpura.

OTHER: Exacerbation of porphyric symptoms.

Dosage and Administration: The usual dosage of Equagesic-M is one or two tablets, each tablet containing meprobamate, 200 mg, and aspirin, 325 mg, orally 3 to 4 times daily as needed for the relief of pain when tension or anxiety is present.

Equagesic-M is not recommended for patients 12 years of age and under.

Overdosage: Treatment of overdose with Equagesic-M is essentially symptomatic and supportive. Any drug remaining in the stomach should be removed. Induction of vomiting or gastric lavage may be indicated. Activated charcoal may reduce absorption of both aspirin and meprobamate.

Overdosage with aspirin produces the usual symptoms and signs of salicylate intoxication. Observation and treatment should include management of hyperthermia, specific parenteral electrolyte therapy for ketoacidosis and dehydration, watching for evidence of hemorrhagic manifestations due to hypoprothrombinemia which, if it occurs, usually requires whole-blood transfusions.

Suicidal attempts with meprobamate have resulted in drowsiness, lethargy, stupor, ataxia, coma, shock, vasomotor and respiratory collapse. Some suicidal attempts have been fatal.

The following data have been reported in the literature and from other sources. These data are not expected to correlate with each case (considering factors such as individual susceptibility and length of time from ingestion to treatment), but represent the usual ranges reported.

Acute simple overdose (meprobamate alone): Death has been reported with ingestion of as little as 12 gram meprobamate and survival with as much as 40 gram.

BLOOD LEVELS:

0.5–2.0 mg percent represents the usual blood-level range of meprobamate after therapeutic doses. The level may occasionally be as high as 3.0 mg percent.

3–10 mg percent usually corresponds to findings of mild-to-moderate symptoms of overdosage, such as stupor or light coma.

10–20 mg percent usually corresponds to deeper coma, requiring more intensive treatment. Some fatalities occur.

At levels greater than 20 mg percent, more fatalities than survivals can be expected.

Acute combined overdose (meprobamate with other psychotropic drugs or alcohol): Since effects can be additive, a history of ingestion of a low dose of meprobamate plus any of these compounds (or of a relatively low blood or tissue level) cannot be used as a prognostic indicator.

In cases where excessive doses have been taken, sleep ensues rapidly and blood pressure, pulse, and respiratory rates are reduced to basal levels. Any drug remaining in the stomach should be removed and symptomatic treatment given. Should respiration or blood pressure become compromised, respiratory assistance, central-nervous-system stimulants, and pressor agents should be administered cautiously as indicated. Diuresis, osmotic (mannitol) diuresis, peritoneal dialysis, and hemodialysis have been used successfully in removing both aspirin and meprobamate. Alkalinization of the urine increases the excretion of salicylates. Careful monitoring of urinary output is necessary, and caution should be taken to avoid overhydration. Relapse and death, after initial recovery, have been attributed to incomplete gastric emptying and delayed absorption.

How Supplied: Equagesic®-M (meprobamate with aspirin) tablets are packaged in bottles of 50 scored tablets.

[Shown in Product Identification Section]

EQUANIL® Ⓒ ℞
(meprobamate)
Capsules • Tablets

How Supplied: Tablets (white, scored)—200 mg and 400 mg, bottles of 50, 100, 500, 1000, and REDIPAK® (Strip Pack), boxes of 25; REDIPAK® (Unit Dose Medication), boxes of 100 (individually wrapped). WYSEALS® EQUANIL (meprobamate), especially coated for easy swallowing, sealed yellow tablets—400 mg, bottles of 50 and 500. Capsules—400 mg, bottles of 50.

For prescribing information write to Professional Service, Wyeth Laboratories, Box 8299, Philadelphia, PA, 19101, or contact your local Wyeth representative.

[Shown in Product Identification Section]

FUROSEMIDE ℞
Injection, USP

How Supplied: Furosemide Injection, USP, Wyeth®, is available in the following dosage strength in packages of 25 ampuls and in TUBEX® Sterile Cartridge-Needle Units, packaged in boxes of 10 TUBEX.

10 mg per ml, NDC 0008-0628; 2 ml, 4 ml, and 10 ml ampuls and 2 ml TUBEX.

Store at Controlled Room Temperature, 15°–30° C (59°–86° F).

Protect TUBEX from light.

HEPARIN Lock Flush Solution, USP ℞
anticoagulant for clearing intermittent infusion sets

Description: Wyeth's TUBEX® Heparin Lock Flush Solution, USP, is a sterile solution. Each ml contains either 10 or 100 USP units heparin sodium derived from porcine intestinal mucosa (standardized for use as an anticoagulant) in normal saline solution, and not more than 10 mg benzyl alcohol as a preservative.

The potency is determined by biological assay using a USP reference standard based upon units of heparin activity per milligram.

How Supplied: Heparin Lock Flush Solution, USP, anticoagulant for clearing intermittent infusion sets, is available as 1 ml TUBEX® Sterile Cartridge-Needle Units, each ml containing 10 USP units or 100 USP units of Heparin Sodium, in packages of 50 TUBEX.

For prescribing information write to Professional Service, Wyeth Laboratories, Box 8299, Philadelphia, PA, 19101, or contact your local Wyeth representative.

HEPARIN ℞
Sodium Injection, USP

Description: Wyeth's TUBEX® Heparin Sodium Injection, USP, is a sterile solution. Each ml contains 1,000, 2,500, 5,000, 7,500, 10,000, 15,000, or 20,000 USP units heparin sodium, derived from porcine intestinal mucosa (standardized for use as an anticoagulant), in water for injection, and not more than 10 mg benzyl alcohol as a preservative.

The potency is determined by biological assay using a USP reference standard based upon units of heparin activity per milligram.

How Supplied: TUBEX® Heparin Sodium Injection, USP, is supplied as follows:

Each TUBEX® Sterile Cartridge-Needle Unit (1 ml size) contains one of the following concentrations of heparin sodium:

1,000 USP Units per ml (22 gauge x 1-1/4 inch needle)

2,500 USP Units per ml (25 gauge x 5/8 inch needle)

5,000 USP Units per 0.5 ml (10,000 USP Units per ml) (25 gauge x 5/8 inch needle)

5,000 USP Units per ml (22 gauge x 1-1/4 inch needle)

5,000 USP Units per ml (25 gauge x 5/8 inch needle)

7,500 USP Units per ml (25 gauge x 5/8 inch needle)

10,000 USP Units per ml (25 gauge x 5/8 inch needle)

15,000 USP Units per ml (25 gauge x 5/8 inch needle)

20,000 USP Units per ml (25 gauge x 5/8 inch needle)

in packages of ten TUBEX®.

For prescribing information write to Professional Service, Wyeth Laboratories, Box 8299, Philadelphia, PA, 19101, or contact your local Wyeth representative.

LO/OVRAL® ℞
Tablets

Description: Each LO/OVRAL® tablet contains 0.3 mg of norgestrel (dl-13-beta-ethyl-17-

alpha-ethinyl-17-beta-hydroxygon- 4-en-3-one), a totally synthetic progestogen, and 0.03 mg of ethinyl estradiol (19-Nor-17α-pregna-1,3,5 (10)-trien-20-yne-3,17-diol).

Clinical Pharmacology: Combination oral contraceptives act primarily through the mechanism of gonadotropin suppression due to the estrogenic and progestational activity of the ingredients. Although the primary mechanism of action is inhibition of ovulation, alterations in the genital tract, including changes in the cervical mucus (which increase the difficulty of sperm penetration) and the endometrium (which reduce the likelihood of implantation), may also contribute to contraceptive effectiveness.

Indications and Usage: LO/OVRAL® is indicated for the prevention of pregnancy in women who elect to use oral contraceptives as a method of contraception.

Oral contraceptives are highly effective. The pregnancy rate in women using conventional combination oral contraceptives (containing 35 mcg or more of ethinyl estradiol or 50 mcg or more of mestranol) is generally reported as less than one pregnancy per 100 woman-years of use. Slightly higher rates (somewhat more than 1 pregnancy per 100 woman-years of use) are reported for some combination products containing 35 mcg or less of ethinyl estradiol, and rates on the order of 3 pregnancies per 100 woman-years are reported for the progestogen-only oral contraceptives.

These rates are derived from separate studies conducted by different investigators in several population groups and cannot be compared precisely. Furthermore, pregnancy rates tend to be lower as clinical studies are continued, possibly due to selective retention in the longer studies of those patients who accept the treatment regimen and do not discontinue as a result of adverse reactions, pregnancy, or other reasons.

In clinical trials with LO/OVRAL®, 1,700 patients completed 22,489 cycles, and a total of two pregnancies were reported. This represents a pregnancy rate of 0.12 per 100 woman-years.

Table 1 gives ranges of pregnancy rates reported in the literature[1] for other means of contraception. The efficacy of these means of contraception (except the IUD) depends upon the degree of adherence to the method.

TABLE 1

PREGNANCIES PER 100 WOMAN-YEARS

IUD, less than 1–6; Diaphragm with spermicidal products (creams or jellies), 2–20; Condom, 3–36; Aerosol foams, 2–29; Jellies and creams, 4–36;

Periodic abstinence (rhythm) all types, less than 1–47:

1. Calendar method, 14–47;
2. Temperature method, 1–20;
3. Temperature method—intercourse only in postovulatory phase, less than 1–7;
4. Mucus method, 1–25;

No contraception, 60–80.

Dose-Related Risk of Thromboembolism from Oral Contraceptives: Two studies have shown a positive association between the dose of estrogens in oral contraceptives and the risk of thromboembolism.[2,3] For this reason, it is prudent and in keeping with good principles of therapeutics to minimize exposure to estrogen. The oral-contraceptive product prescribed for any given patient should be that product which contains the least amount of estrogen that is compatible with an acceptable pregnancy rate and patient acceptance. It is recommended that new acceptors of oral contraceptives be started on preparations containing 0.05 mg or less of estrogen.

Contraindications: Oral contraceptives should not be used in women with any of the following conditions:

1. Thrombophlebitis or thromboembolic disorders.
2. A past history of deep-vein thrombophlebitis or thromboembolic disorders.
3. Cerebral-vascular or coronary-artery disease.
4. Known or suspected carcinoma of the breast.
5. Known or suspected estrogen-dependent neoplasia.
6. Undiagnosed abnormal genital bleeding.
7. Known or suspected pregnancy (see Warning No. 5).
8. Benign or malignant liver tumor which developed during the use of oral contraceptives or other estrogen-containing products.

Warnings:

Cigarette smoking increases the risk of serious cardiovascular side effects from oral-contraceptive use. This risk increases with age and with heavy smoking (15 or more cigarettes per day) and is quite marked in women over 35 years of age. Women who use oral contraceptives should be strongly advised not to smoke.

The use of oral contraceptives is associated with increased risk of several serious conditions, including thromboembolism, stroke, myocardial infarction, hepatic adenoma, gallbladder disease, hypertension. Practitioners prescribing oral contraceptives should be familiar with the following information relating to these risks.

1. *Thromboembolic Disorders and Other Vascular Problems:* An increased risk of thromboembolic and thrombotic disease associated with the use of oral contraceptives is well-established. Three principal studies in Great Britain[4–6] and three in the United States[7–10] have demonstrated an increased risk of fatal and nonfatal venous thromboembolism and stroke, both hemorrhagic and thrombotic.

These studies estimate that users of oral contraceptives are 4 to 11 times more likely than nonusers to develop these diseases without evident cause (Table 2).

CEREBROVASCULAR DISORDERS

In a collaborative American study[9,10] of cerebrovascular disorders in women with and without predisposing causes, it was estimated that the risk of hemorrhagic stroke was 2.0 times greater in users than nonusers and the risk of thrombotic stroke was 4 to 9.5 times greater in users than in nonusers (Table 2).

TABLE 2

SUMMARY OF RELATIVE RISK OF THROMBOEMBOLIC DISORDERS AND OTHER VASCULAR PROBLEMS IN ORAL-CONTRACEPTIVE USERS COMPARED TO NONUSERS

	Relative risk, times greater
Idiopathic thromboembolic disease	4–11
Postsurgery thromboembolic complications	4–6
Thrombotic stroke	4–9.5
Hemorrhagic stroke	2
Myocardial infarction	2–12

MYOCARDIAL INFARCTION

An increased risk of myocardial infarction associated with the use of oral contraceptives has been reported,[11,12,13] confirming a previously suspected association. These studies, conducted in the United Kingdom, found, as expected, that the greater the number of underlying risk factors for coronary-artery disease (cigarette smoking, hypertension, hypercholesterolemia, obesity, diabetes, history of preeclamptic toxemia) the higher the risk of developing myocardial infarction, regardless of whether the patient was an oral-contraceptive user or not. Oral contraceptives, however, were found to be a clear additional risk factor.

In terms of relative risk, it has been estimated[52] that oral-contraceptive users who do not smoke (smoking is considered a major predisposing condition to myocardial infarction) are about twice as likely to have a fatal myocardial infarction as nonusers who do not smoke. Oral-contraceptive users who are also smokers have about a 5-fold increased risk of fatal infarction compared to users who do not smoke, but about a 10- to 12-fold increased risk compared to non-users who do not smoke. Furthermore, the amount of smoking is also an important factor. In determining the importance of these relative risks, however, the baseline rates for various age groups, as shown in Table 3, must be given serious consideration. The importance of other predisposing conditions mentioned above in determining relative and absolute risks has not as yet been quantified; it is quite likely that the same synergistic action exists, but perhaps to a lesser extent.

TABLE 3

Estimated annual mortality rate per 100,000 women from myocardial infarction by use of oral contraceptives, smoking habits, and age (in years):

	Myocardial infarction			
	Women aged 30–39		Women aged 40–44	
Smoking habits	Users	Non-users	Users	Non-users
All smokers	10.2	2.6	62.0	15.9
Heavy*	13.0	5.1	78.7	31.3
Light	4.7	0.9	28.6	5.7
Nonsmokers	1.8	1.2	10.7	7.4
Smokers and nonsmokers	5.4	1.9	32.8	11.7

*Heavy smoker: 15 or more cigarettes per day.

From JAIN, A.K., *Studies in Family Planning, 8*:50, 1977

RISK OF DOSE

In an analysis of data derived from several national adverse-reaction reporting systems,[2] British investigators concluded that the risk of thromboembolism, including coronary thrombosis, is directly related to the dose of estrogen used in oral contraceptives. Preparations containing 100 mcg or more of estrogen were associated with a higher risk of thromboembolism than those containing 50–80 mcg of estrogen. Their analysis did suggest, however, that the quantity of estrogen may not be the sole factor involved. This finding has been confirmed in the United States.[3] Careful epidemiological studies to determine the degree of thromboembolic risk associated with progestogen-only oral contraceptives have not been performed. Cases of thromboembolic disease have been reported in women using these products, and they should not be presumed to be free of excess risk.

ESTIMATE OF EXCESS MORTALITY FROM CIRCULATORY DISEASES

A large prospective study[53] carried out in the U.K. estimated the mortality rate per 100,000 women per year from diseases of the circulatory system for users and nonusers of oral contraceptives according to age, smoking habits, and duration of use. The overall excess death rate annually from circulatory diseases for oral-contraceptive users was estimated to be 20 per 100,000 (ages 15–34—5/100,000; ages 35–44—33/100,000; ages 45–49—140/100,000), the risk being concentrated in older women, in those with a long duration of use, and in cigarette smokers. It was not possible, however, to examine the interrelationships of age, smoking, and duration of use, nor to compare the effects of continuous vs. intermittent use. Although the study showed a 10-fold increase in death due to circulatory diseases in users for 5 or more years, all of these deaths occurred in women 35 or older. Until larger numbers of women under 35 with continuous use for 5 or more years are available, it is not possible to

Continued on next page

Wyeth—Cont.

assess the magnitude of the relative risk for this younger age group.

The available data from a variety of sources have been analyzed[14] to estimate the risk of death associated with various methods of contraception. The estimates of risk of death for each method include the combined risk of the contraceptive method (e.g., thromboembolic and thrombotic disease in the case of oral contraceptives) plus the risk attributable to pregnancy or abortion in the event of method failure. This latter risk varies with the effectiveness of the contraceptive method. The findings of this analysis are shown in Figure 1 below.[14] The study concluded that the mortality associated with all methods of birth control is low and below that associated with childbirth, with the exception of oral contraceptives in women over 40 who smoke. (The rates given for Pill only/smokers for each age group are for smokers as a class. For "heavy" smokers (more than 15 cigarettes a day), the rates given would be about double; for "light" smokers (less than 15 cigarettes a day), about 50 percent. The lowest mortality is associated with the condom or diaphragm backed up by early abortion. The risk of thromboembolic and thrombotic disease associated with oral contraceptives increases with age after approximately age 30 and, for myocardial infarction, is further increased by hypertension, hypercholesterolemia, obesity, diabetes, or history of preeclamptic toxemia and especially by cigarette smoking.

Based on the data currently available, the following chart gives a gross estimate of the risk of death from circulatory disorders associated with the use of oral contraceptives:

SMOKING HABITS AND OTHER PREDISPOSING CONDITIONS—
RISK ASSOCIATED WITH USE OF ORAL CONTRACEPTIVES

Age	Below 30	30–39	40+
Heavy smokers	C	B	A
Light smokers	D	C	B
Nonsmokers (no predisposing conditions)	D	C,D	C
Nonsmokers (other predisposing conditions)	C	C,B	B,A

A—Use associated with very high risk.
B—Use associated with high risk.
C—Use associated with moderate risk.
D—Use associated with low risk.

The physician and the patient should be alert to the earliest manifestations of thromboembolic and thrombotic disorders (e.g., thrombophlebitis, pulmonary embolism, cerebrovascular insufficiency, coronary occlusion, retinal thrombosis, and mesenteric thrombosis). Should any of these occur or be suspected, the drug should be discontinued immediately.

A four- to six-fold increased risk of postsurgery thromboembolic complications has been reported in oral-contraceptive users.[15,16]

If feasible, oral contraceptives should be discontinued at least 4 weeks before surgery of a type associated with an increased risk of thromboembolism or prolonged immobilization.

2. *Ocular Lesions:*
There have been reports of neuro-ocular lesions such as optic neuritis or retinal thrombosis associated with the use of oral contraceptives. Discontinue oral-contraceptive medication if there is unexplained, sudden or gradual, partial or complete loss of vision; onset of proptosis or diplopia; papilledema; or retinal-vascular lesions, and institute appropriate diagnostic and therapeutic measures.

3. *Carcinoma:*
Long-term continuous administration of either natural or synthetic estrogen in certain animal species increases the frequency of carcinoma of the breast, cervix, vagina, and liver. Certain synthetic progestogens, none currently contained in oral contraceptives, have been noted to increase the incidence of mammary nodules, benign and malignant, in dogs.

In humans, three case-control studies have reported an increased risk of endometrial carcinoma associated with the prolonged use of exogenous estrogen in postmenopausal women.[17,18,19] One publication[20] reported on the first 21 cases submitted by physicians to a registry of cases of adenocarcinoma of the endometrium in women under 40 on oral contraceptives. Of the cases found in women without predisposing risk factors for adenocarcinoma of the endometrium (e.g., irregular bleeding at the time oral contraceptives were first given, polycystic ovaries), nearly all occurred in women who had used a sequential oral contraceptive. These products are no longer marketed. No evidence has been reported suggesting an increased risk of endometrial cancer in users of conventional combination or progestogen-only oral contraceptives.

Several studies[8,21–24] have found no increase in breast cancer in women taking oral contraceptives or estrogen. One study,[25] however, while also noting no overall increased risk of breast cancer in women treated with oral contraceptives, found an excess risk in the subgroups of oral-contraceptive users with documented benign breast disease. A reduced occurrence of benign breast tumors in users of oral contraceptives has been well-documented.[8,21,25,26,27]

Figure 1. Estimated annual number of deaths associated with control of fertility and no control per 100,000 nonsterile women, by regimen of control and age of woman.

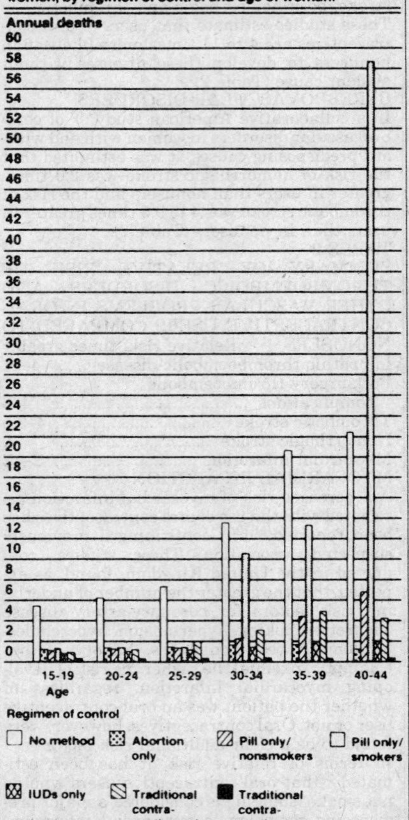

In summary, there is at present no confirmed evidence from human studies of an increased risk of cancer associated with oral contraceptives. Close clinical surveillance of all women taking oral contraceptives is, nevertheless, essential. In all cases of undiagnosed persistent or recurrent abnormal vaginal bleeding, appropriate diagnostic measures should be taken to rule out malignancy. Women with a strong family history of breast cancer or who have breast nodules, fibrocystic disease, or abnormal mammograms should be monitored with particular care if they elect to use oral contraceptives instead of other methods of contraception.

4. *Hepatic Tumors:*
Benign hepatic adenomas have been found to be associated with the use of oral contraceptives.[28,29,30,46] One study[46] showed that oral contraceptive formulations with high hormonal potency were associated with a higher risk than lower potency formulations. Although benign, hepatic adenomas may rupture and may cause death through intra-abdominal hemorrhage. This has been reported in short-term as well as long-term users of oral contraceptives. Two studies relate risk with duration of use of the contraceptive, the risk being much greater after 4 or more years of oral-contraceptive use.[30,46] While hepatic adenoma is a rare lesion, it should be considered in women presenting abdominal pain and tenderness, abdominal mass or shock. A few cases of hepatocellular carcinoma have been reported in women taking oral contraceptives. The relationship of these drugs to this type of malignancy is not known at this time.

5. *Use in or Immediately Preceding Pregnancy, Birth Defects in Offspring, and Malignancy in Female Offspring:*
The use of female sex hormones—both estrogenic and progestational agents—during early pregnancy may seriously damage the offspring. It has been shown that females exposed in utero to diethylstilbestrol, a nonsteroidal estrogen, have an increased risk of developing in later life a form of vaginal or cervical cancer that is ordinarily extremely rare.[31,32] This risk has been estimated to be of the order of 1 in 1,000 exposures or less.[33,47] Although there is no evidence at the present time that oral contraceptives further enhance the risk of developing this type of malignancy, such patients should be monitored with particular care if they elect to use oral contraceptives instead of other methods of contraception. Furthermore, a high percentage of such exposed women (from 30 to 90%) have been found to have epithelial changes of the vagina and cervix.[34–38] Although these changes are histologically benign, it is not known whether this condition is a precursor of vaginal malignancy. Male children so exposed may develop abnormalities of the urogenital tract.[48,49,50] Although similar data are not available with the use of other estrogens, it cannot be presumed that they would not induce similar changes.

An increased risk of congenital anomalies, including heart defects and limb defects, has been reported with the use of sex hormones, including oral contraceptives, in pregnancy.[39–42,51] One case-control study[42] has estimated a 4.7-fold increase in risk of limb-reduction defects in infants exposed in utero to sex hormones (oral contraceptives, hormonal withdrawal tests for pregnancy, or attempted treatment for threatened abortion). Some of these exposures were very short and involved only a few days of treatment. The data suggest that the risk of limb-reduction defects in exposed fetuses is somewhat less than one in 1,000 live births.

In the past, female sex hormones have been used during pregnancy in an attempt to treat threatened or habitual abortion. There is considerable evidence that estrogens are ineffective for these indications, and there is no evidence from well-controlled studies that progestogens are effective for these uses.

There is some evidence that triploidy and possibly other types of polyploidy are increased among abortuses from women who become pregnant soon after ceasing oral contraceptives.[43] Embryos with these anomalies are virtually always aborted spontaneously. Whether there is an overall increase in spontaneous abortion of pregnancies conceived soon after stopping oral contraceptives is unknown.

It is recommended that, for any patient who has missed two consecutive periods, pregnancy should be ruled out before continuing the contraceptive regimen. If the patient has not adhered to the prescribed schedule, the possibility of pregnancy should be considered at the time of the first missed period (or after 45 days from the last menstrual period if the progestogen-only oral contraceptives are used), and further use of oral contraceptives should be withheld until pregnancy has been ruled out. If pregnancy is confirmed, the patient should be apprised of the potential risks to the fetus, and the advisability of continuation of the pregnancy should be discussed in the light of these risks.

It is also recommended that women who discontinue oral contraceptives with the intent of becoming pregnant use an alternate form of contraception for a period of time before attempting to conceive.

Many clinicians recommend 3 months, although no precise information is available on which to base this recommendation.

The administration of progestogen-only or progestogen-estrogen combinations to induce withdrawal bleeding should not be used as a test of pregnancy.

6. *Gallbladder Disease:*

Studies [8,23,26] report an increased risk of surgically confirmed gallbladder disease in users of oral contraceptives and estrogens. In one study, an increased risk appeared after 2 years of use and doubled after 4 or 5 years of use. In one of the other studies, an increased risk was apparent between 6 and 12 months of use.

7. *Carbohydrate and Lipid Metabolic Effects:*

A decrease in glucose tolerance has been observed in a significant percentage of patients on oral contraceptives. For this reason, prediabetic and diabetic patients should be carefully observed while receiving oral contraceptives.

An increase in triglycerides and total phospholipids has been observed in patients receiving oral contraceptives.[44] The clinical significance of this finding remains to be defined.

8. *Elevated Blood Pressure:*

An increase in blood pressure has been reported in patients receiving oral contraceptives.[26] In some women, hypertension may occur within a few months of beginning oral-contraceptive use. In the first year of use, the prevalence of women with hypertension is low in users and may be no higher than that of a comparable group of nonusers. The prevalence in users increases, however, with longer exposure, and in the fifth year of use is two-and-a-half to three times the reported prevalence in the first year. Age is also strongly correlated with the development of hypertension in oral-contraceptive users. Women who previously have had hypertension during pregnancy may be more likely to develop elevation of blood pressure when given oral contraceptives. Hypertension that develops as a result of taking oral contraceptives usually returns to normal after discontinuing the drug.

9. *Headache:*

The onset or exacerbation of migraine or development of headache of a new pattern which is recurrent, persistent, or severe, requires discontinuation of oral contraceptives and evaluation of the cause.

10. *Bleeding Irregularities:*

Breakthrough bleeding, spotting, and amenorrhea are frequent reasons for patients discontinuing oral contraceptives. In breakthrough bleeding, as in all cases of irregular bleeding from the vagina, nonfunctional causes should be borne in mind. In undiagnosed persistent or recurrent abnormal bleeding from the vagina, adequate diagnostic measures are indicated to rule out pregnancy or malignancy. If pathology has been excluded, time or a change to another formulation may solve the problem. Changing to an oral contraceptive with a higher estrogen content, while potentially useful in minimizing menstrual irregularity, should be done only if necessary, since this may increase the risk of thromboembolic disease.

Women with a past history of oligomenorrhea or secondary amenorrhea or young women without regular cycles may have a tendency to remain anovulatory or to become amenorrheic after discontinuation of oral contraceptives. Women with these preexisting problems should be advised of this possibility and encouraged to use other contraceptive methods. Post-use anovulation, possibly prolonged, may also occur in women without previous irregularities.

11. *Ectopic Pregnancy:*

Ectopic as well as intrauterine pregnancy may occur in contraceptive failures. However, in progestogen-only oral contraceptive failures, the ratio of ectopic to intrauterine pregnancies is higher than in women who are not receiving oral contraceptives, since the drugs are more effective in preventing intrauterine than ectopic pregnancies.

12. *Breast-feeding:*

Oral contraceptives given in the postpartum period may interfere with lactation. There may be a decrease in the quantity and quality of the breast milk. Furthermore, a small fraction of the hormonal agents in oral contraceptives has been identified in the milk of mothers receiving these drugs.[45] The effects, if any, on the breast-fed child have not been determined. If feasible, the use of oral contraceptives should be deferred until the infant has been weaned.

Precautions:

GENERAL

1. A complete medical and family history should be taken prior to initiation of oral contraceptives. The pretreatment and periodic physical examinations should include special reference to blood pressure, breasts, abdomen and pelvic organs, including Papanicolaou smear and relevant laboratory tests. As a general rule, oral contraceptives should not be prescribed for longer than 1 year without another physical examination being performed.
2. Under the influence of estrogen-progestogen preparations, pre-existing uterine leiomyomata may increase in size.
3. Patients with a history of psychic depression should be carefully observed and the drug discontinued if depression recurs to a serious degree. Patients becoming significantly depressed while taking oral contraceptives should stop the medication and use an alternate method of contraception in an attempt to determine whether the symptom is drug-related.
4. Oral contraceptives may cause some degree of fluid retention. They should be prescribed with caution, and only with careful monitoring, in patients with conditions which might be aggravated by fluid retention, such as convulsive disorders, migraine syndrome, asthma, or cardiac or renal insufficiency.
5. Patients with a past history of jaundice during pregnancy have an increased risk of recurrence of jaundice while receiving oral-contraceptive therapy. If jaundice develops in any patient receiving such drugs, the medication should be discontinued.
6. Steroid hormones may be poorly metabolized in patients with impaired liver function and should be administered with caution in such patients.
7. Oral-contraceptive users may have disturbances in normal tryptophan metabolism which may result in a relative pyridoxine deficiency. The clinical significance of this is yet to be determined.
8. Serum folate levels may be depressed by oral-contraceptive therapy. Since the pregnant woman is predisposed to the development of folate deficiency and the incidence of folate deficiency increases with increasing gestation, it is possible that if a woman becomes pregnant shortly after stopping oral contraceptives, she may have a greater chance of developing folate deficiency and complications attributed to this deficiency.
9. The pathologist should be advised of oral-contraceptive therapy when relevant specimens are submitted.
10. Certain endocrine- and liver-function tests and blood components may be affected by estrogen-containing oral contraceptives:

a. Increased sulfobromophthalein retention.
b. Increased prothrombin and factors VII, VIII, IX, and X; decreased antithrombin 3; increased norepinephrine-induced platelet aggregability.
c. Increased thyroid-binding globulin (TBG) leading to increased circulating total-thyroid hormone, as measured by protein-bound iodine (PBI), T4 by column, or T4 by radioimmunoassay. Free T3 resin uptake is decreased, reflecting the elevated TBG; free T4 concentration is unaltered.
d. Decreased pregnanediol excretion.
e. Reduced response to metyrapone test.

Information for the Patient: (See Patient Labeling Printed Below.)

Drug Interactions: Reduced efficacy and increased incidence of breakthrough bleeding have been associated with concomitant use of rifampin. A similar association has been suggested with barbiturates, phenylbutazone, phenytoin sodium, ampicillin, and tetracycline.

Carcinogenesis: See Warnings section for information on the carcinogenic potential of oral contraceptives.

Pregnancy: Pregnancy category X. See Contraindications and Warnings.

Nursing Mothers: See Warnings.

Adverse Reactions: An increased risk of the following serious adverse reactions has been associated with the use of oral contraceptives (see Warnings):

- Thrombophlebitis.
- Pulmonary embolism.
- Coronary thrombosis.
- Cerebral thrombosis.
- Cerebral hemorrhage.
- Hypertension.
- Gallbladder disease.
- Benign hepatomas.
- Congenital anomalies.

There is evidence of an association between the following conditions and the use of oral contraceptives, although additional confirmatory studies are needed:

- Mesenteric thrombosis.
- Neuro-ocular lesions, e.g., retinal thrombosis and optic neuritis.

The following adverse reactions have been reported in patients receiving oral contraceptives and are believed to be drug-related:

- Nausea and/or vomiting, usually the most common adverse reactions, occur in approximately 10% or less of patients during the first cycle. Other reactions, as a general rule, are seen much less frequently or only occasionally.
- Gastrointestinal symptoms (such as abdominal cramps and bloating).
- Breakthrough bleeding.
- Spotting.
- Change in menstrual flow.

Continued on next page

Wyeth—Cont.

Dysmenorrhea.
Amenorrhea during and after treatment.
Temporary infertility after discontinuance of treatment.
Edema.
Chloasma or melasma which may persist.
Breast changes: tenderness, enlargement, and secretion.
Change in weight (increase or decrease).
Change in cervical erosion and cervical secretion.
Possible diminution in lactation when given immediately post-partum.
Cholestatic jaundice.
Migraine.
Increase in size of uterine leiomyomata.
Rash (allergic).
Mental depression.
Reduced tolerance to carbohydrates.
Vaginal candidiasis.
Change in corneal curvature (steepening).
Intolerance to contact lenses.

The following adverse reactions have been reported in users of oral contraceptives, and the association has been neither confirmed nor refuted:

Premenstrual-like syndrome.
Cataracts.
Changes in libido.
Chorea.
Changes in appetite.
Cystitis-like syndrome.
Headache.
Nervousness.
Dizziness.
Hirsutism.
Loss of scalp hair.
Erythema multiforme.
Erythema nodosum.
Hemorrhagic eruption.
Vaginitis.
Porphyria.

Acute Overdose: Serious ill effects have not been reported following acute ingestion of large doses of oral contraceptives by young children. Overdosage may cause nausea, and withdrawal bleeding may occur in females.

Dosage and Administration: To achieve maximum contraceptive effectiveness, LO/OVRAL® must be taken exactly as directed and at intervals not exceeding 24 hours. The dosage of LO/OVRAL® is one tablet daily for 21 consecutive days per menstrual cycle according to prescribed schedule. Tablets are then discontinued for 7 days (three weeks on, one week off).

It is recommended that LO/OVRAL® tablets be taken at the same time each day, preferably after the evening meal or at bedtime.

During the first cycle of medication, the patient is instructed to take one LO/OVRAL® tablet daily for twenty-one consecutive days beginning on day five of her menstrual cycle. (The first day of menstruation is day one.) The tablets are then discontinued for one week (7 days). Withdrawal bleeding should usually occur within three days following discontinuation of LO/OVRAL®.

(If LO/OVRAL® is first taken later than the fifth day of the first menstrual cycle of medication or postpartum, contraceptive reliance should not be placed on LO/OVRAL® until after the first seven consecutive days of administration. The possibility of ovulation and conception prior to initiation of medication should be considered.)

The patient begins her next and all subsequent 21-day courses of LO/OVRAL® tablets on the same day of the week that she began her first course, following the same schedule: 21 days on—7 days off. She begins taking her tablets on the 8th day after discontinuance regardless of whether or not a menstrual period has occurred or is still in progress. Any time a new cycle of LO/OVRAL® is started later than the 8th day the patient should be protected by another means of contraception until she has taken a tablet daily for seven consecutive days.

If spotting or breakthrough bleeding occurs, the patient is instructed to continue on the same regimen. This type of bleeding is usually transient and without significance; however, if the bleeding is persistent or prolonged the patient is advised to consult her physician.

Although the occurrence of pregnancy is highly unlikely if LO/OVRAL® is taken according to directions, if withdrawal bleeding does not occur, the possibility of pregnancy must be considered. If the patient has not adhered to the prescribed schedule (missed one or more tablets or started taking them on a day later than she should have) the probability of pregnancy should be considered at the time of the first missed period and appropriate diagnostic measures taken before the medication is resumed. If the patient has adhered to the prescribed regimen and misses two consecutive periods, pregnancy should be ruled out before continuing the contraceptive regimen.

The patient should be instructed to take a missed tablet as soon as it is remembered. If two consecutive tablets are missed they should both be taken as soon as remembered. The next tablet should be taken at the usual time.

Any time the patient misses one or two tablets she should also use another method of contraception until she has taken a tablet daily for seven consecutive days. If breakthrough bleeding occurs following missed tablets it will usually be transient and of no consequence.

While there is little likelihood of ovulation occurring if only one or two tablets are missed, the possibility of ovulation increases with each successive day that scheduled tablets are missed. If three consecutive tablets are missed, all medication should be discontinued and the remainder of the package discarded. A new tablet cycle should be started on the 8th day after the last tablet was taken, and an alternate means of contraception should be prescribed during the seven days without tablets and until the patient has taken a tablet daily for seven consecutive days. In the nonlactating mother LO/OVRAL® may be prescribed in the postpartum period either immediately or at the first postpartum examination whether or not menstruation has resumed.

How Supplied: LO/OVRAL® tablets (0.3 mg norgestrel + 0.03 mg ethinyl estradiol) are available in containers of 21 tablets.

Also Available: LO/OVRAL®-28 tablets in containers of 28 tablets, consisting of 21 white LO/OVRAL® tablets (0.3 mg norgestrel + 0.03 mg ethinyl estradiol) and 7 pink inert tablets.

References:

1. "Population Reports," Series H, Number 2, May 1974; Series I, Number 1, June 1974; Series B, Number 2, January 1975; Series H, Number 3, 1975; Series H, Number 4, January 1976 (published by the Population Information Program, The George Washington University Medical Center, 2001 S St. NW., Washington, D.C.).
2. Inman, W. H. W., Vessey, M. P., Westerholm, B., and Engelund, A., "Thromboembolic disease and the steroidal content of oral contraceptives. A report to the Committee on Safety of Drugs," Brit Med J *2*:203–209, 1970.
3. Stolley, P. D., Tonascia, J. A., Tockman, M. S., Sartwell, P. E., Rutledge, A. H., and Jacobs, M. P., "Thrombosis with low-estrogen oral contraceptives," Am J Epidemiol *102*:197–208, 1975.
4. Royal College of General Practitioners, "Oral contraception and thromboembolic disease," J Coll Gen Pract *13*:267–279, 1967.
5. Inman, W. H. W., and Vessey, M. P., "Investigation of deaths from pulmonary, coronary and cerebral thrombosis and embolism in women of childbearing age," Brit Med J *2*:193–199, 1968.
6. Vessey, M. P., and Doll, R., "Investigation of relation between use of oral contraceptives and thromboembolic disease. A further report," Brit Med J *2*:651–657, 1969.
7. Sartwell, P. E., Masi, A. T., Arthes, F. G., Greene, G. R., and Smith, H. E., "Thromboembolism and oral contraceptives: an epidemiological case control study," Am J Epidemiol *90*:365–380, 1969.
8. Boston Collaborative Drug Surveillance Program, "Oral contraceptives and venous thromboembolic disease, surgically confirmed gallbladder disease and breast tumors," Lancet *1*:1399–1404, 1973.
9. Collaborative Group for the Study of Stroke in Young Women, "Oral contraception and increased risk of cerebral ischemia or thrombosis," N Engl J Med *288*:871–878, 1973.
10. Collaborative Group for the Study of Stroke in Young Women, "Oral contraceptives and stroke in young women: associated risk factors," JAMA *231*:718–722, 1975.
11. Mann, J. I., and Inman, W. H. W., "Oral contraceptives and death from myocardial infarction," Brit Med J *2*:245–248, 1975.
12. Mann, J. I., Inman, W. H. W., and Thorogood, M., "Oral contraceptive use in older women and fatal myocardial infarction," Brit Med J *2*:445–447, 1976.
13. Mann, J. I., Vessey, M. P., Thorogood, M., and Doll, R., "Myocardial infarction in young women with special reference to oral contraceptive practice," Brit Med J *2*:241–245, 1975.
14. Tietze, C., "New Estimates of Mortality Associated with Fertility Control," Family Planning Perspectives, *9*:74–76, 1977.
15. Vessey, M. P., Doll, R., Fairbairn, A. S., and Glober, G., "Post-operative thromboembolism and the use of oral contraceptives," Brit Med J *3*:123–126, 1970.
16. Greene, G. R., Sartwell, P. E., "Oral contraceptive use in patients with thromboembolism following surgery, trauma, or infection," Am J Pub Health *62*:680–685, 1972.
17. Smith, D. C., Prentice, R., Thompson, D. J., and Herrmann, W. L., "Association of exogenous estrogen and endometrial carcinoma," N Engl J Med *293*:1164–1167, 1975.
18. Ziel, H. K., and Finkle, W. D., "Increased risk of endometrial carcinoma among users of conjugated estrogens," N Engl J Med *293*:1167–1170, 1975.
19. Mack, T. N., Pike, M. C., Henderson, B. E., Pfeffer, R. I., Gerkins, V. R., Arthur, M., and Brown, S. E., "Estrogens and endometrial cancer in a retirement community," N Engl J Med *294*:1262–1267, 1976.
20. Silverberg, S. G., and Makowski, E. L., "Endometrial carcinoma in young women taking oral contraceptive agents," Obstet Gynecol *46*:503–506, 1975.
21. Vessey, M. P., Doll, R., and Sutton, P. M., "Oral contraceptives and breast neoplasia: a retrospective study," Brit Med J *3*:719–724, 1972.
22. Vessey, M. P., Doll, R., and Jones K., "Oral contraceptives and breast cancer. Progress report of an epidemiological study," Lancet *1*:941–943, 1975.
23. Boston Collaborative Drug Surveillance Program, "Surgically confirmed gallbladder disease, venous thromboembolism and breast tumors in relation to postmenopausal estrogen therapy," N Engl J Med *290*:15–19, 1974.
24. Arthes, F. G., Sartwell, P. E., and Lewison, E. F., "The pill, estrogens, and the breast. Epidemiologic aspects," Cancer *28*:1391–1394, 1971.
25. Fasal, E., and Paffenbarger, R. S., "Oral contraceptives as related to cancer and benign lesions of the breast," J Natl Cancer Inst *55*:767–773, 1975.
26. Royal College of General Practitioners, "Oral Contraceptives and Health," London, Pitman, 1974.
27. Ory, H., Cole P., MacMahon, B., and Hoover, R., "Oral contraceptives and reduced

risk of benign breast diseases," N Engl J Med *294*:419–422, 1976.
28. Baum, J., Holtz, F., Bookstein, J. J., and Klein, E. W., "Possible association between benign hepatomas and oral contraceptives," Lancet *2*:926–928, 1973.
29. Mays, E. T., Christopherson, W. M., Mahr, M. M., and Williams, H. C., "Hepatic changes in young women ingesting contraceptive steroids. Hepatic hemorrhage and primary hepatic tumors," JAMA *235*:730–732, 1976.
30. Edmondson, H. A., Henderson, B., and Benton, B., "Liver-cell adenomas associated with use of oral contraceptives," N Engl J Med *294*:470–472, 1976.
31. Herbst, A. L., Ulfedler, H., and Poskanzer, D. C., "Adenocarcinoma of the vagina," N Engl J Med *284*:878–881, 1971.
32. Greenwald, P., Barlow, J. J., Nasca, P. C., and Burnett, W., "Vaginal cancer after maternal treatment with synthetic estrogens," N Engl J Med *285*:390–392, 1971.
33. Lanier, A. P., Noller, K. L., Decker, D. G., Elveback, L., and Kurland, L. T., "Cancer and stilbestrol. A follow-up of 1719 persons exposed to estrogens in utero and born 1943–1959," Mayo Clin Pro *48*:793–799, 1973.
34. Herbst, A. L., Kurman, R. J., and Scully, R. E., "Vaginal and cervical abnormalities after exposure to stilbestrol in utero," Obstet Gynecol *40*:287–298, 1972.
35. Herbst, A. L., Robboy, S. J., Macdonald, G. J., and Scully, R. E., "The effects of local progesterone on stilbestrol-associated vaginal adenosis," Am J Obstet Gynecol *118*:607–615, 1974.
36. Herbst, A. L., Poskanzer, D. C., Robboy, S. J., Friedlander, L., and Scully, R. E., "Prenatal exposure to stilbestrol: a prospective comparison of exposed female offspring with unexposed controls," N Engl J Med *292*:334–339, 1975.
37. Stafl, A., Mattingly, R. F., Foley, D. V., Fetherston, W., "Clinical diagnosis of vaginal adenosis," Obstet Gynecol *43*:118–128, 1974.
38. Sherman, A. I., Goldrath, M., Berlin, A., Vakhariya, V., Banooni, F., Michaels, W., Goodman, P., and Brown, S., "Cervical-vaginal adenosis after in utero exposure to synthetic estrogens," Obstet Gynecol *44*:531–545, 1974.
39. Gal, I., Kirman, B., and Stern, J., "Hormone pregnancy tests and congenital malformation," Nature *216*:83, 1967.
40. Levy, E. P., Cohen, A., and Fraser, F. C., "Hormone treatment during pregnancy and congenital heart defects," Lancet *1*:611, 1973.
41. Nora, J. J., and Nora, A. H., "Birth defects and oral contraceptives," Lancet *1*:941–942, 1973.
42. Janerich, D. T., Piper, J. M., and Glebatis, D. M., "Oral contraceptives and congenital limb-reduction defects," N Engl J Med *291*:697–700, 1974.
43. Carr, D. H., "Chromosome studies in selected spontaneous abortions: I. Conception after oral contraceptives," Canad Med Assoc J *103*:343–348, 1970.
44. Wynn, V., Doar, J. W. H., and Mills, G. L., "Some effects of oral contraceptives on serum-lipid and lipoprotein levels," Lancet *2*:720–723, 1966.
45. Laumas, K. R., Malkani, P. K., Bhatnagar, S., and Laumas, V., "Radioactivity in the breast milk of lactating women after oral administration of 3 H-norethynodrel," Amer J Obstet Gynecol *98*:411–413, 1967.
46. Center for Disease Control, "Increased Risk of Hepatocellular Adenoma in Women with Long-term use of Oral Contraceptives," Morbidity and Mortality Weekly Report, *26*:293–294, 1977.
47. Herbst, A. L., Cole, P., Colton, T., Robboy, S. J., Scully, R. E., "Age-incidence and Risk of Diethylstilbestrol-related Clear Cell Adenocarcinoma of the Vagina and Cervix," Am. J. Obstet. Gynecol., *128*:43–50, 1977.
48. Bibbo, M., Al-Naqeeb, M., Baccarini, I., Gill, W., Newton, M., Sleeper, K. M., Sonek, M., Wied, G. L., "Follow-up Study of Male and Female Offspring of DES-treated Mothers. A Preliminary Report," Jour. of Repro. Med., *15*:29–32, 1975.
49. Gill, W. B., Schumacher, G. F. B., Bibbo, M., "Structural and Functional Abnormalities in the Sex Organs of Male Offspring of Mothers Treated with Diethylstilbestrol (DES)," Jour. of Repro. Med., *16*:147–153, 1976.
50. Henderson, B. E., Senton, B., Cosgrove, M., Baptista, J., Aldrich, J., Townsend, D., Hart, W., Mack, T., "Urogenital Tract Abnormalities in Sons of Women Treated with Diethylstilbestrol," Pediatrics, *58*:505–507, 1976.
51. Heinonen, O. P., Slone, D., Nonson, R. R., Hook, E. B., Shapiro, S., "Cardiovascular Birth Defects and Antenatal Exposure to Female Sex Hormones," N. Engl. J. Med., *296*:67–70, 1977.
52. Jain, A. K., "Mortality Risk Associated with the Use of Oral Contraceptives," Studies in Family Planning, *8*:50–54, 1977.
53. Beral, V., "Mortality Among Oral Contraceptive Users," Lancet, *2*:727–731, 1977.

The patient labeling for oral-contraceptive drug products is set forth below:

Brief Summary Patient Package Insert

Cigarette smoking increases the risk of serious adverse effects on the heart and blood vessels from oral-contraceptive use. This risk increases with age and with heavy smoking (15 or more cigarettes per day) and is quite marked in women over 35 years of age. Women who use oral contraceptives should not smoke.

Oral contraceptives taken as directed are about 99% effective in preventing pregnancy. (The mini-pill, however, is somewhat less effective.) Forgetting to take your pills increases the chance of pregnancy. Women who have or have had clotting disorders, cancer of the breast or sex organs, unexplained vaginal bleeding, a stroke, heart attack, angina pectoris, or who suspect they may be pregnant should not use oral contraceptives. Various drugs, such as some antibiotics, may also decrease the effectiveness of oral contraceptives.

Most side effects of the pill are not serious. The most common side effects are nausea, vomiting, bleeding between menstrual periods, weight gain, and breast tenderness. However, proper use of oral contraceptives requires that they be taken under your doctor's continuous supervision, because they can be associated with serious side effects which may be fatal. Fortunately, these occur very infrequently. The serious side effects are:

1. Blood clots in the legs, lungs, brain, heart, or other organs, and hemorrhage into the brain due to bursting of a blood vessel.
2. Liver tumors, which may rupture and cause severe bleeding.
3. Birth defects if the pill is taken while you are pregnant.
4. High blood pressure.
5. Gallbladder disease.

The symptoms associated with these serious side effects are discussed in the detailed leaflet given you with your supply of pills. Notify your doctor if you notice any unusual physical disturbance while taking the pill.

The estrogen in oral contraceptives has been found to cause breast cancer and other cancers in certain animals. These findings suggest that oral contraceptives may also cause cancer in humans. However, studies to date in women taking currently marketed oral contraceptives have not confirmed that oral contraceptives cause cancer in humans.

The detailed leaflet describes more completely the benefits and risks of oral contraceptives. It also provides information on other forms of contraception. Read it carefully. If you have any questions, consult your doctor.

Caution: Oral contraceptives are of no value in the prevention or treatment of venereal disease.

DETAILED PATIENT LABELING

WHAT YOU SHOULD KNOW ABOUT ORAL CONTRACEPTIVES

Oral contraceptives ("the pill") are the most effective way (except for sterilization) to prevent pregnancy. They are also convenient and, for most women, free of serious or unpleasant side effects. Oral contraceptives must always be taken under the continuous supervision of a physician.

It is important that any woman who considers using an oral contraceptive understand the risks involved. Although the oral contraceptives have important advantages over other methods of contraception, they have certain risks that no other method has. Only you can decide whether the advantages are worth these risks. This leaflet will tell you about the most important risks. It will explain how you can help your doctor prescribe the pill as safely as possible by telling him about yourself and being alert for the earliest signs of trouble. And it will tell you how to use the pill properly, so that it will be as effective as possible. There is more detailed information available in the leaflet prepared for doctors. Your pharmacist can show you a copy; you may need your doctor's help in understanding parts of it.

WHO SHOULD NOT USE ORAL CONTRACEPTIVES

A. If you have any of the following conditions, you should not use the pill:

1. Clots in the legs or lungs.
2. Angina pectoris.
3. Known or suspected cancer of the breast or sex organs.
4. Unusual vaginal bleeding that has not yet been diagnosed.
5. Known or suspected pregnancy.

B. If you have had any of the following conditions, you should not use the pill:

1. Heart attack or stroke.
2. Clots in the legs or lungs.

C. Cigarette smoking increases the risk of serious adverse effects on the heart and blood vessels from oral-contraceptive use. This risk increases with age and with heavy smoking (15 or more cigarettes per day) and is quite marked in women over 35 years of age. Women who use oral contraceptives should not smoke.

D. If you have scanty or irregular periods or are a young woman without a regular cycle, you should use another method of contraception because, if you use the pill, you may have difficulty becoming pregnant or may fail to have menstrual periods after discontinuing the pill.

DECIDING TO USE ORAL CONTRACEPTIVES

If you do not have any of the conditions listed above and are thinking about using oral contraceptives, to help you decide, you need information about the advantages and risks of oral contraceptives and of other contraceptive methods as well. This leaflet describes the advantages and risks of oral contraceptives. Except for sterilization, the IUD, and abortion, which have their own exclusive risks, the only risks of other methods of contraception are those due to pregnancy should the method fail. You doctor can answer questions you may have with respect to other methods of contraception. He can also answer any questions you may have after reading this leaflet on oral contraceptives.

1. What Oral Contraceptives Are and How They Work. Oral contraceptives are of two types. The most common, often simply called "the pill," is a combination of an estrogen and

Continued on next page

Wyeth—Cont.

a progestogen, the two kinds of female hormones. The amount of estrogen and progestogen can vary, but the amount of estrogen is most important because both the effectiveness and some of the dangers of oral contraceptives are related to the amount of estrogen. This kind of oral contraceptive works principally by preventing release of an egg from the ovary. When the amount of estrogen is 50 micrograms or more, and the pill is taken as directed, oral contraceptives are more than 99% effective (i.e., there would be less than 1 pregnancy if 100 women used the pill for 1 year). Pills that contain 20 to 35 micrograms of estrogen vary slightly in effectiveness, ranging from 98% to more than 99% effective.

The second type of oral contraceptive, often called the "mini-pill", contains only a progestogen. It works in part by preventing release of an egg from the ovary but also by keeping sperm from reaching the egg and by making the uterus (womb) less receptive to any fertilized egg that reaches it. The mini-pill is less effective than the combination oral contraceptive, about 97% effective. In addition, the progestogen-only pill has a tendency to cause irregular bleeding which may be quite inconvenient, or cessation of bleeding entirely. The progestogen-only pill is used despite its lower effectiveness in the hope that it will prove not to have some of the serious side effects of the estrogen-containing pill (see below), but it is not yet certain that the mini-pill does in fact have fewer serious side effects. The discussion below, while based mainly on information about the combination pills, should be considered to apply as well to the mini-pill.

2. Other Nonsurgical Ways to Prevent Pregnancy. As this leaflet will explain, oral contraceptives have several serious risks. Other methods of contraception have lesser risks or none at all. They are also less effective than oral contraceptives, but, used properly, may be effective enough for many women.

The following table gives reported pregnancy rates (the number of women out of 100 who would become pregnant in 1 year) for these methods.

PREGNANCIES PER 100 WOMEN PER YEAR

Intrauterine device (IUD), less than 1-6; Diaphragm with spermicidal products (creams or jellies), 2-20; Condom (rubber), 3-36; Aerosol foams, 2-29; Jellies and creams, 4-36;

Periodic abstinence (rhythm) all types, less than 1-47:

1. Calendar method, 14-47;
2. Temperature method, 1-20;
3. Temperature method—intercourse only in postovulatory phase, less than 1-7;
4. Mucus method, 1-25;

No contraception, 60-80.

The figures (except for the IUD) vary widely because people differ in how well they use each method. Very faithful users of the various methods obtain very good results, except for users of the calendar method of periodic abstinence (rhythm). Except for the IUD, effective use of these methods requires somewhat more effort than simply taking a single pill every day, but it is an effort that many couples undertake successfully. Your doctor can tell you a great deal more about these methods of contraception.

3. The Dangers of Oral Contraceptives.

a. *Circulatory disorders (abnormal blood clotting and stroke due to hemorrhage)*

Blood clots (in various blood vessels of the body) are the most common of the serious side effects of oral contraceptives. A clot can result in a stroke (if the clot is in the brain), a heart attack (if the clot is in a blood vessel of the heart), or a pulmonary embolus (a clot which forms in the legs or pelvis, then breaks off and travels to the lungs). Any of these can be fatal. Clots also occur rarely in the blood vessels of the eye, resulting in blindness or impairment of vision in that eye. There is evidence that the risk of clotting increases with higher estrogen doses. It is therefore important to keep the dose of estrogen as low as possible, so long as the oral contraceptive used has an acceptable pregnancy rate and doesn't cause unacceptable changes in the menstrual pattern. Furthermore, cigarette smoking by oral-contraceptive users increases the risk of serious adverse effects on the heart and blood vessels. This risk increases with age and with heavy smoking (15 or more cigarettes per day) and begins to become quite marked in women over 35 years of age. For this reason, women who use oral contraceptives should not smoke. The risk of abnormal clotting increases with age in both users and nonusers of oral contraceptives, but the increased risk from the contraceptive appears to be present at all ages. For oral-contraceptive users in general, it has been estimated that in women between the ages of 15 and 34 the risk of death due to a circulatory disorder is about 1 in 12,000 per year, whereas for nonusers the risk is about 1 in 50,000 per year. In the age group 35 to 44, the risk is estimated to be about 1 in 2,500 per year for oral-contraceptive users and about 1 in 10,000 per year for nonusers.

Figure 1. Estimated annual number of deaths associated with control of fertility and no control per 100,000 nonsterile women, by regimen of control and age of woman.

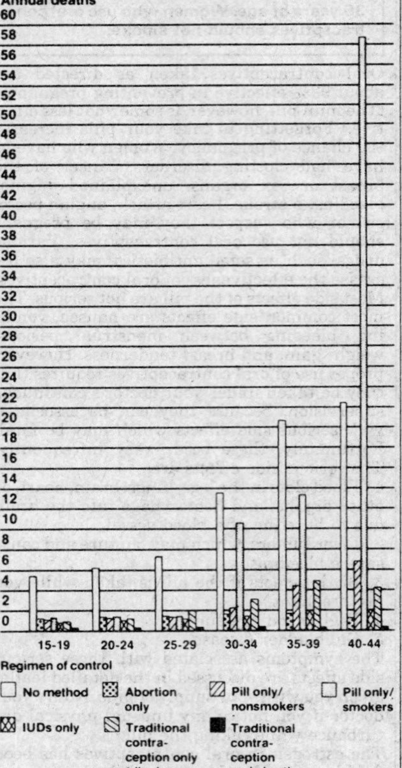

Even without the pill the risk of having a heart attack increases with age and is also increased by such heart attack risk factors as high blood pressure, high cholesterol, obesity, diabetes, and cigarette smoking. Without any risk factors present, the use of oral contraceptives alone may double the risk of heart attack. However, the combination of cigarette smoking, especially heavy smoking, and oral contraceptive use greatly increases the risk of heart attack. Oral-contraceptive users who smoke are about 5 times more likely to have a heart attack than users who do not smoke and about 10 times more likely to have a heart attack than nonusers who do not smoke. It has been estimated that users between the ages of 30 and 39 who smoke have about a 1 in 10,000 chance each year of having a fatal heart attack compared to about a 1 in 50,000 chance in users who do not smoke, and about a 1 in 100,000 chance in nonusers who do not smoke. In the age group 40 to 44, the risk is about 1 in 1,700 per year for users who smoke compared to about 1 in 10,000 for users who do not smoke and to about 1 in 14,000 per year for nonusers who do not smoke. Heavy smoking (about 15 cigarettes or more a day) further increases the risk. If you do not smoke and have none of the other heart attack risk factors described above, you will have a smaller risk than listed. If you have several heart attack risk factors, the risk may be considerably greater than listed.

In addition to blood-clotting disorders, it has been estimated that women taking oral contraceptives are twice as likely as nonusers to have a stroke due to rupture of a blood vessel in the brain.

b. *Formation of tumors.* Studies have found that when certain animals are given the female sex hormone, estrogen, which is an ingredient of oral contraceptives, continuously for long periods, cancers may develop in the breast, cervix, vagina, and liver.

These findings suggest that oral contraceptives may cause cancer in humans. However, studies to date in women taking currently marketed oral contraceptives have not confirmed that oral contraceptives cause cancer in humans. Several studies have found no increase in breast cancer in users, although one study suggested oral contraceptives might cause an increase in breast cancer in women who already have benign breast disease (e.g., cysts).

Women with a strong family history of breast cancer or who have breast nodules, fibrocystic disease, or abnormal mammograms or who were exposed to DES (Diethylstilbestrol), an estrogen, during their mother's pregnancy must be followed very closely by their doctors if they choose to use oral contraceptives instead of another method of contraception. Many studies have shown that women taking oral contraceptives have less risk of getting benign breast disease than those who have not used oral contraceptives. Recently, strong evidence has emerged that estrogens (one component of oral contraceptives), when given for periods of more than one year to women after the menopause, increase the risk of cancer of the uterus (womb). There is also some evidence that a kind of oral contraceptive which is no longer marketed, the sequential oral contraceptive, may increase the risk of cancer of the uterus. There remains no evidence, however, that the oral contraceptives now available increase the risk of this cancer. Oral contraceptives do cause, although rarely, a benign (nonmalignant) tumor of the liver. These tumors do not spread, but they may rupture and cause internal bleeding, which may be fatal. A few cases of cancer of the liver have been reported in women using oral contraceptives, but it is not yet known whether the drug caused them.

c. *Dangers to a developing child if oral contraceptives are used in or immediately preceding pregnancy.* Oral contraceptives should not be taken by pregnant women because they may damage the developing child. An increased risk of birth defects, including heart defects and limb defects, has been associated with the use of sex hormones, including oral contraceptives, in pregnancy. In addition, the developing female child whose mother has received DES (diethylstilbestrol), an estrogen, during pregnancy has a risk of getting cancer of the vagina or cervix in her teens or young adulthood. This risk is estimated to be about 1 in 1,000 exposures or less. Abnormalities of the urinary and sex organs have been reported in male offspring so exposed. It is possible that other estrogens, such as the estrogens in oral contraceptives, could have the same effect in the child if the mother takes them during pregnancy.

If you stop taking oral contraceptives to become pregnant, your doctor may recommend that you use another method of contraception for a short while. The reason for this is that there is evidence from studies in women who have had "miscarriages" soon after stopping the pill, that the lost fetuses are more likely to be abnormal. Whether there is an overall increase in "miscarriage" in women who become pregnant soon after stopping the pill as compared with women who do not use the pill is not known, but it is possible that there may be. If, however, you do become pregnant soon after stopping oral contraceptives, and do not have a miscarriage, there is no evidence that the baby has an increased risk of being abnormal.

d. *Gallbladder disease.* Women who use oral contraceptives have a greater risk than nonusers of having gallbladder disease requiring surgery. The increased risk may first appear within 1 year of use and may double after 4 or 5 years of use.

e. *Other side effects of oral contraceptives.* Some women using oral contraceptives experience unpleasant side effects that are not dangerous and are not likely to damage their health. Some of these may be temporary. Your breasts may feel tender, nausea and vomiting may occur, you may gain or lose weight, and your ankles may swell. A spotty darkening of the skin, particularly of the face, is possible and may persist. You may notice unexpected vaginal bleeding or changes in your menstrual period. Irregular bleeding is frequently seen when using the mini-pill or combination oral contraceptives containing less than 50 micrograms of estrogen.

More serious side effects include worsening of migraine, asthma, epilepsy, and kidney or heart disease because of a tendency for water to be retained in the body when oral contraceptives are used. Other side effects are growth of preexisting fibroid tumors of the uterus; mental depression, and liver problems with jaundice (yellowing of the skin). Your doctor may find that levels of sugar and fatty substances in your blood are elevated; the long-term effects of these changes are not known. Some women develop high blood pressure while taking oral contraceptives, which ordinarily returns to the original levels when the oral contraceptive is stopped.

Other reactions, although not proved to be caused by oral contraceptives, are occasionally reported. These include more frequent urination and some discomfort when urinating, nervousness, dizziness, some loss of scalp hair, an increase in body hair, an increase or decrease in sex drive, appetite changes, cataracts, and a need for a change in contact lens prescription, or inability to use contact lenses.

After you stop using oral contraceptives, there may be a delay before you are able to become pregnant or before you resume having menstrual periods. This is especially true of women who had irregular menstrual cycles prior to the use of oral contraceptives. As discussed previously, your doctor may recommend that you wait a short while after stopping the pill before you try to become pregnant. During this time, use another form of contraception. You should consult your physician before resuming use of oral contraceptives after childbirth, especially if you plan to nurse your baby. Drugs in oral contraceptives are known to appear in the milk, and the long-range effect on infants is not known at this time. Furthermore, oral contraceptives may cause a decrease in your milk supply as well as in the quality of the milk.

4. Comparison of the Risks of Oral Contraceptives and Other Contraceptive Methods. The many studies on the risks and effectiveness of oral contraceptives and other methods of contraception have been analyzed to estimate the risk of death associated with various methods of contraception. This risk has two parts: (a) the risk of the method itself (e.g., the risk that oral contraceptives will cause death due to abnormal clotting), and (b) the risk of death due to pregnancy or abortion in the event the method fails. The results of this analysis are shown in the bar graph p2168. The height of the bars is the number of deaths per 100,000 women each year. There are six sets of bars, each set referring to a specific age group of women. Within each set of bars, there is a single bar for each of the different contraceptive methods. For oral contraceptives, there are two bars—one for smokers and the other for nonsmokers. The analysis is based on present knowledge, and new information could, of course, alter it. The analysis shows that the risk of death from all methods of birth control is low and below that associated with childbirth, except for oral contraceptives in women over 40 who smoke. It shows that the lowest risk of death is associated with the condom or diaphragm (traditional contraception) backed up by early abortion in case of failure of the condom or diaphragm to prevent pregnancy. Also, at any age the risk of death (due to unexpected pregnancy) from the use of traditional contraception, even without a backup of abortion, is generally the same as or less than that from use of oral contraceptives.

HOW TO USE ORAL CONTRACEPTIVES AS SAFELY AND EFFECTIVELY AS POSSIBLE, ONCE YOU HAVE DECIDED TO USE THEM

1. What to Tell your Doctor.

You can make use of the pill as safely as possible by telling your doctor if you have any of the following:

a. Conditions that mean you should not use oral contraceptives:

Clots in the legs or lungs.
Clots in the legs or lungs in the past.
A stroke, heart attack, or angina pectoris.
Known or suspected cancer of the breast or sex organs.
Unusual vaginal bleeding that has not yet been diagnosed.
Known or suspected pregnancy.

b. Conditions that your doctor will want to watch closely or which might cause him to suggest another method of contraception:

A family history of breast cancer.
Breast nodules, fibrocystic disease of the breast, or an abnormal mammogram.

Diabetes.	Heart or kidney disease.
High blood pressure.	Epilepsy.
High cholesterol.	Mental depression.
Cigarette smoking.	Fibroid tumors of the uterus.
Migraine headaches.	Gallbladder disease.

c. Once you are using oral contraceptives, you should be alert for signs of a serious adverse effect and call your doctor if they occur.

Sharp pain in the chest, coughing blood, or sudden shortness of breath (indicating possible clots in the lungs).
Pain in the calf (possible clot in the leg).
Crushing chest pain or heaviness (indicating possible heart attack).
Sudden severe headache or vomiting, dizziness or fainting, disturbance of vision or speech, or weakness or numbness in an arm or leg (indicating a possible stroke).
Sudden partial or complete loss of vision (indicating a possible clot in the eye).
Breast lumps (you should ask your doctor to show you how to examine your own breasts).
Severe pain in the abdomen (indicating a possible ruptured tumor of the liver).
Severe depression.
Yellowing of the skin (jaundice).

2. How to Take the Pill So That It is Most Effective.

Reduced effectiveness and an increased incidence of breakthrough bleeding have been associated with the use of oral contraceptives with antibiotics such as rifampin, ampicillin, and tetracycline or with certain other drugs such as barbiturates, phenylbutazone or phenytoin sodium. You should use an additional means of contraception during any cycle in which any of these drugs are taken.

To achieve maximum contraceptive effectiveness, oral contraceptives must be taken exactly as directed and at intervals not exceeding 24 hours. It is recommended that tablets be taken at the same time each day, preferably after the evening meal or at bedtime. Taking them on a definite schedule will decrease the chance of forgetting a tablet and also help keep the proper amount of medication in your system. See detailed instructions below for Ovral® and Lo/Ovral®, Ovral®-28 and Lo/Ovral®-28, and for Ovrette®.

OVRAL®, LO/OVRAL®

The dosage of Ovral® and Lo/Ovral® is one tablet daily for 21 days in a row per menstrual cycle. Tablets are then discontinued for 7 days. The basic schedule is 21 days on—7 days off.

During the first month, you should begin taking Ovral® or Lo/Ovral® on Day 5 of your menstrual cycle whether or not you still have your period. (Day 1 is the first day of menstruation, even if it is almost midnight when you start.) Note: During your first month on Ovral® or Lo/Ovral®, if you start taking tablets later than Day 5 of your menstrual cycle, you should protect yourself by also using another method of birth control until you have taken a tablet daily for seven consecutive days. Thereafter, if you follow directions carefully you will obtain the full contraceptive benefit. If you begin taking tablets later than the proper day, the possibility of ovulation and pregnancy occurring before beginning medication should be considered.

Take one tablet every day until you finish all 21 tablets. No tablets are then taken for one week (7 days). Your period will usually begin about three days after you take the last tablet. Don't be alarmed if the amount of bleeding is not the same as before. On the 8th day, start a new Pilpak®, even if you still have your period. If, for example, you took Ovral® or Lo/Ovral® for the first time on a Tuesday, the 8th day will also be a Tuesday. Thus, you will always begin a new cycle on the same day of the week as long as you do not interrupt your original schedule. If you start taking tablets later than the 8th day, you should protect yourself by also using another method of birth control until you have taken a tablet daily for seven days in a row.

OVRAL®-28, LO/OVRAL®-28

The dosage of Ovral®-28 and Lo/Ovral®-28 is one white active tablet daily for 21 consecutive days followed by one pink inactive tablet daily for 7 consecutive days. The basic schedule is 21 days on white active tablets—7 days on pink inactive tablets. Always take all 21 white tablets in each Pilpak® before taking the pink tablets.

You should begin taking Ovral®-28 or Lo/Ovral®-28 on the first Sunday after your menstrual period begins, whether or not you are still bleeding. If your period begins on a Sunday, take your first tablet that very same day. Your first white tablet is marked with a large arrow and the word "Start". Note: During your first month on Ovral®-28 or Lo/Ovral®-28, you should protect yourself by also using another method of birth control until you have taken a white tablet daily for seven consecutive days. Thereafter, if you follow directions carefully, you will obtain the full contraceptive benefit. If you begin taking tablets later than the proper day, the possibility of ovulation and pregnancy occurring be-

Continued on next page

Wyeth—Cont.

fore beginning medication should be considered. Take one tablet every day until you finish all 21 white tablets in a Pilpak®, followed by all seven pink tablets. Your period will usually begin about three days after you take the last white tablet, which will be during the time you are taking the pink tablets. Don't be alarmed if the amount of bleeding is not the same as before. The day after you have taken your last pink tablet, begin a new Pilpak® of tablets (taking all 21 white tablets first, just as you did before) so that you will take a tablet every day without interruption. The starting day for each new Pilpak® will always be Sunday. If in any cycle you start tablets later than the proper day, you should also use another method of birth control until you have taken a white tablet daily for 7 days in a row.
Spotting or Breakthrough Bleeding:
Spotting is slight staining between menstrual periods which may not even require a pad. Breakthrough bleeding is a flow much like a regular period, requiring sanitary protection. Spotting is more common than breakthrough bleeding, and both occur more often in the first few cycles than in later cycles. These types of bleeding are usually temporary and without significance. It is important to continue taking your pills on schedule. If the bleeding persists for more than a few days, consult your doctor.
Forgotten Pills:
Ovral® and Lo/Ovral® each contain 21 active white tablets per Pilpak®. Ovral®-28 and Lo/Ovral®-28 each contain 21 active white tablets plus 7 pink inactive tablets per Pilpak®.
The chance of becoming pregnant is probably quite small if you miss only one white tablet in a cycle. Of course, with each additional one you skip, the chance increases. If you miss one or more pink tablets (Ovral®-28, Lo/Ovral®-28) you are still protected against pregnancy as long as you begin taking your next white tablet on the proper day. It is important to take a missed white tablet as soon as it is remembered. If two consecutive white tablets are missed they should both be taken as soon as remembered. The next tablet should then be taken at the usual time. Any time you miss one or two white tablets, or begin a new Pilpak® after the proper starting day, you should also use another method of birth control until you have taken a white tablet daily for seven consecutive days. If breakthrough bleeding occurs following missed tablets, it will usually be temporary and of no consequence. While there is little likelihood of pregnancy occurring if only one or two white tablets are missed, the possibility of pregnancy increases with each successive day that scheduled white tablets are missed.
If you are taking Ovral® or Lo/Ovral® and forget to take three white tablets in a row, do not take them when you remember. Wait four more days—which makes a whole week without tablets. Then begin a new Pilpak® on the 8th day after the last tablet was taken. During the seven days without tablets, and until you have taken a white tablet daily for seven consecutive days, you should protect yourself from pregnancy by also using another method of birth control.
If you are taking Ovral®-28 or Lo/Ovral®-28 and forget to take three white tablets in a row, do not take them when you remember. Stop taking all medication until the first Sunday following the last missed tablet. Then, whether or not you have had your period, and even if you are still bleeding, start a new Pilpak®. During the days without tablets, and until you have taken a white tablet daily for seven consecutive days, you should protect yourself from pregnancy by also using another method of birth control.

OVRETTE®
Ovrette® is administered on a continuous daily dosage schedule, one tablet each day, every day of the year. Take the first tablet on the first day of your menstrual period. Tablets should be taken at the same time every day, without interruption, whether bleeding occurs or not. If bleeding is prolonged (more than 8 days) or unusually heavy, you should contact your doctor.
Forgotten Pills:
The risk of pregnancy increases with each tablet missed. Therefore, it is very important that you take one tablet daily as directed. If you miss one tablet, take it as soon as you remember and also take your next tablet at the regular time. If you miss two tablets, take one of the missed tablets as soon as you remember, as well as your regular tablet for that day at the proper time. Furthermore, you should use another method of birth control in addition to taking Ovrette® until you have taken fourteen days (2 weeks) of medication.
If more than two tablets have been missed, Ovrette® should be discontinued immediately and another method of birth control used until the start of your next menstrual period. Then you may resume taking Ovrette®.

At times there may be no menstrual period after a cycle of pills.
Therefore, if you miss one menstrual period but have taken the pills *exactly as you were supposed to,* continue as usual into the next cycle. If you have not taken the pills correctly and miss a menstrual period, or if you are taking mini-pills and it is 45 days or more from the start of your last menstrual period, you may be pregnant and should stop taking oral contraceptives until your doctor determines whether or not you are pregnant. Until you can get to your doctor, use another form of contraception. If two consecutive menstrual periods are missed, you should stop taking pills until it is determined whether you are pregnant. If you do become pregnant while using oral contraceptives, you should discuss the risks to the developing child with your doctor.
3. Periodic Examination.
Your doctor will take a complete medical and family history before prescribing oral contraceptives. At that time and about once a year thereafter, he will generally examine your blood pressure, breasts, abdomen, and pelvic organs (including a Papanicolaou smear, i.e., test for cancer).
SUMMARY
Oral contraceptives are the most effective method, except sterilization, for preventing pregnancy. Other methods when used conscientiously, are also very effective and have fewer risks. The serious risks of oral contraceptives are uncommon, and the "pill" is a very convenient method of preventing pregnancy.
If you have certain conditions or have had these conditions in the past, you should not use oral contraceptives, because the risk is too great. These conditions are listed in the leaflet. If you do not have these conditions, and decide to use the "pill", please read the leaflet carefully so that you can use the "pill" most safely and effectively.
Based on his or her assessment of your medical needs, your doctor has prescribed this drug for you. Do not give the drug to anyone else.

[*Shown in Product Identification Section*]

MAZANOR® Ⓒ ℞
(mazindol)

Description: Mazanor (mazindol) is an imidazoisoindole anorectic agent. It is chemically designated as 5-p-chloro-phenyl-5-hydroxy-2,3-dihydro-5H-imidazo (2,1-a)isoindole, a tautomeric form of 2- [2'-(p-chlorobenzoyl)phenyl]-2-imidazoline.
Actions: Mazanor (mazindol), although an isoindole, has pharmacologic activity similar in many ways to the prototype drugs used in obesity, the amphetamines. Actions include central-nervous-system stimulation in humans and animals, as well as such amphetamine-like effects in animals as the production of stereotyped behavior. Animal experiments also suggest certain differences from phenethylamine anorectic drugs, e.g., amphetamine, with respect to site and mechanism of action; for example, mazindol appears to exert its primary effects on the limbic system. The significance of these differences for humans is uncertain. It does not cause brain norepinephrine depletion in animals; on the other hand, it does appear to inhibit storage-site uptake of norepinephrine as is suggested by its marked protentiation of the effect of exogenous norepinephrine on blood pressure in dogs (see "Warnings") and on smooth-muscle contraction *in vitro.*
Tolerance has been demonstrated with all drugs of this class in which this phenomenon has been studied.
Drugs used in obesity are commonly known as "anorectics" or "anorexigenics." It has not been established, however, that the action of such drugs in treating obesity is exclusively one of appetite suppression. Other central-nervous-system actions or metabolic effects may be involved as well.
Adult obese subjects, instructed in dietary management and treated with anorectic drugs, lose more weight on the average than those treated with placebo and diet, as determined in relatively short-term clinical trials.
The average magnitude of increased weight loss of drug-treated patients over placebo-treated patients in studies of anorectics in general is ordinarily only a fraction of a pound a week. The rate of weight loss is greatest in the first weeks of therapy for both drug and placebo subjects and tends to decrease in succeeding weeks.
The amount of weight loss associated with the use of Mazanor (mazindol), as with other anorectic drugs, varies from trial to trial, and the increased weight loss appears to be related in part to variables other than the drugs prescribed, such as the interaction between physician-investigator and the patient, the population treated, and the diet prescribed. The importance of non-drug factors in such weight loss has not been elucidated.
The natural history of obesity is measured in years, whereas, most studies cited are restricted to a few weeks duration; thus, the total impact of drug-induced weight loss over that of diet alone must be considered clinically limited.
Indication: Mazanor (mazindol) is indicated in the management of exogenous obesity as a short-term (a few weeks) adjunct in a regimen of weight reduction based on caloric restriction. The limited usefulness of agents of this class (see "Actions") should be measured against possible risk factors inherent in their use, such as those described below.
Contraindications: Glaucoma, hypersensitivity or idiosyncrasy to Mazanor (mazindol).
Agitated states.
Patients with a history of drug abuse.
During or within 14 days following the administration of monoamine oxidase inhibitors (hypertensive crises may result).
Warnings: Tolerance to the effect of many anorectic drugs may develop within a few weeks; if this occurs, the recommended dose should not be exceeded in an attempt to increase the effect; rather, the drug should be discontinued.
Mazanor (mazindol) may impair the ability of the patient to engage in potentially hazardous activities, such as operating machinery or driving a motor vehicle; the patient should therefore be cautioned accordingly.
DRUG INTERACTIONS
Mazanor (mazindol) may decrease the hypotensive effect of guanethidine; patients should be monitored accordingly.

Mazanor (mazindol) may markedly potentiate the pressor effect of exogenous catecholamines. If it should be necessary to give a pressor amine agent (e.g., levarterenol or isoproterenol) to a patient in shock (e.g., from a myocardial infarction) who has recently been taking Mazanor (mazindol), extreme care should be taken in monitoring blood pressure at frequent intervals and initiating pressor therapy with a low initial dose and careful titration.

DRUG DEPENDENCE

Mazanor (mazindol) shares important pharmacologic properties with amphetamines. Amphetamines and related stimulant drugs have been extensively abused and can produce tolerance and severe psychologic dependence. In this regard, the manifestations of chronic overdosage or withdrawal of Mazanor (mazindol) have not been determined in humans. Abstinence effects have been observed in dogs after abrupt cessation for prolonged periods. There was some self-administration of the drug in monkeys. EEG studies and "liking" scores in human studies yielded equivocal results. While the abuse potential of Mazanor (mazindol) has not been further defined, the possibility of dependence should be kept in mind when evaluating the desirability of including Mazanor (mazindol) as part of a weight-reduction program.

USAGE IN PREGNANCY

Mazanor (mazindol) was studied in reproduction experiments in rats and rabbits, and an increase in neonatal mortality and a possible increased incidence of rib anomalies in rats were observed at relatively high doses. Although these studies have not indicated important adverse effects, use of mazindol by women who are or may become pregnant requires that the potential benefit be weighed against the possible hazard to mother and infant.

USAGE IN CHILDREN

Mazanor (mazindol) is not recommended for use in children under 12 years of age.

Precautions: Insulin requirements in diabetes mellitus may be altered in association with the use of mazindol and the concomitant dietary regimen.

The least amount feasible should be prescribed or dispensed at one time in order to minimize the possibility of overdosage.

Use only with caution in hypertension with monitoring of blood pressure, since evidence is insufficient to rule out a possible adverse effect on blood pressure in some hypertensive patients. The drug is not recommended in severely hypertensive patients. The drug is not recommended for patients with symptomatic cardiovascular disease including arrhythmias.

Adverse Reactions: The most common adverse effects of Mazanor (mazindol) are: dry mouth, tachycardia, constipation, nervousness, and insomnia.

Cardiovascular: Palpitation, tachycardia.

Central Nervous System: Overstimulation, restlessness, dizziness, insomnia, dysphoria, tremor, headache, depression, drowsiness, weakness.

Gastrointestinal: Dryness of the mouth, unpleasant taste, diarrhea, constipation, nausea, other gastrointestinal disturbances.

Skin: Rash, excessive sweating, clamminess.

Endocrine: Impotence, changes in libido have rarely been observed with Mazanor (mazindol).

Eye: Treatment of dogs with high doses of Mazanor (mazindol) for long periods resulted in some corneal opacities, reversible on cessation of medication. No such effect has been observed in humans.

Dosage and Administration: Usual dosage is 1 mg three times daily, one hour before meals, or 2 mg once daily, one hour before lunch. The lowest effective dose should be used. To determine the lowest effective dose, therapy with Mazanor may be initiated at 1 mg once a day, and adjusted to the need and response of the patient. Should G.I. discomfort occur, Mazanor may be taken with meals.

Overdosage: There are no data as yet on acute overdosage with Mazanor (mazindol) in humans.

Manifestations of acute overdosage with amphetamines and related substances include restlessness, tremor, rapid respiration, dizziness. Fatigue and depression may follow the stimulatory phase of overdosage. Cardiovascular effects include tachycardia, hypertension, and circulatory collapse. Gastrointestinal symptoms include nausea, vomiting, and abdominal cramps. While similar manifestations of overdosage may be seen with Mazanor (mazindol), their exact nature has yet to be determined. The management of acute intoxication is largely symptomatic. Data are not available on the treatment of acute intoxication with Mazanor (mazindol) by hemodialysis or peritoneal dialysis, but the substance is poorly soluble except at very acid pH.

How Supplied: Mazanor® (mazindol) Tablets, Wyeth®, are available in the following dosage strength in bottles of 30 tablets:

1 mg, NDC 0008-0071, white, round, scored tablet marked "WYETH" and "71".

Keep bottles tightly closed.
Store below 25° C (77° F).
Dispense in tight containers.

[*Shown in Product Identification Section*]

MEPERGAN® ℂ ℞

(meperidine HCl and promethazine HCl) Injection

Description: This product is available in concentration providing 25 mg each of meperidine hydrochloride and promethazine hydrochloride per ml with 0.1 mg edetate disodium, 0.04 mg calcium chloride, and not more than 0.75 mg sodium formaldehyde sulfoxylate, 0.25 mg sodium metabisulfite, and 5 mg phenol with sodium acetate buffer.

Actions: Meperidine hydrochloride is a narcotic analgesic with multiple actions qualitatively similar to those of morphine. Phenergan® (promethazine HCl) is a phenothiazine derivative that has several different pharmacologic properties including antihistaminic, sedative, and antiemetic actions.

Indications: As a preanesthetic medication when analgesia and sedation are indicated. As an adjunct to local and general anesthesia.

Contraindications: Hypersensitivity to meperidine or promethazine.

Under no circumstances should Mepergan be given by intra-arterial injection, due to the likelihood of severe arteriospasm and the possibility of resultant gangrene (see Warnings).

Mepergan should not be given by the subcutaneous route; evidence of chemical irritation has been noted and necrotic lesions have resulted on rare occasions following subcutaneous injection. The preferred parenteral route of administration is by deep intramuscular injection.

Meperidine is contraindicated in patients who are receiving monoamine oxidase inhibitors (MAOI) or those who have received such agents within 14 days.

Therapeutic doses of meperidine have inconsistently precipitated unpredictable, severe, and occasionally fatal reactions in patients who have received such agents within 14 days. The mechanism of these reactions is unclear. Some have been characterized by coma, severe respiratory depression, cyanosis, and hypotension, and have resembled the syndrome of acute narcotic overdose. In other reactions the predominant manifestations have been hyperexcitability, convulsions, tachycardia, hyperpyrexia, and hypertension. Although it is not known that other narcotics are free of the risk of such reactions, virtually all of the reported reactions have occurred with meperidine. If a narcotic is needed in such patients, a sensitivity test should be performed in which repeated, small, incremental doses of morphine are administered over the course of several hours while the patient's condition and vital signs are under careful observation.

(Intravenous hydrocortisone or prednisolone have been used to treat severe reactions, with the addition of intravenous chlorpromazine in those cases exhibiting hypertension and hyperpyrexia. The usefulness and safety of narcotic antagonists in the treatment of these reactions is unknown.)

Warnings: Tolerance and Addiction Liability

Warning—may be habit forming

DRUG DEPENDENCE: Meperidine can produce drug dependence of the morphine type and therefore has the potential for being abused. Psychic dependence, physical dependence, and tolerance may develop upon repeated administration of meperidine, and it should be prescribed and administered with the same degree of caution appropriate to the use of morphine. Like other narcotics, meperidine is subject to the provisions of the Federal narcotic laws.

INTERACTION WITH OTHER CENTRAL-NERVOUS-SYSTEM DEPRESSANTS: Meperidine should be used with great caution and in reduced dosage in patients who are concurrently receiving other narcotic analgesics, general anesthetics, phenothiazines, other tranquilizers, sedative-hypnotics, tricyclic antidepressants, and other CNS depressants (including alcohol). Respiratory depression, hypotension, and profound sedation or coma may result.

The sedative action of promethazine hydrochloride is additive to the sedative effects of central-nervous-system depressants; therefore, agents such as alcohol, barbiturates, and narcotic analgesics should either be eliminated or given in reduced dosage in the presence of promethazine hydrochloride. When given concomitantly with promethazine hydrochloride the dose of barbiturates should be reduced by at least one-half and the dose of analgesic depressants, such as morphine or meperidine, should be reduced by one-quarter to one-half.

HEAD INJURY AND INCREASED INTRACRANIAL PRESSURE: The respiratory depressant effects of meperidine and its capacity to elevate cerebrospinal-fluid pressure may be markedly exaggerated in the presence of head injury, other intracranial lesions, or a preexisting increase in intracranial pressure. Furthermore, narcotics produce adverse reactions which may obscure the clinical course of patients with head injuries. In such patients, meperidine must be used with extreme caution and only if its use is deemed essential.

INADVERTENT INTRA-ARTERIAL INJECTION: Due to the close proximity of arteries and veins in the areas most commonly used for intravenous injection, extreme care should be exercised to avoid perivascular extravasation or inadvertent intra-arterial injection of Mepergan. Reports compatible with inadvertent intra-arterial injection suggest that pain, severe chemical irritation, severe spasm of distal vessels, and resultant gangrene requiring amputation is likely under such circumstances. Intravenous injection was intended in all the cases reported, but perivascular extravasation or arterial placement of the needle is now suspect. There is no proven successful management of this condition after it occurs, although sympathetic block and heparinization are commonly employed during the acute management because of the results of animal experiments with other known arteriolar irritants. Aspiration of dark blood does not preclude intra-arterial needle placement, because blood is discolored upon contact with promethazine. Use of syringes with rigid plungers or of small bore needles might obscure typical arterial backflow if this is relied upon alone.

Continued on next page

Wyeth—Cont.

INTRAVENOUS USE: If necessary, meperidine may be given intravenously, but the injection should be given very slowly, preferably in the form of a diluted solution. Rapid intravenous injection of narcotic analgesics, including meperidine, increases the incidence of adverse reactions; severe respiratory depression, apnea, hypotension, peripheral circulatory collapse, and cardiac arrest have occurred. Meperidine should not be administered intravenously unless a narcotic antagonist and the facilities for assisted or controlled respiration are immediately available. When meperidine is given parenterally, especially intravenously, the patient should be lying down.

When used intravenously, Mepergan® (meperidine hydrochloride and promethazine hydrochloride) should be given at a rate not to exceed 1 ml (25 mg of each component) per minute. When administering any irritant drug intravenously it is usually preferable to inject it through the tubing of an intravenous infusion set that is known to be functioning satisfactorily. In the event that a patient complains of pain during intended intravenous injection of Mepergan, the injection should immediately be stopped to provide for evaluation of possible arterial placement or perivascular extravasation.

ASTHMA AND OTHER RESPIRATORY CONDITIONS: Meperidine should be used with extreme caution in patients having an acute asthmatic attack, patients with chronic obstructive pulmonary disease or cor pulmonale, patients having a substantially decreased respiratory reserve, and patients with preexisting respiratory depression, hypoxia, or hypercapnia. In such patients, even usual therapeutic doses of narcotics may decrease respiratory drive while simultaneously increasing airway resistance to the point of apnea.

HYPOTENSIVE EFFECT: The administration of meperidine may result in severe hypotension in an individual whose ability to maintain his blood pressure has already been compromised by a depleted blood volume or concurrent administration of drugs such as the phenothiazines or certain anesthetics.

USAGE IN AMBULATORY PATIENTS: Meperidine may impair the mental and/or physical abilities required for the performance of potentially hazardous tasks such as driving a car or operating machinery. The patient should be cautioned accordingly.

Meperidine, like other narcotics, may produce orthostatic hypotension in ambulatory patients.

USAGE IN PREGNANCY AND LACTATION: Meperidine should not be used in pregnant women prior to the labor period, unless in the judgment of the physician the potential benefits outweigh the possible hazards, because safe use in pregnancy prior to labor has not been established relative to possible adverse effects on fetal development.

When used as an obstetrical analgesic, meperidine crosses the placental barrier and can produce respiratory depression in the newborn; resuscitation may be required (see section on Overdosage).

Meperidine appears in the milk of nursing mothers receiving the drug.

Precautions: SUPRAVENTRICULAR TACHYCARDIAS: Meperidine should be used with caution in patients with atrial flutter and other supraventricular tachycardias because of a possible vagolytic action which may produce a significant increase in the ventricular response rate.

CONVULSIONS: Meperidine may aggravate preexisting convulsions in patients with convulsive disorders. If dosage is escalated substantially above recommended levels because of tolerance development, convulsions may occur in individuals without a history of convulsive disorders.

ACUTE ABDOMINAL CONDITIONS: The administration of meperidine or other narcotics may obscure the diagnosis or clinical course in patients with acute abdominal conditions.

SPECIAL-RISK PATIENTS: Meperidine should be given with caution and the initial dose should be reduced in certain patients such as the elderly or debilitated, and those with severe impairment of hepatic or renal function, hypothyroidism, Addison's disease, and prostatic hypertrophy or urethral stricture.

Antiemetics may mask the symptoms of an unrecognized disease and thereby interfere with diagnosis.

Patients in pain who have received inadequate or no analgesia have been noted to develop "athetoid-like" movements of the upper extremities following the parenteral administration of promethazine. These symptoms usually disappear upon adequate control of the pain.

Ambulatory patients should be cautioned against driving automobiles or operating dangerous machinery until it is known that they do not become drowsy or dizzy from promethazine hydrochloride therapy.

Adverse Reactions: The major hazards of meperidine, as with other narcotic analgesics, are respiratory depression and, to a lesser degree, circulatory depression; respiratory arrest, shock, and cardiac arrest have occurred. The most frequently observed adverse reactions include light-headedness, dizziness, sedation, nausea, vomiting, and sweating. These effects seem to be more prominent in ambulatory patients and in those who are not experiencing severe pain. In such individuals, lower doses are advisable. Some adverse reactions in ambulatory patients may be alleviated if the patient lies down.

Other adverse reactions include:

CENTRAL NERVOUS SYSTEM: Euphoria, dysphoria, weakness, headache, agitation, tremor, uncoordinated muscle movements, transient hallucinations and disorientation, visual disturbances and, rarely, extrapyramidal reactions.

GASTROINTESTINAL: Dry mouth, constipation, biliary-tract spasm.

CARDIOVASCULAR: Flushing of the face, tachycardia, bradycardia, palpitation, faintness, syncope.

Cardiovascular effects from promethazine have been rare. Minor increases in blood pressure and occasional mild hypotension have been reported. Venous thrombosis at the injection site has been reported. Intra-arterial injection of Mepergan may result in gangrene of the affected extremity (see Warnings).

GENITOURINARY: Urinary retention.

ALLERGIC: Pruritus, urticaria, other skin rashes, wheal and flare over the vein with IV injection.

Photosensitivity, although extremely rare, has been reported. Occurrence of photosensitivity may be a contraindication to further treatment with promethazine or related drugs.

OTHER: Pain at injection site; local tissue irritation and induration following subcutaneous injection, particularly when repeated; antidiuretic effect.

Patients may occasionally complain of autonomic reactions such as dryness of the mouth, blurring of vision and, rarely, dizziness following the use of promethazine.

Very rare cases have been reported where patients receiving promethazine have developed leukopenia. In one instance agranulocytosis has been reported. In nearly every instance reported, other toxic agents known to have caused these conditions have been associated with the administration of promethazine.

Dosage and Administration: WARNING—BARBITURATES ARE NOT CHEMICALLY COMPATIBLE IN SOLUTION WITH MEPERGAN® (MEPERIDINE HYDROCHLORIDE AND PROMETHAZINE HYDROCHLORIDE), AND SHOULD NOT BE MIXED IN THE SAME SYRINGE.

The TUBEX® (Sterile Cartridge-Needle Unit) is designed for single-dose use. VIALS should be used when required doses are fractions of a milliliter, as indicated below.

Mepergan® is usually administered intramuscularly. However, in certain specific situations, the intravenous route may be employed. INADVERTENT INTRA-ARTERIAL INJECTION CAN RESULT IN GANGRENE OF THE AFFECTED EXTREMITY (see Warnings). SUBCUTANEOUS ADMINISTRATION IS CONTRAINDICATED, AS IT MAY RESULT IN TISSUE NECROSIS (see Contraindications). INJECTION INTO OR NEAR PERIPHERAL NERVES MAY RESULT IN PERMANENT NEUROLOGICAL DEFICIT.

When used intravenously, the rate should not be greater than 1 ml of Mepergan (25 mg of each component) per minute; it is preferable to inject through the tubing of an intravenous infusion set that is known to be functioning satisfactorily.

ADULT DOSE: 1-2 ml (25-50 mg of each component) per single injection, which can be repeated every 3 to 4 hours.

CHILDREN 12 YEARS OF AGE AND UNDER: 0.5 mg of each component per pound of body weight. The dosage may be repeated every 3 to 4 hours as necessary. For preanesthetic medication the usual adult dose is 2 ml (50 mg of each component) intramuscularly with or without appropriate atropine-like drug. Atropine sulfate 0.3 to 0.4 mg or scopolamine hydrobromide 0.25 to 0.4 mg in sterile solution may be mixed in the same syringe with Mepergan. Repeat doses of 50 mg or less of both promethazine and meperidine may be administered by either route at 3- to 4-hour intervals, as necessary. As an adjunct to local or general anesthesia the usual dose is 2 ml (50 mg each of meperidine and promethazine).

Overdosage: SYMPTOMS: Serious overdose with meperidine is characterized by respiratory depression (a decrease in respiratory rate and/or tidal volume, Cheyne-Stokes respiration, cyanosis), extreme somnolence progressing to stupor or coma, skeletal muscle flaccidity, cold and clammy skin, and sometimes bradycardia and hypotension. In severe overdosage, particularly by the intravenous route, apnea, circulatory collapse, cardiac arrest, and death may occur.

TREATMENT: Primary attention should be given to the reestablishment of adequate respiratory exchange through provision of a patent airway and institution of assisted or controlled ventilation. The narcotic antagonists, naloxone hydrochloride, nalorphine hydrochloride, and levallorphan tartrate, are specific antidotes against respiratory depression which may result from overdosage or unusual sensitivity to narcotics, including meperidine. Therefore, an appropriate dose of one of these antagonists should be administered, preferably by the intravenous route, simultaneously with efforts at respiratory resuscitation.

An antagonist should not be administered in absence of clinically significant respiratory or cardiovascular depression.

Oxygen, intravenous fluids, vasopressors, and other supportive measures should be employed as indicated.

NOTE: In an individual physically dependent on narcotics, the administration of the usual dose of a narcotic antagonist will precipitate an acute withdrawal syndrome. The severity of this syndrome will depend on the degree of physical dependence and the dose of antagonist administered. The use of narcotic antagonists in such individuals should be avoided if possible. If a narcotic antagonist must be used to treat serious respiratory depression in the physically dependent patient, the antagonist should be administered with extreme care and only one-fifth to one-tenth the usual initial dose administered.

Attempted suicides with promethazine have resulted in deep sedation, coma, rarely convulsions and cardiorespiratory symptoms compatible with the depth of sedation present. Extrapyramidal reactions may be treated with anticholinergic antiparkinson agents, diphenhydramine, or barbiturates.

If severe hypotension occurs, levarterenol or phenylephrine may be indicated. Epinephrine is probably best avoided, since it has been suggested that promethazine overdosage could produce a partial alpha-adrenergic blockade.

A paradoxical reaction, characterized by hyperexcitability and nightmares, has been reported in children receiving large single doses of promethazine.

How Supplied: Mepergan® (meperidine hydrochloride and promethazine hydrochloride) is supplied in 10 ml vials and TUBEX® Sterile Cartridge-Needle Units.

Subject to Regulations of Federal Bureau Narcotics and Dangerous Drugs.

	Myocardial infarction			
	Women aged 30-39		Women aged 40-44	
Smoking habits	Users	Nonusers	Users	Nonusers
All smokers	10.2	2.6	62.0	15.9
Heavy*	13.0	5.1	78.7	31.3
Light	4.7	0.9	28.6	5.7
Nonsmokers	1.8	1.2	10.7	7.4
Smokers and nonsmokers	5.4	1.9	32.8	11.7

* Heavy smoker: 15 or more cigarettes per day.
From JAIN, A.K., *Studies in Family Planning*, 8:50, 1977

NORDETTE® ℞
TABLETS
(levonorgestrel and ethinyl estradiol tablets)

Description:
ORAL CONTRACEPTIVE
Each Nordette® tablet contains 0.15 mg of levonorgestrel (*d*(-)-13 beta-ethyl-17-alpha-ethinyl-17-beta-hydroxygon-4-en-3-one), a totally synthetic progestogen, and 0.03 mg of ethinyl estradiol (19-nor-17α-pregna-1,3,5 (10)-trien-20-yne-3,17-diol).

Clinical Pharmacology: Combination oral contraceptives act primarily through the mechanism of gonadotropin suppression due to the estrogenic and progestational activity of the ingredients. Although the primary mechanism of action is inhibition of ovulation, alterations in the genital tract, including changes in the cervical mucus (which increase the difficulty of sperm penetration) and the endometrium (which reduce the likelihood of implantation), may also contribute to contraceptive effectiveness.

Indications and Usage: Nordette® is indicated for the prevention of pregnancy in women who elect to use oral contraceptives as a method of contraception.

Oral contraceptives are highly effective. The pregnancy rate in women using conventional combination oral contraceptives (containing 35 mcg or more of ethinyl estradiol or 50 mcg or more of mestranol) is generally reported as less than one pregnancy per 100 woman-years of use. Slightly higher rates (somewhat more than 1 pregnancy per 100 woman-years of use) are reported for some combination products containing 35 mcg or less of ethinyl estradiol, and rates on the order of 3 pregnancies per 100 woman-years are reported for the progestogen-only oral contraceptives.

These rates are derived from separate studies conducted by different investigators in several population groups and cannot be compared precisely. Furthermore, pregnancy rates tend to be lower as clinical studies are continued, possibly due to selective retention in the longer studies of those patients who accept the treatment regimen and do not discontinue as a result of adverse reactions, pregnancy, or other reasons.

In clinical trials with Nordette®, 1,084 patients completed 8,186 cycles, and a total of three pregnancies were reported. This represents a pregnancy rate of 0.48 per 100 woman-years.

Table 1 gives ranges of pregnancy rates reported in the literature[1] for other means of contraception. The efficacy of these means of contraception (except the IUD) depends upon the degree of adherence to the method.

TABLE 1
PREGNANCIES PER 100 WOMAN-YEARS
IUD, less than 1–6; Diaphragm with spermicidal products (creams or jellies), 2–20; Condom, 3–36; Aerosol foams, 2–29; Jellies and creams, 4–36;
Periodic abstinence (rhythm) all types, less than 1–47:
1. Calendar method, 14–47;
2. Temperature method, 1–20;
3. Temperature method—intercourse only in postovulatory phase, less than 1–7;
4. Mucus method, 1–25;
No contraception, 60–80.

Dose-Related Risk of Thromboembolism from Oral Contraceptives: Two studies have shown a positive association between the dose of estrogens in oral contraceptives and the risk of thromboembolism.[2,3] For this reason, it is prudent and in keeping with good principles of therapeutics to minimize exposure to estrogen. The oral-contraceptive product prescribed for any given patient should be that product which contains the least amount of estrogen that is compatible with an acceptable pregnancy rate and patient acceptance. It is recommended that new acceptors of oral contraceptives be started on preparations containing 0.05 mg or less of estrogen.

Contraindications: Oral contraceptives should not be used in women with any of the following conditions:
1. Thrombophlebitis or thromboembolic disorders.
2. A past history of deep-vein thrombophlebitis or thromboembolic disorders.
3. Cerebral-vascular or coronary-artery disease.
4. Known or suspected carcinoma of the breast.
5. Known or suspected estrogen-dependent neoplasia.
6. Undiagnosed abnormal genital bleeding.
7. Known or suspected pregnancy (see Warning No. 5).
8. Benign or malignant liver tumor which developed during the use of oral contraceptives or other estrogen-containing products.

Warnings:

Cigarette smoking increases the risk of serious cardiovascular side effects from oral-contraceptive use. This risk increases with age and with heavy smoking (15 or more cigarettes per day) and is quite marked in women over 35 years of age. Women who use oral contraceptives should be strongly advised not to smoke.
The use of oral contraceptives is associated with increased risk of several serious conditions, including thromboembolism, stroke, myocardial infarction, hepatic adenoma, gallbladder disease, hypertension. Practitioners prescribing oral contraceptives should be familiar with the following information relating to these risks.

1. *Thromboembolic Disorders and Other Vascular Problems:* An increased risk of thromboembolic and thrombotic disease associated with the use of oral contraceptives is well-established. Three principal studies in Great Britain[4–6] and three in the United States[7–10] have demonstrated an increased risk of fatal and nonfatal venous thromboembolism and stroke, both hemorrhagic and thrombotic. These studies estimate that users of oral contraceptives are 4 to 11 times more likely than nonusers to develop these diseases without evident cause (Table 2).

CEREBROVASCULAR DISORDERS
In a collaborative American study[9,10] of cerebrovascular disorders in women with and without predisposing causes, it was estimated that the risk of hemorrhagic stroke was 2.0 times greater in users than nonusers and the risk of thrombotic stroke was 4 to 9.5 times greater in users than in nonusers (Table 2).

TABLE 2
SUMMARY OF RELATIVE RISK OF THROMBOEMBOLIC DISORDERS AND OTHER VASCULAR PROBLEMS IN ORAL-CONTRACEPTIVE USERS COMPARED TO NONUSERS

	Relative risk, times greater
Idiopathic thromboembolic disease	4-11
Postsurgery thromboembolic complications	4-6
Thrombotic stroke	4-9.5
Hemorrhagic stroke	2
Myocardial infarction	2-12

MYOCARDIAL INFARCTION
An increased risk of myocardial infarction associated with the use of oral contraceptives has been reported,[11,12,13] confirming a previously suspected association. These studies, conducted in the United Kingdom, found, as expected, that the greater the number of underlying risk factors for coronary-artery disease (cigarette smoking, hypertension, hypercholesterolemia, obesity, diabetes, history of preeclamptic toxemia) the higher the risk of developing myocardial infarction, regardless of whether the patient was an oral-contraceptive user or not. Oral contraceptives, however, were found to be a clear additional risk factor.

In terms of relative risk, it has been estimated[52] that oral-contraceptive users who do not smoke (smoking is considered a major predisposing condition to myocardial infarction) are about twice as likely to have a fatal myocardial infarction as nonusers who do not smoke. Oral-contraceptive users who are also smokers have about a 5-fold increased risk of fatal infarction compared to users who do not smoke, but about a 10- to 12-fold increased risk compared to nonusers who do not smoke. Furthermore, the amount of smoking is also an important factor. In determining the importance of these relative risks, however, the baseline rates for various age groups, as shown in Table 3, must be given serious consideration. The importance of other predisposing conditions mentioned above in determining relative and absolute risks has not as yet been quantified; it is quite likely that the same synergistic action exists, but perhaps to a lesser extent.

TABLE 3
Estimated annual mortality rate per 100,000 women from myocardial infarction by use of oral contraceptives, smoking habits, and age (in years):
[See table above].

RISK OF DOSE
In an analysis of data derived from several national adverse-reaction reporting systems,[2] British investigators concluded that the risk of

Continued on next page

Wyeth—Cont.

thromboembolism, including coronary thrombosis, is directly related to the dose of estrogen used in oral contraceptives. Preparations containing 100 mcg or more of estrogen were associated with a higher risk of thromboembolism than those containing 50-80 mcg of estrogen. Their analysis did suggest, however, that the quantity of estrogen may not be the sole factor involved. This finding has been confirmed in the United States.[3] Careful epidemiological studies to determine the degree of thromboembolic risk associated with progestogen-only oral contraceptives have not been performed. Cases of thromboembolic disease have been reported in women using these products, and they should not be presumed to be free of excess risk.

ESTIMATE OF EXCESS MORTALITY FROM CIRCULATORY DISEASES

A large prospective study[53] carried out in the U.K. estimated the mortality rate per 100,000 women per year from diseases of the circulatory system for users and nonusers of oral contraceptives according to age, smoking habits, and duration of use. The overall excess death rate annually from circulatory diseases for oral-contraceptive users was estimated to be 20 per 100,000 (ages 15-34—5/100,000; ages 35-44—33/100,000; ages 45-49—140/100,000), the risk being concentrated in older women, in those with a long duration of use, and in cigarette smokers. It was not possible, however, to examine the interrelationships of age, smoking, and duration of use, nor to compare the effects of continuous vs. intermittent use. Although the study showed a 10-fold increase in death due to circulatory diseases in users for 5 or more years, all of these deaths occurred in women 35 or older. Until larger numbers of women under 35 with continuous use for 5 or more years are available, it is not possible to assess the magnitude of the relative risk for this younger age group.

The available data from a variety of sources have been analyzed[14] to estimate the risk of death associated with various methods of contraception. The estimates of risk of death for each method include the combined risk of the contraceptive method (e.g., thromboembolic and thrombotic disease in the case of oral contraceptives) plus the risk attributable to pregnancy or abortion in the event of method failure. This latter risk varies with the effectiveness of the contraceptive method. The findings of this analysis are shown in Figure 1 above.[14]

The study concluded that the mortality associated with all methods of birth control is low and below that associated with childbirth, with the exception of oral contraceptives in women over 40 who smoke. (The rates given for Pill only/smokers for each age group are for smokers as a class. For "heavy" smokers (more than 15 cigarettes a day), the rates given would be about double; for "light" smokers (less than 15 cigarettes a day), about 50 percent. The lowest mortality is associated with the condom or diaphragm backed up by early abortión. The risk of thromboembolic and thrombotic disease associated with oral contraceptives increases with age after approximately age 30 and, for myocardial infarction, is further increased by hypertension, hypercholesterolemia, obesity, diabetes, or history of preeclamptic toxemia and especially by cigarette smoking.

Based on the data currently available, the following chart gives a gross estimate of the risk of death from circulatory disorders associated with the use of oral contraceptives:

(See table above)

The physician and the patient should be alert to the earliest manifestations of thromboembolic and thrombotic disorders (e.g., thrombophlebitis, pulmonary embolism, cerebrovascular insufficiency, coronary occlusion, retinal thrombosis, and mesenteric thrombosis).

SMOKING HABITS AND OTHER PREDISPOSING CONDITIONS—RISK ASSOCIATED WITH USE OF ORAL CONTRACEPTIVES

Age	Below 30	30-39	40+
Heavy smokers	C	B	A
Light smokers	D	C	B
Nonsmokers (no predisposing conditions)	D	C,D	C
Nonsmokers (other predisposing conditions)	C	C,B	B,A

A—Use associated with very high risk.
B—Use associated with high risk.
C—Use associated with moderate risk.
D—Use associated with low risk.

Should any of these occur or be suspected, the drug should be discontinued immediately.

A four- to six-fold increased risk of postsurgery thromboembolic complications has been reported in oral-contraceptive users.[15,16] If feasible, oral contraceptives should be discontinued at least 4 weeks before surgery of a type associated with an increased risk of thromboembolism or prolonged immobilization.

2. *Ocular Lesions:*
There have been reports of neuro-ocular lesions such as optic neuritis or retinal thrombosis associated with the use of oral contraceptives. Discontinue oral-contraceptive medication if there is unexplained, sudden or gradual, partial or complete loss of vision; onset of proptosis or diplopia; papilledema; or retinal-vascular lesions, and institute appropriate diagnostic and therapeutic measures.

3. *Carcinoma:*
Long-term continuous administration of either natural or synthetic estrogen in certain animal species increases the frequency of carcinoma of the breast, cervix, vagina, and liver. Certain synthetic progestogens, none currently contained in oral contraceptives, have been noted to increase the incidence of mammary nodules, benign and malignant, in dogs.

In humans, three case-control studies have reported an increased risk of endometrial carcinoma associated with the prolonged use of exogenous estrogen in postmenopausal women.[17,18,19] One publication[20] reported on the first 21 cases submitted by physicians to a registry of cases of adenocarcinoma of the endometrium in women under 40 on oral contraceptives. Of the cases found in women without predisposing risk factors for adenocarcinoma of the endometrium (e.g., irregular bleeding at the time oral contraceptives were first given, polycystic ovaries), nearly all occurred in women who had used a sequential oral contraceptive. These products are no longer marketed. No evidence has been reported suggesting an increased risk of endometrial cancer in users of conventional combination or progestogen-only oral contraceptives.

Several studies[8,21–24] have found no increase in breast cancer in women taking oral contraceptives or estrogens. One study,[25] however, while also noting no overall increased risk of breast cancer in women treated with oral contraceptives, found an excess risk in the subgroups of oral-contraceptive users with documented benign breast disease. A reduced occurrence of benign breast tumors in users of oral contraceptives has been well-documented.[8,21,25,26,27]

In summary, there is at present no confirmed evidence from human studies of an increased risk of cancer associated with oral contraceptives. Close clinical surveillance of all women taking oral contraceptives is, nevertheless, essential. In all cases of undiagnosed persistent or recurrent abnormal vaginal bleeding, appropriate diagnostic measures should be taken to rule out malignancy. Women with a strong family history of breast cancer or who have breast nodules, fibrocystic disease, or abnormal mammograms should be monitored with particular care if they elect to use oral contraceptives instead of other methods of contraception.

Figure 1. Estimated annual number of deaths associated with control of fertility and no control per 100,000 nonsterile women, by regimen of control and age of woman.

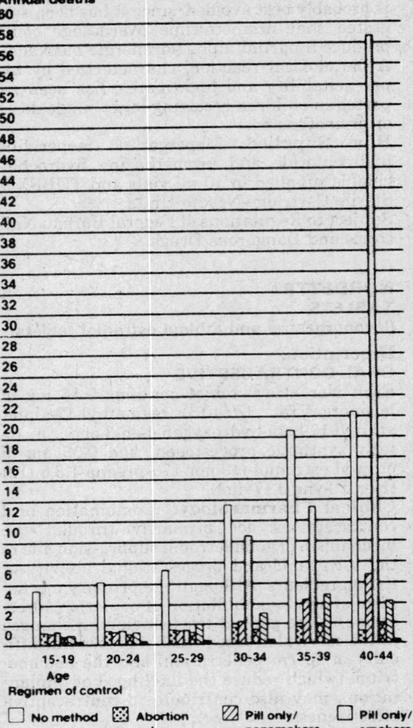

4. *Hepatic Tumors:*
Benign hepatic adenomas have been found to be associated with the use of oral contraceptives.[28,29,30,46] One study[46] showed that oral traceptive formulations with high hormonal potency were associated with a higher risk than lower potency formulations. Although benign, hepatic adenomas may rupture and may cause death through intra-abdominal hemorrhage. This has been reported in short-term as well as long-term users of oral contraceptives. Two studies relate risk with duration of use of the contraceptive, the risk being much greater after 4 or more years of oral-contraceptive use.[30,46] While hepatic adenoma is a rare lesion, it should be considered in women presenting abdominal pain and tenderness, abdominal mass or shock. A few cases of hepatocellular carcinoma have been reported in women taking oral contraceptives. The relationship of these drugs to this type of malignancy is not known at this time.

5. *Use in or Immediately Preceding Pregnancy, Birth Defects in Offspring, and Malignancy in Female Offspring:*
The use of female sex hormones—both estrogenic and progestational agents—during early pregnancy may seriously damage the offspring. It has been shown that females exposed in utero to diethylstilbestrol, a nonsteroidal estrogen, have an increased risk of developing in later life a form of vaginal or cervical cancer that is ordinarily extremely rare.[31,32] This risk has been estimated to be of the order of 1 in 1,000 exposures or less.[33,47] Although there is

no evidence at the present time that oral contraceptives further enhance the risk of developing this type of malignancy, such patients should be monitored with particular care if they elect to use oral contraceptives instead of other methods of contraception. Furthermore, a high percentage of such exposed women (from 30 to 90%) have been found to have epithelial changes of the vagina and cervix.[34–38] Although these changes are histologically benign, it is not known whether this condition is a precursor of vaginal malignancy. Male children so exposed may develop abnormalities of the urogenital tract.[48,49,50] Although similar data are not available with the use of other estrogens, it cannot be presumed that they would not induce similar changes.

An increased risk of congenital anomalies, including heart defects and limb defects, has been reported with the use of sex hormones, including oral contraceptives, in pregnancy.[39–42,51] One case-control study[42] has estimated a 4.7-fold increase in risk of limb-reduction defects in infants exposed in utero to sex hormones (oral contraceptives, hormonal withdrawal tests for pregnancy, or attempted treatment for threatened abortion). Some of these exposures were very short and involved only a few days of treatment. The data suggest that the risk of limb-reduction defects in exposed fetuses is somewhat less than one in 1,000 live births.

In the past, female sex hormones have been used during pregnancy in an attempt to treat threatened or habitual abortion. There is considerable evidence that estrogens are ineffective for these indications, and there is no evidence from well-controlled studies that progestogens are effective for these uses.

There is some evidence that triploidy and possibly other types of polyploidy are increased among abortuses from women who become pregnant soon after ceasing oral contraceptives.[43] Embryos with these anomalies are virtually always aborted spontaneously. Whether there is an overall increase in spontaneous abortion of pregnancies conceived soon after stopping oral contraceptives is unknown. It is recommended that, for any patient who has missed two consecutive periods, pregnancy should be ruled out before continuing the contraceptive regimen. If the patient has not adhered to the prescribed schedule, the possibility of pregnancy should be considered at the time of the first missed period (or after 45 days from the last menstrual period if the progestogen-only oral contraceptives are used), and further use of oral contraceptives should be withheld until pregnancy has been ruled out. If pregnancy is confirmed, the patient should be apprised of the potential risks to the fetus, and the advisability of continuation of the pregnancy should be discussed in the light of these risks.

It is also recommended that women who discontinue oral contraceptives with the intent of becoming pregnant use an alternate form of contraception for a period of time before attempting to conceive. Many clinicians recommend 3 months, although no precise information is available on which to base this recommendation.

The administration of progestogen-only or progestogen-estrogen combinations to induce withdrawal bleeding should not be used as a test of pregnancy.

6. *Gallbladder Disease:*
Studies[8,23,26] report an increased risk of surgically confirmed gallbladder disease in users of oral contraceptives and estrogens. In one study, an increased risk appeared after 2 years of use and doubled after 4 or 5 years of use. In one of the other studies, an increased risk was apparent between 6 and 12 months of use.

7. *Carbohydrate and Lipid Metabolic Effects:*
A decrease in glucose tolerance has been observed in a significant percentage of patients on oral contraceptives. For this reason, prediabetic and diabetic patients should be carefully observed while receiving oral contraceptives. An increase in triglycerides and total phospholipids has been observed in patients receiving oral contraceptives.[44] The clinical significance of this finding remains to be defined.

8. *Elevated Blood Pressure:*
An increase in blood pressure has been reported in patients receiving oral contraceptives.[26] In some women, hypertension may occur within a few months of beginning oral-contraceptive use. In the first year of use, the prevalence of women with hypertension is low in users and may be no higher than that of a comparable group of nonusers. The prevalence in users increases, however, with longer exposure, and in the fifth year of use is two-and-a-half to three times the reported prevalence in the first year. Age is also strongly correlated with the development of hypertension in oral-contraceptive users. Women who previously have had hypertension during pregnancy may be more likely to develop elevation of blood pressure when given oral contraceptives. Hypertension that develops as a result of taking oral contraceptives usually returns to normal after discontinuing the drug.

9. *Headache:*
The onset or exacerbation of migraine or development of headache of a new pattern which is recurrent, persistent, or severe, requires discontinuation of oral contraceptives and evaluation of the cause.

10. *Bleeding Irregularities:*
Breakthrough bleeding, spotting, and amenorrhea are frequent reasons for patients discontinuing oral contraceptives. In breakthrough bleeding, as in all cases of irregular bleeding from the vagina, nonfunctional causes should be borne in mind. In undiagnosed persistent or recurrent abnormal bleeding from the vagina, adequate diagnostic measures are indicated to rule out pregnancy or malignancy. If pathology has been excluded, time or a change to another formulation may solve the problem. Changing to an oral contraceptive with a higher estrogen content, while potentially useful in minimizing menstrual irregularity, should be done only if necessary, since this may increase the risk of thromboembolic disease.

Women with a past history of oligomenorrhea or secondary amenorrhea or young women without regular cycles may have a tendency to remain anovulatory or to become amenorrheic after discontinuation of oral contraceptives. Women with these preexisting problems should be advised of this possibility and encouraged to use other contraceptive methods. Post-use anovulation, possibly prolonged, may also occur in women without previous irregularities.

11. *Ectopic Pregnancy:*
Ectopic as well as intrauterine pregnancy may occur in contraceptive failures. However, in progestogen-only oral contraceptive failures, the ratio of ectopic to intrauterine pregnancies is higher than in women who are not receiving oral contraceptives, since the drugs are more effective in preventing intrauterine than ectopic pregnancies.

12. *Breast-feeding:*
Oral contraceptives given in the postpartum period may interfere with lactation. There may be a decrease in the quantity and quality of the breast milk. Furthermore, a small fraction of the hormonal agents in oral contraceptives has been identified in the milk of mothers receiving these drugs.[45,54,55] The effects, if any, on the breast-fed child have not been determined. If feasible, the use of oral contraceptives should be deferred until the infant has been weaned.

Precautions:

GENERAL

1. A complete medical and family history should be taken prior to initiation of oral contraceptives. The pretreatment and periodic physical examinations should include special reference to blood pressure, breasts, abdomen and pelvic organs, including Papanicolaou smear and relevant laboratory tests. As a general rule, oral contraceptives should not be prescribed for longer than 1 year without another physical examination being performed.
2. Under the influence of estrogen-progestogen preparations, preexisting uterine leiomyomata may increase in size.
3. Patients with a history of psychic depression should be carefully observed and the drug discontinued if depression recurs to a serious degree. Patients becoming significantly depressed while taking oral contraceptives should stop the medication and use an alternate method of contraception in an attempt to determine whether the symptom is drug-related.
4. Oral contraceptives may cause some degree of fluid retention. They should be prescribed with caution, and only with careful monitoring, in patients with conditions which might be aggravated by fluid retention, such as convulsive disorders, migraine syndrome, asthma, or cardiac or renal insufficiency.
5. Patients with a past history of jaundice during pregnancy have an increased risk of recurrence of jaundice while receiving oral-contraceptive therapy. If jaundice develops in any patient receiving such drugs, the medication should be discontinued.
6. Steroid hormones may be poorly metabolized in patients with impaired liver function and should be administered with caution in such patients.
7. Oral-contraceptive users may have disturbances in normal tryptophan metabolism which may result in a relative pyridoxine deficiency. The clinical significance of this is yet to be determined.
8. Serum folate levels may be depressed by oral-contraceptive therapy. Since the pregnant woman is predisposed to the development of folate deficiency and the incidence of folate deficiency increases with increasing gestation, it is possible that if a woman becomes pregnant shortly after stopping oral contraceptives, she may have a greater chance of developing folate deficiency and complications attributed to this deficiency.

INFORMATION FOR THE PATIENT
(See Patient Labeling Printed p. 2177)

LABORATORY TESTS

1. The pathologist should be advised of oral-contraceptive therapy when relevant specimens are submitted.
2. Certain endocrine- and liver-function tests and blood components may be affected by estrogen-containing oral contraceptives:
a. Increased sulfobromophthalein retention.
b. Increased prothrombin and factors VII, VIII, IX, and X; decreased antithrombin 3; increased norepinephrine-induced platelet aggregability.
c. Increased thyroid-binding globulin (TBG) leading to increased circulating total-thyroid hormone, as measured by protein-bound iodine (PBI), T4 by column, or T4 by radioimmunoassay. Free T3 resin uptake is decreased, reflecting the elevated TBG; free T4 concentration is unaltered.
d. Decreased pregnanediol excretion.
e. Reduced response to metyrapone test.

DRUG INTERACTIONS

Reduced efficacy and increased incidence of breakthrough bleeding have been associated with concomitant use of rifampin. A similar association has been suggested with barbiturates, phenylbutazone, phenytoin sodium, ampicillin, and tetracycline.

CARCINOGENESIS, MUTAGENESIS, IMPAIRMENT OF FERTILITY

Continued on next page

Wyeth—Cont.

See WARNINGS section #3, 4, and 5 for information on carcinogenesis, mutagenesis, and impairment of fertility.

PREGNANCY

Pregnancy category X. See Contraindications and Warnings.

NURSING MOTHERS

See WARNINGS. Because of the potential for adverse reactions in nursing infants from oral-contraceptive tablets, a decision should be made whether to discontinue the drug, taking into account the importance of the drug to the mother.

Adverse Reactions: An increased risk of the following serious adverse reactions has been associated with the use of oral contraceptives (see Warnings):

Thrombophlebitis
Pulmonary embolism.
Coronary thrombosis.
Cerebral thrombosis.
Cerebral hemorrhage.
Hypertension.
Gallbladder disease.
Benign hepatomas.
Congenital anomalies.

There is evidence of an association between the following conditions and the use of oral contraceptives, although additional confirmatory studies are needed:

Mesenteric thrombosis.
Neuro-ocular lesions, e.g., retinal thrombosis and optic neuritis.

The following adverse reactions have been reported in patients receiving oral contraceptives and are believed to be drug-related:

Nausea and/or vomiting, usually the most common adverse reactions, occur in approximately 10 percent or less of patients during the first cycle. Other reactions, as a general rule, are seen much less frequently or only occasionally.
Gastrointestinal symptoms (such as abdominal cramps and bloating).
Breakthrough bleeding.
Spotting.
Change in menstrual flow.
Dysmenorrhea.
Amenorrhea during and after treatment.
Temporary infertility after discontinuance of treatment.
Edema.
Chloasma or melasma which may persist.
Breast changes: tenderness, enlargement, and secretion.
Change in weight (increase or decrease).
Change in cervical erosion and cervical secretion.
Possible diminution in lactation when given immediately postpartum.
Cholestatic jaundice.
Migraine.
Increase in size of uterine leiomyomata.
Rash (allergic).
Mental depression.
Reduced tolerance to carbohydrates.
Vaginal candidiasis.
Change in corneal curvature (steepening).
Intolerance to contact lenses.

The following adverse reactions have been reported in users of oral contraceptives, and the association has been neither confirmed nor refuted:

Premenstrual-like syndrome.
Cataracts.
Changes in libido.
Chorea.
Changes in appetite.
Cystitis-like syndrome.
Headache.
Nervousness
Dizziness.
Hirsutism.
Loss of scalp hair.
Erythema multiforme.
Erythema nodosum.
Hemorrhagic eruption.
Vaginitis.
Porphyria.

Acute Overdose: Serious ill effects have not been reported following acute ingestion of large doses of oral contraceptives by young children. Overdosage may cause nausea, and withdrawal bleeding may occur in females.

Dosage and Administration: To achieve maximum contraceptive effectiveness, Nordette® must be taken exactly as directed and at intervals not exceeding 24 hours. The dosage of Nordette® is one tablet daily for 21 consecutive days per menstrual cycle according to prescribed schedule. Tablets are then discontinued for 7 days (three weeks on, one week off). It is recommended that Nordette® tablets be taken at the same time each day, preferably after the evening meal or at bedtime.

During the first cycle of medication, the patient is instructed to take one Nordette® tablet daily for twenty-one consecutive days beginning on day five of her menstrual cycle. (The first day of menstruation is day one.) The tablets are then discontinued for one week (7 days). Withdrawal bleeding should usually occur within three days following discontinuation of Nordette®.

(If Nordette® is first taken later than the fifth day of the first menstrual cycle of medication or postpartum, contraceptive reliance should not be placed on Nordette® until after the first seven consecutive days of administration. The possibility of ovulation and conception prior to initiation of medication should be considered.)

The patient begins her next and all subsequent 21-day courses of Nordette® tablets on the same day of the week that she began her first course, following the same schedule: 21 days on—7 days off.

She begins taking her tablets on the 8th day after discontinuance regardless of whether or not a menstrual period has occurred or is still in progress. Any time a new cycle of Nordette® is started later than the 8th day the patient should be protected by another means of contraception until she has taken a tablet daily for seven consecutive days.

If spotting or breakthrough bleeding occurs, the patient is instructed to continue on the same regimen. This type of bleeding is usually transient and without significance; however, if the bleeding is persistent or prolonged the patient is advised to consult her physician. Although the occurrence of pregnancy is highly unlikely if Nordette® is taken according to directions, if withdrawal bleeding does not occur, the possibility of pregnancy must be considered. If the patient has not adhered to the prescribed schedule (missed one or more tablets or started taking them on a day later than she should have) the probability of pregnancy should be considered at the time of the first missed period and appropriate diagnostic measures taken before the medication is resumed. If the patient has adhered to the prescribed regimen and misses two consecutive periods, pregnancy should be ruled out before continuing the contraceptive regimen.

The patient should be instructed to take a missed tablet as soon as it is remembered. If two consecutive tablets are missed they should both be taken as soon as remembered. The next tablet should be taken at the usual time.

Any time the patient misses one or two tablets she should also use another method of contraception until she has taken a tablet daily for seven consecutive days. If breakthrough bleeding occurs following missed tablets it will usually be transient and of no consequence. While there is little likelihood of ovulation occurring if only one or two tablets are missed, the possibility of ovulation increases with each successive day that scheduled tablets are missed. If three consecutive tablets are missed, all medication should be discontinued and the remainder of the package discarded. A new tablet cycle should be started on the 8th day after the last tablet was taken, and an alternate means of contraception should be prescribed during the seven days without tablets and until the patient has taken a tablet daily for seven consecutive days. In the nonlactating mother Nordette® may be prescribed in the postpartum period either immediately or at the first postpartum examination whether or not menstruation has resumed.

How Supplied: Nordette® Tablets (0.15 mg levonorgestrel + 0.03 mg ethinyl estradiol tablets), Wyeth®, are available in Pilpak® dispensers of 21 tablets: NDC 0008-0075, light-orange, round tablet marked "WYETH" and "75".

References:

1. "*Population Reports,*" Series H, Number 2, May 1974; Series I, Number 1, June 1974; Series B, Number 2, January 1975; Series H, Number 3, 1975; Series H, Number 4, January 1976 (published by the Population Information Program, The George Washington University Medical Center, 2001 S St. NW., Washington, D.C.).
2. Inman, W. H. W., Vessey, M. P., Westerholm, B., and Engelund, A., "Thromboembolic disease and the steroidal content of oral contraceptives. A report to the Committee on Safety of Drugs," Brit Med J *2:*203-209, 1970.
3. Stolley, P. D., Tonascia, J. A., Tockman, M. S., Sartwell, P. E., Rutledge, A. H., and Jacobs, M. P., "Thrombosis with low-estrogen oral contraceptives," Am J Epidemiol *102:*197-208, 1975.
4. Royal College of General Practitioners, "Oral contraception and thromboembolic disease," J Coll Gen Pract *13:*267-279, 1967.
5. Inman, W. H. W., and Vessey, M. P., "Investigation of deaths from pulmonary, coronary and cerebral thrombosis and embolism in women of childbearing age," Brit Med J *2:*193-199, 1968.
6. Vessey, M. P., and Doll, R., "Investigation of relation between use of oral contraceptives and thromboembolic disease. A further report," Brit Med J *2:*651-657, 1969.
7. Sartwell, P. E., Masi, A. T., Arthes, F. G., Greene, G. R., and Smith, H. E., "Thromboembolism and oral contraceptives: an epidemiological case control study," Am J Epidemiol *90:*365-380, 1969.
8. Boston Collaborative Drug Surveillance Program, "Oral contraceptives and venous thromboembolic disease, surgically confirmed gallbladder disease and breast tumors," Lancet *1:*1399-1404, 1973.
9. Collaborative Group for the Study of Stroke in Young Women, "Oral contraception and increased risk of cerebral ischemia or thrombosis," N Engl J Med *288:*871–878, 1973.
10. Collaborative Group for the Study of Stroke in Young Women, "Oral contraceptives and stroke in young women: associated risk factors," JAMA *231:*718-722, 1975.
11. Mann, J. I., and Inman, W. H. W., "Oral contraceptives and death from myocardial infarction," Brit Med J *2:*245-248, 1975.
12. Mann, J. I., Inman, W. H. W., and Thorogood, M., "Oral contraceptive use in older women and fatal myocardial infarction," Brit Med J *2:*445-447, 1976.
13. Mann, J. I., Vessey, M. P., Thorogood, M., and Doll, R., "Myocardial infarction in young women with special reference to oral contraceptive practice," Brit Med J *2:*241-245, 1975.
14. Tietze, C., "New Estimates of Mortality Associated with Fertility Control," Family Planning Perspectives, *9:*74-76, 1977.
15. Vessey, M. P., Doll, R., Fairbairn, A. S., and Glober, G., "Post-operative thromboembolism and the use of oral contraceptives," Brit Med J *3:*123-126, 1970.
16. Greene, G. R., Sartwell, P. E., "Oral contraceptive use in patients with thromboembolism following surgery, trauma, or infection," Am J Pub Health *62:*680-685, 1972.

17. Smith, D. C., Prentice, R., Thompson, D. J., and Herrmann, W. L., "Association of exogenous estrogen and endometrial carcinoma," N Engl J Med *293:*1164-1167, 1975.
18. Ziel, H. K., and Finkle, W. D., "Increased risk of endometrial carcinoma among users of conjugated estrogens," N Engl J Med *293:*1167-1170, 1975.
19. Mack, T. N., Pike, M. C., Henderson, B. E., Pfeffer, R. I., Gerkins, V. R., Arthur, M., and Brown, S. E., "Estrogens and endometrial cancer in a retirement community," N Engl J Med *294:*1262-1267, 1976.
20. Silverberg, S. G., and Makowski, E. L., "Endometrial carcinoma in young women taking oral contraceptive agents," Obstet Gynecol *46:*503-506, 1975.
21. Vessey, M. P., Doll, R., and Sutton, P. M., "Oral contraceptives and breast neoplasia: a retrospective study," Brit Med J *3:*719-724, 1972.
22. Vessey, M. P., Doll, R., and Jones K., "Oral contraceptives and breast cancer. Progress report of an epidemiological study," Lancet *1:*941-943, 1975.
23. Boston Collaborative Drug Surveillance Program, "Surgically confirmed gallbladder disease, venous thromboembolism and breast tumors in relation to postmenopausal estrogen therapy," N Engl J Med *290:*15-19, 1974.
24. Arthes, F. G., Sartwell, P. E., and Lewison, E. F., "The pill, estrogens, and the breast. Epidemiologic aspects," Cancer *28:*1391-1394, 1971.
25. Fasal, E., and Paffenbarger, R. S., "Oral contraceptives as related to cancer and benign lesions of the breast," J Natl Cancer Inst *55:*767-773, 1975.
26. Royal College of General Practitioners, "Oral Contraceptives and Health," London, Pitman, 1974.
27. Ory, H., Cole, P., MacMahon, B., and Hoover, R., "Oral contraceptives and reduced risk of benign breast diseases," N Engl J Med *294:*419-422, 1976.
28. Baum, J., Holtz, F., Bookstein, J. J., and Klein, E. W., "Possible association between benign hepatomas and oral contraceptives," Lancet *2:*926-928, 1973.
29. Mays, E. T., Christopherson, W. M., Mahr, M. M., and Williams, H. C., "Hepatic changes in young women ingesting contraceptive steroids. Hepatic hemorrhage and primary hepatic tumors," JAMA *235:*730-732, 1976.
30. Edmondson, H. A., Henderson, B., and Benton, B., "Liver-cell adenomas associated with use of oral contraceptives," N Engl J Med *294:*470-472, 1976.
31. Herbst, A. L., Ulfedler, H., and Poskanzer, D. C., "Adenocarcinoma of the vagina," N Engl J Med *284:*878-881, 1971.
32. Greenwald, P., Barlow, J. J., Nasca, P. C., and Burnett, W., "Vaginal cancer after maternal treatment with synthetic estrogens," N Engl J Med *285:*390-392, 1971.
33. Lanier, A. P., Noller, K. L., Decker, D. G., Elveback, L., and Kurland, L. T., "Cancer and stilbestrol. A follow-up of 1719 persons exposed to estrogens in utero and born 1943-1959," Mayo Clin Pro *48:*793-799, 1973.
34. Herbst, A. L., Kurman, R. J., and Scully, R. E., "Vaginal and cervical abnormalities after exposure to stilbestrol in utero," Obstet Gynecol *40:*287-298, 1972.
35. Herbst, A. L. Robboy, S. J., Macdonald, G. J., and Scully, R. E., "The effects of local progesterone on stilbestrol-associated vaginal adenosis." Am J Obstet Gynecol *118:*607:615, 1974.
36. Herbst, A. L., Poskanzer, D. C., Robboy, S. J., Friedlander, L., and Scully, R. E., "Prenatal exposure to stilbestrol: a prospective comparison of exposed female offspring with unexposed controls," N Engl J Med *292:*334-339, 1975.
37. Stafl, A., Mattingly, R. F., Foley, D. V., Fetherston, W., "Clinical diagnosis of vaginal adenosis," Obstet Gynecol *43:*118-128, 1974.
38. Sherman, A. I., Goldrath, M., Berlin, A., Vakhariya, V., Banooni, F., Michaels, W., Goodman, P., and Brown S., "Cervical-vaginal adenosis after in utero exposure to synthetic estrogens," Obstet Gynecol *44:*531-545, 1974.
39. Gal, I., Kirman, B., and Stern, J., "Hormone pregnancy tests and congenital malformation," Nature *216:*83, 1967.
40. Levy, E. P., Cohen, A., and Fraser, F. C., "Hormone treatment during pregnancy and congenital heart defects," Lancet *1:*611, 1973.
41. Nora, J. J., and Nora, A. H., "Birth defects and oral contraceptives," Lancet *1:*941-942, 1973.
42. Janerich, D. T., Piper, J. M., and Glebatis, D. M., "Oral contraceptives and congenital limb-reduction defects," N Engl J Med *291:*697-700, 1974.
43. Carr, D. H., "Chromosome studies in selected spontaneous abortions: I. Conception after oral contraceptives," Canad Med Assoc J *103:*343-348, 1970.
44. Wynn, V., Doar, J. W. H., and Mills, G. L., "Some effects of oral contraceptives on serum-lipid and lipoprotein levels," Lancet *2:*720-723, 1966.
45. Laumas, K. R., Malkani, P. K., Bhatnagar, S., and Laumas, V., "Radioactivity in the breast milk of lactating women after oral administration of 3 H-norethynodrel," Amer J Obstet Gynecol *98:*411-413, 1967.
46. Center for Disease Control, "Increased Risk of Hepatocellular Adenoma in Women with Long-term use of Oral Contraceptives," Morbidity and Mortality Weekly Report, *26:*293-294, 1977.
47. Herbst, A. L., Cole, P., Colton, T., Robboy, S. J., Scully, R. E., "Age-incidence and Risk of Diethylstilbestrol-related Clear Cell Adenocarcinoma of the Vagina and Cervix," Am J Obstet Gynecol, *128:*43-50, 1977.
48. Bibbo, M., Al-Naqeeb, M., Baccarini, I., Gill, W., Newton, M., Sleeper, K. M., Sonek, M., Wied, G. L., "Follow-up Study of Male and Female Offspring of DES-treated Mothers. A Preliminary Report," Jour of Repro Med, *15:*29-32, 1975.
49. Gill, W. B., Schumacher, G. F. B., Bibbo, M., "Structural and Functional Abnormalities in the Sex Organs or Male Offspring of Mothers Treated with Diethylstilbestrol (DES)," Jour of Repro Med, *16:*147-153, 1976.
50. Henderson, B. E., Senton, B., Cosgrove, M., Baptista, J., Aldrich, J., Townsend, D., Hart, W., Mack, T., "Urogenital Tract Abnormalities in Sons of Women Treated with Diethylstilbestrol," Pediatrics, *58:*505-507, 1976.
51. Heinonen, O. P., Slone, D., Nonson, R. R., Hook, E. B., Shapiro, S., "Cardiovascular Birth Defects and Antenatal Exposure to Female Sex Hormones," N Engl J Med *296:*67-70, 1977.
52. Jain, A. K., "Mortality Risk Associated with the Use of Oral Contraceptives," Studies in Family Planning, *8:*50-54, 1977.
53. Beral, V., "Mortality Among Oral Contraceptive Users," Lancet, *2:*727-731, 1977.
54. Nilsson, S., Nygren, K., and Johansson, E., "Ethinyl Estradiol in Human Milk and Plasma after Oral Administration," Contraception *17:*131-139, 1978.
55. Nilsson, S., Nygren, K., and Johansson, E., "d-Norgestrel Concentrations in Maternal Plasma, Milk and Child Plasma During Administration of Oral Contraceptives to Nursing Women," Am J Obstet Gynecol, *129:*178, 1977.

The patient labeling for oral-contraceptive drug products is set forth below:

Brief Summary Patient Package Insert

Cigarette smoking increases the risk of serious adverse effects on the heart and blood vessels from oral-contraceptive use. This risk increases with age and with heavy smoking (15 or more cigarettes per day) and is quite marked in women over 35 years of age. Women who use oral contraceptives should not smoke.

Oral contraceptives taken as directed are about 99% effective in preventing pregnancy. (The mini-pill, however, is somewhat less effective.) Forgetting to take your pills increases the chance of pregnancy. Women who have or have had clotting disorders, cancer of the breast or sex organs, unexplained vaginal bleeding, a stroke, heart attack, angina pectoris, or who suspect they may be pregnant should not use oral contraceptives. Various drugs, such as some antibiotics, may also decrease the effectiveness of oral contraceptives.

Most side effects of the pill are not serious. The most common side effects are nausea, vomiting, bleeding between menstrual periods, weight gain, and breast tenderness. However, proper use of oral contraceptives requires that they be taken under your doctor's continuous supervision, because they can be associated with serious side effects which may be fatal. Fortunately, these occur very infrequently. The serious side effects are:

1. Blood clots in the legs, lungs, brain, heart, or other organs, and hemorrhage into the brain due to bursting of a blood vessel.
2. Liver tumors, which may rupture and cause severe bleeding.
3. Birth defects if the pill is taken while you are pregnant.
4. High blood pressure.
5. Gallbladder disease.

The symptoms associated with these serious side effects are discussed in the detailed leaflet given you with your supply of pills. Notify your doctor if you notice any unusual physical disturbance while taking the pill.

The estrogen in oral contraceptives has been found to cause breast cancer and other cancers in certain animals. These findings suggest that oral contraceptives may also cause cancer in humans. However, studies to date in women taking currently marketed oral contraceptives have not confirmed that oral contraceptives cause cancer in humans.

The detailed leaflet describes more completely the benefits and risks of oral contraceptives. It also provides information on other forms of contraception. Read it carefully. If you have any questions, consult your doctor.

Caution: Oral contraceptives are of no value in the prevention or treatment of venereal disease.

DETAILED PATIENT LABELING

WHAT YOU SHOULD KNOW ABOUT ORAL CONTRACEPTIVES

Oral contraceptives ("the pill") are the most effective way (except for sterilization) to prevent pregnancy. They are also convenient and, for most women, free of serious or unpleasant side effects. Oral contraceptives must always be taken under the continuous supervision of a physician.

It is important that any woman who considers using an oral contraceptive understand the risks involved. Although the oral contraceptives have important advantages over other methods of contraception, they have certain risks that no other method has. Only you can decide whether the advantages are worth these risks. This leaflet will tell you about the most important risks. It will explain how you can help your doctor prescribe the pill as safely as possible by telling him about yourself and being alert for the earliest signs of trouble. And it will tell you how to use the pill properly, so that it will be as effective as possible. There is more detailed information available in the leaflet prepared for doctors. Your pharmacist can show you a copy; you may need your doctor's help in understanding parts of it.

WHO SHOULD NOT USE ORAL CONTRACEPTIVES

Continued on next page

Wyeth—Cont.

A. If you have any of the following conditions, you should not use the pill:
1. Clots in the legs or lungs.
2. Angina pectoris.
3. Known or suspected cancer of the breast or sex organs.
4. Unusual vaginal bleeding that has not yet been diagnosed.
5. Known or suspected pregnancy.

B. If you have had any of the following conditions, you should not use the pill:
1. Heart attack or stroke.
2. Clots in the legs or lungs.

C. Cigarette smoking increases the risk of serious adverse effects on the heart and blood vessels from oral-contraceptive use. This risk increases with age and with heavy smoking (15 or more cigarettes per day) and is quite marked in women over 35 years of age. Women who use oral contraceptives should not smoke.

D. If you have scanty or irregular periods or are a young woman without a regular cycle, you should use another method of contraception because, if you use the pill, you may have difficulty becoming pregnant or may fail to have menstrual periods after discontinuing the pill.

DECIDING TO USE ORAL CONTRACEPTIVES

If you do not have any of the conditions listed above and are thinking about using oral contraceptives, to help you decide, you need information about the advantages and risks of oral contraceptives and of other contraceptive methods as well. This leaflet describes the advantages and risks of oral contraceptives. Except for sterilization, the IUD, and abortion, which have their own exclusive risks, the only risks of other methods of contraception are those due to pregnancy should the method fail. Your doctor can answer questions you may have with respect to other methods of contraception. He can also answer any questions you may have after reading this leaflet on oral contraceptives.

1. What Oral Contraceptives Are and How They Work. Oral contraceptives are of two types. The most common, often simply called "the pill," is a combination of an estrogen and a progestogen, the two kinds of female hormones. The amount of estrogen and progestogen can vary, but the amount of estrogen is most important because both the effectiveness and some of the dangers of oral contraceptives are related to the amount of estrogen. This kind of oral contraceptive works principally by preventing release of an egg from the ovary. When the amount of estrogen is 50 micrograms or more, and the pill is taken as directed, oral contraceptives are more than 99% effective (i.e., there would be less than 1 pregnancy if 100 women used the pill for 1 year). Pills that contain 20 to 35 micrograms of estrogen vary slightly in effectiveness, ranging from 98% to more than 99% effective.

The second type of oral contraceptive, often called the "mini-pill", contains only a progestogen. It works in part by preventing release of an egg from the ovary but also by keeping sperm from reaching the egg and by making the uterus (womb) less receptive to any fertilized egg that reaches it. The mini-pill is less effective than the combination oral contraceptive, about 97% effective. In addition, the progestogen-only pill has a tendency to cause irregular bleeding which may be quite inconvenient, or cessation of bleeding entirely. The progestogen-only pill is used despite its lower effectiveness in the hope that it will prove not to have some of the serious side effects of the estrogen-containing pill (see below), but it is not yet certain that the mini-pill does in fact have fewer serious side effects. The discussion below, while based mainly on information about the combination pills, should be considered to apply as well to the mini-pill.

2. Other Nonsurgical Ways to Prevent Pregnancy. As this leaflet will explain, oral contraceptives have several serious risks. Other methods of contraception have lesser risks or none at all. They are also less effective than oral contraceptives, but, used properly, may be effective enough for many women.

The following table gives reported pregnancy rates (the number of women out of 100 who would become pregnant in 1 year) for these methods.

PREGNANCIES PER 100 WOMEN PER YEAR

Intrauterine device (IUD), less than 1–6; Diaphragm with spermicidal products (creams or jellies), 2–20; Condom (rubber), 3–36; Aerosol foams; 2–29; Jellies and creams, 4–36;

Periodic abstinence (rhythm) all types, less than 1–47:
1. Calendar method, 14–47;
2. Temperature method, 1–20;
3. Temperature method—intercourse only in postovulatory phase, less than 1–7;
4. Mucus method, 1–25;

No contraception, 60–80.

The figures (except for the IUD) vary widely because people differ in how well they use each method. Very faithful users of the various methods obtain very good results, except for users of the calendar method of periodic abstinence (rhythm). Except for the IUD, effective use of these methods requires somewhat more effort than simply taking a single pill every day, but it is an effort that many couples undertake successfully. Your doctor can tell you a great deal more about these methods of contraception.

3. The Dangers of Oral Contraceptives.

a. *Circulatory disorders (abnormal blood clotting and stroke due to hemorrhage).*

Blood clots (in various blood vessels of the body) are the most common of the serious side effects of oral contraceptives. A clot can result in a stroke (if the clot is in the brain), a heart attack (if the clot is in a blood vessel of the heart), or a pulmonary embolus (a clot which forms in the legs or pelvis, then breaks off and travels to the lungs). Any of these can be fatal. Clots also occur rarely in the blood vessels of the eye, resulting in blindness or impairment of vision in that eye. There is evidence that the risk of clotting increases with higher estrogen doses. It is therefore important to keep the dose of estrogen as low as possible, so long as the oral contraceptive used has an acceptable pregnancy rate and doesn't cause unacceptable changes in the menstrual pattern. Furthermore, cigarette smoking by oral-contraceptive users increases the risk of serious adverse effects on the heart and blood vessels. This risk increases with age and with heavy smoking (15 or more cigarettes per day) and begins to become quite marked in women over 35 years of age. For this reason, women who use oral contraceptives should not smoke. The risk of abnormal clotting increases with age in both users and nonusers of oral contraceptives, but the increased risk from the contraceptive appears to be present at all ages. For oral-contraceptive users in general, it has been estimated that in women between the ages of 15 and 34 the risk of death due to a circulatory disorder is about 1 in 12,000 per year, whereas for nonusers the rate is about 1 in 50,000 per year. In the age group 35 to 44, the risk is estimated to be about 1 in 2,500 per year for oral-contraceptive users and about 1 in 10,000 per year for nonusers.

Even without the pill the risk of having a heart attack increases with age and is also increased by such heart attack risk factors as high blood pressure, high cholesterol, obesity, diabetes, and cigarette smoking. Without any risk factors present, the use of oral contraceptives alone may double the risk of heart attack. However, the combination of cigarette smoking, especially heavy smoking, and oral-contraceptive use greatly increases the risk of heart attack. Oral-contraceptive users who smoke are about 5 times more likely to have a heart attack than users who do not smoke and about 10 times more likely to have a heart attack than nonusers who do not smoke. It has been estimated that users between the ages of 30 and 39 who smoke have about a 1 in 10,000 chance each year of having a fatal heart attack compared to about a 1 in 50,000 chance in users who do not smoke, and about a 1 in 100,000 chance in nonusers who do not smoke. In the age group 40 to 44, the risk is about 1 in 1,700 per year for users who smoke compared to about 1 in 10,000 for users who do not smoke and to about 1 in 14,000 per year for nonusers who do not smoke. Heavy smoking (about 15 cigarettes or more a day) further increases the risk. If you do not smoke and have none of the other heart attack risk factors described above, you will have a smaller risk than listed. If you have several heart attack risk factors, the risk may be considerably greater than listed.

In addition to blood-clotting disorders, it has been estimated that women taking oral contraceptives are twice as likely as nonusers to have a stroke due to rupture of a blood vessel in the brain.

Figure 1. Estimated annual number of deaths associated with control of fertility and no control per 100,000 nonsterile women, by regimen of control and age of woman.

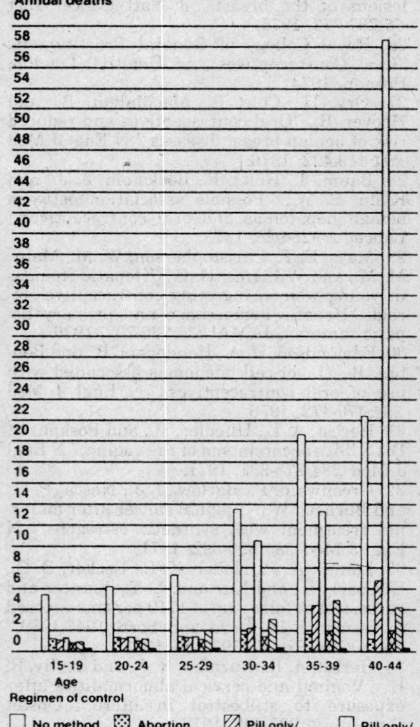

b. *Formation of tumors.* Studies have found that when certain animals are given the female sex hormone, estrogen, which is an ingredient of oral contraceptives, continuously for long periods, cancers may develop in the breast, cervix, vagina, and liver.

These findings suggest that oral contraceptives may cause cancer in humans. However, studies to date in women taking currently marketed oral contraceptives have not confirmed that oral contraceptives cause cancer in humans. Several studies have found no increase in breast cancer in users, although one study suggested oral contraceptives might cause an increase in breast cancer in women who already have benign breast disease (e.g., cysts).

Women with a strong family history of breast cancer or who have breast nodules, fibrocystic disease, or abnormal mammograms or who were exposed to DES (Diethylstilbestrol), an estrogen, during their mother's pregnancy must be followed very closely by their doctors if they choose to use oral contraceptives instead of another method of contraception. Many studies have shown that women taking oral contraceptives have less risk of getting benign breast disease than those who have not used oral contraceptives. Recently, strong evidence has emerged that estrogens (one component of oral contraceptives), when given for periods of more than one year to women after the menopause, increase the risk of cancer of the uterus (womb). There is also some evidence that a kind of oral contraceptive which is no longer marketed, the sequential oral contraceptive, may increase the risk of cancer of the uterus. There remains no evidence, however, that the oral contraceptives now available increase the risk of this cancer. Oral contraceptives do cause, although rarely, a benign (nonmalignant) tumor of the liver. These tumors do not spread, but they may rupture and cause internal bleeding, which may be fatal. A few cases of cancer of the liver have been reported in women using oral contraceptives, but it is not yet known whether the drug caused them.

c. *Dangers to a developing child if oral contraceptives are used in or immediately preceding pregnancy.* Oral contraceptives should not be taken by pregnant women because they may damage the developing child. An increased risk of birth defects, including heart defects and limb defects, has been associated with the use of sex hormones, including oral contraceptives, in pregnancy. In addition, the developing female child whose mother has received DES (diethylstilbestrol), an estrogen, during pregnancy has a risk of getting cancer of the vagina or cervix in her teens or young adulthood. This risk is estimated to be about 1 in 1,000 exposures or less. Abnormalities of the urinary and sex organs have been reported in male offspring so exposed. It is possible that other estrogens, such as the estrogens in oral contraceptives, could have the same effect in the child if the mother takes them during pregnancy.

If you stop taking oral contraceptives to become pregnant, your doctor may recommend that you use another method of contraception for a short while. The reason for this is that there is evidence from studies in women who have had "miscarriages" soon after stopping the pill, that the lost fetuses are more likely to be abnormal. Whether there is an overall increase in "miscarriage" in women who become pregnant soon after stopping the pill as compared with women who do not use the pill is now known, but it is possible that there may be.

If, however, you do become pregnant soon after stopping oral contraceptives, and do not have a miscarriage, there is no evidence that the baby has an increased risk of being abnormal.

d. *Gallbladder disease.* Women who use oral contraceptives have a greater risk than nonusers of having gallbladder disease requiring surgery. The increased risk may first appear within 1 year of use and may double after 4 or 5 years of use.

e. *Other side effects of oral contraceptives.* Some women using oral contraceptives experience unpleasant side effects that are not dangerous and are not likely to damage their health. Some of these may be temporary. Your breasts may feel tender, nausea and vomiting may occur, you may gain or lose weight, and your ankles may swell. A spotty darkening of the skin, particularly of the face, is possible and may persist. You may notice unexpected vaginal bleeding or changes in your menstrual period. Irregular bleeding is frequently seen when using the mini-pill or combination oral contraceptives containing less that 50 micrograms of estrogen.

More serious side effects include worsening of migraine, asthma, epilepsy, and kidney or heart disease because of a tendency for water to be retained in the body when oral contraceptives are used. Other side effects are growth of preexisting fibroid tumors of the uterus; mental depression; and liver problems with jaundice (yellowing of the skin). Your doctor may find that levels of sugar and fatty substances in your blood are elevated; the long-term effects of these changes are not known. Some women develop high blood pressure while taking oral contraceptives, which ordinarily returns to the original levels when the oral contraceptive is stopped.

Other reactions, although not proved to be caused by oral contraceptives, are occasionally reported. These include more frequent urination and some discomfort when urinating, nervousness, dizziness, some loss of scalp hair, an increase in body hair, an increase or decrease in sex drive, appetite changes, cataracts, and a need for a change in contact lens prescription, or inability to use contact lenses.

After you stop using oral contraceptives, there may be a delay before you are able to become pregnant or before you resume having menstrual periods. This is especially true of women who had irregular menstrual cycles prior to the use of oral contraceptives. As discussed previously, your doctor may recommend that you wait a short while after stopping the pill before you try to become pregnant.

During this time, use another form of contraception. You should consult your physician before resuming use of oral contraceptives after childbirth, especially if you plan to nurse your baby. Drugs in oral contraceptives are known to appear in the milk, and the long-range effect on infants is not known at this time. Furthermore, oral contraceptives may cause a decrease in your milk supply as well as in the quality of the milk.

4. Comparison of the Risks of Oral Contraceptives and Other Contraceptive Methods. The many studies on the risks and effectiveness of oral contraceptives and other methods of contraception have been analyzed to estimate the risk of death associated with various methods of contraception. This risk has two parts: (a) the risk of the method itself (e.g., the risk that oral contraceptives will cause death due to abnormal clotting), and (b) the risk of death due to pregnancy or abortion in the event the method fails. The results of this analysis are shown in the bar graph below. The height of the bars is the number of deaths per 100,000 women each year. There are six sets of bars, each set referring to a specific age group of women. Within each set of bars, there is a single bar for each of the different contraceptive methods. For oral contraceptives, there are two bars—one for smokers and the other for nonsmokers. The analysis is based on present knowledge, and new information could, of course, alter it. The analysis shows that the risk of death from all methods of birth control is low and below that associated with childbirth, except for oral contraceptives in women over 40 who smoke. It shows that the lowest risk of death is associated with the condom or diaphragm (traditional contraception) backed up by early abortion in case of failure of the condom or diaphragm to prevent pregnancy. Also, at any age the risk of death (due to unexpected pregnancy) from the use of traditional contraception, even without a backup of abortion, is generally the same as or less than that from use of oral contraceptives.

HOW TO USE ORAL CONTRACEPTIVES AS SAFELY AND EFFECTIVELY AS POSSIBLE, ONCE YOU HAVE DECIDED TO USE THEM

1. What to Tell your Doctor.

You can make use of the pill as safely as possible by telling your doctor if you have any of the following:

a. Conditions that mean you should not use oral contraceptives:
   - Clots in the legs or lungs.
   - Clots in the legs or lungs in the past.
   - A stroke, heart attack, or angina pectoris.
   - Known or suspected cancer of the breast or sex organs.
   - Unusual vaginal bleeding that has not yet been diagnosed.
   - Known or suspected pregnancy.

b. Conditions that your doctor will want to watch closely or which might cause him to suggest another method of contraception:
   - A family history of breast cancer.
   - Breast nodules, fibrocystic disease of the breast, or an abnormal mammogram.

Diabetes.	Heart or kidney disease.
High blood pressure.	Epilepsy.
High cholesterol.	Mental depression.
Cigarette smoking.	Fibroid tumors of the uterus.
Migraine headaches.	Gallbladder disease.

c. Once you are using oral contraceptives, you should be alert for signs of a serious adverse effect and call your doctor if they occur:
   - Sharp pain in the chest, coughing blood, or sudden shortness of breath (indicating possible clots in the lungs).
   - Pain in the calf (possible clot in the leg).
   - Crushing chest pain or heaviness (indicating possible heart attack).
   - Sudden severe headache or vomiting, dizziness or fainting, disturbance of vision or speech, or weakness or numbness in an arm or leg (indicating a possible stroke).
   - Sudden partial or complete loss of vision (indicating a possible clot in the eye).
   - Breast lumps (you should ask your doctor to show you how to examine your own breasts).
   - Severe pain in the abdomen (indicating a possible ruptured tumor of the liver).
   - Severe depression.
   - Yellowing of the skin (jaundice).

2. How to Take the Pill So That It is Most Effective.

Reduced effectiveness and an increased incidence of breakthrough bleeding have been associated with the use of oral contraceptives with antibiotics such as rifampin, ampicillin, and tetracycline or with certain other drugs such as barbiturates, phenylbutazone or phenytoin sodium. You should use an additional means of contraception during any cycle in which any of these drugs are taken.

To achieve maximum contraceptive effectiveness, oral contraceptives must be taken exactly as directed and at intervals not exceeding 24 hours. It is recommended that tablets be taken at the same time each day, preferably after the evening meal or at bedtime. Taking them on a definite schedule will decrease the chance of forgetting a tablet and also help keep the proper amount of medication in your system. See detailed instructions below for Nordette®, Ovral® and Lo/Ovral®, Nordette®-28, Ovral®-28 and Lo/Ovral®-28, and for Ovrette®.

NORDETTE®, OVRAL®, LO/OVRAL®

The dosage of Nordette®, Ovral® and Lo/Ovral® is one tablet daily for 21 days in a row per menstrual cycle. Tablets are then discontinued for 7 days. The basic schedule is 21 days on —7 days off.

During the first month, you should begin taking Nordette®, Ovral® or Lo/Ovral® on Day 5 of your menstrual cycle whether or not you still have your period. (Day 1 is the first day of menstruation, even if it is almost midnight

Continued on next page

Wyeth—Cont.

when you start.) Note: During your first month on Nordette®, Ovral® or Lo/Ovral®, if you start taking tablets later than Day 5 of your menstrual cycle, you should protect yourself by also using another method of birth control until you have taken a tablet daily for seven consecutive days. Thereafter, if you follow directions carefully you will obtain the full contraceptive benefit. If you begin taking tablets later than the proper day, the possibility of ovulation and pregnancy occurring before beginning medication should be considered.

Take one tablet every day until you finish all 21 tablets. No tablets are then taken for one week (7 days). Your period will usually begin about three days after you take the last tablet. Don't be alarmed if the amount of bleeding is not the same as before. On the 8th day, start a new Pilpak®, even if you still have your period. If, for example, you took Nordette®, Ovral® or Lo/Ovral® for the first time on a Tuesday, the 8th day will also be a Tuesday. Thus, you will always begin a new cycle on the same day of the week as long as you do not interrupt your original schedule. If you start taking tablets later than the 8th day, you should protect yourself by also using another method of birth control until you have taken a tablet daily for seven days in a row.

NORDETTE®-28, OVRAL®-28, LO/OVRAL®-28

The dosage of Nordette®-28, Ovral®-28 and Lo/Ovral®-28 is one white or light-orange active tablet daily for 21 consecutive days followed by one pink inactive tablet daily for 7 consecutive days. The basic schedule is 21 days on white or light-orange active tablets—7 days on pink inactive tablets. Always take all 21 white or light-orange tablets in each Pilpak® before taking the pink tablets.

You should begin taking Nordette®-28, Ovral®-28 or Lo/Ovral®-28 on the first Sunday after your menstrual period begins, whether or not you are still bleeding. If your period begins on a Sunday, take your first tablet that very same day. Your first white or light-orange tablet is marked with a large arrow and the word "Start". Note: During your first month on Nordette®-28, Ovral®-28 or Lo/Ovral®-28, you should protect yourself by also using another method of birth control until you have taken a white or light-orange tablet daily for seven consecutive days. Thereafter, if you follow directions carefully, you will obtain the full contraceptive benefit. If you begin taking tablets later than the proper day, the possibility of ovulation and pregnancy occurring before beginning medication should be considered. Take one tablet every day until you finish all 21 white or light-orange tablets in a Pilpak®, followed by all seven pink tablets. Your period will usually begin about three days after you take the last white or light-orange tablet, which will be during the time you are taking the pink tablets. Don't be alarmed if the amount of bleeding is not the same as before. The day after you have taken your last pink tablet, begin a new Pilpak® of tablets (taking all 21 white or light-orange tablets first, just as you did before) so that you will take a tablet every day without interruption. The starting day for each new Pilpak® will always be Sunday. If in any cycle you start tablets later than the proper day, you should also use another method of birth control until you have taken a white or light-orange tablet daily for 7 days in a row.

Spotting or Breakthrough Bleeding:

Spotting is slight staining between menstrual periods which may not even require a pad. Breakthrough bleeding is a flow much like a regular period, requiring sanitary protection. Spotting is more common than breakthrough bleeding, and both occur more often in the first few cycles than in later cycles. These types of bleeding are usually temporary and without significance. It is important to continue taking your pills on schedule. If the bleeding persists for more than a few days, consult your doctor.

Forgotten Pills:

Nordette®, Ovral® and Lo/Ovral® each contain 21 active white or light-orange tablets per Pilpak®. Nordette®-28, Ovral®-28 and Lo/Ovral®-28 each contain 21 active white or light-orange tablets plus 7 pink inactive tablets per Pilpak®.

The chance of becoming pregnant is probably quite small if you miss only one white or light-orange tablet in a cycle. Of course, with each additional one you skip, the chance increases. If you miss one or more pink tablets (Nordette®-28, Ovral®-28, Lo/Ovral®-28) you are still protected against pregnancy as long as you begin taking your next white or light-orange tablet on the proper day. It is important to take a missed white or light-orange tablet as soon as it is remembered. If two consecutive white or light-orange tablets are missed they should both be taken as soon as remembered. The next tablet should then be taken at the usual time. Any time you miss one or two white or light-orange tablets, or begin a new Pilpak® after the proper starting day, you should also use another method of birth control until you have taken a white or light-orange tablet daily for seven consecutive days. If breakthrough bleeding occurs following missed tablets, it will usually be temporary and of no consequence. While there is little likelihood of pregnancy occurring if only one or two white or light-orange tablets are missed, the possibility of pregnancy increases with each successive day that scheduled white or light-orange tablets are missed.

If you are taking Nordette®, Ovral® or Lo/Ovral® and forget to take three white or light-orange tablets in a row, do not take them when you remember. Wait four more days—which makes a whole week without tablets. Then begin a new Pilpak® on the 8th day after the last tablet was taken. During the seven days without tablets, and until you have taken a white or light-orange tablet daily for seven consecutive days, you should protect yourself from pregnancy by also using another method of birth control.

If you are taking Nordette®-28, Ovral®-28 or Lo/Ovral®-28 and forget to take three white or light-orange tablets in a row, do not take them when you remember. Stop taking all medication until the first Sunday following the last missed tablet. Then, whether or not you have had your period, and even if you are still bleeding, start a new Pilpak®. During the days without tablets, and until you have taken a white or light-orange tablet daily for seven consecutive days, you should protect yourself from pregnancy by also using another method of birth control.

OVRETTE®

Ovrette® is administered on a continuous daily dosage schedule, one tablet each day, every day of the year. Take the first tablet on the first day of your menstrual period. Tablets should be taken at the same time every day, without interruption, whether bleeding occurs or not. If bleeding is prolonged (more than 8 days) or unusually heavy, you should contact your doctor.

Forgotten Pills:

The risk of pregnancy increases with each tablet missed. Therefore, it is very important that you take one tablet daily as directed. If you miss one tablet, take it as soon as you remember and also take your next tablet at the regular time. If you miss two tablets, take one of the missed tablets as soon as you remember, as well as your regular tablet for that day at the proper time. Furthermore, you should use another method of birth control in addition to taking Ovrette® until you have taken fourteen days (2 weeks) of medication. If more than two tablets have been missed, Ovrette® should be discontinued immediately and another method of birth control used until the start of your next menstrual period. Then you may resume taking Ovrette®.

At times there may be no menstrual period after a cycle of pills. Therefore, if you miss one menstrual period but have taken the pills *exactly as you were supposed to,* continue as usual into the next cycle. If you have not taken the pills correctly and miss a menstrual period, or if you are taking mini-pills and it is 45 days or more from the start of your last menstrual period, you may be pregnant and should stop taking oral contraceptives until your doctor determines whether or not you are pregnant. Until you can get to your doctor, use another form of contraception. If two consecutive menstrual periods are missed, you should stop taking pills until it is determined whether you are pregnant. If you do become pregnant while using oral contraceptives, you should discuss the risks to the developing child with your doctor.

3. Periodic Examination.

Your doctor will take a complete medical and family history before prescribing oral contraceptives. At that time and about once a year thereafter, he will generally examine your blood pressure, breasts, abdomen, and pelvic organs (including a Papanicolaou smear, i.e., test for cancer).

SUMMARY

Oral contraceptives are the most effective method, except sterilization, for preventing pregnancy. Other methods, when used conscientiously, are also very effective and have fewer risks. The serious risks of oral contraceptives are uncommon, and the "pill" is a very convenient method of preventing pregnancy.

If you have certain conditions or have had these conditions in the past, you should not use oral contraceptives, because the risk is too great. These conditions are listed in the leaflet. If you do not have these conditions, and decide to use the "pill", please read the leaflet carefully so that you can use the "pill" most safely and effectively.

Based on his or her assessment of your medical needs, your doctor has prescribed this drug for you. Do not give the drug to anyone else.

NORDETTE®-28 ℞
TABLETS
(levonorgestrel and ethinyl estradiol tablets)

Description:
ORAL CONTRACEPTIVE

21 light-orange Nordette® tablets, each containing 0.15 mg of levonorgestrel (*d*(-)-13 beta-ethyl -17- alpha-ethinyl -17- beta-hydroxygon-4-en-3-one), a totally synthetic progestogen, and 0.03 mg of ethinyl estradiol (19-nor-17α-pregna-1,3,5 (10)-trien-20-yne-3,17-diol), and 7 pink inert tablets.

Clinical Pharmacology: See NORDETTE®
Indications and Usage: See NORDETTE
Dose-Related Risk of Thromboembolism from Oral Contraceptives: See NORDETTE
Contraindications: See NORDETTE
Warnings: See NORDETTE
Precautions: See NORDETTE
Adverse Reactions: See NORDETTE
Acute Overdosage: See NORDETTE

Dosage and Administration: To achieve maximum contraceptive effectiveness, Nordette®-28 must be taken exactly as directed and at intervals not exceeding 24 hours. The dosage of Nordette®-28 is one light-orange tablet daily for 21 consecutive days followed by one pink inert tablet daily for 7 consecutive days according to prescribed schedule. It is recommended that tablets be taken at the same time each day, preferably after the evening meal or at bedtime.

During the first cycle of medication, the patient is instructed to begin taking Nordette®-28 on the first Sunday after the onset of menstruation. If menstruation begins on a Sunday, the first tablet (light-orange) is taken that day. One light-orange tablet should be taken daily for 21 consecutive days followed by one pink inert tablet daily for 7 consecutive days. Withdrawal bleeding should usually occur within three days following discontinuation of light-orange tablets.

During the first cycle, contraceptive reliance should not be placed on Nordette®-28 until a light-orange tablet has been taken daily for 7 consecutive days. The possibility of ovulation and conception prior to initiation of medication should be considered.

The patient begins her next and all subsequent 28-day courses of tablets of the same day of the week (Sunday) on which she began her first course, following the same schedule: 21 days on light-orange tablets—7 days on pink inert tablets. If in any cycle the patient starts tablets later than the proper day, she should protect herself by using another method of birth control until she has taken a light-orange tablet daily for 7 consecutive days.

If spotting or breakthrough bleeding occurs, the patient is instructed to continue on the same regimen. This type of bleeding is usually transient and without significance; however, if the bleeding is persistent or prolonged, the patient is advised to consult her physician. Although the occurrence of pregnancy is highly unlikely if Nordette®-28 is taken according to directions, if withdrawal bleeding does not occur, the possibility of pregnancy must be considered. If the patient has not adhered to the prescribed schedule (missed one or more tablets or started taking them on a day later than she should have), the probability of pregnancy should be considered at the time of the first missed period and appropriate diagnostic measures taken before the medication is resumed. If the patient has adhered to the prescribed regimen and misses two consecutive periods, pregnancy should be ruled out before continuing the contraceptive regimen. The patient should be instructed to take a missed light-orange tablet as soon as it is remembered. If two consecutive light-orange tablets are missed, they should both be taken as soon as remembered. The next tablet should be taken at the usual time. Any time the patient misses one or two light-orange tablets she should also use another method of contraception until she has taken a light-orange tablet daily for seven consecutive days. If the patient misses one or more pink tablets, she is still protected against pregnancy *provided* she begins taking light-orange tablets again on the proper day.

If breakthrough bleeding occurs following missed light-orange tablets, it will usually be transient and of no consequence. While there is little likelihood of ovulation occurring if only one or two light-orange tablets are missed, the possibility of ovulation increases with each successive day that scheduled light-orange tablets are missed. (If three consecutive light-orange Nordette® tablets are missed, all medication should be discontinued and the remainder of the 28-day package discarded. A new tablet cycle should be started on the first Sunday following the last missed tablet, and an alternate means of contraception should be prescribed during the days without tablets and until the patient has taken a light-orange tablet daily for 7 consecutive days.) In the nonlactating mother, Nordette® may be prescribed in the postpartum period either immediately or at the first postpartum examination whether or not menstruation has resumed.

How Supplied: Nordette®-28 Tablets (0.15 mg levonorgestrel + 0.03 mg ethinyl estradiol tablets), Wyeth®, NDC 0008-2533, are available in Pilpak® dispensers of 28 tablets, consisting of 21 light-orange, round, active tablets marked "WYETH" and "75" and 7 pink, round, inert tablets marked "WYETH" and "486".

References: See NORDETTE

Brief Summary Patient Package Insert: See NORDETTE

DETAILED PATIENT LABELING: See NORDETTE

NURSOY®

Soy protein formula
READY-TO-FEED
CONCENTRATED LIQUID

Nursoy® milk free formula is intended to meet the nutritional needs of infants and children who are not breast feeding and are allergic to cow's milk protein or intolerant to lactose. Professional advice should be followed.

Ingredients: (in normal dilution supplying 20 calories per fluidounce): 87% water; 6.7% sucrose; 3.4% oleo, coconut, oleic (safflower) and soybean oils; 2.3% soy protein isolate; 0.10% potassium citrate; 0.09% monobasic sodium phosphate; 0.04% calcium carbonate; 0.04% dibasic calcium phosphate; 0.03% magnesium chloride; 0.03% calcium chloride; 0.03% soy lecithin; 0.03% calcium carrageenan; 0.03% calcium hydroxide; 0.03% l-methionine; 0.01% sodium chloride; 0.01% potassium bicarbonate; ferrous, zinc, manganese and cupric sulfates; (68ppb) potassium iodide; ascorbic acid; choline chloride; alpha tocopheryl acetate; niacinamide; calcium pantothenate; riboflavin; vitamin A palmitate; thiamine hydrochloride; pyridoxine hydrochloride; beta-carotene; phytonadione; folic acid; biotin; activated 7-dehydrocholesterol; cyanocobalamin.

PROXIMATE ANALYSIS

at 20 calories per fluidounce

READY-TO-FEED and CONCENTRATED LIQUID:

	(W/V)
Protein	2.1%
Fat	3.6%
Carbohydrate	6.9%
Ash	0.35%
Water	87.0%
Crude fiber	not more than 0.01%
Calories/fl. oz.	20

Vitamins, Minerals: In normal dilution, each quart contains:

A	2,500	IU
D_3	400	IU
E	9	IU
K_1	0.1	mg
C (ascorbic acid)	55	mg
B_1 (thiamine)	0.67	mg
B_2 (riboflavin)	1	mg
B_6	0.4	mg
B_{12}	2	mcg
Niacin mg equivalents	9.5	
Pantothenic acid	3	mg
Folic acid	50	mcg
Choline	85	mg
Inositol	26	mg
Biotin	35	mcg
Calcium	600	mg
Phosphorus	420	mg
Sodium	190	mg
Potassium	700	mg
Chloride	355	mg
Magnesium	65	mg
Manganese	0.2	mg
Iron	12	mg
Copper	0.45	mg
Zinc	3.5	mg
Iodine	65	mcg

Preparation: *Ready-to-Feed* (32 fl. oz. cans of 20 calories per fluidounce formula)—shake can, open and pour into previously sterilized nursing bottle; attach nipple and feed. Cover opened can and immediately store in refrigerator. Use contents of can within 48 hours of opening.

Concentrated Liquid—For normal dilution supplying 20 calories per fluidounce, use equal amounts of Nursoy® liquid and cooled, previously boiled water. *Note: Prepared formula should be used within 24 hours.*

How Supplied: *Ready-to-Feed*—presterilized and premixed, 32 fluidounce (1 quart) cans, cases of 6; *Concentrated Liquid*—13 fluidounce cans, cases of 24.

Also available to hospitals only:

Ready-to-Feed 4 oz. disposable bottles (48 bottles/case) as part of the Wyeth Hospital Infant Feeding System.

OMNIPEN® ℞

(ampicillin)
CAPSULES

How Supplied: Omnipen® (ampicillin) Capsules—250 mg ampicillin anhydrous, bottles of 100 and 500 capsules; 500 mg, bottles of 100 and 500 capsules. Redipak® Unit Dose Medication, 250 mg and 500 mg, boxes of 100 capsules (individually wrapped).

For prescribing information write to Professional Service, Wyeth Laboratories, Box 8299, Philadelphia, PA, 19101, or contact your local Wyeth representative.

[*Shown in Product Identification Section*]

OMNIPEN® ℞

(ampicillin)
ORAL SUSPENSION

How Supplied: Omnipen® (ampicillin) for Oral Suspension in bottles of powder for reconstitution. When reconstituted with water they will make a palatable suspension containing 125 mg, 250 mg, or 500 mg ampicillin per 5 ml.

For prescribing information write to Professional Service, Wyeth Laboratories, Box 8299, Philadelphia, PA, 19101, or contact your local Wyeth representative.

OMNIPEN® Pediatric Drops ℞

(ampicillin)
ORAL SUSPENSION

How Supplied: One bottle of powder for reconstitution with water to make 20 ml suspension. When reconstituted according to instructions on label, each ml contains 100 mg of ampicillin.

For prescribing information write to Professional Service, Wyeth Laboratories, Box 8299, Philadelphia, PA, 19101, or contact your local Wyeth representative.

OMNIPEN®-N ℞

(ampicillin sodium)
INJECTION

How Supplied: Omnipen®-N (ampicillin sodium) for Injection: Ampicillin sodium equivalent to 125 mg, 250 mg, 500 mg, 1 gram, or 2 gram ampicillin per standard vial; 10 gram per pharmacy bulk vial. Piggyback Units: Supplied in single units equivalent to 500 mg, 1 gram or 2 gram ampicillin per unit, packed in 10 vials per package.

For prescribing information write to Professional Service, Wyeth Laboratories, Box 8299, Philadelphia, PA, 19101, or contact your local Wyeth representative.

OVRAL® TABLETS ℞

Description: Each Ovral® tablet contains 0.5 mg of norgestrel (dl-13-beta-ethyl-17-alpha-ethinyl-17-beta-hydroxygon-4-en-3-one), a totally synthetic progestogen, and 0.05 mg of ethinyl estradiol (19-Nor-17α-pregna-1,3,5 (10)-trien-20-yne-3,17-diol).

Clinical Pharmacology: See LO/OVRAL®.

Indications and Usage: Ovral® is indicated for the prevention of pregnancy in women who elect to use oral contraceptives as a method of contraception.

Oral contraceptives are highly effective. The pregnancy rate in women using conventional combination oral contraceptives (containing 35 mcg or more of ethinyl estradiol or 50 mcg or

Continued on next page

Wyeth—Cont.

more of mestranol) is generally reported as less than one pregnancy per 100 woman-years of use. Slightly higher rates (somewhat more than 1 pregnancy per 100 woman-years of use) are reported for some combination products containing 35 mcg or less of ethinyl estradiol, and rates on the order of 3 pregnancies per 100 woman-years are reported for the progestogen-only oral contraceptives.

These rates are derived from separate studies conducted by different investigators in several population groups and cannot be compared precisely. Furthermore, pregnancy rates tend to be lower as clinical studies are continued possibly due to selective retention in the longer studies of those patients who accept the treatment regimen and do not discontinue as a result of adverse reactions, pregnancy, or other reasons.

In clinical trials with Ovral®, 6,806 patients completed 127,872 cycles, and a total of 19 pregnancies were reported. This represents a pregnancy rate of 0.19 per 100 woman-years. All of the pregnancies reported in these trials were the result of patient failure.

Table 1 gives ranges of pregnancy rates reported in the literature[1] for other means of contraception. The efficacy of these means of contraception (except the IUD) depends upon the degree of adherence to the method.

TABLE 1
PREGNANCIES PER 100 WOMAN-YEARS

IUD, less than 1–6; Diaphragm with spermicidal products (creams or jellies), 2–20; Condom, 3–36; Aerosol foams, 2–29; Jellies and creams, 4–36;

Periodic abstinence (rhythm) all types, less than 1–47:

1. Calendar method, 14–47;
2. Temperature method, 1–20;
3. Temperature method—intercourse only in postovulatory phase, less than 1–7;
4. Mucus method, 1–25;

No contraception, 60–80.

Dose-Related Risk of Thromboembolism from Oral Contraceptives: See LO/OVRAL.
Contraindications: See LO/OVRAL.
Warnings: See LO/OVRAL.
Precautions: See LO/OVRAL.
Information for the Patient: See LO/OVRAL.
Drug Interactions: See LO/OVRAL.
Carcinogenesis: See LO/OVRAL.
Pregnancy: See LO/OVRAL.
Nursing Mothers: See LO/OVRAL.
Adverse Reactions: See LO/OVRAL.
Acute Overdose: See LO/OVRAL.
Dosage and Administration: To achieve maximum contraceptive effectiveness, Ovral® must be taken exactly as directed and at intervals not exceeding 24 hours. The dosage of Ovral® is one tablet daily for 21 consecutive days per menstrual cycle according to prescribed schedule. Tablets are then discontinued for 7 days (three weeks on, one week off). It is recommended that Ovral® tablets be taken at the same time each day, preferably after the evening meal or at bedtime.

During the first cycle of medication, the patient is instructed to take one Ovral® tablet daily for twenty-one consecutive days beginning on day five of her menstrual cycle. (The first day of menstruation is day one.) The tablets are then discontinued for one week (7 days). Withdrawal bleeding should usually occur within three days following discontinuation of Ovral®. (If Ovral® is first taken later than the fifth day of the first menstrual cycle of medication or postpartum, contraceptive reliance should not be placed on Ovral® until after the first seven consecutive days of administration. The possibility of ovulation and conception prior to initiation of medication should be considered.) The patient begins her next and all subsequent 21-day courses of Ovral® tablets on the same day of the week that she began her first course, following the same schedule: 21 days on—7 days off.

She begins taking her tablets on the 8th day after discontinuance regardless of whether or not a menstrual period has occurred or is still in progress. Any time a new cycle of Ovral® is started later than the 8th day the patient should be protected by another means of contraception until she has taken a tablet daily for seven consecutive days.

If spotting or breakthrough bleeding occurs, the patient is instructed to continue on the same regimen. This type of bleeding is usually transient and without significance; however, if the bleeding is persistent or prolonged the patient is advised to consult her physician. Although the occurrence of pregnancy is highly unlikely if Ovral® is taken according to directions, if withdrawal bleeding does not occur, the possibility of pregnancy must be considered. If the patient has not adhered to the prescribed schedule (missed one or more tablets or started taking them on a day later than she should have) the probability of pregnancy should be considered at the time of the first missed period and appropriate diagnostic measures taken before the medication is resumed. If the patient has adhered to the prescribed regimen and misses two consecutive periods, pregnancy should be ruled out before continuing the contraceptive regimen.

The patient should be instructed to take a missed tablet as soon as it is remembered. If two consecutive tablets are missed they should both be taken as soon as remembered. The next tablet should be taken at the usual time.

Any time the patient misses one or two tablets she should also use another method of contraception until she has taken a tablet daily for seven consecutive days. If breakthrough bleeding occurs following missed tablets it will usually be transient and of no consequence. While there is little likelihood of ovulation occurring if only one or two tablets are missed, the possibility of ovulation increases with each successive day that scheduled tablets are missed. If three consecutive tablets are missed, all medication should be discontinued and the remainder of the package discarded. A new tablet cycle should be started on the 8th day after the last tablet was taken, and an alternate means of contraception should be prescribed during the seven days without tablets and until the patient has taken a tablet daily for seven consecutive days. In the nonlactating mother Ovral® may be prescribed in the postpartum period either immediately or at the first postpartum examination whether or not menstruation has resumed.

How Supplied: Ovral® tablets (0.5 mg norgestrel + 0.05 mg ethinyl estradiol) are available in containers of 21 tablets.
Also Available: Ovral®-28 tablets in containers of 28 tablets, consisting of 21 white Ovral® tablets (0.5 mg norgestrel + 0.05 mg ethinyl estradiol) and 7 pink inert tablets.
References: See LO/OVRAL®.
Brief Summary Patient Package Insert: See LO/OVRAL®.
DETAILED PATIENT LABELING: See LO/OVRAL®.

[*Shown in Product Identification Section*]

OVRETTE® ℞
(norgestrel)
TABLETS

Each OVRETTE® tablet contains 0.075 mg of norgestrel (dl-13-beta-ethyl-17-alpha-ethinyl-17-beta-hydroxygon-4-en-3-one).

Description: Each OVRETTE® tablet contains 0.075 mg of a single active steroid ingredient, norgestrel, a totally synthetic progestogen. The available data suggest that the *d*-enantiomeric form of norgestrel is the biologically active portion. This form amounts to 0.0375 mg per OVRETTE® tablet.

Clinical Pharmacology: The primary mechanism through which OVRETTE® prevents conception is not known, but progestogen-only contraceptives are known to alter the cervical mucus, exert a progestational effect on the endometrium, interfering with implantation, and, in some patients, suppress ovulation.

Indications and Usage: OVRETTE® is indicated for the prevention of pregnancy in women who elect to use oral contraceptives as a method of contraception. Oral contraceptives are highly effective. The pregnancy rate in women using conventional combination oral contraceptives (containing 35 mcg or more of ethinyl estradiol or 50 mcg or more of mestranol) is generally reported as less than one pregnancy per 100 woman-years of use. Slightly higher rates (somewhat more than 1 pregnancy per 100 woman-years of use) are reported for some combination products containing 35 mcg or less of ethinyl estradiol, and rates on the order of 3 pregnancies per 100 woman-years are reported for the progestogen-only oral contraceptives.

These rates are derived from separate studies conducted by different investigators in several population groups and cannot be compared precisely. Furthermore, pregnancy rates tend to be lower as clinical studies are continued, possibly due to selective retention in the longer studies of those patients who accept the treatment regimen and do not discontinue as a result of adverse reactions, pregnancy, or other reasons.

In clinical trials with OVRETTE®, 2,752 patients completed 38,245 cycles, and a total of 78 pregnancies were reported. This represents a pregnancy rate of 2.45 per 100 woman-years. Approximately one-half of the pregnancies reported in these trials were due to method failure, and the other half were due to patient failure.

Table 1 gives ranges of pregnancy rates reported in the literature[1] for other means of contraception. The efficacy of these means of contraception (except the IUD) depends upon the degree of adherence to the method.

TABLE 1
PREGNANCIES PER 100 WOMAN-YEARS

IUD, less than 1–6; Diaphragm with spermicidal products (creams or jellies), 2–20; Condom, 3–36; Aerosol foams, 2–29; Jellies and creams, 4–36;

Periodic abstinence (rhythm) all types, less than 1–47:

1. Calendar method, 14–47;
2. Temperature method, 1–20;
3. Temperature method—intercourse only in postovulatory phase, less than 1–7;
4. Mucus method, 1–25;

No contraception, 60–80.

Dose-Related Risk of Thromboembolism from Oral Contraceptives: Two studies have shown a positive association between the dose of estrogens in oral contraceptives and the risk of thromboembolism.[2,3] For this reason, it is prudent and in keeping with good principles of therapeutics to minimize exposure to estrogen. The oral-contraceptive product prescribed for any given patient should be that product which contains the least amount of estrogen that is compatible with an acceptable pregnancy rate and patient acceptance. It is recommended that new acceptors of oral contraceptives be started on preparations containing 0.05 mg or less of estrogen.

Contraindications: Oral contraceptives should not be used in women with any of the following conditions:

1. Thrombophlebitis or thromboembolic disorders.
2. A past history of deep-vein thrombophlebitis or thromboembolic disorders.
3. Cerebral-vascular or coronary-artery disease.

4. Known or suspected carcinoma of the breast.
5. Known or suspected estrogen-dependent neoplasia.
6. Undiagnosed abnormal genital bleeding.
7. Known or suspected pregnancy (see Warning No. 5).
8. Benign or malignant liver tumor which developed during the use of oral contraceptives or other estrogen-containing products.

Warnings

Cigarette smoking increases the risk of serious cardiovascular side effects from oral-contraceptive use. This risk increases with age and with heavy smoking (15 or more cigarettes per day) and is quite marked in women over 35 years of age. Women who use oral contraceptives should be strongly advised not to smoke. The use of oral contraceptives is associated with increased risk of several serious conditions, including thromboembolism, stroke, myocardial infarction, hepatic adenoma, gallbladder disease, hypertension. Practitioners prescribing oral contraceptives should be familiar with the following information relating to these risks.

1. *Thromboembolic Disorders and Other Vascular Problems:* An increased risk of thromboembolic and thrombotic disease associated with the use of oral contraceptives is well-established. Three principal studies in Great Britain[4–6] and three in the United States[7–10] have demonstrated an increased risk of fatal and nonfatal venous thromboembolism and stroke, both hemorrhagic and thrombotic. These studies estimate that users of oral contaceptives are 4 to 11 times more likely than nonusers to develop these diseases without evident cause (Table 2).

CEREBROVASCULAR DISORDERS

In a collaborative American study[9,10] of cerebrovascular disorders in women with and without predisposing causes, it was estimated that the risk of hemorrhagic stroke was 2.0 times greater in users than nonusers and the risk of thrombotic stroke was 4 to 9.5 times greater in users than in nonusers (Table 2).

TABLE 2

SUMMARY OF RELATIVE RISK OF THROMBOEMBOLIC DISORDERS AND OTHER VASCULAR PROBLEMS IN ORAL-CONTRACEPTIVE USERS COMPARED TO NONUSERS

	Relative risk, times greater
Idiopathic thromboembolic disease	4–11
Postsurgery thromboembolic complications	4–6
Thrombotic stroke	4–9.5
Hemorrhagic stroke	2
Myocardial infarction	2–12

MYOCARDIAL INFARCTION

An increased risk of myocardial infarction associated with the use of oral contraceptives has been reported,[11,12,13] confirming a previously suspected association. These studies, conducted in the United Kingdom, found, as expected, that the greater the number of underlying risk factors for coronary-artery disease (cigarette smoking, hypertension, hypercholesterolemia, obesity, diabetes, history of preeclamptic toxemia) the higher the risk of developing myocardial infarction, regardless of whether the patient was an oral-contraceptive user or not. Oral contraceptives, however, were found to be a clear additional risk factor.

In terms of relative risk, it has been estimated[52] that oral-contraceptive users who do not smoke (smoking is considered a major predisposing condition to myocardial infarction) are about twice as likely to have a fatal myocardial infarction as nonusers who do not smoke. Oral-contraceptive users who are also smokers have about a 5-fold increased risk of fatal infarction compared to users who do not smoke, but about a 10- to 12-fold increased risk compared to nonusers who do not smoke. Furthermore, the amount of smoking is also an important factor. In determining the importance of these relative risks, however, the baseline rates for various age groups, as shown in Table 3, must be given serious consideration. The importance of other predisposing conditions mentioned above in determining relative and absolute risks has not as yet been quantified; it is quite likely that the same synergistic action exists, but perhaps to a lesser extent.

TABLE 3

Estimated annual mortality rate per 100,000 women from myocardial infarction by use of oral contraceptives, smoking habits, and age (in years):

	Myocardial infarction			
	Women aged 30–39		Women aged 40–44	
Smoking habits	Users	Non-users	Users	Non-users
All smokers	10.2	2.6	62.0	15.9
Heavy*	13.0	5.1	78.7	31.3
Light	4.7	0.9	28.6	5.7
Nonsmokers	1.8	1.2	10.7	7.4
Smokers and nonsmokers	5.4	1.9	32.8	11.7

*Heavy smoker: 15 or more cigarettes per day.

From JAIN, A.K., *Studies in Family Planning, 8*:50, 1977

RISK OF DOSE

In an analysis of data derived from several national adverse-reaction reporting systems,[2] British investigators concluded that the risk of thromboembolism, including coronary thrombosis, is directly related to the dose of estrogen used in oral contraceptives. Preparations containing 100 mcg or more of estrogen were associated with a higher risk of thromboembolism than those containing 50–80 mcg of estrogen. Their analysis did suggest, however, that the quantity of estrogen may not be the sole factor involved. This finding has been confirmed in the United States.[3] Careful epidemiological studies to determine the degree of thromboembolic risk associated with progestogen-only oral contraceptives have not been performed. Cases of thromboembolic disease have been reported in women using these products, and they should not be presumed to be free of excess risk.

ESTIMATE OF EXCESS MORTALITY FROM CIRCULATORY DISEASES

A large prospective study[53] carried out in the U.K. estimated the mortality rate per 100,000 women per year from diseases of the circulatory system for users and nonusers of oral contraceptives according to age, smoking habits, and duration of use. The overall excess death rate annually from circulatory diseases for oral-contraceptive users was estimated to be 20 per 100,000 (ages 15–34—5/100,000; ages 35–44—33/100,000; ages 45–49—140/100,000), the risk being concentrated in older women, in those with a long duration of use, and in cigarette smokers. It was not possible, however, to examine the interrelationships of age, smoking, and duration of use, nor to compare the effects of continuous vs. intermittent use. Although the study showed a 10-fold increase in death due to circulatory diseases in users for 5 or more years, all of these deaths occurred in women 35 or older. Until larger numbers of women under 35 with continuous use for 5 or more years are available, it is not possible to assess the magnitude of the relative risk for this younger age group.

The available data from a variety of sources have been analyzed[14] to estimate the risk of death associated with various methods of contraception. The estimates of risk of death for each method include the combined risk of the contraceptive method (e.g., thromboembolic and thrombotic disease in the case of oral contraceptives) plus the risk attributable to pregnancy or abortion in the event of method failure. This latter risk varies with the effectiveness of the contraceptive method. The findings of this analysis are shown in Figure 1 below.[14] The study concluded that the mortality associated with all methods of birth control is low and below that associated with childbirth, with the exception of oral contraceptives in women over 40 who smoke. (The rates given for Pill only/smokers for each age group are for smokers as a class. For "heavy" smokers (more than 15 cigarettes a day), the rates given would be about double; for "light" smokers (less than 15 cigarettes a day), about 50 percent. The lowest mortality is associated with the condom or diaphragm backed up by early abortion. The risk of thromboembolic and thrombotic disease associated with oral contraceptives increases with age after approximately age 30 and, for myocardial infarction, is further increased by hypertension, hypercholesterolemia, obesity, diabetes, or history of preeclamptic toxemia and especially by cigarette smoking.

Based on the data currently available, the following chart gives a gross estimate of the risk of death from circulatory disorders associated with the use of oral contraceptives:

SMOKING HABITS AND OTHER PREDISPOSING CONDITIONS— RISK ASSOCIATED WITH USE OF ORAL CONTRACEPTIVES

Age	Below 30	30–39	40+
Heavy smokers	C	B	A
Light smokers	D	C	B
Nonsmokers (no predisposing conditions)	D	C,D	C
Nonsmokers (other predisposing conditions)	C	C,B	B,A

A—Use associated with very high risk.
B—Use associated with high risk.
C—Use associated with moderate risk.
D—Use associated with low risk.

The physician and the patient should be alert to the earliest manifestations of thromboembolic and thrombotic disorders (e.g., thrombophlebitis, pulmonary embolism, cerebrovascular insufficiency, coronary occlusion, retinal thrombosis, and mesenteric thrombosis). Should any of these occur or be suspected, the drug should be discontinued immediately.

A four- to six-fold increased risk of postsurgery thromboembolic complications has been reported in oral-contraceptive users.[15,16] If feasible, oral contraceptives should be discontinued at least 4 weeks before surgery of a type associated with an increased risk of thromboembolism or prolonged immobilization.

2. *Ocular Lesions:*

There have been reports of neuro-ocular lesions such as optic neuritis or retinal thrombosis associated with the use of oral contraceptives. Discontinue oral-contraceptive medication if there is unexplained, sudden or gradual, partial or complete loss of vision; onset of proptosis or diplopia; papilledema; or retinal-vascular lesions, and institute appropriate diagnostic and therapeutic measures.

3. *Carcinoma:*

Long-term continuous administration of either natural or synthetic estrogen in certain animal species increases the frequency of carcinoma of the breast, cervix, vagina, and liver. Certain synthetic progestogens, none currently contained in oral contraceptives, have been noted

Continued on next page

Wyeth—Cont.

to increase the incidence of mammary nodules, benign and malignant, in dogs.

In humans, three case-control studies have reported an increased risk of endometrial carcinoma associated with the prolonged use of exogenous estrogen in postmenopausal women.[17,18,19] One publication[20] reported on the first 21 cases submitted by physicians to a registry of cases of adenocarcinoma of the endometrium in women under 40 on oral contraceptives. Of the cases found in women without predisposing risk factors for adenocarcinoma of the endometrium (e.g, irregular bleeding at the time oral contraceptives were first given, polycystic ovaries), nearly all occurred in women who had used a sequential oral contraceptive. These products are no longer marketed. No evidence has been reported suggesting an increased risk of endometrial cancer in users of conventional combination or progestogen-only oral contraceptives.

Figure 1. Estimated annual number of deaths associated with control of fertility and no control per 100,000 nonsterile women, by regimen of control and age of woman.

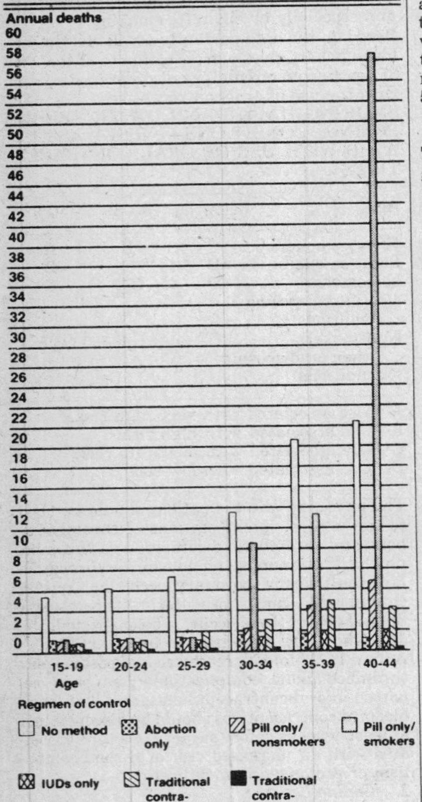

Several studies[8,21–24] have found no increase in breast cancer in women taking oral contraceptives or estrogens. One study,[25] however, while also noting no overall increased risk of breast cancer in women treated with oral contraceptives, found an excess risk in the subgroups of oral-contraceptive users with documented benign breast disease. A reduced occurrence of benign breast tumors in users of oral contraceptives has been well-documented.[8,21,25,26,27] In summary, there is at present no confirmed evidence from human studies of an increased risk of cancer associated with oral contraceptives. Close clinical surveillance of all women taking oral contraceptives is, nevertheless, essential. In all cases of undiagnosed persistent or recurrent abnormal vaginal bleeding, appropriate diagnostic measures should be taken to rule out malignancy. Women with a strong family history of breast cancer or who have breast nodules, fibrocystic disease, or abnormal mammograms should be monitored with particular care if they elect to use oral contraceptives instead of other methods of contraception.

4. *Hepatic Tumors:*

Benign hepatic adenomas have been found to be associated with the use of oral contraceptives.[28,29,30,46] One study[46] showed that oral contraceptive formulations with high hormonal potency were associated with a higher risk than lower potency formulations. Although benign, hepatic adenomas may rupture and may cause death through intra-abdominal hemorrhage. This has been reported in short-term as well as long-term users of oral contraceptives. Two studies relate risk with duration of use of the contraceptive, the risk being much greater after 4 or more years of oral-contraceptive use.[30,46] While hepatic adenoma is a rare lesion, it should be considered in women presenting abdominal pain and tenderness, abdominal mass or shock. A few cases of hepatocellular carcinoma have been reported in women taking oral contraceptives. The relationship of these drugs to this type of malignancy is not known at this time.

5. *Use in or Immediately Preceding Pregnancy, Birth Defects in Offspring, and Malignancy in Female Offspring:*

The use of female sex hormones—both estrogenic and progestational agents—during early pregnancy may seriously damage the offspring. It has been shown that females exposed in utero to diethylstilbestrol, a nonsteroidal estrogen, have an increased risk of developing in later life a form of vaginal or cervical cancer that is ordinarily extremely rare.[31,32] This risk has been estimated to be of the order of 1 in 1,000 exposures or less.[33,47] Although there is no evidence at the present time that oral contraceptives further enhance the risk of developing this type of malignancy, such patients should be monitored with particular care if they elect to use oral contraceptives instead of other methods of contraception. Furthermore, a high percentage of such exposed women (from 30 to 90%) have been found to have epithelial changes of the vagina and cervix.[34–38] Although these changes are histologically benign, it is not known whether this condition is a precursor of vaginal malignancy. Male children so exposed may develop abnormalities of the urogenital tract.[48,49,50] Although similar data are not available with the use of other estrogens, it cannot be presumed that they would not induce similar changes.

An increased risk of congenital anomalies, including heart defects and limb defects, has been reported with the use of sex hormones, including oral contraceptives, in pregnancy.[39–42,51] One case-control study[42] has estimated a 4.7-fold increase in risk of limb-reduction defects in infants exposed in utero to sex hormones (oral contraceptives, hormonal withdrawal tests for pregnancy, or attempted treatment for threatened abortion). Some of these exposures were very short and involved only a few days of treatment. The data suggest that the risk of limb-reduction defects in exposed fetuses is somewhat less than one in 1,000 live births.

In the past, female sex hormones have been used during pregnancy in an attempt to treat threatened or habitual abortion. There is considerable evidence that estrogens are ineffective for these indications, and there is no evidence from well-controlled studies that progestogens are effective for these uses.

There is some evidence that triploidy and possibly other types of polyploidy are increased among abortuses from women who become pregnant soon after ceasing oral contraceptives.[43] Embryos with these anomalies are virtually always aborted spontaneously. Whether there is an overall increase in spontaneous abortion of pregnancies conceived soon after stopping oral contraceptives is unknown.

It is recommended that, for any patient who has missed two consecutive periods, pregnancy should be ruled out before continuing the contraceptive regimen. If the patient has not adhered to the prescribed schedule, the possibility of pregnancy should be considered at the time of the first missed period (or after 45 days from the last menstrual period if the progestogen-only oral contraceptives are used), and further use of oral contraceptives should be withheld until pregnancy has been ruled out. If pregnancy is confirmed, the patient should be apprised of the potential risks to the fetus, and the advisability of continuation of the pregnancy should be discussed in the light of these risks.

It is also recommended that women who discontinue oral contraceptives with the intent of becoming pregnant use an alternate form of contraception for a period of time before attempting to conceive. Many clinicians recommend 3 months, although no precise information is available on which to base this recommendation.

The administration of progestogen-only or progestogen-estrogen combinations to induce withdrawal bleeding should not be used as a test of pregnancy.

6. *Gallbladder Disease:*

Studies[8,23,26] report an increased risk of surgically confirmed gallbladder disease in users of oral contraceptives and estrogens. In one study, an increased risk appeared after 2 years of use and doubled after 4 or 5 years of use. In one of the other studies, an increased risk was apparent between 6 and 12 months of use.

7. *Carbohydrate and Lipid Metabolic Effects:*

A decrease in glucose tolerance has been observed in a significant percentage of patients on oral contraceptives. For this reason, prediabetic and diabetic patients should be carefully observed while receiving oral contraceptives.

An increase in triglycerides and total phospholipids has been observed in patients receiving oral contraceptives.[44] The clinical significance of this finding remains to be defined.

8. *Elevated Blood Pressure:*

An increase in blood pressure has been reported in patients receiving oral contraceptives.[26] In some women, hypertension may occur within a few months of beginning oral-contraceptive use. In the first year of use, the prevalence of women with hypertension is low in users and may be no higher than that of a comparable group of nonusers. The prevalence in users increases, however, with longer exposure, and in the fifth year of use is two-and-a-half to three times the reported prevalence in the first year. Age is also strongly correlated with the development of hypertension in oral-contraceptive users. Women who previously have had hypertension during pregnancy may be more likely to develop elevation of blood pressure when given oral contraceptives. Hypertension that develops as a result of taking oral contraceptives usually returns to normal after discontinuing the drug.

9. *Headache:*

The onset or exacerbation of migraine or development of headache of a new pattern which is recurrent, persistent, or severe, requires discontinuation of oral contraceptives and evaluation of the cause.

10. *Bleeding Irregularities:*

Breakthrough bleeding, spotting, and amenorrhea are frequent reasons for patients discontinuing oral contraceptives. In breakthrough bleeding, as in all cases of irregular bleeding from the vagina, nonfunctional causes should be borne in mind. In undiagnosed persistent or recurrent abnormal bleeding from the vagina, adequate diagnostic measures are indicated to rule out pregnancy or malignancy. If pathology has been excluded, time or a change to another formulation may solve the problem. Changing to an oral contraceptive with a higher estrogen content, while potentially useful in minimizing menstrual irregularity, should be done only if necessary, since this may increase the risk of thromboembolic disease.

An alteration in menstrual patterns is likely to occur in women using progestogen-only oral contraceptives. The amount and duration of flow, cycle length, breakthrough bleeding, spotting, and amenorrhea will probably be quite variable. Bleeding irregularities occur more frequently with the use of progestogen-only oral contraceptives than with the combinations, and the dropout rate due to such conditions is higher.

Women with a past history of oligomenorrhea or secondary amenorrhea or young women without regular cycles may have a tendency to remain anovulatory or to become amenorrheic after discontinuation of oral contraceptives. Women with these preexisting problems should be advised of this possibility and encouraged to use other contraceptive methods. Post-use anovulation, possibly prolonged, may also occur in women without previous irregularities.

11. *Ectopic Pregnancy:*
Ectopic as well as intrauterine pregnancy may occur in contraceptive failures. However, in progestogen-only oral contraceptive failures, the ratio of ectopic to intrauterine pregnancies is higher than in women who are not receiving oral contraceptives, since the drugs are more effective in preventing intrauterine than ectopic pregnancies.

12. *Breast-feeding:*
Oral contraceptives given in the postpartum period may interfere with lactation. There may be a decrease in the quantity and quality of the breast milk. Furthermore, a small fraction of the hormonal agents in oral contraceptives has been identified in the milk of mothers receiving these drugs.[45] The effects, if any, on the breast-fed child have not been determined. If feasible, the use of oral contraceptives should be deferred until the infant has been weaned.

Precautions

GENERAL

1. A complete medical and family history should be taken prior to initiation of oral contraceptives. The pretreatment and periodic physical examinations should include special reference to blood pressure, breasts, abdomen and pelvic organs, including Papanicolaou smear and relevant laboratory tests. As a general rule, oral contraceptives should not be prescribed for longer than 1 year without another physical examination being performed.
2. Under the influence of estrogen-progestogen preparations, preexisting uterine leiomyomata may increase in size.
3. Patients with a history of psychic depression should be carefully observed and the drug discontinued if depression recurs to a serious degree. Patients becoming significantly depressed while taking oral contraceptives should stop the medication and use an alternate method of contraception in an attempt to determine whether the symptom is drug-related.
4. Oral contraceptives may cause some degree of fluid retention. They should be prescribed with caution, and only with careful monitoring, in patients with conditions which might be aggravated by fluid retention, such as convulsive disorders, migraine syndrome, asthma, or cardiac or renal insufficiency.
5. Patients with a past history of jaundice during pregnancy have an increased risk of recurrence of jaundice while receiving oral-contraceptive therapy. If jaundice develops in any patient receiving such drugs, the medication should be discontinued.
6. Steroid hormones may be poorly metabolized in patients with impaired liver function and should be administered with caution in such patients.
7. Oral-contraceptive users may have disturbances in normal tryptophan metabolism which may result in a relative pyridoxine deficiency. The clinical significance of this is yet to be determined.
8. Serum folate levels may be depressed by oral-contraceptive therapy. Since the pregnant woman is predisposed to the development of folate deficiency and the incidence of folate deficiency increases with increasing gestation, it is possible that if a woman becomes pregnant shortly after stopping oral contraceptives, she may have a greater chance of developing folate deficiency and complications attributed to this deficiency.
9. The pathologist should be advised of oral-contraceptive therapy when relevant specimens are submitted.
10. Certain endocrine- and liver-function tests and blood components may be affected by estrogen-containing oral contraceptives:

a. Increased sulfobromophthalein retention.
b. Increased prothrombin and factors VII, VIII, IX, and X; decreased antithrombin 3; increased norepinephrine-induced platelet aggregability.
c. Increased thyroid-binding globulin (TBG) leading to increased circulating total-thyroid hormone, as measured by protein-bound iodine (PBI), T4 by column, or T4 by radioimmunoassay. Free T3 resin uptake is decreased, reflecting the elevated TBG; free T4 concentration is unaltered.
d. Decreased pregnanediol excretion.
e. Reduced response to metyrapone test.

This product contains FD&C Yellow No. 5 (tartrazine) which may cause allergic-type reactions (including bronchial asthma) in certain susceptible individuals. Although the overall incidence of FD&C Yellow No. 5 (tartrazine) sensitivity in the general population is low, it is frequently seen in patients who also have aspirin hypersensitivity.

Information for the Patient: See LO/OVRAL®.

Drug Interactions: Reduced efficacy and increased incidence of breakthrough bleeding have been associated with concomitant use of rifampin. A similar association has been suggested with barbiturates, phenylbutazone, phenytoin sodium, ampicillin, and tetracycline.

Carcinogenesis: See Warnings section for information on the carcinogenic potential of oral contraceptives:

Pregnancy: Pregnancy category X. See Contraindications and Warnings.

Nursing Mothers: See Warnings.

Adverse Reactions: An increased risk of the following serious adverse reactions has been associated with the use of oral contraceptives (see Warnings):

Thrombophlebitis.
Pulmonary embolism.
Coronary thrombosis.
Cerebral thrombosis.
Cerebral hemorrhage.
Hypertension.
Gallbladder disease.
Benign hepatomas.
Congenital anomalies.

There is evidence of an association between the following conditions and the use of oral contraceptives, although additional confirmatory studies are needed;

Mesenteric thrombosis.
Neuro-ocular lesions, e.g., retinal thrombosis and optic neuritis.

The following adverse reactions have been reported in patients receiving oral contraceptives and are believed to be drug-related:

Nausea and/or vomiting, usually the most common adverse reactions, occur in approximately 10% or less of patients during the first cycle. Other reactions, as a general rule, are seen much less frequently or only occasionally.
Gastrointestinal symptoms (such as abdominal cramps and bloating).
Breakthrough bleeding.
Spotting.
Change in menstrual flow.
Dysmenorrhea.
Amenorrhea during and after treatment.
Temporary infertility after discontinuance of treatment.
Edema
Chloasma or melasma which may persist.
Breast changes: tenderness, enlargement, and secretion.
Change in weight (increase or decrease)
Change in cervical erosion and cervical secretion.
Possible diminution in lactation when given immediately postpartum.
Cholestatic jaundice.
Migraine.
Increase in size of uterine leiomyomata.
Rash (allergic).
Mental depression.
Reduced tolerance to carbohydrates.
Vaginal candidiasis.
Change in corneal curvature (steepening).
Intolerance to contact lenses.

The following adverse reactions have been reported in users of oral contraceptives, and the association has been neither confirmed nor refuted:

Premenstrual-like syndrome.
Cataracts.
Changes in libido.
Chorea.
Changes in appetite.
Cystitis-like syndrome.
Headache.
Nervousness.
Dizziness.
Hirsutism.
Loss of scalp hair.
Erythema multiforme.
Erythema nodosum.
Hemorrhagic eruption.
Vaginitis.
Porphyria.

Acute Overdose: Serious ill effects have not been reported following acute ingestion of large doses of oral contraceptives by young children. Overdosage may cause nausea, and withdrawal bleeding may occur in females.

Dosage and Administration: To achieve maximum contraceptive effectiveness, OVRETTE® must be taken exactly as directed and at intervals not exceeding 24 hours. OVRETTE® is administered on a continuous daily dosage regimen starting on the first day of menstruation, i.e., one tablet each day, every day of the year.

Tablets should be taken at the same time each day and continued daily, without interruption, whether bleeding occurs or not. The patient should be advised that, if prolonged bleeding occurs, she should consult her physician. In the non-nursing mother, OVRETTE® may be prescribed in the postpartum period either immediately or at the first postpartum examination whether or not menstruation has resumed.

The risk of pregnancy increases with each tablet missed. If the patient misses one tablet, she should be instructed to take it as soon as she remembers and to also take her next tablet at the regular time. If she misses two tablets, she should take one of the missed tablets as soon as she remembers, as well as taking her regular tablet for that day at the proper time. Furthermore, she should use a method of non-hormonal contraception in addition to taking OVRETTE® until fourteen tablets have been taken. If more than 2 tablets have been missed, OVRETTE® should be discontinued immedi-

Continued on next page

Wyeth—Cont.

ately and a method of nonhormonal contraception should be used until menses has appeared or pregnancy has been excluded. If menses does not appear within 45 days from the last period, a method of nonhormonal contraception should be substituted until the start of the next menstrual period or an appropriate diagnostic procedure is performed to rule out pregnancy.

How Supplied: OVRETTE® (as yellow, round tablets) is available in 28-tablet dispensers.

References:

1. "*Population Reports*," Series H, Number 2, May 1974; Series I, Number 1, June 1974; Series B, Number 2, January 1975; Series H, Number 3, 1975; Series H, Number 4, January 1976 (published by the Population Information Program, The George Washington University Medical Center, 2001 S St. NW., Washington, D.C.).
2. Inman, W. H. W., Vessey, M. P., Westerholm, B., and Engelund, A., "Thromboembolic disease and the steroidal content of oral contraceptives. A report to the Committee on Safety of Drugs," Brit Med J *2*:203-209, 1970.
3. Stolley, P. D., Tonascia, J. A., Tockman, M. S., Sartwell, P. E., Rutledge, A. H., and Jacobs, M. P., "Thrombosis with low-estrogen oral contraceptives," Am J Epidemiol *102*:197–208, 1975.
4. Royal College of General Practitioners, "Oral contraception and thromboembolic disease," J Coll Gen Pract *13*:267–279, 1967.
5. Inman, W. H. W., and Vessey, M. P., "Investigation of deaths from pulmonary, coronary and cerebral thrombosis and embolism in women of childbearing age," Brit Med J *2*:193–199, 1968.
6. Vessey, M.P., and Doll, R., "Investigation of relation between use of oral contraceptives and thromboembolic disease. A further report," Brit Med J *2*:651–657, 1969.
7. Sartwell, P.E., Masi, A. T., Arthes, F. G., Greene, G. R., and Smith, H. E., "Thromboembolism and oral contraceptives: an epidemiological case control study," Am J Epidemiol *90*:365–380, 1969.
8. Boston Collaborative Drug Surveillance Program, "Oral contraceptives and venous thromboembolic disease, surgically confirmed gallbladder disease and breast tumors," Lancet *1*:1399–1404, 1973.
9. Collaborative Group for the Study of Stroke in Young Women, "Oral contraception and increased risk of cerebral ischemia or thrombosis," N Engl J Med *288*:871–878, 1973.
10. Collaborative Group for the Study of Stroke in Young Women. "Oral contraceptives and stroke in young women: associated risk factors," JAMA *231*:718–722, 1975.
11. Mann, J. I., and Inman, W. H. W., "Oral contraceptives and death from myocardial infarction," Brit Med J *2*:245–248, 1975.
12. Mann, J. I., Inman, W. H. W., and Thorogood, M., "Oral contraceptive use in older women and fatal myocardial infarction," Brit Med J *2*:445–447, 1976.
13. Mann, J. I., Vessey, M. P., Thorogood, M., and Doll, R., "Myocardial infarction in young women with special reference to oral contraceptive practice," Brit Med J *2*:241–245, 1975.
14. Tietze, C., "New Estimates of Mortality Associated with Fertility Control," Family Planning Perspectives, *9*:74–76, 1977.
15. Vessey, M. P., Doll, R., Fairbairn, A. S., and Glober, G., "Post-operative thromboembolism and the use of oral contraceptives," Brit Med J *3*:123–126, 1970.
16. Greene, G. R., Sartwell, P. E., "Oral contraceptive use in patients with thromboembolism following surgery, trauma, or infection," Am J Pub Health *62*:680–685, 1972.
17. Smith, D. C., Prentice, R., Thompson, D. J., and Herrmann, W. L., "Association of exogenous estrogen and endometrial carcinoma," N Eng J Med *293*:1164–1167, 1975.
18. Ziel, H. K., and Finkle, W. D., "Increased risk of endometrial carcinoma among users of conjugated estrogens," N Engl J Med *293*:1167–1170, 1975.
19. Mack, T. N., Pike, M. C., Henderson, B. E., Pfeffer, R. I., Gerkins, V. R., Arthur, M., and Brown, S. E., "Estrogens and endometrial cancer in a retirement community,"N Engl J Med *294*:1262–1267, 1976.
20. Silverberg, S. G., and Makowski, E. L., "Endometrial carcinoma in young women taking oral contraceptive agents," Obstet Gynecol *46*:503–506, 1975.
21. Vessey, M. P., Doll, R., and Sutton, P. M., "Oral contraceptives and breast neoplasia: a retrospective study," Brit Med J *3*:719–724, 1972.
22. Vessey, M.P., Doll, R., and Jones, K., "Oral contraceptives and breast cancer. Progress report of an epidemiological study," Lancet *1*:941–943, 1975.
23. Boston Collaborative Drug Surveillance Program, "Surgically confirmed gallbladder disease, venous thromboembolism and breast tumors in relation to postmenopausal estrogen therapy," N Engl J Med *290*:15–19, 1974.
24. Arthes, F. G., Sartwell, P. E., and Lewison, E. F., "The pill, estrogens, and the breast. Epidemiologic aspects," Cancer *28*:1391–1394, 1971.
25. Fasal, E., and Paffenbarger, R. S., "Oral contraceptives as related to cancer and benign lesions of the breast," J Natl Cancer Inst *55*:767–773, 1975.
26. Royal College of General Practitioners, "Oral Contraceptives and Health," London, Pitman, 1974.
27. Ory, H., Cole, P., MacMahon, B., and Hoover, R., "Oral contraceptives and reduced risk of benign breast diseases," N Engl J Med *294*:419–422, 1976.
28. Baum, J., Holtz, F., Bookstein, J. J., and Klein, E. W., "Possible association between benign hepatomas and oral contraceptives," Lancet *2*:926–928, 1973.
29. Mays, E. T., Christopherson, W. M., Mahr, M. M., and Williams, H. C., "Hepatic changes in young women ingesting contraceptive steroids. Hepatic hemorrhage and primary hepatic tumors," JAMA *235*:730–732, 1976.
30. Edmondson, H. A., Henderson, B., and Benton, B., "Liver-cell adenomas associated with use of oral contraceptives," N Engl J Med *294*:470–472, 1976.
31. Herbst, A. L., Ulfedler, H., and Poskanzer, D. C., "Adenocarcinoma of the vagina," N Engl J Med *284*:878–881, 1971.
32. Greenwald, P., Barlow, J. J., Nasca, P. C., and Burnett, W., "Vaginal cancer after maternal treatment with synthetic estrogens," N Engl J Med *285*:390–392, 1971.
33. Lanier, A. P., Noller, K. L., Decker, D. G., Elveback, L., and Kurland, L. T., "Cancer and stilbestrol. A follow-up of 1719 persons exposed to estrogens in utero and born 1943–1959," Mayo Clin Pro *48*: 793–799, 1973.
34. Herbst, A. L., Kurman, R. J., and Scully, R. E., "Vaginal and cervical abnormalities after exposure to stilbestrol in utero," Obstet Gynecol *40*:287–298, 1972.
35. Herbst, A. L., Robboy, S. J., Macdonald, G. J., and Scully, R. E., "The effects of local progesterone on stilbestrol-associated vaginal adenosis," Am J Obstet Gynecol *118*:607–615, 1974.
36. Herbst, A. L., Poskanzer, D. C., Robboy, S. J., Friedlander, L., and Scully, R. E., "Prenatal exposure to stilbestrol: a prospective comparison of exposed female offspring with unexposed controls," N Engl J. Med *292*:334–339, 1975.
37. Stafl, A., Mattingly, R. F., Foley, D. V., Fetherston, W., "Clinical diagnosis of vaginal adenosis," Obstet Gynecol *43*:118–128, 1974.
38. Sherman, A. I., Goldrath, M., Berlin, A., Vakhariya, V., Banooni, F., Michaels, W., Goodman, P., and Brown, S., "Cervical-vaginal adenosis after in utero exposure to synthetic estrogens," Obstet Gynecol *44*:531–545, 1974.
39. Gal, I., Kirman, B., and Stern, J., "Hormone pregnancy tests and congenital malformation," Nature *216*:83, 1967.
40. Levy, E. P., Cohen, A., and Fraser, F. C., "Hormone treatment during pregnancy and congenital heart defects," Lancet *1*:611, 1973.
41. Nora, J. J., and Nora, A. H., "Birth defects and oral contraceptives," Lancet *1*:941–942, 1973.
42. Janerich, D. T., Piper, J. M., and Glebatis, D. M., "Oral contraceptives and congenital limb-reduction defects," N Engl J Med *291*:697–700, 1974.
43. Carr, D. H., "Chromosome studies in selected spontaneous abortions: I. Conception after oral contraceptives," Canad Med Assoc J *103*:343–348, 1970.
44. Wynn, V., Doar, J. W. H., and Mills, G. L., "Some effects of oral contraceptives on serum-lipid and lipoprotein levels," Lancet *2*:720–723, 1966.
45. Laumas, K. R., Malkani, P. K., Bhatnager, S., and Laumas, V., "Radioactivity in the breast milk of lactating women after oral administration of 3 H-norethynodrel," Amer J Obstet Gynecol *98*:411–413, 1967.
46. Center for Disease Control, "Increased Risk of Hepatocellular Adenoma in Women with Long-term use of Oral contraceptives," Morbidity and Mortality Weekly Report, *26*:293–294, 1977.
47. Herbst, A. L., Cole, P., Colton, T., Robboy, S. J., Scully, R. E., "Age-incidence and Risk of Diethylstilbestrol-related Clear Cell Adenocarcinoma of the Vagina and Cervix," Am. J. Obstet. Gynecol., *128*:43–50, 1977.
48. Bibbo, M., Al-Naqeeb, M., Baccarini, I., Gill, W., Newton, M., Sleeper, K. M., Sonek, M., Wied, G. L., "Follow-up Study of Male and Female Offspring of DES-treated Mothers. A Preliminary Report," Jour. of Repro. Med., *15*:29–32, 1975.
49. Gill, W. B., Schumacher, G. F. B., Bibbo, M., "Structural and Functional Abnormalities in the Sex Organs of Male Offspring of Mothers Treated with Diethylstilbestrol (DES)," Jour. of Repro. Med., *16*:147–153, 1976.
50. Henderson, B. E., Senton, B., Cosgrove, M., Baptista, J., Aldrich, J., Townsend, D., Hart, W., Mack., T., "Urogenital Tract Abnormalities in Sons of Women Treated with Diethylstilbestrol," Pediatrics, *58*:505–507, 1976.
51. Heinonen, O. P., Slone, D., Nonson, R. R., Hook, E. B., Shapiro, S., "Cardiovascular Birth Defects and Antenatal Exposure to Female Sex Hormones," N. Eng. J. Med., *296*:67–70, 1977.
52. Jain, A. K., "Mortality Risk Associated with the Use of Oral Contraceptives," Studies in Family Planning, *8*:50–54, 1977.
53. Beral, V., "Mortality Among Oral Contraceptive Users," Lancet, *2*:727–731, 1977.

Brief Summary Patient Package Insert: See LO/OVRAL®

DETAILED PATIENT LABELING: See LO/OVRAL®.

OXYTOCIN ℞

Injection, USP
(synthetic)

Description: TUBEX® Injection Oxytocin is a sterile aqueous solution containing in each ml an oxytocic activity equivalent to 10 USP Posterior Pituitary Units. The solution contains 0.5% chlorobutanol (a chloroform derivative) as preservative, and acetic acid to adjust pH.

Action: Oxytocin acts on smooth muscle of the uterus to stimulate contractions. It also has a stimulant effect on the mammary gland. Oxytocin largely avoids the elevation of blood pressure caused by the pressor factor in posterior pituitary injection. Oxytocin can initiate uterus contraction or increase the force of contractions when administered during pregnancy. It is more effective at term as the uterus becomes progressively more sensitive to oxytocic activity.

Indications:

IMPORTANT NOTICE
Oxytocin is indicated for the medical rather than the elective induction of labor. Available data and information are inadequate to define the benefits-to-risks considerations in the use of the drug product for elective induction. Elective induction of labor is defined as the initiation of labor for convenience in an individual with a term pregnancy who is free of medical indications.

ANTEPARTUM: Oxytocin is indicated for the initiation or improvement of uterine contractions, where this is desirable and considered suitable, in order to achieve early vaginal delivery for fetal or maternal reasons. It is indicated for (1) induction of labor in patients with a medical indication for the initiation of labor, such as Rh problems, maternal diabetes, preeclampsia at or near term, when delivery is in the best interest of mother and fetus or when membranes are prematurely ruptured and delivery is indicated; (2) stimulation or reinforcement of labor, as in selected cases of uterine inertia; (3) as adjunctive therapy in the management of incomplete or inevitable abortion. In the first trimester curettage is generally considered primary therapy. In second trimester abortion, oxytocin infusion will often be successful in emptying the uterus. Other means of therapy, however, may be required in such cases.

POSTPARTUM: Oxytocin is indicated to produce uterine contractions during the third stage of labor and to control postpartum bleeding or hermorrhage.

Contraindications: Oxytocin is contraindicated in any of the following conditions:
significant cephalopelvic disproportion;
unfavorable fetal positions or presentations which are undeliverable without conversion prior to delivery, i.e., transverse lies;
in obstetrical emergencies where the benefit-to-risk ratio for either the fetus or the mother favors surgical intervention;
in cases of fetal distress where delivery is not imminent;
prolonged use in uterine inertia or severe toxemia;
hypertonic uterine patterns;
patients with hypersensitivity to the drug;
induction or augmentation of labor in those cases where vaginal delivery is contraindicated, such as cord presentation or prolapse, total placenta previa, and vasa previa.

Warnings: Oxytocin, when given for induction or stimulation of labor, must be administered only by intravenous infusion (drip method) and with adequate medical supervision in a hospital.

Precautions:

1. All patients receiving intravenous oxytocin must be under continuous observation by trained personnel with a thorough knowledge of the drug and qualified to identify complications. A physician qualified to manage any complications should be immediately available.

2. When properly administered, oxytocin should stimulate uterine contractions similar to those seen in normal labor. Overstimulation of the uterus by improper administration can be hazardous to both mother and fetus. Even with proper administration and adequate supervision, hypertonic contractions can occur in patients whose uteri are hypersensitive to oxytocin.

3. Except in unusual circumstances, oxytocin should not be administered in the following conditions: prematurity, borderline cephalopelvic disproportion, previous major surgery on the cervix or uterus, including cesarean section, overdistention of the uterus, grand multiparity, or invasive cervical carcinoma. Because of the variability of the combinations of factors which may be present in the conditions listed above, the definition of "unusual circumstances" must be left to the judgment of the physician. The decision can only be made by carefully weighing the potential benefits which oxytocin can provide in a given case against rare but definite potential for the drug to produce hypertonicity or tetanic spasm.

4. Maternal deaths due to hypertensive episodes, subarachnoid hemorrhage, rupture of the uterus, and fetal deaths due to various causes have been reported associated with the use of parenteral oxytocic drugs for induction of labor or for augmentation in the first and second stages of labor.

5. Oxytocin has been shown to have an intrinsic antidiuretic effect, acting to increase water reabsorption from the glomerular filtrate. Consideration should, therefore, be given to the possibility of water intoxication, particularly when oxytocin is administered continuously by infusion and the patient is receiving fluids by mouth.

Adverse Reactions: The following adverse reactions have been reported:
fetal bradycardia
neonatal jaundice
anaphylactic reaction
postpartum hemorrhage
cardiac arrhythmia
fatal afibrinogenemia
nausea
vomiting
premature ventricular contractions
pelvic hematoma

Excessive dosage or hypersensitivity to the drug may result in uterine hypertonicity, spasm, tetanic contraction, or rupture of the uterus.

The possibility of increased blood loss and afibrinogenemia should be kept in mind when administering the drug.

Severe water intoxication with convulsions and coma has occurred, associated with a slow oxytocin infusion over a 24-hour period. Maternal death due to oxytocin-induced water intoxication has been reported.

Dosage and Administration: Dosage of oxytocin is determined by uterine response. The following dosage information is based upon the various regimens and indications in general use.

A. INDUCTION OR STIMULATION OF LABOR

Intravenous infusion (drip method) is the only acceptable method of administration for the induction or stimulation of labor.

Accurate control of the rate of infusion flow is essential. An infusion pump or other such device and frequent monitoring of strength of contractions and fetal heart rate are necessary for the safe administration of oxytocin for the induction or stimulation of labor. If uterine contractions become too powerful, the infusion can be abruptly stopped, and oxytocic stimulation of the uterine musculature will soon wane.

1. An intravenous infusion of non-oxytocin-containing solution should be started. Physiologic electrolyte solution should be used except under unusual circumstances.

2. To prepare the usual solution for infusion, the contents of one 1-ml TUBEX® (10 units) is combined aseptically with 1,000 ml of nonhydrating diluent (physiologic electrolyte solution). The combined solution, rotated in the infusion bottle to insure thorough mixing, contains 10 mU/ml. Add the container with dilute oxytocic solution to the system through use of a constant infusion pump or other such device, to control accurately the rate of infusion.

3. The initial dose should be no more than 1–2 mU/min. The dose may be gradually increased in increments of no more than 1 to 2 mU/min. until a contraction pattern has been established which is similar to normal labor.

4. The fetal heart rate, resting uterine tone, and the frequency, duration, and force of contractions should be monitored.

5. The oxytocin infusion should be discontinued immediately in the event of uterine hyperactivity or fetal distress. Oxygen should be administered to the mother. The mother and the fetus must be evaluated by the responsible physician.

B. CONTROL OF POSTPARTUM UTERINE BLEEDING

1. Intravenous infusion (Drip Method)

To control postpartum bleeding, 10 to 40 units of oxytocin may be added to 1,000 ml of a nonhydrating diluent (physiologic electrolyte solution) and run at a rate necessary to control uterine atony.

2. Intramuscular Administration

1 ml (10 units) of oxytocin can be given after delivery of the placenta.

C. TREATMENT OF INCOMPLETE OR INEVITABLE ABORTION

Intravenous infusion with physiologic saline solution, 500 ml, or 5% dextrose in physiologic saline solution to which 10 units of oxytocin have been added should be infused at a rate of 20 to 40 drops per minute.

How Supplied: Oxytocin Injection, USP (synthetic), 10 USP units in 1 ml TUBEX® (Sterile Cartridge-Needle Units) supplied in packages of 10 TUBEX®.

Keep in a refrigerator, do not freeze.

When stored out of refrigeration at temperatures of up to 26° C (79° F), this product has exhibited acceptable data for a period not exceeding three (3) months.

PATHOCIL® ℞

(dicloxacillin sodium monohydrate)
CAPSULES • ORAL SUSPENSION

Description: Dicloxacillin sodium monohydrate is an isoxazolyl penicillin which resists destruction by the enzyme penicillinase (beta-lactamase). It is the monohydrate sodium salt of 6-[3-(2,6- Dichlorophenyl) -5- methyl-4-isoxazolecarboxamido]-3, 3-dimethyl-7-oxo-4-thia-1-azabicyclo [3.2.0] heptane-2-carboxylic acid.

Actions:

Pharmacology

Dicloxacillin sodium monohydrate is resistant to destruction by acid and is exceptionally well absorbed from the gastrointestinal tract. Oral administration of dicloxacillin sodium monohydrate gives blood levels considerably higher than those obtained with equivalent doses of any other presently available oral penicillin.

Microbiology

In vitro dicloxacillin is active against certain gram-positive cocci, including most strains of beta-hemolytic streptococci, pneumococci, penicillin G-sensitive staphylococci and, because of its resistance to penicillinase, penicillin G-resistant staphylococci. Dicloxacillin has less intrinsic antibacterial activity and a narrower spectrum than penicillin G.

Disc Susceptibility Tests

Quantitative methods that require measurement of zone diameters give the most precise estimates of antibiotic susceptibility. One such procedure* has been recommended for use with discs for testing susceptibility to penicillinase-resistant penicillin-class antibiotics. Interpretations correlate diameters on the disc test with MIC values for penicillinase-resistant penicillins. With this procedure, a report from the laboratory of "susceptible" indicates that the infecting organism is likely to respond to therapy. A report of "resistant" indicates that the infecting organism is not likely to respond to therapy. A report of "intermediate susceptibility" suggests that the organism would be susceptible if high dosage is used, or if the in-

Continued on next page

Wyeth—Cont.

fection is confined to tissues and fluids (e.g., urine), in which high antibiotic levels are attained.

Indications: Although the principal indication for dicloxacillin is in the treatment of infections due to penicillinase-producing staphylococci, it may be used to initiate therapy in such patients in whom a staphylococcal infection is suspected. (See Important Note.)

Bacteriologic studies to determine the causative organisms and their sensitivity to dicloxacillin should be performed.

In serious, life-threatening infections, oral preparations of the penicillinase-resistant penicillins should not be relied on for initial therapy.

Important Note: When it is judged necessary that treatment be initiated before definitive culture and sensitivity results are known, the choice of dicloxacillin should take into consideration the fact that it has been shown to be effective only in the treatment of infections caused by pneumococci, Group A beta-hemolytic streptococci, and penicillin G-resistant and penicillin G-sensitive staphylococci. If the bacteriology report later indicates the infection is due to an organism other than a penicillin G-resistant staphylococcus sensitive to dicloxacillin, the physician is advised to continue therapy with a drug other than dicloxacillin or any other penicillinase-resistant penicillin.

Recent studies have reported that the percentage of staphylococcal isolates resistant to penicillin G outside the hospital is increasing, approximating the high percentage of resistant staphylococcal isolates found in the hospital. For this reason, it is recommended that a penicillinase-resistant penicillin be used as initial therapy for any suspected staphylococcal infection until culture and sensitivity results are known.

Dicloxacillin acts through a mechanism similar to that of methicillin against penicillin G-resistant staphylococci. Strains of staphylococci resistant to methicillin have existed in nature and it is known that the number of these strains reported has been increasing. Such strains of staphylococci have been capable of producing serious disease, in some instances resulting in fatality. Because of this, there is concern that widespread use of the penicillinase-resistant penicillins may result in the appearance of an increasing number of staphylococcal strains which are resistant to these penicillins.

Methicillin-resistant strains are almost always resistant to all other penicillinase-resistant penicillins (cross-resistance with cephalosporin derivatives also occurs frequently). Resistance to any penicillinase-resistant penicillin should be interpreted as evidence of clinical resistance to all in spite of the fact that minor variations in *in vitro* sensitivity may be encountered when more than one penicillinase-resistant penicillin is tested against the same strain of staphylococcus.

Contraindications: A history of a previous hypersensitivity reaction to any of the penicillins is a contraindication.

Warnings: Serious and occasionally fatal hypersensitivity (anaphylactoid) reactions have been reported in patients on penicillin therapy. Although anaphylaxis is more frequent following parenteral therapy, it has occurred in patients on oral penicillins. These reactions are more apt to occur in individuals with a history of sensitivity to multiple allergens.

There have been reports of individuals with a history of penicillin hypersensitivity reactions who experienced severe hypersensitivity reactions when treated with cephalosporins. Before therapy with a penicillin, careful inquiry should be made concerning previous hypersensitivity reactions to penicillins, cephalosporins, and other allergens. If an allergic reaction occurs, appropriate therapy should be instituted and discontinuance of dicloxacillin therapy considered. The usual agents (antihistamines, pressor amines, corticosteroids) should be readily available.

Usage in pregnancy

Safety for use in pregnancy has not been established.

Precautions: As with any potent drug, periodic assessment of organ-system function, including renal, hepatic, and hematopoietic, should be made during prolonged therapy.

The possibility of bacterial and fungal superinfection should be kept in mind during long-term therapy. If overgrowth of resistant organisms occurs, appropriate measures should be taken.

This oral preparation should not be relied upon in patients with severe illness or with nausea, vomiting, gastric dilatation, cardiospasm or intestinal hypermotility.

Since experience in neonates is limited, a dose for the newborn is not recommended at this time.

Adverse Reactions: Gastrointestinal disturbances such as nausea, vomiting, epigastric discomfort, flatulence, and loose stools have been noted in some patients receiving dicloxacillin. As with other penicillins, pruritus, urticaria, skin rashes, eosinophilia, anaphylactic reactions, and other allergic symptoms have been occasionally encountered.

Minor changes in the results of liver-function tests such as transient elevation of SGOT and changes in cephalin flocculation tests have been reported. The clinical significance of these changes is unknown.

Dosage and Administration: For mild-to-moderate upper respiratory and localized skin and soft tissue infections due to sensitive organisms:

Adults and children weighing 40 Kg (88 lbs.) or more: 125 mg q. 6h.

Children weighing less than 40 Kg (88 lbs.): 12.5 mg/Kg/day in equally-divided doses q. 6h.

For more severe infections such as those of the lower respiratory tract or disseminated infections:

Adults and children weighing 40 Kg (88 lbs.) or more: 250 mg q. 6h or higher.

Children weighing less than 40 Kg (88 lbs.): 25 mg/Kg/day or higher in equally-divided doses q. 6h.

Since experience in neonates is limited, a dose for the newborn is not recommended at this time.

Dicloxacillin sodium monohydrate is best absorbed when taken on an empty stomach, preferably one to two hours before meals.

N.B.: INFECTIONS CAUSED BY GROUP A BETA-HEMOLYTIC STREPTOCOCCI SHOULD BE TREATED FOR AT LEAST 10 DAYS TO HELP PREVENT THE OCCURRENCE OF ACUTE RHEUMATIC FEVER OR ACUTE GLOMERULONEPHRITIS.

How Supplied: Capsules equivalent to 250 mg. dicloxacillin, bottles of 100.

Powder for Oral Suspension containing dicloxacillin sodium monohydrate equivalent to 62.5 mg. dicloxacillin per 5 ml, bottles to yield 100 ml.

---

*Bauer, A.W., Kirby, W.M.M., Sherris, J.C., and Turck, M.: Antibiotic Testing by a Standardized Single Discs Method, Am. J. Clin. Pathol., 45:493, 1966; Standardized Disc Susceptibility Test, FEDERAL REGISTER 37:20527-29, 1972.

[*Shown in Product Identification Section*]

PEN • VEE® K ℞

(penicillin V potassium)
TABLETS • FOR ORAL SOLUTION

How Supplied: Pen·Vee® K (penicillin V potassium) is supplied in tablets containing 125 mg (200,000 units), 250 mg (400,000 units), and 500 mg (800,000 units); and as powders for reconstitution which provide oral solutions containing 125 mg (200,000 units) or 250 mg (400,000 units) per 5 ml.

For prescribing information write to Professional Service, Wyeth Laboratories, Box 8299, Philadelphia, PA, 19101, or contact your local Wyeth representative.

[*Shown in Product Identification Section*]

PHENERGAN® ℞

(promethazine hydrochloride)
INJECTION

Description: Each ml of TUBEX® (Sterile Cartridge-Needle Unit) contains either 25 or 50 mg promethazine hydrochloride with 0.1 mg edetate disodium, 0.04 mg calcium chloride, not more than 5 mg monothioglycerol and 5 mg phenol with sodium acetate-acetic acid buffer. Each Ampul of injection contains either 25 mg or 50 mg promethazine hydrochloride with 0.1 mg edetate disodium, 0.04 mg calcium chloride, not more than 0.25 mg sodium metabisulfite and 5 mg phenol with sodium acetate-acetic acid buffer.

Actions: Promethazine hydrochloride, a phenothiazine derivative, possesses antihistaminic, sedative, antimotion-sickness, antiemetic, and anticholinergic effects. The duration of action is generally from four to six hours. The major side reaction of this drug is sedation. As an antihistamine it acts by competitive antagonism, but does not block the release of histamine. It antagonizes in varying degrees most but not all of the pharmacological effects of histamine.

Indications: The injectable form of promethazine hydrochloride is indicated for the following conditions:

1. Amelioration of allergic reactions to blood or plasma.
2. In anaphylaxis as an adjunct to epinephrine and other standard measures after the acute symptoms have been controlled.
3. For other uncomplicated allergic conditions of the immediate type when oral therapy is impossible or contraindicated.
4. Active treatment of motion sickness.
5. Preoperative, postoperative, and obstetric (during labor) sedation.
6. Prevention and control of nausea and vomiting associated with certain types of anesthesia and surgery.
7. As an adjunct to analgesics for the control of postoperative pain.
8. For sedation and relief of apprehension and to produce light sleep from which the patient can be easily aroused.
9. Intravenously in special surgical situations, such as repeated bronchoscopy, ophthalmic surgery, and poor-risk patients, with reduced amounts of meperidine or other narcotic analgesic as an adjunct to anesthesia and analgesia.

Contraindications: Promethazine is contraindicated in comatose states, in patients who have received large amounts of central-nervous-system depressants (alcohol, barbiturates, narcotics, etc.) and in patients who have demonstrated an idiosyncrasy or hypersensitivity to promethazine.

Under no circumstances should promethazine be given by intra-arterial injection due to the likelihood of severe arteriospasm and the possibility of resultant gangrene (see Warnings). Phenergan injection should not be given by the subcutaneous route; evidence of chemical irritation has been noted and necrotic lesions have resulted on rare occasions following subcutaneous injection. The preferred parenteral route of administration is by deep intramuscular injection.

Warnings: Promethazine may impair the mental and/or physical abilities required for the performance of potentially hazardous tasks such as driving a vehicle or operating machinery. The concomitant use of alcohol or other central-nervous-system depressants may have an additive effect. Patients should be warned accordingly.

USAGE IN PREGNANCY: The safe use of promethazine has not been established with respect to the possible adverse effects upon fetal development. Therefore, the need for the use of this drug during pregnancy should be weighed against the possible but unknown hazards to the developing fetus.

USE IN CHILDREN: Excessively large dosages of antihistamines, including promethazine, in children may cause hallucinations, convulsions, and sudden death. In children who are acutely ill associated with dehydration, there is an increased susceptibility to dystonias with the use of promethazine hydrochloride injection.

CAUTION SHOULD BE EXERCISED WHEN ADMINISTERING PHENERGAN TO CHILDREN. ANTIEMETICS ARE NOT RECOMMENDED FOR TREATMENT OF UNCOMPLICATED VOMITING IN CHILDREN, AND THEIR USE SHOULD BE LIMITED TO PROLONGED VOMITING OF KNOWN ETIOLOGY. THE EXTRAPYRAMIDAL SYMPTOMS WHICH CAN OCCUR SECONDARY TO PHENERGAN® ADMINISTRATION MAY BE CONFUSED WITH THE CNS SIGNS OF UNDIAGNOSED PRIMARY DISEASE, e.g., ENCEPHALOPATHY OR REYE'S SYNDROME. THE USE OF PHENERGAN SHOULD BE AVOIDED IN CHILDREN WHOSE SIGNS AND SYMPTOMS MAY SUGGEST REYE'S SYNDROME, OR OTHER HEPATIC DISEASES.

USE IN THE ELDERLY (APPROXIMATELY 60 YEARS OR OLDER): Since therapeutic requirements for sedative drugs tend to be less in elderly patients, the dosage of Phenergan should be reduced for these patients.

OTHER CONSIDERATIONS: Drugs having anticholinergic properties should be used with caution in patients with asthmatic attack, narrow-angle glaucoma, prostatic hypertrophy, stenosing peptic ulcer, pyloroduodenal obstruction, and bladder-neck obstruction.

Phenergan should be used with caution in patients with bone-marrow depression. Leukopenia and agranulocytosis have been reported, usually when Phenergan has been used in association with other known toxic agents.

INADVERTENT INTRA-ARTERIAL INJECTION: Due to the close proximity of arteries and veins in the areas most commonly used for intravenous injection, extreme care should be exercised to avoid perivascular extravasation or inadvertent intra-arterial injection. Reports compatible with inadvertent intra-arterial injection of promethazine, usually in conjunction with other drugs intended for intravenous use, suggest that pain, severe chemical irritation, severe spasm of distal vessels, and resultant gangrene requiring amputation are likely under such circumstances. Intravenous injection was intended in all the cases reported but perivascular extravasation or arterial placement of the needle is now suspect. There is no proven successful management of this condition after it occurs, although sympathetic block and heparinization are commonly employed during the acute management because of the results of animal experiments with other known arteriolar irritants. Aspiration of dark blood does not preclude intra-arterial needle placement, because blood is discolored upon contact with promethazine. Use of syringes with rigid plungers or of small bore needles might obscure typical arterial backflow if this is relied upon alone.

When used intravenously promethazine hydrochloride should be given in a concentration no greater than 25 mg per ml and at a rate not to exceed 25 mg per minute. When administering any irritant drug intravenously it is usually preferable to inject it through the tubing of an intravenous infusion set that is known to be functioning satisfactorily. In the event that a patient complains of pain during intended intravenous injection of promethazine, the injection should immediately be stopped to provide for evaluation of possible arterial placement or perivascular extravasation.

Precautions: Promethazine may significantly affect the actions of other drugs. It may increase, prolong, or intensify the sedative action of central-nervous-system depressants, such as anesthetics, barbiturates, or alcohol. When given concomitantly with promethazine hydrochloride, the dose of barbiturates should be reduced by at least one-half, and the dose of narcotics should be reduced by one-quarter to one-half. Dosage must be individualized. Excessive amounts of promethazine relative to a narcotic may lead to restlessness and motor hyperactivity in the patient with pain; these symptoms usually disappear with adequate control of the pain. Promethazine should be used cautiously in persons with cardiovascular disease or impairment of liver function.

Although reversal of the vasopressor effect of epinephrine has not been reported with promethazine, the possibility should be considered in case of promethazine overdose.

Adverse Reactions: CNS EFFECTS: Drowsiness is the most prominent CNS effect of this drug. Extrapyramidal reactions may occur with high doses; this is almost always responsive to a reduction in dosage. Other reported reactions include dizziness, lassitude, tinnitus, incoordination, fatigue, blurred vision, euphoria, diplopia, nervousness, insomnia, tremors, convulsive seizures, oculogyric crises, excitation, catatonic-like states, and hysteria.

CARDIOVASCULAR EFFECTS: Tachycardia, bradycardia, faintness, dizziness, and increases and decreases in blood pressure have been reported following the use of promethazine hydrochloride injection. Venous thrombosis at the injection site has been reported. INTRA-ARTERIAL INJECTION MAY RESULT IN GANGRENE OF THE AFFECTED EXTREMITY (see Warnings).

GASTROINTESTINAL: Nausea and vomiting have been reported, usually in association with surgical procedures and combination drug therapy.

ALLERGIC REACTIONS: These include urticaria, dermatitis, asthma, and photosensitivity. Angioneurotic edema has been reported.

OTHER REPORTED REACTIONS: Leukopenia and agranulocytosis, usually when Phenergan® has been used in association with other known toxic agents, have been reported. Thrombocytopenic purpura and jaundice of the obstructive type have been associated with the use of promethazine. The jaundice is usually reversible on discontinuation of the drug. Subcutaneous injection has resulted in tissue necrosis. Nasal stuffiness may occur. Dry mouth has been reported.

LABORATORY TESTS: The following laboratory tests may be affected in patients who are receiving therapy with promethazine hydrochloride:

Pregnancy Tests—Diagnostic pregnancy tests based on immunological reactions between HCG and anti-HCG may result in false-negative or false-positive interpretations.

Glucose Tolerance Test—An increase in glucose tolerance has been reported in patients receiving promethazine hydrochloride.

PARADOXICAL REACTIONS (OVERDOSAGE): Hyperexcitability and abnormal movements which have been reported in children following a single administration of promethazine may be manifestations of relative overdosage, in which case, consideration should be given to the discontinuation of the promethazine and to the use of other drugs. Respiratory depression, nightmares, delirium, and agitated behavior have also been reported in some of these patients.

Drug Interactions: NARCOTICS AND BARBITURATES: The CNS depressant effects of narcotics and barbiturates are additive with promethazine hydrochloride.

MAO INHIBITORS: Drug interactions, including an increased incidence of extra-pyramidal effects, have been reported when some MAO inhibitors and phenothiazines are used concomitantly. Although such a reaction has not been reported with promethazine, the possibility should be considered.

Dosage and Administration: The preferred parenteral route of administration for promethazine hydrochloride is by deep intramuscular injection. The proper intravenous administration of this product is well-tolerated, but use of this route is not without some hazard.

INADVERTENT INTRA-ARTERIAL INJECTION CAN RESULT IN GANGRENE OF THE AFFECTED EXTREMITY (see Warnings). SUBCUTANEOUS INJECTION IS CONTRAINDICATED AS IT MAY RESULT IN TISSUE NECROSIS (see Contraindications). When used intravenously, promethazine hydrochloride should be given in concentration no greater than 25 mg/ml at a rate not to exceed 25 mg per minute; it is preferable to inject through the tubing of an intravenous infusion set that is known to be functioning satisfactorily.

ALLERGIC CONDITIONS: The average adult dose is 25 mg. This dose may be repeated within two hours if necessary, but continued therapy, if indicated, should be via the oral route as soon as existing circumstances permit. After initiation of treatment, dosage should be adjusted to the smallest amount adequate to relieve symptoms. The average adult dose for amelioration of allergic reactions to blood or plasma is 25 mg.

SEDATION: In hospitalized adult patients, nighttime sedation may be achieved by a dose of 25 to 50 mg of promethazine hydrochloride.

PRE-AND POST-OPERATIVE USE:

As an adjunct to pre- or post-operative medication, 25 to 50 mg of promethazine hydrochloride in adults may be combined with appropriately reduced doses of analgesics and atropine-like drugs as desired. Dosage of concomitant analgesic or hypnotic medication should be reduced accordingly.

NAUSEA AND VOMITING: For control of nausea and vomiting the usual adult dose is 12.5 to 25 mg, not to be repeated more frequently than every four hours. When used for control of post-operative nausea and vomiting, the medication may be administered either intramuscularly or intravenously and dosage of analgesics and barbiturates reduced accordingly.

OBSTETRICS: Phenergan® in doses of 50 mg will provide sedation and relieve apprehension in the early stages of labor. When labor is definitely established, 25 to 75 mg (average dose, 50 mg) promethazine hydrochloride may be given intramuscularly or intravenously with an appropriately reduced dose of any desired narcotic. Amnesic agents may be administered as necesssary. If necessary, Phenergan with a reduced dose of analgesic may be repeated once or twice at four-hour intervals in the course of a normal labor. A maximum total dose of 100 mg of Phenergan may be administered during a 24-hour period to patients in labor.

CHILDREN: In children under the age of 12 years the dosage should not exceed half that of the suggested adult dose. As an adjunct to premedication the suggested dose is 0.5 mg per lb.

Continued on next page

Wyeth—Cont.

of body weight in combination with an equal dose of narcotic or barbiturate and the appropriate dose of an atropine-like drug. Antiemetics should not be used in vomiting of unknown etiology in children.

Management of Overdosage: Signs and symptoms of overdosage range from mild depression of the central nervous system and cardiovascular system, to profound hypotension, respiratory depression, and unconsciousness. Stimulation may be evident, especially in children and geriatric patients. Atropine-like signs and symptoms—dry mouth, fixed, dilated pupils, flushing, etc., as well as gastrointestinal symptoms, may occur. The treatment of overdosage is essentially symptomatic and supportive. Early gastric lavage may be beneficial if promethazine has been taken orally. Centrally acting emetics are of little use.

Avoid analeptics, which may cause convulsions. Severe hypotension usually responds to the administration of levarterenol or phenylephrine. EPINEPHRINE SHOULD NOT BE USED, since its use in a patient with partial adrenergic blockade may further lower the blood pressure. Extrapyramidal reactions may be treated with anticholinergic antiparkinson agents, diphenhydramine, or barbiturates. Additional measures include oxygen and intravenous fluids. Limited experience with dialysis indicates that it is not helpful.

How Supplied: Phenergan® (promethazine hydrochloride) Injection as TUBEX® (Sterile Cartridge-Needle Unit), either 25 or 50 mg per ml, in packages of 10 TUBEX, and Ampuls of 1 ml, either 25 or 50 mg per ml, in packages of 5 and 25 Ampuls.

PHENERGAN® ℞
(promethazine hydrochloride)
TABLETS • SYRUP •
RECTAL SUPPOSITORIES

Description: Each tablet contains 12.5 mg., 25 mg., or 50 mg. promethazine hydrochloride; the syrup contains 6.25 mg. or 25 mg. promethazine hydrochloride per 5 ml.; each rectal suppository contains 12.5 mg., 25 mg. or 50 mg. promethazine hydrochloride with ascorbyl palmitate, silicon dioxide, white wax and cocoa butter.

Actions: Phenergan® is a phenothiazine derivative that has several different types of pharmacologic properties. In addition to its antihistaminic action, which is of marked potency and prolonged duration, it also provides antiemetic as well as sedative actions, so that it is useful in a variety of clinical situations.

Indications: Phenergan, either orally or by suppository, is useful in the management of the following conditions:

Perennial and seasonal allergic rhinitis.

Vasomotor rhinitis.

Allergic conjunctivitis due to inhalant allergens and foods.

Mild, uncomplicated allergic skin manifestations of urticaria and angioedema.

Amelioration of allergic reactions to blood or plasma.

Dermographism.

As therapy for anaphylactic reactions adjunctive to epinephrine and other standard measures after the acute manifestations have been controlled.

Preoperative, postoperative, or obstetric sedation.

Prevention and control of nausea and vomiting associated with certain types of anesthesia and surgery.

Therapy adjunctive to meperidine or other analgesics for control of postoperative pain.

Sedation in both children and adults as well as relief of apprehension and production of light sleep from which the patient can be easily aroused.

Active and prophylactic treatment of motion sickness.

Antiemetic effect in postoperative patients.

Contraindications: Phenergan is contraindicated in individuals with a known hypersensitivity to the drug.

Warnings: The sedative action of promethazine hydrochloride is additive to the sedative effects of central-nervous-system depressants; therefore, agents such as alcohol, barbiturates and narcotic analgesics should either be eliminated or given in reduced dosage in the presence of promethazine hydrochloride. When given concomitantly with promethazine hydrochloride the dose of barbiturates should be reduced by at least one-half and the dose of analgesic depressants, such as morphine or meperidine, should be reduced by one-quarter to one-half.

Precautions: Ambulatory patients should be cautioned against driving automobiles or operating dangerous machinery until it is known that they do not become drowsy or dizzy from promethazine hydrochloride therapy.

Antiemetics may mask the symptoms of an unrecognized disease and thereby interfere with diagnosis.

Adverse Reactions: Patients may occasionally complain of autonomic reactions such as dryness of the mouth, blurring of vision and, rarely, dizziness.

Very rare cases have been reported where patients receiving promethazine have developed leukopenia. In one instance agranulocytosis has been reported. In nearly every instance reported, other toxic agents known to have caused these conditions have been associated with the administration of promethazine.

Cardiovascular by-effects from promethazine have been rare. Minor increases in blood pressure and occasional mild hypotension have been reported.

Photosensitivity, although extremely rare, has been reported. Occurrence of photosensitivity may be a contraindication to further treatment with promethazine or related drugs. In the presence of abraded or denuded rectal lesions the patient may experience initial local discomfort following administration of promethazine hydrochloride suppositories.

Attempted suicides with promethazine have resulted in deep sedation, coma, rarely convulsions and cardiorespiratory symptoms compatible with the depth of sedation present. A paradoxical reaction has been reported in children receiving single doses of 75 mg. to 125 mg. orally, characterized by hyperexcitability and nightmares.

Dosage and Administration: Allergy: The average oral dose is 25 mg. taken before retiring; however, 12.5 mg. may be taken before meals and on retiring, if necessary. Children tolerate this product well. Single 25 mg. doses at bedtime or 6.25 to 12.5 mg. taken three times daily will usually suffice. After initiation of treatment, in children or adults, dosage should be adjusted to the smallest amount adequate to relieve symptoms. When the oral route is not feasible, Phenergan HCl Rectal Suppositories in 25 mg. doses may be used. The dose may be repeated within two hours if necessary, but oral therapy should be resumed if indicated and existing circumstances permit.

The administration of promethazine hydrochloride in 25 mg. doses will control minor transfusion reactions of an allergic nature.

Motion Sickness: The average adult dose is 25 mg. taken twice daily. The initial dose should be taken one-half to one hour before anticipated travel and be repeated eight to twelve hours later if necessary. On succeeding days of travel, it is recommended that 25 mg. be given on arising and again before the evening meal. For children, Phenergan Tablets, Syrup, or Rectal Suppositories, 12.5 to 25 mg., twice daily, may be administered.

Nausea and Vomiting: The average effective dose of Phenergan for the active therapy of nausea and vomiting in children or adults is 25 mg. When oral medication cannot be tolerated, the dose should be given parenterally (cf. Phenergan Injection) or by rectal suppository. 12.5 to 25 mg. doses may be repeated as necessary at four- to six-hour intervals.

For nausea and vomiting in children the dose should be adjusted to the age and weight of the patient and the severity of the condition being treated.

For prophylaxis of nausea and vomiting, as during surgery and the postoperative period, the average dose is 25 mg. repeated at four- to six-hour intervals as necessary.

Sedation: This product relieves apprehension and induces a quiet sleep from which the patient can be easily aroused. Administration of 12.5 to 25 mg. Phenergan by the oral route or by rectal suppository at bedtime will provide sedation in children. Adults usually require 25 to 50 mg. for nighttime, presurgical or obstetrical sedation.

Pre- and Postoperative Use: Phenergan in 12.5 to 25 mg. doses for children and 50 mg. doses for adults the night before surgery relieves apprehension and produces a quiet sleep.

For preoperative medication, children require doses of 0.5 mg. per pound of body weight in combination with an equal dose of meperidine and the appropriate dose of an atropine-like drug. Phenergan Suppositories, 25 mg., in children up to three years, and 50 mg. suppositories in older children, may be used in lieu of oral or parenteral medication. Usual adult dosage is 50 mg. Phenergan with an equal amount of meperidine and the required amount of a belladonna alkaloid.

Postoperative sedation and adjunctive use with analgesics may be obtained by the administration of 12.5 to 25 mg. in children and 25 to 50 mg. doses in adults.

How Supplied: *Tablets*—**12.5 mg.** (orange, scored), bottles of 100 and 1000, and REDIPAK® Unit Dose Medication, boxes of 100 (individually wrapped); **25 mg.** (white, scored), bottles of 100 and 1000, REDIPAK® Strip Pack, boxes of 25, and REDIPAK® Unit Dose Medication, boxes of 100 (individually wrapped); **50 mg.** (pink), bottles of 100. *Syrup*—6.25 mg. per 5 ml. (alcohol 1.5%), pint bottles. *Syrup Fortis*—25 mg. per 5 ml. (alcohol 1.5%), pint bottles. *Rectal Suppositories*—12.5 mg., 25 mg. and 50 mg., boxes of 12; 25 mg. and 50 mg. also available in REDIPAK® (Unit of Use Suppository Pack), boxes of 25.

[Shown in Product Identification Section]

PHENERGAN® Expectorant with Codeine ℂ ℞

PHENERGAN® Expectorant PLAIN (without Codeine) ℞

PHENERGAN® VC Expectorant with Codeine ℂ ℞

PHENERGAN® VC Expectorant PLAIN (without Codeine) ℞

PHENERGAN® Expectorant with Dextromethorphan PEDIATRIC ℞

For prescribing information write to Professional Service, Wyeth Laboratories, Box 8299, Philadelphia, Pa., 19101, or contact your local Wyeth representative.

SMA®
Iron fortified
infant formula
READY–TO–FEED
CONCENTRATED LIQUID
POWDER

Breast milk is the preferred feeding for newborns. Infant formula is intended to replace or supplement breast milk when breast feeding is not possible or is insufficient, or when mothers elect not to breast feed.

Good maternal nutrition is important for the preparation and maintenance of breast feeding. Extensive or prolonged use of partial bottle feeding, before breast feeding has been well established, could make breast feeding difficult to maintain. A decision not to breast feed could be difficult to reverse.

Professional advice should be followed on all matters of infant feeding. Infant formula should always be prepared and used as directed. Unnecessary or improper use of infant formula could present a health hazard. Social and financial implications should be considered when selecting the method of infant feeding.

SMA® is unique among prepared formulas for its fat blend, whey-dominated protein composition, amino acid pattern and mineral content. SMA®, utilizing a hybridized safflower (oleic) oil, became the first infant formula offering fat and calcium absorption equal to that of human milk, with a physiologic level of linoleic acid. Thus, the fat blend in SMA® provides a ready source of energy, helps protect infants against neonatal tetany and produces a ratio of Vitamin E to polyunsaturated fatty acids (linoleic acid) more than adequate to prevent hemolytic anemia.

By combining reduced minerals whey with skimmed cow's milk, SMA® adjusts the protein content to within the range of human milk, reverses the whey-protein to casein ratio of cow's milk so that it is like that of human milk, and reduces the mineral content to a physiologic level.

The resultant 60:40 whey-protein to casein ratio provides protein nutrition superior to a casein-dominated formula. In addition, the essential amino acids, including cystine, are present in amounts close to those of human milk. So the protein in SMA® is of high biologic value.

The physiologic mineral content makes possible a low renal solute load which helps protect the functionally immature infant kidney, increases expendable water reserves and helps protect against dehydration.

Use of lactose as the carbohydrate results in a physiologic stool flora and a low stool pH, decreasing the incidence of perianal dermatitis.

Ingredients: SMA® Concentrated Liquid or Ready-to-Feed. Water; nonfat milk; reduced minerals whey; lactose; oleo, coconut, oleic (safflower), and soybean oils; soy lecithin; calcium carrageenan. *Minerals:* Potassium bicarbonate; calcium chloride and citrate; potassium chloride; sodium citrate; ferrous sulfate; sodium bicarbonate; zinc, cupric, and manganese sulfates. *Vitamins:* Ascorbic acid, alpha tocopheryl acetate, niacinamide, vitamin A palmitate, calcium pantothenate, thiamine hydrochloride, riboflavin, pyridoxine hydrochloride, beta-carotene, folic acid, phytonadione, activated 7-dehydrocholesterol, biotin, cyanocobalamin.

SMA® Powder. Nonfat milk; reduced minerals whey; lactose; oleo, coconut, oleic (safflower), and soybean oils; soy lecithin.

Minerals: Calcium chloride; sodium bicarbonate; calcium hydroxide; ferrous sulfate; potassium hydroxide and bicarbonate; potassium chloride; zinc, cupric, and manganese sulfates.

Vitamins: Ascorbic acid, alpha tocopheryl acetate, niacinamide, vitamin A palmitate, calcium pantothenate, thiamine hydrochloride, riboflavin, pyridoxine hydrochloride, beta-carotene, folic acid, phytonadione, activated 7-dehydrocholesterol, biotin, cyanocobalamin.

PROXIMATE ANALYSIS
at 20 calories per fluidounce
READY-TO-FEED, POWDER, and CONCENTRATED LIQUID:

	(w/v)
Fat	3.6%
Carbohydrate	7.2%
Protein	1.5%
60% Lactalbumin (whey protein)	0.9%
40% Casein	0.6%
Ash	0.25%
Crude Fiber	None
Total Solids	12.6%
Calories/fl. oz.	20

Vitamins, Minerals: In normal dilution, each quart contains 2500 IU vitamin A, 400 IU vitamin D_3, 9 IU vitamin E, 55 mcg vitamin K_1, 0.67 mg vitamin B_1 (thiamine), 1 mg vitamin B_2 (riboflavin), 55 mg vitamin C (ascorbic acid), 0.4 mg vitamin B_6 (pyridoxine hydrochloride), 1 mcg vitamin B_{12}, 9.5 mg equivalents niacin, 2 mg pantothenic acid, 50 mcg folic acid, 14 mcg biotin, 100 mg choline, 420 mg calcium, 312 mg phosphorus, 50 mg magnesium, 142 mg sodium, 530 mg potassium, 355 mg chloride, 12 mg iron, 0.45 mg copper, 3.5 mg zinc, 150 mcg manganese, 65 mcg iodine.

Preparation: *Ready-to-Feed* (8 and 32 fl. oz. cans of 20 calories per fluidounce formula)—shake can, open and pour into previously sterilized nursing bottle; attach nipple and feed. Cover opened can and immediately store in refrigerator. Use contents of can within 48 hours of opening.

Powder—(1 pound can)—For normal dilution supplying 20 calories per fluidounce, use 1 scoop (or 1 standard tablespoonful) of powder, packed and leveled, to 2 fluidounces of cooled, previously boiled water. For larger amount of formula, use ¼ standard measuring cup of powder, packed and leveled, to 8 fluidounces (1 cup) of water. Three of these portions make 26 fluidounces of formula.

(Unit-of-Use Packets)—For normal dilution supplying 20 calories per fluidounce, use 1 packet of SMA powder to 7 fluidounces of cooled, previously boiled water.

Concentrated Liquid—For normal dilution supplying 20 calories per fluidounce, use equal amounts of SMA® liquid and cooled, previously boiled water.

Note: Prepared formula should be used within 24 hours.

How Supplied: *Ready-to-Feed*—presterilized and premixed, 32 fluidounce (1 quart) cans, cases of 6; 8 fluidounce cans, cases of 24 (4 carriers of 6 cans). *Powder*—1 pound cans with measuring scoop, cases of 12; Unit-of-Use Packets, 1.06 oz. packet, 48 packets/case (12 cartons of 4 packets each). *Concentrated Liquid*— 13 fluidounce cans, cases of 24.

For Hospital Nursery Use—an infant feeding system which provides premixed, presterilized, ready-to-feed items, thus saving space, time and equipment. It eliminates washing, measuring, mixing, sterilizing, refrigerating and heating.

The system is offered in a choice of two forms:

1. Prefilled and presterilized 4 oz. glass bottles for which sterile nipple assemblies are available, to be attached before feeding. These units may be used again after resterilizing or may be discarded, as desired.
2. The E-Z NURSER® (single unit nurser), also prefilled and presterilized, consists of a 4 oz. glass bottle with sterile nipple already attached; the entire unit is designed to be discarded after use.

The following items are supplied in both the forms described above:

SMA® Ready-to-Feed	
13 calories/oz.	48 bottles of 4 fl. oz.
20 calories/oz.	48 bottles of 4 fl. oz.
24 calories/oz.	48 bottles of 4 fl. oz.
27 calories/oz.	48 bottles of 4 fl. oz.
SMA® lo-iron Ready-to-Feed	
20 calories/oz.	48 bottles of 4 fl. oz.
"preemie" SMA® Ready-to-Feed	
24 calories/oz.	48 bottles of 4 fl. oz.
(Not available in the E-Z NURSER®)	
Distilled Water	48 bottles of 4 fl. oz.
Glucose, 5% in Distilled	
Water, 6 calories/oz.	48 bottles of 4 fl. oz.
Glucose, 10% in Distilled	
Water, 12 calories/oz.	48 bottles of 4 fl. oz.
NURSOY® (soy protein formula)	
20 calories/oz.	48 bottles of 4 fl. oz.
(Not available in the E-Z NURSER®)	

Supplied in 8 oz. bottles, to which sterile nipple assemblies must be attached before feeding, are the following:

SMA® Ready-to-Feed	
20 calories/oz.	24 bottles of 8 fl. oz.
Oral Electrolyte Solution	24 bottles of 8 fl. oz.
Distilled Water	24 bottles of 8 fl. oz.
Homogenized Milk	24 bottles of 8 fl. oz.
Skim Milk	24 bottles of 8 fl. oz.

NIPPLE ASSEMBLIES—presterilized, for both premature and term infants, single-hole and cross-cut, suitable for use with all ready-to-feed products requiring them, cartons of 288 nipple units.

ACCUFEED™, Wyeth Graduated Nursers—presterilized, disposable nursers (60 ml capacity) for accurately measured feedings, packages of 200.

Also Available: SMA® lo-iron. For those who appreciate the particular advantages of SMA®, the infant formula closest in composition nutritionally to mother's milk, but who sometimes need or wish to recommend a formula that does not contain a high level of iron, now there is SMA® lo-iron with all the benefits of regular SMA® but with a reduced level of iron of 1.4 mg per quart. Infants should receive supplemental dietary iron from an outside source to meet daily requirements.

Concentrated Liquid, 13 fl. oz. cans, cases of 24. Powder, 1 pound cans with measuring scoop, cases of 12. Ready-to-Feed, 32 fl. oz. cans, cases of 6.

Preparation of the standard 20 calories per fluidounce formula of SMA® lo-iron is the same as SMA® iron fortified given above.

SERAX® Ⓒ ℞
(oxazepam)
CAPSULES • TABLETS

Description: A therapeutic agent providing versatility and flexibility in control of common emotional disturbances, this product exerts prompt action in a wide variety of disorders associated with anxiety, tension, agitation and irritability, and anxiety associated with depression. In tolerance and toxicity studies on several animal species, this product reveals significantly greater safety factors than related compounds (chlordiazepoxide and diazepam) and manifests a wide separation of effective doses and doses inducing side effects.

Serax is 7 chloro-1,3-dihydro-3-hydroxy-5-phenyl-2*H*-1,4-benzodiazepin-2-one.

Animal Pharmacology and Toxicology: In mice, SERAX exerts an anticonvulsant (anti-Metrazol®) activity at 50 percent effective doses of about 0.6 mg. per kg. orally. (Such anticonvulsant activity of benzodiazepines correlates with their tranquilizing properties.) To produce ataxia (rotabar test) and sedation (abolition of spontaneous motor activity), the 50 percent effective doses of this product are greater than 5 mg. per kg. orally. Thus about ten times the therapeutic (anticonvulsant) dose must be given before ataxia ensues, indicating a wide separation of effective doses and doses inducing side effects.

In evaluation of antianxiety activity of compounds, conflict behavioral tests in rats differentiate continuous response for food in the presence of anxiety-provoking stress (shock) from drug-induced motor incoordination. This product shows significant separation of doses required to relieve anxiety and doses producing sedation or ataxia. Ataxia-producing doses exceed those of related CNS-acting drugs.

Continued on next page

Wyeth—Cont.

Acute oral LD_{50} in mice is greater than 5000 mg. per kg., compared to 800 mg. per kg. for a related compound (chlordiazepoxide).
Subacute toxicity studies in dogs for four weeks at 480 mg. per kg. daily showed no specific changes; at 960 mg. per kg. two out of eight died with evidence of circulatory collapse. This wide margin of safety is significant compared to chlordiazepoxide HCl, which showed non-specific changes in six dogs at 80 mg. per kg. On chlordiazepoxide, two out of six died with evidence of circulatory collapse at 127 mg. per kg., and six out of six died at 200 mg. per kg. daily. Chronic toxicity studies of Serax in dogs at 120 mg. per kg. per day for 52 weeks produced no toxic manifestation.
Fatty metamorphosis of the liver has been noted in six-week toxicity studies in rats given this product at 0.5% of the diet. Such accumulations of fat are considered reversible as there is no liver necrosis or fibrosis.
Breeding studies in rats through two successive litters did not produce fetal abnormality.
This product has a single major metabolite in man, a glucuronide excreted in the urine.
Indications: Serax (oxazepam) is indicated for the management of anxiety disorders or for the short-term relief of the symptoms of anxiety. Anxiety or tension associated with the stress of everyday life usually does not require treatment with an anxiolytic.
Anxiety associated with depression is also responsive to Serax (oxazepam) therapy.
This product has been found particularly useful in the management of anxiety, tension, agitation and irritability in older patients.
Alcoholics with acute tremulousness, inebriation, or with anxiety associated with alcohol withdrawal are responsive to therapy.
The effectiveness of Serax in long-term use, that is, more than 4 months, has not been assessed by systematic clinical studies. The physician should reassess periodically the usefulness of the drug for the individual patient.
Contraindications: History of previous hypersensitivity reaction to oxazepam. Oxazepam is not indicated in psychoses.
Warnings: As with other CNS-acting drugs, patients should be cautioned against driving automobiles or operating dangerous machinery until it is known that they do not become drowsy or dizzy on oxazepam therapy.
Patients should be warned that the effects of alcohol or other CNS-depressant drugs may be additive to those of Serax, possibly requiring adjustment of dosage or elimination of such agents.

USE IN PREGNANCY

An increased risk of congenital malformations associated with the use of minor tranquilizers (chlordiazepoxide, diazepam, and meprobamate) during the first trimester of pregnancy has been suggested in several studies. Serax, a benzodiazepine derivative, has not been studied adequately to determine whether it, too, may be associated with an increased risk of fetal abnormality. Because use of these drugs is rarely a matter of urgency, their use during this period should almost always be avoided. The possibility that a woman of childbearing potential may be pregnant at the time of institution of therapy should be considered. Patients should be advised that if they become pregnant during therapy or intend to become pregnant they should communicate with their physician about the desirability of discontinuing the drug.
Precautions: Although hypotension has occurred only rarely, oxazepam should be administered with caution to patients in whom a drop in blood pressure might lead to cardiac complications. This is particularly true in the elderly patient.
In some patients exhibiting drug dependency through chronic overdose with Serax (oxazepam) withdrawal symptoms have been noted on discontinuance of drug administration. Withdrawal symptoms have also been reported following abrupt discontinuance of benzodiazepines taken continuously at therapeutic levels for several months. Careful supervision of dose and amounts prescribed for patients is advised, especially with those patients with a known propensity for taking excessive quantities of drugs. Excessive and prolonged use in susceptible persons, for example, alcoholics, former addicts, and others, may result in dependence on or habituation to the drug. Where excessive dosage is continued for weeks or months, dosage should be reduced gradually rather than abruptly stopped. Abrupt discontinuance of doses in excess of the recommended dose may result in some cases in the occurrence of epileptiform seizures. Withdrawal symptoms following abrupt discontinuance are similar to those seen with barbiturates.
Serax 15 mg tablets, *but none of the other available dosage forms of this product,* contain FD&C Yellow No. 5 (tartrazine) which may cause allergic-type reactions (including bronchial asthma) in certain susceptible individuals. Although the overall incidence of FD&C Yellow No. 5 (tartrazine) sensitivity in the general population is low, it is frequently seen in patients who also have aspirin hypersensitivity.
Adverse Reactions: The necessity for discontinuation of therapy due to undesirable effects has been rare. Transient mild drowsiness is commonly seen in the first few days of therapy. If it persists, the dosage should be reduced. In few instances, dizziness, vertigo, headache and rarely syncope have occurred either alone or together with drowsiness. Mild paradoxical reactions, i.e., excitement, stimulation of affect, have been reported in psychiatric patients; these reactions may be secondary to relief of anxiety and usually appear in the first two weeks of therapy.
Other side effects occurring during oxazepam therapy include rare instances of minor diffuse skin rashes—morbilliform, urticarial and maculopapular—nausea, lethargy, edema, slurred speech, tremor and altered libido. Such side effects have been infrequent and are generally controlled with reduction of dosage.
Although rare, leukopenia and hepatic dysfunction including jaundice have been reported during therapy. Periodic blood counts and liver function tests are advisable.
Ataxia with oxazepam has been reported in rare instances and does not appear to be specifically related to dose or age.
Although the following side reactions have not as yet been reported with oxazepam, they have occurred with related compounds (chlordiazepoxide and diazepam): paradoxical excitation with severe rage reactions, hallucinations, menstrual irregularities, change in EEG pattern, blood dyscrasias including agranulocytosis, blurred vision, diplopia, incontinence, stupor, disorientation, fever and euphoria.
Dosage and Administration: Because of the flexibility of this product and the range of emotional disturbances responsive to it, dosage should be individualized for maximum beneficial effects.
[See table below].

This product is not indicated in children under 6 years of age. Absolute dosage for children 6–12 years of age is not established.
How Supplied: Capsules—10 mg. (pink and white), 15 mg. (red and white), 30 mg. (maroon and white), bottles of 100 and 500, and Redi-pak® (Strip Pack), boxes of 25; 15 and 30 mg. capsules also in Redipak® Unit Dose Medication, boxes of 100, (individually wrapped).
Tablets—15 mg. (yellow), bottles of 100.
[*Shown in Product Identification Section*]

SERAX (oxazepam)

	Usual Dose
Mild to moderate anxiety, with associated tension, irritability, agitation or related symptoms of functional origin or secondary to organic disease.	10 to 15 mg, 3 or 4 times daily
Severe anxiety syndromes, agitation or anxiety associated with depression.	15 to 30 mg, 3 or 4 times daily
Older patients with anxiety, tension, irritability and agitation.	Initial dosage: 10 mg, 3 times daily. If necessary, increase cautiously to 15 mg, 3 or 4 times daily
Alcoholics with acute inebriation, tremulousness, or anxiety on withdrawal.	15 to 30 mg, 3 or 4 times daily

SIMECO® OTC
(aluminum hydroxide gel, magnesium hydroxide, simethicone)
SUSPENSION

Composition: Each teaspoonful (5 ml) contains aluminum hydroxide gel equivalent to 365 mg of dried gel, USP, 300 mg of magnesium hydroxide and 30 mg of simethicone. Sodium content is 0.3 mEq-0.6 mEq per teaspoonful. High potency and low dose are provided by high concentration of antacid per teaspoonful.
Indications: For the symptomatic relief of hyperacidity associated with the diagnosis of peptic ulcer, gastritis, peptic esophagitis, gastric hyperacidity and hiatal hernia. To relieve the symptoms of gas.
Dosage and Administration: Usually: 1 or 2 teaspoonfuls undiluted or with a little water to be taken 3 or 4 times daily between meals and at bedtime. 5 ml SIMECO suspension neutralizes 22 mEq of acid.
Drug Interaction Precautions: Alumina-containing antacids should not be used concomitantly with any form of tetracycline therapy.
How Supplied: Suspension—Cool mint flavor available in 12 fl. oz. plastic bottles.

TUBEX® Closed Injection System

The Tubex® closed injection system delivers injectable medication in accurately machine-measured doses with each sterile, prefilled cartridge-needle unit permanently identified up to the moment of injection. Precisely calibrated single-use cartridge-needle units eliminate cross contamination and minimize dosage errors. Super-sharp, siliconized needles minimize penetration pressure. Medication is easily delivered via the sturdy, stainless Tubex® hypodermic syringe.
Tubex sterile cartridge-needle units are ready for instant use, fit easily into the physician's bag, and are readily stored and inventoried in the office.
Tamp-r-tel® (tamper resistant package) — a clear, sturdy plastic package for all Tubex narcotics and barbiturates — adds a new dimension to the handling and record keeping of these controlled drugs. In Tamp-r-tel, each Tubex® sterile cartridge-needle unit is locked

into an individual slot within the package by its own end-lock tab, which is easily broken to release the unit for use. Once the end-lock tab is broken, it is almost impossible to replace it. TAMP-R-TEL thus enhances package integrity, discourages pilferage and facilitates "at a glance" drug count.

The following products are currently available in TUBEX® closed injection system. *For prescribing information on products listed write to Professional Service, Wyeth Laboratories, P.O. Box 8299, Philadelphia, PA, 19101, or contact your local Wyeth representative.*

Product and Needle Size
Units Per Pkg — NDC 0008-

NARCOTICS in TAMP-R-TEL®
(tamper resistant package)

CODEINE PHOSPHATE, USPⒸ●
30 mg (1/2 gr.) (25 G × 5/8") 10—1 ml — 0608-01
60 mg (1 gr.) (25 G × 5/8") 10—1 ml — 0609-01

HYDROMORPHONE HYDROCHLORIDE, USP Ⓒ●
1 mg (1/60 gr.) (25 G × 5/8") 10—1 ml fill in 2 ml — 0387-01
1 mg (1/60 gr.) (22 G × 1 1/4") 10—1 ml fill in 2 ml — 0387-03
2 mg (1/30 gr.) (25 G × 5/8") 10—1 ml fill in 2 ml — 0295-02
2 mg (1/30 gr.) (22 G × 1 1/4") 10—1 ml fill in 2 ml — 0295-01
3 mg (1/20 gr.) (25 G × 5/8") 10—1 ml fill in 2 ml — 0388-01
4 mg (1/15 gr.) (25 G × 5/8") 10—1 ml fill in 2 ml — 0296-02
4 mg (1/15 gr.) (22 G × 1 1/4") 10—1 ml fill in 2 ml — 0296-01

MEPERGAN® (Meperidine HCl and Promethazine HCl) 25 mg each/ml Ⓒ●
(22 G × 1 1/4") 10—2 ml — 0235-01

MEPERIDINE HYDROCHLORIDE, USP Ⓒ●
25 mg (25 G × 5/8") 10—1 ml fill in 2 ml — 0601-03
25 mg (22 G × 1 1/4") 10—1 ml fill in 2 ml — 0601-02
50 mg (25 G × 5/8") 10—1 ml fill in 2 ml — 0602-03
50 mg (22 G × 1 1/4") 10—1 ml fill in 2 ml — 0602-02
75 mg (25 G × 5/8") 10—1 ml fill in 2 ml — 0605-03
75 mg (22 G × 1 1/4") 10—1 ml fill in 2 ml — 0605-02
100 mg (25 G × 5/8") 10—1 ml fill in 2 ml — 0613-03
100 mg (22 G × 1 1/4") 10—1 ml fill in 2 ml — 0613-02

MORPHINE SULFATE, USP Ⓒ●
2 mg (1/30 gr.) (25 G × 5/8") 10—1 ml — 0532-01
4 mg (1/15 gr.) (25 G × 5/8") 10—1 ml — 0533-01
8 mg (1/8 gr.) (25 G × 5/8") 10—1 ml — 0205-02
8 mg (1/8 gr.) (25 G × 5/8") 10—1 ml fill in 2 ml — 0205-01
8 mg (1/8 gr.) (22 G × 1 1/4") 10—1 ml fill in 2 ml — 0205-03
10 mg (1/6 gr.) (25 G × 5/8") 10—1 ml — 0206-03
10 mg (1/6 gr.) (25 G × 5/8") 10—1 ml fill in 2 ml — 0206-02
10 mg (1/6 gr.) (22 G × 1 1/4") 10—1 ml fill in 2 ml — 0206-01
15 mg (1/4 gr.) (25 G × 5/8") 10—1 ml — 0207-03
15 mg (1/4 gr.) (25 G × 5/8") 10—1 ml fill in 2 ml — 0207-02
15 mg (1/4 gr.) (22 G × 1 1/4") 10—1 ml fill in 2 ml — 0207-01

BARBITURATES in TAMP-R-TEL®

PENTOBARBITAL SODIUM, USP Ⓒ●
50 mg (3/4 gr.) (22 G × 1 1/4") 10—1 ml — 0303-01
100 mg (1 1/2 gr.) (22 G × 1 1/4") 10—2 ml — 0303-02

PHENOBARBITAL SODIUM, USP Ⓒ
30 mg (1/2 gr.) (22 G × 1 1/4") 10—1 ml — 0499-01
60 mg (1 gr.) (22 G × 1 1/4") 10—1 ml — 0457-01
130 mg (2 gr.) (22 G × 1 1/4") 10—1 ml — 0304-01

SECOBARBITAL SODIUM, USP Ⓒ●
50 mg (3/4 gr.) (22 G × 1 1/4") 10—1 ml — 0305-01
100 mg (1 1/2 gr.) (22 G × 1 1/4") 10—2 ml — 0305-02

● Narcotic order blank required.

ANTIBIOTICS

BICILLIN® C-R (Penicillin G Benzathine and Penicillin G Procaine Suspension) 300,000 U each/ml
600,000 U (20 G × 1 1/4") 10—1 ml — 0026-17
600,000 U (20 G × 1 1/4") 50—1 ml — 0026-13
600,000 U (20 G × 1") 10—1 ml — 0026-18
1,200,000 U (20 G × 1 1/4") 10—2 ml — 0026-16
1,200,000 U (20 G × 1 1/4") 50—2 ml — 0026-14
1,200,00 U (20 G × 1") 10—2 ml — 0026-19
1,200,000 U (20 G × 1 1/4 ") 10—2 ml (disposable syringe) — 0026-21
2,400,000 U (18 G × 2") 10—4 ml (disposable syringe) — 0026-22

BICILLIN C-R 900/300
(900,000 units Penicillin G Benzathine and 300,000 units Penicillin G Procaine in suspension)
1,200,000 U (20 G × 1 1/4") 10—2 ml — 0079-01

BICILLIN LONG-ACTING (Sterile Penicillin G Benzathine Suspension)
600,000 U (20 G × 1 1/4") 10—1 ml — 0021-08
900,000 U (20 G × 1 1/4") 10—1.5 ml fill in 2 ml — 0021-13
1,200,000 U (20 G × 1 1/4") 10—2 ml — 0021-07
1,200,000 U (20 G × 1 1/4") 10—2 ml (disposable syringe) — 0021-11
2,400,000 U (18 G × 2") 10—4 ml (disposable syringe) — 0021-12

WYCILLIN® (Sterile Penicillin G Procaine Suspension)
300,000 U (22 G × 1 1/4") 10—1 ml — 0134-02
600,000 U (20 G × 1 1/4") 10—1 ml — 0018-10
600,000 U (20 G × 1 1/4") 50—1 ml — 0018-07
1,200,000 U (20 G × 1 1/4") 10—2 ml — 0018-08
2,400,000 U (18 G × 2") 10—4 ml (disposable syringe) — 0018-12

WYCILLIN Injection and PROBENECID Tablets
(Sterile Penicillin G Procaine Suspension and Probenecid Tablets)
2,400,000 U (18 G × 2") 2—4 ml — 2517-01
(package contains two disposable syringes and two 0.5 gram Probenecid tablets)

BIOLOGICALS

DIPHTHERIA and TETANUS TOXOIDS ADSORBED (PEDIATRIC)
(25 G × 5/8") 10—0.5 ml — 0338-01

IMMUNE SERUM GLOBULIN (HUMAN), USP
(20 G × 1 1/4") 1—2 ml — 0437-02

INFLUENZA VIRUS VACCINE
(purified sub-virion)
1982-1983 Formula
(25 G × 5/8") 10—0.5 ml — 0633-02

TETANUS and DIPHTHERIA TOXOIDS ADSORBED (ADULT)
(25 G × 5/8") 10—0.5 ml — 0341-01

TETANUS IMMUNE GLOBULIN (HUMAN)
250 U (20 G × 1 1/4") 10—1 ml — 0408-03

TETANUS TOXOID ADSORBED
(25 G × 5/8") 10—0.5 ml — 0339-01

TETANUS TOXOID FLUID
(25 G × 5/8") 10—0.5 ml — 0340-01

TRIPLE ANTIGEN (Diphtheria and Tetanus Toxoids and Pertussis Vaccine Adsorbed)
(25 G × 5/8") 10—0.5 ml — 0358-01

Continued on next page

Wyeth—Cont.

VITAMINS

CYANOCOBALAMIN, USP
100 mcg (22 G × 1¼″)
10—1 ml 0265-01

1,000 mcg (25 G × ⅝″)
10—1 ml 0264-03

1,000 mcg (22 G × 1¼″)
10—1 ml 0264-01

1,000 mcg (22 G × 1¼″)
10—1 ml fill in 2 ml 0264-02

THIAMINE HYDROCHLORIDE, USP
100 mg (22 G × 1¼″)
10—1 ml fill in 2 ml 0302-01

CARDIOVASCULAR AGENTS

DIGOXIN, USP
0.25 mg (22 G × 1¼″)
10—1 ml 0480-02

0.5 mg (22 G × 1¼″)
10—2 ml 0480-01

EPINEPHRINE, USP (1:1000)
(25 G × ⅝″)
10—1 ml 0263-01

FUROSEMIDE, USP
20 mg (22 G × 1¼″)
10—2 ml 0628-04

HEPARIN SODIUM, USP
1,000 USP units (22 G × 1¼″)
10—1 ml 0275-01

2,500 USP units (25 G × ⅝″)
10—1 ml 0482-01

5,000 USP units (25 G × ⅝″)
10—0.5 ml 0277-02

5,000 USP units (25 G × ⅝″)
10—1 ml 0278-02

5,000 USP units (22 G × 1¼″)
10—1 ml 0278-01

7,500 USP units (25 G × ⅝″)
10—1 ml 0293-01

10,000 USP units (25 G × ⅝″)
10—1 ml 0277-01

15,000 USP units (25 G × ⅝″)
10—1 ml 0279-01

20,000 USP units (25 G × ⅝″)
10—1 ml 0276-01

WYAMINE® SULFATE (Mephentermine Sulfate)
30 mg (22 G × 1¼″)
10—1 ml 0239-01

SPECIAL AGENTS

ATIVAN® (Lorazepam)Ⓒ
2 mg/ml (22 G × 1¼″)
10—1 ml fill in 2 ml 0581-02

4 mg/ml (22 G × 1¼″)
10—1 ml fill in 2 ml 0570-02

CHLORPROMAZINE HYDROCHLORIDE, USP
25 mg (22 G × 1¼″)
10—1 ml 0435-01

50 mg (22 G × 1¼″)
10—2 ml 0435-03

DEXAMETHASONE SODIUM PHOSPHATE, USP
4 mg (22 G × 1¼″)
10—1 ml 0546-01

DIMENHYDRINATE, USP
50 mg (22 G × 1¼″)
10—1 ml 0485-01

DIPHENHYDRAMINE HYDROCHLORIDE, USP
50 mg (22 G × 1¼″)
10—1 ml 0384-01

ERGONOVINE MALEATE, USP
0.2 mg (1/300 gr.) (22 G × 1¼″)
10—1 ml 0307-01

HEPARIN LOCK FLUSH Solution, USP
10 USP units (25 G × ⅝″)
50—1 ml 0523-01

100 USP units (25 G × ⅝″)
50—1 ml 0487-01

HYDROXYZINE HCl, USP
25 mg (22 G × 1¼″)
10—1 ml 0540-01

50 mg (22 G × 1¼″)
10—1 ml 0541-01

100 mg (22 G × 1¼″)
10—2 ml 0541-02

LARGON® (Propiomazine HCl) (1678CB)
20 mg (22 G × 1¼″)
10—1 ml 0260-01

LIDOCAINE HYDROCHLORIDE, USP
1% 10 mg/ml (25 G × ⅝″)
10—2.5 ml 0454-01

2% 20 mg/ml (25 G × ⅝″)
10—2.5 ml 0460-01

OXYTOCIN, USP (Synthetic)
10 USP units (22 G × 1¼″)
10—1 ml 0406-01

PHENERGAN® (Promethazine HCl)
25 mg (22 G × 1¼″)
10—1 ml 0416-01

50 mg (22 G × 1¼″)
10—1 ml 0417-01

PROCHLORPERAZINE EDISYLATE, USP
5 mg (22 G × 1¼″)
10—1 ml 0542-01

10 mg (22 G × 1¼″)
10—2 ml 0542-02

SPARINE® (Promazine HCl)
25 mg (22 G × 1¼″)
10—1 ml 0232-01

50 mg (22 G ×1¼″)
10—1 ml 0236-01

100 mg (22 G × 1¼″)
10—2 ml 0236-02

SODIUM CHLORIDE, USP (Bacteriostatic)
(22 G × 1¼″)
50—2.5 ml 0333-05

(25 G × ⅝″)
50—2.5 ml 0333-02

TUBEX, EMPTY, STERILE CARTRIDGE-NEEDLE UNITS
(25 G × ⅝″)
50—1 ml 9103-02

(22 G × 1¼″)
50—1 ml 9103-01

(25 G × ⅝″)
50—2 ml 9103-04

(22 G × 1¼″)
50—2 ml 9103-03

UNIPEN® ℞

(nafcillin sodium) as the monohydrate
INJECTION • CAPSULES • POWDER FOR ORAL SOLUTION • TABLETS

Description: Unipen (nafcillin sodium) is a semisynthetic penicillin developed by Wyeth research. Although primarily designed as an antistaphylococcal penicillin, in limited clinical trials it has been shown to be effective in the treatment of infections caused by pneumococci and Group A beta-hemolytic streptococci. Because of this wide gram-positive spectrum, this product is particularly suitable for *Initial Therapy* in severe or potentially severe infections before definitive culture results are known and in which staphylococci are suspected.

This product is readily soluble and can be conveniently administered in both oral and parenteral dosage forms. It is resistant to inactivation by staphylococcal penicillinase. Following intramuscular administration in humans, it rapidly appears in the plasma, penetrates body tissues in high concentration, and diffuses well into pleural, pericardial, and synovial fluids.

NOTE: Unipen contains 2.9 milliequivalents of sodium per gram of nafcillin as the sodium salt.

Microbiology: Unipen is a bactericidal penicillin which has shown activity *in vitro* against both penicillin G-sensitive and penicillin G-resistant strains of *Staphylococcus aureus* as well as against pneumococcus, beta-hemolytic streptococcus, and alpha streptococcus (viridans).

In experimental mouse infections induced with pneumococci, beta-hemolytic streptococci, and both penicillin G-susceptible and penicillin G-resistant strains of *Staph. aureus*, nafcillin sodium was compared with methicillin and oxacillin. Regardless of the route of drug administration (intramuscular or oral), nafcillin sodium was consistently and significantly more effective than the other two penicillins. The fate of a penicillin G-resistant strain of *Staph. aureus* was determined in the kidneys of mice treated with penicillin G, methicillin, and nafcillin sodium. Animals injected with the nafcillin sodium showed negative cultures after the fourteenth day, whereas positive kidney cultures were obtained during the entire 28-day period from mice treated with penicillin G and methicillin.

Pharmacology: Unipen is relatively nontoxic for animals. The acute LD_{50} of this product by oral administration in rats and mice was greater than 5 g/kg; by intramuscular administration in rats 2800 mg/kg; by intraperitoneal administration in rats, 1240 mg/kg; and by intravenous administration in mice, 1140 mg/kg. The intraperitoneal LD_{50} in dogs is 600 mg/kg. Animal studies indicated that local tissue responses following intramuscular administration of 25% solutions were minimal and resembled those of penicillin G rather than methicillin.

Animal studies indicate that antibacterial amounts are concentrated in the bile, kidney, lung, heart, spleen, and liver. Eighty-four percent of an intravenously administered dose can be recovered by biliary cannulation and 13 percent by renal excretion in 24 hours. High and prolonged tissue levels can be demonstrated by both biological activity assays and C^{14} distribution patterns.

At comparable dosage, intramuscular absorption of this product is nearly equivalent to that of intramuscular methicillin, and oral absorption to that of oral oxacillin. Blood concentrations may be tripled by the concurrent use of probenecid. Clinical studies with nafcillin sodium monohydrate in infants under three days of age and prematures have revealed higher blood levels and slower rates of urinary excretion than in older children and adults.

Studies of the effect of this product on reproduction in rats and rabbits have been completed and reveal no fetal or maternal abnormalities. These studies include the observation of the effects of administration of the drug before conception and continuously through weaning (one generation).

Disc Susceptibility Tests: Quantitative methods that require measurement of zone diameters give the most precise estimates of antibiotic susceptibility. One such procedure* has been recommended for use with discs for testing susceptibility to penicillinase-resistant penicillin-class antibiotics. Interpretations correlate diameters on the disc test with MIC values for penicillinase-resistant penicillins. With this procedure, a report from the laboratory of "susceptible" indicates that the infecting organism is likely to respond to therapy. A report of "resistant" indicates that the infecting organism is not likely to respond to therapy. A report of "intermediate susceptibility" suggests that the organism would be susceptible if high dosage is used, or if the infection is confined to tissues and fluids (e.g., urine) in which high antibiotic levels are attained.

*Bauer, A.W., Kirby, W.M.M., Sherris, J.C., and Turck, M.: Antibiotic Testing by a Standardized Single-Disc Method, Am. J. Clin. Pathol., *45*:493, 1966; Standardized Disc Susceptibility Test, FEDERAL REGISTER *37*:20527–29, 1972.

Indications: Although the principal indication for nafcillin sodium is in the treatment of infections due to penicillinase-producing staphylococci, it may be used to initiate therapy in such patients in whom a staphylococcal infection is suspected. (See Important Note below.)

Bacteriologic studies to determine the causative organisms and their sensitivity to nafcillin sodium should be performed.

In serious, life-threatening infections, oral preparations of the penicillinase-resistant penicillins should not be relied on for initial therapy.

Important Note: When it is judged necessary that treatment be initiated before definitive culture and sensitivity results are known, the choice of nafcillin sodium should take into consideration the fact that it has been shown to be effective only in the treatment of infections caused by pneumococci, Group A beta-hemolytic streptococci, and penicillin G-resistant and penicillin G-sensitive staphylococci. If the bacteriology report later indicates the infection is due to an organism other than a penicillin G-resistant staphylococcus sensitive to nafcillin sodium, the physician is advised to continue therapy with a drug other than nafcillin sodium or any other penicillinase-resistant, semisynthetic penicillin.

Recent studies have reported that the percentage of staphylococcal isolates resistant to penicillin G outside the hospital is increasing, approximating the high percentage of resistant staphylococcal isolates found in the hospital. For this reason, it is recommended that a penicillinase-resistant penicillin be used as initial therapy for any suspected staphylococcal infection until culture and sensitivity results are known.

Methicillin is a compound that acts through a mechanism similar to that of nafcillin sodium against penicillin G-resistant staphylococci. Strains of staphylococci resistant to methicillin have existed in nature, and it is known that the number of these strains reported has been increasing. Such strains of staphylococci have been capable of producing serious disease, in some instances resulting in fatality. Because of this there is concern that widespread use of the penicillinase-resistant penicillins may result in the appearance of an increasing number of staphylococcal strains which are resistant to these penicillins.

Methicillin-resistant strains are almost always resistant to all other penicillinase-resistant penicillins (cross-resistance with cephalosporin derivatives also occurs frequently). Resistance to any penicillinase-resistant penicillin should be interpreted as evidence of clinical resistance to all, in spite of the fact that minor variations in *in vitro* sensitivity may be encountered when more than one penicillinase-resistant penicillin is tested against the same strain of staphylococcus.

Contraindications: A history of allergic reaction to any of the penicillins is a contraindication.

Warnings: Serious and occasionally fatal hypersensitivity (anaphylactoid) reactions have been reported in patients on penicillin therapy. Although anaphylaxis is more frequent following parenteral therapy, it has occurred in patients on oral penicillins. These reactions are more apt to occur in individuals with a history of sensitivity to multiple allergens.

There have been reports of individuals with a history of penicillin hypersensitivity reactions who have experienced severe hypersensitivity reactions when treated with a cephalosporin. Before therapy with a penicillin, careful inquiry should be made concerning previous hypersensitivity reactions to penicillins, cephalosporins, and other allergens. If an allergic reaction occurs, appropriate therapy should be instituted, and discontinuation of nafcillin therapy considered. The usual agents (antihistamines, pressor amines, corticosteroids) should be readily available.

Precautions: As with any potent drug, periodic assessment of organ-system function, including renal, hepatic and hematopoietic, should be made during prolonged therapy.

The possibility of bacterial and fungal overgrowth should be kept in mind during long-term therapy. If overgrowth of resistant organisms occurs, appropriate measures should be taken.

The oral route of administration should not be relied upon in patients with severe illness, or with nausea, vomiting, gastric dilatation, cardiospasm, or intestinal hypermotility.

Safety for use in pregnancy has not been established.

Particular care should be taken with intravenous administration because of the possibility of thrombophlebitis.

Adverse Reactions: Reactions to nafcillin sodium have been infrequent and mild in nature. As with other penicillins, the possibility of an anaphylactic reaction or serum-sickness-like reactions should be considered. A careful history should be taken. Patients with histories of hay fever, asthma, urticaria, or previous sensitivity to penicillin are more likely to react adversely.

Transient leukopenia, neutropenia with evidence of granulocytopenia or thrombocytopenia are infrequent and usually associated with prolonged therapy with high doses of penicillin. These alterations have been noted to return to normal after cessation of therapy.

The few reactions associated with the intramuscular use of nafcillin sodium have been skin rash, pruritus, and possible drug fever. As with other penicillins, reactions from oral use of the drug have included nausea, vomiting, diarrhea, urticaria, and pruritus.

Dosage and Administration: It is recommended that parenteral therapy be used initially in severe infections. The patient should be placed on oral therapy with this product as soon as the clinical condition warrants. Very severe infections may require very high doses.

Intravenous route: 500 mg every 4 hours; double the dose if necessary in very severe infections.

The required amount of drug should be diluted in 15 to 30 ml of Sterile Water for Injection, U.S.P., or Sodium Chloride Injection, U.S.P., and injected over a 5- to 10-minute period. This may be accomplished through the tubing of an intravenous infusion if desirable.

Stability studies on nafcillin sodium at concentrations of 2 mg/ml to 40 mg/ml in the following intravenous solutions indicate the drug will lose less than 10% activity at room temperature (70°F.) or, if kept under refrigeration, during the time period stipulated:

STABILITY OF	ROOM TEMPERATURE	REFRIGERATED
Sterile Water for Injection	24 hours	96 hours
Isotonic sodium chloride	24 hours	96 hours
5% dextrose in water	24 hours	96 hours
5% dextrose in 0.4% sodium chloride solution	24 hours	96 hours
Ringer's solution	24 hours	96 hours
M/6 sodium lactate solution	24 hours	96 hours

Discard any unused portions of intravenous solutions after 24 hours if kept at room temperature or after 96 hours if kept under refrigeration.

Only those solutions listed above should be used for the intravenous infusion of UNIPEN (nafcillin sodium). The concentration of the antibiotic should fall within the range of 2 to 40 mg/ml. The drug concentrate and the rate and volume of the infusion should be adjusted so that the total dose of nafcillin is administered before the drug loses its stability in the solution in use.

There is no clinical experience available on the use of this agent in neonates or infants for this route of administration.

This route of administration should be used for relatively short-term therapy (24-48 hours) because of the occasional occurrence of thrombophlebitis, particularly in elderly patients.

PIGGYBACK UNITS (for Intravenous Drip Use)—

As diluents, use the following solutions: Sterile Water for Injection, Isotonic Sodium Chloride, 5% dextrose in water, 5% dextrose in 0.4% sodium chloride solution, Ringer's solution, or M/6 sodium lactate solution.

1-GRAM BOTTLE:

Add a minimum of 49 ml diluent, and shake well. If lower concentrations are desired, the solution could be further diluted with up to a total of 99 ml of diluent.

Amount of Diluent	Concentration of Solution
49 ml	20 mg/ml
99 ml	10 mg/ml

1.5-GRAM BOTTLE:

Add a minimum of 49 ml diluent, and shake well. If lower concentrations are desired, the solution could be further diluted with up to a total of 99 ml of diluent.

Amount of Diluent	Concentration of Solution
49 ml	30 mg/ml
99 ml	15 mg/ml

2-GRAM BOTTLE:

Add a minimum of 49 ml diluent, and shake well. If lower concentrations are desired, the solution could be further diluted with up to a total of 99 ml of diluent.

Amount of Diluent	Concentration of Solution
49 ml	40 mg/ml
99 ml	20 mg/ml

Continued on next page

Wyeth—Cont.

4-GRAM BOTTLE:
Add 97 ml diluent, and shake well. The resulting solution will contain 40 mg/ml.
The resulting solutions may then be administered alone or with the intravenous solutions listed above. Discard unused solution after 24 hours at room temperature (70°F) or 96 hours if kept under refrigeration. Administer piggyback through an IV tubing very slowly (at least 30–60 minutes) to avoid vein irritation.
At times it may be desired to use the contents of the piggyback bottles for addition to large-volume IV fluids. In this case the entire vial contents should be dissolved in not less than 25 ml of Sterile Water for Injection. Use the resulting concentration within 24 hours when kept at room temperature or within 96 hours when kept under refrigeration.

Intramuscular Route: 500 mg every 6 hours in adults; decrease the interval to 4 hours if necessary in severe infections. In infants and children a dose of 25 mg/kg (about 12 mg per pound) twice daily is usually adequate.
For neonates, 10 mg/kg is recommended twice daily.
To reconstitute, see directions and table below. The clear solution should be administered by deep intragluteal injection immediately after reconstitution. After reconstitution, keep refrigerated (2°–8° C) and use within 7 days, keep at room temperature (25° C) and use within 3 days, or keep frozen (−20° C) for up to 3 months.

Oral Route: In adults a dose of 250 to 500 mg every 4 to 6 hours is sufficient for mild-to-moderate infections. In severe infections 1 gram every 4 to 6 hours may be necessary.
In children, streptococcal pharyngitis cases have responded to a dosage of 250 mg t.i.d. Beta-hemolytic streptococcal infections should be treated for at least ten days to prevent development of acute rheumatic fever or glomerulonephritis.
Children and infants with scarlet fever and pneumonia should receive 25 mg/kg/day in four divided doses. For staphylococcal infections, 50 mg/kg/day in four divided doses is recommended. For neonates, 10 mg/kg three to four times daily is recommended. If inadequate, resort to parenteral UNIPEN® (nafcillin sodium) Wyeth.
To reconstitute the powder for oral solution, add the water in two separate portions. Shake well after each addition. After reconstitution the solution must be refrigerated. Discard any unused portion after one week.

How Supplied:
FOR ORAL ADMINISTRATION—
CAPSULES: containing nafcillin sodium, as the monohydrate, equivalent to 250 mg. nafcillin buffered with calcium carbonate, bottles of 100, and REDIPAK® Unit Dose Medication boxes of 100 (individually wrapped).
TABLETS (film-coated): containing nafcillin sodium, as the monohydrate, equivalent to 500 mg. nafcillin buffered with calcium carbonate, bottles of 50.
ORAL SOLUTION: Supplied as a powder for oral solution. When reconstituted with water each 5 ml will contain nafcillin sodium equivalent to 250 mg nafcillin, bottle to make 100 ml.
FOR PARENTERAL ADMINISTRATION—(intravenous or intramuscular)
VIALS: Supplied in vial sizes of 500 mg, 1 gram, and 2 gram nafcillin sodium as the monohydrate, buffered. When reconstituted as recommended (see table below) with Sterile Water for Injection, USP, Sodium Chloride Injection, USP, Bacteriostatic Water for Injection, USP (Tubex®), or Bacteriostatic Water for Injection, USP, with parabens or with benzyl alcohol, each vial contains, respectively, 2, 4, or 8 ml of solution. Each ml contains nafcillin sodium equivalent to 250 mg nafcillin buffered with 10 mg sodium citrate.

Vial Size	Amount of Diluent	Nafcillin Sodium Solution
500 mg	1.7 ml	2 ml
1 gram	3.4 ml	4 ml
2 gram	6.8 ml	8 ml

Also Available: 10 gram pharmacy bulk vial.
FOR INTRAVENOUS USE ONLY—
PIGGYBACK UNITS: Supplied in single units equivalent to 1, 1.5, 2, or 4 gram nafcillin per unit buffered with 40 mg sodium citrate per gram.
[*Shown in Product Identification Section*]

WYAMYCIN® E ℞
Liquid
(erythromycin ethylsuccinate oral suspension)

Description: Erythromycin is produced by a strain of *Streptomyces erythraeus* and belongs to the macrolide group of antibiotics. It is basic and readily forms salts with acids. The base, the stearate salt, and the esters are poorly soluble in water. Erythromycin ethylsuccinate is an ester of erythromycin suitable for oral administration.
The pleasant-tasting, fruit-flavored liquids are supplied ready for oral administration.
The ready-made suspensions are intended primarily for pediatric use but can also be used in adults.
Actions: The mode of action of erythromycin is by inhibition of protein synthesis without affecting nucleic acid synthesis. Resistance to erythromycin of some strains of *Hemophilus influenzae* and staphylococci has been demonstrated. Culture and susceptibility testing should be done. If the Kirby-Bauer method of disc susceptibility is used, a 15 mcg erythromycin disc should give a zone diameter of at least 18 mm when tested against an erythromycin-susceptible organism.
Orally administered erythromycin ethylsuccinate suspensions are readily and reliably absorbed. Serum levels are comparable when the drug is administered in either the fasting or nonfasting state.
After absorption, erythromycin diffuses readily into most body fluids. In the absence of meningeal inflammation low concentrations are normally achieved in the spinal fluid, but passage of the drug across the blood-brain barrier increases in meningitis. In the presence of normal hepatic function, erythromycin is concentrated in the liver and excreted in the bile; the effect of hepatic dysfunction on excretion of erythromycin by the liver into the bile is not known. After oral administration, less than 5 percent of the activity of the administered dose can be recovered in the urine.
Erythromycin crosses the placental barrier, but fetal plasma levels are generally low.
Indications: *Streptococcus Pyogenes* (Group A beta-hemolytic streptococcus):
Upper- and lower-respiratory-tract, skin, and soft tissue infections of mild-to-moderate severity.
Injectable penicillin G benzathine is considered by the American Heart Association to be the drug of choice in the treatment and prevention of streptococcal pharyngitis and in long-term prophylaxis of rheumatic fever.
When oral medication is preferred for treatment of the above conditions, penicillin G, V, or erythromycin are alternate drugs of choice.
When oral medication is given, the importance of strict adherence by the patient to the prescribed dosage regimen must be stressed. A therapeutic dose should be administered for at least 10 days.
Although no controlled clinical efficacy trials have been conducted, oral erythromycin has been suggested by the American Heart Association and American Dental Association for use in a regimen for prophylaxis against bacterial endocarditis in patients hypersensitive to penicillin who have congenital heart disease or rheumatic or other acquired valvular heart disease when they undergo dental procedures and surgical procedures of the upper respiratory tract.[1] Erythromycin is not suitable prior to genitourinary or gastrointestinal tract surgery.
NOTE: When selecting antibiotics for the prevention of bacterial endocarditis the physician or dentist should read the full joint statement of the American Heart Association and the American Dental Association.[1]
Staphylococcus Aureus: Acute infections of skin and soft tissue of mild-to-moderate severity. Resistant organisms may emerge during treatment.
Streptococcus Pneumoniae (Diplococcus pneumoniae): Upper-respiratory-tract infections (e.g., otitis media, pharyngitis) and lower-respiratory-tract infections (e.g., pneumonia) of mild-to-moderate degree.
Mycoplasma Pneumoniae (Eaton agent, PPLO): For respiratory infections due to this organism.
Hemophilus Influenzae: For upper-respiratory-tract infections of mild-to-moderate severity when used concomitantly with adequate doses of sulfonamides. Not all strains of this organism are susceptible at the erythromycin concentrations ordinarily achieved (see appropriate sulfonamide labeling for prescribing information).
Treponema Pallidum: Erythromycin is an alternate choice of treatment for primary syphilis in patients allergic to the penicillins. In treatment of primary syphilis, spinal-fluid examinations should be done before treatment and as part of follow-up after therapy.
Corynebacterium Diphtheriae and *C. Minutissimum:* As an adjunct to antitoxin, to prevent establishment of carriers, and to eradicate the organism in carriers.
In the treatment of erythrasma.
Entamoeba Histolytica: In the treatment of intestinal amebiasis only. Extra-enteric amebiasis requires treatment with other agents.
Listeria Monocytogenes: Infections due to this organism.
Legionnaires' Disease: Although no controlled clinical efficacy studies have been conducted, *in vitro* and limited preliminary clinical data suggest that erythromycin may be effective in treating Legionnaires' Disease.
Contraindications: Erythromycin is contraindicated in patients with known hypersensitivity to this antibiotic.
Warnings: USAGE IN PREGNANCY: Safety for use in pregnancy has not been established.
Precautions: Erythromycin is principally excreted by the liver. Caution should be exercised in administering the antibiotic to patients with impaired hepatic function. There have been reports of hepatic dysfunction, with or without jaundice, occurring in patients receiving oral erythromycin products.
Recent data from studies of erythromycin reveal that its use in patients who are receiving high doses of theophylline may be associated with an increase of serum theophylline levels and potential theophylline toxicity. In case of theophylline toxicity and/or elevated serum theophylline levels, the dose of theophylline should be reduced while the patient is receiving concomitant erythromycin therapy.
Surgical procedures should be performed when indicated.
Adverse Reactions: The most frequent side effects of erythromycin preparations are gastrointestinal, such as abdominal cramping and discomfort, and are dose-related. Nausea, vomiting, and diarrhea occur infrequently with usual oral doses.
During prolonged or repeated therapy, there is a possibility of overgrowth of nonsusceptible bacteria or fungi. If such infections occur, the drug should be discontinued and appropriate therapy instituted.

Mild allergic reactions such as urticaria and other skin rashes have occurred. Serious allergic reactions, including anaphylaxis, have been reported.

Dosage and Administration: Erythromycin ethylsuccinate suspensions may be administered without regard to meals.

Children: Age, weight, and severity of the infection are important factors in determining the proper dosage. In mild-to-moderate infections the usual dosage of erythromycin ethylsuccinate for children is 30 to 50 mg/kg/day in divided doses. For more severe infections this dosage may be doubled.

The following dosage schedule is suggested for mild-to-moderate infections:

Body Weight	Total Daily Dose
Under 10 lbs.	30-50 mg/kg/day 15-25 mg/lb/day
10 to 15 lbs.	200 mg
16 to 25 lbs.	400 mg
26 to 50 lbs.	800 mg
51 to 100 lbs.	1200 mg
over 100 lbs.	1600 mg

The total daily dosage must be administered in divided doses.

Adults: 400 mg erythromycin ethylsuccinate every 6 hours is the usual dose. Dosage may be increased up to 4 gram per day according to the severity of the infection.

If twice-a-day dosage is desired in either adults or children, one-half of the total daily dose may be given every 12 hours.

In the treatment of streptococcal infections, a therapeutic dosage of erythromycin ethylsuccinate should be administered for at least 10 days. In continuous prophylaxis against recurrences of streptococcal infections in persons with a history of rheumatic heart disease, the usual dosage is 400 mg twice a day.

For prophylaxis against bacterial endocarditis[1] in patients with congenital heart disease or rheumatic or other acquired valvular heart disease when undergoing dental procedures or surgical procedures of the upper respiratory tract, give 1.0 gm (20 mg/kg for children) orally 1-½ to 2 hours before the procedure, and then 500 mg (10 mg/kg for children) orally every 6 hours for 8 doses.

For Treatment of Primary Syphilis:
Adults—48 to 64 gram, given in divided doses over a period of 10 to 15 days.

For Intestinal Amebiasis:
Adults—400 mg four times daily for 10 to 14 days.
Children—30 to 50 mg/kg/day in divided doses for 10 to 14 days.

For treatment of Legionnaires' Disease:
Although optimal doses have not been established, doses utilized in reported clinical data were those recommended above, 1.6 to 4 gram daily in divided doses.

How Supplied: Wyamycin® E 200 (erythromycin ethylsuccinate oral suspension) is supplied in 1-pint bottles. Each 5 ml teaspoonful of fruit-flavored suspension contains activity equivalent to 200 mg of erythromycin.

Wyamycin® E 400 (erythromycin ethylsuccinate oral suspension) is supplied in 1-pint bottles. Each 5 ml teaspoonful of fruit-flavored suspension contains activity equivalent to 400 mg of erythromycin.

Also Available: Wyamycin® S (erythromycin stearate) tablets, containing the equivalent of 250 mg erythromycin, are available in bottles of 100 and 500 film-coated tablets. Wyamycin® S (erythromycin stearate) tablets, containing the equivalent of 500 mg erythromycin, are available in bottles of 100 film-coated tablets.

Reference:

1. American Heart Association. 1977. Prevention of bacterial endocarditis. Circulation. 56:139A-143A.

[*Shown in Product Identification Section*]

WYANOIDS® OTC
Hemorrhoidal Suppositories

Description: Each suppository contains 15 mg extract belladonna (0.19 mg equiv. total alkaloids), 3 mg ephedrine sulfate, zinc oxide, boric acid, bismuth oxyiodide, bismuth subcarbonate, and peruvian balsam in cocoa butter and beeswax. Wyeth Wyanoids have an unusual "torpedo" design which facilitates insertion and insures retention.

Indications: For the temporary relief of pain and itching of hemorrhoidal tissue in many cases.

Warning: Not to be used by persons having glaucoma or excessive pressure within the eye, by elderly persons (where undiagnosed glaucoma or excessive pressure within the eye occurs most frequently), or by children under 6 years of age, unless directed by a physician. Discontinue use if blurring of vision, rapid pulse, or dizziness occurs. Do not exceed recommended dosage. Not for frequent or prolonged use. If dryness of the mouth occurs, decrease dosage. If eye pain occurs, discontinue use and see your physician immediately as this may indicate undiagnosed glaucoma. In case of rectal bleeding, consult physician promptly.

Usual Dosage: One suppository twice daily for six days.

Directions: Remove wrapper of suppository and insert suppository rectally with gentle pressure, pointed end first. Use preferably upon arising and at bedtime.

How Supplied: Boxes of 12.

Also Available: Wyanoid® Hemorrhoidal Ointment.

The ointment contains zinc oxide, boric acid, ephedrine sulfate, benzocaine and peruvian balsam in a soothing emollient base. Tubes of 1 ounce with applicator.

[*Shown in Product Identification Section*]

WYANOIDS® HC ℞
Rectal Suppositories
(with hydrocortisone)

Description: Each suppository contains 10 mg. hydrocortisone acetate, 15 mg. extract belladonna (0.19 mg. equiv. total alkaloids), 3 mg. ephedrine sulfate, 176 mg. zinc oxide, 543 mg. boric acid, 30 mg. bismuth oxyiodide, 146 mg. bismuth subcarbonate, 30 mg. peruvian balsam in cocoa butter and beeswax.

Action: Hydrocortisone, an active adrenal cortical hormone and the chief corticosteroid in human plasma, appears to act directly on the tissues of the body and reduces the tissue response to acute inflammation. In the management of severe inflammatory anorectal disorders, it has proved to be a significant advance over spasmolytics, astringents, and emollients which formerly were often the only therapy available.

The combination of hydrocortisone and the soothing ingredients of the Wyanoids base relieves itching, burning, and soreness and tends to reduce inflammation and edema.

Indications

Based on a review of this drug by the National Academy of Sciences—National Research Council and/or other information, FDA has classified the indication as follows:

"Possibly" effective: Treatment of proctitis secondary to ulcerative colitis.

Final classification of the less-than-effective indications requires further investigation.

Dosage: One suppository inserted rectally twice daily for six days or as required.

WARNING: Hydrocortisone should not be used until an adequate proctologic examination is completed and a diagnosis made. Other specific measures against infections, allergy, and other causal factors must not be neglected.

Belladonna should not be used in patients with glaucoma or organic pyloric stenosis. It should be used with caution in prostatism, urinary retention, elderly persons, and children under six years of age. If eye pain occurs, the drug should be discontinued since this may indicate undiagnosed glaucoma.

Patients should be cautioned not to exceed the prescribed dose, to decrease dose if dryness of the mouth occurs, and to discontinue use if rapid pulse, blurring of vision, or dizziness occurs.

Frequent or prolonged use of preparations containing belladonna should be avoided.

How Supplied: Wyanoids® HC Suppositories are available in boxes of 12 suppositories; and Redipak®, Unit of Use Suppository Pack, as combination packages of one Wyanoids HC Suppository, one finger cot, and one 0.5 gram packet of lubricant (White Petrolatum, U.S.P.) in packages of 25 combination packages.

[*Shown in Product Identification Section*]

WYCILLIN® ℞
(sterile penicillin G procaine suspension)
INJECTION

FOR DEEP INTRAMUSCULAR INJECTION ONLY

Description: This product is designed to provide a stable aqueous suspension of sterile penicillin G procaine, ready for immediate use. This eliminates the necessity for addition of any diluent, required for the usual dry formulation of injectable penicillin.

Each TUBEX® (Sterile Cartridge-Needle Unit, Wyeth), 1,200,000 units (2 ml size) or 600,000 units (1 ml size) or disposable syringe 2,400,000 units (4 ml size) contains penicillin G procaine in a stabilized aqueous suspension with sodium citrate buffer; and as w/v, approximately 0.5% lecithin, 0.5% carboxymethylcellulose, 0.5% povidone, 0.1% methylparaben and 0.01% propylparaben.

Each TUBEX, 300,000 units (1 ml size), contains penicillin G procaine in a stabilized aqueous suspension with sodium citrate buffer; and as w/v, approximately 0.3% lecithin, 0.9% carboxymethylcellulose, 0.9% povidone, 0.14% methylparaben, and 0.015% propylparaben.

Wycillin (sterile penicillin G procaine suspension) must be stored in a refrigerator. Keep from freezing. This will prevent deterioration and assure that no significant loss of potency occurs within the expiration date.

Wycillin suspension in the TUBEX and disposable syringe formulations is viscous and opaque. Read "Contraindications," "Warnings," "Precautions," and "Dosage and Administration" sections prior to use.

Actions and Pharmacology: Penicillin G exerts a bactericidal action against penicillin-sensitive microorganisms during the stage of active multiplication. It acts through the inhibition of biosynthesis of cell-wall mucopeptide. It is not active against the penicillinase-producing bacteria, which include many strains of staphylococci. Penicillin G exerts high *in vitro* activity against staphylococci (except penicillinase-producing strains), streptococci (Groups A, C, G, H, L, and M), and pneumococci. Other organisms sensitive to penicillin G are *Neisseria gonorrhoeae, Corynebacterium diphtheriae, Bacillus anthracis,* Clostridia, *Actinomyces bovis, Streptobacillus moniliformis, Listeria monocytogenes,* and Leptospira. *Treponema pallidum* is extremely sensitive to the bactericidal action of penicillin G.

Continued on next page

Wyeth—Cont.

Sensitivity plate testing: If the Kirby-Bauer method of disc sensitivity is used, a 10-unit penicillin disc should give a zone greater than 28 mm when tested against a penicillin-sensitive bacterial strain.
Penicillin G procaine is an equimolecular compound of procaine and penicillin G, administered intramuscularly as a suspension. It dissolves slowly at the site of injection, giving a plateau type of blood level at about 4 hours which falls slowly over a period of the next 15–20 hours.
Approximately 60% of penicillin G is bound to serum protein. The drug is distributed throughout the body tissues in widely varying amounts. Highest levels are found in the kidneys with lesser amounts in the liver, skin, and intestines. Penicillin G penetrates into all other tissues to a lesser degree with a very small level found in the cerebrospinal fluid. With normal kidney function the drug is excreted rapidly by tubular excretion. In neonates and young infants and in individuals with impaired kidney functions, excretion is considerably delayed. Approximately 60–90 percent of a dose of parenteral penicillin G is excreted in the urine within 24–36 hours.

Indications: Penicillin G procaine is indicated in the treatment of moderately severe infections due to penicillin-G-sensitive microorganisms that are sensitive to the low and persistent serum levels common to this particular dosage form. Therapy should be guided by bacteriological studies (including sensitivity tests) and by clinical response.
NOTE: When high, sustained serum levels are required, aqueous penicillin G, either IM or IV, should be used.
The following infections will usually respond to adequate dosages of intramuscular penicillin G procaine:
Streptococcal infections (Group A—without bacteremia). Moderately severe to severe infections of the upper respiratory tract, skin and soft-tissue infections, scarlet fever, and erysipelas.
NOTE: Streptococci in Groups A, C, G, H, L, and M are very sensitive to penicillin G. Other groups, including Group D (enterococcus), are resistant. Aqueous penicillin is recommended for streptococcal infections with bacteremia.
Pneumococcal infections. Moderately severe infections of the respiratory tract.
NOTE: Severe pneumonia, empyema, bacteremia, pericarditis, meningitis, peritonitis, and arthritis of pneumococcal etiology are better treated with aqueous penicillin G during the acute stage.
Staphylococcal infections—penicillin-G-sensitive. Moderately severe infections of the skin and soft tissues.
NOTE: Reports indicate an increasing number of strains of staphylococci resistant to penicillin G, emphasizing the need for culture and sensitivity studies in treating suspected staphylococcal infections.
Indicated surgical procedures should be performed.
Fusospirochetosis (Vincent's gingivitis and pharyngitis). Moderately severe infections of the oropharynx respond to therapy with penicillin G procaine.
NOTE: Necessary dental care should be accomplished in infections involving the gum tissue.
Treponema pallidum (syphilis); all stages.
N. gonorrhoeae; acute and chronic (without bacteremia).
Yaws, Bejel, Pinta.
C. diphtheriae—penicillin G procaine as an adjunct to antitoxin for prevention of the carrier stage.
Anthrax.
Streptobacillus moniliformis and *Spirillum minus* infections (rat-bite fever).
Erysipeloid.
Subacute bacterial endocarditis (Group A streptococcus), only in extremely sensitive infections.
Although no controlled clinical efficacy studies have been conducted, aqueous crystalline penicillin G for injection and penicillin G procaine suspension have been suggested by the American Heart Association and the American Dental Association for use as part of a combined parenteral-oral regimen for prophylaxis against bacterial endocarditis in patients who have congenital heart disease or rheumatic or other acquired valvular heart disease when they undergo dental procedures and surgical procedures of the upper respiratory tract.[1]
Since it may happen that *alpha* hemolytic streptococci relatively resistant to penicillin may be found when patients are receiving continuous oral penicillin for secondary prevention of rheumatic fever, prophylactic agents other than penicillin may be chosen for these patients and prescribed in addition to their continuous rheumatic fever prophylactic regimen.
NOTE: When selecting antibiotics for the prevention of bacterial endocarditis, the physician or dentist should read the full joint statement of the American Heart Association and the American Dental Association.[1]

Contraindications: A previous hypersensitivity reaction to any penicillin is a contraindication.
Do not inject into or near an artery or nerve.

Warnings: Serious and occasionally fatal hypersensitivity (anaphylactoid) reactions have been reported in patients on penicillin therapy.
Serious anaphylactoid reactions require immediate emergency treatment with epinephrine. Oxygen and intravenous corticosteroids should also be administered as indicated.
Although anaphylaxis is more frequent following parenteral therapy, it has occurred in patients on oral penicillins. These reactions are more apt to occur in individuals with a history of sensitivity to multiple allergens.
There have been well-documented reports of individuals with a history of penicillin hypersensitivity reactions who have experienced severe hypersensitivity reactions when treated with a cephalosporin. Before therapy with a penicillin, careful inquiry should be made concerning previous hypersensitivity reactions to penicillins, cephalosporins, and other allergens. If an allergic reaction occurs, the drug should be discontinued and the patient treated with the usual agents, e.g., pressor amines, antihistamines, and corticosteroids.
Immediate toxic reactions to procaine may occur in some individuals, particularly when a large single dose is administered in the treatment of gonorrhea (4.8 million units). These reactions may be manifested by mental disturbances, including anxiety, confusion, agitation, depression, weakness, seizures, hallucinations, combativeness, and expressed "fear of impending death." The reactions noted in carefully controlled studies occurred in approximately one in 500 patients treated for gonorrhea. Reactions are transient, lasting from 15–30 minutes.
Inadvertent intravascular administration, including inadvertent direct intraarterial injection or injection immediately adjacent to arteries, of Wycillin (sterile penicillin G procaine suspension) and other penicillin preparations has resulted in severe neurovascular damage, including transverse myelitis with permanent paralysis, gangrene requiring amputation of digits and more proximal portions of extremities, and necrosis and sloughing at and surrounding the injection site. Such severe effects have been reported following injections into the buttock, thigh, and deltoid areas. Other serious complications of suspected intravascular administration which have been reported include immediate pallor, mottling or cyanosis of the extremity both distal and proximal to the injection site followed by bleb formation; severe edema requiring anterior and/or posterior compartment fasciotomy in the lower extremity. The above described severe effects and complications have most often occurred in infants and small children. Prompt consultation with an appropriate specialist is indicated if any evidence of compromise of the blood supply occurs at, proximal to, or distal to the site of injection.[2-10] See "Contraindications," "Precautions," and "Dosage and Administration" sections.
Quadriceps femoris fibrosis and atrophy have been reported following repeated intramuscular injections of penicillin preparations into the anterolateral thigh.
Injection into or near a nerve may result in permanent neurological damage.

Precautions: Penicillin should be used with caution in individuals with histories of significant allergies and/or asthma.
Care should be taken to avoid intravenous or intraarterial administration, or injection into or near major peripheral nerves or blood vessels, since such injections may produce neurovascular damage. See "Contraindications," "Warnings," and "Dosage and Administration" sections.
In suspected staphylococcal infections, proper laboratory studies, including sensitivity tests, should be performed.
A small percentage of patients are sensitive to procaine. If there is a history of sensitivity make the usual test: Inject intradermally 0.1 ml of a 1 to 2 percent procaine solution. Development of an erythema, wheal, flare, or eruption indicates procaine sensitivity. Sensitivity should be treated by the usual methods, including barbiturates, and procaine penicillin preparations should not be used. Antihistaminics appear beneficial in treatment of procaine reactions.
The use of antibiotics may result in overgrowth of nonsusceptible organisms. Constant observation of the patient is essential. If new infections due to bacteria or fungi appear during therapy, the drug should be discontinued and appropriate measures taken.
Whenever allergic reactions occur, penicillin should be withdrawn unless, in the opinion of the physician, the condition being treated is life-threatening and amenable only to penicillin therapy.
In prolonged therapy with penicillin, and particularly with high-dosage schedules, periodic evaluation of the renal and hematopoietic systems is recommended.
When treating gonococcal infections in which primary or secondary syphilis may be suspected, proper diagnostic procedures, including dark-field examinations, should be done. In all cases in which concomitant syphilis is suspected, monthly serological tests should be made for at least four months.

Adverse Reactions: Penicillin is a substance of low toxicity but does possess a significant index of sensitization. The following hypersensitivity reactions associated with use of penicillin have been reported: Skin rashes, ranging from maculopapular eruptions to exfoliative dermatitis; urticaria; serum-sicknesslike reactions, including chills, fever, edema, arthralgia, and prostration. Severe and often fatal anaphylaxis has been reported (see "Warnings"). As with other treatments for syphilis, the Jarisch-Herxheimer reaction has been reported.
Procaine toxicity manifestations have been reported (see "Warnings"). Although procaine hypersensitivity reactions have not been reported with this drug, there are patients who are sensitive to procaine (see "Precautions").

Dosage and Administration: **Shake TUBEX cartridge and disposable syringe vigorously before injecting contents.**

Penicillin G procaine (aqueous) is for intramuscular injection only.

Administer by DEEP INTRAMUSCULAR INJECTION in the upper, outer quadrant of the buttock. In infants and small children, the midlateral aspect of the thigh may be preferable. When doses are repeated, vary the injection site.

When using the TUBEX cartridge:

The Wyeth Tubex® cartridge for this product incorporates several features that are designed to facilitate the visualization of blood on aspiration if a blood vessel is inadvertently entered.

The design of this cartridge is such that blood which enters its needle will be quickly visualized as a red or dark-colored "spot." This "spot" will appear on the barrel of the glass cartridge immediately proximal to the blue hub. Prior to injection, in order to determine where this "spot" can be seen, the operator should first insert and secure the cartridge in the Tubex syringe in the usual fashion. The needle cover should then be removed and the cartridge and syringe held in one hand with the needle pointing away from the operator. If the 2 ml metal syringe is used the glass cartridge should then be rotated by turning the plunger of the syringe clockwise until the flat bevel at the tip of the needle is pointing upward and is horizontal when viewed directly from above. An imaginary straight line then drawn from the middle of the flat bevel to the back edge of the blue hub where it joins the glass will point to the area on the glass cartridge where the "spot" can be visualized. If the 1 ml metal syringe is used it will not be possible to continue to rotate the glass cartridge clockwise once it is properly engaged and fully threaded; it can, however, then be rotated counterclockwise as far as necessary to properly orient the bevel of the needle and locate the observation area. (In this same area in some cartridges a dark spot may sometimes be visualized prior to injection. This is the proximal end of the needle and does not represent a foreign body in, or other abnormality of, the suspension.)

Thus, before the needle is inserted into the selected muscle, it is important for the operator to orient the flat bevel of the needle so that any blood which might enter after its insertion and during aspiration can be visualized in the area of the cartridge where it will appear and not be obscured by the metal syringe or other obstructions.

After selection of the proper site and insertion of the needle into the selected muscle, aspirate by pulling back on the plunger. While maintaining negative pressure for 2–3 seconds, carefully observe the barrel of the cartridge in the area previously identified (see above) for the appearance of a red or dark-colored "spot." Blood or "typical blood color" may not be seen if a blood vessel has been entered—only a mixture of blood and Wycillin. The appearance of *any* discoloration is reason to withdraw the needle and discard the glass Tubex cartridge. If it is elected to inject at another site, a new cartridge should be used. If no blood or discoloration appears, inject the contents of the cartridge slowly. Discontinue delivery of the dose if the subject complains of severe immediate pain at the injection site or if, especially in infants and young children, symptoms or signs occur suggesting onset of severe pain.

When using the disposable syringe:

The Wyeth disposable syringe for this product incorporates several new features that are designed to facilitate its use.

A single small indentation, or "dot", has been punched into the metal ring that surrounds the neck of the syringe near the base of the needle. It is important that this "dot" be placed in a position so that it can be easily visualized by the operator following the intramuscular insertion of the syringe needle.

After selection of the proper site and insertion of the needle into the selected muscle, aspirate by pulling back on the plunger. While maintaining negative pressure for 2–3 seconds, carefully observe the barrel of the syringe immediately proximal to the location of the "dot" for appearance of blood or any discoloration. Blood or "typical blood color" may *not* be seen if a blood vessel has been entered—only a mixture of blood and Wycillin. The appearance of any discoloration is reason to withdraw the needle and discard the syringe. If it is elected to inject at another site, a new syringe should be used. If no blood or discoloration appears, inject the contents of the syringe slowly. Discontinue delivery of the dose if the subject complains of severe immediate pain at the injection site or if in infants and young children symptoms or signs occur suggesting onset of severe pain.

Pneumonia (pneumococcal), moderately severe (uncomplicated): 600,000–1,000,000 units daily.

Streptococcal infections (Group A), moderately severe to severe tonsillitis, erysipelas, scarlet fever, upper respiratory tract, skin and soft tissue: 600,000–1,000,000 units daily for 10-day minimum.

Staphylococcal infections, moderately severe to severe: 600,000–1,000,000 units daily.

In pneumonia, streptococcal (Group A) and staphylococcal infections in children under 60 pounds: 300,000 units daily.

Bacterial endocarditis (Group A streptococci) only in extremely sensitive infections: 600,000–1,000,000 units daily.

For prophylaxis against bacterial endocarditis[1] in patients with congenital heart disease or rheumatic or other acquired valvular heart disease when undergoing dental procedures or surgical procedures of the upper respiratory tract, use a combined parenteral-oral regimen. One million units of aqueous crystalline penicillin G (30,000 units/kg in children) intramuscularly mixed with 600,000 units penicillin G procaine (600,000 units for children) should be given one-half to one hour before the procedure. Oral penicillin V (phenoxymethyl penicillin), 500 mg for adults or 250 mg for children less than 60 lbs., should be given every 6 hours for 8 doses. Doses for children should not exceed recommendations for adults for a single dose or for a 24-hour period.

Syphilis—

Primary, secondary, and latent with a negative spinal fluid in adults and children over 12 years of age: 600,000 units daily for 8 days—total 4,800,000 units.

Late (tertiary, neurosyphilis, and latent syphilis with positive spinal-fluid examination or no spinal-fluid examination): 600,000 units daily for 10–15 days—total 6–9 million units.

Congenital syphilis under 70-lb. body weight: 10,000 units/kg/day for 10 days.

Yaws, Bejel, and Pinta: Treatment as syphilis in corresponding stage of disease.

Although some isolates of *Neisseria gonorrhoeae* have decreased susceptibility to penicillin, this inherent resistance is relative, not absolute, and penicillin in large doses remains the drug of choice for these strains. Strains producing penicillinase, however, are resistant to penicillin G, and a drug other than penicillin G should be used. Physicians are cautioned not to use less than the recommended doses.

Gonorrheal infections (uncomplicated)—Men or Women: Aqueous penicillin G procaine, 4.8 million units intramuscularly, divided into at least two doses and injected at different sites at one visit, together with 1 gram of oral probenecid, preferably given just before the injection.

NOTE: Treatment of severe complications of gonorrhea should be individualized, using large amounts of short-acting penicillin.

Gonorrheal endocarditis should be treated intensively with aqueous penicillin G. Prophylactic or epidemiologic treatment for gonorrhea (male and female) is accomplished with the same treatment schedules as for the uncomplicated gonorrhea.

Retreatment

The National Center for Disease Control, Venereal Disease Branch, U.S. Department of Health, Education and Welfare, Atlanta, Georgia, recommends:

Test of cure procedures at approximately 7–14 days after therapy. In the male, a gram-stained smear is adequate if positive; otherwise, a culture specimen should be obtained from the anterior urethra. In the female, culture specimens should be obtained from both the endocervical and anal canal sites.

Retreatment in the male is indicated if the urethral discharge persists for three or more days following initial therapy and the smear or culture remains positive. Follow-up treatment consists of 4,800,000 units of aqueous penicillin G procaine intramuscularly, divided in two injection sites at a single visit.

In uncomplicated gonorrhea in the female, retreatment is indicated if follow-up cervical or rectal cultures remain positive for *N. gonorrhoeae.* Follow-up treatment consists of 4,800,000 units of aqueous penicillin G procaine daily on two successive days.

Syphilis: All gonorrhea patients should have a serologic test for syphilis at the time of diagnosis. Patients with gonorrhea who also have syphilis should be given additional treatment appropriate to the stage of syphilis.

Diphtheria—adjunctive therapy with antitoxin: 300,000–600,000 units daily.

Diphtheria carrier state: 300,000 units daily for 10 days.

Anthrax-cutaneous: 600,000–1,000,000 units/day.

Vincent's infection (fusospirochetosis): 600,000–1,000,000 units/ day.

Erysipeloid: 600,000–1,000,000 units/day.

Streptobacillus moniliformis and *Spirillum minus* (rat-bite fever): 600,000–1,000,000 units/day.

How Supplied: *300,000 units per ml*—1 ml TUBEX® sterile cartridge-needle unit, packages of 10; *600,000 units per ml*—1 ml TUBEX sterile cartridge-needle unit, packages of 10 and 50; *1,200,000 units in 2 ml* TUBEX packages of 10; *2,400,000 units in 4 ml* single-dose disposable syringe, packages of 10.

References:

1. American Heart Association: Prevention of bacterial endocarditis. *Circulation. 56:*139A-143A, 1977.

2. SHAW, E.: Transverse myelitis from injection of penicillin. *Am. J. Dis. Child.. 11:*548, 1966.

3. KNOWLES, J.: Accidental intra-arterial injection of penicillin. *Am. J. Dis. Child.. 111:*552, 1966.

4. DARBY, C., et al: Ischemia following an intragluteal injection of benzathine-procaine penicillin G mixture in a one-year-old boy. *Clin. Pediatrics, 12:*485, 1973.

5. BROWN, L. & NELSON, A.: Postinfectious intravascular thrombosis with gangrene. *Arch. Surg., 94:*652, 1967.

6. BORENSTINE, J.: Transverse myelitis and penicillin (Correspondence). *Am. J. Dis. Child., 112:*166, 1966.

7. ATKINSON, J.: Transverse myelopathy secondary to penicillin injection. *J. Pediatrics. 75:*867, 1969.

8. TALBERT, J. et al: Gangrene of the foot following intramuscular injection in the lateral thigh: A case report with recommendations for prevention. *J. Pediatrics. 79:*110, 1967.

9. FISHER, T.: Medicolegal affairs. *Canad. Med. Assoc. J., 112:*395, 1975.

10. SCHANZER, H. et al: Accidental intraarterial injection of penicillin G. *JAMA. 242:*1289, 1979.

Continued on next page

Wyeth—Cont.

WYCILLIN® and PROBENECID ℞

(sterile penicillin G procaine suspension and probenecid tablets)
Disposable Syringe and Tablets
Wycillin is for deep IM injection only.

Description: The Wycillin disposable syringe is designed to provide a stable aqueous suspension of sterile penicillin G procaine, ready for immediate use. This eliminates the necessity for addition of any diluent, required for the usual dry formulation of injectable penicillin.

Each syringe, 2,400,000 units (4 ml size), contains penicillin G procaine in a stabilized aqueous suspension with sodium citrate buffer; and as w/v, approximately 0.5% lecithin, 0.5% carboxymethylcellulose, 0.5% povidone, 0.1% methylparaben, and 0.01% propylparaben.

Wycillin must be stored in a refrigerator. Keep from freezing. This will prevent deterioration and assure that no significant loss of potency occurs within the expiration date.

Probenecid is a uricosuric and renal tubular-blocking agent.

Wycillin suspension in the disposable syringe formulation is viscous and opaque. Read "Contraindications," "Warnings," "Precautions," and "Dosage and Administration" sections prior to use.

Actions and Pharmacology: Penicillin G exerts a bactericidal action against penicillin-sensitive microorganisms during the stage of active multiplication. It acts through the inhibition of biosynthesis of cell-wall mucopeptide. It is not active against the penicillinase-producing bacteria, which include many strains of staphylococci. Neisseria gonorrhoeae are included among the various organisms which are sensitive to penicillin G. Penicillin G procaine is an equimolecular salt of procaine and penicillin G, administered intramuscularly as a suspension. It dissolves slowly at the site of injection, giving a plateau type of blood level at about 4 hours which falls slowly over a period of the next 15–20 hours. Approximately 60% to 90% of a dose of penicillin G is excreted in the urine within 24 to 36 hours.

Approximately 60% of penicillin G is bound to serum protein. The drug is distributed throughout the body tissues in widely varying amounts, with highest levels found in the kidneys and lesser amounts in the liver, skin, and intestines. Penicillin G penetrates into all other tissues to a lesser degree, with a very small level found in the cerebrospinal fluid. With normal kidney function the drug is excreted rapidly by tubular excretion. In neonates and young infants and in individuals with impaired kidney function, excretion is considerably delayed.

Probenecid inhibits the tubular reabsorption of urate, thus increasing the urinary excretion of uric acid and decreasing serum uric acid levels. It also inhibits the tubular excretion of penicillin and usually increases penicillin plasma levels, regardless of the route by which the antibiotic is given. A 2-fold to 4-fold elevation has been demonstrated for various penicillins. Probenecid does not influence plasma concentrations of salicylates, nor the excretion of streptomycin, chloramphenicol, chlortetracycline, oxytetracycline, or neomycin.

Indications: Wycillin and Probenecid is indicated for the single-dose treatment of uncomplicated (without bacteremia) urethral, cervical, rectal, or pharyngeal infections caused by *Neisseria gonorrhoeae* (gonorrhea) in men and women.

Susceptibility studies should be performed when recurrent infections or resistant strains are encountered. Urethritis and the presence of gram-negative diplococci in urethral smears are strong presumptive evidence of gonorrhea. Culture or fluorescent antibody studies will confirm the diagnosis. Therapy may be instituted prior to obtaining results of susceptibility testing.

Contraindications: A history of a previous hypersensitivity reaction to any of the penicillins or to Probenecid is a contraindication.

Probenecid is not recommended in persons with known blood dyscrasias or uric kidney stones or during an acute attack of gout. It is not recommended in conjunction with penicillin G procaine suspension in the presence of known renal impairment.

Do not inject into or near an artery or nerve.

Warnings: PENICILLIN G PROCAINE: Serious and occasionally fatal hypersensitivity (anaphylactoid) reactions have been reported in patients on penicillin therapy. Serious anaphylactoid reactions require immediate emergency treatment with epinephrine. Oxygen and intravenous corticosteroids should also be administered as indicated. Although anaphylaxis is more frequent following parenteral therapy, it has occurred in patients on oral penicillins. These reactions are more apt to occur in individuals with a history of sensitivity to multiple allergens.

There have been well-documented reports of individuals with a history of penicillin-hypersensitivity reactions who have experienced severe hypersensitivity reactions when treated with a cephalosporin. Before therapy with a penicillin, careful inquiry should be made concerning previous hypersensitivity reactions to penicillins, cephalosporins, and other allergens. If an allergic reaction occurs, the drug should be discontinued and the patient treated with the usual agents, e.g., pressor amines, antihistamines, and corticosteroids.

Immediate toxic reactions to procaine may occur in some individuals, particularly when a large single dose is administered in the treatment of gonorrhea (4.8 million units). These reactions may be manifested by mental disturbances, including anxiety, confusion, agitation, depression, weakness, seizures, hallucinations, combativeness, and expressed "fear of impending death." The reactions noted in carefully controlled studies occurred in approximately one in 500 patients treated for gonorrhea. Reactions are transient, lasting from 15–30 minutes.

Inadvertent intravascular administration, including inadvertent direct intraarterial injection or injection immediately adjacent to arteries, of Wycillin (sterile penicillin G procaine suspension) and other penicillin preparations has resulted in severe neurovascular damage, including transverse myelitis with permanent paralysis, gangrene requiring amputation of digits and more proximal portions of extremities, and necrosis and sloughing at and surrounding the injection site. Such severe effects have been reported following injections into the buttock, thigh, and deltoid areas. Other serious complications of suspected intravascular administration which have been reported include immediate pallor, mottling or cyanosis of the extremity both distal and proximal to the injection site followed by bleb formation; severe edema requiring anterior and/or posterior compartment fasciotomy in the lower extremity. The above-described severe effects and complications have most often occurred in infants and small children. Prompt consultation with an appropriate specialist is indicated if any evidence of compromise of the blood supply occurs at, proximal to, or distal to the site of injection.[1-9] See "Contraindications," "Precautions," and "Dosage and Administration" sections.

Quadriceps femoris fibrosis and atrophy have been reported following repeated intramuscular injections of penicillin preparations into the anterolateral thigh.

Injection into or near a nerve may result in permanent neurological damage.

PROBENECID: Exacerbation of gout following therapy with Probenecid may occur; in such cases colchicine therapy is advisable.

In patients on Probenecid, the use of salicylates in either small or large doses is not recommended because it antagonizes the uricosuric action of Probenecid. Patients on Probenecid who require a mild analgesic agent should receive acetaminophen rather than salicylates, even in small doses.

USAGE IN PREGNANCY: The safety of these drugs for use in pregnancy has not been established.

Precautions: PENICILLIN G PROCAINE: When treating gonococcal infections in which primary or secondary syphillis may be suspected, proper diagnostic procedures, including dark-field examinations, should be done. In all cases in which concomitant syphilis is suspected, monthly serological tests should be made for at least four months. Patients with gonorrhea, who also have syphilis, should be given additional appropriate parenteral penicillin treatment.

Penicillin should be used with caution in individuals with histories of significant allergies and/or asthma. When administering Wycillin, care should be taken to avoid intravenous or intraarterial administration, or injection into or near major peripheral nerves or blood vessels, since such injections may produce neurovascular damage. See "Contraindications," "Warnings," and "Dosage and Administration" sections.

A small percentage of patients are sensitive to procaine. If there is a history of sensitivity, make the usual test: Inject intradermally 0.1 ml of a 1- to 2-percent procaine solution. Development of an erythema, wheal, flare, or eruption indicates procaine sensitivity. Sensitivity should be treated by the usual methods, including barbiturates, and procaine penicillin preparations should not be used. Antihistaminics appear beneficial in treatment of procaine reactions.

PROBENECID: Use Probenecid with caution in patients with a history of peptic ulcer. A reducing substance may appear in the urine of patients receiving Probenecid. Although this disappears with discontinuance of therapy, a false diagnosis of glycosuria may be made because of a false-positive Benedict's test.

Adverse Reactions: WYCILLIN: Penicillin is a substance of low toxicity but does possess a significant index of sensitization. The following hypersensitivity reactions associated with use of penicillin have been reported: Skin rashes, ranging from maculopapular eruptions to exfoliative dermatitis; urticaria; serum-sickness-like reactions, including chills, fever, edema, arthralgia, and prostration. Severe and often fatal anaphylaxis has been reported (see "Warnings"). As with other treatments for syphilis, the Jarisch-Herxheimer reaction has been reported.

Procaine toxicity manifestations have been reported (see "Warnings"). Although procaine hypersensitivity reactions have not been reported with this drug, there are patients who are sensitive to procaine (see "Precautions").

PROBENECID: The following are the principal adverse reactions which have been reported as associated with the use of Probenecid, generally with more prolonged or repeated administration: Hypersensitivity reactions (including anaphylaxis), nephrotic syndrome, hepatic necrosis, aplastic anemia; also other anemias, including hemolytic anemia related to genetic deficiency of glucose-6-phosphate dehydrogenase.

Dosage and Administration:

Shake disposable syringe well before using.

Penicillin G procaine (aqueous) is for intramuscular injection only.

Administer by DEEP INTRAMUSCULAR INJECTION in the upper, outer quadrant of the buttock. When doses are repeated, vary the injection site.

The Wyeth disposable syringe for this product incorporates several new features that are designed to facilitate its use.

A single small indentation, or "dot", has been punched into the metal ring that surrounds the neck of the syringe near the base of the needle. It is important that this "dot" be placed in a position so that it can be easily visualized by the operator following the intramuscular insertion of the syringe needle.

After selection of the proper site and insertion of the needle into the selected muscle, aspirate by pulling back on the plunger. While maintaining negative pressure for 2–3 seconds, carefully observe the barrel of the syringe immediately proximal to the location of the "dot" for appearance of blood or any discoloration. Blood or "typical blood color" may *not* be seen if a blood vessel has been entered—only a mixture of blood and Wycillin.

The appearance of any discoloration is reason to withdraw the needle and discard the syringe. If it is elected to inject at another site, a new syringe should be used. If no blood or discoloration appears, inject the contents of the syringe slowly. Discontinue delivery of the dose if the subject complains of severe immediate pain at the injection site or if in infants and young children symptoms or signs suggesting onset of severe pain.

Although some isolates of *Neisseria gonorrhoeae* have decreased susceptibility to penicillin, this inherent resistance is relative, not absolute, and penicillin in large doses remains the drug of choice for these strains. Strains producing penicillinase, however, are resistant to penicillin G, and a drug other than penicillin G should be used.

GONORRHEAL INFECTIONS (UNCOMPLICATED) MEN OR WOMEN: Aqueous penicillin G procaine, 4.8 million units intramuscularly, divided into at least two doses and injected at different sites at one visit, together with 1 gram (2 tablets, 0.5 gram each) of Probenecid orally, given just before the injections. Physicians are cautioned to use no less than the recommended dosages.

NOTE: Treatment of severe complications of gonorrhea should be individualized, using large amounts of short-acting penicillin. Gonorrheal endocarditis should be treated intensively with aqueous penicillin G. Prophylactic or epidemiologic treatment for gonorrhea (male and female) is accomplished with the same treatment schedules as for the uncomplicated gonorrhea.

RETREATMENT: The National Center for Disease Control, Venereal Disease Branch, U.S. Department of Health, Education and Welfare, Atlanta, Georgia, recommends:

Test of cure procedures at approximately 7–14 days after therapy. In the male, a gram-stained smear is adequate if positive; otherwise, a culture specimen should be obtained from the anterior urethra. In the female, culture specimens should be obtained from both the endocervical and anal canal sites.

Retreatment in the male is indicated if the urethral discharge persists for three or more days following initial therapy and the smear or culture remains positive. Follow-up treatment consists of 4,800,000 units of aqueous penicillin G procaine, intramuscular, divided in two injection sites at a single visit.

In uncomplicated gonorrhea in the female, retreatment is indicated if follow-up cervical or rectal cultures remains positive for *N. gonorrhoeae*. Follow-up treatment consists of 4,800,000 units of aqueous penicillin G procaine daily on two successive days.

Syphilis: All gonorrhea patients should have a serologic test for syphilis at the time of diagnosis. Patients with gonorrhea who also have syphilis should be given additional treatment appropriate to the stage of syphilis.

How Supplied: Supplied as a combination package containing two disposable syringes of Wycillin® (sterile penicillin G procaine suspension) (2,400,000 units each) and two tablets Probenecid, Benemid® (0.5 gram each).

Wycillin® Disposable Syringes manufactured by **Wyeth Laboratories Inc.,** Philadelphia, PA 19101

Probenecid Tablets (Benemid®) manufactured by **Merck, Sharp and Dohme,** Division of Merck & Co., West Point, PA 19486

References:

1. SHAW, E.: Transverse myelitis from injection of penicillin, *Am. J. Dis. Child., 111:*548, 1966.
2. KNOWLES, J.: Accidental intra-arterial injection of penicillin. *Am. J. Dis. Child., 111:*552, 1966.
3. DARBY, C., et al: Ischemia following an intragluteal injection of benzathine-procaine penicillin G mixture in a one-year-old boy. *Clin. Pediatrics, 12:*485, 1973.
4. BROWN, L. & NELSON, A.: Postinfectious intravascular thrombosis with gangrene, *Arch. Surg., 94:*652, 1967.
5. BORENSTINE, J.: Transverse myelitis and penicillin (Correspondence), *Am. J. Dis. Child., 112:*166, 1966.
6. ATKINSON, J.: Transverse myelopathy secondary to penicillin injection. *J. Pediatrics, 75:*867, 1969.
7. TALBERT, J. et al: Gangrene of the foot following intramuscular injection in the lateral thigh: A case report with recommendations for prevention. *J. Pediatrics, 70:*110, 1967.
8. FISHER, T.: Medicolegal affairs, *Canad. Med. Assoc. J., 112:*395, 1975.
9. SCHANZER, H. et al: Accidental intraarterial injection of penicillin G. *JAMA, 242:*1289, 1979.

WYDASE® (hyaluronidase) INJECTION ℞

Description: This product, a preparation of highly purified bovine testicular hyaluronidase, is available in two dosage forms, as follows: WYDASE LYOPHILIZED: Hyaluronidase, dehydrated in the frozen state under high vacuum, with lactose and thimerosal (mercury derivative).

Reconstitute with Sodium Chloride Injection, USP, before use, usually in the proportion of one milliliter per 150 USP units of hyaluronidase (WYDASE LYOPHILIZED).

Each vial of 1500 USP units contains 1.0 mg thimerosal (mercury derivative), added as a preservative, and 13.3 mg lactose. Each vial of 150 USP units contains 0.075 mg thimerosal (mercury derivative), added as a preservative, and 2.66 mg lactose.

WYDASE SOLUTION (Stabilized): An injection solution ready for use, containing 150 USP units of hyaluronidase per milliliter with 8.5 mg. sodium chloride, 1 mg. edetate disodium, 0.4 mg. calcium chloride, sodium biphosphate buffer, and not more than 0.1 mg. thimerosal (mercury derivative).

The USP hyaluronidase unit is equivalent to the turbidity-reducing (TR) unit and the International Unit.

Action: The enzymatic action of hyaluronidase hydrolyzes hyaluronic acid, a viscous polysaccharide found in the interstices of the tissues, where it normally obstructs diffusion of invasive substances. Thus hyaluronidase promotes diffusion and consequently absorption of fluids in the tissues, and has the action of the spreading factor of Duran-Reynals. When no spreading factor is present, material injected subcutaneously spreads very slowly; but hyaluronidase causes rapid spreading, provided local interstitial pressure is adequate to furnish the necessary mechanical impulse. Such an impulse is normally initiated by injected solutions. The rate of diffusion is proportionate to the amount of enzyme, and the extent is proportionate to the volume of solution.

Intravenous administration of even 75,000 USP units (500 times the maximal therapeutic dose) of hyaluronidase in animals causes no significant change in blood pressure, respiration, body temperature, or kidney function, and no histological changes in the tissues. Results from an experimental study on the influence of hyaluronidase in bone repair supports the conclusion that this enzyme alone, in the usual clinical dosage, does not deter bone healing. Hyaluronidase has no effect on the spread of localized infection provided it is not injected into the infected area, and seems to have no deleterious effect on bacterial or viral infections. But when crude testicular extracts which contained tissue irritants as well as "spreading factor" were used, an increase in area and virulence of the infection was observed.

Indications: This drug is indicated as an adjuvant to increase the absorption and dispersion of other injected drugs, for hypodermoclysis, and as an adjunct in subcutaneous urography for improving resorption of radiopaque agents.

Contraindications: Do not inject hyaluronidase into acutely inflamed or cancerous areas.

Precautions: Discontinue hyaluronidase if sensitization occurs. Sensitivity to hyaluronidase occurs infrequently. A preliminary test for sensitivity should be conducted. The skin test is made by an intradermal injection of approximately 0.02 ml. of the solution. A positive reaction consists of a wheal with pseudopods appearing within five minutes and persisting for 20 to 30 minutes and accompanied by localized itching. Transient vasodilation at the site of the test, i.e., erythema, is not a positive reaction.

When epinephrine is injected along with hyaluronidase the usual precautions for the use of epinephrine in cardiovascular disease, thyroid disease, diabetes, digital nerve block, ischemia of the fingers and toes, etc., should be observed.

Dosage and Administration: WYDASE® (hyaluronidase) should be administered only as discussed below, since its effects relative to the absorption and dispersion of other drugs are not produced when it is administered intravenously.

ABSORPTION AND DISPERSION OF INJECTED DRUGS. Absorption and dispersion of other injected drugs may be enhanced by adding 150 units hyaluronidase to the menstruum containing the other medication.

HYPODERMOCLYSIS. Insert needle with aseptic precautions. With tip lying free and movable between skin and muscle, begin clysis; fluid should start in readily without pain or lump. Then inject Solution Wydase into rubber tubing close to needle. An alternate method is to inject Wydase under skin prior to clysis. 150 units will facilitate absorption of 1000 ml. or more of solution. As with all parenteral fluid therapy, observe effect closely, with same precautions for restoring fluid and electrolyte balance as in intravenous injections. The dose, the rate of injection, and the type of solution (saline, glucose, Ringer's, etc.) must be adjusted carefully to the individual patient. When solutions devoid of inorganic electrolytes are given by hypodermoclysis, hypovolemia may occur. This may be prevented by using solutions containing adequate amounts of inorganic electrolytes and/or controlling the volume and speed of administration.

Hyaluronidase may be added to small volumes of solution (up to 200 ml.), such as a small clysis for infants or solutions of drugs for subcutaneous injection. **For children less than 3 years old the volume of a single clysis should be limited to 200 ml.; and in premature infants or during the neonatal period, the daily dosage should not exceed 25 ml. per kilogram of body weight; the rate of administration should not be greater than 2 ml. per minute. For older patients the rate and volume of administration**

Continued on next page

Wyeth—Cont.

should not exceed those employed for intravenous infusion.
SUBCUTANEOUS UROGRAPHY. The subcutaneous route of administration of urographic contrast media is indicated when intravenous administration cannot be successfully accomplished, particularly in infants and small children. With the patient prone, 75 units of Wydase® (hyaluronidase) Wyeth is injected subcutaneously over each scapula, followed by injection of the contrast medium at the same sites.
How Supplied:
WYDASE® LYOPHILIZED:
150 USP (TR) units, vials of 1 ml.;
1500 USP (TR) units, vials of 10 ml.
WYDASE® SOLUTION (Stabilized):
150 USP (TR) units per ml., vials of 1 ml. and 10 ml.

WYGESIC® Ⓒ ℞

Each tablet contains:
65 mg propoxyphene HCl
and 650 mg acetaminophen.
Description: Propoxyphene hydrochloride is an odorless white crystalline powder with a bitter taste. It is freely soluble in water. Chemically, it is alpha-(+)-4-(Dimethylamino)-3-methyl-1,2-diphenyl-2-butanol Propionate Hydrochloride.
Acetaminophen is a white, crystalline powder, possessing a slightly bitter taste. It is soluble in boiling water and freely soluble in alcohol. Chemically, it is N-Acetyl-p-aminophenol.
Clinical Pharmacology: Propoxyphene is a centrally acting narcotic analgesic agent.
Repeated doses of propoxyphene at 6-hour intervals lead to increasing plasma concentrations, with a plateau after the ninth dose at 48 hours.
Propoxyphene is metabolized in the liver to yield norpropoxyphene. Propoxyphene has a half-life of 6 to 12 hours, whereas that of norpropoxyphene is 30 to 36 hours.
Norpropoxyphene has substantially less central-nervous-system-depressant effect than propoxyphene, but a greater local anesthetic effect, which is similar to that of amitriptyline and antiarrhythmic agents, such as lidocaine and quinidine.
In animal studies in which propoxyphene and norpropoxyphene were continuously infused in large amounts, intracardiac conduction time (P-R and QRS intervals) was prolonged. Any intracardiac conduction delay attributable to high concentrations of norpropoxyphene may be of relatively long duration.
Actions: Propoxyphene is a mild narcotic analgesic structurally related to methadone.
The combination of propoxyphene and acetaminophen produces greater analgesia than that produced by either propoxyphene or acetaminophen administered alone.
Indications: These products are indicated for the relief of mild-to-moderate pain, either when pain is present alone or when it is accompanied by fever.
Contraindications: Hypersensitivity to propoxyphene or to acetaminophen.
Warnings

Do not prescribe propoxyphene for patients who are suicidal or addiction-prone.
Prescribe propoxyphene with caution for patients taking tranquilizers or antidepressant drugs and patients who use alcohol in excess.
Tell your patients not to exceed the recommended dose and to limit their intake of alcohol.
Propoxyphene products in excessive doses, either alone or in combination with other CNS depressants, including alcohol, are a major cause of drug-related deaths. Fatalities within the first hour of overdosage are not uncommon. In a survey of deaths due to overdosage conducted in 1975, in approximately 20% of the fatal cases, death occurred within the first hour (5% occurred within 15 minutes). Propoxyphene should not be taken in doses higher than those recommended by the physician. The judicious prescribing of propoxyphene is essential to the safe use of this drug. With patients who are depressed or suicidal, consideration should be given to the use of nonnarcotic analgesics. Patients should be cautioned about the concomitant use of propoxyphene products and alcohol because of potentially serious CNS-additive effects of these agents. Because of its added depressant effects, propoxyphene should be prescribed with caution for those patients whose medical condition requires the concomitant administration of sedatives, tranquilizers, muscle relaxants, antidepressants, or other CNS-depressant drugs. Patients should be advised of the additive depressant effects of these combinations.
Many of the propoxyphene-related deaths have occurred in patients with previous histories of emotional disturbances or suicidal ideation or attempts as well as histories of misuse of tranquilizers, alcohol, and other CNS-active drugs. Some deaths have occurred as a consequence of the accidental ingestion of excessive quantities of propoxyphene alone or in combination with other drugs. Patients taking propoxyphene should be warned not to exceed the dosage recommended by the physician.

DRUG DEPENDENCE: Propoxyphene, when taken in higher-than-recommended doses over long periods of time, can produce drug dependence characterized by psychic dependence and, less frequently, physical dependence and tolerance. Propoxyphene will only partially suppress the withdrawal syndrome in individuals physically dependent on morphine or other narcotics. The abuse liability of propoxyphene is qualitatively similar to that of codeine although quantitatively less, and propoxyphene should be prescribed with the same degree of caution appropriate to the use of codeine.
USAGE IN AMBULATORY PATIENTS: Propoxyphene may impair the mental and/or physical abilities required for the performance of potentially hazardous tasks, such as driving a car or operating machinery. The patient should be cautioned accordingly.
Precautions
DRUG INTERACTIONS: The CNS-depressant effect of propoxyphene is additive with that of other CNS depressants, including alcohol.
USAGE IN PREGNANCY: Safe use in pregnancy has not been established relative to possible adverse effects on fetal development. Instances of withdrawal symptoms in the neonate have been reported following usage during pregnancy. Therefore, propoxyphene should not be used in pregnant women unless, in the judgment of the physician, the potential benefits outweigh the possible hazards.
USAGE IN NURSING MOTHERS: Low levels of propoxyphene have been detected in human milk. In postpartum studies involving nursing mothers who were given propoxyphene, no adverse effects were noted in infants receiving mother's milk.
USAGE IN CHILDREN: Propoxyphene is not recommended for use in children, because documented clinical experience has been insufficient to establish safety and a suitable dosage regimen in the pediatric age group.
Adverse Reactions: In a survey conducted in hospitalized patients, less than 1% of patients taking propoxyphene hydrochloride at recommended doses experienced side effects. The most frequently reported have been dizziness, sedation, nausea, and vomiting. Some of these adverse reactions may be alleviated if the patient lies down.
Other adverse reactions include constipation, abdominal pain, skin rashes, light-headedness, headache, weakness, euphoria, dysphoria, and minor visual disturbances.
Cases of liver dysfunction have been reported.
Dosage and Administration: This product is given orally. The usual dose is 65 mg propoxyphene HCl and 650 mg acetaminophen every 4 hours as needed for pain. The maximum recommended dose of propoxyphene HCl is 390 mg per day.
Management of Overdosage: Initial consideration should be given to the management of the CNS effects of propoxyphene overdosage. Resuscitative measures should be initiated promptly.
SYMPTOMS OF PROPOXYPHENE OVERDOSAGE: The manifestations of acute overdosage with propoxyphene are those of narcotic overdosage. The patient is usually somnolent, but may be stuporous or comatose and convulsing. Respiratory depression is characteristic. The ventilatory rate and/or tidal volume is decreased, which results in cyanosis and hypoxia. Pupils, initially pinpoint, may become dilated as hypoxia increases. Cheyne-Stokes respiration and apnea may occur. Blood pressure and heart rate are usually normal initially, but blood pressure falls and cardiac performance deteriorates, which ultimately results in pulmonary edema and circulatory collapse unless the respiratory depression is corrected and adequate ventilation is restored promptly. Cardiac arrhythmias and conduction delay may be present. A combined respiratory-metabolic acidosis occurs, owing to retained CO_2 (hypercapnea) and to lactic acid formed during anaerobic glycolysis. Acidosis may be severe if large amounts of salicylates have also been ingested. Death may occur.
TREATMENT OF PROPOXYPHENE OVERDOSAGE: Attention should be directed first to establishing a patent airway and to restoring ventilation. Mechanically assisted ventilation, with or without oxygen, may be required, and positive-pressure respiration may be desirable if pulmonary edema is present. The narcotic antagonist naloxone will markedly reduce the degree of respiratory depression and should be administered promptly, preferably intravenously, 0.4 to 0.8 mg, and carefully repeated as necessary at 20- to 30-minute intervals.
The duration of action of the antagonist may be brief. If no response is observed after 10 mg of naloxone have been administered, the diagnosis of propoxyphene toxicity should be questioned. (Nalorphine and levallorphan may be used if naloxone is not available, but these agents are not as satisfactory as naloxone).
Blood gases, pH, and electrolytes should be monitored in order that acidosis and any electrolyte disturbance present may be corrected promptly. Acidosis, hypoxia, and generalized CNS depression predispose to the development of cardiac arrhythmias. Ventricular fibrillation or cardiac arrest may occur and necessitate the full complement of cardiopulmonary resuscitation (CPR) measures. Respiratory acidosis rapidly subsides as ventilation is restored and hypercapnea eliminated, but lactic acidosis may require intravenous bicarbonate for prompt correction.
Electrocardiographic monitoring is essential. Prompt correction of hypoxia, acidosis, and electrolyte disturbance (when present) will help prevent these cardiac complications and will increase the effectiveness of agents administered to restore normal cardiac function.
In addition to the use of a narcotic antagonist, the patient may require careful titration with an anticonvulsant to control convulsions. Ana-

leptic drugs (for example, caffeine or amphetamine) should not be used because of their tendency to precipitate convulsions.
General supportive measures, in addition to oxygen, include, when necessary, intravenous fluids, vasopressor-inotropic compounds, and, when infection is likely, anti-infective agents. Gastric lavage may be useful, and activated charcoal can adsorb a significant amount of ingested propoxyphene. Dialysis is of little value in poisoning due to propoxyphene. Efforts should be made to determine whether other agents, such as alcohol, barbiturates, tranquilizers, or other CNS depressants, were also ingested, since these increase CNS depression as well as cause specific toxic effects.
SYMPTOMS OF ACETAMINOPHEN OVERDOSAGE: Symptoms of massive overdosage with acetaminophen may include nausea, vomiting, anorexia, and abdominal pain, beginning shortly after ingestion and lasting for a period of 12 to 24 hours.
Evidence of liver damage is usually delayed, appearing during the next 24 to 48 hours. However, early recognition may be difficult since early symptoms may be mild and nonspecific. After the initial symptoms, the patient may feel less ill; however, laboratory determinations are likely to show a rapid rise in liver enzymes including serum transaminase and lactic dehydrogenase and bilirubin. In case of serious hepatotoxicity, jaundice, coagulation defects, hypoglycemia, encephalopathy, and coma may follow.
Death from hepatic failure may result 3 to 7 days after overdosage.
TREATMENT OF ACETAMINOPHEN OVERDOSAGE: Acetaminophen is rapidly absorbed, and efforts to remove the drug from the body should not be delayed. Subject to primary consideration of the CNS-depressant effects of propoxyphene, gastric lavage should be instituted.
Activated charcoal is probably ineffective unless administered almost immediately after acetaminophen ingestion.
Neither forced diuresis nor hemodialysis appear to be effective in removing acetaminophen. Since acetaminophen in overdose may have an antidiuretic effect and may produce renal damage, administration of fluids should be carefully monitored to avoid overload.
It has been reported that mercaptamine (cysteamine) or other thiol compounds may protect against liver damage if given soon after overdosage (8-10 hours). N-acetyl-cysteine is under investigation as a less toxic alternative to mercaptamine, which may cause anorexia, nausea, vomiting, and drowsiness. A Poison Control Center should be consulted for the latest antidote information.
Clinical and laboratory evidence of hepatotoxicity may be delayed up to one week. Acetaminophen plasma levels and half-life may be useful in assessing the likelihood of hepatotoxicity. Serial hepatic enzyme determinations are also recommended.
How Supplied: Wygesic® tablets, containing 65 mg propoxyphene hydrochloride and 650 mg acetaminophen per scored tablet, are supplied in bottles of 100 and 500 tablets and in Redipak® Strip Pack, Wyeth®, boxes of 100 (10 strips of 10).

PATIENT INFORMATION

YOUR PRESCRIPTION FOR A PROPOXYPHENE PRODUCT
Your doctor has chosen to prescribe a medicine containing propoxyphene. Propoxyphene is used for the relief of pain.
It is important that you read and understand the information in this leaflet. If you have any questions, ask your doctor or pharmacist.

GENERAL CAUTIONS

OTHER DRUGS: Combinations of excessive doses of propoxyphene, alcohol, and tranquilizers may be dangerous. Make sure your doctor knows that you are taking tranquilizers, sleep aids, antidepressant drugs, antihistamines, or any other drugs that make you sleepy. The use of these drugs with propoxyphene increases their sedative effects and may lead to overdosage symptoms, including death (see "Overdosage" below).
ALCOHOL: Heavy use of alcohol with propoxyphene is hazardous and may lead to overdosage symptoms (see "Overdosage" below). THEREFORE, LIMIT YOUR INTAKE OF ALCOHOL WHILE TAKING PROPOXYPHENE.
REGULAR ACTIVITIES: Propoxyphene may cause drowsiness or impair your mental and/or physical abilities; therefore, use caution when driving a vehicle or operating dangerous machinery. DO NOT perform any hazardous task until you have seen your response to this drug.
PREGNANCY: Do not take propoxyphene or other drugs during pregnancy unless your doctor knows you are pregnant and specifically recommends their use.
CHILDREN: Propoxyphene is not recommended for use in children under 12 years of age.
ALLERGY: Do not take propoxyphene if you have had an allergic reaction to any drug containing propoxyphene.
DEPENDENCE: Propoxyphene, when taken in higher-than-recommended doses over a long period of time, has produced physical and psychologic dependence (a craving for the drug or an inability to function normally without the drug).
Side Effects: When propoxyphene is taken as directed, side effects are infrequent. Among those reported are drowsiness, dizziness, nausea, and vomiting. If these effects occur, some of them may go away if you lie down.
Less frequently reported side effects include constipation, abdominal pain, skin rashes, light-headedness, headache, weakness, minor visual disturbances, and feelings of elation or discomfort.
If one of these side effects occurs and becomes severe, contact your physician.
Dosage: Your prescription should be taken as directed by your doctor. Do not exceed the maximum daily dose shown below. Always follow dosage recommendations carefully—do *not* increase the dosage without your doctor's approval. If you miss a dose of the drug, do *not* take twice as much the next time.

Propoxyphene HCl with Acetaminophen	
65 mg	650 mg
MAXIMUM DAILY DOSE	
6	

Overdosage: An overdosage of propoxyphene, alone or in combination with other drugs, including alcohol, may cause weakness, difficulty in breathing, confusion, anxiety, and more severe drowsiness and dizziness. Extreme overdosage may lead to unconsciousness and death.
In *any* suspected overdosage situation, GET EMERGENCY HELP IMMEDIATELY.
Other Information: This medication was prescribed specifically for you. It should not be given to anyone else even if his/her condition appears to be similar to yours. If you want more information or have any questions about propoxyphene, ask your doctor or pharmacist. There is a more detailed leaflet available from them. You may need their help in understanding parts of the detailed leaflet.
Keep this and all other drugs out of the reach of children.

[*Shown in Product Identification Section*]

WYMOX® ℞
(amoxicillin)
Capsules and Oral Suspension

How Supplied: Capsules contain 250 mg or 500 mg amoxicillin as the trihydrate, and are supplied in bottles of 100 and 500 for the 250 mg capsules and bottles of 50 and 500 for the 500 mg capsules. WYMOX Oral Suspension is supplied in bottles of powder for reconstitution. When reconstituted with water, it will make a palatable suspension containing amoxicillin trihydrate equivalent to 125 mg or 250 mg amoxicillin per 5 ml.
For prescribing information write to Professional Service, Wyeth Laboratories, Box 8299, Philadelphia, PA, 19101, or contact your local Wyeth representative.

[*Shown in Product Identification Section*]

WYTENSIN® ℞
(guanabenz acetate)

Description: Wytensin (guanabenz acetate), an antihypertensive agent for oral administration, is an aminoguanidine derivative, 2,6-dichlorobenzylideneaminoguanidine acetate, and its structural formula is:

[Structural formula: 2,6-dichlorobenzylidene–C(H)=N–N(H)–C(=NH)NH_2 · CH_3COOH]

It is an odorless, white to off-white, crystalline substance, sparingly soluble in water and soluble in alcohol, with a molecular weight of 291.14. Each tablet of Wytensin is equivalent to 4 mg or 8 mg of free guanabenz base.
Wytensin is available as 4 or 8 mg tablets for oral administration.
Clinical Pharmacology: Wytensin is an orally active central alpha-2 adrenergic agonist. Its antihypertensive action appears to be mediated via stimulation of central alpha adrenergic receptors, resulting in a decrease of sympathetic outflow from the brain at the bulbar level to the peripheral circulatory sytem.
PHARMACOKINETICS
In human studies, about 75% of an orally administered dose of Wytensin is absorbed and metabolized with less than 1% of unchanged drug recovered from the urine. Peak plasma concentrations of unchanged drug occur between two and five hours after a single oral dose. The average half-life for Wytensin is about 6 hours. The site or sites of metabolism of Wytensin and the consequences of renal or hepatic insufficiency on excretion of Wytensin or its metabolites have not been determined. The effect of meals on the absorption of Wytensin has not been studied.
PHARMACODYNAMICS
The onset of the antihypertensive action of Wytensin begins within 60 minutes after a single oral dose and reaches a peak effect within two to four hours. The effect of an acute single dose is reduced appreciably six to eight hours after administration, and blood pressure approaches baseline values within 12 hours of administration.
The acute antihypertensive effect of Wytensin occurs without major changes in peripheral resistance, but its chronic effect appears to be a decrease in peripheral resistance. A decrease in blood pressure is seen in both the supine and standing positions without alterations of normal postural mechanisms, so that postural hypotension has not been observed. Wytensin decreases pulse rate by about 5 beats per minute. Cardiac output and left ventricular ejection fraction are unchanged during long-term therapy.
With effective control of blood pressure in hypertensive patients, Wytensin has not demonstrated any significant effect on glomerular filtration rate, renal blood flow, renal sodium or potassium excretion, renal concentrating ability, body fluid volume, or body weight. In clinical trials of six to thirty months, hypertensive patients whose blood pressure was con-

Continued on next page

Wyeth—Cont.

trolled with Wytensin lost one to four pounds of body weight. The mechanism of this weight loss has not been established. Tolerance to the antihypertensive effect of Wytensin has not been observed.

During long-term administration of Wytensin, there is a small decrease in serum cholesterol and total triglycerides without any change in the high-density lipoprotein fraction. Plasma norepinephrine, serum dopamine beta-hydroxylase and plasma renin activity are decreased during chronic administration of Wytensin. No changes in serum electrolytes, uric acid, blood-urea nitrogen, calcium, or glucose have been observed.

Wytensin and hydrochlorothiazide have been shown to have at least partially additive effects in patients not responding adequately to either drug alone.

Indications and Usage: Wytensin is indicated in the treatment of hypertension. It may be employed alone or in combination with a thiazide diuretic.

Contraindication: Wytensin is contraindicated in patients with a known sensitivity to the drug.

Precautions:

1. Sedation: Wytensin causes sedation or drowsiness in a large fraction of patients. When Wytensin is used with centrally active depressants, such as phenothiazines, barbiturates, and benzodiazepines, the potential for additive sedative effects should be considered.
2. Patients with vascular insufficiency: Wytensin, like other antihypertensive agents, should be used with caution in patients with severe coronary insufficiency, recent myocardial infarction, cerebrovascular disease, or severe hepatic or renal failure.
3. Rebound: Sudden cessation of therapy with central alpha agonists like Wytensin may rarely result in "overshoot" hypertension and more commonly produces an increase in serum catecholamines and subjective symptomatology.

INFORMATION FOR PATIENTS

Patients who receive Wytensin should be advised to exercise caution when operating dangerous machinery or driving motor vehicles until it is determined that they do not become drowsy or dizzy from the medication. Patients should be warned that their tolerance for alcohol and other CNS depressants may be diminished. Patients should be advised not to discontinue therapy abruptly.

LABORATORY TESTS

In clinical trials, no clinically significant laboratory test abnormalities were identified during either acute or chronic therapy with Wytensin. Tests carried out included CBC, urinalysis, electrolytes, SGOT, bilirubin, alkaline phosphatase, uric acid, BUN, creatinine, glucose, calcium, phosphorus, total protein, and Coombs' test. During long-term administration of Wytensin, there was a small decrease in serum cholesterol and total triglycerides without any change in the high-density lipoprotein fraction. In rare instances on occasional nonprogressive increase in liver enzymes has been observed. However, no clinical evidence of hepatic disease has been found.

DRUG INTERACTIONS

Wytensin has not been demonstrated to cause any drug interactions when administered with other drugs, such as digitalis, diuretics, analgesics, anxiolytics, and antiinflammatory or antiinfective agents, in clinical trials. However, the potential for increased sedation when Wytensin is administered concomitantly with CNS depressant drugs should be noted.

DRUG/LABORATORY TEST INTERACTIONS

No laboratory test abnormalities were identified with the use of Wytensin.

CARCINOGENESIS, MUTAGENESIS, IMPAIRMENT OF FERTILITY

No evidence of carcinogenic potential emerged in rats during a two-year oral study with Wytensin at doses up to 9.5 mg/kg/day, i.e., about 10 times the maximum recommended human dose. In the Salmonella microsome mutagenicity (Ames) test system, Wytensin at 200-500 mcg per plate or at 30-50 mcg/ml in suspension gave dose-related increases in the number of mutants in one (TA 1537) of five *Salmonella typhimurium* strains with or without inclusion of rat liver microsomes. No mutagenic activity was seen at doses up to those which inhibit growth in the eukaryotic microorganism, *Schizosaccharomyces pombe*, or in Chinese hamster ovary cells at doses up to those which were lethal to the cells in culture. In another eukaryotic system, *Saccharomyces cerevisiae*, Wytensin produced no activity in an assay measuring induction of repairable DNA damage. Reproductive studies showed a decreased pregnancy rate in rats administered high oral doses (9.6 mg/kg) of Wytensin, suggesting an impairment of fertility. The fertility of treated males (9.6 mg/kg) may also have been affected, as suggested by the decreased pregnancy rate of their mates, even though the females received Wytensin only during the last third of pregnancy.

PREGNANCY

Pregnancy Category C

WYTENSIN MAY HAVE ADVERSE EFFECTS ON THE FETUS WHEN ADMINISTERED TO PREGNANT WOMEN. A teratology study in mice has indicated a possible increase in skeletal abnormalities when Wytensin is given orally at doses of 3 to 6 times the maximum recommended human dose of 1.0 mg/kg. These abnormalities, principally costal and vertebral, were not noted in similar studies in rats and rabbits. However, increased fetal loss has been observed after oral Wytensin administration to pregnant rats (14 mg/kg) and rabbits (20 mg/kg). Reproductive studies of Wytensin in rats have shown slightly decreased live-birth indices, decreased fetal survival rate, and decreased pup body weight at oral doses of 6.4 and 9.6 mg/kg. There are no adequate, well-controlled studies in pregnant women. Wytensin should be used during pregnancy only if the potential benefit justifies the potential risk to the fetus.

NURSING MOTHERS

Because no information is available on the excretion of Wytensin in human milk, it should not be administered to nursing mothers.

PEDIATRIC USE

The safety and effectiveness of Wytensin in children less than 12 years of age have not been demonstrated. Therefore, its use in this age group cannot be recommended at this time.

Adverse Reactions: The incidence of adverse effects has been ascertained from controlled clinical studies conducted in the United States and is based on data from 859 patients who received Wytensin for up to 3 years. There is some evidence that the side effects are dose-related.

The following table shows the incidence of adverse effects occurring in at least 5% of patients in a study comparing Wytensin to placebo, at a starting dose of 8 mg b.i.d.

Adverse Effect	Placebo (%) n=102	Wytensin (%) n=109
Dry mouth	7	28
Drowsiness or sedation	12	39
Dizziness	7	17
Weakness	7	10
Headache	6	5

In other controlled clinical trials at the starting dose of 16 mg/day in 476 patients, the incidence of dry mouth was slightly higher (38%) and that of dizziness was slightly lower (12%), but the incidence of the most frequent adverse effects was similar to the placebo-controlled trial. Although these side effects were not serious, they led to discontinuation of treatment about 15% of the time. In more recent studies using an initial dose of 8 mg/day in 274 patients, the incidence of drowsiness or sedation was lower, about 20%.

Other adverse effects were reported during clinical trials with Wytensin but are not clearly distinguished from placebo effects and occurred with a frequency of 3% or less:

Cardiovascular—chest pain, edema, arrhythmias, palpitations.

Gastrointestinal—nausea, epigastric pain, diarrhea, vomiting, constipation, abdominal discomfort.

Central nervous system—anxiety, ataxia, depression, sleep disturbances.

ENT disorders—nasal congestion.

Eye disorders—blurring of vision.

Musculoskeletal—aches in extremities, muscle aches.

Respiratory—dyspnea.

Dermatologic—rash, pruritus.

Urogenital—urinary frequency, disturbances of sexual function.

Other—gynecomastia, taste disorders.

Drug Abuse and Dependence: No reported dependence or abuse has been associated with the administration of Wytensin.

Overdosage: Accidental ingestion of Wytensin caused hypotension, somnolence, lethargy, irritability, miosis, and bradycardia in two children aged one and three years. Gastric lavage and administration of pressor substances, fluids, and oral activated charcoal resulted in complete and uneventful recovery within 12 hours in both patients.

Since experience with accidental overdosage is limited, the suggested treatment is mainly supportive while the drug is being eliminated from the body and until the patient is no longer symptomatic. Vital signs and fluid balance should be carefully monitored. An adequate airway should be maintained and, if indicated, assisted respiration instituted. There are no data available on the dialyzability of Wytensin.

Dosage and Administration: Dosage with Wytensin should be individualized. A starting dose of 4 mg twice a day is recommended, whether Wytensin is used alone or with a thiazide diuretic. Dosage may be increased in increments of 4 to 8 mg per day every one to two weeks, depending on the patient's response. The maximum dose studied to date has been 32 mg twice daily, but doses as high as this are rarely needed.

How Supplied: Wytensin® (guanabenz acetate) Tablets, Wyeth®, are available in the following dosage strengths:

4 mg, NDC 0008-0073, white, round tablet marked "WYETH" and "73", in bottles of 100.

8 mg, NDC 0008-0074, white, round, scored tablet marked "WYETH" and "74", in bottles of 100.

Keep bottles of Wytensin Tablets tightly closed.

Dispense in tight containers.

Protect from light.

[*Shown in Product Identification Section*]

Products are cross-indexed

by product classifications

in the

BLUE SECTION

Youngs Drug Products Corp.

P.O. Box 385
865 CENTENNIAL AVENUE
PISCATAWAY, NJ 08854

Sole Distributors for products manufactured by HOLLAND-RANTOS COMPANY, INC.

KORO-FLEX® ℞
ARCING SPRING DIAPHRAGM

Composition: Improved contouring spring; natural latex diaphragm.
Action and Uses: Half-moon shape when compressed, facilitates introduction along vaginal floor beyond cervix for easy, correct placement.
Administration and Dosage: As directed.
How Supplied: Available as a kit containing trial size tubes of KOROMEX^{II} CONTRACEPTIVE JELLY and KOROMEX^{II} CONTRACEPTIVE CREAM (Stock #136). Also available in a set (Plastic Compact Bag) containing regular size KOROMEX^{II} CONTRACEPTIVE JELLY, trial size KOROMEX^{II} CONTRACEPTIVE CREAM. AND Jelly/Cream Applicator (stock #536). Sizes 60 mm.–95 mm. at gradations of 5 mm.

KOROMEX® COIL SPRING DIAPHRAGM ℞

Action and Uses: The KOROMEX COIL SPRING DIAPHRAGM is made of pure latex rubber. The cadmium plated coil spring is tension - adjusted. The diaphragm is used with KOROMEX^{II} CONTRACEPTIVE JELLY or KOROMEX^{II} CONTRACEPTIVE CREAM for conception control.
How Supplied: Available as a kit containing trial size tubes of KOROMEX^{II} CONTRACEPTIVE JELLY and KOROMEX^{II} CONTRACEPTIVE CREAM (Stock #131). Also available in a set (plastic compact bag) containing an INTRODUCER, regular size KOROMEX^{II} CONTRACEPTIVE JELLY, trial size KOROMEX^{II} CONTRACEPTIVE CREAM and Jelly/Cream Applicator (Stock #541). Sizes 50 mm.–100 mm. at gradations of 5 mm.

KOROMEX® CONTRACEPTIVE FOAM OTC

(See PDR For Nonprescription Drugs)

KOROMEX^{II} CONTRACEPTIVE CREAM OTC

(See PDR For Nonprescription Drugs)

KOROMEX^{II} CONTRACEPTIVE JELLY OTC

(See PDR For Nonprescription Drugs)

KOROMEX^{II}–A CONTRACEPTIVE JELLY OTC

(See PDR For Nonprescription Drugs)

KOROSTATIN VAGINAL TABLETS ℞
(nystatin vaginal tablets)
Nystatin

Description: KOROSTATIN nystatin Vaginal Tablets U.S.P. is an oblong shaped vaginal tablet, each containing 100,000 units Nystatin, U.S.P.
Nystatin is a polyene antibiotic of undetermined structural formula that is obtained from Streptomyces noursei.
Clinical Pharmacology: Nystatin is an antifungal antibiotic which is both fungistatic and fungicidal in vitro against a wide variety of yeasts and yeast-like fungi. It probably acts by binding to sterols in the cell membrane of the fungus with a resultant change in membrane permeability allowing leakage of intracellular components. It exhibits no appreciable activity against bacteria or trichomonads.
No detectable blood levels are obtained following topical or vaginal application.
Indications and Usage: Nystatin Vaginal Tablets are effective for the local treatment of vulvovaginal candidiasis (moniliasis). The diagnosis should be confirmed, prior to therapy by KOH smears and/or cultures. Other pathogens commonly associated with vulvovaginitis (Trichomonas and Haemophilus vaginalis) do not respond to nystatin and should be ruled out by appropriate laboratory methods.
Contraindications: This preparation is contraindicated in patients with a history of hypersensitivity to any of its components.

Precautions:
General
Discontinue treatment if sensitization or irritation is reported during use.
Laboratory Tests
If there is a lack of response to Nystatin Vaginal Tablets, appropriate microbiological studies should be repeated to confirm the diagnosis and rule out other pathogens, before instituting another course of antimycotic therapy.
Usage in Pregnancy
No adverse effects or complications have been attributed to nystatin in infants born to women treated with nystatin vaginal tablets.

Adverse Reactions: Nystatin U.S.P. is virtually nontoxic and nonsensitizing and is well tolerated by all age groups, even on prolonged administration. Rarely, irritation or sensitization may occur (see PRECAUTIONS).

Dosage and Administration: The usual dosage is one tablet (100,000 units nystatin) daily for two weeks. The tablets should be deposited high in the vagina by means of the applicator. "Instructions for the Patient" are printed on each package.
Even though symptomatic relief may occur within a few days, treatment should be continued for the full course.
It is important that therapy be continued during menstruation. Adjunctive measures such as therapeutic douches are unnecessary and sometimes inadvisable. Cleansing douches may be used by nonpregnant women, if desired, for esthetic purposes.
How Supplied: In packages of 15 and 30 individual foil wrapped tablets with applicator. Refrigeration is not required for these tablets. KOROSTATIN Vaginal Tablets should be stored below 30°C. (86°F.).

KORO–SULF® Vaginal Cream ℞
(sulfisoxazole)

Description: Koro-Sulf (Sulfisoxazole) Vaginal Cream is a non-staining water dispersible, absorptive cream containing 10% Sulfisoxazole in a base of stearic acid, polysorbate 60, sorbitan monostearate, boric acid, glycerin, methyl paraben, propyl paraben and water.
Actions: The 4.5 pH of Koro-Sulf Cream is approximately that of the normal, healthy vaginal tract. The mechanism of action is that of an antibacterial sulfonamide.
Indications: Koro-Sulf Cream is indicated for treatment of *Hemophilus vaginalis* vaginitis.
Contraindications: Koro-Sulf Cream is contraindicated in patients with known hypersensitivity to any of its components.
Warnings: If the patient develops local irritation to the drug, treatment should be discontinued.
Adverse Reactions: In addition to local irritation, the following reactions have been reported rarely: allergic reaction, pruritus, urticaria and vulvitis.
Dosage and Administration: From 2.5 ml to 5 ml (½ to 1 applicatorful) of Koro-Sulf Cream should be introduced into the vagina twice daily, in the morning and upon retiring. Therapy should be continued up to two weeks, and may be repeated if necessary.
How Supplied: Three-ounce (85 grams) tubes, with 5 ml reusable applicator.

NYLMERATE^{II}® Solution Concentrate OTC

(See PDR For Nonprescription Drugs)

TRIPLE X

(See PDR For Nonprescription Drugs)

(Continued from page 448)

New York
N.Y. City Poison Center 340-4494
Dept. of Health 764-7667
Bureau of Laboratories
455 First Ave. 10016
Nyack
Hudson Valley Poison Center 353-1000
Nyack Hospital (Pharmacy)
North Midland Ave. 10960
Rochester
Finger Lakes Poison Control Center 275-5151
Life Line, Univ. of Rochester Medical Center 14642
Schenectady
Ellis Hospital Poison Control 382-4039
1101 Nott Street 12308 382-4121
382-4039
Syracuse
Syracuse Poison Inf. Ctr. 476-7529
750 E. Adams St. 13210
Troy
St. Mary's Hospital 272-5792
Poison Control Center
1300 Massachusetts Ave. 12180
Utica
St. Luke's Memorial Hospital Center 798-6200
P.O. Box 479 13502
Watertown
House of the Good Samaritan Hospital 788-8700
Corner Washington & Pratt Sts. 13602

NORTH CAROLINA

STATE COORDINATOR
Duke University Medical Center (919)684-8111
Durham 27710 (800)672-1697 (Statewide)
Asheville
Western N.C. Poison Control Center
Memorial Mission Hospital 255-4490
509 Biltmore Ave. 28801
Charlotte
Mercy Hospital 379-5827
2001 Vail Ave. 28207
Durham
Duke University Medical Center 684-8111
Poison Center
P.O. Box 3007 27710
Greensboro
Triad Poison Center
Moses H. Cone Hospital 379-4105
1200 N. Elm St. 27420
Hendersonville
Margaret R. Pardee Memorial Hospital 693-6522 Ext. 555
Fleming St. 28739
Hickory
Catawba Memorial Hospital 322-6649
Fairgrove-Church Rd. 28601
Jacksonville
Onslow Memorial Hospital 577-2555
Western Blvd. 28540
Wilmington
New Hanover Memorial Hosp. 343-7046
2131 S. 17th St. 28401

NORTH DAKOTA

STATE COORDINATOR
Department of Health (701) 224-2388
Bismarck 58505
Bismarck
Bismarck Hospital 223-4357
300 N. 7th St. 58501
Fargo
St. Luke's Hospital 280-5575
Fifth St. at Mills Ave. 58122
Grand Forks
United Hospital 780-5282
1200 S. Columbia Rd. 58201
Minot
St. Joseph's Hospital 857-2553
Third St. & Fourth Ave., S.E. 58701
Williston
Mercy Hospital 572-7661
1301 15th Ave. W. 58801

OHIO

STATE COORDINATOR
Department of Health (614)466-5190
Columbus 43216
Akron
Children's Hospital Medical Center of Akron 379-8562 (800) 362-9922 (Ohio)
281 Locust 44308
Canton
Aultman Hospital 452-9911
Emergency Room 438-6203
2600 Sixth St., S.W. 44710
Cincinnati
Drug & Poison Inf. Ctr.
Bridge Medical Science Bldg.
Univ. of Cincinnati 872-5111
Rm. 7701
231 Bethesda Ave. 45267
Cleveland
Greater Cleveland Poison Control Center 228-1323
2119 Abington Rd. 44106
Columbus
Central Ohio Poison Center 228-1323
Children's Hospital of Ohio
700 Children's Dr. 43205
Dayton
Children's Medical Center 222-2227
One Children's Plaza 45404 (800) 762-0727 (Statewide)
Lorain
Lorain Community Hospital 282-2220
3700 Kolbe Rd. 44053
Mansfield
Mansfield General Hospital 522-3411
335 Glessner Ave. 44903 Ext. 2545
Springfield
Community Hospital 325-1255
2615 E. High St. 44505
Toledo
Poison Information Center 381-3897
Medical College Hospital
P.O. Box 6190 43679
Youngstown
Mahoning Valley Poison Control Center
St. Elizabeth Hospital & Med Ctr. 746-2222
1044 Belmont Ave. 44501
Zanesville
Bethesda Hospital 454-4221
Bethesda Poison Control Center
2951 Maple Ave. 43701

OKLAHOMA

STATE COORDINATOR
Oklahoma Poison Control Ctr (405) 271-5454
Oklahoma Children's Memorial Hospital 800-522-4611
P.O. Box 26307
Oklahoma City 73126
Ada
Valley View Hospital 332-2323
1300 E. 6th St. 74820 Ext. 200
Lawton
Comanche County Memorial Hospital 355-8620 Ext. 296
3401 Gore Blvd. 73501
McAlester
McAlester General Hospital, West 426-1800
P.O. Box 669 74501 Ext. 240
Oklahoma City
Oklahoma Poison Control Center 271-5454
Oklahoma Children's Memorial Hospital 800-522-4611 (Statewide)
P.O. Box 26307
73126
Ponca City
St. Joseph Medical Center 765-0584
14th & Hartford 74601
Tulsa
Hillcrest Medical Center 560-5755
1120 S. Utica

OREGON

Portland
Oregon Poison Control and Drug Info. Center
University of Oregon (503) 225-8968
Health Sciences Center 97201 1-800-452-7165 (Statewide)

PANAMA

Ancon
U.S.A. Meddac Panama 252-7500
Gorgas U.S. Army Hospital
APO Miami 34004

PENNSYLVANIA

STATE COORDINATOR
Director, Division of Drugs Devices and Cosmetics (717) 787-2307
Department of Health
P.O. Box 90
Harrisburg 17108
Allentown
Lehigh Valley Poison Center 433-2311
Allentown General Hospital
17th & Chew St. 18102
Altoona
Keystone Region Poison Center 946-3711
Mercy Hospital
2500 Seventh Ave. 16603
Bloomsburg
The Bloomsburg Hospital 784-4241
549 E. Fair St. 17815
Chester
Sacred Heart General Hosp. 494-4400
9th and Wilson St. 19013
Danville
Susquehanna Poison Center 275-6116
Geisinger Medical Center 271-6116
North Academy Ave. 17821
East Stroudsburg
Pocono Hospital 421-4000
206 E. Brown St. 18301
Easton
Easton Hospital 250-4000
21st & Lehigh St. 18042
Erie
Doctors Osteopathic 454-2120
252 W. 11th St. 16502
Hamot Medical Center 452-4242
201 State St. 16550
Millcreer Community Hospital 864-4031
5515 Peach St. 16509
St. Vincent's Health Center 452-3232
232 W. 25th St. 16544

Gettysburg
Annie M. Warner Hospital 334-9155
S. Washington St. 17325

Hanover
Hanover General Hospital 637-3711
300 Highland Ave. 17331

Hershey
Capital Area Poison Center 534-6111
Milton S. Hershey Medical Center
University Dr. 17033

Jersey Shore
Jersey Shore Hospital 398-0100
Thompson St. 17740

Johnstown
Conemaugh Valley Memorial Hospital 535-5351
1086 Franklin St. 15905

Laurel Highlands Poison Center 535-8255
320 Main St. 15901

Mercy Hospital 535-5353
1020 Franklin St. 15905

Lancaster
Lancaster General Hospital 295-8322
555 North Duke St. 17604

St. Joseph's Hospital 299-4546
250 College Ave. 17604

Lehighton
Gnaden-Huetten Memorial Hospital 377-1300
11th & Hamilton St. 18235

Lewiston
Lewiston Hospital 248-5411
Highland Ave. 17044

Nanticoke
Nanticoke State Hospital 735-5000
N. Washington St. 18634

Paoli
Paoli Memorial Hospital 19301 648-1043

Philadelphia
Philadelphia Poison Information 922-5523
922-5524
321 University Ave. 19104

Philipsburg
Philipsburg State General Hospital 342-3320
Loch Lomond Rd. 16866

Pittsburgh
Pittsburgh Poison Center
Children's Hospital 681-6669
647-5600
125 DeSoto St. 15214

Pottsville
Good Samaritan Hospital 622-3400
E. Norwegian and Tremont St. 17901

Reading
Community General Hospital 375-9115
145 N. 6th St. 19601

Sayre
The Robert Packer Hospital 888-6666
Guthrie Square 18840

Sellersville
Grandview Hospital 18960 257-3611

Somerset
Somerset Community Hospital 443-2626
225 South Center Ave. 15501 443-1877
(Hotline)

State College
Centre Community Hospital 238-4351
Orchard Rd. 16801

York
Memorial Osteopathic Hospital 843-8623
325 S. Belmont St. 17403 Ext. 123

York Hospital 771-2311
1001 S. George St. 17405

PUERTO RICO

STATE COORDINATOR
University of Puerto Rico (809) 765-4880
Rio Piedras (809) 765-0615

Arecibo
District Hospital 878-3535
of Arecibo 00613 (Info. Only) Ext. 707

Fajardo
District Hospital 863-0505
of Fajardo 00649

Mayaguez
Mayaguez Medical Center 832-8686
Dept. of Health Ext. 1816, 1514
P.O. Box 1868 00709

Ponce
District Hospital of Ponce 00731 842-2550

Rio Piedras
Children's Hospital 754-8535
Center of Puerto Rico 00936

San Juan
Pharmacy School 753-4849
Medical Sciences (809) 763-0196
Campus 00936

RHODE ISLAND

STATE COORDINATOR
Rhode Island Poison Control Center
Rhode Island Hospital (401) 277-5727
593 Eddy St.
Providence 02902

Providence
Rhode Island Poison Center 277-5727
Rhode Island Hospital
Annex Bldg. 442
593 Eddys 02902

SOUTH CAROLINA

STATE COORDINATOR
Department of Health & Environmental Control (803) 758-5654
Columbia 29201

Charleston
National Pesticide Telecommunications Network 792-4201

Medical University of South Carolina (800) 922-0193
171 Ashley Ave. 29403

Columbia
Palmetto Poison Center 765-7359
College of Pharmacy (800) 922-1117
University of S.C. 29208

SOUTH DAKOTA

STATE COORDINATOR
Department of Health (605) 773-3361
Pierre 57501

Aberdeen
The Dakota Midland Poison Control Center 225-1880
(800) 592-1889
1400 15th Ave., N.W. 57401

Rapid City
Rapid City Regional Poison Control 341-8222
800-742-8925
P.O. Box 6000
353 Fairmont Blvd. 57709

Sioux Falls
McKennan Hospital Poison Center 336-3894
800 East 21st St. 57101 (800) 952-0123
(Statewide)

TENNESSEE

STATE COORDINATOR
Department of Public Health (615) 741-2407
Division of Emergency Serices
Nashville 37216

Chattanooga
T.C. Thompson Children's Hospital 755-6100
910 Blackford St. 37403

Columbia
Maury County Hospital 381-4500
1224 Trotwood Ave. Ext. 110
38401

Cookeville
Cookeville General Hospital 526-4818
142 W. 5th St. 38501

Jackson
Madison General Hospital 424-0424
708 W. Forest 38301 Ext. 525

Johnson City
Medical Center Hospital 461-6572
Emergency Department
400 State of Franklin Rd. 37601

Knoxville
Memorial Research Center and Hospital 971-3261
1924 Alcoa Highway 37920

Memphis
Southern Poison Center 528-6048
LeBonheur Children's Medical Center
848 Adams Ave. 38103

Nashville
Vanderbilt University Hospital 322-6435
21st & Garland 37232

TEXAS

STATE COORDINATOR
Texas Department of Health (512) 458-7254
Div. of Occupational Health
Austin 78756

Abilene
Hendrick Hospital 677-7762
19th & Hickory Sts. 79601

Amarillo
Amarillo Hospital District 376-4292
Amarillo Emergency Receiving Center
P.O. Box 1110
1501 Coulter Dr. 79175

Austin
Brackenridge Hospital 478-4490
14th & Sabine Sts. 78701

Beaumont
Baptist Hospital of Southeast Texas 833-7409
P.O. Box 1591
College & 11th St. 77701

Corpus Christi
Memorial Medical Center 881-4559
P.O. Box 5280
2606 Hospital Blvd. 78405

El Paso
El Paso Poison Control Center 533-1244
R.E. Thomason General Hospital
P.O Box 20009
4815 Alameda Ave. 79905

Fort Worth
W.I. Cook Children's Hospital 336-6611
1212 W. Lancaster 76102

Galveston
Southeast Texas Poison Control Center 765-1420
8th & Mechanic Sts. 77550

Harlingen
Valley Baptist Hospital 421-1859
P.O. Box 2588
2101 S. Commerce St.
78550

Houston
Southeast Texas Poison Control Center 654-1701
8th and Mechanic St.
Galveston, Tex. 77550

Laredo
Mercy Hospital 724-6247
1515 Logan St. 78040

Lubbock
Methodist Hospital 793-4366
3615 19th St. 79410

Odessa
Medical Center Hospital 333-1231
Poison Control
P.O. Box 7239 79760

Plainview
Central Plains Regional Hospital 296-9601
2601 Dimmitt Rd. 79072

San Angelo
Shannon West Texas Memorial Hospital 653-6741 Ext. 318
120 E. Harris 76901

San Antonio
Department of Pediatrics 223-6361
Univ. of Texas Health Science Center at San Antonio Ext. 473
7703 Floyd Curl Dr. 78284

Tyler
Medical Center Hospital 597-0351
1000 S. Beckham St. 75701

Waco
Hillcrest Baptist Hosp. 753-1412
3000 Herring Ave. 76708

Wichita Falls
Wichita Falls General Hospital 322-6771
Emergency Room
1600 8th St. 76301

UTAH

STATE COORDINATOR
Utah Department of Health (801) 533-6161
Division Family Health Services
Salt Lake City 84113

Salt Lake City
Intermountain Regional Poison Control Center 581-2151
50 N. Medical Drive 84132

VERMONT

STATE COORDINATOR
Department of Health (802) 862-5701
Burlington 05401

Burlington
Vermont Poison Control 658-3456
Medical Center Hospital 05401

VIRGINIA

STATE COORDINATOR
Division of Emergency Medical Services (804) 786-5188
Room 1102, 109 Governor St.
Richmond 23219

Alexandria
Alexandria Hospital 379-3070
4320 Seminary Rd. 22314

Arlington
Arlington Hospital 558-6161
5129 N. 16th St. 22205

Blacksburg
Montgomery County Community Hospital 951-1111 Ext. 140
Rt. 460, S. 24060

Charlottesville
Blue Ridge Poison Center 924-5543
Univ. of Virginia Hospital 22903
(800) 446-9876 (Deaf Out-of-State)
(800) 552-3723 (Deaf VA Only)

Falls Church
Fairfax Hospital 698-3600
3300 Gallows Rd. 22046

Hampton
Hampton General Hospital 722-1131
3120 Victoria Blvd. 23661

Harrisonburg
Rockingham Memorial Hospital 433-9706
738 S. Mason St. 22801

Lexington
Stonewall Jackson Hosp. 463-9141
22043 Ext. 219

Lynchburg
Lynchburg Gen. Marshall Lodge Hosp., Inc. 528-2066
Tate Springs Rd. 24504

Nassawadox
Northampton-Accomack Memorial Hospital 23413 442-8700

Newport News
Riverside Hospital 599-2050
500 J. Clyde Morris Blvd. 23601

Norfolk
DePaul Hospital 489-5288
Granby St. at Kingsley
Lane 23505

Petersburg
Petersburg General Hospital 861-2992
Mt. Erin & Adams Sts. 23803

Portsmouth
U.S. Naval Hospital 398-5898
23708

Richmond
Central Virginia Poison Center 786-9123
Medical College of Virginia
Virginia Commonwealth University
Box 522 MCV Station 23298

Roanoke
Southwest Virginia Poison Center
Roanoke Memorial Hospital 981-7336
Belleview at Jefferson St.
P.O. Box 13367 24033

Staunton
King's Daughters' Hospital 885-6848
P.O. Box 3000 24401

Waynesboro
Waynesboro Community Hospital 942-4096
501 Oak Ave. 22980

Williamsburg
Williamsburg Community Hosp. 253-6005
1238 Mt. Vernon Ave.
Drawer H 23185

VIRGIN ISLANDS

STATE COORDINATOR
Dept. of Health (809) 774-6097
St. Thomas 00801 774-0117

ST. CROIX

Charles Harwood Memorial Christiansted Hospital 00820 773-8331

ST. JOHN

Morris F. DeCastro Clinic 776-6252
Cruz Bay 00830

ST. THOMAS

Knud-Hansen Memorial Hospital 774-9000 Ext. 224
00801 Ext. 225

WASHINGTON

STATE COORDINATOR
Department of Social & Health Services (206) 522-7478
Seattle 98115

Seattle
Seattle Poison Center 634-5254
Children's Orthopedic Hosp. & Med. Center (800) 732-6985
4800 Sandpoint Way, N.E.
98105

Spokane
Deaconess Hospital 747-1077
W. 800 5th Ave. 99210 (800) 572-5842 (Statewide)

Tacoma
Mary Bridge Poison Information Center
Mary Bridge Children's Hospital 272-1281
311 S. L St. 98405

Yakima
Central Washington Poison Center 248-4400
Yakima Valley Memorial Hospital (800) 572-9176 (Statewide)
2811 Tieton Dr. 98902

WEST VIRGINIA

STATE COORDINATOR
Department of Health (304) 348-2971
Charleston 25305

Charleston
West Virginia Poison System (800) 642-3625
3110 MacCorkle Ave. SE 384-4211
Charleston 25304

WISCONSIN

STATE COORDINATOR
Department of Health & Social Services, Div. of Health (608) 267-7174
Madison 53701

Eau Claire
Eau Claire Poison Center 835-1515
Luther Hospital
1225 Whipple 54701

Green Bay
Green Bay Poison Control Center 433-8100
St. Vincent Hospital
835 S. Van Buren St. 54305

LaCrosse
St. Francis Hospital 784-3971
700 West Ave. N 54601

Madison
Madison Area Poison Center 262-3702
University Hospital and Clinic
600 Highland Ave. 53792

Milwaukee
Milwaukee Poison Center 931-4114
Milwaukee Children's Hospital
1700 W. Wisconsin 53233

WYOMING

STATE COORDINATOR
Office of Emergency Medical Services (307) 777-7955
Department of Health & Social Services
Cheyenne 82002

Cheyenne
Wyoming Poison Center 635-9256
De Paul Hospital (800) 442-2704
2600 East 18th St. 82001

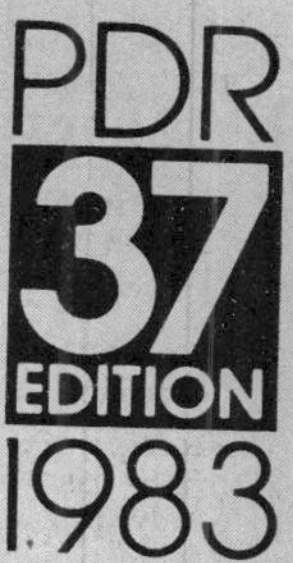

SECTION 7

Diagnostic Product Information

This section is intended to reflect the increased use of diagnostic products in the practice of medicine. It is intended for the use of all practitioners and is included in this format to make it easier for the physician to find the information which he seeks about these products.

Products described in PHYSICIANS' DESK REFERENCE® which have official package circulars must be in full compliance with Food & Drug Administration regulations pertaining to labeling for prescription drugs. These regulations require that for PDR copy, "indications and usage, dosages, routes, methods, and frequency and duration of administration, description, clinical pharmacology and supply and any relevant warnings, hazards, contraindications, adverse reactions, potential for drug abuse and dependence, overdosage and precautions" must be the *"same in language and emphasis"* as the approved labeling for the product. FDA regards the words *"same in language and emphasis"* as requiring VERBATIM use of the approved labeling providing such information. Furthermore, the information in the approved labeling that is emphasized by the use of type set in a box or in capitals, bold face, or italics must be given the same emphasis in PDR. For products which do not have official package circulars, the Publisher emphasized to manufacturers the necessity of describing such products comprehensively so that physicians would have access to all information essential for intelligent and informed prescribing. In organizing and presenting the material in PHYSICIANS' DESK REFERENCE, the Publisher is providing all the information made available to PDR by manufacturers.

This edition of PHYSICIANS' DESK REFERENCE contains the latest product information available at press-time. During the year, however, new and revised information about the products described herein may be furnished us. This information will be published in the PDR Supplement. Therefore, before prescribing or administering any product described in the following pages, you should first consult the PDR Supplement.

In presenting the following material to the medical profession, the Publisher is not necessarily advocating the use of any product listed.

Abbott Laboratories
DIAGNOSTICS DIVISION
ABBOTT PARK 6C4, DEPT. 49B
NORTH CHICAGO, IL 60064

THYPINONE® ℞
(Protirelin)

Description: Chemically, Thypinone (protirelin) is identified as 5-oxo-L-prolyl-L-histidyl-L-proline amide. It is a synthetic tripeptide which is believed to be structurally identical with the naturally-occurring thyrotropin-releasing hormone produced by the hypothalamus.

Thypinone (protirelin) is supplied as 1 ml ampules. Each ampule contains 500 mcg protirelin in a sterile non-pyrogenic isotonic saline solution having a pH of 5.5 to 7.5. In addition, each ampule contains sodium chloride, 9.0 mg, water for injection, and hydrochloric acid as needed to adjust pH. Thypinone (protirelin) is intended for intravenous administration.

Clinical Pharmacology: Pharmacologically, Thypinone increases the release of the thyroid stimulating hormone (TSH) from the anterior pituitary. Prolactin release is also increased. It has recently been observed that approximately 65% of acromegalic patients tested respond with a rise in circulating growth hormone levels, the clinical significance is as yet not clear. Following intravenous administration, the mean plasma half-life of protirelin in normal subjects is approximately five minutes. TSH levels rise rapidly and reach a peak at 20 to 30 minutes. The decline in TSH levels takes place more slowly, approaching baseline levels after approximately three hours.

Indications and Usage: Thypinone (protirelin) is indicated as an adjunctive agent in the diagnostic assessment of thyroid function. As an adjunct to other diagnostic procedures, testing with Thypinone may yield useful information in patients with pituitary or hypothalamic dysfunction.

Thypinone (protirelin) is indicated as an adjunct to evaluate the effectiveness of thyrotropin suppression with a particular dose of T4 in patients with nodular or diffuse goiter. A normal TSH baseline value and a minimal difference between the 30 minute and baseline response to Thypinone (protirelin) injection would indicate adequate suppression of the pituitary secretion of TSH.

Thypinone (protirelin) may be used, adjunctively, for adjustment of thyroid hormone dosage given to patients with primary hypothyroidism. A normal or slightly blunted TSH response, thirty minutes following Thypinone (protirelin) injection, would indicate adequate replacement therapy.

Warnings: Transient changes in blood pressure, either increases or decreases, frequently occur immediately following administration of Thypinone (protirelin). BLOOD PRESSURE SHOULD THEREFORE BE MEASURED BEFORE THYPINONE (PROTIRELIN) IS ADMINISTERED AND AT FREQUENT INTERVALS DURING THE FIRST 15 MINUTES AFTER ITS ADMINISTRATION. Increases in systolic pressure (usually less than 30 mm Hg) and/or increases in diastolic pressure (usually less than 20 mm Hg) have been observed more frequently than decreases in pressure. These changes have not ordinarily persisted for more than 15 minutes nor have they required therapy. MORE SEVERE DEGREES OF HYPERTENSION OR HYPOTENSION WITH OR WITHOUT SYNCOPE HAVE BEEN REPORTED IN A FEW PATIENTS.

To minimize the incidence and/or severity of hypotension, THE PATIENT SHOULD BE SUPINE BEFORE, DURING AND AFTER THYPINONE (PROTIRELIN) ADMINISTRATION. IF A CLINICALLY IMPORTANT CHANGE IN BLOOD PRESSURE OCCURS, MONITORING OF BLOOD PRESSURE SHOULD BE CONTINUED UNTIL IT RETURNS TO BASELINE LEVELS.

THYPINONE (PROTIRELIN) SHOULD NOT BE ADMINISTERED TO PATIENTS IN WHOM MARKED RAPID CHANGES IN BLOOD PRESSURE WOULD BE DANGEROUS UNLESS THE POTENTIAL BENEFIT CLEARLY OUTWEIGHS THE POTENTIAL RISK.

Precautions: Thyroid hormones reduce the TSH response to Thypinone (protirelin). Accordingly, patients in whom Thypinone is to be used diagnostically should be taken off liothyronine (T3) approximately seven days prior to testing and should be taken off thyroid medications containing levothyroxine (T4), e.g., desiccated thyroid, thyroglobulin, or liotrix, at least 14 days before testing. Hormone therapy is NOT to be discontinued when the test is used to evaluate the effectiveness of thyroid suppression with a particular dose of T4 in patients with nodular or diffuse goiter, or for adjustment of thyroid hormone dosage given to patients with primary hypothyroidism.

Chronic administration of levodopa has been reported to inhibit the TSH response to Thypinone.

It is not advisable to withdraw maintenance doses of adrenocortical drugs used in the therapy of known hypopituitarism. Several published reports have shown that prolonged treatment with glucocorticoids at physiologic doses has no significant effect on the TSH response to thyrotropin releasing hormone, but that the administration of pharmacologic doses of steroids reduces the TSH response.

Therapeutic doses of acetylsalicylic acid (2 to 3.6 g/day) have been reported to inhibit the TSH response to protirelin. The ingestion of acetylsalicylic acid caused the peak level of TSH to decrease approximately 30% as compared to values obtained without acetylsalicylic acid administration. In both cases, the TSH peak occurred 30 minutes post-administration of protirelin.

Pregnancy

Reproduction studies have been performed in rats and rabbits. At doses 1-½ and 6 times the human dose, there was an increase in the number of resorption sites in the pregnant rabbit. There are no studies in pregnant women which bear on the safety of Thypinone for the human fetus. Thypinone should be used in pregnant women only when clearly needed.

Adverse Reactions: Side effects have been reported in about 50% of the patients tested with Thypinone (protirelin). Generally, the side effects were minor, have occurred promptly, and have persisted for only a few minutes following injection.

Cardiovascular Reactions

MARKED CHANGES IN BLOOD PRESSURE INCLUDING BOTH HYPERTENSION AND HYPOTENSION WITH OR WITHOUT SYNCOPE, HAVE BEEN REPORTED IN A SMALL NUMBER OF PATIENTS.

Endocrine Reaction

Breast enlargement and leakage in lactating women for up to two or three days.

Other Reactions

Nausea; urge to urinate; flushed sensation; lightheadedness; bad taste; abdominal discomfort; headache; and dry mouth. Less frequently reported were: anxiety; sweating; tightness in the throat; pressure in the chest; tingling sensation; and drowsiness.

Dosage and Administration: Thypinone (protirelin) is intended for intravenous administration with the patient in the supine position. The drug is administered as a bolus over a period of 15 to 30 seconds, with the patient remaining supine for an additional 15 minutes during which time the blood pressure is monitored.

Dosage

Adults: 500 mcg. Doses between 200 and 500 mcg have been used. 500 mcg is considered the optimum dose to give the maximum response in the greatest number of patients. Doses greater than 500 mcg are unlikely to elicit a greater TSH response.

Children age 6 to 16 years: 7 mcg/kg body weight up to 500 mcg.

Infants and children up to 6 years: Experience is limited in this age group; doses of 7 mcg/kg have been administered.

One blood sample for TSH assay should be drawn immediately prior to the injection of Thypinone, and a second sample should be obtained 30 minutes after injection.

The TSH response to Thypinone (protirelin) is reduced by repetitive administration of the drug. Accordingly, if the Thypinone test is repeated, an interval of seven days before testing is recommended.

Elevated serum lipids may interfere with the TSH assay. Thus, fasting (except in patients with hypopituitarism) or a low-fat meal is recommended prior to the test.

Interpretation of Test Results: Interpretation of the TSH response to Thypinone (protirelin) requires an understanding of thyroid-pituitary-hypothalamic physiology and knowledge of the clinical status of the individual patient. Because the TSH test results may vary with the laboratory, the physician should be familiar with the TSH assay method used and the normal range for the laboratory performing the assay.

TSH response 30 minutes after Thypinone administration in normal subjects and in patients with hyperthyroidism and hypothyroidism are presented in Figure 1. The diagnoses were established prior to the administration of Thypinone on the basis of the clinical history, physical examination, and the results of other thyroid and/or pituitary function tests.

Among the normal euthyroid subjects, women and children were found to have higher levels of TSH at 30 minutes than men. Among the patients with hyperthyroidism or primary (thyroidal), secondary (pituitary) or tertiary (hypothalamic) hypothyroidism, no significant differences in TSH levels by age or sex were found.

Normal: Baseline TSH levels of less than 10 microunits/ml (μU/ml) were observed in 97% of euthyroid normal subjects tested. Thirty minutes after Thypinone (protirelin), the

Figure 1
Mean ± One Standard Deviation of TSH levels Observed at Baseline and 30 Minutes After Thypinone (μU/ml)

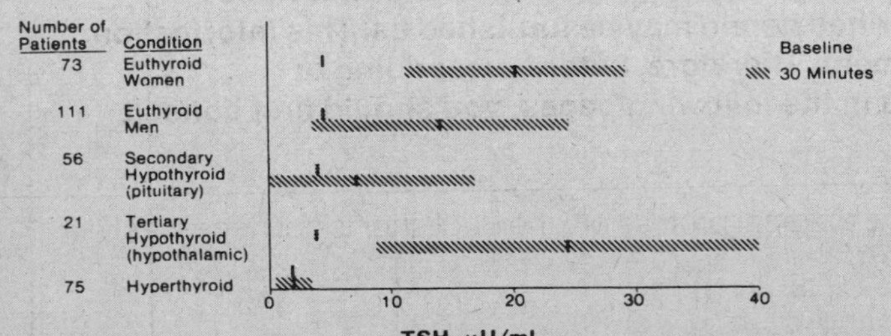

serum TSH increased by 2.0 μU/ml or more in 95% of euthyroid subjects.
Hyperthyroidism: All hyperthyroid patients tested had baseline TSH levels of less than 10 μU/ml and a rise of less than 2 μU/ml 30 minutes after Thypinone.
Primary (thyroidal) hypothyroidism: The diagnosis of primary hypothyroidism is frequently supported by finding clearly elevated baseline TSH levels; 93% of patients tested had levels above 10 μU/ml. Thypinone (protirelin) administration to these patients generally would not be expected to yield additional useful information. Ninety-four percent of patients with primary hypothyroidism given Thypinone in clinical trials responded with a rise in TSH of 2.0 μU/ml or greater; since this response is also found in normal subjects, Thypinone testing does not differentiate primary hypothyroidism from normal.
Secondary (pituitary) and tertiary (hypothalamic) hypothyroidism: In the presence of clinical and other laboratory evidence of hypothyroidism, the finding of a baseline TSH level less than 10 μU/ml should suggest secondary or tertiary hypothyroidism. In this situation, a response to Thypinone of less than 2 μU/ml suggests secondary hypothyroidism since this response was observed in about 60% of patients with secondary hypothyroidism and only approximately 5% of patients with tertiary hypothyroidism. A TSH response to Thypinone greater than 2 μU/ml is not helpful in differentiating between secondary and tertiary hypothyroidism since this response was noted in about 40% of the former and about 95% of the latter.
Establishing the diagnosis of secondary or tertiary hypothyroidism requires a careful history and physical examination along with appropriate tests of anterior pituitary and or target gland function. The Thypinone test should not be used as the only laboratory determinant for establishing these diagnoses.
[See table above].
How Supplied: As 1 ml ampules—boxes of 5 (NDC 0074-8971-05). Each ml contains Thypinone (protirelin) 0.50 mg (500 mcg), sodium chloride 9.0 mg for isotonicity, and pH adjusted with hydrochloric acid.

Table 1
Characterization Based on Serum TSH Levels at Baseline and 30 Minutes after Thypinone

	Baseline Serum TSH (μU/ml)	Change of Serum TSH (μU/ml) at 30 Minutes
Euthyroidism (normal thyroid function)	10 or less (usually 6 or less; 20% have < 1.5 μU/ml)	2 or more (usually 6 to 30)
Hyperthyroidism	10 or less (usually 4 or less)	less than 2
Primary Hypothyroidism (thyroidal)	more than 10 (usually 15 to 200)	2 or more (usually 20 or more)
Secondary Hypothyroidism (pituitary)	10 or less (usually 6 or less)	less than 2 (59%) 2 to 50 (41%)
Tertiary Hypothyroidism (hypothalamic)	10 or less (often less than 2)	2 or more

Adria Laboratories Inc.
5000 POST ROAD
DUBLIN, OH 43017

TYMTRAN® Injection ℞
(Ceruletide Diethylamine)

Description: TYMTRAN (ceruletide diethylamine) is a sterile nonpyrogenic solution of a synthetic decapeptide for injection. Ceruletide is related chemically and pharmacologically to the natural intestinal hormone cholecystokinin. Each 2 ml ampul contains 40 mcg of the ceruletide free acid (as the diethylamine salt) and 2 mg sodium thiomalate as an antioxidant in water. The pH is adjusted to 7.0 with sodium hydroxide. The air space in the ampul is filled with nitrogen. Ceruletide free acid is L-pyroglutamyl-L-glutaminyl-L-aspartyl-L-tyrosyl-(0-sulfate) -L- threonylglycyl -L- tryptophanyl-L-methionyl-L- aspartyl-L-phenylalaminamide.

```
                 SO3H
                  |
Pyr-Gln-Asp-Tyr-Thr-Gly-Trp-Met-Asp-Phe-NH2
```

The empirical formula is $C_{58}H_{73}N_{13}O_{21}S_2$ and the molecular weight is 1352.
Clinical Pharmacology: The effects of TYMTRAN are qualitatively identical to the effects of cholecystokinin. TYMTRAN contracts the gallbladder, stimulates pancreatic exocrine and gastric secretions, delays gastric emptying, inhibits motility of the proximal duodenum, and stimulates motility of the distal duodenum, jejunum, ileum, and to a lesser extent the colon. It also increases coordinated propulsion in the small bowel, as evidenced by decreased transit time of barium from the jejunum to the cecum. TYMTRAN exerts an initial inhibitory effect followed by an excitatory effect on the motility and electrical activity of the gastric antrum. It also delays gastric emptying, an action related in part to partial pylorospasm. Increased gastric acid and pancreatic exocrine secretions have also been reported following TYMTRAN administration.
TYMTRAN produces a contraction of the gallbladder when injected intramuscularly. The resulting evacuation of bile is similar to the physiological response to endogenous cholecystokinin. Gallbladder contraction is evident within 10 minutes after intramuscular TYMTRAN injection and contraction exceeding 40% usually occurs within 15 to 20 minutes. In some patients, contraction of the gallbladder and consequent expulsion of contrast materials into the cystic duct allows clear visualization of the cystic and/or common bile ducts. TYMTRAN causes a greater, more consistent contraction of the gallbladder than a fatty meal.
Indications and Usage:
Cholecystokinetic Cholecystography—TYMTRAN is indicated as an aid in oral cholecystography whenever contraction of the gallbladder would facilitate diagnostic visualization. It may aid diagnosis by:
1. Detecting small stones in cases where initial views of the gallbladder are negative, particularly when the gallbladder is very densely opacified or in any way obscured.
2. Freeing the gallbladder from overlying gas shadows where repositioning does not help.
3. Differentiating stones from polyps.
4. Confirming the presence of cholesterolosis or adenomyomatosis.
5. Contracting a distended gallbladder.
6. Causing evacuation of radiopaque bile into the bile ducts to improve visualization of the common bile and cystic ducts.

TYMTRAN-assisted cholecystography does not interfere with a subsequent upper gastrointestinal series when performed 45 minutes after the administration of TYMTRAN.
Radiological Examination of the Small Bowel—TYMTRAN is indicated for adjunctive use in radiological examination of the small bowel in patients with slow interim transit of barium beyond the distal jejunum. (See DOSAGE AND ADMINISTRATION section below for specific directions on proper use of TYMTRAN during a small bowel study; failure to follow these directions can lead to inadequate visualization of the small bowel.)
Contraindications: TYMTRAN is contraindicated in patients known to be hypersensitive to it and in patients with intestinal obstruction.
Precautions: Theoretically, stimulation of the gallbladder by a cholecystokinetic agent could dislodge a stone into the cystic duct or common duct. Although no such event has occurred to date in patients given TYMTRAN, TYMTRAN should not be given to a patient with known gallstones or to a patient whose gallbladder is not visualized. TYMTRAN should not be employed in small bowel radiography in a patient with known gallstones.
Although there is no known evidence of deleterious effects of TYMTRAN in patients with the problems listed below, the possibility of adverse consequences should be considered: acute pancreatitis, appendicitis, hollow visceral perforation, peritonitis, gastrointestinal bleeding or bowel ulceration, penetrating or bleeding peptic ulcer, pyloric stenosis, obstruction of the common bile duct, infection of the gallbladder, non-visualizing gallbladder (such as in acute cholecystitis, cystic duct obstruction and empyema of the gallbladder), and acute abdomen due to any other causes.
Drug/Laboratory Test Interactions—TYMTRAN administration does not confound the results of any of the most common laboratory tests. It is, however, not advisable to do a TYMTRAN-assisted cholecystographic or small bowel examination during a glucose tolerance test because TYMTRAN is capable of increasing the insulin release in glucose-loaded subjects. TYMTRAN administration may also cause a transient rise in serum amylase or serum bilirubin levels consequent to a pharmacological stimulation of pancreatic exocrine secretions or to a choleretic effect, respectively.
Carcinogenesis, Mutagenesis and Impaired Fertility—No information is available in laboratory animals or man.
Pregnancy—Category C. TYMTRAN has been shown to increase slightly the incidence of resorptions in rabbits when given at 80 times the recommended dose. There are no adequate and well-controlled studies in pregnant women. TYMTRAN should be used during pregnancy only if the potential benefit justifies the potential risk to the fetus.
Labor/Delivery—TYMTRAN, due to its effects on smooth muscle, should not be administered to pregnant women near term because of the possibility of inducing labor prematurely.
Nursing Mothers—It is not known whether this drug is excreted in human milk. Because many drugs are excreted in human milk, caution should be exercised when TYMTRAN is administered to a nursing woman.
Pediatric Use—Safety and effectiveness in children have not been established.
Adverse Reactions: In most cases, reactions to TYMTRAN are mild or moderate and brief in duration. The two most frequently encountered systemic adverse reactions to TYMTRAN are abdominal pain or cramps and nausea. Each of these reactions occurs in about 1 in 10 patients.

Continued on next page

Adria—Cont.

Vomiting is experienced in about 1 out of 100 cases. The incidence of other systemic reactions has been low (less than 1 in 100 cases). These reactions include eructation, regurgitation, weakness, flushing, dizziness, hypotension, diarrhea, sweating, an urge to defecate, an urge to urinate, hiccoughs and gas. The gastrointestinal symptoms are probably manifestations of the pharmacologic actions of TYMTRAN, i.e., delayed gastric emptying and increased intestinal motility. Reactions such as dizziness and hypotension might be secondary to other reactions, such as nausea and abdominal cramps, although the possibility of a direct TYMTRAN effect cannot be excluded. Reactions such as hypotension and dizziness are seldom seen and, when they occur, are transient and self-limited.

Isolated instances of clinically significant rises in alkaline phosphatase and serum aminotransferases have been observed after administration of TYMTRAN, but a causal relationship between these changes and TYMTRAN has not been established. Elevation in serum amylase has been observed and is related to the administration of TYMTRAN, an effect also produced by cholecystokinin. Transient elevation of serum bilirubin has also been noted and is probably due to a choleretic effect of TYMTRAN.

Overdosage: No clinically significant overdose incidents have been reported. However, overdosage can be expected to lead to nausea, vomiting, diarrhea, abdominal cramps and a fall in systemic arterial blood pressure accompanied by dizziness and/or fainting. Symptoms of overdosage should be treated symptomatically. These symptoms, however, can be expected to be short-lasting and self-limited. Laboratory findings could possibly include a) hyperamylasemia, b) hypoglycemia, and c) a rise in total serum bilirubin levels.

Dosage and Administration: For contraction of the gallbladder during cholecystography or roentgenological study of the small bowel, 0.3 mcg/kg intramuscular dose of TYMTRAN is recommended. For convenience, the table below can be used:

Dosage Table

BODY WEIGHT		VOLUME OF TYMTRAN
kg	lb	ml
40-60	88-133	0.8
61-80	134-177	1.0
81-100	178-221	1.3
101-120	222-254	1.6

Injection site pain has been reported in many patients following TYMTRAN administration. Pain is transient and is mild or moderate in most cases. Dilution of the TYMTRAN dose with 0.5 ml of Sodium Chloride Injection USP (0.9%) is recommended to reduce pain on injection.

For cholecystography, roentgenograms should be taken at 10 and 30 minutes after injection of TYMTRAN. When visualization of the cystic and common bile ducts is of particular importance, an additional film 5 minutes after injection is recommended.

For adequate visualization during small bowel studies, the following procedure has been found to produce good results: 1) the total volume of barium given should be at least 16 ounces (480 ml), and 2) TYMTRAN should be injected when the head of the barium column has reached the distal jejunum or proximal ileum, and there is adequate filling of at least four jejunal loops with a significant amount of barium in the free lumen, as well as between folds. Since TYMTRAN retards gastric emptying, it is essential that enough barium suspension be in the small bowel before TYMTRAN is administered. If filling of the small intestine is insufficient after administration of TYMTRAN, the standard type of small bowel examination can be resumed about one hour after the drug has been given, since its effect will be minimal by that time.

How Supplied: TYMTRAN is supplied in 2 ml glass ampuls containing 40 mcg (20 mcg/ml) of ceruletide free acid as the diethylamine salt. There are five 2 ml ampuls in each carton (NDC 0013-7406-94).

TYMTRAN conforms to specifications for two years if stored in a cool dark place (8–15°C) or under refrigeration (2–8°C).

Ames Division

Miles Laboratories, Inc.
P.O. BOX 70
ELKHART, IN 46515

N–MULTISTIX®
Reagent Strips

Designed for testing of urine specimens for protein, glucose, ketones, bilirubin, occult blood, urobilinogen, nitrite, and to indicate urinary pH. N-MULTISTIX provides significant information in 45 seconds which relates to urinary tract status, renal function, carbohydrate metabolism, liver function, biliary tract status, and is an aid in differential diagnosis of liver disease.

No. 2829—N-MULTISTIX Reagent Strips, bottles of 100.

Ordering/Pricing Information:
(219) 264-8645
Customer Services: (219) 264-8901

N-MULTISTIX® SG
Reagent Strips

N-MULTISTIX® SG is a firm plastic strip to which are affixed nine separate reagent areas which test for specific gravity, pH, protein, glucose, ketone (acetoacetic acid), bilirubin, blood, nitrite, and urobilinogen in urine. Test results may provide information regarding the status of carbohydrate metabolism, kidney and liver function, acid-base balance and bacteriuria.

OTHER AVAILABLE REAGENT STRIPS AND/OR TABLETS

	Glucose	Protein	pH	Blood	Ketones	Bilirubin	Urobilinogen	Phenylketones (PKU)	Nitrite	Specific Gravity
CLINISTIX®	X									
*CLINITEST®	X									
DIASTIX®	X									
URISTIX®	X	X								
ALBUSTIX®		X								
BUMINTEST®		X								
COMBISTIX®	X	X	X							
HEMA-COMBISTIX®	X	X	X	X						
HEMASTIX®				X						
LABSTIX®	X	X	X	X	X					
KETO-DIASTIX®	X				X					
KETOSTIX®					X					
ACETEST®					X					
BILI-LABSTIX®	X	X	X	X	X	X				
ICTOTEST®						X				
MULTISTIX®	X	X	X	X	X	X	X			
N-MULTISTIX®	X	X	X	X	X	X	X		X	
N-MULTISTIX®SG	X	X	X	X	X	X	X		X	X
UROBILISTIX®							X			
PHENISTIX®								X		
N-URISTIX®	X	X							X	
MICROSTIX®-NITRITE (test for Nitrite)									X	

*Available as 5-drop or 2-drop methods.

No. 2740—N-MULTISTIX® SG Reagent Strips, bottles of 100
No. 2741—MULTISTIX® SG Reagent Strips, bottles of 100

CHEK-STIX®
Urinalysis Control Strips

CHEK-STIX® Urinalysis Control Strips are Reactive Controls for Specific Gravity, pH, Protein, Glucose, Ketone (Acetoacetic Acid), Bilirubin, Blood, Nitrite and Urobilinogen for Use with Ames Visual Reagent Strips.
Each CHEK-STIX® Urinalysis Control Strip is a firm plastic strip to which are affixed six separate analyte areas. These each contain one or more natural or synthetic ingredients which, when dissolved out of the analyte areas in a measured quantity of distilled or deionized water, provide positive or defined results with Ames Visual Reagent Strips used in urinalysis.
No. 1360K—CHEK-STIX bottles of 25

DIASTIX®
Reagent Strips
KETO-DIASTIX®
Reagent Strips

DIASTIX is a clear, flexible plastic strip to which is affixed a reagent area for the quantitative, 30-second determination of glucose in urine. KETO-DIASTIX is designed for the determination of ketone and glucose in urine. Results are read by comparison with color chart (on containers): ketone in 15 seconds, glucose in 30 seconds.
No. 2806–DIASTIX Reagent Strips, plastic vials of 50.
No. 2803—DIASTIX Reagent Strips, bottles of 100.
No. 2882—KETO-DIASTIX Reagent Strips, bottles of 100.
No. 2883—KETO-DIASTIX Reagent Strips, bottles of 50.

TEK-CHEK®
Controls for Routine Urinalysis

A convenient quality control system to help determine if AMES urinalysis tests are properly performed and interpreted. Particularly valuable in instituting a quality control system, or making an existing system more convenient by the use of ready-made controls.
No. 1301—TEK-CHEK #1, package of 4 vials, negative reactions for all AMES urine tests.*
No. 1302—TEK-CHEK #2, package of 4 vials, positive for protein and nitrite; all other AMES tests negative.*
No. 1303—TEK-CHEK #3, package of 4 vials, positive for glucose all other AMES tests negative.*
No. 1304—TEK-CHEK #4, package of 4 vials, positive reactions for protein, glucose, ketones, bilirubin, and blood.*

*pH and specific gravity values specified in package insert.

AMES TDA™
Therapeutic Drug Assays
Fluorescent Immunoassays for the Quantitative Determination of Therapeutic Drugs in Serum

Ames TDA Tests are used to monitor patient serum drug levels. The data provided assists in establishing and maintaining serum drug levels in the therapeutic range.
Description: Ames TDA™/Therapeutic Drug Assays are a convenient series of non-radioisotopic assays for the quantitative determination of specific therapeutic drugs in serum or plasma. The series utilize a unique homogeneous substrate-labeled fluorescent immunoassay which is both easy to perform and requires no separation steps. Results can be read in any standard fluorometer.
Ames TDA/Therapeutic Drug Assays are available in kits of 100 tests each.
No. 3770—Ames TDA/GENTAMICIN
No. 3771—Ames TDA/TOBRAMYCIN
No. 3774—Ames TDA/AMIKACIN
No. 3775—Ames TDA/THEOPHYLLINE
No. 3772—Ames TDA/PHENYTOIN
No. 3773—Ames TDA/PHENOBARBITAL
No. 3776—Ames TDA/CARBAMAZEPINE
No. 3777—Ames TDA/PRIMIDONE
No. 3798—Ames TDA/QUINIDINE

DEXTROSTIX®
Reagent Strips

Descriptions: DEXTROSTIX is a firm plastic strip with an impregnated paper area that provides a reagent system for determination of blood glucose levels with the use of one drop of fingertip or venous blood. DEXTROSTIX is a convenient 60-second test which can be read semiquantitatively against a comparison color chart on bottle label or quantitatively with the EYETONE® Reflectance Colorimeter or DEXTROMETER™ Reflectance Colorimeter.
No. 2888—DEXTROSTIX Reagent Strips, bottles of 25.
No. 2893—DEXTROSTIX Reagent Strips, individually foil-wrapped, package of 10.
No. 2895—DEXTROSTIX Reagent Strips, bottles of 100.
Product Descriptions
#5537 DEXTRO-CHECK Calibrator—For use with Ames DEXTROSTIX® Reagent Strips to calibrate either the EYETONE® Reflectance Colorimeter or the DEXTROMETER® Reflectance Colorimeter. The vial cap of this calibrator is color-coded white and each product contains two 5 mL vials of solution.
#5593 DEXTRO-CHEK® Calibrators for GLUCOMETER® Reflectance Photometer—For use in calibrating GLUCOMETER using DEXTROSTIX. Since GLUCOMETER incorporates a two point calibration procedure, this product package contains one 5 mL vial each of Low Calibrator and High Calibrator solution. The vial caps are color-coded blue (Low) and red (High).
#5591 DEXTRO-CHEK® NORMAL Control—For use with all Ames blood glucose instruments/reagent strip systems and for Ames blood glucose reagent strips read visually. The vial cap is color-coded brown and each package contains two 5 mL vials of NORMAL Control Solution. The package insert gives complete directions for use and expected ranges of the test results using the various meters and reagent strips. The ranges of test results have been individually established for each reagent strip/instrument system. This product is for use by those individuals wanting to run a control test in the euglycemic (normal) range of blood glucose values.
#5538 DEXTRO-CHEK HIGH Control—For use with all Ames reagent strip/instrument systems. For visual reading, a range of test results is only given for DEXTROSTIX. The vial cap is color-coded orange and each package contains two 5 mL vials of HIGH Control Solution. The package insert gives complete directions for use and expected ranges of test results. The ranges of test results have been individually established for each reagent strip/instrument system. This product is for use by those individuals wanting to run a control test in the hyperglycemic (elevated) range of blood glucose values.
#5589 DEXTRO-CHEK® LOW Control—For use with the DEXTROMETER/DEXTROSTIX System and the GLUCOMETER/DEXTROSTIX System. The vial cap is color-coded light green and each package contains two 5 mL vials of LOW Control Solution. The package insert gives complete directions for use and expected ranges of test results. The ranges of test results have been individually established for each reagent strip/instrument system. This product is for use by those individuals wanting to run a control test in the hypoglycemic (low) range of blood glucose values.

HEMA-CHEK™
Slide Test for the Qualitative Determination of Fecal Occult Blood

HEMA-CHEK™ is a slide test for the qualitative determination of occult blood in feces. When a specimen containing occult blood is placed on the HEMA-CHEK impregnated paper, hemoglobin will come in contact with the guaiac reagent. When HEMA-CHEK Developer is added, the presence of hemoglobin is indicated by a blue color. HEMA-CHEK is a simple, convenient and economical test by which results can be obtained within thirty seconds.
No. 2592—HEMA-CHEK Slide Test, 100 Tests, 1 × 25 mL Developer and Applicators
No. 2593—HEMA-CHEK Patient Dispensing Pak, 300 Tests, 3 × 25 mL Developer, Applicators, and 100 Patient Envelopes
No. 2594—HEMA-CHEK, 1000 Tests, 10 × 25 mL Developer, and Applicators

MICROCULT®–GC
Miniaturized Culture Test for the Detection of Neisseria Gonorrhoeae

MICROCULT-GC test system consists of a plastic Culture Slide containing two dry culture areas, a bottle of Rehydration Fluid, a CO_2-Generating Tablet to provide the proper environment during incubation, and Cytochrome Oxidase Detection Strips to visualize growth locations after culture.
MICROCULT-GC culture tests are available in kits of 25 culture slides (#3026). Also available Ames MICROSTIX® Incubator (#3056).

MICROSTIX®–3
Reagent Strips

Description:
Test for Nitrite, total bacteria and gram negative bacteria in urine
A firm, plastic strip containing A separate areas—a chemical test area for immediate recognition of nitrite in urine, and two culture areas for semiquantitation of bacterial growth after 18 hours. One culture area supports total bacterial growth (both gram-positive and gram-negative) the other, only gram negative organisms. The dry-reagent microbiologic technology provides a unique culture medium which does not require refrigeration and is more stable than agar plates. A compact MICROSTIX Incubator is available.
No. 3009 — Box of 25 foil-wrapped MICROSTIX-3 Reagent Strips, with 25 incubation pouches and 25 labels.

MICROSTIX®–CANDIDA
Miniaturized Culture Test for the Detection of Candida Species in Vaginal Specimens

MICROSTIX®-CANDIDA is a culture test which contains a selective growth medium for *Candida* species and is intended as an aid to diagnosis of *Candida*.
The MICROSTIX-CANDIDA test system consists of a firm, plastic strip to which is affixed a dry culture area, a bottle of water for rehydration, and a plastic pouch which provides a suitable environment for the strip during incubation. The test area uses a modified Nickerson's medium which contains a support nutrient along with agents to inhibit bacterial growth, and is a selective isolation medium for *Candida* species. The dry-reagent microbiological technology provides a unique culture vehicle which does not require refrigeration, and possesses much longer stability than conventional agar plates or slide tests.

Continued on next page

Ames—Cont.

No. 3004—MICROSTIX-CANDIDA culture tests are available in kits of 25 strips.
No. 3056—MICROSTIX Incubator.

MICROSTIX®-Nitrite
Reagent Strip Kit
Indicator of Urinary Tract Infection

MICROSTIX®-Nitrite is a home test kit containing plastic strips with an impregnated reagent area that will determine the presence of nitrite in urine, an indicator of Urinary Tract Infection. MICROSTIX®-Nitrite is a convenient 30-second test that, after being dipped in urine, is read by comparison with a color chart. Any shade of pink color is a positive test result. The test is run on three consecutive first morning specimens. MICROSTIX®-Nitrite Kit No. 3014 contains 3 foil wrapped strips, 3 urine collection cups and patient instructions. Designed for patient home use.

N-URISTIX®
Reagent Strips
Dip-and Read Test for Nitrite, Glucose and Protein in Urine

N-URISTIX® is a firm, plastic strip to which three separate reagent areas are affixed for testing for nitrite, glucose and protein in urine. When considered along with other clinical and biochemical tests, N-URISTIX results may provide clinically meaningful information on the status of a number of metabolic and physiological states, such as kidney function, carbohydrate metabolism and urinary tract infection.
No. 2854-N-URISTIX Reagent Strips, bottles of 100 strips.

VISIDEX™ Reagent Strips
Visual Test for Glucose in Whole Blood

VISIDEX Reagent Strips are disposable plastic strips with two reagent pads for determining the concentration of glucose in whole blood. A semipermeable membrane serves as a barrier to blood cell migration into the reagent area. The reagent strip is for visual interpretation only.
No. 2651—VISIDEX bottles of 25
No. 2652—VISIDEX bottles of 100

AMES INSTRUMENTS

AMES FLUORO-COLORIMETER

Description: Ames Fluoro-Colorimeter is a compact, solid-state instrument for use with fluorometric, turbidimetric, or colorimetric assays. The instrument incorporates a large, easy-to-read meter with relative intensity scales of 0–100% and 0–32% and an optical density scale of 0–2A. A recorder outlet is provided for use with any 50mv potentiometric recorder. Filters necessary to perform Ames TDA™ Therapeutic Drug Assays are included with the instrument.
No. 3378—Ames Fluoro-Colorimeter

CLINI-TEK®
Reflectance Photometer

Description: The CLINI-TEK® Reflectance Photometer is a semiautomated bench-top instrument designed to read CLINI-TEK® Reagent Strips for routine urine chemistries and to display results in clinically meaningful units. A CLINI-TEK Form Printer is available as an option to provide a hard copy record of urinalysis results.
CLINI-TEK Reagent Strips utilize chemistries identical to those on visually read Ames Reagent Strips but incorporate an identification area which enables the CLINI-TEK instrument to identify the reagent strip it is reading.
No. 5500—CLINI-TEK® Instrument
No. 5150—CLINI-TEK® Tape Printer
No. 5501—CLINI- TEK® Foot switch
No. 5156—CLINI-TEK Form Printer
No. 5163—CLINI-TEK Report Form (3-part)
No. 5164—CLINI-TEK Report Form (5-part)
No. 5166—CLINI-TEK Form Printer Ribbon
Reagent strips for use with CLINI-TEK are No. 5429 N-MULTISTIX® for CLINI-TEK®, No. 5420 MULTISTIX® for CLINI-TEK®, No. 5414 BILILABSTIX For CLINI-TEK, and 5410 LABSTIX for CLINI-TEK

DEXTROMETER™
Reflectance Colorimeter with Digital Display

Description: DEXTROMETER quantitatively measures whole blood glucose when it is used with DEXTROSTIX® Reagent Strips. It is compact and portable for on-site glucose screening, testing, and monitoring. Operation is simple—a one-step calibration procedure is all that is necessary for routine testing. DEXTRO-CHEK™ Standard and Controls are also available to assure the user of the system's reliability.
No. 5570—DEXTROMETER Reflectance Colorimeter.
No. 5576—DEXTROMETER Rechargeable Battery Pack, (optional—must be ordered separately).

GLUCOMETER®
Battery-Powered Reflectance Photometer with Digital Display and Built-In Timer

GLUCOMETER® quantitatively measures whole blood glucose when it is used with DEXTROSTIX® Reagent Strips. Battery-operated and with a built-in timer, it is compact and portable for on-site glucose testing and monitoring. Operation is simple, with easy calibration procedures using either the DEXTRO-CHEK® Calibrators or Calibration Chips.
No. 5580—GLUCOMETER Reflectance Photometer (41.5 V AA Alkaline Batteries; Operating Manual; one pkg. Calibration Chips, one Wash Bottle; Leatherette Carrying Case)

SERALYZER®
Reflectance Photometer and Solid Phase Reagent Strips

The SERALYZER® System for blood chemistries consists of a Reflectance Photometer, a series of solid-phase Reagent Strips and Test Modules, plus an Accessory Kit for specimen preparation.
No. 5110—SERALYZER Instrument Package: (includes No. 5136 below) SERALYZER Reflectance Photometer, Power Cord, Hex Wrenches (2), Strip Guide Clamps (2), Spare Fuses (2), and Operating Manual
No. 5136—SERALYZER Accessory Kit: PIP-DIL™ Diluter, PIP-DIL Pipette Tips (200), MLA® Pipette, MLA Pipette Tips (1,000), Module Rack, and Foot Switch

Reagent Strips

2710 Seralyzer Glucose Reagent Strips—bottles of 25
2711 Seralyzer BUN Reagent Strips—bottles of 25
2712 Serlyzer Uric Acid Reagent Strips—bottles of 25
2713 Seralyzer LDH Reagent Strips—bottles of 25
2703 Seralyzer T. Bilirubin Reagent Strips—bottles of 25
2715 Seralyzer Cholesterol Reagent Strips—bottles of 25
2719 Seralyzer Creatinine Reagent Strips—bottles of 25
2721 Seralyzer CK Reagent Strips—bottles of 25

URIN-TEK®
System for Urine Specimen Collection

The system consists of a disposable plastic tube (15 ml. capacity) with an easy-on, easy-off plastic cap, a self-adhesive identification label, a flat-bottom 3 oz. paper collection cup, and a 10-tube disposable tube holder for easy specimen collection, transport and testing.
No. 4202—URIN-TEK System with 5 twist-top plastic bags, each containing 100 tubes, caps, labels, and collection cups, and 1 disposable tube holder.
No. 4204—URIN-TEK Tubes Only (500).
No. 4205—URIN-TEK Caps Only (500).
No. 4221—URIN-TEK Urine Tube Rack-each.

Ayerst Laboratories
Division of American Home Products Corporation
685 THIRD AVE.
NEW YORK, NY 10017

FACTREL® ℞
(gonadorelin hydrochloride)
Synthetic Luteinizing Hormone Releasing Hormone (LH-RH)
DIAGNOSTIC USE ONLY

Description: An agent for use in evaluating hypothalamic-pituitary gonadotropic function. FACTREL (gonadorelin hydrochloride) injectable is available as a sterile lyophylized powder for reconstitution and administration by subcutaneous or intravenous routes.
Chemical Name: 5-oxo-L-prolyl-L-histidyl-L-tryptophyl-L-seryl-L-tyrosyl-glycyl-L-leucyl-L-arginyl-L-prolyl glycinamide hydrochloride [See formula below].
FACTREL is $C_{55}H_{75}N_{17}O_{13}HCl$, as the mono- or dihydrochloride, or their mixture. The gonadorelin base has a molecular weight of 1182.33. It is a white powder, soluble in alcohol and water, hygroscopic and moisture-sensitive, and stable at room temperature. The synthetic decapeptide, FACTREL, has a chemical composition and structure identical to the natural hor-

Structural Formula:

mone, identified from porcine or ovine hypothalami.

Each vial of FACTREL contains 100 or 500 mcg gonadorelin as the hydrochloride, with 100 mg lactose, U.S.P. Each ampul of sterile diluent contains 2% benzyl alcohol and Water for Injection, U.S.P.

Clinical Pharmacology: FACTREL has been shown to have gonadotropin-releasing effects upon the anterior pituitary. The range for normal baseline LH levels, as determined from the literature, is 5–25 mIU/ml in postpubertal males, and postpubertal and premenopausal females. The standard used is the Second International Reference Preparation—HMC. This range may not correspond in each laboratory performing the assay since the concentration of LH in normal individuals varies with different assay methods. The normal responses to FACTREL analyzed from the results of clinical studies included:

(1) LH peak mIU/ml)
(highest LH value post-FACTREL administration)

(2) Maximum LH increase (mIU/ml)
(peak LH value—LH baseline value)

(3) LH percent response

$$\frac{\text{peak LH—baseline LH}}{\text{baseline LH}} \times 100\%$$

(4) Time to peak (minutes)
(time required to reach LH peak value)

Normal adult subjects were shown to have these LH responses following FACTREL administration by subcutaneous or intravenous routes.

I. MALE ADULTS:

A) Subcutaneous Administration

The results are based on 18 tests in males between the ages of 18–42 years, inclusive:

(1) LH peak: mean 60.3 ± 26.2 mIU/ml
100% ≥ 24.0 mIU/ml
90% ≥ 32.8 mIU/ml

(2) Maximum LH increase: mean 46.7 ± 20.8 mIU/ml
100% ≥ 12.3 mIU/ml
90% ≥ 20.9 mIU/ml

(3) LH percent response: mean 437 ± 243% range: 66–1853%
90% ≥ 188%

(4) Time to peak: mean 34 ± 13 min.

B) Intravenous Administration

The results are based on 26 tests in males between the ages of 19–58 years, inclusive:

(1) LH peak: mean 63.8 ± 40.3 mIU/ml
100% ≥ 12.6 mIU/ml
90% ≥ 26.0 mIU/ml

(2) Maximum LH increase: mean 51.3 ± 35.2 mIU/ml
100% ≥ 7.4 mIU/ml
90% ≥ 14.8 mIU/ml

(3) LH percent response: mean 481 ± 184% range: 67–2139%
90% ≥ 142%

(4) Time to peak: mean 27 ± 14 min.

In males older than 50 years, the LH baseline and peak levels tend to be higher; however, the maximum LH increases do not differ in regard to age.

II. FEMALE ADULTS:

A) Subcutaneous Administration

The results are based on 38 tests in females between the ages of 19–36 years, inclusive:

(1) LH peak: mean 67.9 ± 27.5 mIU/ml
100% ≥ 12.5 mIU/ml
90% ≥ 39.0 mIU/ml

(2) Maximum LH increase: mean 52.8 ± 26.4 mIU/ml
100% ≥ 7.5 mIU/ml
90% ≥ 23.8 mIU/ml

(3) LH percent response: mean 374 ± 221% range: 108–981%
90% ≥ 185%

(4) Time to peak: mean 71.5 ± 49.6 min.

B) Intravenous Administration

The results are based on 31 tests in females between the ages of 20–35 years inclusive:

(1) LH peak: mean 57.6 ± 36.7 mIU/ml
100% ≥ 20.0 mIU/ml
90% ≥ 24.6 mIU/ml

(2) Maximum LH increase: mean 44.5 ± 31.8 mIU/ml
100% ≥ 7.5 mIU/ml
90% ≥ 16.2 mIU/ml

(3) LH percent response: mean 356 ± 282% range: 60–1300%
90% ≥ 142%

(4) Time to peak: mean 36 ± 24 min.

The FACTREL tests on which the normal female responses are based were performed in the early follicular phase of the menstrual cycle (Days 1–7).

In menopausal and postmenopausal females, the baseline LH levels are elevated and the maximum LH increases are exaggerated when compared with the premenopausal levels.

Patients with clinically diagnosed or suspected pituitary and/or hypothalamic dysfunction were often shown to have subnormal or no LH responses following FACTREL administration. For example, in clinical tests of 6 patients with known postpubertal panhypopituitarism, and 11 patients with Prader-Willi Syndrome, 100% showed subnormal responses or no rise in LH. Subnormal responses to the FACTREL test also were observed in 21 (95%) of 22 patients with prepubertal panhypopituitarism. In 19 patients with Sheehan Syndrome, 16 (84%) had a subnormal response. In the FACTREL test in 44 patients with Kallmann Syndrome, 33 (77%) had subnormal LH responses.

Indications and Usage: FACTREL as a single injection is indicated for evaluating the functional capacity and response of the gonadotropes of the anterior pituitary. This single injection test does not measure pituitary gonadotropic reserve for which more prolonged or repeated administration may be required. The LH response is useful in testing patients with suspected gonadotropin deficiency, whether due to the hypothalamus alone or in combination with anterior pituitary failure. FACTREL is also indicated for evaluating residual gonadotropic function of the pituitary following removal of a pituitary tumor by surgery and/or irradiation. In clinical studies to date, however, the single injection test has not been useful in differentiating pituitary disorders from hypothalamic disorders. The FACTREL test can be performed concomitantly with other post-treatment evaluations.

The results of the FACTREL test complement the clinical examination and other laboratory tests used to confirm or substantiate hypogonadotropic hypogonadism.

In cases where there is a normal response, it indicates the presence of functional pituitary gonadotropes. The single injection test does not measure pituitary gonadotropic reserve.

Contraindications: Hypersensitivity to gonadorelin hydrochloride or any of the components.

Precautions: Although allergic and hypersensitivity reactions have been observed with other polypeptide hormones, to date no such reactions have been encountered following the administration of a single 100 mcg dose of FACTREL. Antibody formation has been rarely reported after chronic administration of large doses of FACTREL.

The FACTREL test should be conducted in the absence of other drugs which directly affect the pituitary secretion of the gonadotropins. These would include a variety of preparations which contain androgens, estrogens, progestins, or glucocorticoids. The gonadotropin levels may be transiently elevated by spironolactone, minimally elevated by levodopa, and suppressed by oral contraceptives and digoxin. The response to FACTREL may be blunted by phenothiazines and dopamine antagonists which cause a rise in prolactin.

Pregnancy Category B. Reproduction studies have been performed in mice, rats, and rabbits at doses up to 50 times the human dose, and have revealed no evidence of harm to the fetus due to FACTREL. There are, however, no adequate and well-controlled studies in pregnant women. Because animal reproduction studies are not always predictive of human response, this drug should be used during pregnancy only if clearly needed.

Appropriate precautions should be taken because the effects of LH-RH on the fetus and developing offspring have not been adequately evaluated. Repetitive, high doses of FACTREL may cause luteolysis and inhibition of spermatogenesis.

Adverse Reactions: Systemic complaints such as headaches, nausea, lightheadedness, abdominal discomfort and flushing have been reported rarely following administration of 100 mcg of FACTREL. Local swelling, occasionally with pain and pruritus, at the injection site may occur if FACTREL is administered subcutaneously. Local and generalized skin rash have been noted after chronic subcutaneous administration.

Overdosage: FACTREL has been administered parenterally in doses up to 3 mg BID for 28 days without any signs or symptoms of overdosage. In case of overdosage or idiosyncrasy, symptomatic treatment should be administered as required.

Dosage and Administration: Adults: 100 mcg dose, subcutaneously or intravenously. In females for whom the phase of the menstrual cycle can be established, the test should be performed in the early follicular phase (Days 1–7).

Test Methodology: To determine the status of the gonadotropin secretory capacity of the anterior pituitary, a test procedure requiring seven venous blood samples for LH is recommended.

PROCEDURE:

1. Venous blood samples should be drawn at -15 minutes and immediately prior to FACTREL administration. The LH baseline is obtained by averaging the LH values of the two samples.
2. Administer a bolus of 100 mcg of FACTREL subcutaneously or intravenously.
3. Draw venous blood samples at 15, 30, 45, 60, and 120 minutes after administration.
4. Blood samples should be handled as recommended by the laboratory that will determine the LH content. It must be emphasized that the reliability of the test is directly related to the inter-assay and intra-assay reliability of the laboratory performing the assay.

Interpretation of Test Results: Interpretation of the LH response to FACTREL requires an understanding of the hypothalamic-pituitary physiology, knowledge of the clinical status of the individual patient, and familiarity with the normal ranges and the standards used in the laboratory performing the LH assays.

Figures 1 through 4 represent the LH response curves after FACTREL administration in normal subjects. The normal LH response curves were established between the 10th percentile (B line) and 90th percentile (A line) of all LH responses in normal subjects analyzed from the results of clinical studies. LH values are reported in units of mIU/ml and time is displayed in minutes. Individual patient responses should be plotted on the appropriate curve. A subnormal response in patients is defined as three or more LH values which fall below the B line of the normal LH response curve.

Continued on next page

Ayerst—Cont.

In cases where there is a blunted or borderline response, the FACTREL test should be repeated.

Fig. 1:
Normal Male LH Response After FACTREL 100 mcg, Subcutaneous Administration 10th and 90th percentiles.

LH (mIU/ml)

Minutes post-dose

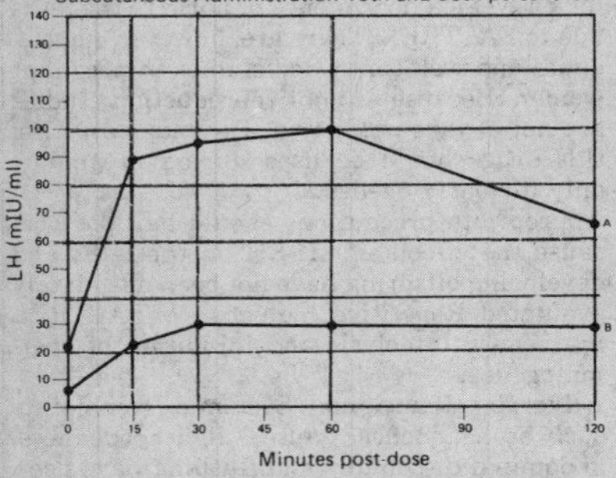

Fig. 2:
Normal Male LH Response After FACTREL 100 mcg, Intravenous Administration 10th and 90th percentiles.

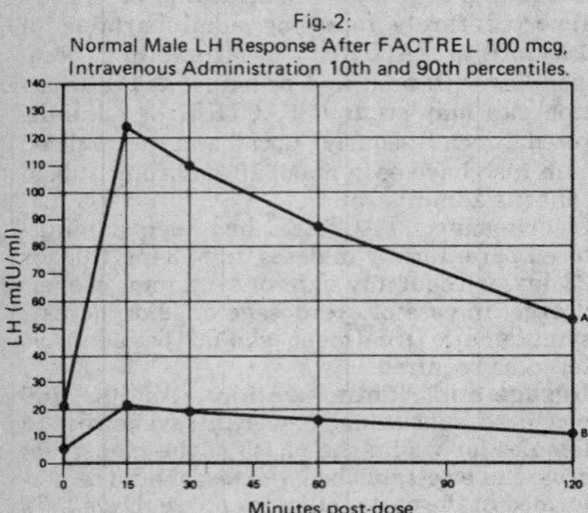

Fig. 3
Normal Female LH Response After FACTREL 100 mcg, Subcutaneous Administration 10th and 90th percentiles.

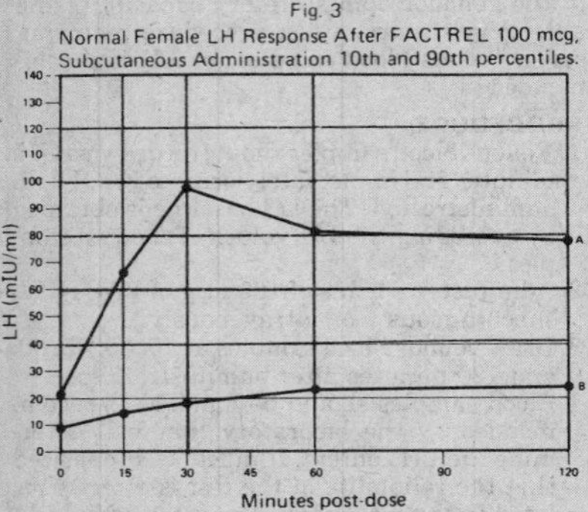

Fig. 4:
Normal Female LH Response After FACTREL 100 mcg, Intravenous Administration 10th and 90th percentiles.

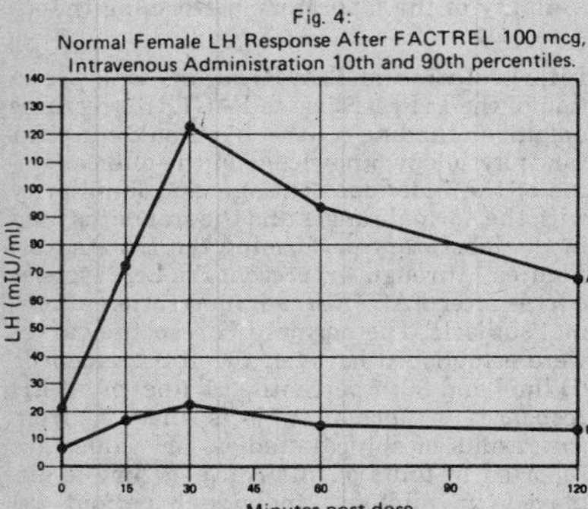

The FACTREL test complements the clinical assessment of patients with a variety of endocrine disorders involving the hypothalamic-pituitary axis. In cases where there is a normal response, it indicates the presence of functional pituitary gonadotropes. The single injection test does not determine the pathophysiological cause for the subnormal response and does not measure pituitary gonadotropic reserve.

How Supplied: LYOPHILIZED POWDER in single-dose vials containing 100 mcg (NDC 0046-0507-05) and 500 mcg (NDC 0046-0509-05) gonadorelin as the hydrochloride with 100 mg lactose, U.S.P. Each vial is accompanied by one ampul containing 2 ml sterile diluent of 2% benzyl alcohol in Water for Injection, U.S.P.

Directions: Store at room temperature (approximately 25°C).
Reconstitute 100 mcg vial with 1.0 ml of the accompanying sterile diluent.
Reconstitute 500 mcg vial with 2.0 ml of the accompanying sterile diluent.
Prepare solution immediately before use.
After reconstitution, store at room temperature and use within 1 day.
Discard unused reconstituted solution and diluent.
Diagnostic Method of Use Patent 3,947,569

PEPTAVLON® ℞

Brand of pentagastrin
A diagnostic agent for evaluation of gastric acid secretory function.

Actions: PEPTAVLON (pentagastrin) contains the C-terminal tetrapeptide responsible for the actions of the natural gastrins and, therefore, acts as a physiologic gastric acid secretagogue. The recommended dose of 6 mcg/kg subcutaneously produces a peak acid output which is reproducible when used in the same individual.
PEPTAVLON stimulates gastric acid secretion approximately ten minutes after subcutaneous injection, with peak responses occurring in most cases twenty to thirty minutes after administration. Duration of activity is usually between sixty and eighty minutes.

Indications: PEPTAVLON (pentagastrin) is used as a diagnostic agent to evaluate gastric acid secretory function. It is useful in testing for:
Anacidity:—as a diagnostic aid in patients with suspected pernicious anemia, atrophic gastritis, or gastric carcinoma.
Hypersecretion:—as a diagnostic aid in patients with suspected duodenal ulcer or postoperative stomal ulcer, and for the diagnosis of Zollinger-Ellison tumor.
PEPTAVLON (pentagastrin) is also useful in determining the adequacy of acid-reducing operations for peptic ulcer.

Contraindications: Hypersensitivity or idiosyncrasy to pentagastrin.

Warnings: *Use in Pregnancy*—The use of pentagastrin in pregnancy has NOT been studied, and the benefit of administration of the drug must be weighed against any possible risk to the mother and/or fetus.
Use in Children—There are insufficient data to recommend the use of, or establish a dosage, in children.

****

In amounts in excess of the recommended dose, pentagastrin may cause inhibition of gastric acid secretion.

Precautions: Use with caution in patients with pancreatic, hepatic, or biliary disease. Like gastrin, pentagastrin could, in some cases, have the physiologic effect of stimulating pancreatic enzyme and bicarbonate secretion, as well as biliary flow.

Adverse Reactions: Pentagastrin causes fewer and less severe cardiovascular and other adverse reactions than histamine or betazole. The majority of reactions to pentagastrin are related to the gastrointestinal tract.
The following reactions associated with the use of pentagastrin have been reported.
Gastrointestinal: abdominal pain, desire to defecate, nausea, vomiting, borborygmi, blood-tinged mucus
Cardiovascular: flushing, tachycardia
Central Nervous System: dizziness, faintness or lightheadedness, drowsiness, sinking feeling, transient blurring of vision, tiredness, headache
Allergic and Hypersensitivity Reactions: May occur in some patients.
Miscellaneous: shortness of breath, heavy sensation in arms and legs, tingling in fingers, chills, sweating, generalized burning sensation, warmth, pain at site of injection, bile in collected specimens

Dosage and Administration: *Adults:* 6 mcg/kg subcutaneously. Effect begins in about ten minutes; peak response usually occurs in twenty to thirty minutes. (For discussion of the test and explicit directions, consult Baron, J.H.: Gastric Function Tests, in Wastell, C.: Chronic Duodenal Ulcer, New York, Appleton-Century-Crofts, 1972, pp. 82–114.)
Note: Data are inadequate to recommend the use of, or establish a dosage, in children.

Overdosage: In case of overdosage or idiosyncrasy, symptomatic treatment should be administered as required.

How Supplied: PEPTAVLON—In 2 ml ampuls. Each ml contains 0.25 mg (250 mcg) pentagastrin. Also contains 0.88% sodium chloride, and Water for Injection U.S.P. The pH is adjusted with ammonium hydroxide. Cartons of 10 (NDC 0046-3290-10).

Bio-Dynamics

A Boehringer Mannheim Company
9115 HAGUE ROAD
INDIANAPOLIS, IN 46250

CHEMSTRIP bG™ BLOOD GLUCOSE TEST

Dip-and-Read Test Strips for Semi-Quantitative Determination of Glucose in Whole Blood

Summary and Explanation: CHEMSTRIP bG is a sensitive and specific test strip which facilitates accurate semi-quantitative determination of blood glucose within 2 minutes.
CHEMSTRIP bG is a glucose test strip with 2 separate test zones whose different reagent concentrations optimize sensitivity and colorimetric accuracy of semi-quantitative values from 20 mg/dl to 800 mg/dl. A wide range of test values permits wide use of CHEMSTRIP bG—for **stat** semi-quantitative assays of hypo- and hyperglycemia in neonatal, surgical, and cardiac care, as well as in emergency diagnosis of coma, mass screening of metabolic status, monitoring of diabetes mellitus and in home blood glucose monitoring programs.

Specimen Collection and Preparation: CHEMSTRIP bG is free from interference when used with fresh capillary blood. It is specific for D-glucose in whole blood and nonreactive to fructose, lactose, galactose, and pentose sugars. Hematocrit values between 30–70% have no significant effect, and neither physiologic concentrations of uric or ascorbic acid, nor therapy with heparin, EDTA or the usual plasma expanders, affect test results with CHEMSTRIP bG.

Procedure for *In Vitro* Diagnostic Use: Two-minute test procedure with CHEMSTRIP bG requires only 3 steps: (1) Place a large enough drop of whole blood on the reagent area to cover both test zones completely. (2) After 60 seconds, wipe off the blood with a dry cotton ball and then rewipe the strip 2 more times. **Do not use water;** unlike other strips, CHEMSTRIP bG needs no washing. (3) After another 60 seconds, read test results by comparing test-zone colors with the vial label's color values for 20, 40, 80, 120, 180, and 240 mg/dl. (For colors **darker** than those for 240 mg/dl, wait an extra minute before reading 400 or 800 mg/dl.) The 8 clearly separate, precalibrated color values

Chemstrip Test Parameters

	Nitrite	pH	Protein	Glucose	Ketones	Urobilinogen	Bilirubin	Blood	Leukocytes	Catalog No.	Strips Per Vial
CHEMSTRIP™ 9	X	X	X	X	X	X	X	X	X	398438	100
CHEMSTRIP™ 8	X	X	X	X	X	X	X	X		200697	100
CHEMSTRIP™ 7L		X	X	X	X	X	X	X	X	416240	100
CHEMSTRIP™ 7		X	X	X	X	X	X	X		200719	100
CHEMSTRIP™ 6L		X	X	X	X		X	X	X	416258	100
CHEMSTRIP™ 6		X	X	X	X		X	X		200727	100
CHEMSTRIP™ 5L		X	X	X	X			X	X	416266	100
CHEMSTRIP™ 5		X	X	X	X			X		200735	100
CHEMSTRIP™ 4		X	X	X				X		203840	100
CHEMSTRIP™ 3		X	X	X						274232	100
CHEMSTRIP™ GP			X	X						200743	100
CHEMSTRIP™ uGK				X	X					00513	100
CHEMSTRIP™ K					X					00515	100
CHEMSTRIP™ uG				X						00511	100
CHEMSTRIP™ L									X	398403	100

facilitate reproducible reading and permit practical estimation of intermediate values.

How Supplied: Nonbreakable aluminum vials of 25 test strips, moisture-protected by drying agent in vial cap. Cat. No. 00501. Vial of 50 test strips, Cat. No. 00503.

Complete self-testing system also available. Kit includes 25 test strips, lancets, cotton balls, alcohol wipes, illustrated "How-to-Use" card and diabetic information guide. Cat. No. 00505.

Ordering/Pricing/Technical Information: Call (317) 845-2000 or toll-free (800) 428-4674.

CHEMSTRIP™ URINE TESTING SYSTEM

Dip and Read Test Strips for Nitrite-pH-Protein-Glucose-Ketones-Urobilinogen-Bilirubin-Blood-Leukocytes in Urine

Summary and Explanation: CHEMSTRIP is a uniquely constructed test strip of inert plastic to which a nylon mesh bonds, without glue, 1 to 9 reagent papers to determine nitrite, pH, protein, glucose, ketones, urobilinogen, bilirubin, blood and leukocytes in urine. The nylon mesh holds each reagent paper in place, protects it and promotes rapid and even urine-diffusion in each complete test area. To prevent the "run-over" phenomenon, certain test papers also have an inert absorbent paper between the reagent paper and the plastic strip. [See table above].

CHEMSTRIPS are packaged in an aluminum vial with a tight-fitting cap which contains a drying agent. Each CHEMSTRIP is stable and ready for use when removed from the vial. No additional equipment or instrumentation is required.

Specimen Collection and Preparation: CHEMSTRIPS may be used on any freshly voided urine specimen or on urines collected under special conditions, such as first-morning specimens and postprandial urines. The urine must be collected in a clean container and should be tested as soon as possible after collection (do not centrifuge). It is of particular importance to use fresh urine to obtain the best results with the test for urine bilirubin because this compound is very unstable when exposed to room temperature and daylight. If testing cannot be performed within an hour after collection, the specimen should be refrigerated immediately at 2 to 8° C and returned to room temperature before testing. Mix thoroughly before use.

Procedure for *In Vitro* Diagnostic Use. For convenience, all values on the strip may be read at 60 seconds (during the second minute) after immersion in the urine. Color changes occurring more than 2 minutes after strip immersion are not of diagnostic value. (Semi-quantitative assay of abnormally high glucose concentrations may require 4–5 minutes, however.) Color changes that occur only along the edge of the test area should be ignored. Careful removal of excess urine should eliminate this effect.

Calibration of the CHEMSTRIP during use is not required. Color blocks on vial label are previously calibrated by use of precise standards during the manufacturing process.

Ordering/Pricing/Technical Information: Call (317) 845-2000 or toll free (800) 428-4674.

Products are cross-indexed by

generic and chemical names

in the

YELLOW SECTION

Lederle Laboratories

A Division of American Cyanamid Co.
ONE CYANAMID PLAZA
WAYNE, NJ 07470

TUBERCULIN, OLD, TINE TEST® ℞

Description: The TUBERCULIN, OLD, TINE TEST® is a sterile, simple, multiple-puncture, disposable intradermal test device for the detection of tuberculin reactivity. These convenient devices are especially useful in mass tuberculosis screening programs.

Each test unit consists of a stainless steel disc attached to a plastic handle. Projecting from the disk are four triangular-shaped prongs (tines) which are 2 mm long and approximately 4 mm apart. The tines have been mechanically dipped in a solution of Old Tuberculin, containing 7% Acacia (Gum Arabic) and 8.5% Lactose as stabilizers, and then dried. The entire unit has been sterilized by ethylene oxide gas. No preservative has been added. The unit is disposable and there is no need for syringes, needles, and other equipment necessary for the standard intradermal tests.

TUBERCULIN, OLD, TINE TEST® UNITS have been standardized by clinical evaluation in human subjects to give reactions equivalent to or more potent than 5 T.U.* of standard old tuberculin administered intradermally in the Mantoux test. However, all multiple puncture-type devices must be regarded as screening tools and other appropriate diagnostic procedures such as the Mantoux test should be utilized for retesting reactors.

*U.S. (International) tuberculin units.

Indications and Usage: TUBERCULIN, OLD, TINE TEST® is indicated to detect tuberculin-sensitive individuals. Tine Test units are also useful in programs to determine priorities for additional testing (i.e., chest x-rays) and in epidemiological surveys to identify those areas having high levels of infection.

In clinical studies covering various geographical areas of the U.S. and all age groups, with a total of 30,588 test subjects, there were 911 (4%) false positive reactors among 26,236 subjects who were Mantoux negative, and 342 (8%) false negative reactors among 4,352 subjects who were Mantoux positive.

The frequency of repeated tuberculin tests depends on the risk of exposure of the child and on the prevalence of tuberculosis in the population group. For the pediatrician's office or outpatient clinic, an annual or biennial tuberculin test, unless local circumstances clearly indicate otherwise, is appropriate. The initial test should be done at the time of, or preceding, the measles immunization.[1] The repeated testing of uninfected individuals does not sensitize to tuberculin. Among individuals with waning sensitivity to homologous or heterologous mycobacterial antigens, however, the stimulus of a tuberculin test may "boost" or increase the size of the reaction to a second test, even causing an apparent development of sensitivity in some cases.[2]

Precautions: Tuberculin testing should be done with caution in individuals with active tuberculosis. Although activation of quiescent lesions is rare, if a patient has a history of occurrence of vesiculation and necrosis with a previous tuberculin test by any method, tuberculin testing should be avoided.

Although clinical allergy to acacia is very rare, this product contains some acacia as stabilizer and should be used with caution in patients with known allergy to this component.

Reactivity to the test may be suppressed in patients who are receiving corticosteroids or immunosuppressive agents, or those who have recently been vaccinated with live virus vaccines such as measles, mumps, rubella, polio, etc.

With a positive reaction further diagnostic procedures must be considered. These may include x-ray of the chest, microbiologic examinations of sputa and other specimens, and confirmation of the positive Tine Test reaction (except vesiculation reactions) using the Mantoux method. In general, the Tine Test does not need to be repeated. Antituberculous chemotherapy should not be instituted solely on the basis of a single positive Tine Test.

When vesiculation occurs, the reaction is to be interpreted as strongly positive and a repeat test by the Mantoux method must not be attempted. Similar or more severe vesiculation with or without necrosis is likely to occur.

Pregnancy Category C. Animal reproduction studies have not been conducted with Tuberculin, Old, TINE TEST®. It is also not known whether Tuberculin, Old, TINE TEST can cause fetal harm when administered to a pregnant woman or can affect reproduction capacity. Tuberculin, Old, TINE TEST, should be given to a pregnant woman only if clearly needed.

During pregnancy, known positive reactors may demonstrate a negative response to a Tuberculin Tine Test.

Adverse Reactions: Vesiculation (positive reaction), ulceration, or necrosis may occur at

Continued on next page

The information on each product appearing here is based on labelling effective in August, 1982 and is either the entire official brochure or an accurate condensation therefrom. Official brochures are enclosed in product packages. Information concerning all Lederle products may be obtained from the Professional Services Department, Lederle Laboratories, Pearl River, New York, 10965.

Lederle—Cont.

the test site in highly sensitive persons. Pain, pruritis, and discomfort at the test site may be relieved by cold packs or by topical glucocorticoid ointment or cream. Transient bleeding may be observed at a puncture site and is of no significance.

Dosage and Administration: TUBERCULIN, OLD, TINE TEST® UNITS have been standardized by clinical evaluation in human subjects to give reactions equivalent to or more potent than 5 T.U.* of standard old tuberculin administered intradermally in the Mantoux test. However, all multiple puncture-type devices must be regarded as screening tools and other appropriate diagnostic procedures such as the Mantoux test should be utilized for retesting reactors.

*U.S. (International) tuberculin units.

The volar surface of the upper one-third of the forearm, over a muscle belly, is the preferred site. Hairy areas, and areas without adequate subcutaneous tissue, e.g., concavities over a tendon or bone should be avoided.

Alcohol, acetone, ether, or soap and water may be used to cleanse the skin. The area must be clean and thoroughly dry before application of the TUBERCULIN, OLD, TINE TEST®.

Expose the four coated tines by removing the protective cap while holding the plastic handle. Grasp the patient's forearm firmly, since the sharp momentary sting may cause the patient to jerk his or her arm, resulting in scratching. Stretch the skin of the forearm tightly and apply the disc with the other hand. **Hold at least one second.** Release tension grip on forearm. Withdraw tine unit.

Sufficient pressure should be exerted so that the four puncture sites, and circular depression of the skin from the plastic base are visible.

Local care of the skin is not necessary.

TUBERCULIN, OLD, TINE TEST® Unit must never be re-used.

Reading Reactions: Tests should be read at 48-72 hours. Vesiculation or the extent of induration are the determining factors; erythema without induration is of no significance. Readings should be made in good light with the forearm slightly flexed. The size of the induration in millimeters should be determined by inspection, measuring, and palpation with gentle finger stroking. Indentification of the application site is usually easy because of the distinct four-point pattern. The diameter of the largest single reaction around one of the puncture sites should be measured. With pronounced reactions, the areas of induration around the puncture sites may coalesce.

Interpretation:

Positive Reactions

A. **Vesiculation.** If vesiculation is present, the test may be interpreted as positive, in which case the management of the patient is the same as that for one classified as positive to the Mantoux test.[3]

B. **Induration, 2mm or Greater**
The test may be interpreted as positive but further diagnostic procedures must be considered. These may include x-ray of the chest, microbiologic examination of sputa and other specimens, and confirmation of the positive Tine Test reaction using the Mantoux Method.

Negative Reaction

Induration Less Than 2mm. With a negative reaction there is no need for retesting unless the person is a contact of a patient with tuberculosis or there is clinical evidence suggestive of the disease.[3]

Descriptive literature illustrating typical reactions is available upon request.

How Supplied: TUBERCULIN, OLD, TINE TEST® is supplied as follows:

25 individual tests in a jar
100 individual tests
250 individual tests

Storage: TUBERCULIN, OLD, TINE TEST® UNITS should be stored unrefrigerated below 30° C (86° F).

References:

1. Report of the Committee on the Control of Infectious Diseases. American Academy of Pediatrics, 1977.
2. Comstock, G.W., et al, The Tuberculin Skin Test, Amer. Rev. Respiratory Disease 104:769-775, No. 5 (Nov) 1971.
3. Committee on Diagnostic Skin Testing of the American Thoracic Society, The Tuberculin Test (Revised 1974). New York, American Lung Association, 1974.

Military Depot and USPHS Depots
NSN 6505-00-890-1534, 25 Tests

TUBERCULIN PURIFIED PROTEIN DERIVATIVE TINE TEST® (PPD) ℞

Description: THE TUBERCULIN, PURIFIED PROTEIN DERIVATIVE (PPD) TINE TEST® is a sterile, simple, multiple-puncture, disposable intradermal test device for the detection of tuberculin reactivity. These convenient devices are especially useful in mass tuberculosis screening programs.

Each test unit consists of a stainless steel disc attached to a light blue plastic handle. Projecting from the disc are four triangular-shaped prongs (tines) which are 2 mm long and approximately 4 mm apart. The tines have been mechanically dipped into a concentrated solution of PPD. The PPD concentrate is prepared by the Seibert Process[1,2] and is stabilized with seven percent acacia (gum Arabic), thirty percent dextrose and five percent glycerol. The glycerol also acts as a humectant preventing the film on the tines from becoming brittle-dry. The final PPD concentrate is standardized against U.S. Standard PPD. The tines are dipped into concentrated PPD, capped and sterilized with ethylene oxide. The Tine Test (PPD) unit is disposable, and there is no need for syringes, needles, and other equipment necessary for the standard intradermal tests.

The Tine Test (PPD) units have been standardized by clinical evaluation in human subjects to give reactions equivalent to or more potent than 5 T.U.* of standard PPD administered intradermally in the Mantoux test. However, all multiple puncture-type devices must be regarded as screening tools and other appropriate diagnostic procedures such as the Mantoux test should be utilized for retesting reactors.

*(International) tuberculin units.

Indications and Usage: TUBERCULIN, PURIFIED PROTEIN DERIVATIVE TINE TEST® PPD is indicated to detect tuberculin-sensitive individuals. Tine Test units are also useful in programs to determine priorities for additional testing (i.e., chest x-rays) and in epidemiological surveys to identify those areas having high levels of infection.

Data obtained from clinical studies with a total of 3,062 volunteer subjects (males and females), ranging in age from 4 to 96 years, of which 47.5% (1,443) were Mantoux positive, clearly demonstrates that Tine Test PPD, when used as a screening test to determine tuberculin reactivity is associated with very little, if any, adverse reactivity. Other than the skin test reaction itself, slight vesiculation and slight ulceration were the only adverse experiences reported. The slight to mild vesiculation was equally divided between the two tests (Tine Test, 54/3062, 1.78%, and PPD-T Mantoux, 55/3062, 1.81%). The slight ulceration observed with one subject at 72 hours was associated with the Tine Test site. Of the subjects classified as positive or intermediate by PPD-T Mantoux, 93.8% were classified similarly with the Tine Test. The results of the clinical trials revealed a 72-hour false positive rate of 10.9% and a false negative rate of 6.2%.

In clinical studies of more than 1,800 PPD-S Mantoux positive subjects only 6.3% gave negative Tine Test PPD reactions at 72 hours; of more than 1,900 Tine Test PPD positive tests, less than 11% gave negative Mantoux results. The frequency of repeated tuberculin tests depends on risk of exposure of the child and on the prevalence of tuberculosis in the population group. For the pediatrician's office or outpatient clinic, an annual or biennial tuberculin test, unless local circumstances clearly indicate otherwise, is appropriate. The initial test should be done at the time of, or preceding, the measles immunization.[3] The repeated testing of uninfected individuals does not sensitize to tuberculin. Among individuals with waning sensitivity to homologous or heterologous mycobacterial antigens, however, the stimulus of a tuberculin test may "boost" or increase the size of the reaction to a second test, even causing an apparent development of sensitivity in some cases.[4]

Precautions: Tuberculin testing should be done with caution in individuals with active tuberculosis. However, activation of quiescent lesions is rare. If a patient has a history of occurrence of vesiculation and necrosis with a previous tuberculin test by any method, tuberculin testing should be avoided.

Although clinical allergy to acacia is very rare, this product contains some acacia as stabilizer and should be used with caution in patients with known allergy to this component.

Reactivity to the test may be suppressed in patients who are receiving corticosteroids or immunosuppressive agents, or those who have recently been vaccinated with live virus vaccines such as measles, mumps, rubella, polio, etc.

With a positive reaction, further diagnostic procedures must be considered. These may include x-ray of the chest, microbiologic examinations of sputa and other specimens, and confirmation of the positive Tine Test reaction (except vesiculation reactions) using the Mantoux method. In general, the Tine Test does not need to be repeated. Antituberculous chemotherapy should not be instituted solely on the basis of a single positive Tine Test.

When vesiculation occurs, the reaction is to be interpreted as strongly positive and a repeat test by the Mantoux method must not be attempted. Similar or more severe vesiculation with or without necrosis is likely to occur.

Pregnancy Category C. Animal reproduction studies have not been conducted with Tuberculin, Purified Protein Derivative [PPD] TINE TEST®. It is also not known whether Tuberculin, Purified Protein Derivative [PPD] TINE TEST can cause fetal harm when administered to a pregnant woman or can affect reproduction capacity. Tuberculin, Purified Protein Derivative [PPD] TINE TEST should be given to a pregnant woman only if clearly needed.

During pregnancy, known positive reactors may demonstrate a negative response to a Tuberculin [PPD] Tine Test.

Adverse Reactions: Vesiculation (positive reaction), ulceration, or necrosis may occur at the test site in highly sensitive persons. Pain, pruritis, and discomfort at the test site may be relieved by cold packs or by topical glucocorticoid ointment or cream. Transient bleeding may be observed at a puncture site and is of no significance.

Dosage and Administration: The Tine Test (PPD) units have been standardized by clinical evaluation in human subject to give reactions equivalent to or more potent that 5 T.U.* of standard PPD administered intradermally in the Mantoux test. However, all multiple puncture-type devices must be regarded as screening tools and other appropriate diagnostic procedures such as the Mantoux test should be utilized for retesting reactors.

*U.S. (International) tuberculin units.

The volar surface of the upper one-third of the

forearm, over a muscle belly, is the preferred site. Hairy areas, and areas without adequate subcutaneous tissue, e.g., concavities over a tendon or bone should be avoided.
Alcohol, acetone, ether, or soap and water may be used to cleanse the skin. The area must be clean and thoroughly dry before application of the Tine Test PPD.
Expose the four coated tines by removing the protective cap while holding the plastic handle. Grasp the patient's forearm firmly, since the sharp momentary sting may cause the patient to jerk his or her arm, resulting in scratching. Stretch the skin of the forearm tightly and apply the disc with the other hand. ***Hold at least one second.*** Release tension grip on forearm. Withdraw tine unit.
Sufficient pressure should be exerted so that the four puncture sites, and a circular depression of the skin from the plastic base are visible.
Local care of the skin is not necessary.
TUBERCULIN, PURIFIED PROTEIN DERIVATIVE TINE TEST® PPD Unit *must never be re-used.*
Reading Reactions: Tests should be read at *72 hours.* Vesiculation or the extent of induration are the determining factors; erythema without induration is of no significance. Readings should be made in good light with the forearm slightly flexed. The size of the induration in millimeters should be determined by inspection, measuring, and palpation with gentle finge stroking. Identification of the application site is usually easy because of the distrinct four-point pattern. The diameter of the largest single reaction around one of the puncture sites should be measured. With pronounced reactions, the areas of induration around the puncture sites may coalesce.
Interpretation:
Positive Reactions
A. **Vesiculation.** If vesiculation is present, the test may be interpreted as positive, in which case the management of the patient is the same as that for one classified as positive to the Mantoux Test.[5]
B. **Induration, 2mm or Greater**
The test may be interpreted as positive but further diagnostic procedures must be considered. These may include x-ray of the chest, microbiologic examination of sputa and other specimens, and confirmation of the positive Tine Test reaction using the Mantoux Method.

Negative Reaction
Induration Less Than 2mm. With a negative reaction there is no need for retesting unless the person is a contact of a patient with tuberculosis or there is clinical evidence suggestive of the disease.[5]
Descriptive literature illustrating typical reactions is available upon request.
How Supplied: Tuberculin, Purified Protein Derivative Tine Test® PPD is supplied as follows:
25 Individual tests in a jar
100 Individual tests
Storage: Tine Test PPD Units should be stored unrefrigerated below 30° C (86° F.)
References:
1. Seibert, F. B. "Isolation and Properties of Purified Protein Derivatives of Tuberculin." *Am. Rev. Tuberc.*, 30 (1934) 713.
2. Seibert, F.B., and Glenn, J.F. "Tuberculin Purified Protein Derivative—Preparation and Analysis of a Large Quantity for Standard." *Amer. Rev. Tuberc.*, 44 (1941) 9.
3. Report of the Committee on the Control of Infectious Diseases. American Academy of Pediatrics, 1977.
4. Comstock, G.W., et al., The Tuberculin Skin Test, *Amer. Rev. Respiratory Disease* 104:769–775, No. 5 (Nov) 1971.
5. Committee on Diagnostic Skin Testing of the American Thoracic Society, The Tuberculin Test (Revised 1974), New York, American Lung Association 1974.

Eli Lilly and Company
**307 E. McCARTY ST.
INDIANAPOLIS, IN 46285**

HISTAMINE PHOSPHATE ℞
Injection, USP
For Gastric Histamine Test

Description: Histamine is a basic substance which may be obtained by decarboxylation of the amino acid histidine. It is usually administered as the stable, water-soluble acid phosphate. Two molecules of phosphoric acid are attached to each molecule of histamine.
Since the molecular weight of histamine phosphate is 307.15 and that of histamine itself is 111.15, 2.75 mg of the salt are required to obtain 1 mg of the active principle.

Actions: Histamine acts on the vascular system, smooth muscle, and exocrine glands. Histamine increases the volume and acidity of the gastric juice.

Indication: Histamine phosphate solution is intended for subcutaneous administration to test the ability of the gastric mucosa to produce hydrochloric acid.

Contraindications: The gastric histamine test is contraindicated in patients with a history of hypersensitivity to histamine products. It is contraindicated in patients with hypotension, severe hypertension, vasomotor instability, bronchial asthma (past or present), urticaria (past or present), or severe cardiac, pulmonary, or renal disease.

Warnings: Attacks of severe asthma or other serious allergic conditions may be precipitated by the administration of histamine phosphate. The possible benefit that may be derived from the gastric histamine test should be carefully weighed against the serious untoward reactions that may develop in patients with allergic diseases. Small doses by any route of administration may precipitate asthma in patients with bronchial disease. The utmost caution is advised in using histamine in such patients.

When histamine phosphate is administered, pull back on the syringe plunger before the injection is made to be sure the end of the needle is not in a blood vessel. Care should be taken to avoid accidental introduction into a vein or artery. Epinephrine, 1:1000, should be immediately available to counteract the effects of histamine.

Usage in Pregnancy—The safety of this agent for use during pregnancy or lactation has not been established; therefore, the benefits must be weighed against its possible hazards to the mother and child.

The physician must carefully weigh the risk/benefit ratio when considering the use of the gastric histamine test in patients with pheochromocytoma.

Precautions: Average or large doses of histamine may cause flushing, dizziness, headache, nervousness, local or generalized allergic manifestations, marked hypertension or hypotension, tachycardia, and abdominal cramps. These reactions may be alarming and are potentially dangerous. Local reactions at the site of injection may include erythema and edema. Histamine increases the acid of the gastric juice and may cause symptoms of peptic ulcer. A large subcutaneous dose of histamine may cause severe occipital headache, blurred vision, anginal pain, a rapid drop in blood pressure, and cyanosis of the face. Overdosage may cause severe symptoms, including circulatory collapse, shock, and even death. The blood pressure and pulse should be carefully monitored during injection of histamine.
Use with caution in patients with any cardiac abnormality.

Adverse Reactions: Following the injection of an average or large dose of histamine, side effects may include such local reactions as erythema and edema and/or such systemic reactions as flushing, dizziness, headache, bronchial constriction, dyspnea, visual disturbances, faintness, syncope, urticaria, asthma, marked hypertension or hypotension, weakness, palpitation, tachycardia, nervousness, abdominal cramps, diarrhea, nausea, vomiting, metallic taste, local or generalized allergic manifestations, or collapse with convulsions.
Administration and Dosage—Gastric Histamine Test: *Histamine Test*—After the basal gastric secretion has been collected, histamine phosphate is given subcutaneously. The dose is 0.0275 mg of histamine phosphate (or 0.01 mg of the histamine base) per kg of body weight. The gastric contents are then collected in four 15-minute specimens for one hour and analyzed for volume, acidity, pH. and acid output.
Augmented Histamine Test—Initially, a suitable dose of antihistamine is administered intramuscularly, e.g., 10 mg chlorpheniramine maleate, 50 mg pyrilamine maleate, or 50 mg diphenhydramine hydrochloride.
After the conclusion of the basal secretion study, histamine phosphate is given subcutaneously in a dose of 0.04 mg/kg of body weight.
Before undertaking these procedures, the physician should thoroughly familiarize himself with the technique or methodology of performing the gastric histamine test or the augmented histamine test and with the interpretation of the results from standard reference texts.
Overdosage: Overdosage of Histamine Phosphate Injection may cause severe symptoms, including circulatory collapse, shock, and even death (*see* Warnings, Precautions, and Adverse Reactions). If accidental overdosage is discovered early, temporary application of a tourniquet proximally to the injection site may be tried to slow down the absorption of the drug.
Antidotes to histamine are the following:
Epinephrine hydrochloride, 0.1–0.5 ml of a 1:1000 aqueous solution, given subcutaneously in case of emergency due to severe reactions.
An antihistamine preparation may be given intramuscularly to prevent or ameliorate systemic reactions to the drug.
How Supplied: (℞) *Histamine Phosphate Injection, USP: Vials No. 328.* 2.75 mg (equivalent to 1 mg histamine base) in 5 ml, 5 ml, rubber-stoppered, in singles (10 per carton) (NDC 0002-1635-01); 1 ml contains 0.55 mg histamine phosphate (equivalent to 0.2 mg histamine base), with 16 mg glycerin and 2 mg phenol. Phosphoric acid may have been added to adjust the pH. *Ampoules No. 269.* 2.75 mg (equivalent to 1 mg histamine base), 1 ml, in packages of 6 (NDC 0002-1622-16) and 100 (NDC 0002-1622-02).

[032482]

HISTAMINE PHOSPHATE ℞
Injection, USP
Histamine Test for Pheochromocytoma

Description: Histamine is a basic substance which may be obtained by decarboxylation of the amino acid histidine. It is usually administered as the stable, water-soluble acid phosphate. Two molecules of phosphoric acid are attached to each molecule of histamine.
Since the molecular weight of histamine phosphate is 307.15 and that of histamine itself is 111.15, 2.75 mg of the salt are required to obtain 1 mg of the active principle.
Each ml of Ampoules No. 338, Histamine Phosphate Injection, USP (histamine test for pheochromocytoma), contains 0.275 mg hista-

Continued on next page

Lilly—Cont.

mine phosphate (equivalent to 0.1 mg histamine) and 9 mg sodium chloride.

Indication: Histamine Phosphate Injection may be used intravenously for the presumptive diagnosis of pheochromocytoma.

Contraindications: The histamine test for pheochromocytoma is contraindicated in the elderly or in the presence of severe hypertension.

Warnings: Attacks of severe asthma or other serious allergic conditions may be precipitated by the administration of histamine phosphate. The possible benefit that may be derived from the histamine test for pheochromocytoma should be carefully weighed against the serious untoward reactions that may develop in patients with severe allergic diseases.

Precautions: Average or large doses of histamine may cause flushing, dizziness, headache, nervousness, local or generalized allergic manifestations, marked hypertension or hypotension, tachycardia, and abdominal cramps. These reactions may be alarming and are potentially dangerous. Histamine increases the acid of the gastric juice and may cause symptoms of peptic ulcer. Small doses by any route of administration may precipitate asthma in patients with bronchial disease. The utmost caution is advised in using histamine in such patients and in those with a history of bronchial asthma.

Frequent checks of the blood pressure and pulse should be made during intravenous injections of histamine. If there is a dangerous fall in blood pressure, a prompt injection of epinephrine should be given.

A large dose of histamine may cause severe occipital headache, blurred vision, anginal pain, a rapid drop in blood pressure, and cyanosis of the face. Overdosage by the intravenous route may cause severe symptoms, including vasomotor collapse, shock, and even death.

Adverse Reactions: Following the injection of an average or large dose of histamine, side effects may include such systemic reactions as flushing, dizziness, headache, bronchial constriction, dyspnea, visual disturbances, faintness, syncope, urticaria, asthma, marked hypertension or hypotension, palpitation, tachycardia, nervousness, abdominal cramps, diarrhea, vomiting, metallic taste, local or generalized allergic manifestations, or collapse with convulsions.

Administration and Dosage—Histamine Test for Pheochromocytoma: Antihypertensive drugs, sympathomimetic agents, sedatives, and narcotics should be withheld from the patient for at least 24 hours, preferably 72 hours, before the histamine test is performed. *Food should not be withheld.*

The histamine test for pheochromocytoma is a provocative test and, therefore, is indicated only for the occasional patient who has paroxysmal signs of excessive catecholamine secretion and who has normal urinary values for assays of catecholamines and metabolites during periods when he is asymptomatic.

A well-conducted test provides information on the symptomatic and physiologic responses and changes in urinary catecholamine levels. This test is to be used only in patients in whom resting blood pressure does not exceed 150/110.

Epinephrine should be available in case a severe hypotensive response is produced. Phentolamine should be on hand to depress any alarming increase in blood pressure.

The patient rests in bed while a slow intravenous infusion of either 5% dextrose or isotonic saline solution is established. The blood pressure is recorded until it is stable. At that time, a two-hour period of urine collection for catecholamine assay is started. At the end of this period, histamine is rapidly administered through the infusion, and another two-hour urine collection is started.

The first dose of histamine should be 0.01 mg, or 10 mcg. This dose is provided in 0.1 ml of Ampoules No. 338 (0.275 mg histamine phosphate, or 0.1 mg histamine, in 1 ml of solution). If no response is observed within five minutes, a dose of 0.05 mg (50 mcg) should be administered. The blood pressure and pulse are to be recorded every 30 seconds for 15 minutes. The expected responses in both positive and negative tests are headache, flushing, and a decrease in blood pressure followed within two minutes by an increase.

Positive tests have been defined as—

1. An increase in blood pressure of at least 20/10 mm Hg greater than that obtained with the cold pressor test.
2. An increase in blood pressure of at least 60/40 mm Hg above the base line and greater than that with the cold pressor test.

An increase in urinary catecholamine levels from normal during the pretest control period to abnormally high during the test lessens the possibility of false-positive tests.

How Supplied: (℞) *Ampoules No. 338, Histamine Phosphate Injection, USP,* 0.275 mg (equivalent to 0.1 mg histamine), 1 ml, in packages of 6.
(NDC 0002-1639-16) [050182]

TES-TAPE® OTC
(glucose enzymatic test strip) USP

For In Vitro Diagnostic Use in Testing for the Presence and Semiquantitative Measurement of Glucose in Human Urine

Tes-Tape has been used since 1956, when Dr. A. S. Keston described the novel idea of using two enzymes simultaneously to test for glucose and Dr. J. P. Comer published data on the specificity and accuracy of Tes-Tape for the semiquantitative analysis of urine glucose.

During the development and testing of this urine test method, Tes-Tape was found to be an accurate and reliable semiquantitative method for determining urine glucose. To date, relatively few instances of faulty results have occurred with the use of Tes-Tape. Problems associated with the product are usually due to improper techniques or exposure of the tape to adverse conditions or due to drugs which have an inhibitory effect on the enzyme reaction. Considerable data may be found in the published scientific documents.

Tes-Tape is impregnated with the enzymes glucose oxidase and peroxidase and an oxidizable substrate, orthotolidine. When the tape is dipped into urine containing glucose, the glucose oxidase catalyzes the reaction of glucose in the urine with oxygen from the air to form gluconic acid and hydrogen peroxide. The enzyme peroxidase (from horseradish) then catalyzes the reaction of hydrogen peroxide and orthotolidine to form a blue color. With the addition of a yellow dye (FDC Yellow No. 5) to the paper, the possible color range of the test is extended from yellow to light green to deep blue. If no glucose is present, the tape maintains its yellow color.

Reactive Ingredient	Approximate Amount per 1.5 Inches of Tape
Glucose oxidase	3.78 units
Horseradish peroxidase	2.82 PZ units
O-tolidine	0.136 mg

Nonreactive ingredients include filter paper, FDC Yellow No. 5 coloring, buffers, stabilizers, and wetting agents.

For in vitro diagnostic use. Store below 86°F (30°C). Protect from high humidity and light. Do not use if the tape becomes dark yellow or yellowish-brown or if a 2 percent reading is not obtained when the reliability is tested, as described under the heading **Important**.

The urine should be collected in a container free of chemicals and glucose.

If the freshly voided specimen is not to be tested within four hours, it should be refrigerated.

Drugs that are known to have an inhibitory effect on the enzyme reactions include ascorbic acid (vitamin C), dipyrone, gentisic acid (a metabolite of aspirin), homogentisic acid (present in alkaptonuria), levodopa, meralluride injection, and methyldopa. The inhibiting effect is notable on the dipped part of the tape, but accurate readings may be obtained by observing the narrow band of color at the junction of the dry and wet portions. A separation of glucose from the inhibitory substances occurs as the urine travels along the dry portion of the tape. Ingestion of more than 1.5 g of ascorbic acid may produce urine with inhibitory action on Tes-Tape.

Specimens for storage or shipment should be refrigerated or preserved with up to 0.37 percent formaldehyde.

All materials are provided for the test and include dispenser, tape, and color chart.

Results on the color chart are expressed in percent of glucose (urine sugar) and by a corresponding arbitrary system of 0, +, + +, + + +, + + + +, representing 0, $\frac{1}{10}$, $\frac{1}{4}$, $\frac{1}{2}$, 2 (or more) percent of glucose respectively.

When testing, do not place the tape on the lavatory or on paper or allow moistened portion to contact fingers. Contamination of the tape by glucose from other sources (e.g., perspiration, tears, and saliva) or with a residue of chlorine from lavatory cleansing agents can cause false-positive results.

Patients who are receiving high doses of ascorbic acid or whose urine contains dipyrone, meralluride, homogentisic acid, gentisic acid, levodopa, or methyldopa should read only the very narrow band of color in the moist portion of the tape above the level to which it was dipped into the specimen.

Very high doses of ascorbic acid may cause a false-negative test even with the above precaution. (Urinary levels of ascorbic acid in excess of 0.1 percent are necessary to block the test completely. This concentration is most likely to appear within three to seven hours after a single dose of 1.5 g or more.)

Normal urine should test 0 percent with Tes-Tape. Persons using Tes-Tape for a screening test should report all values above 0 percent to their physician. Diabetic urine values in the range of the color chart should also be recorded and reported to the patient's physician. Measured values of 2 percent should be reported as 2 percent or more.

The overall semiquantitative accuracy of Tes-Tape originally reported in 1956 on 1000 determinations was 96 percent. This was confirmed in 1973 on 14,000 determinations over a two-year period. These data were obtained on urine samples containing concentrations of glucose at each increment shown to be measurable on the color chart. The color chart provided is based on the average color perception of many observers. Patients who have difficulty in differentiating color should seek the advice of their physician before using Tes-Tape.

Numerous other clinical and laboratory studies have shown that Tes-Tape is accurate in qualitative and semiquantitative determination of urine sugar. Tes-Tape is specific for glucose in urine sugar testing. Except for instances involving contamination of the tape or urine receptacle with glucose from other sources (e.g., perspiration, tears, and saliva) or with a residue of chlorine from cleansing agents, there is no known clinical situation in which a false-positive test for glucose occurs with Tes-Tape. The sensitivity of Tes-Tape is such that it will react with concentrations of 0.05 percent glucose or more. Trace reactions shown by the development of a very light yellow-green color may be observed with less than this amount of glucose.

After opening plastic wrapper, use tape within four months. It must be used prior to expiration date.

Important: The reliability of a roll of Tes-Tape may easily be checked by dipping a piece into a properly prepared glucose solution.* The tape should be removed immediately, as one would when testing a urine specimen. After two minutes have elapsed, the reading obtained when the tape is compared with the color chart should be approximately + + + + (2 percent). If such a reading is not obtained, the tape has apparently deteriorated and should not be used.

Measurements for the amount of glucose present (semiquantitative) should not be made after two minutes because the colors gradually change as the tape dries. Screening tests for the presence of glucose (qualitative) in urine may be made for several hours after the tape has dried.

The patient should consult the package insert in regard to Procedure, What to Do If Tape Breaks, and a record chart for urine sugar tests with Tes-Tape.

*If a properly prepared glucose solution is not available, any nationally known *sugar (glucose)-containing* beverage from a freshly opened bottle or can is satisfactory. (Diet cola beverages would not be satisfactory.)

How Supplied: *M-73, Tes-Tape® (Glucose Enzymatic Test Strip, USP),* dispenser package, approximately 100 tests, in single packages. (NDC 0002-2344-41) [021182]

M-73—100 tests—6505-00-559-6859A

Merieux Institute, Inc.

1200 N.W. 78TH AVENUE
SUITE 109
MIAMI, FL 33126

TUBERCULIN, MONO-VACC® TEST ℞
(old tuberculin)
Multiple Puncture Device

NDC 50361-772425 25 test per box

Norwich Eaton Pharmaceuticals, Inc.

Professional Products Group
(formerly Eaton Laboratories)
Consumer Products Group
(formerly Norwich Products)
NORWICH, NY 13815

SARENIN® ℞
(saralasin acetate)

The following text is based on official labeling in effect August 1, 1982.

Description: Sarenin (saralasin acetate), an angiotensin II antagonist which has partial agonist action, represents a new class of pharmacologic agents. Sarenin is 1-(N-methylglycine)-5-L-valine-8-L-alanine angiotensin II acetate (salt) hydrate. The lyophilized peptide powder, saralasin acetate, is synthesized from amino acids and contains both water of hydration and acetic acid (as acetate salt).

The acetic-acid-free anhydrous peptide, saralasin, has a molecular weight of 912.07. Saralasin acetate is highly soluble in water (about 150 g/liter at 25°C) and in 90% and 95% aqueous alcohol (35 and 15 g/liter, respectively). It is available as a sterile aqueous solution for intravenous infusion in ampuls containing saralasin acetate equivalent to a total of 18 mg saralasin.

Clinical Pharmacology: Sarenin (saralasin acetate) is an angiotensin II analog that binds to angiotensin II tissue receptors, but is a less effective vasoconstrictive agonist than angiotensin II. It therefore has a dual action depending on the circulating levels of angiotensin II. In the presence of high levels of circulating angiotensin II, Sarenin competitively inhibits the binding of angiotensin II to the receptor sites and acts as an antagonist of angiotensin II, lowering blood pressure. In the presence of low levels of circulating angiotensin II, Sarenin behaves as an agonist, raising the blood pressure.

The response to Sarenin is highly dependent on fluid and electrolyte status. Thus, in a normal person who is severely sodium depleted, maintenance of blood pressure can become angiotensin-dependent and Sarenin can cause a fall in blood pressure. On the other hand, in hypertensive patients with high levels of circulating angiotensin, the degree of angiotensin dependence can be decreased by excessive salt intake or increased by salt depletion. Moreover, since systemic vasoconstriction and plasma volume are interdependent, all antihypertensive medications may affect the Sarenin response.

THE USEFULNESS OF SARENIN AS A DIAGNOSTIC AGENT REQUIRES CAREFUL ATTENTION TO THE CONDITIONS OF ADMINISTRATION and the test procedure described under DOSAGE AND ADMINISTRATION should be followed carefully.

Sarenin has been studied in patients with hypertension as well as in non-hypertensive subjects. Among the persons tested, the following Sarenin-induced blood pressure responses have occurred:

1. Initial Transient Pressor Effect: Most patients tested have had a pressor response beginning within a minute after starting infusion, peaking in about 2 to 3 minutes and then evolving into one of the responses listed below. THE TRANSIENT RESPONSE IS IGNORED WITH RESPECT TO DIAGNOSTIC CRITERIA but has approached changes of 30 mm Hg systolic and 30 mm Hg diastolic in some patients. The transient pressor response may be related to Sarenin-induced release of catecholamines from the adrenal medulla or nerve endings or to the agonist effects of Sarenin on vascular smooth muscle.

2. Depressor Response: This response, which has lasted in some patients for up to 30 minutes following the discontinuance of Sarenin administration, is an indicator of blood-pressure dependence on angiotensin II. It results from competitive inhibition of angiotensin II, by Sarenin, at the level of the vascular receptor. Although it is most commonly observed in angiotensin II-dependent hypertensives, it has also been observed in some sodium-depleted normal subjects. A depressor response, although highly dependent upon past drug history and the sodium-balance of the patient, has been correlated with such variables as elevated peripheral vein renin, lateralizing renal vein renin, and the favorable clinical outcome of those patients who have undergone corrective surgery.

3. Pressor Response: Sarenin administration has caused a sustained increase of blood pressure, usually small, but as great as 40 mm Hg systolic and 40 mm Hg diastolic in some hypertensive patients. This response, which has lasted in some patients longer than 30 minutes following the discontinuance of Sarenin administration, is most likely to occur in patients with low circulating levels of angiotensin II but is not a reliable indicator of low-renin hypertension. The sustained pressor response may be attributed to Sarenin-induced release of catecholamines from the adrenal medulla or nerve endings or to the angonistic effects of Sarenin on vascular muscle.

4. Neutral Response: In other patients, Sarenin administration has elicited no sustained changes in blood pressure. The neutral response is suggestive of a noncontributory role for angiotensin II in blood pressure maintenance.

Sarenin is metabolized in the body by aminopeptidases. It has a mean plasma half-life of about 3 minutes, and a mean pharmacologic half-life of about 8 minutes, although its biological effects, once attained, have lasted longer than 30 minutes.

Indications and Usage: Sarenin is indicated for the detection of angiotensin II-dependent hypertension. It is intended to be used as one of several tests, such as peripheral plasma renin activity (PRA), intravenous pyelogram (IVP), renal arteriogram, and renal vein renin (RVR) tests to help detect a renal cause of hypertension. Like other tests of the renin-angiotensin system; the Sarenin test has a demonstrated error rate (false positive and false negative) and the test accuracy is highly dependent upon fluid and electrolyte status, use of antihypertensive drugs, and precise techniques of testing (see DOSAGE AND ADMINISTRATION). The use of Sarenin in conjunction with results of IVP and/or PRA determinations can aid in determining which patients might profit from more invasive procedures such as renal vein renins or renal arteriography.

There is agreement between the Sarenin test and other tests for renovascular hypertension when all are properly performed. The addition of Sarenin to the standard diagnostic regimen, however, reduces the false negative rate of the test battery as shown by the following bar graph. This summary, based on clinical studies of 90 patients with surgically-proven renovascular hypertension, shows the false negative rates of the Sarenin test (S), the peripheral plasma renin activity assay (PRA), the renal vein renin activity assay (RVR), and the intravenous pyelogram (IVP), alone and in combination.

[See table above].

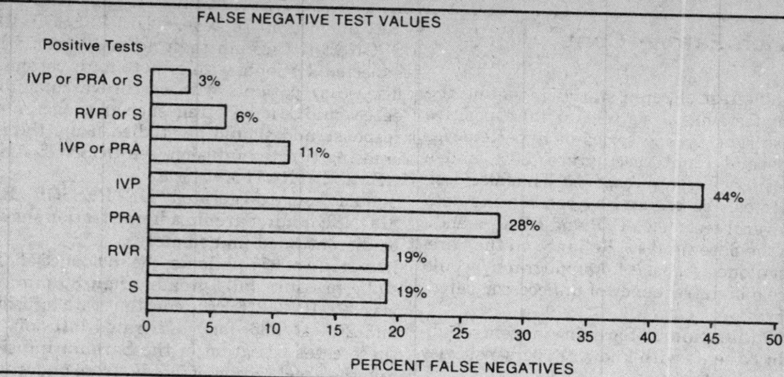

Addition of the Sarenin test thus reduces but does not eliminate the chance that renovascular hypertension will remain undetected by any test.

A negative Sarenin test in the face of a clinical history or physical findings suggesting renal artery disease or other renal disorders should not lead to termination of the search for a renal etiology of hypertension.

Continued on next page

Norwich Eaton—Cont.

Any single test of renin status, including the Sarenin test, has a significant false positive response rate. In one series of hypertensives with normal renal vasculature, 30% had a false positive Sarenin response. The false positive rate can be reduced by considering data from several tests (e.g., IVP and PRA, in addition to the Sarenin test). Reliance on the Sarenin test alone as a basis for angiography would produce a high frequency of unnecessary angiography.

Contraindications: Sarenin is contraindicated in patients with known hypersensitivity to the drug.

Warnings: *The PRESSOR and DEPRESSOR RESPONSES to Sarenin constitute its expected pharmacologic activity; exaggerated responses may occur, however, and can be precipitated by certain conditions, such as improper sodium depletion and concomitant drug therapy. Therefore, thorough review of the CONTRAINDICATIONS, WARNINGS, and PRECAUTIONS, and strict adherence to the procedure (see DOSAGE AND ADMINISTRATION) is advised. Sarenin testing should be undertaken in a hospital setting either on an inpatient or outpatient basis.*

It is desirable to stop all antihypertensive medication for one to two weeks prior to the Sarenin test in order to obtain a valid result, and potentially significant elevations in blood pressure may occur during this period. If necessary for blood pressure control, the use of a diuretic during the two-week pretest period is acceptable; but the likelihood of a false positive Sarenin test is enhanced under these conditions. The known rates of false positive and false negative tests were based on patients who had been taking no medications, including diuretics, for two weeks prior to Sarenin testing.

A. Hypertensive Effects:

1. Initial Transient Pressor Effect. An initial but transient pressor effect, which usually peaks within the first 2 to 3 minutes after the beginning of the Sarenin test and lasts about 5 minutes, has been observed in 90% of all patients. This effect should not be confused with the more sustained PRESSOR RESPONSE.

2. Exaggerated Pressor Response. This pressor response to Sarenin, in theory indicative of a low level of angiotensin II dependency, may be artifically induced or enhanced by factors which suppress peripheral renin activity, such as inadequate sodium depletion and certain antihypertensive drugs. In clinical trials on 877 patients, the incidence of sustained diastolic pressure rises greater than 20 mm Hg was 2% (7/342) for the constant rate infusion and 0.6% (3/535) for the titrated infusion. In patients in whom a PRESSOR RESPONSE may constitute a significant risk (particularly in those with grade III or grade IV retinopathy Keith-Wagener-Barker classification), the increasing titration infusion test method should be used. (See DOSAGE AND ADMINISTRATION).

3. Rebound Hypertension. In rare instances, patients who experience a marked DEPRESSOR RESPONSE or those with very severe hypertension may exhibit a rebound hypertension 1 to 3 hours after the test. Patients should be monitored at 15 minute intervals for at least 3 hours following cessation of the infusion. In cases of rebound hypertension which is characterized by blood pressures significantly above baseline levels, Sarenin may be reinstituted at the previously effective infusion level and then withdrawn very gradually. Usual therapy for hypertension should then be employed if necessary.

B. Hypotensive Effects:

Patients with a marked angiotensin II dependency, as well as those on antihypertensive therapy or who are markedly sodium-depleted, may have a more severe DEPRESSOR RESPONSE to Sarenin than normally would be expected. Patients with symptomatic coronary disease or patients with cerebrovascular disease would be at risk from such an exaggerated response and should be studied using the increasing titrated infusion (see DOSAGE AND ADMINISTRATION).

Should an exaggerated DEPRESSOR RESPONSE occur, Sarenin administration should be discontinued immediately.

In a group of 877 patients, the incidence of diastolic pressure falls greater than 30 mm Hg was 3% (10/342) for the constant rate infusion, and 2% (11/535) for the titrated infusion. In these cases cessation of the Sarenin infusion and the acceleration of 5% dextrose and water infusion successfully restored blood pressure.

Precautions: One case has been reported in which a patient with pheochromocytoma experienced a precipitous rise in blood pressure following Sarenin infusion.

The partial agonist effects of Sarenin on the renal vasculature may be reflected by a reduction in renal blood flow generally similar to that induced by increased physical activity or postural change.

Pregnancy Category B. Reproduction studies have been performed in rats and rabbits at doses up to 550 times the human dose and have revealed no evidence of harm to the fetus due to Sarenin. There are, however, no adequate and well-controlled studies in pregnant women. Because animal reproduction studies are not always predictive of human response, this drug should be used during pregnancy only if clearly needed.

Pediatric Use:

The Sarenin test has been administered to detect the renin-dependency of various forms of pediatric hypertension on 65 occasions in 60 patients ranging in age from 2½ years to 14 years. No serious adverse reactions to Sarenin occurred in these children although two patients complained of localized discomfort at the injection site, and a third developed anal pruritus. The conditions ceased following discontinuation of the drug. The Sarenin test appears to be safe for pediatric use, and, as in adults, there appears to be agreement between the Sarenin test and other tests for renovascular hypertension when all are properly performed.

Adverse Reactions:

Exaggerated depressor response (see WARNINGS)

Exaggerated pressor response (see WARNINGS)

Extrasystoles: In patients with pre-existing EKG abnormalities (either transient or persistent) occasional extrasystoles during Sarenin infusion have been reported. It is not known whether these were drug related, or, if so, were caused by the drug or the blood pressure change.

The following adverse reactions occurred in less than 10% of the patients:

Headache
Malaise
Nausea
Light-headedness
Local discomfort at injection site

Dosage and Administration: Patient Preparation: Thoroughly review the WARNINGS and PRECAUTIONS. Mildly deplete the patient of sodium by one of these means: 80 mg furosemide p.o. in the evening before the Sarenin test; or 40 mg furosemide i.v. 3 to 4 hours prior to the test; or a low sodium diet (10 mEq) for 3 to 5 days prior to the test. Withhold all antihypertensive medications (except diuretics when necessary) for at least one week and preferably 2 weeks prior to Sarenin testing. *Either inadequate or severe sodium depletion as well as concomitant antihypertensive medications may precipitate an exaggerated PRESSOR or DEPRESSOR RESPONSE. (See WARNINGS.)*

Procedure:

1. Keep the patient at rest in the supine position throughout the test, preferably in a quiet setting.
2. Begin an i.v. infusion of 5% dextrose in water at a rate sufficient to keep the vein open.
3. Begin monitoring blood pressure every 2 minutes, delaying Sarenin infusion until blood pressure is stable for at least four successive readings.
4. Continue monitoring and recording blood pressure at 2-minute intervals and begin Sarenin administration (preferably without alerting the patient) by one of the following methods (all calculations are based on the saralasin content, 18 mg per 30 ml, of the Sarenin (saralasin acetate) solution):

a. Constant Rate Infusion. Infuse 30 ml Sarenin via the i.v. line over a period of 20 to 30 minutes.

b. Increasing Titrated Infusion. *The increasing titrated infusion is particularly suited for those patients in whom an exaggerated PRESSOR or DEPRESSOR RESPONSE may constitute a significant risk. (See WARNINGS.)*

Infuse Sarenin via the i.v. line beginning at a rate of 0.05 micrograms saralasin per kilogram body weight per minute. If no response is noted after 10 to 15 minutes, the dosage should be increased at 10-minute intervals, according to the following recommended schedule, until either a PRESSOR or DEPRESSOR RESPONSE occurs or the maximum dose is achieved:

Beginning dose:
0.05 micrograms/kg/min.
5.0 micrograms/kg/min.
10.0 micrograms/kg/min.
20.0 micrograms/kg/min.

With either method, the infusion should be stopped if a sustained (more than 8 minutes) PRESSOR or DEPRESSOR RESPONSE is observed.

Continue to monitor and record blood pressure at 2-minute intervals throughout the infusion and for 15 minutes postinfusion or until the blood pressure returns to pretest level, WHICHEVER IS LONGER.

Patients who experience a marked DEPRESSOR RESPONSE, especially those with very severe hypertension and a history of hypertensive encephalopathy, may exhibit a rebound hypertension 1 to 3 hours after test. Therefore, patients of this nature should be monitored at 15-minute intervals for 3 hours following cessation of the infusion. (See WARNINGS.)

Sarenin should be prepared immediately before use. Any remaining product should be discarded upon completion of the test.

Parenteral drug products should be inspected visually for particulate matter and discoloration prior to administration whenever solution and container permit.

Definition of Sarenin Test Results: The response to a Sarenin test should be defined as either a:

1. DEPRESSOR RESPONSE
2. PRESSOR RESPONSE
3. NEUTRAL RESPONSE

The assessment of the Sarenin test response is based on the observed change in mean diastolic pressure calculated from blood pressure values recorded before and during Sarenin administration.

A. Control Pressure—the average of the last four diastolic pressure readings obtained just before the start of the Sarenin test.

B. Sarenin Pressure—that diastolic pressure which demonstrates the maximum sustained change from Control Pressure. The Sarenin Pressure is calculated as the average of the four consecutive diastolic blood pressures that differ most from Control Pressure. Outlier blood pressure readings should be excluded.

It is important that both the Control Pressure and Sarenin Pressure be based on four consecutive blood pressure readings, and that outlier values be excluded from the calculations.

Interpretation of Sarenin Test Results:
1. Depressor Response (probably high angiotensin II) is signified by a sustained decrease in diastolic pressure of at least 7 mm Hg. Those patients exhibiting a DEPRESSOR RESPONSE to a Sarenin test, along with other suggestive clinical features, should undergo further evaluation for a possible correctable renal cause of hypertension.
2. Pressor Response (probably low angiotensin II) is signified by an increase in diastolic pressure of at least 10 mm Hg. In theory, this response indicates low angiotensin II dependency, but in fact these responses give poor guidance as to whether the renin levels are low or normal.
3. Neutral Response is signified by a change in diastolic pressure which lies between the above two criteria (7 mm Hg decrease; 10 mm Hg increase).
A NEUTRAL or PRESSOR RESPONSE may not always exclude the diagnosis of angiotensin II dependency, especially when inadequate diuresis has failed to minimize the contribution of the volume factor to the hypertensive state. If a NEUTRAL or PRESSOR RESPONSE is attributed to inadequate diuresis, or if other observations continue to point toward renovascular hypertension, consideration should be given to repeating the Sarenin test after more vigorous diuretic preparation. (See CLINICAL PHARMACOLOGY and DOSAGE AND ADMINISTRATION.)
How Supplied: Sarenin is available as a sterile aqueous solution, supplied in ampuls of 30 ml containing saralasin acetate equivalent to 18 mg saralasin. The NDC number is 0149-0722-31.

Distributed by:
Norwich Eaton Pharmaceuticals, Inc.
Norwich, New York 13815
Manufactured by:
Sterling Drug, Inc.
New York, New York 10016
72231-P3

Parke-Davis
DIVISION OF WARNER-LAMBERT COMPANY
201 TABOR ROAD
MORRIS PLAINS, NEW JERSEY 07950

Parke-Davis
DIV WARNER-LAMBERT INC
SANTURCE, PR 00911

APLISOL® ℞
(tuberculin purified protein derivative, diluted [Stabilized Solution])

Description: Aplisol (tuberculin PPD, diluted) is an aqueous solution of a purified protein fraction isolated from culture filtrates of human-type strains of *Mycobacterium tuberculosis* by the method of F B Seibert. This product is made from a single master lot (No. 974777) to eliminate lot-to-lot variation inherent in manufacturing. The solution is stabilized with polysorbate (Tween) 80, buffered with potassium and sodium phosphates, and contains approximately 0.35% phenol as a preservative.
The product is clinically equivalent in potency to the standard PPD-S* (5 TU† per 0.1 ml) of the U S Public Health Service, National Center for Disease Control, and is ready for immediate use without further dilution. The 5-TU dose of tuberculin PPD intradermally (Mantoux) is recommended as the standard tuberculin test, and tuberculin PPD is recommended by the American Lung Association as an aid in the detection of infection with *Mycobacterium tuberculosis.* Reactions to the Mantoux test are interpreted on the basis of a quantitative measurement of the response to a specific dose (5 TU PPD-S or equivalent) of tuberculin PPD. Other dosages are regarded as having no demonstrable usefulness in ordinary practice. Accordingly, Aplisol is available in only one potency (5 TU equivalent) and the use of this potency only is recommended. The selection of 5 TU as the test dose is based upon data indicating that (1) the 5-TU dose gives measurable reactions in over 95 percent of the known tuberculous infected; (2) doses larger than 5 TU might elicit reactions not caused by tuberculous infection; and (3) nonreactors to doses considerably less than 5 TU are not accepted as negative but are retested with a stronger dose.
This product meets all applicable standards.
Indications: Tuberculin PPD is recommended by the American Lung Association as an aid in the detection of infection with *Mycobacterium tuberculosis.* The standard tuberculin test recommended employs the intradermal (Mantoux) test using a 5-TU dose of tuberculin PPD. The 0.1-ml test dose of Aplisol (tuberculin PPD, diluted) is equivalent to the 5-TU dose recommended as clinically established and standardized with PPD-S.
Warnings: Tuberculin should not be administered to known tuberculin-positive reactors because of the severity of reactions (eg, vesiculation, ulceration, or necrosis) that may occur at the test site in very highly sensitive individuals.
Avoid injecting tuberculin subcutaneously. If this occurs, no local reaction develops, but a general febrile reaction and/or acute inflammation around old tuberculous lesions may occur in highly sensitive individuals.
Precautions: A separate, heat-sterilized syringe and needle, or a sterile, disposable unit should be used for each individual patient to prevent possible transmission of homologous serum hepatitis virus and other infectious agents from one person to another.
Syringes that have previously been used with histoplasmin, blastomycin, and other antigens should not be used for tuberculin.
As with any biological product, epinephrine should be immediately available in case an anaphylactoid or acute hypersensitivity reaction occurs.
Adverse Reactions: In highly sensitive individuals, strongly positive reactions including vesiculation, ulceration, or necrosis may occur at the test site. Cold packs or topical steroid preparations may be employed for symptomatic relief of the associated pain, pruritus, and discomfort.
Strongly positive test reactions may result in scarring at the test site.
Dosage and Administration:
Standard Method (Mantoux Test)
The Mantoux test is performed by intradermally injecting with a syringe and needle exactly 0.1 ml of tuberculin PPD, diluted. The result is read 48 to 72 hours later and induration only is considered in interpreting the test. The standard test is performed as follows.

1. The site of the test is usually the flexor or dorsal surface of the forearm about 4 inches below the elbow. Other skin sites may be used, but the flexor surface of the forearm is preferred.
2. The skin at the injection site is cleansed with 70% alcohol and allowed to dry.
3. The test material is administered with a tuberculin syringe (0.5 or 1.0 ml) fitted with a short (½ inch) 26- or 27-gauge needle.
4. The syringe and needle should be of a sterile, disposable, single-use type or should have been sterilized by autoclaving, boiling, or by the use of dry heat. A separate, sterile unit should be used for each person tested.
5. The diaphragm of the vial stopper should be wiped with 70% alcohol.
6. The needle is inserted through the stopper diaphragm of the inverted vial. Exactly 0.1 ml is filled into the syringe, with care being taken to exclude air bubbles and to maintain the lumen of the needle filled.
7. The point of the needle is inserted into the most superficial layers of the skin with the needle bevel pointing upward. As the tuberculin solution is injected, a pale bleb 6 to 10 mm in size (⅜ inch) will rise over the point of the needle. This is quickly absorbed and no dressing is required.

In the event the injection is delivered subcutaneously (ie, no bleb will form), or if a significant part of the dose leaks from the injection site, the test should be repeated immediately at another site at least 5 cm (2 inches) removed.
The Mantoux test is the standard of comparison for all other tuberculin tests.
Aplisol is a stabilized solution of tuberculin PPD. Data indicate that Aplisol is stable when prefilled into syringes and stored in a refrigerator for up to 30 days.
However, the practice of storing such prefilled syringes is not recommended as good practice because of the increased potential for contamination.
Interpretation of Tuberculin Reaction
Readings of Mantoux reactions should be made during the period from 48 to 72 hours after the injection. Induration only should be considered in interpreting the test. The diameter of induration should be measured transversely to the long axis of the forearm and recorded in millimeters. Erythema of less than 10 mm should be disregarded. If the area of erythema is greater than 10 mm and induration is absent, the injection may have been made too deeply and retesting is indicated.
Reactions should be interpreted as follows.
Positive—Induration measuring 10 mm or more. This indicates hypersensitivity to tuberculoprotein and should be interpreted as positive for past or present infection with *M tuberculosis.*
Doubtful—Induration measuring 5 to 9 mm. Retesting is indicated using a different site of injection. Evaluation to rule out cross-reaction from other mycobacterial infection should be considered.
Negative—Induration of less than 5 mm. This indicates a lack of hypersensitivity to tuberculoprotein and tuberculosis infection is highly unlikely.
It should be noted that reactivity to tuberculin may be depressed or suppressed for as long as four weeks by viral infections, live virus vaccines (ie, measles, smallpox, polio, rubella, and mumps), or by the administration of corticosteroids. Malnutrition may also have a similar effect. When of diagnostic importance, a negative test should be accepted as proof that hypersensitivity is absent only after normal reactivity to nonspecific irritants has been demonstrated.
A child who is known to have been exposed to a tuberculous adult must not be adjudged free of infection until he has a negative tuberculin reaction at least 10 weeks after contact with the tuberculous person has ceased.
A positive tuberculin reaction does not necessarily signify the presence of active disease. Further diagnostic procedures should be carried out before a diagnosis of tuberculosis is made.
How Supplied:
N 0071-4525-03 (Bio 1525)
1 ml (10 tests)—rubber
diaphragm-capped vial

Continued on next page

This product information was prepared in October, 1982. On these and other Parke-Davis Products, information may be obtained by addressing PARKE-DAVIS, Division of Warner-Lambert Company, Morris Plains, New Jersey 07950.

Parke-Davis—Cont.

N 0071-4525-08 (Bio 1607)
5 ml (50 tests)—rubber diaphragm-capped vial
This product should be stored at 2 to 8 C (36 to 46 F), and protected from light.
AHFS 36:84 **4525 G030**
121 876100/ZF

*PPD-S (No. 49608) World Health Organization International PPD-Tuberculin Standard (PPD-S is a dried powder from which WHO and U S Standard tuberculin solutions are made.)
†U S Tuberculin Unit

APLITEST® ℞
(tuberculin purified protein derivative)
Multiple-Puncture Device

Description: Aplitest (tuberculin PPD) is a sterile, single-use, multiple-puncture type device for use in determining the tuberculin sensitivity status of individuals. These convenient, disposable devices are especially useful in mass tuberculosis screening programs. The product packaging also facilitates the use of Aplitest units for testing of individual patients in office, ward, or clinic settings.
Each Aplitest unit consists of a cylindrical plastic holder bearing four equally spaced stainless steel tines at one end. The tines have been coated by dipping in a solution of tuberculin PPD and dried.
These devices are designed so that the narrow (tine-bearing) end of each unit fits into the hollow, handle portion of the adjacent unit (or into a protective cap) to protect the tines and maintain their sterility.
The purified tuberculin protein fraction is isolated from culture filtrates of human-type strains of *Mycobacterium tuberculosis* by the method of Florence B Seibert. Purified tuberculin protein solution is prepared from a single master lot (No. 975302) to eliminate lot-to-lot variation.
The tuberculin solution which is applied to the tines is buffered with potassium and sodium phosphates and contains approximately 0.5% phenol as a preservative.
Tuberculin PPD is employed as the diagnostic reagent because, in studies by Parke-Davis, it was demonstrated to offer greater negative and overall test agreement with the Mantoux tests than did Old Tuberculin. In clinical trials comparing multiple-puncture devices with Old Tuberculin-coated tines to those coated with tuberculin PPD, the Old Tuberculin devices engendered a significantly greater incidence of false-positive reactions than did the tuberculin PPD devices.
Aplitest has been standardized by clinical studies in human subjects against 5 TU* of PPD-S administered intradermally by the Mantoux test and guidelines relating response to the two treatments have been formulated. (See Interpretation of Response section.)
The incidence of false-positive reactions engendered by Aplitest is significantly reduced relative to the rate associated with the OT-coated tine. However, all multiple-puncture type devices should be regarded as screening tools and appropriate diagnostic procedures (eg, Mantoux test with tuberculin PPD diluted, Aplisol®), should be employed for retesting "doubtful" reactors.
Indications: Aplitest is indicated to detect tuberculin-sensitive individuals. Aplitest units are also useful in programs to establish priorities for additional testing (ie, chest x-rays) and in epidemiological surveys to identify areas with high levels of infection.
Regular periodic (annual) testing of tuberculin-negative persons is recommended and is especially valuable because the conversion of an individual from negative to positive is highly indicative of recent tuberculosis infection. Repeated testing of the uninfected individual does not sensitize to tuberculin. In persons with waning sensitivity to homologous or heterologous mycobacterial antigens, however, the stimulus of a tuberculin test may boost or increase the size of reaction to a second test, even causing an apparent development of sensitivity in some instances.
Warning: Tuberculin should not be administered to known tuberculin-positive reactors because of the severity of reactions (eg, vesiculation, ulceration, or necrosis) that may occur at the test site in very highly sensitive individuals.
Precautions: A separate, sterile unit must be used for each individual patient and disposed of after use.
As with any biological product, epinephrine should be immediately available in case an anaphylactoid or acute hypersensitivity reaction occurs.
Sensitivity may decrease or disappear temporarily during or immediately following severe febrile illness, measles, and other exanthemas, live virus vaccination, sarcoidosis, overwhelming miliary or pulmonary tuberculosis, and the administration of corticosteroids or immunosuppressive drugs. Severe malnutrition may also have a similar effect.
A positive tuberculin reaction does not necessarily signify the presence of active disease. Further diagnostic procedures should be carried out before a diagnosis of tuberculosis is made.
Adverse Reactions: In highly sensitive individuals, strongly positive reactions including vesiculation, ulceration, or necrosis may occur at the test site. Cold packs or topical steroid preparations may be employed for symptomatic relief of the associated pain, pruritus, and discomfort.
Strongly positive test reactions may result in scarring at the test site.
Minimal bleeding may be experienced at a puncture site. This occurs infrequently and does not affect the interpretation of the test.
Dosage and Administration: Each Aplitest unit provides for the intradermal administration of one test-dose of tuberculin PPD.
Method of Application
1. The preferred site of the test is the flexor surface of the forearm about 4 inches below the elbow. Other suitable skin sites, such as the dorsal surface of the forearm, may be used. Areas without adequate subcutaneous tissue, such as over a tendon, should be avoided.
2. The skin at the test site should be cleansed with 70% alcohol, or other suitable agents, and allowed to dry thoroughly.
3. To expose the four impregnated tines, grasp the device (top one if stacked) and twist to break the perforated label seal. To prevent loss of sterility of the other units in a stack, the top unit must always be removed first and the remaining ones in sequence. Care should be taken to avoid breaking the seals on the remaining units when the end unit is removed.
4. Grasp the patient's forearm firmly to stretch the skin taut at the test site and to prevent any jerking motion of the arm that could cause scratching with the tines.
5. Apply the Aplitest unit firmly and without twisting to the test area for approximately one second. Sufficient pressure should be exerted to assure that all four tines have penetrated the skin of the test area.
6. Dispose of used units in a manner to avoid accidents. Do not re-use.
Interpretation of Response: Reading of reactions should be made during the period from 48 to 72 hours after application of Aplitest and should be conducted under good lighting conditions. Induration only should be considered in interpreting the test. Erythema should be disregarded. The diameter of the induration of the greatest response at any of the four puncture points should be determined by visual inspection and palpation. If there is coalescence of reaction, the largest diameter of coalescent induration should be measured and recorded.
The American Thoracic Society recommends that responses to all multiple-puncture tuberculin skin test devices be interpreted as follows. If vesiculation is present, the test may be interpreted as positive. If vesiculation is not present, induration of 2 mm or more is considered as a doubtful reaction and should be confirmed by Mantoux testing. Induration of less than 2 mm and/or erythema of any size is a negative test and there is no need for re-testing.
In clinical studies with Aplitest, it has been determined that coalescence of the induration around two or more puncture sites corresponds more than 90% of the time to 10 mm or more of induration in the same individual tested by Mantoux at the 5-TU level with PPD-S.†
Thus, the following criteria of interpretation have been established.
Vesiculation—Positive Reaction
The test should be interpreted as positive and the management of the subject is the same as that for one classified as positive by Mantoux test.
Coalescence of induration from two or more puncture points—Doubtful Reaction
A subject with a coalescent reaction may be considered for Mantoux retest.
However, more than 90% of the time this reaction was equivalent to a reaction of 10 mm or more of induration with PPD-S (5 TU) administered by Mantoux test. Other criteria, such as contact with tuberculosis patients and case history, should be considered to determine the likelihood that such a reaction is considered positive.
2 mm or more of induration without coalescence—Doubtful Reaction
Reactions of this size range reflect sensitivity that can result from infection with either atypical mycobacteria or *M tuberculosis;* hence, they are classified as doubtful.
A standard Mantoux test should be done on all subjects in this group. Management should be based on the reaction to the Mantoux test, as well as other clinical considerations.
Less than 2 mm of induration—Negative Reaction
There is no need for retesting unless the individual is in contact with a case of tuberculosis or there is clinical evidence suggestive of the disease.
Selection of the appropriate criteria for interpretation of response to the tuberculin PPD Aplitest should be made in accordance with the objectives of the specific testing program and with consideration of the history and clinical status of the individuals.
How Supplied:
N 0071-4589-13 (Bio 1589) 25-test package, five stacks of five Aplitest units
Aplitest (tuberculin PPD, multiple-puncture device) units should be stored at no warmer than 30 C (86 F).
AHFS 36:84 **ZD**

*US (International) Tuberculin Units

†Purified Protein Derivative (Seibert). Lot No. 49608, the standard adopted by the World Health Organization in 1952 as International PPD Tuberculin and used to prepare the official US Public Health Service 5-TU solution of tuberculin for skin testing known as PPD-S.

Products are
listed alphabetically in the
PINK SECTION.

Roche Laboratories
Division of Hoffmann-La Roche Inc.
NUTLEY, NJ 07110

TENSILON®
(edrophonium chloride/Roche) ℞
Injectable Solution
ampuls • vials

The following text is complete prescribing information based on official labeling in effect August 1, 1982.

Description: Tensilon is a short and rapid-acting cholinergic drug. Chemically, edrophonium chloride is ethyl (*m*-hydroxyphenyl)-dimethylammonium chloride.

10-ml vials: Each ml contains, in a sterile solution, 10 mg edrophonium chloride/Roche compounded with 0.45% phenol and 0.2% sodium sulfite as preservatives, buffered with sodium citrate and citric acid, and pH adjusted to approximately 5.4.

1-ml ampuls: Each ml contains, in a sterile solution, 10 mg edrophonium chloride/Roche compounded with 0.2% sodium sulfite, buffered with sodium citrate and citric acid, and pH adjusted to approximately 5.4.

Actions: Tensilon is an anticholinesterase drug. Its pharmacological action is due primarily to the inhibition or inactivation of acetylcholinesterase at sites of cholinergic transmission. Its effect is manifest within 30 to 60 seconds after injection and lasts an average of 10 minutes.

Indications: Tensilon is recommended for the differential diagnosis of myasthenia gravis and as an adjunct in the evaluation of treatment requirements in this disease. It may also be used for evaluating emergency treatment in myasthenic crises. Because of its brief duration of action, it is not recommended for maintenance therapy in myasthenia gravis.

Tensilon is also useful whenever a curare antagonist is needed to reverse the neuromuscular block produced by curare, tubocurarine, gallamine triethiodide or dimethyl-tubocurarine. It is *not* effective against decamethonium bromide and succinylcholine chloride. It may be used adjunctively in the treatment of respiratory depression caused by curare overdosage.

Contraindications: Known hypersensitivity to anticholinesterase agents; intestinal and urinary obstructions of mechanical type.

Warnings: Whenever anticholinesterase drugs are used for testing, a syringe containing 1 mg of atropine sulfate should be immediately available to be given in aliquots intravenously to counteract severe cholinergic reactions which may occur in the hypersensitive individual, whether he is normal or myasthenic. Tensilon should be used with caution in patients with bronchial asthma or cardiac dysrhythmias. The transient bradycardia which sometimes occurs can be relieved by atropine sulfate. Isolated instances of cardiac and respiratory arrest following administration of Tensilon have been reported. It is postulated that these are vagotonic effects.

Usage in Pregnancy: The safety of Tensilon during pregnancy or lactation in humans has not been established. Therefore, use of Tensilon in women who may become pregnant requires weighing the drug's potential benefits against its possible hazards to mother and child.

Precautions: Patients may develop "anticholinesterase insensitivity" for brief or prolonged periods. During these periods the patients should be carefully monitored and may need respiratory assistance. Dosages of anticholinesterase drugs should be reduced or withheld until patients again become sensitive to them.

Adverse Reactions: Careful observation should be made for severe cholinergic reactions in the hyperreactive individual. The myasthenic patient in crisis who is being tested with Tensilon should be observed for bradycardia or cardiac standstill and cholinergic reactions if an overdose is given. The following reactions common to anticholinesterase agents may occur, although not all of these reactions have been reported with the administration of Tensilon, probably because of its short duration of action and limited indications: **Eye:** Increased lacrimation, pupillary constriction, spasm of accommodation, diplopia, conjunctival hyperemia. **CNS:** Convulsions, dysarthria, dysphonia, dysphagia. **Respiratory:** Increased tracheobronchial secretions, laryngospasm, bronchiolar constriction, paralysis of muscles of respiration, central respiratory paralysis. **Cardiac:** Arrhythmias (especially bradycardia), fall in cardiac output leading to hypotension. **G.I.:** Increased salivary, gastric and intestinal secretion, nausea, vomiting, increased peristalsis, diarrhea, abdominal cramps. **Skeletal Muscle:** Weakness, fasciculations. **Miscellaneous:** Increased urinary frequency and incontinence, diaphoresis.

Dosage and Administration: *Tensilon Test in the Differential Diagnosis of Myasthenia Gravis:*[1-8]

Intravenous Dosage (Adults): A tuberculin syringe containing 1 ml (10 mg) of Tensilon is prepared with an intravenous needle, and 0.2 ml (2 mg) is injected intravenously within 15 to 30 seconds. The needle is left *in situ. Only* if no reaction occurs after 45 seconds is the remaining 0.8 ml (8 mg) injected. If a cholinergic reaction (muscarinic side effects, skeletal muscle fasciculations and increased muscle weakness) occurs after injection of 0.2 ml (2 mg), the test is discontinued and atropine sulfate 0.4 mg to 0.5 mg is administered intravenously. After one-half hour the test may be repeated.

Intramuscular Dosage (Adults): In adults with inaccessible veins, dosage for intramuscular injection is 1 ml (10 mg) of Tensilon. Subjects who demonstrate hyperreactivity to this injection (cholinergic reaction), should be retested after one-half hour with 0.2 ml (2 mg) of Tensilon intramuscularly to rule out false-negative reactions.

Dosage (Children): The intravenous testing dose of Tensilon in children weighing up to 75 lbs is 0.1 ml (1 mg); above this weight, the dose is 0.2 ml (2 mg). If there is no response after 45 seconds, it may be titrated up to 0.5 ml (5 mg) in children under 75 lbs, given in increments of 0.1 ml (1 mg) every 30 to 45 seconds and up to 1 ml (10 mg) in heavier children. In infants, the recommended dose is 0.05 ml (0.5 mg). Because of technical difficulty with intravenous injection in children, the intramuscular route may be used. In children weighing up to 75 lbs, 0.2 ml (2 mg) is injected intramuscularly. In children weighing more than 75 lbs, 0.5 ml (5 mg) is injected intramuscularly. All signs which would appear with the intravenous test appear with the intramuscular test except that there is a delay of two to ten minutes before a reaction is noted.

Tensilon Test for Evaluation of Treatment Requirements in Myasthenia Gravis: The recommended dose is 0.1 ml to 0.2 ml (1 mg to 2 mg) of Tensilon, administered intravenously one hour after oral intake of the drug being used in treatment.[1-5] Response will be myasthenic in the undertreated patient, adequate in the controlled patient, and cholinergic in the overtreated patient. Responses to Tensilon in myasthenic and nonmyasthenic individuals are summarized in the accompanying chart.[2]

Responses to Tensilon in Myasthenic and Nonmyasthenic Individuals

	Myasthenic*	Adequate**	Cholinergic***
Muscle Strength . . . (ptosis, diplopia, dysphonia, dysphagia, dysarthria, respiration, limb strength)	Increased	No change	Decreased
Fasciculations . . . (orbicularis oculi, facial muscles, limb muscles)	Absent	Present or absent	Present or absent
Side reactions . . . (lacrimation, diaphoresis, salivation, abdominal cramps, nausea, vomiting, diarrhea)	Absent	Minimal	Severe

*Myasthenic Response—occurs in untreated myasthenics and may serve to establish diagnosis; in patients under treatment, indicates that therapy is inadequate.
**Adequate Response—observed in treated patients when therapy is stabilized; a typical response in normal individuals. In addition to this response in nonmyasthenics, the phenomenon of forced lid closure is often observed in psychoneurotics.[1]
***Cholinergic Response—seen in myasthenics who have been overtreated with anticholinesterase drugs.

Tensilon Test in Crisis: The term *crisis* is applied to the myasthenic whenever severe respiratory distress with objective ventilatory inadequacy occurs and the response to medication is not predictable. This state may be secondary to a sudden increase in severity of myasthenia gravis (myasthenic crisis), or to overtreatment with anticholinesterase drugs (cholinergic crisis).

When a patient is apneic, controlled ventilation must be secured immediately in order to avoid cardiac arrest and irreversible central nervous system damage. No attempt is made to test with Tensilon until respiratory exchange is adequate. *Dosage used at this time is most important:* If the patient is cholinergic, Tensilon will cause increased oropharyngeal secretions and further weakness in the muscles of respiration. If the crisis is myasthenic, the test clearly improves respiration and the patient can be treated with longer-acting intravenous anticholinesterase medication. When the test is performed, there should not be more than 0.2 ml (2 mg) Tensilon in the syringe. An intravenous dose of 0.1 ml (1 mg) is given initially. The patient's heart action is carefully observed. If, after an interval of one minute, this dose does not further impair the patient, the remaining 0.1 ml (1 mg) can be injected. If no clear improvement of respiration occurs after 0.2 ml (2 mg) dose, it is usually wisest to discontinue all anticholinesterase drug therapy and secure controlled ventilation by tracheostomy with assisted respiration.[5]

For Use as a Curare Antagonist: Tensilon should be administered by intravenous injection in 1 ml (10 mg) doses given slowly over a period of 30 to 45 seconds so that the onset of cholinergic reaction can be detected. This dosage may be repeated whenever necessary. The maximal dose for any one patient should be 4 ml (40 mg). Because of its brief effect, Tensilon should not be given prior to the administration of curare, tubocurarine, gallamine triethiodide or dimethyl-tubocurarine; it should be used at the time when its effect is needed. When given to counteract curare overdosage, the effect of each dose on the respiration should be carefully observed before it is repeated, and assisted ventilation should always be employed.

Drug Interactions: Care should be given when administering this drug to patients with symptoms of myasthenic weakness who are

Continued on next page

Roche—Cont.

also on anticholinesterase drugs. Since symptoms of anticholinesterase overdose (cholinergic crisis) may mimic underdosage (myasthenic weakness), their condition may be worsened by the use of this drug. (See OVERDOSAGE section for treatment.)

Overdosage: With drugs of this type, muscarine-like symptoms (nausea, vomiting, diarrhea, sweating, increased bronchial and salivary secretions and bradycardia) often appear with overdosage (cholinergic crisis). An important complication that can arise is obstruction of the airway by bronchial secretions. These may be managed with suction (especially if tracheostomy has been performed) and by the use of atropine. Many experts have advocated a wide range of dosages of atropine *(for Tensilon, see atropine dosage below)*, but if there are copious secretions, up to 1.2 mg intravenously may be given initially and repeated every 20 minutes until secretions are controlled. Signs of atropine overdosage such as dry mouth, flush and tachycardia should be avoided as tenacious secretions and bronchial plugs may form. A total dose of atropine of 5 to 10 mg or even more may be required. The following steps should be taken in the management of overdosage of Tensilon:

1. Adequate respiratory exchange should be maintained by assuring an open airway, and the use of assisted respiration augmented by oxygen.
2. Cardiac function should be monitored until complete stabilization has been achieved.
3. Atropine sulfate in doses of 0.4 to 0.5 mg should be administered intravenously. This may be repeated every 3 to 10 minutes. Because of the short duration of action of Tensilon the total dose required will seldom exceed 2 mg.
4. Pralidoxime chloride (a cholinesterase reactivator) may be given intravenously at the rate of 50 to 100 mg per minute; usually the total dose does not exceed 1000 mg. Extreme caution should be exercised in the use of pralidoxime chloride when the cholinergic symptoms are induced by double-bond phosphorous anticholinesterase drugs.[9]
5. If convulsions or shock is present, appropriate measures should be instituted.

How Supplied: *Multiple Dose Vials,* 10 ml. *Ampuls,* 1 ml, boxes of 10.

References:

1. Osserman, K.E. and Kaplan, L.I., *J.A.M.A., 150:*265, 1952.
2. Osserman, K.E., Kaplan, L.I. and Besson, G., *J. Mt. Sinai Hosp., 20:*165, 1953.
3. Osserman, K.E. and Kaplan, L.I., *Arch. Neurol. & Psychiat., 70:*385, 1953.
4. Osserman, K.E. and Teng, P., *J.A.M.A., 160:*153, 1956.
5. Osserman, K.E. and Genkins, G., *Ann. N.Y. Acad. Sci., 135:*312, 1966.
6. Tether, J.E., Second International Symposium Proceedings, Myasthenia Gravis, 1961, p. 444.
7. Tether, J.E., in H.F. Conn: *Current Therapy 1960,* Philadelphia, W. B. Saunders Company, p. 551.
8. Tether, J.E., in H.F. Conn: *Current Therapy 1965,* Philadelphia, W. B. Saunders Company, p. 556.
9. Grob, D. and Johns, R.J., *J.A.M.A., 166:*1855, 1958.

Products are cross-indexed by generic and chemical names in the **YELLOW SECTION**

Sclavo Inc.

5 MANSARD COURT
WAYNE, NJ 07470

SclavoTest®–PPD ℞

Tuberculin Purified Protein Derivative (PPD) Multiple Puncture Device

Composition/Description: SclavoTest-PPD is a sterile multiple-puncture device containing a tuberculin PPD used for the identification of individuals who have a delayed hypersensitivity to tuberculin. SclavoTest-PPD is an easy-to-use, self-contained, unit-dose disposable system which minimizes waste and can be stored at room temperature. No needles, syringes, or vials are needed.

The SclavoTest-PPD device is composed of a plastic handle with four sharp stainless steel points to which has been affixed and dried a tuberculin PPD solution. The retracted points are projected, after the device is placed upon the skin, by gentle pressure applied through a spring inside the handle. SclavoTest-PPD is stored at room temperature until the moment of use in a hermetically sealed unit-dose blister pack, which is designed to impede the passage of moisture and maintain sterility.

Adverse Reactions: Vesiculation, occasionally necrosis, ulceration.

How Supplied: 1, 20 or 250 units individually blister-sealed in strips of 1.

E.R. Squibb & Sons, Inc.

GENERAL OFFICES
P.O. BOX 4000
PRINCETON, NJ 08540

CARDIOGRAFIN® ℞

(Diatrizoate Meglumine Injection USP 85%)

Description: Cardiografin is a radiopaque contrast agent for use in roentgenography of the heart and major vessels, including the aorta. It is supplied as a sterile, aqueous solution for intravascular administration. Each ml. provides 850 mg. diatrizoate meglumine, 3.2 mg. sodium citrate as a buffer and 0.4 mg. edetate disodium as a sequestering agent. *Each ml. of solution also contains approximately 0.91 mg. (0.04 mEq.) sodium (45.5 mg./50 ml.)* and 400 mg. (20 g./50 ml.) organically bound iodine. At the time of manufacture, the air in the container is replaced by nitrogen.

Actions: Following introduction into a vessel or directly into the heart, diatrizoate meglumine is rapidly diffused through the vascular system and is excreted by the kidneys. As the contrast medium enters the cardiac chambers, the vessels and the aorta, lesions or malformations of the heart and obstruction or anomalies of the major thoracic vessels are visualized.

Indications: Cardiografin (Diatrizoate Meglumine Injection USP 85%) is indicated for adult angiocardiography and thoracic aortography.

Contraindications: This preparation is contraindicated in patients with a hypersensitivity to salts of diatrizoic acid or with advanced uremia.

Warnings: A definite risk exists in the use of intravascular contrast agents in patients who are known to have multiple myeloma. In such instances there has been anuria resulting in progressive uremia, renal failure, and eventually death. Although neither the contrast agent nor dehydration has separately proved to be the cause of anuria in myeloma, it has been speculated that the combination of both may be the causative factor. The risk in myelomatous patients is not a contraindication to the procedures; however, partial dehydration in the preparation of these patients for the examination is not recommended since this may predispose for the precipitation of myeloma protein in the renal tubules. No form of therapy, including dialysis, has been successful in reversing this effect. Myeloma, which occurs most commonly in persons over age 40, should be considered before instituting intravascular administration of contrast agents.

Administration of radiopaque materials to patients known or suspected to have pheochromocytoma should be performed with extreme caution. If, in the opinion of the physician, the possible benefits of such procedures outweigh the considered risks, the procedures may be performed; however, the amount of radiopaque medium injected should be kept to an absolute minimum. The blood pressure should be assessed throughout the procedure and measures for treatment of a hypertensive crisis should be available.

The inherent risks of *angiocardiography* in patients with chronic pulmonary emphysema must be weighed against the necessity for performing the procedure.

Contrast media have been shown to promote the phenomenon of sickling in individuals who are homozygous for sickle cell disease when the material is injected intravenously or intra-arterially.

Since iodine-containing contrast agents may alter the results of thyroid function tests, such tests, if indicated, should be performed prior to the administration of this preparation.

A history of sensitivity to iodine *per se* or to contrast media other than salts of diatrizoic acid is not an absolute contraindication to the use of diatrizoate meglumine, but calls for extreme caution in administration.

Precautions: Diagnostic procedures which involve the use of radiopaque contrast agents should be carried out under the direction of personnel with the prerequisite training and with a thorough knowledge of the particular procedure to be performed (see ADVERSE REACTIONS).

Severe, life-threatening reactions suggest hypersensitivity to the radiopaque agent, which has prompted the use of several pretesting methods, none of which can be relied upon to predict severe reactions. Many authorities question the value of any pretest. A history of bronchial asthma or allergy, a family history of allergy, or a previous reaction to a contrast agent warrant special attention. Such a history, by suggesting histamine sensitivity and a consequent proneness to reactions, may be more accurate than pretesting in predicting the likelihood of a reaction, although not necessarily the severity or type of reaction in the individual case.

The sensitivity test most often performed is the slow injection of 0.5 to 1.0 ml. of the radiopaque medium, administered intravenously, prior to injection of the full diagnostic dose. It should be noted that the absence of a reaction to the test dose does not preclude the possibility of a reaction to the full diagnostic dose. If the test dose causes an untoward response of any kind, the necessity for continuing with the examination should be carefully reevaluated and, if it is deemed essential, the examination should be conducted with all possible caution. In rare instances, reactions to the test dose itself may be extremely severe; therefore, close observation of the patient and facilities for emergency treatment appear indicated.

Renal toxicity has been reported in a few patients with liver dysfunction who were given oral cholecystographic agents followed by intravascular contrast agents. Administration of Cardiografin (Diatrizoate Meglumine Injection USP 85%) should therefore be postponed in any patient with a known or suspected hepatic or biliary disorder who has recently taken a cholecystographic contrast agent.

Caution should be exercised with the use of radiopaque media in severely debilitated pa-

tients, in those with marked hypertension, and in cases of congestive heart failure.
When any percutaneous technique is employed the possibility of thrombosis or of other complications due to the mechanical trauma of the procedure should be borne in mind.
Consideration must be given to the functional ability of the kidneys before injecting this preparation. Decreased excretion of the contrast material due to impaired renal function increases the possibility of renal damage or other adverse reactions. Combined renal and hepatic disease present an additional hazard.
Acute renal failure has been reported with the use of contrast agents in patients with diabetic nephropathy and susceptible nondiabetic patients (often elderly with preexisting renal disease).
Contrast agents may interfere with some chemical determinations made on urine specimens; therefore, urine should be collected before administration of the contrast medium or two or three days afterwards.
Repeated intra-aortic injections may be hazardous.
Usage in Pregnancy: The safety of diatrizoate meglumine for use during pregnancy has not been established with respect to adverse effects upon fetal development; therefore, this preparation should be used in pregnant patients only when, in the judgment of the physician, its use is deemed essential to the welfare of the patient.
Adverse Reactions: Adverse reactions accompanying the use of iodine-containing intravascular contrast agents are usually mild and transient although severe and life-threatening reactions, including fatalities, have occurred. Because of the possibility of severe reactions to the procedure and/or the radiopaque medium, appropriate emergency facilities and well-trained personnel should be available to treat both conditions. Emergency facilities and personnel should remain available for 30 to 60 minutes following the procedure since severe delayed reactions have been known to occur.
Nausea, vomiting, flushing, or a generalized feeling of warmth are the reactions seen most frequently with intravascular injection. Symptoms which may occur are chills, fever, sweating, headache, dizziness, pallor, weakness, severe retching and choking, wheezing, a rise or fall in blood pressure, ventricular fibrillation, cardiac arrest, facial or conjunctival petechiae, urticaria, pruritus, rash and other eruptions, edema, cramps, tremors, itching, sneezing, lacrimation, etc. Antihistaminic agents may be of benefit; rarely such reactions may be severe enough to require discontinuation of dosage. Pulmonary edema, spasm, seizures, hemiparesis, and impairment of vision have occurred with parenteral injection of diatrizoates.
Severe reactions which may require emergency measures may take the form of a cardiovascular reaction characterized by peripheral vasodilatation with resultant hypotension and reflex tachycardia, apnea, dyspnea, agitation, confusion, and cyanosis progressing to unconsciousness. Or, the histamine-liberating effect of these compounds may induce an allergic-like reaction which may range in severity from rhinitis or angioneurotic edema to laryngeal or bronchial spasm or anaphylactoid shock.
Temporary renal shutdown or other nephropathy may occur.
Although local tissue tolerance is usually good, there have been a few reports of a burning or stinging sensation or numbness and of venospasm or venous pain, and partial collapse of the injected vein. Neutropenia or thrombophlebitis may occur.
Adverse reactions may also occur as a consequence of the procedure for which the contrast agent is used. Adverse reactions due to *angiocardiography* in adults have included arrhythmia and death. In *thoracic aortography,* the risks of the procedure include injury to the aorta and neighboring organs, pleural puncture, renal damage including infarction and acute tubular necrosis with oliguria and anuria, accidental selective filling of the right renal artery during the translumbar procedure in the presence of preexistent renal disease, retroperitoneal hemorrhage from the translumbar approach, spinal cord injury and pathology associated with the syndrome of transverse myelitis, generalized petechiae, and death following hypotension, arrhythmia and anaphylactoid reactions.
Dosage and Administration: The vial should be warmed in a water bath to 37° to 40° C. before use, thereby minimizing the viscosity of the solution. Since the contrast medium is given by rapid injection, the patient should be watched for untoward reactions during the injection.
In the preparation of the patient, preanesthetic medication should be given.
Angiocardiography: Normally, patients not under general anesthesia experience a feeling of bodily warmth in the area injected. This sensation is of short duration. Transient nausea and vomiting, tightness of the chest, or headache may occur in some patients. The contrast agent may be administered by injection into a large peripheral vein or, to increase the density, by catheter, approximating the catheter tip to the right heart or other area where pathology is suspected. Mechanical injectors permit a faster injection rate and greater bolus density.
The suggested dose for adults is 40 to 50 ml. This dose may be repeated once if necessary.
A preliminary control film may be made in the usual manner. After the medium has been injected, serial films are usually taken in rapid sequence and continued until the desired information is obtained.
Thoracic Aortography: The contrast agent may be injected into the aorta by translumbar or retrograde methods of administration. Unless general anesthesia is employed, patients should be warned that they may feel some transient pain or burning during the injection followed by a feeling of warmth immediately afterward.
The suggested adult dose is 15 to 20 ml. as a single injection and repeated if indicated.
A scout film may be made before the preparation is administered.
How Supplied: Cardiografin (Diatrizoate Meglumine Injection USP 85%) is available in 50 ml. single-dose vials. An excess volume (1 ml.) is available in each container for sensitivity testing.
Storage: When kept in the syringe for prolonged periods of time prior to injection, the preparation should be protected from exposure to strong light.
Note: Prolonged standing may result in the separation of solids. To obtain a clear solution, place vial in boiling water and shake gently until solids redissolve. Allow solution to cool to 37° to 40° C. before use. The preparation should be injected promptly after withdrawal into the syringe, and the syringe should be rinsed as soon as possible after injection to prevent freezing of the plunger.

CHOLOGRAFIN® MEGLUMINE ℞
(Iodipamide Meglumine Injection USP 52%)
FOR INTRAVENOUS USE ONLY

Description: Cholografin Meglumine is a radiopaque contrast agent for rapid intravenous cholangiography and cholecystography supplied as a sterile, aqueous solution. Each ml. provides 520 mg. iodipamide meglumine with 3.2 mg. sodium citrate as a buffer and 0.4 mg. edetate disodium as a sequestering agent; pH has been adjusted between 6.5 and 7.7 with meglumine. *Each ml. of solution also contains approximately 0.91 mg. (0.039 mEq.) sodium [18.2 mg./20 ml.]* and 257 mg. organically bound iodine (5.2 g./20 ml.). At the time of manufacture, the air in the container is replaced by nitrogen.
The appearance of the solution may vary from essentially colorless to light amber. Solutions which have become substantially darker, however, should not be used.
Clinical Pharmacology: Following intravenous administration of Cholografin Meglumine, iodipamide is carried to the liver where it is rapidly secreted. The contrast medium appears in the bile within 10 to 15 minutes after injection, thus permitting visualization of the hepatic and common bile ducts, even in cholecystectomized patients. The biliary ducts are readily visualized within about 25 minutes after administration, except in patients with impaired liver function. The gallbladder begins to fill within an hour after injection; maximum filling is reached after two to two and one-half hours. The contrast medium is finally eliminated in the feces without passing through the enterohepatic circulation, except for approximately 10 percent of the intravenously administered dose which is excreted through the kidneys.
The LD_{50} for intravenous administration of a 52% iodipamide meglumine solution in mice is 6.2 plus or minus 0.3 ml./kg. (equivalent to 3224 plus or minus 156 mg. iodipamide meglumine/kg.).
Indications and Usage: Cholografin Meglumine (Iodipamide Meglumine Injection USP 52%) is indicated for intravenous cholangiography and cholecystography as follows: (a) visualization of the gallbladder and biliary ducts in the differential diagnosis of acute abdominal conditions, (b) visualization of the biliary ducts, especially in patients with symptoms after cholecystectomy, and (c) visualization of the gallbladder in patients unable to take oral contrast media or to absorb contrast media from the gastrointestinal tract.
Contraindications: Iodipamide meglumine is contraindicated in patients with a hypersensitivity to salts of iodipamide or who exhibit sensitivity reactions to the test dose. It is also contraindicated in patients with concomitant severe impairment of renal and liver function.
Warnings: Administration of radiopaque materials to patients known or suspected to have pheochromocytoma should be performed with extreme caution. If, in the opinion of the physician, the possible benefits of such procedures outweigh the considered risks, the procedures may be performed; however, the amount of radiopaque medium injected should be kept to an absolute minimum. The blood pressure should be assessed throughout the procedure and measures for treatment of a hypertensive crisis should be available.
Contrast media have been shown to promote the phenomenon of sickling in individuals who are homozygous for sickle cell disease when the material is injected intravenously or intra-arterially.
Since iodine-containing contrast agents may alter the results of thyroid function tests, such tests, if indicated, should be performed prior to the administration of this preparation.
A history of sensitivity to iodine *per se* or to other contrast agents is not an absolute contraindication to the use of iodipamide meglumine, but calls for extreme caution in administration.
Precautions: Diagnostic procedures which involve the use of radiopaque contrast agents should be carried out under the direction of personnel with the prerequisite training and with a thorough knowledge of the particular procedure to be performed. Appropriate facilities should be available for coping with situations which may arise as a result of the procedure, as well as for emergency treatment of severe reactions to the contrast agent itself.

Continued on next page

Squibb—Cont.

After intravascular administration of a radiopaque agent, competent personnel and emergency facilities should be available for at least 30 to 60 minutes, since severe delayed reactions have been known to occur.
These severe, life-threatening reactions suggest hypersensitivity to the radiopaque agent, which has prompted the use of several pretesting methods, none of which can be relied upon to predict severe reactions. Many authorities question the value of any pretest. A history of bronchial asthma or allergy, a family history of allergy, or a previous reaction to a contrast agent warrant special attention. Such a history, by suggesting histamine sensitivity and a consequent proneness to reactions, may be more accurate than pretesting in predicting the likelihood of a reaction, although not necessarily the severity or type of reaction in the individual case.
The sensitivity test most often performed is the slow injection of 0.5 to 1.0 ml. of the radiopaque medium, administered intravenously, prior to injection of the full diagnostic dose. It should be noted that the absence of a reaction to the test dose does not preclude the possibility of a reaction to the full diagnostic dose. If the test dose causes an untoward response of any kind, the neccessity for continuing with the examination should be carefully reevaluated and, if it is deemed essential, the examination should be conducted with all possible caution. In rare instances reactions to the test dose itself may be extremely severe; therefore, close observation of the patient, and facilities for emergency treatment, appear indicated.
Caution should be exercised with the use of radiopaque media in severely debilitated patients and in those with marked hypertension. The possibility of thrombosis should be borne in mind when intravenous techniques are employed.
Contrast agents may interfere with some chemical determinations made on urine specimens; therefore, urine should be collected before administration of the contrast medium or two or more days afterwards.
Some clinicians feel it may be advisable to have a continuous intravenous infusion running prior to and during administration of the drug. ***The admixture of Benadryl® (Diphenhydramine Hydrochloride Injection) with Cholografin Meglumine (Iodipamide Meglumine Injection USP 52%) may cause a precipitate which may form in the syringe or tubing. If antihistamines are administered concomitantly, they should not be mixed with the contrast agent but administered at another site.***
Usage in Pregnancy: The safety of iodipamide meglumine for use during pregnancy has not been established; therefore, it should be used in pregnant patients only when, in the judgment of the physician, its use is deemed essential to the welfare of the patient.
Adverse Reactions: Local reactions at the site of injection are not observed, unless excessive amounts are extravasated during injection. After too rapid administration, mild transient symptoms such as restlessness, sensations of warmth, sneezing, perspiration, salivation, flushing, pressure in the upper abdomen, dizziness, nausea, vomiting, chills, fever, headache, pallor and tremors may occur. These symptoms disappear when the injection has been completed. Rarely, swollen eyelids, laryngospasm, respiratory difficulties, hypotension, cardiac reactions and cyanosis have been reported. Hypersensitivity reactions may occur. In rare instances, despite the most careful sensitivity testing, anaphylactoid reactions may occur.
Renal function tests may be altered and renal failure may occur.

Dosage and Administration: Cholografin Meglumine is for intravenous use only.
Directions for Use: *Preparation of the Patient:* For best results, the usual preliminary measures for cholecystography are recommended, particularly in cholecystectomized patients, i.e., a low residue diet on the day before examination and administration of castor oil the night before or neostigmine at the time of examination to dispel excess intestinal gas. Cholecystography is preferably carried out in the morning with the patient fasting.
Dose: The usual adult dose is 20 ml. For infants and children, the suggested dose is 0.3 to 0.6 ml./kg. of body weight; the dosage for infants and children should not exceed 20 ml.
Note: The dose should not be repeated for 24 hours.
Administration: After warming to body temperature, Cholografin Meglumine (Iodipamide Meglumine Injection USP 52%) should be given by slow intravenous injection, following the usual precautions of intravenous administration. *It is important that the preparation be injected slowly over a period of 10 minutes.* Use of a narrow bore hypodermic needle will ensure a slow rate of injection. During the injection, the patient should be watched for untoward reactions such as a feeling of warmth, flushing and occasionally nausea. Nausea indicates that the injection rate is too rapid.
Radiography: A scout film should be exposed routinely before the intravenous injection is made.
Position of the patient: With the patient prone and right side elevated, radiographs are made in the posterior-anterior projection. Some radiologists prefer the supine position with the left side elevated. Serial 10-minute exposures should be started 10 minutes after the injection is made and continued until optimal visualization of the *biliary ducts* is obtained. Wet films should be examined immediately by the radiologist. In some cases a 15-degree rotation or the upright position may prove helpful. Depending on the situation revealed by the roentgenograms in which the duct is first seen, the position of the subject should be changed to displace the shadow of the common bile duct from that of the spine. Tomography is a useful technique for enhancing bile duct visualization after administration of the radiopaque medium.
Examination of the *gallbladder* should be started about two hours after administration. The standard positions in routine examination of the gallbladder should be used unless otherwise indicated. There is no need for the patient to remain quiet awaiting the time for the gallbladder film to be exposed. Moderate activity on the part of the patient will, in most cases, preclude "stratification" of the contrast agent in the gallbladder. If the contrast medium should stratify in the gallbladder, decubitus as well as upright films should be obtained. Additional exposures may be made after the ingestion of a fatty meal.
If visualization is not achieved after two and one-half hours, the patient should be returned for a 24-hour film, whenever possible. Occasionally, delayed opacification of the gallbladder will occur in 24 hours.
In infants and children, gallbladder visualization may be expected to occur 30 minutes to four hours after administration.
Note: In the presence of liver disease (BSP retention greater than 30 to 40 percent), the contrast medium is not excreted efficiently by the liver and visualization is usually not achieved. Visualization is rarely achieved in the presence of a serum bilirubin of 3.0 mg. per 100 ml. if the elevated bilirubin level is due to mechanical obstruction or hepatocellular damage. In the presence of severe liver damage, the contrast agent is excreted by the kidneys.
Interpretation: When intravenous cholecystography and cholangiography are used as an aid in the differential diagnosis of acute abdominal conditions, visualization of the gallbladder is considered strong evidence against a diagnosis of acute cholecystitis, while nonvisualization of the gallbladder two and one-half hours after administration *with* visualization of the bile ducts is considered strong evidence in favor of a diagnosis of acute cholecystitis (if the bile ducts are only faintly visualized, gallbladder films four hours after administration may occasionally show visualization of the gallbladder). When neither the bile ducts nor the gallbladder is visualized, the study provides no definitive information with regard to determining the presence or absence of acute cholecystitis.
How Supplied: In single dose vials of 20 ml. An excess volume (1 ml.) is available in each container for sensitivity testing. (Military Depot Item, NSN6505-00-926-9109; V.A. Depot Item, NSN6505-00-926-9109A.)
Storage: Protect from light; store at room temperature; avoid excessive heat.
In the event that crystallization occurs, the solution may be clarified by placing the vial in hot water and shaking gently for several minutes or until the solids redissolve. If cloudiness persists, discard the preparation. Allow the solution to cool to body temperature before administering.

CHOLOGRAFIN® MEGLUMINE FOR INFUSION ℞

(Iodipamide Meglumine Injection USP 10.3%)
FOR INTRAVENOUS USE ONLY

Description: Cholografin Meglumine for Infusion (Iodipamide Meglumine Injection USP 10.3%) is a radiopaque contrast agent for slow intravenous cholangiography and cholecystography supplied as a sterile, aqueous solution. Each ml. provides 103 mg. iodipamide meglumine with 3.2 mg. sodium citrate as a buffer and 0.4 mg. edetate disodium as a sequestering agent; pH has been adjusted between 6.5 and 7.7 with meglumine. *Each ml. of solution also contains approximately 0.91 mg. (0.039 mEq) sodium [91 mg./100 ml.]* and 51 mg. organically bound iodine (5.1 g./100 ml.). At the time of manufacture, the air in the container is replaced by nitrogen.
The appearance of the solution may vary from essentially colorless to pale yellow. Solutions which have become substantially darker, however, should not be used.
Clinical Pharmacology: Following intravenous administration of Cholografin Meglumine for Infusion (Iodipamide Meglumine Injection USP 10.3%), iodipamide is carried to the liver where it is rapidly excreted. The contrast medium appears in the bile, thus permitting visualization of the hepatic and common bile ducts, even in cholecystectomized patients. The biliary ducts are readily visualized after administration, except in patients with impaired liver function; visualization may be apparent from 20 to 40 minutes after the infusion is started with optimum visualization usually occurring after 40 to 80 minutes. The gallbladder begins to fill within an hour after the infusion is completed; maximum filling is reached after three hours. The contrast medium is finally eliminated in the feces without passing through the enterohepatic circulation, except for approximately 10 percent of the intravenously administered dose which is excreted through the kidneys.
Indications and Usage: Cholografin Meglumine for Infusion (Iodipamide Meglumine Injection USP 10.3%) is indicated for intravenous cholangiography and cholecystography as follows: (a) visualization of the gallbladder and biliary ducts in the differential diagnosis of acute abdominal conditions, (b) visualization of the biliary ducts, especially in patients with symptoms after cholecystectomy, and (c) visualization of the gallbladder in patients unable to take oral contrast media or to absorb contrast media from the gastrointestinal tract.

Contraindications: Iodipamide meglumine is contraindicated in patients with a hypersensitivity to salts of iodipamide or who exhibit sensitivity reactions to the test dose. It is also contraindicated in patients with concomitant severe impairment of renal and liver function.

Warnings: Administration of radiopaque materials to patients known or suspected to have pheochromocytoma should be performed with extreme caution. If, in the opinion of the physician, the possible benefits of such procedures outweigh the considered risks, the procedures may be performed; however, the amount of radiopaque medium injected should be kept to an absolute minimum. The blood pressure should be assessed throughout the procedure and measures for treatment of a hypertensive crisis should be available.

Contrast media have been shown to promote the phenomenon of sickling in individuals who are homozygous for sickle cell disease when the material is injected intravenously or intra-arterially.

Since iodine-containing contrast agents may alter the results of thyroid function tests, such tests, if indicated, should be performed prior to the administration of this preparation.

A history of sensitivity to iodine *per se* or to other contrast agents is not an absolute contraindication to the use of iodipamide meglumine, but calls for extreme caution in administration.

Precautions: Diagnostic procedures which involve the use of radiopaque contrast agents should be carried out under the direction of personnel with the prerequisite training and with a thorough knowledge of the particular procedure to be performed. Appropriate facilities should be available for coping with situations which may arise as a result of the procedure, as well as for emergency treatment of severe reactions to the contrast agent itself.

After intravascular administration of a radiopaque agent, competent personnel and emergency facilities should be available for at least 30 to 60 minutes, since severe delayed reactions have been known to occur.

These severe, life-threatening reactions suggest hypersensitivity to the radiopaque agent, which has prompted the use of several pretesting methods, none of which can be relied upon to predict severe reactions. Many authorities question the value of any pretest. A history of bronchial asthma or allergy, a family history of allergy, or a previous reaction to a contrast agent warrant special attention. Such a history, by suggesting histamine sensitivity and a consequent proneness to reactions, may be more accurate than pretesting in predicting the likelihood of a reaction, although not necessarily the severity or type of reaction in the individual case.

The sensitivity test most often performed is the slow injection of 0.5 to 1.0 ml. of the radiopaque medium, administered intravenously prior to infusion of the full diagnostic dose. It should be noted that the absence of a reaction to the test dose does not preclude the possibility of a reaction to the full diagnostic dose. If the test dose causes an untoward response of any kind, the necessity for continuing with the examination should be carefully reevaluated and, if it is deemed essential, the examination should be conducted with all possible caution. In rare instances reactions to the test dose itself may be extremely severe; therefore, close observation of the patient, and facilities for emergency treatment, appear indicated.

Caution should be exercised with the use of radiopaque media in severely debilitated patients and in those with marked hypertension. The possibility of thrombosis should be borne in mind when intravenous techniques are employed.

Contrast agents may interfere with some chemical determinations made on urine specimens; therefore, urine should be collected before administration of the contrast medium or two or three days afterwards.

The admixture of Benadryl® (Diphenhydramine Hydrochloride Injection) with Cholografin Meglumine for Infusion (Iodipamide Meglumine Injection USP 10.3%) may cause a precipitate which may form in the syringe or tubing. If antihistamines are administered concomitantly, they should not be mixed with the contrast agent but administered at another site.

Usage in Pregnancy: The safety of iodipamide meglumine for use during pregnancy has not been established; therefore, it should be used in pregnant patients only when, in the judgment of the physician, its use is deemed essential to the welfare of the patient.

Adverse Reactions: Local reactions at the site of infusion are not observed, unless excessive amounts are extravasated during infusion. After too rapid administration, mild transient symptoms such as restlessness, sensations of warmth, sneezing, perspiration, salivation, flushing, pressure in the upper abdomen, dizziness, nausea, vomiting, chills, fever, headache, pallor and tremors may occur. These symptoms disappear when the infusion has been completed. Rarely, swollen eyelids, laryngospasm, respiratory difficulties, hypotension, cardiac reactions and cyanosis have been reported. Hypersensitivity reactions may occur. In rare instances, despite the most careful sensitivity testing, anaphylactoid reactions may occur.

Renal function tests may be altered and renal failure may occur.

Dosage and Administration: Cholografin Meglumine for Infusion (Iodipamide Meglumine Injection USP 10.3%) is for intravenous use only.

Directions for Use: *Preparation of the Patient:* For best results, the usual preliminary measures for cholecystography are recommended, particularly in cholecystectomized patients, i.e., a low residue diet on the day before examination and administration of castor oil the night before or neostigmine at the time of examination to dispel excess intestinal gas. Cholecystography is preferably carried out in the morning with the patient fasting.

Dose: The usual adult dose is 100 ml.

Note: The dose should not be repeated for 24 hours.

Administration: After warming to body temperature, Cholografin Meglumine for Infusion (Iodipamide Meglumine Injection USP 10.3%) should be given by slow intravenous infusion, following the usual precautions of intravenous administration. *It is preferable that the preparation be infused slowly over a period of 30 to 45 minutes.* During the infusion, the patient should be watched for untoward reactions such as a feeling of warmth, flushing and occasionally nausea. Nausea indicates that the infusion rate is too rapid.

Radiography: A scout film should be exposed routinely before the intravenous infusion is made.

Position of the Patient: With the patient prone and the right side elevated, radiographs are made in the posterior-anterior projection. Some radiologists prefer the supine position with the left side elevated. Serial exposures should begin 20 minutes after the infusion is started and be continued every 20 minutes until optimal visualization of the *biliary ducts* is obtained. Wet films should be examined immediately by the radioloist. In some cases a 15-degree rotation or the upright position may prove helpful. Depending on the situation revealed by the roentgenograms in which the duct is first seen, the position of the subject should be changed to displace the shadow of the common bile duct from that of the spine. Tomography is a useful technique for enhancing bile duct visualization after administration of the radiopaque medium.

Examination of the *gallbladder* should be started about two hours after the infusion is completed. The standard positions in routine examination of the gallbladder should be used unless otherwise indicated. There is no need for the patient to remain quiet awaiting the time for the gallbladder film to be exposed. Moderate activity on the part of the patient will, in most cases, preclude "stratification" of the contrast agent in the gallbladder. If the contrast medium should stratify in the gallbladder, decubitus as well as upright films should be obtained. Additional exposures may be made after the ingestion of a fatty meal.

If visualization is not achieved after two and one-half hours, the patient should be returned for a 24-hour film, whenever possible. Occasionally, delayed opacification of the gallbladder will occur in 24 hours.

Note: In the presence of liver disease (BSP retention greater than 30% to 40%), the contrast medium is not excreted efficiently by the liver and visualization is usually not achieved. Visualization is rarely achieved in the presence of a serum bilirubin of 3.0 mg. per 100 ml. if the elevated bilirubin level is due to mechanical obstruction or hepatocellular damage. In the presence of severe liver damage, the contrast agent is excreted by the kidneys.

Interpretation: When intravenous cholecystography and cholangiography are used as an aid in the differential diagnosis of acute abdominal conditions, visualization of the gallbladder is considered strong evidence against a diagnosis of acute cholecystitis, while nonvisualization of the gallbladder two and one-half hours after administration *with* visualization of the bile ducts is considered strong evidence in favor of a diagnosis of acute cholecystitis (if the bile ducts are only faintly visualized, gallbladder films four hours after administration may occasionally show visualization of the gallbladder). When neither the bile ducts nor the gallbladder is visualized, the study provides no definite information with regard to determining the presence or absence of acute cholecystitis.

How Supplied: Cholografin Meglumine for Infusion (Iodipamide Meglumine Injection USP 10.3%) is available in single-dose bottles of 100 ml. An excess volume (1 ml.) is available in each container for sensitivity testing.

Storage: Protect from light. Store at room temperature; avoid excessive heat.

CHOLOVUE® ℞

(Iodoxamate Meglumine Injection 40.3%)
For Cholecystocholangiography
FOR INTRAVENOUS USE ONLY

Description: Cholovue (Iodoxamate Meglumine Injection 40.3%) is a radiopaque medium for intravenous cholecystocholangiography supplied as a sterile, nonpyrogenic, aqueous solution. Each ml. provides 403 mg. iodoxamate meglumine with 0.4 mg edetate disodium as a sequestering stabilizing agent. The pH of the clear, colorless to pale yellow solution has been adjusted to 6.5 to 7.7 with meglumine and iodoxamic acid.

The solution contains approximately 0.05 mg (0.002 mEq) sodium and 183 mg. organically bound iodine per ml. At the time of manufacture, the air in the container is replaced by nitrogen.

Chemically, iodoxamate meglumine is 3,3′-[(1, 16-dioxo-4, 7, 10, 13-tetraoxahexadecane-1,16-diyl)-diimino]bis[2,4,6-triiodobenzoic acid],bis [N-methylglucamine] salt.

Clinical Pharmacology: Following intravenous administration, iodoxamate is carried to the liver where it is rapidly excreted. The contrast agent appears in the bile within 10 to 15 minutes after injection and permits visualization of the subhepatic, hepatic, and common bile ducts, even in cholecystectomized patients.

Continued on next page

Squibb—Cont.

Visualization may be impaired, delayed, or poor in patients with impaired liver function. The contrast agent is eliminated primarily in the feces; less than 15 percent of the administered dose is excreted by the kidneys.

Indications and Usage: Cholovue (Iodoxamate Meglumine Injection 40.3%) is indicated for intravenous cholecystocholangiography for: (a) rapid visualization of the gallbladder and biliary ducts in the differential diagnosis of acute abdominal conditions, (b) visualization of the biliary ducts, especially in patients with symptoms after cholecystectomy, and (c) visualization of the gallbladder in patients unable to take or tolerate an oral contrast medium or to absorb a contrast agent from the gastrointestinal tract.

Contraindications: Iodoxamate Meglumine Injection 40.3% is contraindicated in patients with concomitant severe impairment of hepatic and renal function.

Warnings: Administration of radiopaque contrast media to patients known or suspected to have pheochromocytoma should be performed only if the physician deems that the possible benefits outweigh the considered risks; the procedure should then be performed with extreme caution and the volume of the contrast medium to be injected should be kept to an absolute minimum. The blood pressure should be assessed throughout the procedure and measures for treatment of a hypertensive crisis should be available.

Since the use of contrast agents excreted by the kidneys has caused renal failure in patients with multiple myeloma, the physician should carefully consider the benefit/risk ratio in such cases.

Thyroid storm associated with the administration of radiopaques in hyperthyroid patients has been reported.

Contrast media which are administered intravenously have been shown to promote the phenomenon of sickling in individuals who are homozygous for sickle cell disease.

A history of sensitivity to iodine *per se* or to any contrast agent is not an absolute contraindication to the use of iodoxamate meglumine, but calls for extreme caution in administration.

Radiopaque drugs should be used under the direction of personnel with a thorough knowledge and appropriate training in the radiographic procedure being performed.

All procedures utilizing contrast media carry a definite risk or producing adverse reactions. While most reactions may be minor, life-threatening and fatal reactions may occur without warning. The risk-benefit factor should always be carefully evaluated before such a procedure is undertaken. At all times a fully equipped emergency cart, or equivalent supplies and equipment, and personnel competent in recognizing and treating adverse reactions of all severity (or situations which may arise as a result of the procedure) should be immediately available. If a serious reaction should occur, administration should be discontinued immediately.

Since severe delayed reactions have been known to occur, emergency facilities and competent personnel should be available for at least 30 to 60 minutes after administration.

Epinephrine, corticosteroids, antihistamines and/or other agents may be of benefit in the event of an adverse reaction.

In case of collapse due to anaphylactoid reaction, appropriate resuscitative measures should be begun immediately.

Precautions: General: Caution should be exercised with the use of a contrast medium in severely debilitated or dehydrated patients and in those with marked hypertension.

Renal toxicity has been reported in patients with liver dysfunction who were given oral cholecystographic agents followed by urographic agents. Administration of urographic agents should therefore be postponed in any patient with a known or suspected hepatic or biliary disorder who has recently had a cholecystographic contrast agent.

When any intravenous technique is employed, the possibility of thrombosis or other complications due to the mechanical trauma of the procedure should be borne in mind.

Sensitivity Testing: Severe, life-threatening reactions to radiopaque agents often resemble hypersensitivity phenomena. This has prompted the use of several pretesting methods, none of which can be relied on to predict severe reactions. Many authorities question the value of any pretest. A history of bronchial asthma or allergy, a family history of allergy, or a previous reaction to a contrast agent warrant special attention. Such a history, by suggesting histamine sensitivity and a consequent proneness to reactions may be more accurate than pretesting in predicting the likelihood of a reaction, although it will not necessarily indicate the severity or type of reaction in the individual case.

The sensitivity test most often performed is the slow intravenous injection of 0.5 to 1.0 ml. of the contrast medium prior to injection of the full diagnostic dose. It should be noted that the absence of a reaction to the test dose does not preclude the possibility of a reaction to the full diagnostic dose. If the test dose causes an untoward reaction of any kind, the necessity for continuing with the examination should be carefully reevaluated and, if it is deemed essential to continue, the examination should be conducted with all possible caution. In rare instances reactions to the test dose itself may be extremely severe; therefore, close observation of the patient and facilities for emergency treatment are essential.

Laboratory Test Interactions: Contrast agents may interfere with some chemical determinations made on urine specimens; therefore, urine should be collected before administration of the contrast medium or two or more days afterwards.

Since iodine-containing contrast agents may alter the results of thyroid function tests which depend on iodine estimations (e.g., PBI and radioactive iodine uptake studies), such tests, if indicated, should be performed prior to the administration of this preparation. However, measurements of serum thyroxine concentration involving use of tests such as the Resin Triiodothyronine Uptake test, "RT_3U," or the Thyroxine (Displacement) assay, "$T_4(D)$," are not affected.

Pregnancy: Teratogenic Effects—Pregnancy Category B. Reproduction studies have been performed in rats and rabbits at repeat doses up to 12 times the human dose and have revealed no evidence of teratogenic effects; however, in rabbits, at repeat doses eight times higher than the human dose there was evidence of loss of litter, increased resorptions, and reduced weight gain of dams and newborn pups. There are, however, no adequate and well-controlled studies in pregnant women. Because animal reproduction studies are not always predictive of human response, this drug should be used during pregnancy only if clearly needed.

Nursing Mothers: It is not known whether this drug is excreted in human milk. Because many drugs are excreted in human milk, caution should be exercised when Iodoxamate Meglumine Injection 40.3% is administered to a nursing mother.

Pediatric Use: Safety and effectiveness in children have not been established.

Adverse Reactions: Most reactions have been mild and transient. In clinical studies with iodoxamate meglumine, reactions occurred in approximately 11.5 to 14.8 percent of patients.

The most frequent adverse reactions to iodoxamate meglumine are nausea and/or vomiting, blood pressure changes, hives or rash, pruritus, headache, and abdominal pain or discomfort; these occur in approximately one to seven of 200 patients.

Less frequent adverse reactions are tachycardia, premature atrial contraction, palpitation, tachypnea, blurred vision, burning or itching eyes, photophobia, erythema, facial edema, dizziness, weakness, drowsiness, lightheadedness, midsternal tightness, fever, sensation of warmth, chills, sneezing, coughing, diarrhea, and retching which occur in approximately one to four of 1000 patients.

Additional reactions reported in the literature for iodoxamate meglumine include shock, collapse, severe renal impairment, paresthesia, precordial pain, dyspnea, confusion, difficulty in urination, constriction of throat, general malaise, fatigue, and bitter and metallic taste.

Other reactions to intravenous iodinated contrast agents may occur; the histamine-liberating effect of these compounds may induce a reaction which may range in severity from anaphylactoid shock (rarely) to bronchial or laryngeal spasm to angioneurotic edema or rhinitis.

Severe reactions to intravenous iodinated contrast agents, which may require emergency measures (see WARNINGS), may take the form of a cardiovascular reaction characterized by peripheral vasodilatation with resultant hypotension and reflex tachycardia, dyspnea, agitation, confusion, and cyanosis progressing to unconsciousness. Rare cases of cardiac arrest, cardiac arrhythmias (including ventricular fibrillation), hypertension, temporary renal shutdown or other nephropathy may occur.

An adverse reaction may be severe enough to require discontinuation of the injection.

Dosage and Administration: Cholovue (Iodoxamate Meglumine Injection 40.3%) is for intravenous use only.

Parenteral drug products should be inspected visually for particulate matter and discoloration prior to administration, whenever solution and container permit.

If precipitation or solidification has occurred due to storage in the cold, immerse the container in warm water and shake intermittently to dissolve any solids. If this warming procedure does not produce a clear solution, do not use the preparation.

Preparation of the Patient: For best results the usual preliminary measures for cholecystocholangiography are recommended, i.e., a low residue diet on the day before examination and administration of a laxative the night before. Radiography is preferably carried out in the morning with the patient fasting. Water should be allowed *ad lib* to prevent dehydration.

Dose: The recommended adult dose is 20 ml. *This dose should not be repeated before four days have elapsed.*

Administration: After bringing to body temperature, Cholovue (Iodoxamate Meglumine Injection 40.3%) should be given by slow intravenous injection, following the usual precautions for intravenous administration. *It is important that the dose be injected slowly over a period of 10 minutes.* Use of a narrow-bore hypodermic needle will ensure a slow rate of injection, During the injection, the patient should be watched for untoward reactions such as a feeling of warmth, flushing, and occasionally nausea. Nausea indicates that the injection rate is too rapid. If an adverse reaction occurs, the injection should be slowed or temporarily discontinued. If the adverse reaction persists, the injection should be discontinued and, if necessary, appropriate treatment or emergency measures undertaken (see WARNINGS).

Drug Incompatabilities: The admixture of Benadryl® (Diphenhydramine Hydrochloride Injection) with Cholovue (Iodoxamate Meglumine Injection 40.3%) may cause a precipitate to form in the syringe. If antihistamines are administered concomitantly, they should **not** be mixed with the contrast medium but should be administered at another site.

Roentgenographic Procedure: A scout film should be exposed before the intravenous injection is made.

Position of the Patient: With the patient prone and right side elevated, radiographs are made in the posterior-anterior projection. Some radiologists prefer the supine position with the left side elevated. Serial exposures at 10-minute intervals should be started 10 minutes after injection is completed and continued until optimal visualization of the biliary ducts is obtained. Wet films should be examined immediately by the radiologist. In some patients, a 15-degree rotation or the upright position may prove helpful. Depending on the situation revealed by the roentgenograms in which the ducts are first seen, the position of the subject should be changed to displace the shadow of the common bile duct from that of the spine. Tomography is a useful technique for enhancing bile duct visualization after administration of a radiopaque contrast medium.

Visualization of the biliary ducts as well as the gallbladder occurs in some patients as early as 10 minutes after completion of administration.

Visualization of ducts occurs most frequently from *40 to 60 minutes* after administration.

Examination of the gallbladder should be started about *30 minutes* after administration is completed; *visualization of the gallbladder* occurs most frequently at *60 to 90 minutes.* If opacification is absent, radiographs should be taken hourly for *two to three hours* after drug administration. The standard position for routine examination of the gallbladder should be used unless otherwise indicated. Moderate activity on the part of the patient, while waiting for the gallbladder film to be exposed, will in most cases preclude "stratification" of the contrast agent in the gallbladder. If the contrast agent should stratify in the gallbladder, decubitus as well as upright films should be obtained. Additional exposures may be made after the administration of a cholecystogogic agent such as Kinevac® (Sincalide for Injection) [see package insert accompanying that product for complete information] or ingestion of a fatty meal.

If visualization is not achieved after two to three hours, the patient should return for a 24-hour film whenever possible since, occasionally, delayed opacification of the gallbladder will occur.

Note: In the presence of liver disease (serum bilirubin greater than 3.0 mg%), contrast agents are not excreted efficiently by the liver and satisfactory visualization may not be achieved, although some diagnostic films have been obtained in patients with serum bilirubin above 4.0 mg%, especially when the elevation in serum bilirubin is not due to mechanical obstruction or severe hepatocellular damage. The extent of renal excretion of the contrast agent is directly proportional to the degree of hepatic impairment. Although the kidney normally excretes less than 15 percent of an administered dose within 72 hours, this percentage probably increased with the severity of hepatic dysfunction.

Interpretation: When intravenous cholecystocholangiography is used as an aid in the differential diagnosis of acute abdominal conditions, visualization of the gallbladder is considered evidence against a diagnosis of acute cholecystitus, while nonvisualization of the gallbladder two to three hours after administration, *with* visualization of the bile ducts, is considered evidence supporting a diagnosis of acute cholecystitis. (If the bile ducts are only faintly visualized, gallbladder films four hours after administration may occasionally show visualization of the gallbladder.) When neither the bile ducts nor the gallbladder are visualized, the study provides no definitive information with regard to determining the presence or absence of acute cholecystitis.

How Supplied: Cholovue (Iodoxamate Meglumine Injection 40.3%) is available in 20 ml. single-dose vials. Each vial contains an excess volume (1 ml.) for sensitivity testing.

Storage: Store at room temperature; avoid excessive heat; protect from light.

CHOLOVUE® FOR INFUSION ℞

(Iodoxamate Meglumine Injection 9.9%)
For Drip Infusion Cholecystocholangiography
FOR INTRAVENOUS USE ONLY

Description: Cholovue for Infusion (Iodoxamate Meglumine Injection 9.9%) is a radiopaque contrast medium for intravenous cholecystocholangiography supplied as a sterile, nonpyrogenic, aqueous solution. Each ml. provides 99 mg. iodoxamate meglumine with 0.1 mg. edetate disodium as a sequestering stabilizing agent. The pH of the clear, colorless to light amber solution has been adjusted to 6.5 to 7.7 with meglumine and iodoxamic acid. *The solution contains approximately 0.012 mg. (0.0005 mEq) sodium* and 45 mg. organically bound iodine per ml. At the time of manufacture, the air in the container is replaced with nitrogen.

Chemically, iodoxamate meglumine is 3,3'-[(1,16-dioxo-4, 7, 10, 13-tetraoxahexadecane-1, 16-diyl)-diimino]bis[2,4,6-triiodobenzoic acid], bis[N-methylglucamine]salt.

Clinical Pharmacology: Following intravenous infusion, iodoxamate is carried to the liver where it is rapidly excreted. The contrast agent appears in the bile before completion of the infusion and permits visualization of the subhepatic, hepatic, and common bile ducts, even in cholecystectomized patients. The biliary ducts are readily visualized at the completion of the infusion, except in patients with impaired liver function in whom visualization may be impaired, delayed, or poor. The gallbladder begins to fill by the time the infusion is complete; maximal filling is reached after one hour.

The contrast agent is eliminated primarily in the feces. Less than 15 percent of the administered dose is excreted by the kidneys.

Indications and Usage: Cholovue for Infusion (Iodoxamate Meglumine Injection 9.9%) is indicated for intravenous cholecystocholangiography for: (a) rapid visualization of the gallbladder and biliary ducts in the differential diagnosis of acute abdominal conditions, (b) visualization of the biliary ducts, especially in patients with symptoms after cholecystectomy, and (c) visualization of the gallbladder in patients unable to take or tolerate an oral contrast medium or to absorb a contrast agent from the gastrointestinal tract.

Contraindications: Iodoxamate Meglumine Injection 9.9% is contraindicated in patients with concomitant severe impairment of hepatic and renal function.

Warnings: Administration of radiopaque contrast media to patients known or suspected to have pheochromocytoma should be performed only if the physician deems that the possible benefits outweigh the considered risks; the procedure should then be performed with extreme caution and the volume of the contrast medium to be injected should be kept to an absolute minimum. The blood pressure should be assessed throughout the procedure and measures for treatment of a hypertensive crisis should be available.

Since the use of contrast agents excreted by the kidneys has caused renal failure in patients with multiple myeloma, the physician should carefully consider the benefit/risk ratio in such cases.

Thyroid storm associated with the administration of radiopaques in hyperthyroid patients has been reported.

Contrast media which are administered intravenously have been shown to promote the phenomenon of sickling in individuals who are homozygous for sickle cell disease.

A history of sensitivity to iodine *per se* or to any contrast agent is not an absolute contraindication to the use of iodoxamate meglumine, but calls for extreme caution in administration.

Radiopaque drugs should be used under the direction of personnel with a thorough knowledge and appropriate training in the radiographic procedure being performed.

All procedures utilizing contrast media carry a definite risk of producing adverse reactions. While most reactions may be minor, life-threatening and fatal reactions may occur without warning. The risk-benefit factor should always be carefully evaluated before such a procedure is undertaken. At all times a fully equipped emergency cart, or equivalent supplies and equipment, and personnel competent in recognizing and treating adverse reactions of all severity (or situations which may arise as a result of the procedure) should be immediately available. If a serious reaction should occur, administration should be discontinued immediately.

Since severe delayed reactions have been known to occur, emergency facilities and competent personnel should be available for at least 30 to 60 minutes after administration.

Epinephrine, corticosteroids, antihistamines and/or other agents may be of benefit in the event of an adverse reaction.

In case of collapse due to anaphylactic reaction, appropriate resuscitative measures should be begun immediately.

Precautions: General: Caution should be exercised with the use of a contrast medium in severely debilitated or dehydrated patients and in those with marked hypertension. The increased osmotic load associated with drip infusion cholecystocholangiography should also be considered in patients with congestive heart failure.

Renal toxicity has been reported in patients with liver dysfunction who were given oral cholecystographic agents followed by urographic agents. Administration of urographic agents should therefore be postponed in any patient with a known or suspected hepatic or biliary disorder who has recently had a cholecystographic contrast agent.

When any intravenous infusion technique is employed, the possibility of thrombosis or other complications due to the mechanical trauma of the procedure should be borne in mind.

The recommended rate of infusion should not be exceeded.

Sensitivity Testing: Severe, life-threatening reactions to radiopaque agents often resemble hypersensitivity phenomena. This has prompted the use of several pretesting methods, none of which can be relied on to predict severe reactions. Many authorities question the value of any pretest. A history of bronchial asthma or allergy, a family history of allergy, or a previous reaction to a contrast agent warrant special attention. Such a history, by suggesting histamine sensitivity and a consequent proneness to reactions may be more accurate than pretesting in predicting the likelihood of a reaction, although it will not necessarily indicate the severity or type of reaction in the individual case.

The sensitivity test most often performed is the slow intravenous injection of 0.5 to 1.0 ml. of the contrast medium prior to infusion of the full diagnostic dose. It should be noted that the absence of a reaction to the test dose does not preclude the possibility of a reaction to the full

Continued on next page

Squibb—Cont.

diagnostic dose. If the test dose causes an untoward reaction of any kind, the necessity for continuing with the examination should be carefully reevaluated and, if it is deemed essential to continue, the examination should be conducted with all possible caution. In rare instances reactions to the test dose itself may be extremely severe; therefore, close observation of the patient, and facilities for emergency treatment, are essential.

Laboratory Test Interactions: Contrast agents may interfere with some chemical determinations made on urine specimens; therefore, urine should be collected before administration of the contrast medium or two or more days afterwards.

Since iodine-containing contrast agents may alter the results of thyroid function tests which depend on iodine estimations (e.g., PBI and radioactive iodine uptake studies), such tests, if indicated, should be performed prior to the administration of this preparation. However, measurements of serum thyroxine concentration involving use of tests such as the Resin Triiodothyronine Uptake test, "RT3 U," or the Thyroxine (Displacement) assay, "T4 (D)," are not affected.

Pregnancy: Tetratogenic Effects—Pregnancy Category B. Reproduction studies have been performed in rats and rabbits at repeat doses up to 12 times the human dose and have revealed no evidence of teratogenic effects; however, in rabbits, at repeat doses eight times higher than the human dose there was evidence of loss of litter, increased resorptions, and reduced weight gain of dams and newborn pups. There are, however, no adequate and well-controlled studies in pregnant women. Because animal reproduction studies are not always predictive of human response, this drug should be used during pregnancy only if clearly needed.

Nursing Mothers: It is not known whether this drug is excreted in human milk. Because many drugs are excreted in human milk, caution should be exercised when Iodoxamate Meglumine Injection 9.9% is administered to a nursing mother.

Pediatric Use: Safety and effectiveness in children have not been established.

Adverse Reactions: Most reactions have been mild and transient. In clinical studies with iodoxamate meglumine, reactions occurred in approximately 11.5 to 14.8 percent of patients.

The most frequent adverse reactions to iodoxamate meglumine are nausea and/or vomiting, blood pressure changes, hives or rash, pruritis, headache, and abdominal pain or discomfort; these occur in approximately one to seven of 200 patients.

Less frequent adverse reactions are tachycardia, premature atrial contraction, palpitation, tachypnea, blurred vision, burning or itching eyes, photophobia, erythema, facial edema, dizziness, weakness, drowsiness, lightheadedness, midsternal tightness, fever, sensation of warmth, chills, sneezing, coughing, diarrhea, and retching which occur in approximately one to four of 1000 patients.

Additional reactions reported in the literature for iodoxamate meglumine include shock, collapse, severe renal impairment, paresthesia, precordial pain, dyspnea, confusion, difficulty in urination, constriction of throat, general malaise, fatigue, and bitter and metallic taste.

Other reactions to intravenous iodinated contrast agents may occur; the histamine-liberating effect of these compounds may induce a reaction which may range in severity from anaphylactoid shock (rarely) to bronchial or laryngeal spasm to angioneurotic edema or rhinitis.

Severe reactions to intravenous iodinated contrast agents, which may require emergency measures (see WARNINGS), may take the form of a cardiovascular reaction characterized by peripheral vasodilatation with resultant hypotension and reflex tachycardia, dyspnea, agitation, confusion, and cyanosis progressing to unconsciousness. Rare cases of cardiac arrest, cardiac arrhythmias (including ventricular fibrillation), hypertension, temporary renal shutdown or other nephropathy may occur.

An adverse reaction may be severe enough to require discontinuation of the infusion.

Dosage and Administration: Cholovue for Infusion (Iodoxamate Meglumine Injection 9.9%) is for intravenous use only.

Parenteral drug products should be inspected visually for particulate matter and discoloration prior to administration, whenever solution and container permit.

If precipitation or solidification has occurred due to storage in the cold, immerse the container in warm water and shake intermittently to dissolve any solids. If this warming procedure does not produce a clear solution, do not use the preparation.

Preparation of the Patient: For best results the usual preliminary measures for cholecystocholangiography are recommended, i.e., a low residue diet on the day before examination and administration of a laxative the night before. Radiography is preferably carried out in the morning with the patient fasting. Water should be allowed *ad lib* to prevent dehydration.

Dose: The recommended adult dose is 100 ml. *This dose should not be repeated before four days have elapsed.*

Administration: After bringing to body temperature, Cholovue for Infusion (Iodoxamate Meglumine Injection 9.9%) should be given by slow intravenous drip infusion, following the usual precautions for intravenous drip administration. *It is important that the dose be injected slowly over a period of approximately 30 minutes (3 ml./min.).* During the infusion, the patient should be watched for untoward reactions such as a feeling of warmth, flushing, and occasionally nausea. Nausea indicates that the infusion rate is too rapid. If an adverse reaction occurs, the infusion should be slowed or temporarily discontinued. If the adverse reaction persists, the infusion should be discontinued and, if necessary, appropriate treatment or emergency measures undertaken (see WARNINGS).

Drug Incompatibilities: The admixture of Benadryl® (Diphenhydramine Hydrochloride Injection) with Cholovue for Infusion (Iodoxamate Meglumine Injection 9.9%) may cause a precipitate to form in the infusion bottle or tubing. If antihistamines are administered concomitantly, they should **not** be mixed with the contrast medium but should be administered at another site.

Roentgenographic Procedure: A scout film should be exposed before the intravenous infusion is made.

Position of the Patient: With the patient prone and right side elevated, radiographs are made in the posterior-anterior projection. Some radiologists prefer the supine position, with the left side elevated. Serial exposures may be started immediately after infusion is completed and continued until optimal visualization of the biliary ducts is obtained. Wet films should be examined immediately by the radiologist. In some patients, a 15-degree rotation or the upright position may prove helpful. Depending on the situation revealed by the roentgenograms in which the ducts are first seen, the position of the subject should be changed to displace the shadow of the common bile duct from that of the spine. Tomography is a useful technique for enhancing bile duct visualization after administration of a radiopaque contrast medium. Visualization of the biliary ducts as well as the gallbladder occurs in some patients before the completion of infusion. *Visualization of ducts* occurs most frequently from *30 to 60 minutes* after infusion.

Examination of the gallbladder should be started about *20 minutes* after administration is completed; *visualization of the gallbladder* occurs most frequently at *one to two hours.* If opacification is absent, radiographs should be taken hourly for *four hours* after drug administration. The standard position for routine examination of the gallbladder should be used unless otherwise indicated. Moderate activity on the part of the patient, while waiting for the gallbladder film to be exposed, will in most cases preclude "stratification" of the contrast agent in the gallbladder. If the contrast agent should stratify in the gallbladder, decubitus as well as upright films should be obtained. Additional exposures may be made after the administration of a cholecystogogic agent such as Kinevac® (Sincalide for Injection) [see package insert accompanying that product for complete information] or ingestion of a fatty meal. If visualization is not achieved after four hours, the patient should return for a 24-hour film whenever possible since, occasionally, delayed opacification of the gallbladder will occur.

Note: In the presence of liver disease (serum bilirubin greater than 3.0 mg%), contrast agents are not excreted efficiently by the liver and satisfactory visualization may not be achieved although some diagnostic films have been obtained in patients with serum bilirubin above 4.0 mg%, especially when the elevation in serum bilirubin is not due to mechanical obstruction or severe hepatocellular damage. The extent of renal excretion of the contrast agent is directly proportional to the degree of hepatic impairment. Although the kidney normally excretes less than 15 percent of an administered dose within 72 hours, this percentage probably increases with the severity of hepatic dysfunction.

Interpretation: When intravenous cholecystocholangiography is used as an aid in the differential diagnosis of actue abdominal conditions, visualization of the gallbladder is considered evidence against a diagnosis of acute cholecystitis, while nonvisualization of the gallbladder four hours after administration *with* visualization of the bile ducts is considered evidence supporting a diagnosis of acute cholecystitis. (If the bile ducts are only faintly visualized, gallbladder films four hours after administration may occasionally show visualization of the gallbladder.) When neither the bile ducts nor the gallbladder are visualized, the study provides no definitive information with regard to determining the presence or absence of acute cholecystitis.

How Supplied: Cholovue for Infusion (Iodoxamate Meglumine Injection 9.9%) is available in calibrated single-dose 100 ml. infusion bottles (designed to be suspended from an I.V. stand). Each bottle contains an excess volume (1 ml.) for sensitivity testing.

Storage: Store at room temperature; avoid excessive heat; protect from light.

CYSTOGRAFIN® ℞

(Diatrizoate Meglumine Injection USP 30%)
For retrograde cystourethrography
Not intended for intravascular injection

Description: Cystografin is a radiopaque contrast agent supplied as a sterile, aqueous solution. Each ml. provides 300 mg. diatrizoate meglumine with 0.4 mg. edetate disodium as a sequestering agent. Each ml. of solution also contains approximately 141 mg. organically bound iodine. At the time of manufacture, the air in the container is replaced by nitrogen. The preparation should be protected from strong light.

Indication: Cystografin (Diatrizoate Meglumine Injection USP 30%) is indicated for retrograde cystourethrography.

Contraindications: This preparation is contraindicated in patients with a hypersensitivity to salts of diatrizoic acid.

Warnings: Severe sensitivity reactions are more likely to occur in patients with a personal or family history of bronchial asthma, significant allergies, or previous reactions to contrast agents.

A history of sensitivity to iodine *per se* or to other contrast agents is not an absolute contraindication to the use of diatrizoate meglumine, but calls for extreme caution in administration.

Precautions: Safe and effective use of this preparation depends upon proper dosage, correct technique, adequate precautions, and readiness for emergencies.

Retrograde cystourethrography should be performed with caution in patients with a known active infectious process of the urinary tract. Sterile technique should be employed in administration. During administration, care should be taken to avoid excessive pressure, rapid or acute distention of the bladder, and trauma.

Contrast agents may interfere with some chemical determinations made on urine specimens; therefore, urine should be collected before administration of the contrast medium or two or more days afterwards.

Pregnancy—Teratogenic Effects: Pregnancy Category C

Animal reproduction studies have not been conducted with diatrizoate meglumine injection. It is also not known whether diatrizoate meglumine injection can cause fetal harm when administered to a pregnant woman or can affect reproduction capacity. Cystografin should be administered to a pregnant woman only if clearly needed.

Adverse Reactions: Retrograde genitourinary procedures may cause such complications as hematuria, perforation of the urethra or bladder, introduction of infection into the genitourinary tract, and oliguria or anuria.

If intravasation of this drug occurs, the reactions which may be associated with intravenous administration may possibly be encountered. Hypersensitivity or anaphylactoid reactions may occur. Severe reactions may be manifested by edema of the face and glottis, respiratory distress, convulsions or shock; such reactions may prove fatal unless promptly controlled by such emergency measures as maintenance of a clear airway and immediate use of oxygen and resuscitative drugs.

Dosage and Administration: Preparation of the patient—Appropriate preparation is desirable for optimal results. A laxative the night before the examination and a low residue diet the day before the procedure are recommended.

Dosage—The dose for retrograde use in cystography and voiding cystourethrography ranges from 25 to 300 ml. depending on the age of the patient and the degree of bladder irritability; amounts greater than 300 ml. may be used if the bladder capacity allows. Best results are obtained when the bladder is filled with the contrast agent. If desired, the preparation may be diluted with sterile water or sterile saline as indicated below.

Administration—After sterile catheterization, the bladder should be filled to capacity with Cystografin (Diatrizoate Meglumine Injection USP 30%) using a suitable sterile administration set. Care should be taken to avoid using excessive pressure. The presence of bladder discomfort or reflux and/or spontaneous voiding usually indicates that the bladder is full.

Radiography—The commonly employed radiographic techniques should be used. A scout film is recommended before the contrast agent is administered.

Dilution directions—USE DILUTED SOLUTIONS IMMEDIATELY. Use sterile water or sterile saline as a diluent.

Using the **100 ml. bottle:** For a 30% (w/v) diatrizoate meglumine solution, use the 100 ml. bottle undiluted [100 ml. total volume, 14.1% (w/v) organically bound iodine]; for a 24% (w/v) diatrizoate meglumine solution, add 25 ml. diluent to the 100 ml. bottle [125 ml. total volume, 11.3% (w/v) organically bound iodine]; for a 20% (w/v) diatrizoate meglumine solution, add 50 ml. diluent to the 100 ml. bottle [150 ml. total volume, 9.4% (w/v) organically bound iodine]; for an 18% (w/v) diatrizoate meglumine solution, add 67 ml. diluent to the 100 ml. bottle [167 ml. total volume, 8.5% (w/v) organically bound iodine].

Using the **300 ml. bottle:** For a 30% (w/v) diatrizoate meglumine solution, use the 300 ml. bottle undiluted [300 ml. total volume, 14.1% (w/v) organically bound iodine]; for a 25.7% (w/v) diatrizoate meglumine solution, add 50 ml. diluent to the 300 ml. bottle [350 ml. total volume, 12.1% (w/v) organically bound iodine]; for a 22.5% (w/v) diatrizoate meglumine solution, add 100 ml. diluent to the 300 ml. bottle [400 ml. total volume, 10.6% (w/v) organically bound iodine]; for a 20% (w/v) diatrizoate meglumine solution, add 150 ml. diluent to the 300 ml. bottle [450 ml. total volume, 9.4% (w/v) organically bound iodine]; for an 18% (w/v) diatrizoate meglumine solution, add 200 ml. diluent to the 300 ml. bottle [500 ml. total volume, 8.5% (w/v) organically bound iodine].

How Supplied: Cystografin (Diatrizoate Meglumine Injection USP 30%) is available in 200 ml. and 500 ml. bottles containing 100 ml. and 300 ml. diatrizoate meglumine respectively with sufficient capacity for dilution up to 167 ml. and 500 ml. respectively.

Storage: Store at room temperature; protect from light.

DIATRIZOATE MEGLUMINE INJECTION USP 76% ℞

Not Indicated for Use in Selective Coronary Arteriography.

Description: Diatrizoate Meglumine Injection USP 76% is a radiopaque contrast agent supplied in vials as a sterile, aqueous solution for parenteral administration. Each ml. provides 760 mg. diatrizoate meglumine with 3.2 mg. sodium citrate as a buffer and 0.4 mg. edetate disodium as a sequestering agent. *Each ml. of solution also contains approximately 0.91 mg. (0.04 mEq.) sodium* and 358 mg. organically bound iodine. At the time of manufacture, the air in the container is replaced by nitrogen.

Clinical Pharmacology: Following intravascular injection, Diatrizoate Meglumine Injection USP 76% is rapidly transported through the bloodstream to the kidneys and is excreted unchanged in the urine by glomerular filtration. When urinary tract obstruction is severe enough to block glomerular filtration, the agent appears to be excreted by the tubular epithelium.

Renal accumulation is sufficiently rapid so that the period of maximal opacification of the renal passages may begin as early as 5 minutes after injection. In infants and small children excretion takes place somewhat more promptly than in adults, so that maximal opacification occurs more rapidly and is less sustained. The normal kidney eliminates the contrast medium almost immediately. In nephropathic conditions, particularly when excretory capacity has been altered, the rate of excretion varies unpredictably, and opacification may be delayed for 30 minutes or more after injection; with severe impairment opacification may not occur. Generally, however, the medium is concentrated in sufficient amounts and promptly enough to permit a thorough evaluation of the anatomy and physiology of the urinary tract. After intramuscular injection, the contrast agent is promptly absorbed and normally reaches the renal passages within 20 to 60 minutes.

Intravascular injection of diatrizoate meglumine also opacifies those vessels in the path of flow of the medium, permitting visualization until the circulating blood dilutes the concentration of the medium. Thus selective angiography may be performed following injection directly into veins or arteries.

Indications: Diatrizoate Meglumine Injection USP 76% is indicated in excretion urography, aortography, pediatric angiocardiography, and peripheral arteriography.

Contraindications: This preparation is contraindicated in patients with a hypersensitivity to salts of diatrizoic acid. Urography is contraindicated in patients with anuria.

Warnings: A definite risk exists in the use of intravascular contrast agents in patients who are known to have multiple myeloma. In such instances there has been anuria resulting in progressive uremia, renal failure and eventually death. Although neither the contrast agent nor dehydration has separately proved to be the cause of anuria in myeloma, it has been speculated that the combination of both may be the causative factor. The risk in myelomatous patients is not a contraindication to the procedures; however, partial dehydration in the preparation of these patients for the examination is not recommended since this may predispose to the precipitation of myeloma protein in the renal tubules. No form of therapy, including dialysis, has been successful in reversing this effect. Myeloma, which occurs most commonly in persons over age 40, should be considered before intravascular administration of a contrast agent.

Administration of radiopaque materials to patients known or suspected to have pheochromocytoma should be performed with extreme caution. If, in the opinion of the physician, the possible benefits of such procedures outweigh the considered risks, the procedures may be performed; however, the amount of radiopaque medium injected should be kept to an absolute minimum. The blood pressure should be assessed throughout the procedure and measures for treatment of a hypertensive crisis should be available.

The inherent risks of angiocardiography in cyanotic infants and patients with chronic pulmonary emphysema must be weighed against the necessity for performing this procedure. In pediatric angiocardiography, a dose of 10 to 20 ml. may be particularly hazardous in infants weighing less than 7 kg. This risk is probably significantly increased if these infants have preexisting right heart "strain," right heart failure, and effectively decreased or obliterated pulmonary vascular beds.

Contrast media have been shown to promote the phenomenon of sickling in individuals who are homozygous for sickle cell disease when the material is injected intravenously or intra-arterially.

Urography can be performed with extreme caution in patients with severe concomitant hepatic and renal disease.

Since iodine-containing contrast agents may alter the results of thyroid function tests, such tests, if indicated, should be performed prior to the administration of this preparation.

A history of sensitivity to iodine *per se* or to other contrast agents is not an absolute contraindication to the use of diatrizoate meglumine, but calls for extreme caution in administration.

Precautions: Diagnostic procedures which involve the use of radiopaque contrast agents should be carried out under the direction of

Continued on next page

Squibb—Cont.

personnel with the prerequisite training and with a thorough knowledge of the particular procedure to be performed (see ADVERSE REACTIONS).

Severe, life-threatening reactions suggest hypersensitivity to the radiopaque agent, which has prompted the use of several pretesting methods, none of which can be relied upon to predict severe reactions. Many authorities question the value of any pretest. A history of bronchial asthma or allergy, a family history of allergy, or a previous reaction to a contrast agent warrant special attention. Such a history, by suggesting histamine sensitivity and a consequent proneness to reactions, may be more accurate than pretesting in predicting the likelihood of a reaction, although not necessarily the severity or type of reaction in the individual case.

The sensitivity test most often performed is the slow injection of 0.5 to 1.0 ml. of the radiopaque medium, administered intravenously, prior to injection of the full diagnostic dose. It should be noted that the absence of a reaction to the test dose does not preclude the possibility of a reaction to the full diagnostic dose. If the test dose causes an untoward response of any kind, the necessity for continuing with the examination should be carefully reevaluated, and if it is deemed essential, the examination should be conducted with all possible caution. In rare instances reactions to the test dose itself may be extremely severe; therefore, close observation of the patient and facilities for emergency treatment appear indicated.

Renal toxicity has been reported in a few patients with liver dysfunction who were given oral cholecystographic agents followed by urographic agents. Administration of Diatrizoate Meglumine Injection USP 76% should therefore be postponed in any patient with a known or suspected hepatic or biliary disorder who has recently taken a cholecystographic contrast agent.

Caution should be exercised with the use of radiopaque media in severely debilitated patients and in those with marked hypertension. The possibility of thrombosis should be borne in mind when percutaneous techniques are employed.

Consideration must be given to the functional ability of the kidneys before injecting diatrizoate meglumine.

Contrast agents may interfere with some chemical determinations made on urine specimens; therefore, urine should be collected before administration of the contrast medium or two or more days afterwards.

The following precautions pertain to specific procedures:

Excretion urography: Adequate visualization may be difficult or impossible to attain in uremic patients or others with severely impaired renal function (see CONTRAINDICATIONS).

Acute renal failure has been reported in diabetic patients with diabetic nephropathy and susceptible nondiabetic patients (often elderly with preexisting renal disease) following excretion urography. Therefore, careful consideration should be given before performing this procedure in these patients.

Aortography: Repeated intra-aortic injections may be hazardous.

Pediatric angiocardiography: Repeated injections may be hazardous particularly in infants weighing less than 7 kg. (see WARNINGS).

Peripheral arteriography: Hypotension or moderate decreases in blood pressure seem to occur frequently with intra-arterial (brachial) injections; therefore, the blood pressure should be monitored during the immediate ten minutes after injection; this blood pressure change is transient and usually requires no treatment.

Usage in Pregnancy: The safety of diatrizoate meglumine for use during pregnancy has not been established; therefore, this preparation should be used in pregnant patients only when, in the judgment of the physician, its use is deemed essential to the welfare of the patient.

Adverse Reactions: Adverse reactions accompanying the use of iodine-containing intravascular contrast agents are usually mild and transient although severe and life-threatening reactions, including fatalities, have occurred. Because of the possibility of severe reactions to the procedure and/or the radiopaque medium, appropriate emergency facilities and well-trained personnel should be available to treat both conditions. Emergency facilities and personnel should remain available for 30 to 60 minutes following the procedure since severe delayed reactions have been known to occur.

Nausea, vomiting, flushing, or a generalized feeling of warmth are the reactions seen most frequently with intravascular injection. Symptoms which may occur are chills, fever, sweating, headache, dizziness, pallor, weakness, severe retching and choking, wheezing, a rise or fall in blood pressure, facial or conjunctival petechiae, urticaria, pruritus, rash and other eruptions, edema, cramps, tremors, itching, sneezing, lacrimation, etc. Antihistaminic agents may be of benefit; rarely such reactions may be severe enough to require discontinuation of dosage.

Although local tissue tolerance is usually good, there have been a few reports of a burning or stinging sensation or numbness and of venospasm or venous pain, and partial collapse of the injected vein. Neutropenia or thrombophlebitis may occur.

Severe reactions which may require emergency measures, may take the form of a cardiovascular reaction characterized by peripheral vasodilatation with resultant hypotension and reflex tachycardia, dyspnea, agitation, confusion, and cyanosis progressing to unconsciousness. Or, the histamine-liberating effect of these compounds may induce an allergic-like reaction which may range in severity from rhinitis or angioneurotic edema to laryngeal or bronchial spasm or anaphylactoid shock.

Temporary renal shutdown or other nephropathy may occur.

Adverse reactions may sometimes occur as a consequence of the procedure for which the contrast agent is used. Adverse reactions in **excretion urography** have included cardiac arrest, ventricular fibrillation, anaphylaxis with severe asthmatic reaction, and flushing due to generalized vasodilatation In **aortography**, the risks of procedures include injury to the aorta and neighboring organs, pleural puncture, renal damage including infarction and acute tubular necrosis with oliguria and anuria, accidental selective filling of the right renal artery during the translumbar procedure in the presence of preexistent renal disease, retroperitoneal hemorrhage from the translumbar approach, spinal cord injury and pathology associated with the syndrome of transverse myelitis, generalized petechiae, and death following hypotension, arrhythmia, and anaphylactoid reactions. Adverse reactions in **pediatric angiocardiography** have included arrhythmia and death. During **peripheral arteriography,** complications have occurred including hemorrhage from the puncture site, thrombosis of the vessel, and brachial plexus palsy following axillary artery injections.

Dosage and Administration: Diatrizoate Meglumine Injection USP 76% should be at body temperature when injected, and may need to be warmed before use. If kept in a syringe for prolonged periods before injection, it should be protected from exposure to strong light. Syringes should be rinsed as soon as possible after injection to prevent freezing of the plunger.

Withdrawal of the contrast agent should be accomplished under aseptic conditions with sterile needle and syringe.

Excretion Urography: Appropriate preparation of the patient is desirable for optimal results. A laxative the night before the examination, a low residue diet the day before, and low liquid intake for 12 hours prior to the procedure may be used to clear the gastrointestinal tract and to induce a partial dehydration which is believed to increase the urinary concentration of the contrast medium. Enemas are to be avoided to prevent rehydration.

Preparatory partial dehydration is not recommended in infants, young children, the elderly, or azotemic patients (especially those with polyuria, oliguria, diabetes, advanced vascular disease, or preexisting dehydration). The undesirable dehydration in these patients may be accentuated by the osmotic action of the medium.

In uremic patients partial dehydration is not necessary and maintenance of adequate fluid intake is particularly desirable.

The usual intravenous dose for patients aged 16 years or more is 20 ml., but 30 ml. and 40 ml. have been used. Children require less in proportion to weight: Under 6 months of age — 4 ml.; 6 to 12 months — 6 ml.; 1 to 2 years — 8 ml.; 2 to 5 years — 10 ml.; 5 to 7 years — 12 ml.; 8 to 10 years — 14 ml.; 11 to 15 years — 16 ml.

The preparation is given by intravenous injection. If flushing or nausea occurs during administration, injection should be slowed or briefly interrupted until the side effects have disappeared.

A scout film should be made before the contrast medium is administered. To allow for individual variation, several films should be exposed beginning approximately 5 minutes after injection. In patients with renal dysfunction, optimal visualization may be delayed until 30 minutes or more after injection.

NOTE: In infants and children and in certain adults, the medium may be injected intramuscularly. The suggested dose is the same as the intravenous dose, divided and given bilaterally in the gluteal muscles. Radiographs should be taken at 20, 40, and 60 minutes after the medium is injected.

Aortography: Diatrizoate Meglumine Injection USP 76% injected into the aorta by the translumbar or retrograde method of administration permits radiographic visualization of the aorta, its major branches and the abdominal arteries. An incidental nephrogram is obtained as the contrast medium travels through the renal vasculature, provided it has been injected above the renal artery.

Patients should be prepared in a manner similar to that used for intravenous urography. Premedication with a suitable barbiturate is generally indicated.

As in any form of surgery, certain hazards accompany aortographic procedures (see ADVERSE REACTIONS).

For adults and children over 16 years of age, the usual dose is 15 to 40 ml. as a single injection, repeated if indicated. Children require less in proportion to weight. Doses up to a total of 160 ml. have been given safely.

Since the medium is given by rapid injection in this procedure, patients should be watched for untoward reactions during the injection. Unless general anesthesia is employed, patients should be warned that they may feel some transient pain or burning during the injection followed by a feeling of warmth immediately afterward.

A scout film should be made before the contrast agent is administered. The first radiogram should be taken as the last few ml. of the contrast medium are being injected.

Pediatric Angiocardiography: Angiocardiography with Diatrizoate Meglumine Injection USP 76% may be performed by injection into a large peripheral vein or by direct catheterization of the heart. An excretory urogram can be obtained 10 to 15 minutes after injection of the contrast medium since it is concentrated in and eliminated by the kidneys.

Patients should be prepared in a manner similar to that used for intravenous urography. Appropriate preanesthetic medication should be given.

Clinical studies in man, and related animal experiments, have suggested that the hypertonicity of diatrizoate contrast agents produces significant hemodynamic effects, especially in right-sided injections. Large volumes of such agents cause a drop in peripheral arterial and systemic pressures and cardiac output, a rise in pulmonary arterial and right-heart pressures, bradycardia, and regular ectopic beats. Resulting effects on peripheral arterial and pulmonary arterial pressures are postulated to be due to mechanical blockage of the pulmonary vascular bed and clumping of red cells.

Hypertonic solutions cause a decrease in hematocrit *in vitro* and *in vivo* and shrinkage of red blood cells.

It is suggested that hemodynamic changes be monitored and that pressures considered abnormal under roentgenographic conditions be allowed to return to a preangiographic level before continuation of radiopaque injection; this usually takes 15 minutes.

The suggested single dose for children *under* 5 years of age is 10 to 20 ml., depending on the size of the child. For children 5 to 10 years of age, single doses of 20 to 30 ml. are recommended. Doses up to a total of 100 ml. have been given safely.

Since the contrast medium is given by rapid injection, the patient should be watched for untoward reactions during the injection. Some patients not under general anesthesia may experience a feeling of bodily warmth, tightness of the chest and throbbing headache. All these sensations are of short duration. Transient nausea and vomiting may occur in some patients.

A preliminary control film should be made in the usual manner.

Peripheral Arteriography: Appropriate preparation of the patient is indicated, including suitable premedication. For visualization of an entire extremity, a single dose of 20 to 40 ml. is suggested; for the upper or lower half of the extremity only, 10 to 20 ml. is usually sufficient.

Injection is made into the femoral or subclavian artery by the percutaneous or operative method. Because the contrast agent is given by rapid injection, flushing of the skin may occur. Patients not under general anesthesia may experience nausea and vomiting or a transient feeling of warmth. Vascular spasm is not likely to occur.

A scout film should be made routinely before administering the contrast medium. Radiograms of the upper half of the extremity are taken while the last few ml. are being injected, followed by radiograms of the lower half of the extremity a few seconds later.

How Supplied: Diatrizoate Meglumine Injection USP 76% is available in 20 ml. and 50 ml. single-dose vials. An excess volume (1 ml.) is available in each container for sensitivity testing.

Storage: The preparation should be stored at room temperature, protected from light. If precipitation or solidification has occurred due to storage in the cold, immerse the container in hot water and shake intermittently to redissolve any solids.

GASTROGRAFIN® ℞

(Diatrizoate Meglumine and Diatrizoate Sodium Solution USP)

Description: Gastrografin is a water-soluble, oral radiopaque medium for radiographic examination of the gastrointestinal tract. Each ml. contains 660 mg. diatrizoate meglumine and 100 mg. diatrizoate sodium. Each 30 ml. contains approximately 11 g. organically bound iodine (367 mg./ml.).

Clinical Pharmacology: Gastrografin is an oral contrast medium for the radiographic examination of the gastrointestinal tract; it is water-soluble, of medium viscosity, and provides uniform radiopacity; it is not absorbed from the gastrointestinal tract in significant amounts; it is nonirritating, well tolerated and, unlike barium, it is relatively nontoxic when accidentally introduced into body cavities; it is palatable, readily miscible with gastrointestinal fluids and with blood and it is not affected by retained food particles. Because it is not particulate, there is no hazard of inspissation.

Indications and Usage: Gastrografin is indicated for radiography of the gastrointestinal tract following oral or rectal administration. The preparation is particularly indicated where the use of barium is not feasible or is potentially dangerous.

Contraindications: This preparation is contraindicated in patients with a hypersensitivity to salts of diatrizoic acid.

Warnings: A history of sensitivity to iodine *per se* or to contrast media other than salts of diatrizoic acid is not an absolute contraindication to the use of Gastrografin but calls for extreme caution in administration.

Iodine-containing contrast agents may alter the results of thyroid function tests; therefore, if such tests are indicated, they should be performed prior to the administration of Gastrogafin (Diatrizoate Meglumine and Diatrizoate Sodium Solution USP).

Precautions: Oral administration in children may cause a decrease in circulating plasma volume due to osmosis when the contrast agent passes through the stomach and small intestine. In the very young child (weighing less than 21 lbs.) and the debilitated child, the loss of plasma fluid may be sufficient to cause a shock-like state which, if left untreated, could be life-threatening. This hazard can be avoided by dilution of the contrast medium with water before administration, and by the adequate hydration of the child before and after the procedure. The same considerations may possibly apply in elderly cachectic individuals as well.

The possibility of accidental aspiration into the trachea or into a tracheoesophageal fistula following ingestion or instillation, which could result in serious pulmonary complications (e.g., pulmonary edema or pneumonitis) even though the medium may be promptly expectorated, should be kept in mind.

Consideration should be given to the potential for precipitation of water-soluble contrast agents under conditions that may promote hyperacidity (i.e., fasting, emotional upset, or stress). Harmful effects directly attributable to precipitate formation have not been reported. However, the possibility of interpreting the precipitate radiologically as an anatomical abnormality (i.e., ulceration of the stomach or small intestine) or injury, should be kept in mind.

Usage in Pregnancy—Safety for use during pregnancy has not been established; therefore, the preparation should be used in pregnant patients only when, in the judgment of the physician, its use is deemed essential to the welfare of the patient.

Adverse Reactions: Orally administered salts of diatrizoic acid are usually well tolerated.

Occasionally, some degree of diarrhea may be encountered due to the osmotic activity of the preparation when it is used as an enema. In young children fluids should be administered intravenously or by clysis to prevent dehydration.

Dosage and Administration: Not for parenteral use.

Preparation of the patient: The routine preparatory measures employed for barium studies are also indicated for Gastrografin. Adequate preparation is desirable for optimal results.

Dosage: Adult oral dosage may range from 30 to 90 ml., depending on the nature of the examination and the size of the patient. For infants and children up to 5 years of age, 30 ml. are usually adequate; for children 5 to 10 years of age, the suggested dose is 60 ml.

For the very young child (weighing less than 21 lbs.) and the debilitated child, *the dose should be diluted:* 1 part Gastrografin in 3 parts water is recommended. For other infants and children, the dose may be diluted 1:1, if desired, with water, carbonated beverages, milk or mineral oil. A 1:1 dilution is also recommended when the contrast medium is used in elderly cachectic individuals.

The preparation should also be diluted when it is used for enemas and enterostomy instillations. When used as an enema, the suggested dilution for adults is 240 ml. in 1,000 ml. of tap water. For children under 5 years of age, a 1:5 dilution in tap water is suggested; for children over 5 years of age, 90 ml. in 500 ml. of tap water is a suitable dilution.

Administration: Gastrografin (Diatrizoate Meglumine and Diatrizoate Sodium Solution USP) may be ingested directly or given by tube. When used in infants, it may be given in a nursing bottle.

How Supplied: As an aqueous, flavored solution in bottles of 120 ml. [V.A. Depot Item, NSN6505-01-008-3323A.]

Storage: Store at room temperature; avoid excessive heat.

KINEVAC® ℞

(Sincalide for Injection)

Description: Kinevac is a sterile, lyophilized, white powder of the synthetic C-terminal octapeptide of cholecystokinin. Each vial provides 5 mcg. sincalide with 45 mg. sodium chloride as a carrier; sodium hydroxide or hydrochloric acid may be added during manufacture to adjust the pH to 5.5 to 6.5. When reconstituted with 5 ml. of Sterile Water for Injection USP, each ml. contains 1 mcg. sincalide and 9 mg. sodium chloride. At the time of manufacture, the air in the vial is replaced by nitrogen.

Actions: When injected intravenously, sincalide produces a substantial reduction in gallbladder size by causing this organ to contract. The evacuation of bile that results is similar to that which occurs physiologically in response to endogenous cholecystokinin. The intravenous (bolus) administration of sincalide causes a prompt contraction of the gallbladder that becomes maximal in 5 to 15 minutes, as compared with the stimulus of a fatty meal which causes a progressive contraction that becomes maximal after approximately 40 minutes. Generally, a 40 percent reduction in radiographic area of the gallbladder is considered satisfactory contraction.

Like cholecystokinin, sincalide, when given in conjunction with secretin stimulates pancreatic secretion; concurrent administration increases the volume of pancreatic secretion and the output of bicarbonate and protein (enzymes) by the gland. This combined effect of secretin and sincalide permits the assessment of specific pancreatic function through measurement and analysis of the duodenal aspirate. The parameters usually determined are: volume of the secretion; bicarbonate concentration; and amylase content (which parallels the content of trypsin and total protein).

Indications: Kinevac (Sincalide for Injection) is a diagnostic agent which may be used: (1) to provide a sample of gallbladder bile that may be aspirated from the duodenum for analysis of its composition, e.g., to determine the degree of cholesterol saturation, (2) in conjunction with secretin (see DOSAGE AND ADMINISTRATION) to stimulate pancreatic secretion

Continued on next page

Squibb—Cont.

for analysis of its composition and examination of cytology, e.g., in suspected cancer of the pancreas, (3) for postevacuation cholecystography, where the physician deems this procedure indicated but wishes to avoid the fatty meal.

Contraindications: The preparation is contraindicated in patients sensitive to sincalide.

Warnings:

Usage in Pregnancy: Although no teratogenic or antifertility effects were seen in animal studies, data are inadequate to determine the safety of sincalide in human pregnancy. Accordingly, sincalide should be used in pregnant women only when, in the judgment of the physician, the benefits outweigh the possible risk to the fetus.

Usage in Children: The safety of sincalide for use in children has not been established.

Precautions: The possiblity exists that stimulation of gallbladder contraction in patients with small gallbladder stones could lead to the evacuation of the stones from the gallbladder, resulting in their lodging in the cystic duct or in the common bile duct. The risk of such an event is considered to be minimal because sincalide, when given as directed, does not ordinarily cause complete contraction of the gallbladder.

Adverse Reactions: Gastrointestinal symptoms such as abdominal discomfort or pain, and an urge to defecate, frequently accompany the injection of sincalide. These phenomena are usually manifestations of the physiologic action of the drug, which include delayed gastric emptying and increased intestinal motility, and are not to be construed as necessarily indicating an abnormality of the biliary tract unless there is other clinical or radiologic evidence of disease. Nausea, dizziness, and flushing occur occasionally.

Dosage and Administration: For prompt contraction of the gallbladder, a dose of 0.02 mcg. sincalide per kg. (1.4 mcg. per 70 kg.) is injected intravenously over a 30- to 60-second interval; if satisfactory contraction of the gallbladder does not occur in 15 minutes, a second dose, 0.04 mcg. sincalide per kg., may be administered. When Kinevac (Sincalide for Injection) is used in cholecystography, roentgenograms are usually taken at five-minute intervals after the injection. For visualization of the cystic duct, it may be necessary to take roentgenograms at one-minute intervals during the first five minutes after the injection.

For the Secretin-Kinevac test of pancreatic function, the patient receives a dose of 0.25 units secretin per kg. infused intravenously over a 60-minute period. Thirty minutes after the initiation of the secretin infusion, a separate I.V. infusion of Kinevac at a total dose of 0.02 mcg. per kg. is administered over a 30-minute interval. For example, the total dose for a 70 kg. patient is 1.4 mcg. of sincalide; therefore, dilute 1.4 ml. of reconstituted Kinevac solution to 30 ml. with Sodium Chloride Injection USP and administer at a rate of 1 ml. per minute.

Reconstitution and Storage: Kinevac (Sincalide for Injection) may be stored at room temperature prior to reconstitution.

To reconstitute, aseptically add 5 ml. of Sterile Water for Injection USP to the vial; the solution may be kept at room temperature and should be used within 24 hours of reconstitution, after which time any unused portion should be discarded.

How Supplied: In vials containing 5 mcg. of sincalide.

MEDOTOPES® ℞
(Radiopharmaceuticals)

Medotopes represent the latest developments in nuclear medicine. They are available only to those physicians who are qualified by training and experience in the safe use and handling of radionuclides and whose experience and training have been approved by the appropriate government agency authorized to license the use of radionuclides. Medotopes are supplied in a variety of forms intended for diagnostic or therapeutic use. (For a partial list of available radiopharmaceutical products see Alphabetical Index by Manufacturer Section of the PDR.)

All Medotopes have appropriate packaging safeguard to protect against unnecessary exposure.

Each order is custom-handled, each delivery custom-routed by Squibb Traffic Service.

For information on preparations currently available, write Medotopes Customer Services. P.O. Box 4000, Princeton, N.J. 08540

ORAGRAFIN® CALCIUM GRANULES ℞
(Ipodate Calcium for Oral Suspension USP)

ORAGRAFIN® SODIUM CAPSULES ℞
(Ipodate Sodium Capsules USP)

Description: Oragrafin Calcium Granules (Ipodate Calcium for Oral Suspension USP) and Oragrafin Sodium Capsules (Ipodate Sodium Capsules USP) are oral radiopaque media for cholangiography and cholecystography. Ipodate *calcium* is available in single-dose foil packets providing 3 g. ipodate calcium as granules dispersed in flavored sucrose. When mixed with water, the granules produce a pleasantly-flavored suspension. Ipodate *sodium* is available in capsules providing 500 mg. ipodate sodium per capsule. The capsules contain FD&C Yellow No. 5 (tartrazine).

The organically bound iodine content of ipodate calcium and ipodate sodium is 61.7% (approximately 1.85 g./packet) and 61.4% (approximately 307 mg./capsule), respectively.

Clinical Pharmacology: Ipodate calcium and ipodate sodium are absorbed from the gastrointestinal tract, excreted by the liver into the bile, and stored and concentrated in the gallbladder. The calcium salt, which is absorbed somewhat faster than the sodium salt, appears in the ducts as early as 30 minutes after ingestion. Optimal concentration of either salt in the hepatic and biliary ducts occurs within one to three hours after ingestion in nearly all cases; rarely, maximal opacification may be delayed for as much as five hours. Adequate opacification of the ducts usually persists for about 45 minutes. The ducts may be visualized in patients who have undergone cholecystectomy.

The gallbladder is optimally opacified approximately 10 hours after ingestion of either salt. Diagnostically adequate filling, however, often takes place within five hours or less after ingestion, particularly with the calcium salt. Thus, studies of ducts and gallbladder may be carried out in as little as five hours when necessary or desirable. In this connection, it should be pointed out that both salts have been administered to unprepared patients as well as to previously prepared patients, with no significant difference in results.

Indications and Usage: Ipodate calcium and ipodate sodium are indicated for cholecystography. They may also be used for cholangiography, although they are not considered the drugs of choice.

Contraindications: Both preparations are contraindicated in patients who are hypersensitive to ipodate salts.

Warnings: A history of sensitivity to iodine *per se* or to other iodinated compounds is not an absolute contraindication to the use of these preparations, but calls for extreme caution in administration.

Usage in Pregnancy—The safety of these preparations for use during pregnancy has not been established; therefore, they should be used in pregnant patients only when, in the judgment of the physician, their use is deemed essential to the welfare of the patient.

Precautions: Increasing the dosage above that recommended increases the possibility of hypotension.

Anuria may result when these preparations are administered to patients with combined renal and hepatic disease or severe renal impairment.

Renal toxicity has been reported in a few patients with liver dysfunction who were given oral cholecystographic agents followed by urographic agents. Administration of urographic agents should therefore be postponed in any patient with a known or suspected hepatic or biliary disorder who has recently taken a cholecystographic contrast agent.

Gastrointestinal disorders which interfere with absorption, liver disorders which interfere with excretion, or obstruction of the biliary duct may result in nonvisualization of the hepatic and biliary ducts and the gallbladder.

Contrast agents may interfere with some chemical determinations made on urine specimens; therefore, urine should be collected before administration of the contrast medium or two or more days afterwards.

Thyroid function tests, if indicated, should be performed prior to the administration of these preparations since iodine-containing contrast agents may alter the results of these tests.

Oragrafin Sodium Capsules (Ipodate Sodium Capsules USP) contain FD&C Yellow No. 5 (tartrazine) which may cause allergic-type reactions (including bronchial asthma) in certain susceptible individuals. Although the overall incidence of FD&C Yellow No. 5 (tartrazine) sensitivity in the general population is low, it is frequently seen in patients who also have aspirin hypersensitivity.

Adverse Reactions: Ipodate calcium and ipodate sodium are usually well tolerated. Unwanted effects such as mild and transient nausea, vomiting, or diarrhea sometimes occur but the incidence can be reduced by restricting the dosage to 3 g. and administering only the granules to patients who may be prone to gastrointestinal reactions. Headache, dysuria, or abdominal pains may occur infrequently as transient disturbances.

Hypersensitivity reactions may include urticaria, serum sickness-like reactions (fever, rash, arthralgia), other skin rashes, and, rarely, anaphylactoid shock. They are more likely to occur in individuals with a history of allergy, asthma, hay fever, or urticaria, and in those who have previously demonstrated hypersensitivity to iodine compounds.

Dosage and Administration: The capsules should be taken with as little water as possible. They may be swallowed in rapid succession or slowly over the course of ½ hour or more, depending on patient preference.

The granules should be stirred vigorously into a small amount of water (¼ glass or less) and swallowed immediately. If lukewarm rather than cold water is used, the patient will find the suspension quite palatable and there will be less likelihood of nausea.

A total dose of 6 g. (12 capsules or two packets of granules) per 24 hour period should not be exceeded.

When an upper gastrointestinal barium study is scheduled, prior administration of either salt will not interfere. Either salt may also be used in conjunction with an intravenous cholangiographic agent.

The recommended dosage and patient preparation for cholangiography and/or cholecystography are as follows:

Routine Cholecystography: On the day before the examination, the patient may, if feasible, eat a high-fat lunch so that the gallbladder will evacuate and refill with opacified bile. The evening meal should be eaten two hours before the contrast medium is taken; there is no need to change the patient's customary diet, whether low-fat or routine. The contrast agent should be administered 10 to 12 hours before the roentgenologic examination. The usual dose is six capsules (providing 3 g. ipodate sodium), although up to 12 capsules may be given; one to two packets of granules may be used instead. No other food or drink except small amounts of water should be taken before the examination. A mild laxative or other cathartic may be given, but is not generally necessary.

Roentgenologic examination of the gallbladder is performed the next morning in the usual manner, employing the standard positions. An immediate study of the wet films will determine any need for repositioning of the patient. Administration of a fat meal or other cholecystokinetic agent provides good dynamic studies of gallbladder function. If a barium meal examination is also to be performed, the fat meal may be given simultaneously with or following the barium meal. Gallbladder function studies are then made after the barium meal examination is completed.

Repeat Examination: To minimize the possibility of diagnostic error, it may be desirable to repeat the study when the initial examination results in nonvisualization or is nondiagnostic. If the repeat examination also results in nonvisualization, gallbladder disease may be inferred although it should be recognized that nonvisualization may be due to other factors (see PRECAUTIONS); also, a small proportion of normal gallbladders may fail to visualize.

Reexamination can be performed on the same day if the usual dose (3 g.) was administered initially; administer 3 g. (one packet) of the granules or, alternatively, 3 g. ipodate sodium (six capsules).

At least five days should intervene between the initial and repeat examinations when the total dose will exceed 6 g.

A total dose of 6 g. per 24-hour period should not be exceeded.

Cholangiography: No prior preparation of the patient is necessary. For this procedure, the granules should be used. They are administered one hour before cholangiography. Although only one packet (providing 3 g. ipodate calcium) may suffice, two packets (6 g.) are usually necessary for visualization of the ducts.

Beginning one hour after ingestion of the granules, and at 15-minute intervals thereafter, films should be taken, preferably with the aid of tomography or laminography. With proper positioning of the patient, residual contrast medium in the gastrointestinal tract is not likely to be a problem, particularly with the more rapidly absorbed calcium salt. Optimal visualization of the ducts is generally achieved between 1½ and 2½ hours after ingestion of the medium.

Combined Cholangiography and Cholecystography: Preparation of the patient and administration of dosage should be as outlined under *Routine Cholecystography*, with a dose of six capsules or, if preferred, one packet of granules taken on the evening before examination. On the following morning, one hour before the examination, one additional packet of granules should be administered.

Beginning one hour after the morning dose, and at 15-minute intervals thereafter, films should be made, preferably with the use of tomography or laminography. While the gallbladder will have concentrated the evening dose of the medium, the additional morning dose will provide opacification of the ducts, and simultaneous visualization may be achieved. When satisfactory films have been obtained, a fat meal may be administered to provide gallbladder function studies.

Rapid Combined Cholangiography and Cholecystography: No prior preparation of the patient is necessary. On the day of examination, the patient should be given two packets of granules. Beginning one hour later, examination of the ducts should be performed as described above under *Cholangiography*. If the gallbladder has not opacified sufficiently by the time the cholangiographic examination is completed, further cholecystograms may be taken after two or three hours. Dynamic studies of gallbladder function may be carried out in the usual manner.

How Supplied: Oragrafin Calcium Granules (Ipodate Calcium for Oral Suspension USP) are supplied in single-dose foil packets providing 3 g. ipodate calcium per packet; boxes of 25 packets.

*Oragrafin Sodium Capsules (Ipodate Sodium Capsules USP) are available for oral use providing 500 mg. ipodate sodium per capsule; boxes of 24 cards (6 capsules per card), bottles of 100, and Unimatic® cartons of 100.

Storage: Store the Granules at room temperature. Store the Capsules at room temperature; avoid excessive heat.

*[*Shown in Product Identification Section*]

RENOGRAFIN®-60 ℞

(Diatrizoate Meglumine and Diatrizoate Sodium Injection USP)

Description: Renografin-60 is a radiopaque contrast agent supplied as a sterile, aqueous solution. Each ml. provides 520 mg. diatrizoate meglumine and 80 mg. diatrizoate sodium with 3.2 mg. sodium citrate, and 0.4 mg. edetate disodium; pH has been adjusted between 7.0 and 7.6 with sodium hydroxide. *Each ml. of solution also contains approximately 3.76 mg. (0.16 mEq.) sodium* and 292.5 mg. organically bound iodine. At the time of manufacture, the air in the container is replaced by nitrogen.

Clinical Pharmacology: Following intravascular injection, Renografin-60 (Diatrizoate Meglumine and Diatrizoate Sodium Injection USP) is rapidly transported through the bloodstream to the kidneys and is excreted unchanged in the urine by glomerular filtration. When urinary tract obstruction is severe enough to block glomerular filtration, the agent appears to be excreted by the tubular epithelium.

Certain applications of the contrast agent make use of the natural physiologic mechanism of excretion. Thus, the intravenous injection of the agent permits visualization of the kidneys and urinary passages.

Renal accumulation is sufficiently rapid that the period of maximal opacification of the renal passages may begin as early as five minutes after injection. In infants and small children excretion takes place somewhat more promptly than in adults, so that maximal opacification occurs more rapidly and is less sustained. The normal kidney eliminates the contrast medium almost immediately. In nephropathic conditions, particularly when excretory capacity has been altered, the rate of excretion varies unpredictably, and opacification may be delayed for 30 minutes or more after injection; with severe impairment opacification may not occur. Generally, however, the medium is concentrated in sufficient amounts and promptly enough to permit a thorough evaluation of the anatomy and physiology of the urinary tract.

After intramuscular injection, the contrast agent is promptly absorbed and normally reaches the renal passages within 20 to 60 minutes.

Intravascular injection of diatrizoate also opacifies those vessels in the path of flow of the medium, permitting visualization until the circulating blood dilutes the concentration of the medium. Thus selective angiography may be performed following injection directly into veins or arteries such as the carotid, the vertebral, or the vessels of the extremities.

Under certain circumstances, specific parts of the body which do not concentrate the contrast agent physiologically may be visualized by injecting the agent directly into the region to be studied. The biliary tract is one organ system which may be visualized in this manner. In operative cholangiography, injection of the radiopaque medium into the cystic duct or choledochal lumen, at laparotomy, opacifies the intra- and extra-hepatic biliary ductal system, revealing the nature and location of obstructions such as stones or strictures. Injection of the medium through an in-place T-tube, immediately after exploration of the common duct, permits the visualization of retained stones. A repetition of "T-tube cholangiography," performed as part of the postoperative follow-up, insures the patency of the ductal system before removal of the T-tube. The biliary ductal system may also be opacified by the percutaneous-transhepatic route. In relatively long-standing biliary obstruction, the biliary ducts are usually enlarged sufficiently to be located promptly by percutaneous transhepatic probing, permitting injection of the contrast agent directly into the biliary ductal system.

If the contrast agent is injected directly into the splenic pulp, significant opacification of the splenic and portal veins is obtained. Because of gravity, the dependent portions of the portal system are better opacified than the superior portions. The agent is carried from the portal vein into the hepatic veins, and a diffuse opacification of the liver results. In patients with portal hypertension, collateral pathways caused by the change in portal blood flow may be visualized and esophageal varices are often delineated. The procedure may reveal the site of portal obstruction.

Injection of Renografin-60 (Diatrizoate Meglumine and Diatrizoate Sodium Injection USP) directly into a joint space provides visual information about joint derangements.

A small amount of the radiopaque agent injected into a normal cervical or lumbar disk will, under optimal conditions, concentrate within the nucleus pulposus. In the presence of disk pathology the injected agent may reveal significant bulging or disruption of the annulus beyond its normal confines and may identify disk degeneration, retropulsion, or rupture.

Computed Tomography—Renografin-60 enhances computed tomographic brain scanning through augmentation of radiographic efficiency. The degree of enhancement of visualization of tissue density is directly related to the iodine content in an administered dose; peak iodine blood levels occur immediately following rapid injection of the dose. These levels fall rapidly within five to ten minutes. This can be accounted for by the dilution in the vascular and extracellular fluid compartments which causes an initial sharp fall in plasma concentration. Equilibration with the extracellular compartments is reached in about ten minutes; thereafter, the fall becomes exponential. Maximum contrast enhancement frequently occurs after peak blood iodine levels are reached. The delay in maximum contrast enhancement can range from five to forty minutes, depending on the peak iodine levels achieved and the cell type of the lesion. This lag suggests that radiographic contrast enhancement is at least in part dependent on the accumulation of iodine within the lesion and outside the blood pool although the mechanism by which this occurs is not clear. The radiographic enhancement of nontumoral lesions, such as arteriovenous malformations and aneurysms, is probably dependent on the iodine content of the circulating blood pool.

Indications: Renografin-60 is indicated in excretion urography (by direct I.V. or drip infusion); cerebral angiography; peripheral arteriography; venography; operative, T-tube, or percutaneous transhepatic cholangiography; splenoportography; arthrography; and discography.

Computed Tomography: Renografin-60 (Diatrizoate Meglumine and Diatrizoate Sodium Injection USP) is also indicated for radiographic contrast enhancement in computed

Continued on next page

Squibb—Cont.

tomography (CT) of the brain. Contrast enhancement is advantageous in delineating or ruling out disease in suspicious areas which may otherwise not have been satisfactorily visualized.

Tumors—Renografin-60 may be useful to demonstrate the presence and extent of certain malignancies such as: gliomas including malignant gliomas, glioblastomas, astrocytomas, oligodendrogliomas and gangliomas; ependymomas; medulloblastomas; meningiomas; neuromas; pinealomas; pituitary adenomas; craniopharyngiomas; germinomas; and metastatic lesions.

The usefulness of contrast enhancement for the investigation of the retrobulbar space and in cases of low grade or infiltrative glioma has not been demonstrated. In cases where lesions have calcified, there is less likelihood of enhancement. Following therapy, tumors may show decreased or no enhancement.

Non-Neoplastic Conditions—The use of Renografin-60 may be beneficial in the enhancement of images of lesions not due to neoplasms. Cerebral infarctions of recent onset may be better visualized with the contrast enhancement, while some infarctions are obscured if a contrast medium is used. The use of Renografin-60 (Diatrizoate Meglumine and Diatrizoate Sodium Injection USP) improved the contrast enhancement in approximately 60 percent of cerebral infarctions studied from one week to four weeks from the onset of symptoms.

Sites of active infection also will produce contrast enhancement following contrast medium administration.

Arteriovenous malformations and aneurysms will show contrast enhancement. In the case of these vascular lesions, the enhancement is probably dependent on the iodine content of the circulating blood pool.

Hematomas and intraparenchymal bleeders seldom demonstrate any contrast enhancement. However, in cases of intraparenchymal clot, for which there is no obvious clinical explanation, contrast medium administration may be helpful in ruling out the possibility of associated arteriovenous malformation.

The opacification of the inferior vermis following contrast medium administration has resulted in false-positive diagnoses in a number of normal studies.

Contraindications: This preparation is contraindicated in patients with a hypersensitivity to salts of diatrizoic acid.

Urography is contraindicated in patients with anuria.

Specific contraindications to **percutaneous transhepatic cholangiography** include a prothrombin time below 50 percent and evidence of coagulation defects.

Splenoportography should not be performed on any patient for whom splenectomy is contraindicated, since complications of the procedure at times make splenectomy necessary. Other contraindications include prothrombin time below 50 percent, significant thrombocytopenia or coagulation defect, and any condition which may increase the possibility of rupture of the spleen.

Arthrography should not be performed if infection is present in or near the joint.

Discography should not be performed in patients with an infection or open injury near the region to be examined.

Warnings: A definite risk exists in the use of intravascular contrast agents in patients who are known to have multiple myeloma. In such instances there has been anuria resulting in progressive uremia, renal failure and eventually death. Although neither the contrast agent nor dehydration has separately proved to be the cause of anuria in myeloma, it has been speculated that the combination of both may be the causative factor. The risk in myelomatous patients is not a contraindication to the procedures; however, partial dehydration in the preparation of these patients for the examination is not recommended since this may predispose to the precipitation of myeloma protein in the renal tubules. No form of therapy, including dialysis, has been successful in reversing this effect. Myeloma, which occurs most commonly in persons over age 40, should be considered before intravascular administration of a contrast agent.

Administration of radiopaque materials to patients known or suspected to have pheochromocytoma should be performed with extreme caution. If, in the opinion of the physician, the possible benefits of such procedures outweigh the considered risks, the procedures may be performed; however, the amount of radiopaque medium injected should be kept to an absolute minimum. The blood pressure should be assessed throughout the procedure and measures for treatment of a hypertensive crisis should be available.

Cerebral angiography should be undertaken with special caution in extreme age, poor clinical condition, advanced arteriosclerosis, severe arterial hypertension, cardiac decompensation, recent cerebral embolism, or thrombosis.

Urography should be performed with extreme caution in patients with severe concomitant hepatic and renal disease.

Contrast media have been shown to promote the phenomenon of sickling in individuals who are homozygous for sickle cell disease when the material is injected intravenously or intra-arterially.

Since iodine-containing contrast agents may alter the results of thyroid function tests, such tests, if indicated, should be performed prior to the administration of this preparation.

A history of sensitivity to iodine *per se* or to other contrast agents is not an absolute contraindication to the use of diatrizoate, but calls for extreme caution in administration.

Avoid accidental introduction of this preparation into the subarachnoid space since even small amounts may produce convulsions and possible fatal reactions.

Precautions: Diagnostic procedures which involve the use of radiopaque contrast agents should be carried out under the direction of personnel with the prerequisite training and with a thorough knowledge of the particular procedure to be performed (see ADVERSE REACTIONS).

Severe, life-threatening reactions suggest hypersensitivity to the radiopaque agent, which has prompted the use of several pretesting methods, none of which can be relied upon to predict severe reactions. Many authorities question the value of any pretest. A history of bronchial asthma or allergy, a family history of allergy, or a previous reaction to a contrast agent warrant special attention. Such a history, by suggesting histamine sensitivity and a consequent proneness to reactions, may be more accurate than pretesting in predicting the likelihood of a reaction, although not necessarily the severity or type of reaction in the individual case.

The sensitivity test most often performed is the slow injection of 0.5 to 1.0 ml. of the radiopaque medium, administered intravenously, prior to injection of the full diagnostic dose. It should be noted that the absence of a reaction to the test dose does not preclude the possibility of a reaction to the full diagnostic dose. If the test dose causes an untoward response of any kind, the necessity for continuing with the examination should be carefully reevaluated and, if it is deemed essential, the examination should be conducted with all possible caution. In rare instances, reactions to the test dose itself may be extremely severe; therefore, close observation of the patient, and facilities for emergency treatment, appear indicated.

Renal toxicity has been reported in a few patients with liver dysfunction who were given oral cholecystographic agents followed by urographic agents. Administration of Renografin-60 (Diatrizoate Meglumine and Diatrizoate Sodium Injection USP) should therefore be postponed in any patient with a known or suspected hepatic or biliary disorder who has recently taken a cholecystographic contrast agent.

Caution should be exercised with the use of radiopaque media in severely debilitated patients and in those with marked hypertension. The possibility of thrombosis should be borne in mind when percutaneous techniques are employed.

Consideration must be given to the functional ability of the kidneys before injecting this preparation.

Contrast agents may interfere with some chemical determinations made on urine specimens; therefore, urine should be collected before administration of the contrast medium or two or more days afterwards.

The following precautions pertain to specific procedures:

Peripheral arteriography: Hypotension or moderate decreases in blood pressure seem to occur frequently with intra-arterial (brachial) injections; therefore, the blood pressure should be monitored during the immediate ten minutes after injection; this blood pressure change is transient and usually requires no treatment.

Excretion urography: Adequate visualization may be difficult or impossible to attain in uremic patients or others with severely impaired renal function (see CONTRAINDICATIONS). The increased osmotic load associated with drip infusion pyelography should be considered in patients with congestive heart failure. The diuretic effect of the drip infusion pyelography procedure may hinder assessment of residual urine in the bladder. The recommended rate of infusion should not be exceeded.

Acute renal failure has been reported in diabetic patients with diabetic nephropathy and susceptible nondiabetic patients (often elderly with preexisting renal disease) following excretion urography. Therefore, careful consideration should be given before performing this procedure in these patients.

Operative and T-tube cholangiography: Injection should be made slowly to prevent extravasation of the medium into the peritoneal cavity, and to minimize reflux flow into the pancreatic duct which may result in pancreatic irritation.

Percutaneous transhepatic cholangiography: To reduce the possibility of bile leakage and consequent peritonitis, as much of the contrast agent as possible should be aspirated on completion of successful films. All patients should be carefully and constantly monitored for 24 hours after the procedure for signs of internal hemorrhage or bile leakage; if these complications are recognized immediately, remedial measures can be instituted promptly with minimal increase in morbidity. Percutaneous transhepatic cholangiography is not without risk and should therefore be reserved for special circumstances when ordinary studies of the biliary system have failed to provide the requisite information in jaundiced patients who are not good candidates for surgery. The procedure should only be attempted when competent surgical intervention can be promptly obtained if needed.

Splenoportography: It is best to avoid manipulations which would prolong the time the needle is in the spleen since they may contribute to subcapsular extravasation of the contrast agent and also to postpuncture bleeding. Following splenoportography, the patient should lie on his left side for several hours and should be closely observed for 24 hours for signs of internal bleeding, which is the most common complication of the procedure. Fatal hemorrhage has occurred on rare occasion, but leakage of up to 300 ml. of blood from the spleen is apparently not uncommon. Blood transfusions may be required, and rarely splenectomy.

Discography: To minimize the possibility of introducing infection, discography should be postponed in any patient with an infection or open injury near the region to be examined, including upper respiratory infections in the case of cervical discography. All possible care should be taken to preclude contamination and resultant infection of the disk, which has been reported after discography. In cervical discography, particular care is needed to avoid puncturing the esophagus and thereby introducing contamination into the disk. Rupture of the disk is highly unlikely if care in performance is observed, but may occur if the point of the needle has been barbed by contact with bone; use of the two-needle technique should help reduce this hazard.

Usage in Pregnancy: Safety for use during pregnancy has not been established; therefore, the preparation should be used in pregnant patients only when, in the judgment of the physician, its use is deemed essential to the welfare of the patient.

Adverse Reactions: Adverse reactions accompanying the use of iodine-containing intravascular contrast agents are usually mild and transient although severe and life-threatening reactions, including fatalities, have occurred. Because of the possibility of severe reactions to the procedure and/or the radiopaque medium, appropriate emergency facilities and well-trained personnel should be available to treat both conditions. Emergency facilities and personnel should remain available for 30 to 60 minutes following the procedure since severe delayed reactions have been known to occur.

Nausea, vomiting, flushing, or a generalized feeling of warmth are the reactions seen most frequently with intravascular injection. Symptoms which may occur are chills, fever, sweating, headache, dizziness, pallor, weakness, severe retching and choking, wheezing, a rise or fall in blood pressure, facial or conjunctival petechiae, urticaria, pruritus, rash and other eruptions, edema, cramps, tremors, itching, sneezing, lacrimation, etc. Antihistaminic agents may be of benefit; rarely such reactions may be severe enough to require discontinuation of dosage.

Severe reactions which may require emergency measures may take the form of a cardiovascular reaction characterized by peripheral vasodilatation with resultant hypotension and reflex tachycardia, dyspnea, agitation, confusion, and cyanosis progressing to unconsciousness. Or, the histamine-liberating effect of these compounds may induce an allergic-like reaction which may range in severity from rhinitis or angioneurotic edema to laryngeal or bronchial spasm or anaphylactoid shock.

Temporary renal shutdown or other nephropathy may occur. Temporary neurologic effects of varying severity have occurred in a few instances, particularly when the medium was used for angiography in the diagnosis of cerebral pathology. Although local tissue tolerance is usually good, there have been a few reports of a burning or stinging sensation or numbness and of venospasm or venous pain, and partial collapse of the injected vein. Neutropenia or thrombophlebitis may occur.

Adverse effects may sometimes occur as a consequence of the procedure for which the contrast agent is used. Adverse reactions in **excretion urography** have included cardiac arrest, ventricular fibrillation, anaphylaxis with severe asthmatic reaction, and flushing due to generalized vasodilation. **Cerebral angiography** has been known to cause temporary neurologic complications such as induction of seizures, particularly in patients with convulsive disorders; confusional states or drowsiness; transient paresis; coma; temporary disturbances in vision; or seventh nerve weakness. During **peripheral arteriography,** complications have occurred including hemorrhage from the puncture site, thrombosis of the vessel, and brachial plexus palsy following axillary artery injections.

Complications of **percutaneous transhepatic cholangiography** have been estimated to occur in four to six percent of cases and have included bile leakage and biliary peritonitis, gallbladder perforation, internal bleeding, septicemia involving gram-negative organisms, and tension pneumothorax from inadvertent puncture of the diaphragm and lung. Bile leakage may be more likely in patients with complete obstruction due to carcinoma.

During **splenoportography,** intraperitoneal extravasation of the contrast medium may cause transient diaphragmatic irritation or mild to moderate transient pain which may sometimes be referred to the shoulder, the periumbilical region, or other areas. Because of the proximity of the pleural cavity, accidental pneumothorax has been known to occur. Inadvertent injection of the medium into other nearby structures is not likely to cause untoward consequences.

Arthrography may induce joint pain or increase existing pain, particularly if a large dose is used and the medium extravasates into surrounding soft tissue. Pain or discomfort is usually immediate and transient but may be delayed or of extended duration (up to 24 hours). Lipid-filled histiocytes have been found in tissue removed following arthrography. The technique of **discography** may be painful, particularly when disk pathology exists. Pain on injection may also be related to the volume of the dose. The nature of the disk pathology or extravasation of contrast agent may cause referred pain.

When any percutaneous technique is employed, the possibility of thrombosis or of other complications due to the mechanical trauma of the procedure should be borne in mind.

Dosage and Administration: Renografin-60 (Diatrizoate Meglumine and Diatrizoate Sodium Injection USP) should be at body temperature when injected and may need to be warmed before use. If kept in a syringe for prolonged periods before injection, it should be protected from exposure to strong light.

Dilution and withdrawal of the contrast agent should be accomplished under aseptic conditions with sterile needle and syringe.

Excretion Urography—Appropriate preparation of the patient is desirable for optimal results. In adults and older children, a laxative the night before the examination, a low residue diet the day before, and low liquid intake for 12 hours prior to the procedure may be used to clear the gastrointestinal tract and to induce a partial dehydration which is believed to increase the urinary concentration of the contrast medium. Preparatory partial dehydration is not recommended in infants, young children, the elderly, or azotemic patients (especially those with polyuria, oliguria, diabetes, advanced vascular disease, or preexisting dehydration). The undesirable dehydration in these patients may be accentuated by the osmotic diuretic action of the medium.

In uremic patients partial dehydration is not necessary and maintenance of adequate fluid intake is particularly desirable.

Direct I.V. Injection—The dose range for adults is 25 to 50 ml.; the usual dose is 25 ml.; children require proportionately less. Suggested dosages are as follows: Under 6 months—5 ml.; 6 to 12 months—8 ml.; 1 to 2 years—10 ml.; 2 to 5 years—12 ml.; 5 to 7 years—15 ml.; 8 to 10 years—18 ml.; 11 to 15 years—20 ml.; adults (16 years and older)—25 to 50 ml. In adults, when the smaller dose has provided inadequate visualization, or when poor visualization is anticipated, the 50 ml. dose may be given. Drip infusion may be used when direct I.V. pyelography is not expected to be or has not been satisfactory (see below).

The preparation is given by intravenous injection. If flushing or nausea occurs during administration, injection should be slowed or briefly interrupted until the side effects have disappeared.

A scout film should be made before the contrast medium is administered. To allow for individual variation, several films should be exposed beginning approximately five minutes after injection. In patients with renal dysfunction, optimal visualization may be delayed until 30 minutes or more after injection.

NOTE: In infants and children and in certain adults, the medium may be injected intramuscularly. The suggested dose is 25 ml. for adults and proportionately less for children, divided and given bilaterally in the gluteal muscles. Radiographs should be taken at 20, 40, and 60 minutes after the medium is injected.

Drip Infusion Pyelography—In drip infusion pyelography, the recommended dose of Renografin-60 is calculated on the basis of 1 ml. of Renografin-60 (Diatrizoate Meglumine and Diatrizoate Sodium Injection USP) per pound of body weight diluted with an equal volume of Sterile Water for Injection USP. The diluted preparation (30%) is given by I.V. infusion through a large bore (17- to 18-gauge) needle at a rate of 40 ml. per minute. The recommended rate of infusion should not be exceeded and the total volume administered should generally not exceed 300 ml. In older patients and in patients with known or suspected cardiac decompensation, a slower rate of infusion is probably wise.

If nausea or flushing occurs during administration, the infusion should be slowed or briefly interrupted.

Films are taken before the onset of the infusion and at the desired intervals following its completion. When renal function is normal, a nephrogram may be taken as soon as the infusion is completed, and films of the collecting system at 10 and 20 minutes thereafter. Voiding cystourethrograms are usually optimal at 20 minutes after the infusion is completed. In hypertensive patients, early minute sequence films may be taken during the course of infusion, in addition to subsequent pyelograms. In patients with renal dysfunction, optimal visualization is usually delayed, and late films are taken as indicated.

The nephrogram obtained by the drip infusion procedure may be dense enough to obscure the pelvocalyceal system in some cases. The presence of gas in the bowel may hamper early visualization of the renal collecting system. Tomographic "cuts" may help to overcome such difficulties.

Nephrotomography may begin when the infusion is completed. The sustained contrast achieved by the drip infusion technique eliminates the need for precise timing and teamwork that is necessary with ordinary nephrotomography. Thus, if nephrograms taken after infusion of the medium suggest the need for sectional films, or if preselected tomographic "cuts" are not sufficient, additional tomograms may be obtained at once, and without repetition of dosage.

Cerebral Angiography—Appropriate preparation of the patient is indicated, including suitable premedication. The average single dose for adults is 10 ml. repeated as indicated. Children require less in proportion to weight.

Either the percutaneous or operative method of administration may be used. For visualization of the cerebral vessels, the contrast medium is injected into the common carotid artery; for angiography of the vessels in the posterior fossa or the occipital lobes, the medium is injected into the vertebral artery. Since the

Continued on next page

Squibb—Cont.

medium is given by rapid injection, the patient should be watched for untoward reactions. Unless general anesthesia is used, patients should be warned that the medium may provoke movement and that they may feel transient pain, flushing, or burning during the injection.
A scout film should be made routinely before the contrast medium is injected. Serial films begun while the last few ml. are being injected should permit visualization of the arterial, intermediate, and venous phases.
Peripheral Arteriography—Appropriate preparation of the patient is indicated, including suitable premedication. For visualization of an entire extremity, a single dose of 20 to 40 ml. is suggested; for the upper or lower half of the extremity only, 10 to 20 ml. is usually sufficient.
Injection is made into the femoral or subclavian artery by the percutaneous or operative method. Because the contrast agent is given by rapid injection, flushing of the skin may occur. Patients not under general anesthesia may experience nausea and vomiting or a transient feeling of warmth. Vascular spasm is not likely to occur.
A scout film should be made routinely before administering the contrast medium. Radiograms of the upper half of the extremity are taken while the last few ml. are being injected, followed by radiograms of the lower half of the extremity a few seconds later.
Venography—For visualization of veins in the upper extremities, a single dose of 10 ml. per extremity is suggested. For veins in the lower extremities, doses of 20 to 40 ml. per extremity are suggested. In exceptional circumstances, larger doses may be necessary; visualization of the iliac vein, extensive varicosities or large veins may require 50 ml. or more. Total doses up to 100 ml. per lower extremity have been used safely.
For visualization of an upper extremity, the medium may be given by percutaneous injection into any convenient superficial vein of the forearm or hand. For the visualization of a lower extremity it should be injected into a superficial vein on the lateral side of the foot. The medium is injected rapidly; patients should be observed for untoward reactions.
Radiograms are taken when injection is completed; sufficient time should be allowed to permit diffusion of the contrast medium.
Operative and Postoperative Cholangiography—Operative cholangiography is performed as soon as the gallbladder and ducts have been exposed surgically. The usual dose is 10 ml. but as much as 25 ml. may be needed, depending on the caliber of the ducts. If desired, the contrast agent may be diluted 1:1 with Sodium Chloride Injection USP under strict aseptic procedures. The contrast medium is instilled slowly through the stump of the cystic duct or directly into the choledochal lumen. Following surgical exploration of the ductal system, repeat studies may be performed before closure of the abdomen, using the same dose as before.
Postoperatively, the ductal system may be examined by injection of the contrast agent through an in-place T-tube. "T-tube cholangiography" is usually performed eight to ten days after operation; the usual dose is the same as for operative cholangiography.
For each procedure, films are taken immediately after instillation of the medium and are read immediately. Additional films are then taken if necessary.
Percutaneous Transhepatic Cholangiography—Facilities for emergency surgery should be available whenever this examination is performed. Appropriate premedication of the patient is recommended; drugs which are likely to cause spasm, such as morphine, should be avoided.
Depending on the caliber of the biliary tree, a dose of 20 to 40 ml. is generally sufficient to opacify the entire ductal system. The contrast agent may be diluted 1:1 with Sodium Chloride Injection USP, if desired, under strict aseptic procedures.
Injection is made into a biliary duct by the percutaneous transhepatic method. Before the dose is administered, as much bile as possible is aspirated. The medium is then slowly injected into the duct under very slight pressure. If a duct is not located promptly, successive small doses of 1 to 2 ml. are injected into the liver as the needle is gradually withdrawn, until a duct is visualized by x-ray. If no duct can be located after three or four attempts, the procedure is abandoned.
Serial films are taken rapidly during and after injection of the medium into the biliary ducts. Repositioning of the patient, if necessary, should be done with care.
In hepatocellular disease, the biliary ducts are generally not enlarged and cannot successfully be opacified by this method. Thus, in the presence of long-standing jaundice, failure to obtain a successful percutaneous transhepatic cholangiogram by a person experienced in the technique is generally considered to be strongly suggestive of nonobstructive or hepatocellular-type jaundice.
Splenoportography—Prior gastrointestinal x-ray examination should include particular attention to the lower esophageal area. A hematologic survey, including prothrombin time and platelet count, should be performed. The patient should have no food for several hours and should be mildly sedated. Splenoportography is usually performed under local anesthesia.
Approximately 20 to 25 ml. of the contrast agent is usually adequate. The dose is injected rapidly, following radiologic location and percutaneous puncture of the spleen.
Preliminary films are taken to locate the spleen before the injection is begun. Rapid serial films are then started simultaneously with injection of the dose. Serial films are necessary since the entire portal system cannot be captured on a single film and also because of individual variations in portal circulation time.
Arthrography—The amount of contrast agent required is dependent on the size of the joint to be injected. For an adult, the following doses are generally suitable: Knee—5 to 15 ml.; shoulder or hip—5 to 10 ml.; other joints—1 to 4 ml. Dosage for children should be suitably reduced.
The injection site should be prepared aseptically. Excessive synovial fluid should be aspirated to minimize pain and to reduce intra-articular dilution of the contrast agent. If indicated, the agent may be administered under local anesthesia. After injection of the medium, the joint should be manipulated gently in order to spread the medium throughout the joint space. In some instances, double contrast arthrography, injecting both air and contrast medium, has been of value.
Films are taken from several angles; stereoscopic films may be advantageous.
When the contrast agent is used to opacify a joint space, much of the agent may be aspirated at the end of the procedure.
Discography—No prior preparation of the patient is required although administration of an analgesic or sedative 20 minutes before the procedure may be helpful. Discography is performed under local anesthesia using the usual aseptic precautions.
Dosage is generally determined by the amount of contrast agent which can easily be injected into the disk without force. A cervical disk will normally accept up to 0.5 ml. and a lumbar disk 1 or 2 ml. The amount may vary, and injection should be discontinued when resistance is felt. The rate of injection may influence the amount which can be injected. To reduce the probability of extravasation and to minimize unnecessary pain, injection should be made slowly and not more than 2 ml. should be injected into any one disk.
A two-needle technique may be used to administer the contrast medium, with a large-gauge needle to locate the disk and a small-gauge needle within the larger one to puncture the disk and administer the medium. The correct position of the two needles is established radiologically before the medium is injected.
Spot roentgenograms should be taken anteroposteriorly, obliquely, and laterally as soon as disks have been injected.
When the contrast agent is used for discography, it need not be aspirated at the end of the procedure.
Computed Tomography—The suggested dose range is 50 to 100 ml. by intravenous administration; scanning may be performed immediately after completion of administration. Doses for children should be proportionately less, depending on age and weight.
Patient Preparation—No special patient preparation is required for contrast enhancement of CT brain scanning. However, it is advisable to insure that patients are well hydrated prior to examination.
How Supplied: Single dose vials of 10, 30, 50, and 100 ml., and in single dose bottles of 100 ml. An excess volume (1 ml.) is available in each container for sensitivity testing. [50 ml. vials—Military Depot Item, NSN6505-00-135-2600, V.A. Depot Item, NSN6505-00-135-2600A.]
Storage: The preparation should be stored at room temperature, protected from light. If precipitation or solidification has occurred due to storage in the cold, immerse the container in hot water and shake intermittently to redissolve any solids.

RENOGRAFIN®-76 ℞
(Diatrizoate Meglumine and Diatrizoate Sodium Injection USP)

Description: Renografin-76 is a radiopaque contrast agent for parenteral use supplied as a sterile, aqueous solution. Each ml. provides 660 mg. diatrizoate meglumine and 100 mg. diatrizoate sodium with 3.2 mg. sodium citrate as a buffer and 0.4 mg. edetate disodium as a sequestering agent; pH has been adjusted to 7.0 to 7.6 with sodium hydroxide. *Each ml. of solution also contains approximately 4.48 mg. (0.19 mEq.) sodium* and 370 mg. organically bound iodine. At the time of manufacture, the air in the container is replaced by nitrogen
Clinical Pharmacology: Following intravascular injection, Renografin-76 is rapidly transported through the bloodstream to the kidneys and is excreted unchanged in the urine by glomerular filtration. When urinary tract obstruction is severe enough to block glomerular filtration, the agent appears to be excreted by the tubular epithelium.
Renal accumulation is sufficiently rapid so that the period of maximal opacification of the renal passages may begin as early as five minutes after injection. In infants and small children, excretion takes place somewhat more promptly than in adults, so that maximal opacification occurs more rapidly and is less sustained. The normal kidney eliminates the contrast medium almost immediately. In nephropathic conditions, particularly when excretory capacity has been altered, the rate of excretion varies unpredictably, and opacification may be delayed for 30 minutes or more after injection; with severe impairment opacification may not occur. Generally, however, the medium is concentrated in sufficient amounts and promptly enough to permit a thorough evaluation of the anatomy and physiology of the urinary tract.
After intramuscular injection, the contrast agent is promptly absorbed and normally reaches the renal passages within 20 to 60 minutes.

Intravascular injection of diatrizoate also opacifies those vessels in the path of flow of the medium, permitting visualization until the circulating blood dilutes the concentration of the medium. Thus selective angiography may be performed following injection directly into veins or arteries.

Computed Tomography—Renografin-76 (Diatrizoate Meglumine and Diatrizoate Sodium Injection USP) enhances computed tomographic brain scanning through augmentation of radiographic efficiency. The degree of enhancement of visualization of tissue density is directly related to the iodine content in an administered dose; peak iodine blood levels occur immediately following rapid injection of the dose. These levels fall rapidly within five to ten minutes. This can be accounted for by the dilution in the vascular and extracellular fluid compartments which causes an initial sharp fall in plasma concentration. Equilibration with the extracellular compartments is reached in about ten minutes; thereafter, the fall becomes exponential. Maximum contrast enhancement frequently occurs after peak blood iodine levels are reached. The delay in maximum contrast enhancement can range from five to forty minutes, depending on the peak iodine levels achieved and the cell type of the lesion. This lag suggests that radiographic contrast enhancement is at least in part dependent on the accumulation of iodine within the lesion and outside the blood pool although the mechanism by which this occurs is not clear.
The radiographic enhancement of nontumoral lesions, such as arteriovenous malformations and aneurysms, is probably dependent on the iodine content of the circulating blood pool.

Indications: Renografin-76 is indicated in excretion urography, aortography, pediatric angiocardiography, peripheral arteriography, selective renal arteriography, selective visceral arteriography, selective coronary arteriography, and selective coronary arteriography combined with left ventriculography.

Computed Tomography—Renografin-76 is also indicated for radiographic contrast enhancement in computed tomography (CT) of the brain. Contrast enhancement is advantageous in delineating or ruling out disease in suspicious areas which may otherwise not have been satisfactorily visualized.

Tumors—Renografin-76 may be useful to demonstrate the presence and extent of certain malignancies such as: gliomas including malignant gliomas, glioblastomas, astrocytomas, oligodendrogliomas and gangliomas; ependymomas; medulloblastomas; meningiomas; neuromas; pinealomas; pituitary adenomas; craniopharyngiomas; germinomas; and metastatic lesions.

The usefulness of contrast enhancement for the investigation of the retrobulbar space and in cases of low grade or infiltrative glioma has not been demonstrated.

In cases where lesions have calcified, there is less likelihood of enhancement. Following therapy, tumors may show decreased or no enhancement.

Non-Neoplastic Conditions—The use of Renografin-76 (Diatrizoate Meglumine and Diatrizoate Sodium Injection USP) may be beneficial in the enhancement of images of lesions not due to neoplasms. Cerebral infarctions of recent onset may be better visualized with the contrast enhancement, while some infarctions are obscured if a contrast medium is used. The use of Renografin-76 (Diatrizoate Meglumine and Diatrizoate Sodium Injection USP) improved the contrast enhancement in approximately 60 percent of cerebral infarctions studied from one week to four weeks from the onset of symptoms.

Sites of active infection also will produce contrast enhancement following contrast medium administration.

Arteriovenous malformations and aneurysms will show contrast enhancement. In the case of these vascular lesions, the enhancement is probably dependent on the iodine content of the circulating blood pool.

Hematomas and intraparenchymal bleeders seldom demonstrate any contrast enhancement. However, in cases of intraparenchymal clot, for which there is no obvious clinical explanation, contrast medium administration may be helpful in ruling out the possibility of associated arteriovenous malformation.

The opacification of the inferior vermis following contrast medium administration has resulted in false-positive diagnoses in a number of normal studies.

Contraindications: This preparation is contraindicated in patients with a hypersensitivity to salts of diatrizoic acid.

Urography is contraindicated in patients with anuria.

Warnings: A definite risk exists in the use of intravascular contrast agents in patients who are known to have multiple myeloma. In such instances there has been anuria resulting in progressive uremia, renal failure and eventually death. Although neither the contrast agent nor dehydration has separately proved to be the cause of anuria in myeloma, it has been speculated that the combination of both may be the causative factor. The risk in myelomatous patients is not a contraindication to the procedures; however, partial dehydration in the preparation of these patients for the examination is not recommended since this may predispose to the precipitation of myeloma protein in the renal tubules. No form of therapy, including dialysis, has been successful in reversing this effect. Myeloma, which occurs most commonly in persons over age 40, should be considered before intravascular administration of a contrast agent.

Administration of radiopaque materials to patients known or suspected to have pheochromocytoma should be performed with extreme caution. If, in the opinion of the physician, the possible benefits of such procedures outweigh the considered risks, the procedures may be performed; however, the amount of radiopaque medium injected should be kept to an absolute minimum. The blood pressure should be assessed throughout the procedure and measures for treatment of a hypertensive crisis should be available.

The inherent risks of *angiocardiography* in cyanotic infants and patients with chronic pulmonary emphysema must be weighed against the necessity for performing this procedure. In *pediatric angiocardiography,* a dose of 10 to 20 ml. may be particularly hazardous in infants weighing less than 7 kg. This risk is probably significantly increased if these infants have preexisting right heart "strain," right heart failure, and effectively decreased or obliterated pulmonary vascular beds.

Urography should be performed with extreme caution in patients with severe concomitant hepatic and renal disease.

Selective visceral arteriography should be performed with extreme caution in patients with severe generalized atherosclerosis, specifically with plaques or aneurysms at the level of the iliac or femoral arteries.

Selective coronary arteriography should be performed only in selected patients and those in whom the expected benefits outweigh the procedural risk.

Contrast media have been shown to promote the phenomenon of sickling in individuals who are homozygous for sickle cell disease when the material is injected intravenously or intra-arterially.

Since iodine-containing contrast agents may alter the results of thyroid function tests, such tests, if indicated, should be performed prior to the administration of this preparation.

A history of sensitivity to iodine *per se* or to other contrast agents is not an absolute contraindication to the use of diatrizoate, but calls for extreme caution in administration.

Precautions: Diagnostic procedures which involve the use of radiopaque contrast agents should be carried out under the direction of personnel with the prerequisite training and with a thorough knowledge of the particular procedure to be performed (see ADVERSE REACTIONS).

Severe, life-threatening reactions suggest hypersensitivity to the radiopaque agent, which has prompted the use of several pretesting methods, none of which can be relied upon to predict severe reactions. Many authorities question the value of any pretest. A history of bronchial asthma or allergy, a family history of allergy, or a previous reaction to a contrast agent warrant special attention. Such a history, by suggesting histamine sensitivity and a consequent proneness to reactions, may be more accurate than pretesting in predicting the likelihood of a reaction although not necessarily the severity or type of reaction in the individual case.

The sensitivity test most often performed is the slow injection of 0.5 to 1.0 ml. of the radiopaque medium, administered intravenously, prior to injection of the full diagnostic dose. It should be noted that the absence of a reaction to the test dose does not preclude the possibility of a reaction to the full diagnostic dose. If the test dose causes an untoward response of any kind, the necessity for continuing with the examination should be carefully reevaluated and, if it is deemed essential, the examination should be conducted with all possible caution. In rare instances, reactions to the test dose itself may be extremely severe; therefore, close observation of the patient and facilities for emergency treatment appear indicated.

Renal toxicity has been reported in a few patients with liver dysfunction who were given oral cholecystographic agents followed by urographic agents. Administration of Renografin-76 (Diatrizoate Meglumine and Diatrizoate Sodium Injection USP) should therefore be postponed in any patient with a known or suspected hepatic or biliary disorder who has recently taken a cholecystographic contrast agent.

Caution should be exercised with the use of radiopaque media in severely debilitated patients and in those with marked hypertension. The possibility of thrombosis should be borne in mind when percutaneous techniques are employed.

Consideration must be given to the functional ability of the kidneys before injecting this preparation.

Contrast agents may interfere with some chemical determinations made on urine specimens; therefore, urine should be collected before administration of the contrast medium or two or more days afterwards.

The following precautions pertain to specific procedures:

Excretion urography: Adequate visualization may be difficult or impossible to attain in uremic patients or others with severely impaired renal function (see CONTRAINDICATIONS).

Acute renal failure has been reported in diabetic patients with diabetic nephropathy and susceptible nondiabetic patients (often elderly with preexisting renal disease) following excretion urography. Therefore, careful consideration should be given before performing this procedure in these patients.

Aortography: Repeated intra-aortic injections may be hazardous.

Pediatric angiocardiography: Repeated injections may be hazardous particularly in infants weighing less than 7 kg. (see WARNINGS).

Peripheral arteriography: Hypotension or moderate decreases in blood pressure seem to

Continued on next page

Squibb—Cont.

occur frequently with intra-arterial (brachial) injections; therefore, the blood pressure should be monitored during the immediate ten minutes after injection; this blood pressure change is transient and usually requires no treatment.

Selective coronary arteriography: It is recommended that the procedure should not be performed for approximately four weeks following the diagnosis of myocardial infarction. Mandatory prerequisites to the procedure are experienced personnel, ECG monitoring apparatus, and adequate facilities for immediate resuscitation and cardioversion.

Usage in Pregnancy: Safety for use during pregnancy has not been established; therefore, this preparation should be used in pregnant patients only when, in the judgment of the physician, its use is deemed essential to the welfare of the patient.

Adverse Reactions: Adverse reactions accompanying the use of iodine-containing intravascular contrast agents are usually mild and transient although severe and life-threatening reactions, including fatalities, have occurred. Because of the possibility of severe reactions to the procedure and/or the radiopaque medium, appropriate emergency facilities and well-trained personnel should be available to treat both conditions. Emergency facilities and personnel should remain available for 30 to 60 minutes following the procedure since severe delayed reactions have been known to occur.

Nausea, vomiting, flushing, or a generalized feeling of warmth are the reactions seen most frequently with intravascular injection. Symptoms which may occur are chills, fever, sweating, headache, dizziness, pallor, weakness, severe retching and choking, wheezing, a rise or fall in blood pressure, facial or conjunctival petechiae, urticaria, pruritus, rash and other eruptions, edema, cramps, tremors, itching, sneezing, lacrimation, etc. Antihistaminic agents may be of benefit; rarely, such reactions may be severe enough to require discontinuation of dosage.

Although local tissue tolerance is usually good, there have been a few reports of a burning or stinging sensation or numbness and of venospasm or venous pain, and partial collapse of the injected vein. Neutropenia or thrombophlebitis may occur.

Severe reactions which may require emergency measures may take the form of a cardiovascular reaction characterized by peripheral vasodilatation with resultant hypotension and reflex tachycardia, dyspnea, agitation, confusion, and cyanosis progressing to unconsciousness. Or, the histamine-liberating effect of these compounds may induce an allergic-like reaction which may range in severity from rhinitis or angioneurotic edema to laryngeal or bronchial spasm or anaphylactoid shock.

Temporary renal shutdown or other nephropathy may occur.

Adverse reactions may sometimes occur as a consequence of the procedure for which the contrast agent is used. Adverse reactions in *excretion urography* have included cardiac arrest, ventricular fibrillation, anaphylaxis with severe asthmatic reaction, and flushing due to generalized vasodilatation. In *aortography,* the risks of procedures include injury to the aorta and neighboring organs, pleural puncture, renal damage including infarction and acute tubular necrosis with oliguria and anuria, accidental selective filling of the right renal artery during the translumbar procedure in the presence of preexistent renal disease, retroperitoneal hemorrhage from the translumbar approach, spinal cord injury and pathology associated with the syndrome of transverse myelitis, generalized petechiae, and death following hypotension, arrhythmia, and anaphylactoid reactions. Adverse reactions in *pediatric angiocardiography* have included arrhythmia and death. During *peripheral arteriography,* complications have occurred including hemorrhage from the puncture site, thrombosis of the vessel, and brachial plexus palsy following axillary artery injections. During *selective coronary arteriography* and *selective coronary arteriography combined with left ventriculography,* most patients will have transient ECG changes. Transient arrhythmias may occur infrequently. Ventricular fibrillation may result from manipulation of the catheter during the procedure or administration of the medium. Other reactions may include hypotension, chest pain, and myocardial infarction. Transient elevation of CPK (creatine phosphokinase) has occurred in approximately 30 percent of the patients tested. Fatalities have been reported. Complications due to the procedure include hemorrhage, thrombosis, pseudoaneurysms at the puncture site, and dislodgment of arteriosclerotic plaques. Dissection of the coronary vessels and transient sinus arrest have occurred rarely.

Adverse reactions in *selective renal arteriography* include nausea, vomiting, hypotension and hypertension. Post-arteriographic changes in laboratory studies include transient elevations in BUN, serum creatinine and glucose.

Complications due to the procedure during *selective visceral arteriography* include hematomas, thrombosis, pseudoaneurysms at injection site, and dislodgment of arteriosclerotic plaques. Other reactions may include urticaria, hypotension, hypertension, and insignificant changes in renal function and liver chemistry tests.

Dosage and Administration: Renografin-76 (Diatrizoate Meglumine and Diatrizoate Sodium Injection USP) should be at body temperature when injected, and may need to be warmed before use. Syringes should be rinsed as soon as possible after injection to prevent freezing of the plunger.

Withdrawal of the contrast agent should be accomplished under aseptic conditions with sterile needle and syringe.

Excretion Urography

Appropriate preparation of the patient is desirable for optimal results. A laxative the night before the examination, a low residue diet the day before, and low liquid intake for 12 hours prior to the procedure may be used to clear the gastrointestinal tract and to induce a partial dehydration which is believed to increase the urinary concentration of the contrast medium. Enemas are to be avoided to prevent rehydration.

Preparatory partial dehydration is not recommended in infants, young children, the elderly, or azotemic patients (especially those with polyuria, oliguria, diabetes, advanced vascular disease, or preexisting dehydration). The undesirable dehydration in these patients may be accentuated by the osmotic diuretic action of the medium.

In uremic patients partial dehydration is not necessary and maintenance of adequate fluid intake is particularly desirable.

The usual intravenous dose for patients aged 16 years or more is 20 ml., but 30 or 40 ml. have been used. Children require less in proportion to weight: Under 6 months of age—4 ml.; 6 to 12 months—6 ml.; 1 to 2 years—8 ml.; 2 to 5 years—10 ml.; 5 to 7 years—12 ml.; 8 to 10 years—14 ml.; 11 to 15 years—16 ml.

The preparation is given by intravenous injection. If flushing or nausea occurs during administration, injection should be slowed or briefly interrupted until the side effects have disappeared.

A scout film should be made before the contrast medium is administered. To allow for individual variation, several films should be exposed beginning approximately five minutes after injection. In patients with renal dysfunction, optimal visualization may be delayed until 30 minutes or more after injection.

NOTE: In infants and children and in certain adults, the medium may be injected intramuscularly. The suggested dose is the same as the intravenous dose divided and given bilaterally in the gluteal muscles. Radiographs should be taken at 20, 40, and 60 minutes after the medium is injected.

Aortography

Renografin-76 (Diatrizoate Meglumine and Diatrizoate Sodium Injection USP) injected into the aorta by the translumbar or retrograde method of administration permits radiographic visualization of the aorta, its major branches and the abdominal arteries. An incidental nephrogram is obtained as the contrast medium travels through the renal vasculature, provided it has been injected above the renal artery.

Patients should be prepared in a manner similar to that used for intravenous urography. Premedication with a suitable barbiturate is generally indicated.

As in any form of surgery, certain hazards accompany aortographic procedures (see ADVERSE REACTIONS).

For adults and children over 16 years of age, the usual dose is 15 to 40 ml. as a single injection, repeated if indicated. Children require less in proportion to weight. Doses up to a total of 160 ml. have been given safely.

Since the medium is given by rapid injection in this procedure, patients should be watched for untoward reactions during the injection. Unless general anesthesia is employed, patients should be warned that they may feel some transient pain or burning during the injection followed by a feeling of warmth immediately afterward.

A scout film should be made before the contrast agent is administered. The first radiogram should be taken as the last few ml. of the contrast medium are being injected.

Pediatric Angiocardiography

Angiocardiography with Renografin-76 (Diatrizoate Meglumine and Diatrizoate Sodium Injection USP) may be performed by injection into a large peripheral vein or by direct catheterization of the heart. An excretory urogram can be obtained 10 to 15 minutes after injection of the contrast medium since it is concentrated in and eliminated by the kidneys.

Patients should be prepared in a manner similar to that used for intravenous urography. Appropriate preanesthetic medication should be given.

Clinical studies in man and related animal experiments have suggested that the hypertonicity of diatrizoate contrast agents produces significant hemodynamic effects, especially in right-sided injections. Large volumes of such agents cause a drop in peripheral arterial and systemic pressures and cardiac output, a rise in pulmonary arterial and right-heart pressures, bradycardia, and regular ectopic beats. Resulting effects on peripheral arterial and pulmonary arterial pressures are postulated to be due to mechanical blockage of the pulmonary vascular bed and clumping of red cells.

Hypertonic solutions cause a decrease in hematocrit *in vitro* and *in vivo,* and shrinkage of red blood cells.

It is suggested that hemodynamic changes be monitored and that pressures considered abnormal under roentgenographic conditions be allowed to return to a preangiographic level before continuation of radiopaque injection; this usually takes 15 minutes.

The suggested single dose for children *under* five years of age is 10 to 20 ml., depending on the size of the child. For children 5 to 10 years of age, single doses of 20 to 30 ml. are recommended. Doses up to a total of 100 ml. have been given safely.

Since the contrast medium is given by rapid injection, the patient should be watched for untoward reactions during the injection. Some

patients not under general anesthesia may experience a feeling of bodily warmth, tightness of the chest and throbbing headache. All these sensations are of short duration. Transient nausea and vomiting may occur in some patients.
A preliminary control film should be made in the usual manner.

Peripheral Arteriography
Appropriate preparation of the patient is indicated, including suitable premedication. For visualization of an entire extremity, a single dose of 20 to 40 ml. is suggested; for the upper or lower half of the extremity only, 10 to 20 ml. is usually sufficient.
Injection is made into the femoral or subclavian artery by the percutaneous or operative method. Because the contrast agent is given by rapid injection, flushing of the skin may occur. Patients not under general anesthesia may experience nausea and vomiting or a transient feeling of warmth. Vascular spasm is not likely to occur.
A scout film should be made routinely before administering the contrast medium. Radiograms of the upper half of the extremity are taken while the last few ml. are being injected, followed by radiograms of the lower half of the extremity a few seconds later.

Selective Renal Arteriography
The usual dose is 5 to 10 ml. injected into either or both renal arteries via femoral artery catheterization. This dose may be repeated as necessary; doses up to 60 ml. have been given.

Selective Visceral Arteriography
The usual dose is 30 to 50 ml. injected into the appropriate visceral artery (celiac axis and its branches, superior mesenteric artery, or inferior mesenteric artery) via femoral artery catheterization. This may be repeated as necessary. It is recommended that the combined total dose not exceed 250 ml.

Selective Coronary Arteriography
The usual dose is 4 to 10 ml. injected into a coronary artery. This dose, repeated as necessary, may be administered into each coronary artery; doses up to a total of 150 ml. have been given. Patients should be monitored continuously by ECG throughout the procedure.

Selective Coronary Arteriography Combined with Left Ventriculography
For left ventriculography the usual dose is 35 to 50 ml. injected into the left ventricle. This may be repeated as necessary. It is recommended that the total dose for combined selective coronary arteriography and left ventriculography not exceed 200 ml.

Computed Tomography
The suggested dose is 50 to 125 ml. by intravenous administration; scanning may be performed immediately after completion of administration. Doses for children should be proportionately less, depending on age and weight.
Patient Preparation—No special patient preparation is required for contrast enhancement of CT brain scanning. However, it is advisable to insure that patients are well hydrated prior to examination.
How Supplied: Single dose vials of 20 ml. and 50 ml. and single dose bottles of 100 ml. and 200 ml. An excess volume (1 ml.) is available in each container for sensitivity testing. [50 ml. vials—Military Depot Item, NSN6505-01-103-8583 and V.A. Depot Item, NSN6505-00-159-5008A; 200 ml. bottle—V.A. Depot Item, NSN6505-00-138-7344A].
Storage: The preparation should be stored at room temperature, protected from light. If precipitation or solidification has occurred due to storage in the cold, immerse the container in hot water and shake intermittently to redissolve any solids.

RENO-M-30® ℞
(Diatrizoate Meglumine Injection USP 30%)
For retrograde pyelography
Not intended for intravascular injection

Description: Reno-M-30 is a radiopaque contrast agent for retrograde pyelography supplied as a sterile, aqueous solution. Each ml. provides 300 mg. diatrizoate meglumine with 3.2 mg. sodium citrate as a buffer, 0.4 mg. edetate disodium as a sequestering agent, and 1 mg. methylparaben and 0.3 mg. propylparaben as preservatives. Each ml. of solution also contains approximately 141 mg. organically bound iodine. At the time of manufacture, the air in the container is replaced by nitrogen.
Indications: Reno-M-30 (Diatrizoate Meglumine Injection USP 30%) is intended for retrograde or ascending pyelography. This procedure may be used if intravenous excretion urography is contraindicated and it is also useful in complementing other diagnostic information.
Contraindications: Contraindications pertain to the procedure of retrograde pyelography rather than to the administration of the medium *per se.* Retrograde pyelography should not be performed in those conditions which do not allow for the successful catheterizaton of the ureters such as extensive urinary tuberculosis, tumors of the bladder, impassable obstructions of the ureters, or marked enlargement of the prostate gland.
Warning: Apart from the possible adverse effects of diatrizoate meglumine, the hazards of the performance of a retrograde genitourinary procedure exist. These include such complications as hematuria, perforation of the ureter or bladder, introduction of infection into the genitourinary tract, and oliguria or anuria.
Precautions: Because of the possibility of inducing temporary suppression of urine, it is wise to avoid repetition of retrograde pyelography within 48 hours in patients with reduced renal function.
Retrograde pyelography should be performed with caution in patients with a known active infectious process of the urinary tract.
Contrast agents may interfere with some chemical determinations made on urine specimens; therefore, urine should be collected before administration of the contrast medium or two or more days afterwards.
Adverse Reactions: The incidence of adverse reactions with diatrizoate meglumine is very low. Costovertebral angle tenderness, elevated temperature and flank pain have been reported in a few patients following use of the preparation for retrograde pyelography, as have nausea, sweating and flushing.
Irritation of the urinary tract mucosa attributable to the contrast agent itself is not likely to occur. However, the technique of retrograde pyelography may be painful and may initiate pelvic, caliceal, or ureteral spasms with consequent renal colic.
Since retrograde pyelography does not involve systemic administration of a contrast agent, the risk of severe reactions, which may occur with intravenous administration, is extremely remote. However, they should be kept in mind whenever a contrast agent is administered. Severe reactions may be manifested by edema of the face and glottis, respiratory distress, convulsions, or shock; such reactions may prove fatal unless promptly controlled by such emergency measures as maintenance of a clear airway and immediate use of oxygen and resuscitative drugs. Like other sensitivity phenomena, severe reactions are more likely to occur in patients with a personal or family history of bronchial asthma, significant allergies, drug reactions, or previous reactions to contrast agents.
Dosage and Administration: Preparation of the patient: Appropriate preparation is desirable for optimal results. A laxative the night before the examination and a low residue diet the day before the procedure are recommended.
Dosage: The usual dose for patients aged 16 years or more is 15 ml. for unilateral and appropriately increased volumes for bilateral pyelograms. Approximately 5 to 6 ml. will generally be required for each exposure. The dosage for children should be proportionately smaller than the adult dose.
As supplied, the preparation provides maximum opacification. If a lesser contrast is desired, it may be diluted with sterile distilled water.
Administration: Reno-M-30 (Diatrizoate Meglumine Injection USP 30%) may be introduced by a gravity flow system or by syringe. When the syringe method is used, the injection should be made slowly and care should be exercised to use as little manual pressure as possible. Regardless of the system used, injection of the contrast medium should be terminated as soon as the patient complains of a sense of fullness or pain in the renal region.
Radiography: The commonly employed radiographic techniques should be used. A scout film is recommended before the contrast agent is administered.
How Supplied: Available in multiple-dose vials of 50 ml. and 100 ml.
Storage: The preparation should be protected from strong light and stored at room temperature; avoid freezing.

RENO-M-60® ℞
(Diatrizoate Meglumine Injection USP 60%)

Description: Reno-M-60 is a radiopaque contrast agent supplied as a sterile, aqueous solution for parenteral use. Each ml. provides 600 mg. diatrizoate meglumine with 3.2 mg. sodium citrate as a buffer and 0.4 mg. edetate disodium as a sequestering agent; pH has been adjusted between 6.5 and 7.7 with meglumine or diatrizoic acid. *Each ml. of solution also contains appoximately 0.91 mg. (0.04 mEq.) sodium* and 282 mg. organically bound iodine. At the time of manufacture, the air in the container is replaced by nitrogen.
Clinical Pharmacology: Following intravascular injection, Reno-M-60 (Diatrizoate Meglumine Injection USP 60%) is rapidly transported through the bloodstream to the kidneys and is excreted unchanged in the urine by glomerular filtration. When urinary tract obstruction is severe enough to block glomerular filtration, the agent appears to be excreted by the tubular epithelium.
Certain applications of the contrast agent make use of the natural physiologic mechanism of excretion. Thus, the intravenous injection of the agent permits visualization of the kidneys and urinary passages.
Renal accumulation is sufficiently rapid that the period of maximal opacification of the renal passages may begin as early as five minutes after injection. In infants and small children excretion takes place somewhat more promptly than in adults, so that maximal opacification occurs more rapidly and is less sustained. The normal kidney eliminates the contrast medium almost immediately. In nephropathic conditions, particularly when excretory capacity has been altered, the rate of excretion varies unpredictably, and opacification may be delayed for 30 minutes or more after injection; with severe impairment opacification may not occur. Generally, however, the medium is concentrated in sufficient amounts and promptly enough to permit a thorough evaluation of the anatomy and physiology of the urinary tract.
After intramuscular injection, the contrast agent is promptly absorbed and normally reaches the renal passages within 20 to 60 minutes.
Intravascular injection of diatrizoate meglumine also opacifies those vessels in the path of

Continued on next page

Squibb—Cont.

flow of the medium, permitting visualization until the circulating blood dilutes the concentration of the medium. Thus selective angiography may be performed following injection directly into veins or arteries such as the carotid, the vertebral, or the vessels of the extremities.

Under certain circumstances, specific parts of the body which do not concentrate the contrast agent physiologically may be visualized by injecting the agent directly into the region to be studied. The biliary tract is one organ system which may be visualized in this manner. In operative cholangiography, injection of the radiopaque medium into the cystic duct or choledochal lumen, at laparotomy, opacifies the intra- and extra-hepatic biliary ductal system, revealing the nature and location of obstructions such as stones or strictures. Injection of the medium through an in-place T-tube, immediately after exploration of the common duct, permits the visualization of retained stones. A repetition of "T-tube cholangiography," performed as part of the postoperative follow-up, insures the patency of the ductal system before removal of the T-tube. The biliary ductal system may also be opacified by the percutaneous-transhepatic route. In relatively long-standing biliary obstruction, the biliary ducts are usually enlarged sufficiently to be located promptly by percutaneous transhepatic probing, permitting injection of the contrast agent directly into the biliary ductal system.

If the contrast agent is injected directly into the splenic pulp, significant opacification of the splenic and portal veins is obtained. Because of gravity, the dependent portions of the portal system are better opacified than the superior portions. The agent is carried from the portal vein into the hepatic veins, and a diffuse opacification of the liver results. In patients with portal hypertension, collateral pathways caused by the change in portal blood flow may be visualized and esophageal varices are often delineated. The procedure may reveal the site of portal obstruction.

Injection of Reno-M-60 (Diatrizoate Meglumine Injection USP 60%) directly into a joint space provides visual information about joint derangements.

A small amount of the radiopaque agent injected into a normal cervical or lumbar disk will, under optimal conditions, concentrate within the nucleus pulposus. In the presence of disk pathology the injected agent may reveal significant bulging or disruption of the annulus beyond its normal confines and may identify disk degeneration, retropulsion, or rupture.

Indications: Reno-M-60 (Diatrizoate Meglumine Injection USP 60%) is indicated in excretion urography (by direct I.V. or drip infusion); cerebral angiography; peripheral arteriography; venography; operative, T-tube, or percutaneous transhepatic cholangiography; splenoportography; arthrography; and discography.

Contraindications: This preparation is contraindicated in patients with a hypersensitivity to salts of diatrizoic acid.

Urography is contraindicated in patients with anuria.

Specific contraindications to **percutaneous transhepatic cholangiography** include a prothrombin time below 50 percent and evidence of coagulation defects.

Splenoportography should not be performed on any patient for whom splenectomy is contraindicated since complications of the procedure at times make splenectomy necessary. Other contraindications include prothrombin time below 50 percent, significant thrombocytopenia or coagulation defect, and any condition which may increase the possibility of rupture of the spleen.

Arthrography should not be performed if infection is present in or near the joint.

Discography should not be performed in patients with an infection or open injury near the region to be examined.

Warnings: A definite risk exists in the use of intravascular contrast agents in patients who are known to have multiple myeloma. In such instances there has been anuria resulting in progressive uremia, renal failure, and eventually death. Although neither the contrast agent nor dehydration has separately proved to be the cause of anuria in myeloma, it has been speculated that the combination of both may be the causative factor. The risk in myelomatous patients is not a contraindication to the procedures; however, partial dehydration in the preparation of these patients for the examination is not recommended since this may predispose to the precipitation of myeloma protein in the renal tubules. No form of therapy, including dialysis, has been successful in reversing this effect. Myeloma, which occurs most commonly in persons over age 40, should be considered before intravascular administration of a contrast agent.

Administration of radiopaque materials to patients known or suspected to have pheochromocytoma should be performed with extreme caution. If, in the opinion of the physician, the possible benefits of such procedures outweigh the considered risks, the procedures may be performed; however, the amount of radiopaque medium injected should be kept to an absolute minimum. The blood pressure should be assessed throughout the procedure and measures for treatment of a hypertensive crisis should be available.

Cerebral angiography should be undertaken with special caution in extreme age, poor clinical condition, advanced arteriosclerosis, severe arterial hypertension, cardiac decompensation, recent cerebral embolism, or thrombosis.

Urography should be performed with extreme caution in patients with severe concomitant hepatic and renal disease.

Contrast media have been shown to promote the phenomenon of sickling in individuals who are homozygous for sickle cell disease when the material is injected intravenously or intra-arterially.

Since iodine-containing contrast agents may alter the results of thyroid function tests, such tests, if indicated, should be performed prior to the administration of this preparation.

A history of sensitivity to iodine *per se* or to other contrast agents is not an absolute contraindication to the use of diatrizoate meglumine, but calls for extreme caution in administration.

Avoid accidental introduction of this preparation into the subarachnoid space since even small amounts may produce convulsions and possible fatal reactions.

Precautions: Diagnostic procedures which involve the use of radiopaque contrast agents should be carried out under the direction of personnel with the prerequisite training and with a thorough knowledge of the particular procedure to be performed (see ADVERSE REACTIONS).

Severe, life-threatening reactions suggest hypersensitivity to the radiopaque agent, which has prompted the use of several pretesting methods, none of which can be relied upon to predict severe reactions. Many authorities question the value of any pretest. A history of bronchial asthma or allergy, a family history of allergy, or a previous reaction to a contrast agent warrant special attention. Such a history, by suggesting histamine sensitivity and a consequent proneness to reactions, may be more accurate than pretesting in predicting the likelihood of a reaction, although not necessarily the severity or type of reaction in the individual case.

The sensitivity test most often performed is the slow injection of 0.5 to 1.0 ml. of the radiopaque medium, administered intravenously, prior to injection of the full diagnostic dose. It should be noted that the absence of a reaction to the test dose does not preclude the possibility of a reaction to the full diagnostic dose. If the test dose causes an untoward response of any kind, the necessity for continuing with the examination should be carefully reevaluated and, if it is deemed essential, the examination should be conducted with all possible caution. In rare instances, reactions to the test dose itself may be extremely severe; therefore, close observation of the patient, and facilities for emergency treatment, appear indicated.

Renal toxicity has been reported in a few patients with liver dysfunction who were given oral cholecystographic agents followed by urographic agents. Administration of Reno-M-60 (Diatrizoate Meglumine Injection USP 60%) should therefore be postponed in any patient with a known or suspected hepatic or biliary disorder who has recently taken a cholecystographic contrast agent.

Caution should be exercised with the use of radiopaque media in severely debilitated patients and in those with marked hypertension. The possibility of thrombosis should be borne in mind when percutaneous techniques are employed.

Consideration must be given to the functional ability of the kidneys before injecting diatrizoate meglumine.

Contrast agents may interfere with some chemical determinations made on urine specimens; therefore, urine should be collected before administration of the contrast medium or two or more days afterwards.

The following precautions pertain to specific procedures:

Peripheral arteriography: Hypotension or moderate decreases in blood pressure seem to occur frequently with intra-arterial (brachial) injections; therefore, the blood pressure should be monitored during the immediate ten minutes after injection; this blood pressure change is transient and usually requires no treatment.

Excretion urography: Adequate visualization may be difficult or impossible to attain in uremic patients or others with severely impaired renal function (see CONTRAINDICATIONS). The increased osmotic load associated with drip infusion pyelography should be considered in patients with congestive heart failure. The diuretic effect of the drip infusion pyelography procedure may hinder assessment of residual urine in the bladder. The recommended rate of infusion should not be exceeded.

Acute renal failure has been reported in diabetic patients with diabetic nephropathy and susceptible nondiabetic patients (often elderly with preexisting renal disease) following excretion urography. Therefore, careful consideration should be given before performing this procedure in these patients.

Operative and T-tube cholangiography: Injection should be made slowly to prevent extravasation of the medium into the peritoneal cavity, and to minimize reflux flow into the pancreatic duct which may result in pancreatic irritation.

Percutaneous transhepatic cholangiography: To reduce the possibility of bile leakage and consequent peritonitis, as much of the contrast agent as possible should be aspirated on completion of successful films. All patients should be carefully and constantly monitored for 24 hours after the procedure for signs of internal hemorrhage or bile leakage; if these complications are recognized immediately, remedial measures can be instituted promptly with minimal increase in morbidity. Percutaneous transhepatic cholangiography is not without risk and should therefore be reserved for special circumstances when ordinary studies of the biliary system have failed to provide the requisite information in jaundiced patients who are not good candidates for surgery. The procedure should only be attempted when competent surgical intervention can be promptly obtained if needed.

Splenoportography: It is best to avoid manipulations which would prolong the time the needle is in the spleen since they may contribute to subcapsular extravasation of the contrast agent and also to postpuncture bleeding. Following splenoportography, the patient should lie on his left side for several hours and should be closely observed for 24 hours for signs of internal bleeding, which is the most common complication of the procedure. Fatal hemorrhage has occurred on rare occasion, but leakage of up to 300 ml. of blood from the spleen is apparently not uncommon. Blood transfusions may be required, and rarely splenectomy.

Discography: To minimize the possibility of introducing infection, discography should be postponed in any patient with an infection or open injury near the region to be examined, including upper respiratory infections in the case of cervical discography. All possible care should be taken to preclude contamination and resultant infection of the disk, which has been reported after discography. In cervical discography, particular care is needed to avoid puncturing the esophagus and thereby introducing contamination into the disk. Rupture of the disk is highly unlikely if care in performance is observed, but may occur if the point of the needle has been barbed by contact with bone; use of the two-needle technique should help reduce this hazard.

Usage in Pregnancy: The safety of diatrizoate meglumine for use during pregnancy has not been established; therefore, this preparation should be used in pregnant patients only when, in the judgment of the physician, its use is deemed essential to the welfare of the patient.

Adverse Reactions: Adverse reactions accompanying the use of iodine-containing intravascular contrast agents are usually mild and transient although severe and life-threatening reactions, including fatalities, have occurred. Because of the possibility of severe reactions to the procedure and/or the radiopaque medium, appropriate emergency facilities and well-trained personnel should be available to treat both conditions. Emergency facilities and personnel should remain available for 30 to 60 minutes following the procedure since severe delayed reactions have been known to occur.

Nausea, vomiting, flushing, or a generalized feeling of warmth are the reactions seen most frequently with intravascular injection. Symptoms which may occur are chills, fever, sweating, headache, dizziness, pallor, weakness, severe retching and choking, wheezing, a rise or fall in blood pressure, facial or conjunctival petechiae, urticaria, pruritus, rash and other eruptions, edema, cramps, tremors, itching, sneezing, lacrimation, etc. Antihistaminic agents may be of benefit; rarely such reactions may be severe enough to require discontinuation of dosage.

Severe reactions which may require emergency measures may take the form of a cardiovascular reaction characterized by peripheral vasodilatation with resultant hypotension and reflex tachycardia, dyspnea, agitation, confusion, and cyanosis progressing to unconsciousness. Or, the histamine-liberating effect of these compounds may induce an allergic-like reaction which may range in severity from rhinitis or angioneurotic edema to laryngeal or bronchial spasm or anaphylactoid shock.

Temporary renal shutdown or other nephropathy may occur. Temporary neurologic effects of varying severity have occurred in a few instances, particularly when the medium was used for angiography in the diagnosis of cerebral pathology. Although local tissue tolerance is usually good, there have been a few reports of a burning or stinging sensation or numbness and of venospasm or venous pain, and partial collapse of the injected vein. Neutropenia or thrombophlebitis may occur.

Adverse effects may sometimes occur as a consequence of the procedure for which the contrast agent is used. Adverse reactions in **excretion urography** have included cardiac arrest, ventricular fibrillation, anaphylaxis with severe asthmatic reaction, and flushing due to generalized vasodilation. **Cerebral angiography** has been known to cause temporary neurologic complications such as induction of seizures, particularly in patients with convulsive disorders; confusional states or drowsiness; transient paresis; coma; temporary disturbances in vision; or seventh nerve weakness. During **peripheral arteriography,** complications have occurred including hemorrhage from the puncture site, thrombosis of the vessel, and brachial plexus palsy following axillary artery injections.

Complications of **percutaneous transhepatic cholangiography** have been estimated to occur in four to six percent of cases and have included bile leakage and biliary peritonitis, gallbladder perforation, internal bleeding, septicemia involving gram-negative organisms, and tension pneumothorax from inadvertent puncture of the diaphragm and lung. Bile leakage may be more likely in patients with complete obstruction due to carcinoma.

During **splenoportography,** intraperitoneal extravasation of the contrast medium may cause transient diaphragmatic irritation or mild to moderate transient pain which may sometimes be referred to the shoulder, the periumbilical region, or other areas. Because of the proximity of the pleural cavity, accidental pneumothorax has been known to occur. Inadvertent injection of the medium into other nearby structures is not likely to cause untoward consequences.

Arthrography may induce joint pain or increase existing pain, particularly if a large dose is used and the medium extravasates into surrounding soft tissue. Pain or discomfort is usually immediate and transient but may be delayed or of extended duration (up to 24 hours). Lipid-filled histiocytes have been found in tissue removed following arthrography. The technique of **discography** may be painful, particularly when disk pathology exists. Pain on injection may also be related to the volume of the dose. The nature of the disk pathology or extravasation of contrast agent may cause referred pain.

When any percutaneous technique is employed, the possibility of thrombosis or of other complications due to the mechanical trauma of the procedure should be borne in mind.

Dosage and Administration: Reno-M-60 (Diatrizoate Meglumine Injection USP 60%) should be at body temperature when injected and may need to be warmed before use. If kept in a syringe for prolonged periods before injection, it should be protected from exposure to strong light.

Dilution and withdrawal of the contrast agent should be accomplished under aseptic conditions with sterile needle and syringe.

Excretion Urography—Appropriate preparation of the patient is desirable for optimal results. In adults and older children, a laxative the night before the examination, a low residue diet the day before, and low liquid intake for 12 hours prior to the procedure may be used to clear the gastrointestinal tract and to induce a partial dehydration which is believed to increase the urinary concentration of the contrast medium. Preparatory partial dehydration is not recommended in infants, young children, the elderly, or azotemic patients (especially those with polyuria, oliguria, diabetes, advanced vascular disease, or preexisting dehydration). The undesirable dehydration in these patients may be accentuated by the osmotic diuretic action of the medium.

In uremic patients partial dehydration is not necessary and maintenance of adequate fluid intake is particularly desirable.

Direct I.V. Injection—The dose range for adults is 25 to 50 ml.; the usual dose is 25 ml.; children require proportionately less. Suggested dosages are as follows: Under 6 months—5 ml.; 6 to 12 months—8 ml.; 1 to 2 years—10 ml.; 2 to 5 years—12 ml.; 5 to 7 years—15 ml.; 8 to 10 years—18 ml.; 11 to 15 years—20 ml.; adults (16 years and older)—25 to 50 ml. In adults, when the smaller dose has provided inadequate visualization or when poor visualization is anticipated, the 50 ml. dose may be given. Drip infusion may be used when direct I.V. pyelography is not expected to be or has not been satisfactory (see below).

The preparation is given by intravenous injection. If flushing or nausea occurs during administration, injection should be slowed or briefly interrupted until the side effects have disappeared.

A scout film should be made before the contrast medium is administered. To allow for individual variation, several films should be exposed beginning approximately five minutes after injection. In patients with renal dysfunction, optimal visualization may be delayed until 30 minutes or more after injection.

NOTE: In infants and children and in certain adults, the medium may be injected intramuscularly. The suggested dose is 25 ml. for adults and proportionately less for children, divided and given bilaterally in the gluteal muscles. Radiographs should be taken at 20, 40, and 60 minutes after the medium is injected.

Drip Infusion Pyelography—In drip infusion pyelography, the recommended dose of Reno-M-60 is calculated on the basis of 1 ml. of Reno-M-60 (Diatrizoate Meglumine Injection USP 60%) per pound of body weight diluted with an equal volume of Sterile Water for Injection USP. The diluted preparation (30%) is given by I.V. infusion through a large bore (17- to 18-gauge) needle at a rate of 40 ml. per minute. The recommended rate of infusion should not be exceeded and the total volume administered should generally not exceed 300 ml. In older patients and in patients with known or suspected cardiac decompensation, a slower rate of infusion is probably wise.

If nausea or flushing occurs during administration, the infusion should be slowed or briefly interrupted.

Films are taken before the onset of the infusion and at the desired intervals following its completion. When renal function is normal, a nephrogram may be taken as soon as the infusion is completed, and films of the collecting system at 10 and 20 minutes thereafter. Voiding cystourethrograms are usually optimal at 20 minutes after the infusion is completed. In hypertensive patients, early minute sequence films may be taken during the course of infusion, in addition to subsequent pyelograms. In patients with renal dysfunction, optimal visualization is usually delayed, and late films are taken as indicated.

The nephrogram obtained by the drip infusion procedure may be dense enough to obscure the pelvocalyceal system in some cases. The presence of gas in the bowel may hamper early visualization of the renal collecting system. Tomographic "cuts" may help to overcome such difficulties.

Nephrotomography may begin when the infusion is completed. The sustained contrast achieved by the drip infusion technique eliminates the need for precise timing and teamwork that is necessary with ordinary nephrotomography. Thus, if nephrograms taken after infusion of the medium suggest the need for sectional films, or if preselected tomographic

Continued on next page

Squibb—Cont.

"cuts" are not sufficient, additional tomograms may be obtained at once, and without repetition of dosage.

Cerebral Angiography—Appropriate preparation of the patient is indicated, including suitable premedication. The average single dose for adults is 10 ml., repeated as indicated. Children require less in proportion to weight.

Either the percutaneous or operative method of administration may be used. For visualization of the cerebral vessels, the contrast medium is injected into the common carotid artery; for angiography of the vessels in the posterior fossa or the occipital lobes, the medium is injected into the vertebral artery. Since the medium is given by rapid injection, the patient should be watched for untoward reactions. Unless general anesthesia is used, patients should be warned that the medium may provoke movement and that they may feel transient pain, flushing, or burning during the injection.

A scout film should be made routinely before the contrast medium is injected. Serial films begun while the last few ml. are being injected should permit visualization of the arterial, intermediate, and venous phases.

Peripheral Arteriography—Appropriate preparation of the patient is indicated, including suitable premedication. For visualization of an entire extremity, a single dose of 20 to 40 ml. is suggested; for the upper or lower half of the extremity only, 10 to 20 ml. is usually sufficient.

Injection is made into the femoral or subclavian artery by the percutaneous or operative method. Because the contrast agent is given by rapid injection, flushing of the skin may occur. Patients not under general anesthesia may experience nausea and vomiting or a transient feeling of warmth. Vascular spasm is not likely to occur.

A scout film should be made routinely before administering the contrast medium. Radiograms of the upper half of the extremity are taken while the last few ml. are being injected, followed by radiograms of the lower half of the extremity a few seconds later.

Venography—For visualization of veins in the upper extremities, a single dose of 10 ml. per extremity is suggested. For veins in the lower extremities, doses of 20 to 40 ml. per extremity are suggested. In exceptional circumstances, larger doses may be necessary; visualization of the iliac vein, extensive varicosities or large veins may require 50 ml. or more. Total doses up to 100 ml. per lower extremity have been used safely.

For visualization of an upper extremity, the medium may be given by percutaneous injection into any convenient superficial vein of the forearm or hand. For the visualization of a lower extremity, it should be injected into a superficial vein on the lateral side of the foot. The medium is injected rapidly; patients should be observed for untoward reactions.

Radiograms are taken when injection is completed; sufficient time should be allowed to permit diffusion of the contrast medium.

Operative and Postoperative Cholangiography—Operative cholangiography is performed as soon as the gallbladder and ducts have been exposed surgically. The usual dose is 10 ml., but as much as 25 ml. may be needed, depending on the caliber of the ducts. If desired, the contrast agent may be diluted 1:1 with Sodium Chloride Injection USP under strict aseptic procedures.

The contrast medium is instilled slowly through the stump of the cystic duct or directly into the choledochal lumen. Following surgical exploration of the ductal system, repeat studies may be performed before closure of the abdomen, using the same dose as before.

Postoperatively, the ductal system may be examined by injection of the contrast agent through an in-place T-tube. "T-tube cholangiography" is usually performed eight to ten days after operation; the usual dose is the same as for operative cholangiography.

For each procedure, films are taken immediately after instillation of the medium and are read immediately. Additional films are then taken if necessary.

Percutaneous Transhepatic Cholangiography—Facilities for emergency surgery should be available whenever this examination is performed. Appropriate premedication of the patient is recommended; drugs which are likely to cause spasm, such as morphine, should be avoided.

Depending on the caliber of the biliary tree, a dose of 20 to 40 ml. is generally sufficient to opacify the entire ductal system. The contrast agent may be diluted 1:1 with Sodium Chloride Injection USP, if desired, under strict aseptic procedures.

Injection is made into a biliary duct by the percutaneous transhepatic method. Before the dose is administered, as much bile as possible is aspirated. The medium is then slowly injected into the duct under very slight pressure. If a duct is not located promptly, successive small doses of 1 to 2 ml. are injected into the liver as the needle is gradually withdrawn, until a duct is visualized by x-ray. If no duct can be located after three or four attempts, the procedure is abandoned.

Serial films are taken rapidly during and after injection of the medium into the biliary ducts. Repositioning of the patient, if necessary, should be done with care.

In hepatocellular disease, the biliary ducts are generally not enlarged and cannot successfully be opacified by this method. Thus, in the presence of long-standing jaundice, failure to obtain a successful percutaneous transhepatic cholangiogram by a person experienced in the technique is generally considered to be strongly suggestive of nonobstructive or hepatocellular-type jaundice.

Splenoportography—Prior gastrointestinal x-ray examination should include particular attention to the lower esophageal area. A hematologic survey, including prothrombin time and platelet count, should be performed. The patient should have no food for several hours and should be mildly sedated. Splenoportography is usually performed under local anesthesia.

Approximately 20 to 25 ml. of the contrast agent is usually adequate. The dose is injected rapidly, following radiologic location and percutaneous puncture of the spleen.

Preliminary films are taken to locate the spleen before the injection is begun. Rapid serial films are then started simultaneously with injection of the dose. Serial films are necessary since the entire portal system cannot be captured on a single film and also because of individual variations in portal circulation time.

Arthrography—The amount of contrast agent required is dependent on the size of the joint to be injected. For an adult, the following doses are generally suitable: Knee—5 to 15 ml.; shoulder or hip—5 to 10 ml.; other joints—1 to 4 ml. Dosage for children should be suitably reduced.

The injection site should be prepared aseptically. Excessive synovial fluid should be aspirated to minimize pain and to reduce intraarticular dilution of the contrast agent. If indicated, the agent may be administered under local anesthesia. After injection of the medium, the joint should be manipulated gently in order to spread the medium throughout the joint space. In some instances, double contrast arthrography, injecting both air and contrast medium, has been of value.

Films are taken from several angles; stereoscopic films may be advantageous.

When the contrast agent is used to opacify a joint space, much of the agent may be aspirated at the end of the procedure.

Discography—No prior preparation of the patient is required, although administration of an analgesic or sedative 20 minutes before the procedure may be helpful. Discography is performed under local anesthesia using the usual aseptic precautions.

Dosage is generally determined by the amount of contrast agent which can easily be injected into the disk without force. A cervical disk will normally accept up to 0.5 ml. and a lumbar disk 1 or 2 ml. The amount may vary, and injection should be discontinued when resistance is felt. The rate of injection may influence the amount which can be injected. To reduce the probability of extravasation and to minimize unnecessary pain, injection should be made slowly and not more than 2 ml. should be injected into any one disk.

A two-needle technique may be used to administer the contrast medium, with a large-gauge needle to locate the disk and a small-gauge needle within the larger one to puncture the disk and administer the medium. The correct position of the two needles is established radiologically before the medium is injected.

Spot roentgenograms should be taken anteroposteriorly, obliquely, and laterally as soon as disks have been injected.

When the contrast agent is used for discography, it need not be aspirated at the end of the procedure.

How Supplied: Single dose vials of 10 ml., 30 ml., 50 ml., and 100 ml., and single dose bottles of 100 ml. An excess volume (1 ml.) is available in each container for sensitivity testing.

Storage: The preparation should be stored at room temperature, protected from light. If precipitation or solidification has occurred due to storage in the cold, immerse the container in hot water and shake intermittently to redissolve any solids.

RENO-M-DIP® ℞

(Diatrizoate Meglumine Injection USP 30%)
For Intravenous Drip Infusion

Description: Reno-M-DIP is a radiopaque contrast agent supplied as a sterile, aqueous solution for intravenous drip infusion, in 300 ml. bottles. Each ml. provides 300 mg. diatrizoate meglumine with 0.4 mg. edetate disodium as a sequestering agent; pH has been adjusted between 6.5 and 7.7 with meglumine or diatrizoic acid. *Each ml. of solution also contains approximately 0.054 mg. (0.002 mEq.) sodium (16.2 mg./300 ml.)* and 141 mg. (42.3 g./300 ml.) organically bound iodine.

Clinical Pharmacology: Following intravenous administration, diatrizoate meglumine is rapidly transported through the bloodstream to the kidneys and is excreted unchanged in the urine by glomerular filtration. When urinary tract obstruction is severe enough to block glomerular filtration, the agent appears to be excreted by the tubular epithelium.

Diuresis commonly occurs, due primarily to the osmotic effects of the contrast agent.

Drip Infusion Pyelography—When a large volume of the contrast agent is administered in dilute form by intravenous drip infusion, the nephrographic phase of renal excretion is enhanced, and a dense, sustained nephrogram is usually obtained.

Following drip infusion of the contrast agent, the upper and lower urinary tract is opacified. Anatomically complete pyelograms and voiding cystograms may be obtained, and the entire course of the ureter may be seen on a single film. Filling defects may be visualized and the site of an obstruction may be clearly localized. Renal accumulation is sufficiently rapid that optimal opacification of the kidney normally is reached by the time the infusion is completed, while filling of the collecting system is maximal within 20 or 30 minutes after the start of the infusion. Impairment of renal function commonly delays accumulation and excretion of the contrast agent, so that opacification may be delayed until three or more hours after the infusion; with severe impairment adequate opacification may not occur.

Because transport of the contrast agent is slowed by renal dysfunction, the ischemic kidney of renal vascular hypertension may be distinguished from the normal kidney. Renal ischemia produces a nephrogram which is slower to appear, less dense, and sustained for a markedly prolonged period of time.

Computed Tomography—Reno-M-DIP (Diatrizoate Meglumine Injection USP 30%) enhances computed tomographic brain scanning through augmentation of radiographic efficiency. The degree of enhancement of visualization of tissue density is directly related to the iodine content in an administered dose; peak iodine blood levels occur immediately following rapid infusion of the dose. These levels fall rapidly within five to ten minutes. This can be accounted for by the dilution in the vascular and extracellular fluid compartments which causes an initial sharp fall in plasma concentration. Equilibration with the extracellular compartments is reached in about ten minutes; thereafter, the fall becomes exponential. Maximum contrast enhancement frequently occurs after peak blood iodine levels are reached. The delay in maximum contrast enhancement can range from five to forty minutes, depending on the peak iodine levels achieved and the cell type of the lesion. This lag suggests that radiographic contrast enhancement is at least in part dependent on the accumulation of iodine within the lesion and outside the blood pool although the mechanism by which this occurs is not clear. The radiographic enhancement of nontumoral lesions, such as arteriovenous malformations and aneurysms, is probably dependent on the iodine content of the circulating blood pool.

Indications and Usage:

Drip Infusion Pyelography—Reno-M-DIP is indicated for use in those patients in whom routine pyelography would not be expected to be, or has not been, satisfactory for diagnosis. It is not intended to replace retrograde pyelography where this procedure is indicated.

Computed Tomography—Reno-M-DIP is also indicated for radiographic contrast enhancement in computed tomography (CT) of the brain. Contrast enhancement is advantageous in delineating or ruling out disease in suspicious areas which may otherwise not have been satisfactorily visualized.

Tumors—Reno-M-DIP may be useful to demonstrate the presence and extent of certain malignancies such as: gliomas including malignant gliomas, glioblastomas, astrocytomas, oligodendrogliomas and gangliomas; ependymomas; medulloblastomas; meningiomas; neuromas; pinealomas; pituitary adenomas; craniopharyngiomas; germinomas; and metastatic lesions.

The usefulness of contrast enhancement for the investigation of the retrobulbar space and in cases of low grade or infiltrative glioma has not been demonstrated. In cases where lesions have calcified, there is less likelihood of enhancement. Following therapy, tumors may show decreased or no enhancement.

Non-Neoplastic Conditions—The use of Reno-M-DIP (Diatrizoate Meglumine Injection USP 30%) may be beneficial in the enhancement of images of lesions not due to neoplasms. Cerebral infarctions of recent onset may be better visualized with the contrast enhancement, while some infarctions are obscured if a contrast medium is used. The use of Reno-M-DIP (Diatrizoate Meglumine Injection USP 30%) improved the contrast enhancement in approximately 60 percent of cerebral infarctions studied from one week to four weeks from the onset of symptoms.

Sites of active infection also will produce contrast enhancement following contrast medium administration.

Arteriovenous malformations and aneurysms will show contrast enhancement. In the case of these vascular lesions, the enhancement is probably dependent on the iodine content of the circulating blood pool.

Hematomas and intraparenchymal bleeders seldom demonstrate any contrast enhancement. However, in cases of intraparenchymal clot, for which there is no obvious clinical explanation, contrast medium administration may be helpful in ruling out the possibility of associated arteriovenous malformation.

The opacification of the inferior vermis following contrast medium administration has resulted in false-positive diagnoses in a number of normal studies.

Contraindications: This preparation is contraindicated in patients with a hypersensitivity to salts of diatrizoic acid.

The administration of diatrizoate meglumine is contraindicated in patients with anuria.

Warnings: A definite risk exists in the use of intravascular contrast agents in patients who are known to have multiple myeloma. In such instances there has been anuria resulting in progressive uremia, renal failure and eventually death. Although neither the contrast agent nor dehydration has separately proved to be the cause of anuria in myeloma, it has been speculated that the combination of both may be the causative factor. The risk in myelomatous patients is not a contraindication to the procedures; however, partial dehydration in the preparation of these patients for the examination is not recommended since this may predispose to the precipitation of myeloma protein in the renal tubules. No form of therapy, including dialysis, has been successful in reversing this effect. Myeloma, which occurs most commonly in persons over age 40, should be considered before intravascular administration of a contrast agent.

Administration of radiopaque materials to patients known or suspected to have pheochromocytoma should be performed with extreme caution. If, in the opinion of the physician, the possible benefits of such procedures outweigh the considered risks, the procedures may be performed; however, the amount of radiopaque medium injected should be kept to an absolute minimum. The blood pressure should be assessed throughout the procedure and measures for treatment of a hypertensive crisis should be available.

Contrast media have been shown to promote the phenomenon of sickling in individuals who are homozygous for sickle cell disease when the material is injected intravenously or intraarterially.

Diatrizoate meglumine should be used with extreme caution in patients with severe concomitant hepatic and renal disease.

Since iodine-containing contrast agents may alter the results of thyroid function tests, such tests, if indicated, should be performed prior to the administration of this preparation.

A history of sensitivity to iodine *per se* or to other contrast media is not an absolute contraindication to the use of diatrizoate meglumine but calls for extreme caution in administration.

Precautions: Diagnostic procedures which involve the use of radiopaque contrast agents should be carried out under the direction of personnel with the prerequisite training and with a thorough knowledge of the particular procedure to be performed (see ADVERSE REACTIONS).

Severe, life-threatening reactions suggest hypersensitivity to the radiopaque agent, which has prompted the use of several pretesting methods, none of which can be relied upon to predict severe reactions. Many authorities question the value of any pretest. A history of bronchial asthma or allergy, a family history of allergy, or a previous reaction to a contrast agent warrant special attention. Such a history, by suggesting histamine sensitivity and a consequent proneness to reactions, may be more accurate than pretesting in predicting the likelihood of a reaction, although not necessarily the severity or type of reaction in the individual case.

The sensitivity test most often performed is the slow injection of 0.5 to 1.0 ml. of the radiopaque medium, administered intravenously, prior to injection of the full diagnostic dose. It should be noted that the absence of a reaction to the test dose does not preclude the possibility of a reaction to the full diagnostic dose. If the test dose causes an untoward response of any kind, the necessity for continuing with the examination should be carefully reevaluated and, if it is deemed essential, the examination should be conducted with all possible caution. In rare instances, reactions to the test dose itself may be extremely severe; therefore, close observation of the patient and facilities for emergency treatment appear indicated.

The recommended rate of infusion should not be exceeded.

Renal toxicity has been reported in a few patients with liver dysfunction who were given oral cholecystographic agents followed by urographic agents. Diagnostic infusion studies should therefore be postponed in any patient with a known or suspected hepatic or biliary disorder who has recently taken a cholecystographic contrast agent.

The diuretic effect of the drip infusion procedure may hinder an assessment of residual urine in the bladder.

Consideration must be given to the functional ability of the kidneys before injecting diatrizoate meglumine. Adequate visualization may be difficult or impossible to attain in uremic patients or others with severely impaired renal function.

Acute renal failure has been reported with the use of contrast agents in patients with diabetic nephropathy and susceptible nondiabetic patients (often elderly with preexisting renal disease).

Contrast agents may interfere with some chemical determinations made on urine specimens; therefore, urine should be collected before administration of the contrast medium or two or more days afterwards.

Usage in Pregnancy: The safety of diatrizoate meglumine for use during pregnancy has not been established; therefore, it should be used in pregnant patients only when, in the judgment of the physician, its use is deemed essential to the welfare of the patient.

Adverse Reactions: Adverse reactions accompanying the use of iodine-containing intravascular contrast agents are usually mild and transient although severe and life-threatening reactions, including fatalities, have occurred.

Because of the possibility of severe reactions to the procedure and/or the radiopaque medium, appropriate emergency facilities and well-trained personnel should be available to treat both conditions. Emergency facilities and personnel should remain available for 30 to 60 minutes following the procedure since severe delayed reactions have been known to occur.

Nausea and urticaria have been the reactions most frequently encountered with administration of contrast agents by drip infusion. Such symptoms as chills, metallic taste, vomiting, dizziness, a rise or fall in blood pressure, itching, flushing, or generalized feeling of warmth, sneezing, etc., may occur. Rarely, such reactions may be severe enough to require discontinuation of dosage.

Severe reactions which may require emergency measures may take the form of a cardio-

Continued on next page

Squibb—Cont.

vascular reaction characterized by peripheral vasodilatation with resultant hypotension and reflex tachycardia, dyspnea, and confusion and cyanosis progressing to unconsciousness. Or, the histamine-liberating effect of these compounds may induce an allergic-like reaction which may range in severity from rhinitis or angioneurotic edema to laryngeal or bronchial spasm or anaphylactoid shock.

Temporary renal shutdown or other nephropathy may occur.

Although local tissue tolerance to diatrizoate meglumine is usually good, intravenous injection of the medium in a more concentrated formulation has produced a few instances of a burning or stinging sensation and of venospasm or venous pain.

Dosage and Administration:
Reno-M-DIP (Diatrizoate Meglumine Injection USP 30%) should be at body temperature when infused and may need to be warmed before use.

Drip Infusion Pyelography—While preparation of the patient is not essential for drip infusion pyelography, it is advocated by some investigators. If desired, adults and older children may be given a laxative the night before the examination and a low residue diet the day before, to clear the gastrointestinal tract. Clinicians who feel that partial dehydration enhances radiographic contrast recommend a low liquid intake for 12 hours prior to the procedure; however, adequate hydration has improved the quality of films for other investigators. Preparatory partial dehydration is not recommended in infants, young children, the elderly, or azotemic patients (especially those with polyuria, oliguria, diabetes, advanced vascular disease, or preexisting dehydration). The undesirable dehydration in these patients may be accentuated by the osmotic diuretic action of the medium.

In uremic patients partial dehydration is not necessary and maintenance of adequate fluid intake is particularly desirable.

Cleansing enemas are not recommended since they may increase residual gas in the bowel.

The recommended dose is 2 ml. per pound of body weight. The preparation is given by continuous intravenous infusion, over a period of 8 minutes or longer (see PRECAUTIONS), through a needle with a large bore, usually a 17- or 18-gauge needle. In older patients and in patients with known or suspected cardiac decompensation, a slower rate of infusion is probably wise.

If nausea or flushing occurs during administration, the infusion should be slowed or briefly interrupted.

Films are taken before the onset of the infusion and at the desired intervals following its completion. When renal function is normal, a nephrogram may be taken as soon as the infusion is completed, and films of the collecting system at 10 and 20 minutes thereafter. Voiding cystourethrograms are usually optimal at 20 minutes after the infusion is completed. In hypertensive patients, early minute sequence films may be taken during the course of infusion, in addition to subsequent pyelograms. In patients with renal dysfunction, optimal visualization is usually delayed, and the late films are taken as indicated.

The nephrogram obtained by the drip infusion procedure may be dense enough to obscure the pelvocalyceal system in some cases. The presence of gas in the bowel may hamper early visualization of the renal collecting system. Tomographic "cuts" may help to overcome such difficulties.

Nephrotomography may begin when the infusion is completed. The sustained contrast achieved by the drip infusion technique eliminates the need for precise timing and teamwork that is necessary with ordinary nephrotomography. Thus, if nephrograms taken after infusion of the medium suggest the need for sectional films, or if preselected tomographic "cuts" are not sufficient, additional tomograms may be obtained at once, and without repetition of dosage.

Computed Tomography—The suggested dose is 2 ml. per pound of body weight by intravenous drip over a period of eight minutes or longer; scanning may be performed during administration and/or immediately afterwards.

Patient Preparation—No special patient preparation is required for contrast enhancement of CT brain scanning. However, it is advisable to insure that patients are well hydrated prior to examination.

How Supplied: Available in single-dose bottles of 300 ml. and in single-dose bottles of 300 ml. with Solution Administration Set. An excess volume (1 ml.) is available in each container for sensitivity testing.

Storage: The preparation should be protected from strong light and stored at room temperature.

RENOVIST® ℞
(Diatrizoate Meglumine and Diatrizoate Sodium Injection USP)

Description: Renovist is a radiopaque contrast agent supplied in vials as a sterile, aqueous solution. Each ml. provides 343 mg. diatrizoate meglumine and 350 mg. diatrizoate sodium with 3.2 mg. sodium citrate and 0.4 mg. edetate disodium; pH has been adjusted to 6.5 to 7.7 with sodium hydroxide. *Each ml. of solution also contains approximately 13.5 mg. (0.58 mEq.) sodium (675 mg./50 ml.)* and 370.5 mg. (18.5 g./50 ml.) organically bound iodine. At the time of manufacture, the air in the container is replaced by nitrogen.

Clinical Pharmacology: Following intravascular injection, Renovist is rapidly transported through the bloodstream to the kidneys and is excreted unchanged in the urine by glomerular filtration. When urinary tract obstruction is severe enough to block glomerular filtration, the agent appears to be excreted by the tubular epithelium.

Renal accumulation is sufficiently rapid so that the period of maximal opacification of the renal passages may begin as early as five minutes after injection. In infants and small children, excretion takes place somewhat more promptly than in adults, so that maximal opacification occurs more rapidly and is less sustained. The normal kidney eliminates the contrast medium almost immediately. In nephropathic conditions, particularly when excretory capacity has been altered, the rate of excretion varies unpredictably, and opacification may be delayed for 30 minutes or more after injection; with severe impairment opacification may not occur. Generally, however, the medium is concentrated in sufficient amounts and promptly enough to permit a thorough evaluation of the anatomy and physiology of the urinary tract.

After intramuscular injection, the contrast agent is promptly absorbed and normally reaches the renal passages within 20 to 60 minutes.

Intravascular injection of diatrizoate also opacifies those vessels in the path of the flow of the medium, permitting visualization until the circulating blood dilutes the concentration of the medium. Thus selective angiography may be performed following injection directly into veins or arteries.

Indications: Renovist (Diatrizoate Meglumine and Diatrizoate Sodium Injection USP) is indicated for use in excretion urography, aortography, angiocardiography, peripheral arteriography, peripheral venography, and venocavography.

Contraindications: This preparation is contraindicated in patients with a hypersensitivity to salts of diatrizoic acid.

Urography is contraindicated in patients with anuria.

Warnings: A definite risk exists in the use of intravascular contrast agents in patients who are known to have multiple myeloma. In such instances there has been anuria resulting in progressive uremia, renal failure, and eventually death. Although neither the contrast agent nor dehydration has separately proved to be the cause of anuria in myeloma, it has been speculated that the combination of both may be the causative factor. The risk in myelomatous patients is not a contraindication to the procedures; however, partial dehydration in the preparation of these patients for the examination is not recommended since this may predispose to the precipitation of myeloma protein in the renal tubules. No form of therapy, including dialysis, has been successful in reversing this effect. Myeloma, which occurs most commonly in persons over age 40, should be considered before intravascular administration of a contrast agent.

Administration of radiopaque materials to patients known or suspected to have pheochromocytoma should be performed with extreme caution. If, in the opinion of the physician, the possible benefits of such procedures outweigh the considered risks, the procedures may be performed; however, the amount of radiopaque medium injected should be kept to an absolute minimum. The blood pressure should be assessed throughout the procedure and measures for treatment of a hypertensive crisis should be available.

The inherent risks of angiocardiography in cyanotic infants and patients with chronic pulmonary emphysema must be weighed against the necessity for performing this procedure. In pediatric angiocardiography, a dose of 10 to 20 ml. may be particularly hazardous in infants weighing less than 7 kg. This risk is probably significantly increased if these infants have preexisting right heart "strain," right heart failure, and effectively decreased or obliterated pulmonary vascular beds.

Contrast media have been shown to promote the phenomenon of sickling in individuals who are homozygous for sickle cell disease when the material is injected intravenously or intra-arterially.

Urography should be performed with extreme caution in patients with severe concomitant hepatic and renal disease.

Since iodine-containing contrast agents may alter the results of thyroid function tests, such tests, if indicated, should be performed prior to the administration of this preparation.

A history of sensitivity to iodine *per se* or to other contrast agents is not an absolute contraindication to the use of diatrizoate, but calls for extreme caution in administration.

Precautions: Diagnostic procedures which involve the use of radiopaque contrast agents should be carried out under the direction of personnel with the prerequisite training and with a thorough knowledge of the particular procedure to be performed (see ADVERSE REACTIONS).

Severe, life-threatening reactions suggest hypersensitivity to the radiopaque agent, which has prompted the use of several pretesting methods, none of which can be relied upon to predict severe reactions. Many authorities question the value of any pretest. A history of bronchial asthma or allergy, a family history of allergy, or a previous reaction to a contrast agent warrant special attention. Such a history, by suggesting histamine sensitivity and a consequent proneness to reactions, may be more accurate than pretesting in predicting the likelihood of a reaction, although not necessarily the severity or type of reaction in the individual case.

The sensitivity test most often performed is the slow injection of 0.5 to 1.0 ml. of the radiopaque medium, administered intravenously, prior to injection of the full diagnostic dose. It should be noted that the absence of a reaction to the test dose does not preclude the possibility of a reaction to the full diagnostic dose. If the test dose causes an untoward response of any kind, the necessity for continuing with the examination should be carefully reevaluated and, if it is deemed essential, the examination should be conducted with all possible caution. In rare instances, reactions to the test dose itself may be extremely severe; therefore, close observation of the patient, and facilities for emergency treatment, appear indicated.

Renal toxicity has been reported in a few patients with liver dysfunction who were given oral cholecystographic agents followed by urographic agents. Administration of Renovist (Diatrizoate Meglumine and Diatrizoate Sodium Injection USP) should therefore be postponed in any patient with a known or suspected hepatic or biliary disorder who has recently taken a cholecystographic contrast agent.

Caution should be exercised with the use of radiopaque media in severely debilitated patients and in those with marked hypertension. The possibility of thrombosis should be borne in mind when percutaneous techniques are employed.

Consideration must be given to the functional ability of the kidneys before injecting this preparation.

Contrast agents may interfere with some chemical determinations made on urine specimens; therefore, urine should be collected before administration of the contrast medium or two or more days afterwards.

The following precautions pertain to specific procedures:

Excretion urography: Adequate visualization may be difficult or impossible to obtain in uremic patients or others with severely impaired renal function (see CONTRAINDICATIONS).

Acute renal failure has been reported in diabetic patients with diabetic nephropathy and susceptible nondiabetic patients (often elderly with preexisting renal disease) following excretion urography. Therefore, careful consideration should be given before performing this procedure in these patients.

Aortography: Repeated intra-aortic injections may be hazardous.

Angiocardiography: Repeated injections may be hazardous particularly in infants weighing less than 7 kg. (see WARNINGS).

Peripheral arteriography: Hypotension or moderate decreases in blood pressure seem to occur frequently with intra-arterial (brachial) injections; therefore, the blood pressure should be monitored during the immediate ten minutes after injection; this blood pressure change is transient and usually requires no treatment.

Peripheral venography: Caution should be exercised in the presence of thrombosis or phlebitis.

Usage in Pregnancy: Safety for use during pregnancy has not been established with respect to adverse effects upon fetal development; therefore, this preparation should be used in pregnant patients only when, in the judgment of the physician, its use is deemed essential to the welfare of the patient.

Adverse Reactions: Adverse reactions accompanying the use of iodine-containing intravascular contrast agents are usually mild and transient although severe and life-threatening reactions, including fatalities, have occurred. Because of the possibility of severe reactions to the procedure and/or the radiopaque medium, appropriate emergency facilities and well-trained personnel should be available to treat both conditions. Emergency facilities and personnel should remain available for 30 to 60 minutes following the procedure since severe delayed reactions have been known to occur.

Nausea, vomiting, flushing, or a generalized feeling of warmth are the reactions seen most frequently with intravascular injection. Symptoms which may occur are chills, fever, sweating, headache, dizziness, pallor, weakness, severe retching and choking, wheezing, a rise or fall in blood pressure, ventricular fibrillation, cardiac arrest, facial or conjunctival petechiae, urticaria, pruritus, rash and other eruptions, edema, cramps, tremors, itching, sneezing, lacrimation, etc. Antihistaminic agents may be of benefit; rarely, such reactions may be severe enough to require discontinuation of dosage. Pulmonary edema, spasm, seizures, hemiparesis, and impairment of vision have occurred.

Although local tissue tolerance is usually good, there have been a few reports of a burning or stinging sensation or numbness and of venospasm or venous pain, and partial collapse of the injected vein. Neutropenia or thrombophlebitis may occur.

Severe reactions are a possibility. Such reactions which may require emergency measures may take the form of a cardiovascular reaction characterized by peripheral vasodilatation with resultant hypotension and reflex tachycardia, apnea, dyspnea, agitation, confusion, and cyanosis progressing to unconsciousness. Or, the histamine-liberating effect of these compounds may induce an allergic-like reaction which may range in severity from rhinitis or angioneurotic edema to laryngeal or bronchial spasm or anaphylactoid shock.

Temporary renal shutdown or other nephropathy may occur.

Adverse reactions may sometimes occur as a consequence of the procedure for which the contrast agent is used. Adverse reactions in **excretion urography** have included cardiac arrest, ventricular fibrillation, anaphylaxis with severe asthmatic reaction, and flushing due to generalized vasodilatation. In **aortography,** the risks of procedures include injury to the aorta and neighboring organs, pleural puncture, renal damage including infarction and acute tubular necrosis with oliguria and anuria, accidental selective filling of the right renal artery during the translumbar procedure in the presence of preexistent renal disease, retroperitoneal hemorrhage from the translumbar approach, spinal cord injury and pathology associated with the syndrome of transverse myelitis, generalized petechiae, and death following hypotension, arrhythmia, and anaphylactoid reactions. Adverse reactions in **angiocardiography** have included arrhythmia and death. During **peripheral arteriography,** complications have occurred including hemorrhage from the puncture site, thrombosis of the vessel, and brachial plexus palsy following axillary artery injections.

Dosage and Administration: Renovist (Diatrizoate Meglumine and Diatrizoate Sodium Injection USP) should be at body temperature when injected, and may need to be warmed before use. The preparation should be used as promptly as possible following withdrawal into the syringe, and syringes should be rinsed as soon as possible after injection to prevent freezing of the plunger.

Note: In the event crystallization occurs, the solution may be clarified by placing the vial in a water bath at 40° to 50° C. and shaking gently for two to three minutes or until the solids redissolve.

Withdrawal of the contrast agent should be accomplished under aseptic conditions with sterile needle and syringe.

Excretion Urography: Appropriate preparation of the patient is desirable for optimal results. A laxative the night before the examination, a low residue diet the day before, and low liquid intake for 12 hours prior to the procedure are recommended. The partial dehydration so induced is believed to effect a greater urinary concentration of the contrast medium. Enemas are to be avoided to prevent rehydration.

Preparatory partial dehydration is not recommended in infants, young children, the elderly, or azotemic patients (especially those with polyuria, oliguria, diabetes, advanced vascular disease, or preexisting dehydration). The undesirable dehydration in these patients may be accentuated by the osmotic action of the medium.

For many patients aged 16 years or older, an intravenous dose of 25 ml. is sufficient; alternatively, in instances where inadequate visualization may be anticipated, a higher dose may be administered on a weight basis (0.36 to 0.45 ml./lb.). Children under 16 require proportionately less: Under 6 months of age—5 ml.; 6 to 12 months—8 ml.; 1 to 2 years—10 ml.; 2 to 5 years—12 ml.; 5 to 7 years—15 ml.; 7 to 10 years—18 ml.; 10 to 15 years—20 ml.

Use of a 20- or 21-gauge needle is recommended. During the injection, the patient should be watched for untoward reactions. If flushing or nausea occurs, the rate of injection should be slowed or administration briefly interrupted until the side effects have disappeared.

A scout film should be made before Renovist is administered. Since maximal opacification of the urinary tract usually occurs between 5 to 15 minutes after injection of the contrast agent, radiographs are best taken during this period. To allow for individual variation, several films should be exposed. In infants and children maximal opacification occurs more rapidly after injection and is sustained over a shorter period of time. In patients with renal dysfunction, optimal opacification may be delayed for 30 minutes or more after injection.

Aortography: Renovist (Diatrizoate Meglumine and Diatrizoate Sodium Injection USP) injected into the aorta by the translumbar or retrograde method of administration permits radiographic visualization of the aorta, its major branches, and the abdominal arteries. An incidental nephrogram is obtained as the contrast medium travels through the renal vasculature, provided it has been injected above the renal artery.

Patients should be prepared in a manner similar to that used for intravenous urography. Premedication with a suitable barbiturate is generally indicated.

As in any form of surgery, certain hazards accompany aortographic procedures (see ADVERSE REACTIONS).

For adults and children over 16 years of age, the usual dose is 15 to 25 ml. as a single injection, repeated if indicated. Children require less in proportion to age and weight.

Since the medium is given by rapid injection in this procedure, patients should be watched for untoward reactions during the injection. Unless general anesthesia is employed, patients should be warned that they may feel some transient pain or burning during the injection followed by a feeling of warmth immediately afterward.

A scout film should be made before the contrast agent is administered. The first radiogram should be taken as the last few ml. of the contrast medium are being injected.

Angiocardiography: Angiocardiography with Renovist (Diatrizoate Meglumine and Diatrizoate Sodium Injection USP) may be performed by injection into a large peripheral vein or by direct catheterization of the heart. An excretory urogram can be obtained 10 to 15 minutes after injection of the contrast medium since it is concentrated in and eliminated by the kidneys.

Patients should be prepared in a manner similar to that used for intravenous urography. Appropriate preanesthetic medication should be given.

Continued on next page

Squibb—Cont.

Clincal studies in man, and related animal experiments, have suggested that the hypertonicity of diatrizoate contrast agents produces significant hemodynamic effects, especially in right-sided injections. Large volumes of such agents cause a drop in peripheral arterial and systemic pressures and cardiac output, a rise in pulmonary arterial and right-heart pressures, bradycardia, and regular ectopic beats. Resulting effects on peripheral arterial and pulmonary arterial pressures are postulated to be due to mechanical blockage of the pulmonary vascular bed and clumping of red cells.

Hypertonic solutions cause a decrease in hematocrit *in vitro* and *in vivo*, and shrinkage of red blood cells.

It is suggested that hemodynamic changes be monitored and that pressures considered abnormal under roentgenographic conditions be allowed to return to a preangiographic level before continuation of radiopaque injection; this usually takes 15 minutes.

For adults the suggested single dose is 50 ml.; doses up to a total of 200 ml. have been given safely. Children under 16 require proportionally less. The suggested single dose for children under 2 years of age is 10 to 15 ml., depending upon the weight of the child; the smallest amount necessary to obtain adequate visualization should be used. For children 2 to 4 years of age, single doses of 15 to 20 ml. are recommended; for children 4 to 10 years of age, 20 to 30 ml. Doses up to 100 ml. have been given safely. For children 10 to 15 years of age, dosage depends on the size of the patient.

Since the contrast medium is given by rapid injection, the patient should be watched for untoward reactions during the injection. Some patients not under general anesthesia may experience a feeling of bodily warmth, tightness of the chest, and throbbing headache. All these sensations are of short duration. Transient nausea and vomiting may occur in some patients.

The roentgenograms should be taken immediately at the beginning of the injection and continued for 5 to 10 seconds or longer, depending upon the desired roentgenographic information.

Peripheral Arteriography: Renovist is injected into the femoral or subclavian artery by the percutaneous or operative method. If only the lower half of the extremity is to be studied, Renovist is injected into the brachial or popliteal artery.

Appropriate preparation of the patient is indicated, including suitable premedication.

For visualization of an entire extremity, a single dose of 20 to 40 ml. is suggested. For arteriography of the upper half or the lower half of the extremity only, a single dose of 10 to 20 ml. is sufficient.

Because the contrast medium is given by rapid injection, flushing of the skin may occur. Patients not under general anesthesia may experience a feeling of warmth and, rarely, nausea and vomiting.

A scout film should be made routinely before administering the contrast medium. Radiograms of the upper half should be taken while the last 2 ml. of Renovist (Diatrizoate Meglumine and Diatrizoate Sodium Injection USP) are being injected, followed by radiograms of the lower half of the extremity a few seconds later.

Peripheral Venography: For visualization of an upper extremity, Renovist may be given by percutaneous injection into any convenient superficial vein of the forearm or hand. For visualization of a lower extremity, it should be injected into a superficial vein on the lateral side of the foot.

Appropriate preparation of the patient is indicated, including suitable premedication.

For the visualization of an upper extremity in adults, a single dose of 20 ml. is suggested; a single dose of 20 ml. is sufficient for the visualization of a lower extremity. Children require less in proportion to age and weight.

The contrast medium is administered rapidly in this procedure.

The radiographs are taken at the termination of the injection.

Venocavography: Inferior venocavography may be performed with Renovist injected into the saphenous, femoral, or iliac veins by percutaneous injection, either directly or by catheterization procedures.

Appropriate preparation of the patient is indicated, including suitable premedication.

For adults the suggested average single dose is 30 to 60 ml. The dosage for children depends upon age and weight.

Renovist (Diatrizoate Meglumine and Diatrizoate Sodium Injection USP) is injected as rapidly as possible via the saphenous vein and roentgenograms are taken immediately. A repeat injection is given if an additional view is desired. An alternate technique is to catheterize both femoral veins and to place the catheter in each common iliac vein immediately caudad to their junction. Bilateral injection gives better filling than the unilateral injection.

Roentgenograms are taken immediately after injection of the medium. They are taken in a supine position and in the right posterior oblique or lateral position.

How Supplied: Available in 50 ml. single-dose vials. An excess volume (1 ml.) is available in each container for sensitivity testing.

Storage: Protect from light. Store at room temperature.

RENOVIST® II ℞

(Diatrizoate Meglumine and Diatrizoate Sodium Injection USP)

Description: Renovist II is a radiopaque contrast agent supplied in vials as a sterile, aqueous solution. Each ml. provides 285 mg. diatrizoate meglumine and 291 mg. diatrizoate sodium with 3.2 mg. sodium citrate as a buffer, and 0.4 mg. edetate disodium as a sequestering agent; pH has been adjusted between 6.5 and 7.7 with sodium hydroxide. *Each ml. of solution also contains approximately 11.39 mg. (0.49 mEq.) sodium* and 309 mg. organically bound iodine. At the time of manufacture, the air in the container is replaced by nitrogen.

Clinical Pharmacology: Following intravascular injection, Renovist II is rapidly transported through the bloodstream to the kidneys and is excreted unchanged in the urine by glomerular filtration. When urinary tract obstruction is severe enough to block glomerular filtration, the agent appears to be excreted by the tubular epithelium.

Renal accumulation is sufficiently rapid so that the period of maximal opacification of the renal passages may begin as early as 5 minutes after injection. In infants and small children excretion takes place somewhat more promptly than in adults, so that maximal opacification occurs more rapidly and is less sustained. The normal kidney eliminates the contrast medium almost immediately. In nephropathic conditions, particularly when excretory capacity has been altered, the rate of excretion varies unpredictably, and opacification may be delayed for 30 minutes or more after injection; with severe impairment, opacification may not occur. Generally, however, the medium is concentrated in sufficient amounts and promptly enough to permit a thorough evaluation of the anatomy and physiology of the urinary tract.

After intramuscular injection, the contrast agent is promptly absorbed and normally reaches the renal passages within 20 to 60 minutes.

Intravascular injection of diatrizoate also opacifies those vessels in the path of the flow of the medium, permitting visualization until the circulating blood dilutes the concentration of the medium. Thus, selective angiography may be performed following injection directly into veins or arteries.

Indications: Renovist II (Diatrizoate Meglumine and Diatrizoate Sodium Injection USP) is indicated for use in excretion urography, aortography, angiocardiography, peripheral arteriography, peripheral venography, and venocavography.

Contraindications: This preparation is contraindicated in patients with a hypersensitivity to salts of diatrizoic acid.

Urography is contraindicated in patients with anuria.

Warnings: A definite risk exists in the use of intravascular contrast agents in patients who are known to have multiple myeloma. In such instances there has been anuria resulting in progressive uremia, renal failure, and eventually death. Although neither the contrast agent nor dehydration has separately proved to be the cause of anuria in myeloma, it has been speculated that the combination of both may be the causative factor. The risk in myelomatous patients is not a contraindication to the procedures; however, partial dehydration in the preparation of these patients for the examination is not recommended since this may predispose to the precipitation of myeloma protein in the renal tubules. No form of therapy, including dialysis, has been successful in reversing this effect. Myeloma, which occurs most commonly in persons over age 40, should be considered before intravascular administration of a contrast agent.

Administration of radiopaque materials to patients known or suspected to have pheochromocytoma should be performed with extreme caution. If, in the opinion of the physician, the possible benefits of such procedures outweigh the considered risks, the procedures may be performed; however, the amount of radiopaque medium injected should be kept to an absolute minimum. The blood pressure should be assessed throughout the procedure and measures for treatment of a hypertensive crisis should be available.

The inherent risks of angiocardiography in cyanotic infants and patients with chronic pulmonary emphysema must be weighed against the necessity for performing this procedure. In pediatric angiocardiography, a dose of 10 to 20 ml. may be particularly hazardous in infants weighing less than 7 kg. This risk is probably significantly increased if these infants have preexisting right heart "strain," right heart failure, and effectively decreased or obliterated pulmonary vascular beds.

Contrast media have been shown to promote the phenomenon of sickling in individuals who are homozygous for sickle cell disease when the material is injected intravenously or intra-arterially.

Urography should be performed with extreme caution in patients with severe concomitant hepatic and renal disease.

Since iodine-containing contrast agents may alter the results of thyroid function tests, such tests, if indicated, should be performed prior to the administration of this preparation.

A history of sensitivity to iodine *per se* or to other contrast agents is not an absolute contraindication to the use of diatrizoate, but calls for extreme caution in administration.

Precautions: Diagnostic procedures which involve the use of radiopaque contrast agents should be carried out under the direction of personnel with the prerequisite training and with a thorough knowledge of the particular procedure to be performed (see ADVERSE REACTIONS).

Severe, life-threatening reactions suggest hypersensitivity to the radiopaque agent, which has prompted the use of several pretesting methods, none of which can be relied upon to predict severe reactions. Many authorities question the value of any pretest. A history of bronchial asthma or allergy, a family history of allergy, or a previous reaction to a contrast agent warrant special attention. Such a history, by suggesting histamine sensitivity and a consequent proneness to reactions, may be more accurate than pretesting in predicting the likelihood of a reaction, although not necessarily the severity or type of reaction in the individual case.

The sensitivity test most often performed is the slow injection of 0.5 to 1.0 ml. of the radiopaque medium, administered intravenously, prior to injection of the full diagnostic dose. It should be noted that the absence of a reaction to the test dose does not preclude the possibility of a reaction to the full diagnostic dose. If the test dose causes an untoward response of any kind, the necessity for continuing with the examination should be carefully reevaluated and, if it is deemed essential, the examination should be conducted with all possible caution. In rare instances, reactions to the test dose itself may be extremely severe; therefore, close observation of the patient, and facilities for emergency treatment, appear indicated.

Renal toxicity has been reported in a few patients with liver dysfunction who were given oral cholecystographic agents followed by urographic agents. Administration of Renovist II (Diatrizoate Meglumine and Diatrizoate Sodium Injection USP) should therefore be postponed in any patient with a known or suspected hepatic or biliary disorder who has recently taken a cholecystographic contrast agent.

Caution should be exercised with the use of radiopaque media in severely debilitated patients and in those with marked hypertension.

The possibility of thrombosis should be borne in mind when percutaneous techniques are employed.

Consideration must be given to the functional ability of the kidneys before injecting this preparation.

Contrast agents may interfere with some chemical determinations made on urine specimens; therefore, urine should be collected before administration of the contrast medium or two or more days afterwards.

The following precautions pertain to specific procedures:

Excretion urography: Adequate visualization may be difficult or impossible to obtain in uremic patients or others with severely impaired renal function (see CONTRAINDICATIONS).

Acute renal failure has been reported in diabetic patients with diabetic nephropathy and susceptible nondiabetic patients (often elderly with preexisting renal disease) following excretion urography. Therefore, careful consideration should be given before performing this procedure in these patients.

Aortography: Repeated intra-aortic injections may be hazardous.

Angiocardiography: Repeated injections may be hazardous particularly in infants weighing less than 7 kg. (see WARNINGS).

Peripheral arteriography: Hypotension or moderate decreases in blood pressure seem to occur frequently with intra-arterial (brachial) injections; therefore, the blood pressure should be monitored during the immediate ten minutes after injection; this blood pressure change is transient and usually requires no treatment.

Peripheral venography: Caution should be exercised in the presence of thrombosis or phlebitis.

Usage in Pregnancy: Safety for use during pregnancy has not been established with respect to adverse effects upon fetal development; therefore, this preparation should be used in pregnant patients only when, in the judgment of the physician, its use is deemed essential to the welfare of the patient.

Adverse Reactions: Adverse reactions accompanying the use of iodine-containing intravascular contrast agents are usually mild and transient although severe and life-threatening reactions, including fatalities, have occurred. Because of the possibility of severe reactions to the procedure and/or the radiopaque medium, appropriate emergency facilities and well-trained personnel should be available to treat both conditions. Emergency facilities and personnel should remain available for 30 to 60 minutes following the procedure since severe delayed reactions have been known to occur.

Nausea, vomiting, flushing, or a generalized feeling of warmth are the reactions seen most frequently with intravascular injection. Symptoms which may occur are chills, fever, sweating, headache, dizziness, pallor, weakness, severe retching and choking, wheezing, a rise or fall in blood pressure, ventricular fibrillation, cardiac arrest, facial or conjunctival petechiae, urticaria, pruritus, rash and other eruptions, edema, cramps, tremors, itching, sneezing, lacrimation, etc. Antihistaminic agents may be of benefit; rarely, such reactions may be severe enough to require discontinuation of dosage. Pulmonary edema, spasm, seizures, hemiparesis, and impairment of vision have occurred.

Although local tissue tolerance is usually good, there have been a few reports of a burning or stinging sensation or numbness and of venospasm or venous pain, and partial collapse of the injected vein. Neutropenia or thrombophlebitis may occur.

Severe reactions which may require emergency measures may take the form of a cardiovascular reaction characterized by peripheral vasodilatation with resultant hypotenson and reflex tachycardia, apnea, dyspnea, agitation, confusion, and cyanosis progressing to unconsciousness. Or, the histamine-liberating effect of these compounds may induce an allergic-like reaction which may range in severity from rhinitis or angioneurotic edema to laryngeal or bronchial spasm or anaphylactoid shock.

Temporary renal shutdown or other nephropathy may occur.

Adverse reactions may sometimes occur as a consequence of the procedure for which the contrast agent is used. Adverse reactions in **excretion urography** have included cardiac arrest, ventricular fibrillation, anaphylaxis with severe asthmatic reaction, and flushing due to generalized vasodilatation. In **aortography,** the risks of procedures include injury to the aorta and neighboring organs, pleural puncture, renal damage including infarction and acute tubular necrosis with oliguria and anuria, accidental selective filling of the right renal artery during the translumbar procedure in the presence of preexistent renal disease, retroperitoneal hemorrhage from the translumbar approach, spinal cord injury and pathology associated with the syndrome of transverse myelitis, generalized petechiae, and death following hypotension, arrhythmia and anaphylactoid reactions. Adverse reactions in **angiocardiography** have included arrhythmia and death. During **peripheral arteriography,** complications have occurred including hemorrhage from the puncture site, thrombosis of the vessel, and brachial plexus palsy following axillary artery injections.

Dosage and Administration: Renovist II (Diatrizoate Meglumine and Diatrizoate Sodium Injection USP) should be at body temperature when injected, and may need to be warmed before use. Renovist II should be used as promptly as possible following withdrawal into the syringe, and syringes should be rinsed as soon as possible after injection to prevent freezing of the plunger.

Since Renovist II does not usually crystallize in storage even at low temperatures, the need for heating of the preparation to effect re-solution is reduced.

Note: In the event crystallization does occur, the solution may be clarified by placing the vial in a water bath at 40° to 50° C. and shaking gently for two to three minutes or until the solids redissolve.

Withdrawal of the contrast agent should be accomplished under aseptic conditions with sterile needle and syringe.

Excretion Urography: Appropriate preparation of the patient is desirable for optimal results. A laxative the night before the examination, a low residue diet the day before, and low liquid intake for 12 hours prior to the procedure are recommended. The partial dehydration so induced is believed to effect a greater urinary concentration of the contrast medium. Enemas are to be avoided to prevent rehydration.

Preparatory partial dehydration is not recommended in infants, young children, the elderly, or azotemic patients (especially those with polyuria, oliguria, diabetes, advanced vascular disease, or preexisting dehydration). The undesirable dehydration in these patients may be accentuated by the osmotic action of the medium.

The usual intravenous dose for patients aged 16 or more is 30 ml. Children under 16 require proportionately less: Under 6 months of age—6 ml.; 6 to 12 months—10 ml.; 1 to 2 years—12 ml.; 2 to 5 years—15 ml.; 5 to 7 years—18 ml.; 7 to 10 years—22 ml.; 10 to 15 years—24 ml.; 16 years and over—30 ml.

Use of a 20- or 21-gauge needle is recommended. During the injection, the patient should be watched for untoward reactions. If flushing or nausea occurs, the rate of injection should be slowed or administration briefly interrupted until the side effects have disappeared.

A scout film should be made before Renovist II is administered. Since maximal opacification of the urinary tract usually occurs between 5 to 15 minutes after injection of this contrast agent, radiographs are best taken during this period. To allow for individual variation, several films should be exposed. In infants and children, maximal opacification occurs more rapidly after injection and is sustained over a shorter period of time. In patients with renal dysfunction, optimal opacification may be delayed for 30 minutes or more after injection.

Aortography: Renovist II injected into the aorta by the translumbar or retrograde method of administration permits radiographic visualization of the aorta, its major branches and the abdominal arteries. An incidental nephrogram is obtained as the contrast medium travels through the renal vasculature, provided it has been injected above the renal artery.

Patients should be prepared in a manner similar to that used for intravenous urography. Premedication with a suitable barbiturate is generally indicated.

As in any form of surgery, certain hazards accompany aortographic procedures (see ADVERSE REACTIONS).

For adults and children over 16 years of age, the usual dose is 20 to 30 ml. as a single injection, repeated if indicated. Chidren require less in proportion to age and weight.

Since the medium is given by rapid injection in this procedure, patients should be watched for untoward reactions during the injection. Unless general anesthesia is employed, patients should be warned that they may feel some transient pain or burning during the injection followed by a feeling of warmth immediately afterward.

A scout film should be made before the contrast agent is administered. The first radiogram should be taken as the last few ml. of the contrast medium are being injected.

Angiocardiography: Angiocardiography with Renovist II (Diatrizoate Meglumine and Diatrizoate Sodium Injection USP) may be performed by injection into a large peripheral

Continued on next page

Squibb—Cont.

vein or by direct catheterization of the heart. An excretory urogram can be obtained 10 to 15 minutes after injection of the contrast medium since it is concentrated in and eliminated by the kidneys.
Patients should be prepared in a manner similar to that used for intravenous urography. Appropriate preanesthetic medication should be given.
Clinical studies in man, and related animal experiments, have suggested that the hypertonicity of diatrizoate contrast agents produces significant hemodynamic effects, especially in right-sided injections. Large volumes of such agents cause a drop in peripheral arterial and systemic pressures and cardiac output, a rise in pulmonary arterial and right-heart pressures, bradycardia, and regular ectopic beats. Resulting effects on peripheral arterial and pulmonary arterial pressures are postulated to be due to mechanical blockage of the pulmonary vascular bed and clumping of red cells.
Hypertonic solutions cause a decrease in hematocrit *in vitro* and *in vivo*, and shrinkage of red blood cells.
It is suggested that hemodynamic changes be monitored and that pressures considered abnormal under roentgenographic conditions be allowed to return to a preangiographic level before continuation of radiopaque injection; this usually takes 15 minutes.
For adults the suggested single dose is 50 ml.; doses up to a total of 200 ml. have been given safely. Children under 16 require proportionally less. The suggested single dose for children under 2 years of age is 10 to 20 ml., depending upon the weight of the child; the smallest amount necessary to obtain adequate visualization should be used. For children 2 to 4 years of age, single doses of 20 to 30 ml. are recommended; for children 4 to 10 years of age, 30 to 40 ml. Doses up to 100 ml. have been given safely. For children 10 to 15 years of age, dosage depends on the size of the patient.
Since the contrast medium is given by rapid injection, the patient should be watched for untoward reactions during the injection. Some patients not under general anesthesia may experience a feeling of bodily warmth, tightness of the chest and throbbing headache. All these sensations are of short duration. Transient nausea and vomiting may occur in some patients.
The roentgenograms should be taken immediately at the beginning of the injection and continued for 5 to 10 seconds or longer, depending upon the desired roentgenographic information.
Peripheral Arteriography: Renovist II is injected into the femoral or subclavian artery by the percutaneous or operative method. If only the lower half of the extremity is to be studied, Renovist II is injected into the brachial or popliteal artery.
Appropriate preparation of the patient is indicated, including suitable premedication.
For visualization of an entire extremity, a single dose of 30 to 50 ml. is suggested. For arteriography of the upper half or the lower half of the extremity only, a single dose of 20 to 30 ml. is sufficient.
Because the contrast medium is given by rapid injection, flushing of the skin may occur. Patients not under general anesthesia may experience a feeling of warmth and, rarely, nausea and vomiting.
A scout film should be made routinely before administering the contrast medium. Radiograms of the upper half should be taken while the last 2 ml. of Renovist II are being injected, followed by radiograms of the lower half of the extremity a few seconds later.
Peripheral Venography: For visualization of an upper extremity, Renovist II (Diatrizoate Meglumine and Diatrizoate Sodium Injection USP) may be given by percutaneous injection into any convenient superficial vein of the forearm or hand. For visualization of a lower extremity, it should be injected into a superficial vein on the lateral side of the foot.
Appropriate preparation of the patient is indicated, including suitable premedication.
For the visualization of an upper extremity in adults, a single dose of 20 ml. is suggested; a single dose of 20 ml. is sufficient for the visualization of a lower extremity. Children require less in proportion to age and weight.
The contrast medium is administered rapidly in this procedure.
The radiographs are taken at the termination of the injection.
Venocavography: Inferior venocavography may be performed with Renovist II injected into the saphenous, femoral or iliac veins by percutaneous injection, either directly or by catheterization procedures.
Appropriate preparation of the patient is indicated, including suitable premedication.
For adults the suggested average single dose is 30 to 60 ml. The dosage for children depends upon age and weight.
Renovist II (Diatrizoate Meglumine and Diatrizoate Sodium Injection USP) is injected as rapidly as possible via the saphenous vein and roentgenograms are taken immediately. A repeat injection is given if an additional view is desired. An alternate technique is to catheterize both femoral veins and to place the catheter in each common iliac vein immediately caudad to their junction. Bilateral injection gives better filling than the unilateral injection.
Roentgenograms are taken immediately after injection of the medium. They are taken in a supine position and in the right posterior oblique or lateral position.
How Supplied: Available in 30 ml. and 60 ml. single-dose vials. An excess volume (1 ml.) is available in each container for sensitivity testing.
Storage: Protect from light. Store at room temperature.

RENOVUE®-65 ℞
(Iodamide Meglumine Injection)

Description: Renovue-65 is a radiopaque urographic contrast agent supplied as a sterile, nonpyrogenic, aqueous, intravenous solution providing 65% iodamide meglumine with approximately 30% (300 mg./ml.) organically bound iodine; the solution also contains 0.01% edetate disodium as a sequestering stabilizing agent. The clear, colorless to pale yellow solution has a viscosity of 6.4 cps. at 37° C. and 8.6 cps. at 25° C.; the pH has been adjusted to 6.5 to 7.7 with iodamide. The solution has an osmolarity of approximately 1.59 mOsm per ml. at 37° C. *Renovue-65 contains approximately 0.0124 mg. (0.0005 mEq.) sodium per ml.* At the time of manufacture, the air in the container is replaced with nitrogen.
Chemically, iodamide meglumine is 3-(acetylamino)-5 [(acetylamino)methyl] -2,4,6-triiodobenzoic acid, N-methylglucamine salt.
Clinical Pharmacology: Following intravenous injection, Renovue-65 is rapidly transported through the bloodstream to the kidneys and is excreted essentially unchanged in the urine, principally by glomerular filtration. However, at least one-third of the intravenous dose is secreted by the renal tubules.
After injection, the contrast agent permits visualization of the kidneys and urinary passages through the natural physiologic mechanism of excretion.
Renal accumulation is sufficiently rapid so that the period of maximal opacification of the renal passages may begin as early as one minute after injection. Normal kidneys rapidly eliminate the contrast medium. In nephropathic conditions, particularly when excretory capacity has been altered, the rate of excretion varies unpredictably, and opacification may be delayed for 30 minutes or more after injection; with severe renal impairment, opacification may not occur. Generally the medium is concentrated sufficiently and promptly enough to permit satisfactory visualization of the urinary tract.
Indications and Usage: Renovue-65 is a diagnostic agent for intravenous excretory urography.
Contraindications: There are no absolute contraindications to the use of Renovue-65 (Iodamide Meglumine Injection) (see WARNINGS).
Warnings: A definite risk exists in the performance of excretion urography in patients who are known to have multiple myeloma, because of the great possibility of producing transient to fatal renal failure. The risk of excretion urography in myelomatous patients is not a contraindication to the procedure; however, dehydration in the preparation of these patients should be avoided, since this may predispose to the precipitation of protein in the renal tubules.
Administration of radiopaque materials to patients known or suspected to have pheochromocytoma should be performed only if the physician deems that the possible benefits outweigh the considered risks; the procedure should then be performed with extreme caution and the volume of radiopaque medium injected should be kept to an absolute minimum. The blood pressure should be assessed throughout the procedure and measures for treatment of a hypertensive crisis should be available.
Contrast media administered intravenously have been shown to promote the phenomenon of sickling in individuals who are homozygous for sickle cell disease.
Urography should be performed with extreme caution in patients with severe concomitant hepatic and renal disease, or anuria.
A history of sensitivity to iodine *per se* or to any contrast agent is not an absolute contraindication to the use of iodamide meglumine, but calls for extreme caution in administration.
Precautions: *General*—All procedures utilizing contrast media carry a definite risk of producing adverse reactions. While most reactions may be minor, life-threatening and fatal reactions may occur without warning. The risk-benefit factor should always be carefully evaluated before such a procedure is undertaken. At all times a fully equipped emergency cart, or equivalent supplies and equipment, and personnel competent in recognizing and treating adverse reactions of all severity or situations which may arise as a result of the procedure should be immediately available. If a serious reaction should occur, administration should be discontinued immediately.
Since severe delayed reactions have been known to occur, emergency facilities and competent personnel should be available for at least 30 to 60 minutes after administration.
Renal toxicity has been reported in a few patients with liver dysfunction who were given oral cholecystographic agents followed by urographic agents. Administration of Iodamide Meglumine Injection should therefore be postponed in any patient with a known or suspected hepatic or biliary disorder who has recently taken a cholecystographic contrast agent.
Caution should be exercised with the use of radiopaque media in severely debilitated patients and in those with marked hypertension.
Consideration must be given to the functional ability of the kidneys before injecting this preparation.
When any intravenous injection technique is employed, the possibility of thrombosis or of other complications due to the mechanical trauma of the procedure should be borne in mind.

Contrast agents may interfere with some chemical determinations made on urine specimens; therefore, urine should be collected before administration of the contrast medium or two or more days afterwards.
Since iodine-containing contrast agents may alter the results of thyroid function tests depending on iodine estimations (e.g., PBI and radioactive iodine uptake studies), such tests, if indicated, should be performed prior to administration of this preparation. However, measurements of serum thyroxine concentration involving use of tests such as the Resin Triiodothyronine Uptake test, "RT_3U," or the Thyroxine (Displacement) assay, "$T_4(D)$," are not affected.
Premedication with antihistamines to avoid or minimize possible allergic reactions, or their use in the management of adverse reactions, may be considered; however, admixture of an antihistamine with a contrast agent may result in a precipitate (see DOSAGE AND ADMINISTRATION).
Use of a diuretic prior to the examination in order to increase the urinary concentration of the contrast medium is not desirable (see DOSAGE AND ADMINISTRATION); dehydration may predispose to a greater incidence of, or more severe, reactions.
Sensitivity Testing—Severe, life-threatening reactions to radiopaque agents often resemble hypersensitivity phenomena. This has prompted the use of several pretesting methods, none of which can be relied on to predict severe reactions. Many authorities question the value of any pretest. A history of bronchial asthma or allergy, a family history of allergy, or a previous reaction to a contrast agent warrant special attention. Such a history, by suggesting histamine sensitivity and a consequent proneness to reactions may be more accurate than pretesting in predicting the likelihood of a reaction, although it will not necessarily indicate the severity or type of reaction in the individual case.
The sensitivity test most often performed is the slow intravenous injection of 0.5 to 1.0 ml. of the radiopaque medium prior to injection of the full diagnostic dose. It should be noted that the absence of a reaction to the test dose does not preclude the possibility of a reaction to the full diagnostic dose. If the test dose causes an untoward response of any kind, the necessity for continuing with the examination should be carefully reevaluated and, if it is deemed essential, the examination should be conducted with all possible caution. In rare instances reactions to the test dose itself may be extremely severe; therefore, close observation of the patient and facilities for emergency treatment are essential.
Usage in Pregnancy—No teratogenic effects attributable to the Iodamide Meglumine Injection have been observed in reproduction studies performed in mice, rats, and rabbits. Safety for use during pregnancy in humans has not been established. Although there is no clearly defined risk, the possibility of infrequent or subtle damage to the fetus cannot be excluded. Iodamide Meglumine Injection should be used in pregnant women only when clearly needed.
Adverse Reactions: In clinical studies with iodamide meglumine, adverse reactions occurred in approximately 9.5 to 13 percent of patients. The most frequently seen reactions were nausea and/or vomiting, urticaria, pruritus, a rise or fall in blood pressure, sneezing, and sensation of warmth, individually occurring at a frequency of approximately one to five percent. Reactions were usually mild. Reactions occurring less frequently are: generalized flushing, lacrimation, headache, edema of the eyelids, coughing, retching, bitter or metallic taste, pharyngeal burning sensation, nasal congestion, hoarseness, sweating and weakness, malaise, perianal burning sensation, pain and erythema around the injection site due to faulty technique, bradycardia, hyperpnea, and shock.
Other reactions to iodinated contrast media may occur including chills, fever, pulse rate increase, shortness of breath, dizziness, syncope, restlessness, lightheadedness, pallor, choking, chest pain, tachycardia, laryngeal or pulmonary edema, dysphagia, facial or conjunctival petechiae, rash and other eruptions, wheezing, asthmatic reaction, cramps, tremors, anxiety, hemiparesis, hematomas and ecchymoses due to technique, vein cramp, partial collapse of the injected vein, thrombophlebitis and cellulitis following injection, neutropenia, transient proteinuria, hysterical reaction and numbness of head and neck, and convulsions. "Iodism" (salivary gland swelling) has been reported infrequently; immediate or delayed rigors sometimes with hyperpyrexia has occurred rarely.
Antihistaminic agents may be of benefit in the event of adverse reactions. Adverse reactions may be severe enough to require discontinuation of injection.
Severe reactions to contrast agents, which may require emergency measures (see PRECAUTIONS), may take the form of a cardiovascular reaction characterized by peripheral vasodilatation with resultant hypotension and reflex tachycardia, dyspnea, agitation, confusion, and cyanosis progressing to unconsciousness. Rare cases of cardiac arrest, ventricular fibrillation, cardiac arrhythmias, and hypertension may occur. The histamine-liberating effect of these compounds may induce an allergic-like reaction which may range in severity from rhinitis or angioneurotic edema to laryngeal or bronchial spasm and, rarely, anaphylactoid shock.
Rarely, temporary renal shutdown or other nephropathy may occur.
Dosage and Administration: Renovue-65 (Iodamide Meglumine Injection) should be at body temperature when injected, and may need to be warmed before use. If kept in a syringe for prolonged periods before injection, it should be protected from exposure to strong light.
Appropriate preparation of the patient is desirable for optimal results. A laxative the night before the examination and a low residue diet the day before the procedure may be used to clear the gastrointestinal tract. However, a normal liquid intake during this time is desirable. Partial dehydration, although it is believed to increase the urinary concentration of the contrast medium, is not recommended in infants or young children, in whom the injection represents an osmotic load superimposed upon the increased serum osmolality obtained by partial dehydration.
Renovue-65 is administered by intravenous injection. In both adults and children the dosage should be administered within 1 to 2 minutes.
Adults—The recommended adult dose is 0.8 ml. per kg. body weight, up to a maximum total dose of 50 ml.
Infants and Children—Pediatric patients require proportionately less and suggested dosages are as follows: Under 6 months—5 ml.; 6 to 12 months—8 ml.; 1 to 2 years—10 ml.; 3 to 5 years—12 ml.; 6 to 7 years—15 ml.; 8 to 10 years—18 ml.; 11 to 12 years—20 ml.; over 12 years—0.8 ml. per kg. body weight, up to a maximum total dose of 50 ml.
If flushing or nausea occurs during administration, injection should be slowed or briefly interrupted until the side effects have disappeared. If a serious reaction should occur, administration should be discontinued immediately.
The admixture of Benadryl® (Diphenhydramine Hydrochloride Injection) with Renovue-65 may cause a precipitate to form in the syringe. If antihistamines are administered concomitantly (see PRECAUTIONS), they should *not* be mixed with the contrast agent and should be administered at another site.
Roentgenographic Procedure: A scout film should be made before the contrast medium is administered. Several films should be exposed after injection to allow for individual variation and to insure visualization of the desired sites of the urinary tract. Times at which optimal opacification may be observed in most patients are as follows: renal parenchyma at 1 minute after injection; calyces, pelves, and ureters at 10 minutes; and urinary bladder at 20 minutes. In patients with renal dysfunction, optimal visualization may be delayed until 30 minutes or more after injection.
How Supplied: Available in 50 ml. single-dose vials containing sufficient excess for sensitivity testing.
Storage: The preparation should be stored at room temperature, protected from light and excessive heat. If precipitation or solidification has occurred due to storage in the cold, immerse the container in hot water and shake intermittently to dissolve any solids.

RENOVUE®-DIP ℞
(Iodamide Meglumine Injection 24%)
For Drip Infusion Pyelography

Description: Renovue-DIP is a radiopaque contrast agent for drip infusion pyelography supplied as a sterile, nonpyrogenic, aqueous, intravenous solution providing 24% iodamide meglumine with approximately 11.1% (111 mg./ml.) organically bound iodine. The solution also contains 0.00368% edetate disodium as a sequestering agent. The clear, colorless to pale yellow solution has a viscosity of 1.8 cps. at 37° C. and 2.0 cps. at 25° C.; the pH has been adjusted to 6.5 to 7.7 with iodamide. The solution has an osmolarity of approximately 0.5 mOsm per ml. at 37° C. *Renovue-DIP contains approximately 0.0046 mg. (0.0002 mEq.) sodium per ml.* At the time of manufacture, the air in the container is replaced with nitrogen.
Chemically, iodamide meglumine is 3-(acetylamino)-5 [(acetylamino)methyl] -2,4,6-triiodobenzoic acid, N-methylglucamine salt.
Clinical Pharmacology: Following intravenous infusion, Renovue-DIP is rapidly transported through the bloodstream to the kidneys and is excreted essentially unchanged in the urine, principally by glomerular filtration. However, at least one-third of the intravenous dose is secreted by the renal tubules.
After infusion, the contrast agent permits visualization of the kidneys and urinary passages through the natural physiologic mechanism of excretion.
Renal accumulation is sufficiently rapid so that the period of maximal opacification of the renal passages may begin within five minutes after start of infusion. Normal kidneys rapidly eliminate the contrast medium. In nephropathic conditions, particularly when excretory capacity has been altered, the rate of excretion varies unpredictably, and opacification may be delayed for 60 minutes or more after start of infusion; with severe renal impairment, opacification may not occur. Generally the medium is concentrated sufficiently and promptly enough to permit satisfactory visualization of the urinary tract.
Indications and Usage: Renovue-DIP is a diagnostic agent for excretion urography by intravenous infusion.
Contraindications: There are no absolute contraindications to the use of Renovue-DIP (Iodamide Meglumine Injection 24%) (see WARNINGS).
Warnings: A definite risk exists in the performance of excretion urography in patients who are known to have multiple myeloma, because of the great possibility of producing transient to fatal renal failure. The risk of ex-

Continued on next page

Squibb—Cont.

cretion urography in myelomatous patients is not a contraindication to the procedure; however, dehydration in the preparation of these patients should be avoided, since this may predispose to the precipitation of protein in the renal tubules.

Administration of radiopaque materials to patients known or suspected to have pheochromocytoma should be performed only if the physician deems that the possible benefits outweigh the considered risks; the procedure should then be performed with extreme caution and the volume of radiopaque medium injected should be kept to an absolute minimum. The blood pressure should be assessed throughout the procedure and measures for treatment of a hypertensive crisis should be available.

Contrast media administered intravenously have been shown to promote the phenomenon of sickling in individuals who are homozygous for sickle cell disease.

Urography should be performed with extreme caution in patients with severe concomitant hepatic and renal disease, or anuria.

A history of sensitivity to iodine *per se* or to any contrast agent is not an absolute contraindication to the use of iodamide meglumine, but calls for extreme caution in administration.

Precautions: *General*—All procedures utilizing contrast media carry a definite risk of producing adverse reactions. While most reactions may be minor, life-threatening and fatal reactions may occur without warning. The risk-benefit factor should always be carefully evaluated before such a procedure is undertaken. At all times a fully equipped emergency cart, or equivalent supplies and equipment, and personnel competent in recognizing and treating adverse reactions of all severity (or situations which may arise as a result of the procedure) should be immediately available. If a serious reaction should occur, administration should be discontinued immediately.

Since severe delayed reactions have been known to occur, emergency facilities and competent personnel should be available for at least 30 to 60 minutes after administration.

Renal toxicity has been reported in a few patients with liver dysfunction who were given oral choleystographic agents followed by urographic agents. Administration of Iodamide Meglumine Injection 24% should therefore be postponed in any patient with a known or suspected hepatic or biliary disorder who has recently taken a cholecystographic contrast agent.

Caution should be exercised with the use of radiopaque media in severely debilitated patients and in those with marked hypertension.

The increased osmotic load associated with drip infusion pyelography should also be considered in patients with congestive heart failure.

Consideration must be given to the functional ability of the kidneys before infusing this preparation.

The diuretic effect of the drip infusion pyelography procedure may hinder assessment of residual urine in the bladder.

When any intravenous infusion technique is employed, the possibility of thrombosis or of other complications due to the mechanical trauma of the procedure should be borne in mind.

The recommended rate of infusion should not be exceeded.

Contrast agents may interfere with some chemical determinations made on urine specimens; therefore, urine should be collected before administration of the contrast medium or two or more days afterwards.

Since iodine-containing contrast agents may alter the results of thyroid function tests which depend on iodine estimations (e.g., PBI and radioactive iodine uptake studies), such tests, if indicated, should be performed prior to the administration of this preparation. However, measurements of serum thyroxine concentration involving use of tests such as the Resin Triiodothyronine Uptake test, "RT_3U," or the Thyroxine (Displacement) assay, "$T_4(D)$," are not affected.

Premedication with antihistamines to avoid or minimize possible allergic reactions, or their use in the management of adverse reactions, may be considered; however, admixture of an antihistamine with a contrast agent may result in a precipitate (see DOSAGE AND ADMINISTRATION).

Use of a diuretic prior to the examination in order to increase the urinary concentration of the contrast medium is not desirable (see DOSAGE AND ADMINISTRATION); dehydration may predispose to a greater incidence of, or more severe, reactions.

Sensitivity Testing: Severe, life-threatening reactions to radiopaque agents often resemble hypersensitivity phenomena. This has prompted the use of several pretesting methods, none of which can be relied on to predict severe reactions. Many authorities question the value of any pretest. A history of bronchial asthma or allergy, a family history of allergy, or a previous reaction to a contrast agent warrant special attention. Such a history, by suggesting histamine sensitivity and a consequent proneness to reactions may be more accurate than pretesting in predicting the likelihood of a reaction, although it will not necessarily indicate the severity or type of reaction in the individual case.

The sensitivity test most often performed is the slow intravenous injection of 0.5 to 1.0 ml. of the radiopaque medium, prior to infusion of the full diagnostic dose. It should be noted that the absence of a reaction to the test dose does not preclude the possibility of a reaction to the full diagnostic dose. If the test dose causes an untoward response of any kind, the necessity for continuing with the examination should be carefully reevaluated and, if it is deemed essential, the examination should be conducted with all possible caution. In rare instances reactions to the test dose itself may be extremely severe; therefore, close observation of the patient, and facilities for emergency treatment, are essential.

Usage in Pregnancy: No teratogenic effects attributable to Iodamide Meglumine Injection 24% have been observed in reproduction studies performed in mice, rats, and rabbits. Safety for use during pregnancy in humans has not been established. Although there is no clearly defined risk, the possibility of infrequent or subtle damage to the fetus cannot be excluded. Iodamide Meglumine Injection 24% should be used in pregnant women only when clearly needed.

Pediatric Use: Administration of iodamide meglumine by infusion has not been evaluated in pediatric patients; however, Renovue-65 (Iodamide Meglumine Injection), the less dilute formulation, is available for use in infants and children. See the package insert accompanying that product for complete information.

Adverse Reactions: In clinical studies with iodamide meglumine, adverse reactions occurred in approximately 9.5 to 13 percent of patients. The most frequently seen adverse reactions were nausea and/or vomiting, urticaria, pruritus, and a rise or fall in blood pressure, individually occurring at a frequency of approximately one to five percent. Reactions were usually mild. Reactions occurring less frequently are generalized flushing, retching, nasal congestion, sneezing, flank tenderness, chills, syncope, pulse rate increase, hyperpnea, shortness of breath, chest pain, tachycardia, and hemiparesis.

Other reactions to iodinated contrast media may occur including fever; dizziness; headache; lacrimation; sweating and weakness; lightheadedness; restlessness; pallor; coughing; choking; hoarseness; laryngeal or pulmonary edema; dysphagia; malaise; edema of the eyelids; bitter or metallic taste; pharyngeal burning sensation; facial or conjunctival petechiae; rash and other eruptions; perianal burning sensation; wheezing; asthmatic reaction; cramps; tremors; anxiety; pain, erythema, hematomas, and ecchymoses around injection site due to faulty technique; warmth or burning sensation; vein cramp; partial collapse of the injected vein; thrombophlebitis and cellulitis following injection; neutropenia; transient proteinuria; hysterical reaction and numbness of head and neck; bradycardia; shock; and convulsions. "Iodism" (salivary gland swelling) has been reported infrequently; immediate or delayed rigors sometimes with hyperpyrexia has occurred rarely.

Antihistaminic agents may be of benefit in the event of adverse reactions. Adverse reactions may be severe enough to require discontinuation of infusion.

Severe reactions to contrast agents, which may require emergency measures (see PRECAUTIONS), may take the form of a cardiovascular reaction characterized by peripheral vasodilatation with resultant hypotension and reflex tachycardia, dyspnea, agitation, confusion, and cyanosis progressing to unconsciousness. Rare cases of cardiac arrest, ventricular fibrillation, cardiac arrhythmias, and hypertension may occur. The histamine-liberating effect of these compounds may induce an allergic-like reaction which may range in severity from rhinitis or angioneurotic edema to laryngeal or bronchial spasm and, rarely, anaphylactoid shock.

Rarely, temporary renal shutdown or other nephropathy may occur.

Dosage and Administration: Renovue-DIP (Iodamide Meglumine Injection 24%) should be at body temperature when infused, and may need to be warmed before use.

Appropriate preparation of the patient is desirable for optimal results. A laxative the night before the examination and a low residue diet the day before the procedure may be used to clear the gastrointestinal tract. However, a normal liquid intake during this time is desirable.

The recommended adult dose is 4.5 ml. per kg. of body weight, administered intravenously by continuous infusion, with a maximum total dose of 300 ml.; the appropriate volume should be infused in approximately 10 minutes (about 30 ml. per minute for a 147 lb. or heavier patient), through a large-bore (usually 17- or 18-gauge) needle. In older patients and in patients with known or suspected cardiac decompensation, a slower rate of infusion is probably wise. If flushing or nausea occurs during administration, infusion should be slowed or briefly interrupted until the side effects have disappeared. If a serious reaction should occur, administration should be discontinued immediately.

The admixture of Benadryl® (Diphenhydramine Hydrochloride Injection) with Renovue-DIP may cause a precipitate to form in the tubing. If antihistamines are administered concomitantly (see PRECAUTIONS), they should *not* be mixed with the contrast agent and should be administered at another site.

Roentgenographic Procedure: A scout film should be made before the contrast medium is administered. Several films should be exposed after infusion to allow for individual variation and to insure visualization of the desired sites of the urinary tract. Times at which optimal opacification may be first observed in the majority of patients are as follows: renal parenchyma at 10 minutes after start of infusion, calyces and pelves at 20 minutes, and ureters and bladder at 30 minutes. In patients with renal dysfunction, optimal visualization may be delayed until 60 minutes or more after the start of infusion.

How Supplied: Available in packages of 10 single-dose 300 ml. infusion bottles and packages of 10 single-dose 300 ml. infusion bottles with solution administration sets. The bottles are calibrated, designed to be suspended from an I.V. stand, and contain sufficient excess for sensitivity testing.
Storage: The preparation should be stored at room temperature, protected from light and excessive heat. If precipitation or solidification has occurred due to storage in the cold, immerse the container in hot water and shake intermittently to dissolve any solids.

SINOGRAFIN® ℞
(Diatrizoate Meglumine and Iodipamide Meglumine Injection)

Description: Sinografin is available as a sterile, aqueous solution for intrauterine instillation. Each ml. provides 527 mg. diatrizoate meglumine and 268 mg. iodipamide meglumine with 3.2 mg. sodium citrate as a buffer, and 0.4 mg. edetate disodium. Each vial contains approximately 3.8 g. organically bound iodine (380 mg./ml.). At the time of manufacture, the air in the container is replaced by nitrogen.
Actions: Following intrauterine administration, immediate visualization of the uterus and tubes is achieved. Present evidence indicates that any medium spilled into the peritoneal cavity as a result of the procedure is absorbed within 20 to 60 minutes. A 24-hour film has shown complete absorption even in cases of large hydrosalpinx.
Indications: Sinografin is indicated for use in hysterosalpingography.
Contraindications: This preparation is contraindicated during pregnancy or in the presence of acute pelvic inflammatory disease. Hysterosalpingography should not be attempted within 30 days following curettage or conization. Sinografin should not be administered to patients with a hypersensitivity to iodipamide or salts of diatrizoic acid.
Warnings: Since iodine-containing contrast agents may alter the results of thyroid function tests, such tests, if indicated, should be performed prior to the administration of this drug.
A history of sensitivity to iodine *per se* or to contrast media other than iodipamide or salts of diatrizoic acid is not an absolute contraindication to the use of Sinografin but calls for extreme caution in administration.
Precautions: Hypersensitivity reactions have occurred and are more likely in patients with a personal or familial history of allergy. These may be manifested by reactions such as urticaria, respiratory symptoms and circulatory collapse. Facilities for treatment of circulatory collapse and respiratory distress should be immediately available, and patients should be carefully observed during performance of the examination and for at least 30 to 60 minutes thereafter.
When performing radiography, serial x-ray pictures should be taken where possible in preference to fluoroscopic visualization to minimize radiation exposure.
Adverse Reactions: Hypersensitivity reactions, which include sweating, flushing, pruritus, urticaria, skin rashes, arthralgia, respiratory distress, and circulatory collapse have occurred. Chills, fever, nausea, vomiting, and abdominal pain and tenderness are occasionally seen following instillation of the contrast material.
Dosage and Administration: *Dosage:* 3 to 4 ml. of Sinografin are usually adequate to visualize the uterus, and an additional 3 to 4 ml. will demonstrate the tubes. Total dosage varying from 1.5 to 10 ml. has been employed with satisfactory results.
Preparation of the patient: Hysterosalpingography should be performed three to five days after the cessation of the patient's menstrual period as a precautionary measure. An enema and vaginal douche one hour before the examination are helpful, but not essential. The patient should empty her bladder before the examination. Since the procedure is remarkably free of pain when Sinografin is used, the use of a narcotic or anesthesia is unnecessary.
Administration: The patient is placed in the lithotomy position and the vulva is cleansed with a suitable antiseptic solution. A Graves-type vaginal speculum is introduced, the cervix is exposed, and the vaginal vault is sponged with antiseptic solution.
A tenaculum is placed on the cervical lip, usually the anterior lip. A sterile sound may be passed to determine the position of the uterus and the direction of the cervical canal, and, when necessary, the cervical canal may be dilated. (Sounding the uterine cavity and dilatation of the canal are not usually required when a flexible cannula tip is used.)
A sterile syringe containing the Sinografin is attached by Luer-Lok to a uterine cannula. The two-way cannula valve is opened and all air bubbles in the cannula and syringe are expressed. About 1.5 to 2 ml. of Sinografin are required to fill the cannula. (If preferred, a tubal insufflator under controlled pressure with a salpingogram attachment may be used instead of the syringe.)
The cannula tip is inserted into the cervical canal so that the adjustable rubber acorn obturator fits snugly at the external os. Careful placement of the cannula is important to avoid trauma and pain. Squeezing the trigger of the cannula to provide simultaneous traction on the tenaculum and forward pressure on the cannula should give a nonleaking cervical seal. Sinografin flows freely so that only gentle pressure on the plunger is necessary.
The connection at the external os is checked for leakage. If the acorn obturator is inadequate, an inflatable balloon-obturator may be used to seal the cervical canal. When the equipment has been positioned satisfactorily, the tenaculum and cannula may be fixed in position until the procedure is terminated.
Radiography: Sinografin is administered in fractional doses of approximately 1 ml. A scout film may be made before the medium is administered. After the initial injection, a film should be made using a Bucky diaphragm. After each successive injection of 1 ml., a film is taken, developed immediately, and inspected in the dark room before the next fractional dose of Sinografin is given, until the procedure is completed. Further injection and subsequent films can be made as required using posterior-anterior or oblique angles.
Clinical experience indicates that tubal patency, if present, will be demonstrable at the time of the injection and delayed films have not been required. The medium is completely absorbed within one hour, unless there is an obstruction and dilatation of the tubes, in which case absorption is generally complete within 24 hours. Any residual Sinografin within the uterine cavity is usually expelled immediately upon removal of the cannula.
How Supplied: Available in single-dose vials of 10 ml.
Storage: Store at room temperature (20° to 25°C.) and protect against exposure to strong light. The Sinografin solution may vary in color from essentially colorless to light amber; however, solutions which have become strongly discolored should not be used. Sinografin should be used as promptly as possible following withdrawal into the syringe, and the syringe should be rinsed as soon as possible after injection to prevent freezing of the plunger.

For information on Squibb products, write to: Squibb Professional Services Department, Lawrenceville-Princeton Road, Princeton, N.J. 08540.

Winthrop Laboratories
90 PARK AVENUE
NEW YORK, NY 10016

AMIPAQUE® ℞
brand of metrizamide

Description: Metrizamide, 2-[3-Acetamido-2, 4, 6-triiodo-5-(N-methylacetamido) benzamido]-2-deoxy-D-glucopyranose, is a compound derived from metrizoic acid and glucosamine. It is a nonionic water-soluble contrast medium with a molecular weight of 789 (iodine content: 48.25%).
The viscosity in centipoise of the "use" concentration ranges from 2.9 at 170 mgI/ml to 12.7 at 300 mgI/ml at room temperature (20 C) and from 1.8 to 6.2 at body temperature (37 C) respectively. Osmolality in mOsm/kg at 37 C ranges from 300 at 170 mgI/ml concentration to 484 at 300 mgI/ml. CSF is approximately 301. Specific gravity ranges from 1.184 at 170 mgI/ml to 1.329 at 300 mgI/ml. (CSF normal range is 1.005 to 1.009.) The pH of the solution reconstituted from the diluent is approximately 7.4.
AMIPAQUE is provided as a sterile, white lyophilized powder under vacuum. Each 3.75 g/20 ml vial contains 3.75 g metrizamide (1.81 g organically-bound iodine) and 1.2 mg edetate calcium disodium. Each 6.75 g/50 ml vial contains 6.75 g metrizamide (3.26 g organically-bound iodine) and 2.16 mg edetate calcium disodium.
Each 20 ml vial of sterile aqueous diluent contains 0.05 mg/ml sodium bicarbonate in water for injection. pH is adjusted with carbon dioxide, USP, if necessary.
AMIPAQUE solution and powder is sensitive to heat or light and, therefore, should be protected from exposure.
Clinical Pharmacology: AMIPAQUE is absorbed from cerebrospinal fluid into the bloodstream. Approximately 60 percent of the administered dose is excreted unchanged through the kidneys within 48 hours.
The initial concentration and volume of the medium, in conjunction with appropriate patient manipulation, will determine the extent of the diagnostic contrast that can be achieved. This can be monitored by fluoroscopy.
Following subarachnoid injection conventional radiography will continue to provide good diagnostic contrast for at least 30 minutes. At about 1 hour diagnostic degree of contrast will not usually be available. However, sufficient contrast for CT myelography will be available for several hours. CT myelography, following conventional myelography, should be deferred for at least 4 hours to reduce the degree of contrast.
Following subarachnoid placement, irrespective of the position in which the patient is later maintained, slow upward diffusion of AMIPAQUE takes place through the CSF. After introduction into the lumbar subarachnoid space, without special positioning of the patient, computerized tomography (CT) shows CSF contrast enhancement in the thoracic region in about 1 hour, in the cervical region in about 2 hours, and in the basal cisterns in 3 to 4 hours.
When low doses (4 to 6 ml of 170 to 190 mgI/ml) of AMIPAQUE are introduced into the lumbar CSF and moved cephalad under gravity control and examined by CT scanning, they will pro-

This product information was effective as of November 19, 1982. On these and other products of Winthrop Laboratories, detailed information may be obtained on a current basis by direct inquiry to the Professional Services Department, 90 Park Avenue, New York, NY 10016 (212) 907-2525.

Winthrop—Cont.

vide immediate CSF contrast in the basal cisterns. Depending on the specific technique used, the lateral, third, and fourth ventricles may also be visualized. The contrast in this area will markedly diminish at 6 hours and disappear by 24 hours. CSF enhancement will be evident at the cortical sulci and interhemispheric fissures at 6 hours.

Between 12 and 24 hours the surfaces of the cerebrum and cerebellum, in contact with the subarachnoid spaces, will develop a "blush" effect on the scan which will normally disappear in 36 to 48 hours. The rate, time, extent of diffusion, and the disappearance or stasis of AMIPAQUE as demonstrated with CT scanning, can be used to detect or infer the presence of CNS or CSF circulation abnormalities.

Indications and Usage: AMIPAQUE is indicated for lumbar, thoracic, cervical, and total columnar myelography and for use in computerized tomography of the intracranial subarachnoid spaces following spinal subarachnoid injection.

Contraindications: AMIPAQUE, brand of metrizamide, should not be administered to patients with a known hypersensitivity to metrizamide.

Intrathecal administration of corticosteroids with AMIPAQUE is contraindicated.

Immediate repeat myelography, in the event of technical failure, is contraindicated because of overdosage considerations. (See interval recommendation under DOSAGE AND ADMINISTRATION.)

Lumbar puncture should not be performed in the presence of significant local or systemic infection where bacteremia is likely.

Warnings: If grossly bloody CSF is encountered, the possible benefits of a myelographic procedure should be considered in terms of the risk to the patient.

Fatal reactions have been associated with the administration of water-soluble contrast media. Therefore, it is of utmost importance that a course of action be carefully planned in advance for the immediate treatment of serious reactions, and that adequate and appropriate facilities and personnel be readily available in case of a severe reaction.

Caution is advised in patients with a history of epilepsy, severe cardiovascular disease, chronic alcoholism or multiple sclerosis.

Elderly patients may present a greater risk following myelography. The need for the procedure in these patients should be evaluated carefully. Special attention must be paid to dose and concentration of the medium, hydration, and technique used.

Patients who are receiving anticonvulsants should be maintained on this therapy. Should a seizure occur, intravenous diazepam or phenobarbital sodium is recommended. In patients with a history of seizure activity who are not on anticonvulsant therapy, premedication with barbiturates or phenytoin should be considered.

Prophylactic anticonvulsant treatment with barbiturates should be considered in patients with evidence of inadvertent intracranial entry of a large or concentrated bolus of the contrast medium since there is an increased risk of seizures in such cases.

Drugs which lower the seizure threshold, especially phenothiazine derivatives, including those used for their antihistamine properties should not be used with AMIPAQUE. Others include MAO inhibitors, tricyclic antidepressants, CNS stimulants, psychoactive drugs described as analeptics, major tranquilizers, or antipsychotic drugs. Such medication should be discontinued at least 48 hours before myelography, should not be used for the control of nausea and vomiting, and should not be resumed for at least 24 hours postprocedure.

Care is required in patient management to prevent inadvertent intracranial entry of a large dose or concentrated bolus of the medium. Also, effort should be directed to avoid rapid dispersion of the medium causing inadvertent rise to intracranial levels (eg, by active patient movement). Direct intracisternal or ventricular administration for standard radiography (not CT) is not recommended.

In most reported cases of major motor seizures one or more of the following factors were present. Therefore avoid:

- Deviations from recommended procedure or in myelographic management.
- Use in patients with a history of epilepsy.
- Inadvertent overdosage.
- Intracranial entry of a bolus or premature diffusion of a high concentration of the medium.
- Medication with neuroleptic drugs or phenothiazine antinauseants.
- Failure to maintain elevation of the head during the procedure, on the stretcher, or in bed.
- Excessive and particularly active patient movement or straining.

At concentrations of 200 mgI/ml or less, these seizures have been noted only very rarely.

Treatment with intravenous diazepam or administration of phenobarbital sodium has provided rapid control of seizures. (See PATIENT MANAGEMENT.)

Precautions: Before a contrast medium is injected, the patient should be questioned for a history of allergy. Although a history of allergy, including asthma, may imply a greater than usual risk, it does not arbitrarily contraindicate the use of the medium. No conclusive relationship between severe reactions and antigen-antibody reactions or other manifestations of allergy has been established.

In patients with severe renal insufficiency or failure, the drug is excreted by the liver into the bile at a much slower rate. Patients with hepatorenal insufficiency should not be examined unless the possibility of benefit clearly outweighs the additional risk.

Repeat Procedure: See DOSAGE AND ADMINISTRATION.

If nondisposable equipment is used, scrupulous care should be taken to prevent residual contamination with traces of cleansing agents.

Pregnancy Category B. Reproduction studies have been performed in rats and rabbits up to 70 times the human dose and have revealed no evidence of impaired fertility or harm to the fetus due to AMIPAQUE. There are, however, no adequate and well controlled studies in pregnant women. Because animal reproduction studies are not always predictive of human response, this drug should be used during pregnancy only if clearly needed.

Nursing Mothers. It is not known whether the contrast medium is excreted in human milk, many are. Though there is no sufficient information on the excretion of AMIPAQUE in breast milk, the potential for adverse reaction in nursing infants exists. As with all drugs and procedures, the physician must assess the expected benefits for the procedure for the mother against the potential for risk to the infant, as well as taking into account whether to discontinue nursing.

Pediatric Use. Until further experience is gained in children younger than 12 years, administration of AMIPAQUE, brand of metrizamide, in this age group is not recommended.

Adverse Reactions: The most frequently occurring adverse reactions are headache, nausea, and vomiting. These reactions occur 3 to 8 hours postinjection, almost all occurring within 24 hours. They are usually mild to moderate in degree lasting for a few hours and usually disappearing within 24 hours. Rarely, headaches may be severe or persist for days. The reported incidence of headaches varies from 20 to over 60 percent and they are often accompanied by nausea and vomiting. Headaches tend to be more frequent and persistent in patients not optimally hydrated. (See PATIENT MANAGEMENT.)

Backache, neck stiffness, numbness and paresthesias, leg or sciatic-type pain occurred less frequently, often in the form of a transient exacerbation of preexisting symptomatology. Temperature elevations and dizziness have also been reported.

Cardiovascular: Chest pain, tachycardia, bradycardia and other arrhythmias, hypertension or hypotension.

Transient alterations in **vital signs** may occur. Their significance must be assessed on an individual basis.

Other rarely occurring adverse reactions include the following:

Major motor seizures: Focal or generalized grand mal seizures have occurred with an incidence reported between 0.1 and 0.3 percent. They have usually occurred 4 to 12 hours following injection, and have consisted of one or two episodes 1 or more hours apart, which have responded promptly to the intravenous injection of diazepam. For prolonged prophylaxis barbiturates have been recommended.

Early onset of seizures (less than 2 hours) is indicative of early substantial intracranial entry.

Transitory EEG changes are frequent and usually take the form of slow wave activity.

An **aseptic meningitis** syndrome, has been reported rarely (less than 0.1%). It was usually preceded by pronounced headaches, nausea and vomiting. Onset usually occurred about 12 to 18 hours postprocedure. Prominent features were meningismus, fever, sometimes with oculomotor signs and mental confusion. Lumbar puncture revealed a high white cell count, high protein content often with a low glucose level and with absence of organisms. The condition usually started to clear spontaneously about 10 hours after onset, with complete recovery over 2 to 3 days.

Allergy or Idiosyncrasy: Chills, pruritus, urticaria, nasal congestion, dyspnea, and a case of Guillain-Barre syndrome.

CNS Irritation: Mild and transitory perceptual aberrations such as hallucinations, depersonalization, anxiety, depression, hyperesthesia, visual, auditory or speech disturbances, confusion and disorientation. In addition, malaise, weakness, EEG changes, meningismus, hyperreflexia or areflexia, hypertonia or flaccidity, restlessness, tremor, echoacousia, echolalia, asterixis or dysphasia have occurred.

Profound mental disturbances have also rarely been reported. They have usually consisted of various forms and degrees of aphasia, mental confusion or disorientation. The onset is usually at 8-10 hours and lasts for about 24 hours, without aftereffects. However, occasionally they have been manifest as apprehension, agitation, or progressive withdrawal in several instances to the point of stupor. In a few cases these have been accompanied by transitory hearing loss or other auditory symptoms and visual disturbances (believed subjective or delusional). In one case persistent cortical loss of vision has been reported in association with convulsions. Ventricular block has been reported in two cases.

Rarely, persistent though transitory weakness in the leg or ocular muscles has been reported.

Peripheral neuropathies have been rare and transitory. They include sensory and/or motor or nerve root disturbances, myelitis, persistent leg muscle pain or weakness, or 6th nerve palsy, or cauda equina syndrome. Muscle cramps, fasciculation or myoclonia, spinal convulsion, or spasticity are unusual and have responded promptly to a small intravenous dose of diazepam.

Overdosage: There is clinical evidence that reactions, particularly seizures and mental aberrations, following the administration of myelographic doses in excess of those recommended tend to be dose related. Even use of a

recommended dose can produce effects tantamount to overdosage, if incorrect management of the patient during or immediately following the procedure permits inadvertent early intracranial entry of a large portion of the medium.
Treatment: See ADVERSE REACTIONS—Major motor seizures.
The subarachnoid LD_{50} in mice is greater than 1,500 mgI/kg.

Dosage and Administration: See also PATIENT MANAGEMENT. The dosage and concentration of AMIPAQUE, brand of metrizamide, will depend on the degree and extent of contrast required in the area(s) under examination and on the equipment and technique employed. Concentrations which are approximately isotonic (170 to 190 mgI/ml) are recommended for examination in the lumbar region. For movement of the medium to distant target areas, higher concentrations are recommended to compensate for dilution of AMIPAQUE with CSF.
A total dose of 3000 mg iodine or a concentration of 300 mgI/ml should not be exceeded. As in all diagnostic procedures, the least amount to produce adequate visualization should be used. Most procedures do not require either maximum dose or concentration. The incidence of serious adverse reactions is considerably less with concentrations of 200 mgI/ml or less. The dose and concentration used in the spinal area influence ultimate intracranial concentrations.
Anesthesia is not necessary. Premedication sedatives or tranquilizers are usually not needed (see PRECAUTIONS). Patients should be well hydrated. Epileptic patients should be maintained on their anticonvulsant medication.
As with any lumbar puncture, sterile technique must be employed. The lumbar puncture is usually made between L3 and L4, but if pathology is suspected at this level the interspace immediately above or below may be selected. A lateral cervical puncture may also be used.

Rate of Injection: To avoid excessive mixing with CSF and consequent loss of contrast as well as premature dispersion upward, injection must be made slowly over 1 to 2 minutes. The lumbar puncture needle is removed immediately following injection since it is not necessary to remove AMIPAQUE after injection into subarachnoid spaces.
An interval of at least 48 hours should be allowed before repeat examination; however, whenever possible 5 to 7 days is recommended. The recommended usual and maximum doses of AMIPAQUE are summarized in the table above.

DOSAGE TABLE—Iodine Content

Procedure	Conc. of Solution (mgI/ml)	Usual Recommended Dose* (ml)	Max. Dose Total (mgI)
Lumbar myelogram	170–190	10–15	2850
Thoracic myelogram	220	12	2640
Cervical myelogram (via lumbar injection)	250–300	10	3000
Cervical myelogram (via lateral cervical injection)	220	10	2200
Total columnar myelography	250–280	10	2800
CT cisternography (via lumber injection)	170–190	4–6	1140

* Refer to RECONSTITUTION TABLE for preparation of Solution.

PREPARATION OF THE SOLUTION:
1. Select the correct iodine concentration recommended for the procedure in the DOSAGE TABLE.
2. The volume of diluent required to obtain that iodine concentration can be obtained from the RECONSTITUTION TABLE.
3. Using a sterile technique with a small gauge transfer needle (approximately 22 gauge to help prevent coring), withdraw the required amount of diluent.
4. Insert this volume of diluent into the lyophil vial also using the fine needle. Contents under vacuum. Use only if vacuum is present as evidenced by diluent being drawn into vial when stopper is punctured. Leave syringe and needle in place.
5. Gently swirl the vial (without shaking) until its contents are dissolved (approximately 3 to 10 minutes) to insure complete dissolution of the lyophil. The resulting solution should be clear and colorless to slightly yellow. Do not use if undissolved particulate matter or bubbles are present.
6. Withdraw the volume of AMIPAQUE, brand of metrizamide, recommended for the procedure in the DOSAGE TABLE.
7. Detach syringe and attach to myelographic injection unit. Use immediately after reconstitution. Discard any unused portion.
[See table below].

Patient Management:
Suggestions for Usual Patient Management
Preprocedure
- Discontinue neuroleptic drugs (including phenothiazines, eg, chlorpromazine, prochlorperazine, and promethazine) 48 hours beforehand.
- Maintain normal diet up to 2 hours before.
- Ensure hydration—fluids up to procedure.

During Procedure
- Use minimum dose and concentration required for satisfactory contrast. (See DOSAGE AND ADMINISTRATION.)
- In all positioning techniques keep the patient's head elevated above highest level of spine.
- Do not lower head of table more than 15° during thoraco-cervical procedures.
- In patients with excessive lordosis consider lateral position for injection and movement of the medium cephalad.
- Avoid intracranial entry of a bolus.
- Avoid early and high cephalad dispersion of the medium.
- Inject slowly over 1 to 2 minutes to avoid excessive mixing.
- Abrupt or active patient movement causes excessive mixing with CSF. Instruct patient to remain passive. Move patient slowly and only as necessary.
- To maintain as a bolus, move medium to distal area very slowly under fluoroscopic control.
- At completion of direct cervical or lumbo-cervical procedures, raise head of table steeply (45°) for about 2 minutes to restore medium to lower levels.

Postprocedure
- Raise head of stretcher to at least 15° before moving patient onto it.
- Movement onto stretcher, and off the stretcher to bed, should be done slowly with patient completely passive, maintaining head up position.
- Before moving patient onto bed, raise head of bed 15° to 30°.
- Advise patient to remain still in bed, in head up position, especially in first few hours.
- Maintain close observation for at least 12 hours after myelogram.
- After 8 hours, patient may be lowered to a horizontal position for further 16 hours.
- Obtain visitors cooperation in keeping the patient quiet and in head up position, especially in first few hours.
- Encourage oral fluids and diet as tolerated.
- If nausea or vomiting occurs, do not use phenothiazine antinauseants. Persistent nausea and vomiting will result in dehydration. Therefore, prompt consideration of replacement by intravenous fluids is recommended.

RECONSTITUTION TABLE

Conc. of Solution (mgI/ml)	Volume of Diluent to be Added: 3.75 g Vial (ml)	6.75 g Vial (ml)
170	8.9	16.1
180	8.3	15.0
190	7.8	14.0
220	6.5	11.7
250	5.5	10.0
260	5.2	9.4
270	5.0	9.0
280	4.7	8.5
290	4.5	8.1
300	4.3	7.8
	The volume of the final solution will equal the volume of the diluent + 1.7 ml	The volume of the final solution will equal the volume of the diluent + 3.1 ml

The volume of the final solution will exceed the amount required to achieve the recommended dosage. For precise volume for injection refer to DOSAGE TABLE.

Continued on next page

This product information was effective as of November 19, 1982. On these and other products of Winthrop Laboratories, detailed information may be obtained on a current basis by direct inquiry to the Professional Services Department, 90 Park Avenue, New York, NY 10016 (212) 907-2525.

Winthrop—Cont.

How Supplied:
Kits, each containing
One-3.75 g/20 ml single-dose vial of AMIPAQUE with 1 vial of diluent (NDC 0024-0044-01); or
One-6.75 g/50 ml single-dose vial of AMIPAQUE with 1 vial of diluent (NDC 0024-0046-01).
Combination packs, each containing
Five-3.75 g/20 ml single-dose vials of AMIPAQUE with 5 vials of diluent (NDC 0024-0044-12); or
Five-6.75 g/50 ml single-dose vials of AMIPAQUE with 5 vials of diluent (NDC 0024-0046-12).
Protect vials of AMIPAQUE, brand of metrizamide, from heat or light.

Distributed by
Winthrop Laboratories
Division of Sterling Drug Inc
New York, NY 10016
Manufactured by
Nyegaard & Co • AS
Nycoveien 2, Oslo 4, Norway

BILOPAQUE® SODIUM ℞
brand of tyropanoate sodium, USP

ORAL CHOLECYSTOGRAPHIC MEDIUM

Description: BILOPAQUE sodium, brand of tyropanoate sodium, is sodium 2-(3-butyramido-2,4, 6- triiodobenzyl)- butanoate. BILOPAQUE sodium is an off-white, odorless, hygroscopic solid containing 57.4 percent iodine. The molecular weight is 663.1. BILOPAQUE sodium is soluble in water to 14.7 percent.
Clinical Pharmacology: After ingestion, BILOPAQUE is absorbed from the duodenum into the bloodstream. The liver converts it primarily into radiopaque glucuronic acid conjugates, which are concentrated by the functioning gallbladder. These conjugates provide visualization of the gallbladder and may, upon contraction of the gallbladder, provide visualization of the extrahepatic ducts.
Indication and Usage: BILOPAQUE is indicated for radiographic delineation of the gallbladder.
Contraindications: BILOPAQUE should not be administered to patients with advanced hepatorenal disease, severe impairment of renal function, or severe gastrointestinal disorders that prevent absorption.
Warnings: **Usage in Pregnancy.** Although no teratogenic effects attributable to BILOPAQUE have been observed in animals, safe use of the agent in pregnant women has not been established. Before cholecystography with BILOPAQUE is performed in women of childbearing potential, the benefit should be weighed against the possible risk to the patient or child. In addition, most authorities consider elective contrast radiography of the abdomen contraindicated during pregnancy.
The use of BILOPAQUE in children under 12 years is not recommended, since no clinical trials have been performed in this age group.
Elevation of protein-bound iodine for several months and false-positive urine albumin tests for several days may occur after ingestion of cholecystographic media.
Precautions: Caution should be exercised in administration of BILOPAQUE to patients with known iodine sensitivity.
Severe, advanced liver disease may interfere with metabolism of the radiopaque medium, and therefore, a greater amount of unchanged BILOPAQUE may be diverted to the kidney. Renal function in patients with severe, advanced liver disease should be assessed before cholecystography, and renal output and hepatic function should be observed for a few days after the procedure.
The recommended dose of BILOPAQUE should not be exceeded in patients with preexisting renal disease. Possible renal irritation in susceptible individuals could result in reflex vascular spasm with partial or complete renal shutdown.
Patients with renal or hepatic diseases should not be dehydrated beforehand and should drink liberal amounts of fluids after taking the capsules.
The uricosuric effect of BILOPAQUE should be considered when it is administered to patients with evidence of impaired renal function.
Caution is advised in patients with symptoms of coronary artery disease.
Adverse Reactions: The most common reactions after administration of BILOPAQUE have been mild and transient *gastrointestinal disturbances* including nausea, abdominal cramps, diarrhea, vomiting, and weakness and abdominal discomfort. *Allergic type reactions affecting* skin, mucous membrane, and systemic hypersensitivity reactions are unusual and include urticaria with or without pruritus, erythema, morbilliform rash, and localized areas of edema. Very rarely a systemic serum sickness-type reaction with fever, rash, and arthralgia has been reported. *Other reactions,* which have occurred infrequently, include dysuria, dyspnea, difficulty in swallowing, headache, perspiration, dizziness, fatigue, lightheadedness, pain or cramps in limbs, and rarely, laryngotracheal edema.
Very rarely disturbances in hepatic, renal, or cardiovascular function have been reported with cholecystographic media, usually in patients with preexisting disease (see Precautions).
Dosage and Administration: A single oral dose of 3 g (4 capsules) is recommended for adults. The optimal time interval between administration of BILOPAQUE and cholecystography is 10 to 12 hours, although satisfactory results have been reported as early as 4 to 6 hours.
The use of BILOPAQUE in children under 12 years is not recommended, since no clinical trials have been performed in this age group.
If no visualization occurs after administration of BILOPAQUE, repeat examination with a 3 g dose may be performed the following day. *Increasing the amount of the repeat dose is not recommended.*
Cholestasis is a common cause of nonvisualization in patients who have been on almost completely fat-free diets. To reduce the incidence of false-negative nonvisualization, such patients should eat a diet containing some fat for one or two days before cholecystographic examination. Fat is a long-acting cholecystagogue, and will stimulate emptying of the gallbladder and prepare it to receive the radiopaque medium. *The meal immediately before ingestion of the BILOPAQUE capsules should be fat free.*
Preparatory dehydration is unnecessary and undesirable, especially in elderly patients. After the fat-free evening meal, the patient should swallow 4 BILOPAQUE capsules (3 g) with water. Between ingestion of BILOPAQUE and cholecystographic examination, the patient should take nothing by mouth except water, and should not smoke or chew gum.
Many physicians believe that the quality of gallbladder visualization is enhanced when the intestine is relatively free of residue. This may be achieved with an enema the morning of the examination, or a laxative the day before.
For observation of gallbladder contractility, the patient may be given a fatty meal or a cholecystagogue after the initial x-ray examination. Additional exposures may be made 5 to 30 minutes later.
Nonvisualization
Nonvisualization in routine cholecystography with BILOPAQUE, brand of tyropanoate sodium, usually implies substantial loss of gallbladder function. However, nonvisualization may also result on occasion from other factors not related to disease of the biliary tract.
Repeat Examination
When adequate visualization is not obtained initially, repeat cholecystography with the recommended dose of 3 g helps reduce the possibility of diagnostic error. A larger dose is not recommended. Disease may be inferred with reasonable certainty if the gallbladder does not visualize on repeat examination.
How Supplied: Capsules of 750 mg—Envelopes of 4 capsules (3 g, the recommended dose), in boxes of 25 (NDC 0024-0134-03).
[*Shown in Product Identification Section*]

HYPAQUE® SODIUM ℞
brand of diatrizoate sodium, USP
ORAL POWDER
HYPAQUE® SODIUM ORAL SOLUTION
brand of diatrizoate sodium solution, USP

For Examination of the Gastrointestinal Tract

Description: HYPAQUE sodium, brand of diatrizoate sodium, is sodium 3,5-diacetamido-2,4,6-triiodobenzoate ($C_{11}H_8I_3N_2NaO_4$) and contains 59.87 per cent iodine. It is available as a powder and a liquid. The powder (for preparing radiopaque solutions) provides about 600 mg organically-bound iodine per gram of powder and contains caramel as a coloring agent. The 41.66 per cent oral solution is supplied as a thin, slightly viscous, colorless to light brown solution of diatrizoate sodium in water. Each ml contains 249 mg of organically-bound iodine.
Clinical Pharmacology: When administered orally or given as an enema, the medium produces excellent opacification and delineation of the upper and lower gastrointestinal tract; however, because of dilution, contrast in the small bowel may be unsatisfactory. HYPAQUE solutions are particularly valuable when a more viscous agent, such as barium sulfate which is not water soluble, is unsuitable or potentially harmful.
From 0.04 to 1.2 per cent of the medium may be absorbed from the gastrointestinal tract after oral administration. In some patients, particularly in infants and patients with engorgement of the intestinal mucosa, sufficient absorption to cause some visualization of the urinary tract may occur occasionally. HYPAQUE is also absorbed across the peritoneum and pleura.
Indications and Usage: This medium is indicated for radiographic examination of the gastrointestinal tract following oral or rectal administration.
Warnings: Serious or fatal reactions have been associated with the parenteral administration of radiopaque media. It is important that a course of action be carefully planned in advance for the treatment of possible serious reactions with oral use of HYPAQUE solutions. (See Precautions.)
Usage in Pregnancy. The safety of orally administered HYPAQUE solutions during pregnancy has not been established. Therefore, before administration of the drug to women of childbearing potential, the benefit to the patient should be carefully weighed against the possible risk to the fetus. In addition, most authorities consider elective contrast radiography of the abdomen contraindicated during pregnancy.
Precautions: A 10 per cent solution of the medium in water is isotonic. Hence, the solutions generally employed clinically (ie, from 15 to 40 per cent) are hypertonic. Highly hypertonic solutions may draw excessive amounts of fluid into the intestine and may lead to hypovolemia. In very young or debilitated children, and in elderly cachectic persons, the loss of plasma fluid may be sufficient to cause a shock-like state which, if untreated, could be dangerous to the patient. Wherever possible, the use of the lower concentrations is advised for in-

fants and young children (under 10 kg) and for dehydrated or debilitated patients. The higher concentrations should be used in such patients only when necessary and with great caution. It is advisable to correct any electrolyte disturbances before using solutions that are extremely hypertonic.
Bronchial entry of the medium causes a copious osmotic effusion. Therefore, pulmonary entry by aspiration or by use in patients with esophagotracheal fistula should be avoided.
Caution is also advised in patients with severe renal or hepatic disease.
Adverse Reactions: There have been few reported cases of adverse reactions with orally administered solutions of water-soluble contrast agents. Because of their osmotic effect, such solutions tend to exert cathartic action, but this is generally considered an advantage. Nausea, vomiting, or slight diarrhea may occasionally occur, particularly when the medium is used in a high concentration or large volume. Urticaria has been observed in a few patients; presumably the condition was caused by allergy to the contrast medium and it was readily alleviated by antihistamine therapy.
Because small amounts of the medium may be absorbed, the possibility of systemic reactions should be considered, particularly in cases of perforation.
Dosage and Administration:
Adults: ***Oral,*** from 90 to 180 ml of a 25 to 40 per cent solution.
Enema, from 500 to 1000 ml of a 15 to 25 per cent solution.
Infants and Children: ***Oral,*** from 30 to 75 ml of a 20 to 40 per cent solution.
Enema, from 100 to 500 ml of a 10 to 15 per cent solution, depending on weight of patient.
Warning: Neither the powder nor the liquid is to be used for the preparation of solutions for parenteral injection. [See table.]

Directions for Measurement and Dilution

A. *Using powder*

Solution (%)	Measuring spoons* of powder (per 100 ml diluent†)
10	1
15	1½
20	2
25	2½
40	4

* One level measuring spoon is equal to approximately 10 g of powder.
† Solutions may be sweetened or flavored (eg, with vanilla, lemon, chocolate); the diluent may be water, milk, or a carbonated drink.

B. *Using liquid* (Approximate Values)

Solution (%)	Dilution Required
40	Use undiluted
25	Dilute each 60 ml to 100 ml
20	Dilute each 50 ml to 100 ml
15	Dilute each 40 ml to 100 ml
10	Dilute each 25 ml to 100 ml

How Supplied: **Powder**—*cans* of 250 g with measuring spoon (approximately 10 g capacity), NDC 0024-0769-01
bottles of 10 g, NDC 0024-0769-10
Liquid—*bottles* of 120 ml, each containing 50 g of diatrizoate sodium, NDC 0024-0768-01

HYPAQUE® SODIUM 20% ℞
brand of diatrizoate sodium injection, USP
Sterile Aqueous Solution

For Retrograde Pyelography Only
Not for Intravascular injection

Description: HYPAQUE sodium, brand of diatrizoate sodium, is sodium 3,5-diacetamido-2,4,6-triiodobenzoate containing 59.87 per cent iodine. HYPAQUE sodium 20 per cent (w/v) is a sterile, clear, colorless or nearly colorless aqueous solution containing 120 mg of organically-bound iodine per ml. It also contains edetate calcium disodium 0.01 per cent as stabilizer and benzyl alcohol 1 per cent as antiseptic preservative. The pH is adjusted between 6.5 and 7.7 with sodium hydroxide or hydrochloric acid. The medium can be sterilized by heat in the customary manner without decomposition but should be protected from strong light.
Action: HYPAQUE sodium 20 per cent is a radiopaque medium used to delineate the renal pelvis and ureters.
Indication: HYPAQUE sodium 20 per cent is indicated for use in retrograde pyelography.
Warnings: Serious or fatal reactions have been associated with the administration of radiopaque media. It is of utmost importance that a course of action be carefully planned in advance for the immediate treatment of serious reactions, and that adequate and appropriate facilities be readily available in case a severe reaction occurs.
Usage in Pregnancy. Safe use of HYPAQUE sodium 20 per cent during pregnancy has not been established. Therefore, before administration of the drug to women of childbearing potential, the benefit to the patient should be carefully weighed against the possible risk to the fetus. In addition, most authorities consider elective contrast radiography of the abdomen contraindicated during pregnancy.
Precautions: It has long been known that oliguria or anuria may rarely follow bilateral retrograde pyelography or uncomplicated cystoscopic ureteral manipulation. Various mechanisms have been proposed to explain this occurrence, such as reflex anuria, edema, and occlusion of the ureteral orifices from local trauma, pressure, manipulation, sensitivity to the radiopaque medium or to residual disinfecting antiseptic on ureteral catheters, pyelotubular backflow, transient interstitial renal edema with increased pressure, and reduced renal blood flow. Because of the possibility of acute renal failure following bilateral retrograde pyelography, some authors conclude that retrograde pyelography should be done on only one side at a time.
Adverse Reactions: Minor side reactions are nausea, vomiting, excessive salivation, and sweating. Discomfort and colic because of ureteropelvic spasm occasionally may follow the examination.
With HYPAQUE sodium, brand of diatrizoate sodium injection, 20 per cent, reflux into the bloodstream or lymphatics (pyelovenous or pyelolymphatic backflow) as a result of undue pressure of administration is not apt to result in a generalized reaction.
Dosage and Administration: Considerable variations in renal pelvic capacity account for differences in the quantities of radiopaque medium suggested for retrograde pyelography. The solution is introduced slowly, avoiding force, and is immediately stopped at the first evidence of renal or abdominal discomfort to avoid overdistention or injury. The procedure is not carried out unless the patient is conscious enough to react to pain. Introduction of the medium by gravity from an elevated buret is considered the best procedure, but injection by syringe is suitable, particularly in small children.
The renal pelvis is relatively nondistensible. The usual volumes of the 20 per cent solution suggested for unilateral introduction are:

Infants under 1 year	Less than 1.5 ml
Children 5 years of age and under	1.5 to 3.0 ml
Children over 5 years of age	4.0 to 5.0 ml
Adults	6.0 to 10.0 ml

The volume needed will vary according to the individual and the disorder under examination. Twenty milliliters or more may be necessary for diagnostic pyelograms in patients with hydronephrosis.
When the diagnostic information required warrants a bilateral examination in one procedure, a double volume of the "use" solution is required. The bilateral procedure may be employed, usually without untoward effects. (See Precautions.)
Intravascular administration is not recommended since the multiple-dose vials contain an antiseptic preservative.
How Supplied: Multiple-dose vials of 100 ml

HYPAQUE® Sodium 25% ℞
brand of diatrizoate sodium injection, USP
Sterile Aqueous Solution

INTRAVENOUS INFUSION FOR UROGRAPHY AND CT SCAN ENHANCEMENT

Description: HYPAQUE sodium, brand of diatrizoate sodium, is monosodium 3, 5-diacetamido-2, 4, 6-triiodobenzoate ($C_{11}H_8I_3N_2NaO_4$), which contains 59.87 per cent organically-bound iodine.
The 25 per cent solution (w/v) contains 150 mg iodine per ml and 0.4 mEq (9.05 mg) sodium per ml. It has an osmolarity of approximately 657 mOs per liter (0.657 mOs per ml) at 25 C and is, therefore, hypertonic. The viscosity (cps) is about 1.59 at 25 C and 1.19 at 37 C. Sodium carbonate or hydrochloric acid has been added to adjust pH between 6.5 and 7.7. The sterile, aqueous solution is clear and nearly colorless. It is relatively thermostable and may be autoclaved once. It does not contain an antibacterial preservative, and *unused portions remaining in the container should be discarded.* The solution should be protected from strong light. The 25 per cent solution contains edetate calcium disodium 1:10,000 as a sequestering stabilizing agent.
Clinical Pharmacology: HYPAQUE sodium 25 per cent is a diagnostic radiopaque medium which provides visualization of internal structures. In urography, the infusion technique facilitates the administration of the larger dose of contrast medium for improved diagnostic visualization of the entire urinary system.
Infusion of HYPAQUE sodium 25 per cent will increase density differentials of intracranial structures during computed tomographic scanning, often providing additional diagnostic information.
Infusion urography. Infusion urography is a method of excretion urography utilizing a relatively large volume of HYPAQUE sodium 25 per cent by rapid intravenous infusion. The medium is carried rapidly to the kidneys where it is excreted unchanged in the urine. If renal function is normal, excretion begins almost immediately.
Intravenous infusion of a large volume of dilute contrast material has been shown to give

Continued on next page

This product information was effective as of November 19, 1982. On these and other products of Winthrop Laboratories, detailed information may be obtained on a current basis by direct inquiry to the Professional Services Department, 90 Park Avenue, New York, NY 10016 (212) 907-2525.

Winthrop—Cont.

consistently excellent pyelograms, dense nephrograms, and satisfactory cystograms and voiding urethrograms.
A more anatomically complete visualization of the urinary tract is generally attainable with the infusion technique than with conventional urographic techniques. It may be particularly useful when indeterminate or unsatisfactory results have been obtained with conventional urographic studies. The infusion technique may be utilized prior to retrograde pyelography when this procedure is being considered as it may obviate the need for a retrograde study.
Nephrotomography following infusion urography will frequently provide an accurate differential diagnosis between renal tumors and cysts. Infusion nephrotomography has also been successfully utilized in the localization of adrenal tumors. Nephrotomographic sections are usually made immediately following the completion of the infusion urogram. However, adequate tomograms may be obtained for as long as 40 minutes following the completion of the infusion.

Indications and Usage: HYPAQUE sodium 25 per cent is indicated for use in intravenous urography and contrast enhancement of computerized axial tomography for cerebral imaging.

Warnings: Serious or fatal reactions have been associated with the administration of radiopaque media. It is of utmost importance that a course of action be carefully planned in advance for the immediate treatment of serious reactions, and that adequate and appropriate facilities and personnel be readily available in case a severe reaction occurs.
Intravascular administration of contrast media may promote sickling in patients who are homozygous for sickle cell disease. Therefore, fluid restriction is not advised.
The results of PBI and RAI uptake studies, which depend on iodine estimations, will not reflect thyroid function for up to 16 days following administration of iodinated urographic media. However, function tests not depending on iodine estimations, eg, T_3 resin uptake or free thyroxine assays, are not affected.

Precautions: Before injecting a contrast medium, the patient should be questioned for a history of allergy. Although a history of allergy may imply a greater than usual risk, it does not arbitrarily contraindicate the use of the medium. Premedication with antihistamines to avoid or minimize possible allergic reactions may be considered. **Benadryl®, brand of diphenhydramine hydrochloride, however, may cause precipitation when mixed with HYPAQUE sodium.** The intravenous injection of a test dose of 0.5 to 1 ml of the contrast agent before injection of the full dose has been employed in an attempt to predict severe or fatal adverse reactions. The preponderance of recent scientific literature, however, now demonstrates that this provocative test procedure is not reliably predictive of serious or fatal reactions. Severe reactions and fatalities have occurred with the test dose alone, with the full dose after a nonreactive test dose, and with or without a history of allergy. No conclusive relationship between severe or fatal reactions and antigen-antibody reactions or other manifestations of allergy has been established. A history of allergy may be useful in predicting reactions of a mild or intermediate nature.

Usage in pregnancy. Safe use of HYPAQUE sodium, brand of diatrizoate sodium injection, 25 per cent during pregnancy has not been established. Therefore, before administration of the drug to women of childbearing potential, the benefit to the patient should be carefully weighed against the possible risk to the fetus. In addition, most authorities consider elective contrast radiography of the abdomen contraindicated during pregnancy.
Caution is advised in patients with severe cardiovascular disease and in patients with a history of bronchial asthma or other allergic manifestations or of sensitivity to iodine.
In myelomatosis, urography should only be performed with caution. If a weak protein-binding agent such as a diatrizoate is used for the procedure, it is essential to omit preparatory dehydration, administer fluids, and attempt to alkalinize the urine.
Immediate adverse reactions to infusion urography have not been reported to occur at a higher frequency or greater severity than with routine excretory urography. However, sequelae of this procedure are possible some hours after the examination. The infusion imposes not only a sudden osmotic load, but also may present as much as 160 mEq of sodium (3.7 g) to patients with established, decreased glomerular filtration and renal tubular damage. In addition, these patients may also have coexisting or associated cardiovascular disease. Therefore, the possibility of the development of congestive heart failure hours after the procedure should be considered.
Because of the possibility of inducing temporary suppression of urine, it is wise to allow an interval of at least 48 hours to pass before repeating infusion urography in patients with unilateral or bilateral reduction of normal renal function.
Preparatory dehydration or abdominal compression may not be necessary in infusion urography. Preparatory dehydration may be dangerous in infants, young children, the elderly, and azotemic patients (especially those with polyuria, oliguria, diabetes, advanced vascular disease, or preexisting dehydration). The undesirable dehydration in these patients may be accentuated by the osmotic diuretic action of the medium.

Adverse Reactions: Reactions accompanying the use of contrast media may vary directly with the concentration of the substance, the amount used, the technique used, and the underlying pathology.
The following adverse reactions, usually of a minor nature, have occurred in 10 to 14 per cent of patients who have received diatrizoate solutions and similar contrast media. *Cardiovascular reactions:* rare cases of cardiac arrhythmias (including ventricular fibrillation), hypertension, hypotension, shock, and cardiac arrest; vein cramp, thrombophlebitis, vasodilatation with flushing. *Renal reactions:* occasionally, transient proteinuria, and rarely, oliguria and anuria which may be secondary to hypotension. *Allergic reactions:* asthmatic attacks, nasal and conjunctival symptoms, dermal reactions such as urticaria, and rarely, anaphylactic shock, sometimes with fatal outcome. Infrequently, immediate or delayed chills can occur, sometimes accompanied by fever. *Respiratory reactions:* pulmonary or laryngeal edema, bronchospasm, laryngospasm, dyspnea, cyanosis, coughing. *CNS reactions:* restlessness, confusion, convulsions. *Other reactions:* pain on injection, hematomas, ecchymoses, warmth, fever, nausea, vomiting, anxiety, headache, dizziness, excessive salivation. Infrequently, "iodism" (salivary gland swelling) from organic iodinated compounds appears two days after exposure and subsides by the sixth day. Rarely, disseminated intravascular coagulation has occurred.

Dosage and Administration:
Infusion urography. The recommended dose is calculated on the basis of 2 ml of HYPAQUE sodium, brand of diatrizoate sodium injection, 25 per cent per pound of body weight. The average dose of the solution for adults is 300 ml; for optimum results, a minimum dose of 250 ml should be used. A maximum dose of 400 ml is generally sufficient for the largest of subjects. The solution is administered intravenously through an 18-gauge needle over a period of three to ten minutes. Pyelographic films are taken at 10, 20, and 30 minutes from the beginning of the infusion. Early 2, 3, 4, and 5 minute films are obtained when indicated for the evaluation of hypertension. Nephrotomographic sections are best taken just at the end of the infusion, and voiding cystourethrograms when desired are usually made at 30 minutes.
CT scanning. The dose and administration will depend on the technique and equipment used. The usual dose in adults is 300 ml of HYPAQUE sodium 25 per cent, infused over 10 to 20 minutes.

How Supplied:
Cartons of 10 calibrated bottles of 300 ml (NDC 0024-0758-03)
Cartons of 10 calibrated bottles of 300 ml with 10 intravenous infusion sets (NDC 0024-0757-03)
The solution should be protected from strong light. *Discard any unused portion remaining in the container.*

HYPAQUE-CYSTO® ℞

brand of diatrizoate meglumine injection, USP
Sterile Aqueous Solution

FOR RETROGRADE CYSTOURETHROGRAPHY

Description: HYPAQUE-CYSTO is a radiopaque medium which contains approximately 141 mg organically-bound iodine per ml. It is a 30 per cent (weight/volume) sterile aqueous solution of the meglumine salt of 3, 5-diacetamido-2, 4, 6-triiodobenzoic acid ($C_{18}H_{26}I_3N_3O_9$). The viscosity is 1.94 cps at 25 C and 1.42 cps at 37 C. The pH is adjusted with hydrochloric acid, or diatrizoic acid, or meglumine. HYPAQUE-CYSTO is clear and colorless to pale yellow. It should be protected from strong light. The solution is relatively thermostable and may be autoclaved. Edetate calcium disodium 1:10,000 has been added as a sequestering stabilizing agent.

Action: HYPAQUE-CYSTO is a diagnostic radiopaque medium which provides visualization of the lower urinary tract.

Indication: HYPAQUE-CYSTO is indicated for retrograde cystourethrography.

Adverse Reactions: No irritation or other undesirable effects have been reported following the administration of HYPAQUE-CYSTO in clinical investigations.

Dosage and Administration: After the bladder is emptied, HYPAQUE-CYSTO is gently instilled without force, often beyond the first desire to micturate, but not beyond the point of urgency or mild discomfort. The volume required to fill the bladder to slightly less than capacity may vary from patient to patient.
Bladder capacity in normal adults is generally 200 to 300 ml, and rarely, up to 600 ml. Capacity at birth is 20 to 50 ml, and increases about 400 per cent in the first year. In children 3 to 5 years old, bladder capacity is 150 to 180 ml. In children older than 8 years, it is in the low adult range.
In disease, bladder capacity in adults may vary from 50 ml in a hypertonic reflex bladder to over 1000 ml in an atonic or sensory paralytic bladder or chronic lower urinary tract obstruction.
Repeat examination may be required to detect reflux, or in function studies.
The concentration varies with technique and equipment used. HYPAQUE-CYSTO may be diluted with sterile water or 5 per cent dextrose solution, as indicated in the following tables.
STANDARD PACKAGE
(250 ml of HYPAQUE-CYSTO in 500 ml bottle)

TO MAKE		ADD	FINAL SOLUTION CONTAINS
Final conc.	Final volume	Sterile water or 5% dextrose solution	Iodine
30 %	250 ml	—	141 mg/ml
25 %	300 ml	50 ml	118 mg/ml
21.4%	350 ml	100 ml	101 mg/ml
20 %	375 ml	125 ml	94 mg/ml
18.8%	400 ml	150 ml	88 mg/ml
16.7%	450 ml	200 ml	78 mg/ml
15 %	500 ml	250 ml	71 mg/ml

PEDIATRIC PACKAGE
(100 ml of HYPAQUE-CYSTO in 300 ml bottle)

TO MAKE		ADD	FINAL SOLUTION CONTAINS
Final conc.	Final volume	Sterile water or 5% dextrose solution	Iodine
30%	100 ml	—	141 mg/ml
24%	125 ml	25 ml	113 mg/ml
20%	150 ml	50 ml	94 mg/ml
15%	200 ml	100 ml	71 mg/ml
12%	250 ml	150 ml	56 mg/ml
10%	300 ml	200 ml	47 mg/ml

How Supplied:
STANDARD PACKAGE—Calibrated 500 ml dilution bottles containing 250 ml HYPAQUE-CYSTO; rubber stoppered, with inner removable seal and screw neck. Boxes of 10 (NDC 0024-0734-01)
PEDIATRIC PACKAGE—Calibrated 300 ml dilution bottles containing 100 ml HYPAQUE-CYSTO, brand of diatrizoate meglumine injection; rubber stoppered, with inner removable seal and screw neck.

HYPAQUE® MEGLUMINE 30% ℞

brand of diatrizoate meglumine injection, USP
Sterile Aqueous Solution

INTRAVENOUS INFUSION FOR UROGRAPHY AND CT SCAN ENHANCEMENT

Description: HYPAQUE meglumine 30 per cent is a solution of 1-Deoxy-1-(methylamino)-D-glucitol 3, 5-diacetamido-2, 4, 6-triiodobenzoate (salt), with a molecular formula of $C_7H_{17}NO_5 \cdot C_{11}H_9I_3N_2O_4$.
The 30 per cent solution (w/v) contains approximately 141 mg of organically-bound iodine per ml. It has a viscosity of 1.94 cps at 25 C and 1.42 cps at 37 C. The pH is adjusted with hydrochloric acid, or diatrizoic acid, or meglumine. Edetate calcium disodium 1:10,000 has been added as a sequestering stabilizing agent. The sterile aqueous solution is clear and colorless to pale yellow. HYPAQUE meglumine 30 per cent is relatively thermostable and may be autoclaved once. It does not contain an antibacterial preservative, and *unused portions remaining in the container should be discarded.* The solution should be protected from the strong light.
Clinical Pharmacology: HYPAQUE meglumine 30 per cent is a diagnostic radiopaque medium which provides visualization of internal structures. In urography, the infusion technique facilitates the administration of the larger dose of contrast medium for improved diagnostic visualization of the entire urinary system.
Infusion of HYPAQUE meglumine 30 per cent will increase density differentials of intracranial structures during computed tomographic scanning, often providing additional diagnostic information.
Indications and Usage: HYPAQUE meglumine 30 per cent is indicated for use in intravenous urography and contrast enhancement of computerized axial tomography for cerebral imaging.
Warnings: Serious or fatal reactions have been associated with the administration of radiopaque media. It is of utmost importance that a course of action be carefully planned in advance for the immediate treatment of serious reactions, and that adequate and appropriate facilities and personnel be readily available in case a severe reaction occurs.
Intravascular administration of contrast media may promote sickling in patients who are homozygous for sickle cell disease. Therefore, fluid restriction is not advised.
The results of PBI and RAI uptake studies, which depend on iodine estimations, will not reflect thyroid function for up to 16 days following administration of iodinated urographic media. However, function tests not depending on iodine estimations, eg, T_3 resin uptake or free thyroxine assays, are not affected.
Precautions: Before injecting a contrast medium, the patient should be questioned for a history of allergy. Although a history of allergy may imply a greater than usual risk, it does not arbitrarily contraindicate the use of the medium. Premedication with antihistamines to avoid or minimize possible allergic reactions may be considered. **Benadryl®, brand of diphenhydramine hydrochloride, however, may cause precipitation when mixed with HYPAQUE meglumine 30 per cent.** The intravenous injection of a test dose of 0.5 to 1 ml of the contrast agent before infusion of the full dose has been employed in an attempt to predict severe or fatal adverse reactions. The preponderance of recent scientific literature, however, now demonstrates that this provocative test procedure is not reliably predictive of serious or fatal reactions. Severe reactions and fatalities have occurred with the test dose alone, with the full dose after a nonreactive test dose, and with or without a history of allergy. No conclusive relationship between severe or fatal reactions and antigen-antibody reactions or other manifestations of allergy has been established. A history of allergy may be useful in predicting reactions of a mild or intermediate nature.
Usage in pregnancy. No teratogenic effects attributable to a 60 per cent solution of HYPAQUE meglumine have been observed in reproduction studies in animals. However, before administration of HYPAQUE meglumine, brand of diatrizoate meglumine injection, 30 per cent to women of childbearing potential, the benefit to the patient should be carefully weighed against the possible risk to the fetus. In addition, most authorities consider elective contrast radiography of the abdomen contraindicated during pregnancy.
Caution is advised in patients with severe cardiovascular disease and in patients with a history of bronchial asthma or other allergic manifestations, or of sensitivity to iodine. Transient ECG changes have been reported in older patients with evidence of heart disease. In myelomatosis, urography should only be performed with caution. If a weak protein-binding agent such as a diatrizoate is used for the procedure, it is essential to omit preparatory dehydration, to administer fluids, and attempt to alkalinize the urine.
Immediate adverse reactions to infusion urography have not been reported to occur at a higher frequency or with greater severity than with routine excretory urography. However, sequelae of this procedure are possible some hours after the examination. The infusion imposes a sudden osmotic load. This should be considered in patients with established, decreased glomerular filtration and renal tubular damage. In addition, these patients may also have coexisting or associated cardiovascular disease. Therefore, there is a possibility of the development of congestive heart failure hours after the procedure.
Because of the possibility of inducing temporary suppression of urine, it is wise to allow an interval of at least 48 hours to pass before repeating infusion urography in patients with unilateral or bilateral reduction of normal renal function.
Preparatory dehydration or abdominal compression may not be necessary in infusion urography. Preparatory dehydration may be dangerous in infants, young children, the elderly, and azotemic patients (especially those with polyuria, oliguria, diabetes, advanced vascular disease, or preexisting dehydration). The undesirable dehydration in these patients may be accentuated by the osmotic diuretic action of the medium.
Adverse Reactions: Reactions accompanying the use of contrast media may vary directly with the concentration of the substance, the amount used, the technique used, and the underlying pathology.
The following adverse reactions, usually of a minor nature, have occurred in 10 to 14 per cent of patients who have received diatrizoate solutions and similar iodinated contrast media. *Cardiovascular reactions:* rare cases of cardiac arrhythmias (including ventricular fibrillation), hypertension, hypotension, shock, and cardiac arrest; vein cramp, thrombophlebitis, vasodilatation with flushing. *Renal reactions:* occasionally, transient proteinuria, and rarely, oliguria and anuria which may be secondary to hypotension. *Allergic reactions:* asthmatic attacks, nasal and conjunctival symptoms, dermal reactions such as urticaria, and rarely, anaphylactic shock, sometimes with fatal outcome. Infrequently, immediate or delayed chills can occur, sometimes accompanied by fever. *Respiratory reactions:* pulmonary or laryngeal edema, bronchospasm, laryngospasm, dyspnea, cyanosis, coughing. *CNS reactions:* restlessness, confusion, convulsions. *Other reactions:* pain on injection, hematomas, ecchymoses, warmth, fever, nausea, vomiting, anxiety, headache, dizziness, excessive salivation. Infrequently, "iodism" (salivary gland swelling) from organic iodinated compounds appears two days after exposure and subsides by the sixth day. Rarely, disseminated intravascular coagulation has occurred.
Dosage and Administration:
Infusion urography. The recommended dose for infusion urography is calculated on the basis of 2 ml of HYPAQUE meglumine 30 per cent per pound of body weight. The average dose of the solution for adults is 300 ml; for optimal results, a minimum dose of 250 ml should be used. A maximum dose of 400 ml is generally sufficient for the largest of subjects.
The solution is infused over a period of three to ten minutes. Radiographs are usually taken at 10, 20, and 30 minutes from the beginning of the infusion. Earlier films may be obtained for the evaluation of hypertension. Nephrograms are usually obtained at the end of the infusion, and voiding cystourethrograms are usually obtained 30 minutes after the beginning of the infusion.
CT scanning. The dose and administration will depend on the technique and equipment used. The usual dose in adults is 300 ml of HYPAQUE meglumine, brand of diatrizoate meglumine injection, 30 per cent, infused over 10 to 20 minutes.

This product information was effective as of November 19, 1982. On these and other products of Winthrop Laboratories, detailed information may be obtained on a current basis by direct inquiry to the Professional Services Department, 90 Park Avenue, New York, NY 10016 (212) 907-2525.

Continued on next page

Winthrop—Cont.

How Supplied:
Cartons of 10 calibrated bottles of 300 ml
(NDC 0024-0739-03)
Cartons of 10 calibrated bottles of 300 ml with 10 intravenous infusion sets
(NDC 0024-0740-03)
The solution should be protected from strong light. *Discard any unused portion remaining in the container.*

HYPAQUE® SODIUM 50% ℞
brand of diatrizoate sodium injection, USP
Sterile Aqueous Injection

Description: HYPAQUE sodium, brand of diatrizoate sodium, is monosodium 3, 5-diacetamido-2, 4, 6-triiodobenzoate ($C_{11}H_8I_3N_2NaO_4$), that contains 59.87 percent iodine. HYPAQUE sodium 50 percent (w/v) contains 300 mg iodine per ml, 0.8 mEq (18.1 mg) sodium per ml, and has an osmolarity of approximately 1270 mOs per liter (1.27 mOs per ml) with a viscosity (cps) of about 3.25 at 25 C and 2.34 at 37 C. All dilutions of HYPAQUE sodium are hypertonic. Sodium carbonate and either sodium hydroxide or hydrochloric acid have been added to adjust the pH between 6.5 and 7.7. If a solution of this medium is chilled, crystals may form but readily dissolve if the vial is placed in moderately hot water before use; cool to body temperature before injecting. The sterile aqueous solution is clear and nearly colorless. It is relatively thermostable and may be autoclaved without harmful effects. It should be protected from strong light. The 50 percent solution contains edetate calcium disodium 1:10,000 as a sequestering stabilizing agent.
Action: A radiopaque medium used to delineate internal structures.
Indications: HYPAQUE sodium 50 percent is indicated for excretory urography, cerebral and peripheral angiography, aortography, intraosseous venography, direct cholangiography, hysterosalpingography, and splenoportography.
Contraindications, General: Do not use HYPAQUE sodium 50 percent for myelography or for examination of dorsal cysts or sinuses which might communicate with the subarachnoid space. Even a small amount of the medium in the subarachnoid space may produce convulsions and result in fatality. Epidural injection is also contraindicated.
Warnings, General: Serious or fatal reactions have been associated with the administration of radiopaque media. It is of utmost importance that a course of action be carefully planned in advance for the immediate treatment of serious reactions, and that adequate and appropriate facilities be readily available in case a severe reaction occurs.
Selective spinal arteriography or arteriography of trunks providing spinal branches can cause mild to severe muscle spasm. However, serious neurologic sequelae, including permanent paralysis, have occasionally been reported. (See also Aortography, Precautions.)
Usage in Pregnancy. Safe use of HYPAQUE sodium 50 percent during pregnancy has not been established. Therefore, before administration of the drug to women of childbearing potential, the benefit to the patient should be carefully weighed against the possible risk to the fetus. In addition, most authorities consider elective contrast radiography of the abdomen contraindicated during pregnancy.
Since intravascular administration of contrast media may promote sickling in patients who are homozygous for sickle cell disease, fluid restriction is not advised.
The results of PBI and RAI uptake studies, which depend on iodine estimations, will not reflect thyroid function for up to 16 days following administration of iodinated urographic media. However, function tests not depending on iodine estimations, eg, T_3 resin uptake or direct thyroxine assays, are not affected.
Pheochromocytoma: Administer with caution. (See Aortography, Warnings.)
Precautions, General: Before injecting a contrast medium, the patient should be questioned for a history of allergy. Although a history of allergy may imply a greater than usual risk, it does not arbitrarily contraindicate the use of the medium. Premedication with antihistamines to avoid or minimize possible allergic reactions may be considered. **Benadryl®, brand of diphenhydramine hydrochloride, however, may cause precipitation when mixed in the same syringe with HYPAQUE sodium.** The intravenous injection of a test dose of 0.5 ml to 1 ml of the contrast agent before injection of the full dose has been employed in an attempt to predict severe or fatal adverse reactions. The preponderance of recent scientific literature, however, now demonstrates that this provocative test procedure is not reliably predictive of serious or fatal reactions. Severe reactions and fatalities have occurred with the test dose alone, with the full dose after a nonreactive test dose, and with or without a history of allergy. No conclusive relationship between severe or fatal reactions and antigen-antibody reactions or other manifestations of allergy has been established. A history of allergy may be useful in predicting reactions of a mild or intermediate nature.
Caution is advised in patients with severe cardiovascular disease and in patients with a history of bronchial asthma or other allergic manifestations, or of sensitivity to iodine.
Adverse Reactions, General: Reactions accompanying the use of contrast media may vary directly with the concentration of the substance, the amount used, the technique used, and the underlying pathology.
Adverse reactions, usually of a minor nature, have occurred in 10 to 14 percent of patients who have received HYPAQUE sodium, brand of diatrizoate sodium, intravenously. Rarely, atheromatous or other embolic phenomena can occur in angiography. *Cardiovascular reactions* include vasodilatation with flushing, hypotension, and vein cramp (occasionally thrombosis or rarely, thrombophlebitis) in the injected vein. Serious reactions include rare cases of cardiac arrhythmias (eg, ventricular fibrillation), shock, and cardiac arrest. Transient proteinuria may occur occasionally following the injection of radiopaques and, rarely, oliguria and anuria (renal shutdown) have been reported as a secondary effect of a hypotensive reaction. *Allergic reactions* include asthmatic attacks, nasal and conjunctival symptoms, dermal reactions such as urticaria and, rarely, anaphylactoid shock. Rare fatalities have been reported, due to this or unknown causes. Severe reactions may also be manifested by signs and symptoms relating to the *respiratory system* (dyspnea, cyanosis, pulmonary or laryngeal edema), or to the *nervous system* (restlessness, confusion, or convulsions). Infrequently, immediate or delayed rigors can occur, sometimes accompanied by hyperpyrexia. *Other reactions* include nausea, vomiting, excessive salivation, anxiety, headache, and dizziness. Infrequently, "iodism" (salivary gland swelling) from organic compounds appears two days after exposure and subsides by the sixth day. Rarely, disseminated intravascular coagulation has occurred.
Subcutaneous extravasation, chiefly because of hypertonicity of the medium, causes transitory stinging. If the volume is small, ill effects are very unlikely. However, if subcutaneous extravasation is extensive, especially in the foot, the physician should consider infiltration with Sterile Water for Injection, USP, or injection of spreading agents. (See also Subcutaneous and Intramuscular Dosage in section on Excretory Urography.)
Diffuse petechiae have been described and, in several instances, were traced to contamination of syringes, gloves with talc, or fine lint.

EXCRETORY UROGRAPHY

When injected intravenously, the medium is carried rapidly to the kidneys where it is eliminated unchanged in the urine. If the kidneys are functioning normally, the substance is excreted almost immediately.
Precautions: Because of the possibility of inducing temporary suppression of urine, it is wise to allow an interval of at least 48 hours to pass before repeating excretory or retrograde pyelography in patients with unilateral or bilateral reduction of normal renal function.
In myelomatosis, urography should only be performed with caution. If a weak protein-binding agent such as a diatrizoate is used for the procedure, it is essential to omit preparatory dehydration, administer fluids, and attempt to alkalinize the urine.
Preparatory dehydration may be dangerous in infants, young children, the elderly, and azotemic patients (especially those with polyuria, oliguria, diabetes, advanced vascular disease, or preexisting dehydration). The undesirable dehydration in these patients may be accentuated by the osmotic diuretic action of the medium.
Dosage and Administration:
Preliminary Preparation of Patient
Clear shadows are often obtained with the radiopaque medium in patients who have had no preliminary preparation for urography. However, the largest precentage of satisfactory films is secured by following a routine that assures the highest possible concentration of the opaque material in the urinary tract at the time of the x-ray exposure. This is accomplished by directing the patient to abstain from fluids for 12 to 15 hours before the intravenous injection so that partial dehydration results. (See Precautions concerning dehydration.) Unless contraindicated, a laxative is taken at bedtime to eliminate gas from the intestine.
Intravenous Dosage. Adults: A dose of 30 ml of the 50 percent solution administered intravenously with or without compression produces diagnostic shadows in the majority of adults subjected to partial dehydration and to effective purgation. If the administration of 30 ml does not provide satisfactory visualization, this dose may be repeated in 15 to 30 minutes. In persons of slight build, 20 ml may produce adequate shadows.
Larger doses ranging from 50 ml to 60 ml of the 50 percent solution may be used for routine excretory urography in adults. The increased dosage offers better and more complete visualization of the urinary tract. This technique requires neither compression nor dehydration and is more effective in obese patients. Adverse reactions to the larger dose are similar to those encountered with lower doses without an increase in incidence, severity, or type of reaction. Voiding cystourethrograms may be obtained when desired. For the best results and minimal side effects, it is advisable to inject the total amount of solution intravenously in one to three minutes.
Children: The dosage of the 50 percent solution for children under 6 months of age is 5 ml; for children 6 to 12 months of age, 6 ml to 8 ml; for children 1 to 2 years of age, 8 ml to 10 ml; for children 2 to 5 years of age, 10 ml to 12 ml; for children 5 to 7 years of age, 12 ml to 15 ml; for children 7 to 11 years of age, 15 ml to 18 ml, and for children 11 to 15 years of age, 18 ml to 20 ml.
Subcutaneous Dosage. The compound may be given subcutaneously, diluted with equal quantities of sterile water for injection. Although not necessary, hyaluronidase (150 turbidity units) may be given simultaneously if desired. The total volume is divided into two

equal doses and injected over each scapula. A large, rounded mass appears after the injection has been completed. A piece of cotton saturated with collodion may be applied over each injection point to prevent seepage of the contrast medium.

Adults and older children: The usual dose is 20 ml to 30 ml of the 50 percent solution diluted with equal quantities of sterile water for injection.

Infants and young children: The dose ranges from 5 ml of the 50 percent solution for smaller infants up to 15 ml for older children and should be diluted with equal quantities of sterile water for injection.

Intramuscular Dosage. The 50 percent solution may also be injected intramuscularly undiluted or diluted with an equal quantity of sterile water for injection. Generally, the total volume is introduced into the gluteal muscles in two separate, equal doses. Hyaluronidase also may be injected if desired.

Generally, doses of 5 ml to 15 ml of the 50 percent solution may be administered to **children;** the usual 20 ml to 30 ml dose is suggested for **adults.**

Roentgenography

Intravenous Technique. A film should be exposed routinely before the intravenous injection is made. If the plain film shows evidence of gas accumulation, it may be best to defer the examination to some other day.

Excellent shadows can often be obtained immediately after administration of the radiopaque medium (within a five-minute period). If preliminary preparation has been carried out, the urinary organs are usually best visualized on films exposed 5, 10, or 15 minutes after intravenous injection. If a film of the bladder is required, it generally is taken 25 or 35 minutes after injection.

In patients with impaired renal function, the best shadows may not be obtainable until later (30 minutes or more) because of delayed excretion, and additional film may have to be exposed.

Subcutaneous Technique. The excretion of the drug occurs promptly so that films may be exposed at intervals of 10, 20, and 30 minutes.

Intramuscular Technique. Diagnostically, visualization of the upper urinary tract following the intramuscular administration of the 50 percent solution has been found almost to equal that achieved with intravenous injections. Since excretion of the medium is rapid, it may be evident within five minutes after intramuscular injection. The time for obtaining the best filling and contrast varies, but the first exposure is generally made after a 10-minute interval.

CEREBRAL ANGIOGRAPHY

Inasmuch as cerebral angiography is a highly specialized procedure requiring the use of special techniques, it is recommended that HYPAQUE sodium, brand of diatrizoate sodium, be used for this purpose only by persons skilled and experienced in carrying out the procedure.

Contraindication: Carotid angiography should be avoided during the progressive period of a stroke because of the increased risk of cerebral complications.

Precautions: Patients on whom cerebral angiography is to be employed should be selected with care. The 50 percent solution should be used with caution in instances of extreme senility (but not old age per se), advanced arteriosclerosis, severe hypertension, and cardiac decompensation. Although cerebral angiography has been considered contraindicated in patients who have recently experienced cerebral embolism or thrombosis (stroke syndrome), many experts now believe that the diagnostic value of the procedure, when employed early as an aid in locating lesions amenable to operation, outweighs any added risk to the patient. Furthermore, a small number of postangiographic fatalities, including progressive thrombosis already evident clinically before angiography, have occurred in which the procedure did not appear to play any direct role. Patients with severe cerebrovascular disease may be examined primarily by indirect methods of angiography.

Care should be exercised to avoid contaminating catheters, syringes, needles, and contrast media with glove powder or cotton fibers.

In subarachnoid hemorrhage, angiography is expected to be hazardous. In migraine, the procedure can be hazardous because of ischemic complications, particularly if performed during or soon after an attack.

Adverse Reactions: Defects in arteriographic technique, the presence of occlusive atherosclerotic vascular disease, repeated injections of the contrast media, or doses higher than those recommended constitute the major sources of arteriographic complications.

Untoward reactions during cerebral angiography are for the most part mild and temporary although permanent visual field defects and deaths have been reported.

Vascular reactions include flushing, vessel spasm, thrombosis, and cutaneous petechiae. Neurologic complications include transient cerebral blindness, neuromuscular disorders, convulsions, coma, hemiparesis, unilateral dysesthesias, visual field defects, aphasia, amnesia, and respiratory difficulties.

Dosage and Administration: For carotid and vertebral angiography, depending upon the method used, most clinicians generally employ doses of 8 ml to 12 ml. Additional injections may be made as indicated. In the retrograde (brachial) method, a single injection of 35 ml to 50 ml is generally used.

Depending upon the vessel injected and the method employed, other dosages may be used as indicated.

PERIPHERAL ANGIOGRAPHY

The 50 percent solution may be administered to establish the peripheral vascular status of the patient by means of arteriography and venography and to delineate the vascularity of bone tumors, etc through intraosseous injection. Angiographically visualized detail has proved helpful in the determination of the nature and severity of vascular disease, the site or sites of organic obstruction or vessel occlusion, and the extent of collateral circulation.

Precautions: Extreme caution is advised in considering peripheral arteriography in patients suspected of having thromboangiitis obliterans (Buerger's disease) since any procedure (even insertion of a needle or catheter) may induce a severe arterial or venous spasm. Caution is also advisable in patients with severe ischemia associated with ascending infection.

Adverse Reactions: Adverse reactions observed during peripheral arteriography may sometimes be due to arterial trauma during the procedure (ie, insertion of needle or catheter, subintimal injection, perforation, etc) as well as to the hypertonicity or effect of the medium. Reported adverse reactions include transient arterial spasm, extravasation, hemorrhage, hematoma formation with tamponade, injury to nerves in close proximity to artery, thrombosis, dissecting aneurysm, arteriovenous fistula (eg, with accidental perforation of femoral artery and vein during the needling), and transient leg pain from contraction of calf muscles in femoral arteriography. Transient hypotension has been reported after intraarterial (brachial) injection of the medium. Also, brachial plexus injury has been reported with axillary artery injections.

During venography in the presence of venous stasis, inflammatory changes and thrombosis may occur. Thrombosis is rare if the vein is irrigated following the injection.

Dosage and Administration: Diagnostic arteriograms may be obtained with 25 ml to 35 ml of HYPAQUE sodium, brand of diatrizoate sodium injection, 50 percent introduced into the brachial artery in the upper extremity or the femoral artery in the lower extremity.

The presence and location of venous obstructions in the vessels of the extremities may also be demonstrated by the injection of 15 ml to 40 ml of the 50 percent solution. For visualization of the great saphenous vein, the upper femoral or the iliac veins, the medium is generally injected into the great saphenous vein in the lower leg at a rate of 1 ml per second. When demonstration of the small saphenous vein, the popliteal vein, or the lower femoral vein is necessary, injection is performed in a superficial vein of the outer aspect of the foot. The axillary and subclavian veins are best delineated by introducing the medium into the median basilic vein at the rate of 1 ml per second and exposing films during the process of injection.

AORTOGRAPHY

HYPAQUE sodium, brand of diatrizoate sodium injection, 50 percent may be administered intravenously or intraarterially by accepted techniques to visualize the aorta and its major branches.

Warnings: *Pheochromocytoma:* Administration of angiographic media to patients known or suspected to have pheochromocytoma can cause dangerous changes in blood pressure. A minimum dose should be injected. The blood pressure should be carefully monitored and measures for controlling major fluctuations should be available.

During aortography by the translumbar technique, extreme care is advised to avoid inadvertent intrathecal injection since the injection of even small amounts (5 ml to 7 ml) of the contrast medium may cause convulsions, permanent sequelae, or fatality. Should the accident occur, the patient should be placed upright to confine the hyperbaric solution to a low level, anesthesia may be required to control convulsions, and if there is evidence of a large dose having been administered, a careful cerebrospinal fluid exchange-washout should be considered.

Precautions: The presence of a vigorous pulsatile flow should be established before using a catheter or pressure injection technique. A small "pilot" dose (about 2 ml) should be administered to locate the exact site of needle or catheter tip to help prevent injection of the main dose into a branch of the aorta or intramurally. In the translumbar technique, severe pain during injection may indicate intramural placement and abdominal or back pain afterwards may indicate hemorrhage from the injection site. Following catheter procedures, gentle pressure hemostasis for 5 to 10 minutes is advised, followed by observation for 30 to 60 minutes and immobilization of the limb for several hours to prevent hemorrhage from the site of arterial puncture.

The care and experience with which the procedure is performed, the amount and type of medium used, the age and condition of the patient, and the premedication and anesthesia employed, influence the incidence and severity

Continued on next page

This product information was effective as of November 19, 1982. On these and other products of Winthrop Laboratories, detailed information may be obtained on a current basis by direct inquiry to the Professional Services Department, 90 Park Avenue, New York, NY 10016 (212) 907-2525.

Winthrop—Cont.

of reactions or complications that may be encountered. Since aortography is not without some danger, it should be employed only by persons experienced in the technique.
Repeated injections of the solution during a single study should be avoided whenever possible.
Under conditions of slowed aortic circulation there is an increased likelihood of aortography causing muscle spasm. Occasional serious neurologic complications, including paraplegia, have also been reported in patients with aortic-iliac or even femoral artery bed obstruction, abdominal compression, hypotension, hypertension, spinal anesthesia, injection of vasopressors to increase contrast, and low injection sites (L2-3). In these patients the concentration, dose, and number of repeat injections of the medium should be maintained at a minimum with appropriate intervals between injections. The position of the patient and catheter tip should be carefully evaluated.
Aortic Branches: Since serious neurologic complications, including quadriplegia, have occasionally been reported following spinal arteriography or selective injection of arterial trunks providing spinal artery branches (usually the thyrocervical, costocervical, subclavian, vertebral, bronchial, intercostal), great care is necessary to avoid entry of a large concentrated bolus of the medium. Thus, a "pilot" dose may establish correct position of the catheter tip. The concentration of the medium should not be over 50 percent. The carefully individualized dose is usually under 5 ml but preferably 3 ml to 4 ml and the number of repeat injections held to a minimum with appropriate intervals between injections. Pain or muscle spasm during the injection may require reevaluation of the procedure.
Adverse Reactions: The most common reaction to the medium is a mild burning sensation on injection. In addition to the reactions described in the general section, the following have been reported: mesenteric and intestinal necrosis, acute pancreatitis, renal shutdown (usually transitory), and neurologic complications following inadvertent injection of a large part of the aortic dose into a branch of the aorta. Entry of the large aortic dose into the renal artery can cause, even in the absence of symptoms, albuminuria, cylindruria, and hematuria, and an elevated BUN. Rapid and complete return of function usually follows. Also reported are coronary occlusion, hemorrhage from puncture site, arterial perforation by catheter or needle, thrombosis, embolism, and subintimal injection with aortic dissection by the medium.
Dosage and Administration: The amount of each individual dose is a more important consideration than the total dosage used. Sufficient time should elapse between each injection to allow for subsidence of hemodynamic disturbances.
Retrograde (catheter) aortography—For **adults** and **children,** 0.5 ml to 1 ml per kg of body weight.
Intravenous aortography —For **adults** and **children,** 1 ml per kg of body weight.
Translumbar aortography—For **adults,** 10 ml to 30 ml. For **children** under 12 years, the dose is proportionate to age.
Selective renal arteriography—For **adults** and **children** over 14 years of age. 5 ml to 8 ml with repeat injections as indicated. For **younger children,** the dose is proportionate to age.

INTRAOSSEOUS VENOGRAPHY

The 50 percent solution may be injected directly into the bone marrow in the study of venous circulation of the bone and extraosseous tissue in the immediate drainage area.
A general anesthetic is sometimes necessary since the method is painful. Occasionally, extravasation of the contrast medium from the needle into the soft tissue may occur.
Dosage and Administration: After aspiration of 4 ml of marrow, 10 ml to 20 ml of the medium are injected.
To visualize the pterygoid venous plexus, 5 ml to 8 ml of the contrast medium are injected into the medullary cavity of the mandible.

DIRECT CHOLANGIOGRAPHY

Precaution: In the presence of acute pancreatitis, direct cholangiography, if necessary, should be employed with caution, injecting no more than 5 ml to 10 ml without undue pressure.
Adverse Reactions: Adverse reactions may often be attributed to injection pressure or excessive volume of the medium, resulting in overdistention. Such pressure may produce a sensation of epigastric fullness, followed by moderate pain in the back or right upper abdominal quadrant, which will subside when injection is stopped.
Some of the medium may enter the pancreatic duct and cause a transient serum amylase elevation 6 to 18 hours later, without apparent ill effects. Occasionally, nausea, vomiting, fever, and tachycardia have been observed. Pancholangitis resulting in liver abscess or septicemia has been reported.
Dosage and Administration: The solution should be warmed to body temperature before administration. The injection is made slowly without undue pressure, taking great care to avoid introducing bubbles.
Operative—If no resistance is encountered, from 10 to 15 ml of a 25 to 50 percent solution is injected or instilled into the cystic duct or common bile duct, as indicated. In patients with obstructive jaundice, 40 ml to 50 ml of the medium may be injected directly into the gallbladder after aspiration of its contents.
Postexploratory or completion T-tube cholangiography may also be performed after exploration of the common bile duct.
Postoperative—Delayed cholangiograms are usually made from the fifth to the tenth postoperative day prior to removal of the T-tube. In case of a dilated ductal tract, a larger volume (up to 100 ml) of radiopaque medium may be required for complete filling and visualization.

PERCUTANEOUS TRANSHEPATIC CHOLANGIOGRAPHY

Percutaneous transhepatic cholangiography is recommended for carefully selected patients for the differential diagnosis of jaundice due to extrahepatic biliary obstruction or parenchymal disease. The procedure is only employed where oral or intravenous cholangiography and other procedures have failed to provide the necessary information. In obstructive cases, percutaneous transhepatic cholangiography is used to determine the cause and site of the obstruction to help plan surgery. The technique may also be of value in avoiding laparotomy in poor risk jaundice patients since failure to enter a duct suggests hepatocellular disease. Careful attention to technique is essential for the success and safety of the procedure. The procedure is usually performed under local anesthesia following analgesic premedication (eg, 100 mg meperidine intramuscularly).
Contraindications: Percutaneous transhepatic cholangiography is contraindicated in patients with coagulation defects and prolonged prothrombin times until normal, or near normal, coagulation is achieved, eg, with vitamin K.
Precautions: Percutaneous transhepatic cholangiography should only be attempted when compatible blood for potential transfusions is in readiness and emergency surgical measures are available. The patient should be carefully monitored for at least 24 hours to insure prompt detection of bile leakage and hemorrhage. Cholespastic premedication, as with morphine, should be avoided. Respiratory movements should be controlled during introduction of the needle.
Adverse Reactions: In percutaneous transhepatic cholangiography, some discomfort is common, but severe pain is unusual. Complications of the procedure are often serious and have been reported in four to six percent of patients. These reactions have included bile leakage and peritonitis, which are more likely to occur in patients with obstructions that cause unrelieved high biliary pressure. Bleeding (sometimes massive with exsanguination) may occur, especially in patients with clotting abnormalities. Blood-bile fistula, manifested by an early urogram (within 2 minutes), has been reported. Hypotension with fever and chills, as manifestations of septicemia, have occurred. Tension pneumothorax, cholangitis, and bacteremia have been reported.
Dosage and Administration: As the needle is advanced or withdrawn, a bile duct may be located by frequent aspiration for bile or mucus into a syringe filled with normal saline. As much bile as possible is aspirated. The usual dose of HYPAQUE sodium, brand of diatrizoate sodium injection, 50 percent is 20 ml to 40 ml but the range can be from 10 ml to 60 ml depending on degree of biliary dilatation present. The injection may be repeated for exposures in different planes. If a duct is not readily located by aspiration, entry may be established by the injection of succesive small doses of 1 ml or 2 ml of the medium under x-ray observation as the needle is withdrawn. If a duct is not located after three or four attempts, the procedure should be abandoned. Inability to enter a duct strongly suggests hepatocellular disease.

HYSTEROSALPINGOGRAPHY

Hysterosalpingography may be performed with either the 50 percent solution, or if a somewhat more viscous solution is preferred, diatrizoate meglumine and diatrizoate sodium, 90 percent.
Contraindications: The procedure should not be performed during the menstrual period or when menstrual flow is imminent, nor should it be performed when infection is present in any portion of the genital tract, including the external genitalia. The procedure is also contraindicated for pregnant women or for those in whom pregnancy is suspected. Its use is not advised for six months after termination of pregnancy, or 30 days after conization or curettage.
Precaution: In patients with carcinoma or in those in whom the condition is suspected, caution should be exercised to avoid possible spread of the lesion by the procedure.
Adverse Reactions: Cramping may occur during the injection and sometimes mild lower abdominal pain may be present for an hour or two afterwards. Even when the medium gains entrance into venous or lymphatic channels, systemic effects are rare. Generalized urticaria or slight transient hyperpyrexia, however, has been reported.
Dosage and Administration:
Preparation of the Patient
It is preferable to perform the procedure approximately 10 days after the patient's menstrual period. The patient should empty the bladder before the examination. An enema and vaginal douche are not essential but may be given one hour before the study. Premedication is not necessary.
Approximately 4 ml will suffice to fill a normal uterine cavity, with an additional 3 ml or 4 ml for the fallopian tubes. These amounts may vary depending on the nature of the disease.

SPLENOPORTOGRAPHY

Splenoportography is usually performed under mild preoperative sedation and under local anesthesia.
Contraindications: Splenoportography should not be performed on any patient for whom splenectomy is contraindicated, since complications of the procedure at times make splenectomy necessary. Other contraindications include prolonged prothrombin time or other coagulation defects, significant thrombocytopenia, and any condition which may increase the possibility of rupture of the spleen.
Precautions: Prior gastrointestinal x-ray examination should include particular attention to the lower esophageal area. A hematologic survey, including prothrombin time and platelet count, should be performed. To minimize risk of bleeding, manipulation during or after entry of the needle should be avoided. Caution is advised in patients whose spleen has recently become tender and palpable.
Following splenoportography, the patient should lie on his left side for several hours and should be closely observed for 24 hours for signs of internal bleeding.
Adverse Reactions: Internal bleeding is the most common serious complication of splenoportography. Although leakage of up to 300 ml of blood is apparently not uncommon, sometimes blood transfusion and rarely, splenectomy, may be required to control hemorrhage. Peritoneal extravasation may cause transient diaphragmatic irritation or mild to moderate transient pain which may sometimes be referred to the shoulder, the periumbilical region, or other areas. Because of the proximity of the pleural cavity, accidental pneumothorax has been known to occur. Inadvertent injection of the medium into other nearby structures is not likely to cause untoward consequences.
Dosage and Administration: A preliminary small "pilot" dose is injected to confirm splenic entry, followed usually by rapid injection of 20 ml to 25 ml of HYPAQUE sodium, brand of diatrizoate sodium injection, 50 percent. Rapid serial exposures are started with the injection of the dose and continued until contrast is observed in the entire portal system.
How Supplied: Vials of 20 ml, rubber stoppered,boxes of 25 (NDC 0024-0764-04).
Vials of 30 ml, rubber stoppered, boxes of 25 (NDC 0024-0765-04).
Vials of 50 ml, rubber stoppered, boxes of 25 (NDC 0024-0766-04).
Boxes of 10 calibrated 200 ml dilution bottles with hanger containing 100 ml HYPAQUE sodium 50%; rubber stoppered, with 10 intravenous infusion sets (NDC 0024-0767-02).
Boxes of 10 calibrated 200 ml dilution bottles with hanger containing 150 ml HYPAQUE sodium 50%; rubber stoppered, with 10 intravenous infusion sets (NDC 0024-0770-01).
Boxes of 10 calibrated 200 ml bottles with hanger containing 200 ml HYPAQUE sodium 50%; rubber stoppered (NDC 0024-0771-02).

HYPAQUE® MEGLUMINE 60% ℞
brand of diatrizoate meglumine injection, USP
Sterile Aqueous Injection

FOR EXCRETORY UROGRAPHY, CEREBRAL ANGIOGRAPHY, PERIPHERAL ARTERIOGRAPHY, VENOGRAPHY, DIRECT CHOLANGIOGRAPHY, SPLENOPORTOGRAPHY, ARTHROGRAPHY, AND DISCOGRAPHY

Description: HYPAQUE meglumine, brand of diatrizoate meglumine, is meglumine 3, 5-diacetamido-2, 4, 6-triiodobenzoate ($C_{18}H_{26}I_3N_3O_9$), which contains 47.06 percent iodine. It is a colorless, microcrystalline solid that is readily soluble in water.
HYPAQUE meglumine 60 percent (w/v) is a sterile aqueous solution containing 60 g of the meglumine salt of diatrizoic acid per 100 ml of solution. It was specifically designed for those indications in which the physician does not desire to use a sodium-containing radiopaque medium. The solution is a clear, colorless to pale yellow liquid, and the pH is adjusted between 6.5 and 7.7 with diatrizoic acid or meglumine solution. It is a relatively thermostable solution and may be autoclaved without harmful effects, although it should be protected from strong light. The 60 percent solution contains edetate calcium disodium 1:10,000 as a sequestering stabilizing agent. Each 1 ml contains approximately 282 mg of organically bound iodine. The viscosity of the solution is 6.17 cps at 25 C and 4.12 cps at 37 C.
Action: A radiopaque medium used to delineate internal structures.
Indications: HYPAQUE meglumine 60 percent is indicated for excretory urography; cerebral angiography; peripheral arteriography; venography; operative, T-tube, or percutaneous transhepatic cholangiography; splenoportography; arthrography; and discography.
Contraindications, General: **Do not use HYPAQUE meglumine 60 percent solution for myelography or for examination of dorsal cysts or sinuses which might communicate with the subarachnoid space.** Injection of even a small amount into the subarachnoid space may produce convulsions and result in fatality. Epidural injection is also contraindicated.
Warnings, General: Serious or fatal reactions have been associated with the administration of radiopaque media. It is of utmost importance that a course of action be carefully planned in advance for the immediate treatment of serious reactions, and that adequate and appropriate facilities be readily available in case a severe reaction occurs.
Selective spinal arteriography or arteriography of trunks providing spinal branches can cause mild to severe muscle spasm. However, serious neurologic sequelae, including permanent paralysis, have occasionally been reported. (See also Angiography, Precaution.)
Usage in Pregnancy. No teratogenic effects attributable to HYPAQUE meglumine 60 percent have been observed in reproduction studies in animals. However, before administration of HYPAQUE meglumine 60 percent to women of childbearing potential, the benefit to the patient should be carefully weighed against the possible risk to the fetus. In addition, most authorities consider elective contrast radiography of the abdomen contraindicated during pregnancy.
Administration of radiopaque materials to patients known or suspected to have **pheochromocytoma** should be performed with extreme caution. If, in the opinion of the physician, the possible benefits of such procedures outweigh the considered risk, the amount of radiopaque material injected should be kept to an absolute minimum. The blood pressure should be assessed throughout the procedure, and measures for treatment of a hypertensive crisis should be available.
Contrast media have been shown to promote the phenomenon of sickling in individuals who are homozygous for sickle cell disease when the material is injected intravenously or intraarterially.
Precautions, General: Before a contrast medium is injected, the patient should be questioned for a history of allergy. Although a history of allergy may imply a greater than usual risk, it does not arbitrarily contraindicate the use of the medium. Premedication with antihistamines to avoid or minimize possible allergic reactions may be considered. **Benadryl®, brand of diphenhydramine hydrochloride, however, may cause precipitation when mixed in the same syringe with HYPAQUE meglumine, brand of diatrizoate meglumine.**
The intravenous injection of a test dose of 0.5 ml to 1 ml of the contrast agent before injection of the full dose has been employed in an attempt to predict severe or fatal adverse reactions. The preponderance of recent scientific literature, however, now demonstrates that this provocative test procedure is not reliably predictive of serious or fatal reactions. Severe reactions and fatalities have occurred with the test dose alone, with the full dose after a nonreactive test dose, and with or without a history of allergy. No conclusive relationship between severe or fatal reactions and antigen-antibody reactions or other manifestations of allergy has been established. A history of allergy may be useful in predicting reactions of a mild or intermediate nature.
Caution is advised in patients with severe cardiovascular disease, hyperthyroidism, extreme senility (but not old age per se), and in patients with a history of bronchial asthma or other allergic manifestations, or of sensitivity to iodine.
The results of PBI and RAI uptake studies, which depend on iodine estimations, will not reflect thyroid function for up to 16 days following administration of iodinated urographic media. However, function tests not depending on iodine estimations, eg, T_3 resin uptake or direct thyroxine assays, are not affected.
Adverse Reactions, General: Reactions accompanying the use of contrast media may vary directly with the concentration of the substance, the amount used, the technique used, and the underlying pathology.
The following have been reported after administration of diatrizoates and other iodinated contrast media. *Reactions due to technique:* hematomas and ecchymoses. *Hemodynamic reactions:* vein cramp and thrombophlebitis following intravenous injection. *Cardiovascular reactions:* rare cases of cardiac arrhythmias, hypertension, hypotension and shock, and cardiac arrest. Occasionally, transient proteinuria, and rarely, oliguria or anuria. *Allergic reactions:* asthmatic attacks, nasal and conjunctival symptoms, dermal reactions such as urticaria, and rarely, anaphylactic reactions. Signs and symptoms related to the *respiratory system:* pulmonary or laryngeal edema, bronchospasm; or to the *nervous system:* restlessness, convulsions. *Other reactions:* flushing, pain, warmth, nausea, vomiting, anxiety, headache, and dizziness. Rarely, immediate or delayed rigors can occur, sometimes accompanied by hyperpyrexia. Infrequently, "iodism" (salivary gland swelling) from organic iodinated compounds appears two days after exposure and subsides by the sixth day. Rarely, disseminated intravascular coagulation has occurred.
Subcutaneous extravasation, chiefly because of hypertonicity of the medium, causes transitory stinging. If the volume is small, ill effects are very unlikely. However, if subcutaneous extravasation is extensive, especially in the foot, the physician should consider infiltration with Sterile Water for Injection, USP, or injection of spreading agents.
Diffuse petechiae have been described and, in several instances, were traced to contamination of syringes, gloves with talc, or fine lint.

Continued on next page

This product information was effective as of November 19, 1982. On these and other products of Winthrop Laboratories, detailed information may be obtained on a current basis by direct inquiry to the Professional Services Department, 90 Park Avenue, New York, NY 10016 (212) 907-2525.

Winthrop—Cont.

EXCRETORY UROGRAPHY

Indication: Since HYPAQUE meglumine, brand of diatrizoate meglumine injection, 60 percent is rapidly eliminated by the kidneys in radiopaque concentration, its use is indicated for excretory urography.
Precautions: See section on Precautions, General.
Some clinicians consider multiple myeloma a contraindication to excretory urography because of the great possibility of producing transient to fatal renal failure. Others believe that the risk of causing anuria is definite but small. If excretory urography is performed in the presence of multiple myeloma, dehydration should be avoided since it favors protein precipitation in renal tubules.
Because of the possibility of temporary suppression of urine, it is wise to allow an interval of at least 48 hours before excretory urography is repeated in patients with unilateral or bilateral reduction of normal renal function.
Preparatory dehydration may be dangerous in infants, young children, the elderly, and azotemic patients (especially those with polyuria, oliguria, diabetes, advanced vascular disease, or preexisting dehydration). The undesirable dehydration in these patients may be accentuated by the osmotic diuretic action of the medium.
Adverse Reactions: See section on Adverse Reactions, General.
Dosage and Administration:
Intravenous Dosage
Adults. A dose of 30 ml to 60 ml produces excellent shadows in the majority of adults subjected to partial dehydration and effective purgation. In persons of slight build, 20 ml produces adequate shadows. For best results and minimal reactions, the total 30 ml to 60 ml should be injected in one to three minutes and compression may be used. A small intravenous test dose may be administered as a possible aid in determining sensitivity to the medium. (See Precautions, General.)
Children. The suggested dosage for children up to 12 years old is presented in the table. Children older than 12 years may be given an adult dose.
[See table below].
Preliminary Preparation of Patient
Although clear shadows are often seen in patients who have had no preliminary preparation for urography, the largest percentage of satisfactory films is obtained in patients who abstain from fluids for 12 to 15 hours before the intravenous injection so that partial dehydration results. (See Precautions concerning dehydration.) Unless contraindicated, a laxative may be taken at bedtime to eliminate gas from the intestine.
Roentgenographic Technique
A preliminary scout film may be obtained before the intravenous injection. Excellent shadows can often be obtained immediately after administration of the radiopaque medium (within a five-minute period). If preliminary preparation has been carried out, the urinary organs are usually best visualized on films exposed 5, 10, or 15 minutes after intravenous injection. If a film of the bladder is required, it is generally taken 25 or 35 minutes after injection.
In patients with impaired renal function, the best shadows may not be obtainable until later (30 minutes or more) because of delayed excretion, and additional film may have to be exposed.
Most urologists and roentgenologists believe that compression immediately above the symphysis (obtained by application of a small hollow rubber ball about the size of a grapefruit or by the rolled bed sheet technique) assures adequate filling of the pelves and ureters, and hence is of great value. Although compression undoubtedly improves the urogram, it also seems to increase the possibility of pyelorenal backflow or reflux by raising the pressure within the urinary tract.

ANGIOGRAPHY

Precaution: Since serious neurologic complications, including quadriplegia, have occasionally been reported following spinal arteriography or selective injection of arterial trunks providing spinal artery branches (usually the thyrocervical, costocervical, subclavian, vertebral, bronchial, intercostal), great care is necessary to avoid entry of a large concentrated bolus of the medium. Thus, a "pilot" dose may establish correct position of the catheter tip. The concentration of the medium should not be over 60 percent. The carefully individualized dose is usually under 5 ml but preferably 3 ml to 4 ml and the number of repeat injections held to a minimum with appropriate intervals between injections. Pain or muscle spasm during the injection may require reevaluation of the procedure.

CEREBRAL ANGIOGRAPHY

Indication: HYPAQUE meglumine, brand of diatrizoate meglumine injection, 60 percent may be administered for visualization of the cerebral vessels. Inasmuch as cerebral angiography is a highly specialized procedure requiring the use of special techniques, it is recommended that HYPAQUE meglumine 60 percent be used for this purpose only by persons skilled and experienced in carrying out the procedure.
Contraindication: Carotid angiography during the progressive period of a stroke should be avoided, particularly on the left side because of the increased risk of cerebral complications.
Precautions: See Section on Precautions, General.
Patients in whom cerebral angiography is to be performed should be selected with care.
Although cerebral angiography has been considered contraindicated in patients who have recently experienced cerebral embolism or thrombosis (stroke syndrome), many experts now believe that the diagnostic value of the procedure, when employed early as an aid in locating lesions amenable to operation, outweighs any added risk to the patient. Furthermore, a small number of postangiographic fatalities have been reported, including progressive thrombosis already clinically evident before angiography, in which the procedure did not appear to play any direct role. Patients with severe cerebrovascular disease should be examined primarily by indirect methods of angiography.
In cerebral angiography, every precaution must be taken to prevent untoward reactions. Reactions may vary directly with the concentration of the substance, the amount used, the speed and frequency of injections, and the interval between injections.
In subarachnoid hemorrhage, angiography is expected to be hazardous. In migraine, the procedure can be hazardous because of ischemic complications, particularly if performed during or soon after an attack.
Adverse Reactions: See Section on Adverse Reactions, General.
With any contrast medium introduced into the cerebral vasculature, neurologic complications, including neuromuscular disorders, seizures, loss of consciousness, hemiplegia, unilateral dysesthesias, visual field defects, language disorders (aphasia), amnesia, and respiratory difficulties may occur, particularly when the extent of the intrinsic lesion is unknown. Such untoward reactions are for the most part temporary, although permanent visual field defects have been reported. Some investigators who are experienced in angiographic procedure emphasize the fact that they tend to occur after repeated injections or higher doses of the contrast medium. Other clinicians find that they occur most frequently in elderly patients. Inasmuch as the procedure itself is attended by technical difficulties regardless of the risk the patient presents (eg, mechanical catheter obstruction of the vertebral artery can cause transient blindness), the more experienced the radiologic team, the fewer the complications of any degree that are apt to arise.
Dosage and Administration: A dose of 8 ml to 12 ml injected at a rate not exceeding the normal flow in the carotid artery (about 5 ml per second) is suggested. The dose may be repeated as indicated; however, an increased risk attends each repeat injection. Children require a smaller dose in proportion to weight. Light anesthesia may be required in these procedures.

PERIPHERAL ARTERIOGRAPHY AND VENOGRAPHY

Indication: HYPAQUE meglumine, brand of diatrizoate meglumine injection, 60 percent may be administered for peripheral arteriography and for venography.
Precautions: See Section on Precautions, General.
Extreme caution is advised in considering peripheral arteriography in patients suspected of having thromboangiitis obliterans (Buerger's disease) since any procedure (even insertion of a needle or catheter) may induce a severe arterial or venous spasm. Caution is also advisable in patients with severe ischemia associated with ascending infection.
Adverse Reactions: See Section on Adverse Reactions, General. Soreness in extremities has also been reported.
Adverse reactions observed during peripheral arteriography may sometimes be due to arterial trauma during the procedure (ie, insertion of needle or catheter, subintimal injection, perforation, etc) as well as to the hypertonicity or effect of the medium. Reported adverse reactions include transient arterial spasm, extravasation, hemorrhage, hematoma formation with tamponade, injury to nerves in close proximity to artery, thrombosis, dissecting aneurysm, arteriovenous fistula (eg, with accidental perforation of femoral artery and vein during the needling), and transient leg pain from contraction of calf muscles in femoral arteriography. Transient hypotension has been reported after intraarterial (brachial) injection of the medium. Also, brachial plexus injury has been reported with axillary artery injections.
During venography in the presence of venous stasis, inflammatory changes and thrombosis may occur. Thrombosis is rare if the vein is irrigated following the injection.
Dosage and Administration: Diagnostic arteriograms may be obtained with 20 ml to 40 ml of HYPAQUE meglumine, brand of diatrizoate meglumine injection, 60 percent intro-

Pediatric Dosage for Excretory Urography

Age	Body Weight	Dosage
Under 2 years	up to 10 lb	5 ml to 10 ml
	10 to 30 lb	10 ml to 15 ml
2 to 12 years	30 to 60 lb	15 ml to 30 ml
	over 60 lb	30 ml

duced into the larger peripheral arteries by percutaneous or operative methods. Visualization of veins in the extremities may be accomplished with 10 ml to 20 ml.

DIRECT CHOLANGIOGRAPHY

Contraindications: Percutaneous transhepatic cholangiography is contraindicated in patients with coagulation defects and prolonged prothrombin times until normal, or near normal, coagulation is achieved (eg, with vitamin K).

Precautions: In the presence of acute pancreatitis, direct cholangiography, if necessary, should be employed with caution, injecting no more than 5 ml to 10 ml without undue pressure.

Percutaneous transhepatic cholangiography should only be attempted when compatible blood for potential transfusions is in readiness and emergency surgical measures are available. The patient should be carefully monitored for at least 24 hours to insure prompt detection of bile leakage and hemorrhage. Cholespastic premedication, as with morphine, should be avoided. Respiratory movements should be controlled during introduction of the needle.

Adverse Reactions: Adverse reactions may often be attributed to injection pressure or excessive volume of the medium, resulting in overdistention. Such pressure may produce a sensation of epigastric fullness, followed by moderate pain in the back or right upper abdominal quadrant, which will subside when injection is stopped.

Some of the medium may enter the pancreatic duct and cause a transient serum amylase elevation 6 to 18 hours later, without apparent ill effects. Occasionally, nausea, vomiting, fever, and tachycardia have been observed. Pancholangitis resulting in liver abscess or septicemia has been reported.

In percutaneous transhepatic cholangiography, some discomfort is common, but severe pain is unusual. Complications of the procedure are often serious and have been reported in four to six per cent of patients. These reactions have included bile leakage and peritonitis, which are more likely to occur in patients with obstructions that cause unrelieved high biliary pressure. Bleeding (sometimes massive with exsanguination) may occur, especially in patients with clotting abnormalities. Blood-bile fistula, manifested by an early urogram (within 2 minutes) has been reported. Hypotension with fever and chills, as manifestations of septicemia, have occurred. Tension pneumothorax, cholangitis, and bacteremia have been reported.

Dosage and Administration: The solution should be warmed to body temperature before administration. The injection is made slowly without undue pressure, taking great care to avoid introducing bubbles.

Operative—If no resistance is encountered, from 10 ml to 15 ml (sometimes up to 25 ml) of a 30 to 60 percent solution is injected or instilled into the cystic duct or common bile duct, as indicated. In patients with obstructive jaundice, 40 ml to 50 ml of the medium may be injected directly into the gallbladder after aspiration of its contents.

Postexploratory or completion T-tube cholangiography may also be performed after exploration of the common bile duct.

Postoperative—Delayed cholangiograms are usually made from the fifth to the tenth postoperative day prior to removal of the T-tube.

Percutaneous transhepatic cholangiography is recommended for carefully selected patients for the differential diagnosis of jaundice due to extrahepatic biliary obstruction or parenchymal disease. The procedure is only employed where oral or intravenous cholangiography and other procedures have failed to provide the necessary information. In obstructive cases, percutaneous transhepatic cholangiography is used to determine the cause and site of the obstruction to help plan surgery. The technique may also be of value in avoiding laparotomy in poor risk jaundice patients since failure to enter a duct suggests hepatocellular disease. Careful attention to technique is essential for the success and safety of the procedure. The procedure is usually performed under local anesthesia following analgesic premedication (eg, 100 mg meperidine intramuscularly).

As the needle is advanced or withdrawn, a bile duct may be located by frequent aspiration for bile or mucus into a syringe filled with normal saline. As much bile as possible is aspirated. The usual dose of HYPAQUE meglumine, brand of diatrizoate meglumine injection, 60 percent is 20 ml to 40 ml but the range can be from 10 ml to 60 ml depending on degree of biliary dilatation present. The injection may be repeated for exposures in different planes. If a duct is not readily located by aspiration, entry may be established by the injection of successive small doses of 1 ml or 2 ml of the medium under x-ray observation as the needle is withdrawn. If a duct is not located after three or four attempts, the procedure should be abandoned. Inability to enter a duct strongly suggests hepatocellular disease.

SPLENOPORTOGRAPHY

Indication: Splenoportography is usually performed under mild preoperative sedation and under local anesthesia.

Contraindications: Splenoportography should not be performed on any patient for whom splenectomy is contraindicated, since complications of the procedure at times make splenectomy necessary. Other contraindications include prolonged prothrombin time or other coagulation defects, significant thrombocytopenia, and any condition which may increase the possibility of rupture of the spleen.

Precautions: Prior gastrointestinal x-ray examination should include particular attention to the lower esophageal area. A hematologic survey, including prothrombin time and platelet count, should be performed. To minimize risk of bleeding, manipulation during or after entry of the needle should be avoided. Caution is advised in patients whose spleen has recently become tender and palpable.

Following splenoportography, the patient should lie on his left side for several hours and should be closely observed for 24 hours for signs of internal bleeding.

Adverse Reactions: Internal bleeding is the most common serious complication of splenoportography. Although leakage of up to 300 ml of blood is apparently not uncommon, sometimes blood transfusions and, rarely, splenectomy, may be required to control hemorrhage. Peritoneal extravasation may cause transient diaphragmatic irritation or mild to moderate transient pain which may sometimes be referred to the shoulder, the periumbilical region, or other areas. Because of the proximity of the pleural cavity, accidental pneumothorax has been known to occur. Inadvertent injection of the medium into other nearby structures is not likely to cause untoward consequences.

Dosage and Administration: A preliminary small "pilot" dose is injected to confirm splenic entry, followed usually by rapid injection of 20 ml to 25 ml of HYPAQUE meglumine, brand of diatrizoate meglumine injection, 60 percent. Rapid serial exposures are started with the injection of the dose and continued until contrast is observed in the entire portal system.

ARTHROGRAPHY

Indications: Arthrography may be helpful in the diagnosis of posttraumatic or degenerative joint diseases, synovial rupture, the visualization of communicating bursae or cysts, and in meniscography. However, the technique is of little value unless the arthrograms are interpreted by well-trained personnel.

Contraindication: Arthrography is contraindicated when there is infection in or near the joint.

Precautions: See section on Precautions, General.

A strict, aseptic technique is required to avoid introducing infection.

Adverse Reactions: See section on Adverse Reactions, General.

Injection of HYPAQUE meglumine 60 percent into the joint usually causes immediate but transient discomfort. However, delayed, severe, or persistent pain may occur occasionally. Severe pain often results from undue use of pressure or the injection of large volumes. Joint swelling after injection is rare. Effusion, occasionally requiring aspiration, can occur in patients with rheumatoid arthritis.

Dosage and Administration: The procedure is usually performed with analgesic premedication and under local anesthesia. The amount of HYPAQUE meglumine 60 percent injected depends solely on the capacity of the joint. The damaged joint may require doses greatly exceeding those for normal joints. As much fluid as possible should first be aspirated from the joint; then, the medium should be injected gently to avoid overdistention of the joint capsule. Passive manipulation is sometimes used to disperse the medium in the joint. Sometimes, a 1 ml or 2 ml test dose is injected; immediate pain may indicate extravasation or extracapsular injection which, if confirmed by x-ray, requires relocation of the needle.

A single injection is usually adequate for multiple exposures. Contrast is good during the first 10 minutes after injection, adequate at 10 to 15 minutes, and begins to fade at 15 to 25 minutes.

The following approximate volumes have been used in normal adult joints:

Knee, shoulder, hip—5 ml to 15 ml
Temporomandibular—0.5 ml
Other—1 ml to 4 ml

"Double contrast arthrography," using a mixture of the medium and air or a dilution of HYPAQUE meglumine, brand of diatrizoate meglumine injection, 60 percent to a 30 percent concentration, has been employed.

DISCOGRAPHY

Indications: Cervical discography is a more hazardous procedure than lumbar discography, and the interpretation of the cervical discograms is more difficult.

The injected medium gradually diffuses throughout the disc and is absorbed rapidly. In a normal disc, good contrast is evident for 10 to 15 minutes. In a ruptured disc, the medium is absorbed more rapidly. Aspiration of the medium on completion of discography is considered unnecessary.

Continued on next page

This product information was effective as of November 19, 1982. On these and other products of Winthrop Laboratories, detailed information may be obtained on a current basis by direct inquiry to the Professional Services Department, 90 Park Avenue, New York, NY 10016 (212) 907-2525.

Winthrop—Cont.

Contraindications: Discography is contraindicated when there is infection or open injury near the region to be examined.
Warning: Inadvertent subarachnoid injection must be avoided since even the small dose of the medium used in discography might result in convulsions and death. The onset of signs of pain, cramps, or convulsions (requiring anesthesia) may occur within minutes to an hour.
Precautions: A strict, aseptic technique is required to avoid introducing infection. The examination should be postponed if local or systemic infection is present. In cervical discography, care should be taken to avoid contamination of the disc by inadvertent puncture of the esophagus. Laceration of the disc by use of a needle that has become barbed by forceful impingement on a vertebra, should be avoided. The patient should be cautioned not to move during introduction of the needle.
Adverse Reactions: In the normal disc, only minor discomfort will occur during injection. More discomfort will result if excessive pressure or volume is used. Pain is unusual and may indicate extravasation.
In the damaged disc, however, the injection can cause pain, sometimes severe, which mimics the symptoms. Transient backache or headache, as in lumbar puncture, often occurs. Extravasation from the disc into the lateral recesses and extradurally into the spinal canal or local soft tissue does not usually cause adverse effects.
Dosage and Administration: Discography is usually performed with parenteral analgesia or sedation, and under local anesthesia. To minimize disc and tissue trauma, a two-needle technique is usually employed. An 18 to 20 gauge needle is used to penetrate to the disc and then a very fine (25 or 26 gauge) lumbar puncture-type needle is inserted through the needle to penetrate the disc.
Because of the resistance encountered, it is difficult to inject more than 0.2 ml to 0.3 ml of HYPAQUE meglumine, brand of diatrizoate meglumine injection, 60 percent into a normal disc. Occasionally, however, a cervical disc can accept up to 0.5 ml and a lumbar disc, 1 ml (rarely, 2 ml) before resistance is encountered. Mild discomfort with little or no frank pain may indicate a normal disc.
In ruptured and some abnormal discs, 1 ml to 2 ml or more can be introduced without resistance; and, particularly if only one disc has pathology, the patient usually experiences pain, sometimes severe, with distribution characteristic of his symptoms. To minimize the amount of HYPAQUE extravasated, no more than 2 ml is injected in any one disc.
The procedure should be planned so that the duration of the discogram allows multiple exposures with a single dose. It has been recommended for diagnostic reasons that the procedure (injection and discogram) be performed on one disc at a time. Injection of a number of discs under suspicion, however, may be performed as part of one procedure.
How Supplied:
Vials of 20 ml, rubber stoppered, boxes of 25 (NDC 0024-0744-04).
Vials of 30 ml, rubber stoppered, boxes of 25 (NDC 0024-0745-04).
Vials of 50 ml, rubber stoppered, boxes of 25 (NDC 0024-0746-04).
Vials of 100 ml, rubber stoppered, boxes of 10 (NDC 0024-0747-02).
Boxes of 10 calibrated 200 ml dilution bottles with hanger containing 100 ml HYPAQUE meglumine 60%; rubber stoppered, with 10 intravenous infusion sets (NDC 0024-0748-02).
Boxes of 10 calibrated 200 ml dilution bottles with hanger containing 150 ml HYPAQUE meglumine 60%; rubber stoppered, with 10 intravenous infusion sets (NDC 0024-0749-01).
Boxes of 10 calibrated 200 ml dilution bottles with hanger containing 200 ml HYPAQUE meglumine 60%; rubber stoppered, (NDC 0024-0750-02).

HYPAQUE®-M, 75% ℞

brand of diatrizoate meglumine and diatrizoate sodium injection, USP
Sterile Aqueous Injection

A Radiopaque Medium for Angiocardiography, Aortography, Angiography, and Urography

Description: HYPAQUE-M, 75 per cent is a sterile aqueous solution containing 25 per cent (w/v) of the sodium salt and 50 per cent (w/v) of the meglumine salt of 3,5-diacetamido-2,4,6-triiodobenzoic acid. Each ml contains approximately 385 mg of organically-bound iodine and 0.39 mEq (or 9 mg) sodium per ml. The solution is hypertonic and has a viscosity of approximately 8.3 cps at 37 C. The final pH is adjusted between 6.5 and 7.7 with sodium hydroxide, or hydrochloric acid, or sodium carbonate. Edetate calcium disodium 1:10,000 has been added as a sequestering stabilizing agent. The solution may be autoclaved once. Discard any unused portion remaining in the container. It should be protected from strong light. At body temperature the solution is clear and colorless to pale straw color. Crystals may form in the solution on cooling; they are readily redissolved on warming; the solution, however, should be administered at body temperature.
Indications, General: HYPAQUE-M, 75 per cent is indicated for angiocardiography, aortography, angiography, and urography.
Contraindications, General: Do not use HYPAQUE-M, 75 per cent for myelography or for examination of dorsal cysts or sinuses which might communicate with the subarachnoid space. Injection of even a small amount into the subarachnoid space may produce convulsions and result in fatality. Epidural injection is also contraindicated. (See also Abdominal Aortography, Warnings.)
HYPAQUE-M, 75 per cent should not be injected directly into the carotid or vertebral arteries.
Warnings, General: Serious or fatal reactions have been associated with the administration of radiopaque media. It is of utmost importance that a course of action be carefully planned in advance for the immediate treatment of serious reactions, and that adequate and appropriate facilities and personnel be readily available in case a severe reaction occurs.
Selective spinal arteriography or arteriography of trunks providing spinal branches (usually the thyrocervical, costocervical, subclavian, vertebral, bronchial, intercostal) can cause mild to severe muscle spasm. However, serious neurologic sequelae, including permanent paralysis, could occur. Therefore, the advisability of using less concentrated solutions, as diatrizoate 50 per cent or 60 per cent solutions, should be considered although the complication has been reported with these lower concentrations.
Usage in Pregnancy. Safe use of HYPAQUE-M, 75 per cent during pregnancy has not been established. Therefore, before administration of the drug to women of childbearing potential, the benefit to the patient should be carefully weighed against the possible risk to the fetus. In addition, most authorities consider elective contrast radiography of the abdomen contraindicated during pregnancy.
Since intravascular administration of contrast media may promote sickling in patients who are homozygous for sickle cell disease, fluid restriction is not advised.
The results of PBI and RAI uptake studies, which depend on iodine estimations, will not reflect thyroid function for up to 16 days following administration of urographic media. However, function tests not depending on iodine estimations, eg, T_3 resin uptake or free thyroxine assays, are not affected.
Pheochromocytoma: Administer with caution. (See Abdominal Aortography, Warnings.)
Precautions, General: Before injecting a contrast medium, the patient should be questioned for a history of allergy. The intravenous injection of a test dose of 0.5 to 1 ml of the contrast agent before injection of the full dose has been employed in an attempt to predict severe or fatal adverse reactions. The preponderance of recent scientific literature, however, now demonstrates that this provocative test procedure is not reliably predictive of serious or fatal reactions. Severe reactions and fatalities have occurred with the test dose alone, with the full dose after a nonreactive test dose, and with or without a history of allergy. No conclusive relationship between severe or fatal reactions and antigen-antibody reactions or other manifestations of allergy has been established. A history of allergy may be useful in predicting reactions of a mild or intermediate nature. The drug should be used with great care in patients with advanced renal destruction associated with severe uremia.
Due to the transitory increase in circulatory osmotic load, HYPAQUE-M, brand of diatrizoate meglumine and diatrizoate sodium injection, 75 per cent should be used with caution in patients with congestive heart failure and such patients should be observed for several hours to detect delayed hemodynamic disturbances. In angiographic procedures dehydration of the patient is unnecessary and undesirable, especially if large doses of the medium are to be used.
Caution is advised in patients with severe cardiovascular disease, hyperthyroidism, extreme senility (but not old age *per se*), and in patients with a history of bronchial asthma or other allergic manifestations, or of sensitivity to iodine.
Adverse Reactions, General: Adverse effects are usually mild and transient and occur during or very shortly after injection. Some may be delayed for 15 to 20 minutes and occasionally, even hours. These reactions may be caused directly by the medium or by an abrupt hemodynamic change induced by the medium. During or immediately following injection, a facial flush or a feeling of body warmth, faintness, sweating, headache, chest tightness or pain, tingling of the lips, tongue, mouth, or extremities, and a metallic taste may occur and usually have little significance. Reactions attributable to allergy or idiosyncrasy have been sneezing, coughing, generalized urticaria or pruritus, angioneurotic edema, laryngospasm, bronchospasm, nasal stuffiness, rhinitis anxiety, dyspnea, and dizziness. Infrequently, immediate or delayed chills can occur, sometimes accompanied by hyperpyrexia. Rarely, disseminated intravascular coagulation has occurred. Serious reactions are more prone to occur in patients with severe congenital defects in whom hypoxia is present.
Cardiovascular Changes: These disturbances are usually mild and transitory but at times may proceed to heart failure or aggravate an existing failure. Peripheral vasodilatation is often evident as a feeling of warmth or flushing. Arrhythmias due to the medium or manipulation of the catheter may occur. They are usually mild and brief, although ventricular fibrillation and arrest have occurred. EKG changes may occur, particularly with good filling of the coronary arteries. Severe hypotension, coronary insufficiency, or rarely, shock and peripheral-vascular collapse have been reported. Red blood cell sludging and agglutin-

ation, crenation, and transitory (two- to three-hour) changes in coagulation mechanism may occur.

Complications due to technical factors include brachial plexus injury (usually transient), often due to injection technique (patient will complain of pain or paresthesia), extravasation of the medium, or prolonged incorrect placement of the arm. Hematomas, ecchymoses, and rarely atheromatous or other embolic phenomena can occur. Subcutaneous extravasation causes transitory stinging, chiefly because of the hypertonicity of the medium. If the volume is small, ill effects are very unlikely. However, if subcutaneous extravasation is extensive, especially in the foot, the physician should consider infiltration with Sterile Water for Injection, USP, or injection of spreading agents. Diffuse petechiae have been described and, in several instances, were traced to contamination of syringes, gloves with talc, or fine lint. Loss or weakness of pulse and fall in blood pressure in a catheterized artery may occur in about 5 per cent of patients and usually require no treatment. Intramural injection or pericardial placement (with tamponade, requiring pericardiocentesis) has occurred.

Urinary Response: Changes in renal function rarely occur, although diuresis and dehydration can follow large or repeated doses.

Nervous system disturbances may include mental confusion, visual or speech disturbances, vertigo, or rarely, convulsions.

Angiocardiography

Pharmacology—Hemodynamic Changes: Due to its physical characteristics (chiefly tonicity and viscosity) and the volume administered, HYPAQUE-M, brand of diatrizoate meglumine and diatrizoate sodium injection, 75 per cent may cause a number of transitory hemodynamic changes. When the medium is ejected from the left ventricle or introduced at the root of the ascending aorta, a brief (three seconds) hypertensive response is usually induced, followed immediately by a decrease in aortic and peripheral blood pressures below normal levels, lasting for at least two minutes. This hypotensive phase may be followed by a 15- to 20-minute period of fluctuating blood pressure.

Clinical doses (up to 1 ml per kg) injected into the vena cava or right heart outflow tract usually cause an irregular rise in right ventricular blood pressure, a slight increase in pulmonary artery blood pressure, and delayed signs of peripheral hypotension.

Other changes reported clinically include an increase in cardiac output and atrial pressure, a decrease in myocardial contractile force, and at the peak of postinjection hypotension, a marked rise in aortic and carotid blood flow, and elevation of central venous pressure. At dosage levels used in angiocardiography, the hematocrit and hemoglobin level may fall about 10 to 15 per cent and serum osmolality may rise 10 to 12 per cent. Blood carbon dioxide, pH, and BUN levels may fall. These changes commence immediately after injection, reach a maximum in two to five minutes, and return to normal values in 10 to 15 minutes. However, after the initial rise, plasma volume may decrease and continue to fall below control levels, even beyond 30 minutes, probably due to diuresis. If repeat injections are made in rapid succession, these changes are likely to be more pronounced. (See also Dosage and Administration.) HYPAQUE-M, 75 per cent is not metabolized. It is eliminated unchanged, rapidly and completely, in the urine by glomerular filtration.

Precautions: During administration of large doses of HYPAQUE-M, brand of diatrizoate meglumine and diatrizoate sodium injection, 75 per cent, continuous monitoring of vital signs is desirable. Caution is advised in the administration of large doses to patients with incipient heart failure because of the possibility of aggravation of the preexisting condition. Hypotension should be corrected promptly since it may induce serious arrhythmias.

Because of the hemodynamic changes which may occur on injection into the right heart outflow tract, special care, especially regarding dosage, should be observed in patients with right ventricular failure, pulmonary hypertension, or obliterated pulmonary vascular beds.

Precautions in Infants

Apnea, bradycardia and other arrhythmias, cerebral effects (lethargy and depression), and a tendency to acidosis are more likely to occur in cyanotic infants. It is desirable that vital signs be monitored on an intensive care basis afterwards to detect delayed adverse effects (arrhythmia, electrolyte and hemodynamic disturbances). Infants are more likely than adults to respond with convulsions, particularly after repeated injections. Unlike in the adult, the amount of the total dosage in young infants is of particular importance. (See Dosage and Administration.)

Adverse Reactions: See Adverse Reactions, General.

Dosage and Administration: The individual dose is determined by the size of the structure to be visualized, the anticipated degree of hemodilution, and valvular competence. Weight is a minor consideration in adults. The size of each individual dose is a more important consideration than the total dosage used. When large individual doses are administered, as for contrast in the cardiac chambers and thoracic aorta, it has been suggested that 20 minutes be permitted to elapse between each injection to allow for subsidence of hemodynamic disturbances.

Adult Dosage: Adult dose of HYPAQUE-M, 75 per cent is usually 35 to 50 ml into either left or right chamber, outflow tracts, or aorta. The individual dose for intravenous angiocardiography ranges from 70 to 100 ml often injected simultaneously bilaterally by pressure injection, half of the dose into each antecubital vein.

Pediatric Dosage: The usual dose is 0.5 to 1 ml per kg for a subject with heart of normal size and intact valves and septum. For patients with stenotic lesions, 0.5 ml per kg is recommended. Doses up to 1.5 ml per kg may be required in cardiomegaly, large volume shunts, or where right cardiac injection is also intended to opacify left chambers.

Young Infant Dosage: The individual dose is similar to that described under Pediatric Dosage. It has been suggested, however, that the total dosage administered should be maintained below 3 ml per kg in infants under two months of age in any one procedure.

ARTERIOGRAPHY

CORONARY ARTERIOGRAPHY

Coronary arteriography should only be used in carefully selected patients when the value of the anticipated information outweighs the risk involved.

Contraindication: Routine coronary arteriography should be deferred for four weeks in patients with clinically apparent myocardial infarction.

Precaution: Continuous EKG monitoring for early detection of arrhythmias is desirable.

Adverse Reactions: Transitory EKG changes occur almost inevitably with good filling. Transient arrhythmia may occur. (See also Adverse Reactions, General.) Serum enzymes may be elevated for 24 hours.

Dosage and Administration: The usual dose for adults is 50 ml of HYPAQUE-M, brand of diatrizoate meglumine and diatrizoate sodium injection, 75 per cent delivered into the **root of the aorta** for simultaneous bilateral angiograms. For injection at the **sinus of Valsalva**, the usual dose is 15 to 25 ml on either side. For **selective coronary procedures**, as by the Sones technique, the individual dose recommended is 3 to 5 ml into either artery. This dose may be injected alternately into the right and left coronary artery, and repeated.

ABDOMINAL AORTOGRAPHY

HYPAQUE-M, 75 per cent solution may be injected by commonly accepted techniques, such as translumbar, retrograde catheter, retrograde pressure injection (by cannula) or by antegrade (brachial) catheter for examination of the aorta and its major branches.

Warnings: During aortography by the translumbar technique, extreme care is advised to avoid inadvertent intrathecal injection since the injection of even small amounts (5 to 7 ml) of the contrast medium may cause convulsions, permanent sequelae, or fatality. Should the accident occur, the patient should be placed upright to confine the hyperbaric solution to a low level, anesthesia may be required to control convulsions, and if there is evidence of a large dose having been administered, a careful cerebrospinal fluid exchange-washout should be considered.

Pheochromocytoma: Administration of angiographic media to patients known or suspected to have pheochromocytoma can cause dangerous changes in blood pressure. A minimum dose should be injected. The blood pressure should be carefully monitored and measures for controlling major fluctuations should be available.

Precautions: The presence of a vigorous pulsatile flow should be established before using a catheter or pressure injection technique. A small "pilot" dose (about 2 ml) should be administered to locate the exact site of needle or catheter tip to help prevent injection of the main dose into a branch of the aorta or intramurally. In the translumbar technique, severe pain during injection may indicate intramural placement and abdominal or back pain afterwards may indicate hemorrhage from the injection site. Following catheter procedures, gentle pressure hemostasis for 5 to 10 minutes is advised, followed by observation for 30 to 60 minutes and immobilization of the limb for several hours to prevent hemorrhage from the site of arterial puncture.

Under conditions of slowed aortic circulation there is an increased likelihood of aortography causing muscle spasm. Occasional serious neurologic complications, including paraplegia, have also been reported in patients with aortic-iliac or even femoral artery bed obstruction, abdominal compression, hypotension, hypertension, spinal anesthesia, injection of vasopressors to increase contrast, and low injection sites (L2-3). In these patients the concentration, dose, and number of repeat injections of the medium should be maintained at a minimum with appropriate intervals between injections. The position of the patient and catheter tip should be carefully evaluated.

Adverse Reactions: The only adverse reaction expected is a mild burning sensation on injection. Unusual reactions can occur, as in angiocardiography. An abrupt hypertensive episode can occur following entry of the medium into the renal artery in patients with pheochromocytoma. Mesenteric necrosis, acute pancreatitis, and renal shutdown (usually transitory) and neurologic complications have been reported following inadvertent in-

Continued on next page

This product information was effective as of November 19, 1982. On these and other products of Winthrop Laboratories, detailed information may be obtained on a current basis by direct inquiry to the Professional Services Department, 90 Park Avenue, New York, NY 10016 (212) 907-2525.

Winthrop—Cont.

jection of a large part of the aortic dose into a branch of the aorta. Entry of the large aortic dose into the renal artery can cause, even in the absence of symptoms, albuminuria, cylindruria, and hematuria, and an elevated BUN. Rapid and complete return of function usually follows.

Dosage and Administration: The average adult dose range of HYPAQUE-M, brand of diatrizoate meglumine and diatrizoate sodium injection, 75 per cent is 10 to 15 ml by translumbar technique and by retrograde catheter, 15 to 25 ml. In infants and children and thin adults, the use of a less concentrated medium for aortography, such as diatrizoate sodium 50 per cent, is advised in doses of 0.5 ml per kg. For retrograde pressure injection (cannula) the usual adult dose is 35 to 40 ml of HYPAQUE-M, brand of diatrizoate meglumine and diatrizoate sodium injection, 75 per cent solution.

RENAL ARTERIOGRAPHY

Renal arteriography by aortography or by selective catheterization of the renal artery may be used to establish renal vascular status in the diagnosis of renal and immediate extrarenal pathology.

Precaution: In the selective renal procedure, inadvertent entry into a lumbar artery can be avoided by using a test dose.

Adverse Reactions: Transitory increase in resistance of the renovascular bed can occur with a slight disturbance in function. Renal damage is rare even in azotemic patients. Inadvertent entry of a large dose (as in aortography) into the renal artery can cause, even in the absence of symptoms, albuminuria, cylindruria, and hematuria, and an elevated BUN. Rapid and complete return of function usually follows.

Dosage and Administration: By aortography, 10 to 25 ml. By selective renal arteriography, 5 to 8 ml. The dose may be repeated as indicated.

PERIPHERAL ARTERIOGRAPHY

The use of HYPAQUE-M, 75 per cent is sometimes preferred over less concentrated media in selected cases for femoral and brachio-axillary arteriography in adults.

Precautions: Pulsation should be present in the artery to be injected. In thromboangiitis obliterans, or ascending infection associated with severe ischemia, angiography should be performed with extreme caution, if at all.

Adverse Reactions: Pain or a burning sensation with some spasm may occur, and is more marked in patients with arterial insufficiency. Therefore, the procedure is more satisfactorily performed under general or, for the lower extremity, spinal anesthesia.

Arterial thrombosis, displacement of arterial plaques, and ipsilateral venous thrombosis are very rare complications.

Dosage and Administration: The usual dose of HYPAQUE-M, 75 per cent is 10 to 25 ml, which may be repeated. Appropriate dosage in infants and children of a less concentrated medium, such as diatrizoate sodium 50 per cent, will usually provide adequate contrast.

UROGRAPHY

NEPHROTOMOGRAPHY AND "ADEQUATE" OR HIGH DOSE UROGRAPHY

HYPAQUE-M, 75 per cent solution may be used for excretory urography in selected patients. It may be used when prior urography has failed to provide diagnostic contrast and f... preliminary excretory tract study to detect ...ction in azotemic patients or to avoid ...de instrumentation. It may also be ... high dosage medium to intensify and ...he nephrographic effect when the prime purpose is examination of the renal parenchyma, especially with tomography. When combined with a urea "washout" technique, HYPAQUE-M, 75 per cent provides the necessary increased pyelographic contrast and diuresis required for screening or special examination of patients with suspected renal hypertension.

Contraindication: Urography is contraindicated in patients with anuria.

Precautions: Although azotemia is not considered a contraindication, care is required in patients with advanced renal failure. The usual preparatory dehydration should be omitted, and urinary output should be observed for one to two days in these patients.

Preparatory dehydration is dangerous in infants, young children, the elderly, and azotemic patients (especially those with polyuria, oliguria, diabetes, advanced vascular disease, or preexisting dehydration). The undesirable dehydration in these patients may be accentuated by the osmotic diuretic action of the medium.

When HYPAQUE-M, brand of diatrizoate meglumine and diatrizoate sodium injection, 75 per cent is used with a urea "washout" procedure, the patient should also be observed for a few hours to detect signs of undue dehydration caused by increased diuresis induced by both the medium and the urea. Ingestion of water may be required for rehydration.

In myelomatosis, urography should only be performed with caution. If a weak protein-binding agent such as a diatrizoate is used for the procedure, it is essential to omit preparatory dehydration, administer fluids, and attempt to alkalinize the urine.

Adverse Reactions: Side effects following this relatively high dose urography are usually mild and transitory and do not appear to occur more frequently or severely than those induced by "standard dose" urography. Nausea, facial flushing, and emesis are not uncommon reactions. (See also Adverse Reactions, General.)

Dosage and Administration: In adults, the single dose of HYPAQUE-M, 75 per cent is usually 50 ml. The dose in infants and children is 0.5 to 1 ml/kg (not to exceed 50 ml). It is injected rapidly intravenously.

How Supplied: HYPAQUE-M, 75 per cent is supplied in vials of 20 ml (NDC 0024-0785-04) and 50 ml (NDC 0024-0786-04), boxes of 25.

HYPAQUE®-76 ℞

brand of diatrizoate meglumine and diatrizoate sodium injection, USP
Sterile Aqueous Injection

For Excretory Urography, Aortography, Angiocardiography (Ventriculography, Pulmonary Angiography, Selective Coronary Arteriography), Peripheral Angiography (Peripheral Arteriography and Peripheral Venography), Intravenous Digital Arteriography, Selective Renal Arteriography, Selective Visceral Arteriography, Central Venography, Renal Venography.

Description: HYPAQUE-76 is a diagnostic radiopaque medium and is supplied as a 76 percent sterile aqueous solution providing 66 percent (w/v) diatrizoate meglumine and 10 percent (w/v) diatrizoate sodium. Each ml contains approximately 370 mg iodine and 0.16 mEq (3.68 mg) sodium. The solution is hypertonic and has a viscosity of approximately 9 cps at 37 C. The pH is adjusted between 7.0 and 7.6 with Na_2CO_3 and HCl or NaOH. Edetate calcium disodium 0.01 percent has been added as a sequestering stabilizing agent. The solution is clear and colorless to pale straw color. The solution may be autoclaved once. Discard any unused portion remaining in the container. The solution should be stored at room temperature and protected from strong light. Crystals may form in the solution on cooling; they are readily redissolved on warming; the solution, however, should be administered at body temperature.

Diatrizoate meglumine is 1-deoxy-1-(methylamino)-D-glucitol 3, 5-diacetamido-2, 4, 6-triiodobenzoate (salt).

Diatrizoate sodium is monosodium 3,5-diacetamido-2,4,6-triiodobenzoate.

Clinical Pharmacology, General: Following intravascular injection, HYPAQUE-76 is rapidly transported through the bloodstream to the kidneys and is excreted unchanged in the urine by glomerular filtration. When urinary tract obstruction is severe enough to block glomerular filtration, the agent appears to be excreted by the tubular epithelium.

Renal accumulation is sufficiently rapid that the period of maximal opacification of the renal passages may begin as early as five minutes after injection. In infants and small children excretion takes place somewhat more promptly than in adults, so that maximal opacification occurs more rapidly and is less sustained. The normal kidney eliminates the contrast medium almost immediately. In nephropathic conditions, particularly when excretory capacity has been altered, the rate of excretion varies unpredictably, and opacification may be delayed for 30 minutes or more after injection; with severe impairment opacification may not occur. Generally, however, the medium is concentrated in sufficient amounts and promptly enough to permit a thorough evaluation of the anatomy and physiology of the urinary tract. While circulating in tissue fluids, the compound remains ionized. However, it is not metabolized but excreted unchanged in the urine, each diatrizoate molecule remaining "obligated" to its sodium or meglumine moiety.

In patients with normal kidneys, a nephrogram, in the vascular phase, becomes apparent in 30 to 60 seconds, followed by an excretory phase. Urograms become apparent in about 2 minutes, with optimum contrast starting in 5 minutes. (See also Pharmacology-Hemodynamic Changes in section on ANGIOCARDIOGRAPHY.)

Indications and Usage, General:

HYPAQUE-76 is indicated for excretory urography, aortography, angiocardiography (ventriculography, pulmonary angiography, selective coronary arteriography), peripheral angiography (peripheral arteriography and peripheral venography), intravenous digital arteriography, selective renal arteriography, selective visceral arteriography, central venography, and renal venography.

Contraindications, General: Do not use HYPAQUE-76 for myelography or for examination of dorsal cysts or sinuses which might communicate with the subarachnoid space.

Injection of even a small amount into the subarachnoid space may produce convulsions and result in fatality. Epidural injection is also contraindicated. (See also Aortography, Warnings.)

HYPAQUE-76 should not be injected directly into the carotid or vertebral arteries.

HYPAQUE-76 is contraindicated in patients with a hypersensitivity to salts of diatrizoic acid.

Urography is contraindicated in patients with anuria.

Warnings, General: Serious or fatal reactions have been associated with the administration of radiopaque media. It is of utmost importance that a course of action be carefully planned in advance for the immediate treatment of serious reactions, and that adequate and appropriate facilities and personnel be readily available in case a severe reaction occurs. (See also Adverse Reactions, General.)

Selective spinal arteriography or arteriography of trunks providing spinal branches (usually the thyrocervical, costocervical, subclavian, vertebral, bronchial, intercostal) can cause mild to severe muscle spasm. However, serious neurologic sequelae, including permanent paralysis, could occur. Therefore, the advisability of using less concentrated solutions, as diatrizoate 50 per cent or 60 per cent solutions, should be considered although the complication has been reported with these lower concentrations.

Since intravascular administration of contrast media may promote sickling in patients who are homozygous for sickle cell disease, fluid restriction is not advised.

Pheochromocytoma: Administer with caution. (See Aortography, Warnings.)

Myelomatosis: A definite risk exists in the use of intravascular contrast agents in patients who are known to have multiple myeloma. In such instances there has been anuria resulting in progressive uremia, renal failure, and eventually death. Although neither the contrast agent nor dehydration has separately proved to be the cause of anuria in myeloma, it has been speculated that the combination of both may be the causative factor. The risk in myelomatous patients is not a contraindication to the procedures; however, partial dehydration in the preparation of these patients for the examination is not recommended since this may predispose to the precipitation of myeloma protein in the renal tubules. No form of therapy, including dialysis, has been successful in reversing this effect. Myeloma, which occurs most commonly in persons over age 40, should be considered before intravascular administration of a contrast agent. (See also Excretory Urography, Precautions.)

Cyanotic Infants: See Angiocardiography, Precautions.

Hepatorenal Disease: See Excretory Urography, Precautions.

Precautions, General: Before injecting a contrast medium, the patient should be questioned for a history of allergy. The intravenous injection of a test dose of 0.5 ml to 1 ml of the contrast agent before injection of the full dose has been employed in an attempt to predict severe or fatal adverse reactions. The preponderance of recent scientific literature, however, now demonstrates that this provocative test procedure is not reliably predictive of serious or fatal reactions. Severe reactions and fatalities have occurred with the test dose alone, with the full dose after a nonreactive test dose, and with or without a history of allergy. No conclusive relationship between severe or fatal reactions and antigen-antibody reactions or other manifestations of allergy has been established. A history of allergy may be useful in predicting reactions of a mild or intermediate nature. However, a history of sensitivity to iodine per se or to other contrast agents is not an absolute contraindication to the use of diatrizoate, but calls for extreme caution in administration. Although azotemia is not a contraindication, the medium should be used with great care in patients with advanced renal destruction associated with severe uremia. (See also Excretory Urography, Precautions.)

Due to the transitory increase in circulatory osmotic load, HYPAQUE-76 should be used with caution in patients with congestive heart failure. Blood pressure should be monitored and patients observed for several hours to detect delayed hemodynamic disturbances.

In angiographic procedures dehydration of the patient is unnecessary and undesirable, especially if large doses of the medium are to be used.

Caution is advised in patients with severe cardiovascular disease, hyperthyroidism, extreme senility (but not old age per se), and in patients with a history of bronchial asthma or other allergic manifestations, or of sensitivity to iodine.

Renal toxicity has been reported in a few patients with liver dysfunction who were given oral cholecystographic agents followed by urographic agents. Administration of HYPAQUE-76, brand of diatrizoate meglumine and diatrizoate sodium injection, should therefore be postponed in any patient with a known or suspected hepatic or biliary disorder who has recently taken a cholecystographic contrast agent.

Caution should be exercised with the use of radiopaque media in severely debilitated patients and in those with marked hypertension. The possibility of thrombosis should be borne in mind when percutaneous techniques are employed.

Repeat doses: The size of each individual dose is a more important consideration than the total dosage used. However, each repeat dose may be an additional hazard. When large individual doses are administered, as in the cardiac chambers and thoracic aorta, it has been suggested that an adequate time be permitted to elapse between each injection to allow for subsidence of hemodynamic disturbances.

Drug Interactions—Benadryl®, brand of diphenhydramine hydrochloride, may cause precipitation when mixed in the same syringe with HYPAQUE-76.

Drug/Laboratory Test Interactions—The results of PBI and RAI uptake studies, which depend on iodine estimations, will not reflect thyroid function for up to 16 days following administration of urographic media. However, function tests not depending on iodine estimations, eg, T_3 resin uptake or free thyroxine assays, are not affected.

Contrast agents may interfere with some physical and chemical determinations made on urine specimens; therefore, urine should be collected before administration of the contrast medium or two or more days afterwards.

Carcinogenesis, Mutagenesis, Impairment of Fertility: No long-term animal studies have been performed to evaluate the potential of diatrizoate meglumine or diatrizoate sodium in these areas.

Pregnancy Category C. Animal reproduction studies have not been conducted with HYPAQUE-76. It is also not known whether HYPAQUE-76 can cause fetal harm when administered to a pregnant woman or can affect reproduction capacity. HYPAQUE-76 should be given to a pregnant woman only if clearly needed.

Nursing Mothers. It is not known whether this drug is excreted in human milk. Because many drugs are excreted in human milk, caution should be exercised when HYPAQUE-76 is administered to a nursing woman.

Pediatric Use. See specific Dosage and Administration section under individual Indications and Usage sections.

Adverse Reactions, General: Reactions accompanying the use of contrast media may vary directly with the concentration of the substance, the amount used, the technique used, and the underlying pathology. Most reactions occur during, or in the first five minutes after injection. Therefore, a physician should be immediately available and the patient constantly observed during this time. It is also advised that a physician be generally available for at least the next 30 minutes.

The following have been reported after administration of diatrizoates and other iodinated contrast media. *Reactions due to technique:* hematomas and ecchymoses. *Hemodynamic reactions:* vein cramp and thrombophlebitis following intravenous injection. *Cardiovascular reactions:* rare cases of cardiac arrhythmias, reflex tachycardia, chest pain, cyanosis, hypertension, hypotension, peripheral vasodilatation, shock, and cardiac arrest. *Renal reactions:* occasionally, transient proteinuria, and rarely, oliguria or anuria. *Allergic reactions:* asthmatic attacks, nasal and conjunctival symptoms, dermal reactions such as urticaria with or without pruritus, as well as pleomorphic rashes, sneezing and lacrimation, and rarely anaphylactic reactions. Rare fatalities have occurred, due to this or unknown causes. Signs and symptoms related to the *respiratory system:* pulmonary or laryngeal edema, bronchospasm, dyspnea; or to the *nervous system:* restlessness, tremors, convulsions. *Other reactions:* flushing, pain, warmth, metallic taste, nausea, vomiting, anxiety, headache, confusion, pallor, weakness, sweating, localized areas of edema, especially facial cramps, neutropenia, and dizziness. Rarely, immediate or delayed rigors can occur, sometimes accompanied by hyperpyrexia. Infrequently, "iodism" (salivary gland swelling) from organic iodinated compounds appears two days after exposure and subsides by the sixth day.

Subcutaneous extravasation, chiefly because of hypertonicity of the medium, causes transitory stinging. If the volume is small, ill effects are very unlikely. However, if subcutaneous extravasation is extensive, especially in the foot, the physician should consider infiltration with Sterile Water for Injection, USP, or injection of spreading agents.

Diffuse petechiae have been described and, in several instances, were traced to contamination of syringes, gloves with talc, or fine lint.

Additional warnings, precautions, and directions are included in the following sections on special procedures.

Overdosage: At dosage levels of 1 ml/lb, the incidence of unpleasant side effects increases. At total dosage of 2 ml/lb, administered over a short period of time (eg, 30 minutes), clinical signs of systemic intolerance appear (mostly related to hyperosmolar effects) and are manifest as tremors, irritability, and tachycardia. Acute intravenous LD_{50} in mice is about 12,000 mg/kg.

The diatrizoates are dialyzable.

Dosage and Administration, General: See specific individual Indications and Usage sections.

Parenteral drug products should be inspected visually for particulate matter and discoloration prior to administration, whenever solution and container permit.

Individual Indications and Usage:

EXCRETORY UROGRAPHY

Nephrotomography and "Adequate" or High Dose Urography

HYPAQUE-76 solution may be used for excretory urography in selected patients. It may be used when prior urography has failed to provide diagnostic contrast and for preliminary excretory tract study to detect obstruction in azotemic patients or to avoid retrograde instrumentation. It may also be used as a high dosage medium to intensify and prolong the nephrographic effect when the prime purpose is examination of the renal parenchyma, especially with tomography. When combined with the urea "washout" technique, HYPAQUE-76 provides the necessary increased pyelographic contrast and diuresis required for screening or special examination of patients with suspected renal hypertension.

Contraindication: Urography is contraindicated in patients with anuria.

Precautions: Although azotemia is not considered a contraindication, care is required in patients with advanced renal failure. The usual preparatory dehydration should be omitted, and urinary output should be observed for one to two days in these patients. Adequate visualization may be difficult or impossible to attain in patients with severely impaired renal and/or hepatic function. Use with extreme caution in patients with concomitant hepatore-

Continued on next page

This product information was effective as of November 19, 1982. On these and other products of Winthrop Laboratories, detailed information may be obtained on a current basis by direct inquiry to the Professional Services Department, 90 Park Avenue, New York, NY 10016 (212) 907-2525.

Winthrop—Cont.

nal disease. Preparatory dehydration is dangerous in infants, young children, the elderly, and azotemic patients (especially those with polyuria, oliguria, diabetes, advanced vascular disease, or preexisting dehydration). The undesirable dehydration in these patients may be accentuated by the osmotic diuretic action of the medium.

When HYPAQUE-76, brand of diatrizoate meglumine and diatrizoate sodium injection, is used with a urea "washout" procedure, the patient should also be observed for a few hours to detect signs of undue dehydration caused by increased diuresis induced by both the medium and the urea. Ingestion of water may be required for rehydration.

In myelomatosis, urography should only be performed with caution. If a weak protein-binding agent such as a diatrizoate is used for the procedure, it is essential to omit preparatory dehydration, administer fluids, and attempt to alkalinize the urine.

Adverse Reactions: Side effects following this relatively high dose urography are usually mild and transitory and do not appear to occur more frequently or severely than those induced by "standard dose" urography. Nausea, facial flushing, and emesis are not uncommon reactions. (See also Adverse Reactions, General.)

Dosage and Administration: The usual intravenous dose for adults is 50 ml, with a range of 40 ml to 100 ml. Children require less in proportion to weight: Under 6 months of age—4 ml; 6 to 12 months—6 ml; 1 to 2 years—8 ml; 2 to 5 years—10 ml; 5 to 7 years—12 ml; 8 to 10 years—14 ml; 11 to 15 years—16 ml.

AORTOGRAPHY

HYPAQUE-76, brand of diatrizoate meglumine and diatrizoate sodium injection, solution may be injected by commonly accepted techniques, such as translumbar, retrograde catheter, retrograde pressure injection (by cannula) or by antegrade (brachial) catheter for examination of the aorta and its major branches.

Warnings: During aortography by the translumbar technique, extreme care is advised to avoid inadvertent intrathecal injection since the injection of even small amounts (5 ml to 7 ml) of the contrast medium may cause convulsions, permanent sequelae, or fatality. Should the accident occur, the patient should be placed upright to confine the hyperbaric solution to a low level, anesthesia may be required to control convulsions, and if there is evidence of a large dose having been administered, a careful cerebrospinal fluid exchange-washout should be considered.

Pheochromocytoma: Administration of angiographic media to patients known or suspected to have pheochromocytoma can cause dangerous changes in blood pressure. A minimum dose should be injected. The blood pressure should be carefully monitored and measures for controlling major fluctuations should be available.

Precautions: The presence of a vigorous pulsatile flow should be established before using a catheter or pressure injection technique. A small "pilot" dose (about 2 ml) should be administered to locate the exact site of needle or catheter tip to help prevent injection of the main dose into a branch of the aorta or intramurally. In the translumbar technique, severe pain during injection may indicate intramural placement and abdominal or back pain afterwards may indicate hemorrhage from the injection site. Following catheter procedures, gentle pressure hemostasis for 5 to 10 minutes is advised, followed by observation for 30 to 60 minutes and immobilization of the limb for several hours to prevent hemorrhage from the site of arterial puncture.

Under conditions of *slowed aortic circulation* there is an increased likelihood of aortography causing muscle spasm. Occasional serious neurologic complications, including paraplegia, have also been reported in patients with aortic-iliac or even femoral artery bed obstruction, abdominal compression, hypotension, hypertension, spinal anesthesia, injection of vasopressors to increase contrast, and low injection sites (L2–3). In these patients the concentration, dose, and number of repeat injections of the medium should be maintained at a minimum with appropriate intervals between injections. The position of the patient and catheter tip should be carefully evaluated.

Adverse Reactions: The only adverse reaction expected is a mild burning or painful sensation on injection. Unusual reactions can occur, as in angiocardiography. An abrupt hypertensive episode can occur following entry of the medium into the renal artery in patients with pheochromocytoma. Mesenteric necrosis, acute pancreatitis, and renal shutdown (usually transitory) and neurologic complications have been reported following inadvertent injection of a large part of the aortic dose into a branch of the aorta. Entry of the large aortic dose into the renal artery can cause, even in the absence of symptoms, albuminuria, cylindruria, and hematuria, and an elevated BUN. Rapid and complete return of function usually follows.

Additional procedural reactions include injury to the aorta and neighboring organs, pleural puncture, renal damage including infarction and acute tubular necrosis with oliguria and anuria, accidental selective filling of the right renal artery during the translumbar procedure in the presence of preexistent renal disease, retroperitoneal hemorrhage from the translumbar approach.

Dosage and Administration: *Adult:* The usual adult dose as a single injection is 40 ml to 50 ml, repeated if indicated, to a total of 160 ml.

Pediatric: The usual single dose ranges from 0.3 ml/kg to 0.9 ml/kg. The total dose should not exceed 1 ml/kg.

ANGIOCARDIOGRAPHY

Pharmacology-Hemodynamic Changes

Due to its physical characteristics (chiefly tonicity and viscosity) and the volume administered, HYPAQUE-76 may cause a number of transitory hemodynamic changes. When the medium is ejected from the left ventricle or introduced at the root of the ascending aorta, a brief (three seconds) hypertensive response is usually induced, followed immediately by a decrease in aortic and peripheral blood pressures below normal levels, lasting for at least two minutes. This hypotensive phase may be followed by a 15- to 20-minute period of fluctuating blood pressure.

Clinical doses (up to 1 ml per kg) injected into the vena cava or right heart outflow tract usually cause an irregular rise in right ventricular blood pressure, a slight increase in pulmonary artery blood pressure, and delayed signs of peripheral hypotension.

Other changes reported clinically include an increase in cardiac output and atrial pressure, a decrease in myocardial contractile force, and at the peak of postinjection hypotension, a marked rise in aortic and carotid blood flow, and elevation of central venous pressure. At dosage levels used in angiocardiography, the hematocrit and hemoglobin level may fall about 10 to 15 percent and serum osmolality may rise 10 to 12 percent. Blood carbon dioxide, pH, and BUN levels may fall. These changes commence immediately after injection, reach a maximum in two to five minutes, and return to normal values in 10 to 15 minutes. However, after the initial rise, plasma volume may decrease and continue to fall below control levels, even beyond 30 minutes, probably due to diuresis. If repeat injections are made in rapid succession these changes are likely to be more pronounced. (See also Dosage and Administration.) HYPAQUE-76 is not metabolized. It is eliminated unchanged, rapidly and completely, in the urine by glomerular filtration.

Precautions: During administration of large doses of HYPAQUE-76, brand of diatrizoate meglumine and diatrizoate sodium injection, continuous monitoring of vital signs is desirable. Caution is advised in the administration of large doses to patients with incipient heart failure because of the possibility of aggravation of the preexisting condition. Hypotension should be corrected promptly since it may induce serious arrhythmias.

Because of the hemodynamic changes which may occur on injection into the right heart outflow tract, special care, especially regarding dosage, should be observed in patients with right ventricular failure, pulmonary hypertension, or obliterated pulmonary vascular beds.

Precautions in Infants

Apnea, bradycardia and other arrhythmias, cerebral effects (lethargy and depression), and a tendency to acidosis are more likely to occur in cyanotic infants. It is desirable that vital signs be monitored on an intensive care basis afterwards to detect delayed adverse effects (arrhythmia, electrolyte and hemodynamic disturbances). Infants are more likely than adults to respond with convulsions, particularly after repeated injections. Unlike in the adult, the amount of the total dosage in young infants is of particular importance. (See Dosage and Administration.)

Adverse Reactions: See Adverse Reactions, General.

Dosage and Administration: The individual dose is determined by the size of the structure to be visualized, the anticipated degree of hemodilution, and valvular competence. Weight is a minor consideration in adults. The size of each individual dose is a more important consideration than the total dosage used. When large individual doses are administered, as for contrast in the cardiac chambers and thoracic aorta, it has been suggested that 20 minutes be permitted to elapse between each injection to allow for subsidence of hemodynamic disturbances.

Ventriculography

Adult: The usual adult dose in a single injection is 45 ml, with a range of 40 ml to 50 ml. This may be repeated as necessary. However, when combined with selective coronary arteriography, the total dose should not exceed 225 ml.

Pediatric: The usual single dose is 0.2 ml/kg to 0.3 ml/kg. The total dose should not exceed 50 ml.

Pulmonary Angiography or Arch Study Used Alone

Adult: The usual single adult dose is 30 ml, with a range of 10 ml to 56 ml.

Pediatric: The dose ranges from 0.3 ml/kg to 0.9 ml/kg. The total dose should not exceed 1 ml/kg.

Combined Angiocardiographic Procedures Multiple Procedures

With continuing advances in radiologic techniques and the development of more sophisticated equipment as well as more versatile and reliable radiopaque media, it is possible to examine multiple vascular systems and target organs during a single radiographic examination of the patient.

Multiple procedures of selective angiography require multiple injections of the contrast medium into several specific target organs and result in a greater dosage. Large doses of HYPAQUE-76 were well tolerated in multiple injections and multiple procedures of angiography.

See general sections for Contraindications, Warnings, Precautions, Adverse Reactions, and Dosage and Administration recommendations as well as those sections pertinent to the specific procedures.

Adult: The maximum total dose for multiple procedures should not exceed 225 ml.

Pediatric: When multiple procedures are required in pediatric use, the total dose administered should be maintained below 4 ml/kg, or especially in young infants below 3 ml/kg.

Selective Coronary Arteriography

Adult: The usual adult dose for right or left coronary arteriography is 8 ml (range 4 ml to 10 ml) repeated as required up to a total dose of 120 ml for coronary arteriography alone.

PERIPHERAL ANGIOGRAPHY

The use of HYPAQUE-76, brand of diatrizoate meglumine and diatrizoate sodium injection, is sometimes preferred over less concentrated media in selected cases for femoral and brachio-axillary arteriography in adults.

Precautions: Pulsation should be present in the artery to be injected. In thromboangiitis obliterans, or ascending infection associated with severe ischemia, angiography should be performed with extreme caution, if at all.

Adverse Reactions: Pain or a burning sensation with some spasm may occur, and is more marked in patients with arterial insufficiency. Therefore, the procedure is more satisfactorily performed under general or, for the lower extremity, spinal anesthesia.

Technical complications have included hemorrhage from the puncture site, and brachial plexus palsy following axillary artery injections.

Arterial thrombosis, displacement of arterial plaques, and ipsilateral venous thrombosis are very rare complications.

Dosage and Administration

Arteriography (aorto-iliac runoff and peripheral)

Adult: The single adult dose for femoral arteriography varies from 20 ml to 60 ml, depending on the site of placement, ie, aorto-iliac runoff, iliofemoral, femoral. For the upper limb, 20 ml to 40 ml is usually sufficient. These doses may be repeated up to three times.

VENOGRAPHY

Dosage and Administration

Central Venography: *Adult:* For central venography (inferior or superior vena cava), the total adult dose is 40 ml to 50 ml, repeated up to two times.

Renal Venography: *Adult:* The usual adult dose is 20 ml to 40 ml.

Peripheral Venography: *Adult:* The usual single adult dose is 40 ml, with a range of 40 ml to 60 ml.

SELECTIVE RENAL ARTERIOGRAPHY

Dosage and Administration: *Adult:* The usual adult dose is 8 ml, repeated up to three times. The dose ranges from 5 ml to 10 ml.

SELECTIVE VISCERAL ARTERIOGRAPHY

Dosage and Administration

Celiac Axis: The usual adult dose ranges from 30 ml to 40 ml with subselective arteriography of its branches, eg, hepatic, usual dose of 25 ml with a range of 15 ml to 30 ml; mesenteric, usual dose of 30 ml with a range of 20 ml to 40 ml; splenic, usual dose of 20 ml with a range of 20 ml to 50 ml.

Superior Mesenteric: The usual adult dose is 30 ml with a range of 20 ml to 40 ml.

The maximum total dose should not exceed 175 ml.

INTRAVENOUS DIGITAL ARTERIOGRAPHY

Arteriograms of diagnostic quality can be obtained following the intravenous administration of HYPAQUE-76 employing digital subtraction and computer imaging enhancement equipment. The intravenous route of administration using these techniques has the advantage of being less invasive than the corresponding selective catheter placement of the medium. The dose is administered into a peripheral vein usually by mechanical injection although sometimes by rapid manual injection. The technique has been used most frequently to visualize the ventricles, the aorta and most of its larger branches including carotid, cerebral, vertebral, renal, celiac, mesenterics, and the major peripheral vessels of the limbs.

Precautions: Since the dose is usually administered mechanically under high pressure, rupture of smaller peripheral veins has occurred. It has been suggested that this can be avoided by using an intravenous catheter threaded proximally beyond larger tributaries or in the case of the antecubital vein, into the superior vena cava. Sometimes the femoral vein is used.

Dosage and Administration: The usual dose of HYPAQUE-76 per injection by the intravenous digital technique is 30 ml to 60 ml with a range of 0.5 ml/kg to 1 ml/kg administered as a bolus 7.5 ml/second to 30 ml/second using a pressure injector. The dose and rate of injection will depend primarily on the type of equipment and technique used, with first exposures made on calculated circulation time.

How Supplied: Vials of 30 ml, rubber stoppered, boxes of 25 (NDC 0024-0775-04)

Vials of 50 ml, rubber stoppered, boxes of 25 (NDC 0024-0776-04)

Vials of 100 ml, rubber stoppered, boxes of 10 (NDC 0024-0777-02)

Calibrated bottles of 200 ml, rubber stoppered, boxes of 10 (NDC 0024-0778-02)

Calibrated 200 ml dilution bottles with hanger containing 100 ml HYPAQUE-76; rubber stoppered, boxes of 10 (NDC 0024-0779-02)

HYPAQUE®-M, 90% ℞

brand of diatrizoate meglumine and diatrizoate sodium injection, USP
Sterile Aqueous Injection

A Radiopaque Medium for Angiocardiography, Aortography, Angiography, Urography, and Hysterosalpingography

Description: HYPAQUE-M, 90 per cent is a sterile aqueous solution containing 30 per cent (w/v) of the sodium salt and 60 per cent (w/v) of the meglumine salt of 3,5-diacetamido-2,4,6-triiodobenzoic acid. Each ml contains approximately 462 mg of organically-bound iodine and 0.47 mEq (or 10.9 mg) sodium. The solution is hypertonic and has a viscosity of approximately 18.7 cps at 37 C. The final pH is adjusted between 6.5 and 7.7 with sodium hydroxide, or hydrochloric acid, or sodium carbonate. Edetate calcium disodium 1:10,000 has been added as a sequestering stabilizing agent. The solution may be autoclaved once. Discard any unused portion remaining in the container. It should be protected from strong light. At body temperature the solution is clear and colorless to pale straw color. Crystals may form in the solution on cooling; they are readily redissolved on warming; the solution, however, should be administered at body temperature.

Indications, General: HYPAQUE-M, 90 per cent is indicated for angiocardiography, aortography, angiography, urography, and hysterosalpingography.

Contraindications, General: Do not use HYPAQUE-M, 90 per cent for myelography or for examination of dorsal cysts or sinuses which might communicate with the subarachnoid space. Injection of even a small amount into the subarachnoid space may produce convulsions and result in fatality. Epidural injection is also contraindicated. (See also Abdominal Aortography, Warnings.)

HYPAQUE-M, 90 per cent should not be injected directly into the carotid or vertebral arteries.

Warnings, General: Serious or fatal reactions have been associated with the administration of radiopaque media. It is of utmost importance that a course of action be carefully planned in advance for the immediate treatment of serious reactions, and that adequate and appropriate facilities and personnel be readily available in case a severe reaction occurs.

Selective spinal arteriography or arteriography of trunks providing spinal branches (usually the thyrocervical, costocervical, subclavian, vertebral, bronchial, intercostal) can cause mild to severe muscle spasm. However, serious neurologic sequelae, including permanent paralysis, could occur. Therefore, the advisability of using less concentrated solutions, as diatrizoate 50 per cent or 60 per cent solutions, should be considered although the complication has been reported with these lower concentrations.

Usage in Pregnancy. Safe use of HYPAQUE-M, 90 per cent during pregnancy has not been established. Therefore, before administration of the drug to women of childbearing potential, the benefit to the patient should be carefully weighed against the possible risk to the fetus. In addition, most authorities consider elective contrast radiography of the abdomen contraindicated during pregnancy.

Since intravascular administration of contrast media may promote sickling in patients who are homozygous for sickle cell disease, fluid restriction is not advised.

The results of PBI and RAI uptake studies, which depend on iodine estimations, will not reflect thyroid function for up to 16 days following administration of urographic media. However, function tests not depending on iodine estimations, eg, T_3 resin uptake or free thyroxine assays, are not affected.

Pheochromocytoma: Administer with caution. (See Abdominal Aortography, Warnings.)

Precautions, General: Before injecting a contrast medium, the patient should be questioned for a history of allergy. The intravenous injection of a test dose of 0.5 to 1 ml of the contrast agent before injection of the full dose has been employed in an attempt to predict severe or fatal adverse reactions. The preponderance of recent scientific literature, however, now demonstrates that this provocative test procedure is not reliably predictive of serious or fatal reactions. Severe reactions and fatalities have occurred with the test dose alone, with the full dose after a nonreactive test dose, and with or without a history of allergy. No conclusive relationship between severe or fatal reactions and antigen-antibody reactions or other manifestations of allergy has been established. A history of allergy may be useful in predicting reactions of a mild or intermediate nature. The drug should be used with great care in patients with advanced renal destruction associated with severe uremia.

Due to the transitory increase in circulatory osmotic load, HYPAQUE-M, brand of diatrizoate meglumine and diatrizoate sodium injection, 90 per cent should be used with caution in patients with congestive heart failure and such patients should be observed for several hours to detect delayed hemodynamic disturbances.

In angiographic procedures dehydration of the patient is unnecessary and undesirable, especially if large doses of the medium are to be used.

Caution is advised in patients with severe cardiovascular disease, hyperthyroidism, extreme senility (but not old age *per se*), and in patients with a history of bronchial asthma or other

Continued on next page

This product information was effective as of November 19, 1982. On these and other products of Winthrop Laboratories, detailed information may be obtained on a current basis by direct inquiry to the Professional Services Department, 90 Park Avenue, New York, NY 10016 (212) 907-2525.

Winthrop—Cont.

allergic manifestations, or of sensitivity to iodine.

Adverse Reactions, General: Adverse effects are usually mild and transient and occur during or very shortly after injection. Some may be delayed for 15 to 20 minutes and occasionally, even hours. These reactions may be caused directly by the medium or by an abrupt hemodynamic change induced by the medium. During or immediately following injection, a facial flush or a feeling of body warmth, faintness, sweating, headache, chest tightness or pain, tingling of the lips, tongue, mouth, or extremities, and a metallic taste may occur and usually have little significance. Reactions attributable to allergy or idiosyncrasy have been sneezing, coughing, generalized urticaria or pruritus, angioneurotic edema, laryngospasm, bronchospasm, nasal stuffiness, rhinitis, anxiety, dyspnea, and dizziness. Infrequently, immediate or delayed chills can occur, sometimes accompanied by hyperpyrexia. Rarely, disseminated intravascular coagulation has occurred. Serious reactions are more prone to occur in patients with severe congenital defects in whom hypoxia is present.

Cardiovascular Changes: These disturbances are usually mild and transitory but at times may proceed to heart failure or aggravate an existing failure. Peripheral vasodilatation is often evident as a feeling of warmth or flushing. Arrhythmias due to the medium or manipulation of the catheter may occur. They are usually mild and brief, although ventricular fibrillation and arrest have occurred. EKG changes may occur, particularly with good filling of the coronary arteries. Severe hypotension, coronary insufficiency, or rarely, shock and peripheral-vascular collapse have been reported. Red blood cell sludging and agglutination, crenation, and transitory (two- to three-hour) changes in coagulation mechanism may occur.

Complications due to technical factors include brachial plexus injury (usually transient), often due to injection technique (patient will complain of pain or paresthesia), extravasation of the medium, or prolonged incorrect placement of the arm. Hematomas, ecchymoses, and rarely atheromatous or other embolic phenomena can occur. Subcutaneous extravasation causes transitory stinging, chiefly because of the hypertonicity of the medium. If the volume is small, ill effects are very unlikely. However, if subcutaneous extravasation is extensive, especially in the foot, the physician should consider infiltration with Sterile Water for Injection, USP, or injection of spreading agents. Diffuse petechiae have been described and, in several instances, were traced to contamination of syringes, gloves with talc, or fine lint. Loss or weakness of pulse and fall in blood pressure in a catheterized artery may occur in about 5 per cent of patients and usually require no treatment. Intramural injection or pericardial placement (with tamponade, requiring pericardiocentesis) has occurred.

Urinary Response: Changes in renal function rarely occur, although diuresis and dehydration can follow large or repeated doses.

Nervous system disturbances may include mental confusion, visual or speech disturbances, vertigo, or rarely, convulsions.

ANGIOCARDIOGRAPHY

Pharmacology—Hemodynamic Changes: Due to its physical characteristics (chiefly tonicity and viscosity) and the volume administered, HYPAQUE-M, brand of diatrizoate meglumine and diatrizoate sodium injection, 90 per cent may cause a number of transitory hemodynamic changes. When the medium is ejected from the left ventricle or introduced at the root of the ascending aorta, a brief (three seconds) hypertensive response is usually induced, followed immediately by a decrease in aortic and peripheral blood pressures below normal levels, lasting for at least two minutes. This hypotensive phase may be followed by a 15- to 20-minute period of fluctuating blood pressure.

Clinical doses (up to 1 ml per kg) injected into the vena cava or right heart outflow tract usually cause an irregular rise in right ventricular blood pressure, a slight increase in pulmonary artery blood pressure, and delayed signs of peripheral hypotension.

Other changes reported clinically include an increase in cardiac output and atrial pressure, a decrease in myocardial contractile force, and at the peak of postinjection hypotension, a marked rise in aortic and carotid blood flow, and elevation of central venous pressure. At dosage levels used in angiocardiography, the hematocrit and hemoglobin level may fall about 10 to 15 per cent and serum osmolality may rise 10 to 12 per cent. Blood carbon dioxide, pH, and BUN levels may fall. These changes commence immediately after injection, reach a maximum in two to five minutes, and return to normal values in 10 to 15 minutes. However, after the initial rise, plasma volume may decrease and continue to fall below control levels, even beyond 30 minutes, probably due to diuresis. If repeat injections are made in rapid succession, these changes are likely to be more pronounced. (See also Dosage and Administration.) HYPAQUE-M, 90 per cent is not metabolized. It is eliminated unchanged, rapidly and completely, in the urine by glomerular filtration.

Precautions: During administration of large doses of HYPAQUE-M, brand of diatrizoate meglumine and diatrizoate sodium injection, 90 per cent, continuous monitoring of vital signs is desirable. Caution is advised in the administration of large doses to patients with incipient heart failure because of the possibility of aggravation of the preexisting condition. Hypotension should be corrected promptly since it may induce serious arrhythmias.

Because of the hemodynamic changes which may occur on injection into the right heart outflow tract, special care, especially regarding dosage, should be observed in patients with right ventricular failure, pulmonary hypertension, or obliterated pulmonary vascular beds.

Precautions in Infants

Apnea, bradycardia and other arrhythmias, cerebral effects (lethargy and depression), and a tendency to acidosis are more likely to occur in cyanotic infants. It is desirable that vital signs be monitored on an intensive care basis afterwards to detect delayed adverse effects (arrhythmia, electrolyte and hemodynamic disturbances). Infants are more likely than adults to respond with convulsions, particularly after repeated injections. Unlike in the adult, the amount of the total dosage in young infants is of particular importance. (See Dosage and Administration.)

Adverse Reactions: See Adverse Reactions, General.

Dosage and Administration: The individual dose is determined by the size of the structure to be visualized, the anticipated degree of hemodilution, and valvular competence. Weight is a minor consideration in adults. The size of each individual dose is a more important consideration than the total dosage used. When large individual doses are administered, as for contrast in the cardiac chambers and thoracic aorta, it has been suggested that 20 minutes be permitted to elapse between each injection to allow for subsidence of hemodynamic disturbances.

Adult Dosage: Adult dose of HYPAQUE-M, brand of diatrizoate meglumine and diatrizoate sodium injection, 90 per cent is usually 35 to 50 ml into either left or right chamber, outflow tracts, or aorta. The individual dose for intravenous angiocardiography ranges from 70 to 100 ml often injected simultaneously bilaterally by pressure injection, half of the dose into each antecubital vein.

Pediatric Dosage: The usual dose is 0.5 to 1 ml per kg for a subject with heart of normal size and intact valves and septum. For patients with stenotic lesions, 0.5 ml per kg is recommended. Doses up to 1.5 ml per kg may be required in cardiomegaly, large volume shunts, or where right cardiac injection is also intended to opacify left chambers.

Young Infant Dosage: The individual dose is similar to that described under Pediatric Dosage. It has been suggested, however, that the total dosage administered should be maintained below 3 ml per kg in infants under two months of age in any one procedure.

ARTERIOGRAPHY

CORONARY ARTERIOGRAPHY

Coronary arteriography should only be used in carefully selected patients when the value of the anticipated information outweighs the risk involved.

Contraindication: Routine coronary arteriography should be deferred for four weeks in patients with clinically apparent myocardial infarction.

Precaution: Continuous EKG monitoring for early detection of arrhythmias is desirable.

Adverse Reactions: Transitory EKG changes occur almost inevitably with good filling. Transient arrhythmia may occur. (See also Adverse Reactions, General.) Serum enzymes may be elevated for 24 hours.

Dosage and Administration: The usual dose for adults is 50 ml of HYPAQUE-M, 90 per cent delivered into the **root of the aorta** for simultaneous bilateral angiograms. For injection at the **sinus of Valsalva,** the usual dose is 15 to 25 ml on either side. For **selective coronary procedures,** as by the Sones technique, the individual dose recommended is 3 to 5 ml into either artery. This dose may be injected alternately into the right and left coronary artery, and repeated.

ABDOMINAL AORTOGRAPHY

HYPAQUE-M, brand of diatrizoate meglumine and diatrizoate sodium injection, 90 per cent solution may be injected by commonly accepted techniques, such as translumbar, retrograde catheter, retrograde pressure injection (by cannula) or by antegrade (brachial) catheter for examination of the aorta and its major branches.

Warnings: During aortography by the translumbar technique, extreme care is advised to avoid inadvertent intrathecal injection since the injection of even small amounts (5 to 7 ml) of the contrast medium may cause convulsions, permanent sequelae, or fatality. Should the accident occur, the patient should be placed upright to confine the hyperbaric solution to a low level, anesthesia may be required to control convulsions, and if there is evidence of a large dose having been administered, a careful cerebrospinal fluid exchange-washout should be considered.

Pheochromocytoma: Administration of angiographic media to patients known or suspected to have pheochromocytoma can cause dangerous changes in blood pressure. A minimum dose should be injected. The blood pressure should be carefully monitored and measures for controlling major fluctuations should be available.

Precautions: The presence of a vigorous pulsatile flow should be established before using a catheter or pressure injection technique. A small "pilot" dose (about 2 ml) should be administered to locate the exact site of needle or catheter tip to help prevent injection of the main dose into a branch of the aorta or intramurally. In the translumbar technique, severe pain during injection may indicate intramural placement and abdominal or back pain afterwards may indicate hemorrhage from the injection site. Following catheter procedures, gentle pressure hemostasis for 5 to 10 minutes is advised, followed by observation for 30 to 60 minutes and immobilization of the limb for several hours to prevent hemorrhage from the site of arterial puncture.

Under conditions of slowed aortic circulation there is an increased likelihood of aortography causing muscle spasm. Occasional serious neurologic complications, including paraplegia, have also been reported in patients with aorticiliac or even femoral artery bed obstruction, abdominal compression, hypotension, hypertension, spinal anesthesia, injection of vasopressors to increase contrast, and low injection sites (L2-3). In these patients the concentration, dose, and number of repeat injections of the medium should be maintained at a minimum with appropriate intervals between injections. The position of the patient and catheter tip should be carefully evaluated.

Adverse Reactions: The only adverse reaction expected is a mild burning sensation on injection. Unusual reactions can occur, as in angiocardiography. An abrupt hypertensive episode can occur following entry of the medium into the renal artery in patients with pheochromocytoma. Mesenteric necrosis, acute pancreatitis, and renal shutdown (usually transitory) and neurologic complications have been reported following inadvertent injection of a large part of the aortic dose into a branch of the aorta. Entry of the large aortic dose into the renal artery can cause, even in the absence of symptoms, albuminuria, cylindruria, and hematuria, and an elevated BUN. Rapid and complete return of function usually follows.

Dosage and Administration: The average adult dose range of HYPAQUE-M, 90 per cent is 10 to 15 ml by translumbar technique and by retrograde catheter, 15 to 25 ml. In infants and children and thin adults, the use of a less concentrated medium for aortography, such as diatrizoate sodium 50 per cent, is advised in doses of 0.5 ml per kg. For retrograde pressure injection (cannula) the usual adult dose is 35 to 40 ml of HYPAQUE-M, 90 per cent solution.

PERIPHERAL ARTERIOGRAPHY

The use of HYPAQUE-M, 90 per cent is sometimes preferred over less concentrated media in selected cases of femoral and brachio-axillary arteriography in adults.

Precaution: Pulsation should be present in the artery to be injected. In thromboangiitis obliterans, or ascending infection associated with severe ischemia, angiography should be performed with extreme caution, if at all.

Adverse Reactions: Pain or a burning sensation with some spasm may occur, and is more marked in patients with arterial insufficiency. Therefore, the procedure is more satisfactorily performed under general or, for the lower extremity, spinal anesthesia.

Arterial thrombosis, displacement of arterial plaques, and ipsilateral venous thrombosis are very rare complications.

Dosage and Administration: The usual dose of HYPAQUE-M, brand of diatrizoate meglumine and diatrizoate sodium injection, 90 per cent is 10 to 25 ml, which may be repeated. Appropriate dosage in infants and children of a less concentrated medium, such as diatrizoate sodium 50 per cent, will usually provide adequate contrast.

UROGRAPHY

NEPHROTOMOGRAPHY AND "ADEQUATE" OR HIGH DOSE UROGRAPHY

HYPAQUE-M, 90 per cent solution may be used for excretory urography in selected patients. It may be used when prior urography has failed to provide diagnostic contrast and for preliminary excretory tract study to detect obstruction in azotemic patients or to avoid retrograde instrumentation. It may also be used as a high dosage medium to intensify and prolong the nephrographic effect when the prime purpose is examination of the renal parenchyma, especially with tomography. When combined with a urea "washout" technique, HYPAQUE-M, 90 per cent provides the necessary increased pyelographic contrast and diuresis required for screening or special examination of patients with suspected renal hypertension.

Contraindication: Urography is contraindicated in patients with anuria.

Precautions: Although azotemia is not considered a contraindication, care is required in patients with advanced renal failure. The usual preparatory dehydration should be omitted, and urinary output should be observed for one to two days in these patients.

Preparatory dehydration is dangerous in infants, young children, the elderly, and azotemic patients (especially those with polyuria, oliguria, diabetes, advanced vascular disease, or preexisting dehydration). The undesirable dehydration in these patients may be accentuated by the osmotic diuretic action of the medium.

When HYPAQUE-M, 90 per cent is used with a urea "washout" procedure, the patient should also be observed for a few hours to detect signs of undue dehydration caused by increased diuresis induced by both the medium and the urea. Ingestion of water may be required for rehydration.

In myelomatosis, urography should only be performed with caution. If a weak protein-binding agent such as a diatrizoate is used for the procedure, it is essential to omit preparatory dehydration, administer fluids, and attempt to alkalinize the urine.

Adverse Reactions: Side effects following this relatively high dose urography are usually mild and transitory and do not appear to occur more frequently or severely than those induced by "standard dose" urography. Nausea, facial flushing, and emesis are not uncommon reactions. (See also Adverse Reactions, General.)

Dosage and Administration: In adults, the single dose of HYPAQUE-M, 90 per cent is usually 50 ml. The dose in infants and children is 0.5 to 1 ml per kg (not to exceed 50 ml). It is injected rapidly intravenously.

HYSTEROSALPINGOGRAPHY

HYPAQUE-M, brand of diatrizoate meglumine and diatrizoate sodium injection, 90 per cent may be selected when a viscous medium of high density is required. Otherwise, a less dense and less viscous medium, such as diatrizoate sodium 50 per cent, may be used.

Contraindications: The procedure should not be performed during the menstrual period or when menstrual flow is imminent. It should not be performed when infection is present in any portion of the genital tract. The procedure is also contraindicated for pregnant women or for those in whom pregnancy is suspected. Its use is not advised for six months after termination of pregnancy, or for thirty days after conization or curettage.

Precautions: In patients with carcinoma or in those in whom the condition is suspected, caution should be exercised to avoid possible spread of the lesion by the procedure. The effect on PBI or RAI studies is similar to that in Angiography. (See Warnings, General.)

Adverse Reactions: Cramping may occur during the injection and sometimes mild lower abdominal pain may be present for an hour or two afterwards. Even when the medium gains entrance into venous or lymphatic channels, systemic effects are rare. Generalized urticaria or slight transient hyperpyrexia, however, has been reported.

Dosage and Administration: Approximately 4 ml of HYPAQUE-M, 90 per cent will fill the uterine cavity and an additional 3 to 4 ml will fill the fallopian tubes in normal subjects. A larger volume may be required in some disease states. Slow injection is advisable.

How Supplied: HYPAQUE-M, 90 per cent is supplied in vials of 50 ml, boxes of 25 (NDC 0024-0788-04).

TELEPAQUE® ℞

brand of iopanoic acid tablets, USP

Description: TELEPAQUE, brand of iopanoic acid tablets, is 3-amino-α-ethyl-2,4,6-triiodohydrocinnamic acid ($C_{11}H_{12}I_3NO_2$). It is a cream-colored solid which is insoluble in water. It contains 66.68 percent organically-bound iodine and has a molecular weight of 570.93. TELEPAQUE is an oral radiopaque medium for cholecystography and cholangiography. Each off-white, scored tablet contains 500 mg iopanoic acid.

Clinical Pharmacology: TELEPAQUE is absorbed from the duodenum, excreted by the liver as a glucuronide, and stored and concentrated in the gallbladder. This conjugate provides visualization of the gallbladder and may, upon contraction of the gallbladder, provide visualization of the extrahepatic ducts. Approximately 50 percent of the administered dose is excreted within 24 hours, and each day thereafter, 50 percent of the remainder; excretion is complete in about five days. Partition of excretion is approximately two thirds through the gastrointestinal tract and one third through the kidneys. The glucuronide of TELEPAQUE is not reabsorbed to any extent; thus, there is no enterohepatic recycling. The glucuronide is visible in the intestinal tract as discrete radiopacities.

The healthy gallbladder concentrates TELEPAQUE; faint contrast becomes apparent in about four hours, and maximum contrast in about 14 hours. In substantial gallbladder disease, concentration does not take place and no contrast is apparent.

Indications and Usage: TELEPAQUE is indicated for use in oral cholecystography. It may also be used for oral cholangiography, although it is not considered the method of choice.

Contraindications: Administration of TELEPAQUE is contraindicated in severe impairment of renal function and particularly in advanced hepatorenal disease. It is also contraindicated in severe gastrointestinal disorders that prevent absorption, and in some patients sensitive to iodinated compounds.

Warning: **Usage in Pregnancy**. Reproduction studies have not been performed in animals. Before cholecystography in women who are of childbearing potential, the benefits should be weighed against the possible risk to the fetus.

Precautions: *Cholecystography in Liver Disease.* TELEPAQUE is generally well tolerated by patients with impaired liver function, and adequate gallbladder visualization can often be achieved in the presence of hepatic disease. However, severe, advanced liver disease (eg,

Continued on next page

This product information was effective as of November 19, 1982. On these and other products of Winthrop Laboratories, detailed information may be obtained on a current basis by direct inquiry to the Professional Services Department, 90 Park Avenue, New York, NY 10016 (212) 907-2525.

Winthrop—Cont.

bilirubin exceeding 5 mg per 100 ml) very frequently results in nonvisualization of the gallbladder.
Severe, advanced liver disease may interfere with metabolism of the radiopaque medium, and therefore, a greater amount of unchanged TELEPAQUE will be diverted for renal excretion, increasing the load on the kidneys. Although renal difficulty has rarely been attributed to TELEPAQUE, renal function in patients with severe, advanced liver disease should be assessed before cholecystography, and renal output and hepatic function should be observed for a few days after the procedure.
Renal Disease. Patients with preexisting renal disease should not receive high doses of cholecystographic media. Possible renal irritation in susceptible individuals could result in reflex vascular spasm with partial or complete renal shutdown.
Dehydration. Patients with renal or hepatic diseases should not be dehydrated beforehand and should drink liberal amounts of fluids after taking the tablets.
Uricosuric Effect. It has been shown that TELEPAQUE has uricosuric activity. This fact should be taken into consideration when the product is administered to patients with evidence of impaired renal function.
Coronary Disease. Caution is advised in patients with coronary disorders, especially those with recent symptoms of coronary artery disease. Blood pressure should be observed after administration of cholecystographic media to these patients.
Elderly Patients. For elderly patients, see Dosage.

Effect on Laboratory Tests

Thyroid Function Tests. The results of PBI and RAI uptake studies, which depend on iodine estimations, will not reflect thyroid function for several months following administration of cholecystographic media. However, function tests not depending on iodine estimations, eg, T_3 resin uptake or free thyroxine assays, are not affected.
Liver Function Tests. Bilirubin, thymol turbidity, cephalin flocculation, and serum enzyme values are unaffected but TELEPAQUE may delay BSP clearance values for up to two days.
Pseudoalbuminuria may be present for three days in response to certain chemical protein precipitation tests. Positive reactions should be verified by the heat-and-acetic acid or colorimetric dip-strip methods.
Uricosuric Effect. TELEPAQUE may increase the rate of excretion of uric acid, lowering blood levels and raising urinary excretion values for a few days.

Adverse Reactions: Most reactions are mild and transitory; a very low incidence of serious side effects has been attributed to TELEPAQUE.
Most frequently reported have been mild and transitory nausea, vomiting, cramps, and diarrhea (usually occurring as a few loose stools). Frank diarrhea and cramps have been noted in only a small number of patients, and severe diarrhea with prostration is rare. A mild stinging sensation during urination may occur. Skin, mucous membrane, and systemic hypersensitivity reactions are unusual and include urticaria with or without pruritus, erythema, morbilliform rash, and localized areas of edema. Very rarely a systemic serum sickness-type reaction with fever, rash, and arthralgia has been reported. A few cases of transitory thrombocytopenia with petechiae have been reported. Miscellaneous subjective complaints are dryness of the throat, burning on swallowing, heartburn, sore throat, dizziness, and headache.
Very rarely disturbances in hepatic, renal, or cardiovascular function have been reported, usually in patients with preexisting disease (see Precautions).

Dosage and Administration:

Adult Dosage

The standard adult dose of 3 g (six tablets) is usually ingested with water in the evening after a fat-free dinner, about 14 hours before the cholecystography. In some instances, double doses of 6 g (12 tablets) may be ingested, eg, for duct visualization or for some repeat examinations made over 7 days later. Many radiologists prefer that the patient take a laxative (eg, castor oil) about four to six hours before ingesting TELEPAQUE, brand of iopanoic acid tablets. (See also Repeat Examination.) Preparatory dehydration is unnecessary and undesirable, especially in elderly patients.
The use of large or repeated doses over a number of days to force visualization of a poorly functioning gallbladder *in elderly patients* is not recommended.

Diet before Cholecystography

A normal diet (containing some fat) is advised at least one or two days before TELEPAQUE cholecystography. The meal immediately before ingestion of TELEPAQUE, however, should be *strictly fat free:* eg, fruit or fruit juice; vegetables *cooked without fat;* bread with jelly; coffee or tea with sugar but *no milk or cream. No meats are permitted.*
During the interval between ingestion of TELEPAQUE and the morning of cholecystographic examination the patient should take *nothing by mouth* except water, and should not smoke or chew gum. In the morning, before the radiologic examination, the patient may take an enema in order to remove accumulated gas which might interfere with visualization.

Fatty Meal after Cholecystography

After the gallbladder has been visualized the patient may be given a fat-containing meal or a commercially available cholecystagogue, for determining the extent and duration of gallbladder contractility (thus, the degree of function), to help identify small radiolucent stones or to visualize the bile ducts.

Duct Visualization

Occasionally, the bile ducts may be visualized on the original film during cholecystography. However, in a substantial percentage of patients, administration of a fat is necessary. The more frequent the roentgenographic exposures, the greater the probability of visualization of the ducts; however, the best time intervals are usually 20 and 30 minutes after the fatty meal. Some investigators believe contrast in the ducts is enhanced by an increased dose of TELEPAQUE (up to 6 g).

Repeat Examination

Most radiologists consider repeat examination desirable when the gallbladder does not visualize initially, in order to reduce the possibility of false diagnosis. If the second cholecystographic examination also results in nonvisualization, gallbladder disease may be inferred with reasonable certainty.
For repeat examination on the same day as the initial cholecystographic procedure, an additional 3 g (six tablets) may be given. However, if repeat cholecystography is to be performed with a double dose, a period of at least five to seven days should intervene between the first and the repeat examinations. No more than a total of 6 g (12 tablets) should be ingested during a 24-hour period.

How Supplied:
Tablets of 500 mg,
envelopes of 6 tablets, boxes of 25
(NDC 0024-1931-03)
[*Shown in Product Identification Section*]

GUIDE TO MANAGEMENT OF DRUG OVERDOSE

Prepared by:
Eric G. Comstock, M.D.
and
Eugene V. Boisaubin, M.D.
Department of Medicine
Baylor College of Medicine
Houston, Texas

INTRODUCTION: The following discussion is designed for use in adult patients. In the pediatric age group, general principles apply, but the volumes of fluid or suggested medication must be adjusted for body size. Symptomatic and supportive care is the basis for treatment of drug overdose. All other approaches are secondary. Procedures directed toward the offending substance, such as the performance of gastric lavage or the administration of a specific pharmacologic antagonist, should be undertaken only after adequate vital function has been assured. Procedures to facilitate excretion of toxic substances, such as peritoneal or extracorporeal dialysis and forced diuresis are required infrequently, and should never be relied upon as the primary approach to treatment. For sedative, hypnotic, and tranquilizer drugs, alone or in combination, supportive care is sufficient as outlined in the following discussion.

INITIAL ASSESSMENT: If the patient is symptomatic, determine the adequacy of respiration and cardiac function and note reflex activity, such as pupillary, corneal, gag and deep tendon. If vital function is compromised, or consciousness is impaired, proceed immediately to supportive measures.

THE ASYMPTOMATIC PATIENT: The drug overdosed patient may be asymptomatic because he has not ingested a sufficient dose of the drugs, or because a sufficient quantity has not been absorbed to produce symptoms. After the ingestion of a life threatening quantity of drugs, symptoms may be delayed as long as six hours, although ordinarily symptoms are manifested within thirty (30) minutes to two (2) hours. Ingestion of alcohol simultaneoulsy with drugs may shorten the time for symptoms to appear. Vomiting should be induced only during the asymptomatic interval. If significant central nervous system depression intervenes between the administration of emetic and the occurrence of vomiting, then the airway should be protected by insertion of a cuffed endotracheal tube. Fluids must be forced orally to obtain satisfactory results from any effort to induce vomiting. An alternate approach to the asymptomatic patient alleged to have ingested drugs, is the administration by mouth of a slurry of no less than 100 grams of activated charcoal powder (USP) in water. Gastric lavage with a large caliber tube (34 French) may be performed in the asymptomatic patient. Any patient whose consciousness is impaired to the point where a cuffed endotracheal tube will be tolerated should be intubated prior to the performance of gastric lavage.

THE SYMPTOMATIC PATIENT: If the patient is symptomatic all treatment procedures directed toward the toxic substance are secondary to the support of vital function. If the patient is in coma, attention to respiratory support and cardiac function should proceed immediately.

RESPIRATORY SUPPORT: Examine the mouth. Remove all foreign material including dentures. Position the head so that respiration is not sonorous and so that regurgitated stomach contents are not readily aspirated. If respiration is not present, provide ventilation by mouth-to-mouth, ambu bag, or positive pressure respirator until the patient is adequately oxygenated. Insert an oropharyngeal airway and suction excess secretions while preparing to insert an endotracheal tube. A cuffed endotracheal tube should be inserted and inflated. Bronchial suction should be administered to clear mucus and foreign material. Determine that the chest is being inflated symmetrically and that breath sounds are audible bilaterally. After the acute emergency, determine placement of the endotracheal tube by x-ray. Monitor adequacy of ventilation using arterial blood gases.

IV ACCESS AND CARDIAC FUNCTION: While one member of the treatment team is assuring adequate ventilation, a second member of the team should be assuring adequate IV access by insertion of an 18 gauge venous catheter and initiation of IV fluid administration such as Ringers Lactate or ½ normal saline at a maintenance rate in adults of 150 ml. per hour. Since hypotension from sedative drug intoxication results from relative hypovolemia complicated frequently by dehydration, the rate of intravenous infusion should be increased to 10-20 cc per minute if the systolic pressure is under 80 mm of mercury. Placing the patient in the Trendelenburg position may quickly correct small to moderate degrees of hypotension. A central venous pressure catheter or a Swan-Ganz catheter is required if the continuous high rate infusion reaches one (1) liter within one hour or if the positive fluid balance exceeds two (2) liters during the first two hours. Intermittent monitoring of central venous pressure should continue throughout the period of intensive supportive care. A baseline electrocardiogram should be obtained as soon as vital functions have been supported. The appearance of conduction defects should lead to suspicion of drugs with direct cardiac effects, such as the tricyclic antidepressants. In uncomplicated sedative drug overdose, the central venous pressure will be under ten centimeters of water and will not change appreciably with high volume fluid infusion. If the central venous pressure increases abruptly in excess of five centimeters of water, or if the CVP exceeds 16 centimeters of water, high rate fluid infusion should be stopped pending evaluation of cardiac status. Adequate tissue perfusion is obtained with a systolic pressure in the range of 80 to 100 milliliters of mercury. A systolic pressure higher than this is required only in the patient with pre-existing hypertension. The formation of urine is an indication that tissue perfusion is adequate.

URINARY CATHETERIZATION: An in-dwelling urinary catheter should be inserted early in the course of treatment of any unconscious drug overdose patient. Upon insertion of the catheter, the volume of residual urine should be measured and the specimen should be saved separately for urinalysis including specific gravity, labeled for drug analysis, and sent to the laboratory to be retained for 24 hours. Recording of urine output hourly is necessary to maintain fluid balance records. Abrupt cessation of urine output most frequently is due to an obstructed catheter, but deserves immediate appraisal. Anuria for a period in excess of one hour should lead to reduction of high rate intravascular volume infusion until cardiac and renal status has been reappraised. Failure to achieve adequate urinary output after initial emptying of the bladder may reflect uncompensated dehydration and relative hypovolemia, each of which must be corrected before balanced fluid intake and output plus insensible loss can be achieved. The immediate or automatic use of diuretics at this stage only aggravates the basic defect and may result in intractable hypotension. Addition of vasopressor drugs at this stage may precipitate renal failure. Electrolyte solutions as transient volume expanders are preferred to whole